KU-281-436

STROKE

A Practical Guide to Management

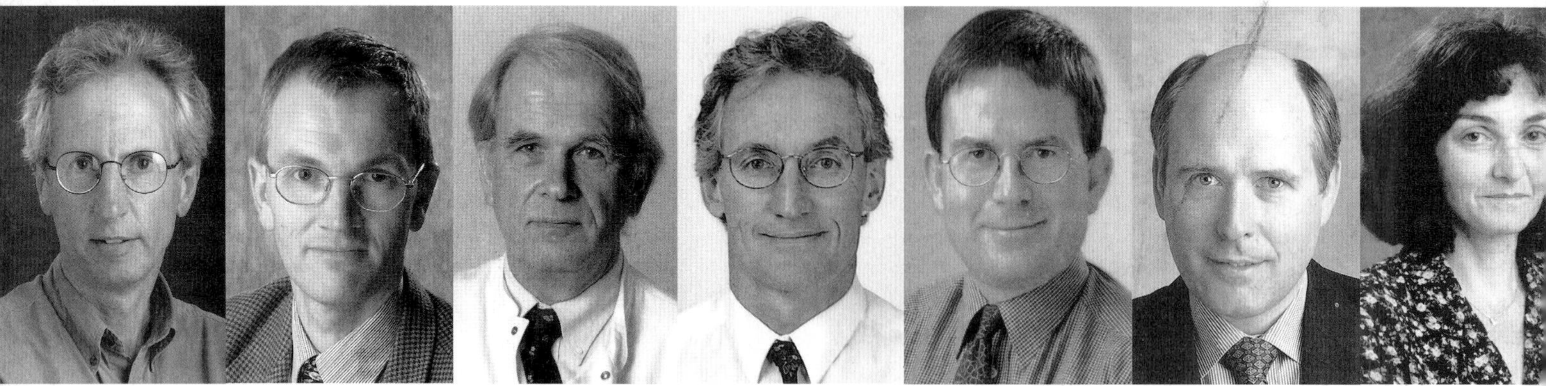

From left to right: C.P. Warlow, M.S. Dennis, J. van Gijn, G.J. Hankey, P.A.G. Sandercock, J.M. Bamford, J.M. Wardlaw

Dedication

We would like to dedicate the second edition of this book to all patients with stroke and transient ischaemic attacks who, over the years, have agreed to be observed or entered into randomized controlled trials. Without their help, there would have been no therapeutic progress.

STROKE

A practical guide to management

C.P. Warlow, M.S. Dennis, J. van Gijn, G.J. Hankey, P.A.G. Sandercock, J.M. Bamford, J.M. Wardlaw

Foreword by H.J.M. Barnett

Second Edition

U.W.E.L.
LEARNING RESOURCES
ACC. No. 2273494
CLASS 616.81 WAR
CONTROL 0632054182
DATE 15 JUL 2002
SITE UW

Blackwell
Science

© 1996, 2001 by
Blackwell Science Ltd
Editorial Offices:
Osney Mead, Oxford OX2 0EL
25 John Street, London WC1N 2BS
23 Ainslie Place, Edinburgh EH3 6AJ
350 Main Street, Malden
MA 02148-5018, USA
54 University Street, Carlton
Victoria 3053, Australia
10, rue Casimir Delavigne
75006 Paris, France

Other Editorial Offices:
Blackwell Wissenschafts-Verlag GmbH
Kurfürstendamm 57
10707 Berlin, Germany

Blackwell Science KK
MG Kodenmacho Building
7–10 Kodenmacho Nihombashi
Chuo-ku, Tokyo 104, Japan

First published 1996
Reprinted 1997
Second edition 2001
Reprinted 2002

Set by Sparks Computer Solutions Ltd,
Oxford, UK (www.sparks.co.uk)
Printed in Great Britain at the Alden Press,
Oxford and Northampton, and bound by
MPG Books Ltd, Bodmin, Cornwall

The Blackwell Science logo is a
trade mark of Blackwell Science Ltd,
registered at the United Kingdom
Trade Marks Registry

The right of the Authors to be
identified as the Authors of this Work
has been asserted in accordance
with the Copyright, Designs and
Patents Act 1988.

All rights reserved. No part of
this publication may be reproduced,
stored in a retrieval system, or
transmitted, in any form or by any
means, electronic, mechanical,
photocopying, recording or otherwise,
except as permitted by the UK
Copyright, Designs and Patents Act
1988, without the prior permission
of the copyright owner.

A catalogue record for this title
is available from the British Library

ISBN 0-632-05418-2

Library of Congress
Cataloging-in-publication Data

Stroke: a practical guide to management/
C.P. Warlow ... [*et al.*]; foreword by
H.J.M. Barnett.—2nd ed.
p. ; cm
Includes bibliographical references
and index
ISBN 0-632-05418-2
1. Cerebrovascular disease. I. Warlow,
Charles.
[DNLM: 1. Cerebrovascular Accident
—therapy. 2. Intracranial
Haemorrhages—therapy. 3. Ischaemic
Attack, Transient—therapy.
WL355 S9208 2000]
RC388.5 .S847 2000
616.8'1—dc21

00-059905

DISTRIBUTORS

Marston Book Services Ltd
PO Box 269
Abingdon, Oxon OX14 4YN
(*Orders*: Tel: 01235 465500
Fax: 01235 465555)

The Americas
Blackwell Publishing
c/o AIDC
PO Box 20
50 Winter Lane
Williston, VT 05495-0020
(*Orders*: Tel: 800 216 2522
Fax: 802 864 7626)

Australia
Blackwell Science Pty Ltd
54 University Street
Carlton, Victoria 3053
(*Orders*: Tel: 3 9347 0300
Fax: 3 9347 5001)

For further information on
Blackwell Science, visit our website:
www.blackwell-science.com

Contents

Website of the book

We have cited websites as well as publications. The Universal Resources Locators (URLs) for these websites are given in the text. The book has an associated website (http://www.dcn.ed.ac.uk/spgm) and in it you will find all of the URLs cited in the book, listed by chapter. To go to the website you want, just click on the link provided. The website also contains links to materials which were not available at the time of going to press but have since been published or made publicly available.

List of Contributors

J.M. Bamford MD FRCP
Consultant Neurologist
St James' University Hospital
Beckett Street
Leeds, UK

M.S. Dennis MD FRCP
Reader in Stroke Medicine
Department of Clinical Neurosciences
Western General Hospital
Crewe Road
Edinburgh, UK

G.J. Hankey MD FRCPE FRACP
Consultant Neurologist
Department of Neurology
Royal Perth Hospital
Wellington Street
Perth
Western Australia
Australia

P.A.G. Sandercock DM FRCP
Professor of Medical Neurology
Department of Clinical Neurosciences
Western General Hospital
Crewe Road
Edinburgh, UK

J. van Gijn MD FRCP FRCPE
Professor and Chairman
Department of Neurology
University Medical Centre of Utrecht
Utrecht
The Netherlands

J.M Wardlaw MD FRCP FRCR
Reader in Neuroradiology
Department of Clinical Neurosciences
Western General Hospital
Crewe Road
Edinburgh, UK

C.P. Warlow MD FRCP
Professor of Medical Neurology
Department of Clinical Neurosciences
Western General Hospital
Crewe Road
Edinburgh, UK

Foreword

Stroke neurology during the first half of the 20th century was for the academic specialist. As mentioned in the Foreword to the First Edition of this book, studies on cerebral localization and correlation with functional anatomy were pursuits of keen interest to the scientist, but not of immediate value applicable to the individual patient. The first big breakthrough came when Moniz introduced angiography of the cerebral arteries. Not long after that came the concept of large artery disease in the extracranial cerebral circulation as a cause of stroke. The stage was set for the equally important identification of transient ischaemic attack, the warning symptoms of stroke. Endarterectomy and antithrombotics followed, pursued at first on a case-by-case basis. Then randomized controlled trials attempting to prevent stroke or reduce its progression by antithrombotics and by endarterectomy were carried out. They were negative partly because of flawed design. Meanwhile the heart, aorta and penetrating arteries emerged as equal in importance to the large arteries causing stroke. The age of neurochemistry was dawning and knowledge was accumulating about the changes brought about by cerebral ischaemia. The pharmaceutical industry took up the challenge of possible post-ischaemic neuroprotection. Revolutionary improvement in brain and vascular imaging and the evolution of good methodology for clinical trials seeking preventive and treatment strategies combined to make evidence-based stroke neurology a credible reality.

According to World Health statistics, stroke is still the world's second most common cause of death, behind only heart disease. This continued heavy burden of stroke is partly explained by longer survival because of improved health in the developed and in some parts of the developing world. Larger numbers of people are reaching the later decades of life when the occurrence of stroke reaches its peak. The World Health statistics signal the need for redoubling of research efforts in the prevention and treatment field. The previous despair and hopelessness, which permeated the thinking about stroke, have become things of the past. Furthermore, there is great need to ensure wide dissemination of knowledge about the meritorious prevention measures which have evolved. The reality of benefit from early treatment, despite the fact that the ischaemic event has occurred, must be accepted and the profession made fully aware of the implications of this knowledge. Surely, there will be more to come.

The greatest stimulus to advancing research and dissemination of evidence-based knowledge is good literature. At long last we are being well served here. Some books on stroke deal in monograph form with particular aspects of the field. Others are encyclopaedic and combine basic and clinical knowledge designed for exhaustive coverage of disorders of the blood supply of the brain and the consequences of its disorder. Both have important roles. The present volume is designed differently. It is meant to cover the field but to do so in a practical manner. First, the manifestations of disturbances of the blood supply to the brain are defined for the readers. Having achieved this, what can and should be done for the individual patient is set out. Practitioners who care for patients threatened with or already afflicted by a cerebral vascular disorder are part of the expected audience. Recent major advances are brought into focus for the practitioner in clear and readable language. The providers of healthcare cannot ignore these revolutionary changes.

British, Dutch and Australian pioneers in the emerging practical science came together as friends to produce a reader-friendly but scientifically accurate multi-authored first edition of this book in 1996. The first edition was so well received and so much has happened since then that a second edition is obligatory. There are 18 chapters carefully organized in as many subdivisions as the particular topic requires. This makes for considerable ease for the reader to turn quickly to the appropriate part of the book when faced with a particular problem in the clinic or at the bedside. The authors adopted a rather unique *modus operandi* in the creation of the first edition and this is continued. Obviously, they divide the writing between the seven co-authors, but the final version of each chapter and each section is completed around the editorial table. This ensures a seamless work which reads smoothly and avoids the repetition and even the contradictions which may detract from the pleasure of reading some large works from recognized authorities. The authority of this volume is ensured because seven leaders in the field present the reader with their combined wisdom.

Practitioners of medicine, patients at risk of stroke and patients who have had a stroke are indebted to the team who produced this book. Politicians and public health bureaucrats should know its contents.

H.J.M. Barnett MD

Acknowledgements

We have had invaluable help and advice from many people in the preparation of this second edition. So thank you all, including:

Judi Clarke
Carl Counsell
Alice Emmott
Hazel Fraser
Paut Greebe
Gord Gubitz
Alistair Lammie
Peter Langhorne
Rob Larbalestier
Richard Lindley
Mike McDowell
Michael Mackie
Nick Morgan
Ross Naylor
David Perry
David Prentice
Peter Rothwell
Mark Smith
Ian Starkey
Cathie Sudlow
Stuart Taylor
Brenda Thomas
Theo vanVroonhoven
Nic Weir

Also, thank you to our teachers and colleagues from whom we have learned so many worthwhile things over the years:

Henry Barnett
Lou Caplan
David Chadwick
Iain Chalmers
Rory Collins
Hans van Crevel
Richard Doll
Geoff Donnan
Stuart Douglas
Shah Ebrahim
Barbara Farrell
C. Miller Fisher
Chris Foote
John Fry
Mike Gent
Michael Harrison
Jim Heron
Bryan Matthews
Richard Peto
Gabriel Rinkel
Geoffrey Rose
David Sackett
David Shepherd
Jim Slattery
Rien Vermeulen
Ted Stewart-Wynne
Derick Wade
Eelco Wijdicks

Abbreviations

We don't care much for abbreviations. They are not literate (Oliver Twist was not abbreviated to OT each time Dickens mentioned his name!), they don't look good on the printed page, and they make things more difficult to read and understand, particularly for non-experts. But they do save space and so we have to use them. However, we will avoid them as far as we can in tables, figures and the practice points. We will try to define any abbreviations the first time they are used in each chapter, or even in each section if they are not very familiar. But, if we fail to be comprehensible, then here is a rather long list to refer to.

ACA	Anterior cerebral artery
ACE	Angiotensin converting enzyme
AChA	Anterior choroidal artery
ACoA	Anterior communicating artery
ACST	Asymptomatic Carotid Surgery Trial
ADH	Antidiuretic hormone
ADL	Activities of daily living
ADP	Adenosine diphosphate
ADPKD	Autosomal dominant polycystic kidney disease
AF	Atrial fibrillation
AFx	Amaurosis fugax
AH	Ataxic hemiparesis
AICA	Anterior inferior cerebellar artery
AIDS	Acquired immune deficiency syndrome
ANCA	Antineutrophil cytoplasmic antibody
ANF	Antinuclear factor
APS	Antiphospholipid syndrome
APT	Antiplatelet Trialists' Collaboration
APTT	Activated partial thromboplastin time
ARAS	Ascending reticular activating system
ARD	Absolute risk difference
ASA	Atrial septal aneurysm
ASD	Atrial septal defect
ATIII	Antithrombin III
ATP	Adenosine triphosphate
ATT	Antithrombotic Trialists' Collaboration
AVF	Arteriovenous fistula
AVM	Arteriovenous malformation
BA	Basilar artery
BIH	Benign intracranial hypertension
BMI	Body mass index
BP	Blood pressure
C	Celsius
CAA	Cerebral amyloid angiopathy
CADASIL	Cerebral autosomal dominant arteriopathy with subcortical infarcts and leukoencephalopathy
CAST	Chinese Acute Stroke Trial
CAVATAS	Carotid and Vertebral Artery Translumenal Angioplasty Study
CBF	Cerebral blood flow
CBFV	Cerebral blood flow velocity
CBV	Cerebral blood volume
CCA	Common carotid artery
CEA	Carotid endarterectomy
CHD	Coronary heart disease
CI	Confidence interval
CK	Creatine kinase
$CMRO_2$	Cerebral metabolic rate of oxygen
CMRglu	Cerebral metabolic rate of glucose
CNS	Central nervous system
CPP	Cerebral perfusion pressure
CPSP	Central post-stroke pain
CSF	Cerebrospinal fluid
CT	Computed tomography
CTA	Computed tomographic angiography
CVR	Cerebrovascular resistance
DBP	Diastolic blood pressure
DCHS	Dysarthria clumsy-hand syndrome
DIC	Disseminated intravascular coagulation
DNA	Deoxyribose nucleic acid
DSA	Digital subtraction angiography
DSM	Diagnostic and statistical manual of mental disorders
DVT	Deep venous thrombosis (in the legs or pelvis)
DWI	Diffusion weighted (MR) imaging
EACA	Epsilon-aminocaproic acid
EADL	Extended activities of daily living
EAFT	European Atrial Fibrillation Trial
ECA	External carotid artery
ECASS	European Cooperative Acute Stroke Study
ECG	Electrocardiogram
EC-IC	Extracranial-intracranial
ECST	European Carotid Surgery Trial
EEG	Electroencephalogram
EMG	Electromyography
ESR	Erythrocyte sedimentation rate
FDA	Food and Drug Administration
FIM	Functional independence measure

FLAIR	Fluid attenuated inversion recovery
FMD	Fibromuscular dysplasia
fMRI	Functional magnetic resonance imaging
GCS	Glasgow Coma Scale
GEF	Glucose extraction fraction
GKI	Glucose, potassium and insulin
HACP	Homolateral ataxia and crural paresis
Hg	Mercury
HITS	High intensity transient signals
HIV	Human immunodeficiency virus
HTI	Haemorrhagic transformation of an infarct
HU	Hounsfield units
IAA	Internal auditory artery
ICA	Internal carotid artery
ICIDH	International classification of impairments, disabilities and handicaps
ICP	Intracranial pressure
ICVT	Intracranial venous thrombosis
IADSA	Intra-arterial digital subtraction angiography
INR	International normalized ratio
IST	International Stroke Trial
IVDSA	Intravenous digital subtraction angiography
IVM	Intracranial vascular malformation
kPa	Kilopascals
L	Litre
LACI	Lacunar infarction
LACS	Lacunar syndrome
LGN	Lateral geniculate nucleus
LP	Lumbar puncture
LSA	Lenticulostriate artery
M	Molar
MAC	Mitral annulus calcification
MAOI	Monoamine oxidase inhibitor
MAST-I	Multicentre Acute Stroke Trial—Italy
MCA	Middle cerebral artery
MCTT	Mean cerebral transit time
MES	Microembolic signals
MI	Myocardial infarction
MLF	Medial longitudinal fasciculus
MMSE	Mini mental state examination
MR	Magnetic resonance
MRA	Magnetic resonance angiography
MRC	Medical Research Council
MRI	Magnetic resonance imaging
MRS	Magnetic resonance spectroscopy
MRV	Magnetic resonance venogram
MVP	Mitral valve prolapse
NASCET	North American Symptomatic Carotid Endarterectomy Trial
NELH	National Electronic Library for Health
NG	Nasogastric
NINDS	National Institute of Neurological Disorders and Stroke
NNT	Numbers-needed-to-treat
OCSP	Oxfordshire Community Stroke Project
OEF	Oxygen extraction fraction
OHS	Oxford Handicap Scale
OR	Odds ratio
PACI	Partial anterior circulation infarction
$Pa\text{CO}_2$	Arterial partial pressure of carbon dioxide
$Pa\text{O}_2$	Arterial partial pressure of oxygen
PACS	Partial anterior circulation syndrome
PCA	Posterior cerebral artery
PChA	Posterior choroidal artery
PCoA	Posterior communicating artery
PCV	Packed cell volume
PE	Pulmonary embolism
PEG	Percutaneous endoscopic gastrostomy
PET	Positron emission tomography
PFO	Patent foramen ovale
PICA	Posterior inferior cerebellar artery
PICH	Primary intracerebral haemorrhage
PMS	Pure motor stroke
PNH	Paroxysmal nocturnal haemoglobinuria
POCI	Posterior circulation infarction
POCS	Posterior circulation syndrome
PD	Proton density
PSE	Present state examination
PSS	Pure sensory stroke
PTA	Percutaneous translumenal angioplasty
PVD	Peripheral vascular disease
PWI	Perfusion weighted (MR) imaging
RAH	Recurrent artery of Heubner
RCT	Randomized controlled trial
RIND	Reversible ischaemic neurological deficit
RNA	Ribonucleic acid
ROR	Relative odds reduction
RR	Relative risk
RRR	Relative risk reduction
rt-PA	Recombinant tissue plasminogen activator

SADS	Schedule for affective disorders and schizophrenia
SAH	Subarachnoid haemorrhage
SBP	Systolic blood pressure
SCA	Superior cerebellar artery
SD	Standard deviation
SEPIVAC	Studio epidemiologico sulla incidenza delle vasculopathie acute cerebrali
SF36	Short form 36
SIADH	Syndrome of inappropriate secretion of antidiuretic hormone
SK	Streptokinase
SLE	Systemic lupus erythematosus
SMS	Sensorimotor stroke
SPAF	Stroke prevention in atrial fibrillation
SPECT	Single photon emission computed tomography
SVD	Small vessel disease
TACI	Total anterior circulation infarction
TACS	Total anterior circulation syndrome
TCD	Transcranial Doppler
TENS	Transcutaneous electrical nerve stimulation
TGA	Transient global amnesia
TIA	Transient ischaemic attack
TMB	Transient monocular blindness
TOAST	Trial of ORG 10 172 in Acute Stroke Therapy
TEA	Tranexamic acid
TTP	Thrombotic thrombocytopenic purpura
VA	Vertebral artery
VB	Vertebrobasilar
WHO	World Health Organization
WFNS	World Federation of Neurological Surgeons

CHAPTER ONE

Introduction

1.1 Introduction to the first edition

1.1.1 Aims and scope of the book

We, the authors of this book, regard ourselves as practising—and practical—doctors who look after stroke patients in very routine day-to-day practice. The book is for people like us: neurologists, geriatricians, stroke physicians, radiologists and general internal physicians. But it is not just for doctors. It is also for nurses, therapists, managers and anyone else who wants practical guidance about all and any of the problems to do with stroke—from aetiology to organization of services, from prevention to occupational therapy and from any facet of cure to any facet of care. In other words, it is for anyone who has to deal with stroke in clinical practice. It is not a book for armchair theoreticians, who usually have no sense of proportion as well as difficulty in seeing the wood from the trees. Or, maybe, it is particularly for them so that they can be led back into the real world.

The book takes what is known as a problem-orientated approach. The problems posed by stroke patients are discussed in the sort of order that they are likely to present themselves. Is it a stroke? What sort of stroke is it? What caused it? What can be done about it? How can the patient and carer be supported in the short term and long term? How can any recurrence be prevented? How can stroke services be better organized? Unlike traditional textbooks, which linger on dusty shelves, there are no '-ology' chapters. Aetiology, epidemiology, pathology and the rest represent just the tools to solve the problems—so they are used when they are needed, and not discussed in isolation. For example, to prevent strokes one needs to know how frequent they are (epidemiology), what types of stroke there are (pathology), what causes them (aetiology) and what evidence there is to support therapeutic intervention (randomized controlled trials). Clinicians mostly operate on a need-to-know basis, and so when a problem arises they need the information to solve it at that moment, from inside their head, from a colleague—and we hope from a book like this.

1.1.2 General principles

To solve a problem one obviously needs relevant information. Clinicians, and others, should not be making decisions based on whim, dogma or the last case, although most do, at least some of the time—ourselves included. It is better to search out the reliable information based on some reasonable criterion for what is meant by reliable, get it into a sensible order, review it and make a summary that can be used at the bedside. If one does not have the time to do this—and who does for every problem?—then one has to search out someone else's systematic review. Or find the answer in this book. Good clinicians have always done all this intuitively, although recently the process has been blessed with the title of 'evidence-based medicine', and now even 'evidence-based patient-focused medicine'! In this book we have used the evidence-based approach, at least where it is possible to do so. Therefore, where a systematic review of a risk factor or a treatment is available we have cited it, and not just emphasized single studies done by us or our friends and with results to suit our prejudices. But so often there is no good evidence or even any evidence at all available, and certainly no systematic reviews. What to do then? Certainly not what most doctors are trained to do: 'Never be wrong, and if you are, never admit it!' If we do not know something, we will say so. But, like other clinicians, we may have to make decisions even when we do not know what to do, and when nobody else does either. One cannot always adopt the policy of 'if you don't know what to do, don't do it'. Throughout the book we will try to indicate where there is no evidence, or feeble evidence, and describe what *we* do and will continue to do until better evidence becomes available; after all, it is these murky areas of practice that need to be flagged up as requiring further research. Moreover, in clinical practice, all of us ask respected colleagues for advice, not because they may know something that we do not but because we want to know what they would do in a difficult situation.

1.1.3 Methods

We were all taught to look at the 'methods' section of a scientific paper before anything else. If the methods are no good, then there is no point in wasting time and reading further. In passing, we do regard it as most peculiar that some medical journals still print the methods section in smaller letters than the rest of the paper. Therefore, before anyone reads further, perhaps we should describe the methods we have adopted.

It is now impossible for any single person to write a comprehensive book about stroke that has the feel of having been written by someone with hands-on experience of the whole subject. The range of problems is far too wide. Therefore, the sort of stroke book that we as practitioners want—and we hope others do too—has to be written by a group of people. Rather than putting together a huge multiauthor book, we thought it would be better and more informative, for ourselves as well as readers, to write a book together that would take a particular approach (evidence-based, if you will) and end up with a coherent message. After all, we have all worked together over many years, our views on stroke are more convergent than divergent, and so it should not be too terribly difficult to write a book together.

Like many things in medicine, and in life, this book started over a few drinks to provide the initial momentum to get going, on the occasion of a stroke conference in Geneva in 1993. At that time, we decided that the book was to be comprehensive (but not to the extent of citing every known reference), that all areas of stroke must be covered, and who was going to start writing which section. A few months later, the first drafts were then commented on in writing and in detail by all the authors before we got back together for a general discussion—again over a few drinks, but on this occasion at the Stockholm stroke conference in 1994. Momentum restored, we went home to improve what we had written, and the second draft was sent round to everyone for comments in an attempt to improve the clarity, remove duplication, fill in gaps and expunge as much remaining neurodogma, neurofantasy and neuroastrology as possible. Our final discussion was held at the Bordeaux stroke meeting in 1995, and the drinks that time were more in relief and celebration that the end was in sight. Home we all went to update the manuscript and make final improvements before handing over the whole lot to the publisher in January 1996.

This process may well have taken longer than a conventional multiauthor book in which all the sections are written in isolation. But it was surely more fun, and hopefully the result will provide a uniform and coherent view of the subject. It is, we hope, a 'how to do it' book, or at least a 'how we do it' book.

1.1.4 Using the book

This is not a stroke encyclopaedia. Many very much more comprehensive books and monographs are available now, or soon will be. Nor is this really a book to be read from cover to cover. Rather, it is a book that we would like to be used on stroke units and in clinics to help illuminate stroke management at various different stages, both at the level of the individual patient and for patients in general. So we would like it to be kept handy and referred to when a problem crops up: how should swallowing difficulties be identified and managed? Should an angiogram be done? Is raised plasma fibrinogen a cause of stroke? How many beds should a stroke unit have? And so on. If a question is not addressed at all, then we would like to know about it so that it can be dealt with in the next edition, if there is to be one, which will clearly depend on sales, the publisher, and enough congenial European stroke conferences to keep us going.

It should be fairly easy to find one's way around the book from the chapter headings and the contents list at the beginning of each chapter. If that fails, then the index will do instead. We have used a lot of cross-referencing to guide the reader from any starting point and so avoid constant reference to the index.

As mentioned earlier, we have tried to be as selective as possible with the referencing. On the one hand, we want to allow readers access to the relevant literature, but on the other hand we do not want the text to be overwhelmed by references—particularly by references to unsound work. To be selective, we have tried to cite recent evidence-based systematic reviews and classic papers describing important work. Other references can probably mostly be found by those who want to dig deeper in the reference lists of the references we have cited.

Finally, we have liberally scattered what some would call practice points and other maxims throughout the book. These we are all prepared to sign up to, at least in early 1996. Of course, as more evidence becomes available, some of these practice points will become out of date.

1.1.5 Why a stroke book now?

Stroke has been somewhat of a Cinderella area of medicine, at least with respect to the other two of the three most common fatal disorders in the developed world—coronary heart disease and cancer. But times are gradually changing, particularly in the last decade when stroke has been moving up the political agenda, when research has been expanding perhaps in the slipstream of coronary heart disease research, when treatments to prevent, if not treat, stroke have become available and when the pharmaceutical industry has taken more notice. It seems that there is now so much information about stroke that many practitioners are beginning to be overwhelmed. Therefore, now is a good time to try to capture all this information, digest it and then write down a practical approach to stroke management based on the best available evidence and research. This is our excuse for putting together what we know and what we do not know, what we do and why we do it.

1.2 Introduction to the second edition

Whether we enjoyed our annual 'stroke book' dinners at the European Stroke Conference too much to abandon them, or whether we thought there really was a lot of updating to do, we found ourselves working on this second edition four short years after the first. It has certainly helped to have been so much encouraged by the many people who seemed to like the book, and find it useful. We have kept to the same format, authors, and principles outlined above in the introduction to the first edition. The first step was for all of us to read the whole book again and collect together any new comments and criticisms for each of the other authors. We then rewrote our respective sections and circulated them to all the other authors for their further comments (and they were not shy in giving them). We prepared our final words in early 2000.

A huge technical advance since writing the first edition has been the widespread availability of e-mail and the use of the Internet. Even more than before, we have genuinely been able to write material together; one author does a first draft, sends it as an attachment across the world in seconds, the other author appends ideas and e-mails the whole attachment back to the first author, copying to other authors for comments perhaps, and so on until it is perfect. Of course, we still do not all agree about absolutely everything all of the time. After all, we want readers to have a feel for the rough and ragged growing edge of stroke research, where there is bound to be disagreement. If we all knew what to do for stroke patients there would be no need for randomized controlled trials to help us do better—an unrealistic scenario if ever there was one. So where there is uncertainty, and where we disagree, we have tried to make that plain. But, on the whole, we are all still prepared to sign up to the practice points.

In this second edition, we have been able to correct the surprising number of minor typographical errors and hope not to have introduced any more, get all the X-rays the right way up, improve on some of the figures, remove some duplication, reorder a few sections, put in some more subheadings to guide the readers, make the section on acute ischaemic stroke more directive, improve the index, and generally tidy the whole thing up. It should now be easier to keep track of intracranial venous thrombosis and, in response to criticism, we have extended the section on leukoaraiosis, even though it is not strictly either a cause or a consequence of stroke. We have also introduced citations to what we have called 'floating references'—in other words, published work that is constantly being changed and updated as new information becomes available. An obvious example is the Cochrane Library, which is updated every 3 months and available on CD-ROM and the Internet. There are no page numbers, and the year of publication is always the present one. We have therefore cited such 'floating references' as being in the present year 2000. But we know that this book will not be read much until the year 2001 and subsequent years, when readers will have to look at the contemporary Cochrane Library, not the one published in 2000. The same applies to the new *British Medical Journal* series called 'Clinical Evidence' which is being updated every 6 months, and to any websites that may be updated at varying intervals and are still very much worth directing readers towards.

Rather to our surprise, there is a lot of new information to get across on stroke. Compared with 4 years ago, the concept of organized stroke services staffed by experts in stroke care has taken root and has allowed the increasingly rapid assessment of patients with 'brain attacks'. It is no longer good enough to sit around waiting 24 h or more to see if a patient is going to have a transient ischaemic attack or a stroke, and then another 24 h for a CT brain scan to exclude intracerebral haemorrhage. These days we have to assess and scan stroke patients as soon as they arrive in hospital, perhaps give thrombolysis to a few, and enter many more into clinical trials, start aspirin in ischaemic stroke, and get the multidisciplinary team involved—and all of this well within 24 h of symptom onset. Through the Cochrane Library, which was in its infancy when the first edition was published, there is now easy, regularly updated electronic access to systematic reviews of most of the acute interventions and secondary prevention strategies for stroke, although the evidence base for rehabilitation techniques is lagging behind. Catheter angiography is giving way to non-invasive imaging. MR techniques are racing ahead of the evidence as to how they should be used in routine clinical practice. For better or worse, coiling cerebral aneurysms is replacing clipping. The pharmaceutical industry is still tenaciously hanging on to the hope of 'neuroprotection' in acute ischaemic stroke, despite numerous disappointments. Hyperhomocysteinaemia and infections are the presently fashionable risk factors for ischaemic stroke, and they may or may not stand the test of time. So, in this second edition, we have tried to capture all these advances—and retreats—and set them in the context of an up-to-date understanding of the pathophysiology of stroke and the best available evidence of how to manage it. Of course, it is an impossible task, because something new is always just around the corner. But then 'breakthroughs' in medicine take time to mature—maybe years until the evidence becomes unassailable and is gradually accepted by front-line clinicians. And then we can all sit back doing what we believe to be 'the right thing' for a few more years until the next 'breakthrough' changes our view of the world yet again.

We hope that the ideas and recommendations in this book will be sufficient 99% of the time—at least for the next 4 years, when we will have to see about a third edition.

CHAPTER TWO

Development of knowledge concerning cerebrovascular disease

'Our knowledge of disorders of the cerebral circulation and their manifestations is deficient in all aspects' was the opening sentence of the chapter on cerebrovascular diseases in a popular German textbook of neurology at the beginning of the 20th century (Oppenheim 1913). Almost 90 years later, this lament still holds true, despite the considerable advances that have been made since then. In fact, the main reason for Oppenheim suggesting this deficiency—the limitations of pathological anatomy—is almost equally valid today. True, our methods of observation nowadays are no longer confined to the dead, as they were then, and they have been greatly expanded, first by catheter angiography, then by brain imaging and measurement of cerebral blood flow and metabolism, and most recently by non-invasive methods of vascular imaging such as ultrasound and magnetic resonance angiography. None the less, our observations are still mostly anatomical, and after the event. It is only in rare instances that are we able to reconstruct the dynamics of a stroke—even less for ischaemic than haemorrhagic stroke, in which brain computed tomography (CT) or magnetic resonance imaging (MRI) in the acute phase gives an indication of where a blood vessel has ruptured (although not why exactly there, and why at that time) and how far the extravasated blood has invaded the brain parenchyma or the subarachnoid space. With ischaemic stroke, one may find a source of embolism in the heart or a large artery, but the embolus itself usually escapes detection except by ultra-early angiography (Fieschi *et al.* 1989) or transcranial ultrasound techniques (Zanette *et al.* 1995). Only too often, the physician is left with a dead piece of brain, without even the faintest clue about either the malefactor or the weapon. The few instances in which a stroke is caught red-handed are made up of fatal events, e.g. massive infarction when an embolus is mechanically dislodged from the internal carotid artery (Beal *et al.* 1981), or haemorrhages occurring during a scanning procedure, such as rupture of an aneurysm during angiography (Hayakawa *et al.* 1978; Saitoh *et al.* 1995), or haemorrhagic transformation in several areas of an infarct at the same time in a patient on anticoagulants (Franke *et al.* 1990).

So it is with modesty, rather than in triumph, that we look back on the past. In each epoch, the problems of stroke have been approached by the best minds, with the best tools available. Of course many ideas in the past were wrong, but so presumably are many of our own. Even though we are firm believers in what is now called 'evidence-based medicine', some of our notions may well be based on paradigms that will not survive the test of time. Our knowledge may have vastly increased in the recent past, but it is still a mere island in an ocean of ignorance.

2.1 Ideas change slowly

The history of medicine, like that of kings and queens in world history, is usually described by a string of dates and names, by which we leapfrog from one discovery to another. The interval between such identifiable advances is measured in centuries when we describe the art of medicine at the beginning of civilization, but in mere years where our present times are chronicled. This leads to the impression that we are witnessing a dazzling explosion of knowledge. Some qualifications of this view are needed, however. First of all, any generation of mankind takes a myopic view of history, in that the importance of recent developments is overestimated. The Swedish Academy of Sciences therefore often waits for years—sometimes even decades—before awarding Nobel prizes, until scientific discoveries have withstood the test of time. When exceptions were made for the prize in medicine, the early accolades were often not borne out: Wagner-Jauregg's malaria treatment of neurosyphilis (1927) is no longer regarded as a landmark, and Moniz's prize (1949) for prefrontal leucotomy seems no longer justified, but at least he also introduced contrast angiography of the brain, although this procedure may again not survive beyond the end of this century. We can only hope that the introduction of X-ray CT by Hounsfield (Nobel prize for medicine in 1979; Fig. 2.8) will be judged as equally momentous by future generations as by ourselves.

Another important caveat in reviewing progress in medicine is that most discoveries gain ground only slowly. Even if new insights were quickly accepted by peer scientists, which was often not the case, it could still be decades before these had trickled down to the rank and file of medical practitioners. The mention of a certain date for a discovery may create the false impression that this change in medical thinking occurred almost overnight, like the introduction of a single European currency. In most instances, this was far from the truth. An apt example is the extremely slow rate at which the concept of lacunar infarction became accepted by the medical community, despite its profound implications in terms of pathophysiology, treatment and prognosis. The first pathological descriptions date from around 1840 (Dechambre 1838; Durand-Fardel 1842), but it took the clinicopathological correlations of C. Miller Fisher (Fig. 2.6) in the 1960s before the neurological community and its textbooks started to take any notice (Fisher & Curry 1965; Fisher 1965; Fisher 1969). However, it was not until the instantaneous clinicoanatomical correlations provided by high-resolution techniques for brain imaging in the 1980s that no practising neurologist could avoid knowing about lacunar infarcts—some 150 years after the first description! It is best to become reconciled to the idea that a slow rate of diffusion of new knowledge is unavoidable. A contemporary survey amongst primary care physicians in the US, in which they were asked about their use of recent clinical advances (such as the determination of glycosylated haemoglobin as a measure for the control of diabetes) showed that between 20% and 50% of them were not aware of these advances, or were not using them (Williamson *et al.* 1989). The problem is one of all times. Biumi, one of the early pathologists, lamented in 1765: 'Sed difficile est adultis novas opiniones inserere, evellere insitas' ('But it is difficult to insert new opinions into adults and to remove rooted ones'). How slowly new ideas were accepted and acted upon, against the background of contemporary knowledge, can often be inferred from textbooks, particularly if written by full-time clinicians rather than by research-minded neurologists. An American textbook from 1923 even cites some observations of Morgagni, dating from 1761 (Jelliffe & White 1923)! None the less, we shall occasionally quote old textbooks to illustrate the development of thinking about stroke, particularly important landmarks.

Conversely, a new discovery or even a new fashion may be interpreted beyond its proper limits and linger on as a distorted idea for decades. Take the discovery of vitamin B_1 deficiency as the cause of a tropical polyneuropathy almost a century ago; the notion that a neurological condition, considered untreatable almost by definition, could be cured by a simple nutritional supplement made such an impact on the medical community that even in some Western countries vitamin B_1 is still widely used as a panacea for almost any neurological symptom.

Therefore, there are at least two kinds of medical history—at the front line and that of the medical profession as a whole. The landmarks are easy to identify only with the hindsight of present knowledge. In reality, new ideas often only gradually dawned on consecutive scientists, instead of the popular notion of a blinding flash of inspiration occurring in a single individual. For this reason, interpretations of the history of stroke are not always identical (Schiller 1970; McHenry 1981). A related problem, and one that we have only partly solved in this chapter, is that many important primary sources are not only scarce, but also not easily accessible, having been written in Latin.

2.2 The anatomy of the brain and its blood supply

From at least the time of Hippocrates (460–370 BC), the brain was credited with intelligence and thought, and also with movements of the opposite side of the body, judging from the occurrence of unilateral convulsions after head wounds on the contralateral side (McHenry 1969). Yet stroke, or 'apoplexy' (being struck down), was defined as a sudden but mostly general, rather than focal, disorder of the brain. The pathogenesis was explained according to the humoral theory, based on the balance between the four humours: blood, phlegm, black bile and yellow bile. Anatomy played almost no part in these explanations. Apoplexy was often attributed to accumulation of black bile in the arteries of the brain, obstructing the passage of animated spirits from the ventricles (Clarke 1963). Galen of Pergamon (131–201), a prolific writer and animal experimenter, further popularized the knowledge and tradition accumulated at the end of the Greek culture. Galen distinguished 'karos' from 'apoplexy', in that respiration was unaffected in the former condition (Galenus, edition of 1824). His texts (there are no known drawings of his observations) were to become axiomatic throughout the Dark and Middle Ages. Rearrangement and abridgement of the classical masters, particularly Galen, became the essence of medical knowledge (Karenberg & Hort 1998a). Leading Islamic physicians such as Avicenna (980–1037) tried to reconcile Galenic tenets with the Aristotelian view of the heart as the seat of the mind (Karenberg &

Hort 1998b). In Western Europe, mostly deprived of Greek learning until the fall of Constantinople in 1453 prompted the Renaissance, these Arabic texts were translated into Latin before those of Galen and Hippocrates (Jardine 1996; Karenberg & Hort 1998c). But all this was theory, without anatomical counterpart; dissection of the human body was precluded by its divine connotations. Any illustrations of the brain that are known from the 13th century (Albertus Magnus) or the following one (Mundinus) are crude and schematic representations of Galenic theories, rather than attempts at copying the forms of nature. As a consequence, many other disease conditions with sudden onset must have been misclassified as 'apoplexy'.

In 1543, Andries van Wesele (1514–64), the great Renaissance anatomist who Latinized his name to Andreas Vesalius, produced the first accurate drawings of the brain in his famous book *De humani corporis fabrica libri septem*, with the help of the draughtsman Johan Stephaan van Calcar and the printer Oporinus in Basle (Vesalius 1543). It was the same year in which Copernicus published *De revolutionibus*, proclaiming the sun and not the earth as the centre of the universe. Vesalius largely ignored the blood vessels of the brain, although he retracted an earlier drawing (Fig. 2.1) depicting a '*rete mirabile*', a network of blood vessels at the base of the brain that Galen had found in pigs and oxen and that had been extrapolated to the human brain ever since (Vesalius

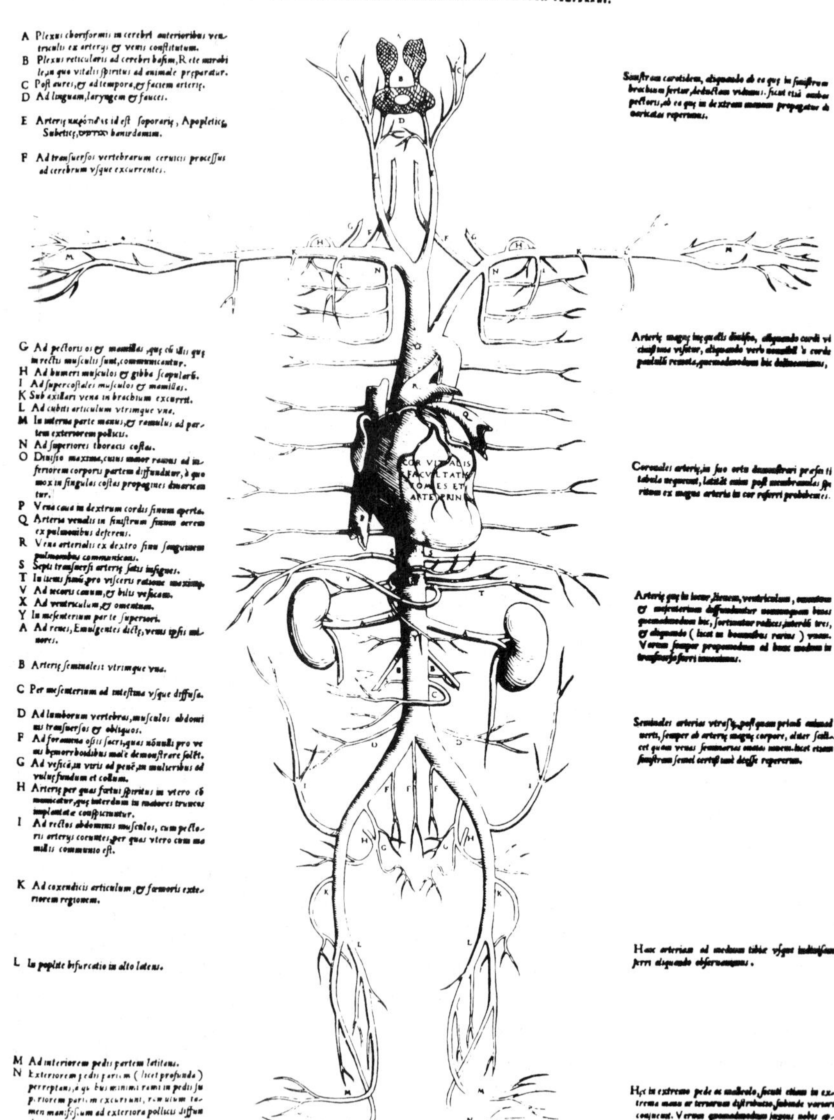

Fig. 2.1 Plate depicting the blood vessels, from Vesalius' *Tabulae Anatomicae Sex*, of 1538. This shows the carotid arteries ending up in a network (B) at the base of the brain; the structures marked (A) represent the choroid plexus in the lateral ventricles. The network of blood vessels (*rete mirabile*) is found in oxen; Galen had assumed it was found also in the human brain—a belief perpetuated throughout the Dark and Middle Ages, up to the early Renaissance. Leonardo da Vinci also drew a (human?) brain with a '*rete mirabile*' at its base (Todd 1991). Vesalius retracted the existence of a network in his atlas of 1543.

1538; Clarke & Dewhurst 1972). Before him, Berengario da Carpi had also denied the existence of the *rete* (Berengario da Carpi 1523). Vesalius was vehemently attacked by traditionally minded contemporaries as an iconoclast of Galenic dogmas, but at first he did not go as far as outright opposition to the central Galenic tenet that the blood could pass through the septum between the right and left ventricle of the heart, allowing the mixture of blood and air and the elimination of 'soot'. Instead, he praised the Creator for having made the openings so small that nobody could detect them—another striking example of how the power of theories may mislead even the most inquisitive minds. Only later, in the 1555 edition of his *De humani corporis fabrica*, did he firmly state that the interventricular septum was tightly closed. The decisive blow to the humoral theory came in 1628, through the description of the circulation by William Harvey (1578–1657), although it need no longer surprise us that it took many decades before his views were widely accepted. Harvey's work formed the foundation for the recognition of the role of blood vessels in the pathogenesis of stroke.

Thomas Willis (1641–75) is remembered not so much for having coined the term 'neurology', or for his iatrochemical theories, a modernized version of humoral medicine, or for his part in the successful resuscitation of Ann Green after judicial hanging (Dewhurst 1980), as he is for his work on the anatomy of the brain, first published in 1664 (Meyer & Hierons 1962), and especially for his description of the vascular interconnections at the base of the brain (Fig. 2.2). Before him, others had observed at least part of the circle (Fallopius 1561; Casserio 1627; Vesling 1647; Wepfer 1658), in the case of Casserio and Vesling even with an illustration. But, undisputedly, it was Willis who most clearly grasped the functional implications of these anastomoses, in a passage illustrating his proficiency in performing necropsies as well as post-mortem experiments (from a posthumous translation) (Willis 1684):

> We have elsewhere shewed, that the *Cephalick* Arteries, viz. the *Carotides*, and the *Vertebrals*, do so communicate with one another, and all of them in different places, are so ingraffed one in another mutually, that if it happen, that many of them should be stopped or pressed together at once, yet the blood being admitted to the Head, by the passage of one Artery only, either the *Carotid* or the *Vertebral*, it would presently pass thorow all those parts exterior and interior: which indeed we have sufficiently proved by an experiment, for that Ink being squirted in the trunk of one Vessel, quickly filled all the sanguiferous passages, and every where stained the Brain it self. I once opened the dead Carcase of one wasted away, in which the right Arteries, both the *Carotid* and the *Vertebral*, within the Skull, were become bony and impervious, and did shut forth the blood from that side, notwithstanding the sick person was not troubled with the astonishing Disease.

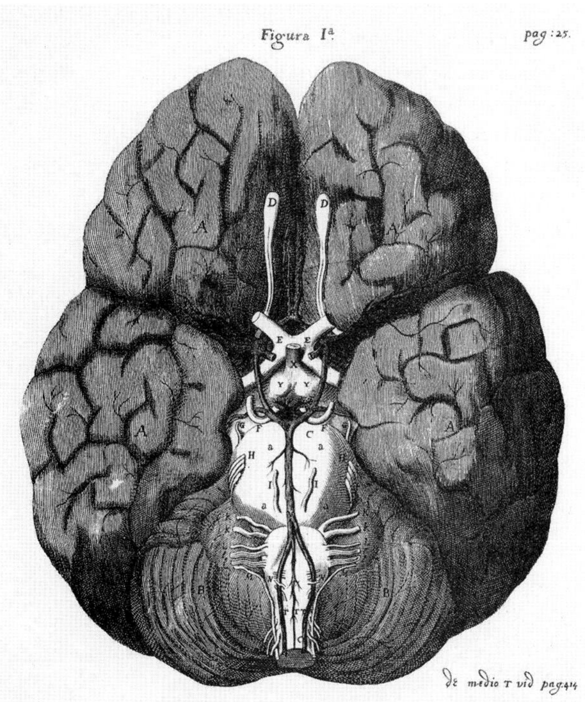

Fig. 2.2 Illustration of the base of the brain from Willis's *Cerebri Anatome* (1664), showing the interconnections between the right and left carotid systems, and also between these two and the posterior circulation (drawing by Christopher Wren).

It seems that the idea of infusing coloured liquids into blood vessels, practised from 1659 onwards, had come from Christopher Wren (1632–1723) (Dewhurst 1980). He also made the etchings for Willis's book; after the great fire of London in 1666, Wren was the architect of St. Paul's cathedral and numerous other churches.

2.3 What happens in 'apoplexy'?

Willis's 'astonishing Disease', apoplexy, had of old intuitively been attributed to some ill-defined obstruction, whether from want of 'animal spirits' via the nerves in the tradition of Greek medicine, or, after Harvey's time, by deprivation of blood flow. Yet it should be remembered that the notion of an intrinsic 'nervous energy' only slowly lost ground. Even the great 18th-century physician Boerhaave, though clearly recognizing the role of blood vessels and the heart in the development of apoplexy, also invoked obstruction of the cerebrospinal fluid (Boerhaave 1715). In Table 2.1 we have provided a schematic representation of the development of ideas about apoplexy, and their relationship to arterial lesions, through the ages. That Willis had found 'bony' and 'impervious' arteries in patients who actually had not died from a stroke was probably the reason that he was not outspoken on the pathogenesis of apoplexy. His contemporaries, Wepfer (1620–95) in Schaffhausen, and Bayle (1622–1709)

Table 2.1 The development of ideas about 'apoplexy' and its relationship with arterial lesions.

Medical scientist	Ideas about 'apoplexy'		Medical scientist	Observations on arterial lesions	Historical events
	Haemorrhagic	Non-haemorrhagic			
Hippocrates (Kos) (460–370 BC)	Sudden loss of consciousness, as a result of brain disease				0 Birth of Jesus Christ
Galenus (Pergamum and Rome) (131–201)	Sudden loss of consciousness, as a result of brain disease				
Wepfer (Schaffhausen) (1620–95)	Extravasation of blood in brain tissue (1658)		Wepfer (Schaffhausen) (1620–1695)	'Corpora fibrosa' (1658)	1642 Rembrandt paints *Night Watch*
Bayle (Toulouse) (1622–1709)			Bayle (Toulouse) (1622–1709)	Calcifications (1677)	1682 Peter I ascends Russian throne
Willis (Oxford) (1621–75)			Willis (Oxford) (1621–1675)	'Bony, impervious arteries' (1684)	
Mistichelli (Pisa) (1675–1715)	Paralysis is unilateral, and crossed with respect to lesion (1709)				1707 Union between England and Scotland
Boerhaave (Leiden) (1668–1738)	'Stoppage of the spirits'		Boerhaave (Leiden) (1668–1735)	Narrowing due to cartilaginous change (1735)	1729 Bach writes *St Matthew's Passion*
Morgagni (Padua) (1682–1771)	'Sanguineous apoplexy' (1761)	'Serous apoplexy', extravasation of serum? (1761)			1776 US Declaration of Independence
Baillie (London) (1761–1823)			Baillie (London) (1761–1823)	Hardening of arteries associated with haemorrhage? (1795)	
Rostan (Paris) (1790–1866)		'Ramollissement' (1820): —softening more frequent than haemorrhage —condition not inflammatory?	Rostan (Paris) (1790–1866)	Ossification of cerebral arteries (1820)	1815 Battle of Waterloo; Schubert writes *Erlkönig*

Lallemand (Montpellier) (1790–1853)	Cerebral softening is definitely inflammatory in nature (1824)			
Lobstein (Strasburg) (1777–1835)		Lobstein (Strasburg) (1777–1835)	'Arteriosclerosis' (1829)	1829 Stephenson builds the railway steam engine 'The Rocket'
Abercrombie (Edinburgh) (1780–1844)	Cerebral softening analogous to gangrene of limb? (1836)	Abercrombie (Edinburgh) (1780–1844)	Due to ossification of of arteries?	1837 Queen Victoria ascends throne of British Empire
Carswell (London) (1793–1857)	Cerebral softening caused by obliteration of arteries? (one of possible causes, 1838)			1848 Year of revolutions; Louis-Napoléon elected President of France
Rokitansky (Vienna) (1804–78)	'Encephalomalacia' (1844): —white, or serous (congestion) —red (inflammatory) —yellow (frequent; unexplained)			1859 Darwin publishes *The Origin of Species*
Cruveilhier (Paris) (1791–1874)	Cerebral softening caused by capillary congestion, secondary to 'irritation' (1862)			1863 Manet paints *Le Déjeuner sur l'herbe*
Virchow (Berlin) (1821–1902)	'Yellow softening'of the brain is secondary to arterial obliteration (Carswell); any inflammation is secondary	Virchow (Berlin) (1821–1902)	Arteriosclerosis leads to thrombosis; thrombi may be torn off and lodge distally ('embolism') (1856)	1869 Opening of the Suez Canal
Cohnheim (Berlin) (1839–1884)	'Infarction' (stuffing) is haemorrhagic by definition, as opposed to ischaemic necrosis (1872)	Cohnheim (Berlin) (1839–1884)	End-arteries most vulnerable; paradoxical embolism	1871 Stanley meets Livingstone at Ujiji 1877 Bell invents telephone, Edison the phonograph
		Chiari (Prague) (1851–1916)	Thrombosis at the carotid bifurcation may cause secondary embolization to the brain (1905)	1895 Röntgen discovers X-rays in Würzburg 1907 Ehrlich introduces arsphenamine as treatment for syphilis

in Toulouse, only tentatively associated apoplexy with 'corpora fibrosa' (Wepfer 1658) or with calcification of cerebral arteries (Bayle 1677).

Wepfer not only recognized arterial lesions, but he also made one of the great advances in the knowledge about stroke by distinguishing between, on the one hand, arterial obstruction preventing the influx of blood and, on the other, extravasation of blood into the substance of the brain or the ventricular cavities, which were traditionally seen as an important source of mental energy. What still largely escaped him was the focal nature of apoplexia, which instead he mainly regarded as a process of global stunning. The four cases of haemorrhage Wepfer described were massive, at the base of the brain or deep in the parenchyma. In cases with obvious hemiplegia—incidentally a term dating back to Byzantine medicine in the 7th century (Paulus Aegineta (625–690); edition of 1844)—Wepfer suspected dysfunction of the ipsilateral rather than the contralateral side. He also observed patients who had recovered from apoplectic attacks, and he noted that those most liable to apoplexy were 'the obese, those whose face and hands are livid, and those whose pulse is constantly unequal'.

That the paralysis was on the opposite side of the apoplectic lesion was clearly predicted by Domencio Mistichelli (1675–1715) from Pisa (Mistichelli 1709) on the basis of his observation of the decussation of the pyramids (Fig. 2.3). A landmark in the recognition of the anatomical substrate of stroke was the work of Morgagni (1682–1771); he was professor of medicine and subsequently of pathological anatomy in Padua. In 1761, Morgagni published an impressive series of clinicopathological observations collected over a lifetime (he was 79 at the time of publication), in which he not only confirmed the notion of crossed paralysis but also firmly divided apoplexy into 'sanguineous apoplexy' and 'serous apoplexy' (and a third form that was neither serous nor sanguineous) (Morgagni 1761). A decade later, Portal (1742–1832) rightly emphasized that it was impossible to distinguish between these two forms during life (Portal 1781). It would be a grave anachronism, however, to assume that 'serous' (non-haemorrhagic) apoplexy was recognized as being the result of impaired blood flow, let alone of mechanical obstruction of blood vessels. Some even linked the arterial hardening with brain haemorrhages and not with the serous apoplexies (Baillie 1793). Although we have seen that 17th-century scientists such as Bayle and Wepfer associated some non-haemorrhagic cases of apoplexy with obstruction of blood flow, in the 18th century medical opinion swayed towards 'vascular congestion', a kind of prehaemorrhagic state. That explanation was propounded not only by Morgagni (Morgagni 1761), but also by many of his contemporaries and followers (Portal 1781; Hall 1836; Burrows 1846). Cheyne (1777–1836) pointed out that, in patients who had survived a 'stroke of apoplexy' for a considerable time, post-mortem examination might show a brain cavity filled with serum which was rusty yellow in colour and which may have stained the substance of the adjacent brain tissue; but he may have been describing a residual lesion after cerebral haemorrhage rather than infarction (Cheyne 1812).

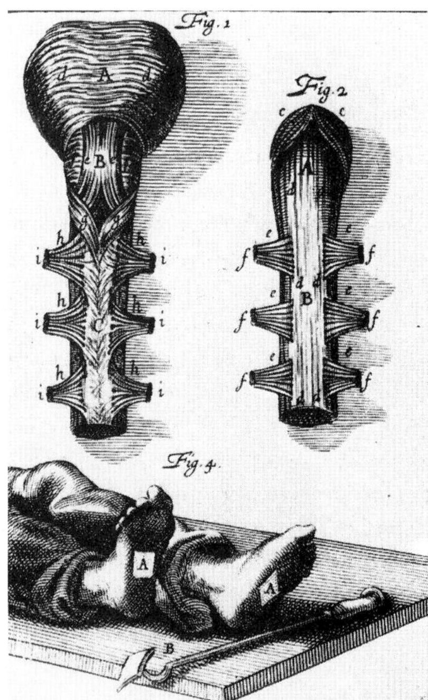

Fig. 2.3 Illustration from Mistichelli's book on apoplexy (1709), in which he shows the decussation of the pyramids and also the outward rotation of the leg on the paralysed side.

The anatomical, organ-based approach exemplified by Morgagni reflected the Italian practice, in which the separation between physicians and surgeons was much less strict than in northern Europe with its more theoretical framework of medicine. The proponents of the latter school of thinking were Boerhaave (1668–1738) in Leiden and later Cullen (1710–90) in Edinburgh, both the most influential clinical teachers of their time. They established a nosological classification that was based much more on holistic theory, in terms of a disturbed system, than on actual observations at the level of the organ, at least with 20th-century hindsight (King 1991). Probably our own time will be branded as the era of exaggerated reductionism! In the intellectual tradition of the Dutch–Scottish school, purely clinical classifications of apoplexy were proposed in the early 19th century by Serres (with and without paralysis), by Abercrombie (primary apoplexy, with deprivation of sense and motion, and sometimes with convulsions; a second type beginning with headache; and a third type with loss of power on one side of the body and of speech, often with recovery) and by Hope and Bennett (transient apoplexy, primary apoplexy with death or slow recovery, ingravescent apoplexy with partial recovery and relapse, and paraplexic apoplexy with paralysis) (Serres 1819; Abercrombie 1828; Hope *et al.* 1840).

There are several reasons why the brain lesion in what we now call cerebral infarction was not actually identified until the middle of the 19th century. Firstly, it was impossible to recognize ischaemic softening in patients who had usually died not long after their stroke. Fixation methods were not available until the end of the 18th century; Vicq d'Azyr, Marie Antoinette's physician, was the first to use alcohol as a tissue fixative (Vicq d'Azyr 1786), and formaldehyde fixation was not employed until a century later (Blum 1893). Secondly, it is probable that many patients diagnosed as having died from apoplexy in fact had suffered from other conditions. If in our time the diagnosis can be wrong in as many as 13% of patients referred and subsequently admitted to hospital with a presumed stroke (Norris & Hachinski 1982), the diagnostic accuracy was presumably no better in centuries past.

2.4 Cerebral infarction (ischaemic stroke)

The organ-based approach to medicine quickly spread from Italy to other countries. In France, the first proponents were surgeons. After the French revolution, the strict distinction between medicine and surgery disappeared, driven by the reorganization of hospital care (no longer managed by the church but by the state) and by the need to train a large number of new doctors for military as well as civilian duties ('peu lire, beaucoup voir, beaucoup faire') (Foucault 1963; Bynum 1994). It was Léon Rostan (1790–1866) (Fig. 2.4), a physician at the Salpêtrière in Paris, who clearly recognized softening of the brain as a separate lesion, distinct from haemorrhage, although the pathogenesis still escaped him. He published his findings in an unillustrated monograph, the first edition of which appeared in 1820 (Rostan 1820). The lesions were most commonly found in the corpus striatum, thalamus and centrum semiovale, but they also occurred in the cerebral cortex, brainstem and cerebellum. Old cases showed a yellowish-green discoloration, whereas if the patients had died soon after the event, the colour of the lesion was chestnut or reddish. The softening might be so exteme as to lead to the formation of a cyst. In other patients, it was difficult to detect any change in firmness or in colour. Rostan distinguished softening of the brain from 'apoplexy', a term he no longer used for stroke in general, but which he regarded as being synonymous with haemorrhagic stroke. He supposed that softening of the brain was more frequent than brain haemorrhage, although some haemorrhages were secondary to softening. The clinical manifestations were thought to occur in two stages: first "fugitive" disturbances in the use of a limb, in speech, or in visual or auditory perception, sooner or later followed by hemiplegia and coma, in a slowly progressive fashion.

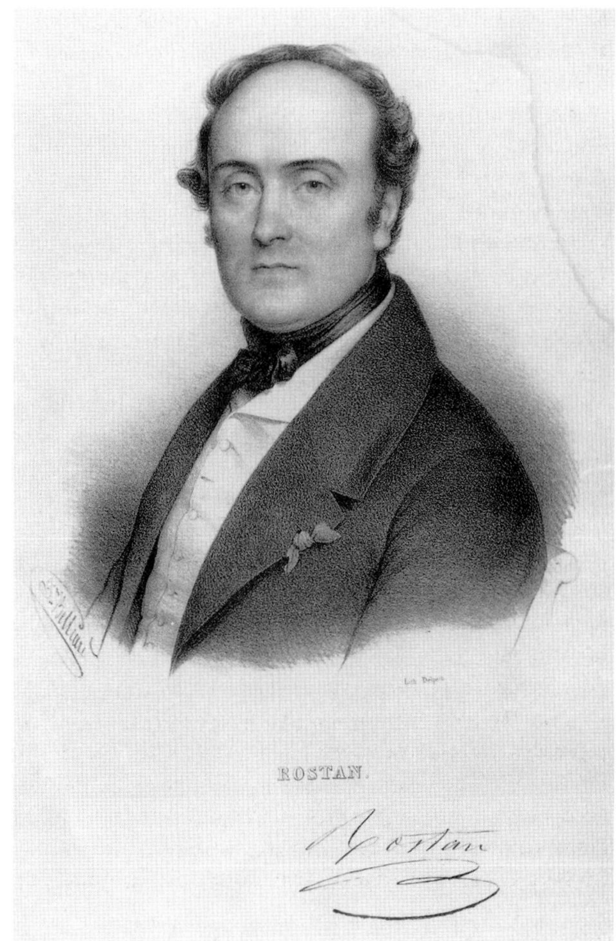

Fig. 2.4 Léon Rostan (1790–1866).

Although Rostan recognized 'ossification' of the cerebral arteries, he did not associate these lesions with cerebral softening via obstruction of the arterial system. That 'paradigm', in 20th-century terminology, had not yet entered medicine (Kuhn 1962). But at least he doubted the prevailing opinion that the lesion was some kind of inflammatory response. After all, there was redness and swelling (*rubor*, *tumor*), if not warmth and pain (*calor*, *dolor*), to complete the cardinal signs of inflammation delineated by Celsus in the first century AD. Rostan's contemporary Lallemand (1790–1853) was much more outspoken, and had little doubt that inflammation was at the root of cerebral softening (Lallemand 1824). Twentieth-century doctors who find this difficult to understand should understand that inflammation was one of the overriding medical paradigms from the middle of the 18th century until the middle of the 19th (King 1991). Just as in our time some poorly understood disease conditions are explained in terms of slow virus infections or autoimmune disease, perhaps erroneously, inflammation seemed for a long time the most logical explanation for liquefaction of brain tissue.

The first suspicion of a relationship between arterial disease and *'ramollissement'*, as many English writers continued to call brain softening in deference to Rostan, was voiced by Abercrombie, in a late edition of his textbook (Abercrombie 1836). He drew an analogy with gangrene, caused by 'failure of circulation', this in turn being secondary to 'ossification of arteries'. The role of arterial obstruction as a primary cause of softening of the brain was confirmed by others (Bright 1831; Carswell 1838), but the theory of inflammation continued to be defended by a few adherents (Cruveilhier 1842; Durand-Fardel 1843). Some were aware that apoplexy could be caused by 'cerebral anaemia' (as opposed to congestion), not only through loss of blood but also by reduced vascular pressure, particularly in the case of heart disease (Burrows 1846).

Other missing links in the understanding of cerebral infarction were clarified by Rokitansky (1804–78) in Vienna and Virchow (1821–1902) in Berlin. Rokitansky divided cerebral softening (which he termed 'encephalomalacia') into three varieties: red (haemorrhagic) softening, inflammatory in nature; white softening (synonymous with 'serous apoplexy'), caused by congestion and oedema; and, the most common variety, yellow softening, of which the pathogenesis was unknown. Virchow (Fig. 2.5) revolutionized medical thinking about vascular disease by firmly putting the emphasis on changes in the vessel wall rather than in the blood; Schiller called this the victory of 'solidism' over 'humoralism' (Schiller 1970). Virchow also firmly established that thrombosis of arteries was caused not by inflammation but by fatty metamorphosis of the vessel wall, even if he had to found his own journal before his papers were published (Virchow 1847; Virchow 1856). For these changes in the arterial wall, Virchow revived the term 'arteriosclerosis', first used by Lobstein (Lobstein 1829). Virchow's disciple, Julius Cohnheim, introduced the word 'infarction' in a medical context, but strictly reserved it for haemorrhagic necrosis ('stuffing', by seeping of blood into ischaemic tissue, through damaged walls of capillaries) as opposed to ischaemic necrosis (Cohnheim 1872).

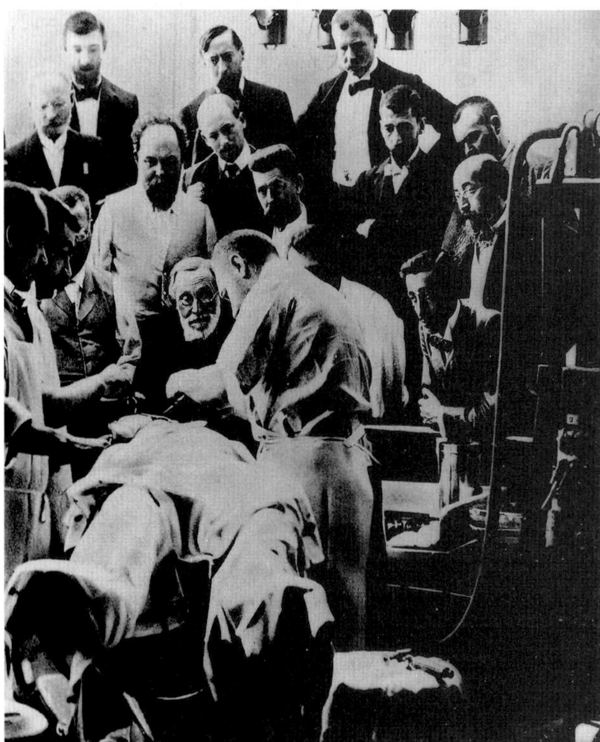

Fig. 2.5 Rudolph Virchow (1821–1902), teaching at a post-mortem in the Charité Hospital in Berlin.

2.5 Thrombosis and embolism

Virchow observed thrombosis secondary to atherosclerosis, and also embolism (a term newly coined by him, at least in medical parlance) in patients with gangrene of the lower limbs caused by clots from the heart. He extrapolated these events to the cause of cerebral softening (Virchow 1847): 'Here there is either no essential change in the vessel wall and its surroundings, or this is ostensibly secondary. I feel perfectly justified in claiming that these clots never originated in the local circulation but that they are torn off at a distance and carried along in the blood stream as far as they can go.'

The relationship between vegetations on the heart valves and stroke had in fact been suggested a century earlier by Boerhaave's pupil Gerard van Swieten, personal physician to the Austrian empress Maria Theresa and founder of the Viennese school of medicine (van Swieten 1755):

> It has been established by many observations that these polyps occasionally attach themselves as excrescences to the columnae carneae of the heart, and perhaps then separate from it and are propelled, along with the blood, into the pulmonary artery or the aorta, and its branches ... were they thrown into the carotid or vertebral arteries, could disturb—or if they completely blocked all approach of arterial blood to the brain—utterly abolish the functions of the brain.

For more than a century after Virchow's accurate pathological descriptions of arterial occlusions, the term 'cerebral embolism' was almost synonymous with embolism from the heart (parenthetically, it still is in many contemporary textbooks and papers—another illustration of how slowly ideas change). Sources of embolism in the extracranial arteries were hardly considered until the 1960s, at least in teaching. By the same token, the term 'cerebral thrombosis' remained firmly entrenched in clinical thinking as being more or less synonymous with cerebral infarction without associated heart disease, the implication being that in these cases the site of the atheromatous occlusion was in the intracranial vessels. For example, this is what the sixth edition of Brain's *Diseases of the Nervous System* says on the subject (Brain 1968):

> Progressive occlusion of cerebral blood vessels impairs the circulation in the regions they supply. The effects of this depend upon the size and situation of the vessel, and the rate of onset of the occlusion particularly in relation to the collateral circulation. Actual obstruction

of an artery by atheroma, with or without subsequent thrombosis, causes softening of the region of the brain supplied by the vessel.

That the notion of 'local atherosclerosis = *in situ* thrombosis' has persisted for such a long time must have been because of its appealing simplicity, not because there were no observations to the contrary. As long ago as 1905, Chiari had drawn attention to the frequency of atherosclerosis in the region of the carotid bifurcation and had suggested that embolization of atheromatous material might be a cause of cerebral softening (Chiari 1905), and not much later Hunt had described the relationship between carotid occlusion and stroke (Hunt 1914). But the general acceptance of *extracranial* atherosclerosis as an important cause of cerebral ischaemia came only after two further developments. The first was the attention generated by Miller Fisher's studies, in which he re-emphasized the role of atherosclerosis at the carotid bifurcation, at least in white patients (Fisher 1951). He clinically correlated these lesions not only with contralateral hemiplegia but also with attacks of monocular blindness in the ipsilateral eye (Fisher 1952). The second development was imaging. Cerebral angiography by direct puncture of the carotid artery had been introduced in Portugal by Moniz in 1927 (Moniz 1927; Moniz 1940), but imaging of the carotid bifurcation in patients with stroke became common only after the advent of catheter angiography (Seldinger 1953), and later of ultrasound techniques. These methods often showed abnormalities of the internal carotid artery near its origin, at least in patients with transient or permanent deficits from presumed ischaemia in the territory of the mainstem of the middle cerebral artery, or one of its branches. If these patients are investigated early—within 6 h of the attack—the site where the embolus has become impacted can be demonstrated even more often than its source, in about 75% of patients, by means of angiography (Fieschi *et al.* 1989) or with transcranial Doppler monitoring (Zanette *et al.* 1995). The therapeutic implications of identifying lesions in the extracranial carotid artery in symptomatic patients became clear through the two large randomized controlled trials of carotid endarterectomy in the 1980s and 1990s, which showed overall benefit from the operation for severe degrees of stenosis, in the first few years after symptom onset (Barnett *et al.* 1998; European Carotid Surgery Trial Collaborative Group 1998).

In some 40% of patients with temporary or permanent occlusion of large intracranial vessels, no source of embolism can be found in the neck or in the heart. Pathological observations suggesting that the aorta may harbour atherosclerotic lesions (Soloway & Aronson 1964) were recently confirmed in a large post-mortem series (Amarenco *et al.* 1992). During life, transoesophageal echocardiography may similarly detect sources of embolism in the aorta more often in stroke patients than in controls, or in patients with known atheromatous lesions elsewhere in the cerebral circulation (Amarenco *et al.* 1994). Of course, there is more to ischaemic stroke than thromboembolism from large vessels, but the history of small vessel disease and non-atheromatous causes of ischaemia is rather recent, and these subjects will be taken up in Chapters 6 and 7.

Before concluding the sections on cerebral infarction, thrombosis and embolism, we should like briefly to draw attention to the term 'cerebrovascular accident' ('CVA') which enjoyed some undeserved popularity in the middle half of the 20th century. One problem was that sometimes it was used as synonymous with cerebral infarction, at other times as denoting stroke in general. In this day and age, the term is a highly specific sign of woolly thinking. We can do no better than quote Schiller (Schiller 1970):

> That rather blurry and pompous piece of nomenclature must have issued from the well-meant tendency to soften the blow to patients and their relatives, also from a desire to replace 'stroke', a pithy term that may sound unscientific and lacking gentility. 'Cerebrovascular accident (CVA)' can be traced to the early 1930s—between 1932, to be exact, when it was still absent from the 15th edition of *Dorland's Medical Dictionary*, and the following edition of 1936 where it first appeared.

The occasional medical student or junior doctor who still takes recourse to the term 'CVA' in an attempt to cover up ignorance about the precise type of stroke in a given patient (while avoiding sharing terms with the laity) should either find out or come clean about not knowing. Anyway, there is nothing 'accidental' about most strokes; there are different types of strokes and there are many causes that are anything but accidental.

2.6 Transient ischaemic attacks

It is difficult to trace the first descriptions of what we now call transient ischaemic attacks (TIAs) of the brain or eye, because symptoms representing focal deficits were not clearly distinguished from non-specific symptoms of a more global nature such as fainting or headache (Hachinski 1982). Wepfer recorded that he had seen patients who recovered from hemiplegia in one day or less (Wepfer 1658). An 18th-century account has been retrieved in the patient's own words, not muddled by medical interpretation (Kraaijeveld *et al.* 1984), and therefore it is as lucid as it would have been today. The subject is Jean Paul Grandjean de Fouchy, writing in 1783, at the age of 76 years (Benton & Joynt 1960):

> Toward the end of dinner, I felt a little increase of pain above the left eye and in that very instant I became unable to pronounce the words that I wanted. I heard what was said, and I thought of what I ought to reply, but I spoke other words than those which would express my thoughts, or if I began them I did not complete them, and I substituted other words for them.

> I had nevertheless all movements as freely as usual ... I saw all objects clearly, I heard distinctly what was being said; and the organs of thought were, it seemed to me, in a natural state. This sort of paroxysm lasted almost a minute.

Once it had become established, in the middle of the 19th century, that cerebral softening was not caused by an inflammatory process but by occlusion of cerebral arteries, temporary episodes of ischaemia were recognized increasingly often (Wood 1852; Jackson 1875; Hammond 1881; Gowers 1893; Osler 1911; Oppenheim 1913). In the course of time, three main theories have been invoked to explain the pathophysiology of TIAs, at least in relation to atherosclerosis: the vasospasm theory, the haemodynamic theory, and the thromboembolic theory (Hachinski 1982).

2.6.1 The vasospasm theory

Arterial spasm as a cause of gangrene of the extremities was described by Raynaud (1834–81) in his doctoral thesis of 1862 (Raynaud 1862). His theory of vasospasm was then extrapolated to the cerebral circulation (Peabody 1891; Russel 1909). The latter, writing about a 50-year-old farmer who had suffered three attacks of tingling and numbness in the right arm and the right side of the face, dismissed thrombosis ('Thrombus, once formed, does not break up and disappear in some mysterious way') and instead invoked a phenomenon of 'local syncope', analogous to Raynaud's disease, or some cases of migraine: 'There must be some vessel constriction, local in site, varying in degree and in extent, coming and going, intermittent' (Russel 1909). Even the great Osler mounted the bandwagon of the vasospastic theory to explain transient attacks of aphasia and paralysis: 'We have plenty of evidence that arteries may pass into a state of spasm with obliteration of the lumen and loss of function in the parts supplied' (Osler 1911). Vasospasm remained the most popular theory to explain transient ischaemic attacks (TIAs) in the first half of the 20th century, and provided the rationale for so-called cerebral vasodilators. Up to the 1980s, this class of presumably useless drugs was still widely prescribed in some European countries, not only for TIAs but for 'senility' in general, and in France these drugs were the third most commonly prescribed category in 1982 (Payer 1989).

In the front line of medicine, however, the vasospastic theory has gone into decline, firstly because the cerebral arteries are amongst the least reactive in the body (Pickering 1948; Denny-Brown 1951), and secondly because more plausible theories have emerged (see below). Only under strictly defined conditions can vasospasm be a causal factor in the pathogenesis of cerebral ischaemia—namely after subarachnoid haemorrhage or in association with migraine—and even in these conditions its role is arguable. Nevertheless, vasospasm has recently resurfaced as a possible cause of episodes of transient monocular blindness that are frequent and stereotyped and have no altitudinal distribution (Burger *et al.* 1991), or even of transient motor or sensory deficits not related to migraine (Call *et al.* 1988). Such events must be extremely rare.

2.6.2 The haemodynamic theory

The notion of 'low flow' as a cause of cerebral ischaemia should perhaps be attributed to Ramsay Hunt, who drew an analogy between the symptoms of carotid stenosis or occlusion and the symptoms of intermittent claudication in patients with severe peripheral arterial disease (Hunt 1914). But it was especially after 1951, when Denny-Brown suggested that transient ischaemic attacks (TIAs) might be caused by 'episodic insufficiency in the circle of Willis', that interest in the haemodynamic aspects of TIAs was fully aroused (Denny-Brown 1951). Indeed, it was mainly the surgical community for which the concept of 'cerebral intermittent claudication' continued to have great appeal, despite the incongruity of the relatively constant blood flow to the brain, and the large fluctuations in flow that occur in the legs, dependent on the level of activity, and despite the lack of support from clinical studies. When the blood pressure was artificially lowered, by means of hexamethonium and postural tilting, in 35 patients who had either experienced TIAs or who had known carotid artery disease, only one of the patients developed symptoms of focal cerebral ischaemia before non-focal syncopal symptoms which signified global rather than focal ischaemia of the brain (Kendell & Marshall 1963). Similarly, cerebral ischaemia with naturally occurring attacks of hypotension, such as cardiac dysrhythmias, is almost always syncopal and not focal in nature (Reed *et al.* 1973), and cardiac dysrhythmias do not occur more often in patients with TIAs than in controls (De Bono & Warlow 1981). Once the first successful carotid reconstruction had been reported (Eastcott *et al.* 1954), the intuitive belief in the haemodynamic theory led to an ever-increasing number of carotid endarterectomies being performed (indeed, often called 'carotid disobstruction') in patients with and even without TIAs, despite the absence of any formal proof of efficacy. These developments caused understandable concern in the neurological community (Barnett *et al.* 1984; Warlow 1984) and fortunately ended in well-designed clinical trials, which have served to define to a large extent the place of this operation (section 16.8).

That the haemodynamic theory does not apply to the majority of patients with TIAs is not to say that the exceptional patient cannot suffer from 'misery perfusion' (Klijn *et al.* 1997). In the presence of multiple occlusions or stenoses of the extracranial arteries, the haemodynamic reserve may be so poor that minor changes in systolic blood pressure cannot be compensated for (section 6.6.5). Such triggering events include a change from a sitting to a standing position, turning the head, heating of the face or looking into bright light (Caplan & Sergay 1976; Bogousslavsky & Regli 1983; Ross Russell & Page 1983). Perhaps for this small group of patients, extracranial–intracranial bypass surgery has something to offer after all, despite the negative results of the randomized controlled trial in a large but relatively unselected group of patients with occlusion of the internal carotid or middle cerebral artery (EC-IC Bypass Study Group 1985).

2.6.3 The thromboembolic theory

In the 1950s, C. Miller Fisher (Fig. 2.6) not only gave new impetus to some older observations about the relationship between stroke and atheromatous lesions of the carotid bifurcation, but also provided evidence that the pathogenesis was more complex than could be explained by fixed arterial narrowing. Firstly, he saw a patient in whom hemiplegia had been preceded by attacks of transient monocular blindness in the contralateral eye, 'the wrong eye' (Fisher 1952). Secondly, through patient and extensive ophthalmoscopic observations, he saw white bodies passing slowly through the retinal arteries during an attack of transient monocular blindness (Fig. 2.7), the whitish appearance and friability of the moving material suggesting they were emboli, largely made up of platelets (Fisher 1959). These findings were confirmed by Ross Russell (Ross Russell 1961), whilst others saw atheromatous emboli in the retinal vessels, which did not move but had become impacted (Witmer & Schmid 1958; Hollenhorst 1961).

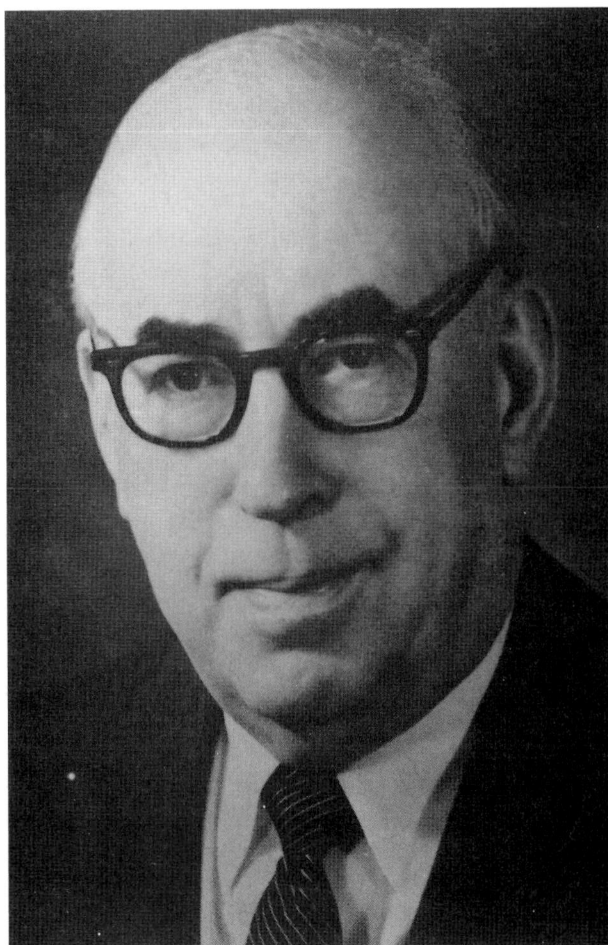

Fig. 2.6 C. Miller Fisher.

After these direct observations of the ocular fundus, additional—but more indirect—arguments corroborated the notion of artery-to-artery embolism as an important cause of transient ischaemic attacks (TIAs):

- in many patients with attacks involving the cortical territory of the middle cerebral artery there is an associated lesion of the internal carotid artery, but in only very few of them is the stenosis severe enough, with a residual lumen of 1–2 mm, for blood flow to be impaired below critical levels, even assuming there is no collateral circulation (Archie & Feldtman 1981). In addition, the stenosis is constant but the episodes of ischaemia transient, without evidence for cardiac dysrhythmias as an additional factor;
- during carotid endarterectomy, fresh and friable thrombi are seen adherent to atheromatous plaques at the carotid bifurcation, especially in those patients who had experienced recent TIAs (Gunning *et al.* 1964);
- in patients with ocular as well as cerebral TIAs, the two kinds of attack occur separately and almost never at the same time (Gunning *et al.* 1964);
- manual compression of the carotid artery may lead to dislodgement of atheromatous emboli to the cerebral circulation (Beal *et al.* 1981);
- if patients continue to have TIAs after occlusion of the ipsilateral internal carotid artery, there is often an additional atheromatous lesion in the common carotid or external carotid artery, these vessels at the same time being important collateral channels, supplying the cerebral hemisphere via retrograde flow in the ophthalmic artery (Bogousslavsky & Regli 1983);
- asymptomatic emboli have been seen to flash up during angiography (Watts 1982), and fibrin thrombi have been seen to pass through a cortical artery during craniotomy for a bypass procedure (Barnett 1979). The recently developed technique of transcranial Doppler monitoring has uncovered an ongoing stream of high-intensity transient signals, probably small emboli, in patients with symptomatic carotid lesions (Markus 1993). These signals disappear after carotid endarterectomy (Siebler *et al.* 1993), their rate depending on the interval since operation (van Zuilen *et al.* 1995).

Whilst artery-to-artery thromboembolism from atheromatous plaques may seem the most important factor in explaining TIAs and ischaemic strokes, it is not necessarily the only one, not even in single patients. For example, it is probable that emboli have especially damaging effects in vascular beds that are chronically underperfused.

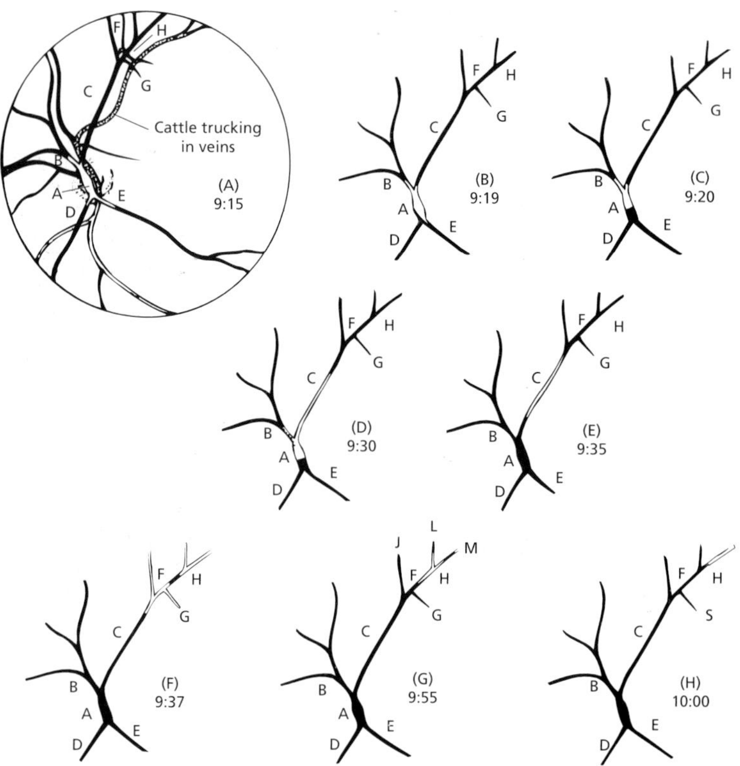

Fig. 2.7 Diagrams of observations in a patient with an attack of transient monocular blindness in the left eye (except the upper temporal quadrant); the attack had started at 8.55 a.m., 20 min before the beginning of the observations. The column of blood in the retinal arteries was in some places interrupted by white segments, initially at the stems of the superior and inferior retinal arteries (A); also the column of blood in at least six venous branches of the superior half of the retina was broken into transverse bands. The white segments in the retinal arteries slowly passed through the superior temporal artery (B–H). At (C), the vision in the upper half of the visual field had returned. At (D), a fine trickle of erythrocytes moved slowly along one side of white segment AB to the superior nasal artery, and at (E), vision had also returned in the inferior temporal quadrant. After (H), when the column of blood had been completely restored, vision returned to normal (with permission from C.M. Fisher 1959).

2.7 Intracerebral haemorrhage

As pointed out above, extravasation of blood into the brain parenchyma was first recognized by Wepfer (Wepfer 1658) and subsequently by Morgagni (Morgagni 1761). The cause remained obscure, and to a large extent still is (Adams & vander Eecken 1953). In 1855, before blood pressure could be measured, Kirkes observed hypertrophy of the heart in 17 of 22 patients with fatal brain haemorrhage (Kirkes 1855). In 1868, Charcot and Bouchard examined the brains of patients who had died from intracerebral haemorrhage and immersed them in running water; they found multiple, minute outpouchings of small blood vessels, so-called miliary aneurysms (Charcot & Bouchard 1868). The irony of these two names being joined is that Bouchard, once Charcot's pupil, in later years generated much hostility between himself and his former chief, because he wanted to found a school of his own and to be considered the most influential man in the faculty of medicine (Satran 1974; Iragui 1986). It was in this adversarial atmosphere that in 1892 Bouchard, as president of the jury that had to judge the competition for the rank of *professeur agrégé*, did not admit Charcot's pupil Babinski. Babinski subsequently left academic medicine by becoming chief of the Pitié hospital, where he devoted much time to the study of clinical signs, including the now famous 'toe sign' (van Gijn 1996). The aneurysms described by Charcot and Bouchard were white or brownish-coloured nodules about 0.5–2.0 mm in diameter, attached to a small arteriole, most often in the basal ganglia (Fig. 8.1). At the beginning of the present century, the theory of Charcot and Bouchard came under attack, and some proposed that most of these dilatations were not aneurysms at all but occlusive thrombi at the site of rupture (Ellis 1909); in Chapter 8 it is explained that some other 'miliary aneurysms' may in fact have been clots in perivascular (Virchow–Robin) spaces.

Alternative explanations for the pathogenesis of primary intracerebral haemorrhage included preceding necrosis of brain tissue, including its vessels. The frequent co-existence of hypertension led Rosenblath to postulate that a renal toxin caused necrosis of vessel walls (Rosenblath 1918), and Westphal to assume that arterial spasm was an intermediate factor (Westphal 1932). Another theory was that arteries dilate and rupture only when a previous infarct has occurred, thus depriving the feeding vessel of its normal support (Schwartz 1930; Hiller 1935; Globus *et al.* 1949)—and the notion of 'haemorrhagic transformation of an infarct' is very much alive today in the era of thrombolysis for acute ischaemic stroke (section 11.5). In the 1960s, injection techniques revived the notion of microaneurysms (Ross Russell 1963; Cole & Yates 1967), although some still suspect that the injection pressures can artifactually distend or rupture vessel walls (Challa *et al.* 1992).

Cerebral amyloid angiopathy was first recognized as a cause of primary intracerebral haemorrhage at the begin-

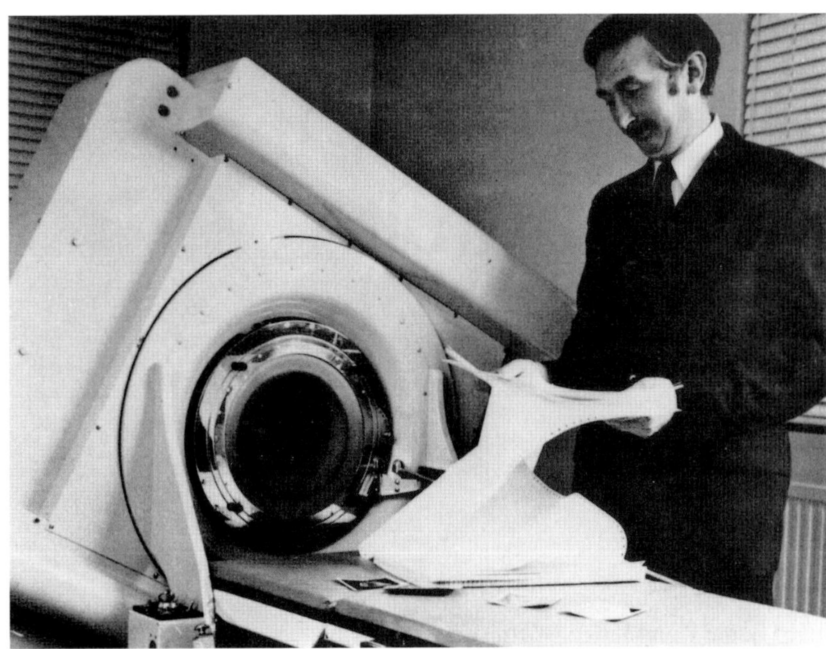

Fig. 2.8 Godfrey N. Hounsfield, the British engineer who received the Nobel prize in medicine in 1979 for the development of computed tomography (together with the American physicist A.M. Cormack).

ning of the 20th century (Fischer 1910; Scholz 1938; Pantelakis 1954). This type of haemorrhage occurs especially at the border of white and grey matter and not in the deep regions of the brain that are the most common sites of haemorrhages associated with microaneurysms. The first series of such patients appeared in the 1970s (Torack 1975; Jellinger 1977) (section 8.2.2).

The invention of computed tomography by Hounsfield (Fig. 2.8) in the 1970s made it possible to distinguish intracerebral haemorrhage quickly and reliably from cerebral infarction (Hounsfield 1973; Hayward & O'Reilly 1976) (Fig. 2.9).

2.8 Subarachnoid haemorrhage

'Meningeal apoplexy' has intrigued not only practising physicians and anatomists but also medical historians (Ljunggren *et al.* 1993). The disorder was not recognized until 3 years before the battle of Waterloo, and in the next 125 years numerous accounts appeared that combined a few personal cases with attempts to review the entire world literature up to that time, the last being a heroic overview of 1125 patients (McDonald & Korb 1939).

2.8.1 Diagnosis

The first unequivocal description of an aneurysm, although unruptured, was by Biumi in 1765, who saw it not on the circle of Willis but in the cavernous sinus (at the time called 'Vieussens' receptacle') (Biumi 1765). Morgagni had also mentioned dilatations of arteries that may have been aneurysms (Morgagni 1761). In 1812, Cheyne provided the first illustration of lethal subarachnoid haemorrhage at the base of the brain (Fig. 2.10), but the aneurysm that must have been the source of the haemorrhage was not recognized at the time (Cheyne 1812). One year later, Blackall reported a post-mortem observation in which the haemorrhage as well as the offending aneurysm (of the basilar artery) were

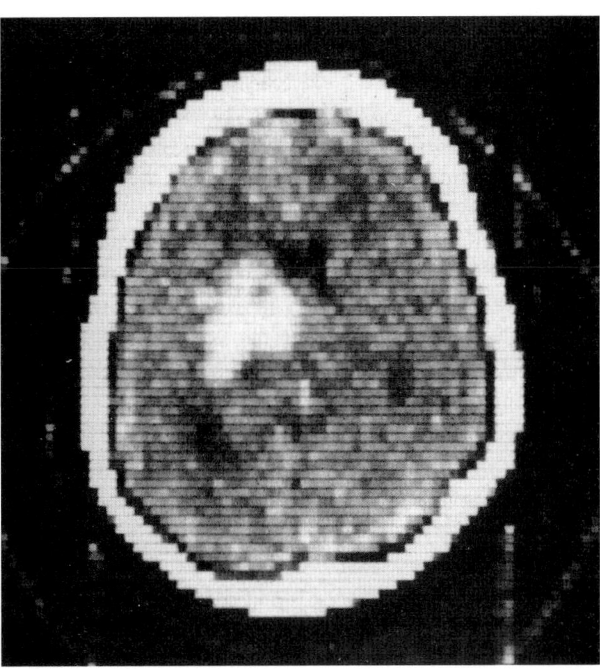

Fig. 2.9 Computed tomography scan of an intracerebral haemorrhage, made in the early 1970s (with permission from New & Scott 1975).

both identified (Blackall 1813). Soon afterwards, Hodgson emphasized that the extravasated blood was contained under the arachnoid membrane (Hodgson 1815). Serres, not aware of these publications, published two similar observations in a French periodical (Serres 1826). In England, Richard Bright, one of the champions of the movement of 'organ-based medicine' that had started in Italy and France (Berry & Mackenzie 1992), added some further case reports in 1831, including an illustration of a pea-sized aneurysm on a branch of the middle cerebral artery (Bright 1831) (Fig. 2.11). The erroneous notion that aneurysms are congenital malformations, caused by a defect in the muscular layer of the arterial wall (Chapter 9), was first put forward in 1887 (Eppinger 1887) and subsequently adopted by other writers (Wichern 1912; Turnbull 1914), to be perpetuated in contemporary textbooks and students' minds. Turnbull also pointed out, correctly, that syphilis was an extremely rare cause of aneurysms.

It took a long time before the clinical features were sorted out. Brinton pointed out that fatal rupture was not the only possible presentation of aneurysms, and that other manifestations were local pressure, convulsive attacks, or inflammation (here he probably referred to cerebral infarction, which was barely recognized at the time; section 2.4); he also found that patients could harbour aneurysms without any symptoms at all (Brinton 1852). The sudden onset of the headache and the accompanying paralysis of the third cranial nerve in some patients with aneurysms at the origin of the posterior communicating artery from the internal carotid artery led Lebert to suppose that the diagnosis might be made during life (Lebert 1866)—a feat that was only rarely achieved before the advent of vascular imaging (Bull 1877; Cushing 1923; Symonds 1923).

Of the technical developments that would make it so much easier to establish the diagnosis of aneurysmal subarachnoid haemorrhage during life, the first was the lumbar puncture, introduced for therapeutic purposes in hydrocephalic patients (Quincke 1891). Froin, in his thesis of 1904, analysed the cerebrospinal fluid for the presence of blood cells as well as of blood pigments, after haemolysis. The next advances were neuroradiological. The first angiographic visualization of a cerebral aneurysm during life was reported in 1933 (Moniz 1933), 6 years after the technique had been first applied (Moniz 1927). In those days, angiography was a hazardous procedure (involving surgical dissection of the artery), to such an extent that someone like Cushing only rarely exposed his patients to it before neurosurgical exploration. Even today, in the era of selective catheterization, the risks are far from negligible. Fortunately, the technique of magnetic resonance angiography is making rapid advances and may soon replace the invasive techniques, at least for diagnostic purposes (Atlas *et al.* 1994; Korogi *et al.* 1994). The greatest leap in our times was the advent of CT (Hounsfield 1973); this technique made it pos-

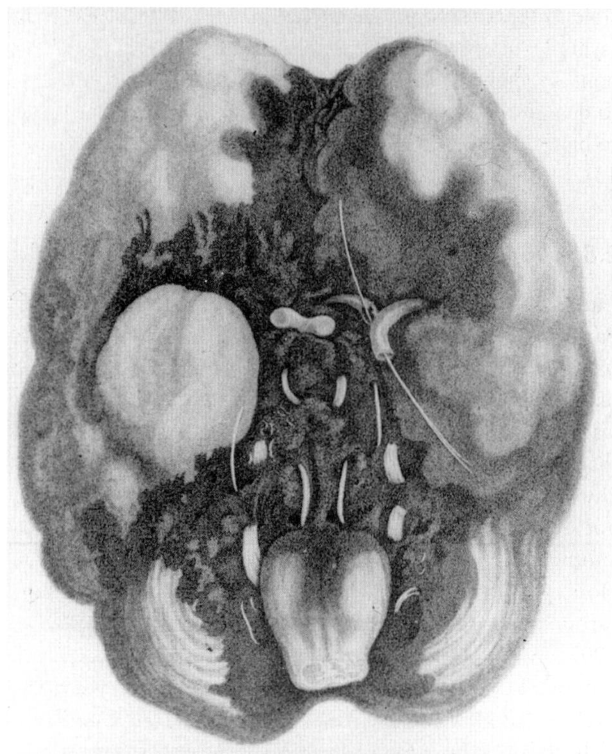

Fig. 2.10 The first anatomical illustration of subarachnoid haemorrhage, from Cheyne (1812). A probe has been passed into the proximal end of the internal carotid artery, and it emerges at the presumed site of rupture; the offending aneurysm was not recognized at the time, but presumably it was at the origin of the posterior communicating artery from the carotid artery, or at the anterior communicating artery complex.

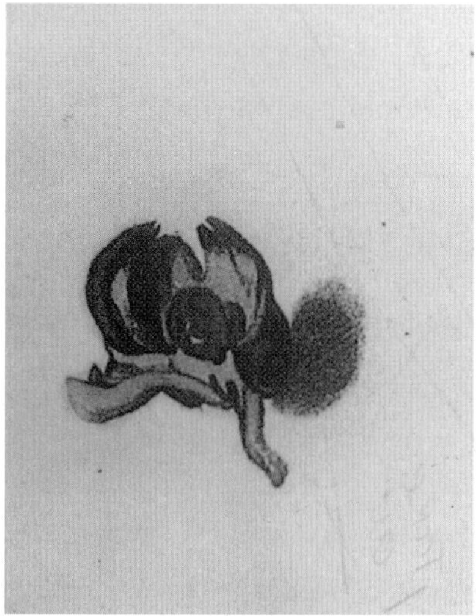

Fig. 2.11 Pea-sized aneurysmal dilatation of one of the branches of the middle cerebral artery (opened), containing a clot; the abnormality was surrounded by a large, fresh haemorrhage, which had caused the death of the 19-year-old patient, 8 days after a first episode with sudden headache (from Bright 1831).

sible to localize the extent of the haemorrhage in a precise fashion, to largely separate aneurysmal haemorrhage from non-aneurysmal haemorrhage and, by serial investigations, to detect and distinguish the most important complications: re-bleeding, delayed ischaemia and hydrocephalus (Chapter 13).

2.8.2 Surgical treatment

Carotid ligation was practised since the times of Ambroise Paré (1510–90) as a method to staunch arterial bleeding in patients with neck wounds, and once aneurysms were recognized as the cause of subarachnoid haemorrhage it was a logical step to consider this procedure as a method to decrease the risk of re-bleeding (Bull 1877). Hutchinson would actually have carried out the operation in 1875 had the patient not declined at the last moment, going on to survive for another 11 years (Hutchinson 1875). Around 1886, it was Horsley who was one of the first who ligated the (common) carotid artery in the neck, for a tumorous aneurysm (Beadles 1907). For decades, this remained the only surgical intervention possible, but most patients were managed conservatively because the complications of surgery were considerable (Schorstein 1940).

In 1931, the Edinburgh neurosurgeon Norman Dott (1897–1973) (Fig. 2.12), at that time only a 33-year-old, carried out the first intracranial operation for a ruptured aneurysm (Todd *et al.* 1990). It was a more or less desperate attempt, because the aneurysm had already re-bled twice, leaving the patient comatose for some hours after the last episode and with some degree of right-sided hemiparesis and aphasia. To complicate matters further, the 53-year-old patient was a well-known Edinburgh solicitor and chairman of the board of governors of the Royal Hospital for Sick Children. But both the patient and the young neurosurgeon were prepared to take the risk (Rush & Shaw 1990). About the operation, Dott wrote (Dott 1932):

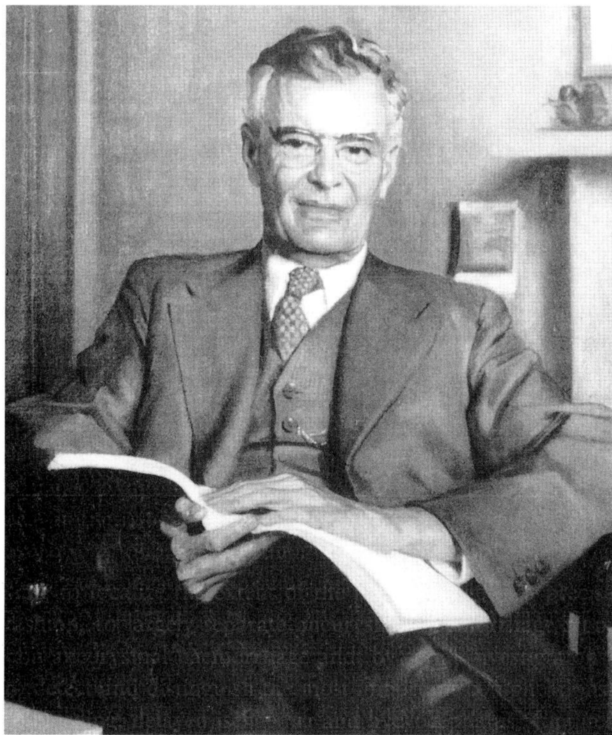

Fig. 2.12 Norman Dott (1897–1973).

> A left frontal approach was employed and it was a difficult matter to elevate the tense and oedematous brain and identify the basal structures, which were bloodstained and largely embedded in clot. The left optic nerve was found and the internal carotid artery was defined at its outer side. This vessel was closely followed upwards, outwards and backwards to its bifurcation into the middle and anterior cerebral arteries. As this point was being cleared of tenacious clot a formidable arterial haemorrhage filled the wound. With the aid of suction apparatus, held closely to the bleeding point, we were able to see the aneurysm. It sprang from the upper aspect of the bifurcation junction; it was about 3 mm in diameter; blood spurted freely from its semidetached fundus. Meanwhile a colleague was obtaining fresh muscle from the patient's leg. A small fragment of muscle was accurately applied to the bleeding point and held firmly in place so that it checked the bleeding and compressed the thin walled aneurysmal sac. Thus it was steadily maintained for 12 minutes. As the retaining instrument was then cautiously withdrawn, no further bleeding occurred. The vessel was further cleared and thin strips of muscle were prepared and wound around it until a thick collar of muscle embedded the aneurysm and adjacent arterial trunks (Fig. 2.13).

The patient recovered well, and a few weeks later Dott wrote, his sense of triumph carefully hidden: 'Mr Colin Black's tibialis anticus seems to have stuck well to his internal carotid—he has gone for a holiday' (Rush & Shaw 1990). In later years, Dott and his patient went fishing together on a number of occasions, and Mr Black's neurological condition remained good until he died from myocardial infarction 11 years after the momentous operation. Unfortunately, on later occasions the outcome with a direct approach to the aneurysm was often disappointing, if not fatal, and Dott reverted to ligating the internal carotid artery in the neck, or the proximal anterior cerebral artery intracranially.

In 1937, Dandy was the first to use a clip to occlude the neck of the aneurysm that had bled (Dandy 1938). But in some patients, a clip could not be secured, and in those cases he often had to have recourse to so-called trapping, by clipping the parent vessel on either side of the aneurysm. Drake devised a technique for approaching basilar artery aneurysms, notoriously difficult until then, and managed

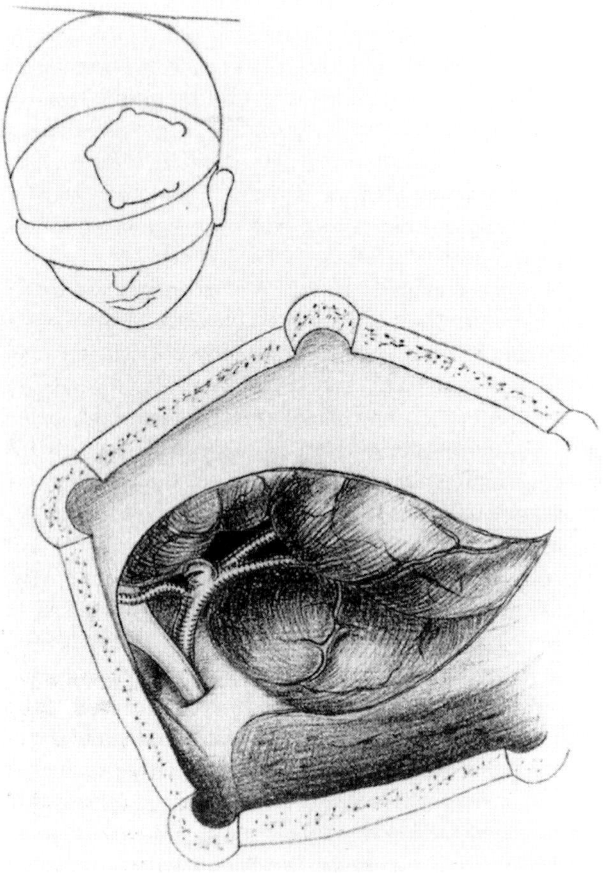

Fig. 2.13 Norman Dott's drawing of the first intracranial operation for aneurysm. The proximal middle cerebral artery aneurysm was exposed and wrapped with muscle through a left frontal flap (with permission from Todd *et al.* 1990).

to apply clips to them (Drake 1961). In the 1960s, spring clips, which could be removed when placement was less than optimal, came into use and replaced the silver clips used by Dandy. Nevertheless, the direct operation of aneurysms remained dangerous, and randomized controlled trials of the efficacy of surgery were equivocal (Chapter 13). Attempts to make the operation safer included temporary cardiac arrest, hypotension and deep hypothermia, all without much success, although no formal trials were done.

In the 1980s, a consensus developed amongst neurosurgeons that direct operation of the aneurysm should best be delayed until 12–14 days after the initial haemorrhage. This regimen meant, of course, that a proportion of patients rebled or suffered other complications in the meantime. The gradual introduction of the operating microscope for aneurysm surgery in the 1970s made early operation (within 3 days) not only feasible but also fashionable, despite the dearth of evidence from randomized controlled trials (Chapter 13). The medical management of patients with ruptured aneurysms has also improved in the last decade, especially with regard to the prevention of delayed cerebral ischaemia. While the question of the optimal time for operating on ruptured aneurysms has not been definitively resolved, endovascular methods for occluding aneurysms ('coiling') are rapidly gaining ground.

2.9 Treatment and its pitfalls

Doctoring has always implied treatment. In the past, medical management was almost invariably based on erroneous pathophysiological concepts, and the treatments were almost invariably ineffective, if not actually harmful—a situation often repeated in present times, and much more often than physicians and surgeons care to admit. Anyone who finds it amusing to read about 19th-century regimens, including measures such as bleeding, mustard poultices, castor oil and turpentine enemas as treatments for apoplexy, should read post-1950 treatises about the efficacy of vasodilator drugs or about transplantation of omentum to the intracranial cavity, as a chastening experience.

2.9.1 The numerical method

Before different treatments could ever be compared, it was necessary to find methods for grouping patients together, and therefore trying somehow to convert disease outcomes into numbers. The Paris physician Pierre Charles Alexandre Louis (1787–1872; he survives eponymously in the *angulus Ludovici* of the sternum) is generally credited with the introduction of the numerical method in medicine. In fact, his contribution was more a credo than a practical method (Matthews 1995). True enough, there is the famous example of his empirical criticism of bloodletting: of 47 patients with pneumonia treated with bloodletting, 18 died, against only nine of the 36 patients in the untreated group (Louis 1835). But Louis did not have the mathematical training to estimate the likelihood that a difference of this magnitude might arise by chance. The mathematician Jules Gavarret (1809–90) criticized the analysis and conclusions of Louis' studies, although he agreed with the design. Even more purely mathematical was the notion of the 'average human', an approach proposed by Adolphe Quetelet (1796–1874).

Groups and averages—these were notions that evoked not merely resistance, but outright revulsion in the ranks of the established medical professionals. How on earth could one ever ignore the unique characteristics of each single individual by forcing these together into an artificial 'mean'? And how could one ever believe in a standard treatment, any more than in a standard shoe? The advent of experimental physiology intensified the opposition. The famous Claude Bernard (1813–78) warned that one will never encounter an 'average' in nature, and that grouping of observations will obscure the true relationships between natural phenomena (Bernard 1865). And the equally legendary Lord Lister

(1827–1912) relied more on the theoretical basis of his antiseptic method than on the actual death rates (Lister 1870).

Until the 20th century, counting disease events was limited to population studies (Stolley & Lasky 1995). The beginnings of epidemiology can be traced to Sir William Petty (1623–87), one of the founders of the Royal Society, and John Graunt (1620–74). They worked together collecting numerical data to describe patterns of mortality. A century and a half later, E. Blackmore reported not only on deaths but also on incident cases of disease in Plymouth (Blackmore 1829a; Blackmore 1829b). Victorian counterparts took this further. William Farr (1807–83), who had trained under Louis in Paris, linked self-devised classifications of diseases and occupations to population statistics at the General Registry Office. John Snow (1813–58) mapped the occurrence of cholera cases in the streets of London and related them to the positions of the local water pumps; these studies culminated in Snow's famous act of removing the handle from the Broad Street pump, during the 1854 cholera epidemic.

The first epidemiological studies of stroke were not performed until after the second world war. An early study of incidence in the community was done in the UK (Acheson *et al.* 1968). Population-based studies, addressing risk factors specifically for stroke, were subsequently reported from the US (the Framingham cohort), Japan, and Finland (Kannel *et al.* 1965; Hirota *et al.* 1975; Salonen *et al.* 1979).

2.9.2 Clinical trials

The era of rational treatment dawned with the introduction of the randomized controlled trial. The principle slowly gained acceptance after the landmark UK Medical Research Council trial of streptomycin in pulmonary tuberculosis with random assignment to treatment groups (Medical Research Council 1948). Some forerunners had already used parallel control groups. Louis (1787–1872) (section 2.9.1) had been preceded by James Lind (1716–94), who in 1753 found that lemons and oranges prevented scurvy in sailors (see Controlled Trials from History—http://www.rcpe.ac.uk/controlled_trials/index.html). A further step was the introduction of chance to obtain an equal balance between the experimental group and the control group. Fibiger (1867–1928) in 1898 (serum for diphtheria) used assignment on alternate days (Fibiger 1898; Hróbjartsson *et al.* 1998), and in 1931 Amberson *et al.* flipped a coin to divide patients with pulmonary tuberculosis into those who received gold treatment and controls (Amberson *et al.* 1931). Blinding of patients was also practised by Amberson *et al.*, as had been done 4 years earlier by Ferguson *et al.* in 1927, in a test of vaccines for the common cold (Ferguson *et al.* 1927). Blinding of those who were to assess outcome was advocated in 1944 by the chest physicians Hinshaw and Feldman (Hinshaw & Feldman 1944), and eventually carried out in the MRC streptomycin trial of 1948. Allocation in that historic trial took place by means of randomization. An important advantage of random allocation, applied by R.A. Fisher in agriculture in the 1920s, is that it favours equal and unbiased balancing between the two groups (Fisher 1926). But the main reason why Sir Austin Bradford Hill (1897–1991), the trial's principal investigator, chose randomization was that it ensured concealment of the allocation schedule from those involved in entering patients in the trial; there could be no foreknowledge of what the next patient was going to get (Doll 1998; Chalmers 1999).

Clinical trials in cerebrovascular disease were no exception to the rule that most methodological errors have to be committed before they are recognized, because the correct solutions are often counter-intuitive. In the 1950s, anticoagulant drugs seemed a rational form of treatment to prevent further strokes in survivors of (presumed) brain infarction. The same Bradford Hill who had pioneered the tuberculosis trial took the initiative for two such trials, the first in 142 and the second, with exclusion of hypertensives, in 131 patients (Hill *et al.* 1960; Hill *et al.* 1962). There was no significant difference in the rate of non-fatal stroke between the treatment groups and controls, while there was some excess of fatal strokes, possibly haemorrhages, in patients on anticoagulants. From that time onwards, anticoagulants were largely abandoned in the prevention of stroke, unless for specific indications such as a source of embolism in the heart. It took at least two decades before it dawned on the neurological community that trials of anticoagulants in brain ischaemia had been too small, separately as well as collectively, to detect even large protective effects, apart from other shortcomings (Jonas 1988). The same applied to an early secondary prevention trial with dipyridamole (Acheson *et al.* 1969).

A pioneer trial of medical treatment in acute stroke was with corticosteroids, by Dyken and White in 1956. They stratified rather than randomized, found a trend towards a higher death rate in the treated group (13/17 against 10/19 in controls), and ended up by identifying many of the methodological problems in this type of trial (Dyken & White 1956). The first trial of carotid endarterectomy excluded surgical mishaps from the analysis (Fields *et al.* 1970); subsequently the operation boomed to worrying levels, until restrained by methodologically sound trials (section 16.8.5). The first large trial of aspirin in stroke prevention evoked much controversy (Canadian Cooperative Study Group 1978), for one thing because its initiators had chosen 'stroke or death' as the outcome event instead of stroke alone (Kurtzke 1979); it took time for neurologists to realize that they treat whole patients rather than only their brains. Also, the initial conclusion that aspirin was ineffective for women is now a classical example of the dangers of subgroup analysis.

2.9.3 Measuring outcome: the ghost of Gall

One of the greatest stumbling-blocks in trials of acute stroke is the babel of tongues with regard to the measurement of outcome (van Gijn 1992). Traditionally, so-called 'stroke scales' have been applied for this aim, analogous to scales for other neurological conditions, such as Parkinson's disease or multiple sclerosis. But, although the stated purpose of 'stroke scales' is to measure outcome, these scales are nothing but codifications of the neurological examination, developed for no other purpose than that of localizing lesions within the nervous system. With such a diagnostic approach, different functions of the nervous system are separately assessed: power of limbs, speech, visual fields, etc. This reductionist, mechanistic notion of brain function reflects the localizationists' position in the scientific battle that raged in the second half of the 19th century, the opposing party being that of equipotentiality.

The equipotentialists believed that the brain worked as a unitary system, brain tissue being omnipotent and flexible in its function. Consequently, brain damage would result in a decrease in the overall level of performance, not in loss of specific functions. The champion of the equipotentialists was the French physiologist Flourens, who supported his views with experiments on dogs and pigeons (Flourens 1824). The opposing concept, that of localization of specific functions, was propounded in a somewhat bizarre fashion by the anatomists Gall and Spurzheim (Gall & Spurzheim 1819). They believed that every intellectual and moral property had its own position on the surface of the brain (Fig. 2.14) and that the degree of development of these dispositions could be identified by locating overlying protuberances on the skull (Blakemore 1977) (Fig. 2.15). However, the theory of localization gained respectability after the stimulation experiments of Fritsch and Hitzig on anaesthetized dogs, in which they found that weak electrical currents applied through platinum electrodes to the anterior regions of the brain surface produced muscle contractions in the opposite half of the body (Fritsch & Hitzig 1870). The clash between the adherents of the two theories culminated in 1881 at the Third International Congress of Medicine, held in London (Thorwald 1957). The equipotentialists were represented by the German physiologist Goltz, who showed the audience a dog in which a substantial portion of the brain had been removed by means of a hose, but who could still move all limbs, trunk and tail, and who had retained all his senses. Later, it would turn out that the lesions were less extensive than had been claimed, and on the same afternoon Ferrier showed two chimpanzees, one deaf after removal of the auditory cortex, the other limping with a hemiplegic gait after extirpation of the contralateral motor area (the sight of which led Charcot to exclaim: '*Mais c'est un malade!*').

Fig. 2.14 Phrenology head (1916); each region of the skull is supposed to represent a mental faculty, such as 'mirthfulness', 'perception of form', or 'ideality'.

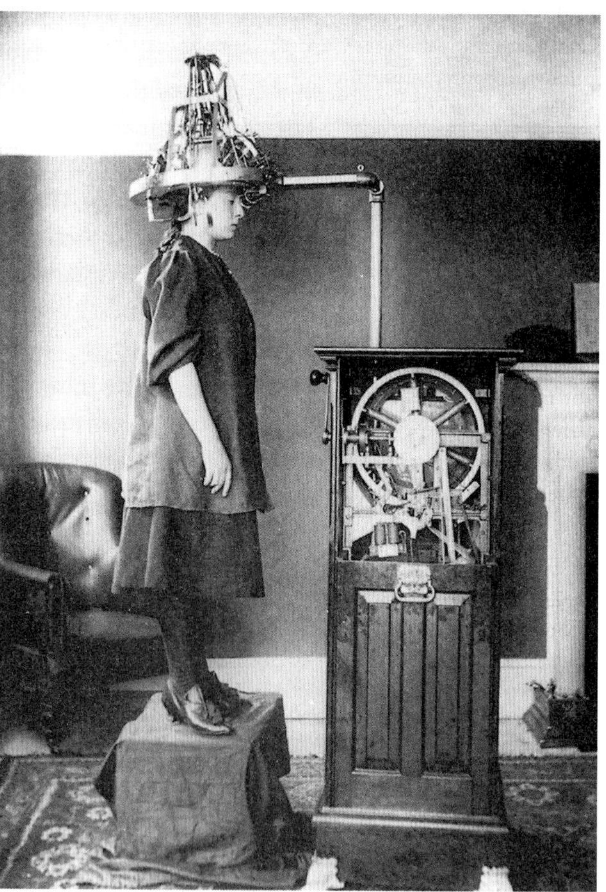

Fig. 2.15 The pseudoscience of phrenology lived on well beyond the 19th century. The Lavery Electric Phrenometer of 1907 was intended to lend modern accuracy to the measurements of bumps on the skull (with permission from Blakemore 1977).

The localizationists had won the day, but they won too completely. The greater part of the brain has no 'primary' motor, sensory, or cognitive tasks, and serves to connect and integrate the separate 'functions'. Similarly, everyday life consists of a multitude of tasks that are integrated and difficult to separate. Mood, initiative and speed of thinking are some of the essential features of human life that can be severely affected by stroke but are sadly ignored in 'stroke scales'. It is therefore naïve to try and rebuild an entire human being from separate 'functions', even apart from the insoluble problem of how to add up the different items to something meaningful (Table 2.2). Patients are more than the sum of their signs (van Gijn & Warlow 1992). A higher, more integrated level of measurement is needed—that is, scales should measure function not at the level of the organ, but at the level of the person (disability scales), or even at the level of social interaction (handicap scales). What really counts for patients is what they can do in life, compared with what they want to do or were once able to do.

2.9.4 Meta-analysis

In the 1970s and 1980s, Richard Peto and colleagues Tom Chalmers and Iain Chalmers developed a method to overcome the problem that single trials may or may not show a significant difference in treated patients compared with controls, and that the exact magnitude of the difference, expressed as a confidence interval, was usually uncertain. They proposed a simple statistical method to overview the results of all related trials in a given field by which the differences between the treatment group and the control group in each trial are combined (Yusuf *et al.* 1985). The key assumption is that, if a given treatment has any material effect on the incidence or outcome of disease, then the direction, although not necessarily the size, of this effect tends to be similar in different circumstances, i.e. in different trials. If all available studies are combined, the confidence interval around the estimate of the treatment effect can be narrowed considerably, and so the estimate is more precise. Reviewer bias is avoided as well, because meta-analysis requires the presentation and synthesis of the results of *all* relevant trials, not just the trial that happens to provide the result one wants. There is a pressing need for up-to-date systematic reviews of all the available evidence regarding the various aspects of care of stroke patients—indeed, of all medical interventions. This need has led to the Cochrane Collaboration, which includes a stroke review group (Counsell *et al.* 1995) (http://www.dcn.ed.ac.uk/csrg).

Table 2.2 The state of an individual cannot be constructed from separate components: imagine you meet 'the boy next door' from your childhood, after an interval of 30 years, and that your question 'How are you?' is answered with a list of details, instead of a general statement ('fine', for example).

Profession	Dentist	For 15 years
Civil state	Married	Wife 1.68 m, 59 kg
Bank account	Positive	9634.92
Car	Volvo	240S
Holidays	Tuscany	3 weeks
Sport	Golf	Handicap 8
		Grand total?

2.10 Epilogue

Despite the many advances in the knowledge about stroke that we have highlighted, our story could not but remain anachronistic and fragmented. It is extremely difficult to try and stand in the shoes of one's forebears, because one has to erase all newly acquired knowledge (Temkin 1971). For those of us who can think back as short a time span as three decades, what diagnosis did we make, in those times, in patients we now know to have survived carotid dissection or intracranial venous thrombosis—to name but two examples? Heaven only knows. In the same way, not so much longer ago, it was impossible to distinguish cerebral haemorrhage from infarction; or haemorrhage from some mysterious other condition that mimicked haemorrhage but in which the brain looked practically normal; or stroke from other brain diseases; or even stroke from heart disease. Also, our account has been anecdotal. In reality, the progress of science is slow and continuous, not a succession of breakthroughs. This also applies to the few decades we have witnessed during our own careers. We do not expect a sensational novelty when we walk into the hospital tomorrow, or when we open this week's *Lancet,* but a lot has changed since we were medical students. This refers not only to the body of medical knowledge, but also to the methods of medical research. Empirical testing has gained ascendancy over pathophysiological theory, and the aim of benefit just for the individual patient has been complemented by the population perspective. The rate of change is a bit like the shifting position of the sun across the skies: one cannot see it move, but there is a dramatic difference between dawn and sunset. We expect to see many more dawns in stroke research.

References

Please note that all references taken from *The Cochrane Library* are given a current date as this database is updated on a quarterly basis. Please refer to the current *Cochrane Library* article for the latest review. The same applies to the *British Medical Journal* 'Clinical Evidence' series which is updated every six months.

Abercrombie, J. (1828) *Pathological and Clinical Researches on Diseases of the Brain and Spinal Cord.* Waugh & Innes, Edinburgh.

Abercrombie, J. (1836) *Pathological and Practical Researches on Diseases of the Brain and Spinal Cord.* 2nd (corresponding to 3rd Brit.). Carey, Lea & Blanchard, Philadelphia.

Acheson, J., Acheson, H.W. & Tellwright, J.M. (1968) The incidence and pattern of cerebrovascular disease in general practice. *Journal of the Royal College of General Practitioners* **16**, 428–436.

Acheson, J., Danta, G. & Hutchinson, E.C. (1969) Controlled trial of dipyridamole in cerebral vascular disease. *British Medical Journal* **1**, 614–615.

Adams, R.D. & vander Eecken, H.M. (1953) Vascular diseases of the brain. *Annual Review of Medicine* **4**, 213–252.

Amarenco, P., Cohen, A., Tzourio, C. *et al.* (1994) Atherosclerotic disease of the aortic arch and the risk of ischemic stroke. *New England Journal of Medicine* **331**, 1474–1479.

Amarenco, P., Duyckaerts, C., Tzourio, C., Henin, D., Bousser, M.G. & Hauw, J.J. (1992) The prevalence of ulcerated plaques in the aortic arch in patients with stroke. *New England Journal of Medicine* **326**, 221–225.

Amberson, J.B., McMahon, B.T. & Pinner, M. (1931) A clinical trial of sanocrysin in pulmonary tuberculosis. *American Review of Tuberculosis* **24**, 401–435.

Archie, J.P. & Feldtman, J.P. (1981) Critical stenosis of the internal carotid artery. *Surgery* **89**, 67–70.

Atlas, S.W., Listerud, J., Chung, W. & Flamm, E.S. (1994) Intracranial aneurysms: depiction on MR angiograms with a multifeature-extraction, ray-tracing postprocessing algorithm. *Radiology* **192**, 129–139.

Baillie, M. (1793) The morbid anatomy of some of the most important parts of the human body. J. Johnson & G. Nicol, London.

Barnett, H.J.M. (1979) The pathophysiology of transient cerebral ischemic attacks: therapy with antiplatelet antiaggregants. *Medical Clinics of North America* **63**, 649–680.

Barnett, H.J.M., Plum, F. & Walton, J.N. (1984) Carotid endarterectomy—an expression of concern. *Stroke* **15**, 941–943.

Barnett, H.J.M., Taylor, W., Eliasziw, M. *et al.* (1998) Benefit of carotid endarterectomy in patients with symptomatic moderate or severe stenosis. *New England Journal of Medicine* **339**, 1415–1425.

Bayle, F. (1677) *Tractatus de Apoplexia*. B. Guillemette, Toulouse.

Beadles, C.F. (1907) Aneurisms of the larger cerebral arteries. *Brain* **30**, 285–336.

Beal, M.F., Park, T.S. & Fisher, C.M. (1981) Cerebral atheromatous embolism following carotid sinus pressure. *Archives of Neurology* **38**, 310–312.

Benton, A.L. & Joynt, R.J. (1960) Early descriptions of aphasia. *Archives of Neurology* **3**, 205–222.

Berengario da Carpi, J. (1523) *Isagogae Breves, Perlucide ac Uberrime, in Anatomiam Humani Corporis*. Benedictum Hectoris, Bologna.

Bernard, C. (1865) *Introduction à l'Etude de la Médicine Expérimentale*. J.-B. Baillière, Paris.

Berry, D. & Mackenzie, C. (1992) *Richard Bright (1789–1858)—Physician in an Age of Revolution and Reform*. Royal Society of Medicine, London.

Biumi, F. (1765) Observatio V: Carotis ad receptaculum Vieusenii aneurysmatica etc. In: *Observationes anatomicae, Scholiis illustratae*. S. & J. Lichtmans, Milan. pp. 373–379.

Blackall, J. (1813) *Observations on the Nature and Cure of Dropsies*, 5th edn. Longman & Co., London. pp. 132–135.

Blackmore, E. (1829a) Reports on the diseases of Plymouth, I. *Edinburgh Medical & Surgical Journal* **31**, 266–287.

Blackmore, E. (1829b) Reports on the diseases of Plymouth, II. *Edinburgh Medical & Surgical Journal* **32**, 1–20.

Blakemore, C. (1977) *Mechanics of the Mind*. Cambridge University Press, Cambridge.

Blum, F. (1893) Der Formaldehyd als Härtungsmittel—vorläufige Mitteilung. *Zeitschrift für Wissenschaftliche Mikroskopie und Mikroskopische Technik* **10**, 314–315.

Boerhaave, H. (1715) *Aphorismi de Cognoscendis et Curandis Morbis*, 2nd edn. J. van der Linden, Leiden.

Bogousslavsky, J. & Regli, F. (1983) Delayed TIAs distal to bilateral occlusion of carotid arteries—evidence for embolic and hemodynamic mechanisms. *Stroke* **14**, 58–61.

Brain, R. (1968) *Diseases of the Nervous System*. 6th edn, p. 261. Oxford University Press, Oxford.

Bright, R. (1831) *Reports of Medical Cases, Selected with a View of Illustrating the Symptoms and Cure of Diseases by a Reference to Morbid Anatomy*. Longman, Rees, Orme, Brown & Green, London.

Brinton, W. (1852) Report on cases of cerebral aneurism. *Transactions of the Pathological Society of London* **3**, 47–49.

Bull, E. (1877) Akut Hjerneaneurisma-Okulomotoriusparalyse-Meningealapoplexi. *Norsk Magasin for Laegevidenskapen* **7**, 890–895.

Burger, S.K., Saul, R.F., Selhorst, J.B. & Thurston, S.E. (1991) Transient monocular blindness caused by vasospasm. *New England Journal of Medicine* **325**, 870–873.

Burrows, G. (1846) *On Disorders of Cerebral Circulation and on the Connection between Affections of the Brain and Disease of the Heart*. Longman, Brown, Green & Longmans, London.

Bynum, W.F. (1994) *Science and the Practice of Medicine in the Nineteenth Century*. Cambridge University Press, Cambridge.

Call, G.K., Fleming, M.C., Sealfon, S., Levine, H., Kistler, J.P. & Fisher, C.M. (1988) Reversible cerebral segmental vasoconstriction. *Stroke* **19**, 1159–1170.

Canadian Cooperative Study Group (1978) A randomized trial of aspirin and sulfinpyrazone in threatened stroke. *New England Journal of Medicine* **299**, 53–59.

Caplan, L.R. & Sergay, S. (1976) Positional cerebral ischaemia. *Journal of Neurology, Neurosurgery and Psychiatry* **39**, 385–391.

Carswell, R. (1838) *Pathological Anatomy: Illustrations of the Elementary Forms of Disease.*

Casserio, G. (1627) *Tabulae anatomicae* (ed. D. Bucretius). E. Deuchinum, Venice.

Challa, V.L., Moody, D.M. & Bell, M.A. (1992) The Charcot–Bouchard aneurysm controversy: impact of a new histologic technique. *Journal of Neuropathology and Experimental Neurology* **51**, 264–271.

Chalmers, I. (1999) Why transition from alternation to randomisation in clinical trials was made. *British Medical Journal* **319**, 1372.

Charcot, J.M. & Bouchard, C. (1868) Nouvelles recherches sur la pathogénie de l'hémorrhagie cérébrale. *Archives de Physiologie Normale et Pathologique* **1**, 110–127, 643–665, 725–734.

Cheyne, J. (1812) *Cases of Apoplexy and Lethargy with Observations on Comatose Patients*. Underwood, London.

Chiari, H. (1905) Über das Verhalten des Teilungswinkels des Carotis communis bei der Endarteritis chronica deformans. *Verhandlungen der Deutschen Pathologischen Gesellschaft* **9**, 326–330.

Clarke, E. (1963) Apoplexy in the Hippocratic writings. *Bulletin of the History of Medicine* **37**, 301–314.

Clarke, E. & Dewhurst, K. (1972) *An Illustrated History of Brain Function*, pp. 56–59. Sandford Publications, Oxford.

Cohnheim, J. (1872) *Untersuchungen über die embolischen Processe*. Hirschwald, Berlin.

Cole, F.M. & Yates, P.O. (1967) The occurrence and significance of intracerebral micro-aneurysms. *Journal of Pathology and Bacteriology* **93**, 393–411.

Counsell, C., Warlow, C., Sandercock, P., Fraser, H. & van Gijn, J. (1995) The Cochrane Collaboration Stroke Review Group: meeting the need for systematic reviews in stroke care. *Stroke* **26**, 498–502.

Cruveilhier, J. (1842) *Anatomie pathologique du corps humain; descriptions avec figures lithographiés et coloriés; des diverses altérations morbides dont le corps humain est susceptible*. J.-B. Baillière, Paris.

Cushing, H. (1923) Contributions to the clinical study of cerebral aneurysms. *Guy's Hospital Report* **73**, 159–163.

Dandy, W.E. (1938) Intracranial aneurysm of internal carotid artery, cured by operation. *Annals of Surgery* **107**, 654–657.

De Bono, D.P. & Warlow, C.P. (1981) Potential sources of emboli in patients with presumed transient cerebral or retinal ischaemia. *Lancet* **i**, 343–346.

Dechambre, A. (1838) Mémoire sur la curabilité du ramollissement cérébral. *Gazette Médicale de Paris* **6**, 305–314.

Denny-Brown, D. (1951) The treatment of recurrent cerebrovascular symptoms and the question of 'vasospasm'. *Medical Clinics of North America* **35**, 1457–1474.

Dewhurst, K. (1980) *Thomas Willis's Oxford Lectures*. Sandford Publications, Oxford.

Doll, R. (1998) Controlled trials: the 1948 watershed. *British Medical Journal* **317**, 1217–1220.

Dott, N. (1932) Intracranial aneurysms: cerebral arterio-radiography: surgical treatment. *Transactions of the Medical and Chirurgical Society of Edinburgh* **47**, 219–240.

Drake, C.G. (1961) Bleeding aneurysms of the basilar artery: direct surgical management in four cases. *Journal of Neurosurgery* **18**, 230–238.

Durand-Fardel, C.L.M. (1842) Mémoire sur une altération particulière de la substance cérébrale. *Gazette Médicale de Paris* **10**, 23–38.

Durand-Fardel, C.L.M. (1843) *Traité du ramollissement du cerveau*. J.-B. Baillière, Paris.

Dyken, M.L. & White, P.T. (1956) Evaluation of cortisone in treatment of cerebral infarction. *Journal of the American Medical Association* **162**, 1531–1534.

Eastcott, H.H.G., Pickering, G.W. & Robb, C.G. (1954) Reconstruction of internal carotid artery in a patient with intermittent attacks of hemiplegia. *Lancet* **ii**, 994–996.

EC–IC Bypass Study Group (1985) Failure of extracranial–intracranial arterial bypass to reduce the risk of ischemic stroke: results of an international randomized trial. *New England Journal of Medicine* **313**, 1191–1200.

Ellis, A.G. (1909) The pathogenesis of spontaneous intracerebral hemorrhage. *Proceedings of the Pathological Society of Philadelphia* **12**, 197–235.

Eppinger, H. (1887) Pathogenesis (Histogenesis und Aetiologie) der Aneurysmen einschliesslich des Aneurysma equi verminosum. *Archiv klinischer Chirurgie* **35** (Suppl. 1), 1–563.

European Carotid Surgery Trial Collaborative Group (1998) Randomised trial of endarterectomy for recently symptomatic carotid stenosis: final results of the MRC European carotid surgery trial (ECST). *Lancet* **351**, 1379–1387.

Fallopius, G. (1561) *Observationes anatomicae*. Marcus Antonius Ulmus, Venice.

Ferguson, F.R., Davey, A.F.C. & Topley, W.W.C. (1927) The value of mixed vaccines in the prevention of the common cold. *Journal of Hygiene* **26**, 98–109.

Fibiger, J. (1898) Om Serumbehandling af Difteri. *Hospitalstidende* **6** (309–25), 337–350.

Fields, W.S., Maslenikov, V., Meyer, J.S., Hass, W.K., Remington, R.D. & Macdonald, M. (1970) Joint study of extracranial arterial occlusion, V: progress report of prognosis following surgery or nonsurgical treatment for transient ischemic attacks and cervical carotid artery lesions. *Journal of the American Medical Association* **211**, 1993–2003.

Fieschi, C., Argentino, C., Lenzi, G.L., Sacchetti, M.L., Toni, D. & Bozzao, L. (1989) Clinical and instrumental evaluation of patients with ischemic stroke within the first six hours. *Journal of Neurological Sciences* **91**, 311–321.

Fischer, O. (1910) Die presbyophrene Demenz, deren anatomische Grundlage und klinische Abgrenzung. *Zeitschrift für die gesamte Neurologie und Psychiatrie* **3**, 371–471.

Fisher, C.M. (1951) Occlusion of the internal carotid artery. *Archives of Neurology and Psychiatry* **65**, 346–377.

Fisher, C.M. (1952) Transient monocular blindness associated with hemiplegia. *Archives of Ophthalmology* **47**, 167–203.

Fisher, C.M. (1959) Observations on the fundus oculi in transient monocular blindness. *Neurology* **9**, 333–347.

Fisher, C.M. (1965) Lacunes: small, deep cerebral infarcts. *Neurology* **15**, 774–784.

Fisher, C.M. (1969) The arterial lesions underlying lacunes. *Acta Neuropathologica (Berlin)* **12**, 1–15.

Fisher, C.M. & Curry, H.B. (1965) Pure motor hemiplegia of vascular origin. *Archives of Neurology* **13**, 30–44.

Fisher, R.A. (1926) The arrangement of field experiments. *Journal of the Ministry of Agriculture* **33**, 503–513.

Flourens, M.J.P. (1824) *Recherches expérimentales sur les propriétés et les fonctions du système nerveux, dans les animaux vertébrés*. Crevot, Paris.

Foucault, M. (1963) *Naissance de la Clinique*. Presses Universitaires de France, Paris.

Franke, C.L., Ramos, L.M.P. & van Gijn, J. (1990) Development of multifocal haemorrhage in a cerebral infarct during computed tomography [letter]. *Journal of Neurology, Neurosurgery and Psychiatry* **53**, 531–532.

Fritsch, G.T. & Hitzig, E. (1870) Ueber die elektrische Erregbarkeit des Grosshirns. *Archiv für Anatomie, Physiologie und wissenschaftliche Medizin* **37**, 300–332.

Galenus (edition of 1824) *Opera Omnia*. Translated and edited by G.G. Kühn. Cnobloch, Leipzig.

Gall, F.J. & Spurzheim, J.C. (1819) *Anatomie et physiologie du système nerveux en général, et du cerveau en particulier, avec des observations sur la possibilité de reconnaître plusieurs dispositions intellectuelles et morales de l'homme et des animaux, par la configurations de leurs têtes*. Schoell, Paris.

van Gijn, J. (1992) Measurement of outcome in stroke prevention trials. *Cerebrovascular Diseases* **2** (Suppl. 1), 23–34.

van Gijn, J. (1996) *The Babinski Sign—a Centenary*. Utrecht University, Utrecht.

van Gijn, J. & Warlow, C.P. (1992) Down with stroke scales! *Cerebrovascular Diseases* **2**, 244–246.

Globus, J.H., Epstein, J.A., Green, M.A. & Marks, M. (1949) Focal cerebral hemorrhage experimentally induced. *Journal of Neuropathology and Experimental Neurology* **8**, 113–116.

Gowers, W.R. (1893) *A Manual of Diseases of the Nervous System*, Vol. **2**, p. 432. J. & A. Churchill, London.

Gunning, A.J., Pickering, G.W., Robb-Smith, A.H.T. & Ross Russell, R.W. (1964) Mural thrombosis of the internal carotid artery and subsequent embolism. *Quarterly Journal of Medicine* **33**, 155–195.

Hachinski, V.M. (1982) Transient cerebral ischemia: a historical sketch. In: *Historical Aspects of the Neurosciences (Festschrift for M. Critchley)* (eds F. Clifford Rose & W.F. Bynum), pp. 185–193. Raven Press, New York.

Hall, M. (1836) *Lectures on the nervous system and its diseases*. Sherwood, Gilbert & Piper, London.

Hammond, W.A. (1881) *Diseases of the Nervous System*. D. Appleton, New York.

Hayakawa, I., Watanabe, T., Tsuchida, T. & Sasaki, A. (1978) Perangiographic rupture of intracranial aneurysms. *Neuroradiology* **16**, 293–295.

Hayward, R.D. & O'Reilly, G.V. (1976) Intracerebral haemorrhage: accuracy of computerised transverse axial scanning in predicting the underlying aetiology. *Lancet* **1**, 1–4.

Hill, A.B., Marshall, J. & Shaw, D.A. (1960) A controlled clinical trial of long-term anticoagulant therapy in cerebrovascular disease. *Quarterly Journal of Medicine* **29**, 597–609.

Hill, A.B., Marshall, J. & Shaw, D.A. (1962) Cerebrovascular disease: a trial of long-term anticoagulant tharapy. *British Medical Journal* **ii**, 1003–1006.

Hiller, F. (1935) Zirkulationsstörungen im Gehirn. Eine klinische und pathologisch-anatomische Studie. *Archiv für Psychiatrie und Nervenkrankheiten* **103**, 1–53.

Hinshaw, H.C. & Feldman, W.H. (1944) Evaluation of chemotherapeutic agents in clinical tuberculosis. *American Review of Tuberculosis* **50**, 202–213.

Hirota, Y., Katsuki, S. & Asano, C. (1975) A multivariate analysis of risk factors for cerebrovascular disease in Hisayama, Kyushu Island, Japan. *Behaviormetrika* **2**, 1–11.

Hodgson, J. (1815) *A Treatise on the Diseases of Arteries and Veins, Containing the Pathology and Treatment of Aneurisms and Wounded Arteries*. T. Underwood, London.

Hollenhorst, R.W. (1961) Significance of bright plaques in the retinal arterioles. *Journal of the American Medical Association* **178**, 23–29.

Hope, J., Bennett, J.H., Pritchard, J.C., Taylor, R.H. & Thomson, T. (1840) *Dissertations on nervous diseases*. In: *Library of Practical Medicine* (ed. A. Tweedie). Lea & Blanchard, Philadelphia.

Hounsfield, G.N. (1973) Computerised transverse axial scanning (tomography), I: description of system. *British Journal of Radiology* **46**, 1016–1022.

Hróbjartsson, A., Gotsche, P.C. & Gluud, C. (1998) The controlled clinical trial turns 100 years: Fibiger's trial of serum treatment of diphtheria. *British Medical Journal* **317**, 1243–1245.

Hunt, J.R. (1914) The role of the carotid arteries in the causation of vascular lesions of the brain, with remarks on special features of the symptomatology. *American Journal of Medical Science* **147**, 704–713.

Hutchinson, J. (1875) Aneurism of the internal carotid artery within the skull diagnosed eleven years before the patient's death: spontaneous cure. *Transactions of the Clinical Society of London* **8**, 127–131.

Iragui, V.J. (1986) The Charcot–Bouchard controversy. *Archives of Neurology* **43**, 290–295.

Jackson, J.H. (1875) A lecture on softening of the brain. *Lancet* **ii**, 335–338.

Jardine, L. (1996) *Worldly Goods—a New History of the Renaissance*. Macmillan, London.

Jelliffe, S.E. & White, W.A. (1923) *Diseases of the Nervous System—a Text-Book of Neurology and Psychiatry*. H. & K. Lewis, London.

Jellinger, K. (1977) Cerebrovascular amyloidosis with cerebral hemorrhage. *Journal of Neurology* **214**, 195–206.

Jonas, S. (1988) Anticoagulant therapy in cerebrovascular disease: a review and meta-analysis. *Stroke* **19**, 1043–1048.

Kannel, W.B., Dawber, T.R., Cohen, M.E. & McNamara, P.M. (1965) Vascular disease of the brain—epidemiological aspects: the Framingham study. *American Journal of Public Health* **55**, 1355–1366.

Karenberg, A. & Hort, I. (1998a) Medieval descriptions and doctrines of stroke: preliminary analysis of select sources. Part I: The struggle for terms and theories—late antiquity and early middle ages (300–800). *Journal of the History of Neuroscience* 7, 162–173.

Karenberg, A. & Hort, I. (1998b) Medieval descriptions and doctrines of stroke: preliminary analysis of select sources. Part II: Between Galenism and Aristotelism—Islamic theories of apoplexy (800–1200). *Journal of the History of Neuroscience* 7, 174–185.

Karenberg, A. & Hort, I. (1998c) Medieval descriptions and doctrines of stroke: preliminary analysis of select sources. Part III: Multiplying speculations—the high and late middle ages (1000–1450). *Journal of the History of Neuroscience* 7, 186–200.

Kendell, R.E. & Marshall, J. (1963) Role of hypotension in the genesis of transient focal cerebral ischaemic attacks. *British Medical Journal* **2**, 344–348.

King, L.S. (1991) *Transformations in American Medicine—from Benjamin Rush to William Osler*. Johns Hopkins University Press, Baltimore.

Kirkes, W.S. (1855) On apoplexy in relation to chronic renal disease. *Medical Times Gazette* **11**, 515–516.

Klijn, C.J.M., Kappelle, L.J., Tulleken, C.A.F. & van Gijn, J. (1997) Symptomatic carotid artery occlusion—a reappraisal of hemodynamic factors. *Stroke* **28**, 2084–2093.

Korogi, Y., Takahashi, M., Mabuchi, N. *et al.* (1994) Intracranial aneurysms: diagnostic accuracy of three-dimensional, Fourier transform, time-of-flight MR angiography. *Radiology* **193**, 181–186.

Kraaijeveld, C.L., van Gijn, J., Schouten, H.J. & Staal, A. (1984) Interobserver agreement for the diagnosis of transient ischemic attacks. *Stroke* **15**, 723–725.

Kuhn, T.S. (1962) *The Structure of Scientific Revolutions*. Chicago University Press, Chicago.

Kurtzke, J.F. (1979) Controversy in neurology: the Canadian study on TIA and aspirin—a critique of the Canadian TIA study. *Annals of Neurology* **5**, 597–599.

Lallemand, F. (1824) *Recherches anatomo-pathologiques sur l'encéphale et ses dépendances*. Béchet, Paris.

Lebert, H. (1866) Über die Aneurysmen der Hirnarterien. Eine Abhandlung in Briefen an Herrn Geheimrat Professor Dr. Frerichs. *Berliner klinische Wochenschrift* **3**, 209–405 (8 instalments).

Lister, J. (1870) Effect of the antiseptic system of treatment on the salubrity of a surgical hospital. *Lancet* **i** (4–6), 40–42.

Ljunggren, B., Sharma, S. & Buchfelder, M. (1993) Intracranial aneurysms. *Neurosurgical Quarterly* **3**, 120–152.

Lobstein, J.F.M. (1829) *Traité d'anatomie pathologique*. Levrault, Paris.

Louis, P.C.A. (1835) *Recherches sur les effets de la saignée*. de Mignaret, Paris.

Markus, H. (1993) Transcranial Doppler detection of circulating cerebral emboli: a review. *Stroke* **24**, 1246–1250.

Matthews, J.R. (1995) *Quantification and the Quest for Medical Certainty*. Princeton University Press, Princeton.

McDonald, C.A. & Korb, M. (1939) Intracranial aneurysms. *Archives of Neurology and Psychology* **42**, 298–328.

McHenry, L.C. (1969) *Garrison's History of Neurology*. Charles C. Thomas, Springfield.

McHenry, L.C. (1981) A history of stroke. *International Journal of Neurology* **15**, 314–326.

Medical Research Council (1948) Streptomycin treatment of pulmonary tuberculosis. *British Medical Journal* **ii**, 769–782.

Meyer, A. & Hierons, R. (1962) Observations on the history of the 'Circle of Willis'. *Medical History* **6**, 119–130.

Mistichelli, D. (1709) *Trattato dell'apoplessia*. A. de Rossi, Rome.

Moniz, E. (1927) L'encéphalographie artérielle, son importance dans la localisation des tumeurs cérébrales. *Revue Neurologique (Paris)* **48**, 72–90.

Moniz, E. (1933) Anévrysme intra-cranien de la carotide interne droite rendu visible par l'artériographie cérébrale. *Revue d'Oto-Neuro-Ophthalmologie* **11**, 198–203.

Moniz, E. (1940) *Die cerebrale Arteriographie und Phlebographie*. Julius Springer, Berlin.

Morgagni, G.B. (1761) *De Sedibus et Causis Morborum per Anatomen Indigatis Libri Quinque*. ex typographica Remondiana, Vienna.

New, P.J.F. & Scott, W.R. (1975) *Computed Tomography of the Brain and Orbit (EMI Scanning)*. Williams & Wilkins, Baltimore.

Norris, J.W. & Hachinski, V.C. (1982) Misdiagnosis of stroke. *Lancet* **1**, 328–331.

Oppenheim, H. (1913) *Lehrbuch der Nervenkrankheiten für Ärtzte und Studierende*. S. Karger, Berlin.

Osler, W. (1911) Transient attacks of aphasia and paralysis in states of high blood pressure and arteriosclerosis. *Canadian Medical Association Journal* **1**, 919–926.

Pantelakis, S. (1954) Un type particulier d'angiopathie sénile du système nerveux central: l'angiopathie congophile—topographie et fréquence. *Monatsschrift für Psychiatrie und Neurologie* **128**, 219–256.

Paulus Aegineta (625–690) (1844) *The Seven Books* (translated by Francis Adams). The Sydenham Society, London.

Payer, L. (1989) *Medicine and Culture—Notions of Health and Sickness in Britain, the US, France and West Germany*. V. Gollancz, London.

Peabody, G.L. (1891) Relation between arterial disease and visceral changes. *Transactions of the Association of American Physicians* **6**, 154–178.

Pickering, G.W. (1948) Transient cerebral paralysis in hypertension and in cerebral embolism, with special reference to the pathogenesis of chronic hypertensive encephalopathy. *Journal of the American Medical Association* **137**, 423–430.

Portal, A. (1781) Observations sur l'apoplexie. *Histoire de l'Académie des Sciences* **83**, 623–630.

Quincke, H. (1891) Die Lumbalpunktion des Hydrocephalus. *Berliner klinische Wochenschrift* **28**, 965–968.

Raynaud, M. (1862) *De l'asphyxie locale et de la gangrène symmétrique des extrémités*. L. Leclerc, Paris.

Reed, R.L., Siekert, R.G. & Merideth, J. (1973) Rarity of transient focal cerebral ischemia in cardiac dysrhythmia. *Journal of the American Medical Association* **223**, 893–895.

Rosenblath, L. (1918) Über die Entstehung der Hirnblutung bei dem Schlaganfall. *Deutsche Zeitschrift für Nervenkrankheiten* **61**, 10–143.

Ross Russell, R.W. (1961) Observations on the retinal blood-vessels in monocular blindness. *Lancet* **11**, 1422–1428.

Ross Russell, R.W. (1963) Observations on intracerebral aneurysms. *Brain* **86**, 425–442.

Ross Russell, R.W. & Page, N.G.R. (1983) Critical perfusion of the brain and retina. *Brain* **106**, 434.

Rostan, L. (1820) *Recherches sur le ramollissement du cerveau. Ouvrage dans lequel on s'efforce de distinguer les diverses affections de ce viscère par des signes caractéristiques*. Béchet, Paris.

Rush, C. & Shaw, J.F. (1990) *With Sharp Compassion: Norman Dott—Freeman Surgeon of Edinburgh*. Aberdeen University Press, Aberdeen.

Russel, W. (1909) A post-graduate lecture on intermittent closing of the cerebral arteries: its relation to temporary and permanent paralysis. *British Medical Journal* **2**, 1109–1110.

Saitoh, H., Hayakawa, K., Nishimura, K. *et al.* (1995) Rerupture of cerebral aneurysms during angiography. *AJNR: the American Journal of Neuroradiology* **16**, 539–542.

Salonen, J.T., Puska, P. & Mustaniemi, H. (1979) Changes in morbidity and mortality during comprehensive community programme to control cardiovascular diseases during 1972–7 in North Karelia. *British Medical Journal* **2**, 1178–1183.

Satran, R. (1974) Joseph Babinski in the competitive examination (agrégation) of 1892. *Bulletin of the New York Academy of Medicine* **50**, 626–635.

Schiller, F. (1970) Concepts of stroke before and after Virchow. *Medical History* **14**, 115–131.

Scholz, W. (1938) Studien zur Pathologieder Hirngefässe, II. Die drusige Entartung der Hirnarterien und -capillaren. *Zeitschrift für die gesamte Neurologie und Psychiatrie* **162**, 694–715.

Schorstein, J. (1940) Carotid ligation in saccular intracranial aneurysms. *British Journal of Surgery* **28**, 50–70.

Schwartz, P. (1930) *Arten der Schlaganfälle des Gehirns*. Julius Springer, Berlin.

Seldinger, S.I. (1953) Catheter replacement of the needle in percutaneous arteriography. *Acta Radiologica* **39**, 368–378.

Serres, E.R.A. (1819) Nouvelle division des apoplexies. *Annales de Médicine et de Chirurgie* **1**, 246–363.

Serres, E.R.A. (1826) Observations sur la rupture des anévrysmes des artères du cerveau. *Archives générales de Médicine* **10**, 419–431.

Siebler, M., Sitzer, M., Rose, G., Bendfeldt, D. & Steinmetz, H. (1993) Silent cerebral embolism caused by neurologically symptomatic high-grade carotid stenosis. Event rates before and after carotid endarterectomy. *Brain* **116**, 1005–1015.

Soloway, H.B. & Aronson, S.M. (1964) Atheromatous emboli to central nervous system. *Archives of Neurology* **11**, 657–667.

Stolley, P.D. & Lasky, T. (1995) *Investigating disease patterns—the science of epidemiology*. W.H. Freeman and Comp., New York.

van Swieten, G.L.B. (1755) *Commentaria in Hermanni Boerhaave Aphorismos De Cognoscendis et Curandis Morbis*, Vol. 3. J. & H. Verbeek, Leiden.

Symonds, C.P. (1923) Contributions to the clinical study of intracranial aneurysms. *Guy's Hospital Report* 73, 139–158.

Temkin, O. (1971) The historiography of ideas in medicine. In: *Modern Methods in the History of Medicine* (ed. E. Clarke), pp. 1–21. The Athlone Press, London.

Thorwald, J. (1957) *Das Weltreich der Chirurgen*. Steingrüben, Stuttgart.

Todd, E.M. (1991) *The Neuroanatomy of Leonardo da Vinci*. American Association of Neurological Surgeons, Park Ridge.

Todd, N.V., Howie, J.E. & Miller, J.D. (1990) Norman Dott's contribution to aneurysm surgery. *Journal of Neurology, Neurosurgery and Psychiatry* **53**, 455–458.

Torack, R.M. (1975) Congophilic angiopathy complicated by surgery and massive hemorrhage. A light and electron microscopic study. *American Journal of Pathology* **81**, 349–365.

Turnbull, H.M. (1914) Alterations in arterial structure, and their relation to syphilis. *Quarterly Journal of Medicine* **8**, 201–254.

Vesalius, A. (1538) *Tabulae anatomicae*. D. Bernardini, Venice.

Vesalius, A. (1543) *De humani corporis fabrica*. J. Oporini, Basle.

Vesling, J. (1647) *Syntagma Anatomicum, Locis Pluribus Actum, Emendatum, Novisque Iconibus Diligenter Exornatum*. Pauli Frombotti Bibliopolae, Padua.

Vicq d'Azyr, F. (1786) *Traité d'anatomie et de physiologie*. F. A. Didot, Paris.

Virchow, R.L.K. (1847) Ueber die akute Entzündung der Arterien. *Archiv für Pathologie und Anatomie* **1**, 272–378.

Virchow, R.L.K. (1856) Thrombose und embolie: gefässentzündung und septische infektion. In: *Gesammelte Abhandlungen zur Wissenschaftlichen Medizin* (ed. R.L.K. Virchow), pp. 219–735. Meidinger, Frankfurt.

Warlow, C. (1984) Carotid endarterectomy: does it work? *Stroke* **15**, 1068–1076.

Watts, C. (1982) External carotid artery embolus from the internal carotid artery 'stump' during angiography—case report. *Stroke* **13**, 515–517.

Wepfer, J.J. (1658) *Observationes Anatomicae, ex Cadaveribus Eorum, Quos Sustulit Apoplexia, cum Exercitatione de Ejus Loco Affecto*. J.C. Suteri, Schaffhausen.

Westphal, K. (1932) Über die Entstehung und Behandlung der Apoplexia sanguinea. *Deutsche medizinische Wochenschrift* **58**, 685–690.

Wichern, H. (1912) Klinische Beiträge zur Kenntnis der Hirnaneurysmen. *Deutsche Zeitschrift für Nervenheilkunde* **44**, 220–263.

Williamson, J.W., German, P.S., Weiss, R., Skinner, E.A. & Bowes, F (1989) Health science information management and continuing education of physicians. A survey of U.S. primary care practitioners and their opinion leaders. *Annals of Internal Medicine* **110**, 151–160.

Willis, T. (1684) *Dr. Willis's practice of physick*. Dring, Harper & Leigh, London.

Witmer, R. & Schmid, A. (1958) Cholesterinkristall als retinaler arterieller Embolus. *Ophthalmologica* **135**, 432–433.

Wood, G.B. (1852) *Treatise on the practice of medicine*. Lippincott, Philadelphia.

Yusuf, S., Peto, R., Lewis, J., Collins, R. & Sleight, P. (1985) Beta blockade during and after myocardial infarction: an overview of the randomized trials. *Progress in Cardiovascular Disease* **27**, 335–371.

Zanette, E.M., Roberti, C., Mancini, G., Pozzilli, C., Bragoni, M. & Toni, D. (1995) Spontaneous middle cerebral artery reperfusion in ischemic stroke. A follow-up study with transcranial Doppler. *Stroke* **26**, 430–433.

van Zuilen, E.V., Moll, F.L., Vermeulen, F.E., Mauser, H.W., van Gijn, J. & Ackerstaff, R.G. (1995) Detection of cerebral microemboli by means of transcranial Doppler monitoring before and after carotid endarterectomy. *Stroke* **26**, 210–213.

CHAPTER THREE

Is it a vascular event and where is the lesion? Identifying and interpreting the symptoms and signs of cerebrovascular disease

3.1 Introduction

If one is to produce a complete diagnostic formulation in a patient presenting with a possible cerebrovascular event, a series of questions need to be answered using information from the history, examination and appropriate investigations (Table 3.1). Although we will describe the process in what we hope seems to be an orderly sequence, in real-life practice new pieces of information that are relevant to different parts of the diagnostic process keep appearing all the time, and the physician always needs to be alert to this. In this chapter, we will work systematically through the process required to determine whether or not the event was vascular in origin, and where the lesion is in the brain. At the same time, one should be trying to relate this to an identifiable vascular territory and recognizable clinical syndrome (Chapter 4). Then, usually with the help of suitably planned investigations, one should try and determine the pathological type of that event (Chapter 5) and the cause (Chapters 6, 7, 8 and 9). Finally, the resulting impairments, disabilities and handicaps experienced by patients and their carers need to be assessed (Chapter 15).

The diagnosis of a cerebrovascular vs. a non-vascular event is something that continues to be based primarily on clinical information, even in an increasingly technological environment. By definition, all patients with a transient ischaemic attack (TIA) or stroke will have had focal neurological symptoms, although depending on the timing of the assessment, these may have resolved, and the patient may or may not have abnormal physical signs (section 3.2). This emphasizes the crucial importance of the first contact between clinician and patient whilst taking a history and performing a physical examination. It is also very important to obtain information from any observers, family and friends, combined with a review of the patient's medical records, particularly when

Table 3.1 The diagnostic process.

Is it a stroke, a transient ischaemic attack, or a brain attack?	Chapter 3
Which part of the brain has been affected?	Chapter 3
Which arterial territory has been affected?	Chapter 4
Is there a recognizable clinical syndrome?	Chapter 4
What pathological type of cerebrovascular event is it?	Chapter 5
What disease process caused the cerebrovascular event?	Chapters 6–8
What, if any, are the functional consequences?	Chapter 15

the patient is unable to communicate clearly. Even with the arrival of hyper-acute stroke treatments, when there is pressure to assess and treat patients as quickly as possible, it remains vitally important to take a detailed history of the presenting symptoms from all available sources. Although in this context it may actually be detrimental to the patients to spend time chasing details that are not of immediate relevance to the diagnosis (e.g. smoking history, family history), continued efforts should nevertheless be made to obtain the relevant information over the subsequent few days.

A record in the notes such as 'no history available' probably reflects laziness on the part of a doctor who has not tried fully to obtain it, rather than the real lack of any information.

The examination may not only confirm the presence of focal neurological signs anticipated from the history but also alert the clinician to relevant yet unanticipated disorders (e.g. malignant hypertension); possible aetiological explanations for the event (e.g. atrial fibrillation, carotid bruits, cardiac murmurs, etc.; section 6.6.7); contraindications to investigation (e.g. a pacemaker and magnetic resonance examination); and nursing and rehabilitation needs (e.g. impaired swallowing, pre-existing reduced visual or auditory acuity). A sophisticated knowledge of neurology is not needed to elicit and recognize the clinical features of a cerebrovascular event, but it should go without saying that physicians must continually make efforts to refine their clinical abilities if the symptoms and signs are to be documented accurately. It is surprising how rarely one sees this mentioned in textbooks; yet, for example, if radiologists were beginning to use a new imaging modality, it would be accepted that they need to be trained and, even after that, there would be a continuous learning and auditing process. Failure to recognize or, conversely, a tendency to over-interpret a clinical symptom or sign, is no different from failing to report an infarct on computed tomography (CT) or reporting incorrectly a Virchow–Robin space as a lacunar infarct on magnetic resonance imaging (MRI). It has been shown that the accuracy of the clinical diagnosis of lacunar stroke (section 4.3.2)—albeit when judged against neuroimaging—is significantly better when the clinician has a specific interest in cerebrovascular disease, and there is no reason to believe that this would not be the same for other types of stroke (Lodder *et al.* 1994). The importance of clinical signs in medicine is now being investigated by the CARE (Clinical Assessment of the Reliability of the Examination) international collaborative group (McAlister *et al.* 1999).

A sophisticated knowledge of neurology is not needed to elicit and recognize the clinical features of a cerebrovascular event, but physicians must continually make efforts to refine their clinical abilities if the symptoms and signs are to be documented accurately.

There are many texts devoted to the honing of clinical skills and the recognition and interpretation of the many subtle and interesting facets of disturbed function of the nervous system (e.g. Duus 1989; Patten 1995). The following section is therefore not intended to give a comprehensive account of the subject. However, there are some aspects that seem particularly relevant to the diagnosis and management of patients with cerebrovascular disease, and we will concentrate on these. It is worth remembering that the art of diagnosis is to assign the symptoms and signs their due degree of importance.

3.2 Transient ischaemic attack, stroke or 'brain attack'—what's in a name?

In the first edition of this book, we accepted without much comment the traditional definitions of transient ischaemic attack (TIA) and stroke. Because a great deal of research and clinical practice is based around these definitions, we will continue to use them as a basic framework. However, we recognize that with the increasing focus on hyper-acute treatments and patients being assessed within a few hours of the onset of symptoms, the question must be asked whether the arbitrary distinction between TIA and stroke based on a 24-h cut-off, which was developed primarily for epidemiological purposes, remains valid and useful. Ideally, when writing a textbook, one would have liked any new or controversial issues to have been the subject of considerable professional discussion. But when it comes to the definition of cerebrovascular events, so far at least any such discussion has not been very extensive. Therefore, we can only offer our own thoughts on how the area might develop over the next few years.

3.2.1 The diagnosis of transient ischaemic attack

A standard definition of a TIA is 'a clinical syndrome characterized by an acute loss of focal cerebral or monocular function with symptoms lasting less than 24 h and which is thought to be due to inadequate cerebral or ocular blood supply as a result of low blood flow, arterial thrombosis or embolism associated with disease of the arteries, heart or blood' (adapted from Hankey & Warlow 1994).

Because the diagnosis of TIA is clinical and not based on any specific diagnostic test, we have to rely on a certain constellation of clinical features that are thought to have a similar pathophysiological background (i.e. caused by focal cerebral or ocular ischaemia) and to be associated with similar outcomes (i.e. an increased risk of stroke and other major vascular events). Focal neurological symptoms are those that arise from a disturbance in an identifiable and localized area of the brain—for example, unilateral weakness or sensory loss from lesions of the motor and sensory pathways (Table 3.2). However, there are some focal neurological symptoms which, when they occur in isolation (such as rotational vertigo, transient amnesia, deafness, dysarthria or diplopia) should probably not be considered as TIAs, because they all occur more commonly in non-vascular conditions.

Localized cerebral ischaemia causes focal neurological symptoms, i.e. the symptoms of a transient ischaemic attack or stroke.

On the other hand, non-focal symptoms are not usually caused by localized cerebral ischaemia; for example, faintness, non-specific dizziness, light-headedness, confusion, mental deterioration, incontinence, drop attacks, or loss of consciousness (Table 3.3). Such symptoms are common, especially in the elderly population, and although they may be caused by cerebral ischaemia, there are many other more common non-vascular causes. Therefore, it is generally accepted that they should not be interpreted as TIAs—not least because when they occur in isolation, they do not seem to predict future serious vascular events. There is a serious risk that if non-focal symptoms, particularly when they are short-lived, are regarded as being due to TIA, then the term will become a 'diagnostic dustbin', with consequent inappropriate and potentially hazardous investigation, treatment and advice to patients.

Non-focal symptoms such as faintness, dizziness or generalized weakness are seldom, if ever, due to focal cerebral ischaemia (i.e. seldom a transient ischaemic attack or stroke), but may be due to generalized brain ischaemia (e.g. syncope) as well as non-vascular causes (e.g. hyperventilation or anxiety).

Table 3.2 Focal neurological and ocular symptoms.

Motor symptoms
Weakness or clumsiness of one side of the body, in whole or in part (hemiparesis, monoparesis)
Simultaneous bilateral weakness (paraparesis, quadriparesis)*
Difficulty in swallowing (dysphagia)*
Imbalance (ataxia)*

Speech/language disturbances
Difficulty in understanding or expressing spoken language (aphasia)
Difficulty in reading (dyslexia) or writing (dysgraphia)
Difficulty in calculating (dyscalculia)
Slurred speech (dysarthria)*

Sensory symptoms
Altered feeling on one side of the body, in whole or in part (hemisensory disturbance)

Visual symptoms
Loss of vision in one eye, in whole or in part (transient monocular blindness)
Loss of vision in half or quarter of the visual field (hemianopia, quadrantanopia)
Bilateral blindness
Double vision (diplopia)*

Vestibular symptoms
A spinning sensation (vertigo)*

Behavioural/cognitive symptoms
Difficulty in dressing, combing hair, cleaning teeth; geographical disorientation (visuospatial–perceptual dysfunction)
Forgetfulness (amnesia)*

* As an isolated symptom, this may not necessarily indicate a focal brain lesion (e.g. due to focal cerebral ischaemia or haemorrhage).

Table 3.3 Non-focal neurological symptoms.

Generalized weakness and/or sensory disturbance
Light-headedness
Faintness
'Blackouts' with altered or loss of consciousness or fainting, with or without impaired vision in both eyes
Incontinence of urine or faeces
Confusion
Ringing in ears (tinnitus)

Additionally, transient global amnesia (section 3.4.3) and migraine (section 3.4.1) are not considered to be TIAs, because their prognosis is on average much better than that in TIA patients (Hodges & Warlow 1990a, b; Dennis & Warlow 1992).

TIAs fulfilling the above definition are usually presumed to be due to ischaemia. Primary intracerebral haemorrhage almost invariably causes more prolonged or permanent focal neurological dysfunction, although there are isolated reports of neurological deficits that have resolved within a few days (Scott & Miller 1985; Dennis *et al.* 1987), and even 24 h (Gunatilake 1998; Ivo 1999). However, one sometimes needs to probe quite hard to be sure about the duration of symptoms from the history. For example, 'I got better in 24 h' does not necessarily mean 'I got completely back to normal', and it is the latter to which we are referring when defining a TIA. The majority of TIAs, and particularly ocular attacks, last less than an hour, and only about 5% last more than 12 h (Fig. 3.1).

A 77-year-old man, whilst standing in his garden, suddenly developed weakness of the right arm and unsteadiness on walking. He had no headache or vomiting. He sat down and within 3 h was 'better', although on closer questioning it emerged that his arm had not returned to normal for about 3 days. A CT brain scan 8 days later showed a small haemorrhage in the left putamen. This was not a TIA in either its duration or pathology

3.2.2 The diagnosis of stroke

The most widely accepted definition of a stroke is 'a clinical syndrome characterized by rapidly developing clinical symptoms and/or signs of focal, and at times global (applied to patients in deep coma and those with subarachnoid haemorrhage), loss of cerebral function, with symptoms lasting more than 24 h or leading to death, with no apparent cause other than that of vascular origin' (Hatano 1976). This definition embraces stroke due to cerebral infarction, primary intracerebral haemorrhage (PICH), intraventricular haemorrhage and most cases of subarachnoid haemorrhage (SAH). By convention, it does not include subdural haemorrhage, epidural haemorrhage, or intracerebral haemorrhage or infarction caused by trauma, infection or tumour; nor does this definition embrace patients with SAH who are conscious and have a headache but no abnormal neurological signs (neck stiffness is not invariable and does not occur for several hours). It also excludes patients with retinal infarction. Since the clinical and research implications for the diagnosis, investigation, treatment and prognosis of SAH are, for the most part, quite distinct from those of other forms of stroke, we think it would be better to have a completely separate definition for SAH (Chapter 9). The definition of stroke could then become 'a clinical syndrome characterized by an acute loss of focal cerebral function with symptoms lasting more than 24 h or leading to death, and which is thought to be due to either spontaneous haemorrhage into the brain substance or inadequate cerebral blood supply to a part of the brain as a result of low blood flow, thrombosis, or embolism associated with diseases of the blood vessels, heart, or blood'.

The clinical differentiation of 'stroke' from 'not a stroke' has been reported to be accurate more than 95% of the time if there is a clear history (from the patient or carer) of focal brain dysfunction of sudden onset (or first noticed on waking), with symptoms persisting for more than 24 h (Allen 1983; Sandercock *et al.* 1985). This is particularly true if the patient is elderly or has other vascular diseases or risk factors, because the prevalence—i.e. the prior (or pretest) probability of stroke—is greater in elderly people with vascular disease than in younger people who have no evidence of vascular disease. However, the accuracy of the diagnosis of stroke also depends on the timing of the assessment.

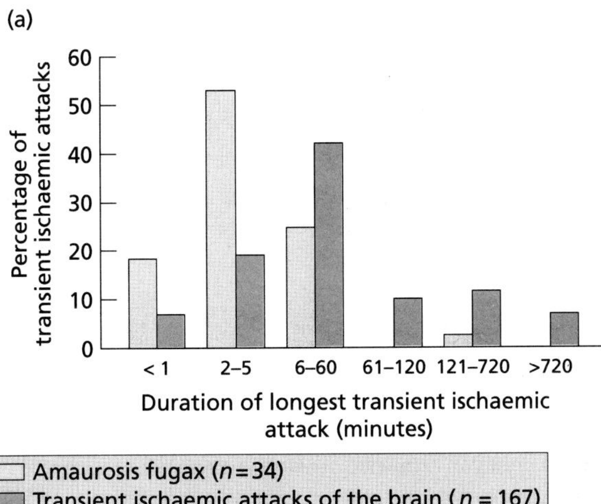

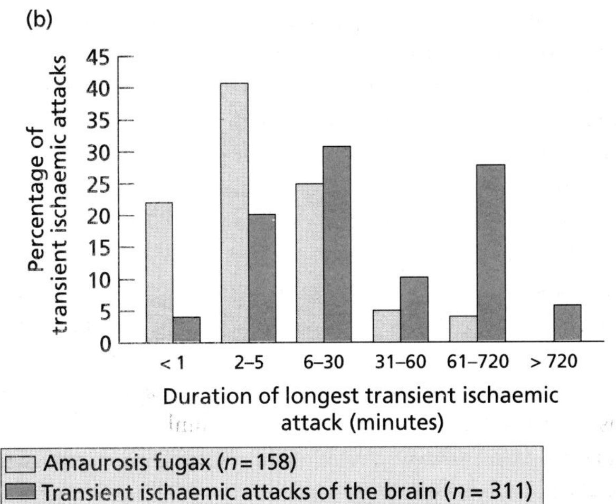

Fig. 3.1 Histogram of the duration of the longest transient ischaemic attack (TIA) before presentation amongst: (a) 184 TIA patients in the Oxfordshire Community Stroke Project; (b) 469 TIA patients in a hospital-referred series (with permission from Hankey & Warlow 1994).

Sandercock *et al.* (1985) were assessing patients at a mean of 4 days after onset of symptoms, rather than during the first few hours as is often the case in current clinical practice. It is important to remember that as time passes, other bits of the history or physical signs emerge and are likely to improve diagnostic accuracy. On the other hand, it can also be difficult if patients are first seen a long time after the onset of their stroke, particularly when they are elderly, because they may not remember clearly the onset and nature of their symptoms, and any clinical signs may have resolved.

As with TIA, it is sometimes not possible to obtain a clear history of the onset, or even the nature of the symptoms, although the reasons are likely to be somewhat different—e.g. because the patient is unconscious, confused, demented or dysphasic. In these patients in particular, the presence of a persistent focal neurological deficit may not be due to stroke but to head trauma, encephalitis, brain abscess, brain tumour or a chronic subdural haematoma (section 3.4). The presence of symptoms or signs that are unusual in uncomplicated stroke, such as papilloedema and unexplained fever, should call into question the clinical diagnosis. Also, a persistent focal neurological deficit may be due to a previous stroke, and the new clinical presentation may be due to a non-vascular problem such as pneumonia (section 15.12). In the absence of information about the rate of onset and progression of symptoms, it is crucial to search for indirect clues to their cause in the past history and physical examination, and to continue to assess the patient over time for the development of new signs such as fever, and for the improvement that characterizes most non-fatal strokes.

The diagnosis of a cerebrovascular event is usually made at the bedside, not in the laboratory or in the X-ray department. It depends on the history of the sudden onset of focal neurological symptoms in the appropriate clinical setting (usually an older patient with vascular risk factors) and the exclusion of other conditions that can present in a similar way.

It is worth mentioning that the absence of an obvious focal neurological deficit by no means excludes a stroke in patients who have suffered a *sudden* decline in neurological function. It may simply be a consequence of a delay in presentation, so that the signs have resolved, or it may be that the signs are rather subtle (but nevertheless functionally important to the patient) and have been missed. Commonly overlooked problems include patients who have a visuospatial or perceptual disorder (e.g. dressing apraxia, geographical disorientation) but no weakness in the limbs due to a non-dominant parietal lesion (section 3.3.3); subtle cognitive dysfunction (section 3.3.3); or truncal and gait ataxia due to a cerebellar stroke, which is only apparent (or elicitable) if the patient is sat up, got out of bed and asked to walk (Dunne *et al.* 1986; Mori & Yamadori 1987) (section 3.3.7). These are the types of deficit that may be missed (but should not be) on busy ward rounds, during a hurried post-carotid endarterectomy or coronary artery bypass surgery assessment, or indeed any time.

3.2.3 The overlap between transient ischaemic attack and stroke, and the concept of 'brain attack'

The standard definition of TIA allows abnormal but functionally unimportant focal neurological signs such as reflex asymmetry or an extensor plantar response to persist for longer than 24 h, provided the *symptoms* have resolved—this occurs in about 5% of patients (Hankey *et al.* 1991). Furthermore, on CT or standard MR imaging, evidence of infarction may be present in an area of the brain relevant to the transient symptoms in at least 25% of patients (Awad *et al.* 1986; Dennis *et al.* 1990a; Hankey & Warlow 1994). In the past, this led some authors to suggest that patients with transient focal neurological symptoms lasting less than 24 h, but with an anatomically appropriate area of presumed infarction on the scan, should not be classified as having TIAs but as having 'cerebral infarction with transient signs' (CITS) (Waxman & Toole 1983; Bogousslavsky & Regli 1984; Murros *et al.* 1989). In the first edition of this book, we identified the following problems with such a scheme:

- a CT or MRI scan becomes essential for the diagnosis of TIA, and as technology advances the definition of a TIA would be constantly changing (e.g. diffusion-weighted MRI has been reported to show abnormalities that were not present on T2-weighted MRI in a third of patients with clinical TIAs (Bryan *et al.* 1991; Kidwell *et al.* 1999);
- there is a gradual increase in the percentage of patients with a 'relevant' abnormality on brain imaging as the duration of symptoms increases, with no distinct change at 24 h (Fig. 3.2)—arguing against there being significantly different underlying pathophysiology (Awad *et al.* 1986; Koudstaal *et al.* 1989; Kidwell *et al.* 1999);
- the 'relevant' abnormality on CT or MRI may not represent infarction occurring at the time of the TIA (it may be an old infarct or even an old haemorrhage). To some extent, this argument may be countered by the use of diffusion-weighted MR techniques, but in that case the imaged abnormalities may only be present for a short time (Kidwell *et al.* 1999; Lecouvet *et al.* 1999);
- a new diagnostic category would have to be made for patients with a clinically definite stroke (i.e. symptoms for more than 24 h) who have a normal CT or MRI, which could hardly be called a 'TIA' (Hankey & Warlow 1994).

In the early 1990s, the most important clinical issue was whether the presence or absence of presumed brain infarction in TIA patients had any meaning as an independent predictor of subsequent important vascular events, such as stroke. There appeared to be no significant differences in the

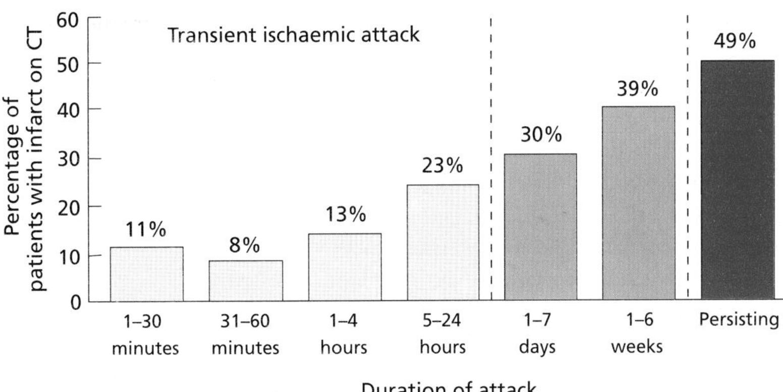

Fig. 3.2 Duration of ischaemic attack and percentage of patients with an appropriately sited low-density area on a CT brain scan (with permission from Koudstaal *et al.* 1992).

clinical features, prevalence of vascular risk factors and characteristics of the TIA in patients with and without a relevant infarct on CT, and it remains uncertain whether the presence of such a 'TIA scar' is associated with an increased risk of future stroke (Dennis *et al.* 1989c; Dennis *et al.* 1990a; Koudstaal *et al.* 1991a; Dutch TIA Trial Study Group 1993; Eliasziw *et al.* 1995) (section 16.1.1). Therefore, we concluded that patients with clinically definite TIAs who had an appropriately sited and presumably ischaemic lesion on CT or MRI should have the fact noted, but should still be classified as having had a TIA and not a stroke.

The presence of a presumed ischaemic lesion in the relevant part of the brain on CT or MR scan in a patient who presents with transient symptoms lasting less than 24 h should not change the diagnosis of transient ischaemic attack to stroke.

It is still important to distinguish TIA from minor ischaemic stroke when conducting incidence and case–control studies of cerebrovascular disease for several reasons. Complete case ascertainment is much less likely to be obtained for TIA than for stroke, since patients who experience brief attacks (i.e. TIA) are more likely to ignore or forget them, and are less likely to report them to a doctor than patients who suffer more prolonged or disabling events (i.e. stroke). However, when performing such studies, it is important to check up on any TIAs that are reported, because sometimes a mild stroke is incorrectly labelled by the non-specialist as a 'TIA'. Another point that is relevant for case–control studies is that there is less change in 'acute phase' haemostatic factors related to thrombosis and there is, by definition, no survival bias amongst TIA patients. There are also good reasons to continue making the distinction in everyday practice. The differential diagnosis of focal neurological symptoms lasting minutes (e.g. epileptic seizures, migraine) is somewhat different from that of attacks lasting several hours to days (e.g. intracranial tumour, intracerebral haemorrhage), and the reliability of the clinical diagnosis of stroke is much better than for TIA (section 3.4). It can aid assessment of casemix in individual units (section 17.6.3) and also audits of management (section 17.6.2).

On the other hand, patients with TIA and mild ischaemic stroke have many similarities: they have a similar age and sex distribution, a similar prevalence of vascular risk factors (and probably therefore pathogenesis; section 6.2) and they share the same long-term risk of serious vascular events (Whisnant *et al.* 1999) (section 16.1.1). Thus, from the point of view of secondary prevention, there seems no pressing need to distinguish them, and indeed many clinical trials of secondary prevention have focused on patients with reversible ischaemic attacks (who recover in minutes, days, or weeks) rather than those with major disabling ischaemic stroke and permanent handicap.

The problem—which was always inherent, but which has become much more apparent in the era of increasingly rapid assessment and treatment of patients with acute cerebrovascular disease—is how to use these time-based definitions of stroke and TIA in patients who are being seen, and in some cases treated with potentially dangerous drugs, within a few hours of the onset of symptoms. If one takes a scenario such as that of the hemiparetic patient being assessed 2 h after the onset of symptoms, one of the most common questions asked by students and residents is 'but how do you know whether this attack will turn out to be a TIA or a stroke'? At this point, it is instructive to return to the origins of these definitions. In one of the first attempts to define various aspects of cerebrovascular disease (Advisory Council for the National Institute of Neurological Diseases and Blindness 1958), attacks of 'transient cerebral ischaemia without infarction' were considered to last '10 seconds, 10 minutes or even an hour'. This definition was reflected in early epidemiological studies such as that of Acheson *et al.* (1968), who used a definition of stroke that included patients with symptoms lasting more than 1 h. As can be seen from Fig. 3.1, the majority of patients who are ultimately classified as having a TIA have symptoms that last minutes rather than hours—a fact that makes the original definition of TIA look very sensible! However, in 1975 the Advisory Council produced a further statement, which described 'transient ischemic attacks ... commonly lasting from two to 15 min but occasionally lasting as long as a day (24 h)' and 'completed stroke ... duration more than 24 hours' (Advisory Council for the National Institute of Neurological Diseases and Blindness 1975), a distinction that was then carried over to the widely used WHO definition (Hatano 1976).

Looked at from the perspective of physicians seeing patients acutely (i.e. within 24 h from onset of symptoms), there are basically two groups of patients: those whose symptoms have resolved at the time of assessment and therefore can be correctly referred to as having TIAs, and those who still have symptoms with or without relevant physical signs. It would seem inappropriate (and potentially confusing) to use the term 'stroke' in this situation, and we can see that there may be value in using a new term such as 'brain attack', not least because it would remind clinicians about issues such as the accuracy of diagnosis and the scope of the differential diagnosis (sections 3.4 and 3.5), which almost certainly differ somewhat from patients with completed stroke (i.e. a patient being seen with symptoms after 24 h have passed). At present, there are few data concerning in-hospital diagnostic accuracy in this particular clinical group. Allder *et al.* (1999) reported an 8.6% rate of clinical misdiagnosis in a study of 70 patients who were imaged at a mean of 11.4 h post-onset. However, data have been reported for the prehospital diagnosis of hyper-acute cerebrovascular disease by paramedical personnel using a variety of protocols, with positive predictive values of about 70–80% (Kothari *et al.* 1995; Harbison *et al.* 1999; Kidwell *et al.* 2000).

3.3 The clinical approach to the diagnosis of a cerebrovascular event

When a patient presents with a suspected transient ischaemic attack, 'brain attack' or stroke, the first question to answer is whether it really is a vascular event or not. This begins with and depends on a sound, carefully taken clinical history.

Initially, it is important to take the patient and/or eyewitness back to the onset of symptoms—recording their own words and not just your interpretation of them. This can usually be achieved by asking the three questions: 'When did it happen?' 'Where were you when it happened?' and 'What were you doing when it happened?' For clarification, it is always worth asking patients to describe their symptoms in an alternative way, particularly if the terms they use are rather vague, e.g. 'dizziness'. Also it can sometimes be useful to ask patients whether they would have been able to do a specific task at the time of symptom onset; for example, if the patient describes an arm as being 'dead', asking whether they could lift the arm above their head would at least give a pointer as to whether the use of the word 'dead' was referring to a motor or just a sensory deficit.

The use of certain terms is often culturally determined, and you must not assume that your interpretation of the term is the same as the patient's. The most appropriate response if you are unsure is 'what do you mean by that?' or 'try and describe what you mean in another way'.

Whilst taking the history, it is always worth bearing in mind that you are trying to obtain information about the following:

- The nature of the symptoms and signs (sections 3.3.1–3.3.7):
  Which modalities were involved (e.g. motor, sensory, visual)?
  Which anatomical areas were involved (e.g. face, arm, leg and was it the whole of the limb, one or both eyes)?
  Were the symptoms focal or non-focal (Tables 3.2 and 3.3)?
  What was their quality (i.e. 'negative', causing loss of sensory, motor or visual function; or 'positive', causing limb jerking, tingling, hallucinations)?
  What were the functional consequences (e.g. unable to stand, unable to lift arm)?
- The speed of onset and temporal course of the neurological symptoms (section 3.3.8):
  What time of day did they begin?
  Was the onset sudden?
  Were the symptoms more or less maximal at onset; did they spread or progress in a stepwise, remitting, or progressive fashion over minutes/hours/days; or were there fluctuations between normal and abnormal function?
- Were there any possible precipitants (section 3.3.9)?
  What was the patient doing at the time and immediately preceding the onset?
- Were there any accompanying symptoms (section 3.3.10)?
  Headache, epileptic seizures, panic and anxiety, vomiting, hiccups, chest pain.
- Is there any relevant past history (section 3.3.11)?
  Have there been any previous attacks of TIA or stroke?
  Is there a history of hypertension, hypercholesterolaemia, diabetes mellitus, angina, myocardial infarction, intermittent claudication, or arteritis?
  Is there a family history of vascular or thrombotic disorders?
- Are there any relevant lifestyle habits/behaviours (section 3.3.12)?
  Cigarette-smoking, alcohol consumption, diet, physical activity, medications (especially the oral contraceptive pill, antithrombotic drugs, anticoagulants, and recreational drugs such as amphetamine).

3.3.1 The nature of the symptoms and signs

The natural starting-point when taking the history is the neurological symptoms themselves. In order to interpret them correctly, the physician needs to be clear about the definitions of terms used, have a working knowledge of simple neuroanatomy, be aware of common clinical patterns caused by cerebrovascular disease, and also be able to recognize when symptoms are not likely to be due to a vascular event. The physician also needs to be able to elicit relevant clinical signs. In the next sections, we will describe the most important aspects of each of these components of the clinical assessment.

The functional modalities that are affected by transient ischaemic attack (TIA) and stroke reflect the areas of the brain that are involved by the ischaemia or haemorrhage. In patients with cerebrovascular disease, these can be considered under the headings of disturbance of conscious level, higher cerebral function, motor function, somatic sensory function, visual function and hearing, balance and coordination. It is important to remember that, particularly during a brief episode of ischaemia, the neurological symptoms can only reflect the activities in which the patient was engaged during the attack—another reason to ask carefully about the activities at symptom onset. For example, if the patient was not speaking or did not try to speak or read during the event, it is impossible to know whether aphasia or alexia was present or not. Similarly, a weak leg may well not be noticed if the patient was not standing. As many hours of wakefulness are spent in an alert state with eyes open, with a keen sensorium, an upright posture and often speaking or reading, it is not surprising that most of the symptoms that TIA patients experience are of motor, somatosensory, visual or language function (Table 3.4). Other more transient activities such as swallowing and calculation are, not surprisingly, less frequently reported. Presumably TIAs, like strokes, can start during sleep, but the patient will be unaware of them if they have resolved before waking.

3.3.2 Disturbance of conscious level

(see also section 15.3)

Consciousness may be defined as 'the state of awareness of the self and the environment', whilst coma is the total absence of such awareness (Plum & Posner 1985). Vascular diseases are probably the second most common cause of non-traumatic coma after metabolic/toxic disorders, and up to 20% of patients with stroke—but not with transient ischaemic attacks (TIAs)—may have some impairment of consciousness (Bogousslavsky *et al.* 1988; Melo *et al.* 1992a). One reason for starting with a discussion of consciousness is that it is an assessment that appears on nearly all emergency paramedical documentation. Furthermore, the evaluation of all other functional modalities is much more difficult (and probably less reliable) if there is a reduced conscious level, and it is also a very important predictor of survival and functional outcome (section 10.2.7). Consciousness is usually considered to have two components: alertness (or arousal) and content (or the sum of cognitive and affective mental functions), but when dealing with a predominantly focal disorder such as stroke, where there are frequently cognitive deficits, one tends to consider the 'conscious level' in the more restricted sense of level of alertness.

Table 3.4 Neurological symptoms during transient ischaemic attacks.

	% (total = 184)
Unilateral weakness, heaviness or clumsiness	50
Unilateral sensory symptoms	35
Slurred speech (dysarthria)	23
Transient monocular blindness	18
Difficulty in speaking (aphasia)	18
Unsteadiness (ataxia)	12
Dizziness (vertigo)	5
Homonymous hemianopia	5
Double vision (diplopia)	5
Bilateral limb weakness	4
Difficulty in swallowing (dysphagia)	1
Crossed motor and sensory loss	1

From a series of 184 patients with a definite transient ischaemic attack (TIA) in the Oxfordshire Community Stroke Project (Dennis 1988). Many patients had more than one symptom (e.g. weakness as well as sensory loss) and no patient had isolated dysarthria, ataxia, vertigo, diplopia or dysphagia. Lone bilateral blindness was excluded from this analysis but later considered to be a TIA (Dennis *et al.* 1989a).

Clinical anatomy

Consciousness is dependent on the proper functioning of the ascending reticular activating system (ARAS). This is a complex functional rather than anatomical grouping of neural structures in the upper brainstem, the subthalamic region and the thalamus (mainly the intralaminar nuclei) (Brodal 1981a). Focal lesions that impair consciousness tend to either disrupt the ARAS directly (i.e. mainly infratentorial lesions), or are large supra-tentorial lesions, which cause secondary brainstem compression (Fig. 3.3).

Clinical assessment

Although terms such as 'drowsy', 'obtunded' and 'stuporous' are used by clinicians, they are imprecise and therefore liable to variable interpretation, and they fail to reflect the continuum of alertness between coma and normality. Relatives

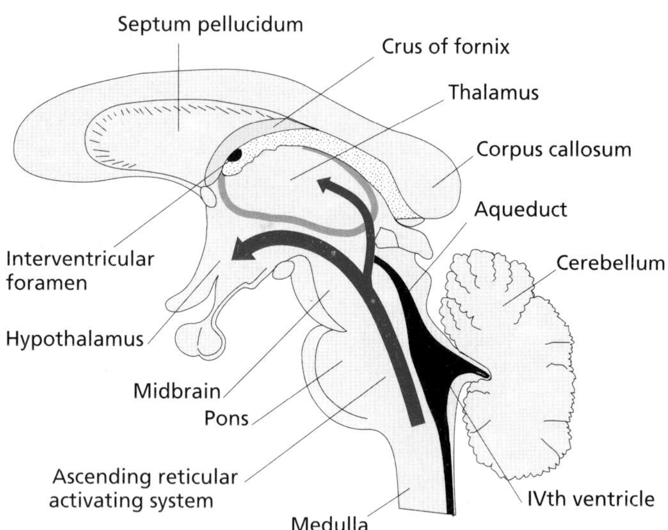

Fig. 3.3 Diagrammatic representation in the sagittal plane of the subcortical areas involved in consciousness (especially the ascending reticular activating system).

may use the term 'unconscious' to describe any state of impaired awareness, and it is very important to ascertain just how rousable the patient was—did the relatives try stimulating them, etc.? Some of the above terms have been used in 'stroke scales' (section 17.6.3), but in that situation operational definitions are described in the relevant manuals (remember that most of these scales were originally developed for use in clinical trials). Thus, it is perhaps not surprising that in this context there is reasonable inter-observer reliability—e.g. for the conscious level questions in the Scandinavian Stroke Scale, the weighted kappa value is 0.74 (Lindenstrom *et al.* 1991).

Once a patient comes into contact with paramedical personnel, the Glasgow Coma Scale (GCS) provides a structured way of describing conscious level, and it is often part of the standard ambulance and nursing observation forms (Table 3.5) (Teasdale & Jennett 1974). It was developed for patients with head injury, and some care is needed when applying it to patients with stroke. It should be stressed to staff that the motor deficit must be assessed in the 'normal' side and not on the side with the motor deficit, and in the arm and not the leg, where the motor responses may be largely of spinal origin. One should probably take more note of each subscore than of the total, since specific focal deficits, and particularly global aphasia, depress the overall score disproportionately to the level of alertness. Prasad and Menon (1998) reported that, in patients with acute stroke, the prediction of outcome was as accurate when using only the eye and motor subscales of the GCS as it was using the full scale. Any deterioration in the GCS should prompt the clinician to consider whether it is because of the progression of the neurological deficit or because of non-vascular factors, such as infection, metabolic disturbance, or the effect of drugs (section 15.5).

Clinical practice

Loss of consciousness during a TIA is extremely unusual and should always prompt a search for alternative explanations, of which syncope is probably the most common (section 3.4.12). Even when transient loss of consciousness is followed by a hemiparesis, it is more commonly caused by an epileptic seizure resulting in a Todd's paresis (section 3.4.2). Although brief episodes of loss of consciousness, sometimes during paroxysms of coughing (Linzer *et al.* 1992), are recognized to occur in some patients with vertebrobasilar occlusive disease and, rarely, in patients with bilateral carotid

Table 3.5 The Glasgow Coma Scale.

Eye opening	
E1	None
E2	To painful stimuli
E3	To command/voices
E4	Spontaneously with blinking
Motor response (best response in unaffected limb)	
M1	None
M2	Arm extension to painful stimulus
M3	Arm flexion to painful stimulus
M4	Arm withdraws from painful stimulus
M5	Hand localizes painful stimulus in the face (reaches at least chin level).
M6	Obeys commands
Verbal response	
V1	None
V2	Sounds but no recognizable words
V3	Inappropriate words/expletives
V4	Confused speech
V5	Normal

The score should be reported as 'Ex, My, Vz, total score $= x+y+z/15$'

occlusive disease (Yanagihara *et al.* 1989), they are far more frequently due to hypotension, systemic disorders and generalized epileptic seizures (Kapoor 1991). When loss of consciousness does occur during a TIA, it seems to be associated with brainstem or bihemispheric ischaemia caused by either vertebrobasilar or bilateral carotid occlusive disease (Yanagihara *et al.* 1989). A few cases may be due to ischaemia in the territory of small, perforating arteries which supply the upper brainstem including components of the reticular activating system. Sometimes elderly patients are found, usually early in the morning or in the afternoon, profoundly unresponsive without other neurological signs and they recover completely within 12 h (Haimovic & Beresford 1992). These episodes may recur, and all diagnostic tests are unremarkable; the electroencephalogram (EEG) usually shows only diffuse slowing of the background rhythm. Whether or not this is a sleep disorder is unknown (Rao *et al.* 1994).

Loss of consciousness during a transient ischaemic attack is extremely unusual.

Almost instantaneous loss of consciousness caused by a stroke suggests either a subarachnoid haemorrhage or an intrinsic brainstem haemorrhage. Later depression of the conscious level is most likely to occur in patients with displacement of midline structures (Ropper 1986, 1989). Transtentorial herniation is an almost invariable, but later, accompaniment (Reich *et al.* 1993). A large intracerebral haematoma, and particularly a cerebellar haematoma, may result in loss of consciousness within a few hours of stroke onset, due to secondary brainstem compression. Early impairment of consciousness from a supratentorial infarct is most unusual. This is probably because the associated cerebral oedema responsible for the mass effect, and so the midline shift, usually takes 1–3 days to develop, although evidence of transtentorial herniation may be present within 24 h (Shaw *et al.* 1959; Silver *et al.* 1984). In post-mortem studies, Torvik & Jorgensen (1964, 1966) and Greenhall (1977) showed that infarction of the complete middle cerebral artery (MCA) territory is needed before significant lateral and caudal displacement of midline structures occurs. Not surprisingly, level of consciousness is one of the best predictors of survival after stroke (section 10.2.7).

There are a number of relatively rare clinical syndromes in which patients have severely impaired responsiveness, but not impairment of consciousness. The neuroanatomical and management implications of these states are important:

• *the 'locked-in' syndrome* is probably the most important to recognize. This is a state of motor de-efferentation, where there is usually severe paralysis not only of the limbs but also of the neck, jaw and face. Indeed, the only muscles remaining under voluntary control may be those concerned with vertical eye movements and the ability to blink. All this occurs with clear, and often extremely distressing, retention of awareness. The patient is unable to communicate by word or movement other than by blinking or moving the eyes up and down, but is fully aware of the surroundings and attempts to respond to them. Hearing, vision and often sensation are retained (Bauby 1997). There is usually an extensive, bilateral lesion in the ventral pons, which interrupts the descending motor tracts as well as the centre for horizontal eye movements in the pons, but the oculomotor nuclei and descending pathways for vertical eye movements are spared together with the ascending reticular activating system (Fig. 3.4). In this condition, cognitive functions must be considered normal and so the patients must be given a full explanation of their predicament. One often needs to reiterate this to other staff and take appropriate account of the normal cognition and sensation when planning long-term care, since prolonged survival in this state is possible (Katz *et al.* 1992).

The relatives and staff caring for patients with the locked-in syndrome need reminding regularly that sensation, cognitive functions and awareness are all normal.

• *akinetic mutism* and *abulia* are states where there is limited responsiveness to the environment, although the patients appear alert (or at least wakeful) in that their eyes are open and they follow objects. However, in contrast to the locked-in syndrome, the physical examination does not reveal evidence of a major lesion of the descending motor pathways. At its most extreme, patients with akinetic mutism may lie with open eyes, follow objects and become agitated or even say the occasional appropriate word following noxious stimuli (thus distinguishing this state from that of coma or the persistent vegetative state); but otherwise they do not respond to their environment. Occasionally, catatonic posturing may occur (Cairns *et al.* 1941; Plum & Posner 1985). If patients recover from this state, they have no recollection of it. 'Abulia' is a term used to describe a less severe presentation of reduced spontaneous movement and speech (Fisher 1995). Such patients often appear to have a marked flatness of affect, but with adequate stimulation they can be shown to be conscious and have relatively preserved cognition. Both akinetic mutism and abulia occur with bilateral damage to the cingulum, caudate nuclei and anterior limb of the internal capsule. Although these states are most commonly seen after head injury, following anterior communicating artery aneurysmal subarachnoid haemorrhage, or in multi-infarct states, they can occur with unilateral infarction of the caudate nucleus or occlusion of the recurrent artery of Heubner (Fig. 4.12). Akinetic mutism can also occur with severe hydrocephalus. It has been suggested that the clinical features arise because of an alteration of dopaminergic extrapyramidal modulatory signals from the caudate to the frontal lobe. Treatment with dopamine agonists has been reported to be of benefit in individual cases or small series, but there

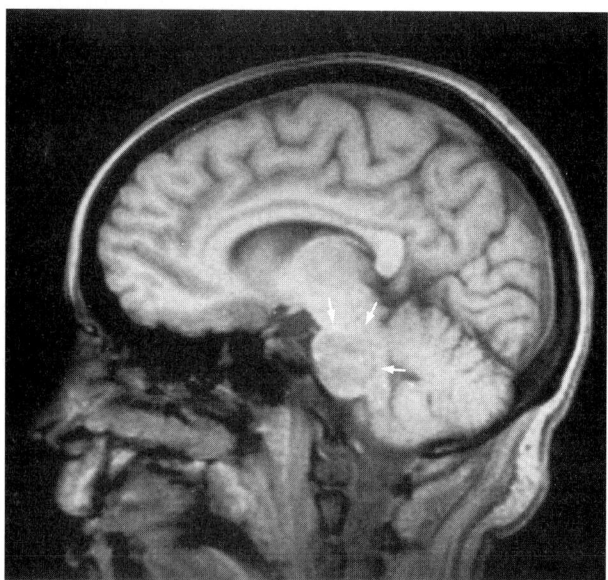
(a)

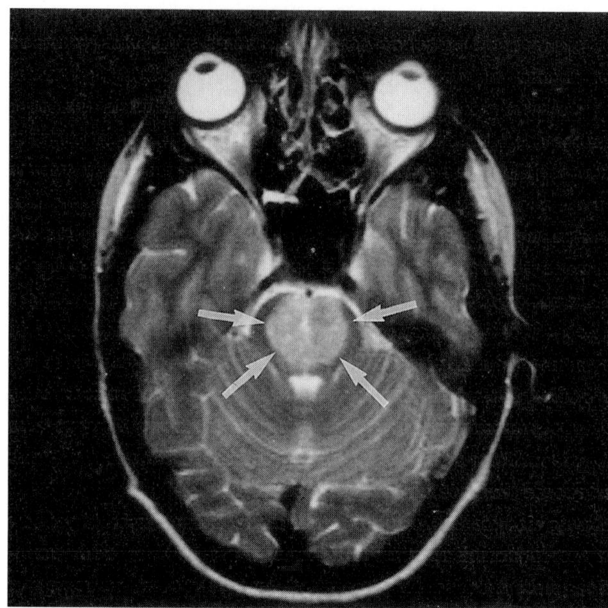
(b)

Fig. 3.4 (a) A T1-weighted, sagittal magnetic resonance (MR) scan showing a ventral pontine infarct (arrows) in a patient with the locked-in syndrome. (b) An axial T2-weighted MR scan of the same patient, showing the infarct as a large hyperintense lesion involving the whole of the pons (arrows).

have not been any randomized controlled trials (Ross & Stewart 1981; Barrett 1991).

• *the persistent vegetative state* is mentioned here for completeness. In this state, there appears to be wakefulness and preserved autonomic function, but total lack of cognition. It rarely occurs because of a focal vascular event, and is usually the result of a diffuse insult to the cerebral cortex (e.g. trauma, hypoxia) but with relative sparing of the brainstem. The diagnosis should not be made until 12 months have elapsed from the time of onset (Jennett & Plum 1972; Spudis 1991; American Neurological Association 1993; Howard & Miller 1995; Wade & Johnston 1999).

• *brainstem death*, on the other hand, is caused quite frequently by vascular disease. The detailed issues surrounding this condition are beyond the scope of this text, but have been reviewed extensively (Conference of Medical Royal Colleges and their Faculties in the United Kingdom 1976, 1979, 1995).

All these states of altered responsiveness should be distinguished from other physical disorders such as extreme extrapyramidal bradykinesia and bradyphrenia, paralysis from neuromuscular disorders, and also from psychiatric conditions, such as catatonia, depression or hysteria (Table 3.6).

All staff must take care when standing near an apparently unresponsive patient to talk and behave as though the patient was fully conscious.

Table 3.6 Causes of impaired consciousness after stroke.

Primary damage to subcortical structures (e.g. thalamus) or to the reticular activating system in the brainstem (e.g. brainstem haemorrhage)
Secondary damage to the reticular activating system in the brainstem (e.g. large supratentorial haemorrhage or infarct with transtentorial herniation and midline shift due to oedema)
Co-existing metabolic derangement (e.g. hypoglycaemia, hypoxia, renal or hepatic failure)
Drugs (e.g. sedatives)
To be distinguished from normal consciousness but with impaired responsiveness due to:
Locked-in syndrome
Akinetic mutism
Abulia
Severe extrapyramidal bradykinesia
Severe depression
Catatonia
Hysterical conversion syndrome
Paralysis from neuromuscular disorders

3.3.3 Disturbance of higher cerebral function

Because of its sheer complexity, higher cerebral function (by which we mean those mental activities exceeding elementary functions), whilst being one of the most fascinating aspects of neurological practice, is often perceived as one of the most difficult areas for the clinician. This need not be so if one remembers that the roles (and information needs) of clinicians, neuropsychologists and remedial therapists are very different. It is perfectly respectable for the clinician dealing with stroke patients to be able to identify disorders of higher cerebral function in general terms to facilitate diagnosis, lesion localization and basic management. This does not require the use of the detailed assessment batteries that may help the neuropsychologist to investigate specific neural mechanisms or the therapist to monitor the rehabilitation process. In this section, we will therefore concentrate on the bedside or clinical assessment of disturbances of higher cerebral function.

The clinician dealing with stroke patients should be able to identify cognitive disorders in general terms, without resorting to detailed assessment batteries, in order to facilitate diagnosis, lesion localization and basic management. Few cognitive functions are absolutely specific for a single area of the brain, and few tests are absolutely specific for a single aspect of higher cerebral function.

There is continuing debate amongst neuropsychologists about how localized (or not) certain cerebral functions are. In general, it is useful to distinguish those functions that are 'distributed'—i.e. involve several areas of the cortex, such as attention, concentration, memory and higher-order social behaviour—from more 'localized' functions such as speech and language, and visuospatial function and praxis (Hodges 1994). However, it must be remembered that few tests are absolutely specific for a single aspect of higher cerebral function. Clearly, it is important for the physician to determine the handedness of an individual patient, but the descriptions below assume left-hemisphere dominance.

Attention and concentration

Attention and concentration are the ability to maintain a coherent stream of thought or action. They are not synonymous with wakefulness. There are a number of terms used to describe disordered attention. Perhaps the most common is 'confusion', which in general means an inability to think with customary clarity, coherence and speed. However, the definition of 'thinking' is also imprecise, because this is a term that refers variably to problem-solving or to coherence of ideas about a subject. 'Delirium' is a term that is often used interchangeably with 'confusion', although it does have an operational definition (American Psychiatric Association 1987) and is often used to refer to instances in which there is, additionally, increased psychomotor activity or perceptual disturbances (e.g. agitation, hallucinations, thrashing about). 'Disorientation' may be used to describe a more severe disorder of attention.

Clinical anatomy

Attention and concentration depend on the integrated activity of the neocortex (predominantly the prefrontal, posterior parietal and ventral temporal lobes), the thalamus and brainstem. The reticular formation and other brainstem nuclei receive input from both ascending and descending pathways and there are then major ascending tracts to the thalamus, particularly the intralaminar nuclei.

Clinical assessment

Failure of attention results in patients being unable to sustain concentration, and they are often reported to lack interest in things around them or to be tired or distractible. Another common complaint is that they have problems with memory. This may or may not be true, but from a practical point of view, if there is a significant disorder of attention, then extreme care is required when interpreting the results of testing other higher-order functions such as memory. Attention and concentration can be assessed at the bedside using the tests shown in Table 3.7.

Clinical practice

Acute stroke patients, particularly the elderly, are often described as being confused, but this should not be considered as a focal neurological symptom *per se* (it tends to be a symptom of systemic upset resulting in a metabolic/toxic encephalopathy, for which appropriate investigations and treatment may be needed). However, patients who appear confused should be assessed carefully, because in fact they may have an underlying focal neurological disturbance such as aphasia, visuospatial or perceptual disturbance, hemianopia, or amnesia.

Inattentiveness is rarely reported as an isolated phenomenon in patients with stroke. It is more often a component of syndromes originating from lesions in a wide range of sites, but most frequently right parietal lesions, when there may be few if any motor and somatic sensory symptoms and signs. Pedersen *et al.* (1998) reported that 23% of patients in the Copenhagen Stroke Study had evidence of impaired orientation at the time of admission, and this was still present in 12% of survivors at the completion of rehabilitation.

Table 3.7 Bedside testing of attention and concentration.

Orientation (in person, time and place)
Digit span forwards and backwards*
Recite months of the year, or days of the week, backwards
Serial subtraction of 7s (although note that calculative ability needs to be intact)

* The normal range would be forwards: 6 ± 1; backwards: 5 ± 1.

Memory

The nomenclature of memory and theories about memory processing are changing (Hodges 1994). One method of dividing memory function is into 'explicit' memory (that which is available to conscious access) and 'implicit' memory (that which relates to learned responses and conditioned reflexes). Explicit memory may be 'episodic' (dealing with specific events and episodes that have been personally experienced, e.g. Australia winning the world cup in cricket and rugby), or 'semantic' (dealing with knowledge of facts, concepts and the meaning of words, e.g. 'stroke is a clinical syndrome'). The terms 'short-term memory' and 'long-term memory' are used loosely by clinicians and often rather differently by neuropsychologists. The current prevailing opinion is that there is a 'working memory' for very short-term or immediate recall of verbal and spatial material and a number of systems that work in parallel dealing with long-term memory for different types of material. However, for the clinician, who will know more or less precisely the time of the stroke, it is probably easier to distinguish anterograde amnesia (failure to acquire new memories) from retrograde amnesia (failure to recall previously learnt material).

The terms 'short-term memory' and 'long-term memory' are used loosely by clinicians and often rather differently by neuropsychologists. In patients with stroke, it may be easier to distinguish anterograde amnesia from retrograde amnesia.

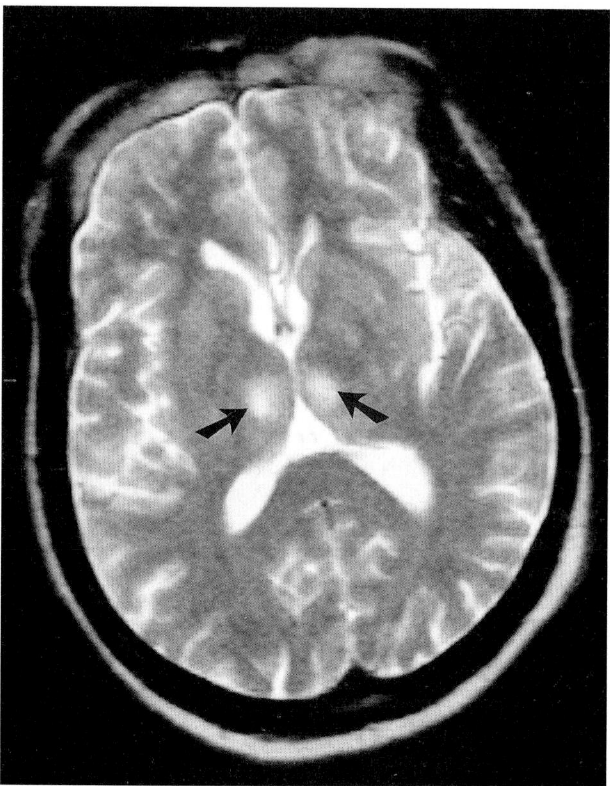

Fig. 3.5 A T2-weighted axial magnetic resonance (MR) scan, showing bilateral thalamic infarction (arrows) in a patient with a major cardiac source of embolism (atrial fibrillation plus left atrial thrombus). The patient also sustained infarction in both cerebellar hemispheres at the same time as the thalamic infarction. There was a severe, global amnesia.

Clinical anatomy

The important structures for memory are the medial temporal lobes and thalamus (particularly the dorsomedial nuclei), i.e. structures usually supplied by the posterior circulation (section 4.2.3), although disorders of the frontal lobes may also influence memory. Severe amnesia is usually the result of bilateral lesions (particularly of the thalamus; Fig. 3.5). Verbal memory is affected predominantly by left hemisphere lesions, and non-verbal memory by right hemisphere lesions—although the latter often has less impact on functional abilities.

Clinical assessment

A complaint of impaired memory should not just be taken at face value. As mentioned above, it can occur because of a problem with attentiveness and concentration resulting in failure of registration of new information. Not infrequently, patients with nominal aphasia are reported as having memory problems as are patients with geographical disorientation. Patients with stroke are generally of an age when there is a natural decline in memory. Therefore, although many patients complain of memory problems, it may be difficult to identify those that are the direct result of the vascular disease. Relatives often have quite disparate views about a patient's pre-stroke memory and it is therefore often difficult to quantify the problem unless it was severe. A suggested method for assessing memory is set out in Table 3.8.

Clinical practice

Since lesions in many parts of the cerebral hemispheres can cause some disturbance of memory, there are few syndromes that are absolutely typical of stroke disease. With most memory disorders caused by a vascular lesion, new information may be registered but will not be retained for more than a few minutes. Additionally, there will usually be a degree of retrograde amnesia. Perhaps the most frequent stroke lesion causing amnesia is infarction of the medial temporal lobe. Visual disorders (e.g. hemianopia or upper quadrantanopia, colour anomia, visual agnosia) should be looked for carefully, because they are also caused by occlusion of the posterior cerebral artery (section 4.2.3). If there is particularly severe amnesia, always consider paramedian thalamic infarction, which is frequently bilateral because a significant number of people have both paramedian arteries arising from one stem (Fig. 3.5) (section 4.2.3).

Table 3.8 Bedside testing of memory.

First check that patient is attentive (Table 3.7) and that language function is adequate (Table 3.9).

Anterograde verbal memory
Give patient a name, address and name of a flower
Ensure that they have registered the information (repeat three times)
Test the patient 3, 5 and possibly 10 min later

Anterograde visual memory
Show the patient faces in a magazine.
Ensure they have recognized them.
Retest after 5 min

Retrograde memory
Ask the patient to describe recent events on the ward, or visits from relatives
Ask about important historical events and major events in the patient's life, e.g. date of marriage

The syndrome of transient global amnesia is described in detail in section 3.4.3. Most episodes are not due to degenerative vascular disease and are unlikely to recur, and this syndrome should therefore not be considered as a transient ischaemic attack. A stroke may cause a pure amnesic syndrome by involvement of either the dorsomedial nucleus or the mammillothalamic tract (Hankey & Stewart-Wynne 1988; Ott & Saver 1993; Bogousslavsky 1995). However, in most cases of thalamic amnesia there are also signs of midbrain or temporal lobe dysfunction, such as somnolence, vertical gaze palsies and corticospinal and spinothalamic tract signs. In general, there is relative sparing of verbal memory with right thalamic lesions and visuospatial memory with left thalamic lesions, although global amnesia has been reported from unilateral lesions.

Speech and language

Disorders of speech and language are commonly encountered in patients with stroke and transient ischaemic attack (section 15.30). At the outset, it is important to stress that the two are not synonymous, in that reading and writing are also important language functions (language itself is difficult to define, but may be considered as a system for the expression of thoughts, feelings, etc. by the use of sounds and/or conventional symbols). Furthermore, the production (or expression) and comprehension (or reception) of speech should be considered separately. The recognition of specific problems is important for the management and advice given to both patients and their carers.

Traditionally, the primary distinction to be made is between *aphasia* (defined as an acquired disorder of the production and/or comprehension of spoken and/or written language) and *anarthria/dysarthria* (defined as a disorder of articulation of single sounds) or *dysphonia* (defined as a disorder of phonation of language). Many subcategories of each type of disorder have been described. We will use the term 'aphasia' rather than 'dysphasia' to avoid confusion, since in the USA 'dysphasia' is applied to developmental language disorders. *Anomia* is an inability to generate a specific name. In the context of a vascular event, it is usually a manifestation of aphasia, but one needs to remember the possibility of an amnesic disorder. *Speech apraxia* is a syndrome in which there is inconstant misarticulation of single sounds, in the absence of dysarthria (in which there is constant misarticulation).

Alexia is an inability to name or interpret previously learned printed symbols. The patient can see individual letters, but cannot decode a series of letters into a recognizable word. When it occurs in isolation, this is sometimes referred to as 'word blindness'. *Agraphia* is an acquired disorder of writing.

Disorders of speech and language are not synonymous; reading and writing are also important language functions that should be assessed.

Clinical anatomy
In general, non-fluent (expressive) aphasia is likely to be due to a lesion of the dominant frontal lobe, although not necessarily confined to Broca's area (Mohr *et al.* 1978a). Recent work has suggested that Broca's aphasia is a syndrome with elements that range from initial mutism to speech apraxia and the classical pattern of agrammatism, and that the articulatory component is most heavily represented in the left insular region (Dronkers 1996; Donnan *et al.* 1999; Wise *et al.* 1999). Fluent (receptive) aphasia is likely to be due to a more posterior lesion (but not necessarily confined to Wernicke's area). However, most patients with stroke have a combination referred to as 'mixed aphasia' (or, if severe, 'global aphasia'), due to more extensive lesions within the dominant hemisphere. Consequently, there is often an associated right hemiparesis and hemianopia.

Occasionally, one encounters patients with non-fluent aphasia in whom repetition is intact. This is termed *transcortical motor aphasia,* and it is usually caused by lesions restricted to the anterior cerebral artery territory (section 4.2.2). The equivalent fluent aphasia with normal repetition (termed *transcortical sensory aphasia*) occurs with strokes in the left temporo-occipital region. Lesions of the thalamus may also result in predominantly non-fluent aphasia, in which case they may be associated with fluctuating alertness.

The motor dysfunction causing dysarthria may be a result of cerebellar, pyramidal, extrapyramidal, or facial nerve dysfunction. Anarthria may occur as part of a pseudobulbar palsy caused by bilateral lesions of the internal capsule (not necessarily at the same time) or with a single lesion involving both sides of the brainstem.

Alexia, with or without agraphia, may result from strokes that involve the medial aspect of the left occipital lobe and the splenium of the corpus callosum. There is usually a right visual field defect but no hemiparesis, and it is thought that the lesion in the splenium interrupts the transfer of visual information from the normal left visual field (right occipital lobe) to the damaged left hemisphere language areas.

Clinical assessment

Disturbance of speech is a common symptom in patients with cerebrovascular disease. If a patient's speech is described 'as if drunk', and if the ability to understand and express spoken and written language is preserved, then the problem is dysarthria or dysphonia. If the main difficulty is understanding or expressing spoken or written language—such as difficulty in reading (can see the letters but cannot make sense of them); difficulty in writing, even though the use of the hand is otherwise normal (often not the case); or difficulty in producing sentences, with words not being in their proper place or even non-words being used—then the problem is aphasia.

If speech production is so severely affected that the patient is mute, it is important to ascertain whether it is a language deficit (aphasia) or an articulatory deficit (anarthria) that is present. This can be difficult to assess from the history alone, particularly in the acute stage, but as the patient recovers some speech a more accurate assessment can be made. However, care must be taken if the patient is being assessed after the acute phase, since during the recovery from milder forms of aphasia, articulation may be impaired and evidence of language dysfunction can be difficult to detect. An anarthric patient will understand and respond to yes/no questions by nodding and will be able to follow written and verbal commands and write normally, whereas an aphasic patient probably would not normally be able to. *Cortical dysarthria* and *aphemia* are terms used in the (very rare) cases when the patient is mute but comprehension, reading and writing are intact and there are no signs to suggest a bulbar palsy. Of course, aphasia and anarthria may co-exist, and there are other causes of no verbal output such as akinetic mutism (section 3.3.2).

As with other aspects of the examination, the physician has to judge how relevant detailed testing actually is, since in the majority of patients with stroke the language disorders are anything but subtle. Table 3.9 sets out a scheme of bedside testing that will detect most speech and language problems. The moderate inter-observer reliability for the detection of aphasia (Table 3.20) reflects the difficulties of performing detailed testing in many patients with stroke, especially where there may be associated deafness, confusion, etc. However, there is a general tendency in everyday clinical practice to underestimate the receptive component of an aphasia, particularly if the clinician does not go beyond questions requiring a yes/no answer, or simple social conversation.

Table 3.9 Bedside testing of language function.

First ensure any hearing-aid has a battery, is switched on and that appropriate, clean spectacles are worn.
Also check that you are using the patient's native language—if not, use an interpreter.

Spontaneous speech
Consider output (whether fluent or non-fluent), articulation and content: during history-taking and for a structured task (e.g. 'describe your surroundings').

Auditory comprehension
Simple yes/no questions (e.g. is Russia the capital of Moscow? can dogs fly? do you put your shoes on before your socks?).
Give commands (being careful not to use non-verbal cues) of one, two and three steps using common objects, such as the manipulation of three different-coloured pens (care needs to be taken to ensure complex motor tasks do not involve the use of limbs with significant weakness or apraxia).

Naming
Ask the patient to name objects, parts of objects, colours, body parts, famous faces (certain groups, particularly the naming of people, may be more severely affected).
If visual agnosia is present, use auditory/tactile presentation, e.g. bunch of keys.

Repetition
'West Register Street' (difficult if dysarthric)
'No ifs, ands or buts' (difficult if aphasic)

Reading
Aloud, e.g. from a book or newspaper
Comprehension of the same piece

Writing
Spontaneous ('why have you come into hospital?')
Dictation ('the quick brown fox jumped over the lazy black dog')
Copying

Articulation
Ask the patient to say:
p/p/p/p/p/p (labial sounds, which test the orbicularis oris)
t/t/t/t/t/t (lingual sounds, which test the anterior tongue)
k/k/k/k/k/k (palatal sounds, which test the posterior tongue and palate)
p/t/k/p/t/k (tests the overall coordination of sounds)

The assessment of language function may be difficult or impossible in those with severe deafness and/or confusion.

Clinical practice

> *Beware labelling a patient as dysphasic when other symptoms and signs suggest isolated non-dominant hemisphere dysfunction.*

'Crossed' aphasia is a disturbance of language which occurs from a right hemisphere lesion in a right-hand dominant patient and is seen in about 4% of such patients (Pedersen *et al.* 1995; Bakar *et al.* 1996). It is presumed that some right-handed patients have mixed cerebral dominance for language, but other causes include bilateral strokes (including the thalamus), previous strokes, and possibly diaschisis (areas of cerebral hypometabolism remote from the site of injury, presumed to be due to trans-synaptic functional deactivation), although this latter mechanism is contentious (Bowler *et al.* 1995). It is worth noting that many dextral patients with right hemisphere strokes show subtle alterations in the affective aspects of speech, such as intonation (aprosody).

It is important not to assume that dysarthria is always due to a brainstem lesion. It can occur with facial weakness in a hemispheric stroke, and it can be very severe indeed with bilateral hemispheric or capsular lesions (Helgason *et al.* 1988). *Isolated dysarthria* can be the only manifestation of a lacune at the genu of the internal capsule or in the corona radiata. In such cases, there is specific impairment of corticolingual fibres (Urban *et al.* 1999). However, because there are many more common causes, isolated dysarthria should not generally be considered to be a cerebrovascular event unless there is an appropriately sited acute infarct or haemorrhage.

Foreign accent syndrome is a rare, acquired disorder of speech in which native speakers listening to a patient speaking their language describe hearing a foreign-sounding accent—yet the patient may never have been exposed to any other language or dialect before the stroke. It is probably due to an inability to make the normal phonetic and phonemic contrasts of the native language. The syndrome has most often been associated with small, subcortical infarcts in the left cerebral hemisphere (Monrad-Krohn 1947; Graff-Radford *et al.* 1986; Gurd *et al.* 1988).

Visuospatial dysfunction

Many patients with stroke fail to respond to stimulation of, or to report information from, the side contralateral to the cerebral lesion. The underlying causes of such 'neglect' are much debated, but currently most authorities consider it to be a modality-specific disorder of attention rather than a primary defect of sensory processing. There are two broad categories of neglect: intrapersonal (i.e. with respect to the patient's own body) and extrapersonal or topographical (i.e. with respect to the surrounding environment). A number of different types and/or degrees of severity of neglect occur in patients with stroke, and in many, a combination of somatic sensory deficits and disturbed visual perception, as well as conceptual negation of deficits, contribute to the clinically apparent 'neglect': hence the use of the broader term 'visuospatial dysfunction'. Table 3.10 provides a glossary of the terms that are used. Visuospatial problems are a major cause of disability and handicap, and they impede the patient's functional recovery (section 15.28).

Clinical anatomy

Visuospatial dysfunction is almost always more severe in

Table 3.10 Glossary of terms describing disorders of visuospatial function.

Hemi-inattention: where the patient's behaviour during examination suggests an inability to respond appropriately to environmental stimuli on one side, e.g. people approaching, noises or activity in the ward.

Sensory or tactile extinction: where the patient fails to register a tactile stimulus (light touch) on one side of their body when both sides are stimulated simultaneously (i.e. double simultaneous stimulation) but where the patient has registered the stimulus when each side was stimulated separately.

Visual inattention or extinction: where the patient fails to register a visual stimulus (e.g. finger movement) in one homonymous visual field when the same stimulus is presented to both fields simultaneously, but where the patient had no field defect on normal testing.

Allaesthesia: where the patient consistently attributes sensory stimulation on one side to stimulation of the other. This is related to right/left confusion, where the patient consistently moves the limbs on one side when requested to move the limbs on the other.

Anosognosia: where the patient denies the presence of a neurological impairment on one side, most often weakness.

Non-belonging: where the patient denies ownership of the limbs on one side of their body, or even attributes the limb to another person.

Related phenomena seen in parietal lobe dysfunction:

Anosodiaphoria: refers to an indifference to a perceived weakness, or other impairment.

Astereognosis: where the patient is unable to recognize objects placed in the affected hand yet has preserved cutaneous sensation.

Agraphaesthesia: where the patient is unable to identify a number drawn on the palm of the affected hand yet has preserved cutaneous sensation.

Geographical disorientation: where the patient becomes lost in familiar surroundings despite being able to see.

Dressing apraxia: where the patient is unable to dress, or dresses inappropriately, despite having no apparent weakness, sensory loss, visual or neglect problems. This is occasionally seen in a pure form and probably occurs because of a combination of disordered body image, and sensory and visual inattention rather than being a true apraxia.

posterior parietal lesions of the non-dominant hemisphere, particularly those that extend to the visual association areas. Although it can occur with left hemisphere lesions, when it does so detection is often hindered by co-existent language disturbances and inability to use the dominant hand.

Clinical assessment

Relatives may report little more than 'confusion' or 'difficulty in dressing' (Hier *et al.* 1983; Devinsky *et al.* 1988). If visuospatial problems are suspected from the history, they should therefore be carefully and systematically sought in the examination. By simply observing how patients respond to their environment and carry out tasks, one can often deduce the presence of visuospatial problems (Fig. 3.6). An obvious example would be if a patient (without a hemianopia) does not register the doctor's presence when approached from one side, even when spoken to. Alternatively, they might be unable to find their way back to their hospital bed after being taken to the toilet, suggesting geographical disorientation. The nurses and therapists are often better placed than the doctor to identify visuospatial problems, so it is important that these staff are trained to recognize and report them to other members of the team.

An elderly man who lived alone reported that he woke one morning and thought that there was 'something in bed with me'. He said it felt warm, and was pressing against the left side of his body. He thought his cat had got into bed with him, but when he touched it with his right hand he realized that it was his left arm. He had had a right parietal infarct during the night.

One can often deduce the presence of visuospatial problems by simply observing how the patient responds to the environment and carries out tasks around the ward.

Table 3.11 sets out a bedside examination that should detect significant visuospatial dysfunction, and Fig. 3.7 shows the type of abnormal drawing of a flower that may occur when there has been a non-dominant parietal stroke. Drawing a clock face is a commonly used test (Fig. 3.8), although this may not be specific for visual neglect but rather reflect other cognitive problems (Ishiai *et al.* 1993; Watson *et al.* 1993). Of the many cancellation tasks available, the star cancellation test is probably the most sensitive, and it is easy to use (Fig. 3.9), although it is only one component of the Behavioural Inattention Test (Halligan *et al.* 1989). There is evidence that using two or three different tests increases the sensitivity and specificity of detecting visual neglect, but this may not always be practical in the setting of acute stroke (Jehkonen *et al.* 1998). Many aspects of these assessments of visuospatial function require subjective judgements to be made by the physician—which probably accounts for the relatively poor inter-observer reliability (Table 3.20).

Although many other tests to identify and quantify visuospatial dysfunction have been described, the 'gold standard' against which the tests are evaluated is often regarded as the opinion of an occupational therapist (Stone *et al.* 1991, 1992). Therefore, although test batteries may be more objective and repeatable, they may not be any more valid than a bedside assessment. Also, one could reasonably argue that these test batteries are not particularly relevant, because they do not test functionally important tasks such as washing, dressing and feeding. Despite their limitations in routine clinical practice, test batteries are undoubtedly useful in further characterizing deficits in selected patients with difficult or persistent problems, in helping to explain a patient's functional problems, and in research.

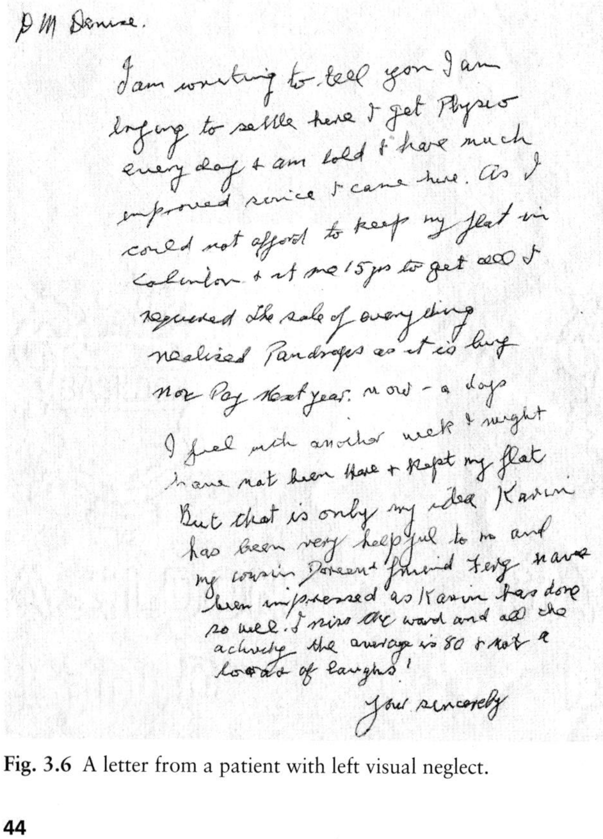
D M Denise.
I am writing to tell you I am
longing to settle here & get Physio
every day & am told I have much
improved since I came here. As I
could not afford to keep my flat in
Colindale & it me 15 yrs to get all I
required the sale of everything
realised Pandrops as it is big
nor Pay next year. now - a days
I feel with another week I might
have not been there & kept my flat
But that is only my idea Karin
has been very helpful to me and
my cousin Doreen & friend Terry have
been impressed as Karin has done
so well. I miss the ward and all the
activity the average is 80 & not a
loads of laughs!
Yours sincerely

Fig. 3.6 A letter from a patient with left visual neglect.

Table 3.11 Bedside tests of visuospatial function.

Is the patient aware, and reacting appropriately to their deficit?
Observe the patient's response to the environment.
Observe the patient's ability to carry out a specific task.
Check for sensory and visual extinction.
Copy a simple picture, e.g. a flower (Fig. 3.7).
Draw a clock face and put the numbers in (Fig. 3.8).
Perform the star cancellation test (Fig. 3.9).

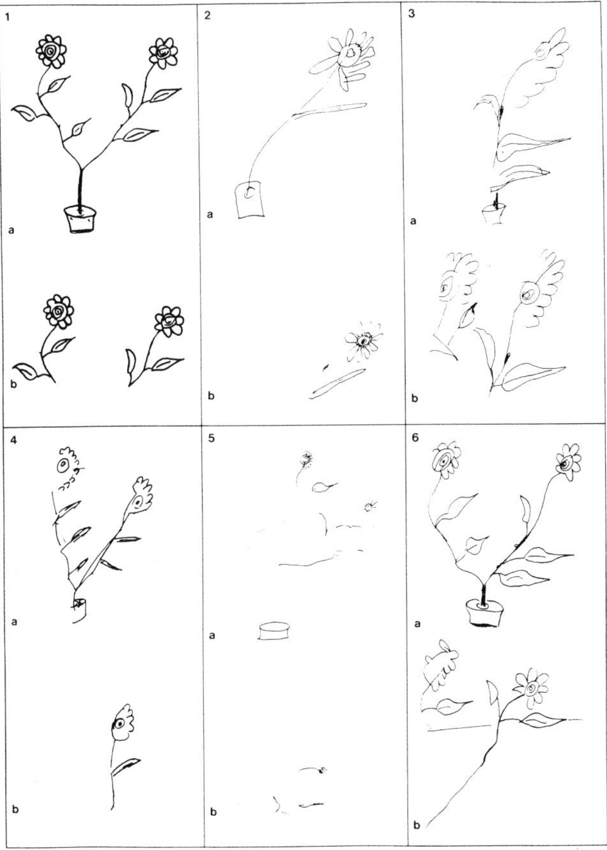

Fig. 3.7 Abnormalities on copying flowers. Five patients with damage to the right hemisphere were asked to copy pictures (a) and (b) in panel 1. The figures illustrate the variations seen in copying tasks. 2: This patient has mainly neglected the information on the left side of the page. 3: This patient has omitted the left-hand components of the objects, but has shifted attention to the right-hand side of another object placed to the left of the neglected space. 4: This patient has drawn the right side of both flowers in the pot, but has completely neglected the left of the two separate flowers. 5: This patient has transposed objects in the left field to the right field, i.e. both flowers are drawn on a single stem. This phenomenon has been likened to allaesthesia, which has been reported for tactile and visual modalities. 6: This patient has produced a 'hallucinatory' rabbit in the left field when copying the separate flowers. This has been termed a 'metamorphopsia', and when it is restricted to one visual field it has been likened to lateralized confabulations, which may occasionally be seen in patients with neglect (with permission from Marshall & Halligan 1993).

Clinical practice

When there is an isolated problem with visuospatial function—i.e. when it is not accompanied by a more easily recognized 'stroke' deficit such as weakness—the behaviour of the person may seem extremely bizarre. We have seen examples such as:

An elderly man who drove his car along a street unaware that he was scraping the sides of a whole row of other cars on the left hand side. A prosecution for dangerous driving was being considered after he had been shown to have normal visual fields (when each eye was tested in turn but not together) and not to have been under the influence of alcohol, until a neurologist asked him to draw a clock face. The result was very similar to Fig. 3.8a, and the CT scan showed a small right parietal haematoma.

The unusual behaviour can be interpreted as being due to psychiatric disease:

A middle-aged single lady was flying home from a holiday in Spain when she became 'confused'. On disembarking from the aircraft, she was staggering to the left, appeared unable to follow the signs to the customs point, and could not find her passport in her left-hand jacket pocket. She was held initially by the police on suspicion of alcohol or drug intoxication, but was then admitted to a psychiatric hospital. It was only a week later, when she had a transient ischaemic attack affecting power in her left hand, that a right parietal infarct and severe stenosis of the right internal carotid artery were discovered.

Perhaps not surprisingly, there is some evidence that patients who have varying degrees of indifference to their stroke are more likely to delay seeking medical attention (Ghika-Schmid *et al.* 1999)

Disorders of praxis

Apraxia is defined as the loss of ability to perform learned movements that cannot be explained by weakness, sensory loss, incoordination, inattention and other perceptual disorders, or by failure to understand the command. Dressing and constructional apraxias are best considered as disorders of visuospatial function rather than true apraxias (see above). Although the terms 'verbal apraxia' or 'speech apraxia' may be used by speech and language therapists when there are repeated phonemic substitutions, in practice such patients usually also have evidence of aphasia and/or dysarthria.

Clinical anatomy

It is thought that the programmes of learned movements (engrams) reside predominantly in the basal ganglia of the left hemisphere, although clearly the left superior temporal region (Wernicke's area) will be required for interpretation of the command. Messages then pass to the left premotor frontal cortex and finally, via the anterior corpus callosum, to the right premotor frontal cortex (Fig. 3.10). Lesions in the posterior left hemisphere may result in bilateral apraxia (because the message is not transmitted); those in the premotor areas are usually associated with a hemiparesis and therefore apraxia may only be apparent in the non-paralysed limbs; and finally, a lesion of the corpus callosum may cause

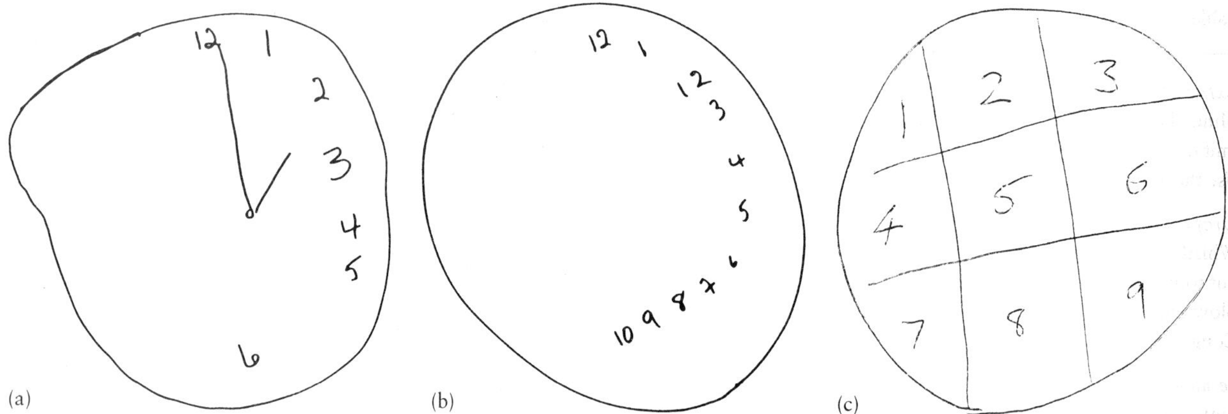

Fig. 3.8 (a) A drawing of a clock face by a patient with left visuospatial disturbance after a stroke, showing crowding of the digits on the right and neglect of the left side of the clock face. (b) A drawing of a clock face by a confused, elderly patient who had not had a stroke. The crowding of digits on the right occurs because of a failure of planning. Many normal people insert 12, 3, 6 and 9 before the other numbers. (c) A rather bizarre drawing of a clock face by a patient with strokes affecting both cerebral hemispheres.

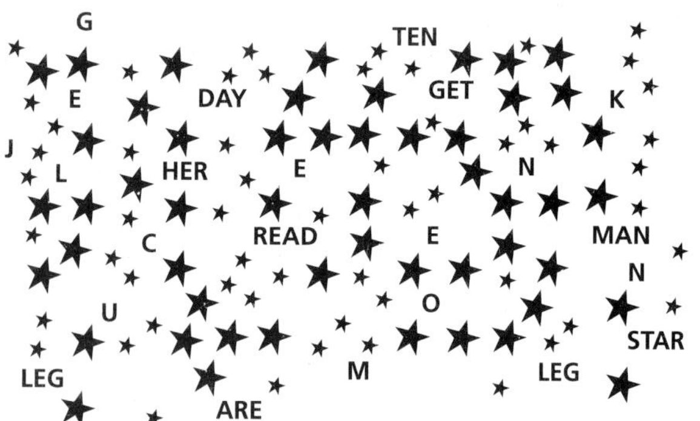

Fig. 3.9 Star cancellation test. The chart is placed in front of the patient, who is asked to cross out all the small stars whilst ignoring the large stars and letters (with permission from Thames Valley Test Company, 7–9 The Green, Flempton, Bury St Edmunds, Suffolk IP28 6EL, UK).

isolated apraxia of the left limbs, with normal function of the right limbs (Kazui & Sawada 1993).

Clinical assessment

Apraxia should always be considered as a potential explanation where there seems to be a disparity between the degree of deficit as tested on the bed (when one often gives the patient relatively simple commands) and much more severely impaired functional abilities when the patient is observed around the ward. Patients have difficulty with, or are incapable of, miming actions, imitating how an object is used, or even making symbolic gestures, even though at other times they may be observed making the individual movements that would be needed to perform the action. In general, they will have most difficulty in miming the action, less difficulty in imitating the examiner, and least difficulty when actually

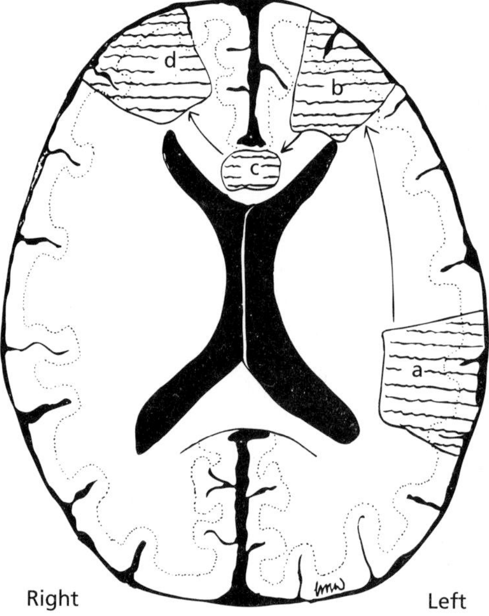

Fig. 3.10 Diagrammatic representation of the lesions that can result in apraxia. (a) The dominant temporoparietal cortex is the probable site of the programmes of learned movements (engrams). Lesions here result in bilateral apraxias, due to failure to transmit the motor information to both frontal lobes, although the clinical signs may be difficult to identify because the interpretation of the command may also be affected by receptive aphasia. (b) Although lesions of the dominant frontal lobe will often be associated with expressive aphasia, comprehension is usually relatively spared. The apraxia may only be apparent in the left limbs, since there will usually be a right hemiparesis. (c) Lesions in the anterior corpus callosum may result in isolated apraxia of the left limbs, because of failure of transmission of the motor information to the right frontal lobe, whilst the right arm and leg move normally. (d) Lesions of the non-dominant frontal lobe are not usually associated with clinically apparent apraxias, because there will usually be a left hemiparesis.

Table 3.12 Bedside testing of praxis.

Extremities. Ask the patient to:
Mime the use of a pen, comb and toothbrush
Imitate the examiner's use of the same objects
Use the actual objects

Orofacial. Ask the patient to:
Whistle
Put tongue out
Blow out cheeks
Cough

*Serial actions.** Ask the patient to mime:
Putting the address on a letter
Then seal it
Then put a stamp on it

* Traditionally, in less politically correct days, the test was to mime taking out, lighting and smoking a pipe or cigarette. This would almost constitute a reflex action in many stroke patients and should not be encouraged!

given the object to use. The more sequences there are to the action, the more difficult it is and so the more sensitive the test. These relatively common problems are sometimes referred to as 'ideomotor apraxias', and they can be distinguished from ideational apraxias when the patient has difficulty in performing a sequence of movements even though the individual movements can be performed normally. However, the latter probably occurs very rarely in a pure form, and the distinction between ideomotor and ideational apraxias is of little value to clinicians. Table 3.12 suggests ways of screening for apraxia. We are not aware of any data to indicate the inter-observer reliability for detecting apraxias, but suspect it might not be very high.

Clinical practice
In patients with stroke, the main problem is being sure that they have understood the command, because lesions of the relevant areas will often result in aphasia. Nevertheless, De Renzi *et al.* (1980) reported that with an imitation test (i.e. no verbal command), 80% of patients with aphasia also had evidence of apraxia. It is very important to be aware that apraxic patients may perform actions reflexly that they are unable to do when asked. This should not be misinterpreted as a sign of a hysterical conversion disorder. In some patients, orofacial apraxia may contribute to post-stroke dysphagia and dysarthria.

3.3.4 Disturbance of the motor system

To most people, motor deficits are the most characteristic manifestation of a stroke or TIA. Monoplegia is the complete paralysis of one arm or leg, whilst hemiplegia refers to complete paralysis of one side of the body. The terms 'monoparesis' and 'hemiparesis' (which have a different derivation from Greek) strictly refer to a partial paralysis of the relevant body parts, although the terms are often used interchangeably with 'monoplegia' and 'hemiplegia'.

Clinical anatomy
Particular areas of the motor cortex, when stimulated, result in movement of a particular body part. This localization of function is traditionally portrayed by the homunculus (or manikin) (Penfield & Boldrey 1937). Although the absolute neuroanatomical relationships may be incorrect (Schott 1993), in cerebrovascular practice it remains useful as an *aide-mémoire* (Fig. 3.11).

The corticospinal tract (Fig. 3.12) descends from the primary and supplementary motor cortex, the fibres converging in the corona radiata. There is evidence from primates, however, that the corticospinal tracts contain a significant number of fibres (perhaps as many as 40%) from cortical areas other than the primary and supplementary motor areas, particularly the parietal lobe (Russell & DeMeyer 1961). The fibres then pass through the internal capsule. The traditional view is that those fibres relating to the head pass through the anterior limb; those relating to the mouth, larynx and pharynx are in the genu; those relating to the arm are in the anterior part of the posterior limb; whilst those relating to the leg lie more posteriorly. In fact, the fibres almost certainly follow an oblique course through the capsule, becoming progressively more posteriorly placed in the caudal segments of the capsule (Ross 1980). The fibres then pass into the brainstem. Here, the fibres that originate in the precentral gyrus lie in the cerebral peduncles of the midbrain and the base of the pons before entering the medullary pyramids (i.e. the pyramidal tracts). Fibres that originate outside the precentral gyrus mostly do not synapse with motor neurones, but rather with various structures rostral to the pyramids. It is a clinical observation that severe spasticity may be seen with small lesions of the internal capsule, whereas the degree of spasticity from cortical lesions is more variable. It is thought that muscle tone is normally moderated by the inhibitory effect of corticoreticular fibres (Brown 1994) (section 15.20).

The majority of fibres in the corticospinal tract decussate in the lower medulla and come to lie in an anterolateral position in the spinal cord, although a variable proportion remain uncrossed; this may be of some clinical relevance in the recovery of certain voluntary motor activities after stroke, although as yet there is no neurophysiological support for this hypothesis (Chollet *et al.* 1991; Palmer *et al.* 1992). These uncrossed fibres project to motor neurones in the medial part of the ventral horns, subserving axial and proximal muscles, corresponding with movements of the trunk, or of two limbs together. The uncrossed corticospinal

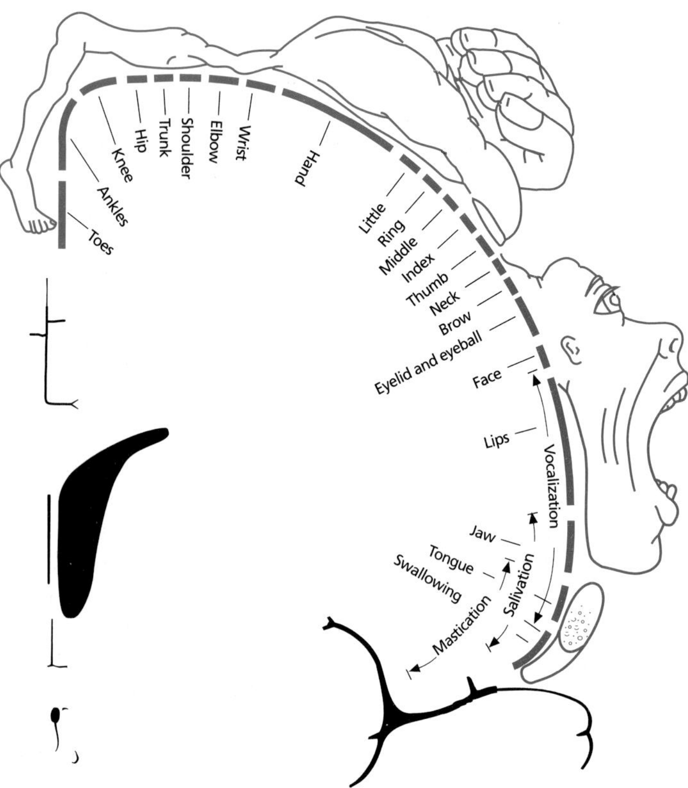

Fig. 3.11 Topographical organization of the motor cortex in the cerebral hemisphere, coronal view (the motor homunculus) (after Penfield & Rasmussen 1950).

fibres cannot be invoked to explain residual function in distal parts of an otherwise plegic limb, nor deficits in contralateral limbs.

The facial nerve nucleus has a rostral portion from which fibres innervate the muscles of the upper face, whilst the more caudal portion of the nucleus supplies fibres to the muscles of the lower face. It was thought previously that the typical upper motor neurone pattern of facial weakness (i.e. weakness of the lower face with preservation of movement of the upper face) came about because of bi-hemispheric input to the rostral part of the nucleus. However, it seems that most of the corticobulbar fibres terminate in the caudal part of the nucleus whilst the rostral part has direct input from the reticular formation (Jenny & Saper 1987). It is also worth remembering that the caudal loop of the descending fibres to the facial nerve descends as far as the medulla and explains why lesions of the medullary pyramid or medial medulla can be associated with contralateral upper motor neurone-type facial weakness (Chokroverty *et al.* 1975; Leestma & Noronha 1976; Ropper *et al.* 1979; Cavazos *et al.* 1996; Terao *et al.* 1997).

Clinical assessment

Motor symptoms are usually described as 'weakness', 'heaviness' and 'clumsiness', and are the most common symptoms described by TIA and stroke patients (Table 3.4). They are often accompanied by sensory symptoms of some sort, which can lead to diagnostic confusion because a purely weak limb may be described by the patient as 'numb' or 'dead'. Descriptions such as 'heaviness' and 'numbness' should not simply be accepted as evidence of motor and sensory disturbance, respectively. In our experience, the terms are used interchangeably (and are often culturally determined), and a little more interrogation is often rewarding. Once again, it can be valuable to ask patients to describe the symptom in an alternative way and also to have them explain what the functional consequences of the symptom were.

> *Patients use terms such as 'heaviness' and 'numbness' interchangeably; further questioning is needed to distinguish between motor and sensory deficits.*

In patients with suspected TIA, unilateral facial weakness is probably under-reported, because they do not realize they have had facial weakness unless they have seen themselves in the mirror, or the attack was witnessed by an observer. If there is a clear history of slurred speech, but no symptoms of cerebellar or bulbar dysfunction, it is reasonable to suspect facial weakness, because this may cause dysarthria if the patient attempts to speak. However, care should be taken before accepting a patient's or relative's description of the lateralization of a facial weakness. They should be asked, 'Which side dropped?', and 'Did saliva trickle from one side of the mouth?' Typically, an upper motor neurone facial

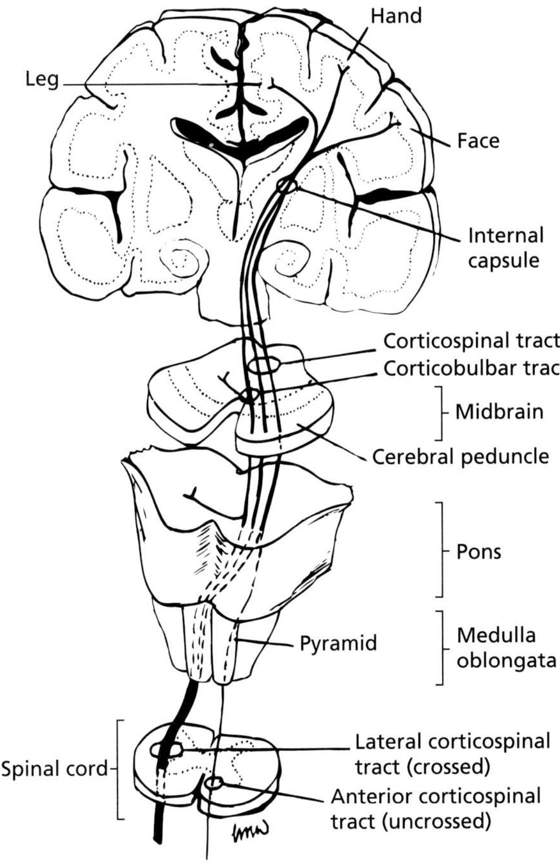

Fig. 3.12 Diagrammatic representation of the corticospinal and corticobulbar tracts.

weakness affects the lower half of the face, whilst function of the forehead muscles is preserved. Mild weakness may only be apparent by observing asymmetry of the nasolabial folds. If the examiner is uncertain whether a facial weakness is present, or whether it is simply the normal side-to-side asymmetry, it may be useful to ask the patient to attempt to whistle, an action that requires fine control of the facial muscles. A mild upper motor neurone facial weakness can be overcome during emotionally generated movements, e.g. a smile (Hopf *et al.* 1992).

Patients sometimes complain of being 'generally weak'. This should be viewed as a non-focal neurological symptom, as it is rarely described by patients when they strictly mean motor weakness. It is sometimes used as a term for fatigue, tiredness, lethargy and just occasionally loss of balance.

For the clinician, the difficulties with the physical examination lie not with the densely hemiplegic patient with increased tone, brisk deep tendon reflexes and an extensor plantar response, but rather with the patient with a mild deficit. Subtle abnormalities of motor function may be detectable in the hand at a time when there is no objective weakness. It has been shown that impairment of fine finger movements (or rapid alternating hand movements) is the most sensitive clinical test of corticospinal function (Louis *et al.* 1995). This equates with functional problems reported by patients who, in the face of normal power, often have difficulty with delicate motor tasks such as doing up buttons or controlling pens and may describe the problem as 'clumsiness'. Of course, they are much more likely to notice this in their normally dominant hand. This is probably due to a subtle increase in co-contraction of antagonist muscles secondary to the reduced input to the spinal motor neurones.

The impairment of fine finger or rapid hand movements is probably the most sensitive clinical test of corticospinal function.

Drift from the horizontal of the outstretched arm with the eyes closed is often suggested as a good screening test of motor function (Fig. 3.13). However, it must be remembered that there are several other potential causes for this, although the patterns of drift may be subtly different. These include loss of proprioception, when the fingers tend to move independently—so-called 'piano-playing' or 'pseudoathetosis'; neglect, when there tend to be much larger-amplitude movements, including upwards; or cerebellar dysfunction, when there tend to be larger-amplitude oscillations,

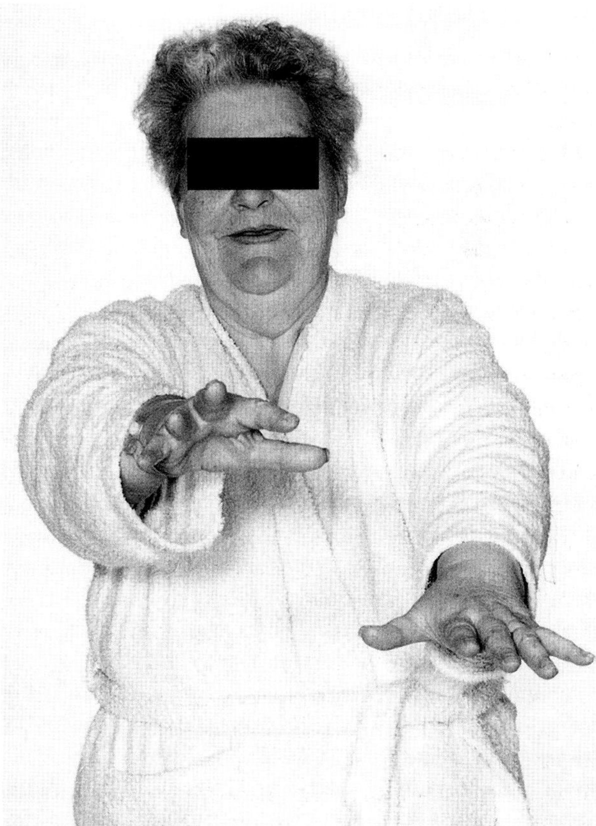

Fig. 3.13 Downward drift of the outstretched left arm in a patient with a mild corticospinal motor deficit.

particularly if sharp downward pressure is applied to the arm. Thus, as a screening test for motor dysfunction, it is quite sensitive but not very specific and should be used in conjunction with the examination of fine finger movements. Some clinicians favour performing the test with the patient's palms facing upwards, and if asymmetrical internal rotation occurs without downward drift this is taken as a sign of very subtle motor dysfunction.

Minor motor deficits affecting the leg are probably best detected by rapid tapping of the foot against the examiner's hand, when striking asymmetry of the rate or rhythm may be present. Additionally, the patient's gait should be observed carefully.

Drift from the horizontal of the outstretched arm with the eyes closed and rapid tapping of the foot against the examiner's hand are good screening tests of motor function in the arm and leg, respectively, but neither test is very specific.

The pattern of weakness within an individual limb is traditionally taught to be of localizing value. In particular, when the ratio of flexor to extensor strength is high at the elbow and wrist but low at the knee, this is often described as a 'pyramidal distribution' of weakness, and the presence of a central (rather than peripheral) lesion is inferred. Thijs *et al.* (1998) have suggested that this pattern is simply a function of the intrinsically greater strength in antigravity muscles together with the effects of hypertonia—the actual pattern of weakness being equally common in patients with peripheral lesions. Perhaps not surprisingly, the authors commented that the deep tendon reflexes were of more value as a localizing feature, although it is sobering to remember that the inter-observer reliability of two standard notation scales for grading tendon reflexes is probably no better than 'fair' (kappa < 0.35) (Manschot *et al.* 1998).

Although there is moderate inter-observer agreement about the presence or absence of weakness (Table 3.20), the standard methods of grading power (e.g. the Medical Research Council [MRC] system) are of limited value in patients with stroke (section 15.21). As with assessment of conscious level, stroke scales such as the Scandinavian Neurological Stroke Scale, which have an operational definition of the grades of weakness, can be shown to have moderately good inter-observer reliability (Lindenstrom *et al.* 1991). However, as will be seen in Chapter 4, it is the anatomical extent rather than the severity of the motor deficit that is of most importance for clinicoanatomical correlation, and from a functional point of view, a description of some action the patient cannot perform is often of more value (e.g. holding a cup of water, combing hair)—both when trying to understand the problems that the patient is having and also for appropriate goal setting during rehabilitation.

More attention should be focused on the anatomical extent of the weakness and the functional consequences, rather than trying to grade the severity using a motor scale.

An extensor plantar response is only one part of a nociceptive spinal flexion reflex, which in its complete form (the sign of Babinski) involves flexion at the hip, knee and ankle as well as extension of the great toe (van Gijn 1995) (Fig. 3.14). Failure to appreciate this perhaps explains, in part, the rather poor reliability of the sign (Louis *et al.* 1995). Whilst the presence of a Babinski response signifies a lesion of the corticospinal tract, it is not an invariable accompaniment of such lesions, particularly if there is no weakness of the foot.

Although swallowing involves both the motor and sensory systems, mention will be made of it here. The gag reflex alone does not constitute an adequate examination of the ninth and tenth cranial nerves, nor is it a good indicator of swallowing ability (section 15.17). Sensation on the two sides of the soft palate should be tested individually with an orange-stick, elevation of the palate should be observed, and the patient should be asked to cough. Failure to oppose the vocal cords adequately will result in some air escaping, and such a finding should alert the physician that the patient may have swallowing difficulties.

Clinical practice

In most epidemiological studies, over 80% of patients have had motor symptoms or signs. Weakness usually affects one side of the body: the face, arm, or leg in isolation (brachial or crural monoparesis or monoplegia); each limb as a whole or in part; or a combination of these (hemiparesis or hemiplegia). Lesions in the internal capsule tend to result in a hemiparesis/hemiplegia that is equally severe (proportional) in the arm and leg and is often not accompanied by other neurological symptoms and signs—a pure motor stroke (section 4.3.2). When there is a brachial monoparesis, or the weakness affects predominantly the hand and face, it is more likely to be due to a cortical rather than a subcortical lesion (Boiten & Lodder 1991; Timsit *et al.* 1997). When weakness involves the hand only, it is often referred to as the 'cortical hand syndrome'. This is often attributed initially to a peripheral nerve lesion by the referring doctor, but closer analysis reveals that this would require simultaneous involvement of the median, ulnar and radial nerves, a most unlikely occurrence. It is generally considered to occur because of the large cortical representation of the hand. Of course, cortical infarcts causing such a deficit are often not visualized on CT scanning. Isolated upper motor neurone facial weakness, however, seems to be of less localizing value, and it can certainly occur with very small infarcts in the genu of the internal capsule and in the pons (Bogousslavsky & Regli 1990a; Hopf *et al.* 1990).

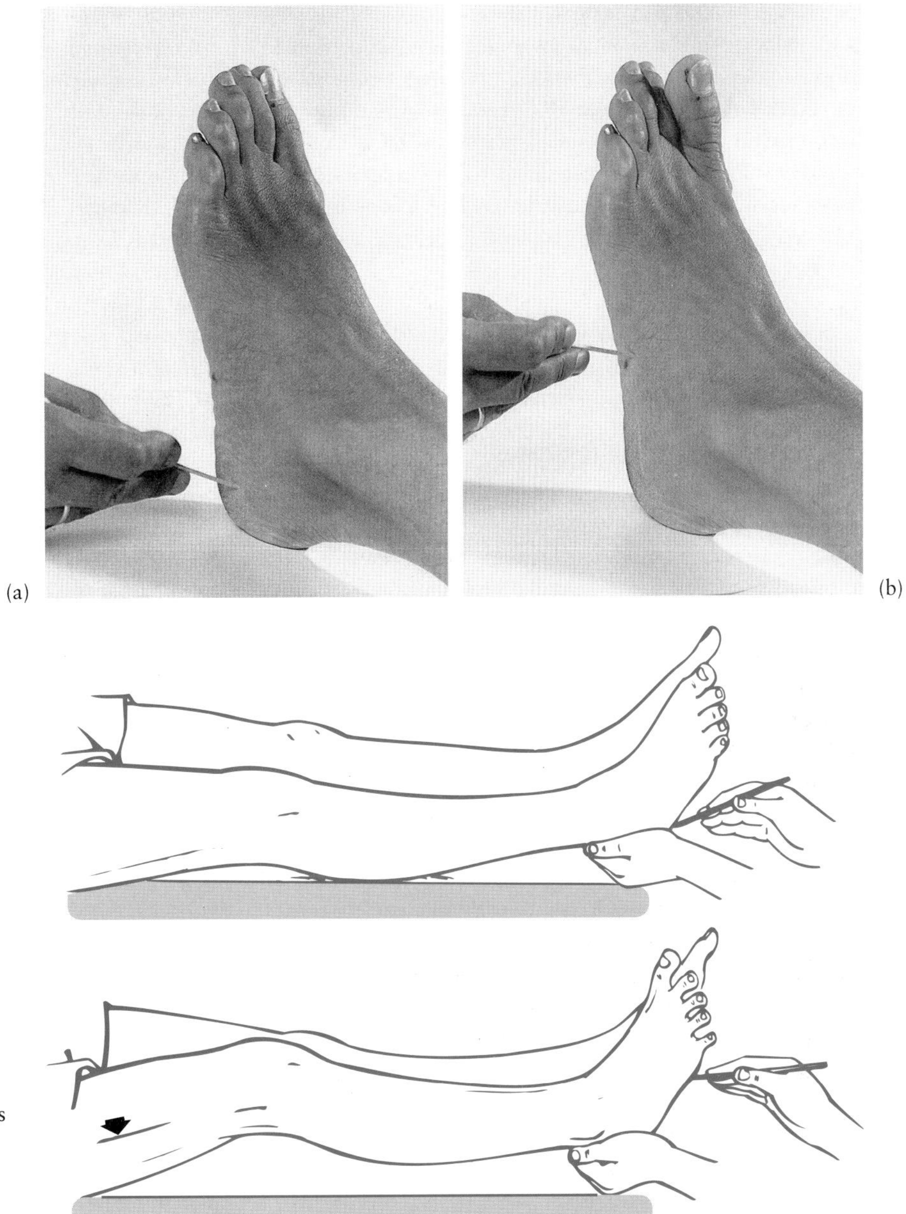

Fig. 3.14 The Babinski sign, evoked in this case by stroking the lateral part of the dorsum rather than the sole of the foot, in order to avoid voluntary withdrawal (a, b). The tendon of extensor hallucis longus can be seen on the dorsum of the hallux and the foot. (c) The Babinski sign involves contraction of the extensor hallucis longus simultaneously with other muscles that shorten the leg: tibialis anterior, the hamstrings (arrow), and the tensor fasciae latae (with permission from van Gijn 1995).

When weakness is confined to, or predominates in, the leg, the lesion is most likely to involve the territory of the anterior cerebral artery (Bogousslavsky & Regli 1990b) (section 4.2.2). Remember that if such a deficit is accompanied by headache or seizures, then a sagittal sinus thrombosis is a possible explanation (section 5.5.2). The occurrence of crossed weakness (i.e. weakness of one side of the face and the contralateral limbs) indicates a brainstem or multifocal disturbance. Paraplegia, triplegia and tetraplegia all occur more commonly from spinal than cerebrovascular disorders (although see 'locked-in syndrome', section 3.3.2).

When bilateral motor signs develop simultaneously—particularly if a cranial nerve palsy or crossed sensory disturbance (pointing to a brainstem lesion) are not present—and there is no sensory or reflex level to suggest a spinal cord lesion, one must consider cardiogenic embolism (i.e. causing two or more lesions), abnormalities of the circle of Willis (section 4.2.2), or systemic hypotension (resulting in bilateral boundary-zone infarcts, section 4.2.4) as potential causes. Very rarely the latter condition results in paralysis predominantly of both arms (the 'man in the barrel' syndrome), with bilateral infarction in the area of cortex at the boundary between the anterior and middle cerebral arteries (Sage & van Uitert 1986).

Although most strokes causing facial weakness result in a typical upper motor neurone pattern, there are some exceptions, which can lead to the erroneous diagnosis of Bell's palsy if there is minimal associated limb weakness. The most obvious exception is that of a brainstem stroke affecting the facial nerve nucleus. However, one should always bear in mind that interindividual variation in facial innervation does mean that, occasionally, patients with very severe lower facial weakness from a supranuclear lesion also have some weakness of the upper face as well, particularly in the first few days after a stroke.

Remember that vascular lesions of the seventh cranial nerve nucleus will involve both the upper and lower parts of the face; this pattern is not always due to idiopathic Bell's palsy.

One sometimes encounters patients who at one moment seem to have (or are reported to have) a dense hemiplegia (usually left-sided) and yet, very soon afterwards, are observed to move the 'paralysed' limbs. Staff may attribute such a sequence of events to a hysterical conversion disorder. However, this pattern can be seen with the so-called capsular warning syndrome, or crescendo small vessel TIAs (Donnan *et al.* 1993, 1995), although in such cases the episodes seem much more discrete (section 6.6.3). It can also occur in patients with a haemodynamically significant internal carotid artery (ICA) stenosis, presumably due to subtle changes in distal perfusion pressure. However, the majority are patients in whom this seems to be a manifestation of an inattention/neglect syndrome, or even apraxia. In patients who are recovering from what appears to be an extensive non-dominant hemisphere stroke, what seems to be a dense hemiplegia may improve very rapidly as the inattention/neglect begins to resolve—a fact that needs to be borne in mind when predicting the eventual functional outcome. It has been suggested that these phenomena may be responsible for the excess of left over right hemiplegia that has been reported in some large series of stroke cases (Sterzi *et al.* 1993).

It is always important to see whether a patient can sit up, get off the bed and walk, provided there is no risk to the patient or physician, whatever the motor deficit when tested on the bed. A severe deficit may be due to neglect and not weakness, whilst no motor deficit at all may be associated with profound ataxia of gait.

Dysphagia is a common feature of acute stroke, either as a focal sign of the direct effects of the stroke on corticobulbar pathways or as a non-focal sign of the secondary effects of cerebral oedema, brain herniation, or altered consciousness. However, it is commonly not recognized, because it is not assessed particularly well and aspiration may be 'silent' (Kidd *et al.* 1993, 1995) (section 15.17). In patients who are persistently dysphagic, the cortical representation of the pharynx in the unaffected hemisphere increases (as assessed by transcranial magnetic stimulation) compared with those patients whose dysphagia recovers (Hamdy *et al.* 1998). Dysphagia is rarely reported by TIA patients, probably because any transient deficit is unlikely to coincide with eating or drinking.

Movement disorders such as hemiballismus, unilateral asterixis, hemichorea and focal dystonia are uncommon but well-recognized manifestations of contralateral, and also possibly ipsilateral, small deep vascular lesions of the subthalamic nucleus, striatum and thalamus (Kase *et al.* 1981; Russo 1983; Stell *et al.* 1994; Crozier *et al.* 1996; Krystkowiak *et al.* 1998). Also, involuntary tonic limb spasms may arise contralateral to ventral pontine brainstem infarction (Kaufman *et al.* 1994). About 1% of patients with acute stroke will have a hyperkinetic movement disorder at some point, but the abnormal movements usually regress spontaneously (Ghika-Schmid *et al.* 1997). Transient cerebral ischaemia may also masquerade as paroxysmal dyskinesia; Hess *et al.* (1991) described repetitive, stereotyped, involuntary left arm movements (painless flexion and pronation of the wrist and elbow followed by abduction of the shoulder and hand behind the head) lasting 1–5 min in a patient with distal right ICA occlusion and poor intracranial collateral circulation who suffered a right hemisphere ischaemic stroke soon after.

Occasionally, one encounters patients who describe jerking movements of the limbs just before the onset of a stroke or TIA (Baquis *et al.* 1985; Yanagihara *et al.* 1985; Tatemichi *et al.* 1990). The distinction from focal motor epilepsy may be difficult (section 3.4.2). In contrast to epileptic seizures, these attacks may be provoked by postural change (from lying to sitting or standing up), hyperextension of the neck, walking, coughing, or starting or increasing antihypertensive therapy, and they may be alleviated promptly by sitting or lying down, all of which suggest they are due to low flow rather than embolism (section 6.6.5). There is certainly an association with severe ICA stenosis or occlusion (Fig. 3.15), and in some cases the attacks have stopped after carotid endarterectomy (Stark 1985; Baquis *et al.* 1985; Baumgartner & Baumgartner 1998; Zaidat *et al.* 1999). The pattern has also been reported with internal boundary-zone infarcts (Chambers & Bladin 1995) (section 4.2.4). However, such a syndrome should always be an indication for brain imaging, even if a patient has had other episodes that have been considered to be due to cerebrovascular disease, since tumours may present in this manner, i.e. with focal epileptic seizures (Coleman *et al.* 1993). Previous strokes may also be complicated by focal epileptic seizures (section 15.8).

Another situation in which a patient may move an apparently paralysed limb is as part of certain reflex movements, e.g. yawning, coughing, or crying. These associated reactions or synkinesias are not voluntary, but anxious relatives may see them and become overly optimistic about the patient's recovery. Additionally, movements of the normal limb may

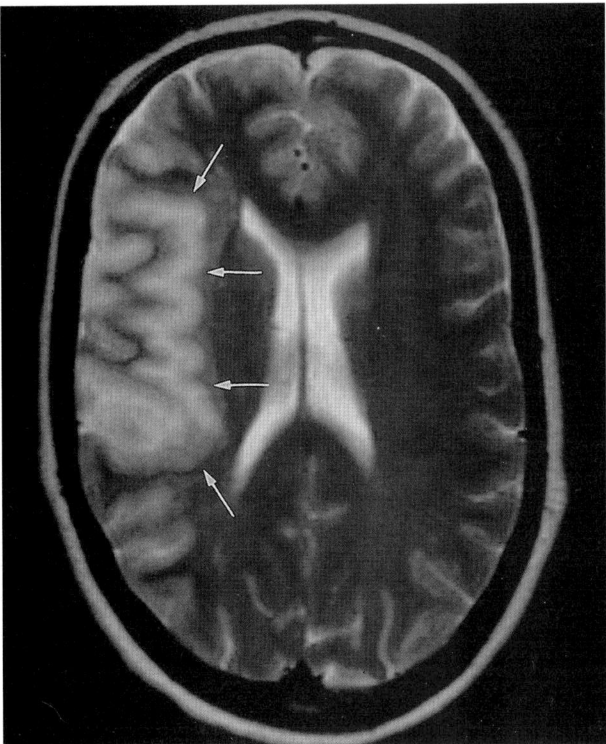
(a)

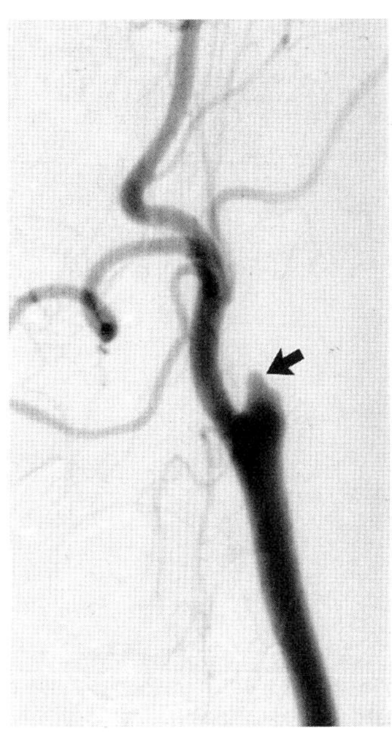
(b)

Fig. 3.15 A patient presented with several episodes of jerking of the left arm, which were initially thought to be epileptic. A CT brain scan was normal. Three days later, he awoke with a left hemiparesis. A T2-weighted axial magnetic resonance scan (a) showed an extensive area of infarction in an area usually supplied by the middle cerebral artery (arrows), and a catheter angiogram (b) showed occlusion of the ipsilateral internal carotid artery (arrow).

evoke mirror movements in the paralysed limb. Anxious relatives should be counselled concerning involuntary movements or associated reactions that they may witness and to which they might attach too much prognostic significance.

Other conditions that sometimes need to be considered in the differential diagnosis of motor dysfunction are drop attacks, cataplexy and motor neurone disease (section 3.4.12).

3.3.5 Disturbance of the somatic sensory system

There are broadly two types of sensory message passing from the periphery to the brain. *Superficial sensation* (also known as cutaneous or exteroceptive) includes light touch, pain and temperature modalities. *Deep (or proprioceptive) sensation* refers to joint position sense and deep pressure. Synthesis and appreciation of these sensory inputs occur at a cortical level. *Discriminative sensation* refers to stereognosis, two-point discrimination and graphaesthesia (section 3.3.3).

Paraesthesiae are positive sensory phenomena (e.g. pins and needles) that are presumed to occur because of partial damage to the sensory tracts or posterior horn cells, which become hyperexcitable (perhaps akin to brisk reflexes), such that ectopic impulses are generated either spontaneously or after a normal stimulus-evoked volley of impulses.

Clinical anatomy

The main sensory pathways are shown in Fig. 3.16. The traditional view is that impulses for superficial sensation are conveyed in the spinothalamic tracts, which synapse in the dorsal horn, cross the midline at spinal level and then ascend through the lateral spinal cord and brainstem. Fibres from sacral areas lie laterally in the tract, whereas those from the arm lie more medially. Fibres carrying similar sensory impulses from the face enter the ipsilateral, descending (or spinal) trigeminal nucleus and cross the midline in the upper cervical spinal cord. They then ascend through the medulla, close to the medial lemniscus, and separate to join the medial part of the spinothalamic tract in the pons.

The relevant fibres for deep sensation are primarily in the ipsilateral posterior columns of the spinal cord, synapsing in the gracile and cuneate nuclei. Decussation occurs in the caudal medulla, after which the fibres ascend through the brainstem in the medial lemniscus. Fibres from the legs lie more medially in the dorsal columns and anteriorly in the medial lemniscus than those from the arms. Fibres carrying similar sensory impulses from the face enter the primary trigeminal nucleus in the pons and cross the midline at this level to form the trigeminal lemniscus, which lies adjacent to the medial lemniscus.

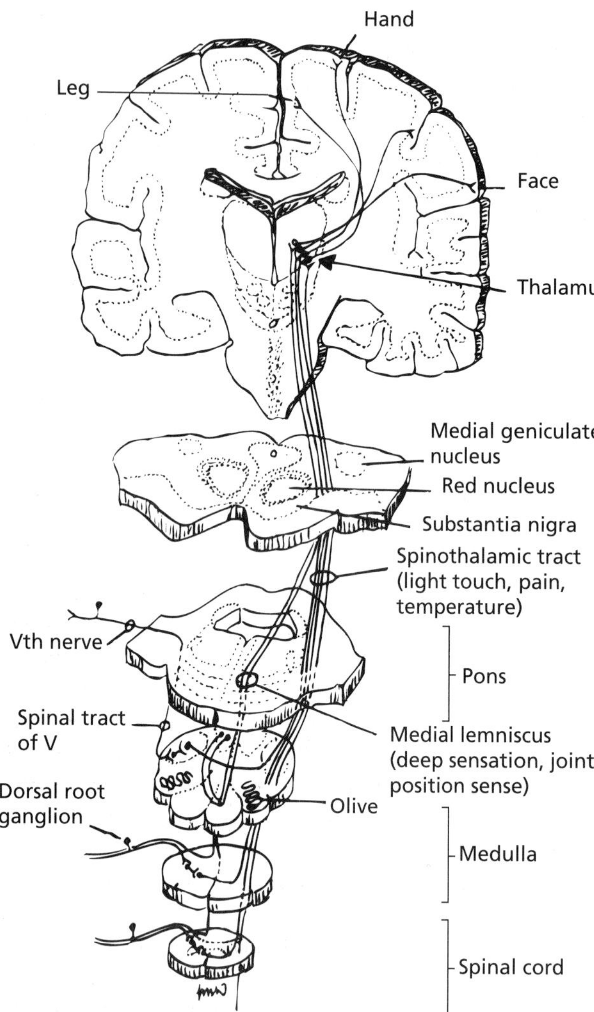

Fig. 3.16 Diagrammatic representation of the main sensory pathways between the entry of the dorsal root to the spinal cord and the sensory cortex.

All these ascending fibres converge towards the midbrain and project, in the main, to the posterior group of thalamic nuclei and in particular to the ventro-postero-lateral (VPL) nuclei (trunk and legs) and ventro-postero-medial (VPM) nuclei (face, tongue, fingers). Lesions of the thalamus often involve all sensory modalities, although deep sensation may be more affected than somatic sensation (Brodal 1981b; Sacco *et al.* 1987). From the thalamus there are probably two main projections. The first is to the postcentral or primary somatic cortex. Here there is somatotopic representation, with the leg uppermost and the face lowermost. The afferent projection is mainly from the dorsal column/medial lemniscus via the VPL and VPM nuclei, and is concerned with sensory discrimination. The areas of sensory representation resemble those of the motor homunculus (Fig. 3.11). A second projection is to the area adjacent to the upper part of the Sylvian fissure and insula. Here there is less discrete localization, but in general, the face is rostral and the leg caudal. Interestingly, stimulation of this area may result in bilateral symptoms. Lesions confined to the parietal lobe are generally regarded as affecting higher-level 'discriminatory' functions (i.e. proprioception, two-point discrimination, stereognosis) rather than primary modalities, although there are cases in the literature (referred to as 'pseudothalamic') in which the opposite pattern has occurred (Bowsher 1995).

Clinical assessment

Somatosensory symptoms due to stroke are usually described by the patient as numbness ('like the numbness I have after going to the dentist'), tingling, or a dead sensation; occasionally as loss of temperature sensation when in the bath or shower; and very rarely as pain. Additionally, patients often lack the ability to describe unusual sensations in a manner that allows accurate classification, and the descriptions that are used seem to vary between cultures. It is widely recognized that the formal testing of the sensory system is one of the most unreliable parts of the neurological examination (Table 3.20). Quite frequently there will be no detectable sensory loss. In general, therefore, one should take due note of sensory symptoms even in the absence of a deficit on examination. Indeed, assuming the patients are able to communicate and do not have neglect, the only situation in which they will have sensory loss without sensory symptoms is when there is a restricted problem of discriminatory rather than primary sensory function (due to a parietal lesion)—something that is uncommon in clinical practice. Conversely, care needs to be taken over the interpretation of very transient sensory symptoms, which can be within the range of normal experience, although the clinician should not accept uncritically the patients' common interpretation of sensory symptoms as being due to a 'trapped nerve' or 'lying in a draught'.

Formal testing of the sensory system is the most unreliable part of the neurological examination. However, the physician should always take due note of sensory symptoms, even when there is no deficit on examination.

Somatic sensation should be tested in the standard manner, using a wisp of cotton wool and an appropriate pin (i.e. not a hat pin, or hypodermic needle) or other sharp object that can be disposed of after it has been used. Proprioception may be assessed with the patient's arms outstretched, the fingers spread and the eyes closed. The examiner should look for drift of the patient's arm in a 'pseudoathetoid' or 'piano-playing' manner. This can be amplified by asking the patient to touch the tip of his or her nose with the forefinger whilst the eyes remain closed, when those with disturbed proprioception will repeatedly miss the target. This screening test will assess proprioception around proximal as well as distal joints, but as mentioned above, drift can also be due to a motor deficit or neglect/inattention. Therefore, if possible, one should always attempt the traditional method of testing joint position sense of the distal interphalangeal joints. If there is aphasia, it is sometimes worth asking the patient to indicate with gesture the direction of movement. Romberg's test is rarely of value unless lower limb motor function is entirely normal, in which case it is a sensitive measure of position sense in the legs.

As with other aspects of examination, the physician dealing with stroke patients needs to have a repertoire of tests allowing adjustment to particular circumstances, since it will be impossible to conduct the 'standard' examination of sensation in the presence of drowsiness, aphasia, or dementia. However, in most cases there will at least be a 'normal' side to permit comparison of response. The physician should always remember that patient (and doctor) fatigue will impair the reliability of results, and tired patients become increasingly suggestible. In such cases, one may have to rely on identifying a difference in response between the patient's right and left side to predominantly somatic sensory stimuli, such as pin-prick or deep pressure, e.g. squeezing the Achilles tendon. The presence of severe visuospatial disturbance may make meaningful sensory testing impossible.

Clinical practice

The lacunar syndrome of *pure sensory stroke* is typically caused by a lateral thalamic infarct or haemorrhage. The deficit may involve all modalities, or may spare pain and temperature sensation (Sacco *et al.* 1987; Paciaroni & Bogousslavsky 1998). If there is extension to the internal capsule, a sensorimotor stroke may occur (Mohr *et al.* 1977) (section 4.3.2).

The *Déjerine–Roussy syndrome* (Déjerine & Roussy 1906; Caplan *et al.* 1988) is caused by more extensive lateral thalamic infarction, and consists of a mild contralateral hemiparesis, marked hemianaesthesia, hemiataxia, astereognosis and frequently paroxysmal pain/hyperaesthesia and choreoathetotic movements. The original cases had extension of the infarcts into the internal capsule and towards the putamen, although most of the features of this syndrome result from involvement of the ventroposterior nucleus (VPN) and VPL nuclei of the thalamus (section 4.2.3). *Central pain* alone may be caused by lesions at any level of the somatosensory pathways (Bowsher *et al.* 1998). In our experience, patients with a diffuse pain in the body at the onset of the event often turn out to have a non-organic/functional disorder, and patients with severe localized limb pain tend to have other disorders, such as nerve root compression in the neck or low back, or even myocardial infarction if the pain is down the arm or in the hand.

Some patients have restricted sensory syndromes that affect unusual combinations of body parts. The most frequently encountered is the *cheiro-oral syndrome*, where there is a sensory abnormality over the perioral area (sometimes bilaterally) and ipsilateral palm. In some patients, the foot may be involved (the *cheiro-oral–pedal syndrome*) and, in both the hand and foot, certain digits may be affected whilst others are spared (a pseudoradicular distribution). Although lesions at most levels of the sensory pathways can give these patterns, lesions in the VPN of the thalamus are the most likely (Kim 1994; Kim & Lee 1994). It is thought that sensory projections from the face (with a particularly large representation for the lips), hand and foot are somatotopically arranged in the ventral portion of the nucleus, and the fingertips have particularly large representation areas, with that for the thumb more medial and the little finger more laterally. The projection areas for the trunk and proximal limbs are relatively small and sited more dorsally. Deficits restricted to these areas are very infrequent (Kim 1996). However, a similar proximity of projection areas through the corona radiata and in the sensory cortex may also occur, and consequently lesions in these areas may also result in the cheiro-oral syndrome. An isolated deficit in a *pseudoradicular distribution* (most often involving the thumb and forefinger) is probably more often caused by a cortical lesion, because a stroke of any given size would affect fibres from a more restricted anatomical area in the cortex than in the thalamus. Bilateral symptoms may occur from midpontine lesions, because the sensory fibres from the mouth, arm and leg are once again arranged somatotopically in the medial lemnisci. Other theories that may account for these syndromes have been discussed by Kim (1994).

A *pseudospinal* sensory disturbance, i.e. a defect of pain and temperature sensation below a certain level on the trunk, is usually a sign of spinal cord disease, but this may occur from ischaemic lesions in the lateral medulla (Matsumoto *et al.* 1988). This is thought to be due to the orientation of fibres from different body parts within the lateral spinothalamic tract. Although patients usually have a contralateral facial sensory loss as well, during the recovery phase this can disappear, leaving only the pseudospinal sensory loss. It is also worth noting that infarction of the cervical spinal cord causing a partial Brown–Séquard syndrome can be due to bilateral vertebral artery dissection (Weidauer *et al.* 1999)

A study of 82 patients who were investigated for unilateral motor or sensory symptoms, or both, without 'hard' neurological signs, found that a physical disorder was considerably more likely if the symptoms were on the right side of the body than on the left (Rothwell 1994), supporting previous work suggesting that hyperventilation and conversion hysteria are associated with symptoms predominantly on the left side of the body (Galin *et al.* 1977; Stern 1977; Blau *et al.* 1983; Perkin & Joseph 1986) (section 3.4.8). The reason is uncertain, although it may be related to asymmetrical hemispheric function during altered mood; during anxiety states, perception of left-sided visual and auditory stimuli is increased, whereas in depression perception is greatest for right-sided stimuli (Liotti *et al.* 1991). Alternatively, if someone subconsciously 'chooses' to have impaired function in a limb, it is inconvenient to choose the dominant side. Occasionally, one encounters patients who report a sensory disturbance (usually numbness) affecting either the whole of their body or sometimes all the body except the face. In the absence of any hard neurological signs, such a pattern is not likely to be due to organic disease.

3.3.6 Disturbance of the visual system

When trying to assess the visual disturbances that occur in patients with cerebrovascular disease, one needs to consider: the reception of visual stimuli by the eyes; the transmission of the visual information from the eyes to the occipital cortex; and the interpretation of the visual information in the occipital cortex. Additionally, we have included in this section information about pupillary reactions and eye movements.

Vision

Clinical anatomy

Lesions at different sites in the visual pathway give highly characteristic abnormalities. The various patterns of visual loss related to specific anatomical lesions are shown in Fig. 3.17. *Amaurosis fugax* (AFx) (meaning literally 'fleeting blindness') and *transient monocular blindness* (TMB) are terms used interchangeably to describe temporary loss of vision in *one* eye. TMB may be caused by transient ischaemia in the distribution of the ophthalmic, posterior ciliary, or central retinal artery. Vascular lesions affecting the optic chiasm symmetrically (when one might detect a bitemporal hemianopia) are rare. Indeed, the only vascular lesion of note would be a large aneurysm of the circle of Willis.

Homonymous visual field deficits (i.e. loss of vision in the corresponding part of the visual fields in both eyes) signify a retrochiasmal lesion. Lesions of the lateral geniculate nucleus (LGN) may result in homonymous horizontal sectoranopia (i.e. a segmental defect that respects the vertical but not the horizontal meridian), but these rarely occur in isolation (Frisén 1979). The optic radiations pass from the LGN as the most posterior structures of the internal capsule. Involvement at this level is probably one of the causes of hemianopia in extensive middle cerebral artery (MCA) territory infarction, but the radiations do not seem to be affected by occlusion of a single perforating artery. Restricted lesions of the inferior optic radiation between the LGN and the calcarine cortex, where the fibres swing over the temporal horn of the lateral ventricle and deep into the temporal lobe (Meyer's loop), result in a homonymous superior quadrantanopia, whilst lesions of the superior optic radiation in the parietal lobe result in a homonymous inferior quadrantanopia.

On purely anatomical grounds, one might anticipate encountering an inferior quadrantanopia fairly frequently, because the MCA is traditionally considered to supply the area through which the superior but not the inferior optic

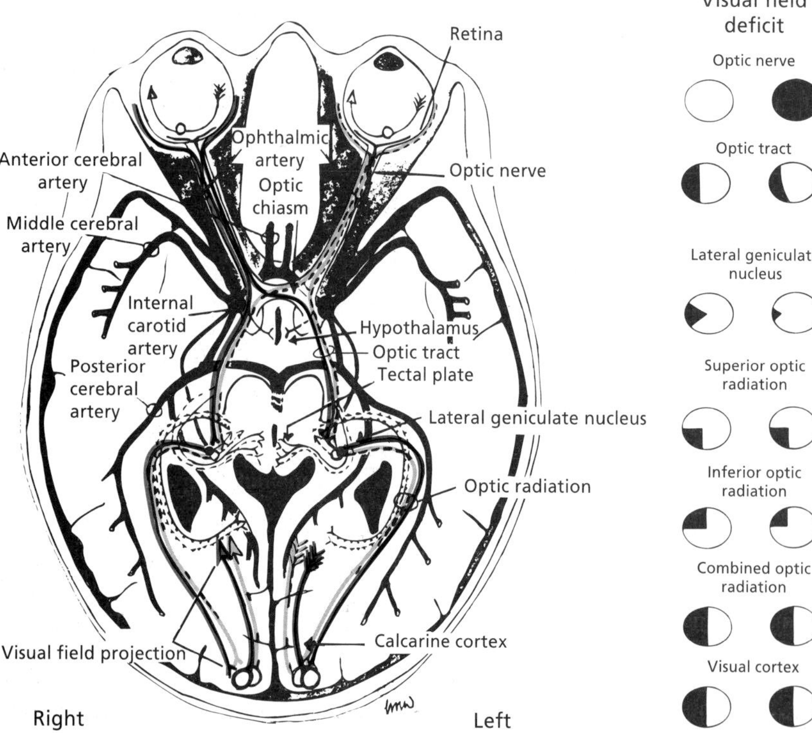

Fig. 3.17 Diagram of the visual pathways and their vascular supply, and the visual field deficits that may result from vascular lesions at various sites along the visual pathway. Note that the visual fields represented by the arrows on the retina correspond with the arrowheads and tails superimposed on the visual cortex. The dark green represents visual pathways originating in the right eye (R) and the light green those from the left eye (L). Arteries are shown in solid black.

radiation passes. However, in some patients, the territory area of supply of the MCA extends much more posteriorly than is apparent on standard 'maps' (section 4.2.2), and an MCA lesion thus produces a homonymous hemianopia by interrupting the converging optic radiations. Also, perforating arteries from the carotid system supply the optic tracts and LGN (section 4.2.2). In other patients, the posterior cerebral artery (PCA) may derive its blood supply via the posterior communicating artery, and therefore, like the MCA, be affected by embolism from the internal carotid artery. Perhaps the most likely explanation, however, is that in many patients there is a mixture of a true visual field loss and either visual inattention or aphasia.

If the entire calcarine cortex or optic tract on one side is damaged, there will be a complete homonymous hemianopia, including macular vision. When this is an isolated feature, it is most likely to be due to a lesion in the occipital lobe, and when this is an infarct it will most often be due to occlusion of the PCA (Trobe *et al.* 1973). Embolism is probably the most frequent cause, but giant-cell arteritis and migraine are other aetiologies that need to be considered. Sparing of macular vision with an otherwise complete hemianopia does occur in PCA territory infarction. The conventional explanation is that the infarction is confined to the lateral cortical surface and that the macular cortex is spared because it receives sufficient collateral supply from the terminal branches of the MCA (section 4.2.2). In theory, if the deficit in the two eyes is incongruous, it is most likely to be due to lesions of the optic tracts, whereas if the deficits are entirely congruous, the lesion is likely to be in the calcarine cortex. However, it can be difficult to make this distinction in routine clinical practice.

Visual agnosia is when primary visual perception is intact but the patient is unable to identify an object without resorting to the use of other sensory modalities such as touch. *Prosopagnosia* is a syndrome in which patients cannot recognize familiar faces, even though they can describe them. In its pure form it is very rare, but it can result in enormous distress if patients deny recognizing their close family. Most lesions causing visual agnosia are in the anterior part of the dominant occipital lobe (the so-called visual association areas) and the angular gyrus, although the majority of cases of prosopagnosia have occurred with bilateral lesions (Hodges 1994).

Clinical assessment

Many patients have great difficulty in describing visual symptoms, particularly when they have resolved. It is therefore very important to be clear what a patient means. For example, the term 'blackout' may be used to mean bilateral blindness but also loss of consciousness, and some patients who report 'blurred vision' in both eyes are actually trying to describe double vision. We find it useful to establish the functional severity of the visual disturbance—e.g. were they unable to find their way around, or unable to recognize faces (neither of which would occur with either TMB or an homonymous hemianopia).

In cases of vascular TMB the symptoms usually occur without provocation, but they may occasionally be precipitated by bright or white light, a change in posture, exercise, a hot bath or a heavy meal, particularly in patients with severe ipsilateral carotid disease (section 6.6.5). Generally, the visual loss during vascular TMB is painless (although some patients do complain of a dull ache or numbness in or above the eye) and usually very rapid. It is often described by the patient as if a blind or shutter had come down from above or, less often, up from below. The visual loss may be restricted to either the upper or lower half of the visual field and, less frequently, to the peripheral nasal and/or temporal field (in which case, be suspicious that the visual loss is or was binocular). A pattern of diffuse, constricting or patchy loss may also occur (Bogousslavsky *et al.* 1986; Bruno *et al.* 1990). It has been reported that the prognosis for subsequent stroke, myocardial infarction, or vascular death is worse for those with complete rather than partial loss of vision, and with blurred rather than blackened vision (Donders *et al.* 1996). TMB may recur, usually in a stereotyped fashion, but the area of visual impairment may vary from one episode to the next, depending on which part of the retina is ischaemic.

A frequent and, from a vascular anatomical point of view, very important clinical problem is trying to differentiate a transient homonymous hemianopia from TMB. The single most important question is to ask whether the patient covered each eye in turn during the episode. For patients without any residual visual disturbance, it can be useful to cover one eye and ask the patient whether that reproduces the previously experienced effect. After covering the 'good eye', patients with TMB (of the 'bad eye') will have seen nothing, whereas patients with a homonymous hemianopia will have still seen something in the remaining half of the visual field. On the other hand, when patients cover the affected eye during TMB, they tend not to notice any visual disturbance because of normal vision from the other eye. In our experience, asking patients whether they saw half of everything often seems to cause confusion, and it may be better to ask them to look at your face and describe what they might have seen if they had been having an attack (but don't be offended!).

When a patient complains of transient loss of vision in one eye, do not assume that the visual loss was monocular; it may have been a homonymous hemianopia.

Patients may not recognize an isolated homonymous hemianopia, or they may simply describe it as 'blurred vision' or 'a shadow'. Even if they covered each eye in turn during the symptoms, it still may not be possible to be really confident, because homonymous hemianopia does not necessarily split macular vision and may be interpreted by the patient as loss of vision in one eye only. The presence of other symptoms may be helpful—for example, if there are ipsilateral visual and brain symptoms the visual problem is likely to be a hemianopia, whereas if they are contralateral it points to TMB.

It may be difficult to test *visual acuity* formally (e.g. with a Snellen chart) in patients with acute stroke, because of drowsiness, aphasia, or the fact that they are bed-bound, but at least testing with a hand-held acuity chart or simply using everyday written material should be attempted. Many stroke patients are elderly, and concomitant eye diseases such as glaucoma, senile macular degeneration, cataracts and diabetic retinopathy are therefore common. It is important to identify these conditions at an early stage, because they may make rehabilitation significantly more difficult. Indeed, the improved visual acuity that follows a cataract extraction may make the difference between being able to live independently (and safely) or not, for a patient who has residual disability from a stroke. Because of the very large representation of the macula area in the occipital cortex, even patients who have a complete homonymous hemianopia do not have significantly reduced visual acuity *per se*.

One should be surprised if elderly patients attempt, never mind accomplish, tests of visual acuity without clean spectacles.

If the visual loss is persistent (i.e. beyond several hours) and ophthalmoscopy reveals pallor of all or a section of the retina (due to cloudy swelling of the retinal ganglion cells), then the diagnosis is retinal infarction (Fig. 3.18). Additional findings may include an afferent pupillary defect, embolic material in the retinal arteries or arterioles, and a cherry-red spot over the fovea (due to accentuation of the normal fovea, which is devoid of ganglion cells, by the opalescent halo) in cases of central retinal artery occlusion (Fig. 3.19).

If the eye is red and painful with a fixed, semidilated, oval pupil and cloudy/steamy cornea, then acute glaucoma is the likely diagnosis (section 3.5.1) (Fig. 3.20). Finding episcleral vascular congestion, a cloudy cornea, neo-vascularization of the iris (rubeosis iridis) and a sluggishly reactive mid-dilated pupil indicates chronic anterior segment ocular ischaemia which may be due to carotid occlusive disease, or small vessel disease, particularly in a diabetic. This is so-called *ischaemic oculopathy* (section 6.6.7) (Fig. 3.21).

If there is a visual field defect, such as an absolute or relative inferior altitudinal hemianopia, inferior nasal segmental loss, or central scotoma, and if ophthalmoscopy reveals swelling of a segment or all of the optic disc (which may be indistinguishable from that seen with raised intracranial pressure), pallor of the disc, flame-shaped haemorrhages near the disc and distended veins (Fig. 3.22), then the diagnosis is likely to be *anterior ischaemic optic neuropathy* (section 3.5.2).

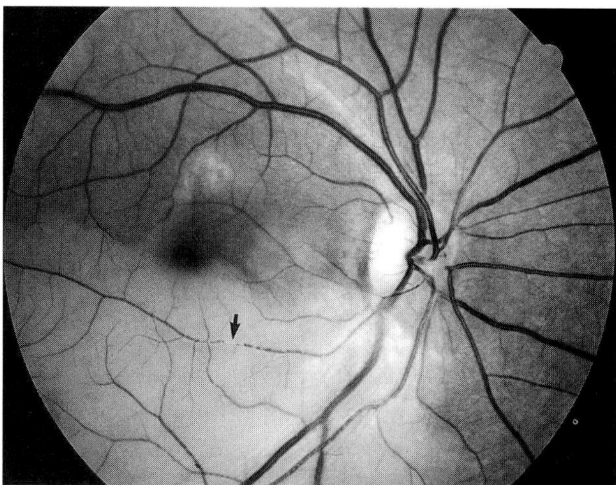

Fig. 3.18 An ocular fundus photograph of a patient with inferior temporal branch retinal artery occlusion, showing pallor of the inferior half of the retina due to cloudy swelling of the retinal ganglion cells caused by retinal infarction. The inferior temporal branch arteriole is attenuated and contains embolic material (arrow) (courtesy of Mr Matthew Wade, Department of Medical Illustrations, Royal Perth Hospital). Also reproduced in colour; see colour plate facing p. 84.

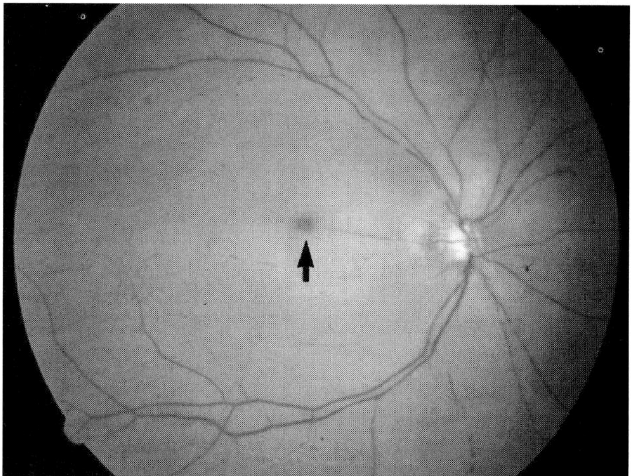

Fig. 3.19 Central retinal artery occlusion. An ocular fundus photograph, showing a cherry-red spot over the fovea (arrow) due to accentuation of the normal fovea (which is devoid of ganglion cells) by the opalescent halo of infarction of the retina (courtesy of Mr Matthew Wade, Department of Medical Illustrations, Royal Perth Hospital). Also reproduced in colour; see colour plate facing p. 84.

Ophthalmoscopy may reveal emboli of varying composition, although it is worth remembering that between 1% and 2% of the population over the age of 50 have asymptomatic retinal emboli (Mitchell *et al.* 1997; Klein *et al.* 1999). The most common type are the bright orange or yellow crystals of cholesterol that originate from ulcerated atheroma in

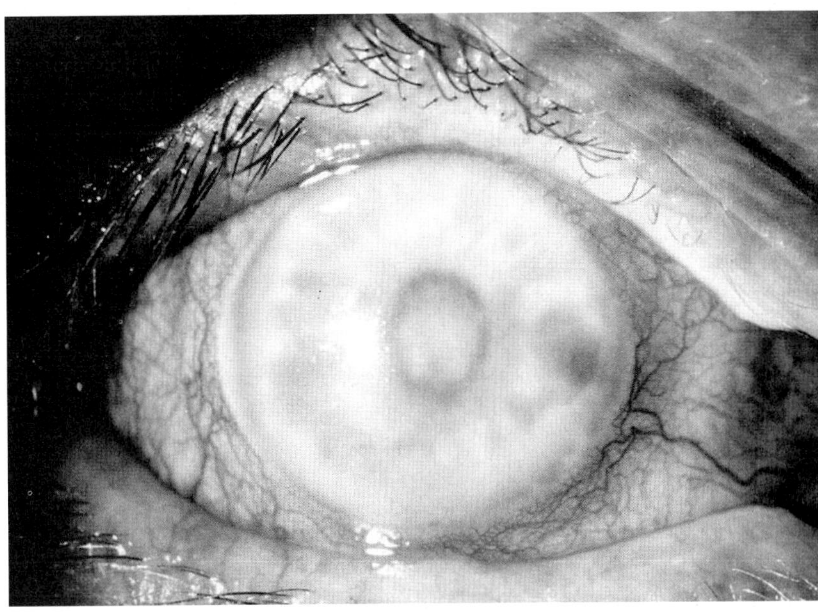

Fig. 3.20 A photograph of the eye of a patient with acute glaucoma. Note the congested sclera, cloudy cornea and oval pupil (courtesy of Mr Matthew Wade, Department of Medical Illustrations, Royal Perth Hospital). Also reproduced in colour; see colour plate facing p. 84.

(a) 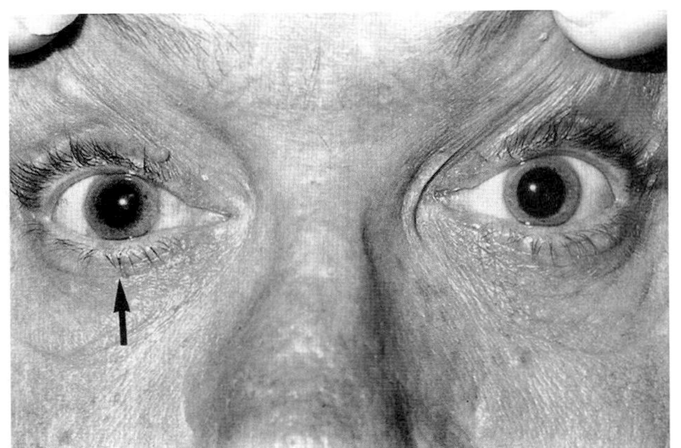

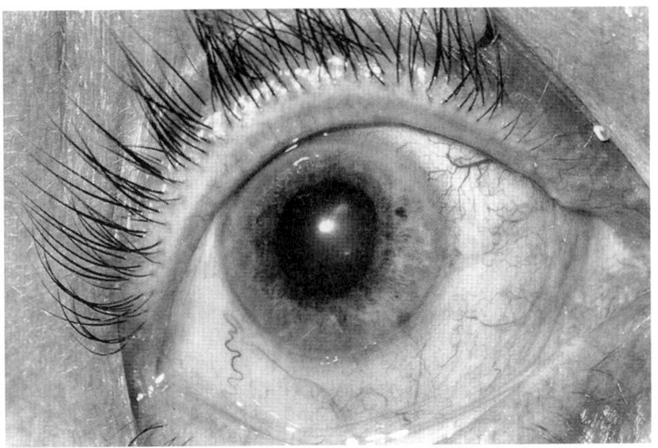 (b)

Fig. 3.21 (a) Ischaemic oculopathy of the right eye. (b) Note the episcleral vascular congestion, cloudy cornea, neovascularization of the iris (rubeosis of the iris) and mid-dilated pupil on external examination of the eye, which indicate chronic anterior segment ocular ischaemia due to carotid occlusive disease (with permission from Hankey & Warlow 1994). Also reproduced in colour; see colour plate facing p. 84.

proximal arteries. Although cholesterol crystals are actually white, they appear orange or golden because their thin, fish-scale contour permits blood to pass above and below them and thus produce their characteristic refractile appearance (Fig. 3.23). Most of the crystals, because of their small size, thin flat structure and lack of adhesiveness, pass through the retinal arterioles rapidly and rarely occlude the larger vessels, although it is probable that large clumps of crystals briefly occlude the central artery of the retina, producing TMB, before breaking up and being flushed away.

White plugs of fibrin, platelets, or fatty material are less common. They occur in all sizes and are more likely to be symptomatic. Calcium emboli are chalky white angular crystals that tend to occur in patients with calcific aortic stenosis, and they may permanently occlude the central retinal artery (behind the cribriform plate), or one of the branch retinal arterioles near the optic disc. Other less common types of emboli include microorganisms (septic), fat and tumour cells. Roth spots, which are very small white infarcts encircled by haemorrhage, were thought to be caused by septic emboli, but it now seems more likely that they are due to rupture of retinal capillaries and the extrusion of whole blood (Ling & James 1998). Sharma *et al.* (1997; 1998) reported that whilst the inter-observer and intra-observer agreement for the detection of retinal emboli was quite high (kappa = 0.73 and 0.63, respectively) the agreement on a range of qualitative assessments of emboli type was much poorer.

The presence of narrowing, focal irregularity/constriction and tortuosity of retinal arterioles, arteriovenous nipping and fluffy white patches of transudate ('cotton-wool patches'),

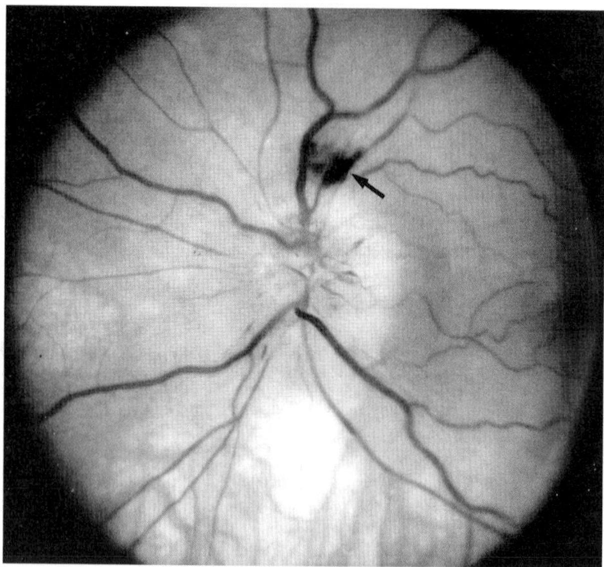

Fig. 3.22 An ocular fundus photograph of a patient with anterior ischaemic optic neuropathy due to occlusion of the posterior ciliary arteries as a result of giant cell arteritis. Note the oedema of the optic disc and flame-shaped haemorrhages (arrow) (courtesy of Mr Matthew Wade, Department of Medical Illustrations, Royal Perth Hospital). Also reproduced in colour; see colour plate facing p. 84.

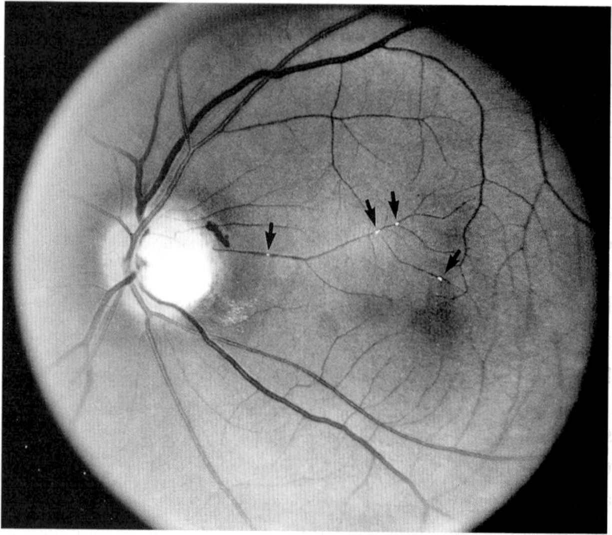

Fig. 3.23 An ocular fundus photograph, showing golden orange cholesterol crystals (Hollenhorst plaques) in the cilioretinal artery (arrows). The cilioretinal artery is present in only about one-third of the population. It originates from a branch of the short posterior ciliary artery and supplies the macula (courtesy of Mr Matthew Wade, Department of Medical Illustrations, Royal Perth Hospital). Also reproduced in colour; see colour plate facing p. 84.

which are thought to be small focal infarcts in the inner layers of the retina, indicate long-standing hypertension. If papilloedema and retinal haemorrhages are also present, this indicates malignant hypertension, but this is much less common these days (Fig. 3.24). The presence of retinal haemorrhages without the other changes of hypertensive or diabetic retinopathy in a patient with a non-traumatic, acute neurological event is strong evidence of a haemorrhagic stroke. They are usually caused by a very sudden increase in intracranial pressure, which is transmitted to the distal optic nerve sheath, where it causes a temporary obstruction of retinal venous outflow. The subsequent rise in retinal venous pressure leads to secondary bleeding from retinal veins and capillaries (Fahmy 1973). The appearance of the haemorrhage depends on its site. Small dot and blot haemorrhages lie in the deep retinal layers; linear haemorrhages in the superficial (nerve fibre) layer; 'thumbprint' haemorrhages with frayed borders are preretinal or superficial retinal; and large subhyaloid haemorrhages lie between the retina and the internal limiting membrane. Subhyaloid haemorrhages (large round haemorrhages with a fluid level) and other types of retinal haemorrhage can be seen in some patients with subarachnoid haemorrhage (see Fig. 5.43) (Keane 1979). Other possible causes of subhyaloid haemorrhage in a patient with suspected stroke include conditions that cause a rapid increase in intracranial pressure (such as acute hydrocephalus and sudden expansion of a massive intracerebral haemorrhage), bleeding diatheses, intravenous drug abuse, haemorrhagic retinal infarction due to embolism from infective endocarditis, carbon monoxide poisoning and high-altitude stress (Keane 1979).

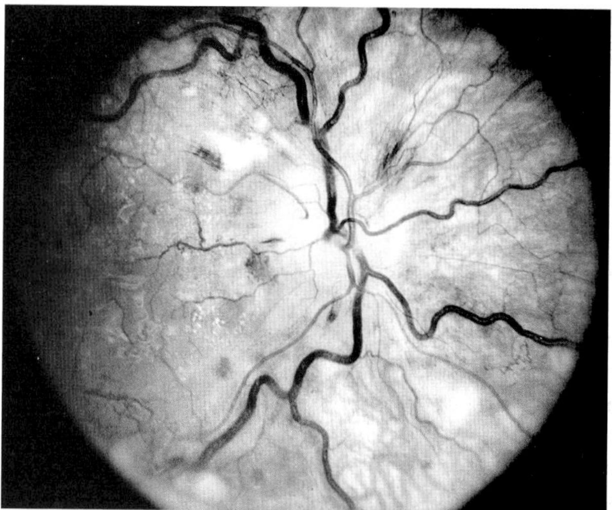

Fig. 3.24 An ocular fundus photograph, showing narrowing and tortuosity of retinal arterioles, arteriovenous nipping, retinal haemorrhages and papilloedema. These are the features of hypertensive retinopathy seen in malignant hypertension (courtesy of Mr Matthew Wade, Department of Medical Illustrations, Royal Perth Hospital). Also reproduced in colour; see colour plate facing p. 84.

Assessment of the visual fields must be tailored to the patient's overall condition, and it is important that the physician has a repertoire of methods and does not give up simply because 'formal' testing by confrontation is impossible in a patient who is drowsy, aphasic, cognitively impaired, or just cannot sit up. It is important to remember that kinetic testing (i.e. using moving objects, waggling fingers, etc.) is a less sensitive way of detecting deficits than static methods such as counting fingers or comparing colours in each hemifield (i.e. there is a dissociation between the visual perception of form and of movement). Furthermore, although standard texts suggest that it should be easy to distinguish a true hemianopia from visual inattention, the reality with many patients with stroke is that one is left saying that there is probably 'an abnormality' of the visual field.

If the patients can understand and communicate, one should first ask them to describe what they see in front of them, perhaps using the same text as for testing visual acuity, and ideally testing each eye individually. After that, hold up fingers sequentially in each quadrant of vision in each eye and ask the patient to count them or, for greater sensitivity, use a pin with a red tip. This will detect a hemianopia or quadrantanopia. Following this, try to perform bilateral, simultaneous finger movement to detect evidence of visual inattention. Testing of the visual fields with automated perimetry is extremely tiring and of little value in the acute situation. Indeed, it may produce bizarre deficits that are normally associated with non-organic disorders. However, it may be necessary later when there is doubt about eligibility for driving (section 15.32.2).

Although testing of the visual fields using conventional confrontation methods is often impossible because the patient is drowsy, dysphasic, cognitively impaired, or cannot sit up, one can usually use other methods to determine whether or not there is an abnormality.

If, for whatever reason, the patient cannot follow commands, one will need to use quite gross stimuli to be sure of eliciting and identifying a response if the visual fields are intact. Examples include seeing if there is any response to moving a brightly coloured object in one hemifield, getting a colleague to approach the patient from one side, or seeing whether the patient blinks when a threatening stimulus (e.g. a quickly moving finger) is brought towards the eye (although one needs to be careful that the associated air current is not simply stimulating a corneal reflex). A hemianopia is almost always associated with an ipsilateral loss of this blink reflex, although the reverse is not always true. If the patient is not aphasic and there are members of the team around the bed, ask the patient to point to each one of the team in turn. An asymmetrical response to any of these tests suggests that a field defect, inattention, neglect or a combination of these is present. It is not surprising, given these difficulties, that the inter-observer reliability of the assessment of visual fields is relatively poor (Table 3.20).

Clinical practice

Some patients with severe stenosis or occlusion of one or both internal carotid arteries (ICAs) may experience a visual disturbance in one or both eyes on exposure to bright sunlight or white light. Blurring, dimming, or constriction of the visual field from the periphery to the centre of vision of the involved eye develops over minutes rather than seconds. Objects appear bleached like a photographic negative, or there may be a scotoma or complete visual loss; an altitudinal defect is most unusual (section 6.6.5) (Furlan *et al.* 1979; Wiebers *et al.* 1989; Sempere *et al.* 1992). Such transient episodes of monocular or binocular blindness are presumed to be due to low flow in the choroidal circulation. They are typically less rapid in onset than the brief transient attacks of embolic origin, and sight returns more gradually. Sunglasses may be an effective symptomatic treatment.

Cortical blindness is a syndrome in which the patient has no vision despite having normally functioning eyes and anterior visual pathways. Cases of sudden, spontaneous and simultaneous dimming or loss of vision in all of the visual field of both eyes are presumed to be due to bilateral occipital lobe (visual cortices and optic radiations) ischaemia/infarction. If the visual symptoms occur in isolation (without associated symptoms of focal cerebral ischaemia, seizures, or reduction in consciousness) in an elderly patient and if they resolve within 24 h, they are probably due to a transient ischaemic attack (TIA) of the occipital lobes, because the prognosis for subsequent stroke and other serious vascular events is similar to the prognosis in other elderly TIA patients (Dennis *et al.* 1989a). However, when the same symptom occurs in adolescents and young adults, investigations are unlikely to reveal a cause, and the long-term prognosis appears benign (Bower *et al.* 1994).

Occasionally, when the deficit persists, true cortical blindness has to be distinguished from non-organic visual loss. This is best detected with an optokinetic drum or a long piece of material with vertical stripes (e.g. a scarf or tape measure), since it is impossible to suppress nystagmus voluntarily if there is visual function. Sometimes, genuine bilateral blindness is denied by the patient (*Anton's syndrome*). The denial of blindness signifies involvement of the association areas adjacent to the primary visual cortex, but otherwise the pathogenesis is as unclear as that of the denial of left hemiplegia or anosognosia in general. Perhaps the right hemisphere component is crucial.

Visual hallucinations can occur in patients with stroke involving the occipital, temporal and parietal cortices as well as the eye, optic pathways and cerebral peduncle (section 15.27.3). Visual hallucinations secondary to occipital lesions most commonly consist of elementary (unformed) visual perceptions, sensations of light and colours, simple geometric figures and movements. Posterior temporal lesions, involving the association cortex, result in more complex (formed) visual hallucinations, consisting of faces and scenes that may include objects, pictures and people (Kolmel 1985; Cohen *et al.* 1992; Martin *et al.* 1992). Lesions in the high midbrain, particularly the pars reticulata of the substantia nigra, may give rise to the so-called 'peduncular hallucinosis' of Lhermitte, in which the hallucinations are purely visual, appear natural in form and colour, move about as in an animated cartoon, and are usually considered to be unreal, abnormal phenomena (i.e. insight is preserved) (McKee *et al.* 1990). More commonly, however, visual hallucinations are due to non-vascular disorders such as migraine or partial seizures (in which case, the hallucinations are usually unformed), psychosis, or an adverse effect of a drug such as levodopa. *Micropsia,* which is the illusion of objects appearing smaller than normal, and *palinopsia,* which is the persistence or recurrence of visual images after the stimulus has been removed, can occur with parietal lobe lesions (Critchley 1951).

Flashing lights, shooting stars, scintillations, or other positive phenomena in the area of impaired vision occasionally arise during retinal or optic nerve ischaemia, but are far more commonly encountered during migraine or glaucoma (Goodwin *et al.* 1987).

Pupils

Clinical anatomy

The size of the pupil is determined by the balance of tonic impulses from the pupillodilator fibres, which receive input from the sympathetic nervous system, and from the pupilloconstrictor fibres, which receive input from the parasympathetic nervous system.

The sympathetic fibres descend ipsilaterally from the hypothalamus, through the lateral brainstem adjacent to the spinothalamic tract. They occupy a more central position in the lateral grey column of the cervical spinal cord and exit via the first thoracic root. The fibres then pass across the apex of the lung to enter the sympathetic chain, which ascends through the neck in association with the carotid artery. The fibres associated with sweating separate in the superior cervical ganglion and then travel in association with branches of the external carotid artery. The other fibres enter the cranial cavity on the surface of the internal carotid artery. The fibres innervate the pupil via the long ciliary nerves, whilst those with a supply to the tarsal muscles are carried in the third cranial nerve.

Following reception of light by the retina, impulses are conveyed in the optic nerve. After the optic chiasm, they are conducted in both optic tracts to both Edinger–Westphal nuclei (a distinct part of the third nerve nuclear complex). The parasympathetic nerves exit alongside the third nerve and travel with it to the orbit (Fig. 3.25). There, they synapse in the ciliary ganglion, which gives rise to the short ciliary nerves that innervate the sphincter pupillae and the ciliary muscle. Lesions anterior to the lateral geniculate body result in loss of the pupillary light reflex.

Clinical assessment

It is very uncommon for a patient to be aware of pupillary abnormalities. Just occasionally, they will notice that the pupils are unequal—they will usually think one is dilated, rather than the more common abnormality of one being constricted. With a truly dilated pupil, the patient may be distressed by abnormal brightness. The response of the pupils to

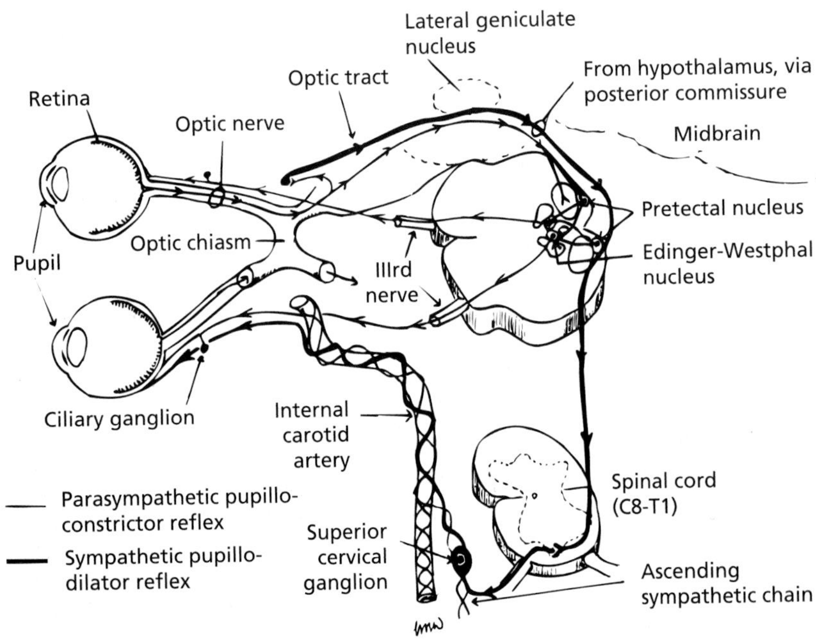

Fig. 3.25 The neurogenic control of pupil size: an outline of the parasympathetic and sympathetic pathways involved in pupilloconstriction (—) and pupillodilatation (**—**). The third cranial nerve nuclear complex consists of: the Edinger–Westphal nuclei concerned with parasympathetic innervation of the pupils; the midline nucleus of Perlia, concerned with convergence and accommodation; and the lateral nuclei, which innervate the levator palpebrae, superior recti, inferior obliques, medial recti and inferior recti. It is possible for vascular lesions to result in ischaemia of the lateral nuclei (resulting in an extraocular palsy) but spare the pupilloconstrictor fibres from the Edinger–Westphal nuclei.

light—both direct and consensual—should be tested, as well as accommodation, if possible.

Interruption of the descending sympathetic pathway in the brainstem and at other sites before the carotid bifurcation results in a complete ipsilateral *Horner's syndrome*, i.e. miosis, ptosis and loss of sweating on the side of the face. Lesions of the internal carotid artery (e.g. carotid dissection, section 7.2.1) generally spare facial sweating. Sometimes a transient Horner's syndrome is the only clue to a carotid dissection (Leira *et al.* 1998).

Clinical practice

There are many causes of *anisocoria* (unequal pupils) in the elderly, and most of them are not vascular. Perhaps the commonest is the use of pupilloconstrictor drops to treat glaucoma, but any local inflammatory condition (e.g. iritis) can cause anisocoria. Physiological anisocoria may occur in up to 20% of the normal population.

In elderly patients with stroke, always remember that they may be using pupilloconstrictor drops for glaucoma.

Because of the functional separation of fibres within the third nerve nuclear complex, it is possible for third nerve palsies from midbrain vascular lesions to spare the pupillary reaction, which remains normal to light (Breen *et al.* 1992; Saeki *et al.* 1996). On the other hand, in an unconscious patient with extensive damage to the midbrain (either due to intrinsic disease or secondary to pressure from above), the pupils will both be fixed and either dilated or in a mid-position (4–5 mm), depending on whether the sympathetic as well as the parasympathetic fibres are involved. Bilateral 'pinpoint' pupils in an unconscious patient suggest an extensive lesion in the pons if there is no evidence of drug overdose. This is thought to be due to a combination of damage to the sympathetic fibres and irritation of the parasympathetic fibres (lesions solely of sympathetic fibres do not usually result in such intense pupilloconstriction). Despite this, the pupils will react to a bright light, although this may be difficult to observe (Plum & Posner 1980).

External ocular movements and eyelids

Clinical anatomy

The function of the external ocular muscles is to maintain fusion of the images from each retina. The oculomotor (third nerve) complex in the midbrain innervates the medial, superior and inferior recti and inferior oblique muscles. The trochlear nerve (fourth nerve), also originating in the midbrain, innervates the superior oblique muscles, and the abducens nerve (sixth nerve) in the pons innervates the lateral rectus muscles. Other structures of importance include the medial longitudinal fasciculus (MLF), which effectively links the nuclei; the paramedian pontine reticular formation, sometimes known as the pontine lateral gaze centre; and the rostral interstitial nucleus of the MLF in the midbrain, which generates the vertical and torsional components of eye movement (Fig. 3.26). The cerebellum and vestibular nuclei are also important for the control of eye movements.

The supranuclear control of conjugate eye movement is of relevance to patients with stroke. Voluntary eye movements are initiated in the frontal eye field, which is anterior to the precentral gyrus, whilst the reflex visual pursuit movements

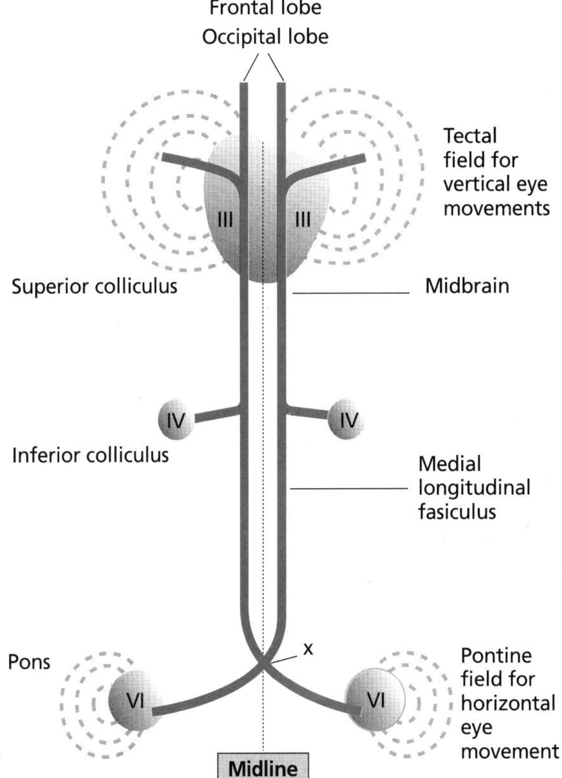

Fig. 3.26 The role of the medial longitudinal fasciculus (MLF) in the control of conjugate gaze. Conjugate gaze requires coordinated action of the third, fourth and sixth cranial nerve nuclei in the brainstem. The MLF links these nuclei and also provides the pathway for inputs from the frontal eye field (for voluntary movements) and the occipital lobe (for reflex movements), as well as the tectal field for vertical eye movements and the pontine field for horizontal eye movements. 'X' indicates the site of the lesion that results in the classical bilateral internuclear ophthalmoplegia often associated with multiple sclerosis. Vascular lesions more often result in a unilateral internuclear ophthalmoplegia, presumably because they are more likely to respect the midline than a plaque of demyelination. Following a cortical lesion, there may be reduced ipsilateral input to the MLF/pontine field for lateral gaze, resulting in conjugate deviation of the eyes towards the lesion. Conversely, a lesion of the lateral pons may prevent ipsilateral lateral gaze, and there may be conjugate deviation of the eyes away from the side of the lesion.

involve the occipital cortex and visual association areas. The fibres from these areas do not directly innervate the oculomotor nuclei, but rather their input is integrated by the reticular system and the MLF. Although both cerebral hemispheres contribute to the control of eye movement, clinical observation suggests that the right hemisphere may have more influence on voluntary movements (De Renzi *et al.* 1982; Pierrot-Deseilligny *et al.* 1987).

The levator palpebrae are innervated by the superior division of the oculomotor nerves, as are the superior rectus muscles, with which they have a common embryological origin. Because of this, movement of the eyelids is closely linked to vertical eye movements (Schmidtke & Buttner-Ennever 1992). The superior and inferior tarsal muscles receive sympathetic innervation via the third cranial nerve. They assist eye opening, and when they are paralysed (as in Horner's syndrome), the palpebral fissure is narrowed.

Nystagmus is an involuntary, biphasic ocular oscillation that can occur with lesions of the vestibular pathway and cerebellum. In patients with vascular disease, there may be either ischaemia of the end organs or of the vestibular nuclei in the brainstem, and the pattern of associated signs may therefore be of more use in localizing the lesions than attempts to analyse the nystagmus itself—i.e. with nuclear lesions, there are likely to be other signs of brainstem disturbance.

Clinical assessment

When patients have an acute, extensive hemispheric stroke (more often in the right hemisphere) that involves the frontal eye field, a conjugate deviation of gaze towards the side of the cerebral lesion can be observed (De Renzi *et al.* 1982). This normally settles over a period of 1–2 weeks. The patients are usually drowsy so that reflex pursuit movements cannot be assessed, although if the lesion was confined to the frontal lobe one might expect such movements to be retained. If patients have an acute pontine lesion, conjugate deviation away from the side of the lesion may occur, but this is less likely to recover.

When a patient complains of double vision, the following questions help to identify the site of the problem: is the double vision present when one eye is closed (monocular diplopia), or only when both eyes are open (binocular diplopia)? Are the images separated side by side (horizontal), one above the other (vertical), or at an angle to one another (oblique)? And in which direction of gaze are the images separated maximally? If the patient is conscious, communicative and cooperative, the eye movements can be tested in the normal way. However, it is difficult to do this if patients cannot follow commands. In such cases, spontaneous movements in each direction should be observed to confirm the absence of a gaze palsy. One can also stimulate patients to look in each direction by doing something 'interesting' in different fields of vision—so that they follow the examiner's face, for example, rather than a finger or a pen. This also has the advantage that the examiner can continually reinforce the command 'watch my nose'. Always look at the head posture, since patients may tilt or turn their head in the direction of action of the weak muscle.

The patient may be stimulated to look in each direction by doing something 'interesting' in different fields of vision—so that they follow the examiner's face, for example, rather than a finger or a pen.

Nystagmus of brainstem or cerebellar origin is probably best appreciated by asking the patient to fixate on, and then follow, a moving target. Remember that a few irregular 'jerks' of the eyes are often seen in normal people when they move their eyes, particularly at the extremes of lateral gaze. Acquired pendular nystagmus (i.e. where there is a sinusoidal waveform) is associated with lesions of the tegmentum of the pons and medulla (Lopez *et al.* 1996). Upbeat nystagmus is associated with pontine or cerebellar lesions, and downbeat nystagmus with lesions in the medulla or craniocervical junction. A torsional or rotatory component can occur from both central and peripheral lesions. Convergence retraction nystagmus is considered indicative of midbrain disease; this is actually a disorder of horizontal eye movement rather than true nystagmus (Plum & Posner 1980).

A number of related disorders, which are probably due to a disturbance of saccadic eye movements, are associated with cerebellar disease. These include ocular dysmetria (where there is overshoot of the eyes on attempted fixation), ocular flutter (where there are occasional bursts of rapid horizontal oscillations) and so-called square wave jerks (Kennard *et al.* 1994).

Clinical practice

Transient diplopia in isolation may or may not be an indication of a brainstem ischaemic event (it could be due to myasthenia gravis, for example). However, transient diplopia in association with other symptoms of brainstem or cerebellar dysfunction—such as unilateral or bilateral motor or sensory disturbances, vertigo, ataxia or dysarthria—usually signifies a transient ischaemic attack in the vertebrobasilar circulation.

Monocular diplopia is usually due to intra-ocular disease causing light rays to be dispersed onto the retina (e.g. corneal disease, cataract, vitreous haemorrhage) or to functional (non-neurological) disturbance. It has been reported rarely after occipital lesions but it is not due to paralysis of extraocular muscles.

Even though it is sometimes claimed to be a pathognomonic sign of multiple sclerosis, vascular disease can cause an *internuclear ophthalmoplegia* (failure of adduction in the adducting eye, with nystagmus in the abducting eye), due to involvement of the MLF on the side of the adducting eye;

however, this tends to be unilateral rather than bilateral, as is the case in multiple sclerosis (Fig. 3.26) (Chadwick 1993). A failure of conjugate horizontal gaze to one side can occur with ischaemia of the ipsilateral paramedian pontine reticular formation. Additional involvement of the ipsilateral MLF (with failure of adduction of the ipsilateral eye on attempted gaze to the other side) may result in the so-called '*one-and-a-half syndrome*', where the only remaining horizontal eye movement is abduction of the contralateral eye.

Just occasionally, one encounters patients who are unable to open their eyes. If *bilateral ptosis* is associated with a vertical gaze palsy and there is no suggestion of conditions such as myasthenia gravis, then it is probably due to a nuclear third nerve palsy or a right hemisphere lesion (Lepore 1987; Averbuch-Heller *et al.* 1996). It must be distinguished from *apraxia of eyelid opening*, in which patients are unable to open their eyes on command but can do so spontaneously, and also blepharospasm.

Ocular bobbing is a sign that is usually only present with an impaired conscious level and extensive pontine disease. The spontaneous rapid downward movement of the eyes is followed by a slow drift back to the original position (Fisher 1964). It is thought to occur because of the tendency of such patients to have roving eye movements but, without any horizontal gaze, the only observable movements are in the vertical plane.

Oscillopsia is an illusion of movement, or oscillation of the environment. The patient may complain that static objects are oscillating either from side to side or up and down. This can occur with nystagmus or any of the other tonic abnormalities of eye movement, but these can sometimes be difficult to demonstrate. The symptom, although uncommon, can be extremely distressing and disabling.

Tortopia is the illusion of transient tilting or inversion of the environment. This can occur with cerebellar ischaemia.

3.3.7 Disturbance of hearing, balance and coordination

Clinical anatomy

Vertigo may be defined as any subjective or objective illusion of motion (usually rotation) or position. It may be a symptom of dysfunction of the labyrinth in the inner ear, the vestibular nerve, the vestibular nucleus in the lateral medulla, or the pathways from the vestibular nucleus to the vestibular cortex, which is probably at the posterior end of the insula (Grad & Baloh 1989; Oas & Baloh 1992; Brandt *et al.* 1995; Hotson & Baloh 1998).

Dysequilibrium is a sensation of imbalance when standing or walking due to impairment of vestibular, sensory, cerebellar, visual, or motor function, and consequently it may be due to lesions in many parts of the nervous system.

Ataxia (derived from the Greek meaning 'lack of order') may be considered as either disordered coordination of the extremities (limb ataxia) or imbalance of gait (truncal ataxia). It is typically associated with disorders of the cerebellum or the cerebellar connections in the brainstem. However, lesions of the thalamus, particularly within the thalamogeniculate territory, may present with isolated ataxia—although more often there is an additional motor and/or sensory deficit (Melo *et al.* 1992b; Solomon *et al.* 1994). The most likely explanation is that the ventrolateral nucleus receives input from the cerebellar, vestibular and spinothalamic systems (e.g. dentato-rubro-thalamic tract). A related condition in which patients are unable to stand or even sit unsupported, in the absence of significant motor deficit, has been termed *astasia* and is associated with lesions in the posterolateral thalamus (Masdeu & Gorelick 1988).

Sudden unilateral hearing impairment, with or without ipsilateral tinnitus, is a symptom of dysfunction of the cochlea, vestibulocochlear nerve, or cochlear nucleus.

The relationship between the ascending and descending fibre tracts and the cranial nerve nuclei in the brainstem is shown in Fig. 3.27.

Clinical assessment

When patients complain of an illusory sense of movement, the first step is to distinguish rotatory vertigo or tilting of the visual axis from less specific symptoms, and then to localize the disturbance to the brainstem (central) or to the vestibulocochlear nerve or labyrinth (peripheral) (Halmagyi & Cremer 2000). It is not so much the character of the vertigo that helps to localize the disorder as the associated features of the attacks. For example, vertigo accompanied by features of brainstem dysfunction such as diplopia and face and limb sensory disturbance, with normal hearing, points to a central cause; whereas vertigo associated with auditory or ear symptoms points to a peripheral cause. A determined attempt must be made to define as closely as possible the patient's actual sensations, and direct questions must be asked; for example, 'is it a spinning feeling or just a light-headedness?' (Matthews 1975). Descriptions that include a subjective or objective illusion of motion, such as spinning or whirling, which is usually so unpleasant that it makes the patient feel nauseated and also unable to stand, denote what is meant by vertigo. Feelings of 'light-headedness, swaying, a swimming feeling, walking on air, queer head or faintness' (often with accompanying feelings of panic, palpitations or breathlessness), without a feeling of motion, are non-specific symptoms that may be caused by a wide variety of systemic disturbances (usually hypotension or overbreathing). Precipitating factors and premonitory symptoms may be of diagnostic value, as also may be the mode of onset (whether sudden or gradual), the duration, and the presence of any associated symptoms such as deafness, tinnitus and ear pain or fullness (Ahmad *et al.* 1992).

Unsteadiness is a fairly common symptom in stroke/transient ischaemic attack (TIA) patients, but unless it is associated with clearly focal symptoms or residual neuro-

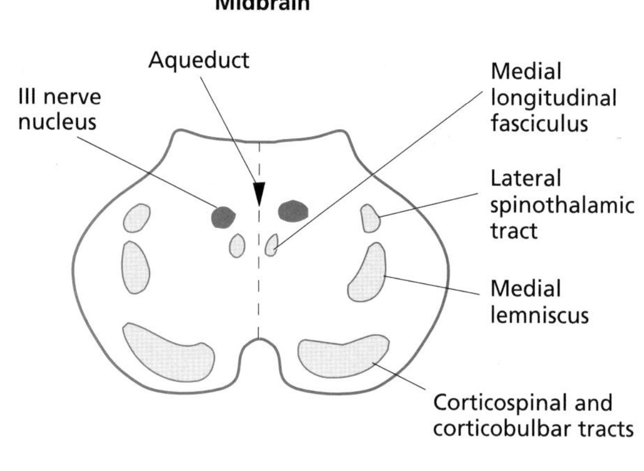

(a)

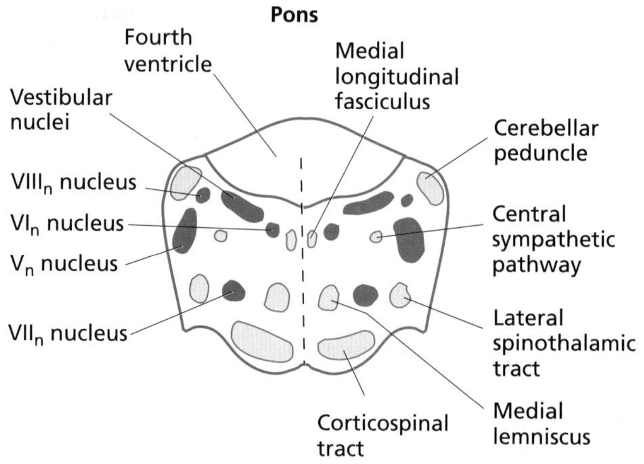

(b)

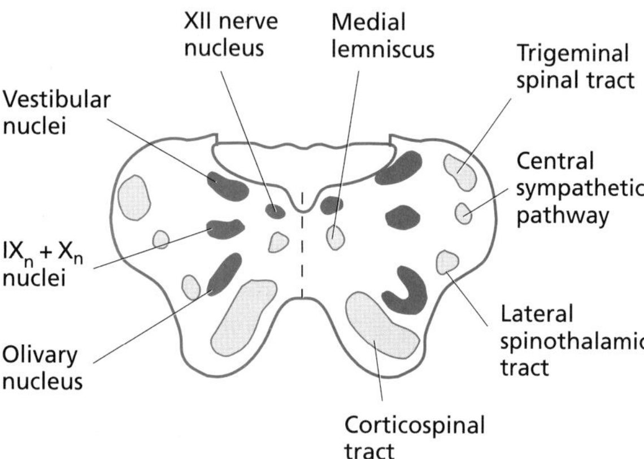

(c)

Fig. 3.27 Diagrammatic representation of the main anatomical structures within the brainstem: (a) midbrain, (b) pons, (c) medulla.

logical signs of weakness or ataxia, it can be difficult to decide whether the patient means weakness, incoordination, vertigo, presyncope or anxiety, or indeed a combination of these. Sometimes it is helpful to ask patients whether they felt unsteady in the head or in the legs, or whether it was a visual problem. Patients often complain of being unsteady when they have rotational vertigo, but it is useful to ask quite specifically if there was persisting unsteadiness *after* the vertigo had stopped—a positive response being suggestive of a central rather than a peripheral problem.

The most common manifestation of cerebrovascular disease involving the cerebellum or its connections is truncal ataxia. Signs in the limbs are traditionally considered to need involvement of the ipsilateral cerebellar hemisphere rather than the midline structures, and thus there are often no cerebellar signs when the limbs are examined on the bed. Consequently, the problem may be overlooked if the patient's gait is not examined. If the disorder is mild, asking the patient to turn round quickly may be the most sensitive way of detecting an abnormality. It is also worth asking about the impact of loss of visual fixation, e.g. in the dark, in a shower, or performing Romberg's test. Most ataxic syndromes are somewhat worse when visual fixation is lost, but a marked loss of balance should make one think of disordered proprioception (i.e. sensory ataxia). Nystagmus has been discussed earlier.

Cerebellar disorders may not be identified if the patient's gait is not examined.

Care must be taken when faced with a resolving hemiparesis, since at this time cerebellar-like signs can be elicited that are probably just a manifestation of impaired corticospinal control. This is most relevant when trying to distinguish the lacunar syndromes of pure motor stroke and ataxic hemiparesis (section 4.3.2).

Clinical practice

Many patients complain of 'dizziness', either around the onset of a stroke or at other times, but this term is too imprecise to be of localizing value, even between carotid and vertebrobasilar territories, although it is probably more frequent in the latter. Other sensory experiences, such as giddiness, light-headedness, swimminess, or a feeling of passing out may be caused by diffuse cerebral ischaemia due to postural hypotension, vasoactive medication, cardiac dysrhythmias (all common in the elderly), and they may also occur with anxiety states, panic attacks and hyperventilation. These symptoms are of no localizing value and should not be considered to be indicative of a stroke/TIA.

The tendency to label any episode of 'dizziness', especially in the elderly, as 'vertebrobasilar ischaemia or insufficiency' should be strongly resisted. All too frequently, one sees patients who have complained of 'dizziness' when turning their neck, and have then had a cervical spine X-ray that shows some degenerative changes (extremely common in the elderly population), and who are then told that they are 'trapping the blood supply to the brain'. What little work there is to support this theory is mainly based on post-mortem studies (Toole & Tucker 1960; Koskas *et al.* 1992) or dynamic arteriography in highly selected patients (Ruotolo *et al.* 1992) (section 7.1). Furthermore, many of the patients initially described under this banner had clear focal disturbances of brainstem and occipital lobe function (Williams & Wilson 1962). There is thought to be a considerable proprioceptive input from structures in and around the cervical spine to the vestibular system, and therefore for the vast majority of patients with these non-focal symptoms, the terms simply engender undue anxiety about impending strokes and divert attention from more likely and potentially treatable explanations of their dizziness. A recent community-based controlled study has stressed the role of the clinical assessment in the diagnosis of these patients (Colledge *et al.* 1996).

When vertigo is an isolated phenomenon, and particularly when it is induced by head movement, it has long been viewed as a symptom of peripheral rather than central dysfunction. The relatively common condition of benign paroxysmal positional vertigo is described in section 3.4.7. However, there are reports that some cerebellar strokes and even lesions of more central pathways may mimic these 'peripheral' symptoms (Huang & Yu 1985; Gomez *et al.* 1996). Indeed, one study reported that in elderly patients with isolated vertigo that had lasted more than 48 h, 25% had evidence of cerebellar infarction on MRI (Norrving *et al.* 1995). Halmagyi and Cremer (2000) suggest that multidirectional nystagmus that is not suppressed by visual fixation, an inability to stand without support and a negative 'head impulse test' in a patient with a first-ever attack of acute, spontaneous vertigo points to a central rather than a peripheral process. Vomiting is a common accompaniment of severe rotational vertigo, which is usually peripheral in origin.

Sudden hearing loss may be caused by trauma, tympanic membrane rupture, viral and other infections, or toxic and metabolic disorders. How often sudden unilateral hearing loss in isolation (without vertigo or other brainstem dysfunction) is due to vascular disease is unknown, because histopathological examination of the temporal bone and labyrinth at post-mortem is not performed routinely and, if it is, it is usually carried out so long after the onset of hearing loss that the clinical details are unclear. Nevertheless, there is some histopathological evidence of labyrinthine infarction due to vascular disease (Kimura & Perlman 1958; Gussen 1976; Belal 1980; Kim *et al.* 1999). Even greater uncertainty prevails as to whether transient deafness in isolation is ever due to a TIA in the internal auditory artery territory.

Acute cerebellar syndromes that can mimic strokes may be caused by drug toxicity, Wernicke's encephalopathy and Creutzfeldt–Jakob disease (sections 3.4.5 and 3.4.6).

3.3.8 The speed of onset of the symptoms and temporal course

Patients with a transient ischaemic attack (TIA) or stroke usually describe their neurological symptoms as coming on abruptly, without warning, and as being more or less maximal at onset. It is worth remembering, however, that patients are often frightened by their symptoms and are probably not very accurate about the exact time (seconds vs. minutes) they take to develop. If several parts of the body (e.g. face, arm and leg) are affected, the symptoms usually start in each part almost simultaneously rather than intensifying or spreading ('marching') from one part to another—a pattern more typical of either focal epilepsy or a migrainous aura.

Because it is the suddenness of onset that stamps the event as vascular, it is useful to ask patients what they were doing at the time; if they were awake and do not remember, the onset was probably not that sudden.

Less commonly, other patterns are encountered: the symptoms may evolve steadily over minutes or hours, they may develop in a saltatory (stuttering/stepwise) fashion over several hours, and occasionally they may continue to increase over a few days. In the last case, it can be virtually impossible to decide whether this is due to the primary condition continuing to evolve, or due to other factors such as the development of cerebral oedema, infection, or metabolic upset. Not surprisingly, there is no agreed definition of the widely used term 'stroke-in-progression' (section 15.5), but it is an area of current interest given the increasing use of thrombolysis (Nakamura *et al.* 1999; Dávalos *et al.* 1999; DeGrabba *et al.* 1999). Of course, in the face of a progressing deficit, it may not be possible to be absolutely certain whether the diagnosis is actually that of stroke/TIA, and the degree of diagnostic uncertainty will influence the extent of the investigations needed to firm up the clinical diagnosis.

3.3.9 Possible precipitants

In addition to giving an impression of the suddenness of onset of the symptoms, asking the patients (or witnesses) what they were doing at the time of symptom onset can also give useful circumstantial support to a diagnosis of a vascular event. More ischaemic and haemorrhagic strokes occur during the morning (between 6 a.m. and noon) than at other times of the day (an increased risk of about 50%) (Wroe *et al.* 1992; Elliott 1998). The cause of the circadian variation in stroke onset is unexplained.

Vigorous physical activity and coitus have been associated with haemorrhagic stroke, particularly subarachnoid haemorrhage (section 5.6.1) However, apart from isolated case reports, there is no evidence that such activities precipitate TIAs and ischaemic stroke (Teman *et al.* 1995; Friberg *et al.* 1995).

A change in posture (section 6.6.6), neck turning (section 7.1), exposure to bright or white light (Furlan *et al.* 1979), bending, straining, or sneezing (Harrison 1999), exercise, a hot bath, or a heavy meal (Kamata *et al.* 1994) may provoke cerebral and ocular ischaemic symptoms in people with severe carotid and vertebrobasilar occlusive disease and with a compromised collateral cerebral and ocular circulation (section 6.6.5). Of course, some of these stimuli may also provoke non-vascular symptoms, such as those due to hypoglycaemia (after a large carbohydrate meal) and seizures (after exposure to bright flashing lights).

Certain circumstances may predispose to arterial dissection. These include chiropractic and neck manipulation, road traffic accidents and head injuries. There can often be a delay of days or weeks between the trauma and the first neurological symptoms (sections 7.2.1 and 8.2.13).

Drug abuse is increasingly common, and it is not confined to the very youngest age groups. Both ischaemic and haemorrhagic strokes may be caused by such substances (section 7.15), and one should therefore have a relatively low threshold for specific questioning and toxicology screening.

Symptoms beginning shortly after starting or increasing the dose of hypotensive drugs or vasodilators should raise the possibility of a so-called 'low-flow' stroke/TIA due to the combination of systemic hypotension, focal arterial stenosis/occlusion/compression and poor collateral circulation (section 6.6.5). A similar argument might also apply to symptoms present on waking from a general anaesthetic, although other factors such as intravascular thrombosis may be present, particularly if the symptoms are referable to the posterior circulation (Tettenborn *et al.* 1993). Obviously, patients undergoing cardiac or carotid surgery are at special risk, and this should be explained to them prior to surgery (section 7.18).

Pregnancy and the puerperium are times when otherwise healthy young women may be predisposed to stroke as a result of paradoxical embolism from the venous system of the legs or pelvis, intracranial haemorrhage due to eclampsia, a ruptured arteriovenous malformation, or intracranial venous sinus thrombosis (section 7.14).

There is a complex relationship between migraine and cerebrovascular disease, and this is discussed in detail in sections 3.4.1 and 7.8.

There is some evidence that significant 'life events' in the preceding year may increase the risk of a stroke (House *et al.* 1990) (section 6.3.3). Everson *et al.* (1997) have reported an association between workplace stress-induced blood pressure reactivity and the progression of carotid atherosclerosis.

3.3.10 Accompanying symptoms

The presence of accompanying symptoms may be useful in sorting out whether the pathogenesis is vascular.

Headache

Headache occurs in about one-sixth of patients at the onset of a transient ischaemic attack of the brain or eye, about 25% of patients with acute ischaemic stroke, about 50% of patients with primary intracerebral haemorrhage and nearly all patients with subarachnoid haemorrhage. Cortical ischaemia causes headache more often than small, deep, lacunar infarcts (Koudstaal *et al.* 1991b; Vestergaard *et al.* 1993; Arboix *et al.* 1994; Jorgensen *et al.* 1994; Kumral *et al.* 1995) (sections 6.6.6 and 15.9). Given that ischaemic strokes are four times as common as haemorrhagic strokes, the predictive value of headache for the presence of haemorrhagic stroke is about 33%, while the predictive value of 'no headache' for ischaemic stroke is about 86%. The cause of the headache associated with ischaemic events is unknown. As cerebral ischaemia activates platelets (Lane *et al.* 1983; Shah *et al.* 1985), Edmeads (1979, 1983) has suggested that the headache is due to the release of vasoactive substances such as serotonin and prostaglandins from platelets activated by cortical cerebral ischaemia. Other possibilities include distortion or dilatation of collateral blood vessels and mechanical stimulation of intracranial nociceptive afferents (Kumral *et al.* 1995). Just occasionally, external carotid artery territory emboli can result in ischaemia of the scalp, and so pain. Of course, some of the headaches are probably due to anxiety and muscle tension.

One must remember that the headache may not only be a consequence of the vascular event, but also a marker of the underlying cause of the event. Headache in anyone presenting with ischaemia of the brain or eye demands immediate exclusion of giant-cell arteritis (section 7.3). Similarly, the presence of severe pain on one side of the head, face, eye, or neck around the time of onset is highly suggestive of carotid or vertebral arterial dissection (section 7.2.1). Other causes of headache with focal neurological signs include migrainous stroke, meningitis and intracranial venous thrombosis, but usually there are other clues to these diagnoses.

Epileptic seizures (see also sections 3.4.2, 6.6.6 and 15.8)

About 3% of patients with acute stroke have a past history

of epileptic seizures, one-third of these occurring for the first time in the previous year (Burn *et al.* 1997). About 2% of patients have an epileptic seizure at the onset of the stroke; about half are generalized and half are partial seizures. Seizures at stroke onset are more common in patients presenting with intracerebral or subarachnoid haemorrhage rather than arterial ischaemic stroke. They are, however, a characteristic feature of intracranial venous infarction. Onset seizures are associated with an increased risk of further seizures.

Todd's paresis refers to a focal deficit that may follow a seizure (Todd 1856). It is presumed to occur because of depletion of energy stores during repetitive depolarization and repolarization of a particular area of the brain. In general, the deficit usually resolves very quickly (within minutes), but in patients with prior cerebral damage, e.g. an earlier stroke, the deficit can last for several days, or there may be permanent deterioration, making the distinction from a recurrent stroke very difficult (Bogousslavsky *et al.* 1992).

Vomiting

Vomiting is very rare during TIA and is uncommon even in patients with stroke. When it does occur, it suggests either a posterior fossa stroke (because of vertigo in some cases, and presumably because of direct involvement of the 'vomiting centre' in the area postrema in the floor of the fourth ventricle in other cases), or a large supratentorial stroke causing raised intracranial pressure (Mohr *et al.* 1978b). Vomiting within 2 h of stroke onset is highly predictive of intracranial haemorrhage (Allen 1983). Occasionally, patients with brainstem ischaemia can have profuse vomiting with little or no vertigo and few other clinical signs (Fisher 1996).

Hiccups and abdominal pain

Hiccups consist of brief bursts of intense inspiratory activity, involving the diaphragm and inspiratory intercostal muscles, with reciprocal inhibition of the expiratory intercostal muscles. Glottic closure occurs almost immediately after the onset of diaphragmatic contraction, generating the characteristic sound and sense of discomfort. Hiccups usually resolve spontaneously after a few minutes. If they persist for days, they may indicate underlying structural or functional disturbances of the medulla (affecting the region of the vagal nuclei and the tractus solitarius), or of afferent or efferent nerves to the respiratory muscles (Howard 1992). Hiccups are a well-recognized phenomenon in patients with lateral medullary infarction, but may occur with a lesion of any part of the medullary region that is associated with respiratory control. Neurogenic hiccup rarely occurs in isolation, and associated brainstem or long tract signs are usually evident (section 15.10).

If patients who have presented with a stroke also complain of abdominal pain, they may have ischaemia of the bowel or viscera—particularly if there are pointers to cardiogenic embolism being the underlying cause of the stroke (such as atrial fibrillation).

Chest pain, palpitations and shortness of breath

It is always worth enquiring specifically about the occurrence of chest pain and/or palpitations at the time of onset of the stroke/TIA, because of the frequent co-existence of cerebral and coronary atheroma and the potential for cardiac dysrhythmias to precipitate embolism (section 6.5). Other relevant causes of chest pain and/or shortness of breath include aortic dissection, pulmonary embolism and atypical pneumonia.

Panic and anxiety

The sudden loss of limb, speech, or eye function is a frightening experience, which often evokes considerable anxiety and panic in patients and carers. Patients may consequently hyperventilate and in turn develop presyncopal or sensory symptoms. These include perioral and distal limb paraesthesia bilaterally, and even unilateral sensory symptoms (left-sided more than right-sided) (Rothwell 1994). Under these circumstances, it is important to try and distinguish between the primary (stroke/TIA) and secondary (panic/anxiety) symptoms. It is also important to be clear about the timing of the symptoms; for example, palpitations occurring immediately before or concurrently with stroke/TIA are less likely to be a consequence of panic and anxiety than similar symptoms that clearly follow the onset of the neurological symptoms.

Not infrequently, one encounters patients who are recovering from a stroke that has caused a hemisensory disturbance. There comes a point during the recovery process when they are not aware of the residual symptoms when they are engrossed in other activities. But when they are resting, and particularly at night, the sensory disturbance is once again apparent. If at this stage they begin to panic and hyperventilate because they think that they have had a recurrent stroke, the symptoms can be amplified, but by taking a careful history and giving a clear explanation of why the symptoms have become more prominent, the patients can be reassured without the need for further investigations.

3.3.11 Past medical history

It is important to ask more than once about previous neurological symptoms. Many patients have told us several days after their transient ischaemic attack (TIA) or stroke about prior TIAs, having not recalled them for a number of reasons at the time of their first consultation. Sometimes this is because of anxiety, and of course a few patients are affected by altered awareness or amnesia during the event. Others

Table 3.13 Checklist of symptoms of cerebrovascular disease.

Have you ever been told that you have had a stroke, mini-stroke, transient ischaemic attack or brain attack?
If so, when did this occur and can you describe what happened?

Have you ever suddenly:
- Lost vision or gone blind in one eye?
- Had double vision for more than a few seconds?
- Had jumbled speech, slurred speech or difficulty in talking?
- Had weakness or loss of feeling in the face, arm or leg?
- Had clumsiness of the arm or leg?
- Had unsteadiness walking?
- Had a spinning (dizzy) sensation?
- Lost consciousness?

How long did the symptoms last?

Do you still have these symptoms?

Did you see a doctor about the episode and, if so, who was it and what were you told, and were you admitted to hospital?

What medications/drugs are you taking? (Particularly aspirin, warfarin)

may not wish to disclose such information for fear of potential repercussions for their employment or driving status. It is the doctor's responsibility to explore these possibilities with insight, sensitivity and confidentiality, using all available sources of information. Sometimes a detailed history of previous episodes helps confirm an alternative diagnosis such as focal epilepsy or migraine, whilst a detailed drug history may identify previous use of aspirin, or warfarin given after an otherwise forgotten event. We would recommend working through a checklist of focal neurological symptoms such as those in Table 3.13.

It is also important to ask specifically about the presence of common vascular risk factors (e.g. hypertension, diabetes, smoking); other manifestations of vascular disease (e.g. coronary heart disease, peripheral vascular disease); heart disease (e.g. valvular heart disease or cardiomyopathy—also remembering that many lay people think a stroke is a form of heart attack); pointers to a thrombotic tendency (e.g. prior unexplained deep venous thrombosis); and clues to vasculitis (e.g. arthralgia, skin rashes, renal problems (sections 6.6.6, 6.6.7 and 7.3).

3.3.12 Lifestyle habits and behaviour

It is important to ask about potentially relevant (and modifiable) lifestyle factors. The most important is tobacco consumption. It is also useful to get an idea about other habits such as the amount of exercise that the patient takes, the type of diet, consumption of alcohol and also other 'recreational' drugs.

3.4 Differential diagnosis of focal cerebral symptoms of sudden onset

The differential diagnosis of focal cerebral symptoms of sudden onset is very dependent on the time at which the patient is being assessed. In the previous edition of this book, we discussed patients with transient ischaemic attack (TIA) and stroke separately. This is still appropriate for patients who are seen more than 24 h after the onset of their symptoms. However, in an era of increasingly acute assessment and treatment of patients with cerebrovascular disease, 'real-life' medicine is highlighting the fact that this dichotomy is rather artificial. As discussed earlier, it is not so much that the terms TIA and stroke are redundant, but rather that one needs a term for those patients who will go on to have persisting symptoms, but when they are assessed less than 24 h after the onset. We have used the term 'brain attack' for this group and have included it in Table 3.14, which lists those conditions that we think it is important to be aware of when assessing a patient with focal cerebral symptoms of sudden or recent onset. In the sections that follow, where appropriate, the discussion continues to describe those features that are of particular relevance to patients with TIA, or with stroke. At the moment, there is virtually no information about these issues that is specific to 'brain attack' patients, i.e. those seen within a few hours of symptom onset.

3.4.1 Migraine

Transient ischaemic attack

Classical migraine (migraine with aura) differs from TIA in that it usually starts in younger patients who may have a family history of migraine. It begins with an aura that commonly consists of positive symptoms of focal cerebral dysfunction that develop gradually over 5–20 min and last less than 60 min (Olesen 1988; Welch & Levine 1990; Blau 1991, 1992). The most common aura consists of homonymous, unilateral or central visual symptoms, such as flashes of light, zigzag lines, scintillations, or fortification spectra, which gradually 'build up', expand and migrate across the visual field. Somatosensory or motor disturbances, such as paraesthesias or heaviness in one or more limbs, may also occur, evolving and spreading over a period of minutes in a 'marching' fashion (e.g. spread of tingling from hand to arm to face to tongue over several minutes). The serial progression from one accompaniment to another without delay, such as from visual symptoms to paraesthesias and then to aphasia, is quite characteristic. Sometimes, however, the symptoms are negative and consist of 'blind patches' (often a homonymous hemianopia) and, rarely, even loss of colour vision (Lawden & Cleland 1993). Headache and nausea usually follow the focal neurological symptoms immediately or after an interval of less than an hour, but in some patients

Table 3.14 The differential diagnosis of focal neurological symptoms: the conditions that can be confused with transient ischaemic attack, brain attack, and stroke.

	Transient ischaemic attack	Brain attack	Stroke
Migraine	+++	++	+
Epilepsy			
Partial seizures	+++	++	+
Todd's paresis	+++	++	+
Transient global amnesia	+++	++	–
Structural intracranial lesions			
Subdural haematoma	++	++	++
Tumour	+	++	++
Arteriovenous malformation/aneurysm	++	++	+
Metabolic/toxic disorders			
Hypoglycaemia	+++	++	+
Hyperglycaemia	+++	++	+
Hyponatraemia	++	++	+
Hypercalcaemia	++	++	+
Hepatic encephalopathy	+	++	++
Wernicke's encephalopathy	+	++	++
Hypertensive encephalopathy	+	++	++
Posterior leukoencephalopathy syndrome	+	++	++
CNS infections			
Encephalitis	+	++	++
Brain abscess	+	++	++
Subdural empyema	+	++	++
Creutzfeldt–Jakob disease	–	–	+
Progressive multifocal leukoencephalopathy	–	–	+
Labyrinthine disorders			
Vestibular neuronitis	+	++	++
Ménière's disease	++	–	–
Benign paroxysmal positional vertigo	++	–	–
Benign recurrent vertigo	++	+	–
Vestibular epilepsy	+	–	–
Psychological disorders			
Hyperventilation	+++	–	–
Panic attacks	+++	–	–
Somatisation/conversion disorder	+++	++	++
Head injury	+	+	++
Multiple sclerosis	+	+	++
Neuromuscular disorders			
Mononeuropathy	++	++	++
Radiculopathy	++	++	++
Myasthenia gravis	++	++	+
Motor neurone disease	–	–	+

+++ Common or frequent; ++ encountered regularly in a busy practice or important, treatable condition; + infrequent; – rare.

they precede the neurological symptoms and in others they occur simultaneously. Often there is associated photophobia and phonophobia, which clearly help distinguish migraine attacks from TIAs. The headache usually lasts 4–72 h.

It is not unusual for patients who have experienced classical migraine to suffer identical auras at other times, but without headache, particularly as they get older. This should not cause confusion with TIAs. However, diagnostic difficulty arises when an older patient (over 40 years) with no previous history of classical migraine presents following a first-ever episode of transient symptoms of focal neurological dysfunction that are typical of a migraine aura, but without any associated headache (Peatfield 1987). Several series of older patients with presumed acephalgic migraine (otherwise referred to as 'migraine aura without headache' or 'late-life migraine accompaniments'), have been described (Whitty 1967; Fisher 1971, 1980, 1986). In our study, 50 patients diagnosed as having a migrainous visual aura without headache and 50 age-matched and sex-matched patients from the same neurology clinic diagnosed as having definite TIAs were followed up prospectively for up to 10 years (Dennis & Warlow 1992). Only one migraine patient suffered a subsequent serious vascular event (a myocardial infarction), compared with three TIA patients who suffered a stroke and two others who died from vascular disease. The relative odds of a stroke occurring in a TIA patient compared with a 'migraine aura without headache' patient were 7.6 (95% confidence interval [CI], 0.8–74), and the relative odds of any serious vascular event (stroke, myocardial infarction, or vascular death) was 3.8 (95% CI, 0.8–19). Similar outcomes have been reported from the Framingham study, in which about 0.5% of the study population had had migraine-like visual symptoms without headache, or a history of migraine coming on for the first time over the age of 50 years (Wijman *et al.* 1998). Whilst one could infer from these results that the causes of the symptoms in patients with TIA and acephalgic migraine are different, Meyer *et al.* (1998) have suggested that it may be a consequence of differences in the age-related cerebral vasodilator capacitance secondary to atherosclerosis.

A 69-year-old former general practitioner was referred by a cardiologist for suspected ocular TIAs, a diagnosis that caused some alarm. He had unexpectedly suffered a myocardial infarction at the age of 59, and had been receiving betablocker and aspirin treatment since then. The attacks in question, of which he had now had nine, first occurred more than 2 years previously, but had increased in frequency. Each attack began with a small, bright spot on the left or right side of the centre of vision. He verified that it occurred in both eyes by covering each eye in turn. In the course of 1–3 min, the bright spot would gradually enlarge and change into a cloudy area, until the centre of vision became obscured; the border of the opaque zone consisted of intensely bright and flickering shapes: zigzag lines, stars and sparks (Fig. 3.28). This phenomenon would remain for about 15 min; if he tried to read, he could not make out the words in the centre. Finally, it would disappear over a few minutes. He never had headache or other symptoms with the attacks, and was able to resume his normal activities afterwards. He could not recall that he had suffered similar attacks, or migraine, earlier in his life. This was migraine, not TIAs.

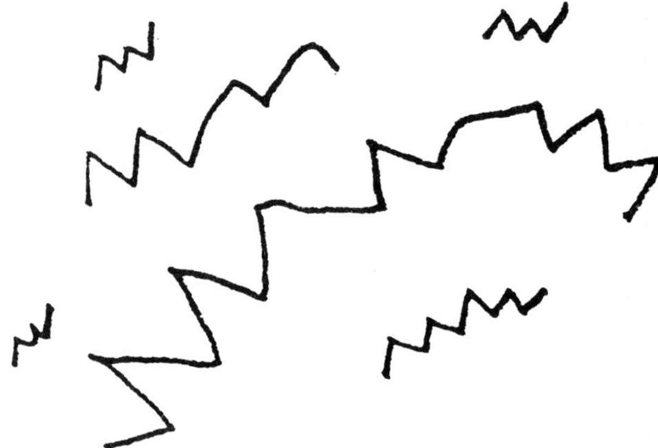

Fig. 3.28 A drawing made by a physician who experienced 'late-life migraine accompaniments'. He wrote the following caption: 'These zigzag lines appear during an attack in both eyes, more often to the left than to the right of the centre of vision, sometimes on both sides. The lines flicker on and off, about six times per second; they are colourless. Sometimes a dazzling white spot will appear within a line, which also turns on and off.'

A detailed history eliciting the slow onset, and spread and intensification of neurological symptoms—particularly if positive and visual or referable to both hemispheres—would point towards the diagnosis of migraine. Careful questioning about headaches or abdominal symptoms in childhood, or menstrually related headaches, may suggest a prior migrainous tendency even if the label was not used at the time. A positive family history of migraine would also be additional circumstantial evidence. Of course, if the patient is young (i.e. less than about 40 years of age), with a normal heart and no other clinical manifestations of arterial disease, it is most unlikely that the symptoms are those of a TIA caused by atherothrombosis. Perhaps this explains why young female patients with suspected TIA, with or without a family history of migraine, do not seem to have any higher risk of stroke than other women of the same age (Holt Larsen *et al.* 1990). In this group, one does need to keep in mind the remote possibility of thrombophilic and vasculitic disorders, and many believe these women should not be prescribed the combined oral contraceptive pill (section 7.13.1). But, for the most part, these patients need reassurance that they have not 'had a stroke' and therefore do not require any potentially hazardous investigations or treatments.

There is really no convincing evidence that arteriovenous malformations (AVMs) or aneurysms occur more frequently than can be accounted for by chance in patients with migraine aura. There can be particular concern when these symptoms occur for the first time during pregnancy, because of the recognized propensity for meningiomas and possibly AVMs to become symptomatic at this time (Mas & Lamy 1998; Carroll *et al.* 1999). In this group of patients, we would suggest very careful and repeated clinical examinations looking for residual focal signs following a single attack, and a low threshold for MR scanning if the attacks are multiple and stereotyped, particularly if the same side of the brain is always involved.

In older patients, particularly those with their first attack of acephalgic migraine and if the neurological symptoms are other than positive visual ones, the distinction from TIAs can be much more difficult. From a purely pragmatic point of view, it seems prudent to modify any vascular risk factors and recommend aspirin in this group of patients. However, aspirin is a good antimigraine drug, and one needs to be careful that the cessation of attacks following its use is not taken as a sign that the patient has definitely had TIAs (Buring *et al.* 1990). In some patients, particularly those with no circumstantial evidence to support a diagnosis of migraine, it is probably reasonable to consider both brain imaging and carotid ultrasound.

Stroke

Occasionally, the aura of a previously experienced and otherwise unremarkable attack of migraine persists for days or longer—a so-called migrainous stroke (section 7.8.1). The simultaneous occurrence of a stroke and a migraine attack may be (Easton 1993; Welch 1994):

• coincidental (both conditions are common; the prevalence of migraine in the general population is about 10% and ischaemic cerebrovascular disease about 0.8%);

• causal (either migraine may predispose to cerebral ischaemia by leading to platelet activation, arteriolar constriction and dehydration, or cerebral ischaemia may trigger a migraine attack) (Olesen *et al.* 1993);

• a misdiagnosis (e.g. arterial dissection may cause headache and a neurological deficit due to thromboembolism that is misinterpreted as migraine);

• or both may be a manifestation of a disease such as mitochondrial encephalomyopathy with lactic acidosis and stroke-like episodes (MELAS) (Gubbay *et al.* 1989) (section 7.19) or an arteriovenous malformation (section 8.2.4).

The 69-year-old wife of a general practitioner had suffered from classical migraine since she was a teenager. Her attacks always began with visual fortification spectra, progressing to a hemianopia (either left or right) over the next 10 min. The visual disturbance would resolve after about 30 min, and she would then get a severe throbbing headache, nausea and vomiting. She had always recognized bright light as a potential trigger factor. Because of a family history of glaucoma, an optician recommended that she have her visual fields tested using a Humphrey perimeter. She found the flashes of white light uncomfortable, and by the end of the examination she was aware that she had her typical migrainous visual disturbance in her right visual field. The headache was unusually severe and she went straight to bed. When she woke 6 h later, the headache had resolved but the right hemianopia was still present. A brain CT scan later that day showed a recent left occipital infarct. No other explanation for the stroke was found despite detailed investigation. The hemianopia persisted, and it was presumed that this had been a true migrainous stroke.

3.4.2 Epilepsy

Transient ischaemic attack

Partial (focal) seizures can be distinguished from TIAs because they usually cause sudden positive sensory or motor phenomena that spread or 'march' fairly quickly to adjacent body parts. Although positive sensory phenomena, such as tingling, can occur in TIAs, they tend to arise in all affected body parts at the same time (i.e. in the face, arm and leg together), whereas the symptoms of focal seizures spread from one body part to another over a minute or so (cf. migraine aura, where any spread is usually over several minutes; section 3.4.1). Negative motor symptomatology, such as postictal or Todd's paresis, is a well-recognized phenomenon that may follow a partial motor seizure or a generalized seizure with focal onset, but this should be obvious from the history unless the patient was asleep or is aphasic and there is no witness (Todd 1856) (section 3.3.10). Difficulty arises in the very rare patient in whom epileptic seizures actually cause transient 'negative' symptoms during the electrical discharge (Globus *et al.* 1982; Lee & Lerner 1990). One then has to rely on other factors, such as the patient's age, any past history of seizures and the nature of the symptoms. For example, transient speech arrest (as opposed to aphasia with muddled language output), which is characterized by the sudden onset of cessation of speech, often accompanied by aimless staring and subsequent amnesia for the details of the episode, is usually epileptic in origin rather than ischaemic (Cascino *et al.* 1991). Transient aphasia (Suzuki *et al.* 1992) and rarely bilateral blindness (Bauer *et al.* 1991) or amnesia (Hodges & Warlow 1990a, b; Kopelman *et al.* 1994; Zeman *et al.* 1998) can also be epileptic.

Distinguishing between seizures and TIAs can occasionally be very difficult. Sometimes it requires prolonged and careful observation of and interaction with the patient (and witnesses) over several visits. The diagnosis should not be rushed, as patients may have several types of attack with different causes. Initially, it is important to explain the diagnostic uncertainty to the patient and the reasons why it is necessary to establish the precise diagnosis; to exclude a structural intracranial lesion (with brain imaging); and to advise the patient not to drive or put themselves in a position in which they would be a danger to themselves or others if they were to have another attack. Clues to the diagnosis of epilepsy can be obtained by taking a careful, targeted history, particularly with respect to previous epileptic seizures and any symptoms that immediately preceded the onset of the neurological deficit (e.g. epigastric discomfort and olfactory or gustatory hallucinations due to an initial partial sensory seizure). The interictal EEG can be misleading (except that a patient having several episodes a day is unlikely to have an entirely normal EEG if the attacks really are seizures). Ambulatory or telemetered EEG examination requires skilled and careful analysis because of the potential for a false-positive diagnosis of epilepsy. Nevertheless, concomitant video recording of an attack can be very useful. The serum prolactin is often, but not always, raised after generalized tonic–clonic seizures (peaking at 15–20 min after the seizure and declining to baseline levels by 60 min). However, a less convincing rise occurs after partial seizures, which unfortunately is exactly where the confusion with TIA usually arises (Rao *et al.* 1989). Also, the predictive value of prolactin levels in the diagnosis of epilepsy depends on the population under study, the interval since the seizure, and the criteria chosen to define an abnormal level (Yerby *et al.* 1987; Fisher *et al.* 1991). For example, there may be problems with interpretation after repetitive seizures that have a seizure-free interval of less than 24 h (Malkowicz *et al.* 1995). If recurrent partial seizures are suspected, brain MR should be performed to seek a focal structural lesion too small to be seen on CT, such as mesial temporal sclerosis, a hamartoma, or a tumour, usually in the frontal or temporal lobe. However, transient abnormalities that might be mistaken for areas of ischaemia on brain MR have been reported in patients with partial status epilepticus, although the abnormalities tend not to respect normal vascular distributions (Lansberg *et al.* 1999).

A 64-year-old woman described about 20 attacks of pins and needles in her right arm and leg over a period of 6 weeks. Each attack lasted for about 5 min, and there were no associated symptoms. On closer interrogation, she said that the sensation started in the right foot and then over a period of about 1 min spread 'like water running up my leg' to involve the whole leg and arm. Each attack was identical. A brain CT scan showed a glioma in the left parietal lobe. A diagnosis of partial sensory seizures secondary to the glioma was made.

Stroke

Epileptic seizures are one of the most common causes of misdiagnosis of stroke. In a series of 821 consecutive patients admitted to an acute stroke unit, the initial diagnosis of 'stroke' proved to be epileptic seizures in 4% (Norris & Hachinski 1982). The usual scenario is a patient with postictal confusion, stupor, coma, or hemiparesis in whom the preceding seizure was unwitnessed or unrecognized. Recurrent partial epileptic seizures that are secondary to a previous stroke can sometimes cause a prolonged exacerbation of the initial neurological deficit and so be mistaken for a recurrent stroke (Bogousslavsky *et al.* 1992; Hankey 1993). Topiramate, one of the new generation of antiepileptic drugs, has been reported to cause hemiparesis in patients with preexisting brain damage (Stephen *et al.* 1999).

3.4.3 Transient global amnesia

Transient global amnesia (TGA) is a very characteristic clinical syndrome that typically occurs in a middle-aged or elderly person. There is a sudden disorder of memory, which is often reported as confusion (Fisher & Adams 1964; Hodges 1991). For some hours, the patient cannot memorize any current information (anterograde amnesia) and often cannot recall more distant events over the past weeks or years (retrograde amnesia) (Hodges & Ward 1989; Evans *et al.* 1993). There is no loss of personal identity, personality, problem-solving, language or visuospatial function, and the patient can perform complex activities such as driving a motor car. The patient seems healthy, but repetitively asks the same questions and has to be reminded continually of what he or she has just done. There are no other symptoms, apart from perhaps headache. After the attack, anterograde memory returns to normal, but the patient cannot remember anything that happened during the amnesic period. The retrograde amnesia tends to diminish with recovery, but probably leaves a short retrograde gap in all cases. Recurrences are not very common, about 3% per year (Hodges & Warlow 1990a, b; Melo *et al.* 1992c; Easton 1995).

The early reports tended to view TGA as a type of TIA, and of course one does encounter patients with pure amnestic strokes (section 3.3.3). However, careful case–control studies have shown that both the prevalence of vascular risk factors and the rates of subsequent stroke or myocardial infarction are much lower in the TGA group and are indeed approximately similar to those in the age-matched general population (Hodges & Warlow 1990a, b; Lauria *et al.* 1998). Although this does not exclude the possibility of a thromboembolic mechanism in an individual patient, overall it seems inappropriate to consider TGA as a form of TIA. The suggestion of an increased prevalence of patent foramen ovale (diagnosed using transcranial Doppler ultrasound) in patients with TGA should be viewed with caution unless replicated in larger series (Klotzsch *et al.* 1996).

There is no difference in the prevalence of epilepsy between TGA patients and control groups, but an important minority (7%) of TGA patients go on to develop epilepsy, usually within 1 year of presentation (Hodges & Warlow

1990a; Zeman *et al.* 1998). These patients tend to have had shorter attacks of 'TGA', lasting less than 1 h, and have already experienced more than one attack at the time of presentation. It must be presumed that in this minority of cases with 'TGA', the cause was temporal lobe epileptic seizures from the beginning. Because of this, driving is generally allowed after a single episode of TGA but not after multiple attacks (Cartlidge 1991).

Migraine is more common in TGA patients than in control groups, and there are some theoretical reasons to implicate migraine in its pathogenesis (Hodges & Warlow 1990a, b; Melo *et al.* 1992c). Studies have reported marked bilateral hypoperfusion of the medial temporal lobes during the TGA attack, which resolved several weeks afterwards (Evans *et al.* 1993). However, it is not known whether the perfusion defect is a primary event or secondary to a reduction in cerebral metabolic activity in these areas, or due to other factors. A recent study of 10 patients with TGA using diffusion-weighted MRI reported transient signal abnormalities bilaterally in three patients and in the left medial temporal lobe in another four patients. The signal abnormality was considered compatible with cellular oedema, although the authors could not be certain about the underlying cause (Strupp *et al.* 1998). Hodges (1991) has hypothesized that diverse stressful precipitants may trigger a release of an excitotoxic neurotransmitter (such as glutamate), which then temporarily shuts down normal memory function in the medial temporal regions via spreading depression, leading in turn to a fall in cerebral perfusion.

3.4.4 Structural intracranial lesions

Although structural intracranial lesions often cause focal brain dysfunction, the onset of symptoms and signs is usually gradual over several days or weeks, not abrupt like strokes or transient ischaemic attacks (TIAs). Possible explanations for transient neurological symptoms in patients with a structural intracranial lesion are listed in Table 3.15. In the past, about 5% of patients who were initially diagnosed as having an acute stroke on the basis of the history and examination turned out to have a structural intracranial lesion on brain imaging such as a subdural haematoma, tumour or arteriovenous malformation (AVM) (Sandercock *et al.* 1985). In such cases, there has usually been some doubt about the rate of onset of the focal neurological deficit. Little is known about the rates of false-positive clinical diagnosis for patients with a 'brain attack', but of course most of these patients will be having early brain imaging.

Table 3.15 Possible explanations for transient focal neurological symptoms in patients with a structural intracranial lesion.

Partial epileptic seizures
Spreading depression of Leao (as some suppose occurs in migraine)
Vascular 'steal', leading to focal brain ischaemia adjacent to the tumour
A sudden change in intracranial pressure, as may occur following haemorrhage into a tumour
Vessel encasement or direct compression by the tumour mass
Indirect compression of vessels by herniating tissue or coning (usually a preterminal event)

Subdural haematoma (SDH) (see also section 8.10)

Transient focal neurological symptoms such as hemiparesis, aphasia and speech arrest may occur as a consequence of a chronic SDH (Melamed *et al.* 1975; Williams 1979; Noda *et al.* 1981; Moster *et al.* 1983). SDH may rarely present with the abrupt onset of focal neurological signs, which then persist and so mimic a stroke (Luxon & Harrison 1979). In one series, three of the 821 patients admitted with a diagnosis of stroke were eventually shown to have an SDH (Norris & Hachinski 1982). However, each patient had a confusional state and minor neurological signs starting 3 days to 3 weeks previously. Therefore, SDH should be suspected if there is evidence of subacute onset of focal neurological symptoms and signs; persistent headache; more confusion and drowsiness than expected from the neurological deficit; or a progressive or fluctuating clinical course. Although SDHs occur in all age groups, they are more frequent amongst the elderly, in chronic alcoholics and in patients receiving anticoagulants or who have another bleeding diathesis. About 50% of patients recall sustaining a head injury, which may have been mild. SDH is a rare complication of lumbar puncture (Whiteley *et al.* 1993).

In the acute phase, the brain CT scan usually shows a unilateral area of hyperdensity in the subdural space, ipsilateral effacement of sulci, and a mass effect causing shift of the midline and distortion of the ventricular system (Fig. 3.29). There is a transitional stage between seven and 21 days, during which clotted blood evolves on the CT scan from a region of hyperintensity to one of isointensity. This can easily be missed, particularly if the subdural haematomas are bilateral, when there is little if any midline shift or asymmetrical ventricular compression (Davenport *et al.* 1994). Thereafter, the haematoma becomes hypodense and thus more easily visible. MRI is more sensitive than CT for detecting subdural haematomas. The EEG may show focal delta activity, but this is non-specific (Nicoli *et al.* 1990). In a few cases, a subdural haematoma may prove to be an incidental finding, and the TIA can be attributed to more commonly recognized factors such as carotid artery disease (Moster *et al.* 1983).

Tumour

Occasionally—perhaps if there is bleeding into a tumour—

(a) 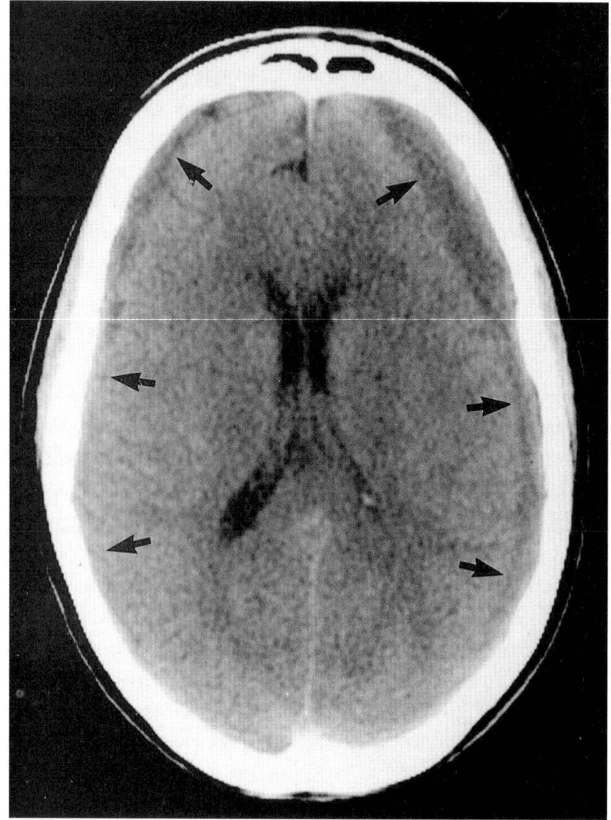

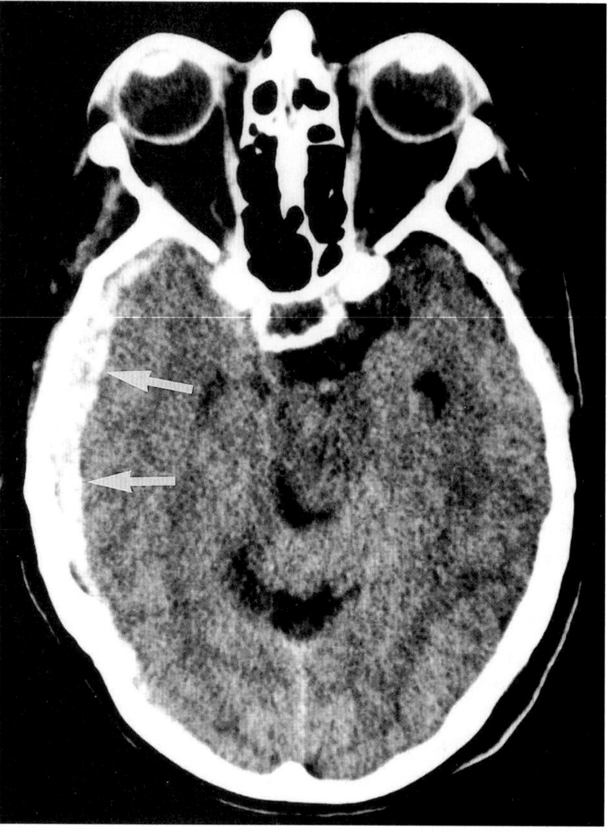 (b)

Fig. 3.29 (a) A CT brain scan, showing bilateral subdural haematomas (arrows) in a patient in atrial fibrillation who was taking warfarin and who presented with a week-long history of intermittent headache on waking and three episodes of weakness, each lasting about 5 min. The first attack affected her left hand, the others her right leg. No drainage procedure was carried out, but the warfarin was stopped, and her symptoms and the subdurals resolved. (b) A plain (non-contrast) CT brain scan, showing a unilateral area of hyperdensity in the subdural space (arrows) due to an acute subdural haematoma, with ipsilateral effacement of sulci and mass effect causing shift of the midline and distortion of the ventricular system. (c) A plain CT brain scan, showing an isodense left frontal subacute subdural haematoma (arrows)—illustrating the difficulty of identifying subdurals on CT at this stage of their evolution.

(c) 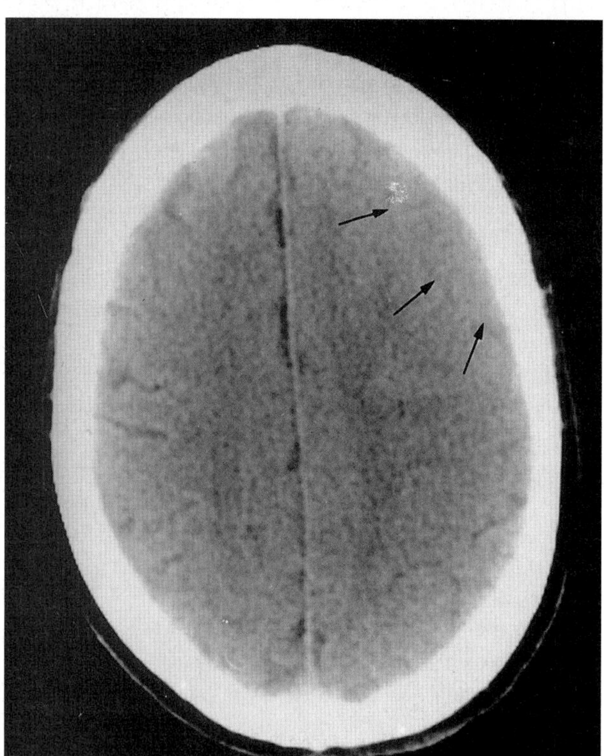

there can be a sudden focal neurological deficit, although this usually lasts longer than 24 h. Greater diagnostic difficulty arises when a structural lesion causes a partial and non-convulsive seizure, with or without postictal (Todd's) paresis, or intermittent focal neurological symptoms (so-called 'tumour attacks') that do not seem to be epileptic in origin (Daly *et al.* 1961; Fowler 1970; Weisberg & Nice 1977; Fritz *et al.* 1983; Ross 1983; Davidovitch & Gadoth 1988). Amongst

2449 patients suspected strongly enough by their neurologist of having had a TIA or mild stroke to be randomized in the UK-TIA aspirin trial, 11 (0.4%) were found later to have an intracranial neoplasm (glioma or meningioma), while one had a vascular malformation (Coleman *et al.* 1993). The clinical features associated with these 'tumour attacks' were focal jerking or shaking, pure sensory phenomena, loss of consciousness and isolated aphasia or speech arrest. With time, a more obvious epileptic syndrome often declares itself.

A 78-year-old woman complained of many attacks of weakness and clumsiness of the left arm over a period of 4 months. The weakness came on suddenly, lasted for between 10 and 45 min, and was not associated with any other symptoms. In between attacks, she had no symptoms. A diagnosis of transient ischaemic attack was made by both her general practitioner and the neurologist, and she was started on aspirin. A brain CT scan was performed later because the attacks continued, and this showed a meningioma involving the right frontal lobe (Fig. 3.30). A final diagnosis of 'tumour attacks' was made, but in view of the patient's age, the neurosurgeon thought an operation was not advisable.

It is important to consider intracranial tumours in the differential diagnosis of a patient with progressing neurological deficit, particularly if the rate of progression is relatively slow (over several days, weeks, or months) and there is a history of recent headache or epileptic seizures, signs of papilloedema, or any evidence of a primary extracranial source of malignancy. All nine (1%) of the 821 patients with suspected stroke studied by Norris & Hachinski (1982) who turned out to have a cerebral tumour had a hemiparesis gradually evolving over several weeks to several months. Three of these patients presented with seizures and five had papilloedema on admission—a finding that is most uncommon in acute stroke.

Papilloedema is very uncommon in acute stroke.

The brain tumours that tend to bleed are glioblastoma, choroid plexus papilloma, meningioma, neuroblastoma, melanoma, hypernephroma, lymphoma, endometrial carcinoma, bronchial carcinoma, and choriocarcinoma (section 8.5.1). The CT scan may then disclose intracerebral haemorrhage in an unusual location or associated with a lot of oedema, or multiple haemorrhages, or it may show other metastatic deposits (Fig. 3.31). If there has been no haemorrhage into the tumour, the CT scan usually shows a region of low attenuation (due to cerebral oedema) with imprecise

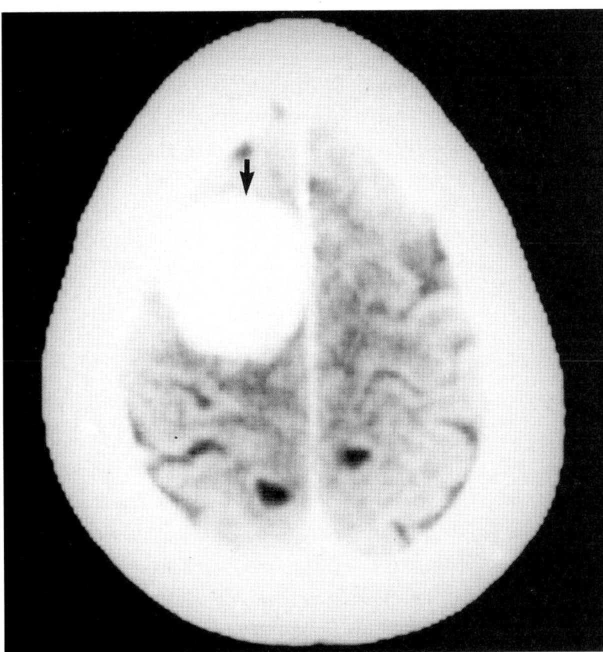

Fig. 3.30 A CT brain scan after intravenous injection of contrast, showing a meningioma involving the posterior part of the right frontal lobe (arrow) in a patient who presented with a history suggestive of transient ischaemic attacks. Over 3 months, this elderly lady had had eight attacks of sudden onset of weakness affecting the left arm, each lasting a few minutes. Between attacks, the neurological examination was entirely normal.

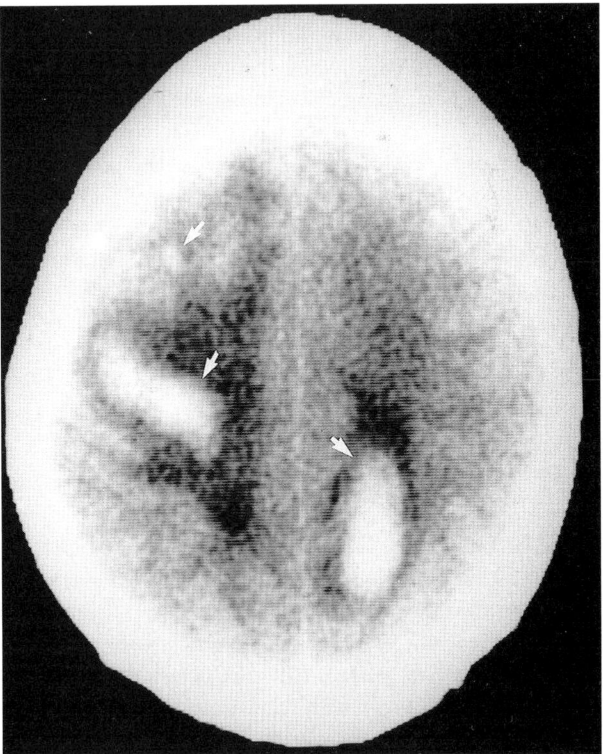

Fig. 3.31 An unenhanced CT brain scan, showing multiple areas of high density (arrows) due to spontaneous intracerebral haemorrhage into what turned out at post-mortem to be metastases from choriocarcinoma.

boundaries and some mass effect, causing effacement of sulci or ventricular compression. If there is a breakdown of the blood–brain barrier, as commonly occurs in patients with cerebral tumours, then intravenous injection of iodinated contrast material leaks into the tumour and is seen on CT as an area of diffuse or peripheral enhancement (Fig. 3.32). A similar, but nevertheless distinctive, appearance of enhancement of the gyri, which may be seen within 1–2 weeks of a recent cerebral infarct, is also due to breakdown of the blood–brain barrier (Fig. 3.33). This can make interpretation difficult, particularly if only a contrast-enhanced scan is performed. If the clinical examination and CT are ambiguous, patients should be followed up clinically (because with a tumour they usually deteriorate), and a follow-up CT or MRI should be performed within a few weeks to a few months (depending on the patient's progress) to see if the lesion has resolved or, if it is a tumour, continued to grow.

Aneurysms and arteriovenous malformations
(sections 8.2.3, 8.2.4 and 9.1.1)

Intracranial aneurysms and cerebral AVMs can cause transient focal neurological deficits mimicking a TIA, and even transient monocular blindness (Fisher *et al.* 1980; Ross 1983; Bogousslavsky *et al.* 1985; Abe *et al.* 1989; Anon. 1989). Possible explanations are embolization of thrombus from within an aneurysm (section 7.6), vascular steal around an AVM, a partial seizure, or a small intraparenchymal haemorrhage. Aneurysms and AVMs are one of the more common causes of intracerebral haemorrhage (sections 8.2.3 and 8.2.4), but they may also cause focal neurological symptoms and signs as a direct consequence of their mass effect and compression of surrounding structures, e.g. a third cranial nerve palsy from a posterior communicating artery aneurysm.

Brain CT, with and without contrast, MRI or intra-arterial cerebral angiography, may be required to make the diagnosis. Just occasionally, AVMs can be suspected clinically, e.g. if there is cutaneous evidence of the Sturge–Weber syndrome or hereditary haemorrhagic telangiectasia, a past history of subarachnoid haemorrhage, or, reputedly, a cranial bruit.

3.4.5 Metabolic and toxic disorders

Encephalopathies due to metabolic or toxic disturbances generally present with either epileptic seizures or a subacute alteration in consciousness, and few if any focal neurological signs (perhaps only generalized hyperreflexia, with or without extensor plantar responses). However, occasionally the presentation may be acute, with focal neurological symptoms and signs, and it can therefore mimic a stroke or transient ischaemic attack. Amongst 1460 consecutive patients admitted to an acute stroke unit, Berkovic *et al.* (1984) found that in 10 (0.7%) the cause was a metabolic encephalopathy such as hypoglycaemia (three cases), hyperglycaemia (three), hyponatraemia (three) and hypoxia (one). The usual symptoms and signs of the metabolic disorders were frequently minimal or absent. In a similar study by Norris and Hachinski (1982), out of 23 patients (2.8%) who were misdiagnosed as having an acute stroke, seven patients were intoxicated with drugs or alcohol and three had a metabolic encephalopathy. Amongst the other patients, seven had psychogenic disorders, three had senile confusional states, and three had subdural haematoma.

Hypoglycaemia

Hypoglycaemia may cause both transient and permanent focal neurological symptoms and signs, which can occur without the characteristic adrenergic symptoms (Montgomery & Pinner 1964; Hoeldtke *et al.* 1982; Malouf & Brust 1985; Wallis *et al.* 1985; Foster & Hart 1987; Amiel 1993; Brierley *et al.* 1995) (section 7.16). The patient is almost always being treated with hypoglycaemic agents, but one needs to remember factitious hypoglycaemia, insulinoma, Addison's disease, hypopituitarism, hypothyroidism, sepsis, terminal malignancy or liver failure, starvation, or that the patient may be on drugs whose adverse effects include hypoglycaemia (Rother *et al.* 1992). The symptoms tend to be stereotyped in an individual, and are most likely to occur before meals (i.e. before breakfast or during the night, after fasting for some time), after exercise, or 2–3 h after the ingestion of sugars and starch; they are relieved by glucose administration. The blood glucose is usually less than 2.5 mmol/L at the onset of an attack, but it may have normalized spontaneously or with glucose administration by the time the patient is seen. Particularly if a diabetic patient presents with a suspected stroke early in the morning, it is imperative that hypoglycaemia be considered and appropriate treatment given rapidly, although a blood glucose estimation should be mandatory for all patients with suspected stroke (Silas *et al.* 1981).

A 63-year-old man was admitted to a surgical ward because of abdominal pain, diarrhoea and signs of intestinal obstruction, 2 months after a partial gastrectomy for a gastric ulcer. He received only intravenous fluids and nothing by mouth. Five days after admission, he became restless and confused. Two hours later, left-sided weakness was noted. The neurology resident found a left hemiplegia and hypaesthesia, including the face, with a completely normal level of consciousness. The provisional diagnosis was ischaemic stroke, but the next morning the nurses found him unresponsive. On repeated examination, there was no eye opening to pain, extension of the arm was the best motor response, and there was no verbal response. The pupils were normal, but no oculocephalic responses could be elicited. The glucose level was 1.5 mmol/L. After administration of 100 mL of 50% glucose, there was a rapid restitution of consciousness and limb power.

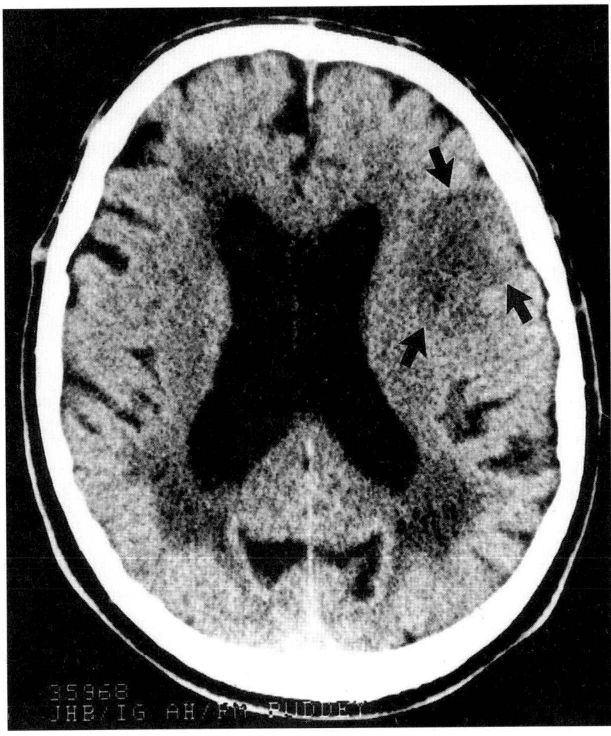

(a)

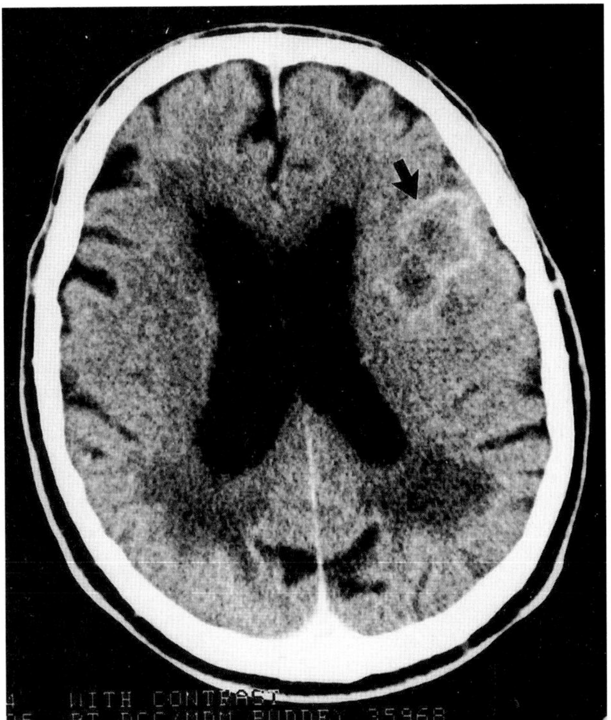

(b)

Fig. 3.32 A CT brain scan of a cerebral tumour, showing: (a) a region of low attenuation (due to cerebral oedema), with imprecise boundaries (arrows) and some mass effect, causing effacement of sulci. (b) After intravenous injection, iodinated contrast material leaks into the tumour and is seen as an area of diffuse or peripheral enhancement (arrow).

Hyperglycaemia

The hyperosmolarity of hyperglycaemia can itself cause regional reduction of cerebral blood flow, focal neurological deficits, focal epilepsy, stroke-like syndromes and cerebral infarction (Maccario 1968; Duckrow *et al.* 1985; Lin & Chang 1994) (section 7.16). These deficits usually resolve as the blood glucose returns to normal.

Hyponatraemia

The most frequent neurological manifestation of hyponatraemia is a reduced level of attention or consciousness. Tremor, myoclonus and seizures may also occur. Focal symptoms such as a hemiparesis are infrequent. The reason for the appearance of focal symptoms is unclear; possibly the metabolic disturbance 'unmasks' a previously subclinical cerebral lesion (Faris & Poser 1964). The deficits usually respond to correction of the hyponatraemia, but this should be done cautiously to minimize the risk of developing central pontine myelinolysis (Ruby & Burton 1977). Of course, a stroke and in particular subarachnoid haemorrhage may be the cause of the hyponatraemia (section 15.18.2) and many cases are iatrogenic (e.g. use of intravenous fluids, diuretics and carbamazepine). Given that many patients with stroke have been smokers, always look for evidence of a bronchial carcinoma if the pattern of serum and urine osmolalities suggests the syndrome of inappropriate ADH secretion.

Hypercalcaemia

The usual neurological manifestations of hypercalcaemia are either psychiatric symptoms or an encephalopathy, often accompanied by headache and sometimes seizures. Occasionally, cerebral infarction occurs, and it has been postulated that the underlying cause is vasospasm (Longo & Witherspoon 1980; Walker *et al.* 1980).

Hepatic encephalopathy

It is most unlikely that an acute or subacute portosystemic encephalopathy would be mistaken for a stroke or TIA. One case report in the literature describes a woman who developed a left hemiparesis following a general anaesthetic for manipulation of her left shoulder and at the time of transfer to the rehabilitation hospital was found to have a mild hepatic encephalopathy (Atchison *et al.* 1992). Acquired (non-Wilsonian) hepatocerebral degeneration can present with dysarthria, ataxia and intention tremor as well as upper motor neurone signs in the limbs, although there is usually a history of progressive deterioration (Victor *et al.* 1965; Lewis *et al.* 2000). The catch is that routine liver

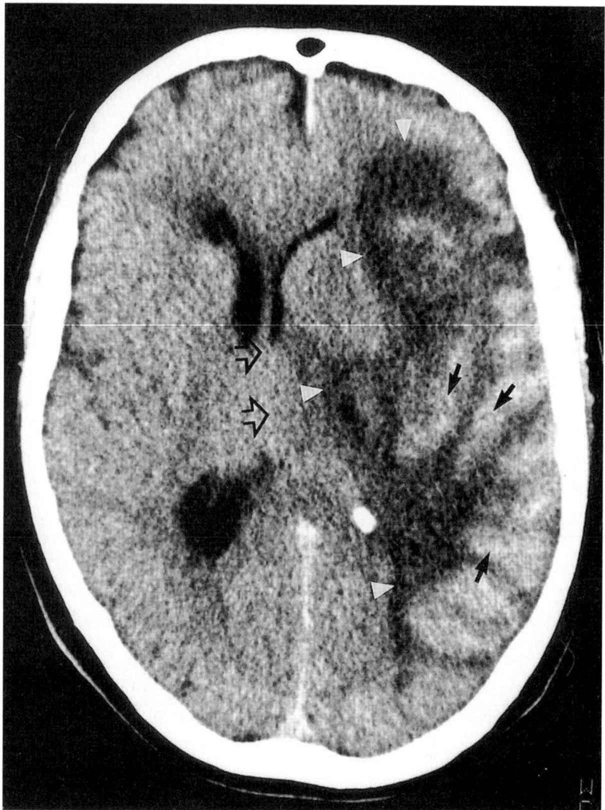

Fig. 3.33 A CT brain scan (with contrast) 8 days after stroke onset, showing a region of low attenuation consistent with infarction (white arrowheads) in the territory of the middle cerebral artery, and a serpiginous gyral pattern of high attenuation due to breakdown of the blood–brain barrier (black arrows). There is a considerable mass effect, with displacement of midline structures (open arrows), effacement of the lateral ventricle, and obliteration of sulci.

function tests may be normal although the serum ammonia is raised.

Wernicke's encephalopathy

Wernicke's disease (thiamine-deficient encephalopathy) can sometimes be mistaken for a stroke because of an unusually sudden onset of diplopia (due to abducens and conjugate gaze palsies and nystagmus), ataxia and mental confusion, either singly or, more often, in various combinations (Harper *et al.* 1986; Victor *et al.* 1989). It is due to thiamine deficiency and is seen mainly, although not exclusively, in alcoholics and the malnourished elderly (Vortmeyer *et al.* 1992). It may also be a symptom of other disorders that cause lesions in the temporal lobes or diencephalon (e.g. infarction, surgical resection, herpes simplex virus infection, hypoxic encephalopathy, Alzheimer's disease, tumours of the third ventricle).

The diagnosis can be difficult, because the history of symptom onset may be unclear due to recent alcohol intoxication or the presence of Korsakoff's psychosis, a mental disorder in which retentive memory is impaired out of all proportion to other cognitive functions in an otherwise alert and responsive patient. Pointers to the diagnosis on examination are: signs of peripheral neuropathy (present in more than 80% of patients), postural hypotension (autonomic neuropathy), disordered cardiovascular function (tachycardia, exertional dyspnoea, minor ECG abnormalities), and impaired capacity to discriminate between odours (in the chronic stage of the disease due to a lesion of the medial dorsal nucleus of the thalamus). The diagnosis is supported by showing a marked reduction in red cell transketolase activity (one of the enzymes of the hexose monophosphate shunt that requires thiamine pyrophosphate as a cofactor) and a striking improvement in the oculomotor disorders (but not other disorders such as amnesia, polyneuropathy, and blindness) within hours of the administration of thiamine; completely normal values of transketolase are usually attained within 24 h. Failure of the ocular palsies to respond to thiamine within a few days should raise doubts about the diagnosis of Wernicke's disease. The medial thalamic and periaqueductal lesions may be demonstrated on MRI of the brain. If Wernicke's disease is a diagnostic possibility, take blood (for red cell transketolase, thiamine and glucose levels) and then treat immediately with thiamine and glucose (since hypoglycaemia can precipitate Wernicke's disease); do not waste time waiting for the results to come back.

Hypertensive encephalopathy

Although hypertensive encephalopathy associated with malignant or accelerated phase hypertension is now rare, it occurs most commonly in patients with an established history of hypertension, although only when the diastolic blood pressure exceeds about 150 mmHg. However, it is also seen in previously normotensive patients whose cerebral autoregulation is normal and so easily exceeded by a rapid rise in blood pressure, sometimes with a diastolic blood pressure of no more than 100 mmHg (i.e. associated with conditions such as pre-eclampsia, acute nephritis, phaeochromocytoma, renin-secreting tumour, ingestion of sympathomimetic drugs and tricyclic antidepressants, ingestion of tyramine in conjunction with a monoamine oxidase inhibitor, head injury, autonomic hyperactivity in patients with the Guillain–Barré syndrome or spinal cord disorders, and with baroreceptor reflex failure after bilateral carotid endarterectomy) (Calhoun & Oparil 1990; Ille *et al.* 1995). The cause is thought to be widespread cerebral oedema resulting from a breakdown of cerebral blood flow autoregulation. The pathological hallmark of accelerated or malignant hypertension is fibrinoid necrosis in resistance vessels in the retina and kidneys. The clinical picture is usually dominated by the subacute onset of headache, nausea, vomiting, confusion, declining conscious state, blurred vision, seizures and focal or generalized weakness (Healton *et al.* 1982). There may be focal neurological signs, generalized or focal seizures and hypertensive retinopathy (including papilloedema) (Fig. 3.24). Hypertensive encephalopathy can sometimes be mistaken for intracranial venous thrombosis (particularly in pregnancy) or an arterial stroke, especially if there is doubt about the onset of symptoms (i.e. if the patient is confused or obtunded) and if the blood pressure is only moderately elevated; even a severely elevated blood pressure can be a consequence of stroke as well as a cause of stroke, but in these cases there is unlikely to be evidence of end-organ damage such as retinopathy (section 15.7.1).

The aim of treatment should be a smooth reduction in blood pressure over hours rather than minutes; indeed precipitous falls in blood pressure can cause boundary-zone infarcts (section 4.2.4).

Posterior leukoencephalopathy syndrome (PLES)

PLES is a recently recognized syndrome that has many similarities to hypertensive encephalopathy except that there is usually no evidence of hypertensive end-organ damage, and the prognosis is generally very good (Hinchey *et al.* 1996). Patients present with cortical blindness, headaches, vomiting and seizures, and brain MR shows very extensive white matter abnormalities typical of oedema in the posterior regions of both hemispheres (Fig. 3.34). The onset is often associated with a sudden rise in blood pressure (e.g. associated with pregnancy, renal disease including the use of erythropoietin, or blood transfusion) but it has also been associated with a number of immunosuppressive therapies (section 7.12). There is usually fairly rapid improvement of both the clinical and MR abnormalities.

3.4.6 Central nervous system infections

Encephalitis, brain abscess and subdural empyema

If a patient with a focal neurological deficit has an altered conscious state and a fever, then localized infection (meningoencephalitis, brain abscess or subdural empyema) needs to be considered (and perhaps even treated empirically), particularly if there is no other cause for the fever (such as pneumonia, urinary tract infection or deep venous thrombosis). There may also be a history of subacute evolution of systemic upset (fever, malaise, lethargy) and focal neurological symptoms, as well as seizures, meningism or a predisposing condition such as sinusitis, mastoiditis, otitis, pneumonia, or congenital heart disease. Of course, it is conceivable that the diagnosis of stroke is correct, and the cause of the stroke is an infection (section 7.11).

(a)

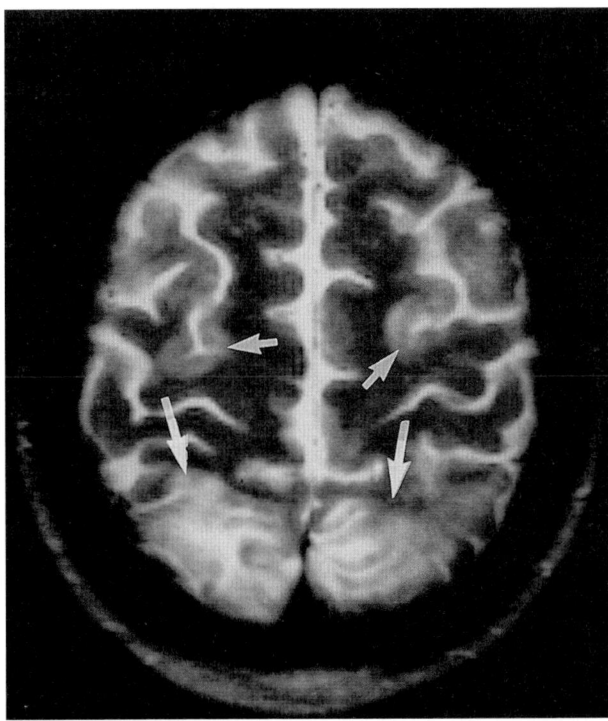

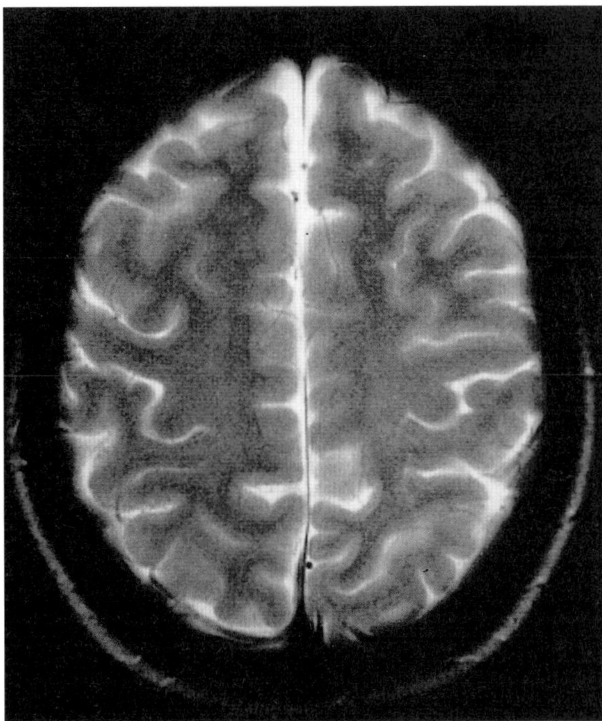

(b)

Fig. 3.34 T2-weighted brain magnetic resonance (MR) scans of a patient with the posterior leukoencephalopathy syndrome (PLES), which occurred following a rapid blood transfusion after placental abruption. On the day of onset (a), the patient suddenly became cortically blind in association with a severe headache. She also had several seizures. On T2 MR, there were areas of increased signal in both occipital cortices (long arrows). Note also the areas of increased cortical signal in the parietal regions (short arrows). All her symptoms resolved over 7 days. Three months later, there was no residual visual field deficit, and the scan was normal (b).

The EEG, brain CT, MR scan and cerebrospinal fluid (CSF) are usually characteristically abnormal (Mauser *et al.* 1986; Saul *et al.* 1986; Khan *et al.* 1995). For example, the parasitic infection cysticercosis may present like a stroke, but the patient will probably have lived in an endemic area and the CT scan often shows an area of calcification within a cyst, as well as scattered foci of parenchymal calcification (McCormick *et al.* 1982). In unilateral subdural empyema, the EEG shows extensive unilateral depression of cortical activity and focal delta waves lasting up to 2 s (Mauser *et al.* 1986), and the CT shows a non-homogeneous lenticular or semilunar extracerebral lesion with mass effect. However, the CT can be normal early on, and repeated (sometimes daily) scanning may be required to identify the subdural empyema. Likewise, brain CT or MRI of a cerebral abscess usually shows a low-density lesion that is not in a specific vascular territory and has peripheral ring enhancement following intravenous contrast; but sometimes the presentation can be acute and the typical CT findings of an abscess can be delayed for several weeks after the onset of the focal neurological deficit (Kong *et al.* 1993; Hogan 1994). It can also be difficult to distinguish radiologically between herpes simplex encephalitis of the frontotemporal lobes and a middle cerebral artery territory infarct (Fig. 3.35). If the patient has focal neurological signs, is systemically unwell with fever and has what looks like a normal CT scan, then an abscess, subdural empyema, and meningoencephalitis therefore need to be excluded by MR scan, EEG and CSF examination.

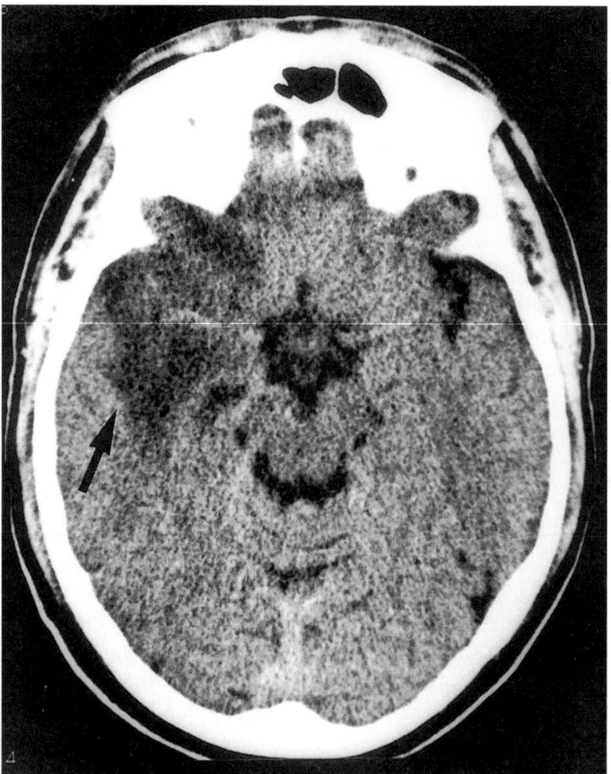

Fig. 3.35 A CT brain scan (with intravenous contrast), showing a region of low intensity in the right temporal lobe (arrow) due to herpes simplex encephalitis. Note how it can sometimes be difficult to distinguish encephalitis in the frontotemporal lobes from a middle cerebral artery territory infarct radiologically. Usually, however, the site of the encephalitis does not conform to a specific vascular territory, and the radiological characteristics of the lesion are different: low density with patchy high density (due to haemorrhagic necrosis) and oedema (see also Fig. 5.22).

Creutzfeldt–Jakob disease (CJD)

Sporadic CJD typically presents with a combination of rapidly progressive (over weeks) dementia and myoclonus, which may be accompanied by symptoms and signs of visual, pyramidal and cerebellar dysfunction. However, CJD may occasionally present acutely with a stroke-like syndrome. Amongst a series of 532 patients with 'definite' or 'probable' CJD, the onset was sufficiently abrupt to be diagnosed as a stroke in 30 cases (5.6%); the diagnosis was made by a consultant physician or neurologist in 28 cases and even fulfilled the standard WHO criteria for stroke in two (McNaughton & Will 1994). Of 29 patients who had a CT scan, five (17%) were reported to have a low-density lesion like an 'infarct' that was appropriate to the clinical signs, and a further five showed 'other' infarct-like areas. This type of presentation has not been reported in new variant CJD.

It is difficult to understand how the pathological changes in CJD could lead to a sudden onset of focal neurological dysfunction. However, unlike most strokes, the symptoms evolve over hours to days to weeks, and continued observation and follow-up of the patient reveals progressive cognitive impairment, multifocal neurological deficits and, in particular, myoclonus. The EEG changes that are more specific for CJD often occur late in the disorder.

If a 'stroke' patient deteriorates and develops myoclonus or dementia, think of sporadic Creutzfeldt–Jakob disease and order one or more EEGs.

3.4.7 Labyrinthine disorders

Vestibular neuronitis (labyrinthitis)

This is probably the commonest cause of severe acute vertigo. There is associated nausea, vomiting, nystagmus and ataxia, but no deafness or tinnitus. The acute symptoms usually last for several days and may be followed by positional vertigo for some weeks (Buchele & Brandt 1988; Hotson & Baloh 1998). The evidence for a viral involvement of the superior part of the trunk of the vestibular nerve is scanty. A very similar, if not identical, clinical syndrome can clearly be caused by minor cerebellar strokes, and the diagnosis is only revealed by MR imaging (section 3.3.7).

Ménière's disease

Ménière's disease is characterized by repeated crises of quite severe rotatory or whirling vertigo, which can be acute in onset and last from several minutes to a few days. Varying degrees of nausea and vomiting, unilateral (initially) low-pitched tinnitus, sensorineural deafness and a feeling of fullness or pressure in the ear are almost always present as well (Ludman 1990). It usually begins in middle age. The diagnostic difficulty may come with the first attack, when the auditory symptoms may be mild or non-existent and caloric tests may be normal. In these cases, cerebellar infarction is a possible differential diagnosis (section 3.3.7).

Benign paroxysmal positional vertigo

Benign paroxysmal positional vertigo is characterized by recurrent episodes of vertigo and nystagmus that occur only after suddenly changing the position of the head—for example, when looking up, rolling over in bed and turning the head toward the affected ear, lying down, bending over and straightening up (Baloh 1987; Baloh *et al.* 1993; Denholm 1993; Lempert *et al.* 1995). The vertigo is usually severe but very brief in duration, certainly less than 1 min, and usually less than 15 s. Hearing is normal. There may be a history of recent head trauma, viral illness, stapes surgery or chronic middle ear disease, but many cases are idiopathic. The cause in most cases is otolith debris in the posterior semicircular canal (Gresty *et al.* 1992; Lempert *et al.* 1995; Strupp *et al.* 1995). The diagnosis is established from the history and using the Dix–Hallpike manoeuvre (Dix & Hallpike 1952). The patient is moved quickly from a sitting to a supine position, and the head is tilted over the end of the examination couch until it has been lowered about 30° below the level of the couch; simultaneously, the head is turned 30–40° to one side. If the test is positive, there is a latent interval of a few seconds before the patient experiences a paroxysm of vertigo accompanied by rotatory/torsional nystagmus, with the upper pole of the eye beating towards the floor and the undermost ear, usually lasting less than 15 s and no more than 30–40 s. The vertigo and nystagmus then stop, a phenomenon known as adaptation. If the patient sits up again, the direction of vertigo and nystagmus often reverse direction. If the manoeuvre is repeated, the vertigo and nystagmus become less apparent and 'fatigue'. The treatment of choice is a positioning manoeuvre such as the Epley, which improves symptoms in about 80% of cases (Hotson & Baloh 1998).

Benign recurrent vertigo

Attacks of spontaneous vertigo not accompanied by cochlear or other neurological symptoms in young or middle-aged adults, lasting from 20 min to a few hours, have been called 'benign recurrent vertigo' (Slater 1979). The demographics and precipitants of this condition are very similar to those of migraine, and the attacks may respond to standard migraine prophylactic drugs, suggesting that it is a migraine variant—but the exact pathophysiology remains uncertain.

Vestibular epilepsy

Very rarely, vertigo may occur as part of a seizure disorder. The focus can be in either the temporal lobe or parietal association cortex, both of which receive bilateral vestibular projections from the thalamus (Kogeorgos *et al.* 1981; Brandt 1991).

3.4.8 Psychological disorders

Many patients have recurrent attacks of transient, focal (or non-focal) neurological symptoms, which after appropriate medical assessment cannot be explained in terms of a conventionally defined medical disease, and which have been termed 'functional somatic syndromes' (Wessely *et al.* 1999). An alternative term is 'somatization disorder', which has been defined as 'the tendency to experience and communicate psychological distress in the form of physical symptoms and to seek medical help for them' (Samuels 1995).

Attacks that are emotionally based take several forms, such as hyperventilation attacks, panic attacks, anxiety attacks, swoons, tantrums and deliberate simulation (Betts 1990). Functional overbreathing (hyperventilation) usually causes bilateral limb and perioral sensory symptoms, but occasionally the symptoms are confusingly unilateral and usually it is the left limbs that are affected (Blau *et al.* 1983). Features distinguishing these attacks from transient ischaemic attacks include the patient's age (usually young) and sex (usually female), the circumstances of the attack, the lack of underlying vascular risk factors, the presence of other inexplicable symptoms often over many years, and often the emotional context (anxiety, indifference or ambivalence). The history tends to be vague and inconsistent and may disclose social disruption or personality disturbance.

Patients can also present with persisting impairment of neurological function (e.g. loss of power or sensation in their limbs, disordered speech or vision, or inability to walk). Such hysterical conversion (unconscious) or malingering (conscious) can, superficially, be difficult to distinguish from stroke. The patient usually has some or all of the characteristics described above, but these problems do occur in older as well as younger patients, although it is very common for there to be a past psychiatric history of some sort. There may or may not be some evidence of potential for gain and, if so, the gain is almost always 'primary' (solution of emotional conflict) rather than 'secondary' (financial compensation). Sometimes there is a 'model' with a real illness (e.g. a friend or family member with a stroke).

On examination, for those with apparent weakness, there are no hard signs of upper or lower motor neurone dysfunction (such as abnormal reflexes, extensor plantar response) and no pressure sores. Voluntary effort may be intermittent, with simultaneous contraction of agonist and antagonist muscles along with excessive effort in irrelevant muscle groups and prominent verbal grunts (the wrestler's sign). With encouragement, it is usually possible to elicit full muscle power, even though this may only be momentary and interspersed with episodes of apparent 'collapsing weakness'. There is also inconsistency in what the patient can and cannot do and between examinations; for example, the patient may be unable to lift either leg off the bed, but can still sit up from the supine position and walk (Norris & Hachinski 1982). The area of reported sensory loss tends to be inconsistent and more frequently involves the left side of the body (Rothwell 1994). Other suggestive features are signs that are not reproducible, inconsistent with function (e.g. absent joint position sense but normal gait with eyes closed), or incompatible with normal sensory anatomy (e.g. with eyes shut, the patient responds normally to the examiner touching the tip of the index finger and asking the patient to touch the tip of their nose with it, but later the patient appears to have loss of sensation to formal light touch or position sense testing in the same finger). Other clues to functional sensory loss include nonsense behaviour (e.g. patient responds 'no' to being touched in the numb area), vibration sense being lost on just one side of the sternum, numbness with circular borders in the limbs, sensory loss on the trunk that changes side when the patient is turned over, and the observation of patients deftly palpating a small object between their fingers followed by a statement that they are unable to feel what it is. Peripheral sensory nerve action potentials, nerve conduction studies, somatosensory and motor evoked potentials are all normal, but it is often not necessary to resort to these.

Visual function in patients complaining of bilateral blindness who have a normal neuro-ophthalmological examination and who are suspected of malingering can be inferred by testing for optokinetic nystagmus, which cannot be suppressed voluntarily.

Finally, it is important to be very careful when diagnosing focal neurological symptoms and signs as functional, and to do so only after repeated observation, because sometimes conditions such as carotid or vertebral artery dissection, and myasthenia gravis in young people, can produce variable neurological signs and have a normal series of baseline investigations (McCormick & Halbach 1993). Furthermore, it is not uncommon for patients with an organic disorder to have functional overlay as well, as if to try and draw attention to their real underlying problem.

3.4.9 Head injury

Head injury and stroke can co-exist, or predispose to each other. For example, head injury may cause intracranial haemorrhage, which can be mistaken for a primary stroke if the patient is amnesic for the injury and has no external scalp evidence of injury. Head injury can also lead to ischaemic stroke as a result of arterial dissection in the neck or head (section 7.1). On the other hand, stroke can precipitate a fall, causing head injury and, if the CT scan shows intracranial haemorrhage, the primary stroke event may be missed (Berlit *et al.* 1991; Sakas *et al.* 1995). An accurate history from relevant people (the patient, witnesses, family members, ambulance officers and family doctor) is essential to try and sort all this out. The radiological findings can also shed some light on the cause; intracranial haemorrhage from head injury tends to be more common in the frontal and anterior temporal regions, superficial and multiple, and there may be accompanying extension into the subarachnoid space and associated skull fractures (Fig. 3.36) (section 9.1.4). One can often see soft tissue swelling of the scalp on the CT scan.

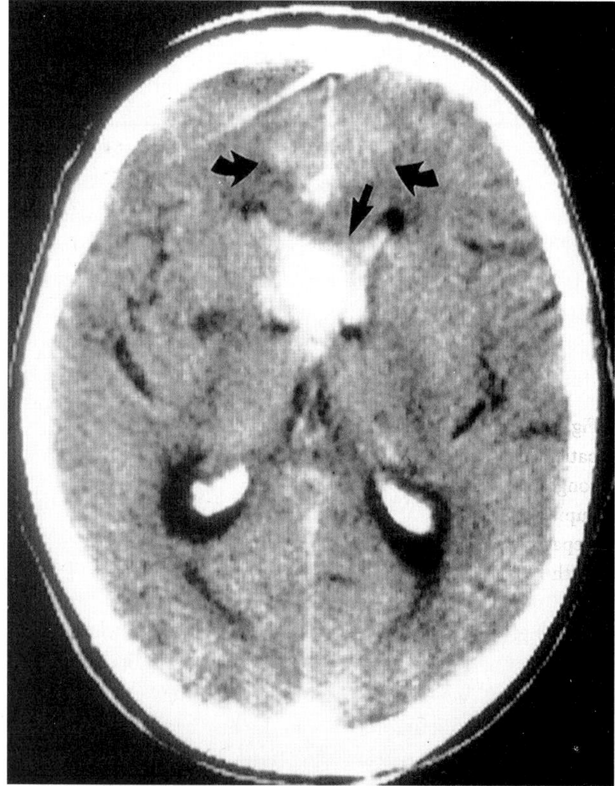

Fig. 3.36 A CT brain scan, showing blood in the subarachnoid space in a patient who presented with confusion following a head injury. There is blood in the anterior interhemispheric fissure (arrow), in a pattern suggestive of spontaneous subarachnoid haemorrhage. However, the presentation apparently following a head injury and the suggestion of frontal haemorrhagic contusions (curved arrows) clouded the interpretation of the CT scan and delayed recognition of the true pathology (anterior communicating artery aneurysmal haemorrhage).

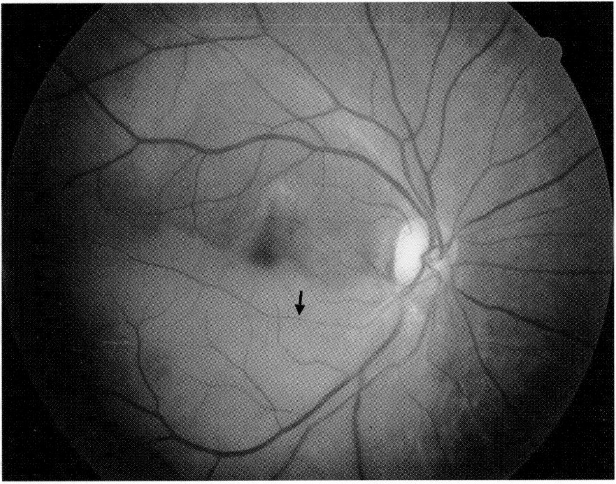

Fig. 3.18 An ocular fundus photograph of a patient with inferior temporal branch retinal artery occlusion, showing pallor of the inferior half of the retina due to cloudy swelling of the retinal ganglion cells caused by retinal infarction. The inferior temporal branch arteriole is attenuated and contains embolic material (arrow) (courtesy of Mr Matthew Wade, Department of Medical Illustrations, Royal Perth Hospital).

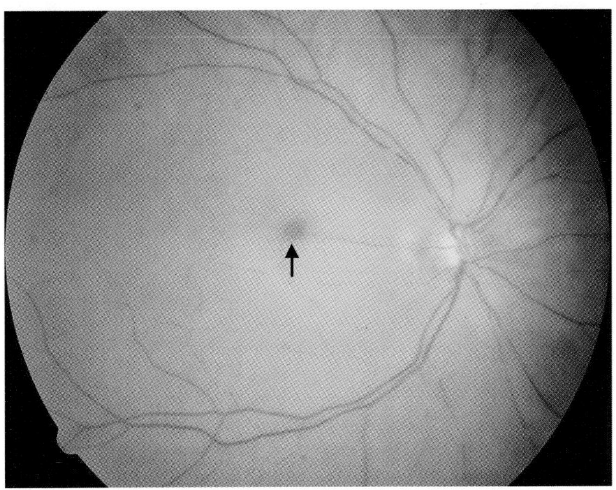

Fig. 3.19 Central retinal artery occlusion. An ocular fundus photograph, showing a cherry-red spot over the fovea (arrow) due to accentuation of the normal fovea (which is devoid of ganglion cells) by the opalescent halo of infarction of the retina (courtesy of Mr Matthew Wade, Department of Medical Illustrations, Royal Perth Hospital).

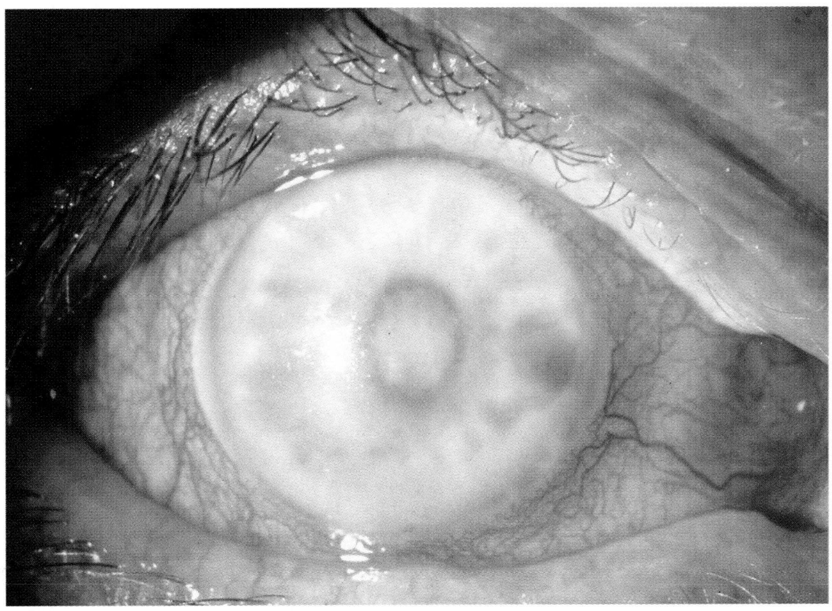

Fig. 3.20 A photograph of the eye of a patient with acute glaucoma. Note the congested sclera, cloudy cornea and oval pupil (courtesy of Mr Matthew Wade, Department of Medical Illustrations, Royal Perth Hospital).

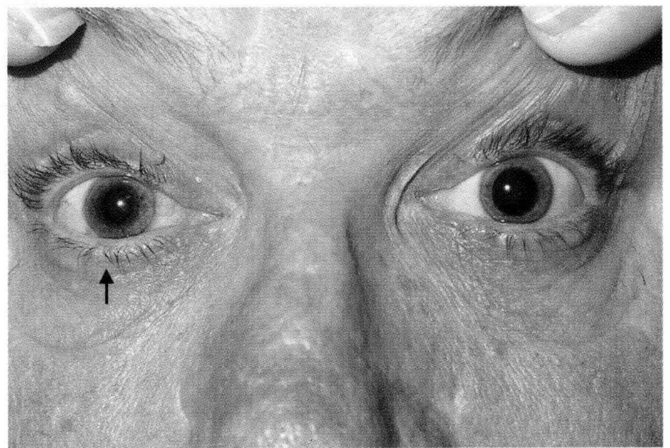

(a)

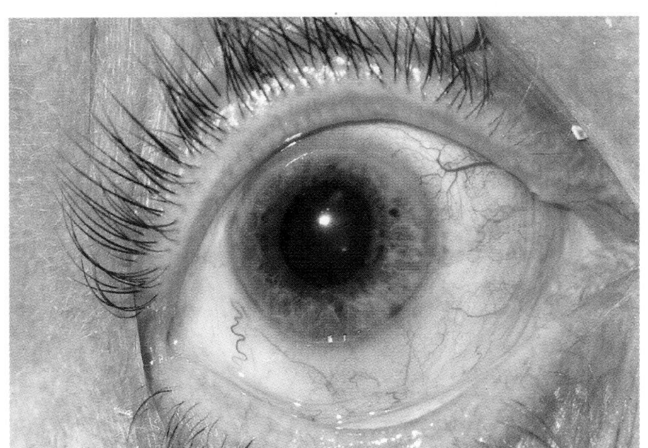

(b)

Fig. 3.21 (a) Ischaemic oculopathy of the right eye. (b) Note the episcleral vascular congestion, cloudy cornea, neovascularization of the iris (rubeosis of the iris) and mid-dilated pupil on external examination of the eye, which indicate chronic anterior segment ocular ischaemia due to carotid occlusive disease (with permission from Hankey & Warlow 1994).

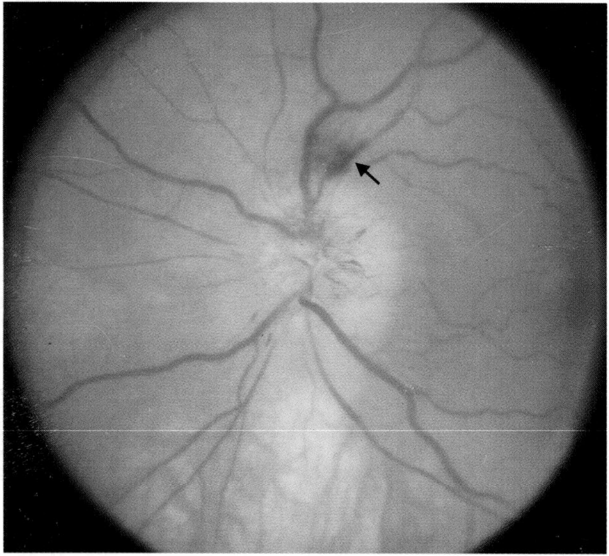

Fig. 3.22 An ocular fundus photograph of a patient with anterior ischaemic optic neuropathy due to occlusion of the posterior ciliary arteries as a result of giant cell arteritis. Note the oedema of the optic disc and flame-shaped haemorrhages (arrow) (courtesy of Mr Matthew Wade, Department of Medical Illustrations, Royal Perth Hospital).

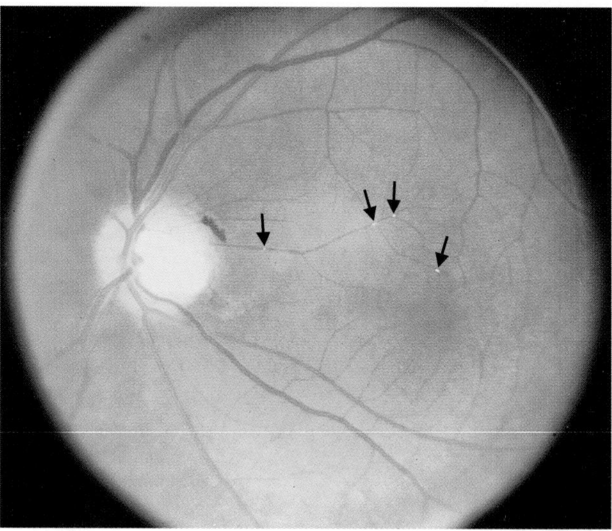

Fig. 3.23 An ocular fundus photograph, showing golden orange cholesterol crystals (Hollenhorst plaques) in the cilioretinal artery (arrows). The cilioretinal artery is present in only about one-third of the population. It originates from a branch of the short posterior ciliary artery and supplies the macula (courtesy of Mr Matthew Wade, Department of Medical Illustrations, Royal Perth Hospital).

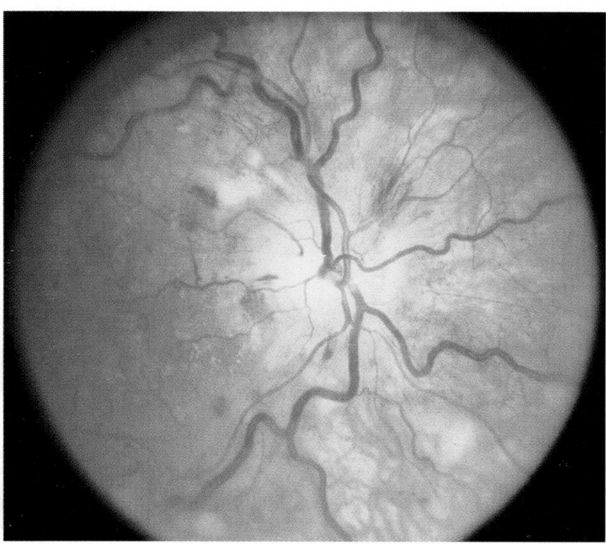

Fig. 3.24 An ocular fundus photograph, showing narrowing and tortuosity of retinal arterioles, arteriovenous nipping, retinal haemorrhages and papilloedema. These are the features of hypertensive retinopathy seen in malignant hypertension (courtesy of Mr Matthew Wade, Department of Medical Illustrations, Royal Perth Hospital).

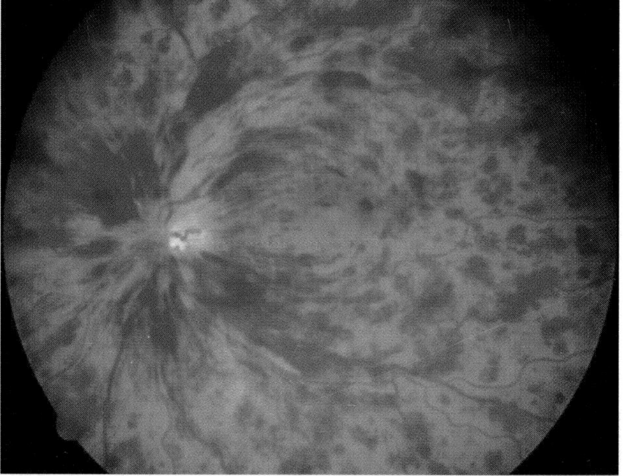

Fig. 3.38 An ocular fundus photograph, showing engorged retinal veins and multiple retinal haemorrhages due to central retinal vein thrombosis (courtesy of Mr Matthew Wade, Department of Medical Illustrations, Royal Perth Hospital).

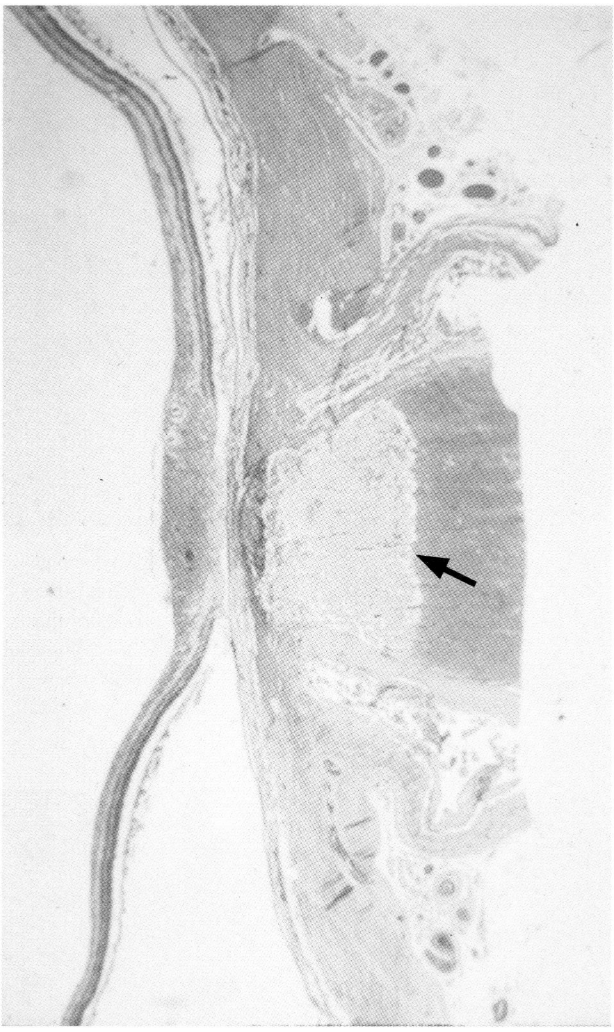

Fig. 3.39 A photomicrograph of anterior ischaemic optic neuropathy caused by giant-cell arteritis. The arrow indicates the infarcted optic nerve head (courtesy of Dr J.F. Cullen, Western General Hospital, Edinburgh).

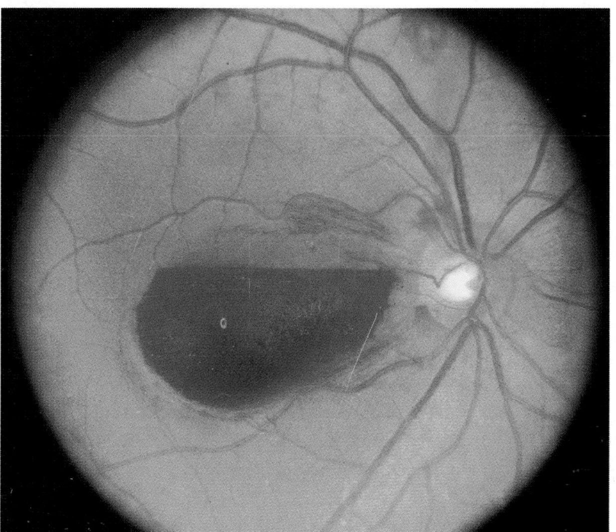

Fig. 5.43 Ocular fundus of a patient with subhyaloid haemorrhage, appearing as sharply demarcated linear streaks of brick red-coloured blood or flame-shaped haemorrhage in the preretinal layer, adjacent to the optic disc and spreading out from the optic disc (courtesy of Mr Matthew Wade, Department of Medical Illustrations, Royal Perth Hospital).

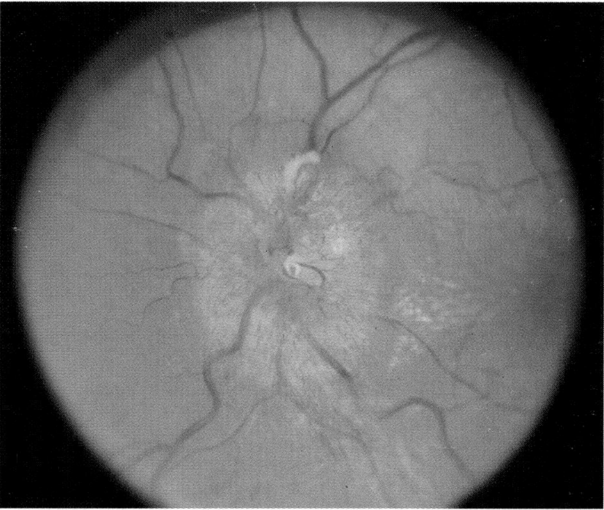

Fig. 3.40 An ocular fundus photograph, showing papilloedema. Note the congested, swollen disc, with loss of the physiological cup, a blurred disc margin and congested retinal veins (courtesy of Mr Matthew Wade, Department of Medical Illustrations, Royal Perth Hospital).

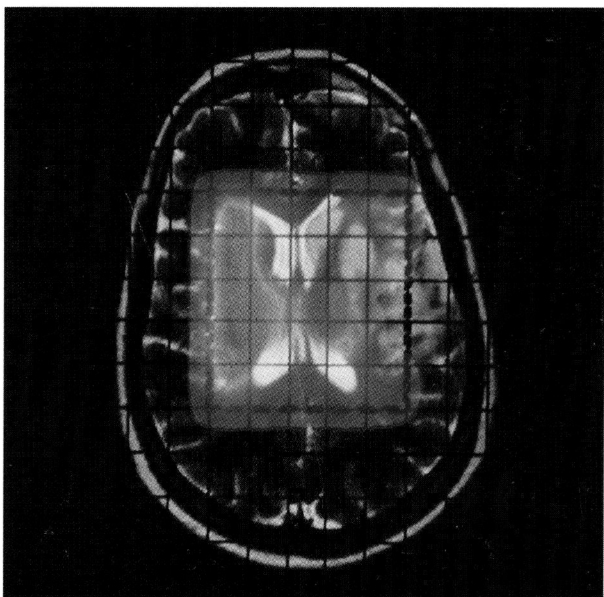

Fig. 5.36 Magnetic resonance spectroscopic chemical shift imaging at 2 days after stroke in a patient with an extensive left middle cerebral artery infarct. The T2 image is in the background and the spectroscopic colour image of the distribution of the normal neuronal metabolite *N*-acetyl aspartate is superimposed. Red indicates normal amounts of the normal metabolite and greens and blues indicate progressive absence of this metabolite. Note that the area of increased T2 signal of the infarct corresponds with the area of blue in keeping with neuronal loss.

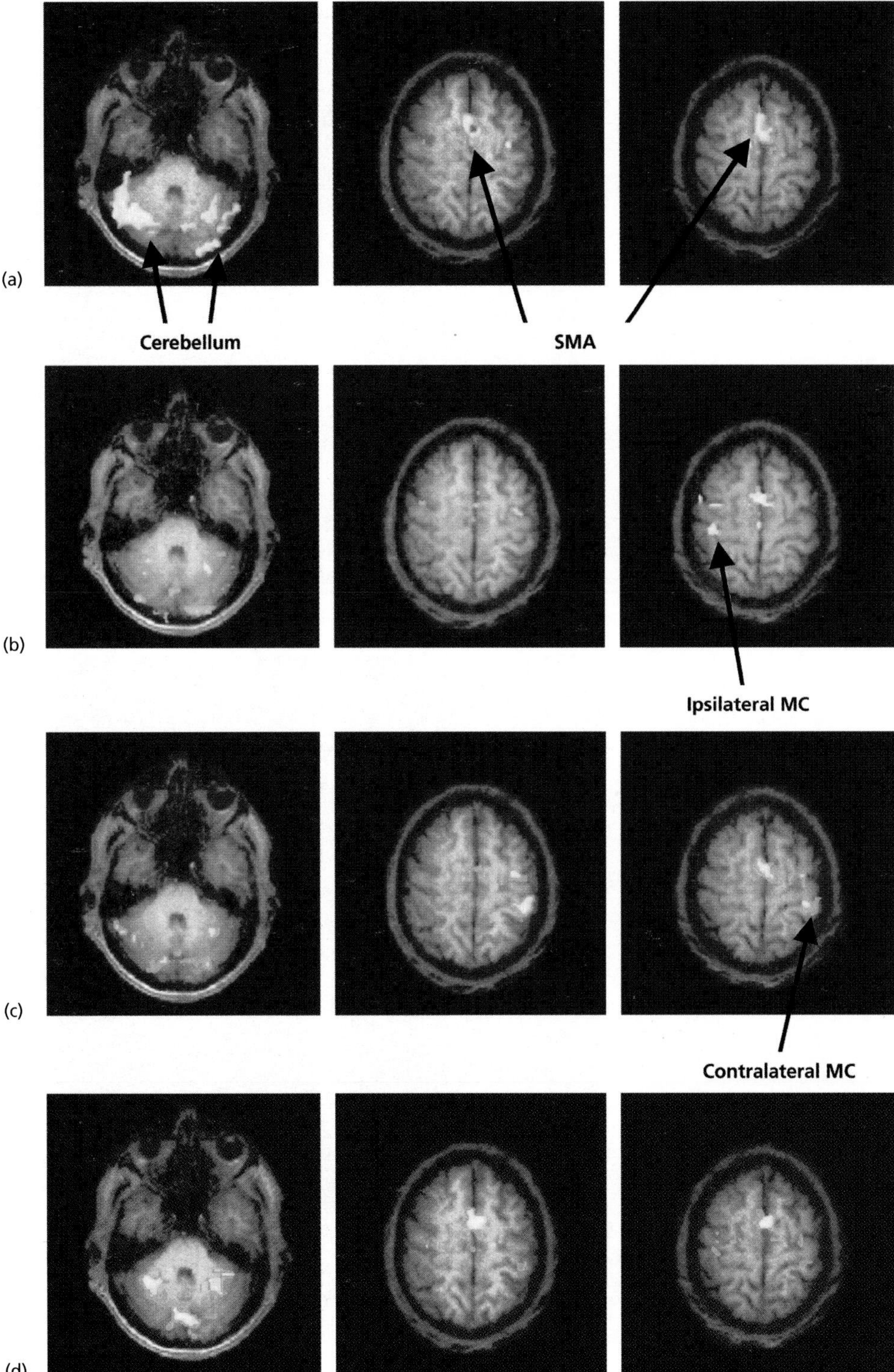

Fig. 10.7 Functional magnetic resonance imaging (fMRI) studies of dynamic changes in patterns of brain activation associated with hand movement accompanying recovery from an ischaemic stroke. The panels show the blood oxygenation level-dependent (BOLD) fMRI activations in the cerebral cortex and cerebellum accompanying flexion–extension of digits in one hand at about 1.5 Hz. These activation volumes show local areas of increased blood flow with task-specific neuronal activation. The right hemisphere is represented on the left side of the images. Activation of the supplementary motor cortex (SMA), primary sensorimotor cortex (MC), and cerebellum are easily identified. From 2 weeks after the infarct (a) to 5 weeks after the infarct (b), there was functional improvement in the paretic left hand associated with increased activation of contralateral MC and decreased activation in SMA and the cerebellum. In contrast, movements of the unaffected right hand do not show clearly significant changes in the patterns of brain activation between the 2-week scan (c) and 5-week scan (d). (Images courtesy of H. Johannsen-Berg, S. Pendlebury and P.M. Matthews, Centre for Functional Magnetic Resonance Imaging of the Brain, University of Oxford).

3.4.10 Multiple sclerosis

Patients with multiple sclerosis (MS) usually develop focal neurological symptoms in their third or fourth decade (as opposed to the seventh and eighth decades for stroke). The onset is typically subacute, with the condition coming on over days or even weeks. The diagnosis is seldom difficult, because these patients are usually young women without any vascular diseases or risk factors, the symptoms are as often positive as negative, there are usually more neurological signs than symptoms (compared with TIA and stroke, in which there are often more symptoms than signs), and some may have evidence of disease in other parts of the central nervous system that is asymptomatic but readily detected by clinical examination or MRI. Also, there may be a history of previous episodes of focal neurological dysfunction that are more typical of MS, such as optic neuritis or transverse myelitis. However, sometimes symptoms start abruptly and so can mimic a transient ischaemic attack or stroke, particularly if the initial presentation is one of optic neuritis, a restricted spinal cord syndrome, or a dystonic limb attack (Twomey & Espir 1980; Harper *et al.* 1981; Galer *et al.* 1990; Drulovic *et al.* 1993).

The location and shape of the lesions on brain CT or MRI are usually fairly characteristic (Fig. 3.37) (i.e. discrete round or oval lesions in the white matter of the cerebral or cerebellar hemispheres and brainstem, in the corpus callosum, and adjacent to the temporal horns of the lateral ventricles, not corresponding to territories supplied by specific cerebral arteries); the CSF usually shows raised immunoglobulin G (IgG) and oligoclonal bands, which are not present in the serum (Drulovic *et al.* 1993). However, none of these features is specific; for example, oligoclonal bands may also be found in patients with acute stroke, particularly if due to vasculopathies associated with Behçet's disease, systemic lupus erythematosus and sarcoidosis, although in many of these cases oligoclonal bands will also be present in the serum (Markowitz & Kokmen 1983; McLean *et al.* 1995) (section 7.3).

3.4.11 Neuromuscular disorders

Mononeuropathy and radiculopathy

It is surprising how often transient ischaemic attack and stroke affecting the hand or arm have to be distinguished from a median neuropathy at the wrist (carpal tunnel syndrome), an ulnar neuropathy at the elbow, or cervical radiculopathy (Dawson *et al.* 1990). Peripheral nerve lesions, e.g. radial nerve palsy (Norris & Hachinski 1982), or nerve root lesions may occasionally give rise to the sudden onset (or sudden awareness, on waking up from sleep) of persisting focal sensory or motor symptoms, which can be confused with 'pseudoradicular' strokes (these being due to small lesions confined to the contralateral precentral or postcentral gyrus, corona radiata, or thalamus (Omae *et al.* 1992; Kim 1994) (section 3.3.5). However, the physical signs of a peripheral nerve lesion (i.e. lower motor neurone signs and/or sensory loss to pain in a dermatomal or nerve distribution) are different from those of an intracranial cortical/subcortical lesion, which tend to be associated with upper motor neurone signs and/or loss of discriminative/'cortical' sensations, such as joint position sense and two-point discrimination ability. However, there are patients with the 'cortical hand syndrome' (section 3.3.4) in whom such distinguishing features are not present. Nerve conduction studies will usually be able to identify a peripheral mononeuropathy unless the problem is very acute, but they are less helpful for more proximal radicular problems unless there are clearly absent F waves.

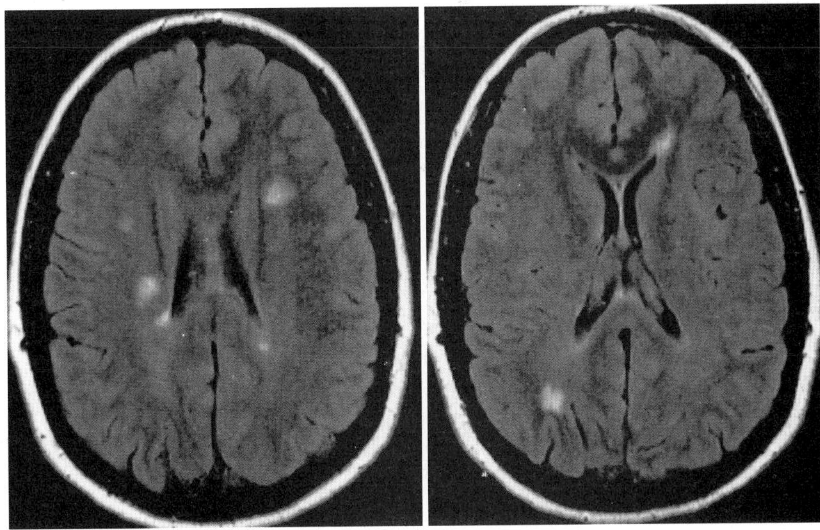

Fig. 3.37 A fluid-attenuated inversion recovery (FLAIR) magnetic resonance brain scan, showing the typical 'flame-shaped' periventricular white matter lesions (white areas) in a patient with multiple sclerosis (see also Fig. 7.3).

Myasthenia gravis

Although the symptoms of myasthenia gravis usually come on gradually, there are instances of fairly rapid development, sometimes precipitated by infection (usually respiratory), drugs, or emotional upset. The muscles of the eyes (levator palpebrae and extraocular muscles) and less often the face, jaw, throat and neck are the first to be affected (causing ptosis, diplopia, dysarthria or dysphagia), but in rare cases the initial complaint may be of limb weakness. The subsequent clinical course of a fluctuating oculofaciobulbar palsy can then be mistaken for a brainstem vascular event, but the weakness tends to persist (if left untreated) and to increase as the day wears on. Fatigability can be demonstrated by asking the patient to sustain the activity of the symptomatically involved muscles; ask the patient to look at the ceiling for 2–3 min without blinking (increasing ptosis) or to fixate in lateral or vertical gaze (increasing diplopia). Conversely, muscle power improves after a brief rest, or in response to a 10-mg test dose of edrophonium (Tensilon) intravenously, or neostigmine (1.5 mg) intramuscularly. A preceding dose of atropine 0.5 mg not only counteracts parasympathetic overstimulation but also serves as a placebo control for the motor effects. The diagnosis is supported by a positive antiacetylcholine receptor antibody assay, electromyography, and the presence of either a thymoma or thymic hyperplasia on a CT scan of the mediastinum.

Motor neurone disease (MND)

It is surprising how often patients with bulbar MND are said to have a vascular pseudobulbar palsy. Early on, when there may be little more than a subtle dysarthria, the typical features of MND, i.e. the presence of upper and motor neurone signs in the same limb and fasciculation of the tongue, are usually absent. What then tends to happen is that a brain CT or MRI is performed, which may show evidence of leukoaraiosis—and the two are linked, despite the latter being a quite common asymptomatic finding in this age group. The more useful investigation is electromyography (EMG), which may reveal subclinical evidence of denervation (in at least three limbs and possibly the tongue), which could not be caused by vascular disease.

3.4.12 Important non-focal disorders

Syncope

This is probably the most important *non-focal* syndrome of impaired consciousness to recognize. Syncope has been defined as a loss of consciousness and postural tone due to a sudden fall in blood flow to the brain (Kapoor 1991). Sometimes the loss of consciousness may occur abruptly, without any warning (e.g. syncope due to aortic stenosis, complete heart block), but more commonly there is history of a preceding feeling of light-headedness, faintness or 'dizziness' (not rotational vertigo), bilateral dimming or loss of vision (not to be confused with lone bilateral blindness), sounds seeming to be distant, generalized weakness, and symptoms of adrenergic activity such as nausea, hot and cold feelings and sweating. During the attack, the patient is pale, sweaty/clammy and floppy, rather than cyanosed and rigid as in an epileptic seizure. The pulse may be absent or difficult to feel (but this cannot be relied on) and the patient may be incontinent of urine. If the patient is lying flat and is not held upright (by someone or by an obstacle), then consciousness is regained within seconds, and there is very little mental confusion or difficulty in recalling the warning symptoms (unless there has been head trauma). Additional clinical features during unconsciousness may include multifocal, arrhythmic, myoclonic jerks (in up to 90% of cases, particularly in patients who are held upright), head turns, oral automatisms, righting movements (sustained head-raising or sitting up), eye movements (upward or lateral deviation of the eyes) and visual and auditory hallucinations, all of which are likely to lead to an erroneous diagnosis of epilepsy (Lempert *et al.* 1994). There are usually no focal neurological symptoms unless the drop in blood pressure occurs in the presence of severe occlusive arterial disease in the neck, or impaired cerebral autoregulation due to a previous stroke (section 6.6.5). The key to the diagnosis of syncope is a sound clinical history (Hoefnagels *et al.* 1991). Making a correct diagnosis is important, because some causes are quite serious (e.g. Stokes–Adams attacks) and if misdiagnosed as a transient ischaemic attack may lead to the patient being denied an effective and possibly life-saving treatment (e.g. pacemaker implantation).

Drop attacks

An important non-focal motor syndrome to recognize is that of 'drop attacks'. These are caused by a sudden loss of postural tone not induced by change of posture or movement of the head, causing the patient to fall to the ground without loss of consciousness, and not accompanied by vertigo or other sensation. The patient may be unable to rise immediately after the fall, despite being uninjured, because of weakness or ataxia, and the symptoms are sometimes precipitated by a change in head or body posture. The most common differential diagnosis is vertebrobasilar ischaemia, but here there is usually some warning that the patient is going to fall. Additionally, there are brainstem symptoms, such as vertigo or diplopia.

Drop attacks have been attributed to epilepsy, tumours in the region of the foramen magnum or third ventricle, vestibular disease, myxoedema, old age and even subconscious guilt, but in the vast majority of cases no cause is found and the episode is called a 'cryptogenic drop attack'. Amongst

40 patients evaluated by Stevens and Matthews (1973), all were women and the average age at onset was 44 years. The fall occurred whilst walking in all but one patient and could not be attributed to wearing high-heeled shoes. During follow-up, drop attacks continued to occur as an isolated symptom for many years, and although distressing were not associated with any serious prognostic implications. Meissner *et al.* (1986) reported that amongst 108 patients with drop attacks, the overall stroke rate was approximately 0.5% per annum—not significantly different from that in a normal age-matched and sex-matched population. The sex ratio, circumstances of the falls and favourable prognosis suggest that the cause reflects differences between the two sexes in the mechanism of walking rather than in any central neurological disturbance.

Cataplexy

This is another condition in which there is sudden loss of muscle tone, which is virtually unique to the narcolepsy syndrome (Aldrich 1990). Laughter is the most common precipitant, but other forms of emotion and athletic activities can induce cataplexy. Severe attacks cause complete paralysis except for the respiratory muscles, whereas the more common partial episodes cause patients to drop objects or to sit down or stop walking. Less than 1% of attacks involve unilateral weakness. Momentary attacks are the usual pattern, and they generally last less than a minute. Prolonged episodes may be associated with hallucinations. Rarely, cataplexy that is almost continuous ('status cataplecticus') may occur. Although the excessive daytime sleepiness usually begins several months before the onset of episodes of cataplexy, up to 10% of patients with the narcolepsy syndrome have cataplexy first. The multiple sleep latency test is a useful diagnostic technique; more than 80% of patients with the narcolepsy syndrome have a mean sleep latency of less than 5 min and at least two rapid eye movement periods at the onset of sleep during the procedure (Amira *et al.* 1985). More than 95% of patients with the narcolepsy syndrome will be positive for the HLA antigens DR2 or DQ1, but so will 10–20% of the normal population (Mignot 1998).

3.4.13 Neuroimaging in the differential diagnosis of focal neurological symptoms of sudden onset

(see also section 5.3)

Transient ischaemic attacks (TIAs)

The main purpose of brain CT or MRI in patients with a suspected TIA is to detect an underlying structural intracranial lesion which may present like a TIA. It is not to detect low-density lesions (presumed infarcts) or to exclude primary intracerebral haemorrhage (PICH), as it is in patients with stroke or 'brain attacks', because definite PICH only exceptionally causes focal neurological symptoms lasting less than 24 h (section 3.2.1).

Limited data indicate that the yield of CT for detecting structural lesions is about 1% in patients with suspected TIA (Hankey & Warlow 1992, 1994). With such a low yield, the routine examination of every patient who has had a single TIA with CT must be very carefully considered (section 6.7.3). The small minority of 'TIA' patients with structural intracranial lesions who will be missed by not performing a CT scan are likely to continue to have symptoms (and so return to the doctor), and their outcome is unlikely to be altered by a short delay in diagnosis. It is our impression that the small yield of structural brain lesions from CT is almost always in patients with carotid distribution cerebral TIAs, and there is some evidence to suggest that performing CT in patients with vertebrobasilar territory TIAs and transient monocular blindness is a waste of resources (Kingsley *et al.* 1980). But the data on the cost-effectiveness of CT and MRI in TIA patients are very poor, and there is a need for a methodologically sound prospective, multicentre study of this question, particularly in view of the considerable cost implications of a policy of 'CT or MRI for all suspected TIA patients'.

At present, we believe that CT should be reserved for patients with more than one TIA of the brain (and not at all if the attacks affect the eye only), particularly if they are in the carotid territory, and for those being considered for carotid endarterectomy (to avoid operating on someone with a symptomatic meningioma, for example), but we acknowledge that this is controversial (Martin *et al.* 1991). The CT scan should initially be a non-contrast study. Contrast should be used subsequently if a meningioma, giant aneurysm or vascular malformation is suspected, or alternatively MRI and MR angiography should be performed. For patients who continue to have vertebrobasilar TIAs despite optimal medical therapy, and in whom a brain CT scan is unhelpful and an abnormality in the posterior fossa is still suspected, an MRI study should be done because, although more expensive, MR images of the posterior fossa (and also the cerebral hemispheres) are superior to CT for detecting infarcts as well as demyelinating and structural lesions (Davis *et al.* 1989; Hommel *et al.* 1990; Edelman & Warach 1993). However, even MRI is not 100% sensitive in detecting brainstem infarcts (Besson *et al.* 1992).

Brain attack

If a patient is seen within 24 h of onset, and has persisting symptoms at that time, then from the point of view of neuroimaging they should be considered as having a stroke rather than a TIA. In the acute stage—within about 5 h of symptom onset—of clinically definite ischaemic stroke, CT will show abnormalities consistent with the diagnosis in about 50% of cases, assuming that the casemix is similar to that in the clinical trial that reported these figures (Von Kummer *et al.* 1997). Also, of course, CT will rule out intracranial haemorrhage.

Stroke

The diagnosis of stroke remains primarily clinical, and the main role of imaging studies such as CT and MRI is to assist in establishing the underlying brain pathology (Chapter 5) and cause (Chapters 6 and 8). There may be doubt about the clinical diagnosis of stroke in up to 20% of patients with suspected stroke (Sandercock *et al.* 1985; Wardlaw 1994), particularly when:

- the history of the onset is unclear (? sudden) because of coma, aphasia, confusion, or lack of a witness;
- when the clinical features are atypical for stroke (e.g. gradual onset, seizures, no clear focal neurological signs);
- when the clinical course is atypical (e.g. failure of the neurological deficit to slowly improve);
- when the patient is young (age less than 50 years) with no vascular risk factors (i.e. low pretest probability of stroke);
- and when subarachnoid haemorrhage (SAH) is suspected (Table 3.16).

The choice of CT or MRI will depend on local availability; how ill, confused or restless the patient is; and cost and effectiveness. If CT is available, it should be performed as soon as possible in all patients, because it is the best technique for diagnosing or excluding early intracranial haemorrhage (ICH) (section 5.3.4) and it is essential to image suspected SAH (section 5.6.3). MRI is no substitute and can fail to detect SAH. CT will not show an infarct in a variable proportion of ischaemic strokes, particularly small deep infarcts and posterior fossa infarcts, and if it is performed within 24 h of onset. MRI will more often confirm the site of cerebral infarction suspected clinically, but as yet this is rarely necessary for clinical management; the immediate priority is to exclude ICH. So MRI is not necessarily better than CT (Mohr *et al.* 1995). Furthermore, CT is an excellent technique for ill, confused patients—as many stroke patients are—and MRI is a more difficult technique to apply (Table 3.17).

Table 3.16 Indications for immediate brain CT (or MRI) in suspected stroke (also section 6.7.3).

To help distinguish 'stroke' from 'not-stroke':
- Unclear history of sudden onset of focal neurological symptoms (i.e. because of coma, aphasia, confusion, no witness)
- Atypical clinical features (i.e. gradual onset, seizures, no clear focal neurological signs)
- Atypical progression/worsening of 'stroke' after onset
- Young patient (age < 50 years) with no vascular risk factors

To distinguish intracranial haemorrhage from ischaemic stroke (section 5.3)

Subarachnoid haemorrhage suspected (CT prior to lumbar puncture where possible, not MRI, section 5.6.3)

To establish whether a patient fulfils the eligibility criteria for thrombolysis (section 11.5.3)

Note: the sudden onset of a focal neurological deficit is, by definition, a stroke syndrome (or a transient ischaemic attack if the deficit resolves within 24 h), even if the CT scan is normal, provided that other non-vascular possibilities, such as multiple sclerosis and a somatization disorder, have been excluded.

3.4.14 Electroencephalography in the differential diagnosis of focal neurological symptoms of sudden onset (see also section 6.7.12)

With the increasing availability of neuroimaging, the indications for an electroencephalogram (EEG) in patients with suspected transient ischaemic attack (TIA) or stroke are now very limited. An EEG is often requested when the clinical diagnosis of TIA is in doubt and partial (focal or localization-related) seizures are a possibility (Faught 1993). However, whilst about 35% of all patients with clinically definite epilepsy consistently have epileptiform discharges on the waking interictal EEG, and 50% do so on some occasions with repeated recording sleep-deprived recordings, we know very little about the sensitivity and specificity of the test when the diagnosis is in doubt (Chadwick 1990). Further difficulty arises as a result of the poor specificity of EEG abnormalities (all too frequently, patients with non-epileptic events such as TIAs are reported to have an abnormal EEG).

The role of the EEG in patients with persisting neurological signs is to help exclude a number of conditions that may mimic stroke, particularly when the brain imaging is normal. For example, patients with non-convulsive status epilepticus

Table 3.17 Circumstances in which brain MRI is preferable to CT (also section 5.3.6).

More than 10 days have elapsed since stroke onset, CT scan may show a low-density area that could have been infarction or resolving haemorrhage, and it is essential to know whether the stroke was ischaemic or haemorrhagic.

When the CT scan is negative and it is crucial to be able to localize the infarct (this is only very occasionally necessary), MRI is more likely to image the lesion.

Arterial dissection is a suspected cause of ischaemic stroke, in which case both axial imaging and MR angiography may provide diagnostic information (section 7.2.1).

may present with the sudden onset of a confusional state, and in both Creutzfeldt–Jakob disease and herpes simplex encephalitis, where there can be clinical deterioration with new focal neurological signs, the EEG can have characteristic abnormalities (although not in all the patients all the time). The EEG is not useful for confirming stroke; in other words, stroke is a clinical diagnosis and there are no specific EEG features. The usual EEG findings in acute stroke are a localized reduction of normal cortical rhythms and a major surrounding slow-wave abnormality with individual waves of less than 1 Hz (Binnie & Prior 1994). Focal EEG slowing, however, is not specific, and only indicates the presence and side of a lesion (Faught 1993). Although it has been suggested that the EEG may help distinguish between small deep (lacunar) and cortical infarction, the clinical features and brain CT or MRI scan are more effective tools for doing this (MacDonnell *et al.* 1988; Kappelle *et al.* 1990). A normal EEG can help to confirm the diagnosis of 'locked-in syndrome' from a lesion in the ventral pons (section 3.3.2), and can also lend support to a diagnosis of a somatization disorder.

3.5 Differential diagnosis of transient monocular blindness

Transient monocular blindness (TMB) and amaurosis fugax are two different terms for describing the same symptom—blurring or loss of vision in the whole or part of the visual field of one eye. It is commonly caused by ischaemia of the retina (usually as a result of embolism from the origin of the ipsilateral internal carotid artery or from the heart), and sometimes by ischaemia of the anterior optic nerve (usually due to disease of the posterior ciliary artery). However, there are other causes of TMB which it is important to differentiate because the prognosis and treatments differ (Table 3.18). Many are uncommon and frequently go unrecognized if the patient is not examined during the acute episode.

Patients with transient monocular blindness must have a competent ophthalmological examination to exclude primary disorders of the eye before one jumps to the conclusion that the explanation is vascular disease.

Table 3.18 Causes of transient monocular blindness.

Retinal disorders (section 3.5.1)
Vascular
- Atherothromboembolism or other arterial disorders (e.g. dissection, etc., affecting the proximal arteries, particularly the internal carotid artery origin) (Table 6.2)
- Embolism from the heart (section 6.5)
- Low retinal artery perfusion
- Retinal migraine

High resistance to retinal perfusion
- Intracranial vascular malformation (section 8.2.4)
- Central or branch retinal vein thrombosis
- Raised intraocular pressure (glaucoma)
- Raised intracranial pressure
- Increased blood viscosity (section 7.9)
- Malignant arterial hypertension (section 3.4.5)

Retinal haemorrhage

Non-vascular
- Retinal detachment
- Paraneoplastic retinopathy
- Phosphenes
- Lightning streaks of Moore
- Chorioretinitis

Optic nerve disorders (section 3.5.2)
Vascular
- Anterior ischaemic optic neuropathy
- Systemic hypotension
- Arteritis (e.g. giant cell) (section 7.3)
- Malignant arterial hypertension (section 3.4.5)

Non-vascular
- Papilloedema
- Optic neuritis and Uhthoff's symptom
- Dysplastic coloboma

Eye/orbital disorders (section 3.5.3)
Vitreous haemorrhage
Reversible diabetic cataract
Lens subluxation
Orbital tumour (e.g. optic nerve-sheath meningioma)

3.5.1 Retinal disorders

Retinal migraine or 'vasospasm'

Migraine with aura (classical migraine) is usually ushered in by 'positive' binocular visual symptoms. Transient monocular visual symptoms followed by pulsatile headache have occasionally been described in patients with known migraine, and this is classified as 'retinal migraine' (Hedges & Lackman 1976). Retinal migraine is much more difficult to diagnose if there is no headache associated with the attacks. TMB as a result of thromboembolism and retinal migraine are distinguished on the basis of the patient's symptoms; the former is characterized by the abrupt onset of 'negative' monocular visual phenomena (blindness), which is painless and usually lasts only a few minutes, whilst the latter is characterized by the gradual build-up of transient monocular visual impairment (i.e. scotoma or blindness), which is usually incomplete and may be associated with 'positive' visual symptoms (e.g. scintillations) lasting for up to an hour, as well as a pulsatile headache or orbital pain (Blau 1992; Blau & MacGregor 1993). Sometimes it can be very difficult to distinguish between retinal ischaemia and retinal migraine, particularly in older patients. Attacks of positive visual phenomena lasting longer than the 5 min or so expected for retinal ischaemia not infrequently turn out to be associated with angiographic evidence of ipsilateral internal carotid artery (ICA) stenosis (Goodwin *et al.* 1987). It has been suggested that the results of non-invasive investigations, such as carotid ultrasound, may help distinguish between the two—i.e. the presence of tight stenosis of the ICA on the symptomatic side is suggestive of retinal ischaemia (due to artery-to-artery embolism), and the absence of carotid disease favours retinal migraine (Sandercock & Smart 1990). However, this is only circumstantial evidence.

Patients have been described with frequent (one to 30 episodes per day), stereotyped episodes of brief (lasting less than 3 min) unilateral visual loss caused by presumed vasospasm (Burger *et al.* 1991). Fundus examination during the episodes of blindness showed constriction of the retinal arteries and segmentation in a thin and slowly moving column of blood. The calibre of the retinal vessels was restored with the return of vision. Another patient has been reported in whom multiple daily episodes of brief unilateral visual loss stopped when the patient was treated with a calcium channel blocker, suggesting that vasospasm may have been the underlying cause (Winterkorn & Teman 1991). The same authors have also reported another patient with recurrent episodes of TMB associated with sexual intercourse, which stopped after he began to take 20 mg of nifedipine by mouth half an hour before anticipated intercourse (Teman *et al.* 1995). However, as there is really no proof of vasospasm, we have to be very cautious in the interpretation of these observations.

The results of prognostic studies showing that patients with TMB have a better prognosis than patients with TIA of the brain suggest that a considerable proportion of these patients may have been cases of retinal migraine, or something else benign (Dennis *et al.* 1990b; Hankey *et al.* 1991, 1992; Dutch TIA Trial Study Group 1993; Rothwell *et al.* 1999). Those who proceeded to subsequent vascular events, such as stroke or retinal infarction, were presumably true cases of retinal ischaemia due to carotid stenosis, heart disease, or other less common conditions such as arteritis and procoagulant states (Tippin *et al.* 1989; Gutrecht *et al.* 1991; O'Sullivan *et al.* 1992).

The question therefore arises, how do we define retinal migraine? Is it a diagnosis based on the clinical symptoms and signs, the results of investigations, the response to treatment, or the prognosis? It has been traditionally diagnosed on the basis of the clinical history, but this may be non-specific, and it is seldom possible to examine the patient during the episode to see if 'vasospasm' is present. The presence of carotid disease may be coincidental, and of course the response to treatment and the prognosis are hardly helpful at the time the diagnosis has to be made. For practical purposes, if it is not possible to confidently distinguish retinal ischaemia and migraine from the history, the patient should be assessed, investigated and treated as having a case of retinal ischaemia.

Dural arteriovenous malformation (AVM)

Anterior and middle fossa dural AVMs may very rarely cause TMB, probably because of transient lowering of retinal arterial pressure associated with shunting of blood away from the ophthalmic artery (Bogousslavsky *et al.* 1985).

Central or branch retinal vein thrombosis

Thrombosis of the central retinal vein, or branch retinal vein, sometimes presents with attacks of TMB. The visual loss tends to be patchy rather than complete. The fundoscopic appearance is characteristic, and consists of engorged retinal veins and multiple retinal haemorrhages (Hayreh 1976) (Fig. 3.38).

Glaucoma

In narrow-angle (closed-angle, angle-closure) glaucoma, there is apposition of the peripheral iris to the trabecular meshwork. The extent of angle closure determines the decrease in outflow and in turn the increase in intra-ocular pressure. Elevated intra-ocular pressure reduces perfusion pressure of the eye and so reduces blood flow to the choroid, retina and disc (Best *et al.* 1969). Transient monocular visual disturbance may occur, particularly in poor light when the pupil is dilated (Fisher 1967; Ravits & Seybold 1984). The onset is usually subacute. Vision may be decreased, blurred, foggy, or smoke-like, and the patient may see haloes around lights. Some patients complain of light sensitivity during the attack and most, but not all, have eye pain, which may radiate to the side of the head. The symptoms may last from a few minutes to hours. The presence of eye pain and the stereotyped

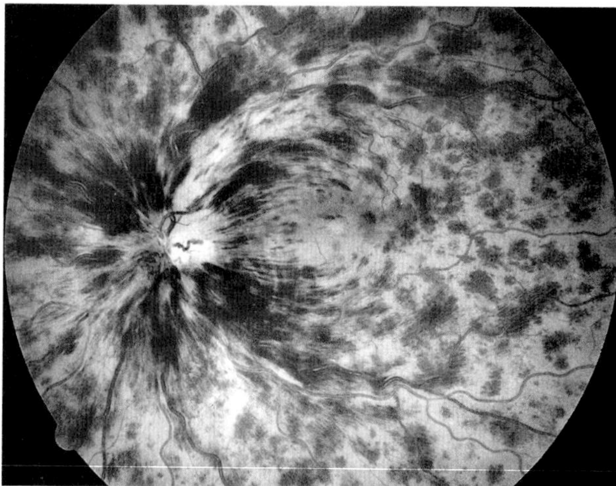

Fig. 3.38 An ocular fundus photograph, showing engorged retinal veins and multiple retinal haemorrhages due to central retinal vein thrombosis (courtesy of Mr Matthew Wade, Department of Medical Illustrations, Royal Perth Hospital). Also reproduced in colour; see colour plate facing p. 84.

recurrence of attacks under certain lighting conditions can be useful clues to the diagnosis, particularly if the eye is red, the cornea cloudy and the pupil oval in shape (Fig. 3.20). The intra-ocular pressure should be checked in most, if not all, patients with TMB, but in those who have glaucoma it is not always raised between attacks.

Retinal and other intra-ocular haemorrhage

A small retinal haemorrhage may cause sudden reduced vision in one eye that resolves within hours. The diagnosis should be evident on ophthalmoscopy, particularly if the pupil is dilated. Similarly, vitreous and anterior chamber haemorrhage may cause TMB (Amaurosis Fugax Study Group 1990). The cause may be evident from the history; for example, sudden visual loss caused by preretinal haemorrhages within the macula may occur during physical exertion, sexual activity, or Valsalva manoeuvre (Friberg *et al.* 1995).

Paraneoplastic retinopathy

Transient episodes, lasting seconds to minutes, of painless monocular dimming of the central field of vision and overwhelming visual glare and photosensitivity when exposed to bright light are suggestive of not only photoreceptor dysfunction due to transient retinal ischaemia, but also paraneoplastic retinopathy (Jacobsen *et al.* 1990). Patients may also experience transient bizarre entoptic symptoms (alterations in normal light perception resulting from intraoptic phenomena, akin to the subjective perception of light resulting from mechanical compression of the eyeball) (Keltner *et al.* 1983; Jacobsen *et al.* 1990). Ophthalmoscopy usually reveals attenuated retinal arterioles, electroretinography demonstrates abnormal cone and rod-mediated responses, and antiretinal antibodies may be identified in the serum (Grunwald *et al.* 1985). Over the subsequent months, progressive visual loss occurs, during which time a small-cell carcinoma of the lung often declares itself.

Phosphenes

Phosphenes are flashes of light and coloured spots that are induced by eye movement in a dark environment and occur in the absence of luminous stimuli. They may occur with disease of the visual system at many different sites, such as optic neuritis in the recovery phase, perhaps as a result of the mechanical effects of movement of the optic nerve. However, mechanical pressure on the normal eyeball may also induce a phosphene, as every child discovers, by stimulating the retina. Phosphenes may also occur in a healthy dark-adapted closed eye after a saccade (flick phosphene).

Lightning streaks of Moore

In a dark environment, elderly people frequently experience recurrent, brief, stereotypic, vertical flashes of light in the temporal visual field of one eye, which are elicited by eye movement. These are known as Moore's lightning streaks and are benign. It is believed that, with advanced age, the posterior vitreous may collapse and detach from the retina, leading to persistent vitreoretinal adhesions. The mechanical forces associated with eye movement exert traction on the macula and retina, and induce the photopsias (subjective sensations of sparks or flashes of light) (Zaret 1985).

Chorioretinitis

Macular disease due to chorioretinitis or retinal pigmentary degeneration can sometimes lead to loss of vision in bright light (Severin *et al.* 1967; Glaser *et al.* 1977).

3.5.2 Optic nerve disorders

Anterior ischaemic optic neuropathy

Anterior ischaemic optic neuropathy (AION) is due to ischaemia in the territory of supply of the posterior ciliary arteries, branches of the ophthalmic artery which supply the anterior part of the optic nerve, the choroid and outer retina (Hayreh 1975). Because the optic disc is close to an arterial border zone between the territories of the two major posterior ciliary arteries, it is particularly liable to ischaemia when the systemic blood pressure falls, when the intra-ocular pressure rises, or when there is occlusive disease of local small arteries (Anon. 1984). Less often, AION is caused by thrombotic or embolic occlusion of the posterior ciliary arteries or of the arterioles feeding the anterior part of the optic nerve, e.g. by giant-cell arteritis (Fig. 3.39) and other types of vasculitis, such as polyarteritis nodosa (Hayreh 1975; Reich *et al.* 1990) (section 7.3). Atherosclerosis is another presumed cause, given that patients with AION have an increased prevalence of hypertension and diabetes and an increased risk of subsequent cerebrovascular and cardiovascular events, but we are not aware of any histological proof of atheromatous occlusion of these arteries (Boghen & Glaser 1975; Goodwin 1985; Guyer *et al.* 1985). Embolic occlusion does occur, although much less frequently than thrombotic occlusion; however, this impression may be based partly on our inability to see the emboli in these vessels on ophthalmoscopy, as compared with the easily seen emboli in the retinal arteries (Lieberman *et al.* 1978). The usual source of embolism is presumably the carotid bifurcation, but this remains uncertain.

Ischaemia of the optic disc is characterized clinically by the sudden onset of painless visual loss in one eye. This may

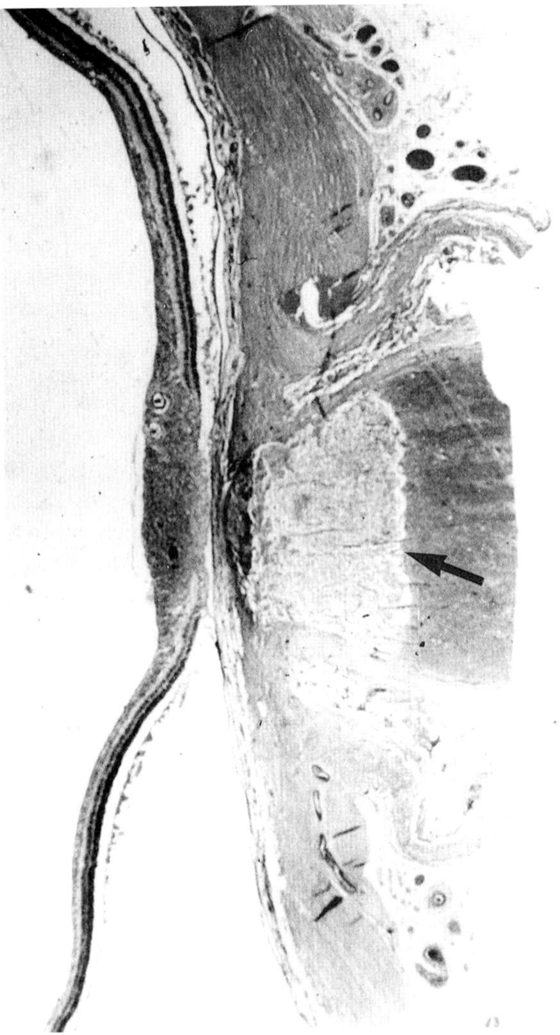

Fig. 3.39 A photomicrograph of anterior ischaemic optic neuropathy caused by giant-cell arteritis. The arrow indicates the infarcted optic nerve head (courtesy of Dr J.F. Cullen, Western General Hospital, Edinburgh). Also reproduced in colour; see colour plate facing p. 84.

involve the whole field, but it tends to be more severe in the lower quadrants because the upper segment of the optic disc is more vulnerable to ischaemia (Hayreh 1981). In the early stages, the circulation may be so precariously balanced that minor postural change may have profound effects on the degree of visual loss. The visual loss is often severe, non-progressive and prolonged, but it can be brief (and present as transient monocular blindness), or it can progress over several hours or days. In AION due to giant-cell arteritis, the visual loss may develop in both eyes within a few days and, rarely, almost simultaneously. Normal visual acuity does not exclude AION, and almost any part of the visual field can be affected. The common patterns of visual loss are an altitudinal hemifield defect (loss of either the upper or, more frequently, the lower half of the field in one eye), an inferior nasal segmental loss, and a central scotoma. The disc may appear normal at first, but within a few days it becomes pale and swollen, often with small flame-shaped haemorrhages radiating from the disc margin (ischaemic papillopathy), distended veins and, occasionally, cotton-wool spots due to ischaemic change in the surrounding retina (Fig. 3.22). The swelling may involve only one segment of the disc, or may be more marked in one segment than in another. The disc swelling is attributed partly to leakage of plasma from damaged blood vessels and partly to arrest of axoplasmic transport along damaged nerve fibres. The disc swelling itself may be indistinguishable from that seen with raised intracranial pressure, but the vision is usually normal in the latter condition. In about 50% of eyes with AION due to giant-cell arteritis, the disc swelling has a chalky white appearance (Hayreh 1981). Later, the swelling subsides, to be succeeded by optic atrophy with attenuation of the small blood vessels on the disc surface. The prognosis for recovery of vision is variable. Many patients recover good central vision, but are left with arcuate and sectorial visual field defects corresponding to loss of bundles of nerve fibres. In other patients, visual loss may be complete and permanent.

Malignant arterial hypertension

Some patients with malignant hypertension experience transient monocular blindness due to ischaemia of the optic nerve head (Hayreh *et al.* 1986). Associated headache, seizures, encephalopathy, renal impairment, high blood pressure and the characteristic ophthalmoscopic features of hypertension point to the diagnosis (Fig. 3.24).

Papilloedema

Patients with papilloedema (Fig. 3.40) from any cause may experience transient visual blurring or obscurations, with or without photopsias (Hayreh 1977). The visual loss in chronic papilloedema is often postural, occurring as patients get up from a chair (or bend over), and may involve either eye alone, or both eyes together. The explanation may be transient optic nerve ischaemia secondary to a relative decrease in orbital blood flow, as a result of raised cerebrospinal fluid pressure in the subarachnoid space around the optic nerve, and so increased pressure in the veins draining the optic nerve head. A history of episodes of visual blurring or blindness in someone with papilloedema should lead to urgent investigation and appropriate action, because permanent visual loss will eventually follow, gradually or suddenly.

Optic neuritis and Uhthoff's symptom

Patients with acute and chronic optic nerve demyelination due to multiple sclerosis may experience transiently decreased vision in one or both eyes during exercise (Uhthoff's symp-

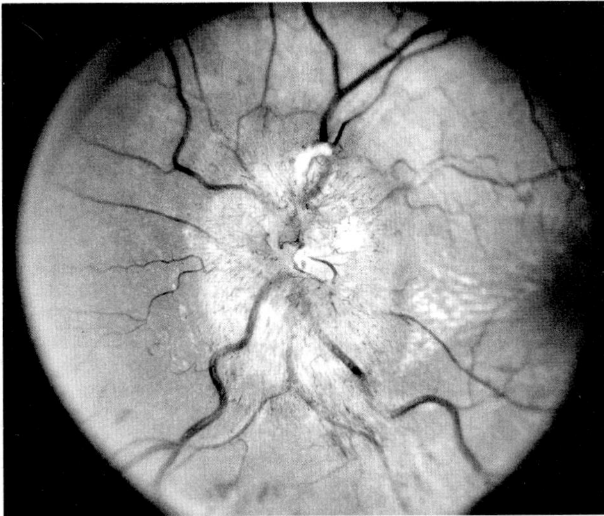

Fig. 3.40 An ocular fundus photograph, showing papilloedema. Note the congested, swollen disc, with loss of the physiological cup, a blurred disc margin and congested retinal veins (courtesy of Mr Matthew Wade, Department of Medical Illustrations, Royal Perth Hospital). Also reproduced in colour; see colour plate facing p. 84.

tom), or in association with other causes of increased temperature, emotional stress, increased illumination, eating, drinking, smoking and menstruation. The pathophysiology of Uhthoff's symptom is unknown, although reversible conduction block in demyelinated nerve fibres secondary to an increase in body temperature or to changes in blood electrolyte levels or pH is believed to play a role (Scholl *et al.* 1991). Ophthalmoscopy may be normal, but if the optic nerve head is inflamed, the optic disc may be swollen and look similar to papilloedema.

Optic disc anomalies

Transient monocular visual obscurations are occasionally associated with an elevated optic disc without increased intracranial pressure. Examples include congenital anomalies of the optic disc, such as drüsen or posterior staphyloma (Seybold & Rosen 1977).

3.5.3 Orbital disorders

Transient changes in the ocular media or intra-ocular pressure, such as vitreous floaters, vitreous haemorrhage, anterior chamber haemorrhage, lens subluxation, reversible cataract (in a diabetic) and glaucoma may cause transient monocular visual disturbance (Ravits & Seybold 1984; Paylor *et al.* 1985). The uveitis–glaucoma–hyphaema syndrome may follow cataract extraction and intra-ocular lens implantation (Cates & Newman 1998). Most of these conditions can be excluded by a competent ophthalmological examination. Intraorbital masses, such as an optic nerve sheath meningioma, may produce gaze-evoked transient monocular blindness; the blindness is limited to the duration of gaze in the affected direction and the visual acuity usually returns to normal about 30 s after the eye moves back to the primary position. The loss of vision is possibly caused by a reduction in flow to the blood vessels surrounding the optic nerve itself (Wilkes *et al.* 1979; Brown & Sheilds 1981; Bradbury *et al.* 1987).

3.6 Improving the reliability of the clinical diagnosis of a cerebrovascular event

For every patient who presents to their family doctor with a definite transient ischaemic attack (TIA), there are many more who present with transient neurological symptoms due to other disorders. For example, in the Oxfordshire Community Stroke Project (OCSP), 512 patients were referred by their family doctor or a hospital doctor with a diagnosis of 'possible TIA', of whom 317 (62%) were considered by the OCSP neurologists not to have had a TIA (Table 3.19). In

Table 3.19 Final diagnosis of all 512 patients with suspected transient ischaemic attacks notified to the Oxfordshire Community Stroke Project *(modified from* Dennis *et al.* 1989b).

Confirmed transient ischaemic attacks	209
Incident (i.e. first-ever)	184
Prevalent (i.e. had previous attacks)	11
Lone bilateral blindness*	14
Not transient ischaemic attacks	303
Migraine	52
Syncope	48
Possible TIA†	46
'Funny turn'‡	45
Isolated vertigo	33
Epilepsy	29
Transient global amnesia	17
Isolated diplopia	4
Drop attack	3
Intracranial meningioma	2
Miscellaneous	24

* Lone bilateral blindness was classified as a transient ischaemic attack after following up these patients and noting their similar prognosis to patients with definite transient ischaemic attack (Dennis *et al.* 1989a).

† Possible transient ischaemic attack was diagnosed in patients with transient focal neurological symptoms in whom the clinical features were not sufficiently clear to make a diagnosis of definite transient ischaemic attack or of anything else.

‡ 'Funny turn' was used to describe transient episodes of only non-focal symptoms not due to any identifiable condition (e.g. isolated and transient confusion).

another study, 30% of the patients originally classified by their doctors as having TIAs were reclassified as not having TIAs when their records were reviewed by a stroke specialist (Calanchini *et al.* 1977). This problem is not unique to family doctors and junior hospital doctors. Kraaijeveld *et al.* (1984) investigated the inter-observer agreement for the diagnosis of TIA of the brain amongst eight senior and interested neurologists from the same department, who interviewed 56 patients in alternating pairs. Both neurologists agreed that 36 patients had a TIA and 12 had not, but they disagreed about eight (kappa = 0.65; for perfect agreement kappa would be 1.0).

Even experienced neurologists with an interest in cerebrovascular disease show considerable inter-observer variability in the diagnosis of transient ischaemic attack. This variability does not imply lack of skill, but rather it is inherent in the clinical assessment of symptoms and signs. Sometimes the available information does not allow one to come to a 'right answer' as to whether the event was a transient ischaemic attack or not—in which case one ends up working on the basis of probability.

We are all familiar with the scenario of the junior doctor describing the physical signs in a particular patient (whom he had gone back to check just before the ward round), only for the consultant to examine the patient and find that some are not present. Various reasons are muttered under the junior doctor's breath, including the passage of time, clinical experience, or just plain senility, but in fact inter-observer agreement for physical signs, even between consultants, is not very impressive in stroke patients (Table 3.20). Making the diagnosis of a cerebrovascular event shares many similarities with the diagnostic process in other areas of medicine. Much information about the reasons for clinical disagreement, and strategies to reduce it that can usefully be applied to the diagnosis of cerebrovascular disease, are available from the general literature.

3.6.1 Reasons for clinical disagreement

There are several factors that can increase the chance of clinical disagreement (Sackett *et al.* 1991). The main one is difficulty in eliciting and interpreting the history of the event. For example, since the symptoms of most TIAs resolve within about 15–60 min, the diagnosis is almost always based entirely on the clinical history, which for a number of reasons may not be very clear: the patient may have forgotten the symptoms (because of either poor memory or delay in presenting to medical attention); the symptoms may have been remembered, but are difficult to describe (e.g. transient homonymous hemianopia); or the patient may have been so frightened by the attack that he or she was more preoccupied with the immediate outcome than the exact nature of the deficit. All of these problems are more common in the elderly.

Several studies have shown that clinicians can differ in the interpretation of even isolated elements of the history, such as 'blurred or foggy vision' (Sisk *et al.* 1970; Calanchini *et*

Table 3.20 Inter-observer agreement for neurological signs in stroke patients.

	Kappa value	
Signs examined	Lindley *et al.* (1993)	Shinar *et al.* (1985)
Conscious level	0.60	0.38
Confusion	0.21	NS
Dementia	NS	0.34
Weakness of arm	0.77	NS
Weakness of hand	0.68	0.58 (right) 0.49 (left)
Weakness of leg	0.64	NS
Weakness of face	0.63	0.51 (right) 0.66 (left)
Sensory loss on hand	0.19	0.50 (right) 0.32 (left)
Sensory loss on arm	0.15	NS
Aphasia/language	0.70	0.54
Dysarthria	0.51	0.53
Visuospatial dysfunction	0.44	NS
Hemianopia	0.39	0.40
Cerebellar signs/ataxia	0.46	0.45
Cranial nerve palsy	0.34	NS
Extraocular movement disorder	0.30	0.77

NS, not stated.

al. 1977; Shinar *et al.* 1985; Koudstaal *et al.* 1986, 1989). Of course, patients also use similar terms to describe widely differing experiences (e.g. the term 'dizziness' may be used to describe rotational vertigo, ataxia, bilateral dimming of vision, or light-headedness).

Another problem is that the generally accepted definitions of stroke and TIA lack specific detail about which 'focal' symptoms are not acceptable (? isolated vertigo). In the context of TIAs, what is an acceptable lower time limit for the duration of symptoms? Is a sudden focal neurological deficit, particularly a sensory deficit, of less than 5 s duration a TIA? (Hankey & Warlow 1994). Diagnostic conformity can only be achieved if precise criteria are available that are valid, reliable and generally accepted (Kessler *et al.* 1991). In the particular case of TIA, it is difficult to determine the validity of any single diagnostic criterion, because there is no 'gold standard' against which to judge it. Kraaijeveld *et al.* (1984) used more explicit criteria for the diagnosis of TIA, and these have been modified (Sandercock 1991) (Table 3.21).

More widespread and consistent consideration, discussion and application of these criteria could enhance diagnostic accuracy and inter-observer agreement, and it has been suggested that this might improve patient management and care (Shinar *et al.* 1985). However, it must be remembered that as the diagnostic criteria become more specific, sensitivity is sacrificed and so an increasing number of genuine TIAs may be discarded and left untreated. Conversely, if the criteria become less specific, there may be a tendency to overdiagnose TIA, and this can also have adverse consequences such as the loss of a job, driver's or pilot's licence, money and self-esteem, as well as resulting in inappropriate investigation and treatment.

3.6.2 Strategies to reduce inter-observer variation in the diagnosis of a cerebrovascular event

Sackett *et al.* (1991) highlighted the clinical skills required to obtain an accurate and useful history (Table 3.22), and six strategies for preventing or minimizing clinical disagreement (Table 3.23). If these principles are applied with a knowledge of the diagnostic criteria (e.g. Table 3.21), then diagnostic inconsistency should be minimized. If there is still uncertainty about the diagnosis at the end of the history, then the general examination and special investigations aimed at detecting vascular diseases and risk factors may provide useful circumstantial evidence (Table 3.24). The odds of an event being due to cerebrovascular disease are going to be substantially less if the patient is young and has no vascular risk factors, compared with an elderly patient who has several vascular risk factors, clinical evidence of established vascular disease (e.g. carotid or femoral bruits, absent peripheral pulses) or symptomatic vascular disease elsewhere (e.g. angina, intermittent claudication)—i.e. make sure that you use all the clinical evidence available to you.

We would recommend that in patients who present with symptoms that might suggest a stroke or TIA, but who have

Table 3.21 Diagnostic criteria for transient ischaemic attack.

Nature of symptoms
Focal neurological or monocular symptoms

Quality of symptoms
'Negative' symptoms, representing loss of focal neurological or monocular function (e.g. weakness, numbness, asphasia, loss of vision)
Rarely, 'positive' symptoms occur (e.g. pins and needles, limb shaking, scintillating visual field abnormality)

Time course of symptoms
Onset: abrupt, starting in different parts of the body (e.g. face, arm, leg) at more or less the same time, without intensification or spread ('march'); deficit maximal usually within a few seconds
Offset: symptoms resolve more gradually but completely, usually within an hour and, by definition, always within 24 h. Very brief attacks, lasting only seconds, are unusual except for transient monocular blindness (TMB) (note: we do not know how brief an attack of TMB can be and still be classified as TMB due to transient ischaemia; perhaps 10 s or so?)

Associated symptoms
Transient ischaemic attacks usually occur without warning
Antecedent symptoms are rare, but may reflect the cause (e.g. neck and face pain due to carotid dissection, headache due to giant-cell arteritis). Otherwise, antecedent symptoms (e.g. headache, nausea or epigastric discomfort) usually suggest migraine or epilepsy
Headache may occur during and after a transient ischaemic attack; it must be distinguished from migraine headache
Loss of consciousness is almost never due to a transient ischaemic attack; it usually suggests syncope or epilepsy

Neurological signs
Following symptomatic recovery, a few physical signs, such as reflex asymmetry or an extensor plantar response, which are not functionally significant, may be elicited

Brain CT or MR scan
The scan may show small areas of low density, consistent with brain infarction, in a relevant part of the brain, or may have areas of hypodensity (on CT) or increased signal (on T2 weighted MR) remote from the symptomatic area

Frequency of attacks
Transient ischaemic attacks often recur, but very frequent stereotyped attacks raise the possibility of partial epileptic seizures (sometimes due to an underlying structural abnormality such as an arteriovenous malformation, chronic subdural haematoma or cerebral tumour) or hypoglycaemia

Table 3.22 Clinical skills required to obtain an accurate and useful history (adapted from Sackett *et al.* 1991).

The ability to:
Establish understanding
Establish information
Interview logically
Listen
Interrupt only when necessary
Observe non-verbal cues
Establish a good relationship
Interpret the interview
Tell the story in plain language
Tell the story in chronological order
Make the story 'human'

Like this:
This 85-year-old widow was standing up at the kitchen table peeling potatoes at 7 p.m. on 26 July 2000, with her daughter, when she suddenly stopped talking, dropped the potato peeler she was holding in her right hand and fell to the floor. She was unable to get up and has not been able to speak or move her right arm or leg since

Not like this:
This lady developed sudden dysphasia and right hemiparesis

Table 3.23 Strategies for preventing or minimizing clinical disagreement (adapted from Sackett *et al.* 1991).

Assess the patient in a suitable consulting environment, i.e. quiet room, minimal interruptions
Necessary equipment available: ophthalmoscope, sphygmomanometer, etc., telephone to call witnesses (to clarify history) or colleagues (to obtain advice)
Clarify and confirm key points
Repeat key elements of the history or examination
Corroborate important findings with witnesses, documents and, if necessary, appropriate tests
Ask 'blinded' colleagues to see the patient also (i.e. at ward teaching sessions)
Report evidence as well as inference, making a clear distinction between the two, reporting exactly what the patient said and then your interpretation (e.g. 'the patient complained of heaviness of the right arm and leg' and not 'the patient complained of right-sided weakness' or 'the patient complained of right hemiparesis')
Apply the art and social sciences of medicine, as well as the biological sciences of medicine
Make sure you have enough time for the entire consultation

symptoms that are too vague, uncharacteristic or occurred in unusual circumstances, the diagnosis of 'possible stroke or TIA' should be made and further evidence sought by talking to witnesses of the event and by reassessing the patients

Table 3.24 Clinical features (i.e. the milieu) influencing the probability that the event was a stroke or transient ischaemic attack.

Very likely to be vascular, almost definite
Atrial fibrillation and rheumatic heart disease
Frequent carotid-distribution transient ischaemic attacks and focal, long, loud bruit over the carotid bifurcation on the symptomatic side
History and physical signs suggestive of infective endocarditis (i.e. fever, splinter haemorrhages, cardiac murmur)
Recent myocardial infarction (in last 3–4 weeks)

Likely to be vascular, but less definite
Atrial fibrillation and non-rheumatic primary valvular heart disease (but remember that 10% of fibrillating stroke patients have primary intracerebral haemorrhage as the cause of the stroke)
Arterial bruits anywhere (e.g. carotid, orbital, cardiac, aortic, femoral)
Prosthetic heart valve, taking anticoagulants (but some strokes are haemorrhagic, and some transient ischaemic attacks are related to co-existent carotid artery disease)

Unlikely to be vascular (particularly if neurological symptoms are transient)
Less than 40 years of age, no symptomatic vascular disease, no vascular risk factors, no family history of thrombosis or premature vascular disease

after any further symptoms (Whisnant *et al.* 1990). Premature labelling of an event as being due to cerebrovascular disease may prevent the correct diagnosis being considered as events unfold (Coleman *et al.* 1993). This does not prevent one identifying and managing vascular risk factors, and even considering the use of low-dose aspirin, but we think that invasive investigations should usually be avoided.

> *When coming to a view about whether an event was a transient ischaemic attack or stroke, always make use of all the clinical evidence, both general and neurological, that is available after a detailed history and examination.*

If the history is elicited independently by a second physician, a subsequent comparison of the symptoms as well as their interpretation may lead to a greatly increased reliability of the diagnosis (Koudstaal *et al.* 1986). Teaching hospitals in particular are in a privileged position to apply this powerful but expensive diagnostic 'instrument', but even so, it is still unrealistic except for the occasional very difficult case. What is often available to those in hospitals, however, is an account by the referring physician who saw the patient at an earlier time after the onset of symptoms—be sure to read it carefully and go over any symptoms described that were not reported to yourself by the patient. Implicit within this is the responsibility for all clinicians who take a history to document it in the patient's or witness's own words and not simply record their own interpretation.

The use of checklists written in simple language has been shown to be improve inter-observer reliability, and is likely to be useful for computer-aided diagnosis and further research studies (Koudstaal *et al.* 1986). But although checklists may encourage more thorough history-taking, the symptoms still have to be interpreted correctly. Very short checklists have been used successfully by paramedical personnel for diagnosing cerebrovascular events hyper-acutely (Harbison *et al.* 1999; Kidwell *et al.* 2000).

The difficulties of establishing a uniform consensus between clinicians about the diagnosis of TIA in particular has led some investigators to develop and evaluate computer-based systems to reduce the intra-observer and inter-observer variation in the diagnosis (Reggia *et al.* 1984). If validated, these systems could have a role beyond research studies, provided they were practical enough to be programmed into a hospital or primary care computerized network.

The relatively poor inter-observer agreement for physical signs (Table 3.20) is not peculiar to patients with stroke. It is to be hoped that proposed large-scale multicentre studies to evaluate rigorously the clinical examination will provide information that can improve this situation (McAlister *et al.* 1999).

References

Please note that all references taken from *The Cochrane Library* are given a current date as this database is updated on a quarterly basis. Please refer to the current *Cochrane Library* article for the latest review. The same applies to the *British Medical Journal* 'Clinical Evidence' series which is updated every six months.

Abe, M., Kjellberg, R.N. & Adams, R.D. (1989) Clinical presentations of vascular malformations of the brainstem: comparison of angiographically positive and negative types. *Journal of Neurology, Neurosurgery and Psychiatry* **52**, 167–175.

Acheson, J., Acheson, H.W.K. & Tellwright, J.M. (1968) The incidence and pattern of cerebrovascular disease in general practice. *Journal of the Royal College of General Practitioners* **16**, 428–436.

Advisory Council for the National Institute of Neurological Diseases and Blindness (1958) A classification and outline of cerebrovascular diseases. *Neurology* **8**, 395–434.

Advisory Council for the National Institute of Neurological Diseases and Blindness (1975) A classification and outline of cerebrovascular diseases. *Stroke* **6**, 564–616.

Ahmad, N., Wilson, J.A., Barr-Hamilton, R.M., Kean, D.M. & MacLennan, W.J. (1992) The evaluation of dizziness in elderly patients. *Postgraduate Medical Journal* **68**, 558–561.

Aldrich, M.S. (1990) Narcolepsy. *New England Journal of Medicine* **323**, 389–394.

Allder, S.J., Moody, A.R., Martel, A.L. *et al.* (1999) Limitations of clinical diagnosis in acute stroke. *Lancet* **354**, 1523.

Allen, C.M.C. (1983) Clinical diagnosis of the acute stroke syndrome. *Quarterly Journal of Medicine* **208**, 515–523.

Amaurosis Fugax Study Group (1990) Current management of amaurosis fugax. *Stroke* **21**, 201–208.

American Neurological Association (1993) Persistent vegetative state: report of the American Neurological Association Committee on Ethical Affairs. *Annals of Neurology* **33**, 386–391.

American Psychiatric Association (1987) *Diagnostic and Statistical Manual of Mental Disorders*. 3rd edn, revised (DSM-III-R), pp. 100–103. American Psychiatric Association, Washington, D.C.

Amiel, S. (1993) Reversal of unawareness of hypoglycaemia. *New England Journal of Medicine* **329**, 876–877.

Amira, S.A., Johnson, T.S. & Logowitz, N.B. (1985) Diagnosis of narcolepsy using multiple sleep latency test: analysis of current laboratory criteria. *Sleep* **8**, 325–331.

Anonymous (1984) Ischaemia of the optic disc. *Lancet* **ii**, 1391–1392.

Anonymous (1989) Vascular malformations in the brainstem. *Lancet* **ii**, 720–721.

Arboix, A., Massons, J., Oliveres, M., Arribas, M.P. & Titus, F. (1994) Headache in acute cerebrovascular disease: a prospective clinical study in 240 patients. *Cephalgia* 14: 37–40.

Atchison, J.W., Pellegrino, M., Herbers, P., Tipton, B. & Matkovic, V. (1992) Hepatic encephalopathy mimicking stroke: a case report. *American Journal of Physical Medicine and Rehabilitation* **71**, 114–118.

Averbuch-Heller, L., Stahl, J.S., Remler, B.F. & Leigh, R.J. (1996) Bilateral ptosis and upgaze palsy with right hemispheric lesions. *Annals of Neurology* **40**, 465–468.

Awad, I., Modic, M., Little, J.R., Furlan, A.V. & Weinstein, M. (1986) Focal parenchymal lesions in transient ischaemic attacks: correlation of computed tomography and magnetic resonance imaging. *Stroke* **17**, 399–402.

Bakar, M., Kirshner, H.S. & Wertz, R.T. (1996) Crossed aphasia: functional brain imaging with PET or SPECT. *Archives of Neurology* **53**, 1026–1032.

Baloh, R.W. (1987) Benign positional vertigo: clinical and oculographic features in 240 cases. *Neurology* **37**, 371–378.

Baloh, R.W., Jacobsen, K. & Honrubia, V. (1993) Horizontal semicircular canal variant of benign positional vertigo. *Neurology* **43**, 2542–2549.

Baquis, G.D., Pessin, M.S. & Scott, R.M. (1985) Limb shaking: a carotid TIA. *Stroke* **16**, 444–448.

Barrett, K. (1991) Treating organic abulia with bromocriptine and lisuride: four case studies. *Journal of Neurology, Neurosurgery and Psychiatry* **54**, 718–721.

Bauby, J.-D. (1997) *The Diving-bell and the Butterfly*. Fourth Estate, London.

Bauer, J., Schuler, P., Feistel, H., Hilz, M.J. & Stefan, H. (1991) Blindness as an ictal phenomenon: investigations with EEG and SPECT in two patients suffering from epilepsy. *Journal of Neurology* **238**, 44–46.

Baumgartner, R.W. & Baumgartner, I. (1998) Vasomotor reactivity is exhausted in transient ischaemic attacks with limb shaking. *Journal of Neurology, Neurosurgery and Psychiatry* **65**, 561–564.

Belal, A. Jr (1980) Pathology of vascular sensorineural hearing impairment. *Laryngoscope* **90**, 1831–1839.

Berkovic, S.F., Bladin, P.F. & Darby, D.G. (1984) Metabolic disorders presenting as stroke. *Medical Journal of Australia* **140**, 421–424.

Berlit, P., Rakicky, J. & Tornow, K. (1991) Differential diagnosis of spontaneous and traumatic intracranial haemorrhage. *Journal of Neurology, Neurosurgery and Psychiatry* **54**, 1118.

Besson, G., Hommel, M., Clavier, I. & Perret, J. (1992) Failure of magnetic resonance imaging in the detection of pontine lacune. *Stroke* **23**, 1535.

Best, M., Blumenthal, M., Futterman, H.A. & Galin, M.A. (1969) Critical closure of intraocular blood vessels. *Archives of Ophthalmology* **82**, 385–392.

Betts, T. (1990) Pseudoseizures: seizures that are not epilepsy. *Lancet* **ii**, 163–164.

Binnie, C.D. & Prior, P.F. (1994) Electroencephalography. *Journal of Neurology, Neurosurgery and Psychiatry* **57**, 1308–1319.

Blau, J.N. (1991) The clinical diagnosis of migraine: the beginning of therapy. *Journal of Neurology* **238**, S6–S11.

Blau, J.N. (1992) Classical migraine: symptoms between visual aura and headache onset. *Lancet* **340**, 355–356.

Blau, J.N. & MacGregor, E.A. (1993) Retinal migraine. *Lancet* **342**, 1185.

Blau, J.N., Wiles, C.M. & Solomon, F.S. (1983) Unilateral somatic symptoms due to hyperventilation. *British Medical Journal* **286**, 1108.

Boghen, D.R. & Glaser, J.S. (1975) Ischaemic optic neuropathy: the clinical profile and natural history. *Brain* **98**, 689–708.

Bogousslavsky, J. (1995) Thalamic infarcts. In: *Lacunar and Other Subcortical Infarctions* (eds G.A. Donnan, B. Norrving, J.M. Bamford, & J. Bogousslavsky), pp. 149–170. Oxford University Press, Oxford.

Bogousslavsky, J. & Regli, F. (1984) Cerebral infarction with transient signs

(CITS): do TIAs correspond to small deep infarcts in internal carotid artery occlusion? *Stroke* **15**, 536–539.

Bogousslavsky, J. & Regli, F. (1990a) Capsular genu syndrome. *Neurology* **40**, 1499–1502.

Bogousslavsky, J. & Regli, F. (1990b) Anterior cerebral artery territory infarction in the Lausanne Stroke Registry: clinical and etiologic patterns. *Archives of Neurology* **47**, 144–150.

Bogousslavsky, J., Vinuela, F., Barnett, H.J.M. & Drake, C.G. (1985) Amaurosis fugax as the presenting manifestation of dural arteriovenous malformation. *Stroke* **16**, 891–893.

Bogousslavsky, J., Hachinski, V.C., Boughner, D.R., Fox, A.J., Vinuela, F. & Barnett, H.J.M. (1986) Clinical predictors of cardiac and arterial lesions in carotid transient ischaemic attacks. *Archives of Neurology* **43**, 229–233.

Bogousslavsky, J., van Melle, G. & Regli, F. (1988) The Lausanne Stroke Registry: Analysis of 1000 consecutive patients with first stroke. *Stroke* **19**, 1083–1092.

Bogousslavsky, J., Martin, R., Regli, F., Despland, P.-A. & Bolyn, S. (1992) Persistent worsening of stroke sequelae after delayed seizures. *Archives of Neurology* **49**, 385–388.

Boiten, J. & Lodder, J. (1991) Isolated monoparesis is usually caused by superficial infarction. *Cerebrovascular Diseases* **1**, 337–340.

Bower, S., Dennis, M., Warlow, C., Jordan, N. & Sagar, H. (1994) Long term prognosis of transient lone bilateral blindness in adolescents and young adults. *Journal of Neurology, Neurosurgery and Psychiatry* **57**, 734–736.

Bowler, J.V., Wade, J.P., Jones, B.E. *et al.* (1995) Contribution of diaschisis to the clinical deficit in human cerebral infarction. *Stroke* **26**, 1000–1006.

Bowsher, D. (1995) The management of central post-stroke pain. *Postgraduate Medical Journal* **71**, 598–604.

Bowsher, D., Leijon, G. & Thuomas, K.A. (1998) Central poststroke pain: correlation of MRI with clinical pain characteristics and sensory abnormalities. *Neurology* **51**, 1352–1358.

Bradbury, P.G., Levy, I.S. & McDonald, W.I. (1987) Transient uniocular visual loss on deviation of the eye in association with intraorbital tumours. *Journal of Neurology, Neurosurgery and Psychiatry* **50**, 615–619.

Brandt, T. (1991) Vestibular epilepsy. In: *Vertigo: its Multisensory Syndromes,* pp. 91–97. Springer-Verlag, London.

Brandt, T., Botzel, K., Yousry, T., Dieterich, M. & Schulze, S. (1995) Rotational vertigo in embolic stroke of the vestibular and auditory cortices. *Neurology* **45**, 42–44.

Breen, L.A., Hopf, H.C., Farris, B.K. & Gutmann, L. (1992) Pupil-sparing oculomotor nerve palsy due to midbrain infarction. *Archives of Neurology* **49**, 348.

Brierley, E.J., Broughton, D.L., James, O.F.W. & Alberti, K.G.M.M. (1995) Reduced awareness of hypoglycaemia in the elderly despite an intact counter-regulatory response. *Quarterly Journal of Medicine* **88**, 439–445.

Brodal, A. (1981a) The reticular formation. In: *Neurological Anatomy in Relation to Clinical Medicine,* 3rd edn, pp. 394–447. Oxford University Press, Oxford.

Brodal, A. (1981b) The somatic afferent pathways. In: *Neurological Anatomy in Relation to Clinical Medicine,* 3rd edn, pp. 46–147. Oxford University Press, Oxford.

Brown, G.C. & Sheilds, J.A. (1981) Amaurosis fugax secondary to presumed cavernous haemangioma of the orbit. *Annals of Ophthalmology* **13**, 1205–1209.

Brown, P. (1994) Pathophysiology of spasticity. *Journal of Neurology, Neurosurgery and Psychiatry* **57**, 773–777.

Bruno, A., Corbett, J.J., Biller, J., Adams, H.P. Jr & Qualls, C. (1990) Transient monocular visual loss patterns and associated vascular abnormalities. *Stroke* **21**, 34–39.

Bryan, R.N., Levy, L.M., Whitlow, W.D., Killian, J.M., Preziosi, T.J. & Rosario, J.A. (1991) Diagnosis of acute cerebral infarction: comparison of CT and MR imaging. *American Journal of Roentgenology* **157**, 585–594.

Buchele, W. & Brandt, Th. (1988) Vestibular neuritis: a horizontal semicircular canal paresis? *Advances in Oto-Rhino-Laryngology* **42**, 157–161.

Burger, S.K., Saul, R.F., Selhorst, J.B. & Thurston, S.E. (1991) Transient monocular blindness caused by vasospasm. *New England Journal of Medicine* **325**, 870–873.

Buring, J.E., Peto, R. & Hennekens, C.H. (1990) Low-dose aspirin for migraine prophylaxis. *Journal of the American Medical Association* **264**, 1711–1713.

Burn, J., Dennis, M., Bamford, J., Sandercock, P., Wade, D. & Warlow, C. (1997) Epileptic seizures after a first stroke: the Oxfordshire Community Stroke Project. *British Medical Journal* **315**, 1582–1587.

Cairns, H., Oldfield, R.C., Pennybacker, J.B. & Whitteridge, D. (1941) Akinetic mutism with an epidermoid cyst of the 3rd ventricle. *Brain* **64**, 273–290.

Calanchini, P.R., Swanson, P.D., Gotshall, R.A. *et al.* (1977) Cooperative study of hospital frequency and character of transient ischaemic attacks, 4: the reliability of diagnosis. *Journal of the American Medical Association* **238**, 2029–2033.

Calhoun, D.A. & Oparil, S. (1990) Treatment of hypertensive crisis. *New England Journal of Medicine* **323**, 1177–1183.

Caplan, L.R., Dewitt, L.D., Pessin, M.S., Gorelick, P.B. & Adelman, L.S. (1988) Lateral thalamic infarcts. *Archives of Neurology* **45**, 959–964.

Carroll, R.S., Zhang, J. & Black, P.M. (1999) Expression of estrogen receptors alpha and beta in human meningiomas. *Journal of Neuro-oncology* **42**, 109–116.

Cartlidge, N.E.F. (1991) Transient global amnesia: recurrences are rare and patients may drive. *British Medical Journal* **302**, 62–63.

Cascino, G.D., Westmoreland, B.F., Swanson, T.H. & Sharbrough, F.W. (1991) Seizure-associated speech arrest in elderly patients. *Mayo Clinic Proceedings* **66**, 254–258.

Cates, C.A. & Newman, D.K. (1998) Transient monocular visual loss due to uveitis–glaucoma–hyphaema (UGH) syndrome. *Journal of Neurology, Neurosurgery and Psychiatry* **65**, 131–132.

Cavazos, J.E., Bulsara, K., Caress, J., Osumi, A. & Glass, J.P. (1996) Pure motor hemiplegia including the face induced by an infarct of the medullary pyramid. *Clinical Neurology and Neurosurgery* **98**, 21–23.

Chadwick, D. (1990) Diagnosis of epilepsy. *Lancet* **336**, 291–295.

Chadwick, D. (1993) The cranial nerves and special senses. In: *Brain's Diseases of the Nervous System,* 10th edn, pp. 77–126. Oxford University Press, Oxford.

Chambers, B.R. & Bladin, C.F. (1995) Internal watershed infarction. In: *Lacunar and Other Subcortical Infarctions* (eds G.A. Donnan, B. Norrving, J.M. Bamford, & J. Bogousslavsky), pp. 139–148. Oxford University Press, Oxford.

Chokroverty, S., Rubino, F.A. & Haller, C. (1975) Pure motor hemiplegia due to pyramidal infarction. *Archives of Neurology* **32**, 647–648.

Chollet, F., DiPiero, V., Wise, R.J.S., Brooks, D.J., Dolan, R.J. & Frackowiak, R.S.J. (1991) The functional anatomy of motor recovery after stroke in humans: a study with positron emission tomography. *Annals of Neurology* **29**, 63–71.

Cohen, L., Verstichel, P. & Pierrot-Deseilligny, C. (1992) Hallucinatory vision of a familiar face following right temporal haemorrhage. *Neurology* **42**, 2052.

Coleman, R.J., Bamford, J.M. & Warlow, C.P. (for the UK TIA Study Group) (1993) Cerebral tumours that mimic transient cerebral ischaemia: lessons from a large multi-centre trial. *Journal of Neurology, Neurosurgery and Psychiatry* **56**, 563–566.

Colledge, N.R., Barr-Hamilton, R.M., Lewis, S.J., Sellar, R.J. & Wilson, J.A. (1996) Evaluation of investigations to diagnose the cause of dizziness in elderly people: a community based controlled study. *British Medical Journal* **313**, 788–792.

Conference of Medical Royal Colleges and their Faculties in the United Kingdom (1976) Diagnosis of brain death. *British Medical Journal* **ii**, 1187–1188.

Conference of Medical Royal Colleges and their Faculties in the United Kingdom (1979) Diagnosis of brain death. *British Medical Journal* **i**, 332.

Conference of Medical Royal Colleges and their Faculties in the United Kingdom (1995) Criteria for the diagnosis of brain stem death. *Journal of the Royal College of Physicians* **29**, 381–382.

Critchley, M. (1951) Types of visual perseveration: palinopsia and illusory visual spread. *Brain* **74**, 267–299.

Crozier, S., Lehéricy, S., Verstichel, P., Masson, C. & Masson, M. (1996) Transient hemiballism/hemichorea due to an ipsilateral subthalamic nucleus infarction. *Neurology* 47: 267–268.

Daly, D.D., Svien, H.J. & Yoss, R.E. (1961) Intermittent cerebral symptoms with meningiomas. *Archives of Neurology* **5**, 287–293.

Dávalos, A., Toni, D., Iweins, F. *et al.* (1999) Neurological deterioration in acute ischemic stroke: potential predictors and associated factors in the European Cooperative Acute Stroke study (ECASS) I. *Stroke* **30**, 2631–2636.

Davenport, R.J., Statham, P.F.X. & Warlow, C.P. (1994) Detection of bilateral isodense subdural haematomas. *British Medical Journal* **309**, 792–794.

Davidovitch, S. & Gadoth, N. (1988) Neurological deficit simulating transient ischaemic attacks due to intracranial meningioma. *European Neurology* **28**, 24–26.

Davis, S.M., Tress, B.M., Dowling, R., Donnan, G.A., Kiers, L. & Rossiter, S.C. (1989) Magnetic resonance imaging in posterior circulation infarction: impact on diagnosis and management. *Australian and New Zealand Journal of Medicine* **19**, 219–225.

Dawson, D.M., Hallett, M. & Millender, L.H. (1990) *Entrapment Neuropathies*, 2nd edn, p. 38. Little, Brown, Boston.

De Renzi, E., Motti, F. & Nichelli, P. (1980) Imitating gestures: a quantitative approach to ideomotor apraxia. *Archives of Neurology* **37**, 6–10.

De Renzi, E., Colombo, A., Faglioni, P. & Gilbertoni, M. (1982) Conjugate gaze paresis in stroke patients with unilateral damage. *Archives of Neurology* **39**, 482–486.

DeGrabba, T.J., Hallenbeck, J.M., Pettigrew, K.D., Dutka, A.J. & Kelly, B.J. (1999) Progression in acute stroke: value of the initial NIH stroke scale score on patient stratification in future trials. *Stroke* **30**, 1208–1212.

Déjerine, J. & Roussy, G. (1906) Le syndrome thalamique. *Revue Neurologique (Paris)* **14**, 521–532.

Denholm, S.W. (1993) Benign paroxysmal positional vertigo. *British Medical Journal* **307**, 1507–1508.

Dennis, M.S. (1988) *Transient Ischaemic Attacks in the Community* [MD dissertation]. University of London, London.

Dennis, M.S., Bamford, J.M., Molyneux, A.J. & Warlow, C.P. (1987) Rapid resolution of signs of primary intracerebral haemorrhage in computed tomograms of the brain. *British Medical Journal* **295**, 379–381.

Dennis, M.S., Bamford, J.M., Sandercock, P.A.G. & Warlow, C.P. (1989a) Lone bilateral blindness: a transient ischaemic attack. *Lancet* **i**, 185–188.

Dennis, M.S., Bamford, J.M., Sandercock, P.A.G. & Warlow, C.P. (1989b) Incidence of transient ischaemic attacks in Oxfordshire, England. *Stroke* **20**, 333–339.

Dennis, M.S., Bamford, J.M., Sandercock, P.A.G. & Warlow, C.P. (1989c) A comparison of risk factors and prognosis for transient ischaemic attacks and minor ischaemic strokes: the Oxfordshire Community Stroke Project. *Stroke* **20**, 1494–1499.

Dennis, M.S., Bamford, J.M., Sandercock, P.A.G., Molyneux, A. & Warlow, C.P. (1990a) Computerised tomography in patients with transient ischaemic attacks: when is a transient ischaemic attack not a transient ischaemic attack but a stroke? *Journal of Neurology* **237**, 257–261.

Dennis, M.S., Bamford, J., Sandercock, P. & Warlow, C. (1990b) Prognosis of transient ischaemic attacks in the Oxfordshire Community Stroke Project. *Stroke* **21**, 848–853.

Dennis, M.S. & Warlow, C.P. (1992) Migraine aura without headache: transient ischaemic attack or not? *Journal of Neurology, Neurosurgery and Psychiatry* **55**, 437–440.

Devinsky, O., Bear, D. & Volpe, B.T. (1988) Confusional states following posterior cerebral artery infarction. *Archives of Neurology* **45**, 160–163.

Dix, M. & Hallpike, C. (1952) The pathology, symptomatology and diagnosis of certain common disorders of the vestibular system. *Annals of Otology, Rhinology and Laryngology* **32**, 364.

Donders, R.C.J.M., Kappelle, L.J., Algra, A. *et al.* (1996) Subtypes of transient monocular blindness and subsequent risk of vascular complications. *Cerebrovascular Diseases* **6**, 241–247.

Donnan, G.A., O'Malley, H.M., Quang, L., Hurley, S. & Bladin, P.F. (1993) The capsular warning syndrome: pathogenesis and clinical features. *Neurology* **43**, 957–962.

Donnan, G.A., O'Malley, H.M., Quang, L., Hurley, S. & Bladin, P.F. (1995) The capsular warning syndrome and lacunar transient ischaemic attacks. In: *Lacunar and Other Subcortical Infarctions* (eds G.A. Donnan, B. Norrving, J.M. Bamford, & J. Bogousslavsky), pp. 47–55. Oxford University Press, Oxford.

Donnan, G.A., Carey, L.M. & Saling, M.M. (1999) More (or less) on Broca. *Lancet* **353**, 1031.

Dronkers, N.F. (1996) A new brain region for coordinating speech articulation. *Nature* **384**, 159–161.

Drulovic, B., Ribaric-Jankes, K., Kostic, V.S. & Sternic, N. (1993) Sudden hearing loss as the initial monosymptom of multiple sclerosis. *Neurology* **43**, 2703–2705.

Duckrow, R.B., Beard, D.C. & Brennan, R.W. (1985) Regional cerebral blood flow decreases during hyperglycaemia. *Annals of Neurology* **17**, 267–272.

Dunne, J.W., Leedman, P.J. & Edis, R.H. (1986) Inobvious stroke: a cause of delirium and dementia. *Australian and New Zealand Journal of Medicine* **16**, 771–778.

Dutch TIA Trial Study Group (1993) Predictors of major vascular events in patients with a transient ischaemic attack or nondisabling stroke. *Stroke* **24**, 527–531.

Duus, P. (1989) *Topical Diagnosis in Neurology*. Georg Thieme Verlag, Stuttgart.

Easton, J.D. (1993) Treatment for preventing migraine-related stroke. *Cerebrovascular Diseases* **3**, 244–247.

Easton, J.D. (1995) The diagnostic evaluation of transient global amnesia. *Cerebrovascular Diseases* **5**, 212–216.

Edelman, R. & Warach, S. (1993) Magnetic resonance imaging. *New England Journal of Medicine* **328**, 708–716.

Edmeads, J. (1979) The headaches of ischaemic cerebrovascular disease. *Headache* **19**, 345–349.

Edmeads, J. (1983) Complicated migraine and headache in cerebrovascular disease. *Neurological Clinics* **1**, 385–397.

Eliasziw, M., Streifler, J.Y., Spence, J.D. *et al.* (1995) Prognosis for patients following a transient ischaemic attack with and without a cerebral infarction on brain CT. *Neurology* **45**, 428–431.

Elliott, W.J. (1998) Circadian variation in the timing of stroke onset: a meta-analysis. *Stroke* **29**, 992–996.

Evans, J., Wilson, B., Wraight, P. & Hodges, J.R. (1993) Neuropsychological and SPECT scan findings during and after transient global amnesia: evidence for the differential impairment of remote episodic memory. *Journal of Neurology, Neurosurgery and Psychiatry* **56**, 1227–1230.

Everson, S.A., Lynch, J.W., Chesney, M.A. *et al.* (1997) Interaction of workplace demands and cardiovascular reactivity in progression of carotid atherosclerosis: population based study. *British Medical Journal* **314**, 553–558.

Fahmy, J.A. (1973) Fundal haemorrhages in ruptured intracranial aneurysms, 1: material, frequency, and morphology. *Acta Ophthalmologica* **51**, 189–198.

Faris, A.A. & Poser, C.M. (1964) Experimental production of focal neurological deficit by systemic hyponatraemia. *Neurology* **14**, 206–211.

Faught, E. (1993) Current role of electroencephalography in cerebral ischaemia. *Stroke* **24**, 609–613.

Fisher, C.M. (1964) Ocular bobbing. *Archives of Neurology* **11**, 543–546.

Fisher, C.M. (1967) Some neuro-ophthalmological observations. *Journal of Neurology, Neurosurgery and Psychiatry* **30**, 383–392.

Fisher, C.M. (1971) Cerebral ischaemia: less familiar types. *Clinical Neurosurgery* **18**, 267–336.

Fisher, C.M. (1980) Late-life migraine accompaniments as a cause of unexplained transient ischaemic attacks. *Canadian Journal of Neurological Sciences* **7**, 9–17.

Fisher, C.M. (1986) Late-life migraine accompaniments: further experience. *Stroke* **17**, 1033–1042.

Fisher, C.M. (1995) Abulia. In: *Stroke Syndromes* (eds J. Bogousslavsky & L.R. Caplan), pp. 182–187. Cambridge University Press, Cambridge.

Fisher, C.M. (1996) Vomiting out of proportion to dizziness in ischemic brainstem strokes. *Neurology* **47**, 267.

Fisher, C.M. & Adams, R.D. (1964) Transient global amnesia. *Acta Neurologica Scandinavica* **40** (Suppl. 9), 1–83.

Fisher, M., Davidson, R.I. & Marcus, E.M. (1980) Transient focal cerebral ischaemia as a presenting manifestation of unruptured cerebral aneurysms. *Annals of Neurology* **8**, 367–372.

Fisher, R.S., Chan, D.W., Bare, M. & Lesser, R.P. (1991) Capillary prolactin measurement for diagnosis of seizures. *Annals of Neurology* **29**, 187–190.

Foster, J.W. & Hart, R.G. (1987) Hypoglycaemic hemiplegia: two cases and a clinical review. *Stroke* **18**, 944–946.

Fowler, G.W. (1970) Meningioma and intermittent aphasia of 44 years' duration. *Journal of Neurosurgery* **3**, 100–102.

Friberg, T.R., Braunstein, R.A. & Bressler, N.M. (1995) Sudden visual loss associated with sexual activity. *Archives of Ophthalmology* **113**, 738–742.

Frisén, L. (1979) Quadruple sectoranopia and sectorial optic atrophy: a syndrome of the distal anterior choroidal artery. *Journal of Neurology, Neurosurgery and Psychiatry* **42**, 590–594.

Fritz, V.U., Levien, L.J. & Hagen, D.J. (1983) Cerebral tumours mimicking transient cerebral events. *South African Journal of Surgery* **21**, 243–250.

Furlan, A.J., Whisnant, J.P. & Kerns, T.P. (1979) Unilateral visual loss in bright light: an unusual symptom of carotid artery occlusive disease. *Archives of Neurology* **36**, 675–676.

Galer, B.S., Lipton, R.B., Weinstein, S., Bello, L. & Solomon, S. (1990) Apoplectic headache and oculomotor palsy: an unusual presentation of multiple sclerosis. *Neurology* **40**, 1465–1466.

Galin, D., Diamond, R. & Braff, D. (1977) Lateralization of conversion symptoms: more frequent on the left. *American Journal of Psychiatry* **134**, 578–580.

Ghika-Schmid, F., Ghika, J., Regli, F. & Bogousslavsky, J. (1997) Hyperkinetic movement disorders during and after acute stroke: the Lausanne Stroke Registry [published erratum appears in *Journal of Neurological Sciences* (1997) **152**, 234–235]. *Journal of Neurological Sciences* **146**, 109–116.

Ghika-Schmid, F., van Melle, G., Guex, P. & Bogousslavsky, J. (1999) Subjective experience and behavior in acute stroke: the Lausanne Emotion in Acute Stroke Study. *Neurology* **52**, 22–28.

van Gijn, J. (1995) The Babinski reflex. *Postgraduate Medical Journal* **71**, 645–648.

Glaser, J.S., Savino, P.J., Sumers, K.D., McDonald, S.A. & Knighton, R.W. (1977) The photostress recovery test in the clinical assessment of visual function. *American Journal of Ophthalmology* **83**, 255–260.

Globus, M., Lavi, E., Alexander, F. & Oded, A. (1982) Ictal hemiparesis. *European Neurology* **21**, 165–168.

Gomez, C.R., Cruz-Flores, S., Malkoff, M.D., Sauer, C.M. & Burch, C.M. (1996) Isolated vertigo as a manifestation of vertebrobasilar ischaemia. *Neurology* **47**, 94–97.

Goodwin, J.A. (1985) Acute ischaemic optic neuropathy. *Journal of the American Medical Association* **254**, 951–952.

Goodwin, J.A., Gorelick, P.B. & Helgason, C.M. (1987) Symptoms of amaurosis fugax in atherosclerotic carotid artery disease. *Neurology* **37**, 829–832.

Grad, A. & Baloh, R.W. (1989) Vertigo of vascular origin: clinical and electronystagmographic features in 84 cases. *Archives of Neurology* **46**, 281–284.

Graff-Radford, N.R., Cooper, W.E., Colsher, P.L. & Damasio, A.R. (1986) An unlearned foreign accent in a patient with aphasia. *Brain Language* **28**, 86–94.

Greenhall, R.C.D. (1977) *Pathological Findings in Acute Cerebrovascular Disease and Their Clinical Implications* [MD dissertation]. University of Oxford, Oxford.

Gresty, M.A., Bronstein, A.M., Brandt, T. & Dieterich, M. (1992) Neurology of otolith function: peripheral and central disorders. *Brain* **115**, 647–673.

Grunwald, G.B., Klein, R., Simmonds, M.A. & Kornguth, S.E. (1985) Autoimmune basis for visual paraneoplastic syndrome in patients with small cell lung carcinoma. *Lancet* **i**, 658–661.

Gubbay, S.S., Hankey, G.J., Tan, N.T.S. & Fry, J.M. (1989) Mitochondrial encephalomyopathy with steroid dependence. *Medicine Journal of Australia* **151**, 100–107.

Gunatilake, S.B. (1998) Rapid resolution of symptoms and signs of intracerebral haemorrhage: case reports. *British Medical Journal* **316**, 1495–1496.

Gurd, J.M., Bessell, N.J., Bladon, R.A.W. & Bamford, J.M. (1988) A case of foreign accent syndrome, with follow-up clinical, neuropsychological and phonetic descriptions. *Neuropsychologia* **26**, 237–251.

Gussen, R. (1976) Sudden deafness of vascular origin: a human temporal bone study. *Annals of Otology, Rhinology and Laryngology* **85**, 94–100.

Gutrecht, J.A., Kattwinkel, N. & Stillman, M.J. (1991) Retinal migraine, chorea, and retinal artery thrombosis in a patient with primary antiphospholipid antibody syndrome. *Journal of Neurology* **238**, 55–56.

Guyer, D.R., Miller, N.R., Auer, C.L. & Fine, S.L. (1985) The risk of cerebrovascular and cardiovascular disease in patients with anterior ischaemic optic neuropathy. *Archives of Ophthalmology* **103**, 1136–1142.

Haimovic, I.C. & Beresford, H.R. (1992) Transient unresponsiveness in the elderly: report of five cases. *Archives of Neurology* **49**, 35–37.

Halligan, P.W., Marshall, J.C. & Wade, D.T. (1989) Visuospatial neglect: underlying factors and test sensitivity. *Lancet* **ii**, 908–911.

Halmagyi, G.M. & Cremer, P.D. (2000) Assessment and treatment of dizziness. *Journal of Neurology, Neurosurgery and Psychiatry* **68**, 129–136.

Hamdy, S., Aziz, Q., Rothwell, J.C. *et al.* (1998) Recovery of swallowing after dysphagic stroke relates to functional reorganization in the intact motor cortex. *Gastroenterology* **115**, 1104–1112.

Hankey, G.J. (1993) Prolonged exacerbation of the neurological sequelae of stroke by post-stroke partial epileptic seizures. *Australian and New Zealand Journal of Medicine* **23**, 306.

Hankey, G.J. & Stewart-Wynne, E.G. (1988) Amnesia following thalamic haemorrhage: another stroke syndrome. *Stroke* **19**, 776–778.

Hankey, G.J. & Warlow, C.P. (1992) Cost-effective investigation of patients with suspected transient ischaemic attacks. *Journal of Neurology, Neurosurgery and Psychiatry* **55**, 171–176.

Hankey, G.J. & Warlow, C.P. (1994). *Transient Ischaemic Attacks of the Brain and Eye*. W.B. Saunders, London.

Hankey, G.J., Slattery, J.M. & Warlow, C.P. (1991) The prognosis of hospital-referred transient ischaemic attacks. *Journal of Neurology, Neurosurgery and Psychiatry* **54**, 793–802.

Hankey, G.J., Slattery, J.M. & Warlow, C.P. (1992) Transient ischaemic attacks: which patients are at high (and low) risk of serious vascular events? *Journal of Neurology, Neurosurgery and Psychiatry* **55**, 640–652.

Harbison, J., Massey, A., Barnett, L., Hodge, D. & Ford, G.A. (1999) Rapid ambulance protocol for acute stroke. *Lancet* **353**, 1935.

Harper, C.G., Bajada, S., Chakera, T. & Cook, R. (1981) Acute central nervous system disorder mimicking stroke. *Medical Journal of Australia* **1**, 136–138.

Harper, C.G., Giles, M. & Finlay-Jones, R. (1986) Clinical signs in the Wernicke–Korsakoff complex: a retrospective analysis of 131 cases diagnosed at necropsy. *Journal of Neurology, Neurosurgery and Psychiatry* **49**, 341–345.

Harrison, M.J.G. (1999) Transient ischaemic attacks related to carotid stenosis precipitated by straining, bending, and sneezing. *Postgraduate Medical Journal* **75**, 145–146.

Hatano, S. (1976) Experience from a multicentre stroke register: a preliminary report. *Bulletin of the World Health Organization* **54**, 541–553.

Hayreh, S.S. (1975). *Anterior Ischaemic Optic Neuropathy*. Springer-Verlag, New York.

Hayreh, S.S. (1976) So-called 'central retinal vein occlusion', 1: pathogenesis, terminology, clinical features. *Ophthalmologica* **172**, 1–13.

Hayreh, S.S. (1977) Optic disc oedema in raised intracranial pressure, 4: associated visual disturbances and their pathogenesis. *Archives of Ophthalmology* **95**, 1566–1579.

Hayreh, S.S. (1981) Anterior ischaemic optic neuropathy. *Archives of Neurology* **38**, 675–678.

Hayreh, S.S., Servais, G.E. & Virdi, P.S. (1986) Fundus lesions in malignant hypertension, 5: hypertensive optic neuropathy. *Ophthalmology* **93**, 74–87.

Healton, E.B., Brust, J.C., Feinfeld, D.A. & Thomson, G.E. (1982) Hypertensive encephalopathy and the neurologic manifestations of malignant hypertension. *Neurology* **32**, 127–132.

Hedges, T.R. & Lackman, R.D. (1976) Isolated ophthalmic migraine in the differential diagnosis of cerebro-ocular ischaemia. *Stroke* **7**, 379–381.

Helgason, C., Wilbur, A., Weiss, A., Redmond, K.J. & Kingsbury, N.A. (1988) Acute pseudobulbar mutism due to discrete bilateral capsular infarction in the territory of the anterior choroidal artery. *Brain* **111**, 507–524.

Hess, D.C., Nichols, F.T., Sethi, K.D. & Adams, R.J. (1991) Transient cerebral ischaemia masquerading as paroxysmal dyskinesia. *Cerebrovascular Diseases* **1**, 54–57.

Hier, D.B., Mondlock, J. & Caplan, L.R. (1983) Behavioural abnormalities after right hemisphere stroke. *Neurology* **33**, 337–344.

Hinchey, J., Chaves, C., Appignani, B. *et al.* (1996) A reversible posterior leukoencephalopathy syndrome. *New England Journal of Medicine* **334**, 494–500.

Hodges, J.R. (1991) *Transient Global Amnesia: Clinical and Neuropsychological Aspects*. W.B. Saunders, London.

Hodges, J.R. (1994) *Cognitive Assessment for Clinicians*. Oxford University Press, Oxford.

Hodges, J.R. & Ward, C.D. (1989) Observations during transient global amnesia. *Brain* **112**, 595–620.

Hodges, J.R. & Warlow, C.P. (1990a) The aetiology of transient global amnesia: a case–control study of 114 cases with prospective follow-up. *Brain* **113**, 639–657.

Hodges, J.R. & Warlow, C.P. (1990b) Syndromes of transient amnesia: towards a classification: a study of 153 cases. *Journal of Neurology, Neurosurgery and Psychiatry* **53**, 834–843.

Hoefnagels, W.A.J., Padberg, G.W., Overweg, J., van der Velde, E.A. & Roos, R.A.C. (1991) Transient loss of consciousness: the value of the history for distinguishing seizure from syncope. *Journal of Neurology* **238**, 39–43.

Hoeldtke, R.D., Boden, G., Shuman, C.R. & Owen, O.E. (1982) Reduced epinephrine secretion and hypoglycaemia in diabetic autonomic neuropathy. *Annals of Internal Medicine* **96**, 459–463.

Hogan, R.E. (1994) Sudden 'stroke-like' onset of hemiparesis due to bacterial brain abscess. *Neurology* **44**, 569–570.

Holt Larsen, B., Soelberg Sorensen, P. & Marquardsen, J. (1990) Transient ischaemic attacks in young patients: a thromboembolic or migrainous manifestation? A 10 year follow up study of 46 patients. *Journal of Neurology, Neurosurgery and Psychiatry* **53**, 1029–1033.

Hommel, M., Besson, G., Le Bas, J.F. *et al.* (1990) Prospective study of lacunar infarction using magnetic resonance imaging. *Stroke* **21**, 546–554.

Hopf, H.C., Tettenborn, B. & Kramer, G. (1990) Pontine supranuclear facial palsy. *Stroke* **21**, 1754–1757.

Hopf, H.C., Muller-Forell, W. & Hopf, N.J. (1992) Localization of emotional and volitional facial paresis. *Neurology* **42**, 1918–1923.

Hotson, J.R. & Baloh, R.W. (1998) Acute vestibular syndrome. *New England Journal of Medicine* **339**, 680–685.

House, A., Dennis, M., Mogridge, L., Hawton, K. & Warlow, C. (1990) Life events and difficulties preceding stroke. *Journal of Neurology, Neurosurgery and Psychiatry* **53**, 1024–1028.

Howard, R.S. (1992) Persistent hiccups. *British Medical Journal* **305**, 1237–1238.

Howard, R.S. & Miller, D.H. (1995) The persistent vegetative state. *British Medical Journal* **310**, 341–342.

Huang, C.Y. & Yu, Y.L. (1985) Small cerebellar strokes may mimic labyrinthine lesions. *Journal of Neurology, Neurosurgery and Psychiatry* **48**, 263–265.

Ille, O., Woimant, F., Pruna, A., Corabianu, O., Idatte, J.M. & Haguenau, M. (1995) Hypertensive encephalopathy after bilateral carotid endarterectomy. *Stroke* **26**, 488–491.

Ishiai, S., Sugishita, M., Ichikawa, T., Gono, S. & Watabiki, S. (1993) Clock-drawing test and unilateral spatial neglect. *Neurology* **43**, 106–110.

Ivo, J. (1999) CT scanning can differentiate between ischaemic attack and haemorrhage. *British Medical Journal* **319**, 1197.

Jacobsen, D.M., Thirkill, C.E. & Tipping, S.J. (1990) A clinical triad to diagnose paraneoplastic retinopathy. *Annals of Neurology* **28**, 162–167.

Jehkonen, M., Ahonen, J.-P., Dastidar, P., Koivisto, A.-M., Laippala, P. & Vilkki, J. (1998) How to detect visual neglect in acute stroke. *Lancet* **351**, 727–728.

Jennett, B. & Plum, F. (1972) Persistent vegetative state after brain damage: a syndrome in search of a name. *Lancet* **i**, 734–737.

Jenny, A.B. & Saper, C.B. (1987) Organization of the facial nucleus and cortico-facial projection in the monkey: a reconsideration of the upper motor neurone facial palsy. *Neurology* **37**, 930–939.

Jorgensen, H.S., Jespersen, H.F., Nakayama, H., Raaschou, H.O. & Olsen, T.S. (1994) Headache in stroke: the Copenhagen Stroke Study. *Neurology* **44**, 1793–1797.

Kamata, T., Yokota, T., Furukawa, T. & Tsukagoshi, H. (1994) Cerebral ischaemic attack caused by postprandial hypotension. *Stroke* **25**, 511–513.

Kapoor, W.N. (1991) Diagnostic evaluation of syncope. *American Journal of Medicine* **90**, 91–106.

Kappelle, L.J., van Huffelen, A.C. & van Gijn, J. (1990) Is the EEG really normal in lacunar stroke? *Journal of Neurology, Neurosurgery and Psychiatry* **53**, 63–66.

Kase, C.S., Maulsby, G.O., deJuan, E. & Mohr, J.P. (1981) Hemichorea–hemiballism and lacunar infarction in the basal ganglia. *Neurology* **31**, 452–455.

Katz, R.T., Haig, A.J., Clark, B.B. & DiPaola, R.J. (1992) Long-term survival, prognosis and life-care planning for 29 patients with chronic locked-in syndrome. *Archives of Physical Medicine and Rehabilitation* **73**, 403–408.

Kaufman, D.K., Brown, R.D. & Karnes, W.E. (1994) Involuntary tonic spasms of a limb due to a brainstem lacunar infarction. *Stroke* **25**, 217–219.

Kazui, S. & Sawada, T. (1993) Callosal apraxia without agraphia. *Annals of Neurology* **33**, 401–403.

Keane, J.R. (1979) Retinal haemorrhage: its significance in 100 patients with acute encephalopathy of unknown cause. *Archives of Neurology* **36**, 691–694.

Keltner, J.L., Roth, A.M. & Chang, R.S. (1983) Photoreceptor degeneration: possible autoimmune disorder. *Archives of Ophthalmology* **101**, 564–569.

Kennard, C., Crawford, T.J. & Henderson, C. (1994) A pathophysiological approach to saccadic eye movements in neurological and psychiatric disease. *Journal of Neurology, Neurosurgery and Psychiatry* **57**, 881–885.

Kessler, C., Freyberger, H.J., Dittmann, V. & Ringelstein, E.B. (1991) Interrater reliability in the assessment of neurovascular diseases. *Cerebrovascular Diseases* **1**, 43–48.

Khan, S., Yaqub, B.A., Poser, C.M., Al Deeb, S.M. & Bohlega, S. (1995) Multiphasic disseminated encephalomyelitis presenting as alternating hemiplegia. *Journal of Neurology, Neurosurgery and Psychiatry* **58**, 467–470.

Kidd, D., Lawson, J., Nesbitt, R. & MacMahon, J. (1993) Aspiration in acute stroke: a clinical study with videofluoroscopy. *Quarterly Journal of Medicine* **86**, 825–829.

Kidd, D., Lawson, J., Nesbitt, R. & MacMahon, J. (1995) The natural history and clinical consequences of aspiration in acute stroke. *Quarterly Journal of Medicine* **88**, 409–413.

Kidwell, C.S., Alger, J.R., Di Salle, F. *et al.* (1999) Diffusion MRI in patients with transient ischemic attacks. *Stroke* **30**, 1174–1180.

Kidwell, C.S., Starkman, S., Eckstein, M., Weems, K. & Saver, J.L. (2000) Identifying stroke in the field: prospective validation of the Los Angeles Prehospital Stroke Screen (LAPSS). *Stroke* **31**, 71–76.

Kim, J.S. (1994) Restricted acral sensory syndrome following minor stroke: further observation with special reference to differential severity of symptoms among individual digits. *Stroke* **25**, 2497–2502.

Kim, J.S. (1996) Restricted nonacral sensory syndrome. *Stroke* **27**, 988–990.

Kim, J.S. & Lee, M.C. (1994) Stroke and restricted sensory syndromes. *Neuroradiology* **36**, 258–263.

Kim, J.S., Lopez, I., DiPatre, P.L., Liu, F., Ishiyama, A. & Baloh, R.W. (1999) Internal auditory artery infarction: clinicopathologic correlation. *Neurology* **52**, 40–44.

Kimura, R. & Perlman, H.B. (1958) Arterial obstruction of the labyrinth: cochlear changes. *Annals of Otology, Rhinology and Laryngology* **67**, 5–24.

Kingsley, D.P.E., Radue, E.W. & Du Boulay, E.P.G.H. (1980) Evaluation of computed tomography in vascular lesions of the vertebrobasilar territory. *Journal of Neurology, Neurosurgery and Psychiatry* **43**, 193–197.

Klein, R., Klein, B.E., Jensen, S.C., Moss, S.E. & Meuer, S.M. (1999) Retinal emboli and stroke: the Beaver Dam eye study. *Archives of Ophthalmology* **117**, 1063–1068.

Klotzsch, C., Sliwka, U., Berlit, P. & Noth, J. (1996) An increased frequency of patent foramen ovale in patients with transient global amnesia: analysis of 53 consecutive patients. *Archives of Neurology* **53**, 504–508.

Kogeorgos, J., Scott, D.F. & Swash, M. (1981) Epileptic dizziness. *British Medical Journal* **282**, 687–689.

Kolmel, H. (1985) Complex visual hallucinations in the hemianopic field. *Journal of Neurology, Neurosurgery and Psychiatry* **48**, 29–38.

Kong, H.L., Ong, B.K.C., Lee, T.K.Y. & Cheah, J.S. (1993) Melioidosis of the brain presenting with a stroke syndrome. *Australian and New Zealand Journal of Medicine* **23**, 413–414.

Kopelman, M.D., Panaayiotopoulos, C.P. & Lewis, P. (1994) Transient epileptic amnesia differentiated from psychogenic 'fugue': neuropsychological, EEG, and PET findings. *Journal of Neurology, Neurosurgery and Psychiatry* **57**, 1002–1004.

Koskas, F., Comizzoli, I., Gobin, Y.P. *et al.* (1992) Effects of spinal mechanics on the vertebral artery. In: *Vertebrobasilar Arterial Disease* (eds R. Berguer, L.R. Caplan), pp. 15–28. QMP, St Louis.

Kothari, R., Barsan, W., Brott, T., Broderick, J. & Ashbrock, S. (1995) Frequency and accuracy of prehospital diagnosis of acute stroke. *Stroke* **26**, 937–941.

Koudstaal, P.J., van Gijn, J., Staal, A., Duivenvoorden, H.J., Gerritsma, J.G.M. & Kraaijeveld, C.L. (1986) Diagnosis of transient ischaemic attacks: improvement of interobserver agreement by a check-list in ordinary language. *Stroke* **17**, 723–728.

Koudstaal, P.J., Gerritsma, J.G.M. & van Gijn, J. (1989) Clinical disagreement on the diagnosis of transient ischaemic attack: is the patient or the doctor to blame? *Stroke* **20**, 300–301.

Koudstaal, P.J., van Gijn, J., Lodder, J. *et al.* (1991a) Transient ischaemic attacks with and without a relevant infarct on computed tomographic scans cannot be distinguished clinically. *Archives of Neurology* **48**, 916–920.

Koudstaal, P.J., van Gijn, J., Kappelle, L.J. *et al.* (1991b) Headache in transient or permanent cerebral ischaemia. *Stroke* **22**, 754–759.

Koudstaal, P.J., van Gijn, J., Frenken, C.W. *et al.* (1992) TIA, RIND, minor stroke: a continuum, or different subgroups? *Journal of Neurology, Neurosurgery and Psychiatry* **55**, 95–97.

Kraaijeveld, C.L., van Gijn, J., Schouten, H.J.A. & Staal, A. (1984) Interobserver agreement for the diagnosis of transient ischaemic attacks. *Stroke* **15**, 723–725.

Krystkowiak, P., Martinat, P., Defebvre, L., Pruvo, J.P., Leys, D. & Destée, A. (1998) Dystonia after striatopallidal and thalamic stroke: clinicoradiological correlations and pathophysiological mechanisms. *Journal of Neurology, Neurosurgery and Psychiatry* **65**, 703–708.

Kumral, E., Bogousslavsky, J., Van Melle, G., Regli, F. & Pierre, P. (1995) Headache at stroke onset: the Lausanne Stroke Registry. *Journal of Neurology, Neurosurgery and Psychiatry* **58**, 490–492.

Lane, D.A., Wolff, S., Ireland, H., Gawel, M. & Foadi, M. (1983) Activation of coagulation and fibrinolytic systems following stroke. *British Journal of Haematology* **53**, 655–658.

Lansberg, M.G., O'Brien, M.W., Norbash, A.M., Moseley, M.E., Morrell, M. & Albers, G.W. (1999) MRI abnormalities associated with partial status epilepticus. *Neurology* **52**, 1021–1027.

Lauria, G., Gentile, M., Fassetta, G., Casetta, I. & Caneve, G. (1998) Transient global amnesia and transient ischaemic attack: a community-based case–control study. *Acta Neurologica Scandinavica* **97**, 381–385.

Lawden, M.C. & Cleland, P.G. (1993) Achromatopsia in the aura of migraine. *Journal of Neurology, Neurosurgery and Psychiatry* **56**, 708–709.

Lecouvet, F.E., Duprez, T.P.J., Raymackers, J.M., Peeters, A. & Cosnard, G. (1999) Resolution of early diffusion-weighted and FLAIR MRI abnormalities in a patient with TIA. *Neurology* **52**, 1085–1087.

Lee, H. & Lerner, A. (1990) Transient inhibitory seizures mimicking crescendo TIAs. *Neurology* **40**, 165–166.

Leestma, J.E. & Noronha, A. (1976) Pure motor hemiplegia, medullary pyramid lesion, and olivary hypertrophy. *Journal of Neurology, Neurosurgery and Psychiatry* **39**, 877–884.

Leira, E.C., Bendixen, B.H., Kardon, R.H. & Adams, H.P. Jr (1998) Brief, transient Horner's syndrome can be a hallmark of carotid artery dissection. *Neurology* **50**, 289–290.

Lempert, T., Bauer, M. & Schmidt, D. (1994) Syncope: a videometric analysis of 56 episodes of transient cerebral hypoxia. *Annals of Neurology* **36**, 233–237.

Lempert, T., Gresty, M.A. & Bronstein, A.M. (1995) Benign positional vertigo: recognition and treatment. *British Medical Journal* **311**, 489–491.

Lepore, F.E. (1987) Bilateral cerebral ptosis. *Neurology* **37**, 1043–1046.

Lewis, M.B., MacQuillan, G., Bamford, J.M. & Howdle, P.D. (2000) Delayed myelopathic presentation of the acquired hepatocerebral syndrome. *Neurology* **54**, 1011.

Lieberman, M.F., Shahi, A. & Green, W.R. (1978) Embolic ischaemic optic neuropathy. *American Journal of Ophthalmology* **86**, 206–210.

Lin, J.-J. & Chang, M.-K. (1994) Hemiballism–hemichorea and non-ketotic hyperglycaemia. *Journal of Neurology, Neurosurgery and Psychiatry* **57**, 748–750.

Lindenstrom, E., Boysen, G., Christiansen, L.W., Hansen B.R. & Nielsen, P.W. (1991) Reliability of the Scandinavian Neurological Stroke Scale. *Cerebrovascular Diseases* **1**, 103–107.

Lindley, R.I., Warlow, C.P., Wardlaw, J.M., Dennis, M.S., Slattery, J. & Sandercock, P.A.G. (1993) Interobserver reliability of a clinical classification of acute cerebral infarction. *Stroke* **24**, 1801–1804.

Ling, R. & James, B. (1998) White-centred retinal haemorrhages (Roth spots). *Postgraduate Medical Journal* **74**, 581–582.

Linzer, M., McFarland, T.A., Belkin, M. & Caplan, L. (1992) Critical carotid and vertebral arterial occlusive disease and cough syncope. *Stroke* **23**, 1017–1020.

Liotti, M., Sava, D., Rizzolatti, G. & Carrarra, P.I. (1991) Differential hemispheric asymmetries in depression and anxiety: a reaction time study. *Biological Psychiatry* **29**, 887–899.

Lodder, J., Bamford, J., Kappelle, J. & Boiten, J. (1994) What causes false clinical prediction of small deep infarcts? *Stroke* **25**, 86–91.

Longo, D.L. & Witherspoon, J.M. (1980) Focal neurological symptoms in hypercalcaemia. *Neurology* **30**, 200–201.

Lopez, L.I., Gresty, M.A., Bronstein, A.M., du Boulay, E.P. & Rudge, P. (1996) Clinical and MRI correlations in 27 patients with acquired pendular nystagmus. *Brain* **119**, 465–472.

Louis, E.D., King, D., Sacco, R. & Mohr, J.P. (1995) Upper motor neuron signs in acute stroke: prevalence, interobserver reliability, and timing of initial examination. *Journal of Stroke Cerebrovascular Diseases* **5**, 49–55.

Ludman, H. (1990) Menière's disease. *British Medical Journal* **301**, 1232–1233.

Luxon, L.M. & Harrison, M.J. (1979) Chronic subdural haematoma. *Quarterly Journal of Medicine* **48**, 43–53.

McAlister, F.A., Straus, S.E., & Sackett, D.L., on behalf of the CARE-COAD1 Group (1999) Why we need large, simple studies of the clinical examination: the problem and a proposed solution. *Lancet* **354**, 1721–1724.

Maccario, M. (1968) Neurological dysfunction associated with nonketotic hyperglycaemia. *Archives of Neurology* **19**, 535–536.

McCormick, G.F. & Halbach, V.V. (1993) Recurrent ischaemic events in two patients with painless vertebral artery dissection. *Stroke* **24**, 598–602.

McCormick, G.F., Zee, C. & Heiden, J. (1982) Cysticercosis cerebri: review of 127 cases. *Archives of Neurology* **39**, 534.

MacDonnell, R.A.L., Donnan, G.A., Bladin, P.F., Berkovic, S.F. & Wriedt, C.H.R. (1988) The electroencephalogram and acute ischaemic stroke: distinguishing cortical from lacunar infarction. *Archives of Neurology* **45**, 520–524.

McKee, A.C., Levine, D., Kowall, N.W. & Richardson, E.P. Jr (1990) Peduncular hallucinosis associated with isolated infarction of the substantia nigra pars reticulata. *Annals of Neurology* **27**, 500.

McLean, B.N., Miller, D. & Thompson, E.J. (1995) Oligoclonal banding of IgG in CSF, blood–brain barrier function, and MRI findings in patients with sarcoidosis, systemic lupus erythematosus, and Behçet's disease involving the nervous system. *Journal of Neurology, Neurosurgery and Psychiatry* **58**, 548–554.

McNaughton, H.K. & Will, R.G. (1994) Creutzfeldt–Jakob disease presenting acutely as stroke: an analysis of 30 cases. *Annals of Neurology* **36**, 313.

Malkowicz, D.E., Legido, A., Jackel, R.A., Sussman, N.M., Eskin, B.A. & Harner, R.N. (1995) Prolactin secretion following repetitive seizures. *Neurology* **45**, 448–452.

Malouf, R. & Brust, J.C.M. (1985) Hypoglycaemia: causes, neurological manifestations and outcome. *Annals of Neurology* **17**, 421–430.

Manschot, S., van Passel, L., Buskens, E., Algra, A. & van Gijn, J. (1998) Mayo and NINDS scales for assessment of tendon reflexes: between observer agreement and implications for communication. *Journal of Neurology, Neurosurgery and Psychiatry* **64**, 253–255.

Markowitz, H. & Kokmen, E. (1983) Neurologic diseases and the cerebrospinal fluid immunoglobulin profile. *Mayo Clinic Proceedings* **58**, 273–274.

Marshall, J.C. & Halligan, P.W. (1993) Visuo-spatial neglect: a new copying test to assess perceptual parsing. *Journal of Neurology* **240**, 37–40.

Martin, J.D., Valentine, J., Myers, S.I., Rossi, M.B., Patterson, C.B. & Clagett, G.P. (1991) Is routine CT scanning necessary in the preoperative evaluation of patients undergoing carotid endarterectomy? *Journal of Vascular Surgery* **14**, 267–270.

Martin, R., Bogousslavsky, J. & Regli, F. (1992) Striatocapsular infarction and 'release' visual hallucinations. *Cerebrovascular Diseases* **2**, 111–113.

Mas, J.L. & Lamy, C. (1998) Stroke in pregnancy and the puerperium. *Journal of Neurology* **245**, 305–313.

Masdeu, J.C. & Gorelick, P.B. (1988) Thalamic astasia: inability to stand after unilateral thalamic lesions. *Annals of Neurology* **23**, 596–603.

Matsumoto, S., Okuda, B., Imai, T. & Kameyama, M. (1988) A sensory level on the trunk in lower lateral brainstem lesions. *Neurology* **38**, 1515–1519.

Matthews, W.B. (1975). *Practical Neurology*. 3rd edn, p. 76. Blackwell Scientific Publications, London.

Mauser, H.W., van Huffelen, A.C. & Tulleken, C.A.F. (1986) The EEG in the diagnosis of subdural empyema. *Electroencephalography and Clinical Neurophysiology* **64**, 511–516.

Meissner, I., Wiebers, D.O., Swanson, J.W. & O'Fallon, W.M. (1986) The natural history of drop attacks. *Neurology* **36**, 1029–1034.

Melamed, E., Lavy, S. & Reches, A. (1975) Chronic subdural haematoma simulating transient cerebral ischaemic attacks: case report. *Journal of Neurosurg* **42**, 101–103.

Melo, T.P., de Mendonca, A., Crespo, M., Carvalho, M. & Ferro, J.M. (1992a) An emergency room based study of stroke coma. *Cerebrovascular Diseases* **2**, 93–101.

Melo, T.P., Bogousslavsky, J., Moulin, T., Nader, J. & Regli, F. (1992b) Thalamic ataxia. *Journal of Neurology* **239**, 331–337.

Melo, T.P., Ferro, J.M. & Ferro, H. (1992c) Transient global amnesia: a case–control study. *Brain* **115**, 261–270.

Meyer, J.S., Terayama, Y., Konno, S. *et al.* (1998) Age-related cerebrovascular disease alters the symptomatic course of migraine. *Cephalgia* **18**, 202–208.

Mignot, E. (1998) Genetic and family aspects of narcolepsy. *Neurology* **50** (Suppl. 1), S16–S22.

Mitchell, P., Wang, J.J., Li, W., Leeder, S.R. & Smith, W. (1997) Prevalence of asymptomatic retinal emboli in an Australian urban community. *Stroke* **28**, 63–66.

Mohr, J.P., Kase, C.S., Meckler, R.J. & Fisher, C.M. (1977) Sensorimotor stroke due to thalamocapsular ischemia. *Archives of Neurology* **34**, 734–741.

Mohr, J.P., Pessin, M.S., Finkelstein, S., Funkenstein, H.H., Duncan, G.W. & Davis, K.R. (1978a) Broca aphasia: pathologic and clinical. *Neurology* **28**, 311–324.

Mohr, J.P., Caplan, L.R., Melski, J. *et al.* (1978b) The Harvard Cooperative Stroke Registry: a prospective registry. *Neurology* **28**, 754–762.

Mohr, J.P., Biller, J., Hilal, S.K. *et al.* (1995) Magnetic resonance versus computed tomographic imaging in acute stroke. *Stroke* **26**, 807–812.

Monrad-Krohn, G.H. (1947) Dysprosody or altered melody of language. *Brain* **70**, 405–415.

Montgomery, B.M. & Pinner, C.A. (1964) Transient hypoglycaemic hemiplegia. *Archives of Internal Medicine* **114**, 680–684.

Mori, E. & Yamadori, A. (1987) Acute confusional state and acute agitated delirium: occurrence after infarction in the right middle cerebral artery territory. *Archives of Neurology* **44**, 1139–1143.

Moster, M.L., Johnston, D.E. & Reinmuth, O.M. (1983) Chronic subdural haematoma with transient neurological deficits: a review of 15 cases. *Annals of Neurology* **14**, 539–542.

Murros, K.E., Evans, G.W., Toole, J.F., Howard, G. & Rose, L.A. (1989) Cerebral infarction in patients with transient ischaemic attacks. *Journal of Neurology* **236**, 182–184.

Nakamura, K., Saku, Y., Ibayashi, S. & Fujishima, M. (1999) Progressive motor deficits in lacunar infarction. *Neurology* **52**, 29–33.

Nicoli, F., Milandre, L., Lemarquis, P., Bazan, M. & Jau, P. (1990) Hématomes sous-duraux chroniques et déficits neurologiques transitoires. *Revue Neurologique (Paris)* **146**, 256–263.

Noda, S., Kawada, M. & Umezaki, H. (1981) A case of chronic subdural haematoma simulating transient cerebral ischaemic attacks. *Clinical Neurology* **21**, 271–273.

Norris, J.W. & Hachinski, V.C. (1982) Misdiagnosis of stroke. *Lancet* **i**, 328.

Norrving, B., Magnusson, M. & Holtas, S. (1995) Isolated acute vertigo in the elderly: vestibular or vascular disease? *Acta Neurologica Scandinavica* **91**, 43–48.

Oas, J.G. & Baloh, R.W. (1992) Vertigo and the anterior inferior cerebellar artery syndrome. *Neurology* **42**, 2274–2279.

Olesen, J. (1988) Classification and diagnostic criteria for headache disorders, cranial neuralgias and facial pain. *Cephalgia* **8** (Suppl. 7), 19–28.

Olesen, J., Friberg, L., Olsen, T.K. *et al.* (1993) Ischaemia-induced (symptomatic) migraine attacks may be more frequent than migraine-induced ischaemic insults. *Brain* **116**, 187–202.

Omae, T., Tsuchiya, T. & Yamaguchi, T. (1992) Cheiro-oral syndrome due to lesions in the corona radiata. *Stroke* **23**, 599–601.

O'Sullivan, F., Rossor, M. & Elston, J.S. (1992) Amaurosis fugax in young people. *British Journal of Ophthalmology* **76**, 660–662.

Ott, B.R. & Saver, J.L. (1993) Unilateral amnesic stroke. *Stroke* **24**, 1033–1042.

Paciaroni, M. & Bogousslavsky, J. (1998) Pure sensory syndromes in thalamic stroke. *European Neurology* **39**, 211–217.

Palmer, E., Ashly, P. & Hajek, V.E. (1992) Ipsilateral fast corticospinal pathways do not account for recovery in stroke. *Annals of Neurology* **32**, 519–525.

Patten, J. (1995) *Neurological Differential Diagnosis*. Springer-Verlag, London.

Paylor, R.R., Selhorst, J.B. & Weinberg, R.S. (1985) Reversible monocular cataract simulating amaurosis fugax. *Annals of Opththalmology* **17**, 423–425.

Peatfield, R.C. (1987) Can transient ischaemic attacks and classical migraine always be distinguished? *Headache* **27**, 240–243.

Pedersen, P.M., Jorgensen, H.S., Nakayama, H., Raaschou, H.O. & Olsen, T.S. (1995) Aphasia in acute stroke: incidence, determinants, and recovery. *Annals of Neurology* **38**, 659–666.

Pedersen, P.M., Jorgensen, H.S., Nakayama, H., Raaschou, H.O. & Olsen, T.S. (1998) Impaired orientation in acute stroke: frequency, determinants, and time-course of recovery. *Cerebrovascular Diseases* **8**, 90–96.

Penfield, W. & Boldrey, E. (1937) Somatic motor and sensory representation in the cerebral cortex of man as studied by electrical stimulation. *Brain* **60**, 389–443.

Penfield, W. & Rasmussen, T. (1950). *The Cerebral Cortex of Man*. Macmillan, New York.

Perkin, G.D. & Joseph, R. (1986) Neurological manifestations of the hyperventilation syndrome. *Journal of Royal Society of Medicine* **79**, 448–450.

Pierrot-Deseilligny, C., Rivaud, S., Penet, C. & Rigolet, M.-H. (1987) Latencies of visually guided saccades in unilateral hemispheric cerebral lesions. *Annals of Neurology* **21**, 138–148.

Plum, F. & Posner, J.B. (1985) *Diagnosis of Stupor and Coma*. 3rd edn. Philadephia. FA Davis.

Prasad, K. & Menon, G.R. (1998) Comparison of three strategies of verbal scoring of the Glasgow Coma Scale in patients with stroke. *Cerebrovascular Diseases* **8**, 79–85.

Rao, M.L., Stefan, H. & Bauer, J. (1989) Epileptic but not psychogenic seizures are accompanied by simultaneous elevation of serum pituitary hormones and cortisol levels. *Neuroendocrinology* **49**, 33–39.

Rao, T.H., Schneider, L.B. & Lupyan, Y. (1994) Transient unresponsiveness in the elderly. *Archives of Neurology* **51**, 644.

Ravits, J. & Seybold, M.E. (1984) Transient monocular visual loss from narrow angle glaucoma. *Archives of Neurology* **41**, 991–993.

Reggia, J.A., Tabb, R., Price, T.R., Banko, M. & Hebel, R. (1984) Computer-aided assessment of transient ischaemic attacks: a clinical evaluation. *Archives of Neurology* **41**, 1248–1254.

Reich, J.B., Sierra, J., Camp, W., Zanzonico, P., Deck, M.D.F. & Plum, F. (1993) Magnetic resonance imaging measurements and clinical changes accompanying transtentorial and foramen magnum brain herniation. *Annals of Neurology* **33**, 159–170.

Reich, K.A., Giansiracusa, D.F. & Strongwater, S.L. (1990) Neurologic manifestations of giant cell arteritis. *American Journal of Medicine* **89**, 67–72.

Ropper, A. (1986) Lateral displacement of the brain and level of consciousness in patients with acute hemispheral mass. *New England Journal of Medicine* **314**, 953–958.

Ropper, A.H. (1989) A preliminary MRI study of the geometry of brain displacement and level of consciousness with acute intracranial masses. *Neurology* **39**, 622–627.

Ropper, A.H., Fisher, C.M. & Kleinman, G.M. (1979) Pyramidal infarction in the medulla: a cause of pure motor hemiplegia sparing the face. *Neurology* **29**, 91–95.

Ross, E.D. (1980) Localization of the pyramidal tract in the internal capsule by whole brain dissection. *Neurology* **30**, 59–64.

Ross, E.D. & Stewart, R.M. (1981) Akinetic mutism from hypothalamic damage: successful treatment with dopamine agonists. *Neurology* **31**, 1435–1439.

Ross, T.R. (1983) Transient tumour attacks. *Archives of Neurology* **40**, 633–636.

Rother, J., Schreiner, A., Wentz, K.-U. & Hennerici, M. (1992) Hypoglycaemia presenting as basilar artery thrombosis. *Stroke* **23**, 112–113.

Rothwell, P.M. (1994) Investigation of unilateral sensory or motor symptoms: frequency of neurological pathology depends on side of symptoms. *Journal of Neurology, Neurosurgery and Psychiatry* **57**, 1401–1402.

Rothwell, P.M. & Warlow, C.P. on behalf of the European Carotid Surgery Trialists' Collaborative Group (1999) Prediction of benefit from carotid endarterectomy in individual patients: a risk-modelling study. *Lancet* **353**, 2105–2110.

Ruby, R.J. & Burton, J.R. (1977) Acute reversible hemiparesis and hyponatraemia. *Lancet* **i**, 1212.

Ruotolo, C., Hazan, H., Rancurel, G. & Kieffer, E. (1992) Dynamic arteriography. In: *Vertebrobasilar Arterial Disease* (eds R. Berguer & L.R. Caplan), pp. 116–123. Quality Medical Publishing, St Louis.

Russell, J.R. & DeMeyer, W. (1961) The quantitative cortical origin of pyramidal axons of *Macaca rhesus*, with some remarks on the slow rate of axolysis. *Neurology* **11**, 96–108.

Russo, L.S. (1983) Focal dystonia and lacunar infarction of the basal ganglia: a case report. *Archives of Neurology* **40**, 61–62.

Sacco, R.L., Bello, J.A., Traub, R. & Brust, J.C.M. (1987) Selective proprioceptive loss from a thalamic lacunar stroke. *Stroke* **18**, 1160–1163.

Sackett, D.L., Haynes, R.B., Guyatt, G.H. & Tugwell, P. (1991). *Clinical Epidemiology: a Basic Science for Clinical Medicine*, 2nd edn, pp. 19–49. Little, Brown, Boston.

Saeki, N., Murai, N. & Sunami, K. (1996) Midbrain tegmental lesions affecting or sparing the pupillary fibres. *Journal of Neurology, Neurosurgery and Psychiatry* **61**, 401–406.

Sage, J.I. & van Uitert, R.L. (1986) Man-in-the-barrel syndrome. *Neurology* **36**, 1102–1103.

Sakas, D.E., Dias, L.S. & Beale, D. (1995) Subarachnoid haemorrhage presenting as head injury. *British Medical Journal* **310**, 1186–1187.

Samuels, A.H. (1995) Somatisation disorder: a major public health issue. *Medical Journal of Australia* **163**, 147–149.

Sandercock, P.A.G. (1991) Recent developments in the diagnosis and management of patients with transient ischaemic attacks and minor ischaemic stroke. *Quarterly Journal of Medicine* **286** (78), 101–112.

Sandercock, P.A.G. & Smart, S.E. (1990) Migraine or amaurosis fugax? The value of ultrasound. *Scottish Medical Journal* **35**, 147.

Sandercock, P.A.G., Molyneux, A. & Warlow, C. (1985) Value of computed tomography in patients with stroke: Oxfordshire Community Stroke Project. *British Medical Journal* **290**, 193–197.

Saul, R.F., Gallagher, J.G. & Mateer, J.E. (1986) Sudden hemiparesis as the presenting sign in cryptococcal meningitis. *Stroke* **17**, 753–754.

Schmidtke, K. & Buttner-Ennever, J.A. (1992) Nervous control of eyelid function: a review of clinical, experimental and pathological data. *Brain* **115**, 227–247.

Scholl, G.B., Song, H.-S. & Wray, S.H. (1991) Uhthoff's symptom in optic neuritis: relationship to magnetic resonance imaging and development of multiple sclerosis. *Annals of Neurology* **30**, 180–184.

Schott, G.D. (1993) Penfield's homunculus: a note on cerebral cartography. *Journal of Neurology, Neurosurgery and Psychiatry* **56**, 329–333.

Scott, W.R. & Miller, B.R. (1985) Intracerebral haemorrhage with rapid recovery. *Archives of Neurology* **42**, 133–136.

Sempere, A.P., Duarte, J., Coria, F. & Claveria, L.E. (1992) Loss of vision by the colour white: a sign of carotid occlusive disease. *Stroke* **23**, 1179.

Severin, S.L., Tour, R.L. & Kershaw, R.H. (1967) Macular function and the photostress test 2. *Archives of Ophthalmology* **77**, 163–167.

Seybold, M.E. & Rosen, P.N. (1977) Peripapillary staphyloma and amaurosis fugax. *Annals of Ophthalmology* **9**, 1139–1141.

Shah, A.B., Beamer, N. & Coull, B.M. (1985) Enhanced *in vivo* platelet activation in subtypes of ischaemic stroke. *Stroke* **16**, 643–647.

Sharma, S., ten Hove, M.W., Pinkerton, R.M. & Cruess, A.F. (1997) Interobserver agreement in the evaluation of acute retinal artery occlusion. *Canadian Journal of Ophthalmology* **32**, 441–444.

Sharma, S., Pater, J.L., Lam, M. & Cruess, A.F. (1998) Can different types of retinal emboli be reliably differentiated from one another? An inter- and intraobserver agreement study. *Canadian Journal of Ophthalmology* **33**, 144–148.

Shaw, C.M., Alvord, E.C. & Berry, R.G. (1959) Swelling of the brain following ischaemic infarction with arterial occlusion. *Archives of Neurology* **1**, 161–177.

Shinar, D., Gross, C.R., Mohr, J.P. *et al.* (1985) Interobserver variability in the assessment of neurologic history and examination in the Stroke Data Bank. *Archives of Neurology* **42**, 557–565.

Silas, J.H., Grant, D.S. & Maddocks, J.L. (1981) Transient hemiparetic attacks due to unrecognised nocturnal hypoglycaemia. *British Medical Journal* **282**, 132–133.

Silver, F.L., Norris, J.W., Lewis, A.J. & Hachinski, V.C. (1984) Early mortality following stroke: a prospective view. *Stroke* **3**, 492–496.

Sisk, C., Ziegler, D.K. & Zileli, T. (1970) Discrepancies in recorded results from duplicate neurological history and examination in patients studied for prognosis in cerebrovascular disease. *Stroke* **1**, 14–18.

Slater, R. (1979) Benign recurrent vertigo. *Journal of Neurology, Neurosurgery and Psychiatry* **42**, 363–367.

Solomon, D.H., Barohn, R.J., Bazan, C. & Grissom, J. (1994) The thalamic ataxia syndrome. *Neurology* **44**, 810–814.

Spudis, E.V. (1991) The persistent vegetative state, 1990. *Journal of Neurological Sciences* **102**, 128–136.

Stark, S.R. (1985) Transient dyskinesia and cerebral ischaemia. *Neurology* **35**, 445.

Stell, R., Davis, S. & Carroll, W.M. (1994) Unilateral asterixis due to a lesion of the ventrolateral thalamus. *Journal of Neurology, Neurosurgery and Psychiatry* **57**, 878–880.

Stephen, L.J., Maxwell, J.E. & Brodie, M.J. (1999) Transient hemiparesis with topiramate. *British Medical Journal* **318**, 845.

Stern, D.B. (1977) Lateral distribution of conversion reactions. *Journal of Nervous and Mental Disease* **164**, 122–128.

Sterzi, R., Bottini, G. & Celani, M.G. (1993) Hemianopia, hemianaesthesia, and hemiplegia after right and left hemisphere damage: a hemispheric difference. *Journal of Neurology, Neurosurgery and Psychiatry* **56**, 308–310.

Stevens, D.L. & Matthews, W.B. (1973) Cryptogenic drop attacks: an affliction of women. *British Medical Journal* **1**, 439–442.

Stone, S.P., Wilson, B., Wroot, A. *et al.* (1991) The assessment of visuo-spatial neglect after acute stroke. *Journal of Neurology, Neurosurgery and Psychiatry* **54**, 345–350.

Stone, S.P., Patel, P., Greenwood, R.J. & Halligan, P.W. (1992) Measuring visual neglect in acute stroke and predicting its recovery: the visual neglect recovery index. *Journal of Neurology, Neurosurgery and Psychiatry* **55**, 431–436.

Strupp, M., Brandt, T. & Steddin, S. (1995) Horizontal canal benign paroxysmal positional vertigo: reversible ipsilateral caloric hypoexcitability caused by canalolithiasis? *Neurology* **45**, 2072–2076.

Strupp, M., Bruning, R., Wu, R.H., Deimling, M., Reisser, M. & Brandt, T. (1998) Diffusion-weighted MRI in transient global amnesia: signal intensity in the left mesial temporal lobe in 7 of 10 patients. *Annals of Neurology* **43**, 164–170.

Suzuki, I., Shimizu, H., Ishijima, B., Tani, K., Sugishita, M. & Adachi, N. (1992) Aphasic seizure caused by focal epilepsy in the left fusiform gyrus. *Neurology* **42**, 2207–2210.

Tatemichi, T.K., Young, W.L., Prohovnik, I., Gitelman, D.R., Correll, J.W. & Mohr, J.P. (1990) Perfusion insufficiency in limb-shaking transient ischaemic attacks. *Stroke* **21**, 341–347.

Teasdale, G. & Jennett, B. (1974) Assessment of coma and impaired consciousness: a practical scale. *Lancet* **ii**, 81–84.

Teman, A.J., Winterkorn, J.M.S. & Weiner, D. (1995) Transient monocular blindness associated with sexual intercourse. *New England Journal of Medicine* **333**, 393.

Terao, S., Takatsu, S., Izumi, M. *et al.* (1997) Central facial weakness due to medial medullary infarction: the course of facial corticobulbar fibres. *Journal of Neurology, Neurosurgery and Psychiatry* **63**, 391–393.

Tettenborn, B., Caplan, L.R., Sloan, M.A. *et al.* (1993) Postoperative brainstem and cerebellar infarcts. *Neurology* **43**, 471–477.

Thijs, R.D., Notermans, N.C., Wokke, J.H.J., van der Graaf, Y. & van Gijn, J. (1998) Distribution of muscle weakness of central and peripheral origin. *Journal of Neurology, Neurosurgery and Psychiatry* **65**, 794–796.

Timsit, S., Logak, M., Manai, R. & Rancurel, G. (1997) Evolving isolated hand palsy: a parietal lobe syndrome associated with carotid artery disease. *Brain* **120**, 2251–2257.

Tippin, J., Corbett, J.J., Kerber, R.E., Schroeder, E. & Thompson, H.S. (1989) Amaurosis fugax and ocular infarction in adolescents and young adults. *Annals of Neurology* **26**, 69–77.

Todd, R.B. (1856). *Clinical Lectures on Paralysis*. Churchill, London.

Toole, J.F. & Tucker, S.H. (1960) Influence of head position upon cerebral circulation. *Archives of Neurology* **2**, 616–623.

Torvik, A. & Jorgensen, L. (1964) Thrombotic and embolic occlusions of the carotid arteries in an autopsy series, 1: prevalence, location and associated disease. *Journal of Neurological Sciences* **1**, 24–39.

Torvik, A. & Jorgensen, L. (1966) Thrombotic and embolic occlusions of the carotid arteries in an autopsy series, 2: cerebral lesions and clinical course. *Journal of Neurological Sciences* **3**, 410–432.

Trobe, J.D., Lorber, M.L. & Schlezinger, N.S. (1973) Isolated homonymous hemianopia. *Archives of Ophthalmology* **89**, 377–381.

Twomey, J.A. & Espir, M.L.E. (1980) Paroxysmal symptoms as the first manifestations of multiple sclerosis. *Journal of Neurology, Neurosurgery and Psychiatry* **43**, 296–304.

Urban, P.P., Wicht, S., Hopf, N.C., Fleischer, S. & Nickel, O. (1999) Isolated dysarthria due to extracerebellar lacunar stroke: a central monoparesis of the tongue. *Journal of Neurology, Neurosurgery and Psychiatry* **66**, 495–501.

Vestergaard, K., Andersen, G., Nielsen, M.I. & Jensen, T.S. (1993) Headache in stroke. *Stroke* **24**, 1621–1624.

Victor, M., Adams, R.D. & Cole, M. (1965) The acquired hepatocerebral degeneration. *Medicine (Baltimore)* **44**, 345–396.

Victor, M., Adams, R.D. & Collins, G.H. (1989). *The Wernicke–Korsakoff Syndrome and Related Neurologic Disorders Due to Alcoholism and Malnutrition*, 2nd edn. Davis, Philadelphia.

Von Kummer, R., Allen, K.L., Holle, R. *et al.* (1997) Acute stroke: usefulness of early CT findings before thrombolytic therapy. *Radiology* **205**, 327–333.

Vortmeyer, A.O., Hagel, C. & Laas, R. (1992) Haemorrhagic thiamine deficient encephalopathy following prolonged parenteral nutrition. *Journal of Neurology, Neurosurgery and Psychiatry* **55**, 826–829.

Wade, D.T. & Johnston, C. (1999) The permanent vegetative state: practical guidance on diagnosis and management. *British Medical Journal* **319**, 841–844.

Walker, G.L., Williamson, P.M., Ravich, R.B. & Roche, J. (1980) Hypercalcaemia associated with cerebral vasospasm causing infarction. *Journal of Neurology, Neurosurgery and Psychiatry* **43**, 464–467.

Wallis, W.E., Donaldson, I., Scott, R.S. & Wilson, J. (1985) Hypoglycaemia masquerading as cerebrovascular disease (hypoglycaemic hemiplegia). *Annals of Neurology* **18**, 510–512.

Wardlaw, J.M. (1994) Is routine computed tomography in strokes unnecessary? *British Medical Journal* **309**, 1498–1500.

Watson, Y.I., Arfken, C.L. & Birge, S.J. (1993) Clock completion: an objective screening test for dementia. *Journal of the American Geriatrics Society* **41**, 1235–1240.

Waxman, S.G. & Toole, J.F. (1983) Temporal profile resembling TIA in the setting of cerebral infarction. *Stroke* **14**, 433–437.

Weidauer, S., Claus, D. & Gartenschlager, M. (1999) Spinal sulcal artery syndrome due to spontaneous bilateral vertebral artery dissection. *Journal of Neurology, Neurosurgery and Psychiatry* **67**, 550–551.

Weisberg, L.A. & Nice, C.N. (1977) Intracranial tumour simulating the presentation of cerebrovascular syndromes: early detection with cerebral computed tomography. *American Journal of Medicine* **63**, 517–524.

Welch, K.M.A. (1994) Relationship of stroke and migraine. *Neurology* **44** (Suppl. 7), S33–S36.

Welch, K.M.A. & Levine, S.R. (1990) Migraine-related stroke in the context of the International Headache Society Classification of Head Pain. *Archives of Neurology* **47**, 458–462.

Wessely, S., Nimnuan, C. & Sharpe, M. (1999) Functional somatic syndromes: one or many? *Lancet* **354**, 936–939.

Whisnant, J.P. & Colleagues for the National Institute of Neurological Disorders and Stroke (1990) Classification of cerebrovascular diseases, 3. *Stroke* **21**, 637–676.

Whisnant, J.P., Brown, R.D., Petty, G.W., O'Fallon, W.M., Sicks, J.D. & Wiebers, D.O. (1999) Comparison of population-based models of risk factors for TIA and ischemic stroke. *Neurology* **53**, 532–536.

Whiteley, S.M., Murphy, P.G., Kirollos, R.W. & Swindells, S.R. (1993) Headache after dural puncture. *British Medical Journal* **306**, 917–918.

Whitty, C.W.M. (1967) Migraine without headache. *Lancet* **ii**, 283–285.

Wiebers, D.O., Swanson, J.W., Cascino, T.L. & Whisnant, J.P. (1989) Bilateral loss of vision in bright light. *Stroke* **20**, 554–558.

Wijman, C.A., Wolf, P.A., Kase, C.S., Kelly-Hayes, M. & Beiser, A.S. (1998) Migrainous visual accompaniments are not rare in late life: the Framingham study. *Stroke* **29**, 1539–1543.

Wilkes, S.R., Troutmann, J.C., DeSanto, L.W. & Campbell, R.J. (1979) Osteoma: an unusual cause of amaurosis fugax. *Mayo Clinical Proceedings* **54**, 258–260.

Williams, D. & Wilson, T.G. (1962) The diagnosis of the major and minor syndromes of basilar insufficiency. *Brain* **85**, 741–774.

Williams, R.S. (1979) Chronic subdural haematoma simulating transient cerebral ischaemic attacks. *Annals of Neurology* **5**, 597.

Winterkorn, J.M.S. & Teman, A.J. (1991) Recurrent attacks of amaurosis fugax treated with calcium channel blocker. *Annals of Neurology* **30**, 423–425.

Wise, R.J.S., Greene, J., Büchel, C. & Scott, S.K. (1999) Brain regions involved in articulation. *Lancet* **353**, 1057–1061.

Wroe, S.J., Sandercock, P., Bamford, J., Dennis, M., Slattery, J. & Warlow, C. (1992) Diurnal variation in incidence of stroke: Oxfordshire community stroke project. *British Medical Journal* **304**, 155–157.

Yanagihara, T., Piepgras, D.G. & Klass, D.W. (1985) Repetitive involuntary movements associated with episodic cerebral ischaemia. *Annals of Neurology* **18**, 244–250.

Yanagihara, T., Klass, D.W., Piepgras, D.G. & Houser, O.W. (1989) Brief loss of consciousness in bilateral carotid occlusive disease. *Archives of Neurology* **46**, 858–861.

Yerby, M.S., van Belle, G., Friel, P.N. & Wilensky, A.J. (1987) Serum prolactins in the diagnosis of epilepsy: sensitivity, specificity, and predictive value. *Neurology* **37**, 1224–1226.

Zaidat, O.O., Werz, M.A., Landis, D.M.D. & Selman, W. (1999) Orthostatic limb shaking from carotid hypoperfusion. *Neurology* **53**, 650.

Zaret, B.S. (1985) Lightning streaks of Moore: a cause of recurrent stereotypic visual disturbance. *Neurology* **35**, 1078–1081.

Zeman, A.Z.J., Boniface, S.J. & Hodges, J.R. (1998) Transient epileptic amnesia: a description of the clinical and neuropsychological features in 10 cases and a review of the literature. *Journal of Neurology, Neurosurgery and Psychiatry* **64**, 435–443.

CHAPTER FOUR

Which arterial territory is involved? Developing a clinically-based method of subclassification

4.1 General introduction

Once the clinical diagnosis of a cerebrovascular (vs. non-vascular) event has been made, one should then consider how extending the diagnostic process (i.e. further subclassification) might help in the subsequent investigation and management of patients and their relatives. Table 4.1 lists the reasons for subclassifying patients with cerebrovascular disease, which, whilst not all of immediate value to the individual patient, may be helpful when considering the general management of cerebrovascular disease and overall burden to the community.

Table 4.1 Potential benefits of subclassifying patients with symptomatic cerebrovascular disease (strokes and transient ischaemic attacks).

Aid cost-effective and timely search for the cause of the stroke and associated risk factors
Aid planning of immediate supportive care and rehabilitation programme
Improve prognostication for survival, functional outcome, and recurrence
Stratify entry to clinical trials to reduce heterogeneity and therefore have the best chance of demonstrating treatment benefit if it is present
Help put the results of clinical trials into the context of an individual physician's own practice
Provide more sensitive assessment of casemix in individual units, for comparative audit and contracting purposes
Aid audit of management

It is stating the obvious to say that there is still no uniformity of subclassification either between or within countries, or often even amongst different patients of an individual physician. There are undoubtedly many reasons for this, and indeed, since the first edition of this book, the extra dimension of new hyper-acute treatments and the developing concept of 'brain attack' have added further complexity.

In the era before computed tomography (CT), considerable interest was focused on time-based subclassification. However, we have seen already that the distinction between stroke and transient ischaemic attack (TIA) (i.e. whether symptoms persist for more or less than 24 h) is arbitrary, does not have any rational pathophysiological basis (section 3.2), and is of little value to the physician seeing a patient with persisting symptoms a few hours after onset. Similarly, there is no evidence to suggest that a distinction between 'major stroke' and 'minor stroke' (defined as symptoms lasting more or less than 1 week, respectively (Royal College of Physicians 1989), or reversible ischaemic neurological deficit (RIND)—variously defined as cases in which symptoms resolve in less than 1 week or 3 weeks—conveys any useful pathophysiological information. Setting aside for one moment the fact that any stroke (major or minor) may be caused by cerebral haemorrhage or infarction, an identical vascular lesion (of which carotid occlusion would be a good example) might give any of these temporal patterns, or even be asymptomatic. To the physician seeing patients with stroke acutely (even if that is not within the first 24 h), the fact that the complete time-based classification may not be made in all cases until at least a week has elapsed means that the system is only of value in retrospect. Furthermore, contrary to what one might think, it does not impart any useful information about residual disability, since a patient with persistent tingling in one hand for more than 1 week would be classified technically as having a 'major stroke' in just the same way as a patient who had a dense hemiplegia. Additionally, the tendency for some physicians to use the terms 'minor' and 'major' as a type of shorthand to describe the level of residual disability simply leads to confusion. Consequently, we will not be using these terms, except in a few places where we will define exactly what we mean by 'major', 'minor', etc.

There are now a number of well known and somewhat similar schemes of subclassification (usually only applicable to ischaemic stroke) that focus on the underlying cause of the stroke (e.g. Kunitz *et al.* 1984; Bogousslavsky *et al.* 1988; Foulkes *et al.* 1988; Adams *et al.* 1993). Most of these were developed for specific research projects in specialist institutions—a quite different situation from routine clinical practice. Inherent in most of them is an entirely understandable desire to establish the pathophysiological factors underlying every individual stroke, since it is with this knowledge that rational treatments aimed both at limiting the acute damage and at secondary prevention will be developed and deployed. However, even with the most intensive investigation protocols, such diagnostic certainty remains elusive in up to 40% of patients (Sacco *et al.* 1989; Lindgren *et al.* 1994a). Furthermore, such classifications have only moderate inter-observer reliability (Gross *et al.* 1986; Gordon *et al.* 1993; Berger *et al.* 1996). A further problem is that of trying to classify the mechanism of stroke when patients are assessed in the hyper-acute phase. Using the detailed protocol of the TOAST study, Madden *et al.* (1995) reported that the initial (< 24 h from onset) impression of stroke subtype of the physicians involved in this trial based on clinical, CT, electrocardiographic and initial laboratory results was confirmed in only 62% of cases when the classification was reviewed at three months in the light of all available investigational results (carotid duplex was performed in 73%, echocardiography in 69%, brain magnetic resonance imaging (MRI) in 28% and angiography in 10%). Bogousslavsky *et al.* (1993) reported a series of 100 patients from a single institution with symptoms of less than 12 h duration who were assessed by a dedicated stroke team (a stroke neurologist, a stroke fellow and a neurology resident) by means of a standard protocol (Table 4.2). In this group, the initial clinical diagnosis of stroke aetiology was confirmed by subsequent investigations in 70%, although in a further 24%—initially diagnosed as having large artery disease (16%) or cardioembolism (8%)—the 'error' of the clinical diagnosis occurred only because they were unable to allocate the patients to any specific group according to their protocol after the investigations, i.e. they were finally classified as having infarcts of uncertain origin. It is not known, however, whether this degree of clinical accuracy can be replicated outside the confines of specialist stroke centres.

Table 4.2 Definitions of aetiological subtypes of ischaemic stroke in the Lausanne Stroke Registry (Bogousslavsky *et al.* 1993).

Large artery atherosclerosis

Atherosclerosis with stenosis: narrowing of > 50% of the lumen diameter or occlusion of the corresponding extracranial artery or large intracranial artery (middle cerebral, posterior cerebral or basilar arteries) in the absence of another aetiology

Atherosclerosis without stenosis: plaques or < 50% stenosis in the middle cerebral, posterior cerebral or basilar arteries, in the absence of another aetiology and in patients with at least two of the following five risk factors: age > 50 years, hypertension, diabetes mellitus, cigarette smoking, or hypercholesterolaemia

Cardioembolism

Intracardiac thrombus or tumour, rheumatic mitral stenosis, prosthetic mitral or aortic valves, endocarditis, atrial fibrillation, sick sinus syndrome, left ventricular aneurysm or akinesia after myocardial infarct, acute (< 3 months) myocardial infarct, or global cardiac hypokinesia or dyskinesia, in absence of another aetiology

Small artery disease

Infarction in the territory of a deep perforating artery in a patient with known hypertension, in the absence of another aetiology

Other aetiologies

Includes dissection, fibromuscular dysplasia, saccular aneurysm, arteriovenous malformation, cerebral venous thrombosis on angiography, vasculitis, haematological conditions, migraine, or other

Undetermined aetiology

None of the above causes of cerebral infarction could be determined

> *We still do not have the knowledge or the technology to determine the exact cause of stroke in every patient.*

Thus, whilst clues about the likely cause of the event are apparent from the history and examination (e.g. the presence of atrial fibrillation), any classification that places an undue reliance on the results of investigations will be difficult to use for *every* patient in routine clinical practice (as opposed to research) (Woo *et al.* 1999). Factors that may influence the ability to subclassify in this way include:

- the variable availability of such investigations;
- the perceived appropriateness of using a particular investigation for an individual patient (e.g. because of the degree of pre-stroke or post-stroke disability, cost);
- the variability of the results, arising from both observer-dependent and technology-dependent factors (Chapter 5);
- the speed with which any classification needs to be made (e.g. particularly now for acute treatments, Chapter 11).

A review of the literature on aetiological subclassification shows that most schemes approach the problem almost entirely from the point of view of the acute-phase clinician. However, it is worth noting that despite being used quite widely in research practice, there are no long-term, community-based, natural history studies of strokes subdivided in this way, although incidence rates have been reported recently (Petty *et al.* 1999). What tends to be overlooked is that the process of subclassification of stroke has the potential to refine the practice of many other medical and paramedical professionals, as well as health-care purchasers and planners, and they are often more interested in the clinical deficits and functional consequences resulting from the parenchymal lesion (section 4.3) rather than in the underlying pathogenesis. In view of this, it is perhaps surprising that relatively little attention has been paid to developing classifications based on the site and size of the parenchymal brain lesion. To some extent, this may be because it was anticipated that the advances in neuroimaging would make any clinically based classification redundant, and also the tendency to concentrate on 'scales' that purport to quantify individual neurological deficits, but fail to take a broad view of the effect on the patient as a whole (section 17.6.3). Superficially, a method of subclassification based on the imaged site of parenchymal infarction or ischaemia (i.e. a topographical classification) and then describing this in terms of the likely vascular territory involved would be attractive, and indeed is quite often referred to in the literature (e.g. Bogousslavsky *et al.* 1993). But although imaging has certainly aided our understanding of the anatomical substrate underlying some of the deficits and is of undoubted benefit in the subclassification of primary intracerebral haemorrhage (PICH) and subarachnoid haemorrhage (Chapters 5, 8 and 9), it has so far failed to provide a useful framework for classification of ischaemic stroke and TIA, let alone the entity of 'brain attack'. The reasons for this include the following:

- the enormous inter-individual and intra-individual variability of the vascular supply to the brain (section 4.2);
- the current limitations of even the most sophisticated imaging technology in producing reliable results in *all* patients with stroke—particularly within hours of onset of ischaemic stroke (sections 5.3.5 and 5.3.8);
- the constantly changing technology—even different researchers have different machines;
- the problems with generalizability of such a system, even if appropriate images were available (as they may well be in the future), given current problems with the funding of health care worldwide;
- the current lack of data correlating cross-sectional imaging with outcome;
- the illogicality of basing a system on imaging 'holes in the brain', when the current thrust of acute treatments is to prevent such holes appearing. However, recent developments in diffusion weighted MR imaging are perhaps more promising (section 5.3.9).

One can argue that a basic method of subclassification should, if possible, be applicable to *all* patients during life, irrespective of age, disability and geographical location—and in practical terms, this means having a clinical rather than an investigation-based classification. Further support comes from the many recent community-based studies of stroke that have provided data on the prognosis and have used some form of clinical examination (which can be applied almost universally), supplemented in some studies by ancillary investigations (which may be applied to a subset of patients, selected according to individual circumstances). The conclusions of such studies are much more likely to relate to everyday clinical practice worldwide than those from hospital-based data banks in academic hospitals.

Whilst it is clearly unrealistic to expect any single method of subclassification to satisfy all the disparate requirements of everyone involved in stroke care, service planning, teaching and research, it would seem logical to try and organize the clinical information derived from the history and examination in a manner that facilitates a modular and hierarchical approach to subclassification—i.e. additional but complementary levels of subclassification can be used in any particular situation to suit individual requirements and facilities. After the clinical history and examination, the clinician will have some information about the site of the parenchymal lesion, the vascular territory affected and possibly some clues to the pathogenesis (e.g. the presence of atrial fibrillation). Thus, a basic scheme of subclassification needs to provide a skeleton on which these fragments of information about an individual patient can be hung in an orderly manner so as to orientate further management. It would seem logical to attempt to identify groups of patients with broadly similar parenchymal lesions, since these are likely to be caused by broadly similar types of vascular disease. Following on from this, such groups might be expected to have a distinctive prognosis. In many ways, this process is simply an extension of the traditional neurological teaching of first determining the site of the lesion, since this nearly always narrows the range of possible underlying disorders. Ideally, such a 'core' clinical skeleton, usable in everyday practice, could be built on both by scientists and clinicians according to their access to, or the applicability of, various investigations. Used in this way, a system of classification should also facilitate the integration and application of research findings from the university centres into everyday practice.

It is very important at this point to recognize the limitations of both clinical and instrumental data; neither will be 100% sensitive and specific, although there is a tendency for the results of investigations to be perceived, almost automatically, as the gold standard. This fact may partially explain the trend for the literature to over-emphasize exceptions to general clinical rules, although even the most sophisticated images have to be interpreted (just like physical symptoms and signs) with the potential for both inter-observer and intra-observer variability and significant numbers of false positives and false negatives (section 5.3.5). Thus, anyone using any classification must be blessed with a healthy dose of realism. There is never going to be complete certainty about issues in clinical medicine, and cerebrovascular disease is no exception. There are always going to be exceptions to the rules, and one definition of clinical acumen might be the ability to sense when such exceptions are likely to occur.

One should not presume that the results of investigations will necessarily be any more sensitive or specific than the clinical findings. Investigations contribute most to the diagnostic process when set in a proper clinical context and when they take the pre-test probability of the disorder into account.

In section 4.2, we will review the relevant vascular anatomy, and then in section 4.3 describe a system linking this with the features of the clinical examination of patients with 'brain attack' or stroke that assist parenchymal localization, as discussed in Chapter 3. Although the discussion below relates primarily to infarcts, the syndromes described may equally be caused by PICH. Since not all physicians worldwide have instantaneous access to CT scanning, there is an advantage in having a method that can subclassify strokes irrespective of their pathological type, at least until the type is known as a result of later CT or MR scanning.

4.2 The cerebral arterial supply

4.2.1 Introduction

In order for the information from the clinical history and examination to be formulated in a manner that will have as much relevance as possible to the underlying vascular lesion, the clinician needs to have a working knowledge of the cerebral blood supply. This will also be required for planning and interpreting the results of investigations and assessing the relevance of possible treatments. However, the general assumption that the vascular supply of the brain parenchyma follows an entirely predictable pattern (as depicted in many textbooks) and that there are patterns of infarction which are 'typical' of a particular pathogenesis (e.g. cardioembolism) certainly should not be accepted without closer scrutiny. Many classifications refer to 'standard' maps of the areas of distribution of individual arteries, especially those that have been produced as cross-sectional templates to correspond with CT/MR sections (e.g. Damasio 1983). The theory goes that if one plots the site and size of the lesion seen on the scan onto these maps, then the occluded artery can be identified. Additionally, certain sites are identified as arterial boundary-zones, and further assumptions are then often made about the underlying pathophysiological process—i.e. low flow rather than thromboembolism (sections 4.2.4 and 6.6.5). However, it is clear that the cerebral circulation is a dynamic system with large inter-individual and intra-individual variability (i.e. between hemispheres and even varying with time) (van der Zwan 1990; van der Zwan *et al.* 1992, 1993), and that atheroma or other arterial disease in one part of the system may have complex and relatively unpredictable effects on the patterns of vascular supply. Not surprisingly, this means that attributing an infarct to a particular underlying pathogenesis on the basis of its site and size is often incorrect (Lang *et al.* 1995; Hennerici & Schwartz 1998; Hennerici *et al.* 1998). More recent publications dealing with the localization of the arterial lesion have begun to take this variability into account (Tatu *et al.* 1996; Tatu *et al.* 1998). But even then, there has to be a lesion on the scan to localize—something that is actually becoming less frequent with very early scanning, unless the latest MR techniques are used; and even when lesions are visible, their size may change with time (Fig. 4.1).

Attributing an infarct to a particular pathogenesis purely on the basis of its site and size is often incorrect.

One important consequence of the above is that at the level of the individual patient, the occlusion of a specific artery may present clinically in different ways. Nevertheless, in this chapter, we have attempted to relate each section of the vascular anatomy to the symptoms and signs *commonly* encountered in clinical practice.

The cerebral vascular anatomy can be described in two main parts: the anterior (carotid) and posterior (vertebrobasilar, VB) systems. For each system, there are three components: the extracranial arteries, the major intracranial arteries, and the small (in terms of diameter) superficial and deep perforating arteries. These component arteries have different structural and functional characteristics, which means that infarction within their territory of distribution is likely to be caused predominantly by different causes (Table 4.3). The extracranial vessels (e.g. the common carotid artery, CCA) have a trilaminar structure (intima, media and adventitia) and act as capacitance vessels (Fig. 4.2a). A limited number of anastomotic channels exist between these arteries. The larger intracranial arteries (e.g. the middle cerebral artery, MCA) have potentially important anastomotic connections over the pial surface (vander Eecken & Adams 1953) and at the base of the brain, via the circle of Willis and choroidal circulation (see below). The adventitia of these large intracranial arteries is thinner than that of the extracranial vessels, with little elastic tissue (Fig. 4.2b). The media is also thinner, although the internal elastic lamina is thicker (such changes occurring gradually as the arterial diameter decreases). Thus, these vessels are more rigid than extracranial vessels of similar size. The small, deep perforating (e.g. the lenticulostriate arteries, LSAs) and superficial perforating arteries from the pial surface are predominantly end-arteries, with very limited anastomotic potential, and are primarily resistance vessels (Fig. 4.2c). The overall resistance in any

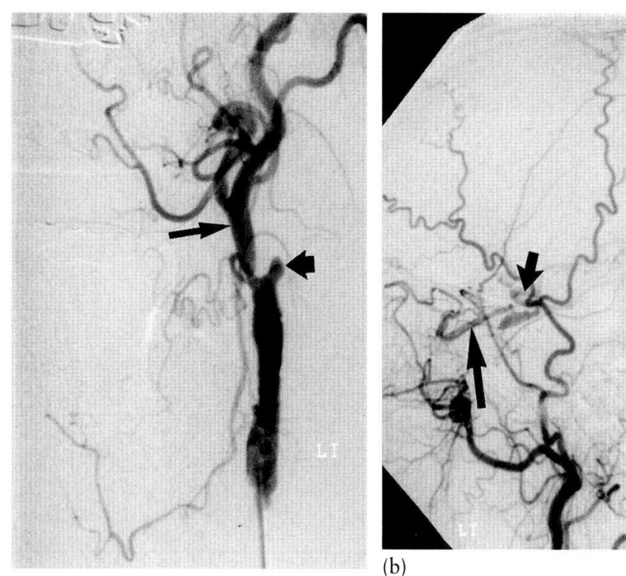

Fig. 4.6 (a) A selective intra-arterial catheter angiogram, showing occlusion of the left internal carotid artery (ICA, short arrow) and filling of the external carotid artery (ECA, long arrow). (b) Intracranial views of the same angiogram (lateral projection), showing retrograde filling of the ophthalmic artery (long arrow) from the ECA, which provides a collateral supply to the distal ICA (short arrow, showing the carotid siphon) (courtesy of Dr M. Weston, St James's University Hospital, Leeds).

Posterior communicating artery (PCoA)

The next branch of the ICA is usually the PCoA. Arising from the dorsal aspect of the ICA, it tracks caudally to join the posterior cerebral artery (PCA) (Fig. 4.7). The PCoA may give off small branches, which contribute to the blood supply of the basal ganglia.

Aneurysms at the origin of the PCoA may present with a painful third nerve palsy with pupillary involvement, or subarachnoid haemorrhage (section 9.3.5). In a few patients, both PCoAs are absent. This may result in much more marked deficits from lesions of the posterior circulation than in patients with a functionally intact circle of Willis (see below).

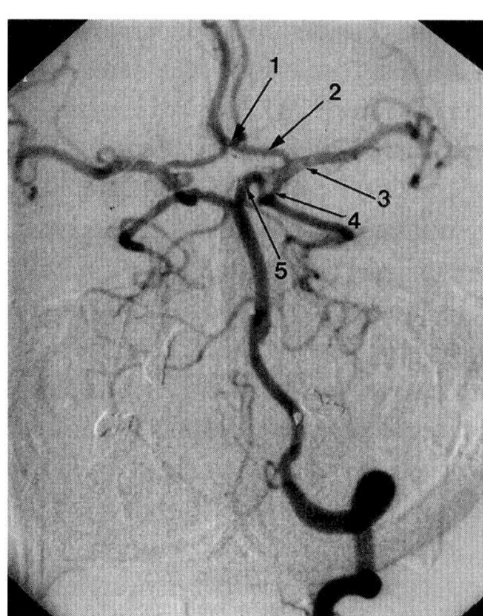

Fig. 4.7 Demonstration of the components of the circle of Willis by intra-arterial catheter angiography (anteroposterior projection). The whole of the circle is filled from a selective left vertebral artery injection in a patient who had bilateral internal carotid artery occlusions. The components are: 1, anterior communicating artery; 2, anterior cerebral artery; 3, middle cerebral artery; 4, posterior communicating artery; 5, posterior cerebral artery (P_1 segment) (courtesy of Dr M. Weston, St James's University Hospital, Leeds).

Anterior choroidal artery (AChA)

Just before its terminal bifurcation into the anterior cerebral artery and middle cerebral artery (MCA), the ICA usually gives rise to the AChA (Fig. 4.8), although just occasionally it can arise from either the proximal stem of the MCA or the PCoA. It is a relatively small branch which gains its name because of supplying the choroid plexus, but it may also supply the globus pallidus, anterior hippocampus, uncus, lower part of the posterior limb of the internal capsule and rostral portions of the midbrain, including the cerebral peduncle (Marinkovic *et al.* 1999). It accompanies the optic tract and sends branches to the lateral geniculate nucleus (LGN) and the rostral part of the optic radiation. It may anastomose with the posterior choroidal artery (a branch of the posterior cerebral artery).

Isolated occlusion of the AChA may be more often due to intrinsic disease of the artery complicated by *in situ* thrombosis than embolism from more proximal sources (section 6.6.2). Also, the AChA may be particularly susceptible to the effects of intracarotid chemotherapy (Tamaki *et al.* 1997). AChA territory infarcts typically produce a contralateral hemiparesis and hemisensory deficit, the latter often sparing proprioception. Higher cortical modalities such as language and visuospatial function may be affected, and are attributed to extension of the ischaemia to the lateral thalamus. Large AChA territory infarcts have an additional visual field defect. This can be a homonymous hemianopia (due to ischaemia of using any classification must be blessed with a healthy dose of realism. There is never going to be complete certainty about issues in clinical medicine, and cerebrovascular disease is no exception. There are always going to be exceptions to the rules, and one definition of clinical acumen might be the ability to sense when such exceptions are likely to occur.

One should not presume that the results of investigations will necessarily be any more sensitive or specific than the clinical findings. Investigations contribute most to the diagnostic process when set in a proper clinical context and when they take the pre-test probability of the disorder into account.

In section 4.2, we will review the relevant vascular anatomy, and then in section 4.3 describe a system linking this with the features of the clinical examination of patients with 'brain attack' or stroke that assist parenchymal localization, as discussed in Chapter 3. Although the discussion below relates primarily to infarcts, the syndromes described may equally be caused by PICH. Since not all physicians worldwide have instantaneous access to CT scanning, there is an advantage in having a method that can subclassify strokes irrespective of their pathological type, at least until the type is known as a result of later CT or MR scanning.

4.2 The cerebral arterial supply

4.2.1 Introduction

In order for the information from the clinical history and examination to be formulated in a manner that will have as much relevance as possible to the underlying vascular lesion, the clinician needs to have a working knowledge of the cerebral blood supply. This will also be required for planning and interpreting the results of investigations and assessing the relevance of possible treatments. However, the general assumption that the vascular supply of the brain parenchyma follows an entirely predictable pattern (as depicted in many textbooks) and that there are patterns of infarction which are 'typical' of a particular pathogenesis (e.g. cardioembolism) certainly should not be accepted without closer scrutiny. Many classifications refer to 'standard' maps of the areas of distribution of individual arteries, especially those that have been produced as cross-sectional templates to correspond with CT/MR sections (e.g. Damasio 1983). The theory goes that if one plots the site and size of the lesion seen on the scan onto these maps, then the occluded artery can be identified. Additionally, certain sites are identified as arterial boundary-zones, and further assumptions are then often made about the underlying pathophysiological process—i.e. low flow rather than thromboembolism (sections 4.2.4 and 6.6.5). However, it is clear that the cerebral circulation is a dynamic system with large inter-individual and intra-individual variability (i.e. between hemispheres and even varying with time) (van der Zwan 1990; van der Zwan *et al.* 1992, 1993), and that atheroma or other arterial disease in one part of the system may have complex and relatively unpredictable effects on the patterns of vascular supply. Not surprisingly, this means that attributing an infarct to a particular underlying pathogenesis on the basis of its site and size is often incorrect (Lang *et al.* 1995; Hennerici & Schwartz 1998; Hennerici *et al.* 1998). More recent publications dealing with the localization of the arterial lesion have begun to take this variability into account (Tatu *et al.* 1996; Tatu *et al.* 1998). But even then, there has to be a lesion on the scan to localize—something that is actually becoming less frequent with very early scanning, unless the latest MR techniques are used; and even when lesions are visible, their size may change with time (Fig. 4.1).

Attributing an infarct to a particular pathogenesis purely on the basis of its site and size is often incorrect.

One important consequence of the above is that at the level of the individual patient, the occlusion of a specific artery may present clinically in different ways. Nevertheless, in this chapter, we have attempted to relate each section of the vascular anatomy to the symptoms and signs *commonly* encountered in clinical practice.

The cerebral vascular anatomy can be described in two main parts: the anterior (carotid) and posterior (vertebrobasilar, VB) systems. For each system, there are three components: the extracranial arteries, the major intracranial arteries, and the small (in terms of diameter) superficial and deep perforating arteries. These component arteries have different structural and functional characteristics, which means that infarction within their territory of distribution is likely to be caused predominantly by different causes (Table 4.3). The extracranial vessels (e.g. the common carotid artery, CCA) have a trilaminar structure (intima, media and adventitia) and act as capacitance vessels (Fig. 4.2a). A limited number of anastomotic channels exist between these arteries. The larger intracranial arteries (e.g. the middle cerebral artery, MCA) have potentially important anastomotic connections over the pial surface (vander Eecken & Adams 1953) and at the base of the brain, via the circle of Willis and choroidal circulation (see below). The adventitia of these large intracranial arteries is thinner than that of the extracranial vessels, with little elastic tissue (Fig. 4.2b). The media is also thinner, although the internal elastic lamina is thicker (such changes occurring gradually as the arterial diameter decreases). Thus, these vessels are more rigid than extracranial vessels of similar size. The small, deep perforating (e.g. the lenticulostriate arteries, LSAs) and superficial perforating arteries from the pial surface are predominantly end-arteries, with very limited anastomotic potential, and are primarily resistance vessels (Fig. 4.2c). The overall resistance in any

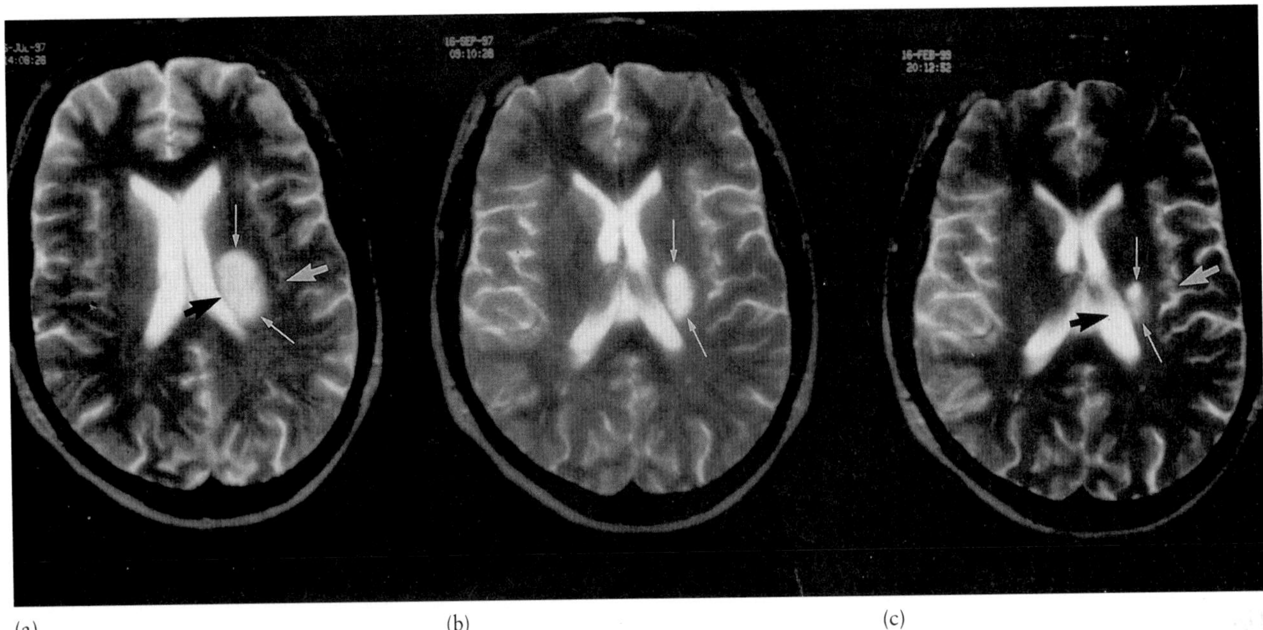

(a) (b) (c)

Fig. 4.1 Sequential T2-weighted magnetic resonance brain scans of a patient with a pure motor stroke affecting the right arm and leg, showing the decreasing size of the small, left deep infarct over time (thin white arrows). (a) Day 1, (b) 2 months, (c) 19 months post-stroke. Note that there is some swelling of the lesion in the acute phase (there is slight compression of the adjacent left lateral ventricle (black arrow) and of the Sylvian fissure (thick white arrow), which decreases with time, so that at 19 months, there is an *ex-vacuo* effect—the left lateral ventricle is now larger (black arrow) and the Sylvian fissure more visible (thick white arrow).

Table 4.3 Functional characteristics of arteries.

Main arteries
Anastomotic potential via circle of Willis, extracranial connections and pial collaterals
Thus, marked variability in the area of ischaemia
Embolism or *in situ* thrombosis is the most likely cause of occlusion
Cortical branch arteries
Anastomotic potential via pial collaterals
Thus, moderate variability in the area of ischaemia
Embolism is the most likely cause of occlusion
Deep perforating arteries
Limited anastomotic potential
Thus, very restricted areas of ischaemia
Intrinsic small vessel disease is the most likely cause of occlusion

section of the arterial tree is inversely proportional to the vascular density, which, on average, is approximately four times greater in grey matter (cortical and subcortical) than in white matter (van der Zwan *et al.* 1993).

4.2.2 The anterior (carotid) system

Common carotid artery (CCA)

The left CCA usually arises directly from the left side of the aortic arch, whereas the right CCA arises from the innominate (brachiocephalic) artery (Figs 4.3 & 6.2). The CCAs ascend through the anterior triangle of the neck, and at the level of the thyroid cartilage divide into the internal carotid artery (ICA) and the external carotid artery (ECA). Throughout, the CCA is intimately associated with the ascending sympathetic fibres. Thus, lesions of the CCA (trauma, dissection or sometimes thrombotic occlusion) may cause an ipsilateral oculosympathetic palsy (Horner's syndrome) with involvement of sudomotor fibres to the face. Damage to the CCA, or thrombus within it, may also result in carotidynia, a syndrome characterized by tenderness over the artery and pain referred to the ipsilateral frontotemporal region. It may also be the site of radiotherapy-induced damage (section 7.12).

Carotid bifurcation

The carotid bifurcation is usually at the level of the thyroid cartilage, but the exact site may vary by several centimetres (Fig. 4.4). It contains the carotid body (see below). The ICA is usually posterior to the ECA. The carotid body and carotid sinus nerve receive their blood supply from the ECA. The bifurcation is one of the most common sites for atheroma to develop in whites, and it is over this area that bruits can be heard (section 6.6.7). However, there is no way of telling on auscultation whether a bruit arises from the ICA, ECA or both. One practical point relates to carotid duplex scan-

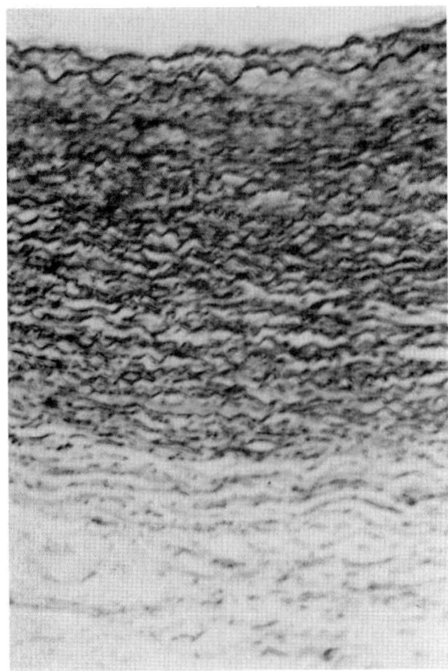
(a)

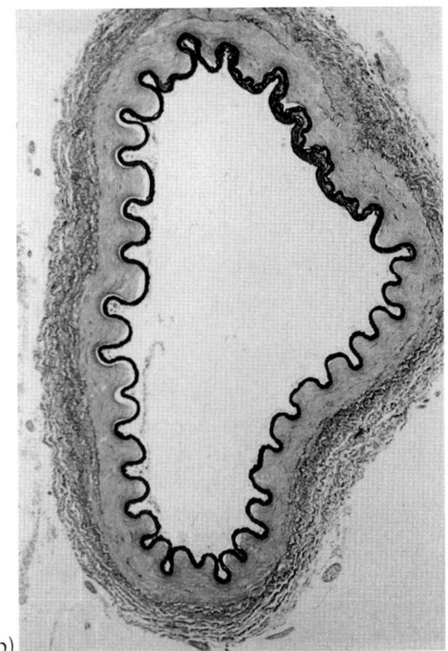
(b)

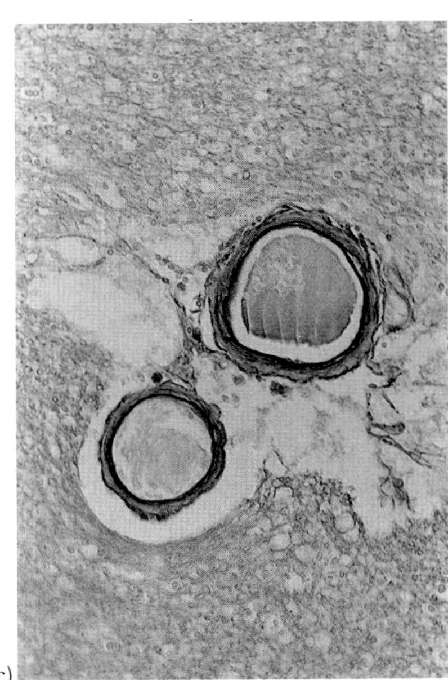
(c)

Fig. 4.2 (a) Internal carotid artery just above the common carotid bifurcation (elastic van Gieson (EVG) × 120). The intima at the top of the photograph is barely visible, lying inside an ill-defined internal elastic lamina. The relatively thick media is rich in elastic tissue. The adventitia is thin and poorly defined. (b) Cross-section of the middle cerebral artery (EVG × 50). The intima is barely visible, and lies internal to the folded internal elastic lamina, which shows mild focal reduplication. Both media and adventitia are thinner than in extracranial arteries of comparable size. The media is virtually devoid of elastic tissue. There is no definite external elastic lamina. (c) A pair of basal ganglionic perforating vessels (EVG × 250). Each of these vessels has an indistinct internal elastic lamina, and a media composed of two to three layers of smooth muscle cells; arterioles are devoid of an internal elastic lamina (photographs courtesy of Dr Alistair Lammie, Department of Neuropathology, University of Wales College of Medicine).

ning. In general, duplex images the bifurcation and ICA/ECA for a few centimetres distal to the bifurcation. However, in patients with a high bifurcation, technical difficulties may be encountered, and only the CCA may be imaged.

The carotid body responds to increases in the arterial partial pressure of oxygen ($Pa\text{O}_2$), blood flow and arterial pH, and to decreases in $Pa\text{CO}_2$ or blood temperature. It has a modulatory role on pulse rate, blood pressure and hypoxic ventilatory drive (Calverley 1999). Increased discharges in the carotid sinus nerve can be caused by stretching of the wall of the carotid sinus, and will increase the depth and rate of respiration and increase peripheral vascular resistance. Carotid sinus hypersensitivity is probably an under-recognized cause of collapse in the elderly, but is not necessarily associated with structural disease of the bifurcation (Parry *et al.* 2000).

External carotid artery (ECA)

In patients with cerebrovascular disease, the branches of the ECA (ascending pharyngeal, superior thyroid, lingual, occipital, facial, posterior auricular, internal maxillary and superficial temporal) are mainly of interest because of the potential for anastomoses with branches of the intracranial ICA in patients with a proximal ICA occlusion, and their involvement in giant-cell arteritis (section 7.3). In the presence of an extracranial ICA occlusion or severe stenosis, blood flow may be maintained to the ipsilateral intracranial circulation by ECA–ICA collaterals (see below). It has been suggested that transient monocular blindness can occur due to intermittent failure of perfusion through ECA–ICA collaterals because of stenosis of the ECA origin, particularly when there is ipsilateral ICA occlusion or severe stenosis. Palpable pulsation of the temporal artery may be reduced or absent with ipsilateral CCA or ECA occlusion and, conversely, may be increased when there is ipsilateral ICA occlusion. The presence of extracranial branches distinguishes the ECA from the ICA on arterial studies (Fig. 4.4).

Internal carotid artery (ICA)

The ICA on both sides arises from the carotid bifurcation and ascends through the foramen lacerum in the skull base. Along the petrosal section, it gives off small branches to the tympanic cavity and the artery of the pterygoid canal, which may anastomose with the internal maxillary artery, a branch of the ECA.

Torvik and Jorgensen (1964, 1966) demonstrated in a series of 994 consecutive autopsies (which represented 76% and 40% of in-hospital and total deaths, respectively, during the time period) that in 42 of 54 (78%) cases with an ICA occlusion there was evidence of ipsilateral infarction,

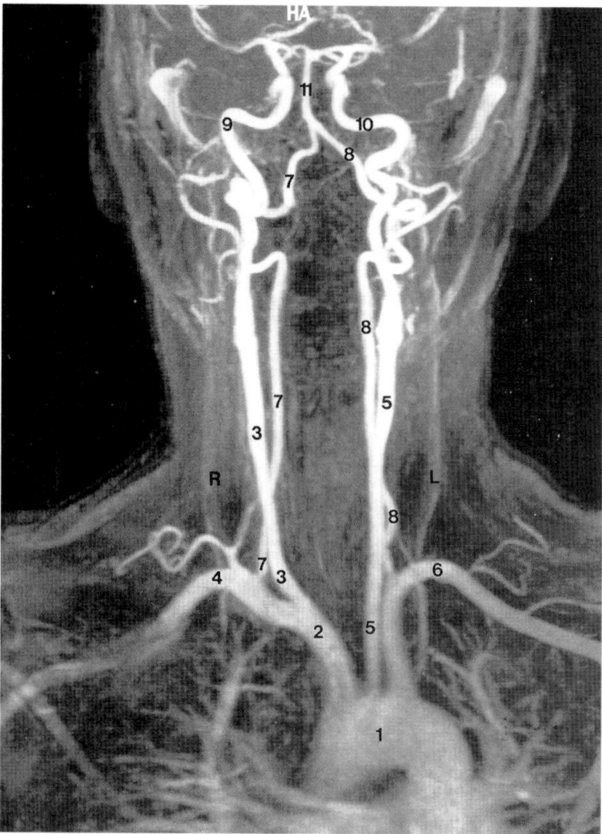

Fig. 4.3 A contrast-enhanced magnetic resonance angiogram, showing the origins of the major vessels from the aorta, the cervical course of the carotid and vertebral arteries, and the intracranial connections of the anterior and posterior arterial systems. R, right; L, left; 1, aortic arch; 2, innominate artery; 3, right common carotid artery; 4, right subclavian artery; 5, left common carotid artery; 6, left subclavian artery; 7, right vertebral artery; 8, left vertebral artery; 9, right internal carotid artery; 10, left internal carotid artery; 11, basilar artery (courtesy of Dr J.A. Guthrie, St James's University Hospital, Leeds).

although in about 20% the occlusion had not caused any symptoms, at least as far as could be established from retrospective case-note review. When neurological symptoms do occur from disease of the ICA, they may be due to artery-to-artery embolism, low distal flow, or occlusion due to local arterial thrombosis. The clinical picture may range from a transient disturbance of ipsilateral cortical or ocular function to the 'full house' of hemiplegia, hemianaesthesia, hemianopia and profound disturbance of higher cortical function.

The proximal extracranial ICA is commonly affected by atheroma and when occlusion occurs it is probably most often due to rupture and instability of an atherosclerotic plaque (Lammie *et al.* 1999) (section 6.3.2). Other conditions involving the extracranial ICA include trauma causing arterial dissection (when the neck is hyperextended and/or rotated and the artery stretched over the transverse process of C1/2) or pseudoaneurysms, which may be a source of emboli (section 7.1); spontaneous arterial dissection with little or no such trauma (section 7.2.1); or a local arteritis secondary to paratonsillar infections (section 7.11). The sympathetic chain lies on the surface of the ICA and can be affected by any of the above processes. The resulting oculosympathetic palsy should spare the sudomotor fibres to the face because they are associated with the branches of the ECA. Around the origin of the ICA are the superior laryngeal and hypoglossal nerves, which may be affected by operative procedures (section 16.8.4 and Fig. 16.21).

Carotid siphon

The S-shaped carotid siphon lies within the venous plexus of the cavernous sinus adjacent to cranial nerves III, IV, V^1, V^2 and VI, which run in the lateral wall of the sinus. There are several small branches (the most important of which is the meningohypophyseal trunk), which may anastomose with branches of the ECA. One congenital variant worth noting is the persistence of the trigeminal artery, which may arise from the ICA as it enters the cavernous sinus and links with the basilar artery, usually between the superior cerebellar artery (SCA) and the anterior inferior cerebellar artery.

Atheroma may affect the ICA in the siphon. Although it may be a cause of embolism, flow restriction and, in a few cases, complete occlusion, the resulting symptoms are similar to those originating from more proximal ICA disease. The degree of atheroma is not necessarily related to that at the carotid bifurcation and when occlusion occurs in the siphon it is more likely to be due to impaction of an embolus from a proximal site than *in situ* thrombosis (Lammie *et al.* 1999).

Cavernous sinus thrombosis classically presents with varying degrees of ophthalmoplegia, chemosis and proptosis (sometimes bilateral, because the venous plexus communicates across the midline) in a patient with evidence of facial or sinus sepsis (Fig. 4.5) (DiNubile 1988). Aneurysms at the level of the cavernous sinus are relatively common and may present with third nerve dysfunction. If there is rupture of the artery that is confined by the sinus, then a *caroticocavernous fistula* may develop. The typical picture is of pulsatile proptosis, with ophthalmoplegia and reduced visual acuity (section 8.2.14).

Supraclinoid internal carotid artery

The short supraclinoid portion of the ICA lies in the subarachnoid space and is related to the third cranial nerve. The most important branch is the ophthalmic artery, which enters the orbit through the optic foramen. This, and the other branches of the ophthalmic artery (lacrimal, supraorbital, ethmoidal, palpebral), is probably the most important anastomotic link with the ECA (Fig. 4.6).

Transient monocular blindness (amaurosis fugax) may be due to emboli passing from the ICA to the ophthalmic artery

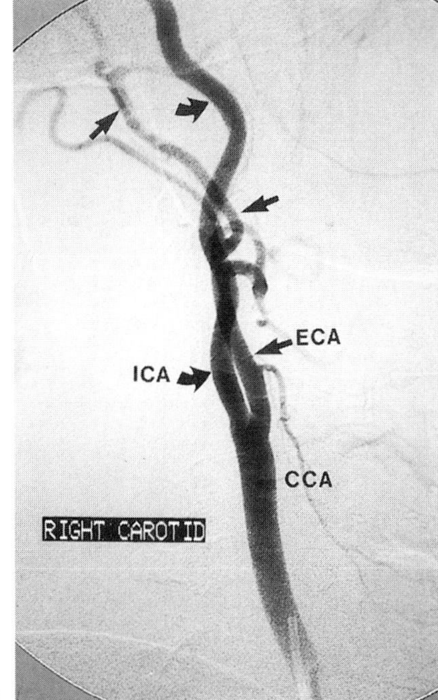

(a)

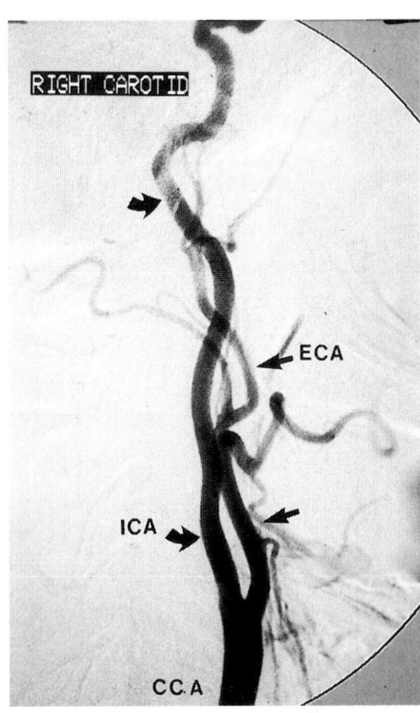

(b)

Fig. 4.4 Catheter carotid angiograms; (a) anteroposterior projection, (b) lateral projection. ECA, external carotid artery and its branches (straight arrows); ICA, internal carotid artery (curved arrows); CCA, common carotid artery.

Fig. 4.5 A T1-weighted, gadolinium-enhanced, coronal magnetic resonance scan, showing thrombosis within the left cavernous sinus. The thrombus (long arrow) is seen separate from the flow void in the left internal carotid artery (short arrow). Enhancement is seen in the sphenoid sinus (broad arrow), which is due to infection. The patient had a fever, chemosis and a partial third nerve palsy.

(Fisher 1959) (section 3.3.6). However, a large proportion of such patients have no evidence of ICA disease, nor for that matter cardiac or aortic sources of embolism, and therefore local atheroma within the ophthalmic arterial system remains a possibility. Fixed deficits come from retinal artery occlusion (usually considered to be embolic) and ischaemic optic neuropathy (section 3.5.2), although the latter is surprisingly infrequent with ICA occlusion, presumably because of collateral flow. The combination of ocular and cerebral hemisphere ischaemic attacks on the same side is a strong pointer towards severe ICA stenosis or occlusion, although the symptoms rarely occur simultaneously. When ICA occlusion occurs, the distal extent of the thrombus may end at the level of the ophthalmic artery. The supraclinoid ICA may be involved by inflammatory/infective processes, such as tuberculous meningitis, in the basal subarachnoid space. Severe stenosis or occlusion of the distal part of the supraclinoid and more distal ICA is always present in cases of the moyamoya syndrome (section 7.5).

The combination of ocular and cerebral hemisphere ischaemic attacks on the same side is a strong pointer towards severe internal carotid artery stenosis or occlusion.

There are also a number of small perforating branches that supply the hypophysis, hypothalamus and optic chiasm. Other branches may pass through the anterior perforated substance to supply the genu and part of the posterior limb of the internal capsule, and the globus pallidus.

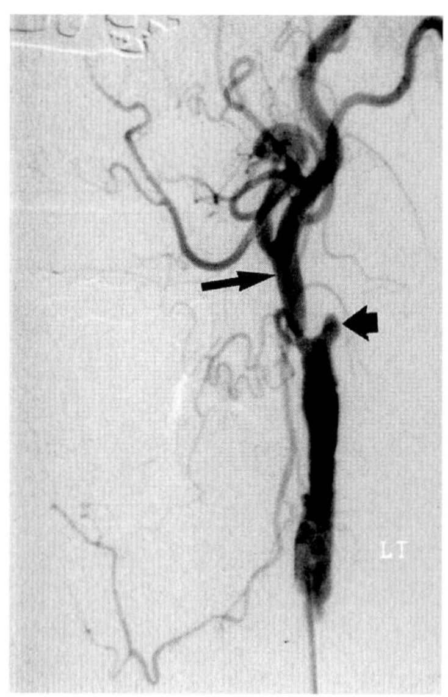

(a)

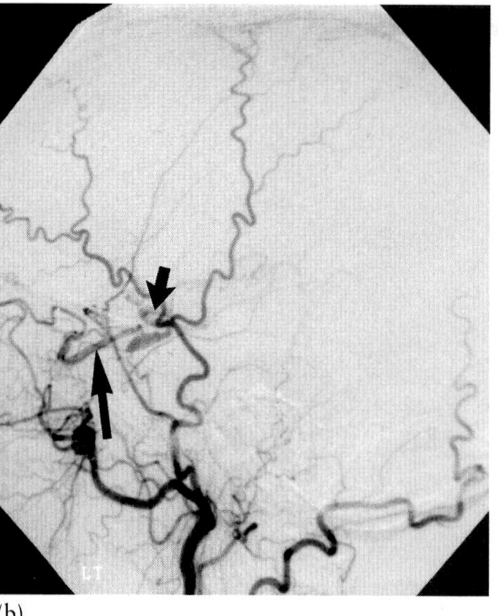

(b)

Fig. 4.6 (a) A selective intra-arterial catheter angiogram, showing occlusion of the left internal carotid artery (ICA, short arrow) and filling of the external carotid artery (ECA, long arrow). (b) Intracranial views of the same angiogram (lateral projection), showing retrograde filling of the ophthalmic artery (long arrow) from the ECA, which provides a collateral supply to the distal ICA (short arrow, showing the carotid siphon) (courtesy of Dr M. Weston, St James's University Hospital, Leeds).

Posterior communicating artery (PCoA)

The next branch of the ICA is usually the PCoA. Arising from the dorsal aspect of the ICA, it tracks caudally to join the posterior cerebral artery (PCA) (Fig. 4.7). The PCoA may give off small branches, which contribute to the blood supply of the basal ganglia.

Aneurysms at the origin of the PCoA may present with a painful third nerve palsy with pupillary involvement, or subarachnoid haemorrhage (section 9.3.5). In a few patients, both PCoAs are absent. This may result in much more marked deficits from lesions of the posterior circulation than in patients with a functionally intact circle of Willis (see below).

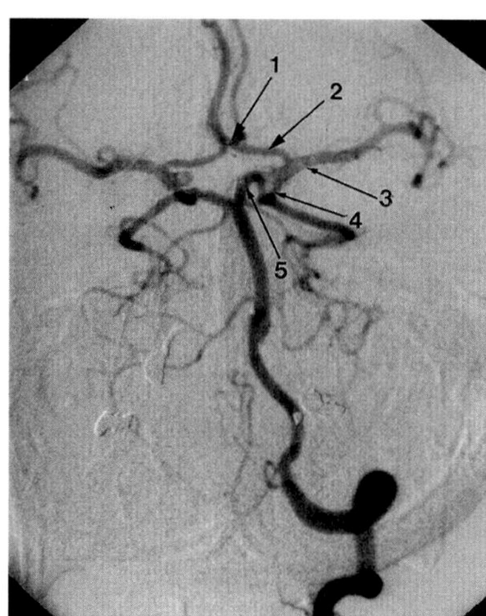

Fig. 4.7 Demonstration of the components of the circle of Willis by intra-arterial catheter angiography (anteroposterior projection). The whole of the circle is filled from a selective left vertebral artery injection in a patient who had bilateral internal carotid artery occlusions. The components are: 1, anterior communicating artery; 2, anterior cerebral artery; 3, middle cerebral artery; 4, posterior communicating artery; 5, posterior cerebral artery (P_1 segment) (courtesy of Dr M. Weston, St James's University Hospital, Leeds).

Anterior choroidal artery (AChA)

Just before its terminal bifurcation into the anterior cerebral artery and middle cerebral artery (MCA), the ICA usually gives rise to the AChA (Fig. 4.8), although just occasionally it can arise from either the proximal stem of the MCA or the PCoA. It is a relatively small branch which gains its name because of supplying the choroid plexus, but it may also supply the globus pallidus, anterior hippocampus, uncus, lower part of the posterior limb of the internal capsule and rostral portions of the midbrain, including the cerebral peduncle (Marinkovic *et al.* 1999). It accompanies the optic tract and sends branches to the lateral geniculate nucleus (LGN) and the rostral part of the optic radiation. It may anastomose with the posterior choroidal artery (a branch of the posterior cerebral artery).

Isolated occlusion of the AChA may be more often due to intrinsic disease of the artery complicated by *in situ* thrombosis than embolism from more proximal sources (section 6.6.2). Also, the AChA may be particularly susceptible to the effects of intracarotid chemotherapy (Tamaki *et al.* 1997). AChA territory infarcts typically produce a contralateral hemiparesis and hemisensory deficit, the latter often sparing proprioception. Higher cortical modalities such as language and visuospatial function may be affected, and are attributed to extension of the ischaemia to the lateral thalamus. Large AChA territory infarcts have an additional visual field defect. This can be a homonymous hemianopia (due to ischaemia of

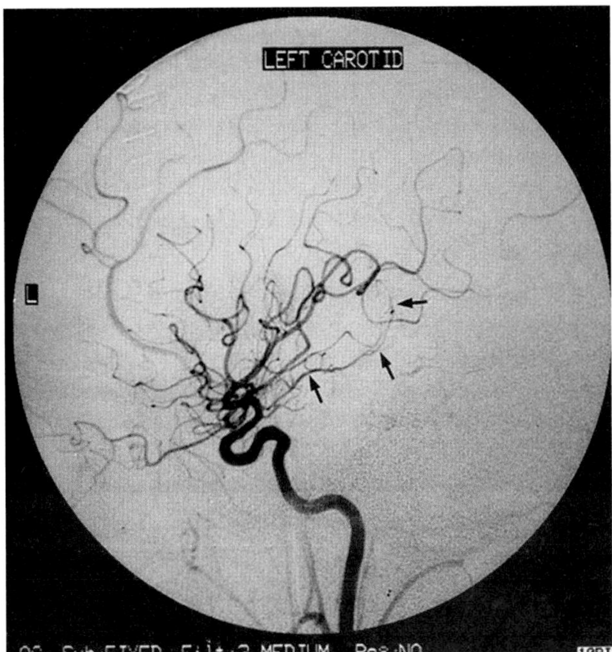

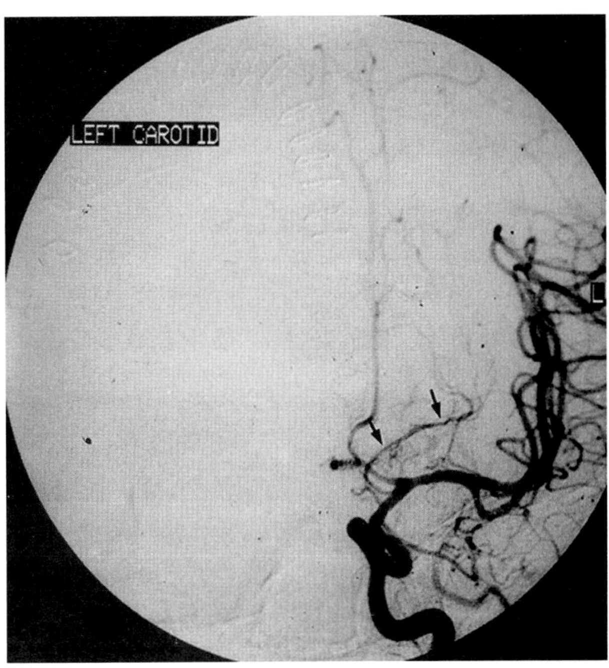

(a) (b)

Fig. 4.8 Left carotid catheter angiogram, showing the anterior choroidal artery (arrows); (a) lateral view, (b) anteroposterior view.

the optic tract), but the pathognomonic pattern is considered to be a homonymous horizontal sectoranopia due to involvement of the LGN (Frisén 1979; Helgason 1995).

Distal internal carotid artery

At the bifurcation of the ICA, the main continuing branch is usually the middle cerebral artery, whilst the smaller anterior cerebral artery and the PCoA form the anterior portion of the circle of Willis (Fig. 4.7). This is not a common site for atheroma, but can be the superior extent of a carotid dissection (section 7.2.1). It is also a site of aneurysm formation (section 9.1.1).

Circle of Willis

In the embryo, a large branch from the ICA provides most of the blood supply to the occipital lobes. From this branch, the future PCoA and postcommunicating (P2) segment of the posterior cerebral artery (PCA) will develop and, in general, will link with the precommunicating (P1) segment of the PCA, which develops from the basilar artery. According to Padget (1948), the arterial components of the circle of Willis and the origins of its branches (i.e. the anterior cerebral arteries (ACAs), the PCAs, the anterior communicating artery (ACoA) and the PCoAs) are formed by 6–7 weeks of gestation. At this stage, the PCoA and the P1 segment of the PCA are usually of approximately similar diameter and contribute equally to the supply of the P2 segment of the PCA. Van Overbeeke *et al.* (1991) showed that this 'transitional' configuration is present in nearly 80% of fetuses under 20 weeks' gestation, but over the next 20 weeks (and particularly between the 21st and 29th weeks of gestation, which coincides with the period of most rapid growth of the occipital lobes) there is a change. In the majority, the P1 segment of the PCA becomes larger than the PCoA, resulting in the 'adult' configuration, where the occipital lobes are supplied primarily by the posterior circulation. However, in a minority, the PCoA becomes larger and the occipital lobes then obtain most of their blood supply from the carotid circulation, a situation which is referred to as a 'fetal' configuration. The 'transitional configuration' persists in less than 10% of adults (Riggs & Rupp 1963) although the exact proportions of the different configurations are difficult to estimate from the literature, because of the very variable selection criteria that have been used (van Overbeeke *et al.* 1991).

Anomalies of the circle of Willis are reported in between half and four-fifths of cases, depending on selection criteria, and certainly seem to be more prevalent in patients with cerebrovascular disease (Alpers & Berry 1963; Riggs & Rupp 1963). The distribution of the abnormalities found in Riggs and Rupp's (1963) study of 994 cases is shown in Fig. 4.9. In this study, hypoplasia of part of the anterior part of the circle of Willis was found in 13%, of the posterior part in 32%, and of both parts in 36%. They noted that when there was maldevelopment of either the P1 segment of the PCA or the precommunicating (A1) segment of the ACA, there was usually an ectopic origin of the distal branches. Taken alongside the haemodynamic consequences of the hypoplastic segments of the circle of Willis, these anatomical factors are likely to result in considerable variation in the area of supply of the major intracerebral arteries and the ability of the cerebral

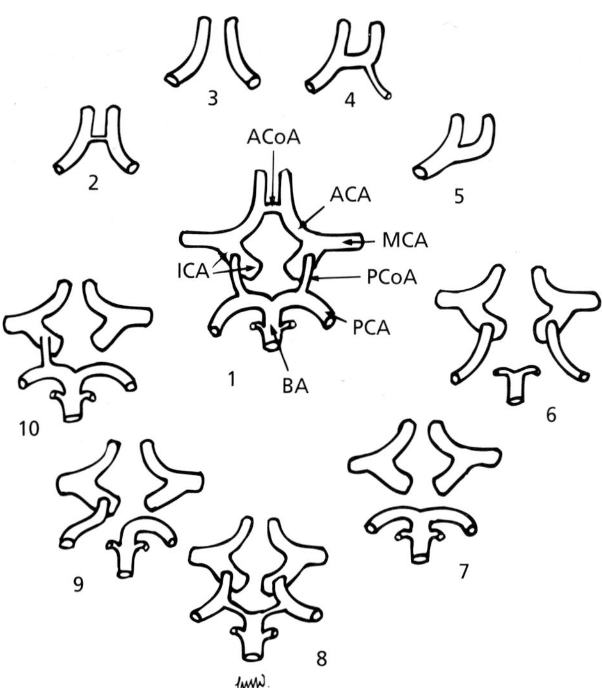

Fig. 4.9 Anomalies of the circle of Willis. In the centre is a complete circle of Willis (1). There are 21 possible variants. Those involving the anterior cerebral arteries (ACA) and anterior communicating artery (ACoA) are shown at the top (2–5) and some of those involving the posterior communicating arteries (PCoA) below (6–10). The anterior part of the circle provides poor collateral supply in 24% of people and no collateral supply in 7%. The most common anomaly of the PCoA is direct origin from the internal carotid artery (ICA) (6 and 9 above), which occurs in 30% of people (BA, basilar artery; PCA, posterior cerebral artery; MCA, middle cerebral artery).

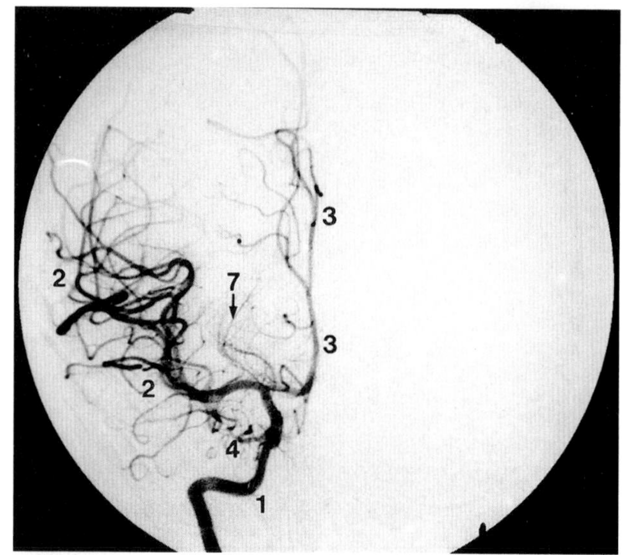

(a)

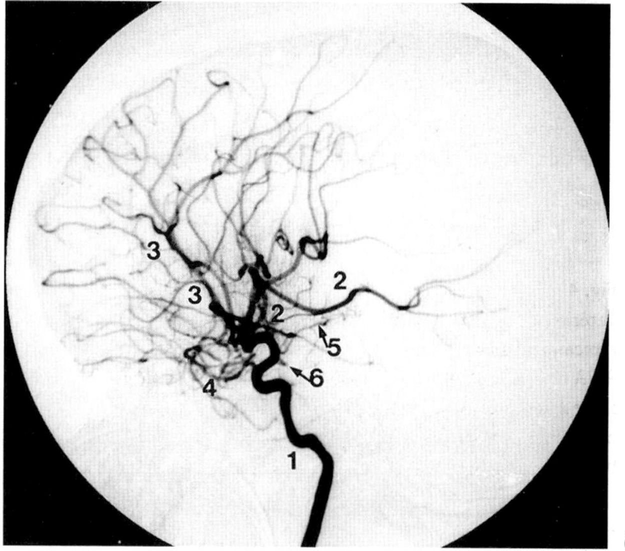

(b)

Fig. 4.10 Selective carotid catheter angiogram of the anterior intracranial circulation; (a) anteroposterior projection (b) lateral projection. 1, internal carotid artery; 2, middle cerebral artery and its branches; 3, anterior cerebral artery and its branches; 4, ophthalmic artery; 5, anterior choroidal artery; 6, vestigial stump of the posterior communicating artery (normal variant); 7, lenticulostriate arteries.

circulation to respond to changes in perfusion pressure when more proximal arteries are diseased (Hillen 1986; van der Zwan *et al.* 1993). Not surprisingly, one cannot identify any particular clinical syndrome related to the anomalies of the circle of Willis.

Anterior cerebral artery (ACA)

The ACA arises as the medial branch of the bifurcation of the ICA, at the level of the anterior clinoid process. The proximal, precommunicating A1 segments of the ACAs pass medially and forward over the optic nerve or chiasm and corpus callosum to enter the interhemispheric fissure, where they are linked by the anterior communicating artery (ACoA) (Fig. 4.10). The distal, postcommunicating A2 segments run together in the interhemispheric fissure and then continue backwards as the anterior pericallosal and callosomarginal arteries. Other branches include the orbitofrontal, frontopolar, anterior, middle and posterior internal frontal, paracentral and superior and inferior parietal arteries. The anterior pericallosal arteries may form anastomoses with the posterior pericallosal arteries from the posterior cerebral artery. The potential minimum and maximum areas of supply are shown in Fig. 4.11 (van der Zwan *et al.* 1992).

Isolated infarction of the ACA territory is comparatively rare, other than when due to 'vasospasm' complicating subarachnoid haemorrhage (section 13.6.1). Part of the explanation may be that if the proximal ACA is occluded, the distal ACA obtains a blood supply from the other ACA, via

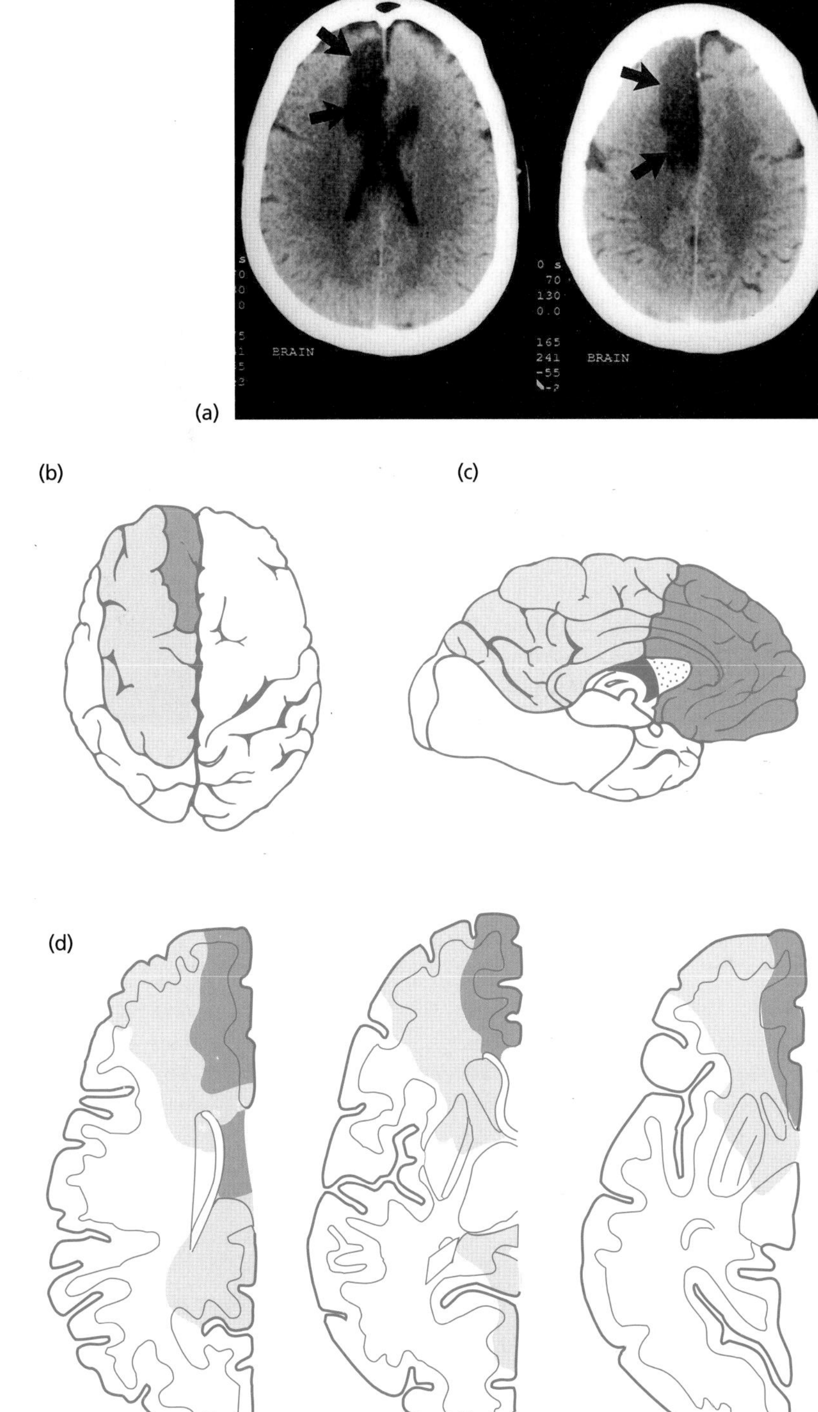

Fig. 4.11 Ischaemia in the territory of the anterior cerebral artery (ACA). (a) The typical appearance on a CT brain scan of ACA territory infarction (arrows). However, there is great inter-individual and inter-hemispheric variability in the area supplied by the ACA (b, c). The dark green areas show the only part of the cortex on the superolateral surface (b) and the medial surface (c) of the hemisphere, which was *always* supplied by the ACA in a large pathological study (van der Zwan 1991). The pale green areas represent the maximum extent of the area that may be supplied by the ACA in some patients. (d) A similar degree of variability exists for the subcortical territory supplied by the ACA. The figure shows the minimum (dark green) and maximum (pale green) areas of supply at three levels in the same pathological study (with permission from Dr A. van der Zwan).

the ACoA. Bilateral ACA territory infarction should always prompt a search for an ACoA aneurysm which may have bled recently, although it may also be caused by thromboembolism in patients where both ACAs receive their supply from the same carotid artery via the ACoA, or more rarely when the distal branches cross the midline in the interhemispheric fissure. The majority of cases of ACA territory infarction are probably due to either cardiogenic embolism or artery-to-artery embolism from an occluded or stenosed internal carotid artery (Bogousslavsky & Regli 1990).

Bilateral anterior cerebral artery territory infarction should always prompt a search for an anterior communicating artery aneurysm which may have bled recently.

The motor deficit in the leg usually predominates over that in the arm and is often most marked distally, in contrast to that from cortical middle cerebral artery infarcts (Critchley 1930). When the arm is affected, this is usually attributed to extension of the ischaemic area to the internal capsule (Bogousslavsky & Regli 1990), although in some cases it may also be a form of motor 'neglect' through involvement of the supplementary motor area. There is often no sensory deficit, but when present it is usually mild. When the motor deficit is bilateral, ACA territory infarction needs to be distinguished from a lesion in the spinal cord or brainstem. The same applies to sensory deficits, but these are usually mild. Other frontal lobe features may be present, including urinary incontinence, lack of motivation or, paradoxically, agitation and social disinhibition. Abulia and akinetic mutism (section 3.3.2) may occur, usually with bilateral lesions. A grasp reflex may be elicited if the motor deficit in the hand is not too great. Various aphasic syndromes have been described, and these are usually attributed to involvement of the dominant supplementary motor area (rather than Broca's area). Typically, there will be reduced spontaneous output but preserved repetition. These patients may be mute immediately after the onset of the stroke. Occlusion of the ACA can result in apraxias and other disconnection syndromes (Kazui & Sawada 1993) (section 3.3.3). Interruption of frontocerebellar tracts can result in incoordination of the contralateral limbs which may mimic cerebellar dysfunction, a fact which in the pre-CT era resulted occasionally in suboccipital explorations looking for cerebellar tumours (Gado *et al.* 1979). When there is also a corticospinal deficit, it may mimic the lacunar syndrome of homolateral ataxia and crural paresis (see below, and Bogousslavsky *et al.* 1992). Amnesic disorders are also encountered, particularly after rupture of an ACoA aneurysm. The 'alien-hand sign' refers to a variety of dissociative movements between right and left hands due to a lesion of the mesial frontal lobe and/or corpus callosum (McNabb *et al.* 1988).

Recurrent artery of Heubner (RAH)

The RAH is an inconstant branch of the ACA, which, if present, usually arises just beyond the level of the ACoA. It may supply the head of the caudate, the inferior portion of the anterior limb of the internal capsule, and the hypothalamus (Fig. 4.12). The deficit from unilateral occlusion of the RAH depends on the extent of the capsular supply. Weakness of the face and arm, often with dysarthria, is said to be characteristic (Critchley 1930). The syndromes of akinetic mutism or abulia (section 3.3.2) may occur but are usually associated with bilateral lesions.

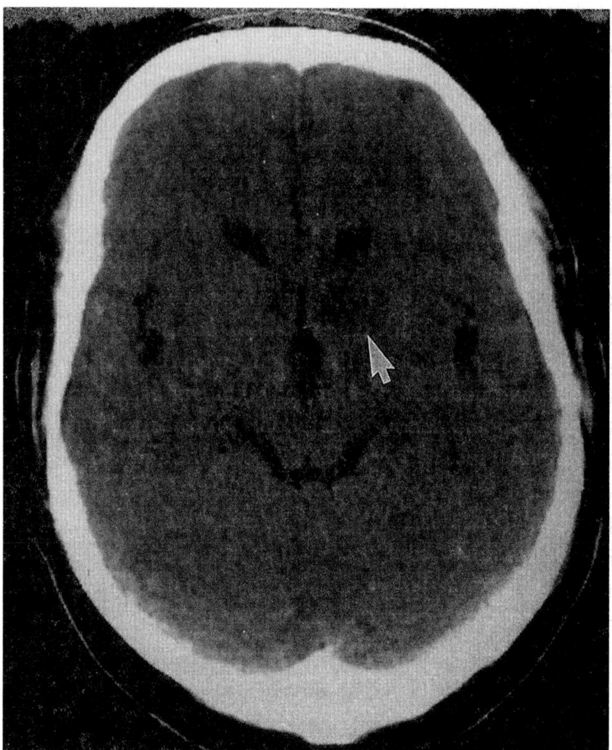

Fig. 4.12 A CT brain scan showing the typical area of infarction (arrow) resulting from occlusion of the recurrent artery of Heubner.

Deep perforating arteries (medial striate)

A variable number of small branches from the A1 segment of the ACA and ACoA enter the anterior perforated substance and may supply the anterior striatum, the ventral anterior limb of the internal capsule and the anterior commissure. They may also supply the optic chiasm and tract (Perlmutter & Rhoton 1976). As with the RAH, if the medial striate arteries contribute to the vascular supply of the internal capsule, weakness of the face and arm may occur.

Middle cerebral artery (MCA)—mainstem

The first segment of the MCA tracks laterally between the upper surface of the temporal lobe and the inferior surface of the frontal lobe until it reaches the lateral part of the Sylvian fissure (Fig. 4.10). The lenticulostriate arteries (LSAs) mostly arise from the proximal part of the MCA mainstem (see below).

Atheroma may develop *in situ*, but this is uncommon in whites and perhaps more frequent in Orientals (section 6.3.3). Therefore, in whites the mechanism of occlusion tends to be either impaction of an embolus, extension of a more proximal thrombus (e.g. from the internal carotid artery), or less commonly intracranial dissection (Olsen *et al.* 1985; Fieschi *et al.* 1989; Heinsius *et al.* 1998). As far as we know, occlusion of the MCA mainstem is nearly always symptomatic, although some young patients with very good cortical collateral supply may have remarkably few symptoms. In most cases, the occlusion occurs in the proximal mainstem, thereby involving the LSAs, and consequently there is ischaemia of both the deep and superficial territory of the MCA. Typically, this presents as a contralateral hemimotor and sensory deficit, hemianopia and disturbance of the relevant higher cortical functions (e.g. aphasia if in the dominant hemisphere). If the cortical collateral supply from the ACA and PCA is good, the brunt of the ischaemia may fall on the subcortical structures, resulting in a striatocapsular infarct, because thrombus occludes the origins of the deep perforating arteries, which are functional end-arteries (see below). Nevertheless, there is often a degree of cortical ischaemia without infarction and consequently the clinical deficits can be very similar (see below). If the occlusion is more distal in the mainstem and there is no ischaemia in the LSA territory, the leg may be relatively spared, because most fibres will originate in cortical areas usually supplied by the ACA, and will descend medially in the corona radiata adjacent to the lateral ventricle (Ueda *et al.* 1992).

Middle cerebral artery—deep perforating arteries

From the main MCA mainstem, there are a variable number of lenticulostriate arteries (LSAs), usually 6–12, most of which emerge at right angles to the parent artery and enter the anterior perforated substance. Three groups can be identified—medial, middle and lateral. The LSAs may supply the lentiform nucleus, lateral head of the caudate nucleus, anterior limb of the internal capsule, part of the globus pallidus and dorsal parts of the internal capsule (Fig. 4.13). Some of the LSAs, particularly those in the lateral group, have their origin from either a cortical branch of the MCA, or from either the superior or inferior divisions of the MCA (Marinkovic *et al.* 1985).

When a thrombus in the MCA mainstem lies over the origins of all of the LSAs, a 'comma'-shaped infarct (when viewed in the axial plane) may develop—a so-called *striatocapsular infarct* (Fig. 4.14) (section 6.6.2). About one-third to one-half of cases will have a potential cardiac source of embolism, one-third will have stenotic or occlusive disease of the ICA and one-third will have stenosis or occlusion confined to the MCA mainstem (Weiller 1995; Horowitz & Tuhrim 1997). Angiographic studies have shown that MCA mainstem occlusion of this type may often be relatively short-lived, presumably due to fragmentation of the embolus (Olsen *et al.* 1985; Fieschi *et al.* 1989). The deficit in the limbs tends to be motor rather than sensory and is often similar in the arm and leg. In about 70% there are symptoms of cortical dysfunction, although these may be mild and resolve rapidly. The pathogenesis of the cortical symptoms is much debated but seems most likely to be due to actual cortical

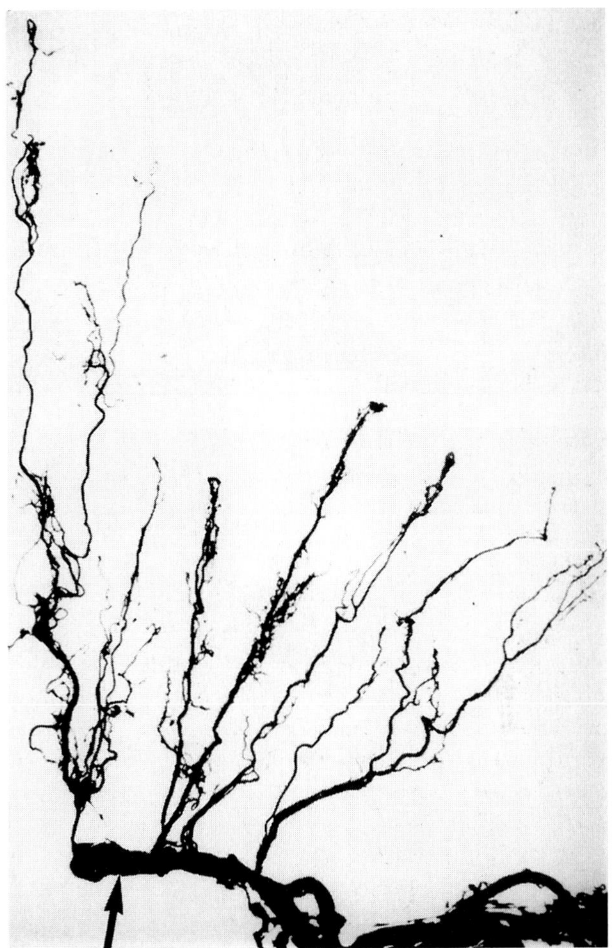

Fig. 4.13 Post-mortem demonstration of the deep perforating arteries arising from the mainstem of the middle cerebral artery (arrow).

ischaemia, which is not imaged by CT or MR, although it may be detected by functional imaging, such as positron emission tomography (PET) and single-photon emission CT (SPECT) (Weiller 1995). The alternative explanations include deafferentation of the cortex, direct interruption of subcortical–cortical pathways, or involvement of subcortical structures which subserve language functions. Hemianopia is an unusual feature.

Occlusion of a *single* LSA results in a 'lacunar infarct' (Fig. 4.15), there being no functional anastomoses between adjacent perforating arteries (Marinkovic *et al.* 1985). It should be stressed that 'lacunar infarction' is a pathological term, and for clarity the radiological equivalent should probably be referred to as a 'small, deep infarct' (Donnan *et al.* 1993). Most occlusions of single, deep perforating arteries from the MCA mainstem are probably caused by local *in situ* small vessel disease rather than embolism, although the number of pathologically verified cases is very small (section 6.4). There is considerable inter-individual variation in

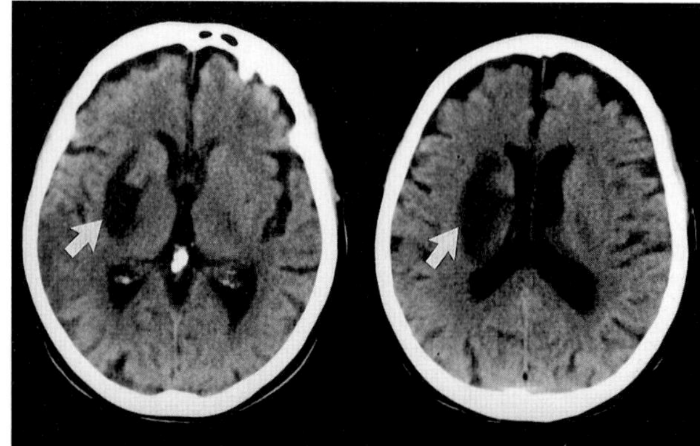

(a)

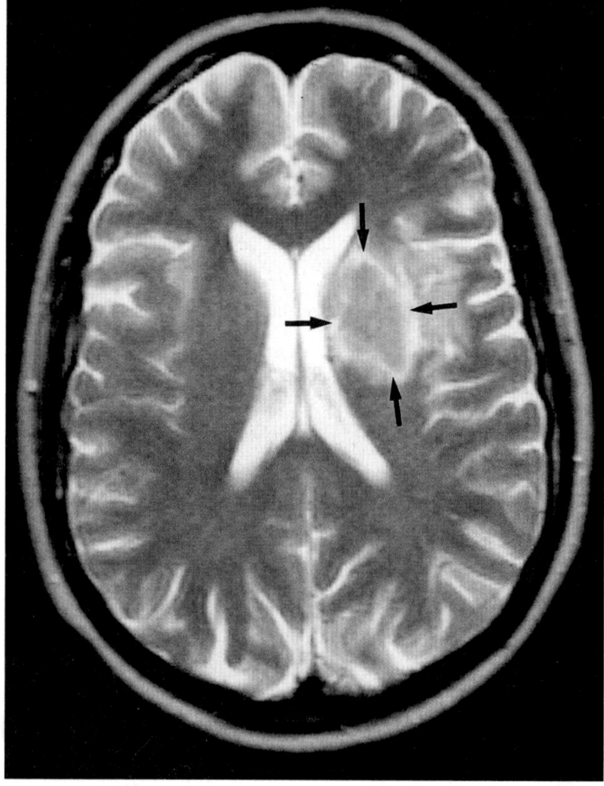

(b)

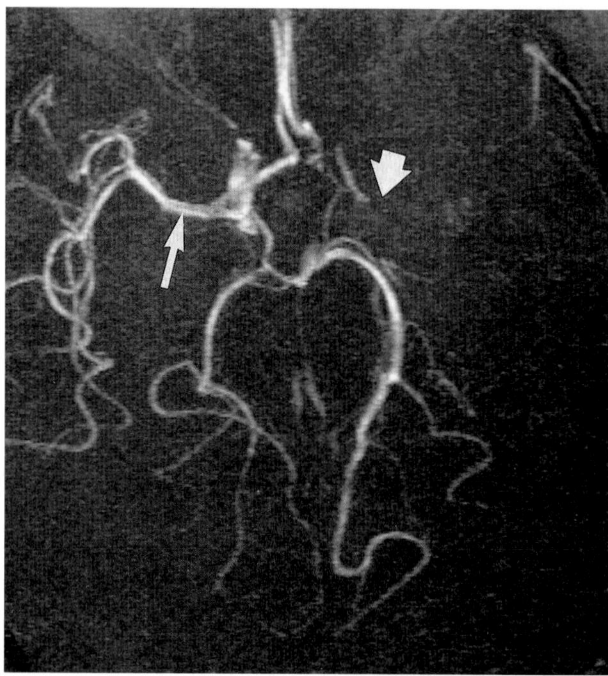

(c)

Fig. 4.14 Striatocapsular infarction (a) The typical appearance of a right striatocapsular infarct on a CT brain scan (arrows). (b) A T2-weighted axial magnetic resonance (MR) scan, showing a left striatocapsular infarct (arrows), and (c) an MR angiogram from the same patient, showing lack of flow in the proximal segment of the left middle cerebral artery (broad arrow). Normal flow is seen in the right middle cerebral artery (narrow arrow). The patient had had a recent anterior myocardial infarction, and it was presumed that an embolus had lodged in the proximal left middle cerebral artery (see also Fig. 6.20e).

the number of LSAs, and in general the largest area is supplied by the most lateral branch. Additionally, the volume of an individual infarct will depend on the actual site of occlusion—i.e. the more proximal the occlusion in the LSA, the larger the lacune. The tendency for studies not to consider imaged lesions greater than 1.5 cm diameter as the radiological equivalent of lacunes probably leads to underreporting, the figure emanating originally from pathological studies (Fisher 1965a). When the results of acute imaging and subsequent autopsy have been compared directly, the lesion at autopsy was significantly smaller (Donnan *et al.* 1982). Single lacunes *may* present with one of the classical 'lacunar syndromes' (section 4.3.2) or with isolated movement disorders, such as hemiballismus. However, the majority of lacunes (80%) are clinically silent (or at least clinically unrecognized), occurring most frequently in the lentiform nucleus (Fisher 1965a).

Lacunar infarction is a pathological term, and for clarity the radiological equivalent should probably be referred to as a 'small, deep infarct'.

Multiple supratentorial lacunes, also referred to as *état lacunaire*, may present as a pseudobulbar palsy, with or without *marche à petits pas*. This abnormality of gait superficially resembles that of Parkinson's disease, but debate continues as to whether a true Parkinsonian syndrome can occur from small, deep infarcts in the basal ganglia (Critchley 1929; Eadie & Sutherland 1964; Parkes *et al.* 1974; Friedman *et al.* 1986; Ebersbach *et al.* 1999). It is important to distinguish *état lacunaire* from the dilatations of perivascular spaces (*état criblé*) that are often present in the basal ganglia of hypertensive individuals, which may be difficult to differentiate on MR scans (Hauw 1995) (Fig. 4.16). These are not due to infarction and have not been convincingly associated with any particular clinical presentation (section 5.7.2).

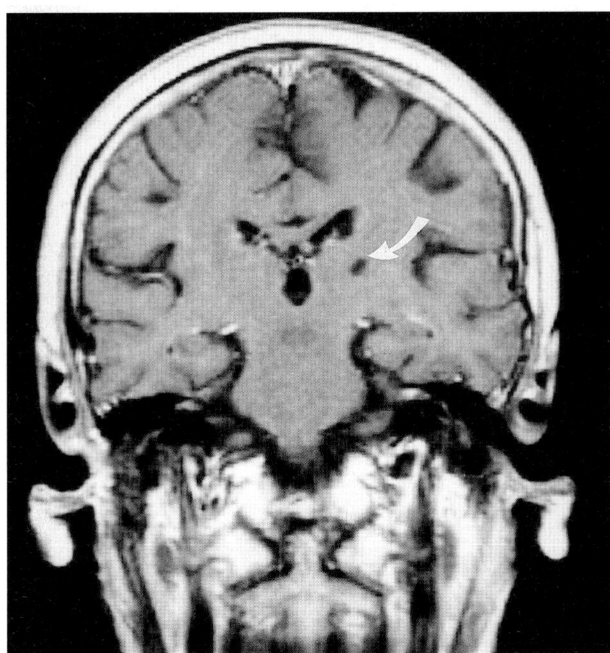

(a)

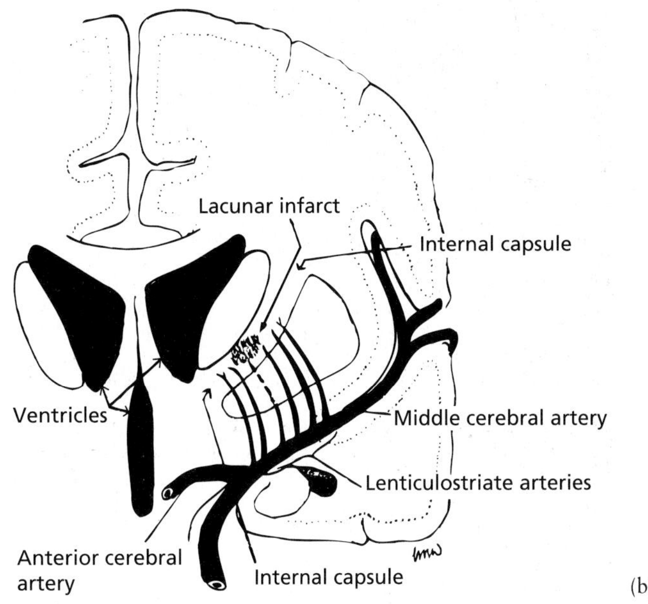

(b)

Fig. 4.15 Lacunar infarction. (a) The typical appearance of a small, deep infarct confined to the territory of a single, deep perforating artery on a T1-weighted, coronal magnetic resonance scan (curved arrow). (b) A diagrammatic representation of the case, demonstrating the likely underlying vascular process (coronal brain section); one of the lenticulostriate arteries is occluded (broken line).

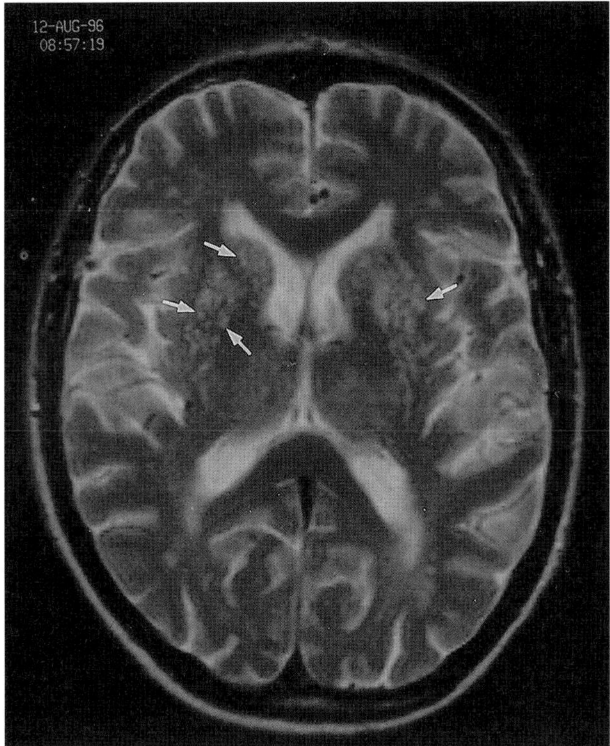

(a)

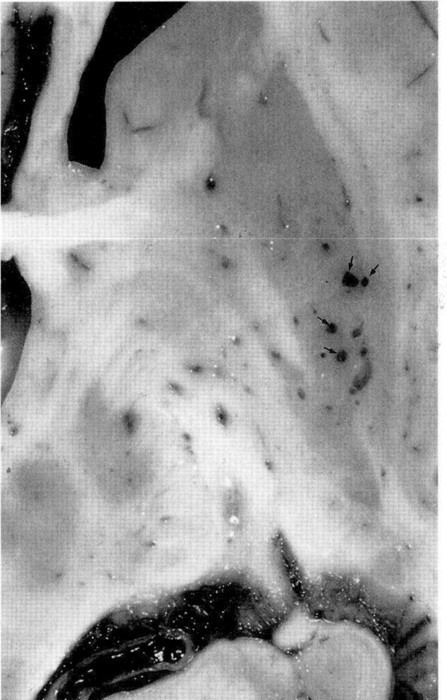

(b)

Fig. 4.16 The appearance of *état criblé* (i.e. dilated perivascular spaces) (a) on a T2-weighted magnetic resonance brain scan (arrows) and (b) in a pathological specimen (tiny arrows).

Middle cerebral artery—cortical branches

In the Sylvian fissure, the MCA usually bifurcates into superior and inferior divisions. The superior division usually gives rise to the orbitofrontal, prefrontal, pre-Rolandic, Rolandic, anterior parietal and posterior parietal branches, whilst the inferior division usually gives rise to the angular, temporo-occipital, posterior temporal, middle temporal, anterior tem-

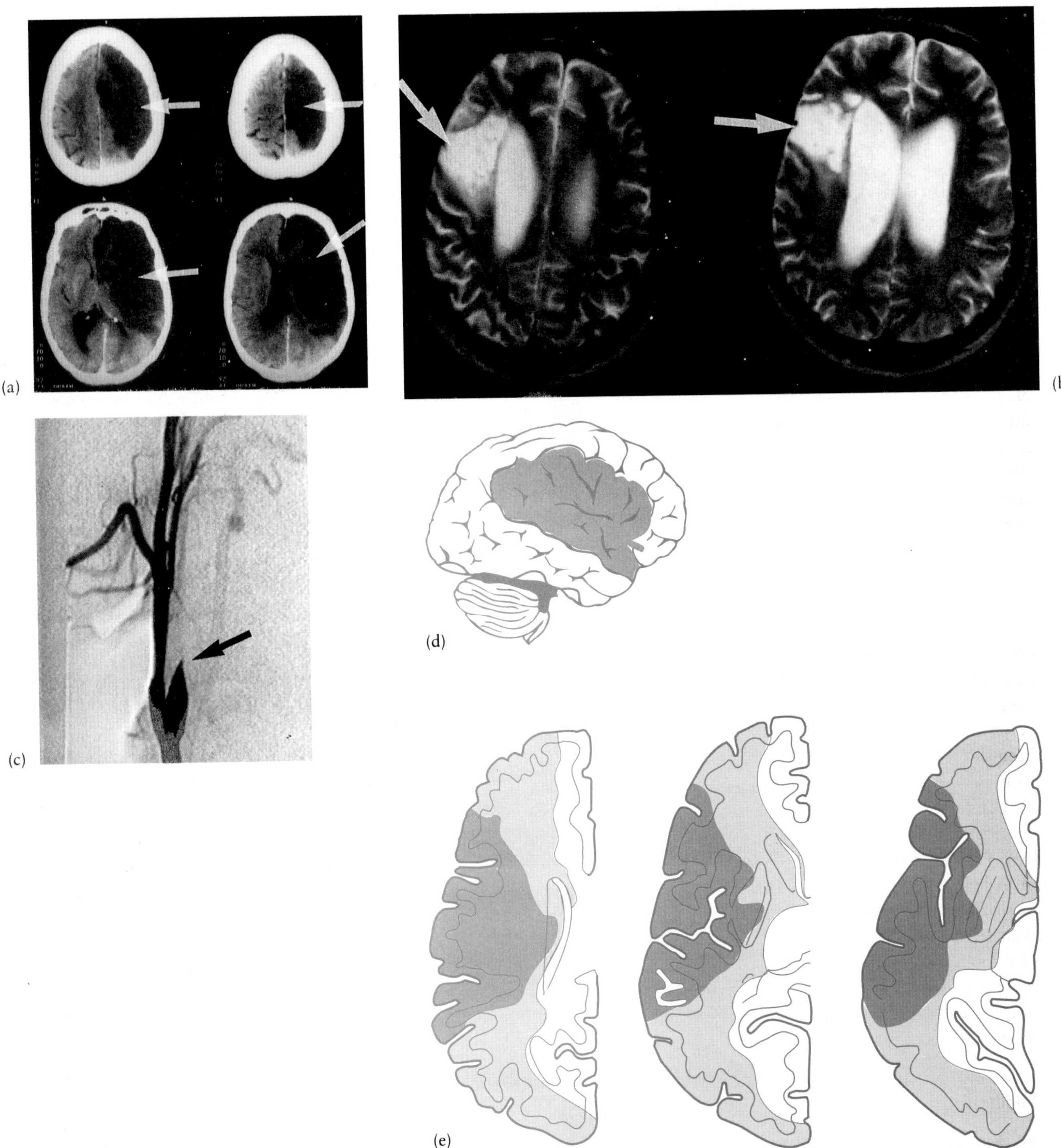

Fig. 4.17 Ischaemia in the territory of the middle cerebral artery (MCA). (a) The typical appearance on a CT brain scan of extensive MCA territory infarction (arrows) in a patient who had an occluded mainstem of the MCA. (b) The typical appearance on a T2-weighted magnetic resonance scan of MCA branch occlusion (arrows). (c) The patient whose scan is shown in (b) was a young man who had dissected the proximal internal carotid artery (ICA) (arrow) in a road accident. The intra-arterial digital subtraction angiogram shows a smooth, tapering, complete occlusion of the proximal ICA, typical of dissection. (d) However, there is great inter-individual and inter-hemispheric variability in the area of brain supplied by the MCA. The dark green area shows the only part of the cortex on the lateral surface of the hemisphere which was *always* supplied by the MCA in a large pathological study (van der Zwan 1991). (e) A similar degree of variability exists for the subcortical territory supplied by the MCA. The figure shows the minimum (pale green) and maximum (dark green) areas of supply at three levels in the same pathological study (with permission of Dr A. van der Zwan).

poral and temporopolar branches. However, there are many variations in this pattern. The potential minimum and maximum area of supply of these branches is shown in Fig. 4.17 (van der Zwan *et al.* 1992). At their origins, the luminal diameter of these vessels is usually about 1 mm, but by the time they anastomose with the cortical branches of the anterior and posterior cerebral arteries, they are usually less than 0.2 mm in diameter (vander Eecken & Adams 1953). There is almost no collateral supply between individual branches of the MCA.

Local atherosclerotic disease of the MCA branches is unlikely although they can be affected by cerebral vasculitis, amyloid angiopathy and mycotic aneurysms. Therefore, the main causes of ischaemia are probably embolism, or low-flow, secondary to more proximal vascular lesions (Olsen *et al.* 1985; Bogousslavsky *et al.* 1990). The usual clinical syndrome resulting from occlusion of the superior division is much the same as for the MCA mainstem, but in general the motor and sensory deficits are greater in the face and arm than in the leg. Occlusion of the inferior division usually causes a homonymous hemianopia or superior quadrantanopia and fluent aphasia (in the dominant hemisphere) but relatively mild problems in the limbs, although higher level discriminatory sensory functions may be affected. A similar pattern can, however, occur with occlusion of the posterior cerebral artery (section 4.2.3). The area of infarcted cortex can be very small. Indeed, the distinction on CT from cortical atrophy can be difficult (section 5.3.5). As a result, some very restricted clinical deficits may occur. For example, it has been shown that isolated arm weakness is much more likely to occur from a cortical than a subcortical lesion (Boiten & Lodder 1991a). Although there is a large volume of classical neurological literature correlating various restricted 'MCA' syndromes (most of which include some disturbance of higher cortical function) with ischaemia or haemorrhage in specific areas of brain parenchyma (Foix & Levy 1927; Waddington & Ring 1968), the inter-individual variability of the vascular anatomy means that it is virtually impossible to link them reliably with occlusions of particular MCA branches. Furthermore, many of the reports do not deal with deficits in the acute phase of stroke.

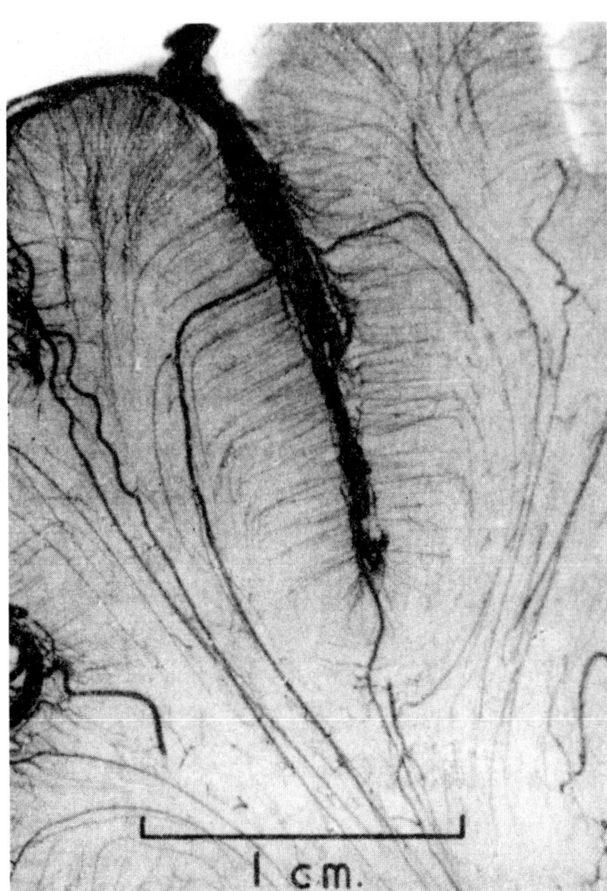

Fig. 4.18 Pathological demonstration of the medullary perforating arteries arising from branches of the middle cerebral artery on the cortical surface (courtesy of Dr Nigel Hyman, Radcliffe Infirmary, Oxford, UK).

Middle cerebral artery—medullary perforating arteries

MCA medullary perforating arteries arise from the cortical arteries on the surface of the hemispheres. They are usually 20–50 mm in length and descend to supply the subcortical white matter (i.e. centrum semiovale), converging centripetally towards the lateral ventricle (De Reuck 1971) (Fig. 4.18). These are functional end-arteries, and their distal fields are part of the internal boundary-zone (section 4.2.4).

Isolated infarcts of the centrum semiovale are rare (Uldry & Bogousslavsky 1995; Read *et al.* 1998). The majority are small (< 1.5 cm in diameter) and probably arise from occlusion of a single medullary perforating artery, although this has never been verified pathologically. The spectrum of clinical presentation is similar to that of single deep MCA perforating artery (i.e. lenticulostriate artery) occlusions, with the classical lacunar syndromes of pure motor stroke, sensorimotor stroke and ataxic hemiparesis predominating. In such cases, there is rarely evidence of large vessel disease or cardioembolism. Larger infarcts in this area present with a syndrome similar to more extensive MCA cortical infarction, with weakness/sensory loss which is more marked in the face and arm than leg, aphasia or visuospatial disturbance and, if the optic radiation is involved, a visual field defect. These are more often associated with large vessel disease (ICA/MCA occlusion or stenosis). However, such infarcts may in fact be in the internal boundary-zone (Read *et al.* 1998). The potential explanations for deficits of 'cortical' modalities are similar to those for striatocapsular infarction, i.e. ischaemia without necrosis, deafferentation of the cortex, or involvement of subcortical structures subserving 'cortical' functions, but there is little evidence to support any of these explanations.

4.2.3 The posterior (vertebrobasilar) system

The vertebrobasilar (VB) system develops quite separately from the carotid system and is subject to many more changes during fetal development. It is this that probably accounts for the much greater variation in arterial configuration within the VB than in the carotid system and it may contribute to the development of ischaemia (Chaturvedi *et al.* 1999).

Precerebral vertebral artery

The right vertebral artery (VA) arises as the first branch of the right subclavian artery (which arises from the innominate artery), whilst the left VA arises as the first branch of the left subclavian artery (which arises directly from the aortic arch) (Figs 4.3 and 4.19). The course of the VA is traditionally divided into segments. The first segment is from the origin to the transverse foramen at either C5 or C6. The next segment is within the transverse foramina from this level to C2. The third segment circles the arch of C1 and passes between the atlas and occiput. The major branch outside the skull is the single, midline anterior spinal artery, formed by a contribution from both VAs.

The origin of the VA can be affected by atheroma, either within the VA itself or by overlying plaque in the larger parent vessel, and may be the site of occlusion or source of emboli (Caplan & Tettenborn 1992b; Crawley *et al.* 1998). It may also be involved in inflammatory disorders, such as Takayasu's arteritis (section 7.3). The extracranial VA may also be the site of arterial dissection (Caplan & Tettenborn 1992a) (section 7.2.1). Trapping of the VA by cervical spondylosis is frequently cited as a cause of symptoms attributed to 'vertebrobasilar insufficiency', but in reality, both the symptoms (which are generally non-focal) and the X-ray changes of cervical spondylosis are common in the vascular age group and rarely is there a convincing cause-and-effect relationship (section 7.1). However, thrombus may form in the VA after prolonged or unusual neck posturing (Caplan & Tettenborn 1992a; Tettenborn *et al.* 1993).

Intracranial vertebral artery

The fourth segment of the VA is intracranial, until the two arteries unite to form the basilar artery (BA) at the pontomedullary junction (Fig. 4.19). As the VAs pierce the dura, there is a decrease in the adventitial and medial layer, with

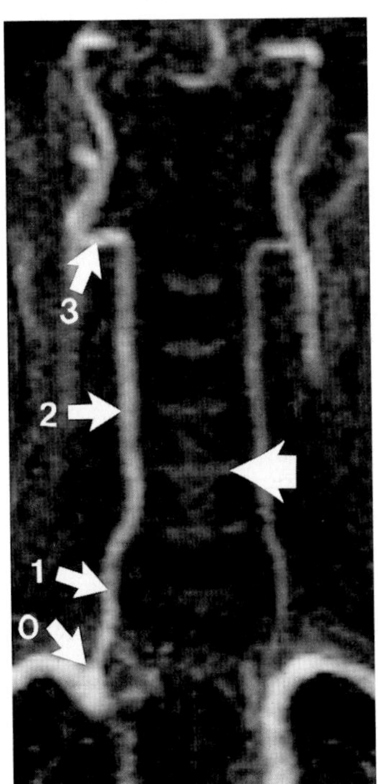

(a)

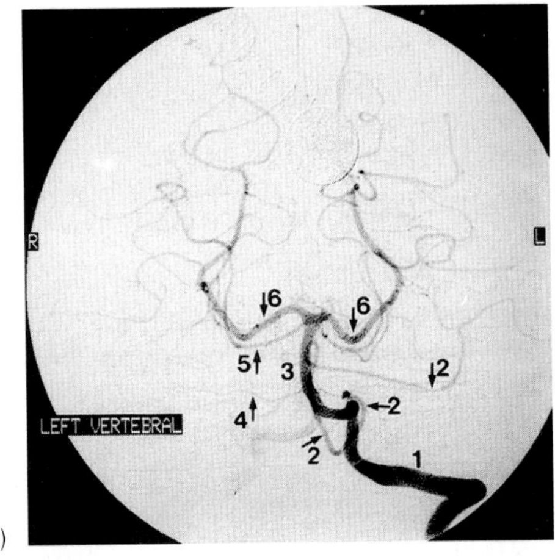

(b)

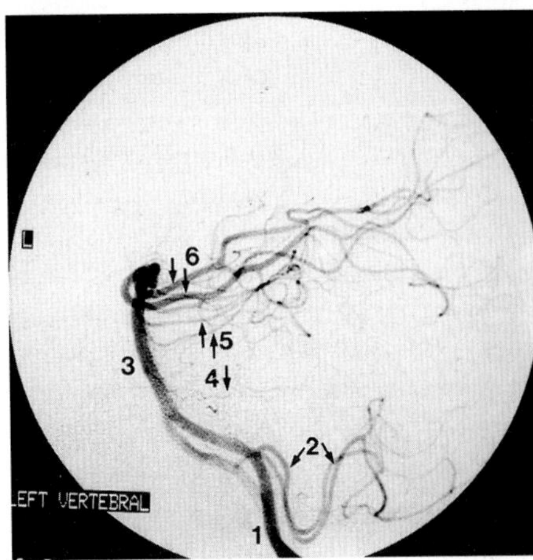

(c)

Fig. 4.19 Angiographic demonstration of the vertebrobasilar arterial system. (a) Anteroposterior projection of a magnetic resonance angiogram, showing the extracranial vertebral arteries. The numbers refer to the segments of the artery; 0, the origin; 1, the precanal portion; 2, the intracanalicular part; and 3, the horizontal part. The large arrow shows an intravertebral disc. (b) Anteroposterior projection of an intra-arterial catheter angiogram, showing (1) the distal vertebral artery; (2) the posterior inferior cerebellar artery; (3) the basilar artery; (4) the anterior inferior cerebellar artery; (5) the superior cerebellar artery; (6) the posterior cerebral arteries. (c) Lateral projection of an intra-arterial angiogram, showing the arteries as numbered above.

marked reduction in both medial and external elastic laminae. There may be branches which supply the medulla.

As with the internal carotid artery, occlusion of the VA may be asymptomatic. At the other extreme, there may be extensive infarction of the lateral medulla and inferior cerebellar hemisphere. Atheroma remains a common cause of stenosis or occlusion (Shin *et al.* 1999). Dissection of the intracranial VA may present with subarachnoid haemorrhage (Caplan & Tettenborn 1992a). The subclavian steal syndrome occurs when there is haemodynamically significant stenosis of the subclavian artery proximal to the origin of the VA. In this situation, the direction of blood flow is normal in the contralateral VA but reversed in the ipsilateral VA, with blood passing into the axillary artery from the VA. The blood pressure will be lower in the affected arm. Exercise of the ipsilateral arm increases the flow away from the brainstem, which may cause neurological symptoms. However, it is noteworthy that reversed flow in VA is a common finding on ultrasound and angiographic studies in patients with no neurological symptoms (Hennerici *et al.* 1988) (section 6.7.6).

Reversed flow in one vertebral artery is a common finding in patients with no neurological symptoms.

Posterior inferior cerebellar artery (PICA)

The PICAs usually arise from the intracranial vertebral artery (VA), although one may be absent in up to 25% of patients (Fig. 4.19). Also, the VA may terminate in the PICA. Small branches from the PICA may supply the lateral medulla, but more frequently it is supplied by direct branches from the VA originating between the ostium of PICA and the origin of the BA (Duncan *et al.* 1975). There are medial and lateral branches of the PICA, the medial branch usually supplying the cerebellar vermis and adjacent hemisphere and the lateral branch the cortical surface of the cerebellar tonsil and suboccipital cerebellar hemisphere.

Historically, occlusion of the PICA has been linked to lateral medullary infarcts, causing Wallenberg's syndrome. This consists of an ipsilateral Horner's syndrome (descending sympathetic fibres), loss of spinothalamic function over the contralateral limbs (spinothalamic tract) and ipsilateral face (descending trigeminal tract), vertigo, nausea, vomiting and nystagmus (vestibular nuclei), ipsilateral ataxia of limbs (inferior cerebellar peduncle) and ipsilateral paralysis of palate, larynx and pharynx (nucleus ambiguus), resulting in dysarthria, dysphonia and dysphagia. As with other 'classical' eponymous brainstem syndromes, the complete form of Wallenberg's syndrome is relatively infrequent in clinical practice. Indeed, syndromes which do not involve the lateral medulla but only the cerebellum are now recognized as being more frequent. They usually present with vertigo, headache, ataxia (of gait and limbs) and nystagmus. Another striking symptom is ipsilateral axial lateropulsion, which seems to the patient like lateral displacement of their centre of gravity (Amarenco *et al.* 1991). Isolated vertigo has been reported in cases of PICA territory infarction (Duncan *et al.* 1975; Huang & Yu 1985), although overall this is best considered to be a non-focal symptom (section 3.2.1). Infarcts restricted to either the medial or lateral branches of the PICA usually cause less impairment (Kase *et al.* 1993).

Basilar artery (BA)

The general pattern of branches from the BA is of short paramedian (perforating) branches, which supply the base of the pons to either side of the midline and also the paramedian aspects of the pontine tegmentum. As with the anterior circulation, the frequency of infarction from occlusion of such perforating arteries has probably been underestimated, although infarcts arising from BA disease are less well documented, partly because of the difficulty of imaging such infarcts with CT and also because catheter angiography of the VB system so seldom has any clinical utility that it is not often performed. The lateral aspects of the base of the pons and the tegmentum are supplied by pairs of short and long circumferential arteries, which also supply the cerebellar hemispheres.

Occlusion of a single paramedian artery, resulting in a restricted infarct in the brainstem, can present with any of the classical lacunar syndromes (section 4.3.2). Disturbances of eye movement (either nuclear or internuclear) may also occur from such lesions, either in isolation or in addition to pure motor deficits (e.g. Weber's syndrome) (Hommel *et al.* 1990a; Fisher 1991). Unlike the anterior circulation, where intrinsic disease of the anterior cerebral or middle cerebral artery mainstem is uncommon, occlusion of the mouth of a single perforating artery by a plaque of atheroma in the parent artery (BA) needs to be considered alongside intrinsic small vessel disease as the underlying mechanism (Caplan 1989). The 'locked-in syndrome' occurs with bilateral infarction, or haemorrhage, of the base of the pons (section 3.3.2).

The *'top of the basilar syndrome'* is a constellation of symptoms and signs that may occur when an embolus impacts in the rostral BA, resulting in bilateral ischaemia of rostral brainstem structures and of the posterior cerebral artery territories (Caplan 1980). The syndrome consists of variable pupillary responses, supranuclear paresis of vertical gaze, ptosis or lid retraction, somnolence, hallucinations, involuntary movements such as hemiballismus (from involvement of rostral brainstem structures), visual abnormalities such as cortical blindness (from involvement of the occipital lobes), and an amnesic state (from involvement of the temporal lobes or thalamus).

Sometimes the BA becomes elongated (and therefore tortuous) and dilated (Figs 4.20 and 6.5). This is known as dolichoectasia, and the importance of this may have been

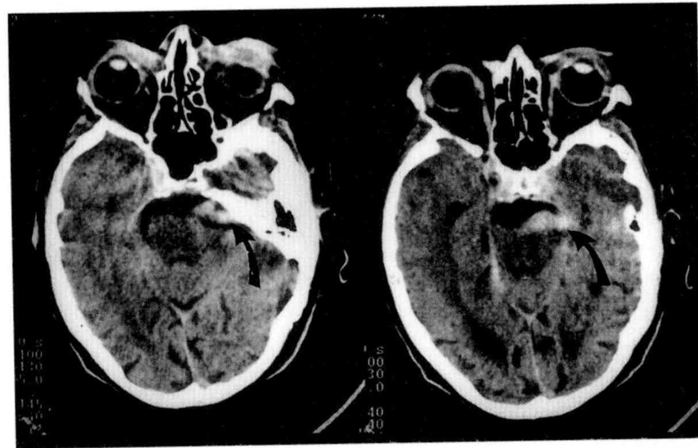

(a)

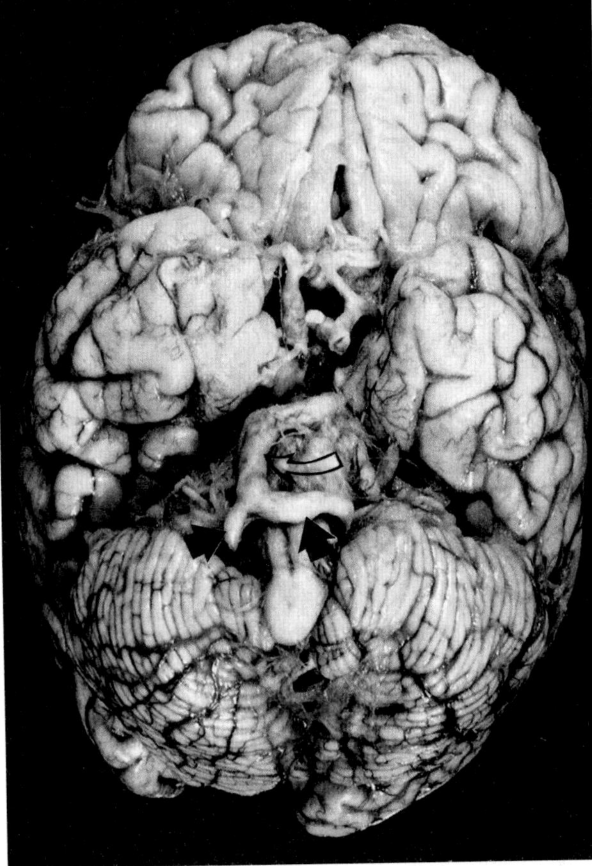

(b)

Fig. 4.20 (a) An axial CT brain scan, showing dolichoectasia of the basilar artery extending into the cerebellopontine angle (curved arrow). At this stage, the patient presented with trigeminal neuralgia. (b) Post-mortem demonstration of the vertebral artery (closed arrows) and basilar artery (open arrow) in the same patient two years later, after massive infarction of the brainstem and cerebellum (courtesy of Dr L. Bridges, University of Leeds).

underestimated (Schwartz *et al.* 1993; Ince *et al.* 1998) (section 6.3.2). There are four potential consequences:

• the dilated artery may directly compress the brainstem, resulting in a mixture of cranial nerve and longtract signs;

• the disruption of laminar flow predisposes to *in situ* thrombosis, which may occlude the origins of the paramedian or long circumferential branches;

• there may be distal embolization from the areas of *in situ* thrombosis;

• the changes in contour of the BA may result in distortion around the origins of the perforating arteries.

Anterior inferior cerebellar artery (AICA)

The AICAs originate from the caudal basilar artery (Fig. 4.19) and give off branches to the rostral medulla and base of the pons before supplying the rostral cerebellar structures. In most cases, they also give rise to the internal auditory arteries (IAA), but these may come directly from the BA or, occasionally, the superior cerebellar artery or PICA. They are effectively end-arteries. The IAA supplies the seventh and eighth cranial nerves within the auditory canal and, on entering the inner ear, divides into the common cochlear and anterior vestibular arteries. The common cochlear artery then divides into the main cochlear artery, which supplies the spiral ganglion, the basilar membrane structures and the stria vascularis, whilst the posterior vestibular artery supplies the inferior part of the saccule and the ampulla of the semicircular canal. The anterior vestibular artery supplies the utricle and ampulla of the anterior and horizontal semicircular canals (Baloh 1992).

Isolated occlusion of the AICA is probably relatively uncommon, but when it does occur there is almost always infarction in both the cerebellum and pons (Amarenco & Hauw 1990a). Symptoms tend to be tinnitus, vertigo and nausea, with an ipsilateral Horner's syndrome, an ipsilateral nuclear facial palsy, dysarthria, nystagmus, ipsilateral trigeminal sensory loss, cerebellar ataxia (in the ipsilateral limbs) and sometimes a contralateral hemiparesis (i.e. similar to the lateral medullary syndrome with the seventh and eighth nerve lesions replacing those of the ninth and tenth nerves and a hemiparesis). Ischaemia in the territory of the internal auditory artery is probably an under-recognized cause of sudden unilateral deafness, which may occur in isolation, as may vertigo (Amarenco *et al.* 1993; Kim *et al.* 1999) (section 3.3.7). Occlusion of the AICA is probably most often secondary to atherothrombosis in the BA, or anomalies such as dolichoectasia.

Superior cerebellar artery (SCA)

The SCA arises from the basilar artery (BA), immediately before its terminal bifurcation (Fig. 4.19). It usually supplies the dorsolateral midbrain and has branches to the superior cerebellar peduncle and superior surface of the cerebellar hemispheres. The 'classical' syndrome of occlusion of the whole territory of the SCA includes an ipsilateral Horner's syndrome, limb ataxia and intention tremor, with contralateral spinothalamic sensory loss, contralateral upper motor neurone type facial palsy and sometimes a contralateral fourth nerve palsy. In its pure form, it is rare. However, it is often associated with other infarcts in the distal territory of the BA, and may have a poor prognosis (Amarenco & Hauw 1990b). Infarcts that only involve the cerebellar territory of the SCA, on the other hand, have a better prognosis (Amarenco *et al.* 1991; Struck *et al.* 1991). In these cases, headache, limb and gait ataxia, dysarthria, vertigo and vomiting are most prominent, but cases with some of these deficits in isolation have been reported, due to occlusion of the distal branches (Amarenco *et al.* 1994). Vertigo is much less common in SCA than PICA or AICA territory infarction (Kase *et al.* 1993). Embolism (either cardiac or artery-to-artery) is considered the most frequent cause of both complete and partial SCA territory infarcts.

The arterial supply of the cerebellum

The cerebellum is supplied by the three long circumferential arteries (PICA, AICA, SCA) described above. The PICA usually supplies the inferior surface, the AICA the rostral surface and the SCA the tentorial surface (Fig. 4.21). Territorial infarction is considered most likely to be caused by thromboembolism, particularly from the heart or the basilar artery. However, these arterial systems also have perforating arteries. Cortical infarction in the cerebellum is of two types: infarction perpendicular to the cortical rim at the boundary-zone between perforating arteries (which lack anastomoses); and infarction that parallels the cortical rim and is the boundary-zone between the SCA and PICA. Small, deep infarcts occur within the deep white matter of the cerebellar hemispheres, usually around the deep boundary-zones. Unlike other small, deep infarcts, the predominant cause may be hypoperfusion secondary to large vessel atherothrombosis (Amarenco 1995) (Fig. 4.22).

Cerebellar infarction may be misdiagnosed as 'labyrinthitis', or even upper gastrointestinal disease if nausea and vomiting are prominent.

Posterior cerebral artery (PCA)

The two PCAs are usually the terminal branches of the basilar artery (BA) (Fig. 4.19). The precommunicating P1 segments of the PCAs pass around the cerebral peduncles and come to lie between the medial surface of the temporal lobe and the upper brainstem. From this portion of the PCA, small paramedian mesencephalic arteries and the thalamic–subthalamic arteries arise to supply the medial midbrain, the thalamus and part of the lateral geniculate body. In about 30% of patients, these vessels arise from a single pedicle and therefore bilateral midbrain infarction can result from a single PCA occlusion. After the posterior communicating

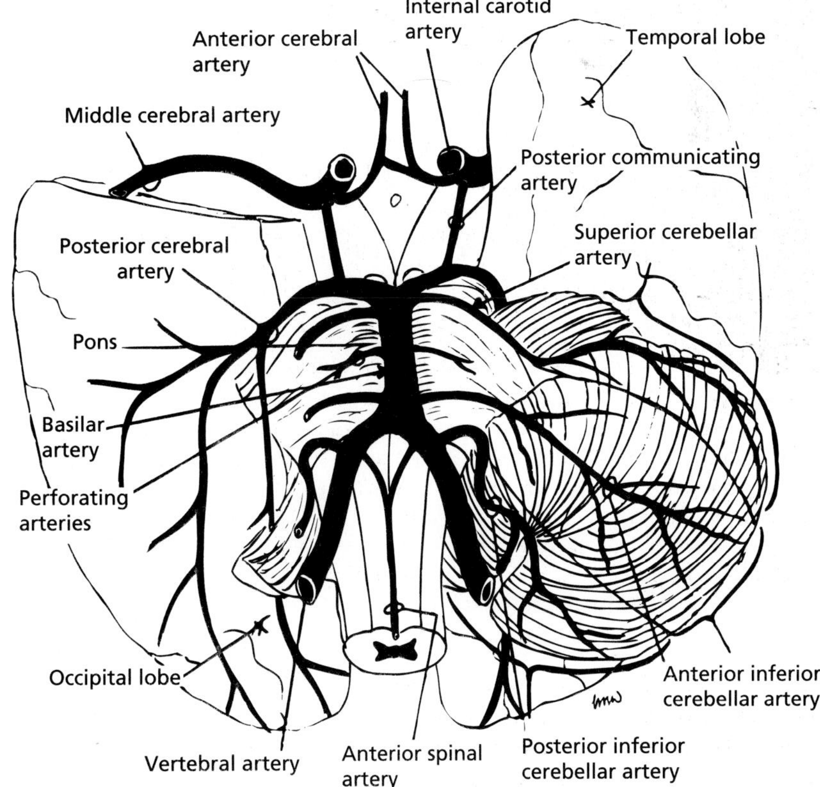

Fig. 4.21 Arterial supply of the cerebellum. The brainstem, cerebellum and inferior surface of the temporal and occipital lobes viewed from anteroinferiorly. The cerebellum, on the left-hand side of the image, has been cut away to reveal the inferior temporal and occipital lobes. Three major pairs of arteries supply the cerebellum: the superior cerebellar, the anterior inferior cerebellar (both branches of the basilar) and the posterior inferior cerebellar arteries (branches of the vertebral arteries). Perforating branches of the basilar artery supply the pons. The medial parts of the medulla are supplied by the anterior spinal artery and the lateral parts by branches of the vertebral arteries. The posterior cerebral arteries supply the posteromedial temporal lobes and the occipital lobes. The superior surface of the cerebellum (not shown) is predominantly supplied by the superior cerebellar arteries.

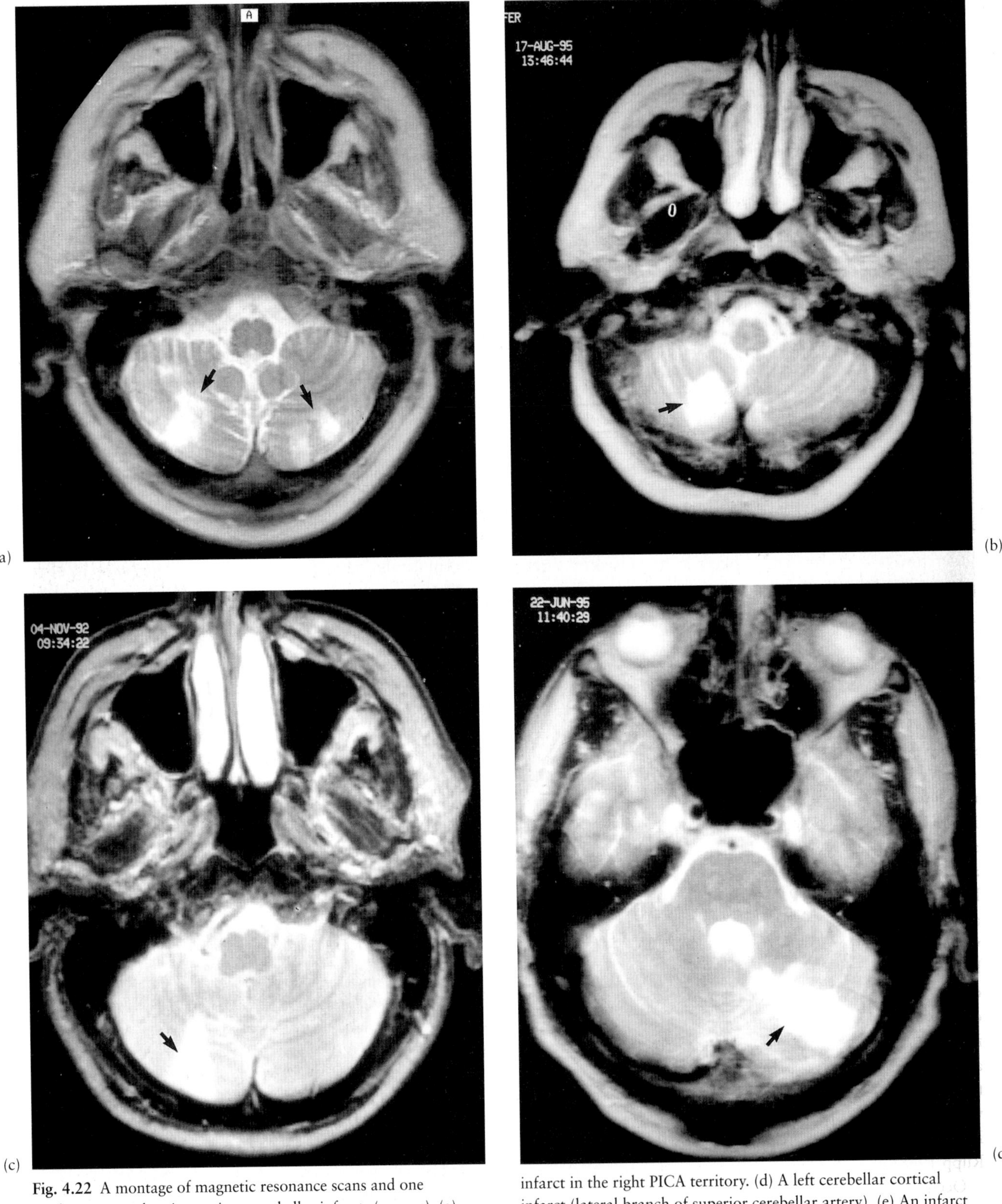

Fig. 4.22 A montage of magnetic resonance scans and one CT brain scan, showing various cerebellar infarcts (arrows). (a) Bilateral small cerebellar cortical infarcts in the posterior inferior cerebellar artery (PICA) territories. (b) A unilateral small right cerebellar cortical infarct (medial branch of PICA). (c) A cortical infarct in the right PICA territory. (d) A left cerebellar cortical infarct (lateral branch of superior cerebellar artery). (e) An infarct in the left brainstem just inferior to the pons (perforating branch of basilar artery). (f) A CT scan, showing a left superior cerebellar infarct (medial branch of the superior cerebellar artery).

(e) 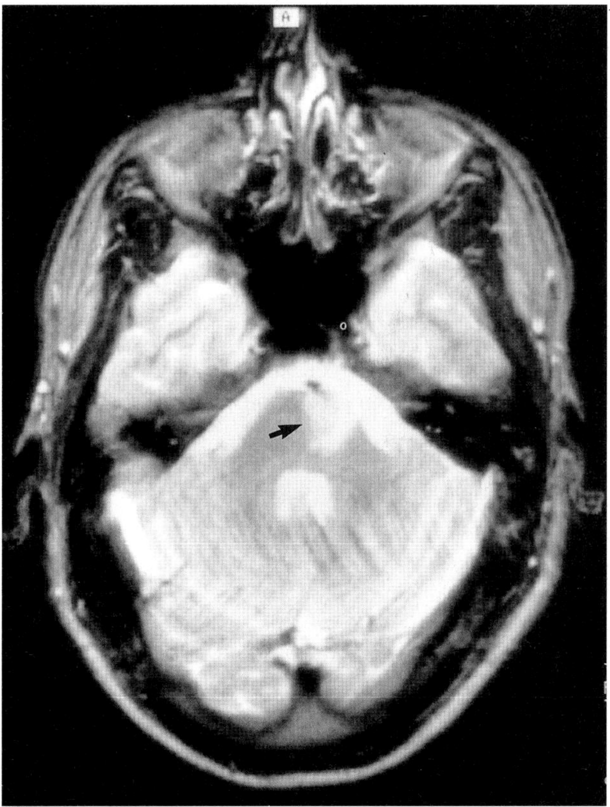

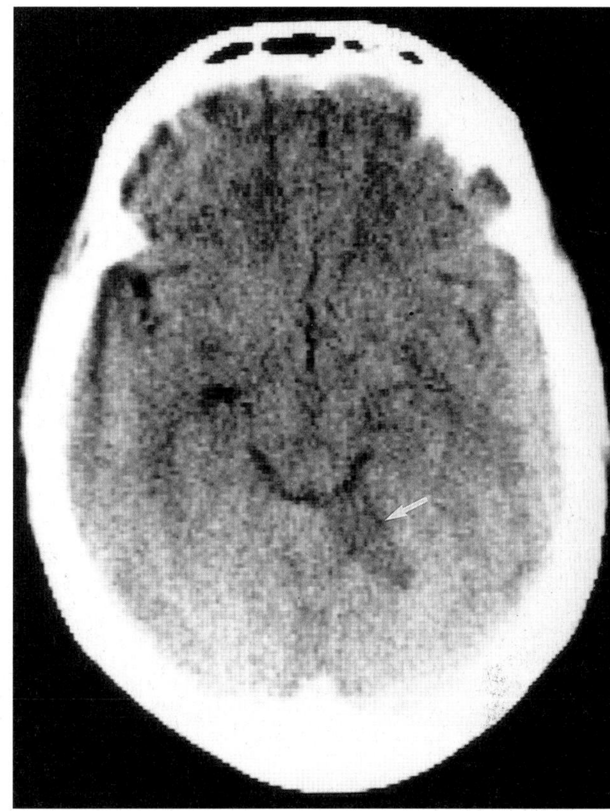 (f)

Fig. 4.22 (*continued*)

artery (PCoA) (from which the polar arteries to the thalamus usually arise), there are usually the thalamogeniculate arteries and the posterior choroidal artery (PChA), both of which supply the thalamus. Once the PCA has passed around the free medial edge of the tentorium, it usually divides into two divisions, with a total of four main branches. The anterior division gives rise to the anterior and posterior temporal arteries, whilst from the posterior division the calcarine and parieto-occipital arteries arise. The posterior pericallosal arteries are usually branches of the parieto-occipital arteries, and pass anteriorly to form a potential anastomosis with the anterior pericallosal arteries from the anterior cerebral artery. The potential minimum and maximum areas of supply of these branches are shown in Fig. 4.23 (van der Zwan *et al.* 1992). During early fetal development, the internal carotid artery (ICA) supplies most of the posterior aspect of the cerebral hemispheres and brainstem through the PCoA. In some adults this pattern persists, with only a vestigial BA–PCA connection and in about 30% one or both PCAs are supplied from the ICA, via the PCoA (Riggs & Rupp 1963; van Overbeeke *et al.* 1991) (section 4.2.2)

Occlusions of the PCA origin are probably most often embolic and may occur subsequent to the arrest of an embolus at the basilar bifurcation (Caplan 1980; Koroshetz & Ropper 1987; Caplan 1993). As with occlusion of the mainstem of the middle cerebral artery (MCA), ischaemia can occur in both the deep and superficial territory of the PCA. Occlusion of the deep perforating branches of the PCA results in ischaemia of the thalamus and upper brainstem, as described below. Such patients may have a hemiparesis in addition to their visual defects and so mimic extensive MCA territory infarction (Hommel *et al.* 1990b, 1991; Chambers *et al.* 1991). Visual field defects are the most commonly encountered syndrome from PCA infarction. A macular-sparing homonymous hemianopia may occur because collateral flow from the MCA supplies the occipital pole, and the optic radiation is not involved (Pessin *et al.* 1987). More restricted infarcts can result in small homonymous sectoranopias. Bilateral occipital infarction may result in cortical blindness. When visual function is less severely affected, disorders of colour vision (discrimination, naming) may be apparent. Transient ischaemia in the PCA territory may give 'positive' visual phenomena which are very similar to those of classical migraine (Fisher 1986). Visual perseverations, such as seeing an object several times despite continued fixation, and continuing to see an object as an after-image (palinopsia) may also occur (Critchley 1951). Disorders of language function may occur from PCA territory infarction, probably due to involvement of the thalamus (see below) or its projection fibres. Alexia, with or without agraphia, may result from left PCA occlusion (section 3.3.3). Amnesic disorders may occur because of direct involvement of the temporal

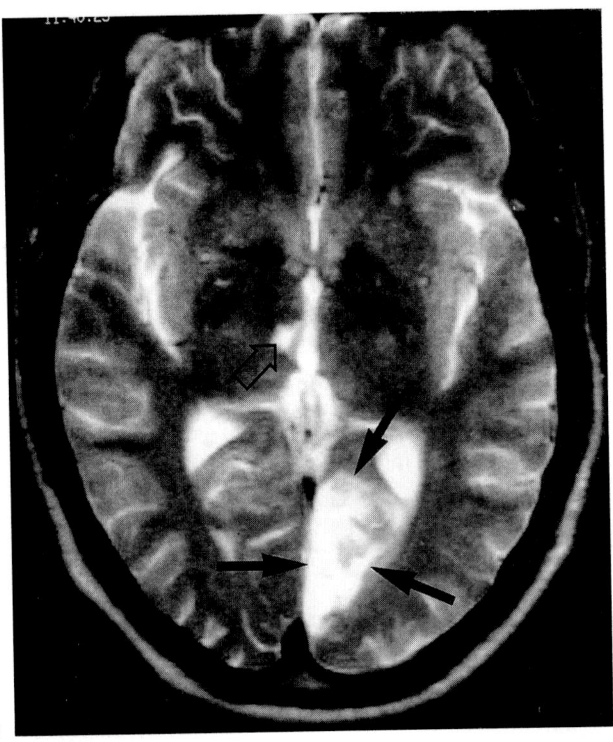

(a)

lobes, the thalamus, or the mamillothalamic tract (Clarke *et al.* 1994) (section 3.3.3). Typically, there is marked amnesia for recent events. Non-dominant hemisphere PCA territory infarcts may result in disorders of visuospatial function.

The arterial supply of the thalamus

The thalamus is involved in about 25% of all posterior circulation strokes (Bogousslavsky 1995), either in isolation following perforating artery occlusion, or in combination with other structures following large artery thrombosis or artery-to-artery embolism. The blood supply to the thalamus comes from four groups of arteries, which over the years have, confusingly, been called by several different names (Fig. 4.24) (Graff-Radford *et al.* 1985). Unlike other small deep infarcts, those in the thalamus produce a wide range of clinical syndromes, which can make clinical localization difficult.

The thalamic–subthalamic arteries (also known as the paramedian, thalamoperforating, and posterior internal optic arteries) arise from the proximal posterior cerebral artery (PCA). They are usually 200–400 μm in luminal diameter. In addition to supplying the thalamus, branches also go to the rostral midbrain. In 30% of people, the branches to the two

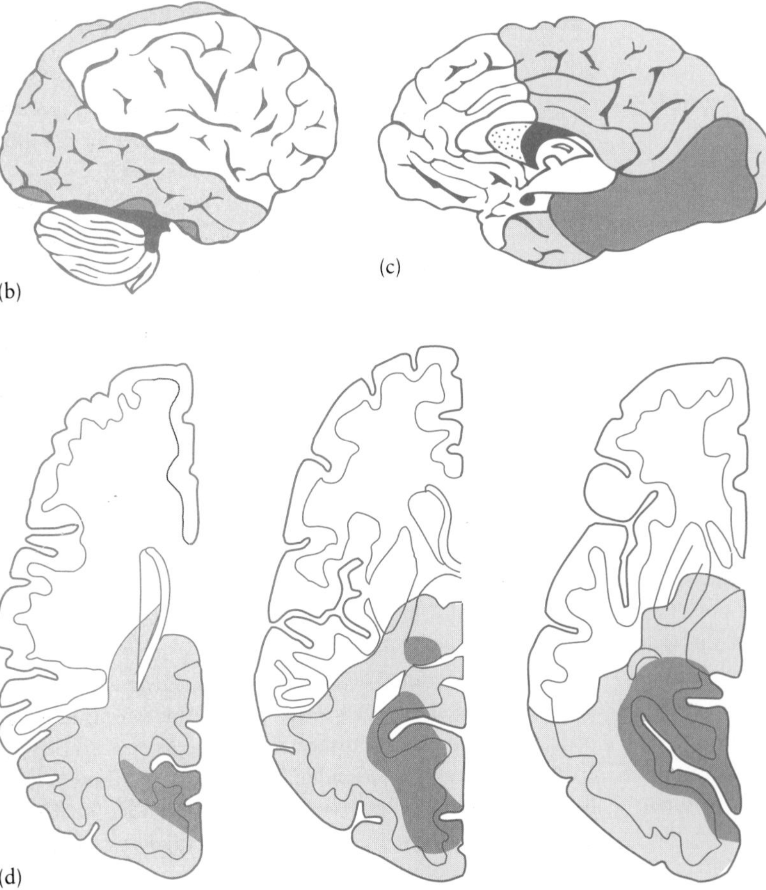

Fig. 4.23 Ischaemia in the territory of the posterior cerebral artery (PCA). (a) The typical appearance on a T2-weighted MR scan of PCA territory infarction (arrows). Note also the small right thalamic infarct (open arrow) in the distribution of a perforating artery from the PCA. However, there is great inter-individual and inter-hemispheric variability in the area supplied by the PCA (b, c). The dark green areas show the only part of the cortex on the lateral surface (b) and the medial surface (c) of the hemisphere, which was *always* supplied by the PCA in a large pathological study (van der Zwan 1991). The pale green represents the maximum extent of the area which may be supplied by the PCA in some patients. (d) A similar degree of variability exists for the subcortical territory supplied by the PCA. The figure shows the minimum (dark green) and maximum (pale green) areas of supply at three levels in the same pathological study (with permission of Dr A. van der Zwan).

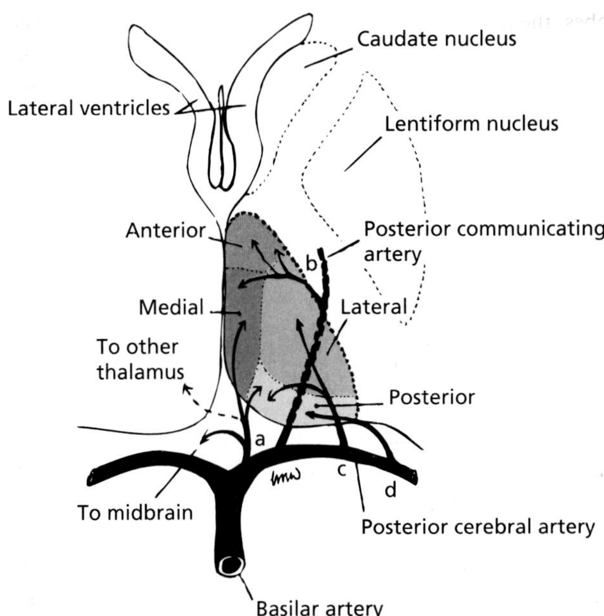

Fig. 4.24 Diagrammatic representation of the arterial supply of the thalamus, showing also the anterior, medial, lateral and posterior nuclei. The branches are: (a) thalamic–subthalamic (paramedian, thalamoperforating, posterior internal optic) arteries. In addition to the thalamus, branches supply the midbrain, and in about 30% the branches to the thalamus in the other hemisphere arise from a common pedicle; (b) polar (tuberothalamic, anterior internal optic) arteries; (c) thalamogeniculate arteries; (d) posterior choroidal arteries.

thalamic hemispheres have a common pedicle from just one PCA (Castaigne *et al.* 1981). They supply the posteromedial thalamus, including the nucleus of the medial longitudinal fasciculus, the posterior dorsomedial nucleus and the intralaminar nuclei. The typical syndrome of unilateral infarction is of acute depression of conscious level, neuropsychological disturbances such as apathy, disorientation and memory dysfunction, and impaired upgaze, with little or no motor or sensory disturbance. The neuropsychological abnormalities are difficult to distinguish from cortical syndromes. The symptoms resulting from bilateral infarcts due to occlusion of a common vascular pedicle are similar to those from unilateral infarction, but are usually much more severe. Hypersomnolence can persist for many weeks, presumably due to involvement of the intralaminar nuclei and rostral fibres of the reticular activating system. Additionally, the syndrome of akinetic mutism can occur (section 3.3.2). Amnesic syndromes are most likely to occur when there is involvement of the dorsomedial nucleus, and mood disturbances may mimic frontal lobe syndromes. Thalamic dementia consists of impaired attention, slowed responses, apathy, poor motivation and amnesia.

The polar arteries (also known as the tuberothalamic, and anterior internal optic arteries) usually arise from the posterior communicating artery, although in about 30% the artery is absent and the vascular supply comes from the thalamic–subthalamic arteries. They supply the anteromedial and anterolateral areas, including the dorsomedial nucleus, the reticular nucleus, the mamillothalamic tract and part of the ventrolateral nucleus. These nuclei have substantial connections with the frontal lobes and the dorsomedial nuclei link with medial temporal lobe structures. The deficits from polar infarcts are mainly neuropsychological; patients tend to be rather apathetic and lack spontaneity. Typically, left-sided infarcts will result in an aphasia that is non-fluent, with poor naming but preserved comprehension and repetition, and impaired learning of verbal material (Bogousslavsky *et al.* 1986). Right-sided infarcts may result in hemineglect syndromes and impaired visuospatial processing. Polar infarcts, particularly if bilateral, may result in acute amnesia (Von Cramon *et al.* 1985).

The thalamogeniculate arteries are five or six small branches arising from the more distal posterior cerebral artery. These are the equivalent of the lenticulostriate arteries of the middle cerebral artery and are usually 400–800 μm in luminal diameter. They supply the ventrolateral thalamus, including the ventro-postero-lateral (VPL) and ventro-postero-medial nuclei (VPM), i.e. the specific relay nuclei for motor and sensory functions. Pure sensory stroke is a typical lateral thalamic deficit due to occlusion of the thalamogeniculate arteries (section 4.3.2). There may be a full hemianaesthesia or there may be partial syndromes such as cheiro-oral, cheiro-podo-oral and pseudoradicular sensory loss (Kim & Lee 1994; Kim 1994) (section 3.3.5). The deficit may involve all modalities or spare pain and temperature sensation (Sacco *et al.* 1987). If there is extension to the internal capsule, a sensorimotor stroke may occur (Mohr *et al.* 1977) (section 4.3.2). Hemiataxia is also a typical feature of involvement of the contralateral ventrolateral nucleus, because of interruption of fibres in the dentato-rubro-thalamic pathway. The clinical features are suggestive of cerebellar dysfunction and are not explained by proprioceptive loss. The Déjerine–Roussy syndrome is caused by more extensive lateral thalamic infarction and is sometimes referred to as the syndrome of the thalamogeniculate pedicle (Déjerine & Roussy 1906; Caplan *et al.* 1988). It consists of a mild hemiparesis, marked hemianaesthesia, hemiataxia, astereognosis and frequently paroxysmal pain/hyperaesthesia (often of delayed onset) and choreoathetotic movements, all contralateral to the lesion. The original cases had extension of the infarcts into the internal capsule and towards the putamen, although most of the features of this syndrome result from involvement of the VPN and ventrolateral nucleus of the thalamus.

Finally, there is the supply from the medial and *lateral posterior choroidal arteries* (PChAs), which also arise from the posterior cerebral artery. These supply the pulvinar and posterior thalamus, the geniculate bodies and the anterior nucleus. Involvement of the PChA presents typically with visual field deficits (upper or lower homonymous quadrantanopia, and rarely homonymous horizontal sectoranopia), with or without hemisensory loss. Some cases will have associated neuropsychological deficits such as transcortical aphasia and disturbance of memory function (Neau & Bogousslavsky 1996).

The thalamic arteries were traditionally considered to be end-arteries, but recent work suggests that functional anastomoses do occur (Bogousslavsky 1995). It is perhaps for this reason that the vascular pathology underlying thalamic infarcts is much more variable than that of other small, deep infarcts.

4.2.4 Arterial boundary-zones

Arterial boundary-zones may be defined as those areas of brain parenchyma where the distal fields of two or more adjacent arteries meet (section 6.6.5). The potential clinical relevance is that one might predict that these areas would be particularly vulnerable to haemodynamic stresses, such as hypotension. There are two types of boundary-zone:

- those where functional anastomoses between the two arterial systems exist, e.g. on the pial surface between the major cerebral arteries (vander Eecken & Adams 1953) and to a lesser extent at the base of the brain between the choroidal circulations;
- those at the junction of the distal fields of two nonanastomosing arterial systems, e.g. deep perforating and pial medullary perforating arteries in the centrum semiovale (Chambers & Bladin 1995).

With the former, the boundary-zone will occur at points of equal pressure between the two arterial systems. Consequently, changes in arterial pressure in one of the systems may result in a shift of the boundary-zone towards the compromised artery (Figs 4.11, 4.17 & 4.23). With the latter, the boundary-zone is likely to be more or less fixed in the individual hemisphere (Fig. 4.25). Both types of boundary-zone are present in the cerebellum.

The impression that might be gained from the clinicoradiological literature is that the major boundary-zones occur at symmetrical, predictable sites in the hemispheres (e.g. Damasio 1983). Consequently, in some classifications of stroke, imaged infarcts in these areas are considered most likely to be haemodynamic rather than embolic in origin, i.e. due to low flow. But, as has been shown in Figs 4.11, 4.17, 4.23 and 4.25, for both types of boundary-zone, there is considerable inter-individual and intra-individual variation (van der Zwan *et al.* 1992). More recent maps of arterial territories have taken account of this work (Tatu *et al.* 1996, 1998). Lang *et al.* (1995) used the minimum and maximum areas of middle cerebral artery supply from van der Zwan *et al.* (1992) to assess whether imaged areas of infarction distal to a haemodynamically significant internal carotid artery lesion would be regarded as being territorial infarcts or boundary-zone infarcts. Using the minimum area of supply, 64% were considered as boundary-zone infarcts, but when the maximum area of supply was considered only 19% were classified in the same way. We do not believe it is always possible to identify 'typical' CT or MR patterns associated with boundary-zone infarction, given the very real difficulty of identifying them *in vivo* (section 6.6.5).

> *We do not believe it always is possible to identify 'typical' CT or MR patterns associated with boundary-zone infarction.*

It has been suggested that whilst cortical boundary-zone infarcts may have many causes (and not just low flow), it is in fact the deep or internal boundary-zone that is most vulnerable to low blood flow factors (Moriwaki *et al.* 1997). However, whereas with cortical infarcts the differential diag-

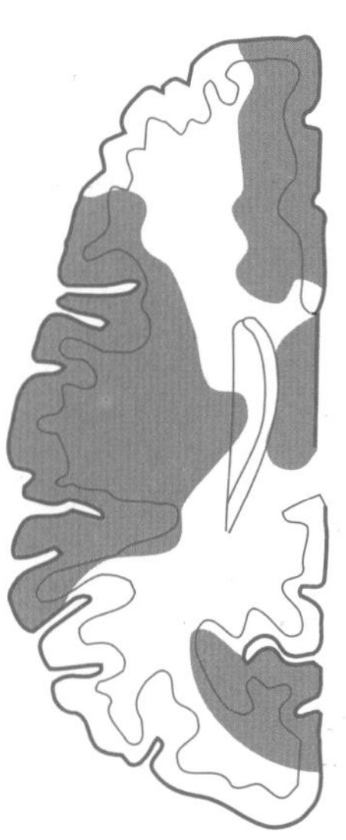
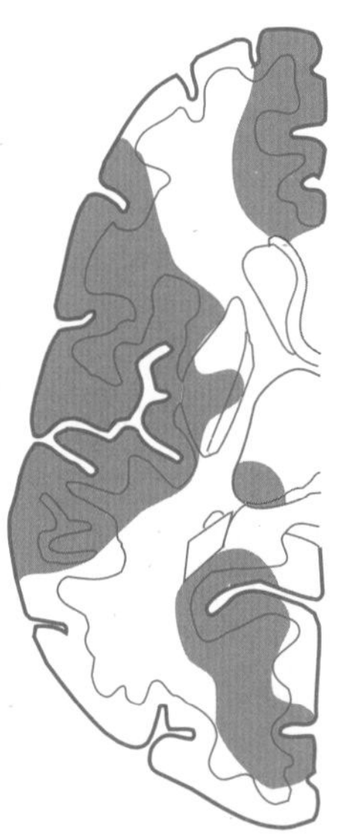
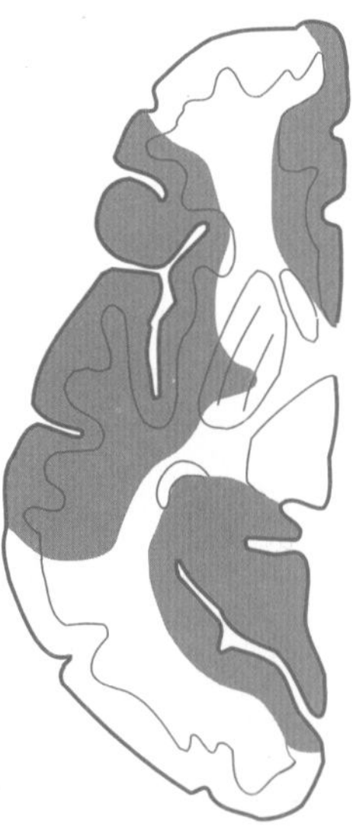

Fig. 4.25 Variability of the boundary-zones. The green shaded areas represent the minimum areas of cerebral supply at three levels of the anterior, middle and posterior cerebral arteries in a large pathological study (van der Zwan 1991), as shown individually in Figs 4.11d, 4.17e and 4.23d. The adjacent unshaded area represents the area of variation within which the boundaries between these territories were found (with permission of Dr A. van der Zwan).

nosis is from distal field embolism, in the subcortical region the differential is from intrinsic disease of the perforating arteries, and there are just as many problems with the anatomical localization of the boundary-zones in individual patients (van der Zwan *et al.* 1992; Read *et al.* 1998).

4.3 The clinical subclassification of cerebrovascular disease

4.3.1 Introduction

The traditional teaching of cerebrovascular neurology is based on the general assumption that particular symptoms and signs arise from restricted areas of damaged brain parenchyma, which, in turn, receive their vascular supply in a predictable manner. This general notion has its origins in the large classical literature describing patterns of neurological deficit which were linked (usually at a later post-mortem) with a particular pattern of vascular lesions, including a myriad of eponymous clinical syndromes. Although these are of value to those interested in exploring the subtleties of cerebral localization, and are the stock in trade of many neurologists' clinical demonstrations, the original descriptions were often of only a handful of cases. Consequently, the sensitivity, specificity and generalizability of many of the clinicoanatomical correlations have rarely been tested on large, unselected groups of patients with stroke. What is clear is that many of these 'classical' vascular syndromes occur infrequently (at least in their pure forms), and even when they do they rarely have a particularly distinctive cause. Thus, they are of limited practical value to the majority of clinicians. Additionally, the descriptions nearly always relate to ischaemic rather than haemorrhagic strokes and, although one might argue that this is perfectly acceptable in the context of a high proportion of patients having brain CT or MR scans, there will remain a large number of clinicians worldwide who do not have ready access to such technology.

Despite being well known, many of the 'classical' vascular syndromes occur rather infrequently in routine clinical practice.

Having taken the history and performed a physical examination, the physician should have established which brain functions have been affected by the stroke. These clinical findings then need to be used to identify groups of patients in a manner which will bring together both the parenchymal anatomy (i.e. the site and size of the parenchymal lesion) and the pathology/aetiology (i.e. the pattern and nature of the vascular lesion). Traditional clinically based classifications have distinguished anterior (carotid) circulation strokes and posterior (vertebrobasilar) circulation strokes (WHO Task Force 1989). It seems reasonable to retain this division, because certain investigations (e.g. carotid duplex) and treatments (e.g. carotid endarterectomy) are only appropriate to one of the vascular territories—whilst recognizing that there can be considerable overlap of symptoms between the two territories (Table 4.4).

In terms of the intracranial circulation (both anterior and posterior), there are striking differences between the structure, anastomotic potential, vascular pathology and functional areas of the brain perfused by: the mainstems of the parent arteries, the cortical branch arteries, and the small, deep perforating arteries (Table 4.3). There is also good evidence that the prognosis of these groups differs (section 10.2.7). A case can therefore be made for further subdividing strokes into those that are restricted to deep, subcortical areas (supplied by small perforating arteries), those that are restricted to superficial cortical areas (supplied by small pial branch arteries) and finally those which involve both deep and cortical structures (implicating the whole area of supply of the cerebral artery), recognizing that this is likely to be easier for anterior rather than posterior circulation events. Next, one needs to consider whether these subgroups can be identified clinically with reasonable reliability. Perhaps rather surprisingly, given their relative obscurity until recent years, the greatest amount of information is available for the group of strokes due to occlusion of a single, deep perforating artery, and these will be considered first.

4.3.2 Lacunar syndromes

The occlusion of a single, deep perforating artery results in a restricted area of infarction known as a 'lacune' (section 6.4) (Fig. 4.26). Technically, it should be described as an ischaemic lacune because similar sized areas of tissue destruction can be caused by haemorrhage, although by common usage an ischaemic cause is presumed (Poirier & Derouesne 1984). The term 'lacune' is a pathological one and if only cross-sectional imaging is available, the term 'small, deep infarct' is preferred, with the presumption that the imaged area of infarction is within the territory of a single perforating artery (Donnan *et al.* 1993). The majority of lacunes occur in areas such as the lentiform nucleus and are thought to be clinically 'silent', or at least unrecognized (Fisher 1969; Tuszynski *et al.* 1989). Although these may be important in some patients with cognitive decline, they are of less relevance when considering patients presenting with a 'stroke'. Other lacunes, however, occur at strategic sites such as in the internal capsule and pons, where clinically eloquent ascending and descending neural tracts are concentrated, with the result that an extensive clinical deficit can occur from an anatomically small lesion (sections 3.3.4 and 3.3.5). If one considers the basic neurovascular pattern described earlier, it should come as no surprise that lesions at such sites are inherently less likely to have a major impact on higher cognitive or visual function than those affecting the cortex.

Table 4.4 Which arterial territory are the neurological problems in?

	Likely arterial territory		
	Anterior	Either	Posterior
Aphasia	+		
Monocular visual loss	+		
Unilateral weakness*		+	
Unilateral sensory disturbance*		+	
Dysarthria †		+	
Ataxia †		+	
Dysphagia †		+	
Diplopia †			+
Vertigo †			+
Bilateral simultaneous visual loss			+
Bilateral simultaneous weakness			+
Bilateral simultaneous sensory disturbance			+
Crossed sensory/motor loss			+

* Usually assumed to be 'anterior', but see under lacunar syndromes (section 4.3.2).

† In isolation, these symptoms are not normally regarded as indicating a cerebrovascular event (section 3.2.1)

Note: whether the neurological symptoms are transient or persistent, and irrespective of whether there are abnormal neurological signs, it can be all but impossible to be sure of which arterial territory is involved, because so often the symptoms are not entirely specific for one particular arterial territory. This is because of individual variation in arterial anatomy and the pattern of any arterial disease affecting the collateral circulation, and because one function can be distributed through both arterial territories (e.g. the corticospinal tract is supplied in the cerebral hemispheres by the anterior circulation and then, in the brainstem, by the posterior circulation). Sometimes brain imaging can help if one particularly recent lesion is found in a relevant place (e.g. if a patient with a hemiplegia has just one infarct in the contralateral pons on MRI, then it is more likely to have been due to posterior than anterior ischaemia). Arterial imaging is unhelpful, because so often a symptomatic lesion in one artery is associated with asymptomatic lesions in other arteries. Arterial bruits are unhelpful for the same reason.

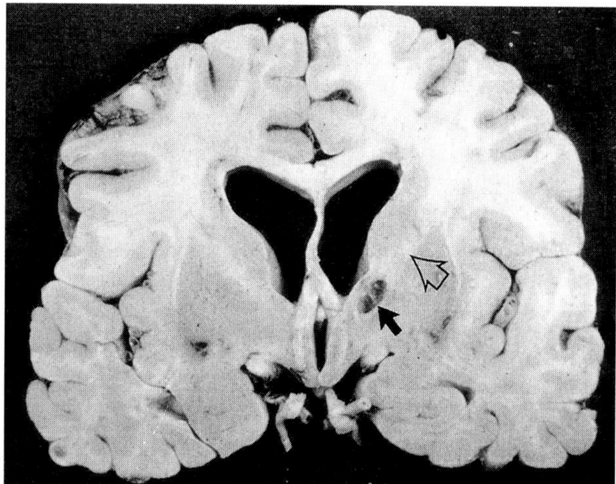

Fig. 4.26 Post-mortem demonstration of a lacune (closed arrow) in the internal capsule (open arrow) of a coronal brain slice.

Initially, a small number of clinical syndromes were correlated with relevant ischaemic lacunes at subsequent post-mortem (Fisher & Cole 1965; Fisher & Curry 1965; Fisher 1965b; Fisher 1967). These came to be regarded as the 'classical' lacunar syndromes (LACS), although before the advent of CT and MR, the sensitivity and specificity of these relationships were impossible to test. The widespread use of CT/MR has resulted in many more syndromes being associated with small, deep infarcts (Fisher 1991). It could be argued that these should all be included as LACS, but rare associations, perhaps due to idiosyncratic variations in the vascular anatomy, whilst of immense interest to researchers, are of little practical use to clinicians (Bamford 1995). Consequently, a recently proposed classification of subcortical infarction suggested that the term 'lacunar syndrome' (LACS) should be restricted to a clinical situation in which the *likely* mechanism of infarction 'involves transient or permanent occlusion of a single perforating artery with a high degree of probability'—i.e. that this mechanism is the *usual* cause of a particular syndrome (Donnan *et al.* 1993) (section 6.6.3). It was also realized that any of the classical LACS could be caused by haemorrhage.

Pure motor stroke (PMS)

PMS is probably the most 'classical' as well as the most frequently encountered of all LACS, and will be described in detail since it exemplifies many of the core features of LACS. The association of pure motor deficits and lacunes was noted early in the 20th century (Besson *et al.* 1991; Hauw 1995), but the clinical 'rules' for diagnosing PMS were not set out until much later, by Fisher and Curry (1965). They defined the syndrome as 'A paralysis complete or incomplete of the face, arm and leg on one side unaccompanied by sensory signs, visual field defect, aphasia, or apractagnosia. In the case of brainstem lesions the hemiplegia will be free of vertigo, deafness, tinnitus, diplopia, cerebellar ataxia, and gross nystagmus.' The definition allowed sensory symptoms but not signs to be present. It was stressed that 'this definition applies to the acute phase of the vascular insult and does not include less recent strokes in which other signs were present to begin with, but faded with the passage of time', e.g. aphasia. This puts into clinical terminology the fundamental neuro-anatomical concepts of LACS (Table 4.5).

For a patient to present with symptoms and signs that fulfil the above criteria, it is most likely that the stroke has been caused by a lesion in an area where the motor tracts are closely packed together, since a lesion of the motor cortex sufficiently extensive to involve the face, arm and leg areas of the homunculus would almost certainly involve neural pathways subserving higher cognitive or visual functions.

Table 4.5 Lacunar syndromes (LACS).

Definition
Maximum deficit from a single vascular event
No visual field deficit
No new disturbance of higher cerebral function
No signs of brainstem disturbance*

Categories of LACS
Pure motor stroke (PMS)
Pure sensory stroke (PSS)
Ataxic hemiparesis (including dysarthria clumsy–hand syndrome and homolateral ataxia and crural paresis) (AH)
Sensorimotor stroke (SMS)

To be acceptable as a PMS, PSS or SMS, the relevant deficit must involve at least two out of three areas of the face, arm and leg, and, with particular reference to the arm, should involve the whole limb and not just the hand.

* In the future, some brainstem syndromes may be reclassified as LACS (section 4.3.2).

Patients with lacunar syndromes should have no aphasia, no visuospatial disturbance, no visual field defect, no clear disturbance of brainstem function and no drowsiness at any time after their stroke, unless caused by a co-existing non-vascular condition.

In the original report of nine autopsied cases, six of the lacunes were in the internal capsule and three in the basis pontis, which emphasizes the point that the same clinical syndrome may occur with occlusion of a perforating artery arising from the middle cerebral artery (anterior circulation) or the basilar artery (posterior circulation). Since then, cases of PMS have been reported with lacunes in other sites along the pyramidal tract, including the corona radiata, the cerebral peduncle and the medullary pyramid (Bamford & Warlow 1988). However, in general, the anatomical distribution in large series seems to be broadly in keeping with the original pathological observations.

In the early 1980s, series of cases with slightly more restricted pure motor deficits (e.g. weakness of just the face and arm, or arm and leg) associated with small, deep infarcts on CT were reported—hence our preference for the term PMS rather than the original pure motor hemiplegia, which implies weakness of the arm and leg (Donnan *et al.* 1982; Rascol *et al.* 1982). The infarcts were in the corona radiata or the junctional zone between it and the internal capsule, where nerve fibres are relatively more dispersed than in the capsule or pons (Donnan *et al.* 1982). Cases with these more restricted deficits are probably best described as 'partial' rather than 'classical' LACS (Bamford 1995), but many large studies that have reported on clinicoanatomical correlations have combined the two groups, and therefore it is not possible to comment separately on the sensitivity and specificity of classical and partial LACS in predicting the site of the lesion. However, it seems that partial LACS are still most likely to be associated with small, deep infarcts, although it should be stressed that the definitions used stated that the *whole* of the arm or leg should be affected, something one suspects is often overlooked. Although one might go even further and include any case with a pure motor deficit no matter how anatomically restricted as a PMS, in practice the more restricted a deficit, the more likely it is to arise from a cortical lesion (Boiten & Lodder 1991a).

Only deficits involving the whole of the face and arm (brachiofacial), or the whole of the arm and leg (brachiocrural), should be accepted as partial lacunar syndromes, and not more restricted deficits that are more likely to be of cortical origin.

Pure sensory stroke (PSS)

The sensory counterpart of pure motor stroke, in terms of the anatomical distribution of the deficit, is encountered much less frequently. Although the definition in the original paper (Fisher 1965b) suggested that there should be objective sensory loss, in a later paper Fisher (1982) noted that there could be cases with persistent sensory symptoms in the absence of objective signs. A case of a partial PSS has been verified pathologically (Fisher 1978a). Most small, deep infarcts causing PSS are in the thalamus, in keeping with the original pathological studies. The lesions causing PSS are the smallest of the symptomatic small, deep infarcts.

Homolateral ataxia and crural paresis, dysarthria–clumsy hand syndrome and ataxic hemiparesis

Unlike the general acceptance of PMS and PSS as 'classical' LACS, this group of syndromes is less accepted as 'lacunar', although they were initially described at about the same time. This may be because of the difficulty of interpreting some physical signs and the fact that they are less common. The original patients with homolateral ataxia and crural paresis (HACP) were described as having weakness of the lower limb, especially the ankle and toes, a Babinski sign and 'striking dysmetria of the arm and leg on the same side' (Fisher & Cole 1965). In the dysarthria–clumsy hand syndrome (DCHS), although the deficit was described as being 'chiefly of dysarthria and clumsiness of one hand', two of the three original patients had signs suggestive of pyramidal dysfunction in the ipsilateral leg, and both had an ataxic gait (Fisher 1967). In his later paper, Fisher (1978b) reported three further patients who had prominent vertical nystagmus as well as pyramidal weakness and cerebellar signs, and suggested that a new term, 'ataxic hemiparesis' (AH) should be used for these cases and those with HACP. The relevant lacunes were all in the basis pontis, and he attributed the variable distribution of the weakness in different cases to the involvement of motor fibres where they are relatively dispersed by the pontine nuclei. It has been reported that if 'rigid' clinical criteria for DCHS are used, the syndrome predicts a lesion in the contralateral basis pontis (Glass *et al.* 1990). On the other hand, Bogousslavsky *et al.* (1992) suggest that true HACP may be caused most frequently by territorial infarcts in the anterior cerebral artery territory. They make the point that many other cases reported with similar-sized infarcts of the corona radiata on CT have had much more extensive deficits. Another possible explanation for the syndromes is that there is a second, non-imaged lesion. The data from detailed MRI studies argue against this being common. In one study, only five of 26 patients (19%) with AH had more than one small, deep infarct on imaging, but the figure for patients with PMS in the same study was similar, with six of 33 (18%) (Hommel *et al.* 1990a). Moulin *et al.* (1995) reported that 10.5% of patients with AH had a 'double lesion'. Additionally, in the Stroke Data Bank study (Chamorro *et al.* 1991), a history of previous, clinically apparent stroke was no more common in the AH/DCHS group than in those with other LACS. Sensory variants of AH have been reported, but there is no evidence that the anatomical and clinical issues raised are significantly different from those between PMS and sensorimotor stroke (see below).

Limb ataxia does not necessarily imply a cerebellar stroke in the presence of ipsilateral pyramidal signs, but may be caused by a lacunar infarct in the basal ganglia or pons.

Sensorimotor stroke

The inclusion of sensorimotor stroke (SMS) as a classical LACS is based on a single patient with a post-mortem, reported almost a decade after the reports of the other classical LACS (Mohr *et al.* 1977). This case was due to a lacune in the ventroposterior nucleus of the thalamus, but there was also pallor of the adjacent internal capsule. Although there were marked sensory and motor signs which persisted, the sensory symptoms preceded the motor ones. There is also post-mortem support for the view that an infarct primarily within the internal capsule can cause an SMS (Tuszynski *et al.* 1989). Groothuis *et al.* (1977) reported a similar syndrome occurring after a small haemorrhage in the same place. The authors made the point that a sensory deficit can occur from lesions of the posterior limb of the internal capsule, presumably by interruption of the thalamocortical pathways. Allen *et al.* (1984) reported 12 patients with SMS who were examined soon after onset, 11 of whom had low-attenuation areas on brain CT. When superimposed, these areas were slightly larger and extended more medially than in patients with PMS, abutting the posterolateral aspect of the thalamus, but were still within the usual territory of a single perforating artery. In an MR study, the infarcts in cases of SMS were larger than in other LACS, although they were still thought to equate with lacunes (Hommel *et al.* 1990a). In the Stroke Data Bank, in which SMS was the most frequent LACS after PMS, 31% had a lesion in the posterior limb of the internal capsule, 22% had a lesion in the corona radiata, 7% in the genu of the capsule, 6% in the anterior limb of the capsule and only 9% in the thalamus (Chamorro *et al.* 1991). The lesions in the corona radiata were on average almost twice as large as those in the capsule, but both were larger than the corresponding values for the PMS group. MR scanning has disclosed that in some CT-negative cases the lesion can be in the medial part of the medulla (Kim *et al.* 1995).

The parenchymal lesion in lacunar syndromes

Table 4.6 summarizes the clinicoradiological correlations for the various LACS and imaged small, deep infarcts in large studies, excluding those studies which specifically studied patients presenting in under 24 h, which will be discussed later (section 4.3.8). Overall, about 10% of patients presenting with a LACS will have a lesion *other* than a small, deep infarct on a scan, which *might* explain the neurological symptoms. The proportion of such 'atypical' patients does seem to be higher for SMS than for the other syndromes, and particular care should therefore be taken with this group.

The vascular lesion in lacunar syndromes

Any of the LACS may be caused by a small haemorrhage, and this accounts for about 5% of cases in community studies (Bamford & Warlow 1988). In the pre-CT era, this fact may have been of some clinical utility, and it may still be in countries with limited access to CT, where therapeutic decisions may have to be made on the basis of probability rather than absolute proof, although it should be noted that the haemorrhage rate of 5% comes mainly from studies of populations of predominantly white European ancestry, and may not be valid in populations in which the prevalence of

Table 4.6 Clinicoradiological correlations of lacunar syndromes.

Syndrome, studies	Setting	Imaging	*n*	Non-lacunar infarct on imaging (*n*, %)
Pure motor stroke (PMS)				
Bamford *et al.* (1987)	Community	CT	49	1 (2)
Hommel *et al.* (1990b)	Hospital	MR	35	0 (0)
Arboix & Marti-Vilalta (1992)	Hospital	CT/MR	137	12 (9)
Melo *et al.* (1992)	Hospital	CT	121	6 (5)
Norrving & Staaf (1991)*	Hospital	CT	123	0 (0)
Norrving & Staaf (1991)†	Hospital	CT	52	5 (9)
Gan *et al.* (1997)	Hospital	CT/MR	101	7 (7)
Pure sensory stroke (PSS)				
Bamford *et al.* (1987)	Community	CT	7	0 (0)
Hommel *et al.* (1990a)	Hospital	MR	12	1 (8)
Arboix & Marti-Vilalta (1992)	Hospital	CT/MR	45	3 (7)
Gan *et al.* (1997)	Hospital	CT/MR	15	0 (0)
Ataxic hemiparesis (AH)				
Bamford *et al.* (1987)	Community	CT	9	0 (0)
Hommel *et al.* (1990a)	Hospital	MR	28	2 (7)
Gan *et al.* (1997)	Hospital	CT/MR	41	1 (1)
Sensorimotor stroke (SMS)				
Bamford *et al.* (1987)	Community	CT	43	2 (5)
Hommel *et al.* (1990a)	Hospital	MR	8	1 (12)
Landi *et al.* (1991)	Hospital	CT	34	3 (11)
Lodder *et al.* (1991)	Hospital	CT	47	5 (11)
Huang *et al.* (1987)	Hospital	CT	37	8 (21)
Arboix & Marti-Vilalta (1992)	Hospital	CT/MR	42	8 (19)
Gan *et al.* (1997)	Hospital	CT/MR	46	1 (2)
All lacunar syndromes				
Wardlaw *et al.* (1996)	Hospital	CT	19	2 (11)
Boiten & Lodder (1991b)	Hospital	CT	109	11 (10)
Ricci *et al.* (1991)	Community	CT	56	2 (4)
Samuelsson *et al.* (1994)	Hospital	MR	91	8 (11)
Anderson *et al.* (1994)‡	Community	CT	69	12 (17)
Kappelle *et al.* (1989)	Hospital	CT	78	5 (6)

* Classical PMS. † Partial PMS. ‡ Retrospective classification from records.

intracranial arterial disease and primary intracerebral haemorrhage is higher.

There is no direct information about the cause of the occlusion of single perforating arteries, except in a handful of cases. Asymptomatic (smaller) lacunes are probably most often the consequence of occlusion by thickened vessel walls, when the usual diameter of the vessel is less than 100 μm (Fisher 1969), although more recently it has been suggested that oedema secondary to the breakdown of the blood–brain barrier may have a role (Lammie 1998). Symptomatic lacunes are probably most often the result of vessel occlusion due to complex small vessel disease or microatheroma, when the vessel diameter is around 400 μm (Fisher 1979) (section 6.4). Some cases, particularly those with basilar perforating artery occlusion, may be caused by obstruction of the mouth of the perforating artery by an atheromatous plaque within the parent artery (Fisher & Caplan 1971). Although an embolic mechanism is possible (Millikan 1995; Ay *et al.* 1999), epidemiological evidence suggests that there is a low frequency of severe carotid stenosis (Kappelle *et al.* 1988; Norrving & Cronqvist 1989; Lindgren *et al.* 1994a; Boiten *et al.* 1996; Mead *et al.* 1997) or any cardiac source of embolism (Lindgren *et al.* 1994a; Boiten & Lodder 1995) (section 6.4).

From the above, it can be seen that a LACS does not reliably distinguish whether the occluded perforating artery arises from the anterior or posterior systems, although in older series (e.g. Rochester, Minnesota: Turney *et al.* 1984) and some schemes of classification (e.g. WHO Task Force 1989), it seems likely that they would always have been considered as anterior circulation strokes. More recently, it has been recognized that small, deep infarcts are the usual cause of certain brainstem syndromes (usually a PMS plus a cranial nerve palsy or eye movement disorder) (Hommel *et al.* 1990a). Before simply accepting these alongside the classical LACS, the even greater paucity of pathological studies should be recognized. As noted above, the vascular lesion may be different, with atheroma overlying the mouth of the perforating artery being more frequent than in the anterior circulation (Fisher & Caplan 1971). Consequently, these types of deficit are not generally included in studies reporting the prognosis of patients with LACS, but this position may need to be reviewed in the light of future MR studies.

4.3.3 Posterior circulation syndromes

Although there are some clinical syndromes due to well-localized lesions within the posterior circulation which, along with their eponymous names, are an integral part of 'classical neurology' (e.g. Weber, Millard–Gubler, Wallenberg), in practice such syndromes are rarely seen in their pure form. Indeed, in many ways, the clinical consequences of a given vascular lesion are probably less predictable than for arteries in the anterior circulation, because of the greater frequency of developmental anomalies and the fact that, instead of a paired system of arteries in which the lumenal diameter decreases as one moves distally, this is the only place in the body where two large arteries join to form a single larger artery. Additionally, until the advent of MRI, clinicoradiological correlation was difficult because of the poorer performance of CT in the posterior fossa compared with the supratentorial compartment. Catheter angiography was also performed much less frequently than for anterior circulation strokes, because it rarely led to any change in the management, such as vascular surgery. A further problem is that, in whites at least, atheroma of the intracranial portion of the vertebral arteries and the basilar artery is more common than in the intracranial carotid or middle cerebral arteries. Thus, whilst small deep infarcts resulting from occlusion of a single perforating artery in the anterior circulation are most likely to be due to intrinsic disease of those vessels, in the posterior circulation the atheromatous disease in the parent artery may cause a similar brain lesion by occluding the origin of a single perforating artery—a process referred to as 'basilar branch occlusion' (section 4.3.2). Consequently, at the present time, one must recognize that the posterior circulation syndromes (POCS) are relatively crude grouping, which from both a topographic and aetiological perspective encompasses a heterogeneous group of strokes (Tei *et al.* 1999) (section 6.6.4).

The clinical syndromes

The clinical deficits that point to the lesion being in the distribution of the posterior circulation are shown in Table 4.7. Other symptoms and signs that may be present in patients with POCS but are not of particular localizing value include Horner's syndrome, nystagmus, vertigo, dysarthria and hearing disturbance. Occasionally, an otherwise typical POCS may be associated with disturbance of higher cerebral function, e.g. aphasia, agnosias. This should not come as a surprise, given the variable supratentorial territory supplied by the posterior cerebral arteries (Hommel *et al.* 1990b, 1991) (section 4.2.3), and these cases should still be considered as POCS.

Table 4.7 Posterior circulation syndromes (POCS).

At time of maximum deficit, any of:
Ipsilateral cranial nerve (III–XII) palsy (single or multiple) with contralateral motor and/or sensory deficit
Bilateral motor and/or sensory deficit
Disorder of conjugate eye movement (horizontal or vertical)
Cerebellar dysfunction without ipsilateral longtract deficit (as seen in ataxic hemiparesis)
Isolated hemianopia or cortical blindness

The parenchymal lesion

In the Oxfordshire Community Stroke Project (OCSP), amongst 109 patients presenting with POCS, of whom 90 had a CT scan within 28 days of stroke onset or post-mortem, nine (10%) were due to primary intracerebral haemorrhage (PICH) (Bamford 1986). In the study from Lund, seven of 39 (18%) patients with POCS had a PICH (Lindgren *et al.* 1994b), and in Perth six of 55 (11%) had PICH (Anderson *et al.* 1994).

The correlation between the clinical syndrome and brain imaging in patients with ischaemic stroke is shown in Table 4.8. The 'inappropriate' lesions included a number of supratentorial small, deep infarcts. Given that most of the studies were based on CT, it is possible that these patients had a further infarct in the brainstem that was not visible. With the increasing use of MRI, it has become clear that certain brainstem syndromes are usually due to small, deep infarcts, compatible with occlusion of a single perforating artery. The two groups that fall into this category are those that generally have a pure motor deficit with, additionally, disorders of eye movement or a single cranial nerve (e.g. Weber's syndrome, pure motor stroke plus third nerve palsy), and those where there is an isolated internuclear ophthalmoplegia. They have been referred to as extended LACS (Bamford 1995). The only detailed study of these patients was reported by Hommel *et al.* (1990a), where all 21 cases presenting with these so-called 'extended LACS' had evidence of a small, deep infarct on MRI. What is not clear at present is the spectrum of clinical syndromes that may be caused by such lesions in the brainstem.

The vascular lesion

Traditionally, pathological series have suggested that within the anterior circulation the ratio of embolism to *in situ* thrombosis is about 3 : 1, whilst in the posterior circulation this ratio is reversed (Escourelle 1978). Recent workers have questioned this, and it seems likely that at least some of the difference is the result of the inevitable selection bias that occurs in pathological series (Caplan & Tettenborn 1992b; Caplan *et al.* 1992; Caplan 1993). Caplan and Tettenborn (1992b) reported that 43% of posterior circulation infarcts were associated with large artery occlusion, 20% were attributed to artery-to-artery emboli, 19% to cardiogenic embolism and 18% to small vessel disease. It seems likely that, because of the shape of the vertebrobasilar system, emboli are most likely to arrest either in the distal portion of the vertebral artery or in the upper portion of the basilar artery. Of 93 cases of isolated homonymous hemianopia associated with a vascular lesion, 80 (96%) were attributed to posterior cerebral artery occlusion (Trobe *et al.* 1973).

The POCS are probably the most heterogeneous group, in terms of both the parenchymal and the vascular lesion, and in the future there is likely to be increasing distinction between those that are due to small and large vessel disease, although it is questionable whether this will be possible on purely clinical grounds. There is a tendency for POCS to be underdiagnosed in non-specialist centres. In our view, this most often results from a failure to appreciate that truncal or gait ataxia is present, because no one bothers to have the patient sit or stand up.

4.3.4 Total anterior circulation syndrome

At the other end of the spectrum of clinical severity from most patients with LACS, hospital clinicians in particular are familiar with the patient who has a complete hemiplegia, hemianopia and evidence of higher cortical dysfunction (especially language or visuospatial function). Additionally, some impairment of consciousness is often present, which can make formal testing of higher cortical function difficult. Such patients are likely to be admitted to hospital more frequently than those with LACS (Bamford *et al.* 1986).

The clinical syndrome

The clinical features of total anterior circulation syndrome

Table 4.8 Correlation between the clinical and imaging findings in patients who presented with posterior circulation syndromes (POCS) due to cerebral ischaemia.

Study	Number	Appropriate infarct	No lesion	Inappropriate infarct
Bamford (1986)*	81	19 (23%)	60 (74%)	2 (2%)
Lindgren *et al.* (1994b)*	32	12 (37%)	20 (62%)	0
Anderson *et al.* (1994)*	36	16 (44%)	16 (44%)	4 (11%)
Wardlaw *et al.* (1996)†	13	8 (62%)	5 (38%)	0
Al-Buhairi *et al.* (1998)†	71	32 (45%)	39 (55%)	0
Mead *et al.* (2000)†	212	105 (50%)	86 (41%)	21 (10%)

* Community-based study, first-ever strokes. † Hospital-based study, first-ever and recurrent strokes.

(TACS) (Table 4.9) are a hemiplegia (usually with an ipsilateral hemisensory loss), a visual field deficit on the same side, and a new disturbance of higher cerebral function referable to the same hemisphere. 'Total' is used in this context to signify that all the major aspects of supratentorial cerebral function have been affected, and it does not imply that there has been infarction in the whole of the anterior circulation territory. Allen *et al.* (1984) used the term 'full house' for the same syndrome. TACS is very much the equivalent of what has been described as the 'complete middle cerebral artery syndrome' in other classifications (WHO Task Force 1989).

The parenchymal lesion

In the Oxfordshire Community Stroke Project (OCSP), amongst 107 patients presenting with TACS, of whom 73 had a CT scan within 28 days of onset, or a post-mortem, 18 cases (25%) were caused by primary intracerebral haemorrhage (PICH) (Bamford 1986). In the study from Lund, 13 of 67 patients with TACS (19%) (Lindgren *et al.* 1994b) and in Perth 28 of 134 (21%) had PICH (Anderson *et al.* 1994).

Up to a quarter of all patients presenting with a total anterior circulation syndrome have an underlying primary intracerebral haemorrhage.

The correlation between the clinical syndrome and brain imaging in patients with ischaemic stroke is shown in Table 4.10. Perhaps the biggest 'catch', as exemplified by the study of Wardlaw *et al.* (1996), is the ability of posterior cerebral artery (PCA) territory ischaemia to produce a TACS. This has been described in detail by Hommel *et al.* (1990b, 1991) and Chambers *et al.* (1991). In general, such patients have a relatively mild hemiparesis but marked aphasia (not always fluent) and a visual field deficit. The motor deficit occurs because of involvement of the small, perforating arteries arising from the proximal PCA, which supply the upper midbrain (section 4.2.3). Although the original definition of TACS simply used the word 'hemiparesis' (Bamford *et al.* 1991), in fact the vast majority of patients in the OCSP who were classified as having TACS were either hemiplegic or had a severe hemiparesis that would certainly have been incompatible with walking. Therefore, it is worth bearing in mind the aphorism 'beware the walking TACS'. Allen (1984) reported that the volume of infarction in patients with TACS, as judged by CT, was significantly greater than for patients with lesser deficits. A similar result was reported by Lindgren *et al.* (1994b) (section 4.3.7).

Table 4.9 Total anterior circulation syndrome (TACS)

At time of maximum deficit, all of:
Hemiplegia or severe hemiparesis contralateral to the cerebral lesion
Hemianopia contralateral to the cerebral lesion
New disturbance of higher cerebral function (e.g. aphasia, visuospatial disturbance)

Occasionally, a total anterior circulation syndrome results from occlusion of the posterior cerebral artery. In such cases, there is often a relatively mild hemiparesis but marked aphasia and visual field loss—'beware the walking TACS'.

The vascular lesion

Foix and Levy (1927) recognized that the TACS pattern of deficit was associated with occlusion of the proximal mainstem of the middle cerebral artery (MCA) and that infarction occurred in both the deep and superficial territories. They also recognized that, on occasion, the extent of infarction in the superficial territory was not as extensive, and they presumed that this reflected functionally effective leptomeningeal collaterals (section 6.6.1). This is a similar argument to that relating to striatocapsular infarction (sec-

Table 4.10 Correlation between the clinical and imaging findings in patients who presented with total anterior circulation syndromes (TACS) due to cerebral ischaemia.

Study	Number	Appropriate infarct	No lesion	Inappropriate infarct
Bamford (1986)*	55	52 (95%)	0	3 (5%)
Lindgren *et al.* (1994b)*	54	35 (65%)	15 (28%)	4 (7%)
Anderson *et al.* (1994)*	68	44 (65%)	10 (15%)	12 (18%)
Wardlaw *et al.* (1996)†	33	31 (94%)	0	2 (6%)
Al-Buhairi *et al.* (1998)†	64	40 (62%)	15 (23%)	9 (14%)
Mead *et al.* (2000)†	94	69 (73%)	7 (7%)	18 (19%)

* Community-based study, first-ever strokes. † Hospital-based study, first-ever and recurrent strokes.

tion 4.2.2). Olsen *et al.* (1985) reported that in 20 patients with extensive hemispheric infarction as judged by CT, 14 had evidence of MCA occlusion and the other six had either occlusion or more than 75% stenosis of the ipsilateral internal carotid artery (ICA). Mead *et al.* (1997) reported that, amongst patients with non-haemorrhagic TACS who had an early carotid duplex examination, 33% had either occlusion or more than 70% ICA stenosis ipsilateral to the cerebral lesion. In a similar Swedish study, Lindgren *et al.* (1994a) reported that 43% of patients with TACS had either ipsilateral ICA occlusion or greater than 80% stenosis, and 57% had a major cardiac source of embolism. In the Lausanne Stroke Registry, in which the topographically defined large MCA territory infarcts would be broadly equivalent to TACS, 41% of patients had occlusion of the ipsilateral ICA and 33% had a major source of cardiac embolism (Heinsius *et al.* 1998).

4.3.5 Partial anterior circulation syndromes

The clinical syndrome

The final group of syndromes have less extensive deficits than TACS and yet do not fulfil the specific criteria for LACS, either because of the presence of higher cortical deficits or because the motor/sensory deficit is too restricted in anatomical terms. These would be broadly similar to a combination of the superficial middle cerebral artery and anterior cerebral artery syndromes in other classifications (WHO Task Force 1989). The clinical features of partial anterior circulation syndromes (PACS) are set out in Table 4.11.

Table 4.11 Partial anterior circulation syndromes (PACS).

At time of maximum deficit, any of:
Motor/sensory deficit + hemianopia
Motor/sensory deficit + new higher cerebral dysfunction
New higher cerebral dysfunction + hemianopia
Pure motor/sensory deficit less extensive than for lacunar syndromes (e.g. monoparesis)
New higher cerebral dysfunction alone (e.g. aphasia)

When more than one type of deficit is present, they must all reflect damage in the same cerebral hemisphere

The parenchymal lesion

In the OCSP, of 135 patients presenting with PACS, of whom 113 had a CT scan within 28 days of stroke onset, or post-mortem, seven (6%) were caused by primary intracerebral haemorrhage (PICH) (Bamford 1986). In the study from Lund, eight of 69 patients with PACS (12%) had a PICH (Lindgren *et al.* 1994b) and in Perth 17 of 126 (13%) (Anderson *et al.* 1994).

The correlation between the clinical syndrome and brain imaging in patients with ischaemic stroke is shown in Table 4.12. Most of the patients with 'inappropriate' infarcts had either multiple small, deep infarcts, or what appeared to be isolated posterior cerebral artery (PCA) territory infarction. Although this is usually considered to be due to embolism from the vertebrobasilar arteries, there will be a few patients whose PCAs are supplied by the carotid system, because of developmental variation in the circle of Willis (section 4.2.2). Allen (1984) showed that patients with the clinical features of PACS had lesions on CT generally extending into the cortex, but significantly smaller than in patients with a 'full house' or TACS. This was confirmed by Lindgren *et al.* (1994b).

The vascular lesion

In an angiographic study of 25 patients with medium (1.5–3.0 cm) areas of infarction on CT, 14 were found to have middle cerebral artery (MCA) occlusion, six had internal carotid artery (ICA) occlusion, and five had no significant angiographic lesion (Olsen *et al.* 1985) (section 6.6.2). Mead *et al.* (1997) reported that 33% of patients with non-

Table 4.12 Correlation between the clinical and imaging findings in patients who presented with partial anterior circulation syndromes (PACS) due to cerebral ischaemia.

Study	Number	Appropriate infarct	No lesion	Inappropriate infarct
Bamford (1986)*	106	47 (44%)	56 (53%)	3 (3%)
Lindgren *et al.* (1994b)*	61	21 (34%)	24 (39%)	16 (26%)
Anderson *et al.* (1994)*	75	25 (33%)	31 (41%)	19 (25%)
Wardlaw *et al.* (1996)†	43	29 (67%)	7 (16%)	7 (16%)
Al-Buhairi *et al.* (1998)†	121	78 (64%)	39 (32%)	4 (3%)
Mead *et al.* (2000)†	441	213 (48%)	143 (32%)	85 (19%)

* Community-based study, first-ever strokes. † Hospital-based study, first-ever and recurrent strokes.

haemorrhagic PACS had either occlusion or more than 70% stenosis of the ICA ipsilateral to the cerebral lesion. In a similar Swedish study, Lindgren *et al.* (1994a) reported that 19% of patients with PACS had either ipsilateral ICA occlusion or greater than 80% stenosis, and 46% had a major cardiac source of embolism. In the Lausanne Stroke Registry, in which the topographically defined limited superficial MCA territory infarcts would be broadly equivalent to the majority of PACS (isolated anterior cerebral artery infarcts being relatively uncommon), 28% of patients had greater than 50% stenosis of the ipsilateral ICA, and 33% had a major source of cardiac embolism (Heinsius *et al.* 1998).

4.3.6 Syndromes of uncertain origin

For a variety of reasons, the physician will occasionally have difficulty allocating cases with confidence on clinical grounds to one of the four stroke syndromes. For example, the patient may have had a previous stroke, be demented, or have had a limb amputated for peripheral vascular disease. In such cases, it may be unclear what *new* neurological deficits have arisen from the current stroke. There are also patients, who are often very elderly, in whom it can be difficult to decide whether they should be classified as having a PACS or a TACS, usually because of uncertainty about the presence of higher cerebral dysfunction or a visual field deficit. If one is not certain about a deficit, it is usually best to consider it absent, and therefore the majority should be considered as having PACS. The exception is if the patient is drowsy, which—if due to the cerebral lesion rather than any metabolic disturbance—would be indicative of an extensive lesion, with the patient being classified as having a TACS. At the other end of the spectrum, one should be quite rigid about applying the rules describing the extent of a motor or sensory deficit which ought to be present before diagnosing an LACS (i.e. only when there is involvement of the face, arm and leg; or the whole of the face and arm; or the whole of the arm and leg). At the end of the day, however, there is some evidence that making a 'best guess' on the basis of the evidence available to you is probably a reasonably accurate strategy (Lindley *et al.* 1993).

Of course, the results of any brain imaging *may* assist the primary classification, i.e. point towards the most likely clinical syndrome (section 4.3.7). This can be of value both in clinical practice and in research, where it will help minimize the risk of bias being introduced, particularly when considering the outcome of various groups of patients.

4.3.7 Using the clinically based Oxfordshire Community Stroke Project (OCSP) classification

Any system of classification will not become widely accepted unless it is easy to use and conveys useful information to the clinician (Table 4.13). How do the clinical syndromes described above measure up to this challenge? The necessary information is, by and large, easy (and inexpensive) to collect from virtually all patients with stroke, and a checklist can be incorporated into stroke clerking or admission forms as an *aide-mémoire*. Each syndrome occurs sufficiently frequently in patients with stroke (Fig. 4.27) to promote pattern recognition, particularly by junior medical staff.

Lindley *et al.* (1993) reported moderately good inter-observer reliability (between a junior and a senior clinician)

Table 4.13 Benefits of using the clinically based Oxfordshire Community Stroke Project classification.

Information is quick, easy and inexpensive to collect on virtually all patients
The syndromes occur frequently enough to promote pattern recognition
Reasonable inter-observer reliability
An indication of the likelihood of the stroke being due to primary intracerebral haemorrhage
Prediction of the volume of ischaemia on CT/MR scan and therefore at an early stage gives an indication of the risk of complications in the acute phase, and longer-term prognosis
An indication of the likely underlying vascular pathology and therefore a guide to appropriate investigations
In the era of acute 'brain attack', it can be used to predict where the 'hole' would have been without effective treatment

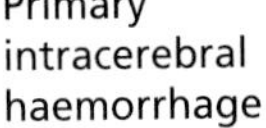

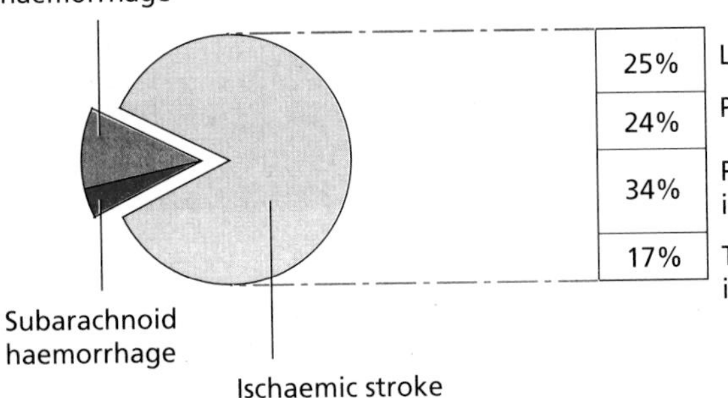

Fig. 4.27 The distribution of clinical subtypes of ischaemic stroke in the Oxfordshire Community Stroke Project.

in the allocation of clinical subtype (kappa = 0.54) and Lindgren *et al.* (1994b) reported that the inter-observer agreement for the allocation of clinical subtypes between the initial 'routine' clinical examination (albeit using a clerking pro forma) and another performed within 1 week by one of the authors was 92% (kappa 0.89). However, it is worth remembering that there is evidence of improved clinicoradiological correlation, for lacunar syndromes (LACS) at least, when the patients are seen by clinicians with a specific interest in stroke (Boiten & Lodder 1991b; Lodder *et al.* 1994).

The syndromes provide the clinician with some indication of the likelihood of a stroke being due to cerebral haemorrhage: unlikely (<5%) with LACS but more likely (25%) with total anterior circulation syndromes (TACS). This in no way obviates the need for CT scanning to make a definitive distinction between infarct and haemorrhage, but unfortunately, many clinicians continue to have restricted access to such facilities (Chapter 5).

The syndromes predict the volume of cerebral infarction in patients with ischaemic stroke (Table 4.14). Thus, very rapidly, clinical staff can predict which patients are at greatest risk of developing impairment of conscious level and may be at risk of aspiration, for example (section 15.17), and the nursing staff and relatives can then be alerted to the possibility. In the study by Pinto *et al.* (1998), amongst patients with ischaemic strokes there was an impaired level of consciousness in 14% of those with TACS, 4% of those with partial anterior circulation syndromes (PACS), 5% of those with posterior circulation syndromes (POCS) and none of those with LACS. Thus, impairment of consciousness developing in a patient with LACS should prompt a search for an alternative explanation, since such patients will not develop significant cerebral oedema. Perhaps not surprisingly, patients with TACS are also more likely to become febrile (often from urinary or respiratory infections) and possibly also hyponatraemic (Pinto *et al.* 1998).

Since the syndromes predict the volume of cerebral infarction, not surprisingly they also predict stroke outcome (section 10.2.7). Not only does this allow more accurate information to be given to the patients and their relatives, it also allows early, realistic discharge planning to begin. More research is required into whether given deficits occurring as part of different syndromes have different patterns of recovery, but certainly clear differences can be predicted for mobility milestones, as well as for the likely length of stay in hospital (Pinto *et al.* 1998; Smith & Baer 1999).

The syndromes provide the clinician with an indication of the most likely underlying vascular lesion (sections 6.6.1–6.6.4). TACS/PACS are likely to be caused by occlusion of the larger cerebral arteries, and the clinician should therefore be thinking about cardiac sources of embolism (Table 4.15), or carotid and aortic atherosclerosis (Tables 4.16 & 4.17). If access to, for example, carotid duplex is restricted, one could argue that patients with PACS—in whom there is a significant chance of finding a more than 70% carotid stenosis in a patient who has a good chance of making an excellent physical recovery, and in whom the risk of early recurrence may be greatest—should take precedence over patients with LACS (Bamford *et al.* 1991; Mead *et al.* 1997; Mead *et al.* 1999a). Conversely, if a patient presents with an LACS, the clinician should not be surprised if there is no lesion on the CT scan, carotid duplex, or echocardiography, and should not 'chase' excessively rare causes of stroke without some good reason.

4.3.8 The Oxfordshire Community Stroke Project (OCSP) classification and acute 'brain attacks'

The OCSP classification was derived primarily for epidemiological purposes from a data set that was based on the clinical examination of patients at a mean of 4 days post-stroke (Bamford *et al.* 1991). Furthermore, the majority of the other data referred to above have come from studies in which a substantial proportion of the patients were assessed more than 24 h after onset of symptoms. It is unlikely, therefore,

Table 4.14 Volume of infarction (in ml) on brain computed tomography according to clinical subtype.

	Total anterior circulation syndromes ($n = 41$)	Partial anterior circulation syndromes ($n = 41$)	Lacunar syndromes ($n = 18$)	Posterior circulation syndromes ($n = 38$)
Lindgren *et al.* (1994b)	91.8	18.8	4.2	8.5
Allen (1984)	134.3	60.2 [a]	3.0	31.8 [e]
		44.5 [b]		7.0 [f]
		40.6 [c]		
		14.0 [d]		

[a] Hemiplegia + hemianopia; [b] hemiplegia + higher cerebral dysfunction; [c] hemianopia + higher cerebral dysfunction; [d] lone higher cerebral dysfunction; [e] brainstem; [f] lone hemianopia.

Table 4.15 Carotid and cardiac findings by clinical subtype of ischaemic stroke (from Lindgren *et al.* 1994a).

	>80% stenosis or occlusion of the ipsilateral carotid artery	Major cardioembolic source
Total anterior circulation syndrome	43%	57%
Partial anterior circulation syndrome	19%	46%
Lacunar syndrome	5%	16%
Posterior circulation syndrome	10%	8%

Table 4.16 Carotid duplex findings by clinical subtype of ischaemic stroke: degree of stenosis ipsilateral to the site of infarction (from Mead *et al.* 1997).

	Stenosis of ipsilateral internal carotid artery			
	0–49%	50–69%	70–99%	Occluded
Total anterior circulation syndrome (*n* = 117)	68 (58%)	6 (5%)	6 (5%)	33 (28%)
Partial anterior circulation syndrome (*n* = 128)	74 (58%)	9 (7%)	25 (20%)	17 (13%)
Lacunar syndrome (*n* = 108)	96 (89%)	8 (7%)	1 (1%)	3 (3%)
Posterior circulation syndrome (*n* = 27)	24 (89%)	2 (7%)	1 (4%)	0 (0%)

Table 4.17 Angiographic findings according to infarct size on brain CT in patients with ischaemic stroke (from Olsen *et al.* 1985).

Infarct size on brain CT	Middle cerebral artery occlusion	Significant internal carotid artery disease	Neither
Large (*n* = 20)	14	6	0
Medium (*n* = 25)	14	6	5
Small (*n* = 15)	0	1	14
None (*n* = 13)	1	1	11

that progression of the neurological deficit occurred in any significant proportion of the patients studied—thereby allowing a key feature of the syndromic diagnosis, i.e. the clinical pattern at the time of *maximum* deficit, to be assessed. We cannot assume, therefore, that the classification remains valid for the hyper-acute examination of patients that is now becoming commonplace—i.e. those with brain attacks that started in the previous few hours. For example, in a recent study of 152 patients with supratentorial ischaemic stroke who were seen within 5 hours of onset of symptoms, 39 (26%) had some neurological deterioration during the subsequent 4 days. (Toni *et al.* 1995). Most of these patients had extensive middle cerebral artery (MCA) territory infarction, and the results would be in keeping with those from the Lausanne Stroke Registry, in which only 159 of 208 (76%) patients with large MCA territory infarcts had a fixed neurological deficit 1 hour after the onset of symptoms (Heinsius *et al.* 1998).

Toni *et al.* (1994) also reported their findings for patients who presented with either a pure motor or sensorimotor stroke, i.e. lacunar syndromes, within 12 h of onset (mean 6.1 h). The results are shown in Table 4.18. It is clear that one can see a patient very early on who would be classified as having a lacunar syndrome (LACS), but who 24 h later would be classified as having a total anterior circulation syndrome (TACS). The pathophysiological basis for this is probably a thrombus in the proximal MCA mainstem, which causes symptoms (and in some cases changes on CT) that are first apparent in this area before the cerebral cortex which may have a better collateral supply. However, Toni *et al.* (1994) also noted that there was another group of patients who presented acutely with non-lacunar syndromes (principally, partial anterior circulation syndromes, PACS) who had small, deep infarcts (equivalent to lacunar infarcts) on the second CT scan. Of these 47 patients, 23 (49%) improved over the following days with resolution of their 'cortical' symptoms and signs—i.e. if they had been examined a few days after the onset and there had been no clear record or history of the clinical pattern at the time of maximum deficit, then they would have been classified (correctly) as having LACS.

All this has led us to question the utility of using the OCSP classification *alone* as a method of stratifying subgroups of patients in hyper-acute intervention trials. How-

Table 4.18 Correlation of early diagnosis of lacunar syndromes with final lesion on CT scan (from Toni *et al.* 1994).

Clinical syndrome at < 12 h	CT at 15 days compatible with lacunar infarction,* or post-mortem	CT at 15 days not compatible with lacunar infarction,* or post-mortem	Positive predictive value
Pure motor stroke (n = 151)	88	63	58%
Sensorimotor stroke (n = 68)	35	33	51%

* i.e. normal scan, or subcortical infarcts < 1.5 cm in diameter.

ever, we think it may still be useful for identifying those patients most likely to have a particular vascular lesion of interest, who might then be targeted for further emergency investigations—e.g. in trials of thrombolysis, it may be logical to distinguish TACS/PACS from LACS as a way of picking out those most likely to have large vessel occlusion. As mentioned at the beginning of this chapter, one rationale of having a clinically based method of subclassification is that if other information is available, then it can be used in a hierarchical manner. For example, Mead *et al.* (1999b) have reported that if patients present with a LACS but have evidence of *new* cortical infarction on CT in a potentially relevant place then they are more likely to have significant disease of the ipsilateral internal carotid artery (odds ratio 3.7, 95% confidence interval [CI], 1.1–12) or a major source of cardiogenic embolism (odds ratio 3.9; 95% CI, 1.2–12) than those patients with small, deep infarcts on CT, i.e. from an aetiological perspective they are more like PACS.

Over the next few years, we can expect to see studies that compare the clinical syndromes with the infarct topography using increasingly sophisticated forms of scanning. Thus, the sequence in the early phase of stroke is likely to be first a clinical (syndromic) diagnosis; followed by a topographical (radiological) diagnosis if the imaging is abnormal and shows a recent, potentially relevant lesion; and then an aetiological diagnosis (Fig. 4.28). Tei *et al.* (1999) describe such a three-step model of subclassification. They studied 250 consecutive patients aged 32–92 years who were seen within 24 h of the onset of symptoms. The first stage of their subclassification was to allocate patients to one of the four clinically defined subgroups. The second stage was to allocate patients to a radiological subgroup, based on CT or MR findings. Then, after completion of all relevant investigations, they allocated patients to an aetiological subgroup. Table 4.19 shows the correlation between the clinical syndromes and the radiological diagnosis, and Table 4.20 shows the correlation between the clinical syndromes and the aetiological diagnosis.

Finally, it is important not to forget that running in parallel with this medically orientated diagnostic model will be a functional diagnosis (of impairment, disability and handicap) and finally a 'social' diagnosis (quality of life, reintegration) (section 10.2).

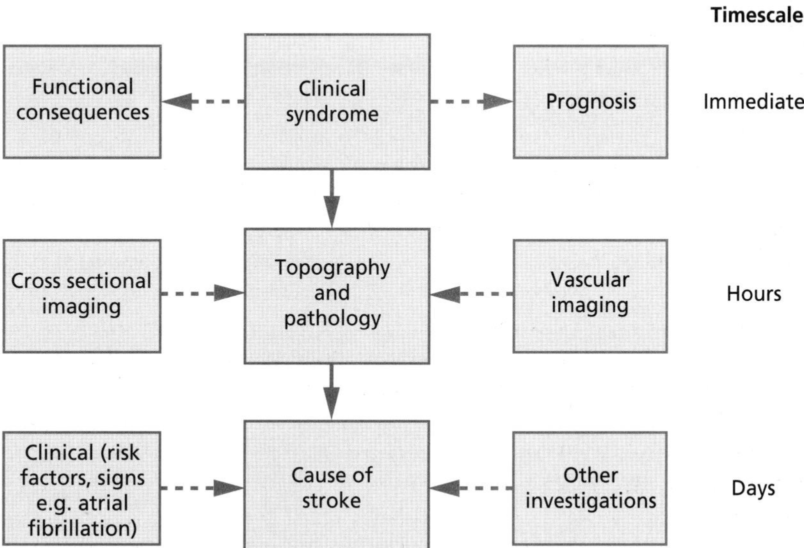

Fig. 4.28 Diagram of the three-step model of acute diagnosis, i.e. syndrome → topography → cause.

Syndrome	*n*	Cortical infarct	Boundary-zone infarct	Lacunar infarct	Posterior circulation infarct	No lesion
Total anterior circulation infarction	55	53 (96%)	1 (2%)	0	1 (2%)	0
Partial anterior circulation infarction	49	36 (73%)	7 (14%)	2 (4%)	1 (2%)	3 (6%)
Lacunar infarction	103	11 (11%)	16 (16%)	70 (68%)	1 (1%)	5 (5%)
Posterior circulation infarction	43	2 (5%)	0	1 (2%)	37 (86%)	3 (6%)
Total	250	102	24	73	40	11

Table 4.19 Correlation of clinical syndrome within first 24 h after onset of ischaemic stroke with CT/MR lesion (from Tei *et al.* 1999).

Syndrome	*n*	Large artery atherosclerosis	Cardioembolic	Small artery disease	Other
Total anterior circulation infarction	55	11 (20%)	34 (62%)	0	10 (18%)
Partial anterior circulation infarction	49	20 (41%)	21 (43%)	0	8 (16%)
Lacunar infarction	103	30 (29%)	0	60 (58%)	13 (13%)
Posterior circulation infarction	43	15 (35%)	9 (21%)	7 (15%)	12 (28%)
Total	250	76	64	67	43

Table 4.20 Correlation of clinical syndrome within first 24 h after onset of ischaemic stroke with final cause of infarction (from Tei *et al.* 1999).

References

Please note that all references taken from *The Cochrane Library* are given a current date as this database is updated on a quarterly basis. Please refer to the current *Cochrane Library* article for the latest review. The same applies to the *British Medical Journal* 'Clinical Evidence' series which is updated every six months.

Adams, H.P. Jr, Bendixen, B.H., Kappelle, L.J. *et al.* (1993) Classification of subtype of acute ischemic stroke: definitions for use in a multicenter clinical trial. *Stroke* 24, 35–41.

Al-Buhairi, A.R., Phillips, S.J., Llewellyn, G. & January, M.M.S. (1998) Prediction of infarct topography using the Oxfordshire Community Stroke Project classification of stroke subtypes. *Journal of Stroke and Cerebrovascular Diseases* 7, 339–343.

Allen, C.M.C. (1984) *The accurate diagnosis and prognosis of acute stroke.* MD thesis, University of Cambridge.

Allen, C.M.C., Hoare, R.D., Fowler, C.J. & Harrison, M.J.G. (1984) Clinicoanatomical correlations of uncomplicated stroke. *Journal of Neurology, Neurosurgery and Psychiatry* 47, 1251–1254.

Alpers, B.J. & Berry, R.G. (1963) Circle of Willis in cerebral vascular disorders. *Archives of Neurology* 8, 398–402.

Amarenco, P. (1995) Small, deep cerebellar infarcts. In: *Lacunar and Other Subcortical Infarctions* (eds G.A. Donnan, B. Norrving, J.M. Bamford & J. Bogousslavsky), pp. 208–213. Oxford University Press, Oxford.

Amarenco, P. & Hauw, J.-J. (1990a) Cerebellar infarction in the territory of the anterior and inferior cerebellar artery. *Brain* **113**, 139–155.

Amarenco, P. & Hauw, J.-J. (1990b) Cerebellar infarction in the territory of the superior cerebellar artery: a clinicopathologic study of 33 cases. *Neurology* **40**, 1383–1390.

Amarenco, P., Roullet, E., Goujon, C., Cheron, F., Hauw, J.-J. & Bousser, M.-G. (1991) Infarction of the anterior part of the rostral cerebellum. *Neurology* **41**, 253–258.

Amarenco, P., Rosengart, A., DeWitt, L.D., Pessin, M.S. & Caplan, L.R. (1993) Anterior inferior cerebellar artery territory infarcts: mechanisms and clinical features. *Archives of Neurology* **50**, 154–161.

Amarenco, P., Levy, C., Cohen, A., Touboul, P.-J., Roullet, E. & Bousser, M.-G. (1994) Causes and mechanisms of territorial and nonterritorial cerebellar infarcts in 115 consecutive cases. *Stroke* **25**, 105–112.

Anderson, C.S., Taylor, B.V., Hankey, G.J., Stewart-Wynne, E.G. & Jamrozik, K.D. (1994) Validation of a clinical classification for subtypes of acute cerebral infarction. *Journal of Neurology, Neurosurgery and Psychiatry* **25**, 1173–1179.

Arboix, A. & Marti-Vilalta, J.L. (1992) Lacunar syndromes not due to lacunar infarcts. *Cerebrovascular Diseases* **2**, 287–292.

Ay, H., Oliveira-Filho, J., Buonanno, F.S. *et al.* (1999) Diffusion-weighted imaging identifies a subset of lacunar infarction associated with embolic source. *Stroke* **30**, 2644–2650.

Baloh, R.W. (1992) Stroke and vertigo. *Cerebrovascular Diseases* **2**, 3–10.

Bamford, J.M. (1986) *The classification and natural history of acute cerebrovascular disease.* MD dissertation, University of Manchester, Manchester.

Bamford, J.M. (1995) Lacunar syndromes: are they still worth diagnosing? In: *Lacunar and Other Subcortical Infarctions* (eds G.A. Donnan, B. Norrving, J.M. Bamford & J. Bogousslavsky), pp. 32–43. Oxford University Press, Oxford.

Bamford, J.M., Sandercock, P.A.G., Warlow, C.P. & Gray, J.M. (1986) Why are acute stroke patients admitted to hospital? The Oxfordshire Community Stroke Project. *British Medical Journal* **292**, 1369–1372.

Bamford, J., Sandercock, P., Jones, L. & Warlow, C. (1987) The natural history of lacunar infarction: the Oxfordshire Community Stroke Project. *Stroke* **18**, 545–551.

Bamford, J.M. & Warlow, C.P. (1988) Evolution and testing of the lacunar hypothesis. *Stroke* **19**, 1074–1082.

Bamford, J., Sandercock, P., Dennis, M., Burn, J. & Warlow, C. (1991) Classification and natural history of clinically identifiable subtypes of cerebral infarction. *Lancet* **337**, 1521–1526.

Berger, K., Kase, C.S. & Buring, J.E. (1996) Interobserver agreement in the classification of stroke in the Physicians' Health Study. *Stroke* **27**, 238–242.

Besson, G., Hommel, M. & Ferret, J. (1991) Historical aspects of the lacunar concept. *Cerebrovascular Diseases* **1**, 306–310.

Bogousslavsky, J. (1995) Thalamic infarcts. In: *Lacunar and Other Subcortical Infarctions* (eds G.A. Donnan, B. Norrving, J.M. Bamford & J. Bogousslavsky), pp. 149–170. Oxford University Press, Oxford.

Bogousslavsky, J. & Regli, F. (1990) Anterior cerebral artery territory infarction in the Lausanne Stroke Registry: clinical and etiologic patterns. *Archives of Neurology* **47**, 144–150.

Bogousslavsky, J., Regli, F. & Assal, G. (1986) The syndrome of unilateral tuberothalamic artery territory infarction. *Stroke* **17**, 434–441.

Bogousslavsky, J., van Melle, G. & Regli, F. (1988) The Lausanne Stroke Registry: analysis of 1000 consecutive patients with first stroke. *Stroke* **19**, 1083–1092.

Bogousslavsky, J., van Melle, G. & Regli, F. (1990) Middle cerebral artery pial territory infarcts: a study of the Lausanne Stroke Registry. *Annals of Neurology* **25**, 555–560.

Bogousslavsky, J., Martin, R. & Moulin, T. (1992) Homolateral ataxia and crural paresis: a syndrome of anterior cerebral artery territory infarction. *Journal of Neurology, Neurosurgery and Psychiatry* **55**, 1146–1149.

Bogousslavsky, J., Regli, F., Besson, G., Melo, T.P. & Nater, B. (1993) Early clinical diagnosis of stroke subtype. *Cerebrovascular Diseases* **3**, 39–44.

Boiten, J. & Lodder, J. (1991a) Isolated monoparesis is usually caused by superficial infarction. *Cerebrovascular Diseases* **1**, 337–340.

Boiten, J. & Lodder, J. (1991b) Lacunar infarcts: pathogenesis and validity of the clinical syndromes. *Stroke* **22**, 1374–1378.

Boiten, J. & Lodder, J. (1995) Risk factors for lacunar infarction. In: *Lacunar and Other Subcortical Infarctions* (eds G.A. Donnan, B. Norrving, J.M. Bamford & J. Bogousslavsky), pp. 56–69. Oxford University Press, Oxford.

Boiten, J., Rothwell, P.M., Slattery, J. & Warlow, C.P. (1996) Ischaemic lacunar stroke in the European Carotid Surgery Trial. *Cerebrovascular Diseases* **6**, 281–287.

Calverley, P. (1999) Blood pressure, breathing, and the carotid body. *Lancet* **354**, 969.

Caplan, L.R. (1980) Top of the basilar syndrome. *Neurology* **30**, 72–79.

Caplan, L.R. (1989) Intracranial branch atheromatous disease: a neglected, understudied, and underused concept. *Neurology* **39**, 1246–1250.

Caplan, L.R. (1993) Brain embolism, revisited. *Neurology* **43**, 1281–1287.

Caplan, L.R. & Tettenborn, B. (1992a) Vertebrobasilar occlusive disease—review of selected aspects, 1: spontaneous dissection of extracranial and intracranial posterior circulation arteries. *Cerebrovascular Diseases* **2**, 256–265.

Caplan, L.R. & Tettenborn, B. (1992b) Vertebrobasilar occlusive disease—review of selected aspects, 2: posterior circulation embolism. *Cerebrovascular Diseases* **2**, 320–326.

Caplan, L.R., Dewitt, L.D., Pessin, M.S., Gorelick, P.B. & Adelman, L.S. (1988) Lateral thalamic infarcts. *Archives of Neurology* **45**, 959–964.

Caplan, L.R., Amarenco, P., Rosengart, A. *et al.* (1992) Embolism from vertebral artery origin occlusive disease. *Neurology* **42**, 1505–1512.

Castaigne, P., Lhermitte, F., Buge, A., Escourolle, R., Hauw, J.J. & Lyon-Caen, O. (1981) Paramedian thalamic and midbrain infarcts: clinical and neuropathological study. *Annals of Neurology* **10**, 127–148.

Chambers, B.R. & Bladin, C.F. (1995) Internal watershed infarction. In: *Lacunar and Other Subcortical Infarctions* (eds G.A. Donnan, B. Norrving, J.M. Bamford & J. Bogousslavsky), pp. 139–148. Oxford University Press, Oxford.

Chambers, B.R., Brooder, R.J. & Donnan, G.A. (1991) Proximal posterior cerebral artery occlusion simulating middle cerebral artery occlusion. *Neurology* **41**, 385–390.

Chamorro, A., Sacco, R.L., Mohr, J.P. *et al.* (1991) Clinical–computed tomographic correlations of lacunar infarction in the Stroke Data Bank. *Stroke* **22**, 175–181.

Chaturvedi, S., Lukovits, T.G., Chen, W. & Gorelick, P.B. (1999) Ischemia in the territory of a hypoplastic vertebrobasilar system. *Neurology* **52**, 980–983.

Clarke, S., Assal, G., Bogousslavsky, J. *et al.* (1994) Pure amnesia after unilateral left polar thalamic infarct: topographic and sequential neuropsychological and metabolic (PET) correlations. *Journal of Neurology, Neurosurgery and Psychiatry* **57**, 27–34.

Crawley, F., Clifton, A. & Brown, M.M. (1998) Treatable lesions demonstrated on vertebral angiography for posterior circulation events. *British Journal of Radiology* **71**, 1266–1270.

Critchley, M. (1929) Arteriosclerotic Parkinsonism. *Brain* **52**, 23–83.

Critchley, M. (1930) The anterior cerebral artery and its syndromes. *Brain* **53**, 120–165.

Critchley, M. (1951) Types of visual perseveration: palinopsia and illusory visual spread. *Brain* **74**, 267–299.

Damasio, H. (1983) A computed tomographic guide to the identification of cerebral vascular territories. *Archives of Neurology* **40**, 138–142.

De Reuck, J. (1971) The human periventricular arterial blood supply and the anatomy of cerebral infarctions. *European Neurology* **5**, 321–334.

Déjerine, J. & Roussy, G. (1906) Le syndrome thalamique. *Revue Neurologique (Paris)* **14**, 521–532.

DiNubile, M.J. (1988) Septic thrombosis of the cavernous sinuses. *Archives of Neurology* **45**, 567–572.

Donnan, G.A., Tress, B.M. & Bladin, P.F. (1982) A prospective study of lacunar infarction using computerized tomography. *Neurology* **32**, 49–56.

Donnan, G.A., Norrving, B., Bamford, J.M. & Bogousslavsky, J. (1993) Subcortical infarction: classification and terminology. *Cerebrovascular Diseases* **3**, 248–251.

Donnan, G.A., O'Malley, H.M., Quang, L., Hurley, S. & Bladin, P.F. (1995) The capsular warning syndrome and lacunar transient ischaemic attacks. In: *Lacunar and Other Subcortical Infarctions* (eds G.A. Donnan, B. Norrving, J.M. Bamford & J. Bogousslavsky), pp. 47–55. Oxford University Press, Oxford.

Duncan, G.W., Parker, S.W. & Fisher, C.M. (1975) Acute cerebellar infarction in the PICA territory. *Archives of Neurology* **32**, 364–368.

Eadie, M.S. & Sutherland, J.M. (1964) Arteriosclerosis and Parkinsonism. *Journal of Neurology, Neurosurgery and Psychiatry* **27**, 237–240.

Ebersbach, G., Sojer, M., Valldeoriola, F. *et al.* (1999) Comparative analysis of gait in Parkinson's disease, cerebellar ataxia and subcortical arteriosclerotic encephalopathy. *Brain* **122**, 1349–1355.

vander Eecken, H.M. & Adams, R.D. (1953) The anatomy and functional significance of the meningeal arterial anastomoses of the human brain. *Journal of Neuropathology and Experimental Neurology* **12**, 132–157.

Escourelle, R. (1978). *Manual of Basic Neuropathology*. Saunders, Philadelphia.

Fieschi, C., Argentino, C., Lenzi, G.L., Sacchetti, M.L., Toni, D. & Bozzao, L. (1989) Clinical and instrumental evaluation of patients with ischemic stroke in the first six hours. *Journal of Neurological Sciences* **91**, 311–322.

Fisher, C.M. (1959) Observations of the fundus occuli in transient monocular blindness. *Neurology* **9**, 333–347.

Fisher, C.M. (1965a) Lacunes: small, deep cerebral infarcts. *Neurology* **15**, 774–784.

Fisher, C.M. (1965b) Pure sensory stroke involving face, arm and leg. *Neurology* **15**, 76–80.

Fisher, C.M. (1967) A lacunar stroke: the dysarthria–clumsy hand syndrome. *Neurology* **17**, 614–617.

Fisher, C.M. (1969) The arterial lesion underlying lacunes. *Acta Neuropathologica (Berlin)* **12**, 1–15.

Fisher, C.M. (1978a) Thalamic pure sensory stroke: a pathologic study. *Neurology* **28**, 1141–1144.

Fisher, C.M. (1978b) Ataxic hemiparesis: a pathologic study. *Archives of Neurology* **35**, 126–128.

Fisher, C.M. (1979) Capsular infarcts: the underlying vascular lesions. *Archives of Neurology* **36**, 65–73.

Fisher, C.M. (1982) Lacunar strokes and infarcts: a review. *Neurology* **32**, 871–876.

Fisher, C.M. (1986) The posterior cerebral artery syndrome. *Canadian Journal of Neurological Sciences* **13**, 232–239.

Fisher, C.M. (1991) Lacunar infarcts: a review. *Cerebrovascular Diseases* **1**, 311–320.

Fisher, C.M. & Caplan, L.R. (1971) Basilar artery branch occlusion: a cause of pontine infarction. *Neurology* **21**, 900–905.

Fisher, C.M. & Cole, M. (1965) Homolateral ataxia and crural paresis: a vascular syndrome. *Journal of Neurology, Neurosurgery and Psychiatry* **28**, 48–55.

Fisher, C.M. & Curry, H.B. (1965) Pure motor hemiplegia from vascular origin. *Archives of Neurology* **13**, 30–44.

Foix, C. & Levy, M. (1927) Les ramollissements sylviens: syndromes des lésions en foyer du territoire de l'artère sylvienne et de ses branches. *Revue Neurologique (Paris)* **11**, 1–51.

Foulkes, M.A., Wolf, P.A., Price, T.R., Mohr, J.P. & Hier, D.B. (1988) The Stroke Data Bank: design, methods, and baseline characteristics. *Stroke* **19**, 547–554.

Friedman, A., Kang, U.J., Tatemichi, T.K. & Burke, R.E. (1986) A case of parkinsonism following striatal lacunar infarction. *Journal of Neurology, Neurosurgery and Psychiatry* **49**, 1087–1088.

Frisén, L. (1979) Quadruple sectoranopia and sectorial optic atrophy: a syndrome of the distal anterior choroidal artery. *Journal of Neurology, Neurosurgery and Psychiatry* **42**, 590–594.

Gado, M., Hanaway, J. & Frank, R. (1979) Functional anatomy of the cerebral cortex by computed tomography. *Journal of Computer Assisted Tomography* **3**, 1–19.

Gan, R., Sacco, R.L., Kargman, J.K., Roberts, J.K., Boden-Albala, B. & Gu, Q. (1997) Testing the validity of the lacunar hypothesis: the Northern Manhattan Stroke Study experience. *Neurology* **48**, 1204–1211.

Glass, J.D., Levey, A.I. & Rothstein, J.D. (1990) The dysarthria–clumsy hand syndrome: a distinct clinical entity related to pontine infarction. *Annals of Neurology* **27**, 487–494.

Gordon, D.L., Bendixen, B.H., Adams, H.P. Jr *et al.* (1993) Interphysician agreement in the diagnosis of subtypes of acute ischemic stroke: implications for clinical trials. *Neurology* **43**, 1021–1027.

Graff-Radford, N.R., Damasio, H., Yamada, T., Eslinger, P.J. & Damasio, A.R. (1985) Nonhaemorrhagic thalamic infarction. *Brain* **108**, 485–516.

Groothuis, D.R., Duncan, G.W. & Fisher, C.M. (1977) The human thalamocortical sensory path in the internal capsule: evidence from a small capsular haemorrhage causing a pure sensory stroke. *Annals of Neurology* **2**, 328–331.

Gross, C.R., Shinar, D., Mohr, J.P. *et al.* (1986) Interobserver agreement in the diagnosis of stroke type. *Archives of Neurology* **43**, 893–898.

Hauw, J.-J. (1995) The history of lacunes. In: *Lacunar and Other Subcortical Infarctions* (eds G.A. Donnan, B. Norrving, J.M. Bamford & J. Bogousslavsky), pp. 3–15. Oxford University Press, Oxford.

Heinsius, T., Bogousslavsky, J. & van Melle, G. (1998) Large infarcts in the middle cerebral artery territory: etiology and outcome patterns. *Neurology* **50**, 341–350 [erratum appears in *Neurology* **50**, 1940–1943].

Helgason, C.M. (1995) Anterior choroidal artery territory infarction. In: *Lacunar and Other Subcortical Infarctions* (eds G.A. Donnan, B. Norrving, J.M. Bamford & J. Bogousslavsky), pp. 131–138. Oxford University Press, Oxford.

Hennerici, M.G. & Schwartz, A. (1998) Acute stroke subtypes: is there a need for reclassification? *Cerebrovascular Diseases* **8** (Suppl. 2), 17–22.

Hennerici, M., Klemm, C. & Rautenberg, W. (1988) The subclavian steal phenomenon: a common vascular disorder with rare neurologic deficits. *Neurology* **38**, 669–673.

Hennerici, M., Daffertshofer, M. & Jakobs, L. (1998) Failure to identify cerebral infarct mechanisms from topography of vascular territory lesions. *American Journal of Neuroradiology* **19**, 1067–1074.

Hillen, L.H. (1986) A mathematical model of the flow in the circle of Willis. *Journal of Biomechanics* **19**, 187–194.

Hommel, M., Besson, G., Le Bas, J.F. *et al.* (1990a) Prospective study of lacunar infarction using magnetic resonance imaging. *Stroke* **21**, 546–554.

Hommel, M., Besson, G., Pollak, P. *et al.* (1990b) Hemiplegia in posterior cerebral artery occlusion. *Neurology* **40**, 1496–1499.

Hommel, M., Moreau, D.O., Besson, G. & Perret, J. (1991) Site of arterial occlusion in the hemiplegic posterior cerebral artery syndrome. *Neurology* **41**, 604–605.

Horowitz, D.R. & Tuhrim, S. (1997) Stroke mechanisms and clinical presentation in large subcortical infarctions. *Neurology* **49**, 1538–1541.

Huang, C.Y. & Yu, Y.L. (1985) Small cerebellar strokes may mimic labyrinthine lesions. *Journal of Neurology, Neurosurgery and Psychiatry* **48**, 263–265.

Huang, C.Y., Woo, E., Yu, Y.L. & Chan, F.L. (1987) When is sensorimotor stroke a lacunar syndrome? *Journal of Neurology, Neurosurgery and Psychiatry* **50**, 720–726.

Ince, B., Petty, G.W., Brown, R.D. Jr, Chu, C.P., Sicks, J.D. & Whisnant, J.P. (1998) Dolichoectasia of the intracranial arteries in patients with first ischemic stroke: a population-based study. *Neurology* **50**, 1694–1698.

Kappelle, L.J., Koudstaal, P.J., van Gijn, J., Ramos, L.M.P. & Keunen, J.E.E. (1988) Carotid angiography in patients with lacunar infarction: a prospective study. *Stroke* **19**, 1093–1096.

Kappelle, L.J., Ramos, L.M.P. & van Gijn, J. (1989) The role of computed tomography in patients with lacunar stroke in the carotid territory. *Neuroradiology* **31**, 316–319.

Kase, C.S., Norrving, B., Levine, S.R. *et al.* (1993) Cerebellar infarction: clinical and anatomical observations in 66 cases. *Stroke* **24**, 76–83.

Kazui, S. & Sawada, T. (1993) Callosal apraxia without agraphia. *Annals of Neurology* **33**, 401–403.

Kim, J.S. (1994) Restricted acral sensory syndrome following minor stroke: further observation with special reference to differential severity of symptoms among individual digits. *Stroke* **25**, 2497–2502.

Kim, J.S. & Lee, M.C. (1994) Stroke and restricted sensory syndromes. *Neuroradiology* **36**, 258–263.

Kim, J.S., Kim, H.G. & Chung, C.S. (1995) Medial medullary syndrome: report of 18 new patients and a review of the literature. *Stroke* **29** (9), 1548–1552.

Kim, J.S., Lopez, I., DiPatre, P.L., Liu, F., Ishiyama, A. & Baloh, R.W. (1999) Internal auditory artery infarction: clinicopathologic correlation. *Neurology* **52**, 40–44.

Koroshetz, W.J. & Ropper, A.H. (1987) Artery-to-artery embolism causing stroke in the posterior circulation. *Neurology* **37**, 292–296.

Kunitz, S.C., Gross, C.R., Heyman, A. *et al.* (1984) The Pilot Stroke Data Bank: definition, design, and data. *Stroke* **15**, 740–746.

Lammie, A. (1998) The role of oedema in lacune formation. *Cerebrovascular Diseases* **8**, 246.

Lammie, G.A., Sandercock, P.A.G. & Dennis, M.S. (1999) Recently occluded intracranial and extracranial carotid arteries. *Stroke* **30**, 1319–1325.

Landi, G., Anzalone, N., Cella, E., Boccardi, E. & Musicco, M. (1991) Are sensorimotor strokes lacunar strokes? A case–control study of lacunar and non-lacunar strokes. *Journal of Neurology, Neurosurgery and Psychiatry* **54**, 1063–1068.

Lang, E.W., Daffertshofer, M., Daffertshofer, A., Wirth, S.B., Chesnut, R.M. & Hennerici, M. (1995) Variability of vascular territory in stroke: Pitfalls and failure of stroke pattern interpretation. *Stroke* **26**, 942–945.

Lindgren, A., Roijer, A., Norrving, B., Wallin, L., Eskilsson, J. & Johansson, B.B. (1994a) Carotid artery and heart disease in subtypes of cerebral infarction. *Stroke* **25**, 2356–2362.

Lindgren, A., Norrving, B., Rudling, O. & Johansson, B.B. (1994b) Comparison of clinical and neuroradiological findings in first-ever stroke: a population-based study. *Stroke* **25**, 1371–1377.

Lindley, R.I., Warlow, C.P., Wardlaw, J.M., Dennis, M.S., Slattery, J. & Sandercock, P.A.G. (1993) Interobserver reliability of a clinical classification of acute cerebral infarction. *Stroke* **24**, 1801–1804.

Lodder, J., Boiten, J., Raak, L. & Heuts van Raak, L. (1991) Sensorimotor syndrome relates to lacunar rather than to non-lacunar cerebral infarction. *Journal of Neurology, Neurosurgery and Psychiatry* **54**, 1097.

Lodder, J., Bamford, J., Kappelle, J. & Boiten, J. (1994) What causes false clinical prediction of small, deep infarcts? *Stroke* **25**, 86–91.

McNabb, A.W., Carol, W.M. & Mastaglia, F.L. (1988) 'Alien-hand' and loss of bimanual co-ordination after dominant anterior cerebral artery territory infarction. *Journal of Neurology, Neurosurgery and Psychiatry* **51**, 218–222.

Madden, K.P., Karanjia, P.N., Adams, H.P. Jr, Clarke, W.R. & the TOAST Investigators. (1995) Accuracy of initial stroke subtype diagnosis in the TOAST study. *Neurology* **45**, 1975–1979.

Marinkovic, S.V., Kovacevic, M.S. & Marinkovic, J.M. (1985) Perforating branches of the middle cerebral artery: microsurgical anatomy of their extracerebral segments. *Journal of Neurosurgery* **63**, 266–271.

Marinkovic, S.V., Gibo, H., Brigante, L., Nikodijevic, I. & Petrovic, P. (1999) The surgical anatomy of the perforating branches of the anterior choroidal artery. *Surgical Neurology* **52**, 30–36.

Mead, G.E., Murray, H., Farrell, A., O'Neill, P.A. & McCollum, C.N. (1997) Pilot study of carotid surgery for acute stroke. *British Journal of Surgery* **84**, 99–992.

Mead, G.E., Wardlaw, J.M., Lewis, S.C., McDowell, M. & Dennis, M.S. (1999a) Can simple clinical features be used to identify patients with severe carotid stenosis on doppler ultrasound? *Journal of Neurology, Neurosurgery and Psychiatry* **66**, 16–19.

Mead, G.E., Lewis, S.C., Wardlaw, J.M., Dennis, M.S. & Warlow, C.P. (1999b) Should computed tomography appearance of lacunar stroke influence patient management? *Journal of Neurology, Neurosurgery and Psychiatry* **67**, 682–684.

Mead, G.E., Lewis, S.C., Wardlaw, J.M., Dennis, M.S. & Warlow, C.P. (2000) How well does the Oxfordshire Community Stroke Project Classification predict the site and size of the infarct on brain imaging? *Journal of Neurological Neurosurg Psychiatry* **68**, 558–562.

Melo, T.P., Bogousslavsky, J., Van Melle, G. & Regli, F. (1992) Pure motor stroke: a reappraisal. *Neurology* **42**, 789–798.

Millikan, C.H. (1995) About lacunes. In: *Lacunar and Other Subcortical Infarctions* (eds G.A. Donnan, B. Norrving, J.M. Bamford & J. Bogousslavsky), pp. 23–28. Oxford University Press, Oxford.

Mohr, J.P., Kase, C.S., Meckler, R.J. & Fisher, C.M. (1977) Sensorimotor stroke due to thalamocapsular ischemia. *Archives of Neurology* **34**, 734–741.

Moriwaki, H., Matsumoto, M., Hashikawa, K. *et al.* (1997) Hemodynamic aspect of cerebral watershed infarction: assessment of perfusion reserve using iodine-123-iodoamphetamine SPECT. *Journal of Nuclear Medicine* **38**, 1556–1562.

Moulin, T., Bogousslavsky, J., Chopard, J.-L. *et al.* (1995) Vascular ataxic hemiparesis: a re-evaluation. *Journal of Neurology, Neurosurgery and Psychiatry* **58**, 422–427.

Neau, J.P. & Bogousslavsky, J. (1996) The syndrome of posterior choroidal artery territory infarction. *Annals of Neurology* **39**, 779–788.

Norrving, B. & Cronqvist, S. (1989) Clinical and radiological features of lacunar versus nonlacunar minor stroke. *Stroke* **20**, 59–64.

Norrving, B. & Staaf, G. (1991) Pure motor stroke from presumed lacunar infarct: incidence, risk factors and initial course. *Cerebrovascular Diseases* **1**, 203–209.

Olsen, T.S., Skriver, E.B. & Herning, M. (1985) Cause of cerebral infarction in the carotid territory: its relations to the size and the location of the infarct and to the underlying vascular lesion. *Stroke* **16**, 459–466.

van Overbeeke, J.J., Hillen, B. & Tulleken, C.A.F. (1991) A comparative study of the circle of Willis in fetal and adult life: the configuration of the posterior bifurcation of the posterior communicating artery. *Journal of Anatomy* **176**, 45–54.

Padget, H. (1948) The development of the cranial arteries in the human embryo. *Contributions to Embryology* **32**, 205–261.

Parkes, J.D., Marsden, C.D., Rees, J.E. *et al.* (1974) Parkinson's disease, cerebral arteriosclerosis, and senile dementia. *Quarterly Journal of Medicine* **43**, 49–61.

Parry, S.W., Richardson, D.A., O'Shea, D., Sen, B. & Kenny, R.A. (2000) Diagnosis of carotid sinus hypersensitivity in older adults: carotid sinus massage in the upright position is essential. *Heart* **83**, 22–23.

Perlmutter, D. & Rhoton, A.L. Jr (1976) Microsurgical anatomy of the anterior cerebral–anterior communicating–recurrent artery complex. *Journal of Neurosurgery* **45**, 259–272.

Pessin, M.S., Lathi, E., Cohen, M.B., Kwan, E.S., Hedges, T.R. III, Caplan, L.R. (1987) Clinical features and mechanism of occipital infarction. *Annals of Neurology* **21**, 290–299.

Petty, G.W., Brown, R.D. Jr, Whisnant, J.P., Sicks, J.D., O'Fallon, W.M. & Wiebers, D.O. (1999) Ischemic stroke subtypes: a population-based study of incidence and risk factors. *Stroke* **30**, 2513–2516.

Pinto, A.N., Melo, T.P., Loureco, M.E. *et al.* (1998) Can a clinical classification of stroke predict complications and treatments during hospitalization? *Cerebrovascular Diseases* **8**, 204–209.

Poirier, J. & Derouesne, C. (1984) Cerebral lacunae: a proposed new classification. *Clinical Neuropathology* **3**, 266.

Rascol, A., Clanet, M., Manelfe, C., Guiraud, B. & Bonafe, A. (1982) Pure motor hemiplegia: CT study of 30 cases. *Stroke* **13**, 11–17.

Read, S.J., Pettigrew, L., Schimmel, L. *et al.* (1998) White matter medullary infarcts: acute subcortical infarction in the centrum ovale. *Cerebrovascular Diseases* **8**, 289–295.

Ricci, S., Celani, M.G. & Caputo, N. (1991) SEPIVAC: a community-based study of stroke incidence in Umbria, Italy. *Journal of Neurology, Neurosurgery and Psychiatry* **54**, 695–698.

Riggs, H.E. & Rupp, C. (1963) Variation in form of circle of Willis. *Archives of Neurology* **8**, 8–14.

Royal College of Physicians (1989) Stroke: towards better management. *Royal College of Physicians of London.*

Sacco, R.L., Bello, J.A., Traub, R. & Brust, J.C.M. (1987) Selective proprioceptive loss from a thalamic lacunar stroke. *Stroke* **18**, 1160–1163.

Sacco, R.L., Ellenberg, J.H., Mohr, J.P. *et al.* (1989) Infarcts of undetermined cause: the NINCDS Stroke Data Bank. *Annals of Neurology* **25**, 382–390.

Samuelsson, M., Lindell, D. & Norrving, B. (1994) Gadolinium-enhanced magnetic resonance imaging in patients with presumed lacunar infarcts. *Cerebrovascular Diseases* **4**, 12–19.

Schwartz, A., Rautenberg, W. & Hennerici, M. (1993) Dolichoectatic intracranial arteries: review of selected aspects. *Cerebrovascular Diseases* **3**, 273–279.

Shin, H.K., Yoo, K.M., Chang, H.M. & Caplan, L.R. (1999) Bilateral intracranial vertebral artery disease in the New England Medical Center, Posterior Circulation Registry. *Archives of Neurology* **56**, 1353–1358.

Smith, M.T. & Baer, G.D. (1999) Achievement of simple mobility milestones after stroke. *Archives of Physical Medicine and Rehabilitation* **80**, 442–447.

Struck, L.K., Biller, J., Bruno, A. *et al.* (1991) Superior cerebellar artery territory infarction. *Cerebrovascular Diseases* **1**, 71–75.

Tamaki, M., Ohno, K., Niimi, Y. *et al.* (1997) Parenchymal damage in the territory of the anterior choroidal artery following supraophthalmic intracarotid administration of CDDP for treatment of malignant gliomas. *Journal of Neuro-oncology* **35**, 65–72.

Tatu, L., Moulin, T., Bogousslavsky, J. & Duvernoy, H. (1996) Arterial territories of human brain: brainstem and cerebellum. *Neurology* **47**, 1125–1135.

Tatu, L., Moulin, T., Bogousslavsky, J. & Duvernoy, H. (1998) Arterial territories of human brain: cerebral hemispheres. *Neurology* **47**, 1699–1708.

Tei, H., Uchiyama, S., Koshimizu, K., Kobayahi, M. & Ohara, K. (1999) Correlation between symptomatic, radiological and etiological diagnosis in acute ischemic stroke. *Acta Neurologica Scandinavica* **99**, 192–195.

Tettenborn, B., Caplan, L.R., Sloan, M.A. *et al.* (1993) Postoperative brainstem and cerebellar infarcts. *Neurology* **43**, 471–477.

Toni, D., Del Duca, R., Fiorelli, M. *et al.* (1994) Pure motor hemiparesis and sensorimotor stroke: accuracy of very early clinical diagnosis of lacunar strokes. *Stroke* **25**, 92–96.

Toni, D., Fiorelli, M., Gentile, M. *et al.* (1995) Progressing neurological deficit secondary to acute ischemic stroke: a study on predictability, pathogenesis, and prognosis. *Archives of Neurology* **52**, 670–675.

Torvik, A. & Jorgensen, L. (1964) Thrombotic and embolic occlusions of the carotid arteries in an autopsy series, 1: prevalence, location and associated disease. *Journal of Neurological Sciences* **1**, 24–39.

Torvik, A. & Jorgensen, L. (1966) Thrombotic and embolic occlusions of the carotid arteries in an autopsy series, 2: cerebral lesions and clinical course. *Journal of Neurological Sciences* **3**, 410–432.

Trobe, J.D., Lorber, M.L. & Schlezinger, N.S. (1973) Isolated homonymous hemianopia. *Archives of Ophthalmology* **89**, 377–381.

Turney, T.M., Garraway, W.M. & Whisnant, J.P. (1984) The natural history of hemispheric and brainstem infarction in Rochester, Minnesota. *Stroke* **15**, 790–794.

Tuszynski, M.H., Petito, C.K. & Levy, D.E. (1989) Risk factors and clinical manifestations of pathologically verified lacunar infarctions. *Stroke* **20**, 990–999.

Ueda, S., Fugitsu, K., Inomori, S. & Kuwabara, T. (1992) Thrombotic occlusion of the middle cerebral artery. *Stroke* **23**, 1761–1766.

Uldry, P.-A. & Bogousslavsky, J. (1995) Acute infarcts in the centrum ovale. In: *Lacunar and Other Subcortical Infarctions* (eds G.A. Donnan, B. Norrving, J.M. Bamford & J. Bogousslavsky), pp. 171–180. Oxford University Press, Oxford.

Von Cramon, D.Y., Hebel, N. & Schuri, U. (1985) A contribution to the anatomical basis of thalamic amnesia. *Brain* **108**, 993–1008.

Waddington, M.M. & Ring, B.A. (1968) Syndromes of occlusions of middle cerebral artery branches: angiographic and clinical correlations. *Brain* **91**, 685–696.

Wardlaw, J.M., Dennis, M.S., Lindley, R.I., Sellar, R.J. & Warlow, C.P. (1996) The validity of a simple clinical classification of acute ischaemic stroke. *Journal of Neurology* **243**, 274–279.

Weiller, C. (1995) Striatocapsular infarcts. In: *Lacunar and Other Subcortical Infarctions* (eds G.A. Donnan, B. Norrving, J.M. Bamford & J. Bogousslavsky), pp. 104–116. Oxford University Press, Oxford.

WHO Task Force on Stroke and Other Cerebrovascular Disorders (1989) Stroke—1989: recommendations on stroke prevention, diagnosis, and therapy. *Stroke* **20**, 1407–1431.

Woo, D., Gebel, J., Miller, R. *et al.* (1999) Incidence rates of first-ever ischemic stroke subtypes among blacks: a population-based study. *Stroke* **30**, 2517–2522.

van der Zwan, A. (1991) *The Variability of the Major Vascular Territories of the Human Brain* [M.D. dissertation]. University of Utrecht, Utrecht.

van der Zwan, A., Hillen, B., Tulleken, C.A.F., Dujovny, M. & Dragovic, L. (1992) Variability of the territories of the major cerebral arteries. *Journal of Neurosurgery* 77, 927–940.

van der Zwan, A., Hillen, B., Tulleken, C.A.F. & Dujovny, M. (1993) A quantitative investigation of the variability of the major cerebral arterial territories. *Stroke* 24, 1951–1959.

CHAPTER FIVE

What pathological type of stroke is it?

5.1 Introduction

Having established the diagnosis of stroke clinically (Chapter 3) and localized the part of the brain and vascular territory involved (Chapter 4), the next step is to identify the pathological nature of the stroke (i.e. infarct or haemorrhage). This is the subject of this chapter, which also covers the diagnosis of intracranial venous thrombosis and leukoaraiosis. Diagnosis of the pathological type of stroke is important because treatment, prognosis and secondary prevention differ for ischaemic and haemorrhagic stroke.

In practical day-to-day terms, most patients have one of the common causes of stroke: ischaemic stroke caused by the complications of atherothrombosis (section 6.3), intracranial small vessel disease (section 6.4) or embolism from the heart (section 6.5); primary (i.e. non-traumatic) intracerebral haemorrhage (PICH) caused by hypertension, for example (section 8.3.1); or subarachnoid haemorrhage (SAH), as a result of a ruptured saccular aneurysm (section 9.1.1). A small minority will have an unusual underlying cause of their PICH: an odd presentation of SAH, a tumour presenting as a 'stroke' or an unusual cause of ischaemic stroke, such as venous infarction. Thus, while most strokes seen clinically, and on imaging, are caused by something which is common, it is important not to assume that all strokes are. Some strokes will result from unusual causes. If there is something odd about either the clinical presentation or the imaging, then it is important to look for an explanation. This point will be illustrated with examples where appropriate.

5.2 Frequency of different pathological types of stroke

It is important to consider the frequency of a condition when evaluating a diagnostic method. The community-based studies of stroke incidence are described in section 17.2.1, and are mentioned here as background to the clinical and imaging diagnosis of stroke type. In a systematic review of these studies, the majority of strokes (about 80%) were said to be caused by cerebral infarction (Sudlow & Warlow 1997) (Fig. 5.1). About 10% were said to be caused by primary intracerebral haemorrhage (PICH), 5% to subarachnoid haemorrhage (SAH) and in 5% the cause was uncertain or a result of non-vascular causes. There was, in general, reasonable agreement between these studies, although older studies from Japan had higher PICH rates, consistent with much anecdotal information that cerebral haemorrhage is considerably more common in Oriental than white populations.

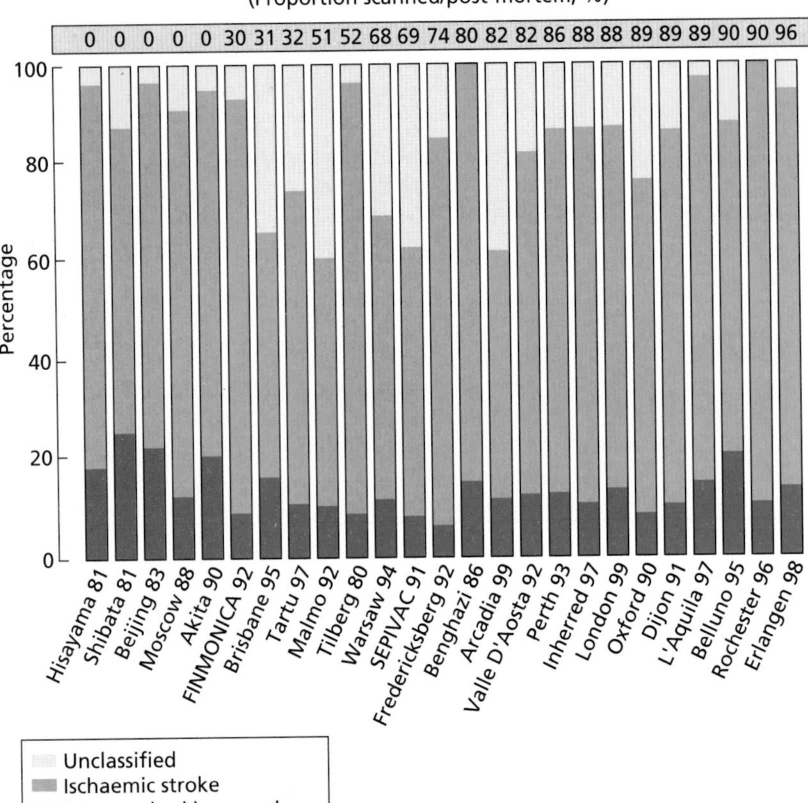

Fig. 5.1 Histogram of the cause of first ever-in-a-lifetime stroke by pathological type ranked according to the proportion of patients who had a CT scan (or a post-mortem) in the community-based studies. Subarachnoid haemorrhage excluded. (The figure was prepared by Dr Sarah Keir, Department of Clinical Neurosciences, The Western General Hospital, Edinburgh, UK.)

However, in none of these studies did the investigators succeed in computed tomography (CT) scanning of *all* the patients soon enough to detect small haemorrhages reliably, i.e. within about a week of stroke onset (section 5.3.4). The best scanning rate achieved was about 90%, but this was within *3 weeks*—not 1 week—of the stroke, even including a more recent study (Kolominsky-Rabas *et al.* 1998; Fig. 5.1). In some studies, the CT scanning rate was either not stated, or was as low as 30%, the diagnosis of infarct or haemorrhage therefore being made on clinical examination. In general, the details of patient scanning (who, when, how many) given in most studies were very patchy. Many studies were carried out before CT scanning was readily available and, in any case, the technology was then less able to demonstrate subtle parenchymal abnormalities. However, nine studies did give details of patients who were or were not scanned (Bamford *et al.* 1990; Jerntop & Berglund 1992; Anderson *et al.* 1993; Jorgensen *et al.* 1995; Carolei *et al.* 1997; Korv *et al.* 1997; Kolominsky-Rabas *et al.* 1998; Stewart *et al.* 1999; Vemmos *et al.* 1999). The patients most likely to be missed from scanning altogether were those with mild strokes, the elderly and patients who died early after the stroke. Most studies were unable to do post-mortems on most patients who died.

In the past therefore it is extremely likely that the frequency of PICH has been underestimated, particularly in the elderly and in patients with mild strokes who may have been managed as out-patients and so did not present to hospital until some days after the stroke. By this time, the features of PICH would have disappeared from the CT scan. It is generally considered that PICH is more frequent in patients with severe and moderate than with mild strokes. However, failure to diagnose small PICHs may have artifactually skewed the distribution curve of PICH towards the severe end of the stroke severity spectrum. Until a community-based incidence study achieves a 100% CT scanning rate within about 5 days of stroke, or uses appropriate magnetic resonance (MR) sequences sensitive to haemorrhage in patients presenting after 5 days (section 5.3.7), the true incidence of PICH and its relationship with stroke severity and patient age will not be known. Support for this notion comes from Rowe *et al.* (1988) who found an apparent increase in the proportion of patients admitted to hospital with PICH, in parallel with the increased use of CT. The increase in PICH was particularly striking for small PICHs, i.e. milder strokes.

In hospital practice, there is a bias towards admitting the more 'severe' strokes, and so perhaps a greater proportion with haemorrhages (perhaps as high as 20%, depending on the speciality) and a greater proportion with large cortical and extensive brainstem–cerebellar infarcts. Thus, fewer patients with minor cortical or brainstem strokes will generally be seen in hospitals.

In both community- and hospital-based studies, a small proportion of 'strokes' turn out to be caused by tumours, infections or some other non-vascular cause presenting as a 'stroke' (section 3.4). There may be clues to a non-vascular cause in that the history or examination is atypical. For example, a recent epileptic seizure, increasing headaches, stuttering onset, or previous malignant disease should all alert the clinician to possible non-vascular conditions. Fortunately, cross-sectional brain imaging can distinguish most of these (Fig. 5.2).

5.3 Differentiating ischaemic stroke from primary intracerebral haemorrhage

From a practical point of view, the first step in classification is the distinction of ischaemic stroke from primary (i.e. non-traumatic) intracerebral haemorrhage (PICH). This distinguishes groups of stroke with differing causes, prospects for survival and recurrence, and will also influence decisions about medical and surgical treatments. While clinical paradigms can be of some assistance (section 5.3.1), the 'gold-standard' for making the distinction is either CT or MR brain scanning (sections 5.3.4 and 5.3.7).

There are three issues to be considered in assessing the reliability of the clinical diagnosis of stroke:

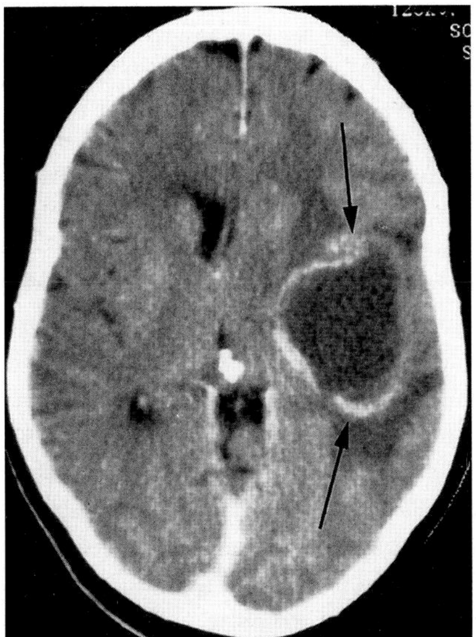

Fig. 5.2 CT brain scan (with intravenous contrast) from a patient who presented with sudden-onset right hemiparesis, but whose scan showed a large primary brain tumour with considerable mass effect (probably a glioblastoma—arrows) to be the cause of symptoms. (Note the scan was performed first without contrast, which was then given to clarify the picture.)

- the diagnosis of stroke itself (i.e. is it a stroke or not?);
- whether the stroke is caused by an infarct or a haemorrhage; and,
- particularly in ischaemic stroke, the site and size of the lesion (i.e. anterior vs. posterior circulation, lacunar vs. cortical, etc.).

The first and third of these have been discussed in Chapters 3 and 4 and will not be mentioned further here. The second is the basis for this chapter and requires the use of CT or MR scanning. However, before proceeding further, there is one key point worth emphasizing which underpins the use of imaging tests generally; it is essential for the correct conduct of the radiological examination that the radiologist has all the relevant information, including time from symptom onset, relevant past history and current background information (such as use of anticoagulants, bleeding disorder, suspected malignancy, trauma). Otherwise the investigation may not be performed in the optimum way to obtain the information required, and misleading (or simply incorrect) reports may be issued (Fig. 5.3).

For the correct conduct and interpretation of diagnostic imaging, the radiologist should receive all relevant information, especially the following:
- *how long ago the stroke occurred;*
- *any previous strokes;*
- *the clinical features of this stroke;*
- *history of malignant disease; and*
- *any concurrent illnesses (e.g. renal failure, diabetes, infection).*

Occasionally it is difficult to differentiate a tumour from an infarct or partially resolved haematoma on the initial CT scan: haematomas may mimic tumours radiologically at certain phases in their evolution (section 5.3.4), and tumours may mimic infarcts (Cameron 1994) (Fig. 5.4). Therefore, it may be necessary to rescan the occasional patient after several weeks, when vascular lesions and tumours can usually be differentiated by the pattern of their evolution with time.

5.3.1 Clinical scoring methods

Before the advent of CT scanning, attempts were made to correlate clinical findings with the pathological type of stroke (confirmed or not at post-mortem). In fatal primary intracerebral haemorrhage (PICH), mostly caused by very large intraparenchymal and intraventricular haemorrhages and subarachnoid haemorrhage (SAHs), the commonly occurring features were drowsiness and severe headache. When CT scanning became available, it was soon clear that many smaller PICHs were not associated with these 'typical' features. Therefore, a number of clinical scoring systems were devised, specifically to differentiate PICH from infarction, for use when CT scanning was less readily available than it

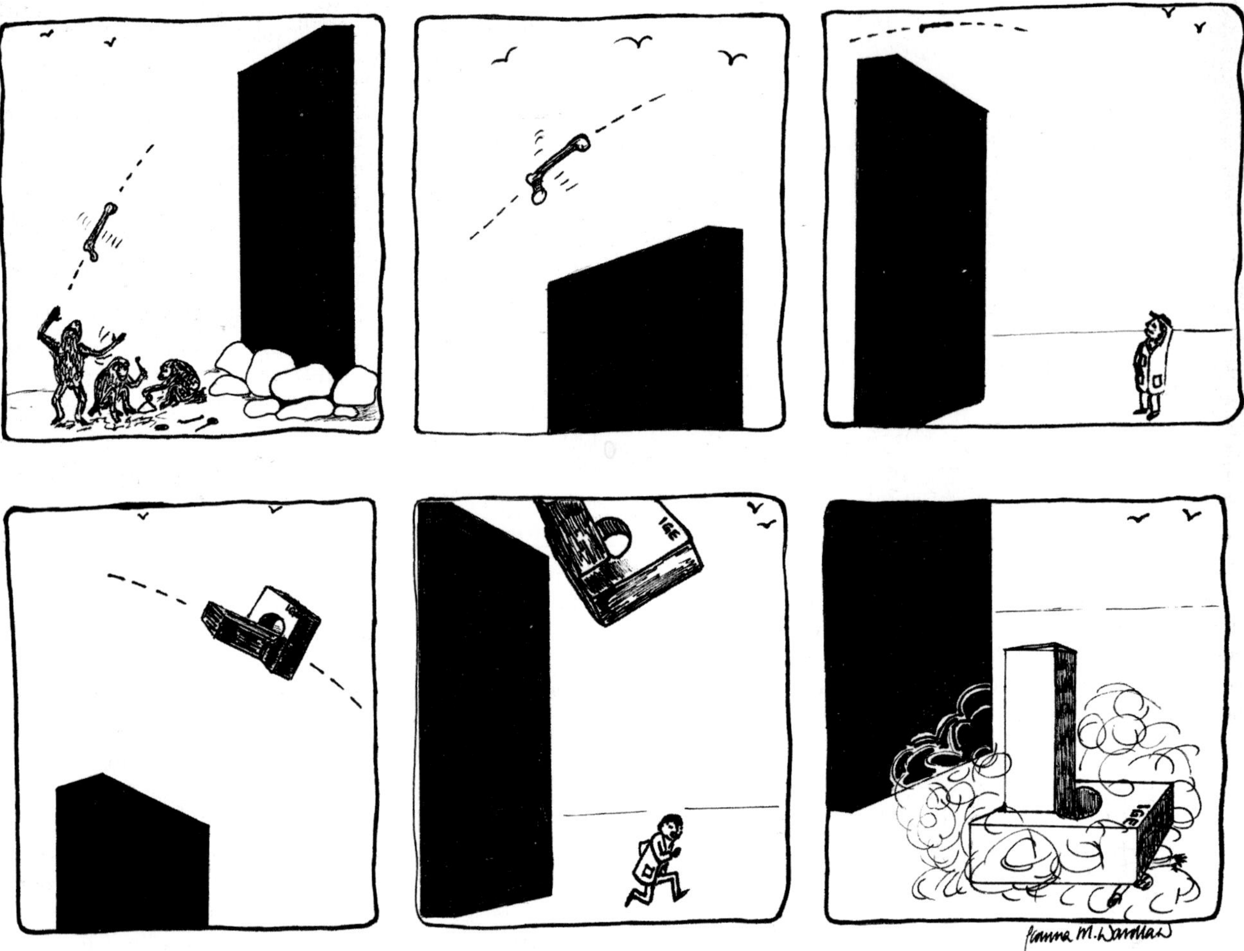

Fig. 5.3 'Beware the double-edged sword of technology.' The cartoon depicts the evolution of the use of 'tools' from the dawn of man to the present day, but tools must be used with intelligence, otherwise our good intentions may backfire. (Adapted from *2001: A Space Odyssey*, with apologies to Stanley Kubrick.)

is now: the Allen (1983) and Siriraj (Poungvarin *et al.* 1991) scores, and a method suggested by Besson *et al.* (1995). Although these systems do increase clinical diagnostic accuracy, prospective studies have shown that, even in patients with a low probability of cerebral haemorrhage on the basis of these scores, at least 7% (with the Allen) and 5% (with the Siriraj) of patients actually had an intracerebral haemorrhage on brain CT (Celani *et al.* 1992, 1994; Lindley *et al.* 1992; Weir *et al.* 1994; Hawkins *et al.* 1995).

Thus, even with a complex and fairly time-consuming clinical scoring method used by physicians experienced in stroke, and even in patients with the lowest a priori probability of haemorrhage (i.e. mild symptoms, European origin rather than Oriental, etc.), the clinical differentiation of ischaemic stroke from haemorrhage will still be wrong, and importantly wrong, in up to 10% of patients. It is likely that less experienced clinicians could be wrong even more often. For example, Fig. 5.5 shows a patient who had less than a 5% chance of haemorrhage according to the Siriraj score, but brain CT showed a thalamic haematoma as the cause of the stroke.

Furthermore, although Hawkins *et al.* (1995) used a population-based registry for their study, only 2% of their patients were out-patients, therefore their results apply to in-patients only. Celani *et al.* (1992) used a community-based registry but did not state what proportion of patients in the scoring study were out-patients and CT was performed up to 30 days after stroke. Only in-patients were studied by Celani *et al.* (1994), Lindley *et al.* (1992) and Weir *et al.* (1994). Thus patients with very mild strokes, who are likely to be seen as out-patients rather than admitted to hospital, were not well represented in any of these studies of scoring systems. As patients with PICH may even, very rarely, present as having a transient ischaemic attack (TIA) (Sohn *et al.* 1991; Aparicio *et al.* 1995; Chen *et al.* 1996; Gunathilake 1998; Ivo 1999), or recover very rapidly (Scott & Miller 1985), it is likely that the frequency of PICH as a cause of minor stroke, or even TIA, has been underestimated. Therefore, clinical scoring methods are very

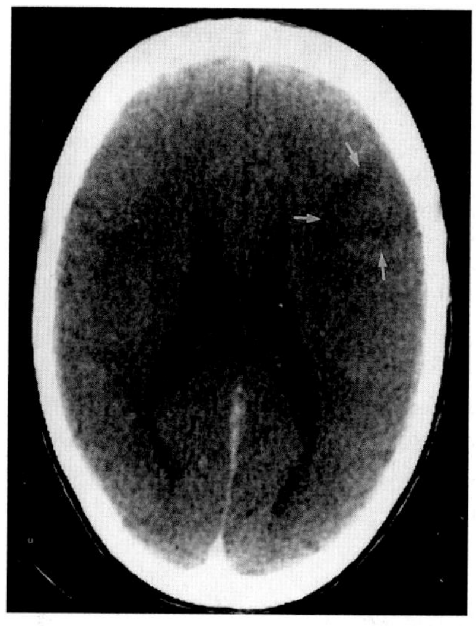
(a)

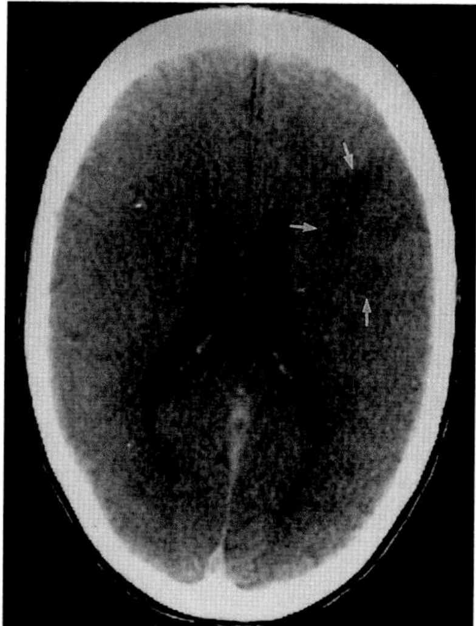
(b)

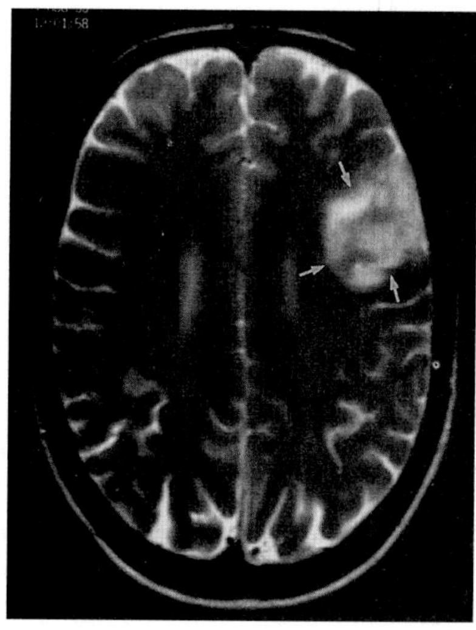
(c)

Fig. 5.4 CT brain scan of a patient with a tumour mimicking an infarct scanned within 12 h of a sudden onset right hemiparesis and dysphasia. (a) Non-contrast CT scan obtained at 12 h after symptom onset. There is a wedge-shaped, relatively ill-defined, low-density area (arrows) involving parietal grey and adjacent white matter, in a distribution consistent with a middle cerebral artery branch occlusion. (b) Repeat CT scan 6 weeks later fails to show any change in the appearance of the lesion. An infarct by this stage would have become atrophied and of the same density as cerebrospinal fluid. (c) T2-weighted MR scan 2 years later shows no change in the shape or size of the lesion, which is entirely consistent with a primary brain tumour. The patient had not received any specific treatment in the interim as her symptoms had not been troublesome.

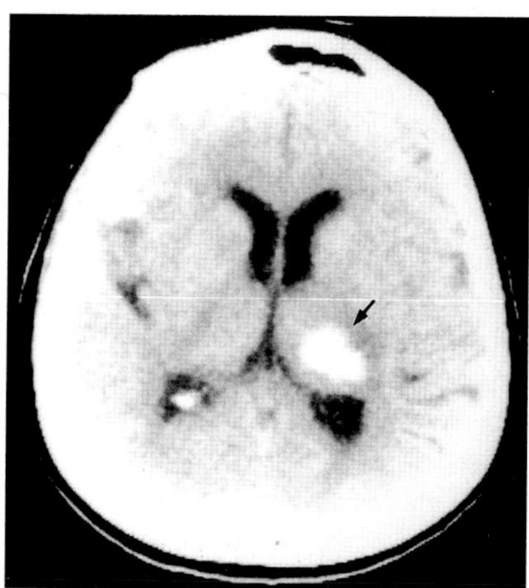

Fig. 5.5 CT brain scan of a patient presenting within 24 h of a stroke, who had less than a 5% chance of having a primary intracerebral haemorrhage (by the Siriraj score). The scan shows a primary thalamic haemorrhage (arrow) to be the cause of the stroke.

unlikely to be able to distinguish minor strokes caused by small haemorrhages from those caused by small infarcts.

> *No clinical scoring method can differentiate, with absolute reliability, ischaemic stroke from primary intracerebral haemorrhage. To do this, brain CT (ideally within a week of stroke) or MRI is required.*

Therefore, the problem with these clinical scoring systems is that they miss small PICHs. Although it may be acceptable to rely on the scores in some circumstances, for example in some aspects of epidemiological work—although this was questioned by Hawkins *et al.* (1995)—and to speed randomization in some acute stroke treatment trials, it may not be in others (e.g. prior to antithrombotic, thrombolytic and anticoagulant treatment). CT and MR scanning are the only methods of distinguishing infarct from haemorrhage reliably, and even then only if they are used appropriately (sections 5.3.4 and 5.3.7).

5.3.2 Cerebrospinal fluid examination

Examination of cerebrospinal fluid (CSF) is clearly important in selected cases with suspected subarachnoid haemorrhage if the CT scan is negative for subarachnoid blood (section 5.6.3). However, it is not required to differentiate ischaemic stroke from primary intracerebral haemorrhage and can be dangerous when there is raised intracranial pressure. In the pre-CT era, CSF examination was more widely used in the diagnosis of all kinds of neurological diseases for which there are now much better diagnostic tests. Abnormalities of the CSF cell and protein content do occur following ischaemic stroke and PICH, but they are so non-specific as to be probably less reliable than clinical features to make the distinction (Fishman 1992) (section 6.7.11).

Examination of the cerebrospinal fluid is useless and potentially hazardous to differentiate ischaemic stroke from primary intracerebral haemorrhage. It only has a role in the diagnosis of CT-negative suspected subarachnoid haemorrhage.

5.3.3 CT scanning

The earliest reports of brain CT scanning in cerebrovascular disease quickly demonstrated its value for differentiating between cerebral haemorrhage and infarction (and other conditions, such as tumours) as the cause of acute focal neurological symptoms. Ambrose (1973) stated that 'in the overall investigation of cerebrovascular disease, computed tomography will, without doubt, come to be an invaluable means of distinguishing between haemorrhage and infarction'. Paxton and Ambrose (1974) reported positive CT findings in all 66 patients with intracerebral haemorrhage and in 27 of 55 patients with ischaemic stroke, and observed density changes in the evolution of the infarcted brain tissue. Kistler *et al.* (1975) and Kinkel and Jacobs (1976) reported CT scans of 111 patients with stroke. The quality of scans was poor by today's standards: pixels were large, scan times long and processing algorithms less sophisticated, all of which limited the visualization of small infarcts and of subtle changes in the early stages of larger infarcts. However, they found that most patients with a permanent neurological deficit had a defect in the appropriate area on brain CT, whereas patients with transient ischaemic attacks did not. They also noted mass effect in the early stages of large cerebral infarcts which, as a result, could be confused with cerebral tumours. In 43% of patients whose scan showed PICH, the clinical diagnosis had been acute ischaemic stroke and the haemorrhage would not have been diagnosed without CT. This was one of the first indications of the unreliability of clinical criteria in differentiating infarct from haemorrhage.

Current CT brain scan technique for stroke

A standard brain CT consists of axial images through the whole brain, starting at the skull base and ending at the vertex, at 1-cm intervals. This usually produces about 10 sequential images. The slices may be contiguous or overlapping, or leave gaps of a few millimetres in between, depending on the age of the scanner. A state-of-the-art mid-1980s scanner performed 10 slices through the whole brain and produced the images in about 10 min. A modern late-1990s spiral CT scanner will produce the same set of images in about 20 s. Images can be acquired at narrower intervals (i.e. less than 1 cm) to show fine detail, or in different planes of section to avoid bone artifacts, and at very fast scan speeds to reduce motion artifact. With modern fast scanners, there is a great temptation to 'do a few extra slices', or to perform brain scans more readily, but it should be noted that an average brain CT scan exposes the patient to the equivalent of 1 year of average background radiation (Royal College of Radiologists 1995). A chest X-ray is equivalent to about 2 days'-worth of background radiation. Pregnancy is a relative contraindication to brain CT, although it can be performed, when really necessary, with careful shielding of the abdomen. As the purpose of CT in acute stroke is largely to differentiate haemorrhage from infarction, contrast is not usually required. Intravenous contrast may be given to help clarify lesions (such as tumours from infarcts, section 5.3.5), but generally is not used in the investigation of stroke, and may cause diagnostic confusion. It is much better to perform a non-enhanced scan first; contrast may be given afterwards if necessary.

A simple routine CT brain scan, i.e. about 10 slices through the whole brain at 1-cm intervals without intravenous contrast, is usually all that is required for acute stroke. This will exclude primary intracerebral haemorrhage, although it may not show the site of any infarction.

The availability of CT scanning varies between hospitals. In areas where CT scanners are scarce (i.e. where the radiology department is very busy), a few simple manoeuvres may help smooth the path of the stroke patient to the CT scanner. Always inform the radiology department of the request for a scan as early as possible in the day; there is nothing more infuriating than being asked to perform a scan at 16.00 h when the patient has been languishing in the hospital since 8.00 h. If the patient is immobile and cannot transfer, send him or her on a trolley; if dependent and the radiology department has few nurses, which applies to most, then send a nurse escort to look after the patient while in the scanning department. Good communication between clinician and radiologist helps their relationship enormously, and so the patients. Later feedback to the radiologist on what has happened to patients is always appreciated.

5.3.4 The appearance of primary intracerebral haemorrhage on brain CT

Recent haemorrhage

Acute parenchymatous haemorrhage is of higher density than normal brain parenchyma, typically about 80 Hounsfield units (HU) compared with 35 HU (Figs 5.5 and 5.6). The density increase occurs, as far as we know, virtually immediately and is thought to be caused by both the haemoglobin content and the matrix of the static blood (or clot). There have been a few reports of cerebral haemorrhages observed while the patient was actually in the CT scanner which confirm the immediacy of the change (Masson *et al.* 1984; Franke *et al.* 1990). As soon as blood stops moving,

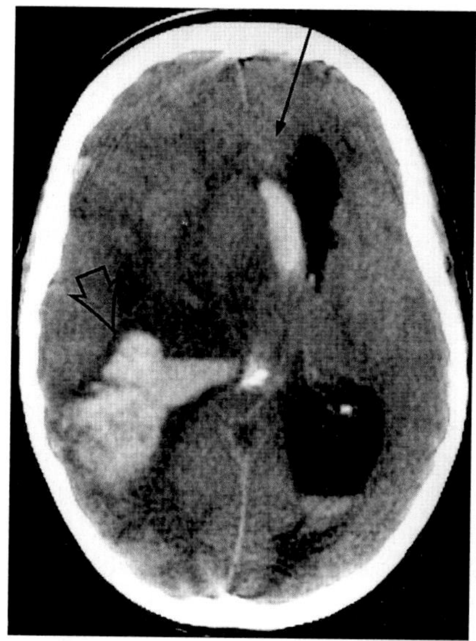

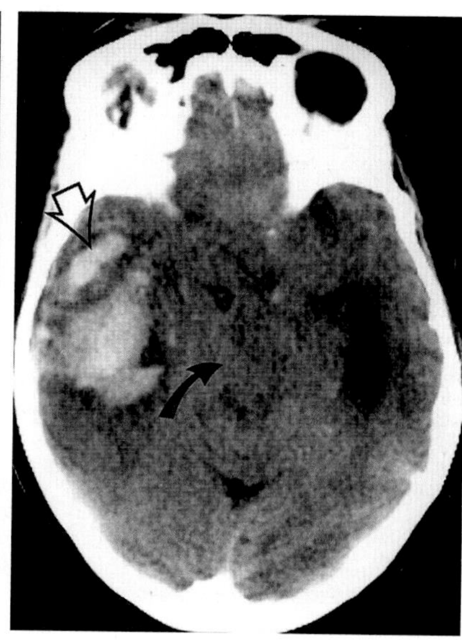

Fig. 5.6 CT brain scan showing a large right temporoparietal primary intracerebral haemorrhage (open arrows) with mass effect causing (a) herniation of the ipsilateral brain under the free edge of the falx (thin arrow); and (b) inferiorly through the tentorial hiatus (curved arrow). There is blood in the lateral ventricles (see blood–cerebrospinal fluid level in occipital pole of left lateral ventricle, and filling the frontal pole of the left lateral ventricle). Note also the dilatation of the left lateral ventricle caused by obstruction of the foramen of Monro. (a) (b)

its density increases to appear 'whiter' on CT. This is true whether the blood is in the subarachnoid space, in the brain parenchyma, or in an embolus or thrombus blocking a large intracranial artery, cortical vein or venous sinus.

The area of high attenuation is usually rather circumscribed (most often rounded or oval) and tends to be of homogeneous density (an exception being the appearance of a blood–fluid level in some large haematomas, see below). The haematoma is surrounded by a variable amount of low attenuation, caused by a combination of oedema and ischaemic necrosis of compressed brain. As well as the increased density, intracerebral haematomas exert mass effect, depending on their size and site, compressing and damaging adjacent structures. If large, supratentorial haematomas cause herniation of the temporal lobe through the tentorial hiatus, with compression of vital brainstem structures, or of the ipsilateral parasagittal cortex under the falx, with compression of the ipsilateral—and dilatation of the contralateral—lateral ventricle (section 11.1.5) (Fig. 5.6).

Haemorrhage in the brain is visible on CT immediately. It does not take a few hours to develop its distinct appearance.

Evolution in appearance of the haematoma with time

The density of the haematoma decreases with time as the haemoglobin breaks down, and it can become isodense with brain and then hypodense within 5 days (Fig. 5.7); larger haematomas take longer to become isodense. Even if isodense, the associated mass effect may still be evident, depending on haematoma size (Fig. 5.8). Later, the haematoma becomes hypodense so that, on CT performed a week or so (Fig. 5.7) to a few months after the stroke, the haematoma appears as a defect of cerebrospinal fluid (i.e. water) density. At this late stage—in fact, at any stage beyond the time when the haematoma becomes isodense—a haematoma may look identical to an old infarct (Dennis *et al.* 1987). The additional problem of distinguishing primary intracerebral haemorrhage from haemorrhagic transformation of an infarct will be discussed in section 5.4. Although large haematomas may remain visible for many weeks, small haematomas become hypodense more quickly. To be sure of differentiating a haematoma from an infarct, the CT scan should be performed as soon as possible, preferably within a week of onset, to be certain of not missing the small bleeds (Dennis *et al.* 1987). This may not be practical in patients who are not admitted to hospital but, in any case, scanning should be performed as soon as it is practical.

Late appearance of the haematoma

After many months the process of haematoma resorption is complete and all that may be left is a small slit-like cavity containing fluid of cerebrospinal fluid density, or no abnormality at all (Franke *et al.* 1991; Sung & Chu 1992; Bradley 1994). Frequently, there is also an *ex vacuo* effect, such as enlargement of the lateral ventricle or sulci adjacent to the site of the former haemorrhage. Dotted or linear high density on brain CT ('pseudocalcification') around the wall of the cavity has been described after large basal ganglia haematomas. This is thought to be caused by visible deposition of haemosiderin and haematoidin (Sung & Chu 1992). In a small proportion of patients, 'pseudocalcification' is the only visible evidence on late CT of previous haemorrhage. In some patients an *ex vacuo* effect may be seen without any cavity (Franke *et al.* 1991).

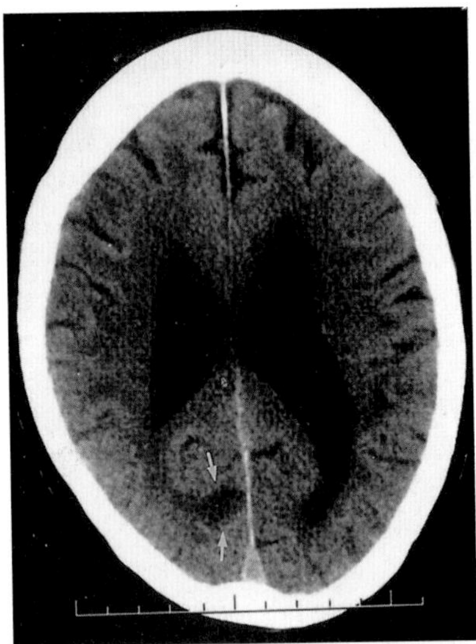
(a)

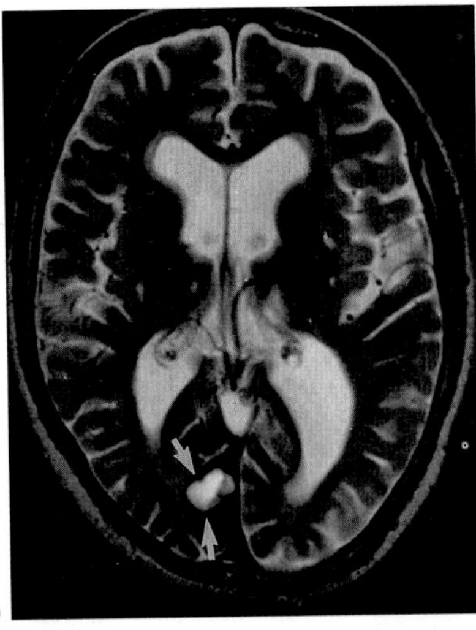
(b)

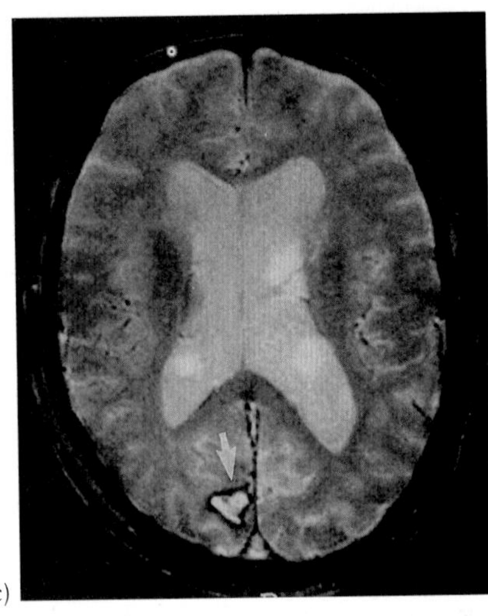
(c)

Fig. 5.7 (a) CT brain scan in an out-patient obtained 8 days after stroke causing left homonymous hemianopia. The arrows point to a low density in the right visual cortex which on CT looks just like a small infarct. (b) Fast spin echo T2, and (c) gradient echo T2 are the corresponding MR images obtained within 1 h of the CT, and which clearly show that the lesion (arrows) was in fact a haemorrhage. Note the dark haemosiderin ring around the edge of the hyperintense area (see also Figs 5.24–5.27).

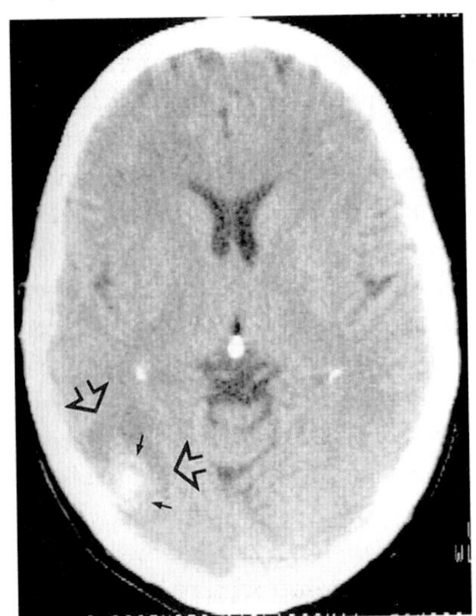
(a)

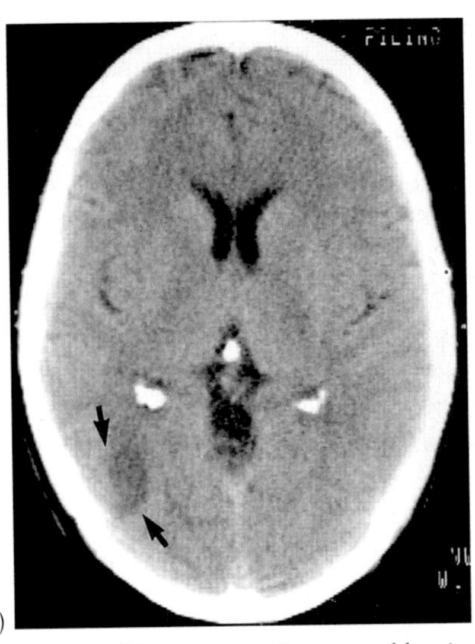
(b)

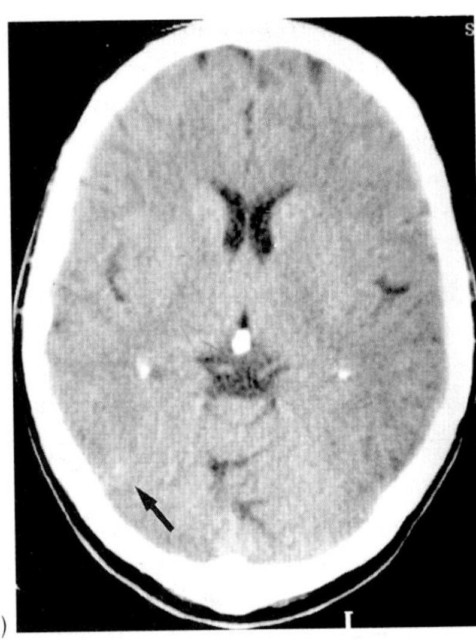
(c)

Fig. 5.8 Sequence showing the change in the appearance of haemorrhage on CT brain scan with time. (a) About 4 days after the stroke there is a hyperdense lesion (fresh blood) in the right occipital cortex (small arrows) with surrounding hypodensity (open arrows) caused by oedema. Scanning sooner after the stroke would have shown slightly more solid hyperdensity (but of similar size) but less hypodense rim (as it takes a day or so for the oedema to develop). Very fresh haemorrhage is seen in Figs 5.5 and 5.6. (b) About 3 weeks after the stroke the hyperdensity has completely disappeared leaving a hypodense lesion with some persistent space-occupying effect (arrows) which could easily be mistaken for an infarct without the prior scan. (c) About 10 weeks after the stroke the lesion has virtually vanished (arrow). The final diagnosis was primary intracerebral haemorrhage—cerebral angiography and follow-up scans did not reveal any underlying structural cause. A larger haemorrhagic lesion would probably have left a residual 'hole' in the brain parenchyma of cerebrospinal fluid density.

To have the maximum chance of excluding a parenchymal haemorrhage, brain CT should be performed within about a week of the stroke, ideally within a few days, otherwise the characteristic 'whiteness' of the fresh haemorrhage will have disappeared.

Does intravenous contrast help?

The use of intravenous contrast in the acute phase can complicate rather than clarify matters, although it may be necessary if an arteriovenous malformation (AVM) or a haemorrhagic metastasis is suspected. In the first few days contrast has very little effect on the appearance of the haematoma, even if an AVM is present, because the haematoma and its mass effect obliterate all visible signs of enhancement. Contrast can be useful if haemorrhage into a metastasis is suspected, because it might show up deposits elsewhere in the brain, not visible on the unenhanced scan, thus establishing the diagnosis. After about a week, enhancement at the edges of the haematoma can be seen (sometimes ring enhancement), similar to the enhancement around tumours and abscesses (Fig. 5.9). Follow-up CT with contrast, preferably allowing a sufficient time delay (possibly several weeks or months depending on the size of the original haematoma) for any mass effect to settle, may be of value in showing tumours or cryptic vascular malformations (which may have been compressed by the acute haematoma, so not visible initially), but MRI is more sensitive and specific (section 5.3.7).

Do all haemorrhages show up on CT?

Given a relatively artifact-free scan and an experienced viewer, all haemorrhages of sufficient volume to cause a clinically apparent stroke will be visualized, assuming the CT scan was performed within the correct time frame, as discussed above. In a small series of anaemic patients, all haematomas were readily visible despite the concern that they might not look 'white' on CT because of their reduced haemoglobin content (Pierce *et al.* 1994). The most difficult area of the brain in which to see haemorrhage is in the posterior fossa, because of frequent artifacts caused by the dense surrounding bone, or movement. Additional thin sections at 0.5-cm slice intervals, instead of the standard 1.0 cm, or use of very rapid scan techniques available on most modern scanners may help. The importance of viewer experience should not be overlooked. In a recent study by Schriger *et al.* (1998), in which CT scans of stroke patients were reviewed by doctors from different disciplines, the admitting physicians only reliably detected 17%, neurologists 40% and general radiologists 52% of intracranial haemorrhages. Errors were to overlook some definite haemorrhages on some scans, and to mistake basal ganglia calcification (a quite frequent finding in the elderly) for haemorrhage.

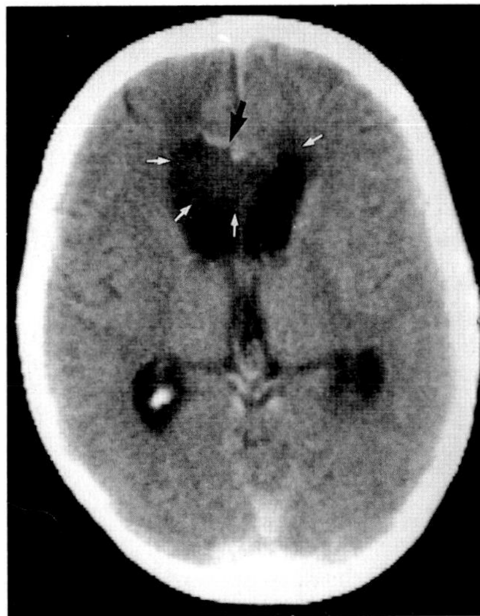

Fig. 5.9 CT brain scan of a patient who presented with a 2-week history of confusion and some headache. The scan shows a hypodense mass in the right frontal lobe and corpus callosum (white arrows), which showed some enhancement with intravenous contrast (black arrow) and was interpreted as being a tumour. However, a biopsy showed only features of resolving haemorrhage, and a subsequent angiogram demonstrated the underlying anterior communicating artery aneurysm. The right frontal mass was simply a 2-week-old haematoma, showing how rapidly even quite sizeable haematomas can lose their 'whiteness' on CT.

Is there any underlying cause of the haematoma?

The underlying cause of the haemorrhage may sometimes be inferred (traumatic, aneurysmal, vascular malformation, or into a tumour, or haemorrhagic transformation of an arterial or venous infarct) from the extent, site and distribution of blood and any associated features (section 8.9.2). One study suggested that a fluid-blood level in an acute intracerebral haematoma on CT occurs more frequently in patients with a coagulopathy, but it was retrospective and a fluid-blood level may simply reflect the age of the haematoma, because many large haematomas go through a phase where there is a fluid level (Pfleger *et al.* 1994). Furthermore, fluid levels have been observed in haematomas associated with cerebral amyloid angiopathy (Miller *et al.* 1999).

Intraparenchymal haematomas secondary to aneurysmal rupture are discussed in greater detail in section 9.4.1. They occur in parts of the brain adjacent to the common sites of aneurysms, and sometimes not in association with visible subarachnoid blood. Absence of subarachnoid blood might be because the patient was scanned late and the blood had cleared from the subarachnoid space, or because there was little leakage of blood into the subarachnoid space at the time of rupture. Typical sites include the inferomedial parts of the frontal lobes (anterior communicating artery aneurysm), the temporal or inferolateral parietal lobe (middle cerebral artery aneurysm), medial temporal lobe (internal carotid–posterior communicating artery aneurysm), and lateral to or in the cerebellar hemisphere (posterior inferior cerebellar artery aneurysm).

In patients with an underlying *arteriovenous malformation* (AVM) (section 8.2.4), abnormal arteries or areas of calcification close to, or in the haematoma may be visible, although in the acute stage a large haematoma can obliterate all signs of the underlying AVM on CT, MR and even catheter angiography. Follow-up imaging several weeks or months later (CT with contrast, MR or contrast intra-arterial angiography, depending on the patient), once the haematoma and its mass effect have resolved, is required to demonstrate small AVMs (section 8.9.4).

Haemorrhage into a tumour is unusual but may be the presenting feature (Fig. 5.10; section 8.5.1). Primary brain tumours associated (occasionally) with haemorrhage include glioblastoma, oligodendroglioma, lymphoma, neuroblastoma, choroid plexus papilloma and meningioma. Secondary brain tumours presenting with haemorrhage are more frequent, although still relatively rare, and include melanoma, choriocarcinoma and thyroid, renal, lung and breast carcinoma. Multiple, mainly peripheral, haemorrhages in a patient with an appropriate past history, and with contrast enhancement, should suggest the diagnosis.

Multiple haematomas can also occur in cerebral amyloid angiopathy, intracranial venous thrombosis and after therapeutic thrombolysis. It seems that 'unusual' causes of intracerebral haemorrhage are being increasingly recognized and, with more experience, more of these should be identified on imaging.

With *cerebral amyloid angiopathy* (section 8.2.2), the haemorrhage tends to be large, rather patchy and diffuse, have a fluid level and occur in multiple sites, either simultaneously or sequentially (Fig. 5.11). The haematoma is typically peripheral (i.e. involves the cortex), and may break through on to the surface of the brain (Miller *et al.* 1999). The patients tend to be elderly, but pathologically proven cerebral amyloid angiopathy has been seen in patients in their 50s.

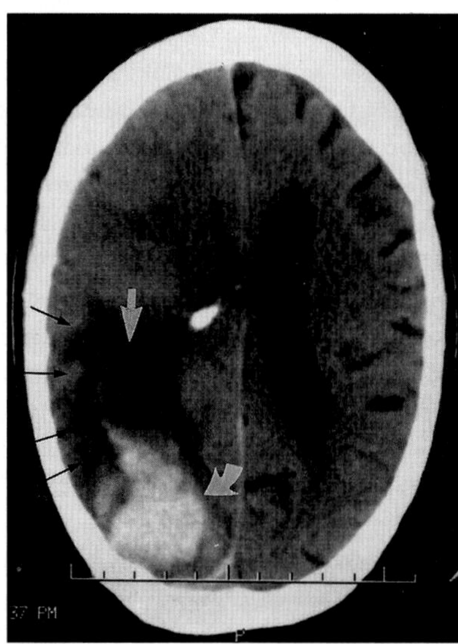

Fig. 5.10 A 74-year-old lady who presented with a sudden-onset left hemiparesis (total anterior circulation syndrome). CT scan at 12 h without contrast shows an extensive right occipitotemporal low density (thick white arrow) with some white matter oedema around it (thin black arrows) and high density of haemorrhage within it (curved white arrow), and much more mass effect than would be expected for a haemorrhage alone. There was little enhancement following intravenous contrast (not shown). At post-mortem there was an underlying glioblastoma. Close questioning of relatives revealed that the patient had behaved increasingly oddly over the previous few months.

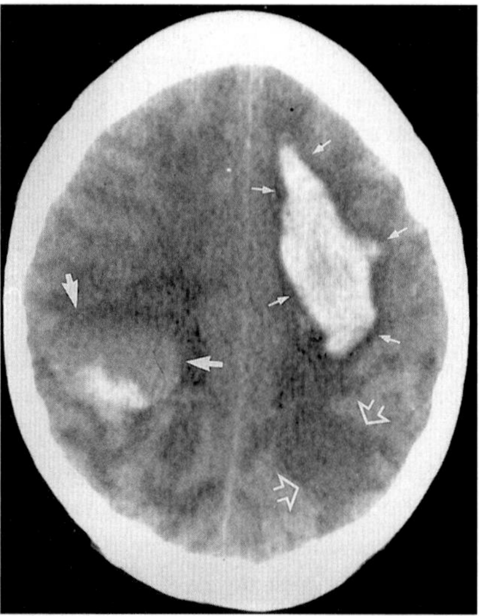

Fig. 5.11 CT brain scan showing typical features of cerebral amyloid angiopathy. There are at least three different haematomas in different parts of the brain (left frontoparietal, right parietal and left occipital lobes) all of different ages (small arrows, thick arrows and open arrows, respectively) (see also Figs 8.6 and 8.7).

Intracranial venous thrombosis will be discussed in more detail below and patients can present with lesions which are mainly haemorrhagic (sections 5.3.5, 5.5.3 and 8.2.10). Deep bilateral haematomas occur in deep cerebral vein occlusion. Cortical haematomas, with a finger-like shape and surrounding low density with excessive mass effect, occur in cortical vein thrombosis (Bakac & Wardlaw 1997). Both may occur with or without signs of sinus thrombosis, such as the 'hyperdense sinus sign' (Figs 5.12, 5.13, 5.40, 5.41 and 5.42).

5.3.5 The appearance of ischaemic stroke on brain CT

Early CT signs of infarction

In the first decade in the development of CT, infarct visibility was limited by the technology. Campbell *et al.* (1978) examined 141 patients admitted to hospital with acute ischaemic stroke as soon after the onset as possible, and again 7 days later, and compared the results with isotope brain scanning. They found that more than 50% of the ischaemic lesions were detected on the first CT scan and 66% on the second scan, compared with 58% on isotope scanning (the only alternative non-invasive diagnostic tool available at the time). It was considered unusual to see changes of infarction on brain CT within 24–48 h of onset, although occasionally

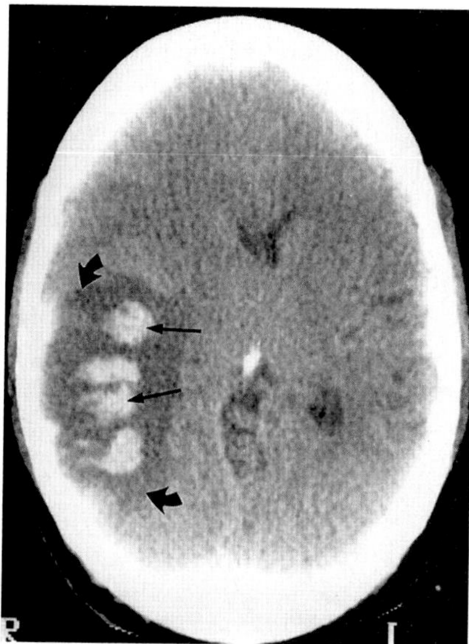

Fig. 5.12 CT brain scan of a right parietal cortical venous infarct taken within 6 h of the onset of symptoms. There is a well-defined hypodense lesion (curved arrows) affecting grey and white matter with some mass effect in the right parietal region. There are finger-like areas of haemorrhage in the centre of the lesion (thin arrows). Note also the rest of the right hemisphere appears slightly swollen, although it is of normal density (note the midline shift). The small midline hyperdensity is the calcified pineal gland. At post-mortem, the thrombosed cortical vein was found overlying the venous infarct. All other cortical veins, venous sinuses and arteries were clear.

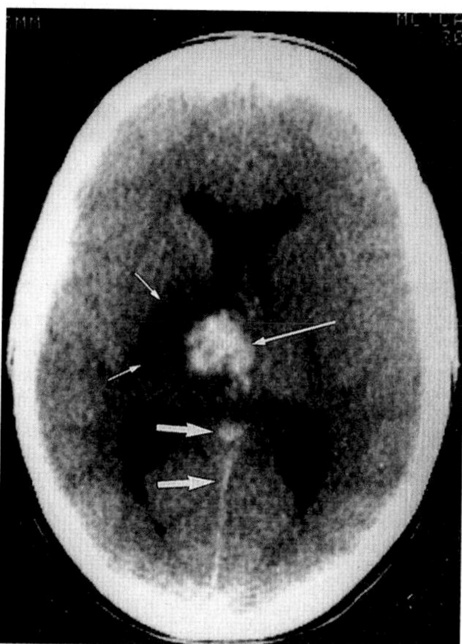

Fig. 5.13 CT brain scan (unenhanced) showing a right thalamic haematoma (long thin arrow) caused by infarction secondary to thrombosis of the deep cerebral veins. Note the increased density in the straight sinus (thick arrows) caused by the thrombus in the sinus (hyperdense sinus sign), and the general brain swelling, and low density around the haemorrhage (short small arrows) indicating the venous infarct (see also Figs 5.12, 5.20, 5.40, 5.41 and 5.42).

ischaemic lesions were seen as early as 3–6 h (Inoue *et al.* 1980; Wall *et al.* 1982).

More recently, with improved CT technology, subtle early signs of cerebral infarction have been recognized. Loss of visualization of the insular ribbon and loss of outline of the lentiform nucleus have been reported within 3 h of onset in ischaemic strokes of the basal ganglia (Tomura *et al.* 1988; Truwit *et al.* 1990; Grond *et al.* 1997; von Kummer *et al.* 1997) (Fig. 5.14). Loss of the normal grey–white matter differentiation (at the cortex–white matter and basal ganglia–white matter interfaces), effacement of the overlying cortical sulci and compression of the lateral ventricle, and hypodensity (i.e. tissue of lower density than the adjacent white and grey matter) are other early signs of infarction. Indeed, some confusion has arisen through use of multiple terms to describe a limited series of signs without good definitions. 'Loss of grey–white matter definition', 'loss of basal ganglia outline' and 'loss of the insular ribbon' are all forms of *hypodensity* in which the ischaemic grey matter first becomes hypodense with respect to normal grey matter. That stage is followed by a greater degree of hypodensity in the infarct where the ischaemic white matter *also* becomes hypodense with respect to normal white matter, as well as the abnormal grey matter becoming *even more* hypodense, so that overall the whole lesion then appears *darker* than the surrounding brain. 'Effacement of the cortical sulci' and 'effacement of the lateral ventricle' are both terms which describe oedema or swelling developing in the infarct. Unfortunately, because hypodensity often accompanies oedema, and because both occur at the same point in the time course after the stroke, these two terms may have been used interchangeably and so caused confusion. It is preferable to use terms which describe what can be seen on the scan (swelling) rather than terms which imply a particular pathological process (oedema) to avoid confusion.

Small infarcts appear later than large ones, because there is less tissue to alter their density. Therefore, lacunar infarcts are less likely to show up in the first 24 h and sometimes do not do so at all (see below) (Donnan *et al.* 1982; Bamford *et al.* 1987; Bonke *et al.* 1989; Lindgren *et al.* 1994) (Fig. 5.15). Small infarcts in the brainstem and cerebellum are particularly difficult to visualize with CT because of artifacts arising from the petrous bones; this is less problematic with modern scanning technology and thinner scan sections (Savoiardo 1986).

Hyperdense artery sign is another early, but indirect, sign of ischaemic stroke (Fig. 5.16). It represents the visualization of acute large cerebral artery occlusion, caused by acute thrombosis or embolism, as an increased density in the artery (Gacs *et al.* 1982; Yang *et al.* 1990; Bastianello *et al.* 1991; Leys *et al.* 1992; Manelf *et al.* 1999) (section 6.7.3). However, the reliability of this sign is uncertain. It may be valid in young patients, in whom the arteries tend to be less calcified, but elderly patients frequently have calcified artery walls,

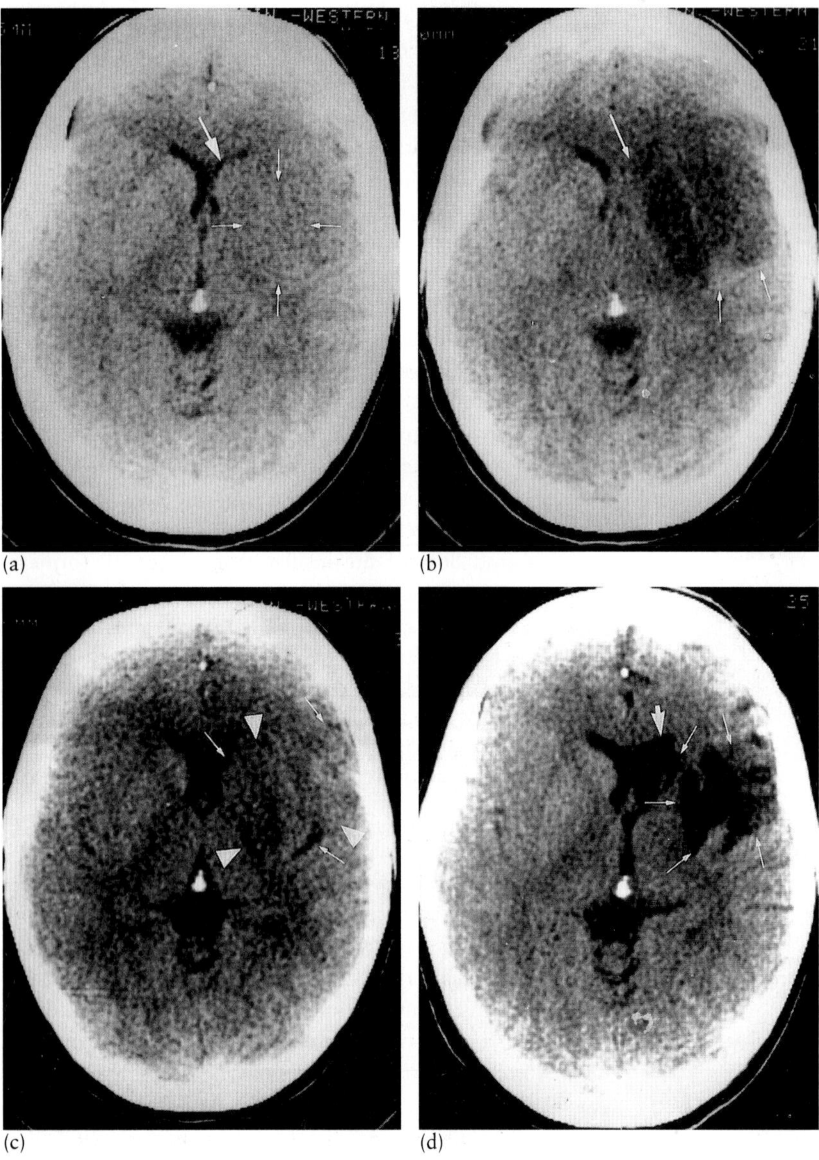

Fig. 5.14 Sequence of CT brain scans to demonstrate the evolution of the appearance of a left middle cerebral artery infarct with time. (a) At 3 h after the stroke there is loss of visibility of the normal basal ganglia and insular cortex (thin arrows indicate where the outline should be—compared with the right basal ganglia which are clearly seen), slight swelling is seen as slight compression of the frontal horn of the left lateral ventricle (thick arrow). (b) At 3 days after the stroke the infarct is more hypodense and clearly demarcated and swollen. There is complete effacement of the left lateral ventricle (thin arrow) and small areas of increased density at the infarct margins suggest petechial haemorrhage (small arrows). The marginal petechial haemorrhage may not be seen—the infarct may simply appear uniformly hypodense with very distinct sharp margins at this stage. Note that the infarct is wedge-shaped and involves cortex and adjacent white matter. (c) At 2 weeks after the stroke the swelling has subsided (the frontal horn of the lateral ventricle and the cortical sulci are clearly seen—arrows), the hypodensity has nearly gone and the lesion has similar density to normal brain as a result of the 'fogging' effect (see Fig. 5.17). At this stage the lesion can be almost impossible to see despite being a sizeable infarct. Arrowheads indicate the margins of the infarct. (d) At 3 months the lesion is a shrunken, cerebrospinal fluid-containing hole (arrows). The surrounding normal structures show an *ex vacuo* effect—the frontal horn of the left lateral ventricle has expanded to take up space vacated by the damaged brain (arrowhead).

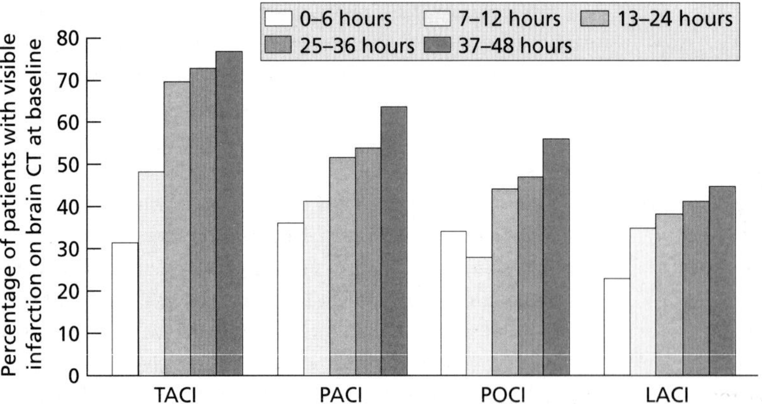

Fig. 5.15 Data from the First International Stroke Trial showing the effect of time and stroke clinical syndrome on the visibility of infarcts on CT scanning. The visibility of infarcts increases with time over the first 2 days from the onset of the stroke, and the larger the infarct the more often it is visible (i.e. total anterior circulation infarcts—TACI—show up more often than lacunar infarcts—LACI). PACI, partial anterior circulation infarct; POCI, posterior circulation infarct. (The figure was prepared by Dr Paul Dorman.)

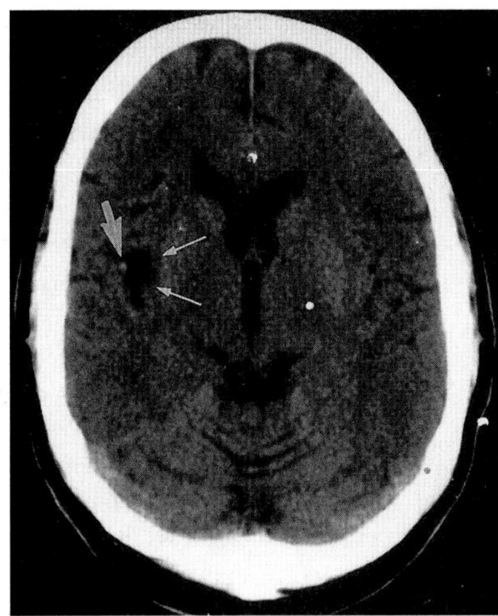

Fig. 5.16 An unenhanced CT brain scan showing a hyperdense middle cerebral artery branch in the right sylvian fissure (thick arrow). Note also the early signs of infarction (hypodensity) in the insular cortex (thin arrows) (see also Fig. 6.24 for a hyperdense middle cerebral artery on CT, and Fig. 5.28 for the equivalent sign on MR).

particularly around the carotid siphon, which can produce a similar appearance. Increased haematocrit can also give the appearance of a hyperdense middle cerebral artery (MCA), although usually bilateral not unilateral (Rauch *et al.* 1993). Evidence of calcification persists on rescanning, but not the hyperdense artery sign, which disappears in a few days. Hankey *et al.* (1988) described a hyperdense basilar artery in four patients with posterior circulation strokes, which disappeared on repeat CT scanning a few days later.

In one series of 36 acute ischaemic stroke patients presenting within 4 h of the onset of MCA territory stroke, the hyperdense artery sign was present in 50% of patients with occlusions proved on angiography within 6 h of onset (Bastianello *et al.* 1991). In a larger series of 272 consecutive patients with first-ever stroke CT-scanned within 12 h of symptom onset, Leys *et al.* (1992) found a hyperdense MCA in 73 (27%) patients, which was 41% of those with an MCA territory infarct. The sign was not dependent on cerebrovascular risk factors and was more likely to occur in cortical and large deep MCA infarcts. It was not an independent predictor of poor outcome; 20% of the patients with the sign recovered within 2 weeks. It disappeared within a few days and was always related to an occlusion of the MCA in patients who had angiography, giving a specificity of 100% but a sensitivity of only 30%. Others have also found the association with larger infarcts (Tomsick *et al.* 1990). However, in more general populations, the hyperdense artery sign was found in only 5% of patients with acute ischaemic stroke (Yang *et al.* 1990). Manelf *et al.* (1999) found the hyperdense artery sign in 107 of 620 patients (18%) randomized in the European Cooperative Acute Stroke Study (ECASS). The initial neurological deficit was more severe, and early infarct oedema more common, in patients with the sign than in those without, but it was not independently associated with poor functional outcome in a multivariate analysis. All these studies were in hospital-admitted patients, who were therefore more likely to have had a 'severe' stroke. In community-based studies it is likely that the hyperdense artery sign is less frequent.

The hyperdense artery sign is a reasonably reliable indicator of an acutely occluded cerebral artery when the hyperdensity is visible at a distance from the carotid siphon, e.g. in the proximal MCA or its branches, and particularly in younger patients. An absent sign is certainly not a reliable indicator of a patent artery. On MR, the equivalent sign is replacement of the arterial signal flow void (black) with a hyperintense signal which is specific for thrombosed blood and therefore less likely to be confused with vessel wall calcification (Mead & Wardlaw 1998) (Fig. 5.28).

The hyperdense artery sign on CT is a reasonably reliable indicator of an occluded cerebral artery when the hyperdensity is visible at a distance from the carotid siphon. An absent sign is certainly not a reliable indicator of a patent artery.

Evolution of the CT appearance of infarction

Evolution of the CT appearance of infarction is illustrated in Fig. 5.14. Initially, the lesion has ill-defined margins and slight swelling and is somewhat hypodense compared with normal brain. The infarct becomes more clearly demarcated and hypodense during the first few days (Hakim *et al.* 1983; Skriver *et al.* 1990). The swelling is usually maximal around the third to fifth days and gradually subsides during the second and third week (Clasen *et al.* 1980; Terent *et al.* 1981; Hakim *et al.* 1983; Skriver *et al.* 1990; Wardlaw *et al.* 1993). Occasionally, however, infarct swelling can occur very rapidly—within the first 24 h—to cause brain herniation, but generally only with very extensive infarcts. The amount of infarct swelling, and the rate at which it appears, varies between patients, for reasons which are not well understood. On balance, swelling is most apparent in large infarcts but presumably also occurs in small ones, although it is difficult to see and is probably clinically less important. Extensive infarct swelling can compress adjacent normal brain and cause brain herniation (section 11.1.5). The presence of recent haemorrhage in the infarct produces areas of increased density relative to both normal brain and the infarcted tissue, and presumably contributes to any swelling (section 5.4).

During the second week, the infarct gradually increases in density, sometimes becoming isodense, so that it is indistinguishable from normal brain. This is the so-called '*fogging effect*' and without close inspection even quite sizeable infarcts may be overlooked (Figs 5.14 and 5.17). The 'fogging

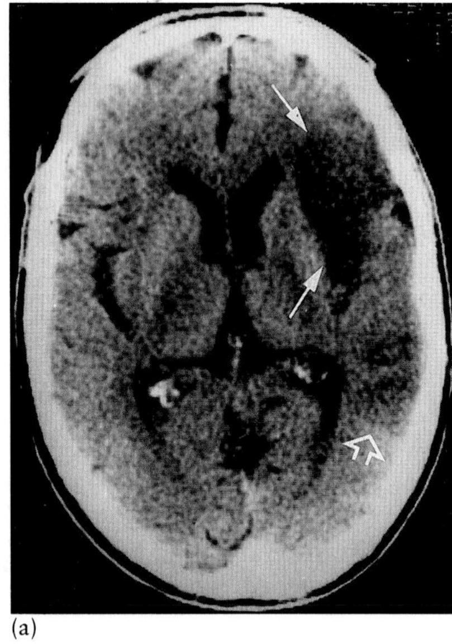
(a)

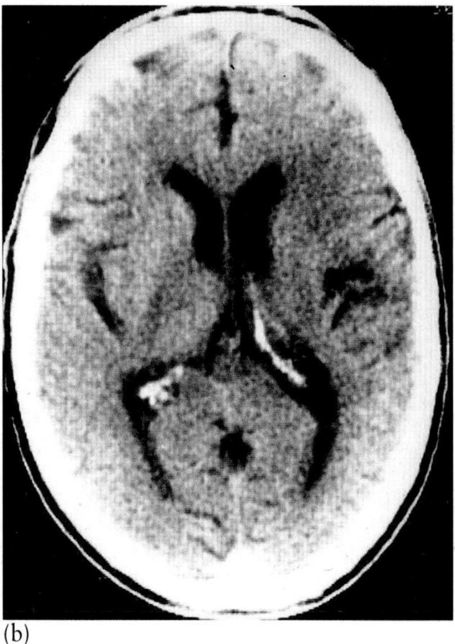
(b)

Fig. 5.17 CT brain scans to demonstrate 'fogging'. (a) Obtained 3 days after onset of a right hemiparesis showing an obvious infarct (hypodense area) in the left parietal cortex and adjacent white matter (thin arrows). The patient had also had a stroke 2 years previously, seen as the small hypodense area in the posterior left temporal region (open arrow). (b) Obtained at 14 days after onset. The recent infarct in the anterior left parietal region is almost invisible—it is now mainly isodense with normal brain and there is no mass effect—as a result of 'fogging' (see also Fig. 5.29).

effect' may make the infarct impossible to see on CT scans performed at this time. It is less pronounced in large infarcts, but may lead to underestimation of infarct size. It does not occur in all infarcts and the rate of occurrence varies between reports. Skriver and Olsen (1981) observed it in 54% of cases scanned 10 days after onset, whereas Becker *et al.* (1979) found it at some time in all cases examined with six consecutive CT scans within 42 days of stroke. The 'fogging effect' may last up to 2 weeks and then the infarct becomes progressively more hypodense (black).

Eventually, a sharply demarcated, atrophic, hypodense (similar to cerebrospinal fluid) defect remains (Fig. 5.14). Although old infarcts usually have sharply demarcated borders, and so it is possible to 'age' infarcts, it is not always possible to tell with absolute certainty how old an infarct is, something that may be overlooked when ascribing particular clinical symptoms to lesions seen on CT.

It is not always possible to tell the age of an infarct on CT, particularly in the case of small deep infarcts. Therefore, do not assume that a particular hypodense area on CT is necessarily relevant to a recent stroke—it could be old and irrelevant.

Effect of intravenous contrast

In the first week intravenous X-ray contrast usually has little effect on the appearance of an infarct, although some enhancement of the gyri may be seen (Wing *et al.* 1976; Davis *et al.* 1977). But, from the end of the first to the third weeks, more striking contrast enhancement occurs, frequently corresponding with the time of maximal blood–brain barrier breakdown and positivity of radioisotope brain scans (Inoue *et al.* 1980; Pullicino & Kendall 1980). The explanation is likely to be a combination of blood–brain barrier breakdown, neovascularization and impaired autoregulation, and the resulting appearance on CT is referred to as 'luxury perfusion' (Sage 1982). The enhancement can be very marked in children and young adults (Fig. 5.18). Hayman *et al.* (1981) suggested that early prominent contrast enhancement in large infarcts correlated strongly with later massive haemorrhagic transformation, as a result of severe early vasogenic oedema. However, most of their patients had large infarcts with a poor prognosis and were therefore probably more likely to develop haemorrhagic transformation anyway (Lodder 1984) (section 5.4). The tendency to enhance with contrast gradually resolves over the following few weeks.

It has been suggested that stroke patients deteriorate as a result of intravenous contrast, although the relationship was not statistically significant (Kendall & Pullicino 1980). It is certainly possible that extravasation of neurotoxic contrast agents could be harmful, but most patients described in the paper had large infarcts with a poor prognosis in any case. Fortunately, in practice, it is rarely necessary to give intravenous contrast as a diagnostic aid. The use of contrast in acute stroke should really be avoided unless absolutely necessary.

Intravenous contrast is rarely required to clarify the CT diagnosis in acute stroke, and should in general be avoided (unless required for CT angiography or perfusion imaging).

How often is an appropriate infarct visible on CT?

In the study by Lindgren *et al.* (1994) an appropriate infarct was seen in 43% of patients with a lacunar infarct (LACI) scanned within 2 days of onset, rising to 75% when scanned

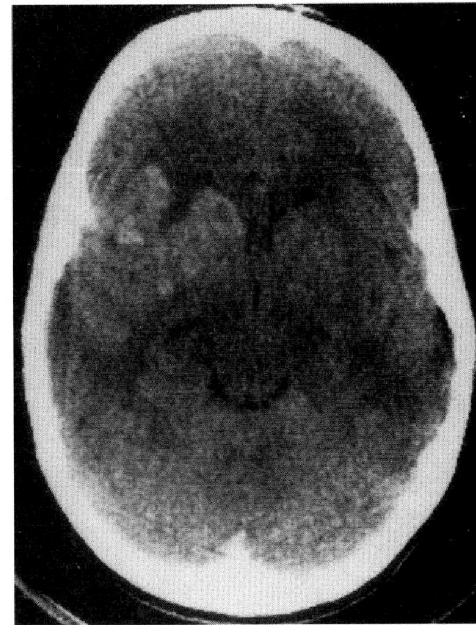

(a)

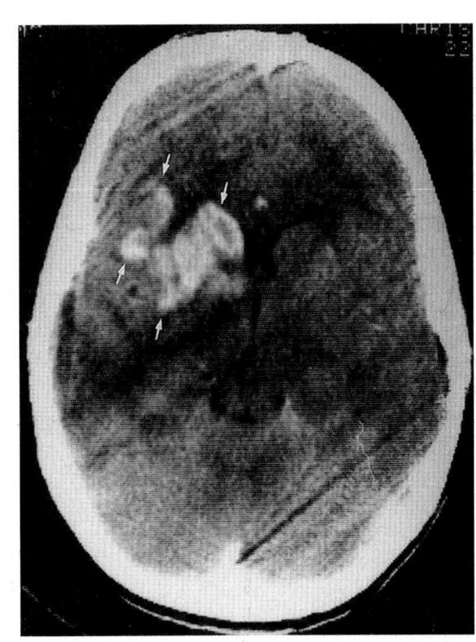

(b)

Fig. 5.18 CT brain scan (a) without, and (b) with intravenous contrast obtained at 10 days after a right basal ganglia infarct in a 10-year-old girl. There is marked serpiginous enhancement of the infarct (arrows) attributed to breakdown of the blood–brain barrier.

more than 16 days after the stroke. The corresponding figures for total anterior circulation infarction (TACI), partial anterior circulation infarction (PACI) and posterior circulation infarction (POCI) patients scanned within 2 days were 44, 41 and 43%, and more than 16 days were 55, 64 and 56%, respectively.

The proportion of patients with a visible infarct depends greatly on local factors, such as casemix, time to first scan, whether or not the scan is repeated, generation of CT scanner, etc. The proportion of TACI patients with a visible infarct was perhaps rather low in the study of Lindgren *et al.* compared with others, including ours (Anderson *et al.* 1994; Mead *et al.* 1996, 2000; Wardlaw *et al.* 1996; Al-Buhairi *et al.* 1998) (Table 5.1). However, the general principle that infarcts tend to become more easily visible with increasing interval from stroke onset is well documented. In a recent study of 993 stroke patients scanned up to 99 days after stroke, 60% had a visible relevant infarct on CT within the first 24 h, rising to 70% by 72 h (Wardlaw *et al.* 1998a). A greater proportion of the TACI patients had a visible infarct than the PACI, LACI or POCI patients, no matter how early or late they were scanned after the stroke. In the International Stroke Trial, the proportion of patients with a visible infarct increased with time from onset to randomization in the first 48 h and the highest proportion of patients with visible infarction was in the TACI group (International Stroke Trials Collaborative Group 1997) (Fig. 5.15). In general, the greater the volume of infarcted tissue, the more often the infarct is visible on CT scanning.

It is uncertain just how many patients with a clinically definite stroke *never* have an appropriate infarct visible on brain CT, but the proportion is probably quite high (up to 50%) and depends on the timing of the scan, the age of the scanner, the thickness of the slices, the cooperation of the patient, the size and age of the infarct, the location (e.g. the brainstem is a difficult area to visualize infarcts on CT), the vigilance of the radiologist, and possibly some pathophysiological characteristic of the lesion itself. However, the main reason for performing the scan is to exclude haemorrhage (or tumour or infection) as the cause of the symptoms and, if the scan is normal, the presumptive diagnosis is of an ischaemic event if the clinical picture is compatible with a stroke.

Brain CT only shows the appropriate infarct in 50–60% of patients with an ischaemic stroke overall. A patient with a clinical diagnosis of stroke, and an early CT scan which is either normal or shows a relevant hypodense lesion, is classified as having an ischaemic stroke. Patients with symptoms of a more extensive stroke are more likely to have a visible relevant infarct than those with symptoms of a minor stroke. Absence of a visible infarct does not mean that the patient has not had a stroke.

How well do the clinical and CT diagnosis of the site of the stroke lesion correspond?

The site of the lesion on brain CT correlates relatively well with the clinical syndrome (Manelfe *et al.* 1981; Damasio 1983; Saito *et al.* 1987; Zeumer & Ringelstein 1987; Anderson *et al.* 1994; Lindgren *et al.* 1994; Mead *et al.* 1996, 2000; Wardlaw *et al.* 1996; Al-Buhairi *et al.* 1998) (Table 5.1). The middle cerebral artery (MCA) territory is the most frequently affected on CT (60%), followed by the posterior cerebral artery (14%), the anterior cerebral artery (5%), the posterior fossa (5%) and the major artery territories combined or boundary-zones (14%) (Savoiardo 1986).

There are six published studies comparing stroke syndrome defined clinically, using the Oxfordshire Community Stroke Project (OCSP) classification (Bamford *et al.* 1991), with the site of the infarct as demonstrated by cross-sectional

Table 5.1 Summary of studies investigating the relationship between the Oxfordshire Community Stroke Project clinical classification of ischaemic stroke and the site of the relevant (i.e. appropriate) infarct on brain CT or MRI.

			Proportion of infarcts appropriate to each of the syndromes					
Study	Number of ischaemic strokes	Recent infarct on CT or MRI (%)	Total anterior circulation infarction	Partial anterior circulation infarction	Lacunar infarction	Posterior circulation infarction	Overall	Comments
Anderson *et al.* (1994)	248	162 (65%)	46/58 (79%)	25/44 (57%)	30/48 (62%)	12/20 (60%)	113/162 (70%)	Community first-ever-in-a-lifetime strokes, retrospectively classified
Lindgren *et al.* (1994)	179	110 (61%)	35/39 (90%)	21/37 (57%)	13/22 (59%)	12/12 (100%)	81/110 (74%)	First-ever-in-a-lifetime stroke. Previously unpublished data provided by personal communication
Wardlaw *et al.* (1996)	108	91 (84%)	30/33 (91%)	30/36 (83%)	12/14 (86%)	8/8 (100%)	80/91 (88%)	Hospital series. Included previous non-disabling strokes
Mead *et al.* (1996)	195	158 (81%)	41/46 (89%)	48/57 (84%)	25/37 (68%)	16/18 (89%)	130/158 (82%)	Hospital series. Only half of CT reports of 378 patients with ischaemic stroke were available
Al-Buhairi *et al.* (1998)	378	239 (63%)	40/49 (82%)	79/82 (94%)	65/66 (98%)	32/32 (100%)	216/228 (95%)	Hospital series of acute ischaemic strokes. Included previous strokes
Mead *et al.* (2000)	1012	655 (65%)	69/87 (79%)	213/298 (71%)	104/144 (73%)	105/126 (83%)	492/655 (76%)	Hospital series. Validity similar for those with and without previous strokes

imaging (section 4.3) (Table 5.1). In each study there was reasonable agreement between the clinical and CT diagnosis of lesion site, despite differences in the study method. In the Perth study the allocation of the stroke clinical syndrome was made retrospectively from the patients' notes and then compared with the lesion site shown by CT or at post-mortem (Anderson *et al.* 1993). In the study by Mead *et al.* (1996) the stroke clinical syndrome was decided prospectively but the radiological diagnosis was obtained from the radiologists' report of the CT scan. These factors may have introduced errors in diagnosis. In the other four studies the stroke clinical syndrome was allocated prospectively and therefore the results are likely to be more reliable. In each study a proportion of the patients had, of course, 'normal' imaging—that is, the imaging did not show an appropriate recent infarct—and these cases were analysed differently in each study. In the Perth study about one-third of the partial anterior circulation infarction (PACI), lacunar infarction (LACI) and posterior circulation infarction (POCI) patients did not show a relevant lesion on CT, and these scans were excluded from the assessment of the accuracy of the clinical diagnosis of lesion site (Anderson *et al.* 1994). Lindgren *et al.* (1994) used multiple CT and MR scans at different times after the stroke and so had fewer patients whose scan did not show a relevant lesion, but it is not clear how they were accounted for in the analysis. It is unlikely that any imaging technique, no matter how sophisticated, will ever be able to demonstrate *all* infarcts.

A problem for comparative studies of imaging (and pathology) with the clinical diagnosis of lesion site is what to do with the 'normal' scans. Should they be discounted from the study and only scans which show a recent lesion included? In that case, a false estimate of the accuracy of the clinical localization might arise, either falsely high or falsely low, because the 'normal' scans, had they shown a lesion, might have displayed it in a different part of the brain from that predicted clinically (e.g. a small deep white matter infarct instead of a predicted cortical infarct in a PACI patient). Therefore, including the 'normal' scans in the analysis is important, and the result can be expressed as the 'best' and 'worst' possible agreement; in the former, one assumes that all the patients with normal scans had a lesion in the area predicted clinically and, in the latter, one assumes that the lesion is elsewhere. In the studies by Wardlaw *et al.* (1996) and Mead *et al.* (2000) 'best' and 'worst' case scenarios were calculated to account for negative scans. In the 'best' case scenario (assuming all patients with a negative CT scan actually had an infarct in the site predicted clinically), the clinical classification agreed with the infarct site demonstrated on CT in 81% of TACIs, 81% of PACIs, 85% of LACIs, and 90% of POCIs (total 84% agreement). In the 'worst' case scenario (assuming all patients with a negative CT scan actually had an infarct in a site other than that predicted clinically), the clinical classification agreed with the CT scan in 73% of TACIs, 48% of PACIs, 40% of LACIs and 50% of POCIs (total 49% agreement). The truth is probably somewhere in between.

In studies of stroke lesion site diagnosed clinically vs. radiologically, and which have used other classifications, the level of agreement between the clinician equipped with the traditional neurological tools of pin and tendon hammer, and the radiologist armed with a scanner, has been no better (Bamford 1992). In the National Institute of Neurological Diseases and Stroke (NINDS) classification, with subdivisions according to the pathological mechanism, the clinical category and the arterial distribution, numerous assumptions must be made for which there is no good evidence; for example, that cardioembolic strokes are of exceptionally rapid onset and not preceded by transient ischaemic attacks (Kittner *et al.* 1990) (section 6.8.3). Using the Trial of ORG 10172 in Acute Stroke Therapy (TOAST) Trial classification, which divides strokes into atherothromboembolic, cardioembolic, small vessel thrombotic, other and unknown, the initial clinical classification agreed with the final diagnosis after diagnostic tests in only 65%, and 15% of patients remained without a clear stroke subtype identification (Madden *et al.* 1994). The Stroke Data Bank classification is also based on the likely pathophysiological cause of the stroke, i.e. large artery atherosclerosis, lacunar, cardiac embolism, tandem arterial pathology, infarct of unknown origin, or other. This classification is heavily dependent on the use of imaging, but it still proved impossible to allocate a likely mechanism for the stroke in 40% of patients (Sacco *et al.* 1989).

In our hospital-based stroke registry, we attempted to assign a cause of stroke in all patients admitted during one sample year (Wardlaw *et al.* 1999a). Amongst 479 patients, those with large cortical infarcts (TACIs) had the greatest proportion of arterial (59%) or cardiac (29%) embolic sources, or both (15%), followed by small cortical infarcts (PACI; 45, 18 and 5%, respectively); lacunar infarcts (33, 8 and 4%, respectively); and posterior circulation infarcts (32, 9 and 4%, respectively) (Fig. 5.19). Thus, while patients with a cardiac source of embolism are at greater risk of having a large cortical than any other type of infarct (if they have a stroke), 74% of patients who *do* have a large cortical infarct have an arterial source of embolism. Patients with small cortical, lacunar or posterior circulation infarcts are less likely to have identifiable cardiac or arterial sources of embolism than patients with large cortical infarcts, but the relative proportions of one to the other are similar. Therefore, not only is it not valid to assume a particular embolic source based solely on ischaemic stroke type, but finding a potential source of embolism does not mean that it was *the* cause of the stroke, and in a large proportion of patients (4–15%) there is more than one potential embolic cause (section 6.8). Thus, the use of a complex classification, or multiple imaging modalities, does not solve the problem.

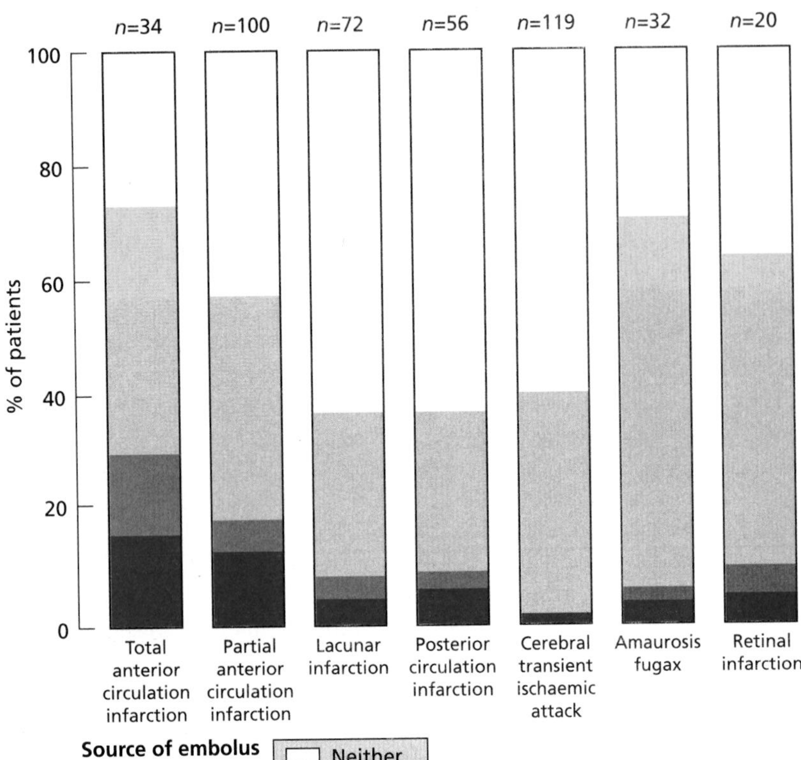

Fig. 5.19 The frequency of sources of emboli in patients with different stroke and transient ischaemic attack types. (The figure was prepared by Dr Stephanie Lewis, Edinburgh, from Wardlaw *et al.* 1999a.)

It is not valid to assume that a particular type of ischaemic stroke was caused by a particular embolic source or in situ thrombosis, and finding a potential source of embolism does not mean that it was the cause of the stroke. In up to 15% of patients (probably a greater proportion the harder one looks) there is more than one potential cause of the stroke.

Does infarct visibility on CT (early or established) have prognostic significance?

How prognostically important is the presence of decreased density in the ischaemic brain tissue within a few hours of stroke onset? It has been suggested that early visualization of an infarct may indicate more profound ischaemia. For example, Higano *et al.* (1990), using positron emission tomography (PET) scanning in nine stroke patients with middle cerebral artery (MCA) occlusion, found that the hypodensity on CT corresponded with the areas of brain with the lowest cerebral blood flow.

There is accumulating evidence that if an infarct is visible early, it carries a worse prognosis than if the patient did not have an infarct visible, although studies so far have not taken account of any relationship between hyper-acute early visible infarction and stroke severity (see below). In the European Cooperative Acute Stroke Study (ECASS), there was a suggestion that patients with an infarct visible on their prerandomization CT scan performed within 6 h of stroke onset, particularly if it involved more than one-third of the MCA territory, had a worse prognosis than those with a normal CT scan (Hacke *et al.* 1995; von Kummer *et al.* 1997). Von Kummer *et al.* (1994) found that early infarct visibility in patients with angiographically proven MCA occlusion was associated with a much worse clinical outcome than patients without early hypodensity. In four other studies examining the prognostic significance of visible infarction within 6–12 h of stroke, hypodensity was associated with a poor outcome (Censori *et al.* 1993; Ceyhan *et al.* 1996; Moulin *et al.* 1996; Toni *et al.* 1997). However, none of the above six studies defined the early infarct signs clearly, it was not clear that the CT scans were read truly blind to the features on follow-up scans or clinical information about the patients, only three used multivariate analysis to adjust for stroke severity, the follow-up was only at 1 month in three studies, 3 months in two studies and 6 months in one study, and the sample size varied from 19 to 620 (median 125). In two studies, some patients received thrombolysis. Thus, while early infarct visibility *may* be associated with more severe strokes and a worse outcome, it is not clear which early infarct signs are important to recognize, nor what effect they may have on prognosis. Also, there are practical problems as a result of the difficulty of recognizing subtle early infarct signs (see below) and the lack of clear operational definitions of those signs.

The effect of *established* visible infarction on prognosis is somewhat clearer; established infarction is easier to recognize, and there are more studies with larger sample sizes. In the International Stroke Trial (IST), patients with an infarct visible on their CT scan performed within 48 h of the stroke onset had a worse prognosis than those with a normal scan and the same clinical stroke syndrome (IST Collaborative Group 1997) (Fig. 5.15). On multiple regression analysis, infarct visibility was an independent adverse prognostic variable, despite quite a lot of 'noise' in the data collection (possibly partly a result of the scans not being reviewed centrally). In our hospital stroke registry study, of 993 patients scanned mostly within the first week of stroke, the presence of a visible infarct was associated with an increased risk of poor functional outcome (OR 2.5; 95% CI, 1.9–3.3) and death (OR 4.5; 95% CI, 2.7–7.5) at 6 months, even after adjusting for time from stroke to scan, and important clinical prognostic variables (Wardlaw *et al.* 1998a). Candelise *et al.* (1991), in a study of 1048 patients, found that visible infarction on CT was associated with an increased risk of death at 6 months (relative risk 2.0; 95% CI, 1.2–3.3) in a multivariate analysis. Heinsius *et al.* (1998) and Finocchi *et al.* (1996) found associations between large infarct size and poor outcome at 1 month in 818 and 351 patients, respectively. Therefore, it seems that a visible established infarct indicates a profound depth of ischaemia, which reflects a marked drop in blood flow to a largish area of brain, which suggests that the outcome will be poor.

Inter-observer reliability in the analysis of CT scans of stroke patients very early after the stroke, and in established infarction

Inter-observer reliability in reporting CT scans in patients with cerebrovascular disease has not been studied extensively. There are two components to the problem: first, being able to recognize the features of very early infarction within the first few hours after the stroke and, secondly, recognition of established infarction on scans obtained perhaps days after the stroke.

Signs of infarction on CT in the first few hours after stroke are subtle (see above) and some signs lack precise definition (e.g. 'a third of the middle cerebral artery territory'). The problem of observer variability of *early* infarct signs has been addressed in six studies (Limburg & Hijdra 1992; von Kummer *et al.* 1996; Dippel *et al.* 1997; von Kummer 1998; Schriger *et al.* 1998; Wardlaw *et al.* 1999b). These used different methods and tested observers with different experience but broadly speaking agreed that the ability of observers to detect early infarct signs on CT was poor. Typical kappa values were in the range 0.14–0.57 (agreement almost no better than chance at all, to moderately better than chance). The more experienced individuals performed slightly better than the less experienced, but with little difference between reading the scans blind to, or with knowledge of the symptoms. Furthermore, only 17% of admitting physicians and 40% of neurologists were even able to recognize intracranial *haemorrhage* with complete reliability (Schriger *et al.* 1998). This is worrying as, in the interests of speed, most stroke CT scans in the very acute phase would likely be read by the admitting neurologist or stroke physician who is probably less experienced than a dedicated neuroradiologist, even after formal training in CT reading (von Kummer 1998).

A further concern is that visible infarction on CT has become a contraindication to thrombolytic therapy in some national guidelines and it may be wrong to base treatment decisions on such an unreliable sign (Adams *et al.* 1996). Our study attempted to understand why observers had such difficulty recognizing early infarct signs, and so what might be done to improve infarct recognition (Wardlaw *et al.* 1999b). Observers often failed to recognize infarct signs which were present, but rarely said they saw signs which were not present. Although they performed very poorly (no better than guessing in some instances), their performance was consistent, i.e. they were recognizing something consistently even if they were describing it incorrectly. If the key signs to recognize could be identified, and their definition simplified, it might be easier for observers to identify early infarction reliably. In the above six studies, and in 11 other studies of various aspects of early infarction (some mentioned above), over 17 different signs of early infarction are mentioned (clearly with some overlap as there are not that many actual signs), very few supplied any definitions, so this is all extremely confusing and unhelpful. Clearly, further work is needed in this area, including examining the possibility of using electronic methods on the CT scanner console to highlight abnormal areas (Lev *et al.* 1999).

In *established* infarction, high levels of agreement (substantial to perfect) were demonstrated in a study of the interpretation of scans in patients with dementia and in another study of patients with stroke (Lee *et al.* 1987; Shinar *et al.* 1987). However, in the study by Shinar *et al.* (1987), all observers had free access to relevant clinical details, so their interpretation of the scans may have been biased. The study by Bonke *et al.* (1989), in which a group of neurologists and radiologists reviewed the same two CT brain scans from patients with a lacunar stroke (camouflaged by an assortment of other scans), accompanied by misleading clinical information, showed that the diagnosis of lacunar infarction did not appear to be biased by informing the observer that the patient was thought clinically to have had a stroke. The lack of bias, even with knowledge of the clinical details, may have been because the study was small and may not be a true reflection of the difficulties encountered in routine practice when faced with a CT scan showing multiple 'holes in the brain' and generalized atrophy. The first makes the diagnosis of recent lacunar infarction difficult, because it is impossible to decide which 'hole' is the relevant one unless serial scans show a new 'hole' developing, and the last makes the diagnosis of a small cortical infarct difficult (when is a large sulcus actually an infarct?).

Inter-observer variation in the interpretation of site of infarction, amount of swelling in the acute stage and haemorrhagic transformation of medium to large infarcts, was evaluated in a study by two experienced neuroradiologists and six trainee radiologists, by using a simple method of classifying stroke CT scans (Wardlaw & Sellar 1994). The agreement was excellent between the two experienced neuroradiologists and good between the trainees and one of the experts. A further study of inter-observer variability in the diagnosis of haemorrhagic transformation on CT showed good agreement for the diagnosis of infarct site and haematomas, but was less good for minor amounts of petechial haemorrhage (Rimdusid *et al.* 1995).

Appearances of established infarction: can we infer anything about the cause of the infarct?

A typical established large artery infarct is wedge-shaped, of decreased density compared with normal brain, sharply demarcated, and occupies a recognizable vascular territory (Damasio 1983; Savoiardo 1986) (Fig. 6.20c). Lacunar infarcts, thought to arise from occlusion of a single perforating artery (section 6.4), are less than 1.5 cm in diameter, usually rounded in shape and sited in the deep white matter, basal ganglia and pons (Donnan *et al.* 1982; Bamford *et al.* 1987; Bamford & Warlow 1988; Bonke *et al.* 1989) (Fig. 6.20d). Boundary-zone infarcts lie in areas of brain at the edge of the large artery vascular territories, i.e. in the parieto-occipital region for the middle–posterior cerebral arteries and over the vertex for the anterior–middle cerebral arteries boundary-zone, or in the internal boundary-zone in the centrum semiovale at the junction of the deep and superficial arterial supply areas (Damasio 1983; Torvik 1984; Graeber *et al.* 1992). However, the boundary-zone areas are potentially more extensive than previously thought, and vary between and within individuals (van der Zwan & Hillen 1991) (sections 4.2.4 and 6.6.5). In our hospital-based stroke registry, the stroke risk factors were compared in 91 patients with presumed boundary-zone and 947 patients with presumed territorial infarction (Mead *et al.* 1998). There were no significant differences in the prevalence of atrial fibrillation, ipsilateral carotid stenosis, hypertension, smoking, angina or breathlessness between the two groups, but contralateral carotid stenosis (> 70%) was more common in patients with boundary-zone infarction (OR 2.2; 95% CI, 1.0–4.7). Thus at least one factor, which may impair cerebral perfusion reserve, may contribute to boundary-zone infarction. However, in any individual patient, it is very difficult to decide on the basis of brain imaging whether an infarct has arisen from occlusion of a cortical branch of the middle cerebral artery (MCA), which might be embolic, or from poor perfusion as a result of established internal carotid artery occlusion (Graeber *et al.* 1992; Lang *et al.* 1995) (section 6.6.5).

Striatocapsular infarcts are larger than lacunae and occur in the deep white matter and basal ganglia, with preservation of the overlying cortex (section 4.2.2). They are thought to arise from transient occlusion of the MCA mainstem, prolonged occlusion of the MCA mainstem with good cortical collaterals, or occlusion of multiple lenticulostriate artery origins from atheroma of the MCA (Weiller *et al.* 1990; Angeloni *et al.* 1991; Donnan *et al.* 1991). This pattern is illustrated in Fig. 6.20e.

Occasionally, ischaemic stroke patients present with a cortical stroke syndrome, either total anterior circulation infarction (TACI) or partial anterior circulation infarction (PACI), but on brain imaging are found to have a recent lacunar infarct in the correct hemisphere without any sign of the expected cortical infarct. Equally, the occasional patient with a lacunar infarct syndrome (LACI) may have a recent cortical infarct on brain imaging with no hint of any subcortical lesion. We reviewed all patients in our hospital-based stroke registry admitted with a LACI or PACI (377 and 637, respectively) from 1990 to 1998, who had brain imaging with CT or MR (Mead *et al.* 1999). In the PACI patients, a recent infarct was seen in 62%, of which 76% were appropriately cortical anterior cerebral artery (ACA) or MCA territory, 16% were lacunar and 8% were in the posterior cerebral artery (PCA) territory. In the LACI patients, a recent infarct was seen in 48%, of which 77% were appropriately lacunar, 19% were cortical ACA or MCA territory, and 4% were PCA territory. Sources of emboli (atrial fibrillation or significant carotid stenosis) were significantly more common in the PACI and LACI patients with cortical infarcts, than in the PACI and LACI patients with lacunar infarcts. There were no significant differences in the proportions of patients with other risk factors. Recurrent stroke was significantly more common in the PACI patients with a cortical infarct than in PACI patients with a lacunar infarct. Morbidity and mortality at 6 months after the stroke was higher in PACI or LACI patients with a cortical infarct than with a lacunar infarct. Thus patients with a cortical infarct on brain imaging behaved like cortical syndromes even if *clinically* they had a lacunar syndrome, and patients with lacunar infarcts on brain imaging behaved like lacunar syndromes even if *clinically* they had a cortical syndrome, in terms of risk factors, recurrent stroke and long-term outcome. This suggests that the syndrome (and so anatomical location of the brain lesion) attributed to an ischaemic stroke patient following clinical examination could usefully be modified by the position of any recent, and likely to be relevant, infarct on brain imaging, as this reflects the underlying vascular lesion and provides practical information to guide clinical management in the hunt for risk factors and determining resource use.

The clinical syndrome attributed to an ischaemic stroke patient following clinical examination may need to be modified if subsequent brain imaging shows a recent and likely to be relevant infarct in a different territory to that expected clinically. For example, a patient with a clinical lacunar syndrome, but whose CT scan shows a recent cortical infarct in the relevant hemisphere, should be regarded as being similar to a patient with a cortical syndrome (i.e. high risk of early recurrent stroke, high probability of ipsilateral carotid stenosis or cardiac source of embolism).

Distinction of arterial infarcts from other conditions on CT

While many infarcts arising from arterial occlusion are easy to diagnose from their site, shape, density and appropriate clinical features, other lesions occasionally produce very similar appearances, which can be confusing.

Venous infarcts (section 5.5) are relatively uncommon and frequently misdiagnosed as arterial infarcts, primary intracerebral haemorrhages, or tumours on CT. It is probable therefore that venous infarcts are a more common cause of infarction and/or haemorrhage than has been previously recognized. In our experience there are often clues on imaging which should point to the correct diagnosis. Many are overlooked simply because the possibility of venous infarction is not even considered (Table 5.2). Further details are given in section 5.5, but the radiology of how to distinguish arterial from venous infarcts is described here.

Cerebral venous disease consists of a spectrum, varying from the effects of sinus thrombosis, without any brain parenchymal change, at one extreme to purely parenchymal lesions, caused by cortical vein thrombosis (infarction with or without haemorrhage) without sinus thrombosis, at the other end. The clinical presentation and radiological appearance in any individual patient depend on the balance of these components. Venous infarcts can usefully be thought of in two parts: the primary features of the parenchymal lesion, and the secondary features of sinus thrombosis, one or both of which may be present. Venous infarcts are typically of low density and may be wedge-shaped, like arterial infarcts, but the key differentiating features are:

- they often do not quite fit the usual site of an arterial infarct;
- they are much more swollen than an equivalent-sized arterial infarct;
- there may be swelling in the hemisphere beyond the low-density area; and
- they often contain haemorrhage (Virapongse *et al.* 1987; Perkin 1995; Bakaç & Wardlaw 1997) (Fig. 5.20). The haemorrhage is typically in the centre of the low-density area and may be patchy and finger-like in distribution, whereas in arterial infarcts the haemorrhage is usually around the edges.

The high density of a thrombosed cortical vein or sinus may also be visible (see hyperdense artery sign above) (Ward-

Table 5.2 Differentiation of arterial from venous infarcts on CT brain imaging.

	Arterial	Venous
Shape	Wedge or rounded	Usually wedge if cortical, rounded if deep
Number occurring simultaneously	Usually single	May be multiple
Density	Early: slightly hypodense Later: more hypodense	Early obvious hypodensity
Margins	Indistinct early, distinct after several days	Distinct early
Swelling	Develops over days	Marked, appears usually very early
Haemorrhage	Infrequent, peripheral finger-like	Frequent, central
Additional signs	Hyperdense artery sign	Hyperdense sinus sign Empty delta sign (after contrast)

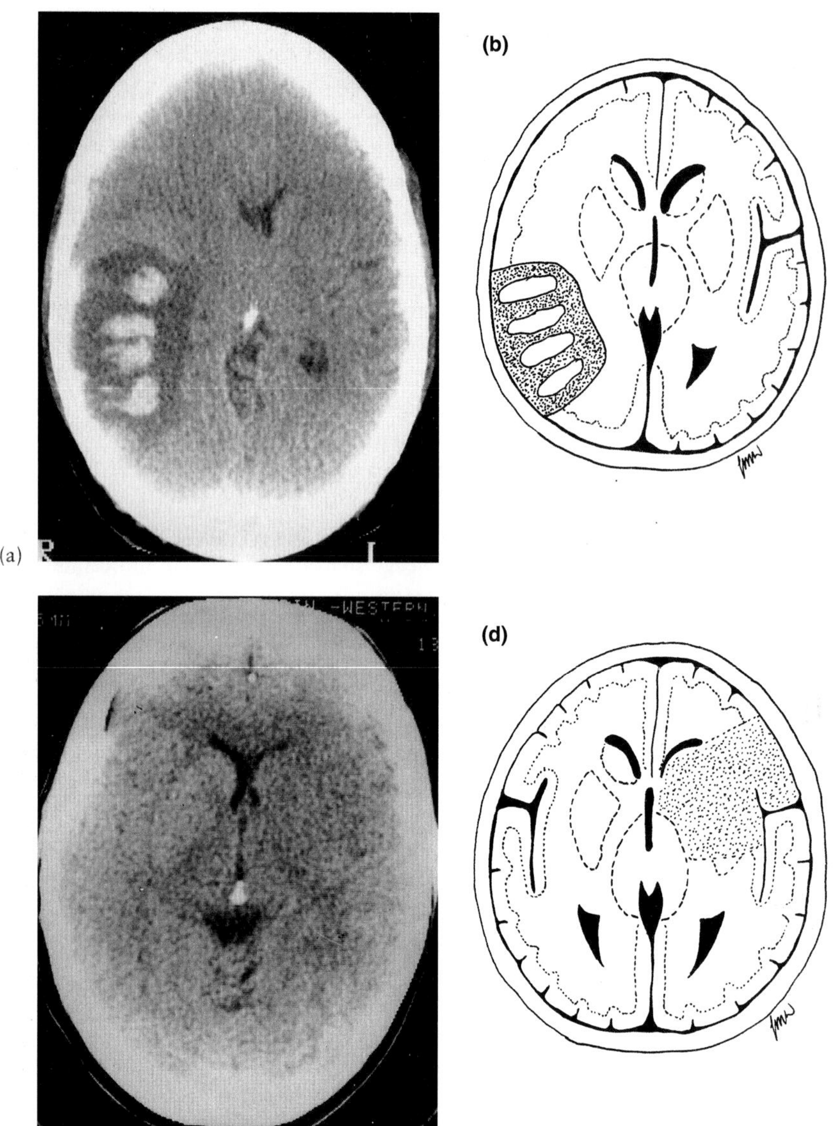

Fig. 5.20 CT brain scans and diagrams to emphasize the differences between typical arterial and venous infarcts. (a) CT brain scan obtained within 6 h of symptom onset showing a right parietal venous infarct. (b) Drawing of (a) to emphasize the key features: the margins are clearly seen and the lesion is very hypodense even at such a short time after onset; there is marked swelling both within the infarct and within the rest of the hemisphere beyond the infarct; and there are central areas of haemorrhage. (c) CT brain scan obtained within 6 h of symptom onset showing a left parietal arterial infarct. (d) Drawing of (c) to emphasize the key features: the margins are ill defined and the lesion is only slightly hypodense compared with normal brain; there is only slight swelling within the infarct and none beyond it; and there is no haemorrhage (see also Figs 5.12, 5.13, 5.14 and 5.21).

law *et al.* 1998c; Miller *et al.* 1999). After intravenous contrast, there may be an 'empty delta' sign in the venous sinus, and serpiginous enhancement at the edges of the infarct (Fig. 5.21).

Viral encephalitis, if relatively focal in distribution, can appear exactly like an infarct, although this is rare. The typical appearance of herpes simplex encephalitis with involvement of the medial temporal lobes should not cause confusion, but we have seen patients with low-density areas in the temporoparietal region associated with rising viral titres, which resolved following treatment with aciclovir (Fig. 5.22). It is vital that the radiology is reviewed with all the clinical information and, if there is any doubt (e.g. fever, subacute onset), other diagnostic tests must be carried out, including an electroencephalogram, MR scan and cerebrospinal fluid examination.

Purulent cerebritis can look like an infarct, although the lesion is usually not wedge-shaped and involves more white matter than cortex, and the clinical picture should allow the distinction to be made.

Tumours. Occasionally, a peripheral metastasis with a large amount of white matter oedema can mimic an infarct on CT, although the density is usually lower than expected in an infarct, and administration of contrast may show up a cortical nodule (Fig. 5.23). If there is still doubt, a repeat CT a few weeks later will usually determine the cause of the abnormality, because infarcts and tumours evolve differently (Fig. 5.4).

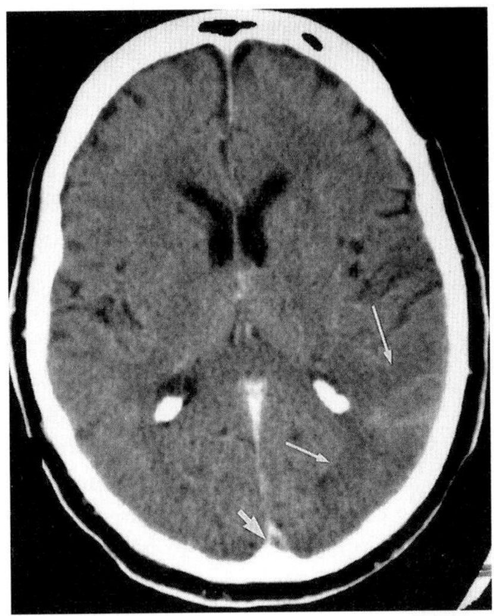

Fig. 5.21 CT brain scan (contrast enhanced) showing a left occipital venous infarct (thin arrows) with a thrombosis of the superior sagittal sinus as shown by the 'empty delta' sign (thick arrow) (see also Figs 5.12, 5.13 and 5.20).

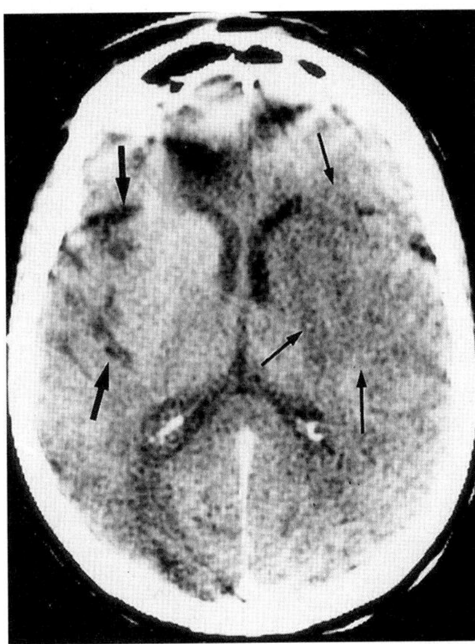

Fig. 5.22 CT brain scan in a 70-year-old woman with a right hemiparesis, confusion and drowsiness, showing an extensive area of low density in the left temporoparietal region including the basal ganglia. The appearance is subtle, but there is loss of the outline of the normal basal ganglia (thin arrows) and loss of the overlying cortical sulci indicating slight swelling (compare with the easily seen right parietal sulci—thick arrows). The initial clinical diagnosis was of a stroke (infarct), but 1 week later the patient deteriorated and the CT scan showed extensive haemorrhage in the left temporoparietal region. Subsequent post-mortem confirmed the diagnosis of herpes simplex encephalitis.

Time is a useful diagnostic tool—'a chronogram'. If in doubt whether a lesion is a tumour or infarct on CT, repeat the scan in a few weeks. Infarcts get smaller (usually), whereas tumours stay the same or get bigger.

5.3.6 Magnetic resonance imaging

Historical note and practical points regarding use of MR

Magnetic resonance (MR) was first used as a clinical tool in the early 1980s. The equipment is expensive, both to purchase and to run, and MR was initially little used in acute stroke. It is not a practical technique for many acutely ill patients because:

- the patient must be placed inside a tube-like structure, which makes access for monitoring and administering anaesthetics difficult;
- the patient must lie still, usually for at least 5 minutes at a time, although recent fast-scanning techniques mean that diagnostic images may be acquired in seconds;
- many acute stroke patients are confused, restless and frightened by the noise and vibration of the scanner, which is rather like being in the engine-room of a very large ship or being near loud machine-gun fire; and
- it is inadvisable for patients with impaired protection of their airway to be placed supine for *any* length of time, regardless of the value of the information so obtained.

Although individual MR image sequences may each take only a minute or so to acquire, there may be prior setting-up time and several sequences have to be carried out, all of which contribute to longer total scanning times with MR than CT. Thus very fast MR image acquisition still cannot compete with the speed or ease of use of a fast CT scanner, so the first-line investigation for stroke patients will probably continue to be CT in the immediate future (Koroshetz & Gonzales 1999), reserving MR for 'difficult cases' with specific questions, and for research (Powers & Zivin 1998; Pritchard & Grossman 1999). However, as MR scanners become less expensive and the access to patients within the scanner becomes easier, and therefore more user-friendly, their use will expand. The great advantages of MR are not only its superior pathoanatomical cross-sectional imaging properties, but that the same machine can image vessels and assess cerebral blood flow non-invasively; provide diffusion and perfusion imaging and spectroscopy to elucidate the pathogenesis of brain damage in ischaemia and how experimental treatments might modify it; and, by functional imaging, elucidate mechanisms of brain recovery.

Many of the general principles of recognizing an infarct by its shape and site, the correlations between clinical findings and infarct site, the time course of infarct swelling and haemorrhagic transformation as have been described for CT are equally relevant to MR and will not be repeated here. Rather, this section highlights where MR imaging provides different information to CT.

Routine brain imaging with MR

A routine MR brain image consists of a midline sagittal

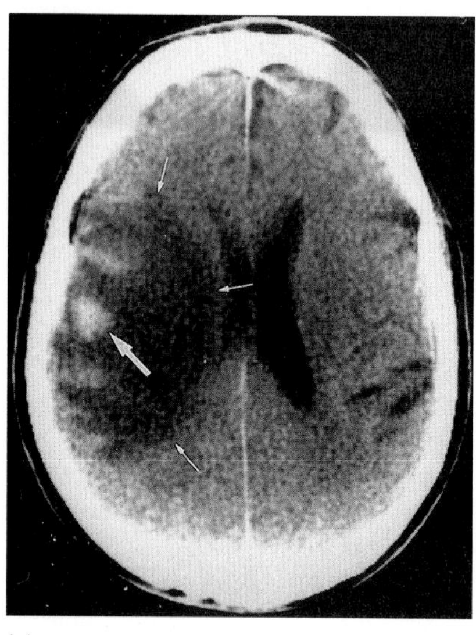

(a)

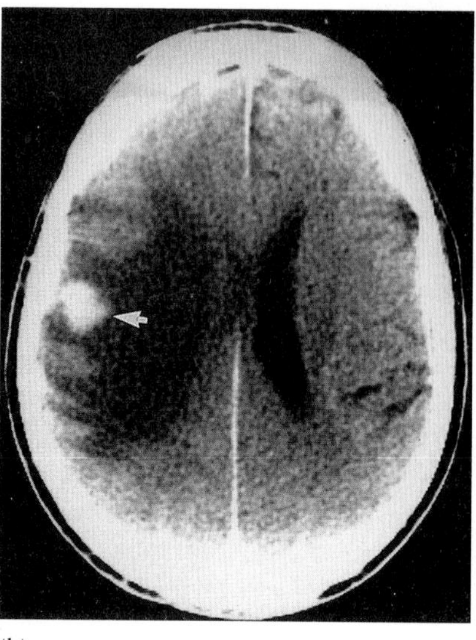

(b)

Fig. 5.23 CT brain scan showing a tumour which looks like an infarct in a 60-year-old man who presented with 'a stroke'. (a) Unenhanced scan shows an extensive right parietal low-density area (thin arrows) with a high-density area in the cortex (thick arrow). This could be misinterpreted as an area of haemorrhage in an infarct. (b) Following intravenous contrast the cortical high-density area enhances (arrow) consistent with a tumour nodule. The low density is therefore caused by oedema. It was in fact a solitary secondary brain tumour, as a subsequent chest X-ray showed a previously undiagnosed primary bronchial carcinoma.

localizing view of the brain, usually T1-weighted, followed by axial T2 and either proton density or fluid attenuated inversion recovery (FLAIR) images covering the whole brain. It is well beyond the scope or intention of this section to describe the differences between these sequences, or indeed what they mean, but in simple terms it is useful to think of T2-weighted images as showing brain water content (so cerebrospinal fluid and areas of oedema will show up as high-signal areas, i.e. white) and proton density and T1-weighted images as showing brain structure. Previously, the sequence routinely used for brain imaging was a spin echo T2 or proton density sequence. Recently, it has become common for manufacturers to supply a fast spin echo T2 and proton density sequence. Fast spin echo sequences take less time to acquire than spin echo, so would generally be the sequences used by radiologists if available. However, it is important to recognize that spin echo and fast spin echo do not produce the same images, the main difference being that fast spin echo is less sensitive to the presence of haemosiderin, a marker of earlier haemorrhage, than spin echo. This, and other MR techniques, are described briefly below.

Contraindications to MR

All patients should be screened for MR compatibility before they enter the magnetic field, but the key contraindications are mentioned here to help avoid inappropriate referrals: pacemakers, intracranial aneurysm clips (all types), and definite metallic intraocular foreign bodies. Metallic prostheses, foreign bodies other than in the eyes or brain, some ventriculoperitoneal shunts, some artificial heart valves and first trimester of pregnancy are all relative contraindications which are useful for the MR department to know about well in advance, so that the individual patient's circumstances can be checked (to see whether MR scanning will be possible without undue risk) and to tailor the scan to the patient.

5.3.7 The appearance of haemorrhage on MRI

The appearance of haemorrhage on MR is governed by the paramagnetic properties of haemoglobin breakdown products and so it changes with time (Bradley 1994) (Fig. 5.24). Freshly extravasated red blood cells contain oxyhaemoglobin, which does not have any paramagnetic properties, so there may be little immediate signal change and, although a lesion may be visible, the differentiation from infarction may be difficult within the first few hours unless specific blind-sensitive sequences are used. In practice, this is not a problem because so few patients are scanned very early and, even when they are, in our experience there has been enough signal change to distinguish haemorrhage from infarct.

Once enough deoxyhaemoglobin has formed (which takes about 24 h), clear changes will be seen and the typical appearance is of a centrally hypointense (dark) T1 image and a markedly hypointense (dark) T2 image. From day one, as methaemoglobin is formed in the red cells, the T1 image becomes hyperintense (bright) while the T2 image remains dark until, following this, as the methaemoglobin becomes extracellular and the haematoma liquefies, the T2 image becomes as hyperintense (bright) as the T1 image. After several weeks, T2 images become bright in the centre with a very dark rim, and T1 images are also bright centrally and moderately dark around the rim. Eventually the dark rim (haemosiderin) around a bright 'hole' on T2 is the only remaining feature. The exact timing and degree of these signal changes vary with the strength of the magnet, which compartment of the brain the haemorrhage lies in, abnormal clotting, haema-

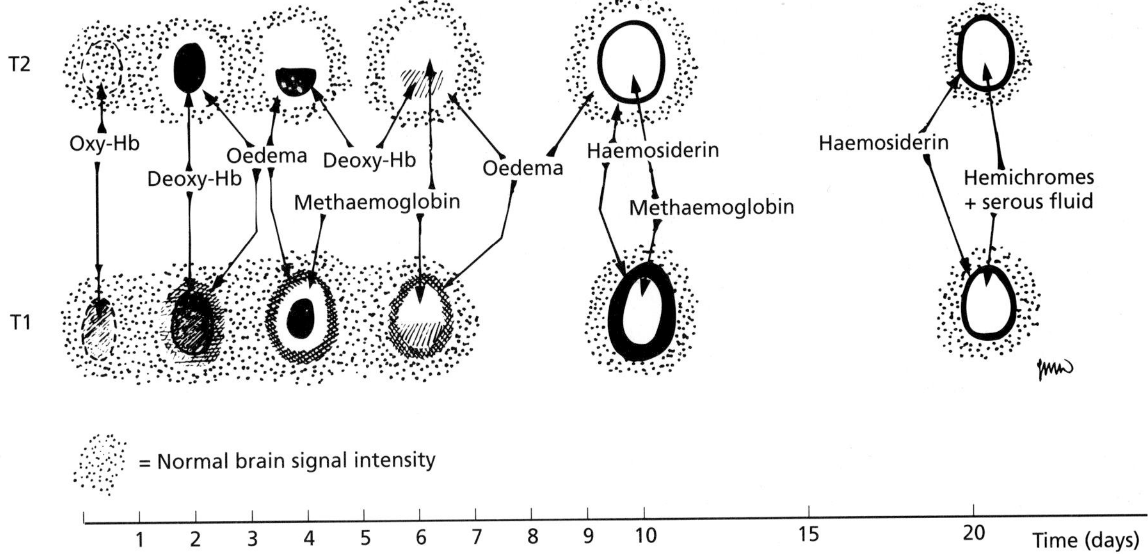

Fig. 5.24 Diagram of the change in the appearance of parenchymal brain haemorrhage on MRI. The top row shows the typical appearance on T2-, and the lower row on T1-weighted imaging. The normal brain is represented by the stippled background. To a certain extent, the exact appearance and timing of the changes depend on the field strength of the magnet. The most important things to remember are that intracellular deoxyhaemoglobin (deoxy-Hb) is dark on T1 and T2, methaemoglobin is bright on T1 and T2, and haemosiderin is dark on T1 and T2. Haemosiderin persists in the margins of a haematoma for years after the original haemorrhage. Oxy-Hb, oxyhaemoglobin.

tocrit, and the exact scan sequence used (Bradley 1994). There are sequences which are very sensitive to the presence of haemoglobin breakdown products, e.g. 'Flash2D' T2 (gradient echo T2), which show petechial haemorrhage in infarcts, previously visible only to the pathologist (Patel *et al.* 1996) (Fig. 5.25). The clinical utility of being able to see such tiny amounts of haemorrhage is uncertain; clinicians may find it less upsetting if they simply do not request this sequence (for fear of finding some blood they wish they had never seen).

Does haemorrhage remain visible indefinitely on MR?

It was once considered that the MR features of haemosiderin persist for life (Fig. 5.26) because, in general, old haematomas are visible pathologically as haemosiderin deposits at post-mortem (Garcia *et al.* 1994). Haemosiderin is one of two major haemoglobin-derived pigments identifiable in tissue sections from around haematomas and represents aggregates of ferritin micelles within lysosomes of phagocytic cells. The other pigment is haematoidin, which is chem-

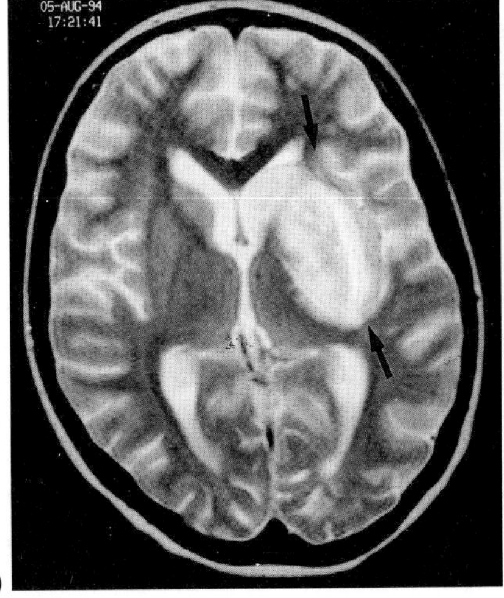

(a)

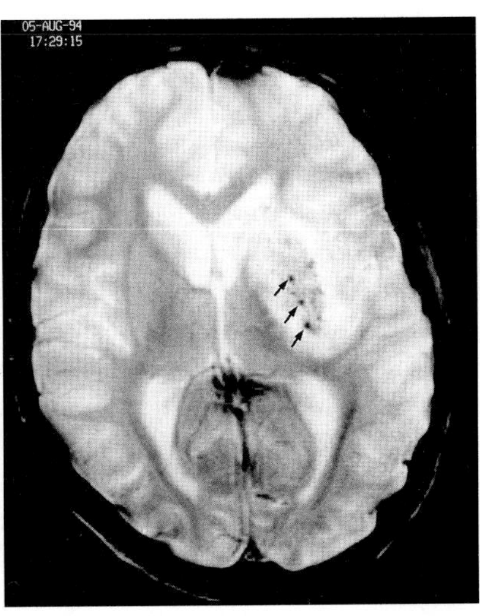

(b)

Fig. 5.25 Magnetic resonance scan of a 5-day-old left striatocapsular infarct to show the extreme sensitivity of appropriate MR sequences to tiny areas of petechial haemorrhage. (a) T2-weighted spin-echo sequence shows the infarct (arrows), but no haemorrhage. (b) T2-weighted gradient-echo 'haem' sequence shows tiny low-signal areas within the infarct caused by tiny amounts of petechial haemorrhage (arrows) such as would normally only be visible to the pathologist. The clinical relevance of this is uncertain.

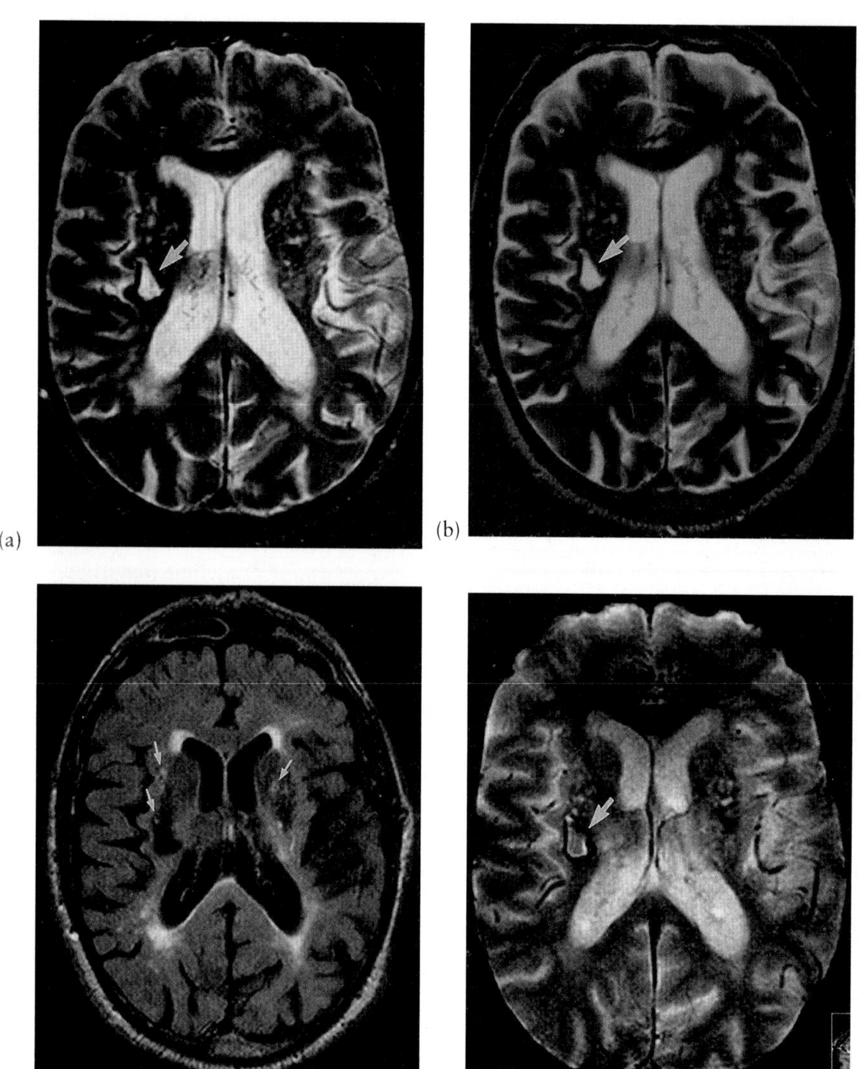

Fig. 5.26 Magnetic resonance scan showing an old parenchymal haemorrhage in the right basal ganglia. (a) T2 spin echo: the lesion has an obvious low signal (dark) area surrounding the high signal centre (arrow). (b) T2 fast spin echo: the lesion is more difficult to identify as an old haemorrhage as the low signal (dark) area is less obvious. (c) Fluid attenuated inversion recovery: several small deep lesions shown (arrows), but no features to identify any of them as haemorrhage. (d) Gradient echo T2: the haemorrhage is obvious.

ically identical to bilirubin, and forms locally as a result of haemoglobin breakdown in a milieu of reduced oxygen tension (Garcia *et al.* 1994). Haemosiderin is ferromagnetic and therefore visible on MR, whereas haematoidin has no particular magnetic properties and is not visible on MR. However, until recently, there had not been a study to determine whether *all* primary intracerebral haemorrhages (PICHs) remain visible for ever, either at post-mortem or on MR imaging. Such a study using post-mortem verification would be virtually impossible to carry out, and studies of the appearance of haemorrhage on MR have focused on the sequence of change in appearance of the haematoma (well covered in Bradley 1994) and not on the basic question of whether all haematomas are visible indefinitely because of their haemosiderin content.

To address the question of long-term haemorrhage visibility on MR, we performed a study in which spin echo T2 and proton density MR (on a 1 Tesla MR scanner) were performed in 116 survivors of moderate to severe head injury, between 1 and 5 years after injury. We used the CT scan from the time of injury to determine the number of patients with intracerebral haemorrhages in the acute stage and reviewed the MR films without being aware of the earlier CT or clinical data. Of the 116 patients, 78 had one or more haemorrhages on their CT scan at the time of injury (total 106 haemorrhages); 96 of these 106 (90%) haemorrhages were visible as haemosiderin on the late MR scan. Of the 10 haemorrhages without haemosiderin on MR, seven were in patients where another haemorrhage *with* haemosiderin was still visible elsewhere in the brain. There were no features of the haemorrhage (site, size, density, sharpness of edges) in the acute stage which correlated with the likelihood of haemosiderin being present at 1 year. Some quite large haematomas showed no trace of haemosiderin. Thus, on routine spin echo imaging, about 10% of former intracerebral haemorrhages (11.5% of patients) showed no trace of haemosiderin and were therefore indistinguishable from other causes of cerebromalacea, such as infarction (Wardlaw & Statham 2000).

This study in head injury was performed on an MR scanner installed in the early 1990s. Many modern scanners provide fast spin echo sequences which are known to be less sensitive to the magnetic effects of haemosiderin than spin echo, and are likely to be used in preference to spin echo as they significantly reduce imaging time (Wehrli & Atlas 1996). Gradient echo sequences are highly sensitive to haemosiderin but would not routinely be performed unless specifically requested, as they add an extra 5 minutes to the scanning time (Patel *et al.* 1996). Furthermore, areas of calcification give a similar appearance to haemosiderin on gradient echo sequences, and so may cause confusion. As traumatic haematomas may resolve differently to spontaneous haematomas presenting as stroke, we undertook a further study in which patients who were known to have had a CT-documented primary intracerebral haemorrhage (PICH) 3 months or more previously were recalled for an MR scan. Twenty-five patients were scanned using spin echo T2, fast spin echo T1, T2 and proton density, FLAIR, and gradient echo sequences on a 2 Tesla MR scanner. Of the 29 former haematomas in 25 patients, all were visible as haemosiderin on spin echo T2, 28 of 29 (96%) on fast spin echo T2, all on gradient echo images and none as haemosiderin on FLAIR. Although the haemosiderin was visible on fast spin echo T2, in some cases it was quite subtle and might readily have been overlooked in the heavy workload of a busy radiologist. Thus, depending on the sequences used and the vigilance of the radiologist, MR will miss a proportion of definite former PICHs. An awareness of this should prompt a request for the most sensitive imaging (a gradient echo sequence) in patients where it is of particular importance not to overlook an earlier PICH. Haemorrhagic transformation of infarction may be recognizable on late MRI as areas of haemosiderin deposition at the margins of an infarct, but there have been no systematic studies to determine how often these features remain detectable on MR.

In general, the characteristic signal changes of parenchymal haemorrhage on MRI persist indefinitely, but only if the appropriate imaging sequences are used; therefore, haematomas can be identified even years after they have occurred. However, not all haematomas will form haemosiderin during their resolution, therefore not all haematomas will be discernible as such on MR performed late after the event.

Is there an underlying cause of the haemorrhage?

Magnetic resonance imaging is probably better than CT at determining the underlying cause of an intracerebral haemorrhage (section 8.9.3). For example, MRI demonstrates venous sinus thrombosis, multiple pinpoint metastases, parenchymal sequelae of vasculitis, primary tumours and arteriovenous malformations, which are all generally less visible on CT. Magnetic resonance venography can confirm sinus occlusion (Dormont *et al.* 1994; Vogl *et al.* 1994; Yuh *et al.* 1994). Magnetic resonance may also have a useful role in determining whether a lesion *was* an infarct or a haematoma in patients who present late after their stroke, too late for CT to make the distinction reliably (see above). However, it is probably better to encourage patients to present as early as possible, through public health and general practitioner education, rather than relying on 'salvage' by MR.

Some patients are found to have evidence on MR of multiple small areas of haemorrhage in their brains, but with no previous relevant symptoms (Fig. 5.27). In one study of 120 consecutive patients aged over 60 years presenting with their first stroke, 33% had previous haemorrhages on MR, either microbleeds or old haematomas (Offenbacher *et al.* 1996).

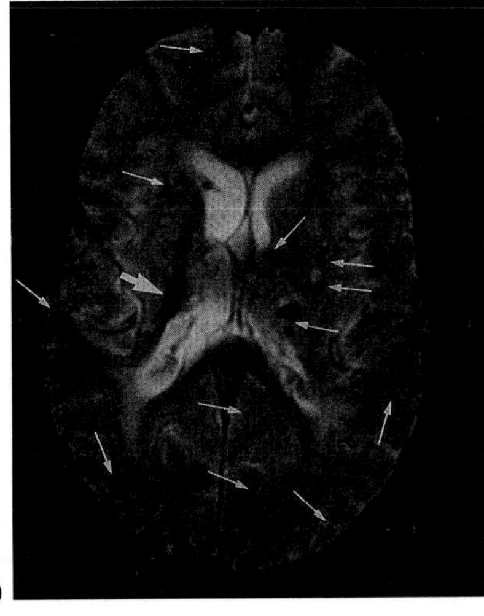

(a)

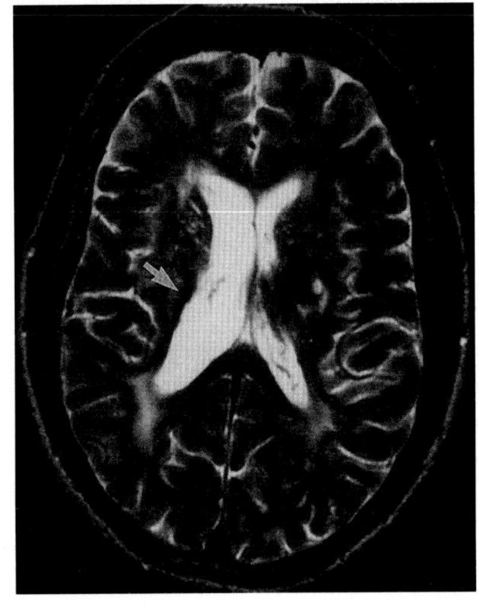

(b)

Fig. 5.27 Magnetic resonance image showing small dots of old haemorrhage all over the brain. (a) Gradient echo sequence shows the old symptomatic lesion was a right basal ganglia–thalamic haemorrhage measuring about 1 cm in diameter (thick arrow), with multiple small low signal dots (dark spots) indicating that tiny asymptomatic haemorrhages have occurred at some point throughout the brain (thin arrows). (b) Fast spin echo T2 demonstrates numerous small deep lesions, but even the old symptomatic right basal ganglia haemorrhage would be difficult to identify as haemorrhagic because of the lack of low signal (dark).

Another study of 72 patients with one previous episode of primary intracerebral haemorrhage found an increased frequency of old haemorrhagic 'holes' in the deep white matter and basal ganglia (in addition to the haemorrhage which had caused the stroke) compared with 137 consecutive patients of similar age with cerebrovascular disease but no known haemorrhage (Scharf *et al.* 1994). The relevance of this is uncertain, but it may be related to the presence of cerebral amyloid angiopathy, and may indicate an increased risk of haemorrhage if the patient is given aspirin, anticoagulants or thrombolytic drugs. Further study is clearly required.

5.3.8 The appearance of ischaemic stroke on MRI

Early MR signs of infarction

The earliest ischaemic changes detectable with *routine* MR (i.e. not with spectroscopy, perfusion or diffusion imaging) are loss of the normal flow void in the symptomatic artery (within minutes of onset), which is the MR equivalent of the hyperdense artery sign on CT (section 5.3.5) (Fig. 5.28); swelling on T1-weighted images without signal change on T2-weighted images (3 h); signal changes on T2-weighted images (8 h); and signal change on T1-weighted images (16 h) (Kertesz *et al.* 1987; Baker *et al.* 1991; Yuh *et al.* 1991; Hasso *et al.* 1994; Ida *et al.* 1994). On routine T1- and T2-weighted imaging large infarcts are often visible within 5 h (Hasso *et al.* 1994; Ida *et al.* 1994) but small cortical and subcortical infarcts may never become visible. In general, infarcts of any size are more often and more quickly visible on fluid attenuated inversion recovery (FLAIR) and diffusion-weighted imaging (DWI), but currently these are not in widespread *routine* use. Diffusion and perfusion MR imaging and spectroscopy are discussed in further detail in section 5.3.9.

It has been said that it is difficult to differentiate between acute cerebral haemorrhage and acute cerebral infarction in the first 24 h (Brant-Zawadski *et al.* 1987; Hayman *et al.* 1991). In our experience, this has not been a problem. Schellinger *et al.* (1999) found no difficulty in identifying parenchymal haemorrhage on MR (DWI, FLAIR, T2) performed within 6 h of stroke onset in nine patients. In any case, after the first few hours MR is much more sensitive to intraparenchymal haemorrhage than CT, because of the paramagnetic effects of deoxyhaemoglobin (section 5.3.7). Tiny areas of haemorrhagic transformation not visible on CT can be identified, which might influence the use of anticoagulants in the future, although at the moment there is insufficient knowledge of their risks and benefits in patients with such minor areas of (petechial) haemorrhage for this information to be of much use (Bryan *et al.* 1991).

Routine MR can sometimes detect signal changes in appropriate areas of the brain lasting up to several days after transient ischaemic attacks (TIAs) (Yuh *et al.* 1991; Hommel *et al.* 1994; Mohr *et al.* 1995). Pronounced brain parenchymal cortical enhancement following intravenous gadolinium injection has been described within the first 24 h after onset in patients with a TIA, partial arterial occlusion and isolated boundary-zone infarcts (Sato *et al.* 1991; Yuh *et al.* 1991; Ida *et al.* 1994).

Evolution of the appearance of infarction on MRI

The general principles of recognition of infarcts from their shape and site in the brain, and any relationship to the underlying cause, are the same as were described for CT scanning (section 5.3.5). Thus, the infarct swells and many of the other features change according to the same time frame (Fig. 5.29). In the second week after infarct onset, diffuse increase

(a)
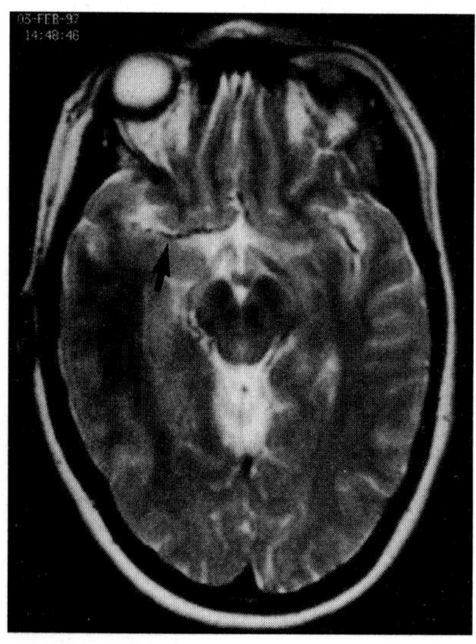

(b)
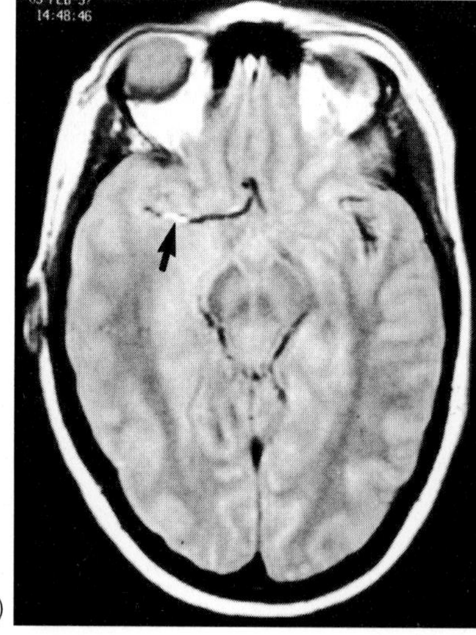

Fig. 5.28 Magnetic resonance image of a thrombosed right middle cerebral artery. Although there appears to be a flow void (dark) signal in the artery on T2 (arrow) (a), on proton density (b) there is an obvious high signal area as a result of the fresh thrombus or embolus (arrow). The examination was undertaken within 12 h of the stroke, but thrombus can appear dark on T2 up to 1–2 days after the stroke.

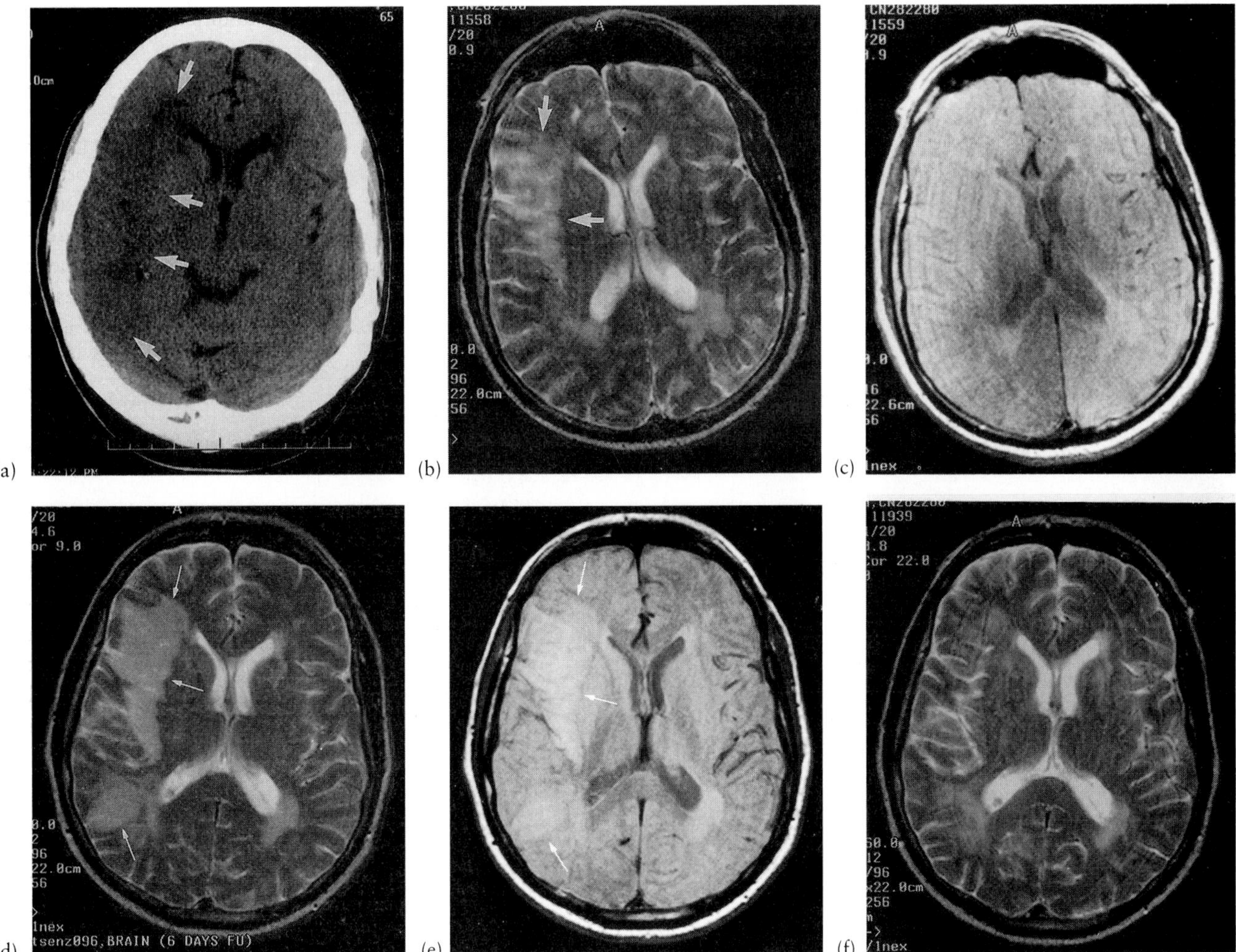

Fig. 5.29 Sequence of scans from a patient with a left hemiparesis (total anterior circulation infarction) to show the typical changes of infarction with time on MR. (a) CT scan at 6 h shows a subtle infarct in the right middle cerebral artery territory (arrows). Note the loss of sulci and the hypodensity. (b) T2 MR image at 12 h shows the infarct in the right frontoparietal region extending to the insula (arrows). (c) Proton density MR image at 12 h on which it is difficult to identify any infarct as there is little signal change and only some mild mass effect. Note the image is degraded by artifact from the patient moving, one of the problems encountered even with fast scan times with MR in stroke. (d) T2 and (e) proton density MR image at 4 days after the stroke. The infarct is much more obvious and there is some swelling in the infarct also. Note the slight effacement of the right lateral ventricle compared with the left. (f) T2 and (g) proton density MR at 10 days after stroke. The infarct is difficult to see because of the effect of 'fogging' which obscures the true extent of the lesion. There is no longer any swelling to alert the viewer to the presence of an abnormality. Not all infarcts disappear with fogging quite so thoroughly, but all do it to a degree. (h) CT at 6 months on which the true extent of the infarct is obvious (arrows). This confirms that the use of MR at 10 days–3 weeks to estimate the final infarct size can result in serious errors. (*continued p. 180*)

in signal (brightness on T2-weighted images) of gyri overlying the infarct is often visible. This is thought to be caused by neovascular capillary proliferation, or loss of autoregulation in leptomeningeal collaterals, and is visible for up to 8 weeks after onset (Brant-Zawadski *et al.* 1987; DeWitt *et al.* 1987). It is mirrored by a similar appearance on CT scanning, attributed to areas of breakdown of the blood–brain barrier corresponding with the gyriform petechial haemorrhages seen at post-mortem (Inoue *et al.* 1980). In the second to third week after onset, some infarcts become isodense with normal brain on CT (fogging effect) and, as they may have lost most of their mass effect by that stage, are difficult to identify. A similar effect has been observed on MR (Pereira *et al.* 1997). Recent MR studies have shown changes in T1 (increased signal) and in T2 (decreased signal) suggestive of diffuse haemorrhage in the second to third week (Fig. 5.30). This is probably a result of leaky capillaries, with diapedesis of red blood cells (Torigoe *et al.* 1990; Bryan *et al.* 1991), and would fit with the 'fogging effect' on CT, as the red blood cells would cause a diffuse increase in Hounsfield

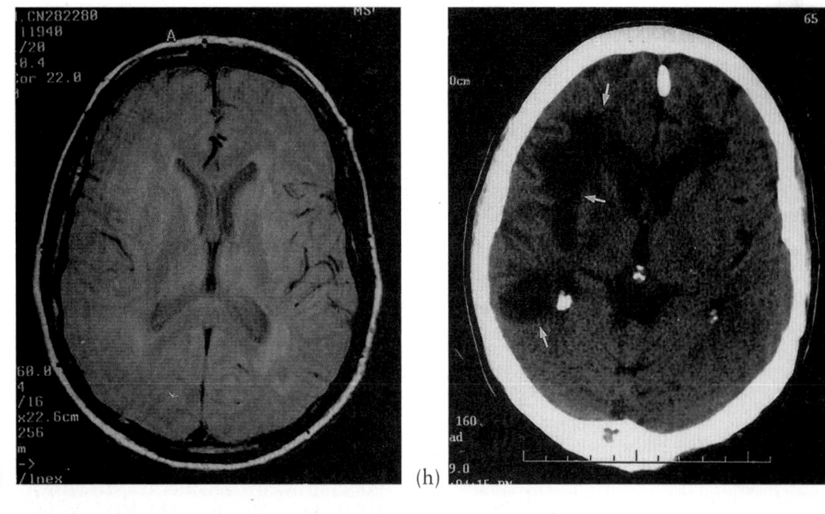

Fig. 5.29 *(continued)*

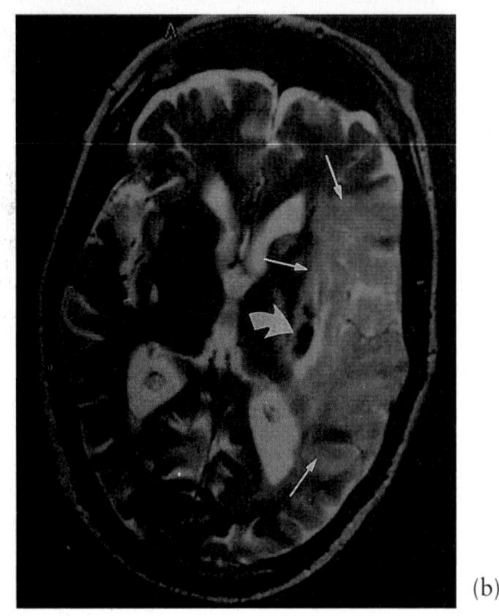

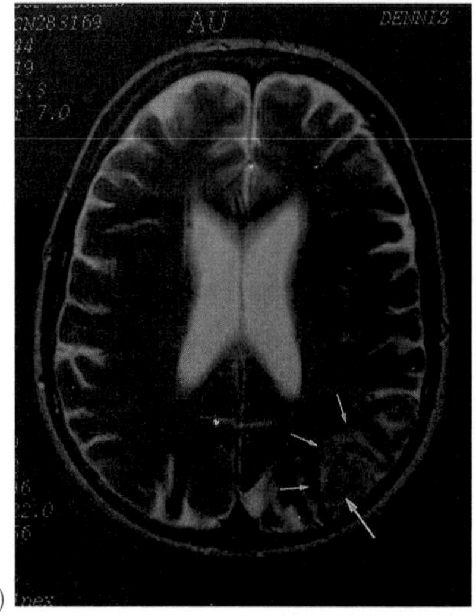

Fig. 5.30 Magnetic resonance T2 images of petechial haemorrhage. (a) A patient with an extensive left middle cerebral artery infarct at 5 days after stroke, with a dark area of haemosiderin (petechial haemorrhage—curved arrow) at the medial margin of the infarcted area (thin arrows). (b) A patient with a left parieto-occipital infarct (short arrows) with tiny areas of dark serpiginous cortical signal caused by gyral petechial haemorrhage (long arrow).

numbers, raising the low density of the lesion to that of normal brain parenchyma.

Infarcts do not usually show enhancement with intravenous contrast with gadolinium until after the first week after stroke onset. Thereafter, they generally show marked contrast enhancement around the edges (and within the infarct if enough contrast is administered) for several weeks (Merten *et al.* 1999). The possible risks of gadolinium in ischaemic brain lesions have not been evaluated, although currently the most widely used method of perfusion imaging requires an injection of gadolinium. Therefore, it would be reasonable to avoid gadolinium if at all possible.

Late appearance of infarction on MRI

After several weeks the infarcted brain appears as an area with similar signal characteristics to cerebrospinal fluid, i.e. bright on T2 and dark on T1, with an *ex vacuo* effect in the surrounding brain. Other long-term effects of ischaemic stroke seen on MR include wallerian degeneration, visible as atrophy and low intensity in the white matter of the brainstem, and the late effects of any haemorrhagic transformation (DeWitt *et al.* 1987) (section 5.4).

How rapidly and how often do infarcts become visible on MRI?

On routine T1- and T2-weighted MR, large infarcts are often visible within 6 h of stroke (Hasso *et al.* 1994; Ida *et al.* 1994). On FLAIR imaging, infarcts may be visible earlier, around 4 h (Noguchi *et al.* 1997). As mentioned above, MR abnormalities may be visible in the brain after as brief an insult as a transient ischaemic attack (TIA) but, on the other hand, not all patients with a clinically definite stroke have a corresponding MR abnormality (Alberts *et al.* 1992), even on diffusion imaging (Ay *et al.* 1999). Of patients who subsequently develop changes on routine T2-weighted MR, about 15% will show abnormalities within 8 h and 90% within

24 h (Kertesz *et al.* 1987). Of note is that 30% of patients showing changes within 24 h on routine MR showed an increase in size of the abnormal signal area on follow-up scan. However, it was not clear if this was a true increase in infarct extent or just the result of infarct swelling. While it is likely that signal changes on routine T2 and proton density MR represent irreversibly damaged brain, this has not yet been conclusively established in patients.

Diffusion-weighted imaging (DWI) can show abnormalities within minutes of the stroke in animals, and presumably also in humans (Yoneda *et al.* 1999), but currently is a less widely available and more cumbersome technique (Chien *et al.* 1992; Warach *et al.* 1995) (section 5.3.9). It certainly shows appropriate lesions when patients have been scanned within 30 min of the stroke (Yoneda *et al.* 1999). However, it is unclear whether this imaged abnormality represents irretrievably damaged brain or whether areas of reversible ischaemia (the ischaemic penumbra) are also being imaged.

Lecouvert *et al.* (1999) described a patient imaged within 4 h of acute ischaemic stroke, with diffusion and FLAIR MR imaging, who had a lesion in the posterior limb of the internal capsule consistent with a lacunar infarct. However, by 24 h the patient had made a full neurological recovery and repeat MR imaging showed no trace of the lacunar lesion. Further follow-up MR imaging at 7 and 30 days remained normal. Four cases of definite ischaemic stroke without a visible lesion on DWI have since been reported (Lefkowitz *et al.* 1999; Wang *et al.* 1999). This suggests that DWI and FLAIR-visible lesions do not always represent irreversibly damaged tissue, and that DWI does not always show damaged brain. Indeed, Ueda *et al.* (1999a) in a study of 18 patients imaged between 6 and 72 h of stroke and not treated with thrombolytic therapy, found abnormalities on diffusion imaging which did not go on to infarction (as demonstrated on follow-up routine CT or T2-weighted MR scanning) in one-quarter of ischaemic lesions (in the absence of clinical follow-up, it is possible that some of these patients actually had TIAs). Abnormalities on diffusion imaging within 24 h of symptom onset, corresponding with the clinical symptoms, have been demonstrated in patients who on clinical follow-up turned out to have TIAs, not strokes (Kidwell *et al.* 1999). Others have documented an increase in the lesion extent on diffusion imaging from the first scan performed within 24 h of stroke to scans some days later (Sorensen *et al.* 1996; Baird *et al.* 1997). Kohno *et al.* (1995), in an experimental model of cerebral infarction, showed abnormal diffusion images in areas of brain when the cerebral blood flow fell below 34–41 mL/100 g/min, which was still well above the threshold considered to represent the ischaemic penumbra (10–20 mL/100 g/min) and of irreversible energy failure (below 9–20 mL/100 g/min). Thus it is clear that diffusion imaging may demonstrate abnormalities in areas of brain which are not yet irreversibly damaged and may recover, and may never show abnormalities in areas of brain which, judging from the patient's symptoms, must be irreversibly damaged. The overall sensitivity and specificity of diffusion imaging (on its own or in combination with other MR techniques) has not yet been precisely defined (Latchaw 1999). More widespread use of MR in ischaemic stroke should make the relevance of early infarct visibility with different MR scanning methods much clearer.

Differentiation of new from old infarcts, and detection of small cortical and subcortical infarcts

Magnetic resonance imaging is able to detect small infarcts well, especially lacunae (Bryan *et al.* 1991). Furthermore, in patients with numerous 'holes in the brain', gadolinium-enhanced MRI often demonstrates which is the recent lacune, because it will enhance whereas older lesions will not (Elster 1992; Samuelsson *et al.* 1994). MRI is more sensitive to small lesions in the brainstem and posterior fossa than CT, because there is no interference from bone artifacts (Simmons *et al.* 1986).

Several studies have demonstrated the usefulness of diffusion-weighted imaging in locating the recent relevant infarct in patients with minor strokes. These patients are likely to have small lesions either in the cortex or subcortical white matter. A small cortical infarct may be difficult to identify on T2 or proton density (PD) MR, or on CT, but is often clearly seen as an area of increased signal on diffusion imaging up to several weeks after the stroke (Wardlaw *et al.* 2000b) (Fig. 5.31). Patients with lacunar infarcts may already have multiple areas of increased signal in the periventricular white matter on T2 or PD MR, or periventricular white matter lucencies on CT, which make it difficult to identify a new lesion amongst established lesions. Diffusion imaging demonstrates the recent lesion as an area of increased signal (Noguchi *et al.* 1998; Ohta *et al.* 1999; Wardlaw *et al.* 2000b (Fig. 5.32). Similarly, in patients with old cortical infarcts, diffusion imaging can also be useful to determine whether there has been a new ischaemic lesion where it is not clear whether any neurological deterioration has been caused by a new ischaemic lesion, or an intercurrent illness making a previous stroke deficit seem worse (Marks *et al.* 1996; Altieri *et al.* 1997; Lindgren *et al.* 1997; Fitzek *et al.* 1998) (section 15.4). On other forms of MR imaging, or on CT, it may be difficult to determine whether a new lesion has formed adjacent to an existing infarct as the cerebromalacic changes sometimes render interpretation difficult.

Fluid attenuated inversion recovery imaging (FLAIR)

Several studies have evaluated FLAIR imaging in acute stroke. Brant-Zawadski *et al.* (1996) retrospectively reviewed 50 patients with suspected stroke imaged with FLAIR and T2 using four blinded observers. Relevant infarcts were visible on the FLAIR sequence and not on T2 in 15 patients, but

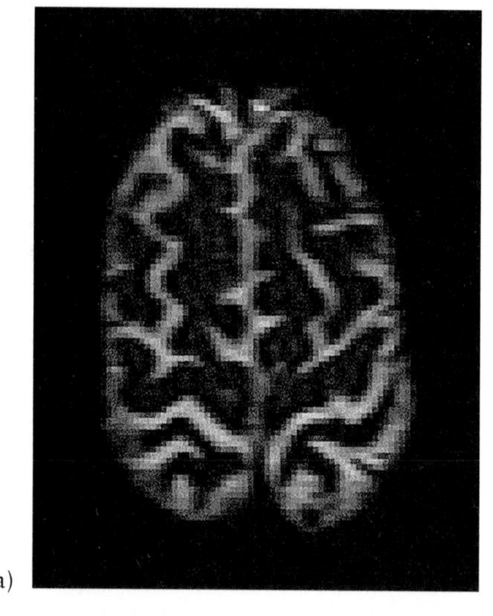
(a)

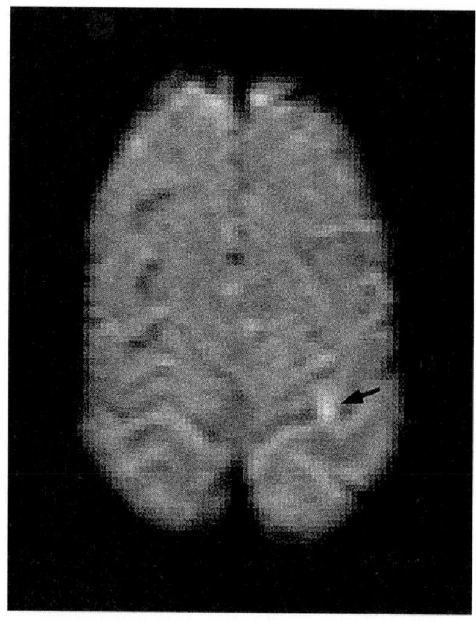
(b)

Fig. 5.31 Magnetic resonance diffusion imaging obtained within 24 h in a patient with symptoms of a minor left cortical infarct. (a) T2 MR does not show any visible lesion, but on diffusion imaging (b) there is a tiny area of high signal in the left parietal cortex (arrow) corresponding with the patient's symptoms. Note the high signal area was visible on all three gradient direction images, confirming that it was 'real' and not just artifact.

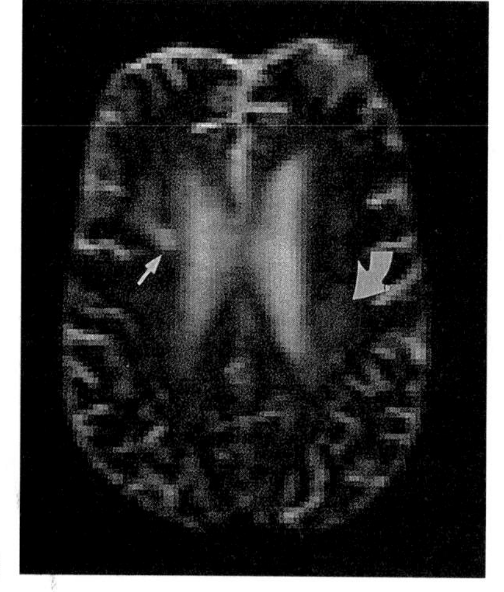
(a)

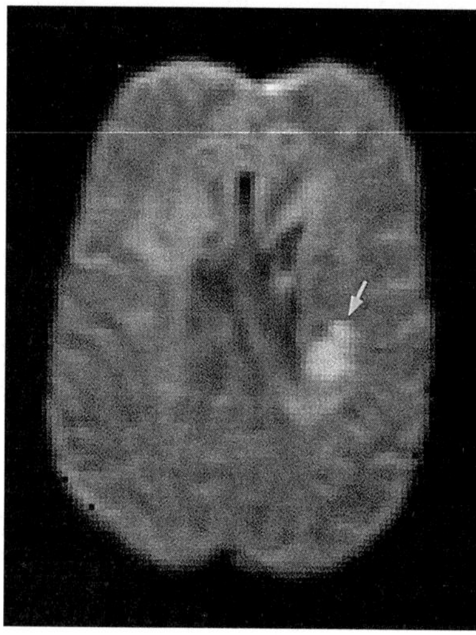
(b)

Fig. 5.32 Diffusion weighted MR images of a patient with a left hemisphere lacunar stroke. (a) T2 MR shows multiple areas of increased signal in the white matter adjacent to the lateral ventricles bilaterally (centrum semiovale). There is an old infarct (discrete high signal—arrow) in the right centrum semiovale, and a slightly prominent 'blotchy' area in the left centrum semiovale more posteriorly (curved arrow), which might be the recent infarct, but with so much other white matter disease it is difficult to be sure. (b) On diffusion imaging the recent infarct is obvious by its increased signal (arrow).

one brainstem infarct was missed by the FLAIR technique. Noguchi *et al.* (1997) found the FLAIR sequence identified acute infarcts earlier than T2-weighted MR in 19 patients scanned within 8 h of stroke onset: 86 vs. 43% within 3 h, 100 vs. 80% between 3 and 6 h, and 100 and 100% by 8 h for the FLAIR and T2 sequences, respectively. Cosnard *et al.* (1999) found the FLAIR sequence useful for identifying the extent of the infarct and was able to demonstrate occluded intracranial arteries (as high signal in place of a flow void) just as well as on MR angiography, in 53 patients studied within 6 h of stroke.

In our experience, FLAIR can demonstrate relevant infarcts days to weeks after the event, helping to locate the lesion in patients presenting late after their stroke. It can be particularly useful for differentiating small cortical and periventricular infarcts which might otherwise be difficult to distinguish from the adjacent cerebrospinal fluid (Fig. 5.33). However, FLAIR also shows more asymptomatic white matter lesions (perhaps as a result of small vessel disease) than does T2 or proton density MR, or CT, which may be more confusing than helpful. It may sometimes be possible to distinguish these old 'holes' from a new 'hole' caused by a lacunar stroke by the slightly less hyperintense (white) signal in the latter—both are hyperintense, but the old lesions are more hyperintense than the new.

5.3.9 Advanced magnetic resonance techniques

Magnetic resonance (MR) permits other useful methods of examining the brain, including MR angiography to demonstrate the arteries and veins; diffusion-weighted imaging (also discussed in section 5.3.8); perfusion-weighted imaging to demonstrate regional cerebral blood flow, volume and transit time, which may complement diffusion-weighted imaging in the demonstration of very early ischaemic changes; MR spectroscopy to show the effect of ischaemia on brain metabo-

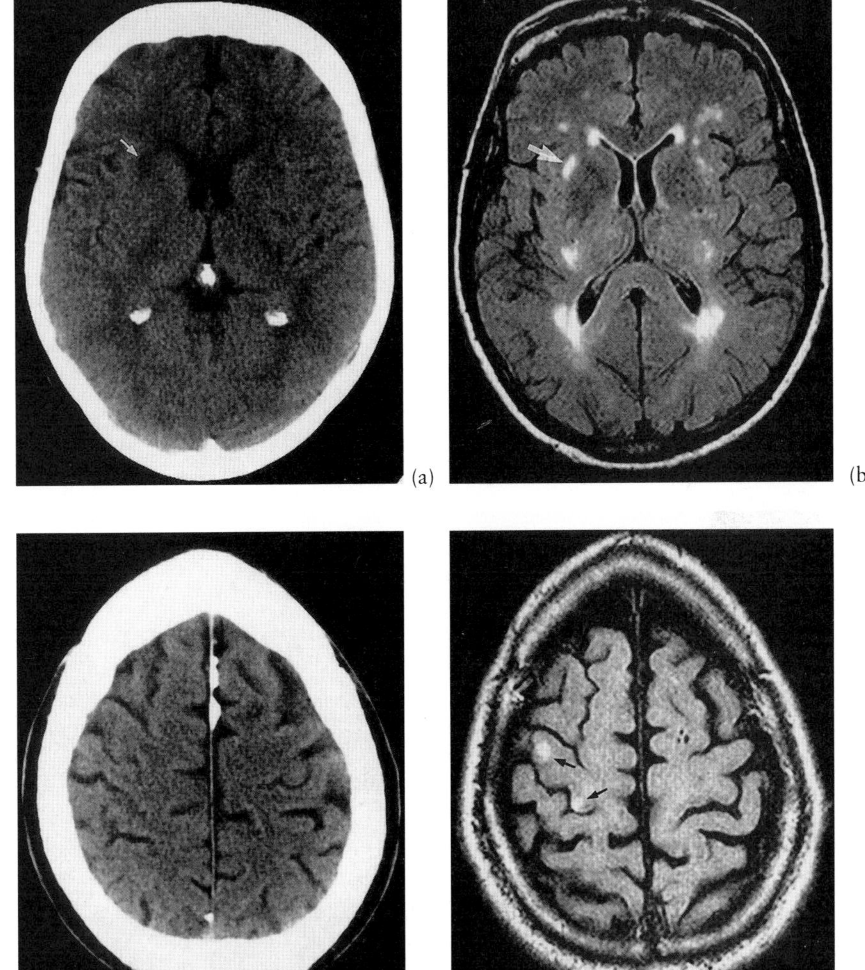

Fig. 5.33 Comparing CT with MR: examples from two patients. Patient 1: (a) on CT one small deep infarct (consistent with the symptoms) is visible in the anterior limb of the right internal capsule (arrow); (b) on MR FLAIR sequence not only is the symptomatic lesion visible (arrow), but numerous other areas of increased signal, a common finding with MR, which can confuse rather than clarify if it is used indiscriminately. Patient 2 had symptoms of a small right cortical infarct: (c) CT was normal, but (d) FLAIR showed high signal in the right parietal cortex (arrows) consistent with recent infarction (T2 was also normal).

lites; and functional MR to identify areas of the brain which control body function. The details of these techniques are beyond the scope of this chapter, but there are excellent reviews describing each technique, as detailed below.

MR angiography

Magnetic resonance angiography allows the acquisition of images of blood vessels, without injection of contrast, by using the signal characteristics of flowing blood (Baker *et al.* 1991; Fisher *et al.* 1992; Warach *et al.* 1992). This technique can be used in acute ischaemic stroke, but the patient must keep very still for the long scanning time so it is not always of practical help (Fig. 5.34). It shows promise for the assessment of carotid stenosis in patients being considered for carotid endarterectomy (section 6.7.5) and is also being evaluated for the detection of intracranial aneurysms (Fisher *et al.* 1992; Huston *et al.* 1993; White *et al.* 2000) (section 9.4.3). It may become a more practical technique for use in patients with ischaemic stroke given the very fast scan times which are now available.

Diffusion-weighted MRI (Figs 5.31, 5.32, 5.35)

Diffusion-weighted MRI (DWI) exploits the Brownian motion of water molecules in the brain and has demonstrated abnormalities in ischaemic tissue within 14 minutes of onset in animal models (Fisher & Sotak 1992). In stroke patients, initial studies have shown alteration of water diffusibility in the suspected infarcted tissue, which varied both within the lesion and with time (Chien *et al.* 1992; Warach *et al.* 1995) (section 5.3.8). Although there has been intense interest in the use of this technique in hyper-acute stroke, resulting in numerous publications, the significance of the changes in relation to clinical outcome, the extent of the ischaemic penumbra, the influence of experimental treatments for ischaemic stroke and the effect of reperfusion, have yet to be fully evaluated (Powers & Zivin 1998; Fisher & Albers

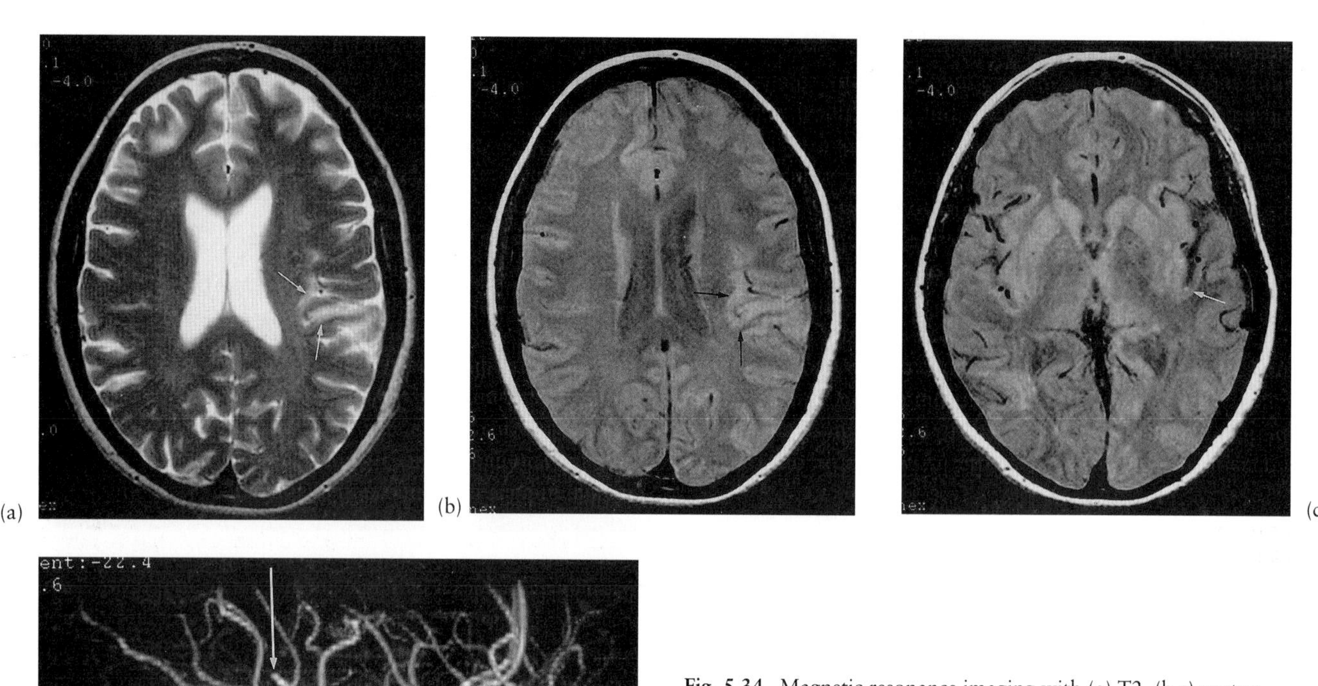

Fig. 5.34 Magnetic resonance imaging with (a) T2, (b,c) proton density and (d) MR angiography of a left middle cerebral artery (MCA) branch occlusion. Note the high signal of recent thrombus is visible on proton density (compare Fig. 5.28) (c, arrow) and the infarct in the insular cortex (a,b, arrows). (a) On T2 only dark signal mimicking a flow void is visible in the MCA branch so the thrombus might be overlooked. (d) The MR angiogram confirms the MCA branch occlusion (arrow).

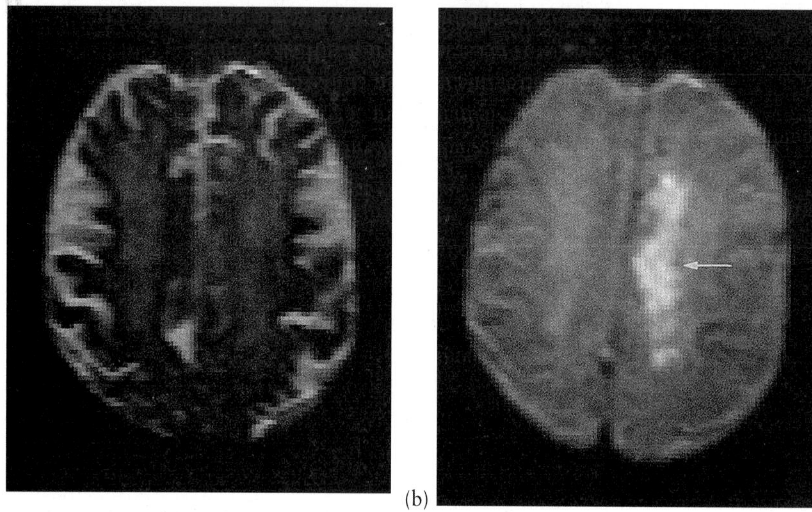

Fig. 5.35 (a) Magnetic resonance T2 and (b) diffusion images of an elderly patient with symptoms of a left cortical infarct. No definite recent lesion is visible on T2, although there is atrophy and white matter increased signal of 'small vessel disease', but on diffusion there is an obvious area of high signal corresponding with the infarct (arrow).

1999; Latchaw 1999; Pritchard & Grossman 1999). In the wave of enthusiasm for diffusion and perfusion MR imaging, it is worth pausing to take a critical look at what the studies have achieved so far, and reflect on the information that is still missing.

The perfect imaging technique for stroke would have most of the characteristics listed in Table 5.3. If, as in the case of DWI, the particular interest is in the use of the technique to diagnose accurately ischaemic stroke, to determine the extent of the lesion, the proportion of still viable brain and the likely clinical outcome, then a study to evaluate the technique would need the features or characteristics outlined in Table 5.4. At the time of writing, 40 studies of DWI in acute ischaemic stroke have been published (too numerous to ref-

Table 5.3 Brain imaging in acute stroke—what would be the ideal technique?

Widely available
Inexpensive
Fast, so as to obtain information quickly while not damaging the patient
Easy to observe the patient in the scanner
Differentiate infarct from haemorrhage from non-vascular lesions
Demonstrate the site of the infarct at any time after the event
Differentiate irreparably damaged brain from salvageable tissue
Demonstrate features which might identify patients at risk of treatment complications
Demonstrate features which identify patients at risk of recurrent stroke
Be repeatable
Not harmful

erence here, and in any case the list would be out of date by the time this book is published). The studies had a mean sample size of only 33. Only four blinded the review of each imaging modality to other imaging results, and to clinical features and outcome. Most had very sketchy details of the clinical state of the patient, such as 'stroke' rather than more detail about the severity of the stroke or the part of the brain affected. Only three had any clinical follow-up, the rest used imaging follow-up. In the 14 studies published to date of diffusion imaging in combination with perfusion imaging, the mean sample size was 18, only two stated that they blinded the imaging interpretation, only four had clinical follow-up (and only two of those at more than 1 month), the rest used imaging follow-up.

Given the small sample sizes, lack of baseline clinical and follow-up information, it is very difficult to extrapolate from these studies, which were conducted in highly specialized centres, to the generality of ischaemic strokes. In particular, to assess what information diffusion imaging might *add* to patient management, e.g. selection of patients for acute stroke treatment, over clinical examination and CT scanning, it is necessary to test diffusion imaging within the context of randomized trials of acute treatments, and so far very little of that has been carried out. Therefore, more information is needed from studies in larger patient populations and ideally in randomized treatment trials to determine whether the information gained from diffusion imaging, with or without perfusion imaging, is worth the effort and leads to improved patient outcome.

Table 5.4 Brain imaging in acute stroke—what would be the ideal study to determine the 'best' imaging modality?

Large sample size
Prospective
Patient population well characterized clinically
Including a broad sample of the type of patients *relevant* to the question being asked and at relevant time point(s) and all *relevant to clinical practice*
Blinded reading of imaging, to clinical and other imaging data
Adequate description of the imaging to allow independent confirmation
Evaluation of complications or difficulties with imaging
Clinical follow-up to relate imaging to long-term outcome

MR diffusion imaging can show abnormal areas corresponding with the clinical symptoms in patients who turn out to have transient ischaemic attacks (TIAs) when imaged within 24 h of onset of symptoms; in 48% of patients in one series (Kidwell *et al.* 1999). Thus diffusion imaging cannot distinguish between patients having TIAs and those who later went on to have definite strokes, although the abnormal areas on DWI in patients who had TIAs were generally smaller and less pronounced than abnormal areas on DWI in patients who had strokes (Kidwell *et al.* 1999).

Diffusion imaging is also non-specific and shows abnormalities that mimic ischaemic stroke such as encephalitis, migraine, vasculitis, brain tumours, following epileptic seizures, abscesses and multiple sclerosis (Bartylla *et al.* 1997; Wang *et al.* 1998). In addition, diffusion imaging does not always show a lesion in patients with definite ischaemic stroke; it was negative in 20% of patients in one series when scanned within 24 h of stroke and about 10% of lesions were never visible (Lovblad *et al.* 1998; Ay *et al.* 1999; Lecouvert *et al.* 1999; Lefkowitz *et al.* 1999; Wang *et al.* 1999). Neither is diffusion imaging good for examining the posterior fossa because of artifacts arising from the bone–air interface which distort the image. Diffusion imaging is very good at identifying small infarcts, which may be helpful in determining subsequent patient management and search for risk factors (Ay *et al.* 1999; Wardlaw *et al.* 2000b). Hence there are problems with sensitivity and specificity and understanding exactly what diffusion imaging means, all of which require further study.

Perfusion-weighted MRI

Perfusion-weighted MRI (PWI) to examine the patency of the cerebral microcirculation can also be performed but, again, information from stroke patients so far is relatively limited (Baker *et al.* 1991; Zigun *et al.* 1993; Rother *et al.* 1994). Perfusion imaging is achieved either by using the magnetic properties of flowing blood ('arterial spin tagging'; Chalela *et al.* 2000), or by injecting an intravenous contrast agent, such as gadolinium, to identify parts of the brain with reduced blood flow through the capillary microcirculation (Rosen *et al.* 1989; Sorensen *et al.* 1999). The former technique is really still in development; the latter has been more widely used, but still only in small numbers of patients. Several parameters can be calculated from the images produced as the contrast passes through the brain (cerebral blood volume, mean transit time, cerebral blood flow) but these are all relative, not absolute. As the other MR techniques mentioned above, perfusion imaging is relatively difficult to apply in confused ischaemic stroke patients, but this problem will lessen with fast scan techniques and experience.

Perfusion imaging has demonstrated areas of reduced perfusion in patients in the expected areas of the brain within 6 h of the stroke when the T1 and T2 images were normal (Rother *et al.* 1994; Sorensen *et al.* 1999). It has been suggested that the difference between the extent of the lesion demonstrated on diffusion imaging and that on perfusion imaging may represent the reversibly damaged, potentially salvageable brain, or penumbra (so called 'perfusion-diffusion mismatch'). Knowledge of the extent of salvageable brain might, in future, be useful to guide the choice of acute stroke treatment, such as thrombolytic therapy. However, at present, the points about diffusion imaging made above suggest that this concept may be an oversimplification of the relatively complex processes taking place in the affected brain (Latchaw 1999). Thus, together with diffusion-weighted imaging, perfusion imaging may be a potentially useful way of identifying the degree of reduction in blood flow and the extent of any ischaemic penumbra in ischaemic stroke, but at present the techniques are relatively impractical, not widely available and insufficiently well understood to provide clear information routinely in stroke (Powers & Zivin 1998). Also, little thought has been given to any adverse effect that might arise from the use of gadolinium.

Magnetic resonance spectroscopy (MRS)

Magnetic resonance spectroscopy can demonstrate metabolic changes in ischaemic tissue *in vivo*, particularly hydrogen, phosphate, carbon, fluorine and sodium metabolism (Bottomley 1989; Baker *et al.* 1991; Howe *et al.* 1993; Ross & Michaelis 1994). *N*-acetyl aspartate (considered to be a marker of 'normal neurones'), creatine and phosphocreatine, choline-containing compounds, lactate and pH have all been measured in preliminary studies in stroke patients, but it is still too early to be certain of the significance of the changes (Howe *et al.* 1993; Saunders *et al.* 1995; Wardlaw *et al.* 1998b). MRS can be performed by either the single voxel (in which a small cubic volume of brain—typically 8 cm^3—is sampled) or by chemical shift imaging techniques (in which spectra from a whole slice of brain are obtained simultaneously) (Fig. 5.36). Both are relatively cumbersome and require the patient to keep still for up to 20 min. Our study, using mainly single voxel spectroscopy, suggested that the greater the reduction in the *N*-acetyl aspartate in the area of signal abnormality on T2, the worse the clinical outcome after the stroke (Wardlaw *et al.* 1998b). It may be possible to study the evolution of metabolite changes in ischaemic stroke and the response to drug treatment *in vivo* using these techniques.

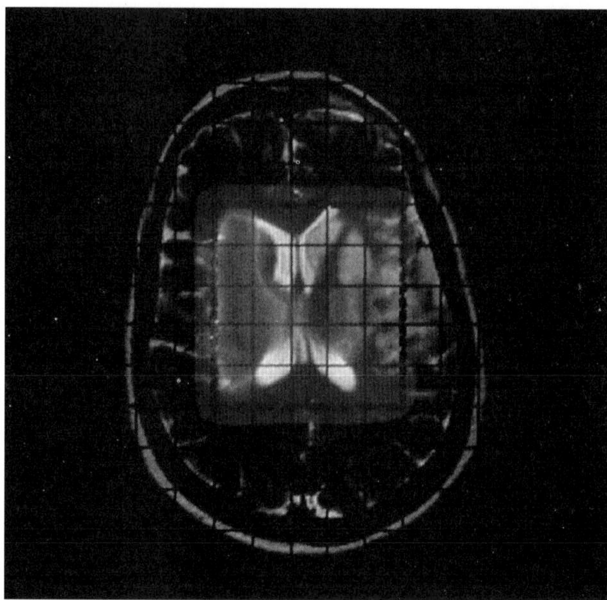

Fig. 5.36 Magnetic resonance spectroscopic chemical shift imaging at 2 days after stroke in a patient with an extensive left middle cerebral artery infarct. The T2 image is in the background and the spectroscopic colour image of the distribution of the normal neuronal metabolite *N*-acetyl aspartate is superimposed. Red indicates normal amounts of the normal metabolite and greens and blues indicate progressive absence of this metabolite. Note that the area of increased T2 signal of the infarct corresponds with the area of blue in keeping with neuronal loss. Also reproduced in colour; see colour plate facing p. 84.

Functional MR imaging (fMRI)

When a part of the cerebral cortex becomes metabolically active its blood flow increases, thereby changing the MR signal obtained from this volume of brain (Ellis 1993; Kwong 1995). For example, if the subject is asked to undertake a task, such as wriggling a finger, while in the MR scanner, and the MR prior to the movement is compared with the image during the task, the difference between the two demonstrates the area of cortex activated by the function. It is thought that areas of the brain which may perhaps be 'taking over'—or at least influencing in some way—the function of damaged areas, can be identified by their activation on fMRI, and the pattern of brain compensation to injury studied during recovery from ischaemic stroke or head injury, or in patients with brain tumours. However, the technique is difficult and great care is required to obtain meaningful results. The subject must keep his or her head very still and only perform (and think about) the requested task, because inadvertent movement of other parts of the body will show up on MR and be misleading. None the less, the technique shows promise by allowing insights into normal brain function as well as into recovery from injury.

5.3.10 Comparative studies of CT and MRI in acute stroke

There have been a few studies comparing the visibility of lesions on brain CT and MRI in acute stroke. Simmons *et al.* (1986), in a retrospective unblinded study, found that infarcts in the posterior fossa were visible in 14 of 14 patients using MR, compared with only seven of 14 on CT. The actual timing of the imaging (i.e. which was performed first) was not stated. Bryan *et al.* (1991), in a blinded study, found a visible relevant infarct in 82% (of 31 patients) on MR but in only 58% on CT within 24 h of stroke. However, the CT was performed on average 4 h *earlier* than the MR, so it is not surprising that MR showed more lesions. An infarct was visible in 88% on both techniques on repeat scan at 1 week. MR showed more areas of haemorrhage on the follow-up scans than CT. Both studies were very small and both technologies have advanced since then.

More recently, Mohr *et al.* (1995), in a prospective blinded study, identified patients within 3 h of stroke onset and compared the infarct visibility on CT and MRI obtained 'concurrently' (actually 8 min–11 h apart, CT usually first). In 80 patients, there were 78 infarcts (35 major and 11 minor hemispheric, 17 brainstem and 15 lacunar) and five haemorrhages. CT (non-contrast) and MR (T2- and proton density-weighted) were equal in their ability to demonstrate early infarction or haematoma despite the CT having the disadvantage of usually being performed first. Some patients with an initially positive CT or MR scan had returned to normal, neurologically, by 24 h, and CT was better than MR at predicting whether or not this neurological improvement occurred. There was a marginally significant correlation between early positive brain imaging by either modality and the severity of the stroke. Thus, although MR is more sensitive for posterior fossa and lacunar infarcts, CT is probably equally good at demonstrating early infarct changes in cortical strokes.

At present, 'routine' CT and MRI are probably equally good at demonstrating early cortical infarcts (except for very small ones) and primary intracerebral haemorrhage, but MRI is superior for lacunar, posterior fossa and probably small cortical infarcts. Whether MRI is 'better' than CT depends on the question being asked of imaging. MRI is certainly less practical and takes longer.

5.3.11 Other 'sophisticated' methods of imaging cerebral ischaemia

Single-photon emission CT (SPECT)

Single-photon emission CT is an isotope technique in which cross-sectional images of the brain are obtained by using either a rotating gamma-camera, or a dedicated SPECT scanner, and computerized reconstruction of the data from the emitted radiation following intravenous administration. Various isotopes are available, such as hexamethyl propylene amine oxime (HMPAO) (Ceretec), which images regional perfusion and therefore can identify areas of abnormal perfusion early, or xenon-133, which can measure regional cerebral blood flow quantitatively (Witt *et al.* 1991). However, the equipment to perform SPECT is not widely available, the scanning times are long (20 minutes or more) and so problems caused by movement artifacts can arise from restless stroke patients, and the isotopes are expensive. A potential source of error, which is particularly relevant to ischaemic stroke, is that blood–brain barrier breakdown alters the behaviour of the isotope and hence the accuracy and interpretation of the images (Merrick 1990).

SPECT can demonstrate appropriate areas of low flow within a few hours of stroke onset. Even in patients with a transient ischaemic attack, up to 60% will have an appropriate abnormality if examined within 24 h of onset (de Bruine *et al.* 1990). In acute ischaemic stroke, SPECT demonstrates an area of relative hypoperfusion corresponding with the ischaemic tissue in most patients studied, although very few if any lacunar stroke patients were included in these studies (Hayman *et al.* 1989; de Bruine *et al.* 1990; Limburg *et al.* 1990; Alexandrov *et al.* 1996; Baird *et al.* 1996; Barber *et al.* 1998). Several studies have indicated that the size of the initial perfusion deficit on SPECT is predictive of the likely clinical outcome—the larger the deficit, the worse the outcome (Limburg *et al.* 1990; Alexandrov *et al.* 1996; Baird *et al.* 1996; Barber *et al.* 1998; Berrouschot *et al.* 2000). Also, that evidence of reperfusion on SPECT is associated with an improved clinical outcome both spontaneously (Baird *et al.* 1996; Barber *et al.* 1998) and in response to thrombolytic therapy (Baird *et al.* 1994; Berrouschot *et al.* 2000; Ueda *et al.* 1999b).

In the first week after the stroke, the relative blood flow in the infarct may be increased or decreased, corresponding with luxury perfusion or persistent hypoperfusion, respectively (Morretti *et al.* 1990). It has also been shown that abnormalities are visible not only in the infarct itself, but also in remote parts of the brain, such as the opposite cerebral hemisphere or the contralateral cerebellum in cerebral cortical infarcts (Raynaud *et al.* 1989; Bowler *et al.* 1995; Infeld *et al.* 1995). This has given rise to the concept of 'diaschisis' or 'shut-down' of areas of the brain not directly involved in the infarct but whose function is in some way influenced, possibly through association fibres. There is some evidence of clinical correlates of 'shut-down' of these areas in terms of symptoms and signs not fully explained by loss of the area of brain directly involved in the infarct (Andrews 1991; Bowler *et al.* 1995).

Positron emission tomography (PET)

Positron emission tomography has the capability to depict a variety of physiological processes, from glucose metabolism to neuroreceptor density, thus allowing study of the normal workings of the brain, as well as the consequences of pathology. The data, derived from collection and analysis of complicated signals from positron-emitting isotopes, can be displayed as colour-coded tomographic pictures (Frackowiak 1985). PET has been available since the 1970s, but the imaging equipment and isotopes are extremely expensive, the scan times are prolonged and the patient must keep very still. Therefore PET is likely to remain a research tool with limited clinical applications for the foreseeable future (Dobkin & Mintun 1993). PET studies in ischaemic stroke have provided evidence that the ischaemic penumbra really does exist in humans and that neural tissue in the penumbra may survive for up to 48 h (Heiss 1992; Heiss *et al.* 1992; Baron *et al.* 1995; Baron 1999; Marchal *et al.* 1999). They have also suggested that neurones in areas of the brain with cerebral blood flow below the threshold traditionally regarded as producing irreversible damage (below 9 mL/100 g brain/min) may be able to recover after successful reperfusion with thrombolysis (Baron *et al.* 1995; Marchal *et al.* 1996; Heiss *et al.* 1997), although probably not below 8.43 mL/100 g brain/min (Marchal *et al.* 1999).

5.4 Differentiating haemorrhagic transformation of an infarct from primary intracerebral haemorrhage

Haemorrhagic transformation of an infarct (HTI) is an aspect of stroke pathophysiology which is particularly difficult to assess and there are many misconceptions about its clinical relevance. The exact frequency of HTI is almost impossible to measure because post-mortem studies are biased towards severe strokes and only give a 'snapshot' of the brain at the point of death, leaving one to speculate on events earlier in the course of the stroke. Imaging offers some improvement, although studies have been small and there has never been a published study where every patient had either a follow-up CT scan or a post-mortem, so they inevitably give a biased estimate of the frequency of HTI and its clinical associations (see below). More information on risk factors, the influence of antithrombotic treatment and the role of reperfusion will become available from the present randomized trials of antithrombotic and thrombolytic treatments (sections 11.3, 11.4 and 11.5).

HTI can usefully be thought of as being either asymptomatic (i.e. picked up on repeat brain imaging but not associated with worsening of symptoms) or symptomatic (definite deterioration in symptoms associated with the appearance of new haemorrhage into an infarct on imaging). HTI is also described as 'petechial' (little areas of patchy haemorrhage without frank haematoma) or as a haematoma, although definitions vary, which accounts for some of the variability of HTI frequency in published studies.

Appearance of haemorrhagic transformation of an infarct on CT or MR

Typically, HTI is distinguished from primary intracerebral haemorrhage (PICH) by the lack of homogeneity of the haemorrhagic area which lies within, or on the edge of an area of low density confined to a single arterial territory, i.e. within a presumed infarct. However, it is clear that some cases which appear radiologically to be parenchymal haematomas are actually caused by HTI occurring within hours of stroke onset, the so-called intra-infarct haematomas (Bogousslavsky *et al.* 1991). Indeed, the HTI can look so like a PICH that, without a prior scan showing no haemorrhage, the patient would have been labelled as PICH. The extent of this problem will become clearer with more experience of early scanning. Currently, however, there are no absolute rules for distinguishing those early HTIs which obliterate the infarct, from a 'true' PICH.

> *Haemorrhagic transformation of an infarct can occur very early after stroke onset and makes the infarct look just like a primary intracerebral haemorrhage on brain CT.*

The more commonly seen forms of HTI consist of serpiginous areas of increased density (whiteness) on CT (or of appropriate signal characteristics on MR) at the margins of the infarct (Fig. 5.37); more obvious patchy areas of increased density throughout the infarct; or frank haematomas exerting mass effect (Fig. 5.38). In large infarcts involving the cortex, curvilinear bands of increased density may be seen at the cortical edge, at the junction of the lesion with white matter and within the lesion in the second and third weeks after the stroke. These areas also enhance markedly when X-ray contrast is given (Davis *et al.* 1977) and are thought to correspond with areas where the capillaries are leaky, where there is blood–brain barrier breakdown and where there is frank petechial haemorrhage at post-mortem (Inoue *et al.* 1980).

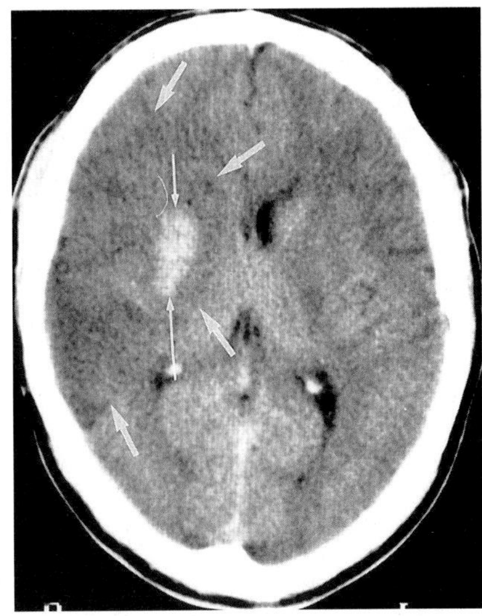

Fig. 5.37 CT brain scan showing petechial haemorrhage (thin arrows) into a right temporoparietal infarct (thick arrows) obtained at 36 h after the stroke. The haemorrhage was not particularly dense, unlike a haematoma (see also Fig. 5.30).

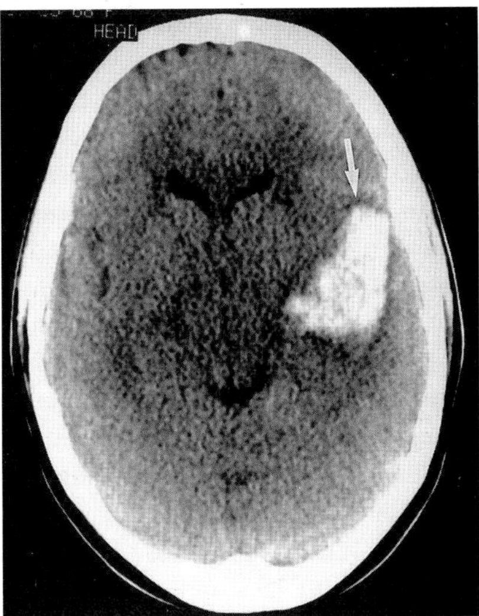

Fig. 5.38 CT brain scan showing very early haemorrhagic transformation of a left temporal arterial infarct. The CT scan was obtained within 3 h of onset of a right hemiparesis and shows a fairly dense haematoma in the left temporal region (arrow). Angiography immediately after the scan showed the proximal left middle cerebral artery mainstem to be occluded by an embolus with dilated lenticulostriate arteries (collateral supply). The source of the embolus was never found. A repeat angiogram at 2 months showed that the left MCA had recanalized.

The influence of observer variability and visual perception

Some of the variability in the reported frequency of petechial haemorrhage must be a result of inter-observer variation, but this is less likely to apply to focal parenchymal haematomas (Wardlaw & Sellar 1994; Rimdusid *et al.* 1995; Motto *et al.* 1997). The visual perception of the density of normal brain is influenced by the density of adjacent tissue; normal brain next to the low density of an infarct looks of higher density than it really is, and so can be mistaken for areas of haemorrhage (Fig. 5.39). To avoid this mistake, the density of the brain can be measured on the CT console to distinguish petechial haemorrhage from normal brain.

Frequency of haemorrhagic transformation of an infarct

Studies using CT and MR scanning have suggested that some degree of petechial haemorrhage occurs in 15–45% of patients and of symptomatic haematoma formation in about 5%, at some point within the 1–2 weeks after stroke (Lodder 1984; Hornig *et al.* 1986, 1993; Okada *et al.* 1989). This may be an under- or overestimate for the following reasons: the studies were all small and few were of consecutive patients or prospective; not all patients were followed-up, only survivors or those who remained in hospital for the study period; the definition of HTI was not stated in all the publications; the influence of inter-observer variability was not taken into account; the generation of scanner used varied

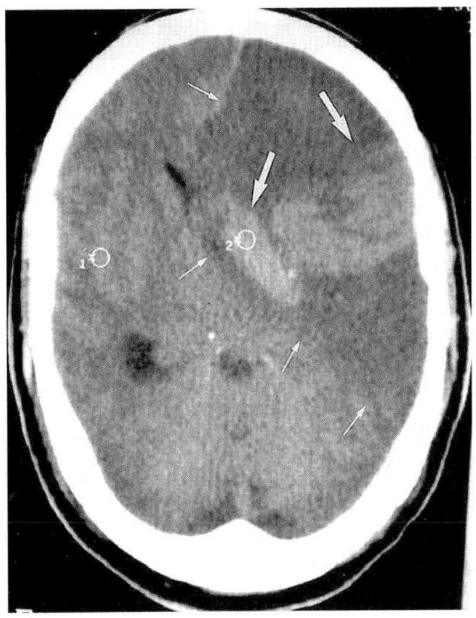

Fig. 5.39 CT brain scan to illustrate the effect of altered brain density on visual perception. The scan was obtained from a 40-year-old man at 24 h after a left middle cerebral artery occlusion causing an extensive left hemispheric infarct (thin arrows). The areas of hyperdensity (thick arrows) within the low density of the infarct were interpreted by the clinician as being caused by haemorrhage because of their apparent brightness. However, the actual density when measured on the CT scanning console was the same as normal grey matter, indicating that the areas of hyperdensity were in fact islands of surviving, i.e. non-infarcted, brain and not haemorrhage at all. Area 1 (normal right insular cortex) was 51 Hounsfield units (HU—the units for measurement of density on CT) and area 2 (apparent increased density within the left infarct) was 46 HU. Blood generally registers at around 70–80 HU.

and hence the sensitivity of the diagnosis of HTI; and the number of patients given antithrombotic drugs was often not stated. Thus, it is very difficult to establish the true frequency of HTI from the published studies.

Some information is available from the control groups of the recent randomized trials of thrombolytic and antithrombotic drugs, such as the Multicentre Acute Stroke Trial—Italy (MAST-I) Group (1995) and the International Stroke Trial (International Stroke Trial Collaborative Group 1997), but even so not all patients had a follow-up scan (or post-mortem). In MAST-I, 69 of the 622 patients randomized died and did not have a second CT scan or post-mortem (MAST-I 1995). In 10% of the control patients the infarct became haemorrhagic but without symptoms by 5 days when follow-up CT was performed, and in 1% the HTI was symptomatic. This finding is reasonably consistent with data from all the control groups of the completed thrombolysis trials (total $n = 2499$) in which symptomatic intracranial haemorrhage occurred in 63/2499 (2.5%) and fatal intracranial haemorrhage in 21/2076 (1%) in patients systematically CT scanned at around 2–5 days after stroke (Wardlaw *et al.* 2000a).

Factors associated with haemorrhagic transformation of an infarct and its clinical relevance

This is also somewhat difficult to establish from published studies, which have so far tended to be small and possibly biased. However, the available evidence suggests that HTI is more frequent in large infarcts (and therefore possibly after cardioembolic stroke) and that its occurrence is associated with a worse clinical outcome (Lodder 1984; Hart & Easton 1986; Hornig *et al.* 1986; Beghi *et al.* 1989; Okada *et al.* 1989; Bozzao *et al.* 1992; Lindley *et al.* 1992; Pessin *et al.* 1992; Rimdusid *et al.* 1995). The relationship with raised blood pressure is uncertain.

Influence of antithrombotic drugs

Haemorrhagic transformation can occur spontaneously in patients treated without anticoagulants (Bogousslavsky & Regli 1985; Ott *et al.* 1986). Patients with HTI have even continued on anticoagulants without any worsening of the haemorrhage, or symptomatic deterioration (Ott *et al.* 1986; Dickmann *et al.* 1988; Pessin *et al.* 1992; Keir *et al.* 2000). Some non-randomized series have found little apparent effect on the risk of haemorrhage with antithrombotic treatment (Chamorro *et al.* 1994; Vemmos *et al.* 1994). The recently updated Cochrane systematic review of antiplatelet drugs in acute ischaemic stroke (which included data from the International and Chinese Acute Stroke Trials) found that aspirin increased the rate of symptomatic intracranial haemorrhage by two per 1000 patients treated, but this was more than offset by a reduction in recurrent ischaemic stroke of seven per 1000 and an increase in patients who were alive and independent at the end of follow-up of 13 per 1000 treated (Gubitz *et al.* 2000b). The recently updated Cochrane systematic review of anticoagulants in acute ischaemic stroke (also including data from the International Stroke Trial) found an increase in symptomatic intracranial haemorrhage of nine per 1000 patients treated, which was not offset by any reduction in recurrent ischaemic strokes (also nine per 1000), nor was there any net benefit in functional outcome (Gubitz *et al.* 2000a).

Possible mechanisms of haemorrhagic transformation of an infarct

Traditionally, HTI was considered to occur when an arterial occlusion, usually cardioembolic in origin, resulted in ischaemia of the distal capillary bed and then, when fragmentation of the embolus occurred, this ischaemic area was subjected to arterial pressure, resulting in rupture of the necrotic arterioles and capillaries (Fisher & Adams 1951). This arose from work with post-mortem brains, but is biased towards patients who die in the early stages of their stroke and who are therefore more likely to have had a large cerebral infarct. The signs of haemorrhage resolve with time so that, in patients dying weeks or months after their stroke, it may no longer be possible to distinguish the relative contribution of infarct and haemorrhage in the residual lesion.

The post-mortem studies of Fisher and Adams (1951) suggested that in most cases of HTI the cause of infarction was an embolus (they did not specify the origin) which had broken up and moved distally, exposing the ischaemic tissue to arterial blood pressure, leading to haemorrhage. Of 373 brains with vascular occlusion (123 with presumed embolism, 89 with presumed *in situ* thrombosis and 161 of uncertain cause), 66 had haemorrhagic infarction and in 63 there was evidence of embolism as the cause of stroke. They did not discuss the possibility that some of their infarcts with open arteries might have been caused by venous thrombosis, nor did they say how the evidence of embolism was obtained.

The idea that embolism is the cause of HTI has become rather entrenched, to the point of HTI being used in some studies as diagnostic of embolic (usually implied cardiac origin) stroke (Lodder *et al.* 1986). Closer examination of the literature on HTI shows that the situation is more complicated than the reperfusion–haemorrhagic transformation hypothesis would suggest (Pessin *et al.* 1992). Shortly before Fisher and Adam's (1951) work became so widely publicized and accepted, Globus and Epstein (1953) published the results of experimental cerebral infarction in monkeys and dogs and some observations on post-mortem brains from stroke patients. They observed that haemorrhage into infarcted tissue was often worse when the occluded symptomatic artery *remained* occluded, and that the haemorrhage seemed to occur around the periphery of the infarct from collateral arterioles and postcapillary venules vasodilating to supply the ischaemic tissue and then leaking. They produced massive intracerebral haemorrhages in dogs by this means, although they noted differences between the species which seemed to depend on the adequacy of the collateral supply. This alternative, but possibly equally attractive, hypothesis has been all but forgotten, although it probably deserves further attention.

There is still debate about the effect of recanalization and so reperfusion of an infarct. Previously, it was accepted that early recanalization, such as might occur with spontaneous lysis of an embolus, increased the risk of haemorrhagic transformation. However, several recent studies have contradicted this, suggesting that haemorrhage is more common into infarcts where the artery remains occluded, as shown by catheter angiography (Ogata 1989; Mori *et al.* 1990, 1992; Bozzao *et al.* 1992; Pessin *et al.* 1992). Berrouschot *et al.* (2000) studied 52 patients, randomized in the second European Cooperative Acute Stroke Study of intravenous recombinant tissue plasminogen activator (rt-PA). Using single photon emission computed tomography (SPECT), they found that patients with major proximal middle cerebral artery occlusion and poor collaterals (i.e. very poor perfusion of the infarct) who did not reperfuse were the most likely to suffer haemorrhagic transformation of the infarct; in those in the placebo group the haemorrhage was less extensive than in those who received rt-PA. Patients with evidence of reperfusion of the infarct on SPECT were *less* likely to have haemorrhagic transformation. Thus it would appear that, contrary to previous thinking, haemorrhagic transformation is more likely to occur in the absence rather than the presence of reperfusion, but there are obviously still many unanswered questions about the causes, associated factors and clinical significance of HTI.

Haemorrhagic transformation of an infarct is more likely in patients who do not recanalize the occluded artery, as opposed to those who do, contrary to previous thinking.

5.5 Intracranial venous thrombosis

The advent of non-invasive brain imaging in the 1980s has resulted in increased recognition of intracranial venous thrombosis (ICVT). Before then, only physicians with a high index of suspicion considered the diagnosis in patients with otherwise unexplained headache, focal deficits, seizures, impaired consciousness, or combinations of these features (Bousser *et al.* 1985).

5.5.1 Predisposing factors

Unlike arterial thrombosis, damage to the vessel wall is a causal factor in only about 10% of patients with ICVT; the underlying disease condition consists of infection, infiltration, or trauma (Bousser & Ross Russell 1997). More important are disorders of coagulation (70%) (Bousser & Ross Russell 1997) (Table 5.5). The most common inherited coagulation defect is factor V Leiden mutation, which is found in some 20% of patients without other obvious causes (Martinelli *et al.* 1996; Zuber *et al.* 1996; Lüdemann *et al.* 1998). The third component of Virchow's triad of causes of thrombosis, stagnant flow, contributes no more than a few per cent (associated with dehydration or with dural puncture, sometimes in combination with hyperosmolar contrast agents). In 20% of patients no contributing factors can be identified and the cause remains shrouded in mystery. Perhaps as yet undiscovered prothrombotic mutations are responsible to some extent.

Often there is no single cause but a combination of contributing factors, for example the post-partum period and protein S deficiency (Galan *et al.* 1995), pregnancy and Behçet's disease (Wechsler *et al.* 1995), oral contraceptives and the factor V Leiden mutation (Dulli *et al.* 1996; de Bruijn *et al.* 1998a), or the same combinations with dural puncture as a third factor (Wilder-Smith *et al.* 1997). The risk of ICVT in the post-partum period increases with maternal age, and with Caesarean section (Lanska & Kryscio 1997, 1998).

In neonates, ICVT is usually associated with acute systemic illness, such as shock or dehydration; in older children the most frequent underlying conditions are local infection (the leading cause until the antibiotic era), coagulopathy (Barron *et al.* 1992; Lancon *et al.* 1999) and—more in Mediterranean countries—Behçet's disease (Saatci *et al.* 1996).

5.5.2 Clinical features

The clinical features consist essentially of headache, focal neurological deficits, epileptic seizures and impairment of consciousness, in different combinations and degrees of severity. The symptoms and signs depend to some extent on which vein is affected, and to an important extent on whether the thrombotic process is limited to the dural sinus or extends to the cortical veins (Bousser & Ross Russell 1997).

In the case of the superior sagittal sinus, which is the one affected in 70–80% of cases, (Ameri & Bousser 1992; Daif *et al.* 1995), sinus thrombosis alone leads to the syndrome of *intracranial hypertension*, i.e. headache and papilloedema. Patients with so-called 'benign intracranial hypertension' (BIH) may in fact have sinus thrombosis; they are more often non-obese or male, but are otherwise indistinguishable from patients with idiopathic BIH (Tehindrazanarivelo *et al.* 1992). Papilloedema can cause transient visual obscurations and sometimes irreversible constriction of the visual fields, beginning in the inferonasal quadrants (Bousser *et al.* 1985). The increased pressure of the cerebrospinal fluid (CSF) may also give rise to VIth nerve palsies, and sometimes to other

Table 5.5 Causal factors in the pathogenesis of intracranial venous thrombosis in adults. (Adapted from Bousser & Ross Russell 1997.)

Prothrombotic states
Pregnancy, puerperium (Cantú & Barinagarrementeria 1993) (section 7.14)

Hereditary coagulopathies
Protein S deficiency (Heistinger *et al.* 1992) (section 7.9)
Antithrombin III deficiency (Sauron *et al.* 1982) (section 7.9)
Factor II (prothrombin) gene mutations (20210 G A) (Biousse *et al.* 1998; Huberfeld *et al.* 1998; Kellett *et al.* 1998; Reuner *et al.* 1998) (section 7.9)
Factor V gene mutations (factor V Leiden) (Martinelli *et al.* 1996; Zuber *et al.* 1996; Lüdemann *et al.* 1998) (section 7.9)
von Willebrand's disease
5,10 methylene tetrahydrofolate reductase (MTHFR) mutation (677 C T) (Hillier *et al.* 1998)
Homocystinuria (Mohamed *et al.* 1991; Cochran & Packman 1992) (section 7.20)
Familial thrombophilia of unknown nature (Kakar *et al.* 1998)

Coagulopathies secondary to blood dyscrasias
Thrombocythaemia (Haan *et al.* 1988) (section 7.9)
Primary polycythaemia (Haan *et al.* 1988; Kyritsis *et al.* 1990) (section 7.9)
Paroxysmal nocturnal haemoglobinuria (Hillmen *et al.* 1995; Hauser *et al.* 1996; Johnson *et al.* 1970) (section 7.9)
Iron deficiency anaemia (Stehle *et al.* 1991) (section 7.9)
Sickle cell disease (Vernant *et al.* 1988) (section 7.9)
Disseminated intravascular coagulation (Bousser & Ross Russell 1997) (section 7.9)
After bone marrow transplantation (Bertz *et al.* 1998) (section 7.12)

Coagulopathies secondary to systemic disease
Behçet's disease (Wechsler *et al.* 1992; Fenwick *et al.* 1997) (section 7.3)
Carcinoma (breast, prostate) (Sigsbee *et al.* 1979; Hickey *et al.* 1982) (section 7.12)
Lymphoma (Bousser *et al.* 1985; Meininger *et al.* 1985)
Systemic lupus erythematosus (Vidailhet *et al.* 1990) (section 7.3)
Nephrotic syndrome (Bousser *et al.* 1985) (section 7.9)
Systemic vasculitis not covered above (section 7.3)
Ulcerative colitis (Das *et al.* 1996), or Crohn's disease (Keller *et al.* 1999) (section 7.17)
Antiphospholipid syndrome (Carhuapoma *et al.* 1997) (section 7.3)

Coagulopathies caused by drugs
Oral contraceptives (3rd generation > 2nd) (de Bruijn *et al.* 1998a,b) (section 7.13.1)
Corticosteroids
Dihydroergotamine (Evans *et al.* 1996)
Androgens (Jaillard *et al.* 1994)
Ecstasy (Rothwell & Grant 1993) (section 7.15)

Coagulopathies secondary to local infection or infiltration
Otitis (Reading & Schurr 1956)
Sinusitis (Southwick *et al.* 1986)
Dental abscess
Tonsillitis
Obstruction by tumour (Plant *et al.* 1991)

Coagulopathies secondary to general infection or infiltration
Uveomeningitis
Sarcoidosis (Byrne & Lawton 1983) (section 7.3)
Chronic meningitis
Subdural empyema
Carcinomatous meningitis

Dural puncture
Epidural anaesthesia
Metrizamide myelography
Diagnostic tap

Trauma (Kinal 1967)

Unknown (20%)

cranial nerve deficits. The onset of the headache is usually gradual, but in up to 15% of patients it is sudden, which may initially suggest the diagnosis of a ruptured aneurysm (de Bruijn *et al.* 1996) (section 5.6.2).

Involvement of *cortical veins* causes one or more areas of venous infarction, with or without haemorrhagic transformation. If the affected veins drain into the sagittal sinus, the venous infarcts are typically located near the midline in the parasagittal and parieto-occipital regions, often on both sides. In the case of the lateral sinus, the venous infarct is usually located in the posterior temporal area (Wardlaw *et al.* 1998c). If the thrombotic process extends to the petrosal sinus, the Vth or VIth cranial nerves may be affected, and with jugular vein thrombosis the IXth to XIth cranial nerves (Bousser & Ross Russell 1997).

Clinically, the infarcts present with epileptic seizures or with focal deficits, such as hemiparesis or aphasia. If unilateral weakness develops (with thrombosis originating in the superior sagittal sinus), it tends to predominate in the leg, in keeping with the parasagittal location of most venous infarcts. Obstruction of cortical veins draining into the posterior part of the superior sagittal sinus, or into the lateral sinus, will relatively often lead to hemianopia, aphasia, or a confusional state. Impairment of consciousness may result from multiple lesions in the cerebral hemispheres, or from transtentorial herniation and compression of the brainstem. Either epilepsy or a focal deficit is a presenting feature in 10–15% of patients (Cantú & Barinagarrementeria 1993); during the course of the illness seizures occur in 10–60% of reported series, and focal deficits in 30–80% (Ameri & Bousser 1992; Cantú & Barinagarrementeria 1993; Daif *et al.* 1995; Tsai *et al.* 1995).

Involvement of the *cortical veins alone*, without sinus thrombosis and its associated signs of increased CSF pressure, is rare but can present as 'stroke' and so may have been under-recognized (Ameri & Bousser 1992; Cantú & Barinagarrementeria 1993). Recently, four such cases have been published together, from different centres (Jacobs *et al.* 1996). Thrombosis of the *deep venous system*, including the great vein of Galen, may lead to bilateral haemorrhagic infarction of the corpus striatum, thalamus, hypothalamus, the ventral corpus callosum, the medial occipital lobe and the upper part of the cerebellum (Ur Rahman & Al Tahan 1993). Needless to say, in those cases the clinical picture is dominated by coma and disturbance of eye movements and pupillary reflexes. Partial syndromes exist and can be survived, sometimes with surprisingly few sequelae (Haley *et al.* 1989; Ameri & Bousser 1992; Baumgartner & Landis 1992). Thrombosis of *cerebellar veins* leads to clinical features resembling those with arterial territory infarcts in the cerebellum (dominated by headache, vertigo, vomiting and ataxia, sometimes followed by impaired consciousness), but with a more gradual onset (Bousser *et al.* 1985; Eng *et al.* 1990; Nayak *et al.* 1994).

5.5.3 Investigations

Non-filling of a sinus, or part of it, on a catheter angiogram is in itself insufficient proof of venous thrombosis. Hypoplasia is an alternative explanation, especially in the case of the left lateral sinus or the anterior third of the superior sagittal sinus. To prove occlusion of a sinus, it is necessary to see delayed emptying or dilatation of collateral veins on the angiogram, or to see evidence of thrombus on CT scanning or MRI (see below and section 5.3.5). In most centres in the western world, MR angiography (MRA) has replaced catheter angiography, especially as MRA in combination with other MR techniques can show the thrombus itself (Lafitte *et al.* 1997) (Fig. 5.40).

Brain CT will readily show 'venous' infarcts: not corresponding with a known arterial territory (Figs 5.20, 5.21); often with haemorrhagic transformation; sometimes bilaterally, in the parasagittal area (Fig. 5.41) or in the deep regions of the brain (Fig. 5.13), or supra- as well as infratentorial (Wardlaw *et al.* 1998c). In addition, CT scanning often provides evidence of the underlying sinus thrombosis: the hyperdense sinus sign or the empty delta sign. Hyperdensity of a venous sinus, on a non-contrast CT scan, through filling with fresh thrombus is seen most clearly in the posterior part of the sagittal sinus ('dense triangle sign') or in the straight sinus (Fig. 5.13). The 'empty delta sign' (Buonanno *et al.* 1978) appears only after injection of intravenous contrast material, through which enhancement occurs of the wall but not in the thrombus in the centre of the (posterior) part of the sagittal sinus that is perpendicularly imaged on an axial CT slice (Fig. 5.42). The name of this sign easily sticks in the mind but it is found in only a small number of patients (Bousser *et al.* 1985).

The way in which evidence of thrombus in dural sinuses appears on MR imaging depends very much on the interval from the time the thrombus began to form (Dormont *et al.* 1994; Isensee *et al.* 1994; Bianchi *et al.* 1998). Three stages can be distinguished in the evolution of thrombus. In the acute stage (days 1–5) it appears strongly hypointense on T2-weighted images and isointense on T1-weighted images (rather as for arterial thrombi, Figs 5.28, 5.40). In the subacute stage (up to day 15) the thrombus signal is strongly hyperintense, initially on T1-weighted images and subsequently also on T2-weighted images. The third stage begins 3–4 weeks after symptom onset: the thrombus signal becomes isointense on T1-weighted images but on T2-weighted images it remains hyperintense, although often non-homogeneous. Recanalization may occur over months in up to one-third of patients, but persistent abnormalities are common and do not signify recurrent thrombosis (Dormont *et al.* 1994; Mas *et al.* 1992). In the brain parenchyma, early changes of venous congestion can be demonstrated on T2-weighted images or with fluid attenuated inversion recovery (FLAIR) techniques, while diffusion-weighted images show only subtle changes, unlike ischaemia from arterial occlusion (Corvol *et al.* 1998; Keller *et al.* 1999).

It is unlikely that many clinicians will rely on ultrasound techniques alone for making the diagnosis of ICVT. Transcranial Doppler with colour coding and contrast enhancement may show decreased, increased or reversed venous flow parallel to the major intracranial sinuses (Wardlaw *et al.* 1994), abnormal flow velocities in the transverse sinus or in the deep venous system (Ries *et al.* 1992; Stolz *et al.* 1999; Valdueza *et al.* 1999), but a normal test far from excludes the diagnosis.

5.6 Subarachnoid haemorrhage

Subarachnoid haemorrhage (SAH) refers to the spontaneous extravasation of blood into the subarachnoid space when a blood vessel near the surface of the brain leaks. It is a condition, not a disease, which has many causes (section 9.1). Although, as described above (section 5.3.1), the clinical distinction of stroke caused by cerebral infarction and intracerebral haemorrhage is unreliable and imaging must be relied upon for diagnosis, the clinical features of SAH are reasonably distinct, and at least this type of stroke can be diagnosed clinically with reasonable confidence. However, confirmatory investigations are needed in almost all cases (section 5.6.3).

5.6.1 Clinical features

Blood in the subarachnoid space is a meningeal irritant and incites a typical clinical response, regardless of aetiology. Patients usually complain of headache, photophobia, stiff neck and nausea, and they may also vomit. Confusion, restlessness and impaired consciousness are also frequent (Table 5.6).

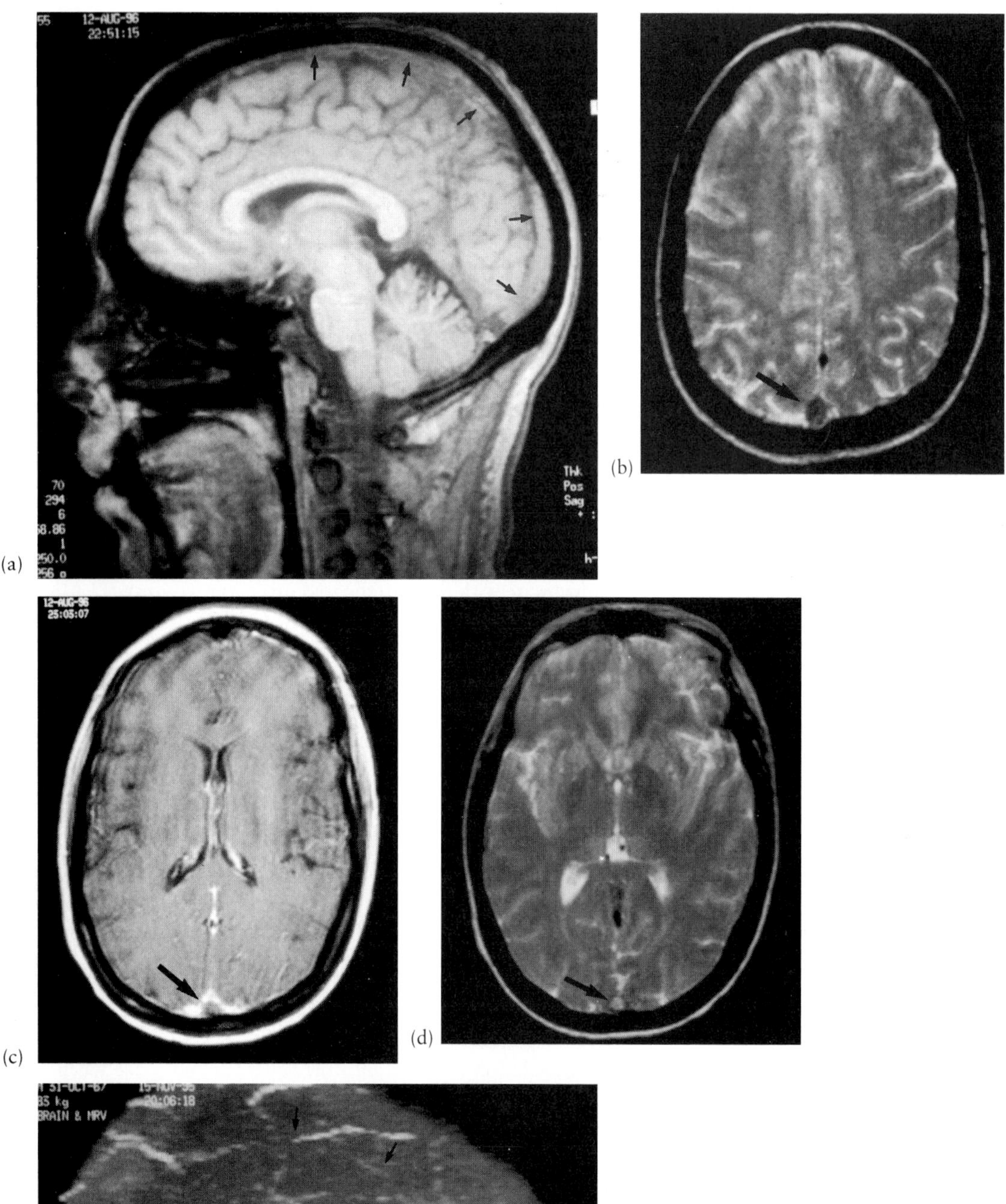

(a) (b) (c) (d) (e)

Fig. 5.40 Magnetic resonance imaging and MR venography of intracranial venous thrombosis. (a) Midline sagittal T1 shows that the normal flow void is replaced by increased signal because of recent venous thrombosis in the sagittal sinus (arrows). (b) Axial T2 shows that the normal flow void in the sagittal sinus (arrow) has been replaced by increased signal (of intermediate intensity) and the sinus appears expanded. (c) T1 image post-intravenous gadolinium shows a filling defect in the sagittal sinus (arrow), the equivalent of the 'empty delta sign' on CT (see also Fig. 5.42). (d) Axial T2 image several days after the image in (b) above, shows that the signal of the thrombus in the sagittal sinus has increased and is now more obvious as the thrombus ages (arrow). (e) MR venography shows some cortical veins and the deep cerebral veins, but the sagittal sinus is completely absent (arrows show the line of where the sinus should be).

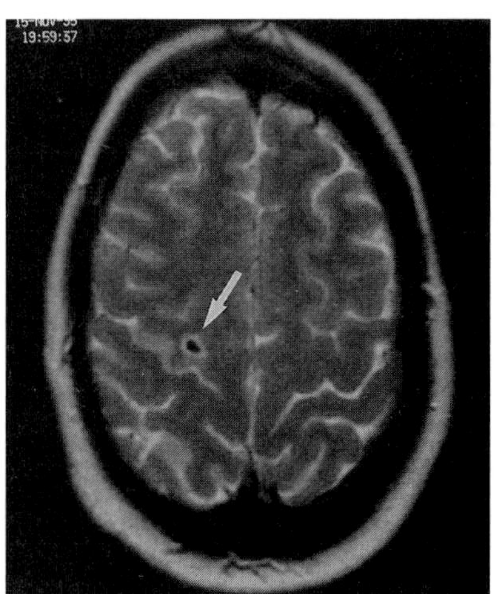

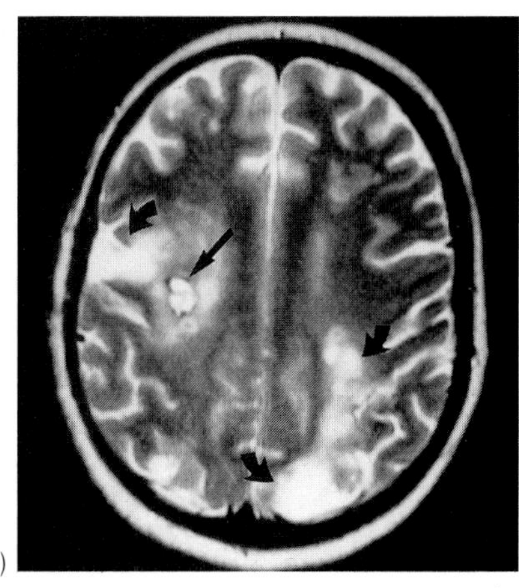

Fig. 5.41 T2 MR images from two different patients to illustrate parasagittal haematomas found in venous sinus thrombosis. (a) A patient with sagittal sinus thrombosis and a small haemorrhage in the right parasagittal parietal cortex (arrow). (b) Another patient with sagittal sinus thrombosis and a right parasagittal haemorrhage (arrow) and infarcts in the left occipital and right parietal regions (curved arrows). Note that in neither case was there an obvious filling defect in the sagittal sinus on T2. (a) (b)

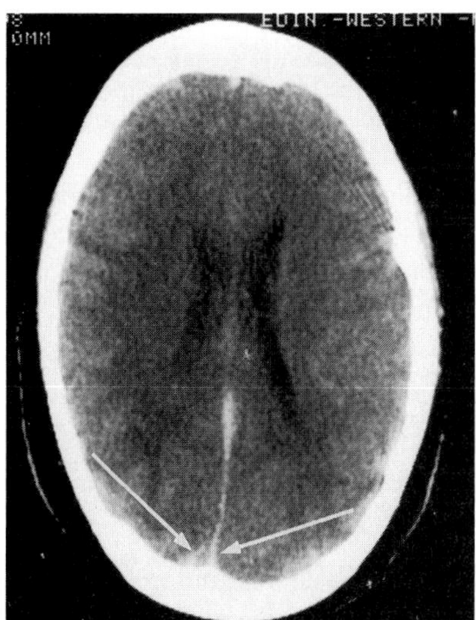

Fig. 5.42 CT brain scan with intravenous contrast shows a triangular filling defect outlined by contrast in the posterior sagittal sinus ('empty delta sign')—arrows (see also Fig. 5.40).

Table 5.6 Diagnosis of subarachnoid haemorrhage.

Principal symptoms
Headache: usually sudden, maximal in seconds, severe, and occipital or retro-orbital; duration: hours (possibly minutes?) to weeks
Nausea
Vomiting
Neck stiffness
Photophobia
Loss of consciousness

Neurological signs
None (very often)
Meningism
Focal neurological signs: IIIrd nerve palsy (posterior communicating artery aneurysm), dysphasia, hemiparesis (arteriovenous malformation, intracerebral haematoma)
Subhyaloid haemorrhages in optic fundi
Fever
Raised blood pressure
Limitation of straight leg raising/Kernig's sign
Altered consciousness

Headache

Headache is the cardinal clinical feature of subarachnoid haemorrhage (SAH). It is the *only* symptom in about one-third of patients (Linn *et al.* 1994, 1998), but a symptom at some stage in 85–100% of patients (Walton 1956; Sarner & Rose 1967; Kopitnik & Samson 1993; Vestergaard *et al.* 1993; Kumral *et al.* 1995). In a consecutive series of 92 patients with SAH caused by ruptured aneurysm, in whom the onset of the headache was recorded, 62 (67%) had headache as the first symptom, the others lost consciousness immediately (van Gijn *et al.* 1985).

The headache arises suddenly, classically in a *split second*, 'like a blow on the head' or 'an explosion inside the head', reaching a maximum within seconds. Of the 62 patients reported above with headache as the first symptom, 54 (87%) had an explosive onset of headache. In the other eight patients, the headache came on more gradually, in minutes rather than seconds. Headache of gradual onset occurs more commonly in patients with non-aneurysmal perimesencephalic SAH, i.e. in about 20% of patients, compared with 13% with aneurysmal SAH (Rinkel *et al.* 1991; Wijdicks *et al.* 1998) (section 9.2.4).

A biphasic headache may occur in patients whose SAH is caused by dissection of a vertebral artery (section 9.1.3): first, a severe occipital headache radiating from the back of the neck, followed after an interval of hours or days by sudden exacerbation of the headache but of a more diffuse type.

In SAH, the headache is generally diffuse and poorly localized but tends to spread over minutes to hours to the back of the head, neck and back as blood tracks down into the spinal subarachnoid space. Sometimes the headache is maximal behind the eyes. The headache is often described by patients as the most severe headache they have ever had, but it can occasionally be milder. It is the suddenness of onset which is most characteristic.

More often than not, there is no obvious precipitating factor (Matsuda *et al.* 1993). Amongst the 33 patients with SAH in the Oxfordshire Community Stroke Project (OCSP), six (18%) occurred while resting (none occurred while asleep), 13 (39%) during moderate activity, and six (18%) during strenuous activity, such as weight-lifting and sexual intercourse; the activity at onset was not known in the other eight patients (Wroe *et al.* 1992). In more recent series, similar and higher proportions (up to 50%) of aneurysmal SAHs have occurred during physical exertion (Ferro & Pinto 1994; Linn *et al.* 1998; Wijdicks *et al.* 1998).

The headache usually lasts 1–2 weeks, sometimes longer. Perhaps it may last only a few hours, or even less, if there has been a small leak of blood, in which case there may be no other associated symptoms, such as neck stiffness. It is not known exactly how short in duration a headache may be and still be a result of SAH. However, we have not encountered anyone with a headache caused by SAH that resolved within an hour. Nevertheless, it is conceivable that this may occur, and so it is perhaps best to consider SAH in anyone with a sudden unusually severe headache, even if it resolves within minutes, particularly if there is any impairment of consciousness.

It is not uncommon in clinical practice to encounter patients who describe having had a severe headache of sudden onset 3 weeks (or more) ago, sounding very much like a SAH, which resolved after a few hours or days. It is then extremely difficult to know what action to take, because decisions about investigation for an aneurysm can then only be based on the patient's history rather than the brain CT or cerebrospinal fluid examination (section 9.4.7).

A history of previous episodes of sudden-onset headache ('sentinel headaches') is generally believed to be common in patients with aneurysmal SAH and is often attributed to a 'warning' leak. However, the notion of frequent 'minor leaks' does not really hold up (section 9.2.3).

> *It is doubtful whether patients with aneurysmal subarachnoid haemorrhage often have preceding and unrecognized 'warning leaks'. Whatever the case, doctors must consider subarachnoid haemorrhage in any patient who reports a sudden severe headache.*

Vomiting

Vomiting (and nausea) is common at the outset, in contrast to other differential diagnoses, such as migraine, in which vomiting more often occurs after the headache starts.

Neck stiffness

Meningism refers to painful resistance to passive or voluntary neck flexion because of irritation of the cervical meninges by subarachnoid blood, or by inflammation. This sign can be elicited in the supine patient by placing both hands behind the patient's head and, as one attempts to lift the head up off the pillow, the patient does not allow the neck to be flexed and so the examiner lifts the patient's head, neck and shoulders off the bed, as if the patient were like a board. In contrast, passive rotation of the neck is achieved with ease.

Neck stiffness caused by meningism is a common symptom and sign of blood in the subarachnoid space, but it does not occur immediately; it takes some 3–12 h and may not develop at all in deeply unconscious patients, or in patients with minor SAH (Vermeulen & van Gijn 1990) (section 9.3.1). Therefore, its absence cannot exclude the diagnosis of SAH in a patient with sudden headache. Brudzinski's sign (flexion at the hip and knee in response to forward flexion of the neck) is also caused by blood in the subarachnoid space but is less reliable.

Pain and stiffness in the back and legs may follow SAH after some hours or days because blood irritates the lumbosacral nerve roots. Kernig's sign (passive extension of the knee with the hip flexed elicits pain in the back and leg and resistance to hamstring stretch) is a sign of inflammation or blood around the lumbosacral nerve roots, but is seldom present without obvious meningism.

Photophobia

Patients are often photophobic and irritable for several days after SAH, presumably as a result of meningeal irritation by the blood.

Loss of consciousness

Loss of consciousness occurred in 50% of patients with presumed aneurysmal SAH who were well enough to be entered into a clinical trial of medical treatment (Vermeulen *et al.* 1984). As these figures do not include the 10–12% of patients with SAH who die at home or during transportation to hospital (Linn *et al.* 1994; Schievink *et al.* 1995), or the 20% who reach hospital and die within the first 24 h (Hijdra & van Gijn 1982), it is likely that at least 60% of all patients with SAH lose consciousness at or soon after onset. The patient may regain alertness and orientation or may remain with various degrees of lethargy, confusion, agitation or obtundation. Bizarre actions, which may be misinterpreted as psychological in origin, include grimacing, spitting, making sucking or kissing sounds, spluttering, singing, whistling, yelling and screaming (Fisher 1975; Reijneveld *et al.* 2000). The altered level of consciousness may be caused by a large amount of blood in the subarachnoid space or to a complication of SAH, such as brain displacement by haematoma or hydrocephalus, reduced cerebral blood flow by the sudden increase in cerebrospinal fluid pressure, or a fall in systemic blood pressure or arterial oxygen concentration.

Epileptic seizures

Epileptic seizures (partial or generalized) may occur at onset or subsequently, as a result of irritation or damage to the cerebral cortex by the subarachnoid and any intracerebral blood. In the Oxfordshire Community Stroke Project, two of the 33 patients (6%, 95% CI, 0%–14%) with SAH had an epileptic seizure at onset, but neither had later seizures (Burn *et al.* 1997) (section 9.2.6). Data from other series indicate that about 10% of patients with SAH develop epileptic seizures, most occurring on the first day of the SAH, but one-third not having their first seizure until 6 months later and one-third of those even more than 1 year later (Sarner & Rose 1967; Hart *et al.* 1981; Hasan *et al.* 1993; Pinto *et al.* 1996). The only independent predictors of epilepsy after SAH are a large amount of cisternal blood on brain CT, and re-bleeding (Hasan *et al.* 1993).

Intra-ocular haemorrhage

Intra-ocular haemorrhage develops in approximately 20% of patients with a ruptured aneurysm and may also complicate non-aneurysmal SAH, or intracranial haemorrhage in general (Manschot 1954). The haemorrhage is caused by a sustained increase in the pressure of the cerebrospinal fluid, with obstruction of the central retinal vein as it traverses the optic nerve sheath, in turn leading to congestion of the retinal veins (Manschot 1954). The haemorrhages mostly appear at the time of aneurysmal rupture, but exceptionally later without evidence of re-bleeding. Linear streaks of blood or flame-shaped haemorrhages appear in the preretinal layer (subhyaloid), usually near the optic disc (Fig. 5.43); one-third lie at the periphery (Fahmy 1973). If large, the preretinal haemorrhage may extend into the vitreous body. Patients may complain of large brown blobs obscuring their vision and, if the haemorrhages do not resolve spontaneously, vitrectomy may be required (section 13.11.1). Patients with ruptured aneurysms and preretinal subhyaloid haemorrhages tend to have a decreased level of consciousness and a worse outcome than patients without (Manschot 1954; Fahmy 1973; Keane 1979; Pfausler *et al.* 1996) (section 13.11.1).

Focal neurological signs

Focal neurological signs at SAH onset suggest an underlying intracerebral structural lesion, such as an arteriovenous malformation (AVM), or an aneurysm which has compressed cranial nerves or has bled into the brain substance, causing an intracerebral haematoma (section 9.3.5). Sometimes the clinical manifestations of a ruptured AVM or aneurysm may be indistinguishable from a stroke syndrome caused by primary intracerebral haemorrhage or cerebral infarction, particularly if little or no blood has entered the subarachnoid space.

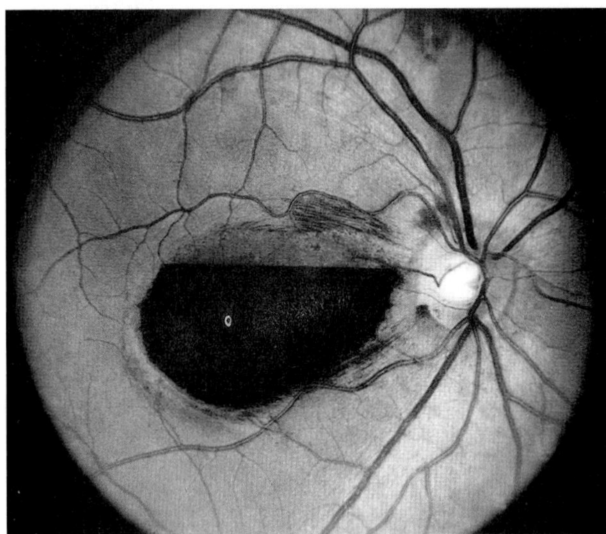

Fig. 5.43 Ocular fundus of a patient with subhyaloid haemorrhage, appearing as sharply demarcated linear streaks of brick red-coloured blood or flame-shaped haemorrhage in the pre-retinal layer, adjacent to the optic disc and spreading out from the optic disc (courtesy of Mr Matthew Wade, Department of Medical Illustrations, Royal Perth Hospital). Also reproduced in colour; see colour plate facing p. 84.

The classic cranial nerve palsy is an oculomotor (IIIrd) nerve palsy which frequently occurs with aneurysms at the origin of the posterior communicating artery from the internal carotid artery (Hyland & Barnett 1954) and less frequently with aneurysms of the carotid bifurcation, the posterior cerebral artery, the basilar bifurcation (Watanabe *et al.* 1982) and the superior cerebellar artery (Vincent & Zimmerman 1980). Third nerve palsy may also occur with unruptured aneurysms (presumably by expansion) or several days after SAH, as a result of swelling of the ipsilateral cerebral hemisphere because of delayed cerebral ischaemia. Most often the pupil is dilated and unreactive but in some patients it is spared (Kissel *et al.* 1983; Nadeau & Trobe 1983). Abducens (VIth) nerve palsies, frequently bilateral in the acute stage, may develop after SAH as a false localizing sign of raised intracranial pressure, because of traction on the nerves against the petrous temporal bone, caused by downward transtentorial herniation of the diencephalon. Occasionally, posterior circulation aneurysms may cause a VIth nerve palsy as a result of direct compression (Fisher 1975).

If a patient presents following a sudden, severe headache and is found to have a IIIrd cranial nerve palsy, rupture of a posterior communicating artery aneurysm is highly likely.

If there are other signs of neurological involvement, such as motor or sensory deficits, visual field defects or aphasia, then it is likely that a haematoma is present, usually within the brain parenchyma but occasionally in the subdural space, extrinsically compressing the brain. Cerebellar and brainstem signs can, however, be caused by the ischaemic effects of vertebral artery dissection (section 9.1.3).

Systemic features

Fever, hypertension, albuminuria, glycosuria and electrocardiographic (ECG) changes may be present in the acute phase. Pyrexia rarely exceeds 38.5°C during the first 2–3 days, but thereafter it may rise to over 39°C, presumably because of the accumulation of breakdown products of blood in the subarachnoid space (Rousseaux *et al.* 1980) (section 9.3.3).

The important distinguishing feature of pyrexia caused by blood in the subarachnoid space and pyrexia caused by intercurrent infection is the pulse rate; it remains disproportionately low in the former and rises with the latter.

About 20–25% of patients with SAH have a history of pre-existing hypertension, but following a SAH about 50% of patients have a markedly raised blood pressure (Artiola *et al.* 1980; Vermeulen *et al.* 1984). In most patients this is a reactive phenomenon, probably serving to counteract the decrease in cerebral perfusion resulting from increased cerebrospinal fluid pressure and later 'vasospasm'. Because the blood pressure returns to normal levels within a few days, antihypertensive drugs are usually not indicated if the patient was previously normotensive (section 9.3.4).

Cardiac dysrhythmias and ECG abnormalities are common after SAH (Brouwers *et al.* 1989; Wijdicks *et al.* 1990) (section 13.10.2). The mechanism is unexplained but is thought to be sustained sympathetic stimulation, perhaps caused by dysfunction of the insular cortex, which results in reversible structural neurogenic damage to the myocardium, such as contraction bands, focal myocardial necrosis and subendocardial ischaemia (Pollick *et al.* 1988; Mayer *et al.* 1994; Svigelj *et al.* 1994). However, there is no correlation between plasma noradrenaline (norepinephrine) concentrations and ECG abnormalities after aneurysmal SAH (Brouwers *et al.* 1995).

Sudden death

Subarachnoid haemorrhage is the major, if not only, stroke type to cause sudden death (within minutes). Sudden (or relatively sudden) death occurs in about 15% of SAH patients, before they receive any medical attention (Bonita & Thomson 1985; Schievink *et al.* 1995). The cause of very sudden death is uncertain but could be the sudden rise in intracranial pressure in cases with a large intracerebral haematoma as well as SAH (it takes some time for SAH to cause raised intracranial pressure sufficient to be fatal unless there is an associated large intracerebral haematoma); intraventricular haemorrhage with acute expansion of the fourth ventricle; cardiac dysrhythmia; and acute pulmonary oedema (Schievink *et al.* 1995).

5.6.2 Differential diagnosis

The abrupt onset of a severe headache may not only be caused by subarachnoid haemorrhage (SAH), but also by several other conditions, such as meningitis or encephalitis, intracerebral haemorrhage (particularly posterior fossa haemorrhage), obstruction of the cerebral ventricles, and a rapid rise in blood pressure (van Gijn 1992, 1999; Edlow & Caplan 2000) (Table 5.7). The most distinctive feature of SAH headache is its sudden onset (maximal within seconds) but, even so, only about 25% of patients with sudden headache in general practice prove to have SAH, falling to 10% if sudden headache is the only symptom (Linn *et al.* 1994). This is because headache with a much more common cause, such as migraine and tension headache, can occasionally arise suddenly. None the less, always be careful; missed SAH can be fatal.

Patients with rare manifestations of common headache syndromes (i.e. sudden onset of migraine) probably outnumber those with common manifestations of rare headache syndromes (i.e. sudden headache in subarachnoid haemorrhage). Therefore, although most people with a sudden severe headache have not had a subarachnoid haemorrhage, they must all be investigated to exclude this diagnosis.

One out of every four patients with sudden, severe headache has a ruptured cerebral aneurysm, or one out of 10 if sudden headache is the only symptom.

Acute painful neck conditions to be distinguished from meningism

Meningism may be a feature of SAH, meningitis, a posterior fossa mass and cerebellar tonsillar coning. However, it characteristically disappears as coma deepens. Other causes of a painful or stiff neck include bony lesions (i.e. trauma or arthritis) and ligamentous strain in the neck, extrapyramidal rigidity, systemic infections, cervical lymphadenitis, parotitis, tonsillitis and upper-lobe pneumonia. However, it is usually quite easy to distinguish meningism from these other acute painful neck conditions. For example, pain arising from the cervical spine may not only be felt in the neck and back of the head but also in the shoulder and arm, it is often

Table 5.7 Differential diagnosis of sudden unexpected headache.

With neck rigidity
Subarachnoid haemorrhage
Acute painful neck conditions
Meningitis
Cerebellar or intraventricular haemorrhage
Pituitary apoplexy
Recent head injury

Without neck rigidity
Migraine
Thunderclap headache
Pressor responses
Benign orgasmic cephalalgia
Benign exertional headache
Reaction while on monoamine oxidase inhibitors
Phaeochromocytoma
Expanding intracranial aneurysm
Carotid or vertebral artery dissection
Intracranial venous thrombosis
Occipital neuralgia
Acute obstructive hydrocephalus

evoked or exacerbated by certain movements or positions of the neck other than flexion, and there is usually tenderness to palpation over segments of the cervical spine.

Meningitis

Meningitis is an acute febrile illness that usually presents subacutely over 1–2 days with generalized headache, meningism, photophobia and fever, but it can be difficult to distinguish from SAH if the patient is found comatose, with neck rigidity and no available history. Clues to the diagnosis of meningitis include a high fever, tachycardia and a purpuric skin rash (meningococcal meningitis). If the patient is fully conscious and has no focal neurological signs and if meningitis is suspected, a lumbar puncture should be performed immediately. However, if the patient is very ill, antibiotics should be given at once, before proceeding to brain CT and then, if indicated because there is no blood seen and no intracranial mass, a cerebrospinal fluid examination.

Cerebellar stroke

Cerebellar stroke often gives rise to sudden severe headache, nausea and vomiting but is usually accompanied by neurological symptoms and signs, such as vertigo and unsteadiness, which help distinguish it from SAH (section 4.2.3). However, if the lesion is large, the patient may present in coma caused by direct brainstem compression or obstruction of cerebrospinal fluid flow from the fourth ventricle, causing hydrocephalus and raised intracranial pressure, or there may be meningism without signs of definite brainstem dysfunction. In a consecutive series of 100 patients with an initial diagnosis of subarachnoid haemorrhage, eight had a cerebellar haematoma (95% CI, 4–16%), and another seven had primary supratentorial brain haemorrhage (see below) (van Gijn & van Dongen 1980). Urgent brain CT is required to confirm the diagnosis of cerebellar haematoma and lumbar puncture should certainly not be performed; indeed, lumbar puncture should almost always be preceded by brain CT in unconscious patients, even if there are no focal signs of a mass lesion and no clinical evidence of raised intracranial pressure (such as papilloedema).

Primary intracerebral haemorrhage

More than 50% of patients with primary intracerebral haemorrhage (PICH) have headache at onset, particularly those with superficial lobar haemorrhages, but the headache is generally not as strikingly sudden in onset as SAH (Melo *et al.* 1996). Furthermore, focal neurological deficits are almost always present in PICH, but they can also occur in about 20–50% of aneurysmal SAHs in which there is intraparenchymal extension of the haemorrhage (Tokuda *et al.* 1995). Conversely, some primary intracerebral haemorrhages, particularly those which are deep, have less prominent focal neurological signs and can easily be mistaken for SAH. CT brain scan is always required.

Intraventricular haemorrhage

Intraventricular haemorrhage, which may be primary (i.e. arising within the ventricles or from immediately beneath the ependymal lining) or secondary to an extension from a parenchymal haemorrhage (i.e. to a caudate haemorrhage or ruptured subependymal vascular malformation with extension into the intraventricular system), may mimic SAH (section 9.1.5). Also, intraventricular haemorrhage may occur together with SAH, usually from a ruptured aneurysm, most frequently at the anterior communicating artery complex. Patients present with sudden severe headache, confusion, vomiting or collapse with loss of consciousness (Darby *et al.* 1988). Brain CT or MR scan is required for diagnosis during life.

Pituitary apoplexy

Haemorrhage into a pituitary tumour (pituitary apoplexy) usually causes a sudden, severe headache, followed by nausea, vomiting, neck stiffness and sometimes a depressed level of consciousness, thus mimicking SAH (Reid *et al.* 1985) (section 9.1.4). Confusingly, the hallmark of pituitary apoplexy, sudden decrease in visual acuity bilaterally (McFadzean *et al.* 1991), may occasionally occur in SAH if there are subhyaloid haemorrhages. However, these should be visible on fundoscopy, and most patients with pituitary apoplexy also have oculomotor palsies because the haemorrhage compresses the oculomotor nerves in the cavernous sinus. CT brain scan is generally required to demonstrate that the pituitary fossa is the source of the haemorrhage.

Migraine

Migraine headache can sometimes arise suddenly ('crash' migraine), be severe and prostrating, unilateral or generalized, and associated with photophobia, irritability, mild confusion, anorexia, mild fever, extraocular muscle palsy (ophthalmoplegic migraine) or symptoms of brainstem disturbance (basilar migraine) and thus be mistaken for SAH. However, migraineurs generally have a past or family history of migraine and the headache is commonly unilateral and throbbing, not so rapid in onset and of shorter duration, and follows the resolution of focal 'positive' neurological symptoms of the migraine aura that arose gradually and spread with intensification over several minutes (Lance 1993). Vomiting tends to start well into the migraine attack, in contrast to SAH, in which it commonly occurs at or soon after onset of the headache.

Benign 'thunderclap' headache

'Thunderclap' headache is characterized by the paroxysmal onset of a severe, generalized pain in the head, sometimes with vomiting, and without obvious precipitant or known cause. It may last up to a day or so. Clinically, the syndrome cannot be reliably distinguished from SAH, but the chances of aneurysmal SAH are increased in the presence of the following features: acute severe headache, female gender, epileptic seizures, a history of loss of consciousness, focal neurological symptoms (e.g. diplopia), and vomiting or exertion preceding the onset of headache (Linn *et al.* 1998). The diagnosis is therefore made by exclusion. If both brain CT and cerebrospinal fluid (performed within 2 weeks after onset (section 5.6.3) are normal, the episode is attributed to an unusually explosive bout of 'ordinary' headache, not SAH. About 50% of these patients have a history of typical migraine or tension-type headache (with gradual onset). Indeed, the prognosis of 'thunderclap' headache is benign; a 3-year follow-up of 71 patients seen in hospital found identical recurrences in 12, again without evidence of SAH, whereas nearly 50% developed episodes of more obvious migraine or tension headache (Wijdicks *et al.* 1988). Of 93 such patients identified in general practice and followed-up for a median period of 5 years, again none suffered SAH; recurrent attacks of 'thunderclap' headache occurred in eight patients, and 13 developed new tension headache or migraine (Linn *et al.* 1999).

> *Headache is common in clinical practice, but 'thunderclap' headache is not.*

Idiopathic stabbing headache

Three specific varieties of sudden, sharp, stabbing headache have been described: ice-pick-like pains, 'jabs and jolts syndrome' and ophthalmodynia (Lance 1993). The pains are mostly at the temples or orbits but on occasions are elsewhere in the head (Raskin & Schwartz 1980). Migraineurs are particularly susceptible (Raskin & Schwartz 1980). Precipitants may be postural change, physical exercise or head motion. As these pains are transient and lancinating, they are unlikely to be confused with the headache of SAH. The mechanism is unknown but the quality of the pain resembles trigeminal neuralgia and suggests paroxysmal neuronal discharge.

'Exploding head' syndrome

Clusters of attacks characterized by a sensation of sudden noise in the head and terror, rather than pain, can strike individuals over the age of 50 years, particularly during the twilight of sleep (Pearce 1989). The aetiology is uncertain.

Post-traumatic headache

Immediately after a head injury there is often headache caused by soft-tissue damage and, if the patient is concussed, intracranial vessels dilate, giving rise to a pulsating headache, which is made worse by head movement, jolting, coughing, sneezing and straining (Lance 1993). Normally the headache gradually disappears as the tissue damage resolves. Tubbs and Potter (1970) found that only 83 of 200 patients admitted to hospital with head injury had a headache by a day or so afterwards, only 22 of those 83 (11%) complained spontaneously (the remainder admitted to headache only on questioning of those 83), and only three required an analgesic.

The diagnosis of post-traumatic headache should not be confused with SAH if there is a history of head injury, but the patient can be amnesic and there may be no witness, in which case acute head injury can be confused with SAH (section 9.1.4). If the CT is suggestive of spontaneous intracranial haemorrhage, the patient should be considered for cerebral angiography to exclude an aneurysm (Sakas *et al.* 1995) (section 5.6.3).

> *If the circumstances of a traumatic head injury are unclear, and there is a reasonable chance that spontaneous intracranial haemorrhage was the cause of the accident and so the head injury, then brain CT should be performed as soon as the patient's condition allows, regardless of the severity of the head injury.*

Benign orgasmic cephalalgia and benign exertional headache

Acute, severe, explosive occipital or generalized headache, usually occurring at the moment of sexual orgasm or during strenuous exercise (benign orgasmic cephalalgia and benign exertional headache, respectively) may mimic SAH (Pascual *et al.* 1996). The history of onset during sexual intercourse (or masturbation) may not be forthcoming without specific and sensitive enquiry. Points in favour of the diagnosis are a history of similar previous sexual or exertional headaches, no alteration in consciousness, short duration of the headache (minutes to hours, although SAH may also possibly cause short-duration headache and it is not known how brief headache caused by SAH can be) and no signs of meningeal irritation, such as neck stiffness, or low back pain, and no sciatica in the ambulant patient (Silbert *et al.* 1991). These headaches can occur at any time in life and do not necessarily occur every time the patient experiences orgasm or exercises strenuously.

If patients present soon after their first-ever sudden orgasmic headache, it is not possible to exclude SAH without brain CT and lumbar puncture. If a patient presents after recurrent attacks, and the history is characteristic, investigation is unnecessary, although some clinicians would perform a CT scan. Diagnostic difficulty also arises in distinguishing benign orgasmic cephalalgia and benign exertional headache of sudden onset from the 'sentinel headache' of SAH, which may be caused by stretching or haemorrhage into the aneurysm wall rather than a minor leak into the subarachnoid space (Wijdicks *et al.* 1988) (section 5.6.1). However, it is not recommended that cerebral angiography be carried out in all cases to distinguish aneurysmal stretch from benign headache.

Reaction while on monoamine oxidase inhibitor drugs

Individuals taking classic monoamine oxidase inhibitors (MAOIs), such as phenelzine, may experience sudden severe headache after ingesting sympathomimetic agents, red wine or foods with a high tyramine content, such as mature cheese, pickled herrings, game and yeast extract. This is because MAOIs irreversibly block the ability of both MAO isoforms (A and B) to metabolize dietary tyramine in the liver (A) and gut wall (B). The combination of a classic MAOI and oral tyramine can provoke dangerous hypertension (section 8.3.1). The headache is often over the occipital region of the head and associated with a rapid rise in blood pressure. It can be relieved by the α-noradrenergic blocking agent, phentolamine. Some cases of intracranial haemorrhage have occurred at the height of a pressor reaction (Lance 1993).

Phaeochromocytoma

Patients with a phaeochromocytoma experience acute pressor reactions and, in about 80% of attacks, complain of headache (Thomas *et al.* 1966). The headache is usually of sudden onset, bilateral, severe and throbbing and often associated with nausea and other symptoms of catecholamine release. It appears to be related to a rapid increase in blood pressure and lasts less than 1 hour in about 75% of patients, but it may last from a few minutes to a few hours. Some patients may collapse with loss of consciousness or develop focal neurological signs during the episode. Attacks may be provoked by exertion, straining, emotional upset, worry or excitement (Lance & Hinterberger 1976).

The diagnosis depends on clinical suspicion being aroused when the history is first taken (which can be difficult because the condition is so rare) and is confirmed by finding increased excretion of catecholamines (metanephrine and vanillylmandelic acid) in three 24-h specimens of urine, or raised plasma-free metanephrine or normetanephrine levels during the attack (Lenders *et al.* 1995). Care must be taken before the urine collection that the patient does not have chronic renal failure and has not been taking anything which can interfere with the assay (such as methyldopa) or confuse the interpretation of finding catecholamines or catecholamine-like substances in the urine (such as sympathomimetic drugs, monoamine oxidase inhibitors or nasal decongestant sprays). Consuming bananas, coffee, tea or chocolate can also interfere with the assay by stimulating the secretion of catecholamines or by producing metabolites similar to catecholamines. The blood sugar is usually raised at the time of the attack, a useful distinction from hypoglycaemic attacks, which may simulate phaeochromocytoma because of secondary release of adrenaline (epinephrine) in response to low blood sugar. The tumour may arise at any point along the line of development of the sympathetic chain from the neck to the pelvis and scrotum. It can be localized by CT and aortic angiography if present in the characteristic suprarenal site.

Expanding intracranial aneurysm

Unruptured aneurysms are not associated with migraine or other recurrent headaches (Lance 1993) but, in extremely rare cases, they may cause a severe headache, even without focal cranial nerve signs; pressure on the IIIrd cranial nerve from a posterior communicating artery aneurysm causes pain behind the eye that can be of fairly sudden onset.

Carotid or vertebral artery dissection

Dissection of the wall of an internal carotid artery may cause a fairly distinctive headache syndrome, which is ipsilateral, involving the forehead, periorbital region, face, teeth or neck, and has a burning or throbbing quality (section 7.2.1). The headache may be associated with an ipsilateral Horner's syndrome or monocular blindness, and contralateral focal neurological symptoms or signs (West *et al.* 1976; Fisher 1982;

Mokri *et al.* 1986; Bogousslavsky *et al.* 1987). Dissection of the wall of a vertebral artery causes pain in the upper posterior neck and occiput, usually on one side, and may be associated with symptoms and signs of posterior circulation ischaemia, such as the lateral medullary syndrome (Caplan *et al.* 1985). Vertebral artery dissection can also cause SAH (section 9.1.3).

Intracranial venous thrombosis (section 5.5)

Thrombosis of the cerebral veins or venous sinuses presents with headache in about 75% of patients (Bousser *et al.* 1985), and can be sudden in onset in about 15% of patients (de Bruijn *et al.* 1996). However, nearly 50% of patients have signs of increased intracranial pressure, one-third have focal neurological signs (such as a hemiparesis or VIth nerve palsy) and one-third also have seizures (section 5.5.2). The brain CT or MRI may show widespread venous infarcts and haemorrhages (sections 5.5.3 and 8.2.10) and the cerebrospinal fluid is normal or contains a modest excess of white blood cells, red blood cells and protein.

Occipital neuralgia

Occipital neuralgia is characterized by an aching or paroxysmal jabbing pain in the posterior neck and occipital region in the distribution of the greater or lesser occipital nerves (Fig. 5.44). It may rarely present quite dramatically, like SAH (Pascual-Leone & Pascual 1992), but is usually characterized by diminished sensation or dysaesthesia of the affected area (C2 distribution), focal tenderness over the point where the greater occipital nerve trunk crosses the superior nuchal line, and a therapeutic response to infiltration of local anaesthetic near the tender area on the nerve trunk.

Acute obstructive hydrocephalus

Any acute obstruction of the flow of cerebrospinal fluid (CSF) causes a rapid increase in intracranial pressure and headache, which is commonly bilateral and exacerbated by coughing, sneezing, straining or head movement. Intermittent obstructive hydrocephalus may therefore cause severe paroxysmal headaches. Tumours in the vicinity of the third ventricle or within it, such as a colloid cyst, may interfere intermittently with CSF outflow or perhaps with the function of the midbrain reticular formation, so that posture cannot be maintained and the patient may fall heavily to the ground because of loss of muscle tone and loss of consciousness. Brain CT or MRI usually identify the offending lesion (Fig. 5.45).

Multiple sclerosis

There is an isolated case report of a 27-year-old man who had been awakened by 'the worst headache' of his life and 2 days later developed an oculomotor nerve palsy, which was considered to be caused by multiple sclerosis. Initial CT, lumbar puncture and cerebral angiogram were unremarkable, but subsequent cerebrospinal fluid examination revealed oligoclonal bands and MRI displayed multiple white matter lesions (Galer *et al.* 1990). It is difficult to be sure whether this patient had multiple sclerosis and whether demyelination was the cause of the symptoms, but the case is nevertheless salutary.

No physical sign can definitely exclude subarachnoid haemorrhage if a sudden onset headache persists for a few hours.

5.6.3 Investigations to confirm the diagnosis of subarachnoid haemorrhage

Investigations are essential in making the diagnosis of subarachnoid haemorrhage (SAH), given that clinical features are usually non-specific (Ramirez-Lassepas *et al.* 1997).

Brain CT

All patients presenting with a suspected recent SAH (i.e.

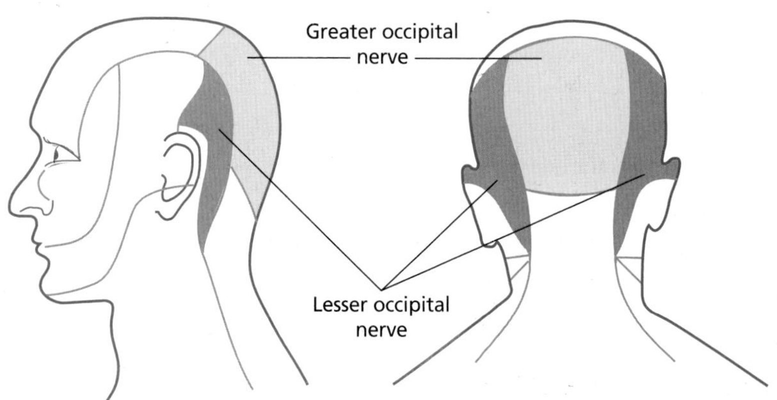

Fig. 5.44 The anatomical distribution of the sensory innervation of the greater and lesser occipital nerves.

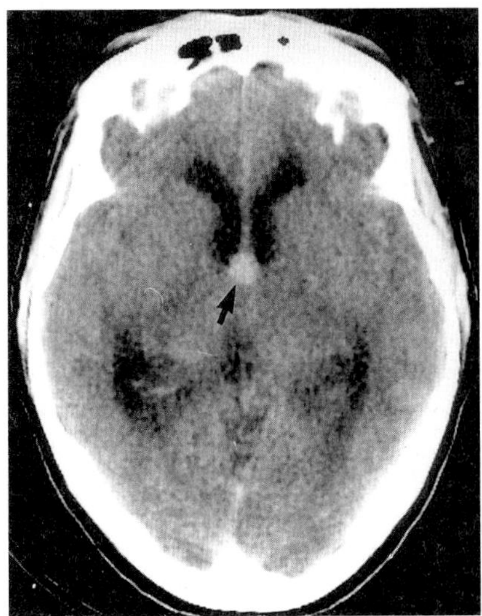

Fig. 5.45 CT brain scan showing a tumour in the third ventricle (arrow) at the foramen of Monro, causing obstructive hydrocephalus.

within the last few days) should initially have an urgent brain CT to determine whether there is blood in the subarachnoid space; the site of any SAH or intracerebral or intraventricular haemorrhage and therefore the likely cause (section 9.4.1); the presence of any complications, such as hydrocephalus; the presence of any contraindications to lumbar puncture, such as cerebral oedema or haematoma with brain shift, or a large cerebellar stroke, in case no blood is evident on CT; and whether there is any other intracranial pathology that may account for the symptoms and signs (Fig. 5.46).

Sensitivity of CT in SAH depends on the amount of subarachnoid blood, the resolution of the scanner, the skill of the radiologist and the timing of the CT after symptom onset. The sensitivity is greatest in the first few days and falls thereafter, as blood in the subarachnoid space is resorbed (Figs 5.47 and 5.48). In fact, the term 'resorption' may not always be appropriate to describe this process; diffusion and sedimentation being alternative explanations. CT evidence of subarachnoid blood can disappear very rapidly. If brain CT (third generation) is performed within 1–2 days after subarachnoid haemorrhage onset, extravasated blood will be demonstrated in more than 95% of patients, but the chance of finding subarachnoid blood on brain CT then decreases sharply, to 50% on day 7, 20% on day 9, and almost nil after 10 days (van Gijn & van Dongen 1982; Brouwers *et al.* 1992).

If brain CT (third generation) is performed within 1–2 days after subarachnoid haemorrhage onset, extravasated blood will be demonstrated in more than 95% of patients.

Of course, minute amounts of subarachnoid blood may be overlooked by the uninitiated (Fig. 5.48). Depending on the amount of blood in the cisterns and the delay before scanning, an 'absent' or 'missing' (isodense) cistern, or absent cortical sulci, may provide the only clue to the presence of subarachnoid blood (Fig. 5.49). Failure to detect SAH with brain CT is particularly likely with an aneurysm of the posterior inferior cerebellar artery (Adams *et al.* 1983; Ruelle *et al.* 1988; Stone *et al.* 1988).

If subarachnoid haemorrhage is suspected but the brain CT scan appears normal, look carefully at the interpeduncular cistern, ambient cisterns, quadrigeminal cistern, the region of the anterior communicating artery and posterior inferior cerebellar artery, the posterior horns of the lateral ventricles and the cortical sulci. If blood is present in these sites, it may be isodense or slightly hyperdense, and hence the normally hypodense cisterns and sulci may be difficult to see and seem 'absent'.

Haemorrhage from an intracranial aneurysm can result not only in SAH but also in an intraparenchymal haematoma.

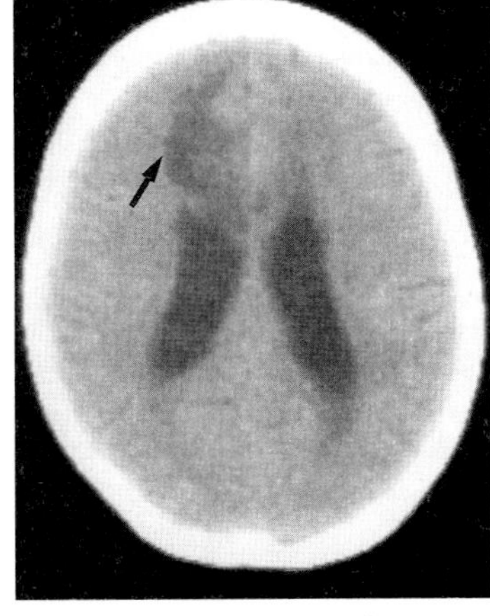

(a)

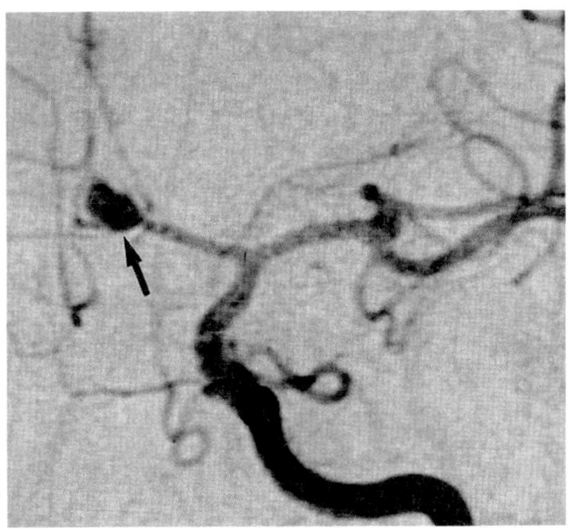

(b)

Fig. 5.46 CT brain scan (a) showing a 2- or 3-week-old intracerebral haemorrhage in the frontal lobes (arrow) of a patient who presented with an acute behavioural disorder and who had been misdiagnosed as being a hysterical alcoholic. (b) Subsequent cerebral angiography revealed an anterior communicating artery aneurysm (arrow) which had ruptured and bled into the frontal lobes.

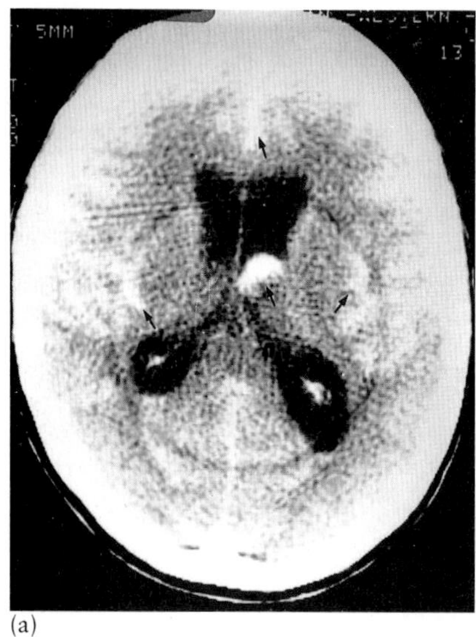

(a)

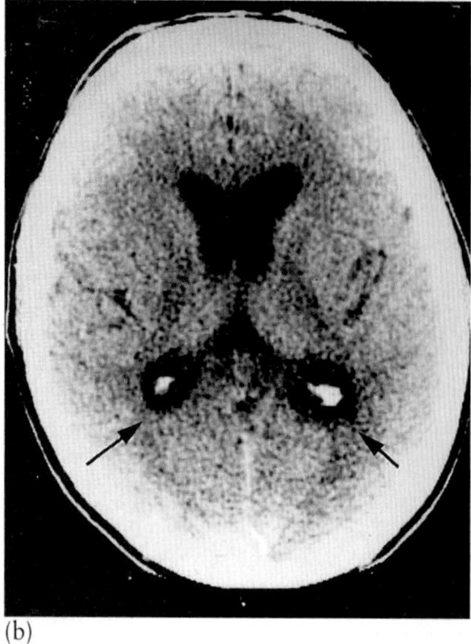

(b)

Fig. 5.47 CT brain scan showing rapid clearance of subarachnoid haemorrhage. (a) CT scan at 12 h after the onset shows extensive subarachnoid blood (hyperdensity—arrows) in all the cortical sulci and the lateral ventricles. (b) At 3 days after onset there is almost complete disappearance of the blood. There is only a tiny amount remaining in the occipital poles of the lateral ventricles (arrows). Note: the large white masses in the posterior horns of the lateral ventricles are calcified portions of the choroid plexus.

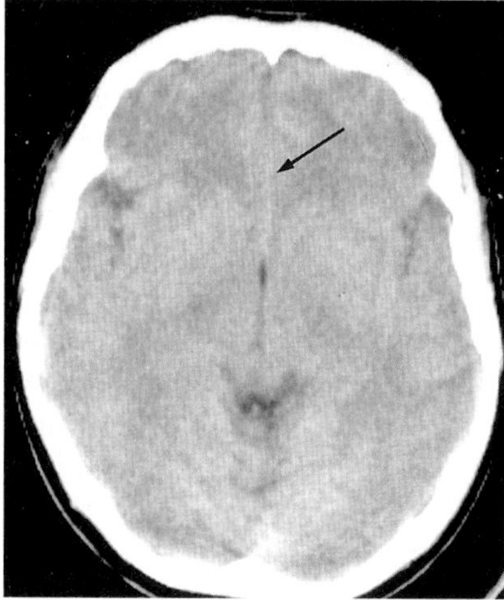

Fig. 5.48 CT brain scan within 24 h of onset of subarachnoid haemorrhage showing only a minute amount of blood in the subarachnoid space. There was a hint of increased density (blood) in the inferior part of the anterior interhemispheric fissure only (arrow).

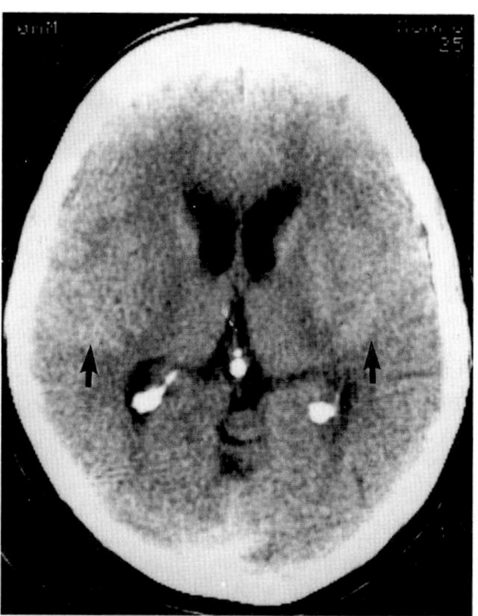

Fig. 5.49 CT brain scan of a patient with subarachnoid haemorrhage showing isodense blood in the cortical sulci giving the appearance of 'absent' sulci. In particular, the Sylvian fissures are not seen because they are filled with just enough blood to raise the density of the cerebrospinal fluid to that of brain parenchyma (arrows).

Intraparenchymal blood is easily seen on plain CT and it generally persists for longer than subarachnoid blood, because the 'resorption' of intraparenchymal blood, as seen on CT, occurs over several days to weeks rather than a few days, which is the case for subarachnoid blood (van Gijn & van Dongen 1982; Brouwers *et al.* 1992). However, small intraparenchymal haematomas can also resolve very quickly, within days (section 5.3.4). The proportion of patients with a haematoma after aneurysmal haemorrhage varies amongst different series because it depends on referral patterns. If patients are admitted to a general neurology service, there is usually little or no selection according to the clinical condition, and moribund patients are included. In these series, the proportion of patients with an intracerebral haematoma is around one-third of all patients with a ruptured aneurysm (van Gijn & van Dongen 1982; Brouwers *et al.* 1992).

Very rarely, a false-positive diagnosis of SAH may be made on the CT brain scan in patients who are comatose and brain dead (i.e. have no cerebral blood flow at the time of the CT scan). The CT scan not only shows cerebral oedema, but hyperdense material in the subarachnoid space which represents blood in congested subarachnoid blood vessels (Opeskin & Silberstein 1998).

A normal CT scan: false-negative, or non-haemorrhagic 'thunderclap' headache? Some patients have a benign type of headache but of sudden onset and of such severity that they are referred to hospital with a provisional diagnosis of SAH. This diagnosis is subsequently excluded by means of early CT and lumbar puncture. The true diagnosis in these patients is 'crash' migraine (section 5.6.2); a sudden exacerbation of tension headache (Pearce & Pearce 1986; Wijdicks *et al.* 1988); benign orgasmic cephalalgia (Lance 1976; Porter & Jankovic 1981) (section 5.6.2); a vascular headache provoked by some other type of exertion (Paulson 1983); or it remains unknown and is called 'thunderclap' headache (section 5.6.2). Investigations are, of course, negative in all these categories of patients, but a CT scan and a lumbar puncture need to be performed before the diagnosis can be made, although only on the first occasion in patients with orgasmic, exertional or other recurrent forms of explosive headache. A normal CT scan alone in such patients leaves a small risk of missing an SAH, or higher if more than 3 days have elapsed. In one consecutive series from the Netherlands, the negative predictive value of CT scanning performed within 12 h of onset of sudden headache was 97% (95% CI, 88–99%). This means that, in this series, 97% of people with a sudden headache who had a normal CT scan (i.e. no subarachnoid blood) within 12 h of onset of headache also had a normal cerebrospinal fluid (CSF) (i.e. negative spectrophotometric analysis of CSF for xanthochromia) more than 12 h after the event, and therefore did not have an SAH (Table 5.8). However, there was an important small minority (3%) with sudden headache and normal CT within 12 h who *did* have xanthochromia in the CSF, and angiography subsequently confirmed a ruptured aneurysm.

A CT brain scan less than 12 h after onset of subarachnoid haemorrhage is normal in about 3% of cases.

Table 5.8 Detection of subarachnoid haemorrhage on early CT brain scan within 12 h of sudden headache in 175 patients with a normal neurological examination and a clinical diagnosis of subarachnoid haemorrhage confirmed by lumbar puncture. (With permission from van der Wee *et al.* 1995.)

Subarachnoid haemorrhage	Yes	No	Total
CT scan positive*	117	0	117
CT scan negative†	2	56	58
Total	119	56	175

*CT scan shows subarachnoid blood.
†CT scan does not show subarachnoid blood.

Sensitivity: 117/119 = 98% (95% CI, 94–99.8%).
Specificity: 56/56 = 100%.
Positive predictive value: 117/117 = 100%.
Negative predictive value: 56/58 = 97% (95% CI, 88–99.6%).

The chance that a lumbar puncture will show evidence of haemorrhage and xanthochromia despite a truly normal CT scan made within hours of a sudden episode of headache depends not only on this small number of early false-negative CT scans in SAH, but also on the relative proportion of patients with non-haemorrhagic, innocuous 'thunderclap' headaches, which in turn depends on local referral patterns.

Always perform a lumbar puncture if the history is suggestive of subarachnoid haemorrhage and the CT scan (performed early, within a few days) is normal. Frequently, the cerebrospinal fluid will be normal too, but occasionally in this setting an abnormal cerebrospinal fluid will be the only objective evidence for the diagnosis of subarachnoid haemorrhage.

Lumbar puncture

Lumbar puncture without prior brain CT is potentially dangerous in patients with an intracerebral haematoma (Duffy 1982). Brain herniation may occur even in patients without focal signs or a decreased level of consciousness (Hillman 1986). If brain CT shows definite evidence of extravasated blood, a lumbar puncture will add no extra information. However, if the CT scan shows no evidence of SAH and there is a convincing history of headache with sudden onset that is still present at the time the patient is seen, then lumbar puncture must be performed to examine the cerebrospinal fluid for blood products (Waserberg & Barlow 1997). In the presence of a negative CT scan, there is a small chance that lumbar puncture will show evidence of SAH (van der Wee *et al.* 1995). After the first day or two, the proportion of false-negative CT scans after SAH becomes increasingly larger, and the importance of lumbar puncture increasingly greater (for the first 2 weeks, at least). Given the proportion of functional, or at least non-SAH, headaches in hospital series, about 30 negative lumbar punctures are needed to find one case of SAH (van der Wee *et al.* 1995).

A lumbar puncture should not be performed until at least 6 h, and preferably 12 h, after headache onset, to enable a reliable distinction to be made between a traumatic tap and haemorrhage in the subarachnoid space. The reason being that it takes up to 12 h for red cells to lyse and for haemoglobin to be broken down into oxyhaemoglobin (pinkish colour) and bilirubin (yellowish colour), which after centrifugation of the CSF results in a yellowish colour of the supernatant (xanthochromia) (Vermeulen & van Gijn 1990). Because xanthochromia is the only reliable proof that haemorrhagic spinal fluid has not resulted from the trauma of the puncture itself (Vermeulen & van Gijn 1990), it is crucial that the CSF is not examined within 12 h of onset of headache; no xanthochromia within 12 h does not exclude SAH and a repeat CSF at a later date may not be able to distinguish xanthochromia caused by SAH from that caused by any trauma from the initial lumbar puncture (Table 5.9).

Lumbar puncture should be performed after a negative CT scan, but not until at least 12 h have elapsed since the onset of headache.

Although a decrease in red blood cell concentration in serial samples, taken at the same procedure, occurs more often in traumatic punctures than in spontaneous intracranial haemorrhage, this *can* still occur after SAH. Conversely, a constant number of red cells can be seen with traumatic taps (Buruma *et al.* 1981; Vermeulen & van Gijn 1990). So the time-honoured 'three-tube method' should be abandoned in favour of looking for xanthochromia. Spinning down any bloodstained CSF should be carried out immediately, otherwise oxyhaemoglobin will form *in vitro*.

Table 5.9 Guidelines for lumbar puncture in patients with suspected subarachnoid haemorrhage but a negative CT brain scan. (Data from Matthews & Frommeyer 1955; Tourtelotte *et al.* 1964.)

If the onset of sudden headache was less than 3 days before

Wait until at least 12 h have elapsed since the onset of symptoms before doing a lumbar puncture.

If the cerebrospinal fluid is not only clear and colourless but also acellular (no more than a few red blood cells/mm^3), a ruptured aneurysm has been excluded and there is no need for further investigation.

If the cerebrospinal fluid is bloodstained:

(a) spin down the cerebrospinal fluid immediately (if it contains red blood cells from a traumatic tap and is allowed to stand, oxyhaemoglobin will be formed *in vitro*, bilirubin will not, but the absence of bilirubin cannot exclude subarachnoid haemorrhage).

(b) perform spectrophotometric analysis of the supernatant for xanthochromia, unless the yellow colour is evident to the naked eye. If spectrophotometry has to be deferred for practical reasons, store the cerebrospinal fluid wrapped in tin foil because daylight may induce breakdown of bilirubin.

If the onset of sudden headache was more than 3 days before

Do a lumbar puncture immediately (after brain CT).

If the cerebrospinal fluid is unequivocally xanthochromic (with or without red cells), no further cerebrospinal fluid tests are necessary.

If the cerebrospinal fluid is clear, colourless and acellular, still do spectrophotometry: the red cells have been lysed and the presence of pigment may not be visible to the naked eye.

If the interval is more than 2 weeks from headache onset, xanthochromia may still be detectable up until 4 weeks, but normal spectrophotometric testing cannot exclude subarachnoid haemorrhage.

It is a widely held myth that the distinction between subarachnoid haemorrhage and a traumatic 'bloody' tap can be made reliably by collecting the cerebrospinal fluid in three consecutive test-tubes and counting the number of red cells in each tube.

Oxyhaemoglobin and bilirubin are the main breakdown products of haemoglobin, at least *in vivo*, and on spectrophotometry they can be recognized by characteristic absorption bands (Barrows *et al.* 1955). However, if the lumbar puncture is performed more than 12 h after the onset of SAH, the yellow colour of the CSF should be visible with the naked eye. If not, competent spectrophotometry should be carried out. At 3 weeks after SAH, xanthochromia can still be found but in only 70% of patients with SAH, confirmed by an earlier positive CT scan, and after 4 weeks in only 40% (Vermeulen *et al.* 1983). Therefore, even if the supernatant seems crystal-clear, the specimen should be stored in darkness until absence of blood pigments is confirmed by spectrophotometric analysis (Vermeulen & van Gijn 1990). There is a view that the predictive value of spectrophotometric analysis of xanthochromia is incompletely established for patients *without* extravasation of blood on CT scanning (Beethan *et al.* 1998). However, there is reasonable evidence that the sudden-headache patients with a normal CT scan and no xanthochromia really do not have an intracranial aneurysm, or at least not one that re-bleeds in the next few years (section 9.4.7).

Bloodstained cerebrospinal fluid should be immediately centrifuged; if the supernatant is yellow this proves haemorrhage. Xanthochromia is almost invariably found between 12 h and 2 weeks after subarachnoid haemorrhage.

It is usually not too difficult to make the clinical distinction between SAH and meningitis, because in most patients with SAH there is an adequate history of an abrupt onset of headache or unconsciousness. The difficulty mainly arises when a patient is found in a confused state with marked neck stiffness and moderate fever; in these cases a lumbar puncture should probably be performed first, unless CT can be carried out very quickly. However, if the diagnosis of meningitis is not sustained and if the CSF is bloodstained, the patient must have an angiogram to exclude an aneurysm or other source of bleeding.

Late presentation with a history of sudden headache

A patient may present a few weeks or more after what sounds like a possible episode of SAH; headache coming on over seconds and having lasted for more than 2 h. If the interval is between 2 and 6 weeks, a lumbar puncture may still show xanthochromia (Vermeulen *et al.* 1989) but a normal

CSF does not exclude SAH. If there has been associated loss of consciousness, or the patient has been severely ill for several days, the probability of a ruptured aneurysm is considerable, and there is a good case for catheter angiography, or at least CT angiography (section 9.4.3). If headache was the only symptom, the probability of SAH is still about 10% (Linn *et al.* 1994). In that case, we would probably perform MR angiography (section 9.4.4). Given that the sensitivity of this technique is in the order of 80–90%, a normal MR angiogram would still leave a 1% risk of an undetected aneurysm in someone whose chance of re-bleeding, at that stage, is steadily decreasing towards an annual rate of about 3%. The disadvantages of catheter angiography in such patients probably outweigh the small residual risk of re-bleeding after an apparently normal MR angiogram.

5.7 Leukoaraiosis

Although leukoaraiosis is not a 'cause' of stroke, it is so closely linked with intracranial small vessel disease that it belongs somewhere in this book. It originated as a radiological concept of more or less symmetrically decreased density of periventricular and subcortical white matter on CT scans, especially in the elderly (Hachinski *et al.* 1986) (Fig. 5.50). A common assumption is that the underlying pathological process is ischaemic demyelination. With the advent of magnetic resonance imaging (MRI), the same reasoning has been applied to hyperintense lesions in the same areas of the white matter on a T2-weighted image, but with the difference that MRI has greater sensitivity (Fig. 5.51). A plethora of studies has shown a correlation between the presence and extent of these lesions and cognitive impairment, ranging from mild slowness of thinking to full-blown subcortical dementia. Even geniuses, such as Haydn, can be affected (Bäzner & Hennerici 1997).

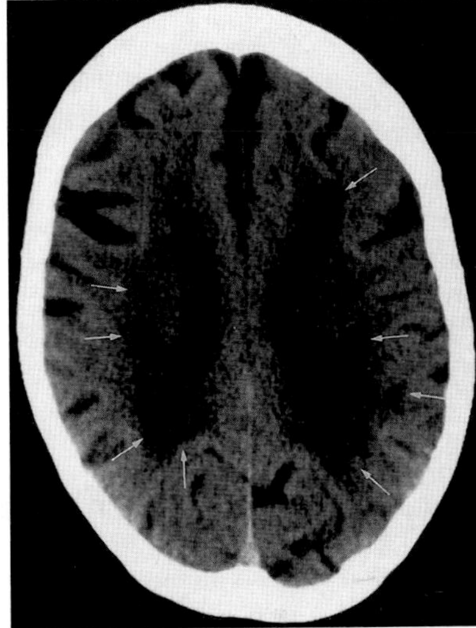

Fig. 5.50 CT brain scan showing leukoaraiosis. Note numerous patchy areas of hypodensity in the periventricular white matter (arrows).

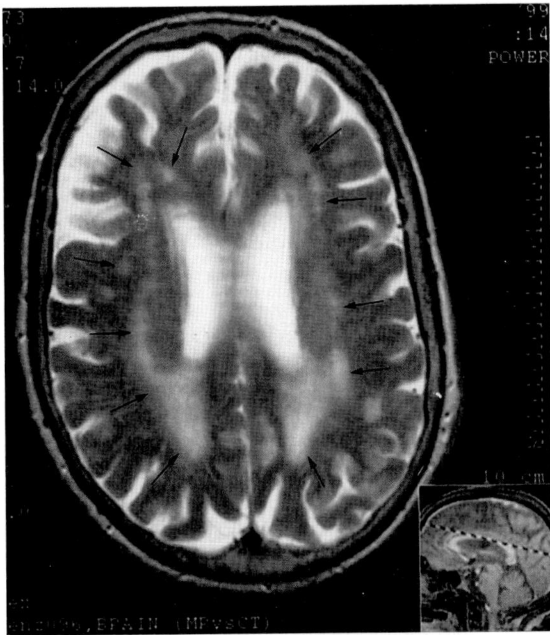

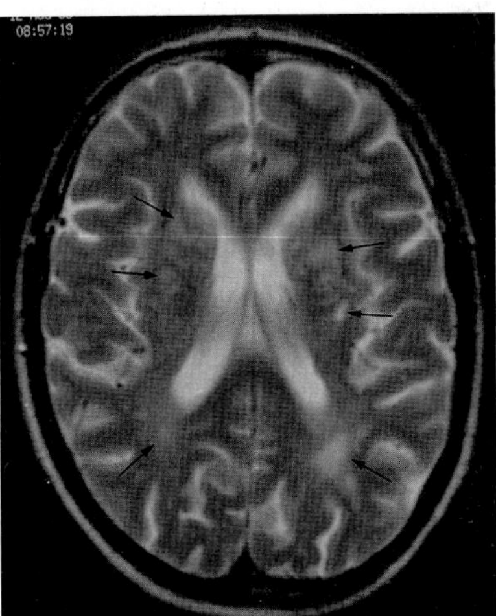

Fig. 5.51 T2-weighted MR to show numerous areas of increased signal in the periventricular white matter—leukoaraiosis. (a) Same patient as in Fig. 5.50, on MR has confluent blotchy hyperintense areas of increased signal throughout the periventricular white matter (arrows). (b) A different patient with milder disease has more discrete hyperintense areas (arrows) in the periventricular white matter (see Fig. 4.16 for an example of enlarged perivascular spaces).

With this concept of mental impairment or even dementia resulting from chronic ischaemia, neurological semeiology has come almost full circle. In this century, at least until the 1960s, gradual deterioration of cognitive function in the elderly was often attributed to atherosclerosis. Netter's then popular textbook on the nervous system has a drawing of a shrivelled brain with fattened arteries (Netter 1964). The pendulum then swung towards the assumption that primary degenerative disease of the Alzheimer type was responsible for all instances of gradual slowing of intellect and loss of memory. According to this line of thinking, vascular causes of dementia could be inferred only through the summation of consecutive strokes, large or small (so-called multi-infarct dementia) (Hachinski *et al.* 1978). Since increasingly sensitive neuroimaging techniques have become available, the concept evolved that ischaemia could affect mentation insidiously, even without overt episodes of stroke. Unlike the older theories, it is now thought that the disease process involves the white instead of the grey matter and that the underlying vascular lesions affect not the large- and medium-sized arteries, but the intracranial small vessels (Esiri *et al.* 1997).

Before this is rejected as yet another untenable simplification, three important qualifications should be mentioned. First, not all cases of cognitive impairment from vascular disease are caused by diffuse changes in the white matter. Secondly, not all mental impairment associated with chronic, progressive demyelination is caused by ischaemia. Thirdly, not all intracranial small vessel disease with chronic demyelination is caused by hypertension. After this qualification, the 'common' type of chronic ischaemia of the white matter, as it is understood today—its risk factors, effects on cognition, and prognostic implications—can be discussed.

5.7.1 Vascular dementia is not synonymous with white matter disease

Not only multiple infarcts but also single, strategically located infarcts may cause dementia. Such instances have been recorded with infarcts in the genu of the internal capsule (Tatemichi *et al.* 1992; Yamanaka *et al.* 1996), thalamus (Wallesch *et al.* 1983; Graff-Radford *et al.* 1984; Van der Werf *et al.* 1999), caudate nucleus (Mendez *et al.* 1989; Bokura & Robinson 1997) and the angular gyrus (Benson & Cummings 1982). Because similarly located infarcts in other patients only rarely cause dementia, the question is, what *additional* factors explain the sudden deterioration of cognitive function? Other than idiosyncratic 'wiring' of an individual patient's brain, the contributing factor may be a co-existing—but until then, subclinical—diffuse disorder of the brain, such as Alzheimer's disease (Pasquier & Leys 1997). Diffuse ischaemia of the brain may also result from systemic hypotension or hypoxia, most often secondary to circulatory arrest, but that situation will not present diagnostic difficulties.

5.7.2 White matter changes with cognitive impairment are not synonymous with ischaemia

Vascular dementia cannot be diagnosed from a scan. Other diseases also cause multifocal or diffuse demyelination in the deep regions of the brain, sometimes in patterns indistinguishable from ischaemic lesions (Table 5.10). Three common categories of white matter changes are discussed separately: those associated with Alzheimer's disease, periventricular gliosis and widening of perivascular spaces.

Alzheimer's disease

Changes in the deep white matter of the brain occur in 25–60% of patients with Alzheimer's disease, although not in the early stages, and perhaps more often in women than in men (Brun & Englund 1986; Wallin *et al.* 1989; Diaz *et al.* 1991; Bennett *et al.* 1992; Erkinjuntti *et al.* 1994). Not surprisingly, patients with Alzheimer's disease and white matter changes have more severe cognitive impairment than those without (Steingart *et al.* 1987; Diaz *et al.* 1991; Starkstein *et al.* 1997). These white matter changes cannot be simply explained away by co-existing vascular disease: vascular risk factors do not sufficiently account for the association (Blennow *et al.* 1991; Bennett *et al.* 1992); cerebral blood flow is less impaired than in patients with vascular dementia and lesions of similar severity (Kawamura *et al.* 1993; DeCarli *et al.* 1996); and the pathological changes in the walls of the small blood vessels are not necessarily 'hypertensive', with thickening of the muscle layer, but may be just non-specific

Table 5.10 Conditions other than small-vessel disease that may cause multifocal or diffuse demyelination of the brain in adults.

Alzheimer's disease (section 5.7.2)
Multiple sclerosis (McQuinn & O'Leary 1987; Fontaine *et al.* 1994)
Progressive multifocal leukoencephalopathy (Steiger *et al.* 1993; Sellal *et al.* 1996)
HIV encephalitis (Miller *et al.* 1997)
Creutzfeldt–Jakob disease (Berciano *et al.* 1991)
Postinfectious demyelination (Kappelle *et al.* 1986)
Trauma (Smith *et al.* 1995)
Radiation therapy (Dropcho 1991)
Chemotherapy (Macdonald 1991; Chen *et al.* 1994)
Treatment with cyclosporin or other immunosuppressants (Hinchey *et al.* 1996; Pullicino *et al.* 1996b; Thyagarajan *et al.* 1997; Nakamura *et al.* 1998) (section 7.12)
Posthypoxic–ischaemic encephalopathy (de Reuck *et al.* 1992; Moroney *et al.* 1996)
Hyperperfusion syndrome (Nencini *et al.* 1993; Hinchey *et al.* 1996; Delanty *et al.* 1997)
Post-transfusion syndrome (Ito *et al.* 1997)
Vitamin B_{12} deficiency (Chatterjee *et al.* 1996; Stojsavljevic *et al.* 1997)
α-Galactosidase deficiency (Fabry's disease) (Grewal 1994; Mendez *et al.* 1997; Crutchfield *et al.* 1998) (section 7.20)
Proximal myotonic myopathy (Hund *et al.* 1997; Mastaglia *et al.* 1998)

hyaline thickening (Rezek *et al.* 1987; Scheltens *et al.* 1995; Tomimoto *et al.* 1999). Cerebral amyloid (congophilic) angiopathy can be found, but in cortical rather than subcortical vessels (Rezek *et al.* 1987; Janota *et al.* 1989; Leys *et al.* 1991; Olichney *et al.* 1995; Tomimoto *et al.* 1999). Finally, extravasation of serum proteins occurs in diseased white matter with vascular determinants, but not with Alzheimer's disease (Tomimoto *et al.* 1996).

If wallerian degeneration secondary to cortical atrophy were the underlying cause of white matter changes in Alzheimer's disease, the severity of the changes in each subcortical brain region should correspond with the density of cortical changes typical of Alzheimer's disease (neurofibrillary tangles and amyloid plaques), but this is not always the case (Brun & Englund 1986; Englund *et al.* 1988; Leys *et al.* 1991). It is therefore by no means certain that the white matter changes in Alzheimer's disease can be explained even by the combined effect of wallerian degeneration and co-existent vascular disease in its usual sense. Given that Alzheimer's disease is more common than vascular dementia, even if one is allowing for differences in criteria (Verhey *et al.* 1996; Wetterling *et al.* 1996), and that diffuse abnormalities of the white matter occur in 25–60% of patients with Alzheimer's disease, vascular dementia in the sense of diffuse leukoencephalopathy cannot be diagnosed just on the basis of radiological criteria (by present standards). The diagnosis of vascular dementia has to be supported by the clinical characteristics of subcortical dementia: slowness of mental processing, apathy and loss of emotional modulation (Cummings & Benson 1984; Filley 1998).

Gliosis and widening of perivascular spaces

Some changes in the white matter visible on MRI do not even represent demyelination. Hyperintense changes immediately adjacent to the wall of the lateral ventricles (caps and rims) correspond to primary gliosis rather than demyelination and are probably secondary to leakage through an ageing ependymal wall (Leifer *et al.* 1990; Chimowitz *et al.* 1992; Fazekas *et al.* 1993). Similarly, widening of the perivascular spaces may produce hyperintensity on T2-weighted images, but these lesions are typically punctate and should not be confused with demyelination (Awad *et al.* 1986; Fazekas *et al.* 1991; Munoz *et al.* 1993) (Fig. 4.16). Dementia in such cases is exceptional and occurs only with widespread dilatation of perivascular spaces (Vital & Julien 1997).

5.7.3 The vascular lesions with leukoaraiosis are not always of the hypertensive type

Some conditions are characterized by intracranial small vessel disease and demyelination of the cerebral white matter, but with morphologic changes in the vessel wall quite distinct from the degenerative type of concentric hyaline wall thickening that is considered typical of chronic hypertension or diabetes mellitus.

Cerebral amyloid angiopathy is the most common alternative condition associated with demyelination of the brain; the amyloid material in the cortical and meningeal vessels can be identified with Congo red staining and is birefringent under polarized light. Although small clusters of familial amyloid angiopathy have been found in the Netherlands and in Iceland, the vast majority of cases are sporadic (Bornebroek *et al.* 1996; Coria & Rubio 1996). It is possible that the vulnerability of the arteriolar wall facilitates the development of intracerebral haemorrhage, which often recurs at different sites in the brain (Gray *et al.* 1985; Vonsattel *et al.* 1991) (section 8.2.2). Transient ischaemic attacks and mild cognitive deterioration may precede the first haemorrhage, but the diagnosis is rarely made at that stage (Greenberg *et al.* 1993). Patients may even be misclassified as having Alzheimer's disease (Lucas *et al.* 1992).

In cerebral autosomal dominant arteriopathy with subcortical infarcts and leukoencephalopathy (CADASIL) (section 7.20) the changes in the arterial wall are distinct, consisting of granular, eosinophilic material. Arterioles of skin, muscle, nerve and other organs may be similarly affected and allow morphological confirmation of the diagnosis from a biopsy of skin or muscle (Goebel *et al.* 1997; Rubio *et al.* 1997; Ruchoux & Maurage 1998).

The archetypal ('hypertensive') form of intracranial small vessel disease associated with demyelination consists of hyaline thickening, collagenous deposits in the media and adventitia, splitting of the elastic lamina, with negative stains for amyloid (Gupta *et al.* 1988; van Swieten *et al.* 1991a; Erkinjuntti *et al.* 1996; Zhang & Olsson 1997). The white matter changes may also affect the pons (Kwa *et al.* 1997); subcortical U-fibres are typically spared. On biochemical analysis, the areas of demyelinated brain tissue show extravasation of serum albumin and immunoglobulins (Wallin *et al.* 1990; Pantoni *et al.* 1993; Tomimoto *et al.* 1996; Akiguchi *et al.* 1998), and on MR spectroscopy an increase in choline-containing metabolites and a decreased signal corresponding to (neuronal) *N*-acetyl aspartate (Constans *et al.* 1995; MacKay *et al.* 1996; Brooks *et al.* 1997). Not surprisingly, functional studies by means of xenon contrast, positron emission tomography or single photon emission computed tomography confirm decreased blood flow and hypometabolism in subcortical regions (Tohgi *et al.* 1991; Yao *et al.* 1992; Miyazawa *et al.* 1997).

5.7.4 Prevalence and determinants of ischaemic leukoaraiosis

The prevalence of leukoaraiosis is highly dependent on age, and on definitions. There are a multitude of rating scales; none have been validated against morphological studies, only a few have been subjected to an inter-observer study and most do not include rating of atrophy and enlarged perivascular spaces (Mäntylä *et al.* 1997; Scheltens *et al.* 1998). In a population-based study of 1077 over-60-year-olds in which a rather sensitive and detailed scale was used, 8% had no lesions in the subcortical region, 20% were free of changes in the deep (periventricular) white matter and only 5% had no lesions at all (de Leeuw *et al.* 1999).

Interestingly, concentric hyaline wall thickening at post-mortem can occasionally be found in patients who are normotensive and not elderly or diabetic (Ma *et al.* 1992; Lammie *et al.* 1997). Furthermore, not all elderly patients with severe hypertension develop severe white matter changes, but only some 25% (van Swieten *et al.* 1991b). This suggests that factors other than age and classical vascular risk factors must be involved in the development of 'hypertensive' small vessel disease, genetic factors being one (Carmelli *et al.* 1998). In case–control and cross-sectional studies of the general population, other factors included the classic vascular risk factors according to the history (hypertension, cigarette-smoking, a history of stroke or heart disease, and diabetes mellitus), and examination or investigation (ankle–arm blood pressure index, carotid plaques and intima-media thickness on ultrasonography) (Schmidt *et al.* 1992; Bots *et al.* 1993; Fukuda & Kitani 1996; Suzuki *et al.* 1997; Goldstein *et al.* 1998). MRI studies in a population cohort in the Netherlands, for which baseline variables had been collected 20 years before, confirmed the influence of long-standing hypertension. For systolic blood pressure the relationship with the extent of the white matter changes was linear, confirming a finding in a US cohort of twins (Swan *et al.* 1998; de Leeuw *et al.* 1999). For diastolic blood pressure, the risk of white matter changes was doubled with a change of 10 mmHg or more, in either direction; the left-hand end of the J-shaped curve is probably explained by the development of heart failure. Previous atrial fibrillation was related to periventricular white matter lesions, but not to more superficial subcortical lesions in the white matter (de Leeuw *et al.* 2000).

> *High blood pressure is neither a sufficient nor a necessary factor for the development of the hyaline intracranial small vessel disorder that is associated with the most common form of white matter changes in the elderly, but together with increasing age it is by far the most important determinant known at present.*

Again, these classical risk factors for vascular disease explain only part of the problem (Ylikoski *et al.* 1993). Fibrinogen has been identified as an additional risk factor in two independent studies (Breteler *et al.* 1994a; Schmidt *et al.* 1997a). Determinants implicated in single studies, without confirmation to date, are serum levels of coagulation factor VIIc (Breteler *et al.* 1994a), levels of vitamin E (Schmidt *et al.* 1997a) and forced expiratory volume (Longstreth *et al.* 1996). Data about associations between apolipoprotein E polymorphisms and white matter changes are conflicting (Schmidt *et al.* 1997b; Kuller *et al.* 1998).

5.7.5 Cognitive correlates of ischaemic leukoaraiosis

Dementia is the end stage of the cognitive changes associated with diffuse thickening of the intracranial small vessels, corresponding with complete rarefaction of the cerebral white matter (except the U-fibres) (de Reuck *et al.* 1980; Román 1987; Mascalchi *et al.* 1989; Revesz *et al.* 1989; Pantoni *et al.* 1996). This so-called subacute arteriosclerotic encephalopathy may represent the same condition that Binswanger described in 1894, but it is uncertain because his original description did not include microscopic studies (Binswanger 1894; Caplan 1995; Pantoni & Garcia 1995). To reiterate, strokes from large artery disease (atheroma) do not necessarily accompany the development of vascular dementia (Pantoni *et al.* 1996).

Even more important, virtually every study to date that has addressed the question, has shown that people with leukoaraiosis have some degree of cognitive impairment. This applies to the elderly in the general population (Breteler *et al.* 1994b; de Groot *et al.* 1997); elderly volunteers (Steingart *et al.* 1986; Schmidt *et al.* 1993; Ylikoski *et al.* 1993); and to patients with hypertension (van Swieten *et al.* 1991b; Schmidt *et al.* 1995). The degree of cognitive impairment is proportional to the degree of white matter changes (Pullicino *et al.* 1996a; de Groot *et al.* 2000). A decrease of blood flow and glucose metabolism on positron emission tomography (PET) scanning are said to reflect the neuropsychological deficits even more closely than the morphological changes themselves (Sabri *et al.* 1999). The impairment of cognitive abilities affects a wide range of functions and is typical of subcortical dementia. Longitudinal studies of brain imaging and neuropsychological tests are still scarce, but provisional reports confirm the progressive nature of the disorder (Martin *et al.* 1997; Veldink *et al.* 1998). Hachinski has coined the term 'dysmentia' to emphasize the fact that any degree of cognitive impairment decreases objective performance as well as subjective quality of life (Hachinski 1992).

There are indications that cognitive impairments are preferentially associated with changes in the deep (periventricular) white matter, whereas changes in the subcortical white matter give rise to depressive symptoms (J.C. de Groot, unpublished observations). An Australian study found that outcome after treatment of depressive symptoms was worse in patients with white matter lesions (O'Brien *et al.* 1998). Apart from cognition, gait is also affected (Briley *et al.* 1997); of course, the combination of gait disturbance and cognitive changes, and ventricular enlargement may suggest normal pressure hydrocephalus, unless MR scanning identifies white matter changes; shunting is rarely successful in patients with vascular risk factors (Boon *et al.* 1999).

Leukoaraiosis is a major challenge in health care, occurring to some degree in almost everyone over the age of 60 years. Full-blown dementia is rare, but many elderly people suffer insidious mental slowing and intellectual decline—not so severe as to compromise independent existence, but often severe enough to drain much of the colour from life.

5.7.6 Prognostic implications for other vascular complications

Ischaemic demyelination of white matter has prognostic implications in that it confers an increased risk of stroke and vascular death, not only among patients with transient ischaemic attacks or non-disabling ischaemic stroke (van Swieten *et al.* 1992; Inzitari *et al.* 1995) but also in the general population (Inzitari *et al.* 1997). In addition, anticoagulants for the secondary prevention of vascular disease in patients with transient ischaemic attacks or non-disabling stroke substantially increase the risk of intracerebral haemorrhage in patients whose baseline CT scan shows leukoaraiosis (Stroke Prevention in Reversible Ischaemia Trial Study Group 1997; Gorter *et al.* 1999).

References

Please note that all references taken from *The Cochrane Library* are given a current date as this database is updated on a quarterly basis. Please refer to the current *Cochrane Library* article for the latest review. The same applies to the *British Medical Journal* 'Clinical Evidence' series which is updated every six months.

Adams, H.P., Jergenson, D.D., Kassell, N.F. & Sahs, A.L. (1980) Pitfalls in the recognition of subarachnoid haemorrhage. *Journal of the American Medical Association* **244**, 794–796.

Adams, H.P., Kassell, N.F., Torner, J.C. & Sahs, A.L. (1983) CT and clinical correlations in recent aneurysmal subarachnoid haemorrhage: a preliminary report of the Cooperative Aneurysm Study. *Neurology* **33**, 981–988.

Adams, H.P. Jr, Brott, T.G., Furlan, A.J. *et al.* (1996) Guidelines for thrombolytic therapy for acute stroke: a supplement to the guidelines for the management of patients with acute ischaemic stroke. A statement for healthcare professionals from a special writing group of the Stroke Council, American Heart Association. *Stroke* **27**, 1711–1718.

Akiguchi, I., Tomimoto, H., Suenaga, T., Wakita, H. & Budka, H. (1998) Blood–brain barrier dysfunction in Binswanger's disease: an immunohistochemical study. *Acta Neuropathologica* **95**, 78–84.

Alberts, M.J., Faulstich, M.E. & Gray, L. (1992) Stroke with negative brain magnetic resonance imaging. *Stroke* **23**, 663–667.

Al-Buhairi, A.R., Phillips, S.J., Llewellyn, G. & January, M.M.S. (1998) Prediction of infarct topography using the Oxfordshire Community Stroke Project classification of stroke subtypes. *Journal of Stroke and Cerebrovascular Diseases* **7**, 339–343.

Alexandrov, A.V., Black, S.E., Ehrlich, L.E. *et al.* (1996) Simple visual analysis of brain perfusion on HMPAO SPECT predicts early outcome in acute stroke. *Stroke* **27**, 1537–1542.

Allen, C.M.C. (1983) Clinical diagnosis of acute stroke syndrome. *Quarterly Journal of Medicine* **43**, 515–523.

Altieri, M., Metz, R., Muller, C., Maeder, P., Meuli, R. & Bogousslavsky, J. (1997) Differentiation of acute versus chronic infarcts by diffusion weighted MRI in patients with multiple ischemic lesions. *Cerebrovascular Diseases* **7** (Suppl. 4), 6.

Ambrose, J. (1973) Computerized transverse axial scanning (tomography): part 2: clinical application. *British Journal of Radiology* **46**, 1023–1047.

Ameri, A. & Bousser, M.G. (1992) Cerebral venous thrombosis. *Neurologic Clinics* **10**, 87–111.

American Nimodipine Study Group (1992) Clinical trial of nimodipine in acute ischemic stroke. *Stroke* **23**, 3–8.

Anderson, C.S., Jamrozik, K., Burvill, P.W. *et al.* (1993) Ascertaining the true incidence of stroke: experience from the Perth Community Stroke Study, 1989–90. *Medical Journal of Australia* **158**, 80–84.

Anderson, C.S., Taylor, B.V., Hankey G.J., Stewart-Wynne, E. & Jamrozik, K.D. (1994) Validation of a clinical classification for subtypes of acute cerebral infarction. *Journal of Neurology, Neurosurgery and Psychiatry* **57**, 1173–1179.

Andreoli, A., di Pasquale, G., Pinelli, G., Grazi, P., Tognetti, F. & Testa, C. (1987) Subarachnoid haemorrhage: frequency and severity of cardiac arhythmias. A survey of 70 cases studied in the acute phase. *Stroke* **18**, 558–564.

Andrews, R.J. (1991) Transhemispheric diaschisis: a review and comment. *Stroke* **22**, 943–949.

Angeloni, U., Bozzao, L., Fantozzi, L.M., Bastianello, S., Kushner, M. & Fieschi, C. (1991) Internal border-zone infarctions following acute middle cerebral artery occlusion. Proceedings of the XIV Symposium Neuroradiologicum 1990. *Neuroradiology* **33** (Suppl.), 232.

Aparicio, A., Sobrino, J., Arboix, A. & Torres, M. (1995) Hematoma intraparenquimatoso que simula un accidente isquemico transitorio. *Medicina Clinica* **104**, 478–479.

Artiola, I., Fortuny, L., Adams, G.B.T. & Briggs, M. (1980) Surgical mortality in an aneurysm population: effects of age, blood pressure and preoperative neurological state. *Journal of Neurology, Neurosurgery and Psychiatry* **43**, 879–882.

Awad, I.A., Johnson, P.C., Spetzler, R.F. & Hodak, J.A. (1986) Incidental subcortical lesions identified on magnetic resonance imaging in the elderly. II: Post-mortem pathological correlations. *Stroke* **17**, 1090–1097.

Ay, H., Buonanna, F.S., Rordorf, G. *et al.* (1999) Normal diffusion-weighted MRI during stroke-like deficits. *Neurology* **52**, 1784–1792.

Baird, A.E., Donnan, G.A., Austin, M.C., Fitt, G.J., Davis, S.M. & McKay, W.J. (1994) Reperfusion after thrombolytic therapy in ischaemic stroke measured by single photon emission computed tomography. *Stroke* **25**, 79–85.

Baird, A.E., Austin, M.C., McKay, W.J. & Donnan, G.A. (1996) Changes in cerebral tissue perfusion during the first 48 hours of ischaemic stroke: relation to clinical outcome. *Journal of Neurology, Neurosurgery and Psychiatry* **61**, 26–29.

Baird, A.E., Benfield, A., Schlaug, G. *et al.* (1997) Enlargement of human cerebral ischaemic lesion volumes measured by diffusion-weighted magnetic resonance imaging. *Annals of Neurology* **41**, 581–589.

Bakac, G. & Wardlaw, J.M. (1997) Problems in the diagnosis of intracranial venous infarction. *Neuroradiology* **39**, 566–570.

Baker, L.L., Kucharczyk, J., Sevick, R.J., Mintorovitsh, J. & Moseley, M.E. (1991) Recent advances in MR imaging/spectroscopy of cerebral ischemia. *American Journal of Roentgenology* **156**, 1133–1143.

Bamford, J. (1992) Clinical examination in diagnosis and subclassification of stroke. *Lancet* **339**, 400–402.

Bamford, J.M. & Warlow, C.P. (1988) Evolution and testing of the lacunar hypothesis. *Stroke* **19**, 1074–1082.

Bamford, J., Sandercock, P.A.G., Jones, L. & Warlow, C.P. (1987) The natural history of lacunar infarction: the Oxfordshire Community Stroke Project. *Stroke* **18**, 545–551.

Bamford, J., Sandercock, P., Dennis, M., Burn, J. & Warlow, C. (1990) A prospective study of acute cerebrovascular disease in the community: the Oxfordshire Community Stroke Project—1981–86. 2: Incidence, case fatality rates and overall outcome at one year of cerebral infarction, primary intracerebral and subarachnoid haemorrhage. *Journal of Neurology, Neurosurgery and Psychiatry* **53**, 16–22.

Bamford, J., Sandercock, P., Dennis, M., Burn, J. & Warlow, C. (1991) Classification and natural history of clinically identifiable subtypes of cerebral infarction. *Lancet* **337**, 1521–1526.

Barber, P.A., Davis, S.M., Infeld, B. *et al.* (1998) Spontaneous reperfusion after ischaemic stroke is associated with improved outcome. *Stroke* **29**, 2522–2528.

Baron, J.-C. (1999) Mapping the ischaemic penumbra with PET: implications for acute stroke treatment. *Cerebrovascular Diseases* **9**, 193–201.

Baron, J.C., von Kummer, R. & del Zoppo, G.J. (1995) Treatment of acute ischaemic stroke: challenging the concept of a rigid and universal time window. *Stroke* **26**, 2219–2221.

Barron, T.F., Gusnard, D.A., Zimmerman, R.A. & Clancy, R.R. (1992) Cerebral venous thrombosis in neonates and children. *Pediatric Neurology* **8**, 112–116.

Barrows, L.J., Hunter, F.T. & Banker, B.Q. (1955) The nature and clinical significance of pigments in the cerebrospinal fluid. *Brain* **78**, 59–80.

Bartylla, K., Hagen, T., Globel, H., Jost, V. & Schneide, G. (1997) Diffusion-weighted magnetic resonance imaging for demonstration of cerebral infarcts. *Radiologie* **37**, 859–864.

Bastianello, S., Pierallini, A., Colonnese, C. *et al.* (1991) Hyperdense middle cerebral artery CT sign. *Neuroradiology* **33**, 207–211.

Baumgartner, R.W. & Landis, T. (1992) Venous thalamic infarction. *Cerebrovascular Diseases* **2**, 353–358.

Bäzner, H.A. & Hennerici, M.G. (1997) What was the reason for Joseph Haydn's mental decline and gait disturbance? A case of subcortical vascular encephalopathy in the early 19th century. *Cerebrovascular Diseases* **7**, 359–366.

Becker, H., Desch, H., Hacker, H. & Pencz, A. (1979) CT fogging effect with ischaemic cerebral infarcts. *Neuroradiology* **18**, 185.

Beetham, R., Fahie-Wilson, M.N. & Park, D. (1998) What is the role of CSF spectrophotometry in the diagnosis of subarachnoid haemorrhage? *Annals of Clinical Biochemistry* **35**, 1–4.

Beghi, E., Bogliun, G., Cavalletti, G. *et al.* (1989) Haemorrhagic infarction: risk factors, clinical and tomographic features and outcome. A case–control study. *Acta Neurologica Scandinavica* **80**, 226–231.

Bennett, D.A., Gilley, D.W., Wilson, R.S., Huckman, M.S. & Fox, J.H. (1992) Clinical correlates of high signal lesions on magnetic resonance imaging in Alzheimer's disease. *Journal of Neurology* **239**, 186–190.

Benson, D.F. & Cummings, J.L. (1982) Angular gyrus syndrome simulating Alzheimer's disease. *Archives of Neurology* **39**, 616–620.

Berciano, J., Diez, C., Polo, J.M., Pascual, J. & Figols, J. (1991) CT appearance of panencephalopathic and ataxic type of Creutzfeldt–Jakob disease. *Journal of Computer Assisted Tomography* **15**, 332–334.

Berrouschot, J., Barthel, H., Hesse, S., Knapp, W.H., Schneider, D. & von Kummer, R. (2000) Reperfusion and metabolic recovery of brain tissue and clinical outcome after ischaemic stroke and thrombolytic therapy. *Stroke* **31**, 1545–1551.

Bertz, H., Laubenberger, J., Steinfurth, G. & Finke, J. (1998) Sinus venous thrombosis: an unusual cause for neurologic symptoms after bone marrow transplantation under immunosuppression. *Transplantation* **66**, 241–244.

Besson, G., Robert, C., Hommel, M. & Perret, J. (1995) Is it clinically possible to distinguish non-hemorrhagic infarct from hemorrhagic stroke? *Stroke* **26**, 1205–1209.

Bianchi, D., Maeder, P., Bogousslavsky, J., Schnyder, P. & Meuli, R.A. (1998) Diagnosis of cerebral venous thrombosis with routine magnetic resonance: an update. *European Neurology* **40**, 179–190.

Binswanger, O. (1894) Die Abgrenzung der allgemeinen progressiven Paralyse. *Berliner Klinische Wochenschrift* **31**, 1102–1105; 1137–1139; 1180–1186.

Biousse, V., Conard, J., Brouzes, C., Horellou, M.H., Ameri, A. & Bousser, M.G. (1998) Frequency of the 20210 G: a mutation in the 3′-untranslated region of the prothrombin gene in 35 cases of cerebral venous thrombosis. *Stroke* **29**, 1398–1400.

Blennow, K., Wallin, A., Uhlemann, C. & Gottfries, C.G. (1991) White-matter lesions on CT in Alzheimer patients: relation to clinical symptomatology and vascular factors. *Acta Neurologica Scandinavica* **83**, 187–193.

Bogousslavsky, J. & Regli, F. (1985) Anticoagulant-induced intracerebral bleeding in brain ischaemia. *Acta Neurologica Scandinavica* **71**, 464–471.

Bogousslavsky, J., Despland, P.-A. & Regli, F. (1987) Spontaneous carotid dissection with acute stroke. *Archives of Neurology* **44**, 137–140.

Bogousslavsky, J., Regli, F., Uske, A. & Maeder, P. (1991) Early spontaneous haematoma in cerebral infarct. *Neurology* **41**, 837–840.

Bokura, H. & Robinson, R.G. (1997) Long-term cognitive impairment associated with caudate stroke. *Stroke* **28**, 970–975.

Bonita, R. & Thomson, S. (1985) Subarachnoid haemorrhage: epidemiology, diagnosis, management and outcome. *Stroke* **16**, 591–594.

Bonke, B., Koudestaal, P.J., Dijkstra, G. *et al.* (1989) Detection of lacunar infarction in brain CT scans: no evidence of bias from accompanying patient information. *Neuroradiology* **31**, 170–173.

Boon, A.J.W., Tans, J.T.J., Delwel, E.J. *et al.* (1999) Dutch Normal-Pressure Hydrocephalus Study: the role of cerebrovascular disease. *Journal of Neurosurgery* **90**, 221–226.

Bornebroek, M., Haan, J., van Buchem, M.A. *et al.* (1996) White matter lesions and cognitive deterioration in presymptomatic carriers of the amyloid precursor protein gene codon 693 mutation. *Archives of Neurology* **53**, 43–48.

Bots, M.L., van Swieten, J.C., Breteler, M.M.B. *et al.* (1993) Cerebral white matter lesions and atherosclerosis in the Rotterdam Study. *Lancet* **341**, 1232–1237.

Bottomley, P.A. (1989) Human *in vivo* NMR spectroscopy in diagnostic medicine: clinical tool or research probe? *Radiology* **170**, 1–15.

Bousser, M.-G. & Ross Russell, R.W. (1997) *Cerebral Venous Thrombosis*. W.B. Saunders, London.

Bousser, M.-G., Chiras, J., Bories, J. & Castaigne, P. (1985) Cerebral venous thrombosis: a review of 38 cases. *Stroke* **16**, 199–213.

Bowler, J.V., Wade, M.D., Jones, B.E. *et al.* (1995) Contribution of diaschisis to the clinical deficit in human cerebral infarction. *Stroke* **26**, 1000–1006.

Bozzao, L., Angeloni, U., Bastianello, S., Fantozzi, L.M., Pierallini, A. & Fieschi, C. (1992) Early angiographic and CT findings in patients with haemorrhagic infarction in the distribution. *American Journal of Neuroradiology* **12**, 1115–1121.

Bradley, W.G. (1994) Haemorrhage and haemorrhagic infections in the brain. In: *Neuroimaging Clinics of North America*, Vol. 4 (Part 4) (eds A.N. Hasso & C.L. Truwit), pp. 707–732. W.B. Saunders, Philadelphia.

Brant-Zawadski, M., Pereira, B., Bartkowski, H. *et al.* (1987) MR imaging and spectroscopy in clinical and experimental cerebral ischaemia: a review of the middle cerebral artery. *American Journal of Neuroradiology* **8**, 39–45.

Brant-Zawadski, M., Atkinson, D., Detrick, M., Bradley, W.G. & Scidmore, G. (1996) Fluid-attenuated inversion recovery (FLAIR) for assessment of cerebral infarction. *Stroke* **27**, 1187–1191.

Breteler, M.M.B., van Swieten, J.C., Bots, M.L. *et al.* (1994a) Cerebral white matter lesions, vascular risk factors, and cognitive function in a population-based study: the Rotterdam Study. *Neurology* **44**, 1246–1252.

Breteler, M.M.B., van Amerongen, N.M., van Swieten, J.C. *et al.* (1994b) Cognitive correlates of ventricular enlargement and cerebral white matter lesions on magnetic resonance imaging: the Rotterdam Study. *Stroke* **25**, 1109–1115.

Briley, D.P., Wasay, M., Sergent, S. & Thomas, S. (1997) Cerebral white matter changes (leukoaraiosis), stroke and gait disturbance. *Journal of the American Geriatrics Society* **45**, 1434–1438.

Bromberg, J.E.C., Rinkel, G.J.E., Algra, A. *et al.* (1995) Subarachnoid haemorrhage in first and second degree relatives of patients with subarachnoid haemorrhage. *British Medical Journal* **311**, 288–289.

Brooks, W.M., Wesley, M.H., Kodituwakku, P.W., Garry, P.J. & Rosenberg, G.A. (1997) ^{1}H-MRS differentiates white matter hyperintensities in subcortical arteriosclerotic encephalopathy from those in normal elderly. *Stroke* **28**, 1940–1943.

Brouwers, P.J.A.M., Wijdicks, E.F.M., Hasan, D. *et al.* (1989) Serial electrocardiographic recording in aneurysmal subarachnoid haemorrhage. *Stroke* **20**, 1162–1167.

Brouwers, P.J.A.M., Wijdicks, E.F.M. & van Gijn, J. (1992) Infarction after aneurysm rupture does not depend on the distribution or clearance rate of blood. *Stroke* **23**, 374–379.

Brouwers, P.J.A.M., Westenberg, H.G.M. & van Gijn, J. (1995) Noradrenaline concentrations and electrocardiographic abnormalities after aneurysmal subarachnoid haemorrhage. *Journal of Neurology, Neurosurgery and Psychiatry* **58**, 614–617.

de Bruijn, S.F.T.M., Stam, J. & Kappelle, L.J. (1996) Thunderclap headache as first symptom of cerebral venous sinus thrombosis. *Lancet* **348**, 1623–1625.

de Bruijn, S.F.T.M., Stam, J., Koopman, M.M.W., Vandenbroucke, J.P. & Cerebral Venous Sinus Thrombosis Study (1998a) Case–control study of risk of cerebral sinus thrombosis in oral contraceptive users who are carriers of hereditary prothrombotic conditions. *British Medical Journal* **316**, 589–592.

de Bruijn, S.F.T.M., Stam, J., Vandenbroucke, J.P. & Cerebral Venous Sinus Thrombosis Study Group (1998b) Increased risk of cerebral venous sinus thrombosis with third-generation oral contraceptives. *Lancet* **351**, 1404.

de Bruine, J., Limburg, M., van Royen, E., Hijdra, A., Hill, T. & van der Schoot, J. (1990) SPET brain imaging with 201 diethyldithiocarbamate in acute ischaemic stroke. *European Journal of Nuclear Medicine* **17**, 248–251.

Brun, A. & Englund, E. (1986) A white matter disorder in dementia of the Alzheimer type: a pathoanatomical study. *Annals of Neurology* **19**,

253–262.

Bryan, R.N., Levy, L.M., Whitlow, W.D., Killian, J.M., Preziosi, T.J. & Rosario, J.A. (1991) Diagnosis of acute cerebral infarction: comparison of CT and MR imaging. *American Journal of Neuroradiology* **12**, 611–620.

Buonanno, F., Moody, D.M., Ball, M.R. & Laster, D.W. (1978) Computed cranial tomographic findings in cerebral sino-venous occlusion. *Journal of Computer Assisted Tomography* **2**, 281–290.

Burn, J., Dennis, M., Bamford, J., Sandercock, P., Wade, D. & Warlow, C. (1997) Epileptic seizures after a first stroke: the Oxfordshire Community Stroke Project. *British Medical Journal* **315**, 1582–1587.

Buruma, O.J.S., Janson, H.L.F., den Bergh F.A.J.T.M. & Bots, G.T.A.M. (1981) Blood-stained cerebrospinal fluid: traumatic puncture or haemorrhage? *Journal of Neurology, Neurosurgery and Psychiatry* **44**, 144–147.

Byrne, J.V. & Lawton, C.A. (1983) Meningeal sarcoidosis causing intracranial hypertension secondary to dural sinus thrombosis. *British Journal of Radiology* **56**, 755–757.

Cameron, E.W. (1994) Transient ischaemic attacks due to meningoma: report of four cases. *Clinical Radiology* **49**, 416–418.

Campbell, J.K., Houser, O.W., Stevens, J.C., Wahner, H.L., Baker, H.L. & Folger, W.N. (1978) Computed tomography and radionuclide imaging in the evaluation of ischaemic stroke. *Radiology* **126**, 695–702.

Candelise, L., Pinardi, G., Morabito, A. & the Italian Acute Stroke Study Group (1991) Mortality in acute stroke with atrial fibrillation. *Stroke* **22**, 169–174.

Cantú, C. & Barinagarrementeria, F. (1993) Cerebral venous thrombosis associated with pregnancy and puerperium: review of 67 cases. *Stroke* **24**, 1880–1884.

Caplan, L.R. (1995) Binswanger's disease: revisited. *Neurology* **45**, 626–633.

Caplan, L.R., Zarins, C.K. & Hemmati, M. (1985) Spontaneous dissection of the extracranial vertebral arteries. *Stroke* **16**, 1030–1038.

Carhuapoma, J.R., Mitsias, P. & Levine, S.R. (1997) Cerebral venous thrombosis and anticardiolipin antibodies. *Stroke* **28**, 2363–2369.

Carmelli, D., DeCarli, C., Swan, G.E. *et al.* (1998) Evidence for genetic variance in white matter hyperintensity volume in normal elderly male twins. *Stroke* **29**, 1177–1181.

Carolei, A., Marini, C., Di Napoli, M. *et al.* (1997) High incidence in the prospective community-based l'Aquila registry (1994–98): first year's results. *Stroke* **28**, 2500–2506.

Chinese Acute Stroke Trial (CAST) Collaborative Group (1997) CAST: randomised placebo-controlled trial of early aspirin use in 20 000 patients with acute ischaemic stroke. *Lancet* **349**, 1641–1649.

Celani, M.G., Ceravolo, M.G., Duca, E. *et al.* (1992) Was it infarction or haemorrhage?: a clinical diagnosis by means of the Allen Score. *Journal of Neurology* **239**, 411–413.

Celani, M.G., Righetti, E., Migliacci, R. *et al.* (1994) Comparability and validity of two clinical scores in the early diagnosis of stroke. *British Medical Journal* **308**, 1674–1676.

Censori, B., Camerlingo, M., Casto, L. *et al.* (1993) Prognostic factors in first-ever stroke in the carotid artery territory seen within six hours after onset. *Stroke* **24**, 532–535.

Ceyhan, A., Ozturk, M., Yalciner, B., Ekit, M., Sozmen, V. & Baybas, S. (1996) Prognostic value of early CT in occlusion of the middle cerebral artery trunk. *Cerebrovascular Diseases* **6** (Suppl. 2), 59.

Chalela, J.A., Alsop, D.C., Maldjian, J.A., Gonzalez-Atavales, J.B., Kasner, S.E. & Detre, J.A. (2000) Magnetic resonance perfusion imaging in acute ischaemic stroke using continuous arterial spin labeling. *Stroke* **31**, 286.

Chamorro, A., Alday, M., Vila, N., Saiz, A. & Tolosa, E. (1994) Safety of anticoagulation following large cerebral infarction. *Neurology* **44**, A287.

Chatterjee, A., Yapundich, R., Palmer, C.A., Marson, D.C. & Mitchell, G.W. (1996) Leukoencephalopathy associated with cobalamin deficiency. *Neurology* **46**, 832–834.

Chen, T.C., Hinton, D.R., Leichman, L., Atkinson, R.D., Apuzzo, M.L. & Couldwell, W.T. (1994) Multifocal inflammatory leukoencephalopathy associated with levamisole and 5-fluorouracil: case report. *Neurosurgery* **35**, 6–42.

Chien, D., Kwong, K.K., Gress, D.R., Buonanno, F.S., Buxton, R.B. & Rosen, B.R. (1992) MR diffusion imaging of cerebral infarction in humans. *American Journal of Neuroradiology* **13**, 1097–1102.

Chimowitz, M.I., Estes, M.L., Furlan, A.J. & Awad, I.A. (1992) Further observations on the pathology of subcortical lesions identified on magnetic resonance imaging. *Archives of Neurology* **49**, 747–752.

Clasen, R.A., Huckman, M.S., Von Roenn, L.A., Pandolfi, S., Laing, I. & Clasen, J.R. (1980) Time course of cerebral swelling in stroke: a correlative autopsy and CT study. *Advances in Neurology* **28**, 395–412.

Cochran, F.B. & Packman, S. (1992) Homocystinuria presenting as sagittal sinus thrombosis. *European Neurology* **32**, 1–3.

Constans, J.M., Meyerhoff, D.J., Gerson, J. *et al.* (1995) H-1 MR spectroscopic imaging of white matter signal hyperintensities: Alzheimer disease and ischemic vascular dementia. *Radiology* **197**, 517–523.

Coria, F. & Rubio, I. (1996) Cerebral amyloid angiopathies. *Neuropathology and Applied Neurobiology* **22**, 216–227.

Corvol, J.C., Oppenheim, C., Manaï, R. *et al.* (1998) Diffusion-weighted magnetic resonance imaging in a case of cerebral venous thrombosis. *Stroke* **29**, 2649–2652.

Cosnard, G., Duprez, T., Grandin, C., Smith, A.M., Munier, T. & Peeters, A. (1999) Fast FLAIR sequence for detecting major vascular abnormalities during the hyperacute phase of stroke: a comparison with MR angiography. *Neuroradiology* **41**, 342–436.

Crutchfield, K.E., Patronas, N.J., Dambrosia, J.M. *et al.* (1998) Quantitative analysis of cerebral vasculopathy in patients with Fabry disease. *Neurology* **50**, 1746–1749.

Cummings, J.L. & Benson, D.F. (1984) Subcortical dementia: review of an emerging concept. *Archives of Neurology* **41**, 874–879.

Daif, A., Awada, A., Al-Rajeh, S. *et al.* (1995) Cerebral venous thrombosis in adults: a study of 40 cases from Saudi Arabia. *Stroke* **26**, 1193–1195.

Damasio, H. (1983) A computed tomographic guide to the identification of cerebral vascular territories. *Archives of Neurology* **40**, 138–142.

Darby, D.G., Donnan, G.A., Saling, M.A., Walsh, K.W. & Bladin, P.F. (1988) Primary intraventricular haemorrhage: clinical and neuropsychological findings in a prospective stroke series. *Neurology* **38**, 68–75.

Das, R., Vasishta, R.K. & Banerjee, A.K. (1996) Aseptic cerebral venous thrombosis associated with idiopathic ulcerative colitis: a report of two cases. *Clinical Neurology and Neurosurgery* **98**, 179–182.

Davis, K.R., Ackerman, R.H., Kistler, J.P. *et al.* (1977) Computed tomography of cerebral infarction: haemorrhage, contrast enhancement and time of appearance. *Computed Tomography* **1**, 71.

DeCarli, C., Grady, C.L., Clark, C.M. *et al.* (1996) Comparison of positron emission tomography, cognition and brain volume in Alzheimer's disease with and without severe abnormalities of white matter. *Journal of Neurology, Neurosurgery and Psychiatry* **60**, 158–167.

Delanty, N., Vaughan, C., Frucht, S. & Stubgen, P. (1997) Erythropoietin-associated hypertensive posterior leukoencephalopathy. *Neurology* **49**, 686–689.

Dennis, M.S., Bamford, J.M., Molyneux, A.J. & Warlow, C.P. (1987) Rapid resolution of signs of primary intracerebral haemorrhage in computed tomograms of the brain. *British Medical Journal* **279**, 379–381.

DeWitt, D., Kistler, P., Miller, D., Richardson, E. & Buonanno, F. (1987) NMR: neuropathologic correlation in stroke. *Stroke* **18**, 342–351.

Diaz, J.F., Merskey, H., Hachinski, V.C. *et al.* (1991) Improved recognition of leukoaraiosis and cognitive impairment in Alzheimer's disease. *Archives of Neurology* **48**, 1022–1025.

Dickmann, U., Voth, E., Schicha, H., Henze, T., Prange, H. & Emrich, D. (1988) Heparin therapy, deep vein thrombosis and pulmonary embolism after intracerebral haemorrhage. *Klinische Wochenschrift* **66**, 1182–1183.

Dippel, D.W.J., Du Ry van Beest Holle, M., van Kooten, F. *et al.* (1997) The validity and reliability of early infarct signs on CT in acute ischaemic stroke. *Cerebrovascular Diseases* **7** (Suppl. 4), 15.

Dobkin, J.A. & Mintun, M.A. (1993) Clinical PET: Aesop's tortoise? *Radiology* **186**, 13–15.

Donnan, G., Tress, B. & Bladin, P. (1982) A prospective study of lacunar infarction using computerised tomography. *Neurology* **32**, 49–56.

Donnan, G.A., Bladin, P.F., Berkovic, S.F., Longley, W.A. & Saling, M.M. (1991) The stroke syndrome of striatocapsular infarction. *Brain* **114**, 51–70.

Dormont, D., Anxionnat, R., Evrad, S., Louaille, C., Chiras, J. & Marsault, C. (1994) MRI in cerebral venous thrombosis. *Journal of Neuroradiology* **21**, 81–99.

Dropcho, E.J. (1991) Central nervous system injury by therapeutic irradiation. *Neurologic Clinics* **9**, 4–88.

Duffy, G.P. (1983) The warning leak in spontaneous subarachnoid haemorrhage. *Medical Journal of Australia* **i**, 514–516.

Dulli, D.A., Luzzio, C.C., Williams, E.C. & Schutta, H.S. (1996) Cerebral venous thrombosis and activated protein C resistance. *Stroke* **27**, 1731–1733.

Edlow, J.A. & Caplan, L.R. (2000) Avoiding pitfalls in the diagnosis of subarachnoid haemorrhage. *New England Journal of Medicine* **342**, 29–36.

Ellis, S.J. (1993) Functional magnetic resonance: neurological enlightenment? *Lancet* **342**, 882.

Elster, A.D. (1992) MR contrast enhancement in the brainstem and deep cerebral infarction. *American Journal of Neuroradiology* **12**, 1127–1132.

Eng, L.J., Longstreth, W.T. Jr, Shaw, C.M., Eskridge, J.M. & Bahls, F.H. (1990) Cerebellar venous infarction: case report with clinicopathologic correlation. *Neurology* **40**, 837–838.

Englund, E., Brun, A. & Alling, C. (1988) White matter changes in dementia of Alzheimer's type: biochemical and neuropathological correlates. *Brain* **111**, 1425–1439.

Erkinjuntti, T., Gao, F., Lee, D.H., Eliasziw, M., Merskey, H. & Hachinski, V.C. (1994) Lack of difference in brain hyperintensities between patients with early Alzheimer's disease and control subjects. *Archives of Neurology* **51**, 260–268.

Erkinjuntti, T., Benavente, O., Eliasziw, M. *et al.* (1996) Diffuse vacuolization (spongiosis) and arteriolosclerosis in the frontal white matter occurs in vascular dementia. *Archives of Neurology* **53**, 325–332.

Esiri, M.M., Wilcock, G.K. & Morris, J.H. (1997) Neuropathological assessment of the lesions of significance in vascular dementia. *Journal of Neurology, Neurosurgery and Psychiatry* **63**, 749–753.

Evans, M.S., Naritoku, D.K., Couch, J.R. & Ghobrial, M.W. (1996) Onset of neurologic deficits after treatment with dihydroergotamine in a patient with sagittal sinus thrombosis. *Clinical Neuropharmacology* **19**, 177–184.

Fahmy, J.A. (1973) Fundal haemorrhages in ruptured intracranial aneurysms. 1: Material, frequency and morphology. *Acta Ophthalmologica* **51**, 189–198.

Fazekas, F., Kleinert, R., Offenbacher, H. *et al.* (1991) The morphologic correlate of incidental punctate white matter hyperintensities on MR images. *American Journal of Neuroradiology* **12**, 915–921.

Fazekas, F., Kleinert, R., Offenbacher, H. *et al.* (1993) Pathologic correlates of incidental MRI white matter signal hyperintensities. *Neurology* **43**, 1683–1689.

Fenwick, S., Goonetilleke, A., Santosh, C.G. & Newman, P.K. (1997) Cerebral venous thrombosis in Behçet's disease. *Journal of Neurology, Neurosurgery and Psychiatry* **63**, 419.

Ferro, J.M. & Pinto, A.N. (1994) Sexual activity is a common precipitant of subarachnoid haemorrhage. *Cerebrovascular Diseases* **4**, 375.

Filley, C.M. (1998) The behavioral neurology of cerebral white matter. *Neurology* **50**, 1535–1540.

Finocchi, C., Gandolfo, F.C., Gasparetto, B., Del Sette, M., Croce, R. & Loeb, C. (1996) Value of early variables as predictors of short-term outcome in patients with acute focal cerebral ischaemia. *Italian Journal of Neurological Science* **17**, 341–346.

Fisher, C.M. (1975) Clinical syndromes in cerebral thrombosis, hypertensive haemorrhage and ruptured saccular aneurysm. *Clinical Neurosurgery* **22**, 117–147.

Fisher, C.M. (1982) The headache and pain of spontaneous carotid dissection. *Headache* **22**, 60–65.

Fisher, M. & Adams, R.D. (1951) Observations on brain embolism with special reference to the mechanism of haemorrhagic infarction. *Journal of Neuropathology and Experimental Neurology* **10**, 92–94.

Fisher, M. & Albers, G.W. (1999) Applications of diffusion–perfusion magnetic resonance imaging in acute stroke. *Neurology* **52**, 1750–1756.

Fisher, M., Sotak, C.H., Minematsu, K. & Li, L. (1992) New magnetic resonance techniques for evaluation cerebrovascular disease. *Annals of Neurology* **32**, 115–122.

Fishman, R.A. (1992) Cerebrospinal fluid in cerebrovascular disorders. In: *Stroke: Pathophysiology, Diagnosis and Management* (eds H.J.M. Barnett, J.P. Mohr, B.M. Stein & F.M. Yatsu), 2nd edn, pp. 103–110. Churchill Livingstone, New York.

Fitzek, C., Tintera, J., Muller-Forell, W. *et al.* (1998) Differentiation of recent and old cerebral infarcts by diffusion-weighted MRI. *Neuroradiology* **40**, 778–782.

Fontaine, B., Seilhean, D., Tourbah, A. *et al.* (1994) Dementia in two histologically confirmed cases of multiple sclerosis: one case with isolated dementia and one case associated with psychiatric symptoms. *Journal of Neurology, Neurosurgery and Psychiatry* **57**, 3–9.

Frackowiak, R.S.J. (1985) *Studies of Energy Metabolism in Human Cerebrovascular Diseases: New Brain Imaging Techniques in Cerebrovascular Diseases.* John Libbey Eurotext, London.

Franke, C.L., Ramos, L.M.P. & van Gijn, J. (1990) Development of multifocal haemorrhage in a cerebral infarct during computed tomography. *Journal of Neurology, Neurosurgery and Psychiatry* **53**, 531–532.

Franke, C.L., van Swieten, J.C. & Van Gijn, J. (1991) Residual lesions after intracerebral haemorrhage. *Stroke* **22**, 1530–1534.

Fukuda, H. & Kitani, M. (1996) Cigarette smoking is correlated with the periventricular hyperintensity grade on brain magnetic resonance imaging. *Stroke* **27**, 645–649.

Gacs, G., Fox, A.J., Barnett, H.J.M. & Vinuela, F. (1982) CT visualisation of intracranial arterial thromboembolism. *Stroke* **14**, 756–762.

Galan, H.L., McDowell, A.B., Johnson, P.R., Kuehl, T.J. & Knight, A.B. (1995) Puerperal cerebral venous thrombosis associated with decreased free protein S: a case report. *Journal of Reproductive Medicine* **40**, 859–862.

Galer, B.S., Lipton, R.B., Weinstein, S., Bello, L. & Solomon, S. (1990) Apoplectic headache and oculomotor palsy: an unusual presentation of multiple sclerosis. *Neurology* **40**, 1465–1466.

Garcia, J.H., Ho, K.-L. & Caccamo, D.V. (1994) Intracerebral haemorrhage: pathology of selected topics. In: *Intracranial Haemorrhage* (eds C.S. Kase & L.R. Caplan), pp. 48–50. Butterworth-Heinemann, Newton, MA.

van Gijn, J. (1992) Subarachnoid haemorrhage. *Lancet* **339**, 653–655.

van Gijn, J. (1999) Pitfalls in the diagnosis of sudden headache. *Proceedings of the Royal College of Physicians (Edinburgh)* **29**, 21–31.

van Gijn, J. & van Dongen, K.J. (1980) Computed tomography in the diagnosis of subarachnoid haemorrhage and ruptured aneurysm. *Clinical Neurology and Neurosurgery* **82**, 11–24.

van Gijn, J. & van Dongen, K.J. (1982) The time course of aneurysmal haemorrhage on computed tomograms. *Neuroradiology* **23**, 153–156.

van Gijn, J., van Dongen, K.J., Vermeulen, M. & Hijdra, A. (1985) Perimesencephalic haemorrhage: a non-aneurysmal and benign form of subarachnoid haemorrhage. *Neurology* **35**, 493–497.

Globus, J.H. & Epstein, J.A. (1953) Massive cerebral haemorrhage: spontaneous and experimentally induced. *Journal of Neuropathology and Experimental Neurology* **12**, 107–131.

Goebel, H.H., Meyermann, R., Rosin, R. & Schlote, W. (1997) Characteristic morphologic manifestation of CADASIL, cerebral autosomal-dominant arteriopathy with subcortical infarcts and leukoencephalopathy, in skeletal muscle and skin. *Muscle and Nerve* **20**, 625–627.

Goldstein, I.B., Bartzokis, G., Hance, D.B. & Shapiro, D. (1998) Relationship between blood pressure and subcortical lesions in healthy elderly people. *Stroke* **29**, 765–772.

Gorter, J.W. & Stroke Prevention in Reversible Ischemia Trial (SPIRIT) Group, European Atrial Fibrillation Trial (EAFT) Group (1999) Major bleeding during anticoagulation after cerebral ischemia: patterns and risk factors. *Neurology* **53**, 1319–1327.

Graeber, M.C., Jordan, E., Mishra, S.K. & Nadeau, S.E. (1992) Watershed infarction on computed tomographic scan: an unreliable sign of hemodynamic stroke. *Archives of Neurology* **49**, 311–313.

Graff-Radford, N.R., Eslinger, P.J., Damasio, A.R. & Yamada, T. (1984) Nonhemorrhagic infarction of the thalamus: behavioral, anatomic and physiologic correlates. *Neurology* **34**, 14–23.

Gray, F., Dubas, F., Roullet, E. & Escourolle, R. (1985) Leukoencephalopathy in diffuse hemorrhagic cerebral amyloid angiopathy. *Annals of Neurology* **18**, 54–59.

Greenberg, S.M., Vonsattel, J.P., Stakes, J.W., Gruber, M. & Finklestein, S.P. (1993) The clinical spectrum of cerebral amyloid angiopathy: presentations without lobar hemorrhage. *Neurology* **43**, 2073–2079.

Grewal, R.P. (1994) Stroke in Fabry's disease. *Journal of Neurology* **241**, 3–6.

Grond, M., von Kummer, R., Sobesky, J., Schmulling, S. & Heiss, W.D. (1997) Early computer-tomography abnormalities in acute stroke. *Lancet* **350**, 1595–1596.

de Groot, J.C., de Leeuw, F.E., Achten, E. *et al.* (1997) Cerebral white matter lesions and cognitive function. *Cerebrovascular Diseases* **7** (Suppl. 4), 6.

de Groot, J.C., de Leeuw, F.E., Oudkerk, M., *et al.* (2000) Cerebral white matter lesions and cognitive function: the Rotterdam Scan Study. *Annals of Neurology* **47**, 145–151.

Gubitz, G., Counsell, C., Sandercock, P. & Signorini, D. (2000a) Anticoagulants for acute ischaemic stroke. In: *The Cochrane Library; Database of Systematic Reviews* Oxford: Update Software.

Gubitz, G., Sandercock, P. & Counsell, C. (2000b) Antiplatelet therapy for acute ischaemic stroke. In: *The Cochrane Library; Database of Systematic Reviews* Oxford: Update Software.

Gunathilake, S.B. (1998) Rapid resolution of symptoms and signs of intracerebral haemorrhage: case reports. *British Medical Journal* **316**, 1495–1496.

Gupta, S.R., Naheedy, M.H., Young, J.C., Ghobrial, M., Rubino, F.A. & Hindo, W. (1988) Periventricular white matter changes and dementia: clinical, neuropsychological, radiological, and pathological correlation. *Archives of Neurology* **45**, 637–641.

Haan, J., Caekebeke, J.F., van der Meer, F.J. & Wintzen, A.R. (1988) Cerebral venous thrombosis as presenting sign of myeloproliferative disorders. *Journal of Neurology, Neurosurgery and Psychiatry* **51**, 1219–1220.

Hachinski, V. (1992) Preventable senility: a call for action against the vascular dementias. *Lancet* **340**, 645–648.

Hachinski, V.C., Lassen, N.A. & Marshall, J. (1978) Multi-infarct dementia: a cause of mental deterioration in the elderly. *Lancet* **ii**, 207–209.

Hachinski, V.C., Potter, P. & Merskey, H. (1986) Leuko-araiosis: an ancient term for a new problem. *Canadian Journal of Neurological Sciences* **13**, 533–534.

Hacke, W., Kaste, M., Fieschi, C. *et al.* for the ECASS Study Group (1995) Intravenous thrombolysis with recombinant tissue plasminogen activator for acute hemispheric stroke: the European Cooperative Acute Stroke Study (ECASS). *Journal of the American Medical Association* **274**, 1017–1025.

Hakim, A.M., Ryder-Cooke, A. & Melanson, D. (1983) Sequential computerised tomographic appearance of strokes. *Stroke* **14**, 893–897.

Haley, E.C. Jr, Brashear, H.R., Barth, J.T., Cail, W.S. & Kassell, N.F. (1989) Deep cerebral venous thrombosis: clinical, neuroradiological and neuropsychological correlates. *Archives of Neurology* **46**, 337–340.

Hankey, G.J., Khangure, M.S. & Stewart-Wynne, E.G. (1988) Detection of basilar artery thrombosis by computed tomography. *Clinical Radiology* **39**, 140–143.

Hart, R.G. & Easton, J.D. (1986) Haemorrhagic infarcts. *Stroke* **17**, 586–589.

Hart, R.G., Byer, J.A., Slaughter, J.L., Hewett, J.E. & Easton, J.D. (1981) Occurrence and implications of seizures in subarachnoid haemorrhage due to ruptured intracranial aneurysms. *Neurosurgery* **8**, 417–421.

Hasan, D., Schonk, R.S.M., Avezaat, C.J.J., Tanghe, H.L.J., van Gijn, J. & van der Lugt, P.J.M. (1993) Epileptic seizures after subarachnoid haemorrhage. *Annals of Neurology* **33**, 286–291.

Hasso, A.N., Stringer, W.A. & Brown, K.D. (1994) Cerebral ischaemia and infarction. In: *Neuroimaging Clinics of North America*, Vol. 4 (Part 4) (eds A.N. Hasso & C.L. Truwit), pp. 733–752. W.B. Saunders, Philadelphia.

Hauser, D., Barzilai, N., Zalish, M., Oliver, M. & Pollack, A. (1996) Bilateral papilledema with retinal hemorrhages in association with cerebral venous sinus thrombosis and paroxysmal nocturnal hemoglobinuria. *American Journal of Ophthalmology* **122**, 592–593.

Hawkins, G.C., Bonita, R., Broad, J.B. & Anderson, N.E. (1995) Inadequacy of clinical scoring systems to differentiate stroke subtypes in population-based studies. *Stroke* **26**, 1338–1342.

Hayman, A.L., Taber, K.H., Jhingran, S.G., Killian, S.M. & Carroll, R.G. (1989) Cerebral infarction: diagnosis and assessment of prognosis by using 123IMP-SPECT and CT. *American Journal of Neuroradiology* **10**, 557–562.

Hayman, A., Taber, K., Ford, J. & Bryan, R. (1991) Mechanisms of MR signal alteration by acute intracerebral blood: old concepts and new theories. *American Journal of Neuroradiology* **12**, 899–907.

Hayman, L.A., Evans, R.A., Bastion, F.O. & Hinck, V.C. (1981) Delayed high dose contrast CT: identifying patients at risk of massive haemorrhagic infarction. *American Journal of Neuroradiology* **2**, 139–146.

Heinsius, T., Bogousslavsky, J. & Van Melle, G. (1998) Large infarcts in the middle cerebral artery territory: aetiology and outcome patterns. *Neurology* **50**, 341–350.

Heiss, W.D. (1992) Experimental evidence of ischaemic thresholds and functional recovery. *Stroke* **23**, 1668–1672.

Heiss, W.-D., Huber, M., Fink, G.R. *et al.* (1992) Progressive derangement of peri-infarct viable tissue in ischaemic stroke. *Journal of Cerebral Blood Flow and Metabolism* **12**, 193–203.

Heiss, W.-D., Grond, M., Thiel, A.V., Stockhausen, H.-M. & Rudolf, J. (1997) Ischaemic brain tissue salvaged from infarction with alteplase. *Lancet* **349**, 159–160.

Heistinger, M., Rumpl, E., Illiasch, H. *et al.* (1992) Cerebral sinus thrombosis in a patient with hereditary protein S deficiency: case report and review of the literature. *Annals of Hematology* **64**, 105–109.

Hickey, W.F., Garnick, M.B., Henderson, I.C. & Dawson, D.M. (1982) Primary cerebral venous thrombosis in patients with cancer—a rarely diagnosed paraneoplastic syndrome. Report of three cases and review of the literature. *American Journal of Medicine* **73**, 740–750.

Higano, S., Uemura, F., Shishido, F. *et al.* (1990) Evaluation of ischaemic threshold for the indication of thrombolytic therapy of embolic stroke in very acute phase. *Stroke* **21** (Suppl. 1), 1–120.

Hijdra, A. & van Gijn, J. (1982) Early death from rupture of an intracranial aneurysm. *Journal of Neurosurgery* **57**, 765–768.

Hillier, C.E.M., Collins, P.W., Bowen, D.J., Bowley, S. & Wiles, C.M. (1988) Inherited prothrombotic risk factors and cerebral venous thrombosis. *QJM—Monthly Journal of the Association of Physicians* **91**, 677–680.

Hillman, J. (1986) Should computed tomography scanning replace lumbar puncture in the diagnostic process in suspected subarachnoid haemorrhage? *Surgical Neurology* **26**, 547–550.

Hillmen, P., Lewis, S.M., Bessler, M., Luzzatto, L. & Dacie, J.V. (1995) Natural history of paroxysmal nocturnal hemoglobinuria. *New England Journal of Medicine* **333**, 1253–1258.

Hinchey, J., Chaves, C., Appignani, B. *et al.* (1996) A reversible posterior leukoencephalopathy syndrome. *New England Journal of Medicine* **334**, 494–500.

Hommel, M., Grand, S., Devoulon, P. & Le Bas, J.-F. (1994) New directions in magnetic resonance in acute cerebral ischemia. *Cerebrovascular Diseases* **4**, 3–11.

Hornig, C.R., Dorndorf, W. & Agnoli, A.L. (1986) Haemorrhagic cerebral infarction: a prospective study. *Stroke* **17**, 179–185.

Hornig, C.R., Bauer, T., Simon, C., Trittmacher, S. & Dorndorf, W. (1993) Haemorrhagic transformation in cardioembolic cerebral infarction. *Stroke* **24**, 465–468.

Howe, F.A., Maxwell, R.J., Saunders, D.E., Brown, M.M. & Griffiths, J.R. (1993) Proton spectroscopy *in vivo*. *Magnetic Resonance Quarterly* **9**, 31–39.

Huberfeld, G., Kubis, N., Lot, G. *et al.* (1998) G20210A prothrombin gene mutation in two siblings with cerebral venous thrombosis. *Neurology* **51**, 316–317.

Hund, E., Jansen, O., Koch, M.C. *et al.* (1997) Proximal myotonic myopathy with MRI white matter abnormalities of the brain. *Neurology* **48**, 33–37.

Huston, J., Lewis, B.D., Wiebers, D.O., Meyer, F.B., Riederer, S.J. & Weaver, A.L. (1993) Carotid artery: prospective blinded comparison of two-dimensional time-of-flight MR angiography with conventional angiograpy and duplex US. *Radiology* **186**, 339–344.

Hyland, H.H. & Barnett, H.J.M. (1954) The pathogenesis of cranial nerve palsies associated with intracranial aneurysms. *Proceedings of the Royal Society of Medicine* **47**, 141–146.

Ida, M., Mizunuma, K. & Tada, S. (1994) Subcortical low intensity in early cortical ischaemia. *American Journal of Neuroradiology* **15**, 1387–1393.

Infeld, B., Davis, S.M., Lichtenstein, M., Mitchell, P.J. & Hopper, J.L. (1995) Crossed cerebellar diaschisis and brain recovery after stroke. *Stroke* **26**, 90–95.

Inoue, Y., Takemoto, K. & Miyamoto, T. (1980) Sequential computed tomography scans in acute cerebral infarction. *Radiology* **135**, 655–662.

International Stroke Trial Collaborative Group (1997) The International Stroke Trial (IST): a randomized trial of aspirin, subcutaneous heparin, both or neither among 19 435 patients with acute ischaemic stroke. *Lancet* **349**, 1569–1581.

Inzitari, D., Di Carlo, A., Mascalchi, M., Pracucci, G. & Amaducci, L. (1995) The cardiovascular outcome of patients with motor impairment and extensive leukoaraiosis. *Archives of Neurology* **52**, 687–691.

Inzitari, D., Cadelo, M., Marranci, M.L., Pracucci, G. & Pantoni, L. (1997) Vascular deaths in elderly neurological patients with leukoaraiosis. *Journal of Neurology, Neurosurgery and Psychiatry* **62**, 177–181.

Isensee, C., Reul, J. & Thron, A. (1994) Magnetic resonance imaging of thrombosed dural sinuses. *Stroke* **25**, 29–34.

Ito, Y., Niwa, H., Iida, T. *et al.* (1997) Post-transfusion reversible posterior leukoencephalopathy syndrome with cerebral vasoconstriction. *Neurology* **49**, 1174–1175.

Ivo, L. (1999) CT scanning can differentiate between ischaemic attack and haemorrhage. *Lancet* **319**, 1197–1198.

Jacobs, K., Moulin, T., Bogousslavsky, J. *et al.* (1996) The stroke syndrome of cortical vein thrombosis. *Neurology* **47**, 376–382.

Jaillard, A.S., Hommel, M. & Mallaret, M. (1994) Venous sinus thrombosis associated with androgens in a healthy young man. *Stroke* **25**, 212–213.

Janota, I., Mirsen, T.R., Hachinski, V.C., Lee, D.H. & Merskey, H. (1989) Neuropathologic correlates of leuko-araiosis. *Archives of Neurology* **46**,

1124–1128.

Jerntop, P. & Berglund, G. (1992) Stroke registry in Malmo, Sweden. *Stroke* **23**, 357–361.

Johnson, R.V., Kaplan, S.R. & Blailock, Z.R. (1970) Cerebral venous thrombosis in paroxysmal nocturnal hemoglobinuria: Marchiafava-Micheli syndrome. *Neurology* **20**, 681–686.

Jorgensen, H.S., Nakayama, H., Raaschou, H.O. & Olsen, T.S. (1995) Intracerebral hemorrhage versus infarction: stroke severity, risk factors and prognosis. *Annals of Neurology* **38**, 45–50.

Kakar, A., Agarwal, C.S. & Arora, A. (1998) Superior sagittal sinus and inferior vena cava thrombosis with acute Budd–Chiari syndrome—superior sagittal sinus thrombosis and inferior vena cava thrombosis with acute Budd–Chiari syndrome due to familial thrombophilia of unknown aetiology. *Postgraduate Medical Journal* **74**, 557–559.

Kappelle, L.J., Wokke, J.H.J., Huynen, C.H. & van Gijn, J. (1986) Acute disseminated encephalitis documented by magnetic resonance imaging and computed tomography: report of a case. *Clinical Neurology and Neurosurgery* **88**, 197–202.

Kawamura, J., Meyer, J.S., Ichijo, M., Kobari, M., Terayama, Y. & Weathers, S. (1993) Correlations of leuko-araiosis with cerebral atrophy and perfusion in elderly normal subjects and demented patients. *Journal of Neurology, Neurosurgery and Psychiatry* **56**, 182–187.

Keane, J.R. (1979) Retinal haemorrhage: its significance in 110 patients with acute encephalopathy of unknown cause. *Archives of Neurology* **36**, 691–694.

Keir, S.L., Lewis, S.C., Wardlaw, J.M., Sandercock, P.A.G., Chen, Z.M. on behalf of the CAST/IST Collaborative Groups (2000) Effects of aspirin or heparin inadvertently given to patients with haemorrhagic stroke. *Stroke* **31**, 314.

Keller, E., Flacke, S., Urbach, H. & Schild, H.H. (1999) Diffusion- and perfusion-weighted magnetic resonance imaging in deep cerebral venous thrombosis. *Stroke* **30**, 1144–1146.

Kellett, M.W., Martin, P.J., Enevoldson, T.P., Brammer, C. & Toh, C.M. (1998) Cerebral venous sinus thrombosis associated with 20210A mutation of the prothrombin gene. *Journal of Neurology, Neurosurgery and Psychiatry* **65**, 611–612.

Kendall, B.E. & Pullicino, P. (1980) Intravascular contrast injection in ischaemic lesions. II: Effect on prognosis. *Neuroradiology* **19**, 241–244.

Kertesz, A., Black, S.E., Nicholson, L. & Carr, T. (1987) The sensitivity and specificity of MRI in stroke. *Neurology* **37**, 1580–1585.

Kidwell, C.S., Alger, J.R., Di Salle, F. *et al.* (1999) Diffusion-weighted magnetic resonance imaging in patients with transient ischaemic attacks. *Stroke* **30**, 1174–1180.

Kinal, M.E. (1967) Traumatic thrombosis of dural venous sinuses in closed head injury. *Journal of Neurosurgery* **27**, 142–145.

Kinkel, W.R. & Jacobs, L. (1976) Computerised axial tomography in cerebrovascular disease. *Neurology* **26**, 924–930.

Kissel, J.T., Burde, R.M., Klingele, T.G. & Zeiger, H.E. (1983) Pupil-sparing oculomotor palsies with internal carotid–posterior communicating artery aneurysms. *Annals of Neurology* **13**, 149–154.

Kistler, J.P., Hochberg, F.H., Brooks, B.R., Richardson, E.P., New, P.F.J. & Schnur, J. (1975) Computerised axial tomography: clinicopathologic correlation. *Neurology* **25**, 201–209.

Kittner, S.J., Sharkness, C.M., Price, T.R. *et al.* (1990) Infarcts with a cardiac source of embolism in the NINCDS Stroke Data Bank: historical features. *Neurology* **40**, 281–284.

Kohno, K., Hoehn-Berlage, M., Mies, G., Back, T. & Hossman, K.A. (1995) Relationship between diffusion-weighted MR images, cerebral blood flow and energy state in experimental brain infarction. *Magnetic Resonance Imaging* **13**, 73–80.

Kolominsky-Rabas, P.L., Sarti, C., Heuschmann, P.U. *et al.* (1998) A prospective community-based study of stroke in Germany—the Erlangen Stroke Project (ESPro): incidence and case fatality at 1, 3 and 12 months. *Stroke* **29**, 2501–2506.

Kopitnik, T.A. & Samson, D.S. (1993) Management of subarachnoid haemorrhage. *Journal of Neurology, Neurosurgery and Psychiatry* **56**, 947–959.

Koroshetz, W.J. & Gonzales, R.G. (1999) Imaging stroke in progress: magnetic resonance advances but computed tomography is poised for counterattack. *Annals of Neurology* **46** (4), 557–558.

Korv, J., Roose, M. & Kaasik, A. (1997) Stroke registry of Tartu, Estonia, from 1991 through 1993. *Cerebrovascular Diseases* 7, 154–162.

Kuller, L.H., Shemanski, L., Manolio, T. *et al.* (1998) Relationship between ApoE, MRI findings, and cognitive function in the Cardiovascular Health Study. *Stroke* **29**, 388–398.

von Kummer, R. (1998) Effect of training in reading CT scans on patient selection for ECASS II. *Neurology* **51** (Suppl. 3), 550–552.

von Kummer, R., Meyding-Lamade, U., Frosting, M. *et al.* (1994) Sensitivity and prognostic value of early CT in occlusion of the middle cerebral artery trunk. *American Journal of Neuroradiology* **15**, 9–15.

von Kummer, R., Holle, R., Grzyska, U. *et al.* (1996) Inter-observer agreement in assessing early CT signs of middle cerebral artery infarction. *American Journal of Neuroradiology* **17**, 1743–1748.

von Kummer, R., Allen, K.L., Holle, R. *et al.* (1997) Acute stroke: usefulness of early CT findings before thrombolytic therapy. *Radiology* **205**, 327–333.

Kumral, E., Bogousslavsky, J., Van Melle, G., Regli, F. & Pierre, P. (1995) Headache at stroke onset: the Lausanne Stroke Registry. *Journal of Neurology, Neurosurgery and Psychiatry* **58**, 490–492.

Kwa, V.I., Stam, J., Blok, L.M. & Verbeeten, B. Jr (1997) T2-weighted hyperintense MRI lesions in the pons in patients with atherosclerosis. *Stroke* **28**, 1357–1360.

Kwong, K.K. (1995) Functional magnetic resonance imaging with echo planar imaging. *Magnetic Resonance Quarterly* **11**, 1–20.

Kyritsis, A.P., Williams, E.C. & Schutta, H.S. (1990) Cerebral venous thrombosis due to heparin-induced thrombocytopenia. *Stroke* **21**, 1503–1505.

Lafitte, F., Boukobza, M., Guichard, J.P. *et al.* (1997) MRI and MRA for diagnosis and follow-up of cerebral venous thrombosis (CVT). *Clinical Radiology* **52**, 672–679.

Lammie, G.A., Brannan, F., Slattery, J. & Warlow, C. (1997) Non-hypertensive cerebral small-vessel disease: an autopsy study. *Stroke* **28**, 2222–2229.

Lance, J.W. (1976) Headache related to sexual activity. *Journal of Neurology, Neurosurgery and Psychiatry* **39**, 1226–1230.

Lance, J.W. (1993) *Mechanism and Management of Headache*, 5th edn. Butterworth-Heinemann, Cambridge University Press, Cambridge.

Lance, J.W. & Hinterberger, H. (1976) Symptoms of phaeochromocytoma, with particular reference to headache, correlated with catecholamine production. *Archives of Neurology* **33**, 281–288.

Lancon, J.A., Killough, K.R., Tibbs, R.E., Lewis, A.I. & Parent, A.D. (1999) Spontaneous dural sinus thrombosis in children. *Pediatric Neurosurgery* **30**, 23–29.

Lang, E.W., Daffertshofer, M., Daffershofer, A., Wirth, S.B., Chesnut, R.M. & Hennerici, M. (1995) Variability of vascular territory in stroke: pitfalls and failure of stroke pattern interpretation. *Stroke* **26**, 942–945.

Lanska, D.J. & Kryscio, R.J. (1997) Peripartum stroke and intracranial venous thrombosis in the National Hospital Discharge Survey. *Obstetrics and Gynecology* **89**, 413–418.

Lanska, D.J. & Kryscio, R.J. (1998) Stroke and intracranial venous thrombosis during pregnancy and puerperium. *Neurology* **51**, 1622–1628.

Latchaw, R.E. (1999) The roles of diffusion and perfusion MR imaging in acute stroke management. *American Journal of Neuroradiology* **20**, 957–959.

Lecouvert, F.E., Duprez, T.P.J., Raymackers, J.M., Peeters, A. & Cosnard, G. (1999) Resolution of early diffusion-weighted and FLAIR MRI abnormalities in a patient with TIA. *Neurology* **52**, 1085–1087.

Lee, D., Vinuela, F., Pelz, D., Lau, C., Donald, A. & Merskey, H. (1987) Interobserver variation in computed tomography of the brain. *Archives of Neurology* **44**, 30–31.

de Leeuw, F.E., de Groot, J.C., Oudkerk, M. *et al.* (1999) A follow-up study of blood pressure and cerebral white matter lesions. *Annals of Neurology* **46**, 827–833.

de Leeuw, F.E., de Groot, J.C., Oudkerk, M. *et al.* (2000) Atrial fibrillation and cerebral white matter lesions: the Rotterdam scan study. *Neurology* **54**, 1795–1800.

Lefkowitz, D., LaBenz, M., Nudo, S.R., Steg, R.E. & Bertoni, J.M. (1999) Hyperacute ischemic stroke missed by diffusion-weighted imaging. *American Journal of Neuroradiology* **20**, 1871–1875.

Leifer, D., Buonanno, F.S. & Richardson, E.P. Jr (1990) Clinicopathologic correlations of cranial magnetic resonance imaging of periventricular white matter. *Neurology* **40**, 911–918.

Lenders, J.W., Keiser, H.R., Goldstein, D.S. *et al.* (1995) Plasma metanephrines in the diagnosis of phaeochromocytoma. *Annals of Internal Medicine* **123**, 101–109.

Lev, M.H., Farkas, J., Gemmete, J.J. *et al.* (1999) Acute stroke: improved nonenhanced CT detection benefits soft-copy interpretation by using variable window width and centre level settings. *Radiology* **213**, 150–155.

Leys, D., Pruvo, J.P., Parent, M. J. *et al.* (1991) Could Wallerian degeneration contribute to 'leuko-araiosis' in subjects free of any vascular disorder? *Journal of Neurology, Neurosurgery and Psychiatry* **54**, 46–50.

Leys, D., Pruvo, J.P., Godefroy, O., Rondepierre, P. & Leclerc, X. (1992) Prevalence and significance of hyperdense middle cerebral artery in acute stroke. *Stroke* **23**, 317–324.

Limburg, M. & Hijdra, A. (1992) The reliability of very early computerised tomography in ischaemic stroke. *Cerebrovascular Diseases* **2**, 206.

Limburg, M., Van Royen, E.A., Hijdra, A., deBruine, J.F. & Verbeeten, B.W.J. (1990) Single photon emission computed tomography and early death in acute ischaemic stroke. *Stroke* **21**, 1150–1155.

Lindgren, A., Norrving, B., Rudling, O. & Johansson, B.O. (1994) Comparison of clinical and neuroradiological findings in first-ever stroke: a population-based study. *Stroke* **25**, 1371–1377.

Lindgren, A., Geijer, B., Brockstedt, S. *et al.* (1997) The use of diffusion-MRI to differentiate acute cerebral infarcts from chronic lesions. *Cerebrovascular Diseases* **7** (Suppl. 4), 60.

Lindley, R.I., Wardlaw, J.M., Ricci, S., Celani, M., Sandercock, P. on behalf of the International Stroke Trial Group (1992) Haemorrhagic transformation of cerebral infarction in acute stroke patients in the International Stroke Trial Pilot. *Cerebrovascular Diseases* **2**, 234.

Linn, F.H.H., Wijdicks, E.F.M., van der Graaf, Y., Weerdesteyn-van Vliet, F.A.C., Bartelds, A.I.M. & van Gijn, J. (1994) Prospective study of sentinel headache in aneurysmal subarachnoid haemorrhage. *Lancet* **344**, 590–593.

Linn, F.H.H., Rinkel, G.J.E., Algra, A. & van Gijn, J. (1998) Headache characteristics in subarachnoid haemorrhage and benign thunderclap headache. *Journal of Neurology, Neurosurgery and Psychiatry* **65**, 791–793.

Linn, F.H.H., Rinkel, G.J.E., Algra, A. & van Gijn, J. (1999) Follow-up of idiopathic thunderclap headache in general practice. *Journal of Neurology* **246**, 946–948.

Lodder, J. (1984) CT detected haemorrhagic infarction: relation with size of infarct and the presence of midline shift. *Acta Neurologica Scandinavica* **70**, 329–335.

Lodder, J., Krijne-Kubat, B. & Broekman, J. (1986) Cerebral haemorrhagic infarction at autopsy: cardiac embolic causes and the relationship to the cause of death. *Stroke* **17**, 626–629.

Longstreth, W.T., Manolio, T.A., Arnold, A. *et al.* (1996) Clinical correlates of white matter findings on cranial magnetic resonance imaging of 3301 elderly people: the cardiovascular health study. *Stroke* **27**, 1274–1282.

Lovblad, K.-O., Laubach, H.-J., Baird, A.E. *et al.* (1998) Clinical experience with diffusion-weighted MR in patients with acute stroke. *American Journal of Neuroradiology* **19**, 1061–1066.

Lucas, C., Parent, M., Delandsheer, E. *et al.* (1992) Hémorragies cérébrales multiples et angiopathie amyloide de la substance blanche dans un cas de maladie d'Alzheimer. [Multiple cerebral hemorrhage and amyloid angiopathy of the white matter in a case of Alzheimer's disease.] *Revue Neurologique* **148**, 218–220 [in French].

Lüdemann, P., Nabavi, D.G., Junker, R. *et al.* (1998) Factor V Leiden mutation is a risk factor for cerebral venous thrombosis—a case-control study of 55 patients. *Stroke* **29**, 2507–2510.

Ma, K.C., Lundberg, P.O., Lilja, A. & Olsson, Y. (1992) Binswanger's disease in the absence of chronic arterial hypertension: a case report with clinical, radiological and immunohistochemical observations on intracerebral blood vessels. *Acta Neuropathologica* **83**, 434–439.

Macdonald, D.R. (1991) Neurologic complications of chemotherapy. *Neurologic Clinics* **9**, 4–67.

McFadzean, R.M., Doyle, D., Rampling, R. *et al.* (1991) Pituitary apoplexy and its effect on vision. *Neurosurgery* **29**, 669–675.

MacKay, S., Meyerhoff, D.J., Constans, J.M., Norman, D., Fein, G. & Weiner, M.W. (1996) Regional gray and white matter metabolite differences in subjects with AD, with subcortical ischemic vascular dementia, and elderly controls with ^{1}H magnetic resonance spectroscopic imaging. *Archives of Neurology* **53**, 167–174.

McQuinn, B.A. & O'Leary, D.H. (1987) White matter lucencies on computed tomography, subacute arteriosclerotic encephalopathy (Binswanger's disease), and blood pressure. *Stroke* **18**, 900–905.

Madden, K., Karanjia, P., Marshfield, W.I., Adams, H., Clarke, W. & the TOAST Investigators (1994) Accuracy of initial stroke subtype diagnosis in the TOAST trial. *Neurology* **44** (Suppl. 2), A271.

Manelfe, C., Clanet, M., Gigaud, M., Bonafe, A., Guiraud, B. & Rascol, A. (1981) Internal capsule: normal anatomy and ischaemic changes demonstrated by computed tomography. *American Journal of Neuroradiology* **2**, 149–155.

Manelfe, C., Larrue, V., von Kummer, R. *et al.* (1999) Association of hyperdense middle cerebral artery sign with clinical outcome in patients treated with tissue plasminogen activator. *Stroke* **30**, 769–772.

Manschot, W.A. (1954) Subarachnoid haemorrhage: intraocular symptoms and their pathogenesis. *American Journal of Ophthalmology* **38**, 501–505.

Mäntylä, R., Erkinjuntti, T., Salonen, O. *et al.* (1997) Variable agreement between visual rating scales for white matter hyperintensities on MRI: comparison of 13 rating scales in a poststroke cohort. *Stroke* **28**, 1614–1623.

Marchal, G., Beaudouin, V., Rioux, P. *et al.* (1996) Prolonged persistence of substantial volumes of potentially viable brain tissue after stroke: a correlative PET-CT study with voxel-based data analysis. *Stroke* **27**, 599–606.

Marchal, G., Benali, K., Iglesias, S., Viader, F., Derlon, J.-M. & Baron, J.-C. (1999) Voxel-based mapping of irreversible ischaemic damage with PET in acute stroke. *Brain* **123**, 2387–2400.

Marks, M.P., de Crespigny, A., Lentz, D., Enzmann, D.R., Albers, G.W. & Moseley, M.E. (1996) Acute and chronic stroke: navigated spin-echo diffusion-weighted MR imaging. *Radiology* **199**, 403–408.

Maroun, F.B., Murray, G.P., Jacob, J.C., Mangan, M.A. & Faridi, M. (1986) Familial intracranial aneurysms: report of three families. *Surgical Neurology* **25**, 85–88.

Martin, C.G.M., van Swieten, J.C., Sever, A.R., Scheltens, Ph., Pieterman, H. & Breteler, M.M.B. (1997) Change in white matter lesions in 60 healthy elderly patients over a 5-year period. *Journal of Neurology* **244** (Suppl. 3), S23.

Martinelli, I., Landi, G., Merati, G., Cella, R., Tosetto, A. & Mannucci, P.M. (1996) Factor V gene mutation is a risk factor for cerebral venous thrombosis. *Thrombosis and Haemostasis* **75**, 393–394.

Mas, J.-L., Meder, J.F. & Meary, E. (1992) Dural sinus thrombosis: long-term follow up by magnetic resonance imaging. *Cerebrovascular Diseases* **2**, 137–144.

Mascalchi, M., Inzitari, D., Dal Pozzo, G., Taverni, N. & Abbamondi, A.L. (1989) Computed tomography, magnetic resonance imaging and pathological correlations in a case of Binswanger's disease. *Canadian Journal of Neurological Sciences* **16**, 214–218.

Masson, M., Prier, S., Desbleds, M.T., Colombani, J.M. & Juliard, J.M. (1984) Transformation d'un infarctus cérébral en hémorragie au cours d'un examen tomodensitométrique, chez un patient sous traitement anticoagulant. *Revue Neurologique* **140**, 502–506.

Mastaglia, F.L., Harker, N., Phillips, B.A. *et al.* (1998) Dominantly inherited proximal myotonic myopathy and leukoencephalopathy in a family with an incidental CLCN1 mutation. *Journal of Neurology, Neurosurgery and Psychiatry* **64**, 543–547.

Matsuda, M., Ohashi, M., Shiino, A., Matsumura, K. & Handa, J. (1993) Circumstances precipitating aneurysmal subarachnoid haemorrhage. *Cerebrovascular Diseases* **3**, 285–288.

Matthews, W.F. & Frommeyer, W.B. (1955) The *in vitro* behaviour of erythrocytes in human cerebrospinal fluid. *Journal of Laboratory and Clinical Medicine* **45**, 508–515.

Mayer, S.A., Fink, M.E., Homma, S. *et al.* (1994) Cardiac injury associated with neurogenic pulmonary oedema following subarachnoid haemorrhage. *Neurology* **44**, 815–820.

Mead, G.E. & Wardlaw, J.M. (1998) Detection of intralumenal thrombus in acute stroke by proton density MR imaging. *Cerebrovascular Diseases* **8**, 133–144.

Mead, G.E., O'Neill, P.A., Farrell, A. & McCollum, C.N. (1996) Does the Oxfordshire Community Stroke project classification predict the site of cerebral infarction? *Cerebrovascular Diseases* **6** (Suppl. 2), 155.

Mead, G.E., Lewis, S.C., Wardlaw, J.M. & Dennis, M.S. (1998) Risk factors for border-zone and territorial infarcts. 7th European Stroke Conference, Edinburgh, UK, May 27–30. *Cerebrovascular Diseases* **8** (Suppl. 4), 28.

Mead, G.E., Wardlaw, J.M., Lewis, S.C., Dennis, M.S. & Warlow, C.P. (1999) Should computed tomography appearance of lacunar stroke influence patient management? *Journal of Neurology, Neurosurgery and Psychiatry* **67**, 682–684.

Mead, G.E., Lewis, S.C., Wardlaw, J.M., Dennis, M.S. & Warlow, C.P. (2000) How well does the Oxfordshire Community Stroke Project classification predict the site and size of infarct on brain imaging? *Journal of Neurology, Neurosurgery and Psychiatry* **68**, 558–562.

Meininger, V., James, J.M., Rio, B. & Zittoun, R. (1985) Occlusions des sinus veineux de la dure-mere au cours des hemopathies. *Revue Neurologique (Paris)* **141**, 228–233.

Melo, T.P., Pinto, A.N. & Ferro, J.M. (1996) Headache in intracerebral haematoma. *Neurology* **47**, 494–500.

Mendez, M.F., Adams, N.L. & Lewandowski, K.S. (1989) Neurobehavioral changes associated with caudate lesions. *Neurology* **39**, 349–354.

Mendez, M.F., Stanley, T.M., Medel, N.M., Li, Z.P. & Tedesco, D.T. (1997) The vascular dementia of Fabry's disease. *Dementia* **8**, 252–257.

Merrick, M.V. (1990) Cerebral perfusion studies. *European Journal of Nuclear Medicine* **17**, 98.

Merten, C.L., Knitelius, H.O., Assheuer, J., Bergmann-Kurz, B., Hedde, J.P. & Bewermeyer, H. (1999) MRI of acute cerebral infarcts: increased contrast enhancement with continuous infusion of gadolinium. *Neuroradiology* **41**, 242–248.

Miller, J., Wardlaw, J.M. & Lammie, G.A. (1999) Intracerebral haemorrhage and cerebral amyloid angiopathy: CT features with pathological correlation. *Clinical Radiology* **54**, 422–429.

Miller, R.F., Lucas, S.B., Hall-Craggs, M.A. *et al.* (1997) Comparison of magnetic resonance imaging with neuropathological findings in the diagnosis of HIV and CMV associated CNS disease in AIDS. *Journal of Neurology, Neurosurgery and Psychiatry* **62**, 346–351.

Miyazawa, N., Satoh, T., Hashizume, K. & Fukamachi, A. (1997) Xenon contrast CT-CBF measurements in high-intensity foci on T2-weighted MR images in centrum semiovale of asymptomatic individuals. *Stroke* **28**, 984–987.

Mohamed, A., McLeod, J.G. & Hallinan, J. (1991) Superior sagittal sinus thrombosis. *Clinical and Experimental Neurology* **28**, 23–36.

Mohr, J.P., Biller, J., Hilal, S.K. *et al.* (1995) Magnetic resonance versus computed tomographic imaging in acute stroke. *Stroke* **26**, 807–812.

Mokri, B., Sundt, T.M., Houser, O.W. & Piepgras, D.G. (1986) Spontaneous dissection of the cervical internal carotid artery. *Annals of Neurology* **19**, 126–138.

Mori, E., Tabuchi, M., Ohsumi, Y. *et al.* (1990) Intra-arterial urokinase infusion therapy in acute thromboembolic stroke. *Stroke* **21**, 1–74.

Mori, E., Yoneda, Y., Tabuchi, M. *et al.* (1992) Intravenous recombinant tissue plasminogen activator in acute carotid artery territory stroke. *Neurology* **42**, 976–982.

Moroney, J.T., Bagiella, E., Desmond, D.W., Paik, M.C., Stern, Y. & Tatemichi, T.K. (1996) Risk factors for incident dementia after stroke: role of hypoxic and ischemic disorders. *Stroke* **27**, 1283–1289.

Morretti, J.-l., Defer, G., Cinotti, L. *et al.* (1990) Luxury perfusion' with ^{99m}Tc-HMPAO and ^{123}I-IMP SPECT imaging during the subacute phase of stroke. *European Journal of Nuclear Medicine* **16**, 17–22.

Motto, C., Aritsu, E., Boccardi, E., De Grandi, C., Piana, A. & Candelise, L. (1997) Reliability of haemorrhagic transformation diagnosis in acute ischaemic stroke. *Stroke* **28**, 302–306.

Moulin, T., Cattin, F., Crepin-Leblond, T. *et al.* (1996) Early CT signs in acute middle cerebral artery infarction: predictive value for subsequent infarct locations and outcome. *Neurology* **47**, 366–375.

Multicentre Acute Stroke Trial—Italy (MAST-I) Group (1995) Randomized controlled trial of streptokinase, aspirin and combination of both in treatment of acute ischaemic stroke. *Lancet* **346**, 1509–1514.

Munoz, D.G., Hastak, S.M., Harper, B., Lee, D. & Hachinski, V.C. (1993) Pathologic correlates of increased signals of the centrum ovale on magnetic resonance imaging. *Archives of Neurology* **50**, 492–497.

Nadeau, S.E. & Trobe, J.D. (1983) Pupil sparing in oculomotor palsy: a brief review. *Annals of Neurology* **13**, 143–148.

Nakamura, M., Fuchinoue, S., Sato, S. *et al.* (1998) Clinical and radiological features of two cases of tacrolimus-related posterior leukoencephalopathy in living related liver transplantation. *Transplantation Proceedings* **30**, 1477–1478.

Nayak, A.K., Karnad, D., Mahajan, M.V., Shah, A. & Meisheri, Y.V. (1994) Cerebellar venous infarction in chronic suppurative otitis media. A case report with review of four other cases. *Stroke* **25**, 1958–1960.

Nencini, P., Inzitari, D., Gibbs, J. & Mangiafico, S. (1993) Dementia with leukoaraiosis and dural arteriovenous malformation: clinical and PET case study. *Journal of Neurology, Neurosurgery and Psychiatry* **56**, 929–931.

Netter, F.H. (1964) The CIBA collection of medical illustrations. I: A compilation of paintings on the normal and pathologic anatomy of the nervous system. CIBA, New York.

Noguchi, K., Ogawa, T., Inugami, A. *et al.* (1997) MRI of acute cerebral infarction: a comparison of FLAIR and T2-weighted fast spin-echo imaging. *Neuroradiology* **39**, 406–410.

Noguchi, K., Nagayoshi, T., Watanabe, N. *et al.* (1998) Diffusion-weighted echo-planar MRI of lacunar infarcts. *Neuroradiology* **40**, 448–451.

O'Brien, J., Ames, D., Chiu, E., Schweitzer, I., Desmond, P. & Tress, B. (1998) Severe deep white matter lesions and outcome in elderly patients with major depressive disorder: follow-up study. *British Medical Journal* **317**, 982–984.

Offenbacher, H., Fazekas, F., Schmidt, R., Koch, M., Fazekas, G. & Kapeller, P. (1996) MR of cerebral abnormalities concomitant with primary intracerebral haematomas. *American Journal of Neuroradiology* **17**, 573–578.

Ogata, J., Yutani, C., Imakita, M. *et al.* (1989) Haemorrhagic infarct of the brain without a reopening of the occluded arteries in cardioembolic stroke. *Stroke* **20**, 876–883.

Ohta, K., Obara, K. & Suzuki, N. (1999) Diagnostic usefulness of echo-planar diffusion-weighted magnetic resonance image in acute phase of lacunar stroke. *Cerebrovascular Diseases* **9** (Suppl. 1), 69.

Okada, Y., Yamaguchi, T., Minematsu, K. *et al.* (1989) Haemorrhagic transformation in cerebral embolism. *Stroke* **20**, 598–603.

Olichney, J.M., Hansen, L.A., Hofstetter, C.R., Grundman, M., Katzman, R. & Thal, L.J. (1995) Cerebral infarction in Alzheimer's disease is associated with severe amyloid angiopathy and hypertension. *Archives of Neurology* **52**, 702–708.

Opeskin, K. & Silberstein, M. (1998) False-positive diagnosis of subarachnoid haemorrhage on computed tomography scan. *Journal of Clinical Neuroscience* **5**, 382–386.

Ott, B.R., Zamani, A., Kleefield, J. & Funkenstein, H.H. (1986) The clinical spectrum of haemorrhagic infarction. *Stroke* **17**, 630–637.

Pantoni, L. & Garcia, J.H. (1995) The significance of cerebral white matter abnormalities 100 years after Binswanger's report: a review. *Stroke* **26**, 1293–1301.

Pantoni, L., Inzitari, D., Pracucci, G. *et al.* (1993) Cerebrospinal fluid proteins in patients with leukoaraiosis: possible abnormalities in blood–brain barrier function. *Journal of Neurological Sciences* **115**, 125–131.

Pantoni, L., Garcia, J.H. & Brown, G.G. (1996) Vascular pathology in three cases of progressive cognitive deterioration. *Journal of Neurological Sciences* **135**, 131–139.

Pascual, J., Iglesias, F., Oterino, A. *et al.* (1996) Cough, exertional and sexual headaches: an analysis of 72 benign and symptomatic cases. *Neurology* **46**, 1520–1524.

Pascual-Leone, A. & Pascual, A.P. (1992) Occipital neuralgia: another benign cause of 'thunderclap' headache. *Journal of Neurology, Neurosurgery and Psychiatry* **55**, 411–415.

Pasquier, F. & Leys, D. (1997) Why are stroke patients prone to develop dementia? *Journal of Neurology* **244**, 135–142.

Patel, M.R., Edelman, R.R. & Warach, S. (1996) Detection of hyperacute primary intraparenchymal haemorrhage by magnetic resonance imaging. *Stroke* **27**, 2321–2324.

Paulson, G.W. (1983) Weightlifter's headache. *Headache* **23**, 193–194.

Paxton, R. & Ambrose, J. (1974) The EMI scanner: a brief review of the first 650 patients. *British Journal of Radiology* **47**, 530.

Pearce, J.M. (1989) Clinical features of the exploding head syndrome. *Journal of Neurology, Neurosurgery and Psychiatry* **52**, 907–910.

Pearce, J.M.S. & Pearce, S.H.S. (1986) Benign paroxysmal cranial neuralgia or cephalgia fugax. *British Medical Journal* **292**, 1015.

Pereira, A.C., Doyle, V.I., Howe, F.A., Griffiths, J.R. & Brown, M.M. (1997) Disappearing cerebral infarcts: a longitudinal MRI study of 16 patients. *Cerebrovascular Diseases* 7 (Suppl. 4), 30.

Perkin, G.D. (1995) Cerebral venous thrombosis: developments in imaging and treatment. *Journal of Neurology, Neurosurgery and Psychiatry* **59**, 1–3.

Pessin, M.S., Teal, P.A. & Caplan, L.R. (1992) Haemorrhagic transformation: guilt by association? *American Journal of Neuroradiology* **12**, 1123–1126.

Pfausler, B., Belcl, R., Metzler, R. *et al.* (1996) Terson's syndrome in spontaneous subarachnoid haemorrhage: a prospective study in 60 consecutive patients. *Journal of Neurosurgery* **85**, 392–394.

Pfleger, M.D., Hardee, E.P., Contant, C.F. & Hayman, A.L. (1994) Sensitivity and specificity of fluid-blood levels for coagulopathy in acute intracerebral haematomas. *American Journal of Neuroradiology* **15**, 217–223.

Pierce, J.N., Taber, K.H. & Hayman, L.A. (1994) Acute intracerebral haemorrhage secondary to thrombocytopenia: CT appearances unaffected by absence of clot retraction. *American Journal of Neuroradiology* **15**, 213–215.

Pinto, A.N., Canhao, P. & Ferro, J.M. (1996) Seizures at the onset of subarachnoid haemorrhage. *Journal of Neurology* **243**, 161–164.

Plant, G.T., Donald, J.J., Jackowski, A., Vinnicombe, S.J. & Kendall, B.E. (1991) Partial, non-thrombotic superior sagittal sinus occlusion due to occipital skull tumours. *Journal of Neurology, Neurosurgery and Psychiatry* **54**, 520–523.

Pollick, C., Cujec, B., Parker, S. & Tator, C. (1988) Left ventricular wall motion abnormalities in subarachnoid haemorrhage: an echocardiographic study. *Journal of the American College of Cardiology* **12**, 600–605.

Porter, M. & Jankovic, J. (1981) Benign coital cephalalgia: differential diagnosis and treatment. *Archives of Neurology* **38**, 710–712.

Poungvarin, N., Viriyavejaku, I.A. & Komontri, C. (1991) Siriraj stroke score and validation study to distinguish supratentorial intracerebral haemorrhage from infarction. *British Medical Journal* **302**, 1565.

Powers, W.J. & Zivin, J. (1998) Magnetic resonance imaging in acute stroke: not ready for prime time. *Neurology* **50**, 842–843.

Pritchard, J.W. & Grossman, R.I. (1999) New reasons for early use of MRI in stroke. *Neurology* **52**, 1733–1736.

Pullicino, P. & Kendall, B.E. (1980) Contrast enhancement in ischaemic lesions. I: Relationship to prognosis. *Neuroradiology* **19**, 235–240.

Pullicino, P., Benedict, R.H.B., Capruso, D.X., Vella, N., Withiam-Leitch, S. & Kwen, P.L. (1996a) Neuroimaging criteria for vascular dementia. *Archives of Neurology* **53**, 723–728.

Pullicino, P., Zimmer, W. & Kwen, P.L. (1996b) Posterior leukoencephalopathy syndrome. *Lancet* **347**, 1557.

Ramirez-Lassepas, M., Espinosa, C.E., Cicero, J.J. *et al.* (1997) Predictors of intracranial pathologic findings in pateints who seek emergency care because of headache. *Archives of Neurology* **54**, 1506–1509.

Raskin, N.H. & Schwartz, R.K. (1980) Icepick-like pain. *Neurology* **30**, 203–205.

Rauch, R.A., Bazan, C., Larsson, E.M. & Jinkins, J.R. (1993) Hyperdense middle cerebral arteries identified on CT as a false sign of vascular occlusion. *American Journal of Neuroradiology* **14**, 669–673.

Raynaud, C., Rancurel, G., Tzourio, N. *et al.* (1989) SPECT analysis of recent cerebral infarction. *Stroke* **20**, 192–204.

Reading, P.V. & Schurr, P. (1956) Thrombosis of the sigmoid sinus. *Lancet* **ii**, 473–476.

Reid, R.L., Quigley, M.E. & Yen, S.S. (1985) Pituitary apoplexy: a review. *Archives of Neurology* **42**, 712–719.

Reijneveld, J.C., Wermer, M., Boonman, Z., van Gijn, J. & Rinkel, G.J.E. (2000) Acute confusional state as a presenting feature in aneurysmal subarachnoid haemorrhage: frequency and characteristics. *Journal of Neurology* **247**, 112–116.

de Reuck, J., Crevits, L., DeCoster, W., Sieben, G. & vander Eecken, H.M. (1980) Pathogenesis of Binswanger's chronic subcortical encephalopathy: a clinical and radiological investigation. *Neurology* **30**, 920–928.

de Reuck, J., Decoo, D., Vienne, J., Strijckmans, K. & Lemahieu, I. (1992) Significance of white matter lucencies in posthypoxic–ischemic encephalopathy: comparison of clinical status and of computed and positron emission tomographic findings. *European Neurology* **32**, 334–339.

Reuner, K.H., Ruf, A., Grau, A. *et al.* (1998) Prothrombin gene G20210→A transition is a risk factor for cerebral venous thrombosis. *Stroke* **29**, 1765–1769.

Revesz, T., Hawkins, C.P., du Boulay, E.P., Barnard, R.O. & McDonald, W.I. (1989) Pathological findings correlated with magnetic resonance imaging in subcortical arteriosclerotic encephalopathy (Binswanger's disease). *Journal of Neurology, Neurosurgery and Psychiatry* **52**, 1337–1344.

Rezek, D.L., Morris, J.C., Fulling, K.H. & Gado, M.H. (1987) Periventricular white matter lucencies in senile dementia of the Alzheimer type and in normal ageing. *Neurology* **37**, 1365–1368.

Ries, S., Steinke, W., Neff, K.W. & Hennerici, M. (1997) Echocontrast-enhanced transcranial color-coded sonography for the diagnosis of transverse sinus venous thrombosis. *Stroke* **28**, 696–700.

Rimdusid, P., Wardlaw, J., Lindley, R.I., Sandercock, P. on behalf of the International Stroke Trial Collaboration Group (1995) Haemorrhagic infarction in acute ischaemic stroke patients: International Stroke Trial Pilot Study. *Cerebrovascular Diseases* **5**, 264.

Rinkel, G.J.E., Wijdicks, E.F.M., Vermeulen, M., Hasan, D., Brouwers, P.J.A.M. & van Gijn, J. (1991) The clinical course of perimesencephalic non-aneurysmal subarachnoid haemorrhage. *Annals of Neurology* **29**, 463–468.

Román, G.C. (1987) Senile dementia of the Binswanger type: a vascular form of dementia in the elderly. *Journal of the American Medical Association* **258**, 1782–1788.

Rosen, B.R., Belliveau, J.W. & Chien, D. (1989) Perfusion imaging by nuclear magnetic resonance. *Magnetic Resonance Quarterly* **5**, 263–281.

Ross, B. & Michaelis, T. (1994) Clinical applications of magnetic resonance spectroscopy. *Magnetic Resonance Quarterly* **10**, 191–247.

Rother, J., Guckel, F., Neff, W., Kuhnen, J., Hennerici, M. & Schwartz, A. (1994) Assessment of cerebral blood volume in acute stroke using dynamic contrast-enhanced magnetic resonance imaging. *Neurology* **44**, A182.

Rothwell, P.M. & Grant, R. (1993) Cerebral venous sinus thrombosis induced by 'ecstasy' [letter]. *Journal of Neurology, Neurosurgery and Psychiatry* **56**, 1035.

Rousseaux, P., Scherpereel, R., Bernard, M.H., Graftieaux, J.P. & Guyot, J.F. (1980) Fever and cerebral vasopsasm in ruptured intracranial aneurysms. *Surgical Neurology* **14**, 459–465.

Rowe, C.C., Donnan, G.A. & Bladin, P.F. (1988) Intracerebral haemorrhage: incidence and use of computed tomography. *British Medical Journal* **297**, 1177–1178.

Royal College of Radiologists (1995) *Making the Best Use of a Department of Clinical Radiology*, 3rd edn. Royal College of Radiologists, London.

Rubio, A., Rifkin, D., Powers, J.M. *et al.* (1997) Phenotypic variability of CADASIL and novel morphologic findings. *Acta Neuropathologica* **94**, 247–254.

Ruchoux, M.M. & Maurage, C.A. (1998) Endothelial changes in muscle and skin biopsies in patients with CADASIL. *Neuropathology and Applied Neurobiology* **24**, 60–65.

Ruelle, A., Cavazzani, P. & Andrioli, G. (1988) Extracranial posterior inferior cerebellar artery aneurysm causing isolated intraventricular haemorrhage: a case report. *Neurosurgery* **23**, 774–777.

Saatci, I., Arslan, S., Topcu, M., Eldem, B., Karagöz, T. & Saatci, Ü. (1996) Case of the month—Behçet disease associated with cerebral venous thrombosis. *European Journal of Pediatrics* **155**, 63–64.

Sabri, O., Ringelstein, E.B., Hellwig, D. *et al.* (1999) Neuropsychological impairment correlates with hypoperfusion and hypometabolism but not with severity of white matter lesions on MRI in patients with cerebral microangiopathy. *Stroke* **30**, 556–566.

Sacco, R.L., Ellenberg, J.H., Mohr, J.P. *et al.* (1989) Infarcts of undetermined cause: the NINDS Stroke Data Bank. *Annals of Neurology* **25**, 382–390.

Sage, M.R. (1982) Blood–brain barrier: a phenomenon of increasing importance to the imaging clinician. *American Journal of Neuroradiology* **3**, 127–138.

Saito, I., Segawa, H., Shiokawa, Y., Taniguchi, M. & Tsutsumi, K. (1987) Middle cerebral artery occlusion: correlation of computed tomography and angiography with clinical outcome. *Stroke* **18**, 863–868.

Sakas, D.E., Dias, L.S. & Beale, D. (1995) Subarachnoid haemorrhage presenting as head injury. *British Medical Journal* **310**, 1186–1187.

Samuelsson, M., Lindell, D. & Norrving, B. (1994) Gadolinium-enhanced magnetic resonance imaging in patients with presumed lacunar infarction. *Cerebrovascular Diseases* **4**, 12–19.

Sarner, M. & Rose, F.C. (1967) Clinical presentation of ruptured intracranial aneurysm. *Journal of Neurology, Neurosurgery and Psychiatry* **30**, 67–70.

Sato, A., Takahashi, S., Soma, Y. *et al.* (1991) Cerebral infarction: early detection by means of contrast enhanced cerebral arteries at MR imaging. *Radiology* **178**, 433–439.

Saunders, D.E., Howe, F.A., van den Boogaart, A., McLean, M.A., Griffiths, J.R. & Brown, M.A. (1995) Continuing ischaemic damage after acute middle cerebral artery infarction in humans demonstrated by short-echo proton spectroscopy. *Stroke* **26**, 1007–1013.

Sauron, B., Chiras, J., Chain, F. & Castaigne, P. (1982) Thrombophlébite cérébelleuse chez un homme porteur d'un déficit familial en antithrombine III. *Revue Neurologique (Paris)* **138**, 685–685.

Savoiardo, M. (1986) CT scanning. In: *Stroke: Pathophysiology, Diagnosis and Management* (eds H.J.M. Barnett, J.P. Mohr, B.M. Stein & F.M. Yatsu), pp. 189–219. Churchill Livingstone, New York.

Scharf, J., Brauherr, E., Forsting, M. & Sartor, K. (1994) Significance of haemorrhagic lacunes on MRI in patients with hypertensive cerebrovascular disease and intracerebral haemorrhage. *Neuroradiology* **36**, 504–508.

Schellinger, P.D., Jansen, O., Fiebach, J.B., Hacke, W. & Sartor, K. (1999) A standardised MRI stroke protocol: comparison with CT in hyperacute intracerebral haemorrhage. *Stroke* **30**, 765–768.

Scheltens, P., Barkhof, F., Leys, D., Wolters, E.C., Ravid, R. & Kamphorst, W. (1995) Histopathologic correlates of white matter changes on MRI in

Alzheimer's disease and normal ageing. *Neurology* **45**, 883–888.

Scheltens, P., Erkinjuntti, T., Leys, D. *et al.* (1998) White matter changes on CT and MRI: an overview of visual rating scales. *European Neurology* **39**, 80–89.

Schievink, W.I., Wijdicks, E.F.M., Parisi, J.E., Piepgras, D.G. & Whisnant, J.P. (1995) Sudden death from aneurysmal subarachnoid haemorrhage. *Neurology* **45**, 871–874.

Schmidt, R., Fazekas, F., Kleinert, G. *et al.* (1992) Magnetic resonance imaging signal hyperintensities in the deep and subcortical white matter: a comparative study between stroke patients and normal volunteers. *Archives of Neurology* **49**, 825–827.

Schmidt, R., Fazekas, F., Offenbacher, H. *et al.* (1993) Neuropsychologic correlates of MRI white matter hyperintensities: a study of 150 normal volunteers. *Neurology* **43**, 2490–2494.

Schmidt, R., Fazekas, F., Koch, M. *et al.* (1995) Magnetic resonance imaging cerebral abnormalities and neuropsychologic test performance in elderly hypertensive subjects: a case–control study. *Archives of Neurology* **52**, 905–910.

Schmidt, R., Fazekas, F., Hayn, M. *et al.* (1997a) Risk factors for microangiopathy-related cerebral damage in the Austrian stroke prevention study. *Journal of Neurological Sciences* **152**, 15–21.

Schmidt, R., Schmidt, H., Fazekas, F. *et al.* (1997b) Apolipoprotein E polymorphism and silent microangiopathy-related cerebral damage: results of the Austrian Stroke Prevention Study. *Stroke* **28**, 951–956.

Schriger, D., Kalafut, M., Starkman, S., Krueger, M. & Saver, J. (1998) Cranial computed tomography interpretation in acute stroke: physician accuracy in determining eligibility for thrombolytic therapy. *Journal of the American Medical Association* **279**, 1293–1297.

Scott, W.R. & Miller, B.R. (1985) Intracerebral haemorrhage with rapid recovery. *Archives of Neurology* **42**, 133–136.

Sellal, F., Mohr, M. & Collard, M. (1996) Dementia in a 58-year-old woman. *Lancet* **347**, 8996.

Shinar, D., Gross, C.R., Hier, D.B. *et al.* (1987) Inter-observer reliability in the interpretation of computed tomographic scans of stroke patients. *Archives of Neurology* **44**, 149–155.

Sigsbee, B., Deck, M.D. & Posner, J.B. (1979) Nonmetastatic superior sagittal sinus thrombosis complicating systemic cancer. *Neurology* **29**, 139–146.

Silbert, P.L., Edis, R.H., Stewart-Wynne, E.G. & Gubbay, S.S. (1991) Benign vascular sexual headache and exertional headache: interrelationships and long-term prognosis. *Journal of Neurology, Neurosurgery and Psychiatry* **54**, 417–421.

Simmons, Z., Biller, J., Adams, H., Dunn, V. & Jacoby, C. (1986) Cerebellar infarction: comparison of computed tomography and magnetic resonance imaging. *Annals of Neurology* **19**, 291–293.

Skriver, E.B. & Olsen, T.S. (1981) Transient disappearance of cerebral infarcts on CT scan, the so-called fogging effect. *Neuroradiology* **22**, 61–65.

Skriver, E.B., Olsen, T.S. & McNair, P. (1990) Mass effect and atrophy after stroke. *Acta Radiologica* **31**, 431–438.

Smith, D.H., Meaney, D.F., Lenkinski, R.E. *et al.* (1995) New magnetic resonance imaging techniques for the evaluation of traumatic brain injury. *Journal of Neurotrauma* **12**, 4–7.

Sohn, Y.H., Kim, S.M., Kim, J.S. & Kim, D.I. (1991) Benign brainstem hemorrhage simulating transient ischemic attack. *Yonsei Medical Journal* **32**, 91–93.

Sorensen, A.G., Buonanno, F.S., Gonzalez, R.G. *et al.* (1996) Hyperacute stroke: evaluation with combined multisection diffusion-weighted and haemodynamically weighted echo-planar MR imaging. *Radiology* **199**, 391–401.

Sorensen, A.G., Copen, W.A., Ostergaard, L. *et al.* (1999) Hyperacute stroke: simultaneous measurement of relative cerebral blood volume, relative cerebral blood flow and mean tissue transit time. *Radiology* **210**, 519–527.

Southwick, F.S., Richardson, E.P. Jr & Swartz, M.N. (1986) Septic thrombosis of the dural venous sinuses. *Medicine (Baltimore)* **65**, 82–106.

Starkstein, S.E., Sabe, L., Vázquez, S. *et al.* (1997) Neuropsychological, psychiatric, and cerebral perfusion correlates of leukoaraiosis in Alzheimer's disease. *Journal of Neurology, Neurosurgery and Psychiatry* **63**, 66–73.

Stehle, G., Buss, J. & Heene, D.L. (1991) Noninfectious thrombosis of the superior sagittal sinus in a patient with iron deficiency anemia [letter]. *Stroke* **22**, 414.

Steiger, M.J., Tarnesby, G., Gabe, S., McLaughlin, J. & Schapira, A.H. (1993) Successful outcome of progressive multifocal leukoencephalopathy with cytarabine and interferon. *Annals of Neurology* **33**, 4–11.

Steingart, A., Lau, K., Fox, A. *et al.* (1986) The significance of white matter lucencies on CT scan in relation to cognitive impairment. *Canadian Journal of Neurological Sciences* **13**, 383–384.

Steingart, A., Hachinski, V.C., Lau, C. *et al.* (1987) Cognitive and neurologic findings in demented patients with diffuse white matter lucencies on computed tomographic scan (leuko-araiosis). *Archives of Neurology* **44**, 36–39.

Stewart, J.A., Dundas, R., Howard, R.S., Rudd, A.G. & Wolfe, C.D.A. (1999) Ethnic differences in incidence of stroke: prospective study with stroke register. *British Medical Journal* **318**, 967–971.

Stojsavljevic, N., Levic, Z., Drulovic, J. & Dragutinovic, G. (1997) A 44-month clinical-brain MRI follow-up in a patient with B_{12} deficiency. *Neurology* **49**, 878–881.

Stolz, E., Kaps, M. & Dorndorf, W. (1999) Assessment of intracranial venous hemodynamics in normal individuals and patients with cerebral venous thrombosis. *Stroke* **30**, 70–75.

Stone, J.L., Crowell, R.M., Gandhi, Y.N. & Jafar, J.J. (1988) Multiple intracranial aneurysms: magnetic resonance imaging for determination of the site of rupture—report of a case. *Neurosurgery* **23**, 97–100.

Stroke Prevention in Reversible Ischemia Trial (SPIRIT) Study Group (1997) A randomized trial of anticoagulants versus aspirin after cerebral ischemia of presumed arterial origin. *Annals of Neurology* **42**, 857–865.

Sudlow, C.L.M. & Warlow, C.P. (1997) Comparable studies of the incidence of stroke and its pathological types: results from an international collaboration. *Stroke* **28**, 491–499.

Sung, C.Y. & Chu, N.S. (1992) Late CT manifestation in spontaneous putaminal haemorrhage. *Neuroradiology* **34**, 200–204.

Suzuki, M., Wada, A., Isaka, Y., Maki, K., Inoue, T. & Fukuhara, Y. (1997) Cerebral magnetic resonance T2 high intensities in end-stage renal disease. *Stroke* **28**, 2528–2531.

Svigelj, V., Grad, A., Tekavcic, I. & Kiauta, T. (1994) Cardiac arrhythmia associated with reversible damage to insula in a patient with subarachnoid haemorrhage. *Stroke* **25**, 1053–1055.

Swan, G.E., DeCarli, C., Miller, B.L. *et al.* (1998) Association of midlife blood pressure to late-life cognitive decline and brain morphology. *Neurology* **51**, 986–993.

van Swieten, J.C., van den Hout, J.H., van Ketel, B.A., Hijdra, A., Wokke, J.H.J. & van Gijn, J. (1991a) Periventricular lesions in the white matter on magnetic resonance imaging in the elderly: a morphometric correlation with arteriolosclerosis and dilated perivascular spaces. *Brain* **114**, 761–774.

van Swieten, J.C., Geyskes, G.G., Derix, M.M. *et al.* (1991b) Hypertension in the elderly is associated with white matter lesions and cognitive decline. *Annals of Neurology* **30**, 825–830.

van Swieten, J.C., Kappelle, L.J., Algra, A., van Latum, J.C., Koudstaal, P.J. & van Gijn, J. (1992) Hypodensity of the cerebral white matter in patients with transient ischemic attack or minor stroke: influence on the rate of subsequent stroke. Dutch TIA Trial Study Group. *Annals of Neurology* **32**, 177–183.

Tatemichi, T.K., Desmond, D.W., Prohovnik, I. *et al.* (1992) Confusion and memory loss from capsular genu infarction: a thalamocortical disconnection syndrome? *Neurology* **42**, 1966–1979.

Tehindrazanarivelo, A., Evrard, S., Schaison, M., Mas, J.-L., Dormont, D. & Bousser, M.-G. (1992) Prospective study of cerebral sinus venous thrombosis in patients presenting with benign intracranial hypertension. *Cerebrovascular Diseases* **2**, 22–27.

Terent, A., Ronquist, G., Bergstrom, K., Hallgren, R. & Aberg, H. (1981) Ischaemic oedema in stroke: a parallel study with computed tomography and cerebrospinal fluid markers of disturbed brain cell metabolism. *Stroke* **12**, 33–40.

Thomas, J.E., Rooke, E. & Kvale, W.F. (1966) The neurologist's experience with phaeochromocytoma: a review of 100 cases. *Journal of the American Medical Association* **197**, 754–758.

Thyagarajan, G.K., Cobanoglu, A. & Johnston, W. (1997) FK506-induced fulminant leukoencephalopathy after single-lung transplantation. *Annals of Thoracic Surgery* **64**, 1461–1464.

Tohgi, H., Chiba, K., Sasaki, K., Hiroi, S. & Ishibashi, Y. (1991) Cerebral perfusion patterns in vascular dementia of Binswanger type compared with senile dementia of Alzheimer type: a SPECT study. *Journal of Neurology* **238**, 365–370.

Tokuda, Y., Inagawa, T., Katoh, Y. *et al.* (1995) Intracerebral haematoma in patients with ruptured cerebral aneurysms. *Surgical Neurology* **43**, 272–277.

Tomimoto, H., Akiguchi, I., Suenaga, T. *et al.* (1996) Alterations of the blood–brain barrier and glial cells in white-matter lesions in cerebrovascular and Alzheimer's disease patients. *Stroke* **27**, 2069–2074.

Tomimoto, H., Akiguchi, I., Akiyama, H. *et al.* (1999) Vascular changes in white matter lesions of Alzheimer's disease. *Acta Neuropathologica* **97**, 629–634.

Tomsick, T., Brott, T., Barsan, W. *et al.* (1990) Thrombus localisation with emergency cerebral computed tomography. *Stroke* **21**, 180.

Tomura, N., Uemura, K., Inugami, A., Fujita, H., Higano, S. & Shishido, F. (1988) Early CT finding in cerebral infarction: obscuration of the lentiform nucleus. *Radiology* **168**, 463–467.

Toni, D., Fiorelli, M., Bastianello, S. *et al.* (1997) Acute ischaemic strokes improving during the first 48 hours of onset: predictability, outcome and possible mechanisms. *Stroke* **28**, 10–14.

Torigoe, R., Harad, K. & Matsuo, H. (1990) Assessment of cerebral infarction by MRI: particularly fogging effect. *No To Shinkei [Brain and Nerve]* **42** (6), 547–552.

Torvik, A. (1984) The pathogenesis of watershed infarcts in the brain. *Stroke* **15**, 221–223.

Tourtelotte, W.W., Metz, L.N., Bryan, E.R. & DeJong, R.N. (1964) Spontaneous subarachnoid hemorrhage: factors affecting the rate of clearing of cerebrospinal fluid. *Neurology* **14**, 301–306.

Truwit, C.L., Barkovitch, A.J., Gean-Marton, A., Hibri, N. & Norman, D. (1990) Loss of the insular ribbon: another sign of acute middle cerebral artery infarction. *Radiology* **176**, 801–806.

Tsai, F.Y., Wang, A.M., Matovich, V.B. *et al.* (1995) MR staging of acute dural sinus thrombosis: correlation with venous pressure measurements and implications for treatment and prognosis. *American Journal of Neuroradiology* **16**, 1021–1029.

Tubbs, O.N. & Potter, J.M. (1970) Early post-concussional headache. *Lancet* **ii**, 128–129.

Ueda, T., Yuh, W.T.C., Maley, J.E., Quets, J.P., Hahn, P.Y. & Magnotta, V.A. (1999a) Outcome of acute ischaemic lesions evaluated by diffusion and perfusion MR imaging. *American Journal of Neuroradiology* **20**, 983–989.

Ueda, T., Sakaki, S., Yuh, W.T.C., Nochide, I. & Ohta, S. (1999b) Outcome in acute stroke with successful intra-arterial thrombolysis and predictive value of initial single photon emission computed tomography. *Journal of Cerebral Blood Flow Metabolism* **19**, 99–108.

Ur Rahman, N. & Al Tahan, A.R. (1993) Computed tomographic evidence of an extensive thrombosis and infarction of the deep venous system. *Stroke* **24**, 744–746.

Valdueza, J.M., Hoffmann, O., Weih, M., Mehraein, S. & Einhäupl, K.M. (1999) Monitoring of venous hemodynamics in patients with cerebral venous thrombosis by transcranial Doppler ultrasound. *Archives of Neurology* **56**, 229–234.

Van der Werf, Y.D., Weerts, J.G.E., Jolles, J., Witter, M.P., Lindeboom, J. & Scheltens, P. (1999) Neuropsychological correlates of a right unilateral lacunar thalamic infarction. *Journal of Neurology, Neurosurgery and Psychiatry* **66**, 36–42.

Veldink, J.H., Scheltens, P., Jonker, C. & Launer, L.J. (1998) Progression of cerebral white matter hyperintensities on MRI is related to diastolic blood pressure. *Neurology* **51**, 319–320.

Vemmos, K.N., Mparmparesou, M., Kontogianni, M., Zis, V., Stranjalis, G. & Moulopoulos, S. (1994) Haemorrhagic transformation in embolic stroke. *Cerebrovascular Diseases* **4**, 230.

Vemmos, K.N., Bots, M.L., Tsibouris, P.K. *et al.* (1999) Stroke incidence and case fatality in southern Greece: the Arcadia Stroke Registry. *Stroke* **30**, 363–370.

Verhey, F.R.J., Lodder, J., Rozendaal, N. & Jolles, J. (1996) Comparison of seven sets of criteria used for the diagnosis of vascular dementia. *Neuroepidemiology* **15**, 166–172.

Vermeulen, M. & van Gijn, J. (1990) The diagnosis of subarachnoid haemorrhage. *Journal of Neurology, Neurosurgery and Psychiatry* **53**, 365–372.

Vermeulen, M., van Gijn, J. & Blijenberg, B.G. (1983) Spectrophotometric analysis of CSF after subarachnoid haemorrhage: limitations in the diagnosis of rebleeding. *Neurology* **33**, 112–114.

Vermeulen, M., Lindsay, K.W., Murray, G.D. *et al.* (1984) Antifibrinolytic treatment in subarachnoid haemorrhage. *New England Journal of Medicine* **311**, 432–437.

Vermeulen, M., Hasan, D., Blijenberg, B.G., Hijdra, A. & van Gijn, J. (1989) Xanthochromia after subarachnoid haemorrhage needs no revisitation. *Journal of Neurology, Neurosurgery and Psychiatry* **52**, 826–828.

Vernant, J.C., Delaporte, J.M., Buisson, G., Bellance, R., Bokor, J. & Loiseau, P. (1988) Complications cerebro-vasculaires de la drepanocytose. *Revue Neurologique (Paris)* **144**, 465–473.

Vestergaard, K., Andersen, G., Nielsen, M.I. & Jensen, T.S. (1993) Headache in stroke. *Stroke* **24**, 1621–1624.

Vidailhet, M., Piette, J.C., Wechsler, B., Busser, M.G. & Brunet, P. (1990) Cerebral venous thrombosis in systemic lupus erythematosus. *Stroke* **21**, 1226–1231.

Vincent, F.M. & Zimmerman, J.E. (1980) Superior cerebellar artery aneurysm presenting as an oculomotor palsy in a child. *Neurosurgery* **6**, 661–664.

Virapongse, C., Cazenave, C., Quisling, R., Sarwar, M. & Hunter, S. (1987) The empty delta sign: frequence and significance in 76 cases of dural sinus thrombosis. *Radiology* **162**, 779–785.

Vital, C. & Julien, J. (1997) Widespread dilatation of perivascular spaces: a leukoencephalopathy causing dementia. *Neurology* **48**, 1310–1313.

Vogl, T.J., Bergman, C., Villringer, A., Einhauple, K., Lissner, J. & Felix, R. (1994) *American Journal of Roentgenology* **162**, 1191–1198.

Vonsattel, J.P., Myers, R.H., Hedley-Whyte, E.T., Ropper, A.H., Bird, E.D. & Richardson, E.P. Jr (1991) Cerebral amyloid angiopathy without and with cerebral hemorrhages: a comparative histological study. *Annals of Neurology* **30**, 637–649.

Wall, S.D., Brant-Zawadzki, M., Jeffrey, R.B. & Barnes, B. (1982) High frequency CT findings within 24 hours after cerebral infarction. *American Journal of Roentgenology* **138**, 307–311.

Wallesch, C.W., Kornhuber, H.H., Kunz, T. & Brunner, R.J. (1983) Neuropsychological deficits associated with small unilateral thalamic lesions. *Brain* **106**, 141–152.

Wallin, A., Blennow, K., Uhlemann, C., Langstrom, G. & Gottfries, C.G. (1989) White matter low attenuation on computed tomography in Alzheimer's disease and vascular dementia: diagnostic and pathogenetic aspects. *Acta Neurologica Scandinavica* **80**, 518–523.

Wallin, A., Blennow, K., Fredman, P., Gottfries, C.G., Karlsson, I. & Svennerholm, L. (1990) Blood–brain barrier function in vascular dementia. *Acta Neurologica Scandinavica* **81**, 318–322.

Walton, J.N. (1956) *Subarachnoid Haemorrhage*. Churchill Livingstone, Edinburgh.

Wang, A.M., Shetty, A.N., Woo, H., Rao, S.K., Manzione, J.V. & Moore, J.R. (1998) Diffusion-weighted MR imaging in evaluation of CNS disease. *Rivista Di Neuroradiologia* **11** (Suppl. 2), 109–112.

Wang, P.Y.-K., Barker, P.B., Wityk, R.J., Ulüg, A.M., van Zijl, P.C.M. & Beauchamp, N.J. (1999) Diffusion-negative stroke: a report of two cases. *American Journal of Neuroradiology* **20**, 1876–1880.

Warach, S., Li, W., Ronthal, M. & Edelman, R.R. (1992) Acute cerebral ischaemia: evaluation with dynamic contrast enhanced MR imaging and MR angiography. *Radiology* **182**, 41–47.

Warach, S., Gaa, J., Siewert, B., Wielopolski, P. & Edelman, R.R. (1995) Acute human stroke studied by whole brain echo planar diffusion-weighted magnetic resonance imaging. *Annals of Neurology* **37**, 231–241.

Wardlaw, J.M. & Sellar, R.J. (1994) A simple practical classification of cerebral infarcts on CT and its inter-observer reliability. *American Journal of Neuroradiology* **15**, 1933–1939.

Wardlaw, J.M. & Statham, P.F.X. (2000) How often is haemosiderin not visible on routine MR following traumatic intracerebral haemorrhage? *Neuroradiology* **42**, 81–84.

Wardlaw, J.M. & White, P.M. (2000) The detection and management of unruptured intracranial aneurysms. *Brain* **123**, 205–221.

Wardlaw, J.M., Dennis, M.S., Lindley, R.I., Warlow, C.P., Sandercock, P.A.G. & Sellar, R.J. (1993) Does early reperfusion of a cerebral infarct influence cerebral infarct swelling in the acute stage or the final clinical outcome? *Cerebrovascular Diseases* **3**, 86–93.

Wardlaw, J.M., Vaughan, G.T., Steers, A.J.W. & Sellar, R.J. (1994) Transcranial Doppler ultrasound findings in cerebral venous sinus thrombosis. *Journal of Neurosurgery* **80**, 332–335.

Wardlaw, J.M., Dennis, M.S., Lindley, R.I., Sellar, R.J. & Warlow, C.P. (1996) The validity of a simple clinical classification of acute ischaemic stroke. *Journal of Neurology* **243**, 274–279.

Wardlaw, J.M., Lewis, S.C., Dennis, M.S., Counsell, C. & McDowall, M. (1998a) Is visible infarction on computed tomography associated with an adverse prognosis in acute ischaemic stroke? *Stroke* **29**, 1315–1319.

Wardlaw, J.M., Marshall, I., Wild, J., Dennis, M.S., Cannon, J. & Lewis, S.C. (1998b) Studies of acute ischaemic stroke with proton magnetic resonance spectroscopy: relation between time from onset, neurological deficit, metabolite abnormalities in the infarct, blood flow and clinical outcome. *Stroke* **29**, 1618–1624.

Wardlaw, J.M., Lammie, G.A. & Whittle, I.R. (1998c) A brain haemorrhage? *Lancet* **351**, 1028.

Wardlaw, J.M., Lewis, S.C., Dennis, M.S. & Warlow, C.P. (1999a) Is it reasonable to assume a particular embolic source from the type of stroke? *Cerebrovascular Diseases* **9** (Suppl. 1), 14.

Wardlaw, J.M., Dorman, P.J., Lewis, S.C. & Sandercock, P.A.G. (1999b) Can stroke physicians and neuroradiologists identify signs of early cerebral infarction on CT? *Journal of Neurology, Neurosurgery and Psychiatry* **67**, 651–653.

Wardlaw, J.M., del Zoppo, G. & Yamaguchi, T. (2000a) Thrombolytic therapy in acute ischaemic stroke. I: Thrombolysis versus control. In: *The Cochrane Library; Database of Systematic Reviews*. Oxford: Update Software.

Wardlaw, J.M., Armitage, P.A., Dennis, M.S., Lewis, S.C., Marshall, I. & Sellar, R. (2000b) The use of diffusion-weighted magnetic resonance imaging to identify infarctions in patients with minor strokes. *Journal of Stroke and Cerebrovascular Disease* **9**, 70–75.

Waserberg, J. & Barlow, P. (1997) Lumbar puncture still has an important role in diagnosing subarachnoid haemorrhage. *British Medical Journal* **315**, 1598–1599.

Watanabe, A., Ishii, R., Tanaka, R., Tokiguchi, S. & Ito, J.C. (1982) Relation of cranial nerve involvement to the location of intracranial aneurysms. *Neurologica Medico-Chirurgica* **22**, 910–916.

Wechsler, B., Vidailhet, M., Piette, J.C. *et al.* (1992) Cerebral venous thrombosis in Behçet's disease: clinical study and long-term follow-up of 25 cases. *Neurology* **42**, 614–618.

Wechsler, B., Génereau, T., Biousse, V. *et al.* (1995) Pregnancy complicated by cerebral venous thrombosis in Behçet's disease. *American Journal of Obstetrics and Gynecology* **173**, 1627–1629.

van der Wee, N., Rinkel, G.J.E., Hasan, D. & Van Gijn, J. (1995) Detection of subarachnoid heamorrhage on early CT: is lumbar puncture still needed after a negative scan? *Journal of Neurology, Neurosurgery and Psychiatry* **58**, 357–359.

Wehrli, F.W. & Atlas, S.W. (1996) Fast imaging: principles, techniques and clinical applications. In: *Magnetic Resonance Imaging of the Brain and Spine* (ed. S.W. Atlas), 2nd edn, pp. 1413–1499. Lippincott-Raven, Philadelphia.

Weiller, C., Ringelstein, E.B., Reiche, W., Thron, A. & Buell, U. (1990) The large striatocapsular infarct: a clinical and pathological entity. *Archives of Neurology* **47**, 1085–1091.

Weir, C.J., Murray, G.D., Adams, F.G., Muir, K.W., Grossett, D.G. & Lees, K.R. (1994) Poor accuracy of scoring systems for differential clinical diagnosis of intracranial haemorrhage and infarction. *Lancet* **344**, 999–1002.

West, T.E.T., Davies, R.J. & Kelly, R.E. (1976) Horner's syndrome and headache due to carotid artery disease. *British Medical Journal* **i**, 818–821.

Wetterling, T., Kanitz, R.D. & Borgis, K.J. (1996) Comparison of different diagnostic criteria for vascular dementia (ADDTC, DSM-IV, ICD-10, NINDS-AIREN). *Stroke* **27**, 30–36.

White, P.M., Wardlaw, J.M. & Easton, V.E. (2000) Can non-invasive imaging tests accurately detect intracranial aneurysms?: a systematic review. *Radiology* (in press).

Wijdicks, E.F.M., Kerkhoff, H. & van Gijn, J. (1988) Long-term follow-up of 71 patients with thunderclap headache mimicking subarachnoid haemorrhage. *Lancet* **ii**, 68–70.

Wijdicks, E.F.M., Vermeulen, M., Murray, G.D., Hijdra, A. & van Gijn, J. (1990) The effect of treating hypertension following aneurysmal subarachnoid haemorrhage. *Clinical Neurology and Neurosurgery* **92**, 111–117.

Wijdicks, E.F.M., Schievink, W.I. & Miller, G.M. (1998) Pretruncal non-aneurysmal subarachnoid hemorrhage. *Mayo Clinic Proceedings* **73**, 745–752.

Wilder-Smith, E., Kothbauer-Margreiter, I., Lämmle, B., Sturzenegger, M., Ozdoba, C. & Hauser, S.P. (1997) Dural puncture and activated protein C resistance: risk factors for cerebral venous sinus thrombosis. *Journal of Neurology, Neurosurgery and Psychiatry* **63**, 351–356.

Wing, S.D., Norman, D., Pollock, J.A. & Newton, T.H. (1976) Contrast enhancement of cerebral infarcts in computed tomography. *Radiology* **121**, 89–92.

Witt, J.-P., Holl, K., Heissler, H.E. & Dietz, H. (1991) Stable xenon CT CBF: effects of blood flow alterations on CBF calculations during inhalation of 33% stable xenon. *American Journal of Neuroradiology* **12**, 973–975.

Wroe, S.J., Sandercock, P., Bamford, J., Dennis, M., Slattery, J. & Warlow, C. (1992) Diurnal variation in incidence of stroke: Oxfordshire Community Stroke Project. *British Medical Journal* **304**, 155–157.

Yamanaka, K., Fukuyama, H. & Kimura, J. (1996) Abulia from unilateral capsular genu infarction: report of two cases. *Journal of Neurological Sciences* **143**, 181–184.

Yang, S.S., Ryu, S.J. & Wu, C.L. (1990) Early CT diagnosis of cerebral ischaemia. *Stroke* **2**, 1–121.

Yao, H., Sadoshima, S., Ibayashi, S., Kuwabara, Y., Ichiya, Y. & Fujishima, M. (1992) Leukoaraiosis and dementia in hypertensive patients. *Stroke* **23**, 1673–1677.

Ylikoski, R., Ylikoski, A., Erkinjuntti, T., Sulkava, R., Raininko, R. & Tilvis, R. (1993) White matter changes in healthy elderly persons correlate with attention and speed of mental processing. *Archives of Neurology* **50**, 818–824.

Yoneda, Y., Tokui, K., Hanihara, T., Kitagaki, H., Tabuchi, M. & Mori, E. (1999) Diffusion-weighted magnetic resonance imaging: detection of ischaemic injury 39 minutes after onset in a stroke patient. *Annals of Neurology* **45**, 794–797.

Yuh, W.T.C., Crain, M.R., Loes, D.J., Greene, G.M., Ryals, T.J. & Sato, Y. (1991) MR imaging of cerebral ischaemia: findings in the first 24 hours. *American Journal of Neuroradiology* **12**, 621–629.

Yuh, W.T.C., Simonson, T.M., Wang, A. *et al.* (1994) Venous occlusive disease: MR findings. *American Journal of Neuroradiology* **15**, 309–316.

Zeumer, H. & Ringelstein, E.B. (1987) Computed tomographic patterns of brain infarctions as a pathogenetic key. In: *New Trends in the Diagnosis and Management of Stroke*, pp. 75–85. Springer Verlag, Heidelberg.

Zhang, W.W. & Olsson, Y. (1997) The angiopathy at subcortical arteriosclerotic encephalopathy (Binswanger's disease): immunohistochemical studies using markers for components of extracellular matrix, smooth muscle actin and endothelial cells. *Acta Neuropathologica* **93**, 219–224.

Zigun, J.R., Frank, J.A., Barrios, F.A. *et al.* (1993) Measurement of brain activity with bolus administration of contrast agents and gradient echo MR imaging. *Radiology* **186**, 353–356.

Zuber, M., Toulon, P., Marnet, L. & Mas, J.L. (1996) Factor V Leiden mutation in cerebral venous thrombosis. *Stroke* **27**, 1721–1723.

van der Zwan, A. & Hillen, B. (1991) Review of the variability of the territories of the major cerebral arteries. *Stroke* **22**, 1078–1084.

CHAPTER SIX

What caused this transient or persisting ischaemic event?

6.1 Introduction

Having decided that a patient has a stroke or transient ischaemic attack (TIA)—or 'brain attack' (Chapter 3), where the brain lesion is (Chapter 3) and its relationship to the vascular supply (Chapter 4), and that the cause is ischaemic rather than haemorrhagic (Chapter 5), the next step is to define the cause of the ischaemia. What caused *this* ischaemic event? If, for whatever reason, it has been impossible to distinguish an ischaemic stroke from primary (i.e. non-traumatic) intracerebral haemorrhage (PICH), then the causes of the latter (Chapter 8) must be considered as well. Naturally, how far one pursues 'the cause' must depend on how much finding it will influence the subsequent management and outcome of an individual patient, and how far an individual patient or their family might want to pursue matters, or even—in some health care systems—how much they can afford.

So often physicians regard stroke as though it was a single disease. A stroke is a clinical syndrome with many causes and the particular cause may determine the immediate outcome (section 10.2), have a substantial impact on the risk of recurrence (section 16.1) and influence the choice of both immediate (Chapters 11 and 12) and long-term treatment (Chapter 16). Moreover, identification of the cause may have unanticipated later relevance; for example, ischaemic stroke caused by carotid dissection as a consequence of a car accident (rather than caused by atherothrombosis) may lead to substantial compensation from an insurance company. Finding the cause is therefore important and may not be very difficult. Indeed, the hunt for the cause makes stroke patients more 'interesting', particularly to some neurologists. The first clue is the clinical syndrome (where and how big is the area of brain ischaemia or infarction, sections 6.6.1–6.6.5), then the general examination—which usually provides more information about the cause than an obsessional neurological examination—and a few well-targeted investigations should complete the picture (section 6.7). A patient may have several competing causes, making it impossible to know which one is *the* cause:

A 70-year-old man suddenly developed weakness of the left arm and leg which recovered in a few days. When he went to his doctor 3 days after onset, there was a left hemiparesis but no visual field defect, nor any obvious sensory inattention or neglect. He was known to be hypertensive, discovered to be in atrial fibrillation and his ECG showed an unsuspected but probably old anterior myocardial infarc-

tion. There was a loud right carotid bruit. Brain CT was normal but MRI showed multiple presumed lacunar infarcts in the periventricular white matter of both cerebral hemispheres. Therefore, the stroke might have been caused by any one of the following:

- *embolism from the heart (either from thrombus in the fibrillating left atrium or from thrombus in the left ventricle as a result of the myocardial infarction) causing a cortical infarct invisible even on MRI (any cortical signs having disappeared by the time the patient went to the doctor);*
- *embolism from atherothrombotic carotid stenosis to cause a cortical infarct invisible even on MRI;*
- *low-flow distal to severe atherothrombotic carotid stenosis or occlusion;*
- *intracranial small vessel disease causing lacunar infarction; or*
- *something unusual, such as thrombocythaemia.*

Focal cerebral or ocular ischaemia is almost always caused by impaired blood flow, usually acutely but sometimes chronically. The question then is: 'Why is, or was, the relevant blood vessel (artery much more often than vein) blocked or narrow?'

6.2 What to expect

There is no *qualitative* difference between an ischaemic stroke and a transient ischaemic attack (TIA); anything which causes an ischaemic stroke may, if less severe or less prolonged, cause a TIA, while anything which causes a TIA may, if more severe or more prolonged, cause an ischaemic stroke. The *quantitative* difference is arbitrary and enshrined in the temporal boundary of symptoms lasting more or less than 24 h. This is, of course, irrelevant if a patient is seen within 24 h and is still symptomatic, where the concept of 'brain attack' is more appropriate (section 3.2.3). It is therefore not surprising that imaging evidence of relevant infarction is more likely the longer the duration of the symptoms (Koudstaal *et al.* 1992; Engelter *et al.* 1999; Kimura *et al.* 1999), that all types of ischaemic stroke are about equally likely to be preceded by TIAs (Petty *et al.* 1999) (Table 6.1) and that the risk factor profiles of ischaemic stroke and TIA are so similar (Whisnant *et al.* 1999). Therefore, there is no great difference between searching for the cause of an ischaemic stroke and searching for the cause of a TIA (Sempere *et al.* 1998).

Anything which causes an ischaemic stroke may, if less severe or less prolonged, cause a transient ischaemic attack, while anything which causes a transient ischaemic attack may, if more severe or more prolonged, cause an ischaemic stroke.

Table 6.1 The frequency of transient ischaemic attacks (TIAs) before various types of ischaemic stroke. (Unpublished data collected by Dr Claudio Sacks from the Oxfordshire Community Stroke Project.)

	Percentage with preceding TIAs
All ischaemic strokes	14
Total anterior circulation infarction	16
Partial anterior circulation infarction	15
Lacunar infarction	12
Posterior circulation infarction	12
Presumed cardioembolic ischaemic stroke	16

In *population*-based studies in white people, about one-half of cerebral ischaemic events, whether permanent or transient, are probably caused by the thrombotic and embolic complications of atheroma, which is a disorder of large and medium-sized arteries, about one-quarter to intracranial small vessel disease causing lacunar infarction, about one-fifth to embolism from the heart, and the rest to rarities (Sandercock *et al.* 1989; Bamford *et al.* 1991) (Fig. 6.1) (Table 6.2). Not surprisingly, where admission rates are low, hospital-referred stroke patients are rather less likely to have lacunar strokes (because they are conscious without any cognitive defect and therefore easier to look after at home) and more likely to have something unusual, particularly if the hospital has a special interest in stroke or one of its causes—hospital-referral bias (Giroud *et al.* 1997) (section 10.2.6). Age will colour expectations too: a 21-year-old female is hardly likely to have atheroma, while an 81-year-old male is relatively very unlikely to have a rare cause of cerebral ischaemia, although this is still possible.

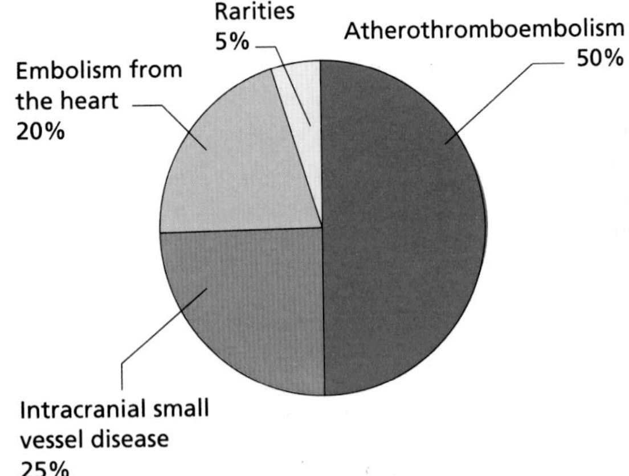

Fig. 6.1 The approximate frequency of the main causes of ischaemic stroke and transient ischaemic attacks in white populations.

Table 6.2 The causes of ischaemia affecting the arterial or venous circulation of the brain and eye.

Atherothromboembolism (section 6.3)
Embolism (section 6.3.2)
Occlusive thrombosis (section 6.3.2)
Low blood flow (section 6.6.5)
Dolichoectasia (section 6.3.2)

Intracranial small vessel disease
'Complex' small vessel disease (section 6.4)
Hyaline arteriosclerosis or 'simple' small vessel disease (section 6.4)
Mural, junctional and microatheroma (section 6.4)
Cerebral amyloid angiopathy (section 8.2.2)
CADASIL (section 7.20)

Connective tissue, inflammatory vascular disorders (and other obscure vasculopathies)
Giant cell arteritis* (section 7.3)
Takayasu's arteritis (section 7.3)
Systemic lupus erythematosus (section 7.3)
Antiphospholipid syndrome* (section 7.3)
Sneddon's syndrome (section 7.3)
Systemic necrotizing vasculitis (section 7.3)
  classic polyarteritis nodosa
  microscopic polyangiitis
  Churg–Strauss syndrome
  Wegener's granulomatosis
Kawasaki's disease (section 7.3)
Henoch–Schoenlein purpura (section 7.3)
Rheumatoid disease (section 7.3)
Sjögren's syndrome (section 7.3)
Behçet's disease (section 7.3)
Relapsing polychondritis (section 7.3)
Progressive systemic sclerosis (scleroderma) (section 7.3)
Essential cryoglobulinaemia (section 7.3)
Malignant atrophic papulosis (Kohlmeier–Degos disease) (section 7.3)
Sarcoidosis (section 7.3)
Primary angiitis of the central nervous system (section 7.3)
Idiopathic reversible cerebral 'vasoconstriction' (section 7.3)
Buerger's disease (thromboangiitis obliterans) (section 7.3)
Paraneoplastic vasculitis (section 7.3)
Vasculitis associated with bone marrow transplantation (section 7.12)
Therapeutic drugs (section 7.3)
Acute posterior multifocal placoid pigment epitheliopathy (section 7.3)
Susac's syndrome (section 7.3)
Eales' disease (section 7.3)
Cogan's syndrome (section 7.3)
Lymphomatoid granulomatosis (section 7.3)

Secondary inflammatory vascular disorders
Infection (section 7.11)
Drugs of abuse* (section 7.15)
Irradiation (section 7.12)
Inflammatory bowel disease (section 7.17)
Coeliac disease (section 7.17)

Congenital
Fibromuscular dysplasia (section 7.4)
Arterial loops (section 7.4)
Ehlers–Danlos syndrome (section 7.4)
Pseudoxanthoma elasticum (section 7.4)
Marfan's syndrome (section 7.4)
Arteriovenous malformations (section 8.2.4)

*Arterial dissection**
Trauma (section 7.1)
Cystic medial necrosis (section 7.2.1)
Fibromuscular dysplasia (section 7.4)
Marfan's syndrome (section 7.4)
Ehlers–Danlos syndrome (section 7.4)
Pseudoxanthoma elasticum (section 7.4)
Inflammatory arterial disease (section 7.3)
Infective arterial disease (e.g. syphilis) (section 7.11)
α-1 antitrypsin deficiency (section 7.2.1)

Trauma
Penetrating neck injury (section 7.1)
  neck laceration/surgery
  missile wounds
  oral trauma
  tonsillectomy
  cerebral catheter angiography
  attempted jugular vein catheterization

Non-penetrating (blunt) neck injury (section 7.1)
  carotid compression
  cervical manipulation
  blow to the neck
  cervical flexion–extension 'whiplash' injury
  minor head movements?
  cervical rib
  fractured clavicle
  bronchoscopy
  endotracheal intubation
  head-banging
  labour
  epileptic seizures
  yoga
  attempted strangulation
  atlanto-occipital instability
  atlanto-axial dislocation
  fractured base of skull
  faulty posture of neck during general anaesthesia, or even a prolonged telephone conversation
  vomiting

Metabolic disorders
Mitochondrial cytopathy (MELAS syndrome) (section 7.19)
Homocystinuria (section 7.20)
Fabry's disease (section 7.20)
Primary oxalosis (section 6.5)

(*Continued p. 226*)

Table 6.2 (*continued*)

Miscellaneous
Cancer (section 7.12)
Irradiation (section 7.12)
Vasospasm (migraine)? (section 7.8)
Pregnancy/oral contraceptives/oestrogens (sections 7.13 and 7.14)
Snake bite (section 7.9)
Fat embolism (section 6.6.6)
Fibrocartilaginous embolism (section 7.1)
Tuberous sclerosis (section 7.20)
Neurofibromatosis (section 7.20)
Aneurysms (section 7.6)
Epidermal naevus syndrome

*The most common 'rare' causes of arterial disease, in total, well under 5% of all patients with ischaemic stroke/TIA.

Haematological causes are listed in Table 7.3.

About 95% of ischaemic strokes and transient ischaemic attacks are caused by the embolic, thrombotic or low-flow consequences of atheroma affecting large and medium-sized arteries, intracranial small vessel disease or embolism from the heart.

This chapter considers the nature of the three main causes of cerebral ischaemia: atherothromboembolism (section 6.3), intracranial small vessel disease (section 6.4) and embolism from the heart (section 6.5). The more unusual causes will be described in Chapter 7.

6.3 Atheroma

Atheroma is by far the most frequent, but certainly not the only, arterial disorder. It is almost universal in the elderly, at least in developed countries. When complicated by thrombosis and embolism, and sometimes by low-flow distal to a severely stenosed artery, it is the most common cause of cerebral ischaemia and infarction. Although very difficult to prove, atheroma itself—uncomplicated by thrombosis and embolism—may *not* have become more prevalent during the first half of the 20th century, despite the rising mortality attributed to stroke and coronary events, nor less prevalent recently as vascular disease mortality has declined (Morris 1951a,b; Joseph *et al.* 1993; Enriquez-Sarano *et al.* 1996). The clinically important consequences of atheroma—ischaemic stroke, myocardial infarction and claudication—are probably more to do with the thrombotic *complications* of atheroma than the atheroma itself. It is, after all, remarkable how widespread atheroma can be at post-mortem in patients with no clinically obvious events. Also, both ischaemic stroke and myocardial infarction can occur even when atheroma is relatively restricted; is this bad atheroma, bad clotting or just bad luck?

6.3.1 The distribution of atheroma

Atheroma affects mainly large and medium-sized arteries, particularly at points of arterial branching (e.g. the carotid bifurcation), curvature (e.g. the aortic arch) and confluence (e.g. the basilar artery) (Fisher 1951, 1954; Hutchinson & Yates 1957; Schwartz & Mitchell 1961; Cornhill *et al.* 1980; Heinzlef *et al.* 1997) (Fig. 6.2). It is remarkable how free of atheroma some arterial sites can be; for example, the internal carotid artery (ICA) between just distal to its origin in the neck (the carotid sinus) and the carotid siphon in the head, and the main cerebral arteries distal to the circle of Willis. Occlusion of the middle cerebral artery (MCA) can sometimes be caused by *in situ* thrombosis complicating an unstable atheromatous plaque, but is much more likely to be caused by embolism from the heart or from a proximal arterial site (Constantinides 1967; Lhermitte *et al.* 1970; Ogata *et al.* 1994). Indeed, even occlusion of the carotid siphon is seldom caused by *in situ* atherothrombosis, but more likely by embolism or a non-atheromatous arterial disorder (Lammie *et al.* 1999). Another unexplained oddity is how the upper limb arteries are far less affected by atheroma than the lower limb arteries.

Atheroma affects large and medium-sized arteries, particularly at places of branching, tortuosity and confluence. It is a multifocal rather than a diffuse disease.

Possible explanations for this multifocal distribution of atheroma are:

- high haemodynamic shear stress and so endothelial trauma, a notion now largely discredited;
- low haemodynamic shear stress, boundary-zone flow separation, directional and stagnation changes in the blood, all leading to intimal proliferation and the accumulation of platelets; and
- turbulence, leading to endothelial damage;

all of which might promote thrombosis, which itself is clearly involved in the progression, if not the very beginnings, of atheroma (Grady 1984; McMillan 1985; Reneman *et al.* 1985; Nicholls *et al.* 1989; Malek *et al.* 1999). Interestingly, there can be very severe atherothrombotic stenosis at a particular site on one side of the body, but none at all at the mirror-image site on the other side, perhaps reflecting intra-individual geometric differences in arterial anatomy (Gnasso *et al.* 1997). Alternatively, perhaps once an atheromatous plaque is established, its growth becomes self-promoting as a result of a positive feedback loop, either biochemical or haemodynamic. This asymmetry clearly cannot be because of asymmetric exposure to vascular risk factors, such as smoking. On the whole, however, individuals with atheroma

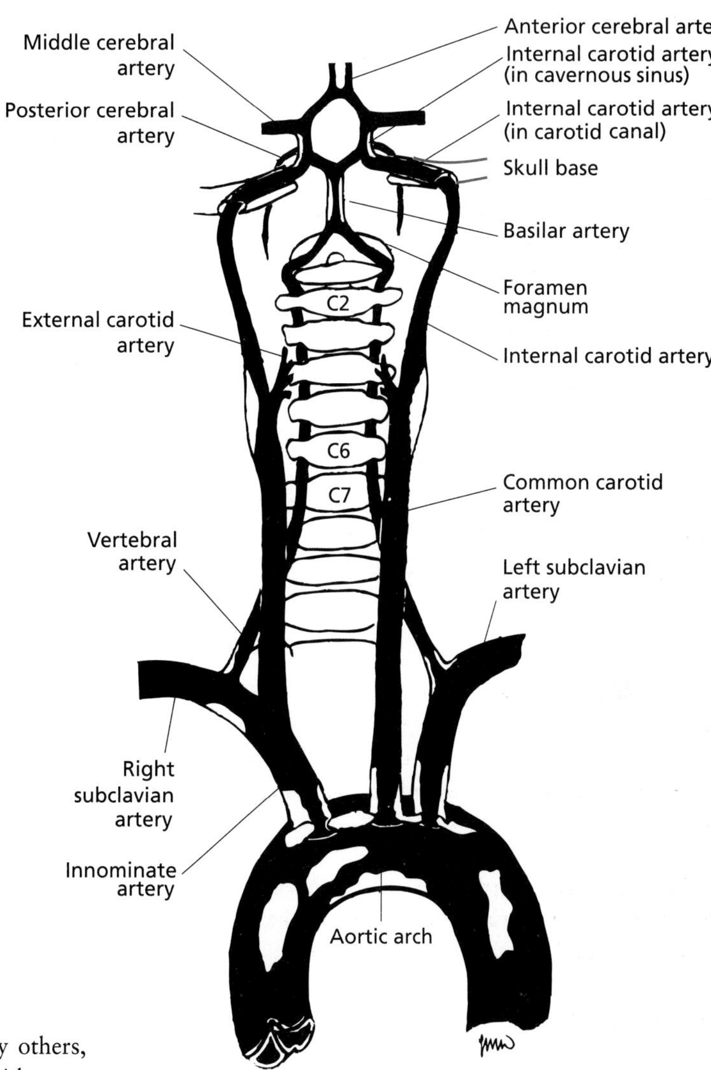

Fig. 6.2 The distribution of atheroma (white indentations of the arterial lumen) in the arteries supplying the brain and eye in white populations. Intracranial atheroma is relatively more severe than extracranial atheroma in Japanese, Chinese and black populations.

affecting one artery tend to have it affecting many others, subclinically if not clinically. Therefore, patients with cerebral ischaemia or carotid disease often already have (Table 6.3) or develop (section 16.1.1) angina, myocardial infarction and claudication (Mitchell & Schwartz 1962; Hertzer *et al.* 1985; Craven *et al.* 1990; Chimowitz *et al.* 1997; O'Leary *et al.* 1999). Presumably, genetic predisposition determines *who* is likely to develop atheroma, or to have particularly extensive or severe atheroma when exposed to causal risk factors, such as hypertension, while the arterial anatomy determines *where* the atheroma occurs. It is, however, notable that black and Oriental people tend to have more intracranial and less extracranial atheroma. However, nowadays, carotid bifurcation stenosis is being more often reported either because the pattern of atheroma is changing in these populations as result of lifestyle changes, or because previous studies were confounded by selection and other biases (Chen *et al.* 1998) (section 6.3.3).

Individuals with atheroma affecting one artery almost always have atheroma affecting many other arteries, with or without clinical manifestations.

6.3.2 The nature, progression and clinical consequences of atheroma

Atheroma begins as intimal fatty streaks in children, it is thought in response to some sort of endothelial injury (Berenson *et al.* 1998; Strong *et al.* 1999; Ross 1999; Napoli *et al.* 1999) (Fig. 6.3). Over many years, circulating monocyte-derived macrophages adhere to and invade the arterial wall. As a result, there is an inflammatory response with cytokine production and T-lymphocyte activation. Intra- and later extracellular cholesterol and other lipids are deposited, particularly in macrophages which are then described as foam cells. Arterial smooth-muscle cells migrate into the lesion and proliferate, fibrosis occurs and so fibrolipid plaques are formed. These plaques, with their lipid core and fibrous cap, encroach upon the media and spread around and along the arterial wall. Some become necrotic, ulcerated and calcified with neovascularization and haemorrhage—so-

	Number	Percentage
Hypertension (blood pressure > 160/90 mmHg, at least twice pre-stroke)	126	52
Angina and/or past myocardial infarction	92	38
Current smoker	66	27
Claudication and/or absent foot pulses	60	25
Major cardiac embolic source	50	20
Transient ischaemic attack	35	14
Cervical arterial bruit	33	14
Diabetes mellitus	24	10
Any of the above	196	80

Table 6.3 The prevalence of vascular risk factors and diseases in 244 patients with a first-ever-in-a-lifetime ischaemic stroke. Data from the Oxfordshire Community Stroke Project (Sandercock *et al.* 1989).

called complicated plaques. The arterial wall thickens, the vessel dilates or the lumen narrows and the artery becomes stiffer and tortuous.

Atheromatous plaques complicated by thrombosis: atherothrombosis

From an early stage, or perhaps even from the very first stage, atheromatous plaques promote platelet adhesion, activation and aggregation, which initiates blood coagulation and thus mural thrombosis (Imparato *et al.* 1979; Gower *et al.* 1987; Fuster *et al.* 1992a,b; Ware & Heistad 1993; Libby 1996) (section 11.1.3). At first, any thrombus may be lysed by fibrinolytic mechanisms in the vessel wall, or incorporated into the plaque which re-endothelializes and so 'heals'. Gradually, the athero- and then atherothrombotic plaque grows, in part because of repeated episodes of mural thrombosis layering one on top of the other, and eventually the lumen may become obstructed. Such occlusive intralumenal thrombus may then propagate proximally or distally in the column of stagnant blood, but usually no further than the next arterial branching point.

Thrombus may also embolize—in whole or in part—to obstruct a smaller distal artery, usually at a branching point; the same one or different ones on several occasions. Emboli consist of any combination of cholesterol crystals and other debris from the plaque, platelet aggregates, and fibrin which may be recently formed and relatively friable or old and well organized. Depending on their size, composition, consistency and age—and presumably the blood flow conditions at the site of impaction—emboli may be lysed, fragment and then be swept on into the microcirculation. Alternatively, they may permanently occlude the distal artery and promote local antero- and retrograde thrombosis which is further encouraged by the release of thromboxane A_2 from platelets, which is also a vasoconstrictor. However, thrombosis is opposed by the release of prostacyclin and nitric oxide, both vasodilators, from the vascular endothelium and by endothelium-derived plasminogen activator. The balance of these pro- and antithrombotic factors may determine whether a thrombus complicating an atheromatous plaque or an occlusive embolus grows, is lysed or becomes incorporated into the arterial wall and so contributes to the gradually enlarging atherothrombotic plaque. Whether acute occlusion of a cerebral vessel leads to infarction depends on not only for how long the blood flow is impaired, but also on the availability and functional capability of the collateral circulation distal to the occlusion (Gunning *et al.* 1964; Castaigne *et al.* 1970; Whisnant 1982; Norris & Bornstein 1986; Vane *et al.* 1990; Caplan & Hennerici 1998) (section 11.1.3).

Embolism from atherothrombotic plaques: atherothromboembolism

Emboli are transmitted to the brain or eye via their normal arterial supply, which itself varies somewhat in distribution between individuals (section 4.2). An embolus from an atherosclerotic carotid bifurcation—usually a plaque at the origin of the internal carotid artery (ICA) but sometimes the distal common or proximal external carotid arteries—normally goes to the eye or the anterior two-thirds of the cerebral hemisphere. But, on occasion, it may go to the occipital cortex if blood is flowing from the ICA via the posterior communicating artery to the posterior cerebral artery. However, if an artery is already occluded, then an embolus may travel via the collateral circulation and impact in an unexpected place. For example, with severe vertebral arterial disease, and therefore poor flow distally into the basilar artery, an embolus from the ICA origin may reach the basilar artery via the circle of Willis. With ICA occlusion, it is still possible to have an ipsilateral middle cerebral artery (MCA) distribution cerebral infarct as a result of:

- an embolus travelling from the *contralateral* ICA origin via the anterior communicating artery;
- an embolus from any blind stump of the occluded ICA, or from disease of the ipsilateral external carotid artery (ECA), via the ECA and orbital collaterals to the MCA;
- an embolus from the tail of thrombus in the ICA distal to the occlusion; or

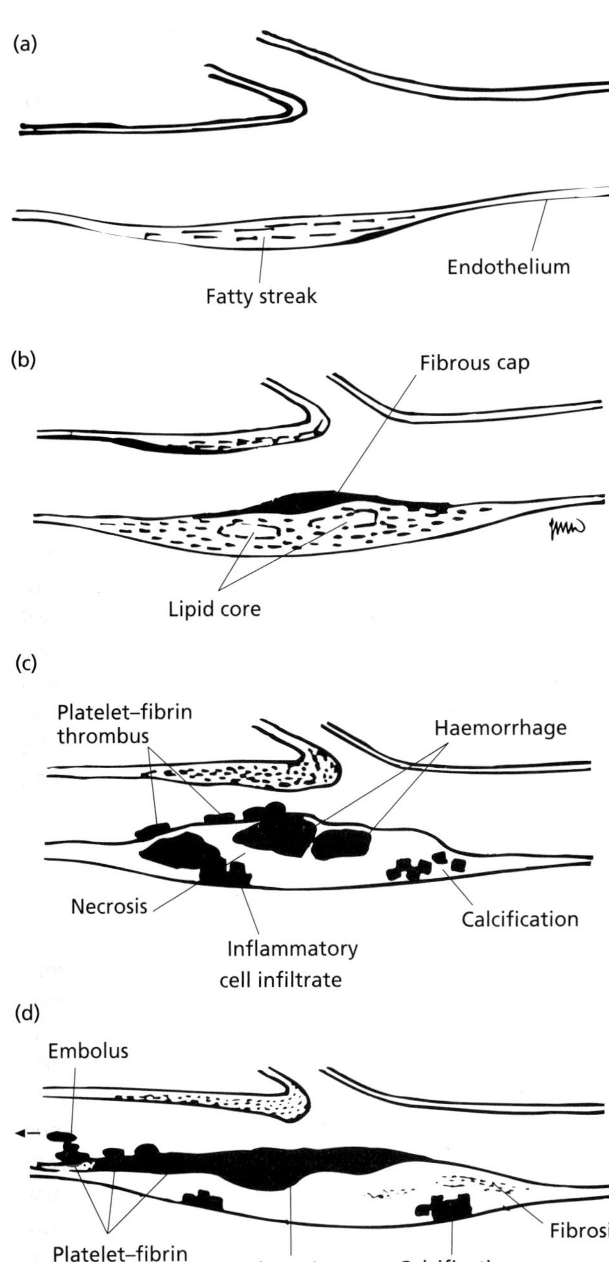

Fig. 6.3 The growth, progression and complications of atheromatous plaques: (a) early deposition of lipid in the artery wall; (b) further build-up of lipid and fibrous material; (c) necrosis, inflammatory cell infiltrate, calcification and new vessel formation, leading to; (d) plaque instability, ulceration and platelet–fibrin thrombus formation on the plaque surface.

• low-flow distal to the ICA occlusion, perhaps within a boundary-zone (section 6.6.5), particularly if the collateral blood supply is poor, cerebrovascular reactivity is impaired and the oxygen extraction ratio high (Countee *et al.* 1981; Hankey & Warlow 1991a; Klijn *et al.* 1997; Grubb *et al.* 1998).

Atherothrombosis affects large and medium-sized arteries and causes about 50% of ischaemic strokes and transient ischaemic attacks, mostly as the result of embolism to the brain, but sometimes as the result of acute thrombotic arterial occlusion or low-flow distal to a severely narrowed or occluded artery.

Curiously, emboli from the neck arteries (or from the heart) seldom seem to enter the small perforating arteries of the brain to cause lacunar infarction (section 6.4).

Symptomatic *in situ* acute atherothrombotic occlusion—rather than artery-to-artery embolism—does not appear to be a very common cause for ischaemic stroke or transient ischaemic attacks (TIAs) in the carotid territory (sections 4.3.4 and 4.3.5). Perhaps this is because atheroma affects the larger arteries (e.g. ICA rather than MCA) and it takes a very large plaque to occlude them, or because the potential for collateral blood flow is better distal to larger arteries (Lhermitte *et al.* 1970; Bogousslavsky *et al.* 1986a). Indeed, once the ICA has occluded, the risk of ipsilateral ischaemic stroke appears to be less than for severe stenosis (Hankey & Warlow 1991a; Klijn *et al.* 1997). On the other hand, symptomatic *in situ* atherothrombotic occlusion may be more common in the posterior circulation (e.g. of the basilar artery) but even here artery-to-artery embolism is well described (Castaigne *et al.* 1973; Caplan & Tettenborn 1992; Koennecke *et al.* 1997; Schwarz *et al.* 1997; Martin *et al.* 1998) (section 4.3.3).

Atherothromboembolism as an acute-on-chronic disorder: plaque instability

Similarly to the coronary arteries, atheromatous plaques in the cerebral circulation—particularly at the carotid bifurcation—probably become 'active' or 'unstable' from time to time with fissuring, cracking or rupture of the fibrous cap, or ulceration. The histological features of plaque instability are a thin fibrous cap, large lipid core, reduced smooth muscle content and high macrophage density (Fuster *et al.* 1999; Lammie *et al.* 1999) (Fig. 6.4a). If the thrombogenic centre of the plaque is exposed to flowing blood, then complicating thrombosis occurs. Plaque instability may even be a 'systemic' tendency because irregularity on angiography—and so presumed instability and ulceration—of symptomatic carotid stenosis is associated with irregularity of the asymptomatic contralateral carotid artery, and with coronary events assumed to be caused by plaque rupture (Rothwell *et al.* 2000a). At other times the plaque is quiescent with a thick fibrous cap or slowly growing without causing any clinical symptoms (Constantinides 1967; Harrison & Marshall 1977; Svindland & Torvik 1988; Torvik *et al.* 1989; Ogata *et al.* 1990, 1994; Davies 1997; Lammie *et al.* 1999) (Fig. 6.4b). In other words, atherothromboembolism is an 'acute-on-chronic disorder'. It is no surprise

(a) 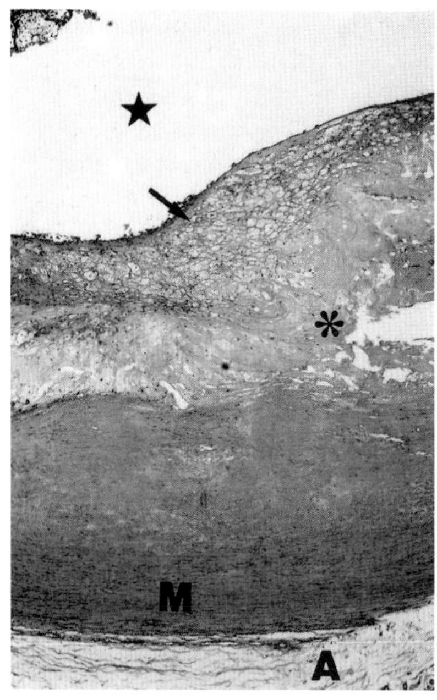

(b)  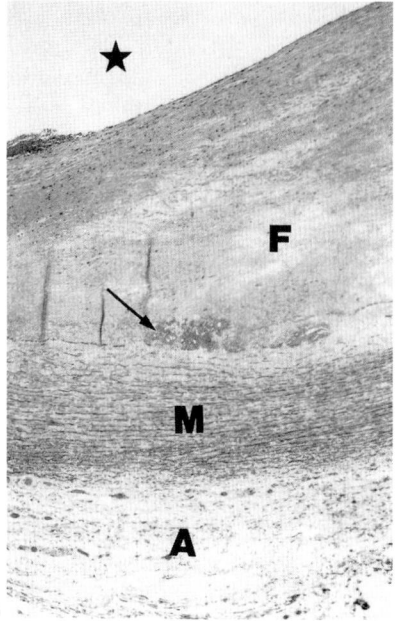

Fig. 6.4 Photomicrographs of transverse sections of the carotid sinus illustrating the pathological features of atherosclerotic plaque stability. (a) An unstable plaque characterized by a large necrotic core (*), and a thin fibrous cap heavily infiltrated by macrophages (arrow). Elsewhere the plaque is ulcerated and the lumen occluded by thrombus, part of which had embolized to the ipsilateral middle cerebral artery causing a fatal ischaemic stroke. (b) A comparable stenotic but stable plaque, comprising largely fibrous tissue (F) with focal calcification (arrow). There is no significant necrotic core or inflammatory cell infiltrate. ★, lumen; A, tunica adventitia; M, tunica media. (Provided by Dr Alistair Lammie.)

therefore that the clinical complications of atheroma reflect this:

- TIAs tend to cluster in time (section 16.1.1);
- stroke tends to occur early after a TIA and affect the same arterial territory (section 16.1.1);
- the risk of ischaemic stroke ipsilateral to severe carotid stenosis is highest soon after symptomatic presentation and then declines, even though the stenosis itself seldom regresses (section 16.8.5);
- presumed artery-to-artery embolic strokes tend to recur particularly early (section 16.1.3);
- emboli are more often detected with transcranial Doppler sonography if carotid stenosis is severe or recently symptomatic (Del Sette *et al.* 1997; Georgiadis *et al.* 1997; Molloy *et al.* 1998; Wijman *et al.* 1998; Droste *et al.* 1999a; Molloy & Markus 1999); and
- the rate of Doppler-detected emboli in the middle cerebral artery tends to decline with time after stroke (Kaposzta *et al.* 1999).

Increasing severity of atherothrombotic stenosis, at least at the origin of the ICA, is undoubtedly a powerful predictor and cause of ischaemic stroke ipsilateral to the lesion (European Carotid Surgery Trialists' Collaborative Group 1998). However, this cannot be the whole explanation because the risk of stroke distal to an asymptomatic stenosis is far less than distal to a recently symptomatic stenosis of the same severity (section 16.9.2); by no means all patients with severe stenosis have a stroke (section 16.8.8); and, relatively mildly stenosed plaques can be complicated by acute carotid occlusion (Lammie *et al.* 1999). Independently of the severity of stenosis, plaque irregularity on the angiogram is associated with increased stroke risk, probably because irregularity represents plaque ulceration and instability with thrombosis and so likely complicating embolism (Molloy & Markus 1999; Rothwell *et al.* 2000b) (section 16.8.8). Curiously, there is not such an obvious relationship between increasing coronary artery stenosis and coronary events. This may be because the coronary arteries are harder to image repeatedly and are more anatomically complicated, because coronary events are more often 'silent' or because the coronary arteries are smaller and more likely to be blocked if a plaque ruptures (Fuster *et al.* 1992a,b).

Atherothromboembolism is an acute-on-chronic disorder, both in its pathology and in its clinical manifestations. Although the formation of atherothrombotic plaques must be a long and gradual process over many years, the clinical manifestations usually occur acutely (e.g. an ischaemic stroke) and tend to cluster in time. For example, stroke tends to occur sooner rather than later after a transient ischaemic attack, perhaps as a result of the breakdown and 'instability' of an atherothrombotic plaque which later 'heals'.

Exactly why a plaque becomes unstable (and then perhaps ulcerates with complicating thrombosis) and another does not, is unknown. Histological comparisons of recently symptomatic vs. asymptomatic carotid plaques—matched for stenosis severity—are not easy to perform. However, it seems as though intraplaque haemorrhage, calcification and the lipid core are similar in both but, crucially, the thickness of the fibrous cap was not assessed in the careful study by Hatsukami *et al.* (1997) and Golledge *et al.* (2000). Similar problems arise with attempts to compare inflammatory processes and the expression of adhesion molecules (DeGraba *et al.* 1998; Jander *et al.* 1998), metalloproteinase expression (Loftus *et al.* 2000), differences in plaque tissue factor (Ardissino *et al.* 1997) and in plaque geometry and motion and so potential stresses on the fibrous cap (Richardson *et al.* 1989; Meairs & Hennerici 1999). Whether infection causes plaque instability is very unclear (section 6.3.3). In all these cross-sectional studies there is always the possibility of reverse causality—that by becoming symptomatic a plaque is changed in its anatomy, motion, biochemistry, etc.

Dolichoectasia

This unusual pattern of arterial disease tends to affect the medium-sized arteries at the base of the brain, particularly the basilar artery, mostly in the elderly but occasionally in children (Little *et al.* 1981; Nishizaki *et al.* 1986; Ince *et al.* 1998) (section 4.2.3). The arteries are widened, tortuous, elongated and are often enlarged enough to be seen as characteristic flow voids on MRI, and as tortuous channels—even without enhancement—or by virtue of calcification in their walls on brain CT (Aichner *et al.* 1993) (Fig. 6.5). When found in an individual, this arterial abnormality is not necessarily the cause of any ischaemic stroke (and very rarely of intracranial haemorrhage, despite the aneurysmal dilatation). However, these vessels can contain thrombus which embolizes, or occludes the origin of small branch arteries of the ectatic vessel, or even occludes the ectatic vessel itself. Cranial nerve and brainstem compression, or hydrocephalus caused by cerebrospinal fluid pathway compression are other occasional complications of basilar ectasia (Pessin *et al.* 1989; Schwartz *et al.* 1993; Passero & Filosomi 1998). Atheroma is the most common cause (Hegedus 1985). Other causes include various types of congenital defect in the vessel wall, Marfan's syndrome (section 7.4) pseudoxanthoma elasticum (section 7.4) and Fabry's disease—both in hemizygotic males and heterozygotic females (section 7.20).

6.3.3 Risk factors and causes of atheroma

The current view is that atheroma is initiated by some sort of endothelial injury and, perhaps in genetically susceptible individuals, is then amplified by lifestyle and environmental factors, already apparent even in children and young adults (Berenson *et al.* 1998). Hypertension, cigarette-smoking, hypercholesterolaemia and social deprivation have their own genetic and other antecedent causes, and interact with each other in complex ways to increase stroke risk (e.g. poor social circumstances, poor diet and smoking are all associated with each other) (Ross 1999). Thrombosis certainly complicates atheroma and may even be involved in its very beginnings (Duguid 1976). Evidence comes from animal models of atheroma, pathological examination of human arteries and epidemiological studies of 'risk factors', although these may be as much risk factors for the complicating thrombosis as for the underlying atheroma itself, if, indeed, the two processes can be separated (Ebrahim & Harwood 1999).

Whatever the exact mechanisms, it is quite clear that certain individual and population characteristics (risk factors) are associated with the *clinical* consequences of atheroma (i.e. ischaemic stroke, myocardial infarction, etc.) (Table 6.4). There is much more information about risk factors for coronary events than for ischaemic stroke, largely because coronary events are more common, patients are more intensively investigated and, it has to be said, the heart is more fashionable with much higher levels of research funding. The tendency for epidemiologists to lump all types of stroke together (haemorrhage with infarct, lacunar infarct with cortical infarct, etc.) might, in part, explain the curious quantitative differences between stroke and coronary heart disease (CHD) risk factors, although qualitatively they are the same. Why are smoking, raised plasma cholesterol and male sex far stronger risk factors for myocardial infarction, while hypertension is a far stronger risk factor for stroke? Could it be that some types of stroke are not to do with cholesterol, smokers and male sex? If these stroke types could be identified and removed from the analysis, together with strokes caused by embolism from the heart, would the remaining ischaemic strokes have a more similar risk factor profile to CHD which, it seems, is less heterogeneous than stroke and mostly to do with atherothrombosis? Furthermore, why is it that some populations, like the Japanese and black Africans, seem to be afflicted far more by stroke than coronary events? During epidemiological transition, does hypertension appear before hypercholesterolaemia, and so stroke before CHD?

It is curious that some risk factors are so much stronger for stroke (e.g. increasing blood pressure) and yet others are so much stronger for coronary heart disease (e.g. increasing plasma cholesterol) if the underlying vascular pathology (atheroma) is much the same.

It is important to be clear that a risk factor merely indicates an *association* between that factor and the disease of interest (Table 6.5). This association may be causal, coincidental or a reflection of reverse causality (i.e. the disease itself changes the risk factor level or prevalence). In some but by no means all instances there is a plausible biological explanation for causal associations, through atherothrombotic arterial disease to the clinical syndrome. A *causal* rather than a coincidental relationship is suggested by a number of rather circumstantial pieces of evidence which on their own may not be very convincing (Glynn 1993):

- a strong association between the risk factor and the disease (i.e. a high relative risk or relative odds);
- consistency of association across several types of studies at different times in different places;

(a) 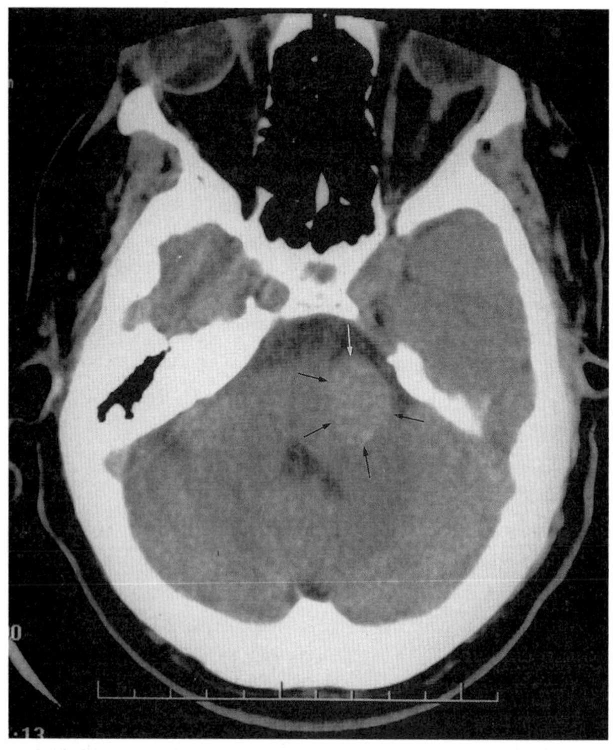

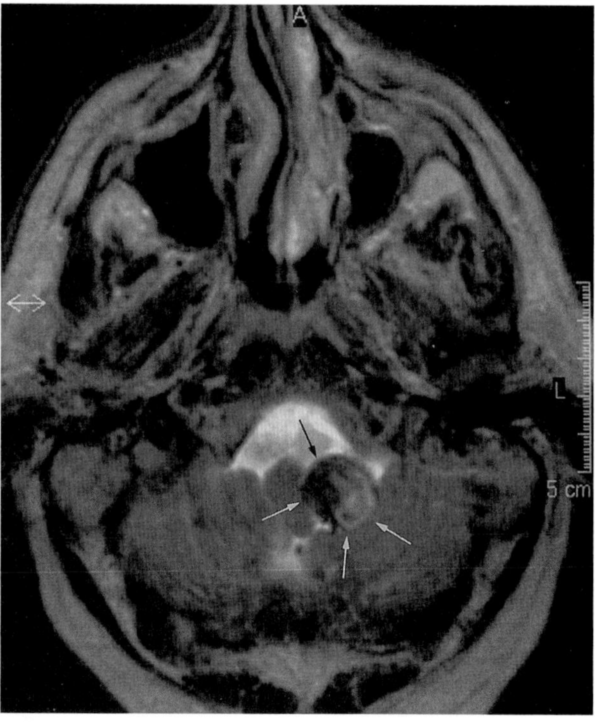 (b)

(c) 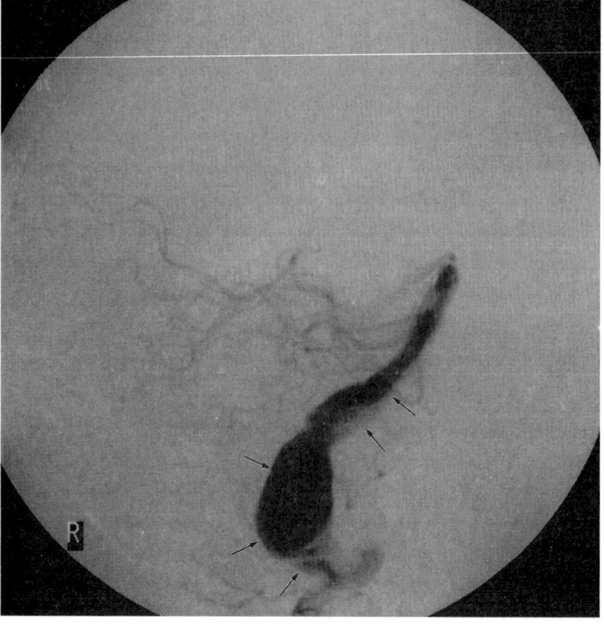

Fig. 6.5 Vertebrobasilar dolichoectasia. (a) On the CT scan there is a 1.5–2 cm rounded mass (arrows) which is of slightly higher density than adjacent brain and sits in the left cerebellopontine angle. The mass is indenting the brainstem. On adjacent sections the mass was obviously longitudinal and contiguous with the vertebral and top end of the basilar arteries. (b) MR examination of the same patient shows the mixed signal mass (arrows). The presence of increased signal indicates either very slowly flowing or partially clotted blood. (c) Intra-arterial angiography shows a lateral projection of the vertebrobasilar circulation. Although the main area of expansion is in the lower basilar artery (arrows), the dolichoectasia actually extends from the upper right vertebral artery almost to the very tip of the basilar artery.

- a dose–response relationship (i.e. the greater the exposure to the risk factor, the greater the risk of the disease);
- independence from confounding variables, particularly age (Fig. 6.6);
- a clear temporal sequence of exposure to the risk factor *before* disease onset, remembering that the onset of atheroma is years before the onset of its clinical manifestations;
- biological and epidemiological plausibility, although there is no end to human ingenuity in constructing plausible hypotheses to explain the natural world; and,
- most convincing of all but not always feasible, demonstration that attenuation of the risk factor leads to a fall in disease incidence, preferably by means of a randomized controlled trial. However, a trial can be negative if the intervention is too

Table 6.4 Factors associated with an increased risk of occlusive vascular disorders (i.e. ischaemic stroke, myocardial infarction, claudication, etc.).

Increasing age
Male sex
Increasing blood pressure
Cigarette-smoking
Diabetes mellitus
Blood lipids* (definite for myocardial infarction but not ischaemic stroke)
Increasing plasma fibrinogen
Raised haematocrit*
High plasma factor VII coagulant activity*
Raised von Willebrand factor antigen*
Low blood fibrinolytic activity*
Raised tissue plasminogen activator antigen*
Hyperhomocysteinaemia
Physical inactivity
Obesity
Diet* (salt, antioxidants, etc.)
Alcohol (none, or heavy drinking)
Race
Social deprivation
Infection*
'Stress'*

*Somewhat uncertain association with ischaemic stroke, perhaps because any association is weak, or has been under-researched in comparison with coronary heart disease, or has been examined in relation to all stroke rather than only ischaemic stroke.

little (i.e. not enough blood pressure lowering), too late (the arterial damage is already done and the clinical consequences are inevitable) or the trial is too small (type II error).

Even if a risk factor is associated with a high relative risk of stroke and the relationship is causal, the factor may still contribute very little to the incidence of stroke if it is rarely present in the population (e.g. rheumatic atrial fibrillation) or if there is a low baseline risk of stroke in the population where the risk factor is acting (e.g. oral contraceptives in young women). In other words, the impact of a risk factor is low if the proportion of stroke cases attributable to that risk factor is low (low population-attributable risk). On the other hand, a causal risk factor with a rather modest relative risk may be of major importance in contributing to stroke incidence if it is very prevalent (e.g. moderate hypertension) and/or the background risk of stroke in the population is high (e.g. in elderly people). The population-attributable risk is then high.

This epidemiological approach to defining risk factors and possible causation has tended to lump all strokes together, more so in prospective cohort than in case–control studies. Therefore, the heterogeneous nature of the pathology and causes of stroke may obscure any relationship between a particular risk factor and, for example, a particular type of stroke, such as haemorrhagic rather than ischaemic, or a lacunar infarct rather than a cardioembolic infarct. Furthermore, stroke itself may:

- change some risk factors, e.g. both blood pressure and blood glucose increase temporarily after acute stroke (sections 15.7 and 15.18.3) while plasma cholesterol falls (section 6.7.1);
- make information of past activities impossible to obtain because of the patient's confusion or aphasia;
- lead to bias in recording risk factors in case–control studies because it is impossible to blind assessors to stroke or control patient status; or
- require treatment which modifies risk factors (e.g. stopping smoking or lowering blood pressure).

Therefore, quick and relatively easy case–control studies based on stroke survivors are fraught with surprising difficulty, especially with hospital-based studies which tend to exclude mild cases and those that die before admission. Using TIA patients as a surrogate for ischaemic stroke, and extracting information from medical records written *before* the TIA, could avoid some of these problems. Studies relating stroke mortality to various risk factors are problematic if the factor itself increases case fatality (such as diabetes mellitus), and also if haemorrhagic and ischaemic strokes are lumped together because haemorrhagic strokes are more likely to cause death. The most unbiased information comes from large prospective community-based cohort studies where all strokes are counted (such as in Framingham). However, these take decades to complete and if a baseline variable has not been collected—or even thought of at the time—it clearly cannot be related to later stroke risk, unless it involves analysis of a baseline stored blood sample.

Studying easily accessible arteries directly with ultrasound, such as the carotid bifurcation, is a relatively recent approach. This gets closer to risk factors for very early changes in the vessel wall (increasing intima-media thickness) and also for atherothrombotic plaque, although ultrasound cannot reliably distinguish atheroma from complicating thrombus (Bonithon-Kopp *et al.* 1996; Crouse *et al.* 1996; O'Leary *et al.* 1996; Wilson *et al.* 1997). This approach is still prone to the familiar problems of observational epidemiology: inadequate sample size, the numerous potential biases in case–control studies, confounding, chance effects in small samples, lack of blinding to case or control status and inappropriate subgroup analyses. Also, in prospective cohort studies, it is not easy to quantify progression or regression of arterial wall thickness or plaques over time. Alterations in a plaque may be as much to do with the difficulty in imaging exactly the same plaque at the same angle, and changes in any complicating thrombus (such as lysis), as with growth or resolution of atheroma in the vessel wall, or as a result of temporary changes in the plaque, such as haemorrhage.

Table 6.5 The association between a risk factor and disease; calculating relative risk and relative odds in cohort and case–control studies.

Cohort studies

A longitudinal study of a cohort of individuals, some of whom have a risk factor for stroke $(a+b)$, and some of whom develop a stroke during follow-up $(a+c)$

		Stroke during follow-up: Yes	No
Risk factor at baseline	Yes	a	b
	No	c	d

The risk of stroke in those with the risk factor $(R+)$ is $\frac{a}{a+b}$

The risk of stroke in those without the risk factor $(R-)$ is $\frac{c}{c+d}$

Therefore: the relative risk (or risk ratio) = $\frac{R+}{R-}$, i.e. $\frac{a}{a+b} \times \frac{c+d}{c} = \frac{ac+ad}{ac+bc}$

and the absolute risk difference = $(R+)-(R-)$

The odds of stroke in those with the risk factor (O+) is $\frac{a}{b}$

The odds of stroke in those without the risk factor (O–) is $\frac{c}{d}$

Therefore: the relative odds (or odds ratio) = $\frac{O+}{O-}$, i.e. $\frac{ad}{bc}$

Note: when stroke is rare (i.e. a and c are small compared with b and d), then the relative risk and relative odds are about the same

Case–control studies

Patients with stroke $(a+c)$ and controls without a stroke $(b+d)$ from the same population are identified and the previous exposure to the risk factor compared using the odds ratio

		Stroke, and non-stroke control patients identified at one point in time: Yes	No
Risk factor present	Yes	a	b
	No	c	d

The odds of a stroke patient having the risk factor are $\frac{a}{c}$

The odds of a control patient having the risk factor are $\frac{b}{d}$

Therefore: the relative odds (or odds ratio) = $\frac{a}{c} \div \frac{b}{d} = \frac{ad}{bc}$

In practice, looking at arteries rather than people has not yet led to any new aetiological insights, perhaps because the sample sizes have been too small and because of other methodological problems.

As can be seen in Table 6.3, the vast majority of ischaemic stroke patients, necessarily taken as a group in most epidemiological studies and therefore including those resulting from small vessel disease and embolism from the heart as well as atheroma, have one or more of the definite vascular risk factors, which will be discussed below.

Age

Increasing age is the strongest risk factor for TIAs and ischaemic stroke, and almost certainly for the various subcategories of ischaemic stroke (Fig. 6.7). For example, an 80-year-old

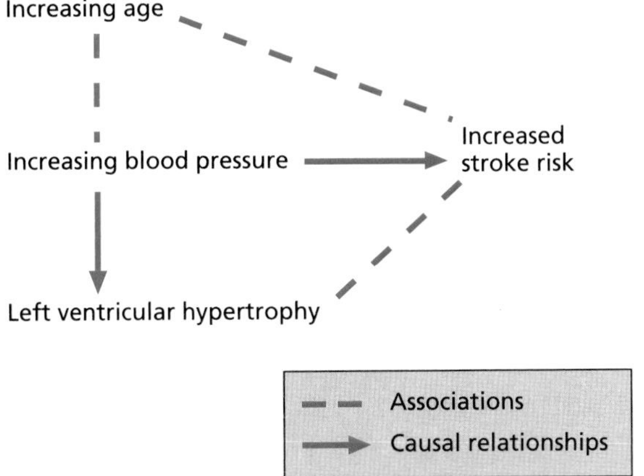

Fig. 6.6 'Confounding' in observational studies which relate a risk factor to a disease such as stroke. In this example, increasing age is associated with both increasing blood pressure and increasing risk of stroke. In fact, age and blood pressure are independent of the confounding effect of one on the other. In other words, for a population of the same age, there is an increasing risk of stroke with increasing blood pressure, and for a population with the same blood pressure, there is an increasing risk of stroke with increasing age. Therefore, irrespective of age, increasing blood pressure is strongly associated with stroke risk. Also, increasing age is associated with increasing stroke risk, not because age and blood pressure are associated, which they are, but because of something else (perhaps increasing prevalence of atrial fibrillation with age, etc.). On the other hand, although left-ventricular hypertrophy is associated with increasing stroke risk, this association more or less disappears if blood pressure is controlled for because, presumably, increasing blood pressure causes *both* stroke and left-ventricular hypertrophy. So hypertension is a confounding factor and explains the left-ventricular hypertrophy–stroke relationship. It is not possible to adjust for confounding factors if they are not measured or even suspected and, when they are, statistical adjustment is not always easy or even possible, so that some associations said to be unconfounded may not be (Davey Smith *et al.* 1992; Datta 1993; Leon 1993; Phillips & Davey Smith 1993).

has about 30 times the risk of ischaemic stroke as a 50-year-old (Bamford *et al.* 1988, 1990).

Sex

There is much less of an excess of ischaemic strokes and TIAs in men than in women compared with coronary events and peripheral arterial disease. What excess there is does not apply in young adults and the very elderly (Lerner & Kannel 1986) (Fig. 6.8). Notwithstanding popular dogma, the equalization of vascular risk in elderly males and females is probably not explained by the natural menopause, although bilateral oophorectomy without oestrogen replacement about doubles the risk of vascular events (van der Schouw *et al.* 1996; Hu *et al.* 1999).

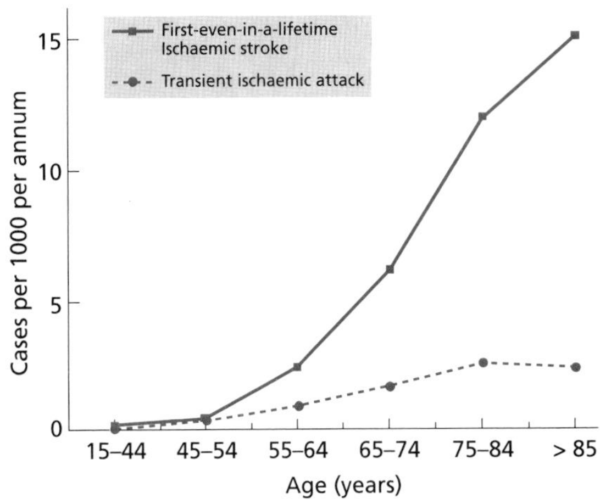

Fig. 6.7 The incidence of first-ever-in-a-lifetime ischaemic stroke and of transient ischaemic attack (TIA) in the Oxfordshire Community Stroke Project. The flattening of TIA and, to some extent, stroke incidence in old age may be because cases did not come to medical attention or, when they did, they were not correctly diagnosed in the elderly (Dennis *et al.* 1989; Bamford *et al.* 1990).

Blood pressure

In healthy populations of both sexes and independently of age, increasing blood pressure is strongly associated with overall stroke risk, and of all the main pathological types, including ischaemic stroke (Whelton 1994). The relationship between usual diastolic blood pressure and subsequent stroke is log–linear with no threshold below which stroke risk becomes stable, at least not within the 'normal' range of 70–110 mmHg (Fig. 6.9). The proportional increase in stroke risk associated with a given increase in blood pressure

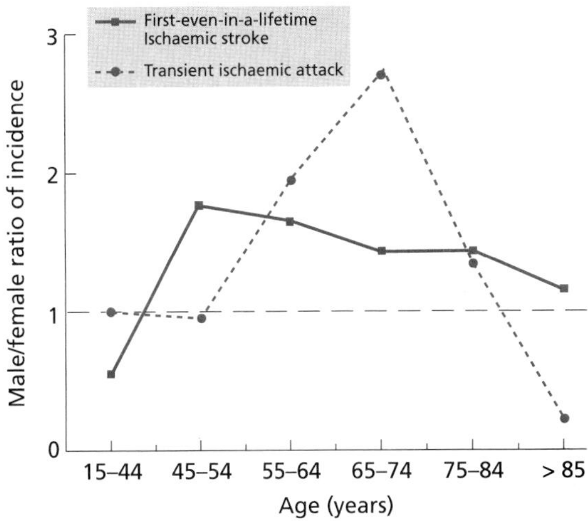

Fig. 6.8 The ratio of male : female incidence of first-ever-in-a-lifetime ischaemic stroke and transient ischaemic attack in the Oxfordshire Community Stroke Project (Dennis *et al.* 1989; Bamford *et al.* 1990).

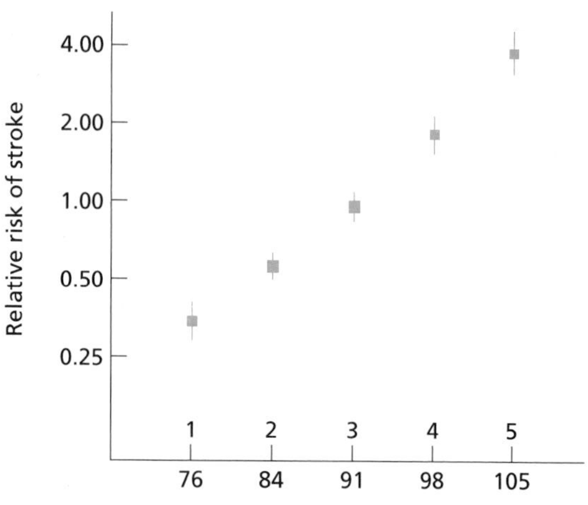

Fig. 6.9 The risk of stroke related to the usual diastolic blood pressure in five categories, defined by usual baseline blood pressure, from a pooled analysis of seven prospective observational studies. Solid squares represent stroke risks relative to risk in the whole study population; their size is proportional to the number of strokes in each blood-pressure category. The vertical lines represent 95% confidence intervals. (With permission from MacMahon *et al.* 1990.)

is similar at all levels of blood pressure. This risk almost doubles with each 7.5 mmHg increase in usual diastolic blood pressure in Western populations, and with each 5.0 mmHg in Japanese and Chinese populations (MacMahon *et al.* 1990; Eastern Stroke and Coronary Heart Disease Collaborative Research Group 1998). However, the strength of the association is attenuated with increasing age, although the absolute risk of stroke in the elderly is far higher than in the young (Prospective Studies Collaboration 1995). It is not clear whether hypertension is still a risk factor in the *very* elderly, where stroke may be associated with low blood pressures, perhaps because low pressures reflect pre-existing cardiovascular disease, such as cardiac failure, and other co-morbid conditions near the time of stroke. However, studies have been small and a systematic overview is required to clarify this issue (Boshuizen *et al.* 1998). Studies which have shown a J-shaped relationship between increasing stroke risk and *low* levels of blood pressure have probably been over-emphasized by publication bias. They have almost certainly included patients with prior vascular disease or treated hypertension, which might explain the higher stroke risks at lower pressures. The relationship between stroke and systolic blood pressure is possibly stronger than with diastolic pressure, and even 'isolated' systolic hypertension with a 'normal' diastolic blood pressure is associated with increased stroke risk (Shaper *et al.* 1991; Keli *et al.* 1992; Sagie *et al.* 1993; Petrovitch *et al.* 1995).

There is no doubt, as confirmed by the results of randomized controlled trials, that the relationship between increasing blood pressure and stroke risk is causal (section 16.3.1). However, it is not clear if all types of stroke are prevented by reducing blood pressure, largely because in the clinical trials they have all been lumped together, haemorrhagic with ischaemic strokes of various types (MacMahon & Rodgers 1993, 1994; Collins & MacMahon 1994; Mulrow *et al.* 1994) (section 16.3.1). Progression of carotid stenosis, at least as assessed by ultrasound, is slowed by treating hypertension (Sutton-Tyrrell *et al.* 1994). Because moderately raised levels of blood pressure are so common in the middle-aged and elderly, increasing blood pressure probably accounts for more ischaemic strokes than anything else.

Hypertension seems to increase the risk of ischaemic stroke by increasing the extent and severity of atheroma (section 6.3), as well as the prevalence of 'simple' and 'complex' intracranial small vessel disease (Ross Russell 1975; Chobanian 1983; Lusiani *et al.* 1987; Reed *et al.* 1988; Sutton-Tyrrell *et al.* 1993; Fine-Edelstein *et al.* 1994) (section 6.4).

Cigarette-smoking

Cigarette-smoking is associated with approximately double the risk of ischaemic stroke in males and females, but less obviously in the elderly, and there is a dose–response relationship (Shinton & Beevers 1989; Donnan *et al.* 1993a; Doll *et al.* 1994; Robbins *et al.* 1994; Haheim *et al.* 1996; Bonita *et al.* 1999). There are not as many data on passive smoking and stroke as there are for coronary events where the association is surprisingly large (Law *et al.* 1997; Jamrozik & Dobson 1999; He *et al.* 1999; You *et al.* 1999). As one would expect, most of the ultrasound and angiogram studies link carotid disease with smoking (Haapanen *et al.* 1989; O'Leary *et al.* 1992; Fine-Edelstein *et al.* 1994; Howard *et al.* 1998). Although cigar-smoking increases the risk of coronary events by about one-quarter, there are insufficient data to link either pipe- or cigar-smoking with stroke, perhaps because there are fewer people who still indulge in this habit (Iribarren *et al.* 1999). The risk of stroke gradually declines after stopping smoking so supporting a causal relationship, but a satisfactory randomized controlled trial proved impossible (Donnan *et al.* 1989; Shinton & Beevers 1989; Rose & Colwell 1992; Kawachi *et al.* 1993; Bonita *et al.* 1999).

Diabetes mellitus

Any studies linking diabetes with *fatal* stroke will exaggerate the association, because diabetics who have a stroke are more likely to die of it than non-diabetics (Jorgensen *et al.* 1994c) (sections 10.2.7 and 15.18.3). In fact, diabetes about doubles the risk of ischaemic stroke over and above confounding with hypertension and other risk factors (Rosengren *et al.* 1989; Manson *et al.* 1991; Burchfiel *et al.* 1994; Qureshi *et al.* 1998; Tuomilehto & Rastenyte 1999; Wannamethee *et al.* 1999). Diabetics also have thicker carotid arterial walls but the relationship with carotid stenosis is less clear, probably because of lack of patient numbers (Fine-Edelstein *et al.* 1994; Niskanen *et al.* 1996; O'Leary *et al.* 1996). So far, randomized trials have not shown that diabetic treatment reduces the risk of stroke (United Kingdom Prospective Diabetes Study Group 1998) (section 16.3.7).

Blood lipids

Increasing plasma total cholesterol, increasing low-density lipoprotein-cholesterol and decreasing levels of high-density lipoprotein-cholesterol are strong risk factors for coronary heart disease, whereas triglyceride levels are not. A long-term reduction of plasma cholesterol by 0.6 mmol/L should and does reduce the relative risk of coronary events by about 25%, perhaps rather more in the young than in the elderly (Law *et al.* 1994; Hokanson & Austin 1996; Downs *et al.* 1998; Long-term Intervention with Pravastatin in Ischaemic Disease (LIPID) Study Group 1998). On the other hand, the relationship with ischaemic stroke is much less clear. Very large systematic reviews of cohort studies have not revealed any association between all stroke types combined and increasing plasma total cholesterol at baseline, except perhaps under the age of 45 years (Prospective Studies Collaboration 1995; Eastern Stroke & Coronary Heart Disease Collaborative Research Group 1998) (Fig. 6.10). Case–control studies provide less reliable measures of association because of their biases, particularly the changes in plasma lipids following stroke (Qizilbash *et al.* 1991) (section 6.7.1). Relating carotid intima-media thickness or stenosis with blood lipids is perhaps too far from the clinical consequences of atheroma to be relevant, or the studies have been too small to be reliable (Reed *et al.* 1988; Homer *et al.* 1991; Fine-Edelstein *et al.* 1994; Willeit *et al.* 1995; Crouse *et al.* 1996; Wilson *et al.* 1997). Any association between plasma lipoprotein (a) and apolipoprotein E genotype with ischaemic stroke is as yet uncertain (van Kooten *et al.* 1996; Margaglione *et al.* 1998; Peng *et al.* 1999).

This marked contrast between coronary disease and ischaemic stroke is even more curious now it is clear that cholesterol lowering reduces the risk of myocardial infarction and stroke, albeit in low-risk of stroke populations, and more obviously for non-fatal than fatal stroke (Di Mascio *et al.* 2000) (section 16.3.2). It is tempting to believe that the observational epidemiology has perhaps missed an ischaemic stroke–lipid connection because:

- the seemingly negative association between increasing plasma cholesterol and intracranial haemorrhage has obscured a positive association with ischaemic stroke in studies where the pathological type of stroke was not accounted for (Fig. 6.11);
- the over-representation of fatal, and therefore more likely to be haemorrhagic, strokes in some studies;
- stroke occurs at a later age than myocardial infarction, so that relatively few strokes have yet occurred in the cohort studies;
- lipids are generally a weaker risk factor in the elderly where most strokes occur;
- the narrow range of cholesterol levels examined in many studies;
- the loss of stroke-susceptible individuals from the study population by prior death from coronary disease;
- uncertainties about the effect of stroke itself on lipid levels in case–control studies; and
- not differentiating ischaemic strokes likely to be caused by intracranial small vessel disease from those caused by large vessel atherothrombosis.

Alternatively, the lack of any plasma cholesterol association with ischaemic stroke may be correct and perhaps the statins reduce stroke risk by some mechanism other than by cholesterol lowering.

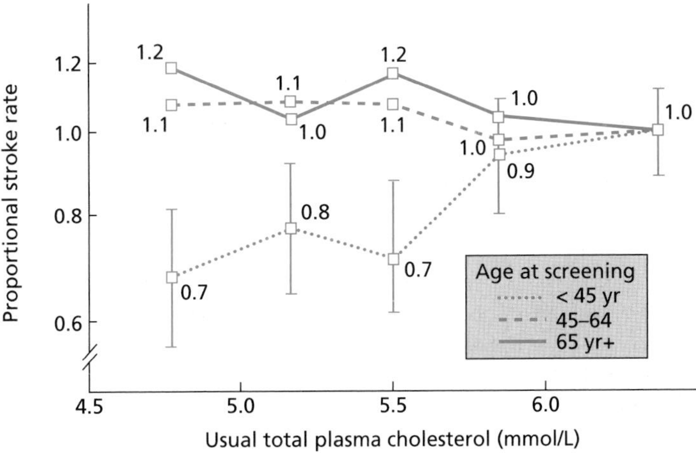

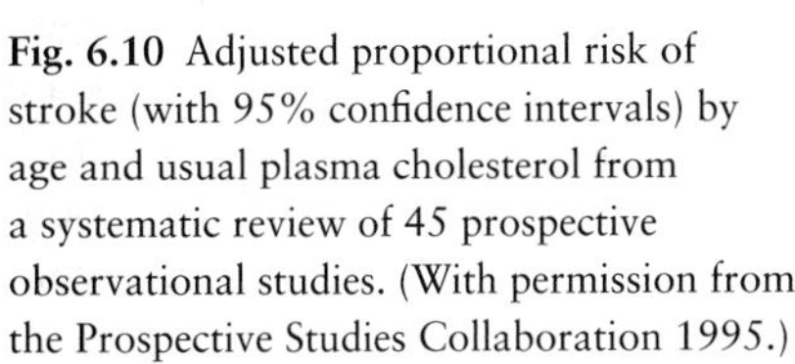
Fig. 6.10 Adjusted proportional risk of stroke (with 95% confidence intervals) by age and usual plasma cholesterol from a systematic review of 45 prospective observational studies. (With permission from the Prospective Studies Collaboration 1995.)

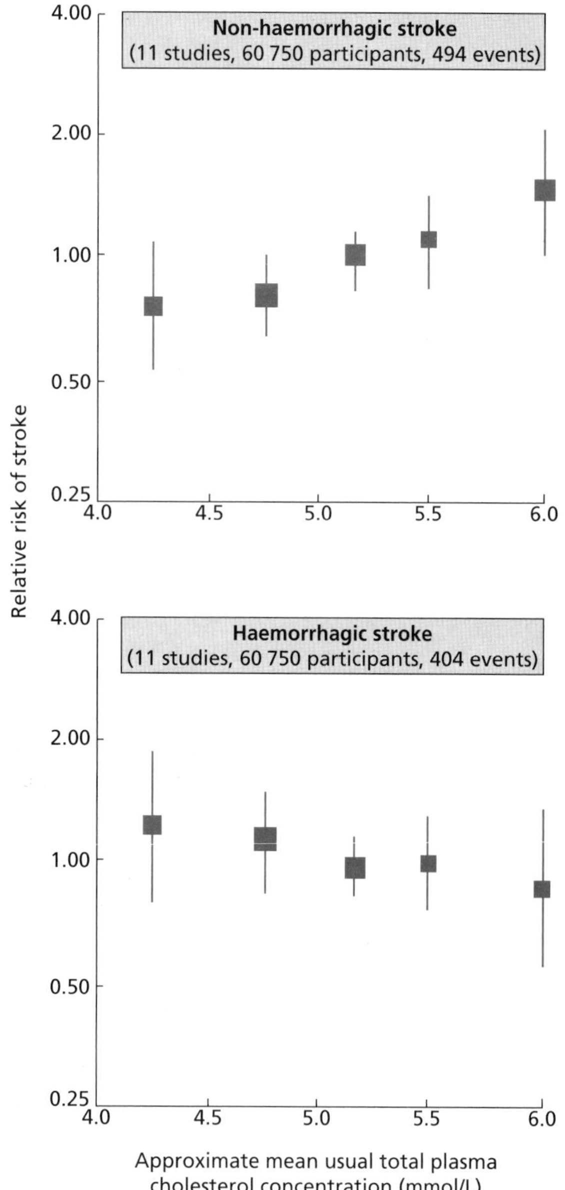

Fig. 6.11 Overall adjusted relative risk (95% confidence intervals) of non-haemorrhagic and haemorrhagic stroke by usual plasma cholesterol from a systematic review of prospective observational studies in China and Japan. The size of the solid squares is proportional to the number of strokes in each cholesterol category and the vertical lines are 95% confidence intervals. (With permission from the Eastern Stroke & Coronary Heart Disease Collaborative Research Group 1998.)

Haemostatic variables

Despite much effort, very few consistent associations have been found between coagulation parameters, fibrinolytic activity, platelet behaviour and vascular disease. Often these variables are altered by acute stroke so that most case–control studies are invalid, and it has not been practical to carry out very many long-term cohort studies.

Plasma fibrinogen has a strong and consistent positive association with stroke and coronary events, but not perhaps with carotid stenosis. Cigarette-smoking is a confounding variable so the effect of cigarette-smoking on stroke may be mediated, at least in part, by increasing the fibrinogen level, thus accelerating thrombosis. Less important but still confusing confounding factors include age, hypertension, diabetes, hyperlipidaemia, lack of exercise, social class, social activity, season of the year, alcohol consumption and stress. It is not yet certain therefore whether increasing plasma fibrinogen really is a causal factor and, if so, whether it acts by increasing plasma viscosity or through promoting thrombosis. The confusion is compounded because there is no standard method for measuring plasma fibrinogen, it tends to rise after acute events including infections, it is not easy to lower plasma fibrinogen, and no satisfactory randomized controlled trials have been reported (Cook & Ubben 1990; Rosengren *et al.* 1990; Qizilbash *et al.* 1991; Ernst & Resch 1993; Fine-Edelstein *et al.* 1994; Brunner *et al.* 1996; Lowe *et al.* 1997; Danesh *et al.* 1998).

Raised haematocrit is an uncertain risk factor for stroke. The association is confounded by the fact that cigarette-smoking, blood pressure and plasma fibrinogen are all positively associated with haematocrit (Welin *et al.* 1987; Gagnon *et al.* 1994; Wannamethee *et al.* 1994). Both raised haematocrit and raised plasma fibrinogen increase *blood viscosity*, another potentially causal risk factor (Lowe *et al.* 1997). No randomized trials are available of lowering haematocrit, viscosity or fibrinogen.

Raised plasma factor VII coagulant activity may be a risk factor for coronary events, and also polymorphisms of the factor VII gene, but there are very few data for stroke (Qizilbash *et al.* 1997; Iacoviello *et al.* 1998).

Raised von Willebrand factor antigen is another possible risk factor for ischaemic stroke (Qizilbash *et al.* 1997).

Low blood fibrinolytic activity and *high plasma plasminogen-activator type I* are coronary risk factors and *raised tissue plasminogen activator antigen* may be associated with both coronary and stroke risk, perhaps because it is a marker of endogenous fibrinolytic activity (Meade *et al.* 1993; Ridker *et al.* 1994; Qizilbash *et al.* 1997; Macko *et al.* 1999; Johansson *et al.* 2000; Kohler & Grant 2000).

Abnormal platelet behaviour has not been convincingly linked with subsequent stroke in cohort studies, and any case–control studies after stroke have great potential for bias as stroke alters platelet function (van Kooten *et al.* 1999). Polymorphisms of platelet membrane glycoprotein IIIa have first been associated with stroke but, as seems to happen so often with genetic studies, then rejected on the basis of larger and more methodologically sound work (Kekomaki *et al.* 1999).

Plasma homocysteine

Because the rare inborn recessive condition of homocystinuria is complicated by arterial and venous thrombosis (section 7.20), it is natural to imagine that mildly raised levels of plasma homocysteine could be a risk factor for or even a cause of vascular disease in general. Elevated plasma homocysteine is positively associated with increasing age, abnormal lipids, smoking, diabetes, chronic renal failure and hypertension, and it is also raised in nutritional deficiencies and probably after stroke and myocardial infarction. None the less, the observational data linking coronary events, stroke, venous thromboembolism and carotid intima-media thickness and stenosis with increasing plasma homocysteine (hyperhomocysteinaemia) are now robust enough for trials of homocysteine-lowering with folic acid and pyridoxine to have been started (Clarke & Collins 1998; Danesh & Lewington 1998; Refsum *et al.* 1998; Welch & Loscalzo 1998; Hankey & Eikelboom 1999; Kittner *et al.* 1999; Perry 1999) (section 16.7.5). It must be remembered that there may be unanticipated risks associated with homocysteine lowering, but the trials will address the balance of any benefits with any risks (Dudman 1999).

Physical exercise

Physical exercise somewhat reduces blood pressure, weight, plasma cholesterol, plasma fibrinogen and the risk of non-insulin-dependent diabetes mellitus and is associated with less cigarette-smoking (Connelly *et al.* 1992; Arroll & Beaglehole 1993). Therefore, not surprisingly, lack of exercise is associated with coronary events and there is also strong evidence of a similar association with stroke (Berlin & Colditz 1990; Evenson *et al.* 1999, Lee *et al.* 1999; Wannamethee & Shaper 1999; Ellekjaer *et al.* 2000; Hu *et al.* 2000). So far there is insufficient evidence from randomized trials to be sure that deliberately increasing exercise levels, in sporting activities or as part of a generally healthy lifestyle, reduces the risk of vascular events, although it should and it would be nice to think that it did (O'Connor *et al.* 1989) (section 16.3.8).

Obesity

Any relationship between obesity and stroke is likely to be confounded by the positive association of obesity with hypertension, diabetes, hypercholesterolaemia and lack of exercise, and the negative association with smoking and concurrent illness. None the less, stroke is more common in the obese and so is overall mortality. How to measure obesity is itself somewhat controversial; a raised waist : hip ratio as a measure of central obesity, and perhaps change in body weight, may be stronger risk factors than the traditional measure of weight compared with height (Walker *et al.* 1996; Rexrode *et al.* 1997; Shaper *et al.* 1997; Calle *et al.* 1999) (section 16.3.5).

Diet

It is technically difficult to measure what people eat and how they cook it, relate any particular diet to events such as stroke which occur years later, and to be sure that any association is not better explained by a confounding variable. For example, people who eat a lot of fruit tend to have a generally 'healthy' lifestyle, not to smoke and they may use less salt (Ness & Powles 1999).

Salt, by increasing systemic blood pressure, is probably associated with increased stroke risk but this issue is still controversial (Frost *et al.* 1991; Law *et al.* 1991a,b; He *et al.* 1999). In observational studies, diets low in the following may be associated with a raised risk of coronary disease and stroke (Diaz *et al.* 1997):

- potassium (Khaw & Barrett-Connor 1987; Iso *et al.* 1999);
- calcium (Iso *et al.* 1999);
- fresh fruit and vegetables (Key *et al.* 1996; Rimm *et al.* 1996; Joshipura *et al.* 1999; Wolk *et al.* 1999);
- fish (Orencia *et al.* 1996; Albert *et al.* 1998); and
- antioxidants such as vitamin E (Steinberg 1993; Hennekens *et al.* 1994), vitamin C (Bulpitt 1995; Nyyssonen *et al.* 1997), beta-carotene (Greenberg *et al.* 1996) and flavonols (Hertog *et al.* 1997).

On the whole, randomized trials of dietary interventions have been disappointing. Either the theory is wrong, or the interventions were too little, too late, for insufficient time or the trials were too small (Steinberg 1995; Stephens 1997; GISSI-Prevenzione Investigators 1999; Heart Outcomes Prevention Evaluation Study Investigators 2000; Hooper *et al.* 2000a,b; Leppala *et al.* 2000). The effect of a vegetarian diet is unclear (Key *et al.* 1996). Despite earlier enthusiasm, it now appears that there is no association between coffee consumption and vascular disease (Kawachi *et al.* 1994; Stensvold *et al.* 1996; Willett *et al.* 1996).

Alcohol

The relationship between alcohol, ischaemic stroke and carotid atheroma is complex and may be U-shaped (van Gijn *et al.* 1993) (section 8.5.2). While heavy alcohol consumption may be an independent and perhaps causal risk factor, it seems that modest consumers are protected to some extent compared with abstainers (Camargo 1989; Marmot & Brunner 1991; Wannamethee & Shaper 1996; Doll 1997; Kiechl *et al.* 1998; Berger *et al.* 1999; Hart *et al.* 1999a; Sacco *et al.* 1999). Whether 'binge' drinking is associated with stroke is uncertain (Gorelick 1987; Hillbom *et al.* 1999). Much of the confusion in relating alcohol consumption with stroke is because (Ben-Shlomo *et al.* 1992):

• people are not always truthful about their alcohol consumption;
• it is difficult to measure alcohol consumption accurately, particularly over time;
• there are varied ways of expressing alcohol consumption (per day, per week, grams, units, number of drinks, regular, binge, etc.);
• different types of alcoholic drinks may have different effects;
• pattern of drinking behaviour may change over time;
• combining ex-drinkers, some of whom may have given up drinking because of symptoms of vascular or other diseases, with lifetime non-drinkers in the analyses;
• the biases inherent in case–control studies;
• publication bias;
• small numbers and so imprecise estimates;
• confounding with cigarette-smoking, hypertension and deprivation which are positively related, and with exercise which is negatively related with alcohol consumption;
• confounding with unknown or unmeasurable factors which might link no drinking or heavy drinking with an excess risk of vascular disease (e.g. healthy vs. risky lifestyle);
• lumping ischaemic and haemorrhagic strokes together; and
• the lack of systematic overviews of all the evidence.

It is also difficult to think of the same biological reason for ischaemic stroke in non-drinkers and heavy drinkers. Possible explanations for the latter are: that alcohol almost certainly increases the blood pressure; traumatic arterial dissection in the neck during an alcohol-related injury; dehydration, hyperviscosity and platelet activation perhaps; sleep apnoea and hypoxia; and that alcohol can cause both atrial fibrillation and cardiomyopathy with embolism to the brain (*Lancet* 1985; MacMahon & Norton 1986; Puddey *et al.* 1987; Marmot *et al.* 1994; Kaplan 1995). Perhaps it would be more productive to ask why modest drinking is protective, if it really is. Increased plasma high-density lipoprotein-cholesterol and lower fibrinogen levels are possibilities (Rimm *et al.* 1999). It is most unlikely that a randomized trial of modest alcohol consumption, in the hope of reducing the risk of vascular disorders without increasing the risk of other disorders, will ever be feasible. Therefore, we are left trying to interpret, with difficulty, the available observational data.

Race

There are no good population-based data on stroke *incidence* in developing countries, with yawning gaps in South and South-East Asia, sub-Saharan Africa and South America (Sudlow and Warlow 1997). None the less, and notwithstanding the difficulty in defining ethnicity, stroke incidence does seem greater in black than white people *living* in Western countries, probably both ischaemic stroke and intracranial haemorrhage (Broderick *et al.* 1998; Sacco *et al.* 1998; Stewart *et al.* 1999). The high prevalence of hypertension, diabetes, sickle cell trait and social deprivation in black people may be part of the explanation (Giles *et al.* 1995; Davey Smith *et al.* 1998; Gorelick 1998). South Asian populations in the UK have a high stroke mortality as well as a high prevalence of coronary disease, central obesity, insulin resistance, diabetes mellitus and other risk factors (Balarajan 1991). This is in part because they are genetically more at risk than white populations by virtue of higher serum lipoprotein (a) concentrations (McKeigue *et al.* 1991; Bhatnagar *et al.* 1995; Winkleby *et al.* 1998; Bhopal *et al.* 1999). Also, Maori and Pacific people living in New Zealand have a higher stroke risk than white New Zealanders (Bonita *et al.* 1997).

The *pattern* of atheroma appears to differ between racial groups. There is probably less extracranial but more intracranial atheroma in black people, Japanese and Chinese compared with white populations. However, the situation is confused by selection bias and small numbers in many studies, and the pattern may be changing (Leung *et al.* 1993; Wityk *et al.* 1996; Chen *et al.* 1998).

Social deprivation

Social deprivation, low socioeconomic status and unemployment are all inextricably linked and associated with increased stroke risk (Kunst *et al.* 1998; van Rossum *et al.* 1999). This association is partly caused by a higher prevalence of vascular risk factors, stress and adverse health behaviours, such as smoking, poor diet and lack of exercise in deprived populations (Davey Smith 1997). Also, it has been suggested that poor health and nutrition *in utero* or infancy are associated with the development of vascular risk factors such as hypertension and adult vascular disease, including stroke (Barker 1994; Martyn *et al.* 1996; Rich-Edwards *et al.* 1997; Forsen *et al.* 1999). It is extremely difficult to disentangle early from later life influences on health and so, not surprisingly, the 'early life' or 'Barker' hypothesis has been refuted by some (Lynch *et al.* 1994; Paneth & Susser 1995; Lucas *et al.* 1999). The possibility of reducing stroke risk by tackling social deprivation is yet another reason to add to the many others to support what has to be political rather than medical action. Randomized trials seem neither necessary nor feasible.

Infection

There has been much recent interest in the notion that infection may in some way contribute to the development of atheroma, the progression of the atherothrombotic plaque and perhaps plaque instability. However, the evidence from observational epidemiological studies of infections in general (Grau *et al.* 1998), and of chronic dental infection (Beck *et al.* 1996), together with serological evidence of specific infectious agents, such as *Chlamydia pneumoniae*, *Helicobacter pylori* and cytomegalovirus, is not very convincing, even for coronary disease where there are—as usual—more data than for stroke (Markus & Mendall 1998; Danesh *et al.* 1999, 2000a; Fagerberg *et al.* 1999; Glader *et al.* 1999; Strachan *et al.* 1999). The generalized inflammatory response in patients with coronary artery disease may be too non-specific to be convincing evidence of infection, and there may well be the familiar problems of confounding and publication bias (Danesh *et al.* 1998, 2000b; Danesh 1999; Ridker *et al.* 2000). None the less, the fact that evidence of chlamydial infection can be found in atherosclerotic plaques is certainly interesting although reverse causality is a possibility, i.e. atheroma *becomes* infected more often than normal arterial wall (Yamashita *et al.* 1998). An early randomized trial to eliminate chlamydia was far too small to be reliable despite being published in a high-impact journal (Gurfinkel *et al.* 1997).

'Stress'

It is part of folklore that stress causes strokes: 'I was so upset, I nearly had a stroke'. Indeed, there are some striking anecdotes.

This 82-year-old lady was admitted for investigation of anaemia and hepatomegaly. She was found to have multiple liver metastases. When she was told the news, she stopped speaking and never spoke again. It took a day or so before the medical staff realized that her mute state was not 'psychological' but that she was aphasic. A brain CT scan showed a left cortical infarct. She died some days later from her malignancy.

However, showing that long-term psychological stressors are associated with stroke, or that shorter term ones precipitate stroke, is not easy. There is some evidence that severely threatening life events (House *et al.* 1990; Rosengren *et al.* 1993), anxiety and depression (Hemingway & Marmot 1999), high levels of anger expression (Everson *et al.* 1999) and psychological stress (Harmsen *et al.* 1990; Everson *et al.* 1997; Hemingway & Marmot 1999) may trigger the onset of stroke, perhaps in people already at risk of stroke.

Non-stroke vascular disease

Because atheroma in one artery is likely to be accompanied by atheroma in others (section 6.3.1), and because embolism from the heart is a common cause of ischaemic stroke (section 6.5), non-stroke vascular disorders are associated with (i.e. are risk factors for) ischaemic stroke and transient ischaemic attack (Table 6.6).

Coronary heart disease (e.g. angina or myocardial infarction) has been repeatedly associated with an increased risk of stroke in post-mortem (Kagan 1976; Stemmermann *et al.* 1984), twin (Brass *et al.* 1996), case–control (Friedman *et al.* 1968; Herman *et al.* 1983; Woo *et al.* 1991; Feigin *et al.* 1998) and cohort studies (Harmsen *et al.* 1990; Shaper *et al.* 1991; Wolf *et al.* 1991). Therefore, it is not surprising that electrocardiogram abnormalities and cardiac failure, because they both so often reflect coronary disease and hypertension, are also associated with increased risk of stroke, as is left-ventricular hypertrophy (Kagan *et al.* 1980; Kannel *et al.* 1983; Knutsen *et al.* 1988; Shaper *et al.* 1991; Pullicino *et al.* 2000). Atrial fibrillation is considered in section 6.5.

Table 6.6 Degenerative vascular disorders outside the head associated with an increased risk of ischaemic stroke and transient ischaemic attack.

Myocardial infarction/angina
Cardiac failure
Left ventricular hypertrophy
Atrial fibrillation
Cervical arterial bruit/stenosis
Peripheral arterial disease

Cervical bruits (carotid or supraclavicular) are usually caused by stenosis of the underlying arteries (section 6.6.7), mostly resulting from atheroma, and so become more common with age; about 5% of asymptomatic people over the age of 75 years have bruits (Sandok *et al.* 1982). Carotid bruits are clearly a risk factor for ischaemic stroke, but not necessarily in the same arterial territory as the bruit, and also for coronary events, because atheroma of one artery is likely to be accompanied by atheroma of other arteries in the same predisposed individual (Wiebers *et al.* 1990). The risk of these various vascular events increases with carotid stenosis severity (section 16.9.2).

Atheroma affecting the leg arteries is associated with cerebrovascular and coronary disease in the same individuals so often that it is not surprising that claudicants have an increased risk of stroke and other serious vascular events (Davey Smith *et al.* 1990; Harmsen *et al.* 1990; Leng *et al.* 1996; Allan *et al.* 1997).

Little seems to be known about the prevalence of *abdominal aortic aneurysms* in ischaemic stroke/TIA patients. It is said to be quite high, about 10–20%, depending on the selection of patients and the size criterion for what constitutes an aneurysm (Carty *et al.* 1993; Karanjia *et al.* 1994).

Other risk factors

Innumerable other associations with coronary heart disease, if not with ischaemic stroke, have been suggested and are supported by varying degrees of evidence. However, there are no 'breakthroughs before breakfast' in observational epidemiology. After all, it was decades after the early reports of the association between hypertension and stroke before increasing blood pressure became generally accepted as being causal. The same slow dawning applied to smoking, and perhaps will come to apply to increasing plasma cholesterol levels. None the less, vascular risk-factorology is clearly alive and well, so much so that the constant revelations—so often in the media first—of yet another 'cause of stroke' have led to a certain amount of cynicism, particularly when the risk factor is so often later found to be nothing of the sort. A few of the 246 risk factors counted by 1981 (Hopkins & Williams 1981), and some of the many others proposed since then, may or may not be important in the causal pathway to stroke (Table 6.7). Even if not, they may still conceivably be helpful in predicting future stroke in individuals and populations. This distinction is important: for example, claudication is clearly not on the causal pathway to stroke but is so strongly associated with stroke risk that it is included in many statistical models which predict later stroke (section 16.1.1).

The most important risk factors for ischaemic stroke and transient ischaemic attack are increasing age, blood pressure and plasma fibrinogen, diabetes mellitus and cigarette-smoking. Of these, raised blood pressure is definitely causal.

6.4 Intracranial small vessel disease

There are a number of pathologies which affect the small (40–400 μm diameter) arteries, arterioles and veins of the meninges and brain: e.g. cerebral amyloid angiopathy (section 8.2.2); vasculitis (section 7.3); atheroma near the origin of the small perforating arteries (see below); and the angiopathy underlying cerebral autosomal dominant arteriopathy with subcortical infarcts and leukoenceophalopathy (CADASIL) (section 7.20). Much more common, however, is what has been termed hyaline arteriosclerosis. This is an almost universal change in the small arteries and arterioles of the aged brain, particularly in the presence of hypertension or diabetes, but sometimes in quite young patients without any of the classical vascular risk factors (Lammie *et al.* 1997) (Fig. 6.12). Important factors in the development of this hyaline arteriosclerosis appear to include not only hypertension and diabetes, but also breakdown of the blood–brain barrier with incorporation of plasma proteins into the vessel wall. The smooth muscle cells in the wall are eventually replaced by collagen which reduces vascular distensibility, and presumably reactivity, but not necessarily the size of the lumen. Unfortunately, over the years, the nomenclature has been very confusing and, as a result, this 'simple' small vessel dis-

Table 6.7 Miscellaneous possible risk factors for vascular disease.

Possible risk factor	References
Snoring and sleep apnoea	Qureshi *et al.* (1997); Young *et al.* (1997)
Corneal arcus	Chambless *et al.* (1990); Menotti *et al.* (1993)
Raised white blood cell count, perhaps because smokers have higher counts than non-smokers	Yarnell *et al.* (1991); Danesh *et al.* (1998)
Raised serum C-reactive protein	Danesh *et al.* (1998)
Large platelets	O'Malley *et al.* (1995)
Type A behaviour	Hemingway & Marmot (1999)
Family history of stroke	Wannamethee *et al.* (1996); Jousilahti *et al.* (1997); Liao *et al.* (1997)
Low serum albumin	Danesh *et al.* (1998)
High body iron stores	Ascherio & Willett (1994)
Impaired ventilatory function	Menotti *et al.* (1993); Wannametheee *et al.* (1995); Hole *et al.* (1996)
Chronic renal failure	Baigent *et al.* (2000)
Dental disease	DeStefano *et al.* (1993); Beck *et al.* (1996)
Low bone density	Browner *et al.* (1993)
Blood group	Whincup *et al.* (1990)
Serum sialic acid	Lindberg *et al.* (1991)
Diagonal ear lobe crease	Patel *et al.* (1992)
Proteinuria	Miettinen *et al.* (1996); Mykkanen *et al.* (1997)
Low serum selenium	Rayman (2000)
Low serum enterolactone	Vanharanta *et al.* (1999)
ACE-genotype	Sharma (1998); Zee *et al.* (1999)
High serum uric acid/gout	Lehto *et al.* (1998); Dobson (1999); Fang & Alderman 2000

(a) 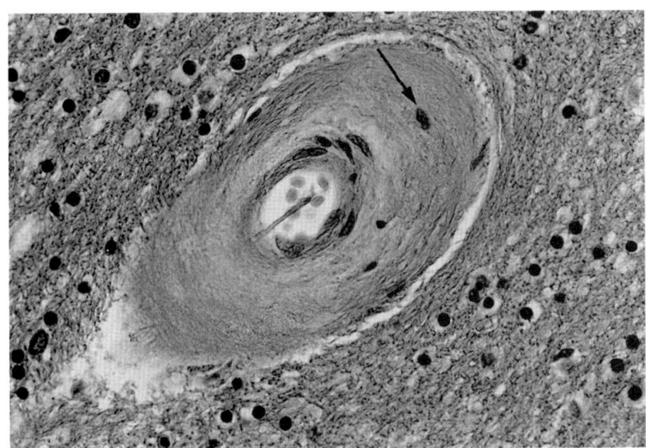 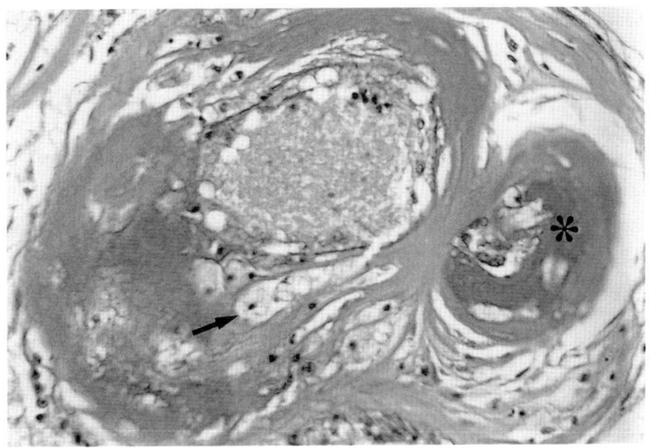 (b)

Fig. 6.12 Photomicrograph of perforating lenticulostriate artery branches in the putamen, illustrating two distinctive patterns of vessel pathology. (a) Concentric hyaline wall thickening with a few remaining vascular smooth-muscle cell nuclei (arrow). The lumen remains patent. Such 'simple' small vessel disease is an almost invariable feature of elderly brains, most prominent in hypertensive and diabetic patients. (b) A complex, disorganized vessel segment showing an asymmetric destructive process with focal fibrinoid material (*) and mural foam cells (arrow). The lumen is visible cut in two planes of section. In this case the vascular lesion was adjacent to and, presumably, the cause of a right striatocapsular lacunar infarct. This 'complex' vessel lesion corresponds with what Fisher termed 'lipohyalinosis'. (Provided by Dr Alistair Lammie.)

ease (SVD) has frequently been confused with a more aggressive-looking disorder of small arteries with disorganization of their walls and foam cell infiltration. It is this 'complex' SVD which Fisher first called 'segmental arterial disorganization' and then 'lipohyalinosis'. The term fibrinoid vessel wall necrosis refers to a different, characteristic, but more acute change in the vessel wall seen, for example, as a consequence of accelerated hypertension and as a reactive phenomenon around acute intracerebral haematomas, spontaneous or traumatic. When healed, this probably takes on the appearance of 'complex' SVD (Lammie 2000) (Fig. 6.12). However, it is by no means certain that 'complex' SVD and acute fibrinoid necrosis are more advanced forms of 'simple' SVD, and there is no evidence that 'simple' SVD is the 'healed' version of complex SVD. None the less, both 'simple' and 'complex' SVD both tend to affect the lenticulostriate perforating branches of the middle cerebral artery, the thalamoperforating branches of the proximal posterior cerebral artery, the perforating branches of the basilar artery to the brainstem, and the vessels in the periventricular white matter.

Because lacunar infarction is seldom fatal (section 10.2.3), and even when post-mortem material becomes available the arterial pathology is hardly likely to be acute, and because it is so difficult and tedious to trace small arteries into previously symptomatic lacunes, very little is known of the nature of the causative vascular lesion. Most of what is known comes from a very small number of careful clinicoanatomical observations by Fisher. He did not describe 'simple' SVD as the underlying vascular pathology of lacunes, but what we prefer to call 'complex' SVD in some cases, and atheroma affecting the origins of the small vessels where they come off the circle of Willis and major cerebral arteries in others (Fisher 1969, 1979, 1991). In theory, one can think of 'mural atheroma' affecting the parent arteries, 'junctional atheroma' affecting the origin of the small perforating arteries where they leave the parent artery, and 'microatheroma' affecting the proximal parts of these small arteries. In practice, at post-mortem these distinctions are more or less impossible to make and the contribution of intracranial atheroma to lacunar infarction has still to be established.

It is conceivable that the same 'complex' SVD causes, in the same or different patients, either arterial occlusion leading to infarction, or rupture leading to intracerebral haemorrhage. Some ruptures may be caused by Charcot–Bouchard microaneurysms, although these may be artifacts of the pathological specimens. In fact, whether they are real or not is semantic, because what matters is not if the vessel wall bulges, but what weakens it in the first place (Fisher 1972; Besson *et al.* 1991; Challa *et al.* 1992; Samuelsson *et al.* 1996; Kwa *et al.* 1998; Roob *et al.* 1999) (section 8.2.1). On the other hand, leukoaraiosis appears to be more associated with 'simple' SVD, and indeed this may be an underlying vascular cause, although it is clearly insufficient on its own, being so common in elderly brains (section 5.7.3).

The current view is that both 'complex' SVD and atheroma at or near the origin of the small perforating vessels arising from the major cerebral arteries cause most, but not all, of the small deep infarcts responsible for lacunar ischaemic strokes (and, by implication, lacunar transient ischaemic attacks) which make up about one-quarter of symptomatic cerebral ischaemic events (Bamford *et al.* 1987; Bamford & Warlow 1988; Besson *et al.* 1991; Hankey & Warlow 1991b; Donnan *et al.* 1995; Sempere *et al.* 1998; Ay *et al.* 1999) (sections 4.3.2 and 6.6.3). However, this hypothesis is not universally accepted (Millikan & Futrell 1990; Horowitz *et al.* 1992). In fact, there is remarkably little *direct* post-mortem evidence of occlusion of these vessels leading to lacunar infarcts, largely because the case fatality of lacunar stroke is so low. The main supporting evidence for a specific small vessel lesion leading to lacunar infarction is much more indirect:

- The relative *lack* of large vessel atheroma or embolic sources in the heart in the vast majority of lacunar patients, compared to those with cortical infarcts (Olsen *et al.* 1985; Lodder *et al.* 1990; Hankey & Warlow 1991b; Landi *et al.* 1993; Mast *et al.* 1994; Gan *et al.* 1997; Mead *et al.* 1999a, 2000a) (Fig. 6.13).
- Emboli are rarely if ever detected in the middle cerebral or common carotid artery by Doppler ultrasound in most studies of patients with lacunar infarction. However, it is not clear at what stage after the onset of stroke it is best to look—too early and an occluded middle cerebral artery might prevent the passage of emboli, too late and any proximal embolic source may have 'healed' (Tegeler *et al.* 1995; Daffertshofer *et al.* 1996; Koennecke *et al.* 1998; Kaposzta *et al.* 1999; Serena *et al.* 2000).
- The lack of an early risk of recurrence also argues against the concept of an active embolic source, either in the heart or an unstable atheromatous plaque (Bamford *et al.* 1991).
- The 'capsular warning syndrome' might suggest that a single perforating vessel is intermittently on the verge of occluding before it finally does so (section 6.6.3).
- The impaired cerebrovascular reactivity in lacunar patients might suggest a specific problem, if not pathology, of the small intracerebral resistance vessels (Molina *et al.* 1999).

Interestingly, 'cortical' (presumed atherothrombotic) and 'lacunar' ischaemic stroke patients probably have a similar vascular risk factor profile, including hypertension (van Gijn & Kraaijeveld 1982; Adams *et al.* 1989; Lodder *et al.* 1990; Sacco *et al.* 1991; Boiten & Lodder 1993; van Zagten *et al.* 1994; Boiten *et al.* 1996; Schmal *et al.* 1998; Petty *et al.* 1999). It is conceivable therefore that the same type of individual (i.e. hypertensive, diabetic, etc.) develops *either* small vessel disease (complex or atheroma) and so lacunar infarcts, *or* large vessel atherothromboembolism and so cortical infarction. The difference in the type of 'degenerative' vascular disease that occurs may perhaps reflect differing genetic susceptibilities. But, on the other hand, many individual patients have these different ischaemic stroke types at different times (Kappelle *et al.* 1995; Samuelsson *et al.* 1996). On balance, we believe it likely that the lacunar hypothesis is correct and so, whatever the exact nature of the underlying small vessel lesion, lacunar infarction is seldom the result of embolization from proximal sites.

About one-quarter of all ischaemic strokes and transient ischaemic attacks are 'lacunar' and many, if not most, lacunar infarcts are caused by disease of the small intracranial perforating arteries, either 'complex' small vessel disease, or atheroma affecting their proximal parts as they arise from their parent cerebral arteries.

One question that has never been answered is whether there is a similar small vessel disease which affects the blood supply to the optic nerve and retina: are there 'lacunar' ocular syndromes equivalent to lacunar cerebral syndromes? What is clear is that a high proportion of patients with ischaemic amaurosis fugax, retinal infarction and anterior ischaemic optic neuropathy do not have any detectable and likely proximal source of embolism (or evidence of low-flow) in the heart, or in the arterial supply to the eye. Perhaps it is these patients who have small vessel disease like patients with ischaemic lacunar strokes (Bogousslavsky *et al.* 1991; Hankey *et al.* 1991a; Fry *et al.* 1993).

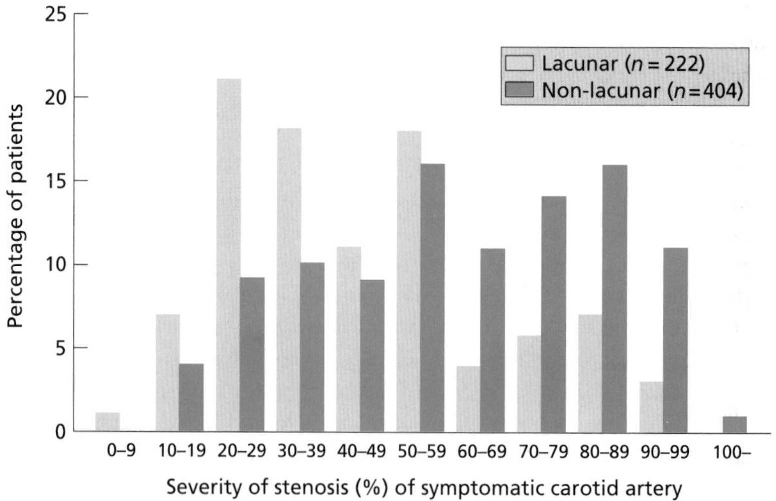

Fig. 6.13 The relationship between the severity of symptomatic carotid stenosis and the likelihood of finding a non-lacunar (territorial) or lacunar infarct on the baseline brain CT in 626 patients in the European Carotid Surgery Trial. Those with severe stenosis are less likely to have lacunar infarcts. (With permission from Boiten *et al.* 1996.)

6.5 Embolism from the heart

The potential for, and fact of, embolism of material from the heart to the brain, and from the venous system through the heart to the brain (paradoxical embolism), as well as to other organs, is undisputed. However, not all cardiac sources of embolism pose equal threats. For example, a mechanical prosthetic valve is much more likely to cause thromboembolism than mitral valve prolapse. In developed countries, embolism from the heart probably causes *about* one-fifth of ischaemic stroke and transient ischaemic attacks (TIAs), although a potential embolic source may be present in nearer one-third (Nishide *et al.* 1983; Cerebral Embolism Task Force 1989; Kittner *et al.* 1991, 1992; Hart 1992; Oppenheimer & Lima 1998) (Fig. 6.1). However, there are two very real and tiresome problems. As technology advances, more and more *potential* cardiac sources of embolism are being identified (Table 6.8), and patients may have two or more competing causes of cerebral ischaemia, such as carotid stenosis and atrial fibrillation. Therefore, it may be unclear whether embolism from the heart is *the* cause in an individual patient, especially when the cardiac lesion is common in normal people (De Bono & Warlow 1981; Bogousslavsky *et al.* 1986a,b, 1990; Caplan 1995).

Not all emboli are of the same size, of the same age, or made of the same thing (fibrin, platelets, calcium, infected vegetations, tumour, etc.). Some are large and impact permanently in the mainstem of the middle cerebral artery to cause total anterior circulation infarction, others impact in a more distal branch of a cerebral artery to cause a partial anterior circulation infarct, others merely cause a TIA, and still others are asymptomatic (Kempster *et al.* 1988; Caplan 1993; Cullinane *et al.* 1998; Nabavi *et al.* 1998). Emboli may also occlude the basilar artery and its branches, and even the internal carotid artery in the neck (Castaigne *et al.* 1973; Caplan 1993). TIAs are about as common before a presumed cardioembolic stroke as before any other (Table 6.1), so supporting the hypothesis that there is no qualitative difference between TIAs and ischaemic strokes. Indeed, embolism from the heart can cause an ischaemic stroke or a TIA, at different times in the same patient.

Embolism from the heart causes about one-fifth of ischaemic strokes and transient ischaemic attacks. The most substantial embolic threats are non-rheumatic and rheumatic atrial fibrillation, infective endocarditis, prosthetic heart valves, recent myocardial infarction, dilated cardiomyopathy, intracardiac tumours and rheumatic mitral stenosis.

Table 6.8 Cardiac sources of embolism in anatomical sequence.

Right-to-left shunt (paradoxical embolism from the venous system or right-atrial thrombus)
Patent foramen ovale
Atrial septal defect
Ventriculoseptal defect
Pulmonary arteriovenous fistula

Left atrium
Thrombus
- atrial fibrillation*
- sinoatrial disease (sick sinus syndrome)
- atrial septal aneurysm

Myxoma and other cardiac tumours*

Mitral valve
Rheumatic endocarditis (stenosis* or regurgitation)
Infective endocarditis*
Mitral annulus calcification
Non-bacterial thrombotic (marantic) endocarditis
Libman–Sacks endocarditis (section 7.3)
Anticardiolipin syndrome (section 7.3)
Prosthetic heart valve*
Papillary fibroelastoma
Mitral valve prolapse (uncertain)
Mitral valve stands (uncertain)

Left ventricle
Mural thrombus
- acute myocardial infarction (within previous few weeks)* (section 7.10)
- left-ventricular aneurysm or akinetic segment (section 7.10)
- dilated or restrictive cardiomyopathy*
- mechanical 'artificial' heart*
- blunt chest injury (myocardial contusion)

Myxoma and other cardiac tumours*
Hydatid cyst
Primary oxalosis (uncertain)

Aortic valve
Rheumatic endocarditis (stenosis or regurgitation)
Infective endocarditis*
Syphilis
Non-bacterial thrombotic (marantic) endocarditis
Libman–Sacks endocarditis (section 7.3)
Anticardiolipin syndrome (section 7.3)
Prosthetic heart valve*
Calcific stenosis/sclerosis/calcification
Aneurysm of the sinus of Valsalva

Congenital heart disease (particularly with right-to-left shunt)

*Cardiac manipulation/surgery/catheterization/valvuloplasty/angioplasty** (section 7.18)

*Substantial risk of embolism.

Atrial fibrillation

Non-rheumatic atrial fibrillation (AF), with clot formed in

the left atrium and then embolizing to the brain, is by far the most common cause of cardioembolic stroke (Table 6.9). However, it cannot cause more than about one-sixth of all strokes at most, because it is present in less than this proportion of ischaemic stroke patients (Sandercock *et al.* 1992). However, AF may be responsible for a greater proportion of ischaemic strokes in the *very* elderly, where its frequency in the population is highest (Wolf *et al.* 1991). The average absolute risk of stroke in unanticoagulated non-rheumatic AF patients without prior stroke is about 4% per year, six times greater than in those in sinus rhythm (Narayan *et al.* 1997; Anderson *et al.* 1998; Hart *et al.* 1999b) (section 16.5.1).

Non-rheumatic atrial fibrillation is the most common cause of embolism from the heart to the brain.

In fibrillating stroke patients, the AF cannot *always* be causal because: some patients have had a primary intracerebral haemorrhage (PICH), although, it is conceivable that PICH has been confused with haemorrhagic transformation of an infarct on computed tomography (CT) (section 5.4); the AF may have been caused by the stroke; perhaps 20% of the fibrillating ischaemic stroke patients have other possible causes, such as carotid stenosis or aortic arch atheroma; and yet others have lacunar (presumed non-embolic) ischaemic strokes (Weinberger *et al.* 1988; Bogousslavsky *et al.* 1990; Sandercock *et al.* 1992; Vingerhoets *et al.* 1993; Kanter *et al.* 1994; Blackshear *et al.* 1999). Also, AF is often caused by either coronary or hypertensive heart disease, both of which may be associated with stroke by mechanisms other than embolism from the left atrium, such as carotid stenosis or intracerebral haemorrhage (Davies & Pomerance 1972). Furthermore, 'only' about 13% or less of non-rheumatic

Table 6.9 Prevalence of potential cardiac sources of embolism in 244 patients with a first-ever-in-a-lifetime ischaemic stroke in the Oxfordshire Community Stroke Project (Sandercock *et al.* 1989).

	Number	Percentage
Any atrial fibrillation	31	13
without rheumatic heart disease	28	11
with rheumatic heart disease	3	1
Mitral regurgitation	15	6
Recent (< 6 weeks) myocardial infarction	12	5
Prosthetic heart valve	3	1
Mitral stenosis	2	1
Paradoxical embolism	1	1
Any of the above	50	20
Other sources of uncertain significance (aortic stenosis/sclerosis, mitral annulus calcification, mitral valve prolapse, etc.)	28	11

atrial fibrillation patients have detectable thrombus in the left atrium by transoesophageal echocardiography (although some thrombi may have completely embolized or be too small to be detected). It is not known whether these patients definitely have a higher stroke risk than those without detectable thrombus (Daniel 1993; Stollberger *et al.* 1998). None the less, AF is clearly *the* cause of ischaemic stroke in many patients, as supported by:

- post-mortem evidence (Aberg 1969; Britton & Gustafsson 1985; Yamanouchi *et al.* 1997a);
- case–control studies (Friedman *et al.* 1968);
- most, but not all, cohort studies (Wolf *et al.* 1978; Davis *et al.* 1987; Flegel *et al.* 1987; Harmsen *et al.* 1990); and
- the lower prevalence of AF in lacunar ischaemic stroke probably caused by small vessel disease (Sandercock *et al.* 1992).

The effective prevention of stroke by anticoagulating fibrillating patients (section 16.5.1) is not a good supporting argument, because it is conceivable that anticoagulation may prevent artery-to-artery as well as heart-to-artery embolic events. As far as it can be established, over half of the strokes in non-rheumatic AF patients are 'cardioembolic' (Hart *et al.* 2000).

Within the fibrillating population, there must be some individuals at particularly high risk and others at particularly low risk of embolization. For example, those with no other detectable cardiac disease (so-called lone AF) have a very low relative and absolute risk of stroke, while those with rheumatic mitral valve disease have a much higher risk (Wolf *et al.* 1978; Close *et al.* 1979; Brand *et al.* 1985; Kopecky *et al.* 1987). Other risk factors include a previous embolic event, increasing age, hypertension, diabetes and—as defined by echocardiography—left-ventricular dysfunction and enlarged left atrium (Atrial Fibrillation Investigators 1994, 1998; Benjamin *et al.* 1995; di Pasquale *et al.* 1995; van Latum *et al.* 1995; Hart *et al.* 1999c). Spontaneous echo contrast in the left atrium, probably a consequence of blood stasis, left-atrial thrombi, left-atrial appendage size and dysfunction, and various haemostatic variables may perhaps be additional risk factors (Chimowitz *et al.* 1993; di Pasquale *et al.* 1995; Lip 1995; Stroke Prevention in Atrial Fibrillation Investigators Committee on Echocardiography 1998; Stollberger *et al.* 1998). What is really needed, however, is not just a list of risk factors predicting stroke, however independent from each other, with slightly different weightings depending on the study, but validated statistical models to predict the probability of stroke in individual fibrillating patients (as is becoming available for symptomatic carotid stenosis, section 16.8.9). A start has been made, but the numbers of strokes are not really large enough for a stable model (Hart *et al.* 1999c).

It is still not clear whether stroke risk is importantly different in those with recent-onset, paroxysmal or thyrotoxic AF compared with chronic persisting AF (Parker & Lawson

1973; Petersen 1990; Lip 1997; Yamanouchi *et al.* 1997b; Stollberger *et al.* 1998; Scardi *et al.* 1999). Without continuous monitoring of the ECG—which is impractical—it is impossible to disentangle patients who are always in sinus rhythm from those with occasional bursts of AF, and those who are usually in AF from those who have occasional episodes of sinus rhythm.

Coronary heart disease

Embolism from left-ventricular mural thrombus complicating acute myocardial infarction, or a chronic left-ventricular aneurysm long after myocardial infarction, is considered in section 7.10, and the complications of cardiac surgery in section 7.18.

Prosthetic heart valves

Prosthetic heart valves, particularly mechanical rather than tissue ones, have long been known to be complicated by thrombosis, followed sometimes by embolism. Furthermore, infective endocarditis is a potential risk for any type of prosthetic valve. Asymptomatic emboli, at least as detected by transcranial Doppler, are surprisingly frequent, but are probably gaseous cavitation bubbles of no clinical consequence and not solid fragments of thrombi (Sliwka & Georgiadis 1998; Georgiadis *et al.* 1999). There is little discernible difference in stroke risk between the different types of mechanical valve, but those in the mitral position are more prone to thrombosis than those in the aortic position. For all valves, the overall risk of embolism is about 2% per year, provided patients with mechanical valves are on anticoagulants (Vongpatanasin *et al.* 1996). Some Bjork–Shiley convexoconcave valves have disintegrated with not only serious cardiac consequences but also embolization of their components to the cerebral circulation (O'Neill *et al.* 1995) (Fig. 6.14). There are some reports of possible embolization of minute metal fragments from apparently normally functioning valves (Naumann *et al.* 1998).

Rheumatic valvular disease

Rheumatic valvular disease, particularly mitral, is a well-recognized cause of embolism to the brain, particularly when the patient is in atrial fibrillation and has thrombosis in the left atrium. Even when the patient is in sinus rhythm and there is no thrombus in the left atrium, degenerate and sometimes calcific fragments of valve can be discharged into the circulation. Infective endocarditis (see below) and intracerebral haemorrhage caused by anticoagulation (section 8.4.1) are other causes of stroke in these patients (Daley *et al.* 1951; Coulshed *et al.* 1970; Swash & Earl 1970).

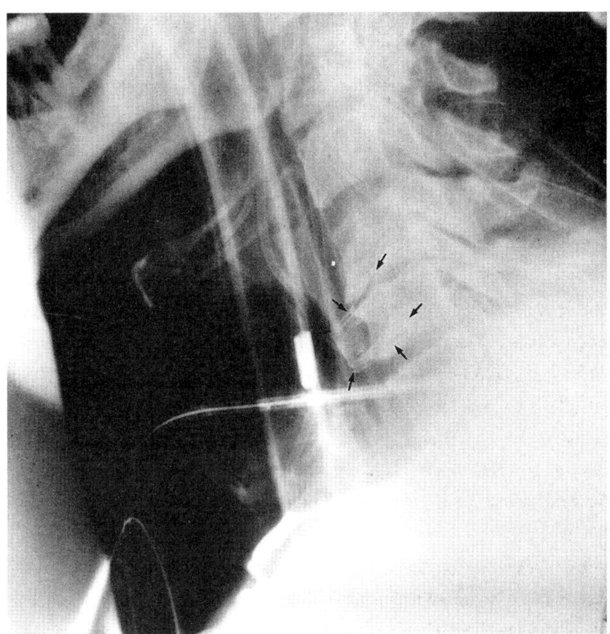

Fig. 6.14 Lateral neck X-ray of a patient whose mechanical heart valve had disintegrated. Part of the valve (arrows) has impacted in the carotid artery.

Non-rheumatic sclerosis and calcification of the aortic and mitral valves

Non-rheumatic sclerosis and particularly calcification of the aortic and mitral valves can occasionally be a source of embolism of thrombotic or calcific material. However, these valvular abnormalities are so common in elderly people that a cause-and-effect relationship is difficult to establish in an individual unless, very unusually, calcific emboli are seen in the retina, on brain CT or at post-mortem. Any associated atrial fibrillation, coronary disease or carotid stenosis compounds the diagnostic problem (Holley *et al.* 1963; Penner & Font 1969; Stein *et al.* 1977; De Bono & Warlow 1979; Brockmeier *et al.* 1981; Nestico *et al.* 1984; Benjamin *et al.* 1992; O'Donoghue *et al.* 1993; Boon *et al.* 1996; Mouton *et al.* 1997; Shanmugam *et al.* 1997; Adler *et al.* 1998).

Mitral valve (or leaflet) prolapse

Mitral valve prolapse (MVP) can be familial and is associated with various inherited disorders of connective tissue (Devereux *et al.* 1982). It is also a common echocardiographic and clinical finding in healthy people but the diagnostic criteria are so variable, and many studies so flawed by referral bias, that there is a wide range of reported prevalence. Almost certainly, MVP has been over-diagnosed in the past (Devereux *et al.* 1987; Freed *et al.* 1999). Therefore, it is all but impossible to pin down MVP as the cause of an ischaemic stroke or transient ischaemic attack (TIA) in an individual unless there is complicating infective endocarditis, atrial fibrillation, gross mitral regurgitation or thrombus in the left atrium.

Uncomplicated mitral valve prolapse should no longer be considered a cause of embolism from the heart to the brain; there must be something additional, such as gross mitral regurgitation, atrial fibrillation or infective endocarditis.

Although MVP may be more common than expected in young TIA patients (Barnett *et al.* 1980), it is odd, if the relationship is causal, that thrombus on the valve cusps is so rare in uncomplicated MVP and that embolism to anywhere other than the brain or eye has never been described (Geyer & Franzini 1979; Chesler *et al.* 1983). Furthermore, MVP does not appear to be more frequent than expected in ischaemic stroke (Cabanes *et al.* 1993; Marini *et al.* 1993; Gilon *et al.* 1999) and there is no definite excess risk of first-ever stroke or recurrent stroke in patients with uncomplicated MVP (Orencia *et al.* 1995a,b). Therefore, in an individual patient, we would not regard uncomplicated MVP as a *definite* cause for ischaemic stroke/TIA, even if no other cause can be found. It is much more likely to be an innocent bystander.

Mitral valve strands

Strands are mobile, thread-like filaments attached to cardiac valves that can nowadays be seen on transoesophageal echocardiography. Although suggested as sources of embolism, or perhaps as increasing the risk of embolism in patients whose valves are abnormal for whatever reason, the evidence so far is not persuasive (Cohen *et al.* 1997).

Infective endocarditis

About one-fifth of patients with acute or subacute infective endocarditis have an ischaemic stroke or transient ischaemic attack as a result of embolism of valvular vegetations. Cerebrovascular symptoms can be the first, but they more often occur in someone who is clearly unwell, perhaps already in hospital, but before the infection has been controlled (Jones & Siekert 1989; Hart *et al.* 1990; Salgado 1991). Haemorrhagic transformation of an infarct, possibly as a consequence of unwise anticoagulation, is fairly common. Primarily haemorrhagic strokes—intracerebral or, rarely, subarachnoid—are as or more commonly caused by a pyogenic vasculitis and vessel wall necrosis as to the more well-known mycotic aneurysms which can be single or multiple and most often affect the distal branches of the middle cerebral artery (Masuda *et al.* 1992; Krapf *et al.* 1999) (section 8.2.11) (Fig. 6.15). These aneurysms do not always rupture and they tend to resolve with time so that, on balance, cerebral angiography to detect unruptured aneurysms with a view to surgery is unnecessary, and so is surgical repair of any asymptomatic aneurysm (van der Meulen *et al.* 1992). Other neurological complications of infective endocarditis include: meningitis; a diffuse encephalopathy, perhaps as a result of showers of small emboli; acute mononeuropathy; rarely, cerebral abscess; discitis; and headache (Jones & Siekert 1989; Kanter & Hart 1991).

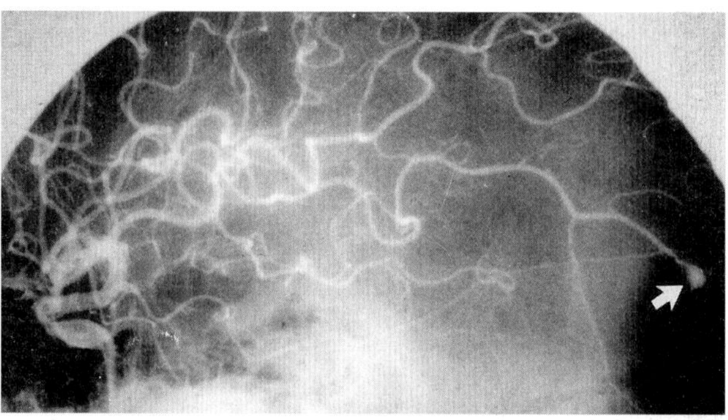

Fig. 6.15 Selective catheter carotid angiogram (lateral skull view) showing a mycotic cerebral aneurysm on a distal branch of the middle cerebral artery (arrow).

It is important to realize that fever, cardiac murmur and vegetations seen on echocardiography are not invariably present in patients with infective endocarditis. Therefore, in an otherwise unexplained ischaemic or haemorrhagic stroke, blood cultures are indicated, particularly if the erythrocyte sedimentation rate is raised, with a mild anaemia, neutrophil leukocytosis and disturbed liver function. The cerebrospinal fluid can be normal, but >100 polymorphs/mm^3 is said to suggest endocarditis. However, as high or higher counts have been described in intracerebral haemorrhage and in haemorrhagic transformation of an infarct, but not in ischaemic stroke (Sornas *et al.* 1972; Powers 1986).

In infective endocarditis the blood cultures can occasionally be negative and the echocardiogram may not show any valvular vegetations. A high index of diagnostic suspicion is required in any unexplained stroke, particularly if there is a cardiac murmur.

Non-bacterial thrombotic (marantic) endocarditis

Small sterile vegetations, consisting of fibrin and platelets, appear on the cardiac valves in cachectic and debilitated patients as a result of cancer (usually adenocarcinomas) and sometimes of disseminated intravascular coagulation, burns and septicaemia, usually but not only in elderly people (Fig. 6.16). Similar vegetations are found in systemic lupus erythematosus and the antiphospholipid syndrome (section 7.3), and possibly protein C deficiency (section 7.9). These vegetations are friable and may embolize to cause ischaemic stroke

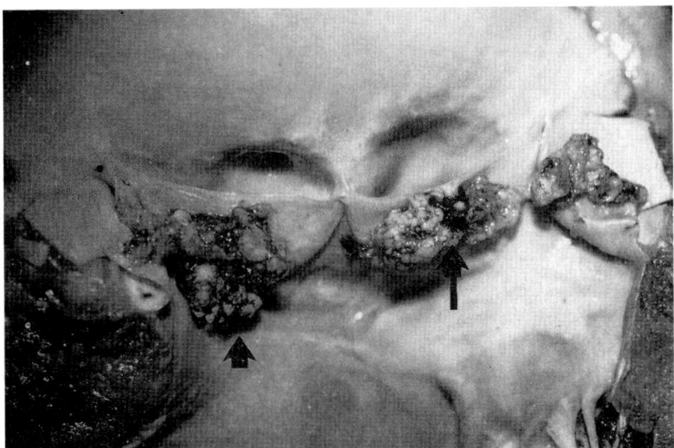

Fig. 6.16 A close-up view of non-infective marantic vegetations (arrows) on the cusps of the aortic valve.

(and sometimes global encephalopathy because of multiple emboli), ischaemia in other organs and pulmonary embolism. The vegetations are so small that they are all but impossible to diagnose during life, although the larger ones can be seen on transoesophageal echocardiography. The diagnosis should be suspected in an ischaemic stroke/transient ischaemic attack patient who is cachectic and who may have additional evidence of systemic embolization without any other cause being found, or if there are antiphospholipid antibodies (Graus *et al.* 1985; Lopez *et al.* 1987; Walz *et al.* 1998).

Non-ischaemic 'primary' cardiomyopathies

Non-ischaemic 'primary' cardiomyopathies are well known to be complicated by intracardiac thrombus and so embolism, particularly if they are of the dilated or restrictive type and there is severe ventricular dysfunction, atrial fibrillation, infective endocarditis or intracardiac thrombus on echocardiography. Hypertrophic cardiomyopathies are most unlikely to be complicated by embolism. Many cardiomyopathies are familial (Fuster *et al.* 1981; Dec & Fuster 1994; Kushwaha *et al.* 1997).

Paradoxical embolism

A number of convincing post-mortem examples (Fig. 6.17) have established that paradoxical embolism can occur from thrombi in the venous system of the legs (or pelvis) through the right to the left side of the heart—and exceptionally from thrombus in the right atrium as a result of cardiac disease or possibly an indwelling venous line—and on to the brain. The right-to-left cardiac conduits for emboli are a patent foramen ovale which, depending as always on the diagnostic criteria, is found in about one-quarter of unselected post-mortems and in almost as many healthy people by using transoesophageal echocardiography; an atrial septal defect; and, rarely, a ventriculoseptal defect (Gautier *et al.* 1991; Jeanrenaud & Kappenberger 1991; Cabanes *et al.* 1993). Although bubbles can frequently be shown to move from the right to the left side of the heart, and appear in the cerebral circulation detected by transcranial Doppler, it is very rare for thrombus to do so, unless the right atrial pressure is raised (section 6.8.3). The risk of recurrent stroke in patients with a patent foramen ovale is probably low and far more information is required from randomized trials before embarking on routine surgical closure (Bogousslavsky *et al.* 1996; Homma *et al.* 1997). Furthermore, surgical closure and no further thought will not prevent embolism from the legs to the lungs in a patient with a treatable cause of deep venous thrombosis (thrombophilias, etc., section 7.9).

Another, but very unusual, route for emboli to reach the brain via the venous system is through or from a pulmonary arteriovenous fistula, either isolated or in patients with hereditary haemorrhagic telangiectasia. Diagnostic clues are finger-clubbing, cyanosis, haemoptysis, bruit over the chest and a 'coin lesion' on the chest X-ray (Dennis 1985) (Fig. 6.18).

> *Although a patent foramen ovale is common in healthy individuals, it is most unusual for cerebral ischaemia to be caused by paradoxical embolism from the right to the left side of the heart, and so to the brain.*

Atrial septal aneurysm

Atrial septal aneurysm, a bulging of the inter-atrial septum into the right or left atrium or both, is an echocardiographic finding in some normal people who seldom have any cardiac signs. The diagnostic criteria are variable which makes it difficult to compare studies and to generalize their results. Perhaps such aneurysms can be complicated by thrombus, embolism and so cerebral ischaemia, perhaps also by atrial fibrillation, but very often they are associated with a patent foramen ovale and so the potential for paradoxical embolism from the venous system (Silver & Dorsey 1978; Nater *et al.* 1992; Cabanes *et al.* 1993; Agmon *et al.* 1999; Berthet *et al.* 2000).

Intracardiac tumours

Myxomas, found in the left atrium much more often than in any other cardiac chamber, are the most common intracardiac tumour but are still extremely rare. Some are familial (Markel *et al.* 1987; Burke & Virmani 1993; Reynen 1995). Tumour or complicating thrombus may embolize to the brain, eye and elsewhere. Myxomatous emboli cause not only focal cerebral ischaemia but also fusiform and irregular aneurysmal dilatations at sites of earlier symptomatic or even asymptomatic embolic occlusions, and these can rupture to cause intracerebral or subarachnoid haemorrhage (Suzuki

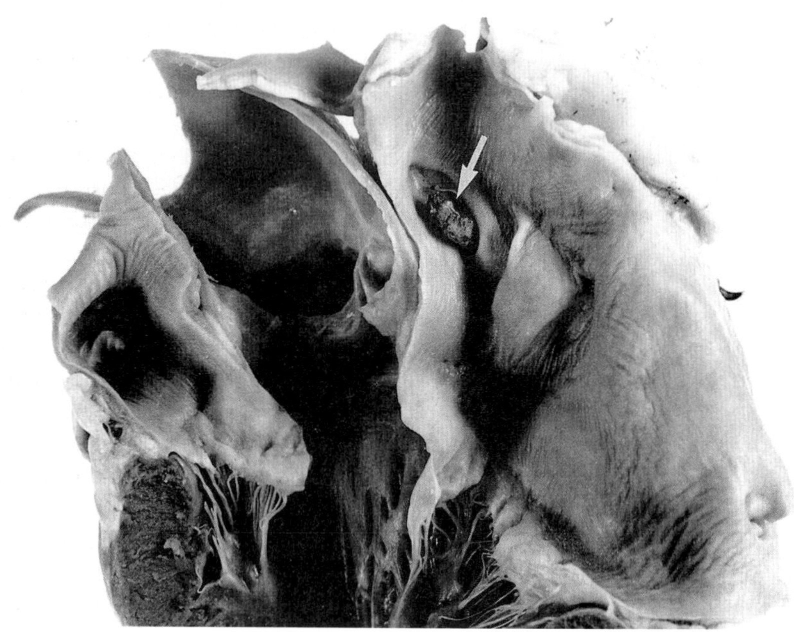
(a)

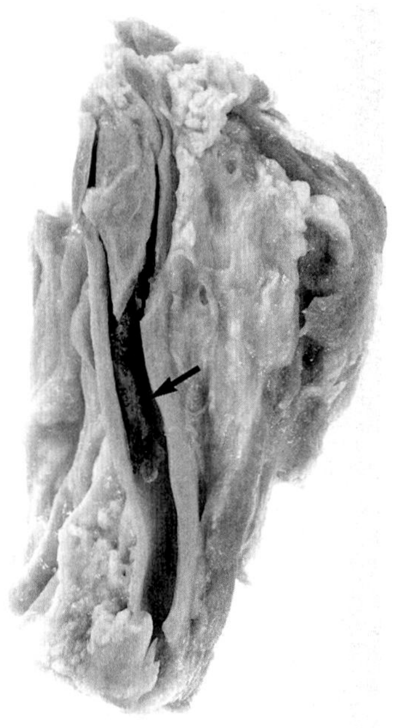
(b)

Fig. 6.17 Paradoxical embolism. A post-mortem specimen showing: (a) a venous thrombus (arrow) protruding through a patent foramen ovale into the left atrium; and (b) part of the same thrombus (arrow) in the right common carotid artery. (Courtesy of Dr John Webb.)

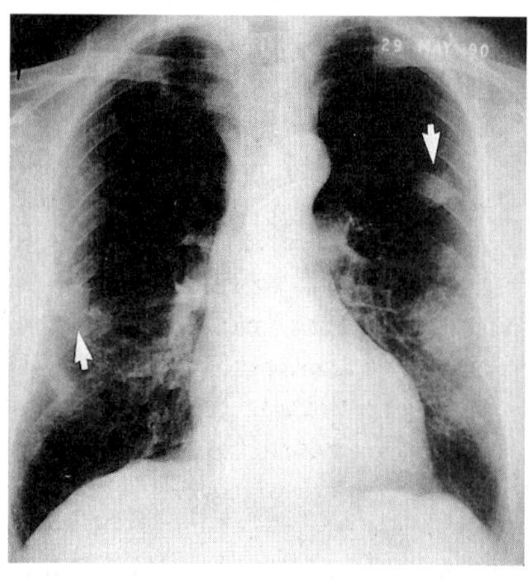
(a)

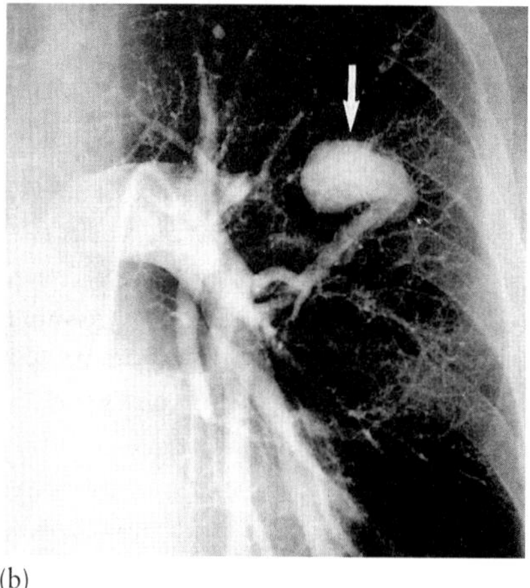
(b)

Fig. 6.18 Pulmonary arteriovenous fistula: (a) chest X-ray showing the fistulae (arrows); (b) pulmonary angiogram showing the fistula on the left more clearly (arrow). (Courtesy of Dr John Reid, Royal Infirmary, Edinburgh.)

et al. 1994) (Fig. 6.19). Brain metastases have also been described (Ng & Poon 1990). Like other cardiac tumours, myxomas can also cause intracardiac obstruction with shortness of breath, palpitations and syncope. They also often cause constitutional problems, such as malaise, fatigue, weight loss, fever, rash, arthralgia, myalgia, anaemia, raised erythrocyte sedimentation rate and hypergammaglobulinaemia. Recurrent neurological problems after resection of the cardiac tumour are very unusual (Roeltgen *et al.* 1981; Mattle *et al.* 1995).

Other even rarer primary and secondary cardiac tumours may embolize, such as valvular fibroelastoma (Joynt *et al.* 1965; Chalmers & Campbell 1987; Giannesini *et al.* 1999).

Sinoatrial disease (sick sinus syndrome)

Sinoatrial disease can be associated with intracardiac thrombus and embolism, particularly if bradycardia alternates with tachycardia or the patient is in atrial fibrillation. It can be familial (Bathen *et al.* 1978; Fisher *et al.* 1988; Pierre *et al.* 1993).

Other unusual causes of embolism from the heart to the brain

Myocardial *hydatid cysts*, thrombus in an *aneurysm of the sinus of Valsalva* and intracardiac calcification caused by *pri-*

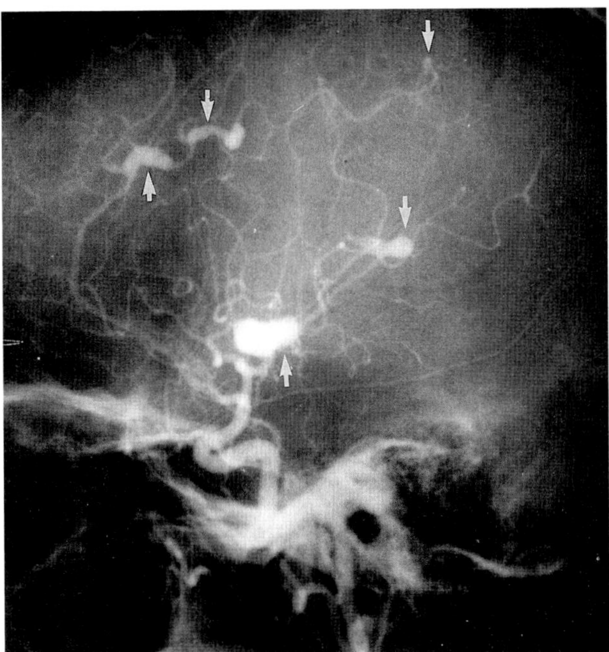

Fig. 6.19 Selective catheter carotid angiogram showing multiple aneurysmal dilatations of cerebral arteries (arrows) as a result of embolism from a cardiac myxoma. (Courtesy of Professor Alastair Compston.)

mary oxalosis are extremely rare causes of embolism to the brain (Shields 1990; Benomar *et al.* 1994; Stollberger *et al.* 1996; Lammie *et al.* 1998). *Myocardial contusion* as a result of blunt chest injury can be associated with left-ventricular thrombus and embolism (Dugani *et al.* 1984).

6.6 From symptoms, signs and clinical syndrome to cause

As emphasized in Chapter 3, the diagnosis of stroke vs. not-stroke, and of transient ischaemic attack (TIA) vs. not-TIA, depends more on the history than on the examination of the nervous system or on brain imaging. The clinical syndrome, based on both the history and examination, reasonably predicts the site and size of the brain lesion which, if ischaemic—haemorrhage having been ruled out by early CT—takes one a long way towards the likely cause of the ischaemic event (Chapter 4) (Fig. 6.20). Clinical localization is easier if the patient has had an established stroke with stable physical signs rather than being in the very early stages when the signs are still evolving (brain attack), or has had a TIA and any signs have disappeared. Using *only* brain CT or MRI to define the site and size of the brain lesion *very* early after stroke or TIA onset, and so to classify the site and size of any infarct, is not helpful because there may be no infarct to be seen. Even later, imaging is not always helpful because it may remain normal even in clinically definite stroke (section 5.3.5 and 5.3.8). Furthermore, CT, and particularly MRI, may not be *immediately* available or even practicable in very ill stroke patients. Brain imaging, however, can *confirm* the site and size of any *visible* ischaemic lesion which has been predicted clinically, and so help towards the likely cause. In about one-quarter of cases where a recent lesion is visible, it is not quite in the expected place to explain the clinical syndrome (Mead *et al.* 1999a). For example, although most pure motor strokes are caused by a lacunar infarct as a result of small vessel disease, in a few cases the CT or MR scan shows striatocapsular infarction which is likely to be caused by middle cerebral artery occlusion with good cortical collaterals (section 6.6.2). The best way to use brain imaging is to *refine* the clinical localization of an infarct, perhaps alerting one to look again for subtle signs that may have been missed if the infarct is not in the expected place, and this helps in finding the underlying cause.

In acute stroke, computed tomography or magnetic resonance imaging should be neither the first nor only way to classify patients on the basis of the size and site of any ischaemic brain lesion. Imaging is used to confirm and refine where the symptoms and neurological signs—in other words the clinical syndrome—suggest the lesion is. From there, it is possible to narrow down the potential causes of the infarct.

6.6.1 Total anterior circulation infarction

The acute ischaemic stroke clinical syndrome of a total anterior circulation infarction (TACI) comprises a hemiparesis, with or without hemisensory loss, homonymous hemianopia; and a new cortical deficit, such as aphasia or neglect. It is a good predictor of infarction of most of the middle cerebral artery (MCA) territory on brain CT, as a consequence of occlusion of either the MCA mainstem (or proximal large branch) or the internal carotid artery (ICA) in the neck (section 4.3.4) (Fig. 6.20c). Occasionally, a TACI can be caused by occlusion of the posterior cerebral artery, but the hemiparesis is usually rather mild. The *cause* of the arterial occlusion therefore is usually in the heart (e.g. embolism as a consequence of atrial fibrillation, recent myocardial infarction, etc.) or it is atherothrombosis (complicated by embolism or occasionally propagating thrombosis) of the ICA or aortic arch. Therefore, if the heart is clinically normal (history, examination, chest X-ray and electrocardiogram) and if there is no evidence of arterial disease in the neck (bruits, palpation perhaps, but mainly duplex sonography), then it is important to consider rarities. For example, infective endocarditis (echocardiogram, blood cultures) and carotid dissection (angiogram possibly, and certainly check for past history of neck trauma). Although transcranial Doppler may confirm an MCA mainstem occlusion (but not if it has already recanalized), it will not help much in the search for a

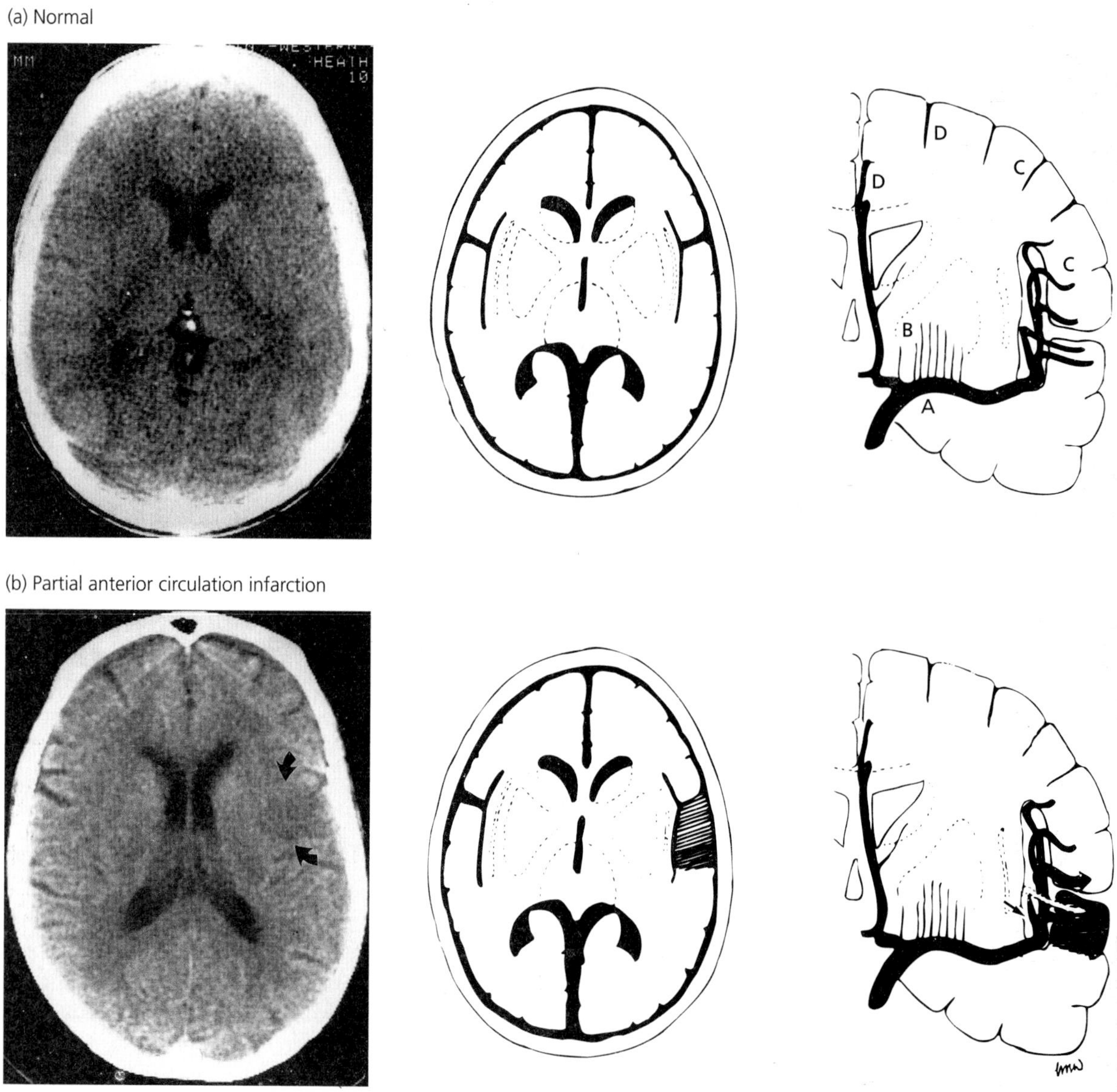

(a) Normal

(b) Partial anterior circulation infarction

Fig. 6.20 Various patterns of arterial occlusion causing different types of ischaemic stroke. Left-hand column: axial CT brain scan through the level of the basal ganglia; middle column, diagram to correspond with the CT brain scan with the area of infarction shaded; right-hand column, diagram of the middle cerebral artery (MCA) and anterior cerebral arteries on a coronal brain section with the area of infarction shaded. A, main trunk of MCA; B, lenticulostriate perforating branches of the MCA; C, cortical branches of the MCA; D, cortical branches of the anterior cerebral arteries. (a) Normal arterial anatomy and CT scan. (b) Occlusion—usually embolic (straight arrow) from heart, aorta or internal carotid artery—of a cortical branch of the MCA and restricted cortical infarct on CT (curved arrows)—partial anterior circulation infarction (PACI). (c) Occlusion—usually embolic (straight arrow) as in (b) above—of MCA mainstem to cause infarction of entire MCA territory (curved arrows)—total anterior circulation infarction (TACI). (d) Occlusion of one lenticulostriate artery to cause a lacunar infarct (arrow); lacunar infarction (LACI). Note that the patient has an old lacunar infarct in the opposite hemisphere. (e) Occlusion of the MCA mainstem (straight arrow) but with good cortical collaterals from the anterior and posterior cerebral arteries to cause a striatocapsular infarct (curved arrows). *(continued)*

cause (Mead *et al.* 2000b). A catheter angiogram *might* if it could be justified on the basis of changing the patient's management (e.g. traumatic carotid dissection could lead to later litigation, fibromuscular dysplasia could stop the search for other explanations, a giant aneurysm with contained thrombus might be surgically treatable, etc.). Increasingly, MRI and MR angiography are replacing catheter angiography to show lesions, such as dissection and aneurysms, but this is not always easily available or particularly practicable in patients in the acute stage of stroke (sections 6.7.3 and 6.7.4).

(c) Total anterior circulation infarction

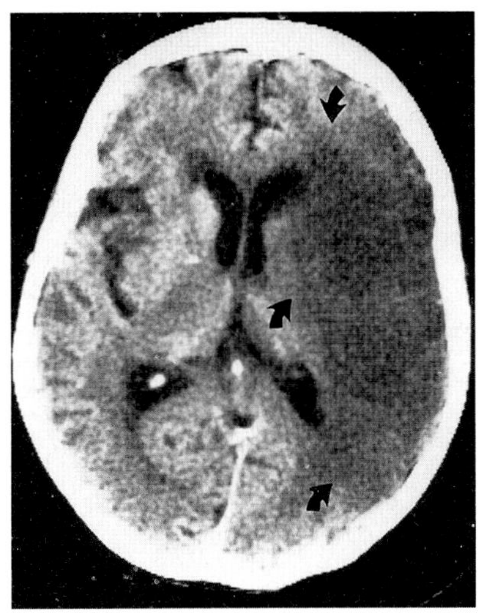
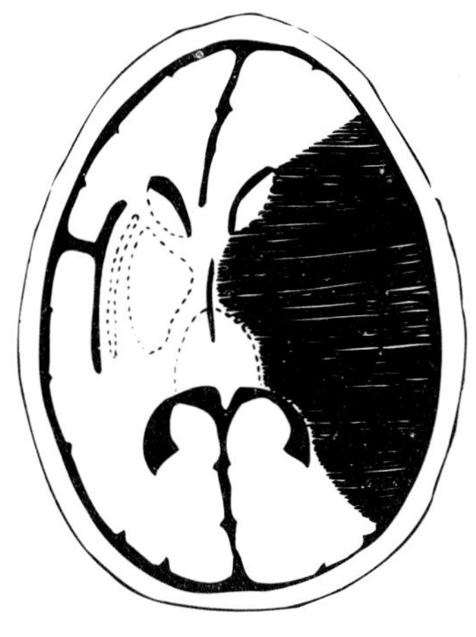
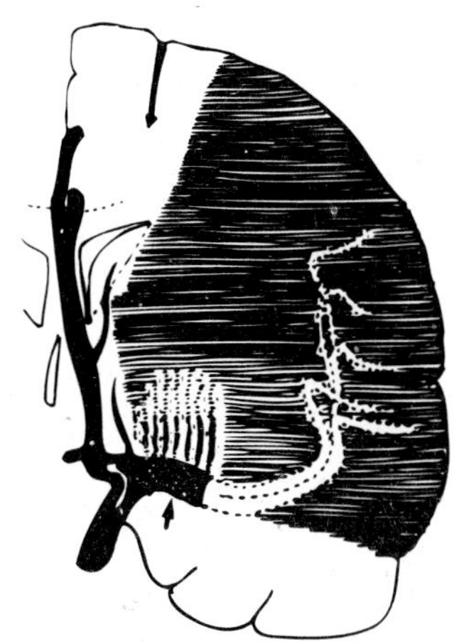

(d) Lacunar infarction

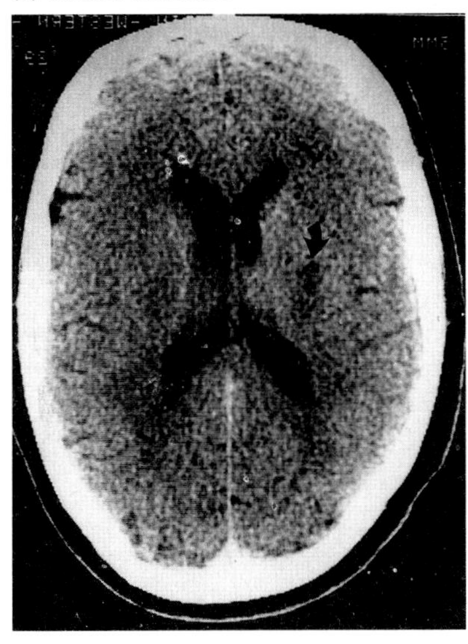
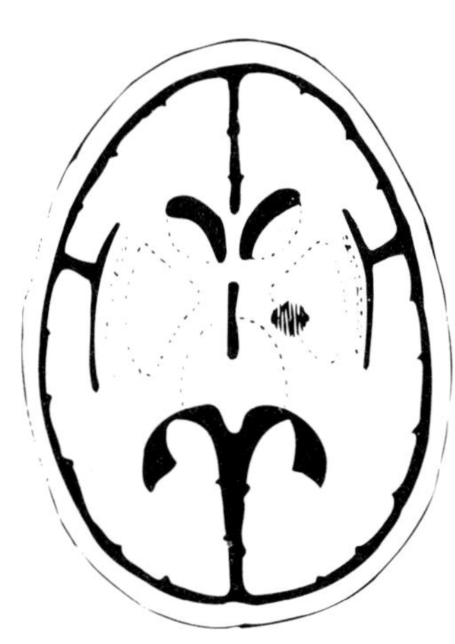
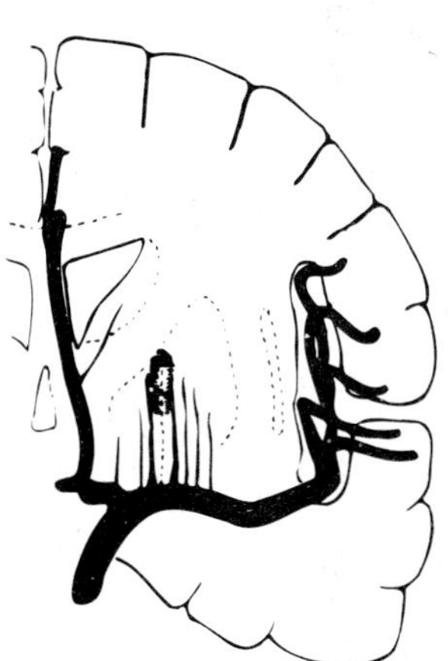

Fig. 6.20 (*continued*)

6.6.2 Partial anterior circulation infarction

A partial anterior circulation infarction (PACI) is a more restricted clinical syndrome with only two out of the three components of the total anterior circulation syndrome (TACS): or a new isolated cortical deficit, such as aphasia; or a predominantly proprioceptive deficit in one limb; or a motor/sensory deficit restricted to one body area or part of one body area (e.g. one leg, one hand, etc.) This syndrome is reasonably predictive of a restricted cortical infarct caused by occlusion of a branch of the middle cerebral artery (MCA) or, much less commonly, of the anterior cerebral artery, as a result of embolism from the heart or from proximal sites of atherothrombosis (usually the carotid bifurcation), or to any other cause of the total anterior circulation infarct (TACI) (sections 4.3.5 and 6.6.1) (Fig. 6.20b).

Investigation is therefore similar to that for the patient with a TACI, except it is usually easier because the patient is fully conscious and less neurologically impaired. However, investigation must be quicker because of the higher risk of early recurrence (section 16.1.2) and because the patient has more to lose from a recurrence which might, next time, be a TACI. The potential for secondary prevention must be considered, particularly eligibility for carotid endarterectomy, and this requires early duplex sonography to find any severe carotid stenosis (section 6.7.5), and eligibility for anticoagulation if the patient is in atrial fibrillation. Transcranial Doppler (TCD) is unlikely to demonstrate the blocked cere-

(e) Striatocapsular infarction

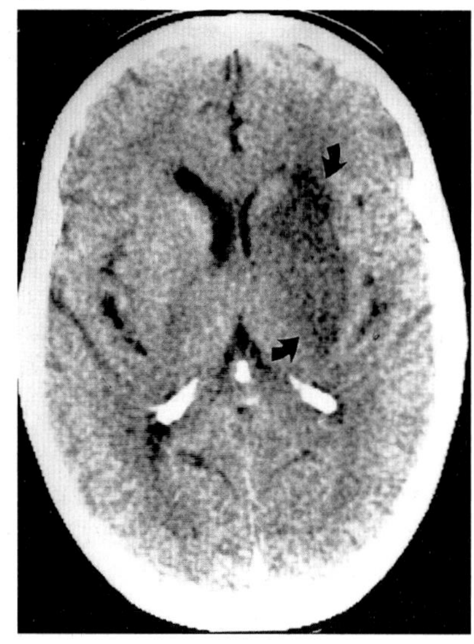

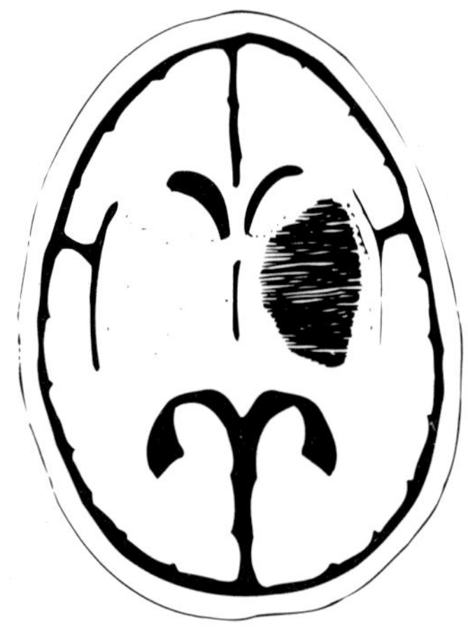

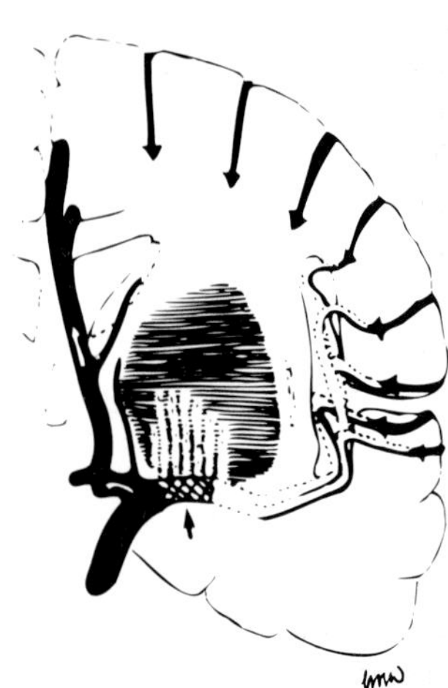

Fig. 6.20 (*continued*)

bral artery because this is almost always distal to the MCA mainstem, at a point where TCD is not particularly sensitive (Mead *et al.* 2000b). Occasionally, however, patients with a large PACI, but falling short of the full definition of a TACI, do have MCA mainstem occlusion, presumably because good collateral flow to the margins of the central infarcted area of brain restricts the clinical syndrome. This is particularly likely with striatocapsular infarction, which usually presents as a PACI (Fig. 4.14). Some PACI syndromes are caused by infarction in the centrum semiovale (section 4.2.2) and in boundary-zones (section 6.6.5). Anterior choroidal artery infarcts may also present as a PACI (or a lacunar syndrome) syndrome and they seem to be caused by either embolism from proximal sites or intracranial small vessel disease (section 4.2.2).

Total and partial anterior circulation infarction/ transient ischaemic attacks are usually caused by occlusion of the mainstem or a branch of the middle cerebral artery, by occlusion of the anterior cerebral artery, or by occlusion of the internal carotid artery. Such occlusions are usually caused by embolism from the heart, to embolism from proximal arterial sites of atherothombosis (the internal carotid artery origin, the aortic arch, etc.) or sometimes to thrombotic occlusion of severe internal carotid artery stenosis.

6.6.3 Lacunar infarction

Lacunar syndromes, the vast majority of which are ischaemic rather than caused by intracerebral haemorrhage, are almost always caused by small, deep, infarcts more likely to be seen on MRI than brain CT (section 4.3.2) (Fig. 6.20d). These small, deep, infarcts are mostly caused by a vasculopathy affecting the small perforating arteries of the brain, and not by embolism from proximal arterial sources or the heart (section 6.4). There is not therefore the same urgency to rule out a cardiac source of embolism or severe carotid stenosis as there is for a partial anterior circulation infarction (PACI) (section 6.6.2). There is some concern that treatment or prevention with antithrombotic drugs *might* be counter-productive if the same underlying vascular disease which causes lacunar infarctions (LACIs) also causes intracerebral haemorrhage (sections 6.4 and 8.2.1). This may be no more than speculation, but most randomized trials did not differentiate different types of likely vascular pathology at randomization, and nor did they categorize the ischaemic stroke outcomes by clinical subtype (Chapters 11 and 16). Also, the presence of leukoaraiosis (section 5.7), which may also be caused by the same small vessel disease, is associated with increased risk of intracerebral haemorrhage in patients in sinus rhythm on long-term anticoagulants after minor cerebrovascular events (Stroke Prevention in Reversible Ischaemia Trial (SPIRIT) Study Group 1997).

The vast majority of lacunar stroke syndromes are caused by ischaemia rather than haemorrhage. Most ischaemic lacunar strokes are the result of a small, deep, not a cortical, infarct. These small, deep infarcts are usually within the distribution of a small, perforating artery. The underlying vascular pathology is probably 'complex' small vessel disease, which differs from atheroma, but sometimes atheroma of the parent artery may occlude the mouth of the perforating artery. Lacunar infarcts are seldom caused by embolism from the heart or from proximal arterial sources.

The *capsular warning syndrome* is a rather characteristic syndrome. Over hours or days, there is cluster of transient ischaemic attacks (TIAs), consisting typically of weakness down the whole of one side of the body without any cognitive or language deficit (i.e. pure motor lacunar TIAs). These are followed within hours or days usually by a lacunar infarct in the internal capsule. This syndrome is presumably caused by intermittent closure of a single lenticulostriate or other perforating artery, followed by complete occlusion, and one is unlikely to find a proximal arterial or cardiac cause, as in any other type of LACI (Donnan *et al.* 1993b).

6.6.4 Posterior circulation infarction

Ischaemia and infarction in the brainstem and/or occipital region is aetiologically more heterogeneous than in the other three main clinical syndromes (Castaigne *et al.* 1973; Caplan & Tettenborn 1992) (section 4.3.3). Emboli from the heart may reach a small artery supplying the brainstem (e.g. superior cerebellar artery) to cause a fairly restricted deficit, block the basilar artery to produce a major brainstem stroke, travel on to block one or both posterior cerebral arteries to cause a homonymous hemianopia or cortical blindness, or any combination of these deficits. Similarly, embolism from the vertebral artery (as a result of atherothrombosis usually but sometimes another disorder, such as dissection) or from atherothrombosis of the basilar artery, aortic arch or innominate or subclavian arteries produces exactly the same neurological features as embolism from the heart (Caplan 1993; Koennecke *et al.* 1997; Yamamoto *et al.* 1999). Even embolism from the carotid territory can, in some individuals with a dominant posterior communicating artery or a persistent trigeminal artery, cause occlusion of the posterior cerebral artery and even brainstem infarction (Zeman *et al.* 1993; Gasecki *et al.* 1994). Basilar occlusion, usually as a result of severe atherothrombotic stenosis, is likely to produce massive brainstem infarction. Obstruction, usually by atherothrombosis, of the origin of the small arteries arising from the basilar artery can produce restricted brainstem syndromes, as can 'complex' small vessel disease within the brainstem; certainly some patients with a lacunar syndrome have a small infarct in the brainstem. A posterior circulation infarction (POCI) does not therefore provide much of a clue to the cause of the ischaemic event. An exception is the patient with simultaneous brainstem signs and a homonymous hemianopia, where embolism from the heart or a proximal artery must be the likely cause and not small vessel disease.

Posterior circulation infarction/transient ischaemic attack can be caused by almost any cause of cerebral ischaemia, which makes it very difficult to be certain of the exact cause in an individual patient.

Cerebellar ischaemic strokes (section 4.2.3) are mostly caused by embolism from the heart, vertebral and basilar arteries, or to atherothrombotic occlusion at the origin of the cerebellar arteries; some are said to result from low blood flow alone (Amarenco & Caplan 1993; Tohgi *et al.* 1993; Chaves *et al.* 1994; Min *et al.* 1999).

Thalamic infarcts (section 4.2.3) can be caused by 'complex' small vessel disease affecting one of the small perforating arteries; atheromatous occlusion of these same arteries where they arise from the posterior cerebral and other medium-sized arteries; and occlusion of these arteries by embolism from the heart, basilar, vertebral and other proximal arterial sites (Castaigne *et al.* 1981; Bogousslavsky & Caplan 1993).

6.6.5 Ischaemic strokes and transient ischaemic attacks caused by low blood flow without acute arterial occlusion: low-flow strokes

The pressure gradient across, and blood flow through large arteries is not affected until their diameter is reduced by more than 50%, often not until by much more (Brice *et al.* 1964; DeWeese *et al.* 1970; Archie & Feldtman 1981). Not surprisingly therefore, even if there is severe disease of the carotid or vertebral arteries, cerebral perfusion pressure is usually normal. However, in some patients, as any stenosis becomes more severe, flow does fall, and eventually cerebral vasodilatation (autoregulation) cannot compensate for the low cerebral perfusion pressure. Cerebral blood flow (CBF) then falls, particularly if the collateral circulation is compromised because the circle of Willis, for example, is incomplete or diseased (Derlon *et al.* 1992; Derdeyn *et al.* 1999; Kluytmans *et al.* 1999) (section 4.2.2). At this stage of exhausted cerebral perfusion reserve, the ratio of cerebral blood flow : cerebral blood volume falls below about 6.0, oxygen extraction fraction starts to rise on positron emission tomography (PET) and stroke risk probably also rises (Gibbs *et al.* 1984; Powers *et al.* 1987; Schumann *et al.* 1998; Grubb *et al.* 1998) (section 11.1.2). Using transcranial Doppler (TCD) to demonstrate impaired cerebrovascular reactivity to a chemical rather than perfusion challenge is an indirect but more practical alternative to PET, but the correlation is not perfect (Derdeyn *et al.* 1999) (section 6.7.9). Isotopic measurement of the mean cerebral transit time (Naylor *et al.* 1994), gradient echo and perfusion weighted MRI (Kleinschmidt *et al.* 1995; Kluytmans *et al.* 1999), MR angiography (Mandai *et al.* 1994) and near-infrared spectroscopy (Smielewski *et al.* 1997) are other possibilities.

Therefore, although the notion that ischaemic strokes are caused by 'hypotension' goes back many years, low CBF alone is not particularly common and cannot easily explain more than a small fraction of strokes. Severe arterial stenosis or occlusion, or good evidence of a fall in systemic blood pressure just before onset, are simply not present in most ischaemic stroke cases (Bladin & Chambers 1994). The majority of ischaemic strokes and transient ischaemic attacks

(TIAs) must be caused, we believe, by embolic or *in situ* acute thrombotic occlusion of an artery to the brain causing blood flow to be suddenly cut off, so causing ischaemia in its territory of supply. Naturally, at times, focal ischaemia *could* also be caused by low-flow without *acute* vessel occlusion but usually only distal to a severely stenosed or occluded internal carotid (ICA) or other artery. This is where the vascular bed is likely to be maximally dilated and therefore where the brain is particularly vulnerable to any fall in perfusion pressure (even more so if arteries carrying collateral blood flow are also diseased). Under these circumstances, a small drop in systemic blood pressure might cause transient or focal ischaemia without any acute occlusive event. Under *normal* circumstances quite a large fall in blood pressure does not cause cerebral symptoms, provided it is transient. This is because of autoregulation of CBF (section 11.1.2). If it does, the symptoms are much more likely to be non-focal (faintness, bilateral blurring of vision, etc.) than focal (Kendell & Marshall 1963) (sections 3.2.1 and 3.4.12).

Boundary-zone ischaemia and infarction

Sometimes, ischaemia occurs not *within* but *between* major arterial territories in their boundary-zones (section 4.2.4). Because this is where perfusion pressure is likely to be most attenuated, it is conceivable that 'low-flow' as a result of low perfusion pressure, as well as acute arterial occlusion caused by embolism, can cause ischaemia in these areas (Torvik 1984; see below). The alternative term of watershed infarction is a misnomer based on geographical ignorance. A watershed is the line separating the water flowing *into* different river basins (i.e. the elevated ground *between* two drainage areas) which differs from the pattern of arterial supply where flow is from larger to smaller vessels.

The evidence that at least some boundary-zone infarcts are caused by low-flow rather than acute arterial occlusion is that sudden, profound and relatively prolonged hypotension (e.g. as a result of cardiac arrest or cardiac surgery) sometimes causes infarction bilaterally in the posterior boundary-zones, between the supply territories of the middle cerebral artery (MCA) and the posterior cerebral artery in the parieto-occipital region. The clinical features include cortical blindness, visual disorientation and agnosia, and amnesia. Unilateral posterior boundary-zone infarction causes contralateral hemianopia, cortical sensory loss and, if in the dominant hemisphere, aphasia. Also, distal to severe carotid stenosis or occlusion, unilateral infarction is well recognized in the anterior boundary-zone between the supply territories of the MCA and anterior cerebral artery in the frontoparasagittal region, but this does not necessarily mean that the cause was low-flow rather than embolism. The clinical features are contralateral weakness of the leg more than the arm and sparing the face, some impaired sensation in the same distribution, and aphasia if in the dominant hemisphere (Bogousslavsky & Regli 1986a,b; Yanagihara *et al.* 1988). Curiously, unilateral boundary-zone infarcts can develop and progress over days and weeks. There is an internal or subcortical boundary-zone in the corona radiata and centrum semiovale, lateral and/or above the lateral ventricle. This lies between the supply of the lenticulostriate perforating branches from the MCA trunk, and the medullary arteries which arise from the cortical branches of the MCA and the anterior and, perhaps, posterior cerebral arteries. Infarction can occur within this internal boundary-zone, usually causing a lacunar or partial anterior circulation syndrome, in association with severe carotid disease and sometimes an obvious haemodynamic precipitating cause (Bladin & Chambers 1993).

The diagnosis of 'low flow' as the cause of ischaemic strokes and TIAs

It would be simplistic to presume that all ischaemic strokes are caused by acute arterial occlusion. However, the definitive diagnosis of stroke resulting from 'low flow' is far from easy. It is probably best inferred from the circumstances surrounding the onset of the symptoms, and to some extent by their nature, and not very much from either the neurological signs or the site of any visible infarct on brain imaging. Naturally, any clinical guidelines to 'low flow' ischaemic episodes cannot be validated against a 'gold standard' because at present there is not one.

Most ischaemic strokes and TIAs occur 'out of the blue' with no precipitating activity. However, on the basis of a number of convincing case reports, a fall in cerebral perfusion pressure—mostly resulting from a fall in systemic blood pressure—should be suspected if the symptoms start under certain circumstances:

- on standing or sitting up quickly, even if postural hypotension cannot be demonstrated in the clinic;
- immediately after a heavy meal;
- in very hot weather;
- after a hot bath or on warming the face;
- with exercise, coughing or hyperventilation;
- during a Valsalva manoeuvre, but paradoxical embolism is another possibility;
- during a clinically obvious episode of cardiac dysrhythmia (chest pain, palpitations, etc.), but embolism from the heart is also possible;
- during operative hypotension (section 7.18); or
- if the patient has recently been started on or increased the dose of any drug likely to cause hypotension, such as calcium blockers or vasodilators.

In addition, there is usually very obvious evidence of severe arterial disease in the neck, i.e. bruits and/or absent pulsations (Caplan & Sergay 1976; Pantin & Young 1980; Raymond *et al.* 1980; Purvin & Dunn 1981; Nobile-Orazio & Sterzi 1981; Stark & Wodak 1983; Milder & Lance 1984; Hankey & Gubbay 1987; Ross Russell 1988; Kamata *et al.*

1994; Gironell *et al.* 1995; Schlingemann *et al.* 1996; Leira *et al.* 1997).

TIAs caused by low flow may be atypical and develop over minutes rather than seconds. Sometimes they consist of jerking and shaking of one arm and/or leg contralateral to the cerebral ischaemia and so are easily confused with focal motor seizures (section 3.3.4), or there is monocular or binocular visual blurring, dimming, fragmentation or bleaching, often only in bright light (section 3.3.6). There may be additional non-focal features, such as faintness, mental vagueness or even loss of consciousness (Furlan *et al.* 1979; Ross Russell & Page 1983; Yanagihara *et al.* 1985; Wiebers *et al.* 1989; Baumgartner & Baumgartner 1998). Low-flow ischaemic oculopathy is discussed in section 6.6.7.

Boundary-zone infarction on brain imaging (or at post-mortem) is *not* necessarily caused by low blood flow (without acute arterial occlusion) but this assumption has bedevilled much of the literature on both the causes of the former and the consequences of the latter. The brain CT/MRI-defined site and size of any visible recent infarction is *not* an accurate way to diagnose a low-flow ischaemic stroke. This is, first, because some boundary-zone infarcts result from embolism (Torvik 1984; Angeloni *et al.* 1990; Belden *et al.* 1999). Secondly, there is much variation between individuals in *where* the boundary-zones are, and they may even change with time in the same individual in response to changes in peripheral resistance (Fig. 6.21). Thirdly, however boundary-zone infarcts are defined on imaging, there is little difference between them and territorial presumed-embolic infarcts in patient demographic characteristics, vascular risk factors and even in the prevalence of arterial disease in the neck severe enough to cause low flow, which is far more often assumed than measured (Hupperts *et al.* 1993, 1996, 1997a,b; Gandolfo *et al.* 1998). However, there have not been many comparative studies, definitions of boundary-zones vary and the numbers of patients have been small. On balance, although some boundary-zone infarcts may have a haemodynamic (i.e. low flow) cause, many others could be caused by embolism or acute occlusive thrombosis. After all, any arterial territory has a terminal zone which forms a boundary with adjacent arterial territories and which is probably particularly vulnerable to ischaemia. There is no reason to suppose that this zone is more susceptible to ischaemia caused by low flow without *acute* arterial occlusion, than as a result of acute arterial occlusion. Another possibility is that boundary-zone infarcts are caused by a combination of embolization to the margins of the territorial supply of a cerebral artery, as well as insufficient perfusion pressure to clear the emboli because of severe arterial disease in the neck, or operative hypotension (Belden *et al.* 1999). Clearly, in view of the diagnostic difficulties, it is quite conceivable that low flow is a more frequent cause of cerebral ischaemia, or less frequent, than currently believed.

The exact sites of the boundary-zones between the territories of supply of the major cerebral arteries are so variable between, and even within, individuals that the diagnosis of infarction in a boundary-zone based on CT/MRI alone is all but impossible. Boundary-zone infarction can be caused by acute arterial obstruction, and low blood flow does not necessarily cause infarction only within boundary-zones.

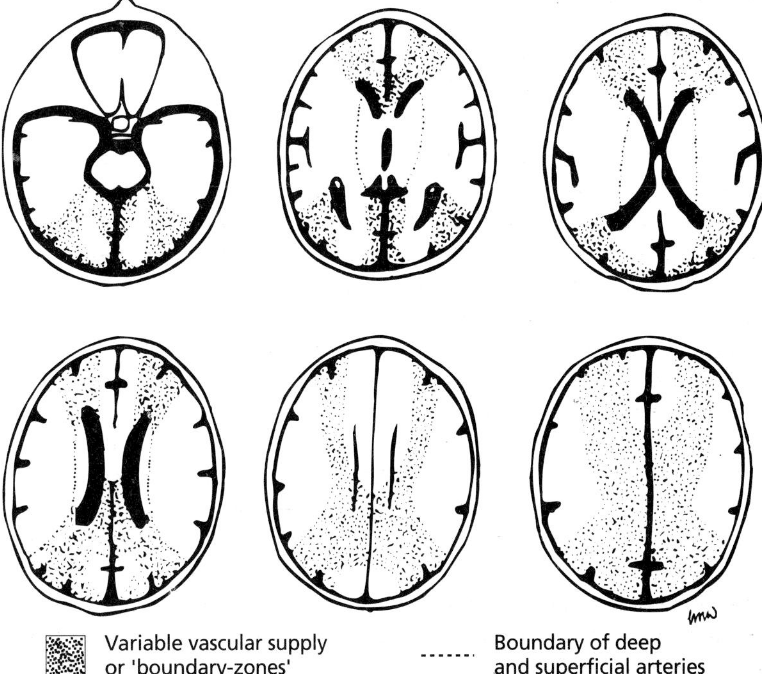

Fig. 6.21 The anterior and posterior boundary-zones between the territories of the middle, anterior and posterior cerebral arteries. The maximum extent of these variable zones is shown on CT templates (see also Figs 4.11, 4.17, 4.23 and 4.25). (Adapted from van der Zwan *et al.* 1992, 1993.)

Implications for treatment

Being certain that an ischaemic episode is caused either by low flow alone, or by acute arterial obstruction, seldom really matters. It makes very little difference if ischaemic stroke or TIA caused by low flow is recognized as such because unless the precipitating factor(s) can be avoided or reversed (particularly over-treatment of hypertension), the management is exactly the same as for presumed embolic causes of ischaemia, i.e. antithrombotic drugs, management of causal vascular risk factors and surgical relief of any obstruction to blood flow if it is practical and safe to do so (section 16.8). However, there is a case for less aggressive treatment of hypertension if there is good evidence of low flow symptoms. It must be acknowledged that in a patient with or without known severe arterial disease, an ischaemic episode may *occasionally* be caused by low flow rather than embolism or some other cause of acute arterial obstruction, and even that different episodes at different times in the same patient are caused by different mechanisms.

6.6.6 Clues from the history

The vast majority of transient ischaemic attacks (TIAs) and ischaemic strokes start suddenly, without any obvious provocation and there are few if any symptoms other than those of a focal neurological or ocular deficit. Sometimes there can be clues to the cause in the history, as well as to whether the patient has had a stroke or TIA in the first place (Chapter 3). These clues may require some tenacity to recognize, or perhaps just an ability to take a history instead of rushing to order lots of tests (Table 6.10).

There will be no clues from the history if no one bothers to take one in the rush to organize a brain scan.

Gradual onset

Gradual onset of ischaemic stroke or TIA over hours or days, rather than seconds or minutes, is unusual but is becoming more recognized now that strokes are being seen much earlier (section 3.3.8). If the onset is gradual, and ischaemic stroke or TIA is not likely to be caused by low flow (section 6.6.5) or migraine (section 7.8), then the diagnosis should be reconsidered and a structural intracranial (or ocular) lesion looked for again, or for the first time if brain imaging has not already been carried out (e.g. intracranial tumour, chronic subdural haematoma, cerebral abscess, section 3.4.4). Under the age of 50 years, multiple sclerosis should also be considered (section 3.4.10). However, a priori, focal neurological deficits which develop over hours, and even over one or two days, in an *elderly* patient are still more likely to have a vascular than a non-vascular cause. This is because the former is so much more common than the latter. It is only when progression occurs over a longer period that the likelihood of a non-vascular cause (such as chronic subdural haematoma) starts to rise.

Precipitating factors

The *exact* activity and *time* of onset may both be important (section 3.3.8). Anything to suggest a drop in cerebral perfusion or blood pressure may be relevant (section 6.6.5), as is pregnancy (section 7.14) and any operative procedure (section 7.18). Head-turning is an occasional cause (section 7.1). Recurrent attacks first thing in the morning or during exercise suggest hypoglycaemia, which is easy to think of in a diabetic patient on hypoglycaemic drugs but more difficult if there is a less obvious cause of hypoglycaemia, such as the very rare insulinoma or drugs, such as pentamidine (sections 3.4.5 and 7.16). Onset during a Valsalva manoeuvre (e.g. lifting a heavy object) suggests a low flow ischaemic stroke (section 6.6.5) or paradoxical embolism (section 6.5), and so sets off a search for deep venous thrombosis if there is evidence on echocardiography of a patent foramen ovale (section 6.8.3).

Headache

Headache at around the onset of ischaemic stroke or TIA occurs in about 25% of patients, is usually mild and, if localized at all, tends to be related to the position of the brain/eye lesion (sections 3.3.10 and 15.9). It is more common with vertebrobasilar than carotid distribution ischaemia, and less common with lacunar ischaemia (Nichols *et al.* 1990; Koudstaal *et al.* 1991; Vestergaard *et al.* 1993; Jorgensen *et al.* 1994a; Kumral *et al.* 1995). Severe pain unilaterally in the head, face, neck or eye at around or before the time of stroke onset is highly suggestive of carotid dissection, while vertebral dissection tends to cause unilateral or sometimes bilateral occipital pain (section 7.2.1). Migrainous stroke may be accompanied by headache (section 7.8.1) and patients with cerebral autosomal dominant arteriopathy with subcortical infarcts and leukoencephalopathy (CADASIL) usually have migraine (section 7.20). In the context of the differential diagnosis of TIAs, migraine should be fairly obvious, unless there is no headache (section 3.4.1). Although intracranial venous thrombosis usually causes either a benign intracranial hypertension syndrome or a subacute encephalopathy, sometimes a focal onset does occur and headache can be a clue (Bousser & Ross Russell 1997) (section 5.5.2). Stroke or TIA in the context of a patient who has had a headache for days or weeks previously must raise the possibility of giant cell arteritis and other inflammatory vascular disorders (section 7.3). Pain in the jaw muscles with chewing, which resolves with rest, strongly suggests claudication, which is caused by external carotid artery disease as a result of giant cell arteritis far more often than atherothrombosis.

Table 6.10 Important clues from the history which may suggest the cause of an ischaemic stroke or transient ischaemic attack, or that the diagnosis of cerebrovascular disease should be reconsidered.

Gradual onset
Low cerebral blood flow (section 6.6.5)
Migraine (section 7.8)
Structural intracranial lesion (section 3.4.4)
Multiple sclerosis (sections 3.4.10)

Precipitating factors
Suspected systemic hypotension or low cerebral perfusion pressure (standing up or sitting up quickly, heavy meal, hot weather, hot bath, warming the face, exercise, coughing, hyperventilation, chest pain or palpitations, starting or changing blood pressure-lowering drugs) (section 6.6.5)
Pregnancy (section 7.14)
Surgery (section 7.18)
Head-turning (section 7.1)
Hypoglycaemia (section 7.16)
Valsalva manoeuvre (paradoxical embolism, section 6.5; or low flow, section 6.6.5)

Recent headache
Carotid/vertebral dissection (section 7.2.1)
Migrainous stroke/transient ischaemic attack (sections 3.4.1 and 7.8)
Intracranial venous thrombosis (section 5.5.2)
Giant cell arteritis (or other inflammatory vascular disorders) (section 7.3)
Structural intracranial lesion (section 3.4.4)

Epileptic seizures
Intracranial venous thrombosis (section 5.0)
Mitochondrial cytopathy (section 7.19)
Non-vascular intracranial lesion (section 3.4.4)

Malaise
Inflammatory arterial disorders (section 7.3)
Infective endocarditis (section 6.5)
Cardiac myxoma (section 6.5)
Cancer (section 7.12)
Thrombotic thrombocytopenic purpura (section 7.9)
Sarcoidosis (section 7.3)

Chest pain
Myocardial infarction (section 7.10)
Aortic dissection (section 7.2.3)
Paradoxical embolism (sections 6.5 and 6.8.3)

Non-stroke vascular disease or vascular risk factors
Heart disease (section 6.5)
Claudication (section 6.3.3)
Hypertension (section 6.3.3)
Smoking (section 6.3.3)

Drugs
Oral contraceptives (section 7.13)
Oestrogens in men (section 7.13)
Blood pressure-lowering/vasodilators (section 6.6.5)
Hypoglycaemic drugs (section 7.16)
Cocaine (section 7.15)
Amphetamines (section 7.15)
Ephedrine (section 7.15)
Phenylpropanolamine (section 7.15)
'Ecstasy' (section 7.15)
Allopurinol (section 7.15)
Interleukin 2 (section 7.3)
Deoxycoformycin (section 7.2)
L-asparaginase (section 7.9)

Injury
Chronic subdural haematoma (section 3.4.4)
Vertebral/carotid artery dissection (section 7.2.1)
Fat embolism (section 6.6.6)

Self-audible bruits
Internal carotid artery stenosis (distal) (section 6.6.7)
Dural arteriovenous fistula (section 8.2.8)
Glomus tumour
Caroticocavernous fistula (section 8.2.14)
Raised intracranial pressure
Intracranial venous thrombosis (section 5.5.2)

Past medical history
Inflammatory bowel disease (section 7.17)
Coeliac disease (section 7.17)
Homocystinuria (section 7.20)
Cancer (section 7.12)
Irradiation of the head or neck (section 7.12)
Recurrent deep venous thrombosis
Recurrent miscarriages
Recent surgery/long distance travel (section 6.8.3)

Family history (Table 6.11)

Epileptic seizures

Epileptic seizures, partial or generalized, within hours of stroke onset are distinctly unusual in adults (<5%) and should lead to a reconsideration of non-stroke brain pathologies (section 3.3.10). They are rather more common in childhood stroke. They are more likely with haemorrhagic than ischaemic strokes and if the infarct is extensive and involves the cerebral cortex (Pohlmann-Eden *et al.* 1996, 1997; Arboix *et al.* 1997; Burn *et al.* 1997). They are also likely with venous infarction (section 5.5.2) and mitochondrial cytopathy (section 7.19). Partial motor seizures can be confused with limb-shaking TIAs, but the former are more clonic and the jerking spreads in a typical jacksonian way from one body part to another (sections 3.3.4 and 6.6.5). Very rarely, transient focal ischaemia seems to cause partial epileptic seizures, but proving a causal relationship is seldom possible (Kaplan 1993). The diagnosis of stroke may be wrong if a tumour on CT is misinterpreted as an infarct, because contrast enhancement can look very similar in both (section 5.3.5). Therefore, partial seizures after a 'stroke' should always be an indication to re-examine the diagnosis. Also, seizures in the presence of a history of a few days malaise, headache and fever should suggest encephalitis and the need for an electroencephalogram to show bilateral diffuse rather than unilateral focal slow waves, and cerebrospinal fluid examination (raised white cell count, but this can also occur in stroke, section 6.7.11).

Malaise

Stroke in the context of a patient who has been generally unwell for days, weeks or months should suggest an inflammatory arterial disorder, particularly giant cell arteritis (section 7.3), infective endocarditis (section 6.5), cardiac myxoma (section 6.5), cancer (section 7.12), thrombotic thrombocytopenic purpura (section 7.9) or even sarcoidosis (section 7.3).

Chest pain

Chest pain may be indicative of a recent myocardial infarction with complicating stroke (section 7.10); aortic dissection, particularly if the pain is also interscapular (section 7.2.3); and pleuritic pain suggests pulmonary embolism and the possibility of paradoxical embolism (section 6.5).

Vascular risk factors

Vascular risk factors (section 6.3.3) and diseases should be sought. It is most unusual for an ischaemic stroke or TIA to occur in someone with *no* vascular risk factors, unless they are very old, or are young with some unusual cause of stroke (Table 6.3). Heart disease of any sort may be relevant (source of embolism to the brain, dysrhythmias causing low-flow ischaemia, etc.) and cardiac symptoms should be specifically sought in the history: angina, shortness of breath, palpitations, etc.

Drugs and drug users

Drugs may well be relevant: oral contraceptives in women and oestrogens in men (section 7.13); anything which lowers the blood pressure (section 6.6.5); hypoglycaemic agents (section 7.16); and drugs of abuse, which seem to be a more common problem in the USA than elsewhere (section 7.15).

Injury

Any injury in the days and weeks before ischaemic stroke or TIA onset is crucial information. A head injury might have caused a chronic subdural haematoma (highly unlikely if more than 3 months previously) and this should have been considered earlier at the stroke vs. non-stroke stage (section 3.4.4). Of possible relevance is an injury to the neck in the hours, days or possibly a few weeks before onset, because this may cause carotid or vertebral dissection (section 7.2.1). After long bone fracture, fat embolism may cause a generalized encephalopathy, but occasionally there are additional focal features (Jacobson *et al.* 1986; Fabian 1993; van Oostenbrugge *et al.* 1996; Forteza *et al.* 1999). It is therefore essential to *ask* about any injury, strangulation, car crash, unusual yoga exercises, neck manipulation, etc., in any unexplained stroke (Table 6.2).

Self-audible bruits

Pulsatile self-audible bruits are rare. They can be differentiated from tinnitus because they are in time with the pulse. They may be audible to the examiner as well. They are unlikely to be caused by carotid bifurcation atherothrombosis because the source of the sound is too far from the ear. They are much more likely to indicate *distal* internal carotid artery stenosis (dissection or, rarely, atherothrombosis), dural arteriovenous fistula near the petrous temporal bone, glomus tumour, caroticocavernous fistula, intracranial venous thrombosis, symptomatic and idiopathic intracranial hypertension, a loop in the internal carotid artery, or just heightened awareness of one's own pulse (Biousse *et al.* 1998; Waldvogel *et al.* 1998).

Past medical history

Past medical history of inflammatory bowel disease (section 7.17), coeliac disease (section 7.17), irradiation of the head and neck (section 7.12), cancer (section 7.12) or even homocystinuria (section 7.20) may be important. Recurrent deep venous thrombosis (DVT) suggests thrombophilia (section 7.9), particularly if there is a family history, or the antiphospholipid syndrome (section 7.3). Recurrent miscarriage is another feature of the antiphospholipid syndrome. *Any* reason for a recent DVT (e.g. a long air journey, or surgery) should raise the question of paradoxical embolism (sections 6.5 and 6.8.3).

> *If a patient has, or has had, deep venous thrombosis in the legs, then consider paradoxical embolism to the brain, a familial clotting factor problem or the antiphospholipid syndrome.*

Previous strokes and/or transient ischaemic attacks

Previous strokes and/or TIAs in different vascular territories are more likely with a proximal embolic source in the heart, or arch of the aorta, than with a single arterial lesion. Attacks going back months or more make certain causes unlikely (e.g. infective endocarditis, arterial dissection).

Family history

There are several rare familial conditions which may be complicated by ischaemic stroke and TIAs (Table 6.11). There is also increasing interest in complex genetic disorders thought to be caused by multiple gene interactions, presumably influenced by environmental factors (Rastenyte *et al.* 1998; Alberts 1999). Genetic factors play at least some part in the development of stroke risk factors, such as hypertension and diabetes. On the other hand, these same risk factors are clearly influenced by the environment (for example, diets rich in fat and in salt tend to raise the plasma cholesterol and blood pressure, respectively). Just how easy it will be to separate out shared genes from shared environment in a disease as common as stroke remains to be seen. Disentangling the interactions and working out the pathway from genotype to phenotype will be monumental tasks.

Table 6.11 Causes of familial stroke (including intracranial haemorrhage) and transient ischaemic attack.

Connective-tissue disorders
Ehlers–Danlos syndrome (section 7.4)
Pseudoxanthoma elasticum (section 7.4)
Marfan's syndrome (section 7.4)
Fibromuscular dysplasia (section 7.4)
Familial mitral valve prolapse (section 6.5)

Haematological disorders
Sickle cell disease/trait (section 7.9)
Antithrombin III deficiency (section 7.9)
Protein C deficiency (section 7.9)
Protein S deficiency (section 7.9)
Plasminogen abnormality/deficiency (section 7.9)
Dysfibrinogenaemia (section 7.9)
Haemophilia and other inherited coagulation factor deficiencies (section 8.4.4)

Others
Familial hypercholesterolaemia
Neurofibromatosis (section 7.20)
Homocystinuria (section 7.20)
Fabry's disease (section 7.20)
Tuberous sclerosis (section 7.20)
Dutch and Icelandic cerebral amyloid angiopathy (section 8.2.2)
Migraine (section 7.8)
Familial cardiac myxoma (section 6.5)
Familial cardiomyopathies (section 6.5)
Mitochondrial cytopathy (section 7.19)
Cerebral autosomal dominant arteriopathy with subcortical infarcts and leukoencephalopathy (CADASIL) (section 7.20)
Sneddon's syndrome (section 7.3)
Arteriovenous malformations (section 8.2.4)
Intracranial saccular aneurysms (sections 8.2.3 and 9.1.1)

6.6.7 Clues from the examination

Neurological examination

Neurological examination is *primarily* to localize the brain lesion, although in patients with transient ischaemic attacks (TIAs), or those seen some days after a minor stroke, there will probably be no signs at all (section 3.3.1). Occasionally, however, there may be a clue to the cause. A Horner's syndrome ipsilateral to a carotid distribution infarct (i.e. not as the result of a brainstem stroke, where it might be expected) suggests dissection of the internal carotid artery (ICA) or sometimes acute atherothrombotic carotid occlusion (section 7.2.1). Lower cranial nerve lesions ipsilateral to a hemispheric cerebral infarct can also occur in carotid dissection and, like Horner's syndrome, are caused by stretching and bulging of the arterial wall in relation to the affected nerves, or ischaemia (section 7.2.1). Ocular ischaemia, as well as III, IV and VI cranial nerve palsies—sometimes with orbital pain—have been described ipsilateral to acute ICA occlusion and stenosis, presumably caused by ischaemia of the nerve trunks (Kapoor *et al.* 1991; Hollinger & Sturzenegger 1999).

In a total anterior circulation infarct or brainstem stroke some drowsiness would be expected, but with more restricted infarcts consciousness is normal. Therefore, if consciousness is impaired and yet the 'stroke' itself seems mild, it is important to:

- reconsider the differential diagnosis (particularly chronic subdural haematoma) (section 3.4.4);
- consider the diffuse encephalopathic disorders which have focal features and which may masquerade as stroke, e.g. cerebral vasculitis of some sort (section 7.3), non-bacterial thrombotic endocarditis (section 6.5), intracranial venous thrombosis (section 5.5.2), mitochondrial cytopathy (section 7.19) and thrombotic thrombocytopenic purpura (section 7.9); and
- remember that co-morbidity, such as pneumonia, sedative drugs, infection and hypoglycaemia, may all make the neurological deficit seem worse than it really is (section 15.4).

If the neurological deficit is mild and yet the patient is drowsy, then consider chronic subdural haematoma, cerebral vasculitis, non-bacterial thrombotic endocarditis, intracranial venous thrombosis, mitochondrial cytopathy, thrombotic thrombocytopenic purpura, sedative drugs, hypoglycaemia, and co-morbidity, such as pneumonia or other infections.

Eyes

The eyes may provide general clues to the cause of a stroke (e.g. diabetic or hypertensive retinopathy), or may reveal papilloedema which would make the diagnosis of ischaemic stroke, or even intracerebral haemorrhage, most unlikely. In addition, it is worth searching thoroughly for evidence of emboli which are very often completely asymptomatic (Arruga & Sanders 1982; Mitchell *et al.* 1997) (section 3.3.6). Fibrin–platelet emboli are dull greyish-white amorphous plugs but are rarely observed, perhaps because they move through the retinal circulation and disperse; they suggest embolism from the heart or proximal sources of atherothrombosis. On the other hand, cholesterol emboli quite often stick at arteriolar branching points, usually without obstructing the blood flow, and appear as glittering orange or yellow bodies reflecting the ophthalmoscope light; obviously these strongly suggest embolization from proximal atheromatous plaques, but they are often asymptomatic. 'Calcific' retinal emboli appear as solid, white and non-reflective bodies and tend to lodge near the edge of the optic disc; they suggest embolism from aortic or mitral valve calcification (section 6.5). Localized areas of periarteriolar sheathing, seen as opaque white obliteration of segments of the retinal arterioles, suggest embolism, usually cholesterol, in the past. Roth spots in the retina are very suggestive of infective endocarditis (section 6.5). Dislocated lenses should suggest Marfan's syndrome (section 7.4) or homocystinuria (section 7.20); angioid streaks in the retina suggest pseudoxanthoma elasticum (section 7.4); and in hyperviscosity syndromes there is a characteristic retinopathy (section 7.9).

Dilated episcleral vessels are a clue to functional anastamoses between branches of the external carotid artery (ECA) and orbital branches of the internal carotid artery (ICA), distal to severe ICA disease (Countee *et al.* 1978). With very severe ICA disease, usually accompanied by severe disease of the ipsilateral ECA, the eye may occasionally become so ischaemic that *venous stasis retinopathy* develops, although arterial disease is not invariable in this condition (Kersemakers *et al.* 1992) (section 3.3.6). Haemorrhages are scattered around the retina with microaneurysms, and the retinal veins are dilatated and irregular. The retinal blood flow is extremely impaired, as demonstrated by lightly compressing the eye with one finger while observing the fundus and noting collapse of the central retinal artery. With more extreme ischaemia, *ischaemic oculopathy* may develop with impaired visual acuity, eye pain, rubeosis of the iris (dilated blood vessels), fixed dilated pupil, 'low-pressure' glaucoma, cataract and corneal oedema (Sturrock & Mueller 1984; Ross Russell & Ikeda 1986) (section 3.3.6). Raised intraocular pressure, i.e. glaucoma, makes the eye more susceptible to low blood flow and ischaemia as a result.

Arterial pulses

It is *always* worth feeling *both* radial pulses simultaneously. Any inequality in timing or volume suggests subclavian or innominate stenosis or occlusion, and this is further supported if there is an ipsilateral supraclavicular bruit or lower blood pressure in the arm with the weak or delayed pulse.

An elderly patient presented with a sudden left-sided hemiparesis and no other symptoms. She had right carotid and supraclavicular bruits. Brain CT was normal. Three days later the duplex examination showed narrowing of the right common carotid artery which appeared to be caused by dissection of the aortic arch. Only then did she admit to some mild chest pain before the stroke, unequal pulses and blood pressures were found in her upper limbs, and chest CT confirmed the aortic dissection. The lessons are that any pain in or around the chest may be relevant and should have been more thoroughly sought, and in all stroke patients both radial pulses must be felt routinely before not after arterial imaging.

Normally, the *internal* carotid artery pulse is too deep and rostral to be felt in the neck. Therefore, any loss of the 'carotid' pulsation reflects common carotid artery (CCA) or innominate occlusion or severe stenosis, both rather rare situations or, perhaps more likely, the artery is too deep to be felt or the neck too thick.

The arterial pulse felt in the neck comes from the common, not the internal carotid artery.

The superficial temporal pulses should be easily felt and symmetrical. If there is unilateral absence or delay, this suggests external carotid artery (ECA) or CCA disease. Tenderness of *any* of the branches of the ECA (occipital, facial, superficial temporal) points towards giant cell arteritis. Tenderness of the carotid artery in the neck (i.e. the CCA) can occur in acute carotid occlusion but is more likely to be a sign of dissection, or possibly arteritis.

Absence of several neck and arm pulses in a young person suggests Takayasu's arteritis (section 7.3). Delayed or absent leg pulses suggests co-arctation of the aorta or, much more commonly, peripheral vascular disease (PVD) which is so common in patients with TIA and ischaemic stroke (section 6.3.3) and may need treating in its own right. Furthermore, PVD is an important predictor of future serious vascular events (section 16.1.1). The state of the femoral artery is important to assess before cerebral angiography via the femoral route (section 6.7.4) and, if after angiography the leg pulses disappear, then it was a complication of the angiography. Other causes of widespread disease of the aortic arch are atheroma, giant cell arteritis, syphilis, subintimal fibrosis, arterial dissection and trauma (Ross & McKusick 1953; Dalal *et al.* 1971; Wickremasinghe *et al.* 1978). Obviously, any evidence of systemic embolism would direct the search towards a source of emboli in the heart (section 6.5).

Finally, while the hand is on the abdomen, aortic aneurysm should be considered while searching for any masses or hepatosplenomegaly. Although the prevalence of aortic aneurysm in these stroke/TIA patients is unknown, it could well be quite high, particularly if the patient has carotid stenosis (section 6.3.3).

Cervical bruits

Listening to the neck is a favourite occupation for inquisitive physicians, and acquisitive surgeons, and can lead to some useful information (Fig. 6.22). A localized bruit, occasionally palpable, over the carotid bifurcation (i.e. high up under the jaw) is predictive of some degree of carotid stenosis, but very tight stenosis (or occlusion) may not cause a bruit at all (Hankey & Warlow 1990) (Fig. 6.23) (Table 6.12). External carotid stenosis can also cause a bruit in the same place. As a sensitive and specific test for severe internal carotid stenosis, a bruit is therefore not particularly useful.

Bruits transmitted from the heart become attenuated as one listens further up the neck towards the angle of the jaw, thyroid bruits are bilateral and more obviously over the gland, a hyperdynamic circulation tends to cause a diffuse bruit, and venous hums are more continuous and roaring and are obliterated by light pressure over the ipsilateral jugular vein (Sandok *et al.* 1982). An arterial bruit in the supraclavicular fossa suggests either subclavian or proximal vertebral arterial disease, but a transmitted bruit from aortic stenosis must also be considered. Normal young adults quite often have a short supraclavicular bruit; the reason is unknown.

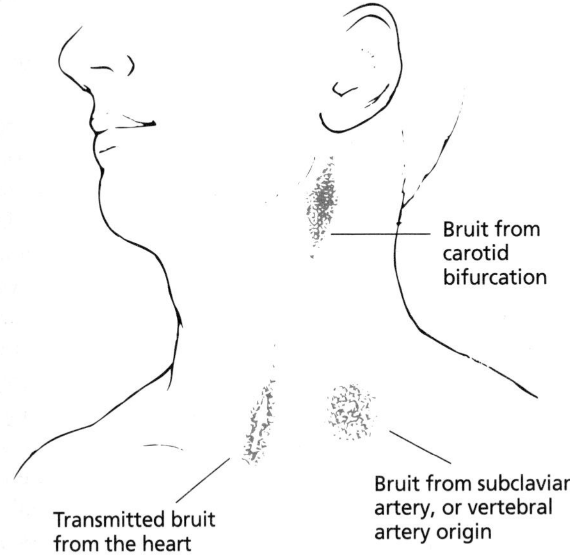

Fig. 6.22 The sites of various cervical bruits. Note that a bruit arising from the carotid bifurcation is high up under the angle of the jaw. Localized supraclavicular bruits are caused either by subclavian or vertebral origin artery stenosis.

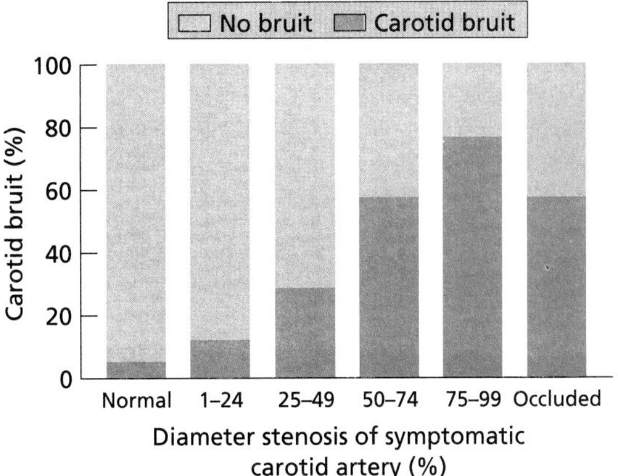

Fig. 6.23 The percentage of patients with a localized bruit over the symptomatic carotid bifurcation for various degrees of stenosis as estimated (using the European Carotid Surgery Trial method) from 298 carotid angiograms. (Adapted with permission from Hankey & Warlow 1990.)

Table 6.12 The source of neck bruits.

Carotid bifurcation arterial bruit
Internal carotid artery origin stenosis
External carotid artery origin stenosis
Supraclavicular arterial bruit
Subclavian artery stenosis
Vertebral artery origin stenosis
Can be normal in young adults
Diffuse neck bruit
Thyrotoxicosis
Hyperdynamic circulation (pregnancy, anaemia, fever, haemodialysis)
Transmitted bruit from the heart and great vessels
Aortic stenosis/regurgitation
Mitral regurgitation
Patent ductus arteriosus
Co-arctation of the aorta
Venous hum

Carotid bruits are neither sufficiently specific nor sensitive to diagnose carotid stenosis severe enough to consider surgery. Physicians and surgeons desperate to use their stethoscopes would do better to measure the blood pressure and listen to the heart.

Cardiac examination

Cardiac examination is important, particularly to look for any cardiac source of embolism (section 6.5). If physicians feel under-confident about their cardiological abilities, then they should get properly trained or a cardiologist will have to be consulted. Atrial fibrillation (AF) will already have been suspected from the radial pulse; left-ventricular hypertrophy suggests hypertension or aortic stenosis, and most *major* cardiac sources of embolism are fairly obvious clinically (e.g. AF, mitral stenosis, prosthetic heart valve).

Fever

Fever is distinctly unusual in the first few hours after stroke onset. Any raised temperature at this time must therefore be taken seriously and endocarditis or other infections, inflammatory vascular disorders or cardiac myxoma considered. Later on, fever is quite common and usually reflects some complication of the stroke (section 15.12).

Skin and nails

The skin and nails occasionally provide clues to the cause of ischaemic stroke or transient ischaemic attack (Table 6.13).

> *Getting to the bottom of the cause of an ischaemic stroke or transient ischaemic attack requires much more than just neurological skills. Stroke medicine, like neurology, is part of general internal medicine. It is important therefore that doctors looking after stroke patients have a good general internal medical training.*

Table 6.13 Clues to the cause of ischaemic stroke/transient ischaemic attack from examination of the skin and nails.

Finger-clubbing	Right-to-left intracardiac shunt (section 6.5) Cancer (section 7.12) Pulmonary arteriovenous malformation (section 6.5) Infective endocarditis (section 6.5) Inflammatory bowel disease (section 7.17)
Splinter haemorrhages	Infective endocarditis (section 6.5) Cholesterol embolization syndrome (section 7.7) Vasculitis (section 7.3)
Scleroderma	Systemic sclerosis (section 7.3)
Livedo reticularis	Sneddon's syndrome (section 7.3) Systemic lupus erythematosus (section 7.3) Polyarteritis nodosa (section 7.3) Cholesterol embolization syndrome (section 7.7)
Lax skin	Ehlers–Danlos syndrome (section 7.4) Pseudoxanthoma elasticum (section 7.4)
Skin colour	Anaemia (section 7.9) Polycythaemia (section 7.9) Cyanosis (right-to-left intracardiac shunt, pulmonary arteriovenous malformation) (section 6.5)
Porcelain-white papules/scars	Kohlmeier–Degos disease (section 7.3)
Skin scars	Ehlers–Danlos syndrome (section 7.4)
Petechiae/purpura/bruising	Thrombotic thrombocytopenic purpura (section 7.9) Fat embolism (section 6.6.6) Cholesterol embolization syndrome (section 7.7) Ehlers–Danlos syndrome (section 7.4)
Orogenital ulceration	Behçet's disease (section 7.3)
Rash	Fabry's disease (section 7.20) Systemic lupus erythematosus (section 7.3) Tuberous sclerosis (section 7.20)
Epidermal naevi	Epidermal naevus syndrome (Dobyns & Garg 1991)
Café-au-lait patches	Neurofibromatosis (section 7.20)
Thrombosed superficial veins, needle marks	Intravenous drug users (section 7.15)

6.7 Investigation

Investigation has little to do with the diagnosis of stroke vs. not-stroke, or of transient ischaemic attack (TIA) vs. not-TIA, which both depend largely on the history in the vast majority of cases (Chapter 3). Investigations are mainly to help unravel the pathological type of stroke (ischaemic stroke vs. intracerebral haemorrhage vs. subarachnoid haemorrhage, as discussed in Chapter 5) and then to determine the cause of the cerebral ischaemia (or intracranial haemorrhage, Chapters 8 and 9), particularly a cause that will influence immediate treatment or long-term management. Investigation may also provide important prognostic information, e.g. left-ventricular hypertrophy on the electrocardiogram (ECG), severe carotid stenosis on ultrasound, etc. (section 16.1.1). In addition, the many patients who also have angina or other cardiac symptoms, claudication or suspected aortic aneurysm may well need specific investigations directed at these problems with a view to appropriate treatment.

Ideally, any investigation should be accurate, non-invasive, accessible, inexpensive and, most importantly, informative in the sense that the result (positive or negative, high or low, etc.) will influence patient management and outcome.

6.7.1 Routine investigations

Although there are no absolute rules, all ischaemic stroke/transient ischaemic attack (TIA) patients, unless they are already heavily dependent or institutionalized, or have already been recently investigated for a previous event, should have basic non-invasive first-line investigations within a few hours of presentation. None of these require hospital admission, although a CT scan does require attendance at hospital (Table 6.14). The chance of picking up a relevant abnormality (yield) may be very low for some tests—e.g. full blood count and erythrocyte sedimentation rate (ESR)—but these are cheap and the consequences of missing a treatable disorder, such as giant cell arteritis, are serious. There is a higher chance of picking up a treatable abnormality with the blood glucose, urine analysis and electrocardiogram (ECG). Depending on the definition, many or even most patients are hypercholesterolaemic, and how this should be acted on is discussed in section 16.3.2; immediately after stroke, but probably not TIA, there is a transient fall in plasma cholesterol, which will underestimate the usual level (Mendez *et al.* 1987; Woo *et al.* 1990). CT brain scanning is discussed in sections 5.3.5 and 6.7.3. If patients have the basic tests and if the results are read, written in the records and acted upon, this may well do more good than the inappropriate ordering of a huge range of further tests and missing some crucial clue from one of the routine investigations (such as an ESR of 100 mm in the first hour).

All patients should have a full blood count, erythrocyte sedimentation rate, plasma glucose, urea, electrolytes and cholesterol, urine analysis, electrocardiogram and perhaps syphilis serology. Most should also have a CT brain scan.

6.7.2 Second-line investigations for selected patients

Second-line investigations (Table 6.15) are usually more costly, invasive and/or dangerous, so they must be targeted on patients most likely to gain from a useful change in management as a consequence of the test result. The likelihood of a relevant result depends on the selection of patients for the investigation, and a balance has to be struck between over-investigation (inconvenience, high cost, possibly high-risk, low yield, false-positive results leading to even more over-investigation) and under-investigation (low cost, low-risk, high yield, but occasional missed diagnosis). This balance depends on the consequences of overlooking a particular diagnosis. For example, missing severe carotid stenosis would be harmful, because carotid endarterectomy reduces the risk of stroke, whereas missing the lupus anticoagulant whose relevance is unknown, and where the effect of any treatment is uncertain, may be of little consequence. Also, the balance will be affected by a reasonable tendency to search particularly hard for a cause in an unusual case without any evidence of atherothromboembolism (section 6.8.1), small vessel disease (section 6.8.2) or embolism from the heart (section 6.8.3), i.e. a patient under the age of about 50 years with no vascular risk factors.

The main indications for the second-line investigations and the disorders likely to be detected are listed in Table 6.15. These will be discussed in further detail in other sections of this chapter and in Chapter 7, although at this stage it will be helpful to discuss imaging the brain, cerebral and coronary circulation, lumbar puncture and the electroencephalogram.

6.7.3 Imaging the brain

Computed tomography

Unenhanced computed tomography (CT) scanning of the brain now really belongs in the category of routine investigation, at least for stroke and brain attack, if not for transient ischaemic attack (TIA). It is the key to distinguishing ischaemic stroke from primary intracerebral haemorrhage (section 5.3.4). This fundamental distinction determines the strategy for looking for the cause of a stroke; it is crucial in decisions about continuing, stopping or starting antithrombotic and inevitably antihaemostatic treatments, such as anticoagulants, aspirin or thrombolysis; and it is also crucial in any later decision which may have to be made about carotid endarterectomy. Increasingly, the appearance of any

Table 6.14 First-line investigations for ischaemic stroke/transient ischaemic attack.

Investigation	Disorders suggested	Yield* (%)
Full blood count	Anaemia, polycythaemia, leukaemia, thrombocythaemia, heparin-induced thrombocytopenia with thrombosis, infections	1
Erythrocyte sedimentation rate	Vasculitis, infections, cardiac myxoma, hyperviscosity, cholesterol embolization syndrome, non-bacterial thrombotic endocarditis	2
Plasma glucose	Diabetes mellitus, hypoglycaemia	5
Urea and electrolytes	Diuretic-induced hypokalaemia, renal failure, hyponatraemia	3
Plasma cholesterol	Hypercholesterolaemia	45
Syphilis serology	Syphilis, anticardiolipin syndrome	< 1†
Urinalysis	Diabetes, renal disease, infective endocarditis, vasculitis, Fabry's disease	5
ECG	Dysrhythmia, left-ventricular hypertrophy, silent myocardial infarction	17
Unenhanced CT brain scan	Intracerebral haemorrhage, non-vascular intracranial cause of transient ischaemic attack stroke-syndrome	20

* The yield represents the proportion of patients in whom a positive test result may lead to a useful change in management (e.g. the diagnosis of diabetes in a previously undiagnosed case). The figures assume that *all* ischaemic stroke/transient ischaemic attack patients have the investigations. Data have been taken from various more or less reliable sources but should not be regarded as precise statements of some universal truth.

† In the Oxfordshire Community Stroke Project, eight of 675 first-ever-in-a-lifetime strokes had positive syphilis serology, of which only one turned out to have previously undiagnosed secondary syphilis (also see Kelley *et al.* 1989). It may be therefore that this investigation should not be routine but only performed in young or middle-aged patients, those likely to have been exposed to infection, and in high-risk populations.

infarction on CT is being used, possibly inappropriately, to determine who gets thrombolysis, but this is not to do with determining the cause of ischaemic stroke (section 11.5.2). The limited, but important, role for CT in excluding intracranial structural lesions that can occasionally present as a TIA or stroke has already been discussed in section 3.4.4. Some would argue that CT is unnecessary in patients with a *single* suspected TIA because it cannot possibly confirm the clinical diagnosis but only rule out intracerebral haemorrhage which has hardly ever been reported to cause focal symptoms lasting less than 24 h (Gunatilake 1998). A structural brain lesion, such as a subdural haematoma, is very unlikely unless the symptoms recur. But, as always, these arguments must be seen in the context of the availability, convenience, risk and cost of the investigation under debate. All agree that transient monocular blindness is certainly one type of TIA where CT is not necessary because examining the eye clinically will exclude any structural cause of the symptoms, and a single brainstem TIA probably does not need a routine brain CT scan either.

It cannot be over-emphasized that very early brain CT is *not* to demonstrate infarcts, it is to exclude haemorrhage. Within the first few hours of stroke onset (i.e. brain attack), the main thrust of management—and indeed research into acute treatment—is to *prevent* the appearance of infarction on CT and so, one hopes, to reduce case fatality and disability. There is therefore usually no need to delay CT in the hope that any infarct will become visible. Nor is there much point in repeating CT in the hope of demonstrating an infarct after an early normal scan, unless the site of any

Table 6.15 Second-line investigations for selected ischaemic stroke/transient ischaemic attack patients.

Investigation	Indications	Possible disorders
Blood		
Liver function	Fever, malaise, raised ESR, suspected malignancy	Giant cell arteritis and other inflammatory arterial disorders, infective endocarditis, non-bacterial thrombotic endocarditis
Calcium	Recurrent focal neurological symptoms very rarely caused by hypercalcaemia	Hypercalcaemia
Thyroid function tests	Atrial fibrillation	Thyrotoxicosis
Activated partial thromboplastin time, dilute Russell's viper time, antinuclear and other autoantibodies	Young (< 50 years) and no other cause found, past or family history of venous thrombosis, especially if unusual sites (cerebral, mesenteric, hepatic veins), recurrent miscarriage, thrombocytopenia, cardiac valve vegetations, livedo reticularis, raised ESR, malaise, positive syphilis serology	Antiphospholipid syndrome, vasculitis, systemic lupus erythematosus
Serum proteins, serum protein electrophoresis, plasma viscosity	Elevated ESR	Paraproteinaemias, nephrotic syndrome, cardiac myxoma
Haemoglobin electrophoresis	Black patients	Sickle cell trait or disease, and other haemoglobinopathies
Protein C and S, antithrombin III, activated protein C resistance, thrombin time*	Personal or family history of thrombosis (usually venous, particularly in unusual sites, such as hepatic vein) at unusually young age	Thrombophilias
Blood cultures	Fever, cardiac murmur, haematuria, deranged liver function, raised ESR, malaise, unexplained stroke	Infective endocarditis
HIV serology	Young (< 40 years), drug addict, homosexual, blood products/transfusion, systemically unwell, lymphadenopathy, pneumonia, cytomegalovirus retinitis, etc.	HIV infection
Lipoprotein fractionation	Elevated cholesterol or strong family history	Hyperlipoproteinaemia
Serum homocysteine	Marfanoid habitus, high myopia, dislocated lenses, osteoporosis, mental retardation, young patient	Homocystinuria
Leucocyte α-galactosidase A	Corneal opacities, cutaneous angiokeratomas, paraesthesias and pain, renal failure	Fabry's disease
Blood/CSF lactate	Young patient, basal ganglia calcification, epilepsy, parieto-occipital ischaemia	Mitochondrial cytopathy
Serum fluorescent treponemal antibody absorption test	Positive screening serology tests	Syphilis
Cardiac enzymes	History or ECG evidence of recent myocardial infarction	Myocardial infarction
Drug screen	Young patient, no other obvious cause	Cocaine/amphetamine, etc.-induced ischaemic stroke
Genetic analysis	Familial stroke with periventricular changes on CT/MRI	CADASIL
Urine		
Amino acids	Marfanoid habitus, high myopia, dislocated, lenses, osteoporosis, mental retardation, young patient	Homocystinuria
Drug screen	Young patient, no other obvious cause	Cocaine/amphetamine, etc.-induced ischaemic stroke

(*continued p. 268*)

Table 6.15 *(continued)*

Investigation	Indications	Possible disorders
Imaging		
Chest X-ray	Hypertension, finger-clubbing, cardiac murmur or abnormal ECG, young patient, ill patient	Enlarged heart, pulmonary arteriovenous malformation, calcified heart valves, baseline in ill patients
MRI	Suggestion of arterial dissection, uncertain diagnosis of stroke	Arterial dissection, loss of flow voids, multiple sclerosis
Carotid ultrasound with a view to carotid surgery	Carotid TIA or mild ischaemic stroke	Extracranial carotid stenosis
Catheter angiography	Carotid ultrasound suggests severe stenosis of recently symptomatic internal carotid artery and patient fit and willing for surgery, suspected arterial dissection, arteriovenous malformation or aneurysm	Arterial dissection, arteriovenous malformation, carotid stenosis
Arch aortography	Symptoms of subclavian steal and unequal brachial pulses and blood pressures	Subclavian or innominate stenosis
Cardiac		
Echocardiography (transthoracic, transoesophageal)	Young (< 50 years), or clinical, ECG or chest X-ray evidence of heart disease likely to cause embolism, aortic arch dissection	Cardiac source of embolism, aortic arch atheroma or dissection
24-hour ECG	Palpitations or loss of consciousness during a suspected TIA, suspicious resting ECG	Intermittent atrial fibrillation or heart block
Others		
Electroencephalogram	Doubt about diagnosis of TIA or stroke: ?epilepsy, ?generalized encephalopathy	Seizure disorder, structural brain lesion, encephalitis, diffuse encephalopathy caused by inflammatory vascular disorders, Creutzfeldt–Jakob disease
CSF	Positive syphilis serology, young patient, ?infective endocarditis, possibility of multiple sclerosis	Vasculitis, syphilis, multiple sclerosis, infective endocarditis
Body red cell mass	Raised haematocrit	Primary polycythaemia
Temporal artery biopsy	Older (> 60 years), jaw claudication, headache, polymyalgia, malaise, anaemia, raised ESR	Giant cell arteritis
Skin biopsy	Familial stroke with periventricular changes on CT/MRI	CADASIL

* Transient falls occur after stroke so any low level must be repeated and family members investigated.

CADASIL, cerebral autosomal dominant arteriopathy with subcortical infarcts and leukoencephalopathy; CSF, cerebrospinal fluid; CT, computed tomography; ECG, electrocardiogram; ESR, erythrocyte sedimentation rate; MRI, magnetic resonance imaging; TIA, transient ischaemic attack.

recent infarct, relevant to the symptoms, may help distinguish carotid from vertebrobasilar distribution attacks. This is relevant when the clinical distinction is difficult; for example, transient hemiparesis in a patient who does not attempt to speak *could* be caused by a cortical, internal capsule or pontine lesion and certainly a patient with the latter would not be considered for carotid surgery (section 4.3.1). Another reason might be if there is a possibility of venous rather than arterial infarction (Table 5.2). On the whole, a *clinically* definite stroke with a normal CT can be assumed to be caused by an infarct. The clinical syndrome is usually predictive enough of the site and size of the brain lesion (sections 4.3.3 and 4.3.8), and so its likely cause (sections 6.6.1–6.6.4), for routine management. In any case, it may not be possible to pinpoint the relevant infarct at all because some patients have so much periventricular low density (leukoaraiosis, section

5.7). Sometimes there are so many small and often asymptomatic infarcts, or so much cortical atrophy, that a small *recently* symptomatic infarct simply cannot be distinguished (section 5.3.5). The problem of reliably detecting boundary-zone infarction has been addressed earlier, and it is looking increasingly likely that many so-called boundary-zone infarcts on CT (or MRI) may not result from low flow but acute arterial occlusion (section 6.6.5).

Occasionally, on an unenhanced CT scan within hours of stroke onset, the middle cerebral or basilar artery is hyperdense, particularly if thin slices are obtained (section 5.3.5) (Fig. 6.24). This is caused by an acute embolus or *in situ* thrombosis in the arterial lumen. Although fairly specific for arterial occlusion, it is not sensitive enough to exclude it. If it is really necessary to know the pattern of intracranial arterial occlusion, then catheter angiography is needed, or possibly MR angiography or transcranial Doppler sonography will do (section 6.7.4). Therefore, in routine practice, the dense artery sign has little impact on determining the cause of cerebral ischaemia, the clinical syndrome being as good or a better predictor of the likely site and size of any infarct, and so of which arterial territory is involved, and of prognosis.

Very early CT brain scanning is mainly to exclude intracerebral haemorrhage and the occasional structural lesion mimicking stroke, it is not to demonstrate infarcts.

In general, therefore, brain CT has little role in determining the *cause* of an ischaemic event, because if one needs to know within hours of the onset, the scan will probably be normal anyway (section 5.3.5). Later on the scan can still be normal and any infarct already reasonably well predicted, both in site and size, on the basis of the neurological symptoms and signs (sections 4.3.7, 4.3.8 and 5.3.5). If there *is* an anatomically relevant and *recent* infarct in a slightly inappropriate place for the clinical syndrome, it is probably best to follow the scan rather than the syndrome (i.e. the infarct is in the correct general area of the brain, such as an internal capsule lacunar infarct on CT/MRI in a patient with a partial anterior circulation clinical syndrome) (Mead *et al.* 1999a). It follows that *repeat* CT scanning, with or without intravenous contrast enhancement, is seldom necessary in the search for the *cause* of an ischaemic event, but it may be needed if there is uncertainty that the patient has had a stroke at all (or even a TIA in some circumstances), or if the patient deteriorates (section 15.5).

The results of brain CT and MRI do not reliably guide early (within hours) decisions in the management of acute ischaemic stroke, but the site and size of any infarct which does eventually appear may, in some cases, help towards finding the cause of the infarct.

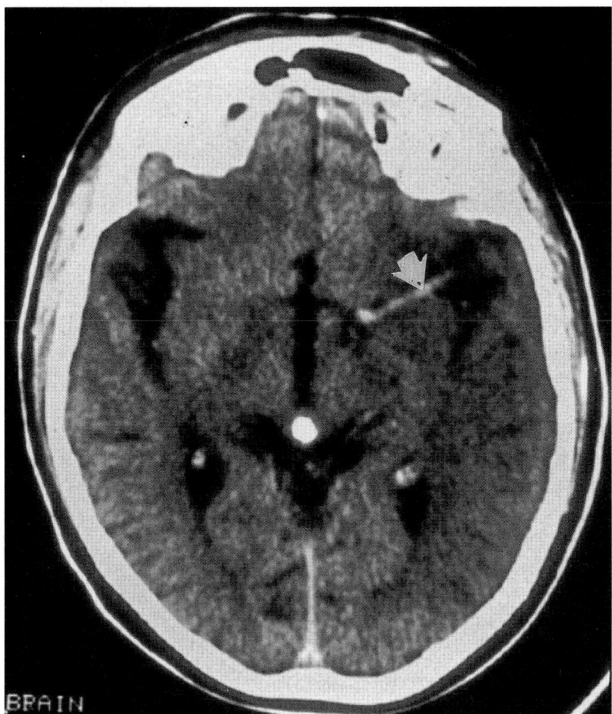

(a)

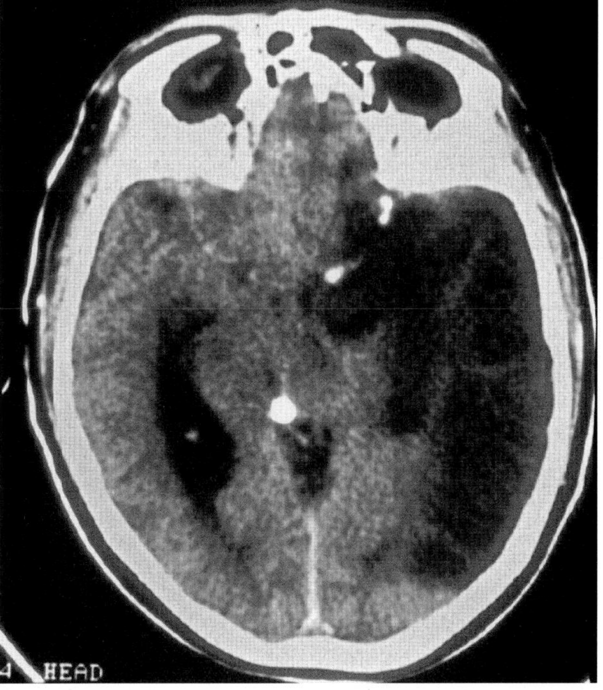

(b)

Fig. 6.24 (a) Hyperdense middle cerebral artery (arrow) on an unenhanced CT brain scan within hours of the onset of a total anterior circulation infarct. At this point the infarct is hardly visible. However, the next day (b) the large left hemisphere infarct is clearly visible and the hyperdense sign has vanished.

Magnetic resonance imaging

Magnetic resonance imaging (MRI) of the brain is more sensitive than CT. It displays smaller infarcts, especially in the brainstem and cerebellum, and is even more sensitive after gadolinium enhancement which may indicate which of several lesions on an unenhanced scan is the recently symptomatic one, even lacunar infarcts sometimes. MRI may also reveal the changes of infarction earlier than CT, but not always (section 5.3.8). It is better at demonstrating small amounts of blood, e.g. petechial haemorrhages at the borders of an infarct (section 5.3.7), but it is not known whether this has any practical impact on stroke management or whether MRI is simply demonstrating what is already suspected from post-mortem studies.

It is still possible to have the clinical syndrome of a stroke, and certainly of a TIA, and yet no relevant lesion on routine and even diffusion-weighted MRI, or at least any relevant lesion that can be differentiated from diffuse or multiple periventricular high-signal areas (Ay *et al.* 1999; Bhadelia *et al.* 1999; Engelter *et al.* 1999; Kidwell *et al.* 1999) (section 5.3.8). Diffusion-weighted MRI can demonstrate extremely early ischaemic lesions before T2- and T1-weighted MRI, but as yet this has little clinical relevance in influencing patient management, or establishing the cause of an ischaemic stroke or TIA (section 5.3.9). However, MRI can certainly help in some ways:

- loss of flow void in a major cerebral vessel may provide direct information about exactly which artery (or vein) is blocked, and where;
- it may be possible to visualize the widening of the arterial wall in cases of cervical artery dissection, but only if the neck as well as the brain is imaged, so making invasive catheter angiography unnecessary (section 7.2.1);
- it may demonstrate arterial ectasia (section 6.3.2);
- it may demonstate the periventricular changes of cerebral autosomal dominant arteriopathy with subcortical infarcts and leukoencephalopathy (CADASIL) (section 7.20); and
- it may come up with surprises, such as the features of multiple sclerosis (section 3.4.10), which can be clinically confused with stroke in young adults, and with small focal infarcts in the cerebellum in some patients with 'isolated vertigo' who in previous times would have been diagnosed as 'acute labyrinthitis', because the less sensitive CT was normal (sections 3.3.7 and 3.4.7).

MRI is considerably less practical than CT in acutely ill, confused, stroke patients, particularly those requiring some form of monitoring, so it is likely that CT will remain the first-line brain imaging investigation for acute stroke for the foreseeable future, reserving MRI for more complicated cases. However, when MR becomes less expensive, even quicker than it is already and less daunting for patients, it will surely replace CT because of its sheer versatility. One short session in one machine should eventually be able to display normal and abnormal brain structure, brain biochemistry with spectroscopy, the pattern of arterial occlusion with angiography, the pattern of cerebral blood flow with perfusion imaging, and brain function with functional MR. Even all this, however, does not do away with the need for a good history and examination first.

'Silent—or unrecognized—cerebral infarction'

Focal low-density areas are often seen on CT (or MRI) in patients with transient ischaemic attack or stroke in areas of the brain that are *clearly irrelevant* to the presenting or any past clinical event; distal to asymptomatic carotid stenosis; in patients with coronary heart disease or atrial fibrillation; and even in apparently normal elderly people (Dennis *et al.* 1990; Herderschee *et al.* 1992; Tanaka *et al.* 1993; Boon *et al.* 1994; Brott *et al.* 1994; Caplan 1994; Jorgensen *et al.* 1994b). These asymptomatic lesions are usually small and deep, rather than large and cortical. The assumption is usually made, but without pathology verification, that the lesions are a result of previous subclinical infarction, or perhaps intracerebral haemorrhage, or that the patient had not recognized or had simply forgotten a previous symptomatic event. The reported frequency of 'silent infarcts' varies enormously, depending on the precise definition of the radiological abnormality, the imaging technique used, how the patients were selected, how certain one can really be about the lack of previous neurological symptoms, whether the observer was blind to any presenting clinical syndrome, and the demographic characteristics of the patients. Also, it is not always easy to differentiate small infarcts from dilated perivascular spaces on MRI (Takao *et al.* 1999).

Perhaps not surprisingly, in view of these methodological difficulties, 'silent infarcts' have no definite relevance in the sense of predicting future strokes but they may be associated with impaired physical and cognitive abilities (EAFT Study Group 1996; Price *et al.* 1997). Also, a very obvious and large cortical infarct, even without previous symptoms, might at least make one reconsider proximal sources of embolism to the brain.

> *'Silent' cerebral infarcts on brain CT/MRI are quite common, but it is unclear whether they have any influence on patient prognosis or management.*

6.7.4 Imaging the cerebral circulation

It would obviously be of interest to image the cerebral circulation repeatedly in everyone with an ischaemic stroke or transient ischaemic attack (TIA) to display which artery is blocked, how quickly recanalization occurs and where any embolus may have originated. However, at present this information does not often influence clinical management and therefore should not be sought *routinely* because of the risk, inconvenience and cost. Indeed, sometimes it simply cannot be sought at all because the technology is either not available (e.g. MRA) or it is difficult to use accurately (e.g. ultrasound). In practice, imaging the cerebral circulation must always be carefully directed to answer a relevant clinical question and any answer must be likely to influence the patient's management (Hankey & Warlow 1992; Sellar 1995).

The main indications for imaging the cerebral circulation are:

- the patient is a potential candidate for carotid surgery (sections 6.7.5 and 16.8.6);
- the possibility of arterial dissection (sections 6.7.7 and 7.2.1);
- acute ischaemic stroke patients under some circumstances (section 6.7.8);
- intracranial venous thrombosis (section 5.5.3);
- frequent vertebrobasilar TIAs, particularly with subclavian steal (sections 6.7.6 and 16.12); and
- research.

6.7.5 Vascular imaging to select patients for carotid surgery

The risks and benefits of carotid endarterectomy are quite finely balanced and so it is essential that imaging the carotid bifurcation to help select patients for surgery is more or less completely risk-free (section 16.8). The critical imaging question is 'how severe is any stenosis at the origin of the internal carotid artery (ICA) ipsilateral to the cerebral or ocular ischaemia?' The 'gold-standard' is intra-arterial selective catheter angiography. However, even this is not a perfect test without any inter-observer variation, but it is reasonably reliable at the severe end of the stenosis spectrum where surgical decisions have to be made (Rothwell *et al.* 1994a; Dippel *et al.* 1997). It is still the 'gold-standard' because it was the first way the whole of the anatomy of the cerebral circulation could be displayed; it has intuitive face validity; and, most importantly, it was the only accurate imaging technique available when the large randomized trials of surgery were recruiting patients. Therefore, any criterion for making the surgery vs. no-surgery decision based on the severity of the stenosis, and then applying the inferences from those trials to routine clinical practice, is implicitly based on catheter angiography. If this decision is now to be based on non-invasive measurement of carotid stenosis, then it must be very certain that what is measured non-invasively can be 'translated' to what would have been measured if angiography had been performed (Rothwell & Warlow 1996).

Performing intra-arterial catheter angiography in everyone with a mild carotid ischaemic event is clearly unacceptable because there is a risk, as well as a cost (see below). Furthermore, less than 20% of these patients actually have severe carotid stenosis; even if only those with 'cortical' rather than 'lacunar' events are selected, the proportion is still less than 30% (Hankey *et al.* 1991b; Hankey & Warlow 1991b; Mead *et al.* 1999b). The rest presumably have an unsuspected source of embolism in the heart, or an arterial embolic source which is not imaged, such as in the aortic arch and common carotid arteries, or intracranial small vessel disease, or less severe carotid bifurcation disease which may still have been the source of embolism but is perhaps unlikely to be so again in the near future, or ischaemia in the vertebrobasilar distribution. Confining angiography to patients with a carotid bifurcation bruit will miss some patients with severe stenosis and still subject too many with mild or moderate stenosis to the risks, but with nothing to gain from carotid surgery (Fig. 6.23). Nor will a combination of a cervical bruit with various clinical features do much better (Mead *et al.* 1999b).

At the time of the first edition of this book we believed that the most cost-effective strategy was to carry out duplex sonography first, followed by catheter angiography if the duplex suggested stenosis or occlusion of the symptomatic ICA (Hankey & Warlow 1990). However, with increasing cost constraints and awareness of angiographic complications, together with improving ultrasound technology and training, it may well now be sensible to omit angiography, *provided* the initial duplex findings are confirmed by an independent observer using duplex again or some other non-invasive technique, such as MRA (see below) (Fig. 6.25).

Catheter angiography

Carotid angiography is inconvenient, invasive, uncomfortable, costly, carries a risk and normally requires hospital admission which may introduce unnecessary delay before carotid endarterectomy and so risk an avoidable stroke in the meantime. About 4% of patients have a transient ischaemic attack (TIA) or stroke—one-quarter of them permanent—as a result of angiography, probably more if the patient has *severe* carotid disease. Indeed, with prior duplex sonography screening, it is *precisely* these severe stenosis patients who are now being selected for angiography (Hankey *et al.* 1990a,b; Davies & Humphrey 1993; Heiserman *et al.* 1994). Clinically 'silent' cerebral ischaemic lesions are apparently more frequent, although this is disputed, and their relevance is very unclear (Bendszus *et al.* 1999; Britt *et al.* 2000). TIAs and strokes complicating angiography occur because, first, the catheter tip dislodges atheromatous plaque or dissects the arterial wall during insertion, injection or flushing; secondly, thrombus may form at the catheter tip or in blood contaminating the contrast-containing syringe; and, finally, exceptionally, as a result of the almost inevitable injection of some air (Gerraty *et al.* 1996). In addition, there are systemic and allergic adverse effects of the contrast material, particularly during intravenous digital subtraction angiography where large quantities are used (bradycardia, hypotension, angina, shortness of breath, nausea, vomiting, headache, epi-

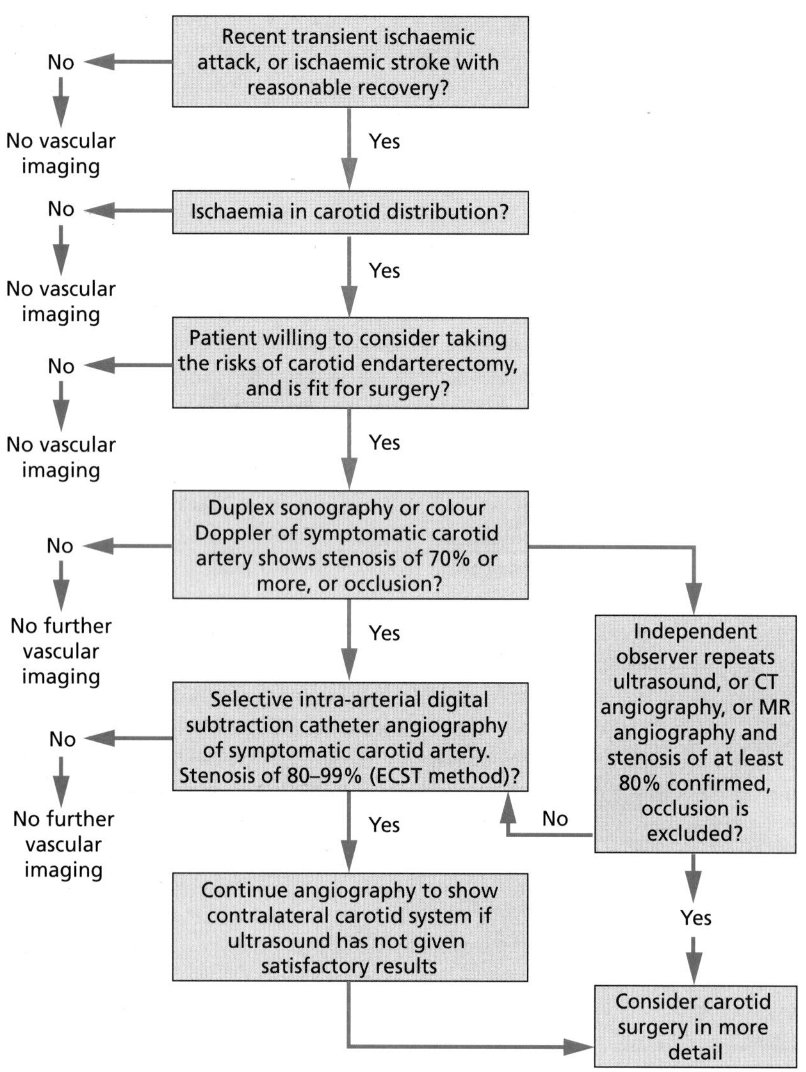

Fig. 6.25 Carotid imaging strategy for patients with ischaemic events to select those suitable for carotid endarterectomy. One strategy exposes the patient to the risks of angiography but may give better measurements of the carotid stenosis as well as details of the intracranial circulation (bottom left-hand side). The other strategy generally avoids angiography (bottom right-hand side).

leptic seizures, transient bilateral cortical blindness, periorbital oedema, urticaria, bronchospasm and renal failure). Some patients develop a haematoma, aneurysm or nerve injury at the site of arterial puncture (which is usually into the femoral artery in the groin), and the occasional patient develops *de novo* or has worsened symptoms of peripheral vascular disease in the leg distal to the puncture site, sometimes even leading to amputation. The cholesterol embolization syndrome is very rare, but it can be fatal (section 7.7).

Compared with cut-film selective intra-arterial catheter angiography recorded directly onto X-ray film, intra-arterial digital subtraction angiography is quicker, the images are easier to manipulate and store, contrast resolution is better although spatial resolution is less, but there is no evidence that less contrast is used or that it is much safer (Warnock *et al.* 1993) (Fig. 6.26). Neither *intravenous* digital subtraction angiography (IVDSA) nor arch aortography is a satisfactory alternative to selective intra-arterial angiography. So often the images are poor and stenoses impossible to measure (particularly with IVDSA), vessels may overlap, there is no accurate information about intracranial vessels and the techniques are not necessarily safer (Pelz *et al.* 1985; Rothwell *et al.* 1998). Even with selective angiography, there can be difficulty distinguishing occlusion from extreme internal carotid artery stenosis, and then late views are needed to see contrast eventually passing up into the head (Fig. 6.27).

Measuring the severity of carotid stenosis on catheter angiograms

Biplanar, but preferably triplanar (Jeans *et al.* 1986), views of the carotid bifurcation are required so that the residual lumen can be seen without overlap of other vessels, measured at the narrowest point, and then compared with a suitable denominator to derive the percentage diameter stenosis. This is the measurement on which decisions concerning carotid endarterectomy have to be made because this is what the randomized controlled trials used (section 16.8.5). The resid-

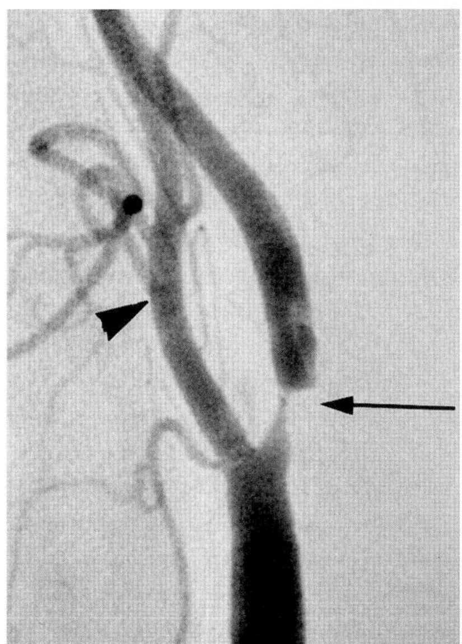

Fig. 6.26 Anteroposterior view of a selective intra-arterial digital subtraction catheter carotid angiogram showing stenosis (arrow) at the origin of the internal carotid artery which can be differentiated easily from the external carotid artery (arrowhead) because the former has no branches in the neck.

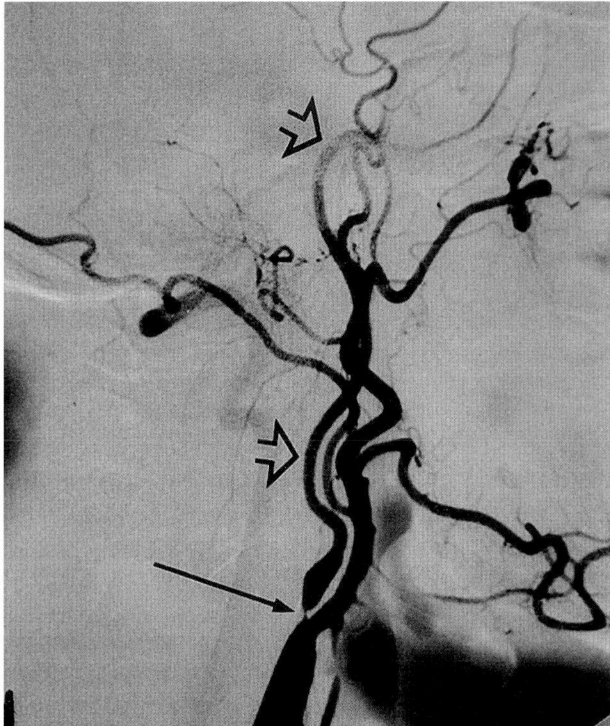

Fig. 6.27 Lateral view of selective catheter carotid angiogram showing almost complete occlusion of the internal carotid artery (arrow) with poor flow distal to the lesion (open arrows) and delayed filling of the carotid siphon. Normally the carotid siphon fills well before the branches of the external carotid artery.

ual lumen *alone* is unsatisfactory, because normal arteries vary in size between individuals and are larger in men than women, and there is also variation in the X-ray magnification factor between different centres. Area stenosis is impossible to measure on catheter angiograms.

The severity of any carotid stenosis must be measured as accurately as possible; guesswork is unacceptable.

There are three possible denominators which can be used (Fig. 6.28). The distal internal carotid artery (ICA)—the North American Symptomatic Carotid Endarterectomy Trial (NASCET)—method tends to underestimate the severity of stenosis at the origin of the ICA because the normal carotid bulb is wider than the distal ICA, and also because distal to severe stenosis the ICA may collapse, increasingly so above a European Carotid Surgery Trial (ECST) measured stenosis of about 50%. On the other hand, at least the denominator to be measured can be seen. The *estimated* diameter at the site of the stenosis, which is usually but not always at the carotid bulb, measures the lesion at the right place but does require some imagination to imagine where the original arterial lumen once *was* (the ECST method). There is least inter-observer variability using the diameter of the normal common carotid artery (the common carotid method). This is almost always seen on selective angiograms, does not vary in size very much in the portion just proximal to the carotid bifurcation, is seldom affected by disease so that a normal part is easy to find, and bears a reasonably constant relationship to the diameter of the normal carotid bulb and distal ICA (Rothwell *et al.* 1994b; Young *et al.* 1996a,b). None the less, it is quite possible for two observers to differ in their assessment of moderate/severe stenosis by 10% and so surgical guidelines or decisions based on a few stenosis percentage points are unrealistic. A rough idea of stenosis in deciles is probably all that can realistically be expected. It would therefore be entirely inappropriate to favour surgery for 71% stenosis and not for 69% stenosis (the patient clearly has *roughly* 70% stenosis), particularly as additional factors are now suspected to weigh in the surgical decision (section 16.8.9).

Increasing stenosis measured by all three methods predicts equally well the risk of ipsilateral ischaemic stroke and they are therefore all valid in this sense (Rothwell *et al.* 1994a). Fortunately, it is easy to convert the measurement by one method to either of the other two because they are all linearly related, at least within the moderate and severe stenosis range (Rothwell *et al.* 1994b). The ECST and common carotid method give essentially identical results and can be converted to the NASCET measurement by the formula:

NASCET % stenosis =
(ECST or common carotid stenosis % − 40)/0.6.

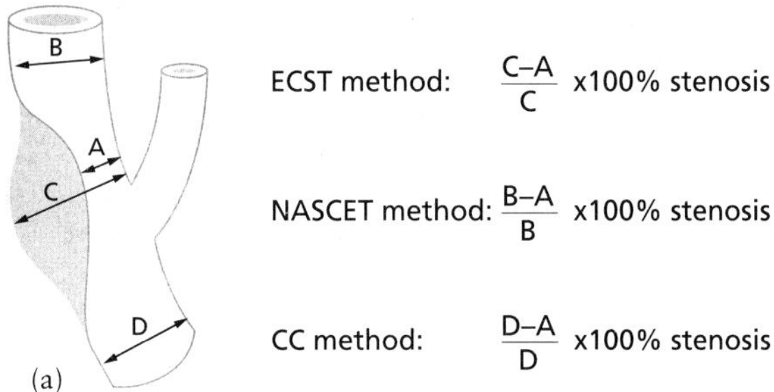

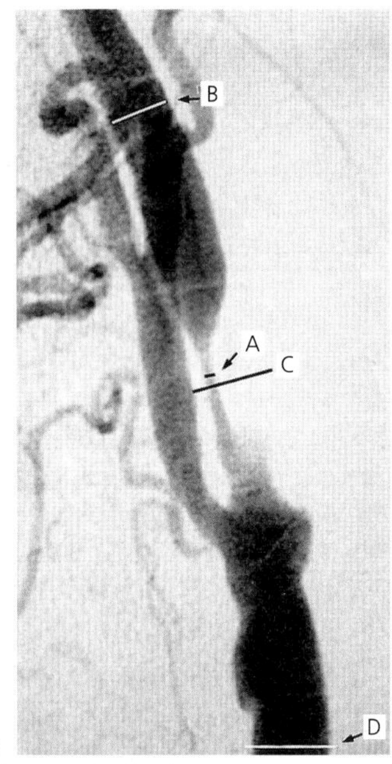

Fig. 6.28 (a) Three methods of measuring percentage diameter stenosis at the origin of the internal carotid artery (ICA) in the neck. All use as the numerator the minimum residual lumen where the stenosis is most severe (A). However, the denominator differs. In the European Carotid Surgery Trial (ECST) method, it is an *estimate* (C) of the normal lumen diameter at the site of the stenosis (whether this is at the bifurcation, more distal in the ICA or in the distal common carotid artery). In the North American Symptomatic Carotid Endarterectomy Trial (NASCET) method, it is the diameter of the ICA lumen when it becomes normal and free of disease, usually well beyond the bulb (B), and in the cases of near occlusion of the ICA an arbitrary 95% stenosis is assigned. In the common carotid method, it is the diameter of the common carotid artery proximal to the bifurcation, where it is free of disease and the diameter is fairly constant (D). (b) An illustrative example from a carotid angiogram in which A–D correspond with the measurements described in (a) above. The stenosis measures 89% by the ECST method, 88% by the common carotid method and 85% by the NASCET method.

It might be imagined that irregularity of an atherothrombotic plaque on an angiogram suggests plaque ulceration, instability, complicating thrombosis and embolism, and therefore predicts what really matters, i.e. ipsilateral ischaemic stroke. However, angiography tends to underestimate the ulceration observed by vascular surgeons and pathologists. It is not clear what the 'gold-standard' of ulceration is supposed to be, either at post-mortem or by imaging, and there is considerable inter-observer variability in the angiographic diagnosis of 'ulceration' (Streifler *et al.* 1994; Rothwell *et al.* 1998). Rather surprisingly perhaps, angiographic irregularity of a stenotic plaque does predict a higher risk of stroke than if the plaque is smooth, given the same degree of stenosis (Eliasziw *et al.* 1994; Rothwell *et al.* 2000b). What effect the angiographic demonstration of a 'floating thrombus' has on the risk of stroke is unknown (Martin *et al.* 1992).

At present therefore the main *angiographic* criteria for the prediction of ipsilateral ischaemic stroke are, despite some inter-observer variability, percentage diameter stenosis, together with plaque irregularity/ulceration. It is mainly on these criteria that the carotid endarterectomy surgery decision is currently made because it was these *angiographic* measurements that the trials used to classify the randomized patients (section 16.8.9).

Duplex sonography

This technique combines real-time ultrasound imaging to display the arterial anatomy combined with pulsed Doppler flow analysis at any point of interest in the vessel lumen (Fig. 6.29). Its accuracy is enhanced and it is technically easier to carry out if the Doppler signals are colour-coded to show the direction of blood flow and its velocity. Power Doppler and intravenous echocontrast may also help (Furst *et al.* 1992; Griewing *et al.* 1996; Droste *et al.* 1999b). The degree of carotid lumenal stenosis is calculated not only from the real-time ultrasound image, which can be inaccurate when the lesion is echolucent or calcification scatters the ultrasound beam, but also from the blood flow velocities derived from the Doppler signal. If colour Doppler is not available, but only grey-scale duplex, it is usually helpful to first insonate the supraorbital artery with a simple continuous-wave Doppler probe, because *inward* flow of blood strongly suggests severe internal carotid artery (ICA) stenosis or occlusion, although not necessarily at the origin.

Although duplex sonography is non-invasive and now widely available, there are some difficulties which any ultrasound service must acknowledge and deal with:

- it is very operator dependent and so requires skill, training and considerable experience to be sure of accurate measurements of stenosis and the avoidance of pitfalls, such as confusing the external with the internal carotid artery;
- it may be difficult to interpret, particularly if there is plaque or periarterial calcification;
- it is not completely reliable in distinguishing very severe (>90%) stenosis (which is operable) from occlusion (which is not), unless used and interpreted with very great care (Furst *et al.* 1999);

(a)

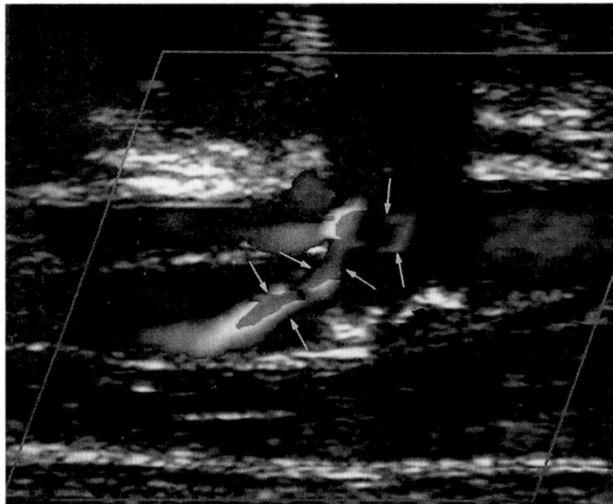

(b)

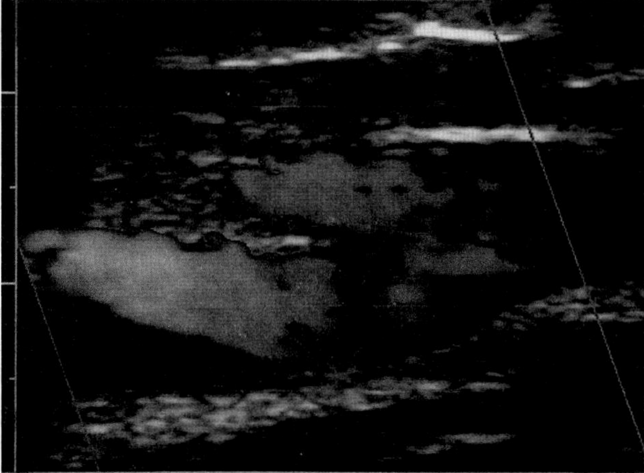

Fig. 6.29 (a) Duplex sonography examination of the carotid bifurcation to show a stenotic plaque (arrows) at the origin of the internal carotid artery. (b) Normal artery for comparison.

• it is not completely sensitive and specific for severe (70–99%) ICA stenosis;
• different machines vary in their accuracy in measuring carotid stenosis (Howard *et al.* 1996); and
• it provides little information about the proximal arterial anatomy, which is seldom affected by disease, relevant to the surgeon, or about distal anatomy. Just how often this is a really important problem is not at all clear (e.g. the position of the upper limit of the stenotic lesion, intracranial stenosis and asymptomatic intracranial aneurysms) (Griffiths *et al.* 1996).

As staff change and machines are updated, constant audit of the results against any subsequent catheter angiography is essential, but this is becoming more and more impractical as fewer angiograms are being performed (Elgersma *et al.* 1998). Another problem is that the technique is still evolving and any conclusions about accuracy in measuring the severity and character of carotid lesions can become dated, and must be applied in the context of the institution (Ringelstein 1995; Carpenter *et al.* 1996). Unfortunately, the literature comparing the accuracy of ultrasound vs. the 'gold-standard' of catheter angiography is bedevilled by poor epidemiological and statistical methods and seldom conforms to standard guidelines for evaluating this kind of diagnostic test (Blakeley *et al.* 1995; Rothwell *et al.* 2000c; P.M. Rothwell, unpublished data) (Table 6.16). None the less, with stringent quality control and confirmation of stenosis by an independent observer (see below), duplex sonography is now the most common way that carotid stenosis severe enough to warrant surgery is diagnosed.

There are no standard and commonly used definitions for the ultrasound appearance of plaques (soft, hard, calcified, etc.) and there is also considerable variation in reporting between and even within the same observers at different times (Arnold *et al.* 1999). Therefore, although unstable and ulcerated plaques are more likely to be symptomatic than stable plaques with fibrous caps (section 6.3.2), the ultrasound inaccuracy compromises any study of the relationship between plaque characteristics on duplex sonography and the risk of later stroke, and so the selection for carotid surgery (Gronholdt 1999). Indeed, the appropriate natural history studies have never been carried out, and now probably never can be, at least not in *symptomatic* patients who mostly require endarterectomy if they have severe ICA stenosis, irrespective of what the plaque looks like on ultrasound. In *asymptomatic* people, there is some evidence that a hypoechoic plaque predicts stroke risk but the numbers were small and this needs to be confirmed (Polak *et al.* 1998). Until it becomes possible to translate carotid plaque irregularity as seen on angiography, which does add to the risk of stroke over and above the degree of stenosis (section 16.8.8), into what is seen on duplex sonography, it will remain tantalis-

Table 6.16 Methodological criteria for comparing a test for measuring carotid stenosis against the 'gold-standard' of intra-arterial catheter angiography.

Prospective study design
Consecutive series of patients, or random sample
Adequate description of the study population
A spectrum of stenosis severity over the clinically relevant range
No exclusion of patients with poor images
Adequate details of the imaging techniques
Images assessed by one technique 'blind' to the images of the other
Adequate detail of exactly how the stenosis is measured by both techniques
Proper statistical methodology for comparing continuous and discontinuous variables
Reproducibility of measurements reported (inter- and intra-observer reliability)
Appropriate sample size for adequate power

ingly difficult to use anything other than stenosis to predict stroke risk if only duplex is being used.

Despite all these limitations, duplex sonography is a remarkably quick and simple investigation in experienced hands, and it is neither unpleasant nor risky. Very rarely, the pressure of the Doppler probe on the carotid bifurcation can dislodge thrombus, or cause enough carotid sinus stimulation to lead to bradycardia or hypotension (Rosario *et al.* 1987; Friedman 1990). The same conceivably applies to the various arterial compression manoeuvres which may be carried out during transcranial Doppler or extracranial Doppler sonography, and such compression should be avoided in patients who may have carotid bifurcation disease (Khaffaf *et al.* 1994; Karnik *et al.* 1995).

Reliable duplex sonography in a laboratory with stringent quality control, with any carotid stenosis confirmed by an independent observer, is now generally the best way to diagnose stenosis that is severe enough for carotid endarterectomy to be worthwhile.

CT angiography

This is a still-evolving non-invasive method used for imaging the carotid arteries (Brink *et al.* 1997). It requires a large dose of intravenous contrast to outline the arterial lumen, there is X-ray exposure, it gives only a limited view of a short segment of the neck arteries usually with no intracranial information, the images obtained depend on the proficiency of the operator in their selection, it tends to under-estimate stenosis, and so far it has not been well evaluated against the 'gold-standard' of selective intra-arterial catheter angiography. However, it does provide multiple viewing angles, three-dimensional reconstruction, and imaging of calcium deposits separately from the vessel lumen outlined by the contrast (Heiken *et al.* 1993; Leclerc *et al.* 1995) (Fig. 6.30).

Magnetic resonance angiography

Although non-invasive and safe, magnetic resonance angiography (MRA) alone is unlikely to be accurate enough in estimating carotid stenosis, at least at the present stage of development (Graves 1997). The pictures are not always adequate to allow measurement of the carotid stenosis (movement and swallowing artifacts are particular problems); the severity of the stenosis tends to be overestimated; there may be a flow gap distal to a stenosis as little as 60%, making precise stenosis measurement impossible, and even in the posterior part of the carotid bulb, in both cases probably because of loss of laminar flow and increased residence times of the blood; irregularity/ulceration are not well seen; and severe stenosis can be confused with occlusion (Siewert *et al.* 1995;

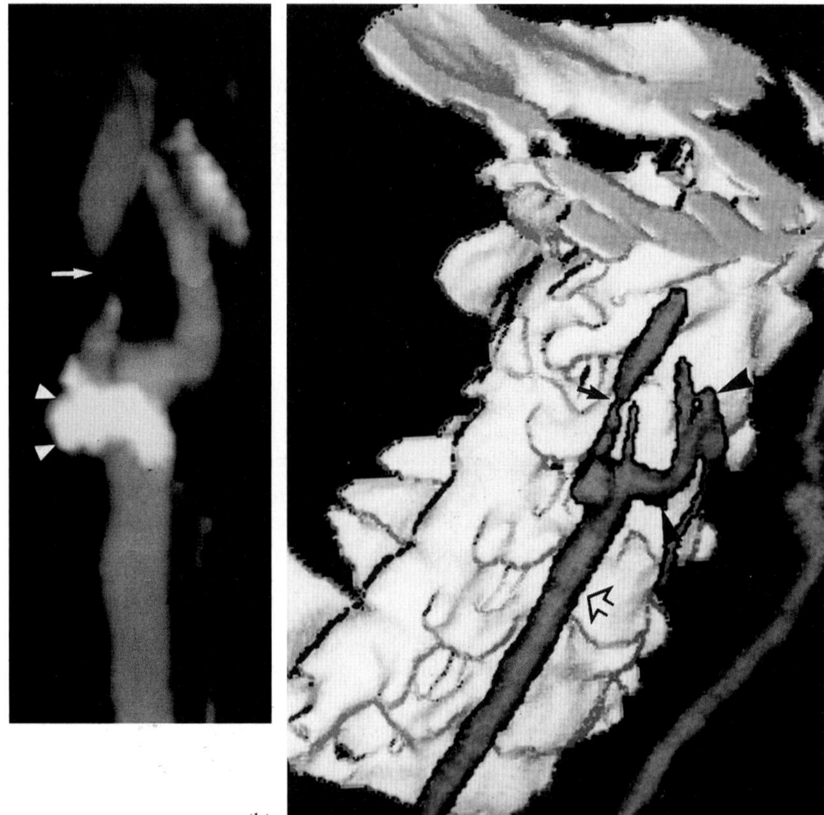

Fig. 6.30 CT angiogram of the carotid bifurcation. (a) Two-dimensional reconstruction to show severe stenosis at the origin of the internal carotid artery (arrow) as well as areas of calcification of the distal common carotid artery (arrow heads). (b) Three-dimensional reconstruction of the same artery to show the relationship with the cervical vertebrae. Common carotid artery (open arrow), internal carotid stenosis (arrow) and external carotid artery and branches (arrowheads).

Levi *et al.* 1996) (Fig. 6.31). So far, there have not been enough methodologically sound comparisons (Table 6.16) of MRA with intra-arterial catheter angiography to distinguish between bias and imprecision over the whole range of stenosis. The comparative studies that have been carried out have been frequently overtaken by changes in MR technology. At present, MRA is expensive, not readily available and claustrophobic for some people, requires the patient to lie still for several minutes, and may be contraindicated if there is any metal in the body (section 5.3.6).

Present policy (Fig. 6. 25)

At present, in all recently symptomatic 'carotid' patients who are fit for and willing to consider carotid endarterectomy, we first perform duplex sonography, if possible blinded to which carotid artery is symptomatic to avoid observer bias. When resources are limited, it may be possible to be a little more selective based on the presence of a carotid bruit and the neurological syndrome (Mead *et al.* 1999b). If the first duplex shows stenosis above about 70% or occlusion, and the patient is still prepared to consider surgery, another observer is asked (blinded to the results of the first duplex) to repeat the duplex (either CT or MR angiography are acceptable non-invasive alternatives if more convenient). From time to time, without their knowledge, it is important to ask the second observer to examine a normal patient to avoid too much a priori bias of severe stenosis during the confirmatory examination. If *both* observers agree that the patient has stenosis, within about 10% points of each other, then the option of surgery is considered further (section 16.8.9). If the observers disagree, then selective catheter angiography is recommended, but usually only of the symptomatic artery to keep any risk to a minimum. However, there are arguments in favour of performing angiography in all patients when a single duplex suggests severe carotid stenosis or occlusion. The difficulty is balancing the risk of catheter angiography and causing a stroke, or a delay during which a stroke occurs, against the risk of missing a surgically treatable stenosis and the patient going on to have a preventable stroke, or of over-diagnosing a severe stenosis with duplex and so exposing the patient to unnecessary surgery.

6.7.6 Frequent vertebrobasilar transient ischaemic attacks

Frequent vertebrobasilar transient ischaemic attacks (TIAs), thought to be caused by atherothromboembolism and unresponsive to antiplatelet drugs or anticoagulants, are unusual. It is not clear that vascular surgery has much to offer other than in the rather special situation of subclavian steal (section 16.12). There is seldom, therefore, a need to visualize the vertebral and basilar arteries. Where this is necessary, ultrasound should be used in the first instance but, because it is more difficult than in the carotid circulation, it may be necessary to use intra-arterial digital subtraction aortography followed by selective catheterization of the vertebral arteries, with intracranial as well as neck views. However, this policy may change with improvements in ultrasound and MR technology. Depending on the surgical approach proposed, it may also be necessary to image the carotid arteries.

Although asymptomatic *subclavian steal* is quite common (reversed vertebral artery flow detected by ultrasound or vertebral angiography), *symptomatic* subclavian steal is rare, presumably because collateral blood flow to the brainstem is enough to compensate for the reversed vertebral artery blood flow distal to ipsilateral subclavian stenosis or occlusion (section 4.2.3). The clinical syndrome is quite easily recognized by unequal blood pressures between the two arms, a supraclavicular bruit and vertebrobasilar TIAs, which may or may not be brought on by exercise of the arm ipsilateral to the subclavian stenosis or occlusion, so increasing blood flow down the vertebral artery from the brainstem to the arm muscles (Fields & Lemak 1972; Bohmfalk *et al.* 1979; Born-

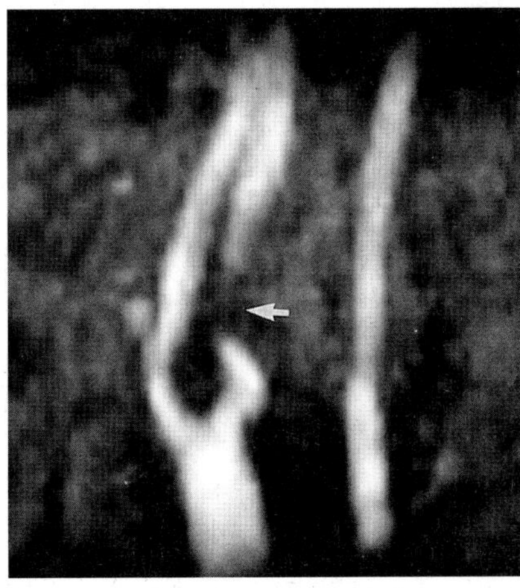
(a)

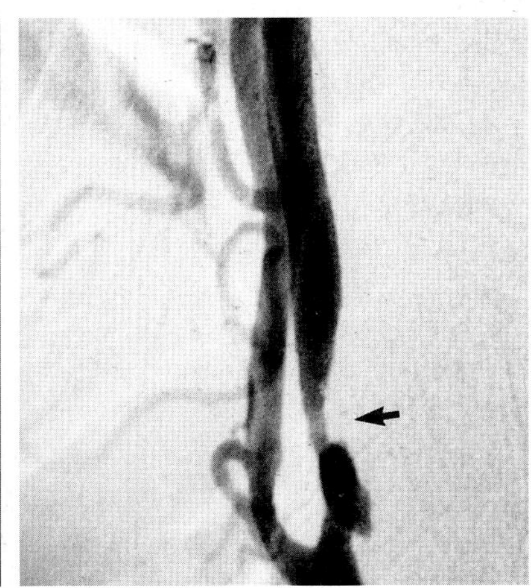
(b)

Fig. 6.31 (a) MR angiogram (three-dimensional time of flight) showing severe internal carotid stenosis. While the stenosis is clearly 'severe', it is not possible to measure its exact severity because of the 'flow gap' (arrow) distal to the lesion. (b) On the other hand, catheter angiography shows the lesion clearly (arrow) so that a stenosis of 82% (by the European Carotid Surgery Trial or common carotid artery method) or 71% (by the North American Symptomatic Carotid Endarterectomy Trial method) can be measured. The marked irregularity of the surface of the stenosis is also clearly visible, whereas this feature was lost on the MRA.

stein & Norris 1986; Hennerici *et al.* 1988). It is only this sort of symptomatic patient who may require surgery and therefore who has to accept the risk of any preceding angiography. *Innominate artery steal* is even rarer, with retrograde vertebral artery flow distal to innominate rather than subclavian artery occlusion (Kempczinski & Hermann 1979; Grosveld *et al.* 1988).

6.7.7 The diagnosis of cervical arterial dissection

Although arterial dissection tends to heal without any treatment, and many physicians do not use anticoagulants or any other specific treatment (section 7.2.1), it is still often necessary to make a definitive diagnosis because this aborts unnecessary further investigation to look for the cause of an ischaemic stroke or transient ischaemic attack; there may be medicolegal issues, such as litigation against some assailant or other person responsible for any trauma; and the patient (and their life insurance company, employers, etc.) can be reassured that the risk of recurrence is more or less zero. The 'gold-standard' imaging was, until recently, intra-arterial catheter angiography because ultrasound was neither specific nor sensitive enough to rely on. However, there is increasing evidence that cross-sectional MRI, to show thrombus within the widened arterial wall, combined with magnetic resonance angiography, is the safer and perhaps now the best option, at least when it is definitively diagnostic (Fig. 7.2).

6.7.8 Vascular imaging in acute ischaemic stroke

Patients with ischaemic stroke may have symptomatic atheromatous stenosis of their extracranial carotid artery and be candidates for carotid endarterectomy. Severe internal carotid artery origin stenosis can be excluded by duplex sonography once there is enough recovery to make surgery a possible option. What possible other reasons are there to take the risk of intra-arterial catheter angiography within the first few hours and days of onset? This issue is much debated and may be resolved, at least the safety aspects, by the further development of MRI, MR angiography, CT angiography and transcranial Doppler sonography. In the current state of knowledge, particularly about interventions to improve stroke outcome, there are not many reasons to want to know the state of the intra- or extracranial circulation outside research protocols:

• In theory, therapeutic thrombolysis should only be effective if a cerebral artery is still blocked by an embolus or thrombus, and so treatment may be not only unnecessary but also dangerous, if the artery is open, by causing haemorrhagic transformation. It therefore makes sense, in theory, to image the cerebral circulation before treatment starts (section 11.5). However, not only is this impractical in most centres but, even with catheter angiography, the small perforating vessels cannot be seen well enough, and none of the trials have addressed whether lacunar ischaemic strokes are as eligible for treatment as those with occlusion of a major cerebral artery (section 11.5.2). Indeed, if 'time is brain', there is almost no time even to exclude intracerebral haemorrhage with CT before starting thrombolysis, and so any intervening arterial imaging is going to have to be extraordinarily quick and widely available 24 h a day, if it is to add anything to management. Transcranial Doppler sonography may become an alternative, but this is insensitive to anything other than occlusion of major cerebral arteries (section 6.7.9).

• Suspicion of traumatic arterial dissection (sections 6.7.7 and 7.2.1).

• An unsuspected aneurysm of the extra- or intracranial circulation large enough to contain thrombus which might embolize to the brain or eye. This is very rare, but surgery may be required to clip or remove an aneurysm, or anticoagulation might be indicated (section 7.6).

• Fibromuscular dysplasia is sometimes found, but whether and how it should be treated is not at all clear (section 7.4).

• The beading and narrowing of cerebral arteries seen in some cases of vasculitis is neither a specific nor sensitive feature. This diagnosis is better made by serological tests, extracranial tissue biopsy (renal, skin, etc.) or by meningeal/cortical biopsy, if clinically justifiable (section 7.3).

• Moyamoya syndrome is exceedingly rare and any treatment possibilities are severely limited (section 7.5).

6.7.9 Transcranial Doppler sonography

Essentially, transcranial Doppler (TCD) sonography provides information on the velocity of blood flow and its direction in relation to the ultrasound probe, in the major intracranial arteries at the base of the brain, and so whether they are occluded or stenosed (Fig. 6.32). It is non-invasive, repeatable on demand, can be performed at the bedside, is not expensive and nor too difficult to perform accurately. It is very safe, although during tests involving compression of the carotid artery it is conceivable that emboli can be released from an underlying atheromatous plaque, and bradycardia can occur (section 6.7.5). However, the patient has to keep reasonably still; the examination can take as long as an hour; the skull is impervious to ultrasound in 5–10% of cases, more with increasing age and in females, but less if intravenous echocontrast is used; exact vessel identification may be difficult, but colour-flow real-time imaging makes this easier; spatial resolution is poor; diagnostic criteria vary; and the technique is not always accurate in comparison with cerebral catheter angiography, although not all that many patients have been compared (Ley-Pozo & Ringelstein 1990; Petty *et al.* 1990; Bornstein & Norris 1994; Baumgartner *et al.* 1997; Baumgartner 1999; Gerriets *et al.* 1999; Markus 1999).

Despite the fact that TCD, like positron emission tomography (PET), has increased our knowledge of the cerebral

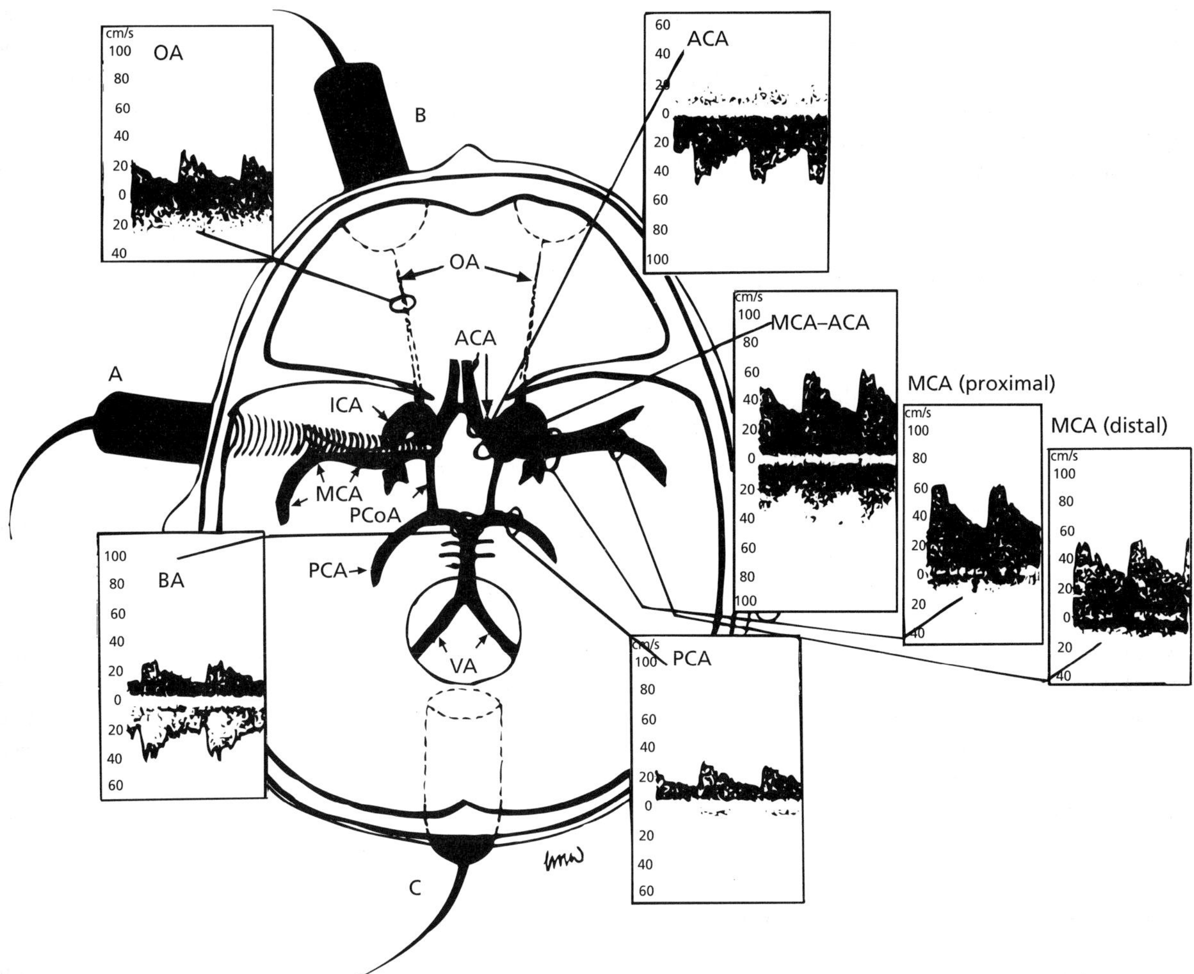

Fig. 6.32 Transcranial Doppler sonography. The base of the skull looked at from above (eyes at top of diagram) to illustrate the cranial sonographic windows (A, temporal; B, orbital; C, foramen magnum) and typical waveforms obtained from the major intracranial arteries. Note that the power output of the transducer must be reduced to 10% of the maximum for the transorbital approach to avoid damage to the eyes. ACA, anterior cerebral artery; BA, basilar artery; ICA, internal carotid artery; MCA, middle cerebral artery; OA, ophthalmic artery; PCA, posterior cerebral artery; PCoA, posterior communicating artery; VA, vertebral artery.

circulation in health and disease, and even though it is inexpensive and quite widely available and repeatable on demand (very unlike PET), it still has rather a minor role in *routine* clinical management. As well as monitoring during carotid endarterectomy (section 16.8.2), the diagnosis of patent foramen ovale (section 6.5) (Table 6.19), sickle cell disease (section 7.9), and perhaps in the future in helping define stroke risk (Babikian *et al.* 1997; Molloy & Markus 1999), there are three other possible indications: display of intracranial arterial occlusion and stenosis; emboli detection; and assessment of cerebrovascular reactivity.

Display of intracranial arterial occlusion and stenosis

Stenosis can be difficult to distinguish from hyperaemia because both increase velocity flow, but TCD can display occlusion of the MCA mainstem if not the branches, of the anterior cerebral artery and, less easily, of the basilar and posterior cerebral arteries. However, at present, this information is of limited *clinical* relevance because it does not really influence management although it might if it was known that thrombolysis, or any other treatment for acute ischaemic stroke, was only indicated if a large artery was *either* open *or* closed (section 11.5.2). It would not help with occlusion of smaller arteries which cannot be seen.

Emboli detection

What may become of more clinical relevance is the detection of emboli as high-intensity transient signals on the sonogram, so-called microembolic signals (MES) (Fig. 6.33). However, there is still controversy surrounding the interpretation of MES and difficulty excluding artifact, distinguishing gaseous from solid material and being sure of the exact

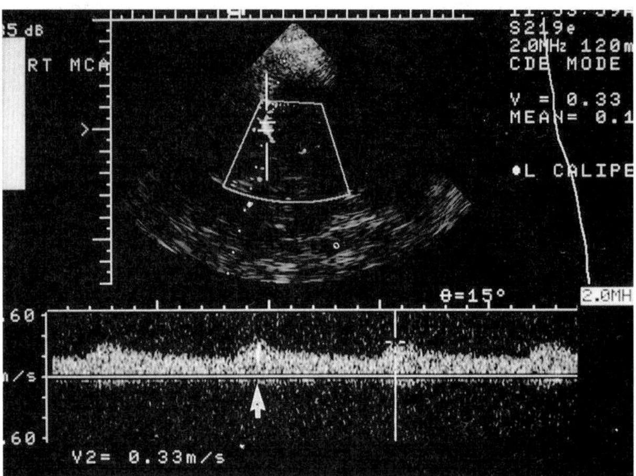

Fig. 6.33 Transcranial Doppler signals from the middle cerebral artery. Arrow shows the high intensity microembolic signal (MES) of an embolus. Note that the embolic signal does not extend beyond the Doppler trace and is of higher intensity (brightness) than the rest of the Doppler signal.

nature of the latter. Also, the methods and criteria for MES detection are not yet standardized (Babikian *et al.* 1994; Ringelstein *et al.* 1998; Smith *et al.* 1998). Although the vast majority of MES appear to be asymptomatic, their detection may help in distinguishing cardiac and aortic arch from carotid emboli, because with the first two, emboli should be detected in several arterial distributions, whereas with the last in only the one arterial distribution distal to the supposed embolic source (Markus *et al.* 1994; Sliwka *et al.* 1997). However, the frequency of MES can be so frustratingly low and variable that their detection requires prolonged monitoring and automation (Markus *et al.* 1999). Conceivably, MES detection might help distinguish organic from hysterical events, be used to monitor acute ischaemic stroke treatment, surgical or medical, and as a surrogate outcome in trials of secondary prevention of stroke.

Assessment of cerebrovascular reactivity

Transcranial Doppler sonography can also be used to assess cerebrovascular reactivity, i.e. the capacity for intracranial vasodilatation in response to acetazolamide, carbon dioxide inhalation or breath-holding, although these three methods do not always produce concordant results (Bishop *et al.* 1986; Markus & Harrison 1992; Dahl *et al.* 1995) (section 11.1.2). However, there is still debate about exactly how to standardize this test (what exactly is 'abnormal'?) and it is not routinely used. It may even be important to recognize normal variation during the day (Ameriso *et al.* 1994). Interestingly, impaired reactivity may have some prognostic significance for identifying individual patients at particularly high risk of stroke from amongst those with carotid stenosis (section 16.8.8) and internal carotid artery occlusion (section 16.11), although the numbers studied have been very small and the situation is far from clear-cut (Derdeyn *et al.* 1999). With time, and presumably increasing collateralization, any impairment of reactivity can return to normal (Kleiser & Widder 1992; Widder *et al.* 1994; Gur *et al.* 1996; Vernieri *et al.* 1999). It is unclear whether the supposed high risk of stroke is because of low cerebral blood flow, or embolism from carotid stenosis or from the distal end of a carotid arterial occlusion, facilitated perhaps by a poor collateral blood supply.

The assessment of cerebrovascular reserve is still not standardized and so far it is unclear whether it has any clinical relevance.

6.7.10 Imaging the coronary circulation

Symptomatic coronary heart disease (CHD) is very common in transient ischaemic attack (TIA) and ischaemic stroke patients; about one-third have angina or have had a myocardial infarction (Table 6.3). It clearly requires the usual cardiological investigation and treatment. In addition, a substantial proportion of patients *without* symptomatic CHD have evidence of subclinical coronary artery lesions, the exact figure depending on how intensively the patients are investigated (section 6.3.1). Therefore, it is hardly surprising that the future risk of serious coronary events is high (section 16.1.1). However, the detection of *asymptomatic* coronary artery disease does not at present influence the long-term management of ischaemic stroke/TIA patients because vascular risk factors will be treated and antithrombotic drugs used anyway, and it is unknown whether coronary artery surgery has any impact on the long-term prognosis in this category of patient. There is no indication therefore for exercise ECG testing, thallium-201 dipyridamole scintigraphy or coronary angiography, unless the patient has cardiac symptoms or other reasons, such as an abnormal resting ECG, to suggest coronary artery disease requiring surgical treatment.

6.7.11 Lumbar puncture

Lumbar puncture is certainly not a routine investigation. It is of no use in differentiating primary intracerebral haemorrhage from ischaemic stroke (section 5.3.2) although it still has an important place in CT scan-negative sudden headache (section 5.6.3). It can be dangerous if there is an infarct or haematoma causing brain shift or obstruction to cerebrospinal fluid (CSF) flow, and in anticoagulated patients it can be complicated by spinal haemorrhage. It is only useful if there is diagnostic doubt and a possibility of encephalitis, meningitis or multiple sclerosis, or if there is concern that any stroke was caused by infectious meningitis, such as syphilis or tuberculosis. Normally, there is no change in the CSF after acute ischaemic stroke but there can be up to 100 white blood cells/mm^3, more if there have been septic emboli to the brain (Powers 1986).

6.7.12 Electroencephalogram

Infarcts, or haemorrhages, involving the cerebral cortex are likely to cause ipsilateral slowing of the electroencephalogram (EEG), but there are better clinical and imaging ways of distinguishing them from deep lesions such as lacunar infarcts. If the diagnosis of stroke is unclear and encephalitis or some other generalized encephalopathy are possibilities, or even Creutzfeldt–Jakob disease, then a bilaterally abnormal EEG would weigh against stroke. Also, when there is confusion between stroke and epilepsy masquerading as stroke, or epilepsy making an old stroke seem worse (sections 15.5 and 15.8), focal seizure activity on the EEG is informative (Faught 1993). An EEG may also help distinguish a transient ischaemic attack from focal epilepsy (section 3.4.2) but a *routine* EEG is not necessary.

6.7.13 Cost-effectiveness

Wherever there is uncertainty, as there certainly is in how far to investigate stroke patients, there is always considerable variation in practice between and within countries—and doctors. Not everyone will agree with our views on the investigation of ischaemic stroke/transient ischaemic attack patients. However, we must emphasize that the criteria for *any* investigation have nothing to do with scientific curiosity or financial profit which can both so easily distort recommendations. We are only interested if the result of an investigation is likely to influence the patient's management in a useful way, without unacceptable risk. What is meant by 'unacceptable' must depend on the *balance* of the risk of investigation and the risk of *not* doing the investigation and so prejudicing a patient's outcome; this balance will surely change as new and safer investigations are developed, and treatments improve. Thus, we are 'minimalist' and should, as a result, be cost-effective. Naturally, we would be the first to acknowledge that the precise *cost* of most investigations is rarely known, although the *charges* may be. The charges do not necessarily reflect the costs, but rather whether the charger wishes to make a profit or is prepared to stand a loss, and also on what the market will bear. However, even this minimalist approach could be seen as over-investigation if, for example, it was decided that carotid endarterectomy was not cost-effective in stroke prevention (section 18.4.1), in which case duplex sonography would hardly ever be needed. On the other hand, those who are more aggressive in their treatments with a view to changing the management of their patients (in our view, very often relying on theory rather than evidence from randomized trials and meta-analysis), would clearly regard our minimalist investigation strategy as sloppy and seriously lacking in detail, perhaps even negligent.

How far a patient is investigated for the cause of their stroke or transient ischaemic attack depends on how the results of any investigation will influence treatment decisions, and these treatment decisions will depend on how far one is driven by theory rather than evidence based on randomized trials and meta-analysis.

What would probably improve cost-effectiveness more than anything else is a quick and efficient method to perform the routine investigations and get the results into the patients' notes without having to repeat tests which go 'missing', as well as minimizing or even abolishing hospital stay. With luck, as more and more hospitals become 'computerized', all the test results for individual patients, and even radiological images, will be available on terminals in the ward, out-patient department and doctor's office. Avoiding one unnecessary day in hospital, because an angiogram has been postponed, could pay for hundreds of full blood counts or serological tests for syphilis. The efficient use of the resources available is likely to be more productive and achievable than complaining about resources that are not available, at least up to a point. A counter-example would be that, without having duplex technology, which is somewhat costly, catheter angiography would either have to be performed for all patients potentially suitable for carotid endarterectomy at considerable risk, or none of them, which would deny stroke prevention to at least some individuals. Therefore, without duplex sonography, one could not possibly have a cost-effective carotid endarterectomy service.

The debate about cost-effectiveness should ideally concentrate on where the real money is (such as MR angiography) and not on inexpensive investigations (such as the erythrocyte sedimentation rate) which, even if performed in extremely large numbers, will have a negligible impact on the overall investigation budget. Moreover, the cost of investigation must be seen within the context of the total hospital costs of stroke. Even in a specialist neuroscience unit, the investigation cost is only about 12% of the budget, while in general internal medical and geriatric units, where the vast majority of strokes are managed, the proportion is less than 2% (section 17.7).

6.8 Identifying the three most common causes of ischaemic stroke and transient ischaemic attack

About 95% of ischaemic strokes and transient ischaemic attacks (TIAs) are caused by atherothromboembolism, small vessel disease or embolism from the heart (Fig. 6.1). The rarities may or may not be reasonably obvious from the clinical history, examination and routine first-line investigations and should be looked for particularly assiduously, with further appropriate investigations, where they are most likely to be present, i.e. in young and middle-aged patients, or if there is no good evidence for one of three main causes of cerebral ischaemia or any of the main stroke risk factors (hypertension, smoking, diabetes mellitus, carotid bruit, and evidence of coronary or peripheral vascular disease). There may the problem of two, three or even four competing causes for cerebral ischaemia in an individual patient. If this is the case, one must concentrate on the treatable. In the region of 10% of patients have evidence of both atherothrombosis and a cardiac source of embolism (De Bono & Warlow 1981; Bogousslavsky *et al.* 1986a), while about two-thirds of patients with an identifiable rare cause of cerebral ischaemia also have one or more of the common vascular risk factors (Table 6.17). Naturally, if a TIA patient definitely has giant cell arteritis then that should be treated, whether or not the patient also has hypertension and atrial fibrillation (AF). As the giant cell arteritis comes under control, one should consider lowering the blood pressure and using anticoagulants or antiplatelet drugs.

In the first minutes of first medical contact, all that is available is the clinical syndrome but this can take one a long way towards establishing the cause, and then a CT brain scan is usually required to rule out cerebral haemorrhage (section 5.3.4). In the next few hours and days, during which further investigations can be carried out, a more precise idea of the cause may be formed which, although useless for influencing any acute treatment, may modify further management. The stroke clinical syndrome is not very helpful in deciding *between* more than one competing cause in an individual patient, although a lacunar event is *unlikely* to be caused by embolism from the heart, aorta or carotid bifurcation, even if one or more of these embolic sources are present. None the less, many physicians feel that severe carotid stenosis should be operated on, and patients with non-rheumatic AF should be anticoagulated, even if the patient has had a recent lacunar ischaemic stroke.

Table 6.17 Non-atheromatous, non-cardioembolic conditions causing or predisposing to ischaemic stroke amongst 244 cases of first-ever-in-a-lifetime ischaemic stroke in the Oxfordshire Community Stroke Project. (Adapted from Sandercock *et al.* 1989.)

	Total number	Percentage
Arteritis	9	4
Migraine	7	3
Major surgery	3	1
Inflammatory bowel disease	3	1
Neck trauma	2	1
Carcinoma of the thyroid	1	< 1
Autoimmune disease*	1	< 1
Leukaemia	1	< 1
Oral contraceptive use (in the past)	1	< 1
Total	28†	12

* One patient with rheumatoid arthritis, glomerulonephritis and myasthenia gravis.

† Eighteen of these 28 patients also had one or more vascular risk factors (hypertension, heart disease, peripheral vascular disease, cervical bruit, diabetes mellitus, etc.), making the exact cause of their ischaemic stroke uncertain. Non-atheromatous, non-embolic conditions were the *only* predisposing factors in 10 of the 244 patients (4%).

Our guidelines to distinguish the three main causes of ischaemic stroke/TIA are based on commonsense and the scientific literature, as far as it goes, but have not and cannot be thoroughly validated, because there is no 'gold-standard' to define the cause in *every* case (Table 6.18). Even for those who die, the post-mortem can still leave uncertainties. Therefore, uncertainty must be accepted and, given the difficulty in defining a precise cause in an individual patient, it is not surprising that in many cases—depending on the diagnostic criteria and how far investigation is taken—no certain cause is found; 40% in the study by Adams *et al.* (1993). However, in clinical practice, the exact cause is less important than deciding what to do next, if anything, i.e. would the result of a particular investigation, and knowing the cause of the stroke, influence the choice of treatment for *this* particular case? For example, one would not anticoagulate a fibrillating stroke patient who was an elderly alcoholic. It then really does not matter whether the infarct was lacunar caused by small vessel disease and so perhaps nothing to do with the AF, or cortical and more likely to be caused by embolism from the heart. Although it is uncertain whether the AF caused the stroke, at least it is certain that anticoagulation is unwise and aspirin could be prescribed instead. If a patient has a patent foramen ovale (PFO) and no other cause of cerebral ischaemia, then paradoxical embolism *might* have been responsible, but because it is unclear what the risk of recurrence is, or whether antithrombotic drugs or surgical closure of the defect influences this risk (section 6.5), then in a sense the PFO is a *clinical* irrelevance. However, it would be of great *scientific* interest if a large number of similar patients were followed-up to study the risk of recurrence so that future clinical practice could be improved.

It is very difficult, and usually impossible, to be sure of the actual cause of an ischaemic stroke or transient ischaemic attack if several potential causes are present in the same individual, and sometimes even if only one is present.

6.8.1 Atherothromboembolism

Although atherothromboembolism is the most common cause of ischaemic stroke/transient ischaemic attack (TIA), about 50% of patients have other causes and so it must not be assumed that every case results from this admittedly common vascular disorder (section 6.3). More positive evi-

Table 6.18 The strength of the evidence for the three main causes of ischaemic stroke and transient ischaemic attack in an individual patient based on a number of clinical variables and investigations.

Variable	Atherothrombo-embolism	Small vessel disease	Embolism from the heart
Age	>50	>50	Any
Total/partial anterior circulation ischaemia (clinical syndrome ± brain imaging)	+++	–	+++
Lacunar ischaemia (clinical syndrome ± brain imaging)	+	+++	+
Boundary-zone ischaemia (brain imaging)	+++	–	–
Posterior cerebral artery ischaemia (clinical syndrome ± brain imaging)	+++	+	+++
Brainstem ischaemia (clinical syndrome ± brain imaging)	++	++	++
Cerebellar ischaemia (clinical syndrome ± brain imaging)	++	+	++
Cholesterol retinal emboli	+++	–	–
Calcific retinal emboli	–	–	++
Recent ischaemic episodes in >one arterial territory, particularly in more than one organ	+	–	+++
Arterial bruits (neck, legs), absent/unequal pulses (neck, arms, legs)	+++	+	–
Duplex sonography/angiogram evidence of severe stenosis/occlusion	+++	+	–
Major cardiac source of embolism	+	–	+++
Clinical evidence of atherothrombosis elsewhere (angina, myocardial infarction, claudication)	++	+	+
Vascular risk factors (hypertension, diabetes, etc.)	++	++	–
Clear evidence of an alternative cause, such as dissection, vasculitis, etc.	–	–	–

+++, Strong supportive evidence; ++, reasonable supportive evidence; +, weak evidence; –, evidence against.

Note: neither the speed of onset of symptoms nor a past history of transient ischaemic attack are helpful.

dence, if possible, is required (Table 6.18). It is not realistic to be precise in every individual, but there are some criteria which make atherothromboembolism more likely:

- a total or partial anterior circulation syndrome without any cardiac embolic source (sections 4.3.4, 4.3.5, 6.6.1 and 6.6.2);
- the presence of vascular risk factors, such as smoking and hypertension;
- absent or diminished pulses or vascular bruits, particularly over the symptomatic artery, together with duplex or angiogram-confirmed severe stenosis;
- cholesterol emboli in the retina;
- boundary-zone infarction on brain imaging.

This problem is more difficult when dealing with vertebrobasilar rather than carotid ischaemia, because there are more causal possibilities and because it is difficult to image the vertebral circulation non-invasively (section 6.7.4). However, a large infarct in the cerebellum or in the territory of the posterior cerebral artery is likely to be atherothromboembolic if there is no cardiac source of embolism.

If possible, it is worth making a positive diagnosis of atherothromboembolism because this stops the fruitless search for alternatives; it directs attention to defining the degree of any symptomatic carotid stenosis and therefore the need for carotid endarterectomy (section 16.8); it also emphasizes the control of vascular risk factors (section 16.3) and the use of antiplatelet drugs (section 16.4). It is impossible to be absolutely precise about whether an event was caused by acute arterial occlusion or low-flow, or either mechanism at different times but, fortunately, this difficulty seldom affects clinical management (section 6.6.5).

6.8.2 Intracranial small vessel disease

That an ischemic stroke or transient ischaemic attack (TIA) was caused by intracranial small vessel disease is highly likely if the clinical syndrome is lacunar—easier in stroke than TIA patients to be sure—and particularly if there is no cardiac source of embolism clinically, no clinical or ultrasound evidence of arterial disease in the neck and no reasonably obvious rare cause of stroke clinically or on the routine investigations (sections 4.3.2 and 6.6.3) (Table 6.18). It is very likely that there will be stroke risk factors but, apart from recent myocardial infarction and atrial fibrillation (AF), these are about as likely as in atherothromboembolic ischaemic stroke (section 6.4). From the *management* point of view, a positive diagnosis of small vessel disease reduces the urgency for the detection of severe carotid stenosis which, if found, is difficult to interpret. Is it really the cause by embolism or low-flow (in which case carotid endarterectomy may be indicated) or is it 'asymptomatic', in which case it probably ought to be left alone? Our view is that, even if the syndrome is lacunar, carotid endarterectomy might be recommended, but only if the patient has severe carotid stenosis on the symptomatic side and other factors in favour of surgery, as perhaps for primary stroke prevention (section 16.8.10). Others may not agree, even though there may be something to be said for carotid surgery and primary stroke prevention. We would be more likely to anticoagulate a lacunar patient in AF, even though the AF *might* not be relevant. At least we could reassure ourselves that worthwhile *primary* stroke prevention is definitely achieved by anticoagulation in patients who are able to handle the treatment (section 16.5.1).

6.8.3 Embolism from the heart

The diagnosis of ischaemic stroke or transient ischaemic attack (TIA) caused by embolism from the heart can only be considered at all if there is an identifiable cardioembolic source, which is the case in about 30% of ischaemic stroke/TIA patients (section 6.5) (Tables 6.8 and 6.9), a higher proportion in recent studies using transoesophageal echocardiography (Mast *et al.* 1994). However, in perhaps one-third the cardiac source is irrelevant, because there is another, perhaps more likely, cause of cerebral ischaemia, such as carotid stenosis (section 6.5).

Other than lacunar syndromes (which are seldom caused by cardiac embolism), the neurological or brain CT/MRI features of any cerebral ischaemic event do not reliably distinguish a cardioembolic from some other cause of ischaemic stroke (Bogousslavsky *et al.* 1986b; Kittner *et al.* 1991, 1992). Fortunately, most cardiac lesions with a substantial embolic threat can be suspected, and even definitively diagnosed, by competent clinical examination, an electrocardiogram (ECG) and a chest X-ray. In addition, *transthoracic* echocardiography may be indicated to refine the clinical diagnosis and guide the management of any suspected lesions (e.g. mitral stenosis, atrial myxoma, etc.). *Transoesophageal* echocardiography, with intravenous echo contrast, is somewhat invasive, uncomfortable, occasionally risky (bronchospasm, hypoxia, angina, cardiac dysrhythmias, vocal cord paresis, bacteraemia, pharyngeal bleeding, oesophageal laceration or perforation, and endocarditis) and perhaps difficult to perform in acute stroke (Daniel *et al.* 1991; Daniel & Mugge 1995). However, it undoubtedly provides more information (e.g. patent foramen ovale, valvular vegetations, thrombus in the left atrium, etc.) and displays atheromatous plaques in at least part of the aortic arch (Tegeler & Downes 1991; Adams & Love 1995; Donnan & Jones 1995; Stollberger *et al.* 1995) (Table 6.19). None the less, *routine* transthoracic, and certainly *routine* transoesophageal echocardiography without preceding transthoracic echocardiography, is not justifiable because the yield in unselected patients is extremely low, particularly in the crucial sense of changing management rather than collecting anatomical information for no very obvious purpose other than research. Putting patients to inconvenience and risk in the search for a diagnosis that does not then lead on to a change—preferably evidence-based—in their management cannot be justifiable (Burnett *et al.* 1984; Good *et al.* 1986; Leung *et al.* 1995; Rauh *et al.* 1996; Censori *et al.* 1998). Transthoracic and then—if necessary—transoesophageal echocardiography may well help if a cardiac source of embolism is suspected on the basis of the history (past rheumatic fever, ischaemic events in more than one vascular territory, etc.), cardiac examination (murmurs, etc.), ECG (atrial fibrillation, recent myocardial infarction), or chest X-ray (enlarged left atrium, valvular calcification), *particularly* if there is no reasonable alternative cause (such as severe symptomatic carotid stenosis, giant cell arteritis, etc.). Moreover, in young patients (<40 years) with no obvious cause of cerebral ischaemia, it is justifiable to examine the heart in considerable detail, even as far as transoesophageal echocardiography (Biller *et al.* 1986; DeRook *et al.* 1992).

It is not clear that transoesophageal echocardiography provides much more information for clinical decision-making than transthoracic echocardiography, although it certainly provides more anatomical information in selected patients.

The presence of intracardiac thrombus on echocardiography does not necessarily mean that embolism has occurred, while the absence of intracardiac thrombus does not necessarily mean that embolism has not occurred. In either case, embolism may recur sooner or later.

The decision whether an identified *potential* embolic source in the heart was *the* cause of the ischaemic stroke or TIA can be quite easy if most of the criteria in Table 6.18 are fulfilled; for example, if the patient is aged 30 years, has a prosthetic heart valve and no vascular disorder or risk factors. Also, some cardiac lesions are much more threatening causes of embolism than others (Table 6.8). On the other hand, it can be impossible; for example, if the patient is a 70-year-old and has both atrial fibrillation and severe carotid stenosis ipsilateral to a cortical infarct, when one might be tempted (correctly perhaps) to recommend anticoagulation as well as carotid endarterectomy. Some cardiac lesions are so common in the normal stroke-free population (e.g. patent foramen ovale, mitral annulus calcification) that their relevance in an individual ischaemic stroke patient is unassessable without additional evidence of embolism. One comes back to treating what is treatable (to prevent stroke recurrence), provided the risks are not thought to outweigh the potential benefits and the patient is prepared to accept the risk of treatment, as well as the benefit. Whether emboli detection with transcranial Doppler becomes helpful in sorting out the origin of emboli remains to be seen, it is certainly not a routinely available investigation as yet (section 6.7.9).

Long-term monitoring of the electrocardiogram

The frequency of cardiac dysrhythmias in transient ischaemic attack (TIA) patients is similar to the frequency in the normal population of the same age (De Bono & Warlow 1981). Therefore, unless a dysrhythmia can be shown to *coincide* with a cerebral ischaemic event (which is unlikely unless the events are occurring, if not daily, at least several times a week), its relevance (in the sense of causing hypotension and so focal cerebral ischaemia) to any neurological symptoms is profoundly uncertain. Hypotensive *focal* cerebral ischaemic events are very uncommon (section 6.6.5). We only monitor the ECG if the ischaemic events are occurring frequently enough to be captured on tape, and particularly if no embolic cause is likely, and the focal neurological symptoms are accompanied by faintness, chest pain, shortness of breath or palpitations. Treatment of the dysrhythmia might then reduce the risk of recurrent symptoms. Other indications are a patient in sinus rhythm, who *might* have paroxysmal atrial fibrillation (history of palpitations or possibly irregular pulse, etc.) and so require anticoagulation (section 16.5), or to check that any treatment to return a fibrillating patient to sinus rhythm has been effective.

Venography

Ultrasound to detect deep venous thrombosis (DVT) of the legs may be required in the rare case where paradoxical embolism is suspected (Kearon *et al.* 1998). If negative, X-ray venography of the legs or MR venography of the pelvic veins is more sensitive (Cramer *et al.* 1998) (section 15.13). Cri-

Table 6.19 Comparison of transthoracic vs. transoesophageal echocardiography for detecting potential cardiac sources of embolism.

Transthoracic echcocardiography preferred	Transoesophageal echocardiography preferred
Left-ventricular thrombus*	Left atrial thrombus*
Left-ventricular dyskinesis	Left atrial appendage thrombus*
Mitral stenosis	Spontaneous echo contrast
Mitral annulus calcification	Intracardiac tumours
Aortic stenosis	Atrial septal defect†
	Atrial septal aneurysm
	Patent foramen ovale†
	Mitral and aortic valve vegetations
	Prosthetic heart valve malfunction
	Aortic arch atherothrombosis/dissection
	Mitral valve prolapse

* The detection of intracardiac thrombus is not *necessarily* relevant, because not all thrombi embolize and the lack of intracardiac thrombus may not be relevant, either because it is too small to be detected or has all embolized already.

† A less invasive alternative is to inject air bubbles or other echocontrast material intravenously and, if there is a right-to-left intracardiac shunt, they can be detected by transcranial Doppler sonography of the middle cerebral artery, particularly with a provocative Valsalva manoeuvre. There is considerable variation in the methods and this influences the diagnostic sensitivity and specificity. It is also uncertain what size of shunt is 'clinically relevant' and some bubbles may pass to the brain through pulmonary rather than cardiac shunts (Droste *et al.* 1999c; Schwarze *et al.* 1999).

teria to suspect paradoxical embolism include (Mas 1991; Ranoux *et al.* 1993; Brogno *et al.* 1994):

• an ischaemic event occurring in the context of a Valsalva manoeuvre (lifting, straining, coughing, trumpet playing, etc.), or anything else likely to increase right-atrial pressure and so encourage blood flow from the right to left atrium;

• a patent foramen ovale identified with contrast echocardiography or transcranial Doppler sonography;

• echocardiographically visible clot in the right atrium or across the inter-atrial septum;

• a reason for DVT or pelvic venous thrombosis (e.g. recent surgery or lengthy travel); and

• no other more likely cause.

However, these clues are far from specific and sensitive for the reliable diagnosis of paradoxical embolism in an individual patient (Petty *et al.* 1997). Furthermore, any venography must be performed early (within 48 h at most) because DVT is so common as a *consequence* of stroke, particularly in a paralysed leg (Warlow 1978; Landi *et al.* 1992) (section 15.13).

References

Please note that all references taken from *The Cochrane Library* are given a current date as this database is updated on a quarterly basis. Please refer to the current *Cochrane Library* article for the latest review. The same applies to the *British Medical Journal* 'Clinical Evidence' series which is updated every six months.

Aberg, H. (1969) Atrial fibrillation. I. A study of atrial thrombosis and systemic embolism in a necropsy material. *Acta Medica Scandinavica* **185**, 373–379.

Adams, H.P. & Love, B.B. (1995) Transoesophageal echocardiography in the evaluation of young adults with ischaemic stroke: promises and concerns. *Cerebrovascular Diseases* **5**, 323–327.

Adams, H.P., Bendixen, B.H., Kappelle, L.J *et al.* (1993) Classification of subtype of acute ischaemic stroke: definitions for use in a multicentre clinical trial. *Stroke* **24**, 35–41.

Adams, R.J., Carroll, R.M., Nichols, F.T. *et al.* (1989) Plasma lipoproteins in cortical versus lacunar infarction. *Stroke* **20**, 448–452.

Adler, Y., Koren, A., Fink, N. *et al.* (1998) Association between mitral annulus calcification and carotid atherosclerotic disease. *Stroke* **29**, 1833–1837.

Agmon, Y., Khandheria, B.K., Meissner, I. *et al.* (1999) Frequency of atrial septal aneurysms in patients with cerebral ischaemic events. *Circulation* **99**, 1942–1944.

Aichner, F.T., Flever, S.R., Birbamer, G.G. & Posch, A. (1993) Magnetic resonance imaging and magnetic resonance angiography of vertebrobasilar dolichoectasia. *Cerebrovascular Diseases* **3**, 280–284.

Albert, C.M., Hennekens, C.H., O'Donnell, C.J. *et al.* (1998) Fish consumption and risk of sudden cardiac death. *Journal of the American Medical Association* **279**, 23–28.

Alberts, M.J. (1999) *Genetics of Cerebrovascular Disease*. Futura, New York.

Allan, P.L., Mowbray, P.I., Lee, A.J. & Fowkes, F.G.R. (1997) Relationship between carotid intima-media thickness and symptomatic and asymptomatic peripheral arterial disease. The Edinburgh Artery Study. *Stroke* **28**, 348–353.

Amarenco, P. & Caplan, L.R. (1993) Vertebrobasilar occlusive disease: review of selected aspects. 3. Mechanisms of cerebellar infarctions. *Cerebrovascular Diseases* **3**, 66–73.

Ameriso, S.F., Mohler, J.G., Suarez, M. & Fisher, M. (1994) Morning reduction of cerebral vasomotor reactivity. *Neurology* **44**, 1907–1909.

Anderson, D.C., Koller, R.L., Asinger, R.W., Bundlie, S.R. & Pearce, L.A. (1998) Atrial fibrillation and stroke: epidemiology, pathophysiology and management. *Neurologist* **4**, 235–258.

Angeloni, U., Bozzao, L., Fantozzi, L., Bastianello, S., Kushner, M. & Fieschi, C. (1990) Internal border-zone infarction following acute middle cerebral artery occlusion. *Neurology* **40**, 1196–1198.

Arboix, A., Garcia-Eroles, L, Massons. J.B., Oliveres, M. & Comes, E. (1997) Predictive factors of early seizures after acute cerebrovascular disease. *Stroke* **28**, 1590–1594.

Archie, J.P. & Feldtman, R.W. (1981) Critical stenosis of the internal carotid artery. *Surgery* **89**, 67–70.

Ardissino, D., Merlini, P.A., Ariens, R., Coppola, R., Bramucci, E. & Mannucci, P.M. (1997) Tissue-factor antigen and activity in human coronary atherosclerotic plaques. *Lancet* **349**, 769–771.

Arnold, J.A., Modaresi, K.B., Thomas, N., Taylor, P.R. & Padayachee, T.S. (1999) Carotid plaque characterization by duplex scanning: observer error may undermine current clinical trials. *Stroke* **30**, 61–65.

Arroll, B. & Beaglehole, R. (1993) Exercise for hypertension. *Lancet* **341**, 1248–1249.

Arruga, J. & Sanders, M.D. (1982) Ophthalmologic findings in 70 patients with evidence of retinal embolism. *Ophthalmology* **89**, 1336–1347.

Ascherio, A. & Willett, W.C. (1994) Are body iron stores related to the risk of coronary heart disease? *New England Journal of Medicine* **330**, 1119–1124.

Atrial Fibrillation Investigators (1994) Risk factors for stroke and efficacy of antithrombotic therapy in atrial fibrillation: analysis of pooled data from five randomised controlled trials. *Archives of Internal Medicine* **154**, 1449–1457.

Atrial Fibrillation Investigators (1998) Echocardiographic predictors of stroke in patients with atrial fibrillation: a prospective study of 1066 patients from 3 clinical trials. *Archives of Internal Medicine* **158**, 1316–1320.

Ay, H., Oliveira-Filho, J., Buonanno, F.S. *et al.* (1999) Diffusion-weighted imaging identifies a subset of lacunar infarction associated with embolic source. *Stroke* **30**, 2644–2650.

Babikian, V.L., Hyde, C., Pochay, V. & Winter, M.R. (1994) Clinical correlates of high-intensity transient signals detected on transcranial Doppler sonography in patients with cerebrovascular disease. *Stroke* **25**, 1570–1573.

Babikian, V.L., Wijman, C.A.C., Hyde, C. *et al.* (1997) Cerebral microembolism and early recurrent cerebral or retinal ischaemic events. *Stroke* **28**, 1314–1318.

Baigent, J., Burbury, K. & Wheeler, D. (2000) Premature cardiovascular disease in chronic renal failure. *Lancet* **356**, 147–152.

Balarajan, R. (1991) Ethnic differences in mortality from ischaemic heart disease and cerebrovascular disease in England and Wales. *British Medical Journal* **302**, 560–564.

Bamford, J.M. & Warlow, C.P. (1988) Evolution and testing of the lacunar hypothesis. *Stroke* **19**, 1074–1082.

Bamford, J., Sandercock, P., Jones, L. & Warlow, C.P. (1987) The natural history of lacunar infarction: the Oxfordshire Community Stroke Project. *Stroke* **18**, 545–551.

Bamford, J., Sandercock, P., Dennis, M. *et al.* (1988) A prospective study of acute cerebrovascular disease in the community: the Oxfordshire Community Stroke Project 1981–86. 1. Methodology, demography and incident cases of first-ever stroke. *Journal of Neurology, Neurosurgery and Psychiatry* **51**, 1373–1389.

Bamford, J., Sandercock, P., Dennis, M.S., Burn, J. & Warlow, C.P. (1990) A prospective study of acute cerebrovascular disease in the community: the Oxfordshire Community Stroke Project 1981–86. 2. Incidence, case fatality rates and overall outcome at one year of cerebral infarction, primary intracerebral and subarachnoid haemorrhage. *Journal of Neurology, Neurosurgery and Psychiatry* **53**, 16–22.

Bamford, J., Sandercock, P., Dennis, M., Burn, J. & Warlow, C. (1991) Classification and natural history of clinically identifiable subtypes of cerebral infarction. *Lancet* **337**, 1521–1526.

Barker, D.J.P. (1994) *Mothers, Babies, and Disease in Later Life*. British Medical Journal Publishing, London.

Barnett, H.J.M., Boughner, D.R., Taylor, D.W., Cooper, P.E., Kostuk, W.J. & Nichol, P.M. (1980) Further evidence relating mitral-valve prolapse to cerebral ischaemic events. *New England Journal of Medicine* **302**, 139–144.

Bathen, J., Sparr, S. & Rokseth, R. (1978) Embolism in sinoatrial disease. *Acta Medica Scandinavica* **203**, 7–11.

Baumgartner, R.W. (1999) Transcranial color-coded duplex sonography. *Journal of Neurology* **246**, 637–647.

Baumgartner, R.W. & Baumgartner, I. (1998) Vasomotor reactivity is exhausted in transient ischaemic attacks with limb shaking. *Journal of Neurology,*

Neurosurgery and Psychiatry **65**, 561–564.

Baumgartner, R.W., Mattle, H.P., Aaslid, R. & Kaps, M. (1997) Transcranial colour-coded duplex sonography in arterial cerebrovascular disease. *Cerebrovascular Diseases* **7**, 57–63.

Beck, J., Garcia, R., Heiss, G., Vokonas, P.S. & Offenbacher, S. (1996) Periodontal disease and cardiovascular disease. *Journal of Periodontology* **67**, 1123–1137.

Belden, J.R., Caplan, L.R., Pessin, M.S. & Kwan, E. (1999) Mechanisms and clinical features of posterior border-zone infarcts. *Neurology* **53**, 1312–1318.

Bendszus, M., Koltzenburg, M., Burger, R., Warmuth-Metz, M., Hofmann, E. & Solymosi, L. (1999) Silent embolism in diagnostic cerebral angiography and neurointerventional procedures: a prospective study. *Lancet* **354**, 1594–1597.

Benjamin, E.J., Plehn, J.F., D'Agostino, R. *et al.* (1992) Mitral annular calcification and the risk of stroke in an elderly cohort. *New England Journal of Medicine* **327**, 374–379.

Benjamin, E.J., D'Agostino, R.B., Belanger, A.J., Wolf, P.A. & Levy, D. (1995) Left atrial size and the risk of stroke and death. The Framingham Heart Study. *Circulation* **92**, 835–841.

Benomar, A., Yahyaoui, M., Birouk, N., Vidailhet, M. & Chkili, T. (1994) Middle cerebral artery occlusion due to hydatid cysts of myocardial and intraventricular cavity cardiac origin: two cases. *Stroke* **25**, 886–888.

Ben-Shlomo, Y., Markowe, H., Shipley, M. & Marmot, M.G. (1992) Stroke risk from alcohol consumption using different control groups. *Stroke* **23**, 1093–1098.

Berenson, G.S., Srinivasan, S.R., Bao, W. *et al.* (1998) Association between multiple cardiovascular risk factors and atherosclerosis in children and young adults. *New England Journal of Medicine* **338**, 1650–1656.

Berger, K., Ajani, U.A., Kase, C.S. *et al.* (1999) Light-to-moderate alcohol consumption and the risk of stroke among US male physicians. *New England Journal of Medicine* **341**, 1557–1564.

Berlin, J.A. & Colditz, G.A. (1990) A meta-analysis of physical activity in the prevention of coronary heart disease. *American Journal of Epidemiology* **132**, 612–628.

Berthet, K., Lavergne, T., Cohen, A. *et al.* (2000) Significant association of atrial vulnerability with atrial septal abnormalities in young patients with ischaemic stroke of unknown cause. *Stroke* **31**, 398–403.

Besson, G., Hommel, M. & Perret, J. (1991) Historical aspects of the lacunar concept. *Cerebrovascular Diseases* **1**, 306–310.

Bhadelia, R.A., Anderson, M., Polak, J.F. *et al.* for the CHS Collaborative Research Group. (1999) Prevalence and associations of MRI-demonstrated brain infarcts in elderly subjects with a history of transient ischaemic attack. The Cardiovascular Health Study. *Stroke* **30**, 383–388.

Bhatnagar, D., Anand, I.S., Durrington, P.N. *et al.* (1995) Coronary risk factors in people from the Indian subcontinent living in West London and their siblings in India. *Lancet* **345**, 405–409.

Bhopal, R., Unwin, N., White, M. *et al.* (1999) Heterogeneity of coronary heart disease risk factors in Indian, Pakistani, Bangladeshi and European origin populations: cross sectional study. *British Medical Journal* **319**, 215–220.

Biller, J., Johnson, M.R., Adams, H.P., Kerber, R.E., Toffol, G.J. & Butler, M.J. (1986) Echocardiographic evaluation of young adults with non-haemorrhagic cerebral infarction. *Stroke* **17**, 608–612.

Biousse, V., Newman, N.J. & Lessell, S. (1998) Audible pulsatile tinnitus in idiopathic intracranial hypertension. *Neurology* **50**, 1185–1186.

Bishop, C.C.R., Powell, S., Insall, M., Rutt, D. & Browse, N.L. (1986) Effect of internal carotid artery occlusion on middle cerebral artery blood flow at rest and in response to hypercapnia. *Lancet* **1**, 710–712.

Blackshear, J.L., Pearce, L.A., Hart, R.G. *et al.* (1999) Aortic plaque in atrial fibrillation: prevalence, predictors and thromboembolic implications. *Stroke* **30**, 834–840.

Bladin, C.F. & Chambers, B.R. (1993) Clinical features, pathogenesis and computed tomographic characteristics of internal watershed infarction. *Stroke* **24**, 1925–32.

Bladin, C.F. & Chambers, B.R. (1994) Frequency and pathogenesis of haemodynamic stroke. *Stroke* **25**, 2179–2182.

Blakeley, D.D., Oddone, E.Z., Hasselblad, V., Simel, D.L. & Matchar, D.B. (1995) Non-invasive carotid artery testing: a meta-analytic review. *Annals of Internal Medicine* **122**, 360–367.

Bogousslavsky, J. & Caplan, L.R. (1993) Vertebrobasilar occlusive disease: review of selected aspects. 3. Thalamic infarcts. *Cerebrovascular Diseases* **3**, 193–205.

Bogousslavsky, J. & Regli, F. (1986a) Unilateral watershed cerebral infarcts. *Neurology* **36**, 373–377.

Bogousslavsky, J. & Regli, F. (1986b) Border-zone infarctions distal to internal carotid artery occlusion: prognostic implications. *Annals of Neurology* **20**, 346–350.

Bogousslavsky, J., Hachinski, V.C., Boughner, D.R., Fox, A.J., Vinuela, F. & Barnett, H.J.M. (1986a) Cardiac and arterial lesions in carotid transient ischaemic attacks. *Archives of Neurology* **43**, 223–228.

Bogousslavsky, J., Hachinski, V.C., Boughner, D.R., Fox, A.R., Vinuela, F. & Barnett, H.J.M. (1986b) Clinical predictors of cardiac and arterial lesions in carotid ischaemic attacks. *Archives of Neurology* **43**, 229–233.

Bogousslavsky, J., van Melle, G., Regli, F. & Kappenberger, L. (1990) Pathogenesis of anterior circulation stroke in patients with non-valvular atrial fibrillations: the Lausanne Stroke Registry. *Neurology* **40**, 1046–1050.

Bogousslavsky, J., Regli, F., Despland, P.A. & Zografos, L. (1991) Optic nerve head infarction: small-artery disease, large-artery disease and cardioembolism. *Cerebrovascular Diseases* **1**, 341–344.

Bogousslavsky, J., Garazi, S., Jeanrenaud, X., Aebischer, N. & van Melle, G. for the Lausanne Stroke with Paradoxal Embolism Study Group (1996) Stroke recurrence in patients with patent foramen ovale: the Lausanne study. *Neurology* **46**, 1301–1305.

Bohmfalk, G.L., Story, J.L., Brown, W.E. & Marlin, A.E. (1979) Subclavian steal syndrome. 1. Proximal vertebral to common carotid artery transposition in three patients and historical review. *Journal of Neurosurgery* **51**, 628–640.

Boiten, J. & Lodder, J. (1993) Prognosis for survival, handicap and recurrence of stroke in lacunar and superficial infarction. *Cerebrovascular Diseases* **3**, 221–226.

Boiten, J., Rothwell, P.M., Slattery, J. & Warlow, C.P. for the European Carotid Surgery Trialists' Collaborative Group (1996) Ischaemic lacunar stroke in the European Carotid Surgery Trial: risk factors, distribution of carotid stenosis, effect of surgery and type of recurrent stroke. *Cerebrovascular Diseases* **6**, 281–287.

Bonita, R., Broad, J.B. & Beaglehole, R. (1997) Ethnic differences in stroke incidence and case fatality in Auckland, New Zealand. *Stroke* **28**, 758–761.

Bonita, R., Duncan, J., Truelson, T., Jackson, R.T. & Beaglehole, R. (1999) Passive smoking as well as active smoking increases the risk of acute stroke. *Tobacco Control* **8**, 156–160.

Bonithon-Kopp, C., Touboul, P.J., Berr, C., Magne, C. & Ducimetiere, P. (1996) Factors of carotid arterial enlargement in a population aged 59–71 years: the EVA study. *Stroke* **27**, 654–660.

Boon, A., Lodder, J., Raak, L.H-V. & Kessels, F. (1994) Silent brain infarcts in 755 consecutive patients with a first-ever supratentorial ischaemic stroke: relationship with index-stroke subtype, vascular risk factors and mortality. *Stroke* **25**, 2384–2390.

Boon, A., Lodder, J., Cheriex, E. & Kessels, F. (1996) Risk of stroke in a cohort of 815 patients with calcification of the aortic valve with or without stenosis. *Stroke* **27**, 847–851.

Bornstein, N.M. & Norris, J.W. (1986) Subclavian steal: a harmless haemodynamic phenomenon? *Lancet* **2**, 303–305.

Bornstein, N.M. & Norris, J.W. (1994) Transcranial Doppler sonography is at present of limited clinical value. *Archives of Neurology* **51**, 1057–1059.

Boshuizen, H.C., Izaks, G.J., van Buuren, S. & Ligthart, G.J. (1998) Blood pressure and mortality in elderly people aged 85) and older: community based study. *British Medical Journal* **316**, 1780–1784.

Bousser, M-G. & Ross Russell, R. (1997) *Cerebral Venous Thrombosis*. Saunders, London.

Brand, F.N., Abbott, R.D., Kannel, W.B. & Wolf, P.A. (1985) Characteristics and prognosis of lone atrial fibrillation: 30-year follow up in the Framingham study. *Journal of the American Medical Association* **254**, 3449–3453.

Brass, L.M., Hartigan, P.M., Page, W.F. & Concato, J. (1996) Importance of cerebrovascular disease in studies of myocardial infarction. *Stroke* **27**, 1173–1176.

Brice, J.G., Dowsett, D.J. & Lower, R.D. (1964) Haemodynamic effects of carotid artery stenosis. *British Medical Journal* **2**, 1363–1366.

Brink, J.A., McFarland, E.G. & Heiken, J.P. (1997) Helical/spiral computed body tomography. *Clinical Radiology* **52**, 489–503.

Britt, P.M., Heiserman, J.E., Snider, R.M., Shill, H.A., Bird, C.R. & Wallace, R.C. (2000) Incidence of postangiographic abnormalities revealed by diffusion-weighted MR imaging. *American Journal of Neuroradiology* **21**, 55–59.

Britton, M. & Gustafsson, C. (1985) Non-rheumatic atrial fibrillation as a risk factor for stroke. *Stroke* **16**, 182–188.

Brockmeier, L.B., Adolph, R.J., Gustin, B.W., Holmes, J.C. & Sacks, J.G. (1981) Calcium emboli to the retinal artery in calcific aortic stenosis. *American Heart Journal* **101**, 32–37.

Broderick, J., Brott, T., Kothari, R. *et al.* (1998) The Greater Cincinnati/Northern Kentucky Stroke Study: preliminary first-ever and total incidence rates of stroke among Blacks. *Stroke* **29**, 415–421.

Brogno, D., Lancaster, G. & Rosenbaum, M. (1994) Embolism interruptus. *New England Journal of Medicine* **330**, 1761–1762.

Brott, T., Tomsick, T., Feinberg, W. *et al.* for the Asymptomatic Carotid Atherosclerosis Study Investigators (1994) Baseline silent cerebral infarction in the asymptomatic carotid atherosclerosis study. *Stroke* **25**, 1122–1129.

Browner, W.S., Pressman, A.R., Nevitt, M.C., Cauley, J.A. & Cummings, S.R. for the Study of Osteoporotic Fractures Research Group (1993) Association between low bone density and stroke in elderly women: the study of osteoporotic fractures. *Stroke* **24**, 940–946.

Brunner, E., Davey Smith, G., Marmot, M., Canner, R., Beksinska, M. & O'Brien, J. (1996) Childhood social circumstances and psychosocial and behavioural factors as determinants of plasma fibrinogen. *Lancet* **347**, 1008–1013.

Bulpitt, C.J. (1995) Vitamin C and vascular disease: be cautious about the association until large randomised trials have been done. *British Medical Journal* **310**, 1548–1549.

Burchfiel, C.M., Curb, J.D., Rodriguez, B.L., Abbott, R.D., Chiu, D. & Yano, K. (1994) Glucose intolerance and 22-year stroke incidence. The Honolulu Heart Program. *Stroke* **25**, 951–957.

Burke, A.P. & Virmani, R. (1993) Cardiac myxoma: a clinicopathologic study. *American Journal of Clinical Pathology* **100**, 671–680.

Burn, J., Dennis, M.S., Bamford, J., Sandercock, P., Wade, D. & Warlow, C.P. (1997) Epileptic seizures after a first ever in a lifetime stroke: the Oxfordshire Community Stroke Project. *British Medical Journal* **315**, 1582–1587.

Burnett, P.J., Milne, J.R., Greenwood, R., Giles, M.R. & Camm, J. (1984) The role of echocardiography in the investigation of focal cerebral ischaemia. *Postgraduate Medical Journal* **60**, 116–119.

Cabanes, L., Mas, J.L., Cohen, A. *et al.* (1993) Atrial septal aneurysm and patent foramen ovale as risk factors for cryptogenic stroke in patients less than 55 years of age: a study using transoesophageal echocardiography. *Stroke* **24**, 1865–1873.

Calle, E.E., Thun, M.J., Petrelli, J.M., Rodriguez, C. & Heath, C.W. (1999) Body-mass index and mortality in a prospective cohort of US adults. *New England Journal of Medicine* **341**, 1097–1105.

Camargo, C.A. (1989) Moderate alcohol consumption and stroke: the epidemiological evidence. *Stroke* **20**, 1611–1626.

Caplan, L.R. (1993) Brain embolism, revisited. *Neurology* **43**, 1281–1287.

Caplan, L.R. (1994) Silent brain infarcts. *Cerebrovascular Diseases* **4** (Suppl. 1), 32–39.

Caplan, L.R. (1995) Clinical diagnosis of brain embolism. *Cerebrovascular Diseases* **5**, 79–88.

Caplan, L.R. & Hennerici, M. (1998) Impaired clearance of emboli (washout) is an important link between hypoperfusion, embolism and ischaemic stroke. *Archives of Neurology* **55**, 1475–1482.

Caplan, L.R. & Sergay, S. (1976) Positional cerebral ischaemia. *Journal of Neurology, Neurosurgery and Psychiatry* **39**, 385–391.

Caplan, L.R. & Tettenborn, B. (1992) Vertebrobasilar occlusive disease: review of selected aspects. 2. Posterior circulation embolism. *Cerebrovascular Diseases* **2**, 320–326.

Carpenter, J.P., Lexa, F.J. & Davis, J.T. (1996) Determination of duplex Doppler ultrasound criteria appropriate to the North American Symptomatic Carotid Endarterectomy Trial. *Stroke* **27**, 695–699.

Carty, G.A., Nachtigal, T., Magyar, R., Herzler, G. & Bays, R. (1993) Abdominal duplex ultrasound screening for occult aortic aneurysm during carotid arterial evaluation. *Journal of Vascular Surgery* **17**, 696–702.

Castaigne, P., Lhermitte, F., Gautier, J-C., Escourolle, R. & Derouesne, C. (1970) Internal carotid artery occlusion: a study of 61 instances in 50 patients with post-mortem data. *Brain* **93**, 231–258.

Castaigne, P., Lhermitte, F., Gautier, J. *et al.* (1973) Arterial occlusions in the vertebro-basilar system: a study of 44 patients with post-mortem data. *Brain* **96**, 133–154.

Castaigne, P., Lhermitte, F., Buge, A., Escourolle, R., Hauw, J.J. & Lyon-Caen, O. (1981) Paramedian thalamic and midbrain infarcts: clinical and neuropathological study. *Annals of Neurology* 10, 127–148.

Censori, B., Colombo, F., Valsecchi, M.G. *et al.* (1998) Early transoesophageal echocardiography in cryptogenic and lacunar stroke and transient ischaemic attack. *Journal of Neurology, Neurosurgery and Psychiatry* **64**, 624–627.

Cerebral Embolism Task Force (1989) Cardiogenic brain embolism: the second report of the cerebral embolism task force. *Archives of Neurology* **46**, 727–743.

Challa, V.R., Moody, D.M. & Bell, M.A. (1992) The Charcot–Bouchard Aneurysm Controversy: impact of a new histologic technique. *Journal of Neuropathology and Experimental Neurology* **51**, 264–271.

Chalmers, N. & Campbell, I.W. (1987) Left atrial metastasis presenting as recurrent embolic strokes. *British Heart Journal* **58**, 170–172.

Chambless, L.E., Fuchs, F.D., Linn, S. *et al.* (1990) The association of corneal arcus with coronary heart disease and cardiovascular disease mortality in the Lipid Research Clinics Mortality Follow-up Study. *American Journal of Public Health* **80**, 1200–1204.

Chaves, C.J., Caplan, L.R., Chung, C-S. *et al.* (1994) Cerebellar infarcts in the New England Medical Center Posterior Circulation Stroke Registry. *Neurology* **44**, 1385–1390.

Chen, W.H., Ho, D.S.W., Ho, S.L., Cheung, R.T.F. & Cheng, S.W.K. (1998) Prevalence of extracranial carotid and vertebral artery disease in Chinese patients with coronary artery disease. *Stroke* **29**, 631–634.

Chesler, E., King, R.A. & Edwards, J.E. (1983) The myxomatous mitral valve and sudden death. *Circulation* **67**, 632–639.

Chimowitz, M.I., DeGeorgia, M.A., Poole, R.M., Hepner, A. & Armstrong, W.M. (1993) Left atrial spontaneous echo contrast is highly associated with previous stroke in patients with atrial fibrillation or mitral stenosis. *Stroke* **24**, 1015–1019.

Chimowitz, M.I., Poole, R.M., Starling, M.R., Schwaiger, M. & Gross, M.D. (1997) Frequency and severity of asymptomatic coronary disease in patients with different causes of stroke. *Stroke* **28**, 941–945.

Chobanian, A.V. (1983) The influence of hypertension and other haemodynamic factors in atherogenesis. *Progress in Cardiovascular Disease* **26**, 177–196.

Clarke, R. & Collins, R. (1998) Can dietary supplements with folic acid or vitamin B6 reduce cardiovascular risk? Design of clinical trials to test the homocystine hypothesis of vascular disease. *Journal of Cardiovascular Risk* **5**, 249–255.

Close, J.B., Evans, D.W. & Bailey, S.M. (1979) Persistent lone atrial fibrillation: its prognosis after clinical diagnosis. *Journal of the Royal College of General Practitioners* **29**, 547–549.

Cohen, A., Tzourio, C., Chauvel, C. *et al.* for the French Study of Aortic Plaques in Stroke (FAPS) Investigators (1997) Mitral valve strands and the risk of ischaemic stroke in elderly patients. *Stroke* **28**, 1574–1578.

Collins, R. & MacMahon, S. (1994) Blood pressure, antihypertensive drug treatment and the risks of stroke and of coronary heart disease. *British Medical Bulletin* **50**, 272–298.

Connelly, J.B., Cooper, J.A. & Meade, T.W. (1992) Strenuous exercise, plasma fibrinogen and factor VII activity. *British Heart Journal* **67**, 351–354.

Constantinides, P. (1967) Pathogenesis of cerebral artery thrombosis in man. *Archives of Pathology* **83**, 422–428.

Cook, N.S. & Ubben, D. (1990) Fibrinogen as a major risk factor in cardiovascular disease. *Trends in Pharmacological Sciences* **11**, 444–451.

Cornhill, J.F., Akins, D., Hutson, M. & Chandler, A.B. (1980) Localisation of atherosclerotic lesions in the human basilar artery. *Atherosclerosis* **35**, 77–86.

Coulshed, N., Epstein, E.J., McKendrick, C.S., Galloway, R.W. & Walker, E. (1970) Systemic embolism in mitral valve disease. *British Heart Journal* **32**, 26–34.

Countee, R.W., Gnanadev, A. & Chavis, P. (1978) Dilated episcleral arteries: a significant physical finding in assessment of patients with cerebrovascular insufficiency. *Stroke* **9**, 42–45.

Countee, R.W., Vijayanathan, T. & Chavis, P. (1981) Recurrent retinal ischaemia beyond cervical carotid lesions: clinical–angiographic correlations and therapeutic implications. *Journal of Neurosurgery* **55**, 532–542.

Cramer, S.C., Rordorf, G., Kaufman, J.A., Buonanno, F., Koroshetz, W.J. & Schwamm, L. (1998) Clinically occult pelvic-vein thrombosis in cryptogenic stroke. *Lancet* **351**, 1927–1928.

Craven, T.E., Ryu, J.E., Espeland, M.A. *et al.* (1990) Evaluation of the associations between carotid artery atherosclerosis and coronary artery stenosis: case–control study. *Circulation* **82**, 1230–1242.

Crouse, J.R., Goldbourt, U., Evans, G. *et al.* for the ARIC Investigators (1996)

Risk factors and segment-specific carotid arterial enlargement in the atherosclerosis risk in communities (ARIC) cohort. *Stroke* **27**, 69–75.

Cullinane, M., Wainwright, R., Brown, A., Monaghan, M. & Markus, H.S. (1998) Asymptomatic embolization in subjects with atrial fibrillation not taking anticoagulants: a prospective study. *Stroke* **29**, 1810–1815.

Daffertshofer, M., Ries, S., Schminke, U. & Hennerici, M. (1996) High-intensity transient signals in patients with cerebral ischaemia. *Stroke* **27**, 1844–1849.

Dahl, A., Russell, D., Rootwelt, K., Nyberg-Hansen, R. & Kerty, E. (1995) Cerebral vasoreactivity assessed with transcranial Doppler and regional cerebral blood flow measurements: dose, serum concentration and time course of the response to acetazolamide. *Stroke* **26**, 2302–2306.

Dalal, P.M., Deshpande, C.K. & Daftary, S.G. (1971) Aortic arch syndrome. *Neurology India* **19**, 155–171.

Daley, R., Mattingly, T.W., Holt, C.L., Bland, E.F. & White, P.D. (1951) Systemic arterial embolism in rheumatic heart disease. *American Heart Journal* **42**, 566–581.

Danesh, J. (1999) Smoldering arteries? Low-grade inflammation and coronary heart disease. *Journal of the American Medical Association* **282**, 2169–2171.

Danesh, J. & Lewington, S. (1998) Plasma homocystine and coronary heart disease: systematic review of published epidemiological studies. *Journal of Cardiovascular Risk* **5**, 229–232.

Danesh, J., Collins, R., Appleby, P. & Peto, R. (1998) Association of fibrinogen, C-reactive protein, albumin or leukocyte count with coronary heart disease: meta-analyses of prospective studies. *Journal of the American Medical Association* **279**, 1477–1482.

Danesh, J., Youngman, L., Clark, S., Parish, S., Peto, R. & Collins, R. (1999) *Helicobacter pylori* infection and early onset myocardial infarction: case–control and sibling pairs study. *British Medical Journal* **319**, 1157–1162.

Danesh, J., Whincup, P., Walker, M. *et al.* (2000a) Low grade inflammation and coronary heart disease: prospective study and updated meta-analyses. *British Medical Journal* **321**, 199–204.

Danesh, J., Whincup, P., Walker, M., *et al.* (2000b) *Chlamydia pneumoniae* IgG titres and coronary heart disease: prospective study and meta-analysis. *British Medical Journal* **321**, 208–213.

Daniel, W.G. (1993) Should transesophageal echocardiography be used to guide cardioversion? *New England Journal of Medicine* **328**, 803–804.

Daniel, W.G. & Mugge, A. (1995) Transoesophageal echocardiography. *New England Journal of Medicine* **332**, 1268–1279.

Daniel, W.G., Erbel, R., Kasper, W. *et al.* (1991) Safety of transesophageal echocardiography: a multicentre survey of 10,419 examinations. *Circulation* **83**, 817–821.

Datta, M. (1993) You cannot exclude the explanation you have not considered. *Lancet* **342**, 345–347.

Davey Smith, G. (1997) Down at heart: the meaning and implications of social inequalities in cardiovascular disease. *Journal of the Royal College of Physicians of London* **31**, 414–424.

Davey Smith, G., Shipley, M.J. & Rose, G. (1990) Intermittent claudication, heart disease risk factors and mortality. The Whitehall Study. *Circulation* **82**, 1925–1931.

Davey Smith, G., Phillips, A.N. & Neaton, J.D. (1992) Smoking as 'independent' risk factor for suicide: illustration of an artifact from observational epidemiology? *Lancet* **340**, 709–712.

Davey Smith, G., Neaton, J.D., Wentworth, D., Stamler, R. & Stamler, J. for the MRFIT Research Group (1998) Mortality differences between black and white men in the USA: contribution of income and other risk factors among men screened for the MRFIT. *Lancet* **351**, 934–939.

Davies, K.N. & Humphrey, P.R. (1993) Complications of cerebral angiography in patients with symptomatic carotid territory ischaemia screened by carotid ultrasound. *Journal of Neurology, Neurosurgery and Psychiatry* **56**, 967–972.

Davies, M.J. (1997) The composition of coronary-artery plaques. *New England Journal of Medicine* **336**, 1312–1314.

Davies, M.J. & Pomerance, A. (1972) Pathology of atrial fibrillation in man. *British Heart Journal* **34**, 520–525.

Davis, P.H., Dambrosia, J.M., Schoenberg, B.S. *et al.* (1987) Risk factors for ischemic stroke: a prospective study in Rochester, Minnesota. *Annals of Neurology* **22**, 319–327.

De Bono, D.P. & Warlow, C.P. (1979) Mitral-annulus calcification and cerebral or retinal ischaemia. *Lancet* **2**, 383–385.

De Bono, D.P. & Warlow, C.P. (1981) Potential sources of emboli in patients with presumed transient cerebral or retinal ischaemia. *Lancet* **1**, 343–346.

December, G.W. & Fuster, V. (1994) Idiopathic dilated cardiomyopathy. *New England Journal of Medicine* **331**, 1564–1575.

DeGraba, T.J., Siren, A-L., Penix, L. *et al.* (1998) Increased endothelial expression of intercellular adhesion molecule-1 in symptomatic versus asymptomatic human carotid atherosclerotic plaque. *Stroke* **29**, 1405–1410.

Del Sette, M., Angeli, S., Stara, I., Finocchi, C. & Gandolfo, C. (1997) Microembolic signals with serial transcranial Doppler monitoring in acute focal ischaemic deficit: a local phenomenon? *Stroke* **28**, 1310–1313.

Dennis, M.S. (1985) Neurological complications of pulmonary arteriovenous malformations. *British Medical Journal* **289**, 1392–1393.

Dennis, M.S., Bamford, J., Sandercock, P. & Warlow, C.P. (1989) Incidence of transient ischaemic attacks in Oxfordshire, England. *Stroke* **20**, 333–339.

Dennis, M., Bamford, J., Sandercock, P., Molyneux, A. & Warlow, C. (1990) Computed tomography in patients with transient ischaemic attacks: when is a transient ischaemic attack not a transient ischaemic attack but a stroke? *Journal of Neurology* **237**, 257–261.

Derdeyn, C.P., Grubb, R.L. & Powers, W.J. (1999) Cerebral haemodynamic impairment: methods of measurements and association with stroke risk. *Neurology* **53**, 251–259.

Derlon, J.M., Bouvard, G., Viader, F. *et al.* (1992) Impaired cerebral hemodynamics in internal carotid occlusion. *Cerebrovascular Diseases* **2**, 72–81.

DeRook, F.A., Comess, K.A., Albers, G.W. & Popp, R.L. (1992) Transoesophageal echocardiography in the evaluation of stroke. *Annals of Internal Medicine* **117**, 922–932.

DeStefano, F., Anda, R.F., Kahn, H.S., Williamson, D.F. & Russell, C.M. (1993) Dental disease and risk of coronary heart disease and mortality. *British Medical Journal* **306**, 688–691.

Devereux, R.B., Brown, W.T., Kramer-Fox, R. & Sachs, I. (1982) Inheritance of mitral valve prolapse: effect of age and sex on gene expression. *Annals of Internal Medicine* **97**, 826–832.

Devereux, R.B., Kramer-Fox, R., Shear, K., Kligfield, P., Pini, R. & Savage, D.D. (1987) Diagnosis and classification of severity of mitral valve prolapse: methodologic, biologic and prognostic considerations. *American Heart Journal* **113**, 1265–1279.

DeWeese, J.A., May, A.G., Lipchik, E.O. & Rob, C.G. (1970) Anatomic and haemodynamic correlations in carotid artery stenosis. *Stroke* **1**, 149–157.

Diaz, M.N., Frei, B., Vita, J.A. & Keaney, J.F. (1997) Antioxidants and atherosclerotic heart disease. *New England Journal of Medicine* **337**, 408–416.

Di Mascio, R., Marchioli, R. & Tognoni, G. (2000) Cholesterol reduction and stroke occurrence: an overview of randomized clinical trials. *Cerebrovascular Diseases* **10**, 85–92.

Dippel, D.W.J., van Kooten, F., Bakker, S.L.M. & Koudstaal, P.J. (1997) Interobserver agreement for 10% categories of angiographic carotid stenosis. *Stroke* **28**, 2483–2485.

Dobson, A. (1999) Is raised serum uric acid a cause of cardiovascular disease or death? *Lancet* **354**, 1578.

Dobyns, W.B. & Garg, B.P. (1991) Vascular abnormalities in epidermal nevus syndrome. *Neurology* **41**, 276–278.

Doll, R. (1997) One for the heart. *British Medical Journal* **315**, 1664–1668.

Doll, R., Peto, R., Wheatley, K., Gray, R. & Sutherland, I. (1994) Mortality in relation to smoking: 40 years' observations on male British doctors. *British Medical Journal* **309**, 901–911.

Donnan, G.A. & Jones, E.F. (1995) Aortic arch atheroma and stroke. *Cerebrovascular Diseases* **5**, 10–13.

Donnan, G.A., McNeil, J.J., Adena, M.A., Doyle, A.E., O'Malley, H.M. & Neill, G.C. (1989) Smoking as a risk factor for cerebral ischaemia. *Lancet* **2**, 643–647.

Donnan, G.A., You, R., Thrift, A. & McNeil, J.J. (1993a) Smoking as a risk factor for stroke. *Cerebrovascular Diseases* **3**, 129–138.

Donnan, G.A., O'Malley, H.M., Quang, L., Hurley, S. & Bladin, P.F. (1993b) The capsular warning syndrome: pathogenesis and clinical features. *Neurology* **43**, 957–962.

Donnan, G.A., Norrving, B., Bamford, J.M. & Bogousslavsky, J. (1995) *Lacunar and Other Subcortical Infarctions*. Oxford University Press, Oxford.

Downs, J.R., Clearfield, M., Weis, S. *et al.* for the AFCAPS/TEXCAPS Research Group (1998) Primary prevention of acute coronary events with lovastatin in men and women with average cholesterol levels: results of AFCAPS/TexCAPS. *Journal of the American Medical Association* **279**, 1615–1622.

Droste, D.W., Dittrich, R., Kemeny, V., Schulte-Altedorneburg, G. & Ringelstein, E.B. (1999a) Prevalence and frequency of microembolic signals in

105 patients with extracranial carotid artery occlusive disease. *Journal of Neurology, Neurosurgery and Psychiatry* **67**, 525–528.

Droste, D.W., Jurgens, R., Nabavi, D.G., Schuierer, G., Weber, S. & Ringelstein, E.B. (1999b) Echocontrast-enhanced ultrasound of extracranial internal carotid artery high-grade stenosis and occlusion. *Stroke* **30**, 2302–2306.

Droste, D.W., Kriete, J-U., Stypmann, J. *et al.* (1999c) Contrast transcranial Doppler ultrasound in the detection of right-to-left shunts: comparison of different procedures and different contrast agents. *Stroke* **30**, 1827–1832.

Dudman, N.P.B. (1999) An alternative view of homocystine. *Lancet* **354**, 2072–2074.

Dugani, B.V., Higginson, L.A.J., Beanlands, D.S. & Akyurekli, Y. (1984) Recurrent systemic emboli following myocardial contusion. *American Heart Journal* **108**, 1354–1357.

Duguid, J.B. (1976) *The Dynamics of Atherosclerosis*. Aberdeen University Press.

EAFT Study Group (1996) Silent brain infarction in non-rheumatic atrial fibrillation. *Neurology* **46**, 159–165.

Eastern Stroke and Coronary Heart Disease Collaborative Research Group (1998) Blood pressure, cholesterol and stroke in eastern Asia. *Lancet* **352**, 1801–1807.

Ebrahim, S. & Harwood, R. (1999) *Stroke: Epidemiology, Evidence and Clinical Practice*. Oxford University Press, Oxford.

Elgersma, O.E.H., Van Leersum, M., Buijs, P.C. *et al.* (1998) Changes over time in optimal duplex threshold for the identification of patients eligible for carotid endarterectomy. *Stroke* **29**, 2352–2356.

Eliasziw, M., Streifler, J.Y., Fox, A.J., Hachinski, V.C., Ferguson, G.G. & Barnett, H.J.M. for the North American Symptomatic Carotid Endarterectomy Trial (1994) Significance of plaque ulceration in symptomatic patients with high-grade carotid stenosis. *Stroke* **25**, 304–308.

Ellekjaer, H., Holmen, J., Ellekjaer, E. & Vatten, L. (2000) Physical activity and stroke mortality in women: ten-year follow-up of the Nord-Trondelag Health Survey, 1984–1986. *Stroke* **31**, 14–18.

Engelter, S.T., Provenzale, J.M., Petrella, J.R. *et al.* (1999) Diffusion MR imaging and transient ischemic attacks [4] (multiple letters). *Stroke* **30**, 2762–2763.

Enriquez-Sarano, M., Klodas, E., Garratt, K.N., Bailey, K.R., Tajik, A.J. & Holmes, D.R. (1996) Secular trends in coronary atherosclerosis-analysis in patients with valvular regurgitation. *New England Journal of Medicine* **335**, 316–322.

Ernst, E. & Resch, K.L. (1993) Fibrinogen as a cardiovascular risk factor: a meta-analysis and review of the literature. *Annals of Internal Medicine* **118**, 956–963.

European Carotid Surgery Trialists' Collaborative Group (1998) Randomised trial of endarterectomy for recently symptomatic carotid stenosis: final results of the MRC European Carotid Surgery Trial (ECST). *Lancet* **351**, 1379–1387.

Evenson, K.R., Rosamond, W.D., Cai, J. *et al.* for the Atherosclerosis Risk in Communities (ARIC) Study Investigators (1999) Physical activity and ischaemic stroke risk. The Atherosclerosis Risk in Communities study. *Stroke* **30**, 1333–1339.

Everson, S.A., Lynch, J.W., Chesney, M.A. *et al.* (1997) Interaction of workplace demands and cardiovascular reactivity in progression of carotid atherosclerosis: population based study. *British Medical Journal* **314**, 553–558.

Everson, S.A., Kaplan, G.A., Goldberg, D.E., Lakka, T.A., Sivenius, J. & Salonen, J.T. (1999) Anger expression and incident stroke: prospective evidence from the Kuopio ischemic heart disease study. *Stroke* **30**, 523–528.

Fabian, T.C. (1993) Unravelling the fat embolism syndrome. *New England Journal of Medicine* **329**, 961–963.

Fagerberg, B., Gnarpe, J., Gnarpe, H., Agewall, S. & Wikstrand, J. (1999) *Chlamydia pneumoniae* but not cytomegalovirus antibodies are associated with future risk of stroke and cardiovascular disease: a prospective study in middle-aged to elderly men with treated hypertension. *Stroke* **30**, 299–305.

Fang, J. & Alderman, M.H. (2000) Serum uric acid and cardiovascular mortality: the NHANES I Epidemiologic Follow-up Study, 1971–1992. *Journal of the American Medical Association* **283**, 2404–2410.

Faught, E. (1993) Current role of electroencephalography in cerebral ischaemia. *Stroke* **24**, 609–613.

Feigin, V.L., Wiebers, D.O., Nikitin, Y.P., O'Fallon, W.M. & Whisnant, J.P. (1998) Risk factors for ischaemic stroke in a Russian community: a population-based case–control study. *Stroke* **29**, 34–39.

Fields, W.S. & Lemak, N.A. (1972) Joint study of extracranial arterial occlusion. VII. Subclavian steal: a review of 168 cases. *Journal of the American Medical Association* **222**, 1139–1143.

Fine-Edelstein, J.S., Wolf, P.A., O'Leary, D.H. *et al.* (1994) Precursors of extracranial carotid atherosclerosis in the Framingham Study. *Neurology* **44**, 1046–1050.

Fisher, C.M. (1951) Occlusion of the internal carotid artery. *Archives of Neurology and Psychiatry* **65**, 346–377.

Fisher, C.M. (1954) Occlusion of the carotid arteries. *Archives of Neurology and Psychiatry* 72, 187–204.

Fisher, C.M. (1969) The arterial lesions underlying lacunes. *Acta Neuropathologica* **12**, 1–15.

Fisher, C.M. (1972) Cerebral miliary aneurysms in hypertension. *American Journal of Pathology* **66**, 313–330.

Fisher, C.M. (1979) Capsular infarcts: the underlying vascular lesions. *Archives of Neurology* **36**, 65–73.

Fisher, C.M. (1991) Lacunar infarcts: a review. *Cerebrovascular Diseases* **1**, 311–320.

Fisher, M., Kase, C.S., Stelle, B. & Mills, R.M. (1988) Ischaemic stroke after cardiac pacemakers implantation in sick sinus syndrome. *Stroke* **19**, 712–715.

Flegel, K.M., Shipley, M.J. & Rose, G. (1987) Risk of stroke in non-rheumatic atrial fibrillation. *Lancet* **1**, 526–529.

Forsen, T., Eriksson, J.G., Tuomilehto, J., Osmond, C. & Barker, D.J.P. (1999) Growth *in utero* and during childhood among women who develop coronary heart disease: longitudinal study. *British Medical Journal* **319**, 1403–1407.

Forteza, A.M., Koch, S., Romano, J.G. *et al.* (1999) Transcranial Doppler detection of fat emboli. *Stroke* **30**, 2687–2691.

Freed, L.A., Levy, D., Levine, J.R.A. *et al.* (1999) Prevalence and clinical outcome of mitral-valve prolapse. *New England Journal of Medicine* **341**, 1–7.

Friedman, G.D., Loveland, D.B. & Ehrlich, S.P. (1968) Relationship of stroke to other cardiovascular disease. *Circulation* **38**, 533–541.

Friedman, S.G. (1990) Transient ischaemic attacks resulting from carotid duplex imaging. *Surgery* **107**, 153–155.

Frost, C.D., Law, M.R. & Wald, N.J. (1991) By how much does dietary salt reduction lower blood pressure? II. Analysis of observational data within populations. *British Medical Journal* **302**, 818.

Fry, C.L., Carter, J.E., Kanter, M.C., Tegeler, C.H. & Tuley, M.R. (1993) Anterior ischaemic optic neuropathy is not associated with carotid artery atherosclerosis. *Stroke* **24**, 539–542.

Furlan, A.J., Whisnant, J.P. & Kearns, T.P. (1979) Unilateral visual loss in bright light: an unusual symptom of carotid artery occlusive disease. *Archives of Neurology* **36**, 675–676.

Furst, G., Saleh, A., Wenserski, F. *et al.* (1999) Reliability and validity of non-invasive imaging of internal carotid artery pseudo-occlusion. *Stroke* **30**, 1444–1449.

Furst, H., Hartl, W.H., Jansen, I., Liepsch, D., Lauterjung, L. & Schildberg, F.W. (1992) Colour-flow Doppler sonography in the identification of ulcerative plaques in patients with high-grade carotid artery stenosis. *American Journal of Neuroradiology* **13**, 1581–1587.

Fuster, V., Gersh, B.J., Giuliani, E.R., Tajik, A.J., Brandenburg, R.O. & Frye, R.L. (1981) The natural history of idiopathic dilated cardiomyopathy. *American Journal of Cardiology* **47**, 525–531.

Fuster, V., Badimon, L., Badimon, J.J. & Chesebro, J.H. (1992a) The pathogenesis of coronary artery disease and the acute coronary syndromes I. *New England Journal of Medicine* **326**, 242–250.

Fuster, V., Badimon, L., Badimon, J.J. & Chesebro, J.H. (1992b) The pathogenesis of coronary artery disease and the acute secondary syndromes II. *New England Journal of Medicine* **326**, 310–318.

Fuster, V., Fayad, Z.A. & Badimon, J.J. (1999) Acute coronary syndromes: biology. *Lancet* **353** (Suppl.), 5–9.

Gagnon, D.R., Zhang, T-J., Brand, F.N. & Kannel, W.B. (1994) Haematocrit and the risk of cardiovascular disease. The Framingham study: a 34-year follow-up. *American Heart Journal* **127**, 674–682.

Gan, R., Sacco, R.L., Kargman, D.E., Roberts, J.K., Boden-Albala, B. & Gu, Q. (1997) Testing the validity of the lacunar hypothesis: the Northern Manhattan Stroke Study experience. *Neurology* **48**, 1204–1211.

Gandolfo, C., Del Sette, M., Finocchi, C., Calautti, C. & Loeb, C. (1998) Internal border-zone infarction in patients with ischaemic stroke. *Cere-*

brovascular Diseases **8**, 255–258.

Gasecki, A.P., Fox, A.J., Lebrun, L.H. & Daneault, N. for the Collaborators of the North American Carotid Endarterectomy Trial (NASCET) (1994) Bilateral occipital infarctions associated with carotid stenosis in a patient with persistent trigeminal artery. *Stroke* **25**, 1520–1523.

Gautier, J.C., Durr, A., Koussa, S., Lascault, G. & Grosgogeat, Y. (1991) Paradoxical cerebral emoblism with a patent foramen ovale: a report of 29 patients. *Cerebrovascular Diseases* **1**, 193–202.

Georgiadis, D., Lindner, A., Manz, M. *et al.* (1997) Intracranial microembolic signals in 500 patients with potential cardiac or carotid embolic source and in normal controls. *Stroke* **28**, 1203–1207.

Georgiadis, D., Baumgartner, R.W., Uhlmann, F., Lindner, A., Zerkowski, H.R. & Zierz, S. (1999) Venous microemboli in patients with artificial heart valves. *Cerebrovascular Diseases* **9**, 238–241.

Gerraty, R.P., Bowser, D.N., Infeld, B., Mitchell, P.J. & Davis, S.M. (1996) Microemboli during carotid angiography: association with stroke risk factors or subsequent magnetic resonance imaging changes? *Stroke* **27**, 1543–1547.

Gerriets, T., Seidel, G., Fiss, I., Modrau, B. & Kaps, M. (1999) Contrast-enhanced transcranial colour-coded duplex sonography: efficiency and validity. *Neurology* **52**, 1133–1137.

Geyer, S.J. & Franzini, D.A. (1979) Myxomatous degeneration of the mitral valve complicated by non-bacterial thrombotic endocarditis with systemic embolisation. *American Journal of Clinical Pathology* **72**, 489–492.

Giannesini, C., Kubis, N., Guyen, A.N., Wassef, M., Mikol, J. & Woimant, F. (1999) Cardiac papillary fibroelastoma: a rare cause of ischaemic stroke in the young. *Cerebrovascular Diseases* **9**, 45–49.

Gibbs, J.M., Wise, R.J.S., Leenders, K.L. & Jones, T. (1984) Evaluation of cerebral perfusion reserve in patients with carotid artery occlusion. *Lancet* **1**, 310–314.

van Gijn, J. & Kraaijeveld, C.L. (1982) Blood pressure does not predict lacunar infarction. *Journal of Neurology, Neurosurgery and Psychiatry* **45**, 147–150.

van Gijn, J., Stampfer, M.J., Wolfe, C. & Algra, A. (1993) The association between alcohol and stroke. In: *Health Issues Related to Alcohol Consumption* (ed. P.M. Verschuren), p. 44. ILSI Press, Washington.

Giles, W.H., Kittner, S.J., Hebel, J.R., Losonczy, K.G. & Sherwin, R.W. (1995) Determinants of black–white differences in the risk of cerebral infarction. The National Health and Nutrition Examination Survey: epidemiologic follow-up study. *Archives of Internal Medicine* **155**, 1319–1324.

Gilon, D., Buonanno, F.S., Joffe, M.M. *et al.* (1999) Lack of evidence of an association between mitral-valve prolapse and stroke in young patients. *New England Journal of Medicine* **341**, 8–13.

Gironell, A., Rey, A. & Marti-Vilalta, J.L. (1995) Positional cerebral ischaemia. *Cerebrovascular Diseases* **5**, 313–314.

Giroud, M., Lemesle, M., Quantin, C. *et al.* (1997) A hospital-based and a population-based stroke registry yield different results: the experience in Dijon, France. *Neuroepidemiology* **16**, 15–21.

GISSI-Prevenzione Investigators (1999) Dietary supplementation with n-3 polyunsaturated fatty acids and vitamin E after myocardial infarction: results of the GISSI-Prevenzione trial. *Lancet* **354**, 447–455.

Glader, C.A., Stegmayr, B., Boman, J. *et al.* (1999) *Chlamydia pneumoniae* antibodies and high lipoprotein (a) levels do not predict ischaemic cerebral infarctions: results from a nested case–control study in northern Sweden. *Stroke* **30**, 2013–2018.

Glynn, J.R. (1993) A question of attribution. *Lancet* **342**, 530–532.

Gnasso, A., Irace, C., Carallo, C. *et al.* (1997) *In vivo* association between low wall shear stress and plaque in subjects with asymmetrical carotid atherosclerosis. *Stroke* **28**, 993–998.

Golledge, J., Greenhalgh, R.M. & Davies, A.H. (2000) The symptomatic carotid plaque. *Stroke* **31**, 774–781.

Good, D.C., Frank, S., Verhulst, S. & Sharma, B. (1986) Cardiac abnormalities in stroke patients with negative arteriograms. *Stroke* **17**, 6–11.

Gorelick, P.B. (1987) Alcohol and stroke. *Stroke* **18**, 268–271.

Gorelick, P.B. (1998) Cerebrovascular disease in African Americans. *Stroke* **29**, 2656–2664.

Gower, D.J., Lewis, J.C., McWhorter, J.M. & Davis, C.H. (1987) Carotid plaque as a source of emboli in humans: a scanning electron microscopic study. *Neurosurgery* **20**, 362–368.

Grady, P.A. (1984) Pathophysiology of extracranial cerebral arterial stenosis: a critical review. *Stroke* **15**, 224–236.

Grau, A.J., Buggle, F., Becher, H. *et al.* (1998) Recent bacterial and viral infection is a risk factor for cerebrovascular ischaemia: clinical and biochemical studies. *Neurology* **50**, 196–203.

Graus, P., Rogers, L.R. & Posner, J.B. (1985) Cerebrovascular complications in patients with cancer. *Medicine* **64**, 16–35.

Graves, M.J. (1997) Magnetic resonance angiography. *British Journal of Radiology* **70**, 6–28.

Greenberg, E.R., Baron, J.A., Karagas, M.R. *et al.* (1996) Mortality associated with low plasma concentration of beta carotene and the effect of oral supplementation. *Journal of the American Medical Association* **275**, 699–703.

Griewing, B., Morgenstern, C., Driesner, F., Kallwellis, G., Walker, M.L. & Kessler, C. (1996) Cerebrovascular disease assessed by colour-flow and power Doppler ultrasonography: comparison with digital subtraction angiography in internal carotid artery stenosis. *Stroke* **27**, 95–100.

Griffiths, P.D., Worthy, S. & Gholkar, A. (1996) Incidental intracranial vascular pathology in patients investigated for carotid stenosis. *Neuroradiology* **38**, 25–30.

Gronholdt, M-L.M. (1999) Ultrasound and lipoproteins as predictors of lipid-rich, rupture-prone plaques in the carotid artery. *Arteriosclerosis, Thrombosis and Vascular Biology* **19**, 2–13.

Grosveld, W.J., Lawson, J.A., Eikelboom, B.C., van der Windt, J.M.V. & Ackerstaff, R.G. (1988) Clinical and haemodynamic significance of innominate artery lesions evaluated by ultrasonography and digital angiography. *Stroke* **19**, 958–962.

Grubb, R.L., Derdeyn, C.P., Fritsch, S.M. *et al.* (1998) Importance of haemodynamic factors in the prognosis of symptomatic carotid occlusion. *Journal of the American Medical Association* **280**, 1055–1060.

Gunatilake, S.B. (1998) Rapid resolution of symptoms and signs of intracerebral haemorrhage: case reports. *British Medical Journal* **316**, 1495–1496.

Gunning, A.J., Pickering, G.W., Robb-Smith, A.H.T. & Ross Russell, R. (1964) Mural thrombosis of the internal carotid artery and subsequent embolism. *Quarterly Journal of Medicine* **33**, 155–195.

Gur, A.Y., Bova, I. & Bornstein, N.M. (1996) Is impaired cerebral vasomotor reactivity a predictive factor of stroke in asymptomatic patients? *Stroke* **27**, 2188–2190.

Gurfinkel, E., Bozovich, G., Daroca, A., Beck, E., Mautner, B. for the ROXIS Study Group (1997) Randomised trial of roxithromycin in non-Q-wave coronary syndromes: ROXIS Pilot Study. *Lancet* **350**, 404–407.

Haapanen, A., Koskenvou, M., Kaprio, J., Kesaniemi, Y.A. & Heikkila, K. (1989) Carotid arteriosclerosis in identical twins discordant for cigarette smoking. *Circulation* **80**, 10–16.

Haheim, L.L., Holme, I., Hjermann, I. & Leren, P. (1996) Smoking habits and risk of fatal stroke: 18) years follow-up of the Oslo Study. *Journal of Epidemiology and Community Health* **50**, 621–624.

Hankey, G.J. & Eikelboom, J.W. (1999) Homocystine and vascular disease. *Lancet* **354**, 407–413.

Hankey, G.J. & Gubbay, S.S. (1987) Focal cerebral ischaemia and infarction due to antihypertensive therapy. *Medical Journal of Australia* **146**, 412–414.

Hankey, G.J. & Warlow, C.P. (1990) Symptomatic carotid ischaemic events: safest and most cost effective way of selecting patients for angiography, before carotid endarterectomy. *British Medical Journal* **300**, 1485–1491.

Hankey, G.J. & Warlow, C.P. (1991a) Prognosis of symptomatic carotid artery occlusion: an overview. *Cerebrovascular Diseases* **1**, 245–256.

Hankey, G.J. & Warlow, C.P. (1991b) Lacunar transient ischaemic attacks: a clinically useful concept? *Lancet* **337**, 335–338.

Hankey, G.J. & Warlow, C.P. (1992) Cost-effective investigation of patients with suspected transient ischaemic attacks. *Journal of Neurology, Neurosurgery and Psychiatry* **55**, 171–176.

Hankey, G.J., Warlow, C.P. & Molyneux, A. (1990a) Complications of cerebral angiography for patients with mild carotid territory ischaemia being considered for carotid endarterectomy. *Journal of Neurology, Neurosurgery and Psychiatry* **53**, 542–548.

Hankey, G.J., Warlow, C.P. & Sellar, R.J. (1990b) Cerebral angiographic risk in mild cerebrovascular disease. *Stroke* **21**, 209–222.

Hankey, G.J., Slattery, J. & Warlow, C.P. (1991a) Prognosis and prognostic factors of retinal infarction: a prospective cohort study. *British Medical Journal* **302**, 499–504.

Hankey, G.J., Slattery, J.M. & Warlow, C.P. (1991b) The prognosis of hospital-referred transient ischaemic attacks. *Journal of Neurology, Neurosurgery and Psychiatry* **54**, 793–802.

Harmsen, P., Rosengren, A., Tsipogiannia, A. & Wilhelmsen, L. (1990) Risk factors for stroke in middle-aged men in Goteborg, Sweden. *Stroke* **21**, 223–229.

Harrison, M.J.G. & Marshall, J. (1977) The finding of thrombus at carotid endarterectomy and its relationship to the timing of surgery. *British Journal of Surgery* **64**, 511–512.

Hart, C.L., Davey Smith, G., Hole, D.J. & Hawthorne, V.M. (1999a) Alcohol consumption and mortality from all causes, coronary heart disease and stroke: results from a prospective cohort study of Scottish men with 21 years of follow up. *British Medical Journal* **318**, 1725–1729.

Hart, R.G. (1992) Cardiogenic embolism to the brain. *Lancet* 339, 589–594.

Hart, R.G., Foster, J.W., Luther, M.F. & Kanter, M.C. (1990) Stroke in infective endocarditis. *Stroke* **21**, 695–700.

Hart, R.G., Benavente, O., McBride, R. & Pearce, L.A. (1999b) Antithrombotic therapy to prevent stroke in patients with atrial fibrillation: a meta-analysis. *Annals of Internal Medicine* **131**, 492–501.

Hart, R.G., Pearce, L.A., McBride, R., Rothbart, R.M. & Asinger, R.W. on behalf of the Stroke Prevention in Atrial Fibrillation (SPAF) Investigators (1999c) Factors associated with ischaemic stroke during aspirin therapy in atrial fibrillation: analysis of 2012 participants in the SPAF I–III clinical trials. *Stroke* **30**, 1223–1229.

Hart, R.G., Pearce, L.A., Miller, V.T. *et al.* on behalf of the SPAF Investigators (2000) Cardioembolic vs. non-cardioembolic strokes in atrial fibrillation: frequency and effect of antithrombotic agents in the Stroke Prevention in Atrial Fibrillation Studies. *Cerebrovascular Diseases* **10**, 39–43.

Hatsukami, T.S., Ferguson, M.S., Beach, K.W. *et al.* (1997) Carotid plaque morphology and clinical events. *Stroke* **28**, 95–100.

He, J., Ogden, L.G., Vupputuri, S., Bazzano, L.A., Loria, C. & Whelton, P.K. (1999) Dietary sodium intake and subsequent risk of cardiovascular disease in overweight adults. *Journal of the American Medical Association* **282**, 2027–2034.

He, J., Vupputuri, S., Allen, K., Prerost, M.R., Hughes, J. & Whelton, P.K. (1999) Passive smoking and the risk of coronary heart disease—a meta-analysis of epidemiologic studies. *New England Journal of Medicine* **340**, 920–926.

Heart Outcomes Prevention Evaluation Study Investigators (2000) Vitamin E supplementation and cardiovascular events in high-risk patients. *New England Journal of Medicine* **342**, 154–160.

Hegedus, K. (1985) Ectasia of the basilar artery with special reference to possible pathogenesis. *Surgical Neurology* **24**, 463–469.

Heiken, J.P., Brink, J.A. & Vannier, M.W. (1993) Spiral (helical) CT. *Radiology* **189**, 647–656.

Heinzlef, O., Cohen, A. & Amarenco, P. (1997) An update on aortic causes of ischaemic stroke. *Current Opinion in Neurology* **10**, 64–72.

Heiserman, J.E., Dean, B.L., Hodak, J.A. *et al.* (1994) Neurologic complications of cerebral angiography. *American Journal of Neuroradiology* **15**, 1401–1407.

Hemingway, H. & Marmot, M. (1999) Psychosocial factors in the aetiology and prognosis of coronary heart disease: systematic review of prospective cohort studies. *British Medical Journal* **318**, 1460–1467.

Hennekens, C.H., Buring, J.E. & Peto, R. (1994) Antioxidant vitamins: benefits not yet proved. *New England Journal of Medicine* **330**, 1080–1081.

Hennerici, M., Klemm, C. & Rautenberg, W. (1988) The subclavian steal phenomenon: a common vascular disorder with rare neurologic deficits. *Neurology* **38**, 669–673.

Herderschee, D., Hijdra, A., Algra, A., Koudstaal, P.J., Kappelle, L.J. & van Gijn, J. for the Dutch TIA Trial Study Group (1992) Silent stroke in patients with transient ischaemic attack or minor ischaemic stroke. *Stroke* **23**, 1220–1224.

Herman, B., Schmitz, P.I.M., Leyten, A.C.M. *et al.* (1983) Multivariate logistic analysis of risk factors for stroke in Tilburg, the Netherlands. *American Journal of Epidemiology* **118**, 514–525.

Hertog, M.G.L., Feskens, E.J.M. & Kromhout, D. (1997) Antioxidant flavonols and coronary heart disease risk. *Lancet* **349**, 699.

Hertzer, N.R., Young, J.R., Beven, E.G. *et al.* (1985) Coronary angiography in 506 patients with extracranial cerebrovascular disease. *Archives of Internal Medicine* **145**, 849–852.

Hillbom, M., Numminen, H. & Juvela, S. (1999) Recent heavy drinking of alcohol and embolic stroke. *Stroke* **30**, 2307–2312.

Hokanson, J.E. & Austin, M.A. (1996) Plasma triglyceride level is a risk factor for cardiovascular disease independent of high-density lipoprotein cholesterol level: a meta-analysis of population-based prospective studies. *Journal of Cardiovascular Risk* **3**, 213–219.

Hole, D.J., Watt, G.C.M., Davey Smith, G., Hart, C.L., Gillis, C.R. & Hawthorne, V.M. (1996) Impaired lung function and mortality risk in men and women: findings from the Renfrew and Paisley prospective population study. *British Medical Journal* **313**, 711–715.

Holley, K.E., Bahn, R.C., McGoon, D.C. & Mankin, H.T. (1963) Spontaneous calcific embolisation associated with calcific aortic stenosis. *Circulation* **27**, 197–202.

Hollinger, P. & Sturzenegger, M. (1999) Painful oculomotor nerve palsy: a presenting sign of internal carotid artery stenosis. *Cerebrovascular Diseases* **9**, 178–181.

Homer, D., Ingall, T.J., Baker, H.L., O'Fallon, W.M., Kottke, B.A. & Whisnant, J.P. (1991) Serum lipids and lipoproteins are less powerful predictors of extracranial carotid artery atherosclerosis than are cigarette smoking and hypertension. *Mayo Clinic Proceedings* **66**, 259–267.

Homma, S., Di Tullio, M.R., Sacco, R.L., Sciacca, R.R., Smith, C. & Mohr, J.P. (1997) Surgical closure of patent foramen ovale in cryptogenic stroke patients. *Stroke* **28**, 2376–2381.

Hooper, L, Capps, N, Clements, G. *et al.* (2000a) Foods or supplements rich in omega-3 fatty acids for preventing cardiovascular disease in patients with ischaemic heart disease (Protocol for a Cochrane Review). In: *The Cochrane Library*. Oxford: Update Software.

Hooper, L, Capps, N, Clements, G. *et al.* (2000b) Anti-oxidant foods or supplements for preventing cardiovascular disease (Protocol for a Cochrane Review). In: *The Cochrane Library*. Oxford: Update Software.

Hopkins, P.N. & Williams, R.R. (1981) A survey of 246 suggested coronary risk factors. *Atherosclerosis* **40**, 1–52.

Horowitz, D.R., Tuhrim, S., Weinberger, J.M. & Rudolp, S.H. (1992) Mechanisms in lacunar infarction. *Stroke* **23**, 325–327.

House, A., Dennis, M.S., Mogridge, L., Hawton, K. & Warlow, C.P. (1990) Life events and difficulties preceding stroke. *Journal of Neurology, Neurosurgery and Psychiatry* **53**, 1024–1028.

Howard, G., Baker, W.H., Chambless, L.E., Howard, V.J., Jones, A.M. & Toole, J.F. for the Asymptomatic Carotid Atherosclerosis Study Investigators (1996) An approach for the use of Doppler ultrasound as a screening tool for haemodynamically significant stenosis (despite heterogeneity of Doppler performance): a multicenter experience. *Stroke* **27**, 1951–1957.

Howard, G., Wagenknecht, L.E., Burke, G.L. *et al.* for the ARIC Investigators (1998) Cigarette smoking and progression of atherosclerosis: the Atherosclerosis Risk in Communities (ARIC) Study. *Journal of the American Medical Association* **279**, 119–124.

Hu, F.B., Grodstein, F., Hennekens, C.H. *et al.* (1999) Age at natural menopause and risk of cardiovascular disease. *Archives of Internal Medicine* **159**, 1061–1066.

Hu, F.B., Stampfer, M.J., Colditz, G.A. *et al.* (2000) Physical activity and risk of stroke in women. *Journal of the American Medical Association* **283**, 2961–2967.

Hupperts, R.M.M., Lodder, J., Heuts-van Raak, E.P.M., Wilmink, J.T. & Kessels, A.G.H. (1996) Border-zone brain infarcts on CT taking into account the variability in vascular supply areas. *Cerebrovascular Diseases* **6**, 294–300.

Hupperts, R.M.M., Warlow, C.P., Slattery, J. & Rothwell, P.M. (1997a) Severe stenosis of the internal carotid artery is not associated with border-zone infarcts in patients randomised in the European Carotid Surgery Trial. *Journal of Neurology* **244**, 45–50.

Hupperts, R.M.M., Lodder, J., Heuts-van Raak, L. & Kessels, F. (1997b) Border-zone small deep infarcts: vascular risk factors and relationship with signs of small- and large-vessel disease. *Cerebrovascular Diseases* **7**, 280–283.

Hutchinson, E.C. & Yates, P.O. (1957) Carotico-vertebral stenosis. *Lancet* **1**, 2–8.

Iacoviello, L., Di Castelnuovo, A., De Knijff, P. *et al.* (1998) Polymorphisms in the coagulation factor VII gene and the risk of myocardial infarction. *New England Journal of Medicine* **338**, 79–85.

Imparato, A.M., Riles, T.S. & Gorstein, F. (1979) The carotid bifurcation plaque: pathologic findings associated with cerebral ischaemia. *Stroke* **10**, 238–245.

Ince, B., Petty, G.W., Brown, R.D., Chu, C-P., Sicks, J.D. & Whisnant, J.P. (1998) Dolichoectasia of the intracranial arteries in patients with first ischaemic stroke: a population-based study. *Neurology* **50**, 1694–1698.

Iribarren, C., Tekawa, I.S., Sidney, S. & Friedman, G.D. (1999) Effect of cigar smoking on the risk of cardiovascular disease, chronic obstructive pulmonary disease and cancer in men. *New England Journal of Medicine* **340**,

1773–1780.

Iso, H., Stampfer, M.J., Manson, J.E. *et al.* (1999) Prospective study of calcium, potassium and magnesium intake and risk of stroke in women. *Stroke* **30**, 1772–1779.

Jacobson, D.M., Terrence, C.F. & Reinmuth, O.M. (1986) The neurologic manifestations of fat embolism. *Neurology* **36**, 847–851.

Jamrozik, K. & Dobson, A. (1999) Please put out that cigarette, grandpa. *Tobacco Control* **8**, 125–126.

Jander, S., Sitzer, M., Schumann, R. *et al.* (1998) Inflammation in high-grade carotid stenosis: a possible role for macrophages and T cells in plaque destabilization. *Stroke* **29**, 1625–1630.

Jeanrenaud, X. & Kappenberger, L. (1991) Patent foramen ovale and stroke of unknown origin. *Cerebrovascular Diseases* **1**, 184–192.

Jeans, W.D., Mackenzie, S. & Baird, R.N. (1986) Angiography in transient cerebral ischaemia using three views of the carotid bifurcation. *British Journal of Radiology* **59**, 135–142.

Johansson, L., Jansson, J., Boman, K., Nilsson, T.K., Stegmayr, B. & Hallmans, G. (2000) Tissue plasminogen activator, plasminogen activator inhibitor-1, and tissue plasminogen activator/plasminogen activator inhibitor-1 complex as risk factors for the development of a first stroke. *Stroke* **31**, 26–32.

Jones, H.R. & Siekert, R.G. (1989) Neurological manifestations of infective endocarditis: review of clinical and therapeutic challenges. *Brain* **112**, 1295–1315.

Jorgensen, H.S., Jespersen, H.F., Nakayama, H., Raaschou, H.O. & Olsen, T.S. (1994a) Headache in stroke: the Copenhagen Stroke Study. *Neurology* **44**, 1793–1797.

Jorgensen, H.S., Nakayama, H., Raaschou, H.O., Gam, J. & Olsen, T.S. (1994b) Silent infarction in acute stroke patients: prevalence, localisation, risk factors and clinical significance. The Copenhagen Stroke Study. *Stroke* **25**, 97–104.

Jorgensen, H.S., Nakayama, H., Raaschou, H.O. & Olsen, T.S. (1994c) Stroke in patients with diabetes. The Copenhagen Stroke Study. *Stroke* **25**, 1977–1984.

Joseph, A., Ackerman, D., Talley, J.D., Johnstone, J. & Kupersmith, J. (1993) Manifestations of coronary atherosclerosis in young trauma victims: an autopsy study. *Journal of the American College of Cardiology* **22**, 459–467.

Joshipura, K.J., Ascherio, A., Manson, J.E. *et al.* (1999) Fruit and vegetable intake in relation to risk of ischaemic stroke. *Journal of the American Medical Association* **282**, 1233–1239.

Jousilahti, P., Rastenyte, D., Tuomilehto, J., Sarti, C. & Vartiainen, E. (1997) Parental history of cardiovascular disease and risk of stroke: a prospective follow-up of 14,371 middle-aged men and women in Finland. *Stroke* **28**, 1361–1366.

Joynt, R.J., Zimmerman, G. & Khalifeh, R. (1965) Cerebral emboli from cardiac tumours. *Archives of Neurology* **12**, 84–91.

Kagan, A.R. (1976) Atherosclerosis and myocardial lesions in subjects dying from fresh cerebrovascular disease. *Bulletin of the World Health Organization* **53**, 597–600.

Kagan, A.R., Popper, J.S. & Rhoads, G.G. (1980) Factors related to stroke incidence in Hawaii Japanese men. The Honolulu Heart Study. *Stroke* **11**, 14–21.

Kamata, T., Yokata, T., Furukawa, T. & Tsukagoshi, H. (1994) Cerebral ischaemic attack caused by postprandial hypotension. *Stroke* **25**, 511–513.

Kannel, W.B., Wolf, P.A. & Verter, J. (1983) Manifestations of coronary disease predisposing to stroke. The Framingham Study. *Journal of the American Medical Association* **250**, 2942–2946.

Kanter, M.C. & Hart, R.G. (1991) Neurologic complications of infective endocarditis. *Neurology* 41, 1015–1020.

Kanter, M.C., Tegeler, C.H., Pearce, L.A. *et al.* on behalf of the Stroke Prevention in Atrial Fibrillation Investigators (1994) Carotid stenosis in patients with atrial fibrillation: prevalence, risk factors and relationship to stroke in the Stroke Prevention in Atrial Fibrillation Study. *Archives of Internal Medicine* **154**, 1372–1377.

Kaplan, N.M. (1995) Alcohol and hypertension. *Lancet* **345**, 1588–1589.

Kaplan, P.W. (1993) Focal seizures resembling transient ischaemic attacks due to subclinical ischaemia. *Cerebrovascular Diseases* **3**, 241–243.

Kapoor, R., Kendall, B.E. & Harrison, M.J.G. (1991) Permanent oculomotor palsy with occlusion of the internal carotid artery. *Journal of Neurology, Neurosurgery and Psychiatry* **54**, 745–746.

Kaposzta, Z., Young, E., Bath, P.M.W. & Markus, H.S. (1999) Clinical application of asymptomatic embolic signal detection in acute stroke: a prospective study. *Stroke* **30**, 1814–1818.

Kappelle, L.J., van Latum, J.C., van Swieten, J.C., Algra, A., Koudstaal, P.J. & van Gijn, J. (1995) Recurrent stroke after transient ischaemic attack or minor ischaemic stroke: does the distinction between small and large vessel disease remain true to type? *Journal of Neurology, Neurosurgery and Psychiatry* **59**, 127–131.

Karanjia, P.N., Madden, K.P. & Lobner, S. (1994) Co-existence of abdominal aortic aneurysm in patients with carotid stenosis. *Stroke* **25**, 627–630.

Karnik, R., Winkler, W-B., Valentin, A., Khaffaf, N. & Slany, J. (1995) Carotid sinus massage and the risk of cerebral embolization. *Stroke* **26**, 1124–1125.

Kawachi, I., Colditz, G.A., Stampfer, M.J. *et al.* (1993) Smoking cessation and decreased risk of stroke in women. *Journal of the American Medical Association* **269**, 232–236.

Kawachi, I., Colditz, G.A. & Stone, C.B. (1994) Does coffee drinking increase the risk of coronary heart disease? Results from a meta-analysis. *British Heart Journal* **72**, 269–275.

Kearon, C., Julian, J.A., Math, M., Newman, T.E. & Ginsberg, J.S. (1998) Non-invasive diagnosis of deep venous thrombosis. *Annals of Internal Medicine* **128**, 663–677.

Kekomaki, S., Hamalainen, L., Kauppinen-Makelin, R., Palomaki, H., Kaste, K. & Kontula, K. (1999) Genetic polymorphism of platelet glycoprotein IIIa in patients with acute myocardial infarction and acute ischaemic stroke. *Journal of Cardiovascular Risk* **6**, 13–17.

Keli, S., Bloemberg, B. & Kromhout, D. (1992) Predictive value of repeated systolic blood pressure measurements for stroke risk. The Zutphen Study. *Stroke* **23**, 347–351.

Kelley, R.E., Bell, L., Kelley, S.E. & Lee, S. (1989) Syphilis detection in cerebrovascular disease. *Stroke* **20**, 230–234.

Kempczinski, R. & Hermann, G. (1979) The innominate steal syndrome. *Journal of Cardiovascular Surgery* **20**, 481–486.

Kempster, P.A., Gerraty, R.P. & Gates, P.C. (1988) Asymptomatic cerebral infarction in patients with chronic atrial fibrillation. *Stroke* **19**, 955–957.

Kendell, R.E. & Marshall, J. (1963) Role of hypotension in the genesis of transient focal cerebral ischaemic attacks. *British Medical Journal* **2**, 344–348.

Kersemakers, P., Beintema, M. & Lodder, J. (1992) Venous stasis retinopathy unlikely results from internal carotid artery obstruction alone. *Cerebrovascular Diseases* **2**, 305–307.

Key, T.J.A., Thorogood, M., Appleby, P.N. & Burr, M.L. (1996) Dietary habits and mortality in 11,000 vegetarians and health conscious people: results of a 17 year follow-up. *British Medical Journal* **313**, 775–779.

Khaffaf, N., Karnik, R., Winkler, W-B., Valentin, A. & Slany, J. (1994) Embolic stroke by compression manoeuvre during transcranial Doppler sonography. *Stroke* **25**, 1056–1057.

Khaw, K-T. & Barrett-Connor, E. (1987) Dietary potassium and stroke-associated mortality: a 12-year prospective population study. *New England Journal of Medicine* **316**, 235–240.

Kidwell, C.S., Alger, J.R., Di Salle, F. *et al.* (1999) Diffusion MRI in patients with transient ischaemic attacks. *Stroke* **30**, 2762–2763.

Kiechl, S., Willeit, J., Rungger, G., Egger, G., Oberhollenzer, F. & Bonora, E. for the Bruneck Study Group (1998) Alcohol consumption and atherosclerosis: what is the relation? Prospective results from the Bruneck Study. *Stroke* **29**, 900–907.

Kimura, K., Minematsu, K., Yasaka, M., Wada, K. & Yamaguchi, T. (1999) The duration of symptoms in transient ischaemic attack. *Neurology* **52**, 976–980.

Kittner, S.J., Sharkness, C.M., Price, T.R. *et al.* (1991) Infarcts with a cardiac source of embolism in the NINCDS Stroke Data Bank: historical features. *Neurology* **40**, 281–284.

Kittner, S.J., Sharkness, C.M., Sloan, M.A. *et al.* (1992) Features on initial computed tomography scan of infarcts with a cardiac source of embolism in the NINDS stroke data bank. *Stroke* **23**, 1748–1751.

Kittner, S.J., Giles, W.H., Macko, R.F. *et al.* (1999) Homocyst(e)ine and risk of cerebral infarction in a biracial population: the stroke prevention in young women study. *Stroke* **30**, 1554–1560.

Kleinschmidt, A., Steinmetz, H., Sitzer, M., Merboldt, K. & Frahm, J. (1995) Magnetic resonance imaging of regional cerebral blood oxygenation changes under acetazolamide in carotid occlusive disease. *Stroke* **26**, 106–110.

Kleiser, B. & Widder, B. (1992) Course of carotid artery occlusions with impaired cerebrovascular reactivity. *Stroke* **23**, 171–174.

Klijn, C.J.M., Kappelle, L.J., Tulleken, C.A.F. & van Gijn, J. (1997) Symptomatic carotid artery occlusion: a reappraisal of haemodynamic factors. *Stroke* **28**, 2084–2093.

Kluytmans, M., van der Grond, J., van Everdingen, K.J., Klijn, C.J.M., Kappelle, L.J. & Viergever, M.A. (1999) Cerebral haemodynamics in relation to patterns of collateral flow. *Stroke* **30**, 1432–1439.

Knutsen, R., Knutsen, S.F., Curb, J.D., Reed, D.M., Dautz, J.A. & Yano, K. (1988) Predictive value of resting electrocardiograms for 12-year incidence of stroke in the Honolulu Heart Program. *Stroke* **19**, 555–559.

Koennecke, H-C., Mast, H., Trocio, S.S., Sacco, R.L., Thompson, J.L.P. & Mohr, J.P. (1997) Microemboli in patients with vertebrobasilar ischaemia: association with vertebrobasilar and cardiac lesions. *Stroke* **28**, 593–596.

Koennecke, H-C., Mast, H., Trocio, S.H. *et al.* (1998) Frequency and determinants of microembolic signals on transcranial Doppler in unselected patients with acute carotid territory ischaemia: a prospective study. *Cerebrovascular Diseases* **8**, 107–112.

Kohler, H.P. & Grant, P.J. (2000) Plasminogen-activator inhibitor type 1 and coronary artery disease. *New England Journal of Medicine* **342**, 1792–1800.

van Kooten, F., van Krimpen, J., Dippel, D.W.J., Hoogerbrugge, N. & Koudstaal, P.J. (1996) Lipoprotein (a) in patients with acute cerebral ischaemia. *Stroke* **27**, 1231–1235.

van Kooten, F., Ciabattoni, G., Koudstaal, P.J., Dippel, D.W.J. & Patrono, C. (1999) Increased platelet activation in the chronic phase after cerebral ischaemia and intracerebral haemorrhage. *Stroke* **30**, 546–549.

Kopecky, S.L., Gersh, B.J., McGoon, M.D. *et al.* (1987) The natural history of lone atrial fibrillation: a population-based study over three decades. *New England Journal of Medicine* **317**, 669–674.

Koudstaal, P.J., van Gijn, J., Kappelle, L.J., for the Dutch TIA Study Group (1991) Headache in transient or permanent cerebral ischaemia. *Stroke* **22**, 754–759.

Koudstaal, P.J., van Gijn, J., Frenken, C.W.G.M. *et al.* for the Dutch TIA Study Group (1992) TIA, RIND, minor stroke: a continuum, or different subgroups? *Journal of Neurology, Neurosurgery and Psychiatry* **55**, 95–97.

Krapf, H., Skalej, M. & Voigt, K. (1999) Subarachnoid hemorrhage due to septic embolic infarction in infective endocarditis. *Cerebrovascular Diseases* **9**, 182–184.

Kumral, E., Bogousslavsky, J., van Melle, G., Regli, F. & Pierre, P. (1995) Headache at stroke onset: the Lausanne Stroke Registry. *Journal of Neurology, Neurosurgery and Psychiatry* **58**, 490–492.

Kunst, A.E., Del Rios, M., Groenhof, F. & Mackenbach, J.P. (1998) Socioeconomic inequalities in stroke mortality among middle-aged men: an international overview. *Stroke* **29**, 2285–2291.

Kushwaha, S.S., Fallon, J.T. & Fuster, V. (1997) Restrictive cardiomyopathy. *New England Journal of Medicine* **336**, 267–276.

Kwa, V.I., Franke, C.L., Verbeeten, B. & Stam, J. for the Amsterdam Vascular Medicine Group (1998) Silent intracerebral microhaemorrhages in patients with ischaemic stroke. *Annals of Neurology* **44**, 372–377.

Lammie, G.A. (2000) Small vessel disease. *Brain* (in press).

Lammie, G.A., Brannan, F., Slattery, J. & Warlow, C. (1997) Non-hypertensive cerebral small-vessel disease: an autopsy study. *Stroke* **28**, 2222–2229.

Lammie, G.A., Wardlaw, J. & Dennis, M. (1998) Thrombo-embolic stroke, moya-moya phenomenon and primary oxalosis. *Cerebrovascular Diseases* **8**, 45–50.

Lammie, G.A., Sandercock, P.A.G. & Dennis, M.S. (1999) Recently occluded intracranial and extracranial carotid arteries: relevance of the unstable atherosclerotic plaque. *Stroke* **30**, 1319–1325.

Lancet (1985) Alcohol and atrial fibrillation. *Lancet* **1**, 1374.

Landi, G., D'Angelo, A., Boccardi, E. *et al.* (1992) Venous thromboembolism in acute stroke: prognostic importance of hypercoagulability. *Archives of Neurology* **49**, 279–283.

Landi, G., Motto, C., Cella, E. *et al.* (1993) Pathogenetic and prognostic features of lacunar transient ischaemic attack syndromes. *Journal of Neurology, Neurosurgery and Psychiatry* **56**, 1265–1270.

van Latum, J.C., Koudstaal, P.J., Venables, G.S., van Gijn, J., Kappelle, L.J. & Algra, A. for the European Atrial Fibrillation Trial (EAFT) Study Group (1995) Predictors of major vascular events in patients with a transient ischaemic attack or minor ischaemic stroke and with non-rheumatic atrial fibrillation. *Stroke* **16**, 801–806.

Law, M.R., Frost, C.D. & Wald, N.J. (1991a) By how much does dietary salt reduction lower blood pressure? I. Analysis of observational data among populations. *British Medical Journal* **302**, 811–815.

Law, M.R., Frost, C.D. & Wald, N.J. (1991b) By how much does dietary salt reduction lower blood pressure? III. Analysis of data from trials of salt reduction. *British Medical Journal* **302**, 819–824.

Law, M.R., Wald, N.J. & Thompson, S.G. (1994) By how much and how quickly does reduction in serum cholesterol concentration lower risk of ischaemic heart disease? *British Medical Journal* **308**, 367–373.

Law, M.R., Morris, J.K. & Wald, N.J. (1997) Environmental tobacco smoke exposure and ischaemic heart disease: an evaluation of the evidence. *British Medical Journal* **315**, 973–980.

Leclerc, X., Godefroy, O., Pruvo, J.P. & Leys, D. (1995) Computed tomographic angiography for the evaluation of carotid artery stenosis. *Stroke* **26**, 1577–1581.

Lee, I-M., Hennekens, C.H., Berger, K., Buring, J.E., Manson, J. & E. (1999) Exercise and risk of stroke in male physicians. *Stroke* **30**, 1–6.

Lehto, S., Niskanen, L., Ronnemaa, T. & Laakso, M. (1998) Serum uric acid is a strong predictor of stroke in patients with non-insulin-dependent diabetes mellitus. *Stroke* **29**, 635–639.

Leira, E.C., Ajax, T. & Adams, H.P. (1997) Limb-shaking carotid transient ischaemic attacks successfully treated with modification of the antihypertensive regimen. *Archives of Neurology* **54**, 904–905.

Leng, G.C., Fowkes, F.G.R., Lee, A.J., Dunbar, J., Housley, E. & Ruckley, C.V. (1996) Use of ankle brachial pressure index to predict cardiovascular events and death: a cohort study. *British Medical Journal* **313**, 1440–1444.

Leon, D.A. (1993) Failed or misleading adjustment for confounding. *Lancet* **342**, 479–481.

Leppala, J.M., Virtamo, J., Fogelholm, R. *et al.* (2000) Controlled trial of alpha-tocopherol and beta-carotene supplements on stroke incidence and mortality in male smokers. *Arteriosclerosis, Thrombosis and Vascular Biology* **20**, 230–235.

Lerner, D.J. & Kannel, W.B. (1986) Patterns of coronary heart disease morbidity and mortality in the sexes: a 26 year follow-up of the Framingham population. *American Heart Journal* **111**, 383–390.

Leung, D.Y., Black, I.W., Cranney, G.B. *et al.* (1995) Selection of patients for transoesophageal echocardiography after stroke and systemic embolic events: role of transthoracic echocardiography. *Stroke* **26**, 1820–1824.

Leung, S.Y., Ng, T.H.K., Yuen, S.T., Lauder, I.J. & Ho, F.C.S. (1993) Pattern of cerebral atherosclerosis in Hong Kong Chinese: severity in intracranial and extracranial vessels. *Stroke* **24**, 779–786.

Levi, C.R., Mitchell, A., Fitt, G. & Donnan, G.A. (1996) The accuracy of magnetic resonance angiography in the assessment of extracranial carotid artery occlusive disease. *Cerebrovascular Diseases* **6**, 231–236.

Ley-Pozo, J. & Ringelstein, E.B. (1990) Non-invasive detection of occlusive disease of the carotid siphon and middle cerebral artery. *Annals of Neurology* **28**, 640–647.

Lhermitte, F., Gautier, J.C. & Derouesne, C. (1970) Nature of occlusions of the middle cerebral artery. *Neurology* **20**, 82–88.

Liao, D., Myers, R., Hunt, S. *et al.* (1997) Familial history of stroke and stroke risk. The Family Heart Study. *Stroke* **28**, 1908–1912.

Libby, P. (1996) Atheroma: more than mush. *Lancet* **348**, S4–S7.

Lindberg, G., Eklund, G.A., Gullberg, B. & Rastam, L. (1991) Serum sialic acid concentration and cardiovascular mortality. *British Medical Journal* **302**, 143–146.

Lip, G.Y.H. (1995) Does atrial fibrillation confer a hypercoagulable state? *Lancet* **346**, 1313–1314.

Lip, G.Y.H. (1997) Does paroxysmal atrial fibrillation confer a paroxysmal thromboembolic risk? *Lancet* **349**, 1565–1566.

Little, J.R., St. Louis, P., Weinstein, M. & Dohn, D.F. (1981) Giant fusiform aneurysm of the cerebral arteries. *Stroke* **12**, 183–188.

Lodder, J., Bamford, J.M., Sandercock, P.A.G., Jones, L.N. & Warlow, C.P. (1990) Are hypertension or cardiac embolism likely causes of lacunar infarction? *Stroke* **21**, 375–381.

Loftus, I.M., Naylor, A.R., Goodall, S. *et al.* (2000) Increased matrix metalloproteinase-9 activity in unstable carotid plaques: a potential role in acute plaque disruption. *Stroke* **31**, 40-47.

Long-term Intervention with Pravastatin in Ischaemic Disease (LIPID) Study Group (1998) Prevention of cardiovascular events and death with pravastatin in patients with coronary heart disease and a broad range of initial cholesterol levels. *New England Journal of Medicine* **339**, 1349–1357.

Lopez, J.A., Ross, R.S., Fishbein, M.C. & Siegel, R.J. (1987) Non-bacterial thrombotic endocarditis: a review. *American Heart Journal* **113**, 773–784.

Lowe, G.D.O., Lee, A.J., Rumley, A., Price, J.F. & Fowkes, F.G.R. (1997) Blood viscosity and risk of cardiovascular events: the Edinburgh Artery Study. *British Journal of Haematology* **96**, 168–173.

Lucas, A., Fewtrell, M.S. & Cole, T.J. (1999) Fetal origins of adult disease: the hypothesis revisited. *British Medical Journal* 319, 245–249.

Lusiani, L., Visona, A., Castellani, V. *et al.* (1987) Prevalence of atherosclerotic involvement of the internal carotid artery in hypertensive patients. *International Journal of Cardiology* 17, 51–56.

Lynch, J.W., Kaplan, G.A., Cohen, R.D. *et al.* (1994) Childhood and adult socioeconomic status as predictors of mortality in Finland. *Lancet* 343, 524–527.

McKeigue, P.M., Shah, B. & Marmot, M.G. (1991) Relation of central obesity and insulin resistance with high diabetes prevalence and cardiovascular risk in South Asians. *Lancet* 337, 971–973.

Macko, R.F., Kittner, S.J., Epstein, A. *et al.* (1999) Elevated tissue plasminogen activator antigen and stroke risk. The stroke prevention in young women study. *Stroke* 30, 7–11.

MacMahon, S. & Norton, R.N. (1986) Alcohol and hypertension: implications for prevention and treatment. *Annals of Internal Medicine* 105, 124–126.

MacMahon, S. & Rodgers, A. (1993) The effects of blood pressure reduction in older patients: an overview of five randomised controlled trials in elderly hypertensives. *Clinical and Experimental Hypertension* 15 (6), 967–978.

MacMahon, S. & Rodgers, A. (1994) Antihypertensive agents and stroke prevention. *Cerebrovascular Diseases* 4 (Suppl. 1), 11–15.

MacMahon, S., Peto, R., Cutler, J. *et al.* (1990) Blood pressure, stroke and coronary heart disease. I. Prolonged differences in blood pressure: prospective observational studies corrected for the regression dilution bias. *Lancet* 335, 765–774.

McMillan, D.E. (1985) Blood flow and the localization of atherosclerotic plaques. *Stroke* 16, 582–587.

Malek, A.M., Alper, S.L. & Izumo, S. (1999) Haemodynamic shear stress and its role in atherosclerosis. *Journal of the American Medical Association* 282, 2035–2042.

Mandai, K., Sueyoshi, K., Fukunaga, R. *et al.* (1994) Evaluation of cerebral vasoreactivity by three-dimensional time-of-flight magnetic resonance angiography. *Stroke* 25, 1807–1811.

Manson, J.E., Colditz, G.A., Stampfer, M.J. *et al.* (1991) A prospective study of maturity-onset diabetes mellitus and risk of coronary heart disease and stroke in women. *Archives of Internal Medicine* 151, 1141–1147.

Margaglione, M., Seripa, D., Gravina, C. *et al.* (1998) Prevalence of apolipoprotein E alleles in healthy subjects and survivors of ischaemic stroke: an Italian case–control study. *Stroke* 29, 399–403.

Marini, C., Carolei, A., Roberts, R.S. *et al.* and the National Research Council Study Group (1993) Focal cerebral ischaemia in young adults: a collaborative case–control study. *Neuroepidemiology* 12, 70–81.

Markel, M.L., Waller, B.F. & Armstrong, W.F. (1987) Cardiac myxoma: a review. *Medicine* 66, 114–125.

Markus, H.S. (1999) Transcranial Doppler ultrasound. *Journal of Neurology, Neurosurgery and Psychiatry* 67, 135–137.

Markus, H.S. & Harrison, M.J.G. (1992) Estimation of cerebrovascular reactivity using transcranial Doppler, including the use of breath-holding as the vasodilatory stimulus. *Stroke* 23, 668–673.

Markus, H.S. & Mendall, M.A. (1998) *Helicobacter pylori* infection: a risk factor for ischaemic cerebrovascular disease and carotid atheroma. *Journal of Neurology, Neurosurgery and Psychiatry* 64, 104–107.

Markus, H.S., Droste, D.W. & Brown, M.M. (1994) Detection of asymptomatic cerebral embolic signals with Doppler ultrasound. *Lancet* 343, 1011–1012.

Markus, H., Cullinane, M. & Reid, G. (1999) Improved automated detection of embolic signals using a novel frequency filtering approach. *Stroke* 30, 1610–1615.

Marmot, M. & Brunner, E. (1991) Alcohol and cardiovascular disease: the status of the U-shaped curve. *British Medical Journal* 303, 565–568.

Marmot, M.G., Elliott, P., Shipley, M.J. *et al.* (1994) Alcohol and blood pressure: the INTERSALT study. *British Medical Journal* 308, 1263–1267.

Martin, P.J., Chang, H.M., Wityk, R. & Caplan, L.R. (1998) Midbrain infarction: associations and aetiologies in the New England Medical Center Posterior Circulation Registry. *Journal of Neurology, Neurosurgery and Psychiatry* 64, 392–395.

Martin, R., Bogousslavsky, J., Miklossy, J. *et al.* (1992) Floating thrombus in the innominate artery as a cause of cerebral infarction in young adults. *Cerebrovascular Diseases* 2, 177–181.

Martyn, C.N., Barker, D.J.P. & Osmond, C. (1996) Mothers' pelvic size, fetal growth and death from stroke and coronary heart disease in men in the UK. *Lancet* 348, 1264–1268.

Mas, J-L. (1991) Patent foramen ovale, stroke and paradoxical embolism. *Cerebrovascular Diseases* 1, 181–183.

Mast, H., Thompson, J.L.P., Voller, H., Mohr, J.P. & Marx, P. (1994) Cardiac sources of embolism in patients with pial artery infarcts and lacunar lesions. *Stroke* 25, 776–781.

Masuda, J., Yutani, C., Waki, R., Ogata, J., Kuriyama, Y. & Yamaguchi, T. (1992) Histopathological analysis of the mechanisms of intracranial haemorrhage complicating infective endocarditis. *Stroke* 23, 843–850.

Mattle, H.P., Maurer, D., Sturzenegger, M., Ozdoba, C., Baumgartner, R.W. & Schroth, G. (1995) Cardiac myxomas: a long-term study. *Journal of Neurology* 242, 689–694.

Mead, G.E., Lewis, S.C., Wardlaw, J.M., Dennis, M.S. & Warlow, C.P. (1999a) Should computed tomography appearance of lacunar stroke influence patient management? *Journal of Neurology, Neurosurgery and Psychiatry* 67, 682–684.

Mead, G.E., Wardlaw, J.M., Lewis, S.C., McDowall, M. & Dennis, M.S. (1999b) Can simple clinical features be used to identify patients with severe carotid stenosis on Doppler ultrasound? *Journal of Neurology, Neurosurgery and Psychiatry* 66, 16–19.

Mead, G.E., Lewis, S.C., Wardlaw, J.M., Dennis, M.S. & Warlow, C.P. (2000a) Severe ipsilateral carotid stenosis in lacunar ischaemic stroke: an innocent bystander? *Journal of Neurology, Neurosurgery and Psychiatry* (in press).

Mead, G.E., Wardlaw, J.M., Dennis, M.S., Lewis, S.C. & Warlow, C.P. (2000b) Relationship between pattern of intracranial artery abnormalities on transcranial Doppler and the Oxfordshire Community Stroke Project clinical classification of ischaemic stroke. *Stroke* 31, 714–719.

Meade, T.W., Ruddock, V., Stirling, Y., Chakrabarti, R. & Miller, G.J. (1993) Fibrinolytic activity, clotting factors and long-term incidence of ischaemic heart disease in the Northwick Park Heart Study. *Lancet* 342, 1076–1079.

Meairs, S. & Hennerici, M. (1999) Four-dimensional ultrasonographic characterization of plaque surface motion in patients with symptomatic and asymptomatic carotid artery stenosis. *Stroke* 30, 1807–1813.

Mendez, I., Hachinski, V. & Wolfe, B. (1987) Serum lipids after stroke. *Neurology* 37, 507–511.

Menotti, A., Lanti, M., Seccareccia, F., Giampaoli, S. & Dima, F. (1993) Multivariate prediction of the first major cerebrovascular event in an Italian population sample of middle-aged men followed up for 25 years. *Stroke* 24, 42–48.

van der Meulen, J.H.P., Weststrate, W., van Gijn, J. & Habbema, J.D.F. (1992) Is cerebral angiography indicated in infective endocarditis? *Stroke* 23, 1662–1667.

Miettinen, H., Haffner, S.M., Lehto, S., Ronnemaa, T., Pyorala, K. & Laakso, M. (1996) Proteinuria predicts stroke and other atherosclerotic vascular disease events in non-diabetic and non-insulin-dependent diabetic subjects. *Stroke* 27, 2033–2039.

Milder, D.G. & Lance, J.W. (1984) Intermittent claudication of one cerebral hemisphere. *Neurology* 34, 692–694.

Millikan, C. & Futrell, N. (1990) The fallacy of the lacune hypothesis. *Stroke* 21, 1251–1257.

Min, W.K., Kim, Y.S., Kim, J.Y., Park, S.P. & Suh, C.K. (1999) Atherothrombotic cerebellar infarction: vascular lesion-MRI correlation of 31 cases. *Stroke* 30, 2376–2381.

Mitchell, J.R.A. & Schwartz, C.J. (1962) Relationship between arterial disease in different sites: a study of the aorta and coronary, carotid and iliac arteries. *British Medical Journal* 1, 1293–1301.

Mitchell, P., Wang, J.J., Li, W., Leeder, S.R. & Smith, W. (1997) Prevalence of asymptomatic retinal emboli in an Australian urban community. *Stroke* 28, 63–66.

Molina, C., Sabin, J.A., Montaner, J., Rovira, A., Abilleira, S. & Codina, A. (1999) Impaired cerebrovascular reactivity as a risk marker for first-ever lacunar infarction: a case–control study. *Stroke* 30, 2296–2301.

Molloy, J. & Markus, H.S. (1999) Asymptomatic embolization predicts stroke and TIA risk in patients with carotid artery stenosis. *Stroke* 30, 1440–1443.

Molloy, J., Khan, N. & Markus, H.S. (1998) Temporal variability of asymptomatic embolization in carotid artery stenosis and optimal recording protocols. *Stroke* 29, 1129–1132.

Morris, J.N. (1951a) Recent history of coronary disease. *Lancet* 1, 1–7.

Morris, J.N. (1951b) Recent history of coronary disease. *Lancet* 1, 69–73.

Mouton, P., Biousse, V., Crassard, I., Bousson, V. & Bousser, M-G. (1997) Ischaemic stroke due to calcific emboli from mitral valve annulus calcification. *Stroke* **28**, 2325–2326.

Mulrow, C.D., Cornell, J.A., Herrera, C.R., Kadri, A., Farnett, L. & Aguilar, C. (1994) Hypertension in the elderly: implications and generalizability of randomised trials. *Journal of the American Medical Association* **272**, 1932–1938.

Mykkanen, L., Zaccaro, D.J., O'Leary, D.H., Howard, G., Robbins, D.C. & Haffner, S.M. (1997) Microalbuminuria and carotid artery intima-media thickness in non-diabetic and NIDDM subjects. The Insulin Resistance Atherosclerosis Study (IRAS). *Stroke* **28**, 1710–1716.

Nabavi, D.G., Arato, S., Droste, D.W. *et al.* (1998) Microembolic load in asymptomatic patients with cardiac aneurysm, severe ventricular dysfunction and atrial fibrillation: clinical and haemorheological correlates. *Cerebrovascular Diseases* **8**, 214–221.

Napoli, C., Glass, C.K., Witztum, J.L., Deutsch, R., D'Armiento, F.P. & Palinski, W. (1999) Influence of maternal hypercholesterolaemia during pregnancy on progression of early atherosclerotic lesions in childhood: Fate of Early Lesions in Children (FELIC) study. *Lancet* **354**, 1234–1241.

Narayan, S.M., Cain, M.E. & Smith, J.M. (1997) Atrial fibrillation. *Lancet* **350**, 943–950.

Nater, B., Bogousslavksy, J., Regli, F. & Stauffer, J. (1992) Stroke patterns with atrial septal aneurysm. *Cerebrovascular Diseases* **2**, 342–346.

Naumann, M., Hofmann, E. & Toyka, K.V. (1998) Multifocal brain MRI hypointensities secondary to embolic metal fragments from a mechanical heart valve prosthesis: a possible source of epileptic seizures. *Neurology* **51**, 1766–1767.

Naylor, A.R., Merrick, M.V., Gillespie, I. *et al.* (1994) Prevalence of impaired cerebrovascular reserve in patients with symptomatic carotid artery disease. *British Journal of Surgery* **81**, 45–48.

Ness, A.R. & Powles, J.W. (1999) The role of diet, fruit and vegetables and antioxidants in the aetiology of stroke. *Journal of Cardiovascular Risk* **6**, 229–234.

Nestico, P.F., Depace, N.L., Morganroth, J., Kotler, M.N. & Ross, J. (1984) Mitral annular calcification: clinical, pathophysiology and echocardiographic review. *American Heart Journal* **107**, 989–996.

Ng, H.K. & Poon, W.S. (1990) Cardiac myxoma metastasizing to the brain: case report. *Journal of Neurosurgery* **72**, 295–298.

Nicholls, S.C., Phillips, D.J., Primozich, J.F. *et al.* (1989) Diagnostic significance of flow separation in the carotid bulb. *Stroke* **20**, 175–182.

Nichols, F.T., Mawad, M., Mohr, J.P., Stein, B., Hilal, S. & Michelsen, W.J. (1990) Focal headache during balloon inflation in the internal carotid and middle cerebral arteries. *Stroke* **21**, 555–559.

Nishide, M., Irino, T., Gotoh, M., Naka, M. & Tsuji, K. (1983) Cardiac abnormalities in ischaemic cerebrovascular disease studied by two-dimensional echocardiography. *Stroke* **14**, 541–545.

Nishizaki, T., Tamaki, N., Takeda, N., Shirakuni, T., Kondoh, T. & Matsumoto, S. (1986) Dolichoectatic basilar artery: a review of 23 cases. *Stroke* **17**, 1277–1281.

Niskanen, L., Rauramaa, R., Miettinen, H., Haffner, S.M., Mercuri, M. & Uusitupa, M. (1996) Carotid artery intima-media thickness in elderly patients with NIDDM and in non-diabetic subjects. *Stroke* **27**, 1986–92.

Nobile-Orazio, E. & Sterzi, R. (1981) Cerebral ischaemia after nifedipine treatment. *British Medical Journal* **283**, 948.

Norris, J.W. & Bornstein, N.M. (1986) Progression and regression of carotid stenosis. *Stroke* **17**, 755–757.

Nyyssonen, K., Parviainen, M.T., Salonen, R., Tuomilehto, J. & Salonen, J.T. (1997) Vitamin C deficiency and risk of myocardial infarction: prospective population study of men from eastern Finland. *British Medical Journal* **314**, 634–638.

O'Connor, G.T., Buring, J.E., Yusuf, S. *et al.* (1989) An overview of randomized trials of rehabilitation with exercise after myocardial infarction. *Circulation* **80**, 234–244.

O'Donoghue, M.E., Dangond, F., Burger, A.J., Suojanen, J.N., Zarich, S. & Tarsy, D. (1993) Spontaneous calcific embolization to the supraclinoid internal carotid artery from a regurgitant bicuspid aortic valve. *Neurology* **43**, 2715–2717.

O'Leary, D.H., Polak, J.F., Kronmal, A. *et al.* on behalf of the CHS Collaborative Research Group (1992) Distribution and correlates of sonographically detected carotid artery disease in the Cardiovascular Health Study. *Stroke* **23**, 1752–1760.

O'Leary, D.H., Polak, J.F., Kronmal, R.A. *et al.* for the Cardiovascular Health Study Collaborative Research Group (1996) Thickening of the carotid wall: a marker for atherosclerosis in the elderly? *Stroke* **27**, 224–231.

O'Leary, D.H., Polak, J.F., Kronmal, R.A., Manolio, T.A., Burke, G.L. & Wolfson, S.K. (1999) Carotid-artery intima and media thickness as a risk factor for myocardial infarction and stroke in older adults for the cardiovascular Health Study Collaborative Research Group. *New England Journal of Medicine* **340**, 14–22.

O'Malley, T., Langhorne, P., Elton, R.A. & Stewart, C. (1995) Platelet size in stroke patients. *Stroke* **26**, 995–999.

O'Neill, W.W., Chandler, J.G., Gordon, R.E. *et al.* (1995) Radiographic detection of strut separations in Bjork–Shiley convexo-concave mitral valves. *New England Journal of Medicine* **333**, 414–419.

Ogata, J., Masuda, J., Yutani, C. & Yamaguchi, T. (1990) Rupture of atheromatous plaque as a cause of thrombotic occlusion of stenotic internal carotid artery. *Stroke* **21**, 1740–1745.

Ogata, J., Masuda, J., Yutani, C. & Yamaguchi, T. (1994) Mechanisms of cerebral artery thrombosis: a histopathological analysis on eight necropsy cases. *Journal of Neurology, Neurosurgery and Psychiatry* **57**, 17–21.

Olsen, T.S., Skriver, E.B. & Herning, M. (1985) Cause of cerebral infarction in the carotid territory: its relation to the size and the location of the infarct and to the underlying vascular lesion. *Stroke* **16**, 459–466.

van Oostenbrugge, R.J., Freling, G., Lodder, J., Lalisang, R. & Twijnstra, A. (1996) Fatal stroke due to paradoxical fat embolism. *Cerebrovascular Diseases* **6**, 313–314.

Oppenheimer, S.M. & Lima, J. (1998) Neurology and the heart. *Journal of Neurology, Neurosurgery and Psychiatry* **64**, 289–297.

Orencia, A.J., Petty, G.W., Khandheria, B.K. *et al.* (1995a) Risk of stroke with mitral valve prolapse in population-based cohort study. *Stroke* **26**, 7–13.

Orencia, A.J., Petty, G.W., Khandheria, B.K., O'Fallon, W.M. & Whisnant, J.P. (1995b) Mitral valve prolapse and the risk of stroke after initial cerebral ischaemia. *Neurology* **45**, 1083–1086.

Orencia, A.J., Daviglus, M.L., Dyer, A.R., Shekelle, R.B. & Stamler, J. (1996) Fish consumption and stroke in men: 30-year findings of Chicago Western Electric Study. *Stroke* **27**, 204–209.

Paneth, N. & Susser, M. (1995) Early origin of coronary heart disease (the 'Barker hypothesis'): hypotheses, no matter how intriguing, need rigorous attempts at refutation. *British Medical Journal* **310**, 411–412.

Pantin, C.F.A. & Young, R.A.L. (1980) Postprandial blindness. *British Medical Journal* **281**, 1686.

Parker, J.L.W. & Lawson, D.H. (1973) Death from thyrotoxicosis. *Lancet* **2**, 894–895.

di Pasquale, G., Urbinati, S. & Pinelli, G. (1995) New echocardiographic markers of embolic risk in atrial fibrillation. *Cerebrovascular Diseases* **5**, 315–322.

Passero, S. & Filosomi, G. (1998) Posterior circulation infarcts in patients with vertebrobasilar dolichoectasia. *Stroke* **29**, 653–659.

Patel, V., Champ, C., Andrews, P.S., Gostelow, B.E., Gunasekara, N.P.R. & Davidson, A.R. (1992) Diagonal earlobe creases and atheromatous disease: a post-mortem study. *Journal of the Royal College of Physicians of London* **26**, 274–277.

Pelz, D.M., Fox, A.J. & Vinuela, F. (1985) Digital subtraction angiography: current clinical applications. *Stroke* **16**, 528–536.

Peng, D-Q., Zhao, S-P. & Wang, J-L. (1999) Lipoprotein (a) and apolipoprotein E epsilon 4 as independent risk factors for ischaemic stroke. *Journal of Cardiovascular Risk* **6**, 1–6.

Penner, R. & Font, R.L. (1969) Retinal embolism from calcified vegetations of aortic valve. *Archives of Ophthalmology* **81**, 565–568.

Perry, I.J. (1999) Homocystine and risk of stroke. *Journal of Cardiovascular Risk* **6**, 235–240.

Pessin, M.S., Chimowitz, M.I., Levine, S.R. *et al.* (1989) Stroke in patients with fusiform vertebrobasilar aneurysms. *Neurology* **39**, 16–21.

Petersen, P. (1990) Thromboembolic complications in atrial fibrillation. *Stroke* **21**, 4–13.

Petrovitch, H., Curb, D. & Bloom-Marcus, E. (1995) Isolated systolic hypertension and risk of stroke in Japanese-American men. *Stroke* **26**, 25–29.

Petty, G.W., Wiebers, W.O. & Meissner, I. (1990) Transcranial Doppler ultrasonography: clinical applications in cerebrovascular disease. *Mayo Clinic Proceedings* **65**, 1350–1364.

Petty, G.W., Khandheria, B.K., Chu, C., Sicks, J.D. & Whisnant, J.P. (1997) Patent foramen ovale in patients with cerebral infarction: a transoesophageal echocardiographic study. *Archives of Neurology* **54**, 819–822.

Petty, G.W., Brown, R.D., Whisnant, J.P., Sicks, J.D., O'Fallon, W.M. & Wiebers, D.O. (1999) Ischaemic stroke subtypes: a population-based study of incidence and risk factors. *Stroke* **30**, 2513–2516.

Phillips, A.N. & Davey Smith, G. (1993) Confounding in epidemiological studies. *British Medical Journal* **306**, 142–143.

Pierre, P., Bogousslavsky, J., Menetrey, R., Regli, F. & Kappenberger, L. (1993) Familial sick sinus disease: another Mendelian aetiology of stroke. *Cerebrovascular Diseases* **3**, 120–122.

Pohlmann-Eden, B., Hoch, D.B., Cochius, J.I. & Henhnerici, M.G. (1996) Stroke and epilepsy: critical review of the literature. I. Epidemiology and risk factors. *Cerebrovascular Diseases* **6**, 332–338.

Pohlmann-Eden, B., Cochius, J.I., Hoch, D.B. & Hennerici, M.G. (1997) Stroke and epilepsy: critical review of the literature. II. Risk factors, pathophysiology and overlap syndrome. *Cerebrovascular Diseases* **7**, 2–9.

Polak, J.F., Shemanski, L., O'Leary, D.H. *et al.* for the Cardiovascular Health Study (1998) Hypoechoic plaque at US of the carotid artery: an independent risk factor for incident stroke in adults aged 65 years or older. *Radiology* **208**, 649–654.

Powers, W.J. (1986) Should lumbar puncture be part of the routine evaluation of patients with cerebral ischaemia? *Stroke* **17**, 332–333.

Powers, W.J., Press, G.A., Grubb, R.L., Gado, M. & Raichle, M.E. (1987) The effect of haemodynamically significant carotid artery disease on the haemodynamic status of the cerebral circulation. *Annals of Internal Medicine* **106**, 27–34.

Price, T.R., Manolio, T.A., Kronmal, R.A. *et al.* for the CHS Collaborative Research Group (1997) Silent brain infarction on magnetic resonance imaging and neurological abnormalities in community-dwelling older adults. The Cardiovascular Health Study. *Stroke* **28**, 1158–1164.

Prospective Studies Collaboration (1995) Cholesterol, diastolic blood pressure and stroke: 13,000 strokes in 450,000 people in 45 prospective cohorts. *Lancet* **346**, 1647–1653.

Puddey, I.B., Beilin, L.J. & Vandongen, R. (1987) Regular alcohol use raises blood pressure in treated hypertensive subjects: a randomised controlled trial. *Lancet* **1**, 647–651.

Pullicino, P.M., Halperin, J.L. & Thompson, J.L.P. (2000) Stroke in patients with heart failure and reduced left ventricular ejection fraction. *Neurology* **54**, 288–294.

Purvin, V.A. & Dunn, D.W. (1981) Nitrate-induced transient ischaemic attacks. *Southern Medical Journal* **74**, 1130–1131.

Qizilbash, N., Jones, L., Warlow, C.P. & Mann, J. (1991) Fibrinogen and lipids as risk factors for transient ischaemic attacks and minor ischaemic strokes. *British Medical Journal* **303**, 605–609.

Qizilbash, N., Duffy, S., Prentice, C.R., Boothby, M. & Warlow, C. (1997) Von Willebrand factor and risk of ischaemic stroke. *Neurology* **49**, 1552–1556.

Qureshi, A.I., Giles, W.H., Croft, J.B. & Bliwise, D.L. (1997) Habitual sleep patterns and risk for stroke and coronary heart disease: a 10-year follow-up from NHANES I. *Neurology* **48**, 904–911.

Qureshi, A.I., Giles, W.H. & Croft, J.B. (1998) Impaired glucose tolerance and the likelihood of non-fatal stroke and myocardial infarction: the Third National Health and Nutrition Examination Survey. *Stroke* **29**, 1329–1332.

Ranoux, D., Cohen, A., Cabanes, L., Amarenco, P., Bousser, M-G. & Mas, J-L. (1993) Patent foramen ovale: is stroke due to paradoxical embolism? *Stroke* **24**, 31–34.

Rastenyte, D., Tuomilehto, J. & Sarti, C. (1998) Genetics of stroke: a review. *Journal of Neurological Sciences* **153**, 132–145.

Rauh, G., Fischereder, M. & Spengel, F.A. (1996) Transoesophageal echocardiography in patients with focal cerebral ischaemia of unknown cause. *Stroke* **27**, 691–694.

Rayman, M.P. (2000) The importance of selenium to human health. *Lancet* **356**, 233–241.

Raymond, L.A., Sacks, J.G., Choromokos, E. & Khodadad, G. (1980) Short posterior ciliary artery insufficiency with hyperthermia (Uhthoff's symptom). *American Journal of Ophthalmology* **90**, 619–623.

Reed, D.M., Resch, J.A., Hayashi, T., MacLean, C. & Yano, K. (1988) A prospective study of cerebral artery atherosclerosis. *Stroke* **19**, 820–825.

Refsum, H., Ueland, P.M., Nygard, O. & Vollset, S.E. (1998) Homocystine and cardiovascular disease. *Annual Review of Medicine* **49**, 31–62.

Reneman, R.S., van Merode, T., Hick, P. & Hoeks, A.P.G. (1985) Flow velocity patterns in and distensibility of the carotid artery bulb in subjects of various ages. *Circulation* **71**, 500–509.

Rexrode, K.M., Hennekens, C.H., Willett, W.C. *et al.* (1997) A prospective study of body mass index, weight change and risk of stroke in women. *Journal of the American Medical Association* **277**, 1539–1545.

Reynen, K. (1995) Cardiac myxomas. *New England Journal of Medicine* **333**, 1610–1617.

Richardson, P.D., Davies, M.J. & Born, G.V.R. (1989) Influence of plaque configuration and stress distribution on fissuring of coronary atherosclerotic plaques. *Lancet* **2**, 941–944.

Rich-Edwards, J.W., Stampfer, M.J., Manson, J.E. *et al.* (1997) Birth weight and risk of cardiovascular disease in a cohort of women followed up since 1976. *British Medical Journal* **315**, 396–400.

Ridker, P.M., Hennekens, C.H., Stampfer, M.J., Manson, J.E. & Vaughan, D.E. (1994) Prospective study of endogenous tissue plasminogen activator and risk of stroke. *Lancet* **343**, 940–943.

Ridker, P.M., Hennekens, C.H., Buring, J.E. & Rifai, N. (2000) C-reactive protein and other markers of inflammation in the prediction of cardiovascular disease in women. *New England Journal of Medicine* **342**, 836–843.

Rimm, E.B., Ascherio, A., Giovannucci, E., Spiegelman, D., Stampfer, M.J. & Willett, W.C. (1996) Vegetable, fruit, and cereal fiber intake and risk of coronary heart disease among men. *Journal of the American Medical Association* **275**, 447–451.

Rimm, E.B., Williams, P., Fosher, K., Criqui, M. & Stampfer, M.J. (1999) Moderate alcohol intake and lower risk of coronary heart disease: meta-analysis of effects on lipids and haemostatic factors. *British Medical Journal* **319**, 1523–1528.

Ringelstein, E.B. (1995) Skepticism toward carotid ultrasonography: a virtue, an attitude or fanaticism? *Stroke* **26**, 1743–1746.

Ringelstein, E.B., Droste, D.W., Babikian, V.L. *et al.* (1998) Consensus on microembolus detection by TCD: International Consensus Group on microembolus detection. *Stroke* **29**, 725–729.

Robbins, A.S., Manson, J.E., Lee, I-M., Satterfield, S. & Hennekens, C.H. (1994) Cigarette smoking and stroke in a cohort of US male physicians. *Annals of Internal Medicine* **120**, 458–462.

Roeltgen, D.P., Weimer, G.R. & Patterson, L.F. (1981) Delayed neurologic complications of left atrial myxoma. *Neurology* **31**, 8–13.

Roob, G., Schmidt, R., Kapeller, P., Lechner, A., Hartung, H-P. & Fazekas, F. (1999) MRI evidence of past cerebral microbleeds in a healthy elderly population. *Neurology* **52**, 991–994.

Rosario, J.A., Hachinski, V.A., Lee, D.H. & Fox, A.J. (1987) Adverse reactions to duplex scanning. *Lancet* **2**, 1023.

Rose, G. & Colwell, L. (1992) Randomised controlled trial of anti-smoking advice: final (20 year) results. *Journal of Epidemiology and Community Health* **46**, 75–77.

Rosengren, A., Welin, L., Tsipogianni, A. & Wilhelmsen, L. (1989) Impact of cardiovascular risk factors on coronary heart disease and mortality among middle-aged diabetic men: a general population study. *British Medical Journal* **299**, 1127–1131.

Rosengren, A., Wilhelmsen, L., Welin, L., Tsipogianni, A., Teger-Nilsson, A. & Wedel, H. (1990) Social influences and cardiovascular risk factors as determinants of plasma fibrinogen concentration in a general population sample of middle-aged men. *British Medical Journal* **300**, 634–638.

Rosengren, A., Orth-Gomer, K., Wedel, H. & Wilhelmsen, L. (1993) Stressful life events, social support and mortality in men born in 1933. *British Medical Journal* **307**, 1102–1105.

Ross, R. (1999) Atherosclerosis: an inflammatory disease. *New England Journal of Medicine* **340**, 115–126.

Ross, R.S. & McKusick, V.A. (1953) Aortic arch syndromes: diminished or absent pulses in arteries arising from arch of aorta. *Archives of Internal Medicine* **92**, 701–740.

Ross Russell, R.W. (1975) How does blood-pressure cause stroke? *Lancet* **2**, 1283–1285.

Ross Russell, R.W. (1988) Cause and treatment of insufficiency in the cerebral circulation. *Clinical Neurology and Neurosurgery* **90**, 19–24.

Ross Russell, R.W. & Ikeda, H. (1986) Clinical and electrophysiological observations in patients with low pressure retinopathy. *British Journal of Ophthalmology* **70**, 651–656.

Ross Russell, R.W. & Page, N.G.R. (1983) Critical perfusion of brain and retina. *Brain* **106**, 149–434.

van Rossum, C.T.M., van de Mheen, H., Breteler, M.M.B., Grobbee, D.E. & Mackenbach, J.P. (1999) Socioeconomic differences in stroke among Dutch elderly women: the Rotterdam Study. *Stroke* **30**, 357–362.

Rothwell, P.M. & Warlow, C.P. (1996) Making sense of the measurement of carotid stenosis. *Cerebrovascular Diseases* **6**, 54–58.

Rothwell, P.M., Gibson, R.J., Slattery, J. & Warlow, C.P. for the European Carotid Surgery Trialists' Collaborative Group (1994a) Prognostic value and reproducibility of measurements of carotid stenosis: a comparison of three methods on 1001 angiograms. *Stroke* **25**, 2440–2444.

Rothwell, P.M., Gibson, R.J., Slattery, J., Sellar, R.J. & Warlow, C.P. for the European Carotid Surgery Trialists' Collaborative Group (1994b) Equivalence of measurements of carotid stenosis: a comparison of three methods on 1001 angiograms. *Stroke* **25**, 2435–2439.

Rothwell, P.M., Gibson, R.J., Villagra, R., Sellar, R. & Warlow, C.P. (1998) The effect of angiographic technique and image quality on the reproducibility of measurement of carotid stenosis and assessment of plaque surface morphology. *Clinical Radiology* **53**, 439–443.

Rothwell, P.M., Villagra, R., Gibson, R., Donders, R.C.J.M. & Warlow, C.P. (2000a) Evidence of a chronic systematic cause of instability of atherosclerotic plaques. *Lancet* **355**, 19–24.

Rothwell, P.M., Gibson, R. & Warlow, C.P. on behalf of the European Carotid Surgery Trialists' Collaborative Group (2000b) Interrelation between plaque surface morphology and degree of stenosis on carotid angiograms and the risk of ischaemic stroke in patients with symptomatic carotid stenosis. *Stroke* **31**, 615–621.

Rothwell, P.M., Pendlebury, S.T., Wardlaw, J. & Warlow, C.P. (2000c) A critical appraisal of the design and reporting of studies of imaging and measurement of carotid stenosis. *Stroke* (in press).

Sacco, R.L., Boden-Albala, B., Gan, R. *et al.* & the North Manhattan Stroke Study Collaborators (1998) Stroke incidence among white, black and hispanic residents of an urban community: the Northern Manhattan Stroke Study. *American Journal of Epidemiology* **147**, 259–268.

Sacco, R.L., Elkind, M., Boden-Albala, B. *et al.* (1999) The protective effect of moderate alcohol consumption on ischaemic stroke. *Journal of the American Medical Association* **281**, 53–60.

Sacco, S.E., Whisnant, J.P., Broderick, J.P., Phillips, S.J. & O'Fallon, W.M. (1991) Epidemiological characteristics of lacunar infarcts in a population. *Stroke* **22**, 1236–1241.

Sagie, A., Larson, M.G. & Levy, D. (1993) The natural history of borderline isolated systolic hypertension. *New England Journal of Medicine* **329**, 1912–1917.

Salgado, A.V. (1991) Central nervous system complications of infective endocarditis. *Stroke* **22**, 1461–1463.

Samuelsson, M., Lindell, D. & Norrving, B. (1996) Presumed pathogenetic mechanisms of recurrent stroke after lacunar infarction. *Cerebrovascular Diseases* **6**, 128–136.

Sandercock, P.A.G., Warlow, C.P., Jones, L.N. & Starkey, I.R. (1989) Predisposing factors for cerebral infarction: the Oxfordshire Community Stroke Project. *British Medical Journal* **298**, 75–80.

Sandercock, P.A.G., Bamford, J., Dennis, M.S. *et al.* (1992) Atrial fibrillation and stroke: prevalence in different stroke types and influence on early and long-term prognosis: the Oxfordshire Community Stroke Project. *British Medical Journal* **305**, 1460–1465.

Sandok, B.A., Whisnant, J.P., Furlan, A.J. & Mickell, J.L. (1982) Carotid artery bruits: prevalence survey and differential diagnosis. *Mayo Clinic Proceedings* **57**, 227–230.

Scardi, S., Mazzone, C., Pandullo, C., Goldstein, D., Poletti, A. & Humar, F. (1999) Lone atrial fibrillation: prognostic differences between paroxysmal and chronic forms after 10 years of follow-up. *American Heart Journal* **137**, 686–691.

Schlingemann, R.O., Smit, A.A.J., Lunel, H.F.E.V. & Hijdra, A. (1996) Amaurosis fugax on standing and angle-closure glaucoma with clomipramine. *Lancet* **347**, 465.

Schmal, M., Marini, C., Carolei, A., Di Napoli, M., Kessels, F. & Lodder, J. (1998) Different vascular risk factor profiles among cortical infarcts, small deep infarcts and primary intracerebral haemorrhage point to different types of underlying vasculopathy: a study from the L'Aquila Stroke Registry. *Cerebrovascular Diseases* **8**, 14–19.

van der Schouw, Y.T., van der Graaf, Y., Steyerberg, E.W., Eijkemans, M.J.C. & Banga, J.D. (1996) Age at menopause as a risk factor for cardiovascular mortality. *Lancet* **347**, 714–718.

Schumann, P., Touzani, O., Young, A.R., Baron, J.C., Morello, R. & MacKenzie, E.T. (1998) Evaluation of the ratio of cerebral blood flow to cerebral blood volume as an index of local cerebral perfusion pressure. *Brain* **121**, 1369–1379.

Schwartz, C.J. & Mitchell, J.R.A. (1961) Atheroma of the carotid and vertebral arterial systems. *British Medical Journal* **2**, 1057–1063.

Schwartz, A., Rautenberg, W. & Hennerici, M. (1993) Dolichoectatic intracranial arteries: review of selected aspects. *Cerebrovascular Diseases* **3**, 273–279.

Schwarz, S., Egelhof, T., Schwab, S. & Hacke, W. (1997) Basilar artery embolism: clinical syndrome and neuroradiologic patterns in patients without permanent occlusion of the basilar artery. *Neurology* **49**, 1346–1352.

Schwarze, J.J., Sander, D., Kukla, C., Wittich, I., Babikian, V.L.J. & Klingelhofer, J. (1999) Methodological parameters influence the detection of right-to-left shunts by contrast transcranial Doppler ultrasonography. *Stroke* **30**, 1234–1239.

Sellar, R.J. (1995) Imaging blood vessels of the head and neck. *Journal of Neurology, Neurosurgery and Psychiatry* **59**, 225–237.

Sempere, A.P., Duarte, J., Cabezas, C. & Claveria, L.E. (1998) Aetiopathogenesis of transient ischaemic attacks and minor ischaemic strokes: a community-based study in Segovia, Spain. *Stroke* **29**, 40–45.

Serena, J., Segura, T., Castellanos, M. & Davalos, A. (2000) Microembolic signal monitoring in hemispheric acute ischaemic stroke: a prospective study. *Cerebrovascular Diseases* **10**, 278–282.

Shanmugam, V., Chhablani, R. & Gorelick, P.B. (1997) Spontaneous calcific cerebral embolus. *Neurology* **48**, 538–539.

Shaper, A.G., Phillips, A.N., Pocock, S.J., Walker, M. & Macfarlane, P.W. (1991) Risk factors for stroke in middle-aged British men. *British Medical Journal* **302**, 1111–1115.

Shaper, A.G., Wannamethee, S.G. & Walker, M. (1997) Body weight: implications for the prevention of coronary heart disease, stroke and diabetes mellitus in a cohort study of middle-aged men. *British Medical Journal* **314**, 1311–1317.

Sharma, P. (1998) Meta-analysis of the ACE gene in ischaemic stroke. *Journal of Neurology, Neurosurgery and Psychiatry* **64**, 227–230.

Shields, D.A. (1990) Multiple emboli in hydatid disease. *British Medical Journal* **301**, 213–214.

Shinton, R. & Beevers, G. (1989) Meta-analysis of relation between cigarette smoking and stroke. *British Medical Journal* **298**, 789–794.

Siewert, B., Patel, M.R. & Warach, S. (1995) Magnetic resonance angiography. *Neurologist* **1**, 167–184.

Silver, M.D. & Dorsey, J.S. (1978) Aneurysms of the septum primum in adults. *Archives of Pathology and Laboratory Medicine* **102**, 62–65.

Sliwka, U. & Georgiadis, D. (1998) Clinical correlations of Doppler microembolic signals in patients with prosthetic cardiac valves: analysis of 580 cases. *Stroke* **29**, 140–143.

Sliwka, U., Lingnau, A., Stohlmann, W-D. *et al.* (1997) Prevalence and time course of microembolic signals in patients with acute stroke: a prospective study. *Stroke* **28**, 358–363.

Smielewski, P., Czosnyka, M., Pickard, J.D. & Kirkpatrick, P. (1997) Clinical evaluation of near-infrared spectroscopy for testing cerebrovascular reactivity in patients with carotid artery disease. *Stroke* **28**, 331–338.

Smith, J.L., Evans, D.H., Bell, P.R. & Naylor, A.R. (1998) A comparison of four methods for distinguishing Doppler signals from gaseous and particulate emboli. *Stroke* **29**, 1133–1138.

Sornas, R., Ostlund, H. & Muller, R. (1972) Cerebrospinal fluid cytology after stroke. *Archives of Neurology* **26**, 489–501.

Stark, R.J. & Wodak, J. (1983) Primary orthostatic cerebral ischaemia. *Journal of Neurology, Neurosurgery and Psychiatry* **46**, 883–891.

Stein, P.D., Sabbah, H.N. & Pitha, J.V. (1977) Continuing disease process of calcific aortic stenosis: role of microthrombi and turbulent flow. *American Journal of Cardiology* **39**, 159–163.

Steinberg, D. (1993) Antioxidant vitamins and coronary heart disease. *New England Journal of Medicine* **328**, 1487–1489.

Steinberg, D. (1995) Clinical trials of antioxidants in atherosclerosis: are we doing the right thing? *Lancet* **346**, 36–38.

Stemmermann, G.N., Hayashi, T., Resch, J.A., Chung, C.S., Reed, D.M. & Rhoads, G.G. (1984) Risk factors related to ischaemic and haemorrhagic cerebrovascular disease at autopsy: the Honolulu Heart Study. *Stroke* **15**, 23–28.

Stensvold, I., Tverdal, A. & Jacobsen, B.K. (1996) Cohort study of coffee intake and death from coronary heart disease over 12 years. *British Medical Journal* **312**, 544–545.

Stephens, N. (1997) Anti-oxidant therapy for ischaemic heart disease: where do we stand? *Lancet* **349**, 1710–1711.

Stewart, J.A., Dundas, R., Howard, R.S., Rudd, A.G. & Wolfe, C.D.A. (1999) Ethnic differences in incidence of stroke: prospective study with stroke register. *British Medical Journal* **318**, 967–971.

Stollberger, C., Brainin, M., Abzieher, F. & Slany, J. (1995) Embolic stroke and transoesophageal echocardiography: can clinical parameters predict the diagnostic yield? *Journal of Neurology* **242**, 437–442.

Stollberger, C., Seitelberger, R., Fenninger, C., Prainer, C. & Slany, J. (1996) Aneurysm of the left sinus of Valsalva: an unusual source of cerebral embolism. *Stroke* **27**, 1424–1426.

Stollberger, C., Chnupa, P., Kronik, G. *et al.* (1998) Transesophageal echocardiography to assess embolic risk in patients with atrial fibrillation. *Annals of Internal Medicine* **128**, 630–647.

Strachan, D.P., Carrington, D., Mendall, M.A. *et al.* (1999) Relation of *Chlamydia pneumoniae* serology to mortality and incidence of ischaemic heart disease over 13 years in the Caerphilly prospective heart disease study. *British Medical Journal* **318**, 1035–1039.

Streifler, J.Y., Eliaziw, M., Fox, A.J. *et al.* for the North American Symptomatic Carotid Endarterectomy Trial (1994) Angiographic detection of carotid plaque ulceration: comparison with surgical observations in a multicentre study. *Stroke* **25**, 1130–1132.

Stroke Prevention in Atrial Fibrillation Investigators Committee on Echocardiography (1998) Transoesophageal echocardiographic correlates of thromboembolism in high-risk patients with non-valvular atrial fibrillation. *Annals of Internal Medicine* **128**, 639–647.

Stroke Prevention in Reversible Ischaemia Trial (SPIRIT) Study Group (1997) A randomised trial of anticoagulants versus aspirin after cerebral ischaemia of presumed arterial origin. *Annals of Neurology* **42**, 857–865.

Strong, J.P., Malcom, G.T., McMahan, C.A. *et al.* (1999) Prevalence and extent of atherosclerosis in adolescents and young adults: implications for prevention from the Pathobiological Determinants of Atherosclerosis in Youth Study. *Journal of the American Medical Association* **281**, 727–735.

Sturrock, G.D. & Mueller, H.R. (1984) Chronic ocular ischaemia. *British Journal of Ophthalmology* **68**, 716–723.

Sudlow, C.L.M. & Warlow, C.P. for the International Incidence Collaboration (1997) Comparable studies on the incidence of stroke and its pathological types: results from an international collaboration. *Stroke* **28**, 491–499.

Sutton-Tyrrell, K., Alcorn, H.G., Wolfson, S.K., Kelsey, S.F. & Kuller, L.H. (1993) Predictors of carotid stenosis in older adults with and without isolated systolic hypertension. *Stroke* **24**, 355–361.

Sutton-Tyrrell, K., Wolfson, S.K. & Kuller, L.H. (1994) Blood pressure treatment slows the progression of carotid stenosis in patients with isolated systolic hypertension. *Stroke* **25**, 44–50.

Suzuki, T., Nagai, R., Yamazaki, T. *et al.* (1994) Rapid growth of intracranial aneurysms secondary to cardiac myxoma. *Neurology* **44**, 570–571.

Svindland, A. & Torvik, A. (1988) Atherosclerotic carotid disease in asymptomatic individuals. *Acta Neurologica Scandinavica* **78**, 506–517.

Swash, M. & Earl, C.J. (1970) Transient visual obscurations in chronic rheumatic heart-disease. *Lancet* **2**, 323–326.

Takao, M., Koto, A., Tanahashi, N., Fukuuchi, Y., Takagi, M. & Morinaga, S. (1999) Pathologic findings of silent, small hyperintense foci in the basal ganglia and thalamus on MRI. *Neurology* **52**, 666–668.

Tanaka, H., Sueyoshi, K., Nishino, M., Ishida, M., Fukunaga, R. & Abe, H. (1993) Silent brain infarction and coronary artery disease in Japanese patients. *Archives of Neurology* **50**, 706–709.

Tegeler, C.H. & Downes, T.R. (1991) Cardiac imaging in stroke. *Stroke* **22**, 1206–1211.

Tegeler, C.H., Knappertz, V.A., Nagaraja, D., Mooney, M. & Dalley, G.M. (1995) Relationship of common carotid artery high intensity transient signals in patients with ischaemic stroke to white matter versus territorial infarct pattern on brain CT scan. *Cerebrovascular Diseases* **5**, 128–132.

Tohgi, H., Takahashi, S., Chiba, K., Hirata, Y. for the Tohoku Cerebellar Infarction Study Group (1993) Cerebellar infarction: clinical and neuroimaging analysis in 293 patients. *Stroke* **24**, 1697–1701.

Torvik, A. (1984) The pathogenesis of watershed infarcts in the brain. *Stroke* **15**, 221–223.

Torvik, A., Svindland, A. & Lindboe, C.F. (1989) Pathogenesis of carotid thrombosis. *Stroke* **20**, 1477–1483.

Tuomilehto, J. & Rastenyte, D. (1999) Diabetes and glucose intolerance as risk factors for stroke. *Journal of Cardiovascular Risk* **6**, 241–249.

UK Prospective Diabetes Study (UKPDS) Group (1998) Intensive blood-glucose control with sulphonylureas or insulin compared with conventional treatment and risk of complications in patients with type 2 diabetes (UKPDS 33). *Lancet* **352**, 837–853.

Vane, J.R., Anggard, E.E. & Botting, R.M. (1990) Regulatory functions of the vascular endothelium. *New England Journal of Medicine* **323**, 27–35.

Vanharanta, M., Voutilainen, S., Lakka, T.A., van der Lee, M., Adlercreutz, H. & Salonen, J.T. (1999) Risk of acute coronary events according to serum concentrations of enterolactone: a prospective populated-based case–control study. *Lancet* **354**, 2112–2115.

Vernieri, F., Pasqualetti, P., Passarelli, F., Rossini, P.M. & Silvestrini, M. (1999) Outcome of carotid artery occlusion is predicted by cerebrovascular reactivity. *Stroke* **30**, 593–598.

Vestergaard, K., Andersen, G., Nielsen, M.I. & Jensen, T.S. (1993) Headache in stroke. *Stroke* **24**, 1621–1624.

Vingerhoets, F., Bogousslavsky, J., Regli, F. & van Melle, G. (1993) Atrial fibrillation after acute stroke. *Stroke* **24**, 26–30.

Vongpatanasin, W., Hillis, L.D. & Lange, R.A. (1996) Prosthetic heart valves. *New England Journal of Medicine* **335**, 407–416.

Waldvogel, D., Mattle, H.P., Sturzenegger, M. & Schroth, G. (1998) Pulsatile tinnitus: a review of 84 patients. *Journal of Neurology* **245**, 137–142.

Walker, S.P., Rimm, E.B., Ascherio, A., Kawachi, I., Stampfer, M.J. & Willett, W.C. (1996) Body size and fat distribution as predictors of stroke among US men. *American Journal of Epidemiology* **144**, 1143–1150.

Walz, E.T., Slivka, A.P., Tice, F.D., Gray, P.C., Orsinelli, D.A. & Pearson, A.C. (1998) Non-infective mitral valve vegetations identified by transoesophageal echocardiography as a cause of stroke. *Journal of Stroke and Cerebrovascular Diseases* **7**, 310–314.

Wannamethee, S.G. & Shaper, A.G. (1996) Patterns of alcohol intake and risk of stroke in middle-aged British men. *Stroke* **27**, 1033–1039.

Wannamethee, S.G. & Shaper, A.G. (1999) Physical activity and the prevention of stroke. *Journal of Cardiovascular Risk* **6**, 213–216.

Wannamethee, G., Perry, I.J. & Shaper, A.G. (1994) Haematocrit, hypertension and risk of stroke. *Journal of Internal Medicine* **235**, 163–168.

Wannamethee, S.G., Shaper, A.G. & Ebrahim, S. (1995) Respiratory function and risk of stroke. *Stroke* **26**, 2004–2010.

Wannamethee, S.G., Shaper, A.G. & Ebrahim, S. (1996) History of parental death from stroke or heart trouble and the risk of stroke in middle-aged men. *Stroke* **27**, 1492–1498.

Wannamethee, S.G., Perry, I.J. & Shaper, A.G. (1999) Non-fasting serum glucose and insulin concentrations and the risk of stroke. *Stroke* **30**, 1780–1786.

Ware, J.A. & Heistad, D.D. (1993) Platelet–endothelium interactions. *New England Journal of Medicine* **328**, 628–635.

Warlow, C.P. (1978) Venous thromboembolism after stroke. *American Heart Journal* **96**, 283–285.

Warnock, N.G., Gandhi, M.R., Bergvall, U. & Powell, T. (1993) Complications of intra-arterial digital subtraction angiography in patients investigated for cerebral vascular disease. *British Journal of Radiology* **66**, 855–858.

Weinberger, J., Rothlauf, E., Materese, E. & Halperin, J. (1988) Non-invasive evaluatuion of the extracranial carotid arteries in patients with cerebrovascular events and atrial fibrillation. *Archives of Internal Medicine* **148**, 1785–1788.

Welch, G.N. & Loscalzo, J. (1998) Homocystine and atherothrombosis. *New England Journal of Medicine* **338**, 1042–1043.

Welin, L., Svardsudd, K., Wilhelmsen, L., Larsson, B. & Tibblin, G. (1987) Analysis of risk factors for stroke in a cohort of men born in 1913. *New England Journal of Medicine* **317**, 521–526.

Whelton, P.K. (1994) Epidemiology of hypertension. *Lancet* **344**, 101–106.

Whincup, P.H., Cook, D.G., Phillips, A.N. & Shaper, A.G. (1990) ABO blood group and ischaemic heart disease in British men. *British Medical Journal* **300**, 1679–1682.

Whisnant, J.P. (1982) Multiple particles injected may all go to the same cerebral artery branch. *Stroke* **13**, 720.

Whisnant, J.P., Brown, R.D., Petty, G.W., O'Fallon, W.M., Sicks, J.D. & Wiebers, D.O. (1999) Comparison of population-based models of risk factors for TIA and ischaemic stroke. *Neurology* **53**, 532–536.

Wickremasinghe, H.R., Peiris, J.B., Thenabadu, P.N. & Sheriffdeen, A.H. (1978) Transient emboligenic aortoarteritis: noteworthy new entity in young stroke patients. *Archives of Neurology* **35**, 416–422.

Widder, B., Kleiser, B. & Krapf, H. (1994) Course of cerebrovascular reactivity in patients with carotid artery occlusions. *Stroke* **25**, 1963–1967.

Wiebers, D.O., Swanson, J.W., Cascino, T.L. & Whisnant, J.P. (1989) Bilateral loss of vision in bright light. *Stroke* **20**, 554–558.

Wiebers, D.O., Whisnant, J.P., Sandok, B.A. & O'Fallon, W.M. (1990) Prospective comparison of a cohort with asymptomatic carotid bruit and a population-based cohort without carotid bruit. *Stroke* **21**, 984–988.

Wijman, C.A.C., Babikian, V.L., Matjucha, I.C.A. *et al.* (1998) Cerebral microembolism in patients with retinal ischaemia. *Stroke* **29**, 1139–1143.

Willeit, J., Kiechl, S., Santer, P. *et al.* (1995) Lipoprotein (a) and asymptomatic carotid artery disease: evidence of a prominent role in the evolution of advanced carotid plaques. The Bruneck Study. *Stroke* **26**, 1582–1587.

Willett, W.C., Stampfer, M.J., Manson, J.E. *et al.* (1996) Coffee consumption and coronary heart disease in women: a ten-year follow-up. *Journal of the American Medical Association* **275**, 458–462.

Wilson, P.W.F., Hoeg, J.M., D'Agostino, R.B. *et al.* (1997) Cumulative effects of high cholesterol levels, high blood pressure and cigarette smoking on carotid stenosis. *New England Journal of Medicine* **337**, 516–522.

Winkleby, M.A., Kraemer, H.C., Ahn, D.K. & Varady, A.N. (1998) Ethnic and socioeconomic differences in cardiovascular disease risk factors: findings for women from the Third National Health and Nutrition Examination Survey 1988–94. *Journal of the American Medical Association* **280**, 356–362.

Wityk, R.J., Lehman, D., Klag, M., Coresh, J., Ahn, H. & Litt, B. (1996) Race and sex differences in the distribution of cerebral atherosclerosis. *Stroke* **27**, 1974–1980.

Wolf, P.A., Dawber, T.R., Thomas, E. & Kannel, W.B. (1978) Epidemiologic assessment of chronic atrial fibrillation and risk of stroke: the Framingham Study. *Neurology* **28**, 973–977.

Wolf, P.A., Abbott, R.D. & Kannel, W.B. (1991) Atrial fibrillation as an independent risk factor for stroke: the Framingham Study. *Stroke* **22**, 983–988.

Wolk, A., Manson, J.E., Stampfer, M.J. *et al.* (1999) Long-term intake of dietary fiber and decreased risk of coronary heart disease among women. *Journal of the American Medical Association* **281**, 1998–2004.

Woo, J., Lam, C.W.K., Kay, R., Wong, H.Y., Teoh, R. & Nicholls, G. (1990) Acute and long term changes in serum lipids after acute stroke. *Stroke* **21**, 1407–1411.

Woo, J., Lau, E., Lam, C.W. *et al.* (1991) Hypertension, lipoprotein (a), and apoliprotein A-I as risk factors for stroke in the Chinese. *Stroke* **22**, 203–208.

Yamamoto, Y., Georgiadis, A.L., Chang, H-M. & Caplan, L.R. (1999) Posterior cerebral artery territory infarcts in the New England Medical Center Posterior Circulation Registry. *Archives of Neurology* **56**, 824–832.

Yamanouchi, H., Nagura, H., Mizutani, T., Matsushita, S. & Esaki, Y. (1997a) Embolic brain infarction in non-rheumatic atrial fibrillation: a clinicopathologic study in the elderly. *Neurology* **48**, 1593–1597.

Yamanouchi, H., Mizutani, T., Matsushita, S. & Esaki, Y. (1997b) Paroxysmal atrial fibrillation: high frequency of embolic brain infarction in elderly autopsy patients. *Neurology* **49**, 1691–1694.

Yamashita, K., Ouchi, K., Shirai, M., Gondo, T., Nakazawa, T. & Ito, H. (1998) Distribution of *Chlamydia pneumoniae* infection in the athersclerotic carotid artery. *Stroke* **29**, 773–778.

Yanagihara, T., Piepgras, D.G. & Klass, D.W. (1985) Repetitive involuntary movement association with episodic cerebral ischaemia. *Annals of Neurology* **18**, 244–250.

Yanagihara, T., Sundt, T., M. & Piepgras, D.G. (1988) Weakness of the lower extremity in carotid occlusive disease. *Archives of Neurology* **45**, 297–301.

Yarnell, J.W.G., Baker, I.A., Sweetnam, P.M. *et al.* (1991) Fibrinogen, viscosity and white blood cell count are major risk factors for ischaemic heart disease. The Caerphilly and Speedwell Collaborative Heart Disease Studies. *Circulation* **83**, 836–844.

You, R.X., Thrift, A.G., McNeil, J.J., Davis, S.M. & Donnan, G.A. (1999) Ischaemic stroke risk and passive exposure to spouses' cigarette smoking. *American Journal of Public Health* **89**, 572–575.

Young, G.R., Humphrey, P.R.D., Nixon, T.E. & Smith, E.T.S. (1996a) Variability in measurement of extracranial internal carotid artery stenosis as displayed by both digital subtraction and magnetic resonance angiography: an assessment of three caliper techniques and visual impression of stenosis. *Stroke* **27**, 467–473.

Young, G.R., Sandercock, P.A.G., Slattery, J., Humphrey, P.R.D., Smith, E.T.S. & Brock, L. (1996b) Observer variation in the interpretation of intra-arterial angiograms and the risk of inappropriate decisions about carotid endarterectomy. *Journal of Neurology, Neurosurgery and Psychiatry* **60**, 152–157.

Young, T., Peppard, P., Palta, M. *et al.* (1997) Population-based study of sleep-disordered breathing as a risk factor for hypertension. *Archives of Internal Medicine* **157**, 1746–1752.

van Zagten, M., Lodder, J., Franke, C., Heuts-van Raak, L., Claassens, C. & Kessels, F. (1994) Different vascular risk factor profiles in primary intracerebral haemorrhage and small deep infarcts do not suggest similar types of underyling small vessel disease. *Cerebrovascular Diseases* **4**, 121–124.

Zee, R.Y., Ridker, P.M., Stampfer, M.J., Hennekens, C.H. & Lindpaintner, K. (1999) Prospective evaluation of the angiotensin-converting enzyme insertion/deletion polymorphism and the risk of stroke. *Circulation* **99**, 340–343.

Zeman, A., Anslow, P. & Greenhall, R. (1993) Persistent trigeminal artery and brain stem stroke. *Cerebrovascular Diseases* **3**, 236–240.

van der Zwan, A., Hillen, B., Tulleken, C.A.F., Dujovny, M. & Dragovic, L. (1992) Variability of the territories of the major cerebral arteries. *Journal of Neurosurgery* **77**, 927–940.

van der Zwan, A., Hillen, B., Tulleken, C.A.F. & Dujovny, M. (1993) A quantitative investigation of the variability of the major cerebral arterial territories. *Stroke* **24**, 1951–1959.

CHAPTER SEVEN

Unusual causes of ischaemic stroke and transient ischaemic attack

Many books devote 95% of any section on the causes of ischaemic stroke and transient ischaemic attacks to the 5% of cases which turn out to have a rare or unusual cause. Although this book aims to be more balanced, it is not unreasonable to discuss rare disorders in detail, particularly if their diagnosis leads to specific early treatment, or the prevention of stroke recurrence. Also, many unusual causes are confusing and require explanation.

7.1 Trauma

Ischaemic strokes and transient ischaemic attacks (TIAs), particularly in young and middle-aged patients, are increasingly found to be caused by arterial trauma, perhaps because physicians are more attuned to the possibility and so ask the right questions, and perhaps because of improved diagnostic technology.

Penetrating neck injury

Penetrating neck injury is more likely to damage the carotid than the better-protected vertebral arteries (Table 6.2). Injury causes laceration, dissection (section 7.2.1), intimal tears and occasionally an arteriovenous fistula, all of which may be complicated by thrombosis occluding the artery, and by embolism to the brain or eye within hours, days or possibly even weeks after the injury. A traumatic aneurysm can gradually develop, perhaps over several years, and any contained thrombus may embolize to the brain or eye (Davis & Zimmerman 1983) (section 7.6).

Non-penetrating (blunt) neck injury

Non-penetrating (blunt) neck injury (Table 6.2) is a more subtle cause of ischaemic stroke and TIA. The injury may have seemed rather trivial at the time, or the cerebrovascular symptoms may be overshadowed by more substantial injuries, and stroke can occur days, weeks or possibly months later (Martin & Humphrey 1998). Blunt trauma causes intimal tearing or dissection with complicating thrombosis and embolism. Traumatic rupture of an atheromatous plaque, vasospasm and delayed aneurysm formation are exceptionally rare (Davis & Zimmerman 1983). The internal carotid artery and, very rarely, the common carotid artery are more vulnerable to a direct blow to the neck or to compression, and the vertebral arteries are more vulnerable to rotational and hyperextension injuries at the level of the atlas and axis (Hughes & Brownell 1968; Sherman *et al.* 1981; Hilton-Jones & Warlow 1985; Pozzati *et al.* 1989; Frisoni & Anzola 1991; Thie *et al.* 1993; Tulyapronchote *et al.* 1994; de Recondo *et al.* 1995; Hufnagel *et al.* 1999).

Subclavian artery injury

The subclavian artery can be damaged distal to the vertebral artery origin by a fractured clavicle or cervical rib, or by clumsy central venous line insertion. This may cause mural thrombosis and, as a result of the normal reversal of subclavian blood flow in diastole, embolization up the vertebral artery, or even up the innominate artery (English & Macaulay 1977; Prior *et al.* 1979). The same flow reversal could also cause spontaneous embolism of atherothrombotic material from the distal subclavian arteries, and even the descending aortic arch, to the brain.

Head injury

In rare instances, ischaemic stroke occurs soon after what appears to be a head injury with no obvious neck problem. However, any associated sudden movement of the neck may have caused extracranial arterial dissection. Other possibilities are intracranial arterial dissection (section 7.2.2); pressure of the distal internal carotid or middle cerebral artery against the bony structures at the base of the skull causing intimal damage and thrombosis; and vasospasm (Sawauchi *et al.* 1999; Zubkov *et al.* 1999). Transient focal neurological episodes can occur minutes after a minor head injury in children, being perhaps in some way 'migrainous' (Haas *et al.* 1975).

Head turning

Turning the head can occlude the vertebral artery against a spondylotic spur of bone. Bearing in mind that the basilar artery usually receives blood from both vertebral arteries, it is hardly surprising that unilateral vertebral occlusion has seldom been convincingly demonstrated to have caused a brainstem ischaemic stroke or TIA, non-specific 'dizziness' being more likely (Sakai *et al.* 1988; Rosengart *et al.* 1993; Sturzenegger *et al.* 1994; Kawaguchi *et al.* 1997; Kuether *et al.* 1997; Strupp *et al.* 2000) (section 4.2.3). Of course, non-specific 'dizziness' or 'light-headedness' during neck extension or head turning is common in the elderly, but the exact cause is very uncertain and may lie in the peripheral vestibular apparatus, as in benign positional vertigo (section 3.4.7). Symptomatic positional occlusion of the carotid artery has hardly ever been reported (Nehls *et al.* 1985). Unusual or forced neck turning or manipulation may cause arterial dissection (section 7.2.1).

Fibrocartilaginous embolism

Fibrocartilaginous embolism is extraordinarily rare in humans, but curiously not so in dogs. Embolic material from a disrupted intervertebral disc, perhaps as a result of trauma, somehow reaches the arterial or venous circulation of the spinal cord, rarely of the brain, to cause infarction. This is all but impossible to diagnose during life (Toro-Gonzalez *et al.* 1993; Tosi *et al.* 1996).

7.2 Arterial dissection in the neck, head and thorax

7.2.1 Cervical arterial dissection

Cervical arterial dissection is usually a result of trauma or coincides with an apparently trivial neck movement. Occasionally, it seems truly spontaneous in patients with cystic medial necrosis, fibromuscular dysplasia, Marfan's syndrome, α-1 antitrypsin deficiency and other less well-characterized, familial, connective tissue disorders (Schievink *et al.* 1998) (Table 6.11). Recent infection has also been suggested (Grau *et al.* 1999). Blood splits the arterial wall to form an intramural haematoma of variable length, and this may extend with time. There may be one or more intimal tears so that the false and true lumen are in communication (Fig. 7.1). Aneurysms sometimes form but seldom become symptomatic (Guillon *et al.* 1999). Dissection can occur anywhere in the extracranial internal carotid artery (ICA), but is unusual at the carotid bifurcation (the most common site for atheroma). In the vertebral artery it tends to affect the distal third. Sometimes it is an extension from dissection proximally in the aorta (see below). The incidence of diagnosed ICA dissection is about 1–4 per 100 000 per annum, but may now be higher with improved awareness and diagnostic imaging, both in stroke patients and in those at particular risk, such as after head and neck trauma (Schievink *et al.* 1993; Rommel *et al.* 1999).

Ischaemic stroke, transient ischaemic attack (TIA), retinal infarction, ischaemic oculopathy—and even spinal cord infarction in the case of vertebral dissection—can be caused by occlusion of the true arterial lumen by the expanded vessel wall; occlusive and propagating thrombosis within the true lumen; and by embolism from thrombosis within the true lumen (O'Connell *et al.* 1985). Usually only one artery is affected, but sometimes two or more appear to be affected more or less simultaneously, perhaps because whatever caused the problem in one artery affected others at the same time (e.g. neck trauma, aortic arch dissection or even infection).

Diagnostic clues, which may be present singly or in combination even without a stroke or TIA, are:

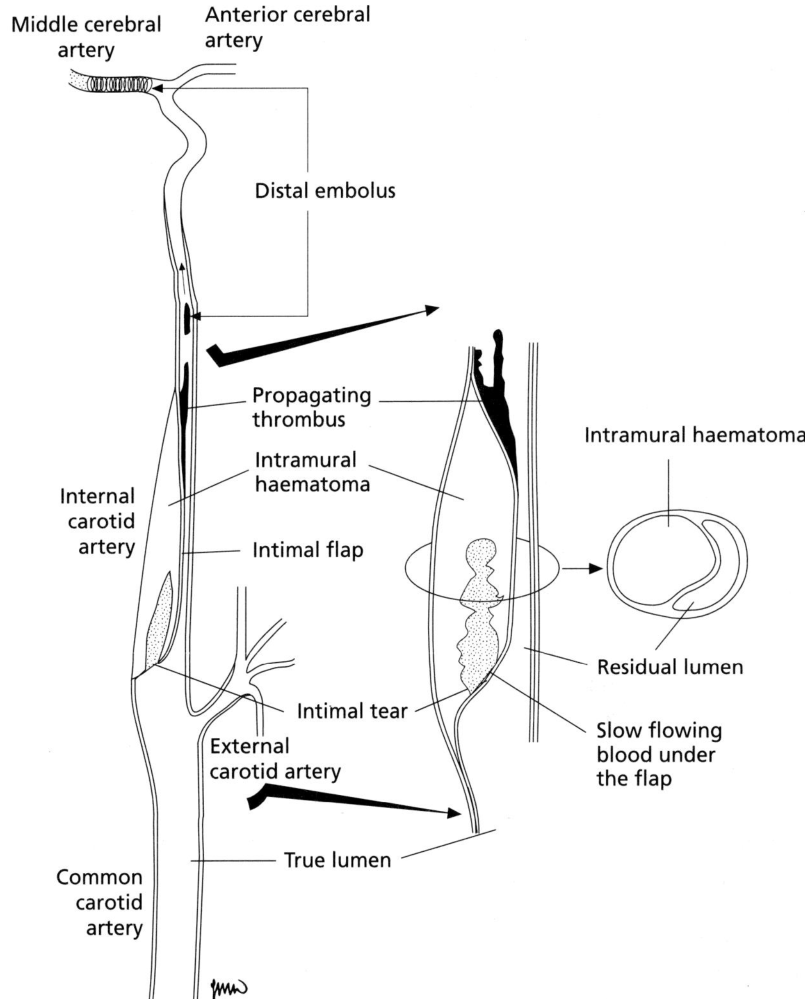

Fig. 7.1 Arterial dissection at the origin of the internal carotid artery showing: intramural thrombus; intimal tear; complicating non-occlusive thrombosis; and embolism causing distal occlusion of the middle cerebral artery.

- pain in the face, around the eye, in the neck or side of the head ipsilateral to ICA dissection, or pain in the back of the head and neck—usually unilaterally—for vertebral dissection;
- a Horner's syndrome as a result of damage to the sympathetic nerve fibres around the ICA;
- a self-audible bruit because carotid dissection tends to spread distally to the base of the skull, or is only present distally;
- occasionally, ipsilateral palsies of one or more lower cranial nerves, particularly the hypoglossal, as a result of pressure from the expanded ICA wall at the base of the skull or, more commonly, of nerve ischaemia, making for false localization of a brainstem stroke. Ocular motor palsies ipsilateral to an ICA dissection are very rare;
- cervical root lesions have recently been described in vertebral dissection, either caused by ischaemia or pressure from the bulging arterial wall.

One or more of these features very often precede, as well as accompany, the onset of cerebral ischaemia by hours or days but, in rare cases, none are present (Mokri *et al.* 1986, 1996; Caplan & Tettenborn 1992; Biousse *et al.* 1995, 1998; Silbert *et al.* 1995; Hetzel *et al.* 1996; de Bray *et al.* 1997; Gout *et al.* 1999).

Cervical arterial dissection is diagnosed by first asking the right question: 'In the last few days or weeks have you injured or damaged your neck, has anyone grabbed or manipulated your neck, have you had a car crash or a recent operation, have you recently been through labour, or done anything to twist your neck?' The correct investigations should then be performed before the dissection heals: duplex ultrasound, magnetic resonance imaging and angiography and, if necessary, selective catheter angiography.

Although ICA (but less often vertebral) dissection can be *suspected* on duplex sonography, the definitive investigation is either catheter angiography or a combination of axial magnetic resonance imaging (MRI) through the lesion to show the mural haematoma, combined with MR angiography (MRA) to display the distribution of the arterial pathology. If one is negative, the other may be positive and so sometimes both catheter angiography and MR are necessary when a correct diagnosis is vital (Mullges *et al.* 1992; Sturzenegger 1995; Auer *et al.* 1998) (Fig. 7.2). Although any imaging modality can show complete arterial occlusion, this is non-specific and does not imply dissection unless there is the typical long tapering 'rat's tail' appearance, a double-lumen, an intimal flap or a haematoma in the arterial wall. Imaging must be performed within days of symptom onset because dissections usually resolve spontaneously, perhaps within days. A completely certain diagnosis which cannot be challenged in court is particularly important when there is a compensation issue after trauma.

Recurrence of dissection, in the same or a different artery, is distinctly unusual; about 1% per annum, except in familial cases where it is more common (Schievink *et al.* 1996; Bassetti *et al.* 1996). This argues against an underlying but as yet unrecognized abnormality of the arterial wall in most patients, and rather favours a 'one off' event such as trauma, although a combination of both is possible (Peters *et al.* 1995).

7.2.2 Intracranial arterial dissection

Intracranial dissection may be caused by a blow on the head, as well as by the other causes of dissection listed in Table 6.2, but very often no cause is found. It is much rarer than extracranial dissection and more often appears to affect the vertebral and basilar arteries than the internal carotid artery and its branches. It is more likely to present with subarachnoid haemorrhage than with cerebral ischaemia. The former is a result of rupture of the aneurysmal bulging of the arterial adventitia, given the lack of external elastic lamina in the intradural section of the arteries, or dissection in the adventitial rather than medial layer of the arterial wall (section 9.1.3).

The diagnosis of unruptured dissections can be suspected by the young age of the patient, often severe headache and the focal neurological features. On cerebral angiography (MRA or, more reliably, by catheter) the findings include a focal area of constriction or dilatation although this can be caused by a clearing embolus; a long tapered occlusion; an intimal flap; an aneurysm; and—probably the only pathognomonic feature—a double lumen which is actually seldom seen (Fig. 9.29). MRI may demonstrate intramural haema-

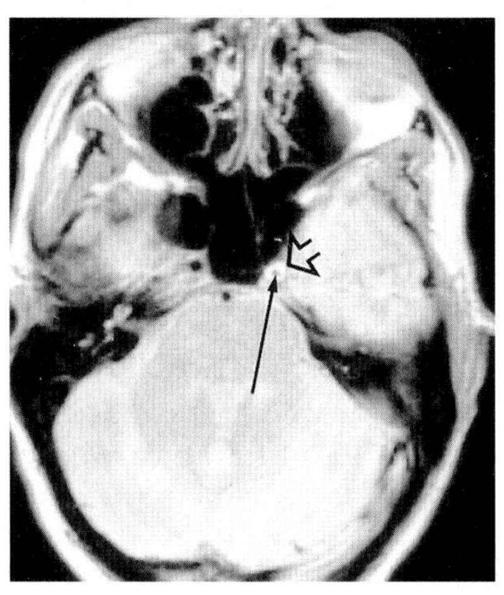

(Ai)

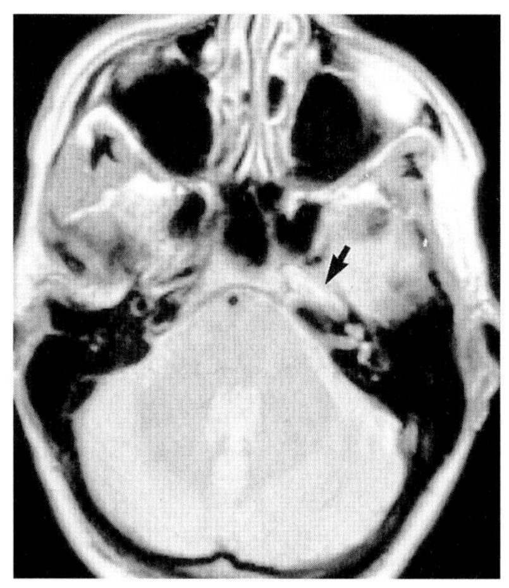

(Aii)

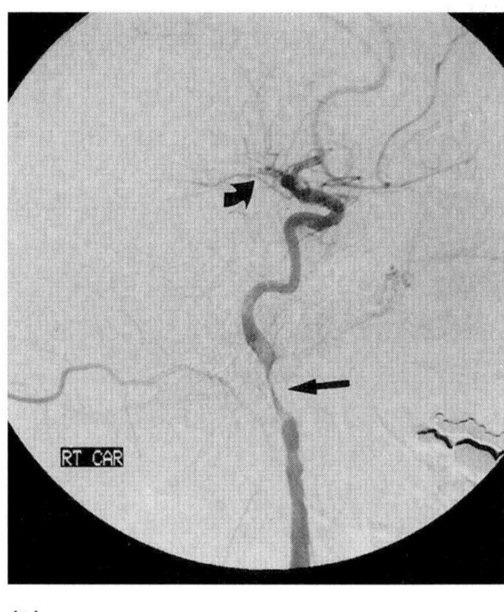

(B)

Fig. 7.2 A carotid dissection on MRI. Expansion of the arterial wall by blood clot is more or less diagnostic but is *not* seen in every case because the lesion may be too small; the MRI cuts are not through the affected part of the artery; there is intralumenal thrombus which cannot be differentiated from intramural haematoma; or perhaps the clot is so fresh that there is not enough methaemoglobin to enhance the signal on T1-weighted images. It is also conceivable that haemorrhage within an atheromatous plaque could be confused with dissection, but atheroma is usually in a different part of the artery. The true lumen is seen as an eccentric signal void on T1- and T2-weighted axial images and is surrounded by semilunar hyperintensity, corresponding with the intramural haematoma, but the signal intensity does depend on the age of the haematoma and the pulse sequence selected. In the example shown (proton density-weighted axial MRI), the dissected distal internal carotid artery is seen passing through the skull base in the carotid canal. Ai, The high signal of the intramural thrombus (open arrow) and central flow void (thin arrow) are clearly seen, rather like a shooting target. Aii, Slice immediately rostral of Ai. B, Carotid dissection on catheter angiography. The diagnostic features include an elongated and tapering stenosis (arrow), often irregular and possibly with complete occlusion of the lumen. Sometimes there is aneurysmal bulging of the adventitial wall, an intimal flap, a floating thrombus or an obviously double lumen. Unlike carotid atheroma, dissection is usually well distal to the internal carotid origin and also it seldom reaches beyond the base of the skull. There may be intracranial distal branch occlusions, presumably as a result of embolism (curved arrow).

toma (Farrell *et al.* 1985; Caplan & Tettenborn 1992; Yoshimoto & Wakai 1997; Mori *et al.* 1998).

7.2.3 Aortic arch dissection

Aortic arch dissection causes *focal* cerebral ischaemia (i.e. ischaemic stroke or transient ischaemic attack) if the dissection extends up one of the major neck arteries to cause occlusion or mural thrombosis and embolism. More often, any cerebral ischaemia is generalized, perhaps causing low-flow infarction, as a result of systemic hypotension caused by cardiac tamponade, acute aortic regurgitation or myocardial infarction. Clues to the diagnosis are:

• sudden and severe anterior chest pain and/or interscapular pain which may move as the dissection extends (very rarely there is no pain at all) (section 6.6.7);
• syncope;
• hypotension;
• diminished, unequal or absent arterial pulses and blood pressures in the arms, neck and sometimes legs;
• acute aortic regurgitation and cardiac failure;
• cardiac tamponade;
• simultaneous or sequential ischaemia in carotid, vertebral, spinal, coronary and other aortic branches if the dissection extends over several centimetres; and
• mediastinal widening and left pleural effusion on the chest X-ray.

The electrocardiogram is normal unless there is complicating acute myocardial infarction. Intra-arterial aortography is diagnostic and allows full evaluation of the extent of the lesion. However, transoesophageal echocardiography and contrast CT or MRI of the aortic arch are safer and perhaps quicker if the expertise is available locally, but give less information about coronary patency (Gerber *et al.* 1986; DeSanctis *et al.* 1987; Carrel *et al.* 1991; Pretre & von Segesser 1997; Hagan *et al.* 2000).

7.3 Connective tissue, inflammatory and other vasculopathies

Most of the autoimmune or collagen vascular and related disorders, such as systemic lupus erythematosus (SLE) and the systemic vasculitides (Table 6.2), can be complicated by, or occasionally present with, various neurological syndromes, including stroke and transient ischaemic attack (TIA) (Sigal 1987; Ferro 1998; Moore & Richardson 1998; Jennekens & Kater 1999; Scolding 1999).

Vasculitic disorders affecting the central nervous system may cause not only thrombosis within arteries and veins, but also rupture of affected vessels with subarachnoid or intracerebral haemorrhage.

Usually—but not always—there is an acute, subacute or chronic inflammatory reaction in the arterial and/or venous wall, with or without granuloma formation, i.e. vasculitis. This mural cellular proliferation, necrosis and subsequent fibrosis may be sufficient to occlude the vessel lumen; precipitate thrombosis, which may be complicated by embolism; and promote aneurysm formation, dissection or even wall rupture. Therefore, these vessel changes may cause not only focal and generalized cerebral ischaemia, either caused by arterial or venous occlusion, but also intracranial haemorrhage. In addition, non-neurological complications (e.g. hypertension caused by renal involvement) and adverse effects of treatment (e.g. opportunistic meningeal and cerebral infections resulting from immunosuppression) may lead to cerebral ischaemia or haemorrhage.

In all cases it is crucial not just to assume that an inflammatory vascular disorder is the cause of the stroke or transient ischaemic attacks, but always to consider the possibilities of the adverse effects of immunosuppression or an opportunistic infection.

Amongst all patients presenting with stroke or TIA there are very few who are already known to have, or who are discovered to have, an inflammatory vascular disorder. In fact, patients with these disorders are more likely to present with a generalized encephalopathy or an aseptic chronic meningitis, with or without focal features, which does not really fit with the 'typical stroke patient' and even less with the 'typical TIA patient'. None the less, these disorders are well worth looking out for, even in stroke and TIA patients, because their presence will require a detailed general evaluation of the patient in terms of renal function, joint problems, etc., and they will certainly change the way the patient is managed. On the other hand, one should not over-react to a moderately raised erythrocyte sedimentation rate (ESR) in a stroke patient who is otherwise well with no clinical features of a systemic disorder. An inflammatory vascular disorder should be considered—or even paraproteinaemia—but as often as not the raised ESR reflects some intercurrent infection before or possibly complicating the stroke, and it soon returns to normal.

Clues to the diagnosis of an inflammatory vascular disorder, unless it is already known, are:

• preceding systemic features, such as weight loss, headache, malaise, skin rash, livedo reticularis, arthropathy, renal failure and fever;
• the lack of any other obvious and more common cause of stroke;
• a raised ESR and C-reactive protein (the latter is usually normal in SLE);
• anaemia, in the routine blood screening tests; and
• when diagnostic suspicion is aroused, more specific immunological tests, such as raised serum anticardiolipin, double-stranded DNA and antineutrophil cytoplasmic antibodies (ANCA).

(a) 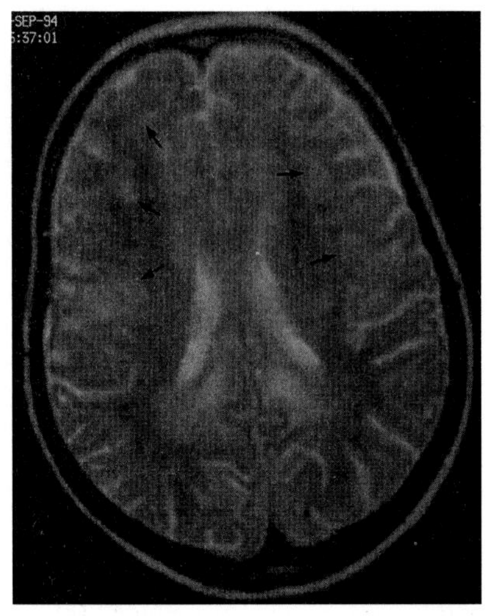

(b) 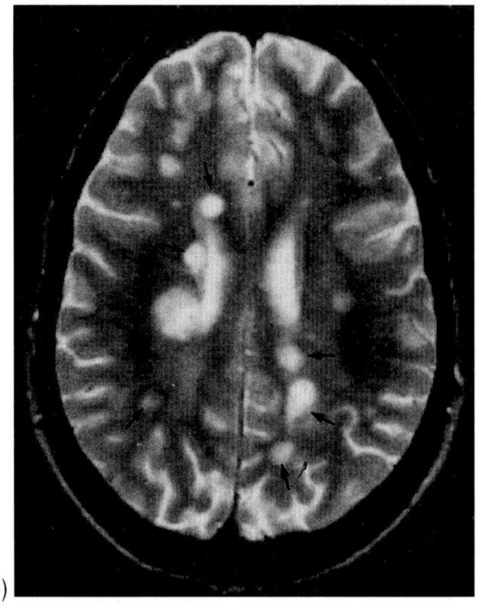

Fig. 7.3 (a) MRI (T2-weighted) of cerebral vasculitis. Note the lesions (infarcts) affect grey as well as white matter (arrows), unlike in multiple sclerosis (b), where only white matter is affected (arrows).

Unless obvious, the diagnosis must usually be confirmed by biopsy of the superficial temporal artery, meninges, cerebral cortex, skin, kidney, etc., as appropriate to the clinical syndrome. However, false-negative biopsies can occur because the vascular lesions can and do heal and they are so often patchy in distribution. Any changes in the cerebrospinal fluid (CSF) are merely a non-specific, lymphocytic, or occasionally neutrophil, inflammatory reaction; oligoclonal bands confined to the CSF do not really help in differentiating vasculitic disorders from multiple sclerosis because this occurs in both (McLean *et al.* 1995). Brain CT and the more sensitive MRI may both show areas of presumed infarction, and sometimes haemorrhage, in both grey and white matter, sometimes with diffuse meningeal and subependymal involvement (Fig. 7.3) (cf. multiple sclerosis where the lesions are confined to the periventricular white matter and corpus callosum, but the distinction is impossible in many cases). There are no *specific* angiographic criteria for cerebral 'vasculitis'; focal narrowing, dilatation and beading of small cerebral arteries, sometimes with aneurysm formation, are seen in many other situations (Table 7.1) (Fig. 7.4). Moreover, angiography is often normal even in biopsy-proven vasculitis. The electroencephalogram may help in the sense that bilateral diffuse slowing in a patient who clinically seems to have only a single focal lesion suggests a diffuse encephalopathic process of some sort, in this context vasculitic.

'Beading' of intracranial arteries on cerebral angiography is neither a specific nor sensitive sign of cerebral vasculitis which cannot be diagnosed reliably without meningeal or cerebral histopathology if there is no safer tissue to biopsy, or if there are no definitely diagnostic serum autoantibodies.

Table 7.1 Some causes of segmental narrowing, dilatation and beading of the cerebral arteries on angiography.

Cerebral vasculitis (section 7.3)
Tumour emboli (section 7.12)
Irradiation (section 7.12)
Malignant meningitis
Chronic meningeal infections (section 7.11)
Drug abuse (cocaine, amphetamines, etc.) (section 7.15)
Multiple emboli
Idiopathic reversible cerebral vasoconstriction (puerperal angiopathy) (sections 7.3 and 7.14)
Intracranial arterial dissection (section 7.2.2)
Intravascular lymphoma
Malignant hypertension
Fabry's disease (section 7.20)
Phaeochromocytoma (section 5.6.2)

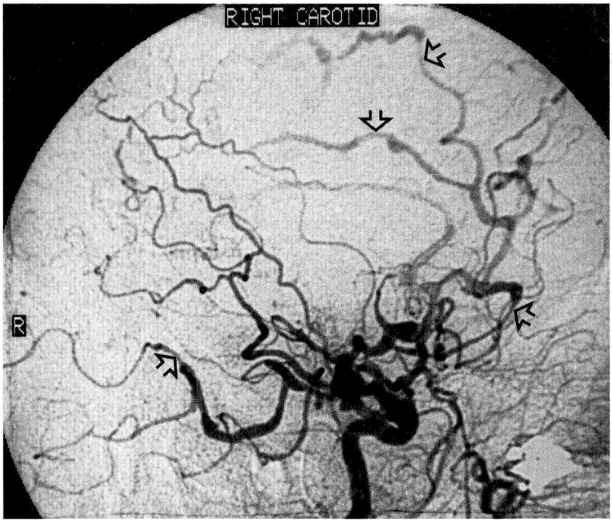

Fig. 7.4 Selective catheter angiogram to show focal dilatations and constrictions (i.e. beading) of branches of the middle and anterior cerebral arteries (arrows).

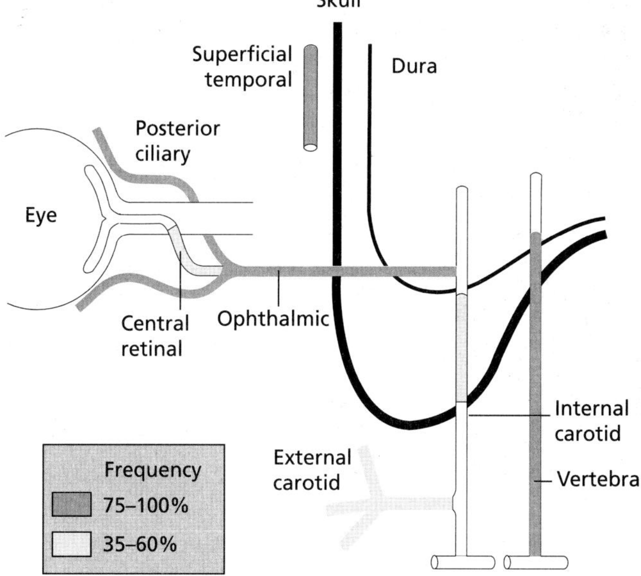

Fig. 7.5 The typical distribution of giant cell arteritis in the arteries of the head and neck. The most frequently affected arteries are the ophthalmic, posterior ciliary, superficial temporal and vertebral. Less often affected are the central retinal, distal internal carotid and other external carotid artery branches. (With permission from Wilkinson & Ross Russell 1972.)

Giant cell arteritis

Giant cell arteritis (temporal arteritis) is probably the most common 'vasculitic' cause of ischaemic stroke. It *should* be easily diagnosed because of the usual accompanying systemic features, such as malaise, polymyalgia, weight loss, low-grade fever and—almost always—an ESR raised well over 50 and often over 100 mm in the first hour, or raised C-reactive protein sometimes even when the ESR is normal (a raised plasma viscosity is probably as informative as a raised ESR). The patients are always elderly, seldom under the age of 60 years and never under the age of 50 years. There is frequently a mild normochromic normocytic anaemia, a raised platelet count and slightly disturbed liver function. Alternative diagnostic possibilities include other inflammatory vascular disorders, infective endocarditis, malignancy, paraproteinaemias and also infections complicating stroke resulting from more usual causes (pneumonia, etc.) (Turnbull 1996; Salvarani *et al.* 1997).

Any medium or large artery may be affected (carotid, vertebral, coronary, femoral, aorta, etc.). The most commonly involved are branches of the external carotid artery (ECA) (superficial temporal, occipital, facial) which cause headache and facial pain, scalp tenderness and sometimes jaw claudication; the ophthalmic, posterior ciliary and central retinal arteries causing infarction of the optic nerve (ischaemic optic neuropathy, section 3.5.2 and Fig. 3.17) more commonly than the retina; and the extradural vertebral more often than the internal carotid arteries causing ischaemic stroke or transient ischaemic attacks (Caselli *et al.* 1988; Hayreh 2000). Curiously, the anterior, middle and posterior cerebral and basilar arteries and their branches are seldom affected (Fig. 7.5).

Biopsy of an affected artery is the definitive investigation to show giant cells and other evidence of chronic inflammation in the vessel wall with destruction of the internal elastic lamina. A clinical diagnosis *alone* is seldom enough to commit elderly patients to months or years of the risks of corticosteroids, nor are ultrasound abnormalities of branches of the ECA (Schmidt *et al.* 1997). If steroid complications occur some months after the start of treatment, the knowledge that a biopsy was positive is immensely reassuring. To maximize the chance of a positive biopsy, it is best to examine an extracranial artery that is *tender*, if possible. Otherwise, at least 2 cm of the superficial temporal artery should be taken and, if negative and the case is still a puzzle, the other superficial temporal artery should be biopsied. Unfortunately, a negative biopsy does not rule out the diagnosis because the arterial lesions can be patchy and a short segment of artery can miss them, particularly if multiple sections have not been examined. Therefore, the clinical diagnosis may have to be accepted, backed up by the complete resolution of the general symptoms (polymyalgia, headache, etc.) within 24–48 h of starting corticosteroids (prednisolone, 80 mg daily) and a normal ESR within about 1 month. The temporal artery biopsy should be performed as soon as the diagnosis is suspected but, if this is impractical, steroids should be started at once as they will not interfere with the histological appearances if the biopsy is performed within a few days. If there is still diagnostic doubt, corticosteroids should be slowly withdrawn and, if symptoms recur or the ESR rises, the diagnostic process must be repeated (Jonasson *et al.* 1979; Huston & Hunder 1980; Hall *et al.* 1983; *Drug & Therapeutics Bulletin* 1993).

If a patient presents with cerebral or ocular ischaemia and is aged over 50 years, and there is a recent history of malaise and headache not likely to be caused by infective endocarditis or other infection, then an erythrocyte sedimentation rate must be performed urgently. If it is raised, high doses of corticosteroids should be started before the results of any temporal artery biopsy are known, and sometimes even before the biopsy is performed.

Takayasu's arteritis

Takayasu's arteritis (pulseless disease) is histologically identical to giant cell arteritis but affects preferentially the aorta and the large arteries arising from it, mainly but not exclusively in young Oriental women. There are multiple regions of smooth stenosis, irregularity, occlusion and aneurysmal bulging (Fig. 7.6). As with giant cell arteritis, there are often systemic problems such as malaise, fever, weight loss, anaemia and a raised ESR, at least in the early stages of the illness.

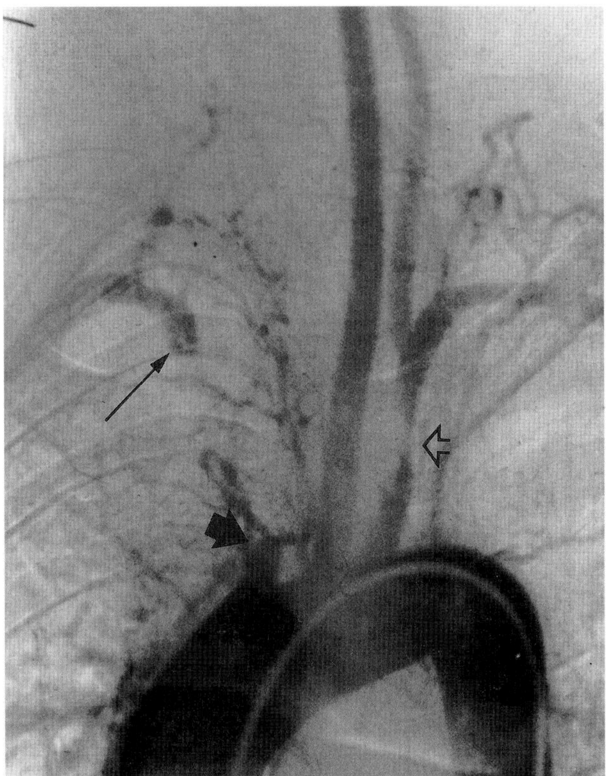

Fig. 7.6 Arch aortogram showing typical features of Takayasu's arteritis. There are long sections of smoothly narrowed lumen affecting several of the major arteries in the neck: the left subclavian artery is *nearly* occluded (open arrow), the innominate and right common carotid artery are occluded (arrow head point to stump) and the right subclavian artery (long arrow) fills via collaterals. (This figure was supplied by Dr Allan Reid, Glasgow Royal Infirmary, UK.)

The neurological features reflect the gradually increasing ischaemia of the tissues as their supplying arteries become stenosed and occluded: claudication of jaw muscles; headache; ischaemic oculopathy (section 6.6.7); syncope, particularly on sitting or standing up; epileptic seizures; confusion; and low-flow cerebral ischaemia with, sometimes, focal ischaemic strokes and transient ischaemic attacks. There may also be ischaemic necrosis of the lips, nasal septum and palate. The arms and hands, and sometimes also the legs, may become ischaemic with unequal or absent pulses and blood pressures, as may the kidneys to cause hypertension (which can be difficult to diagnose if the upper limb arteries are affected). Aortic regurgitation and coronary artery occlusion are further complications (Lupi-Herrera *et al.* 1977; Hall *et al.* 1985).

Systemic lupus erythematosus

This chronic autoimmune multisystem disease more often causes a generalized subacute or chronic encephalopathy than focal ischaemic or haemorrhagic cerebral episodes (Haas 1982; Devinsky *et al.* 1988; Kitagawa *et al.* 1990; Mills 1994; Mitsias & Levine 1994; Hama & Boumpas 1995). Scattered cerebral infarcts and haemorrhages, of varying size, are found in some but by no means all cases at post-mortem. If any vascular lesion *is* found, it is seldom a florid vasculitis but rather bland intimal proliferation involving small vessels, although this may represent healed vasculitis. Why the occasional patient has large artery occlusion is unknown, but embolism from heart valves affected by systemic lupus erythematosus (SLE) is obviously one possibility. Indeed, embolism from non-infective cardiac valvular vegetations to cerebral arteries is probably quite common (Roldan *et al.* 1996).

Most patients have circulating antinuclear antibodies of various sorts, as well as non-neurological features of SLE, such as arthropathy. A raised antinuclear factor is a highly sensitive but not at all specific finding in SLE. Double-stranded DNA and anti-Sm antibodies are much more specific but are found in less than half of cases. A high proportion also have anticardiolipin antibodies (see below) which seem to be particularly associated with cardiac valvular vegetations and arterial thrombosis (Khamashta *et al.* 1990).

Antiphospholipid syndrome

Between 1 and 40% of ischaemic stroke/transient ischaemic attack patients are reported to have raised circulating IgG or, probably less relevant, IgM, anticardiolipin antibodies and/or the lupus anticoagulant detected by the activated partial thromboplastin time or the dilute Russell's viper venom time (Montalban *et al.* 1994; Muir *et al.* 1994; Tuhrim *et al.* 1999a). The exact proportion depends on the selection of patients, the timing of the blood sample after symptom onset, the laboratory methods used, and what level is deemed 'abnormal', bearing in mind spontaneous fluctuations in titre in individuals. However, very few patients have some or all of the constellation of features comprising the antiphospholipid syndrome (APS): recurrent miscarriage, arterial and venous thrombosis in any sized vessel and, variably, livedo reticularis, heart valve vegetations, migraine-like headaches, thrombocytopenia and false-positive non-specific serological tests for syphilis (Feldmann & Levine 1995; Carhuapoma *et al.* 1997; Greaves 1999). If a patient has the typical syndrome but no antibodies, then the test should be repeated after a few weeks because the titres may fall during the acute episode (Drenkard *et al.* 1989). Raised antibodies in a stroke patient without the APS should probably be ignored. Very rarely, and almost always in people already known to have the APS, a catastrophic syndrome occurs with multi-organ failure: adult respiratory distress syndrome, abdominal pain, adrenal failure and a fulminant encephalopathy (Asherson & Piette 1996).

Anticardiolipin antibodies are not specific to the APS, particularly if they are not present in high (> 40 units) titres on *repeated* testing. They can be found in some normal individuals and also in SLE and other collagen vascular disorders, malignancy, lymphoma, paraproteinaemias, human immunodeficiency virus (HIV) and other infections, patients with multiple vascular risk factors, in the elderly, and as a result of a variety of drugs such as phenothiazines, hydralazine, phenytoin, valproate, procainamide and quinidine (Tanne *et al.* 1999). Recently, antiphosphatidyl serine antibodies have been associated with ischaemic stroke but the relevance of this is not clear because patients with and without antibodies are similar (Tuhrim *et al.* 1999b).

The cause of thrombosis, the prognosis for recurrent stroke, the nature of the relationship and overlap with SLE, and what any treatment should be (aspirin, anticoagulants, immunosuppression) are all uncertain (Finazzi *et al.* 1996; Antiphospholipid Antibodies & Stroke Study Group 1997; Levine *et al.* 1997; Verro *et al.* 1998).

The antiphospholipid syndrome cannot be diagnosed on the basis of a single raised titre of anticardiolipin antibody in the serum. The titre must be substantially raised on several occasions and associated not only with cerebral ischaemia but also with some combination of deep venous thrombosis, recurrent miscarriage, livedo reticularis, cardiac valvular vegetations, thrombocytopenia and migraine.

Sneddon's syndrome

Sneddon's syndrome is the rare combination of widespread and prominent livedo reticularis, a very non-specific skin condition (Table 7.2), ischaemic strokes/transient ischaemic attacks, and sometimes autoantibodies associated with SLE (particularly anticardiolipin antibodies and the lupus anticoagulant), if not the full-blown syndrome. It can be familial. This could be one variety of the antiphospholipid syndrome, itself part of the spectrum of SLE (Burton 1988; Stockhammer *et al.* 1993; Kalashnikova *et al.* 1994; Boortz-Marx *et al.* 1995; Geschwind *et al.* 1995; Lossos *et al.* 1995a).

Table 7.2 The causes of livedo reticularis.

Vessel wall disease
Vasculitis (section 7.3)
Atherosclerosis
Intravascular obstruction
Hypercoagulability (section 7.9)
Paraproteinaemia (section 7.9)
Essential cryoglobulinaemia (section 7.3)
Cholesterol embolization syndrome (section 7.7)
Disseminated intravascular coagulation (section 7.9)
Decompression sickness
Infections
Tuberculosis
Meningococcal septicaemia
Endocarditis
Syphilis
Typhus fever
Drugs
Amantadine
Quinine
Catecholamines
Metabolic/endocrine
Cushing's disease
Hypothyroidism
Pellagra
Miscellaneous
Cardiac failure
Lymphoma
Oxalosis
Acute pancreatitis

Primary systemic vasculitis

This is a group of related multisystem disorders, including classic polyarteritis nodosa, Wegener's granulomatosis, the Churg–Strauss syndrome and microscopic polyangiitis (Table 6.2). While involvement of the kidneys, lungs, peripheral nerves and skin is quite common, any cerebrovascular complications are rare. Ischaemia and haemorrhage can affect the brain and eye, with clinical features rather like SLE. However, in contrast, the vascular lesion is a necrotizing vasculitis affecting small and medium-sized arteries, arterioles, venules and capillaries. It is less common to find the serum antibodies characteristic of SLE and more likely to find eosinophilia, raised serum ANCA and haematuria (Moore &

Fauci 1981; Nishino *et al.* 1993; Sehgal *et al.* 1995; Jennette & Falk 1997; Reichhart *et al.* 2000).

Kawasaki disease

This is another systemic vasculitis but more or less confined to infants and children. The illness is acute, with fever, conjunctival injection, fissuring of the lips, cervical lymphadenopathy, rash and reddening of the palms and soles. Although coronary arteritis is the most common serious complication, there are occasionally neurological features: aseptic meningitis, facial palsy, epileptic seizures and encephalopathy (Jennekens & Kater 1999).

Henoch–Schoenlein purpura

This small vessel vasculitis, mainly occurring in children, typically involves the skin, gut and kidneys and is associated with arthritis. Subacute encephalopathy, perhaps with focal features, and peripheral nerve involvement are both rare (Belman *et al.* 1985). Meningoccocal meningitis is an important differential diagnosis.

Rheumatoid disease

Rheumatoid disease is very rarely complicated by a systemic and cerebral necrotizing vasculitis. Atlanto-occipital dislocation can cause symptomatic vertebral artery compression with posterior circulation ischaemia (Watson *et al.* 1977; Beck & Corbett 1983; Howell & Molyneux 1988).

Sjögren's syndrome

Dry eyes and dry mouth as a result of inflammation and destruction of the lacrimal and salivary glands are the defining features of Sjögren's syndrome. Characteristically, serum anti-Ro antibodies are present, and antinuclear and rheumatoid factor are common. Peripheral neuropathy is the most frequent neurological complication of Sjögren's syndrome. Very rarely, there is a systemic and cerebral necrotizing vasculitis, the latter causing transient or permanent focal neurological deficits, aseptic meningitis and global encephalopathy (Alexander *et al.* 1982; de la Monte *et al.* 1983; Bragoni *et al.* 1994; Li *et al.* 1999). Even more rarely, acute tubular necrosis may cause enough hypokalaemia to lead to severe paralysis and neuromuscular respiratory failure (Poux *et al.* 1992).

Behçet's disease

This is an inflammatory relapsing and remitting syndrome of orogenital ulceration and uveitis, often with skin, joint and gut involvement and recurrent venous thrombosis. Both a large and small vessel vasculitis is well described, but florid necrotizing vasculitis appears to be distinctly unusual. Behçet's disease can be complicated by a chronic aseptic meningitis which causes occlusion of cerebral arteries, perhaps more commonly those supplying the brainstem, to cause ischaemic stroke/transient ischaemic attack and primary intracerebral and sometimes subarachnoid haemorrhage. A more global subacute and relapsing encephalopathy is well recognized, as often with low-grade inflammation within the brain as in the vessels, while intracranial venous thrombosis is probably the most commonly recognized neurological complication. The neurological symptoms tend to coincide with flare-ups of the mucocutaneo-ocular symptoms, but can antedate them (Farah *et al.* 1998; Serdaroglu 1998). There are no specific circulating autoantibodies and the diagnosis is usually made by the clinical manifestations and a positive pathergy test (cutaneous needle prick causes an erythematous nodule 24–48 h later).

Relapsing polychondritis

Relapsing polychondritis is a very rare condition characterized by febrile episodes of inflammation affecting the cartilage of the ears, nose, larynx, trachea and ribs. There is often an additional arthropathy, inflammation in the eyes and optic nerve, deafness and vertigo, anaemia and a high ESR. It is sometimes complicated by a systemic and cerebral vasculitis with subacute aseptic meningitis, cranial nerve palsies, global encephalopathy, epileptic seizures and stroke/transient ischaemic attack, aortic arch syndromes and peripheral neuropathy. There are no specific diagnostic tests (Isaak *et al.* 1986; Stewart *et al.* 1988; Ragnaud *et al.* 1996; Kothare *et al.* 1998).

Progressive systemic sclerosis

Progressive systemic sclerosis is characterized by widespread and slowly progressive fibrous sclerosis affecting the skin, lungs, kidneys, gut and heart. It is hardly ever complicated by stroke, but a carotid and cerebral arteritis has been described as well as nondescript intracerebral small vessel disease (Hietaharju *et al.* 1995; Heron *et al.* 1998).

Essential cryglobulinaemia

Peripheral neuropathy is the most common neurological complication of this chronic disease manifested by purpura, Raynaud's phenomenon, arthralgia, hepatic dysfunction, progressive renal failure, plasma cryoglobulins—without any evidence of other causes such as malignancy or infections, and circulating monoclonal and/or polyclonal immunoglobulins. There is a widespread systemic vasculitis with immune complex deposition. There are occasional reports of cerebral vasculitis (Abramsky & Slavin 1974; Gorevic *et al.* 1980; Monti *et al.* 1995).

Malignant atrophic papulosis (Kohlmeier–Degos disease)

Malignant atrophic papulosis is another very rare vasculopathy. There are crops of painless but occasionally itchy, umbilicated, pinkish papules on the trunk, which heal to form distinctive, circular, porcelain-white scars. Intimal endothelial proliferation and thrombosis in small arteries can cause ischaemia and haemorrhage in the brain, spinal cord, gut and other organs. Muscle and nerve are sometimes affected (Subbiah *et al.* 1996).

Sarcoid vasculitis

Sarcoidosis is a systemic, multiorgan, non-caseating, granulomatous disorder which mostly affects the lungs, lymph nodes, eyes and skin. The illness may be subacute and self-limiting, it may recur and is occasionally chronic. As well as intracerebral granulomatous mass lesions, aseptic meningitis and cranial nerve palsies, typically with marked CT or MR contrast enhancement of the leptomeninges, it can cause a vasculitis of the small arteries and veins of the meninges and brain. This may lead to a global encephalopathy (Newman *et al.* 1997; Sharma 1997; Zajicek *et al.* 1999). Focal cerebral ischaemia and haemorrhage causing stroke are much rarer. Because involvement of the nervous system without any systemic features at all is so unusual, the diagnosis should be reasonably obvious from the almost invariable non-neurological features, such as hilar lymphadenopathy, uveitis, etc. A raised serum (or CSF) angiotensin converting enzyme level is neither sensitive nor specific and, as usual with vasculitis, a tissue biopsy is necessary for reliable diagnosis (Sethi *et al.* 1986; Zadra *et al.* 1996; Libman *et al.* 1997).

Primary angiitis of the central nervous system

Primary—or isolated—angiitis of the central nervous system is a rare disorder. Very occasionally it is associated with herpes zoster infection or lymphoma. A granulomatous angiitis, similar to sarcoid, affects the small leptomeningeal, cortical and spinal cord blood vessels to cause a subacute global encephalopathy or dementia, with or without stroke-like episodes caused by ischaemia or sometimes haemorrhage, and sometimes a myelopathy or even radiculopathy. Systemic symptoms are uncommon, but sometimes there is fever, headache, raised ESR and a raised CSF protein with lymphocytosis. The diagnosis can only be made from meningeal/cortical biopsy. Although somewhat risky, a positive biopsy is helpful so that specific immunosuppressive treatment can be given although this is not particularly successful, and sometimes a completely unexpected and yet treatable disorder is discovered (e.g. sarcoidosis) (Hankey 1991; Vollmer *et al.* 1993; Riche *et al.* 1996; Hunn *et al.* 1998; Alrawi *et al.* 1999). So-called benign cases with spontaneous resolution have been described but, unless there is confirmatory histopathology showing vasculitis, the real diagnosis is unclear, particularly if this is based on cerebral angiography which is so non-specific (Woolfenden *et al.* 1998) (Table 7.1).

Idiopathic reversible cerebral 'vasoconstriction'

This is a curious and rather poorly characterized syndrome in which apparently healthy adolescents or young adults suffer severe headache which may start suddenly, nausea and vomiting, fluctuating and sometimes bilateral focal neurological deficits, cortical visual signs, and sometimes seizures (Call *et al.* 1988; Meschia *et al.* 1998). On angiography there is segmental narrowing and dilatation of cerebral arteries which is assumed to be caused by vasoconstriction, notwithstanding the numerous other causes of this (Table 7.1). The arterial changes, if not the neurological impairments, seem to resolve, usually completely, over a matter of weeks. This kind of syndrome has also been described with the use of triptans, in the puerperium, and is presumably similar to that seen in some drug users (section 7.15). It could represent a benign form of primary angiitis of the central nervous system (see above).

Buerger's disease (thromboangiitis obliterans)

Buerger's disease is a rare, but seemingly distinct, inflammatory disorder of mainly distal small and medium arteries and veins, in the lower and upper limbs, causing digital gangrene. It is much more common in men than women, and in smokers. It is often associated with migrating thrombophlebitis and Raynaud's phenomenon but not with the systemic or laboratory disturbances so often seen in other forms of vasculitis. Cerebrovascular complications have very occasionally been described but without a standardized definition of the vasculopathy it is difficult to know if the cases reported were all of the same condition (Biller *et al.* 1981; Drake 1982; Lie 1986; Bischof *et al.* 1999; Larner *et al.* 1999).

Paraneoplastic vasculitis

Vasculitis, sometimes affecting the brain, is recognized as being very rarely associated with various malignant tumours, particularly lymphoproliferative disorders (Wooten & Jasin 1996).

Therapeutic drugs

Various therapeutic drugs have been implicated, with varying levels of proof, in hypersensitivity reactions which may include a cerebral vasculitis, e.g. *allopurinol* (Mills 1971) and *deoxycoformycin* (Steinmetz *et al.* 1989). Non-therapeutic drugs of abuse are discussed in section 7.15.

Acute posterior multifocal placoid pigment epitheliopathy

This is a well defined but rare chorioretinal disorder with bilateral, rapidly deteriorating, central vision which usually recovers in weeks or months. It is occasionally complicated by a systemic, including cerebral, vasculitis with stroke/transient ischaemic attack, aseptic meningitis and global encephalopathy (Comu *et al.* 1996).

Susac's syndrome

The combination of microangiopathy—of unknown nature—of the brain and retina, with bilateral sensorineural hearing loss, is known as Susac's syndrome. Microinfarcts in the brain lead to personality change, dementia and stroke/transient ischaemic attack-like episodes. It is much more common in young women than men (Schwitter *et al.* 1992; Barker *et al.* 1999).

Eales' disease

This rare disorder affects predominantly young men with retinal 'perivasculitis' causing recurrent, bilateral, retinal and vitreous haemorrhage. Stroke and transient ischaemic attack have been described resulting from cerebral and leptomeningeal vasculitis (Herson & Squier 1978; Gordon *et al.* 1988).

Cogan's syndrome

This rare, subacute syndrome is characterized by interstitial keratitis together with vertigo, tinnitus and hearing loss in middle age. There are systemic symptoms, aortic regurgitation, and it is probably caused by a vasculitis. Occasional cases with cerebral vasculitis are found in the literature (Vollertsen *et al.* 1986).

Lymphomatoid granulomatosis

Lymphomatoid granulomatosis is a rare disorder, possibly lymphomatous. It affects mostly the lungs with diffuse infiltration and nodules, but also the skin and the central and peripheral nervous systems with vascular infiltration by abnormal lymphocytes and plasmacytoid cells and a necrotizing vasculitis. The neurological syndrome is of a subacute encephalopathy, cranial neuropathies, seizures and stroke (Liebow 1973; Patton & Lynch 1982; Schmidt *et al.* 1984).

7.4 Congenital arterial anomalies

There are several rather unusual, and sometimes familial, anomalies of the cerebral arteries which are probably congenital, and which may be an occasional cause of cerebral and ocular ischaemia.

Fibromuscular dysplasia

Fibromuscular dysplasia (FMD) is an uncommon, sometimes familial, segmental disorder of small- and medium-sized arteries found at any age, more commonly in females than males and usually affecting more than one artery in an individual (Mettinger 1982; Luscher *et al.* 1987; Chabriat *et al.* 1999). The renal arteries are the most commonly involved, causing hypertension. In the neck, the mid to high cervical portion of the internal carotid artery (ICA) and the vertebral artery at the level of the first two cervical vertebrae are the most common sites, i.e. well away from the usual sites of atheroma. The arterial wall is fibrosed and thickened in segments, alternating with atrophy, so the typical angiographic appearance is of a 'string of beads', or tubular segmental stenosis (Fig. 7.7). Sometimes there is enlargement, and a fibrous 'web' obstructing the proximal ICA, which looks more smooth and regular than typical atherothrombotic stenosis (Kubis *et al.* 1999). FMD is occasionally associated with intracranial vascular malformations and can be complicated by aneurysm formation, dissection and arterio-

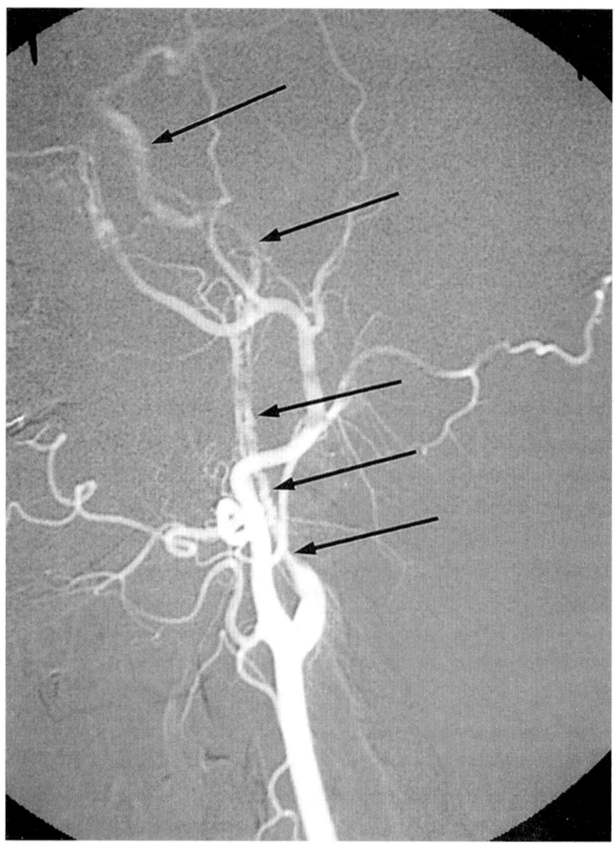

Fig. 7.7 Selective carotid catheter angiogram showing fibromuscular dysplasia of the internal carotid artery. Note the irregular 'beaded' outline of the artery (arrows). (Courtesy of Dr Evelyn Teasdale, Institute of Neurological Sciences, Glasgow, UK.)

venous fistulae. It is unknown how often *uncomplicated* FMD causes thrombosis and embolism. Therefore, when FMD is found on an angiogram, it is not necessarily relevant to any neurological symptoms. It is uncertain whether either antithrombotic drugs or angioplasty are sensible treatments, particularly as the natural history is not really known. The blood pressure should be carefully monitored for life, with a low threshold for investigation for renal artery stenosis.

Hypoplastic carotid arteries

Hypoplastic, or even absent, carotid arteries have been described. Presumably the brain is more likely to become ischaemic, and haemorrhage from fine collaterals can occur. The anomaly is usually an incidental finding when angiography is performed for some unrelated reason, or absent carotid canals are noticed on a CT of the base of the skull (Schlenska 1986; Kubis *et al.* 1996). A hypoplastic, or absent, vertebral artery is quite common, and usually the other vertebral artery is enlarged to compensate. It is important not to confuse these anomalies with the appearances of dissection on imaging.

Internal carotid artery loops

Internal carotid artery loops are probably congenital and of no consequence unless complicated by aneurysmal swelling (section 7.6), hypoglossal nerve palsy or, possibly, pulsatile tinnitus. Focal ischaemia on head movement must be extraordinarily rare (Sarkari *et al.* 1970; Desai & Toole 1975). An association with carotid dissection has been suggested (Barbour *et al.* 1994). Some degree of kinking, buckling and tortuosity of the carotid artery is quite common, becomes more common with increasing age, and is likely to be caused by atheroma or fibromuscular dysplasia, but it can be congenital (Metz *et al.* 1961).

Ehlers–Danlos syndrome type IV, pseudoxanthoma elasticum, Marfan's syndrome and osteogenesis imperfecta

These are all rare inherited disorders of connective or elastic tissue which can affect arteries and so occasionally be complicated by, or present with, arterial dissection or even rupture, aneurysm formation (but not in Marfan's syndrome) and caroticocavernous fistula (Mayer *et al.* 1994; Schievink *et al.* 1994; North *et al.* 1995; Conway *et al.* 1999; van den Berg *et al.* 2000: Pepin *et al.* 2000).

7.5 Moyamoya syndrome

Moyamoya is as rare as the name is memorable. It is not a specific vascular pathology, but a *radiologically* defined pattern of severe stenosis or occlusion of one, or more often both, *distal* internal carotid arteries (ICA), frequently with additional involvement of parts of the circle of Willis and sometimes of the proximal cerebral and basilar arteries (Bruno *et al.* 1988; Chen *et al.* 1988). It may progress. Numerous tiny collaterals develop from the lenticulostriate, thalamoperforating and pial arteries at the base of the brain; orbital and ethmoidal branches of the external carotid artery (ECA); leptomeningeal collaterals from the posterior cerebral artery; and transdural vessels from branches of the ECA. This pattern of collaterals looks like a puff of smoke (moyamoya in Japanese) in the basal ganglia region on the cerebral angiogram (Fig. 7.8). There can be associated intracranial aneurysms (Herreman *et al.* 1994).

The moyamoya syndrome is a radiologically defined pattern of arterial occlusion at the base of the brain displayed by cerebral angiography. There are several causes but often there is no explanation.

This pattern of arterial obstruction is almost, but not entirely, confined to the Japanese and other Asians. It can be familial or congenital, and various acquired causes of arterial occlusion include basal meningeal or nasopharyngeal infection; vasculitis; irradiation; trauma; fibromuscular dysplasia; a generalized fibrous disorder of arteries; sickle cell disease; Down's syndrome; and neurofibromatosis. Atheroma is very rarely responsible, perhaps because it is not usually distrib-

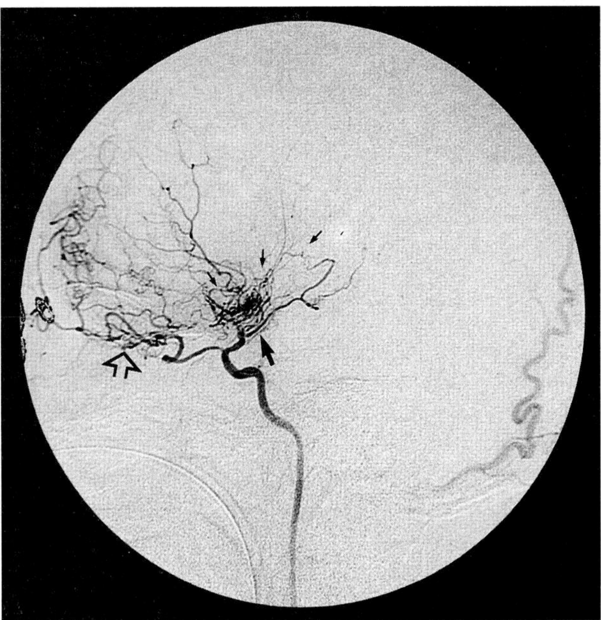

Fig. 7.8 Lateral view of a selective carotid catheter angiogram from a patient with the moyamoya syndrome. The internal carotid artery ends in numerous small dilated lenticulostriate arteries (thin arrows) and meningeal and ophthalmic artery collaterals (fat and open arrows, respectively). (Courtesy of Professor Takenori Yamaguchi, National Cardiovascular Centre, Osaka, Japan.)

uted so distally in the ICA. In most cases, however, no cause is found (Kitahara *et al.* 1979; Ikeda 1991; Bitzer & Topka 1995; Aoyagi *et al.* 1996; Cramer *et al.* 1996).

Children with the syndrome present with recurrent focal cerebral ischaemia and infarction, mental retardation, headache, seizures and, occasionally, involuntary movements, presumably the consequences of low cerebral blood flow. Adults more often present with subarachnoid, intracerebral or ventricular haemorrhage caused by rupture of the collaterals, or of any associated aneurysms (Iwama *et al.* 1997; Chiu *et al.* 1998) (section 8.2.12).

7.6 Embolism from arterial aneurysms

Aneurysms may contain thrombus which can embolize distally, although it is difficult to be certain unless there is no other more likely cause of cerebral ischaemia, and no possibility of vasospasm complicating rupture of an intracranial aneurysm. This course of events has occasionally been described with intracranial saccular and fusiform aneurysms (Steinberger *et al.* 1984; Brownlee *et al.* 1995). It also occurs with extracranial carotid or vertebral aneurysms caused by blunt or penetrating trauma, infection, carotid surgery, irradiation, atheroma, fibromuscular dysplasia or inherited disorders of connective tissue such as Marfan's syndrome and Ehlers–Danlos syndrome type IV (Schwartz *et al.* 1962; Nesbit *et al.* 1979; Mokri & Piepgras 1981; Catala *et al.* 1993). The diagnosis of the aneurysm is made by catheter or magnetic resonance angiography while any thrombus may be seen on CT, magnetic resonance imaging or catheter angiography (Fig. 7.9).

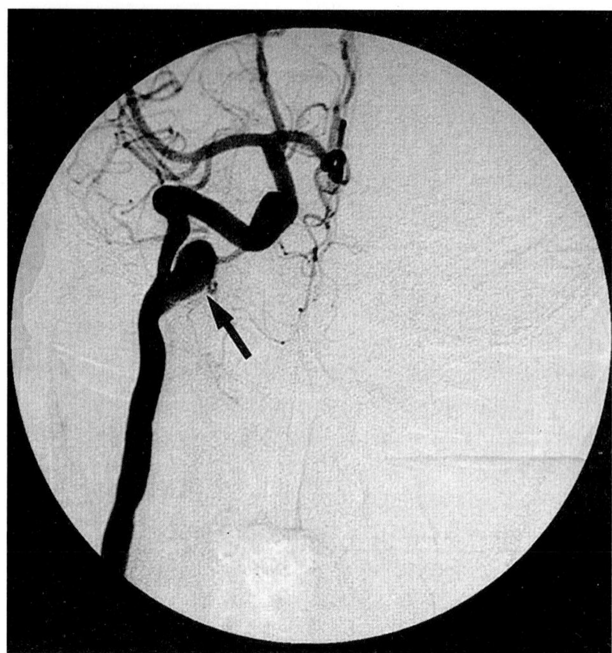

Fig. 7.9 Selective carotid catheter angiogram showing a traumatic extracranial aneurysm of the internal carotid artery (arrow). (Courtesy of Dr Evelyn Teasdale, Institute of Neurological Sciences, Glasgow, UK.)

Extracranial aneurysms should be suspected if there is a pulsatile swelling in the neck or pharynx, dysphagia, a Horner's syndrome or compression of the lower cranial nerves at the base of skull; compression of the spinal cord and roots is exceptional (Dubard *et al.* 1994).

7.7 The cholesterol embolization syndrome

This is a rare syndrome in patients with widespread atheroma. Although it can be spontaneous, it is more often a complication of instrumentation or surgical repair of large atheromatous arteries, such as the aorta, and possibly of anticoagulants or thrombolytic therapy, which releases atheromatous debris and cholesterol crystals into the circulation. Cholesterol emboli are found occluding the microcirculation throughout the body, including the brain and spinal cord. Hours or days after instrumentation or surgery, a subacute syndrome develops rather similar to systemic vasculitis or infective endocarditis. There is malaise, fever, proteinuria, haematuria, renal failure, abdominal pain, gastrointestinal bleeding, drowsiness and confusion, skin petechiae, splinter haemorrhages, livedo reticularis, cyanosis of fingers and toes, peripheral gangrene, raised erythrocyte sedimentation rate, anaemia, thrombocytopenia, neutrophil leukocytosis, eosinophilia, and hypocomplementaemia. The diagnosis is made by finding cholesterol debris in the microcirculation of biopsy material from kidney, skin or muscle. However, the specificity of this finding is uncertain because similar debris can be found in people without the syndrome, albeit rarely (Coppeto *et al.* 1984; Cosio *et al.* 1985; Fine *et al.* 1987; Cross 1991; Blankenship *et al.* 1995; Rhodes 1996; Orr & Banning 1999).

7.8 Migraine

A 'normal' stroke (caused, say, by embolism from severe carotid stenosis) can start during the course of a typical migrainous episode for that particular individual and so appear to have been provoked by migraine—after all, both conditions are common and may coincide by chance. Sometimes a normal stroke, or even asymptomatic low cerebral blood flow, can provoke migrainous episodes with an aura typical for that particular patient, or be followed by typical migraine with an aura which has never been previously experienced (Olesen *et al.* 1993). In practice, it is not always easy to sort out the exact chronological, let alone the exact aetiological, relationship between migraine and stroke in a particular case. It is, however, generally possible, with a careful history, to recognize 'migrainous' strokes.

7.8.1 Migrainous stroke

A *migrainous* stroke should not be a diagnosis of desperation when no other cause for ischaemic stroke can be found, but a *positive* statement to describe a characteristic clinical syndrome (section 3.4.1). The occasional patient, from thousands who have previously had migrainous auras (with or without headache), may one day, for no known reason, experience their typical aura, which then persists as a focal neurological deficit. Brain imaging may or may not show a relevant lesion, presumed infarction. To make the diagnosis, there must not be any reason to suspect that the stroke had been caused by anything else, particularly anything which can be associated or confused with migraine, such as arterial dissection (section 7.2), the antiphospholipid syndrome (section 7.3), cerebral autosomal dominant arteriopathy with subcortical infarcts and leukoencephalopathy (CADASIL) (section 7.20), mitochondrial cytopathy (section 7.19) or even an arteriovenous malformation (section 8.2.4) (Bousser *et al.* 1985; Shuaib 1991). A migrainous stroke often causes a homonymous hemianopia (reflecting the common visual disturbance of migrainous auras), seldom seems to cause persisting and severe disability, and perhaps does not recur very often, although data are sparse (Henrich *et al.* 1986; Hoekstra-van Dalen *et al.* 1996). Arterial occlusion has very rarely been demonstrated and it is not clear why it occurs. 'Vasospasm' is often postulated and is said to have been observed in the retinal circulation during transient monocular blindness in a few patients (Winterkorn *et al.* 1993). Paradoxical embolism is another postulated cause (Del Sette *et al.* 1998).

Migrainous auras lasting the usual 20–30 min can be confused with transient ischaemic attacks, a problem which has been discussed earlier (section 3.4.1). Migraine has very rarely been blamed for intracerebral haemorrhage (section 8.3.2).

A migrainous stroke is a well-defined clinical syndrome. It is not a diagnosis of exclusion or desperation.

7.8.2 Migraine as a risk factor for stroke

Migraine with, and perhaps even without, aura is not a risk factor for ischaemic stroke in general but it may be a risk factor in young women, although this association is based mainly on case–control studies (Becker 1999; Chang *et al.* 1999). Any relationship with myocardial infarction is uncertain (Sternfeld *et al.* 1995). It is not clear if migraine causes stroke in some way, whether factors associated with migraine also cause stroke (perhaps vasospasm, platelet hyperaggregability, etc.) or whether both migraine and stroke reflect some shared underlying factor, possibly genetic.

7.9 Haematological disorders

Occasionally, ischaemic strokes and transient ischaemic attacks (TIAs) complicate an underlying haematological disorder, which itself may be quite common (such as sickle cell disease) or extremely rare (such as protein S deficiency) (Markus & Hambley 1998) (Table 7.3). The diagnosis is not usually difficult because the routine first-line investigations will pick up most of the disorders (full blood count, platelet count and erythrocyte sedimentation rate) and, if there is no obvious other cause, fairly standard haematological tests will pick up the rest (Table 6.15). But, as with cardiac embolism, it can be difficult to know if a diagnosed haematological disorder is *the* cause of an ischaemic stroke if there is also a competing cause. However, as often as not, the haematological disorder needs treating in its own right, so that management decisions are usually fairly straightforward. A haematological disorder may exacerbate any ischaemia caused by co-existent atherothromboembolism, or any other cause of cerebral ischaemia.

Polycythaemia

Polycythaemia is conventionally defined as a haematocrit above 0.50 in males and 0.47 in females, provided the patient is rested and normally hydrated and the blood taken without venous occlusion. Above this level, the exact diagnosis should be refined by measuring the red cell mass.

Polycythaemia rubra vera (primary proliferative polycythaemia) may be complicated by transient ischaemic attacks, ischaemic stroke or intracranial venous thrombosis. The exact risk is unknown because the disease is rare, and no reliable prospective studies are available (Silverstein *et al.* 1962; Wetherley-Mein *et al.* 1987; Gruppo Italiano Studio Policitemia 1995; Zimmermann *et al.* 1999). The increased thrombotic tendency is not just a result of the increased whole-blood viscosity but because also the platelet count is often raised, and platelet activity may be enhanced. Curiously, there can also be a haemostatic defect which is the result of defective platelet function, so causing intracranial haemorrhage. The 'hyperviscosity syndrome' is another complication (see below).

Relative polycythaemia is caused by reduced plasma volume (diuretics, alcohol, dehydration, hypertension, obesity) and *secondary polycythaemia* to a raised red cell mass (chronic hypoxia, smoking, cerebellar haemangioblastoma, renal tumour). Whether the raised haematocrit of relative and secondary polycythaemia is a risk factor for stroke is unclear (section 6.3.3). A direct causal relationship is rather unlikely, although some possible cases have been reported (Doll & Greenberg 1985). Also, increased whole-blood viscosity might have a particularly adverse effect in the microcirculation of a cerebral infarct caused by something else, e.g. embolism from the heart.

Table 7.3 Haematological disorders that may cause or predispose to cerebral and ocular ischaemia.

Quantitative abnormalities of formed blood elements
Polycythaemia rubra vera (section 7.9)
Relative polycythaemia (section 7.9)
Secondary polycythaemia (section 7.9)
Essential thrombocythaemia (section 7.9)
Thrombotic thrombocytopenic purpura and haemolytic–uraemic syndrome (section 7.9)
Iron-deficiency anaemia (section 7.9)

Qualitative abnormalities of formed blood elements
Haemoglobinopathies (e.g. sickle cell disease, haemoglobin SC disease, thalassaemia) (section 7.9)
Paroxysmal nocturnal haemoglobinuria (section 7.9)
Leukaemia (section 7.9)
Intravascular lymphoma (section 7.9)
Abnormalities of platelet secretion, adhesion, aggregation? (section 7.9)

Hyperviscosity
Polycythaemia (section 7.9)
Walldenström's macroglobulinaemia (section 7.9)
Multiple myeloma (section 7.9)

Coagulation disorders (thrombophilias)
Antithrombin III deficiency (Douglas *et al.* 1990; Arima *et al.* 1992) (section 7.9)
Protein S deficiency (Koelman *et al.* 1992; Rich *et al.* 1993; Nighoghossian *et al.* 1994) (section 7.9)
Protein C deficiency (Vieregge *et al.* 1989; Kazui *et al.* 1993; Confavreux *et al.* 1994; van Kuijck *et al.* 1994; Blecic *et al.* 1996) (section 7.9)
Activated protein C resistance most commonly caused by a mutation of the factor V protein (factor V Leiden) (Perry & Pasi 1997; de Bruijn *et al.* 1998; Longstreth *et al.* 1998; Nabavi *et al.* 1998) (section 7.9)
Prothrombin (factor II) mutation (Martinelli *et al.* 1998; Reuner *et al.* 1998) (section 7.9)
Factor VII deficiency (Lefrere *et al.* 1985) (section 7.9)
Elevated factor VIII (Kosik & Furie 1980) (section 7.9)
Plasminogen abnormality or deficiency (Schutta *et al.* 1991; Nagayama *et al.* 1993) (section 7.9)
Elevated concentrations of factors II, VII, VIII (section 6.3.3)
Antifibrinolytic drugs (section 7.9)

Prothrombotic states of uncertain cause
Cancer (section 7.12)
Disseminated intravascular coagulation (section 7.9)
Pregnancy and the puerperium (section 7.14)
Oral contraceptives (section 7.13)
Heparin-associated thrombocytopenia with thrombosis (section 7.9)
Antiphospholipid syndrome (section 7.3)
L-asparaginase (section 7.12)
Nephrotic syndrome (section 7.9)
Desmopressin (section 7.9)
Intravenous immunoglobulin (section 7.9)
Androgens (section 7.9)
Hypereosinophilic syndrome (section 7.9)
Snake bite/scorpion bite/wasp sting (section 7.9)

Essential thrombocythaemia

Essential thrombocythaemia (idiopathic primary thrombocytosis) (sustained platelet count $>600 \times 10^9$/L) causes both arterial and venous thrombosis (Harrison *et al.* 1998). Occasionally, paradoxically, there can be a bleeding tendency because platelet function is defective. Headache, transient focal and non-focal disturbances are the most common neurological symptoms (Preston *et al.* 1979; Murphy *et al.* 1983; Michiels *et al.* 1993; Arboix *et al.* 1995). Before making the diagnosis, other causes of thrombocytosis should be excluded: malignancy, splenectomy or hyposplenism, surgery and other trauma, haemorrhage, iron deficiency, infection, polycythaemia rubra vera, myelofibrosis and leukaemia.

Thrombotic thrombocytopenic purpura

Although rare, thrombotic thrombocytopenic purpura (TTP) is a treatable acute or subacute disease in adults, rather similar to the *haemolytic–uraemic syndrome* in children. Platelet microthrombi cause infarcts in many organs, including the brain, leading to a fluctuating encephalopathic illness, with confusion and epileptic seizures, with or without focal features, rather than a simple stroke syndrome (Kelly *et al.* 1998). Brain CT and MRI may be normal or show infarcts, posterior cerebral oedema, and occasionally intracerebral haemorrhage, possibly caused or exacerbated by therapeutic heparinization or acute hypertension rather than the TTP itself. The patient is ill, with malaise, fever, skin purpura, renal failure, proteinuria and haematuria. The blood film shows thrombocytopenia, haemolytic anaemia and fragmented red cells (Ridolfi & Bell 1981; Sheth *et al.* 1986; Kay *et al.* 1991; Moake 1994; Neild 1994; Oberlander *et al.* 1995; Garrett *et al.* 1996; Bakshi *et al.* 1999).

Leukaemia

Leukaemia is more often the cause of intracranial haemorrhage (section 8.4.5) or the 'hyperviscosity syndrome' (see below) than cerebral arterial or venous occlusion as a result of the increased whole-blood viscosity, a complication of opportunistic infections, or non-bacterial thrombotic endocarditis (Graus *et al.* 1985; Davies-Jones 1995).

Intravascular lymphoma (formerly malignant angioendotheliosis)

Patients with this rare form of B-cell lymphoma, with proliferation of neoplastic lymphocytes within the lumen of small vessels in almost every organ, can present with multifocal stroke and transient ischaemic attack-like episodes, typically in late middle age. But, more often, the cerebral features are diffuse with global dementia. Spinal cord, roots and peripheral nerves can also be involved. Characteristically, there are skin nodules and plaques, malaise and a raised plasma lactate dehydrogenase. Brain imaging is nonspecific with infarct-like and mass lesions, and sometimes meningeal enhancement (Fig. 7.10). Outside the artificial confines of a clinicopathological conference where guesswork and gamesmanship is all important, the diagnosis can only be made by biopsy, typically of the skin or brain.

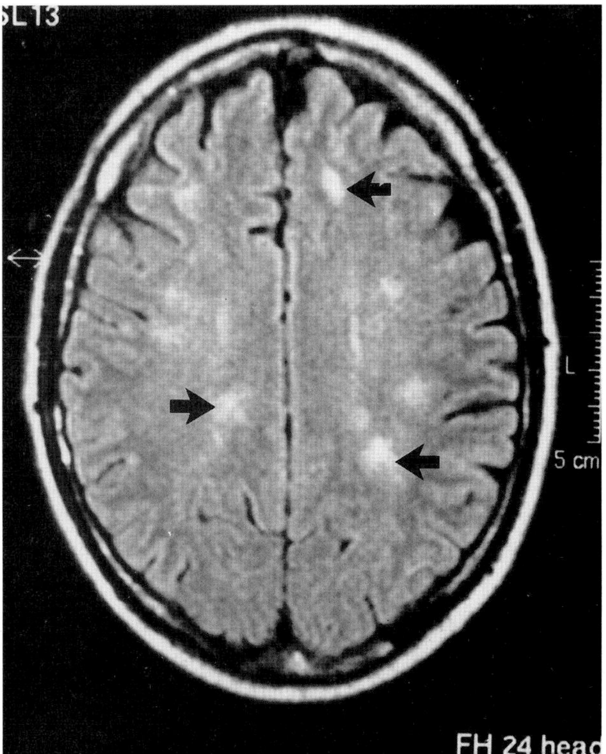

Fig. 7.10 Two MRI (fluid attenuated inversion recovery (FLAIR) sequence) axial views in a patient with histologically proven intravascular lymphoma. Areas of infarction are seen in grey (curved arrow) and white matter (straight arrows).

The course is relentlessly progressive to death within a few months (Glass *et al.* 1993; Chapin *et al.* 1995; Williams *et al.* 1998; Al-Shahi *et al.* in press).

Iron-deficiency anaemia

Iron-deficiency anaemia (and presumably other types as well), if severe, may provoke transient ischaemic attacks, particularly if there is already severe cerebral arterial disease (Siekert *et al.* 1960; Shahar & Sadeh 1991). Anaemia has also been associated with intracranial venous thrombosis and with ischaemic arterial stroke, perhaps because of the associated thrombocythaemia (Saxena *et al.* 1993). In general, anaemia is much more likely to cause non-specific neurological symptoms, such as generalized weakness, poor concentration and faintness (Belman *et al.* 1990; Akins *et al.* 1996). Of course, the anaemia may be symptomatic of some other cause of stroke, such as non-bacterial thrombotic endocarditis in a patient with cancer.

Sickle cell disease

Homozygotic children and young adults often develop ischaemic stroke and, sometimes, intracranial haemorrhage—overall stroke risk about 1% per annum—and perhaps 'silent' cerebral infarction and cognitive decline (Adams *et al.* 1988; Pavlakis *et al.* 1988; DeBaun *et al.* 1998; Earley *et al.* 1998). Stroke is much rarer in heterozygotic adults except in the context of a hypoxia-provoked sickle cell crisis (Greenberg & Massey 1985; Feldenzer *et al.* 1987). Small and large arteries and veins are occluded by thrombi as a result of the rigid red blood cells, raised whole-blood viscosity, thrombocytosis and impaired fibrinolytic activity. There is also fibrous proliferation of the intima which causes arterial stenosis and ectasia, seen on catheter angiography, detectable with MR angiography and inferred from transcranial Doppler of the middle cerebral artery (Rothman *et al.* 1986; Adams *et al.* 1997; Steen *et al.* 1998).

Stroke may complicate *haemoglobin SC disease* (Fabian & Peters 1984). It has also been associated with *thalassaemia*, perhaps as a result of the associated thrombocythaemia, atrial fibrillation, cardiac failure or pseudoxanthoma elasticum (Aessopos *et al.* 1997).

Paroxysmal nocturnal haemoglobinuria

Paroxysmal nocturnal haemoglobinuria is a very rare acquired disorder in which haemopoetic stem cells become peculiarly sensitive to complement-mediated lysis. Venous, and exceptionally arterial, thrombosis occurs in the brain and elsewhere. The patients are almost always anaemic at neurological presentation and there may be a history of abdominal pain, recurrent deep venous thrombosis, dark urine, haemolysis and a low platelet and granulocyte count (Al-Hakim *et al.* 1993; Socie *et al.* 1996).

The paraproteinaemias

Waldenström's macroglobulinaemia and multiple myeloma can both be complicated by arterial or venous cerebral infarction as a result of occlusion of vessels with acidophilic material, thought to be a precipitant of the abnormal plasma proteins. Intracranial haemorrhage also occurs as a result of the reduced number and impaired reactivity of platelets, perhaps as a result of uraemia. However, patients seldom suffer strokes or transient ischaemic attacks, but more often have the '*hyperviscosity syndrome*' of rather uncertain pathology and varying severity: headache, ataxia, diplopia, dysarthria, lethargy, poor concentration, confusion, drowsiness, coma, visual blurring and deafness; the retina shows dilatation and tortuosity of the veins, venous occlusions, papilloedema and haemorrhages. Similar symptoms may also be caused by uraemia, hypercalcaemia or lymphoma complicating the paraproteinaemia (Preston *et al.* 1978; Scheithauer *et al.* 1984; Davies-Jones 1995; Steck 1998).

Thrombophilias and other causes of 'hypercoagulability'

The so-called thrombophilias consist of a number of rare, usually familial, conditions in which spontaneous and recurrent venous thrombosis occurs (usually in the legs but sometimes in the head). Arterial thrombosis is seldom a presenting or complicating feature (Schafer 1994; Munts *et al.* 1998; Ortel 1999) (Table 7.3).

This whole area is both very complex and rapidly evolving. There may be additional causes, or at least precipitants, of stroke in the very small number of cases described (such as oral contraceptives, pregnancy, etc.). Furthermore, although familial deficiencies of antithrombin III, protein C and protein S can undoubtedly cause *venous* thrombosis, as can activated protein C resistance with factor V Leiden mutation, the patients are far more often asymptomatic. Therefore, in patients discovered to have these coagulation abnormalities, it is conceivable that the cause of any *arterial* ischaemic stroke is something quite different (e.g. arterial dissection), so they must be thoroughly investigated. Paradoxical embolism from the venous system is another possible cause, or even that a venous cerebral infarct has been misdiagnosed as an arterial stroke (Table 5.2). Moreover, acute stroke (and pregnancy) may reduce the level of some of these coagulation factors, so the tests must be repeated on several later occasions (with due allowance if the patient is anticoagulated). To make the diagnosis of familial deficiency, the family members must be tested too. The risk of recurrence and what any treatment should be are quite unknown. Therefore, just how relevant these coagulation abnormalities really are, even if an ischaemic stroke is of venous rather than arterial in origin, is uncertain.

> *If a coagulation abnormality is found in a patient with an arterial or venous stroke, then the abnormality must be confirmed weeks or months after the acute event before any persisting and definite 'thrombophilia' can be reliably diagnosed. Even then, the cause of the stroke might be something else and the thrombophilia is either an additional cause, or totally unrelated.*

The *nephrotic syndrome* can be complicated by ischaemic arterial stroke and intracranial venous thrombosis, perhaps as a result of 'hypercoagulability' (Lau *et al.* 1980; Chaturvedi 1993). Hypercoagulability may cause cerebral ischaemia in the *antiphospholipid syndrome* and widespread *malignancy* (sections 7.3 and 7.12). *Immune-mediated heparin-induced thrombocytopenia* is associated with an increased risk of thrombosis in cerebral arteries and veins (Pohl *et al.* 1999, 2000). *Desmopressin*, *intravenous immunoglobulin*, *androgens*, and the *hypereosinophilic syndrome* are other possible causes of hypercoagulability and ischaemic stroke (Weaver *et al.* 1988; Reinhart & Berchtold 1992; Jaillard *et al.* 1994; Steg & Lefkowitz 1994; Grunwald & Sather 1995; Turner & Wills 2000). *Antifibrinolytic drugs* have been reported to cause both cerebral venous and arterial thrombosis (Achiron *et al.* 1990). Defibrination, acute hypertension and bleeding are much more likely consequences of *snake* or *scorpion bite*, but ischaemic stroke has been described (Bashir & Jinkins 1985; Rai *et al.* 1990), as it has after *wasp stings* (Crawley *et al.* 1999).

Despite many attempts to relate *quantitative* abnormalities of platelet behaviour, impaired fibrinolysis and an increase in coagulation factors to ischaemic stroke and transient ischaemic attack in general, no definite cause-and-effect relationship has been demonstrated (section 6.3.3). In most cases, any changes in these haematological variables are a consequence rather than the cause of the cerebral ischaemic event.

Disseminated intravascular coagulation

There are widespread haemorrhagic cerebral infarcts and intracranial haemorrhages which cause an acute or subacute global encephalopathy rather than stroke-like episodes. Because patients are so often critically ill as a result of their primary disease—obstetric disasters, septicaemia, trauma, etc.—it can be very difficult to disentangle any *added* effect of disseminated intravascular coagulation (DIC) on the brain. The diagnosis is supported by a low platelet count, prolonged prothrombin and activated partial thromboplastin times, low plasma fibrinogen, raised fibrin degradation products in plasma, and raised D-dimers (Schwartzman & Hill 1982; Baglin 1996; Levi & ten Cate 1999).

7.10 Stroke in association with acute myocardial infarction

Cerebral and coronary arterial atheroma are so often present in the same patient that it is hardly surprising that there is a past history of myocardial infarction (MI) or current angina in about one-third of ischaemic stroke and transient ischaemic attack (TIA) patients (Table 6.3), and that MI occurs so frequently during their long-term follow-up (section 16.1.1). However, if a stroke (or TIA) occurs within hours or days of an acute MI, it is tempting, and often correct, to suspect a cause-and-effect relationship rather than a coincidence (Table 7.4).

In the prethrombolytic era, left-ventricular mural thrombus, diagnosed by echocardiography, occurred within days of an acute MI in about 20% of patients, mostly in those with large anterior infarcts. Such thrombi may embolize, but most seem to do little harm because *clinically* evident systemic embolism to the brain and elsewhere occurs in less than 5% of all acute MIs (Sloan & Gore 1992; Vaitkus & Barnathan 1993). Furthermore, most patients with emboli detected with transcranial Doppler do not have a stroke (Nadareishvili *et al.* 1999). Ischaemic stroke after an acute MI can have causes other than left ventricular thrombus: emboli as a result of coronary angiography or angioplasty, or atrial fibrillation; low-flow infarction caused by systemic hypotension or cardiac arrest; or paradoxical embolism caused by deep venous thrombosis and a patent foramen ovale. Rarely, some non-atheromatous pathological mechan-

Table 7.4 Causes of stroke and transient ischaemic attacks within hours or days of acute myocardial infarction.

Ischaemic stroke/transient ischaemic attack
Embolism from left-ventricular mural thrombus (section 7.10)
Instrumentation of the aorta/coronary arteries (section 7.18)
Low-flow infarcts caused by hypotension/cardiac arrest (section 6.6.5)
Atrial fibrillation and embolism from the left atrium (section 6.5)
Paradoxical embolism (section 6.5)
Intracerebral haemorrhage
Anticoagulants (section 8.4.1)
Antiplatelet drugs (section 8.4.2)
Thrombolytic drugs (section 8.4.3)
Both myocardial infarction and ischaemic stroke caused by the same disorder
Giant cell arteritis (section 7.3)
Infective endocarditis (section 6.5)
Aortic arch dissection (section 7.2.3)
Embolism from the heart to both cerebral and coronary arteries (e.g. atrial myxoma) (section 6.5)

ism may cause more or less simultaneous brain and heart ischaemia (Table 7.4). It must never be assumed that any stroke is ischaemic unless brain CT has excluded intracerebral haemorrhage, which is more likely in the present age of thrombolytic treatment than it was as a consequence of anticoagulants or aspirin. Haemorrhagic transformation of an infarct is another possibility. However, the overall low stroke risk still seems much the same as ever it was, and is even lower in patients with acute coronary syndromes without persistent ST-segment elevation on the electrocardiogram (ECG) (Fibrinolytic Therapy Trialists' Collaborative Group 1994; Mooe *et al.* 1997; Sloan *et al.* 1997; Gebel *et al.* 1998; Mahaffey *et al.* 1999) (sections 8.4.1–8.4.3).

Stroke complicating acute myocardial infarction is not necessarily caused by embolism from the heart or hypotension. It may be caused by intracerebral haemorrhage, often secondary to thrombolytic treatment. Brain CT scan is always required, as in other stroke patients.

Occasionally, acute MI can be clinically 'silent'. The diagnostic clues are raised cardiac enzymes routinely measured in an ischaemic stroke patient (but these may be unreliable because an increase can occur solely as a result of the stroke) and an ECG showing recent ischaemic changes, such as ST elevation, *particularly* if the changes evolve typically over time (Chin *et al.* 1977; von Arbin *et al.* 1982) (section 15.2.3).

After the acute period, the risk of stroke is much lower, about 8% within 5 years (Tanne *et al.* 1993; Bodenheimer *et al.* 1994; Loh *et al.* 1997). Not all these strokes are caused by embolism from the heart. Many of the patients have disease of their extra- and intracranial arteries as well as other non-cardiac causes of stroke (Martin *et al.* 1993). Whether a left ventricular aneurysm adds to the risk of embolic stroke is unclear.

7.11 Infection

Ischaemic stroke has long been known to complicate chronic meningeal infections which cause inflammation and so secondary thrombosis—and rarely rupture—of arteries and veins on the surface of the brain. Therefore, focal or multifocal ischaemic events in patients with *tuberculous*, *fungal* or *syphilitic meningitis* are not unexpected (Dalal & Dalal 1989; Landi *et al.* 1990; Del Mar Saez de Ocariz *et al.* 1996) (Table 7.5). Occasionally, acute *bacterial meningitis* can be similarly complicated by cerebral infarction (Igarashi *et al.* 1984; Perry *et al.* 1992; Weststrate *et al.* 1996). Some viruses, particularly *herpes zoster*, can cause periarterial inflammation and thrombosis. Middle cerebral artery occlusion with cerebral infarction and, very rarely, intracerebral haemorrhage, has been described a few weeks after ophthalmic zoster (Eidelberg *et al.* 1986; Fukumoto *et al.* 1986; Sigal 1987; Melanson *et al.* 1996) and sometimes after chickenpox (Leopold 1993). The more widespread encephalopathy caused by varicella-zoster results from multiple infarcts and haemorrhages secondary to a large and small artery vasculopathy (Amlie-Lefond *et al.* 1995). *Acquired immune deficiency syndrome* (AIDS) can be complicated by stroke in a variety of *indirect* ways but the small vessel vasculopathy with hyaline change is probably not a direct cause of stroke (Park *et al.* 1990; Kieburtz *et al.* 1993; Dubrovsky *et al.* 1998; Connor *et al.* in press) (Table 7.6). Hepatitis C virus infection can be complicated by a cerebral vasculitis related to essential cryoglobulinaemia (Tembl *et al.* 1999) (section 7.3).

Neurotrichinosis (Fourestie *et al.* 1993), *cysticercosis* (Del Brutto 1992; Bang *et al.* 1997), *mycoplasma* (Mulder & Spierings 1987), *leptospirosis* (Forwell *et al.* 1984), *cytomegalovirus* (Koeppen *et al.* 1981), *cat-scratch disease* (Selby & Walker 1979), *hydatid cysts* (Benomar *et al.* 1994) and, possibly, *borrelia* (Uldry *et al.* 1987; Reik 1993; Oksi *et al.* 1998) are also occasionally complicated by stroke of various sorts. *Infective endocarditis* has been discussed earlier (section 6.5).

Table 7.5 Infections causing ischaemic stroke and transient ischaemic attacks.

Chronic meningitis
Tuberculosis
Fungal (*Cryptococcus*, *Candida*, *Aspergillus*, mucormycosis)
Syphilis

Acute bacterial meningitis
Meningococcal
Pneumococcal
Haemophilus
Borrelia
Leptospirosis

Viral
Herpes zoster
Human immunodeficiency virus (HIV) (Table 7.6)
Cytomegalovirus
Hepatitis C

Mycoplasma

Worms
Neurotrichinosis
Cysticercosis
Hydatid disease

Cat-scratch disease

Carotid inflammation
Pharyngitis
Tonsillitis
Lymphadenitis

Infective endocarditis (section 6.5)

Table 7.6 Causes of stroke in AIDS.

Intracranial haemorrhage
Disseminated intravascular coagulation
Thrombocytopenia
Cerebral infarction
Chronic tuberculous, syphilitic and fungal meningitis
Herpes zoster vasculopathy
Cytomegalovirus vasculopathy
Infective endocarditis
Non-bacterial thrombotic (marantic) endocarditis
Protein S deficiency
Antiphospholipid antibodies
Irradiation
Aneurysms/ectasia

Inflammation of the carotid artery in the neck, with secondary thrombosis, can very occasionally complicate pharyngitis, tonsillitis and lymphadenitis, particularly in children (Bickerstaff 1964). Infection as a risk factor for stroke has been discussed in section 6.3.3.

7.12 Cancer, irradiation and chemotherapy

Stroke and cancer are both so common that any association may be no more than coincidence. Cancer patients may not be fully investigated because of the poor prognosis from their cancer, and so the exact cause of any stroke may be unclear. There are several ways that cancer patients may develop a stroke (Table 7.7) but knowing the exact cause makes little if any difference to the stroke outcome, the risk of recurrence, or the overall prognosis in most cases (Hickey *et al.* 1982; Graus *et al.* 1985; Lefkovitz *et al.* 1986). In any cancer patient, the onset of neurological problems can also be caused by a complication of treatment, radiotherapy or drugs (Keime-Guibert *et al.* 1998).

Irradiation of the head or neck can cause damage not only to the microvasculature but also to intra- and extracranial large- and medium-sized arteries (Fig. 7.11). Months or years after irradiation, a localized, stenotic and accelerated atheromatous lesion in the radiation field may become symptomatic, to cause ischaemic stroke or transient ischaemic attack. Fibrosis of the arterial wall and aneurysm formation with rupture have also been described, as well as the moyamoya syndrome (section 7.5). Ascribing any stroke to irradiation in an individual can be difficult unless the vascular lesion is in an unusual place for atheroma (e.g. terminal carotid artery) or for an aneurysm (e.g. well away from the circle of Willis); the lesion is directly within the radiation field; and there is no other more likely cause (Murros & Toole 1989; Scodary *et al.* 1990; Zuber *et al.* 1993; Bitzer & Topka 1995; Griewing *et al.* 1995; Grill *et al.* 1999).

Table 7.7 Possible causes of stroke in patients with cancer.

Non-bacterial thrombotic (marantic) endocarditis with embolism to the brain (section 6.5)
Tumour embolism, sometimes with intracranial aneurysm formation and rupture to cause intracranial haemorrhage
Opportunistic meningeal infections (herpes zoster, fungi)
Haemorrhage into primary tumours (section 8.5.1)
malignant astrocytoma
oligodendroglioma
medulloblastoma
haemangioblastoma
Haemorrhage into metastases (section 8.5.1)
melanoma
bronchus
germ cell tumours
hypernephroma
choriocarcinoma
Coagulopathy/thrombocytopenia and intracranial haemorrhage
Thrombocythaemia (section 7.9)
Hyperviscosity syndrome (section 7.9)
'Hypercoagulability' (section 7.9)
Paraneoplastic vasculitis (section 7.3)
Neoplastic compression of extra- or intracranial arteries
Irradiation damage to extra- or intracranial arteries (atheroma, fibrosis, aneurysm) (section 7.12)
Intracranial venous thrombosis caused by tumour infiltration or compression, hypercoagulability, etc. (section 5.5.1)
Drugs
cyclosporin (section 7.12)
carboplatin (section 7.12)
L-asparaginase (section 7.12)
methotrexate (section 7.12)
and any causing haemostatic defect

Cyclosporin, usually in transplant recipients, and other chemotherapy drugs, have been associated with headache, nausea, vomiting, cortical blindness, seizures, confusion and coma resulting from a subacute and reversible posterior leukoencephalopathy, perhaps in part a result of a vasculopathy and hypertension. This syndrome may start suddenly enough to be mistaken for a posterior circulation stroke (Reece *et al.* 1991; Hinchey *et al.* 1996; Gijtenbeek *et al.* 1999) (section 3.4.5). *Cisplatin* and *carboplatin* cause similar problems (O'Brien *et al.* 1992). *L-asparaginase* treatment for leukaemia can cause both cerebral ischaemia and haemorrhage (Feinberg & Swenson 1988). High doses of systemic *methotrexate* can be followed a few days later by various transient focal neurological symptoms, rather like a stroke, and merging into a more global encephalopathy with behavioural abnormalities and seizures (Walker *et al.* 1986). Finally, a cerebral

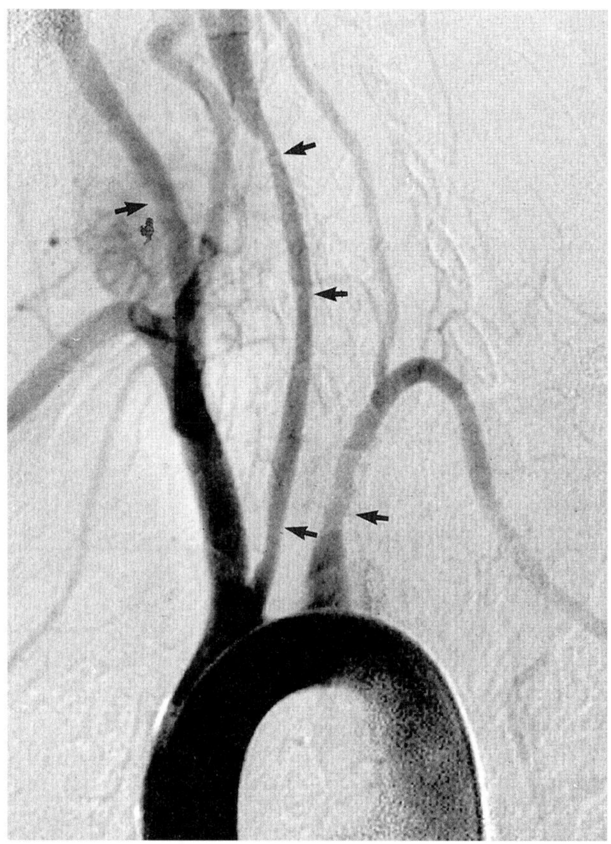

Fig. 7.11 Arch aortogram showing narrowing (arrows) of the large arteries in the neck 20 years after irradiation of cervical lymph nodes affected by Hodgkin's disease.

vasculitis has been reported after bone marrow transplantation for leukaemia (Padovan *et al.* 1999).

7.13 Female sex hormones

High-dose *exogenous oestrogen* given to men increases their risk of vascular death, and presumably also of stroke and other non-fatal vascular events (Coronary Drug Project Research Group 1970; Henriksson & Edhag 1986; Byar & Corle 1988).

7.13.1 Oral contraceptives

Oral contraceptives given to young women may triple their risk of ischaemic stroke, but have less effect on haemorrhagic stroke; the exact mechanisms are unknown (Gillum *et al.* 2000). This excess risk declines rapidly on stopping oral contraceptives. Modern oral contraceptives with a low oestrogen content may carry a negligible risk, but this is difficult to quantify, in part perhaps because women perceived as being of higher risk of stroke may be preferentially prescribed the lowest dose pills. The role of any progestogen component is also difficult to assess, mainly because of small numbers (Becker 1999). Fortunately, the absolute risk of stroke in young women is so low that increasing it by a factor of even 3 makes little difference unless their background risk is raised as a result of smoking, hypertension, by being over the age of about 35 years, or perhaps by having migraine, although it is very unclear whether this applies only to migraine with aura. The blanket recommendation that women with migraine with aura should all avoid oestrogen-containing oral contraceptives seems over-cautious and is based on very weak data (MacGregor & Guillebaud 1998). However, it is commonsense to stop oral contraception if a woman's migraines—with or without aura—become more frequent or severe in some way while on the pill, or perhaps if she develops migraine with aura for the first time. Fortunately, where any stroke risk is deemed unacceptable, there are several alternative contraceptive strategies (Becker 1999). In fact, oral contraceptives probably account for no more than about 10% of strokes in young women, an excess of between 2 and 8 strokes per 100 000 women years (Stampfer *et al.* 1990; World Health Organization Collaborative Study of Cardiovascular Disease and Steroid Hormone Contraception 1996a,b; Heinemann *et al.* 1997; Schwartz *et al.* 1998; Beral *et al.* 1999; Poulter *et al.* 1999). There seems to be an especially high risk of intracranial *venous* thrombosis in women who are both taking oral contraceptives and carrying mutations causing thrombophilia (Vandenbroucke 1998).

Clearly, when advising women on contraception, any small excess risk of stroke or other vascular disorders must be set in the context of the reduced risk of ovarian and other cancers and the risks of pregnancy, both unplanned and planned (Skegg 1999). The lower the oestrogen dose the better it seems, but it is not clear whether progestogen-only pills are safer. If a woman has a stroke while on the pill, either arterial or venous, then oral contraceptives should be stopped indefinitely, even if a plausible alternative cause of stroke emerges. If, despite thorough investigation, no cause is found then it must be assumed that the oral contraceptive was responsible for the stroke although, even in non-pill-takers, strokes of unknown cause occur occasionally.

If a woman on any type of oral contraceptive has a stroke, it is important not to jump to cause-and-effect conclusions. It is important to investigate for all potential causes of stroke in young women. Whether or not a cause is found, it is wise for the woman to avoid oral contraception thereafter.

7.13.2 Hormone replacement therapy

There are endless arguments about the balance of risks and benefits of postmenopausal oestrogen replacement, along with considerable commercial pressure to prescribe. These will never be properly resolved until appropriate randomized trials are carried out. Oestrogen replacement, with or without progestogen, is associated with a favourable lipid profile (higher serum high-density and lower low-density lipoprotein cholesterol) and haemostatic profile (lower plasma fibrinogen, enhanced fibrinolysis) (Nabulsi *et al.* 1993; Writing Group for the PEPI Trial 1995; Koh *et al.* 1997). In theory therefore, hormone replacement should reduce vascular risk, but does it and how can this be set against any other risks and benefits? As far as stroke is concerned, there is no definite hazard or benefit from oestrogens, with or without progestogens, and there may be some benefit for myocardial infarction (Grady *et al.* 1992; Belchetz 1994; Pedersen *et al.* 1997; Petitti *et al.* 1998). On the other hand, there is some increased risk of breast and uterine cancer, and of venous thromboembolism (Davidson 1995; Gutthann *et al.* 1997; Grady *et al.* 2000). However, these conclusions are based only on observational studies which are so easily subject to various forms of bias which cannot easily be corrected, particularly hormone replacement therapy being more likely to be given to women not having vascular risk factors, and requested by women more likely to look after their health (Rodstrom *et al.* 1999). So far the randomized trials, even in aggregate, are too small to be informative, but are hardly encouraging (Hulley *et al.* 1998; Hemminki & McPherson 2000; Herrington *et al.* 2000) (section 16.7.8).

Given the current state of the evidence, if a woman on hormone replacement therapy has a stroke, this by itself is probably not a good reason to stop the treatment.

7.14 Pregnancy and the puerperium

Stroke complicating pregnancy or the puerperium is so rare—perhaps only 1–3 per 10 000 deliveries in developed countries—that it is impossible to estimate the exact risk, and even the size of any excess risk over and above what is expected in non-pregnant females of childbearing age (Grosset *et al.* 1995; Sharshar *et al.* 1995; Kittner *et al.* 1996; Lanska & Kryscio 1998; Mas & Lamy 1998). Amongst the usual causes of strokes in non-pregnant young women, there are some which may be particularly associated with pregnancy (Cantu & Barinagarrementeria 1993; Dyken & Biller 1994; Janssens *et al.* 1995; Comabella *et al.* 1996; Ursell *et al.* 1998; Gasecki *et al.* 1999):

- intracranial venous thrombosis, most often in the puerperium;
- acute middle cerebral or other large artery occlusion, perhaps caused by paradoxical embolism from the legs or pelvic veins;
- cervical arterial dissection during labour;
- low-flow infarction or disseminated intravascular coagulation complicating obstetric disasters;
- ergot-type, bromocriptine and other vasoconstricting drugs causing post-partum cerebral segmental vasoconstriction with headache, seizures, focal infarcts and even haemorrhage, so-called puerperal cerebral angiopathy;
- infective endocarditis;
- peripartum dilating cardiomyopathy and embolism;
- sickle cell crisis; and
- intracranial haemorrhage caused by anticoagulants, disseminated intravascular coagulation or rupture of an aneurysm or vascular malformation.

Eclampsia causes a global encephalopathic syndrome with seizures, headache, cortical blindness and impaired consciousness caused by increasing blood pressure, cerebral oedema, and sometimes vasospasm and haemorrhage, complicated by disseminated intravascular coagulation. Typically, there are bilateral hypodensities on CT and increased T-2 signal on MRI, particularly in the occipital and parietal lobes. It should be distinguished from focal cerebral infarction or haemorrhage, and from intracranial venous thrombosis (Drislane & Wang 1997; Sawle & Ramsay 1998).

Haemorrhagic choriocarcinoma metastases can look exactly like multiple intracerebral haemorrhages, the diagnostic test being a raised serum human chorionic gonadotrophin level (sections 5.3.4 and 8.5.1). There is a curious tendency for migraine auras without headache to occur in pregnancy, and these should be differentiated from transient ischaemic attacks (section 3.4.1).

In general therefore, stroke in pregnancy or the puerperium should be investigated in the same way as any other stroke in a young, otherwise healthy female, but bearing in mind fetal exposure to any diagnostic irradiation. The risk of stroke recurrence in any future pregnancy is unknown, but presumably must be fairly low unless there is a persisting underlying 'cause', such as thrombophilia. The risk of future oral contraception is also unknown, but is perhaps best avoided.

7.15 Drugs of abuse

Cocaine—snorted, smoked or injected—is the most commonly implicated drug of abuse causing stroke (Caplan *et al.* 1982; Sloan *et al.* 1998) (sections 8.5.4 and 9.1.4). Within hours of administration, it can cause ischaemic stroke, transient ischaemic attack, intracerebral, intraventricular and subarachnoid haemorrhage, or paraplegia (Cregler & Mark 1986; Levine *et al.* 1991; Aggarwal *et al.* 1996; Nolte *et al.* 1996). A vasculitis has been rarely described on brain biopsy and inferred much more commonly—probably wrongly—by beading on cerebral angiography (Krendel *et al.* 1990; Fredericks *et al.* 1991). More likely explanations for stroke are an acute rise of systemic blood pressure causing rupture of an unsuspected arteriovenous malformation or aneurysm; vasoconstriction with complicating thrombosis; and possibly cardiac dysrhythmias, myocardial infarction or cardiomyopathy and so cerebral embolism (Daras *et al.* 1991, 1994; Sauer 1991;

Libman *et al.* 1993; Konzen *et al.* 1995; Kaufman *et al.* 1998).

Amphetamines seem to cause a small vessel vasculopathy, leading to intracranial haemorrhage, but acute hypertension is another possible factor; ischaemic stroke is less common (Harrington *et al.* 1983; Rothrock *et al.* 1988; Heye & Hankey 1996) (section 8.5.3). Other sympathomimetic drugs, such as *ephedrine*, *phenylpropanolamine*, *phentermine*, *fenfluramine* and '*Ecstasy*' (methylene dioxymethylamphetamine) may cause stroke in similar ways (Delaney & Estes 1980; Harrington *et al.* 1983; Glick *et al.* 1987; Kase *et al.* 1987; Rothrock *et al.* 1988; Harries & De Silva 1992; Henry *et al.* 1992; Bruno *et al.* 1993; Rothwell & Grant 1993).

Additional causes of stroke, or stroke-like syndromes, likely in young people and particularly in drug-users, should not be forgotten: infective endocarditis (section 6.5); head or neck trauma (section 7.1); embolization of injected particulate foreign matter; contaminating drugs; alcohol abuse (sections 6.3.3 and 8.5.2); and human immunodeficiency virus infection (section 7.11).

7.16 Hypoglycaemia and other metabolic causes of stroke-like syndromes

Hypoglycaemia is the most common 'metabolic' cause of focal cerebral episodes, most of which are probably not ischaemic in origin (Berkovic *et al.* 1984). These episodes are almost always caused by hypoglycaemic drugs rather than an insulinoma, tend to be transient rather than persisting, and consist more often of right- than left-sided weakness. Also, curiously, consciousness is usually normal and there are seldom any of the usual systemic manifestations of hypoglycaemia, such as sweating and tachycardia. The episodes tend to occur soon after waking or after exercise. By the time the patient is seen, the blood glucose may well have returned to normal. Ischaemic stroke is exceptional (Illangasekera 1981; Wallis *et al.* 1985; Pell & Frier 1990; Rother *et al.* 1992; Shintani *et al.* 1993; Service 1995; Shanmugam *et al.* 1997) (section 3.4.5).

Hypercalcaemia, *non-ketotic hyperglycaemia* and *hyponatraemia* have all occasionally been reported to cause transient ischaemic attack and stroke-like episodes but some may actually be partial epileptic seizures (Maccario 1968; Longo & Witherspoon 1980; Walker *et al.* 1980; Daggett *et al.* 1982; Grant & Warlow 1985; Carril *et al.* 1992) (section 3.4.5).

7.17 Gastrointestinal disorders

There are quite a number of case reports of ischaemic stroke, transient ischaemic attacks and intracranial venous thrombosis complicating *ulcerative* and *Crohn's colitis* (Johns 1991; Jorens *et al.* 1991; Jackson *et al.* 1993; Lossos *et al.* 1995b; Wills & Hovel 1996; Jackson *et al.* 1997). The bowel disease is not necessarily active at the time and may even present *after* the stroke. Causal possibilities include thrombocytosis, hypercoagulability, immobility and paradoxical embolism from the legs, vasculitis and dehydration. Curiously, these colitic patients, even without neurological symptoms, are more likely than controls to have what may be 'vasculitic' lesions on brain MRI (Geissler *et al.* 1995). Cerebral vasculitis has also been described with *coeliac disease* but patients with coeliac disease present neurologically more often with encephalopathy than with a focal stroke-like syndrome (Mumford *et al.* 1996).

Food embolism to the brain through an oesophageal–atrial fistula as a complication of oesophageal cancer is a curiosity (Reynolds *et al.* 1997).

7.18 Perioperative stroke

Cardiac surgery

During surgery or within the next few days, about 2% of coronary artery bypass procedures are complicated by stroke, somewhat more often for valve surgery (Rankin *et al.* 1994). A diffuse neurological syndrome with postoperative confusion, soft neurological signs, poor memory and other neuropsychological impairments, is much more common. However, this syndrome mostly resolves in days or weeks, perhaps coinciding with the resolution of the brain swelling which has been demonstrated immediately postoperatively (Harris *et al.* 1993; Roach *et al.* 1996; Selnes *et al.* 1999; Wolman *et al.* 1999). There are numerous possible explanations for these complications, the most common is probably embolism from the heart (Table 7.8). Stroke and neuropsychological complications are more common with increasing age, previous stroke, intraoperative hypotension, severe aortic arch atheroma and lengthy extracorporeal circulation. Bilateral ischaemic optic neuropathy must be distinguished from bilateral occipital infarction; both cause postoperative blindness (*Lancet* 1984).

Whether asymptomatic carotid stenosis or occlusion is causally associated with perioperative stroke is much discussed. Certainly the extent of any association is uncertain because the number of strokes in any study is far too small for precise estimates of *relative* risk even though the *absolute* risk can appear quite high: often patients who might have had a stroke have been excluded from a series by having an elective carotid endarterectomy; the proportion of all operative strokes associated with severe carotid disease is small; most studies have been retrospective; and by no means all patients in the studies have had imaging to assess the severity of stenosis (Hogue *et al.* 1999). With recently symptomatic carotid stenosis the stroke risk may be higher (Dashe *et al.* 1997) (section 16.8.11). Pending a large, prospective and methodologically sound study to clarify this issue, a systematic review of all the available studies is much needed.

Table 7.8 Possible causes of stroke during and soon after cardiac surgery.

Embolization to the brain during surgery (platelet aggregates, fibrin, calcific valvular debris, intracardiac thrombus, endocarditis, atheromatous debris from the aorta, fat, air, and silicone or particulate matter from the pump–oxygenator system)
Embolism after surgery from thrombus on suture lines or on prosthetic material, complicating myocardial infarction, atrial fibrillation or infective endocarditis
Global hypoperfusion and ischaemia resulting from perioperative hypotension (section 6.6.5)
Haemodilution during surgery
A simultaneous carotid endarterectomy under the same anaesthetic (section 16.8.11)
The cholesterol embolization syndrome (section 7.7)
Thrombosis associated with heparin-induced thrombocytopenia (section 7.9)
Intracranial haemorrhage caused by thrombocytopenia, disseminated intravascular coagulation, or antithrombotic drugs
Paradoxical embolism from postoperative deep venous thrombosis (section 6.5)

Instrumentation of the coronary arteries and aorta may very occasionally dislodge valvular, intracardiac or atheromatous aortic and large artery debris and thrombus to cause cerebral ischaemia, but well under 1% of procedures are complicated by stroke of any consequence, although minor events may well have been unnoticed and under-reported (Ayas & Wijdicks 1995; Leker *et al.* 1999). Thrombus may also form on the intra-arterial catheter tip, a fragment of catheter may break off and embolize, there may be systemic hypotension, cerebral air embolism is a possibility, and the cholesterol embolization syndrome is a rare complication (section 7.7). Large doses of intravenous contrast may cause temporary cortical blindness and migrainous auras (Sticherling *et al.* 1998).

General surgery

General surgery is less frequently complicated by stroke than cardiac surgery—less than 2% of cases depending on age—most often in patients with a past history of stroke, widespread vascular disease or chronic obstructive airways disease (Hart & Hindman 1982; Limburg *et al.* 1998). As after cardiac surgery, there is also evidence of postoperative cognitive decline which may persist (Moller *et al.* 1998). There are numerous possible mechanisms (Table 7.9). Sometimes the stroke is coincidental, particularly in elderly people

Table 7.9 Possible causes of stroke during and soon after general surgery.

Intra- or postoperative hypotension causing low-flow infarction, particularly if there are stenotic or occluded arteries supplying the brain (section 6.6.5)
A haemostatic defect resulting from antithrombotic drugs, or disseminated intravascular coagulation, causing intracranial haemorrhage
Occlusion or even dissection of neck arteries caused by faulty handling and positioning during general anaesthesia (section 7.2)
Paradoxical embolism from postoperative deep venous thrombosis (section 6.5)
Penetrating trauma of a neck artery during attempted central venous catheterization or neck surgery (section 7.1)
Perioperative myocardial infarction or atrial fibrillation
Infective endocarditis (section 6.5)
Fat embolism after long bone surgery (section 6.6.6)
The rather nebulous concept of postoperative 'hypercoagulability' (section 7.9)

with multiple vascular risk factors who increasingly are having surgery as anaesthesia becomes safer.

7.19 Mitochondrial cytopathy

A large group of rare multisystem disorders is associated with structural abnormalities of mitochondria, together with biochemical defects in the respiratory chain (Jackson *et al.* 1995; Chinnery & Turnbull 1997a, 1999). Many are now known to be caused by various deletions, duplications and specific mutations in mitochondrial DNA, where inheritance is usually through the maternal line. There are a number of rather characteristic, but often overlapping, clinical phenotypes, one of which is defined by acute focal neurological episodes: mitochondrial encephalomyopathy, lactic acidosis and stroke-like episodes (MELAS).

MELAS almost always presents in children, adolescents or middle-aged adults with recurrent focal cerebral episodes, usually first affecting the occipital lobes, and caused by lesions which were originally regarded as infarcts but not corresponding with the territories of the main cerebral arteries (Ciafaloni *et al.* 1992; Majamaa *et al.* 1997). These episodes tend to be complicated in the acute stage or later, by partial and secondary generalized epileptic seizures. Eventually the patient becomes demented and usually cortically blind. The cause of the brain lesions is uncertain. They are caused either by a defect in brain oxidative metabolism or by the structural changes that can be seen in small cerebral

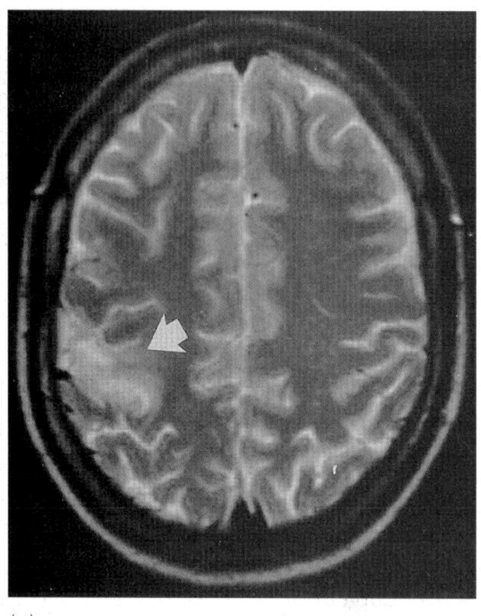
(a)

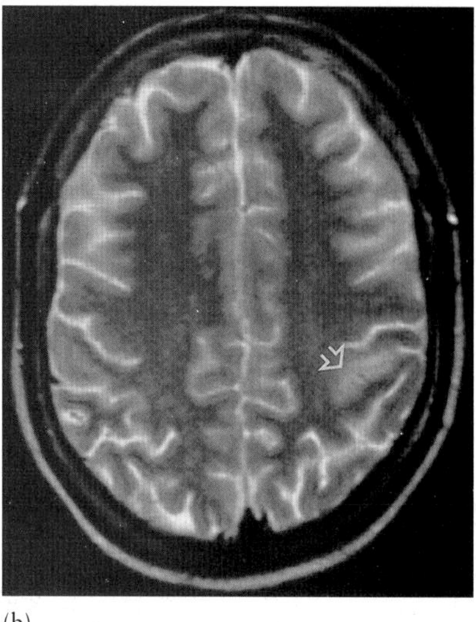
(b)

Fig. 7.12 Mitochondrial encephalomyopathy, lactic acidosis and stroke-like episodes (MELAS): T2-weighted MR scan. The first scan (a) shows an infarct-like hyperintensity in the parieto-occipital cortex (white arrow). The second scan (b) was obtained 2 weeks later and shows a new lesion in the left parieto-occipital cortex (open white arrow); the earlier lesion has vanished.

blood vessels, but not by overt vessel occlusion (Clark *et al.* 1996; Gilchrist *et al.* 1996). MELAS patients are often rather short, with sensorineural deafness, migraine, episodic vomiting, diabetes mellitus and some learning disability. There may be additional features more characteristic of other mitochondrial syndromes, such as proximal muscle weakness, myoclonus, ataxia, exercise intolerance, cardiomyopathy, progressive external ophthalmoplegia, pigmentary retinopathy and ovarian and testicular failure.

The diagnosis of MELAS should be suspected in any young patient with an ischaemic stroke, particularly if it is in the occipital lobe and complicated by epilepsy and if there is no other fairly obvious cause (Chinnery & Turnbull 1997b). CT frequently shows basal ganglia calcification and also areas of low density in the grey and white matter of the cerebral hemispheres, and these may show mass effect and enhancement in the acute stage, and then disappear, eventually to be followed by atrophy (Sue *et al.* 1998) (Fig. 7.12). The fasting plasma and, particularly, cerebrospinal fluid (CSF) lactate is raised, usually at rest. However, CSF lactate may be raised for some days after epileptic seizures, subarachnoid haemorrhage, meningitis and stroke. In most patients, muscle biopsy shows ragged red fibres on Gomori's trichrome staining and, with electron microscopy, large numbers of abnormal mitochondria. The point mutation in mitochondrial DNA (usually at base pair 3243 but occasionally at one of several other sites) can be demonstrated in white blood cells, but sometimes only in muscle. However, not all MELAS patients have known mutations, and sometimes the known mutations can be found in other mitochondrial clinical syndromes, in relatives of MELAS patients who may or may not be symptomatic, and in some normal people (Koo *et al.* 1993; Taylor *et al.* 1996; Chinnery *et al.* 1997). At present, there is no specific treatment.

Children with autosomal recessive cytochrome oxidase deficiency and lactic acidosis have been reported to have stroke-like episodes (Morin *et al.* 1999).

7.20 Miscellaneous genetic conditions

Cerebral autosomal dominant arteriopathy with subcortical infarcts and leukoencephalopathy (CADASIL)

This is a newly and increasingly recognized rare hereditary disorder of small blood vessels caused by mutations of the notch 3 gene on chromosome 19 (Joutel *et al.* 1997). Migraine with aura develops in patients in their 20s, recurrent—mainly lacunar ischaemic—strokes and transient ischaemic attacks in their 30s, progressive subcortical dementia in their 40s, and the patients die in their 50s. Early on, depressive symptoms are common (Chabriat *et al.* 1995; Hutchinson *et al.* 1995; Dichgans *et al.* 1998; Desmond *et al.* 1999). However, the phenotype is constantly being expanded and dementia may be a presenting feature (Filley *et al.* 1999). On CT, and more obviously on MRI, there are very characteristic focal, diffuse and confluent lesions in the periventricular and subcortical cerebral white matter, and sometimes in the brainstem, and these changes very often start before the patients are symptomatic, and they progress with time (Chabriat *et al.* 1998, 1999) (Fig. 7.13). Cerebral angiography should probably be avoided because of the excess risk of neurological complications (Dichgans & Petersen 1997).

The changes in the vessel wall are distinctive. There is a deposit of granular, eosinophilic material in the leptomeningeal and perforating arteries of the brain (Jung *et al.* 1995). The smooth muscle basal lamina of the affected vessels is thickened by granular osmiophilic material which is dense under electron microscopy. Similar changes can be found in

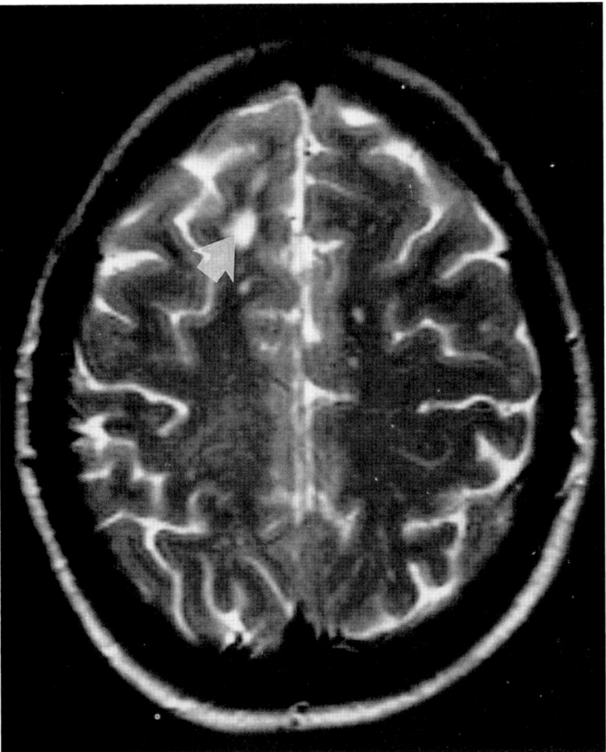

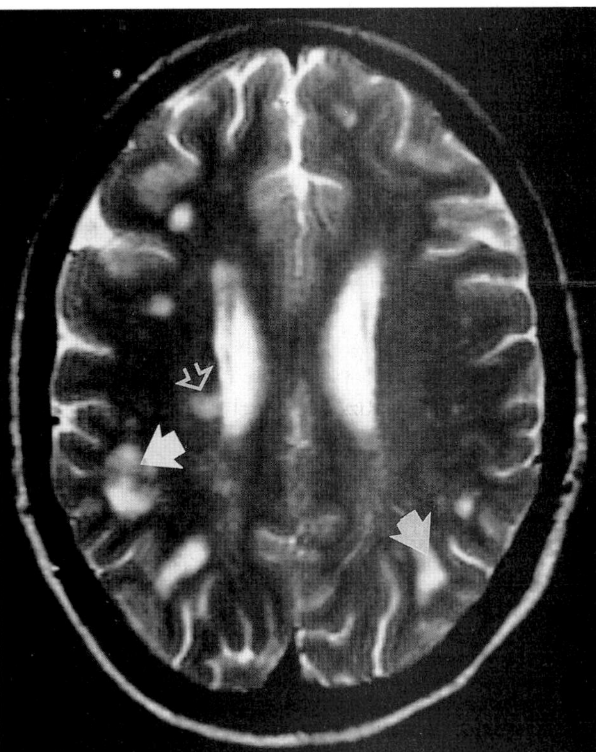

Fig. 7.13 Cerebral autosomal dominant arteriopathy with subcortical infarcts and leukoencephalopathy (CADASIL): T2-weighted MR scan of a 27-year-old woman with frequent migrainous headaches with visual aura. She also had transient episodes of sensory disturbance in her left upper limb, and sometimes weakness. She was both anxious and depressed about her own situation, and about her family where several members had had recurrent strokes and dementia. At the time of the scan there were no abnormal neurological signs. The scan shows numerous abnormal areas in the cerebral white matter just below the cortical ribon (closed white arrows) as well as one or two deep lesions in the cerebral white matter (open white arrow).

the small vessels of the skin, muscle and nerve, which sometimes allows histological, and particularly electron microscopy, confirmation of the diagnosis from skin or muscle biopsy, although this may not always be reliable (Goebel *et al.* 1997; Rubio *et al.* 1997; Furby *et al.* 1998; Ruchoux & Maurage 1998; Mayer *et al.* 1999).

Homocystinuria

This is an autosomal recessive inborn error of metabolism, usually caused by cystathione synthase deficiency. It is complicated by cerebral arterial and intracranial venous thrombosis for reasons that are unclear. The arterial pathology is different from atheroma. The diagnosis should be suspected if there is mental retardation, epileptic seizures, Marfanoid habitus, osteoporosis, high myopia and dislocated lenses (Schimke *et al.* 1965; Mudd *et al.* 1985; Visy *et al.* 1991; Rubba *et al.* 1994). Hyperhomocysteinaemia, insufficiently severe to cause the clinical syndrome of homocystinuria, may be a risk factor for degenerative vascular disease (section 6.3.3).

Fabry's disease

This is a rare, sex-linked, recessive disorder in which there is a deficiency of α-galactosidase A. This results in the accumulation of glycosphingolipids in vascular endothelial and other cells. Clinically evident as well as 'silent' ischaemic strokes, both cortical and subcortical, mostly caused by occlusion of small blood vessels but also larger vessel ectasia, are a common complication whereas intracranial haemorrhage is unusual (Grewal 1994; Mitsias & Levine 1996; Crutchfield *et al.* 1998). The patients are young males (very occasionally heterozygous females) and usually also have skin angiokeratomas in the bathing-trunks area, hypohidrosis, and burning pain and paraesthesia in the hands and feet (but seldom any signs) caused by a small fibre neuropathy. Corneal dystrophy, renal failure and secondary hypertension, myocardial ischaemia and conduction abnormalities are additional complications.

Tuberous sclerosis

This is a multisystem, autosomal dominant disorder which

may possibly be complicated by cerebral emboli from a cardiac rhabdomyosarcoma (Kandt *et al.* 1985). It has also been uncertainly associated with intracranial aneurysms and the moyamoya syndrome (section 7.5).

Neurofibromatosis I

This is another multisystem, autosomal dominant disorder. It may be complicated by: distal carotid occlusion as a result of irradiation for optic nerve glioma and this in turn may cause the moyamoya syndrome (section 7.5); intracranial and extracranial aneurysms; and tumour compression of intracranial arteries (Rizzo & Lessell 1994).

7.21 The young patient

There is nothing very different about the young compared with the elderly ischaemic stroke or transient ischaemic attack patient. The range of causes is similar. However, under the age of about 40 years neither atherothromboembolism (section 6.3) nor 'complex' small vessel disease (section 6.4) are at all likely, although still not impossible, whereas over the age of 60 years these disorders become overwhelmingly more likely than anything other than embolism from the heart (section 6.5).

Young patients attract more than their share of attention and tend to get more intensively investigated, which is not unreasonable because the proportion with an unusual (and often treatable) cause is undoubtedly higher than in the elderly. Innumerable series of 'young stroke patients', meaning anything from younger than 30 years to less than 50 years, probably depending on the age of the author, have been reported. The mix of causes and the proportion with 'no cause' depend on referral bias; investigation intensity; diagnostic criteria differences, and fashion over time; all these can change as more putative causes are discovered. The main causes are embolism from the heart, arterial dissection, inflammatory vascular disorders and migrainous stroke.

7.22 The case with no cause

Even for patients over 50–60 years, ischaemic strokes should not be put down to 'degenerative arterial disease' unless there are clear-cut risk factors (hypertension, smoking) and/or clear-cut evidence of arterial disease (bruits, claudication, angina) and no more obvious cause, such as giant cell arteritis. Nor should they be ascribed to embolism from the heart unless there is a major and threatening cardiac source (e.g. atrial fibrillation, prosthetic heart valve, etc.). There are many other, admittedly rare, possibilities to be considered.

But, after taking an exhaustive history, examining the patient obsessionally and undertaking numerous investigations, there are still some patients where no reasonable explanation for their stroke can be found or in whom any putative cause is somewhat marginal (e.g. mitral leaflet prolapse, oral contraceptives with no prothrombotic or other abnormality, an uncertain diagnosis of migrainous stroke). Naturally, the intensity of the search for a cause must depend on the previous level of dependency and the age of the patient, the severity of the stroke (aggressive investigation is reasonable in milder strokes where there is more to lose from a disabling recurrence), and the consequences of missing the diagnosis. At any age, it is vital to diagnose infective endocarditis as without treatment it can be fatal, whereas traumatic arterial dissection with no medicolegal consequences is not so important because there is no generally accepted treatment and recurrence is unlikely.

In a puzzling case, it is important to go over the history and examination again, and to check not only that the appropriate investigations have been carried out but also that the results have been discussed and are available in the medical records. It may turn out that the diagnosis of stroke or transient ischaemic attack (TIA) has to be revised, particularly if a 'stroke' patient deteriorates or fails to improve in a typical way after the acute stage, taking one back to the 'stroke' vs. 'not-stroke' issues discussed in Chapter 3. It is surprising how often, in young people, multiple sclerosis can be confused with stroke, in elderly patients how the pseudobulbar palsy of motor neurone disease can be called a stroke, and at any age how migraine aura without headache can be confused with TIAs. So 'no cause for a stroke' may simply mean that the patient has not had a stroke in the first place.

If there is no obvious cause for a stroke or transient ischaemic attack, it is important to retake the history, re-examine the patient and check not only that all the relevant investigations have been carried out but that the results have been seen and discussed. If there is still no cause, then follow-up the patient because time, or a recurrence, may provide the crucial clue.

If the ischaemic stroke or TIA diagnosis is secure, all the relevant investigations are negative, the heart is normal, and there are no vascular risk factors or evidence of vascular disease outside the head, then there is little to be done except recommend aspirin as an antithrombotic drug (at least for a while), await events and hope that any recurrence does not bring to light a diagnosis which should have led to an effective treatment at the time of the first stroke. In general, the problem is seldom the lack of a key investigation but more often the lack of a good clinical history. Therefore, other than checking out all the possible investigations in Tables 6.14 and 6.15, it is best to retake the history, re-examine the patient and follow-up the patient carefully. Fortunately, strokes with *truly* no cause seldom seem to recur.

References

Please note that all references taken from *The Cochrane Library* are given a current date as this database is updated on a quarterly basis. Please refer to the current *Cochrane Library* article for the latest review. The same applies to the *British Medical Journal* 'Clinical Evidence' series which is updated every six months.

Abramsky, O. & Slavin, S. (1974) Neurologic manifestations in patients with mixed cryoglobulinaemia. *Neurology* **24**, 245–249.

Achiron, A., Gornish, M. & Melamed, E. (1990) Cerebral sinus thrombosis as a potential hazard of antifibrinolytic treatment in menorrhagia. *Stroke* **21**, 817–819.

Adams, R.J., Nichols, F.T., McKie, V., McKie, K., Milner, P. & Gammal, T.E. (1988) Cerebral infarction in sickle cell anaemia: mechanism based on CT and MRI. *Neurology* **38**, 1012–1017.

Adams, R.J., McKie, V.C., Carl, E.M. *et al.* (1997) Long-term stroke risk in children with sickle cell disease screened with transcranial Doppler. *Annals of Neurology* **42**, 699–704.

Aessopos, A., Farmakis, D., Karagiorga, M., Rombos, I. & Loucopoulos, D. (1997) Pseudoxanthoma elasticum lesions and cardiac complications as contributing factors for strokes in B-thalassemia patients. *Stroke* **28**, 2421–2424.

Aggarwal, S.K., Williams, V., Levine, S.R., Cassin, B.J. & Garcia, J.H. (1996) Cocaine-associated intracranial haemorrhage: absence of vasculitis in 14 cases. *Neurology* **46**, 1741–1743.

Akins, P.T., Glen, S., Nemeth, P.M. & Derdeyn, C.P. (1996) Carotid artery thrombus associated with severe iron-deficiency anaemia and thrombocytosis. *Stroke* **27**, 1002–1005.

Alexander, E.L., Provost, T.T., Stevens, M.B. & Alexander, G.E. (1982) Neurologic complications of primary Sjögren's syndrome. *Medicine* **61**, 247–257.

Al-Hakim, M., Katirji, B., Osorio, I. & Weisman, R. (1993) Cerebral venous thrombosis in paroxysmal nocturnal haemoglobinuria: report of two cases. *Neurology* **43**, 742–746.

Alrawi, A., Trobe, J.D., Blaivas, M. & Musch, D.C. (1999) Brain biopsy in primary angiitis of the central nervous system. *Neurology* **53**, 858–860.

Al-Shahi, R., Warlow, C.P., Jansen, G.H., Frijns, C.J.M. & van Gijn, J. (2001) A 59-year-old man with progressive spinal cord and peripheral nerve dysfunction culminating in encephalopathy. *Journal of Neurology, Neurosurgery and Psychiatry* (in press).

Amlie-Lefond, C., Kleinschmidt-DeMasters, B.K., Mahalingam, R., Davis, L.E. & Gilden, D.H. (1995) The vasculopathy of varicella-zoster virus encephalitis. *Annals of Neurology* **37**, 784–790.

Antiphospholipid Antibodies and Stroke Study Group (APASS) (1997) Anticardiolipin antibodies and the risk of recurrent thrombo-occlusive events and death. *Neurology* **48**, 91–94.

Aoyagi, M., Faukai, N., Yamamoto, M., Nakagawa, K., Matsushima, Y. & Yamamoto, K. (1996) Early development of intimal thickening in superficial temporal arteries in patients with Moyamoya disease. *Stroke* **27**, 1750–1754.

von Arbin, M., Britton, M., de Faire, U., Helmers, C., Miah, K. & Murray, V. (1982) Myocardial infarction in patients with acute cerebrovascular disease. *European Heart Journal* **3**, 136–141.

Arboix, A., Besses, C., Acin, P. *et al.* (1995) Ischaemic stroke as first manifestation of essential thrombocythaemia: report of six cases. *Stroke* **26**, 1463–1466.

Arima, T., Motomura, M., Nishiura, Y. *et al.* (1992) Cerebral infarction in a heterozygote with variant antithrombin III. *Stroke* **23**, 1822–1825.

Asherson, R.A. & Piette. J.-C. (1996) The catastrophic antiphospholipid syndrome 1996. Acute multi-organ failure associated with antiphospholipid antibodies: a review of 31 patients. *Lupus* **5**, 414–417.

Auer, A., Felber, S., Schmidauer, C., Waldenberger, P. & Aichner, F. (1998) Magnetic resonance angiographic and clinical features of extracranial vertebral artery dissection. *Journal of Neurology, Neurosurgery and Psychiatry* **64**, 474–481.

Ayas, N. & Wijdicks, E.F.M. (1995) Cardiac catheterization complicated by stroke: 14 patients. *Cerebrovascular Diseases* **5**, 304–307.

Baglin, T. (1996) Disseminated intravascular coagulation: diagnosis and treatment. *British Medical Journal* **312**, 683–687.

Bakshi, R., Shaikh, Z.A., Bates, V.E. & Kinkel, P.R. (1999) Thrombotic thrombocytopenic purpura: brain CT and MRI findings in 12 patients. *Neurology* **52**, 1285–1288.

Bang, O.Y., Heo, J.H., Choi, S.A. & Kim, D.I. (1997) Large cerebral infarction during praziquantel therapy in neurocysticercosis. *Stroke* **28**, 211–213.

Barbour, P.J., Castaldo, J.E., Rae-Grant, A.D. *et al.* (1994) Internal carotid artery redundancy is significantly associated with dissection. *Stroke* **25**, 1201–1206.

Barker, R.A., Anderson, J.R., Meyer, P., Dick, D.J. & Scolding, N.J. (1999) Microangiopathy of the brain and retina with hearing loss in a 50-year-old woman: extending the spectrum of Susac's syndrome. *Journal of Neurology, Neurosurgery and Psychiatry* **66**, 641–643.

Bashir, R. & Jinkins, J. (1985) Cerebral infarction in a young female following snake bite. *Stroke* **16**, 328–330.

Bassetti, C., Carruzzo, A., Sturzenegger, M. & Tuncdogan, E. (1996) Recurrence of cervical artery dissection: a prospective study of 81 patients. *Stroke* **27**, 1804–1807.

Beck, D.O. & Corbett, J.J. (1983) Seizures due to central nervous system rheumatoid meningovasculitis. *Neurology* **33**, 1058–1061.

Becker, W.J. (1999) Use of oral contraceptives in patients with migraine. *Neurology* **53**, S19–S25.

Belchetz, P.E. (1994) Hormonal treatment of postmenopausal women. *New England Journal of Medicine* **330**, 1062–1071.

Belman, A.L., Leicher, C.R., Moshe, S.L. & Mezey, A.P. (1985) Neurologic manifestations of Schoenlein–Henoch purpura: report of three cases and review of the literature. *Pediatrics* **75**, 687–692.

Belman, A.L., Roque, C.T., Ancona, R., Anand, A.K. & Davis, R.P. (1990) Cerebral venous thrombosis in a child with iron deficiency anaemia and thrombocytosis. *Stroke* **21**, 488–493.

Benomar, A., Yahyaoui, M., Birouk, N., Vidailhet, M. & Chkili, T. (1994) Middle cerebral artery occlusion due to hydatid cysts of myocardial and intraventricular cavity cardiac origin: two cases. *Stroke* **25**, 886–888.

Beral, V., Hermon, C., Kay, C., Hannaford, P., Darby, S. & Reeves, G. (1999) Mortality associated with oral contraceptive use: 25-year follow up of cohort of 46 000 women from Royal College of General Practitioners' oral contraception study. *British Medical Journal* **318**, 96–100.

van den Berg, J.S.P., Hennekam, R.C.M., Cruysberg, J.R.M. *et al.* (2000) Prevalence of symptomatic intracranial aneurysm and ischaemic stroke in pseudoxanthoma elasticum. *Cerebrovascular Diseases* **10**, 315–319.

Berkovic, S.F., Bladin, P.F. & Darby, D.G. (1984) Metabolic disorders presenting as stroke. *Medical Journal of Australia* **140**, 421–424.

Bickerstaff, E.R. (1964) Aetiology of acute hemiplegia in childhood. *British Medical Journal* **2**, 82–87.

Biller, J., Asconape, J., Challa, V.R., Toole, J.F. & McLean, W.T. (1981) A case for cerebral thromboangiitis obliterans. *Stroke* **12**, 686–689.

Biousse, V., d'Anglejan-Chatillon, J., Touboul, P., Amarenco, P. & Bousser, M. (1995) Time course of symptoms in extracranial carotid artery dissections: a series of 80 patients. *Stroke* **26**, 235–239.

Biousse, V., Schaison, M., Touboul, P.-J., D'Anglejan-Chatillon, J. & Bousser, M.-G. (1998) Ischaemic optic neuropathy associated with internal carotid artery dissection. *Archives of Neurology* **55**, 715–719.

Bischof, F., Kuntz, R., Melms, A. & Fetter, M. (1999) Cerebral vein thrombosis in a case with thromboangiitis obliterans. *Cerebrovascular Diseases* **9**, 295–297.

Bitzer, M. & Topka, H. (1995) Progressive cerebral occlusive disease after radiation therapy. *Stroke* **26**, 131–136.

Blankenship, J.C., Butler, M. & Garbes, A. (1995) Prospective assessment of cholesterol embolisation in patients with acute myocardial infarction treated with thrombolytic vs. conservative therapy. *Chest* **107**, 662–668.

Blecic, S., Capel, P., Van Blercom, N., Fery, P., Dhaene, T. & Hildebrand, J. (1996) Bilateral posterior cerebral infarction in a young man with a congenital deficit in protein C. *Cerebrovascular Diseases* **6**, 370–371.

Bodenheimer, M.M., Sauer, D., Shareef, B., Brown, M.W., Fleiss, J.L. & Moss, A.J. (1994) Relation between myocardial infarct location and stroke. *Journal of the American College of Cardiology* **24**, 61–66.

Boortz-Marx, R.L., Clark, B., Taylor, S., Wesa, K.M. & Anderson, D.C. (1995) Sneddon's syndrome with granulomatous leptomeningeal infiltration. *Stroke* **26**, 492–495.

Bousser, M.-G., Baron, J.C. & Chiras, J. (1985) Ischaemic strokes and migraine. *Neuroradiology* **27**, 583–587.

Bragoni, M., Di Piero, V., Priori, R., Valesini, G. & Lenzi, G.L. (1994) Sjögren's syndrome presenting as ischaemic stroke. *Stroke* **25**, 2276–2279.

de Bray, J.M., Penisson-Besnier, I., Dubas, F. & Emile, J. (1997) Extracranial and intracranial vertebrobasilar dissections: diagnosis and prognosis. *Jour-*

nal of Neurology, Neurosurgery and Psychiatry **63**, 46–51.

Brownlee, R.D., Tranmer, B.I., Sevick, R.J., Karmy, G. & Curry, B.J. (1995) Spontaneous thrombosis of an unruptured anterior communicating artery aneurysm: an unusual cause of ischemic stroke. *Stroke* **26**, 1945–1949.

de Bruijn, S.F.T.M., Stam, J., Koopman, M.M.W., Vandenbroucke, J.P. for the Cerebral Venous Sinus Thrombosis Study Group. (1998) Case–control study of risk of cerebral sinus thrombosis in oral contraceptive users who are carriers of hereditary prothrombotic conditions. *British Medical Journal* **316**, 589–592.

Bruno, A., Adams, H.P., Biller, J., Rezai, K., Cornell, S. & Aschenbrener, C.A. (1988) Cerebral infarction due to moyamoya disease in young adults. *Stroke* **19**, 826–833.

Bruno, A., Nolte, K.B. & Chapin, J. (1993) Stroke associated with ephedrine use. *Neurology* **43**, 1313–1316.

Burton, J.L. (1988) Livedo reticularis, porcelain-white scars and cerebral thromboses. *Lancet* **1**, 1263–1265.

Byar, D.P. & Corle, D.K. (1988) Hormone therapy for prostate cancer: results of the Veterans Administration Cooperative Urological Group Studies. *NCI Monographs* **7**, 165–170.

Call, G.K., Fleming, M.C., Sealfon, S., Levine, H., Kistler, J.P. & Fisher, C.M. (1988) Reversible cerebral segmental vasoconstriction. *Stroke* **19**, 1159–1170.

Cantu, C. & Barinagarrementeria, F. (1993) Cerebral venous thrombosis associated with pregnancy and puerperium: review of 67 cases. *Stroke* **24**, 1880–1884.

Caplan, L.R. & Tettenborn, B. (1992) Vertebrobasilar occlusive disease: review of selected aspects. I. Spontaneous dissection of extracranial and intracranial posterior circulation arteries. *Cerebrovasular Diseases* **2**, 256–265.

Caplan, L.R., Hier, D.B. & Banks, G. (1982) Current concepts of cerebrovascular disease—stroke: stroke and drug abuse. *Stroke* **13**, 869–872.

Carhuapoma, J.R., Mitsias, P. & Levine, S.R. (1997) Cerebral venous thrombosis and anticardiolipin antibodies. *Stroke* **28**, 2363–2369.

Carrel, T., Laske, A., Jenny, R., von Segesser, L. & Turina, M. (1991) Neurological complications associated with acute aortic dissection: is there a place for a surgical approach? *Cerebrovascular Diseases* **1**, 296–301.

Carril, J.M., Guijarro, C., Portocarrero, J.S., Solache, I., Jimenez, A. & Valera de Seijas, E. (1992) Speech arrest as manifestation of seizures in non-ketotic hyperglycaemia. *Lancet* 340, 1227.

Caselli, R.J., Hunder, G.G. & Whisnant, J.P. (1988) Neurologic disease in biopsy-proven giant cell (temporal) arteritis. *Neurology* **38**, 352–359.

Catala, M., Rancurel, G., Koskas, F., Martin-Dealassalle, E. & Kiefer, E. (1993) Ischaemic stroke due to spontaneous extracranial vertebral giant aneurysm. *Cerebrovascular Diseases* **3**, 322–326.

Chabriat, H., Vahedi, K., Iba-Zizen, M.T. *et al.* (1995) Clinical spectrum of CADASIL: a study of 7 families. *Lancet* **346**, 934–939.

Chabriat, H., Levy, C., Taillia, H. *et al.* (1998) Patterns of MRI lesions in CADASIL. *Neurology* **51**, 452–457.

Chabriat, H., Tournier-Lasserve, E. & Bousser, M.-G. (1999) Vasculopathies. In: *Genetics of Cerebrovascular Disease* (ed. M.J. Alberts), pp. 195–208. Futura, New York.

Chang, C.L., Donaghy, M., Poulter, N. & World Health Organisation Collaborative Study of Cardiovascular Disease and Steroid Hormone Contraception (1999) Migraine and stroke in young women: case–control study. *British Medical Journal* **318**, 13–18.

Chapin, J.E., Davis, L.E., Kornfeld, M. & Mandler, R.N. (1995) Neurologic manifestations of intravascular lymphomatosis. *Acta Neurologica Scandinavica* **91**, 494–499.

Chaturvedi, S. (1993) Fulminant cerebral infarctions with membranous nephropathy. *Stroke* **24**, 473–475.

Chen, S.T., Liu, Y.H., Hsu, C.Y., Hugan, E.L. & Ryu, S.J. (1988) Moyamoya disease in Taiwan. *Stroke* **19**, 53–59.

Chin, P.L., Kaminski, J. & Rout, M. (1977) Myocardial infarction coincident with cerebrovascular accidents in the elderly. *Age and Ageing* **6**, 29–37.

Chinnery, P.F. & Turnbull, D.M. (1997a) Mitochondrial medicine. *Quarterly Journal of Medicine* 90, 657–667.

Chinnery, P.F. & Turnbull, D.M. (1997b) Clinical features, investigation and management of patients with defects of mitochondrial DNA. *Journal of Neurology, Neurosurgery and Psychiatry* **63**, 559–563.

Chinnery, P.F. & Turnbull, D.M. (1999) Mitochondrial DNA and disease. *Lancet*, 354, S117-S121.

Chinnery, P.F., Howell, N., Lightowlers, R.N. & Turnbull, D.M. (1997) Molecular pathology of MELAS and MERRF: the relationship between mutation load and clinical phenotypes. *Brain* **120**, 1713–1721.

Chiu, D., Shedden, P., Bratina, P. & Grotta, J.C. (1998) Clinical features of moyamoya disease in the United States. *Stroke* **29**, 1347–1351.

Ciafaloni, E., Ricci, E., Shanske, S. *et al.* (1992) MELAS: clinical features, biochemistry and molecular genetics. *Annals of Neurology* **31**, 391–398.

Clark, J.M., Marks, M.P., Adalsteinsson, E. *et al.* (1996) MELAS: clinical and pathologic correlations with MRI, xenon/CT and MR spectroscopy. *Neurology* **46**, 223–227.

Comabella, M., Alvarez-Sabin, J., Rovira, A. & Codina, A. (1996) Bromocriptine and post-partum cerebral angiopathy: a causal relationship? *Neurology* **46**, 1754–1756.

Comu, S., Verstraeten, T., Rinkoff, J.S. & Busis, N.A. (1996) Neurological manifestations of acute posterior multifocal placoid pigment epitheliopathy. *Stroke* **27**, 996–1001.

Confavreux, C., Brunet, P., Petiot, P., Berruyer, M., Trillet, M. & Aimard, G. (1994) Congenital protein C deficiency and superior sagittal sinus thrombosis causing isolated intracranial hypertension. *Journal of Neurology, Neurosurgery and Psychiatry* **57**, 655–657.

Connor, M., Lammie, G.A., Bell, J.E., Warlow, C.P., Simmonds, P. & Brettle, R.D. (2000) Cerebral infarction in adult AIDS patients: observations from the Edinburgh HIV autopsy cohort. *Stroke* (in press).

Conway, J.E., Hutchins, G.M. & Tamargo, R.J. (1999) Marfan syndrome is not associated with intracranial aneurysms. *Stroke* **30**, 1632–1636.

Coppeto, J.R., Lessell, S., Lessell, I.M., Greco, T.P. & Eisenberg, M.S. (1984) Diffuse disseminated atheroembolism: three cases with neuro-ophthalmic manifestation. *Archives of Ophthalmology* **102**, 225–228.

Coronary Drug Project Research Group (1970) The coronary drug project: initial findings leading to modifications of its research protocol. *Journal of the American Medical Association* **214**, 1303–1313.

Cosio, F.G., Zager, R.A. & Sharma, H.M. (1985) Atheroembolic renal disease causes hypocomplementaemia. *Lancet* **1**, 118–121.

Cramer, S.C., Robertson, R.L., Dooling, E.C. & Scott, R.M. (1996) Moyamoya and Down syndrome: clinical and radiological features. *Stroke* **27**, 2131–2135.

Crawley, F., Schon, F. & Brown, M.M. (1999) Cerebral infarction: a rare complication of wasp sting. *Journal of Neurology, Neurosurgery and Psychiatry* **66**, 550–551.

Cregler, L.L. & Mark, H. (1986) Medical complications of cocaine abuse. *New England Journal of Medicine* **315**, 1495–1500.

Cross, S.S. (1991) How common is cholesterol embolism? *Journal of Clinical Pathology* **44**, 859–861.

Crutchfield, K.E., Patronas, N.J., Dambrosia, J.M. *et al.* (1998) Quantitative analysis of cerebral vasculopathy in patients with Fabry disease. *Neurology* **50**, 1746–1749.

Daggett, P., Deanfield, J. & Moss, F. (1982) Neurological aspects of hyponatraemia. *Postgraduate Medical Journal* **58**, 737–740.

Dalal, P.M. & Dalal, K.P. (1989) Cerebrovascular manifestations of infectious disease. In: *Handbook of Clinical Neurology* (eds P.J. Vinken, G.W. Bruyn & H.L. Klawans), p. 411. Elsevier Science, New York.

Daras, M., Tuchman, A.J. & Marks, S. (1991) Central nervous system infarction related to cocaine abuse. *Stroke* **22**, 1320–1325.

Daras, M., Tuchman, A.J., Koppel, B.S., Samkoff, L.M., Weitzner, I. & Marc, J. (1994) Neurovascular complications of cocaine. *Acta Neurologica Scandinavica* **90**, 124–129.

Dashe, J.F., Pessin, M.S., Murphy, R.E. & Payne, D.D. (1997) Carotid occlusive disease and stroke risk in coronary artery bypass graft surgery. *Neurology* **49**, 678–686.

Davidson, N.E. (1995) Hormone replacement therapy: breast versus heart versus bone. *New England Journal of Medicine* **332**, 1638–1639.

Davies-Jones, G.A.B. (1995) Neurological manifestations of haematological disorders. In: *Neurology and General Medicine* (ed. M.J. Aminoff), p. 219. Churchill Livingstone, New York.

Davis, J.M. & Zimmerman, R.A. (1983) Injury of the carotid and vertebral arteries. *Neuroradiology* **25**, 55–69.

DeBaun, M.R., Schatz, J., Siegel, M.J. *et al.* (1998) Cognitive screening examinations for silent cerebral infarcts in sickle cell disease. *Neurology* **50**, 1678–1682.

Del Brutto, O.H. (1992) Cysticercosis and cerebrovascular disease: a review. *Journal of Neurology, Neurosurgery and Psychiatry* **55**, 252–254.

Del Mar Saez de Ocariz, M., Nader, J.A., Del Brutto, O.H. & Santos Zambrano, J.A. (1996) Cerebrovascular complications of neurosyphilis: the return of an old problem. *Cerebrovascular Diseases* **6**, 195–201.

Del Sette, M., Angeli, S., Leandri, M. *et al.* (1998) Migraine with aura and right-to-left shunt on transcranial Doppler: a case–control study. *Cerebrovascular Diseases* **8**, 327–330.

Delaney, P. & Estes, M. (1980) Intracranial haemorrhage with amphetamine abuse. *Neurology* **30**, 1125–1128.

Desai, B. & Toole, J.F. (1975) Kinks, coils and carotids: a review. *Stroke* **6**, 649–653.

DeSanctis, R.W., Doroghazi, R.M., Austen, W.G. & Buckley, M.J. (1987) Aortic dissection. *New England Journal of Medicine* **317**, 1060–1067.

Desmond, D.W., Moroney, J.T., Lynch, T., Chan, S., Chin, S.S. & Mohr, J.P. (1999) The natural history of CADASIL: a pooled analysis of previously published cases. *Stroke* **30**, 1230–1233.

Devinsky, O., Petito, C.K. & Alonso, D.R. (1988) Clinical and neuropathological findings in systemic lupus erythematosus: the role of vasculitis, heart emboli and thrombotic thrombocytopenic purpura. *Annals of Neurology* **23**, 380–384.

Dichgans, M. & Petersen, D. (1997) Angiographic complications in CADASIL. *Lancet* **349**, 776–777.

Dichgans, M., Mayer, M., Uttner, I. *et al.* (1998) The phenotypic spectrum of CADASIL: clinical findings in 102 cases. *Annals of Neurology* **44**, 731–739.

Doll, D.C. & Greenberg, B.R. (1985) Cerebral thrombosis in smokers' polycythaemia. *Annals of Internal Medicine* **102**, 786–787.

Douglas, A.S., Walker, I.D. & Bennett, N.B. (1990) A Scottish Hebridean antithrombin III deficient family: 12 years on. *Scottish Medical Journal* **35**, 108–113.

Drake, M.E. (1982) Winiwarter–Buerger disease ('thromboangiitis obliterans') with cerebral involvement. *Journal of the American Medical Association* **248**, 1870–1872.

Drenkard, C., Sanchez-Guerrero, J. & Alarcon-Segovia, D. (1989) Fall in antiphospholipid antibody at time of thromboocclusive episodes in systemic lupus erythematosus. *Journal of Rheumatology* **16**, 614–617.

Drislane, F.W. & Wang, A. (1997) Multifocal cerebral haemorrhage in eclampsia and severe pre-eclampsia. *Journal of Neurology* **244**, 194–198.

Drug and Therapeutics Bulletin (1993) The management of polymyalgia rheumatica and giant cell arteritis. *Drug and Therapeutics Bulletin* **31**, 65–68.

Dubard, T., Pouchot, J., Lamy, C., Hier, D., Caplan, L.R. & Mas, J.L. (1994) Upper limb peripheral motor deficits due to extracranial vertebral artery dissection. *Cerebrovascular Diseases* **4**, 88–91.

Dubrovsky, T., Curless, R., Scott, G. *et al.* (1998) Cerebral aneurysmal arteriopathy in childhood AIDS. *Neurology* **51**, 560–565.

Dyken, M.E. & Biller, J. (1994) Peripartum cardiomyopathy and stroke. *Cerebrovascular Diseases* **4**, 325–328.

Earley, C.J., Kittner, S.J., Feeser, B.R. *et al.* (1998) Stroke in children and sickle-cell disease: Baltimore–Washington Cooperative Young Stroke Study. *Neurology* **51**, 169–176.

Eidelberg, D., Sotrel, A., Horoupian, D.S., Neumann, P.E., Pumarola-Sune, T. & Price, R.W. (1986) Thrombotic cerebral vasculopathy associated with herpes zoster. *Annals of Neurology* **19**, 7–14.

English, R. & Macaulay, M. (1977) Subclavian artery thrombosis with contralateral hemiplegia. *British Medical Journal* **2**, 1583.

Fabian, R.H. & Peters, B.H. (1984) Neurological complications of hemoglobin SC disease. *Archives of Neurology* **41**, 289–292.

Farah, S., Al-Shubaili, A., Montaser, A. *et al.* (1998) Behçet's syndrome: a report of 41 patients with emphasis on neurological manifestations. *Journal of Neurology, Neurosurgery and Psychiatry* **64**, 382–384.

Farrell, M.A., Gilbert, J.J. & Kaufman, J.C.E. (1985) Fatal intracranial arterial dissection: clinical pathological correlation. *Journal of Neurology, Neurosurgery and Psychiatry* **48**, 111–121.

Feinberg, W.M. & Swenson, M.R. (1988) Cerebrovascular complictions of L-asparaginase therapy. *Neurology* **38**, 127–133.

Feldenzer, J.A., Bueche, M.J., Venes, J.L. & Gebarski, S.S. (1987) Superior sagittal sinus thrombosis with infarction in sickle cell trait. *Stroke* **18**, 656–660.

Feldmann, E. & Levine, S.R. (1995) Cerebrovascular disease with antiphospholipid antibodies: immune mechanisms, significance and therapeutic options. *Annals of Neurology* **37** (Suppl. 1), S114–S130.

Ferro, J.M. (1998) Vasculitis of the central nervous system. *Journal of Neurology* **245**, 766–776.

Fibrinolytic Therapy Trialists' (FTT) Collaborative Group (1994) Indications for fibrinolytic therapy in suspected acute myocardial infarction: collaborative overview of early mortality and major morbidity results from all randomised trials of more than 1000 patients. *Lancet* **343**, 311–322.

Filley, C.M., Thompson, L.L., Sze, C.I., Simon, J.A., Paskavitz, J.F. & Kleinschmidt-DeMasters, B.K. (1999) White matter dementia in CADASIL. *Journal of the Neurological Sciences* **163**, 163–167.

Finazzi, G., Brancaccio, V., Moia, M. *et al.* (1996) Natural history and risk factors for thrombosis in 360 patients with antiphospholipid antibodies: a four-year prospective study from the Italian Registry. *American Journal of Medicine* **100**, 530–536.

Fine, M.J., Kapoor, W. & Falanga, V. (1987) Cholesterol crystal embolisation: a review of 221 cases in the English literature. *Angiology* **38**, 769–784.

Forwell, M.A., Redding, P.J., Brodie, M.J. & Gentleman, D. de R. (1984) Leptospirosis complicated by fatal intracerebral haemorrhage. *British Medical Journal* **289**, 1583.

Fourestie, V., Douceron, H., Brugieres, P., Ancelle, T., Lejonc, J.L. & Gherardi, R.K. (1993) Neurotrichinosis: a cerebrovascular disease associated with myocardial infarction and hypereosinophilia. *Brain* **116**, 603–616.

Fredericks, R.K., Lefkowitz, D.S., Challa, V.R. & Troost, B.T. (1991) Cerebral vasculitis associated with cocaine abuse. *Stroke* **22**, 1437–1439.

Frisoni, G.B. & Anzola, G.P. (1991) Vertebrobasilar ischaemia after neck motion. *Stroke* **22**, 1452–1460.

Fukumoto, S., Kinjo, M., Hokamura, K. & Tanaka, K. (1986) Subarachnoid haemorrhage and granulomatous angiitis of the basilar artery: demonstration of the varicella-zoster-virus in the basilar artery lesions. *Stroke* **17**, 1024–1028.

Furby, A., Vahedi, K., Force, M. *et al.* (1998) Differential diagnosis of a vascular leukoencephalopathy within a CADASIL family: use of skin biopsy electron microscopy study and direct genotypic screening. *Journal of Neurology* **245**, 734–740.

Garrett, W.T., Chang, C.W.J. & Bleck, T.P. (1996) Altered mental status in thrombotic thrombocytopenic purpura is secondary to non-convulsive status epilepticus. *Annals of Neurology* **40**, 245–246.

Gasecki, A.P., Kwiecinski, H., Lyrer, P.A., Lynch, T.G. & Baxter, T. (1999) Dissections after childbirth. *Journal of Neurology* **246**, 712–715.

Gebel, J.M., Sila, C.A., Sloan, M.A. *et al.* for the GUSTO-I Investigators (1998) Thrombolysis-related intracranial haemorrhage: a radiographic analysis of 244 cases from the GUSTO-I trial with clinical correlation. *Stroke* **29**, 563–569.

Geissler, A., Andus, T., Roth, M. *et al.* (1995) Focal white-matter lesions in brain of patients with inflammatory bowel disease. *Lancet* **345**, 897–898.

Gerber, O., Heyer, E.J. & Vieux, U. (1986) Painless dissections of the aorta presenting as acute neurologic syndromes. *Stroke* **17**, 644–647.

Geschwind, D.H., Fitzpatrick, M., Mischel, P.S. & Cummings, J.L. (1995) Sneddon's syndrome is a thrombotic vasculopathy: neuropathologic and neuroradiologic evidence. *Neurology* **45**, 557–560.

Gijtenbeek, J.M.M., van den Bent, M.J. & Vecht, C.H.J. (1999) Cyclosporine neurotoxicity: a review. *Journal of Neurology* **246**, 339–346.

Gilchrist, J.M., Sikirica, M., Stopa, E. & Shanske, S. (1996) Adult-onset MELAS: evidence for involvement of neurons as well as cerebral vasculature in stroke-like episodes. *Stroke* **27**, 1420–1423.

Gillum, L.A., Mamidipudi, S.K. & Johnston, S.C. (2000) Ischaemic stroke risk with oral contraceptives. A meta-analysis. *Journal of the American Medical Association* **284**, 72–78.

Glass, J., Hochberg, F.H. & Miller, D.C. (1993) Intravascular lymphomatosis: a systemic disease with neurologic manifestations. *Cancer* **71**, 3156–3164.

Glick, R., Hoying, J., Cerullo, L. & Perlman, S. (1987) Phenylpropanolamine—an over-the-counter drug causing nervous system vasculitis and intracerebral haemorrhage: case report and review. *Neurosurgery* **20**, 969–974.

Goebel, H.H., Meyermann, R., Rosin, R. & Schlote, W. (1997) Characteristic morphologic manifestation of CADASIL, cerebral autosomal-dominant arteriopathy with subcortical infarcts and leukoencephalopathy, in skeletal muscle and skin. *Muscle Nerve* **20**, 625–627.

Gordon, M.F., Coyle, P.K. & Golub, B. (1988) Eales' disease presenting as stroke in the young adult. *Annals of Neurology* **24**, 264–266.

Gorevic, P.D., Kassab, H.J., Levo, Y. *et al.* (1980) Mixed cryoglobulinaemia: clinical aspects and long-term follow-up of 40 patients. *American Journal of Medicine* **69**, 287–308.

Gout, O., Bonnaud, I., Weill, A. *et al.* (1999) Facial diplegia complicating a bilateral internal carotid artery dissection. *Stroke* **30**, 681–686.

Grady, D., Rubin, S.M., Petitti, D.B. *et al.* (1992) Horomone therapy to prevent disease and prolong life in postmenopausal women. *Annals of Internal Medicine* **117**, 1016–1037.

Grady, D., Wenger, N.K., Herrington, D. *et al.* (2000) Postmenopausal hormone therapy increases risk for venous thromboembolic disease: the heart and estrogen/progestin replacement study. *Annals of Internal Medicine* **132**, 689–696.

Grant, C. & Warlow, C.P. (1985) Focal epilepsy in diabetic non-ketotic hyperglycaemia. *British Medical Journal* **290**, 1204–1205.

Grau, A.J., Brandt, T., Buggle, F. *et al.* (1999) Association of cervical artery dissection with recent infection. *Archives of Neurology* **56**, 851–856.

Graus, P., Rogers, L.R. & Posner, J.B. (1985) Cerebrovascular complications in patients with cancer. *Medicine* **64**, 16–35.

Greaves, M. (1999) Antiphospholipid antibodies and thrombosis. *Lancet* **353**, 1348–1353.

Greenberg, J. & Massey, E.W. (1985) Cerebral infarction in sickle cell trait. *Annals of Neurology* **18**, 354–355.

Grewal, R.P. (1994) Stroke in Fabry's disease. *Journal of Neurology* **241**, 3–6.

Griewing, B., Guo, Y., Doherty, C., Feyerabend, M., Wessel, K. & Kessler, C. (1995) Radiation-induced injury to the carotid artery: a longitudinal study. *European Journal of Neurology* **2**, 379–383.

Grill, J., Couanet, D., Cappelli, C. *et al.* (1999) Radiation-induced cerebral vasculopathy in children with neurofibromatosis and optic pathway glioma. *Annals of Neurology* **45**, 393–396.

Grosset, D.G., Ebrahim, S., Bone, I. & Warlow, C.P. (1995) Stroke in pregnancy and the puerperium: what magnitude of risk? *Journal of Neurology, Neurosurgery and Psychiatry* **58**, 129–131.

Grunwald, Z. & Sather, S.D.C. (1995) Intraoperative cerebral infarction after desmopressin administration in infants in end-stage renal disease. *Lancet* **345**, 1364–1365.

Gruppo Italiano Studio Policitemia (1995) Polycythaemia vera: the natural history of 1213 patients followed for 20 years. *Annals of Internal Medicine* **123**, 656–664.

Guillon, B., Brunereau, L., Biousse, V., Djouhri, H., Levy, C. & Bousser, M.-G. (1999) Long-term follow-up of aneurysms developed during extracranial internal carotid artery dissection. *Neurology* **53**, 117–122.

Gutthann, S.P., Garcia Rodriguez, L.A., Castellsague, J. & Duque Oliart, A. (1997) Hormone replacement therapy and risk of venous thromboembolism: population-based case–control study. *British Medical Journal* **314**, 796–800.

Haas, D.C., Pineda, G.S. & Lourie, H. (1975) Juvenile head trauma syndromes and their relationship to migraine. *Archives of Neurology* **32**, 727–730.

Haas, L.F. (1982) Stroke as an early manifestation of systemic lupus erythematosus. *Journal of Neurology, Neurosurgery and Psychiatry* **45**, 554–556.

Hagan, P.G., Nienaber, C.A., Isselbacher, E.M. *et al.* (2000) The International Registry of Acute Aortic Dissection (IRAD): new insights into an old disease. *Journal of the American Medical Association* **283**, 897–903.

Hall, S., Persellin, S., Lie, J.T., O'Brien, P.C., Kurland, L.T. & Hunder, G.G. (1983) The therapeutic impact of temporal artery biopsy. *Lancet* **2**, 1217–1220.

Hall, S., Barr, W., Lie, J.T., Stanson, A.W., Kazmier, F.J. & Hunder, G.G. (1985) Takayasu arteritis: a study of 32 North American patients. *Medicine* **64**, 89–99.

Hama, N. & Boumpas, D.T. (1995) Cerebral lupus erythematosus: diagnosis and rational drug treatment. *CNS Drugs* **3**, 416–426.

Hankey, G.J. (1991) Isolated angiitis/angiopathy of the central nervous system. *Cerebrovascular Diseases* **1**, 2–15.

Harries, D.P. & De Silva, R. (1992) 'Ecstasy' and intracerebral haemorrhage. *Scottish Medical Journal* **37**, 150–152.

Harrington, H., Heller, A., Dawson, D., Caplan, L. & Rumbaugh, C. (1983) Intracerebral haemorrhage and oral amphetamine. *Archives of Neurology* **40**, 503–507.

Harris, D.N.F., Bailey, S.M., Smith, P.L.C., Taylor, K.M., Oatridge, A. & Bydder, G.M. (1993) Brain swelling in first hour after coronary artery bypass surgery. *Lancet* **342**, 586–587.

Harrison, C.N., Linch, D.C. & Machin, S.J. (1998) Desirability and problems of early diagnosis of essential thrombocythaemia. *Lancet* **351**, 846–847.

Hart, R. & Hindman, B. (1982) Mechanisms of perioperative cerebral infarction. *Stroke* **13**, 766–773.

Hayreh, S.S. (2000) Steroid therapy for visual loss in patients with giant-cell arteritis. *Lancet* **355**, 1572–1573.

Heinemann, L.A., Lewis, M.A., Thorogood, M., Spitzer, W.O., Guggenmoos-Holzmann, I. & Bruppacher, R. (1997) Case–control study of oral contraceptives and risk of thromboembolic stroke: results from International Study on Oral Contraceptives and Health of Young Women. *British Medical Journal* **315**, 1502–1504.

Hemminki, E. & McPherson, K. (2000) Value of drug-licensing documents in studying the effect of postmenopausal hormone therapy on cardiovascular disease. *Lancet* **355**, 566–569.

Henrich, J.B., Sandercock, P.A.G., Warlow, C.P. & Jones, L.N. (1986) Stroke and migraine in the Oxfordshire Community Stroke Project. *Journal of Neurology* **233**, 257–262.

Henriksson, P. & Edhag, O. (1986) Orchidectomy versus oestrogen for prostatic cancer: cardiovascular effects. *British Medical Journal* **293**, 413–415.

Henry, J.A., Jeffreys, K.J. & Dawling, S. (1992) Toxicity and deaths from 3,4-methylenedioxymethamphetamine ('ecstasy'). *Lancet* **340**, 384–387.

Heron, E., Fornes, P., Rance, A., Emmerich, J., Bayle, O. & Fiessinger, J. (1998) Brain involvement in scerloderma: two autopsy cases. *Stroke* **29**, 719–721.

Herreman, F., Nathal, E., Yasui, N. & Yonekawa, Y. (1994) Intracranial aneurysms in Moyamoya disease: report of ten cases and review of the literature. *Cerebrovascular Diseases* **4**, 329–336.

Herrington, D.M., Reboussin, D.M., Brosnihan, K.B. *et al.* (2000) Effects of estrogen replacement on the progression of coronary-artery atherosclerosis. *New England Journal of Medicine* **343**, 522–529.

Herson, R.N. & Squier, M. (1978) Retinal perivasculitis with neurological involvement: a case report with pathological findings. *Journal of the Neurological Sciences* **36**, 111–117.

Hetzel, A., Berger, W., Schumacher, M. & Lucking, C.H. (1996) Dissection of the vertebral artery with cervical nerve root lesions. *Journal of Neurology* **243**, 121–125.

Heye, N. & Hankey, G.J. (1996) Amphetamine-associated stroke. *Cerebrovascular Diseases* **6**, 149–155.

Hickey, W.F., Garnick, M.B., Henderson, I.C. & Dawson, D.M. (1982) Primary cerebral venous thrombosis in patients with cancer—a rarely diagnosed paraneoplastic syndrome: report of three cases and review of the literature. *American Journal of Medicine* **73**, 740–750.

Hietaharju, A., Jaaskelainen, S., Hietarinta, M. & Frey, H. (1995) Central nervous system involvement and psychiatric manifestations in systemic sclerosis (scleroderma): clinical and neurophysiological evaluation. *Acta Neurologica Scandinavica* **87**, 382–387.

Hilton-Jones, D. & Warlow, C.P. (1985) Non-penetrating arterial trauma and cerebral infarction in the young. *Lancet* **1**, 1435–1438.

Hinchey, J., Chaves, C., Appignani, B. *et al.* (1996) A reversible posterior leukoencephalopathy syndrome. *New England Journal of Medicine* **334**, 494–500.

Hoekstra-van Dalen, R.A.H., Cillessen, J.P.M., Kappelle, L.J. & van Gijn, J. (1996) Cerebral infarcts associated with migraine: clinical features, risk factors and follow-up. *Journal of Neurology* **243**, 511–515.

Hogue, C.W., Murphy, S.F., Schechtman, K.B. & Davila-Roman, V.G. (1999) Risk factors for early or delayed stroke after cardiac surgery. *Circulation* **100**, 642–647.

Howell, S.J. & Molyneux, A.J. (1988) Vertebrobasilar insufficiency in rheumatoid atlanto-axial subluxation: a case report with angiographic demonstration of left vertebral artery occlusion. *Journal of Neurology* **235**, 189–190.

Hufnagel, A., Hammers, A., Schonle, P.-W., Bohm, K.-D. & Leonhardt, G. (1999) Stroke following chiropractic manipulation of the cervical spine. *Journal of Neurology* **246**, 683–688.

Hughes, J.T. & Brownell, B. (1968) Traumatic thrombosis of the internal carotid artery in the neck. *Journal of Neurology, Neurosurgery and Psychiatry* **31**, 307–314.

Hulley, S., Grady, D., Bush, T. *et al.* (1998) Randomized trial of estrogen plus progestin for secondary prevention of coronary heart disease in postmenopausal women: Heart and Estrogen/progestin Replacement Study (HERS) Research Group. *Journal of the American Medical Association* **280**, 605–613.

Hunn, M., Robinson, S., Wakefield, L., Mossman, S. & Abernethy, D. (1998) Granulomatous angiitis of the CNS causing spontaneous intracerebral haemorrhage: the importance of leptomeningeal biopsy. *Journal of Neurology, Neurosurgery and Psychiatry* **65**, 956–957.

Huston, K.A. & Hunder, G.G. (1980) Giant cell (cranial) arteritis: a clinical review. *American Heart Journal* **100**, 99–105.

Hutchinson, M., O'Riordan, J., Javed, M. *et al.* (1995) Familial hemiplegic migraine and autosomal dominant ateriopathy with leukoencephalopathy

(CADASIL). *Annals of Neurology* **38**, 817–824.

Igarashi, M., Gilmartin, R.C., Gerald, B., Wilburn, F. & Jabbour, J.T. (1984) Cerebral arteritis and bacterial meningitis. *Archives of Neurology* **41**, 531–535.

Ikeda, E. (1991) Systemic vascular changes in spontaneous occlusion of the circle of Willis. *Stroke* **22**, 1358–1362.

Illangasekera, V.L.U. (1981) Insulinoma masquerading as carotid transient ischaemic attacks. *Postgraduate Medical Journal* **57**, 232–234.

Isaak, B.L., Liesegang, T.J. & Michet, C.J. (1986) Ocular and systemic findings in relapsing polychondritis. *Ophthalmology* **93**, 681–689.

Iwama, T., Hashimoto, N., Murai, B.N., Tsukahara, T. & Yonekawa, Y. (1997) Intracranial rebleeding in moyamoya disease. *Journal of Clinical Neuroscience* **4**, 169–172.

Jackson, L.M., O'Gorman, P.J., O'Connell, J., Cronin, C.C., Cotter, K.P. & Shanahan, F. (1997) Thrombosis in inflammatory bowel disease: clinical setting, procoagulant profile and factor V Leiden. *Quarterly Journal of Medicine* **90**, 183–188.

Jackson, M., Lennox, G., Jaspan, T. & Lowe, J. (1993) Cerebral venous and systemic thrombosis in resolving ulcerative colitis. *Cerebrovascular Diseases* **3**, 178–179.

Jackson, M.J., Schaefer, J.A., Johnson, M.A., Morris, A.A.M., Turnbull, D.M. & Bindoff, L.A. (1995) Presentation and clinical investigation of mitochondrial respiratory chain disease: a study of 51 patients. *Brain* **118**, 339–357.

Jaillard, A.S., Hommel, M. & Mallaret, M. (1994) Venous sinus thrombosis associated with androgens in a healthy young man. *Stroke* **25**, 212–213.

Janssens, E., Hommel, M., Mounier-Vehier, F., Leclerc, X., Guerin du Magenet, B. & Leys, D. (1995) Post-partum cerebral angiopathy possibly due to bromocriptine therapy. *Stroke* **26**, 128–130.

Jennekens, F.G.I. & Kater, L. (1999) *Neurology of the Inflammatory Connective Tissue Diseases*. Saunders, London.

Jennette, J.C. & Falk, R.J. (1997) Small-vessel vasculitis. *New England Journal of Medicine* **337**, 1512–1523.

Johns, D.R. (1991) Cerebrovascular complications of inflammatory bowel disease. *American Journal of Gastroenterology* **86**, 367–370.

Jonasson, F., Cullen, J.F. & Elton, R.A. (1979) Temporal arteritis: a 14-year epidemiological, clinical and prognostic study. *Scottish Medical Journal* **24**, 111–117.

Jorens, P.G., Delvigne, C.R., Hermans, C.R., Haber, I., Holvoet, J. & De Deyn, P.P. (1991) Cerebral arterial thrombosis preceding ulcerative colitis. *Stroke* **22**, 1212.

Joutel, A., Vahedi, K., Corpechot, C. *et al.* (1997) Strong clustering and stereotyped nature of *Notch3* mutations in CADASIL patients. *Lancet* **350**, 1511–1515.

Jung, H.H., Bassetti, C., Tournier-Lasserve, E. *et al.* (1995) Cerebral autosomal dominant arteripathy with subcortical infarcts and leukoencephalopathy: a clinicopathological and genetic study of a Swiss family. *Journal of Neurology, Neurosurgery and Psychiatry* **59**, 138–143.

Kalashnikova, L.A., Nasonov, E.L., Stoyanovich, L.Z., Kovalyov, V.U., Kochel-eva, N.M. & Reshetnyak, T.M. (1994) Sneddon's syndrome and the primary antiphospholipid syndrome. *Cerebrovascular Diseases* **4**, 76–82.

Kandt, R.S., Gebarski, S.S. & Goetting, M.G. (1985) Tuberous sclerosis with cardiogenic cerebral embolism: magnetic resonance imaging. *Neurology* **35**, 1223–1225.

Kase, C.S., Foster, T.E., Reed, J.E., Spatz, E.L. & Girgis, G.N. (1987) Intracerebral haemorrhage and phenylpropanolamine use. *Neurology* **37**, 399–404.

Kaufman, M.J., Levin, J.M., Ross, M.H. *et al.* (1998) Cocaine-induced cerebral vasoconstriction detected in humans with magnetic resonance angiography. *Journal of the American Medical Association* **279**, 376–380.

Kawaguchi, T., Fujita, S., Hosoda, K., Shibata, Y., Iwakura, M. & Tamaki, N. (1997) Rotational occlusion of the vertebral artery caused by transverse process hyperrotation and unilateral apophyseal joint subluxation: case report. *Journal of Neurosurgery* **86**, 1031–1035.

Kay, A.C., Solberg, L.A., Nichols, D.A. & Petitt, R.M. (1991) Prognostic significance of computed tomography of the brain in thrombotic thrombocytopenic purpura. *Mayo Clinic Proceedings* **66**, 602–607.

Kazui, S., Kuriyama, Y., Sakata, T., Hiroki, M., Miyashita, K. & Sawada, T. (1993) Accelerated brain infarction in hypertension complicated by hereditary heterozygous protein C deficiency. *Stroke* **24**, 2097–2103.

Keime-Guibert, F., Napolitano, M. & Delattre, J.-Y. (1998) Neurological complications of radiotherapy and chemotherapy. *Journal of Neurology* **245**, 695–708.

Kelly, P.J., McDonald, C.T.O., Neill, G., Thomas, C., Niles, J. & Rordorf, G. (1998) Middle cerebral artery main stem thrombosis in two siblings with familial thrombotic thrombocytopenic purpura. *Neurology* **50**, 1157–1160.

Khamashta, M.A., Cervera, R., Asherson, R.A. *et al.* (1990) Association of antibodies against phopholipids with heart valve disease in systemic lupus erythematosus. *Lancet* **335**, 1541–1544.

Kieburtz, K.D., Eskin, T.A., Ketonen, L. & Tuite, M.J. (1993) Opportunistic cerebral vasculopathy and stroke in patients with the acquired immunodeficiency syndrome. *Archives of Neurology* **50**, 430–432.

Kitagawa, Y., Gotoh, F., Koto, A. & Okayasu, H. (1990) Stroke in systemic lupus erythematosus. *Stroke* **21**, 1533–1539.

Kitahara, T., Ariga, N., Yamaura, A., Makino, H. & Maki, Y. (1979) Familial occurrence of moyamoya disease: report of three Japanese families. *Journal of Neurology, Neurosurgery and Psychiatry* **42**, 208–214.

Kittner, S.J., Stern, B.J., Feeser, B.R. *et al.* (1996) Pregnancy and the risk of stroke. *New England Journal of Medicine* **335**, 768–774.

Koelman, J.H.T.M., Bakker, C.M., Plandsoen, W.C.G., Peeters, F.L.M. & Barth, P.G. (1992) Hereditary protein S deficiency presenting with cerebral sinus thrombosis in an adolescent girl. *Journal of Neurology* **239**, 105–106.

Koeppen, A.H., Lansing, L.S., Peng, S.-K. & Smith, R.S. (1981) Central nervous system vasculitis in cytomegalovirus infection. *Journal of the Neurological Sciences* **51**, 395–410.

Koh, K.K., Mincemoyer, R., Bui, M.N. *et al.* (1997) Effects of hormone-replacement therapy on fibrinolysis in postmenopausal women. *New England Journal of Medicine* **336**, 683–690.

Konzen, J.P., Levine, S.R. & Garcia, J.H. (1995) Vasospasm and thrombus formation as possible mechanisms of stroke related to alkaloidal cocaine. *Stroke* **26**, 1114–1118.

Koo, B., Becker, L.E., Chuang, S. *et al.* (1993) Mitochondrial encephalopathy, lactic acidosis, stroke-like episodes (MELAS): clinical, radiological, pathological and genetic observations. *Annals of Neurology* **34**, 25–32.

Kosik, K.S. & Furie, B. (1980) Thrombotic stroke associated with elevated plasma factor VIII. *Annals of Neurology* **8**, 435–437.

Kothare, S.V., Chu, C.-C., VanLandingham, K., Richards, K.C., Hosford, D.A. & Radtke, R.A. (1998) Migratory leptomeningeal inflammation with relapsing polychondritis. *Neurology* **51**, 614–617.

Krendel, D.A., Ditter, S.M., Frankel, M.R. & Ross, W.K. (1990) Biopsy-proven cerebral vasculitis associated with cocaine abuse. *Neurology* **40**, 1092–1094.

Kubis, N., Von Langsdorff, D., Petitjean, C. *et al.* (1999) Thrombotic carotid megabulb: fibromuscular dysplasia, septae and ischaemic stroke. *Neurology* **52**, 883–886.

Kubis, N., Zuber, M., Meder, J.F. & Mas, J.-L. (1996) CT scan of the skull base in internal carotid artery hypoplasia. *Cerebrovascular Diseases* **6**, 40–44.

Kuether, T.A., Nesbit, G.M., Clark, W.M. & Barnwell, S.L. (1997) Rotational vertebral artery occlusion: a mechanism of vertebrobasilar insufficiency. *Neurosurgery* **41**, 427–433.

van Kuijck, M.A.P., Rotteveel, J.J., van Oostrom, C.G. & Novakova, I. (1994) Neurological complications in children with protein C deficiency. *Neuropaediatrics* **25**, 16–19.

Lancet (1984) Ischaemia of the optic disc. *Lancet* **1**, 1391–1392.

Landi, G., Villani, F. & Anzalone, N. (1990) Variable angiographic findings in patients with stroke and neurosyphilis. *Stroke* **21**, 333–338.

Lanska, D.J. & Kryscio, R.J. (1998) Stroke and intracranial venous thrombosis during pregnancy and puerperium. *Neurology* **51**, 1622–1628.

Larner, A.J., Kidd, D., Elkington, P., Rudge, P. & Scaravilli, F. (1999) Spatz–Lindenberg disease: a rare cause of vascular dementia. *Stroke* **30**, 687–689.

Lau, S.O., Bock, G.H., Edson, J.R. & Michael, A.F. (1980) Sagittal sinus thrombosis in the nephrotic syndrome. *Journal of Pediatrics* **97**, 948–950.

Lefkovitz, N.W., Roessmann, U. & Kori, S.H. (1986) Major cerebral infarction from tumour embolus. *Stroke* **17**, 555–557.

Lefrere, J.-J., Chaunu, M.-P., Conard, J., Horellou, M.-H. & Samama, M. (1985) Congenital factor VII deficiency and cerebrovascular stroke. *Lancet* **2**, 1006–1007.

Leker, R.R., Pollak, A., Abramsky, O. & Ben-Hur, T. (1999) Abundance of left hemispheric embolic strokes complicating coronary angiography and PTCA. *Journal of Neurology, Neurosurgery and Psychiatry* **66**, 116–117.

Leopold, N.A. (1993) Chickenpox stroke in an adult. *Neurology* **43**,

1852–1853.

Levi, M. & ten Cate, H. (1999) Disseminated intravascular coagulation. *New England Journal of Medicine* **341**, 586–592.

Levine, S.R., Brust, J.C.M., Futrell, N. *et al.* (1991) A comparative study of the cerebrovascular complications of cocaine: alkaloidal versus hydrochloride: a review. *Neurology* **41**, 1173–1177.

Levine, S.R., Salowich-Palm, L., Sawaya, K.L. *et al.* (1997) IgG anticardiolipin antibody titer >40 GPL and the risk of subsequent thrombo-occlusive events and death: a prospective cohort study. *Stroke* **28**, 1660–1665.

Li, J.-Y., Lai, P.-H., Lam, H.-C. *et al.* (1999) Hypertrophic cranial pachymeningitis and lymphocytic hypophysitis in Sjögren's syndrome. *Neurology* **52**, 420–423.

Libman, R.B., Masters, S.R., de Paola, A. & Mohr, J.P. (1993) Transient monocular blindness associated with cocaine abuse. *Neurology* **43**, 228–229.

Libman, R.B., Sharfstein, S., Harrington, W. & Lerner, P. (1997) Recurrent intracerebral haemorrhage from sarcoid angiitis. *Journal of Stroke and Cerebrovascular Diseases* **6**, 373–375.

Lie, J.T. (1986) Thromboangiitis obliterans (Buerger's disease) in women. *Medicine* **65**, 65–72.

Liebow, A.A. (1973) The J. Burns Amberson lecture: pulmonary angiitis and granulomatosis. *American Review of Respiratory Disease* **108**, 1–18.

Limburg, M., Wijdicks, E.F. & Li, H. (1998) Ischemic stroke after surgical procedures: clinical features, neuroimaging and risk factors. *Neurology* **50**, 895–901.

Loh, E., St John Sutton, M.S., Wun, C.C. *et al.* (1997) Ventricular dysfunction and the risk of stroke after myocardial infarction. *New England Journal of Medicine* **336**, 251–257.

Longo, D.L. & Witherspoon, J.M. (1980) Focal neurologic symptoms in hypercalcaemia. *Neurology* **30**, 200–201.

Longstreth, W.T., Rosendaal, F.R., Siscovick, D.S. *et al.* (1998) Risk of stroke in young women and two prothrombotic mutations: factor V Leiden and prothrombin gene variant (G20210A). *Stroke* **29**, 577–580.

Lossos, A., Ben-Hur, T., Ben-Nariah, Z., Enk, C., Gomori, M. & Soffer, D. (1995a) Familial Sneddon's syndrome. *Journal of Neurology* **242**, 164–168.

Lossos, A., River, Y., Eliakim, A. & Steiner, I. (1995b) Neurological aspects of inflammatory bowel disease. *Neurology* **45**, 416–421.

Lupi-Herrera, E., Sanchez-Torres, G., Marcushamer, J., Mispireta, J., Horwitz, S. & Vela, J.E. (1977) Takayasu's arteritis: clinical study of 107 cases. *American Heart Journal* **93**, 94–103.

Luscher, T.F., Lie, J.T., Stanson, A.W., Houser, O.W., Hollier, L.H. & Sheps, S.G. (1987) Arterial fibromuscular dysplasia. *Mayo Clinic Proceedings* **62**, 931–952.

Maccario, M. (1968) Neurological dysfunction associated with nonketotic hyperglycaemia. *Archives of Neurology* **19**, 525–534.

MacGregor, E.A. & Guillebaud, J. (1998) Recommendations for clinical practice: combined oral contraceptives, migraine and ischaemic stroke. *British Journal of Family Planning* **24**, 53–60.

McLean, B.N., Miller, D. & Thompson, E.J. (1995) Oligoclonal banding of OgG in CSF, blood–brain barrier function, and MRI findings in patients with sarcoidosis, systemic lupus erythematosus and Behçet's disease involving the nervous system. *Journal of Neurology, Neurosurgery and Psychiatry* **58**, 548–554.

Mahaffey, K.W., Harrington, R.A., Simoons, M.L. *et al.* for the PURSUIT Investigators (1999) Stroke in patients with acute coronary syndromes: incidence and outcomes in the platelet glycoprotein IIb/IIIa in unstable angina: receptor suppression using integrilin therapy (PURSUIT) trial. *Circulation* **99**, 2371–2377.

Majamaa, K., Turkka, J., Karppa, M., Winqvist, S. & Hassinen, I.E. (1997) The common MELAS mutation A3243G in mitochondrial DNA among young patients with an occipital brain infarct. *Neurology* **49**, 1331–1334.

Markus, H.S. & Hambley, H. (1998) Neurology and the blood: haematological abnormalities in ischaemic stroke. *Journal of Neurology, Neurosurgery and Psychiatry* **64**, 150–159.

Martin, P.J. & Humphrey, P.R.D. (1998) Disabling stroke arising five months after internal carotid artery dissection. *Journal of Neurology, Neurosurgery and Psychiatry* **65**, 136–137.

Martin, R., Bogousslavsky, J. for the Lausanne Stroke Registry Group (1993) Mechanisms of late stroke after myocardial infarct: the Lausanne Stroke Registry. *Journal of Neurology, Neurosurgery and Psychiatry* **56**, 760–764.

Martinelli, I., Sacchi, E., Landi, G., Taioli, E., Duca, F. & Mannucci, P.M. (1998) High risk of cerebral-vein thrombosis in carriers of a prothrombin-gene mutation and in users of oral contraceptives. *New England Journal of Medicine* **338**, 1793–1797.

Mas, J.-L. & Lamy, C. (1998) Stroke in pregnancy and the puerperium. *Journal of Neurology* **245**, 305–313.

Mayer, M., Straube, A., Bruening, R. *et al.* (1999) Muscle and skin biopsies are a sensitive diagnostic tool in the diagnosis of CADASIL. *Journal of Neurology* **246**, 526–532.

Mayer, S.A., Tatemichi, T.K., Spitz, J.L., Desmond, D.W., Gamboa, E.T. & Gropen, T.I. (1994) Recurrent ischaemic events and diffuse white matter disease in patients with pseudoxanthoma elasticum. *Cerebrovascular Diseases* **4**, 294–297.

Melanson, M., Chalk, C., Georgevich, L. *et al.* (1996) Varicella-zoster virus DNA in CSF and arteries in delayed contralateral hemiplegia: evidence for viral invasion of cerebral arteries. *Neurology* **47**, 569–570.

Meschia, J.F., Malkoff, M.D. & Biller, J. (1998) Reversible segmental cerebral arterial vasospasm and cerebral infarction: possible association with excessive use of sumatriptan and midrin. *Archives of Neurology* **55**, 712–714.

Mettinger, K.L. (1982) Fibromuscular dysplasia and the brain. II. Current concept of the disease. *Stroke* **13**, 53–58.

Metz, H., Murray-Leslie, R.M., Bannister, R.G., Bull, J.W.D. & Marshall, J. (1961) Kinking of the internal carotid artery. *Lancet* **1**, 424–426.

Michiels, J.J., Koudstaal, P.J., Mulder, A.H. & van Vliet, H.H.D.M. (1993) Transient neurologic and ocular manifestations in primary thrombocythaemia. *Neurology* **43**, 1107–1110.

Mills, J.A. (1994) Systemic lupus erythematosus. *New England Journal of Medicine* **330**, 1871–1879.

Mills, R.M. (1971) Severe hypersensitivity reactions associated with allopurinol. *Journal of the American Medical Association* **216**, 799–802.

Mitsias, P. & Levine, S.R. (1994) Large cerebral vessel occlusive disease in systemic lupus erythematosus. *Neurology* **44**, 385–393.

Mitsias, P. & Levine, S.R. (1996) Cerebrovascular complications of Fabry's Disease. *Annals of Neurology* **40**, 8–17.

Moake, J.L. (1994) Haemolytic–uraemic syndrome: basic science. *Lancet* **343**, 393–397.

Mokri, B. & Piepgras, D.G. (1981) Cervical internal carotid artery aneurysm with calcific embolism to the retina. *Neurology* **31**, 211–214.

Mokri, B., Sundt, T.M. Jr, Houser, O.W. & Piepgras, D.G. (1986) Spontaneous dissection of the cervical internal carotid artery. *Annals of Neurology* **19**, 126–138.

Mokri, B., Silbert, P.L., Schievink, W.I. & Piepgras, D.G. (1996) Cranial nerve palsy in spontaneous dissection of the extracranial internal carotid artery. *Neurology* **46**, 356–359.

Moller, J.T., Cluitmans, P., Rasmussen, L.S. *et al.* for the ISPOCD Investigators (1998) Long-term postoperative cognitive dysfunction in the elderly ISPOCDI study. *Lancet* **351**, 857–861.

Montalban, J., Rio, J., Khamastha, M. *et al.* (1994) Value of immunologic testing in stroke patients: a prospective multicentre study. *Stroke* **25**, 2412–2415.

de la Monte, S.M., Hutchins, G.M. & Gupta, P.K. (1983) Polymorphous meningitis with atypical mononuclear cells in Sjögren's syndrome. *Annals of Neurology* **14**, 455–461.

Monti, G., Galli, M., Invernizzi, F. *et al.* the GISC. (1995) Cryoglobulinaemias: a multi-centre study of the early clinical and laboratory manifestations of primary and secondary disease. *Quarterly Journal of Medicine* **88**, 115–126.

Mooe, T., Eriksson, P. & Stegmayr, B. (1997) Ischaemic stroke after acute myocardial infarction: a population-based study. *Stroke* **28**, 762–767.

Moore, P.M. & Fauci, A.S. (1981) Neurologic manifestations of systemic vasculitis: a retrospective and prospective study of the clinicopathologic features and responses to therapy in 25 patients. *American Journal of Medicine* **71**, 517–524.

Moore, P.M. & Richardson, B. (1998) Neurology of the vasculitides and connective tissue diseases. *Journal of Neurology, Neurosurgery and Psychiatry* **65**, 10–22.

Mori, K., Nakayama, T., Cho, K., Hirano, A. & Maeda, M. (1998) Dissecting aneurysms limited to the basilar artery: report of two cases and review of the literature. *Journal of Stroke and Cerebrovascular Diseases* **7**, 213–221.

Morin, C., Dube, J., Robinson, B.H. *et al.* (1999) Stroke-like episodes in autosomal recessive cytochrome oxidase deficiency. *Annals of Neurology* **45**, 389–392.

Mudd, S.H., Skovby, F., Levy, H.L. *et al.* (1985) The natural history of homocystinura due to cystathionine β-synthase deficiency. *American Journal of Human Genetics* **37**, 1–31.

Muir, K.W., Squire, I.B., Alwan, W. & Lees, K.R. (1994) Anticardiolipin antibodies in an unselected stroke population. *Lancet* **344**, 452–456.

Mulder, L.J.M.M. & Spierings, E.L.H. (1987) Stroke due to intravascular coagulation in *Mycoplasma pneumoniae* infection. *Lancet* **2**, 1152–1153.

Mullges, W., Ringelstein, E.B. & Leibold, M. (1992) Non-invasive diagnosis of internal carotid artery dissections. *Journal of Neurology, Neurosurgery and Psychiatry* **55**, 98–104.

Mumford, C.J., Fletcher, N.A., Ironside, J.W. & Warlow, C.P. (1996) Progressive ataxia, focal seizures and malabsorption syndrome in a 41-year-old woman. *Journal of Neurology, Neurosurgery and Psychiatry* **60**, 225–230.

Munts, A.G., van Genderen, P.J.J., Dippel, D.W.J., van Kooten, F. & Koudstaal, P.J. (1998) Coagulation disorders in young adults with acute cerebral ischaemia. *Journal of Neurology* **245**, 21–25.

Murphy, M.F., Clarke, C.R.A. & Brearley, R.L. (1983) Superior sagittal sinus thrombosis and essential thrombocythaemia. *British Medical Journal* **287**, 1344.

Murros, K.E. & Toole, J.F. (1989) The effect of radiation on carotid arteries: a review article. *Archives of Neurology* **46**, 449–455.

Nabavi, D.G., Junker, R., Wolff, E. *et al.* (1998) Prevalence of factor V Leiden mutation in young adults with cerebral ischaemia: a case–control study of 225 patients. *Journal of Neurology* **245**, 653–658.

Nabulsi, A.A., Folsom, A.R., White, A. *et al.* for the Atherosclerosis Risk in Communities Study Investigators (1993) Association of hormone-replacement therapy with various cardiovascular risk factors in postmenopausal women. *New England Journal of Medicine* **328**, 1069–1075.

Nadareishvili, Z.G., Choudary, Z., Joyner, C., Brodie, D. & Norris, J.W. (1999) Cerebral microembolism in acute myocardial infarction. *Stroke* **30**, 2679–2682.

Nagayama, T., Shinohara, Y., Nagayama, M., Tsuda, M. & Yamamura, M. (1993) Congenitally abnormal plasminogen in juvenile ischaemic cerebrovascular disease. *Stroke* **24**, 2104–2107.

Nehls, D.G., Marano, S.R. & Spetzler, R.F. (1985) Positional intermittent occlusion of the internal carotid artery: case report. *Journal of Neurosurgery* **62**, 435–437.

Neild, G.H. (1994) Haemolytic–uraemic syndrome in practice. *Lancet* **343**, 398–401.

Nesbit, R.R., Neistadt, A. & May, A.G. (1979) Bilateral internal carotid artery aneurysms. *Archives of Surgery* **114**, 293–295.

Newman, L.S., Rose, C.S. & Maier, L.A. (1997) Sarcoidosis. *New England Journal of Medicine* **336**, 1224–1234.

Nighoghossian, N., Berruyer, M., Getenet, J.-C. & Trouillas, P. (1994) Free protein S spectrum in young patients with stroke. *Cerebrovascular Diseases* **4**, 304–308.

Nishino, H., Rubino, F.A. & Parisi, J.E. (1993) The spectrum of neurologic involvement in Wegener's granulomatosis. *Neurology* **43**, 1334–1337.

Nolte, K.B., Brass, L.M. & Fletterick, C.F. (1996) Intracranial haemorrhage associated with cocaine abuse: a prospective autopsy study. *Neurology* **46**, 1291–1296.

North, K.N., Whiteman, D.A.H., Pepin, M.G. & Byers, P.H. (1995) Cerebrovascular complications in Ehlers–Danlos syndrome Type IV. *Annals of Neurology* **38**, 960–964.

O'Brien, M.E., Tonge, K., Blake, P., Moskovic, E. & Wiltshaw, E. (1992) Blindness associated with high-dose carboplatin. *Lancet* **339**, 558.

O'Connell, B.K., Towfighi, J., Brennan, R.W. *et al.* (1985) Dissecting aneurysms of head and neck. *Neurology* **35**, 993–997.

Oberlander, D.A., Biller, J. & McCarthy, L.J. (1995) Thrombotic thrombocytopenic purpura: a neurological perspective. *Journal of Stroke and Cerebrovascular Disease* **5**, 175–179.

Oksi, J., Kalimo, H., Marttila, R.J. *et al.* (1998) Intracranial aneurysms in three patients with disseminated Lyme borreliosis: cause or chance association? *Journal of Neurology, Neurosurgery and Psychiatry* **64**, 636–642.

Olesen, J., Friberg, L., Olsen, T.S. *et al.* (1993) Ischaemia-induced (symptomatic) migraine attacks may be more frequent than migraine-induced ischaemic insults. *Brain* **116**, 187–202.

Orr, W.P. & Banning, A.P. (1999) Aortic atherosclerotic debris detected by trans-oesophageal echocardiography: a risk factor for cholesterol embolization. *Quarterly Journal of Medicine* **92**, 341–346.

Ortel, T.L. (1999) Genetics of coagulation disorders. In: *Genetics of Cerebrovascular Disease* (ed. M.J. Alberts), pp. 129–156. Futura, New York.

Padovan, C.S., Bise, K., Hahn, J. *et al.* (1999) Angiitis of the central nervous system after allogeneic bone marrow transplantation? *Stroke* **30**, 1651–1656.

Park, Y.D., Belman, A.L., Kim, T.-S. *et al.* (1990) Stroke in paediatric acquired immunodeficiency syndrome. *Annals of Neurology* **28**, 303–311.

Patton, W.F. & Lynch, J.P. (1982) Lymphomatoid granulomatosis: clinicopathologic study of four cases and literature review. *Medicine* **61**, 1–12.

Pavlakis, S.G., Bello, J., Prohovnik, I. *et al.* (1988) Brain infarction in sickle cell anaemia: magnetic resonance imaging correlates. *Annals of Neurology* **23**, 125–130.

Pedersen, A.T., Lidegaard, O., Kreiner, S. & Ottesen, B. (1997) Hormone replacement therapy and risk of non-fatal stroke. *Lancet* **350**, 1277–1283.

Pell, A.C.H. & Frier, B.M. (1990) Restoration of perception of hypoglycaemia after hemiparesis in an insulin-dependent diabetic patient. *British Medical Journal* **300**, 369–370.

Pepin, M., Schwarze, U., Superti-Furga, A. & Byers, P.H. (2000) Clinical and genetic features of Ehlers–Danlos syndrome type IV, the vascular type. *New England Journal of Medicine* **342**, 673–680.

Perry, D.J. & Pasi, K.J. (1997) Resistance to activated protein C and factor V Leiden. *Quarterly Journal of Medicine* **90**, 379–385.

Perry, J.R., Bilbao, J.M. & Gray, T. (1992) Fatal basilar vasculopathy complicating bacterial meningitis. *Stroke* **23**, 1175–1178.

Peters, M., Bohl, J., Thomke, F. *et al.* (1995) Dissection of the internal carotid artery after chiropractic manipulation of the neck. *Neurology* **45**, 2284–2286.

Petitti, D.B., Sidney, S., Quesenberry, C.P. Jr & Bernstein, A. (1998) Ischaemic stroke and use of oestrogen and oestrogen/progestogen as hormone replacement therapy. *Stroke* **29**, 23–28.

Pohl, C., Klockgether, T., Greinacher, A., Hanfland, P. & Harbrecht, U. (1999) Neurological complications in heparin-induced thrombocytopenia. *Lancet* **353**, 1678–1679.

Pohl, C., Harbrecht, U., Greinacher, A. *et al.* (2000) Neurologic complications in immune-mediated heparin-induced thrombocytopenia. *Neurology* **54**, 1240–1245.

Poulter, N.R., Chang, C.L., Farley, T.M.M., Marmot, M.G., Meirik, O. & the WHO Collaborative Study of Cardiovascular Disease and Steroid Hormone Contraception (1999) Effect on stroke of different progestogens in low oestrogen dose oral contraceptives. *Lancet* **354**, 301–302.

Poux, J.M., Peyronnet, P., Le Meur, Y., Favereau, J.P., Charms, J.P. & Leroux-Robert, C. (1992) Hypokalaemic quadriplegia and respiratory arrest revealing primary Sjögren's syndrome. *Clinical Nephrology* **37**, 189–191.

Pozzati, E., Giuliani, G., Poppi, M. & Faenza, A. (1989) Blunt traumatic carotid dissection with delayed symptoms. *Stroke* **20**, 412–416.

Preston, F.E., Cooke, K.B., Foster, M.E., Winfield, D.A. & Lee, D. (1978) Myelomatosis and the hyperviscosity syndrome. *British Journal of Haematology* **38**, 517–530.

Preston, F.E., Martin, J.F., Stewart, R.M. & Davies-Jones, G.A. (1979) Thrombocytosis, circulating platelet aggregates and neurological dysfunction. *British Medical Journal* **2**, 1561–1563.

Pretre, R. & von Segesser, L.K. (1997) Aortic dissection. *Lancet* **349**, 1461–1464.

Prior, A.L., Wilson, L.A., Gosling, R.G., Yates, A.K. & Russell, R.W.R. (1979) Retrograde cerebral embolism. *Lancet* **2**, 1044–1047.

Ragnaud, J.M., Tahbaz, A., Morlat, P., Sire, S., Gin, H. & Aubertin, J. (1996) Recurrent aseptic purulent meningitis in a patient with relapsing polychondritis. *Clinical Infectious Diseases* **22**, 374–375.

Rai, M., Shukla, R.C., Varma, D.N., Bajpai, H.S. & Gupta, S.K. (1990) Intracerebral haemorrhage following scorpion bite. *Neurology* **40**, 1801.

Rankin, J.M., Silbert, P.L., Yadava, O.P., Hankey, G.J. & Stewart-Wynne, E.G. (1994) Mechanism of stroke complicating cardiopulmonary bypass surgery. *Australian and New Zealand Journal of Medicine* **24**, 154–160.

de Recondo, A., Woimant, F., Ille, O., Rougemont, D. & Guichard, J.P. (1995) Post-traumatic common carotid artery dissection. *Stroke* **26**, 705–706.

Reece, D.E., Frei-Lahr, D.A., Shepherd, J.D. *et al.* (1991) Neurologic complications in allogeneic bone marrow transplant patients receiving cyclosporin. *Bone Marrow Transplantation* **8**, 393–401.

Reichhart, M.D., Bogousslavsky, J. & Janzer, R.C. (2000) Early lacunar strokes complicating polyarteritis nodosa: thrombotic microangiopathy. *Neurology* **54**, 883–889.

Reik, L. (1993) Stroke due to Lyme disease. *Neurology* **43**, 2705–2707.

Reinhart, W.H. & Berchtold, P.E. (1992) Effect of high-dose intravenous immunoglobulin therapy on blood rheology. *Lancet* **339**, 662–664.

Reuner, K.H., Ruf, A., Grau, A. *et al.* (1998) Prothrombin gene G_{20210}→A transition is a risk factor for cerebral venous thrombosis. *Stroke* **29**, 1765–1769.

Reynolds, P., Walker, F.O., Eades, J., Smith, J.D. & Lantz, P.E. (1997) Food embolus. *Journal of the Neurological Sciences* **149**, 185–190.

Rhodes, J.M. (1996) Cholesterol crystal embolism: an important 'new' diagnosis for the general physician. *Lancet* **347**, 1641.

Rich, C., Gill, J.C., Wernick, S. & Konkol, R.J. (1993) An unusual cause of cerebral venous thrombosis in a four-year-old child. *Stroke* **24**, 603–605.

Riche, G., Nighoghossian, N., Kopp, N., Froment, J.C. & Trouillas, P. (1996) Pseudobulbar palsy due to isolated angiitis of the central nervous system. *Cerebrovascular Diseases* **6**, 372–373.

Ridolfi, R.L. & Bell, W.R. (1981) Thrombotic thrombocytopenic purpura: report of 25 cases and review of the literature. *Medicine* **60**, 413–428.

Rizzo, J.F. & Lessell, S. (1994) Cerebrovascular abnormalities in neurofibromatosis type 1. *Neurology* **44**, 1000–1002.

Roach, G.W., Kanchuger, M., Mangano, C.M. *et al.* for the Multicenter study of Perioperative Ischaemia Research Group and the Ischemia Research and Education Foundation Investigators (1996) Adverse cerebral outcomes after coronary bypass surgery. *New England Journal of Medicine* **335**, 1857–1863.

Rodstrom, K., Bengtsson, C., Lissner. L. & Bjorkelund, C. (1999) Pre-existing risk factor profiles in users and non-users of hormone replacement therapy: prospective cohort study in Gothenburg, Sweden. *British Medical Journal* **319**, 890–893.

Roldan, C.A., Shively, B.K. & Crawford, M.H. (1996) An echocardiographic study of valvular heart disease associated with systematic lupus erythematosus. *New England Journal of Medicine* **335**, 1424–1430.

Rommel, O., Niedeggen, A., Tegenthoff, M., Kiwitt, P., Botel, U. & Malin, J.-P. (1999) Carotid and vertebral artery injury following severe head or cervical spine trauma. *Cerebrovascular Diseases* **9**, 202–209.

Rosengart, A., Hedges, T.R., Teal, P.A. *et al.* (1993) Intermittent downbeat nystagmus due to vertebral artery compression. *Neurology* **43**, 216–218.

Rother, J., Schreiner, A., Wentz, K. & Hennerici, M. (1992) Hypoglycaemia presenting as basilar artery thrombosis. *Stroke* **23**, 112–113.

Rothman, S.M., Fulling, K.H. & Nelson, J.S. (1986) Sickle cell anaemia and central nervous system infarction: a neuropathological study. *Annals of Neurology* **20**, 684–690.

Rothrock, J.F., Rubenstein, R. & Lyden, P.D. (1988) Ischaemic stroke associated with methamphetamine inhalation. *Neurology* **38**, 589–592.

Rothwell, P.M. & Grant, R. (1993) Cerebral venous sinus thrombosis induced by 'ecstasy'. *Journal of Neurology, Neurosurgery and Psychiatry* **56**, 1035.

Rubba, P., Mercuri, M., Faccenda, F. *et al.* (1994) Premature carotid atherosclerosis: does it occur in both familial hypercholesterolaemia and homocystinuria? Ultrasound assessment of arterial intima-media thickness and blood flow velocity. *Stroke* **25**, 943–950.

Rubio, A., Rifkin, D., Powers, J.M. *et al.* (1997) Phenotypic variability of CADASIL and novel morphologic findings. *Acta Neuropathologica* **94**, 247–254.

Ruchoux, M.M. & Maurage, C.A. (1998) Endothelial changes in muscle and skin biopsies in patients with CADASIL. *Neuropathology and Applied Neurobiology* **24**, 60–65.

Sakai, F., Ishii, K., Igarashi, H. *et al.* (1988) Regional cerebral blood flow during an attack of vertebrobasilar insufficiency. *Stroke* **19**, 1426–1430.

Salvarani, C., Macchioni, P. & Boiardi, L. (1997) Polymyalgia rheumatica. *Lancet* **350**, 43–47.

Sarkari, N.B.S., Holmes, J.M. & Bickerstaff, E.R. (1970) Neurological manifestations associated with internal carotid loops and kinks in children. *Journal of Neurology, Neurosurgery and Psychiatry* **33**, 194–200.

Sauer, C.M. (1991) Recurrent embolic stroke and cocaine-related cardiomyopathy. *Stroke* **22**, 1203–1205.

Sawauchi, S., Terao, T., Tani, S., Ogawa, T. & Abe, T. (1999) Traumatic middle cerebral artery occlusion from boxing. *Journal of Clinical Neuroscience* **6**, 63–67.

Sawle, G.V. & Ramsay, M.M. (1998) The neurology of pregnancy. *Journal of Neurology, Neurosurgery and Psychiatry* **64**, 711–725.

Saxena, V.K., Brands, C., Crols, R., Moens, E., Marien, P. & De Deyn, P.P. (1993) Multiple cerebral infarctions in a young patient with secondary thrombocythaemia due to iron deficiency anaemia. *Acta Neurologica* **15**, 297–302.

Schafer, A.I. (1994) Hypercoagulable states: molecular genetics to clinical practice. *Lancet* **344**, 1739–1742.

Scheithauer, B.W., Rubinstein, L.J. & Herman, M.M. (1984) Leukoencephalopathy in Waldenstrom's macroglobulinemia: immunohistochemical and electron micrscopic observations. *Journal of Neuropathology and Experimental Neurology* **43**, 408–425.

Schievink, W.I., Mokri, B. & Whisnant, J.P. (1993) Internal carotid artery dissection in a community. Rochester, Minnesota, 1987–92. *Stroke* **24**, 1678–1680.

Schievink, W.I., Michels, V.V. & Piepgras, D.G. (1994) Neurovascular manifestations of heritable connective tissue disorders: a review. *Stroke* **25**, 889–903.

Schievink, W.I., Mokri, B., Piepgras, D.G. & Kuiper, J.D. (1996) Recurrent spontaneous arterial dissections: risk in familial versus non-familial disease. *Stroke* **27**, 622–624.

Schievink, W.I., Wijdicks, E.F.M., Michels, V.V., Vockley, J. & Godfrey, M. (1998) Heritable connective tissue disorders in cervical artery dissections: a prospective study. *Neurology* **50**, 1166–1169.

Schimke, R.N., McKusick, V.A., Huang, T. & Pollack, A.D. (1965) Homocystinuria: studies of 20 families with 38 affected members. *Journal of the American Medical Association* **193**, 87–95.

Schlenska, G.K. (1986) Absence of both internal carotid arteries. *Journal of Neurology* **233**, 263–266.

Schmidt, B.J., Meagher-Villemure, K. & Del Carpio, J. (1984) Lymphomatoid granulomatosis with isolated involvement of the brain. *Annals of Neurology* **15**, 478–481.

Schmidt, W.A., Kraft, H.E., Vorpahl, K., Volker, L. & Gromnica-Ihle, E.J. (1997) Colour duplex ultrasonography in the diagnosis of temporal arteritis. *New England Journal of Medicine* **337**, 1336–1342.

Schutta, H.S., Williams, E.C., Baranski, B.G. & Sutula, T.P. (1991) Cerebral venous thrombosis with plasminogen deficiency. *Stroke* **22**, 401–405.

Schwartz, C.J., Mitchell, J.R.A. & Hughes, J.T. (1962) Transient recurrent cerebral episodes and aneurysm of carotid sinus. *British Medical Journal* **1**, 770–771.

Schwartz, S.M., Petitti, D.B., Siscovick, D.S. *et al.* (1998) Stroke and use of low-dose oral contraceptives in young women: a pooled analysis of two US studies. *Stroke* **29**, 2277–2284.

Schwartzman, R.J. & Hill, J.B. (1982) Neurologic complications of disseminated intravascular coagulation. *Neurology* **32**, 791–797.

Schwitter, J., Agosti, R., Ott, P., Kalman, A. & Waespe, W. (1992) Small infarctions of cochlear, retinal and encephalic tissue in young women. *Stroke* **23**, 903–907.

Scodary, D.J., Tew, J.M., Thomas, G.M., Tomsick, T. & Liwnicz, B.H. (1990) Radiation-induced cerebral aneurysms. *Acta Neurochirurgica* **102**, 141–144.

Scolding, N. (1999) *Immunological and Inflammatory Disorders of the Central Nervous System*. Butterworth Heinemann, Oxford.

Sehgal, M., Swanson, J.W., DeRemee, R.A. & Colby, T.V. (1995) Neurologic manifestations of Churg–Strauss syndrome. *Mayo Clinic Proceedings* **70**, 337–341.

Selby, G. & Walker, G.L. (1979) Cerebral arteritis in cat-scratch disease. *Neurology* **29**, 1413–1418.

Selnes, O.A., Goldsborough, M.A., Borowicz, L.M. & McKhann, G.M. (1999) Neurobehavioural sequelae of cardiopulmonary bypass. *Lancet* **353**, 1601–1606.

Serdaroglu, P. (1998) Behçet's disease and the nervous system. *Journal of Neurology* **245**, 197–205.

Service, F.J. (1995) Hypoglycaemic disorders. *New England Journal of Medicine* **332**, 1144–1152.

Sethi, K.D., El Gammal, T., Patel, B.R. & Swift, T.R. (1986) Dural sarcoidosis presenting with transient neurologic symptoms. *Archives of Neurology* **43**, 595–597.

Shahar, A. & Sadeh, M. (1991) Severe anaemia associated with transient neurological deficits. *Stroke* **22**, 1201–1202.

Shanmugam, V., Zimnowodzki, S., Curtin, J. & Gorelick, P.B. (1997) Hypoglycaemic hemiplegia: insulinoma masquerading as stroke. *Journal of Stroke and Cerebrovascular Diseases* **6**, 368–369.

Sharma, O.P. (1997) Neurosarcoidosis: a personal perspective based on the study of 37 patients. *Chest* **112**, 220–228.

Sharshar, T., Lamy, C., Mas, J.L. for the Stroke in Pregnancy Study Group (1995) Incidence and causes of strokes associated with pregnancy and puerperium: a study in public hospitals of Ile de France. *Stroke* **26**, 930–996.

Sherman, D.G., Hart, R.G. & Easton, J.D. (1981) Abrupt change in head position and cerebral infarction. *Stroke* **12**, 2–6.

Sheth, K.J., Swick, H.M. & Haworth, N. (1986) Neurological involvement in haemolytic–uraemic syndrome. *Annals of Neurology* **19**, 90–93.

Shintani, S., Tsuruoka, S. & Shiigai, T. (1993) Hypoglycaemic hemiplegia: a repeat SPECT study. *Journal of Neurology, Neurosurgery and Psychiatry* **56**, 700–701.

Shuaib, A. (1991) Stroke from other aetiologies masquerading as migraine-stroke. *Stroke* **22**, 1068–1074.

Siekert, R.G., Whisnant, J.P. & Millikan, C.H. (1960) Anaemia and intermittent focal cerebral arterial insufficiency. *Archives of Neurology* **3**, 386–390.

Sigal, L.H. (1987) The neurologic presentation of vasculitic and rheumatologic syndromes: a review. *Medicine* **66**, 157–180.

Silbert, P.L., Mokri, B. & Schievink, W.I. (1995) Headache and neck pain in spontaneous internal carotid and vertebral artery dissections. *Neurology* **45**, 1517–1522.

Silverstein, A., Gilbert, H. & Wasserman, L.R. (1962) Neurologic complications of polycythaemia. *Annals of Internal Medicine* **57**, 909–916.

Skegg, D.C.G. (1999) Oral contraception and health. *British Medical Journal* **318**, 69–70.

Sloan, M.A. & Gore, J.M. (1992) Ischaemic stroke and intracranial hemorrhage following thrombolytic therapy for acute myocardial infarction: a risk–benefit analysis. *American Journal of Cardiology* **69**, 21A–38A.

Sloan, M.A., Price, T.R., Terrin, M.L. *et al.* for the TIMI-II Investigators (1997) Ischaemic cerebral infarction after rt-PA and heparin therapy for acute myocardial infarction: the TIMI-II pilot and randomized clinical trial combined experience. *Stroke* **28**, 1107–1114.

Sloan, M.A., Kittner, S.J., Feeser, B.R. *et al.* (1998) Illicit drug-associated ischemic stroke in the Baltimore–Washington Young Stroke Study. *Neurology* **50**, 1688–1693.

Socie, G., Mary, J., de Gramont, A. *et al.* for the French Society of Haematology (1996) Paroxysmal nocturnal haemoglobinuria: long-term follow-up and prognostic factors. *Lancet* **348**, 573–577.

Stampfer, M.J., Willett, W.C., Colditz, G.A., Speizer, F.E. & Hennekens, C.H. (1990) Past use of oral contraceptives and cardiovascular disease: a meta analysis in the context of the Nurses' Health Study. *American Journal of Obstetrics and Gynecology* **163**, 285–291.

Steck, A.J. (1998) Neurological manifestations of malignant and non-malignant dysglobulinaemias. *Journal of Neurology* **245**, 634–639.

Steen, R.G., Langston, J.W., Ogg, R.J., Manci, E., Mulhern, R.K. & Wang, W. (1998) Ectasia of the basilar artery in children with sickle cell disease: relationship to haematocrit and psychometric measures. *Journal of Stroke and Cerebrovascular Diseases* **7**, 32–43.

Steg, R.E. & Lefkowitz, D.M. (1994) Cerebral infarction following intravenous immunoglobulin therapy for myasthenia gravis. *Neurology* **44**, 1180–1181.

Steinberger, A., Ganti, S.R., McMurtry, J.G. & Hilal, S.K. (1984) Transient neurological deficits secondary to saccular vertebrobasilar aneurysms: report of two cases. *Journal of Neurosurgery* **60**, 410–413.

Steinmetz, J.C., DeConti, R. & Ginsburg, R. (1989) Hypersensitivity vasculitis associated with 2-deoxycoformycin and allopurinol therapy. *American Journal of Medicine* **86**, 498–499.

Sternfeld, B., Stang, P. & Sidney, S. (1995) Relationship of migraine headaches to experience of chest pain and subsequent risk for myocardial infarction. *Neurology* **45**, 2135–2142.

Stewart, S.S., Ashizawa, T., Dudley, A.W., Goldberg, J.W. & Lidsky, M.D. (1988) Cerebral vasculitis in relapsing polychondritis. *Neurology* **38**, 150–152.

Sticherling, C., Berkefeld, J., Auch-Schwelk, W. & Lanfermann, H. (1998) Transient bilateral cortical blindness after coronary angiography. *Lancet* **351**, 570.

Stockhammer, G., Felber, S.R., Zelger, B. *et al.* (1993) Sneddon's syndrome: diagnosis by skin biopsy and MRI in 17 patients. *Stroke* **24**, 685–690.

Strupp, M., Planck, J.H., Arbusow, V., Steiger, H., Bruckmann, H. & Brandt, T. (2000) Rotational vertebral artery occlusion syndrome with vertigo due to 'labyrinthine excitation'. *Neurology* **54**, 1376–1379.

Sturzenegger, M. (1995) Spontaneous internal carotid artery dissection: early diagnosis and management of 44 patients. *Journal of Neurology* **242**, 231–238.

Sturzenegger, M., Newell, D.W., Douville, C., Byrd, S. & Schoonover, K. (1994) Dynamic transcranial Doppler assessment of positional vertebrobasilar ischaemia. *Stroke* **25**, 1776–1783.

Subbiah, P., Wijdicks, E., Muenter, M., Carter, J. & Connolly, S. (1996) Skin lesion with a fatal neurologic outcome (Degos' disease). *Neurology* **46**, 636–640.

Sue, C.M., Crimmins, D.S., Soo, Y.S. *et al.* (1998) Neuroradiological features of six kindreds with MELAS tRNA (Leu) A2343G point mutation: implications for pathogenesis. *Journal of Neurology, Neurosurgery and Psychiatry* **65**, 233–240.

Tanne, D., D'Olhaberriague, L., Schultz, L.R., Salowich-Palm, L., Sawaya, K.L. & Levine, S.R. (1999) Anticardiolipin antibodies and their associations with cerebrovascular risk factors. *Neurology* **52**, 1368–1373.

Tanne, D., Goldbourt, U., Zion, M. *et al.* (1993) Frequency and prognosis of stroke/TIA among 4808 survivors of acute myocardial infarction. *Stroke* **24**, 1490–1495.

Taylor, R.W., Chinnery, P.F., Haldane, F. *et al.* (1996) MELAS associated with a mutation in the valine transfer RNA gene of mitochondrial DNA. *Annals of Neurology* **40**, 459–462.

Tembl, J.I., Ferrer, J.M., Sevilla, M.T., Lago, A., Mayordomo, F. & Vilchez, J.J. (1999) Neurologic complications associated with hepatitis C virus infection. *Neurology* **53**, 861–864.

Thie, A., Hellner, D., Lachenmayer, L., Janzen, R.W. & Kunze, K. (1993) Bilateral blunt traumatic dissections of the extracranial internal carotid artery: report of eleven cases and review of the literature. *Cerebrovascular Diseases* **3**, 295–303.

Toro-Gonzalez, G., Navarro-Roman, L., Roman, G.C. *et al.* (1993) Acute ischaemic stroke from fibrocartilaginous emoblism to the middle cerebral artery. *Stroke* **24**, 738–740.

Tosi, L., Rigoli, G. & Beltramello, A. (1996) Fibrocartilaginous embolism of the spinal cord: a clinical and pathogenetic reconsideration. *Journal of Neurology, Neurosurgery and Psychiatry* **60**, 55–60.

Tuhrim, S., Rand, J.H., Wu, X.-X. *et al.* (1999a) Elevated anticardiolipin antibody titre is a stroke risk factor in a multiethnic population independent of isotype or degree of positivity. *Stroke* **30**, 1561–1565.

Tuhrim, S., Rand, J.H., Wu, X.-X. *et al.* (1999b) Antiphosphatidyl serine antibodies are independently associated with ischaemic stroke. *Neurology* **53**, 1523–1527.

Tulyapronchote, R., Selhorst, J.B., Malkoff, M.D. & Gomez, C.R. (1994) Delayed sequelae of vertebral artery dissection and occult cervical fractures. *Neurology* **44**, 1397–1399.

Turnbull, J. (1996) Temporal arteritis and polymyalgia rheumatica: nosographic and nosologic considerations. *Neurology* **46**, 901–906.

Turner, B. & Wills, A.J. (2000) Cerebral infarction complicating intravenous immunoglobulin therapy in a patient with Miller Fisher syndrome. *Journal of Neurology, Neurosurgery and Psychiatry* **68**, 790–791.

Uldry, P.-A., Regli, F. & Bogousslavsky, J. (1987) Cerebral angiopathy and recurrent strokes following *Borrelia burgdorferi* infection. *Journal of Neurology, Neurosurgery and Psychiatry* **50**, 1703–1704.

Ursell, M.R., Marras, C.L., Farb, R., Rowed, D.W., Black, S.E. & Perry, J.R. (1998) Recurrent intracranial haemorrhage due to post-partum cerebral angiopathy: implications for management. *Stroke* **29**, 1995–1998.

Vaitkus, P.T. & Barnathan, E.S. (1993) Embolic potential, prevention and management of mural thrombus complicating anterior myocardial infarction: a meta-analysis. *Journal of the American College of Cardiology* **22**, 1004–1009.

Vandenbroucke, J.P. (1998) Cerebral sinus thrombosis and oral contraceptives: there are limits to predictability. *British Medical Journal* **317**, 483–484.

Verro, P., Levine, S.R. & Tietjen, G.E. (1998) Cerebrovascular ischaemic events with high positive anticardiolipin antibodies. *Stroke* **29**, 2245–2253.

Vieregge, P., Schwieder, G. & Kompf, D. (1989) Cerebral venous thrombosis in hereditary protein C deficiency. *Journal of Neurology, Neurosurgery and Psychiatry* **52**, 135–137.

Visy, J.M., Le Coz, P., Chadefaux, B. *et al.* (1991) Homocystinuria due to 5,10-methylenetetrahydrofolate reductase deficiency revealed by stroke in adult siblings. *Neurology* **41**, 1313–1315.

Vollertsen, R.S., McDonald, T.J., Younge, B.R., Banks, P.M., Stanson, A.W. & Ilstrup, D.M. (1986) Cogan's syndrome: 18 cases and a review of the literature. *Mayo Clinic Proceedings* **61**, 344–361.

Vollmer, T.L., Guarnaccia, J., Harrington, W., Pacia, S.V. & Petroff, O.A.C. (1993) Idiopathic granulomatous angiitis of the central nervous system: diagnostic challenges. *Archives of Neurology* **50**, 925–930.

Walker, G.L., Williamson, P.M., Ravich, R.B.M. & Roche, J. (1980) Hypercalcaemia associated with cerebral vasospasm causing infarction. *Journal of Neurology, Neurosurgery and Psychiatry* **43**, 464–467.

Walker, R.W., Allen, J.C., Rosen, G. & Caparros, B. (1986) Transient cerebral dysfunction secondary to high-dose methotrexate. *Journal of Clinical Oncology* **4**, 1845–1850.

Wallis, W.E., Donaldson, I., Scott, R.S. & Wilson, J. (1985) Hypoglycaemia masquerading as cerebrovascular disease (hypoglycaemic hemiplegia). *Annals of Neurology* **18**, 510–512.

Watson, P., Fekete, J. & Deck, J. (1977) Central nervous system vasculitis in rheumatoid arthritis. *Canadian Journal of Neurological Sciences* **4**, 269–272.

Weaver, D.F., Heffernan, L.P., Purdy, R.A. & Ing, V.W. (1988) Eosinophil-induced neurotoxicity: axonal neuropathy, cerebral infarction and dementia. *Neurology* **38**, 144–146.

Weststrate, W., Hijdra, A. & de Gans, J. (1996) Brain infarcts in adults with bacterial meningitis. *Lancet* **347**, 399.

Wetherley-Mein, G., Pearson, T.C., Burney, P.G.J. & Morris, R.W. (1987) Polycythaemia study: a project of the Royal College of Physicians Research Unit. 1. Objectives, background and design. *Journal of the Royal College of Physicians of London* **21**, 7–16.

Wilkinson, I.M. & Ross Russell, R.W. (1972) Arteries of the head and neck in giant cell arteritis: a pathological study to show the pattern of arterial involvement. *Archives of Neurology* **27**, 378–391.

Williams, R.L., Meltzer, C.C., Smirniotopoulos, J.G., Fukui, M.B. & Inman, M. (1998) Cerebral MR imaging in intravascular lymphomatosis. *American Journal of Neuroradiology* **19**, 427–431.

Wills, A. & Hovell, C.J. (1996) Neurological complications of enteric disease. *Gut* **39**, 501–504.

Winterkorn, J.M.S., Kupersmith, M.J., Wirtschafter, J.D. & Forman, S. (1993) Brief report: treatment of vasospastic amaurosis fugax with calcium-channel blockers. *New England Journal of Medicine* **329**, 396–398.

Wolman, R.L., Nussmeier, N.A., Aggarwal, A. *et al.* for the Ischaemia Research Education Foundation (IREF) Investigators (1999) Cerebral injury after cardiac surgery: identification of a group at extraordinary risk. Multicenter Study of Perioperative Ischemia Research Group (McSPI). *Stroke* **30**, 514–522.

Woolfenden, A.R., Tong, D.C., Marks, M.P., Ali, A.O. & Albers, G.W. (1998) Angiographically defined primary angiitis of the CNS: is it really benign? *Neurology* **51**, 183–188.

Wooten, M.D. & Jasin, H.E. (1996) Vasculitis and lymphoproliferative diseases. *Seminars in Arthritis and Rheumatism* **26**, 564–574.

World Health Organization Collaborative Study of Cardiovascular Disease and Steroid Hormone Contraception (1996a) Ischaemic stroke and combined oral contraceptives: results of an international, multicentre, case–control study. *Lancet* **348**, 498–505.

World Health Organization Collaborative Study of Cardiovascular Disease and Steroid Hormone Contraception (1996b) Haemorrhagic stroke, overall stroke risk and combined oral contraceptives: results of an international, multicentre, case–control study. *Lancet* **348**, 505–510.

Writing Group for the PEPI Trial (1995) Effects of oestrogen or oestrogen/progestin regimens on heart disease risk factors in postmenopausal women: the Postmenopausal Oestrogen/Progestin Interventions (PEPI) Trial. *Journal of the American Medical Association* **273**, 199–208.

Yoshimoto, Y. & Wakai, S. (1997) Unruptured intracranial vertebral artery dissection: clinical course and serial radiographic imagings. *Stroke* **28**, 370–374.

Zadra, M., Brambilla, A., Erli, L.C., Grandi, R. & Finazzi, G. (1996) Neurosarcoidosis, stroke and antiphospholipid antibodies: a case report. *European Journal of Neurology* **3**, 146–148.

Zajicek, J.P., Scolding, N.J., Foster, O. *et al.* (1999) Central nervous system sarcoidosis: diagnosis and management. *Quarterly Journal of Medicine* **92**, 103–117.

Zimmermann, C., Walther, E.U., von Scheidt, W. & Hamann, G.F. (1999) Ischaemic stroke in a 29-year-old man with left atrial spontaneous echoes and polycythaemia vera. *Journal of Neurology* **246**, 1201–1203.

Zuber, M., Khoubesserian, P., Meder, J.F. & Mas, J.L. (1993) A 34-year delayed and focal postirradiation intracranial vasculopathy. *Cerebrovascular Diseases* **3**, 181–182.

Zubkov, A.Y., Pilkington, A.S., Bernanke, D.H., Parent, A.D. & Zhang, J. (1999) Post-traumatic cerebral vasospasm: clinical and morphological presentations. *Journal of Neurotrauma* **16**, 763–770.

CHAPTER EIGHT

What caused this intracerebral haemorrhage?

8.1 Introduction

As a rule, there is no single cause for primary (non-traumatic) intracerebral haemorrhage, but an interaction of several factors. Take the classical example of a so-called hypertensive haemorrhage: a haematoma developing in the region of the basal ganglia, in an elderly patient on anticoagulants for chronic atrial fibrillation and for an even longer period on antihypertensive drugs. Should hypertension or anticoagulants be considered the cause of the intracerebral haemorrhage? Both are major risk factors (Landefeld *et al.* 1989; Juvela *et al.* 1995; Thrift *et al.* 1996). The weight of each of these two factors depends on the degree of damage to the small arteries in the brain as a result of previously raised blood pressure (unknown), on the actual blood pressure immediately before the onset of the haemorrhage (also unknown) and probably also on the intensity of anticoagulation. Even a combination of recognized 'causes', such as hypertension and anticoagulants, does not invariably lead to intracerebral haemorrhage. The presence or absence of other factors, of minor importance by themselves, can be decisive. Examples of such additional factors are age, socioeconomic status (Qureshi *et al.* 1999), alcohol consumption (Thrift *et al.* 1999a) and plasma cholesterol (Segal *et al.* 1999). Not uncommonly, a combination of minor factors may lead to intracerebral haemorrhage, as some patients seem to lack even a single one of the major 'causes'. In general therefore we are dealing with a combination of causal factors rather than with single causes and, even for the major factors, the relationship with intracerebral haemorrhage is neither sufficient nor necessary (Wulff & Gøtzsche 2000).

The major causal factors can be broadly divided into three categories (Table 8.1): anatomical factors (lesions or malformations of the vasculature in the brain), haemodynamic factors (blood pressure) and haemostatic factors (to do with platelet function or the coagulation system). Abnormalities

Table 8.1 Causal factors in primary intracerebral haemorrhage.

Anatomical factors: changes or malformations of the cerebral blood vessels
'Complex' small vessel disease (section 8.2.1)
Amyloid angiopathy (section 8.2.2)
Intracranial saccular aneurysms (section 8.2.3)
Cerebral arteriovenous malformations (section 8.2.4)
Cavernous angiomas (section 8.2.5)
Venous angiomas (section 8.2.6)
Telangiectasias (section 8.2.7)
Dural arteriovenous fistulae (section 8.2.8)
Haemorrhagic transformation of an arterial infarct (sections 5.4 and 8.2.9)
Intracranial venous thrombosis (sections 5.5 and 8.2.10)
Septic arteritis and mycotic aneurysms (section 8.2.11)
Moyamoya syndrome (sections 7.5 and 8.2.12)
Arterial dissection (sections 7.2 and 8.2.13)
Caroticocavernous fistula (section 8.2.14)

Haemodynamic factors
Arterial hypertension, chronic or acute (sections 6.3.3 and 8.3.1)
Migraine (sections 7.8 and 8.3.2)

Haemostatic factors
Anticoagulants (section 8.4.1)
Antiplatelet drugs (section 8.4.2)
Thrombolytic treatment (section 8.4.3)
Clotting factor deficiency (section 8.4.4)
Leukaemia and thrombocytopenia (sections 7.9 and 8.4.5)

Other factors
Intracerebral tumours (section 8.5.1)
Alcohol (sections 6.3.3 and 8.5.2)
Amphetamines (sections 7.15 and 8.5.3)
Cocaine and other sympathomimetic drugs (sections 7.15 and 8.5.4)
Vasculitis (sections 7.3 and 8.5.5)
Trauma ('Spät-Apoplexie') (section 8.5.6)

of the vascular system account for the vast majority of haemorrhages. The type of underlying abnormality varies with age: below the age of 40 years, arteriovenous malformations and cavernomas are the most common single cause of intracerebral haemorrhage, whereas between 40 and 70 years the most frequent lesions are deep haemorrhages from rupture of small perforating arteries, and in the elderly one also finds haemorrhages in the white matter ('lobar' haemorrhages), commonly attributed to amyloid angiopathy (Schutz *et al.* 1990). The exact proportions depend on the age distribution and the prevalence and control of risk factors within a given population. These relative probabilities are discussed in more detail in section 8.6, in relation to the site of the haemorrhage.

8.2 Anatomical factors

8.2.1 Lipohyalinosis ('complex' small vessel disease) and microaneurysms

When Charcot and Bouchard (1868) examined the brains of patients who had died from intracerebral haemorrhage and immersed them in running water to remove not only unclotted blood but also most of the brain tissue, they found multiple, minute out-pouchings of small blood vessels, which they called miliary aneurysms (Charcot & Bouchard 1868). Such miliary aneurysms were most frequent in the thalamus and corpus striatum, and to a somewhat lesser extent in the pons, cerebellum and cerebral white matter (Fig. 8.1). Their view that these microaneurysms were commonly the source of primary bleeding was generally accepted until the beginning of the 20th century, when the lesions they had seen were

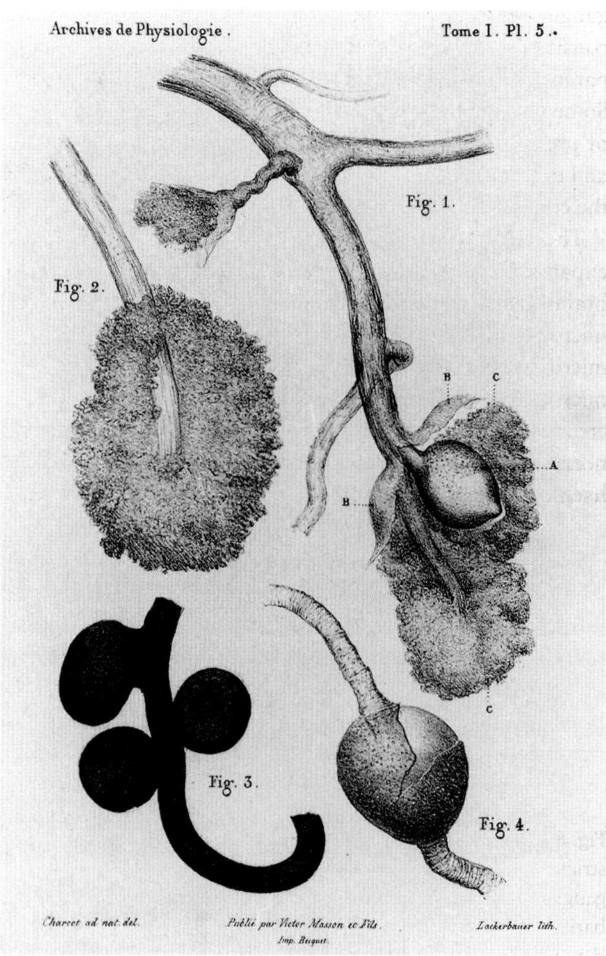

Fig. 8.1 'Miliary aneurysms' (Charcot & Bouchard 1868); (Fig. 1) a microaneurysm within a clot; (Fig. 2) a clot only; (Figs 3 and 4) microaneurysm without surrounding clot.

attributed to nothing more than perivascular collections of blood clot (Ellis 1909; Adams & vander Eecken 1953). Other explanations gained ascendancy, particularly an earlier theory that haemorrhages were in fact secondary to previous brain infarction (sections 2.7 and 5.4). In 1963, Ross Russell not only rediscovered the existence of microaneurysms, but also established a close relationship between these abnormalities and hypertension (Ross Russell 1963). He performed post-mortem studies of the brains of hypertensive and normotensive elderly people, injected barium sulphate into the basal arteries of the brain, and examined brain slices after fixation. Microaneurysms were found in 15 of 16 brains from hypertensive patients, but in only 10 of 38 brains from normotensive people; more than 10 microaneurysms were found only in previously hypertensive patients, with one dubious exception in the control group. The microaneurysms measured 300–900 μm in diameter and were found on small arteries 100–300 μm in diameter, commonly branches of the lateral lenticulostriate arteries in the region of the basal ganglia (Fig. 8.2). On microscopy, the walls of the aneurysm consisted of connective tissue only, the muscle layer of the parent vessel being interrupted at the neck of the aneurysm. Some aneurysms were thrombosed, others showed evidence of previous leakage in the form of iron-laden macrophages, and occasionally a thin-walled aneurysm had ruptured while the contrast agent was being injected.

The rediscovery of microaneurysms was confirmed and expanded in a larger study, by Cole and Yates, of the brains of 100 normotensive patients, seven of whom had microaneurysms, and of 100 hypertensive patients with microaneurysms in 46 cases (Cole & Yates 1967a). Most microaneurysms occurred on vessels below 250 μm in diameter. Twenty of the 100 hypertensive patients and one normotensive patient had died from massive intracerebral haemorrhage, but because of the disruption of brain tissue it was possible on only one occasion to trace the haemorrhage to a specific aneurysm. In 13 of the 46 brains of those hypertensive patients who had microaneurysms, there were also small haemorrhages in the white matter of the cerebral hemispheres, the basal ganglia and the internal capsule; in only four cases were there massive haemorrhages (Cole & Yates 1967b). Apart from hypertension, age was found to be an important determinant for the occurrence of microaneurysms: even in severely hypertensive patients, these lesions were rare under the age of 50 years. The distribution of microaneurysms through the brain paralleled that of small perforating vessels: most densely in the region of the thalamus, basal ganglia and internal capsule, and more sparsely in the pons, cerebellum and cerebral white matter (Fig. 8.3).

Cole and Yates also described two types of pseudoaneurysms, both of which were thought to be the result rather than the cause of intracerebral haemorrhage (Cole & Yates 1967c). One type consisted of globular, often laminated, clots at the site of rupture of an arteriole, varying between 1 mm and 1 cm in diameter. These occlusive thrombi strikingly resembled some of the more ragged aneurysms that had been described by Charcot and Bouchard (1868), and were identical to the 'fibrin globes' reported by Fisher a few years after Cole and Yates' studies (Fisher 1971) (Fig. 8.4). The second type consisted of haemorrhage extending into a short section of the perivascular space of an arteriole, before it entered the main bulk of the haematoma; in this way, the arteriole was covered with an irregular, bullous mantle of clotted blood. These two types of pseudoaneurysms were also found in patients under 40 years with haemorrhages from saccular aneurysms or other specific sources, subjects in whom true microaneurysms are extremely rare.

It is questionable whether microaneurysms are the one and only source of haemorrhage from small perforating vessels. Fisher microscopically examined the border region of

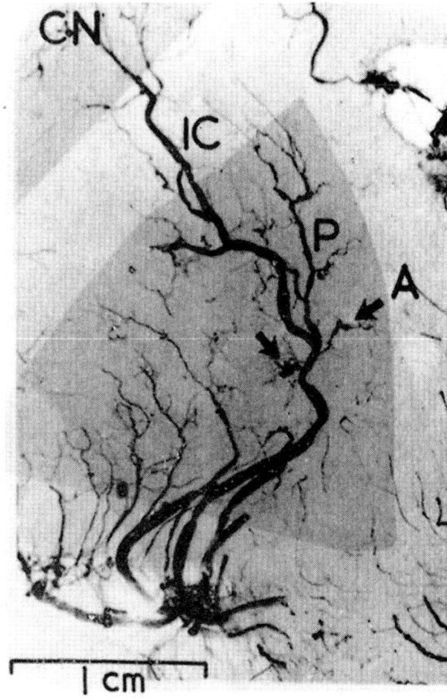

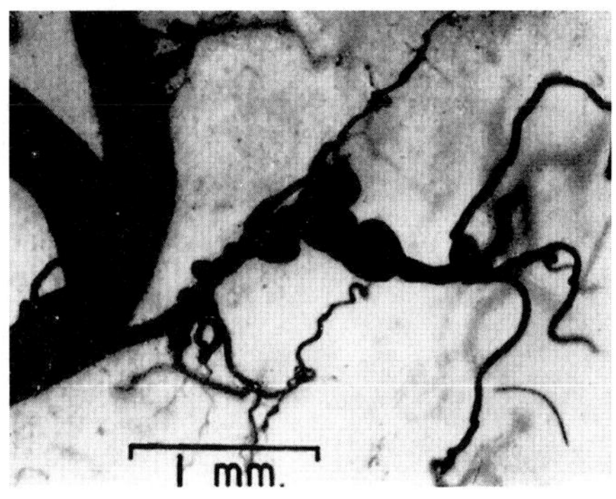

Fig. 8.2 Microaneurysms. Left: X-ray of striate arteries in coronal section of basal ganglia from elderly hypertensive subject; barium sulphate had been injected into the arterial tree before formalin fixation of the brain. Irregularity of main trunks, attenuation of small arteries and a number of microaneurysms (arrows). Right: enlarged view of an area showing multiple aneurysms. (With permission from Ross Russell 1963.)

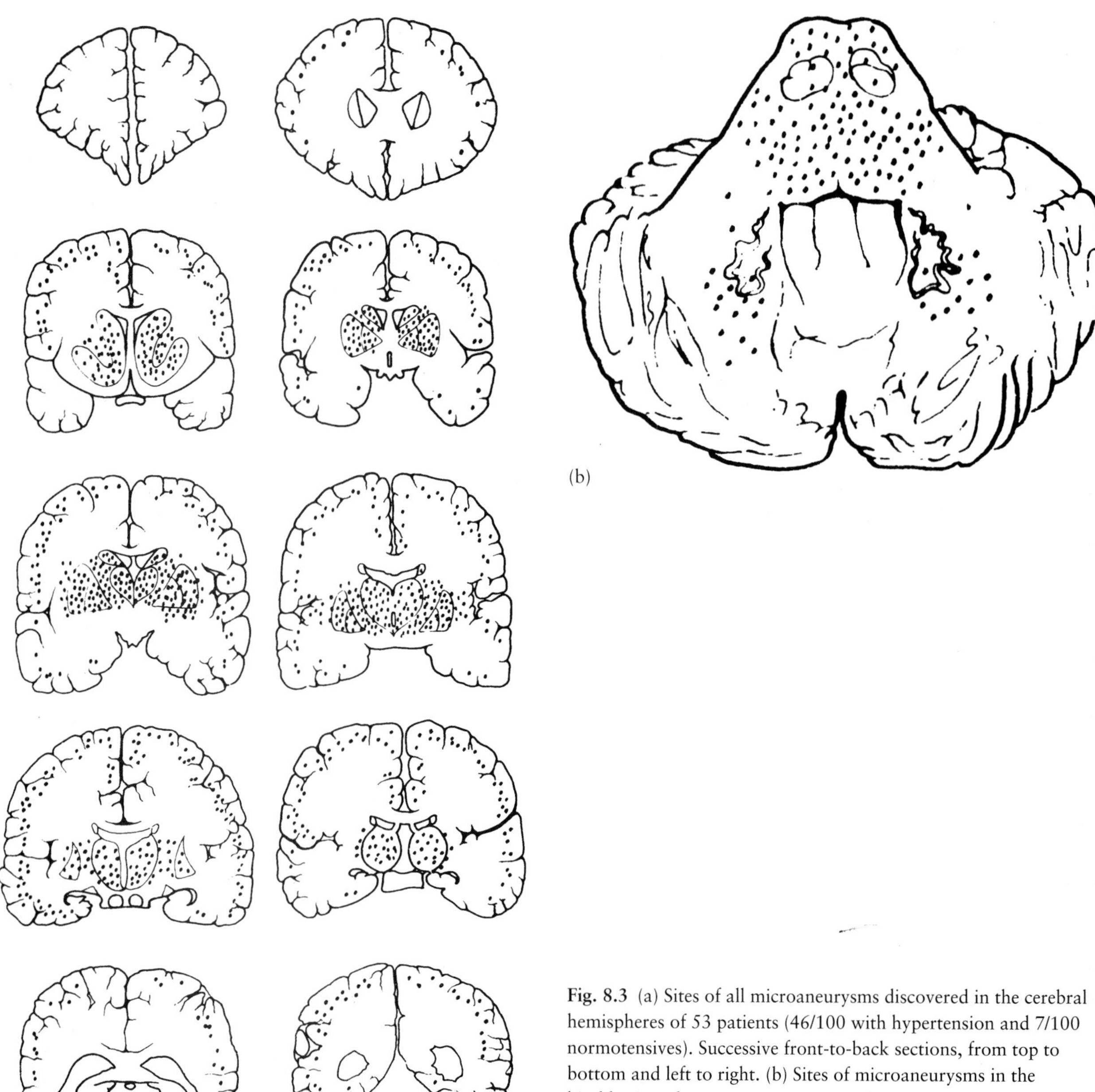

Fig. 8.3 (a) Sites of all microaneurysms discovered in the cerebral hemispheres of 53 patients (46/100 with hypertension and 7/100 normotensives). Successive front-to-back sections, from top to bottom and left to right. (b) Sites of microaneurysms in the hind brains of 53 patients, represented in a single section. (With permission from Cole & Yates 1967b.)

the haematoma in two patients with putaminal haemorrhage and in one patient with a pontine haemorrhage. In all three cases, he found not single but multiple points of bleeding, which were identified as 'fibrin globes', in the margin of the haematoma (Fig. 8.4); the core of each 'fibrin globe' consisted of a plug of platelets, which occluded the lumen of a small artery (Fisher 1971). In the putaminal haemorrhages, he also found the primary source of the haemorrhage, in the form of a clot in the ruptured wall of a relatively large artery. Fisher proposed that rupture of a single small artery might subsequently lead to damage and rupture of other vessels, thus causing an 'avalanche' of secondary haemorrhages. The degenerative changes he found in the walls of the small perforating vessels, consisted of a segmental process of fatty changes and fibrinoid necrosis—what he called lipohyalinosis—but what we would prefer to call 'complex' small vessel disease (section 6.4). These changes were associated with local thinning, spots which might well be vulnerable to microtrauma in the form of an adjacent haemorrhage. Others also found fibrinoid necrosis of the walls of these perforating arterioles as an almost invariable phenomenon in patients with deep intracerebral haemorrhage (Ooneda *et al.* 1973).

Fisher's emphasis on degenerative changes other than microaneurysms was also confirmed by an electron-

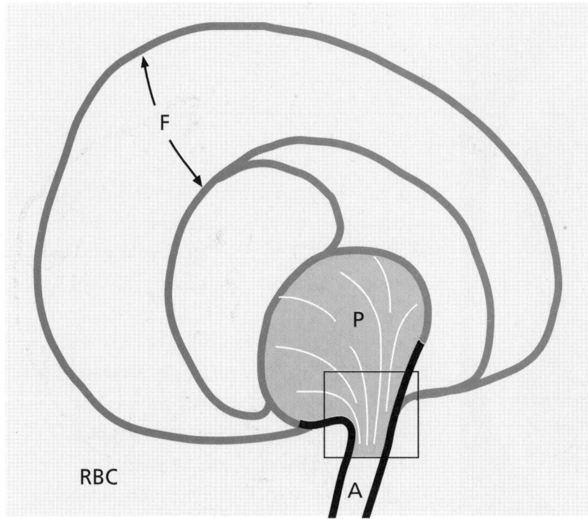

Fig. 8.4 An occlusive thrombus at the site of rupture in a small perforating artery. A, ruptured artery; F, fibrin; P, platelets; RBC, red blood cells. (Redrawn after Fisher 1971, with permission.)

microscopic study of specimens obtained at post-mortem or emergency surgery, which showed the most common site of rupture to be at distal bifurcations of lenticulostriate arteries, and rarely in the wall of a microaneurysm (Takebayashi & Kaneko 1983). The arteries in question were affected by atrophy and fragmentation of smooth-muscle cells. In autopsied cases, the ruptured perforators mostly measured 500–700 μm, in contrast to the smaller size of the arteries previously reported to form microaneurysms. Also, in fatal cases, there were invariably multiple (2–11) sites of rupture.

Some indirect support for the 'avalanche' theory is provided by imaging techniques. Case reports have documented rapid expansion of intracerebral haematomas during a single scanning procedure with CT (Kelley *et al.* 1982; Chen *et al.* 1989), or MRI and angiography (Murai *et al.* 1998). In addition, systematic studies of patients with deep intracerebral haemorrhage in whom the first CT scan was performed within 3 h of the first symptoms, and who underwent a second CT scan 1 h later, showed an increase in size in at least 26% (Broderick *et al.* 1990; Brott *et al.* 1997). If the maximum interval between the first symptoms and the first CT scan is extended to 24 h, a second scan after one to several days shows haematoma enlargement in 14–20% of patients (Fujii *et al.* 1994; Kazui *et al.* 1996). In all these studies, the proportion showing enlargement was greater the earlier the baseline scan was performed after the event; no haematoma progression was documented after 24 h. All this evidence implicates a dynamic process, with a stable phase being reached in a matter of hours. Predisposing baseline factors for haematoma enlargement that have been implicated are liver disease (Fujii *et al.* 1994; Kazui *et al.* 1997), a history of heavy drinking (Fujii *et al.* 1998), the combination of hypertension and poorly regulated diabetes (Kazui *et al.* 1997), an irregular shape of the haematoma (Fujii *et al.* 1994, 1998) and, at a biochemical level, poor activation of the coagulation system (Takahashi *et al.* 1998). Incidentally, clinical deterioration later than 2 days after deep intracerebral haemorrhage is not caused by continued extravasation, but by cerebral oedema (Zazulia *et al.* 1999).

It seems therefore that perforating vessels can tear without preceding aneurysmal dilatation, and that microaneurysms are perhaps as much a marker of degenerative changes in small-calibre arteries as a necessary source of bleeding. The relative proportions of the underlying morphological changes are unknown. Some maintain that even the microaneurysms demonstrated by contemporary studies are artifacts caused by the injection technique, or misinterpretations of arteriolar coils (Challa *et al.* 1992). Not surprisingly, small deep infarcts are relatively common in patients presenting with deep haemorrhages (Tanaka *et al.* 1999). After all, 'complex' small vessel disease is complicated by both occlusion and rupture (section 6.4).

'Hypertensive' intracerebral haemorrhage results from degenerative changes in small perforating vessels, most of which are found in deep regions of the brain: basal ganglia, thalamus, cerebellum and brainstem. Microaneurysms occur on these vessels but are not necessarily the site of rupture.

Deep brain haemorrhages are not always a one-off event (Misra & Kalita 1995; González-Duarte *et al.* 1998) (Fig. 8.5). In consecutive series of patients admitted with haemorrhage in the basal ganglia or cerebellum, 5–6% had had a previous haemorrhage (Chen *et al.* 1995; Neau *et al.* 1997; Bae *et al.* 1999). Because of the design of these studies, some recurrences may have been missed. In the only prospective study on record, the rate in the first year was 7%, against 2% per annum over the subsequent 6 years (Passero *et al.* 1995). At any rate, recurrences of deep haemorrhages are distinctly less common than with haemorrhages at the border between white and grey matter, presumably caused by cerebral amyloid angiopathy (Passero *et al.* 1995) (section 8.2.2). The median interval between the first and second deep haemorrhage is around 2 years (Chen *et al.* 1995; Bae *et al.* 1999); the second site is rarely the same as the first (Bae *et al.* 1999).

8.2.2 Cerebral amyloid angiopathy

It is only in the last few decades that this disorder has been recognized as a cause of primary (non-traumatic) intracerebral haemorrhage (PICH), particularly of lobar haemorrhages. Case reports started to appear at the beginning of the 20th century (Fischer 1910; Vinters 1987), but the first series of patients were not reported until the 1970s (Torack 1975; Jellinger 1977). Interestingly, in the first reports, the condition was usually associated with dementia of the Alzheimer

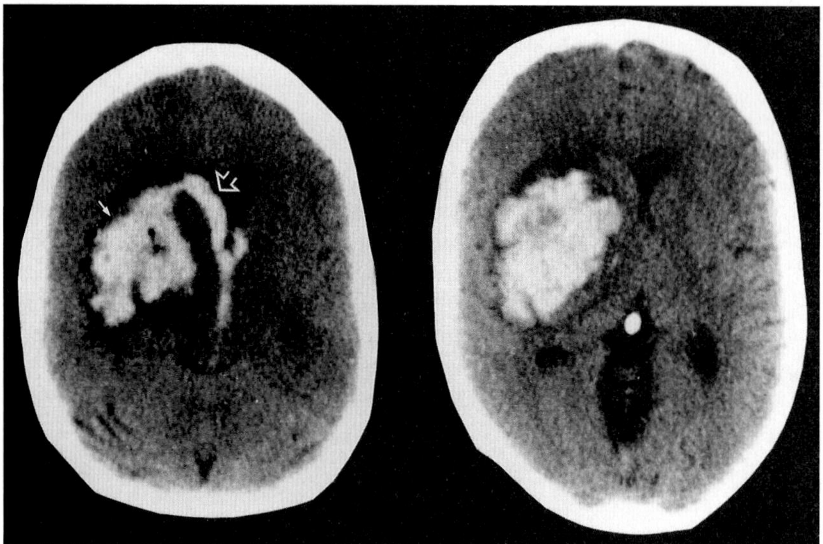

Fig. 8.5 Re-bleeding in a 40-year-old woman with 'hypertensive' intracerebral haemorrhage. Left: CT brain scan showing large haematoma in the right basal ganglia (closed arrow), with rupture into the frontal horn of the right lateral ventricle (open arrow); the haematoma was surgically removed on the same day because of progressive deterioration of consciousness. Right: CT brain scan showing fresh haematoma, indicated by sudden deterioration 4 weeks after the initial episode; angiography was normal.

type, characterized by the presence of amyloid plaques in the brain, but it is now well established that cerebral amyloid angiopathy may occur without clinical evidence of dementia and also without amyloid plaques or any of the other hallmarks of Alzheimer's disease necessarily being present in the brain parenchyma (Gilbert & Vinters 1983; Kalyan Raman & Kalyan Raman 1984). The site of haemorrhages associated with amyloid angiopathy is typically at the border of the grey and white matter of the cerebral hemispheres (Greenberg 1998) (Fig. 8.6). They may rupture towards the surface and spread through the subarachnoid space (Yamada *et al.* 1993). Cerebellar haemorrhages associated with amyloid angiopathy are less common (Masuda *et al.* 1988; Itoh *et al.* 1993). Recurrence of haemorrhage associated with amyloid angiopathy is much more common than with 'hypertensive' small vessel disease (Passero *et al.* 1995) (section 8.2.1); well-documented case histories with 4–8 episodes are on record (Chauveau *et al.* 1990; Weir *et al.* 1999). Serial MR scanning may uncover new haemorrhages, not associated with obvious clinical worsening (Greenberg *et al.* 1999).

The underlying abnormality in cerebral amyloid angiopathy consists of patchy deposits of amyloid in the muscle layer of small and medium-sized cortical arteries (Fig. 8.6). The most common type by far, beta-amyloid, is derived from precursor proteins synthesized *in situ* by smooth muscle cells (Coria & Rubio 1996). Beta-amyloid can also be found in cortical vessels of asymptomatic individuals, the proportion increasing with age, from 5 to 10% in those aged between 60 and 69 years, approximately 25% between ages 70 and 79 years, 40% between 80 and 89 years, to more than 50% in those over 90 years (Tomonaga 1981; Vinters & Gilbert 1983; Masuda *et al.* 1988). Arteries in the occipital, parietal and frontal lobes are most often involved. Beta-amyloid can also be found in the leptomeninges, the cerebral cortex and the subcortical white matter, but not outside the brain (Vinters 1987). Cerebal amyloid angiopathy is not therefore part of a process of generalized amyloidosis. Curiously, amyloid angiopathy of the brain is not limited to humans, as it has also been found in an aged woodpecker (Nakayama *et al.* 1999).

The difference between amyloid angiopathy with or without haemorrhages is twofold. First, amyloid deposition is more extensive in those with haemorrhages, not so much reflected by the proportion of affected cortical vessels but rather by the degree of involvement per vessel (Vonsattel *et al.* 1991; Alonzo *et al.* 1998). Secondly, cortical arteries of patients with amyloid-associated haemorrhages relatively often show evidence of dilatation, disruption and fibrinoid necrosis (Vonsattel *et al.* 1991; Maeda *et al.* 1993).

The genetic background in sporadic cases is largely unknown (for hereditary forms, see below). The only traces of knowledge so far relate to the apolipoprotein E gene. Increasing doses of the 4 allele (0, 1 or 2) are associated with increasing degrees of amyloid deposition (Alonzo *et al.* 1998), whereas the 2 allele predisposes to amyloid-associated damage to the vessel wall, especially fibrinoid necrosis (Greenberg *et al.* 1998; McCarron *et al.* 1999a), and to actual haemorrhages (Nicoll *et al.* 1997; McCarron & Nicoll 1998; McCarron *et al.* 1999b).

The proportion of cerebral haemorrhages related to amyloid angiopathy is probably fairly constant, at least above the age of 50 years, because the steep rise in the incidence of PICH with increasing age applies as much to deep haemorrhages (including those in the cerebellum and pons) as to lobar haemorrhages (Broderick *et al.* 1993a). Given that lobar haemorrhage accounts for approximately 25–40% of all PICH in community-based studies (Broderick *et al.* 1993a; Anderson *et al.* 1994), and that in large post-mortem series 30% of lobar haemorrhages are attributable to amyloid angiopathy (Itoh *et al.* 1993), the proportion of amyloid-related lobar haemorrhages amongst all PICHs would

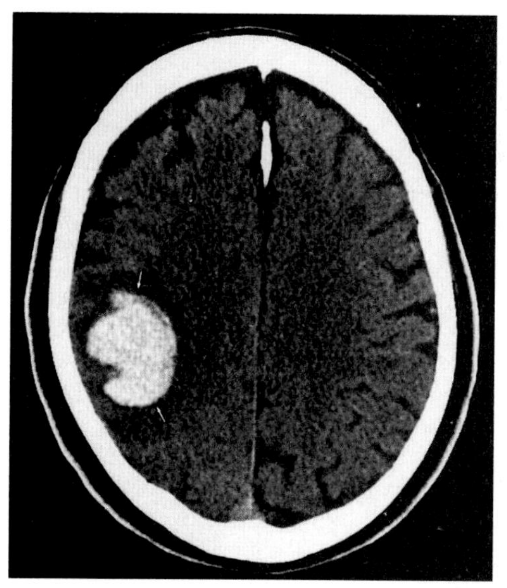
(a)

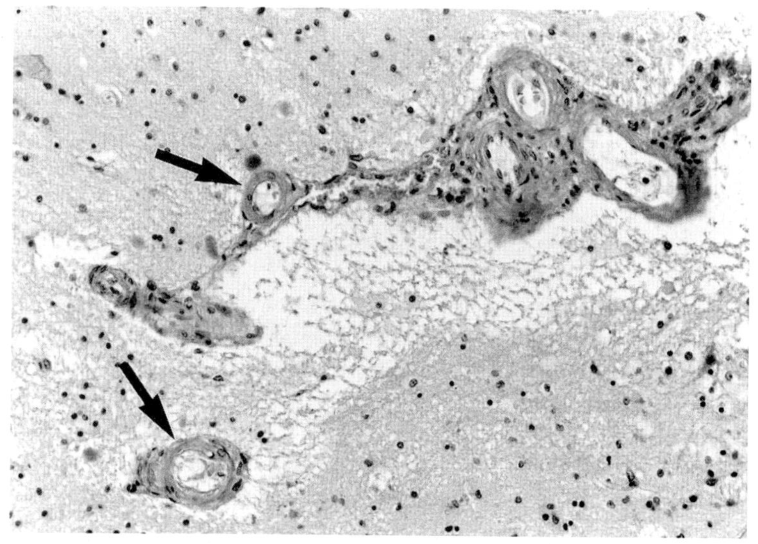
(b)

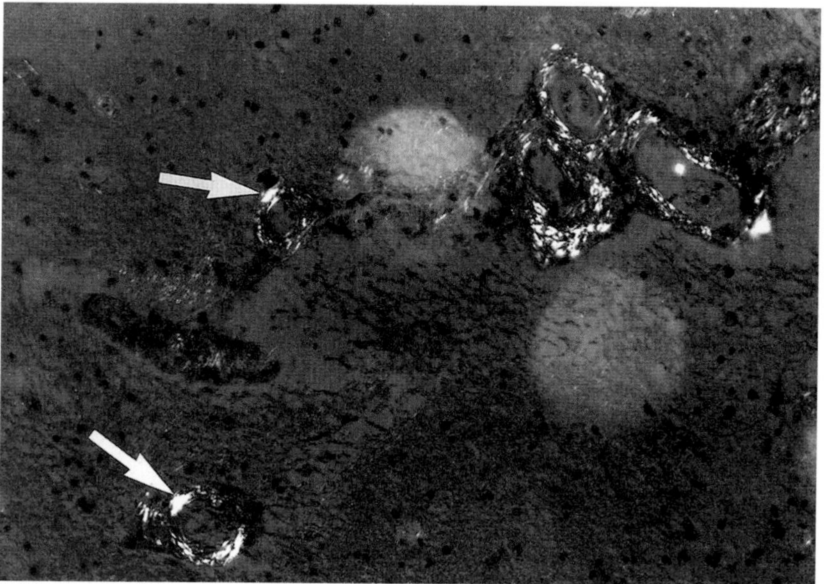
(c)

Fig. 8.6 (a) Lobar haemorrhage (arrows) on CT brain scan, presumably caused by amyloid angiopathy. (b) Histological section of brain with congo-red staining, showing amyloid angiopathy in walls of arterioles (arrows) (magnification ×200). (c) As in (b), showing birefringence under polarized light (arrows).

be about 10%, a rate that was reflected in a small post-mortem series (7/60) from a hospital for chronic care (Ishii *et al.* 1984).

When a single lobar haemorrhage is detected on CT scanning, it is impossible to distinguish between one associated with cerebral amyloid angiopathy and one with arteriolar degeneration; magnetic resonance imaging (MRI) may give a clue to the diagnosis of amyloid angiopathy by showing evidence of previous punctate haemorrhages (Hendricks *et al.* 1990; Kwa *et al.* 1998). If surgery is indicated (Chapter 12), the diagnosis can usually be made from immunohistochemical study of biopsy specimens (Yong *et al.* 1992; Greenberg & Vonsattel 1997). In cerebral amyloid angiopathy, the vessels may be so brittle that even mild head trauma precipitates a haemorrhage (Kalyan Raman & Kalyan Raman 1984). One of our patients was an old lady who bled in both cerebral hemispheres when she tripped getting off a bus, without any direct head injury. Intracranial haemorrhage distant from the site of a previous neurosurgical intervention may also have to be attributed to amyloid angiopathy (Waga *et al.* 1983; Brisman *et al.* 1996). Thrombolytic therapy for myocardial infarction can be another precipitating factor (section 8.4.3).

Two other clinical manifestations of cerebral amyloid angiopathy other than haemorrhages should be briefly mentioned. One consists of recurrent, transient episodes of focal weakness, paraesthesias, numbness with spread and, less often, visual distortion. These attacks may be caused by transient ischaemia (Smith *et al.* 1985; Yong *et al.* 1992). The occurrence of a large cerebral haemorrhage in an area of the brain implicated by the earlier recurrent spells also raises the possibility that partial seizures or small haemorrhages, or a combination of both, may have heralded the larger one (Greenberg *et al.* 1993). For that reason, the occurrence of new-onset, focal seizures followed by intracerebral haemorrhage in the same area of the brain should suggest not only an arteriovenous malformation but also cerebral amyloid angiopathy as a possible underlying cause (Cocito *et al.* 1994). The other non-haemorrhagic clinical syndrome is intellectual deterioration; the underlying lesions may consist not only of multiple haemorrhages, but also diffuse demyelination of the subcortical white matter (Gray *et al.* 1985; Greenberg *et al.* 1993) (leukoaraiosis, section 5.7). In the most common form of diffuse demyelination through chronic ischaemia, the underlying vascular lesion consists of thickening of the walls of the arterioles supplying the white matter, as a result of hypertrophy of the medial layer (van Swieten *et al.* 1991). MR scanning may provide evidence for amyloid angiopathy as the cause for leukoaraiosis if evidence of small, punctate haemorrhages is also found (Hendricks *et al.* 1990).

The occurrence of multiple haemorrhages, either at the same time or separated only by days, is a fairly typical although not unique characteristic of haemorrhages associated with amyloid angiopathy (Gilles *et al.* 1984) (Fig. 8.7). Other causes are listed in Table 8.2 and range from unsuspected head injury to sepsis and diffuse intravascular coagulation. Multifocal haemorrhages are rare (<1%) in patients with PICH and a history of hypertension, in whom the most likely source of haemorrhage is 'complex' small vessel disease with microaneurysms (Weisberg 1981). In the case of simultaneous haemorrhages with cerebral amyloid angiopathy, it is assumed that the arteries affected by amyloid are so fragile that another tear is induced by the initial haemorrhage, even in a distant part of the brain.

Haemorrhages into the cerebral white matter ('lobar' haemorrhages) are most often caused by the same type of 'hypertensive' arteriolar disease that is associated with deep haemorrhages, but in those aged over 70 years cerebral amyloid angiopathy is also a common underlying condition, in approximately 30%. Amyloid angiopathy can be more specifically suspected with multiple or recurrent haemorrhages, preceding episodes of transient neurological deficits or, rarely, a family history of intracerebral haemorrhage.

Autosomal dominant forms of amyloid angiopathy with intracerebral haemorrhages have been reported from the Netherlands (Luyendijk *et al.* 1988; Wattendorff *et al.* 1995) and Iceland (Gudmundsson *et al.* 1972). These are caused by specific mutations of amyloid precursor protein gene and the cystatin-C gene, respectively (Coria & Rubio 1996). In the Dutch type, the intravascular deposits consist of beta-amyloid, similar to the sporadic variant (Coria & Rubio 1996), but the degree of abnormality is not modulated by the apolipoprotein E gene (Bornebroek *et al.* 1997). It is antigenically related to amyloid plaques in Alzheimer's disease (van Duinen *et al.* 1987). The microvascular changes resemble

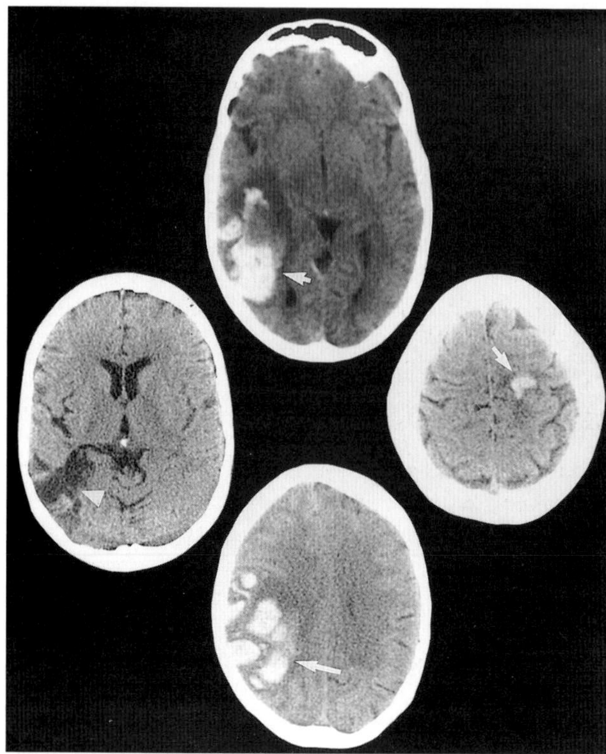

Fig. 8.7 Multiple haemorrhages in a patient with familial amyloid angiopathy (CT scans). Top: haemorrhage in right temporal lobe (arrow), at age 51 years. Left and right: small haemorrhage (arrow) at the convexity of the left hemisphere, at age 54 years; the previous haemorrhage has left a hypodense scar (arrowhead). Bottom: haemorrhage in right parietal lobe (arrow), at age 55 years. The patient died after a fourth episode at the age of 56 years.

Table 8.2 Causes of multiple haemorrhages in brain parenchyma.

Cerebral amyloid angiopathy (section 8.2.2)
Intracranial venous thrombosis (sections 5.5 and 8.2.10)
Thrombolytic treatment (section 8.4.3)
Metastases (melanoma, bronchial carcinoma, renal carcinoma, choriocarcinoma (section 8.5.1)
Cerebral vasculitis (sections 7.3 and 8.5.5)
Diffuse intravascular coagulation (sections 7.9 and 8.4.5) (Wijdicks *et al.* 1994)
Haemostatic disorder (sections 8.4.3 and 8.4.4)
Leukaemia (section 8.4.5)
Eclampsia (Drislane & Wang 1997) (sections 7.14 and 8.3.1)
Unsuspected head injury (section 8.5.6)

those in the sporadic variant (Natté *et al.* 1998; Vinters *et al.* 1998). In the Icelandic form, the amyloid is of the cystatin-C type. It is synthesized not by smooth muscle cells but by astrocytes (Coria & Rubio 1996). The onset of the haemorrhages is at a younger age (median 30 years) than in the Dutch type of hereditary cerebral haemorrhage with amyloidosis (median 55 years) (Jensson *et al.* 1987). A sporadic variant of the cystatin-C mutation has been claimed in a single patient, of Croatian origin, but it is not found in the vast majority of sporadic cases (Graffagnino *et al.* 1995; McCarron *et al.* 2000).

8.2.3 Intracranial saccular aneurysms

In the neurology/neurosurgery service of a large community hospital, approximately one-third of the patients with subarachnoid haemorrhage (SAH) from a ruptured aneurysm have an intracerebral haematoma on CT scanning (van Gijn & van Dongen 1982). Patients with large haematomas often die early, so highly specialized referral centres see a smaller proportion with haematomas. There is no study available, at least not from the CT era, which directly compares the frequency of haematomas from ruptured saccular aneurysms with that of primary intracerebral haematomas. An educated guess can be made from the overall annual incidence per 100 000 in a current Western European population: for first-ever-in-a-lifetime stroke, the rate critically depends on the age distribution (Table 17.3), but overall it is approximately 200 (Bamford *et al.* 1988), some 12%, or 24 per 100 000 consisting of intracerebral haemorrhage, and some 3%, or 6 per 100 000, of SAH (Linn *et al.* 1996). Given that two out of six patients with SAH have a haematoma, as against 24 patients with other types of intracerebral haemorrhage from the population cohort, approximately 1 in 13 of all intracerebral haematomas is secondary to rupture of a saccular aneurysm. However, this is the ratio for all ages combined. Below the age of 65 years, SAH and deep intracerebral haemorrhage are about equally common (Broderick *et al.* 1993b), in which case the proportion of haematomas from aneurysmal haemorrhage will be around 1 in 6.

About 1 in 13 of all intracerebral haematomas is caused by a ruptured saccular aneurysm, but more like 2 in 13 under the age of 65 years.

Haematomas from aneurysmal haemorrhage can be fairly reliably diagnosed on the basis of at least one of two characteristics: the association with cisternal haemorrhage, and the typical location (Hayward & O'Reilly 1976; van Gijn & van Dongen 1980; Laissy *et al.* 1991) (section 9.4.1). It is important to distinguish between an intracerebral haematoma secondary to a ruptured aneurysm and intracerebral haemorrhage originating in the parenchyma, whether deep or lobar, because a patient with a ruptured aneurysm may require more urgent and specific treatment, medical or surgical (section 13.3.1).

If the location of an intracerebral haematoma is compatible with a ruptured aneurysm, the patient should be urgently transferred to a neurosurgical facility for evacuation to at least be considered, even if the patient's clinical condition is poor.

Subdural haematomas may also be caused by aneurysmal rupture. As a rule, there is a tell-tale extravasation of blood in the subarachnoid space as well (section 9.4.1), but occasionally the subdural haematoma is the only manifestation (section 8.10).

8.2.4 Cerebral arteriovenous malformations

Haemorrhage is the initial clinical manifestation in 50–60% of symptomatic arteriovenous malformations (AVMs) (Lobato *et al.* 1992; Brown *et al.* 1996a; Kupersmith *et al.* 1996). Other clinical features include epileptic seizures, headaches (migrainous, related to increased cerebrospinal fluid pressure or non-specific) and progressive neurological deficit (Brown *et al.* 1988; Chimowitz *et al.* 1990; Kupersmith *et al.* 1996). Demonstrable AVMs are the most common single cause of intracerebral haemorrhage in the young, but they underlie no more than about one-third of those cases, at least in a series of 72 patients aged under 45 years referred to a university hospital (Toffol *et al.* 1987). In a population-based study, the annual detection rate of symptomatic AVMs was 1.12 per 100 000 (95% CI, 0.37–1.88) (Brown *et al.* 1996b).

AVMs are tangles of dilated arteries and veins, without a capillary network between them, and are embedded in a stroma devoid of normal brain tissue. On angiography, they are recognizable by the large feeding arteries and the rapid shunting of blood to veins that are enlarged and tortuous, often with a central nidus of dilated vessels, between arteries and veins (section 14.1). Multiple AVMs occur in only 4% of cases if there is no underlying systemic disorder, such as hereditary haemorrhagic telangiectasia (Rendu–Osler–Weber syndrome) (Willinsky *et al.* 1990). Familial occurrence of AVMs is even more exceptional, with 10 families on record in a review from 1991 (Yokoyama *et al.* 1991); of two later reports, one documents a family with three affected generations (Larsen *et al.* 1997; Amin-Hanjani *et al.* 1998).

The larger supratentorial AVMs, about one-third of the total, receive feeding arteries from more than one arterial territory, even up to all three major supratentorial arteries (Parkinson & Bachers 1980). In 10–20% they are associated with thin-walled saccular aneurysms on feeding arteries, but not in the classical sites of saccular aneurysms on the circle of Willis (section 9.1.1). These associated aneurysms are likely sources of bleeding and, with AVMs in which one or more aneurysms have formed, the annual risk of re-bleeding is as high as 7%, against the usual rate of 2–3% per year for AVMs without associated aneurysm, regardless of whether previous rupture has occurred (Aminoff 1987; Heros & Tu 1987; Brown *et al.* 1990; Ondra *et al.* 1990; Marks *et al.* 1992). AVMs are believed to increase in size over the years, but this has rarely been documented (Waltimo 1973; Mendelow *et al.* 1987; Minakawa *et al.* 1989). Spontaneous regression, presumably through thrombosis, does also occur, mostly in patients over 30 years, with AVMs under 2 cm in size and with single feeders (Wakai *et al.* 1983; Minakawa *et al.* 1989)(Fig. 14.4). Spontaneous thrombosis of an AVM is usually preceded by an episode of haemorrhage, but not always (Wharen *et al.* 1982; Guazzo & Xuereb 1994).

Aneurysms are often found on the feeding arteries to arteriovenous malformations, when the risk of bleeding, or re-bleeding, is about double the risk in patients without such aneurysms.

Haemorrhages from AVMs are mostly in the white matter ('lobar') (Fig. 8.20), but they do also occur in the deep nuclei of the cerebral hemisphere (Toffol *et al.* 1987). Subarachnoid haemorrhage results if the haematoma reaches the surface of the brain but, of all haemorrhages secondary to a ruptured AVM, only 4% are purely subarachnoid, without a parenchymal component (Aoki 1991). If there is no associated aneurysm on the arterial side, the site of rupture is mostly on the venous side of the malformation. This is in accordance with the finding that in unruptured AVMs the risk of future bleeding is relatively great if there is only a single draining vein, and even greater if venous drainage is impaired or confined to the deep venous system (Miyasaka *et al.* 1992). Rupture of a vein would also explain the often slower onset of the clinical deficits with haemorrhages from AVMs than with haematomas from rupture of perforating arteries, or saccular aneurysms.

Rupture of an arteriovenous malformation almost invariably results in an intracerebral haematoma, and only exceptionally (4%) in a purely subarachnoid haemorrhage.

Very small vascular malformations may not show up on angiography (Lobato *et al.* 1992). In a series of 72 patients under 45 years with intracerebral haemorrhage, the proportion of unexplained haemorrhages was as high as 25% (Toffol *et al.* 1987). Before neuroimaging techniques, specifically MRI, became widely available, angiographically occult lesions were categorized as 'microangiomas'. In fact these cryptic malformations are mostly cavernous angiomas (Robinson *et al.* 1993a; Tomlinson *et al.* 1994) (section 8.2.5). A small minority consist of small AVMs, venous angiomas, teleangiectasias or mixed lesions (Rapacki *et al.* 1990; Robinson *et al.* 1993a).

8.2.5 Cavernous angiomas (cavernomas)

Cavernous angiomas consist of sharply demarcated areas with widely dilated and thin-walled vascular channels, without intervening brain tissue (Figs 8.8 and 8.9). They are often asymptomatic and are encountered in 0.5% of routine postmortems (Otten *et al.* 1989). It is only after the advent of imaging techniques such as CT, and especially MRI, that these lesions became regularly recognized during life. On T2-weighted MRI, they are characterized by a combination of a reticulated core of mixed signal intensity with a surrounding rim of decreased signal intensity (corresponding to haemosiderin) (Rigamonti *et al.* 1987). Smaller lesions appear as areas of decreased signal intensity (black dots). Cavernous angiomas are located in the white matter or cortex of a cerebral hemisphere in about one-half of all cases, in the posterior fossa in one-third, and in the basal ganglia or thalamus in one-sixth (Kondziolka *et al.* 1995). Exceptional locations include the ventricular system (Reyns *et al.* 1999) and the cerebello-

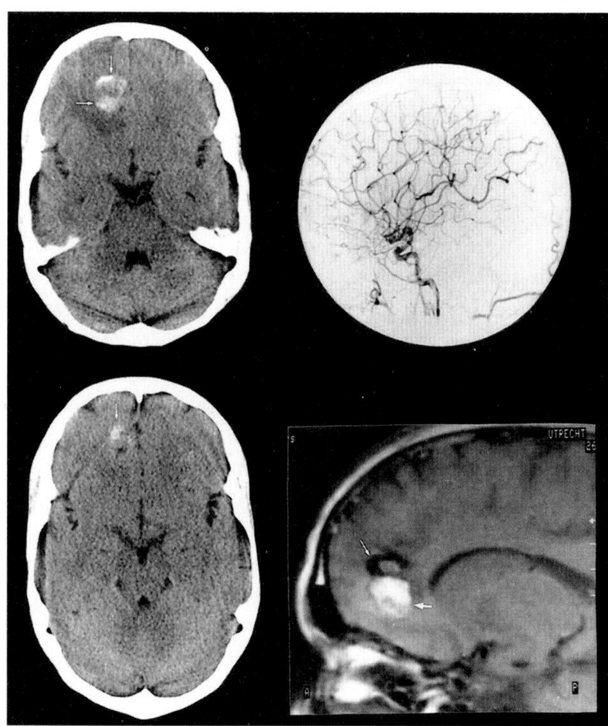

Fig. 8.8 Suspected cavernous angioma in a 25-year-old woman. Top left: CT brain scan showing a parasagittal haemorrhage (arrow) in the right frontal lobe (clinically manifested by sudden headache, followed by a seizure). Top right: normal right carotid angiogram (the left carotid angiogram was also normal). Bottom left: CT brain scan, 3 months after the event; residual lesion with calcification (arrow) and a region of hypodensity. Bottom right: sagittal MRI scan (T1-weighted), 4 months after the event; sharply demarcated, hypodense lesion (thin arrow), with residual, hyperintense region (haemosiderin) at its ventral border (thick arrow).

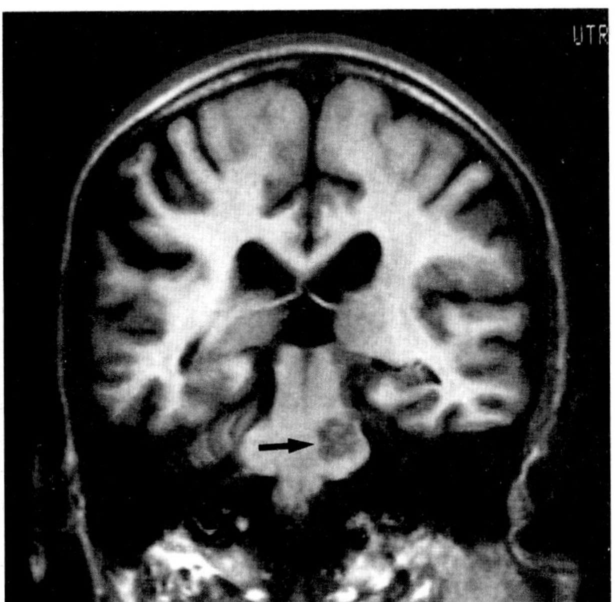

Fig. 8.9 Probable cavernous angioma in the brainstem. MR imaging (T1-weighted scan in the coronal plane) of a 48-year-old woman who had experienced an attack, lasting several hours, of vertigo, tinnitus, a burning feeling around the nose, and pins and needles of the right half of the body below the face. The marginated but rather sharply demarcated border of the abnormality in the left half of the pons and middle cerebellar peduncle in the absence of space-occupying effect suggests a cavernous angioma (arrow). Left vertebral angiography was normal. Three years later, the lesion had not changed.

pontine angle (Kim *et al.* 1997). They can also occur in children as well as adults (Scott *et al.* 1992; Di Rocco *et al.* 1997).

If a cavernous angioma is symptomatic, epileptic seizures are as common a manifestation as haemorrhage, at least in most series (Simard *et al.* 1986; Del Curling *et al.* 1991; Requena *et al.* 1991). Despite the bias that such studies tend to originate from neurosurgical services, the highest proportion with haemorrhage was 50% (Kondziolka *et al.* 1995). The third main clinical syndrome is that of a focal deficit, as cavernomas may grow in size (Pozzati *et al.* 1989, 1996). Understandably, this occurs relatively often with lesions in the brainstem (Robinson *et al.* 1993b; Kondziolka *et al.* 1995). The deficits usually develop in a gradual fashion but may remit, mimicking multiple sclerosis (Vrethem *et al.* 1997; Dougan *et al.* 1998).

The risk of haemorrhage in patients in whom the lesion presents with seizures or focal deficits is rather low, with estimates ranging between 0.25 and 0.6% per annum (Del Curling *et al.* 1991; Kondziolka *et al.* 1995). After a first rupture, re-bleeding is more frequent, at a rate of around 4.5% per annum (Tung *et al.* 1990; Kondziolka *et al.* 1995). Haemorrhages from a cavernous angioma are rarely fatal, as the pressure within these lesions is relatively low (on average less than 40 mmHg) (Little *et al.* 1990). Nevertheless, recurrent haemorrhages may cause progressive neurological deficits (Tung *et al.* 1990; Zimmerman *et al.* 1991).

A familial form of the disorder has been detected, first in Mexican-American families (Rigamonti *et al.* 1988a; Kattapong *et al.* 1995), and more recently in various European countries: Germany (van Schayck *et al.* 1994), the Netherlands (Dellemijn & Vanneste 1993), France (Notelet *et al.* 1997; Labauge *et al.* 1998) and the UK (Stacey *et al.* 1999). Loci for the genes in question have been identified on chromosomes 7q, 7p and 3q, but the genes have not yet been precisely mapped (Gil-Nagel *et al.* 1996; Notelet *et al.* 1997; Polymeropoulos *et al.* 1997; Laberge-le Couteulx *et al.* 1999). Most familial cases have multiple cavernomas; conversely, in a given patient with multiple cavernomas there is a 75% chance that first-degree relatives are affected as well (Labauge *et al.* 1998). New lesions appear in the course of a few years; the annual risk of symptomatic haemorrhage has been estimated at 1.1% per lesion (Zabramski *et al.* 1994).

8.2.6 Venous angiomas

Venous angiomas consist of several dilated veins, without an abnormal input on the arterial side, converging into a single abnormal vein, which in turn drains into the venous system on the surface of the brain or, less commonly, into the deep venous system. The radial orientation of the peripheral veins creates the impression of a *caput medusae* (Fig. 8.10). In a minority there are one or more arterial feeders (Hirata *et al.* 1986; Komiyama *et al.* 1999).Venous angiomas are the most common vascular anomaly incidentally encountered at post-mortem: in a series of over 4000 consecutive post-mortems, 4% of all brains harboured one or more vascular malformations, 63% of which were venous angiomas (Sarwar & McCormick 1978). Most occur in the frontal lobes, followed by the parietal lobes and the cerebellum (Garner *et al.* 1991; Naff *et al.* 1998). The appearance on MR scans is that of a tubular area of decreased signal intensity in the white matter of the brain (Rigamonti *et al.* 1988b) (Fig. 8.11).

As with cavernous angiomas, the most common manifestations of venous angiomas are not haemorrhagic episodes, but seizures or transient focal deficits (Malik *et al.* 1988; Garner *et al.* 1991; McLaughlin *et al.* 1998; Naff *et al.* 1998). Headache is also mentioned in these series, but as a rule this symptom represents the reason for ordering a head scan rather than a true consequence of the lesion. The annual rate of symptomatic haemorrhage in patients with unruptured venous angiomas is very low, between 0.15 and 0.34% (McLaughlin *et al.* 1998; Naff *et al.* 1998). Many regard the abnormal pattern of veins as an anatomical variant rather than as a pathological lesion, and so some have proposed the term 'developmental venous anomaly' (DVA) rather than 'venous angioma' (Goulao *et al.* 1990; Töpper *et al.* 1999).

The enlarged vein, which is the pathognomonic feature of venous angiomas, serves a vital function in drainage of blood

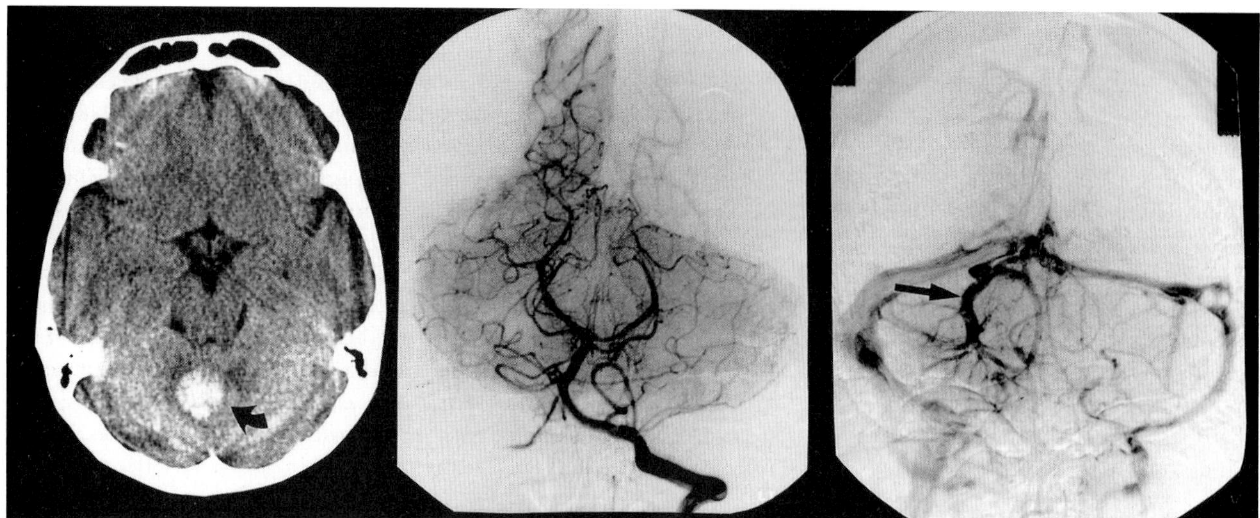

Fig. 8.10 Venous angioma in a 44-year-old man. Left: CT brain scan, showing haematoma in the vermis of the cerebellum (arrow). Middle: left vertebral angiogram, showing normal arterial phase. Right: left vertebral angiogram in the venous phase showing the venous angioma, with abnormal venous structures converging towards a single draining vein (caput medusae, arrow).

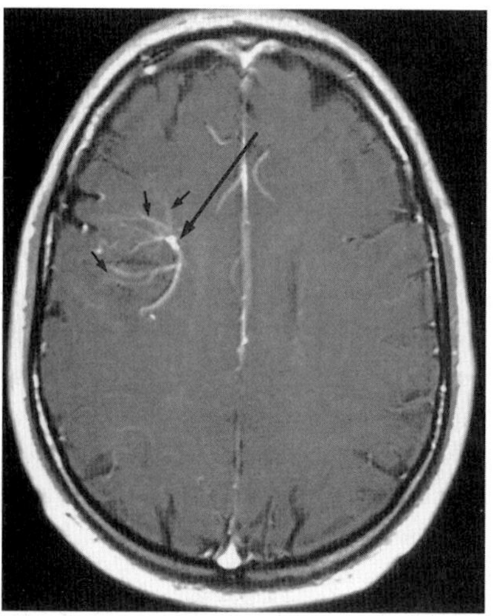

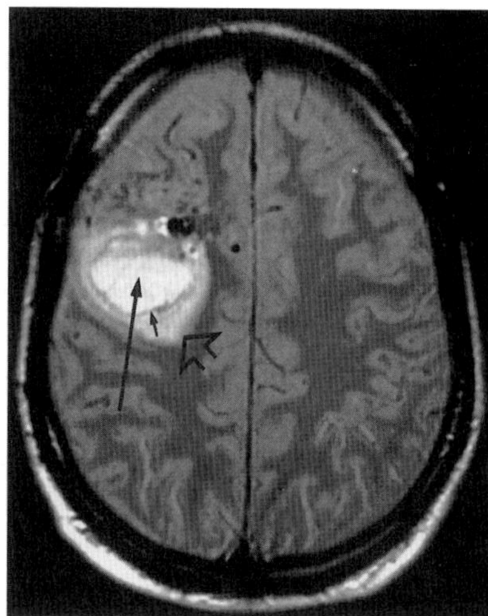

Fig. 8.11 Appearance of ruptured venous angioma on MR scanning, in a 31-year-old man. Left: gadolinium-enhanced T1-weighted MR scan shows the radial orientation of the contributing veins (short arrows), towards a central draining vein (long arrow). Right (early T2-weighted image): haematoma in the right centrum semiovale, represented by a hyperintense core of methaemoglobin (long arrow), surrounded by a hypointense rim of intracellular deoxyhaemoglobin (short arrow) and a hyperintense zone of oedema (open arrow). The central draining vein is represented by a tubular area of hypointensity ('signal void'), caused by the flow of blood.

from structures in the posterior fossa, as the usual drainage pathways are inadequate or absent. Therefore, operative intervention aimed at resection or collapse of such large veins can be disastrous, especially with venous angiomas in the posterior fossa (Senegor *et al.* 1983; Lasjaunias *et al.* 1986). We know of a case history with fatal brain swelling a few days after resection of a venous angioma in the frontal lobe. Operative treatment is therefore rarely indicated (Kondziolka *et al.* 1991). If such lesions do bleed, one should beware of an associated abnormality, such as a cavernous angioma (Rigamonti & Spetzler 1988; Goulao *et al.* 1990; Rigamonti *et al.* 1990; Awad *et al.* 1993; Töpper *et al.* 1999), an arteriovenous malformation (Awad *et al.* 1993; Meyer *et al.* 1995; Mullan *et al.* 1996) or a tumour (Rigamonti *et al.* 1990).

8.2.7 Telangiectasias

Telangiectasias are small lesions where the vessels resemble capillaries but have a widened lumen (20–500 μm), separated by normal brain tissue. They occur most often in the pons. They are mere curiosities, noted in less than 1% of post-mortems, and constituting 17% of all vascular anomalies (Sarwar & McCormick 1978). They have a very low potential for bleeding unless they are multiple, in which case other organs are often affected as well (Rendu–Osler–Weber disease) (Román *et al.* 1978). Two patients with pontine haemorrhage and telangiectasias were described many decades ago (Teilmann 1953). Occasionally, telangiectasias give rise to brainstem deficits without haemorrhage (Farrell & Forno 1970).

8.2.8 Dural arteriovenous fistulae

Dural arteriovenous fistulae are fed by meningeal arteries, most often branches from the middle meningeal or occipital branches of the external carotid artery, more rarely from the internal carotid or vertebral artery themselves (Aminoff 1973). As a rule, drainage is directly into dural sinuses, most often the transverse or sigmoid sinus, less commonly the superior sagittal or cavernous sinus (Fig. 8.12). In exceptional cases, two fistulae occur, draining into different sinuses (Nakamura *et al.* 1997). In a minority, the anomaly communicates with superficial veins of the cerebral convexity or the cerebellum, or with perimesencephalic veins (Aminoff 1973; Obrador *et al.* 1975).

In general, the lesions are acquired, mostly through some occlusive disease of a major sinus, the venous hypertension resulting in abnormal anastomoses between dural arteries and veins (Mironov 1995; Hamada *et al.* 1997). The sinus occlusion may result not only from thrombosis, but also from tumour (Arnautovic *et al.* 1998). Head injury, with or without skull fracture, may cause a dural arteriovenous fistula, presumably through thrombosis of the dural sinus in question (Chaudhary *et al.* 1982). Rarely, a fracture of the anterior skull base underlies the development of a dural fistula (Ishikawa *et al.* 1997) but, altogether, not more than about 1 in 20 cases of dural fistula is associated with head injury (Obrador *et al.* 1975).

Haemorrhage is the presenting event in only 15% of patients with these lesions (Davies *et al.* 1996). It occurs especially with drainage through cortical veins, in which case re-bleeding is not infrequent (Cognard *et al.* 1995; Duffau *et al.* 1999). Extravasation occurs into the subarachnoid space (section 9.1.4) or into the brain parenchyma (Malik *et al.* 1984; Brown *et al.* 1994; Pelz *et al.* 1997). A varix on the draining vein is another risk factor for haemorrhage (Awad *et al.* 1990; Brown *et al.* 1994).

The most common manifestations of dural fistulae are pulsatile tinnitus (if the fistula is near the temporal bone, section 6.6.6), headache and visual symptoms from papilloedema (Brown *et al.* 1994; Cognard *et al.* 1998). The papilloedema reflects increased pressure of cerebrospinal fluid, through increased pressure in the superior sagittal sinus; it causes visual obscurations, inferior nasal field defects or concentric field constriction, and eventually impaired acuity (Wall & George 1987). The annual risk of haemorrhage in patients presenting with non-haemorrhagic symptoms is 1–2% (Brown *et al.* 1994).

8.2.9 Haemorrhagic transformation of an arterial infarct

A fashionable theory at the beginning of the century had it that cerebral infarction preceded *all* instances of primary intracerebral haemorrhage (section 2.7) but now it has become clear that although haemorrhagic transformation occurs in some patients with cerebral infarction—15–45%, depending on patient selection and radiological criteria (Motto *et al.* 1997) (section 5.4)—by no means all cerebral haemorrhages are caused in this way. What concerns us here is that in some cases within this subgroup of patients with haemorrhagic transformation of an infarct the haemorrhage is so dense that it would have been regarded as a primary intracerebral haemorrhage, had not an earlier CT scan after symptom onset shown no haemorrhage (Bogousslavsky *et al.* 1991). Previous transient ischaemic attacks are not a reliable indicator of primary infarction, because they may also precede intracerebral haemorrhage (Gras *et al.* 1993).

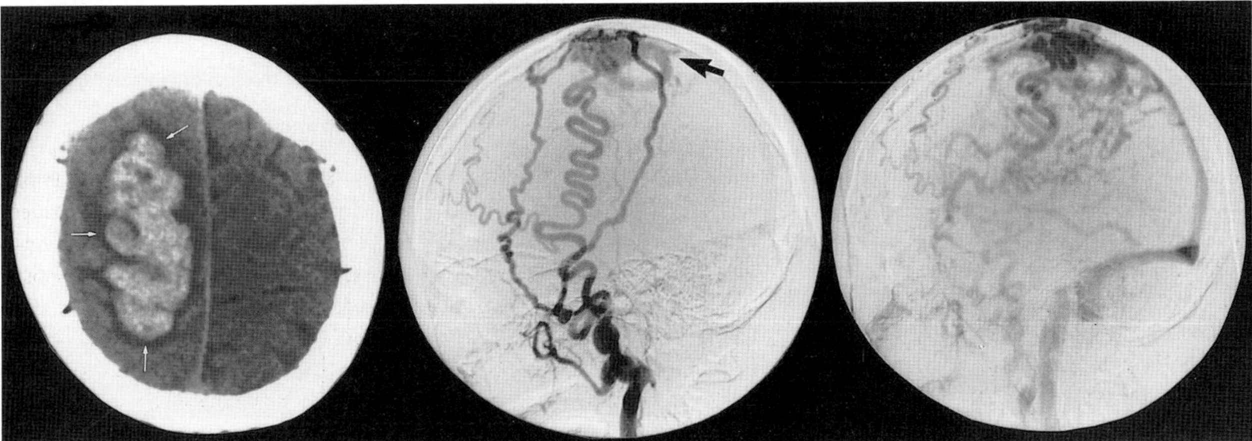

Fig. 8.12 Dural fistula with intraparenchymal haemorrhage. Left: CT brain scan showing a marginated haemorrhage at the convexity of the right hemisphere (arrows); the clinical deficit, a left hemiparesis, had developed gradually over about 1 h. Middle: right external carotid angiogram (arterial phase), showing abnormally large meningeal branches, converging towards the dural fistula (arrow). Right: right external carotid angiogram (venous phase) showing filling of abnormal dilated intracranial veins.

Dense intracerebral haemorrhage secondary to infarction is relatively frequent in patients with ischaemic stroke treated with thrombolytic agents (sections 5.4 and 11.5). This risk is highest with increasing age, severe clinical deficits and early changes of ischaemia on the CT scan (Larrue *et al.* 1997).

8.2.10 Intracranial venous thrombosis

There are many causes of intracranial venous thrombosis (section 5.5). Extensive haemorrhages occur in only a few patients, although the precise proportion depends on referral patterns and also on the assiduousness with which the diagnosis is pursued in patients with the syndrome of benign intracranial hypertension. Haemorrhages are most often secondary to infarction caused by obstruction of cortical veins, i.e. 'venous infarction' (Fig. 8.11). Therefore, the haemorrhage is usually preceded by an ischaemic phase, manifested by focal neurological deficits, epileptic seizures or a global encephalopathy, without radiological evidence of extravasation of blood, the interval being hours or days. Occasionally an intracerebral haematoma may be the presenting feature of intracranial venous thrombosis. In those cases, the diagnosis can be suspected from the location: bilateral and parasagittal with thrombosis of the superior sagittal sinus (Fig. 5.41), and the surface of the temporal lobe with thrombosis of the lateral sinus (Fig. 8.13); in the latter situation the cerebellum may also be involved (Wardlaw *et al.* 1998). Sometimes rupture of a thrombosed vein causes haemorrhage without previous infarction (Krücke 1971).

Intracranial venous thrombosis is an under-diagnosed condition. Apart from other presentations, such as headache, visual symptoms secondary to papilloedema and ischaemic neurological deficits, it should be included in the differential diagnosis of primary intracerebral haemorrhage. The diagnosis should be strongly suspected if the patient is a young woman, if the haemorrhage has been preceded by some of the other neurological manifestations of venous infarction and if the haemorrhage is multiple, in the parasagittal or temporal region.

8.2.11 Septic arteritis and mycotic aneurysms

Infective endocarditis is complicated by intracerebral haemorrhage in about 5% of cases (Kanter & Hart 1991) (section 6.5). It most commonly results not from mycotic aneurysms but from acute, pyogenic necrosis of the arterial wall early in the disease, usually with virulent organisms, such as *Staphylococcus aureus*, and before effective treatment with antibiotics (Hart *et al.* 1987, 1990; Masuda *et al.* 1992). Mycotic aneurysms may develop and rupture later, during antimicrobial therapy, or with less virulent bacteria, such as *Streptococcus viridans*, *Streptococcus sanguis* or *Staphylococcus epidermidis*.

In general, a lobar haemorrhage is only exceptionally associated with endocarditis in a patient without any history of heart disease, recent cerebral ischaemia, recent malaise, fever or loss of weight. This is because the prevalence of 'hypertensive' microangiopathy and amyloid angiopathy is vastly greater than that of infective endocarditis. In addition,

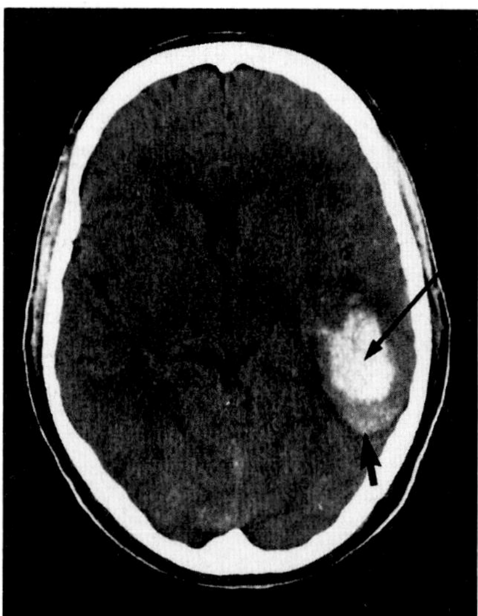
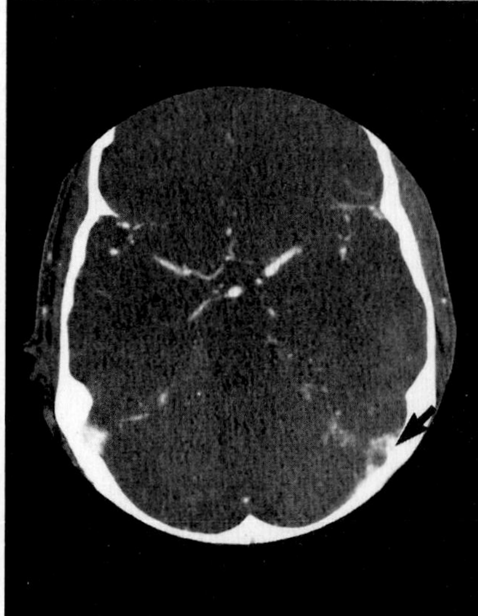
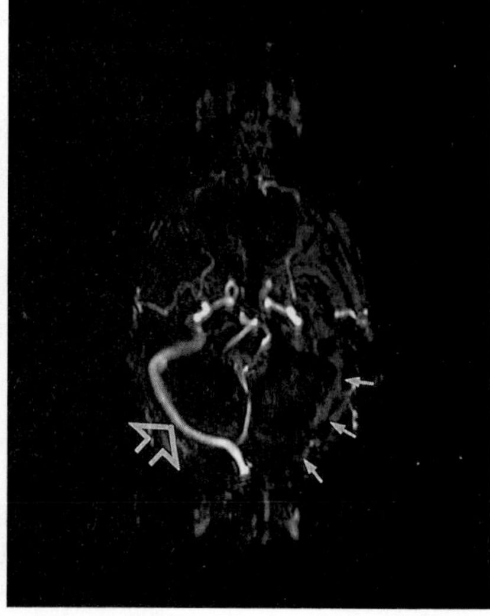

Fig. 8.13 Intracerebral haemorrhage caused by intracranial venous thrombosis, in a 55-year-old man. Left: CT brain scan showing a haemorrhagic lesion in the left temporal lobe; the hyperdense core (long arrow) is surrounded by a rim of slight hyperintensity (short arrow), consistent with haemorrhagic transformation of an infarct. Middle: CT angiogram showing a filling defect in the left sigmoid sinus (arrow) caused by thrombus. Right: MR venogram, with non-filling of the left transverse and sigmoid sinus (short arrows). Note the normal right transverse and sigmoid sinuses (open arrow).

more than 80% of patients with intracerebral haemorrhage from septic emboli have a history of heart disease or intravenous drug abuse, or have had prodromal episodes suggesting embolization, or both (Hart *et al.* 1987; Salgado *et al.* 1987). The combined case fatality of intracerebral haemorrhage and the underlying endocarditis is about 25–50%, higher than that of intracerebral haemorrhage alone in the corresponding age groups (Hart *et al.* 1987; Monsuez *et al.* 1989).

In patients with AIDS, toxoplasmosis or tuberculoma of the brain may lead to intracerebral haemorrhage, presumably through vasculitis (Trenkwalder *et al.* 1992; Roquer *et al.* 1998). In tropical countries, parasitic infections of the brain, such as sparganosis, can be associated with intracerebral haemorrhage (Jeong *et al.* 1998).

8.2.12 Moyamoya syndrome

Intracerebral, subarachnoid or, occasionally, intraventricular haemorrhage is the most common manifestation of the moyamoya syndrome in adults (Nijdam *et al.* 1986; Newman & Al-Memar 1998), whereas in children it is more often encountered as a cause of ischaemic stroke (Bruno *et al.* 1988) (section 7.5). The bleeding is caused by rupture of one of the widened perforating vessels acting as collaterals, or sometimes of an associated dissecting aneurysm (Yamashita *et al.* 1983). Therefore, most haemorrhages occur in the basal ganglia. Without the angiographic diagnosis of the primarily occlusive disorder, these cannot be distinguished from the much more common 'hypertensive' haemorrhages as a result of small vessel disease.

Re-bleeding from dilated collateral pathways has been documented, at a rate of approximately 2% per annum (Houkin *et al.* 1996; Yoshida *et al.* 1999). It is hoped, but not proven, that revascularization procedures decrease the risk of re-bleeding (Houkin *et al.* 1996; Yoshida *et al.* 1999).

8.2.13 Arterial dissection

Haemorrhage is an uncommon complication of arterial dissection, and any extravasation that does occur is almost invariably confined to the subarachnoid space (sections 7.2.2 and 9.1.3).

8.2.14 Caroticocavernous fistula

Pulsating exophthalmos is the most common manifestation of a fistula created by a ruptured aneurysm of the internal carotid artery within the cavernous sinus, or by trauma. Exceptionally, rupture of one of the dilated and congested veins that drain into the cavernous sinus occurs, resulting in an intraparenchymal haematoma (d'Angelo *et al.* 1988; Hiramatsu *et al.* 1991).

8.3 Haemodynamic factors

8.3.1 Arterial hypertension

Chronically raised blood pressure

Chronically raised blood pressure is by far the most powerful risk factor for stroke in general, whether ischaemic or haemorrhagic (section 6.3.3). In many cases, it is chronic hypertension that underlies the degenerative change in small perforating arteries (section 8.2.1) that ultimately leads to their rupture in the basal ganglia, cerebellum or brainstem, or less often in the subcortical white matter. Few prospective studies have assessed the risk of increasing blood pressure for haemorrhagic stroke separately from ischaemic stroke. Those that did found that the risk of haemorrhagic and ischaemic stroke increased to a similar degree with blood pressure, not only in Australia (Jamrozik *et al.* 1994) but also in China and Japan, the stroke rate doubling for each 5 mm increase of diastolic pressure (Rodgers *et al.* 1998). In a case–control study, the relative risk for patients with hypertension (140/90 mmHg or higher) of having intracerebral haemorrhage was 3.9 (95% CI, 2.7–5.7); if the definition of hypertension included evidence of hypertrophy of the left ventricle on the electrocardiogram (ECG), or cardiomegaly on the chest X-ray, the relative risk was 5.4 (95% CI, 3.7–7.9) (Brott *et al.* 1986).

Nevertheless, as pointed out in the introduction to this chapter, hypertension is neither a sufficient nor a necessary cause of intracerebral haemorrhage. Hypertension (as determined by history) was found in only 45% of patients in a consecutive, hospital-based series of patients with intracerebral haemorrhage (Brott *et al.* 1986); this rate was similar for haemorrhages in the thalamus and basal ganglia, where causes other than small vessel disease are unlikely. The proportion of hypertensive patients increased to 56% by adding those with evidence of left-ventricular hypertrophy on the chest X-ray or ECG (Brott *et al.* 1986). In a large and prospective hospital series from the Netherlands, 59% of the patients with intracerebral haemorrhage had a history of hypertension (Franke *et al.* 1992). Similarly, a controlled study of patients who had died from intracerebral haemorrhage showed that only 46% of these fatal cases had been hypertensive, as judged from the heart weight (Bahemuka 1987).

All these pieces of evidence from different sources seem to suggest that, strictly speaking, the term 'hypertensive intracerebral haemorrhage' is a misnomer. On the other hand, the 'normotensive' patients in these series may have had mild degrees of hypertension, without signs of ventricular hypertrophy or end-organ damage. After all, as in any disorder, 'high-risk' patients make up only a small proportion of the patients with the disorder in question, and the majority are patients with only moderate risk: the prevention paradox (Rose 1992) (section 18.5.2).

Factors other than hypertension must contribute to the rupture of small perforating vessels because this occurs in some, but not all, patients with hypertension, and sometimes even without hypertension.

Acutely raised blood pressure

Acutely raised blood pressure can definitely precipitate intracerebral haemorrhage, particularly in previously normotensive individuals whose cerebral blood flow autoregulation is within the normal range, i.e. it can relatively easily be exceeded by raising the blood pressure (Caplan 1988). The rapid increase in perfusion pressure is transmitted to the wall of small arterioles, which are left relatively vulnerable, unlike the hypertrophy associated with long-standing hypertension. Examples of acutely raised blood pressure as a cause of intracerebral haemorrhage are acute renal failure, even after transplantation (Adams *et al.* 1986), and eclampsia (Richards *et al.* 1988) (section 7.14). A rise in blood pressure has also been invoked as an intermediate factor with intracerebral haemorrhage after exposure to severe cold weather (Caplan *et al.* 1984), pain induced by dental procedures (Barbas *et al.* 1987; Cawley *et al.* 1991), electroconvulsive treatment (Weisberg *et al.* 1991a), break dancing (Lee & Clough 1990) and unconventional medical treatments, such as 'coining' (Ponder & Lehman 1994).

After carotid endarterectomy for severe stenosis, there may be relative hypertension in a previously underperfused hemisphere, in some cases resulting in intracerebral haemorrhage (section 16.8.3). Transient but steep rises in blood pressure may also account for at least some of the supratentorial haemorrhages that can occur during or shortly after operations in the posterior fossa, such as microvascular decompression of the Vth cranial nerve for trigeminal neuralgia (Haines *et al.* 1978).

8.3.2 Migraine

Migraine may theoretically be associated with intracerebral haemorrhage in an indirect fashion, through the presence of an arteriovenous malformation which may have precipitated migraine attacks (Weiskrantz *et al.* 1974; Troost *et al.* 1979), but also directly. Three middle-aged women with a long history of migraine attacks suffered lobar haemorrhages after an unusually severe attack, with tenderness of the carotid artery in the neck. On angiography, they had evidence of extensive vasospasm in the ipsilateral internal carotid or intracranial arteries. The density and compactness of the haemorrhages on brain CT did not suggest that they were secondary to infarction (Cole & Aubé 1990). Surgical specimens in two of these patients showed evidence of necrosis in the walls of intracranial vessels, probably as a result of ischaemia, with secondary inflammatory changes. Such events are sufficiently rare to caution against suspecting migraine as a cause of lobar haemorrhage unless severe headache preceded rather than accompanied the stroke, and all other causes have been meticulously excluded.

8.4 Haemostatic factors

8.4.1 Anticoagulants

The anatomical distribution of intracerebral haemorrhage associated with anticoagulants is similar to that of small vessel disease (Kase *et al.* 1985; Franke *et al.* 1990) (section 8.2.1). During treatment with oral anticoagulants, the risk of intracerebral haemorrhage, compared with age-matched control subjects not on anticoagulants, is increased by between seven and 11 times (Wintzen *et al.* 1984; Franke *et al.* 1990; Fogelholm *et al.* 1992). It is unknown what proportion of this excess risk should be attributed to the treatment itself and how much to any small vessel degeneration associated with the vascular condition for which the treatment was given (i.e. confounding by indication). Most of these studies report a disproportionately high risk of intracerebral haemorrhage in the first year of anticoagulant treatment. Intracerebral haemorrhage has also been reported with heparin treatment for non-neurological indications (Babikian *et al.* 1989); perhaps the use of heparin explains at least part of the excess risk of intracerebral haemorrhage in patients on haemodialysis (Onoyama *et al.* 1987; Iseki *et al.* 1993).

Not surprisingly, the risk of intracerebral haemorrhage increases with the intensity of anticoagulation in patients in whom there is a non-neurological indication (Landefeld *et al.* 1989; Cannegieter *et al.* 1995), as well as in patients with cerebral ischaemia (Stroke Prevention In Reversible Ischaemia Trial (SPIRIT) Study Group 1997) (section 16.5.4). Nevertheless, most anticoagulated patients who have an intracerebral haemorrhage are not deeply anticoagulated: the intensity of anticoagulation commonly exceeded the therapeutic range in only a single study (Kase *et al.* 1985), in at most 50% in another (Dawson *et al.* 1993), and only rarely in five larger studies (Wintzen *et al.* 1984; Franke *et al.* 1990; Rådberg *et al.* 1991; Fogelholm *et al.* 1992; SPIRIT Study Group 1997). This is another illustration of the paradox that the absolute number of disease events is greater among patients at moderate risk (representing a small proportion of a very large group) than among patients at high risk (a large proportion of a small group) (section 18.5.2).

Other, independent, risk factors for intracerebral haemorrhage identified in case–control studies of patients with a non-neurological indication for anticoagulation are systolic hypertension, insulin-dependent diabetes, increasing age and a history of stroke (Dawson *et al.* 1993; Hylek & Singer 1994). In patients with cerebral ischaemia, increasing age and leukoaraiosis are the main predictors (SPIRIT Study Group 1997; Gorter *et al.* 1999). Most of these factors probably act through small vessel disease, although intriguingly the presence of a lacunar (rather than cortical) syndrome or infarct before the start of anticoagulant treatment did not seem to be associated with an increased risk of intracerebral bleeding (Gorter *et al.* 1999).

The risk of intracerebral haemorrhage in patients on oral anticoagulants increases with the intensity of anticoagulation, but in most patients with intracerebral haemorrhage while on anticoagulants the international normalized ratio values are within the appropriate range.

A remarkable feature in intracerebral haemorrhage precipitated by anticoagulants is the gradual progression of the clinical deficits, observed in as many as 58% in the only series that systematically addressed this issue (Kase *et al.* 1985). Also, the average volume of the haemorrhage is larger than in intracerebral haemorrhage not associated with anticoagulants, according to studies in which the comparison was not confounded by sampling bias (Franke *et al.* 1990; Rådberg *et al.* 1991). A fluid-blood level within the haematoma (Fig. 8.14), i.e. a horizontal interface between unclotted serum (hypodense) and sedimentated red cells (hyperdense), occurs in 60% of anticoagulant-related intracerebral haemorrhages and only rarely otherwise (Pfleger *et al.* 1994). Cerebral amyloid angiopathy (section 8.2.2) is an example of a condition in which a fluid-blood level within the haematoma may occur with normal clotting.

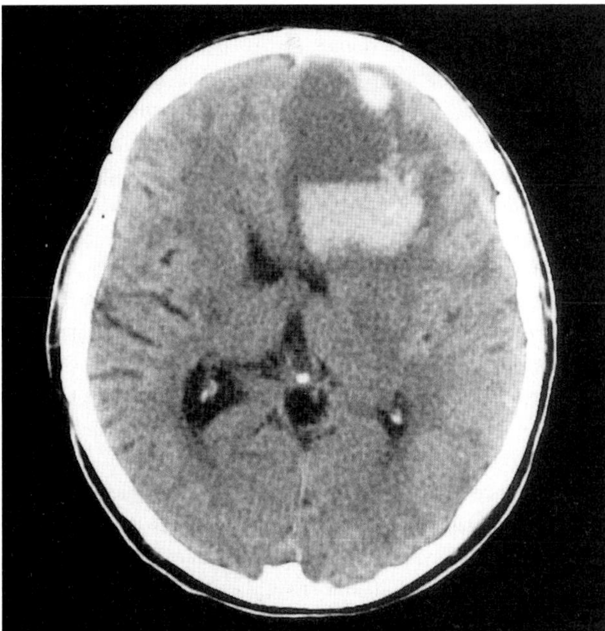

Fig. 8.14 CT brain scan showing a haematoma in the left frontal lobe, with a horizontal border representing the interface between sedimented red blood cells and supernatant plasma, indicating impaired coagulation. There is also distortion of the ventricle and loss of sulci, indicating mass effect.

8.4.2 Antiplatelet drugs

In a complete overview, up to 1991, of all the randomized trials of antiplatelet drugs (mostly aspirin), for any indication, in which at least one haemorrhagic stroke had been recorded as an outcome event, the risk of intracerebral haemorrhage over an average of 2 years was 0.3% in treated patients vs. 0.2% in controls (Antiplatelet Trialists' Collaboration 1994). Although this represents a relative risk of 1.5 (95% CI, 1.1–2.1), the absolute risk is extremely low and can be expressed as one extra haemorrhage for every 1000 treated patients, for a length of time that was around 2 years for most of the trials. For aspirin alone, the risk is similar (He *et al.* 1998). Given the small size of the excess risk, it is no great surprise that a case–control study based on 331 patients with intracerebral haemorrhage found no difference in the use of aspirin (or in use of non-steroidal anti-inflammatory drugs) between cases and controls (Thrift *et al.* 1999b).

Antiplatelet drugs are probably only a relatively minor contributory factor in the pathogenesis of primary intracerebral haemorrhage against a background of much more powerful determinants, most often small vessel disease.

The dosage of aspirin is not an important factor with regard to the rate of intracerebral haemorrhage, at least not according to the few studies in which different dosage was directly compared: 300 vs. 1200 mg (UK-TIA Study Group 1991) and 30 vs. 283 mg (Dutch TIA Trial Study Group 1991). On the other hand, the confidence intervals in these comparisons are wide, as they are in trials comparing different antiplatelet drugs.

8.4.3 Thrombolytic treatment (for non-neurological indications)

Intracerebral haemorrhage is a serious and often fatal complication of thrombolytic therapy for acute myocardial infarction, occurring in 0.5–0.8% of patients, and usually within 24 h (Carlson *et al.* 1988; Kase *et al.* 1990; Gore *et al.* 1991; Uglietta *et al.* 1991; Kase *et al.* 1992; Wijdicks & Jack *et al.* 1993). Factors associated with increased risk are age over 65 years, body weight below 70 kg (in other words, a relatively high dose of the thrombolytic drug), hypertension on admission to hospital and administration of tissue plasminogen activator rather than streptokinase (Anderson *et al.* 1991; Maggioni *et al.* 1992; Simoons *et al.* 1993; Gore *et al.* 1995; Gurwitz *et al.* 1998). Occasionally there is an underlying anatomical anomaly, such as an arteriovenous malformation (Proner *et al.* 1990).

Several clues incriminate cerebral amyloid angiopathy as the most frequent anatomical abnormality underlying this complication. First, a disproportionate number of intracerebral haemorrhages after thrombolysis occur in the white matter of the cerebral hemispheres, and multiple haematomas occur in about one-third (Kase *et al.* 1990; Uglietta *et al.* 1991; Wijdicks & Jack *et al.* 1993; Gebel *et al.* 1998). Secondly, in a few patients in whom brain tissue could be examined after operation or post-mortem, blood vessels showed amyloid changes (Ramsay *et al.* 1990; Pendlebury *et al.* 1991; Leblanc *et al.* 1992; Wijdicks & Jack *et al.* 1993; Sloan *et al.* 1995).

A state of systemically enhanced thrombolysis from these drugs adversely affects the process of haemostasis in the brain, as reflected by fluid levels in lobar haematomas (Wijdicks & Jack *et al.* 1993; Gebel *et al.* 1998) (Fig. 8.14), and by a high case fatality within the first 3 days of 60–80% (Kase *et al.* 1990; Uglietta *et al.* 1991; Wijdicks & Jack *et al.* 1993; Gore *et al.* 1995; Sloan *et al.* 1998; Mahaffey *et al.* 1999). With intracerebral haemorrhage in general, only about one-quarter of patients die within the first 3 days (Franke *et al.* 1992).

8.4.4 Clotting factor deficiency

Spontaneous intracranial bleeding may occur in haemophilia, and with severe deficiency of factors VIII, IX or, rarely, XIII. Head injury may provoke brain haemorrhage in patients, often children, with milder degrees of haemophilia or with von Willebrand's disease (de Tezanos Pinto *et al.* 1992). The interval may be as long as several days (Martinowitz *et al.* 1986). The case fatality is high. Acquired immune deficiency syndrome (AIDS) is sometimes a contributory factor, because factor replacement therapy may be delayed by a patient's impaired judgement (Andes & Wulff 1990). Congenital afibrinogenaemia has also been associated with spontaneous intracerebral haemorrhage (Henselmans *et al.* 1999).

8.4.5 Leukaemia and thrombocytopenia (also section 7.9)

Myeloid leukaemia is complicated by intracerebral haemorrhage in around 20% of cases (Yamauchi & Umeda 1997), whereas this is exceptional in chronic lymphatic leukaemia, or in hairy cell leukaemia (Ng *et al.* 1991). Intracerebral haemorrhage with leukaemia is usually multifocal and part of a generalized bleeding tendency, but occasionally it occurs as an isolated event (Kelly *et al.* 1985). The pathogenesis is diverse. Most often, the direct cause is the formation of aggregates of tumour cells, which obstruct arterioles or capillaries in the cortex or subcortical white matter. This is followed by local proliferation of white cells, with erosion of the vessel wall. Another cause is disseminated intravascular coagulation and consumption coagulopathy. Finally, the underlying cause may be thrombocytopenia, from infiltration of the bone marrow, after transplantation of bone marrow or liver, or as an adverse effect of chemotherapy (Pomeranz *et al.* 1994; Wijdicks *et al.* 1995). Intracerebral haemorrhage should not be attributed to thrombocytopenia unless the platelet count is below 20×10^9/L, because above this value the bleeding time is normal (provided platelet function is intact).

Thrombocytopenia as a cause of intracerebral haemorrhage may also be associated with myelofibrosis (Markel *et al.* 1986), aplastic anaemia, diffuse intravascular coagulation with conditions other than leukaemia, and with idiopathic thrombocytopenic purpura (Werlhof's disease) (Lee & Kim 1998).

8.5 Other factors

8.5.1 Intracerebral tumours

Haemorrhage into an intracerebral tumour accounts for approximately 5% of all intracerebral haemorrhages (Little *et al.* 1979). The connection is not too difficult to make if the patient is already known to have an intracerebral tumour, and it should also come readily to mind with a known extracranial malignant tumour, but the diagnosis may be delayed if intracerebral haemorrhage is the first manifestation of the tumour, which is the case in approximately 50% of all tumour haemorrhages (Little *et al.* 1979). There are various causes for the haemorrhage. Most common is rupture of a fragile vessel in a hypervascular tumour, or necrosis of part of the tumour. An exceptional cause is erosion of normal blood vessels by the tumour, which is characteristic of metastatic choriocarcinoma (van den Doel *et al.* 1985).

On brain CT, several features suggest an underlying tumour (Kase 1986, 1994). These include:

- location of the haemorrhage in other than the deep areas, the corpus callosum being an obvious example, at least if not associated with subarachnoid haemorrhage;
- an irregular, mottled appearance of the haematoma, for instance with a low-density area in the centre, suggesting necrosis (Fig. 8.15);
- occurrence of multiple haemorrhages (a feature shared with some other types of haemorrhage, Table 8.2);
- a disproportionate degree of surrounding oedema or mass effect (also in venous haemorrhagic infarction, section 5.5);
- nodular enhancement of surrounding tissue after intravenous contrast, other than the ring enhancement that represents the inflammatory response to the haemorrhage (section 5.3.4); and
- the appearance of other lesions after intravenous contrast.

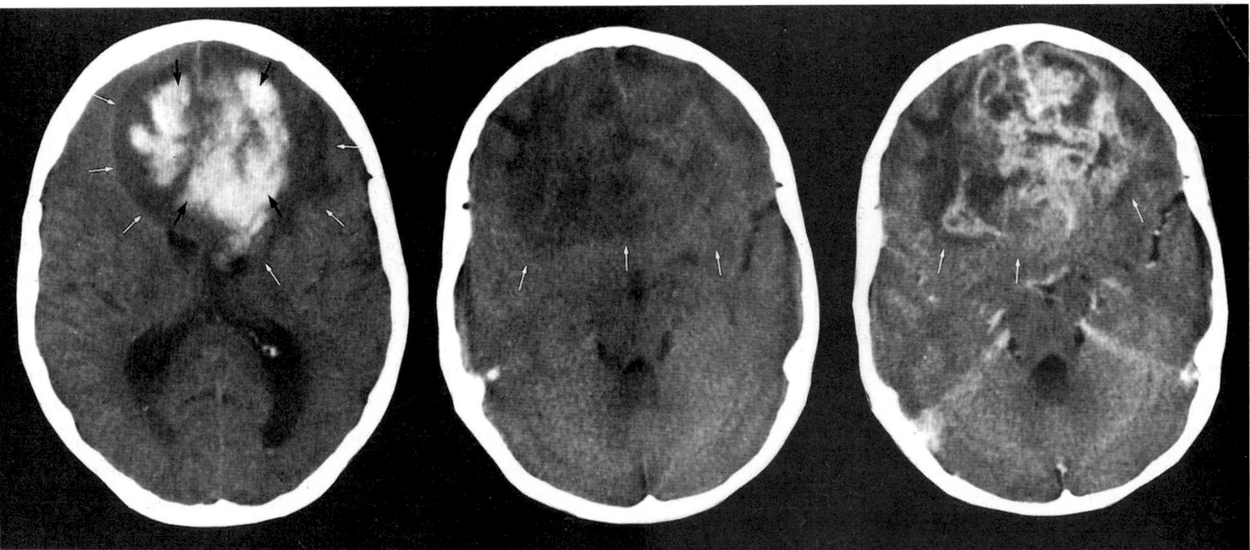

Fig. 8.15 Haemorrhage caused by tumour in a 71-year-old woman. Left: CT brain scan 1 day after sudden loss of consciousness, showing a bifrontal haematoma (black arrows) with irregular shape and disproportionate oedema (hypodense margin around the haematoma; thin arrows). Middle: CT scan 3 months later, after a gradual recovery had been followed by secondary deterioration; diffuse oedema in both frontal lobes with considerable mass effect (arrows). Right: after injection of intravenous contrast a grossly irregular tumour emerges (glioblastoma).

On MRI, the diagnosis of tumour haemorrhage is based on similar characteristics, with the addition that a tumour is less likely (though far from excluded) if haemosiderin is demonstrated as a hypodense rim on T2-weighted images (Destian *et al.* 1989). When doubt remains, e.g. when tumour markers in the serum are negative, as well as investigations of the chest and abdomen, the issue can often be resolved by repeating the scan after an interval of several weeks or months (Fig. 8.15). If for any reason one cannot wait that long, an angiogram of the intracerebral circulation may be helpful by showing pathological vessels.

Metastases are the most common tumours that cause intracerebral haemorrhage, melanoma and bronchial carcinoma being frequent primary tumours, followed by renal carcinoma and choriocarcinoma (Maiuri *et al.* 1985). The last type of tumour is most often associated with pregnancy, but the primary tumour may also be in the testis (Timothy *et al.* 1994). More unusual types of brain metastases to cause haemorrhage are myxoma (Schafhalter-Zoppoth *et al.* 1997), mucinous cancers (Amico *et al.* 1989) and rhabdomyosarcoma (Ahola *et al.* 1998). Gliomas, and particularly glioblastomas, are the next most common group of tumours to bleed (Kase & Louis 1990). Even rarer sources of intracerebral haemorrhage are haemangioblastomas (Matsumura *et al.* 1985), pituitary adenomas (Wakai *et al.* 1995), meningiomas and chondromas (Modesti *et al.* 1976).

8.5.2 Alcohol

Massive intracerebral haemorrhages may occur in alcoholics who have evidence of liver damage, a low platelet count and abnormalities of the clotting system (Weisberg 1988). The haemorrhages may be so extensive that there are no focal deficits but a clinical syndrome suggesting a metabolic encephalopathy. Whether brief spells of excessive drinking ('binge drinking') can precipitate intracerebral haemorrhage, subarachnoid haemorrhage or even stroke in general is controversial, because most of the case–control studies that addressed this issue were subject to bias (van Gijn *et al.* 1993) (section 6.3.3). A regular intake of three or more units of alcohol per day, however, is consistently associated with an increased risk of intracerebral haemorrhage, as well as of subarachnoid haemorrhage (Camargo *et al.* 1989). This effect may be related to the antiplatelet action of alcohol, at least in part (Jakubowski *et al.* 1988). For stroke in general, the increased risk with heavy drinking may be mediated through an increase in blood pressure (Wannamethee & Shaper 1996).

8.5.3 Amphetamines (also section 7.15)

Intracerebral haemorrhages can follow ingestion of amphetamine or methamphetamine, less often dextroamphetamine, with any route of administration and after doses as low as 20 mg (Harrington *et al.* 1983). The interval between ingestion and haemorrhage can be as short as a few minutes and never longer than a few hours. The use of the drug may not be admitted until weeks later (Heye & Hankey 1996). Most of these haemorrhages are lobar, in the subcortical white matter (Caplan 1994). Cerebral angiography shows scattered segments of narrowing and dilatation ('beading') or occlusion. At post-mortem, the lesions correspond with areas of fibrinoid necrosis in small and medium-sized vessels, in the brain as well as in other organs (Citron *et al.* 1970; Shibata *et al.* 1991). There may be underlying anatomical abnormalities which have ruptured, such as an arteriovenous malformation (Lukes 1983; Selmi *et al.* 1995).

8.5.4 *Cocaine and other drugs* (also section 7.15)

As with amphetamines, cocaine-associated haemorrhage may occur after oral ingestion, intravenous injection or inhalation, but relatively more often after inhalation of 'crack' cocaine, a mixture of cocaine hydrochloride and ammonia or baking soda (Levine *et al.* 1991). These haemorrhages occur mostly in the white matter of the cerebral hemispheres. They may be multiple (Green *et al.* 1990). Unlike amphetamines, the proportion with underlying vascular abnormalities, such as aneurysms, is high at about 50%, at least in patients with adequate angiographic or post-mortem studies (Peterson *et al.* 1991). In the remaining group, post-mortem consistently fails to show any vasculopathic changes (Aggarwal *et al.* 1996; Nolte *et al.* 1996). Here the normal blood vessels implicate haemodynamic rather than structural factors, an explanation supported by a higher frequency of pre-existing hypertension than in those with aneurysms (Kibayashi *et al.* 1995). An odd event is bleeding into an acoustic neuroma (Yapor & Gutierrez 1992).

Intracerebral haemorrhage has also been reported in association with the use of ephedrine (Bruno *et al.* 1993) and 'Ecstasy' (Harries & De Silva 1992; Hughes *et al.* 1993). Ergot alkaloids, such as bromocriptine and lisuride, can cause vasoconstriction and probably vessel necrosis in the post-partum period, which can induce parenchymal haemorrhage (Comabella *et al.* 1996; Rob & Park 1998) (section 7.14).

8.5.5 *Vasculitis*

Primary angiitis of the central nervous system is, by definition, not associated with any systemic involvement (section 7.3). The cause is obscure, and it is uncertain whether the condition is a nosological entity (Hankey 1991; Woolfenden *et al.* 1998). Presenting features include chronic headache, mental deterioration, seizures and focal ischaemia. Occasionally, intracerebral haemorrhage may be the first clinical manifestation (Biller *et al.* 1987; Hunn *et al.* 1998). The haemorrhages may recur (Clifford Jones *et al.* 1985) and can be associated with aneurysmal dilatations at changing sites (Nishikawa *et al.* 1998). Other vasculitic disorders affecting the brain can sometimes present with, or be complicated by, intracerebral haemorrhage (section 7.3). These include bacterial meningitis (Gironell *et al.* 1995), HLTV-1 associated myelopathy (Smith *et al.* 1993) and herpes zoster, as a complication of AIDS (Lipton *et al.* 1996), or in isolation (Mossuto Agatiello *et al.* 1987).

8.5.6 *Trauma ('Spät-Apoplexie')*

The antiquity of this notion can be surmised from its exotic ring (Bollinger 1891; DeJong 1942). There is no doubt that even minor trauma may result in rupture of vulnerable arteries, specifically in patients with cerebral amyloid angiopathy (section 8.2.2), or in patients with a deficiency of clotting factors (section 8.4.4). Also there is ample evidence from serial CT scan studies after head injury that a superficial brain contusion may change its aspect within hours or days, from a slightly hypodense, mottled, or even normal appearance to an extensive, space-occupying lesion (Fukamachi *et al.* 1985; Tanaka *et al.* 1988). In all these cases the initial lesion immediately follows the trauma, and is usually accompanied by focal or general neurological deficits. It must therefore be regarded as a medicolegal myth that head trauma can contribute to the development of deep intracerebral haemorrhage after an interval of days or even weeks, without an initial brain lesion. However, it is conceivable that this initial brain lesion may not be severe enough to cause more than rather subtle impairments.

8.6 Relative frequency of causes, according to age and location

As discussed in the introduction to this chapter, age is an important factor in determining the a priori probability of a particular cause of haemorrhage in an individual patient. Arteriovenous malformations are the leading cause in the young and degenerative intracranial small vessel disease in the middle-aged and the elderly, while cerebral amyloid angiopathy is another important cause to consider in the elderly. Some refinements of this rule of thumb are possible, not only by listing causes less common than these three, but also by considering factors other than age, particularly the location of the haematoma. Table 8.3 lists the frequency of the different causes of intracerebral haemorrhage, according to age group and by location (basal ganglia or thalamus, lobar haemorrhages in the cortex or white matter of the cerebral hemispheres, and cerebellum or brainstem). This ranking of the different causes is based partly on three hospital series of young adults (under 45 years) with intracerebral haemorrhage (Toffol *et al.* 1987; Gras *et al.* 1991; Ruíz-Sandoval *et al.* 1999), partly on a large surgical series of lobar haemorrhages with negative angiography, in which thorough histological study of the specimens was carried out (Wakai *et al.* 1992) and, finally, where nothing else is available, on guesswork. The relative importance of the causes depends to some extent also on geographical location, for instance in the case of drug abuse or endocarditis. The order given here reflects the relative frequencies in Europe and should be

Table 8.3 A priori probabilities for structural causes of primary intracerebral haemorrhage (coagulopathies and haemodynamic factors excluded), according to the patient's age and the location of the haematoma.

Age (years)	Basal ganglia/thalamus	Lobar	Cerebellum/brainstem
Below 45	1 AVM or cavernoma 2 Small vessel disease 3 Moyamoya syndrome (4) Amphetamines/cocaine	1 AVM or cavernoma 2 Saccular aneurysm* 3 Tumour 4 Intracranial venous thrombosis† (5) Amphetamines/cocaine 6 Infective endocarditis‡	1 AVM or cavernoma 2 Small vessel disease 3 Tumour
45–69	1 Small vessel disease 2 AVM or cavernoma 3 Atherosclerotic 'moyamoya syndrome' (4) Tumour (5) Cerebral amyloid angiopathy 6 Intracranial venous thrombosis† 7 Infective endocarditis‡	1 Small vessel disease 2 AVM or cavernoma 3 Saccular aneurysm* (4) Cerebral amyloid angiopathy	1 Small vessel disease 2 AVM or cavernoma (3) Tumour
70 or over	1 Small vessel disease (2) Tumour (3) AVM or cavernoma 4 Tumour 5 AVM or cavernoma 6 Intracranial venous thrombosis 7 Infective endocarditis‡	1 Small vessel disease 2 Cerebral amyloid angiopathy 3 Saccular aneurysm* 4 AVM or cavernoma	1 Small vessel disease 2 Cerebral amyloid angiopathy 3 Tumour

* Haematomas in specific locations (see text).

† Haematoma usually in parasagittal area.

‡ With history of valvular heart disease.

AVM, arteriovenous malformation.

Numbers in parentheses: rank order not certain.

adjusted where necessary for cultural and geographical differences.

Arteriovenous malformations are the most common cause of primary intracerebral haemorrhage in the young, degenerative small vessel disease in middle and old age, and cerebral amyloid angiopathy in old age.

8.7 Clues from the history

The cause of intracerebral haemorrhage may occasionally be identified from clues in the history. A past history of intracerebral haemorrhage may indicate a structural lesion, such as an arteriovenous malformation that was not detected on the earlier occasion, especially if the haemorrhage is at the same site in the brain. If the recurrent haemorrhage is distant from the earlier lesion, the underlying condition may be cerebral amyloid angiopathy, especially when there is evidence of associated leukoaraiosis (section 5.7). A family history of intracerebral haemorrhage may indicate a rare hereditary condition, such as cavernoma or a familial variant of amyloid angiopathy. Previous epileptic seizures should raise suspicions about the presence of an arteriovenous malformation, a tumour or, if focal and of recent onset, cerebral amyloid angiopathy (Greenberg *et al.* 1993; Cocito *et al.* 1994). Cerebral amyloid angiopathy should also be suspected with a history of transient ischaemic attacks, intellectual deterioration, or both (Smith *et al.* 1985; Yong *et al.* 1992; Greenberg *et al.* 1993). A record of long-standing hypertension indicates small vessel disease as the most probable underlying condition in a patient with a haematoma in the basal ganglia or in the posterior fossa; on the other hand, hypertension is so common that it may co-exist with other conditions. If the patient is known to have had cancer, especially melanoma, bronchial carcinoma or renal carcinoma, haemorrhage into a brain metastasis is a strong possibility.

The presence of valvular heart disease in a patient with intracerebral haemorrhage must raise the suspicion of septic embolism, although this will not be the cause in the majority of those cases because infective endocarditis is such a rare disease, much rarer than many other causes of intracerebral haemorrhage, such as cerebral amyloid angiopathy. If haemorrhages *at other sites*, such as in the skin, have preceded the haemorrhagic stroke, a disorder of haemostasis is almost too obvious to be missed.

The use of oral anticoagulants is a vital piece of information in patients with intracerebral haemorrhage because, in consultation with the cardiologists, their action should probably be neutralized as soon as possible by intravenous prothrombin complex concentrate and vitamin K (section 12.2.4). It is equally important to know about the use of recreational drugs, particularly cocaine and amphetamines; this information may be withheld for weeks (Heye & Hankey 1996). Finally, the circumstances preceding intracerebral haemorrhage may contribute to identifying its cause: an earlier phase of the illness with a dense neurological deficit (haemorrhagic transformation of an infarct), puerperium (intracranial venous thrombosis, choriocarcinoma), or neck trauma (dissection of the vertebral or carotid artery). In any patient with haemophilia, a 'stroke', unexplained sudden coma or severe headache signifies intracranial bleeding until proved otherwise.

8.8 Clues from the examination

8.8.1 General examination

The general examination provides rather few clues to the cause of an intracerebral haemorrhage, with the exception of petechiae or bruising, indicating a generalized haemostatic disorder, signs of malignant disease (such as cutaneous melanoma), a collapsed lung or enlargement of the liver or spleen, or telangiectasias in the skin and mucous membranes. Auscultating the skull for detecting arteriovenous malformations is useful for impressing naïve readers of textbooks as well as medical students and patients, but is not very rewarding. (We are still waiting for someone, who had no other clues and only by auscultation diagnosed an arteriovenous malformation in an adult, to take up our offer of a free copy of this book.) Cardiac dysrhythmias may reflect compression of the brainstem, especially in patients with an impaired level of consciousness (Stober *et al.* 1988). Finding hypertension on admission is the rule, but only in about one-half of these patients is this a contributing factor (section 8.3.1). In the others it is merely a reactive phenomenon (section 15.7.1). Signs of hypertensive vascular changes in the retina or enlargement of the heart on palpation or percussion will allow the identification of hypertension as a contributing factor, but absence of arteriolar thickening on fundoscopy does not exclude it. Subhyaloid haemorrhages indicate intracranial bleeding in general, most often subarachnoid haemorrhage (Keane 1979) (Fig. 5.43). Heart murmurs may be coincidental but should at least raise the possibility of infective endocarditis as a cause of intracerebral haemorrhage, as should finding needle marks in possible drug addicts.

8.8.2 Neurological examination

The clinical manifestations of intracerebral haemorrhage almost always include focal deficits, with or without a decreased level of consciousness. Coma or a lesser degree of obtundation in general is a non-localizing feature, except with haemorrhages in the posterior fossa.

A *decreased level of consciousness* is one of the classic features of intracerebral haemorrhage as taught to medical students, but it is absent in a sizeable proportion of patients (section 5.3.1). Given that infarcts are four times as common as haemorrhages, and on the assumption that half the patients with intracerebral haemorrhage have a normal level of consciousness along with all those with infarcts, it follows that if the distinction is based only on the level of consciousness, one out of nine times an infarct is diagnosed in a conscious patient it will in fact be an intracerebral haemorrhage. A secondary decrease in the level of consciousness after admission, which occurs in about one-third of all patients, may result from actual enlargement of the haematoma, but also from the formation of oedema around an already large haematoma (especially if the deterioration occurs after 48 h), from obstructive hydrocephalus with posterior fossa haematoma (Fujii *et al.* 1994; Mayer *et al.* 1994; Zazulia *et al.* 1999), or from a medical complication, such as hyponatraemia or neurogenic pulmonary oedema (section 13.10).

The *focal deficits* in intracerebral haemorrhage are determined by the site and size of the haematoma. The pace at which these negative symptoms develop is usually a matter of seconds or minutes, rarely of hours. Rapid resolution of deficits generally indicates ischaemia rather than haemorrhage, but not invariably (Gunatilake 1998).

Table 8.4 lists the variety of clinical syndromes and corresponding locations. Some general comments are appropriate. With thalamic haemorrhages, the nature of the deficits depends on the location within the thalamus, as this conglomerate of nuclei has connections with almost every part of the cerebral cortex. Caudate haemorrhages may produce few focal deficits but a predominance of general symptoms (headache, vomiting and a decrease in the level of consciousness) by rapid extension of the bleed into the ventricular system; these features may mimic subarachnoid haemorrhage (Stein *et al.* 1984). All haemorrhages in the posterior fossa may be complicated by obstructive hydrocephalus, whether in the cerebellum (Gerritsen van der Hoop *et al.* 1988), midbrain (Sand *et al.* 1986) or pons (Masiyama *et al.* 1985). The prognosis of haemorrhages in the pons is not always as bleak as was believed before the CT scan era, when the diag-

Table 8.4 Syndromes of primary intracerebral haemorrhage with corresponding locations. The structure of the table is hierarchical (a given clinical feature will not again be mentioned if that feature appears as a separate heading higher in the table) and parsimonious (combinations of syndromes are possible but have not been separately listed).

Coma
With tetraparesis and lateral gaze palsies: pons (Kushner & Bressman 1985; Masiyama *et al.* 1985; Chung & Park 1992; Murata *et al.* 1999)
With hemiparesis and pupillary abnormalities: posteromedial thalamus (Kawahara *et al.* 1986; Chung *et al.* 1996)
Preceded by vertigo and inability to stand: cerebellum

Hemiparesis
In isolation: frontal lobe (Weisberg & Stazio 1988), putamen (Kim *et al.* 1994; Mori *et al.* 1985) or internal capsule (Kim *et al.* 1994; Mori *et al.* 1985)
Weakness predominating in face and tongue (Kim 1995) or in the arm (Ropper & Davis 1980): frontal lobe
With ipsilateral ataxia: precentral cortex (Tjeerdsma *et al.* 1996), internal capsule; (Kim *et al.* 1994; Mori *et al.* 1985), putamen (Kim *et al.* 1994), unilateral base of pons (Mori *et al.* 1985)
With conjugate deviation to non-paretic side: frontal white matter, putamen or caudate nucleus (Stein *et al.* 1984; Waga *et al.* 1986)
With dysphasia: frontal white matter or putamen of dominant hemisphere (D'Esposito & Alexander 1995)
With hemisensory loss: putamen (Kim *et al.* 1994; Mori *et al.* 1985), internal capsule (Kim *et al.* 1994; Mori *et al.* 1985), dorsal thalamus (Kim *et al.* 1994; Kumral *et al.* 1995; Chung *et al.* 1996) or pons (Mori *et al.* 1985)
With hemisensory loss and dysphasia/neglect (with or without abnormalities of gaze or pupils): posterolateral thalamus (Hirose *et al.* 1985; Kawahara *et al.* 1986; Kumral *et al.* 1995; Chung *et al.* 1996)
With palatal weakness, nystagmus, ipsilateral Horner's syndrome, hypoglossal palsy or cerebellar ataxia: medulla (Barinagarrementeria & Cantú 1994)

Hemisensory loss
In isolation: parietal lobe (Ropper & Davis 1980), internal capsule (Kim *et al.* 1994), midbrain (Tuttle & Reinmuth 1984; Azouvi *et al.* 1989), dorsal pontine tegmentum (Kim *et al.* 1994; Kim & Bae 1997)
Limited to hand and corner of mouth (cheiro-oral syndrome): midbrain tegmentum (Ono & Inoue 1985)
Limited to hand and neck: cheiroretroauricular syndrome: pontine tegmentum (Ferro & Pierre 1998)
With hemiataxia: thalamus (Tatu *et al.* 1996)

Aphasia
Non-fluent: putamen (D'Esposito & Alexander 1995) or caudate nucleus (Kumral *et al.* 1999) of dominant hemisphere
Fluent: posterior temporal lobe of dominant hemisphere (Ropper & Davis 1980; Weisberg *et al.* 1991b)

Hemianopia
Occipital lobe (Ropper & Davis 1980)

Acute behavioural disorder
Posterior temporal lobe of non-dominant hemisphere (Weisberg *et al.* 1991b), anterior thalamus (Chung *et al.* 1996)
With neglect: caudate nucleus of non-dominant hemisphere (D'Esposito & Alexander 1995)

Involuntary movements
Chorea: putamen (Jones *et al.* 1985)

Ataxia
With vertigo: cerebellum (with or without dysarthria, horizontal gaze palsy, facial palsy) (Dunne *et al.* 1987; Kim *et al.* 1994)
With palatal weakness, nystagmus, ipsilateral Horner's syndrome or hypoglossal palsy: medulla (Barinagarrementeria & Cantú 1994)

Oculomotor disorders
Horizontal gaze palsy, unilateral: ventral pontine tegmentum (Kushner & Bressman 1985; Chung & Park 1992)
Horizontal gaze palsy, bilateral: ventral pontine tegmentum (Chung & Park 1992)
Horizontal gaze palsy, unilateral, with contralateral internuclear ophthalmoplegia ('one-and-a-half syndrome'): ventral pontine tegmentum (Fisher 1967; Nakajima 1983)
Upward gaze palsy (with or without Horner's syndrome, IVth nerve palsy): tectum of midbrain (Sand *et al.* 1986)
Total ophthalmoplegia, bilaterally: midbrain tegmentum (Worthington & Halmagyi 1996)
IIIrd nerve palsy, bilaterally: midbrain tegmentum (Getenet *et al.* 1994)
IIIrd nerve palsy, unilaterally, with pupillary involvement: midbrain tegmentum (Shuaib & Murphy 1987) or without (Shuaib & Murphy 1987; Shuaib *et al.* 1989)
Ptosis, bilaterally: midbrain tegmentum (de Mendonca et al. 1990)
Palsy of pupillary constriction, unilaterally: midbrain tegmentum (Shuaib *et al.* 1989)
IVth nerve palsy, bilaterally: midbrain tegmentum (Dussaux *et al.* 1990)

Cranial nerve deficits (other than oculomotor)
Bilateral deafness: pons (Egan *et al.* 1996)

nosis was made only in fatal cases; in prospective series from primary referral centres, the rate of survival is around 40% (Kushner & Bressman 1985; Masiyama *et al.* 1985; Wijdicks & St Louis 1997). In fact, small haemorrhages in the pons, midbrain, thalamus and internal capsule may cause the well-known 'lacunar syndromes', in these cases being caused by small deep haemorrhages rather than by small deep infarcts (Kim *et al.* 1994) (section 4.3.2).

The relative probabilities of intracerebral haemorrhage occurring in the locations shown in Table 8.4 are estimated in Table 8.5. The proportions in this table are only an approximation of the truth, for two reasons. The first is that population-based studies, although unbiased, contain a small proportion of patients with haemorrhages, in which subdivisions are subject to chance effects. Large hospital-based series, on the other hand, suffer from bias in that referral to hospital is less often considered in the case of moribund patients or, at the other extreme, with patients who have only very mild deficits.

8.9 Investigations

8.9.1 Laboratory studies

Routine laboratory investigations (section 6.7.1) should not be forgotten from the point of view of general medical management, but they will seldom uncover the cause of intracerebral haemorrhage (e.g. massive liver damage).

Abnormalities of haemostasis may have contributed to the development of intracerebral haemorrhage, although it should be reiterated that identified and possible causes are not necessarily the only or even the true cause in an individual patient. None the less, haemostatic factors should be considered in every patient with intracerebral haemorrhage. Sometimes the relationship is obvious, such as if the patient is on anticoagulants, but, in other instances, the relationship may be more indirect, such as the haemostatic defect in renal failure. If intracerebral haemorrhage is related to a disorder of haemostasis, this is usually because of impaired clotting, i.e. the secondary phase of haemostasis, which is dependent on adequate levels of coagulation factors. Abnormalities of primary haemostasis have to do with defects of platelet aggregation or from thrombocytopenia; most commonly these result in haemorrhages in the skin and mucous membranes, and much more rarely in haemorrhages in organs such as the brain. The overview of the Antiplatelet Trialists' Collaboration (1994), discussed earlier in section 8.4.2, found an increased rate of intracerebral haemorrhage in patients on antiplatelet drugs, but in absolute terms the excess risk is very small.

The most important screening test of primary haemostatic function is the platelet count. Thrombocytopenia precipitates intracerebral haemorrhage only with values under 20×10^9/L but a normal platelet count is reassuring only if platelet function is normal. If this is uncertain, for example with renal failure or the presence of antiplatelet antibodies, determination of the bleeding time may be helpful, despite its broad normal range. The clotting system (coagulation factors) can be assessed with the partial thromboplastin time, the prothrombin time, the thrombin time or, preferably, the international normalized ratio. Circulating antibodies (usually of the IgG class) may impair the activity of specific coagulation factors (inhibitor syndromes); they develop especially in patients with factor VIII or IX deficiency who have received multiple plasma infusions, but also with autoimmune diseases or in patients being treated with penicillin or streptomycin. Appropriate tests can uncover these specific autoantibodies.

If infective endocarditis is suspected, the diagnosis may be supported by a high erythrocyte sedimentation rate, or C-reactive protein, and blood cultures should also be taken. Leukocytosis up to $12\,500 \times 10^9$/L may result from the intracerebral haemorrhage itself, especially when it is large (Suzuki *et al.* 1995).

Table 8.5 Approximate frequency of the different locations of primary intracerebral haemorrhage.

Location of haemorrhage	Frequency (%)
Putamen or internal capsule	30
Lobar*	30
Thalamus†	15
Cerebellum	10
Entire basal ganglia region	5
Caudate nucleus‡	5
Pons§ or midbrain	5

* Anderson *et al.* 1994; † Kawahara *et al.* 1986; ‡ Stein *et al.* 1984; § Nakajima 1983.

Other sources were the following, all being large (>100 patients) and consecutive hospital series: Schütz *et al.* 1990; Kase *et al.* 1998.

8.9.2 CT scanning of the brain

This is the most important single investigation in patients with suspected intracerebral haematomas. Because of its sensitivity in the recognition of intracerebral blood (section 5.3.4), CT scanning has led to an increased frequency of the diagnosis of intracerebral haemorrhage (Drury *et al.* 1984). The location of the haematoma may to some extent indicate the underlying cause (Figs 8.16–8.19) (Table 8.3). Intraventricular extension of the haemorrhage occurs relatively often with deep haematomas associated with rupture of damaged perforating arteries (section 8.2.1) and carries a relatively poor prognosis, depending on the volume of intraventricular blood (Tuhrim *et al.* 1999). The presence of a fluid-blood level strongly suggests an underlying coagulopathy, either iatrogenic or as a result of haematological disease (Pfleger *et al.* 1994); a fixed clot with a horizontal border may falsely suggest a disorder of coagulation, a problem which can be resolved by repositioning the patient. A grossly irregular margin of a lobar haematoma suggests cerebral amyloid angiopathy, as does extension through the cortex with

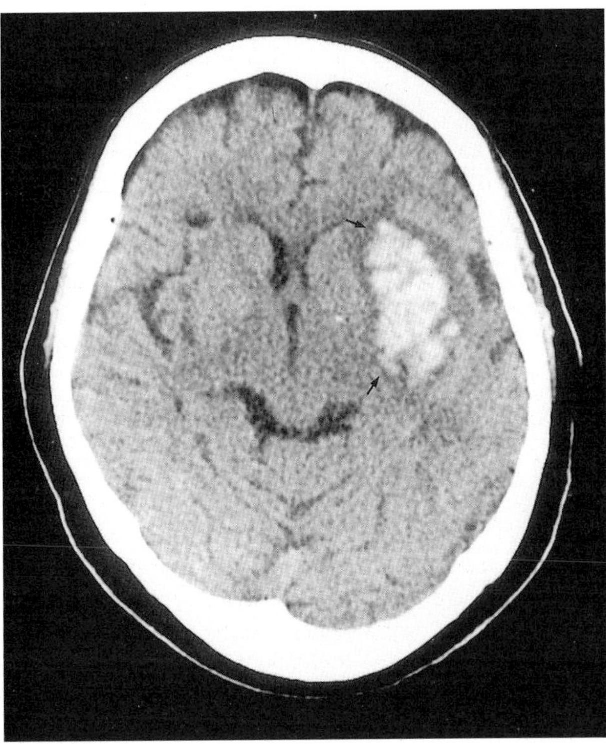

(a)

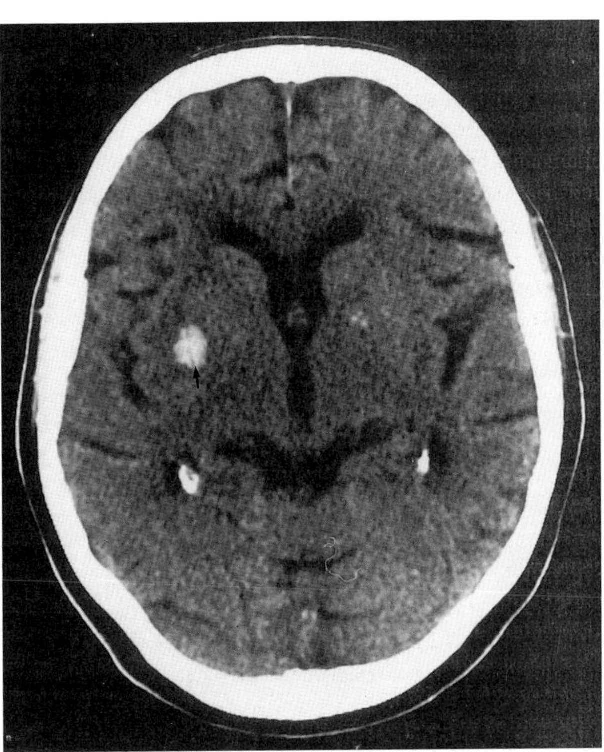

(b)

Fig. 8.16 (a) CT brain scan showing a large haemorrhage in the left basal ganglia (arrows). (b) CT brain scan showing a small haemorrhage in the right internal capsule (arrow).

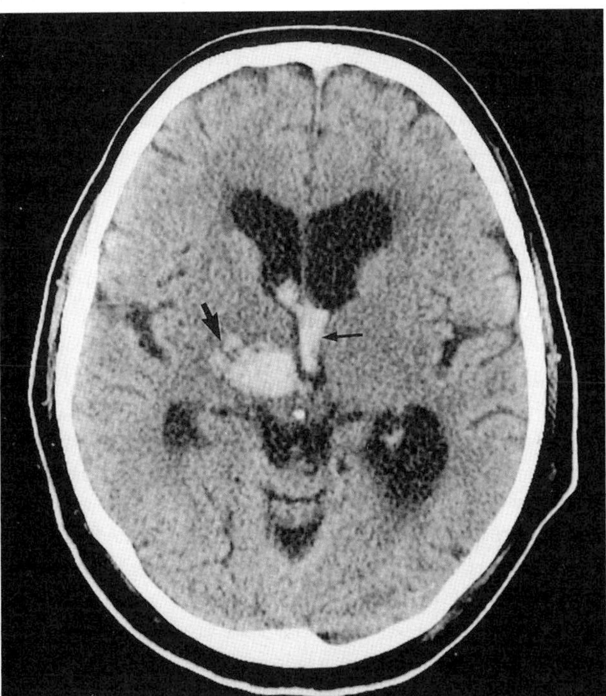

Fig. 8.17 CT brain scan showing a haemorrhage in the right thalamus (thick arrow), with rupture into the third ventricle (thin arrow), resulting in obstructive hydrocephalus with dilatation of the lateral ventricles.

rupture into the subarachnoid space and co-existence of petechial haemorrhages in the cortical or subcortical region (Greenberg *et al.* 1996; Miller *et al.* 1999). If multiple or recurrent haemorrhages are identified on CT (Table 8.2), this should raise the possibility of cerebral amyloid angiopathy in the case of lobar haemorrhages in an elderly patient (Fig. 8.7); of intracranial venous thrombosis if the irregular shape and parasagittal or temporal location suggest infarction as a result of venous congestion, with haemorrhagic transformation (Fig. 8.13); or of metastases if there is a history of malignant disease. A markedly hypodense rim around the clot indicates severe hyperlipidaemia (Hilz *et al.* 1989).

Repeat brain CT before and after injection of contrast may be essential for picking up underlying lesions, such as tumours, arteriovenous malformations or cavernous angiomas. These can be most easily identified weeks or months later, at a stage when the lesion is no longer obscured by mass effect and the haemorrhage has at least partially resolved.

8.9.3 Magnetic resonance imaging

Intraparenchymal haemorrhages can be detected by magnetic resonance imaging (MRI) even a few hours after onset, but special sequences are necessary for an unequivocal diagnosis (Patel *et al.* 1996). MR scanning is especially useful for the demonstration of associated vascular anomalies in patients

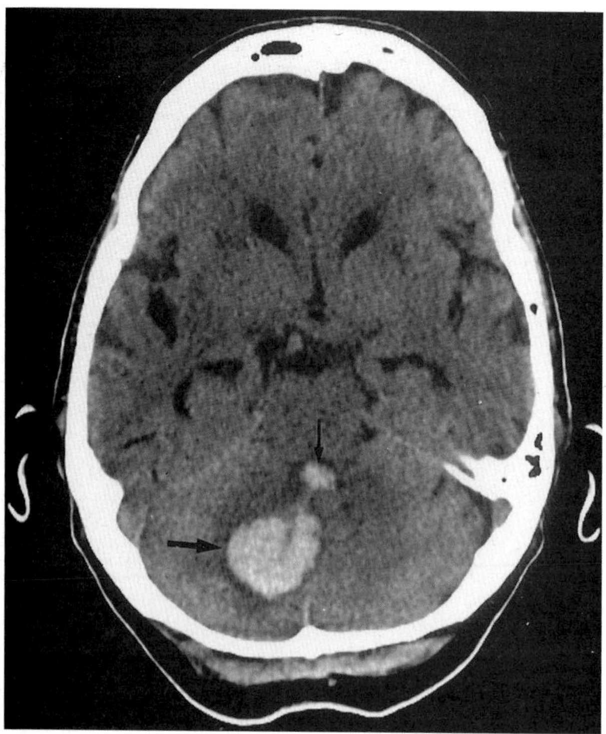

(a)

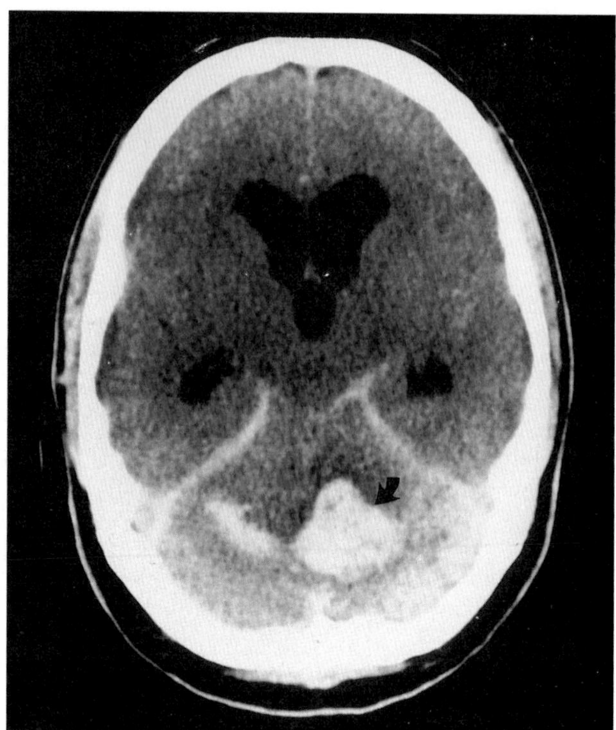

(b)

Fig. 8.18 (a) CT brain scan showing a haemorrhage in the right cerebellar hemisphere (thick arrow), with rupture into the fourth ventricle (thin arrow). (b) CT brain scan showing a large haemorrhage in the left cerebellar hemisphere (arrow) and vermis (and smaller haemorrhage in right cerebellar hemisphere), with compression of the fourth ventricle and obstructive hydrocephalus.

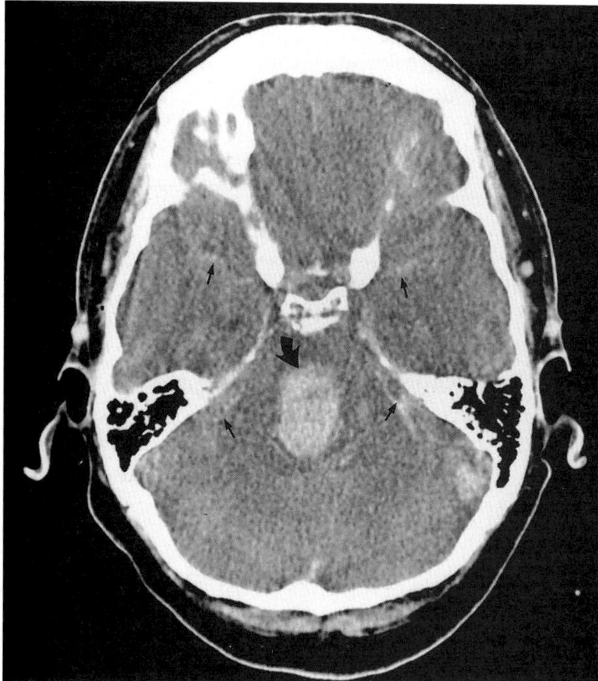

Fig. 8.19 CT scan showing a primary haemorrhage in the pons (thick arrow), with some blood being visible in the subarachnoid space (thin arrows) through rupture into the fourth ventricle (not visible).

with intracerebral haemorrhage (section 5.3.7). As flowing blood is not susceptible in the same way as brain tissue to the changes induced by strong magnetic fields, vascular channels appear as strongly hypointense, 'empty' regions ('signal voids'), representing flowing blood (Figs 8.11 and 8.20). MR scanning can in this way identify arteriovenous malformations and sometimes even saccular aneurysms. Cavernous angiomas are best detected with a gradient echo technique (Brunereau *et al.* 2000). Signs of congestion of pial vessels suggest a dural fistula draining into cortical veins, although most such anomalies communicate with dural sinuses (Willinsky *et al.* 1994) (section 8.2.8). Dedicated techniques for demonstrating moving blood (MR angiography) are even more sensitive for the detection of vascular lesions than MR techniques for structural brain imaging (for aneurysms, see section 9.4.2) (Atlas 1997). The developments of this technique are so rapid that eventually it may replace catheter angiography.

Acute intra-arterial thrombus can be identified through hyperintensity on proton density imaging, whereas on T2-weighted images the thrombus is hypointense and so at that stage cannot be distinguished from flow voids (Mead & Wardlaw 1998) (Fig. 5.28). If intracranial venous thrombosis is suspected as a cause of intracerebral haemorrhage, MRI is a useful tool in showing evidence of thrombi within dural sinuses, but again the abnormalities are time-dependent

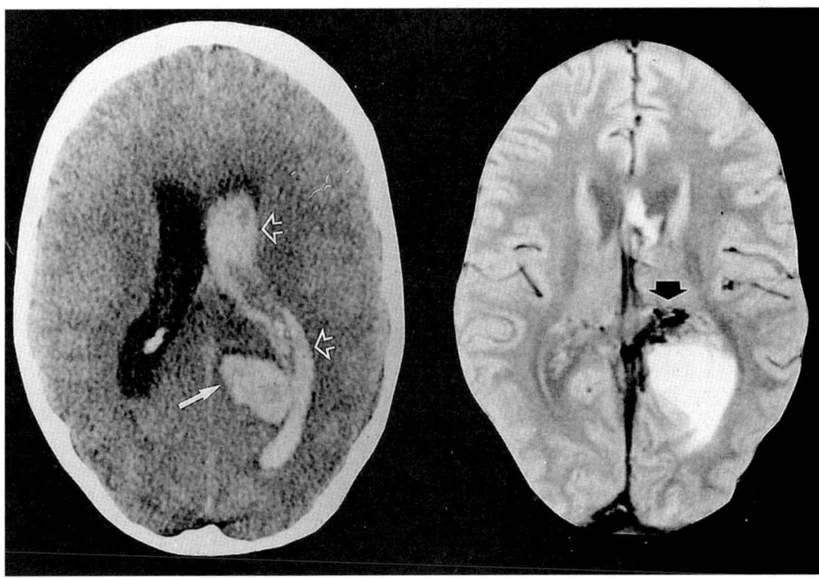

Fig. 8.20 Intracerebral haemorrhage from an arteriovenous malformation. Left: CT brain scan showing a haematoma in the medial part of the left occipital lobe (arrow), with rupture into the left lateral ventricle (open arrows). Right: MR scan (T1-weighted image) shows signal void (black arrow) from the malformation and a large draining vein.

(Isensee *et al.* 1994). In the acute stage (days 1–5), the thrombus appears isointense on T1-weighted images and strongly hypointense on T2-weighted images; in the subacute stage (up to day 15) the thrombus signal is strongly hyperintense on T1- as well as on T2-weighted images; and after the third week the thrombus signal is decreased on all sequences, until normal blood flow is restored (Fig. 5.40).

8.9.4 Cerebral catheter angiography

Introducing a catheter into a peripheral (usually the femoral) artery and guiding it through the aorta to the extracranial vessels and then injecting radio-opaque fluid is not without risk in patients with ischaemic cerebrovascular disease (Hankey *et al.* 1990; Cloft *et al.* 1999) (section 6.7.4). Arterial dissection and contrast hypersensitivity are amongst the greatest dangers. None the less, in patients with intracerebral haemorrhage, catheter angiography is still often indicated to detect underlying vascular lesions that are amenable to specific treatment, particularly arteriovenous malformations, saccular aneurysms and intracranial venous thrombosis (in the last case, only if MR studies are inconclusive). This applies essentially to all patients under 50 years with intracerebral haemorrhage, provided they are fit for surgery. Angiography is especially indicated if the pattern of haemorrhage is compatible with a saccular aneurysm (Griffiths *et al.* 1997). In that situation the angiogram should be performed as quickly as possible, preferably preceded by CT angiography, which may obviate the need for an angiogram (section 9.4.3). Catheter angiography is also needed if MR scanning shows 'flow voids' phenomena consistent with an arteriovenous malformation. The proportion of underlying vascular abnormalities identified by angiography is much greater in normotensive patients with lobar haemorrhages than in deep, 'hypertensive' haemorrhages, especially if there is associated haemorrhage in the subarachnoid space (Toffol *et al.* 1986; Loes *et al.* 1987).

In any patient with intracerebral haemorrhage who is fit for surgery, cerebral catheter angiography should at least be considered, with a view to detecting surgically treatable lesions, particularly saccular aneurysms and arteriovenous malformations. The indication is stronger if the patient is under the age of about 50 years, if the haemorrhage is lobar rather than in the deep regions of the brain, and if the patient is not hypertensive.

The indications for catheter angiography are less clear in patients without any clues to indicate a treatable lesion. It has often been assumed that the probability of finding such a lesion is low in patients over 65 years and in patients with pre-existing hypertension or with haemorrhage in the basal ganglia or the posterior fossa. A unique and prospective study assessed the value of angiography in 42 such 'low-yield' patients, and came up with a surprising number of lesions: eight arteriovenous malformations and two aneurysms (24%; 95% CI, 12–40%) (Halpin *et al.* 1994). The proportion with an angiographically demonstrable lesion was much higher (84%) in a parallel group of 38 patients with lobar haemorrhage who were also relatively young (below a mean of 46 years) and not hypertensive but, conversely, there was still a fair proportion of positive angiograms in the presence of any of the 'negative predictors': 31% in patients above the mean age of 46 years, 13% in those with hypertension, 31% of patients with haemorrhage in the basal ganglia and 18% of those with posterior fossa haemorrhage (McCormick & Rosenfield 1973).

Another study confirmed that normotensive patients under 45 years with deep haemorrhages had angiographic lesions in more than 50% (Zhu *et al.* 1997). Even the combination of high blood pressure and age above the mean was found to be associated with a structural lesion on angiography in 12% (Halpin *et al.* 1994). In summary, the chance of finding a treatable lesion on angiography is greatest in patients with the combined characteristics of age under about 45 years, no history of hypertension, and lobar location. The chance of finding a treatable lesion is progressively lower if one or more of these three features is absent, but a relatively high age should not deter the physician if an aneurysm is suspected; also CT angiography may be useful as an intermediate step (section 9.4.3).

Angiography in search of a vascular anomaly rarely needs to be urgent, because with most lesions re-bleeding occurs only after months or years, if at all. The one and only important exception is when the site of the haematoma suggests a saccular aneurysm. As the sensitivity of MR or CT angiography increases, the need for catheter angiography may disappear, at least for this particular indication. Repeating angiography weeks or months after a negative first study may still uncover small arteriovenous malformations in 10–20%, presumably because in the acute stage the lesion was being compressed by mass effect from the haematoma (Willinsky *et al.* 1993; Halpin *et al.* 1994; Hino *et al.* 1998).

8.10 Primary subdural haematoma

Subdural haematomas without attendant haemorrhage in the subarachnoid space or in the brain parenchyma are traditionally associated with trauma, but they can also occur 'spontaneously' (or, one might speculate, with trauma that is too trivial to be remembered). Although these haematomas are not intraparenchymal, they are still included in this chapter because most of their many possible causes overlap with those of intracerebral haemorrhage (Table 8.6). Anticoagulants are the most common precipitant in urbanized areas of Western Europe, accounting for approximately 25% of all subdural haematomas and 50% of those without obvious trauma (Wintzen & Tijssen 1982). In anticoagulant-associated subdural haematoma, the onset may be very acute and even lethal (Wintzen 1980). In those cases, rapid correction of the coagulation status is mandatory (sections 8.4.1 and 12.2.4), usually followed by craniotomy. A ruptured small pial artery is probably the next most common cause, and sometimes angiography shows the extravasation from a small artery at the surface of the brain into the subdural space (Yasui *et al.* 1995).

If the level of consciousness remains normal, spontaneous resolution may occur, even after an acute onset (Aoki 1990; Kulah *et al.* 1992). On the other hand, patients in whom the onset of symptoms is over days or weeks, and where the haematoma presumably originates from a bridging vein (Wintzen 1980), may deteriorate rather suddenly (Aoki & Tsutsumi 1990). Some chronic subdural haematomas may present with acute headache, mimicking subarachnoid haemorrhage (SAH) (Kotwica & Brzezinski 1985). Most spontaneous subdural haematomas occur over the convexity of the cerebral hemisphere, but they may also be found in the interhemispheric fissure, as a rule with aneurysms (Friedman & Brant Zawadzki 1983; Houtteville *et al.* 1988), or in the posterior fossa (Kanter *et al.* 1984).

A subdural haematoma may also occur together with an intraparenchymal haematoma, from degenerative small vessel disease (Arai 1983; Avis 1993) or an arteriovenous malformation (Ezura & Kagawa 1992), or with SAH, in which case the aneurysmal origin should be obvious (section 9.4.1).

Table 8.6 Causes of spontaneous subdural haematomas without associated intracerebral haemorrhage or subarachnoid haemorrhage.

Rupture of a small pial artery (McDermott *et al.* 1984; Stephenson & Gibson 1989; Bongioanni *et al.* 1991; Borzone *et al.* 1993; Yasui *et al.* 1995)
Saccular aneurysm of major intracerebral artery (Rengachary & Szymanski 1981; Williams *et al.* 1983; O'Leary & Sweeny 1986; Kondziolka *et al.* 1988; Ragland *et al.* 1993)
Arteriovenous malformation (Rengachary & Szymanski 1981; Oikawa *et al.* 1993)
Intracavernous aneurysm of the carotid artery (Hodes *et al.* 1988; McLaughlin *et al.* 1996)
Aneurysm of middle meningeal artery (Korosue *et al.* 1988)
Moyamoya syndrome (Oppenheim *et al.* 1991)
Autosomal dominant polycystic kidney disease (Wijdicks *et al.* 2000)
Anticoagulant treatment (Wintzen & Tijssen 1982)
Thrombolytic treatment (Gore *et al.* 1991; Uglietta *et al.* 1991)
Coagulation defects, also in children (Shih *et al.* 1993)
Dural metastasis (Rothschild & Maxeiner 1990); this may also cause epidural haematoma (Anegawa *et al.* 1989)
Lumbar puncture (Hart *et al.* 1988; Vos *et al.* 1991)

References

Please note that all references taken from *The Cochrane Library* are given a current date as this database is updated on a quarterly basis. Please refer to the current *Cochrane Library* article for the latest review. The same applies to the *British Medical Journal* 'Clinical Evidence' series which is updated every six months.

Adams, H.P. Jr, Dawson, G., Coffman, T.J. & Corry, R.J. (1986) Stroke in renal transplant recipients. *Archives of Neurology* 43, 113–115.

Adams, R.D. & vander Eecken, H.M. (1953) Vascular diseases of the brain. *Annual Review of Medicine* 4, 213–252.

Aggarwal, S.K., Williams, V., Levine, S.R., Cassin, B.J. & Garcia, J.H. (1996) Cocaine-associated intracranial hemorrhage: absence of vasculitis in 14 cases. *Neurology* 46, 1741–1743.

Ahola, D.T., Provenzale, J.M. & Longee, D.C. (1998) Metastatic rhabdomyosarcoma presenting as intracranial hemorrhage: imaging findings. *European Journal of Radiology* **26**, 241–243.

Alonzo, N.C., Hyman, B.T., Rebeck, G.W. & Greenberg, S.M. (1998) Progression of cerebral amyloid angiopathy: accumulation of amyloid-b40 in affected vessels. *Journal of Neuropathology and Experimental Neurology* **57**, 353–359.

Amico, L., Caplan, L.R. & Thomas, C. (1989) Cerebrovascular complications of mucinous cancers. *Neurology* **39**, 522–526.

Amin-Hanjani, S., Robertson, R., Arginteanu, M.S. & Scott, R.M. (1998) Familial intracranial arteriovenous malformations: case report and review of the literature. *Pediatric Neurosurgery* **29**, 208–213.

Aminoff, M.J. (1973) Vascular anomalies in the intracranial dura mater. *Brain* **96**, 601–612.

Aminoff, M.J. (1987) Treatment of unruptured cerebral arteriovenous malformations. *Neurology* **37**, 815–819.

Anderson, C.S., Chakera, T.M., Stewart Wynne, E.G. & Jamrozik, K.D. (1994) Spectrum of primary intracerebral haemorrhage in Perth, Western Australia, 1989–90: incidence and outcome. *Journal of Neurology, Neurosurgery and Psychiatry* **57**, 936–940.

Anderson, J.L., Karagounis, L., Allen, A., Bradford, M.J., Menlove, R.L. & Pryor, T.A. (1991) Older age and elevated blood pressure are risk factors for intracerebral hemorrhage after thrombolysis. *American Journal of Cardiology* **68**, 166–170.

Andes, W.A. & Wulff, K. (1990) Intracranial hemorrhage in hemophiliacs with AIDS [letter]. *Thrombosis and Haemostasis* **63**, 326.

Anegawa, S., Hirohata, S., Tokutomi, T. & Kuramoto, S. (1989) Spontaneous epidural hematoma secondary to dural metastasis from an ovarian carcinoma: case report. *Neurologia Medico-Chirurgica (Tokyo)* **29**, 854–856.

d'Angelo, V.A., Monte, V., Scialfa, G., Fiumara, E. & Scotti, G. (1988) Intracerebral venous hemorrhage in 'high-risk' carotid-cavernous fistula. *Surgical Neurology* **30**, 387–390.

Antiplatelet Trialists' Collaboration (1994) Collaborative overview of randomised trials of antiplatelet therapy. I. Prevention of death, myocardial infarction and stroke by prolonged antiplatelet therapy in various categories of patients. *British Medical Journal* **308**, 81–106.

Aoki, N. (1990) Acute subdural haematoma with rapid resolution. *Acta Neurochirurgica (Wien)* **103**, 76–78.

Aoki, N. (1991) Do intracranial arteriovenous malformations cause subarachnoid haemorrhage? Review of computed tomography features of ruptured arteriovenous malformations in the acute stage. *Acta Neurochirurgica (Wien)* **112**, 92–95.

Aoki, N. & Tsutsumi, K. (1990) Symptomatic subacute subdural haematoma following spontaneous acute subdural haematoma. *Acta Neurochirurgica (Wien)* **102**, 149–151.

Arai, H. (1983) Acute hypertensive subdural hematoma from arterial rupture shortly after the onset of cerebral subcortical hemorrhage: leakage of contrast medium during angiography. *Stroke* **14**, 281–285.

Arnautovic, K.I., Al-Mefty, O., Angtuaco, E. & Phares, L.J. (1998) Dural arteriovenous malformations of the transverse/sigmoid sinus acquired from dominant sinus occlusion by a tumor: report of two cases. *Neurosurgery* **42**, 383–388.

Atlas, S.W. (1997) Magnetic resonance imaging of intracranial aneurysms. *Neuroimaging Clinics of North America* **7**, 709–720.

Avis, S.P. (1993) Non-traumatic acute subdural hematoma: a case report and review of the literature. *American Journal of Forensic Medicine and Pathology* **14**, 130–134.

Awad, I.A., Little, J.R., Akarawi, W.P. & Ahl, J. (1990) Intracranial dural arteriovenous malformations: factors predisposing to an aggressive neurological course. *Journal of Neurosurgery* **72**, 839–850.

Awad, I.A., Robinson, J.R. Jr, Mohanty, S. & Estes, M.L. (1993) Mixed vascular malformations of the brain: clinical and pathogenetic considerations. *Neurosurgery* **33**, 179–188.

Azouvi, P., Tougeron, A., Hussonois, C., Schouman Claeys, E., Bussel, B. & Held, J.P. (1989) Pure sensory stroke due to midbrain haemorrhage limited to the spinothalamic pathway. *Journal of Neurology, Neurosurgery and Psychiatry* **52**, 1427–1428.

Babikian, V.L., Kase, C.S., Pessin, M.S., Norrving, B. & Gorelick, P.B. (1989) Intracerebral hemorrhage in stroke patients anticoagulated with heparin. *Stroke* **20**, 1500–1503.

Bae, H.G., Jeong, D.S., Doh, J.W., Lee, K.S., Yun, I.G. & Byun, B.J. (1999) Recurrence of bleeding in patients with hypertensive intracerebral hemorrhage. *Cerebrovascular Diseases* **9**, 102–108.

Bahemuka, M. (1987) Primary intracerebral hemorrhage and heart weight: a clinicopathologic case–control review of 218 patients. *Stroke* **18**, 531–536.

Bamford, J., Sandercock, P., Dennis, M. *et al.* (1988) A prospective study of acute cerebrovascular disease in the community: the Oxfordshire Community Stroke Project 1981–86. 1. Methodology, demography and incident cases of first-ever stroke. *Journal of Neurology, Neurosurgery and Psychiatry* **51**, 1373–1380.

Barbas, N., Caplan, L., Baquis, G., Adelman, L. & Moskowitz, M. (1987) Dental chair intracerebral hemorrhage. *Neurology* **37**, 511–512.

Barinagarrementeria, F. & Cantú, C. (1994) Primary medullary hemorrhage: report of four cases and review of the literature. *Stroke* **25**, 1684–1687.

Biller, J., Loftus, C.M., Moore, S.A., Schelper, R.L., Danks, K.R. & Cornell, S.H. (1987) Isolated central nervous system angiitis first presenting as spontaneous intracranial hemorrhage. *Neurosurgery* **20**, 310–315.

Bogousslavsky, J., Regli, F., Uske, A. & Maeder, P. (1991) Early spontaneous hematoma in cerebral infarct: is primary cerebral hemorrhage overdiagnosed? *Neurology* **41**, 837–840.

Bollinger, O. (1891) Über traumatische Spät-Apoplexie: ein Beitrag zur Lehre von der Hirnerschütterung. In: *Festschrift, Rudolf Virchow Gewidmed Zur Vollendung Seines 70en Lebensjahres,* pp. 457–470. Hirschwald, Berlin [in German].

Bongioanni, F., Ramadan, A., Kostli, A. & Berney, J. (1991) [Acute subdural hematoma of arteriolar origin. Traumatic or spontaneous?] L'Hématome sous-dural aigu d'origine arteriolaire. Traumatique ou spontane? *Neurochirurgie* **37**, 26–31 [in French].

Bornebroek, M., Haan, J., van Duinen, S.G. *et al.* (1997) Dutch hereditary cerebral amyloid angiopathy: structural lesions and apolipoprotein E genotype. *Annals of Neurology* **41**, 695–698.

Borzone, M., Altomonte, M., Baldini, M. & Rivano, C. (1993) Pure subdural haematomas of arteriolar origin. *Acta Neurochirurgica (Wien)* **121**, 109–112.

Brisman, M.H., Bederson, J.B., Sen, C.N., Germano, I.M., Moore, F. & Post, K.D. (1996) Intracerebral hemorrhage occurring remote from the craniotomy site. *Neurosurgery* **39**, 1114–1121.

Broderick, J.P., Brott, T.G., Tomsick, T., Barsan, W. & Spilker, J. (1990) Ultra-early evaluation of intracerebral hemorrhage. *Journal of Neurosurgery* **72**, 195–199.

Broderick, J.P., Brott, T., Tomsick, T. & Leach, A. (1993a) Lobar hemorrhage in the elderly: the undiminishing importance of hypertension. *Stroke* **24**, 49–51.

Broderick, J.P., Brott, T., Tomsick, T., Miller, R. & Huster, G. (1993b) Intracerebral hemorrhage more than twice as common as subarachnoid hemorrhage. *Journal of Neurosurgery* **78**, 188–191.

Brott, T., Thalinger, K. & Hertzberg, V. (1986) Hypertension as a risk factor for spontaneous intracerebral hemorrhage. *Stroke* **17**, 1078–1083.

Brott, T., Broderick, J., Kothari, R. *et al.* (1997) Early hemorrhage growth in patients with intracerebral hemorrhage. *Stroke* **28**, 1–5.

Brown, R.D. Jr, Wiebers, D.O., Forbes, G. *et al.* (1988) The natural history of unruptured intracranial arteriovenous malformations. *Journal of Neurosurgery* **68**, 352–357.

Brown, R.D. Jr, Wiebers, D.O. & Forbes, G.S. (1990) Unruptured intracranial aneurysms and arteriovenous malformations: frequency of intracranial hemorrhage and relationship of lesions. *Journal of Neurosurgery* **73**, 859–863.

Brown, R.D. Jr, Wiebers, D.O. & Nichols, D.A. (1994) Intracranial dural arteriovenous fistulae: angiographic predictors of intracranial hemorrhage and clinical outcome in non-surgical patients. *Journal of Neurosurgery* **81**, 531–538.

Brown, R.D. Jr, Wiebers, D.O., Torner, J.C. & O'Fallon, W.M. (1996a) Frequency of intracranial hemorrhage as a presenting symptom and subtype analysis: a population-based study of intracranial vascular malformations in Olmsted County, Minnesota. *Journal of Neurosurgery* **85**, 29–32.

Brown, R.D. Jr, Wiebers, D.O., Torner, J.C. & O'Fallon, W.N. (1996b) Incidence and prevalence of intracranial vascular malformations in Olmsted County, Minnesota, 1965–92. *Neurology* **46**, 949–952.

Brunereau, L., Labauge, P., Tournier-Lasserve, E. *et al.* for the French Society of Neurosurgery (2000) Familial form of intracranial cavernous angioma: MR imaging findings in 51 families. *Radiology* **214**, 209–216.

Bruno, A., Adams, H.P. Jr, Biller, J., Rezai, K., Cornell, S. & Aschenbrener, C.A. (1988) Cerebral infarction due to moyamoya disease in young adults. *Stroke* **19**, 826–833.

Bruno, A., Nolte, K.B. & Chapin, J. (1993) Stroke associated with ephedrine use. *Neurology* **43**, 1313–1316.

Camargo, C.A. Jr (1989) Moderate alcohol consumption and stroke: the epidemiologic evidence. *Stroke* **20**, 1611–1626.

Cannegieter, S.C., Rosendaal, F.R., Wintzen, A.R., Van der Meer, F.J.M., Vandenbroucke, J.P. & Briët, E. (1995) Optimal oral anticoagulant therapy in patients with mechanical heart valves. *New England Journal of Medicine* **333**, 11–17.

Caplan, L. (1988) Intracerebral hemorrhage revisited. *Neurology* **38**, 624–627.

Caplan, L.R. (1994) Drugs. In: *Intracerebral Hemorrhage* (eds C.S. Kase & L.R. Caplan), pp. 201–220. Butterworth-Heinemann, Boston.

Caplan, L.R., Neely, S. & Gorelick, P. (1984) Cold-related intracerebral hemorrhage. *Archives of Neurology* **41**, 227.

Carlson, S.E., Aldrich, M.S., Greenberg, H.S. & Topol, E.J. (1988) Intracerebral hemorrhage complicating intravenous tissue plasminogen activator treatment. *Archives of Neurology* **45**, 1070–1073.

Cawley, C.M., Rigamonti, D. & Trommer, B. (1991) Dental chair apoplexy. *Southern Medical Journal* **84**, 907–909.

Challa, V.L., Moody, D.M. & Bell, M.A. (1992) The Charcot–Bouchard aneurysm controversy: impact of a new histologic technique. *Journal of Neuropathology and Experimental Neurology* **51**, 264–271.

Charcot, J.M. & Bouchard, C. (1868) Nouvelles recherches sur la pathogénie de l'hémorrhagie cérébrale. *Archives de Physiologie normale et Pathologique* **1**, 110–127; 643–665; 725–734 [in French].

Chaudhary, M.Y., Sachdev, V.P., Cho, S.H., Weitzner, I. Jr, Puljic, S. & Huang, Y.P. (1982) Dural arteriovenous malformation of the major venous sinuses: an acquired lesion. *American Journal of Neuroradiology* **3**, 13–19.

Chauveau, D., Sirieix, M.E., Schillinger, F., Legendre, C. & Grunfeld, J.P. (1990) Recurrent rupture of intracranial aneurysms in autosomal dominant polycystic kidney disease. *British Medical Journal* **301**, 966–967.

Chen, S.T., Chen, S.D., Hsu, C.Y. & Hogan, E.L. (1989) Progression of hypertensive intracerebral hemorrhage. *Neurology* **39**, 1509–1514.

Chen, S.T., Chiang, C.Y., Hsu, C.Y., Lee, T.H. & Tang, L.M. (1995) Recurrent hypertensive intracerebral hemorrhage. *Acta Neurologica Scandinavica* **91**, 128–132.

Chimowitz, M.I., Little, J.R., Awad, I.A., Sila, C.A., Kosmorsky, G. & Furlan, A.J. (1990) Intracranial hypertension associated with unruptured cerebral arteriovenous malformations. *Annals of Neurology* **27**, 474–479.

Chung, C.S. & Park, C.H. (1992) Primary pontine hemorrhage: a new CT classification. *Neurology* **42**, 830–834.

Chung, C.S., Caplan, L.R., Han, W.C., Pessin, M.S., Lee, K.H. & Kim, J.M. (1996) Thalamic haemorrhage. *Brain* **119**, 1873–1886.

Citron, B.P., Halpern, M., McCarron, M. *et al.* (1970) Necrotizing angiitis associated with drug abuse. *New England Journal of Medicine* **283**, 1003–1011.

Clifford Jones, R.E., Love, S. & Gurusinghe, N. (1985) Granulomatous angiitis of the central nervous system: a case with recurrent intracerebral haemorrhage. *Journal of Neurology, Neurosurgery and Psychiatry* **48**, 1054–1056.

Cloft, H.J., Joseph, G.J. & Dion, J.E. (1999) Risk of cerebral angiography in patients with subarachnoid hemorrhage, cerebral aneurysm and arteriovenous malformation: a meta-analysis. *Stroke* **30**, 317–320.

Cocito, L., Nizzo, R., Bisio, N. & Favale, E. (1994) Epileptic seizures heralding intracerebral hemorrhage [letter]. *Stroke* **25**, 2292–2293.

Cognard, C., Gobin, Y.P., Pierot, L. *et al.* (1995) Cerebral dural arteriovenous fistulas: clinical and angiographic correlation with a revised classification of venous drainage. *Radiology* **194**, 671–680.

Cognard, C., Casasco, A., Toevi, M., Houdart, E., Chiras, J. & Merland, J.J. (1998) Dural arteriovenous fistulas as a cause of intracranial hypertension due to impairment of cranial venous outflow. *Journal of Neurology, Neurosurgery and Psychiatry* **65**, 308–316.

Cole, A.J. & Aubé, M. (1990) Migraine with vasospasm and delayed intracerebral hemorrhage. *Archives of Neurology* **47**, 53–56.

Cole, F.M. & Yates, P.O. (1967a) The occurrence and significance of intracerebral micro-aneurysms. *Journal of Pathology and Bacteriology* **93**, 393–411.

Cole, F.M. & Yates, P. (1967b) Intracerebral microaneurysms and small cerebrovascular lesions. *Brain* **90**, 759–768.

Cole, F.M. & Yates, P.O. (1967c) Pseudo-aneurysms in relation to massive cerebral haemorrhage. *Journal of Neurology, Neurosurgery and Psychiatry* **30**, 61–66.

Comabella, M., Alvarez-Sabin, J., Rovira, A. & Codina, A. (1996) Bromocriptine and post-partum cerebral angiopathy: a causal relationship? *Neurology* **46**, 1754–1756.

Coria, F. & Rubio, I. (1996) Cerebral amyloid angiopathies. *Neuropathology and Applied Neurobiology* **22**, 216–227.

D'Esposito, M. & Alexander, M.P. (1995) Subcortical aphasia: distinct profiles following left putaminal hemorrhage. *Neurology* **45**, 38–41.

Davies, M.A., Terbrugge, K., Willinsky, R., Coyne, T., Saleh, J. & Wallace, M.C. (1996) The validity of classification for the clinical presentation of intracranial dural arteriovenous fistulas. *Journal of Neurosurgery* **85**, 830–837.

Dawson, I., van Bockel, J.H., Ferrari, M.D., van der Meer, F.J., Brand, R. & Terpstra, J.L. (1993) Ischemic and hemorrhagic stroke in patients on oral anticoagulants after reconstruction for chronic lower limb ischemia. *Stroke* **24**, 1655–1663.

DeJong, R.N. (1942) Delayed traumatic intracerebral hemorrhage. *Archives of Neurology and Psychiatry* **48**, 257–266.

Del Curling, O. Jr, Kelly, D.L. Jr, Elster, A.D. & Craven, T.E. (1991) An analysis of the natural history of cavernous angiomas. *Journal of Neurosurgery* **75**, 702–708.

Dellemijn, P.L.I. & Vanneste, J.A.L. (1993) Cavernous angiomatosis of the central nervous system: usefulness of screening the family. *Acta Neurologica Scandinavica* **88**, 259–263.

Destian, S., Sze, G., Krol, G., Zimmerman, R.D. & Deck, M.D. (1989) MR imaging of hemorrhagic intracranial neoplasms. *American Journal of Roentgenology* **152**, 137–144.

Di Rocco, C., Iannelli, A. & Tamburrini, G. (1997) Cavernous angiomas of the brain stem in children. *Pediatric Neurosurgery* **27**, 92–99.

van den Doel, E.M., van Merrienboer, F.J. & Tulleken, C.A.F. (1985) Cerebral hemorrhage from unsuspected choriocarcinoma. *Clinical Neurology and Neurosurgery* **87**, 287–290.

Dougan, C.F., Coulthard, A., Cartlidge, N.E.F. & Burn, D.J. (1998) Familial cavernous angiomas masquerading as multiple sclerosis. *Postgraduate Medical Journal* **74**, 489–491.

Drislane, F.W. & Wang, A.M. (1997) Multifocal cerebral hemorrhage in eclampsia and severe pre-eclampsia. *Journal of Neurology* **244**, 194–198.

Drury, I., Whisnant, J.P. & Garraway, W.M. (1984) Primary intracerebral hemorrhage: impact of CT on incidence. *Neurology* **34**, 653–657.

Duffau, H., Lopes, M., Janosevic, V. *et al.* (1999) Early rebleeding from intracranial dural arteriovenous fistulas: report of 20 cases and review of the literature. *Journal of Neurosurgery* **90**, 78–84.

van Duinen, S.G., Castano, E.M., Prelli, F., Bots, G.T., Luyendijk, W. & Frangione, B. (1987) Hereditary cerebral hemorrhage with amyloidosis in patients of Dutch origin is related to Alzheimer disease. *Proceedings of the National Academy of Sciences of the USA* **84**, 5991–5994.

Dunne, J.W., Chakera, T. & Kermode, S. (1987) Cerebellar haemorrhage. Diagnosis and treatment: a study of 75 consecutive cases. *Quarterly Journal of Medicine* **64**, 739–754.

Dussaux, P., Plas, J. & Brion, S. (1990) [Bilateral paresis of the superior oblique muscle caused by hematoma of the mesencephalic tegmentum] Paresie bilaterale du muscle grand oblique, par hematome de la calotte mesencephalique. *Revue Neurologique* **146**, 45–47 [in French].

Dutch TIA Trial Study Group (1991) A comparison of two doses of aspirin (30 mg vs. 283 mg a day) in patients after a transient ischemic attack or minor ischemic stroke. *New England Journal of Medicine* **325**, 1261–1266.

Egan, C.A., Davies, L. & Halmagyi, G.M. (1996) Bilateral total deafness due to pontine haematoma. *Journal of Neurology, Neurosurgery and Psychiatry* **61**, 628–631.

Ellis, A.G. (1909) The pathogenesis of spontaneous intracerebral hemorrhage. *Proceedings of the Pathological Society of Philadelphia* **12**, 197–235.

Ezura, M. & Kagawa, S. (1992) Spontaneous disappearance of a huge cerebral arteriovenous malformation: case report. *Neurosurgery* **30**, 595–599.

Farrell, D.F. & Forno, L.S. (1970) Symptomatic capillary telangiectasia of the brainstem without hemorrhage: report of an unusual case. *Neurology* **20**, 341–346.

Ferro, J.M. & Pierre, T. (1998) Cheiroretroauricular syndrome: a restricted form of pure sensory stroke due to a pontine hematoma. *Cerebrovascular Diseases* **8**, 51–52.

Fischer, O. (1910) Die presbyophrene Demenz, deren anatomische Grundlage und klinische Abgrenzung. *Zeitschrift für die gesamte Neurologie und Psychiatrie* **3**, 371–471 [in German].

Fisher, C.M. (1967) Some neuro-ophthalmological observations. *Journal of Neurology, Neurosurgery and Psychiatry* **30**, 383–392.

Fisher, C.M. (1971) Pathological observations in hypertensive cerebral hemorrhage. *Journal of Neuropathology and Experimental Neurology* **30**, 536–550.

Fogelholm, R., Eskola, K., Kiminkinen, T. & Kunnamo, I. (1992) Anticoagulant treatment as a risk factor for primary intracerebral haemorrhage. *Journal of Neurology, Neurosurgery and Psychiatry* **55**, 1121–1124.

Franke, C.L., de Jonge, J., van Swieten, J.C., Op de Coul, A.A.W. & van Gijn, J. (1990) Intracerebral hematomas during anticoagulant treatment. *Stroke* **21**, 726–730.

Franke, C.L., van Swieten, J.C., Algra, A. & van Gijn, J. (1992) Prognostic factors in patients with intracerebral haematoma. *Journal of Neurology, Neurosurgery and Psychiatry* **55**, 653–657.

Friedman, M.B. & Brant Zawadzki, M. (1983) Interhemispheric subdural hematoma from ruptured aneurysm. *Computed Radiology* **7**, 129–134.

Fujii, Y., Tanaka, R., Takeuchi, S., Koike, T., Minakawa, T. & Sasaki, O. (1994) Hematoma enlargement in spontaneous intracerebral hemorrhage. *Journal of Neurosurgery* **80**, 51–57.

Fujii, Y., Takeuchi, S., Sasaki, O., Minakawa, T. & Tanaka, R. (1998) Multivariate analysis of predictors of hematoma enlargement in spontaneous intracerebral hemorrhage. *Stroke* **29**, 1160–1166.

Fukamachi, A., Nagaseki, Y., Kohno, K. & Wakao, T. (1985) The incidence and developmental process of delayed traumatic intracerebral haematomas. *Acta Neurochirugica (Wien)* **74**, 35–39.

Garner, T.B., Del Curling, O. Jr, Kelly, D.L. Jr & Laster, D.W. (1991) The natural history of intracranial venous angiomas. *Journal of Neurosurgery* **75**, 715–722.

Gebel, J.M., Sila, C.A., Sloan, M.A. *et al.* (1998) Thrombolysis-related intracranial hemorrhage: a radiographic analysis of 244 cases from the GUSTO-I trial with clinical correlation. *Stroke* **29**, 563–569.

Gerritsen van der Hoop, R., Vermeulen, M. & van Gijn, J. (1988) Cerebellar hemorrhage: diagnosis and treatment. *Surgical Neurology* **29**, 6–10.

Getenet, J.C., Vighetto, A., Nighoghossian, N. & Trouillas, P. (1994) Isolated bilateral third nerve palsy caused by a mesencephalic hematoma. *Neurology* **44**, 981–982.

van Gijn, J. & van Dongen, K.J. (1980) Computed tomography in the diagnosis of subarachnoid haemorrhage and ruptured aneurysm. *Clinical Neurology and Neurosurgery* **82**, 11–24.

van Gijn, J. & van Dongen, K.J. (1982) The time course of aneurysmal haemorrhage on computed tomograms. *Neuroradiology* **23**, 153–156.

van Gijn, J., Stampfer, M.J., Wolfe, C.D.A. & Algra, A. (1993) The association between alcohol and stroke. In: *Health Issues Related to Alcohol Consumption* (ed. P.M. Verschuren), pp. 43–79. ILSI Press, Washington.

Gilbert, J.J. & Vinters, H.V. (1983) Cerebral amyloid angiopathy: incidence and complications in the aging brain. I. Cerebral hemorrhage. *Stroke* **14**, 915–923.

Gilles, C., Brucher, J.M., Khoubesserian, P. & Vanderhaeghen, J.J. (1984) Cerebral amyloid angiopathy as a cause of multiple intracerebral hemorrhages. *Neurology* **34**, 730–735.

Gil-Nagel, A., Dubovsky, J., Wilcox, K.J. *et al.* (1996) Familial cerebral cavernous angioma: a gene localized to a 15-cM interval on chromosome 7q. *Annals of Neurology* **39**, 807–810.

Gironell, A., Domingo, P., Mancebo, J., Coll, P. & Martí-Vilalta, J.L. (1995) Hemorrhagic stroke as a complication of bacterial meningitis in adults: report of three cases and review. *Clinical Infection and Disease* **21**, 1488–1491.

González-Duarte, A., Cantú, C., Ruíz-Sandoval, J.L. & Barinagarrementeria, F. (1998) Recurrent primary cerebral hemorrhage: frequency, mechanisms and prognosis. *Stroke* **29**, 1802–1805.

Gore, J.M., Sloan, M., Price, T.R. *et al.* (1991) Intracerebral hemorrhage, cerebral infarction and subdural hematoma after acute myocardial infarction and thrombolytic therapy in the Thrombolysis in Myocardial Infarction Study: Thrombolysis in Myocardial Infarction, Phase II, pilot and clinical trial. *Circulation* **83**, 448–459.

Gore, J.M., Granger, C.B., Simoons, M.L. *et al.* (1995) Stroke after thrombolysis: mortality and functional outcomes in the GUSTO-I trial. *Circulation* **92**, 2811–2818.

Gorter, J.W. & Stroke Prevention in Reversible Ischemia Trial (SPIRIT) Group, European Atrial Fibrillation Trial (EAFT) Group (1999) Major bleeding during anticoagulation after cerebral ischemia: patterns and risk factors. *Neurology* **53**, 1319–1327.

Goulao, A., Alvarez, H., Garcia Monaco, R., Pruvost, P. & Lasjaunias, P. (1990) Venous anomalies and abnormalities of the posterior fossa. *Neuroradiology* **31**, 476–482.

Graffagnino, C., Herbstreith, M.H., Schmechel, D.E., Levy, E., Roses, A.D. & Alberts, M.J. (1995) Cystatin C mutation in an elderly man with sporadic amyloid angiopathy and intracerebral hemorrhage. *Stroke* **26**, 2190–2193.

Gras, P., Arveux, P., Giroud, M. *et al.* (1991) [Spontaneous intracerebral hemorrhages in young patients. Study of 33 cases] Les hemorragies intracerebrales spontanees du sujet jeune. Etude de 33 cas. *Revue Neurologique* **147**, 653–657 [in French].

Gras, P., Grosmaire, N., Fayolle, H., Vion, P., Giroud, M. & Dumas, R. (1993) [Transient neurologic deficit preceding intracerebral hemorrhage. Physiopathological hypotheses] Deficits neurologiques transitoires precedant les hemorragies intraparenchymateuses. Hypotheses physiopathologiques. *Revue Neurologique* **149**, 224–226 [in French].

Gray, F., Dubas, F., Roullet, E. & Escourolle, R. (1985) Leukoencephalopathy in diffuse hemorrhagic cerebral amyloid angiopathy. *Annals of Neurology* **18**, 54–59.

Green, R.M., Kelly, K.M., Gabrielsen, T., Levine, S.R. & Vanderzant, C. (1990) Multiple intracerebral hemorrhages after smoking 'crack' cocaine. *Stroke* **21**, 957–962.

Greenberg, S.M. (1998) Cerebral amyloid angiopathy: prospects for clinical diagnosis and treatment. *Neurology* **51**, 690–694.

Greenberg, S.M. & Vonsattel, J.P. (1997) Diagnosis of cerebral amyloid angiopathy: sensitivity and specificity of cortical biopsy. *Stroke* **28**, 1418–1422.

Greenberg, S.M., Vonsattel, J.P., Stakes, J.W., Gruber, M. & Finklestein, S.P. (1993) The clinical spectrum of cerebral amyloid angiopathy: presentations without lobar hemorrhage. *Neurology* **43**, 2073–2079.

Greenberg, S.M., Finklestein, S.P. & Schaefer, P.W. (1996) Petechial hemorrhages accompanying lobar hemorrhage: detection by gradient-echo MRI. *Neurology* **46**, 6–4.

Greenberg, S.M., Vonsattel, J.P.G., Segal, A.Z. *et al.* (1998) Association of apolipoprotein E e2 and vasculopathy in cerebral amyloid angiopathy. *Neurology* **50**, 961–965.

Greenberg, S.M., O'Donnell, H.C., Schaefer, P.W. & Kraft, E. (1999) MRI detection of new hemorrhages: potential marker of progression in cerebral amyloid angiopathy. *Neurology* **53**, 1135–1138.

Griffiths, P.D., Beveridge, C.J. & Gholkar, A. (1997) Angiography in non-traumatic brain haematoma: an analysis of 100 cases. *Acta Radiologica* **38**, 797–802.

Guazzo, E.P. & Xuereb, J.H. (1994) Spontaneous thrombosis of an arteriovenous malformation. *Journal of Neurology, Neurosurgery and Psychiatry* **57**, 1410–1412.

Gudmundsson, G., Hallgrimsson, J., Jonasson, T.A. & Bjarnason, O. (1972) Hereditary cerebral haemorrhage with amyloidosis. *Brain* **95**, 387–404.

Gunatilake, S.B. (1998) Rapid resolution of symptoms and signs of intracerebral haemorrhage. *British Medical Journal* **316**, 1495–1496.

Gurwitz, J.H., Gore, J.M., Goldberg, R.J. *et al.* (1998) Risk for intracranial hemorrhage after tissue plasminogen activator treatment for acute myocardial infarction. *Annals of Internal Medicine* **129**, 597–604.

Haines, S.J., Maroon, J.C. & Jannetta, P.J. (1978) Supratentorial intracerebral hemorrhage following posterior fossa surgery. *Journal of Neurosurgery* **49**, 881–886.

Halpin, S.F., Britton, J.A., Byrne, J.V., Clifton, A., Hart, G. & Moore, A. (1994) Prospective evaluation of cerebral angiography and computed tomography in cerebral haematoma. *Journal of Neurology, Neurosurgery and Psychiatry* **57**, 1180–1186.

Hamada, Y., Goto, K., Inoue, T. *et al.* (1997) Histopathological aspects of dural arteriovenous fistulas in the transverse-sigmoid sinus region in nine patients. *Neurosurgery* **40**, 452–457.

Hankey, G.J. (1991) Isolated angiitis/angiopathy of the central nervous sytem. *Cerebrovascular Diseases* **1**, 2–15.

Hankey, G.J., Warlow, C.P. & Sellar, R.J. (1990) Cerebral angiographic risk in mild cerebrovascular disease. *Stroke* **21**, 209–222.

Harries, D.P. & De Silva, R. (1992) 'Ecstasy' and intracerebral haemorrhage. *Scottish Medical Journal* **37**, 150–152.

Harrington, H., Heller, H.A., Dawson, D., Caplan, L. & Rumbaugh, C. (1983) Intracerebral hemorrhage and oral amphetamine. *Archives of Neurology* **40**, 503–507.

Hart, I.K., Bone, I. & Hadley, D.M. (1988) Development of neurological problems after lumbar puncture. *British Medical Journal* **296**, 51–52.

Hart, R.G., Kagan Hallet, K. & Joerns, S.E. (1987) Mechanisms of intracranial hemorrhage in infective endocarditis. *Stroke* **18**, 1048–1056.

Hart, R.G., Foster, J.W., Luther, M.F. & Kanter, M.C. (1990) Stroke in infective endocarditis. *Stroke* **21**, 695–700.

Hayward, R.D. & O'Reilly, G.V. (1976) Intracerebral haemorrhage. Accuracy of computerised transverse axial scanning in predicting the underlying aetiology. *Lancet* **1**, 1–4.

He, J., Whelton, P.K., Vu, B. & Klag, M.J. (1998) Aspirin and risk of hemorrhagic stroke: a meta-analysis of randomized controlled trials. *Journal of the American Medical Association* **280**, 1930–1935.

Hendricks, H.T., Franke, C.L. & Theunissen, P.H. (1990) Cerebral amyloid angiopathy: diagnosis by MRI and brain biopsy. *Neurology* **40**, 1308–1310.

Henselmans, J.M.L., Meijer, K., Haaxma, R., Hew, J. & van der Meer, J. (1999) Recurrent spontaneous intracerebral hemorrhage in a congenitally afibrinogenemic patient: diagnostic pitfalls and therapeutic options. *Stroke* **30**, 2479–2482.

Heros, R.C. & Tu, Y.K. (1987) Is surgical therapy needed for unruptured arteriovenous malformations? *Neurology* **37**, 279–286.

Heye, N. & Hankey, G.J. (1996) Amphetamine-associated stroke. *Cerebrovascular Diseases* **6**, 149–155.

Hilz, M.J., Huk, W., Druschky, K.F. & Erbguth, F. (1989) Fat deposition surrounding intracerebral hemorrhage in a patient suffering from Zieve syndrome. *Neuroradiology* **31**, 102–103.

Hino, A., Fujimoto, M., Yamaki, T., Iwamoto, Y. & Katsumori, T. (1998) Value of repeat angiography in patients with spontaneous subcortical hemorrhage. *Stroke* **29**, 2517–2521.

Hiramatsu, K., Utsumi, S., Kyoi, K. *et al.* (1991) Intracerebral hemorrhage in carotid-cavernous fistula. *Neuroradiology* **33**, 67–69.

Hirata, Y., Matsukado, Y., Nagahiro, S. & Kuratsu, J. (1986) Intracerebral venous angioma with arterial blood supply: a mixed angioma. *Surgical Neurology* **25**, 227–232.

Hirose, G., Kosoegawa, H., Saeki, M. *et al.* (1985) The syndrome of posterior thalamic hemorrhage. *Neurology* **35**, 998–1002.

Hodes, J.E., Fletcher, W.A., Goodman, D.F. & Hoyt, W.F. (1988) Rupture of cavernous carotid artery aneurysm causing subdural hematoma and death: case report. *Journal of Neurosurgery* **69**, 617–619.

Houkin, K., Kamiyama, H., Abe, H., Takahashi, A. & Kuroda, S. (1996) Surgical therapy for adult moyamoya disease can surgical revascularization prevent the recurrence of intracerebral hemorrhage. *Stroke* **27**, 1342–1346.

Houtteville, J.P., Toumi, K., Theron, J., Derlon, J.M., Benazza, A. & Hubert, P. (1988) Interhemispheric subdural haematomas: seven cases and review of the literature. *British Journal of Neurosurgery* **2**, 357–367.

Hughes, J.C., McCabe, M. & Evans, R.J. (1993) Intracranial haemorrhage associated with ingestion of 'ecstasy'. *Archives of Emergency Medicine* **10**, 372–374.

Hunn, M., Robinson, S., Wakefield, L., Mossman, S. & Abernethy, D. (1998) Granulomatous angiitis of the CNS causing spontaneous intracerebral haemorrhage: the importance of leptomeningeal biopsy. *Journal of Neurology, Neurosurgery and Psychiatry* **65**, 956–957.

Hylek, E.M. & Singer, D.E. (1994) Risk factors for intracranial hemorrhage in outpatients taking warfarin. *Annals of Internal Medicine* **120**, 897–902.

Iseki, K., Kinjo, K., Kimura, Y., Osawa, A. & Fukiyama, K. (1993) Evidence for high risk of cerebral hemorrhage in chronic dialysis patients. *Kidney International* **44**, 1086–1090.

Isensee, C., Reul, J. & Thron, A. (1994) Magnetic resonance imaging of thrombosed dural sinuses. *Stroke* **25**, 29–34.

Ishii, N., Nishihara, Y. & Horie, A. (1984) Amyloid angiopathy and lobar cerebral haemorrhage. *Journal of Neurology, Neurosurgery and Psychiatry* **47**, 1203–1210.

Ishikawa, T., Houkin, K., Tokuda, K., Kawaguchi, S. & Kashiwaba, T. (1997) Development of anterior cranial fossa dural arteriovenous malformation following head trauma: case report. *Journal of Neurosurgery* **86**, 291–293.

Itoh, Y., Yamada, M., Hayakawa, M., Otomo, E. & Miyatake, T. (1993) Cerebral amyloid angiopathy: a significant cause of cerebellar as well as lobar cerebral hemorrhage in the elderly. *Journal of Neurological Sciences* **116**, 135–141.

Jakubowski, J.A., Vaillancourt, R. & Deykin, D. (1988) Interaction of ethanol, prostacyclin and aspirin in determining human platelet reactivity *in vitro*. *Arteriosclerosis* **8**, 436–441.

Jamrozik, K., Broadhurst, R.J., Anderson, C.S. & Stewart Wynne, E.G. (1994) The role of lifestyle factors in the etiology of stroke: a population-based case-control study in Perth, Western Australia. *Stroke* **25**, 51–59.

Jellinger, K. (1977) Cerebrovascular amyloidosis with cerebral hemorrhage. *Journal of Neurology* **214**, 195–206.

Jensson, O., Gudmundsson, G., Arnason, A. *et al.* (1987) Hereditary cystatin C (gamma-trace) amyloid angiopathy of the CNS causing cerebral hemorrhage. *Acta Neurologica Scandinavica* **76**, 102–114.

Jeong, S.C., Bae, J.C., Hwang, S.H., Kim, H.C. & Lee, B.C. (1998) Cerebral sparganosis with intracerebral hemorrhage: a case report. *Neurology* **50**, 503–506.

Jones, H.R. Jr, Baker, R.A. & Kott, H.S. (1985) Hypertensive putaminal hemorrhage presenting with hemichorea. *Stroke* **16**, 130–131.

Juvela, S., Hillbom, M. & Palomaki, H. (1995) Risk factors for spontaneous intracerebral hemorrhage. *Stroke* **26**, 1558–1564.

Kalyan Raman, U.P. & Kalyan Raman, K. (1984) Cerebral amyloid angiopathy causing intracranial hemorrhage. *Annals of Neurology* **16**, 321–329.

Kanter, M.C. & Hart, R.G. (1991) Neurologic complications of infective endocarditis. *Neurology* **41**, 1015–1020.

Kanter, R., Kanter, M., Kirsch, W. & Rosenberg, G. (1984) Spontaneous posterior fossa subdural hematoma as a complication of anticoagulation. *Neurosurgery* **15**, 241–242.

Kase, C.S. (1986) Intracerebral hemorrhage: non-hypertensive causes. *Stroke* **17**, 590–595.

Kase, C.S. (1994) Intracranial tumors. In: *Intracerebral Hemorrhage* (eds C.S. Kase & L.R. Caplan), pp. 243–261. Butterworth-Heinemann, Boston.

Kase, C.S. & Louis, D.N. (1990) Case records of the Massachusetts General Hospital. Weekly clinicopathological exercises. Case 26–1990. A 68-year-old man with a right hemiparesis, abulia, and multiple intracerebral hemorrhages. *New England Journal of Medicine* **322**, 1866–1878.

Kase, C.S., Robinson, R.K., Stein, R.W. *et al.* (1985) Anticoagulant-related intracerebral hemorrhage. *Neurology* **35**, 943–948.

Kase, C.S., O'Neal, A.M., Fisher, M., Girgis, G.N. & Ordia, J.I. (1990) Intracranial hemorrhage after use of tissue plasminogen activator for coronary thrombolysis. *Annals of Internal Medicine* **112**, 17–21.

Kase, C.S., Pessin, M.S., Zivin, J.A. *et al.* (1992) Intracranial hemorrhage after coronary thrombolysis with tissue plasminogen activator. *American Journal of Medicine* **92**, 384–390.

Kase, C.S., Mohr, J.P. & Caplan, L.R. (1998) Intracerebral hemorrhage. In: *Stroke—Pathophysiology, Diagnosis, and Management* (eds H.J.M. Barnett, J.P. Mohr, B.M. Stein & F.M. Yatsu), 3rd edn, pp. 649–700. Churchill Livingstone, New York.

Kattapong, V.J., Hart, B.L. & Davis, L.E. (1995) Familial cerebral cavernous angiomas: clinical and radiologic studies. *Neurology* **45**, 492–497.

Kawahara, N., Sato, K., Muraki, M., Tanaka, K., Kaneko, M. & Uemura, K. (1986) CT classification of small thalamic hemorrhages and their clinical implications. *Neurology* **36**, 165–172.

Kazui, S., Naritomi, H., Yamamoto, H., Sawada, T. & Yamaguchi, T. (1996) Enlargement of spontaneous intracerebral hemorrhage: incidence and time course. *Stroke* **27**, 1783–1787.

Kazui, S., Minematsu, K., Yamamoto, H., Sawada, T. & Yamaguchi, T. (1997) Predisposing factors to enlargement of spontaneous intracerebral hematoma. *Stroke* **28**, 2370–2375.

Keane, J.R. (1979) Retinal hemorrhage: its significance in 100 patients with acute encephalopathy of unknown cause. *Archives of Neurology* **36**, 691–694.

Kelley, R.E., Berger, J.R., Scheinberg, P. & Stokes, N. (1982) Active bleeding in hypertensive intracerebral hemorrhage: computed tomography. *Neurology* **32**, 852–856.

Kelly, J.K., Lazo, A., Metes, J., Wilner, H.I. & Watts, F.B. Jr (1985) Intracerebral hemorrhagic dissemination of acute myelocytic leukemia. *American Journal of Neuroradiology* **6**, 113–114.

Kibayashi, K., Mastri, A.R. & Hirsch, C.S. (1995) Cocaine induced intracerebral hemorrhage: analysis of predisposing factors and mechanisms causing hemorrhagic strokes. *Human Pathology* **26**, 659–663.

Kim, J.S. (1995) So-called capsular genu syndrome due to non-capsular strokes. *Cerebrovascular Diseases* **5**, 297–299.

Kim, J.S. & Bae, Y.H. (1997) Pure or predominant sensory stroke due to brain stem lesion. *Stroke* **28**, 1761–1764.

Kim, J.S., Lee, J.H. & Lee, M.C. (1994) Small primary intracerebral hemorrhage: clinical presentation of 28 cases. *Stroke* **25**, 1500–1506.

Kim, M., Rowed, D.W., Cheung, G. & Ang, L.C. (1997) Cavernous malformation presenting as an extra-axial cerebellopontine angle mass: case report. *Neurosurgery* 40, 187–190.

Komiyama, M., Yamanaka, K., Iwai, Y. & Yasui, T. (1999) Venous angiomas with arteriovenous shunts: report of three cases and review of the literature. *Neurosurgery* 44, 1328–1334.

Kondziolka, D., Bernstein, M., ter Brugge, K. & Schutz, H. (1988) Acute subdural hematoma from ruptured posterior communicating artery aneurysm. *Neurosurgery* 22, 151–154.

Kondziolka, D., Dempsey, P.K. & Lunsford, L.D. (1991) The case for conservative management of venous angiomas. *Canadian Journal of Neurological Sciences* 18, 295–299.

Kondziolka, D., Lunsford, L.D. & Kestle, J.R. (1995) The natural history of cerebral cavernous malformations. *Journal of Neurosurgery* 83, 820–824.

Korosue, K., Kondoh, T., Ishikawa, Y., Nagao, T., Tamaki, N. & Matsumoto, S. (1988) Acute subdural hematoma associated with non-traumatic middle meningeal artery aneurysm: case report. *Neurosurgery* 22, 411–413.

Kotwica, Z. & Brzezinski, J. (1985) Chronic subdural hematoma presenting as spontaneous subarachnoid hemorrhage: report of six cases. *Journal of Neurosurgery* 63, 691–692.

Krücke, W. (1971) [Pathology of cerebral vein and sinus thromboses] Pathologie der cerebralen Venen-und Sinusthrombosen. *Radiologe* 11, 370–377 [in German].

Kulah, A., Tasdemir, N. & Fiskeci, C. (1992) Acute spontaneous subdural hematoma in a teenager. *Child's Nervous System* 8, 343–346.

Kumral, E., Kocaer, T., Ertubey, N.O. & Kumral, K. (1995) Thalamic hemorrhage: a prospective study of 100 patients. *Stroke* 26, 964–970.

Kumral, E., Evyapan, D. & Balkir, K. (1999) Acute caudate vascular lesions. *Stroke* 30, 100–108.

Kupersmith, M.J., Vargas, M.E., Yashar, A. *et al.* (1996) Occipital arteriovenous malformations: visual disturbances and presentation. *Neurology* 46, 953–957.

Kushner, M.J. & Bressman, S.B. (1985) The clinical manifestations of pontine hemorrhage. *Neurology* 35, 637–643.

Kwa, V.I.H., Franke, C.L., Verbeeten, B. Jr, Stam, J. & Amsterdam, V.M.G. (1998) Silent intracerebral microhemorrhages in patients with ischemic stroke. *Annals of Neurology* 44, 372–377.

Labauge, P., Laberge, S., Brunereau, L., Levy, C., Tournier-Lasserve, E. & Soc, F.N. (1998) Hereditary cerebral cavernous angiomas: clinical and genetic features in 57 French families. *Lancet* 352, 1892–1897.

Laberge-le Couteulx, S., Jung, H.H., Labauge, P. *et al.* (1999) Truncating mutations in *CCM1*, encoding KRIT1, cause hereditary cavernous angiomas. *Nature Genetics* 23, 189–193.

Laissy, J.P., Normand, G., Monroc, M., Duchateau, C., Alibert, F. & Thiebot, J. (1991) Spontaneous intracerebral hematomas from vascular causes. Predictive value of CT compared with angiography. *Neuroradiology* 33, 291–295.

Landefeld, C.S., Rosenblatt, M.W. & Goldman, L. (1989) Bleeding in outpatients treated with warfarin: relation to the prothrombin time and important remediable lesions. *American Journal of Medicine* 87, 153–159.

Larrue, V., Von Kummer, R., del Zoppo, G. & Bluhmki, E. (1997) Hemorrhagic transformation in acute ischemic stroke: potential contributing factors in the European Cooperative Acute Stroke Study. *Stroke* 28, 957–960.

Larsen, P.D., Hellbusch, L.C., Lefkowitz, D.M. & Schaefer, G.B. (1997) Cerebral arteriovenous malformation in three successive generations. *Pediatric Neurology* 17, 74–76.

Lasjaunias, P., Burrows, P. & Planet, C. (1986) Developmental venous anomalies (DVA): the so-called venous angioma. *Neurosurgical Review* 9, 233–242.

Leblanc, R., Haddad, G. & Robitaille, Y. (1992) Cerebral hemorrhage from amyloid angiopathy and coronary thrombolysis. *Neurosurgery* 31, 586–590.

Lee, K.C. & Clough, C. (1990) Intracerebral hemorrhage after break dancing [letter]. *New England Journal of Medicine* 323, 615–616.

Lee, M.S. & Kim, W.C. (1998) Intracranial hemorrhage associated with idiopathic thrombocytopenic purpura: report of seven patients and a meta-analysis. *Neurology* 50, 1160–1163.

Levine, S.R., Brust, J.C., Futrell, N. *et al.* (1991) A comparative study of the cerebrovascular complications of cocaine: alkaloidal versus hydrochloride—a review. *Neurology* 41, 1173–1177.

Linn, F.H.H., Rinkel, G.J.E., Algra, A. & van Gijn, J. (1996) Incidence of subarachnoid hemorrhage—role of region, year and rate of computed tomography: a meta-analysis. *Stroke* 27, 625–629.

Lipton, S.A., Schaefer, P.W., Adams, R.D. & Ma, M.J. (1996) A 37-year-old man with AIDS, neurologic deterioration and multiple hemorrhagic cerebral lesions—Varicella-zoster leukoencephalitis with hemorrhage and large-vessel vasculopathy—Acquired immunodeficiency syndrome. *New England Journal of Medicine* 335, 1587–1595.

Little, J.R., Dial, B., Belanger, G. & Carpenter, S. (1979) Brain hemorrhage from intracranial tumor. *Stroke* 10, 283–288.

Little, J.R., Awad, I.A., Jones, S.C. & Ebrahim, Z.Y. (1990) Vascular pressures and cortical blood flow in cavernous angioma of the brain. *Journal of Neurosurgery* 73, 555–559.

Lobato, R.D., Rivas, J.J., Gomez, P.A., Cabrera, A., Sarabia, R. & Lamas, E. (1992) Comparison of the clinical presentation of symptomatic arteriovenous malformations (angiographically visualized) and occult vascular malformations. *Neurosurgery* 31, 391–396.

Loes, D.J., Smoker, W.R., Biller, J. & Cornell, S.H. (1987) Non-traumatic lobar intracerebral hemorrhage: CT/angiographic correlation. *American Journal of Neuroradiology* 8, 1027–1030.

Lukes, S.A. (1983) Intracerebral hemorrhage from an arteriovenous malformation after amphetamine injection. *Archives of Neurology* 40, 60–61.

Luyendijk, W., Bots, G.T., Vegter van der Vlis, M., Went, L.N. & Frangione, B. (1988) Hereditary cerebral haemorrhage caused by cortical amyloid angiopathy. *Journal of Neurological Sciences* 85, 267–280.

McCarron, M.O. & Nicoll, J.A.R. (1998) High frequency of apolipoprotein E e2 allele is specific for patients with cerebral amyloid angiopathy-related haemorrhage. *Neuroscience Letters* 247, 45–48.

McCarron, M.O., Nicoll, J.A.R., Stewart, J. *et al.* (1999a) The apolipoprotein E e2 allele and the pathological features in cerebral amyloid angiopathy-related hemorrhage. *Journal of Neuropathology and Experimental Neurology* 58, 711–718.

McCarron, M.O., Nicoll, J.A.R., Ironside, J.W., Love, S., Alberts, M.J. & Bone, I. (1999b) Cerebral amyloid angiopathy-related hemorrhage interaction of APOE e2 with putative clinical risk factors. *Stroke* 30, 1643–1646.

McCarron, M.O., Nicoll, J.A.R., Stewart, J. *et al.* (2000) Absence of cystatin C mutation in sporadic cerebral amyloid angiopathy-related hemorrhage. *Neurology* 54, 242–244.

McCormick, W.F. & Rosenfield, D.B. (1973) Massive brain hemorrhage: a review of 144 cases and an examination of their causes. *Stroke* 4, 946–954.

McDermott, M., Fleming, J.F., Vanderlinden, R.G. & Tucker, W.S. (1984) Spontaneous arterial subdural hematoma. *Neurosurgery* 14, 13–18.

McLaughlin, M.R., Jho, H.D. & Kwon, Y. (1996) Acute subdural hematoma caused by a ruptured giant intracavernous aneurysm: case report. *Neurosurgery* 38, 388–391.

McLaughlin, M.R., Kondziolka, D., Flickinger, J.C., Lunsford, S. & Lunsford, L.D. (1998) The prospective natural history of cerebral venous malformations. *Neurosurgery* 43, 195–200.

Maeda, A., Yamada, M., Itoh, Y., Otomo, E., Hayakawa, M. & Miyatake, T. (1993) Computer-assisted three-dimensional image analysis of cerebral amyloid angiopathy. *Stroke* 24, 1857–1864.

Maggioni, A.P., Franzosi, M.G., Santoro, E., White, H., Van de Werf, F. & Tognoni, G. (1992) The risk of stroke in patients with acute myocardial infarction after thrombolytic and antithrombotic treatment. Gruppo Italiano per lo Studio della Sopravvivenza nell'Infarto Miocardico II (GISSI-2) and the International Study Group. *New England Journal of Medicine* 327, 1–6.

Mahaffey, K.W., Granger, C.B., Sloan, M.A. *et al.* (1999) Neurosurgical evacuation of intracranial hemorrhage after thrombolytic therapy for acute myocardial infarction: experience from the GUSTO-I Trial. *American Heart Journal* 138, 493–499.

Maiuri, F., D'Andrea, F., Gallicchio, B. & Carandente, M. (1985) Intracranial hemorrhages in metastatic brain tumors. *Journal of Neurosurgical Sciences* 29, 37–41.

Malik, G.M., Pearce, J.E., Ausman, J.I. & Mehta, B. (1984) Dural arteriovenous malformations and intracranial haemorrhage. *Neurosurgery* 15, 333–339.

Malik, G.M., Morgan, J.K., Boulos, R.S. & Ausman, J.I. (1988) Venous angiomas: an underestimated cause of intracranial hemorrhage. *Surgical Neurology* 30, 350–358.

Markel, A., Nagler, A., Yoffe, G., Aboud, L. & Brook, G.J. (1986) Acute myelofibrosis with associated intracerebral haemorrhage. *Acta Haematologica (Basel)* 75, 38–39.

Marks, M.P., Lane, B., Steinberg, G.K. & Snipes, G.J. (1992) Intranidal aneurysms in cerebral arteriovenous malformations: evaluation and endovascular treatment. *Radiology* **183**, 355–360.

Martinowitz, U., Heim, M., Tadmor, R. *et al.* (1986) Intracranial hemorrhage in patients with hemophilia. *Neurosurgery* **18**, 538–541.

Masiyama, S., Niizuma, H. & Suzuki, J. (1985) Pontine haemorrhage: a clinical analysis of 26 cases. *Journal of Neurology, Neurosurgery and Psychiatry* **48**, 658–662.

Masuda, J., Tanaka, K., Ueda, K. & Omae, T. (1988) Autopsy study of incidence and distribution of cerebral amyloid angiopathy in Hisayama, Japan. *Stroke* **19**, 205–210.

Masuda, J., Yutani, C., Waki, R., Ogata, J., Kuriyama, Y. & Yamaguchi, T. (1992) Histopathological analysis of the mechanisms of intracranial hemorrhage complicating infective endocarditis. *Stroke* **23**, 843–850.

Matsumura, A., Maki, Y., Munekata, K. & Kobayashi, E. (1985) Intracerebellar hemorrhage due to cerebellar hemangioblastoma. *Surgical Neurology* **24**, 227–230.

Mayer, S.A., Sacco, R.L., Shi, T. & Mohr, J.P. (1994) Neurologic deterioration in non-comatose patients with supratentorial intracerebral hemorrhage. *Neurology* **44**, 1379–1384.

Mead, G.E. & Wardlaw, J.M. (1998) Detection of intraluminal thrombus in acute stroke by proton density MR imaging. *Cerebrovascular Diseases* **8**, 133–134.

Mendelow, A.D., Erfurth, A., Grossart, K. & Macpherson, P. (1987) Do cerebral arteriovenous malformations increase in size? *Journal of Neurology, Neurosurgery and Psychiatry* **50**, 980–987.

de Mendonca, A., Pimentel, J., Morgado, F. & Ferro, J.M. (1990) Mesencephalic haematoma: case report with autopsy study. *Journal of Neurology* **237**, 55–58.

Meyer, B., Stangl, A.P. & Schramm, J. (1995) Association of venous and true arteriovenous malformation: a rare entity among mixed vascular malformations of the brain—case report. *Journal of Neurosurgery* **83**, 141–144.

Miller, J.H., Wardlaw, J.M. & Lammie, G.A. (1999) Intracerebral haemorrhage and cerebral amyloid angiopathy: CT features with pathological correlation. *Clinical Radiology* **54**, 422–429.

Minakawa, T., Tanaka, R., Koike, T., Takeuchi, S. & Sasaki, O. (1989) Angiographic follow-up study of cerebral arteriovenous malformations with reference to their enlargement and regression. *Neurosurgery* **24**, 68–74.

Mironov, A. (1995) Classification of spontaneous dural arteriovenous fistulas with regard to their pathogenesis. *Acta Radiologica* **36**, 582–592.

Misra, U.K. & Kalita, J. (1995) Recurrent hypertensive intracerebral hemorrhage. *American Journal of Medical Science* **310**, 156–157.

Miyasaka, Y., Yada, K., Ohwada, T., Kitahara, T., Kurata, A. & Irikura, K. (1992) An analysis of the venous drainage system as a factor in hemorrhage from arteriovenous malformations. *Journal of Neurosurgery* **76**, 239–243.

Modesti, L.M., Binet, E.F. & Collins, G.H. (1976) Meningiomas causing spontaneous intracranial hematomas. *Journal of Neurosurgery* **45**, 437–441.

Monsuez, J.J., Vittecoq, D., Rosenbaum, A. *et al.* (1989) Prognosis of ruptured intracranial mycotic aneurysms: a review of 12 cases. *European Heart Journal* **10**, 821–825.

Mori, E., Tabuchi, M. & Yamadori, A. (1985) Lacunar syndrome due to intracerebral hemorrhage. *Stroke* **16**, 45–59.

Mossuto Agatiello, L., Iovine, C. & Kniahynicki, C. (1987) Herpes zoster ophthalmicus and delayed ipsilateral intracerebral hemorrhage. *Neurology* **37**, 1264–1265.

Motto, C., Aritzu, E., Boccardi, E., De Grandi, C., Piana, A. & Candelise, L. (1997) Reliability of hemorrhagic transformation diagnosis in acute ischemic stroke. *Stroke* **28**, 302–306.

Mullan, S., Mojtahedi, S., Johnson, D.L. & Macdonald, R.L. (1996) Cerebral venous malformation arteriovenous malformation transition forms. *Journal of Neurosurgery* **85**, 9–13.

Murai, Y., Ikeda, Y., Teramoto, A. & Tsuji, Y. (1998) Magnetic resonance imaging-documented extravasation as an indicator of acute hypertensive intracerebral hemorrhage. *Journal of Neurosurgery* **88**, 650–655.

Murata, Y., Yamaguchi, S., Kajikawa, H., Yamamura, K., Sumioka, S. & Nakamura, S. (1999) Relationship between the clinical manifestations, computed tomographic findings and the outcome in 80 patients with primary pontine hemorrhage. *Journal of Neurological Sciences* **167**, 107–111.

Naff, N.J., Wemmer, J., Hoenig-Rigamonti, K. & Rigamonti, D.R. (1998) A longitudinal study of patients with venous malformations: documentation of a negligible hemorrhage risk and benign natural history. *Neurology* **50**, 1709–1714.

Nakajima, K. (1983) Clinicopathological study of pontine hemorrhage. *Stroke* **14**, 485–493.

Nakamura, M., Tamaki, N., Hara, Y. & Nagashima, T. (1997) Two unusual cases of multiple dural arteriovenous fistulas. *Neurosurgery* **41**, 288–292.

Nakayama, H., Katayama, K.I., Ikawa, A. *et al.* (1999) Cerebral amyloid angiopathy in an aged great spotted woodpecker (*Picoides major*). *Neurobiology of Aging* **20**, 53–56.

Natté, R., Vinters, H.V., Maat-Schieman, M.L.C. *et al.* (1998) Microvasculopathy is associated with the number of cerebrovascular lesions in hereditary cerebral hemorrhage with amyloidosis, Dutch type. *Stroke* **29**, 1588–1594.

Neau, J.P., Ingrand, P., Couderq, C. *et al.* (1997) Recurrent intracerebral hemorrhage. *Neurology* **49**, 106–113.

Newman, P. & Al-Memar, A. (1998) Intraventricular haemorrhage in pregnancy due to Moya-moya disease. *Journal of Neurology, Neurosurgery and Psychiatry* **64**, 686–686.

Ng, M.H., Tsang, S.S., Ng, H.K., Sriskandavarman, V. & Feng, C.S. (1991) An unusual case of hairy cell leukemia: death due to leukostasis and intracerebral hemorrhage. *Human Pathology* **22**, 1298–1302.

Nicoll, J.A., Burnett, C., Love, S. *et al.* (1997) High frequency of apolipoprotein E e2 allele in hemorrhage due to cerebral amyloid angiopathy. *Annals of Neurology* **41**, 716–721.

Nijdam, J.R., Luijten, J.A. & van Gijn, J. (1986) Cerebral haemorrhage associated with unilateral Moyamoya syndrome. *Clinical Neurology and Neurosurgery* **88**, 49–51.

Nishikawa, M., Sakamoto, H., Katsuyama, J., Hakuba, A. & Nishimura, S. (1998) Multiple appearing and vanishing aneurysms: primary angiitis of the central nervous system—case report. *Journal of Neurosurgery* **88**, 133–137.

Nolte, K.B., Brass, L.M. & Fletterick, C.F. (1996) Intracranial hemorrhage associated with cocaine abuse: a prospective autopsy study. *Neurology* **46**, 1291–1296.

Notelet, L., Chapon, F., Khoury, S. *et al.* (1997) Familial cavernous malformations in a large French kindred: mapping of the gene to the CCM1 locus on chromosome 7q. *Journal of Neurology, Neurosurgery and Psychiatry* **63**, 40–45.

O'Leary, P.M. & Sweeny, P.J. (1986) Ruptured intracerebral aneurysm resulting in a subdural hematoma. *Annals of Emergency Medicine* **15**, 944–946.

Obrador, S., Soto, M. & Silvela, J. (1975) Clinical syndromes of arteriovenous malformations of the transverse-sigmoid sinus. *Journal of Neurology, Neurosurgery and Psychiatry* **38**, 436–451.

Oikawa, A., Aoki, N. & Sakai, T. (1993) Arteriovenous malformation presenting as acute subdural haematoma. *Neurological Research* **15**, 353–355.

Ondra, S.L., Troupp, H., George, E.D. & Schwab, K. (1990) The natural history of symptomatic arteriovenous malformations of the brain: a 24-year follow-up assessment. *Journal of Neurosurgery* **73**, 387–391.

Ono, S. & Inoue, K. (1985) Cheiro-oral syndrome following midbrain haemorrhage. *Journal of Neurology* **232**, 304–306.

Onoyama, K., Ibayashi, S., Nanishi, F. *et al.* (1987) Cerebral hemorrhage in patients on maintenance hemodialysis: CT analysis of 25 cases. *European Neurology* **26**, 171–175.

Ooneda, G., Yoshida, Y., Suzuki, K. & Sekiguchi, T. (1973) Morphogenesis of plasmatic arterionecrosis as the cause of hypertensive intracerebral hemorrhage. *Virchows Archiv für Pathologische Anatomie* **361**, 31–38.

Oppenheim, J.S., Gennuso, R., Sacher, M. & Hollis, P. (1991) Acute atraumatic subdural hematoma associated with moyamoya disease in an African-American. *Neurosurgery* **28**, 616–618.

Otten, P., Pizzolato, G.P., Rilliet, B. & Berney, J. (1989) [131 cases of cavernous angioma (cavernomas) of the CNS, discovered by retrospective analysis of 24 535 autopsies] A propos de 131 cas d'angiomes caverneux (cavernomes) du s.n.c., répérés par l'analyse rétrospective de 24 535 autopsies. *Neurochirurgie* **35**, 82–83; 128–31 [in French].

Parkinson, D. & Bachers, G. (1980) Arteriovenous malformations: summary of 100 consecutive supratentorial cases. *Journal of Neurosurgery* **53**, 285–299.

Passero, S., Burgalassi, L., D'Andrea, P. & Battistini, N. (1995) Recurrence of bleeding in patients with primary intracerebral hemorrhage. *Stroke* **26**, 1189–1192.

Patel, M.R., Edelman, R.R. & Warach, S. (1996) Detection of hyperacute primary intraparenchymal hemorrhage by magnetic resonance imaging. *Stroke* **27**, 2321–2324.

Pelz, D.M., Lownie, S.P., Fox, A.J. & Rosso, D. (1997) Intracranial dural arteriovenous fistulae with pial venous drainage: combined endovascular–neurosurgical therapy. *Canadian Journal of Neurological Sciences* **24**,

210–218.

Pendlebury, W.W., Iole, E.D., Tracy, R.P. & Dill, B.A. (1991) Intracerebral hemorrhage related to cerebral amyloid angiopathy and t-PA treatment. *Annals of Neurology* **29**, 210–213.

Peterson, P.L., Roszler, M., Jacobs, I. & Wilner, H.I. (1991) Neurovascular complications of cocaine abuse. *Journal of Neuropsychiatry and Clinical Neurosciences* **3**, 143–149.

Pfleger, M.J., Hardee, E.P., Contant, C.F. Jr & Hayman, L.A. (1994) Sensitivity and specificity of fluid-blood levels for coagulopathy in acute intracerebral hematomas. *American Journal of Neuroradiology* **15**, 217–223.

Polymeropoulos, M.H., Hurko, O., Hsu, F. *et al.* (1997) Linkage of the locus for cerebral cavernous hemangiomas to human chromosome 7q in four families of Mexican-American descent. *Neurology* **48**, 752–757.

Pomeranz, S., Naparstek, E., Ashkenazi, E. *et al.* (1994) Intracranial haematomas following bone marrow transplantation. *Journal of Neurology* **241**, 252–256.

Ponder, A. & Lehman, L.B. (1994) 'Coining' and 'coning': an unusual complication of unconventional medicine. *Neurology* **44**, 774–775.

Pozzati, E., Acciarri, N., Tognetti, F., Marliani, F. & Giangaspero, F. (1996) Growth, subsequent bleeding, and *de novo* appearance of cerebral cavernous angiomas. *Neurosurgery* **38**, 662–669.

Pozzati, E., Giuliani, G., Nuzzo, G. & Poppi, M. (1989) The growth of cerebral cavernous angiomas. *Neurosurgery* **25**, 92–97.

Proner, J., Rosenblum, B.R. & Rothman, A. (1990) Ruptured arteriovenous malformation complicating thrombolytic therapy with tissue plasminogen activator. *Archives of Neurology* **47**, 105–106.

Qureshi, A.I., Giles, W.H. & Croft, J.B. (1999) Racial differences in the incidence of intracerebral hemorrhage: effects of blood pressure and education. *Neurology* **52**, 1617–1621.

Rådberg, J.A., Olsson, J.E. & Rådberg, C.T. (1991) Prognostic parameters in spontaneous intracerebral hematomas with special reference to anticoagulant treatment. *Stroke* **22**, 571–576.

Ragland, R.L., Gelber, N.D., Wilkinson, H.A., Knorr, J.R. & Tran, A.A. (1993) Anterior communicating artery aneurysm rupture: an unusual cause of acute subdural hemorrhage. *Surgical Neurology* **40**, 400–402.

Ramsay, D.A., Penswick, J.L. & Robertson, D.M. (1990) Fatal streptokinase-induced intracerebral haemorrhage in cerebral amyloid angiopathy. *Canadian Journal of Neurological Sciences* **17**, 336–341.

Rapacki, T.F., Brantley, M.J., Furlow, T.W. Jr, Geyer, C.A., Toro, V.E. & George, E.D. (1990) Heterogeneity of cerebral cavernous hemangiomas diagnosed by MR imaging. *Journal of Computer Assisted Tomography* **14**, 18–25.

Rengachary, S.S. & Szymanski, D.C. (1981) Subdural hematomas of arterial origin. *Neurosurgery* **8**, 166–172.

Requena, I., Arias, M., Lopez-Ibor, L. *et al.* (1991) Cavernomas of the central nervous system: clinical and neuroimaging manifestations in 47 patients. *Journal of Neurology, Neurosurgery and Psychiatry* **54**, 590–594.

Reyns, N., Assaker, R., Louis, E. & Lejeune, J.P. (1999) Intraventricular cavernomas: three cases and review of the literature. *Neurosurgery* **44**, 648–654.

Richards, A., Graham, D. & Bullock, R. (1988) Clinicopathological study of neurological complications due to hypertensive disorders of pregnancy. *Journal of Neurology, Neurosurgery and Psychiatry* **51**, 416–421.

Rigamonti, D. & Spetzler, R.F. (1988) The association of venous and cavernous malformations: report of four cases and discussion of the pathophysiological, diagnostic and therapeutic implications. *Acta Neurochirugica (Wien)* **92**, 100–105.

Rigamonti, D., Drayer, B.P., Johnson, P.C., Hadley, M.N., Zabramski, J. & Spetzler, R.F. (1987) The MRI appearance of cavernous malformations (angiomas). *Journal of Neurosurgery* **67**, 518–524.

Rigamonti, D., Hadley, M.N., Drayer, B.P. *et al.* (1988a) Cerebral cavernous malformations: incidence and familial occurrence. *New England Journal of Medicine* **319**, 343–347.

Rigamonti, D., Spetzler, R.F., Drayer, B.P. *et al.* (1988b) Appearance of venous malformations on magnetic resonance imaging. *Journal of Neurosurgery* **69**, 535–539.

Rigamonti, D., Spetzler, R.F., Medina, M., Rigamonti, K., Geckle, D.S. & Pappas, C. (1990) Cerebral venous malformations. *Journal of Neurosurgery* **73**, 560–564.

Rob, J.K. & Park, K.S. (1998) Post-partum cerebral angiopathy with intracerebral hemorrhage in a patient receiving lisuride. *Neurology* **50**, 1152–1154.

Robinson, J.R. Jr, Awad, I.A., Masaryk, T.J. & Estes, M.L. (1993a) Pathological heterogeneity of angiographically occult vascular malformations of the brain. *Neurosurgery* **33**, 547–554.

Robinson, J.R. Jr, Awad, I.A., Magdinec, M. & Paranandi, L. (1993b) Factors predisposing to clinical disability in patients with cavernous malformations of the brain. *Neurosurgery* **32**, 730–735.

Rodgers, A., MacMahon, S., Yee, T. *et al.* (1998) Blood pressure, cholesterol and stroke in eastern Asia. *Lancet* **352**, 1801–1807.

Román, G., Fisher, M., Perl, D.P. & Poser, C.M. (1978) Neurological manifestations of hereditary hemorrhagic teleangiectasis (Rendu–Osler–Weber disease): report of two cases and review of the literature. *Annals of Neurology* **4**, 130–144.

Ropper, A.H. & Davis, K.R. (1980) Lobar cerebral hemorrhages: acute clinical syndromes in 26 cases. *Annals of Neurology* **8**, 141–147.

Roquer, J., Palomeras, E., Knobel, H. & Pou, A. (1998) Intracerebral haemorrhage in AIDS. *Cerebrovascular Diseases* **8**, 222–227.

Rose, G. (1992) *The Strategy of Preventive Medicine*. Oxford Medical Publications, Oxford.

Ross Russell, R.W. (1963) Observations on intracerebral aneurysms. *Brain* **86**, 425–442.

Rothschild, M.A. & Maxeiner, H. (1990) [Spontaneous subdural hemorrhage of natural cause in metastatic renal cell carcinoma] Spontane Subduralblutung aus natürlicher Ursache bei metastasierendem Nierenzellcarcinom. *Beitrage zur Gerichtlichen Medizin* **48**, 223–227.

Ruíz-Sandoval, J.L., Cantú, C. & Barinagarrementeria, F. (1999) Intracerebral hemorrhage in young people: analysis of risk factors, location, causes and prognosis. *Stroke* **30**, 537–541.

Salgado, A.V., Furlan, A.J. & Keys, T.F. (1987) Mycotic aneurysm, subarachnoid hemorrhage and indications for cerebral angiography in infective endocarditis. *Stroke* **18**, 1057–1060.

Sand, J.J., Biller, J., Corbett, J.J., Adams, H.P. Jr & Dunn, V. (1986) Partial dorsal mesencephalic hemorrhages: report of three cases. *Neurology* **36**, 529–533.

Sarwar, M. & McCormick, W.F. (1978) Intracerebral venous angioma: case report and review. *Archives of Neurology* **35**, 323–325.

Schafhalter-Zoppoth, I., Fazekas, F., Kapeller, P. *et al.* (1997) Cardiac myxoma and intracerebral hemorrhage. *Cerebrovascular Diseases* **7**, 239–241.

van Schayck, R., Pantel, J., Faiss, J., Kloss, T., Keidel, M. & Diener, H.D. (1994) Hereditary cavernous angiomas of the brain in a German family [abstract]. *Cerebrovascular Diseases* **4**, 226.

Schutz, H., Bodeker, R.H., Damian, M., Krack, P. & Dorndorf, W. (1990) Age-related spontaneous intracerebral hematoma in a German community. *Stroke* **21**, 1412–1418.

Scott, R.M., Barnes, P., Kupsky, W. & Adelman, L.S. (1992) Cavernous angiomas of the central nervous system in children. *Journal of Neurosurgery* **76**, 38–46.

Segal, A.Z., Chiu, R.I., Eggleston-Sexton, P.M., Beiser, A. & Greenberg, S.M. (1999) Low cholesterol as a risk factor for primary intracerebral hemorrhage: a case–control study. *Neuroepidemiology* **18**, 185–193.

Selmi, F., Davies, K.G., Sharma, R.R. & Neal, J.W. (1995) Intracerebral haemorrhage due to amphetamine abuse: report of two cases with underlying arteriovenous malformations. *British Journal of Neurosurgery* **9**, 93–96.

Senegor, M., Dohrmann, G.J. & Wollmann, R.L. (1983) Venous angiomas of the posterior fossa should be considered as anomalous venous drainage. *Surgical Neurology* **19**, 26–32.

Shibata, S., Mori, K., Sekine, I. & Suyama, H. (1991) Subarachnoid and intracerebral hemorrhage associated with necrotizing angiitis due to methamphetamine abuse: an autopsy case. *Neurologia Medico Chirurgica (Tokyo)* **31**, 49–52.

Shih, S.L., Lin, J.C., Liang, D.C. & Huang, J.K. (1993) Computed tomography of spontaneous intracranial haemorrhage due to haemostatic disorders in children. *Neuroradiology* **35**, 619–621.

Shuaib, A., Israelian, G. & Lee, M.A. (1989) Mesencephalic hemorrhage and unilateral pupillary deficit. *Journal of Clinical Neuro-Ophthalmology* **9**, 47–49.

Shuaib, A. & Murphy, W. (1987) Mesencephalic hemorrhage and third nerve palsy. *Journal of Computer Assisted Tomography* **11**, 385–388.

Simard, J.M., Garcia Bengochea, F., Ballinger, W.E. Jr, Mickle, J.P. & Quisling, R.G. (1986) Cavernous angioma: a review of 126 collected and 12 new clinical cases. *Neurosurgery* **18**, 162–172.

Simoons, M.L., Maggioni, A.P., Knatterud, G. *et al.* (1993) Individual risk assessment for intracranial haemorrhage during thrombolytic therapy. *Lancet* **342**, 1523–1528.

Sloan, M.A., Price, T.R., Petito, C.K. *et al.* (1995) Clinical features and pathogenesis of intracerebral hemorrhage after rt-PA and heparin therapy for acute myocardial infarction: the thrombolysis in myocardial infarction (TIMI) II pilot and randomized clinical trial combined experience. *Neurology* **45**, 649–658.

Sloan, M.A., Sila, C.A., Mahaffey, K.W. *et al.* (1998) Prediction of 30-day mortality among patients with thrombolysis-related intracranial hemorrhage. *Circulation* **98**, 1376–1382.

Smith, D.B., Hitchcock, M. & Philpott, P.J. (1985) Cerebral amyloid angiopathy presenting as transient ischemic attacks: case report. *Journal of Neurosurgery* **63**, 963–964.

Smith, D., Lucas, S. & Jacewicz, M. (1993) Multiple cerebral hemorrhages in HTLV-I-associated myelopathy. *Neurology* **43**, 412–414.

Stacey, R.J., Findlay, G.F.G., Foy, P.M. & Jeffreys, R.V. (1999) Cavernomas in the central nervous system and the relevance of multiple intracranial lesions in the familial form of this disease. *Journal of Neurology, Neurosurgery and Psychiatry* **66**, 117.

Stein, R.W., Kase, C.S., Hier, D.B. *et al.* (1984) Caudate hemorrhage. *Neurology* **34**, 1549–1554.

Stephenson, G. & Gibson, R.M. (1989) Acute spontaneous subdural haematoma of arterial origin. *British Journal of Neurosurgery* **3**, 225–228.

Stober, T., Sen, S., Anstatt, T. & Bette, L. (1988) Correlation of cardiac arrhythmias with brainstem compression in patients with intracerebral hemorrhage. *Stroke* **19**, 688–692.

Stroke Prevention In Reversible Ischemia Trial (SPIRIT) Study Group (1997) A randomized trial of anticoagulants versus aspirin after cerebral ischemia of presumed arterial origin. *Annals of Neurology* **42**, 857–865.

Suzuki, S., Kelley, R.E., Dandapani, B.K., Reyes Iglesias, Y., Dietrich, W.D. & Duncan, R.C. (1995) Acute leukocyte and temperature response in hypertensive intracerebral hemorrhage. *Stroke* **26**, 1020–1023.

van Swieten, J.C., van den Hout, J.H., van Ketel, B.A., Hijdra, A., Wokke, J.H.J. & van Gijn, J. (1991) Periventricular lesions in the white matter on magnetic resonance imaging in the elderly: a morphometric correlation with arteriolosclerosis and dilated perivascular spaces. *Brain* **114**, 761–774.

Takahashi, H., Urano, T., Nagai, N., Takada, Y. & Takada, A. (1998) Progressive expansion of hypertensive intracerebral hemorrhage by coagulopathy. *American Journal of Hematology* **59**, 110–114.

Takebayashi, S. & Kaneko, M. (1983) Electron microscopic studies of ruptured arteries in hypertensive intracerebral hemorrhage. *Stroke* **14**, 28–36.

Tanaka, A., Ueno, Y., Nakayama, Y., Takano, K. & Takebayashi, S. (1999) Small chronic hemorrhages and ischemic lesions in association with spontaneous intracerebral hematomas. *Stroke* **30**, 1637–1642.

Tanaka, T., Sakai, T., Uemura, K., Teramura, A., Fujishima, I. & Yamamoto, T. (1988) MR imaging as predictor of delayed post-traumatic cerebral hemorrhage. *Journal of Neurosurgery* **69**, 203–209.

Tatu, L., Moulin, T., Martin, V., Chavot, D. & Rumbach, L. (1996) Hemiataxia-hypesthesia and small thalamic primary hemorrhages. *Cerebrovascular Diseases* **6**, 166–167.

Teilmann, K. (1953) Hemangiomas of the pons. *Archives of Neurology and Psychiatry* **69**, 208–223.

de Tezanos Pinto, M., Fernandez, J. & Perez Bianco, P.R. (1992) Update of 156 episodes of central nervous system bleeding in hemophiliacs. *Haemostasis* **22**, 259–267.

Thrift, A.G., McNeil, J.J., Forbes, A. & Donnan, G.A. (1996) Risk factors for cerebral hemorrhage in the era of well-controlled hypertension. *Stroke* **27**, 2020–2025.

Thrift, A.G., Donnan, G.A. & McNeil, J.J. (1999a) Heavy drinking, but not moderate or intermediate drinking, increases the risk of intracerebral hemorrhage. *Epidemiology* **10**, 307–312.

Thrift, A.G., McNeil, J.J., Forbes, A. & Donnan, G.A. (1999b) Risk of primary intracerebral haemorrhage associated with aspirin and non-steroidal anti-inflammatory drugs: case–control study. *British Medical Journal* **318**, 759–764.

Timothy, J., Sofat, A., Sharr, M. & Doshi, B. (1994) Unusual presentation of a germ cell neoplasm [letter]. *Journal of Neurology, Neurosurgery and Psychiatry* **57**, 1278–1279.

Tjeerdsma, H.C., Rinkel, G.J.E. & van Gijn, J. (1996) Ataxic hemiparesis from a primary intracerebral haematoma in the precentral area. *Cerebrovascular Diseases* **6**, 45–46.

Toffol, G.J., Biller, J., Adams, H.P. Jr & Smoker, W.R. (1986) The predicted value of arteriography in non-traumatic intracerebral hemorrhage. *Stroke* **17**, 881–883.

Toffol, G.J., Biller, J. & Adams, H.P. Jr (1987) Non-traumatic intracerebral hemorrhage in young adults. *Archives of Neurology* **44**, 483–485.

Tomlinson, F.H., Houser, O.W., Scheithauer, B.W., Sundt, T.M. Jr, Okazaki, H. & Parisi, J.E. (1994) Angiographically occult vascular malformations: a correlative study of features on magnetic resonance imaging and histological examination. *Neurosurgery* **34**, 792–799.

Tomonaga, M. (1981) Cerebral amyloid angiopathy in the elderly. *Journal of the American Geriatrics Society* **29**, 151–157.

Töpper, R., Jürgens, E., Reul, J. & Thron, A. (1999) Clinical significance of intracranial developmental venous anomalies. *Journal of Neurology, Neurosurgery and Psychiatry* **67**, 234–238.

Torack, R.M. (1975) Congophilic angiopathy complicated by surgery and massive hemorrhage: a light and electron microscopic study. *American Journal of Pathology* **81**, 349–365.

Trenkwalder, P., Trenkwalder, C., Feiden, W., Vogl, T.J., Einhäupl, K.M. & Lydtin, H. (1992) Toxoplasmosis with early intracerebral hemorrhage in a patient with the acquired immunodeficiency syndrome. *Neurology* **42**, 436–438.

Troost, B.T., Mark, L.E. & Maroon, J.C. (1979) Resolution of classic migraine after removal of an occipital lobe AVM. *Annals of Neurology* **5**, 199–201.

Tuhrim, S., Horowitz, D.R., Sacher, M. & Godbold, J.H. (1999) Volume of ventricular blood is an important determinant of outcome in supratentorial intracerebral hemorrhage. *Critical Care Medicine* **27**, 617–621.

Tung, H., Giannotta, S.L., Chandrasoma, P.T. & Zee, C.S. (1990) Recurrent intraparenchymal hemorrhages from angiographically occult vascular malformations. *Journal of Neurosurgery* **73**, 174–180.

Tuttle, P.V. & Reinmuth, O.M. (1984) Midbrain hemorrhage producing pure sensory stroke. *Archives of Neurology* **41**, 794–795.

Uglietta, J.P., O'Connor, C.M., Boyko, O.B., Aldrich, H., Massey, E.W. & Heinz, E.R. (1991) CT patterns of intracranial hemorrhage complicating thrombolytic therapy for acute myocardial infarction. *Radiology* **181**, 555–559.

UK Transient Ischaemic Attack (UK-TIA) Study Group (1991) The United Kingdom Transient Ischaemic Attack (UK-TIA) aspirin trial: final results. *Journal of Neurology, Neurosurgery and Psychiatry* **54**, 1044–1054.

Vinters, H.V. (1987) Cerebral amyloid angiopathy: a critical review. *Stroke* **18**, 311–324.

Vinters, H.V. & Gilbert, J.J. (1983) Cerebral amyloid angiopathy: incidence and complications in the aging brain. II. The distribution of amyloid vascular changes. *Stroke* **14**, 924–928.

Vinters, H.V., Natté, R., Maat-Schieman, M.L. *et al.* (1998) Secondary microvascular degeneration in amyloid angiopathy of patients with hereditary cerebral hemorrhage with amyloidosis, Dutch type (HCHWA-D). *Acta Neuropathologica (Berlin)* **95**, 235–244.

Vonsattel, J.P., Myers, R.H., Hedley-Whyte, E.T., Ropper, A.H., Bird, E.D. & Richardson, E.P. Jr. (1991) Cerebral amyloid angiopathy without and with cerebral hemorrhages: a comparative histological study. *Annals of Neurology* **30**, 637–649.

Vos, P.E., de Boer, W.A., Wurzer, J.A. & van Gijn, J. (1991) Subdural hematoma after lumbar puncture: two case reports and review of the literature. *Clinical Neurology and Neurosurgery* **93**, 127–132.

Vrethem, M., Thuomas, K.Å. & Hillman, J. (1997) Cavernous angioma of the brain stem mimicking multiple sclerosis. *New England Journal of Medicine* **336**, 875–876.

Waga, S., Shimosaka, S. & Sakakura, M. (1983) Intracerebral hemorrhage remote from the site of the initial neurosurgical procedure. *Neurosurgery* **13**, 662–665.

Waga, S., Fujimoto, K., Okada, M., Miyazaki, M. & Tanaka, Y. (1986) Caudate hemorrhage. *Neurosurgery* **18**, 445–450.

Wakai, S., Chen, C.H., Wu, K.Y. & Chiu, C.W. (1983) Spontaneous regression of a cerebral arteriovenous malformation: report of a case and review of the literature. *Archives of Neurology* **40**, 377–380.

Wakai, S., Kumakura, N. & Nagai, M. (1992) Lobar intracerebral hemorrhage: a clinical, radiographic and pathological study of 29 consecutive operated cases with negative angiography. *Journal of Neurosurgery* **76**, 231–238.

Wakai, S., Sato, A. & Nagai, M. (1995) Expanding intracerebral hematoma from pituitary adenoma: case report. *Neurosurgery* **37**, 807–808.

Wall, M. & George, D. (1987) Visual loss in pseudotumor cerebri: incidence and defects related to visual field strategy. *Archives of Neurology* **44**, 170–175.

Waltimo, O. (1973) The change in size of intracranial arteriovenous malformations. *Journal of Neurological Sciences* **19**, 21–27.

Wannamethee, S.G. & Shaper, A.G. (1996) Patterns of alcohol intake and risk of stroke in middle-aged British men. *Stroke* **27**, 1033–1039.

Wardlaw, J.M., Lammie, G.A. & Whittle, I.R. (1998) A brain haemorrhage? *Lancet* **351**, 1028.

Wattendorff, A.R., Frangione, B., Luyendijk, W. & Bots, G.T.A.M. (1995) Hereditary cerebral haemorrhage with amyloidosis, Dutch type (HCHWA-D): clinicopathological studies. *Journal of Neurology, Neurosurgery and Psychiatry* **58**, 699–705.

Weir, N.U., van Gijn, J., Lammie, G.A., Wardlaw, J.M. & Warlow, C.P. (1999) Recurrent cerebral haemorrhage in a 65-year-old man: advanced clinical neurology course, Edinburgh, 1997. *Journal of Neurology, Neurosurgery and Psychiatry* **66**, 104–110.

Weisberg, L. (1981) Multiple spontaneous intracerebral hematomas: clinical and computed tomographic correlations. *Neurology* **31**, 897–900.

Weisberg, L.A. (1988) Alcoholic intracerebral hemorrhage. *Stroke* **19**, 1565–1569.

Weisberg, L.A. & Stazio, A. (1988) Non-traumatic frontal lobe hemorrhages: clinical–computed tomographic correlations. *Neuroradiology* **30**, 500–505.

Weisberg, L.A., Elliott, D. & Mielke, D. (1991a) Intracerebral hemorrhage following electroconvulsive therapy. *Neurology* **41**, 1849.

Weisberg, L.A., Shamsnia, M. & Elliott, D. (1991b) Non-traumatic posterior temporal lobe hemorrhage: clinical computed tomographic correlations. *Computerized Medical Imaging and Graphics* **15**, 355–359.

Weiskrantz, L., Warrington, E.K., Sanders, M.D. & Marshall, J. (1974) Visual capacity in the hemianopic field following a restricted occipital ablation. *Brain* **97**, 709–728.

Wharen, R.E., Scheithauer, B.W. & Laws, E.R. (1982) Thrombosed arteriovenous malformations of the brain: an important entity in the differential diagnosis of intractable focal seizure disorders. *Journal of Neurosurgery* **57**, 520–526.

Wijdicks, E.F.M. & Jack, C.R. Jr (1993) Intracerebral hemorrhage after fibrinolytic therapy for acute myocardial infarction. *Stroke* **24**, 554–557.

Wijdicks, E.F.M. & St Louis, E. (1997) Clinical profiles predictive of outcome in pontine hemorrhage. *Neurology* **49**, 1342–1346.

Wijdicks, E.F.M., Silbert, P.L., Jack, C.R. & Parisi, J.E. (1994) Subcortical hemorrhage in disseminated intravascular coagulation associated with sepsis. *American Journal of Neuroradiology* **15**, 763–765.

Wijdicks, E.F.M., De Groen, P.C., Wiesner, R.H. & Krom, R.A.F. (1995) Intracerebral hemorrhage in liver transplant recipients. *Mayo Clinic Proceedings* **70**, 443–446.

Wijdicks, E.F.M., Torres, V.E. & Schievink, W.I. (2000) Chronic subdural hematoma in autosomal dominant polycystic kidney disease. *American Journal of Kidney Disease* **35**, 40–43.

Williams, J.P., Joslyn, J.N., White, J.L. & Dean, D.F. (1983) Subdural hematoma secondary to ruptured intracranial aneurysm: computed tomographic diagnosis. *Journal of Computer Assisted Tomography* **7**, 142–153.

Willinsky, R.A., Lasjaunias, P., Terbrugge, K. & Burrows, P. (1990) Multiple cerebral arteriovenous malformations (AVMs): review of our experience from 203 patients with cerebral vascular lesions. *Neuroradiology* **32**, 207–210.

Willinsky, R.A., Fitzgerald, M., Terbrugge, K., Montanera, W. & Wallace, M. (1993) Delayed angiography in the investigation of intracerebral hematomas caused by small arteriovenous malformations. *Neuroradiology* **35**, 307–311.

Willinsky, R.A., Terbrugge, K., Montanera, W., Mikulis, D. & Wallace, M.C. (1994) Venous congestion: an MR finding in dural arteriovenous malformations with cortical venous drainage. *American Journal of Neuroradiology* **15**, 1501–1507.

Wintzen, A.R. (1980) The clinical course of subdural haematoma: a retrospective study of aetiological, chronological and pathological features in 212 patients and a proposed classification. *Brain* **103**, 855–867.

Wintzen, A.R. & Tijssen, J.G. (1982) Subdural hematoma and oral anticoagulant therapy. *Archives of Neurology* **39**, 69–72.

Wintzen, A.R., de Jonge, H., Loeliger, E.A. & Bots, G.T. (1984) The risk of intracerebral hemorrhage during oral anticoagulant treatment: a population study. *Annals of Neurology* **16**, 553–558.

Woolfenden, A.R., Tong, D.C., Marks, M.P., Ali, A.O. & Albers, G.W. (1998) Angiographically defined primary angiitis of the CNS: is it really benign? *Neurology* **51**, 183–188.

Worthington, J.M. & Halmagyi, G.M. (1996) Bilateral total ophthalmoplegia due to midbrain hematoma [letter]. *Neurology* **46**, 1176–1177.

Wulff, H.R. & Gøtzsche, P. (2000) *Rational Diagnosis and Treatment: Evidence-Based Clinical Decision-Making*, 3rd edn. Blackwell Science, Oxford.

Yamada, M., Itoh, Y., Otomo, E., Hayakawa, M. & Miyatake, T. (1993) Subarachnoid haemorrhage in the elderly: a necropsy study of the association with cerebral amyloid angiopathy. *Journal of Neurology, Neurosurgery and Psychiatry* **56**, 543–547.

Yamashita, M., Tanaka, K., Matsuo, T., Yokoyama, K., Fujii, T. & Sakamoto, H. (1983) Cerebral dissecting aneurysms in patients with moyamoya disease: report of two cases. *Journal of Neurosurgery* **58**, 120–125.

Yamauchi, K. & Umeda, Y. (1997) Symptomatic intracranial haemorrhage in acute nonlymphoblastic leukaemia: analysis of CT and autopsy findings. *Journal of Neurology* **244**, 94–100.

Yapor, W.Y. & Gutierrez, F.A. (1992) Cocaine-induced intratumoral hemorrhage: case report and review of the literature. *Neurosurgery* **30**, 288–291.

Yasui, T., Komiyama, M., Kishi, H. *et al.* (1995) Angiographic extravasation of contrast medium in acute 'spontaneous' subdural hematoma. *Surgical Neurology* **43**, 61–67.

Yokoyama, K., Asano, Y., Murakawa, T. *et al.* (1991) Familial occurrence of arteriovenous malformation of the brain. *Journal of Neurosurgery* **74**, 585–589.

Yong, W.H., Robert, M.E., Secor, D.L., Kleikamp, T.J. & Vinters, H.V. (1992) Cerebral hemorrhage with biopsy-proved amyloid angiopathy. *Archives of Neurology* **49**, 51–58.

Yoshida, Y., Yoshimoto, T., Shirane, R. & Sakurai, Y. (1999) Clinical course, surgical management and long-term outcome of moyamoya patients with rebleeding after an episode of intracerebral hemorrhage: an extensive follow-up study. *Stroke* **30**, 2272–2276.

Zabramski, J.M., Wascher, T.M., Spetzler, R.F. *et al.* (1994) The natural history of familial cavernous malformations: results of an ongoing study. *Journal of Neurosurgery* **80**, 422–432.

Zazulia, A.R., Diringer, M.N., Derdeyn, C.P. & Powers, W.J. (1999) Progression of mass effect after intracerebral hemorrhage. *Stroke* **30**, 1167–1173.

Zhu, X.L., Chan, M.S. & Poon, W.S. (1997) Spontaneous intracranial hemorrhage: which patients need diagnostic cerebral angiography? A prospective study of 206 cases and review of the literature. *Stroke* **28**, 1406–1409.

Zimmerman, R.S., Spetzler, R.F., Lee, K.S., Zabramski, J.M. & Hargraves, R.W. (1991) Cavernous malformations of the brain stem. *Journal of Neurosurgery* **75**, 32–39.

CHAPTER NINE

What caused this subarachnoid haemorrhage?

9.1 Causes of subarachnoid haemorrhage

Approximately 85% of spontaneous haemorrhages into the subarachnoid space arise from rupture of a saccular aneurysm at the base of the brain. This is a serious disorder, not only as a result of the initial haemorrhage, but also because of the potential complications (Chapter 13). In unselected hospital series, the case fatality after 3 months is about 50% (Hijdra *et al.* 1987). Specialized neurosurgical centres tend to publish more optimistic figures, because few patients in poor condition ever reach them (Whisnant *et al.* 1993) (Fig. 9.1). Ten per cent of subarachnoid haemorrhages (SAHs) are non-aneurysmal, idiopathic, and characteristically perimesencephalic in location (section 9.1.2). A small fraction of SAHs are due to arterial dissections or a variety of even rarer conditions (sections 9.1.3 and 9.1.4). In the next sections, we will separately discuss aneurysms, perimesencephalic haemorrhages, arterial dissections, and the rare causes.

> *About 85% of spontaneous subarachnoid haemorrhages are due to the rupture of an intracranial saccular aneurysm, 10% to non-aneurysmal perimesencephalic haemorrhage, and 5% to rarities.*

The presenting features of patients with all these different causes are usually indistinguishable: a severe headache of sudden onset, a depressed level of consciousness, or both; sometimes there are focal deficits, caused by an

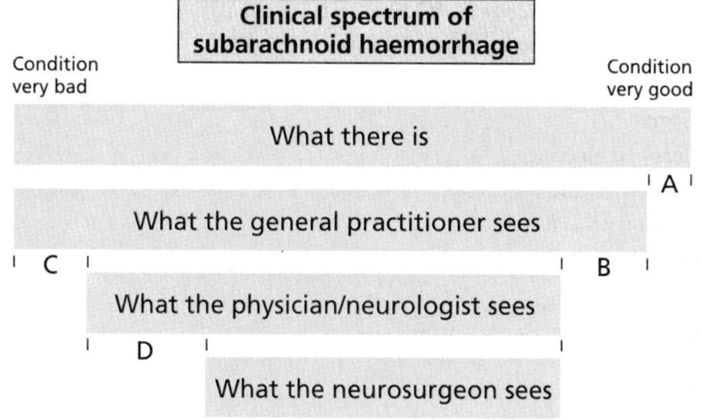

Fig. 9.1 Referral bias in subarachnoid haemorrhage. Patients can fail to reach specialised centres because: A, they do not consult their general practitioner; B, the diagnosis is missed; C, they die before reaching hospital; D, it is assumed that no treatment is possible. (With permission from van Gijn 1992.)

associated intracerebral haematoma or cranial nerve involvement (section 9.3.5). The only exception is non-aneurysmal perimesencephalic haemorrhage, where explosive headache is invariably the only symptom at onset. In the following sections about the pathological and pathophysiological backgrounds to all these causes, we will occasionally run ahead of the story by mentioning the findings on computed tomography (CT) scanning, as this technique—now readily available in many centres as an early adjunct to the history and examination—provides an *in-vivo* picture of the pathology.

9.1.1 Intracranial saccular aneurysms

Although some student textbooks still refer to aneurysms of the cerebral vessels as being congenital, this is wrong: they develop during the course of life. Aneurysms are almost never found in neonates, and they are also rare in children (Rinkel *et al.* 1998). Moreover, in those exceptional childhood aneurysms, there is usually an underlying cause, such as trauma, infection or connective-tissue disorder (Ferry *et al.* 1974; Stehbens 1982) (Table 9.1). Whether Marfan's syndrome belongs with these conditions is debatable: apart from case reports, the relation is supported only by one post-mortem study, in which two of seven patients had one or more aneurysms (Schievink *et al.* 1997a). However, in another post-mortem series the ratio was only one in 25 (Conway *et al.* 1999), and in a clinical cohort of 129 patients with Marfan's syndrome, none had a history of subarachnoid haemorrhage (SAH) (Van den Berg *et al.* 1996).

> *Intracranial aneurysms are not congenital; they develop during life.*

Table 9.1 Hereditary and congenital conditions associated with saccular aneurysms.

Disorders of connective tissue
Ehlers–Danlos syndrome type IV (Schievink *et al.* 1990)
Pseudoxanthoma elasticum (Munyer & Margulis 1981)
α_1-antitrypsin deficiency (Schievink *et al.* 1994b, 1996a)
(Infantile) fibromuscular dysplasia (Cloft *et al.* 1998; Lee *et al.* 1998a)
Neurofibromatosis (Muhonen *et al.* 1991)

Disorders of angiogenesis
Hereditary haemorrhagic telangiectasia (Román *et al.* 1978; Helmchen *et al.* 1995)
Progressive hemifacial atrophy (Parry–Romberg disease) (Schievink *et al.* 1996b)

Associated hypertension
Congenital heart disease (Schievink *et al.* 1996c)
Coarctation of the aorta (Wright 1949; Robinson 1967)
Aortitis syndrome (Asaoka *et al.* 1998)
Autosomal dominant polycystic kidney disease* (Chapman *et al.* 1992; Chauveau *et al.* 1994)

Local haemodynamic stress
Anomalies of the circle of Willis (Kayembe *et al.* 1984)
Arteriovenous malformations (Okamoto *et al.* 1984; Brown *et al.* 1990) (section 9.1.4)
Moyamoya syndrome (Nagamine *et al.* 1981) (section 7.5)

*In polycystic kidney disease, not only hypertension but also developmental factors contribute to the formation of intracranial aneurysms.

Saccular aneurysms arise at sites of arterial branching, usually at the base of the brain, either on the circle of Willis itself or at a nearby branching point (Fig. 9.2, Table 9.2). Aneurysms of the middle cerebral artery tend to have the largest diameter (Qureshi *et al.* 2000). The absolute frequencies depend to some degree on whether fatal cases of SAH have been included and also on the definition of aneurysmal size, and the diligence of the search for unruptured aneurysms. In a systematic review of studies reporting the prevalence of all intracranial aneurysms in patients studied for reasons other than SAH, the best estimate of the frequency for an average adult without specific risk factors was 2.3% (95% confidence interval [CI], 1.7%–3.1%); and this tended to increase with age (Rinkel *et al.* 1998) (section 13.12.1).

On the assumption that up to 5% of people in the population eventually develop at least a single aneurysm in their lifetime, and the knowledge that the annual incidence of

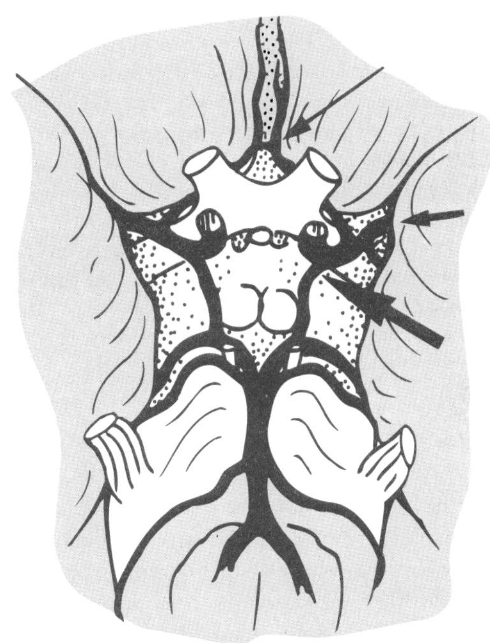

Fig. 9.2 Schematic drawing of the circle of Willis in the suprasellar cistern at the base of the brain. The medial parts of the temporal lobes have been slightly retracted to allow a better view. The anterior communicating artery is at the top of the drawing (long thin arrow), the origin of the posterior communicating artery from the carotid artery is at the lateral border of the suprasellar cistern (thick arrow) and the terminal bifurcation of the basilar artery is found in the most dorsal part of the suprasellar cisterns (bottom part of dotted area), in the interpeduncular fossa. The middle cerebral artery courses laterally, in the horizontal part of the Sylvian fissure (short arrow); aneurysms of this artery are found at the lateral end of the fissure (not visible), where it meets at right angles with the lateral part of the Sylvian fissure and where the artery trifurcates. (With permission from Vermeulen *et al.* 1992.)

Table 9.2 Sites of ruptured aneurysms in 326 consecutive patients (from Vermeulen *et al.* 1984)*.

Site of aneurysm	*n*	%
Anterior communicating artery complex†	134	41
Internal carotid artery‡	101	31
Middle cerebral artery§	60	18
Posterior circulation¶	31	10

*Half the patients were admitted to a general neurology unit and half to a department of neurosurgery; of the 326 aneurysms, 285 were identified on angiography and 41 at post-mortem. In other studies, the distribution is very similar.

† Most aneurysms of the anterior cerebral artery are of the anterior communicating artery, rarely at other sites, such as the pericallosal artery.

‡ Most aneurysms of the internal carotid artery are at the origin of the posterior communicating artery, more rarely at other sites such as the origin of the ophthalmic artery or the terminal bifurcation of the internal carotid artery into the middle and anterior cerebral arteries.

§ Aneurysms of the middle cerebral artery arise in 90% of cases from the point where the mainstem of the artery divides into its main branches, although there is individual variation in whether this point is near the temporal bone or more medially; in the remaining 10%, the aneurysm arises on the proximal segment of the middle cerebral artery, at the origin of lenticulostriate, fronto-orbital or early temporal branches (Hosoda *et al.* 1995).

¶ Most aneurysms of the posterior circulation are at the tip of the basilar artery, less often they are at the origin of the posterior inferior cerebellar artery or at the junction between the posterior cerebral artery and the posterior communicating artery.

aneurysmal SAH is approximately six per 100 000 (Linn *et al.* 1996), which corresponds with a lifetime risk of 0.5%, only about one in 10 cerebral aneurysms ever rupture. The rate at which aneurysms increase in size is often assumed to be gradual, but rapid expansion has been documented and may contribute to the risk of rupture (Barth & De Tribolet 1994).

The notion of 'weak spots'

It is largely unknown why only some adults develop aneurysms at arterial bifurcations and most do not, except in specific, mostly genetically determined conditions (Table 9.1). The once popular notion of a congenital defect in the muscle layer of the wall (tunica media) being a weak spot through which the inner layers of the arterial wall could bulge has been largely dispelled by a number of contradictory observations. Firstly, gaps in the muscle layer of intracranial arteries are equally common in patients with and without aneurysms, and are usually strengthened by densely packed collagen fibrils (Stehbens 1989; Fujimoto 1996; Finlay *et al.* 1998). Secondly, in experimental situations, the internal elastic lamina at the site of such gaps can withstand very high intralumenal pressure without breaking up or bulging out (Glynn 1940). Finally, if an aneurysm has formed, any defect in the muscle layer is located not at the neck of the aneurysm, but somewhere in the wall of the aneurysmal sac (Stehbens 1989). If unruptured aneurysms are operated on, they commonly show an inflammatory reaction, which perhaps heralds impending rupture (Chyatte *et al.* 1999).

Despite aneurysms not being congenital in the strict sense, there is some degree of genetic predisposition for their formation, apart from the specific conditions listed in Table 9.1. It is well known that there are families in which three or more first-degree or second-degree relatives have had an SAH, and at a younger median age than the early 50s, which is the most common age at which sporadic aneurysms rupture (Alberts *et al.* 1995; Bromberg *et al.* 1995a). Patients with a positive family history are younger and more likely to have multiple aneurysms, or aneurysms on the middle cerebral artery, than patients with aneurysms and a negative family history (Norrgard *et al.* 1987; Bromberg *et al.* 1995a; Ronkainen *et al.* 1995a). New aneurysms may form in the course of only a few years (Leblanc 1999). A post-mortem study found degeneration of elastic fibres and increased ground substance in the systemic arteries of two of the three patients with familial aneurysms, but in none of the 25 patients with sporadic aneurysms (Schievink *et al.* 1997b). Such families, with at least two affected first-degree relatives, contribute only a small fraction of all SAHs, accounting for at least 7% but at most 20% of episodes (Schievink 1997) (section 13.12.1).

Some degree of familial clustering also occurs in so-called sporadic subarachnoid haemorrhage (section 13.12.5). Undoubtedly, the familial clustering can to some extent be explained by shared classical vascular risk factors, which are associated with ruptured aneurysms (see next paragraph). Perhaps it is the influence of these factors which leads to local thickening of the intimal layer ('intimal pads') in the arterial wall, distal and proximal to a branching site, findings which some investigators regard as the earliest changes leading to the formation of aneurysms (Walker & Allegre 1954; Hassler 1962). In younger people, these pads consist mainly of smooth-muscle cells, while in older people they are more fibrous (Hassler 1962). It has been suggested that the formation of these pads, in which the intimal layer is inelastic, causes increased strain in the more elastic portions of the vessel wall (Crompton 1966). Nevertheless, classical risk factors such as hypertension explain only part of the familial aggregation of SAH (Bromberg *et al.* 1996). The complementary portion of the genetic factors may well be expressed through minor intrinsic abnormalities of the arterial wall. A variety of studies have offered glimpses of different structural or metabolic abnormalities of this kind:

• myxoid degeneration of connective tissue over the full thickness of the aneurysm wall (O'Boynick *et al.* 1994);
• a decrease in the number and length of reticular fibres in the arterial media of cerebral arteries (Chyatte *et al.* 1990);
• reduced production of collagen type III (Van den Berg *et al.* 1997);
• signs of apoptosis (DNA fragmentation) in the dome and neck of aneurysms (Hara *et al.* 1998);
• elevated levels of proteolytic enzymes, such as elastase in serum (Baker *et al.* 1995; Connolly *et al.* 1997), elastase in aneurysms (Gaetani *et al.* 1998), collagenase in aneurysms (Gaetani *et al.* 1998), or gelatinase produced by cultured skin fibroblasts (Chyatte & Lewis 1997);
• and finally, insertions in the gene for endoglin, a glycoprotein expressed on the surface of human vascular endothelial cells (Takenaka *et al.* 1999).

Acquired risk factors

Some classical risk factors for stroke in general also apply to SAH, but they are not exactly the same as those for intracerebral haemorrhage (Juvela 1996). A systematic review of studies reporting risk factors for SAH included eight longitudinal and 10 case–control studies that fulfilled predefined methodological criteria, such as the diagnosis of SAH being confirmed by CT, and angiography or post-mortem in at least 70% of patients (Teunissen *et al.* 1996). In aggregate, only smoking, hypertension and heavy drinking emerged as significant risk factors, with odds ratios of about two or three. The effect of smoking was confirmed in a later case–control study (Weir *et al.* 1998). Also, smokers have larger aneurysms than non-smokers, and they more often have multiple aneurysms (Juvela 2000; Qureshi *et al.* 2000). For the use of oral contraceptives, the risk was not significantly increased in that general review, but it was in a specific meta-analysis published 2 years later (Johnston *et al.* 1998). The risks were not clear for hormone replacement therapy, or an increased level of plasma cholesterol (Teunissen *et al.* 1996). Seasonal variation does not seem to occur, but circadian variation does, with low rates of rupture at night and high rates during working hours (Schievink *et al.* 1995; Vermeer *et al.* 1997).

Some acquired disease conditions may predispose to the formation of aneurysms: cerebellar haemangioblastoma (Guzman & Grady 1999), metastasis from bronchial carcinoma (Gliemroth *et al.* 1999), and (perhaps) Lyme disease (Oksi *et al.* 1998). Iatrogenic causes include radiation therapy (Jensen & Wagner 1997) (section 7.12), acrylate applied externally for microvascular decompression (Tokuda *et al.* 1998), and superficial temporal artery–middle cerebral artery bypass surgery, with the aneurysm forming at the site of the anastomosis (Sasaki *et al.* 1996).

9.1.2 Non-aneurysmal perimesencephalic haemorrhage

In this radiologically distinct and strikingly harmless variety of subarachnoid haemorrhage (SAH), the extravasated blood is confined to the cisterns around the midbrain, and the centre of the bleeding is immediately anterior to the midbrain (van Gijn *et al.* 1985a; Rinkel *et al.* 1991a; Schwartz & Solomon 1996). In some cases, the only evidence of blood is found anterior to the pons (Zentner *et al.* 1996; Schievink & Wijdicks 1997). Here it is necessary to anticipate in some detail the radiological investigations discussed in section 9.4.1, because this disease entity is defined entirely by the characteristic distribution of the extravasated blood on brain CT, in combination with a normal four-vessel angiogram. The angiographic study is necessary because one in 20–40 patients with a perimesencephalic pattern of haemorrhage has a ruptured aneurysm of the basilar or vertebral artery (Rinkel *et al.* 1991a; Pinto *et al.* 1993; Van Calenbergh *et al.* 1993). By contrast, about 10–20% of ruptured posterior fossa aneurysms have a perimesencephalic pattern of subarachnoid bleeding on CT (Kayama *et al.* 1991; Kallmes *et al.* 1996). The source of these perimesencephalic haemorrhages without an identifiable arterial lesion is obscure. There is no extension of the haemorrhage to the lateral Sylvian fissures or to the anterior part of the interhemispheric fissure. Some sedimentation of blood in the posterior horns of the lateral ventricles may occur, but frank intraventricular haemorrhage or extension of the haemorrhage into the brain parenchyma indicates arterial haemorrhage and rules out this particular condition (Rinkel *et al.* 1991a).

Perimesencephalic haemorrhage constitutes approximately 10% of episodes of SAH and two-thirds of those with a normal angiogram (Rinkel *et al.* 1991a; Farrés *et al.* 1992; Ferbert *et al.* 1992; Kitahara *et al.* 1993; Pinto *et al.* 1993). It can occur in any patient over the age of 20 years, but most patients are in their sixth decade, as with aneurysmal haemorrhage. A history of hypertension is not obtained more often than expected, except in a single study (Canhao *et al.* 1999), and there is no history of 'sentinel headaches' (Rinkel *et al.* 1991b). In one-third of the patients, strenuous activities immediately precede the onset of symptoms, a proportion similar to that found in aneurysmal haemorrhage (van Gijn *et al.* 1985a; Rinkel *et al.* 1991b).

Clinically, there is little to distinguish this idiopathic perimesencephalic haemorrhage from aneurysmal haemorrhage. The headache onset is more often gradual (minutes rather than seconds) than with aneurysmal haemorrhage, but the predictive value of this feature is poor (van Gijn *et al.* 1985a; Linn *et al.* 1998) (section 9.2.4). Loss of consciousness and focal symptoms are exceptional, and then only transient; a seizure at onset virtually rules out the diagnosis (Linn *et al.* 1998). Transient amnesia occurs in about one-third of cases, and is associated with enlargement of the temporal horns on the initial CT scan (Hop *et al.* 1998). On admission, all patients are in perfect clinical condition, apart from their headache (van Gijn *et al.* 1985b; Rinkel *et al.* 1991b). Typically, the early course is uneventful, re-bleeds and delayed cerebral ischaemia simply do not occur. About 20% of patients have acute hydrocephalus on their admission brain CT scan, associated with extravasation of blood in all perimesencephalic cisterns, which probably causes obstruction of the cerebrospinal fluid circulation at the tentorial hiatus (Rinkel *et al.* 1992). But only a few have symptoms from this ventricular dilatation, and even then an excellent outcome can be anticipated (Rinkel *et al.* 1990a, b). The period of convalescence is short, and almost invariably patients are able to resume their previous work and other activities (Rinkel *et al.* 1990a; Brilstra *et al.* 1997). Re-bleeds after the hospital period have not been documented so far, in two series of 77 and 36 patients followed for an average of 4 years and 2 years, respectively (Rinkel *et al.* 1991c; Canhao *et al.* 1995). The quality of life in the long term is excellent (Brilstra *et al.* 1997).

There is a distinct and benign variety of subarachnoid haemorrhage, in which the distribution of extravasated blood on the brain CT scan is different from aneurysmal haemorrhage, in the cisterns around the midbrain or ventral to the pons. The angiogram is completely normal. The long-term outcome is invariably excellent. This condition of non-aneurysmal perimesencephalic subarachnoid haemorrhage accounts for 10% of subarachnoid haemorrhages and two-thirds of subarachnoid haemorrhages with a normal angiogram.

For the time being, the definition of this mild and idiopathic variant of SAH remains a purely descriptive one, based on a combination of radiological and clinical criteria. Some have proposed the term pretruncal rather than perimesencephalic haemorrhage, to include patients in whom the haemorrhage is confined to the prepontine region (Schievink & Wijdicks 1997). However, that term does not take account of cases in which the haemorrhage is confined to the ambient or quadrigeminal cistern (van Gijn *et al.* 1985a; Rinkel & van Gijn 1995). The cause of the bleeding is unknown, largely because post-mortem studies have not been done, the very reason being that the outcome is so good. The mild clinical features, the limited extension of the extravasated blood on brain CT, and the normal angiograms all militate against an aneurysm, or in fact any arterial source of bleeding. Instead, rupture of a vein or a venous malformation in the prepontine or interpeduncular cistern seems a reasonable hypothesis.

We have emphasized above that a perimesencephalic pattern of haemorrhage may *occasionally* (in 2.5–5%) be caused by a ruptured posterior fossa aneurysm. By the same token, even rarer vascular abnormalities may also cause haemorrhage in the cisterns ventral to the lower brainstem: a (possible) capillary telangiectasia in the pons (Wijdicks & Schievink 1997), or lacunar infarction in the vicinity of the haemorrhage, with the conjecture that a small perforating artery had occluded and subsequently ruptured (Tatter *et al.* 1995; Rogg *et al.* 1999). It is rather a shot in the dark to assume that any such rare lesion causes *all* instances of idiopathic perimesencephalic haemorrhage.

9.1.3 Arterial dissection

Dissection in general tends to be recognized more often in the carotid than in the vertebral artery, but subarachnoid haemorrhage from a dissected artery is almost only found with the latter (Kaplan *et al.* 1993; Rinkel *et al.* 1993) (section 7.2.2). Blunt rotational or hyperextension trauma, even if slight, is a common cause of vertebral artery dissection, particularly in the young; iatrogenic causes include not only osteopathic manipulation but also surgery for glioma (Nohjoh *et al.* 1995). In middle-aged patients, dissection may occur more or less spontaneously.

What proportion of SAHs arise from a dissected vertebral artery is unknown. All miscellaneous causes together (including dissection) account for only about 5%, while 85% are aneurysmal haemorrhages and 10% idiopathic perimesencephalic haemorrhages. In a post-mortem study of fatal SAH, dissection was found in five of 110 patients (Sasaki *et al.* 1991a). With vertebral artery dissection in general, the injury to the vessel wall occurs most often in its extracranial course; in about one in eight the intradural portion only is affected, and in a similar proportion both segments of the artery are affected (Mokri *et al.* 1988). If SAH occurs with a dissection starting in the extracranial portion, the plane of cleavage is subadventitial rather than subintimal, and only extension into the intradural portion results in rupture, because there the outer wall of the artery is no longer protected by an external elastic lamina and the muscle layer and the adventitial layer are thinner (Caplan *et al.* 1988). Some propose that an extracranial pseudoaneurysm of the vertebral artery alone may give rise to SAH (Kaplan *et al.* 1993). In that case, one would have to assume—to explain the haemorrhage in the subarachnoid space—that one or more previous haemorrhages had led to adhesions between the outer wall of the artery and the dural sleeve of a cervical root. Sometimes intracranial dissection of the vertebral artery with subarachnoid haemorrhage is associated with anatomical abnormalities such as fenestration at the vertebrobasilar junction (Zhang *et al.* 1994), or a fusiform aneurysm (Yasui *et al.* 1999). It may occur bilaterally (Yasui *et al.* 1998). Dissection with SAH may also affect the posterior inferior cerebellar artery (Fransen & De Tribolet 1994; Jafar *et al.* 1998; Yasui *et al.* 2000), sometimes bilaterally (Shinoda *et al.* 1998), or the basilar artery (Hosoda *et al.* 1991).

Neurological deficits may accompany SAH from vertebral artery dissection (Table 9.3): palsies of cranial nerves IX and X, by subadventitial dissection (Senter & Sarwar 1982), and Wallenberg's syndrome, partial or complete, indicating subintimal dissection with impairment of blood flow in the territory of the posterior inferior cerebellar artery, resulting in ischaemia of the dorsolateral medulla (Caplan *et al.* 1988). Re-bleeds are common—between 30% and 70% in different series; the interval between subsequent bleeding episodes may be as short as a few hours or as long as a few weeks (Caplan *et al.* 1988; Aoki & Sakai 1990; Yamaura *et al.* 1990; Mizutani *et al.* 1995). Repeat rupture may even occur after proximal clipping of the artery (Kawamata *et al.* 1994). Such recurrent events are fatal in approximately half the patients.

Dissection of the intracranial portion of the internal carotid artery, or one of its branches, as a cause of SAH does occur, although it is far less common than dissection of the internal carotid artery in the neck, a condition encountered several times a year in most major neurology services (section 7.2.1). It should especially be suspected if cerebral angiography is negative despite a pattern of haemorrhage on CT that suggests aneurysmal rupture in the anterior circulation (Nakatomi *et al.* 1997). Reported cases have affected the terminal portion of the internal carotid artery (Adams *et al.* 1982; Massoud *et al.* 1992), the middle cerebral artery (Kunze & Schiefer 1971; Sasaki *et al.* 1991b; Piepgras *et al.* 1994) and the anterior cerebral artery (Guridi *et al.* 1993) (Fig. 9.29).

Table 9.3 Clinical features of vertebral artery dissection as the cause of subarachnoid haemorrhage.

- Headache starts low in the neck and then moves up to the head (although this may also occur with ruptured aneurysms)
- Palsies of cranial nerves IX or X occur (compression through subadventitial dissection)
- Symptoms and signs occur that are attributable to ischaemia in the territory of supply of the posterior inferior cerebellar artery:

Lower part of the cerebellar hemisphere
Vertigo
Inability to stand, or even sit
Dysarthria
Seventh nerve palsy, ipsilateral (through secondary compression of pons)
Dysmetria, ipsilateral (often absent)

Dorsolateral medulla oblongata
Horner's syndrome, ipsilateral
Rotatory nystagmus
Numbness of the face, ipsilateral
Numbness of the arm, trunk and leg, contralateral
Dysmetria, ipsilateral
Dysphagia
Hiccups

9.1.4 Rare conditions causing subarachnoid haemorrhage

These are listed in Table 9.4. Some deserve special comment.

Cerebral arteriovenous malformations

Cerebral arteriovenous malformations (AVMs) were formerly believed to cause a substantial proportion of subarachnoid haemorrhages (SAHs), but since the advent of CT it has become clear that haemorrhages from AVMs almost invariably involve the brain parenchyma (section 8.2.4). Subarachnoid bleeding at the convexity of the brain may occur from superficial AVMs, but in less than 5% of ruptured AVMs is the extravasation limited to the subarachnoid space, without intracerebral haematoma (Aoki 1991). Exclusively intraventricular haemorrhage may be associated with an AVM immediately under the ependymal surface (Darby *et al.* 1988) (section 9.1.5). Saccular aneurysms form on feeding arteries of 10–20% of AVMs, presumably because of the greatly increased flow and the attendant strain on the arterial wall. If bleeding occurs in these cases, it is more often from the aneurysm than from the malformation, but the site of the aneurysms is different from the classical sites of saccular aneurysms on the circle of Willis, and again the haemorrhage is more often into the brain itself than into the subarachnoid space (Brown *et al.* 1990; Marks *et al.* 1992).

Very few arteriovenous malformations rupture only into the subarachnoid space. The vast majority form an intracerebral haematoma, with or without extension into the subarachnoid space.

Dural arteriovenous fistulae

Dural arteriovenous fistulae of the tentorium can give rise to a basal haemorrhage that is indistinguishable on CT from aneurysmal haemorrhage (Lasjaunias *et al.* 1986) (section 8.2.8). The anomaly is rare, and can be found from adolescence to old age. Re-bleeding may occur in patients with dural AVMs; in a series of five patients presenting with SAH, three had one or more re-bleeds (Halbach *et al.* 1987).

Spinal arteriovenous malformations

Spinal AVMs, if symptomatic at all, present with SAH in approximately 10% of cases. In more than 50% of these patients, the first haemorrhage occurs before the age of 20 years (Caroscio *et al.* 1980; Kandel 1980). Symptoms may

Table 9.4 Causes of subarachnoid haemorrhage, other than intracranial saccular aneurysms.

Idiopathic perimesencephalic haemorrhage (section 9.1.2)

Lesions of intracranial arteries other than saccular aneurysms
Arterial dissection (section 9.1.3)
Blister-like bulges of the internal carotid artery (Ishikawa *et al.* 1997; Abe *et al.* 1998)
Fusiform aneurysm of basilar artery (Ricolfi *et al.* 1996)
Vertebrobasilar dolichoectasia (Rabb & Barnwell 1998) (section 6.3.2)
Rupture of a circumferential artery in the pontine cistern (Hochberg *et al.* 1974)

Arteriovenous shunts in the brain
Cerebral arteriovenous malformation (section 9.1.4)
Dural arteriovenous fistula (section 9.1.4)
Arteriovenous fistula at the craniocervical junction (Kinouchi *et al.* 1998)

Vascular lesions in the spinal cord
Saccular aneurysm of spinal arteries (section 9.1.4)
Spinal arteriovenous malformation (section 9.1.4)
Cavernous angioma in the cervical cord (Acciarri *et al.* 1992)

Cardiac myxoma (section 9.1.4)

Sickle-cell disease (section 9.1.4)

Vasculitis
Primary angiitis of the central nervous system (Hankey 1991; Kumar *et al.* 1997; Nishikawa *et al.* 1998) (section 7.3)
Polyarteritis (Munn *et al.* 1998) (section 7.3)

Superficial siderosis of the central nervous system (Tomlinson & Walton 1964; Bonito *et al.* 1994; Fearnley *et al.* 1995) (section 9.1.4)

Unsuspected head trauma (section 9.1.4)

Infections
Mycotic cerebral aneurysm (section 9.1.4)
Borreliosis (Chehrenama *et al.* 1997)

Tumours
Pituitary apoplexy (section 9.1.4)
Acoustic neuroma (Yonemitsu *et al.* 1983)
Cervical meningioma (Scotti *et al.* 1987)
Cervical neuroma (Corriero *et al.* 1996;. Caputi *et al.* 1997)

Drugs
Cocaine abuse (section 9.1.4)
Anticoagulants (section 9.1.4)

start with a sudden and excruciating pain in the lower part of the neck, rather than in the head. Pain radiating from the neck to the shoulders or arms points to a cervical origin of the haemorrhage (Acciarri *et al.* 1992). If there are no such clues, the true origin of the haemorrhage emerges only when spinal cord dysfunction develops, after a delay which may be as short as a few hours or as long as a few years (Kandel 1980; Swann *et al.* 1984). Re-bleeds may occur, even repeatedly (Aminoff & Logue 1974). Not only intradural malformations but also dural fistulae in the spinal axis may cause SAH (Willinsky *et al.* 1990). The usual presentation of a dural arteriovenous fistula is that of ascending spinal cord dysfunction (Lee *et al.* 1998b; Van der Meulen *et al.* 1999).

Saccular aneurysms of spinal arteries

Saccular aneurysms of spinal arteries are extremely rare, with approximately 12 patients on record (Handa *et al.* 1992; Mohsenipour *et al.* 1994). As with AVMs of the spinal cord, the clinical features of spinal SAH may be accompanied by those of a transverse lesion of the cord, partial or complete.

Cardiac myxoma

Cardiac myxoma is an extremely rare cause of aneurysm formation; the tumour may metastasize to an intracranial artery, infiltrate the wall and thus cause an aneurysm to develop, even more than a year after operation for the primary tumour (Furuya *et al.* 1995) (section 6.5).

Sickle-cell disease

Sickle-cell disease is commonly complicated by ischaemic stroke, seldom by SAH (Overby & Rothman 1985) (section 7.9). Thirty per cent of patients with sickle-cell disease and SAH are children, and CT scans show blood in the superficial cortical sulci; angiograms reveal no aneurysm but often show multiple distal branch occlusions and a leptomeningeal collateral circulation. The SAH is attributed to rupture of these collaterals (Carey *et al.* 1990). The outcome is poor: only three of 11 recently reviewed children recovered in a good functional state (Carey *et al.* 1990). Most adult patients in whom sickle-cell disease underlies SAH have a ruptured aneurysm at the base of the brain. The haemorrhage is located diffusely in the basal cisterns and the sickle-cell disease could well be coincidental, but the management may include partial exchange transfusions (Love *et al.* 1985).

Superficial siderosis of the central nervous system

This condition is characterized by iron overload of the pial membranes, through chronic oozing of blood from any source in the subarachnoid space. It has been included in this section on subarachnoid haemorrhage for theoretical reasons alone; the clinical picture is completely different and does not include sudden headache (Tomlinson & Walton 1964; Bonito *et al.* 1994; Fearnley *et al.* 1995). The syndrome is almost invariably characterized by subacute sensorineural deafness (95%), cerebellar ataxia (88%) and pyramidal signs (76%). Possible other features include dementia, bladder disturbance, and anosmia. Males are more often affected than females (3 : 1). A source of bleeding has been identified in a little more than half of the cases reported up to 1995 (Fearnley *et al.* 1995). Causes of chronic bleeding include vascular abnormalities of the dura surrounding the spinal cord or cervical roots, a vascular tumour such as an ependymoma of the cauda equina (not really the first place to look if the problem is deafness; Fig. 9.3), as a late complication of a childhood cerebellar tumour (Anderson *et al.* 1999b), or any other vascular abnormality, including rarities such as transthyretin-related amyloidosis of meningeal vessels (Mascalchi *et al.* 1999). Probably the remaining cases are also due to chronic haemorrhage, but it is not clear from where. The high iron content of the pial membranes causes a characteristic signal on magnetic resonance (MR) scanning (Bonito *et al.* 1994; River *et al.* 1994; Uchino *et al.* 1997) (Fig. 9.4).

Head trauma

Trauma and spontaneous SAH are sometimes difficult to disentangle. Patients may be found alone after having been beaten up in a brawl or hit by a drunken driver who drove off. There may be no external wounds to indicate an accident, a decreased level of consciousness (making it impossible to obtain a history), and neck stiffness causing the patient to be worked up for SAH. Conversely, patients who rupture an aneurysm whilst riding a bicycle or driving a car may hit a tree or another vehicle, and the initial diagnosis will be 'traffic accident'. The diagnostic conundrum becomes really difficult when patients after aneurysmal rupture fall, hit their head and sustain a skull fracture (Sakas *et al.* 1995), or when head trauma causes an aneurysm to burst (Sahjpaul *et al.* 1998). Meticulous reconstruction of traffic or sports accidents may therefore be rewarding, especially in patients with disproportionate headache or neck stiffness.

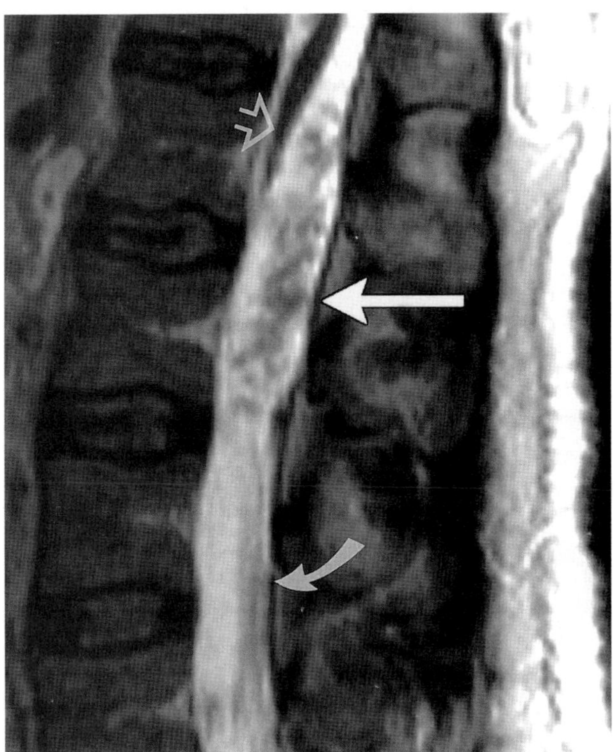

Fig. 9.3 A T2-weighted magnetic resonance scan, showing an ependymoma of the cauda equina (straight arrow) that had caused superficial siderosis of the central nervous system (Fig. 9.4). Note the displacement of the cord anteriorly (open arrow) superior to the ependymoma, and of the nerve roots inferior to the lesion (curved arrow).

Spontaneous subarachnoid haemorrhage may lead to head trauma, whilst head injury may cause superficial contusion of the brain, with accumulation of blood in the subarachnoid space. If there is any doubt, it is vital to disentangle the course of events as accurately as possible.

Fortunately, brain CT may help. If trauma is the cause of SAH, the blood is usually located in the superficial sulci at the convexity of the brain, adjacent to a fracture or to an intracerebral contusion (section 9.4.1).

Mycotic aneurysms

Mycotic aneurysms underlying SAH are most frequently caused by infective endocarditis (section 6.5) or aspergillosis (section 7.11). Of course, most strokes in the context of infective endocarditis are (haemorrhagic) infarcts or intracerebral haemorrhages from pyogenic arteritis (Hart *et al.* 1990; Masuda *et al.* 1992; Krapf *et al.* 1999) (section 8.2.11). Aneurysms associated with infective endocarditis are most often located on distal branches of the middle cerebral artery, because the septic emboli tend to lodge at the periphery of the arterial tree. Consequently, haemorrhages from mycotic aneurysms occur mostly in the cortex and in the underlying white matter, or occasionally in the subarachnoid space at the convexity of the brain (Masuda *et al.* 1992). Sometimes there is an associated subdural haematoma (Barami & Ko 1994). Only approximately 10% of the aneurysms develop at more proximal sites (Brust *et al.* 1990). Therefore, although rupture of a mycotic aneurysm causes an intracerebral haematoma in most patients, some have a basal pattern of haemorrhage on CT that is very similar to that of a ruptured saccular aneurysm. CT-documented re-bleeds have been reported (Steinberg *et al.* 1992).

Most mycotic aneurysms are located superficially in the cerebral hemisphere, in the cortex or underlying white matter.

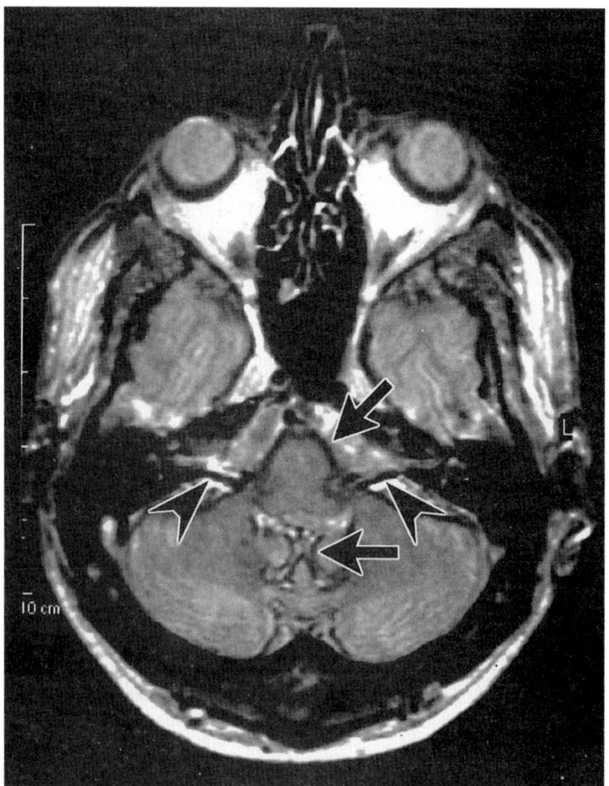

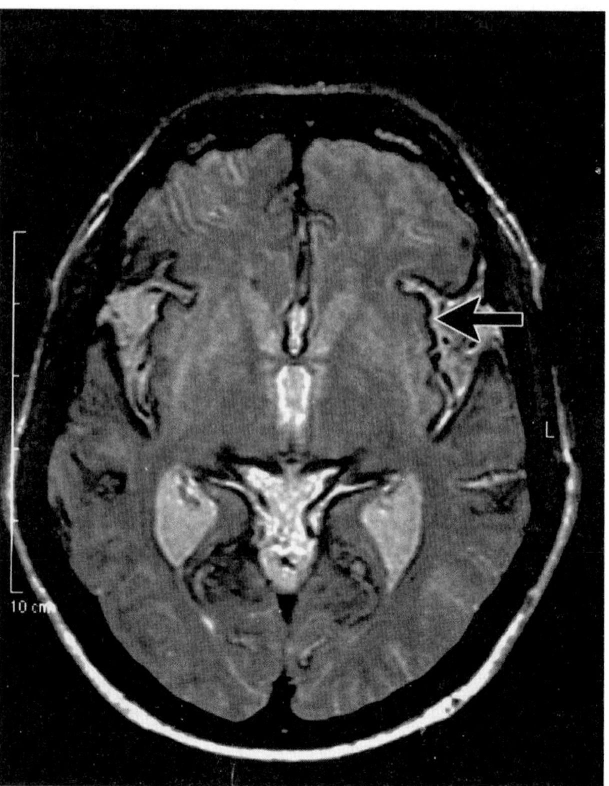

Fig. 9.4 Superficial siderosis of the nervous system. A T2-weighted magnetic resonance image of the brain in a 50-year-old man who presented with bilateral sensorineural hearing loss. The accumulation of ferric ions causes signal loss (black), due to a paramagnetic effect, over the entire pial surface (arrows), and in the acoustic nerves (arrowheads). (With permission from Padberg & Hoogenraad 2000.)

Usually, patients present with clinical features of infected heart valves before SAH occurs, but on rare occasions rupture of a mycotic aneurysm is the initial manifestation of infective endocarditis (Vincent *et al.* 1980; Salgado *et al.* 1987). Mycotic aneurysms may resolve after adequate antibiotic therapy, but at least one patient is on record with late rupture after appropriate treatment (Bamford *et al.* 1986; Brust *et al.* 1990).

Mycotic aneurysms in patients with aspergillosis are usually located on the proximal part of the basilar or carotid artery (Lau *et al.* 1991). Rupture of such an aneurysm causes massive and sometimes fatal SAH in the basal cisterns, indistinguishable from that of a saccular aneurysm (Kowall & Sobel 1988; Lau *et al.* 1991). Aspergillosis is difficult to diagnose, but should particularly be suspected in patients undergoing long-term treatment with antibiotics or immunosuppressive agents. Most patients with haematogenous dissemination have pulmonary lesions, but X-ray films of the chest may be normal early in the course (Young *et al.* 1970; Kowall & Sobel 1988).

Pituitary apoplexy

Pituitary apoplexy has been proposed as one of the causes of SAH of unknown cause (Bjerre *et al.* 1986). The precipitating event of arterial haemorrhage in a pituitary tumour is thought to be tissue necrosis, involving the wall of one or more hypophyseal arteries. The initial features are a sudden and severe headache, with or without nausea, vomiting, neck stiffness and depressed consciousness (Reid *et al.* 1985; Dodick & Wijdicks 1998) (section 5.6.2). The hallmark of pituitary apoplexy is that most patients suffer a sudden decrease in visual acuity: in one series of 15 patients, only two had normal acuity. However, the combination of sudden, severe headache and decreased vision (literally a 'blinding headache') may also occur in patients in whom rupture of an aneurysm is complicated by bilateral subhyaloid haemorrhages, but in most patients with pituitary apoplexy eye movements are disturbed as well, because the haemorrhage compresses the oculomotor, trochlear and abducens nerves in the adjacent cavernous sinus (McFadzean *et al.* 1991). Brain

CT or MR scanning reveals the pituitary fossa as the source of the haemorrhage and in most instances the adenoma itself is visible (Post *et al.* 1980; McFadzean *et al.* 1991).

Cocaine abuse

Cocaine abuse is associated with haemorrhagic as well as with ischaemic stroke (sections 7.15 and 8.5.4). The pattern of haemorrhage on brain CT may be comparable to that of a ruptured saccular aneurysm (Wojak & Flamm 1987), and the diagnosis rests on a confirmatory history or on the results of toxicological tests. In patients with SAH related to the use of the alkaloid form of cocaine, about half have a vascular anomaly, an aneurysm or arteriovenous malformation (Levine *et al.* 1990). Re-bleeds do occur, even in patients with a normal angiogram, and the outcome is often poor (Mangiardi *et al.* 1988). The source of the haemorrhage in patients without an aneurysm is unknown. Although biopsy-proven vasculitis has been found (Krendel *et al.* 1990), changes suggestive of vasculitis often fail to show up on angiograms, admittedly a very poor test (Mangiardi *et al.* 1988; Levine *et al.* 1990) (Table 7.1). Ingestion of *ephedrine* may also precipitate aneurysmal SAH (Bruno *et al.* 1993).

Anticoagulation-related subarachnoid haemorrhage

Anticoagulation-related SAH accounts for some 9% of aneurysmal haemorrhages (Rinkel *et al.* 1997). Less often, anticoagulants cause SAH without an associated aneurysm. In a series of 116 patients with intracranial, extracerebral haemorrhage while on anticoagulant treatment, seven had only SAH, and in only three of these patients was there no cause for the haemorrhage other than anticoagulation (Mattle *et al.* 1989). Severe coagulopathy other than by anticoagulant drugs, for example congenital deficiency of factor VII, is also a rare cause of haemorrhage confined to the subarachnoid space (Papa *et al.* 1994).

9.1.5 Spontaneous intraventricular haemorrhage

Intraventricular haemorrhage is usually associated with either a ruptured aneurysm (most often on the anterior communicating artery complex) or intracerebral haemorrhage. In both situations, the outcome is worse with intraventricular rupture than without, and an intraventricular blood volume of more than 20 mL is invariably fatal without surgical intervention (Brott & Mandybur 1986; Young *et al.* 1990; Fogelholm *et al.* 1992; Roos *et al.* 1995). In contrast, the outcome of 'primary' intraventricular haemorrhage, without detectable cause, is much better than if it is associated with subarachnoid or intraparenchymal haemorrhage; patients may survive even with intraventricular haemorrhages far exceeding 20 mL (Verma *et al.* 1987; Roos *et al.* 1995). The advent of CT scanning proved that intraventricular haemorrhage is not the invariably lethal condition it was once thought to be, when the diagnosis was made only in those who died.

'Primary', or idiopathic, intraventricular haemorrhage is often speculatively attributed to occult vascular malformations in the ependymal wall. But only in exceptional cases can they actually be demonstrated (Waga *et al.* 1985; Darby *et al.* 1988; Nakayama *et al.* 1989; Donnet *et al.* 1992). Specific other causes range from tumours, which are immediately obvious on CT scanning, to small aneurysms at uncommon sites, which only assiduous investigation can uncover (Table 9.5).

Table 9.5 Causes of spontaneous intraventricular haemorrhage.

Uncommon aneurysms
Posterior inferior cerebellar artery (Yeh *et al.* 1985; Osenbach *et al.* 1986; Ruelle *et al.* 1988; Sadato *et al.* 1991)
Anterior inferior cerebellar artery (Oana *et al.* 1991)

Arteriovenous malformations
In the ependymal lining (Waga *et al.* 1985; Darby *et al.* 1988; Nakayama *et al.* 1989; Donnet *et al.* 1992)
Of the choroid plexus (Schmitt 1983; van Rybroek & Moore 1990)
Dural fistula of the superior sagittal sinus (Kataoka & Taneda 1984)

Occlusive arterial disease
Moyamoya syndrome: idiopathic (Ruelle *et al.* 1988), atherosclerotic (Masson *et al.* 1986), or with associated aneurysm (Konishi *et al.* 1985; Hamada *et al.* 1994) (section 7.5)
Lacunar infarction (Gates *et al.* 1986)

Tumours
Pituitary tumour (Tsubota *et al.* 1991)
Ependymoma (Poon & Solis 1985)
Meningioma (Nachanakian *et al.* 1983)

Infectious diseases
Brain abscess (Pascual *et al.* 1987)
Parasitic granuloma (Wong & Ho 1994)

Drugs
Cocaine (Levine *et al.* 1990)
Amphetamines (Imanse & Vanneste 1990)

Wernicke's encephalopathy (Pfister & Von Rosen 1995)

9.2 Clues from the history

The a priori probability of an aneurysm as the cause of subarachnoid haemorrhage (SAH) is so high that other conditions are very unlikely unless there are very strong clues in the history (head trauma, infective endocarditis, sickle-cell disease, pituitary adenoma) or in any antecedent events (violent head movements, cocaine ingestion), or if the first pain was felt in the neck rather than in the head (arterial dissection, or spinal SAH).

9.2.1 Medical history

In patients with a distant history of head injury, and particularly with a skull fracture, a *dural arteriovenous fistula* should be suspected, since healing of the fracture may be accompanied by the development of such a lesion (Chaudhary *et al.* 1982). *Mycotic aneurysms* may give rise to SAH even in patients not known to have a disorder of the heart valves, but this presentation of infective endocarditis is exceptional (Vincent *et al.* 1980; Salgado *et al.* 1987). For practical purposes, the possibility can be safely dismissed in a previously healthy patient in whom the haemorrhage is located at the base of the brain. A diagnosis of a ruptured mycotic aneurysm may well be entertained, however, with a history of malaise and a haemorrhage located at the convexity of the brain. Usually it will not be hard for the physician to get acquainted with the existence of *sickle-cell disease*, a history of *cardiac myxoma*, or the influence of *coagulation disorders*. The use of *anticoagulants* probably does not contribute to the risk of aneurysmal rupture, but it is important to know that in such patients the prognosis is worse than average, and that normal coagulation should be urgently restored by intravenous administration of clotting factors (Rinkel *et al.* 1997). Use of anticoagulants in itself should not be regarded as a sufficient explanation for subarachnoid haemorrhage; the search for an underlying lesion ought to be just as rigorous as in other patients.

Pituitary apoplexy may be difficult to diagnose if an adenoma was not already known about, particularly if a decrease in the level of consciousness precludes a proper assessment of any visual and oculomotor deficits. Usually, the underlying adenoma has insidiously manifested itself before the dramatic occurrence of the haemorrhage, for example by a dull retro-orbital pain, fatigue, a gradual decrease of visual acuity or constriction of the temporal fields, but often these symptoms lead to the diagnosis only in retrospect and not before. There are many contributing conditions and factors that may precipitate haemorrhagic infarction of a pituitary tumour, such as pregnancy, raised intracranial pressure, anticoagulants, cerebral angiography or the administration of gonadotrophin-releasing hormone (Reid *et al.* 1985; Masson *et al.* 1993). On CT scanning the haemorrhage usually remains confined within the tumour capsule, rarely it extends throughout the basal cisterns as with ruptured aneurysms.

9.2.2 Family history

A family history of subarachnoid haemorrhage (SAH) can be a useful clue in patients with sudden headache, although of course that same fact may give rise to false alarms. There are some families in which numerous relatives are struck down by ruptured aneurysms (Bromberg *et al.* 1995a; Schievink 1997). Even in cases of so-called sporadic SAH, the risk in first-degree relatives is increased (Bromberg *et al.* 1995b). Families in which aneurysmal rupture has occurred in two or more first-degree relatives may have an underlying or associated disorder, such as Ehlers–Danlos syndrome type IV, pseudoxanthoma elasticum, hereditary haemorrhagic telangiectasia, polycystic kidney disease, polycystic liver disease, or coarctation of the aorta (Table 9.1), but in most cases of familial aneurysms there is no such overt disorder.

9.2.3 Antecedent events

A *previous episode of sudden headache* hardly increases the likelihood of aneurysmal subarachnoid haemorrhage, despite a widespread belief in the existence of 'sentinel headaches', thought to be 'warning leaks'. Indeed, on specific questioning, 20–40% of patients recall a previous episode of headache that was unusually severe and lasted several hours (Verweij *et al.* 1988; Tolias & Choksey 1996). Many neurosurgeons and neurologists are therefore convinced that important advances in the overall management of ruptured aneurysms can be expected from early recognition of minute episodes of subarachnoid haemorrhage, followed by emergency clipping or coiling of the aneurysm. A major difficulty with the notion of these 'warning leaks' is that almost all studies have been hospital-based, most have been retrospective, and that even prospectively conducted studies are probably biased by hindsight (recall bias). In a prospective study of 148 patients with sudden, severe headache identified in general practice, 37 had subarachnoid haemorrhage (SAH). Other serious neurological conditions were diagnosed in 18. In the remaining 93 patients, no neurological cause of headache was found and after 1 year of follow-up there were no subsequent episodes of SAH, or sudden deaths. Only two of the 37 patients with SAH had had previous episodes of sudden headache on systematic questioning by the general practitioner at the time of presentation with the headache (Linn *et al.* 1994) Also, the amount and distribution of extravasated blood on brain CT, as well as the overall outcome, was similar to that in a previous hospital series of patients with subarachnoid haemorrhage. In other words, first-ever episodes of subarachnoid haemorrhage detected in general practice are not 'small leaks', but the real thing and represent the same spectrum of severity as those seen in hospital.

A second approach to confirm or exclude the existence of 'warning leaks' is to study the clinical and radiological features in a prospective series of patients admitted to hospital with aneurysmal SAH and then to compare the subgroup of patients with a history of preceding episodes of sudden headache, with the others. The distribution of clinical and radiological features is exactly the same in the two groups, and distinctly less severe than in those with a documented rebleed in hospital (Linn *et al.* 2000). In brief, the notion of frequent 'warning leaks' is not supported by epidemiological, clinical and radiological evidence. Notwithstanding the potentially serious consequences for the individual patient, this does not mean that an episode of subarachnoid haemorrhage cannot be missed by primary care physicians—or hospital doctors, for that matter—but avoidance of these errors is unlikely to result in substantial improvement in the overall patient mortality from SAH in the population (Hop J.W., unpublished observations).

A history of even quite minor neck trauma or of sudden, unusual head movements before the onset of headache may provide a clue to the diagnosis of *vertebral artery dissection* as a cause of SAH. Head trauma and primary SAH may be confused (section 9.1.4). Trauma should always be suspected in patients found unconscious in the street, even if there is marked neck stiffness and no superficial wound. Conversely, a traffic accident may sometimes be the result rather than the cause of SAH, and invaluable information obtained from the police or ambulance workers. In a patient known to have swerved from one side of the road to the other before crashing into someone else, the a priori probabilities are rather different (i.e. illness, falling asleep) from those in someone reported to have ignored a red traffic light (i.e. reckless, not paying attention).

Cocaine ingestion as a risk factor may not be immediately obvious in the case of an unconscious patient. Cocaine (or ephedrine) should be considered in young adults with SAH, particularly if the social background is unstable, although in some regions of the world the use of cocaine affects all social strata. Even if many members of the family turn up, one may find that none are aware of illicit drugs being used, or willing to volunteer this information even if they are. In cocaine-associated SAH, there is often an underlying aneurysm (Levine *et al.* 1991; Nolte *et al.* 1996). It is unknown whether cocaine induces not only the rupture but also the development of aneurysms.

9.2.4 Nature of the headache at onset

The key feature in diagnosing subarachnoid haemorrhage (SAH) is the history of sudden, severe and unusual headache. Classically, it comes on in seconds ('a flash', 'just like that', 'a bolt from a blue sky', 'as if I was hit on the head'), or in a few minutes at most. A potential pitfall is that patients may sometimes use the word 'sudden' to describe an episode of headache that came on over half an hour or longer, depending on the interval after which the history is given. And even if the headache really comes on within seconds or minutes, such a history is not specific for ruptured aneurysms, or even for SAH in general. Sudden onset headache may also occur with other intracranial haemorrhages, with non-haemorrhagic brain disease, and especially with innocuous forms of 'thunderclap' headache: variants of vascular headache, migrainous or not, or of muscle contraction headache (Linn *et al.* 1998) (section 5.6.1). Sexual activity may precipitate not only SAH, but also relatively harmless headaches, migrainous or not (Lance 1976; Pascual *et al.* 1996).

In general practice, exceptional forms of common headaches outnumber common forms of a rare disease, in this case a ruptured aneurysm (section 5.6.2). That statement sounds paradoxical, but there are many other examples of this paradox (Rose 1992) (section 18.5.2 and Table 18.6): although high maternal age is a strong risk factor for Down's syndrome, most children with that chromosomal abnormality are born of mothers under 30 years of age. Similarly, most patients with ischaemic stroke are not severely hypertensive, etc. The incidence of aneurysmal haemorrhage is about six per 100 000 population per year (Linn *et al.* 1996). Therefore, a family physician with a practice of 2000 people will, on average, see only one such patient every 8 years. Patients with headache may present not only to general practitioners, but also to an accident and emergency department, where they constitute around 1% of attendances (Fodden *et al.* 1989). The proportion with serious neurological conditions ranges from 16% for all patients with any headache (Fodden *et al.* 1989), to 75% for those with episodes of sudden headache specifically referred to a neurologist (Linn *et al.* 1994; van der Wee *et al.* 1995).

The exact speed of onset of 'sudden' headache, seconds or minutes, in patients without any other deficits, is of little help for the hospital physician in distinguishing aneurysmal haemorrhage from innocuous headaches, or from non-aneurysmal perimesencephalic haemorrhage (section 9.1.2). The predictive value of the speed of onset (seconds vs. 1–5 min) can be calculated from two data sets. Firstly, ruptured aneurysms are nine times as common as non-aneurysmal perimesencephalic haemorrhages (Rinkel *et al.* 1993), and in hospital series these two forms of subarachnoid haemorrhage together are twice as common as innocuous headaches (van der Wee *et al.* 1995). Secondly, headache develops almost instantaneously in 50% of patients with aneurysmal SAH, 35% of patients with non-aneurysmal perimesencephalic haemorrhage, and 68% of patients with benign 'thunderclap' headaches; for an onset within 1–5 min, these proportions are 19%, 35% and 19%, respectively (Linn *et al.* 1998). If, for the sake of simplicity, we ignore patients with sudden headache from other serious (non-haemorrhagic) brain disease, such as intracranial venous thrombosis (de Bruijn *et al.* 1996), calculations on the back of an envelope lead to the disappointing conclusion that an onset within seconds correctly predicts aneurysmal haemorrhage in only 55%, and that headache onset in 5–10 min correctly predicts innocuous headache in only 30%.

In brief, there are no single or combined features of the headache that distinguish reliably, and at an early stage, between SAH and innocuous types of sudden headache (Linn *et al.* 1998). The discomfort and cost of referring the majority of patients for a brief consultation in hospital (which should include CT scanning and a delayed lumbar puncture if this is negative) is probably outweighed by avoidance of the potential disaster of missing a ruptured aneurysm and the patient later being readmitted with re-bleeding, or another secondary complication (van der Wee *et al.* 1995).

It is exceedingly rare for headache at the onset of aneurysmal haemorrhage in an awake patient to be mild or to last less than 2 h, or for the symptoms to consist of non-specific 'dizziness'. If severe headache lasts longer, there is no clinical feature that distinguishes reliably, and at an early stage, between subarachnoid haemorrhage and innocuous types of sudden headache.

Pain at onset in the lower part of the neck (upper neck pain is common also with ruptured intracranial aneurysms), or a sudden and stabbing pain between the shoulder-blades (*coup de poignard* or dagger thrust), with or without radiation to the arms, suggests a *spinal arteriovenous malformation* or *fistula* as the source of SAH. Generally only intradural arteriovenous malformations tend to present with subarachnoid haemorrhage, whereas dural arteriovenous fistulae are associated with a progressive myelopathy and not with haemorrhage, but fistulae at the cervical level can be an exception to this rule (Rosenblum *et al.* 1987; Kinouchi *et al.* 1998). Even if there is severe headache initially, this may evolve into backache or radicular pain, especially if the patient remains up and about.

Sudden pain in the lower neck or between the shoulder-blades is a pointer to spinal subarachnoid haemorrhage, particularly if the pain radiates to the shoulders or arms. Dissection of the thoracic aorta is another possibility.

9.2.5 Loss of consciousness

Loss of consciousness at onset occurs in over half the patients with aneurysmal subarachnoid haemorrhage (SAH) (section 5.6.1). Some patients complain of headache before they lose consciousness, and all patients have severe headache if they regain consciousness. Some patients may enter a confusioned, agitated state (delirium), with or without preceding coma. Bizarre actions may include grimacing, spitting, making sucking or kissing sounds, spluttering, singing, whistling, yelling and screaming (Fisher 1975; Reijneveld *et al.* 2000). More than once, such behaviour has been misinterpreted as psychological in origin. Non-aneurysmal perimesencephalic SAH is typically associated with normal cognitive function; loss of consciousness or altered behaviour practically rules out this diagnosis, but amnesia may occur, mostly in association with an enlarged ventricular system (Hop *et al.* 1998). Head trauma should always be considered in patients who are found unconscious (section 9.1.4).

In patients with an impaired level of consciousness on admission, it is important to ascertain whether this was from the onset, in which case it is the result of global perfusion failure caused by the high cerebrospinal fluid pressure at the time of rupture, or sometimes of an intraparenchymal haematoma. If the level of consciousness decreased only later, a treatable complication should be suspected, such as acute hydrocephalus (section 13.9), or oedema formation around an intraparenchymal haematoma.

9.2.6 Epileptic seizures

Epileptic seizures at the onset of aneurysmal subarachnoid haemorrhage (SAH) occur in approximately 6–16% of patients (Sarner & Rose 1967; Hart *et al.* 1981; Pinto *et al.* 1996). Those with a large amount of cisternal blood on brain CT are relatively often affected (Hart *et al.* 1981) (section 5.6.1). Of course, the majority of patients presenting with *de novo* epilepsy above the age of 25 will have underlying conditions other than subarachnoid haemorrhage, but the diagnosis should be suspected if the postictal headache is unusually severe or prolonged. Seizures have not been documented in patients with perimesencephalic SAH, presumably of venous origin, but they may well complicate haemorrhages from arterial sources other than aneurysms, such as dissection of the vertebral artery, or a vascular malformation.

9.3 Clues from the examination

9.3.1 Neck stiffness

This is a common sign in subarachnoid haemorrhage (SAH) of any cause, but it takes hours to develop and therefore it cannot be used to exclude the diagnosis if a patient is seen soon after the sudden-onset headache. Neck stiffness is also absent in deep coma. If present, the sign does not distinguish between different causes of SAH, and nor between SAH and meningitis (section 5.6.1).

9.3.2 Subhyaloid haemorrhages

The sudden increase in cerebrospinal fluid (CSF) pressure that occurs with rupture of an aneurysm is transmitted to the CSF spaces surrounding the optic nerves and blocks the venous outflow from the retina, which in turn may lead to rupture of retinal veins (Manschot 1954) (section 5.6.1). Such intraocular haemorrhages occur in approximately 17% of patients who survive the acute phase (Pfausler *et al.* 1996; Frizzell *et al.* 1997) (Fig. 5.43); in half of them the blood remains confined to the space between the retina and the vitreous body, in the other half it ruptures into the vitreous body (Terson's syndrome) (section 13.11.1). Exceptionally, the preretinal haemorrhages are the only sign of SAH (Kiriakopoulos *et al.* 1998).

9.3.3 Pyrexia

During the first 2–3 days after subarachnoid haemorrhage,

of aneurysmal or other origin, the body temperature rarely exceeds 38.5°C, but thereafter it may rise to over 39°C (Rousseaux *et al.* 1980) (section 5.6.1).

9.3.4 Hypertension

Hypertension is a well-established risk factor for subarachnoid haemorrhage (SAH) (Teunissen *et al.* 1996), and 20–25% of patients have a history of hypertension (Fortuny *et al.* 1980; Vermeulen *et al.* 1984) (section 5.6.1). On admission, about 50% of patients with aneurysmal SAH have a markedly raised blood pressure. Unfortunately, a high blood pressure is almost the rule in patients presenting to an accident and emergency department for any reason, which makes the predictive value of blood pressure readings in that situation abysmally low. In many patients, this raised blood pressure is a reactive phenomenon, and not a marker of long-standing hypertension; often the blood pressure returns to normal within a few days. The blood pressure changes probably serve to counteract the decrease in cerebral perfusion resulting from increased cerebrospinal fluid pressure and later vasospasm.

9.3.5 Focal neurological deficits

Classically, in the acute phase of aneurysmal subarachnoid haemorrhage, there are no signs other than those of meningeal irritation, but exceptions to this rule can provide useful information about the site or the extent of the haemorrhage (Table 9.6). In the second or third week after rupture, focal deficits are not uncommon, most often representing secondary ischaemia (section 13.8). If the source of the haemorrhage is a giant aneurysm of the circle of Willis (Drake 1979), there may have been focal deficits or other symptoms before rupture, such as multiple cranial nerve palsies, ischaemic deficits through embolism (section 7.6), or epilepsy (Mizobuchi *et al.* 1999).

Table 9.6 Focal neurological signs early after subarachnoid haemorrhage, and their explanation.

Sign	Most common explanation
Hemiparesis	Large subarachnoid clot in Sylvian fissure (middle cerebral artery aneurysm)
Paraparesis	Aneurysm of anterior communicating artery; spinal arteriovenous malformation
Cerebellar ataxia, Wallenberg's syndrome, or both	Dissection of vertebral artery
Third cranial nerve palsy	Aneurysm of the internal carotid artery, at the origin of posterior communicating artery; rarely, aneurysm of the basilar artery or superior cerebellar artery, or pituitary apoplexy
Sixth cranial nerve palsy	Non-specific rise of intracranial cerebrospinal fluid pressure
Cranial nerve IX–XII palsy	Dissection of vertebral artery

Note: intraparenchymal haematomas may give rise to other deficits, depending on their site.

Visual field defects

Anterior communicating artery aneurysms may, in exceptional cases, compress the optic nerve and cause monocular blindness after rupture (Chan *et al.* 1997). They may even penetrate one side of the optic chiasm, and with posterior lesions of the chiasm (optic tract) the visual field defect may be hemianopic (Horiuchi *et al.* 1997). Involvement of the optic chiasm should always raise the possibility of haemorrhage into a pituitary tumour (section 9.1.4).

Third cranial nerve palsy

Complete or partial third nerve palsy is a well-recognized sign after rupture of aneurysms of the internal carotid artery at the origin of the posterior communicating artery (Hyland & Barnett 1954). It can also occur with aneurysms of the basilar tip, or even of the superior cerebellar artery, but these are relatively infrequent sites (Vincent & Zimmerman 1980). Bilateral oculomotor palsies can result from pituitary apoplexy (section 9.1.4). There may be an interval of several days between the oculomotor palsy and then the haemorrhage, presumably by expansion of the wall of the aneurysm first, and later the rupture. Third nerve palsy also occurs with unruptured aneurysms that compress or even fenestrate the nerve (Griffiths *et al.* 1994; Horiuchi *et al.* 1997). Reactive pleocytosis has been reported in aneurysmal third nerve palsies, which erroneously suggests a primary inflammatory process (Keane 1996). The pupil is most often dilated and unreactive, but in some patients the pupil is spared (Kissel *et al.* 1983; Nadeau & Trobe 1983). Oculomotor palsy is relatively common after operative clipping of basilar artery aneurysms (Horikoshi *et al.* 1999).

Parinaud's syndrome

Small, unreactive pupils with impairment of down gaze usually signify hydrocephalus, and rarely a direct impact of the haemorrhage on the midbrain. In a prospective study of 34 patients with acute hydrocephalus after subarachnoid haemorrhage, 30 had an impaired level of consciousness, nine of these 30 had small, non-reactive pupils, and four of these nine also showed persistent downward deviation of the eyes, with otherwise intact brainstem reflexes (van Gijn *et al.* 1985b). The eye signs reflect dilatation of the proximal part of the aqueduct, which causes dysfunction of the pretectal area (Swash 1974). All nine patients with non-reactive pupils had a relative ventricular size of more than 1.2 and were in coma, i.e. they did not open their eyes, obey commands or utter words.

Sixth cranial nerve palsies

Sixth nerve palsies, often bilateral in the acute stage, usually result from the sustained rise of intracranial cerebrospinal fluid pressure, at the time of rupture or later, but occasionally aneurysms of the posterior circulation cause direct compression (Fisher 1975).

Lower cranial nerve palsies

Transmural dissection of the vertebral artery may lead not only to subarachnoid haemorrhage (SAH), but also to compression of cranial nerve IX or X (Senter & Sarwar 1982), and to ischaemia in the territory of the posterior inferior cerebellar artery (Caplan *et al.* 1988). Lower cranial nerve palsies (nerves IX–XII) may also accompany dissection of the carotid artery in the neck, but this is an extremely uncommon cause of SAH (Sturzenegger & Huber 1993) (section 7.2.1).

Hemiparesis

Hemiparesis at onset occurs in approximately 15% of patients with a ruptured aneurysm, usually of the middle cerebral artery (Sarner & Rose 1967). As with other motor symptoms that follow below, the deficit may only be short-lived (for a period of a few minutes). As these deficits may provide a clue to the cause of subarachnoid haemorrhage (SAH), or the site of the aneurysm, they should not be disregarded. Because aneurysms vastly outnumber all other potential causes of SAH, the presence or absence of hemiparesis does not contribute much to the diagnosis of rarer causes, in which hemiparesis may be relatively common, for example with mycotic aneurysms.

Cerebellar signs

Deficits indicating lesions of the cerebellum or brainstem, such as dysmetria, scanning speech, rotatory nystagmus or Horner's syndrome, strongly suggest vertebral artery dissection (Caplan *et al.* 1988).

Paraparesis

Paraparesis may complicate rupture of an aneurysm of the anterior communicating artery complex, as a manifestation of a bifrontal haematoma, or of an intradural arteriovenous malformation of the spinal cord (Rosenblum *et al.* 1987). If paraparesis develops after an interval of several days, it may reflect delayed ischaemia in the territory of both anterior cerebral arteries (Greene *et al.* 1995).

Monoparesis

Weakness of a single leg in the setting of subarachnoid haemorrhage is most often caused by a ruptured aneurysm of the anterior communicating artery, but occasionally and quite unexpectedly the aneurysm is of the posterior inferior cerebellar artery (Ferrante *et al.* 1992). In that case, the deficit is explained by the close proximity of the aneurysm to the corticospinal tract, to the contralateral leg.

9.4 Investigations

The following sections are devoted to investigations aimed at detecting the underlying cause of subarachnoid haemorrhage, with a view to treatment, but of course the investigations needed to assess a patient's general medical condition remain essential: full blood count, glucose, urea, electrolytes, chest X-ray and an electrocardiogram.

9.4.1 Computed tomography (CT)

It was appreciated soon after the advent of CT scanning that the presence and distribution of subarachnoid blood from a ruptured aneurysm could be inferred from radiodense 'white' spots in the subarachnoid space at the base of the brain, which stood out against the much less dense 'black' background of normal cerebrospinal fluid (Kendall *et al.* 1976). CT scanning is still the first-line investigation if subarachnoid haemorrhage (SAH) is suspected because of this characteristic appearance of extravasated blood (section 5.6.3). On MR scanning, the abnormalities are much more subtle, at least in the acute stage. A possible pitfall is the presence of generalized brain oedema, with or without brain death, which causes venous congestion in the subarachnoid space and in this way may mimic SAH (Avrahami *et al.* 1998; Al-Yamany *et al.* 1999). In this section, we shall describe the patterns of bleeding in ruptured aneurysms, according to their site, and also the radiological characteristics of non-aneurysmal sources of haemorrhage.

Patterns of aneurysmal haemorrhage

The distribution of extravasated blood on brain CT is an invaluable though not infallible guide in determining the presence and site of the offending aneurysm, and therefore in planning the order and extent of angiography, particularly in elderly patients, in whom surgical or endovascular repair of

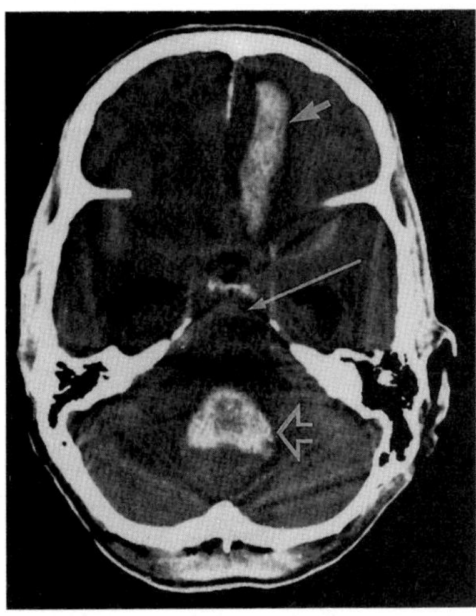

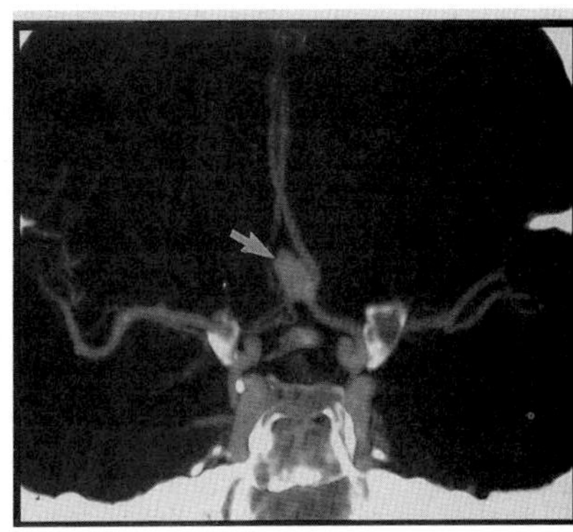

Fig. 9.5 CT brain scans after rupture of an aneurysm of the anterior communicating artery; the haemorrhage extends into the brain parenchyma and the ventricular system. Left: slice through the base of the brain shows a haematoma in the left gyrus rectus (short arrow), blood-filled basal cisterns (long arrow), and a large clot in the distended fourth ventricle (open arrow). Right: CT angiogram (coronal view) shows the aneurysm (arrow).

any additional unruptured aneurysms is not always indicated (Chapter 13). Furthermore, identifying the source of haemorrhage from the scan is helpful if more than one aneurysm is found, because there is a vast difference between the management of a ruptured aneurysm (urgent) (section 13.5) and an unruptured aneurysm (not urgent, if indicated at all) (Lim & Sage 1977) (section 13.12). Even the uncommon event of two aneurysms rupturing at the same time can be correctly diagnosed by CT (Joslyn *et al.* 1985).

Intracerebral haematomas

These are a good indicator of the site of the ruptured aneurysm, whether they are truly intraparenchymal or only distend the subarachnoid space. The prediction of the site of the ruptured aneurysm is correct in at least 90% of haematomas (Laissy *et al.* 1991; Hillman 1993).

Haematomas from an aneurysm of the anterior cerebral artery usually arise near the anterior communicating artery (Fig. 9.2). At least the most proximal part of the haematoma is located near the midline; the distal part may also be paramedian, in the gyrus rectus on one or both sides (Fig. 9.5), or it may split the frontal lobe more laterally (Fig. 9.6). A clot between the frontal horns is a particularly reliable sign of a ruptured anterior communicating artery aneurysm (Jackson *et al.* 1993), although it may be difficult to distinguish between a haematoma in the septum pellucidum (Fig. 9.7) and one in the subarachnoid space (Schulder *et al.* 1987). A haematoma confined to the pericallosal cistern indicates that the aneurysm lies more distally on the anterior cerebral artery, usually at the origin of the pericallosal artery (Fig. 9.8).

Aneurysms arising from the internal carotid artery are most often situated at the origin of the posterior communicating artery, and intracerebral haematomas from rupture at this site are usually found in the medial part of the temporal lobe (Fig. 9.9). Very large haematomas from such aneurysms may also involve the frontal lobe. Haematomas from an aneurysm at the origin of the ophthalmic artery tend to involve the frontal lobe on one side and do not reach the midline, which distinguishes them from intracerebral bleeding from an aneurysm of the anterior communicating artery. If the aneurysm is located at the terminal bifurcation of the internal carotid artery (into the anterior and middle cerebral

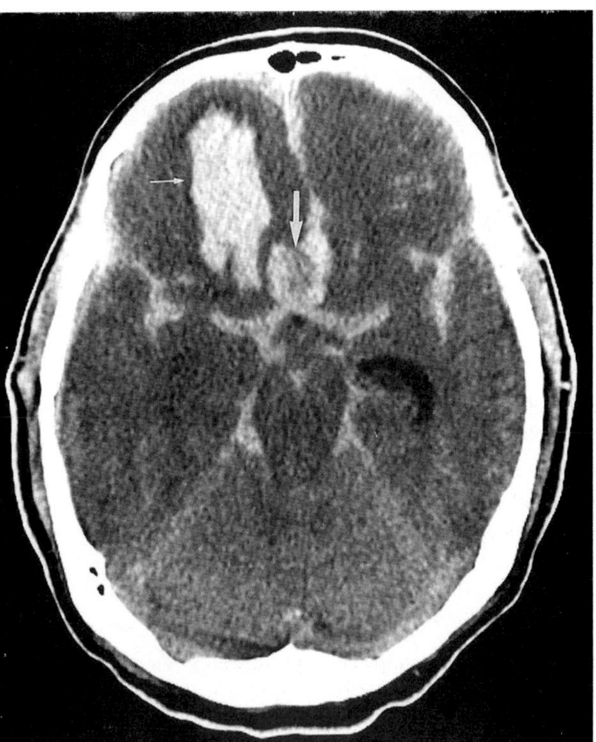

Fig. 9.6 CT brain scan, showing a haematoma (thin arrow) from a large ruptured aneurysm of the anterior communicating artery, in the middle of the right frontal lobe. The aneurysm is visible as a 'filling defect' (thick arrow) within the hyperdense clot of subarachnoid blood.

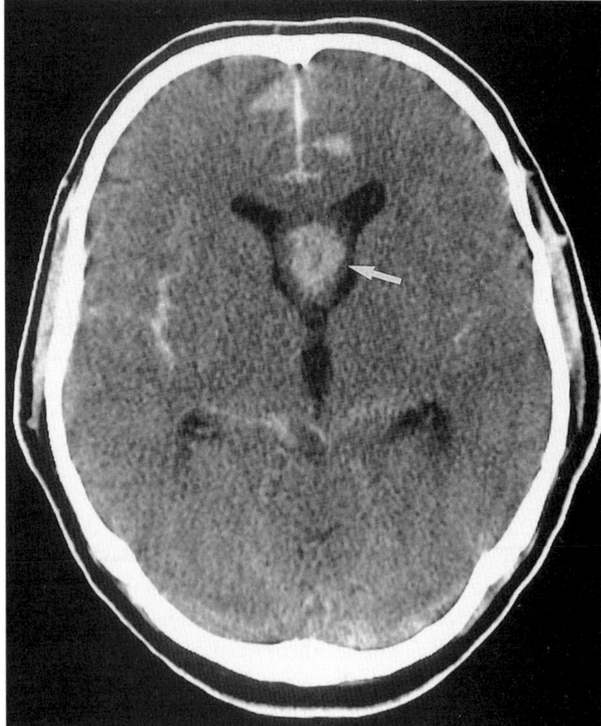

Fig. 9.7 CT brain scan, showing a haematoma in the cavum septum pellucidum (arrow), from a ruptured aneurysm of the anterior communicating artery.

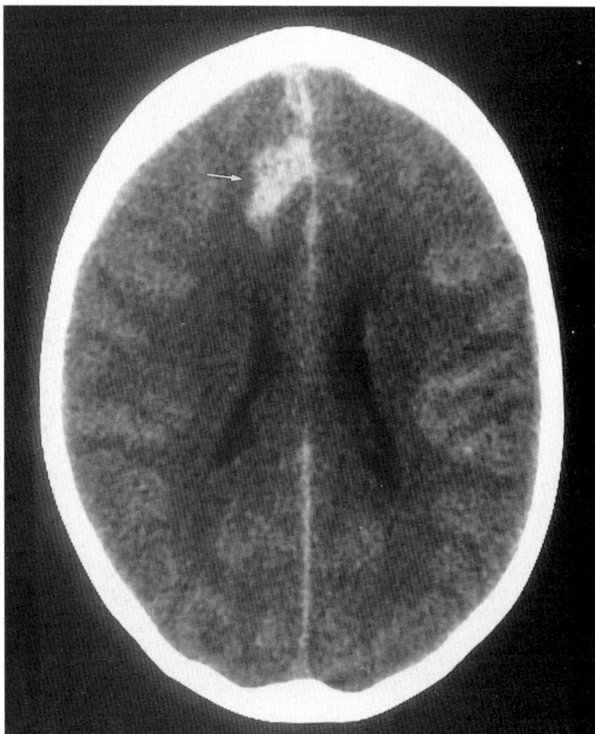

Fig. 9.8 CT brain scan, showing a haematoma in the right cingulate gyrus (arrow), from a ruptured aneurysm of the pericallosal artery.

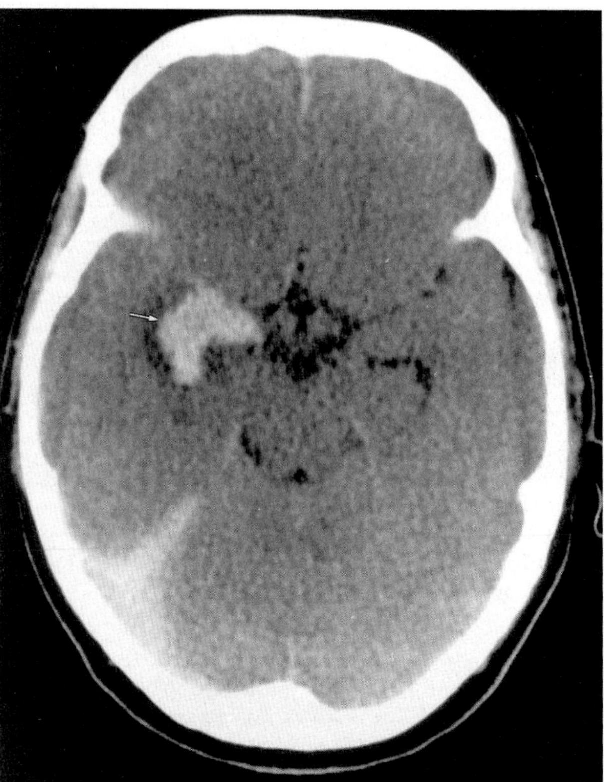

Fig. 9.9 CT brain scan, showing a haematoma in the medial part of the right temporal lobe (arrow), from a ruptured aneurysm of the posterior communicating artery, at its origin from the internal carotid artery.

artery), the haematoma may extend into the head of the caudate nucleus (Hayward & O'Reilly 1976).

Middle cerebral artery aneurysms are almost exclusively located close to the temporal bone, where the mainstem of the artery divides and turns superiorly and posteriorly to enter the lateral part of the Sylvian fissure. Haematomas from aneurysms of this type usually extend from this point posteriorly and superiorly, to follow the course of the lateral fissure (Fig. 9.10). Less often, the haemorrhage is directed medially, in which case it can be distinguished from a haematoma arising in the region of the basal ganglia, from rupture of a small perforating artery, by its lateral border being adjacent to the inner table of the skull (Fig. 9.11).

Aneurysms arising from the posterior circulation rarely give rise to intraparenchymal haematomas. There will always be exceptional situations where physicians are wrong-footed by aneurysms at unusual locations, e.g. the thalamoperforating artery (Kownacki *et al.* 1998) or the middle meningeal artery (Sandin *et al.* 1999). If doubt remains in a deteriorating patient, where rapid evacuation of the haematoma seems indicated, CT angiography may show—or to some extent exclude—an aneurysm (Le Roux *et al.* 1993) (section 9.4.3).

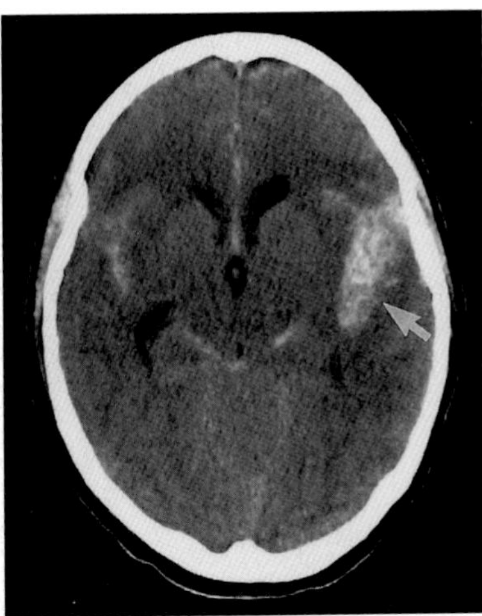

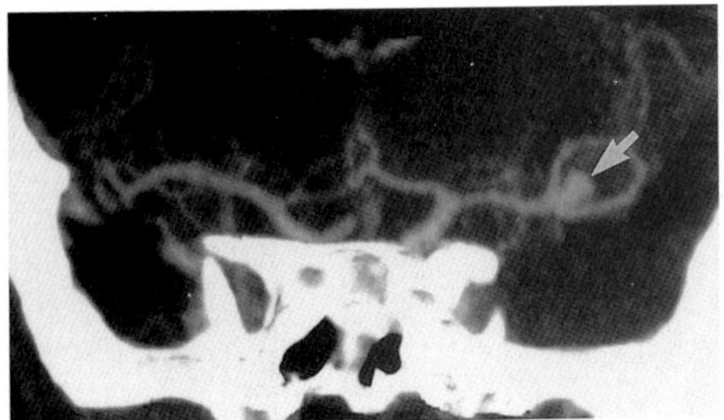

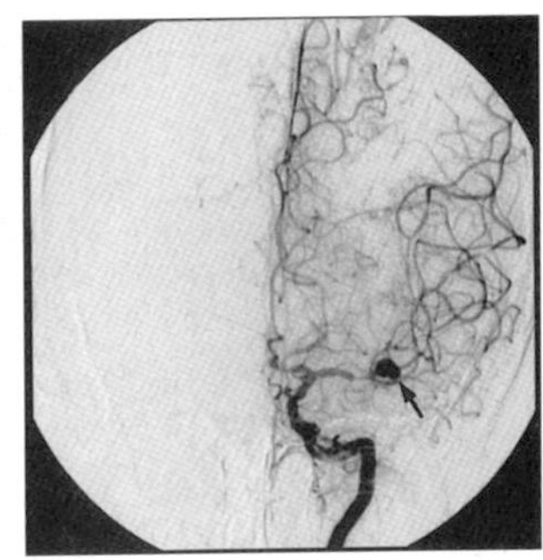

Fig. 9.10 A ruptured aneurysm of the left middle cerebral artery. Left: CT brain scan, showing a haematoma in the lateral part of the left Sylvian fissure (arrow), with diffuse subarachnoid blood also. Middle: CT angiogram (coronal view, detail), showing the aneurysm at the bifurcation of the left middle cerebral artery (arrow). Right: catheter angiogram of the left internal carotid artery, which confirms the presence of the aneurysm (arrow).

Blood in the subarachnoid cisterns

The pattern of haemorrhage is less specific for the site of the aneurysm if the extravasated blood is confined to the subarachnoid cisterns, especially if the haemorrhage is diffuse rather than local (Van der Jagt *et al.* 1999). Moreover, after an interval of 5 days, 50% of patients no longer show cisternal blood on CT (van Gijn & van Dongen 1982). In exceptional cases, the abnormalities have all but disappeared within a single day (Fig. 9.12). The source of subarachnoid haemorrhage can be inferred if the haemorrhage remains confined to, or is most dense in a single cistern, near an arterial branching point site where aneurysms are known to arise (Fig. 9.2). Sometimes the hyperdensity is local but very subtle (Fig. 9.13), which may easily lead to a missed diagnosis in the middle of the night unless at least two physicians have a close look at the scan. With diffuse extravasation, the source of haemorrhage may become clearer on a repeat scan. Aneurysms of the anterior cerebral artery near the anterior communicating artery are the most common site (Table 9.2), and they can be recognized from a region of hyperdensity in the most caudal part of the frontal interhemispheric fissure (Fig. 9.14). Haemorrhage involving the interhemispheric fissure at higher levels, particularly the supracallosal cistern (Fig. 9.15), suggests an aneurysm at the origin of the pericallosal artery, although occasionally haemorrhages from an aneurysm of the anterior communicating artery complex may extend this far (Jackson *et al.* 1993). An asymmetrical distribution of subarachnoid blood in the region of the suprasellar cistern suggests an aneurysm of the internal carotid artery,

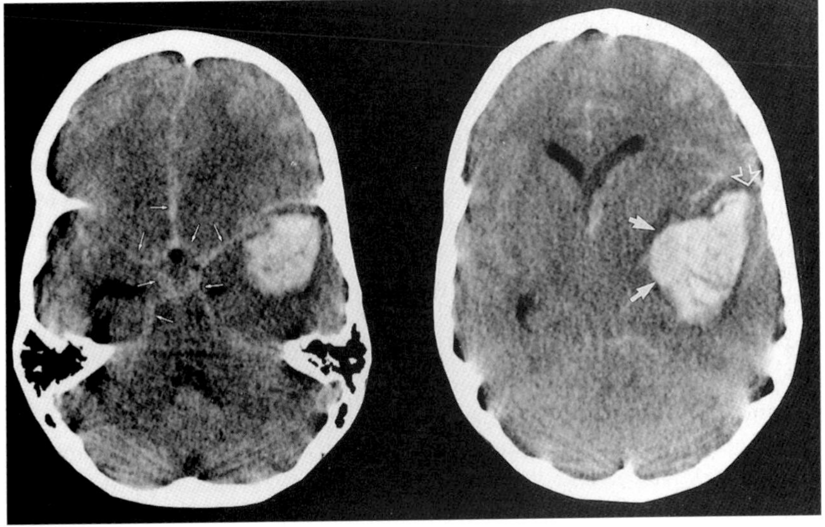

Fig. 9.11 CT brain scan, showing a haematoma from a ruptured aneurysm of the left middle cerebral artery; the haematoma has extended medially from the Sylvian fissure into the subinsular cortex and the putamen (thick arrows), thereby partly mimicking a primary intracerebral haemorrhage from a ruptured perforating artery in the basal ganglia. The characteristic features of aneurysmal bleeding are the concomitant haemorrhage into the basal cisterns (left, thin arrows) and the extreme lateral extension of the haematoma, up to the inner table of the skull (open arrow). Note also the midline brain shift.

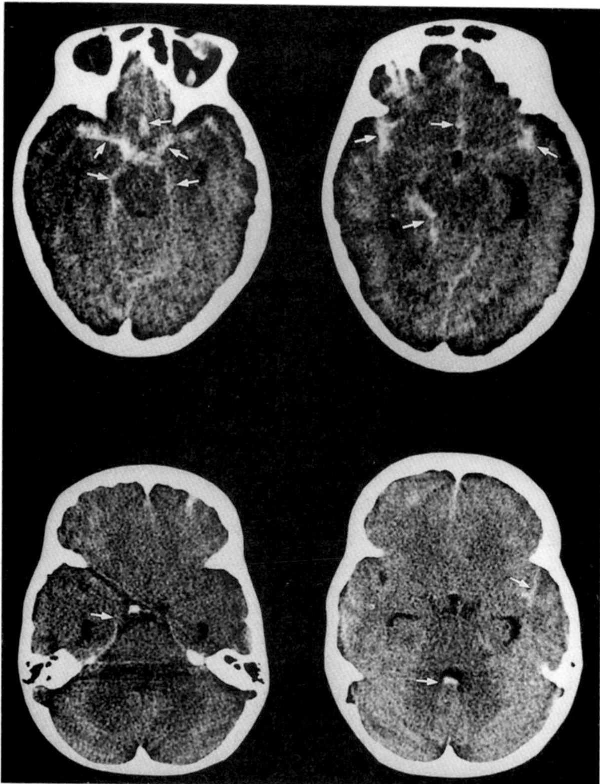

Fig. 9.12 Exceptionally rapid disappearance of subarachnoid blood. Upper row: the CT brain scan 4 h after rupture of an aneurysm of the right posterior communicating artery, at its origin from the carotid artery. Abundant extravasation of blood, throughout the basal cisterns (arrows). Lower row: CT scan 24 h after symptom onset; only a small amount of blood remains (arrows). (With permission from van der Wee *et al.* 1995.)

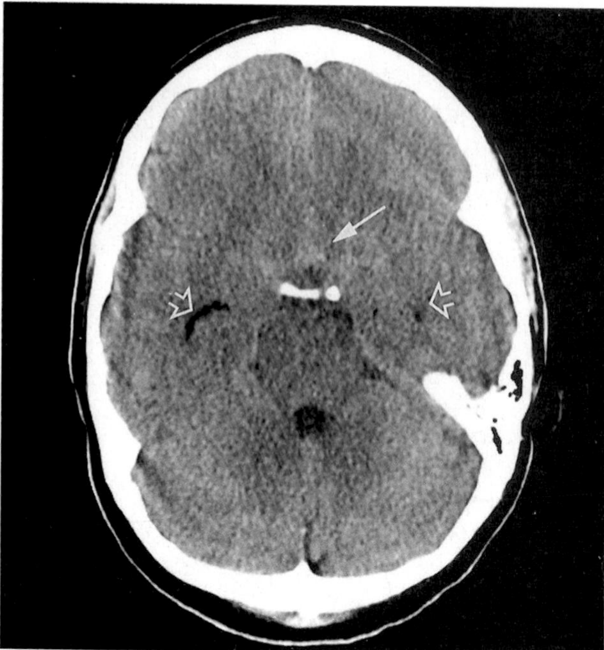

Fig. 9.13 CT brain scan, showing a subtle amount of subarachnoid blood in the anterior part of interhemispheric fissure (arrow), from a ruptured aneurysm of the anterior communicating artery. There is also early hydrocephalus (open arrows point to the slightly dilated temporal horns of the lateral ventricles), and the basal cisterns are not as clearly seen as they should be (due to the presence of a small amount of diffuse subarachnoid blood).

usually at the origin of the posterior communicating artery, which should be suspected when only one side of the suprasellar cisterns is filled with blood, perhaps with some extension to the basal part of the Sylvian fissure (Fig. 9.16). If the patient has an arachnoid cyst of the middle fossa, a posterior communicating artery aneurysm may bleed into the cyst (Barker *et al.* 1998). An aneurysm of the middle cerebral artery can be inferred from extravasation of blood at the junction of the basal and lateral parts of the Sylvian fissure (Fig. 9.17). The haemorrhage may further extend into the lateral fissure. Basilar artery aneurysms are almost invariably found at the terminal bifurcation of the artery; haemorrhages from here are often directed forwards and fill the suprasellar, interhemispheric and (basal) Sylvian cisterns (Fig. 9.18). The posterior inferior cerebellar artery is located near the base of the skull in the posterior fossa, a notoriously difficult region for CT; haemorrhages in this region can be detected only if patients are examined within 3 days of onset, and if the posterior fossa is adequately visualized (Kayama *et al.* 1991) (Fig. 9.19). It is even more difficult if the aneurysm is on a loop below the foramen magnum (Alliez *et al.* 1990).

Intraventricular haemorrhage

This can occur with almost any type of intracranial haemorrhage (section 9.1.5), but most often with aneurysms. In fatal cases, transmission of pressure through the floor of the fourth ventricle can cause acute failure of pontine and medullary functions, this being responsible for 25–50% of early deaths after subarachnoid haemorrhage (Hijdra & van Gijn 1982). Intraventricular haemorrhage occurs mostly with aneurysms of the anterior communicating artery, which bleeds through the lamina terminalis to fill the third and lateral ventricles (Little *et al.* 1977; Weisberg *et al.* 1991). Filling of the third ventricle, but not the lateral ventricles, suggests rupture of a basilar artery aneurysm, especially if the posterior area of the basal cisterns is filled as well (Fig. 9.18). Similarly, rupture of an aneurysm of the posterior inferior cerebellar artery may preferentially fill the fourth ventricle (and sometimes also the third), from the back (Fig. 9.19).

Subdural haematomas

Subdural haematomas develop in 2–3% of cases of aneurysmal rupture (Weir *et al.* 1984; Kamiya *et al.* 1991), most often associated with subarachnoid blood but sometimes as

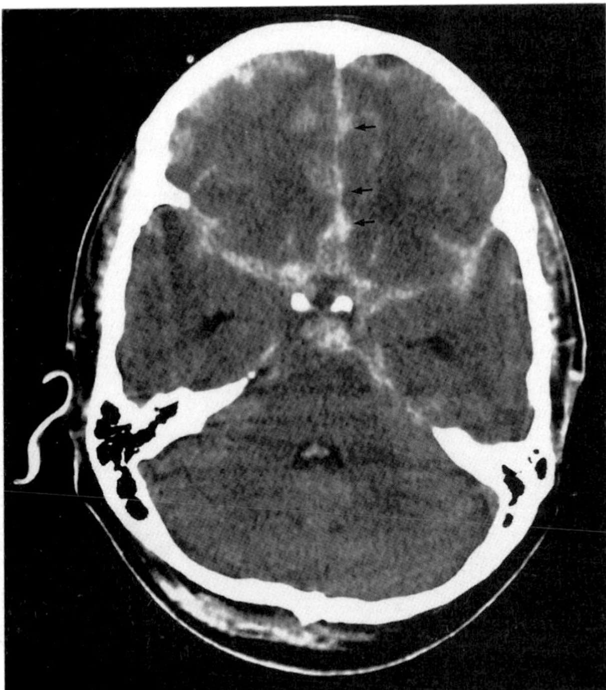

Fig. 9.14 CT brain scan, showing diffuse subarachnoid haemorrhage from a ruptured aneurysm of the anterior communicating artery (the centre of the haemorrhage is in the frontal part of the interhemispheric fissure—arrows).

the only manifestation (Williams *et al.* 1983; O'Leary & Sweeny 1986; Kondziolka *et al.* 1988; Ragland *et al.* 1993). The subdural collection is mostly found at the convexity of the brain, seldom in the interhemispheric fissure (Friedman & Brant Zawadzki 1983). Subdural collections near the skull base are not well visualized on axial CT images. The ruptured aneurysm can be at any of the common sites (Weir *et al.* 1984; Kamiya *et al.* 1991). The most plausible explanation is that the dome of the aneurysmal sac has become adherent to the arachnoid membrane, usually as a result of a previous rupture, recognized or unrecognized (Clarke & Walton 1953). The distinction from subdural haematomas of traumatic origin can be made on the basis of any associated haemorrhage in the subarachnoid space, and also because the haematoma is more often unilateral, hyperdense and crescentic in shape than with trauma (Weir *et al.* 1984) (Fig. 9.20).

Detection of aneurysms

The aneurysm itself is seldom seen on the unenhanced CT scan, and then only when it is very large, or calcified, or both (van Gijn & van Dongen 1980) (Figs 9.6 and 9.21). High-resolution scanning after intravenous contrast, with a slice thickness of 15 mm, is more sensitive (Schmid *et al.* 1987; Teasdale *et al.* 1990), but this technique has now been replaced by CT angiography (section 9.4.3).

Non-aneurysmal (perimesencephalic) patterns of haemorrhage

Fifteen per cent of patients with SAH have a normal angiogram, and two-thirds of these show basal haemorrhages of a distinct kind: mainly or only in the perimesencephalic cisterns, a pattern of haemorrhage seen only rarely in patients with a demonstrable aneurysm (section 9.1.2). Extension to the ambient cisterns or to the basal parts of the Sylvian fissures is common, but the anterior interhemispheric fissure or the lateral Sylvian fissures are never completely filled with blood (Fig. 9.22). No intraventricular haemorrhage ever

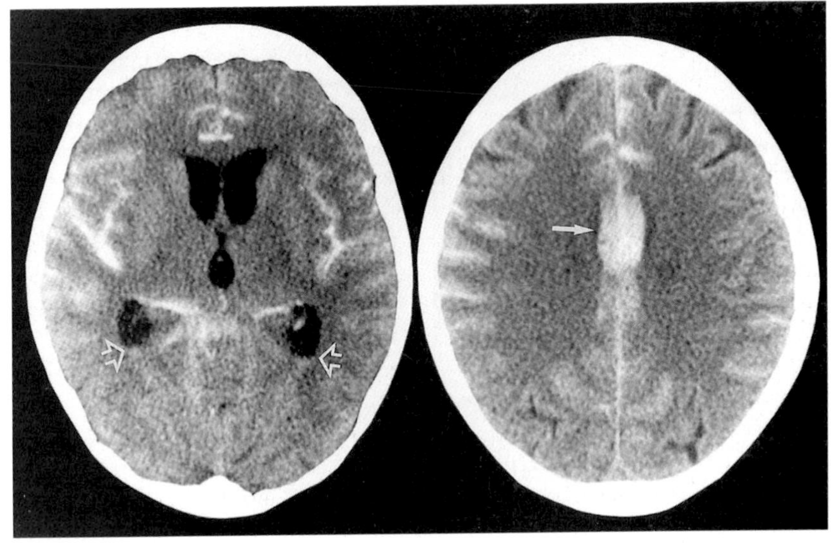

Fig. 9.15 CT brain scan, showing diffuse subarachnoid haemorrhage, with the most dense clot in the pericallosal cistern (arrow), from a ruptured aneurysm of a pericallosal artery. There is also hydrocephalus and a tiny amount of blood layering in the occipital horns of the lateral ventricles (open arrows).

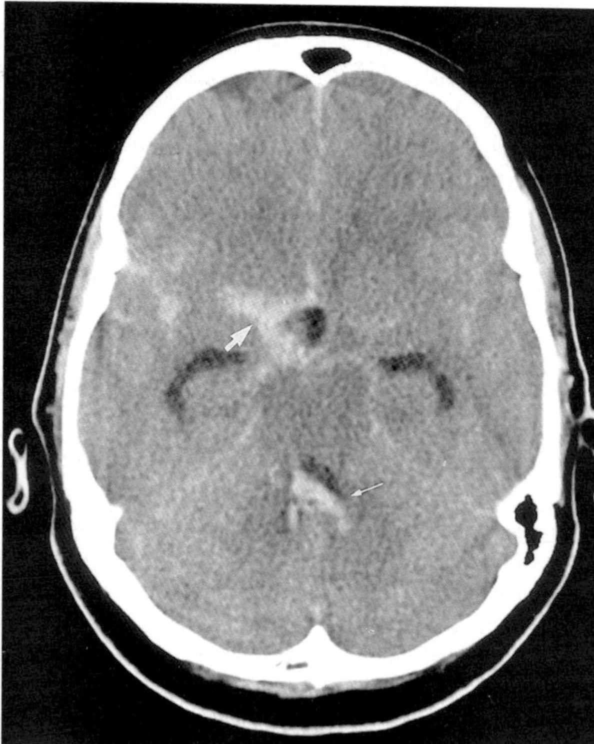

Fig. 9.16 CT brain scan, showing diffuse subarachnoid haemorrhage, most dense in the right half of the suprasellar cistern (arrow) from a ruptured aneurysm of the posterior communicating artery, at its origin from the internal carotid artery. Note also the hydrocephalus and blood in the fourth ventricle (thin arrow).

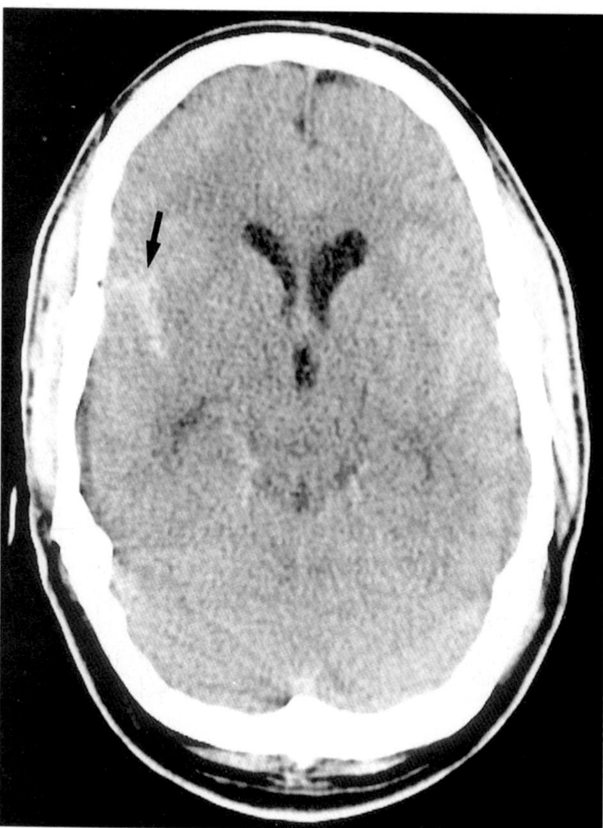

Fig. 9.17 CT brain scan, showing subarachnoid haemorrhage, mainly in the lateral part of the right Sylvian fissure (arrow) from a ruptured aneurysm of the right middle cerebral artery.

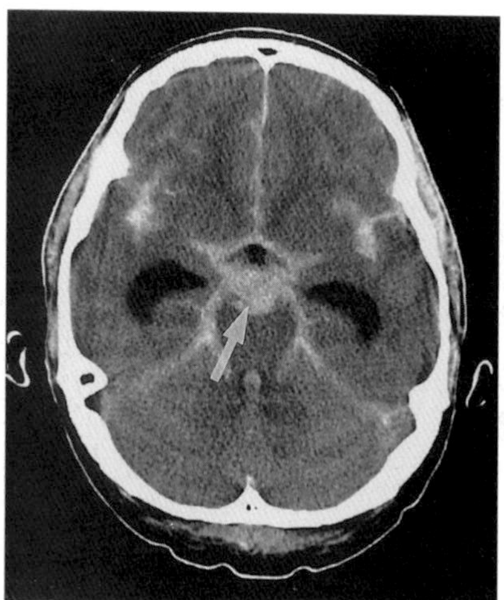

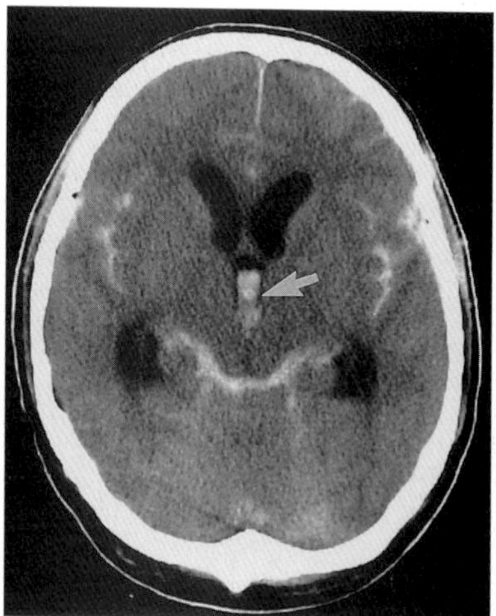

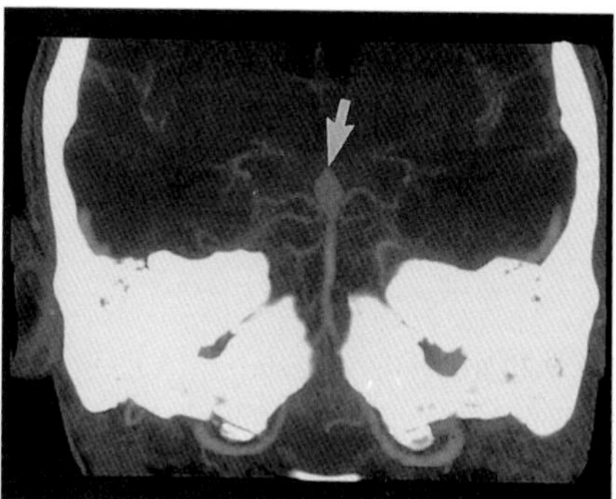

Fig. 9.18 Ruptured aneurysm of the basilar artery. Left and middle: CT brain scan, showing diffuse subarachnoid haemorrhage, most dense in the prepontine cistern (long arrow); there is also rupture into the third ventricle (short arrow). Right: The CT angiogram (coronal view) shows the aneurysm at the apex of the basilar artery (arrow).

occurs, other than some sedimentation of blood in the posterior horns of the lateral ventricles, which probably reflects an abnormal circulation of the cerebrospinal fluid.

The possibility of distinguishing non-aneurysmal perimesencephalic haemorrhage from aneurysmal SAH on early CT scans has been studied in a consecutive series of 221 patients

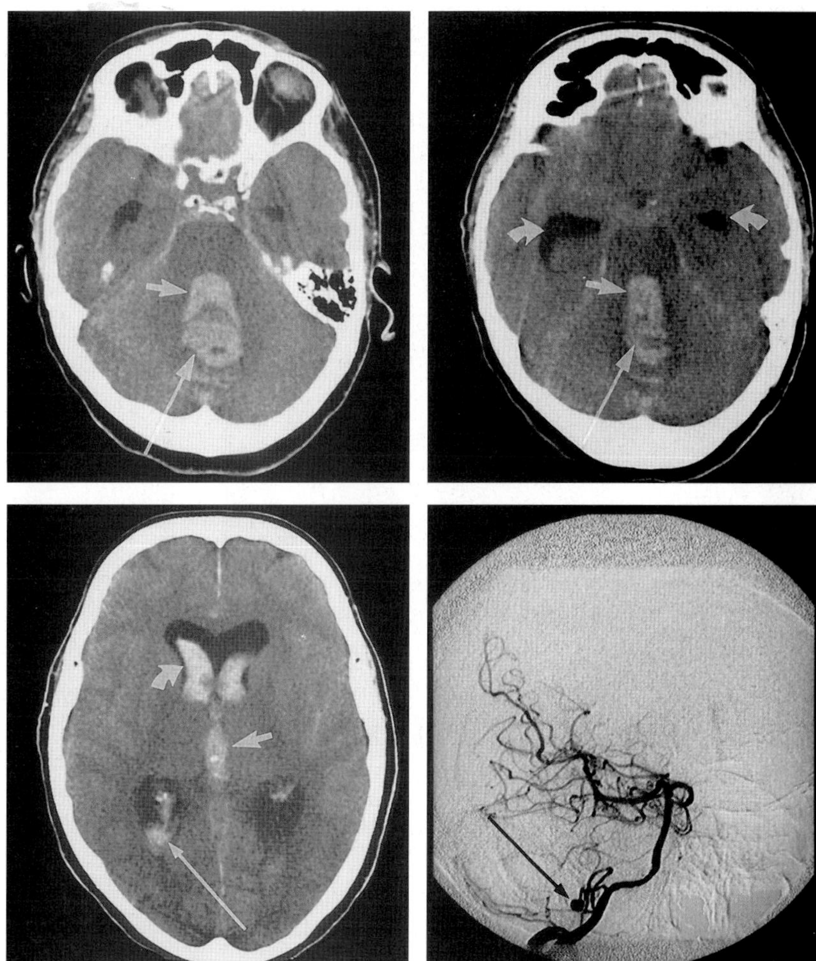

Fig. 9.19 Ruptured aneurysm of the posterior inferior cerebellar artery. Top, left and right: extensive haemorrhage in the fourth ventricle (short arrows), apex of the cisterna magna (dorsal to the fourth ventricle—long arrows), and suprasellar cisterns; dilatation of the temporal horns (curved arrows). Bottom, left: the ventricular haemorrhage extends into the third ventricle (short arrow) and frontal horns of the lateral ventricles (curved arrow); there is some sedimentation of blood in the right posterior horn (long arrow). Bottom, right: catheter angiogram of the right vertebral artery, showing the aneurysm (arrow).

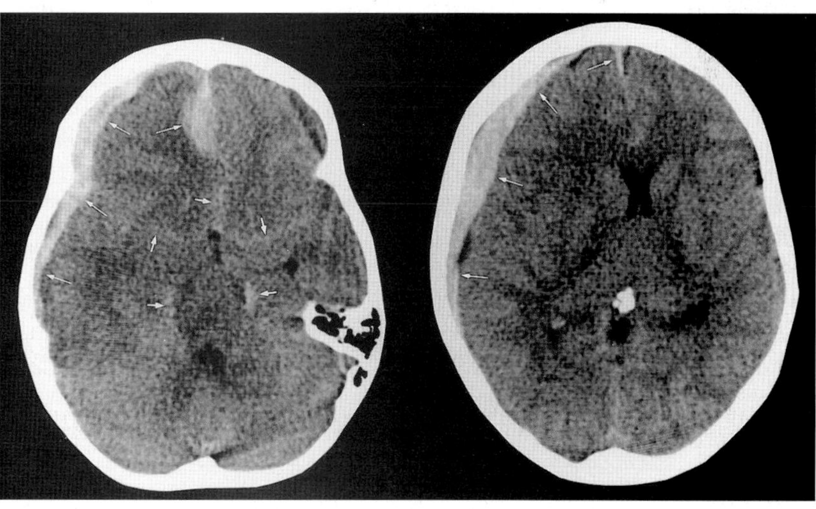

Fig. 9.20 CT brain scan, showing a subdural haematoma at the convexity of the right hemisphere and on the right side of the falx (long arrows), in a 56-year-old woman with spontaneous subarachnoid haemorrhage (site of aneurysm unknown). Diffuse blood is also visible throughout the basal cisterns (short arrows).

who subsequently underwent angiography (Rinkel *et al.* 1991a). Two neuroradiologists tried to predict a normal angiogram among those patients ($n = 37$) in whom blood had predominantly extravasated in the posterior cisterns (15 with an aneurysm and 22 without). Prediction of a normal angiogram was correct in 95% and 94% for the two observers, with excellent interobserver agreement (a kappa value of 0.87, the maximum being 1.0). This shows that non-aneurysmal perimesencephalic haemorrhage can be reliably distinguished in the majority of patients. Nevertheless, these

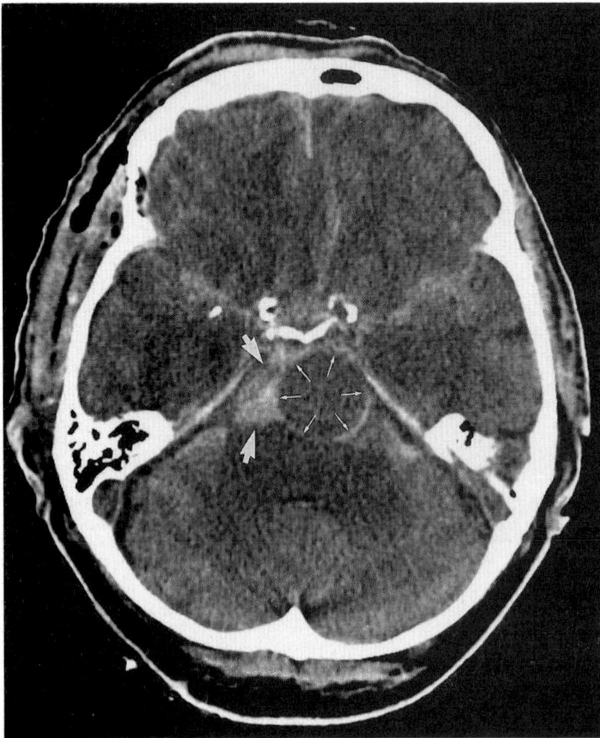

Fig. 9.21 CT brain scan, showing diffuse subarachnoid haemorrhage, most dense in the prepontine cistern (thick arrows) from a giant aneurysm of the basilar artery (the thin arrows delineate the inner margins of the aneurysm).

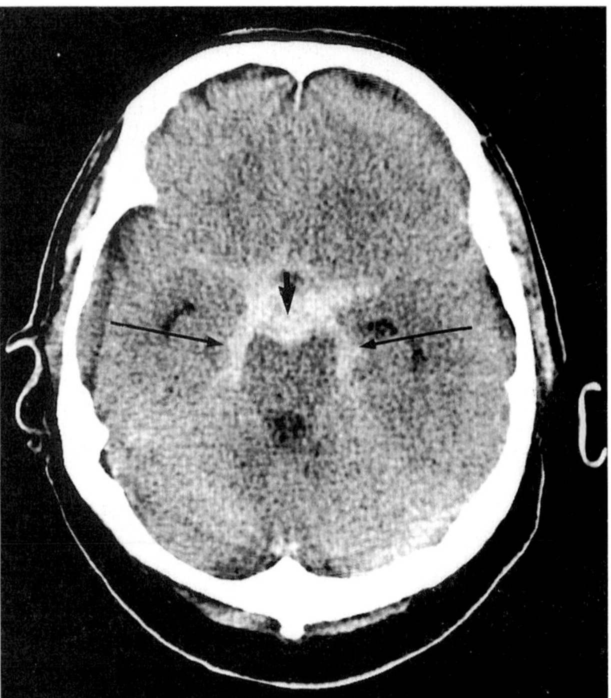

Fig. 9.22 CT brain scan of non-aneurysmal perimesencephalic haemorrhage. The most dense clot is in the interpeduncular (thick arrow) and ambiens (long arrows) cisterns. The anterior part of the interhemispheric fissure and the lateral fissures are not filled, and there is no intraventricular haemorrhage. The angiogram showed no abnormality.

results do not make angiography unnecessary. One patient with a basilar artery aneurysm on angiography (from a total of 15 such patients) was incorrectly classified as a non-aneurysmal pattern of perimesencephalic haemorrhage by both observers (Fig. 9.23). A second study, from another centre, of perimesencephalic patterns of haemorrhage also found a single instance of a patient with a ruptured aneurysm, this time amongst 38 patients (Pinto *et al.* 1993). An estimate of the balance of risks leads to the conclusion that withholding surgical or endovascular treatment in approximately 5% of patients with a perimesencephalic pattern of bleeding, but an undetected basilar artery aneurysm, is more unfavourable than the complications of 'unnecessary' angiographic imaging in the remaining 95%. Later studies have again confirmed that a perimesencephalic pattern of bleeding occasionally arises from posterior circulation aneurysms, sometimes in unusual locations (Schievink *et al.* 1994a). However, there is no need to *repeat* a normal catheter angiogram in a patient with a perimesencephalic pattern of haemorrhage. Even a CT angiogram may be sufficient to exclude a posterior fossa aneurysm, depending on the performance of the local radiological team (Velthuis *et al.* 1999). In contrast, repetition of a negative angiographic study is mandatory with aneurysmal patterns of haemorrhage on the CT scan (section 9.4.6).

Cerebral catheter angiography, or at least CT angiography, is still required in patients with a perimesencephalic subarachnoid pattern of subarachnoid haemorrhage, even though the chance of finding an aneurysm is extremely small. However, unlike with aneurysmal patterns of bleeding, repeating the angiogram after a negative initial angiogram is not required.

Other patterns and sources of haemorrhage

Basal haemorrhages, indistinguishable on CT scanning from those associated with a ruptured aneurysm, may result from vertebral artery dissection, a dural fistula of the tentorium, an arteriovenous malformation in the neck region, cocaine abuse without an associated aneurysm or a mycotic aneurysm with aspergillosis.

Head trauma may result in SAH. If patients are found unconscious, or were seen to have caused an unexplained traffic accident, the question may arise whether the trauma or the SAH was the primary event. With traumatic brain injury, usually the brain CT shows an adjacent contusion at the convexity, different in shape and site from an aneurysmal

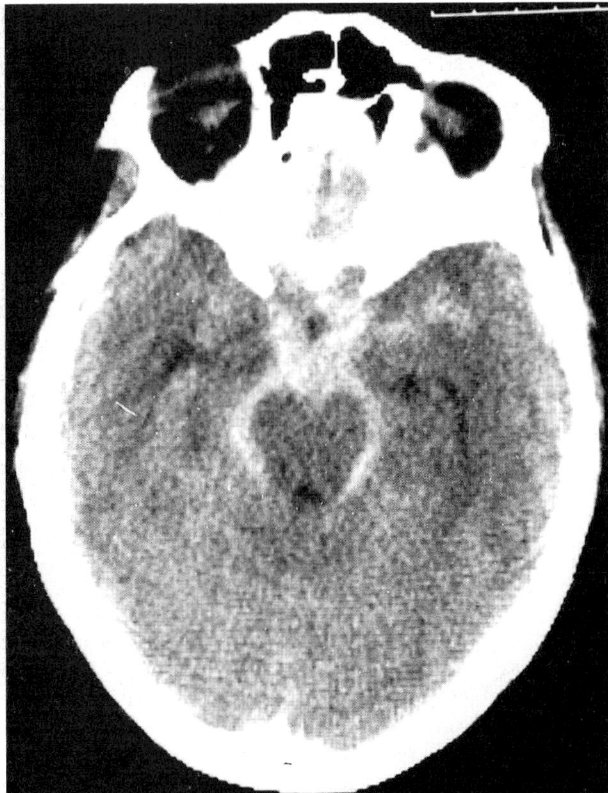

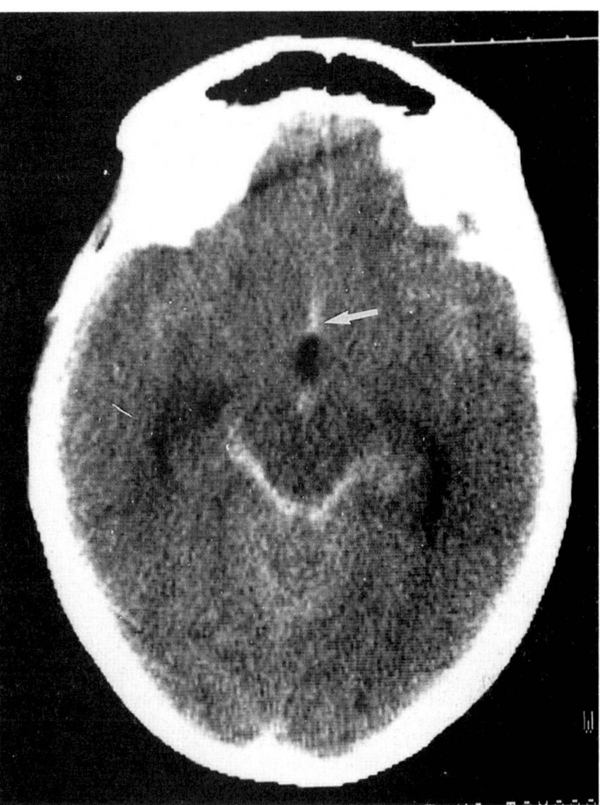

Fig. 9.23 CT brain scan, showing haemorrhage from a basilar artery aneurysm, mistaken by two neuroradiologists for a non-aneurysmal haemorrhage. In retrospect the speck of blood in front of the third ventricle (arrow) might have been a reason for suspecting aneurysmal haemorrhage. (With permission from Rinkel *et al.* 1991c.)

haematoma. Nevertheless, some patients with basal–frontal contusions may show a pattern of haemorrhage resembling that of a ruptured anterior communicating artery aneurysm (Fig. 9.24), and in patients with blood confined to the Sylvian fissure it may also be difficult to distinguish trauma from aneurysmal rupture by the pattern of haemorrhage alone (Fig. 9.25). In some patients with shearing injury, pronounced accumulation of blood can be found in the posterior part of the ambient cistern at the level of the tentorial margin (Takenaka *et al.* 1990). The blood in the ambient cistern may be part of more extensive intracranial haemorrhage, but in some patients with head injury it can be the only site of haemorrhage (Rinkel *et al.* 1993). Blood confined to the ambient cistern has also been reported in a patient on anticoagulants after the relatively mild trauma of a fall in the shower (Lavin & Troost 1984). That site of the haemorrhage makes a ruptured saccular aneurysm as source of the haemorrhage very unlikely. In patients with direct trauma to the neck, or with head injury associated with vigorous neck movement, the trauma can immediately be followed by massive basal haemorrhage resulting from a tear or even a complete rupture of one of the arteries of the posterior circulation, which tends to be rapidly fatal (Harland *et al.* 1983; Dowling & Curry 1988).

9.4.2 Magnetic resonance imaging

In the acute stage of aneurysmal haemorrhage, particularly within the first 24 h, subarachnoid blood can be detected by means of magnetic resonance imaging (MRI) as a region of hyperintensity on spin echo T2-weighted images (Jenkins *et al.* 1988; Satoh & Kadoya 1988) (Fig. 9.26), and even better with the technique of gradient echo T2 sequences (Patel *et al.* 1996), fluid-attenuated inversion recovery (FLAIR) (Noguchi *et al.* 1995), or fluid-attenuated turbo-inversion recovery (FLAT TIRE) (Chrysikopoulos *et al.* 1996). Some studies specifically emphasize the advantages of MRI with aneurysms of the posterior inferior cerebellar artery (Stone *et al.* 1988; Matsumura *et al.* 1990). Undoubtedly there is some publication bias, in that unfavourable performance with MRI in the acute stage of subarachnoid haemorrhage is less likely to have been reported. Also, blinding of observers was at best incomplete, and the number of patients was no more than 20–30 per study. Other workers are more concerned about the balance between sensitivity and specificity of MRI in the acute stage (Atlas 1993). Moreover, the facilities for MRI are much less readily available than CT scans, and when conscious level is impaired the relatively long scanning time increases the problem of movement artifacts. Gadolinium

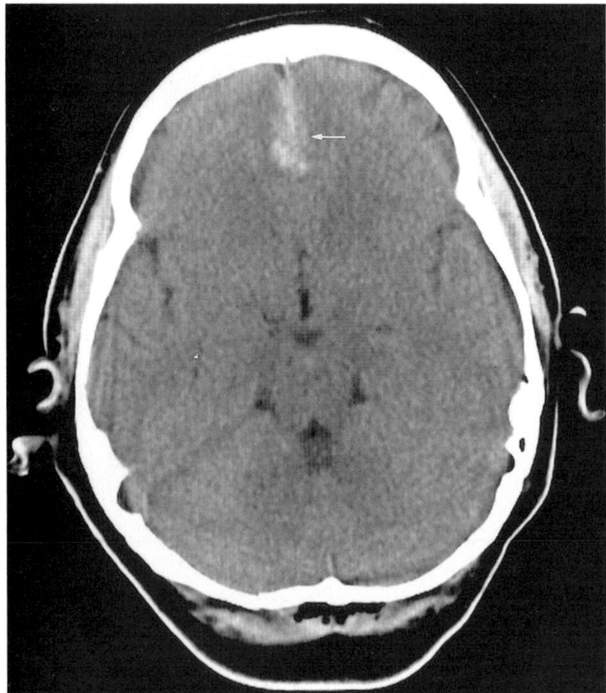

Fig. 9.24 CT brain scan, showing extravasated blood in the frontal interhemispheric fissure (arrow), as a result of trauma (in a 34-year-old woman who had fallen from her horse).

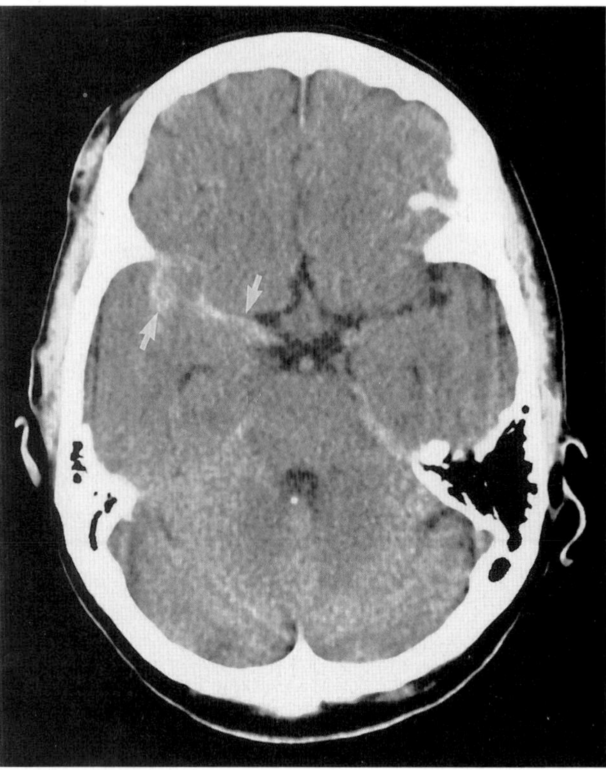

Fig. 9.25 CT brain scan, showing extravasated blood in the horizontal part of the right Sylvian fissure (arrows), as a result of trauma (in a 70-year-old woman who had slipped down stairs).

enhancement may give a false impression of subarachnoid haemorrhage, especially on FLAIR images (Lev & Schaefer 1999).

However, it is especially after the first few days, when the sensitivity of CT scanning for subarachnoid blood rapidly declines, that MRI is most useful (Renowden *et al.* 1994; Ogawa *et al.* 1995). After 4 days, T1-weighted images detect extravasated blood best, owing to the paramagnetic effect of the breakdown products of haemoglobin, i.e. oxyhaemoglobin and methaemoglobin (Di Chiro *et al.* 1986; Spickler *et al.* 1990) (Fig. 9.27). The hyperintensity of 'old' blood may last for at least 2 weeks on T1-weighted images (Matsumura *et al.* 1990), and even longer with the FLAIR technique (Noguchi *et al.* 1997). This makes MRI a unique

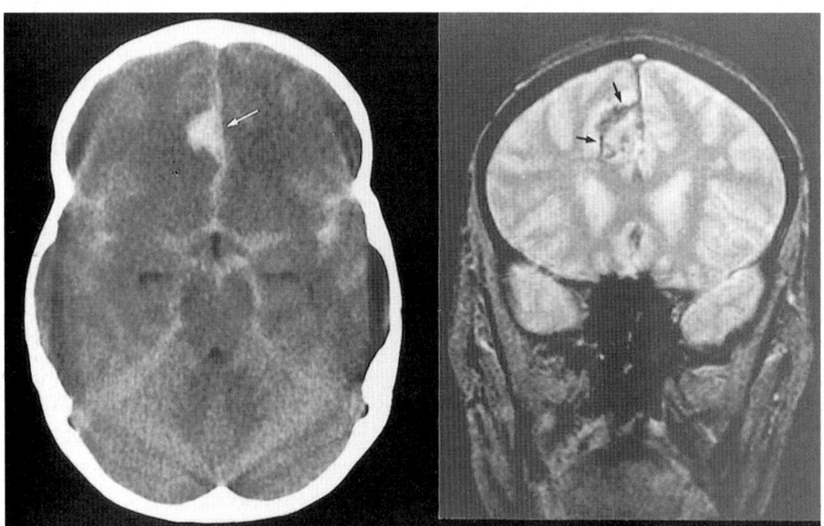

Fig. 9.26 Left: axial CT brain scan after rupture of a pericallosal aneurysm, obtained within 24 h, showing diffuse subarachnoid blood, with local haematoma in the frontal interhemispheric fissure (arrow). Right: coronal magnetic resonance image (T2-weighted) of aneurysmal subarachnoid haemorrhage, on the same day. The rim of the haematoma is hypointense (arrows), corresponding to deoxyhaemoglobin in intact cells, whereas the core is hyperintense (extracellular deoxyhaemoglobin).

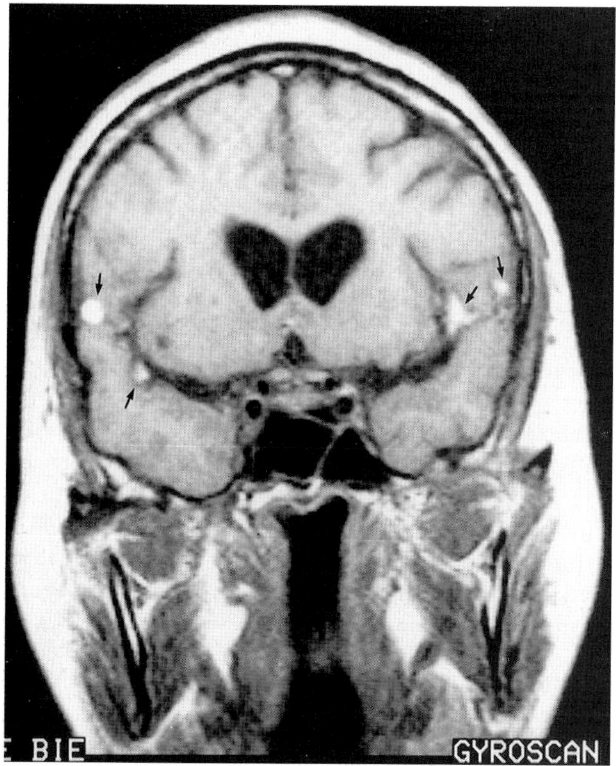

Fig. 9.27 Coronal magnetic resonance scan (T1-weighted) of aneurysmal subarachnoid haemorrhage, after 5 days. Remaining clots of subarachnoid blood in both Sylvian fissures are hyperintense (arrows).

method for identifying the site of the ruptured aneurysm in patients who are not referred until after 1–2 weeks, when brain CT so often no longer shows evidence of subarachnoid blood.

Aneurysms themselves can be identified by MRI as signal-void areas, often associated with focal changes in the brain (Jenkins *et al.* 1988; Matsumura *et al.* 1990). This is most helpful if the angiogram has failed to show an expected aneurysm (Pertuiset *et al.* 1989; Rogg *et al.* 1999). Droplets of Pantopaque (iophendylate) may resemble an aneurysm on MRI (Lidov *et al.* 1996). For the detection of aneurysms, especially in asymptomatic subjects, special MR techniques have been developed that image moving blood (section 9.4.4).

With arterial dissection, MRI (or CT) may detect a thrombus within the dissected wall of the artery (Quint & Spickler 1990; Schwaighofer *et al.* 1990; Woimant & Spelle 1995) (section 7.2). In the case of chronic haemosiderosis, MR scanning shows diffuse deposition of haemosiderin in the subpial layers of the brain and spinal cord (section 9.1.4).

9.4.3 Computed tomographic angiography

Spiral CT scanning is an improved technique that eliminates the problem of 'gaps' between slices, whilst so-called partial-volume phenomena ('dilution' of information within a slice) can be avoided by data-processing techniques such as 'maximal intensity projection', which compress three-dimensional information into a single plane, from many different angles (section 6.7.5). Three-dimensional information can be used most effectively if the observer views the images on a computer screen, where it is possible to rotate the vessels in every possible direction.

In a recent systematic review of the studies published to the end of 1997, which directly compared the results of CT angiography with those of intra-arterial angiography, 26 articles with at least 10 patients were identified (Wardlaw &

(a)

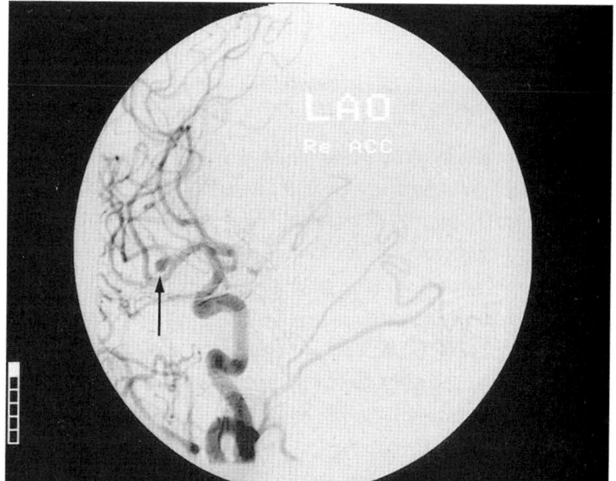

(b)

Fig. 9.28 (a) Magnetic resonance angiogram of the circle of Willis viewed from the front. An aneurysm of the right middle cerebral artery (arrow) is shown in an asymptomatic patient with affected relatives. (b) Confirmation by catheter angiography, in a reversed anterior oblique view (arrow).

White 2000). Only eight of these used blinded-reader review, adequately described techniques, explicitly stated inclusion and exclusion criteria, and provided results from which predictive values (positive or negative) could be derived. All the patients had had a recent subarachnoid haemorrhage (SAH). Overall aneurysm detection rates for CT angiography were in the range of 85–98%. The specificity was also good, at 82–100% (Anderson *et al.* 1999a; Wardlaw & White 2000). In a later study in which CT angiography and catheter angiography were compared in 80 patients with SAH, neurosurgeons assessed CT angiography as equal or superior to catheter angiography in 83% (95% CI, 73%–90%) of 87 aneurysms, and in 74% (95% CI, 63%–82%) they judged that operation could have been based on the CT angiographic findings alone (Velthuis *et al.* 1998). Further technical developments allow three-dimensional reconstruction and virtual endoscopy of the aneurysm and its adjoining vessels (Kato *et al.* 1996; Marro *et al.* 1997).

A great advantage of CT angiography is the speed with which it can be performed, preferably immediately after CT scanning of the brain through which the diagnosis of aneurysmal haemorrhage was suspected, and while the patient is still in the machine. Catheter angiography can generally be omitted if the aneurysm has been adequately visualized by CT angiography and urgent interventions are needed, such as evacuation of an associated haematoma (section 13.3.1). Also, in less urgent situations, CT angiography will probably continue to decrease the need for catheter angiography, unless coiling is the treatment of choice. Whether preoperative catheter angiograms can be omitted depends not only on the resolution of CT angiography, but also on the flexibility of the neurosurgeon.

For the purpose of detecting aneurysms in asymptomatic patients, CT scanning—however sophisticated—is less attractive than magnetic resonance angiography (section 9.4.4), because of the need for intravenous contrast and the small but inevitable risk of allergic reactions.

9.4.4 Magnetic resonance angiography

A recent review of studies comparing MRA with intra-arterial catheter angiography in patients with recent subarachnoid haemorrhage (SAH), under blinded-reader conditions, showed a sensitivity in the range of 76–95% for detecting at least one aneurysm per patient; for the detection of all aneurysms the sensitivity was 75–91%, with specificity in the range 92–100%(Wardlaw & White 2000). An important factor affecting the performance of MRA is the imaging protocol used. A study published in 1990, with satisfactory review methods, found a sensitivity (for identification of at least one aneurysm per patient) of 75% for MRA processed as maximal intensity projection (MIP) alone, but this increased to 95% if axial base and spin echo images were added (Ross *et al.* 1990). Reconstruction in three dimensions allows virtual cisternoscopy (Fellner *et al.* 1998). Aneurysm size is another important factor, with studies consistently indicating sensitivity rates of more than 95% for aneurysms larger than 6 mm, but much less for smaller aneurysms (Atlas *et al.* 1997). For aneurysms smaller than 5 mm, detection rates may be as low as 50% (Korogi *et al.* 1996). Paradoxically, the sensitivity of time-of-flight MRA (the most widely used technique) is also relatively poor for very large aneurysms (Atlas 1997). MRA allows detection of pulsatile increases of aneurysm volume in some cases (Meyer *et al.* 1993), as can ultrasound (section 9.4.5). To sum up, in patients with SAH, MRA is unlikely to replace contrast radiography in the next few years.

Despite its limitations, but thanks to its non-invasive nature, MRA is being used to detect aneurysms in relatives of patients with SAH (Ronkainen *et al.* 1995b; Kojima *et al.* 1998) (Fig. 9.28) (section 13.12). However, the results are poorer because the prevalence of aneurysms is much lower than in SAH. This has serious implications for MRA as a screening method when most of those screened (more than 80%) are unlikely to harbour an aneurysm. Many more of the 'positives' will be 'false-positives' than 'true-positives', and a 'false-positive' diagnosis of aneurysm occurs in 3–8% of normal people in blinded-reader comparisons, even in expert hands (Ronkainen *et al.* 1995b; Raaymakers *et al.* 1999).

Magnetic resonance angiography is without risks and reasonably sensitive (90%), which makes it well suited as an instrument for screening people at risk of intracranial aneurysms, but less suitable for patients with subarachnoid haemorrhage. However, screening of relatives is beneficial only if the probability of an aneurysm is at least 10%.

9.4.5 Ultrasound

The technique of transcranial Doppler (TCD) can be combined with echo imaging (duplex technique) and with colour coding (transcranial colour-coded duplex sonography) (Wardlaw & White 2000). A single study in which the investigator was blinded to the results of angiography (but not to those of CT or MRI) showed that this ultrasound technique detected 23 of 27 aneurysms (Baumgartner *et al.* 1994). A recent modification of colour Doppler, called colour Doppler energy or power Doppler, offers greater sensitivity to flowing blood than standard colour flow imaging. The only study so far that assessed this technique detected 30 of 33 aneurysms (Wardlaw & Cannon 1996). A feature unique to a dynamic technique such as ultrasound, is the potential for assessing the degree to which aneurysms expand during each cardiac cycle (Wardlaw & Cannon 1996), a characteristic depending on intracranial pressure (Wardlaw *et al.* 1998), and flow patterns within the aneurysm (Ujiie *et al.* 1999). Such dynamic features of asymptomatic aneurysms may in the future help predict the risk of rupture. Unfortunately, about 10% of patients will not have an adequate bone window (too thick a skull, to put it bluntly). Also the technique is highly dependent on the skills of the operator. Further interest in TCD for this indication is likely to increase because of the availability of ultrasonic contrast agents and 3-D ultrasound imaging (Bazzocchi *et al.* 1998).

9.4.6 Cerebral catheter angiography

General consideration of risks and benefits

Catheter angiography is not an innocuous procedure. A systematic review of three prospective studies in which patients with subarachnoid haemorrhage (SAH) were distinguished from other indications for catheter angiography found a neurological complication rate (transient or permanent) of 1.8% (Cloft *et al.* 1999). Also, the aneurysm may re-rupture during the procedure, in 1–2% of cases overall (Hayakawa *et al.* 1978; Koenig *et al.* 1979; Saitoh *et al.* 1995). The rupture rate in the 6-h period after angiography has been estimated at 5%, which is higher than the expected rate (Saitoh *et al.* 1995). In certain parts of the world, the aim of making as accurate a diagnosis as possible overrides the balance of risks and benefits for the patient, and an angiogram is felt to be justified in nearly every patient with SAH. By contrast, from a pragmatic point of view, we feel that catheter angiography should be omitted if clipping or coiling of an aneurysm is not a likely therapeutic option, for whatever reason.

In general, catheter angiography in patients with subarachnoid haemorrhage should be performed only with a view to surgical or endovascular treatment or, in exceptional cases, to establish a more firm prognosis.

Timing and extent of angiography

In a patient with an aneurysmal pattern of haemorrhage on CT scanning, the timing of angiography is intricately linked with the timing of operation, or endovascular treatment. Many neurosurgeons advocate early clipping of the aneurysm, within 3 days of the initial bleed, in the belief that not only re-bleeding but also ischaemia might be prevented, in the latter case by washing away extravasated blood. Despite this, the empirical evidence for early intervention is weak (section 13.5.2).

At any rate, angiography with a view to clipping or coiling of the aneurysm should be performed at the earliest opportunity if any intervention is planned within 3 days of SAH onset. If surgery is to be deferred until approximately day 12, the angiogram should be done either before day 4 or on day 10 or 11, to avoid the period of maximum risk for 'cerebral vasospasm'. If the patient is in good condition, early angiography is to be preferred even with late surgery, because intervening complications can often be dealt with more promptly if the site of the offending aneurysm is precisely known.

How extensive should angiography be if CT scanning gives a good indication of the site of the ruptured aneurysm, as is often the case? With aneurysms of the anterior communicating artery, studies of both carotid artery territories are necessary to identify the artery bearing the aneurysm and to determine from which side the distal parts of the anterior cerebral arteries are filled. With aneurysms of the carotid artery at the origin of the posterior communicating artery, the neurosurgeon often finds it useful to know whether the posterior cerebral artery is sufficiently filled via the basilar artery in the event that temporary clipping of the posterior communicating artery is required to control bleeding. In contrast, with aneurysms of the middle cerebral artery it is not usually necessary to have information about any other arterial territory. However, if the patient's age and clinical condition warrant treatment of any unruptured aneurysms as well as the ruptured aneurysm (section 13.12), that is a good reason for performing a four-vessel angiogram, i.e. to display all the branches of both carotid and vertebral arterial systems. An angiogram cannot be termed 'negative' until both vertebral arteries have been visualized, preferably selectively; after all, aneurysms arising from the posterior inferior cerebellar artery or other proximal branches of the vertebral artery will be missed if the posterior circulation is investigated by injection of only a single vertebral artery.

Suspicion of causes other than an aneurysm

In cases of suspected arterial dissection, the diagnosis rests on the angiographic demonstration of narrowing of the artery with signs of an intimal flap, a pseudoaneurysm or a double lumen (sections 7.2.1 and 7.2.2). Catheter angiography may be warranted if CT or MRI fails to confirm the clinical diagnosis of dissection, not with a view to treatment but for excluding other causes (sometimes with a medicolegal background), and for giving a prognosis. Timing of imaging is difficult, because an early angiogram may be normal or show only non-specific arterial narrowing, whereas the abnormalities may have disappeared on a later angiogram (Friedman & Drake 1984) (Fig. 9.29).

In patients in whom CT scanning suggests that the haemorrhage originates near the tentorium, angiography should be directed at the detection of a dural arteriovenous fistula. In that case, it is important to visualize the external carotid artery as well, because branches of this artery can be the main or sole feeders (Aminoff 1973).

In the case of a spinal arteriovenous malformation, brain CT may show blood throughout the basal cisterns and ventricles, which obscures the correct diagnosis (Acciarri *et al.* 1992). Not only negative angiography of the cerebral circulation, but also clinical clues such as sudden backache should form an indication for spinal angiography. However,

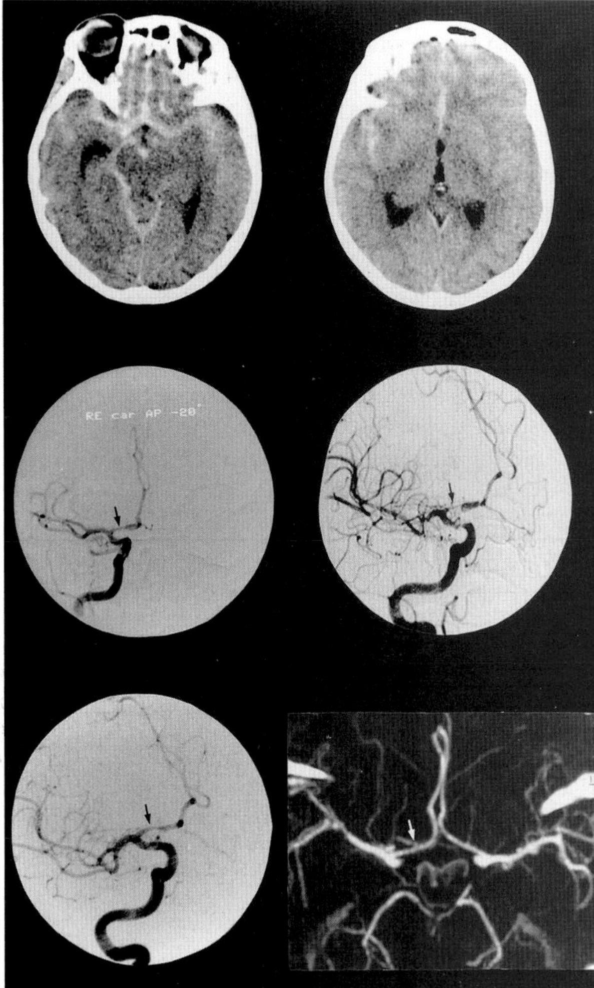

Fig. 9.29 Subarachnoid haemorrhage from dissection of an intracranial artery. Top row: CT brain scan within hours of the haemorrhage, showing diffuse extravasation of blood in the basal cisterns, predominantly on the right side. Middle row, left: right carotid angiogram (anteroposterior view) after one day, showing a narrowed segment in the proximal part of the anterior cerebral artery (arrow). Middle row, right: a second right carotid angiogram (oblique view) after 11 days, showing even more marked narrowing at the same site (arrow). Lower row, left: a third right carotid angiogram (oblique view), 3 months after the haemorrhage; the affected segment has almost returned to normal (arrow). Bottom row, right: a spiral CT scan after intravenous contrast, with maximal intensity projection, 9 months after the haemorrhage; the segment of the proximal right anterior cerebral artery is now completely normal (arrow).

this procedure is not always diagnostic (Kandel 1980; Swann *et al.* 1984). Also, angiography is impractical without localizing signs or symptoms, because so many intercostal arteries have to be catheterized, and the procedure carries a risk of some 5% of a transient or even persisting neurological deficit (Logue 1979; Savader *et al.* 1993). If a vascular malformation of the spinal cord is considered, MRI—particularly in the sagittal plane—is the first-line investigation for detecting the characteristic serpiginous structures, usually on the dorsal aspect of the cord, or at least for detecting an associated extradural or subdural haematoma (D'Angelo *et al.* 1990; Mohsenipour *et al.* 1994). There are no systematic studies available of the usefulness of spinal angiography after a negative MR scan of the spinal cord.

Mycotic aneurysms were missed by angiography in 10% in older series, and even now they may be visible only on repeated studies. A policy of routine angiography in all patients with infective endocarditis is not justified by decision analysis, but after an intracranial haemorrhage, surgical clipping of the ruptured aneurysm, and therefore angiography, should be considered (Van der Meulen *et al.* 1992).

Aneurysmal patterns of haemorrhage but negative catheter angiography

Although non-aneurysmal types of subarachnoid haemorrhage (SAH) were distinguished more than 15 years ago (van Gijn *et al.* 1985a), a steady stream of publications in which SAH patients with a normal angiogram are still treated as a single group has continued to clutter up the scientific literature. That they contribute so little knowledge is to some extent the result of the invariably retrospective design, but the most serious flaw is that they contain a mixed bag of patients (Rinkel *et al.* 1993). The three most common subgroups are:

- patients whose 'SAH' is not real, but in whom a misdiagnosis results from a traumatic lumbar puncture (section 5.6.3);
- patients with non-aneurysmal types of haemorrhage (section 9.2.1);
- patients with a pattern of haemorrhage that is entirely consistent with a ruptured aneurysm, but who nevertheless have a normal angiogram. It is this last category of patients that we shall consider here.

Only two studies have been performed in which patients with an aneurysmal pattern of bleeding on CT were separately distinguished amongst a greater group with SAH and a negative angiogram. In the first, 36 such patients were identified (Rinkel *et al.* 1991c). In the initial hospital period, re-bleeding occurred in three (two of whom died), delayed cerebral ischaemia in one, and symptomatic hydrocephalus in five patients. The patient who survived her re-bleed underwent exploratory craniotomy at the suspected site of the aneurysm (on the middle cerebral artery), and the aneurysm was indeed found and clipped. On long-term follow-up, another patient re-bled and died. One further patient suddenly developed an oculomotor palsy on the side where an aneurysm of the internal carotid artery had been suspected during the initial period of admission, but which had not been found on two angiographic studies. A third angiogram, at the time of the oculomotor palsy, finally showed the expected aneurysm, which was successfully clipped. Thus, not only had three of the 36 patients died, but another four remained incapacitated. Similar results were found in the second study (Canhao *et al.* 1995). Thirty-five patients with a negative angiogram, despite an aneurysmal pattern of haemorrhage on CT, were followed for more than 2 years: three patients re-bled (fatally in one case), two had delayed cerebral ischaemia, and four had hydrocephalus. The occurrence of all these complications is in stark contrast to patients with a non-aneurysmal perimesencephalic pattern of haemorrhage, in whom death and disability from neurological causes do not occur.

The substantial risk of re-bleeding in patients with an aneurysmal pattern of haemorrhage indicates that at least in some patients an aneurysm escapes radiological detection. Other than technical reasons, such as insufficient use of oblique projections, this may have several explanations. Narrowing of blood vessels by 'vasospasm' has been invoked in some cases (Spetzler *et al.* 1974; Bohmfalk & Story 1980; Moritake *et al.* 1981). Thrombosis of the neck of the aneurysm, or of the entire sac, is another possible reason (Edner *et al.* 1978). Obliteration of the aneurysm by pressure of an adjacent haematoma may also prevent visualization, particularly with aneurysms of the anterior communicating artery (Di Lorenzo & Guidetti 1988; Iwanaga *et al.* 1990). Microaneurysms too small to be detected on angiography have also been implicated as a possible source of the haemorrhage, but have rarely been demonstrated (Hayward 1977; Spallone *et al.* 1986).

Given the risk of a later re-bleed, it is in patients with an aneurysmal pattern of haemorrhage on CT that repeat angiography seems most clearly indicated. The combined yield of a second angiogram in eight reported series was 30 aneurysms in 177 patients, or 17% (Ruelle *et al.* 1985; Juul *et al.* 1986; Spallone *et al.* 1986; Suzuki *et al.* 1987; Giombini *et al.* 1988; Cioffi *et al.* 1989; Iwanaga *et al.* 1990; Kaim *et al.* 1996). If it is taken into account that patients with perimesencephalic non-aneurysmal haemorrhage were not excluded from these series, the yield of repeat angiograms in patients with a diffuse or anteriorly located pattern of haemorrhage on CT scanning must be even higher. If a second angiogram again fails to demonstrate the suspected aneurysm, perhaps a third angiogram may be positive, after an interval of several months (Di Lorenzo & Guidetti 1988; Rinkel *et al.* 1991a). In a unique, consecutive series of 14 such patients subjected to a third angiogram, a single aneurysm was found (Suzuki *et al.* 1987). MR imaging has in exceptional cases identified the expected aneurysm, despite a normal catheter angiogram (Pertuiset *et al.* 1989; Renowden *et al.* 1994). CT angiography with three-dimensional projection is an emerging technique, but its value in detecting 'occult' aneurysms has not yet passed the stage of the case report (Dorsch *et al.* 1995).

If a first, as well as a second, catheter angiogram is completely negative (not only both internal carotid arteries but also both vertebral arteries having been injected), despite an aneurysmal pattern of haemorrhage on the CT scan, the search for a vascular lesion should still be doggedly pursued. A reasonable approach is to perform a third investigation some 3 months after SAH onset, the choice (repeat catheter angiography, CT angiography, MRI/MRA) depending on the patient's clinical condition, age, and personal wishes.

Few neurosurgeons perform exploratory craniotomy in patients with a suspected aneurysm, despite repeatedly normal angiograms, but for those who do the rate of aneurysms found and obliterated seems satisfactory: five out of six in one report, the exception probably being a non-aneurysmal perimesencephalic haemorrhage (Jafar & Weiner 1993). Such a course of action is especially indicated in patients with negative angiograms who have nevertheless had, and survived, a re-bleed.

9.4.7 Sudden headache with normal CT and normal CSF: should catheter angiography be done?

If patients present 1–2 weeks after an episode of sudden headache, the diagnostic value of a normal CT scan is very limited, but a lumbar puncture showing crystal-clear cerebrospinal fluid will suffice to exclude subarachnoid haemorrhage (SAH); at least with an initially positive CT scan, the CSF is invariably xanthochromic within this period (Vermeulen *et al.* 1983; Vermeulen *et al.* 1989) (section 5.6.3). The point has been made that xanthochromia may not last as long in the 5% of patients with SAH in whom early CT scanning is negative (Beetham *et al.* 1998) (section 9.4.1). Nevertheless, a hospital-based follow-up study of 71 patients with non-haemorrhagic 'thunderclap' headache, for an average period of 3.3 years, failed to produce a single episode of SAH; 12 patients had identical recurrences, but again without evidence of SAH, and 31 subsequently had regular episodes of tension headache or common migraine (Wijdicks *et al.* 1988). A study of similar design, but based in general practice, again failed to find a single episode of SAH on follow up of patients with sudden headache but negative investigations (Linn *et al.* 1999).

The issue of distinguishing patients with non-haemorrhagic 'thunderclap' headache from those with ruptured aneurysms has been unnecessarily complicated by a few case reports of impressive but rare events. There is one report of fatal aneurysmal rupture in which the presence of iron-containing macrophages was interpreted as evidence of an earlier haemorrhage, in a patient with a preceding episode of headache (Ball 1975). This interpretation is questionable, as the patient survived the second episode for a few days. A second type of case report, exemplified by two patients from different sources, relates how sudden headache and negative findings on CT as well as on lumbar puncture can still be associated with an aneurysm on cerebral angiography, accompanied by arterial narrowing (Day & Raskin 1986; Clarke *et al.* 1988). At operation, no evidence of haemorrhage around the aneurysm was found in either case, but it was claimed that the aneurysm had suddenly enlarged, without rupturing. A more realistic interpretation is that in the course of life a small percentage of adults develop asymptomatic aneurysms, and indiscriminate use of angiography is bound to uncover some of them (section 13.12.1). If it is assumed that the aneurysm was incidental in the two case reports cited above, migraine might explain both the headache and the arterial narrowing ('vasospasm'). Segmental and fully reversible vasospasm has been demonstrated in patients with severe headache but without an aneurysm (Call *et al.* 1988), and even in a patient with benign exertional headache (Silbert *et al.* 1989). Haemorrhage confined to the wall of an aneurysm may indeed have occurred in an occasional patient but must be exceedingly rare amongst all patients with sudden headache. Cerebral catheter angiography carries a risk of transient or permanent ischaemic deficits of approximately one in 30, in patients suspected of an aneurysm or vascular malformation, but without SAH or stroke (Cloft *et al.* 1999). 'Thunderclap' headache does not warrant this potentially dangerous procedure if both the CT scan and the CSF are normal within 2 weeks of the event.

If a patient presents with a sudden severe headache, and the CT scan and lumbar puncture are carried out in less than 2 weeks and are completely normal, with no evidence of intracranial haemorrhage, then cerebral catheter angiography is not indicated.

References

Please note that all references taken from *The Cochrane Library* are given a current date as this database is updated on a quarterly basis. Please refer to the current *Cochrane Library* article for the latest review. The same applies to the *British Medical Journal* 'Clinical Evidence' series which is updated every six months.

Abe, M., Tabuchi, K., Yokoyama, H. & Uchino, A. (1998) Blood blisterlike aneurysms of the internal carotid artery. *Journal of Neurosurgery* **89**, 419–424.

Acciarri, N., Padovani, R., Pozzati, E., Gaist, G. & Manetto, V. (1992) Spinal cavernous angioma: a rare cause of subarachnoid hemorrhage. *Surgical Neurology* **37**, 453–456.

Adams, H.P. Jr, Aschenbrener, C.A., Kassell, N.F., Ansbacher, L. & Cornell, S.H. (1982) Intracranial hemorrhage produced by spontaneous dissecting intracranial aneurysm. *Archives of Neurology* **39**, 773–776.

Alberts, M.J., Quinones, A., Graffagnino, C., Friedman, A. & Roses, A.D. (1995) Risk of intracranial aneurysms in families with subarachnoid hemorrhage. *Canadian Journal of Neurological Sciences* **22**, 121–125.

Alliez, B., Du Lac, P. & Trabulsi, R. (1990) Anevrysme extra-cranien de l'artère cerebelleuse postéro-inférieure. Une observation [Extracranial aneurysm of the posterior inferior cerebellar artery. A case report]. *Neurochirurgie* **36**, 137–140.

Al-Yamany, M., Deck, J. & Bernstein, M. (1999) Pseudo-subarachnoid hemorrhage: a rare neuroimaging pitfall. *Canadian Journal of Neurological Sciences* **26**, 57–59.

Aminoff, M.J. (1973) Vascular anomalies in the intracranial dura mater. *Brain* **96**, 601–612.

Aminoff, M.J. & Logue, V. (1974) Clinical features of spinal vascular malformations. *Brain* **97**, 197–210.

Anderson, G.B., Steinke, D.E., Petruk, K.C., Ashforth, R. & Findlay, J.M. (1999a) Computed tomographic angiography versus digital subtraction angiography for the diagnosis and early treatment of ruptured intracranial aneurysms. *Neurosurgery* **45**, 1315–1320.

Anderson, N.E., Sheffield, S. & Hope, J.K.A. (1999b) Superficial siderosis of the central nervous system: a late complication of cerebellar tumors. *Neurology* **52**, 163–169.

Aoki, N. (1991) Do intracranial arteriovenous malformations cause subarachnoid haemorrhage? Review of computed tomography features of ruptured arteriovenous malformations in the acute stage. *Acta Neurochirurgica (Wien)* **112**, 92–95.

Aoki, N. & Sakai, T. (1990) Rebleeding from intracranial dissecting aneurysm in the vertebral artery. *Stroke* **21**, 1628–1631.

Asaoka, K., Houkin, K., Fujimoto, S., Ishikawa, T. & Abe, H. (1998) Intracranial aneurysms associated with aortitis syndrome: case report and review of the literature. *Neurosurgery* **42**, 157–160.

Atlas, S.W. (1993) MR imaging is highly sensitive for acute subarachnoid hemorrhage ... not! *Radiology* **186**, 319–322.

Atlas, S.W. (1997) Magnetic resonance imaging of intracranial aneurysms. *Neuroimaging Clinics of North America* **7**, 709–720.

Atlas, S.W., Sheppard, L., Goldberg, H.I., Hurst, R.W., Listerud, J. & Flamm, E. (1997) Intracranial aneurysms: detection and characterization with MR angiography with use of an advanced postprocessing technique in a blinded-reader study. *Radiology* **203**, 807–814.

Avrahami, E., Katz, R., Rabin, A. & Friedman, V. (1998) CT diagnosis of non-traumatic subarachnoid haemorrhage in patients with brain edema. *European Journal of Radiology* **28**, 222–225.

Baker, C.J., Fiore, A., Connolly, E.S. Jr, Baker, K.Z. & Solomon, R.A. (1995) Serum elastase and alpha-1-antitrypsin levels in patients with ruptured and unruptured cerebral aneurysms. *Neurosurgery* **37**, 56–62.

Ball, M.J. (1975) Pathogenesis of the 'sentinel headache' preceding berry aneurysm rupture. *Canadian Medical Association Journal* **112**, 78–79.

Bamford, J., Hodges, J. & Warlow, C. (1986) Late rupture of a mycotic aneurysm after 'cure' of bacterial endocarditis. *Journal of Neurology* **233**, 51–53.

Barami, K. & Ko, K. (1994) Ruptured mycotic aneurysm presenting as an intraparenchymal hemorrhage and nonadjacent acute subdural hematoma: case report and review of the literature. *Surgical Neurology* **41**, 290–293.

Barker, R.A., Phillips, R.R., Moseley, I.F., Taylor, W.J., Kitchen, N.D. & Scadding, J.W. (1998) Posterior communicating artery aneurysm presenting with haemorrhage into an arachnoid cyst. *Journal of Neurology, Neurosurgery and Psychiatry* **64**, 558–560.

Barth, A. & De Tribolet, N. (1994) Growth of small saccular aneurysms to giant aneurysms: presentation of three cases. *Surgical Neurology* **41**, 277–280.

Baumgartner, R.W., Mattle, H.P., Kothbauer, K. & Schroth, G. (1994) Transcranial color-coded duplex sonography in cerebral aneurysms. *Stroke* **25**, 2429–2434.

Bazzocchi, M., Quaia, E., Zuiani, C. & Moroldo, M. (1998) Transcranial Doppler: state of the art. *European Journal of Radiology* **27** (Suppl. 2), S141–S148.

Beetham, R., Fahie-Wilson, M.N. & Park, D. (1998) What is the role of CSF spectrophotometry in the diagnosis of subarachnoid haemorrhage? *Annals of Clinical Biochemistry* **35**, 1–4.

Bjerre, P., Videbaek, H. & Lindholm, J. (1986) Subarachnoid hemorrhage with normal cerebral angiography: a prospective study on sellar abnormalities and pituitary function. *Neurosurgery* **19**, 1012–1015.

Bohmfalk, G.L. & Story, J.L. (1980) Intermittent appearance of a ruptured cerebral aneurysm on sequential angiograms: case report. *Journal of Neurosurgery* **52**, 263–265.

Bonito, V., Agostinis, C., Ferraresi, S. & Defanti, C.A. (1994) Superficial siderosis of the central nervous system after brachial plexus injury: case report. *Journal of Neurosurgery* **80**, 931–934.

Brilstra, E.H., Hop, J.W. & Rinkel, G.J.E. (1997) Quality of life after perimesencephalic haemorrhage. *Journal of Neurology, Neurosurgery and Psychiatry* **63**, 382–384.

Bromberg, J.E.C., Rinkel, G.J.E., Algra, A. *et al.* (1995a) Familial subarachnoid hemorrhage: distinctive features and patterns of inheritance. *Annals of Neurology* **38**, 929–934.

Bromberg, J.E.C., Rinkel, G.J.E., Algra, A. *et al.* (1995b) Subarachnoid haemorrhage in first and second degree relatives of patients with subarachnoid haemorrhage. *British Medical Journal* **311**, 288–289.

Bromberg, J.E.C., Rinkel, G.J.E., Algra, A., Van den Berg, U.A.C., Tjin-A-Ton, M.L.R. & van Gijn, J. (1996) Hypertension, stroke, and coronary heart disease in relatives of patients with subarachnoid hemorrhage. *Stroke* **27**, 7–9.

Brott, T. & Mandybur, T.I. (1986) Case–control study of clinical outcome after aneurysmal subarachnoid hemorrhage. *Neurosurgery* **19**, 891–895.

Brown, R.D. Jr, Wiebers, D.O. & Forbes, G.S. (1990) Unruptured intracranial aneurysms and arteriovenous malformations: frequency of intracranial hemorrhage and relationship of lesions. *Journal of Neurosurgery* **73**, 859–863.

de Bruijn, S.F.T.M., Stam, J. & Kappelle, L.J. (1996) Thunderclap headache as first symptom of cerebral venous sinus thrombosis. *Lancet* **348**, 1623–1625.

Bruno, A., Nolte, K.B. & Chapin, J. (1993) Stroke associated with ephedrine use. *Neurology* **43**, 1313–1316.

Brust, J.C., Dickinson, P.C., Hughes, J.E. & Holtzman, R.N. (1990) The diagnosis and treatment of cerebral mycotic aneurysms. *Annals of Neurology* **27**, 238–246.

Call, G.K., Fleming, M.C., Sealfon, S., Levine, H., Kistler, J.P. & Fisher, C.M. (1988) Reversible cerebral segmental vasoconstriction. *Stroke* **19**, 1159–1170.

Canhao, P., Ferro, J.M., Pinto, A.M., Melo, T.P. & Campos, J.G. (1995) Perimesencephalic and nonperimesencephalic subarachnoid haemorrhages with negative angiograms. *Acta Neurochirurgica (Wien)* **132**, 14–19.

Canhao, P., Falcao, F., Melo, T., Ferro, H. & Ferro, J. (1999) Vascular risk factors for perimesencephalic nonaneurysmal subarachnoid hemorrhage. *Journal of Neurology* **246**, 492–496.

Caplan, L.R., Baquis, G.D., Pessin, M.S. *et al.* (1988) Dissection of the intracranial vertebral artery. *Neurology* **38**, 868–877.

Caputi, F., De Sanctis, S., Gazzeri, G. & Gazzeri, R. (1997) Neuroma of the spinal accessory nerve disclosed by a subarachnoid hemorrhage: case report. *Neurosurgery* **41**, 946–950.

Carey, J., Numaguchi, Y. & Nadell, J. (1990) Subarachnoid hemorrhage in sickle cell disease. *Child's Nervous System* **6**, 47–50.

Caroscio, J.T., Brannan, T., Budabin, M., Huang, Y.P. & Yahr, M.D. (1980) Subarachnoid hemorrhage secondary to spinal arteriovenous malformation and aneurysm: report of a case and review of the literature. *Archives of Neurology* **37**, 101–103.

Chan, J.W., Hoyt, W.F., Ellis, W.G. & Gress, D. (1997) Pathogenesis of acute monocular blindness from leaking anterior communicating artery aneurysms: report of six cases. *Neurology* **48**, 680–683.

Chapman, A.B., Rubinstein, D., Hughes, R. *et al.* (1992) Intracranial aneurysms in autosomal dominant polycystic kidney disease. *New England Journal of Medicine* **327**, 916–920.

Chaudhary, M.Y., Sachdev, V.P., Cho, S.H., Weitzner, I. Jr, Puljic, S. & Huang, Y.P. (1982) Dural arteriovenous malformation of the major venous sinuses: an acquired lesion. *American Journal of Neuroradiology* **3**, 13–19.

Chauveau, D., Pirson, Y., Verellen Dumoulin, C., Macnicol, A., Gonzalo, A. & Grunfeld, J.P. (1994) Intracranial aneurysms in autosomal dominant polycystic kidney disease. *Kidney International* **45**, 1140–1146.

Chehrenama, M., Zagardo, M.T. & Koski, C.L. (1997) Subarachnoid hemorrhage in a patient with Lyme disease. *Neurology* **48**, 520–523.

Chrysikopoulos, H., Papanikolaou, N., Pappas, J. *et al.* (1996) Acute subarachnoid haemorrhage: detection with magnetic resonance imaging. *British Journal of Radiology* **69**, 601–609.

Chyatte, D. & Lewis, I. (1997) Gelatinase activity and the occurrence of cerebral aneurysms. *Stroke* **28**, 799–804.

Chyatte, D., Reilly, J. & Tilson, M.D. (1990) Morphometric analysis of reticular and elastin fibers in the cerebral arteries of patients with intracranial aneurysms. *Neurosurgery* **26**, 939–943.

Chyatte, D., Bruno, G., Desai, S. & Todor, R. (1999) Inflammation and intracranial aneurysms. *Neurosurgery* **45**, 1137–1146.

Cioffi, F., Pasqualin, A., Cavazzani, P. & Da Pian, R. (1989) Subarachnoid haemorrhage of unknown origin: clinical and tomographical aspects. *Acta Neurochirurgica (Wien)* **97**, 31–39.

Clarke, C.E., Shepherd, D.I., Chishti, K. & Victoratos, G. (1988) Thunderclap headache [letter]. *Lancet* **2**, 625.

Clarke, E. & Walton, J.N. (1953) Subdural haematoma complicating intracranial aneurysm and angioma. *Brain* **76**, 378–404.

Cloft, H.J., Kallmes, D.F., Kallmes, M.H., Goldstein, J.H., Jensen, M.E. & Dion, J.E. (1998) Prevalence of cerebral aneurysms in patients with fibromuscular dysplasia: a reassessment. *Journal of Neurosurgery* **88**, 436–440.

Cloft, H.J., Joseph, G.J. & Dion, J.E. (1999) Risk of cerebral angiography in patients with subarachnoid hemorrhage, cerebral aneurysm, and arteriovenous malformation: a meta-analysis. *Stroke* **30**, 317–320.

Connolly, E.S. Jr, Fiore, A.J., Winfree, C.J., Prestigiacomo, C.J., Goldman, J.E. & Solomon, R.A. (1997) Elastin degradation in the superficial temporal arteries of patients with intracranial aneurysms reflect changes in plasma elastase. *Neurosurgery* **40**, 903–908.

Conway, J.E., Hutchins, G.M. & Tamargo, R.J. (1999) Marfan syndrome is not associated with intracranial aneurysms. *Stroke* **30**, 1632–1636.

Corriero, G., Iacopino, D.G., Valentini, S. & Lanza, P.L. (1996) Cervical neuroma presenting as a subarachnoid hemorrhage: Case report. *Neurosurgery* **39**, 1046–1049.

Crompton, M.R. (1966) The pathogenesis of cerebral aneurysms. *Brain* **89**, 797–814.

D'Angelo, V., Bizzozero, L., Talamonti, G., Ferrara, M. & Colombo, N. (1990) Value of magnetic resonance imaging in spontaneous extradural spinal hematoma due to vascular malformation: case report. *Surgical Neurology* **34**, 343–344.

Darby, D.G., Donnan, G.A., Saling, M.A., Walsh, K.W. & Bladin, P.F. (1988) Primary intraventricular hemorrhage: clinical and neuropsychological findings in a prospective stroke series. *Neurology* **38**, 68–75.

Day, J.W. & Raskin, N.H. (1986) Thunderclap headache: symptom of unruptured cerebral aneurysm. *Lancet* **2**, 1247–1248.

Di Chiro, G., Brooks, R.A., Girton, M.E. *et al.* (1986) Sequential MR studies of intracerebral hematomas in monkeys. *American Journal of Neuroradiology* **7**, 193–199.

Di Lorenzo, N. & Guidetti, G. (1988) Anterior communicating aneurysm missed at angiography: report of two cases treated surgically. *Neurosurgery* **23**, 494–499.

Dodick, D.W. & Wijdicks, E.F.M. (1998) Pituitary apoplexy presenting as a thunderclap headache. *Neurology* **50**, 1510–1511.

Donnet, A., Balzamo, M., Royere, M.L., Grisoli, F. & Ali Cherif, A. (1992) Syndrome de Korsakoff transitoire au décours d'une hémorragie intraventriculaire [Transient Korsakoff's syndrome after intraventricular hemorrhage]. *Neurochirurgie* **38**, 102–104.

Dorsch, N.W., Young, N., Kingston, R.J. & Compton, J.S. (1995) Early experience with spiral CT in the diagnosis of intracranial aneurysms. *Neurosurgery* **36**, 230–236.

Dowling, G. & Curry, B. (1988) Traumatic basal subarachnoid hemorrhage: report of six cases and review of the literature. *American Journal of Forensic Medicine and Pathology* **9**, 23–31.

Drake, C.G. (1979) Giant intracranial aneurysms: experience with surgical treatment in 174 patients. *Clinics of Neurosurgery* **26**, 12–95.

Edner, G., Forster, D.M., Steiner, L. & Bergvall, U. (1978) Spontaneous healing of intracranial aneurysms after subarachnoid hemorrhage. Case report. *Journal of Neurosurgery* **48**, 450–454.

Farrés, M.T., Ferraz Leite, H., Schindler, E. & Mühlbauer, M. (1992) Spontaneous subarachnoid hemorrhage with negative angiography: CT findings. *Journal of Computer Assisted Tomography* **16**, 534–537.

Fearnley, J.M., Stevens, J.M. & Rudge, P. (1995) Superficial siderosis of the central nervous system. *Brain* **118**, 1051–1066.

Fellner, F., Blank, M., Fellner, C., Böhm-Jurkovic, H., Bautz, W. & Kalender, W.A. (1998) Virtual cisternoscopy of intracranial vessels: a novel visualization technique using virtual reality. *Magnetic Resonance Imaging* **16**, 1013–1022.

Ferbert, A., Hubo, I. & Biniek, R. (1992) Non-traumatic subarachnoid hemorrhage with normal angiogram: long-term follow-up and CT predictors of complications. *Journal of Neurological Sciences* **107**, 14–18.

Ferrante, L., Acqui, M., Mastronardi, L., Celli, P., Lunardi, P. & Fortuna, A. (1992) Posterior inferior cerebellar artery (PICA) aneurysm presenting with SAH and contralateral crural monoparesis: a case report. *Surgical Neurology* **38**, 43–45.

Ferry, P.C., Kerber, C., Peterson, D. & Gallo, A.A. Jr (1974) Arteriectasis, subarachnoid hemorrhage in a three-month-old infant. *Neurology* **24**, 494–500.

Finlay, H.M., Whittaker, P. & Canham, P.B. (1998) Collagen organization in the branching region of human brain arteries. *Stroke* **29**, 1595–1601.

Fisher, C.M. (1975) Clinical syndromes in cerebral thrombosis, hypertensive hemorrhage, and ruptured saccular aneurysm. *Clinics of Neurosurgery* **22**, 117–147.

Fodden, D.I., Peatfield, R.C. & Milsom, P.L. (1989) Beware the patient with a headache in the accident and emergency department. *Archives of Emergency Medicine* **6**, 7–12.

Fogelholm, R., Nuutila, M. & Vuorela, A.L. (1992) Primary intracerebral haemorrhage in the Jyvaskyla region, central Finland. 1985–89: incidence, case fatality rate, and functional outcome. *Journal of Neurology, Neurosurgery and Psychiatry* **55**, 546–552.

Fortuny, L.A., Adams, C.B. & Briggs, M. (1980) Surgical mortality in an aneurysm population: effects of age, blood pressure and preoperative neurological state. *Journal of Neurology, Neurosurgery and Psychiatry* **43**, 879–882.

Fransen, P. & De Tribolet, N. (1994) Dissecting aneurysm of the posterior inferior cerebellar artery. *British Journal of Neurosurgery* **8**, 381–386.

Friedman, A.H. & Drake, C.G. (1984) Subarachnoid hemorrhage from intracranial dissecting aneurysm. *Journal of Neurosurgery* **60**, 325–334.

Friedman, M.B. & Brant Zawadzki, M. (1983) Interhemispheric subdural hematoma from ruptured aneurysm. *Computerized Radiology* **7**, 129–134.

Frizzell, R.T., Kuhn, F., Morris, R., Quinn, C. & Fisher, W.S. III (1997) Screening for ocular hemorrhages in patients with ruptured cerebral aneurysms: a prospective study of 99 patients. *Neurosurgery* **41**, 529–533.

Fujimoto, K. (1996) 'Medial defects' in the prenatal human cerebral arteries: an electron microscopic study. *Stroke* **27**, 706–708.

Furuya, K., Sasaki, T., Yoshimoto, Y., Okada, Y., Fujimaki, T. & Kirino, T. (1995) Histologically verified cerebral aneurysm formation secondary to embolism from cardiac myxoma. Case report. *Journal of Neurosurgery* **83**, 170–173.

Gaetani, P., Tartara, F., Grazioli, V., Tancioni, F., Infuso, L. & Baena, R.R.Y. (1998) Collagen cross-linkage, elastolytic and collagenolytic activities in cerebral aneurysms: a preliminary investigation. *Life Science* **63**, 285–292.

Gates, P.C., Barnett, H.J.M., Vinters, H.V., Simonsen, R.L. & Siu, K. (1986) Primary intraventricular hemorrhage in adults. *Stroke* **17**, 872–877.

van Gijn, J. (1992) Subarachnoid haemorrhage. *Lancet* **339**, 653–655.

van Gijn, J. & van Dongen, K.J. (1980) Computed tomography in the diagnosis of subarachnoid haemorrhage and ruptured aneurysm. *Clinical Neurology and Neurosurgery* **82**, 11–24.

van Gijn, J. & van Dongen, K.J. (1982) The time course of aneurysmal haemorrhage on computed tomograms. *Neuroradiology* **23**, 153–156.

van Gijn, J., van Dongen, K.J., Vermeulen, M. & Hijdra, A. (1985a) Perimesencephalic hemorrhage: a nonaneurysmal and benign form of subarachnoid hemorrhage. *Neurology* **35**, 493–497.

van Gijn, J., Hijdra, A., Wijdicks, E.F.M., Vermeulen, M. & van Crevel, H. (1985b) Acute hydrocephalus after aneurysmal subarachnoid hemorrhage. *Journal of Neurosurgery* **63**, 355–362.

Giombini, S., Bruzzone, M.G. & Pluchino, F. (1988) Subarachnoid hemorrhage of unexplained cause. *Neurosurgery* **22**, 313–316.

Gliemroth, J., Nowak, G., Kehler, U., Arnold, H. & Gaebel, C. (1999) Neoplastic cerebral aneurysm from metastatic lung adenocarcinoma associated with cerebral thrombosis and recurrent subarachnoid haemorrhage. *Journal of Neurology, Neurosurgery and Psychiatry* **66**, 246–247.

Glynn, L.E. (1940) Medial defects in the circle of Willis and their relation to aneurysm formation. *Journal of Pathological Bacteriology* **51**, 213–222.

Greene, K.A., Marciano, F.F., Dickman, C.A. *et al.* (1995) Anterior communicating artery aneurysm paraparesis syndrome: clinical manifestations and pathologic correlates. *Neurology* **45**, 45–50.

Griffiths, P.D., Gholkar, A. & Sengupta, R.P. (1994) Oculomotor nerve palsy due to thrombosis of a posterior communicating artery aneurysm following diagnostic angiography. *Neuroradiology* **36**, 614–615.

Guridi, J., Gallego, J., Monzon, F. & Aguilera, F. (1993) Intracerebral hemorrhage caused by transmural dissection of the anterior cerebral artery. *Stroke* **24**, 1400–1402.

Guzman, R. & Grady, M.S. (1999) An intracranial aneurysm on the feeding artery of a cerebellar hemangioblastoma: case report. *Journal of Neurosurgery* **91**, 136–138.

Halbach, V.V., Higashida, R.T., Hieshima, G.B., Goto, K., Norman, D. & Newton, T.H. (1987) Dural fistulas involving the transverse and sigmoid sinuses: results of treatment in 28 patients. *Radiology* **163**, 443–447.

Hamada, J., Hashimoto, N. & Tsukahara, T. (1994) Moyamoya disease with repeated intraventricular hemorrhage due to aneurysm rupture: report of two cases. *Journal of Neurosurgery* **80**, 328–331.

Handa, T., Suzuki, Y., Saito, K., Sugita, K. & Patel, S.J. (1992) Isolated intramedullary spinal artery aneurysm presenting with quadriplegia: case report. *Journal of Neurosurgery* **77**, 148–150.

Hankey, G.J. (1991) Isolated angiitis/angiopathy of the central nervous system. *Cerebrovascular Diseases* **1**, 2–15.

Hara, A., Yoshimi, N. & Mori, H. (1998) Evidence for apoptosis in human intracranial aneurysms. *Neurological Research* **20**, 127–130.

Harland, W.A., Pitts, J.F. & Watson, A.A. (1983) Subarachnoid haemorrhage due to upper cervical trauma. *Journal of Clinical Pathology* **36**, 1335–1341.

Hart, R.G., Byer, J.A., Slaughter, J.R., Hewett, J.E. & Easton, J.D. (1981) Occurrence and implications of seizures in subarachnoid hemorrhage due to ruptured intracranial aneurysms. *Neurosurgery* **8**, 417–421.

Hart, R.G., Foster, J.W., Luther, M.F. & Kanter, M.C. (1990) Stroke in infective endocarditis. *Stroke* **21**, 695–700.

Hassler, O.L. (1962) Physiological intima cushions in the large cerebral arteries of young individuals, 1: morphological structure and possible significance for the circulation. *Acta Pathologica, Microbiologica, et Immunologica Scandinavica* **55**, 19–27.

Hayakawa, I., Watanabe, T., Tsuchida, T. & Sasaki, A. (1978) Perangiographic rupture of intracranial aneurysms. *Neuroradiology* **16**, 293–295.

Hayward, R.D. (1977) Subarachnoid haemorrhage of unknown aetiology: a clinical and radiological study of 51 cases. *Journal of Neurology, Neurosurgery and Psychiatry* **40**, 926–931.

Hayward, R.D. & O'Reilly, G.V. (1976) Intracerebral haemorrhage: accuracy of computerised transverse axial scanning in predicting the underlying aetiology. *Lancet* **1**, 1–4.

Helmchen, C., Nahser, H.C., Yousry, T., Witt, T.N. & Kuhne, D. (1995) Therapie zerebraler Aneurysmen und arteriovenöser Gefässmalformationen bei der hereditären hämorrhagischen Teleangiektasie (Morbus Rendu–Osler–Weber) [Therapy for cerebral aneurysms and arteriovenous vascular malformations in hereditary hemorrhagic telangiectasia (Rendu–Osler–Weber disease)]. *Nervenarzt* **66**, 124–128.

Hijdra, A. & van Gijn, J. (1982) Early death from rupture of an intracranial aneurysm. *Journal of Neurosurgery* **57**, 765–768.

Hijdra, A., Braakman, R., van Gijn, J., Vermeulen, M. & van Crevel, H. (1987) Aneurysmal subarachnoid hemorrhage: complications and outcome in a hospital population. *Stroke* **18**, 1061–1067.

Hillman, J. (1993) Selective angiography for early aneurysm detection in acute subarachnoid haemorrhage. *Acta Neurochirurgica (Wien)* **121**, 20–25.

Hochberg, F.H., Fisher, C.M. & Roberson, G.H. (1974) Subarachnoid hemorrhage caused by rupture of a small superficial artery. *Neurology* **24**, 319–321.

Hop, J.W., Brilstra, E.H. & Rinkel, G.J.E. (1998) Transient amnesia after perimesencephalic haemorrhage: the role of enlarged temporal horns. *Journal of Neurology, Neurosurgery and Psychiatry* **65**, 590–593.

Horikoshi, T., Nukui, H., Yagishita, T., Nishigaya, K., Fukasawa, I. & Sasaki, H. (1999) Oculomotor nerve palsy after surgery for upper basilar artery aneurysms. *Neurosurgery* **44**, 705–710.

Horiuchi, T., Kyoshima, K., Oya, F. & Kobayashi, S. (1997) Fenestrated oculomotor nerve caused by internal carotid–posterior communicating artery aneurysm: case report. *Neurosurgery* **40**, 397–398.

Hosoda, K., Fujita, S., Kawaguchi, T. *et al.* (1991) Spontaneous dissecting aneurysms of the basilar artery presenting with a subarachnoid hemorrhage: report of two cases. *Journal of Neurosurgery* **75**, 628–633.

Hosoda, K., Fujita, S., Kawaguchi, T., Shose, Y. & Hamano, S. (1995) Saccular aneurysms of the proximal (M1) segment of the middle cerebral artery. *Neurosurgery* **36**, 441–446.

Hyland, H.H. & Barnett, H.J.M. (1954) The pathogenesis of cranial nerve palsies associated with intracranial aneurysms. *Proceedings of the Royal Society of Medicine* **47**, 141–146.

Imanse, J. & Vanneste, J.A.L. (1990) Intraventricular hemorrhage following amphetamine abuse. *Neurology* **40**, 1318–1319.

Ishikawa, T., Nakamura, N., Houkin, K. & Nomura, M. (1997) Pathological consideration of a 'blister-like' aneurysm at the superior wall of the internal carotid artery: case report. *Neurosurgery* **40**, 403–405.

Iwanaga, H., Wakai, S., Ochiai, C., Narita, J., Inoh, S. & Nagai, M. (1990) Ruptured cerebral aneurysms missed by initial angiographic study. *Neurosurgery* **27**, 45–51.

Jackson, A., Fitzgerald, J.B., Hartley, R.W., Leonard, A. & Yates, J. (1993) CT appearances of haematomas in the corpus callosum in patients with subarachnoid haemorrhage. *Neuroradiology* **35**, 420–423.

Jafar, J.J. & Weiner, H.L. (1993) Surgery for angiographically occult cerebral aneurysms. *Journal of Neurosurgery* **79**, 674–679.

Jafar, J.J., Kamiryo, T., Chiles, B.W. & Nelson, P.K. (1998) A dissecting aneurysm of the posteroinferior cerebellar artery: case report. *Neurosurgery* **43**,

353–356.

Jenkins, A., Hadley, D.M., Teasdale, G.M., Condon, B., Macpherson, P. & Patterson, J. (1988) Magnetic resonance imaging of acute subarachnoid hemorrhage. *Journal of Neurosurgery* **68**, 731–736.

Jensen, F.K. & Wagner, A. (1997) Intracranial aneurysm following radiation therapy for medulloblastoma: a case report and review of the literature. *Acta Radiologica* **38**, 37–42.

Johnston, S.C., Colford, J.M. Jr & Gress, D.R. (1998) Oral contraceptives and the risk of subarachnoid hemorrhage: a meta-analysis. *Neurology* **51**, 411–418.

Joslyn, J.N., Williams, J.P., White, J.L. & White, R.L. (1985) Simultaneous rupture of two intracranial aneurysms: CT diagnosis. *Stroke* **16**, 518–521.

Juul, R., Fredriksen, T.A. & Ringkjob, R. (1986) Prognosis in subarachnoid hemorrhage of unknown etiology. *Journal of Neurosurgery* **64**, 359–362.

Juvela, S. (1996) Prevalence of risk factors in spontaneous intracerebral hemorrhage and aneurysmal subarachnoid hemorrhage. *Archives of Neurology* **53**, 734–740.

Juvela, S. (2000) Risk factors for multiple intracranial aneurysms. *Stroke* **31**, 392–397.

Kaim, A., Proske, M., Kirsch, E., von Weymarn, A., Radu, E.W. & Steinbrich, W. (1996) Value of repeat-angiography in cases of unexplained subarachnoid hemorrhage (SAH). *Acta Neurologica Scandinavica* **93**, 366–373.

Kallmes, D.F., Clark, H.P., Dix, J.E. *et al.* (1996) Ruptured vertebrobasilar aneurysms: frequency of the nonaneurysmal perimesencephalic pattern of haemorrhage on CT scans. *Radiology* **201**, 657–660.

Kamiya, K., Inagawa, T., Yamamoto, M. & Monden, S. (1991) Subdural hematoma due to ruptured intracranial aneurysm. *Neurologia Medico-Chirurgica (Tokyo)* **31**, 82–86.

Kandel, E.I. (1980) Complete excision of arteriovenous malformations of the cervical cord. *Surgical Neurology* **13**, 135–139.

Kaplan, S.S., Ogilvy, C.S., Gonzalez, R., Gress, D. & Pile Spellman, J. (1993) Extracranial vertebral artery pseudoaneurysm presenting as subarachnoid hemorrhage. *Stroke* **24**, 1397–1399.

Kataoka, K. & Taneda, M. (1984) Angiographic disappearance of multiple dural arteriovenous malformations. Case report. *Journal of Neurosurgery* **60**, 1275–1278.

Kato, Y., Sano, H., Katada, K. *et al.* (1996) Clinical usefulness of 3-D CT endoscopic imaging of cerebral aneurysms. *Neurological Research* **18**, 98–102.

Kawamata, T., Tanikawa, T., Takeshita, M., Onda, H., Takakura, K. & Toyoda, C. (1994) Rebleeding of intracranial dissecting aneurysm in the vertebral artery following proximal clipping. *Neurological Research* **16**, 141–144.

Kayama, T., Sugawara, T., Sakurai, Y., Ogawa, A., Onuma, T. & Yoshimoto, T. (1991) Early CT features of ruptured cerebral aneurysms of the posterior cranial fossa. *Acta Neurochirurgica (Wien)* **108**, 34–39.

Kayembe, K.N., Sasahara, M. & Hazama, F. (1984) Cerebral aneurysms and variations in the circle of Willis. *Stroke* **15**, 846–850.

Keane, J.R. (1996) Aneurysmal third-nerve palsies presenting with pleocytosis. *Neurology* **46**, 1176.

Kendall, B.E., Lee, B.C. & Claveria, E. (1976) Computerized tomography and angiography in subarachnoid haemorrhage. *British Journal of Radiology* **49**, 483–501.

Kinouchi, H., Mizoi, K., Takahashi, A., Nagamine, Y., Koshu, K. & Yoshimoto, T. (1998) Dural arteriovenous shunts at the craniocervical junction. *Journal of Neurosurgery* **89**, 755–761.

Kiriakopoulos, E.T., Gorn, R.A. & Barton, J.J. (1998) Small retinal hemorrhages as the only sign of an intracranial aneurysm. *American Journal of Ophthalmology* **125**, 401–403.

Kissel, J.T., Burde, R.M., Klingele, T.G. & Zeiger, H.E. (1983) Pupil-sparing oculomotor palsies with internal carotid-posterior communicating artery aneurysms. *Annals of Neurology* **13**, 149–154.

Kitahara, T., Ohwada, T., Tokiwa, K. *et al.* (1993) Clinical study in patients with perimesencephalic subarachnoid hemorrhage of unknown etiology. *No Shinkei Geka* **21**, 903–908.

Koenig, G.H., Marshall, W.H. Jr, Poole, G.J. & Kramer, R.A. (1979) Rupture of intracranial aneurysms during cerebral angiography: report of ten cases and review of the literature. *Neurosurgery* **5**, 314–324.

Kojima, M., Nagasawa, S., Lee, Y.E., Takeichi, Y., Tsuda, E. & Mabuchi, N. (1998) Asymptomatic familial cerebral aneurysms. *Neurosurgery* **43**, 776–781.

Kondziolka, D., Bernstein, M., ter Brugge, K. & Schutz, H. (1988) Acute subdural hematoma from ruptured posterior communicating artery aneurysm. *Neurosurgery* **22**, 151–154.

Konishi, Y., Kadowaki, C., Hara, M. & Takeuchi, K. (1985) Aneurysms associated with moyamoya disease. *Neurosurgery* **16**, 484–491.

Korogi, Y., Takahashi, M., Mabuchi, N. *et al.* (1996) Intracranial aneurysms: diagnostic accuracy of MR angiography with evaluation of maximum intensity projection and source images. *Radiology* **199**, 199–207.

Kowall, N.W. & Sobel, R.A. (1988) Case records of the Massachusetts General Hospital. Weekly clinicopathological exercises. Case 7–1988. A 27-year-old man with acute myelomonocytic leukemia in remission and repeated intracranial hemorrhages. *New England Journal of Medicine* **318**, 427–440.

Kownacki, J.D., Remonda, L., Godoy, N. & Krauss, J.K. (1998) Subependymal thalamic haemorrhage due to a thalamoperforating artery aneurysm. *Journal of Neurology, Neurosurgery and Psychiatry* **65**, 669–678.

Krapf, H., Skalej, M. & Voigt, K. (1999) Subarachnoid hemorrhage due to septic embolic infarction in infective endocarditis. *Cerebrovascular Diseases* **9**, 182–184.

Krendel, D.A., Ditter, S.M., Frankel, M.R. & Ross, W.K. (1990) Biopsy-proven cerebral vasculitis associated with cocaine abuse. *Neurology* **40**, 1092–1094.

Kumar, R., Wijdicks, E.F.M., Brown, R.D. Jr, Parisi, J.E. & Hammond, C.A. (1997) Isolated angiitis of the CNS presenting as subarachnoid haemorrhage. *Journal of Neurology, Neurosurgery and Psychiatry* **62**, 649–651.

Kunze, S. & Schiefer, W. (1971) Angiographic demonstration of a dissecting aneurysm of the middle cerebral artery. *Neuroradiology* **2**, 201–206.

Laissy, J.P., Normand, G., Monroc, M., Duchateau, C., Alibert, F. & Thiebot, J. (1991) Spontaneous intracerebral hematomas from vascular causes. Predictive value of CT compared with angiography. *Neuroradiology* **33**, 291–295.

Lance, J.W. (1976) Headaches related to sexual activity. *Journal of Neurology, Neurosurgery and Psychiatry* **39**, 1226–1230.

Lasjaunias, P., Chiu, M., ter Brugge, K., Tolia, A., Hurth, M. & Bernstein, M. (1986) Neurological manifestations of intracranial dural arteriovenous malformations. *Journal of Neurosurgery* **64**, 724–730.

Lau, A.H.C., Takeshita, M. & Ishii, M. (1991) Mycotic (*Aspergillus*) arteriitis resulting in fatal subarachnoid hemorrhage: a case report. *Angiology* **42**, 251–255.

Lavin, P.J. & Troost, B.T. (1984) Traumatic fourth nerve palsy: clinicoanatomic correlations with computed tomographic scan. *Archives of Neurology* **41**, 679–680.

Le Roux, P.D., Dailey, A.T., Newell, D.W., Grady, M.S. & Winn, H.R. (1993) Emergent aneurysm clipping without angiography in the moribund patient with intracerebral hemorrhage: the use of infusion computed tomography scans. *Neurosurgery* **33**, 189–197.

Leblanc, R. (1999) De novo formation of familial cerebral aneurysms: case report. *Neurosurgery* **44**, 871–876.

Lee, E.K., Hecht, S.T. & Lie, J.T. (1998a) Multiple intracranial and systemic aneurysms associated with infantile-onset arterial fibromuscular dysplasia. *Neurology* **50**, 828–829.

Lee, T.T., Gromelski, E.B., Bowen, B.C. & Green, B.A. (1998b) Diagnostic and surgical management of spinal dural arteriovenous fistulas. *Neurosurgery* **43**, 242–246.

Lev, M.H. & Schaefer, P.W. (1999) Subarachnoid gadolinium enhancement mimicking subarachnoid hemorrhage on FLAIR MR images. *American Journal of Roentgenology* **173**, 1414–1415.

Levine, S.R., Brust, J.C., Futrell, N. *et al.* (1990) Cerebrovascular complications of the use of the 'crack' form of alkaloidal cocaine. *New England Journal of Medicine* **323**, 699–704.

Levine, S.R., Brust, J.C., Futrell, N. *et al.* (1991) A comparative study of the cerebrovascular complications of cocaine: alkaloidal versus hydrochloride: a review. *Neurology* **41**, 1173–1177.

Lidov, M.W., Silvers, A.R., Mosesson, R.E., Stollman, A.L. & Som, P.M. (1996) Pantopaque simulating thrombosed intracranial aneurysms on MRI. *Journal of Computer Assisted Tomography* **20**, 225–227.

Lim, S.T. & Sage, D.J. (1977) Detection of subarachnoid blood clot and other thin, flat structures by computed tomography. *Radiology* **123**, 79–84.

Linn, F.H.H., Wijdicks, E.F.M., van der Graaf, Y., Weerdesteyn-van Vliet, F.A., Bartelds, A.I. & van Gijn, J. (1994) Prospective study of sentinel headache in aneurysmal subarachnoid haemorrhage. *Lancet* **344**, 590–593.

Linn, F.H.H., Rinkel, G.J.E., Algra, A. & van Gijn, J. (1996) Incidence of subarachnoid hemorrhage: role of region, year, and rate of computed tomography: a meta-analysis. *Stroke* **27**, 625–629.

Linn, F.H.H., Rinkel, G.J.E., Algra, A. & van Gijn, J. (1998) Headache characteristics in subarachnoid haemorrhage and benign thunderclap headache. *Journal of Neurology, Neurosurgery and Psychiatry* **65**, 791–793.

Linn, F.H.H., Rinkel, G.J.E., Algra, A. & van Gijn, J. (1999) Follow-up of idiopathic thunderclap headache in general practice. *Journal of Neurology* **246**, 946–948.

Linn, F.H.H., Rinkel, G.J.E., Algra, A. & van Gijn, J. (2000) The notion of 'warning leaks' in subarachnoid haemorrhage: are such patients in fact admitted with a rebleed? *Journal of Neurology, Neurosurgery and Psychiatry* **68**, 332–336.

Little, J.R., Blomquist, G.A. Jr & Ethier, R. (1977) Intraventricular hemorrhage in adults. *Surgical Neurology* **8**, 143–149.

Logue, V. (1979) Angiomas of the spinal cord: review of the pathogenesis, clinical features, and results of surgery. *Journal of Neurology, Neurosurgery and Psychiatry* **42**, 1–11.

Love, L.C., Mickle, J.P. & Sypert, G.W. (1985) Ruptured intracranial aneurysms in cases of sickle cell anemia. *Neurosurgery* **16**, 808–812.

McFadzean, R.M., Doyle, D., Rampling, R., Teasdale, E. & Teasdale, G. (1991) Pituitary apoplexy and its effect on vision. *Neurosurgery* **29**, 669–675.

Mangiardi, J.R., Daras, M., Geller, M.E., Weitzner, I. & Tuchman, A.J. (1988) Cocaine-related intracranial hemorrhage. Report of nine cases and review. *Acta Neurologica Scandinavica* **77**, 177–180.

Manschot, W.A. (1954) Subarachnoid hemorrhage: intraocular symptoms and their pathogenesis. *American Journal of Ophthalmology* **38**, 501–505.

Marks, M.P., Lane, B., Steinberg, G.K. & Snipes, G.J. (1992) Intranidal aneurysms in cerebral arteriovenous malformations: evaluation and endovascular treatment. *Radiology* **183**, 355–360.

Marro, B., Galanaud, D., Valery, C.A. *et al.* (1997) Intracranial aneurysm: inner view and neck identification with CT angiography virtual endoscopy. *Journal of Computer Assisted Tomography* **21**, 587–589.

Mascalchi, M., Salvi, F.P., Pirini, M.G. *et al.* (1999) Transthyretin amyloidosis and superficial siderosis of the CNS. *Neurology* **53**, 1498–1503.

Masson, C., Martin, N., Masson, M. & Cambier, J. (1986) Hémorragie intraventriculaire après endarteriectomie carotidienne. Role des suppléances de type moya moya [Intraventricular hemorrhage after carotid endarterectomy. Role of moyamoya-type collateral circulation]. *Revue Neurologique (Paris)* **142**, 716–719.

Masson, E.A., Atkin, S.L., Diver, M. & White, M.C. (1993) Pituitary apoplexy and sudden blindness following the administration of gonadotrophin releasing hormone. *Clinical Endocrinology (Oxford)* **38**, 109–110.

Massoud, T.F., Anslow, P. & Molyneux, A.J. (1992) Subarachnoid hemorrhage following spontaneous intracranial carotid artery dissection. *Neuroradiology* **34**, 33–35.

Masuda, J., Yutani, C., Waki, R., Ogata, J., Kuriyama, Y. & Yamaguchi, T. (1992) Histopathological analysis of the mechanisms of intracranial hemorrhage complicating infective endocarditis. *Stroke* **23**, 843–850.

Matsumura, K., Matsuda, M., Handa, J. & Todo, G. (1990) Magnetic resonance imaging with aneurysmal subarachnoid hemorrhage: comparison with computed tomography scan. *Surgical Neurology* **34**, 71–78.

Mattle, H., Kohler, S., Huber, P., Rohner, M. & Steinsiepe, K.F. (1989) Anticoagulation-related intracranial extracerebral haemorrhage. *Journal of Neurology, Neurosurgery and Psychiatry* **52**, 829–837.

Meyer, F.B., Huston, J. III & Riederer, S.S. (1993) Pulsatile increases in aneurysm size determined by cine phase contrast MR angiography. *Journal of Neurosurgery* **78**, 879–883.

Mizobuchi, M., Ito, N., Tanaka, C., Sako, K., Sumi, Y. & Sasaki, T. (1999) Unidirectional olfactory hallucination associated with ipsilateral unruptured intracranial aneurysm. *Epilepsia* **40**, 516–519.

Mizutani, T., Aruga, T., Kirino, T., Miki, Y., Saito, I. & Tsuchida, T. (1995) Recurrent subarachnoid hemorrhage from untreated ruptured vertebrobasilar dissecting aneurysms. *Neurosurgery* **36**, 905–913.

Mohsenipour, I., Ortler, M., Twerdy, K., Schmutzhard, E., Attlmayr, G. & Aichner, F. (1994) Isolated aneurysm of a spinal radicular artery presenting as spinal subarachnoid haemorrhage [letter]. *Journal of Neurology, Neurosurgery and Psychiatry* **57**, 767–768.

Mokri, B., Houser, O.W., Sandok, B.A. & Piepgras, D.G. (1988) Spontaneous dissections of the vertebral arteries. *Neurology* **38**, 880–885.

Moritake, K., Handa, H., Ohtsuka, S. & Hashimoto, N. (1981) Vanishing cerebral aneurysm in serial angiography. *Surgical Neurology* **16**, 36–40.

Muhonen, M.G., Godersky, J.C. & VanGilder, J.C. (1991) Cerebral aneurysms associated with neurofibromatosis. *Surgical Neurology* **36**, 470–475.

Munn, E.J., Alloway, J.A., Diffin, D.C. & Arroyo, R.A. (1998) Polyarteritis with symptomatic intracerebral aneurysms at initial presentation. *Journal of Rheumatology* **25**, 2022–2025.

Munyer, T.P. & Margulis, A.R. (1981) Pseudoxanthoma elasticum with internal carotid artery aneurysm. *American Journal of Roentgenology* **136**, 1023–1024.

Nachanakian, A., Gardeur, D., Poisson, M. & Philippon, J. (1983) Hemorragie intra-ventriculaire spontanée secondaire a un méningiome [Spontaneous intraventricular hemorrhage secondary to meningioma]. *Neurochirurgie* **29**, 47–49.

Nadeau, S.E. & Trobe, J.D. (1983) Pupil sparing in oculomotor palsy: a brief review. *Annals of Neurology* **13**, 143–148.

Nagamine, Y., Takahashi, S. & Sonobe, M. (1981) Multiple intracranial aneurysms associated with moyamoya disease: case report. *Journal of Neurosurgery* **54**, 673–676.

Nakatomi, H., Nagata, K., Kawamoto, S. & Shiokawa, Y. (1997) Ruptured dissecting aneurysm as a cause of subarachnoid hemorrhage of unverified etiology. *Stroke* **28**, 1278–1282.

Nakayama, Y., Tanaka, A., Yoshinaga, S., Tomonaga, M., Maehara, F. & Ohkawa, M. (1989) Multiple intracerebral arteriovenous malformations: report of two cases. *Neurosurgery* **25**, 281–286.

Nishikawa, M., Sakamoto, H., Katsuyama, J., Hakuba, A. & Nishimura, S. (1998) Multiple appearing and vanishing aneurysms: primary angiitis of the central nervous system: case report. *Journal of Neurosurgery* **88**, 133–137.

Noguchi, K., Ogawa, T., Inugami, A. *et al.* (1995) Acute subarachnoid hemorrhage: MR imaging with fluid-attenuated inversion recovery pulse sequences. *Radiology* **196**, 773–777.

Noguchi, K., Ogawa, T., Seto, H. *et al.* (1997) Subacute and chronic subarachnoid hemorrhage: diagnosis with fluid-attenuated inversion-recovery MR imaging. *Radiology* **203**, 257–262.

Nohjoh, T., Houkin, K., Takahashi, A. & Abe, H. (1995) Ruptured dissecting vertebral artery aneurysm detected by repeated angiography: case report. *Neurosurgery* **36**, 180–182.

Nolte, K.B., Brass, L.M. & Fletterick, C.F. (1996) Intracranial hemorrhage associated with cocaine abuse: a prospective autopsy study. *Neurology* **46**, 1291–1296.

Norrgard, O., Angquist, K.A., Fodstad, H., Forsell, A. & Lindberg, M. (1987) Intracranial aneurysms and heredity. *Neurosurgery* **20**, 236–239.

Oana, K., Murakami, T., Beppu, T., Yamaura, A. & Kanaya, H. (1991) Aneurysm of the distal anterior inferior cerebellar artery unrelated to the cerebellopontine angle: case report. *Neurosurgery* **28**, 899–903.

O'Boynick, P., Green, K.D., Batnitzky, S., Kepes, J.J. & Pietak, R. (1994) Aneurysm of the left middle cerebral artery caused by myxoid degeneration of the vessel wall. *Stroke* **25**, 2283–2286.

Ogawa, T., Inugami, A., Fujita, H. *et al.* (1995) MR diagnosis of subacute and chronic subarachnoid hemorrhage: Comparison with CT. *American Journal of Roentgenology* **165**, 1257–1262.

Okamoto, S., Handa, H. & Hashimoto, N. (1984) Location of intracranial aneurysms associated with cerebral arteriovenous malformation: statistical analysis. *Surgical Neurology* **22**, 335–340.

Oksi, J., Kalimo, H., Marttila, R.J. *et al.* (1998) Intracranial aneurysms in three patients with disseminated Lyme borreliosis: cause or chance association? *Journal of Neurology, Neurosurgery and Psychiatry* **64**, 636–642.

O'Leary, P.M. & Sweeny, P.J. (1986) Ruptured intracerebral aneurysm resulting in a subdural hematoma. *Annals of Emergency Medicine* **15**, 944–946.

Osenbach, R.K., Blumenkopf, B., McComb, B. & Huggins, M.J. (1986) Ocular bobbing with ruptured giant distal posterior inferior cerebellar artery aneurysm. *Surgical Neurology* **25**, 149–152.

Overby, M.C. & Rothman, A.S. (1985) Multiple intracranial aneurysms in sickle cell anemia: report of two cases. *Journal of Neurosurgery* **62**, 430–434.

Padberg, M. & Hoogenraad, T.U. (2000) Cerebral siderosis by a spinal tumour. *Journal of Neurology* **247**, 473.

Papa, M.L., Schisano, G., Franco, A. & Nina, P. (1994) Congenital deficiency of factor VII in subarachnoid hemorrhage. *Stroke* **25**, 508–510.

Pascual, J., Diez, C., Carda, J.R. & Vazquez Barquero, A. (1987) Intraventricular haemorrhage complicating a brain abscess. *Postgraduate Medical Journal* **63**, 785–787.

Pascual, J., Iglesias, F., Oterino, A., Vazquez-Barquero, A. & Berciano, J. (1996) Cough, exertional, and sexual headaches: an analysis of 72 benign and symptomatic cases. *Neurology* **46**, 1520–1524.

Patel, M.R., Edelman, R.R. & Warach, S. (1996) Detection of hyperacute primary intraparenchymal hemorrhage by magnetic resonance imaging. *Stroke* **27**, 2321–2324.

Pertuiset, B., Haisa, T., Bordi, L., Abou Ouf, S. & Eissa, M. (1989) Detection of a ruptured aneurysmal sac by MRI in a case of negative angiogram—successful clipping of an anterior communicating artery aneurysm: case report. *Acta Neurochirurgica (Wien)* **100**, 84–86.

Pfausler, B., Belcl, R., Metzler, R., Mohsenipour, I. & Schmutzhard, E. (1996) Terson's syndrome in spontaneous subarachnoid hemorrhage: a prospective study in 60 consecutive patients. *Journal of Neurosurgery* **85**, 392–394.

Pfister, H.W. & Von Rosen, F. (1995) Severe intraventricular haemorrhage shown by computed tomography as an unusual manifestation of Wernicke's encephalopathy. *Journal of Neurology, Neurosurgery and Psychiatry* **59**, 555–556.

Piepgras, D.G., McGrail, K.M. & Tazelaar, H.D. (1994) Intracranial dissection of the distal middle cerebral artery as an uncommon cause of distal cerebral artery aneurysm: case report. *Journal of Neurosurgery* **80**, 909–913.

Pinto, A.N., Ferro, J.M., Canhao, P. & Campos, J. (1993) How often is a perimesencephalic subarachnoid haemorrhage CT pattern caused by ruptured aneurysms? *Acta Neurochirurgica (Wien)* **124**, 79–81.

Pinto, A.N., Canhao, P. & Ferro, J.M. (1996) Seizures at the onset of subarachnoid haemorrhage. *Journal of Neurology* **243**, 161–164.

Poon, T.P. & Solis, O.G. (1985) Sudden death due to massive intraventricular hemorrhage into an unsuspected ependymoma. *Surgical Neurology* **24**, 63–66.

Post, M.J., David, N.J., Glaser, J.S. & Safran, A. (1980) Pituitary apoplexy: diagnosis by computed tomography. *Radiology* **134**, 665–670.

Quint, D.J. & Spickler, E.M. (1990) Magnetic resonance demonstration of vertebral artery dissection. Report of two cases. *Journal of Neurosurgery* **72**, 964–967.

Qureshi, A.I., Sung, G.Y., Suri, M.F.K., Straw, R.N., Guterman, L.R. & Hopkins, L.N. (2000) Factors associated with aneurysm size in patients with subarachnoid hemorrhage: Effect of smoking and aneurysm location. *Neurosurgery* **46**, 44–50.

Raaymakers, T.W.M., Buys, P.C., Verbeeten, B. Jr *et al.* (1999) MR angiography as a screening tool for intracranial aneurysms: feasibility, test characteristics, and interobserver agreement. *American Journal of Roentgenology* **173**, 1469–1475.

Rabb, C.H. & Barnwell, S.L. (1998) Catastrophic subarachnoid hemorrhage resulting from ruptured vertebrobasilar dolichoectasia: case report. *Neurosurgery* **42**, 379–382.

Ragland, R.L., Gelber, N.D., Wilkinson, H.A., Knorr, J.R. & Tran, A.A. (1993) Anterior communicating artery aneurysm rupture: an unusual cause of acute subdural hemorrhage. *Surgical Neurology* **40**, 400–402.

Reid, R.L., Quigley, M.E. & Yen, S.S. (1985) Pituitary apoplexy: a review. *Archives of Neurology* **42**, 712–719.

Reijneveld, J.C., Wermer, M., Boonman, Z., van Gijn, J. & Rinkel, G.J.E. (2000) Acute confusional state as presenting feature in aneurysmal subarachnoid hemorrhage: frequency and characteristics. *Journal of Neurology* **247**, 112–116.

Renowden, S.A., Molyneux, A.J., Anslow, P. & Byrne, J.V. (1994) The value of MRI in angiogram-negative intracranial haemorrhage. *Neuroradiology* **36**, 422–425.

Ricolfi, F., Decq, P., Brugieres, P., Blustajn, J., Melon, E. & Gaston, A. (1996) Ruptured fusiform aneurysm of the superior third of the basilar artery associated with the absence of the midbasilar artery: case report. *Journal of Neurosurgery* **85**, 961–965.

Rinkel, G.J.E. & van Gijn, J. (1995) Perimesencephalic haemorrhage in the quadrigeminal cistern. *Cerebrovascular Diseases* **5**, 312–313.

Rinkel, G.J.E., Wijdicks, E.F.M., Vermeulen, M., Hageman, L.M., Tans, J.T. & van Gijn, J. (1990a) Outcome in perimesencephalic (nonaneurysmal) subarachnoid hemorrhage: a follow-up study in 37 patients. *Neurology* **40**, 1130–1132.

Rinkel, G.J.E., Wijdicks, E.F.M., Ramos, L.M.P. & van Gijn, J. (1990b) Progression of acute hydrocephalus in subarachnoid haemorrhage: a case report documented by serial CT scanning. *Journal of Neurology, Neurosurgery and Psychiatry* **53**, 354–355.

Rinkel, G.J.E., Wijdicks, E.F.M., Vermeulen, M. *et al.* (1991a) Nonaneurysmal perimesencephalic subarachnoid hemorrhage: CT and MR patterns that differ from aneurysmal rupture. *American Journal of Neuroradiology* **12**, 829–834.

Rinkel, G.J.E., Wijdicks, E.F.M., Vermeulen, M., Hasan, D., Brouwers, P.J.A.M. & van Gijn, J. (1991b) The clinical course of perimesencephalic nonaneurysmal subarachnoid hemorrhage. *Annals of Neurology* **29**, 463–468.

Rinkel, G.J.E., Wijdicks, E.F.M., Hasan, D. *et al.* (1991c) Outcome in patients with subarachnoid haemorrhage and negative angiography according to pattern of haemorrhage on computed tomography. *Lancet* **338**, 964–968.

Rinkel, G.J.E., Wijdicks, E.F.M., Vermeulen, M., Tans, J.T.J., Hasan, D. & van Gijn, J. (1992) Acute hydrocephalus in nonaneurysmal perimesencephalic hemorrhage: evidence of CSF block at the tentorial hiatus. *Neurology* **42**, 1805–1807.

Rinkel, G.J.E., van Gijn, J. & Wijdicks, E.F.M. (1993) Subarachnoid hemorrhage without detectable aneurysm: a review of the causes. *Stroke* **24**, 1403–1409.

Rinkel, G.J.E., Prins, N.E.M. & Algra, A. (1997) Outcome of aneurysmal subarachnoid hemorrhage in patients on anticoagulant treatment. *Stroke* **28**, 6–9.

Rinkel, G.J.E., Djibuti, M., Algra, A. & van Gijn, J. (1998) Prevalence and risk of rupture of intracranial aneurysms: a systematic review. *Stroke* **29**, 251–256.

River, Y., Honigman, S., Gomori, J.M. & Reches, A. (1994) Superficial hemosiderosis of the central nervous system. *Movement Disorders* **9**, 559–562.

Robinson, R.G. (1967) Coarctation of the aorta and cerebral aneurysm: report of two cases. *Journal of Neurosurgery* **26**, 527–531.

Rogg, J.M., Smeaton, S., Doberstein, C., Goldstein, J.H., Tung, G.A. & Haas, R.A. (1999) Assessment of the value of MR imaging for examining patients with angiographically negative subarachnoid hemorrhage. *American Journal of Roentgenology* **172**, 201–206.

Román, G., Fisher, M., Perl, D.P. & Poser, C.M. (1978) Neurological manifestations of hereditary hemorrhagic teleangiectasis (Rendu–Osler–Weber disease): report of two cases and review of the literature. *Annals of Neurology* **4**, 130–144.

Ronkainen, A., Hernesniemi, J. & Tromp, G. (1995a) Special features of familial intracranial aneurysms: report of 215 familial aneurysms. *Neurosurgery* **37**, 43–47.

Ronkainen, A., Puranen, M.I., Hernesniemi, J.A. *et al.* (1995b) Intracranial aneurysms: MR angiographic screening in 400 asymptomatic individuals with increased familial risk. *Radiology* **195**, 35–40.

Roos, Y.B.W.E.M., Hasan, D. & Vermeulen, M. (1995) Outcome in patients with large intraventricular haemorrhages: a volumetric study. *Journal of Neurology, Neurosurgery and Psychiatry* **58**, 622–624.

Rose, G. (1992) *The Strategy of Preventive Medicine*. Oxford University Press, Oxford.

Rosenblum, B., Oldfield, E.H., Doppman, J.L. & Di Chiro, G. (1987) Spinal arteriovenous malformations: a comparison of dural arteriovenous fistulas and intradural AVM's in 81 patients. *Journal of Neurosurgery* **67**, 795–802.

Ross, J.S., Masaryk, T.J., Modic, M.T., Ruggieri, P.M., Haacke, E.M. & Selman, W.R. (1990) Intracranial aneurysms: evaluation by MR angiography. *American Journal of Roentgenology* **155**, 159–165.

Rousseaux, P., Scherpereel, R., Bernard, M.H., Graftieaux, J.P. & Guyot, J.F. (1980) Fever and cerebral vasospasm in intracranial aneurysms. *Surgical Neurology* **14**, 459–465.

Ruelle, A., Lasio, G., Boccardo, M., Gottlieb, A. & Severi, P. (1985) Long-term prognosis of subarachnoid hemorrhages of unknown etiology. *Journal of Neurology* **232**, 277–279.

Ruelle, A., Cavazzani, P. & Andrioli, G. (1988) Extracranial posterior inferior cerebellar artery aneurysm causing isolated intraventricular hemorrhage: a case report. *Neurosurgery* **23**, 774–777.

van Rybroek, J.J. & Moore, S.A. (1990) Sudden death from choroid plexus vascular malformation hemorrhage: case report and review of the literature. *Clinical Neuropathology* **9**, 39–45.

Sadato, N., Numaguchi, Y., Rigamonti, D., Salcman, M., Gellad, F.E. & Kishikawa, T. (1991) Bleeding patterns in ruptured posterior fossa aneurysms: a CT study. *Journal of Computer Assisted Tomography* **15**, 612–617.

Sahjpaul, R.L., Abdulhak, M.M., Drake, C.G. & Hammond, R.R. (1998) Fatal traumatic vertebral artery aneurysm rupture: case report. *Journal of Neurosurgery* **89**, 822–824.

Saitoh, H., Hayakawa, K., Nishimura, K. *et al.* (1995) Rerupture of cerebral aneurysms during angiography. *American Journal of Neuroradiology* **16**, 539–542.

Sakas, D.E., Dias, L.S. & Beale, D. (1995) Subarachnoid haemorrhage presenting as head injury. *British Medical Journal* **310**, 1186–1187.

Salgado, A.V., Furlan, A.J. & Keys, T.F. (1987) Mycotic aneurysm, subarachnoid hemorrhage, and indications for cerebral angiography in infective endocarditis. *Stroke* **18**, 1057–1060.

Sandin, J.A. III, Salamat, M.S., Baskaya, M. & Dempsey, R.J. (1999) Intracerebral hemorrhage caused by the rupture of a nontraumatic middle meningeal artery aneurysm: case report and review of the literature. *Journal of Neurosurgery* **90**, 951–954.

Sarner, M. & Rose, F.C. (1967) Clinical presentation of ruptured intracranial aneurysm. *Journal of Neurology, Neurosurgery and Psychiatry* **30**, 67–70.

Sasaki, O., Ogawa, H., Koike, T., Koizumi, T. & Tanaka, R. (1991a) A clinicopathological study of dissecting aneurysms of the intracranial vertebral artery. *Journal of Neurosurgery* **75**, 874–882.

Sasaki, O., Koike, T., Tanaka, R. & Ogawa, H. (1991b) Subarachnoid hemorrhage from a dissecting aneurysm of the middle cerebral artery: case report. *Journal of Neurosurgery* **74**, 504–507.

Sasaki, T., Kodama, N. & Itokawa, H. (1996) Aneurysm formation and rupture at the site of anastomosis following bypass surgery. *Journal of Neurosurgery* **85**, 500–502.

Satoh, S. & Kadoya, S. (1988) Magnetic resonance imaging of subarachnoid hemorrhage. *Neuroradiology* **30**, 361–366.

Savader, S.J., Williams, G.M., Trerotola, S.O. *et al.* (1993) Preoperative spinal artery localization and its relationship to postoperative neurologic complications. *Radiology* **189**, 27–28.

Schievink, W.I. (1997) Genetics of intracranial aneurysms. *Neurosurgery* **40**, 651–662.

Schievink, W.I. & Wijdicks, E.F.M. (1997) Pretruncal subarachnoid hemorrhage: an anatomically correct description of the perimesencephalic subarachnoid hemorrhage. *Stroke* **28**, 2572.

Schievink, W.I., Limburg, M., Oorthuys, J.W., Fleury, P. & Pope, F.M. (1990) Cerebrovascular disease in Ehlers–Danlos syndrome type IV. *Stroke* **21**, 626–632.

Schievink, W.I., Wijdicks, E.F.M., Piepgras, D.G., Nichols, D.A. & Ebersold, M.J. (1994a) Perimesencephalic subarachnoid hemorrhage: additional perspectives from four cases. *Stroke* **25**, 1507–1511.

Schievink, W.I., Prakash, U.B., Piepgras, D.G. & Mokri, B. (1994b) Alpha 1-antitrypsin deficiency in intracranial aneurysms and cervical artery dissection. *Lancet* **343**, 452–453.

Schievink, W.I., Wijdicks, E.F.M., Meyer, F.B., Piepgras, D.G., Fode, N.C. & Whisnant, J.P. (1995) Seasons, snow, and subarachnoid hemorrhage: lack of association in Rochester, Minnesota. *Journal of Neurosurgery* **82**, 912–913.

Schievink, W.I., Katzmann, J.A., Piepgras, D.G. & Schaid, D.J. (1996a) Alpha-1-antitrypsin phenotypes among patients with intracranial aneurysms. *Journal of Neurosurgery* **84**, 781–784.

Schievink, W.I., Mellinger, J.F. & Atkinson, J.L.D. (1996b) Progressive intracranial aneurysmal disease in a child with progressive hemifacial atrophy (Parry–Romberg disease): case report. *Neurosurgery* **38**, 1237–1241.

Schievink, W.I., Mokri, B., Piepgras, D.G. & Gittenberger-de Groot, A.C. (1996c) Intracranial aneurysms and cervicocephalic arterial dissections associated with congenital heart disease. *Neurosurgery* **39**, 685–689.

Schievink, W.I., Parisi, J.E., Piepgras, D.G. & Michels, V.V. (1997a) Intracranial aneurysms in Marfan's syndrome: an autopsy study. *Neurosurgery* **41**, 866–870.

Schievink, W.I., Parisi, J.E. & Piepgras, D.G. (1997b) Familial intracranial aneurysms: an autopsy study. *Neurosurgery* **41**, 1247–1251.

Schmid, U.D., Steiger, H.J. & Huber, P. (1987) Accuracy of high resolution computed tomography in direct diagnosis of cerebral aneurysms. *Neuroradiology* **29**, 152–159.

Schmitt, H.P. (1983) Sportunfall oder natürlicher Tod? Haematocephalus internus durch Ruptur eines Plexus-chorioideus-Angioms [Sports accident or natural death? Hematocephalus internus caused by rupture of a choroid plexus angioma]. *Zeitschrift für Rechtsmedizin* **91**, 129–133.

Schulder, M., Hirano, A. & Elkin, C. (1987) 'Caval-septal' hematoma: does it exist? *Neurosurgery* **21**, 239–241.

Schwaighofer, B.W., Klein, M.V., Lyden, P.D. & Hesselink, J.R. (1990) MR imaging of vertebrobasilar vascular disease. *Journal of Computer Assisted Tomography* **14**, 895–904.

Schwartz, T.H. & Solomon, R.A. (1996) Perimesencephalic nonaneurysmal subarachnoid hemorrhage: review of the literature. *Neurosurgery* **39**, 433–440.

Scotti, G., Filizzolo, F., Scialfa, G., Tampieri, D. & Versari, P. (1987) Repeated subarachnoid hemorrhages from a cervical meningioma: case report. *Journal of Neurosurgery* **66**, 779–781.

Senter, H.J. & Sarwar, M. (1982) Nontraumatic dissecting aneurysm of the vertebral artery. *Journal of Neurosurgery* **56**, 128–130.

Shinoda, S., Murata, H., Waga, S. & Kojima, T. (1998) Bilateral spontaneous dissection of the posteroinferior cerebellar arteries: case report. *Neurosurgery* **43**, 357–359.

Silbert, P.L., Hankey, G.J., Prentice, D.A. & Apsimon, H.T. (1989) Angiographically demonstrated arterial spasm in a case of benign sexual headache and benign exertional headache. *Australian and New Zealand Journal of Medicine* **19**, 466–468.

Spallone, A., Ferrante, L., Palatinsky, E., Santoro, A. & Acqui, M. (1986) Subarachnoid haemorrhage of unknown origin. *Acta Neurochirurgica (Wien)* **80**, 12–17.

Spetzler, R.F., Winestock, D., Newton, H.T. & Boldrey, E.B. (1974) Disappearance and reappearance of cerebral aneurysm in serial arteriograms. Case report. *Journal of Neurosurgery* **41**, 508–510.

Spickler, E., Lufkin, R., Teresi, L. *et al.* (1990) MR imaging of acute subarachnoid hemorrhage. *Computerized Medical Imaging and Graphics* **14**, 67–77.

Stehbens, W.E. (1982) Intracranial berry aneurysms in infancy. *Surgical Neurology* **18**, 58–60.

Stehbens, W.E. (1989) Etiology of intracranial berry aneurysms. *Journal of Neurosurgery* **70**, 823–831.

Steinberg, G.K., Guppy, K.H., Adler, J.R. & Silverberg, G.D. (1992) Stereotactic, angiography-guided clipping of a distal, mycotic intracranial aneurysm using the Cosman-Roberts-Wells system: technical note. *Neurosurgery* **30**, 408–411.

Stone, J.L., Crowell, R.M., Gandhi, Y.N. & Jafar, J.J. (1988) Multiple intracranial aneurysms: magnetic resonance imaging for determination of the site of rupture: report of a case. *Neurosurgery* **23**, 97–100.

Sturzenegger, M. & Huber, P. (1993) Cranial nerve palsies in spontaneous carotid artery dissection. *Journal of Neurology, Neurosurgery and Psychiatry* **56**, 1191–1199.

Suzuki, S., Kayama, T., Sakurai, Y., Ogawa, A. & Suzuki, J. (1987) Subarachnoid hemorrhage of unknown cause. *Neurosurgery* **21**, 310–313.

Swann, K.W., Ropper, A.H., New, P.F. & Poletti, C.E. (1984) Spontaneous spinal subarachnoid hemorrhage and subdural hematoma: report of two cases. *Journal of Neurosurgery* **61**, 975–980.

Swash, M. (1974) Periaqueductal dysfunction (the Sylvian aqueduct syndrome): a sign of hydrocephalus? *Journal of Neurology, Neurosurgery and Psychiatry* **37**, 21–26.

Takenaka, K., Sakai, H., Yamakawa, H. *et al.* (1999) Polymorphism of the *endoglin* gene in patients with intracranial saccular aneurysms. *Journal of Neurosurgery* **90**, 935–938.

Takenaka, N., Mine, T., Suga, S. *et al.* (1990) Interpeduncular high-density spot in severe shearing injury. *Surgical Neurology* **34**, 30–38.

Tatter, S.B., Buonanno, F.S. & Ogilvy, C.S. (1995) Acute lacunar stroke in association with angiogram-negative subarachnoid hemorrhage: mechanistic implications of two cases. *Stroke* **26**, 891–895.

Teasdale, E., Statham, P., Straiton, J. & Macpherson, P. (1990) Non-invasive radiological investigation for oculomotor palsy. *Journal of Neurology, Neurosurgery and Psychiatry* **53**, 549–553.

Teunissen, L.L., Rinkel, G.J.E., Algra, A. & van Gijn, J. (1996) Risk factors for subarachnoid hemorrhage: a systematic review. *Stroke* **27**, 544–549.

Tokuda, Y., Inagawa, T., Takechi, A. & Inokuchi, F. (1998) Ruptured de novo aneurysm induced by ethyl 2-cyanoacrylate: case report. *Neurosurgery* **43**, 626–628.

Tolias, C.M. & Choksey, M.S. (1996) Will increased awareness among physicians of the significance of sudden agonizing headache affect the outcome of subarachnoid hemorrhage? Coventry and Warwickshire Study: audit of subarachnoid hemorrhage (Establishing historical controls), hypothesis, campaign layout, and cost estimation. *Stroke* **27**, 807–812.

Tomlinson, B.E. & Walton, J.N. (1964) Superficial haemosiderosis of the central nervous system. *Journal of Neurology, Neurosurgery and Psychiatry* **27**, 332–339.

Tsubota, A., Shishiba, Y., Shimizu, T., Ozawa, Y., Sawano, S. & Yamada, S. (1991) Masked Cushing's disease in an aged man associated with intraventricular hemorrhage and tuberculous peritonitis. *Japanese Journal of Medicine* **30**, 233–237.

Uchino, A., Aibe, H., Itoh, H., Aiko, Y. & Tanaka, M. (1997) Superficial siderosis of the central nervous system: its MRI manifestations. *Clinical Imaging* **21**, 241–245.

Ujiie, H., Tachibana, H., Hiramatsu, O. *et al.* (1999) Effects of size and shape (aspect ratio) on the hemodynamics of saccular aneurysms: a possible index for surgical treatment of intracranial aneurysms. *Neurosurgery* **45**, 119–129.

Van Calenbergh, F., Plets, C., Goffin, J. & Velghe, L. (1993) Nonaneurysmal subarachnoid hemorrhage: prevalence of perimesencephalic hemorrhage in a consecutive series. *Surgical Neurology* **39**, 320–323.

Van den Berg, J.S.P., Limburg, M. & Hennekam, R.C.M. (1996) Is Marfan syndrome associated with symptomatic intracranial aneurysms. *Stroke* **27**, 10–12.

Van den Berg, J.S.P., Limburg, M., Pals, G. *et al.* (1997) Some patients with intracranial aneurysms have a reduced type III type I collagen ratio: a case-control study. *Neurology* **49**, 1546–1551.

Van der Jagt, M., Hasan, D., Bijvoet, H.W.C. *et al.* (1999) Validity of prediction of the site of ruptured intracranial aneurysms with CT. *Neurology* **52**, 34–39.

Van der Meulen, J.H.P., Weststrate, W., van Gijn, J. & Habbema, J.D. (1992) Is cerebral angiography indicated in infective endocarditis? *Stroke* **23**, 1662–1667.

Van der Meulen, M.F.G., Rinkel, G.J.E., Witkamp, T.D. & van Gijn, J. (1999) A man with progressive weakness in his legs. *Lancet* **354**, 830.

Velthuis, B.K., Rinkel, G.J.E., Ramos, L.M.P. *et al.* (1998) Subarachnoid hemorrhage: aneurysm detection and preoperative evaluation with CT angiography. *Radiology* **208**, 423–430.

Velthuis, B.K., Rinkel, G.J.E., Ramos, L.M.P., Witkamp, T.D. & Van Leeuwen, M.S. (1999) Perimesencephalic hemorrhage: exclusion of vertebrobasilar aneurysms with CT angiography. *Stroke* **30**, 1103–1109.

Verma, A., Maheshwari, M.C. & Bhargava, S. (1987) Spontaneous intraventricular haemorrhage. *Journal of Neurology* **234**, 233–236.

Vermeer, S.E., Rinkel, G.J.E. & Algra, A. (1997) Circadian fluctuations in onset of subarachnoid hemorrhage: new data on aneurysmal and perimesencephalic hemorrhage and a systematic review. *Stroke* **28**, 805–808.

Vermeulen, M., van Gijn, J. & Blijenberg, B.G. (1983) Spectrophotometric analysis of CSF after subarachnoid hemorrhage: limitations in the diagnosis of rebleeding. *Neurology* **33**, 112–115.

Vermeulen, M., Lindsay, K.W., Murray, G.D. *et al.*(1984) Antifibrinolytic treatment in subarachnoid hemorrhage. *New England Journal of Medicine* **311**, 432–437.

Vermeulen, M., Hasan, D., Blijenberg, B.G., Hijdra, A. & van Gijn, J. (1989) Xanthochromia after subarachnoid haemorrhage needs no revisitation. *Journal of Neurology, Neurosurgery and Psychiatry* **52**, 826–828.

Vermeulen, M., Lindsay, K.W. & van Gijn, J. (1992) *Subarachnoid Haemorrhage*. W.B. Saunders, London.

Verweij, R.D., Wijdicks, E.F.M. & van Gijn, J. (1988) Warning headache in aneurysmal subarachnoid hemorrhage. A case–control study. *Archives of Neurology* **45**, 1019–1020.

Vincent, F.M. & Zimmerman, J.E. (1980) Superior cerebellar artery aneurysm presenting as an oculomotor nerve palsy in a child. *Neurosurgery* **6**, 661–664.

Vincent, F.M., Zimmerman, J.E., Auer, T.C. & Martin, D.B. (1980) Subarachnoid hemorrhage: the initial manifestation of bacterial endocarditis: report of a case with negative arteriography and computed tomography. *Neurosurgery* **7**, 488–490.

Waga, S., Shimosaka, S. & Kojima, T. (1985) Arteriovenous malformations of the lateral ventricle. *Journal of Neurosurgery* **63**, 185–192.

Walker, A.E. & Allegre, G.W. (1954) The pathology and pathogenesis of cerebral aneurysms. *Journal of Neuropathology and Experimental Neurology* **13**, 248–259.

Wardlaw, J.M. & Cannon, J.C. (1996) Color transcranial 'power' Doppler ultrasound of intracranial aneurysms. *Journal of Neurosurgery* **84**, 459–461.

Wardlaw, J.M. & White, P.M. (2000) The detection and management of unruptured intracranial aneurysms. *Brain* **123**, 205–221.

Wardlaw, J.M., Cannon, J., Statham, P.F.X. & Price, R. (1998) Does the size of intracranial aneurysms change with intracranial pressure? Observations based on color 'power' transcranial Doppler ultrasound. *Journal of Neurosurgery* **88**, 846–850.

van der Wee, N., Rinkel, G.J.E., Hasan, D. & van Gijn, J. (1995) Detection of subarachnoid haemorrhage on early CT: is lumbar puncture still needed after a negative scan? *Journal of Neurology, Neurosurgery and Psychiatry* **58**, 357–359.

Weir, B., Myles, T., Kahn, M. *et al.* (1984) Management of acute subdural hematomas from aneurysmal rupture. *Canadian Journal of Neurological Sciences* **11**, 371–376.

Weir, B.K.A., Kongable, G.L., Kassell, N.F., Schultz, J.R., Truskowski, L.L. & Sigrest, A. (1998) Cigarette smoking as a cause of aneurysmal subarachnoid hemorrhage and risk for vasospasm: a report of the Cooperative Aneurysm Study. *Journal of Neurosurgery* **89**, 405–411.

Weisberg, L.A., Elliott, D. & Shamsnia, M. (1991) Intraventricular hemorrhage in adults: clinical–computed tomographic correlations. *Computerized Medical Imaging and Graphics* **15**, 43–51.

Whisnant, J.P., Sacco, S.E., O'Fallon, W.M., Fode, N.C. & Sundt, T.M. Jr (1993) Referral bias in aneurysmal subarachnoid hemorrhage. *Journal of Neurosurgery* **78**, 726–732.

Wijdicks, E.F.M. & Schievink, W.I. (1997) Perimesencephalic nonaneurysmal subarachnoid hemorrhage: first hint of a cause? *Neurology* **49**, 634–636.

Wijdicks, E.F.M., Kerkhoff, H. & van Gijn, J. (1988) Long-term follow-up of 71 patients with thunderclap headache mimicking subarachnoid haemorrhage. *Lancet* **2**, 68–70.

Williams, J.P., Joslyn, J.N., White, J.L. & Dean, D.F. (1983) Subdural hematoma secondary to ruptured intracranial aneurysm: computed tomographic diagnosis. *Journal of Computed Tomography* **7**, 142–153.

Willinsky, R.A., Terbrugge, K., Lasjaunias, P. & Montanera, W. (1990) The variable presentations of craniocervical and cervical dural arteriovenous malformations. *Surgical Neurology* **34**, 118–123.

Woimant, F. & Spelle, L. (1995) Spontaneous basilar artery dissection: contribution of magnetic resonance imaging to diagnosis. *Journal of Neurology, Neurosurgery and Psychiatry* **58**, 540.

Wojak, J.C. & Flamm, E.S. (1987) Intracranial hemorrhage and cocaine use. *Stroke* **18**, 712–715.

Wong, C.W. & Ho, Y.S. (1994) Intraventricular haemorrhage and hydrocephalus caused by intraventricular parasitic granuloma suggesting cerebral sparganosis. *Acta Neurochirurgica (Wien)* **129**, 205–208.

Wright, C.J.E. (1949) Coarctation of the aorta with death from rupture of a cerebral aneurysm. *Archives of Pathology* **48**, 382–386.

Yamaura, A., Watanabe, Y. & Saeki, N. (1990) Dissecting aneurysms of the intracranial vertebral artery. *Journal of Neurosurgery* **72**, 183–188.

Yasui, T., Sakamoto, H., Kishi, H. *et al.* (1998) Bilateral dissecting aneurysms of the vertebral arteries resulting in subarachnoid hemorrhage: case report. *Neurosurgery* **42**, 162–164.

Yasui, T., Komiyama, M., Nishkawa, M., Nakajima, H., Kobayashi, Y. & Inoue, T. (1999) Fusiform vertebral artery aneurysms as a cause of dissecting aneurysms: report of two autopsy cases and a review of the literature. *Journal of Neurosurgery* **91**, 139–144.

Yasui, T., Komiyama, M., Nishikawa, M. & Nakajima, H. (2000) Subarachnoid hemorrhage from vertebral artery dissecting aneurysms involving the origin of the posteroinferior cerebellar artery: report of two cases and review of the literature. *Neurosurgery* **46**, 196–200.

Yeh, H.S., Tomsick, T.A. & Tew, J.M. Jr (1985) Intraventricular hemorrhage due to aneurysms of the distal posterior inferior cerebellar artery: report of three cases. *Journal of Neurosurgery* **62**, 772–775.

Yonemitsu, T., Niizuma, H., Kodama, N., Fujiwara, S. & Suzuki, J. (1983) Acoustic neurinoma presenting as subarachnoid hemorrhage. *Surgical Neurology* **20**, 125–130.

Young, R.C., Bennett, J.E., Vogel, C.L., Carbone, P.P. & DeVita, V.T. (1970) Aspergillosis: the spectrum of the disease in 98 patients. *Medicine (Baltimore)* **49**, 147–173.

Young, W.B., Lee, K.P., Pessin, M.S., Kwan, E.S., Rand, W.M. & Caplan, L.R. (1990) Prognostic significance of ventricular blood in supratentorial hemorrhage: a volumetric study. *Neurology* **40**, 616–619.

Zentner, J., Solymosi, L. & Lorenz, M. (1996) Subarachnoid hemorrhage of unknown etiology. *Neurological Research* **18**, 220–226.

Zhang, Q.J., Kobayashi, S., Gibo, H. & Hongo, K. (1994) Vertebrobasilar junction fenestration associated with dissecting aneurysm of intracranial vertebral artery. *Stroke* **25**, 1273–1275.

CHAPTER TEN

A practical approach to the management of stroke patients

This chapter introduces the general principles of treating patients with stroke. Because treatment is aimed at improving the patient's outcome, the chapter includes a section on the prognosis of stroke and the factors that may help predict the progress of individual patients. It also introduces a model for treating patients that avoids the pitfalls of the traditional approach, which splits treatment artificially into acute care, rehabilitation and continuing care.

10.1 Aims of treatment

The aims of treatment can be summarized as optimizing the patient's chance of surviving and minimizing the impact of the stroke on the patient and carers. In minimizing the impact of the stroke, one has to think not just about the short-term effects of the stroke on the patient's neurological impairments, but also about its effect on the patient's function (i.e. disability) and role in society (i.e. handicap). Therefore, it is useful to consider the consequences of a stroke in terms of the World Health Organization (WHO) International Classification of Impairments, Disabilities and Handicaps (ICIDH) (WHO 1980). A recent revision of this classification has substituted some new terms (in brackets below) for old ones to emphasize positive aspects (i.e. activity, not disability; participation, not handicap) and highlights the important 'contextual' factors—e.g. personal experiences, physical and social environment—that influence the impact of disease, at each level, on the individual (Duncan *et al.* 2000). The WHO ICIDH divides the consequences of disease into four levels.

Pathology: the underlying pathological substrate of the stroke, e.g. cerebral infarction due to embolic occlusion of a middle cerebral artery from thrombus in the left atrium, resulting from atrial fibrillation due to ischaemic heart disease. Specific medical and surgical treatments (e.g. thrombolytic or neuroprotective drugs) are directed at this level of the disease process (Chapters 11–14).

Impairment: any loss or abnormality of specific psychological, physiological, or anatomical structure or function (e.g. muscle weakness or spasticity, loss of sensation, aphasia) caused by the stroke. Physical therapies, such as physiotherapy or electromyographic biofeedback, are directed at this level (section 15.21).

Disability (activity): any restriction or lack (resulting from an impairment) of ability to perform an activity in the manner or within the range considered normal for a human being (e.g. inability to walk, wash, feed, etc.) due to the stroke. Physical therapies are also used to try to reduce the disability related to impairments.

Handicap (participation): the disadvantage for a given individual, resulting from an impairment or disability, that limits or prevents the fulfilment of a role (depending on age, sex, social and cultural factors) for that individual—e.g. inability to continue the same job. Although more difficult to define and measure than the other levels of disease, handicap is probably the level that best reflects the patient's and carer's perspective. Many aspects of treatment will impact on handicap, but occupational therapy and social work are those most obviously aimed at influencing this level.

Although not included in the WHO ICIDH classification, *quality of life* is obviously an important aspect of a patient's outcome. However, there is no generally accepted definition of quality of life, and it is therefore not surprising that it is difficult to measure (section 17.6.3).

The consequences of a stroke must be considered at five levels: pathology, impairment, disability, handicap and quality of life.

The most obvious effects of a stroke are physical, but in some situations these may not be as important as the cognitive, psychological, social and even financial consequences. Thus, treatment that aims to minimize the impact of a stroke on patients and their carers must be directed at all of these various problems.

10.1.1 Aspects of treatment

Each patient has a unique blend of pathologies, impairments, disabilities and handicaps. Therefore it follows that treatment must be preceded by a comprehensive assessment and should then be tailored to that individual patient. Traditionally, the discussion of the treatment of stroke is split into sections on: general treatment in the acute phase; acute medical and surgical treatments; rehabilitation; and continuing care. However, this structure does not reflect the need for an integrated approach to the management of the patient. For example, patients may develop acute problems (e.g. pneumonia, pulmonary embolism or urinary tract infection) at any stage in their illness, quite often during what is commonly called rehabilitation (Dromerick & Reding 1994; Kalra *et al.* 1995; Davenport *et al.* 1996; Langhorne *et al.* 2000). Conversely, certain aspects of rehabilitation, such as team work and early mobilization, are just as important on the day of the stroke as they are later on.

The term 'rehabilitation' seems to mean different things to different people. Unfortunately, to many physicians who are responsible for the care of stroke patients, the term is synonymous with physical therapy (e.g. physiotherapy, occupational therapy, and speech and language therapy). Having referred the patient to one or more therapists, a physician then mistakenly believes that 'rehabilitation' has been organized. This is far too simplistic. Although there is no universally accepted definition of rehabilitation, most people would view it as a 'goal-orientated' process aimed at minimizing the functional consequences of the stroke, minimizing the impact of the stroke on the lives of the patient and any carers, and maximizing their autonomy. If we include in our definition *all* those components of care that have these aims, it is apparent that rehabilitation must embrace most aspects of care, ranging from the acute medical treatment through to making alterations to the patient's home prior to discharge and providing support later on. Achieving the best possible outcome for the patient requires a broad approach rather than one that just focuses on the primary lesion or just on the resulting impairments.

Rehabilitation is not synonymous with physical therapies such as physiotherapy or occupational therapy—it is a far more complex process.

When the problem is thought of in this way, it becomes artificial—and perhaps even harmful—to separate stroke management into acute care, rehabilitation and continuing care. To compound the problem, these separate components of care may even be provided by different staff in different institutions, which leads to a breakdown in communication and lack of continuity of care. Often, in this modular system of care, one encounters the patient who is 'waiting for rehabilitation', i.e. the patient in the department that normally deals with acute stroke patients for whom there is no immediate place in the rehabilitation facility and who is not progressing. Conversely, one comes across patients in a 'rehabilitation setting' who have developed acute medical problems (e.g. epilepsy or chest pain) and who are denied quick access to the necessary facilities or expertise to ensure optimum management of the problems.

We have therefore abandoned the divisions of treatment into 'acute', 'rehabilitation', etc., and will present an integrated, problem- and goal-orientated approach to optimizing recovery, which we believe overcomes the disadvantages of the traditional approach.

We should abandon the arbitrary division of treatment into acute and rehabilitation phases and adopt an integrated, problem- and goal-orientated approach.

10.1.2 An integrated, problem-orientated and goal-orientated approach

The patient's general management—as distinct from the specific treatment of the stroke pathology (Chapters 11–14)—is primarily aimed at anticipating and preventing potential problems and solving existing ones that are identified at various stages of the illness. One can think of management in terms of many interwoven cycles or loops (Fig. 10.1). The assessment of a problem, or potential problem, includes not only detecting and perhaps measuring it, but also consid-

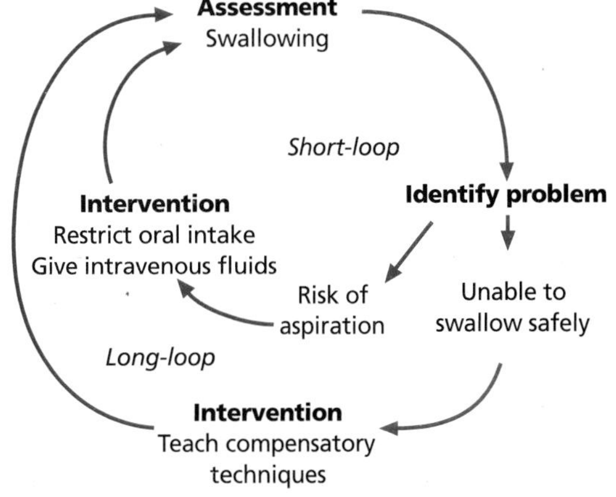

Fig. 10.1 'Short-loop' and 'long-loop' problems.

ering its likely cause and prognosis. This assessment may often have to include the patient's or carer's expectations or wishes (section 10.3.4). Furthermore, we have to remember that assessment is not just a 'once only' activity, but one that should be repeated throughout the illness so that management is tailored to the patient's changing needs.

For some problems, this cycle can be completed in a few minutes (e.g. an obstructed airway is a short-loop problem), whilst for others, the cycle might take weeks to complete (e.g. depression is a long-loop problem). Quite often a problem such as dysphagia will demand both an immediate intervention—e.g. stopping oral intake and giving fluids and perhaps nutrition by an alternative route—and longer-term interventions, such as providing retraining to compensate for swallowing impairment (sections 15.17 and 15.19). Thus, in reality, the general management involves many such cycles layered on top of each other and cycling at different rates, with each having some influence on the others. This model of management applies equally well to acute general care, rehabilitation and continuing care.

10.1.3 A guide to the following sections on management

We have tried to reflect our integrated approach in the structure of the following discussion on management, which is divided into several sections.

What is this patient's prognosis? Section 10.2 deals with the prognosis of stroke with respect to survival and function in groups of patients, and in individual patients. After all, our efforts are aimed at improving the patient's prognosis.

Delivering an integrated management plan: section 10.3 deals with general assessment of the patient, the role of the stroke team and its members, and problem-orientated and goal-orientated care.

Some difficult ethical dilemmas: in section 10.4, we discuss some of the ethical dilemmas that arise in treating stroke patients.

Specific medical and surgical treatments in the acute phase: Chapters 11–14 deal with the pathophysiology of acute stroke and the drug and surgical treatments that aim to reduce the severity of brain injury.

What are the patient's problems? A problem-orientated approach to management: Chapter 15 deals with the problems that may occur after stroke, their assessment, and interventions that may help to prevent or solve these problems.

Preventing recurrent stroke and other serious vascular events: Chapter 16 completes the description of the prognosis of stroke by focusing on the risks of further stroke and other serious vascular events, before moving on to describe various strategies to reduce these risks.

Organizing stroke services: Chapter 17 focuses on the organizational issues that are important when trying to deliver all these various aspects of treatment to large numbers of stroke patients as efficiently and equitably as possible.

10.2 What is this patient's prognosis?

10.2.1 Introduction

It is useful to predict the outcome of individual patients, because this may enable one to:

• have more informed discussions with the patient and/or their carers;

• set more accurate short-term and long-term goals (section 10.3.3);

• weigh the potential risks and benefits of treatment options. For example, one might reserve a particularly hazardous but nevertheless effective treatment for patients in whom the prognosis is poor;

• plan treatment and make early decisions about later discharge and long-term placement to optimize the efficiency of the service;

• make rationing decisions where resources are limited. Thus, if a particular patient is very unlikely to make a good recovery, one could divert resources from that patient to another with a better prognosis who may gain more from the interventions available. It is also wasteful to use resources on patients who will make a good recovery without any intervention at all. Of course, by adopting this approach, one must avoid self-fulfilling prophecies—i.e. if one withdraws treatment from a patient, he or she may do badly because of the lack of input.

Before considering how to predict an *individual's* prognosis, we shall describe the prognosis of the 'average' patient, i.e. the outcome of an unselected cohort of stroke patients. Here, the prognosis with respect to survival and overall functional outcome is described, since this is relevant to all aspects of treatment. The prognosis for particular individual impairments, disabilities and handicaps is dealt with in the appropriate sections of Chapter 15, whilst that relating to the risk of late death, recurrent stroke and other vascular events is dealt with in Chapter 16. The prognosis of subarachnoid haemorrhage is described in detail in Chapter 13.

10.2.2 Collecting reliable information about prognosis

If information concerning the prognosis of stroke is to be useful, it must have been collected using sound methods that minimize bias and maximize precision, accuracy and generalizability (Table 10.1).

Prognosis or natural history?

It is important to distinguish these two terms. Natural history refers to the *untreated* course of an illness from its onset,

Table 10.1 Methodological features that are important in assessing a study of prognosis after stroke (from Sackett *et al.* 1991).

Were the patients identified at an early and uniform point in the course of their disease, and were diagnostic criteria, disease severity, co-morbidity and demographic details for inclusion clearly specified?
If they were, then this is called an 'inception cohort'. When applying data from a study of prognosis, it is important to consider whether the patients studied were similar to one's own patients.

Was the referral pattern described?
Did the study avoid the following:
(a) 'Referral filter bias', which occurs when an inception cohort is assembled on selected cases that are not representative of all cases occurring in the population. This is a particular problem with specialist centres, which attract unusual cases (centripetal bias) or admit or track interesting cases (popularity bias).
(b) 'Diagnostic access bias', which occurs if cases are defined by technology (e.g. intracerebral haemorrhage by brain computed tomography), but the patient's access to the technology is influenced by factors such as their wealth, which may affect their outcome.

Was complete follow-up achieved?
Were all patients who were entered into the study accounted for, and was their clinical status known at the final follow-up? Patients who are lost to follow-up may be systematically different from those who are not. For example, patients with a good recovery may be more mobile or at work and therefore more difficult to follow up, whilst patients may not be followed up because they have died. Therefore, the effect of incomplete follow-up on prognosis is difficult to predict.

Were objective outcome criteria developed and used, and were the criteria reproducible and accurate?
To make sense of prognostic data, it is important to know what the authors meant by terms such as 'recurrent stroke' or 'independent', so that one can apply the data to one's own patients. It is also important that the criteria should be applied consistently.

Was outcome assessment blind?
In other words, were diagnostic suspicion bias and expectation bias avoided in the assessment of patient outcomes? If the observer has a preconceived view that a particular baseline factor is likely to be related to a particular outcome, knowledge of the presence or absence of that factor at the time of follow-up may bias that observer.

Was adjustment for extraneous prognostic factors carried out?
Where authors relate certain baseline factors to the likelihood of specific outcomes, it is important that they should allow for other baseline factors. The most common example of this is age, which partly explains the observed relationships between other factors, e.g. atrial fibrillation and early death. Before applying predictive equations to one's own patients, it is important for the equation to have been tested on an independent test cohort other than the one from which it was developed.

Was the study prospective or retrospective?
In general, prospective studies provide more reliable data than retrospective ones, because cases and events during the follow-up can be defined using strict criteria, complete data are more likely to be available, and they are less prone to biases.

whilst prognosis refers to the probability of a particular outcome occurring either in an individual or a group of patients over a defined period of time after the disease is first identified. The prognosis is likely to be influenced by the severity of illness and any treatment given. Usually, but not always, the prognosis with treatment is better than the natural history, but it may be worse. This section describes the *prognosis* of stroke. No data on the natural history (strictly defined) are available, because even in developing countries, patients with stroke are usually given some treatment, and in those places where minimal or no treatment is given, no studies of prognosis have been reported. Admission to hospital, even without any medical or physical therapy, could be regarded as 'treatment', and may influence outcome.

Sources of prognostic data

No published study of prognosis after stroke fulfils all the criteria summarized in Table 10.1. We have used data from the Oxfordshire Community Stroke Project (OCSP) because it meets, at least partly, most of these criteria (Bamford *et al.* 1987, 1988, 1990a,b, 1991; Dennis *et al.* 1993). Other methodologically sound studies come to broadly similar conclusions, although to compare them directly is difficult because of their different methods, their varying styles of reporting, and because much of the variation in prognosis can be accounted for by differences in casemix and by the play of chance as a result of relatively small sample sizes (Sacco *et al.* 1982; Garraway *et al.* 1983; Turney *et al.* 1984; Kojima *et al.* 1990; Anderson *et al.* 1994) (section 17.6.3). All these studies included predominantly white patients managed in quite well-organized health-care systems during the 1980s—so one must be careful in extrapolating the results to other ethnic groups being cared for in different environments in the early 21st century. There is some evidence that the prognosis of stroke may be improving over time in some populations, although it is unclear whether this is due to improved health of the population, changing severity of stroke, improved treatment, or methodological factors such as improved detection of less severe strokes (Bonita *et al.* 1993; Peltonnen *et al.* 1999) (section 18.2.1).

10.2.3 Prognosis for death

The risk of dying within the first 7 days or within the first 30 days after a first-ever-in-a-lifetime stroke is about 12% and 19%, respectively (Table 10.2). Surprisingly, in the OCSP, the risk of death within 30 days of a second stroke was not significantly greater. However, only small numbers of second strokes occurred, so the confidence intervals around these estimates are wide, and real differences cannot be ruled out (Burn *et al.* 1994). The risk of dying in the years after a stroke remains elevated compared with that in stroke-free individuals (Gresham *et al.* 1998) (Fig. 10.2). Patients with haemorrhagic stroke, either primary intracerebral or subarachnoid, have a much higher early risk of dying than those with ischaemic stroke. Patients with *major* ischaemic strokes, i.e. total anterior circulation infarction (section 4.3.4), also have a very high early risk of death (Fig. 10.3; Table 10.2).

Causes of death

Knowing the causes of these early deaths is important if one is interested in reducing them (Fig. 10.4). In the first few days after stroke, most patients who die do so as a result of the direct effects of the brain damage (Bounds *et al.* 1981; Silver *et al.* 1984; Bamford *et al.* 1990b). In brainstem strokes, the respiratory centre may be affected by the stroke itself, whilst in supratentorial ischaemic or haemorrhagic stroke, dysfunction of the brainstem results from displacement and herniation of oedematous supratentorial brain tissue (Figs 11.14 and 11.15). Deaths occurring within an hour or two of onset are very unusual in ischaemic stroke, because it takes time for cerebral oedema to develop. Almost all such very early deaths after stroke result from intracranial haemorrhage of some sort (Bamford *et al.* 1990a). Some sudden deaths are probably due to co-existing cardiac pathology, or perhaps very rarely cardiac complications of the stroke (section 15.2.3).

Death within a few hours of stroke onset can occur with intracerebral or subarachnoid haemorrhage, or rarely with massive brainstem infarction.

Having survived the first few days, patients may then develop various potentially fatal complications of immobility, the most common being pneumonia (section 15.12) and pulmonary embolism (section 15.13). In addition, pressure sores (section 15.16), dehydration (section 15.18.1) with renal failure, and urinary tract infection (section 15.12) may cause death where basic care is lacking. Because some strokes occur in the context of other serious conditions, e.g. myocardial infarction (section 7.10), cardiac failure (section 6.5) and cancer (section 7.12), some early deaths can, at least in part,

		Case fatality (%)			
Type of stroke	*n*	7 days	30 days	6 months	1 year
All strokes	675	12	19	27	31
Subarachnoid haemorrhage	33	27	46	48	48
Primary intracerebral haemorrhage	66	40	50	58	62
All ischaemic stroke	545	5	10	18	23
Total anterior circulation infarction	92	17	39	57	60
Partial anterior circulation infarction	186	2	4	11	16
Lacunar infarction	138	2	2	7	11
Posterior circulation infarction	129	5	7	14	19

Table 10.2 Death after different pathological types of first-ever-in-a-lifetime stroke. Data from the Oxfordshire Community Stroke Project.

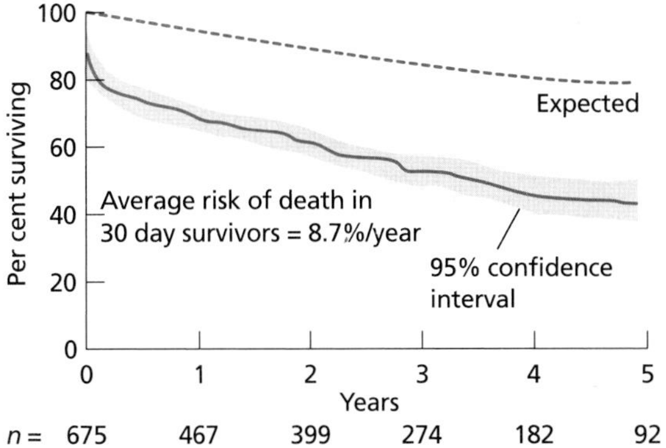

Fig. 10.2 A Kaplan–Meier plot, showing the proportion of patients surviving at increasing intervals after a first-ever-in-a-lifetime stroke compared with the expected survival of people of the same age and sex who have not had a stroke. Data from the Oxfordshire Community Stroke Project. The expected survival was derived from all-cause mortality rates for Oxfordshire (1985) (with permission from Dennis *et al.* 1993).

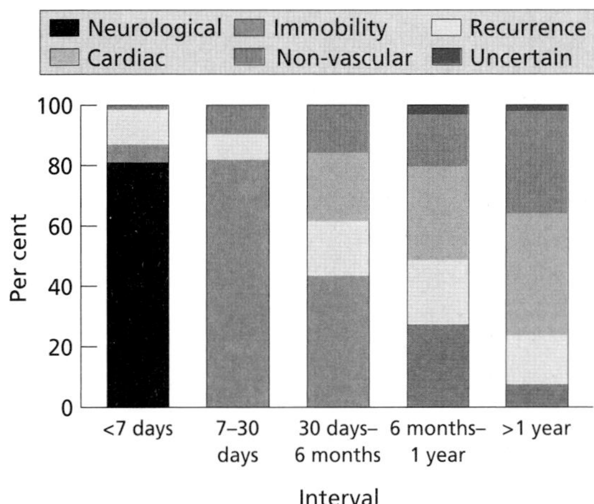

Fig. 10.4 Histogram showing the proportion of patients dying from different causes at increasing intervals after a first-ever-in-a-lifetime stroke (from Bamford *et al.* 1990b; Dennis *et al.* 1993).

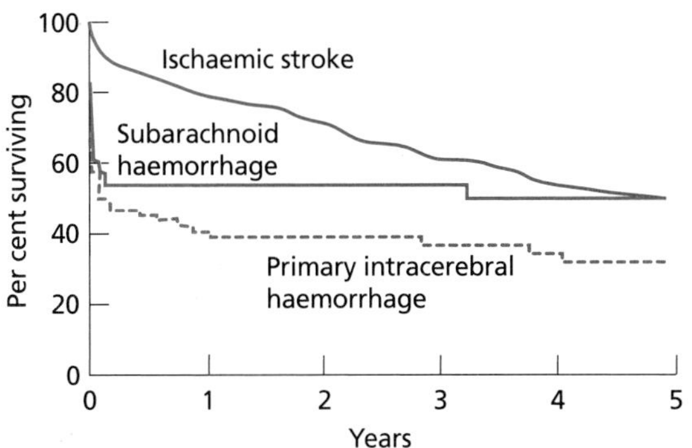

Fig. 10.3 A Kaplan–Meier plot, showing the proportion of patients surviving after a first-ever-in-a-lifetime ischaemic stroke ($n = 545$), primary intracerebral haemorrhage ($n = 66$) and subarachnoid haemorrhage ($n = 33$) (with permission from Dennis *et al.* 1993).

be attributed to these underlying problems. Also, because the risk of stroke recurrence is highest early after the first stroke—about 13% in the first year (section 16.1)—some patients will die from the direct or indirect effects of a recurrent stroke (Burn *et al.* 1994). This is most common in patients with aneurysmal subarachnoid haemorrhage (section 13.5), in whom the recurrence or re-bleed rate is about 30% (without intervention), accounting for the majority of deaths (50% of the total) in the first 30 days (van Gijn 1992). After subarachnoid haemorrhage, clinical worsening frequently results from cerebral ischaemia or obstructive hydrocephalus (sections 13.6 and 13.9).

10.2.4 Prognosis for dependency

Stroke often leaves surviving patients with neurological impairments that prevent them from performing everyday activities and thus make them dependent on others. Figures 10.5 and 10.6 show the proportions of survivors who are independent and dependent in everyday activities at various times after a first-ever-in-a-lifetime stroke and in strokes of different pathologies and clinical subtypes. Other studies have produced similar data (Dombovy *et al.* 1987). It is likely that a greater proportion of patients will become dependent after recurrent strokes. Details of the prognosis with respect to particular impairments, disabilities and handicaps will be discussed in the specific sections dealing with their treatment (Chapter 15), but it is relevant here to discuss the general pattern of recovery after stroke.

10.2.5 Patterns of recovery

Patients who survive an acute stroke almost always improve to a greater or lesser extent. Improvement is reflected not just in a reduction in the neurological impairments but also in any resulting disability and handicap. Various factors have been postulated to explain recovery. In the first few days after a stroke, ischaemic neurones that were not irreversibly damaged during the primary event (i.e those in the ischaemic penumbra), may start to function because of improved blood supply, reversal of metabolic problems, or reduction of cerebral oedema (section 11.1). Resolution of diaschisis (section 5.3.11) is an alternative explanation for early recovery, although this mechanism has not been well established (Seitz *et al.* 1999). Neuroplasticity—the process by which other intact areas of the brain can take over some of the functions of those that have been irreversibly damaged—might explain some of the later improvement (Cohen *et al.* 1998; Weiller 1998; Witte 1998) (Fig. 10.7; see colour plate facing page 84). However, much of the later recovery with respect to disability and handicap is probably due to adaptive changes—i.e. patients learn

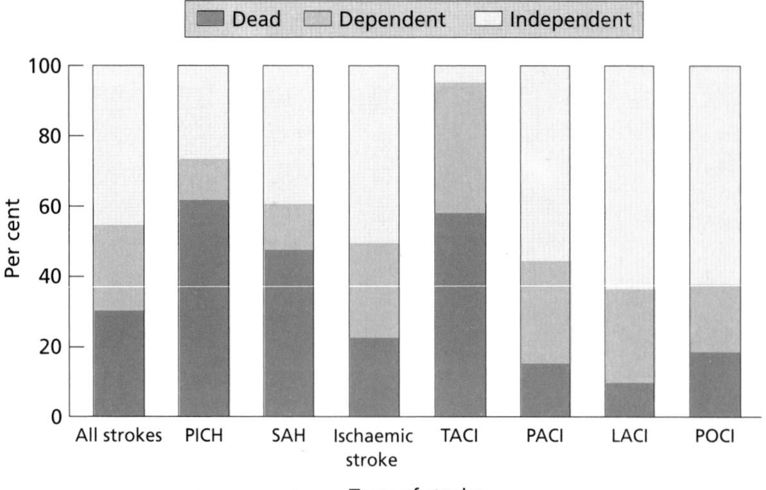

Fig. 10.5 Histogram showing the proportion of patients with different outcomes (i.e. dead, dependent (modified Rankin 3, 4 or 5) or independent (modified Rankin 0, 1 or 2) in activities of daily living) 1 year after their first-ever-in-a-lifetime ischaemic stroke ($n = 545$) and its clinical subtypes (TACI, total anterior circulation infarction; PACI, partial anterior circulation infarction; LACI, lacunar infarction; POCI, posterior circulation infarction), primary intracerebral haemorrhage (PICH; $n = 66$) and subarachnoid haemorrhage (SAH; $n = 33$) (from Bamford *et al.* 1990a, 1991).

techniques to compensate for their remaining impairments, and their environment is altered to maximize their autonomy. The overall 'pattern of recovery' reflects all these processes superimposed upon each other. Because it is so difficult to predict an individual patient's functional outcome, the following general points can be made to patients and their relatives:

- the rate of recovery is usually highest in the first few weeks after the initial stroke;
- functional improvement may continue, albeit at a slower rate, for many months and in some patients for 1–2 years;
- the rate and completeness of recovery varies from patient to patient and is relatively unpredictable, at least in the first few days and weeks after stroke onset.

The pattern of recovery varies among patients and in individuals, and rarely follows that implied by grouped data. Only repeated assessments in individual patients can indicate their pattern of recovery.

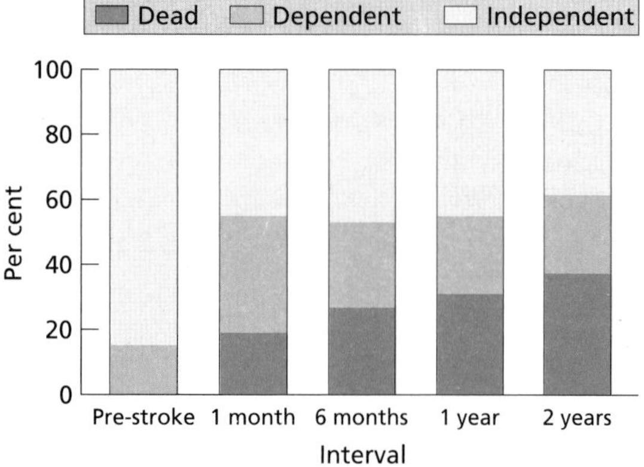

Fig. 10.6 Histogram showing the proportion of patients with different outcomes (i.e. dead, dependent (modified Rankin 3, 4 or 5) or independent (modified Rankin 0, 1 or 2) in activities of daily living) at increasing intervals after their first-ever-in-a-lifetime stroke taking all types together. (Unpublished data from the Oxfordshire Community Stroke Project).

These generalizations are supported by our own experience and also by data from studies in which stroke patients' functional abilities have been repeatedly tested over a period of time (Gray et al. 1990; Duncan et al. 1992; Ashburn 1997). Figure 10.8 shows two graphs which, on the face of it, support the idea that the 'pattern of recovery' follows an almost exponential trajectory. However, one needs to be careful in interpreting such data. These graphs show changes in groups of patients with respect to a particular function over time, which does not mean that all individual patients necessarily follow the same overall pattern. Also, the apparent plateau in recovery after a few months may simply reflect the fact that the tools used to measure the function are often 'ordinal' rather than 'interval' scales (Table 17.20), and also that there is a marked 'ceiling effect'—i.e. the measure is not sensitive to improvements at the upper end of the range of performance (Wellwood et al. 1995; Ashburn 1997). Therefore, the apparent differences in the patterns and duration of recovery for different impairments and disabilities may to some extent reflect the characteristics of the tools used to measure them. For example, it is often said that language function continues to improve for a very long time after a stroke, whilst recovery in arm function does not. This different perception may be due to patients being acutely aware of even small differences in fluency, whilst they may only report an improvement in arm function if they can perform a new function with their hand. Research into the patterns of recovery after stroke that takes these points into account would be helpful.

It is unclear whether patterns of recovery differ among different pathological types of stroke (haemorrhagic versus ischaemic) or subtypes of ischaemic stroke (lacunar versus cortical). Clinical experience suggests that recovery patterns

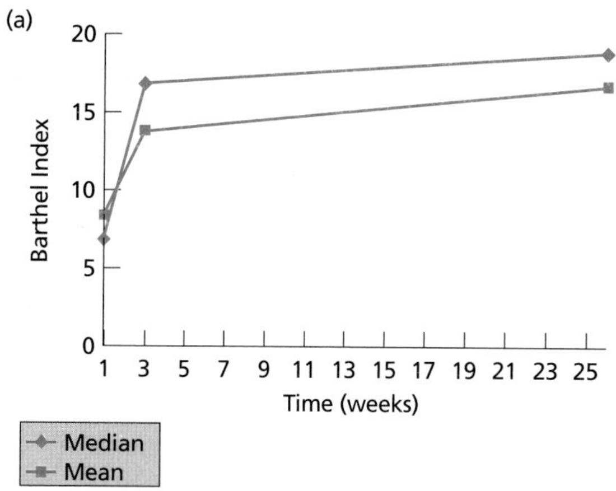

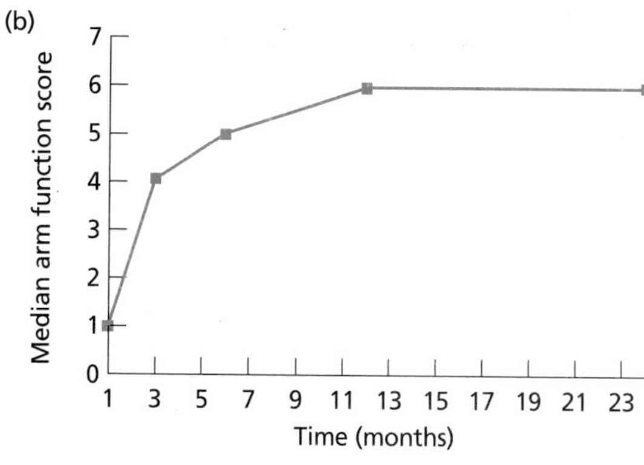

Fig. 10.8 Patterns of recovery after stroke. (a) The graph shows the change in the median and mean Barthel Index over 6 months in the survivors of 976 patients identified in a community-based study with a first-ever or recurrent stroke. (b) The graph shows the change in the median arm function score amongst 84 patients (although not all patients were tested on each occasion) over a follow-up of about 2 years. Although the grouped data suggest an almost exponential recovery, this pattern was rarely observed in individual patients (with permission from Skilbeck *et al.* 1983; Wade & Langton Hewer 1987).

do vary. For instance, we have seen late and dramatic improvements after primary intracerebral haemorrhage, but there are few reliable research data to confirm such observations. Although individual patients may continue to improve for a year or even two, the mean or median (Table 17.20) measure of function in a cohort of stroke patients peaks at about 6 months and then begins to slowly decline (Ashburn 1997). This decline is presumably the result of a combination of subsequent ageing, recurrent strokes, progression of co-morbidity and perhaps withdrawal of physical therapy (section 15.6).

The shape of so-called recovery curves may reflect the properties of the instrument used to measure function as much as the patient's rate of improvement.

10.2.6 Is this the prognosis of your patients?

The prognostic data presented in this section come mainly from the Oxfordshire Community Stroke Project which, over a 4-year period, prospectively registered all patients from a well-defined population who had a first-ever-in-a-lifetime stroke (Bamford *et al.* 1988). After assessment by a study neurologist, as soon after the stroke as possible, patients were prospectively followed for up to 6 years (Dennis *et al.* 1993). Patients were included in the study whether referred to hospital or not, and so provided prognostic data on an unselected community-based cohort of patients with stroke. Studies of prognosis in other community-based series have provided broadly similar results (Sacco *et al.* 1982; Garraway *et al.* 1983; Turney *et al.* 1984; Kojima *et al.* 1990; Anderson *et al.* 1994), although higher case fatality has been reported in other populations, e.g. Siberia (Feigin *et al.* 1996). However, the prognosis of patients in one's own clinical practice may be different because of the following:

- the stroke population is different from that in Oxfordshire during the 1980s; patients may be younger or older, of different racial or ethnic background, have more or less severe strokes, more or less co-morbidity, or a different pattern of stroke pathology. For example, a greater proportion of strokes are attributed to haemorrhage in Japan (Tanaka *et al.* 1981) (section 5.2), and thus one might expect a higher early case fatality (Table 10.2).
- in any hospital, the prognosis of patients will be affected by referral bias (Table 10.1). In general, stroke patients referred to hospital can be expected to have a worse prognosis (i.e. a higher case fatality and worse functional outcome), because a greater proportion of milder cases are looked after by their family doctors at home (Bamford *et al.* 1986). However, this is not always predictable, since in some places younger patients, who have on average a better prognosis (Fig. 10.9), may be referred to hospital more often than older patients. Furthermore, some patients with very severe strokes that are likely to lead to death within a few hours, or who are already living in a nursing home, may not be admitted at all and may therefore be under-represented in a hospitalized cohort. Differences in outcome between hospitals are more likely to reflect the differences in the proportions of patients with severe stroke rather than any differences in treatment given (section 17.6.3).

Hospital admission rates vary considerably from place to place, from country to country, and from time to time. For example, the admission rates in several community-based studies performed over the last couple of decades were: 53% in Siberia, USSR; 55% in Oxfordshire, England; 72% in Auckland, New Zealand; 80% in Perth, Australia and

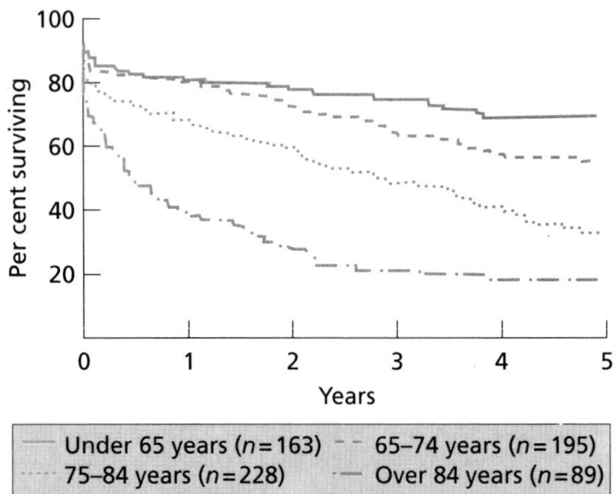

Fig. 10.9 A Kaplan–Meier plot showing the proportion of patients of different ages surviving after a first-ever-in-a-lifetime stroke (with permission from Dennis *et al.* 1993).

Teesside, England; 85% in Perugia, Italy and at least 95% in Umea, Sweden (Bamford *et al.* 1986; Ricci *et al.* 1991; Anderson *et al.* 1993; Bonita *et al.* 1994; Asplund *et al.* 1995; Feigin *et al.* 1996; Rodgers 1999). These data have to be interpreted in the knowledge that definitions of hospital admission vary—e.g. did the patient actually spend a night in a hospital bed? And how were patients who had their stroke whilst in hospital, or who were admitted late after the stroke, handled in the analysis? The type of hospital (e.g. district general, university or tertiary referral hospital) and the specialities represented in it (e.g. neurosurgery, neurology, general medicine, care of the elderly, etc.), will have a major influence on casemix, so that clinicians working in different departments and institutions will form, from their own experience, widely differing views of the prognosis of stroke patients (Horner *et al.* 1995; Petty *et al.* 1998):

- if patients are seen very early after stroke onset (e.g. because the hospital is in a city and has an accident and emergency unit), they are likely to have a worse prognosis than patients who are seen later (such as those referred to a distant tertiary referral centre), because they must survive long enough to be admitted (Table 10.1);
- unless patients are followed up using similar definitions of outcome and for the same time period as those in the published studies, their prognosis will be different (Table 10.1). Also, the reasons why patients are lost to follow-up may be related to their outcome. For example, if dead patients are lost to follow-up, this biases the prognostic data in a favourable direction, and if patients who have made a good recovery (and are mobile) are lost because they move away, this biases the prognostic data in the opposite direction (Table 10.1). Furthermore, if all patients are not followed up, the perceived prognosis is likely to be overly influenced by the outcome of the last few patients, who are remembered most vividly (i.e. recall bias), or perhaps by the patients who had particularly good or particularly bad outcomes;
- if the estimate of the outcome is based on the follow-up of too few patients, it may differ from that in published studies simply by chance alone (the 'good or bad luck effect');
- patients may be managed more or less effectively than those in Oxfordshire and other published studies, and thus the outcomes may be better or worse. However, the likely impact of differences in treatment between centres is likely to be swamped by other factors that have a much greater influence on outcome (e.g. casemix, section 17.6.3).

> *The differences in outcome between your service and those of your colleagues are more likely to reflect differences in the patients you treat than any differences in the quality of care you provide.*

10.2.7 Predicting outcome in individual patients

Unfortunately, it is difficult to predict an *individual* patient's outcome accurately enough for it to be of much value in clinical practice. It is also difficult to define the acceptable accuracy of any predictive tool, because this depends on the consequences, or cost, of getting it wrong. Taking an extreme example, if one was sure that a patient with an apparently severe stroke who was being supported on a ventilator was not going to have an acceptable long-term quality of life, then one might withdraw ventilatory support. However, in this situation one would have to be very confident of one's prediction.

A broad range of factors have been shown to be associated with better than average or worse than average outcomes, including: clinical features shortly after stroke onset; the results of investigations; and the patient's progress over the initial post-stroke period (Table 10.3). Many are interrelated—e.g. conscious level and lesion size on brain computed tomography (CT)—so multiple regression statistical techniques are needed to identify the factors that *independently* predict outcome. Many studies have focused only on factors that are associated with an increased risk of death. However, a growing number also consider those factors that are related to a good or bad functional outcome, and in general these factors are similar to those that predict death. Unfortunately, methodological problems have so far limited the usefulness of these studies (Jongbloed 1990; Hier & Edelstein 1991; Counsell 1998) (Table 10.4). It is useful to have a list of criteria against which one can judge the quality of a study reporting the development of a predictive model to help decide whether it would be 'safe' to use in one's own practice (Table 10.5).

> *At present, it is impossible to predict an individual's outcome early after stroke onset with enough accuracy for it to be of much value in clinical practice.*

Table 10.3 Factors that have been shown to be statistically significant ($P < 0.05$) independent predictors of poor survival and/or poor functional outcome after stroke in at least one study including more than 100 patients (from Counsell 1998).

	Poor survival	Poor survival or poor functional outcome
Demographic features		
Increasing age	+	+
Male sex	+	
Social factors		
Smoking	+	
Excess alcohol	+	+
Unmarried	+	
Living alone	+	
Past history		
Previous stroke/transient ischaemic attack	+	+
Ischaemic heart disease	+	
Peripheral vascular disease		+
Diabetes mellitus	+	
Cancer	+	
General clinical features		
Lost consciousness at onset	+	+
Post-stroke seizures	+	
Atrial fibrillation	+	+
Cardiac failure	+	
Fever	+	
Pneumonia	+	
Obstructive pulmonary disease	+	
Renal disease	+	
Tachycardia	+	
High systolic blood pressure	+	+
High diastolic blood pressure	+	
High pulse pressure		+
Urinary incontinence	+	+
Disability post-stroke	+	+
Neurological signs		
Reduced level of consciousness	+	+
Severe motor deficit	+	+
Bilateral extensor plantars	+	
Pupil abnormality	+	
Impaired proprioception		+
Visuospatial dysfunction		+
Cognitive impairment	+	+
Depression	+	
Poor balance/ataxia		+
Unable to walk	+	
Total anterior circulation syndrome	+	+
Early deterioration	+	
Simple laboratory tests		
High haematocrit	+	
High blood white cell count	+	
High erythrocyte sedimentation rate	+	
Hyperglycaemia	+	
High blood urea/creatinine	+	
High plasma cholesterol	+	
Low arterial Po_2		+
Abnormal electrocardiogram	+	+
Complex tests (CT or MRI brain scan)		
Large stroke lesion (haematoma)	+	+
Site of brain lesion	+	+
Mass effect	+	+
Intraventricular blood (in haemorrhagic stroke)	+	+
Visible infarction		+

CT, computed tomography; MRI, magnetic resonance imaging.

Note: many factors have been identified in just one or two studies, and many of these factors are probably interrelated (e.g. indicating common factors such as frailty, lesion size or stroke severity).

Table 10.4 Methodological problems in studies of prediction of outcome after stroke.

Failure to describe adequately the group of patients in whom the work was done
Use of unrepresentative cohorts of patients, e.g. highly selected patients in rehabilitation settings
Many studies are retrospective, which limits the range and perhaps the reliability of the baseline and outcome data
Failure to define the baseline variables collected adequately
Variation in the timing after stroke of the baseline patient assessments
Failure to measure outcome at a relevant and uniform point after the stroke, i.e. 6 months post-stroke rather than at hospital discharge
Failure to use reliable and valid measures of outcome
Inadequate sample sizes
Failure to use appropriate statistical techniques to adjust for the interactions between baseline variables
Failure to test the accuracy of any predictive model in an independent data set

Table 10.5 Criteria to judge the quality of a study reporting the development of a predictive model for stroke patients (adapted from Counsell 1998).

Is the model externally valid?—i.e. is it applicable to your patients?
Was the model developed in a community-based cohort, i.e. unselected cases?
Were patients with transient ischaemic attack and subarachnoid haemorrhage separated out?
Were there any major exclusion criteria?
Were the age and sex of the patients given?
Were details of any treatment given?
Is the model internally valid?
Was the delay between stroke onset and inclusion given, and was it short?
Were less than 10% of the cohort excluded or lost?
Were baseline and outcome data collected prospectively?
Was outcome measured using valid and reliable instruments?
Was outcome measured at a fixed point after the stroke?
Was follow-up sufficiently long to provide useful data?
Were important predictors included, e.g. stroke severity and age?
Could the predictive variables be collected reliably?
Were statistical analyses appropriate?
Was a stepwise analysis performed?
Were the strengths of correlations between predictive variables assessed (i.e. collinearity). Strong correlations between predictive factors can cause multiple regression techniques to give spurious results.
Was the outcome event per predictive factor ratio (EPV ratio) greater than 10?
Was the ability of the model to discriminate between patients with a good and bad outcome tested? This is best done by establishing the sensitivity and specificity of the model over a full range of probabilities, plotting a receiver operating curve and establishing the area under that curve (Fig. 10.10).
Was the model calibrated to establish any bias of predictions in grouped data? This can be done by plotting the proportions predicted to have a certain outcome against the proportion of patients who actually had that outcome in an independent test data set. Perfect calibration is indicated by the diagonal (Fig. 10.11)
Has the model been validated?
Has the model been tested in the population from which it was derived?
Has the model been tested in an independent population?
Has the model been compared with other predictive systems, including informal clinical judgement?
Has the model been evaluated in a randomized controlled trial, i.e. is its use associated with improved outcomes?
Is the model practical?
Could the predictive variables be collected in practice?
Was the actual model published?
Were confidence intervals for the model given?

Predicting early death

Clinical features which—alone or in combination—indicate severe brainstem dysfunction, whether due to direct damage or as a result of raised intracranial pressure, are highly predictive of early death (Table 10.6). Unfortunately, many patients who die do not show these features, and occasionally patients with more than one of these features make an unexpectedly good recovery (fortunate for the patient, unfortunate for the predictor). Sometimes one sees patients with single predictive factors of a poor outcome, e.g. just periodic respiration (section 15.2.2) but, in isolation, these factors can be associated with a good recovery; it is the *combination* of prognostic factors that is the more powerful predictor.

Predicting longer-term outcomes

It is even more difficult to predict longer-term outcomes. Many of the factors that indicate a high early risk of death also indicate a high risk of long-term dependency if the patient survives (Table 10.3). In general, the patient's age, pre-stroke health status, and indicators of stroke severity (e.g. conscious level, motor impairment, disability, cognitive function) indicate the likelihood of survival free of dependency. In predicting longer-term outcome, one also has the problem that further events—which may be related to the initial stroke (e.g. recurrent strokes and myocardial infarction) or may not (e.g. development of unrelated illness)—can occur and have a major and often quite unpredictable effect on outcome. It is even more difficult to estimate an individual's risk of further vascular events (section 16.1).

Methods of prediction

A variety of different approaches have been taken in predicting outcome after stroke.

The *simplest approach* has been to identify a single factor, the presence or absence of which early after the stroke indi-

Table 10.6 Neurological features that reflect brainstem dysfunction and which in combination are related to a very high risk of early death.

Decreased conscious level (Henon *et al.* 1995)
Conjugate gaze palsy (tonic deviation of gaze) (Tijssen *et al.* 1991)
Severe bilateral motor weakness
Abnormal respiratory pattern (e.g. periodic respiration) (section 15.2.2).
Bilateral extensor plantar responses

cates the likelihood that the patient will have a good or bad outcome. The most widely used examples are reduced level of consciousness and urinary incontinence, which have both been related to a poor survival and functional outcome (Wade & Hewer 1985; Gladman *et al.* 1992; Taub *et al.* 1994). Measures of cognitive function at initial assessment have also been related to poor functional outcomes (Barer 1990; Rose *et al.* 1994; Taub *et al.* 1994). Although such models are simple to use, they are too inaccurate for clinical decision-making (Gladman *et al.* 1992). They have a more obvious use in stratifying patients who are being randomized in clinical trials.

Reduced conscious level and urinary incontinence in the first few days after stroke are both associated, in general, with a poor outcome. Unfortunately, this association is not reliable enough to be useful in managing individual patients.

The *volume of brain damage* is related to outcome. In general, the larger the volume, the worse the clinical outcome, except for critically sited strokes, particularly in the brainstem, where even quite small lesions can be fatal. Many of the clinical indicators of poor prognosis relate quite closely to the size of the brain lesion (Table 10.3). For example, the Oxfordshire Community Stroke Project classification (sections 3.2–4.3.5) reflects the volume of brain damage, and so the prognosis of the different groups varies (Fig. 10.5). Imaging techniques, including CT, single-photon emission CT, and magnetic resonance imaging have so far added little to the accuracy of clinical predictors (Valdimarsson *et al.* 1982; Allen 1984a; Crisi *et al.* 1984; Tuhrim *et al.* 1991; Slattery & Hankey 1992; Wardlaw *et al.* 1998). None of this is at all surprising, because the size of the stroke lesion on brain imaging can so often be predicted from the clinical findings (section 4.3.7). Moreover, a substantial proportion of patients have a normal or near normal CT scan early after even a major ischaemic stroke, which weakens the early predictive utility of any imaging (section 5.3.5). Other technologies, such as transcranial magnetic stimulation, have also been used to predict outcome, although these have not been adequately evaluated (Rapisarda *et al.* 1996).

In general, the larger the stroke lesion, the worse the likely outcome, except for small, critically sited lesions, which may be associated with a poor outcome.

Mathematical models based on regression analyses have been developed by several groups to predict both survival and functional outcome (Prescott *et al.* 1982; Sheikh *et al.* 1983; Wade *et al.* 1983; Allen 1984b; Fullerton *et al.* 1988; Anderson *et al.* 1994; Fiorelli *et al.* 1995; Kwakkel *et al.* 1996; Counsell 1998). Although these are generally a little more accurate than models based on a single variable, any advantage may be offset by the practical difficulties in applying them (Weingarten *et al.* 1990). Also, only one has been tested adequately in independent cohorts of sufficient size (Counsell 1998) (Figs 10.10, 10.11) (Table 10.7). As one would predict, where they have been tested they generally perform less well than in the cohort from which they were developed (Britton *et al.* 1980; Tuhrim *et al.* 1991; Gladman 1992; Gompertz *et al.* 1994). If such models are to be used in routine clinical practice, they need to be further refined, tested prospectively in large independent cohorts of patients, and made more 'user-friendly', so that they do not require the clinician to perform complex calculations. For example, Fig. 10.12 shows a nomogram that allows the user to calculate a patient's probability of being alive and independent 1 year after a stroke. This is based on the mathematical model shown in Table 10.7. Such models are being used to stratify patients by predicted prognosis in large randomized trials, in which complex calculations are easily performed by computer during the randomization process (www.dcn.ed.ac.uk/spgm). Indeed, large randomized trials offer an excellent opportunity to test such predictive models prospectively (Easton *et al.* 2000).

Stroke scales are frequently used to describe the severity of stroke in the acute phase. They are based on the neurological examination, and scores are given depending on the presence, absence, or severity of various impairments. They are used quite reasonably to stratify patients at baseline in acute stroke trials and to monitor change in the acute phase. They are less useful as a measure of long-term outcome (section 17.6.3), although they have been used in this way (Adams *et al.* 1999). The National Institutes of Health Stroke Scale (NIHSS) and other commonly used scales were found to be superior to the Guy's prognostic score, a mathematically derived model (Muir *et al.* 1996.). However, Lai *et al.* (1998) found that the Orpington prognostic scale was both simpler to use and more accurate than the NIHSS in predicting a patient's functional outcome.

Predictions based on measures of function early after a stroke (e.g. the Barthel Index) have been used to predict eventual functional outcome and may be particularly useful for those working in rehabilitation facilities (Granger *et al.* 1989; Lincoln *et al.* 1990; Loewen & Anderson 1990).

The rate of change in some measure of the patient's condition early in the clinical course can be used to predict the likely longer-term outcome (Granger *et al.* 1989; Tilling *et al.* 1999). This might be likened to the growth curves used by paediatricians. Predictions for individuals would then depend on the pattern of recovery observed in large cohorts of patients.

The informal judgements we make about patients during our daily work are the most common method of prediction. Such informal predictions have rarely been evaluated, but their accuracy will clearly depend on the experience of the individual clinician. We demonstrated that judgements made

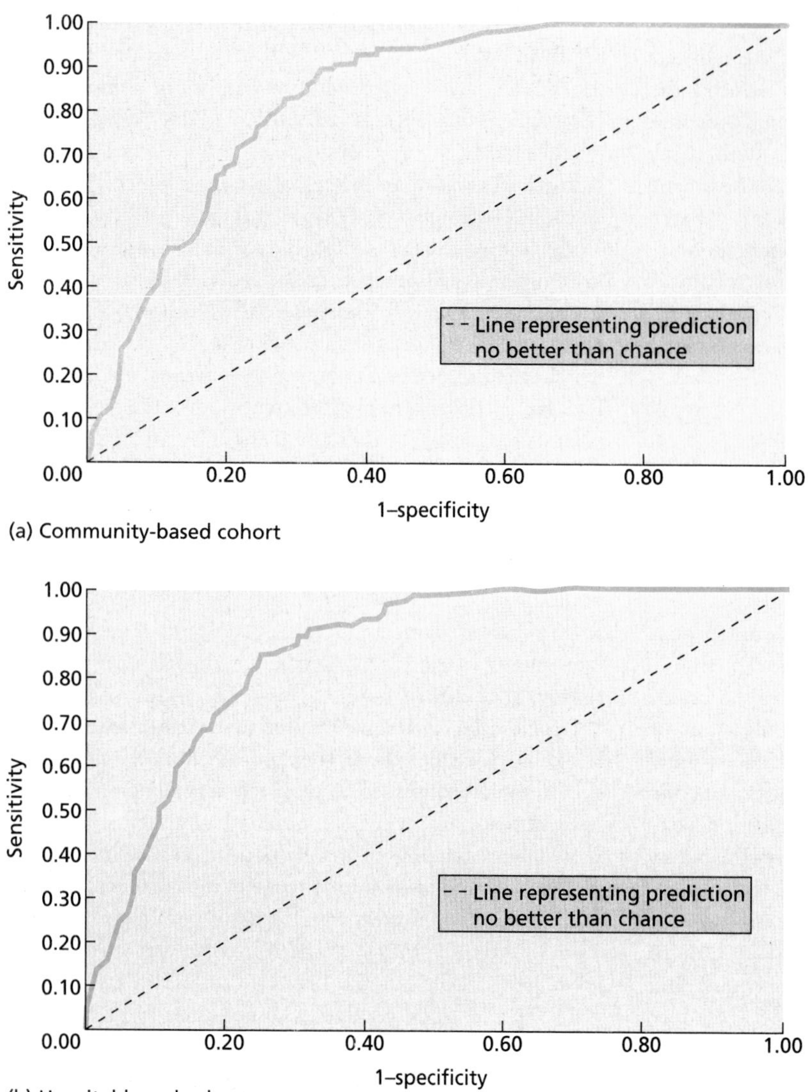

Fig. 10.10 Receiver operating characteristic (ROC) curves for a statistical model (Table 10.7) to predict the probability of survival free of dependency 1 year after stroke. The model was derived from the Oxfordshire Community Stroke Project, and has been tested on two independent cohorts of stroke patients: (a) a community-based cohort derived from the SEPIVAC and Perth Stroke Registries and (b) a hospital-based cohort, the Lothian Stroke Registry. The area under the curves indicates the accuracy of the models—i.e. the larger the area, the more discriminatory the model.

by fairly experienced physicians (i.e. with at least 5 years in practice) about patients' likely level of functional independence were similar to predictions based on a simple mathematical model (Counsell 1998) (Table 10.7). If more formal predictive systems are to be widely adopted, they will need to be shown to be at least as accurate as our informal judgements.

The predictive systems developed so far have not been adequately tested, and are not sufficiently accurate to influence important clinical decisions in individuals. However, they may be useful as tools to guide less experienced clinicians in what to say to patients and carers; choose who to randomize in trials of acute treatment; and to decide which patient is likely to require an extended period of rehabilitation. Predictive systems may prove to be more useful in assessing the quality of care. They can be used to adjust outcome data from different *groups* of patients for differences in casemix, to compare the quality of care given by different hospitals or units (section 17.6.3).

In the future, we expect the fairly crude predictive models currently available to be replaced by more precise, more robust and better validated models. These might be used to predict not only survival and basic functional outcome, but also the rate of recovery of individual impairments, disabilities and handicaps, which is so important in planning treatment. Such models may even be developed by neural networks in addition to the more conventional multiple regression analyses. One might combine several approaches to predicting a patient's outcome, so that one relies on the mathematical modelling in the early stages, but as more data become available from continued observation of the patient, a patient's specific 'recovery curve' might be plotted. One could imagine that these predictive systems could be presented in several forms for clinical use: wall charts; clinical

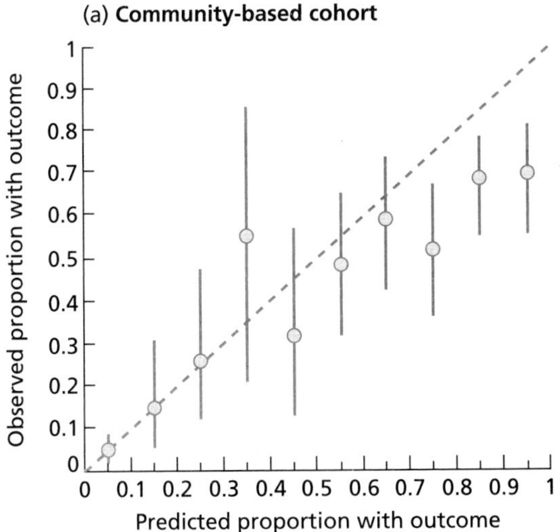

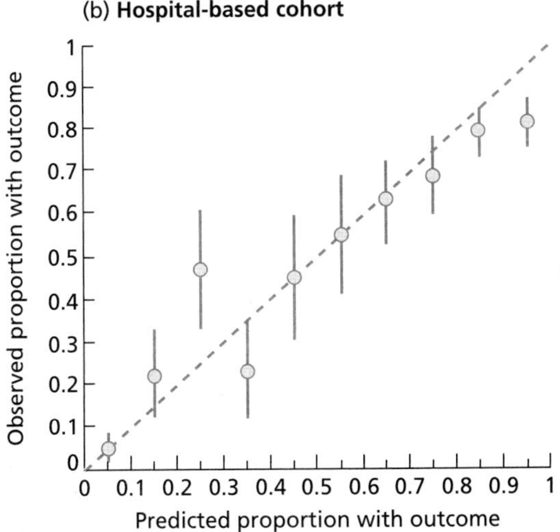

Fig. 10.11 Calibration of a statistical model (Table 10.7) to predict the probability of survival free of dependency 1 year after a stroke. The model was derived from the Oxfordshire Community Stroke Project, and has been tested on two independent cohorts of stroke patients: (a) a community-based cohort derived from the SEPIVAC and Perth Stroke Registries and (b) a hospital based cohort, the Lothian Stroke Registry. The dotted line indicates perfect calibration. The vertical lines indicate the 95% confidence intervals, which depend on the number of patients in each at-risk group. The model calibrates better in the hospital-based than in the community-based cohort, and tends to be optimistic in those with the greatest probability of a good outcome (survival free of dependency).

slide rules; on pocket calculators; palm or desktop computers, or hospital-wide computer networks (www.dcn.ed.ac.uk/spgm). Eventually, any such system, which will inevitably consume resources, will have to be tested to show that it improves the effectiveness and efficiency of stroke services.

Table 10.7 A mathematical model to predict the probability of survival free from dependency in activities of daily living 1 year after a stroke. This was derived from the Oxfordshire Community Stroke Project using logistic regression, and has been externally validated on two independent cohorts of stroke patients (Figs 10.10 and 10.11). Calculating the probability of an outcome is complex (see equation), but easily achieved using a programmable calculator or a nomogram (Fig. 10.12). Health warning—this model should not be used to make firm predictions in individual patients!

Variable†	Parameter coefficient, *b* (SE)	Odds ratio (95% CI)
Constant	15.586 (1.748)	
Age	−0.085 (0.014)	0.92‡ (0.89–0.94)
Living alone	0.384 (0.259)	0.68 (0.41–1.14)
Independent pre-stroke	−3.174 (0.639)	25.00 (6.67–100)
Normal Glasgow Coma Scale verbal	−2.177 (0.504)	9.09 (3.33–25)
Able to lift arms	−2.319 (0.513)	10.00 (3.70–25)
Able to walk	−1.154 (0.402)	3.12 (1.45–7.14)

† Dichotomous variables were coded 1 = yes, 2 = no.
‡ Per year of age.

Probability of outcome is calculated by: $P = e^Y/(1 + e^Y)$, where $Y = a + b_1X_1 + b_2X_2 + \ldots + b_iX_i$.

Y = 15.586 − (0.085 × age) + (0.384 × living alone) − (3.174 × independent pre-stroke) − (2.177 × normal GCS verbal) − (2.319 × able to lift arms) − (1.154 × able to walk), where dichotomous variables have numeric values of 1 or 2 as described above.

10.3 Delivering an integrated management plan

10.3.1 Introduction

The term 'stroke' embraces a very wide spectrum of clinical presentations ranging from neurological deficits lasting just 1 day to those leading rapidly to death or causing lifelong disability. These deficits are layered on a complex mix of pre-existing disease, personality, and social and environmental factors. We have already seen the range of possible pathological types (Chapter 5) and causes (Chapters 6–9), but each patient requires a management plan tailored to his or her own individual needs. In a patient whose symptoms resolve completely within a few days, the emphasis should be on diagnosis and secondary prevention. In a patient with a major disabling stroke, the emphasis must be on treatment of the acute phase, prevention of complications, and rehabilitation. The essential first step in formulating a management plan is a full and detailed assessment.

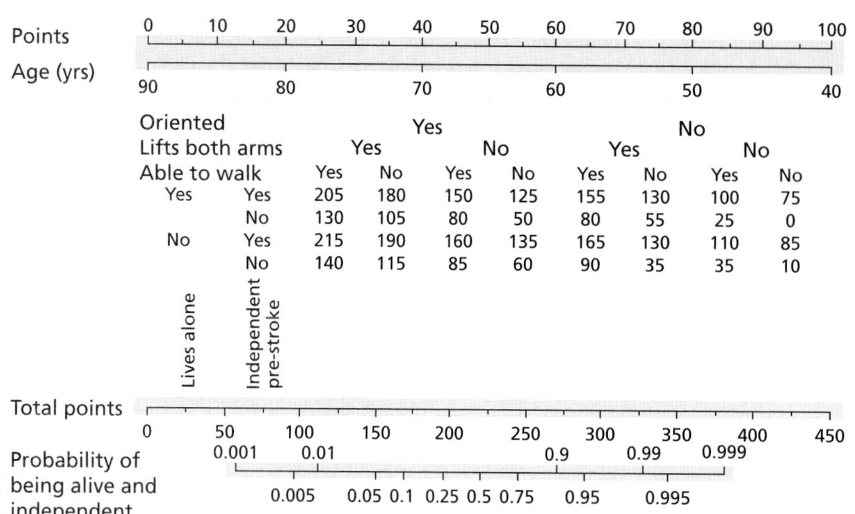

Fig. 10.12 Nomogram for calculating the probability of being alive and independent at 1 year after stroke. To use this chart to predict outcome in a patient: (1) plot the patient's age on the age scale, and mark the points attributable to age on the scale immediately above this; (2) read off the points attributable to the other five variables from the box in the table that fits the patient's condition; (3) add the points for 1 and 2; (4) plot the sum on the 'total points' scale and read off the probability by dropping a perpendicular line to the probability scale below.

10.3.2 Assessment

The assessment should aim to answer the following questions:

• is it a vascular event (transient ischaemic attack or stroke)? (Chapter 3);
• where is the lesion? (Chapters 3 and 4);
• what sort of stroke lesion is it (ischaemic or haemorrhagic)? (Chapter 5);
• what is the likely cause? (Chapters 6–9);
• what is this patient's prognosis? (sections 10.2 and 16.1);
• what are this patient's particular problems? (Chapter 15).

The answers to these questions will determine the management of the patient and which therapeutic interventions are appropriate. The first five questions have been addressed in previous sections, and before proceeding to discuss the assessment of specific problems to complete the diagnostic formulation (Chapter 15), some general principles and the organization of assessment must be considered.

In practice, the patient's first assessment is usually carried out by either a general (family) practitioner in the patient's home, or by a trainee hospital doctor. Neither clinician may have had much training or experience in the assessment of patients with stroke. An average general practitioner with 2000 patients is likely to see only about four new cases of stroke each year. Guidelines, a protocol or, in hospital, a clerking or admission form may be useful tools to ensure that each patient has a thorough and relevant assessment. We, and others, have demonstrated a significant improvement in the completeness of the assessment of stroke patients following the introduction of a stroke clerking or admission form (available on www.dcn.ed.ac.uk/spgm) (Davenport *et al.* 1995; Hancock *et al.* 1997). The use of the form also makes it much easier to access the information subsequently and to identify relevant items that are missing. However, one has to acknowledge the practical difficulties of introducing disease-specific assessment forms in situations—e.g. accident and emergency departments—in which patients with a wide range of medical problems are being assessed. For example, it may not be clear until the end of the assessment what the most likely diagnosis is and therefore which form should have been used. One solution to this might be a 'core form' for all patients, with supplementary sheets for specific common conditions. There is reasonable evidence that patient-specific reminders (e.g. 'if ischaemic stroke, prescribe aspirin'), which can be included in such forms, improve adherence to management guidelines (Effective Health Care 1994; Bero *et al.* 1998). Also, evidence from the field of geriatrics suggests that formal assessment procedures that lead on to appropriate management decisions improve patient outcomes (Wade 1998).

A clerking or admission form will improve the completeness and relevance of the initial assessment and will facilitate communication and audit, but the introduction of diagnosis-specific forms is not without its problems.

Although a physician is often the first person to assess the patient, it is important to emphasize that assessment should often involve other members of the multidisciplinary team (section 10.3.5). It is often very valuable, even on the day of the stroke, to involve the nurse, the physiotherapist and a speech and language therapist. Advice on the patient's risk of pressure sores, lifting, handling and positioning and the patient's ability to swallow safely are all relevant to their care from the moment of hospital admission, or indeed from the moment of assessment at home. The components of the initial assessment and their use are summarized in Table 10.8.

Table 10.8 Types of information that should be collected during the initial assessment of a stroke patient, and their potential value.

Type of information	Diagnosis	Cause	Prognosis	Problems	Secondary prevention
Demographics	+	+	+	+	
History of onset	+	+			
Risk factors	+	+	+	+	+
Co-existing disease		+	+	+	+
Medication		+		+	
Social details			+	+	
Pre-stroke function	+		+	+	+
General examination		+	+	+	+
Neurological examination	+	+	+	+	
Investigations	+	+	+	+	+

It is important to emphasize that assessment is not a 'once only' process, but should continue throughout the course of the patient's recovery from stroke.

Assessment is not a 'once only' process, but should continue throughout the course of the patient's recovery from stroke.

Health professionals involved in the initial assessment of stroke patients learn that, although the patient may be a useful source of information, other people often provide more information that is essential to planning treatment. This is particularly important when the patient, for a variety of reasons, cannot communicate. It is often enormously valuable to spend a little time interviewing the family, neighbours, general practitioner, ambulance technicians, or nursing staff, even if this requires using a telephone (Fig. 10.13).

To complete an assessment it is often essential to talk to family, neighbours, or family doctor; essential information can often be collected by a telephone call to the appropriate person.

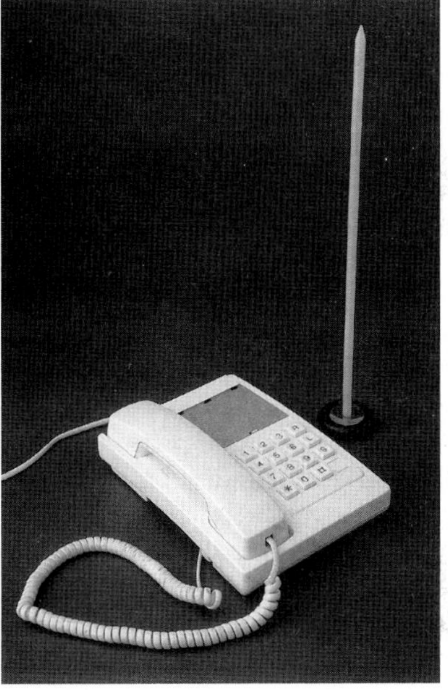

Fig. 10.13 The telephone is a valuable diagnostic tool.

Social environment

The patient's social environment is a very important factor in determining the overall effect that a stroke will have on an individual and his or her family. Accurate knowledge of social networks is therefore critical when setting longer-term goals for rehabilitation and in planning discharge from hospital. Moreover, this allows one to build up a picture of the patient as a person rather than as 'just another stroke' or 'that fibrillating hemiplegic in bed six'. It is so often difficult to see the real person behind the facial weakness, severe aphasia, hemiplegia and incontinence—but that person is usually there and distressed by their predicament. Finding out about the patient's pre-stroke life might encourage members of the team who are caring for the patient to treat them with more understanding and sympathy. Also, it is this background information that allows one to judge the likely effect that the individual's disabilities will have on their role in society, i.e. the likely handicap. This is important, because one of the major aims of rehabilitation is to minimize handicap. For example, it may be more appropriate to put greater energy and resources into occupational therapy for a craftsman than for a schoolteacher, who might require relatively more speech therapy. The patient should, if possible, have a major role in setting such priorities.

It is so often difficult to see the real person behind the facial weakness, severe aphasia, hemiplegia and incontinence—but that person is usually there and distressed by their predicament.

Although a lot of this background information can be collected over a longer period whilst the patient is recovering, it can be useful early on and may be more easily collected at the initial assessment. So often, the family—who may be the only source of this sort of information—disappear within a few hours of the admission and may then not reappear to be asked the relevant questions. It is therefore vital to seize the opportunity when a patient is first admitted, or at least during the next day or two, to obtain as much information from the family and friends as possible. Clearly, this may not be regarded as a medical priority, but professionals other than doctors, in particular the nursing staff, are often well placed to collect it. It is important to remember that a complete picture of the patient's pre-stroke life may be useful when deciding how aggressively to manage a patient (e.g. neurosurgery for obstructive hydrocephalus). Because this background information is so important, but may not be available at the initial assessment, one needs to have some method of identifying which items of data are missing so that they can be sought later on. The clerking or admission form, or a patient record that is shared by the different professions involved (the so-called 'combined' or 'single-patient' record) should fulfil this role. Many stroke units have introduced 'integrated care pathways', which usually include an admission form, multidisciplinary records and guidance on how to manage common problems (for an example see www.dcn.ed.ac.uk/spgm) (section 17.6.4). These have rarely been rigorously evaluated, but one small randomized trial did show improvements in the documentation of assessment, risk factors and patient education (Moloney et al. 1999).

It is just as important to know the home and social circumstances of a stroke patient for early decision-making (such as the desirability of emergency operation) as for later rehabilitation and discharge from hospital.

By the end of the initial assessment, one should have collected enough information to produce a diagnostic formulation, including certainty of stroke diagnosis, site and size of the brain lesion, and the likely causes. This leads on to choices about the intensity of investigation required, and enables the physician to talk to the patient and/or the family about the likely diagnosis, prognosis and management. At this stage, it is valuable to consider, and even list, the particular problems the patient has, to ensure they have all been identified and addressed. It may be useful to use a checklist of the most common ones that occur at this early stage (Table 10.9).

Table 10.9 Some important things to think about during the first day after a patient has had a severe stroke.

- Maintenance of a clear airway
- Treatment of co-existing or underlying disease
- Need to review the patient's usual medication
- Investigation and avoidance of fever
- Adequacy of oxygenation
- Swallowing ability
- Hydration
- Management of urinary incontinence
- Prevention of:
  - Deep venous thrombosis
  - Pressure sores
  - Aspiration
  - Trauma
- Protection of a flaccid shoulder
- Exclusion of fractures
- Obtaining information from and giving information to the patient and family

10.3.3 Identifying problems and setting goals

The patient's assessment, both initially and subsequently, should identify any major problems, and it is these that determine the patient's management. Problems can occur at every level of the patient's illness—i.e. pathology, impairment, disability and handicap. For example, a problem at the pathological level might include 'diagnostic uncertainty' or 'raised erythrocyte sedimentation rate', which should lead on to further investigation if appropriate; whilst a problem at the level of handicap might be that the patient provided the only income for a large family, who now have no money to feed themselves. Having identified a problem, one can then formulate a plan to solve or at least alleviate that problem. Thus, a problem list can be turned into an action plan for the individual patient. Some problems can be dealt with very simply (e.g. antibiotics for a urinary tract infection). These are the 'short-loop problems'. The goal here is simply to remove the problem. Other problems such as immobility—which are more complex, respond more slowly to therapy and may require several different types of intervention—are the 'long-loop problems' (section 10.1.2); here it is useful to set a long-term goal of removing or alleviating the problem, but it is also helpful to set intermediate goals that allow one to judge whether progress is being made towards the long-term goal.

Why a goal-orientated approach has several advantages

Setting goals allows forward planning and provides a useful focus for multidisciplinary team meetings (section 10.3.7). Intermediate goals allow members of the team to coordinate their work, assuming that goals are achieved on time, and so improve efficiency. For example, if patients are to dress the lower half of their body, they must be able to stand. If the physiotherapist can estimate when the patient will be able to stand independently, the occupational therapist can plan when to start working on dressing the lower half. Setting longer-term goals can, for example, allow advanced planning of a pre-discharge home visit and final discharge to the community, which can reduce the patient's length of stay in hospital by the number of days or weeks needed to plan a home visit or to make any necessary adaptations to the patient's home before discharge (e.g. stair rails).

If realistic goals are set, they can then be used to help motivate patients. Recovery from a stroke may be very slow—so slow that the patient and even the therapists are unable to discern any progress being made towards the long-term goal (e.g. to achieve independent mobility). If one sets and achieves intermediate goals (e.g. sitting balance), progress is more easily perceived and morale maintained. The management of patients with stroke in hospital is often allowed to drift without direction or leadership. The responsible clinician waves to the patient on a weekly ward round, in the belief that the therapists are actively rehabilitating the patient. If the head of the multidisciplinary team maintains discipline, and encourages the setting of both intermediate and long-term goals, drift can be avoided. This discipline benefits the patients, the team members and the service as a whole.

Describing goals

Where the goal is simply the removal of a problem, such as a urinary tract infection, it is fairly easy to describe it and then measure progress, e.g. relief of symptoms and sterile urine on a repeat culture. Similarly, long-term goals are often easy to describe, but should take into account the patient's need for accommodation, physical and emotional support, how they might fill their time and what role they play in society (Wade 1992). Judgements about whether these long-term goals have been achieved are relatively straightforward. For example, if the goal is to get a patient home to live with their family, or to return to work, one does not need any complex measures of outcome. In some areas, it is even fairly easy to set intermediate goals. For example, many patients with stroke have problems with mobility, but usually the patient will achieve certain physical milestones on the road to recovery (Fig. 10.14). Further improvement in mobility can be measured by recording the time it takes the patient to walk 10 m (Wade *et al.* 1987). Thus, it is a fairly simple process to set an intermediate goal, which the patient or carer can understand, in terms of the level of function and the date by which it should be achieved.

With other problems, e.g. language and activities of daily living (ADL), intermediate goals are less easily expressed, and thus progress is less easily monitored. Although one could use a score on any one of the huge number of measures of language function or ADL as intermediate goals, these scores are not easily understood by patients and carers, or even by the professionals using them. For example, it is unlikely to mean much to a patient, or even the team members, to aim for a Barthel Index score of 12 out of a maximum of 20 in 2 weeks (section 17.6.3). Despite these difficulties, the team should attempt to identify problems, specify intermediate and long-term goals, and introduce some measures to determine whether progress is being made towards achieving each of them.

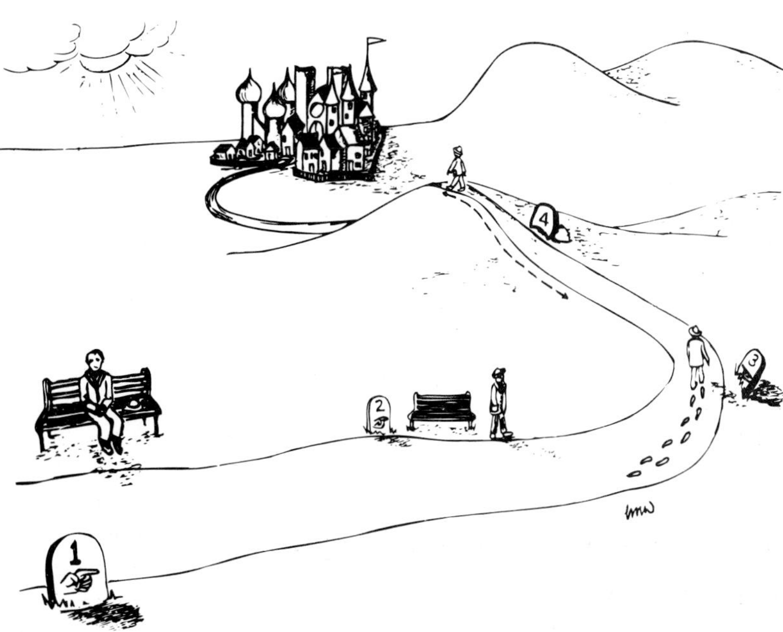

Fig. 10.14 The 'road' to recovery after a hemiplegic stroke, showing some mobility 'milestones': 1, sitting balance for 1 min; 2, standing for 10 s; 3, 10 steps unaided; 4, timed 10-m walk (Smith & Baer 1999).

In every stroke patient, intermediate and long-term goals should be agreed and described so that progress towards them can be measured. Moreover, everyone will feel a sense of achievement when the goals are met.

10.3.4 Goal setting: a diagnostic tool

Goals may also be useful in identifying new or previously unrecognized problems. If a patient is not achieving the goals that have been set, it may be due to a number of causes, which can be divided into team factors, patient factors and carer factors.

Team factors

If the goals are too ambitious because of inaccurate diagnosis, inadequate assessment or uncertainty about the prognosis, then patients will fail to achieve them and this will have a detrimental effect on the patient's and the team's morale. If goals are too easy, then progress may be slower than is, in fact, possible. Also, goal setting must be realistic if one is to use it to coordinate care (section 10.3.3). To set realistic goals in such a way that they are more often achieved than not requires an understanding of the prognosis and of the likely effectiveness of potential interventions. We have already seen that accurate predictions of progress and outcome are difficult in individual patients (section 10.2.7), but informal judgements made by the team may be more accurate, because they are based on observation of the patient's progress over a period of time. Another reason why a patient may not be achieving a goal might be lack of appropriate treatment. Thus, progress may be hampered by too little therapy, or by the wrong sort of therapy. However, since there is currently so little information about the optimum amount or the relative effectiveness of most interventions, it is difficult to sort this out. Team members will much more often have to modify their therapy based on their own experience rather than on evidence from properly conducted randomized controlled trials.

Goals should be meaningful and challenging, but achievable.

Patient and carer factors

New, unrecognized medical or psychological problems (e.g. infection, recurrent stroke or depression) may not present overtly—especially in their early stages—but may develop in a less specific way, causing a patient's progress to slow, stop, or even reverse. One can draw a parallel with the concept of 'failure to thrive' in paediatric practice (Fig. 10.15). If a patient is failing to achieve his or her goals (or milestones), then one needs to identify the cause.

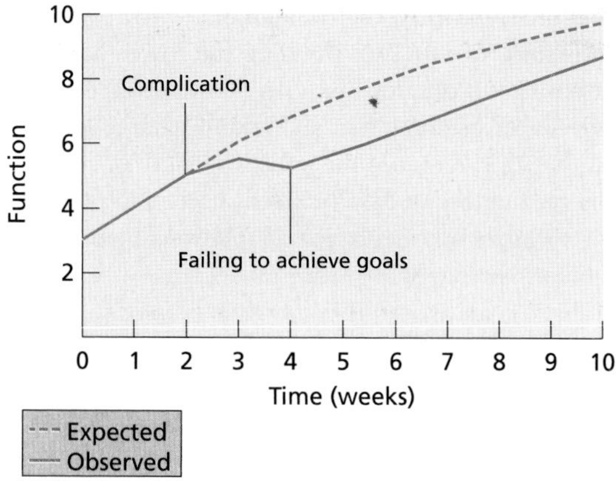

Fig. 10.15 'Failure to thrive' after a stroke. Deviation from the expected recovery pattern might be due to any number of factors, including recurrent stroke, infections, depression, etc.

When a patient is failing to achieve his or her goals (or milestones) then one must identify the cause, and if possible do something about it.

Sometimes the patient or the carer may have different goals from those of the team looking after the patient. This is 'goal mismatch'. For example, a patient who does not want to live alone but would prefer to live with his or her daughter may not achieve the level of independence expected. Therefore, when setting goals it is important to discuss them with the patient and carers—although they may be reticent about discussing such matters openly. It is also important to involve the patient, and perhaps the carer, in setting goals, to ensure that the goals are really relevant to them. Most stroke patients are retired, so that leisure activities may be particularly important to their quality of life (section 15.33.3). The patient may be less interested in a goal aiming at achieving self-care in dressing than in being able to read or do the gardening. In hospital practice, where activities of daily living (ADL) abilities often determine the length of stay, too much emphasis can be placed on ADL-related goals because of the pressures on the team to make beds available for new patients and to minimize costs by discharging the patient as early as possible.

Goal setting may sometimes involve just an individual professional, but more often it needs to involve the rest of the team, the patient, and sometimes the patient's family.

10.3.5 The stroke team

Although a physician usually has overall responsibility for the management of the patient, other members of the multidisciplinary team play an essential part. A systematic review of randomized trials has shown that compared with care on a general medical ward, that on a stroke unit is likely to reduce the mortality, physical dependency and need for institutionalization in patients admitted to hospital with an acute stroke (Stroke Unit Trialists' Collaboration 1997, 2000) (section 17.4.2). The main difference between the two models of care was that stroke unit care is coordinated with a multidisciplinary team. Because stroke patients have such a broad range of problems, their care demands input from several professions. For coordination of the professionals' input, it is important that at least some of them should work as a core team, with regular meetings to discuss the patients' progress and problems (Table 10.10). Other professionals (Table 10.11), who may not be regular members of the team, should be available for consultation about individual patients. Although well established in rehabilitation settings, the team has an important role in all phases of treatment, even on the day of the stroke. Of course, the type and intensity of input from different members of the team will vary at different stages of the patient's illness.

By working closely together and sharing information and skills, some blurring of the boundaries between the roles of the professions becomes possible, and this can provide greater flexibility and efficiency. For example, if the nursing staff are trained by the speech and language therapist to carry out the more straightforward assessments of swallowing, this will provide every patient with a simple and early screening assessment (even at weekends), enabling the speech and language therapist to focus on patients with definite swallowing or communication problems (section 15.17). Some have suggested that we should develop a hybrid therapist who could take on several roles, but this interesting idea has, not surprisingly, met with considerable opposition from the existing professions. This concept may have particular merits in situations in which it is difficult to coordinate the activities of a multidisciplinary team.

Figures 10.16 and 10.17 illustrate two models of how members of the stroke team can provide input to patients and their carers. In the first, each professional predominantly works directly with the patient and/or carer, whilst in the second each professional has less direct patient contact, but influences the care given by a primary nurse. The two models represent the

Table 10.10 The core stroke team.

Physician
Nurse
Physiotherapist
Occupational therapist
Speech and language therapist
Social worker

Table 10.11 Other professionals who may be helpful in the management of particular stroke patients.

Others who may be consulted	Example of problem
Clinical psychologist	Antisocial behaviour
Psychiatrist	Severe depression
Neurosurgeon	Obstructive hydrocephalus
Vascular surgeon	Peripheral artery embolus
Radiologist	Unusual CT scan appearance
Rheumatologist	Painful shoulder
Orthopaedic surgeon	Fractured neck of femur
Optometrist	Refractive problems
Ophthalmologist	Persistent diplopia
Orthotist	Shortened leg, foot drop
Dietician	Weight loss
Pharmacist	Formulations for dysphagia
Dentist	Ill-fitting dentures

CT, computed tomography.

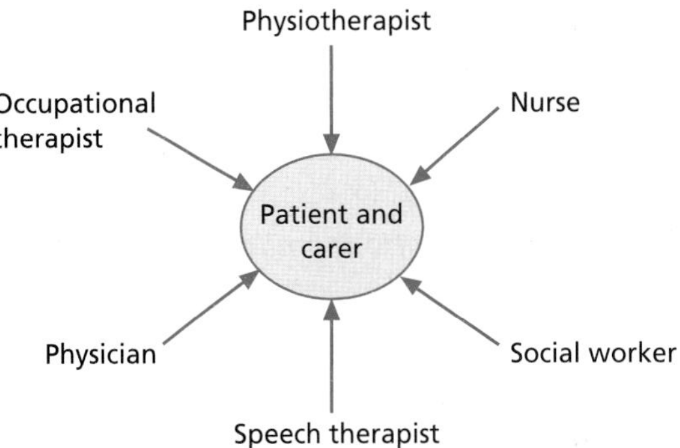

Fig. 10.16 The traditional model of care or rehabilitation, in which each member of the multidisciplinary team interacts independently with the patient and/or carer.

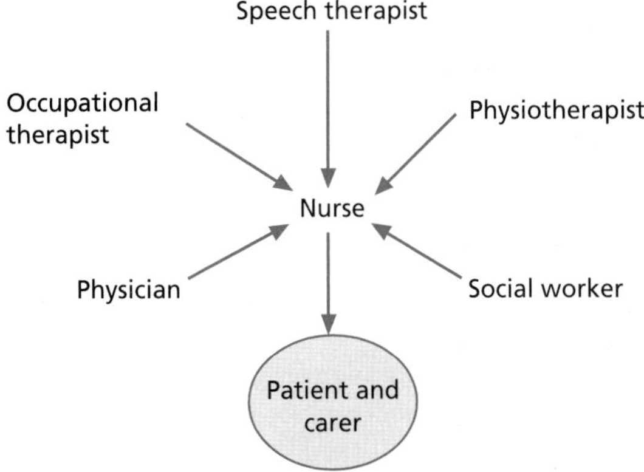

Fig. 10.17 The model of care or rehabilitation that can be adopted on a geographically defined stroke unit, in which each member of the multidisciplinary team influences the nursing input to the patients and carers, as well as having direct interaction with them.

extremes, and it is likely that in the real world care is provided in an intermediate way. Although the model represented in Fig. 10.17 realistically means that patients must be treated in a stroke unit, it has important advantages. Inevitably, because resources are limited, stroke patients receive relatively little time with the therapists. Where this input has been measured, it may amount to less than an hour for each day spent in hospital (Lincoln *et al.* 1996). Training the nurses to practice with the patients the activities initiated by the therapists should encourage consistency and increase the total amount of therapy received by patients. After all, the nurses are caring for patients on a ward throughout the 24-h period. If, for example, the physiotherapists are teaching a patient how to transfer from bed to wheelchair, it is important that the patient should continue to do this in the same way *between* physiotherapy sessions. Without this approach, many of the skills the patient acquires during physiotherapy sessions may not be used during activities on the ward or, more importantly, at home. The same principles apply to input from other therapists. Whether therapy delivered by a non-specialist is as effective as therapy delivered by a highly trained specialist needs to be evaluated in randomized trials. One of the important functions of the team meeting is to harmonize the activity of the therapists and the nurses who provide much of the daily input to the patients. This may be at least one of the reasons why stroke units seem to achieve better outcomes (section 17.4.2).

10.3.6 The roles of the team members

This section outlines the main functions of the core members of the team. In practice, and certainly where a team is functioning well, there will be some blurring of the roles of the team members with each performing the less specialized functions of the others.

Physician

Few doctors really understand the important role that they can play in the care of stroke patients beyond making the initial diagnosis, searching for a treatable cause, giving acute medical therapies and initiating secondary preventative measures. The physician needs to be much more involved in the activities of the team for several reasons:

- usually, rightly or wrongly, political power in health services lies principally with doctors, and therefore if stroke patients are to have access to adequate facilities, the doctor must be involved;
- the physician should be knowledgeable about the pathologies—both stroke and non-stroke—that underlie the patients' functional problems, and should thus understand the prognosis and likely effect of interventions. This is essential for predicting outcome and setting appropriate goals;
- stroke patients commonly have co-existing and complicating medical problems (e.g. diabetes, heart failure, deep venous thrombosis), which need to be identified and treated (Davenport *et al.* 1996; van der Worp & Kappelle 1998; Langhorne *et al.* 2000);
- the physician will often have the broadest knowledge about stroke and is therefore in a good—although not necessarily unique—position to coordinate the team and to chair team meetings. This role is important, because team meetings can become very time-consuming and may lose direction without a strong chairperson (section 10.3.7). Overly long meetings are boring, demoralizing and inefficient;
- the legal responsibility for the patient is the doctor's, and therefore the doctor must be involved at all stages of the patient's care.

Nursing staff

The nursing staff probably have the broadest role in the management of patients with stroke, which includes at least four major components:

- a daily assessment of the patient's problems, both existing and new, and of their abilities and disabilities. Every week, our nurses assess the patients using the Barthel Index (Table 17.19), which focuses their attention on important functional issues. Based on this assessment, they evolve a care plan that aims to meet the individual's needs;
- provision of all the basic needs (e.g. feeding, washing, dressing, toileting, turning and transferring) of dependent patients after a stroke;
- provision of skilled nursing to prevent the development of complications such as pressure sores (section 15.16), painful shoulders (section 15.24), other injuries (section 15.26) and aspiration pneumonia (sections 15.12 and 15.17). This involves correctly positioning and handling the immobile patient (section 15.11). If one adopts a model of team working approximating to that shown in Fig. 10.17, then the nurse's role will include many of the functions of other members of the team;
- supporting the patient and family. With increasing emphasis on improving easily measured clinical outcomes such as case fatality and disability, other aspects of caring for and about patients are easily forgotten, but these are very important to patients and close family members (Pound *et al.* 1995): informing, reassuring, encouraging, advising, supporting and sympathizing. The nurses usually have greatest contact with the patients and family and therefore have an important role in this area. Although in the UK and many other developed countries, we have until now taken our nursing staff for granted, it should be remembered that in some other healthcare systems trained nurses are less available, and much of the patient's day-to-day needs are met by relatives.

Physiotherapist

The physiotherapist has several important roles in caring for stroke patients, depending on their individual needs and the stage of the illness. Soon after a severe stroke, the physiotherapist may be involved in seven functions:

- providing a detailed assessment of the motor and sensory problems of the patient to help estimate the patient's prognosis;
- assessing and treating chest problems, including pneumonia and retention of secretions. Speech and language therapists often find it useful to have a physiotherapist present at swallowing assessments, to help position the patient and to deal promptly with any aspiration (section 15.17);
- advising nurses and other carers on the best way to position patients to prevent changes in tone that may lead ultimately to contractures and further limitation of function (section 15.20);
- teaching the nurses or informal carers the best way to handle the patient to avoid pain or injury to the patient or carer. This will often involve teaching proper methods of transferring, lifting, standing and walking the patient;
- providing therapy to relieve the symptoms associated with painful shoulders or swollen limbs (sections 15.24 and 15.25);
- providing therapy to improve the patient's mobility and arm function (section 15.21);
- advising on walking aids and splints (section 15.32.1) that may sometimes improve a patient's function.

Occupational therapist

Occupational therapists fulfil several roles in the management of stroke patients. These are usually fairly limited in the very early period after a severe stroke, but become more important as the patient recovers and as self-care becomes more relevant. These roles include the following five components:

- an early assessment of the patient to find out how each impairment is likely to restrict the patient's function. This requires an assessment of what the patient was able to do before the stroke and of what their home circumstances are—e.g. ease of access to the front door, bedroom, toilet, or bathroom;
- an assessment of the patient's visuospatial functioning. It is important to remember that many of the objective tests of these aspects of the stroke patient use an occupational therapist's assessment as the gold standard (Stone *et al.* 1991) (section 15.28);
- training the patient and the carer to carry out everyday activities, despite the patient's impairments, is a crucial role (section 15.32). This involves finding the best way of achieving a particular activity for that individual patient. Most input is spent on the activities of daily living (Table 17.19), although in specialized units or those dealing with younger patients, therapy aimed at return to an occupation (section 15.33.2) or leisure activity (section 15.33.3) may be available;
- provision of aids and adaptations to allow patients to function better. In the UK, this includes wheelchair provision, feeding and kitchen aids and bathroom aids, amongst many others (section 15.32);
- assessment of patients' ability to function in their own home. This is often done before discharge in patients who have been admitted to hospital, and is an important element of discharge planning. It is important in identifying problems that are specific to the patient's own home environment and which may have to be solved by further training or by provision of aids or adaptations.

Speech and language therapist

As their title suggests, speech and language therapists have several roles in the care of stroke patients. They include:

- assessment of swallowing safety both initially and as the patient improves, so that their diet and fluid intake matches their swallowing abilities (section 15.17);
- teaching the patient, nurses, or family who are involved with feeding, techniques that help overcome a swallowing impairment and avoid aspiration;
- teaching the patients exercises that *may* increase the rate of recovery of swallowing problems (section 15.17);
- diagnosis and assessment of the patient's communication problems (section 15.30);
- informing both formal and informal carers of the nature of the patient's communication problems. Patients, their families and even the professionals caring for the patient often have great difficulty in understanding what is wrong with a dysphasic patient. They may think the patient is 'confused', 'demented', or simply 'mad'. Because problems with communication so often lead to emotional distress, most therapists take on a counselling role;
- teaching patients, carers or even volunteers strategies to allow the patient to communicate effectively using language (spoken or written), gesture, or communication aids where appropriate;
- providing therapy that *may* enhance the recovery of communication difficulties (section 15.30).

Social worker

The role of the social worker is bound to vary in different societies. In the UK, Australia and the Netherlands (which are the countries we have direct experience of), the social worker is likely to:

- provide patients and their families with practical advice and help at all stages of the patient's illness. For example, arranging subsidized transport for the family to visit the hospital, or extra home care for a dependent relative if the stroke patient was their main carer before admission. Social workers often help with any financial problems that have arisen because the main 'bread-winner' has had a stroke, e.g. by applying for allowances or grants;

• be involved helping to plan the patient's discharge from hospital, or change of accommodation. Social workers often spend a lot of time identifying the wishes and needs of the patient and family and then, with the rest of the team, trying to meet them. Where patients are unable to make decisions for themselves and have no close family, the social worker may need to act as the patient's advocate and make arrangements for financial affairs to be taken care of, perhaps even arranging any change of accommodation (e.g. transfer to a nursing home);

• follow up patients and families after the patient's discharge from hospital, to identify their changing need for support and to make adjustments to any care package;

• provide counselling that *may* be helpful in allowing patients and families to come to terms with the change in circumstances brought about by the stroke. Some organize groups of patients, carers, or both to help solve problems.

One function that should be shared by all members of the team is that of monitoring the patient's condition. Nurses and therapists, in particular, spend a lot of their time handling patients and observing the patient's performance, so they are often in an ideal position to notice the relatively minor changes that may be an early sign of a complication, which might benefit from early treatment.

All members of the team should be alert to changes in the patient's condition that may indicate the development of a complication.

Are the interventions of the team members effective?

It is clear from a systematic review of randomized trials that, compared with the traditional, disorganized pattern of care provided on general medical wards, care coordinated by a well-organized multidisciplinary team results in a better clinical outcome for stroke patients (Stroke Unit Trialists' Collaboration 1997, 2000). However, exactly which specific aspects of this model of care bring about these benefits is unclear (section 17.4.2). Physicians often question the effectiveness of physiotherapy, occupational therapy, speech and language therapy and social work. They point to the lack of research evidence to support the effectiveness of these professionals (but interestingly, without questioning their own effectiveness), or they emphasize particular studies that appear to demonstrate the ineffectiveness of other professions. Unfortunately, these 'negative' studies have, in general, asked the wrong questions, measured the wrong outcomes, been too small, and have not evaluated the intervention in the context of a well-organized stroke team. This has possibly resulted in 'false-negative' studies, with a resulting rejection of valuable team members. Failure to demonstrate a definite effect cannot be taken as proof of a lack of effect (Altman & Bland 1995). There may be uncertainty about the effectiveness, optimum 'dose' and duration of some of the specific therapeutic manoeuvres they use (in common with many medical practices) but, as we have shown, this type of input forms only a small part of their contribution to the care of stroke patients. In fact, there are a number of well conducted randomized trials that have established that interventions by therapists do improve patient outcome (e.g. Walker *et al.* 1999; Gilbertson *et al.* 2000). The evidence for the effectiveness of specific aspects of their work is discussed later (Chapter 15).

10.3.7 Multidisciplinary team meetings

The team must meet regularly if it is to work effectively. All the stroke units included in the recent systematic review of the randomized controlled trials held at least weekly meetings of the multidisciplinary team, separate from conventional ward rounds (Langhorne & Dennis 1998). These meetings have several important functions:

• the entire team can be introduced to new patients and their problems;

• existing patients can be reviewed, and if individual team members have noted a change in their condition or a new problem, this can be communicated to the other members;

• after reviewing each patient's progress and any developing problems, realistic goals can be set jointly, and an appropriate course of action to meet those goals can be agreed (section 10.3.3);

• verbal reports of individual therapist's assessments, and in particular the results of pre-discharge home visits, can be discussed and detailed plans for discharge can be made;

• meetings have an educational role for the team members, students and visitors. For example, we often show the patient's brain CT and discuss the likely pathogenesis of the stroke and any rationale for treatment or therapy.

So that important details are not overlooked, it may be useful to agree a formal structure to the discussions. The structure we have adopted is discussed below. This is not rigidly adhered to, but forms a framework for discussions about individual patients.

Structure of team discussion

The medical details of any new patients are presented by the physician, including a brief account of the patient's symptoms and any relevant past history, including risk factors and the presumed cause of the stroke. The patient's social background is presented briefly by the clinician, but other members of the team are often able to contribute extra details. The patient's neurological impairments are discussed, and the therapists have often identified some that may not have been obvious to the physician. By the time of the meeting, the nursing staff can report on the functional consequences of these impairments (i.e. disability), and using the information about pre-stroke activities, some estimate of the stroke's likely effect on the patient's life after the stroke can be made (i.e. predicted handicap).

At each subsequent meeting, we introduce the patient briefly with a résumé of the date of stroke, stroke pathology, clinical type and presumed cause. We then summarize the problems, goals and actions that were agreed at the last meeting. Each member of the team is then invited to update the rest of the team on the patient's progress, what problems and goals have been solved or achieved, what new goals they plan to set, and how they plan to achieve them. Usually we do this in a set order that tends to reflect the way we think about patients, i.e. pathology, impairment, disability and handicap. The physician starts by updating the team on any changes in the patient's medical condition or the results of any important investigations that may be relevant to other team members. The nurses then give an overall report on the patient's progress, including current performance on the Barthel Index (Table 17.19). This usefully highlights many of the patient's functional problems, as well as giving an objective indication of progress. The therapists follow: first the physiotherapist, then the speech therapist and lastly the occupational therapist. The first two tend to focus more on impairments and the patient's basic functions such as mobility, swallowing and communication, whilst the occupational therapist usually focuses on the broader range of disabilities and how these are likely to affect the patient's everyday life. Lastly, the social worker reports on any problems which close contact with the family may have revealed and any progress regarding discharge planning. This sequence also has the advantage that the occupational therapist and social worker can make use of the information from the others in formulating their own goals and actions.

The discussion is then opened up, and longer-term goals such as timing of home visits, discharges and case (family) conferences are set, and we decide who will do what by the next meeting. This includes deciding who should communicate with the patient and family to ensure that they are involved with the goal-setting process and that their views are taken into account.

Multidisciplinary teams may lack effectiveness if each member is not given an equal chance to contribute. Inevitably, teams will include some more assertive individuals and other less outgoing members, the former tending to dominate discussions. It is important that the team leader—often the physician—ensures that individual members do not monopolize the discussions to the extent that others are not heard. The framework we have adopted lessens the likelihood of this arising, although of course not every member will necessarily have something useful to contribute in each case.

It is important that the person chairing the team meetings should ensure that no individual member, including the chairperson, monopolizes the discussion to the extent that others are not heard.

Involving patients and carers in team meetings

Neither the patient nor the family have been mentioned yet as having a direct input into the team meetings, although their input is obviously crucial in setting goals and planning discharge from hospital. We do not invite them to attend each meeting, but we do try to find out their views on certain issues in advance of the meeting. We also try to ensure that the nature and conclusions of the discussion at the meeting are communicated back to the patient and/or family by the most appropriate team member, most often the nurse. Although it is sometimes vital to involve the patient and families in discussions, we feel that their attendance at each weekly meeting would inhibit the discussion and might be distressing for them. It would also make meetings longer and more unwieldy. Occasionally, we do hold separate team meetings (case conferences or family meetings) to which the patient, family and any other people who are involved—such as the district (community) nurse and home care organizer—are invited. These meetings are useful in planning hospital discharge in complex cases and in resolving differences of opinion between the team members and the patient or family.

Team building

We have found it useful to have separate team meetings at which patients are not discussed. On these occasions, we discuss general management issues, how the team is working, what the problems are, and any changes that might be made in the way we work. These sessions also allow individuals to tell the rest of the team about certain specialized aspects of their jobs. This, we believe, not only encourages some blurring of the distinctions between their functions but also aids team building. Each member can more fully appreciate the contribution made by other members.

We find it useful to have separate team meetings where patients are not discussed. On these occasions, we discuss general management issues, how the team is working, what the problems are, and any changes that might be made in the way we work.

Recording the work of the team

We have not yet found a totally satisfactory method of recording the work of the team. Traditionally, members have each kept their own records so that they may refer to them, but this inevitably leads to much unnecessary duplication. However, a unified record has disadvantages, the main one being that different members of the team require information of varying detail. Thus, the physiotherapist's record contains very detailed notes on the patient's motor functioning that are irrelevant to the social worker. Also, the records may be needed simultaneously by the physiotherapist in the gym and by the occupational therapist on a home visit. In our units, each profession has therefore kept its own records, but they do all make entries in nurses' records. The nurses base their care plans on the discussions at the team meetings. This has been helped by their adoption of a problem-orientated approach, so that the nurses regularly record the patients' problems, the goals and actions aimed at attaining the goals. A compromise in which core details are collected once and shared, whilst more detailed records are kept by each team member, might provide the best and most efficient solution. We also increasingly use structured records in which the results of common assessments and actions taken require only a tick, date and signature, for example www.dcn.ed.ac.uk/spgm. In the future, increased use of information technology may facilitate a combined patient record that avoids some of these problems (Kalra & Fowle 1994). We do ensure that changes in the patient's condition, key decisions and proposed actions (by whom and by when) are recorded in the medical notes. This is important to avoid unnecessary and time-wasting repetition at future meetings and to ensure that decisions lead on to actions.

10.4 Some difficult ethical issues

When patients are judged unlikely to achieve a reasonable quality of life if they survive, many clinicians decide not to strive to ensure survival. This is an extremely difficult decision, since as we have already discussed (section 10.2.7), there are considerable difficulties in predicting outcome reliably. Patients who have had a major stroke are often not in a position to make decisions about their treatment because, due to a depressed conscious level, language or visuospatial problems, they are unable to understand or communicate. Under these circumstances, the family or potential carers should be included in the decision-making process. The family can often provide information allowing judgements to be made about what the patient's likely wishes are. However, some relatives may have their own interests and not just those of the patient to consider. Younger relatives may gain financially from the death of an older relative, and death removes the obligation to care for a severely disabled person. Patients may have even written down what they would like to happen in the event of a life-threatening illness (i.e. a living will). The status of these so called 'living wills' varies from country to country, however. Also, the question arises whether patients' judgements made whilst in good health about the value of life in a dependent state retain their validity. We have encountered people who have become severely disabled and yet have accepted their disability and felt that their quality of life is acceptable or even very good.

It is difficult to know how to react to patients' previously expressed view that they would never, ever want to live in a dependent state or go to a nursing home, when they then seem to cling to life after a major stroke.

One has to be particularly careful in assessing the likely prognosis of an individual patient with an apparently severe stroke. A relatively minor stroke that is complicated by another medical problem (e.g. pneumonia) may be impossible to differentiate from a severe stroke (section 15.4). The complicating medical problem may, if identified, be treated easily to achieve a very satisfactory clinical outcome for the patient.

It is not always easy to distinguish between a patient who has had a catastrophic stroke and one who has had a less severe stroke that is complicated and worsened by infection, epileptic seizures or metabolic problems. The prognosis is much worse for the former patient than the latter one.

Perhaps the most common dilemma is whether or not to give fluids or nutritional support to a patient with an 'apparently severe stroke' who is unable to swallow (Macfie 1997). Few would argue against giving parenteral fluids to a conscious patient to prevent dehydration, thirst and discomfort. However, if the patient is unconscious and thus probably unaware of discomfort, then there is more uncertainty about what to do for the best. Also, if the patient develops an infection very soon after the onset of the stroke, apart from the difficulties mentioned above in assessing the severity of stroke, the question arises as to how aggressively one should treat the patient. Are intravenous antibiotics, physiotherapy or even artificial ventilation and inotropic support appropriate?

There are some facts worth considering before making these difficult decisions. Firstly, most patients who are unconscious after a stroke die in the first few days from the direct neurological effects of the stroke on brainstem function, and not from dehydration or infection (Bounds *et al.* 1981; Silver *et al.* 1984; Bamford *et al.* 1990b) (section 10.2.3). Therefore, by simply giving fluids, it is unlikely that the lives of many patients will be greatly prolonged, but it may give more time to make an accurate assessment of prognosis. If one elects to give a patient fluids, antibiotics or even nutritional support via a feeding tube, this clearly does not have to be continued on a long-term basis. However, in some countries there are laws that prevent clinicians from withdrawing treatment of this kind, and many clinicians feel more uncomfortable about stopping a treatment that they have started than about not starting it in the first place. Apart from worrying about medicolegal issues, one has to consider the reaction of the family. However, in our experience, if the clinician has spent enough time informing the family of the patient's state and likely prognosis, and has involved them in the decisions, then withdrawal of fluids, feeding or antibiotics is usually not a major problem. Unfortunately, in some countries there is a trend for such decisions—especially in severely brain-damaged children and patients in a persistent vegetative state—to be deferred to the legal profession. We cannot hope to have the answers to all these difficult problems, but perhaps it is worth suggesting a general approach that we have found practicable.

Firstly, collect accurate and unbiased information about the patient's life prior to the stroke. It is inadequate to base one's decisions on some measure of the severity of just the stroke, since this may be difficult to estimate accurately, and other factors will influence the prognosis (section 15.4). The patient's pre-stroke functional level and social activity are crucial in making these decisions. Unfortunately, this information is often not collected in sufficient detail during the acute phase, because its relevance to acute care is not recognized (section 10.3.2). One might be less aggressive in treating patient A, who was previously handicapped, miserable and in pain from severe arthritis and living in an institution, than patient B, who has an equally severe stroke but was previously living at home independently with his or her family. Usually, the patient's pre-stroke handicap sets the ceiling on the potential post-stroke outcome, so that these two patients have very different outlooks. It is still a difficult—some would say an impossible—judgement to say whether patient A's life is worth prolonging. Next, it is important to make a detailed assessment of the patient's condition in order to make the best possible judgement about the prognosis. Thirdly, formulate the alternative management plans that might be adopted. These should include those from the most aggressive to the most conservative. Finally, all options must be discussed with other members of the team and any close family members. The family needs to be given accurate information about the diagnosis, problems, likely outcomes and treatment possibilities. It is probably unfair to suggest that the decisions are theirs, but any decision the clinician makes should ideally be compatible with their views. If one does not take the families' wishes into account one is inviting trouble, complaints—and nowadays litigation. It is worth making it clear to them that few decisions are irreversible (except perhaps turning off a ventilator), since circumstances change. One is often in a much better position to make an accurate prognosis having observed the patient's progress over a few days than on the day of the stroke, so that what appeared to be an appropriate intervention on day 1 may appear less appropriate after a few days. The development of better tools to help predict prognosis, and studies that give a better understanding of the effect of our supportive interventions, should make these difficult decisions somewhat easier in the future.

Involve other members of the team and the patient's family in any decisions about how aggressively one should strive to keep a patient alive. Emphasize that most decisions can be reviewed—and reversed—in the light of the patient's progress.

References

Please note that all references taken from *The Cochrane Library* are given a current date as this database is updated on a quarterly basis. Please refer to the current *Cochrane Library* article for the latest review. The same applies to the *British Medical Journal* 'Clinical Evidence' series which is updated every six months.

Adams, H.P. Jr, Davis, P.H., Leira, E.C. *et al.* (1999) Baseline NIH stroke scale score strongly predicts outcome after stroke: a report of the Trial of Org 10172 in Acute Stroke Treatment (TOAST). *Neurology* **53**, 126–131.

Allen, C.M.C. (1984a) Predicting outcome after acute stroke: role of computerised tomography [letter]. *Lancet* **ii**, 25 August, 464–465.

Allen, C.M.C. (1984b) Predicting the outcome of acute stroke: a prognostic score. *Journal of Neurology, Neurosurgery and Psychiatry* **47**, 475–480.

Altman, D.G. & Bland, J.M. (1995) Absence of evidence is not evidence of absence. *British Medical Journal* **311**, 485.

Anderson, C.S., Jamrozik, K.D., Burvill, P.W., Chakera, T.M., Johnson, G.A. & Stewart-Wynne, E.G. (1993) Ascertaining the true incidence of stroke. Experience from the Perth Community Stroke Study, 1989–90. *Medical Journal of Australia* **158**, 80–84.

Anderson, C.S., Jamrozik, K.D., Broadhurst, R.J. & Stewart-Wynne, E.G. (1994) Predicting survival for 1 year among different subtypes of stroke. results from the Perth Community Stroke Study. *Stroke* **25**, 1935–1944.

Ashburn, A. (1997) Physical recovery following stroke. *Physiotherapy* **83**, 480–490.

Asplund, K., Bonita, R., Kuulasmaa, K. *et al.* (1995) Multinational comparisons of stroke epidemiology: evaluation of case ascertainment in the WHO MONICA Stroke Study. *Stroke* **26**, 355–360.

Bamford, J., Sandercock, P., Warlow, C. & Gray, M. (1986) Why are patients with acute stroke admitted to hospital? *British Medical Journal* **292**, 1369–1372.

Bamford, J., Sandercock, P.A.G., Jones, L. & Warlow, C.P. (1987) The natural history of lacunar infarction: the Oxfordshire Community Stroke Project. *Stroke* **18**, 545–551.

Bamford, J., Sandercock, P., Dennis, M. *et al.* (1988) A prospective study of acute cerebrovascular disease in the community: the Oxfordshire Community Stroke Project 1981–86. 1: methodology, demography and incident cases of first-ever stroke. *Journal of Neurology, Neurosurgery and Psychiatry* **51**, 1273–1380.

Bamford, J., Sandercock, P.A.G., Dennis, M.S. & Warlow, C.P. (1990a) A prospective study of acute cerebrovascular disease in the community: the Oxfordshire Community Stroke Project 1981–86, 2: incidence, case fatality rates and overall outcome at one year of cerebral infarction, primary intracerebral and subarachnoid haemorrhage. *Journal of Neurology, Neurosurgery and Psychiatry* **53**, 16–22.

Bamford, J., Dennis, M.S., Sandercock, P., Burn, J. & Warlow, C. (1990b) The frequency, cause and timing of death within 30 days of a first stroke: the Oxfordshire Community Stroke Project. *Journal of Neurology, Neurosurgery and Psychiatry* **53**, 824–829.

Bamford, J., Sandercock, P.A.G., Dennis, M.S., Burn, J. & Warlow, C.P. (1991) Classification and natural history of clinically identifiable subtypes of cerebral infarction. *Lancet* **337**, 1521–1526.

Barer, D.H. (1990) The influence of visual and tactile inattention on predictions for recovery from acute stroke. *Quarterly Journal of Medicine* **273**, 21–32.

Bero, L.A., Grilli, R., Grimshaw, J.M. *et al.* (1998) Closing the gap between research and practice: an overview of systematic reviews of interventions to promote the implementation of research findings. *British Medical Journal* **317**, 465–468.

Bonita, R., Broad, J.B., Beaglehole, R. (1993) Changes in stroke incidence and case-fatality in Auckland, New Zealand, 1981–91. *Lancet* **342**, 1470–1473.

Bonita, R., Anderson, C.S., Broad, J.B. *et al.* (1994) Stroke incidence and case fatality in Australasia: comparison of the Auckland and Perth population-based stroke registers. *Stroke* **25**, 552–557.

Bounds, J.V., Weibers, D.O., Whisnant, J.P. & Okazaki, H. (1981) Mechanisms and timing of deaths from cerebral infarction. *Stroke* **12**, 474–477.

Britton, M., de Faire, U., Helmers, C. & Miah, K. (1980) Prognostication in acute cerebrovascular disease. *Acta Medica Scandinavica* **207**, 37–42.

Burn, J., Dennis, M.S., Bamford, J., Sandercock, P.A.G., Wade, D. & Warlow, C.P. (1994) Long-term risk of recurrent stroke after a first-ever stroke: the Oxfordshire Community Stroke Project. *Stroke* **25**, 333–337.

Cohen, L.G., Ziemann, U., Chen, R. *et al.* (1998) Studies of neuroplasticity with transcranial magnetic stimulation. *Journal of Clinical Neurophysiology* **15**, 305–324.

Counsell, C. (1998) *The prediction of outcome in patients with acute stroke.* DM thesis, Cambridge.

Crisi, G., Colombo, A., de Santis, M., Guerzoni, M.C., Calo, M. & Panzetti, P. (1984) CT and cerebral ischemic infarcts. Correlations between morphological and clinical prognostic findings. *Neuroradiology* **26**, 101–105.

Davenport, R.J., Dennis, M.S. & Warlow, C.P. (1995) Improving the recording of the clinical assessment of stroke patients using a clerking proforma. *Age and Ageing* **24**, 43–48.

Davenport, R.J., Dennis, M.S., Wellwood, I. & Warlow, C.P. (1996) Complications following acute stroke. *Stroke* **27**, 415–420.

Dennis, M.S., Burn, J.P.S., Sandercock, P., Bamford, J.M., Wade, D.T. & Warlow, C.P. (1993) Long term survival after first ever stroke: the Oxfordshire Community Stroke Project. *Stroke* **24**, 796–800.

Dombovy, M.L., Basfird, J.R., Whisnant, J.P. & Bergstalh, E.J. (1987) Disability and use of rehabilitation services following stroke in Rochester, Minnesota, 1975–79. *Stroke* **18**, 830–836.

Dromerick, A. & Reding, M. (1994) Medical and neurological complications during in-patient stroke rehabilitation. *Stroke* **25**, 358–361.

Duncan, P.W., Goldstein, L.B., Matchar, D., Divin, G.W. & Feussner, J. (1992) Measurement of motor recovery after stroke. Outcome assessment and sample size requirements. *Stroke* **23**, 1084–1089.

Duncan, P.W., Jorgensen, H.S. & Wade, D.T. (2000) Outcome measures in acute stroke trials. A systematic review and some recommendations to improve practice. *Stroke* **31**, 1429–1438.

Easton, V. on behalf of the FOOD Trial Collaboration (2000) A tool for stratifying patients by severity in randomised trials of acute stroke treatments. *Cerebrovascular Diseases* **10** (Suppl. 2), 88 [abstract].

Effective Health Care (1994) *Implementing Clinical Practice Guidelines: Can Guidelines Be Used to Improve Practice?* University of Leeds, Leeds.

Feigin, V.L., Wiebers, D.O., Nikitin, Y.P. *et al.* (1996) Epidemiology of stroke in different regions of Siberia, Russia, 1987–88: population-based study in Novosibirsk, Krasnoyarsk, Tynda and Anadyr. *European Journal of Neurology* **3**, 16–22.

Fiorelli, M., Alperovitch, A., Argentino, C. *et al.* (1995) Prediction of long-term outcome in the early hours following acute ischaemic stroke. *Archives of Neurology* **52**, 250–255.

Fullerton, K.J., MacKenzie, G. & Stout, R.W. (1988) Prognostic indices in stroke. *Quarterly Journal of Medicine* **25**, 147–162.

Garraway, W.M., Whisnant, J.P. & Drury, I. (1983) The changing pattern of survival following stroke. *Stroke* **14**, 699–703.

van Gijn, J. (1992) Subarachnoid haemorrhage. *Lancet* **339**, 653–655.

Gilbertson, L., Langhorne, P., Walker, A. & Allen, A. (2000) Domiciliary occupational therapy for stroke patients discharged from hospital: a randomised controlled trial. *British Medical Journal* **320**, 603–606.

Gladman, J.R.F., Harwood, D.M.J. & Barer, D.H. (1992) Predicting the outcome of acute stroke: prospective evaluation of five multivariate models and comparison with simple methods. *Journal of Neurology, Neurosurgery and Psychiatry* **55**, 347–351.

Gompertz, P., Pound, P. & Ebrahim, S. (1994) Predicting stroke outcome: Guy's prognostic score in practice. *Journal of Neurology, Neurosurgery and Psychiatry* **57**, 932–935.

Granger, C.V., Hamilton, B.B., Gresham, G.E. & Kramer, A.A. (1989) The Stroke Rehabilitation Outcome Study, 2: relative merits of the total Barthel Index Score and a four-item subscore in predicting patient outcomes. *Archives of Physical Medicine and Rehabilitation* **70**, 100–103.

Gray, C.S., French, J.M., Bates, D., Cartlidge, N.E.F., James, O.F.W. & Venables, G. (1990) Motor recovery following acute stroke. *Age and Ageing* **19**, 179–184.

Gresham, G.E., Kelly-Hayes, M., Wolf, P.A., Beiser, A.S., Kase, C.S. & D'Agostino, R.B. (1998) Survival and functional status 20 or more years after a first stroke: the Framingham Study. *Stroke* **29**, 793–797.

Hancock, R.J.Y., Oddy, M., Saweirs, W.M. & Court, B. (1997) The RCP stroke audit package in practice. *Journal of the Royal College of Physicians of London* **31**, 74–78.

Henon, H., Godefroy, O., Leys, D. *et al.* (1995) Early predictors of death and disability after acute cerebral ischaemic event. *Stroke* **26**, 392–398.

Hier, D.B. & Edelstein, G. (1991) Deriving clinical prediction rules from stroke outcome research. *Stroke* **22**, 1431–1436.

Horner, R.D., Matchar, D.B., Divine, G.W. & Feussner, J.R. (1995) Relationship between physician specialty and the selection and outcome of ischaemic stroke patients. *Health Service Research* **30** (2), 275–288.

Jongbloed, L. (1990) Problems of methodological heterogeneity in studies predicting disability after stroke. *Stroke* **21** (Suppl. II), 32–4.

Kalra, L. & Fowle, A.J. (1994) An integrated system for multidisciplinary assessments in stroke rehabilitation. *Stroke* **24**, 2210–2214.

Kalra, L., Yu, G., Wilson, K. & Roots, P. (1995) Medical complications during stroke rehabilitation. *Stroke* **26**, 990–994.

Kojima, S., Omura, T., Wakamatsu, W. *et al.* (1990) Prognosis and disability of stroke patients after 5 years in Akita, Japan. *Stroke* **21**, 72–77.

Kwakkel, G., Wagenaar, R.C., Kollen, B.J. & Lankhorst, G.J. (1996) Predicting disability in stroke: a critical review of the literature. *Age and Ageing* **25**, 479–489.

Lai, S.M., Duncan, P.W. & Keighley, J. (1998) Prediction of functional outcome after stroke. Comparison of the Orpington Prognostic Scale and the NIH Stroke Scale. *Stroke* **29**, 1838–1842.

Langhorne, P. & Dennis, M. (1998) Implications for planning stroke services. In: *Stroke Units: an Evidence-Based Approach* (eds P. Langhorne & M. Dennis), pp. 66–79. BMJ Books, London.

Langhorne, P., Stott, D.J., Robertson, L. *et al.* (2000) Medical complications in hospitalised stroke patients: a multicentre study. *Stroke* **31**, 1223–1229.

Lincoln, N.B., Jackson, J.M., Edmans, J.A. *et al.* (1990) The accuracy of predictions about progress of patients on a stroke unit. *Journal of Neurology, Neurosurgery and Psychiatry* **53**, 972–975.

Lincoln, N.B., Willis, D., Philips, S.A., Juby, L.C. & Berman, P. (1996) Comparison of rehabilitation practice on hospital wards for stroke patients. *Stroke* **27**, 18–23.

Loewen, S.C. & Anderson, B.A. (1990) Predictors of stroke outcome using objective measurement scales. *Stroke* **21**, 78–81.

Macfie, J. (1997) Ethics and nutritional support. *Wiener Klinische Wochenschrift* **109**, 850–857.

Moloney, A., Critchelow, B. & Jones, K. (1999) A. multi-disciplinary care pathway in stroke: does it improve care? *Age and Ageing* **28** (Suppl. 1), 42–43.

Muir, K.W., Weir, C.J., Murray, G.D., Povey, C. & Lees, K.R. (1996) Comparison of neurological scales and scoring systems for acute stroke prognosis. *Stroke* **27**, 1817–1820.

Peltonnen, M., Stegmayr, B. & Asplund, K. (1999) Marked improvement since 1985 in short-term and long-term survival after stroke. *Cerebrovascular Diseases* **9** (Suppl. 1), 62.

Petty, B.W., Brown, R.D., Whisnant, J.P., Sicks, J.D., O'Fallon, W.M. & Wiebers, D.O. (1998) Ischemic stroke: outcomes, patient mix, and practice variation for neurologists and generalists in a community. *Neurology* **50**, 1669–1678.

Pound, P., Bury, M., Gompertz, P. & Ebrahim, S. (1995) Stroke patients' views of their admission to hospital. *British Medical Journal* **311**, 18–22.

Prescott, R.J., Garraway, W.M. & Akhtar, A.J. (1982) Predicting functional outcome following acute stroke using a standard clinical examination. *Stroke* **13**, 641–647.

Rapisarda, G., Bastings, E., Maetens de Noorhout, A., Pennisi, G. & Delwaide, P.J. (1996) Can motor recovery in stroke patients be predicted by early transcranial magnetic stimulation? *Stroke* **27**, 2191–2196.

Ricci, S., Celani, M.G., La Rosa, F. *et al.* (1991) Sepivac: a community-based study of stroke incidence in Umbria, Italy. *Journal of Neurology, Neurosurgery and Psychiatry* **54**, 695–698.

Rodgers, H., Thomson, R.G., Gani, A. *et al.* (1999) *Teesside Stroke Register Final Report II: Service Utilization.* Report for NHS R&D Programme.

University of Newcastle.

Rose, L., Bakal, D.A., Fung, T.S., Farn, P. & Weaver, L.E. (1994) Tactile extinction and functional status after stroke: a preliminary investigation. *Stroke* **25**, 1973–1976.

Sacco, R.L., Wolf, P.A., Kannel, W.B. & McNamara, P.M. (1982) Survival and recurrence following stroke: the Framingham Study. *Stroke* **13**, 290–295.

Sackett, D.L., Haynes, R.B., Guyatt, G.H. & Tugwell, M.D. (1991) *Clinical Epidemiology: a Basic Science for Clinical Medicine*, 2nd edn, pp. 173–185. Little, Brown, Boston.

Seitz, R.J., Azari, N.P., Knorr, U., Binkofski, F., Herzog, H. & Freund, H.J. (1999) The role of diaschisis in stroke recovery. *Stroke* **30**, 1844–1850.

Sheikh, K., Brennan, P.J., Meade, T.W., Smith, D.S. & Goldenberg, E. (1983) Predictors of mortality and disability in stroke. *Journal of Epidemiology and Community Health* **37**, 70–74.

Silver, F.L., Norris, J.W., Lewis, A.J. & Hachinski, V.C. (1984) Early mortality following stroke. a prospective view. *Stroke* **15**, 492–496.

Skilbeck, C.E., Wade, D.T., Hewer, R.L. & Wood, V.A. (1983) Recovery after stroke. *Journal of Neurology, Neurosurgery and Psychiatry* **46**, 5–8.

Slattery, J.M. & Hankey, G.J. (1992) Intracerebral haemorrhage: external validation and extension of a model for prediction of 30 day survival. *Annals of Neurology* **32**, 225–226.

Smith, M.T. & Baer, G.D. (1999) Achievement of simple morbidity milestones after stroke. *Archives of Physical Medicine and Rehabilitation* **80**, 442–447.

Stone, S.P., Wilson, B., Wroot, A. *et al.* (1991) The assessment of visuo-spatial neglect after acute stroke. *Journal of Neurology, Neurosurgery and Psychiatry* **54**, 345–350.

Stroke Unit Trialists' Collaboration (1997) Collaborative systematic review of the randomised trials of organised inpatient (stroke unit) care after stroke. *British Medical Journal* **314**, 1151–1159.

Stroke Unit Trialists' Collaboration (2000) Organised inpatient (stroke unit) care for stroke (Cochrane Review). In: *The Cochrane Library, Issue 1.* Update Software, Oxford.

Tanaka, H., Ueda, Y., Date, C. *et al.* (1981) Incidence of stroke in Shibata, Japan: 1976–78. *Stroke* **12**, 460–466.

Taub, N.A., Wolfe, C.D.A., Richardson, E. & Burney, P.G.J. (1994) Predicting the disability of first-time stroke sufferers at 1 year: 12-month follow-up of a population based cohort in Southeast England. *Stroke* **25**, 352–357.

Tijssen, C.C., Bento, P.M., Schulte, M.D., Anton, C.M. & Leyten, M.D. (1991) Prognostic significance of conjugate eye deviation in stroke patients. *Stroke* **22**, 200–202.

Tilling, K.Wolfe, C.D.A., Sdterne, J.A.C. & Rudd, A.G. (1999) Predicting and assessing recovery after stroke: use of the Barthel Index [abstract]. *Cerebrovascular Diseases* **9** (Suppl. 1), 23.

Tuhrim, S., Dambrosia, J.M., Price, T.R. *et al.* (1991) Intracerebral haemorrhage: external validation and extension of a model for prediction of 30 day survival. *Annals of Neurology* **29**, 658–663.

Turney, T.M., Garraway, M. & Whisnant, J.P. (1984) The natural history of hemispheric and brainstem infarction in Rochester, Minnesota. *Stroke* **15**, 790–794.

Valdimarsson, E., Bergvall, U. & Samuelsson, K. (1982) Prognostic significance of cerebral computed tomography results in supratentorial infarction. *Acta Neurologica Scandinavica* **65**, 133–145.

Wade, D.T. (1992) Stroke: rehabilitation and long-term care. *Lancet* **339**, 791–793.

Wade, D.T. (1998) Evidence relating to assessment in rehabilitation. *Clinical Rehabilitation* **12**, 183–186.

Wade, D.T. & Hewer, R.L. (1985) Outlook after an acute stroke: urinary incontinence and loss of consciousness compared in 532 patients. *Quarterly Journal of Medicine* **56**, 601–608.

Wade, D.T. & Langton Hewer, R. (1987) Functional abilities after stroke: measurement, natural history and prognosis. *Journal of Neurology, Neurosurgery and Psychiatry* **50**, 177–182.

Wade, D.T., Skilbeck, C.E. & Hewer, R.L. (1983) Predicting Barthel ADL score at 6 months after an acute stroke. *Archives of Physical Medicine and Rehabilitation* **64**, 24–28.

Wade, D.T., Wood, V.A. & Hewer, R.L. (1985) Recovery after stroke: the first 3 months. *Journal of Neurology, Neurosurgery and Psychiatry* **48**, 7–13.

Wade, D.T., Wood, V.A., Heller, A., Maggs, J. & Hewer, R.L. (1987) Walking after stroke: measurement and recovery over the first 3 months. *Scandinavian Journal of Rehabilitation Medicine* **19**, 25–30.

Walker, M.F., Gladman, J.R., Lincoln, N.B., Siemonsma, P. & Whiteley, T. (1999) Occupational therapy for stroke patients not admitted to hospital: a randomised controlled trial. *Lancet* **354**, 278–280.

Wardlaw, J.M., Lewis, S.C., Dennis, M.S., Counsell, C. & McDowall, M. (1998) Is visible infarction on computed tomography associated with an adverse prognosis in acute ischaemic stroke? *Stroke* **29**, 1315–1319.

Weiller, C. (1998) Imaging recovery from stroke. *Experimental Brain Research* **123**, 13–17.

Weingarten, S., Bolus, R., Riedinger, M.S., Maldonado, L., Stein, S. & Ellrodt, A.G. (1990) The principle of parsimony: Glasgow Coma Scale score predicts mortality as well as the APACHE II score for stroke patients. *Stroke* **21**, 1280–1282.

Wellwood, I., Dennis, M.S. & Warlow, C.P. (1995) A comparison of the Barthel Index and the OPCS disability instrument used to measure outcome after acute stroke. *Age and Ageing* **24**, 54–57.

WHO (1980) *International Classification of Impairments, Disabilities and Handicaps: Conference Papers.* World Health Organization, Geneva.

Witte, O.W. (1998) Lesion-induced plasticity as a potential mechanism for recovery and rehabilitative training. *Current Opinion in Neurology* **11**, 655–662.

van der Worp, H.B. & Kappelle, L.J. (1998) Complications of acute ischaemic stroke. *Cerebrovascular Diseases* **8**, 124–132.

CHAPTER ELEVEN

Specific treatment of acute ischaemic stroke

Focal cerebral ischaemia, caused by acute occlusion of a cerebral blood vessel or sometimes just by low blood flow, initiates a series of events which can lead to irreversible neuronal damage and cell death (i.e. infarction) in the part of the brain supplied by that vessel. Several pathophysiological cascades run in sequence (and in parallel). In the vascular system, rapid changes in platelet and coagulation factors, the vessel wall (particularly the endothelium) and in the thrombus itself interact to produce a very dynamic state, not only at the site of the vessel occlusion, but also more remotely, in both the macro- and microcirculation. In brain tissue, changes occur in neurones, glial cells and other structural components in differing degrees and at different times after the onset of ischaemia, which means that in humans cerebral infarction is a dynamic and highly unstable process, not a discrete 'one-off' event. In other words, infarction is *not* an 'all-or-nothing' episode which is instantaneous in onset, maximal in severity at the moment of onset and irreversibly complete within 6 h (Baron *et al.* 1995; Baron 1999). Specific treatments generally aim to affect one particular point in the pathophysiological cascade.

This chapter begins with a review of pathophysiology, particularly aspects which relate to the specific types of treatment that are described later in the chapter. As far as possible, we base the decision whether or not to use a particular treatment, not merely on its putative physiological effects, but on the evidence from randomized trials in patients which demonstrate the balance of clinical risk and benefit associated with its use. In view of this, the section on each of the specific treatments aims to assess the strength of evidence available and, where possible, to base any recommendations on the results of a systematic review (and meta-analysis) of all the relevant randomized trials of that particular treatment.

11.1 Pathophysiology of acute ischaemic stroke

The pathophysiology of acute ischaemic stroke encompasses two sequential processes: the vascular, haematological or cardiac events that cause the initial reduction (and subsequent change) in local cerebral blood flow; and then the alterations of cellular chemistry that are caused by ischaemia and which lead to necrosis of neurones, glia and other brain cells. This section will discuss cerebral metabolism, regulation of cerebral blood flow, molecular consequences of cerebral ischaemia and how understanding these processes leads on to the development of various treatments for acute ischaemic stroke. The causes of cerebral ischaemia have been described in Chapters 6 and 7.

11.1.1 Cerebral metabolism

Energy demand and cerebral blood flow

The human brain has a high metabolic demand for energy and, unlike other organs, uses glucose (about 75–100 mg/min, or 125 g/day) as its sole substrate for energy metabolism. Glucose is metabolized in the brain entirely via the glycolytic sequence and the tricarboxylic acid cycle (Fig. 11.1).

The brain uses glucose as its only source of energy. During aerobic metabolism each molecule of glucose produces 36 molecules of adenosine triphosphate (ATP), but during anaerobic metabolism only two molecules of ATP are produced along with lactic acid.

Each molecule of glucose is broken down in a series of enzymatic steps (glycolysis) into two molecules (2 M) of pyruvate. During these reactions, the oxidized form of nicotinamide adenine dinucleotide (NAD^+) is reduced (to NADH) and 2 M each of adenosine diphosphate (ADP) and intracellular phosphorus are converted to 2 M of adenosine triphosphate (ATP). In the *presence* of oxygen, pyruvate is metabolized, first by pyruvate dehydrogenase and then by a series of mitochondrial reactions, to carbon dioxide (CO_2) and water (H_2O) with the formation of 36 M of ATP. This is the maximum ATP yield. In the *absence* of oxygen, this sequence of events is blocked or retarded at the stage of pyruvate oxidation, leading to the reduction of pyruvate to lactate by NADH and lactic dehydrogenase. Anaerobic glycolysis therefore still leads to the formation of ATP, as well as lactate, but the energy yield is relatively small (2 M rather than 36 M of ATP from 1 M of glucose). In addition, lactic acid accumulates within and outside cells (hence, the cell is acidified) and mitochondria lose their ability to sequester calcium, so any calcium entering or released within the cell will raise the intracellular calcium level (Siesjö 1992a; Kristián & Siesjö 1998).

ATP is the universal currency for energy. Neurones in the brain require a constant supply of ATP to maintain their integrity and to keep the major intracellular cation, potassium ions (K^+), within the cell, and the major extracellular cations, sodium (Na^+) and calcium ions (Ca^{2+}), outside the cell. As the brain is unable to store energy, it requires a constant supply of oxygenated blood containing an adequate glucose concentration to maintain its function and structural integrity.

The resting brain consumes energy at the same rate as a 20-Watt light bulb.

Global cerebral blood flow (CBF), reflecting both grey and white matter compartments, per unit of brain in a healthy young adult, is about 50–55 mL/100 g of brain per minute, with significantly higher values in those below 20 years of age and lower values in those over 60 years (Leenders *et al.* 1990). For a brain of average weight (1300–1400 g in a 60–65 kg adult), which is only 2% of total adult body weight, the total CBF at rest is disproportionately large at about 800 mL/min, which is 15–20% of the total cardiac output (Kety 1950). At this level of blood flow, whole brain oxygen consumption, usually measured as the cerebral metabolic rate of oxygen ($CMRO_2$), is about 3.3–3.5 mL/100 g of brain per minute, or 45 mL of oxygen per minute, which is 20% of the total oxygen consumption of the body at rest.

11.1.2 Cerebral blood-flow regulation

The fraction of oxygen extracted from the blood, the oxygen extraction fraction (OEF), is fairly constant throughout the brain because CBF, cerebral blood volume (CBV) and $CMRO_2$ as well as the cerebral metabolic rate of glucose (CMRglu) are all coupled (Leenders *et al.* 1990). In the normal resting brain, measurements of CBF are therefore a reliable reflection of cerebral metabolism ($CMRO_2$). If CBF falls, however (down to a level of 20–25 mL/100 g brain per minute), the OEF increases to maintain the $CMRO_2$ (see below).

Over the past 50 years, methods of measuring CBF have become more accurate and reliable and have had a major impact on our understanding of the regulation of CBF and the pathogenesis of cerebral ischaemia (Kety & Schmidt 1945; Baron 1991, 1999; Pulsinelli 1992). Positron emission tomography (PET) now enables CBF, $CMRO_2$, OEF and CMRglu all to be measured in various regions of interest in the brain, both in normal people and after stroke (Baron 1991, 1999).

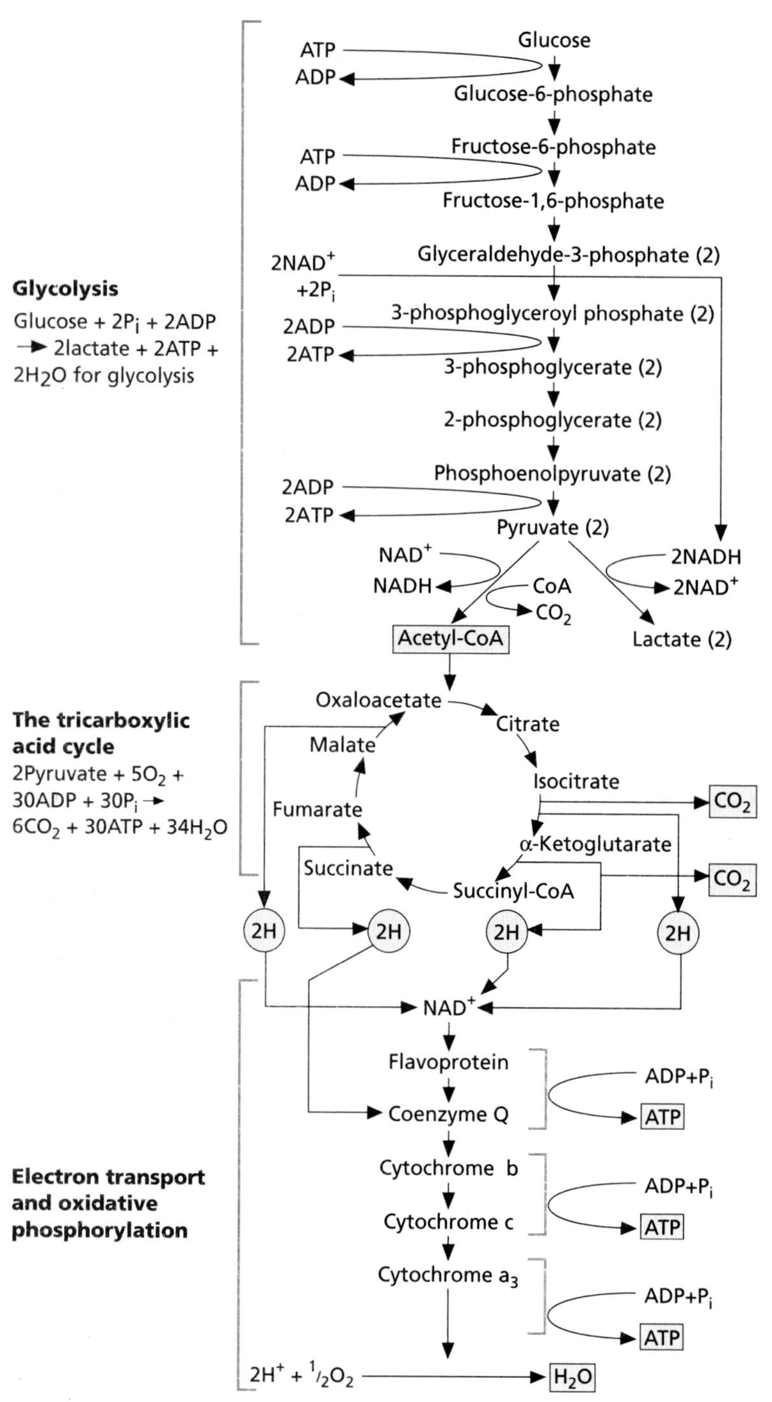

Overall: glucose + $6O_2$ + $36P_i$ + 36ADP → $6CO_2$ + 36ATP + $42H_2O$

Fig. 11.1 The aerobic metabolism of glucose. The stages of the complete aerobic oxidation of glucose to CO_2 and H_2O and the conservation of free energy as ATP. For the glycolytic sequence to pyruvate we have the reaction: glucose + 2ADP + $2P_i$ + $2NAD^+$ → 2pyruvate + 2NADH + $2H^+$ + 2ATP + $2H_2O$, and for the tricarboxylic acid cycle: 2pyruvate + $5O_2$ + 30ADP + $30P_i$ → $6CO_2$ + 30ATP + $34H_2O$. To these are added the equation for the oxidation of two molecules of extramitochondrial NADH formed in the glycolytic conversion of glucose to pyruvate. Oxidation of extramitochondrial NADH may generate either two or three molecules of ATP per pair of electrons, depending on how the electrons from extramitochondrial NADH enter the mitochondria. If we assume that two molecules of ATP are formed in this process, we have 2NADH + $2H^+$ + O_2 + 4ADP + $4P_i$ → $2NAD^+$ + 4ATP + $6H_2O$. The sum of the above three equations is therefore: glucose + $6O_2$ + 36ADP + $36P_i$ → $6CO_2$ + 36ATP + $42H_2O$. The overall equation of anaerobic glycolysis is: glucose + 2ADP + $2P_i$ → 2lactic acid + 2ATP + $2H_2O$.

Cerebral perfusion pressure (CPP)

Under normal conditions, blood flow through the brain is determined by the CPP at the base of the brain and by the cerebrovascular resistance (CVR) imposed by blood viscosity and the size of the intracranial vessels (i.e. flow = pressure/resistance). The CPP represents the difference between arterial pressure forcing blood into the cerebral circulation and the venous pressure. The mean CPP is the mean systemic arterial pressure at the base of the brain when in the recumbent position, which approximates to the diastolic blood pressure (about 80 mmHg), plus one-third of the pulse pressure (one-third of about 40 mmHg) minus the intracranial venous pressure (about 10 mmHg), i.e. 80–85 mmHg.

Cerebrovascular resistance

Under normal conditions, when resting CPP is constant, any change in CBF must be caused by a change in CVR, usually as a result of alteration in the diameter of small intracranial arteries or arterioles. Under these circumstances, there is a direct correlation between CBF and the intravascular CBV. CBF and CBV will both increase as vessels dilate and both decrease as vessels constrict. The CBV : CBF ratio remains relatively constant over a wide range of CBF at normal CPP.

When an artery narrows causing CVR to increase, or when CBF increases, the blood-flow velocity in that segment of artery increases. Although it may seem paradoxical that a reduction in lumenal diameter causes an increase in blood-flow velocity, think of using a hose: putting one's finger over the nozzle generates a high-pressure jet of water. The narrower the lumen at the nozzle, the greater the pressure (and velocity of flow) in the stream of water until the lumen is nearly occluded, at which point velocity becomes substantially reduced and the water dribbles out of the hose. This is one of the principles governing the interpretation of blood-flow velocities in the major basal arteries by transcranial Doppler ultrasound (section 6.7.9). Mean blood-flow velocities within the intracranial arteries vary from 40 to 70 cm/second. As blood-flow velocity is proportional to the second power of the vessel radius, it cannot be equated linearly with volume blood flow (mL/second), which is proportional to the fourth power of the vessel radius (Kontos 1989). If vessel calibre were constant, some assumptions could be made about volume flow from velocity measures, but the calibre of large cerebral arteries varies with changes in blood pressure, partial pressure of arterial carbon dioxide ($Paco_2$), intracranial pressure and age (Markwalder *et al.* 1984).

Metabolic rate of cerebral tissue

In the resting brain with normal CPP, CBF is closely matched to the metabolic demands of the tissue. Therefore, grey matter (which has a high metabolic rate) has higher regional CBF than white matter, which has a relatively low metabolic rate. The ratio between CBF and metabolism is fairly uniform in all areas of the brain and, consequently, the OEF and functional extraction of glucose from the blood are much the same in different areas. Normally, regional OEF is about one-third and the regional glucose extraction fraction is about 10% (Powers 1991). Similarly, local flow varies directly with local brain function by 10–20%, even though global CBF tends to be fairly stable under steady state conditions. For example, during voluntary hand movements, the metabolic activity of the contralateral motor cortex increases over a few seconds and is accompanied by rapid vasodilatation of the local cerebral resistance vessels, leading to an increase in CBF and CBV, rather than any increase in the OEF or the glucose extraction fraction (Lassen *et al.* 1977). Conversely, low regional metabolic activity (as may occur in a cerebral infarct) is associated with reduced metabolic demand and so low CBF. Therefore, low flow does not necessarily mean vessel occlusion but, in this case, non-functioning brain. Although this coupling of flow with metabolism and function has been suspected for over a century (Roy & Sherrington 1890), the mechanism is unknown; it may be that the metabolically active areas of brain produce vasodilatory metabolites, or the resistance vessels may be under neural regulation, or a combination of both (Lou *et al.* 1987).

> *In normal brain, blood flow is closely coupled with metabolic demand. However, if the brain is damaged, blood flow and metabolism become uncoupled and so normal flow no longer necessarily implies normal metabolism and function.*

Arterial carbon dioxide tension ($Paco_2$)

$Paco_2$ has a potent effect on CBF; a 1 mmHg rise in $Paco_2$ within the range of 20–60 mmHg in normal individuals, causes an immediate 3–5% increase in CBF due to dilatation of cerebral resistance vessels (Harper & Bell 1963). In *chronic* respiratory failure, however, causing CO_2 retention, CBF is normal (Fieschi & Lenzi 1983). Changes in arterial oxygen tension (Pao_2) have a modest inverse effect on CBF, unless the Pao_2 falls below about 50 mmHg (6.7 kPa) (Brown *et al.* 1985), when the resultant decline in the oxygen saturation of the blood leads to a fall in CVR and an increase in CBF. Increasing the Pao_2 above the normal level has little effect on CBF.

Whole-blood viscosity

Normally, CBF is inversely related to whole-blood viscosity (Thomas 1982). As the main determinant of whole-blood viscosity (at normal shear rates) is the haematocrit, it follows that CBF and haematocrit are inversely related. But, this relationship is not because the high haematocrit raises viscosity and thereby slows flow (at least not in normal vessels); rather, the higher oxygen content of high haematocrit blood allows CBF to be lower and yet maintain normal oxygen delivery to the tissues in accordance with metabolic demands (Brown & Marshall 1985; Brown *et al.* 1985). A practical example is encountered in patients with leukaemia or paraproteinaemia who have very high blood viscosity but normal CBF (or even high CBF if anaemia co-exists), because CBF depends more on the oxygen content of the blood (which is normal or low) than the viscosity (which is high) (Brown *et al.* 1985). However, at very low shear rates, which might be found in ischaemic brain, for example, because of local vasodilatation, whole-blood viscosity depends more on plasma fibrinogen than haematocrit (Weaver *et al.* 1969). In addition, other local factors such as red cell aggregation, platelet aggregation and perhaps increasing red cell fragility as a result of anoxia, all of which increase blood viscosity, may come into play to reduce flow (Wood & Kee 1985).

Autoregulation

Under normal conditions (i.e. mean systemic arterial blood pressure within 60–160 mmHg), CBF is maintained at a relatively constant level, irrespective of the cerebral perfusion pressure (Fig. 11.2). This capacity to maintain a constant CBF is due to the phenomenon of autoregulation (Powers 1991).

Autoregulation is the ability of cerebral blood flow to remain constant in the face of changes in cerebral perfusion pressure.

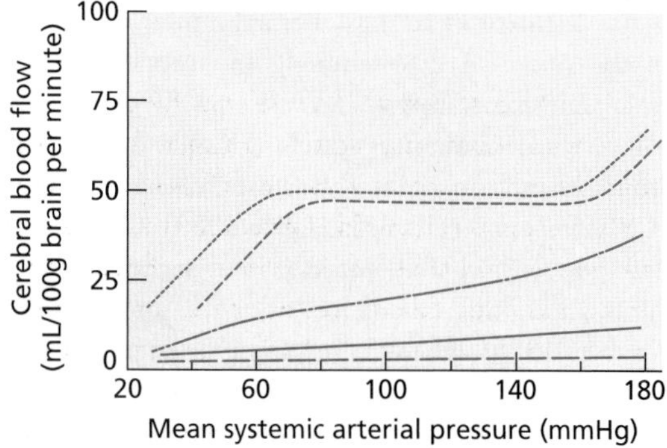

Fig. 11.2 Autoregulation. Relationship between mean systemic arterial blood pressure and cerebral blood flow (CBF) in normal brain tissue and in brain ischaemia. Under normal conditions, CBF is maintained at a relatively constant level, independent of the systemic arterial blood pressure, as long as the mean pressure remains between about 60 and 160 mmHg. This capacity to maintain a constant CBF is due to the phenomenon of autoregulation. In chronic hypertension the curve is shifted to the right. When the brain tissue has been damaged by ischaemia, autoregulation is less effective and CBF follows more closely the changes in systemic arterial pressure. This is particularly important during mild ischaemia when reductions in systemic arterial blood pressure can produce reductions in CBF from above 20 mL/100 g/min, which is sufficient to sustain brain function, to lethal levels below 10 mL/100 g/min (from Strandgaard *et al.* 1973; Dirnagl & Pulsinelli 1990).

Autoregulation is achieved primarily by varying pre-capillary resistance; compensatory vasodilatation of pial and intracerebral arterioles occurs when the blood pressure falls, and compensatory vasoconstriction when the blood pressure rises. Whether myogenic, metabolic or neurogenic processes are responsible for this response is unknown.

If mean arterial pressure falls below about 40–50 mmHg, compensatory vasodilatation and therefore cerebral perfusion reserve is exhausted, and CBF parallels the blood pressure (Harper 1966) (section 6.6.5). Because oxygen delivery to the brain normally far exceeds demand, metabolic activity is maintained at a mean blood pressure of around 40–50 mmHg by increasing the oxygen extraction from the blood (Fig. 11.3). This state of increased OEF has been termed 'misery perfusion' (Baron *et al.* 1981). However, when the OEF is maximal, a state of 'ischaemia' exists; flow is inadequate (< 20 mL/100 g brain per minute) to meet metabolic demands, cellular metabolism is impaired, and so $CMRO_2$ begins to fall (see below) (Powers *et al.* 1984; Pulsinelli 1992). As neuronal activity ceases, the patient usually develops symptoms of neurological dysfunction (if the whole brain is ischaemic, non-focal symptoms such as faintness occur, and if only part of the brain is ischaemic, focal symptoms such as hemiparesis occur).

If the mean arterial pressure rises above the autoregulatory range where compensatory vasoconstriction is maximal (i.e. above about 160 mmHg in normal people), then hyperaemia occurs followed by vasogenic oedema, raised intracranial pressure and the clinical syndrome of hypertensive encephalopathy (section 3.4.5).

The autoregulatory curve is 'set' higher in patients with long-standing hypertension and, consequently, these patients develop symptoms of ischaemia at a relatively higher blood pressure (e.g. mean below about 70 mmHg) than in non-hypertensive patients (e.g. mean below 50 mmHg) (Strandgaard *et al.* 1973; Strandgaard 1978; Barry *et al.* 1982) (Fig. 11.2).

Autoregulation tends to become gradually less effective with increasing age so that elderly people are more likely to develop symptoms of cerebral ischaemia with a fall in blood pressure induced by, for example, postural change (Wollner *et al.* 1979). The reason is not clear but may be related to areas of subclinical cerebral damage where the normal mechanisms of cerebrovascular control may no longer operate. It is also not surprising that autoregulation is impaired in a variety of disease states such as head trauma, diffuse cerebral hypoxia, ischaemic stroke, vasospasm secondary to subarachnoid haemorrhage and in some patients with carotid stenosis or occlusion (Symon *et al.* 1976; Fieschi & Lenzi 1983; Strandgaard & Paulson 1984; Dearden 1985; White & Markus 1997; Dawson *et al.* 2000). Autoregulation is also impaired if the $Paco_2$ is high, presumably because further vasodilatation cannot occur and so the perfusion reserve is exhausted (Aaslid *et al.* 1989). In some patients who have had transient ischaemic attacks or a mild ischaemic stroke,

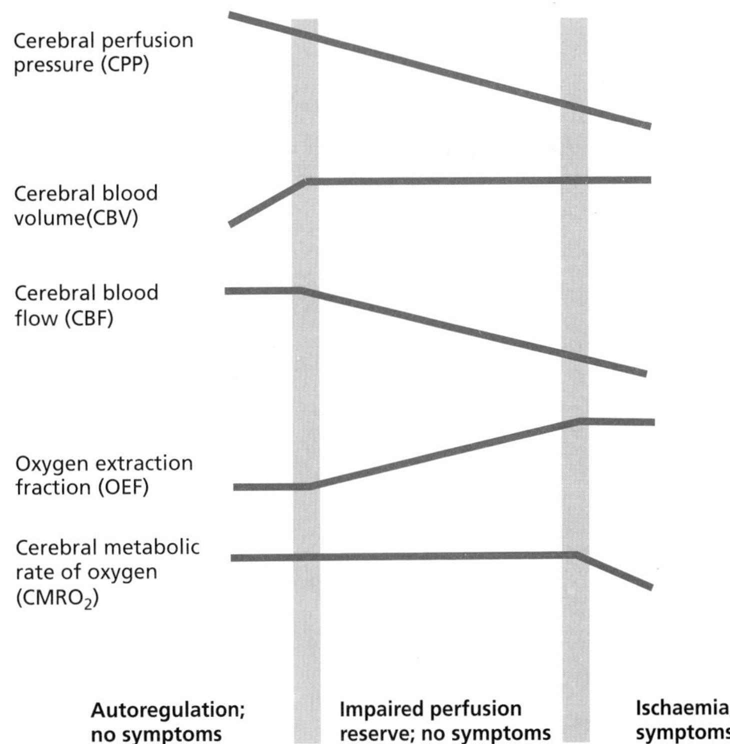

Fig. 11.3 Schematic representation of the protective responses to a progressive fall in cerebral perfusion pressure (CPP). With falling CPP, intracranial arteries dilate to maintain cerebral blood flow (CBF)—autoregulation. This results in an increase in cerebral blood volume (CBV). When vasodilatation (and CBV) is maximal, further falls in CPP result in a fall in CBF and therefore a fall in the CBF : CBV ratio, and an increase in the oxygen extraction fraction (OEF) to maintain tissue oxygenation. This represents a state of impaired cerebral perfusion reserve. When the OEF is maximal, further falls in CPP lead to reduction in the cerebral metabolic rate of oxygen ($CMRO_2$) and the symptoms of cerebral ischaemia.

with subsequently normal angiograms, autoregulation and the cerebrovascular response to $Paco_2$ may be deranged for several weeks (Skinhoj *et al.* 1970; Frackowiak 1985). In all of these situations of impaired autoregulation, CBF varies directly with blood pressure, becoming 'pressure passive', and predisposing to an increased stroke risk, particularly following exposure to hypotensive agents, as occurs perioperatively (Kleiser & Widder 1992).

Measurement of cerebral autoregulation has traditionally been undertaken in animals, and in response to static changes in arterial blood pressure. CBF, or an estimate of CBF such as cerebral blood flow velocity (CBFV), is measured during a large change in blood pressure, usually induced pharmacologically. However, such techniques are not suitable for patients with stroke, or who are at risk of stroke, because the blood pressure change induced could cause or increase brain ischaemia (Lagi *et al.* 1994). Subsequent attempts to safely and non-invasively monitor autoregulation of CBF, or at least the lower limit of autoregulation, have used indirect measures of cerebral autoregulation such as CBFV, as determined by transcranial Doppler (TCD) ultrasound, in response to vasodilatory stimuli such as hypercapnoea (rather than changes in blood pressure) (Aaslid *et al.* 1991; Larsen *et al.* 1994). Although these indirect measures generally correlate with direct measures of cerebral autoregulation (White & Markus 1997), they do measure a slightly different physiological response. Other methods of measuring dynamic autoregulation which are non-invasive, and suitable for use in patients at risk of stroke, aim to evaluate the response of CBF or CBFV to small physiological changes in arterial blood pressure. These include measures of changes in blood pressure induced by the use of bilateral leg cuffs which are inflated suprasystolically and then suddenly deflated to induce a transient fall in blood pressure, and measures of the spontaneous variability in arterial blood pressure by a servo-controlled plethysmograph (Panerai *et al.* 1998). The temporal pattern of the change in blood pressure is correlated with the change in the middle cerebral artery (MCA) CBFV as measured by TCD (Aaslid *et al.* 1989). There is close agreement between these two methods (Panerai *et al.* 1998), and between the thigh method and the classic assessment of static autoregulation (Tiecks *et al.* 1995), despite the fact that TCD measurement of MCA CBFV is only a suitable technique if there is no change in MCA diameter during the change in blood pressure (Dawson *et al.* 2000). Furthermore, TCD measurements of MCA CFBV correlate closely with concurrent measurements of absolute blood flow in the internal carotid artery during this step change in blood pressure (Newell *et al.* 1994).

Cerebral perfusion reserve

The ratio of CBF : CBV (see above) is a measure of cerebral perfusion reserve. A CBF : CBV ratio below about 6.0 indicates maximal vasodilatation and CBV, and exhausted reserve, even if the CBF is still normal. If available, PET scanning will show a rising OEF at this stage, to maintain $CMRO_2$ (Gibbs *et al.* 1984) (Fig. 11.4). If PET is unavailable, the mean cerebral transit time (MCTT), which is the

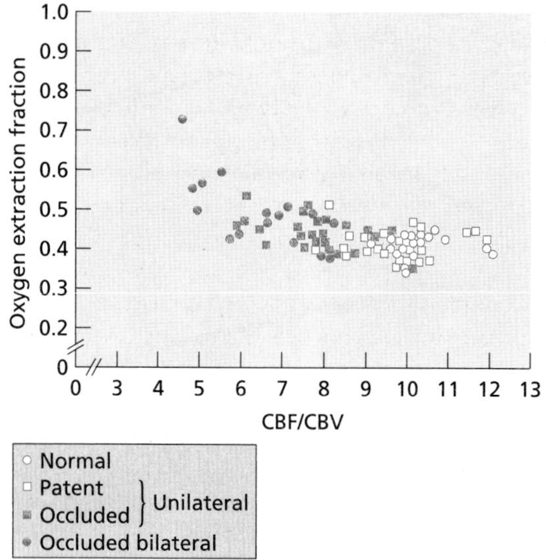

Fig. 11.4 Relationship between the oxygen extraction fraction (OEF) and cerebral blood flow : cerebral blood volume (CBF : CBV) ratio in each of 82 middle cerebral artery regions from 32 patients with varying degrees of carotid artery stenosis and occlusion and nine normal subjects (with permission from Gibbs *et al.* 1984).

reciprocal of CBF : CBV, can be used instead (Merrick *et al.* 1991; Naylor *et al.* 1991).

In clinical practice, cerebral perfusion reserve is more commonly assessed indirectly by measuring the *relative* difference between CBF at baseline and then in response to a vasomotor stimulus such as CO_2 (by inhalation or breath holding) or acetazolamide (by intravenous administration), which increase CBF unless the capacity for cerebral dilatation is exhausted (Markwalder *et al.* 1984; Sullivan *et al.* 1987; Herold *et al.* 1988; Eicke *et al.* 1999). The techniques for measuring relative (not absolute) values of CBF include:

- the xenon-133 (^{133}Xe) inhalation system (Sullivan *et al.* 1987);
- stable Xe computed tomography (CT) (Yamashita *et al.* 1992);
- single-photon emission computed tomography (SPECT) with ^{133}Xe-, iodine-123 (^{123}I)-labelled isopropyliodoamphetamine or technetium-99m (^{99m}Tc)-labelled hexamethylpropyleneamine oxime (HMPAO) (Knop *et al.* 1992; Masdeu *et al.* 1994);
- in theory (but very difficult clinically, particularly in sick patients), three-dimensional time-of-flight magnetic resonance angiography (Mandai *et al.* 1994);
- TCD, which is also used to measure velocity flow in the MCA as a surrogate for CBF, and may be combined with colour duplex M-mode systems to estimate extracranial carotid flow volume (Bishop *et al.* 1986; Markus & Harrison 1992; Newell *et al.* 1994; Eicke *et al.* 1999). Most users of TCD for assessing cerebrovascular reserve prefer CO_2 stimulation to acetazolamide administration (Kleiser *et al.* 1994).

It is important to recognize that these indirect methods of measuring perfusion reserve (i.e. SPECT, TCD, MCTT) are inaccurate when the normal relationships between CBF, CBV, OEF and vascular reactivity are distorted, as occurs in ischaemic and infarcted brain (Powers 1991) (section 6.6.5).

A common clinical scenario of impaired reserve is a patient with stenosis or occlusion of one or both internal carotid arteries, severe enough (at least 50% diameter stenosis) to produce a fall in CPP distally, along with inadequate collateral CBF distally (Powers *et al.* 1987; Schroeder 1988; Powers 1991). Under these circumstances, the brain is vulnerable to any further fall in CPP, as may occur when the patient stands up quickly, when undergoing anaesthesia (e.g. for coronary artery bypass surgery) or starts or increases antihypertensive medication or vasodilators (Kleiser & Widder 1992; Widder *et al.* 1994). Impaired cerebral vasomotor reactivity may be a significant predictor of future stroke. However, correlation of the different methods of measuring autoregulatory vasodilatation, secondary to reduced perfusion pressure, is sufficiently variable to have limited the validity of studies associating haemodynamic impairment with stroke risk (Gur *et al.* 1996; Müller & Schimrigk 1996; Derdeyn *et al.* 1999).

11.1.3 Pathophysiology of cerebral ischaemia

Thrombosis

Acute cerebral ischaemia begins with the occlusion of a cerebral blood vessel, usually by thrombus or embolus, it is rarely due to low flow alone (Raichle 1983). Modern ideas about the pathogenesis of thrombosis began with Rudolph Virchow's dissertation in 1845 in which he enunciated his famous triad that thrombosis was due to changes in the vessel wall, changes in the pattern of blood flow and changes in the constituents of the blood. In fact, this concept had been already hinted at by John Hunter about 50 years earlier (Hunter 1794).

It has since been established that vascular endothelial injury is the most critical event in the formation of a thrombus (Kullo *et al.* 1998; Ross 1999) (section 6.3.2). The most common cause of an abnormal endothelium is atherosclerosis. The initiation, progression and maturation of atherosclerotic plaque has been well documented (Ross 1993, 1999), but it remains uncertain exactly what triggers a 'dormant' atherosclerotic plaque to become unstable and symptomatic. Studies of acute coronary syndromes, at least, indicate that thrombus develops on an atherosclerotic plaque in which the overlying endothelium is eroded or, perhaps more commonly, the plaque has ruptured (Davies 1996, 1997; Burke *et al.* 1997). Ruptured plaques contain a large core of lipid-laden macrophages (foam cells) engorged with oxidized low-density lipoprotein (LDL) cholesterol, and a thin friable overlying fibrous cap devoid of smooth-muscle cells (Davies 1997;

Fuster *et al.* 1997). The oxidized LDL within the lipid core stimulates plaque inflammation, which undermines the structural integrity of the plaque and activates the endothelium to a pro-inflammatory and pro-coagulant state (Nowroth *et al.* 1986; Wilcox *et al.* 1989; Libby 1995; O'Keefe *et al.* 1995; Davies 1996, 1997; Burke *et al.* 1997; DeGraba 1997; McIntyre & Dominiczak 1997; Hunt & Jurd 1998). The plaque may rupture because the large lipid core redistributes the shear stress on the thin fibrous cap and very high loads are imparted upon localized areas of the weakened cap (Cheng *et al.* 1993). This series of events probably also occurs in the cerebral arterial circulation, at least at the carotid bifurcation (section 6.3.2).

Recent epidemiological studies suggest that plaque inflammation (and rupture) may be triggered by exposure (acute or chronic) to an exogenous infectious antigen (section 6.3.3). There is a consistent significant relationship between symptomatic coronary artery disease and moderately elevated markers of inflammation (fibrinogen, C-reactive protein, albumin and leucocyte count) (Danesh *et al.* 1998). There is also a higher than expected incidence of chronic inflammatory conditions, such as chronic dental infection, chronic bronchitis and chronic infection with *Chlamydia pneumoniae*, *Heliobacter pylori* and cytomegalovirus (Cook & Lip 1996; Gurfinkel *et al.* 1997; Ridker *et al.* 1997; Bittner 1998; Ross 1999). Although these associations may be coincidental rather than causal (Danesh *et al.* 1997), a similar, yet less robust, body of evidence is also mounting among patients with ischaemic stroke (Bova *et al.* 1996; Wimmer *et al.* 1996; DeGraba 1997; Grau *et al.* 1997, 1998; Cook *et al.* 1998; DeGraba *et al.* 1998; Markus & Mendall 1998; Yamashita *et al.* 1998; Rothwell *et al.* 2000).

Following plaque rupture or endothelial erosion, blood is exposed to subendothelial structures, particularly fibrillar collagen, which induces platelet adhesion and activation, and blood coagulation. Platelet adhesion is mediated by the interaction of platelet glycoprotein Ib/IX with subendothelial von Willebrand factor under high shear conditions, and by platelet glycoprotein Ia/IIb binding to collagen under low shear conditions. Upon activation, adherent platelets recruit additional platelets into the growing thrombus by three coordinated mechanisms (Hirsh & Weitz 1999):

• firstly, activated platelets release ADP from storage granules, and the ADP binds to the ADP receptor of adjacent platelets, which activates them;

• secondly, activated platelets generate and release arachidonic acid, which is metabolized by the enzyme cyclo-oxygenase to prostaglandin endoperoxide, which in turn is converted by thromboxane synthetase to thromboxane A_2, a very potent vasoconstrictor and platelet agonist which induces further platelet aggregation and secretion. The platelets also release other eicosanoids, such as prostaglandin $F_{2\alpha}$ and serotonin, which induce further vasoconstriction and platelet aggregation (Patrono *et al.* 1990; Schror & Braun 1990; D'Andrea *et al.* 1994; van Kooten *et al.* 1997). The activation of platelets by agonists such as ADP and thromboxane A_2 conformationally activates (and exteriorizes) the final common pathway of platelet activation, the platelet glycoprotein IIb/IIIa, which is the platelet receptor for fibrinogen. Circulating fibrinogen binds to the activated and exteriorized platelet glycoprotein IIb/IIIa receptors on the surface of platelets and leads to platelet aggregation (Coller 1997; Topol *et al.* 1999). Platelet aggregation not only increases the size of the thrombus but it may indirectly lead to vasoconstriction by activating blood leucocytes to induce an acute disturbance in endothelial-dependent relaxation that results in vasoconstriction (Akopov *et al.* 1994). Vascular tone is further modulated by peptides released from endothelial cells, which include the vasoconstrictor endothelin and the vasodilators prostacyclin and nitric oxide (endothelium-derived relaxing factor) (Yanagisawa *et al.* 1988; Faraci & Brian 1994; Levin 1995; Loscalzo 1995);

• thirdly, the modified membrane of activated platelets promotes the assembly of clotting factors on the platelet surface, thereby amplifying thrombin generation (Furie & Furie 1992). The resultant burst of thrombin activates additional platelets and triggers coagulation.

Coagulation is initiated by exposure of blood to tissue factors located in the necrotic core of ruptured atherosclerotic plaques, in the subendothelium of injured vessels, and on the surface of activated leucocytes attracted to the damaged vessel. The original cascade/waterfall hypothesis of blood coagulation is that there are two activating pathways: the tissue factor or extrinsic pathway; and the contact or intrinsic pathway. A revised hypothesis (Broze 1992) maintains there is a single coagulation pathway, triggered by vessel injury and tissue factor (TF) (the factor VIIa/TF complex). TF binds factor VIIa and the resulting factor VIIa/TF complex activates factors IX and X. Factor IXa assembles on the surface of activated platelets as part of the intrinsic tenase complex which comprises factor IXa, factor VIIIa and calcium. Factor Xa, generated through the extrinsic (factor VIIa/TF) and the intrinsic tenase complex, assembles on the surface of activated platelets as part of the prothrombin-activating (prothrombinase) complex, which consists of factor Xa, factor Va, and calcium. When assembled in this way, the prothrombinase complex generates a burst of thrombin activity (Hirsh & Weitz 1999). Thrombin (factor IIa) activates platelets and factors V and VIII, and also converts fibrinogen to fibrin; thrombin then binds to fibrin where it remains active. As a blood clot forms at the site of vessel injury, plasminogen, an inert circulating protein, becomes closely bound to the deposited fibrin and is slowly activated (by tissue plasminogen activator which has been activated by kallikrein) to form plasmin, which digests the fibrin clot to give fibrin degradation products.

Platelets and later fibrin accumulate at, and are limited to, the site of vascular injury. The rest of the vasculature remains free of platelet and fibrin deposits because, in circulating blood, the tendency of the coagulation mechanism to be activated is counterbalanced by inhibitory factors in the blood such as antithrombin III (which inactivates factors IX, X, XI and XII). However, at the point of vessel injury, the activation of the coagulation mechanism is so powerful that the inhibitors are overwhelmed.

There are three major inhibitory systems which modulate the coagulation pathway: the protein C anticoagulant pathway, tissue factor pathway inhibitor (TFPI) and antithrombin. Protein C is activated by the thrombin/thrombomodulin complex on the endothelial cell surface. When thrombin binds to thrombomodulin (an endothelial membrane protein) it undergoes a conformational change at its active site that converts it from a pro-coagulant enzyme to a potent activator of protein C. Activated protein C acts as an anticoagulant, in the presence of protein S, by proteolytic degradation and inactivation of factors Va and VIIIa (Rosenberg & Rosenberg 1984; Furie & Furie 1992). TFPI binds and inactivates factors Xa and the TFPI/factor Xa complex, and then inactivates factor VIIa within the factor VIIa/TF complex. Antithrombin inactivates free thrombin and factor Xa, but these clotting enzymes are protected from inactivation by antithrombin when they are bound to fibrin and activated platelets (Hirsh & Weitz 1999).

Injured endothelium (e.g. as a result of ruptured atherosclerotic plaque) interacts with blood platelets to form nidi of loosely adherent platelets and fibrin that can break off and embolize distally, and also initiate the coagulation cascade that can lead to the formation of an occlusive thrombus.

Pathologists recognize and describe three different types of thrombi (Deykin 1967):

- *red thrombi* are composed mostly of red blood cells and fibrin. They form in areas of slowed blood flow and the vessel wall need not be obviously abnormal (e.g. deep venous thrombosis in the leg veins);
- *white thrombi* are made up of platelets and fibrin and have few red blood cells. They form in areas in which the endothelial surface or vessel wall is abnormal and blood flow is rapid (e.g. thrombosis complicating carotid atheroma);
- *disseminated fibrin deposition* occurs in small blood vessels.

When a major artery is suddenly occluded, arterial blood pressure and blood flow fall distal to the occlusion, and the region of brain supplied by that vessel is acutely deprived of blood supply and is rendered ischaemic. The metabolic and clinical consequences of cerebral ischaemia depend not only on the cascade of events induced by thrombus formation (i.e. biosynthesis of thrombogenic and neurotoxic eicosanoids, breakdown of the blood–brain barrier, diffusion of these products into surrounding brain and reduced microvascular flow in the ischaemic penumbra around the initial focus), but also on the site, severity and duration of cerebral ischaemia and the availability of collateral blood flow (Heiss 1992; Siesjö 1992a).

Availability of collateral blood flow

Occlusion of a cerebral artery reduces but seldom abolishes the delivery of oxygen and glucose to the relevant region of the brain because dense collateral channels partly maintain blood flow in the ischaemic territory. This incomplete ischaemia is responsible for the spatial and temporal dynamics of cerebral infarction (Pulsinelli 1992). Some other areas of the brain, including infarcted tissue, may show relative or absolute hyperaemia (called 'luxury perfusion') due to good collateral blood supply, recanalization of the occluded artery, inflammation or vasodilatation in response to hypercapnia, i.e. flow is in excess of the metabolic demands and so the oxygen extraction fraction is reduced.

Site of cerebral ischaemia

The brain cells which are most vulnerable to ischaemia are neurones, followed in decreasing sensitivity by oligodendroglia, astrocytes and endothelial cells. However, even within the population of neurones, there are many different types that also vary in sensitivity to ischaemia, and in some cases the vulnerability varies with the location of the cells. The most vulnerable neurones to mild ischaemia are the pyramidal neurones in the CA1 and CA4 zones of the hippocampus, followed by neurones in the cerebellum, striatum and neocortex (Brierley 1976; Heros 1994).

Severity and duration of cerebral ischaemia

The transition from normal CBF through to cerebral oligaemia, the ischaemic penumbra and frank tissue infarction occurs in phases, depending on the severity and duration of brain ischaemia (Fig. 11.5). Initially, small declines in perfusion pressure and CBF (< 50 mL/100 g/min) are compensated for by regional vasodilatation to maintain CBF (autoregulation), resulting in a regional increase in CBV (section 11.1.2) (Fig. 11.3). With continued reductions in perfusion pressure and the dilatation of all vessels to capacity, the oxygen extraction fraction (OEF) and glucose extraction fraction (GEF) are increased to maintain a normal cerebral metabolic rate of oxygen ($CMRO_2$) and of glucose (CMRglu). This is a state of 'misery perfusion' which is characterized by reduced CBF, increased OEF (ranging from the normal value of about 30–40% up to the theoretical maximum of 100%), and relatively preserved or even normal oxygen consumption ($CMRO_2$) (Baron 1999). With further cerebral ischaemia (i.e. reduction of CBF to about 50% of normal), several compensatory mechanisms come into play which sacrifice electrophysiological activity; hence, the sup-

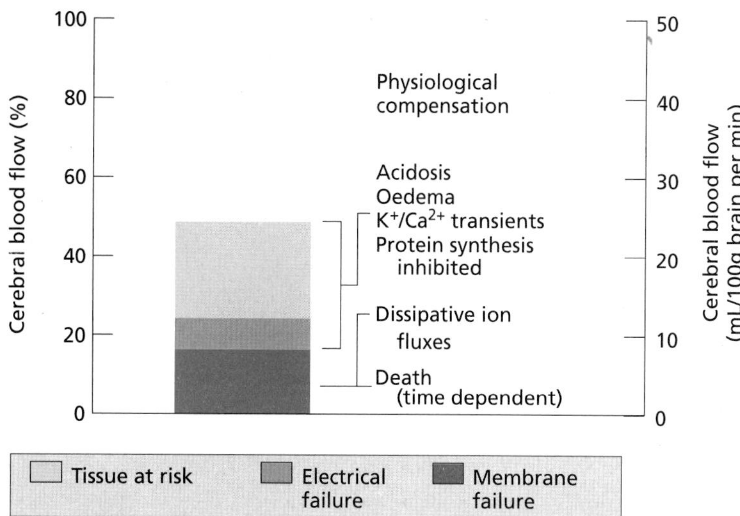

Fig. 11.5 Cerebral blood flow (CBF) thresholds for cell dysfunction and death (from Siesjö 1992a).

pression of neuronal electrical activity as seen on the electroencephalogram (EEG) in order to reduce energy use. This enables near-normal ATP concentrations and membrane ion gradients to be maintained and cell viability to be preserved, at least temporarily. If moderate ischaemia persists, however (i.e. for several hours), cell death occurs.

Critical flow thresholds

Experimental models of focal cerebral ischaemia have identified two critical flow thresholds for certain cell functions: a threshold for electrical failure (loss of neuronal electrical activity) and another threshold for membrane failure (loss of cellular ion homeostasis) (Symon *et al.* 1976; Siesjö 1992a).

The first threshold is reached when the CBF falls below about 20 mL/100 g of brain per minute. At this point, the OEF becomes maximal, the $CMRO_2$ begins to fall (Fig. 11.3), normal neuronal function of the cerebral cortex is affected (Wise *et al.* 1983; Powers *et al.* 1984; Friberg & Olsen 1991), electrical activity in cortical cells ceases (Heiss *et al.* 1976) and evoked cerebral responses from the area of focal ischaemia decrease in amplitude (Heiss 1992). This degree of ischaemia thus represents a threshold for *loss of neuronal electrical activity* (i.e. electrical failure) (Fig. 11.5).

When blood flow falls to about 15 mL/100 g of brain per minute, evoked potentials are lost and the EEG flattens. With further falls in flow, the EEG becomes isoelectric and the water and electrolyte content of ischaemic tissue changes due to cell pump failure (see below). The critical threshold for the beginning of irreversible cell damage is a CBF of about 10 mL/100 g of brain per minute (Siesjö 1992a). For a short period, the neurones may remain viable and recover function if perfusion is restored. At this stage, lack of oxygen inhibits mitochondrial metabolism and activates the inefficient anaerobic metabolism of glucose, causing a local rise in lactate production and so a fall in pH, leading to intra- and extracellular acidosis (Fig. 11.5). The energy-dependent functions of cell membranes to maintain ion homeostasis become progressively impaired; K^+ leaks out of cells into the extracellular space, Na^+ and water enter cells (cytotoxic oedema), and Ca^{2+} also moves into cells (where it causes mitochondrial failure and compromises the ability of intracellular membranes to control subsequent ion fluxes, leading to cytotoxicity) (Harris *et al.* 1981; Cheung *et al.* 1986; Siesjö 1992a). Rapid efflux of K^+ and influx of Ca^{2+} represent a generalized collapse of membrane function. This degree of ischaemia represents a threshold for *loss of cellular ion homeostasis* (i.e. membrane failure) (Siesjö 1992a).

Besides these two major thresholds there is an underlying more complex pattern of thresholds characterized by inhibition of protein synthesis at a threshold of about 45 mL/100 g brain per minute, stimulation of anaerobic glycolysis at 35 mL/100 g/min, the release of neurotransmitters and disturbance of energy metabolism at about 20 mL/100 g/min, and finally anoxic depolarization at less than 15 mL/g/min (Hossmann 1994).

Other than the *degree* of ischaemia, the *duration* of ischaemia also determines whether the thresholds are crossed (Fig. 11.6). With prolonged reductions in CBF below about 10 mL/100 g brain per minute, cellular transport mechanisms and neurotransmitter systems fail; potentially neurotoxic transmitters are released, such as glutamate (Rothman & Olney 1986); free oxygen radicals and lipid peroxides are formed which damage cells further (McCord 1985); and neurones release platelet-activating factor which may be neurotoxic (Lindsberg *et al.* 1991) (see below).

Concept of an ischaemic penumbra

The finding of two separate thresholds, one for cessation of electrical signals and the other for loss of ion homeostasis, which are separated by an intermediate zone characterized

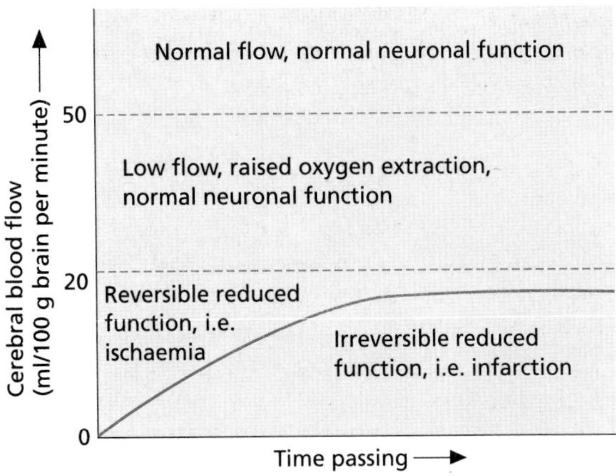

Fig. 11.6 Combined effects of residual cerebral blood flow (CBF) and duration of ischaemia on reversibility of neuronal dysfunction during focal cerebral ischaemia. The solid line delineates the limits of severity and duration of ischaemia that allow survival of any neurones (from Jones *et al.* 1981; Heiss & Rosner 1983).

by cessation of electrical activity of cells with preservation of their membrane potential, led to the concept of an ischaemic penumbra of brain tissue (Astrup *et al.* 1981; Heiss 1992; Siesjö 1992a; Ginsberg & Pulsinelli 1994; Heiss & Graf 1994).

As cerebral blood flow falls, a critical threshold is reached when the electrical activity of neurones is suppressed. As flow falls further, another threshold is reached when cellular integrity begins to break down. Cells falling in between these two thresholds make up the 'ischaemic penumbra': they may not be functioning, but they are still alive and could either recover function or die.

The ischaemic penumbra can be defined as an area of severely ischaemic, functionally impaired, but surviving brain tissue which is at risk of infarction but can be saved, and recover, if it is reperfused before it is irreversibly damaged (hence the concept of 'time is brain') (Baron 1999). Otherwise, it will be progressively recruited into the core of the infarct until maximum infarct extension is reached (Baron 1999). The ischaemic penumbra is not just a topographic locus, but a *dynamic* (time × space) process, characterized by an evolving zone of bioenergetic upheaval (Ginsberg & Pulsinelli 1994; Hakim 1998; Baron 1999).

The most accurate method of measuring the ischaemic penumbra is by positron emmision tomography (PET) using the oxygen-15 steady-state technique. This is a quantitative imaging technique which maps the main physiological variables involved in tissue ischaemia, namely perfusion (or CBF, in mL/100 min), and oxygen consumption ($CMRO_2$, in mL/100 g/min), together with OEF and CBV (in mL/100 g) (Baron 1999). Because PET is not widely available, it has not been possible to apply it in clinical practice to patients with acute ischaemic stroke and determine just how large the ischaemic penumbra is, how long it is likely to remain in this state, how important it is functionally and how much recovery is possible if flow is restored (Lassen *et al.* 1991).

A more widely available and promising potential measure of the ischaemic penumbra is the magnetic resonance imaging (MRI) technique of combined diffusion-weighted imaging (DWI) and perfusion-weighted imaging (PWI), which is currently being evaluated in many acute stroke units (Schlaug *et al.* 1999) (section 5.3.9). DWI is based on the measurement of the diffusion of free water, which is decreased in ischaemic brain tissue. A decrease in the apparent diffusion coefficient, apparent as hyperdensity on diffusion-weighted images, indicates a restriction in the diffusional movement of water and is believed to result from energy failure and subsequent cytotoxic oedema (Hossmann & Hoehn-Berlage 1995). DWI abnormalities typically evolve into infarction in humans, and it has been suggested that the DWI abnormality corresponds to the ischaemic core (Schlaug *et al.* 1999). PWI, on the other hand, provides information on the haemodynamic status of the tissue with the use of paramagnetic contrast agents, for example, gadolinium-based chelates. On the basis of magnetic resonance perfusion imaging data, maps of relative CBF can be calculated, and demonstrate impaired perfusion of both the ischaemic core and the surrounding brain regions, thereby complementing the information derived from DWI (Baird & Warach 1998). During the first hours of stroke evolution, PWI typically demonstrates regions with abnormal perfusion that are larger than the DWI lesions. It has been postulated that this mismatch reflects the ischaemic penumbra (i.e. functionally impaired 'tissue at risk' surrounding the irreversibly damaged ischaemic core) (Karonen *et al.* 1999). Typically, a PWI > DWI lesion is associated with subsequent infarct enlargement but, because PWI is very sensitive in detecting perfusion defects, the PWI/DWI mismatch region may comprise not only tissue at risk but also hypoperfused tissue with CBF values above the critical viability thresholds (Karonen *et al.* 1999; Neumann-Haefelin *et al.* 1999).

Despite the practical difficulties of PET (Baron 1991), and the uncertainty surrounding the validity of DWI/PWI as an accurate measure of the ischaemic penumbra, it is possible to conclude from small but meticulous studies using PET and CT, that there is prolonged persistence of substantial volumes of 'at risk' but potentially viable brain tissue for up to 16–17 h after ischaemic stroke in some patients (Marchal *et al.* 1996; Baron 1999). These data suggest that the time window for effective therapeutic intervention may be longer in humans than predicted from animal studies, but it is unlikely to be a rigid and universal time window for all patients (Heiss & Graf 1994; Baron *et al.* 1995; Baron 1999). As emphasized above, cerebral ischaemia is a dynamic process of fluctuating severity over the first few hours and it may not be possible to predict just how long the time window is to allow successful therapeutic intervention in any one individual (Baron *et al.* 1995). Indeed, we have learnt from randomized trials in acute myocardial infarction (MI), that thrombolysis is still effective in reducing case fatality even when given up to 24 h after the onset of chest pain, despite the widely held belief prior to these studies, mainly based on animal models, that thrombolysis could not possibly be effective if given more than a few hours after acute MI (Fibrinolytic Therapy Trialists' (FTT) Collaborative Group 1994). As PET studies of the brain in humans suggest the 'window' may be as long as 17 h (Marchal *et al.* 1996), we need to keep an open mind about the therapeutic time window and acknowledge that it may vary for different sites of arterial occlusion and brain ischaemia, and for different interventions (Hakim 1998). For example, the time window for thrombolytics may be shorter for neuroprotective agents than for antithrombotic agents; we do not know yet.

In humans it is not clear how long ischaemic brain can survive and still be salvaged by reperfusion or measures to protect neurones from dying. In other words, the duration of the 'time window' for effective therapeutic intervention is unknown.

Reperfusion and brain damage

In the monkey, a middle cerebral artery occlusion that lasts for 30 min or longer often produces some tissue damage, and occlusion periods longer than 60 min frequently cause infarction. However, short-term recovery of electrical and metabolic functions is possible with reperfusion after ischaemic periods as long as 60 min, and reperfusion within 4–8 h can reduce the size of the lesion (Jones *et al.* 1981; Siesjö 1992a). In humans, as stated above, PET studies have demonstrated viable (penumbral) tissue up to 17 h after ischaemic stroke, during which time reperfusion (spontaneously or by treatment) may be effective (Heiss & Graf 1994; Baron 1999). Although reperfusion within the revival times of ischaemic tissues may salvage cells and aid recovery (by restoring oxygen and nutrient delivery to ischaemic brain tissue), it may also be detrimental, causing so-called 'reperfusion injury' due to the resupply of water and osmotic equivalents (which may exacerbate vasogenic oedema), oxygen (which may trigger production of injurious free radicals) and blood-borne cells (such as neutrophils) which may exacerbate ischaemic damage (Ito *et al.* 1979; McCord 1985; Wardlaw *et al.* 1993; Martin 1997). As discussed below, leucocytes migrate into the injured region within hours of reperfusion and may cause tissue injury by occluding the microvasculature, generating oxygen-free radicals, releasing cytotoxic enzymes, altering vasomotor reactivity, and increasing cytokine and chemoattractant release (DeGraba 1998; Prestigiacomo *et al.* 1999). However, in man, the evidence suggests that the benefits of reperfusion can be greater than the hazards (sections 5.4 and 11.5).

11.1.4 Phases and mediators of cell death

With prolonged reductions in cerebral blood flow below about 10 mL/100 g brain per minute, ischaemic necrosis (infarction) occurs. This is a fulminant form of cell death associated with failure of the plasma membrane, swelling of the cell and internal organelles, protein degradation and DNA breakup (Cormio *et al.* 1997; Martin 1997). The mechanisms that give rise to ischaemic cell death have not been determined definitively but considerable evidence from experiments in rodents suggests there are four sequential but overlapping phases in the cascade of cerebral ischaemic damage: excitotoxicity (within minutes), peri-infarct depolarization (minutes to hours), inflammation (hours to days) and apoptosis (days). The major mediators of cell death are: unregulated increases in intracellular cytosolic Ca^{2+} concentration (and perhaps zinc concentration), production of free radicals and acidosis (Fig. 11.7). The induction of immediate early genes and expression of heat shock proteins may modulate the process and facilitate programmed cell death.

Excitotoxicity

Ischaemic neurones deprived of oxygen and glucose rapidly (within minutes) lose ATP and become depolarized, leading to synaptic release of the transmitter glutamate and the electrogenic transport of glutamate from depolarized astrocytes. The resultant build-up of extracellular glutamate results in overstimulation of glutamate receptors. There are five categories of glutamate receptor/channel complex, classified according to the agonist that most efficiently activates them: high- and low-affinity kainate, α-amino-3-hydroxy-5-methyl-4-isoxazole propionic acid (AMPA), *N*-methyl-D-aspartate (NMDA) and quisqualate receptors (Greenamyre & Porter 1994; Muir & Lees 1995).

When glutamate is released from presynaptic endings, it activates the AMPA, kainate and NMDA receptors. The AMPA receptor gates a channel that is permeable to monovalent cations (Na^+, K^+ and H^+). By allowing Na^+ to enter, the opening of this channel leads to depolarization. The NMDA subtype of the glutamate receptor (Fig. 11.8) gates a channel permeable to both monovalent cations and Ca^{2+}. This channel is normally blocked by magnesium (Mg^{2+}) but, since this block is voltage dependent, it is opened when the membrane depolarizes. Therefore, activation of the AMPA receptor leads to Na^+ influx and depolarization, thus overcoming the block and allowing Ca^{2+} to enter via the NMDA channel. Depolarization also allows Ca^{2+} to enter via voltage-sensitive Ca^{2+} channels of the L and T types (Siesjö 1992a).

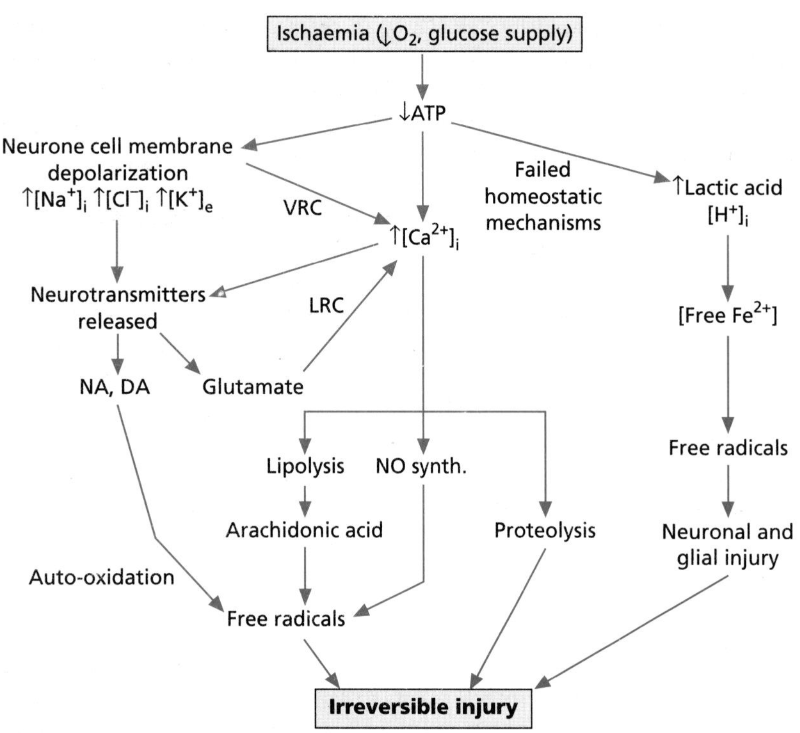

Fig. 11.7 Potential mechanisms of ischaemic brain damage. This diagram illustrates the complexity of the process of ischaemic brain damage with multiple branching pathways and potential sites of interaction when the energy supply to the brain is depleted. $[Ca^{2+}]_i$, intracellular Ca^{2+} concentration; $[Cl^-]_i$, intracellular chloride ion concentration; DA, dopamine; Fe^{2+}, ferrous ions; $[H^+]_i$, intracellular hydrogen ion concentration; $[K^+]_e$, extracellular K^+ concentration; LRC, ligand-regulated Ca^{2+} channels; NA, noradrenaline; $[Na^+]_i$, intracellular Na^+ concentration; NO synth, nitric oxide synthase; VRC, voltage-regulated Ca^{2+} channels (from Pulsinelli 1992).

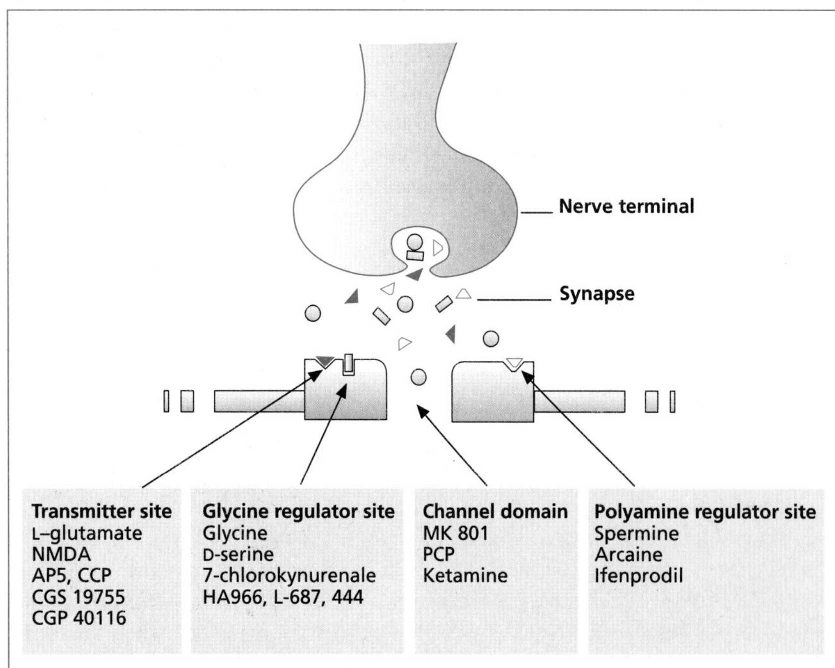

Fig. 11.8 The glutaminergic synapse. Schematic representation showing a presynaptic glutaminergic nerve terminal and a *N*-methyl-D-aspartate (NMDA) receptor in the cell membrane of a postsynaptic neurone. The NMDA receptor and channel complex possess a number of modulatory sites that can be pharmacologically manipulated to either enhance or attenuate glutamate-stimulated ionic fluxes. Interaction of glutamate or a glutamate-like agonist (e.g. NMDA) with the glutamate recognition (transmitter) site leads to activation of inward Ca^{2+} and Na^+ currents that can be damaging when in excess. The glycine and polyamine sites, when acted upon by selective agonists, serve to enhance the effects of glutamate receptor activation. Agents that block any of these sites will attenuate NMDA-receptor-mediated ionic currents. Additionally, within the channel, there are non-competitive and Mg^{2+}-binding sites that attenuate Ca^{2+} influx through the channel when pharmacologically blocked.

Increases in intracellular cytosolic Ca^{2+} concentration

In normal brain tissue, extracellular Ca^{2+} concentration is 10^4–10^5 times greater than its intracellular concentration and most of the mechanisms that maintain this gradient are either directly or indirectly energy dependent. During brain ischaemia, the loss of ATP rapidly leads to a massive influx of Ca^{2+} into the cell as a result of impaired Ca^{2+} pump function, an increase in membrane permeability to Ca^{2+}, release of Ca^{2+} from intracellular compartments, and the release of endogenous excitatory amino acid neurotransmitters such as glutamate from depolarized nerve endings (Lipton & Rosenberg 1994; Kogure & Kogure 1997) (see above) (Fig. 11.9).

The consequence of a non-physiological unregulated rise in intracellular cytoplasmic Ca^{2+} is cell damage. The cell damage is not related to changes in intracellular Ca^{2+} but to changes in total calcium influx (Kristián & Siesjö 1998). The initial calcium load is sequestered, at least in part, by the mitochondria. Mitochondrial calcium accumulation is associated with enhanced production of reactive oxygen species (see below), such as $\cdot O_2^-$, H_2O_2, $\cdot OH$ and nitric oxide. The combination of $\cdot O_2^-$ and nitric oxide can yield peroxynitrate, a metabolite with potentially devastating effects (Kristián & Siesjö 1998). Mitochondrial calcium accumulation and oxidative stress can trigger the assembly (opening) of a high-conductance pore in the inner mitochondrial membrane. The mitochondrial permeability transition (MPT) pore leads to a collapse of the electrochemical potential for H^+, thereby arresting ATP production and triggering production of reactive oxygen species. An increase in total calcium influx also contributes to cell death by activation of Ca^{2+} ATPase (which results in further consumption of cellular ATP); activation of Ca^{2+}-dependent phospholipases, proteases and nucleases; and alteration of protein phosphorylation, which secondarily affects protein synthesis and genome expression (Choi 1995; Lee *et al.* 1999; Zipfel *et al.* 1999).

Thus, there are reasons to believe that excitatory amino acids act by accelerating Ca^{2+} influx into cells, with an ensuing rise in intracellular Ca^{2+}, that calcium is sequestered in mitochondria, and that this sequestration gives rise to the assembly of an MPT pore and production of reactive oxygen species by mitochondria. Clearly this sequence of events could explain the delayed cell death after brief periods of ischaemia, or cell death complicated by persistent hyperglycaemia (Kristián & Siesjö 1998).

Calcium influx is mediated directly and predominantly by NMDA receptors (which gate channels that are highly permeable to Ca^{2+}), but is also triggered secondarily by Na^+ influx through AMPA-, kainate- and NMDA-receptor-gated channels which activate voltage-gated Ca^{2+} channels and reverse operation of the Na^+/Ca^{2+} exchanger. The resultant excessive Ca^{2+} influx leads to elevated intracellular Ca^{2+} concentrations and lethal metabolic derangements, which include calcium-dependent activation of intracellular enzyme systems and the generation of free radicals.

Zinc

Calcium may not be the only divalent cation whose toxic influx contributes to ischaemic brain-cell death. There is increasing evidence that large amounts of the chelatable metal zinc (Zn^{2+}) in excitatory nerve terminals are released upon neuronal stimulation into the synapse (analagous to glutamate) where it can alter the function of various transmitter receptors and voltage-gated ion channels, including inhibiting NMDA receptors (Choi & Koh 1998) (Fig. 11.10). It is postulated that the first step in Zn^{2+}-mediated neuronal death, like Ca^{2+}-mediated neuronal death, is excess entry across the neuronal membrane (probably facilitated by voltage-gated Ca^{2+} channels, transport exchange for intracellular Na^+, NMDA-receptor-gated channels, and any Ca^{2+}-permeable AMPA/kainate channels), triggering prolonged

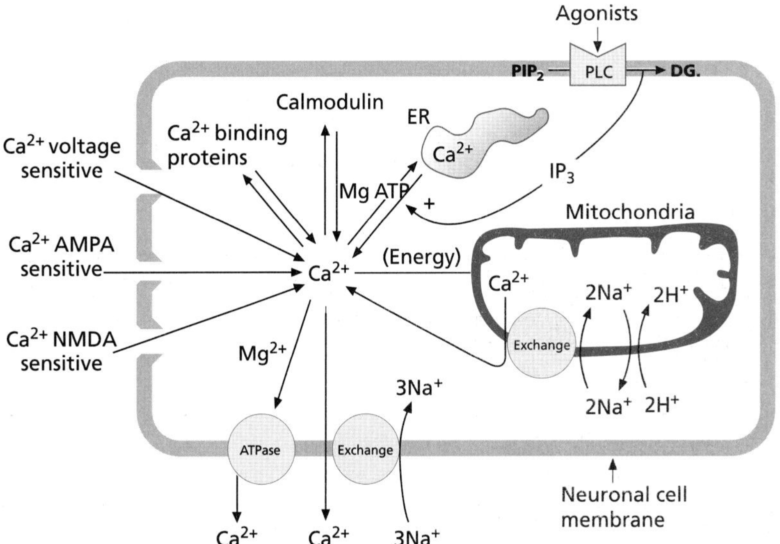

Fig. 11.9 Ca^{2+} homeostasis in neurones. Ca^{2+} influx is regulated by voltage- and ligand (glutamate)-sensitive channels named for their most potent synthetic agonists (*N*-methyl-D-aspartate (NMDA) and amino-3-hydroxy-5-methyl-4-isoxazole propionic acid (AMPA)). Energy-dependent regulation of intracellular Ca^{2+} ($[Ca^{2+}]_i$) is via an ATP-dependent pump, translocation for Na^+ ions and uptake into endoplasmic reticulum (ER) and mitochondria. Energy-dependent Ca^{2+} homeostasis occurs via buffering of Ca^{2+} by calmodulin and other intracellular proteins (calbindin, parvalbumin). DG, diacylglycerol; IP_3, inositol triphosphate; PIP_2, phosphatidyl inositol diphosphate; PLC, phospholipase C. (With permission from Pulsinelli 1992).

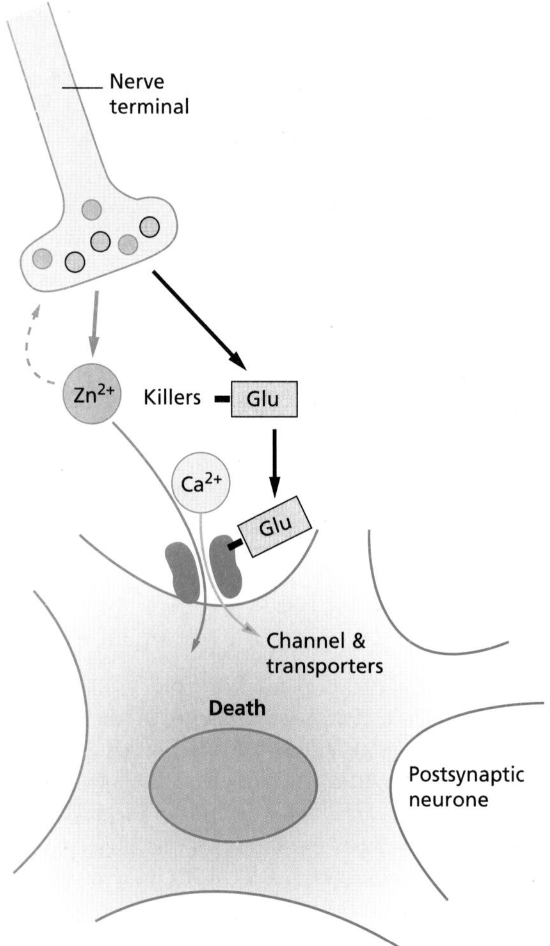

Fig. 11.10 Expanded view of excitotoxicity in ischaemic brain injury, illustrating complex parallels between glutamate (Glu), Zn^{2+} and Ca^{2+}. Glutamate and Zn^{2+} are both neurotransmitters turned killers, as ischaemia triggers their release from excitatory nerve terminals in excessive quantities; Zn^{2+} and Ca^{2+} influx are the second messengers of cell death. Influx of Zn^{2+} and Ca^{2+} probably occurs through voltage-gated Ca^{2+} channels, transport exchange for intracellular Na^+, NMDA-receptor-gated channels and any Ca^{2+}-permeable AMPA receptors (with permission from Lee *et al.* 1999).

mitochondrial superoxide production, and inducing either apoptosis (see below) or necrosis depending on the intensity of exposure (Sensi *et al.* 1999) (Figs 11.11 and 11.12).

Production of free radicals

A free radical is any atom, group of atoms or molecule with an unpaired electron in its outermost orbital (Halliwell 1994; Khan & Butler 1998). Since covalent chemical bonds usually consist of a pair of electrons sharing an orbital, free radicals can be thought of as molecules with an 'open' or 'half' bond, and it is this which accounts for their extreme reactivity (Schmidley 1990). Free radicals are produced in small quantities by normal cellular processes in all aerobic cells; for example, 'leaks' in mitochondrial electron transport allow oxygen to accept single electrons, forming superoxide (O_2^-) (De Bono 1994). However, they are inherently toxic—they can react with and damage proteins, nucleic acids, lipids and other classes of molecules such as the extracellular matrix glycosaminoglycans (e.g. hyaluronic acid). The sulphur-containing amino acids and the polyunsaturated fatty acids (found in high concentrations in the brain) are particularly vulnerable. Fortunately, cells possess appropriate defence mechanisms in the form of free radical scavengers (e.g. vitamins and their analogues such as α-tocopherol and ascorbic acid) and enzymes which metabolize free radicals or their precursors (e.g. superoxide dismutase, catalase and glutathione peroxidase) (De Bono 1994).

During severe ischaemia, insufficient oxygen is available to accept electrons passed along the mitochondrial electron transport chain, leading to eventual reduction ('electron saturation') of the components of this system. In the presence of small amounts of oxygen, these molecules can then autooxidize. The residual oxygen molecules in severely ischaemic brain cannot act as electron acceptors in the 'normal' fashion because oxidation–reduction ('redox') potential sufficient to favour stepwise electron transfer to them cannot be generated by such low concentrations of molecular oxygen.

Free radicals may also be generated during cerebral ischaemia by the release of iron from ferritin stores within ischaemic brain cells (Davalos *et al.* 1994). As the cerebrospinal fluid has a low concentration of ferritin-binding proteins, much of the iron released from damaged brain cells remains unbound and is therefore available to catalyse the generation of radical hydroxyl (OH·), the more malignant free radical species (see below), leading to iron-induced lipid peroxidation (a process that may be inhibited by lazaroids). This process is compounded by the fact that the central nervous system is relatively poorly endowed with superoxide dismutase, an enzyme which scavenges OH· and inhibits iron release from intracellular stores such as ferritin.

The free radical species of potential importance in cerebral ischaemia include O_2^- and OH·. Like other free radicals, they react with and damage proteins, nucleic acids and lipids, particularly the fatty acid component of membrane phospholipids, producing changes in the fluidity and permeability of the cellular membranes (lipid peroxidation) (Halliwell 1994). These, and other mediators of inflammatory reactions such as platelet-activating factor, contribute to ischaemic cell death by targeting the microvasculature and so causing microvascular dysfunction and disruption of the blood–brain barrier.

With reperfusion (section 11.1.3), reactive oxygen radicals may be generated as by-products of the reactions of free arachidonic acid (released from membrane phospholipids during ischaemia) to produce prostaglandins and leukotrienes, and lead to reperfusion injury to the brain and its microvessels.

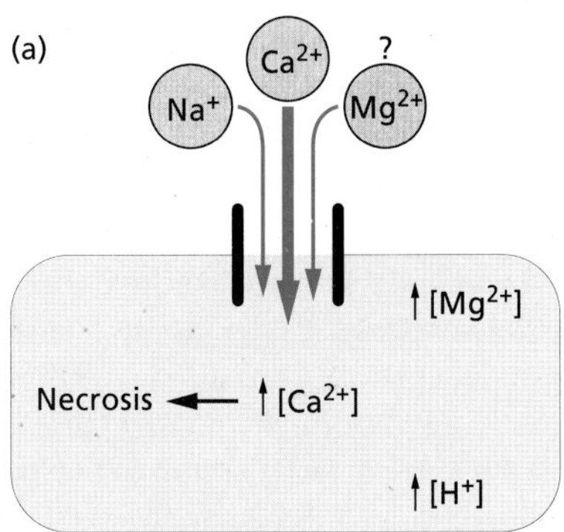

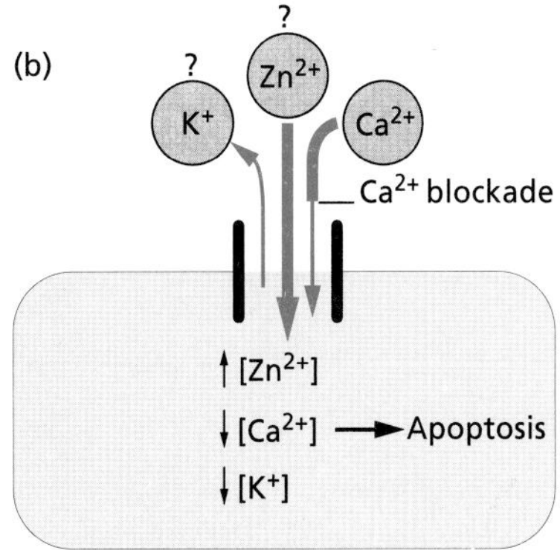

Fig. 11.11 Alterations in neuronal ionic homeostasis contributing to ischaemic neuronal death. (a) Attention has focused primarily on the possibility that excessive Ca^{2+} influx through several channel- and transporter-mediated routes, leading to intracellular Ca^{2+} overload, is a key factor underlying ischaemic neuronal necrosis. Na^+ entry contributes to acute neuronal swelling, and also facilitates Ca^{2+} entry through voltage-gated channels and the Na^+/Ca^{2+} exchanger. Mg^{2+} entry through the NMDA-receptor-gated channel may contribute to acute excitotoxic neuronal swelling and death. The drop in intracellular pH that follows NMDA-receptor-mediated Ca^{2+} influx may contribute to cell injury. (b) Recent evidence indicates that other alterations in cellular ionic homeostasis may also contribute to neuronal death after ischaemic events, in particular under circumstances where programmed cell death is induced. Reduction of intracellular free Ca^{2+} ($[Ca^{2+}]_i$), whether due to diminished entry as depicted or due to alterations in intracellular homeostasis such as diminished release from intracellular stores, favours apoptosis, as does K^+ efflux. Excessive Zn^{2+} entry at lower levels can induce apoptosis, although high levels of toxic Zn^{2+} entry induce necrosis (with permission from Lee *et al.* 1999).

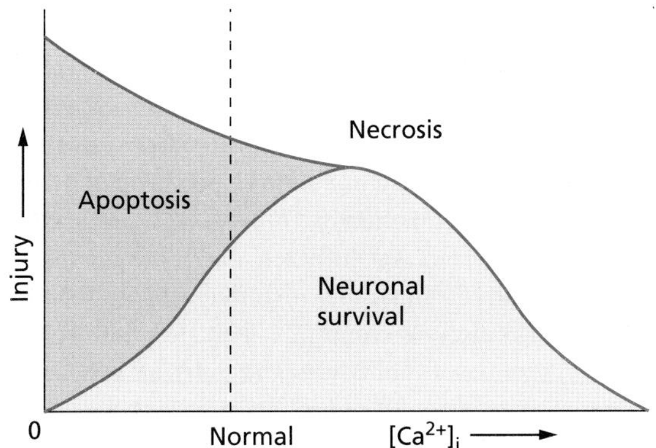

Fig. 11.12 Speculative concept of the relationship between an apoptosis–necrosis continuum, the severity of ischaemic injury and concentration of intracellular free Ca^{2+} ($[Ca^{2+}]_i$). High $[Ca^{2+}]_i$ and more severe injury promote cell death through necrosis, whereas low $[Ca^{2+}]_i$ and milder injury promote cell death through apoptosis (with permission from Lee *et al.* 1999).

Acidosis

Acidosis arises as a result of sustained tissue ischaemia. It may contribute to tissue damage and prevent or retard recovery during reoxygenation by several mechanisms; these include oedema formation, and inhibition of mitochondrial respiration and lactate oxidation (Siesjö 1992b). Cellular acidosis may promote intracellular oedema formation by inducing Na^+ and Cl^- accumulation in the cell via coupled Na^+/H^+ and Cl^-/hydrogen carbonate (HCO_3^-) exchange; acidosis activates the Na^+/H^+ exchange and H^+ leaks back into the cell via the Cl^-/HCO_3^- antiporter causing accumulation of Na^+ and Cl^- in the cell with osmotically obligated water. In other words, the cell tries to regulate intracellular pH at the expense of its own volume regulation (section 11.1.5). Furthermore, extracellular acidosis may outcompete Na^+ at the external site of the Na^+/H^+ antiporter, thereby retarding or preventing H^+ extrusion from acidotic cells. Finally, acidosis may block the lactate oxidase form of the lactate dehydrogenase complex, retarding both oxidation of lactate accumulated during ischaemia and oxidative phosphorylation in isolated mitochondria, thus curtailing ATP production.

Altered gene expression

During early cerebral ischaemia, protein synthesis in virtually all cell types in the brain is generally suppressed. Protein synthesis recovers in regions where cells survive and remains decreased in cells or regions that go on to die. It is unknown whether the decrease in protein synthesis is simply secondary to ischaemic injury or whether it plays some causal role in mediating cell death. Depending on the severity of the ischaemia and the intrinsic nature of the neuronal populations, it is thought that a stress response and changes in gene expression are elicited by ischaemia, which may be vital to cell survival and repair (see apoptosis, below). Specific genes are expressed and their corresponding proteins may be synthesized, such as immediate early genes and their products (c-*fos*, c-*jun* and zinc finger gene), heat shock and other stress genes and proteins, growth factor/receptor genes and amyloid precursor protein. These genes seem likely to be involved in mediating ischaemic injury, or in protection and repair, because they are being selectively transcribed and translated in a cell environment where limited energy availability is suppressing the translation of the majority of genes. Other hypotheses of ischaemic neuronal death, based on a disturbance of mitochondrial gene expression, have also been proposed (Abe *et al.* 1995).

Peri-infarct depolarization

Ischaemia-related and induced repetitive pathological spreading depressions or spreading depression-like depolarizations in the peri-infarct border zone, are believed to contribute to expansion of focal brain infarction (Nedergaard & Astrup 1986; Hossmann 1994; Nedergaard 1996; Takano *et al.* 1996; Koistinaho *et al.* 1999). Spreading depression, as described by Leão (1944, 1947), is characterized by slowly moving, transient and reversible depression of cortical electrical activity that spreads like a wave from the site of onset with a speed of 2–5 mm/min. It represents a propagating disturbance of membrane activity, accompanied by marked alterations in extracellular ion concentrations caused by neuronal depolarization (Siesjö & Bengtsson 1989).

In normal brain, spreading depressions repeatedly elicited over a 5 h period do not lead to neuronal death. However, within minutes to hours of focal brain ischaemia, the failure of energy-dependent membrane pumps that normally maintain ionic homeostasis, the massive presynaptic release of glutamate and activation of NMDA receptors, and the altered membrane permeability, initiate and propagate a wave of ionic transients involving uptake of Ca^{2+}, Na^+ and Cl^- into the cell, and release of K^+ from the cell. It is the elevated extracellular potassium concentration within the evolving infarct region of brain parenchyma that is believed to be a potentially important trigger to promote cortical spreading depressions or spreading depression-like depolarizations in ischaemic tissue (Takano *et al.* 1996). When spreading depression repeatedly collapses ionic gradients, activation of NMDA receptors and gap junctions propagate spreading depressions and trigger a massive Ca^{2+} influx, which in energy-compromised neurones is enough to initiate a cell death cascade (Nedergaard 1996; Koistinaho *et al.* 1999). In other words, when glutamate and potassium are released from ischaemic neurones they diffuse into the extracellular space where they may depolarize neighbouring cells at a rate of several depolarizations per hour, for 3–6 h after energy failure. This results in a spreading wave of depolarization, and energy-consuming repolarization in the stuggling penumbral cells in the peri-infarct region. The size of the core ischaemic lesion increases with each depolarization, until the phase of depolarization passes. This hypothesis is supported by the finding that in focal brain ischaemia, spreading depression increases the ischaemic volume, probably by 23% per spreading depression wave (Nedergaard 1996; Koistinaho *et al.* 1999).

Inflammation

A most important delayed phenomenon, occurring hours to days after onset of ischaemia, is inflammation (Becker 1998; DeGraba 1998). Hitherto considered an epiphenomenon, recent evidence suggests that inflammation contributes to secondary neuronal injury after acute brain ischaemia (DeGraba 1998). Under normal circumstances, the brain does not support a very robust inflammatory response. This is partly because of the relative lack of leucocyte adhesion molecules on the endothelium of the brain microvasculature, e.g. intercellular adhesion molecule (ICAM-1), P-selectin and E-selectin. However, within hours of ischaemic stroke (or infection or injury), as a result of the influx of calcium into cells and production of reactive oxygen metabolites, there is rapid induction of ICAM-1, P-selectin and E-selectin expression on the endothelium of the microvasculature, and upregulation of proinflammatory cytokines, e.g. interleukin (IL)-1β and tumour necrosis factor α (TNF-α) (Lindsberg *et al.* 1996; Shyu *et al.* 1997; Becker 1998). Activated microglia seem to be the main source of early TNF expression, and astrocytes the major source of IL-1β (Becker 1998).

Adhesion of leucocytes to the endothelium may promote ischaemic brain injury in several ways. The leucocytes can impair the flow of erythrocytes through the microvasculature, phospholipase activation in leucocytes may produce substances which cause vasoconstriction and increase platelet aggregation (e.g. leukotrienes, eicosanoids, prostaglandins and platelet-activating factor) and the products of activated leucocytes (e.g. proinflammatory cytokines, toxic oxygen metabolites, proteases, gelatinases and collagenases) can cause tissue injury. Neutrophils also migrate into the ischaemic tissue, reaching a maximum 24–48 h after the stroke, followed by an influx of monocytes and macrophages at about 24 h, which reaches a maximum several days later (Becker 1998).

The expression of inflammatory cytokines stimulates a complex cascade of events involving local endothelial cells, neurones, astrocytes and perivascular cells. A secondary response includes the release of other cytokines, an increase in components of the coagulation system, upregulation of cell adhesion molecule expression, and changes in the expression of components of the immune response. The net effect of these events is transformation of the local endothelium to a prothrombotic/proinflammatory state and induction of leucocyte migration to the site of injury (DeGraba 1998).

Apoptosis

Apoptosis is a mode of programmed cell death in which the cell synthesizes proteins and plays an active role in its own demise (Bredesen 1995; Kuchinsky & Gillardon 2000). It occurs both physiologically and pathologically. For example, during normal human embryonic development, apoptosis results in the loss of the interdigital webs required for normal formation of the fingers and toes. Likewise, tadpoles lose their tails as they develop into frogs. The normal turnover of cells in the intestinal villi is also apoptotic, as is the turnover of normal lymphocytes. Indeed, inhibition of the apoptotic death of lymphocytes may lead to B-cell lymphoma (Bredesen 1995).

Despite the intuitive link between the onset of severe, prolonged ischaemia and ultimate ischaemic neuronal necrosis, mediated by excitotoxicity (as described above), growing evidence indicates that hypoxic/ischaemic cell death continues to some extent hours to days after the onset of ischaemia, particularly within the peri-infarct zone or ischaemic penumbra, by apoptosis as a consequence of a genetically regulated programme that allows cells to die with minimal inflammation or release of genetic material (Kuchinsky & Gillardon 2000). Although ischaemia decreases protein and mRNA synthesis, ischaemia also induces at least 100 genes (and thus protein synthesis), which include immediate early genes (see above), stress proteins, growth factors, adhesion proteins, cytokines, kinases and genes directly regulating apoptosis (Koistinaho & Hokfelt 1997).

Apoptosis is characterized morphologically by coarse, regularly shaped chromatin condensation, loss of cell volume and extrusion of membrane-bound cytoplasmic fragments (apoptotic bodies), and biochemically by DNA fragmentation. These features of apoptosis can be found in neurones and glia after ischaemic injury but frequently with some additional morphological features of necrosis (e.g. swelling of cell and internal organelles). These observations suggest (but do not prove) that excitotoxicity and programmed cell death are triggered in parallel in the ischaemic brain (Choi 1996).

The best evidence implicating apoptosis in ischaemic brain-cell death is the protective action (in animal models) of genetic or pharmacological interventions aimed at selectively blocking the apoptosis cascade (Lee *et al.* 1999). Delivery through a herpesvirus vector, or transgenic overexpression of *bcl-2* which is an antiapoptotic member of a critical family of genes regulating apoptosis (the *bcl-2* proto-oncogene family), reduces infarct volume in mice subjected to focal and transient global brain ischaemia (Linnik *et al.* 1995; Kitagawa *et al.* 1998).

One of the most specific molecular markers and executioners of apoptosis is activation of caspases, a family of cysteine proteases that are critical in the late stages of apoptosis (Schulz *et al.* 1999). During ischaemia, activated caspases dismantle the cell by cleaving multiple substrates including cytoskeletal proteins and enzymes essential for cell repair. Strategies that inhibit caspase activity block cell death in experimental models of mild ischaemia, and preserve neurological function (Ma *et al.* 1998). The therapeutic window for caspase inhibition appears to be substantially longer than for glutamate receptor antagonists, and treatment combinations with both classes of drugs offer a promising approach to decreasing ischaemic injury and expanding the therapeutic window.

Implications for future neuroprotective therapies

Recent advances in our understanding of the mechanism of ischaemic brain injury suggest that future therapeutic directions should aim to refine glutamate-receptor-antagonist therapy, and move beyond the central preoccupation with excitotoxicity and neuronal Ca^{2+} overload, and target other processes and ionic derangements.

Selective blockade of NMDA receptors in cell culture prevents most of the Ca^{2+} influx and neuronal cell death induced by brief intense glutamate exposures, despite not blocking the acute cell swelling mediated by Na^+ influx though unblocked AMPA- or kainate-receptor-gated channels (accompanied by influx of Cl^- and water). NMDA antagonists also markedly attenuate the death of cultured neurones induced by oxygen and/or glucose deprivation (Lee *et al.* 1999). Based on these data, and the association of high concentrations of glutamate in the blood and CSF within 24 h of the onset of acute ischaemic stroke with early neurological deterioration (due to presumed early progression of ischaemic stroke within the first 48 h of stroke) (Castillo *et al.* 1997), several pharmaceutical companies have developed NMDA-antagonist drugs and tested them in human clinical trials. Although some trials are still ongoing, the results from several completed trials have been disappointing (section 11.6). There are many possible reasons: poor trial study design, inadequate sample size and unreliable outcome evaluation; anatomical and aetiological hetereogeneity in the study populations; dose ceilings imposed by adverse effects of the drug; inadequate drug penetration to the site of the lesion; drug delivery after the therapeutic window has closed; publication bias in the basic science literature; and misleading hypotheses from the basic scientific researchers linking NMDA-receptor-mediated excitotoxicity to hypoxic-ischaemic neuronal death. It is more likely, however, that both the pre-clinical and clinical trial data are informative: that is, NMDA receptor overactivation leading to neuronal calcium overload contributes importantly to neuronal cell death after focal brain ischaemia, but is not a predominant mechanism. Perhaps its contribution is masked by the parallel occurrence of other forms of injury (e.g. AMPA/kainate-receptor-mediated toxicity may be the dominant mediator of excitotoxicity on certain cell types), or worse, blocking of NMDA receptors might exacerbate another form of injury altogether (Lee *et al.* 1999). Therefore, the neuroprotective efficacy of NMDA-antagonist therapy might be enhanced by combination with AMPA- or kainate-receptor antagonists, or by blocking excitotoxicity in ways superior to that achievable with unselective (pan-subtype) NMDA antagonists.

There seem to be so many pathways from ischaemia to neuronal cell death that blocking just one of them is probably fruitless; perhaps this is like ligating a feeding artery to an arteriovenous malformation, there are always others that will take over to keep up its blood suppy.

Interference with inflammatory cascades is another approach likely to aid both neuronal and astrocyte survival. Inhibition of the early adherence of leucocytes to blood vessels in the ischaemic region shortly after the insult (by means of antibodies directed against cell-surface ligands such as ICAM-1), may inhibit the release of inflammatory cytokines and limit microvascular occlusion (Zhang *et al.* 1994). Although an initial phase III trial using anti-ICAM antibodies failed (possibly because of murine antibody-induced complications) (Enlimomab Acute Stroke Trial Investigators 1997), a second trial using humanized antibodies directed against the leucocyte integrins, CD11/CD18, is now underway (Goldberg 1997). Alternatively, direct inhibitors of the release or action of proinflammatory cytokines, such as IL-1β or TNF-α, from microglia or astrocytes may prevent the upregulation of leucocyte adhesion molecules on endothelial cells and oedema formation (Betz *et al.* 1995).

If excitotoxic necrosis and apoptosis really are both triggered in parallel in ischaemic brain, the combination of inhibition of excitotoxic necrosis and ischaemic apoptosis may yield greater neuroprotection than either approach alone, and may permit a longer therapeutic time window (Zipfel *et al.* 1999) (Fig. 11.13). Indeed, it is plausible that this combination may be required before approaches directed toward attenuating Ca^{2+} overload, including the use of glutamate-receptor antagonists, produce detectable benefit. Two experimental studies have so far tested the concurrent administration of NMDA antagonists with an antiapoptotic drug.

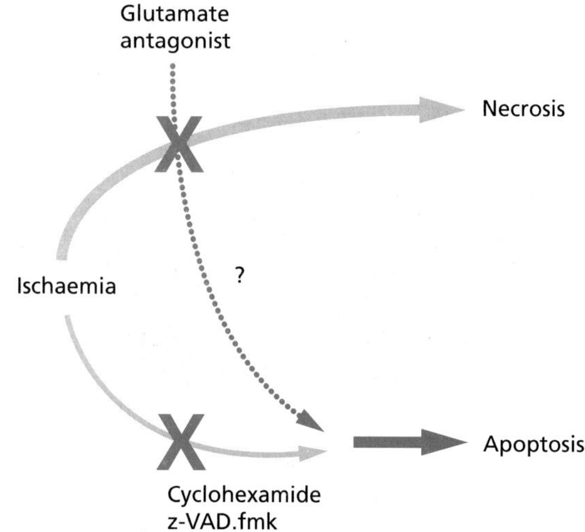

Fig. 11.13 Ischaemia triggers necrosis and apoptosis in parallel. Some antiapoptotic interventions, such as cyclohexamide or z-VAD.fmk, attenuate apoptosis without affecting necrosis. On the other hand, antiexcitotoxic interventions such as glutamate antagonists may exacerbate apoptosis by reducing Ca^{2+} influx and $[Ca^{2+}]_i$ (with permission from Lee *et al.* 1999).

Co-administration of dextrophan with cyclohexamide produced greater than 80% reduction in infarct volume after transient focal brain ischaemia in rats, which was better than either agent alone (Du *et al.* 1996; Ma *et al.* 1998).

Finally, molecular biological techniques are being applied to elucidate further the mechanisms of ischaemic neuronal death and repair and to see if it is possible to switch off, or block, injury-related genes, which programme cell death, and to facilitate protection or repair genes (Kogure & Kato 1993; Sharp 1994). For example, an (antisense) oligonucleotide, complementary to a piece of mRNA, can disrupt or block expression of a gene, the c-*fos* proto-oncogene, that is induced in the intact brain by ischaemia (Liu *et al.* 1994). Since the c-*fos* gene is a transcription factor believed to bind to the promoter of many target genes and regulate their expression, the results pave the way for understanding whether the target genes of the *fos* protein-mediated pathways help cells survive and regenerate, or mediate pathways that lead to cell death following ischaemic injury in brain. If it is shown that c-*fos* is 'bad' for the brain when it is induced in ischaemia, then the finding that ischaemic induction of *fos* protein can be markedly attenuated with the antisense oligonucleotide might have therapeutic implications (Liu *et al.* 1994).

11.1.5 Ischaemic cerebral oedema

Cerebral ischaemia not only causes loss of neuronal function but also cerebral oedema. Within minutes of the onset of ischaemia, cytotoxic cerebral oedema occurs as a result of cell membrane damage allowing intracellular accumulation of water. The grey matter initially tends to be affected more than the white matter (Symon *et al.* 1979). The CT scan appearances are those of well-circumscribed low density involving the cortex and subcortex (section 5.3.5). The blood–brain barrier remains intact according to CT and isotope studies, and endothelial tight junctions are maintained (Bruce & Hurtig 1979). However, after several days of ischaemia, breakdown of the blood–brain barrier leads to vasogenic cerebral oedema as plasma constituents enter the brain extracellular space. The white matter tends to be more affected than the grey matter. The CT scan appearance of vasogenic oedema includes the characteristic finger-like projections of low density in the white matter, which characteristically accompany cerebral tumours.

Animal studies and clinical observations suggest that ischaemic cerebral oedema begins within hours of stroke onset and reaches a maximum volume at 2–4 days and then subsides over 1–2 weeks. On the other hand, CT studies indicate that fluid volume after infarction peaks in 7–10 days and oedema remains detectable for 1 month (Bruce & Hurtig 1979). However, the CT assessment of oedema may be unreliable because of stroke-induced changes in blood volume and tissue density on CT.

In baboons, cerebral oedema can be exacerbated by reperfusion 2 h after stroke onset but it is unknown whether this occurs in humans. Indeed, in the second European–Australasian Acute Stroke Study (ECASS II), fatal cerebral oedema within the first 7 days was more common in the placebo group (4.3% of 391 patients) than in the thrombolytic therapy patients (2.0% of 409 patients) (Bell *et al.* 1985; Hacke *et al.* 1998) (section 11.5.2). Despite some evidence that early spontaneous reperfusion is not associated with a worsening of acute cerebral infarction, and may actually lead to a better clinical outcome (von Kummer & Forsting 1993; Wardlaw *et al.* 1993), the recent thrombolytic trials (section 11.5.2) have reported that presumed reperfusion following thrombolytic therapy may be associated with a higher rate of haemorrhagic transformation of the infarct (section 5.4) and early death (Donnan *et al.* 1995; Hommel *et al.* 1995; Kaste *et al.* 1995).

Cerebral oedema correlates well with mass effect, midline shift, infarct size, neurological status and outcome. Correlation with infarct size perhaps explains why oedema does not seem to be so common or prominent in lacunar and small brainstem infarcts as it is in larger cortical/subcortical infarcts.

The effects of cerebral oedema are to compromise blood flow even further (by increasing pressure in the extravascular space, thus causing vascular congestion and sometimes haemorrhagic transformation) and to cause mass effect, brain shift and eventually brain herniation (Figs 11.14 and 11.15). The main danger of herniation is that it can initiate vascular and obstructive complications which aggravate the original expanding lesion, by compressing important vessels and tissues and causing cerebral ischaemia, congestion and oedema which, in turn, enhances the expanding process. In addition, the herniating brain can compress the aqueduct and subarachnoid spaces and so interfere with cerebrospinal fluid circulation, leading to hydrocephalus and elevated cerebrospinal fluid pressure. There are three patterns of supratentorial brain shift which can be identified by their end stages: cingulate herniation, central transtentorial herniation and uncal herniation (Plum & Posner 1985).

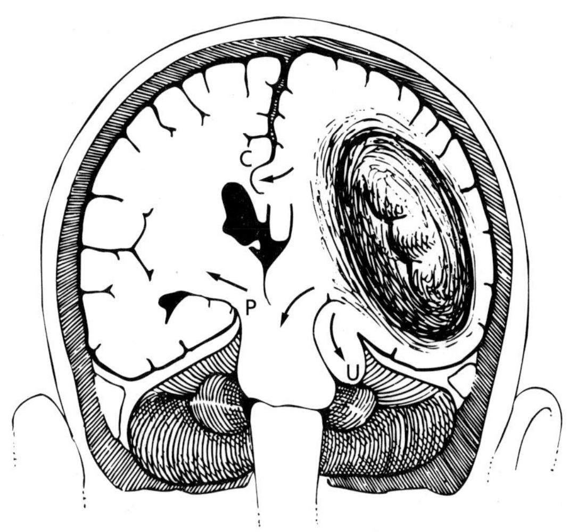

Fig. 11.14 Uncal and cingulate herniation. A mass such as a cerebral haemorrhage, large cerebral infarct or haemorrhagic infarct displaces the diencephalon and mesencephalon horizontally and caudally. The cingulate gyrus (C) on the side of the lesion herniates under the falx cerebri. The uncus (U) of the ipsilateral temporal lobe herniates under the tentorium cerebelli and becomes grooved and swollen and may compress the ipsilateral oculomotor (IIIrd cranial) nerve causing pupillary dilatation (Hutchinson's sign) (Hutchinson 1867). The cerebral peduncle (P) opposite the supratentorial mass becomes compressed against the edge of the tentorium, leading to grooving (Kernohan's notch) and causes a paresis ipsilateral to the cerebral mass lesion (Kernohan & Woltman 1929). Central downward displacement also occurs but is less marked than in Fig. 11.15 (from Plum & Posner 1985).

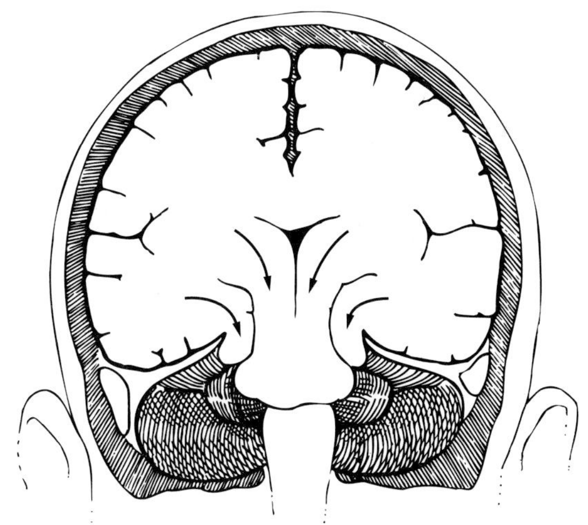

Fig. 11.15 Central transtentorial herniation. Diffuse or multifocal swelling of the cerebral hemispheres (or bilateral subdural or extradural haematomas) compresses and elongates the diencephalon from above. The mammillary bodies are displaced caudally. The cingulate gyrus is not herniated (from Plum & Posner 1985).

Cingulate herniation

Cingulate herniation occurs when the expanding hemisphere shifts across the intracranial cavity, forcing the ipsilateral cingulate gyrus under the falx cerebri, compressing and displacing the internal cerebral vein and the ipsilateral anterior cerebral artery. This may lead to additional infarction in the territory of the anterior cerebral artery (Fig. 11.14).

Central transtentorial herniation

Central transtentorial herniation of the diencephalon is the end result of displacement of the hemispheres and basal nuclei, compressing and eventually displacing the diencephalon and the adjoining midbrain rostro-caudally through the tentorial notch (Fig. 11.15). The great cerebral vein is compressed, which raises the hydrostatic pressure of the entire deep territory it drains. In addition, downward displacement of the midbrain and pons stretches the medial perforating branches of the basilar artery (the artery cannot shift downward because it is tethered to the circle of Willis), leading to paramedian brainstem ischaemia (and haemorrhage if perfusion continues).

Uncal herniation

Uncal herniation characteristically occurs when expanding lesions arising in the temporal fossa or temporal lobe shift the inner, basal edge of the uncus and hippocampal gyrus toward the midline so that they bulge over the incisural edge of the tentorium, and push the adjacent midbrain against the opposite incisural edge (Fig. 11.14). At the same time the IIIrd cranial nerve and the posterior cerebral artery on the side of the expanding temporal lobe are often caught between the overhanging swollen uncus and the free edge of the tentorium or the petroclinoid ligament, leading to a IIIrd nerve palsy and occipital and medial temporal lobe infarction and swelling, which further compounds the problem.

Transtentorial herniation is the most common cause of death during the first week after acute stroke, accounting for about 80% of deaths in cerebral infarction and 90% in cerebral haemorrhage (Hachinski & Norris 1985; Oppenheimer & Hachinski 1992). The risk of death peaks within 24 h for cerebral haemorrhage and at 4–5 days for cerebral infarction. Brainstem compression, with subsequent haemorrhage and infarction within it, accounts for the serious morbidity and mortality associated with herniation.

Transtentorial herniation is the most common cause of death within the first week of onset of both ischaemic stroke and primary intracerebral haemorrhage.

Signs of herniation

The concept of brain herniation being the cause of the neurological signs traditionally associated with herniation (e.g. drowsiness followed by stupor, then coma and pupil dilatation) has evolved from the correlation of clinical symptoms and signs with indirect radiographic studies and the results of post-mortem neuropathology. This concept has been challenged by Ropper (1986, 1989), who acknowledges that central (bilateral diencephalic) and uncal herniation, as described by McNealy and Plum (1962), occurs, but contends that they are a late occurrence and occur *after* the neurological signs of 'so-called' herniation. He believes that coma and other signs attributed to herniation are due to *horizontal* displacement of the brain. He has found that the degree of depressed consciousness correlates linearly with horizontal displacement of the pineal gland (a reference marker), and that there is no correlation between conscious level and concurrent MRI evidence of the vertical displacement of the brain. He has also found, by carefully (and repeatedly) examining 'coning' patients and correlating their clinical signs with the concurrent findings on magnetic resonance brain scans and at post-mortem, that horizontal shift of the brain compresses the contralateral perimesencephalic and ambient cisterns, and *expands* these cisterns on the ipsilateral side of the mass lesion. Only *later* does the brain (uncus and parahippocampal formation) ipsilateral to the mass lesion herniate into this *expanded* space in the ipsilateral ambient and perimesencephalic cisterns, but the uncus does *not compress* the brainstem or the ipsilateral IIIrd cranial nerve. If the ipsilateral pupil dilates, it is because the IIIrd nerve is stretched over the clivus (the clivus bend syndrome). If bilateral pupil dilatation occurs, it is later, and in 95% of cases as a result of a central phenomena (i.e. a nuclear contralateral IIIrd nerve palsy due to brainstem compression ± ischaemia). The contralateral pupil dilates first in about 5% of patients. Ropper therefore contends that:

- the brain moves away from a mass in all directions allowed by dural anatomy;
- herniated medial temporal lobe is not generally the cause of upper brainstem displacement;
- downward movement does not correlate well with consciousness and can occur without coma;
- the degree of horizontal pineal displacement corresponds well with the level of consciousness with acute masses (3–6 mm = drowsiness, 6–9 mm = stupor, > 9 mm = coma);
- impaired consciousness and pineal shift have practical consequences:
  - if the level of consciousness is less than predicted from the degree of pineal shift, another cause for coma can be presumed (e.g. anoxic, metabolic, hydrocephalus);
  - if pineal shift is excessive for the level of consciousness, the mass is chronic;
- precise pineal shift can be used to follow an acute mass and oedema serially with CT brain scans.

Subsequently, however, Reich *et al.* (1993) identified, from midsagittal MRI scans among patients with acute supratentorial mass lesions, that there was downward displacement of the orifice (iter) of the aqueduct below the plane of the tentorial incisura which anticipated or confirmed clinical signs of brain herniation. The respective strengths and weaknesses of the respective hypotheses have been discussed further (Plum *et al.* 1993; Ropper 1993).

11.1.6 Conclusion

Many different mediators have been implicated in brain cell survival and death in cerebral ischaemia. These include platelet-activating factor, platelet adhesion and aggregation, eicosanoids, cytokines, leucocytes, coagulation and fibrinolysis, excitotoxins, Ca^{2+}, acidosis, free radicals, altered gene expression and cellular oedema. It has not been established whether these mediators act in a sequential, hierarchical fashion, or whether they are involved in a network of intricate relationships with overlapping effects. Efforts to treat ischaemic stroke successfully will require an integrated approach to understanding how the ischaemic process is initiated, and how the mediators interact and when.

11.2 General treatment considerations

The primary aims of the specific treatments considered in this chapter are, broadly speaking, to minimize the volume of brain damaged by ischaemia. The assumption is that, if this can be achieved without excess hazard, that neurological impairment, disability and handicap should all correspondingly be reduced in survivors. For patients with a large volume of ischaemic brain, minimizing the volume which infarcts should also reduce the risk of early death, particularly from ischaemic cerebral oedema and transtentorial herniation (section 11.1.5). The pathophysiology of acute cerebral ischaemia is complex (section 11.1.3), and many potential treatments may have more than one mechanism of action; for some, the precise mechanism is unknown. However, the main targets of acute treatment are to: restore and then maintain blood flow, and simultaneously keep alive as much ischaemic brain tissue as possible while the blood supply is being restored.

11.2.1 How to evaluate evidence about different treatments (and other aspects of stroke management)

Evidence-based medicine

We try to base our decisions on whether or not to use a particular treatment in clinical practice on the evidence from randomized trials and from systematic reviews of randomized trials. This approach is part of what is now known as 'evidence-based medicine', a style of medical practice which Sackett described as: 'a life-long process of self-directed learning in which caring for our patients creates the need for clinically important information about diagnosis, prognosis and therapy' (Sackett *et al.* 2000). The book by Sackett and co-authors on the subject is short and clear and provides succinct advice on how to find the best evidence, appraise it critically and then apply it in everyday clinical practice (Sackett *et al.* 2000). This section summarizes what the best forms of evidence are (and why) and where up-to-date evidence can be found.

Why are randomized trials the best way to evaluate treatments?

There is now little disagreement that the randomized controlled trial (RCT) is the best way to evaluate most treatments (Sackett *et al.* 1991) (Table 11.1). It was not always thus. Richard Doll described the approach taken in 1937 when he entered clinical medicine: 'new treatments were almost always introduced on the grounds that in the hands of professor A, or in the hands of a consultant at one of the leading teaching hospitals, the results in a small series of patients (seldom more than 50) had been superior to those recorded by professor B ... or by the same investigator previously' (Doll 1998). Research designs like these, i.e. case series without any controls, series with retrospective controls, and series with concurrent controls but non-random treatment

Table 11.1 Methodological questions in the critical assessment of an article evaluating treatment (modified from Sackett *et al.* 1991).

*Was the assignment of patients to treatment really randomized?**
Was the similarity between groups documented?
Was prognostic stratification used in treatment allocation?
Was foreknowledge of the randomly allocated treatment possible?

Were all clinically relevant outcomes reported?
Was case fatality as well as morbidity reported?
Were deaths from all causes reported?
Were quality-of-life assessments conducted?
Was outcome assessment blind to treatment allocation?

Were the study patients recognizably similar to your own?
Were reproducibly defined exclusion criteria stated?
Was the setting primary, secondary or tertiary care?
Was the type of patient included in the study clearly described?

Were both statistical and clinical significance considered?
If statistically significant, was the difference clinically important?
If not statistically significant, was the study big enough to show a clinically important difference if one really exists?

Is the therapeutic manoeuvre feasible in your practice?
Available, affordable, sensible?
Were contamination† and co-intervention avoided?
Was the manoeuvre administered blind?
Was compliance measured?

Were all patients who entered the study accounted for at its conclusion?
(i.e. were drop-outs, withdrawals, non-compliers and those who crossed over handled appropriately in the analysis?)

* Methods of allocation such as alternation, use of hospital number or date of birth all provide foreknowledge of the next treatment allocation, and so allow the trial allocation process to be subverted and result in selection bias between the two treatment groups.
† In this context, contamination implies that some patients allocated active treatment either do not receive the treatment or are given the treatment which the other treatment group should receive, or some non-trial treatment with similar properties to one of the trial interventions under test.

allocation, may introduce many biases into the assessment of treatment effect (Sackett *et al.* 1991, 2000).

The Medical Research Council trial of streptomycin for pulmonary tuberculosis, designed by the statistician Sir Austin Bradford Hill, is probably the strongest contender for the title 'first clinical trial to use strictly random allocation', although there is some debate about this claim (Medical Research Council 1948; Yoshioka 1998). The trial not only established the benefits of the treatment beyond all reasonable doubt, but also served as the most ethical and equitable way of utilizing the very limited supply of the drug that was available in Britain at the time. It also prevented the treatment 'creeping' into routine clinical practice without being properly evaluated.

We could answer many of the therapeutic questions posed in this book a great deal faster if a larger proportion of stroke patients were entered in appropriate randomized controlled trials.

Strictly random allocation with proper concealment of what the next treatment allocation will be minimizes selection bias. If the doctor can find out what treatment the next patient who enters the trial will be allocated (e.g. by holding the sealed trial allocation envelope up to a bright light), he may be tempted not to enter the patient in the trial. A central telephone randomization system offers complete concealment. The clinician telephones a randomization centre and gives the patient's details over the telephone. These are then recorded on the central computer during the call, and the computer generates the next treatment allocation only after all the baseline data are checked and entered; the patient is then irrevocably in the trial, and selection bias cannot occur.

It is also important to reduce observer bias, if possible, by 'blinding' both the patients and the observers who collect the outcome data (Sackett *et al.* 2000). Random error is reduced by recruiting a sufficiently large sample of patients (Peto *et al.* 1995; Sackett *et al.* 2000). However, RCTs need to be surprisingly large to provide really reliable evidence on the balance of risk and benefit for a particular treatment. If the measure of outcome is an uncommon but serious event, such as death, and the effect of the treatment on that outcome is only moderate, then the trial may need to recruit several tens of thousands of patients (Peto *et al.* 1995). The effort of conducting such large RCTs is substantial, and so many of the 'mega trials' have used a factorial design to assess two or three treatments at the same time without loss of statistical efficiency (Peto *et al.* 1995).

Good trial design seeks to reduce bias and random error in the assessment of treatment effect: strict randomization with concealment reduces selection bias; blinding reduces observer bias; and recruitment of large numbers of patients reduces random error.

Problems with randomized controlled trials in acute stroke from 1956 to the present

Eight years after the streptomycin trial was published in 1948, Dyken and White wrote of the many methodological problems they identified in evaluating treatments for acute stroke; not the least was to know, in an individual patient, whether or not treatment had been effective. They wrote this in the report of the first quasi-randomized study of a medical treatment for acute stroke (Dyken & White 1956). Thirty-six patients were alternately (but not randomly) assigned to cortisone or control. Thirteen of the cortisone patients and 10 of the controls died; a trend against treatment, but an inconclusive result. It is sobering to realize how few large, well-designed and executed trials of treatments for acute stroke there have been, which have reliably answered the questions they set out to address, in the four decades since then. The trials which failed to meet these criteria had weaknesses which included: over-complex eligibility criteria; inadequate sample size; inappropriate measures of outcome; poor standards of execution (i.e. poor trial discipline); and an unacceptably high proportion of patients 'lost' to follow-up. The reports of these studies often gave incomplete descriptions of the methods used (particularly the method of randomization), failed to account for all patients randomized, used inappropriate statistical methods (often with inappropriate subgroup analysis) and provided conclusions that were not supported by the data presented (Bath *et al.* 1998). The picture is now changing and, in general, the design of stroke trials seems to be improving with larger sample sizes, better design and higher standards of execution and reporting (Bath *et al.* 1998). Measures of outcome after stroke are getting simpler, more reliable and valid; complex (and irrelevant) stroke scales to assess outcome (rather than initial stroke severity) may soon be a thing of the past (van Gijn & Warlow 1992) (section 17.6.3). The CONSORT group have produced guidelines to improve the quality of reports of randomized trials (Begg *et al.* 1996), and one can only hope that, in future, stroke trialists will adhere to these guidelines when reporting their trial results.

The ideal would be that the evaluation of new treatments for stroke would be handled in the same way that, for example, new treatments for leukaemia are, i.e. it is normal practice that the great majority of patients with leukaemia in the UK are treated in the context of a randomized trial for at least some aspect of their treatment.

Describing the effects of treatment in numbers

The effects of a treatment can be expressed in a number of ways. *Relative* treatment effects can make a treatment appear to have impressive benefits; 'drug X reduced the risk of event Y by a half'. Table 11.2 describes how the most common

Table 11.2 Describing the numerical results of a clinical trial in different ways.

	Treated	*Control*
No. originally randomized in this group	1000	1000
No. who were dead at the end of the trial	80[a] (8%)	100[b] (10%)
No. alive at the end of the trial	920[c] (92%)	900[d] (90%)

Relative risk of death (RR) = 8%/10% = 0.80*
Relative risk reduction of death
(RRR) = (1 − RR) × 100 = (1 − 0.80) × 100 = 20%

Odds ratio (OR) = (a/c) ÷ (b/d) = ad/bc = 0.78*†
Relative odds reduction = (1 − OR) × 100 = (1 − 0.78) × 100 = 22%†

Absolute risk of death in control group = 100/1000 = 10%
Absolute risk of death in treated group = 80/1000 = 8%
Absolute risk difference in death (ARD) = 10% − 8% = 2%, or 20 deaths avoided or postponed per 1000 patients treated

Number-needed-to-treat to avoid one event (NNT) = 100/ARD = 100/2 = 50†‡ need to be treated to prevent or at least postpone one death

Notes:
* The odds ratio and relative risk both provide an estimate of relative treatment effect. The estimates will be similar if the absolute risk in the Control group is low. However, if the absolute risk in the controls is high, then the odds reduction will be larger than the relative risk reduction (Zhang & Yu 1998). For example, in the Cochrane review of the effect of stroke units, about 62% of patients treated on general medical wards were dead or dependent at the end of follow-up, compared with 58% of patients treated on a stroke unit; this gives an odds ratio of 0.75 and so a relative odds reduction of 25% in favour of stroke units. When the same results are expressed as relative risks, the relative risk of 0.9 and the relative risk reduction of 10% associated with the benefits of stroke units appear more modest. However, the absolute risk difference (calculated with the Metaview programme built into the Cochrane Library software, and making some allowance for the heterogeneity of control rates in the different trials) is an impressive 62 patients per 1000 avoiding death or dependency.
† It is important to calculate the confidence intervals for these estimates of effect. Formulae (and a computer program) are given in Altman *et al.* (2000).
‡ NNTs calculated from a systematic review of several trials must be interpreted with caution and statistical advice on the best method to derive an estimate of NNT is desirable (Smeeth *et al.* 1999).

numerical measures of relative and absolute treatment effects are calculated. The *absolute* benefit is more important for clinical decisions, and is greatly influenced by the frequency of events in the control group. If events are rare in the control group, the absolute benefit will be small and the numbers-needed-to-treat to prevent one event (NNT) will be correspondingly large, so the treatment may have little clinical value in low-risk patients. For example, in a randomized trial, if fatal pulmonary embolism occurred in 0.5% of stroke patients allocated aspirin alone, and in 0.25% of those allocated to the combination of aspirin with a second antithrombotic agent (e.g. low molecular weight heparin) the relative risk reduction (RRR) would be an impressive 50% but the absolute risk difference (ARD) would be only 0.25%. In other words, if we treated 1000 patients, only two or three would avoid fatal pulmonary embolism and the NNT to prevent one person having pulmonary embolism would be 400. However, if fatal pulmonary embolism occurred in 5% of controls, and the RRR was still 50%, the ARD would be 2.5% and the NNT would be just 40 patients.

What are systematic reviews and why do we need them?

The biomedical literature is so enormous that clinicians are faced with an unmanageably large amount of information to assimilate. For example, a search of issue 1, 2000 of the Cochrane Controlled Clinical Trials Register in the Cochrane Library, using the medical subject heading (MESH) term 'cerebrovascular disorders' identified 2600 references to randomized trials, or controlled trials, relevant to the treatment, prevention or rehabilitation of stroke (Cochrane Stroke Group 2000). The literature is growing fast too: on average over 16 new studies under the same term were added each month to the Cochrane Controlled Clinical Trials Register.

Faced with such a confusing and rapidly changing array of information about treatment, what should the busy clinician do? Focus on a few selected reports published in well-known English-language journals? Such selection could easily lead to a biased assessment of the effects of the treatment. Rely on visiting pharmaceutical company representatives and being flown to exotic locations to suffer sponsored symposia? Hopefully not. The best way to minimize bias is to review systematically *all* of the evidence from *all* of the relevant RCTs, both published and unpublished (Peto *et al.* 1995; Sackett *et al.* 2000). The Quality of Reporting of Meta-analyses (QUOROM) Group has stated the views of a panel of experts on what constitues an adequate report of a systematic review (Moher *et al.* 1999). The criteria for assessing a report of a systematic review are outlined in Table 11.3. The last part of this section (p. 467) describes how best to find reports of systematic reviews (see also Hunt & McKibbon 1997; Sackett *et al.* 2000). Briefly, a systematic review:
- defines the question to be addressed;
- uses a defined search strategy to identify relevant studies;
- selects studies and extracts data from them using explicit criteria;
- synthesizes the evidence in a quantitative manner whenever possible (i.e. it can provide an overall estimate of the treatment effect).

Table 11.3 Methodological questions in the critical assessment of a systematic review.

Were the question(s) and methods clearly stated?
Were the search methods used to locate relevant studies comprehensive?
Were explicit methods used to determine which articles to include in the review?
Was the methodological quality of the primary studies assessed?
Were the selection and assessment of the primary studies reproducible and free from bias?
Were differences in individual study results adequately explained?
Were the results of the primary studies combined appropriately?
Were the reviewers' conclusions supported by the data cited?

Note: this is a simple version for 'beginners' (Sackett *et al.* 1991); Cook *et al.* (1995) give more detail; Hunt and McKibbon have written a more detailed review on how to search for and assess reports of systematic reviews (Hunt & McKibbon 1997) and the QUOROM group have reported a consensus group's view of the key features of an adequate report of a meta-analysis (Moher *et al.* 1999).

What is meta-analysis?

Meta-analysis is the numerical technique which derives an overall estimate of the treatment effect from all of the trials included in a systematic (or non-systematic) review. Such overall estimates avoid the selection bias inherent with choosing estimates derived from single trials and are more precise than the estimate from any one trial (i.e. less subject to random error), because they are based on more data.

> *Meta-analysis is not statistical trickery; it is simply the best way to obtain the least biased and most precise estimate of treatment effect from a group of similar trials of the same intervention in the same type of patients and using the same type of outcome measures.*

Hazards of inappropriate subgroup analysis in trials (and systematic reviews)

Subgroup analysis is popular with clinical trialists and people who like to generate hypotheses to explain the 'negative' or 'positive' overall results of particular trials. It is, however, a dangerous sport, since even apparently large effects observed in subgroups can merely be due to the play of chance and not to the treatment itself (Antiplatelet Trialists' Collaboration 1994a; Counsell *et al.* 1994; Peto *et al.* 1995; Sackett *et al.* 2000). Claims for the benefits of a treatment based on a subgroup analysis of a single trial, or of a meta-analysis, need to be viewed with caution and should be seen as hypothesis generating. To test such subgroup hypotheses reliably, generally requires further very large trials with appropriate prespecified hypotheses.

Inappropriate subgroup analyses may have disastrous effects. The report of the Canadian aspirin sulphinpyrazone trial concluded that, overall, among people with threatened stroke, aspirin was associated with a significant 30% reduction in the risk of stroke or death (Gent *et al.* 1980). A subgroup analysis stated that the benefit was confined to males, and was not seen in females. As a result of this analysis, the United States Food and Drug Administration (FDA) licensed aspirin for stroke prevention but only in males, not in females. The results of the Antiplatelet Trialists' Collaboration systematic review in 1994 of all of the relevant randomized trials showed that, among high-risk individuals, the benefits of antiplatelet drugs were similar in males and females, so refuting the results of the Canadian trial aspirin subgroup analysis (Antiplatelet Trialists' Collaboration 1994a).

The FDA did not license aspirin for stroke prevention in women until 1998, so in the years between 1980 and 1998, it seems likely that many women worldwide at high risk of stroke were not treated with aspirin and consequently had strokes which might have otherwise been avoided. Likewise, undue emphasis on the results of a single positive trial in a meta-analysis may result in misleadingly optimistic conclusions. For example, the most widely cited study of therapeutic thrombolysis in acute ischaemic stroke, the NINDS trial, may well have overestimated the benefits of this treatment (National Institute of Neurological Disorders & Stroke (NINDS) rt-PA Stroke Study Group 1995; Wardlaw *et al.* 2000).

Translating the results of trials and systematic reviews into improving clinical practice

There are now many books and articles on how to use the results of trials and systematic reviews to improve one's own clinical practice (Dans *et al.* 1998; Sackett *et al.* 2000). However, it takes a great deal of time and resources to take the next steps, i.e. to develop and implement evidence-based guidelines or policy documents and then consistently apply them to an entire clinical service over a long period. Many strategies to improve clinician performance, ranging from financial incentives, to guidelines, to continuing medical education have all been suggested. The Cochrane Effective Practice and Organization of Care (EPOC) Group is undertaking systematic reviews to identify which interventions have actually achieved an improvement in the clinical practice of health care professionals (Grimshaw 2000). If we are to spend some of our limited health service resources on getting health care professionals to improve their standards of care, it is important that we spend them only on those methods which can bring about a measurable and sustainable change in clinical practice (and do so efficiently and cost-effectively) (Table 17.24). Our efforts to improve standards of care must not be wasted on interventions—such as audit without feedback—that take great effort, but achieve little (Grimshaw & Russell 1993; Thomson O'Brien *et al.* 2000).

Where we look for up-to-date reports of randomized trials, systematic reviews and clinical practice guidelines

Guidance on how to find high-quality, up-to-date evidence in the most efficient way possible is available (Hunt & McKibbon 1997; Sackett *et al.* 2000). Although evidence-based medicine requires one to use up-to-date reports, we have to concede that, with each year that passes after the publication of this book, more and more of the evidence we have cited will be superseded. However, there are now several sources of regularly updated evidence which will fill the information gap until the next edition.

The Cochrane Collaboration Stroke Review Group is coordinating a series of systematic reviews of different forms of health care for the treatment and prevention of stroke which are updated as new information becomes available (Counsell *et al.* 1995; Cochrane Stroke Group 2000). The Cochrane Stroke Group has a website which includes a link to the Cochrane Collaboration website, where abstracts of all the Cochrane systematic reviews are available free of charge (http://www.dcn.ed.ac.uk/csrg).

Where possible therefore we have cited stroke reviews from the Cochrane Database of Systematic Reviews, since they are often of higher quality and are more frequently updated than many corresponding reviews published in conventional paper journals (Jadad *et al.* 1998). Where there was no relevant Cochrane review available, we searched for a high-quality systematic review. The Cochrane Library includes the Database of Abstracts of Reviews of Effectiveness (DARE), a series of quality-assured reviews (and their abstracts) which is a very useful source of such reviews. If we could not find a systematic review, we either resorted to asking a known expert in the field or to a search of the Cochrane Controlled Trials Register; in 2000, this contained over 260 000 references to randomized trials and controlled clinical trials.

Clinical Evidence is a compendium of the best available evidence on effective health care, which is published in book form and will be updated every 6 months (Godlee *et al.* 2000). We have therefore often cited chapters from it rather than the primary sources which were identified, since any recent evidence will be included in the updated chapter; readers must just ensure they are reading the most recent edition.

Furthermore, through the Department of Clinical Neurosciences in Edinburgh, we have established a website which provides links to reliable and regularly updated sources of information relevant to the topics covered in this book (http://www.dcn.ed.ac.uk). Websites of organizations which produce evidence-based guidelines on stroke include: The Royal College of Physicians of London (http://www.rcplondon.ac.uk); the Scottish Intercollegiate Guidelines Network (http://www.show.scot.nhs.uk/sign/clinical.htm); the Cochrane Stroke Group website is building up a list of links to stroke guidelines (http://www.dcn.ed.ac.uk/csrg); the National Electronic Library for Health (NELH) seeks to take this concept further, making relevant up-to-date information on effective forms of health care available to patients and doctors (http://www.nelh.nhs.uk) (Muir Gray & de Lusignan 1999).

11.2.2 Organization of acute stroke services

The way acute stroke services are organized within a particular hospital will depend very much on what resources are available and what treatments are planned. This is discussed in Chapter 17. Clinical and radiological diagnosis of acute stroke is dealt with in Chapters 3, 4 and 5. The other aspects of management in the acute phase, such as how to monitor blood pressure and oxygen saturation, are dealt with in Chapter 15. A number of guideline documents and consensus statements on the acute management of stroke have been published, but each of them makes somewhat different recommendations; this lack of agreement must partly reflect the lack of reliable randomized evidence (Adams *et al.* 1994; European Ad Hoc Consensus Group 1996, 1997; Pan European Consensus Meeting on Stroke 1996; Asia Pacific Consensus Forum on Stroke Management Organising Committees 1998; Royal College of Physicians of Edinburgh 1999).

Many of the recommendations on what monitoring should be done, what action should be taken if abnormalities are detected in physiological parameters (e.g. body temperature, blood glucose level, etc.), and what the essential components of an effective acute stroke service should be, are not based on reliable randomized evidence. However, we aim to provide guidance based on the best available evidence to hand.

11.2.3 Which treatments to use routinely, selectively or not at all (and who should give them)

There is strong evidence to support the routine use of aspirin in almost all patients with acute ischaemic stroke (section 11.3). For anticoagulants, the substantial amounts of available data do not support their routine use, but it may be justifiable to use them in a relatively small proportion of patients for specific reasons (section 11.4). Similarly, there is reasonable evidence (based on relatively small trials) that thrombolytic treatment is probably justifiable in a few, very carefully selected cases; large-scale randomized controlled trials will be needed before its place in routine clinical practice becomes clear (section 11.5). The trials of calcium antagonists and haemodilution have been quite large but do not provide any evidence of benefit; there therefore seems little justification to use these treatments. There are many other interventions which have been tested to some extent, but for which the evidence remains inconclusive. The remainder of this chapter explores these broad conclusions in greater detail. Some treatments, such as intravenous thrombolysis, should only be given in the context of a highly organized specialist acute stroke service, whereas others, such as aspirin, could be used very widely, even where the level of service organization is relatively humble.

There should be no double standards for randomized trials and clinical practice, yet patients given treatments in routine practice are often not given any explanation or information. Many patients refused randomization in the International Stroke Trial when they were told that aspirin and heparin might cause intracranial bleeding, yet how many tens of thousands of patients with acute stroke have been treated with these two drugs (before and since the large-scale trials began) and yet have not been asked for their consent?

11.2.4 Treatments currently in use worldwide

There are enormous variations in the general management of (and outcome after) acute stroke both between and within different countries (Asplund *et al.* 1996; Ebrahim and Redfern 1999; Weir *et al.* 1999). There are also large variations in the use of specific agents such as anticoagulants. A survey of 36 US academic medical centres showed that 29% of a sample of 497 patients with acute ischaemic stroke were treated with intravenous heparin but the proportion treated varied enormously between centres; from 'not at all' in seven centres to 88% in one centre (Moussouttas *et al.* 1999). In the UK, heparin was used much less frequently, and about 10% of physicians said they used low-dose subcutaneous heparin and less than 1% used intravenous heparin *routinely* in patients with acute ischaemic stroke (Lindley *et al.* 1995). In China, although heparin was used routinely by only 1% of doctors, snake venom (which has anticoagulant properties) was used routinely by 32% and there were great variations in use between different centres (Chen *et al.* 1997).

Many agents are used to treat patients with acute stroke, in the mistaken belief that they are effective and safe, yet, for most of them, there is no clear evidence to support their use in routine clinical practice.

There are many possible reasons for these variations, but the lack of really reliable evidence from appropriately large randomized controlled trials and the lack of widely disseminated systematic reviews of existing trial evidence must play at least some part.

11.2.5 Treatment of any specific underlying cause

Although the majority of ischaemic strokes are in one way or another related to atheroma and its thromboembolic complications (section 6.3), intracranial small vessel disease (section 6.4) and embolism from the heart (section 6.5), a small proportion are due to other conditions which are mostly discussed in detail in Chapter 7. The conditions, for which there is at least some evidence about the effect of a treatment to be used in the acute phase, are mentioned individually under that specific treatment.

For the conditions listed below, specific treatments are mentioned briefly and cross references to other relevant sections of the book are given:

- trauma and arterial dissection (section 11.4.2);
- inflammatory vascular disorders (sections 7.3 and 11.8.1);
- congenital arterial anomalies (section 11.11);
- embolism from arterial aneurysms (section 11.11);
- migraine (section 11.11);
- stroke in association with acute myocardial infarction (section 11.4.2);
- infections (section 11.11);
- cancer (section 11.11);
- female sex hormones (sections 11.11 and 16.7.8);
- pregnancy (section 11.11);
- mitochondrial cytopathy (section 11.11);
- cholesterol embolization syndrome (sections 7.7 and 11.11).

It is important to emphasize that, although conditions like vasculitis may be infrequent, failure to recognize and treat them appropriately may lead to a poor outcome or even death. A systematic approach to history taking, examination and investigation will minimize the risk of missing a potentially treatable cause of ischaemic stroke (Chapters 6 and 7).

11.3 Routine use: antiplatelet drugs

11.3.1 Rationale

Potential benefits

On the arterial side, aspirin may act in several ways to reduce the volume of brain tissue damaged by ischaemia. It may prevent distal and proximal propagation of arterial thrombus; prevent re-embolization; prevent platelet aggregation in the microcirculation; reduce the release of thromboxane and other neurotoxic eicosanoids; and, it may even be neuroprotective (Antiplatelet Trialists' Collaboration 1994b; Riepe *et al.* 1997; van Kooten *et al.* 1997; Bednar & Gross 1999) (section 11.1.3). Other agents with antiplatelet actions such as ticlopidine, prostacyclin, nitric oxide, and glycoprotein

IIb/IIIa receptor antagonists or inhibitors may also have beneficial effects (Bednar & Gross 1999). In the venous circulation, among patients at high risk (chiefly as a result of general or orthopaedic surgery) antiplatelet drugs reduce deep venous thrombosis by 39% and pulmonary embolism by 64% (Antiplatelet Trialists' Collaboration 1994c).

Potential risks

However, antiplatelet drugs do have significant antihaemostatic effects. Clark *et al.* (1991) studied the effect of aspirin, heparin and recombinant tissue plasminogen activator (rt-PA) on cerebral bleeding in a rabbit model of acute embolic ischaemic stroke. Aspirin, and to a lesser extent heparin and rt-PA, was associated with an excess of intracerebral haemorrhage. The animals that developed intracerebral haemorrhage all died. In the overview of the randomized trials, antiplatelet drugs were consistently associated with a small but definite excess of both intracranial and extracranial haemorrhages (Antiplatelet Trialists' Collaboration 1994a).

11.3.2 Evidence

Data available

The first randomized trial of antiplatelet drugs in the *prevention* of stroke was reported in 1969 (Acheson *et al.* 1969). A systematic review in 1988 of all of the trials proved that antiplatelet drugs, given long term, reduce the risk of stroke, myocardial infarction and vascular death in high-risk individuals (Antiplatelet Trialists' Collaboration 1988). The benefit of aspirin as treatment for acute myocardial infarction was established in the same year (ISIS-2 Collaborative Group 1988). The lack of data about the effects of antiplatelet drugs as a treatment for the acute phase of stroke led to two large-scale randomized trials of aspirin, the International Stroke Trial (IST) and the Chinese Acute Stroke Trial (CAST), which together randomized over 40 000 patients (Chinese Acute Stroke Trial Collaborative Group 1997; International Stroke Trial Collaborative Group 1997). In the IST, patients were allocated, in an open factorial design, to treatment policies of: 300 mg aspirin daily, heparin, the combination, or to 'avoid both aspirin and heparin' for 14 days. In the CAST, patients were allocated, in a double-blind design, to 1 month of 160 mg aspirin daily or matching placebo.

Two systematic reviews of these data are available. The Cochrane review includes all the completed randomized trials of any antiplatelet drug in acute stroke and examines their effects on a variety of clinical outcomes (Gubitz *et al.* 2000a). The second review is a meta-analysis of individual patient data from CAST and IST to examine the effects of aspirin in particular categories of patient during the scheduled treatment period (Chen *et al.* 2000). Both reviews report the frequency of events during the scheduled treatment period (2–4 weeks), and the Cochrane review also reports effects at the end of the scheduled follow-up (at 6 months in the IST, and 1 month in the CAST) (Gubitz *et al.* 2000a).

Since over 99% of the randomized evidence relates to aspirin, we will refer to aspirin, rather than 'antiplatelet drugs' for the rest of this section.

Recurrent ischaemic stroke during the treatment period

Aspirin significantly reduced the odds of recurrent ischaemic stroke during the treatment period by 30% (95% CI, 20–40%) from 2.3% in controls to 1.6% in treated patients, i.e. avoiding seven events per 1000 patients treated (Chen *et al.* 2000) (Fig. 11.16).

Symptomatic intracranial haemorrhage during the treatment period

There was a small excess of symptomatic intracranial haemorrhages with aspirin (including symptomatic transformation of an infarct). It occurred in 0.8% of controls vs. 1.0% of treated patients, a non-significant 21% relative increase in odds (95% CI, 1% reduction to 49% increase); an excess of about two per 1000 patients treated (Chen *et al.* 2000) (Fig. 11.16).

Death during the treatment period

Aspirin significantly reduced the relative odds of death (without further stroke) during the treatment period by 8% (95% CI, 1–16%) from 5.4% in controls to 5.0% in treated patients, i.e. avoiding four deaths for every 1000 patients treated (Chen *et al.* 2000) (Fig. 11.16).

Recurrent (further) stroke or death during the treatment period

This outcome event summarizes the overall balance of benefit and risk within the treatment period: recurrent ischaemic stroke, recurrent stroke of unknown type, symptomatic intracranial haemorrhage, symptomatic haemorrhagic transformation of the infarct and death from any cause. We refer to this outcome as 'further stroke or death'. Aspirin significantly reduced the relative odds of further stroke or death by 11% (95% CI, 5–15%) from 9.1% to 8.2%; for every 1000 patients treated, nine avoided further stroke or death during the treatment period (Chen *et al.* 2000) (Fig. 11.16).

Death by the end of the scheduled follow-up

The benefit seen during the treatment period was still evident so the difference in deaths from all causes, at the end of follow-up at least a month later, was about eight deaths for every 100 patients treated (Gubitz *et al.* 2000a).

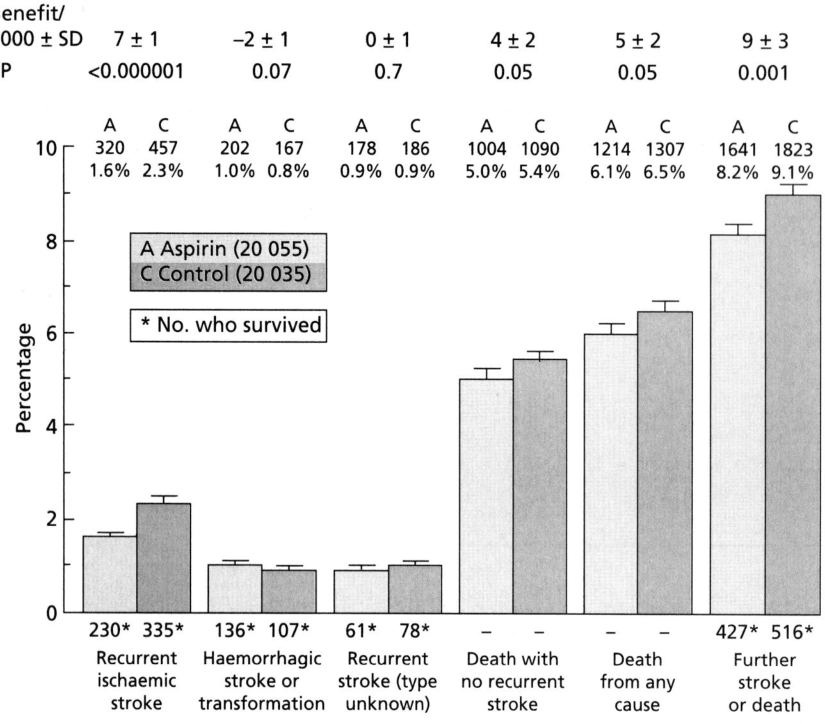

Fig. 11.16 Aspirin in about 40 000 randomized patients with acute ischaemic stroke in the Chinese Acute Stroke Trial (CAST) and International Stroke Trial (IST): absolute effects on different events during the scheduled treatment period. Numbers and percentages of patients are shown with various outcomes during the scheduled treatment period, by allocated treatment. These percentages are plotted as bars with the standard deviation of each bar plotted at the top. The difference between the aspirin (A) and control (C) groups is given as the benefit per 1000 treated, along with its standard deviation and statistical significance (SD and 2*P*); a negative benefit indicates an apparent hazard. The numbers who suffered the relevant event but survived are marked with an asterisk at the foot of each bar (with permission from Chen *et al.* 2000).

Functional outcome at one month or later (dead or dependent, full recovery)

Aspirin significantly reduced the odds of being dead or dependent at final follow-up by 6% (95% CI, 2–8%) from 47.1% in controls to 45.8% in treated patients, i.e. an additional 13 patients alive and independent for every 1000 patients treated. Aspirin also significantly increased the odds of making a complete recovery by 6% (95% CI, 1–11%); an extra 10 patients making a complete recovery for every 1000 patients treated (Gubitz *et al.* 2000a).

Deep venous thrombosis and pulmonary embolism

Two trials including 136 patients reported data on this outcome; only 35 patients developed 'symptomatic or asymptomatic deep venous thrombosis (DVT) during the treatment period'; 29% of those allocated to control and 24% of those allocated to treatment. There was a non-significant 22% relative reduction in the odds of DVT (95% CI, 64% reduction to 67% increase), but it is potentially important; if confirmed, it would imply that for 1000 patients treated about 50 would avoid DVT (Gubitz *et al.* 2000a). However, data for over 40 000 patients were available for the effects of aspirin on pulmonary embolism (PE). Aspirin significantly reduced the relative odds of PE by 29% (95% CI, 4–47%), from 0.5% in controls to 0.3% in treated patients, i.e. for every 1000 patients treated, two avoided PE. Under ascertainment of events in both groups may mean that the *absolute* benefit has been underestimated (the *proportional* reduction is not likely to be biased by under ascertainment); if the true rate of PE were 3% in the controls, and the same proportional reduction applied, then for every 1000 patients given aspirin, 12 might avoid PE (estimate of control PE risk from Davenport *et al.* 1996). These benefits are consistent with those seen in the systematic review of aspirin in the prevention of PE in surgical patients and in the recent Pulmonary Embolism Prevention Trial (Antiplatelet Trialists' Collaboration 1994c; Pulmonary Embolism Prevention Collaborative Group 2000).

These data therefore strengthen the rationale for the routine use of aspirin in the acute phase of a stroke and continuing it long term; aspirin is likely to be adequate thromboprophylaxis for patients at low and moderate risk of DVT and PE. For patients at high risk of DVT, perhaps because of a history of a previous episode of venous thromboembolism or the presence of thrombophilia, then the question is 'what to add to aspirin?' Graded compression stockings are one option and low-dose subcutaneous heparin another; both are supported by reasonable evidence (chiefly from trials in higher risk patients, but not from trials in stroke patients), but both have advantages and disadvantages which are discussed in section 15.13. The Scottish Intercollegiate Guidelines Network (SIGN) guideline on prevention of DVT have recently been updated, and is a useful reference work (Scottish Intercollegiate Guidelines Network 2000; http://www.show.scot.nhs.uk/sign/clinical.htm).

Subgroup analyses

Individual patient data meta-analysis, based on over 40 000 patients with acute ischaemic stroke, did not identify any group in which the benefits—or the risks—were significantly greater than or less than the averages reported above (Chen *et al.* 2000). For the one-third reduction in recurrent ischaemic stroke, the overall treatment effect ($2P < 0.000001$) was large enough for the subgroup analyses to be informative. The recurrence rate among control patients was similar in all 28 subgroups, so the absolute reduction of seven per 1000 did not differ substantially with respect to age, sex, consciousness level, atrial fibrillation, CT findings, blood pressure, stroke subtype or concomitant heparin use. There was no good evidence that the 11% reduction in relative odds of death without further stroke was reversed in any subgroup, or that in any subgroup the increase in haemorrhagic stroke was much larger than the average of about two per 1000, and there was no heterogeneity between the reductions in further stroke or death during the scheduled treatment period (Fig. 11.17).

Aspirin in haemorhagic stroke and in patients without CT or MR brain scans

Among the 9000 patients randomized without a prior CT

Categorization	Recurrent stroke or death during the treatment period: Aspirin	Recurrent stroke or death during the treatment period: Control
Hours from stroke onset to randomization:		
0–6	323 (11.4%)	358 (12.9%)
7–12	379 (11.0%)	367 (10.3%)
13–24	435 (7.7%)	505 (9.1%)
25–48	498 (6.2%)	589 (7.2%)
Age (years):		
<65	411 (5.3%)	441 (5.6%)
65–74	498 (7.4%)	565 (8.5%)
75+	727 (13.2%)	811 (14.7%
Sex:		
Male	872 (7.5%)	997 (8.4%)
Female	769 (9.1%)	826 (10.1%)
Level of consciousness:		
Alert	817 (5.0%)	954 (5.8%)
Drowsy/Coma	820 (23.0%)	865 (24.2%)
Atrial fibrillation:		
Present	421 (18.2%)	420 (18.7%)
Absent	1151 (6.7%)	1337 (7.8%)
CT findings		
Infarct visible	839 (7.7%)	939 (8.6%)
Infarct not visible	408 (8.7%)	457 (9.8%)
No prior CT	385 (8.6%)	421 (9.5%)
Systolic BP (mm Hg):		
<130	216 (9.4%)	249 (10.8%)
130–159	595 (7.8%)	632 (8.5%)
160–189	559 (7.8%)	637 (8.8%)
190+	268 (9.1%)	302 (10.1%)
Stroke syndrome:		
Lacunar	168 (3.1%)	215 (4.0%)
Non-lacunar	1470 (10.0%)	1606 (11.0%)
Allocated trial heparin:		
Yes (IST: A+H vs H)	531 (10.9%)	604 (12.4%)
No (IST: A vs nil)	565 (11.6%)	605 (12.4%)
No (CAST: A vs nil)	545 (5.3%)	614 (5.9%)
Overall prognostic index (3 equal groups):		
Good	167 (2.6%)	189 (2.9%)
Average	336 (5.2%)	404 (6.3%)
Poor	1060 (16.4%)	1155 (17.8%)
Days from randomization to further stroke or death:		
0–1	327 (1.6%)	320 (1.6%)
2–7	757 (3.8%)	884 (4.4%)
+8	557 (2.8%)	619 (3.1%)
Total	1641 (8.2%)	1823 (9.1%)

Fig. 11.17 Aspirin in acute ischaemic stroke: effects on recurrent stroke or death in different subgroups during the scheduled treatment period in the Chinese Acute Stroke Trial (CAST) and International Stroke Trial (IST). Fatal and non-fatal events are included. For each particular subgroup the number of events among aspirin- and no-aspirin-allocated patients, and the odds ratio (dark green square, with area proportional to the total number of patients with an event) are given. A square to the left of the solid vertical line suggests benefit, significant at $2P < 0.01$ only if the whole 99% confidence interval (CI) (horizontal line) is to the left of the solid vertical line. The overall result and its 95% CI is represented by an open diamond. A indicates aspirin; H, heparin. Here and elsewhere, results for those with missing information on particular characteristics are not listed separately (except for computed tomography findings), but numerators and denominators for them can be obtained by subtraction of the subgroup results from the total (e.g. the numbers with no prognostic index calculated were 16/638 aspirin vs. 18/638 control) (with permission from Chen *et al.* 2000).

scan in the IST and CAST, aspirin appeared to be of net benefit, with no unusual excess of haemorrhagic stroke, and among the 800 who had inadvertently been randomized after a haemorrhagic stroke, there was no evidence of net hazard (further stroke or death 67 control vs. 63 aspirin) (Chen *et al.* 2000).

These data are reassuring in that they establish that the patients inadvertently entered in the trials with a haemorrhagic stroke, were not, on average, harmed as a result. However, they do not establish the safety of continued aspirin treatment in patients with primary intracerebral haemorrhage, nor do they establish the safety of giving aspirin to patients who are not CT scanned at all; there is little point CT scanning after a week or so, since, at that stage, CT is decreasingly able reliably to differentiate infarction from haemorrhage (section 5.3.4).

11.3.3 Who to treat

Early aspirin is of benefit for a wide range of patients, so all patients with suspected acute ischaemic stroke should receive it unless there is a clear contraindication. Implementing a hospital policy or guideline of 'immediate aspirin for all patients with acute ischaemic stroke' requires considerable effort; it is of course part of a well-organized stroke service (Chapter 17). Several different strategies may be required to maintain a high level of compliance with the policy (Bero *et al.* 1998; Scottish Intercollegiate Guidelines Network 1999; Woolf *et al.* 1999) (Table 17.24). Such a policy will also reduce the risk of venous thromboembolism.

Atrial fibrillation

The IST and CAST trials included about 4500 patients who were in atrial fibrillation at the time of randomization. In these patients, the risk of recurrent stroke in hospital was 2.9% in the controls and 2.0% in patients allocated aspirin. The one-third reduction in the relative odds of recurrent ischaemic stroke with aspirin was no different to that seen in patients without atrial fibrillation (Chen *et al.* 2000); all such patients should be started on aspirin.

Patients already on antiplatelet drugs

The priority is to perform a brain CT or magnetic resonance (MR) scan to determine whether the stroke is haemorrhagic or ischaemic; if haemorrhagic, antiplatelet drugs should be stopped. In the IST, 4000 patients were already on aspirin or other antiplatelet drugs at randomization. The question of what to do for long-term secondary prevention in patients who have a stroke whilst already on antiplatelet drugs is discussed later (section 16.4.7).

11.3.4 Who not to treat

It should go without saying that a patient with proven primary intracerebral haemorrhage should not have antiplatelet drugs as a treatment for their stroke (Chapter 12). However, patients with intracerebral haemorrhage who have a very clear and pressing indication to continue aspirin (e.g. unstable angina) and are thought—for whatever reason—to have a low risk of further intracerebral bleeding can continue aspirin. The pathophysiology of aneurysmal subarachnoid haemorrhage is rather different and here there have been a few small inconclusive trials in which the primary aim was to prevent ischaemic deficits *after* a ruptured aneurysm had been clipped (Antiplatelet Trialists' Collaboration 1994a) (section 13.6.5).

Patients with a history of definite aspirin sensitivity (e.g. wheeze or skin rash on exposure to aspirin) should not be given aspirin.

11.3.5 When to start

There was no clear evidence of a 'time window' for the benefit of aspirin; the relative benefits among those randomized late (24–48 h after stroke onset) were as great as those randomized early (within the first 0–6 h) (Chen *et al.* 2000). The IST and CAST trials tested a policy of 'start aspirin immediately'; so aspirin should be started as soon as a CT or MR scan has been performed and has excluded intracranial haemorrhage as the cause of the stroke. If the doctor who admits the patient to hospital writes the prescription for aspirin immediately, the patient is more likely to receive long-term aspirin. If writing the aspirin prescription is left until later, it is easily forgotten.

If CT scanning is not immediately available and the clinician feels, on clinical grounds, that the patient is unlikely to have a haemorrhagic stroke (i.e. no 'apoplectic onset', with early headache or vomiting, fully conscious, etc.) (section 5.3.1), then aspirin can be started while the CT or MR scan is being organized. This policy does not appear to reduce the benefits from aspirin (Chen *et al.* 2000).

The risk of intracranial haemorrhage with thrombolysis may be increased if given together with aspirin (Multicentre Acute Stroke Trial Group 1995; Wardlaw *et al.* 2000). In the highly selected few patients to be treated with thrombolysis, it is probably best to delay starting aspirin. Starting aspirin the next day, probably around 24 h after admission and treatment, is unlikely to reduce the benefit of early aspirin (Chen *et al.* 2000).

> *Start aspirin immediately if there is likely to be any delay before a CT or MR scan can be performed and you think intracranial haemorrhage is an unlikely cause*

of the stroke. Delay starting aspirin in patients to be treated with thrombolysis until the day after the treatment has been given.

11.3.6 Agent/dose/route

We use aspirin in a dose of at least 150 mg daily in the acute phase of stroke. The initial dose has to be high (and certainly higher than is required for long-term secondary prevention) to inhibit thromboxane biosynthesis as quickly and completely as possible (Patrono *et al.* 1990; Patrono 1994). For patients who can swallow safely (section 15.17), aspirin can be given by mouth; for the remainder, it can be given rectally by suppository, by nasogastric tube or by intravenous injection (as 100 mg of the lysine salt, infused over 10 min).

11.3.7 Adverse effects

Major extracranial haemorrhage (defined as bleeding serious enough to cause death or require transfusion) is the most frequent serious adverse event. In the trials, the relative increase in odds with aspirin was large (68%; 95% CI, 34–109%), but the absolute excess was small—four additional major extracranial haemorrhages for every 1000 patients treated (Gubitz *et al.* 2000a). The excess was greater among patients allocated heparin (0.9% heparin alone vs. 1.8% allocated aspirin plus heparin; excess nine per 1000) than among other patients (0.5% among those allocated no aspirin and 0.7% allocated aspirin; excess two per 1000) (Chen *et al.* 2000). The risk of adverse events with aspirin can therefore be kept to a minimum by avoiding anticoagulants.

11.4 Selective use: anticoagulants

11.4.1 Rationale

Prevent (or help to reverse) thrombotic occlusion of cerebral arteries, and prevent venous thromboembolism

The rationale for using anticoagulants applies to both the arterial and venous circulations (Hirsh 1991). In large arteries, and in the perforating arteries involved in lacunar infarction, the aim of treatment is to prevent local propagation of the occluding thrombus (or embolus), to tip the balance in favour of spontaneous lysis of the occlusion, and to prevent early re-embolization from any proximal arterial or cardiac sources. In small arteries and the microvessels, anticoagulation might also prevent sludging which may contribute to ischaemia in the penumbral zone around the infarct core. In the venous circulation, anticoagulation should reduce the risk of DVT and PE which are common complications of immobility after stroke (section 15.13).

Problem of haemorrhagic transformation of cerebral infarction

As a cerebral infarct evolves over the first few days, red cells can leak from microvessels. Minor degrees of leakage appear on CT or MR brain scanning as petechiae, but if bleeding is more extensive, a parenchymal haematoma may form (Lyden & Zivin 1993; Larrue *et al.* 1997; del Zoppo 1998). This pathophysiological process is known as haemorrhagic transformation of cerebral infarction (section 5.4). The precise sequence of events is not known. Several factors may contribute to the development of haemorrhagic transformation: augmented collateral flow into the ischaemic area; microvessel damage (and leakiness) and pre-existing cerebral amyloid angiopathy (Lyden & Zivin 1993; del Zoppo 1998). Any anticoagulant, antiplatelet, thrombolytic or defibrinogenating agent could therefore theoretically increase the tendency to intracranial bleeding and this might offset some, or all, of any benefits.

How frequent is haemorrhagic transformation?

The reported frequency of haemorrhagic transformation will depend on many technical factors (section 5.4): the timing of the scan, the sensitivity of the scanning technique, whether or not interpretation of the scan was blinded to clinical features (and to the treatments given) and the classification used (Motto *et al.* 1997). Small degrees of haemorrhagic transformation may not be detected on scanning. In a systematic review of 21 randomized trials of anticoagulants in acute ischaemic stroke, symptomatic intracranial haemorrhage or haemorrhagic transformation during the first 2 weeks was found in 0.5% of the control group (range 0–2.8%) (Gubitz *et al.* 2000b). Asymptomatic transformation, detected by systematically scanning all patients, irrespective of symptoms, was found in 9.4% of controls (range 0–11%) (Gubitz *et al.* 2000b). A non-systematic review of observational series reported frequencies of 15–43% (Lyden & Zivin 1993).

Which infarcts become haemorrhagic?

There are many clinical factors which are said to increase the development of haemorrhagic transformation, including: increased age; clinically major stroke; arterial hypertension; cardioembolic cause; hyperglycaemia; infarction visible on early CT scanning; occlusion of a major cerebral vessel; use of any type of antihaemostatic therapy; and dose of anticoagulant (Lyden & Zivin 1993; Hart *et al.* 1995; Alexandrov *et al.* 1997; International Stroke Trial Collaborative Group 1997; Larrue *et al.* 1997; del Zoppo 1998; Demchuk *et al.* 1999; Wardlaw *et al.* 2000; Gubitz *et al.* 2000b). However, many of the factors are interrelated (e.g. severe stroke, cardioembolic origin and visible infarction on CT scanning all go together) so the *independent* predictors of haemorrhagic transformation have not been sorted out yet (section 5.4).

Clinical impact of haemorrhagic transformation and other intracranial bleeds

The clinical impact of haemorrhagic transformation over and above the effects of the original infarct (i.e. the *independent contribution* of haemorrhagic transformation to the likelihood of a poor outcome) is difficult to assess in an individual patient. Minor degrees of transformation can occur without any clinical deterioration, whereas the development of a large parenchymatous haematoma may be fatal. In a review of the trials of thrombolytic therapy within 6 h of onset, 1.0% of the patients allocated to the control group had a fatal intracranial haemorrhage (Wardlaw *et al.* 2000).

However, even if a specific category of patient were at especially high risk of symptomatic haemorrhagic transformation, which might be exacerbated by an antihaemostatic agent, this does not necessarily mean that the net balance of risk and benefit will be adverse for that type of patient. By analogy with carotid endarterectomy for carotid stenosis, some patients are at high risk of stroke with surgery, but even higher risk without it, so that the net balance of risk and benefit may be favourable, even in high-risk individuals; this may be true for thrombolysis as well (sections 11.5 and 16.8.9).

As well as increasing the risk of haemorrhagic transformation, anticoagulants could both increase the risk of symptomatic intracranial haemorrhage arising *de novo* (as intracerebral, subarachnoid or subdural bleeding) and the risk of bleeding at other, extracranial sites. The key question is therefore whether or not the benefits of treatment outweigh the risks. Randomized trials provide the best means to assess this balance.

11.4.2 Evidence

Data available

By mid-1999, 21 randomized controlled trials comparing anticoagulants with control had been completed and were available for review. The trials tested standard unfractionated heparin, low molecular weight heparin, heparinoid, direct thrombin inhibitors and two tested heparin given for just 24 h followed by oral anticoagulation. Most of the data came from trials in which unfractionated heparin was administered by subcutaneous injection in medium (12 500 IU twice daily) or low dose (5000 IU twice daily). In total, the trials included 23 427 patients with acute presumed ischaemic stroke (Gubitz *et al.* 2000b). Most patients had a CT scan to exclude intracerebral haemorrhage before treatment was started. Patients were generally randomized within 48 h of stroke onset, and treatment continued for about 2 weeks. There were fewer trials directly comparing one agent with another and comparing different doses of the same agent (Counsell & Sandercock 2000; Gubitz *et al.* 2000b). However, a reasonably clear and consistent picture of the effects of anticoagulants in acute ischaemic stroke does emerge.

Recurrent ischaemic stroke during the treatment period

Immediate anticoagulation significantly reduced the relative odds of recurrent ischaemic or unknown stroke (referred to as recurrent ischaemic stroke for simplicity) within the first 2 weeks by 24% (95% CI, 12–35%) from 3.6% in controls to 2.8% in treated patients, i.e. avoiding nine recurrences for every 1000 patients treated. The effects of the different regimens tested were broadly consistent (Fig. 11.18).

Death

There was no significant effect on deaths during the treatment period; 8.7% of controls died compared with 8.5% of treated patients (95% CI, 10% reduction in relative odds to 10% increase) (Fig. 11.18). By the end of the scheduled follow-up at 3–6 months, 20.6% of controls had died compared with 21.4% of treated patients, a non-significant 5% increase in the relative odds of death (95% CI, 2% reduction to 12% increase) (Fig. 11.19).

Symptomatic intracranial haemorrhage during the treatment period

Immediate anticoagulation significantly increased the relative odds of symptomatic intracranial haemorrhage or symptomatic haemorrhagic transformation of the infarct (referred to as symptomatic intracranial haemorrhage for simplicity) by 152% (95% CI, 92–230%), from 0.5% in controls to 1.4% in treated patients, i.e. causing nine symptomatic intracranial haemorrhages for every 1000 patients treated. Each of the regimens tested, when compared to the controls, appeared to increase the risk of symptomatic intracranial haemorrhage. The relative increase was consistent across the different regimens, although (because of small numbers) it was only statistically significant for subcutaneous unfractionated heparin (Fig. 11.18). Indirect comparisons of different dosing regimens showed consistently higher bleeding risks with higher dose regimens (Fig. 11.20a). In the IST, patients allocated to subcutanous unfractionated heparin were randomized to high dose (12 500 IU twice daily) or to low dose (5000 IU twice daily) and the proportions with symptomatic intracranial haemorrhage were 1.8% and 0.7%, respectively—a highly significant 11 per 1000 excess with the higher dose ($2P < 0.00001$) (International Stroke Trial Collaborative Group 1997). A systematic review of all trials directly comparing high- with low-dose anticoagulants in acute stroke supports the finding that the bleeding risks are dose dependent (Gubitz *et al.* 2000c, d).

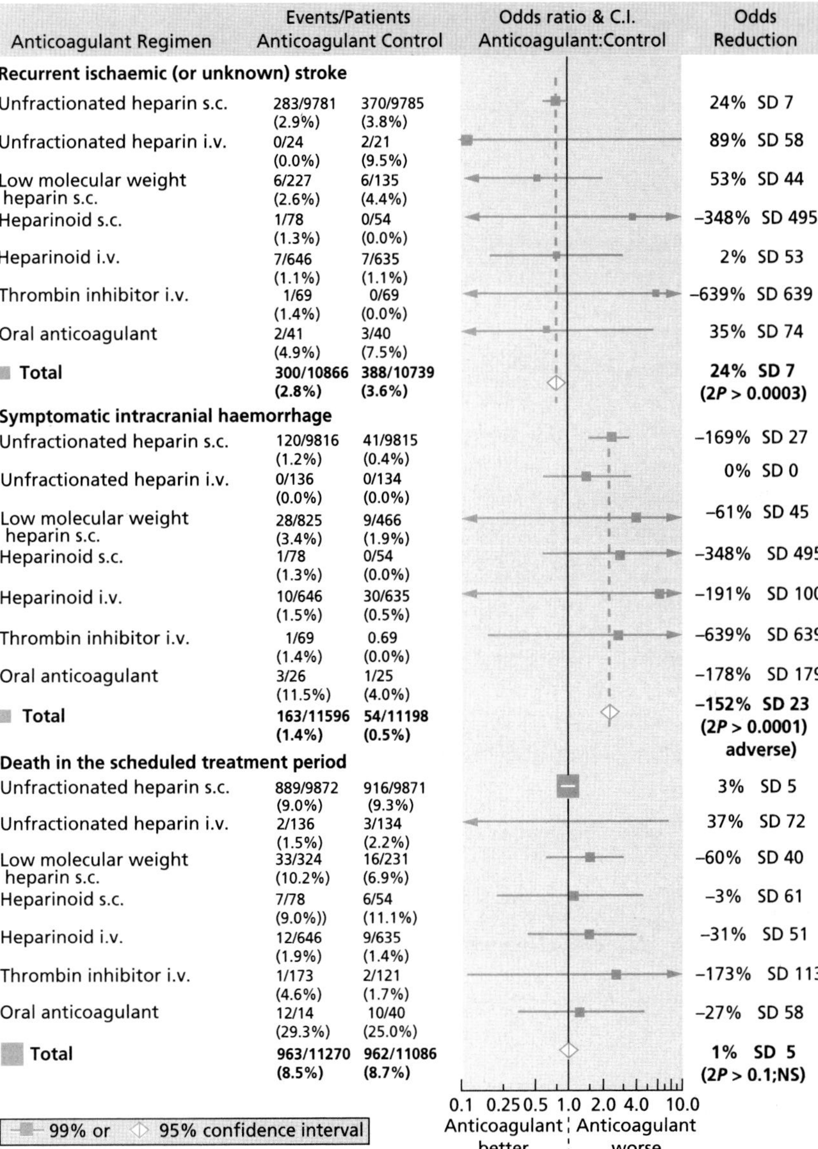

Anticoagulant Regimen
Events/Patients
Anticoagulant Control
Odds ratio & C.I.
Anticoagulant:Control
Odds Reduction
Recurrent ischaemic (or unknown) stroke
Unfractionated heparin s.c. 283/9781 (2.9%) 370/9785 (3.8%) 24% SD 7
Unfractionated heparin i.v. 0/24 (0.0%) 2/21 (9.5%) 89% SD 58
Low molecular weight heparin s.c. 6/227 (2.6%) 6/135 (4.4%) 53% SD 44
Heparinoid s.c. 1/78 (1.3%) 0/54 (0.0%) −348% SD 495
Heparinoid i.v. 7/646 (1.1%) 7/635 (1.1%) 2% SD 53
Thrombin inhibitor i.v. 1/69 (1.4%) 0/69 (0.0%) −639% SD 639
Oral anticoagulant 2/41 (4.9%) 3/40 (7.5%) 35% SD 74
Total 300/10866 (2.8%) 388/10739 (3.6%) 24% SD 7 (2P > 0.0003)
Symptomatic intracranial haemorrhage
Unfractionated heparin s.c. 120/9816 (1.2%) 41/9815 (0.4%) −169% SD 27
Unfractionated heparin i.v. 0/136 (0.0%) 0/134 (0.0%) 0% SD 0
Low molecular weight heparin s.c. 28/825 (3.4%) 9/466 (1.9%) −61% SD 45
Heparinoid s.c. 1/78 (1.3%) 0/54 (0.0%) −348% SD 495
Heparinoid i.v. 10/646 (1.5%) 30/635 (0.5%) −191% SD 100
Thrombin inhibitor i.v. 1/69 (1.4%) 0.69 (0.0%) −639% SD 639
Oral anticoagulant 3/26 (11.5%) 1/25 (4.0%) −178% SD 179
Total 163/11596 (1.4%) 54/11198 (0.5%) −152% SD 23 (2P > 0.0001) adverse)
Death in the scheduled treatment period
Unfractionated heparin s.c. 889/9872 (9.0%) 916/9871 (9.3%) 3% SD 5
Unfractionated heparin i.v. 2/136 (1.5%) 3/134 (2.2%) 37% SD 72
Low molecular weight heparin s.c. 33/324 (10.2%) 16/231 (6.9%) −60% SD 40
Heparinoid s.c. 7/78 (9.0%)) 6/54 (11.1%) −3% SD 61
Heparinoid i.v. 12/646 (1.9%) 9/635 (1.4%) −31% SD 51
Thrombin inhibitor i.v. 1/173 (4.6%) 2/121 (1.7%) −173% SD 113
Oral anticoagulant 12/14 (29.3%) 10/40 (25.0%) −27% SD 58
Total 963/11270 (8.5%) 962/11086 (8.7%) 1% SD 5 (2P > 0.1;NS)
0.1 0.25 0.5 1.0 2.0 4.0 10.0
Anticoagulant better
Anticoagulant worse
99% or 95% confidence interval

Fig. 11.18 Anticoagulants in acute ischaemic stroke: relative effects within the treatment period. Results of a systematic review of the 21 randomized trials comparing heparin with control groups in patients with acute ischaemic stroke: effects on recurrent ischaemic stroke, symptomatic intracranial haemorrhage and death, all within the scheduled treatment period. The estimate of treatment effect is expressed as an odds ratio (solid square) and its 95% confidence interval (horizontal line). The size of the black square is proportional to the amount of information available. An odds ratio of 1.0 corresponds to a treatment effect of zero, an odds ratio of less than 1 suggests treatment is better than control, and an odds ratio of greater than 1 suggests treatment is worse than control. The figures given to the right are relative odds reductions (SD) (with permission from Gubitz *et al.* 2000b).

Functional outcome at 3–6 months (dead or dependent)

The simplest and most robust measure of outcome is the proportion of patients, at the end of follow-up, who are either alive, but need help for everyday activities, or are dead. Overall, 60.1% of controls were dead or dependent compared with 59.7% of treated patients, a non-significant 1% relative odds reduction (95% CI, 6% reduction to 5% increase in the odds of death) (Fig. 11.19).

Extracranial haemorrhage

Haemorrhages into the gastrointestinal tract and elsewhere can occur after stroke (section 15.2.3), and in the trials were reported in 0.4% of controls and 1.3% of treated patients, a significant three-fold increase, i.e. for every 1000 patients treated with anticoagulants, nine have a major extracranial haemorrhage. The indirect comparisons of different agents show that the bleeding risks are higher with higher dose regimens. In the IST, the risk of major extracranial bleeds was 2% among patients allocated high dose and 0.6% among those allocated low dose—a highly significant 14 per 1000 excess with the higher dose ($2P < 0.00001$)(International Stroke Trial Collaborative Group 1997). A systematic review of all trials directly comparing high- with low-dose anticoagulants confirmed this dose dependency (Gubitz *et al.* 2000c, d) (Fig. 11.20b).

Deep venous thrombosis and pulmonary embolism

Data on the effects of anticoagulants on DVT were only available for 916 patients. There was heterogeneity of treatment

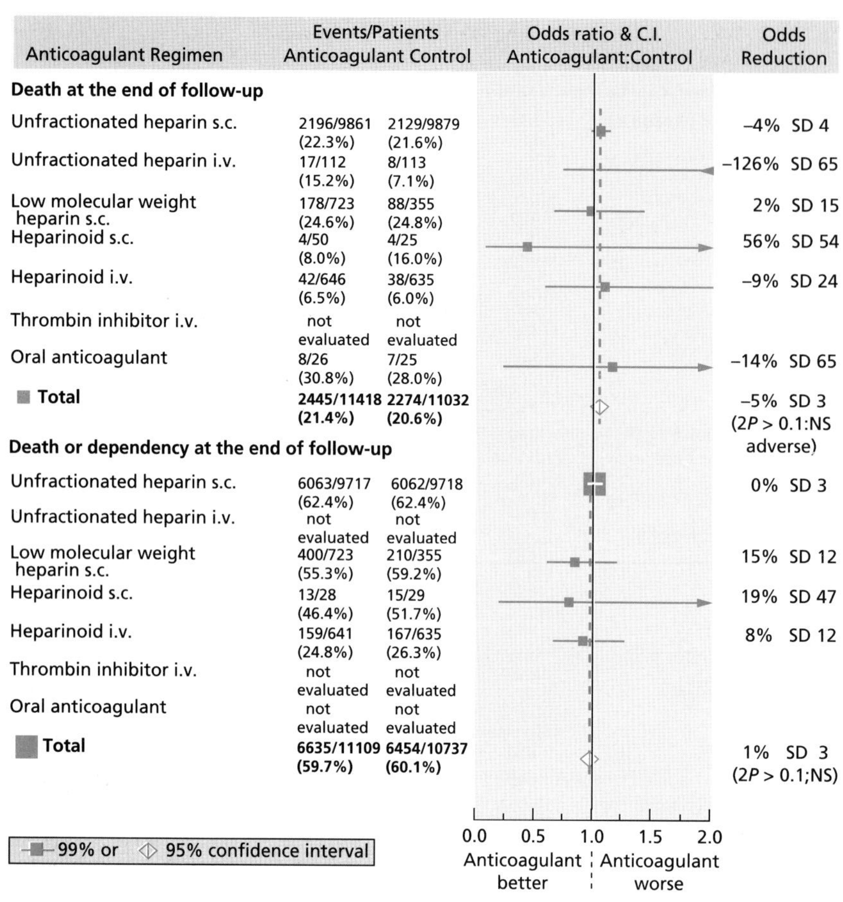

Anticoagulant Regimen
Events/Patients
Anticoagulant Control
Odds ratio & C.I.
Anticoagulant:Control
Odds
Reduction
Death at the end of follow-up
Unfractionated heparin s.c.
2196/9861 (22.3%) 2129/9879 (21.6%)
–4% SD 4
Unfractionated heparin i.v.
17/112 (15.2%) 8/113 (7.1%)
–126% SD 65
Low molecular weight heparin s.c.
178/723 (24.6%) 88/355 (24.8%)
2% SD 15
Heparinoid s.c.
4/50 (8.0%) 4/25 (16.0%)
56% SD 54
Heparinoid i.v.
42/646 (6.5%) 38/635 (6.0%)
–9% SD 24
Thrombin inhibitor i.v.
not evaluated not evaluated
Oral anticoagulant
8/26 (30.8%) 7/25 (28.0%)
–14% SD 65
Total
2445/11418 (21.4%) 2274/11032 (20.6%)
–5% SD 3 (2P > 0.1:NS adverse)
Death or dependency at the end of follow-up
Unfractionated heparin s.c.
6063/9717 (62.4%) 6062/9718 (62.4%)
0% SD 3
Unfractionated heparin i.v.
not evaluated not evaluated
Low molecular weight heparin s.c.
400/723 (55.3%) 210/355 (59.2%)
15% SD 12
Heparinoid s.c.
13/28 (46.4%) 15/29 (51.7%)
19% SD 47
Heparinoid i.v.
159/641 (24.8%) 167/635 (26.3%)
8% SD 12
Thrombin inhibitor i.v.
not evaluated not evaluated
Oral anticoagulant
not evaluated not evaluated
Total
6635/11109 (59.7%) 6454/10737 (60.1%)
1% SD 3 (2P > 0.1;NS)
99% or 95% confidence interval
0.0 0.5 1.0 1.5 2.0
Anticoagulant better
Anticoagulant worse

Fig. 11.19 Anticoagulants in acute ischaemic stroke: relative effects at the end of follow-up. Results of a systematic review of the five randomized trials comparing anticoagulants with control groups in patients with acute ischaemic stroke reporting long-term outcome: effects on death from all causes, and death or dependency. Same conventions as Fig. 11.18 (with permission from Gubitz *et al.* 2000b).

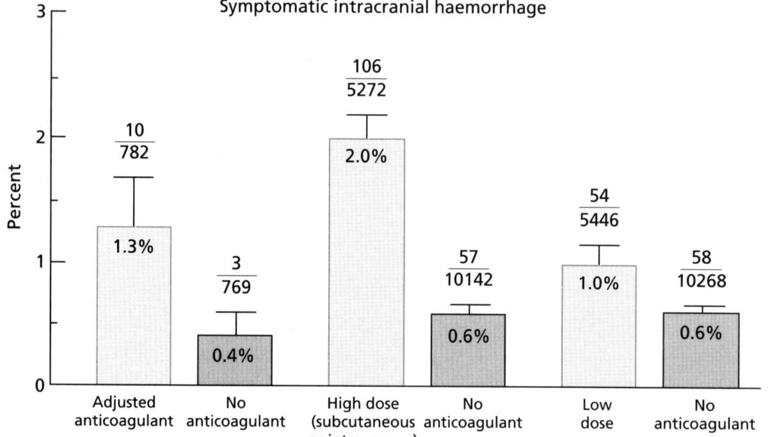

Fig. 11.20 Results of a systematic review of the randomized trials comparing anticoagulants with control groups in patients with acute ischaemic stroke: absolute effects of different regimens on (a) symptomatic intracranial haemorrhage, (b) major extracranial haemorrhage, (c) deep venous thrombosis, and (d) pulmonary embolism (with permission from Gubitz *et al.* 2000b). (*continued*)

effect between the trials, which makes it harder to give a reliable overall estimate of treatment effect. Overall, symptomatic or asymptomatic DVT occurred in 43% of controls and 15% of treated patients, a highly significant 79% reduction in relative odds with anticoagulants (95% CI, 61–85%), i.e. for every 1000 patients treated, 280 avoid DVT. Fatal or non-fatal PE was not systematically sought in the trials. It was reported in only 0.9% of controls and 0.6% of treated patients, a significant 39% reduction in relative odds with anticoagulants (95% CI, 17–55%), i.e. for every 1000 patients treated, three avoid PE. It is difficult to judge whether the reductions in DVT or PE are dose dependent from the indirect comparisons. In the IST, fatal or non-fatal PE occurred in 0.4% of those allocated high dose and 0.7% of those allocated low dose, a non-significant difference (International Stroke Trial Collaborative Group 1997). A

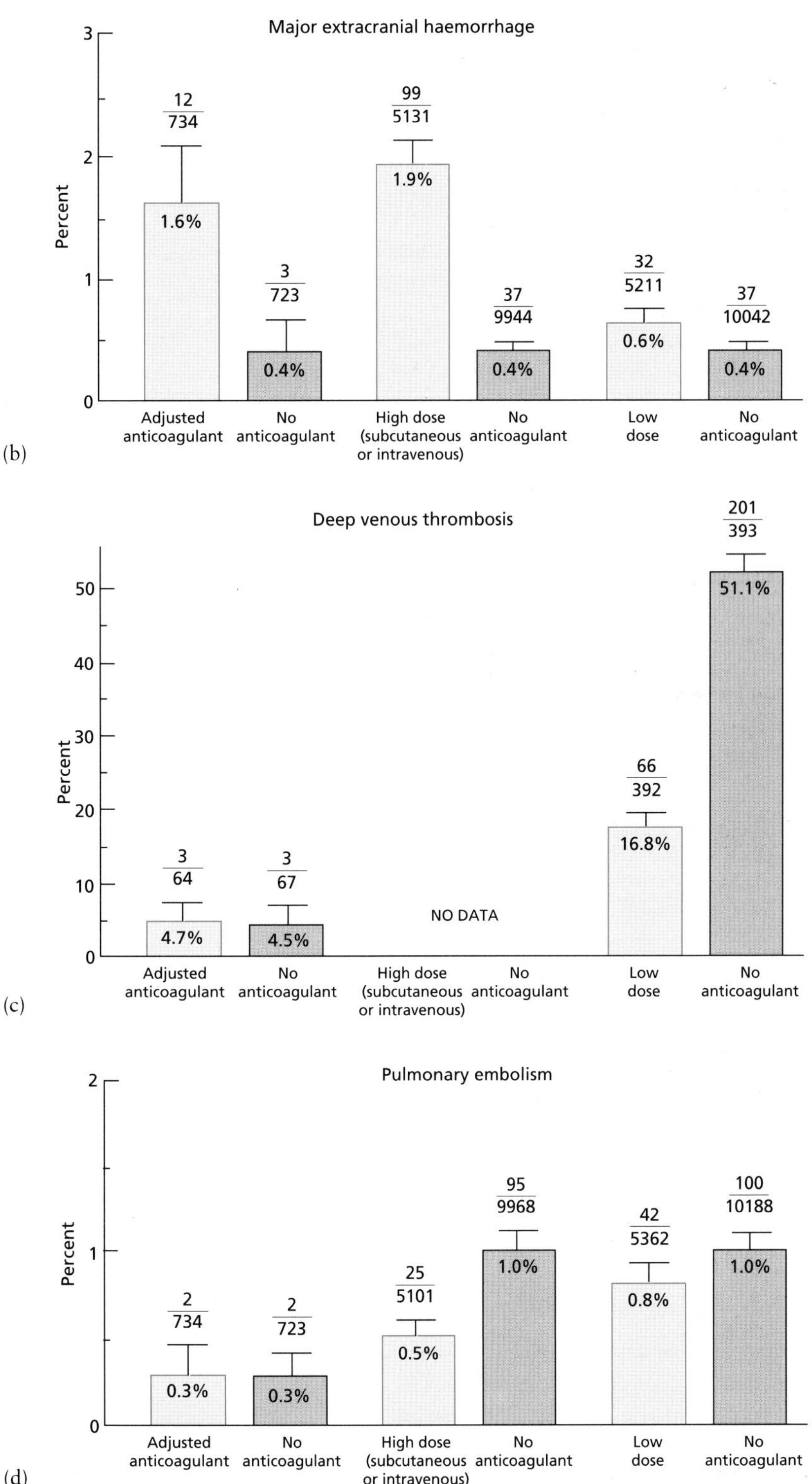

Fig. 11.20 (*continued*)

systematic review of all of the direct randomized comparisons confirmed the greater reduction in PE with higher doses, but the absolute benefit was very small (Gubitz *et al.* 2000c, d) (Fig. 11.20c,d).

If we allow for the likely under ascertainment of pulmonary emboli (section 11.3.2), and assume that the true rate in the controls was 3%, and then apply the same 39% proportional reduction (i.e. from 3% to 1.85%), for every 1000 patients treated about 12 avoid PE. However, even if the benefit is that large, it will still be substantially offset since an extra nine patients will have a major extracranial haemorrhage associated with anticoagulants.

Suspected cardioembolic ischaemic stroke

All patients with atrial fibrillation and ischaemic stroke should have a CT brain scan, since about 5–10% turn out to have primary intracerebral haemorrhage (Sandercock *et al.* 1992). In many centres in the USA, once haemorrhage has been excluded, such patients are treated routinely with intravenous heparin as an emergency (Moussouttas *et al.* 1999). However, there is no evidence to support the use of any intravenous anticoagulant. In the systematic review of all of the available randomized evidence, for all patients with acute ischaemic stroke, any reduction in recurrent ischaemic stroke with heparin, heparinoid or direct thrombin inhibitor given intravenously was offset by a similar-sized increase in symptomatic intracranial haemorrhage (Gubitz *et al.* 2000b) (Figs 11.18–11.20). A sensitivity analysis, restricted to trials of heparin in patients with acute ischaemic stroke of suspected cardioembolic origin, again did not show net benefit from anticoagulants; the analysis included data on over 3200 patients (Gubitz *et al.* 2000b). The small Heparin in Acute Embolic Stroke Trial (HAEST) compared a low molecular weight heparin with aspirin in 449 patients with acute ischaemic stroke of suspected cardioembolic origin and did not show evidence of an advantage to low molecular weight heparin over aspirin (Berge *et al.* 2000).

In patients with suspected acute cardioembolic ischaemic stroke, there is no evidence to support the routine use of immediate anticoagulation with heparin, heparinoid or low molecular weight heparin. Aspirin is a safe and effective alternative to anticoagulants, which substantially reduces the risk of early recurrent stroke in patients with acute ischaemic stroke and atrial fibrillation.

Progressing hemispheric stroke

By far the most important step is to find out why the stroke is 'progressing'. There are numerous causes besides propagating cerebral arterial thrombosis for a worsening neurological deficit (section 15.5) (Tables 15.6 and 15.7). These factors should be identified and treated. For patients in whom all other possible causes for progression have been excluded, many textbooks and reviews recommend immediate intravenous heparin. However, there have not been any trials of intravenous heparin specifically in patients with progressing stroke, and neither the trials of intravenous unfractionated heparin nor of intravenous heparinoid in patients with acute ischaemic stroke showed net benefit overall (Gubitz *et al.* 2000b). There is therefore no direct or indirect evidence to support the use of heparin (either intravenous or subcutaneous) in this particular type of patient.

Basilar thrombosis

The IST included over 2000 patients with posterior circulation ischaemic infarcts, and there was no evidence that the effects of treatment in this subgroup were any different to those seen in the trial overall (International Stroke Trial Collaborative Group 1997). However, it is likely that only a small proportion had occlusion of the basilar artery. Further trials of anticoagulants in 'vertebrobasilar territory infarcts' are probably not warranted; a trial focused on patients with proven basilar occlusion might be justified, but trials which seek to recruit a type of patient only rarely encountered in clinical practice are notoriously difficult to do.

Carotid or vertebral artery dissection

Patients with dissection of the extracranial carotid or vertebral arteries can deteriorate because of arterial occlusion at the site of the dissection, or distally due to artery-to-artery embolization of a thrombus formed at the site of dissection (section 7.2.1). Despite the lack of evidence of benefit from the trials of anticoagulants in ischaemic stroke in general, and the lack of any randomized evidence at all in patients with ischaemic stroke due to arterial dissection, many clinicians are still inclined to use anticoagulants. However, anticoagulants could increase bleeding into the dissected arterial wall, and therefore worsen the situation. A Cochrane systematic review did not identify any randomized trials and a systematic review of the non-randomized studies did not provide any evidence of benefit from anticoagulants (Lyrer & Engelter 2000). In a patient with a confirmed dissection, the factors which might justify the use of anticoagulants are: sudden neurological deterioration presumed due to further embolism (with other, more plausible, causes for deterioration such as cerebral herniation or pneumonia excluded); and the presence of a coincidental prothrombotic state (e.g. acquired thrombophilia). Anticoagulants are probably to be avoided if the patient is clinically stable (or improving) or the cerebral infarct is large (and hence there is a high risk of haemorrhagic transformation).

After the acute phase, remodelling and healing may, within a few months, lead to an arterial lumen which appears virtually normal (Mokri *et al.* 1986; Sturzenegger *et al.* 1995). In other cases, the artery remains occluded, but because the thrombus has probably been covered with endothelium, there is little risk of further thromboembolism. Some clinicians find it helpful to re-image vessels non-invasively with ultrasound or MR angiography a few months after the dissection and, if the vessel has returned to normal, they then stop any antithrombotic therapy. For those few patients with dissection whom we do anticoagulate, most of us do not routinely re-image the vessel before stopping treatment after a few months.

Acute stroke in patients with acute myocardial infarction (see also section 7.10)

The first step in management is to determine if the stroke was due to primary intracerebral haemorrhage, either spontaneous or iatrogenic (e.g. caused by thrombolytic or anticoagulant treatment). Some patients may have iatrogenic ischaemic strokes due to particulate emboli reaching the brain as a complication of some invasive cardiological procedure such as coronary angiography or angioplasty. The value of anticoagulants in these latter patients is not clear, as the embolic material is often atheromatous debris from the large arteries rather than fresh thrombus or platelet aggregates. Patients with full-thickness anterior MI have a higher than average risk of developing left ventricular (LV) thrombus (section 7.10). Although two small trials (SCATI Group 1989; Turpie *et al.* 1989) showed that medium-dose subcutaneous heparin (12 500 IU twice daily) reduced the frequency of LV thrombus, an overview of the 26 trials of anticoagulants in acute MI (including 73 000 patients) found little evidence of any significant further net clinical benefit (in terms of major clinical events) from adding either subcutaneous or intravenous heparin to the treatment of patients who are given aspirin. The value of anticoagulants in a patient with an acute MI complicated by acute ischaemic stroke is unclear (Collins *et al.* 1996; Cairns *et al.* 1998).

Oral anticoagulants, given to stroke-free MI survivors for several months, probably reduce the risk of having a first stroke in the longer term, but given the cost and inconvenience of oral anticoagulants and the uncertainty about the optimal intensity of treatment, aspirin is probably the long-term antithrombotic agent of choice in most patients (Vaitkus *et al.* 1992; Cairns *et al.* 1998). Six months of oral anticoagulants may be worthwhile in patients with MI complicated by acute ischaemic stroke probably due to embolism from the left ventricle, especially if congestive heart failure, atrial fibrillation or extensive LV dysfunction were present (Cairns *et al.* 1998).

11.4.3 Who to treat

Although there is no indication to use anticoagulants *routinely* in patients with acute ischaemic stroke, there are still occasions where they may be appropriate; these are discussed below. The use of heparin after thrombolysis to prevent re-occlusion of the opened cerebral artery is discussed in sections 11.5.2 and 11.5.4.

Heparin, when used for the immediate treatment of patients with acute ischaemic stroke, has risks (haemorrhage in the brain and elsewhere) which exactly cancel out the benefits (fewer recurrent ischaemic strokes and less venous thromboembolism). We therefore do not use this treatment routinely.

Selected patients at high risk of deep venous thrombosis

Factors which increase the risk of DVT and PE after stroke include: the presence of hemiplegia or immobility; dehydration; a history of previous episodes of venous thromboembolism; and the presence of a known thrombophilia (Scottish Intercollegiate Guidelines Network 2000). The management of these factors are further discussed in Chapter 15. Simple, reliable methods to predict which patients are likely to develop DVT would be very useful.

Guidelines vary in their recommendations about whether or not heparin should be used for DVT prevention. Two North American guidelines recommend routine use of heparin for DVT prophylaxis in stroke patients (Adams *et al.* 1994; Albers *et al.* 1998). The Scottish Intercollegiate Guidelines Network document recommended that heparin should only be used in stroke patients at high risk of DVT and PE (Scottish Intercollegiate Guidelines Network 1999; Scottish Intercollegiate Guideines Network 2000). A UK consensus conference was more cautious and noted that the increase in risk of intracranial bleeding was higher than the reduction in risk of PE with heparin and suggested that physical means of preventing DVT should be evaluated (Royal College of Physicians of Edinburgh 1999). Graded compression stockings reduce the risk of DVT after general or orthopaedic surgery after hip fracture (Wells *et al.* 1994; Handoll *et al.* 2000) and intermittent compression devices reduce PE after cardiac surgery (Ramas *et al.* 1996). However, graded compression stockings and other physical means of preventing DVT are costly, uncomfortable for patients, occasionally cause serious complications (in patients with peripheral vascular disease or sensory loss in the legs) and have not been adequately assessed in stroke patients (Chiodo Grandi *et al.* 2000) (section 15.13). The effects of aspirin on DVT and PE are discussed in section 11.3.2. It is not clear whether low-dose subcutaneous heparin can add useful benefit to aspirin for the prevention of DVT and PE without causing an increase in bleeding complications (International Stroke Trial Collaborative Group 1997). This is a controversial area, which is discussed further, along with the management of stroke patients who develop symptoms and signs suggestive of DVT or PE after admission, in section 15.13.

The choice of method for deep venous thrombosis prophylaxis will therefore largely depend on the risk of venous thromboembolism, the likely duration of immobility, and the presence of any predisposing factors. For patients with mild strokes who mobilize within a day or so, and have no other predisposing factors for deep venous thrombosis, aspirin is probably adequate. For immobile patients with predisposing factors (and who do not have bad arterial disease or sensory loss in the legs), graded compression stockings may provide additional protection. If stockings are not acceptable, then low-dose subcutaneous unfractionated heparin is an alternative. There is no evidence that, in stroke patients, low molecular weight heparin or heparinoids offer any clear advantage over unfractionated heparin for venous thromboembolism prophylaxis.

Atrial fibrillation

Patients with atrial fibrillation who have had a stroke or transient ischaemic attack are likely to benefit from long-term oral anticoagulants as secondary prevention, provided there are no contraindications (Table 11.4) (section 16.5 for further details on the selection of patients with atrial fibrillation most likely to benefit). The European Atrial Fibrillation Trial assessed the value of long-term anticoagulants (and aspirin) in secondary prevention after a non-disabling ischaemic stroke or transient ischaemic attack, but did not specifically address the use of anticoagulants during the acute phase to prevent very early re-embolization, so there are few data on the best time to start oral anticoagulants (European Atrial Fibrillation Trial Study Group 1993). To help decide whether or not to use anticoagulants in the acute phase, one should take into account the factors that are likely to increase the risk of haemorrhagic transformation of the infarct (section 11.4.1), the likely risk of recurrent ischaemic stroke within the first week or so, and the severity of the stroke (sections 11.4.5 and 16.5.2).

Ischaemic stroke due to intracranial venous thrombosis

Thrombosis of a cerebral cortical vein or sinus may cause focal cerebral ischaemia resulting in a focal neurological deficit which is indistinguishable from a stroke due to arterial occlusion. Management must be based on accurate diagnosis, confirmed by MR scanning and MR angiography (section 5.5.3), followed by a search for, and treatment of, any underlying cause (e.g. thrombophilia, sepsis, dehydration). Patients with epileptic seizures should be started on anticonvulsants and, if there is clinical or radiological evidence of raised intracranial pressure (and the neuroimaging suggests lumbar puncture is safe), then lumbar puncture—both as a diagnostic test and as a therapeutic manouevre—may be necessary. If lumbar puncture is to be performed, it must be done before antihaemostatic drugs are given.

Two trials have evaluated heparin as a treatment for the whole spectrum of intracranial venous thrombosis (which can present in many different ways, and not just as a mimic of stroke) (Einhaupl *et al.* 1991; de Bruijn *et al.* 1999) (section 5.5.2). A Cochrane systematic review of the randomized trials of anticoagulants is under way (Stam *et al.* 2000). Although the evidence is not strongly in favour of anticoagulants, they do appear safe in these patients. 'Believers' recommend (on the basis of insufficient evidence) anticoagulation with heparin, especially if the patient is deteriorating, and some even suggest local thrombolysis if all else fails (Bousser 1999). In the collaborative European trial, after 3 weeks, patients allocated anticoagulants were put on oral anticoagulants for 3 months (analogous to the treatment of DVT in the leg), which seems sensible (de Bruijn *et al.* 1999).

Table 11.4 Patients with acute ischaemic stroke of suspected cardioembolic origin who should be considered for immediate anticoagulation, and those who should have anticoagulants deferred (or avoided completely).

Immediate anticoagulants worthwhile
Start as soon as possible:
- Transient ischaemic attack or ischaemic stroke with complete recovery within 1–2 days and in atrial fibrillation

Best time to start unclear:
- Non-disabling ischaemic stroke, no haemorrhagic transformation and in atrial fibrillation

Anticoagulants probably worthwhile; best time to start unclear
Acute myocardial infarction within past few weeks and confirmed ischaemic stroke or transient ischaemic attack
Disabling ischaemic stroke and atrial fibrillation

Anticoagulants not worthwhile
Low risk of recurrent cardioembolic stroke without anticoagulants:
- Low-risk cardiac lesion (e.g. hypertrophic cardiomyopathy, uncomplicated mitral valve prolapse)
- Other, non-cardiac lesion, a more likely cause of the ischaemic stroke

Little to gain from long-term anticoagulation:
- Suspected cholesterol embolization syndrome (section 7.7)
- Already severely disabled before the stroke
- Moribund

High risk of cerebral haemorrhage on anticoagulants:
- Infective endocarditis
- Large cerebral infarct with midline shift
- Major haemorrhagic transformation on brain CT
- Likely to comply poorly with anticoagulation therapy
- Severe, uncontrolled hypertension

Absolute or relative contraindication to anticoagulants (sections 11.4.4 and 16,5,3) (Table 11.5)

See Table 16.13 for recommended intensity of anticoagulation.

11.4.4 Who not to treat

Relative contraindications and cautions about the use of anticoagulants are given in Table 11.5. Any patient with acute stroke due to established intracranial haemorrhage, or who has not had a CT brain scan to exclude intracranial

Table 11.5 Contraindications to and cautions with full-dose anticoagulants (these depend on individual circumstances and are seldom absolute) (adapted from Scottish Intercollegiate Guidelines Network 1999).

Uncorrected major bleeding disorder
Thrombocytopenia
Haemophilia
Liver failure
Renal failure

Uncontrolled severe hypertension
Systolic blood pressure over 200 mmHg
Diastolic blood pressure over 120 mmHg

Potential bleeding lesions
Active peptic ulcer
Oesophageal varices
Intracranial aneurysm
Proliferative retinopathy
Recent organ biopsy
Recent trauma or surgery to head, orbit or spine
Recent stroke, but patient has not had CT brain scan or MRI
Recent stroke, with large infarct on CT brain scan or MRI (i.e. high risk of haemorrhagic transformation)
Confirmed intracranial or intraspinal bleeding

History of heparin-induced thrombocytopenia or thrombosis (if heparin planned)

If warfarin planned
Homozygous protein C deficiency (risk of skin necrosis)
History of warfarin-related skin necrosis
Uncooperative/or unreliable patients (long-term therapy)
Risk of falling
Unable to monitor anticoagulation intensity

haemorrhage, should in general not be given anticoagulants. The evidence on the effects of heparin in patients with haemorrhagic stroke is scant but suggests it may indeed be associated with some harm, but the confidence interval is wide (International Stroke Trial Collaborative Group 1997; Gubitz *et al.* 2000b). Warfarin should not be used during pregnancy (sections 11.11 and 16.5).

11.4.5 When to start

The available trial data do not provide reliable evidence on the best time to start anticoagulants. So, in the occasional circumstance where we do feel compelled to use them in acute stroke (section 11.4.3), the decision must be based on the likely risk of events without treatment, and the risk of haemorrhagic transformation with treatment. We are not usually worried about early recurrent ischaemic stroke, because the risk is low (1.2–3.5% within 30 days) and even for patients in atrial fibrillation, the average risk is not much higher (Sandercock *et al.* 1992; International Stroke Trial Collaborative Group 1997; Sandercock & Tanganakul 1997). Symptomatic haemorrhagic transformation of the infarct occurs most commonly during the first 2 weeks and the risk is highest in patients with large infarcts, or uncontrolled hypertension, or in patients given more intensive heparin regimens (Wardlaw & Warlow 1992; Hart *et al.* 1995; International Stroke Trial Collaborative Group 1997; Gubitz *et al.* 2000b).

In patients with transient ischaemic attack or with an ischaemic stroke which resolves within a day or so, the risk of haemorrhagic transformation is probably negligible; if such a patient has a clear indication for the use of long-term anticoagulants (chiefly atrial fibrillation), we would start treatment immediately. In a patient with a major ischaemic stroke and atrial fibrillation, we would wait at least a week or two before starting. We would then consider the relative contraindications listed in Table 11.5 and, if necessary, delay the start of anticoagulants further (or abandon the idea altogether). When oral anticoagulants are started in this way, some time after the acute event, concomitant heparin (to overcome any transient prothrombotic state associated with the start of warfarin) is probably not needed (Scottish Intercollegiate Guidelines Network 1999).

In a patient with a disabling acute ischaemic stroke and atrial fibrillation, the risk of stroke recurrence within the first 2 weeks is low in absolute terms, so we would avoid anticoagulants for the first week or two, or longer if we felt the risk of haemorrhagic transformation of the infarct remained high (i.e. large infarct, uncontrolled hypertension). We would, however, start aspirin immediately. Patients with transient ischaemic attack or very minor ischaemic stroke and atrial fibrillation can be started on aspirin and oral anticoagulants immediately. Aspirin should be stopped once the international normalized ratio is in the therapeutic range.

11.4.6 Agent/dose/route/adverse effects

Agent

Oral anticoagulants do not act sufficiently fast to have a major role within the first few hours of onset of an ischaemic stroke. Anticoagulants must be given by injection if they are to achieve a rapid effect. The majority of the evidence on heparin in acute stroke relates to trials which used unfractionated heparin (Gubitz *et al.* 2000b). Though other agents have been tested, systematic reviews of the direct (Counsell & Sandercock 2000; Gubitz *et al.* 2000b) and indirect comparions (Gubitz *et al.* 2000c) did not provide evidence that any one agent was better than unfractionated subcutaneous heparin. A small trial suggested that fraxiparine was of benefit, but this was not confirmed by a subsequent, larger trial (Kay *et al.* 1995; Hommel 1998).

Dose and route

The risk of bleeding with heparin is clearly dose dependent; the higher the dose, the higher the risk of intracranial and extracranial haemorrhage and there is no evidence to support the use of full-dose adjusted regimens with intravenous unfractionated heparin or heparinoid (International Stroke Trial Collaborative Group 1997; TOAST Investigators 1998; Gubitz *et al.* 2000b, 2000c, 2000d). A further trial is planned, the Rapid Anticoagulation Prevents Ischaemic Damage (RAPID) trial, which will recruit 1000 patients with non-lacunar ischaemic stroke within 12 h of onset to full doses of intravenous unfractionated heparin, or to aspirin 300 mg daily; it aims to start in 2000 (Chamorro 1999).

Until the RAPID trial is complete, there is no indication to use intravenous heparin in acute stroke. If anticoagulants are to be used, low-dose subcutaneous regimens are preferable (e.g. 5000 IU unfractionated heparin two or three times daily) since they are simpler, do not require complex monitoring and are likely to be associated with lower bleeding risks. The options for the treatment of established DVT or PE are discussed in section 15.13.

Adverse effects

Tables 11.6 and 11.7 list the most important adverse effects and cautions to be considered with the use of heparin. The most life-threatening risks are of massive intra- or extracranial haemorrhage. Management of severe extracranial haemorrhage consists of stopping any heparin administration; estimation of the clotting time; and reversal with intravenous protamine sulphate in a dose of 1 mg for every 100 IU of heparin infused in the previous hour (Scottish Intercollegiate Guidelines Network 1999). Protamine should be given slowly over 10 min and the patient monitored for hypotension and bradycardia. Not more than 40 mg of protamine should be administered in any one injection. For advice on reversal of low molecular weight heparin or heparinoids, consult the manufacturer's data sheet. Patients on oral anticoagulants who suffer a head injury or develop any of the neurological symptoms listed in Table 11.7, or who require a diagnostic lumbar puncture, should be investigated and treated as described in Tables 11.7–11.9 (Scottish Intercollegiate Guidelines Network 1999). Reversal of warfarin is often best done in consultation with the local haematology specialist (Table 11.9).

Table 11.6 Adverse effects of heparin.

Local minor complications of subcutaneous heparin at injection site
Discomfort
Bruising

Local complications of intravenous heparin at cannula site (or elsewhere)
Pain at cannula site
Infection at cannula (sometimes with severe systemic infection)
Reduced patient mobility because of infusion lines and pump

Intracranial bleeding
Haemorrhagic transformation of cerebral infarct (potentially disabling or fatal)
Intracerebral haematoma
Subarachnoid haemorrhage
Subdural haematoma

Extracranial haemorrhage
Subcutaneous (can sometimes be massive)
Visceral (haematemesis, melaena, haematuria)

Thrombocytopenia
Type I: dose and duration related, reversible, mild, usually asymptomatic, not serious and often resolves spontaneously
Type II: idiosyncratic, allergic, severe (may be complicated by arterial and venous thrombosis). Affects 3–11% of patients treated with intravenous heparin and less than 1% of patients treated with subcutaneous heparin (Hirsh 1991; Schmitt & Adelman 1993; Aster 1995; Warkentin et al. 1995)

Osteoporosis

Skin necrosis

Alopecia

11.4.7 Acute stroke in a patient already receiving anticoagulants

The first step is, as ever, a CT brain scan. If this shows intracranial haemorrhage then anticoagulants should be stopped and urgently reversed, with vitamin K and administration of clotting factors (with advice of the local haematology specialist) (Hart *et al.* 1995) (section 12.2.4) (Tables 11.7–11.9). Patients with mechanical heart valves are at risk of valve thrombosis and re-embolization if anticoagulants are withdrawn, so the further management of such patients requires careful communication between the stroke physician, the haematologist, and the cardiologist.

If the scan shows an infarct with a slight degree of haemorrhagic transformation, anticoagulants do not necessarily need to be stopped. If the CT is normal or shows bland infarction, the reason for the infarction must be sought. Often, the cause is inadequate warfarin dose, but infective endocarditis must be ruled out; if it has, more careful supervision to maintain the international normalized ratio (INR) above 2.0 (or whatever target range has been chosen for that specific patient) should minimize the risk of further ischaemic strokes (European Atrial Fibrillation Trial Study Group 1995). However, recurrent ischaemic stroke despite an adequate INR may necessitate the addition of low-dose aspirin,

Table 11.7 Advice on management of problems in patients on anticoagulants who have a head injury, develop headaches, neurological symptoms or require a lumbar puncture.

Possible intracranial bleeding

Head injury, headache, drowsiness, confusion or focal neurological symptoms or signs in patients on anticoagulants.

Any patient on anticoagulants who sustains a significant head injury (i.e. any loss of consciousness or amnesia or the presence of a scalp laceration) must undergo CT brain scan to exclude intracranial haemorrhage.

Headache (especially of recent onset, or increasing in severity), impaired consciousness, confusion, or focal neurological symptoms or signs must always arouse the suspicion of intracranial or subdural haemorrhage, and a CT brain scan must be performed (sections 3.3.10 and 5.3)

Need for lumbar puncture or other procedures which may cause intraspinal bleeding

Lumbar puncture, myelography, epidural or spinal anaesthesia, transhepatic percutaneous shunting. All these procedures carry a risk of spinal haemorrhage and paraplegia and should not be performed in any patient on anticoagulants until the anticoagulation has been reversed. The need for lumbar puncture or myelography should be discussed with a neurologist or neurosurgeon before anticoagulants are reversed, since reversal carries a risk of thromboembolism and alternative investigation (e.g. MR scanning) may be preferable

Table 11.8 Strategies for reversal of oral anticoagulation (Scottish Intercollegiate Guidelines Network 1999).

Life-threatening haemorrhage (intracranial or major gastrointestinal bleeding)

Stop warfarin *and*

Give intravenous vitamin K_1 (5 mg, repeated if necessary)

and either intravenous factor IX complex concentrate (also contains factors II and X) (50 IU/kg body weight) *plus* factor VII concentrate (50 IU/kg body weight) (if available) *or* fresh frozen plasma (15 mL/kg—approximately 1 L for adult)

Less severe haemorrhage (e.g. haematuria, epistaxis)

Stop warfarin for 1–2 days

Give vitamin K_1, 0.5–2 mg intravenously or 5–10 mg orally

High international normalized ratio (INR) but no haemorrhage

Stop warfarin, monitor INR, restart warfarin when INR < 5.0

Consider giving vitamin K_1 0.5 mg intravenously or 5 mg orally if INR > 8.0, or other risk factors for bleeding

though this is likely to double the risk of intracranial haemorrhage (Turpie *et al.* 1993; Hart & Benavente 1999) (section 16.5.4).

11.5 Selective use: thrombolysis

11.5.1 Rationale

Restoration of blood flow, to reperfuse the ischaemic brain as soon as possible after a cerebral vessel has been occluded, may lessen the volume of brain damaged by ischaemia, reduce the likelihood of major cerebral oedema and result in a better clinical outcome (section 11.1.3). Therefore, therapeutic attempts to hasten reperfusion by lysing the occluding thrombus with thrombolytic drugs ought to be helpful. However, thrombolytic agents will also lyse haemostatic plugs and thus may increase bleeding. Thrombolytic agents digest fibrinogen, so there may be antithrombotic effects: less fibrin is available to form the fibrin component of the thrombus and anticoagulant fibrin degradation products are formed (Lowe 1998).

11.5.2 Evidence

Data available for thrombolysis in acute stroke

Seventeen trials, including 5216 patients, were included in the most up-to-date systematic review available on the Cochrane Library (Wardlaw *et al.* 2000). The agents tested (proportion of the total data coming from trials of that agent) were: intravenous tissue plasminogen activator (rt-PA) (50%), intravenous streptokinase (42%), intravenous urokinase (3%) and intra-arterial recombinant pro-urokinase (5%). Ninety per cent of the data were derived from trials of intravenous thrombolysis with either rt-PA or streptokinase, given within 6 h of onset of confirmed ischaemic stroke (i.e. CT scan or MRI had ruled out intracranial haemorrhage). Full details of the types of patient randomized, the CT scan criteria, the main design features and results of each trial are given in the Cochrane review (Wardlaw *et al.* 2000).

Fewer data than for acute myocardial infarction

There are less data on the effects of thrombolysis for ischaemic stroke compared with the amount available on the trials of thrombolysis for acute myocardial infarction (MI). Over 58 000 patients with acute MI had been randomized by the time clinicians generally accepted the evidence that thrombolysis saved lives (Fibrinolytic Therapy Trialists' (FTT) Collaborative Group 1994; Peto *et al.* 1995). Furthermore, it required a systematic review of the data from the trials to establish which MI patients were most likely to benefit from treatment, and that the 'time window' for treatment was not a mere 3 h from the onset of chest pain, as predicted from studies in animals, but certainly 12 h in many cases and perhaps as long as 24 h for some specific patients (Fibrinolytic Therapy Trialists' (FTT) Collaborative Group 1994).

Table 11.9 Options for reversal of warfarin therapy (Scottish Intercollegiate Guidelines Network 1999).

Method and dosage	Advantage	Disadvantage
Stop warfarin	Simple	May take several days for INR to normalize, particularly with liver disease
Vitamin K_1	Safe if given slowly	
0.5–5 mg intravenously		2–6 h to take effect
5–10 mg orally		12–24 h to take effect
Factor IX complex concentrate (factors II, IX and X) 50 IU/kg body weight	Acts immediately Small volume Can be given quickly	Exposes patients to pooled blood product which rarely may transmit hepatitis B (but safe from hepatitis C and HIV) Effect is temporary (8–24 h), may need to be repeated Should be combined with vitamin K_1 Risk of thromboembolism
Factor VII concentrate 50 IU/kg body weight	Should be given with factor IX complex concentrate	As for factor IX complex
Fresh frozen plasma 1 L for adult	Acts immediately	Large intravenous volume load Allergic reactions Not as efficacious as factor IX complex concentrate Difficult to give repeat infusions because of large volume Virally inactivated plasma is preferred

Intracranial haemorrhage

There was a very consistent trend across all of the stroke trials for an excess of fatal intracranial haemorrhage and the proportional excess was similar with all the agents. The absolute excess depended on the risk of haemorrhage in the control group, and this risk was somewhat different between trials. However, overall, fatal intracranial haemorrhages increased from 1% in controls to 5.4% in treated patients, a five-fold increase ($P < 0.00001$), equivalent to 44 extra fatal intracranial haemorrhages per 1000 patients treated (Fig. 11.21). Fatal or non-fatal symptomatic intracranial haemorrhages increased from 3% in controls to 10% in treated patients, a three-fold increase ($P < 0.00001$), equivalent to 70 extra symptomatic haemorrhages per 1000 treated (Wardlaw *et al.* 2000).

Death

Overall, thrombolysis significantly increased the odds of death within the first 2 weeks by 85%, from 10% in controls to 17% in treated patients—an excess of 70 deaths per 1000 (Fig. 11.22). However, by the end of follow-up (3 months in most trials), the difference between the two groups was smaller. Sixteen per cent of controls were dead vs. 19% of treated patients, equivalent to 30 extra deaths per 1000 patients treated (Fig. 11.23) (Wardlaw *et al.* 2000). It is not known reliably whether the survival disadvantage from thrombolysis diminishes or increases with longer term follow-up, since only one trial with 624 patients has reported follow-up beyond 6 months (Kwiatkowski *et al.* 1999).

Dead or dependent, or fully recovered at the end of trial follow-up

However, patients who survived the treatment were, on average, less disabled. The majority of the trials reported follow-up at 3 months. Among controls, 59% were dead or dependent at the end of follow-up, compared with 55% among treated patients—a 27% reduction in the relative odds of a bad outcome, equivalent to about 40 patients avoiding death or dependency for every 1000 patients treated within 6 h (Fig. 11.24). The precise definition of dependency did not materially alter these conclusions, i.e. it did not make much difference whether dependent was defined as modified Rankin/Oxford Handicap Score (OHS) 3,4,5 or 2,3,4,5. The proportion of patients making a complete recovery from their stroke (OHS zero) was also increased with thrombolysis (Wardlaw *et al.* 2000). Only three trials, with a total of 1556 patients, reported follow-up data at 6 months and only

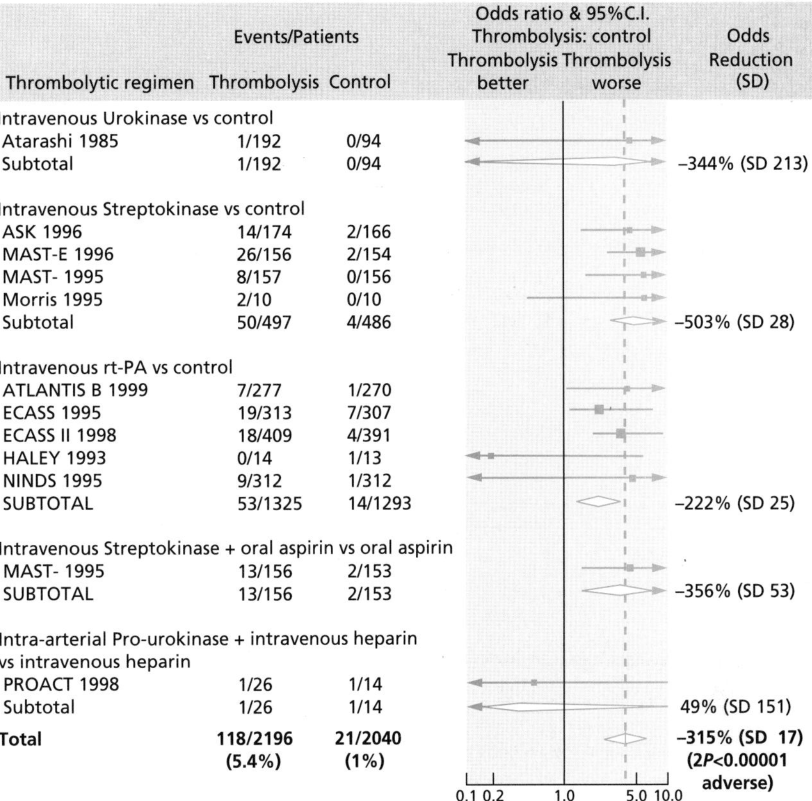

Events/Patients
Odds ratio & 95%C.I.
Thrombolysis: control
Thrombolysis better
Thrombolysis worse
Odds Reduction (SD)
Thrombolytic regimen
Thrombolysis
Control
Intravenous Urokinase vs control
Atarashi 1985 1/192 0/94
Subtotal 1/192 0/94 –344% (SD 213)
Intravenous Streptokinase vs control
ASK 1996 14/174 2/166
MAST-E 1996 26/156 2/154
MAST- 1995 8/157 0/156
Morris 1995 2/10 0/10
Subtotal 50/497 4/486 –503% (SD 28)
Intravenous rt-PA vs control
ATLANTIS B 1999 7/277 1/270
ECASS 1995 19/313 7/307
ECASS II 1998 18/409 4/391
HALEY 1993 0/14 1/13
NINDS 1995 9/312 1/312
SUBTOTAL 53/1325 14/1293 –222% (SD 25)
Intravenous Streptokinase + oral aspirin vs oral aspirin
MAST- 1995 13/156 2/153
SUBTOTAL 13/156 2/153 –356% (SD 53)
Intra-arterial Pro-urokinase + intravenous heparin vs intravenous heparin
PROACT 1998 1/26 1/14
Subtotal 1/26 1/14 49% (SD 151)
Total 118/2196 (5.4%) 21/2040 (1%) –315% (SD 17) (2P<0.00001 adverse)
0.1 0.2 1.0 5.0 10.0

Fig. 11.21 Thrombolysis in acute ischaemic stroke: effects on fatal intracranial haemorrhage. Results of a systematic review of 11 trials. Negative numbers indicate an adverse effect of treatment. Same conventions as Fig. 11.18 except all the confidence intervals are 95% (with permission from Wardlaw *et al.* 2000).

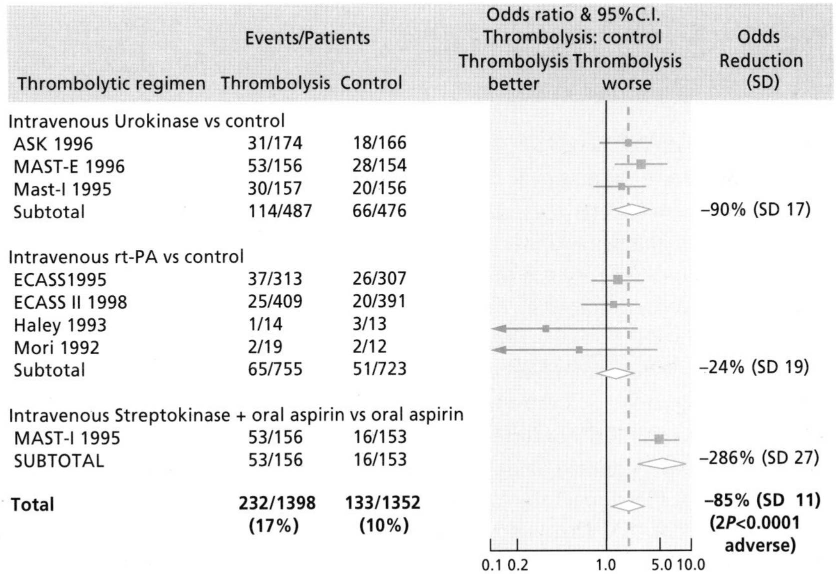

Fig. 11.22 Thrombolysis in acute ischaemic stroke: effects on death within 7–10 days of randomization. Results of a systematic review of seven trials reporting this outcome. Negative numbers indicate an adverse effect of treatment. Same conventions as Fig. 11.18 except all the confidence intervals are 95% (with permission from Wardlaw *et al.* 2000).

one has reported follow-up at 12 months. The benefit seen at 3 months persisted to 12 months in that one trial, but further long-term follow-up data are clearly needed (Kwiatkowski *et al.* 1999).

Subgroups: time since stroke onset

Studies of the pathophysiology of stroke in man suggest that the duration of the therapeutic 'time window' in some types

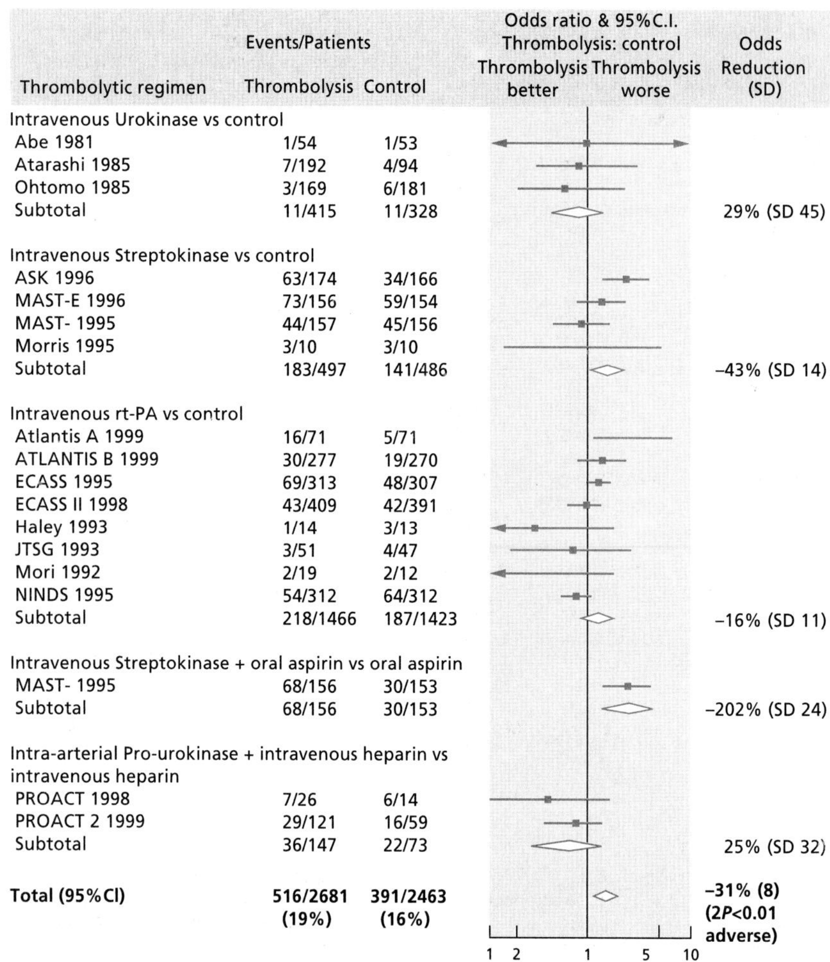

Thrombolytic regimen
Events/Patients
Thrombolysis Control
Odds ratio & 95%C.I.
Thrombolysis: control
Thrombolysis better Thrombolysis worse
Odds Reduction (SD)
Intravenous Urokinase vs control
Abe 1981 1/54 1/53
Atarashi 1985 7/192 4/94
Ohtomo 1985 3/169 6/181
Subtotal 11/415 11/328 29% (SD 45)
Intravenous Streptokinase vs control
ASK 1996 63/174 34/166
MAST-E 1996 73/156 59/154
MAST- 1995 44/157 45/156
Morris 1995 3/10 3/10
Subtotal 183/497 141/486 −43% (SD 14)
Intravenous rt-PA vs control
Atlantis A 1999 16/71 5/71
ATLANTIS B 1999 30/277 19/270
ECASS 1995 69/313 48/307
ECASS II 1998 43/409 42/391
Haley 1993 1/14 3/13
JTSG 1993 3/51 4/47
Mori 1992 2/19 2/12
NINDS 1995 54/312 64/312
Subtotal 218/1466 187/1423 −16% (SD 11)
Intravenous Streptokinase + oral aspirin vs oral aspirin
MAST- 1995 68/156 30/153
Subtotal 68/156 30/153 −202% (SD 24)
Intra-arterial Pro-urokinase + intravenous heparin vs intravenous heparin
PROACT 1998 7/26 6/14
PROACT 2 1999 29/121 16/59
Subtotal 36/147 22/73 25% (SD 32)
Total (95%CI) 516/2681 (19%) 391/2463 (16%) −31% (8) (2P<0.01 adverse)
1 2 1 5 10

Fig. 11.23 Thrombolysis in acute ischaemic stroke: effects on death at the end of follow-up. Results of a systematic review of 16 trials reporting this outcome. Same conventions as Fig. 11.18 except all the confidence intervals are 95% (from Wardlaw *et al.* 2000).

of patient may be quite short (perhaps an hour or less), but much longer (perhaps even 24 h or more) in others (section 11.1.3). The site and size of the infarct, the adequacy of collateral supply and the presence of other factors (e.g. hypotension) may all be important, but in general, the earlier treatment is given the better. Unfortunately, there are too few data available for reliable subgroup analysis to test that hypothesis adequately, or to determine the duration of the therapeutic 'time window' for thrombolysis (Peto *et al.* 1995; Chen *et al.* 2000). A limited analysis suggests that the 'time window' may well be longer than 3 h, but exactly how long is unclear (Fig. 11.25). The analysis is made more difficult because time is just one of four inextricably linked factors: stroke severity (severe strokes arrive quickest at hospital, mild strokes come later); the appearance of the baseline CT scan (the more severe the stroke, the more likely 'infarction' will be visible on an early scan); the time from onset (the longer the time, the more likely infarction will be visible on CT); and reduction in the benefit from treatment with time. There are insufficient data to establish by how much the benefit declines with each extra hour of delay; very large-scale trials with perhaps 10 000 or so patients would be needed to establish the duration of the time window with any precision.

Subgroups: stroke severity, age and baseline CT (or MR) scan

A meta-analysis, using individual patient data from every trial, might go some way to assessing the effect of treatment among subgroups defined by various clinical and radiological features at baseline. However, the data are sparse and multiple subgroup analyses of many small trials are highly likely to generate many false-positive and false-negative associations (Peto *et al.* 1995; Chen *et al.* 2000). For the time being, the data are insufficient to formulate reliable, evidence-based selection criteria to decide which patients should (or should not) be treated.

Subgroups: is any one agent better than another?

Systematic reviews of the indirect (Wardlaw *et al.* 2000) and the direct randomized comparisons of different thrombolytic agents (Liu & Wardlaw 2000), have not established that any

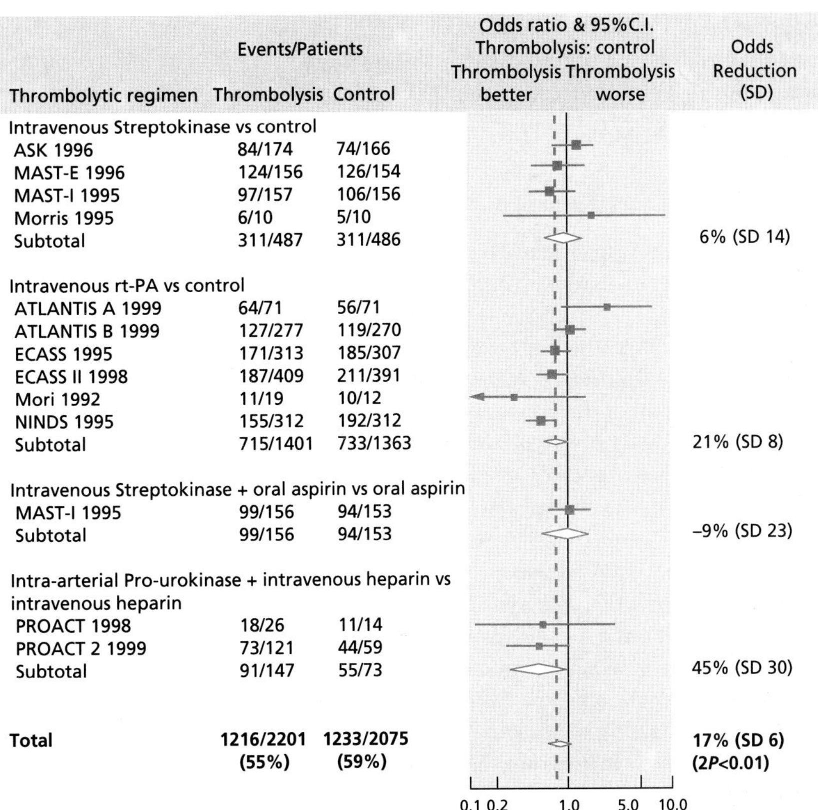

Fig. 11.24 Thrombolysis in acute ischaemic stroke: effects on death or dependency at the end of follow-up. Results of a systematic review of the 12 trials which reported this outcome. Same conventions as Fig. 11.18 except all the confidence intervals are 95% (from Wardlaw *et al.* 2000).

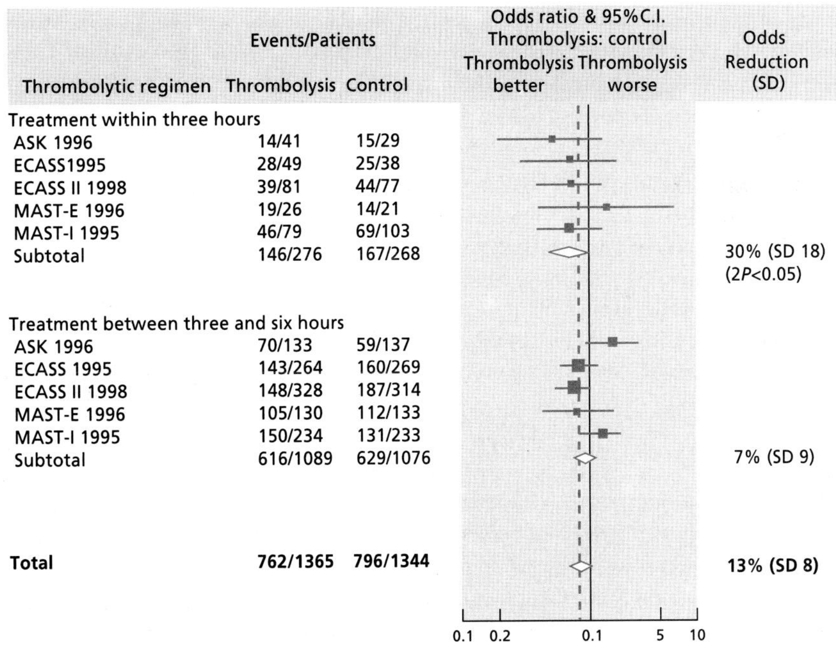

Fig. 11.25 Thrombolysis in acute ischaemic stroke: effects subdivided by time to randomization. Five trials reported their results separately for patients randomized within 3 h of onset, and those randomized within 3–6 h of onset. To minimize the risk of bias, trials only recruiting within 3 h were excluded from this analysis. Same conventions as Fig. 11.18 except all the confidence intervals are 95% (from Wardlaw *et al.* 2000).

one agent is clearly superior to another. In the trials of rt-PA, at the end of follow-up, there were non-significantly more deaths with rt-PA; 13% of the controls died vs. 15% with rt-PA, an absolute excess of 18 per 1000 patients treated (95% CI, reduction of seven to an excess of 43 per 1000). But the estimate is imprecise, and it is not clear whether rt-PA increases or reduces the risk of death. There was, of course, a significant increase in fatal intracranial haemorrhage with rt-PA of about 30 per 1000 (95% CI, 17–41). At 3 months, 57% of controls were dead or dependent vs. 51% of rt-PA treated, a benefit of about 60 per 1000. The guidelines that do recommend the use of thrombolytic therapy suggest that intravenous rt-PA is the agent of choice (European Ad Hoc Consensus Group 1996; Norris *et al.* 1998).

Subgroups: concomitant aspirin or heparin?

In the Multicentre Acute Stroke Trial (MAST-I) there was an interaction of streptokinase with aspirin and the risk of symptomatic intracranial haemorrhage was significantly higher for the combination of aspirin and streptokinase than for either drug separately (Multicentre Acute Stroke Trial (MAST-I) Group 1995). In all of the other trials, aspirin was not randomly allocated, so it is very difficult to determine whether any differences between trials in the frequency of symptomatic intracranial haemorrhage were due to concomitant aspirin treatment or to other factors (such as thrombolytic agent, dose, delay, etc.). However, there was a strong tendency for the effect of thrombolysis to be more favourable in trials where antithrombotic therapy was avoided for the first 24 h (and the more antithrombotic therapy that was given, the less favourable the outcome (Wardlaw *et al.* 2000).

The need for anticoagulants may be different when intra-arterial thrombolysis is used, but there are no trials of intra-arterial thrombolysis which directly randomized patients to 'intravenous heparin' vs. 'no intravenous heparin'. In the Prolyse in Acute Cerebral Thromboembolism (PROACT)-I study of intra-arterial pro-urokinase, at the time of angiography, the first 16 patients were given a 100 IU bolus of unfractionated heparin intravenously, followed by an infusion of 1000 IU/h. However, the Data Monitoring Committee reviewed the data at that stage and, because of the high frequency of intracranial haemorrhage, recommended a reduction in the heparin dose (del Zoppo *et al.* 1998). In the PROACT-II study, all patients received an intravenous bolus of 2000 IU followed by an intravenous infusion of 500 IU/h of unfractionated heparin, and intravenous heparin was given with intra-arterial thrombolysis (Furlan *et al.* 1999).

Intra-arterial thrombolysis for acute, angiographically proven, occlusion of a cerebral artery

There have been four small randomized controlled trials in which occlusion of the relevant cerebral artery was demonstrated before treatment was given. In two of the trials, angiographic confirmation was available in most patients (Mori *et al.* 1992; Yamaguchi *et al.* 1993), and in the two PROACT trials it was a prerequisite for trial entry (del Zoppo *et al.* 1998; Furlan *et al.* 1999). The two PROACT trials compared pro-urokinase plus intravenous heparin vs. intravenous heparin alone. At least one trial comparing intra-arterial thrombolysis plus heparin with heparin alone in basilar thrombosis—the Australian Urokinase Stroke Trial (AUST)—is still underway (Donnan 1999). The benefits of intra-arterial thrombolysis appear to be at least as great as with intravenous rt-PA (Figs 11.23 and 11.24), but the treatment can be given only in a few highly specialized centres, so is only available to a very small proportion of all stroke patients. Treatments which are highly effective, but applicable to only a small proportion of all patients, have almost no effect on reducing the overall burden of stroke (section 18.3). The concomitant heparin treatment used in the PROACT trials was—as might be expected—associated with quite a high risk of symptomatic intracranial haemorrhage in the control groups (14% and 4% of controls in PROACT-1 and -2, respectively), and an even higher rate in the treated patients (15% and 10%, respectively).

Suspected cardioembolic stroke

A small trial comparing rt-PA with controls in 98 patients with suspected cardioembolic ischaemic stroke showed a non-significant trend towards benefit with thrombolysis (Yamaguchi *et al.* 1993). There is some suggestion that an embolus obstructing a cerebral artery may be more susceptible to lysis if it is due to embolism from the heart rather than from a lesion in the extracranial arteries (Chimowitz *et al.* 1994).

Ischaemic stroke following angiography or interventional radiology

There are many possible causes of stroke (both ischaemic and haemorrhagic) after such procedures (sections 6.7.5, 7.18 and 13.5.4). If brain CT has excluded intracranial haemorrhage, and if the intra-arterial catheter is still in place, the radiologist may inject contrast material to see if an occlusive lesion can be visualized. Unfortunately, it may be difficult to ascertain whether the vessel has occluded because of local thrombosis, intimal dissection, arterial spasm or emboli dislodged by the catheter from proximal arterial sites. Even if the vessel is occluded by emboli, it may not be possible to determine whether the emboli consist of atheromatous debris or fresh thrombus. None the less, interventional radiologists like to intervene, and there are several anecdotal reports of thrombolysis to clear the obstruction. A single report of an uncontrolled study in 11 patients who had acute ischaemic strokes during interventional neuroradiological procedures (10 of the 11 were having coils or balloons inserted into inoperable intracranial aneurysms), suggested that thrombolysis within 4 h of symptom onset with an unspecified intra-arterial dose of urokinase was not catastrophic, but then a similar clinical outcome might have been observed without any treatment (Berenstein *et al.* 1994).

The need for further large-scale placebo-controlled trials of intravenous thrombolysis

The available trial data strongly suggest that thrombolysis is potentially a very effective treatment. However, it has been evaluated in a relatively small number of patients treated in specialist centres. This is especially true of intra-arterial thrombolysis. If thrombolysis is to be used more widely, and in less specialized centres, to allow more patients to benefit, then we need reliable answers to a number of important questions: Is there worthwhile net benefit when thrombolysis is given in non-specialist centres? Which patients are most likely to suffer early hazard? Which patients will gain the greatest long-term benefit? How wide is the time window—3, 4, 5, 6, 7, 8 or 9 h? Is the window the same for all subtypes (e.g. is the window for basilar artery thrombosis maybe even 12 h)? How can we overcome organizational and administrative barriers?

To answer these questions reliably, we need to design and conduct appropriately large trials (Peto *et al.* 1995). Large trials are *essential* because if the treatment really works as well as we suspect (or the time window is longer than just 2 or 3 h), it should be used more widely. If, on the other hand, large-scale trials show it to be less effective than expected, we should focus our energies on treatments that are more widely applicable. A trial with at least 10 000 patients would be needed to provide reliable evidence of the sort of effect sizes that we are interested in. The trial would probably have a time window of 6 h, and it would certainly be interesting to think about a wider time window than just 3 h. The eligibility should be based on the uncertainty principle. In some cases the clinician will be certain that they want to treat a patient with thrombolysis; such a patient should be treated. If there is a clear contraindication to treatment, the patient is not treated. If the clinician is uncertain, the most ethical next step is to randomize the patient in a well-conducted trial. The Third International Stroke Trial (IST-3) began randomizing in April 2000 in a limited number of pilot centres (full details of the trial protocol and progress are available at http://www.dcn.ed.ac.uk/ist3).

11.5.3 Who to treat (and in what setting)

The early hazard will rightly deter many neurologists and stroke physicians. But some stroke patients might view the situation differently, especially if they would prefer to die from the stroke than to survive in a disabled state (Solomon *et al.* 1994). Many patients might accept the short-term risk for longer term benefit. Indeed, many patients already accept this kind of trade-off; for example, patients at risk of stroke do seem to be prepared to accept the 5% risk of stroke and/or death complicating carotid surgery in order to reap the long-term benefits (section 16.8.9).

What do we do? Some of us might thrombolyse a young patient presenting within 3 h of an acute ischaemic stroke if the CT was normal. However, such patients are relatively uncommon, and for the generality of patients presenting within 6 h, we would prefer to use thrombolysis within the context of a well-conducted placebo-controlled trial, such as IST-3. This is in line with the recent UK guideline (Wade and the Intercollegiate Working Party for Stroke 2000).

Systematic approach, organization and efficiency

The whole health system will need a new *modus operandi* with a much greater sense of urgency to ensure that stroke patients are admitted, have a CT scan to exclude intracerebral haemorrhage and are randomized (or treated) within a few hours of stroke onset. Chapter 17 provides more detail on the organization of acute stroke services, and Chapter 5 on imaging in acute stroke. There is a minor epidemic of guidelines and websites on acute stroke management; we can vouchsafe for the quality of the SIGN and national guidelines (http://www.show.scot.nhs.uk/sign/clinical.htm and http://www.rcplondon.ac.uk/college/ceeu_stroke_home.htm). A few publications are listed here, but these will become rapidly out of date (Adams *et al.* 1996; European Ad Hoc Consensus Group 1996; Pan European Consensus Meeting on Stroke 1996; European Ad Hoc Consensus Group 1997; Asia Pacific Consensus Forum on Stroke Management Organising Committees 1998; Norris *et al.* 1998; Royal College of Physicians of Edinburgh 1999; Royal College of Physicians of London 2000). The Cochrane Stroke Review Group is assembling a list of relevant websites with stroke guidelines which are more likely to be periodically updated than journal publications (http://www.dcn.ed.ac.uk/csrg).

Changing clinical practice in non-specialist centres by participating in trials

A few highly specialized centres should probably be treating a few very carefully selected patients. However, there is not enough evidence to support the routine use of intravenous thrombolysis in patients with acute ischaemic stroke admitted to non-specialist units. A large-scale collaborative trial, such as IST-3, would provide a mechanism which could enable a wider range of hospitals to use thrombolytic therapy under closely supervised conditions. Experience with thrombolysis for acute myocardial infarction also showed that participation in trials led to better implementation of the trial results; hospitals which had participated in the large-scale trials were more likely to adopt the treatment after the trial was completed (Ketley & Woods 1993).

Essential aspects of thrombolytic therapy (and a caution)

Any protocol for the administration of thrombolytic treatment in a particular hospital must be adapted to local circumstances. Experts cannot agree about the interpretation of the existing data and each of the published guidelines make rather different recommendations, so our own suggestions must be viewed in that context (Table 11.10 and, in more detail, at http://www.dcn.ed.ac.uk/wghstroke).

Table 11.10 Essential aspects of therapeutic thrombolysis.

Preparation and maintenance of service organization:
Audit existing service, identify delays
Draw up 'fast-track' pathway of care in consultation with all relevant disciplines and departments
Train relevant staff
Inform general public and primary care teams

Assess patients immediately:
Ambulance crew perform basic assessment and radio ahead to hospital to warn of arrival
Immediate assessment on arrival at hospital by trained 'triage' nurse or paramedic

Local acute stroke protocol activated including:
Systematic but brief clinical assessment:
  Number of hours since onset of stroke symptoms
  Focal neurological symptoms and signs
  Vital signs (pulse, blood pressure, respiration, temperature)
Intravenous cannula inserted and blood samples taken for basic blood tests (blood glucose measurement essential)
Immediate transfer to neuroimaging
Results of preliminary neuroimaging conveyed to stroke team
Trained stroke physician reviews diagnosis, neuroimaging and other information
Consent/assent sought from patient and/or relative where feasible

Do not give thrombolysis if any of the following are true:
Neuroimaging shows intracranial haemorrhage
Neuroimaging shows a non-stroke lesion as the cause (e.g. cerebral tumour)
On oral anticoagulants and therapeutically anticoagulated (i.e. INR > 1.7)
History of bleeding disorder (e.g. haemophilia)
History of recent bleeding
Arterial puncture at noncompressible site within past 14 days
Major surgery within past 14 days
Previous stroke or serious head injury within past three months
Neurological deficit trivial and likely to recover within next few hours
Evidence of accelerated hypertension
Blood glucose is < 3 or > 22 mmol/L

Decision to give thrombolysis or not must be made by senior member of stroke team

If decision is to give thrombolysis, transfer to place where thrombolysis can be given and monitored closely:
Establish intravenous (IV) infusion if not already done so
Estimate weight, draw up infusion with a dose of 0.9 mg/kg rt-PA
Infuse rt-PA IV: 10% as a bolus over 1–2 min, remainder over 60 min
Monitor pulse and BP:
  Every 15 min during infusion
  Every 30 min for next 2 h, then
  Hourly for 5 h
Neurological observations hourly

Postacute management:
Transfer to stroke unit (if not already there)
Start aspirin 160–300 mg daily 24 h after infusion:
  If able to swallow safely, by mouth
  If not able to swallow safely, per rectum or IV (section 11.3.6)

Note: the Integrated Care Pathway for Acute Stroke at the Western General Hospital is available at http://www.dcn.ed.ac.uk/wghstroke and this gives greater detail on these items.

INR, international normalized ratio; rt-PA, tissue plasminogen activator.

If thrombolysis is to be given safely, a great deal of staff preparation and training is required and efforts must be made to take a very systematic yet efficient approach to assessment and investigation. It is, for example, important to have experienced stroke physicians readily on hand to identify patients with non-stroke disorders. It is wholly inappropriate to expose a person to the risks of thrombolysis if their focal neurological symptoms are due to a non-stroke problem such as a subdural haematoma, an epileptic seizure, migraine or a hysterical conversion disorder (section 3.4). In a wider perspective, there is also the possibility that every patient saved from a nursing home by rt-PA is offset by another patient who never resumed his previous lifestyle because he was rushed to hospital with a presumed diagnosis of stroke, which was erroneous.

11.5.4 Agent/dose/route/concomitant antithrombotic treatment/adverse effects

Agent

The debate about which agent is most effective and safe for patients with acute myocardial infarction continues, though perhaps not as fiercely as it did in 1992 with the suggestion from the third International Study of Infarct Survival (ISIS-3) that streptokinase and rt-PA had similar effects on death, but that the hazard of intracranial bleeding was higher with rt-PA (ISIS-3 Collaborative Group 1992). A systematic review of all the trials directly randomizing between the two agents is badly needed to quell the debate and one is planned (Fibrinolytic Therapy Trialists' Collaborative Group, personal communication). There are no studies which have directly randomized sufficiently large numbers of patients with acute ischaemic stroke between streptokinase, rt-PA and urokinase to allow reliable comparison of the safety and efficacy of these agents. Only indirect comparisons are available and these are not the most reliable way to compare treatment effects; none the less, they did not show major differences in efficacy between the three agents, once the time to treatment is accounted for, so no firm recommendation on the 'best' agent can be made (Wardlaw *et al.* 2000). On the rare occasions when we give a thrombolytic agent outside a trial, we use intravenous rt-PA.

Dose and route

There is a suggestion that low-dose urokinase and low-dose rt-PA are associated with a lower risk of symptomatic intracranial haemorrhage, but the comparisons are confounded by a number of factors, such as baseline severity of stroke, race and time to randomization, so no firm recommendation on the 'best' dose can be given; we use 0.9 mg/kg of rt-PA intravenously (Liu & Wardlaw 2000; Wardlaw *et al.* 2000). Intra-arterial thrombolysis appears to be effective, but criteria for selecting patients for this treatment have not been established. In the PROACT-II trial, patients in the treatment group were given 9 mg of recombinant pro-urokinase intra-arterially (Furlan *et al.* 1999). Patients in both groups received intravenous heparin (see below).

Concomitant antithrombotic treatment

There is no randomized evidence to support the suggestion (Trouillas *et al.* 1998) that patients should receive heparin after intravenous thrombolysis to maintain the patency of the opened artery (Gubitz *et al.* 2000b). If anything, antithrombotic therapy with aspirin or heparin should probably be avoided for at least 24 h (Wardlaw *et al.* 2000). The need for anticoagulants *may* be different when intra-arterial thrombolysis is used. In the PROACT-II study, intravenous heparin was given with intra-arterial thrombolysis (Furlan *et al.* 1999); at the time of angiography, all patients received an intravenous bolus of 2000 IU followed by an intravenous infusion of 500 IU/h of unfractionated heparin. Heparin flush solutions for angiography contained 1 IU/mL of heparin in 0.9% sodium chloride and were infused at 60 mL/h. Otherwise, antithrombotic agents were prohibited for the first 24 h.

Adverse effects

Intracranial haemorrhage is the most feared adverse effect of thrombolytic treatment, and it has been discussed extensively above. Streptokinase infusions can cause hypotension and this was a problem in the Australian Streptokinase (ASK) study (Donnan *et al.* 1995). Tissue plasminogen activator can cause life-threatening upper airway obstruction due to angioneurotic oedema (Pancioli *et al.* 1997).

There is little doubt that successful thrombolytic treatment of carefully selected patients with acute ischaemic stroke can result in much reduced disability in survivors. There is, equally, little doubt that thrombolytic treatment of even carefully selected patients carries a significant early risk of fatal intracranial haemorrhage. The urgent priorities are to establish, by means of appropriate large-scale trials: whether the balance between early hazard and long-term benefit is still favourable when thrombolysis is used in a wider variety of patients and hospital settings; which categories of patient are most likely to benefit; and whether the benefit really persists for more than just a few months.

11.6 Unproven value: neuroprotective agents

Rationale

There are many points in the pathophysiological cascade

between vessel occlusion and irreversible cell death where pharmacological intervention might be beneficial (sections 11.1.3 and 11.1.4), and the pharmaceutical industry has been able to identify a very large number of compounds for clinical development and testing (Muir & Lees 1995; Dorman *et al.* 1996). A list of some of the major agents which are considered to have promising neuroprotective effects in man is given in Table 11.11. There is no generally agreed definition of a neuroprotective drug, but in the context of acute ischaemic stroke, the aim of this class of agents is to limit the volume of brain damaged by ischaemia. There is no doubt that for a number of agents, in a variety of animal models, animals given the agent have smaller volumes of infarcted brain than controls. In animal models, the effect of treatment is generally assessed by pathological examination of the brain, to measure the boundary of the infarcted area and so calculate the infarct volume. Assessed this way, the effects of these agents seem large (Touzani *et al.* 1994). However, the problem comes in assessing neuroprotective drugs in humans where the measure of outcome is clinical, there are many factors which could cloud the assessment of the effect of the drug, and sample sizes must be large (Dorman & Sandercock 1996). Some agents may prove to be effective in patients with primary intracerebral haemorrhage as well as in cerebral infarction (in which case, treatment could be started immediately, whilst brain CT is awaited, or even started before admission to hospital). Some agents are relatively simple to administer, with a short intravenous infusion lasting only a few hours, whereas others may require infusions to be maintained for several days or require careful electrocardiographic monitoring to detect prolongation of the QT interval, which may herald serious cardiac dysrhythmias.

Table 11.11 Neuroprotective agents.

Calcium channel blockers
Nimodipine
Flunarizine

Free radical scavengers—antioxidants
Ebselen
Tirilazad

GABA agonists
Clomethiazole

Glutamate antagonists
AMPA antagonists
  GYKI 52466
  NBQX
    YM90K
    YM872
    ZK-200775 (MPQX)
Kainate antagonist
  SYM 2081
NMDA antagonists
  Competitive NMDA antagonists
    CGS 19755 (Selfotel)
  NMDA channel blockers
    Aptiganel (Cerestat)
    Dextrorphan
    Dextromethorphan
    Magnesium
    Memantine
    MK-801
    NPS 1506
    Remacemide
  Glycine site antagonists
    ACEA 1021
    GV150526
  Polyamine site antagonists
    Eliprodil
    NMDA channel blockers
    Ifenprodil
    Growth factors
    Fibroblast Growth Factor (bFGF)
    Leukocyte adhesion inhibitor
    Anti-ICAM antibody (Enlimomab)
    Hu23F2G
    Nitric oxide inhibitor
    Lubeluzole
    Opioid antagonists
    Naloxone
    Nalmefene
    Phosphatidylcholine precursor
    Citicoline (CDP-choline)
    Serotonin agonists
    Bay x 3072
    Sodium channel blockers
    Fosphenytoin
    619C89
    Potassium channel opener
    BMS-204352

Mechanism unknown, uncertain or multiple actions
  Piracetam
  Lubeluzole

Notes:

Table modified from Stroke Center at Washington University website pages on treatment of acute stroke.

For the most up-to-date information, please see http://www.neuro.wustl.edu/stroke.

This is a list of investigational treatments which have been tested in animals or humans for treatment of stroke.

Methodological considerations

Really reliable evidence about the balance of risk and benefit from these agents in humans will only emerge if some appropriately large simple clinical randomized trials are undertaken (Dorman & Sandercock 1996). The methodological considerations which have been mentioned in relation to other interventions apply equally to neuroprotective agents, but three specific points are worth making. Firstly, there are a number of steps to be taken between first identifying a promising agent during preclinical testing in animals and man before any large-scale clinical trials are mounted; greater attention to achieving these milestones might increase the chances of a successful clinical development and licensing of a neuroprotective drug (Stroke Therapy Academic Industry Round Table (STAIR) 1999). Secondly, these agents should be tested in both ischaemic and haemorrhagic stroke (Dorman & Sandercock 1996). And thirdly, the trials should have sufficient power to detect moderate treatment effects because the effects of these drugs will surely be less striking in humans than they are in experimental animals.

Evidence

Many trials have been completed, but no neuroprotective drug has been licensed for clinical use. Cochrane systematic reviews of two quite widely tested agents, lubeluzole (Gandolfo *et al.* 2000) and tirilazad (Bath 2000) are underway; however, both agents have been withdrawn from further clinical development. The ever increasing number of compounds withdrawn from clinical development in recent years has been a disappointment. These 'failures' of neuroprotective drugs have certainly tempered the opinions of even the diehard optimists who said, just a few years back, that the neuroprotective drugs would make stroke rehabilitation units redundant. However, the situation may change, and it is conceivable that one of the neuroprotective compounds currently undergoing trials may gain a licence for use in acute ischaemic stroke in the next few years.

It is probable that the extremely large reductions in cerebral infarct volumes achieved with neuroprotective agents in experimental animal models will translate into only moderate reductions in disability when used in human acute stroke; neuroprotective therapy is unlikely to prove a panacea for acute stroke.

Adverse effects

Neuroprotective drugs have a wide variety of adverse effects ranging from the minor (e.g. small changes in blood pressure or thrombophlebitis) to major (e.g. severe hallucinations, psychosis, major cardiac problems or severe hypotension) (European Ad Hoc Consensus Group 1998).

Conclusion

In early 2000, none of the agents in Table 11.11 had a product licence for use in acute stroke, and there is no indication to use any of them routinely in clinical practice. The current trials are small and therefore unlikely to define the 'time window' for effective intervention very clearly, and a few 'megatrials' with several tens of thousands of patients may be required to determine, in humans, whether the 'window' is just a few hours or perhaps as long as 24 h or even 48 h. Such megatrials will also help to define which categories of patient are most likely to gain from treatment and which are the most likely to suffer adverse effects (confusion, hallucinations and agitation have been common in the early trials). Even if neuroprotective drugs do become licensed, they are unlikely to be a panacea, and will need to be given in the context of a well-organized acute stroke service (European Ad Hoc Consensus Group 1998).

11.7 Unproven value: other specific agents

11.7.1 Defibrinogenation

Methods used and rationale

There are several defibrinogenating agents. Ancrod is a 234 amino acid glycosylated serine protease derived from the venom of the Malayan pit viper. During Ancrod therapy there is a fall in plasma fibrinogen, plasminogen, plasminogen-activator inhibitor and antiplasmin levels (Lowe 1998). Large quantities of circulating fibrinogen and fibrin degradation products are generated and tissue plasminogen activator is released from the vascular endothelium. In addition to the rapid defibrinogenation, Ancrod reduces plasma and whole-blood viscosity (Lowe 1998). Other defibrinogenating agents are less well characterized (Cerebrovascular Research Group 1982; Hao 1984). Defibrinogenation might improve perfusion in the ischaemic brain and so have a net beneficial effect, provided its use is not associated with a substantial excess of major bleeding.

Evidence

There have been 10 small studies of Ancrod. A systematic review of the three small completed trials of Ancrod which met the inclusion criteria for the review included a total of only 182 patients, showed promising effects, but the number of outcome events was far too small for reliable conclusions (Liu *et al.* 2000). The frequency of intracranial haemorrhage was similar in treated patients and controls, but the included trials had inadequate power to exclude a moderate to substantial hazard of treatment. Since the review was published, the Stroke Treatment with Ancrod Trial (STAT) including 500 patients, has reported promising results (Sherman *et al.* 2000). A further trial is under way in Europe (ESTAT), which aims to recruit over 600 patients.

Conclusion

At present, though the data are promising, there is not enough evidence to justify the use of defibrinogenating agents in routine clinical practice.

11.7.2 Haemodilution

Methods used and rationale

Haemodilution is generally achieved by giving an infusion of dextran, hydroxyethyl starch or albumin (Asplund *et al.* 2000). Such infusions increase blood volume (hypervolaemic haemodilution). In patients with acute stroke in whom an increase in total blood volume may be undesirable, haemodilution can be achieved isovolaemically by simultaneously removing several hundred millilitres of blood. This treatment leads to reduced whole-blood viscosity. If the optimum haematocrit is achieved, any increase in cerebral oxygen delivery achieved in practice might be neuroprotective and so lessen infarct volume.

Evidence

Sixteen trials including 2956 patients have been included in the Cochrane systematic review (Asplund *et al.* 2000). No overall effect on survival was seen (95% CI, 15% reduction in odds to 23% increase in odds of death within 3–6 months). In survivors, neurological outcome was similar in the haemodilution and control groups. The proportion of patients independent in activities of daily living on final follow-up did not differ between the groups. No subgroup could be identified in which treatment was clearly beneficial. Deep venous thrombosis and pulmonary embolism were possibly reduced in the treatment group, but this benefit was partly offset by a trend towards an increase in 'other circulatory events' in the treated group.

Conclusion

Given this information, we can see no reason to use this treatment in routine clinical practice, although it is used quite widely in Austria and in some parts of Eastern Europe.

11.7.3 Calcium antagonists

Rationale

The influx of calcium through voltage-sensitive channels has a role in neuronal death from ischaemia; this influx can be inhibited by a number of agents, so-called calcium channel blockers or antagonists (section 11.1.4).

Evidence

A recent systematic review of 27 randomized trials of different classes of calcium antagonists given as immediate treatment for acute ischaemic stroke included data on 7067 patients (Horn *et al.* 1999, 2000). There was no clear evidence of any effect on death (95% CI, 2% reduction to a 24% increase) or on death or dependency (95% CI, 3% reduction to a 19% increase) (Horn *et al.* 1999, 2000) (Fig. 11.26).

Subgroup analyses: publication bias, the 'time window' and effects of intravenous administration

Regrettably, four of the completed trials remain unpublished. It is interesting to note that their results are almost statistically significantly worse than the estimate of treatment effect derived from the published trials (Fig. 11.27). This is a good example of publication bias (negative or unpromising trials remain unpublished) and emphasizes the importance of including all randomized trials, whether or not they are published. A meta-analysis of nine trials of 120 mg oral nimodipine (trials testing a higher dose were excluded because of adverse effects) suggested, in a subgroup analysis, that patients treated within 12 h of onset had a favourable outcome (Mohr *et al.* 1994). This subgroup finding was not confirmed by the more recent and more comprehensive analyses by Horn *et al.* (Horn *et al.* 1999, 2000). In addition, a trial designed to evalute very early oral nimodipine treatment in acute stroke (the Very Early Nimodipine Use in Stroke—VENUS—study) based in primary care, in which patients were randomized before transfer to hospital to maximize the opportunity for early therapy, again did not provide any evidence of benefit (Horn *et al.* 1999). These data illustrate the hazards of undue emphasis on selective *post hoc* subgroup analyses in trials and meta-analyses which do not show any overall evidence of benefit (Counsell *et al.* 1994).

Again, making due allowance for the exploratory nature of the analysis, the review also suggested that intravenous treatment was associated with a worse outcome than oral treatment (Horn *et al.* 2000). *Post hoc* subgroup analysis of the Intravenous Nimodipine West European Stroke Trial (INWEST) found that high-dose intravenous nimodipine reduced mean systolic blood pressure by 11.4% from its baseline value, and the fall in blood pressure was the most probable explanation for the adverse effects of nimodipine on outcome (Ahmed *et al.* 2000) (section 11.9).

Conclusion

The trials do not provide any evidence to support the routine

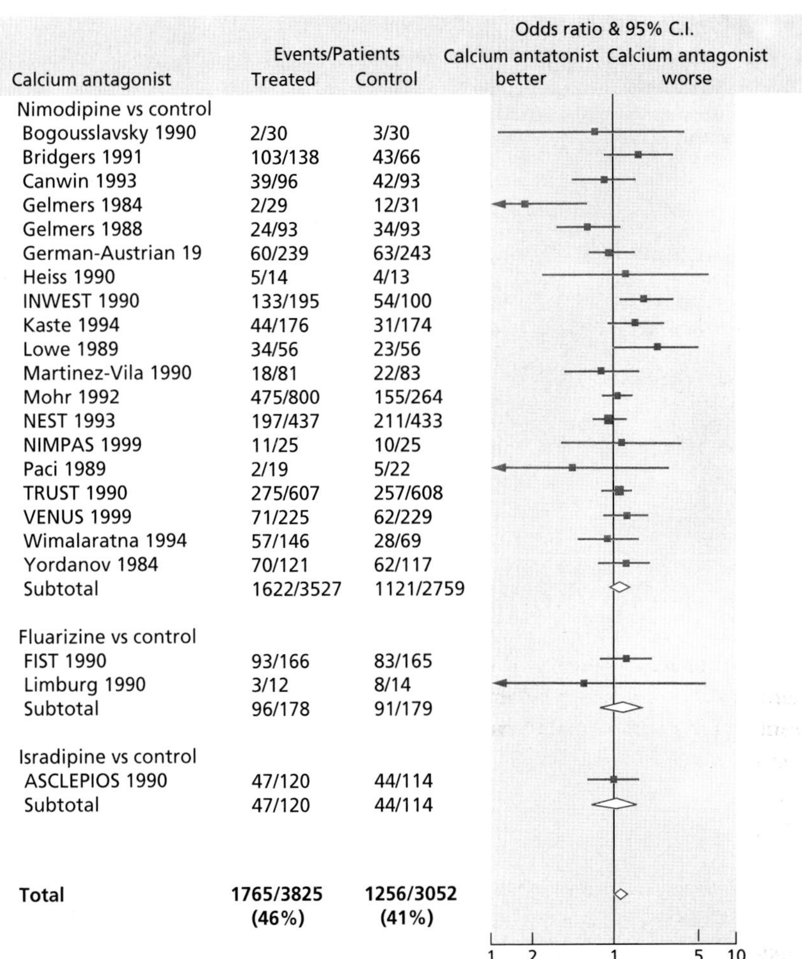

Odds ratio & 95% C.I.
Events/Patients
Calcium antatonist better
Calcium antagonist worse
Calcium antagonist
Treated
Control
Nimodipine vs control
Bogousslavsky 1990 2/30 3/30
Bridgers 1991 103/138 43/66
Canwin 1993 39/96 42/93
Gelmers 1984 2/29 12/31
Gelmers 1988 24/93 34/93
German-Austrian 19 60/239 63/243
Heiss 1990 5/14 4/13
INWEST 1990 133/195 54/100
Kaste 1994 44/176 31/174
Lowe 1989 34/56 23/56
Martinez-Vila 1990 18/81 22/83
Mohr 1992 475/800 155/264
NEST 1993 197/437 211/433
NIMPAS 1999 11/25 10/25
Paci 1989 2/19 5/22
TRUST 1990 275/607 257/608
VENUS 1999 71/225 62/229
Wimalaratna 1994 57/146 28/69
Yordanov 1984 70/121 62/117
Subtotal 1622/3527 1121/2759
Fluarizine vs control
FIST 1990 93/166 83/165
Limburg 1990 3/12 8/14
Subtotal 96/178 91/179
Isradipine vs control
ASCLEPIOS 1990 47/120 44/114
Subtotal 47/120 44/114
Total 1765/3825 (46%) 1256/3052 (41%)
1
2
1
5
10

Fig. 11.26 Calcium antagonists in acute ischaemic stroke: effects on death or dependency at the end of follow-up. Results of a systematic review of 22 trials. Same conventions as Fig. 11.18 except all the confidence intervals are 95% (with permission from Horn & Limburg 2000).

use of oral calcium antagonists in patients presenting within 12 h, or intravenous administration. We do not use calcium antagonists in acute ischaemic stroke patients.

There is no evidence to support the routine use of calcium antagonists in acute ischaemic stroke.

11.7.4 Naftidrofuryl

The mechanism of action of this agent is not entirely clear but it is said to be, broadly speaking, protective to ischaemic neurones (Steiner & Clifford Rose 1986). There have been at least four small trials, none of which provided convincing evidence of benefit (Admani 1978; Steiner & Clifford Rose 1986; Gray *et al.* 1990; Steiner 1996). This treatment cannot be recommended for routine use in patients with acute ischaemic stroke.

11.7.5 Other interventions

A bewildering variety of interventions have been suggested as effective in acute stroke. A reasonably comprehensive list of those which have been tested in randomized controlled trials is given in Table 11.12. None is clearly beneficial. A comprehensive electronic bibliography of controlled trials, the Cochrane Controlled Trials Register (CCTR), is available on CD-ROM and via the internet in the Cochrane Library (which also includes the Cochrane Database of Systematic Reviews). In issue 3, 2000 of *Cochrane Library* the CCTR included 272 130 entries, of which 8248 were indexed as relating to the MESH term 'cerebrovascular-disorders' or the text word 'stroke'. The register also includes the specialized register of trials compiled by the Cochrane Stroke Group (2753 entries from the register were found in issue 3, 2000 with the searchable keyword SR-STROKE).

The Cochrane Controlled Trials Register (CCTR) includes references to reports of trials published in many different places, many of which are not indexed in MEDLINE. A search of CCTR is therefore likely to identify more trials relevant to your therapeutic question than a search of just MEDLINE or EMBASE.

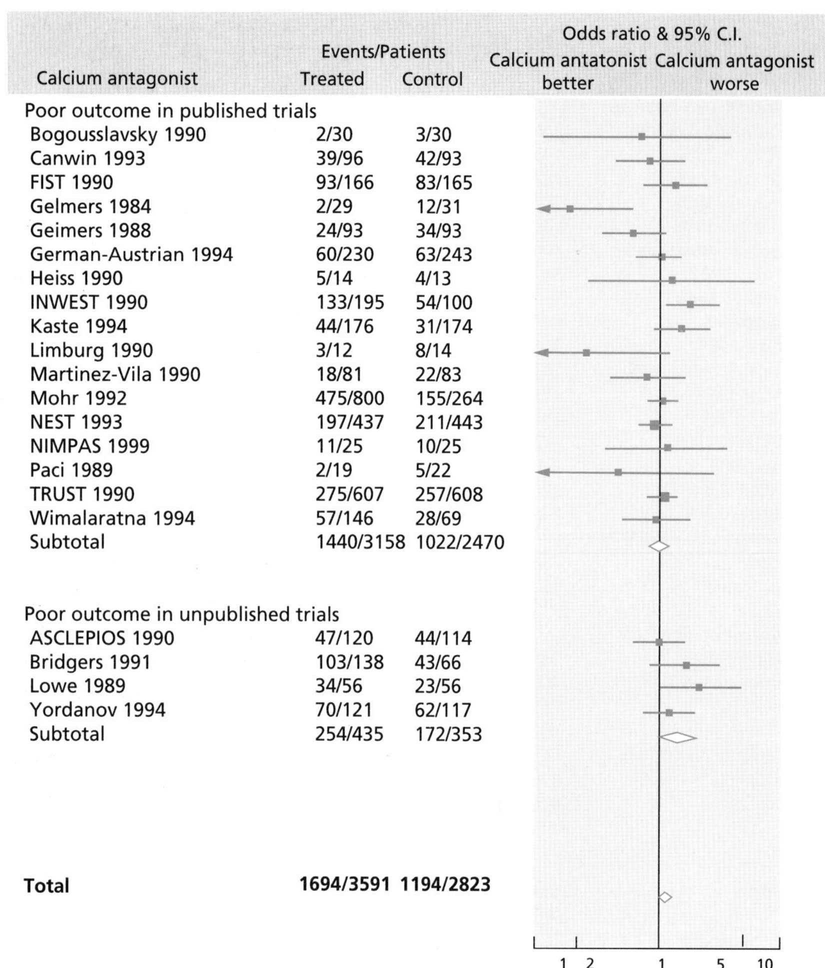

Fig. 11.27 Calcium antagonists in acute ischaemic stroke: effect on death or dependency, subdivided by whether the trial was published or not. Same conventions as in Fig. 11.18 except all the confidence intervals are 95% (Horn & Limburg 2000).

11.8 Unproven value: treatment of cerebral oedema and raised intracranial pressure

11.8.1 Corticosteroids

Rationale

Corticosteroids (such as dexamethasone) reduce *vasogenic* cerebral oedema, which tends to develop about 24–48 h or more after stroke onset, particularly in and around large infarcts (section 11.1.5). Neuroprotective agents which can prevent influx of sodium ions and water into cells should help reduce the *cytotoxic oedema* that develops very early after the onset of ischaemia (section 11.1.5).

Evidence

There have been at least 17 apparently randomized trials in acute stroke. A systematic review of the seven methodologically sound studies (including only 453 patients) showed that treatment was associated with a non-significant 8% increase in the odds of death (95% CI, 32% reduction to 72% increase) (Qizilbash *et al.* 2000). Treatment did not appear to improve outcome in survivors. These data are inadequate to confirm or refute moderate benefit (or moderate hazard). The systematic review was unable to extract data on adverse effects in patients with ischaemic stroke, but the evidence from studies of corticosteroids in patients with primary intracerebral haemorrhage showed a significant excess of adverse effects, such as infections, amongst corticosteroid-treated patients (Poungvarin *et al.* 1987).

Conclusion

We do not use corticosteroids as a routine treatment for unselected patients with ischaemic stroke, nor do we use them in patients who have massive cerebral oedema complicated by transtentorial herniation. Our only indication is in patients with inflammatory vascular disorders (e.g. giant cell arteritis, polyarteritis nodosa, systemic lupus erythematosus; section 7.3). If we suspect the diagnosis of vasculitis, and if the patient is acutely ill or is at high risk of complications

Table 11.12 List of some of the miscellaneous treatments for acute ischaemic stroke, not mentioned in Table 11.11, which have been tested in randomized trials, but no clear evidence of benefit yet demonstrated.

Evaluated in a published Cochrane Systematic Review
Gangliosides
L-Arginine
Nitric oxide donors (nitrates)
Nitric oxide synthase inhibitors
Pentoxifylline, propentofylline and pentifylline
Piracetam
Prostacyclin and analogues
Theophylline, aminophylline, caffeine and analogues
Vinpocetine

Published protocols of ongoing Cochrane Systematic Reviews
Antioxidants
Calcium antagonists
Choline precursors
Cooling therapy

Randomized trials available, but results inconclusive
Acupuncture
Arnica (homeopathic)
Betablocker
Cerebral transplantation of Layton Bioscience (LBS)-neurones
Diaspirin cross-linked haemoglobin
Extracorporeal rheopheresis
Glucose-insulin infusions
Heparin-induced extracorporeal low-density lipoprotein precipitation
Hydergine
Hyperbaric oxygen
Intravenous magnesium
Ornithine alpha-ketoglutarate
Phosphocreatine
Thromboxane A_2 antagonists
Spironolactone
Veinoglobulin
Ventilation therapy

See http://www.dcn.ed.ac.uk/csrg/ to obtain an up-to-date list of Cochrane Stroke Group reviews and protocols.

See http://www.neuro.wustl.edu/stroke/therapy/TherapyIndex_1.html for an up-to-date and more comprehensive list.

without corticosteroids (such as a high risk of blindness in patients with untreated giant cell arteritis), then we start with 60–80 mg oral prednisolone daily. We would arrange a biopsy of the relevant artery (temporal artery for giant cell arteritis or meningeal and brain biopsy for primary angiitis of the central nervous system) to be done as soon as possible after steroids had started; if there is undue delay the biopsy may become non-diagnostic. If primary angiitis is confirmed histologically, cyclophosphamide should probably be added to the corticosteroids (Hankey 1991).

11.8.2 Glycerol and mannitol

Rationale

Glycerol is a hyperosmolar agent which is said to reduce cerebral oedema and possibly increase cerebral blood flow (Righetti *et al.* 2000), and mannitol is an osmotically active agent. These treatments aim to reduce intracranial pressure and thereby improve perfusion in and around infarcts.

Evidence

A systematic review of 11 trials of glycerol in acute stroke, involving 945 patients, showed glycerol was associated with a non-significant 22% relative reduction in the odds of early death (95% CI, 42% reduction to 6% increase) (Righetti *et al.* 2000). At final follow-up, early glycerol treatment was associated with only a non-significant effect on death (95% CI, 27% reduction to 31% increase). The effects of treatment on functional outcome were unclear. There are no large-scale trials of mannitol in acute stroke, but the existing small inconclusive trials are the subject of a current Cochrane review (Bereczki *et al.* 2000).

Conclusion

We do not use glycerol at all in our own clinical practice, although it is often used in Italy; about 50% of patients entered by the 60 Italian centres participating in the International Stroke Trial received glycerol (Ricci 1995). There is no evidence to support either the routine or the selective use of glycerol or mannitol in acute ischaemic stroke.

11.8.3 Surgical decompression

Posterior fossa decompression or shunting for massive cerebellar infarcts

Surgical decompression (or ventricular shunting) of massive cerebellar infarcts may improve cerebral perfusion and also relieve obstructive hydrocephalus. Decompressive surgery has not been evaluated by adequately designed trials, so the selection of patients with cerebellar infarction for decompressive surgery, shunting or medical therapy remains controversial (MacDonell *et al.* 1987; Mathew *et al.* 1995; Jauss *et al.* 1999).

Hemicraniotomy for massive supratentorial infarcts

Some clinicians recommend an aggressive approach to this problem (Kalia & Yonas 1993). A radical procedure removes the cranial bone overlying a massive supratentorial infarct to reduce intracranial pressure. In a non-randomized study 15 (47%) of 32 surgically treated patients were moderately to severely disabled compared with five (24%) of 21 conservatively treated patients, and 11 (34%) of the surgically treated patients died compared with 16 (76%) of the conservatively treated patients. The authors concluded that hemicraniotomy may improve survival in massive hemispheric stroke but the proportion of survivors who remained disabled was still high (Rieke *et al.* 1995; Schwab *et al.* 1998). We do not refer patients for this procedure as part of routine practice, but we would support its use within the context of a randomized trial; such a study is now underway in North America (Frank *et al.* 1999).

11.8.4 Hyperventilation

Hyperventilation is used to lower intracranial pressure (sections 12.2.2 and 15.2.2), but there is no randomized evidence on its effects in patients with stroke available on the Cochrane Controlled Trials Register. Geraci and Geraci (1996) undertook a review of the rather poor data available on the effects of hyperventilation in patients with head injury: one randomized trial (113 patients), six quasi-experimental studies (245 patients) and five descriptive case studies (235 patients). The reviewers concluded that head-injured patients in the prehospital and early phases of care are at *increased* risk of suffering hyperventilation-induced secondary brain injury and that a cautious, highly monitored and selective approach to hyperventilation be adopted.

11.9 Unproven value: blood pressure interventions

Rationale

The observational data relating blood pressure soon after stroke onset with subsequent outcome do not give a clear picture and a systematic review of all the available studies is required (section 15.7). At least one observational study has suggested that higher initial blood pressure is associated with a favourable outcome (Allen 1984), whereas others have suggested that an increasing level of baseline blood pressure in patients with impaired consciousness is associated with a progressively higher probability of a poor outcome (Phillips 1994). However, the data from the IST suggested a U-shaped relationship with early death and poor long-term outcome being more frequent in patients with blood pressures in the highest and lowest quartiles of systolic blood pressure (Signorini *et al.* 1999) (Fig. 11.28). Of course, any relationship between blood pressure and outcome is likely to be confounded by stroke severity and by co-morbid conditions (which may raise or lower blood pressure). These data are all compatible with the hypothesis that adjusting the level of blood pressure to a notional 'optimum' may lead to a better outcome, but do not give a clear rationale to underpin a trial evaluating interventions to alter blood pressure in acute stroke (i.e. is it better to have blood pressure high, and risk breaking through the upper limit of autoregulation if this has not already been impaired by the stroke and so cause cerebral oedema, or better to have it low and risk worsening cerebral ischaemia?) (Bath & Bath 1997; Blood Pressure in Acute Stroke Collaboration (BASC) 2000).

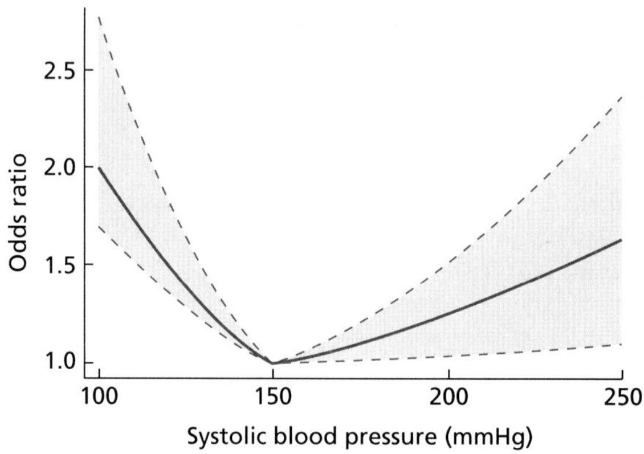

Fig. 11.28 Relationship between baseline systolic blood pressure and death within 14 days among 19 435 patients randomized in the International Stroke Trial (IST). Odds ratio for early death on the *y*-axis for each level of blood pressure compared with 150 mmHg, after adjustment for baseline stroke severity (Signorini *et al.* 1999). The dotted lines and shaded area is the 95% confidence interval for the odds ratio.

Evidence

The blood pressure management algorithms that were used in the NINDS thrombolysis trial have been promoted as the appropriate management strategy for patients with acute ischaemic stroke (particularly those receiving thrombolytic therapy) (Adams *et al.* 1996; Norris *et al.* 1998). However, there is no randomized evidence to support the contention that the recommended manipulations of blood pressure improve outcome. A recent systematic review identified only three small trials of lowering blood pressure in patients with acute stroke, involving just 133 people (Blood Pressure in Acute Stroke Collaboration (BASC) 2000). The trials tested nimodipine (66 patients), nicardipine (five patients), captopril (three patients) and clonidine (two patients). Oral calcium channel blockers reduced systolic blood pressure (weighted mean difference 10.9 mmHg, 95% CI, 2.0–19.7). The greatest fall in blood pressure over the first 24 h was shown in patients given the highest dose of nimodipine. The relationship between change in blood pressure and clinical outcome was not clear in these trials. However, data from the trials of calcium antagonists in acute ischaemic stroke when given as treatment for the stroke (rather than to lower blood pressure) suggest that the larger the fall in blood pressure induced by treatment, the worse the clinical outcome. This is probably because the precipitate fall in blood pressure associated with intravenous nimodipine *increased* the risk of early death and of poor long-term outcome, perhaps by increasing cerebral infarct volume (Wahlgren *et al.* 1994; Ahmed *et al.* 2000; Horn *et al.* 2000). A small trial of betablockers in acute stroke was inconclusive (Barer *et al.* 1988).

Angiotensin-converting enzyme inhibitors maintain cerebral blood flow despite lowering blood pressure in patients with heart failure and otherwise uncomplicated hypertension. In a small phase II study, 24 patients with recent acute ischaemic stroke were randomized to receive 15 days of oral perindopril (4 mg) or placebo. Patients on perindopril had a placebo-corrected reduction in blood pressure of 19/11 mmHg (systolic and diastolic, respectively), but total cerebral blood flow was unaffected (Dyker *et al.* 1997). A further trial is under way of the angiotensin antagonist candesartan cilexetil, in patients with acute ischaemic stroke and an initial blood pressure > 200/100 mmHg or a casual blood pressure > 180/105 mmHg (Schrader & Dominiak 1999).

No studies of interventions to raise blood pressure were found at the time the Cochrane review was last updated, although a small phase II study has since been published which tested the effects of raising blood pressure with diaspirin cross-linked haemoglobin (DCHLb) in 85 patients with acute ischaemic stroke. The treatment caused a significant rise in mean arterial blood pressure. Outcome scores were worse, and there were more deaths and serious adverse events in DCHLb-treated patients compared with controls (Saxena *et al.* 1999).

Conclusion

There is no clear indication to reduce blood pressure routinely in patients with acute ischaemic stroke, so any guidelines are based on observational data and are therefore likely to be unreliable. In our own practice, we do not routinely reduce blood pressure within the first few days, unless there is clear evidence from fundoscopy (or other clinical evidence) of organ damage by accelerated hypertension. Patients who have persistently high blood pressures at 7–14 days after stroke are likely to benefit from long-term antihypertensive drug therapy for secondary prevention (section 16.3.1). There is no reliable evidence on the optimal timing of the start of treatment, but it is convenient to start treatment for patients with sustained hypertension, not previously detected, in long-term secondary prevention about 1 or 2 weeks after stroke onset, before the patient is discharged from hospital (sections 15.7 and 16.3.1).

What to do about the blood pressure in acute ischaemic stroke is unclear: raise it, lower it or leave it alone? We tend to leave it alone unless there is evidence of end-organ damage. We normally start treatment for persisting hypertension about 1 or 2 weeks after stroke onset.

11.10 Unproven value: immediate carotid endarterectomy or interventional radiology

Rationale

For patients with severe carotid stenosis, or occlusion, and an ischaemic stroke in the ipsilateral hemisphere, early restoration of normal vascular anatomy and so flow in the internal carotid artery might improve outcome (Mead & O'Neill 1999). There are undoubtedly a few patients in whom the predominant cerebral problem is low flow in the ipsilateral hemisphere and it is this group that is theoretically most likely to benefit from urgent surgical restoration of flow. For others, the problem is artery-to-artery embolization and, in them, the rationale is removal of the embolic source before a recurrent disabling ischaemic stroke occurs. Some surgeons are prepared to consider surgical removal of an occluding thrombus, but this is likely to be incomplete since a thrombus which has propagated distally into the carotid syphon cannot be extracted.

Evidence

There have been no large-scale randomized controlled trials comparing immediate with deferred carotid surgery (or immediate vs. deferred angioplasty) in patients with acute ischaemic stroke (Pritz 1997; Mead & O'Neill 1999). A randomized pilot study including 25 patients suggested better functional outcome among patients randomized to urgent carotid endarterectomy (i.e. within 1 week), but was too small to be reliable (Welsh *et al.* 1999). The retrospective non-randomized studies suggest that some patients with an acute stroke probably can safely undergo surgery shortly after the diagnosis is made, but do not give reliable evidence on how such patients can be selected, or what the optimum timing of surgery really is (Pritz 1997). Arguments based on non-randomized clinical series of patients do nothing but confuse the issue. Those in favour of surgery (mostly surgeons) cite series showing an apparently low surgical morbidity from operations performed within the first day or two of the onset of stroke, whereas other more conservative people (generally physicians) cite surgical series with prohibitively high morbidity and case fatality. Similarly, enthusiastic proponents of interventional radiology claim that it can be used safely in acute stroke to deal with severe carotid stenosis (Higashida *et al.* 1995).

Conclusion

In theory, it should be straightforward to identify patients with a mild neurological deficit that is either fluctuating or worsening in association with a very severe stenosis of the relevant carotid artery. In practice, such patients are only rarely encountered. We would only advocate the use of any surgical or interventional radiological procedure during the acute phase of ischaemic stroke within the context of a well-organized randomized controlled trial.

11.11 Unproven value: specific treatments for miscellaneous rare causes of acute ischaemic stroke

Congenital arterial anomalies and unruptured aneurysms

Kinks, loop and coils of the carotid or vertebral arteries, suspected as the cause of an ischaemic stroke, should be managed conservatively (section 7.4). If one suspects embolization from an unruptured intracranial aneurysm (section 7.6) the options are to clip the aneurysm surgically, to treat it by endovascular coiling, to give antiplatelet drugs or to do nothing. The balance of risks and benefits for each of these approaches is completely unknown.

Migraine

The pathophysiological relationship between migraine and acute ischaemic stroke is not clear (section 7.8) and there is no sensible clear rationale to use any particular treatment for 'migrainous stroke'. Treatment should follow the same principles as for non-migrainous stroke.

Infections

Infective endocarditis (section 6.5) requires standard treatment with intravenous antibiotics. The choice of antibiotic and duration of treatment should be made in conjunction with microbiologists, and the management of any cardiac complications will require cardiological advice. Other specific infections causing stroke (e.g. syphilis, borrelia and human immunodeficiency virus) should be treated according to the usual protocols.

Cancer

If the malignant lesion happens to be an atrial myxoma, then surgical excision is required (section 6.5). Non-bacterial thrombotic endocarditis (section 6.5) complicating malignancy, even if it can be diagnosed reliably, is not treatable. There is little reliable evidence on the effects of anticoagulants in patients with recurrent arterial thromboembolism associated with cancer, but some guidelines recommend warfarin if events continue despite aspirin (Scottish Intercollegiate Guidelines Network 1999).

Sex hormones

Young women who have an ischaemic stroke whilst taking oral contraceptives should stop them and use an alternative form of contraception (section 7.13). Elderly women on hormone replacement therapy who have a stroke can probably continue safely but many may choose to stop after the stroke (section 7.13).

Pregnancy

If there is a need for anticoagulation during pregnancy, heparin and not warfarin should be used during the first trimester since warfarin may cause fetal abnormalities (Scottish Intercollegiate Guidelines Network 1999). Prolonged heparin therapy can cause osteoporosis in the mother (section 16.5.4).

Mitochondrial cytopathy

No specific treatments are available, although corticosteroids and cofactor therapy may be helpful sometimes (Di Mauro & Moraes 1993; Fox & Dunne 1993; Hammans & Morgan-Hughes 1994) (section 7.19).

Cholesterol embolization syndrome

This condition may be exacerbated by thrombolytic or anticoagulant therapy. If severe, renal failure may develop, requiring haemodialysis (Fine *et al.* 1987; Hyman *et al.* 1987; Anon. 1991) (section 7.7).

References

Please note that all references taken from *The Cochrane Library* are given a current date as this database is updated on a quarterly basis. Please refer to the current *Cochrane Library* article for the latest review. The same applies to the *British Medical Journal* 'Clinical Evidence' series which is updated every six months.

Aaslid, R., Lindegaard, K.F., Sorteberg, W. & Nornes, H. (1989) Cerebral autoregulation dynamics in humans. *Stroke* **20**, 45–52.

Aaslid, R., Newell, D.W., Stooss, R., Sorteberg, W. & Lindegaard, K.F. (1991) Assessment of cerebral autoregulation from simultaneous arterial and venous transcranial doppler recordings in humans. *Stroke* **22**, 1148–1154.

Abe, K., Aoki, M. & Kawagoe, J. (1995) Ischaemic delayed neuronal death. A mitochondrial hypothesis. *Stroke* **26**, 1478–1489.

Acheson, J., Danta, G. & Hutchinson, E.C. (1969) Controlled trial of dipyridamole in cerebral vascular disease. *British Medical Journal* **1**, 614–615.

Adams, H.P., Brott, T.G., Crowell, R.M. *et al.* (1994) Guidelines for the management of patients with acute ischaemic stroke. A Statement for Healthcare Professionals from a Special Writing Group of the Stroke Council, American Heart Association. *Circulation* **90** (3), 1588–1601.

Adams, H.P., Brott, T.G., Furlan, A.J. *et al.* (1996) Guidelines for thrombolytic therapy in stroke: a supplement to the guidelines for the management of patients with acute ischaemic stroke. A Statement for Healthcare Professionals from a Special Writing Group of the Stroke Council, American Heart Association. *Stroke* **27**, 1711–1718.

Admani, A.K. (1978) New approach to treatment of recent stroke. *British*

Medical Journal 2, 1678–1679.

Ahmed, N., Nasman, P. & Wahlgren, N.G. (2000) Effect of intravenous nimodipine on blood pressure and outcome after stroke. *Stroke* **31**, 1250–1255.

Akopov, S.E., Sercombe, R. & Seylaz, J. (1994) Leucocyte-induced acute endothelial dysfunction in middle cerebral artery in rabbits. *Stroke* **25**, 2246–2252.

Albers, G., Easton, J.D., Sacco, R. & Teal, P. (1998) Antithrombotic and thrombolytic therapy for ischemic stroke. *Chest* **114**, 683S–698S.

Alexandrov, A., Black, S., Ehrlich, L., Caldwell, C. & Norris, J. (1997) Predictors of haemorrhagic transformation occurring spontaneously and on anticoagulants in patients with acute ischemic stroke. *Stroke* **28**, 1198–1202.

Allen, C.M. (1984) Predicting the outcome of acute stroke: a prognostic score. *Journal of Neurology, Neurosurgery and Psychiatry* **47**, 475–480.

Altman, D.G., Machin, D., Bryant, T.N. & Gardner, M.J. (eds) (2000) *Statistics with Confidence*, 2nd edn. BMJ Books, London.

Anon. (1991) Cholesterol embolism. *Lancet* **338**, 1365–1366.

Antiplatelet Trialists' Collaboration (1988) Secondary prevention of vascular disease by prolonged antiplatelet treatment. *British Medical Journal* **296**, 320–331.

Antiplatelet Trialists' Collaboration (1994a) Collaborative overview of randomized trials of antiplatelet therapy. I. Prevention of death, myocardial infarction, and stroke by prolonged antiplatelet therapy in various categories of patients. *British Medical Journal* **308**, 81–106.

Antiplatelet Trialists' Collaboration (1994b) Collaborative overview of randomized trials of antiplatelet therapy. II. Maintenance of vascular graft or arterial patency by antiplatelet therapy. *British Medical Journal* **308**, 159–168.

Antiplatelet Trialists' Collaboration (1994c) Collaborative overview of randomized trials of antiplatelet therapy. III. Reduction in venous thrombosis and pulmonary embolism by antiplatelet prophylaxis among surgical and medical patients. *British Medical Journal* **308**, 235–246.

Asia Pacific Consensus Forum on Stroke Management Organising Committees (1998) Asia Pacific Consensus Forum on Stroke Management. *Stroke* **29**, 1730–1736.

Asplund, K., Iraelsson, K. & Schampi, I. (2000) Haemodilution for acute ischaemic stroke. In: *The Cochrane Library*. Oxford: Update Software.

Asplund, K., Ralakangas, A.M., Kuulasmaa, K. *et al.* (1996) Multinational comparison of diagnostic procedures and management of acute stroke: the WHO MONICA study. *Cerebrovascular Diseases* **6**, 66–74.

Aster, R.H. (1995) Heparin-induced thrombocytopenia and thrombosis. *New England Journal of Medicine* **332** (20), 1374–1376.

Astrup, J., Siesjo, B.K. & Symon, L. (1981) Thresholds in cerebral ischaemia — the ischaemic penumbra. *Stroke* **12**, 723–725.

Baird, A.E. & Warach, S. (1998) Magnetic resonance imaging of acute stroke. *Journal of Cerebral Blood Flow and Metabolism* **18**, 583–609.

Barer, D.H., Cruickshank, J.M., Ebrahim, S.B. & Mitchell, J.R. (1988) Low dose beta blockade in acute stroke ('BEST' trial): an evaluation. *British Medical Journal* **296**, 737–741.

Baron, J.C. (1991) Pathophysiology of acute cerebral ischaemia: PET studies in humans. *Cerebrovascular Diseases* **1** (Suppl. 1), 22–31.

Baron, J.C. (1999) Mapping the ischaemic penumbra with PET: implications for acute stroke treatment. *Cerebrovasular Diseases* **9**, 193–201.

Baron, J.C., Bousser, M.G., Rey, A., Guillard, A., Comar, D. & Castaigne, P. (1981) Reversal of focal 'misery–perfusion syndrome' by extra-intracranial arterial bypass in haemodynamic cerebral ischaemia: a case study with ^{15}O positron emission tomography. *Stroke* **12**, 454–459.

Baron, J.C., von Kummer, R. & del Zoppo, G. (1995) Treatment of acute ischaemic stroke: challenging the concept of a rigid time window. *Stroke* **26**, 2219–2221.

Barry, D.I., Strandgaard, S. & Graham, D.I. (1982) Cerebral blood flow in rats with renal and spontaneous hypertension: resetting of the lower limit of autoregulation. *Journal of Cerebral Blood Flow and Metabolism* **2**, 347.

Bath, F. & Bath, P. (1997) What is the correct management of blood pressure in acute stroke? Blood Pressure in Acute Stroke Collaboration. *Cerebrovascular Diseases* **7**, 205–213.

Bath, F., Owen, V. & Bath, P. (1998) Quality of full and final publications reporting acute stroke trials. A systematic review. *Stroke* **29**, 2203–2210.

Bath, P. (2000) Tirilazad for acute ischaemic stroke. In: *The Cochrane Library*. Update Software: Oxford.

Becker, K.J. (1998) Inflammation and acute stroke. *Current Opinion in Neurology* **11**, 45–49.

Bednar, M.M. & Gross, C.E. (1999) Antiplatelet therapy in acute cerebral ischemia. *Stroke* **30**, 887–893.

Begg, C., Cho, M., Eastwood, S. *et al.* (1996) Improving the quality of reporting of randomized controlled trials. The CONSORT statement. *Journal of the American Medical Association* **276**, 637–639.

Bell, B.A., Symon, L. & Branston, N.M. (1985) CBF and time thresholds for the formation of ischaemic cerebral oedema and effect of reperfusion in baboons. *Journal of Neurosurgery* **62**, 31–41.

Bereczki, D., Liu, M., do Prado, G.F. & Fekete, I. (2000) Mannitol for acute ischaemic stroke and cerebral parenchymal haemorrhage. In: *The Cochrane Library*. Oxford: Update Software.

Berenstein, A., Siller, K.A., Setton, A., Nelson, P.K., Levin, D.N. & Kupersmith, M. (1994) Intra arterial urokinase for acute ischaemic stroke during interventional neuroradiological procedures. *Neurology* **44** (Suppl. 2), A356 (Abstract).

Berge, E., Abdelnoor, M., Nakstad, P.H. & Sandset, P.M., on behalf of HAEST study group (2000) Low molecular-weight heparin versus aspirin in patients with acute ischaemic stroke and atrial fibrillation: a double-blind randomised study. *Lancet* **355**, 1205–1210.

Betz, A.L., Yang, G.Y. & Davidson, B.L. (1995) Attenuation of stroke size in rats using an adenoviral vector to induce overexpression of interleukin-1 receptor antagonist in brain. *Journal of Cerebral Blood Flow and Metabolism* **15**, 547–551.

Bishop, C.C.R., Powell, S., Rutt, D. & Browse, N.L. (1986) Transcranial Doppler measurement of middle cerebral artery blood flow velocity: a validation study. *Stroke* **17**, 913–915.

Bittner, V. (1998) Atherosclerosis and the immune system. *Archives of Internal Medicine* **158**, 1395–1396.

Blood Pressure in Acute Stroke Collaboration (BASC) (2000) Interventions for deliberately altering blood pressure in acute stroke. In. *The Cochrane Library*. Oxford: Update Software.

Bousser, M. (1999) Cerebral venous sinus thrombosis. Nothing, heparin or local thrombolysis? *Stroke* **30**, 481–483.

Bova, I.Y., Bornstein, N.M. & Korczyn, A.D. (1996) Acute infection as a risk factor for ischaemic stroke. *Stroke* **27**, 2204–2206.

Bredesen, D.E. (1995) Neural apoptosis. *Annals of Neurology* **38**, 839–851.

Brierley, J. (1976) Cerebral hypoxia. In: *Greenfield's Neuropathology* (eds W. Blackwood & J. Corsellis), pp. 43–85. Arnold, London.

Brown, M.M. & Marshall, J. (1985) Regulation of cerebral blood flow in response to changes in blood viscosity. *Lancet* **i**, 604–609.

Brown, M.M., Wade, J.P.H. & Marshall, J. (1985) Fundamental importance of arterial oxygen content in the regulation of cerebral blood flow in man. *Brain* **108**, 81–93.

Broze, G.J. Jr (1992) The role of tissue factor pathway inhibitor in a revised coagulation cascade. *Seminars in Haematology* **29** (3), 159–169.

Bruce, D.A. & Hurtig, H.I. (1979) Incidence, course, and significance of cerebral oedema associated with cerebral infarction. In: *Cerebrovascular Diseases* (eds T.R. Price & E. Nelson), pp. 191–198. Raven Press, New York.

de Bruijn, S.T.F.M. & Stam, J. for the CVST Group (1999) Randomized, placebo-controlled trial of anticoagulant treatment with low-molecular weight heparin for cerebral sinus thrombosis. *Stroke* **30**, 484–488.

Burke, A.P., Farb, A., Malcolm, G.T., Liang, Y.-H., Smialek, J. & Virmani, R. (1997) Coronary risk factors and plaque morphology in men with coronary disease who died suddenly. *New England Journal of Medicine* **336**, 1276–1282.

Cairns, J., Theroux, P., Lewis, D., Ezekowitz, M., Meade, T.W. & Sutton, G. (1998) Antithrombotic agents in coronary artery disease. *Chest* **114**, 611S–633S.

Castillo, J., Davalos, A. & Noya, M. (1997) Progression of ischaemic stroke and excitotoxic aminoacids. *Lancet* **349**, 79–83.

Cerebrovascular Research Group (1982) China made defibrase in the treatment of cerebral thrombosis: a clinical controlled study. *Bulletin of the Hunan Medicine College* **7** (2), 163–167.

Chamorro, A. (1999) Heparin in acute ischaemic stroke: the case for a new clinical trial. *Cerebrovascular Diseases* **9** (Suppl. 3), 16–23.

Chen, Z.M., Sandercock, P., Xie, J.X., Collins, R., Peto, R. & Liu, L.S. (1997) Hospital management of patients with acute stroke in China. *Journal of Stroke and Cerebrovascular Diseases* **6**, 361–367.

Chen, Z.M., Sandercock, P., Pan, H.C. *et al.* on behalf of the CAST and IST Collaborative Groups (2000) Indications for early aspirin use in acute ischaemic stroke. A combined analysis of 40,000 randomized patients from the Chinese Acute Stroke Trial and the International Stroke Trial. *Stroke*

31, 1240–1249.

Cheng, G.C., Loree, H.M., Kamm, R.D., Fishbein, M.C. & Lee, R.T. (1993) Distribution of circumferential stress in ruptured and stable atherosclerotic lesions. A structural analysis with histopathological correlation. *Circulation* **87**, 1179–1187.

Cheung, J.Y., Bonventre, J.V., Malis, C.D. & Leaf, A. (1986) Calcium and ischaemic injury. *New England Journal of Medicine* **314**, 1670–1676.

Chimowitz, M., Arbor, A., Pessin, M., Furlan, A., Wolpert, S. & del Zoppo, G. (1994) The effect of source of cerebral embolus on susceptibility to thrombolysis. *Neurology* **44** (Suppl. 2), A356 (Abstract).

Chinese Acute Stroke Trial (CAST) Collaborative Group (1997) CAST: randomized placebo-controlled trial of early aspirin use in 20,000 patients with acute ischaemic stroke. *Lancet* **349**, 1641–1649.

Chiodo Grandi, F., Miccio, F., Salvi, R. & Mazzone, C. (2000) Physical means of preventing deep venous thrombosis for patients with stroke. In: *The Cochrane Library*. Oxford: Update Software

Choi, D.W. (1995) Calcium: still center stage in hypoxic-ischemic neuronal death. *Trends in Neurosciences* **18**, 58–60.

Choi, D.W. (1996) Ischaemia-induced neuronal apoptosis. *Current Opinion in Neurobiology* **6**, 667–672.

Choi, D.W. & Koh, J.Y. (1998) Zinc and brain injury. *Annual Review of Neuroscience* **21**, 347–375.

Clark, W.M., Madden, K.P., Lyden, P.D. & Zivin, J.A. (1991) Cerebral haemorrhage risk of aspirin or heparin therapy with thrombolytic treatment in rabbits. *Stroke* **22**, 872–876.

Cochrane Stroke Group (2000) Cochrane Stroke Group module. In: *The Cochrane Library*. Oxford: Update Software.

Coller, B.S. (1997) Platelet GPIIb/IIIa. Antagonists: the first anti-integrin receptor therapeutics. *Journal of Clinical Investigations* **99**, 1467–1471.

Collins, R., MacMahon, S., Flather, M. *et al.* (1996) Clinical effects of anticoagulant therapy in suspected acute myocardial infarction: systematic overview of randomized trials. *British Medical Journal* **313**, 652–659.

Cook, D.J., Sackett, D.L. & Spitzer, W.O. (1995) Methodologic guidelines for systematic reviews of randomized control trials in health care from the Potsdam consultation on meta-analysis. *Journal of Clinical Epidemiology* **48** (1), 167–171.

Cook, P.J. & Lip, G.Y.H. (1996) Infectious agents and atherosclerotic vascular disease. *Quarterly Journal of Medicine* **89**, 727–735.

Cook, P.J., Honeybourne, D., Lip, G.Y.H., Beevers, G., Wise, R. & Davies, P. (1998) *Chlamydia pneumoniae* antibody titers are significantly associated with acute stroke and transient cerebral ischemia. The West Birmingham Stroke Project. *Stroke* **29**, 404–410.

Cormio, M., Robertson, C.S. & Narayan, R.K. (1997) Secondary insults to the injured brain. *Journal of Clinical Neuroscience* **4** (2), 132–148.

Counsell, C. & Sandercock, P. (2000) Low-molecular-weight heparins or heparinoids versus standard unfractionated heparin for acute ischaemic stroke. In: *The Cochrane Library*. Oxford: Update Software.

Counsell, C., Clarke, M.J., Slattery, J. & Sandercock, P. (1994) The miracle of DICE therapy for acute stroke: fact or fictional product of subgroup analysis? *British Medical Journal* **309**, 1677–1681.

Counsell, C., Warlow, C., Sandercock, P., Fraser, H. & van Gijn, J. (1995) The Cochrane Collaboration Stroke Review Group. Meeting the need for systematic reviews in stroke care. *Stroke* **26**, 498–502.

D'Andrea, G., Cananzi, A.R. & Perini, F. (1994) Platelet function in acute ischaemic stroke: relevance of granule secretion. *Cerebrovascular Diseases* **4**, 163–169.

Danesh, J., Collins, R. & Peto, R. (1997) Chronic infections and coronary heart disease: is there a link? *Lancet* **350**, 430–436.

Danesh, J., Collins, R., Appleby, P. & Peto, R. (1998) Association of fibrinogen, C-reactive protein, albumin, or leucocyte count with coronary heart disease. Meta-analysis of prospective studies. *Journal of the American Medical Association* **279**, 1477–1482.

Dans, A.L., Dans, L.F., Guyatt, G.H. & Richardson, S. (1998) Users guide to the medical literature. XIV. How to decide the applicability of clinical trial results to your patient. *Journal of the American Medical Association* **279**, 545–549.

Davalos, A., Fernandez-Real, J.M. & Ricart, W. (1994) Iron-related damage in acute ischaemic stroke. *Stroke* **24**, 1543–1546.

Davenport, R., Dennis, M., Wellwood, I. & Warlow, C. (1996) Complications after acute stroke. *Stroke* **27**, 415–420.

Davies, M.J. (1996) Stability and instability. Two faces of coronary atherosclerosis. *Circulation* **94**, 2013–2020.

Davies, M.J. (1997) The composition of coronary artery plaques. *New England Journal of Medicine* **336**, 1312–1314.

Dawson, S.L., Blake, M.J., Panerai, R.B. & Potter, J.F. (2000) Dynamic but not static cerebral autoregulation is impaired in acute ischaemic stroke. *Cerebrovascular Diseases* **10**, 126–132.

De Bono, D.P. (1994) Free radicals and antioxidants in vascular biology. The roles of reaction kinetics, environment and substrate turnover. *Quarterly Journal of Medicine* **87**, 445–453.

Dearden, N.M. (1985) Ischaemic brain. *Lancet* **ii**, 255–259.

DeGraba, T.J. (1997) Expression of inflammatory mediators and adhesions molecules in human atherosclerotic plaque. *Neurology* **49** (Suppl. 4), S15–S19.

DeGraba, T.J. (1998) The role of inflammation after acute stroke. Utility of pursuing anti-adhesion molecule therapy. *Neurology* **51** (Suppl. 3), S62–S68.

DeGraba, T.J., Siren, A.-L., Penix, L. *et al.* (1998) Increased endothelial expression of intercellular adhesion molecule-1 in symptomatic versus asymptomatic human carotid atherosclerotic plaque. *Stroke* **29**, 1405–1410.

Del Zoppo, G. (1998) Ischaemic damage of brain microvessels: inherent risks for thrombolytic treatment in stroke. *Journal of Neurology, Neurosurgery and Psychiatry* **65**, 1–9.

Del Zoppo, G., Higashida, R.T., Furlan, A.J., Pessin, M.S., Rowley, H.A., Gent, M. & the PROACT Investigators (1998) Prolyse in Acute Cerebral Thromboembolism (PROACT): a phase II randomized trial of recombinant pro-urokinase by direct arterial delivery in acute middle cerebral artery stroke. *Stroke* **29**, 4–11.

Demchuk, A., Morgenstern, L., Krieger, D. *et al.* (1999) Serum glucose level and diabetes predict tissue plasminogen activator-related intracerebral haemorrhage in acute ischemic stroke. *Stroke* **30**, 34–39.

Derdeyn, C.P., Grubb, R.L. Jr & Powers, W.J. (1999) Cerebral haemodynamic impairment. Methods of measurement and association with stroke risk. *Neurology* **53**, 251–259.

Deykin, D. (1967) Thrombogenesis. *New England Journal of Medicine* **276**, 622–628.

Di Mauro, S. & Moraes, C.T. (1993) Mitochondrial encephalomyopathies. *Archives of Neurology* **50**, 1197–1208.

Dirnagl, U. & Pulsinelli, W. (1990) Autoregulation of cerebral blood flow in experimental focal brain ischaemia. *Journal of Cerebral Blood Flow and Metabolism* **10**, 327–336.

Doll, R. (1998) Controlled trials: the 1948 watershed. *British Medical Journal* **317**, 1217–1220.

Donnan, G.A. (1999) Australian Urokinase Stroke Trial (AUST). *Stroke* **30**, 487.

Donnan, G.A., Davis, S.M., Chambers, B.R. *et al.* (1995) Trials of streptokinase in severe acute ischaemic stroke. *Lancet* **345**, 578–579.

Dorman, P. & Sandercock, P. (1996) Considerations in the design of trials of neuroprotective therapy in acute stroke. *Stroke* **27**, 1507–1515.

Dorman, P., Counsell, C. & Sandercock, P. (1996) Recently developed neuroprotective therapies for acute stroke. A qualitative systematic review of clinical trials. *CNS Drugs* **6**, 457–474.

Du, C., Hu, R., Csernansky, C.A., Liu, X.Z., Hsu, C.Y. & Choi, D.W. (1996) Additive neuroprotective effects of dextrorphan and cycloheximide in rats subjected to transient focal cerebral ischaemia. *Brain Research* **718**, 233–236.

Dyken, M.L. & White, P. (1956) Evaluation of cortisone in the treatment of cerebral infarction. *Journal of the American Medical Association* **162**, 1531–1534.

Dyker, A.G., Grosset, D.G. & Lees, K. (1997) Perindopril reduces blood pressure but not cerebral blood flow in patients with recent cerebral ischemic stroke. *Stroke* **28**, 580–583.

Ebrahim, S. & Redfern, J. (1999) *Stroke Care—a Matter of Chance. A National Survey of Stroke Services*. Stroke Association, London.

Eicke, B.M., Buss, E., Bähr, R.R., Hajak, G. & Paulus, W. (1999) Influence of acetazolamide and CO_2 on extracranial flow volume and intracranial blood flow velocity. *Stroke* **30**, 76–80.

Einhaupl, K.M., Villringer, A., Meister, W. *et al.* (1991) Heparin treatment in sinus venous thrombosis [Published erratum appears in *Lancet* 338 (8772), 958]. *Lancet* **338**, 597–600.

Enlimomab Acute Stroke Trial Investigators (1997) The Enlimomab Acute Stroke Trial: final results. *Neurology* **48**, A270.

European Ad Hoc Consensus Group (1996) European strategies for early intervention in stroke. *Cerebrovascular Diseases* **6**, 315–324.

European Ad Hoc Consensus Group (1997) Optimising intensive care in stroke: a European perspective. *Cerebrovascular Diseases* **7**, 113–128.

European Ad Hoc Consensus Group (1998) Neuroprotection as initial therapy in acute stroke. *Cerebrovascular Diseases* **8**, 59–72.

European Atrial Fibrillation Trial Study Group (1993) Secondary prevention in non-rheumatic atrial fibrillation after transient ischaemic attack or minor stroke. *Lancet* **342**, 1255–1262.

European Atrial Fibrillation Trial Study Group (1995) Optimal oral anticoagulant therapy in patients with nonrheumatic atrial fibrillation and recent cerebral ischaemia. *New England Journal of Medicine* **333** (1), 5–10.

Faraci, F.M. & Brian, J.E. (1994) Nitric oxide and the cerebral circulation. *Stroke* **25**, 692–703.

Fibrinolytic Therapy Trialists' (FTT) Collaborative Group (1994) Indications for fibrinolytic therapy in suspected acute myocardial infarction: collaborative overview of early mortality and major morbidity results from all randomized trials of more than 1000 patients. *Lancet* **343**, 311–322.

Fieschi, C. & Lenzi, G.L. (1983) Cerebral blood flow and metabolism in stroke. In: *Vascular Disease of the Central Nervous System* (ed. R.W. Ross Russell), pp. 101–127. Churchill Livingstone, Edinburgh.

Fine, M.J., Kapoor, W. & Falanga, V. (1987) Cholesterol crystal embolisation. a review of 221 cases in the English literature. *Angiology* **38**, 769–784.

Fox, C. & Dunne, J. (1993) Corticosteroid responsive mitochondrial encephalomyopathy. *Australian and New Zealand Journal of Medicine* **23**, 522.

Frackowiak, R.S.J. (1985) The pathophysiology of human cerebral ischaemia: a new perspective obtained with positron emission tomography. *Quarterly Journal of Medicine* **57**, 713–727.

Frank, J.I., Krieger, D., Chyatte, D. & Cancian, S. (1999) HEADDFIRST: hemicraniectomy and durotomy upon deterioration from massive hemispheric infarction. A proposed randomised study. *Stroke* **30**, 243.

Friberg, L. & Olsen, T.S. (1991) Cerebrovascular instability in a subset of patients with stroke and transient ischaemic attack. *Archives of Neurology* **48**, 1026–1031.

Furie, B. & Furie, B.C. (1992) Molecular and cellular biology of blood coagulation. *New England Journal of Medicine* **326**, 800–806.

Furlan, A., Higashida, R., Wechsler, L. *et al.* for the PROACT II Investigators (1999) Recombinant pro-urokinase (r-Pro-UK) in acute ischemic stroke. The PROACT-II study: a randomised controlled trial. *Journal of the American Medical Association* **282**, 2003–2011.

Fuster, V., Fallon, J.T., Badimon, J.J. & Nemerson, Y. (1997) The unstable atherosclerotic plaque: clinical significance and therapeutic intervention. *Thrombosis and Haemostasis* **78** (1), 247–255.

Gandolfo, C. & Conti, M. (2000) Lubeluzole for acute ischaemic stroke. In: *The Cochrane Library*. Oxford: Update Software.

Gent, M., Barnett, H.J., Sackett, D.L. & Taylor, D.W. (1980) A randomized trial of aspirin and sulfinpyrazone in patients with threatened stroke. Results and methodologic issues. *Circulation* **62**, 97–105.

Geraci, E. & Geraci, T. (1996) A look at recent hyperventilation studies: outcomes and recommendations for early use in the head-injured patient. *Journal of Neuroscience Nursing* **28** (4), 222–224, 229–233.

Gibbs, J.M., Wise, R.J.S., Leenders, K.L. & Jones, T. (1984) Evaluation of cerebral perfusion reserve in patients with carotid artery occlusion. *Lancet* **i**, 310–314.

van Gijn, J. & Warlow, C. (1992) Down with stroke scales. *Cerebrovascular Diseases* **2**, 239–247.

Ginsberg, M.D. & Pulsinelli, W.A. (1994) The ischaemic penumbra, injury thresholds and the therapeutic window of acute stroke. *Annals of Neurology* **36**, 553–554.

Godlee, F., Goldmann, D., Donald, A. & Barton, S., eds (2000) *Clinical Evidence*. BMJ Publishing, London.

Goldberg, M.P. (1997) Stroke Trials Database, Internet Stroke Center at Washington University (cited 23 January 2000) <http://www.neuro.wustl.edu/stroke>.

Grau, A.J., Buggle, F., Ziegler, C. *et al.* (1997) Association between acute cerebrovascular ischaemia and chronic and recurrent infection. *Stroke* **28**, 1724–1729.

Grau, A.J., Buggle, F., Becher, H. *et al.* (1998) Recent bacterial and viral infection is a risk factor for cerebrovascular ischaemia: clinical and biochemical studies. *Neurology* **50**, 196–203.

Gray, C.S., French, J.M., Venables, G.S., Cartlidge, N.E., James, O.F. & Bates, D. (1990) A randomised double blind controlled trial of naftidrofuryl in acute stroke. *Age and Ageing* **19**, 356–363.

Greenamyre, J.T. & Porter, R.H.P. (1994) Anatomy and physiology of glutamate in the CNS. *Neurology* **44** (Suppl. 8), S7–S13.

Grimshaw, J. (2000) Effective practice and organisation of care group. In: *The Cochrane Library*. Oxford: Update Software.

Grimshaw, J.M. & Russell, I.T. (1993) Effect of clinical guidelines on medical practice: a systematic review of rigorous evaluations. *Lancet* **342**, 1317–1322.

Gubitz, G., Counsell, C., Sandercock, P. & Signorini, D. (2000a) Antiplatelet agents for acute ischaemic stroke. In: *The Cochrane Library*. Oxford: Update Software.

Gubitz, G., Counsell, C., Sandercock, P. & Signorini, D. (2000b) Anticoagulants for acute ischaemic stroke. In: *The Cochrane Library*. Oxford: Update Software.

Gubitz, G., Counsell, C., Signorini, D. & Sandercock, P. (2000c) Different doses of the same anticoagulant for acute ischaemic stroke. In: *The Cochrane Library*. Oxford: Update Software.

Gubitz, G., Sandercock, P. & Counsell, C. (2000d) Immediate anticoagulant therapy for acute ischaemic stroke: a systematic review of seven randomised trials directly comparing different doses of the same anticoagulant. *Stroke* **31**, 308.

Gur, A.Y., Bova, I. & Bornstein, N.M. (1996) Is impaired cerebral vasomotor reactivity a predictive factor of stroke in asymptomatic patients? *Stroke* **27**, 2188–2190.

Gurfinkel, E., Bozovich, G., Daroco, A., Beck, E. & Mautner B. for the ROXIS Study Group (1997) Randomised trial of roxithromycin in non-Q-wave coronary syndromes: ROXIS Pilot Study. *Lancet* **350**, 404–407.

Hachinksi, V.C. & Norris, J.W. (1985) *The Acute Stroke*. FA David & Company, Philadelphia.

Hacke, W., Kaste, M., Fieschi, C. *et al.* (1998) Randomised double-blind placebo-controlled trial of thrombolytic therapy with intravenous alteplase in acute ischaemic stroke (ECASS II). *Lancet* **352**, 1245–1251.

Hakim, A.M. (1998) Ischemic penumbra. The therapeutic time window. *Neurology* **51** (Suppl. 3), S44–S46.

Halliwell, B. (1994) Free radicals, antioxidants, and human disease: curiosity, cause or consequence? *Lancet* **344**, 721–724.

Hammans, S.R. & Morgan-Hughes, J.A. (1994) Mitochondrial myelopathies: clinical features, investigation, treatment and genetic counselling. In: *Mitochondrial Disorders in Neurology* (eds A.H.V. Shapira & S. DiMauro), pp. 49–74. Butterworth-Heinemann, Oxford.

Handoll, H.H.G., Farrar, M.J., McBirnie, J. *et al.* (2000) Prophylaxis using heparin, low molecular weight heparin and physical methods against deep vein thrombosis and pulmonary embolism in hip fracture surgery. In: *The Cochrane Library*. Oxford: Update Software

Hankey, G.J. (1991) Isolated angiitis/angiopathy of the central nervous system. *Cerebrovascular Diseases* **1**, 2–15.

Hao, W.X. (1984) Effect of antithrombotic enzyme of *Agkistrodon halys* venom in the treatment of cerebral thrombosis. Report of 322 cases. *Chung Hua Shen Ching Ching Shen Ko Tsa Chih* **17** (4), 223–225.

Harper, A.M. (1966) Autoregulation of cerebral blood flow: influence of the arterial blood pressure on the blood flow through the cerebral cortex. *Journal of Neurology, Neurosurgery and Psychiatry* **29**, 398–403.

Harper, A.M. & Bell, R.A. (1963) The effect of metabolic acidosis and alkalosis on the blood flow through the cerebral cortex. *Journal of Neurology, Neurosurgery and Psychiatry* **26**, 341–344.

Harris, R.J., Symon, L. & Branston, N.M. (1981) Changes in extracellular calcium activity in cerebral ischaemia. *Journal of Cerebral Blood Flow and Metabolism* **1**, 203–209.

Hart, R.G. & Benavente, O. (1999) Increased risk of intracranial hemorrhage when aspirin is added to warfarin: a meta-analysis. *Stroke* **30**, 258.

Hart, R.G., Boop, B.S. & Anderson, D.C. (1995) Oral anticoagulants and intracranial haemorrhage. Facts and hypotheses. *Stroke* **26**, 1471–1477.

Heiss, W.D. (1992) Experimental evidence of ischaemic thresholds and functional recovery. *Stroke* **23**, 1668–1672.

Heiss, W.D. & Graf, R. (1994) The ischaemic penumbra. *Current Opinion in Neurology* **7**, 11–19.

Heiss, W.D. & Rosner, G. (1983) Functional recovery of cortical neurones as related to degree and duration of ischaemia. *Annals of Neurology* **14**, 294–301.

Heiss, W.D., Hayakawa, T. & Waltz, A.G. (1976) Cortical neuronal function during ischaemia. Effects of occlusion of one middle cerebral artery on single unit activity in cats. *Archives of Neurology* **33**, 813–820.

Herold, S., Brown, M.M., Frackowiak, R.S.J., Mansfield, A.O., Thomas, D.J. & Marshall, J. (1988) Assessment of cerebral haemodynamic reserve: correlation between PET parameters and CO_2 reactivity measured by intravenous 133 xenon injection technique. *Journal of Neurology, Neurosurgery and Psychiatry* **51**, 1045–1050.

Heros, R.C. (1994) Stroke: early pathophysiology and treatment. *Stroke* **25**, 1877–1881.

Higashida, R.T., Isai, F.Y., Halbach, V.V., Barnwell, S.L., Dourd, C.F. & Hieshima, G.B. (1995) Interventional neurovascular techniques—state of the art therapy. *Journal of Internal Medicine* **237**, 105–115.

Hirsh, J. (1991) Heparin. *New England Journal of Medicine* **324** (22), 1565–1574.

Hirsh, J. & Weitz, J.I. (1999) New antithrombotic agents. *Lancet* **353**, 1431–1436.

Hommel, M. for the FISS-bis Investigators Group (1998) Fraxiparine in Ischaemic Stroke Study (FISS bis). *Cerebrovascular Diseases* 8 (Suppl. 4), 19 (Abstract).

Hommel, M., Boissel, J.P., Cornu, C. *et al.* (1995) Termination of trial of streptokinase in severe acute ischaemic stroke. *Lancet* **345**, 57.

Horn, J., Haan, J., Vermeulen, M. & Limburg, M. (1999) VENUS—very early nimodipine use in stroke. *Stroke* 30, 243.

Horn, J., Limburg, L. & Orgogozo, J.M. (2000) Calcium antagonists for acute ischemic stroke. In: *The Cochrane Library*. Oxford: Update Software

Hossmann, K.-A. (1994) Viability thresholds and the penumbra of focal ischaemia. *Annals of Neurology* **36**, 557–565.

Hossmann, K.-A. & Hoehn-Berlage, M. (1995) Diffusion and perfusion MR imaging of cerebral ischaemia. *Cerebrovascular and Brain Metabolism Reviews* 7, 187–217.

Hunt, B.J. & Jurd, K.M. (1998) Endothelial cell activation. *British Medical Journal* **316**, 1328–1329.

Hunt, D.L. & McKibbon, K.A. (1997) Locating and appraising systematic reviews. *Annals of Internal Medicine* **126**, 532–538.

Hunter, J. (1794) A treatise on the blood, inflammation and gunshot wounds. In: *The Work of John Hunter (1937)* (ed. J.F. Palmer). Longman, London.

Hutchinson, J. (1867) Four lectures on compression of the brain. *Clinical Lecture Reports London Hospital* 4, 10–55.

Hyman, B.T., Landas, S.K., Ashman, R.F., Schelper, R.L. & Robinson, R.A. (1987) Warfarin-related purple toes syndrome and cholesterol microembolisation. *American Journal of Medicine* **82**, 1233–1237.

International Stroke Trial Collaborative Group (1997) The International Stroke Trial (IST): a randomized trial of aspirin, subcutaneous heparin, both, or neither among 19 435 patients with acute ischaemic stroke. *Lancet* **349**, 1569–1581.

ISIS-2 Collaborative Group (1988) Randomised trial of intravenous streptokinase, oral aspirin, both or neither among 17 187 cases of suspected acute myocardial infarction: ISIS-2. *Lancet* **ii**, 349–360.

ISIS-3 Collaborative Group (1992) ISIS-3: a randomised comparison of streptokinase versus tissue plasminogen activator versus anistreplase and of aspirin plus heparin versus aspirin alone among 41 299 cases of suspected acute myocardial infarction. *Lancet* 339, 753–770.

Ito, U., Ohno, K. & Nakamura, R. (1979) Brain oedema during ischaemia and after restoration of blood flow. Measurement of water, sodium, potassium content and plasma protein permeability. *Stroke* **10**, 542–547.

Jadad, A.R., Cook, D.J., Jones, A. *et al.* (1998) Methodology and reports of systematic reviews and meta-analyses: a comparison of Cochrane reviews with articles published in paper-based journals. *Journal of the American Medical Association* **280**, 278–280.

Jauss, M., Krieger, D., Hornig, C., Schramm, J. & Busse, O. for the GASCIS study centers (1999) Surgical and medical management of patients with massive cerebellar infarctions: the German–Austrian Cerebellar Infarction Study. *Journal of Neurology* **246**, 257–264.

Jones, T.H., Morawetz, R.B. & Crowell, R.M. (1981) Thresholds of focal cerebral ischaemia in awake monkeys. *Journal of Neurosurgery* **54**, 773–782.

Kalia, K.K. & Yonas, H. (1993) An. aggressive approach to massive middle cerebral artery infarction. *Archives of Neurology* **50**, 1293–1297.

Karonen, J.O., Vanninen, R.L., Liu, Y. *et al.* (1999) Combined diffusion and perfusion MRI with correlation to single-photon emission CT in acute ischemic stroke. Ischemic penumbra predicts infarct growth. *Stroke* **30**, 1583–1590.

Kaste, M., Hacke, W. & Fieschi, C. (1995) Results of the European Co-operative Acute Stroke Study (ECASS). *Cerebrovascular Diseases* **5**, 255.

Kay, R., Wong, S.K., Yu, L.Y. *et al.* (1995) Low molecular weight heparin for the treatment of acute ischemic stroke. *New England Journal of Medicine* 333, 1588–1593.

Kernohan, J.W. & Woltman, H.W. (1929) Incisura of the crus due to contralateral brain tumour. *Archives of Neurology and Psychiatry* **21**, 274–287.

Ketley, D. & Woods, K.L. (1993) Impact of clinical trials on clinical practice: example of thrombolysis for acute myocardial infarction. *Lancet* **342**, 891–894.

Kety, S.S. (1950) Circulation and metabolism of the human brain in health and disease. *American Journal of Medicine* 8, 205–217.

Kety, S.S. & Schmidt, C.F. (1945) The determination of cerebral blood flow in man by the use of nitrous oxide in low concentrations. *American Journal of Physiology* **143**, 53–66.

Khan, F. & Butler, R. (1998) Free radicals in cardiovascular disease. *Proceedings of the Royal College of Physicians of Edinburgh* **28**, 102–110.

Kitagawa, K., Matsumoto, M., Tsujimoto, Y. *et al.* (1998) Amelioration of hippocampal neuronal damage after global ischaemia by neuronal overexpression of BCL-2 in transgenic mice. *Stroke* **29**, 2616–2621.

Kleiser, B. & Widder, B. (1992) Course of carotid artery occlusions with impaired carbon dioxide reactivity. *Stroke* **23**, 171–174.

Kleiser, B., Scholl, D. & Widder, B. (1994) Assessment of cerebrovascular reactivity by Doppler CO_2 and Diamox testing: which is the appropriate method. *Cerebrovascular Diseases* **4**, 134–138.

Knop, J., Thie, A., Fuchs, C., Siepmann, G. & Zeumer, H. (1992) 99MTC–HMPAO–SPECT with acetazolamide challenge to detect haemodynamic compromise in occlusive cerebrovascular disease. *Stroke* **23**, 1733–1742.

Kogure, K. & Kato, H. (1993) Altered gene expression in cerebral ischaemia. *Stroke* **24**, 2121–2127.

Kogure, T. & Kogure, K. (1997) Molecular and biochemical events within the brain subjected to cerebral ischemia (targets for therapeutic intervention). *Clinical Neuroscience* **4**, 179–183.

Koistinaho, J. & Hokfelt, T. (1997) Altered gene expression in brain ischaemia. *Neuroreport* **8**, i–viii.

Koistinaho, J., Pasonen, S., Yrjanheikki, J. & Chan, P.H. (1999) Spreading depression-induced gene expression is regulated by plasma glucose. *Stroke* **30**, 114–119.

Kontos, H.A. (1989) Validity of cerebral arterial blood flow calculations from velocity measurements. *Stroke* **20**, 1–3.

Kristián, T. & Siesjö, B.K. (1998) Calcium in ischemic cell death. *Stroke* **29**, 705–718.

Kuchinsky, W. & Gillardon, F. (2000) Apoptosis and cerebral ischaemia. *Cerebrovascular Diseases* **10**, 165–169.

Kullo, I.J., Edwards, W.D. & Schwartz, R.S. (1998) Vulnerable plaque: pathobiology and clinical implications. *Annals of Internal Medicine* **129**, 1050–1060.

von Kummer, R. & Forsting, M. (1993) Effects of recanalisation and collateral blood supply on infarct extent and brain oedema after middle cerebral artery occlusion. *Cerebrovascular Diseases* 3, 252–255.

Kwiatkowski, T.G., Libman, R., Frankel, M. *et al.* (1999) Effects of tissue plasminogen activator for acute ischaemic stroke at one year. *New England Journal of Medicine* **340**, 1781–1787.

Lagi, A., Bacalli, S., Cencetti, S., Paggetti, C. & Colzi, L. (1994) Cerebral autoregulation in orthostatic hypotension. A transcranial Doppler study. *Stroke* **25**, 1771–1775.

Larrue, V., von Kummer, R., del Zoppo, G. & Bluhmki, E. (1997) Haemorrhagic transformation in acute ischemic stroke. Potential contributing factors in the European Cooperative Acute Stroke Study. *Stroke* **28**, 957–960.

Larsen, F.S., Olsen, K.S., Hansen, B.A., Paulson, O.B. & Knudsen, G.M. (1994) Transcranial Doppler is valid for determination of the lower limit of cerebral blood flow regulation. *Stroke* **25**, 1985–1988.

Lassen, N.A., Roland, P.E., Larsen, B., Melamed, E. & Soh, K. (1977) Mapping of human cerebral functions: a study of the regional cerebral blood flow pattern during rest, its reproducibility and the activations seen during basic sensory and motor functions. *Acta Neurologica Scandinavica* **64** (Suppl.), 262–263.

Lassen, N.A., Fieschi, C. & Lenzi, G.L. (1991) Ischaemic penumbra and neuronal death: comments on the therapeutic window in acute stroke with particular reference to thrombolytic therapy. *Cerebrovascular Diseases* **1** (Suppl.), 32–35.

Leão, A.A.P. (1944) Spreading depression of activity in the cerebral cortex. *Journal of Neurophysiology* 7, 359–390.

Leão, A.A.P. (1947) Further observations on the spreading depression of activity in the cerebral cortex. *Journal of Neurophysiology* **10**, 409–414.

Lee, J.-M., Zipfel, G.J. & Choi, D.W. (1999) The changing landscape of ischaemic brain injury mechanisms. *Nature* **399** (Suppl. 6738), A7–A14.

Leenders, K.L., Perani, D. & Lammertsma, A.A. (1990) Cerebral blood flow, blood volume and oxygen utilisation. Normal values and effect of age. *Brain* **113**, 27–47.

Levin, E.R. (1995) Endothelins. *New England Journal of Medicine* **333**, 356–361.

Libby, P. (1995) Molecular bases of the acute coronary syndromes. *Circulation* **91**, 2844–2850.

Lindley, R.I., Amayo, E.O., Marshall, J., Sandercock, P. & Warlow, C. (1995) Acute stroke treatment in the UK hospitals: the Stroke Association Survey of Consultant Opinion. *Journal of the Royal College of Physicians* **29**, 479–484.

Lindsberg, P.J., Hallenbeck, J.M. & Feuerstein, G. (1991) Platelet-activating factor in stroke and brain injury. *Annals of Neurology* **30**, 117–129.

Lindsberg, P.J., Carpen, O., Paetau, A., Karjalainen-Lindsberg, M.-L. & Kaste, M. (1996) Endothelial ICAM-1 expression associated with inflammatory cell response in human ischaemic stroke. *Circulation* **94**, 939–945.

Linnik, M.D., Zahos, P., Geschwind, M.D. & Federoff, H.J. (1995) Expression of *bcl-2* from a defective herpes simplex virus-1 vector limits neuronal death in focal cerebral ischaemia. *Stroke* **26**, 1670–1674.

Lipton, S.A. & Rosenberg, P.A. (1994) Excitatory amino acids as a final common pathway for neurologic disorders. *New England Journal of Medicine* **330**, 613–622.

Liu, M. & Wardlaw, J. (2000) Thrombolysis (different doses, routes of administration and agents) for acute ischaemic stroke. In: *The Cochrane Library*. Oxford: Update Software

Liu, M., Counsell, C. & Wardlaw, J. (2000) Fibrinogen depleting agents for acute ischaemic stroke. In: *The Cochrane Library*. Oxford: Update Software

Liu, P.K., Salminen, A. & He, Y.Y. (1994) Suppression of ischaemia-induced Fos expression and AP-1 activity by an antisense oligonucleotide to c-fos mRNA. *Annals of Neurology* **36**, 566–576.

Loscalzo, J. (1995) Nitric oxide and vascular disease. *New England Journal of Medicine* **333**, 251–253.

Lou, H.C., Edvinsson, L. & MacKenzie, E.T. (1987) The concept of coupling blood flow to brain function: revision required? *Annals of Neurology* **22**, 289–297.

Lowe, G. (1998) The pharmacology of thrombolytic and fibrinogen-depleteing agents in the treatment of acute ischaenic stroke. *Cerebrovascular Diseases* **8** (Suppl. 1), 36–42.

Lyden, P. & Zivin, J. (1993) Hemorrhagic transformaton after cerebral ischemia: mechanisms and incidence. *Cerebrovascular and Brain Metabolism Reviews* **5**, 1–16.

Lyrer, P. & Engelter, S. (2000) Antithrombotic drugs for carotid artery dissection. In: *The Cochrane Library*. Oxford: Update Software

Ma, J., Endres, M. & Moskowitz, M.A. (1998) Synergistic effects of caspase inhibitors and MK-801 in brain injury after transient focal cerebral ischaemia in mice. *British Journal of Pharmacology* **124**, 756–762.

McCord, J.M. (1985) Oxygen-derived free radicals in post-ischaemic tissue injury. *New England Journal of Medicine* **312**, 159–163.

MacDonell, R.A.L., Kalnins, R.M. & Donnan, G.A. (1987) Cerebellar infarction: natural history, prognosis and pathology. *Stroke* **18**, 849–855.

McIntyre, M. & Dominiczak, A.F. (1997) Nitric oxide and cardiovascular disease. *Postgraduate Medical Journal* **73**, 630–634.

McNealy, X. & Plum, F. (1962) Brainstem dysfunction with supratentorial mass lesions. *Archives of Neurology* **7**, 10–32.

Mandai, K., Sueyoshi, K. & Fukunaga, R. (1994) Evaluation of cerebral vasoreactivity by three-dimensional time of flight magnetic resonance angiography. *Stroke* **25**, 1807–1811.

Marchal, G., Beaudoin, V., Rioux, P. *et al.* (1996) Prolonged persistence of substantial volumes of potentially viable brain tissue after stroke: a correlative PET–CT study with voxel-based data analysis. *Stroke* **27**, 599–606.

Markus, H.S. & Harrison, M.J.G. (1992) Estimation of cerebrovascular reactivity using transcranial Doppler, include the use of breath-holding as the vasodilatory stimulus. *Stroke* **23**, 668–673.

Markus, H.S. & Mendall, M.A. (1998) *Helicobacter pylori* infection: a risk factor for ischaemic cerebrovascular disease and carotid atheroma. *Journal of Neurology, Neurosurgery and Psychiatry* **64**, 104–107.

Markwalder, T.M., Grolimund, P., Seiler, R.W., Roth, F. & Aaslid, R. (1984) Dependency of blood flow velocity in the middle cerebral artery on end-tidal carbon dioxide partial pressure—a transcranial ultrasound Doppler study. *Journal of Cerebral Blood Flow and Metabolism* **4**, 368–372.

Martin, R.L. (1997) Experimental neuronal protection in cerebral ischaemia. Part 1: Experimental models and pathophysiological responses. *Journal of Clinical Neuroscience* **4** (2), 96–113.

Masdeu, J.C., Brass, L.M., Holman, L. & Kushner, M.J. (1994) Brain single-photon emission computed tomography. *Neurology* **44**, 1970–1977.

Mathew, P., Teasdale, G., Bannan, A. & Oluoch-Olunya, D. (1995) Neurosurgical management of cerebellar haematoma and infarct. *Journal of Neurology, Neurosurgery and Psychiatry* **59**, 287–292.

Mead, G. & O'Neill, P. (1999) Carotid disease in acute stroke: a review. *Journal of Stroke and Cerebrovascular Diseases* **8**, 197–206.

Medical Research Council (1948) Streptomycin treatment of pulmonary tuberculosis. *British Medical Journal* **2**, 769–782.

Merrick, M.V., Ferrington, C.M. & Cowen, S.J. (1991) Parametric imaging of cerebral vascular reserves. 1. Theory, validation and normal values. *European Journal of Medicine* **18**, 171–177.

Moher, D., Cook, D., Eastwood, S., Olkin, I., Rennie, D. & Stroup, D. for the QUOROM Group (1999) Improving the quality of reports of meta-analyses of controlled trials: the QUOROM statement. *Lancet* **354**, 1896–1900.

Mohr, J.P., Orgogozo, J.M. & Hennerici, M. (1994) Meta-analysis of oral nimodipine trials in acute ischaemic stroke. *Cerebrovascular Diseases* **4**, 197–203.

Mokri, B., Sundt, T.M., Houser, W. & Piepgras, D.G. (1986) Spontaneous dissection of the cervical internal carotid artery. *Annals of Neurology* **19**, 126–138.

Mori, E., Yoneda, Y. & Tabuchi, M. (1992) Intravenous recombinant tissue plasminogen activator in acute carotid artery territory stroke. *Neurology* **42**, 976–982.

Motto, C., Aritzu, E., Boccardi, E., de Grandi, C., Piana, A. & Candelise, L. (1997) Reliability of hemorrhagic transformation diagnosis in acute ischemic stroke. *Stroke* **28**, 302–306.

Moussouttas, M.M., Lichtman, J.H., Krumholtz, H.M., Cerese, J. & Brass, L.M. (1999) The use of heparin anticoagulation in acute ischemic stroke among academic medical centers. *Stroke* **30**, 265.

Muir, K.W. & Lees, K.R. (1995) Clinical experience widh excitatory amino acid antagonist drugs. *Stroke* **26** (3), 503–513.

Muir Gray, J.A. & de Lusignan, S. (1999) National Electronic Library for Health (NELH). *British Medical Journal* **319**, 1476–1479.

Müller, M. & Schimrigk, K. (1996) Vasomotor reactivity and pattern of collateral blood flow in severe occlusive carotid artery disease. *Stroke* **27**, 296–299.

Multicentre Acute Stroke Trial (MAST-I) Group (1995) Are thrombolytic and antithrombotic agents safe and useful in acute ischaemic stroke? A randomized controlled trial with streptokinase, aspirin and combination of both treatments. *Lancet* **346**, 1509–1514.

National Institute of Neurological Disorders and Stroke (NINDS) rtPA Stroke Study Group (1995) Tissue plasminogen activator for acute ischemic stroke. *New England Journal of Medicine* **333**, 1581–1587.

Naylor, A.R., Merrick, M.V., Slattery, J.M., Notghi, A., Fennington, C.M. & Miller, J.D. (1991) Parametric imaging of cerebral vascular reserve. 2. Reproducibility, response to CO_2 and comparison with middle cerebral artery velocities. *European Journal of Nucleic Medicine* **18**, 259–264.

Nedergaard, M. (1996) Spreading depression as a contributor to ischaemic brain damage. *Advances in Neurology* **71**, 75–83.

Nedergaard, M. & Astrup, J. (1986) Infarct rim: effect of hyperglycaemia or direct current potential and [^{14}C]2-deoxyglucose phosphorylation. *Journal of Cerebral Blood Flow and Metabolism* **6**, 607–615.

Neumann-Haefelin, T., Wittsack, H.-J., Wenserski, F. *et al.* (1999) Diffusion- and perfusion-weighted MRI. The DWI/PWI mismatch region in acute stroke. *Stroke* **30**, 1591–1597.

Newell, D.W., Aaslid, R., Lam, A.M., Mayberg, T.S. & Winn, R. (1994) Comparison of flow and velocity during dynamic autoregulation testing in humans. *Stroke* **25**, 793–797.

Norris, J.W., Duchan, A., Cote, R. *et al.* (1998) Canadian guidelines for intravenous thrombolytic treatment in acute stroke. *Canadian Journal of the Neurological Sciences* **25**, 257–259.

Nowroth, P.P., Handley, D.A., Esmon, C.T. *et al.* (1986) Interleukin 1 induces endothelial cell procoagulant while suppressing cell-surface anticoagulant activity. *Proceedings of the National Academy of Sciences of the USA* **83**, 3460–3464.

O'Keefe, J.H. Jr, Lavie, C.J. Jr & McCallister, B.D. (1995) Insights into the pathogenesis and prevention of coronary artery disease. *Mayo Clinical Proceedings* **70**, 69–79.

Oppenheimer, S. & Hachinski, V. (1992) Complications of acute stroke. *Lancet* 339, 721–724.

Pan European Consensus Meeting on Stroke (1996) Stroke management in Europe. *Journal of Internal Medicine* **240**, 173–180.

Pancioli, A., Brott, T., Donaldson, V. & Miller, R. (1997) Asymmetric angioneurotic oedema associated with thrombolysis for acute stroke. *Annals of Emergency Medicine* 30 (2), 227–229.

Panerai, R.B., White, R.P., Markus, H.S. & Evans, D.H. (1998) Grading of cerebral dynamic autoregulation from spontaneous fluctuations in arterial blood pressure. *Stroke* **29**, 2341–2346.

Patrono, C. (1994) Aspirin as an antiplatelet drug. *New England Journal of Medicine* 330, 1287–1294.

Patrono, C., Ciabattoni, G. & Davi, G. (1990) Thromboxane biosynthesis in cardiovascular diseases. *Stroke* **21** (Suppl. IV), 130–133.

Peto, R., Collins, R. & Gray, R. (1995) Large-scale randomized evidence: large, simple trials and overviews of trials. *Journal of Clinical Epidemiology* **48** (1), 23–40.

Phillips, S.J. (1994) Pathophysiology and management of hypertension in acute ischaemic stroke. *Hypertension* **23** (1), 131–136.

Plum, F. & Posner, J.B. (1985) *The Diagnosis of Stupor and Coma*, pp. 96–100. F.A. Davis and Co., Philadelphia.

Plum, F., Deck, M. & Reich, J. (1993) Magnetic resonance imaging measurements and clinical changes accompanying transtentorial and foramen magnum brain herniation. *Annals of Neurology* **34**, 748–749.

Poungvarin, N., Bhoopat, W. & Viriyavejakul, A. (1987) Effects of dexamethasone in primary supratentorial intracerebral haemorrhage. *New England Journal of Medicine* **316**, 1229–1233.

Powers, W.J. (1991) Cerebral haemodynamics in ischaemic cerebrovascular disease. *Annals of Neurology* **29**, 231–240.

Powers, W.J., Grabb, R.L. Jr & Raichel, M.E. (1984) Physiological responses to focal cerebral ischaemia in humans. *Annals of Neurology* **16**, 546–552.

Powers, W.J., Press, G.A., Grabb, R.L. Jr, Gado, M. & Raichle, M.E. (1987) The effect of haemodynamically significant carotid artery disease on the haemodynamic status of the cerebral circulation. *Annals of Internal Medicine* **106**, 27–35.

Prestigiacomo, C.J., Kim, S.C., Connolly, S. Jr, Liao, H., Yan, S.-F. & Pinsky, D.J. (1999) CD18-mediated neutrophil recruitment contributes to the pathogenesis of reperfused but not nonreperfused stroke. *Stroke* **30**, 1110–1117.

Pritz, M.B. (1997) Timing of carotid endarterectomy after stroke. *Stroke* **28**, 2563–2567.

Pulmonary Embolism Prevention (PEP) Trial Collaborative Group (2000) Prevention of pulmonary embolism and deep vein thrombosis with low dose aspirin: Pulmonary Embolism Prevention (PEP) trial. *Lancet* **355**, 1295–1302.

Pulsinelli, W. (1992) Pathophysiology of acute ischaemic stroke. *Lancet* **339**, 533–536.

Qizilbash N., Lewington S.L., Lopez-Arrieta J.M. (2000) Corticosteroids for acute ischaemic stroke. In: *The Cochrane Library*. Oxford: Update Software.

Raichle, M (1983) The pathophysiology of brain ischaemia. *Annals of Neurology* **13**, 2–10.

Ramas, R., Salem, B.I., de Pawlikowski, M.P., Goordes, C., Eisenberg, S. & Leidenfrost, R. (1996) The efficacy of pneumatic compression stockings in the prevention of Pulmonary embolism after cardiac surgery. *Chest* **109**, 82–85

Reich, J.B., Sierra, J., Camp, W., Zanzonico, P., Deck, M.D.F. & Plum, F. (1993) Magnetic resonance imaging measurements and clinical changes accompanying transtentorial and foramen magnum brain herniation. *Annals of Neurology* **33**, 159–170.

Ricci, S. (1995) Between country variations in the use of medical treatments for acute stroke. *Cerebrovascular Diseases* **5** (4), 272 (Abstract).

Ridker, P.M, Cushman, M., Stampfer, M.J., Tracy, R.P. & Hennekens, C.H. (1997) Inflammation, aspirin, and the risk of cardiovascular disease in apparently healthy men *New England Journal of Medicine* **336**, 973–979.

Rieke, K., Schwab, S., Krieger, D. *et al.* (1995) Decompressive surgery in space-occupying hemispheric infarction: results of an open, prospective trial. *Critical Care Medicine* **23**, 1576–1587.

Riepe, M.W., Kasischke, K. & Raupach, A. (1997) Acetylsalicylic acid increases tolerance against hypoxic and chemical hypoxia. *Stroke* **28**, 2006–2011.

Righetti, E., Celani, M.G., Cantisani, T., Sterzi, R., Boysen, G. & Ricci, S. (2000) Glycerol for acute ischaemic stroke. In: *The Cochrane Library*. Oxford: Update Software.

Ropper, A.H. (1986) Lateral displacement of the brain and level of consciousness in patients with an acute hemispheral mass. *New England Journal of Medicine* **314**, 953–958.

Ropper, A.H. (1989) A preliminary MRI study of the geometry of brain displacement and level of consciousness with acute intracranial masses. *Neurology* **39**, 622–627.

Ropper, A.H. (1993) Magnetic resonance imaging measurements and clinical changes accompanying transtentorial and foramen magnum brain herniation. *Annals of Neurosurgery* **34**, 748–749.

Rosenberg, R.D. & Rosenberg, J.S. (1984) Natural anticoagulant mechanisms *Journal of Clinical Investigation* **74** (1), 1–6.

Ross, R. (1993) The pathogenesis of atherosclerosis: a perspective for the 1990s. *Nature* **362**, 801–809.

Ross, R. (1999) Atherosclerosis—an Inflammatory disease. *New England Journal of Medicine* **340**, 115–126.

Rothman, S.M. & Olney, J.W. (1986) Glutamate and the pathophysiology of hypoxic–ischaemic brain damage. *Annals of Neurology* **19**, 105–111.

Rothwell, P.M., Villagra, R., Gibson, R., Donders, R.C.J.M. & Warlow, C.P. (2000) Evidence of a chronic systemic cause of instability of atherosclerotic plaques. *Lancet* **355**, 19–24.

Roy, C.S. & Sherrington, C.S. (1890) On the regulation of the blood Supply of the brain. *Journal of Physiology* **11**, 85–108.

Royal College of Physicians of Edinburgh (1999) Consensus conference on medical management of stroke. *Journal of Neurology, Neurosurgery and Psychiatry* **66**, 128–129.

Sackett, D.L., Haynes, R.B., Guyatt, G.H. & Tugwell, P. (1991) *Clinical Epidemiology. A Basic Science for Clinical Medicine*, pp. 173–185. Little, Brown, Toronto.

Sackett, D.L., Strauss, S.E., Richardson, W.S., Rosenberg, W. & Haynes, R.B. (2000) *Evidence Based Medicine. How to Practice and Teach EBM*, 2nd edn. Churchill Livingstone, Edinburgh.

Sandercock, P. & Tanganakul, C. (1997) Very early prevention of stroke recurence. *Cerebrovascular Diseases* **7** (Suppl. 1), 10–15.

Sandercock, P., Bamford, J., Dennis, M. *et al.* (1992) Atrial fibrillation and stroke: prevalence in different types of stroke and influence on early and long term prognosis (Oxfordshire Community Stroke Project). *British Medical Journal* **305**, 1460–1465.

Saxena, R., Wijnhoud, A., Carton, H. & Koudstaal, P. (1999) Controlled safety study of a haemoglobin-based oxygen carrier, DCLHb, in acute ischaemic stroke. *Stroke* **30**, 993–996.

SCATI Group (1989) Randomised controlled trial of subcutaneous calcium–heparin in acute myocardial infarction. The SCATI (Studio sulla Calciparina nell'Angina e nella Trombosi Ventricolare nell'Infarto) Group. *Lancet* **ii**, 182–186.

Schlaug, G., Benfield, A., Baird, A.E. *et al.* (1999) The ischaemic penumbra. Operationally defined by diffusion and perfusion MRI. *Neurology* **53**, 1528–1537.

Schmidley, J.W. (1990) Free radicals in central nervous system ischaemia. *Stroke* **21**, 1086–1090.

Schmitt, B.P. & Adelman, B. (1993) Heparin-associated thrombocytopenia: a critical review and pooled analysis. *American Journal of Medical Science* **305** (4), 208–215.

Schrader, J. & Dominiak, P. (1999) Acute Candesartan Cilexetil Evaluation in Stroke Survivors (ACCESS Study). *Stroke* **30**, 1301.

Schroeder, T (1988) Haemodynamic significance of internal carotid artery disease. *Acta Neurologica Scandinavica* **77**, 353–372.

Schror, K. & Braun, M. (1990) Platelets as a source of vasoactive mediators. *Stroke* **21** (Suppl. IV), 32–35.

Schulz, J.B., Weller, M. & Moskowitz, M.A. (1999) Caspases as treatment targets in stroke and neurodegenerative diseases. *Annals of Neurology* **45**, 421–429.

Schwab, S., Steiner, T., Aschoff, A. *et al.* (1998) Early hemicraniectomy in patients with complete middle cerebral artery occlusion. *Stroke* **29**, 1888–1893.

Scottish Intercollegiate Guidelines Network (1999) *Antithrombotic Therapy. A National Clinical Guideline*. Edinburgh: Scottish Intercollegiate Guidelines Network, Royal College of Physicians. Also available free of charge at: www.show.scot.nhs.uk/sign/clinical.htm.

Scottish Intercollegiate Guidelines Network (2000) *Prevention of Venous Thromboembolism. A National Clinical Guideline*. Edinburgh: Scottish

Intercollegiate Guidelines Network, Royal College of Physicians. Also available at: www.show.scot.nhs.uk/sign/clinical.htm.

Sensi, S.L., Yin, H.Z., Carriedo, S.G., Rao, S.S. & Weiss, J.H. (1999) Preferential Zn^{2+} influx though Ca^{2+} permeable AMPA/kainate channels trigger prolonged mitochondrial superoxide production. *Proceedings of the National Academy of Sciences of the USA* **96**, 2414–2419.

Sharp, F.R. (1994) The sense of antisense fos oligonucleotides. *Annals of Neurology* **36**, 555–556.

Sherman, D.G., Atkinson, R.P., Chippendale, T. *et al.* for the STAT participants (2000) Intravenous Ancrod for treatment of acute ischaemic stroke. The STAT study: a randomized controlled trial. *Journal of the American Medical Association* **283**, 2395–2403.

Shyu, K.G., Chang, J. & Lin, C.C. (1997) Serum levels of intercellular adhesion molecule-1 and E-selectin in patients with acute ischaemic stroke. *Journal of Neurology* **244**, 90–93.

Siesjö, B.K. (1992a) Pathophysiology and treatment of focal cerebral ischaemia. Part I: pathophysiology. *Journal of Neurosurgery* **77**, 169–184.

Siesjö, B.K. (1992b) Pathophysiology and treatment of focal cerebral ischaemia. Part II: mechanisms of damage and treatment. *Journal of Neurosurgery* **77**, 337–354.

Siesjö, B.K. & Bengtsson, F. (1989) Calcium fluxes, calcium antagonists, and calcium-related pathology in brain ischaemia, hypoglycaemia, and spreading depression: a unifying hypothesis. *Journal of Cerebral Blood Flow and Metabolism* **9**, 127–140.

Signorini, D., Sandercock, P. & Warlow, C. for the International Stroke Trial Collaborative Group (1999) Systolic blood pressure on outcome in the international stroke trial. *Cerebrovascular Disorders* **9** (Suppl. 1), 34.

Skinhoj, E., Hoedt-Rasmussen, K., Paulson, O.B. & Lassen, N.A. (1970) Regional cerebral blood flow and its autoregulation in patients with transient focal cerebral ischaemic attacks. *Neurology* **20**, 485–493.

Smeeth, L., Haines, R. & Ebrahim, S. (1999) Numbers needed to treat derived from meta-analyses: sometimes informative, usually misleading. *British Medical Journal* **318**, 1548–1551.

Solomon, N.A., Glick, H.A., Russo, C.J., Lee, J. & Schulman, K.A. (1994) Patient preferences for stroke outcomes. *Stroke* **25**, 1721–1725.

Stam, J., de Bruijn, S.T.F.M. & Deveber, G. (2000) Anticoagulants for cerebral sinus thrombosis. In: *The Cochrane Library*. Oxford: Update Software

Steiner, T. (1996) Naftidrofuryl in the treatment of acute cerebral hemisphere infarction. *Stroke* **27**, 32.

Steiner, T.J. & Clifford Rose, F. (1986) Randomized double blind placebo controlled clinical trial of naftidrofuryl in hemiparetic CT-proven acute cerebral hemisphere infarction. In: *Stroke: Epidemiological, Therapeutic Socio-Economic Aspects* (ed. F. Clifford-Rose), pp. 85–98. Royal Society of Medicine Services International Congress and Symposium Series No 99. London: Royal Society of Medicine Services Ltd.

Strandgaard, S. (1978) Autoregulation of cerebral circulation in hypertension. *Acta Neurologica Scandinavica* **57** (Suppl. 66), 1–82.

Strandgaard, S. & Paulson, O.B. (1984) Cerebral autoregulation. *Stroke* **15**, 413–441.

Strandgaard, S., Olesen, J., Skinhoj, E. & Lassen, N.A. (1973) Autoregulation of brain circulation in severe arterial hypertension. *British Medical Journal* i, 507–510.

Stroke Therapy Academic Industry Round Table (STAIR) (1999) Recommendations for standards regarding pre-clinical testing and restorative drug development. *Stroke* **30**, 2743–2751.

Sturzenegger, M., Mattle, H.P., Rivoir, A. & Baumgartner, R.W. (1995) Ultrasound findings in carotid artery dissection. Analysis of 43 patients. *Neurology* **45**, 691–698.

Sullivan, H.G., Kingsbury, T.B. & Morgan, M.E. (1987) The rCBF response to Diamox in normal subjects and cerebrovascular disease patients. *Journal of Neurosurgery* **67**, 525–534.

Symon, L., Branston, N.M. & Strong, A.J. (1976) Autoregulation in acute focal ischaemia. An experimental study. *Stroke* **7**, 547–554.

Symon, L., Branston, N.M. & Chikovani, O. (1979) Systemic brain oedema following middle cerebral artery occlusion in baboons: relationship between regional cerebral water content and blood flow at 1–2 hours. *Stroke* **2**, 184–191.

Takano, K., Latour, L.L., Formato, J.E. *et al.* (1996) The role of spreading depression in focal ischaemia evaluated by diffusion mapping. *Annals of Neurology* **39**, 308–316.

Thomas, D.J. (1982) Whole blood viscosity and cerebral blood flow. *Stroke* **13**, 285–287.

Thomson O'Brien, M.A., Oxman, A.D., Davis, D.A., Haynes, R.B., Freemantle, N. & Harvey, E.L. (2000) Audit and feedback. effects on professional practice and health care outcomes. In: *The Cochrane Library.* Oxford: Update Software.

Tiecks, F.P., Lam, A.M., Aaslid, R. & Newell, D.W. (1995) Comparison of static and dynamic cerebral autoregulation measurements. *Stroke* **26**, 1014–1019.

TOAST Investigators (1998) Low molecular weight heparinoid, ORG 10172 (Danaparoid), and outcome after acute ischaemic stroke. *Journal of the American Medical Association* **279**, 1265–1272.

Topol, E.J., Byzova, T.V. & Plow, E.F. (1999) Platelet GPIIb-IIIa blockers. *Lancet* **353**, 223–227.

Touzani, O., Young, A.R. & MacKenzie, E.T. (1994) The window of therapeutic opportunity following focal cerebral ischaemia. In: *Pharmacology of Cerebral Ischaemia* (eds J. Krieglstein & H. Oberpichler-Schwenk), pp. 575–588. Medpharm, Stuttgart.

Trouillas, P., Nighoghossian, N., Derex, L. *et al.* (1998) Thrombolysis with intravenous rTPA in a series of 100 cases of acute carotid territory stroke: determination of aetiological, topographic and radiological outcome factors. *Stroke* **29**, 2529–2540.

Turpie, A.G.G., Robinson, J.G. & Doyle, D.J. (1989) Comparison of high-dose with low-dose subcutaneous heparin to prevent left ventricular mural thrombosis in patients with acute transmural anterior myocardial infarction. *New England Journal of Medicine* **320**, 353–357.

Turpie, A.G.G., Gent, M., Laupacis, A., Latour, Y., Gunnstensen, J. & Basile, F. (1993) A comparison of aspirin with placebo in patients treated with warfarin after heart valve replacement. *New England Journal of Medicine* **329**, 524–529.

Vaitkus, P.T., Berllin, J.A., Schwartz, J.S. & Barnathan, E.S. (1992) Stroke complicating acute myocardial infarction. A meta-analysis of risk modification by anticoagulation and thrombolytic therapy. *Archives of Internal Medicine* **152**, 2020–2024.

Van Kooten, F., Ciabattoni, G., Patrono, C., Dippel, D.W. & Koudstaal, P.J. (1997) Platelet activation and lipid peroxidation patients with acute ischemic ischaemic stroke. *Stroke* **28**, 1557–1563.

Wade, D.T. and the Intercollegiate Working Party for Stroke (2000) *National Clinical Guidelines for Stroke.* London: The Royal College of Physicians of London (http://www.rcplondon.ac.uk).

Wahlgren, N.G., MacMahon, D.G., de Keyser, J., Indredavik, B. & Ryman, T. (1994) Intravenous Nimodipine West European Stroke Trial (INWEST) of nimodipine in the treatment of acute ischaemic stroke. *Cerebrovascular Diseases* **4**, 204–210.

Wardlaw, J.M. & Warlow, C. (1992) Thrombolysis in acute ischaemic stroke: does it work? *Stroke* **23**, 1826–1839.

Wardlaw, J.M., Dennis, M., Lindley, R.I., Warlow, C., Sandercock, P. & Sellar, R. (1993) Does early reperfusion of a cerebral infarct influence cerebral infarct swelling in the acute stage or the final clinical outcome? *Cerebrovascular Diseases* **3**, 86–93.

Wardlaw, J., Yamaguchi, T. & del Zoppo, G. (2000) Thrombolysis for acute ischaemic stroke. In: *The Cochrane Library*. Oxford: Update Software

Warkentin, T.E., Levine, M.N., Hirsh, J. *et al.* (1995) Heparin-induced thrombocytopenia in patients treated with low molecular weight heparin or unfractionated heparin. *New England Journal of Medicine* **332** (20), 1330–1335.

Weaver, J.P.A., Evans, A. & Walder, D.N. (1969) The effect of increased fibrinogen content on the viscosity of blood. *Clinical Science* **36**, 1–10.

Weir, N., Signorini, D. & Sandercock, P. (1999) Variations in outcome by country in the International Stroke Trial (IST). *Cerebrovascular Diseases* **9** (Suppl. 1), 36.

Wells, P.S., Lensing, A.W.A. & Hirsh, J. (1994) Graduated compression stockings in the prevention of postoperative venous thromboembolism: a meta analysis. *Archives of Internal Medicine* **154**, 67–72.

Welsh, S., Chant, G., Mead, G., Pole, R., O'Neill, P. & McCollum, C. (1999) Urgent carotid surgery in stroke. *Cerebrovascular Diseases* **9** (Suppl. 1), 43.

White, R.P. & Markus, H.S. (1997) Impaired dynamic cerebral autoregulation in carotid artery stenosis. *Stroke* **28**, 1340–1344.

Widder, B., Kleiser, B. & Krapf, H. (1994) Course of cerebrovascular reactivity in patients with carotid artery occlusion. *Stroke* **25**, 1963–1967.

Wilcox, J.N., Smith, K.M., Schwartz, S.M. & Gordon, D. (1989) Localisation of tissue factor in the normal vessel wall and in the atherosclerotic plaque. *Proceedings of the National Academy of Sciences of the USA* **86**,

2839–2843.

Wimmer, M.L., Sandmann-Strupp, R., Saikku, P. & Haberl, R.L. (1996) Association of chlamydial infection with cerebrovascular disease. *Stroke* **27**, 2207–2210.

Wise, R.J.S., Bernadi, S., Frackowiak, R.J.S., Legg, N.J. & Jones, T. (1983) Serial observations on the pathophysiology of acute stroke. The transition from ischaemia to infarction as reflected in regional oxygen extraction. *Brain* **106**, 197–222.

Wollner, L., McCarthy, S.T., Soper, N.D.W. & Macy, D.J. (1979) Failure of cerebral autoregulation as a cause of brain dysfunction in the elderly. *British Medical Journal* i; 1117–1118.

Wood, J.H. & Kee, D.B. (1985) Haemorrheology of the cerebral circulation in stroke. *Stroke* **16**, 765–772.

Woolf, S.H., Grol, R., Hutchinson, A., Eccles, M. & Grimshaw, J. (1999) Clinical guidelines: potential benefits, limitations and harms of clinical guidelines. *British Medical Journal* **318**, 527–530.

Yamaguchi, T., Hayakawa, T. & Kiuchi, H. (1993) Intravenous tissue plasminogen activator ameliorates the outcome of hyperacute embolic stroke. *Cerebrovascular Diseases* **3**, 269–272.

Yamashita, K., Ouchi, K., Shirai, M., Gondo, T., Makazawa, T. & Ito, H. (1998) Distribution of *Chlamydia pneumoniae* infection in the atherosclerotic carotid artery. *Stroke* **29**, 773–778.

Yamashita, T., Hayashi, M. & Kashiwagi, S. (1992) Cerebrovascular reserve capacity in ischaemia due to occlusion of a major arterial trunk: studies by Xe-CT and the acetazolamide test. *Journal of Computer Assisted Tomography* **16**, 750–755.

Yanagisawa, M., Kurihara, H. & Kimura, S. (1988) A novel potent vasoconstrictor peptide produced by vascular endothelial cells. *Nature* **332**, 411–415.

Yoshioka, A. (1998) Use of randomisation in the Medical Research Council's clinical trial of streptomycin in pulmonary tuberculosis in the 1940s. *British Medical Journal* **317**, 1220–1223.

Zhang, J. & Yu, K.F. (1998) What's the relative risk? A method of correcting the odds ratio in cohort studies of common outcomes. *Journal of the American Medical Association* **280**, 1690–1691.

Zhang, R.L., Chopp, M., Li, Y., Jiang, N. & Rusche, J.R. (1994) Anti-ICAM-1 antibody reduces ischaemic cell damage after transient middle cerebral artery occlusion in the rat. *Neurology* **44**, 1747–1751.

Zipfel, G.J., Lee, J.-M. & Choi, D.W. (1999) Reducing calcium overload in the ischaemic brain. *New England Journal of Medicine* **341**, 1543–1544.

Specific treatment of primary intracerebral haemorrhage

12.1 Pathophysiology

The pathophysiological events following the most common type of primary intracerebral haemorrhage—rupture of one or more deep perforating arteries—are surprisingly complex. Rupture of a blood vessel inevitably causes immediate disruption of white matter tracts, and irreversible damage to neurones in the deep nuclei or cortex. The protective encasement of the skull may become a disadvantage with sudden increases in volume within the intracranial cavity, as is the case with intracerebral haemorrhage. Apart from the brain tissue destroyed by the haemorrhage itself, the attendant increase in intracranial pressure threatens the other parts of the brain, particularly—but not exclusively—when the intracranial pressure reaches levels of the same order of magnitude as the arterial pressure, bringing the cerebral perfusion pressure close to zero. Direct mechanical compression of the brain tissue surrounding the haematoma and, to some extent, vasoconstrictor substances in extravasated blood, also lead to impaired local blood supply (Mendelow 1993). Cellular ischaemia leads to further swelling from oedema, which is initially cytotoxic and later vasogenic (section 11.1.5).

Hydrocephalus may be an additional space-occupying factor. This complication is especially likely to occur with cerebellar haematomas. However, a large haematoma in the region of the basal ganglia may also cause enlargement of the ventricular system, by rupture into the third ventricle, or through dilatation of the opposite lateral ventricle, with midline shift and obstruction of the third ventricle, whilst the ipsilateral ventricle is compressed (Ropper 1986). The zone of ischaemia around the haematoma may extend and swell through systemic factors such as hypotension or hypoxia. Often there is also loss of cerebral autoregulation in the vasculature supplying the region of the haematoma. Some perifocal ischaemic damage occurs at the time of bleeding and cannot be prevented, but the question to be considered here is whether the vicious cycle of ongoing ischaemia causing steadily increasing pressure can be interrupted in its early stages.

12.2 Management

12.2.1 Initial management

Once the patient's ventilation and circulation have been secured and the diagnosis of intracerebral haematoma confirmed by computed tomography (CT) scanning or magnetic resonance imaging (MRI), the next step is often to identify the cause before any specific treatment is initiated (Chapter 8). For example, if surgical evacuation of a life-threatening haematoma is considered, medical measures may have to be taken first (such as substitution of clotting factors in patients with liver failure or on anticoagulants). The surgeon should think twice if cerebral amyloid angiopathy is a likely cause, despite occasional reports in favour of surgical intervention (Izumihara *et al.* 1999). The danger is that the operation provokes new haemorrhages at distant sites (Waga *et al.* 1983; Brisman *et al.* 1996).

Repeated CT scanning is indicated if there is clinical deterioration, which may be caused by re-bleeding at the same or sometimes at a distant site, or by hydrocephalus; if there are no changes, the search for systemic causes of worsening should be intensified (section 15.5).

It is important to know when intervention is useless, i.e. when the outlook is either very good, or very bad. In both cases, only supportive care is called for. Nine separate studies have identified several factors with independent prognostic value for survival (Table 12.1). One group found that a predictive model with four factors (age, level of consciousness, pulse pressure and intraventricular extension of blood), applied to a different series of patients than that from which the model had been derived, correctly predicted the survival status in 94% of patients (Tuhrim *et al.* 1991). For example, a fatal outcome can be anticipated when there is no motor or other response to pain in a patient over 65 years of age with a large intracerebral haemorrhage, even if it is supratentorial. As these patients are invariably ventilated, it is important to exclude any effect of sedative drugs and neuromuscular blocking agents; in general, in patients who

Table 12.1 Factors associated with a poor prognosis in primary intracerebral haemorrhage.

Age (Daverat *et al.* 1991; Lisk *et al.* 1994; Juvela 1995; Fogelholm *et al.* 1997; Hårdemark *et al.* 1999)
Decreased level of consciousness (Portenoy *et al.* 1987; Tuhrim *et al.* 1988; 1994; Lisk *et al.* 1994; Juvela 1995; Hårdemark *et al.* 1999)
Alcohol ingestion in the previous week (Juvela 1995)
Pulse pressure (Tuhrim *et al.* 1988; Fogelholm *et al.* 1997; Terayama *et al.* 1997)
Haematoma volume (Portenoy *et al.* 1987; Tuhrim *et al.* 1988; Daverat *et al.* 1991; Lisk *et al.* 1994)
Intraventricular extension of the haemorrhage (Portenoy *et al.* 1987; Daverat *et al.* 1991; Lisk *et al.* 1994; Juvela 1995)
Hydrocephalus (Diringer *et al.* 1998)

require mechanical ventilation, the case fatality is more than 50% (Gujjar *et al.* 1998). Volumetric analysis alone may also guide prognosis: with supratentorial haemorrhages, the prognosis is poor when the volume of the haematoma exceeds 50 mL, or if the volume of intraventricular haemorrhage exceeds 20 mL (Franke *et al.* 1990; Young *et al.* 1990; Fogelholm *et al.* 1992). Extravasation of contrast material during CT scanning is another relatively bad prognostic sign, probably reflecting ongoing haemorrhage (Becker *et al.* 1999).

Factors predicting the prognosis for survival of patients with primary intracerebral haemorrhage are:
- *level of consciousness (Glasgow Coma Scale)*
- *age*
- *volume of haematoma (poor prognosis if supratentorial haematoma > 50 mL)*
- *intraventricular extension of haemorrhage (poor prognosis if volume > 20 mL)*

The blood pressure is usually increased in patients with intracerebral haematoma, through pre-existing hypertension, a response to a sudden increase in intracranial pressure, or both. There are theoretical arguments in favour of decreasing the blood pressure (in the hope of stopping ongoing bleeding from ruptured small arteries), as well as in favour of increasing it further (in the hope of salvaging marginally perfused areas of brain that are compressed around the haematoma). In the absence of even the flimsiest evidence supporting one or other point of view, the only rational course is to leave the blood pressure alone in the acute phase, unless it is elevated to such a degree that end-organ damage develops (especially in the retina and kidney). This is essentially the same advice as for patients with ischaemic stroke (sections 11.9 and 15.7.1). That is not to say that the patient should be discharged with an elevated blood pressure; a single observational study supports the notion that the long-term risk not only of cardiovascular events in general, but also of rebleeding, may be lowered by adequate blood pressure control (Arakawa *et al.* 1998) (section 16.3.1).

12.2.2 Reduction of intracranial pressure

It is usually assumed that the zone of brain tissue surrounding an intracerebral haematoma is ischaemic, but a unique study using positron emission tomography provided little support for this notion (Hirano *et al.* 1999). There are often factors other than the local effects of the haematoma itself that contribute to raised intracranial pressure. Frequently, these can be treated more directly than the intracerebral lesion, so it is important to be aware of them. They include fever, hypoxia, hypertension, seizures and elevations of intrathoracic pressure (Ropper 1993). A vexing and unsolved question is whether it is useful to measure the actual intracranial pressure by the introduction of an intraventricular catheter or other device, at least in patients with a decreased level of consciousness. Such regimens can certainly be rationalized (Ropper & King 1984; Broderick *et al.* 1999). On the other hand, any invasive procedure can give rise to complications, and the presumed advantages in terms of outcome have not been subjected to controlled studies. Therefore, we prefer to err on the side of caution and base management on clinical and radiological features. Raised intracranial pressure may also be a problem in some patients with ischaemic stroke (section 11.8).

Cerebrospinal fluid drainage

Insertion of a ventricular catheter may be a definitive measure in patients with cerebellar haemorrhage and no signs of direct compression of the brainstem (section 12.2.6). In patients with supratentorial haemorrhage and hydrocephalus, the benefits of cerebrospinal fluid (CSF) diversion are decidedly uncertain. In a series of 22 patients with supratentorial intracerebral haemorrhage and hydrocephalus who were treated with ventriculostomy, intracranial pressure was controlled at < 20 mmHg in 20, but only a single patient had any improvement in hydrocephalus as well as level of consciousness (Adams & Diringer 1998). Only three patients, with small haematoma volumes, survived to 3 months.

In patients with extensive intraventricular haemorrhage secondary to deep intraparenchymal or aneurysmal rupture, drainage of CSF is also performed in some centres, in an attempt to improve the dismal prognosis (section 12.2.1). A review of 22 observational studies suggested that this procedure may be especially helpful when it is combined with instillation of fibrinolytic drugs, but only direct comparisons in randomized controlled trials can establish the true value of these therapeutic measures, in other words the balance of risk and benefit (Nieuwkamp *et al.* 2000).

Hyperventilation

There is no doubt that hyperventilation decreases intracranial pressure, but at the same time there is no controlled evidence to allay concerns that the cure may be worse than the disease. The intracranial pressure goes down because hypocapnia (usually down to about 4 kPa) causes cerebral vasoconstriction; in other words, ischaemia by compression is exchanged for ischaemia by vasoconstriction. Moreover, experimental evidence suggests that the effect on the vessel diameter is short lived, of the order of 6 h; in patients with head injury, hypocapnia affects mainly normal brain vasculature, with a paradoxical increase of blood flow in the injured parts, which may be followed by increased oedema (Darby *et al.* 1988). A randomized controlled trial of prolonged hyperventilation in head-injured patients showed a worse outcome in the treatment group, although the numbers were small and the difference was statistically significant only after 3 and 6 months, but not at 1 year (Muizelaar *et al.* 1991). For patients with intracerebral haematomas, no randomized controlled trials of hyperventilation have been done, but the experience with head trauma is not encouraging. Provisionally, it seems best to reserve this treatment for bridging a few hours in patients for whom surgical evacuation is planned (sections 12.2.5 and 12.2.6).

Osmotic agents

Osmotic agents include mannitol, urea and glycerol, in doses between 0.5 and 2 g/kg. Iodide-containing contrast agents for angiography may have the same effect, although they are used for a different purpose. Osmotic agents extract water from the extracellular into the intravascular compartment of the brain, provided the blood–brain barrier between these two compartments is still intact. Shrinking of the brain therefore occurs especially in oedematous, but otherwise intact regions that surround a lesion with profoundly damaged tissue; the magnitude of the reduction in intracranial pressure parallels the amount of brain with preserved autoregulation (Muizelaar *et al.* 1984; Bell *et al.* 1987). The interval between the infusion and the decrease of intracranial pressure is usually less than an hour, but the effect of a single dose lasts no more than 4–6 h, because the concentration of the solute becomes equilibrated between the intravascular and extracellular compartments. Potential dangers of this treatment include hypotension, hypokalaemia, renal failure from hyperosmolality, haemolysis and congestive heart failure (Yu *et al.* 1992).

Small controlled trials of intravenous glycerol have claimed benefit for patients with acute stroke in general, of course mostly ischaemic (Bayer *et al.* 1987) (section 11.8.2). A somewhat larger trial (more than 100 patients in each group) specifically included patients with intracerebral haemorrhage, and showed no benefit (Yu *et al.* 1992).

Despite the lack of evidence from controlled studies, mannitol (20–25% solution) has become the mainstay of osmotic therapy in many centres. The correct dose cannot be predicted, but a safe regimen is 0.75–1 g/kg initially, then 0.25–0.5 kg every 3–5 h, depending on clinical findings and osmolality (the aim being 295–305 mosm/L initially; if needed, 310–320 mosm/L) (Ropper 1993). With such regimens, the central venous pressure should be monitored, and kept between 5 and 12 mmHg, to prevent hypovolaemia.

Mannitol is widely used in patients with primary intracerebral haemorrhage and a depressed level of consciousness, to decrease intracranial pressure and to alleviate the space-occupying effect of the haematoma in a deteriorating patient, although this custom is not backed up by randomized controlled trials that have clinical effect rather than pressure as the outcome. With corticosteroids, it has not yet been shown that the benefits outweigh the disadvantages.

Corticosteroids

Corticosteroids reduce peritumoral oedema and at first sight it seems rational to expect a similar effect on oedematous brain tissue around an intracerebral haematoma. There have been two small trials, the first undertaken in the early 1970s, before the advent of CT (Tellez & Bauer 1973), and a more recent study in Thailand (Poungvarin *et al.* 1987). Neither trial showed any difference in case fatality between the treated and control groups. The pooled odds ratio for the effect of steroids within the first 2–3 weeks is 1.0 (95% confidence interval [CI], 0.5–2.1). As in acute ischaemic stroke, there was no clear evidence that steroids reduced case fatality, and the confidence interval included the possibilities that steroids could have substantially reduced case fatality or substantially increased it. Only the trial by Poungvarin *et al.* (1987) reported on the proportion of patients making a complete recovery by the 21st day, and although there was a non-significant trend in favour of treatment (odds ratio 0.7; 95% CI, 0.2–2.4), any modest benefits in terms of functional improvement were, in this trial at least, outweighed by the complications of steroid treatment. Almost 50% of the steroid-treated group developed some complication (such as infection, diabetes or bleeding) compared with 13% amongst controls; this difference was highly significant. The trial included patients with all levels of consciousness, in a stratified design. On the basis of a subgroup analysis it might be argued that corticosteroids might, after all, do some good in patients with a Glasgow Coma Scale score of eight or more, but—quite apart from the pitfalls of data-dependent subgroup analyses in general—an advantage emerged only for the case fatality on day 7, and was lost on subsequent days. Thus, any benefit in terms of neurological function is moderate at best, whereas the adverse effects of corticosteroids in these patients are clearly substantial.

12.2.3 Prevention of deep venous thrombosis and pulmonary embolism (section 15.13)

Patients with intracerebral haemorrhage have a substantial risk of deep venous thrombosis (DVT): between 30% and 70%, depending on the severity of the stroke and the degree of immobilization, and on how hard one looks. The risk of pulmonary embolism is 1–5%, possibly higher (Dickmann *et al.* 1988). Of course, physicians are intuitively cautious in using antithrombotic drugs in patients with intracerebral haematomas. On the other hand, drug regimens that prevent clotting as a consequence of venous stasis do not necessarily increase the risk that a small artery in the brain will rupture for a second time. The definitive answer should of course come from clinical trials, not from theoretical considerations.

Subcutaneous heparin

Subcutaneous heparin, usually given as 5000 U two or three times a day, reduces the relative frequency of DVT by 68%, at least after general, orthopaedic and urologic surgery (Collins *et al.* 1988) (section 15.13). In a small, but so far unique, trial in 46 patients with intracerebral haematoma, this regimen was applied 4 days after the haemorrhage in the active treatment group and 10 days after the haemorrhage in the control group (Dickmann *et al.* 1988). Forty per cent (nine of 23) of the patients in the control group developed some evidence of pulmonary embolism (as detected by isotope perfusion lung scanning), against 22% (five of 22) in the treated group. The number of deaths was far too small to exclude the possibility that routine heparin prophylaxis for such patients could substantially increase the risk of fatal intracerebral re-bleeding. In a subsequent non-randomized study, in 68 patients with intracerebral haematoma, treatment was started on day 2, 4, or 10 after the haemorrhage (Boeer *et al.* 1991). For what it is worth, the rate of pulmonary embolism was significantly lower in the group with treatment started on day 2 compared with the other two groups, without a concomitant increase in re-bleeding. But because the group with early treatment was studied after the two other dosage groups, the results may well have been influenced by factors other than the interval before the initiation of treatment.

Aspirin

Aspirin is effective in preventing DVT (approximately 39% relative risk reduction) as well as pulmonary embolism in an overview of all trials in the perioperative period and in medical patients at increased risk (section 11.3.2). Its safety in patients with intracerebral haemorrhage has not been studied, but it is unlikely that the risk of re-bleeding with aspirin is greater than with subcutaneous heparin.

Compression stockings

These are of course the safest method of prophylaxis in patients with intracerebral haematoma, although occasionally pressure sores may be induced (section 15.13). The efficacy of this measure was studied in 12 methodologically sound clinical trials, mostly in patients with moderate risk (after abdominal, gynaecological and intracranial operations), the collective evidence pointing towards a relative risk reduction in DVT of the order of 70% (Wells *et al.* 1994). The occurrence of pulmonary embolism was not included in the 1994 systematic review, but a positive effect emerged from a large trial in patients who underwent cardiothoracic operations (Ramas *et al.* 1996). Thus, unless the disadvantages of heparin are proved to be merely theoretical, application of graduated compression stockings seems to offer the greatest protection and the smallest risk, although the method is fairly labour-intensive and the stockings can be uncomfortable after a time.

Subcutaneous heparin and graduated compression stockings both decrease the risk of deep venous thrombosis in bedridden patients by approximately 70%, and aspirin by approximately 39%, as judged from clinical trials in a variety of postoperative conditions. Because the safety of heparin and aspirin is largely unknown in patients with primary intracerebral haemorrhage, compression stockings are the preferred method of prophylaxis, despite being labour-intensive, and despite the lack of any direct randomized trial evidence in patients with primary intracerebral haemorrhage.

12.2.4 Iatrogenic intracerebral haemorrhage

Anticoagulants

Anticoagulants are associated with an increased risk of intracerebral haemorrhage, although it is difficult to estimate the actual risk, because the underlying condition for which the treatment is being given also contributes to the risk (confounding by indication) (section 8.4.1). It seems rational to reverse the deficiency of clotting factors as quickly as possible, especially in view of the frequent progression of neurological deficits that occurs in these patients, but the validity of this reasoning has never been put to the test in a randomized trial (Kase *et al.* 1985). The first step is intravenous injection of 10–20 mg of vitamin K, at not more than 5 mg/min, followed by infusion of a concentrate of the coagulation factors II, VII, IX and X, or of fresh frozen plasma. Infusion of the factors alone restores the coagulation system more rapidly than whole plasma, and is safer from the point of view of transmission of virus particles (Fredriksson *et al.* 1992) (section 11.4.7). Others advocate prothrombin complex concentrates to antagonize anticoagulants in patients with intracranial haemorrhage, but again only on theoretical grounds (Butler & Tait 1998).

When to resume anticoagulants in patients with a strong indication for this treatment (e.g. those with artificial heart valves) is a problem many clinicians will recognize, but for which only anecdotal experience is available. The essential issue is probably not when evidence of blood has disappeared from the CT scan (that may take weeks or months), but when the ruptured vessel can be assumed to have sufficiently healed. One or two weeks is probably not a bad guess, unless an untreated aneurysm underlies the haemorrhage, as no re-bleeds were reported with such a regimen, although the numbers were small (Leker & Abramsky 1998; Wijdicks *et al.* 1998).

Thrombolytic therapy

Thrombolytic therapy after myocardial infarction is complicated by intracerebral haemorrhage in only a small proportion, but the case fatality is high (section 8.4.3). This grim prognosis warrants attempts at intervention, even without the benefits of randomized trials (Eleff *et al.* 1990; Mahaffey *et al.* 1999). These measures include control of any hypertension and infusion of coagulation factors; the use of antifibrinolytic drugs is controversial even from a theoretical point of view. Life-threatening dysrhythmias may occur as a complication of the myocardial infarct for which the treatment was given, often before the onset of the neurological symptoms, and these should be promptly treated (Sloan *et al.* 1995).

There is no evidence about what to do in patients who develop major intracerebral haemorrhage after thrombolytic treatment for ischaemic stroke (section 11.5). In view of the little we know about operative treatment for primary intracerebral haemorrhage in general (section 12.2.5), it seems best to leave well alone. Also the use of fresh frozen plasma and other measures to reverse the anticoagulant/thrombolytic state may only result in further complications.

Aspirin

Aspirin treatment is associated with a small risk of intracerebral haemorrhage (section 8.4.2). It is reasonable to stop the drug once the diagnosis is made, although no disasters have been documented in instances in which aspirin was continued, or even instituted. At any rate, the antiplatelet effect lasts for several days after discontinuing the drug (Patrono *et al.* 1985). In most trials of aspirin for the secondary prevention of stroke, a handful with small intracerebral haemorrhages have inadvertently been included, before CT scanning established the true diagnosis. However, on balance, aspirin is still effective in preventing stroke overall (section 16.4.1). In the International Stroke Trial, there were more than 700 such patients, in 65% of whom the treatment was discontinued after the CT scan result became available; there were no obviously untoward effects, but the confidence interval was still wide (Sandercock *et al.* 1997; Keir *et al.* 2000). Nobody knows when it is safe to restart aspirin. If there is a very strong indication, then perhaps after a week is reasonable on the assumption that any ruptured blood vessel will be sufficiently healed by then.

12.2.5 Surgery for supratentorial haemorrhage

The frequency of surgical intervention for intracerebral haematoma varies from practically nil, even in developed countries (Franke *et al.* 1992), to 20% of all patients in a metropolitan community of the United States (Greater Cincinnati) (Broderick *et al.* 1994), or even 50% or more of patients in some centres in Germany and Japan (Niizuma *et al.* 1989; Mohadjer *et al.* 1992). This variation must reflect clinical uncertainty, or lack of appropriate evidence from randomized controlled trials (RCTs). It is a great anomaly in medicine and society that surgical methods of treatment are allowed if they are plausible and generally accepted by the surgical community, whereas the introduction of new drugs is safeguarded by a multitude of laws and regulations.

There are four possible surgical procedures to treat intracerebral haematoma: simple aspiration, craniotomy with open surgery, endoscopic evacuation and stereotactic aspiration (Kaufman 1993). Four RCTs have been performed in this area; these have been subjected to a Cochrane review, the results of which are included below (Prasad & Shrivastava 2000). Unless specifically indicated otherwise, the assumption is that we are dealing with deep haemorrhages, from degenerative small vessel disease.

Simple aspiration

Simple aspiration was attempted mainly in the 1950s, but was abandoned because only small amounts of clot could be obtained, and because the procedure could precipitate 'blind' re-bleeding (McKissock *et al.* 1959; Mitsuno *et al.* 1966).

Craniotomy

Open surgery has been the method for removing haematomas in three trials, one of them dating from the pre-CT era (McKissock *et al.* 1961; Juvela *et al.* 1989; Batjer *et al.* 1990). The combined results show that craniotomy is definitely harmful (Fig. 12.1), because of a statistically significant increase in the odds of death or dependency of 2.00 (95% CI, 1.11–3.60). For death alone, the odds ratio with operation was 1.44, with a 95% confidence interval of 0.87–2.37. The largest of the three trials was reported in 1961, but the

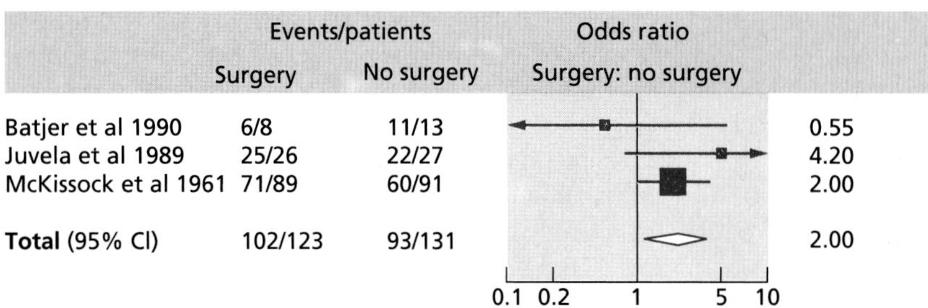

Events/patients
Odds ratio
Surgery
No surgery
Surgery: no surgery
Batjer et al 1990 6/8 11/13 0.55
Juvela et al 1989 25/26 22/27 4.20
McKissock et al 1961 71/89 60/91 2.00
Total (95% CI) 102/123 93/131 2.00
0.1 0.2 1 5 10

Fig. 12.1 The results of a systematic review of three randomized trials that examined the effect of surgery for supratentorial haematoma. Auer *et al.* (1989) evaluated endoscopic evacuation, so their results have not been included in the figure. The boxes show the odds ratio for patients who were dead or dependent at final follow-up. The horizontal bars indicate the 95% confidence intervals. An odds ratio of greater than 1.0 indicates that more patients were dead or dependent in the surgically treated group (reproduced with permission from Prasad & Shrivastava 2000).

two trials with CT (Juvela *et al.* 1989; Batjer *et al.* 1990) also showed a non-significant trend towards an increase in death or dependency (Prasad & Shrivastava 2000). After this Cochrane review, two small single-centre randomized trials were published, with 54 patients altogether; the results were entirely within the range of the overview (Morgenstern *et al.* 1998; Zuccarello *et al.* 1999).

Endoscopic evacuation

Endoscopic evacuation by stereotactic methods was studied in an RCT involving two groups of 50 patients (Auer *et al.* 1989). The authors' interpretation was that surgery had no effect in putaminal and thalamic haemorrhage, but that it was beneficial in subcortical haematomas, provided the patients were aged 60 years or less, and were alert or only drowsy. The problem with this analysis is that not only does it depend on subgroups, but also no overall analysis was reported, and some outcome categories were not reported at all. Recalculation of the results for all patients, according to the proportion who were dead or dependent, showed that surgery reduced this proportion by 24%, which just missed being statistically significant (relative risk 0.76; 95% CI, 0.56–1.02). The effect appears stronger in patients under 60 years and with haematoma volumes exceeding 50 mL. The point estimate of the absolute risk difference was 18% (death or dependency is avoided for 18 out of 100 surgically treated patients), but the true effect may well be anywhere between a benefit of 36 patients avoiding death or dependency and a hazard of three extra patients being dead or dependent per 100 patients surgically treated (Prasad & Shrivastava 2000). In conclusion, stereotactic endoscopic evacuation is a promising technique, but its benefits and specific indications remain to be confirmed by well-conducted and large randomized controlled trials.

Stereotactic aspiration

Stereotactic aspiration without endoscopy, usually combined with instillation of fibrinolytic agents, has been reported in more than 400 patients with supratentorial haemorrhage, either intraparenchymal (Matsumoto & Hondo 1984; Niizuma *et al.* 1989; Mohadjer *et al.* 1992; Miller *et al.* 1993) or intraventricular (Rohde *et al.* 1995). The time has now come for randomized controlled trials of this technique before it is adopted in routine clinical practice, or perhaps rejected.

12.2.6 Surgery for infratentorial haemorrhage

Cerebellar haematomas

Cerebellar haematomas (Figs 8.18 & 12.2) have fairly characteristic clinical features (section 8.8.2), with the exception of massive haemorrhages, which are clinically indistinguishable from brainstem strokes (Gerritsen van der Hoop *et al.* 1988; Ogata *et al.* 1988), and very small haemorrhages, which may mimic a peripheral vestibular disorder (Dunne *et al.* 1987; Gerritsen van der Hoop *et al.* 1988) (section 3.3.7). For decades, there has been a strong impression that surgical evacuation saves lives in patients with cerebellar haematomas who have clinical evidence of progressive compression of the brainstem (Fisher *et al.* 1965). So strong is this impression that a randomized trial in this category of patients is as unlikely to be mounted as it would be in acute appendicitis. But that is not to say there are no areas of controversy.

Firstly, there is no doubt that some patients can be managed conservatively, but there is uncertainty about the selection criteria (Ott *et al.* 1974). In general, an impaired level of consciousness (that is, a Glasgow Coma Scale Score of 13/15 or less) seems a good indication for surgery, provided the brainstem reflexes have not been lost for hours, in which case the outcome is invariably fatal (Kobayashi *et al.* 1994). Some neurosurgeons advocate surgery with large haematomas (> 3–4 cm in diameter), even in alert patients, based on the experience that delayed deterioration of consciousness may be so rapid that the patient cannot be salvaged at this later stage (Brillman 1979; Lui *et al.* 1985; Kobayashi *et*

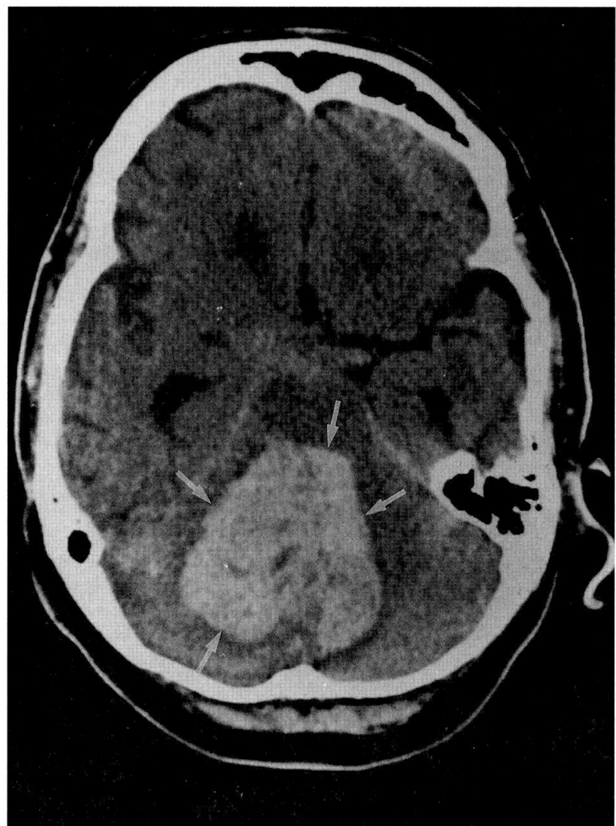

Fig. 12.2 CT brain scan, showing a large cerebellar haematoma (arrows).

al. 1994). Especially haematomas in the vermis, and those associated with distortion of the quadrigeminal cistern, may give rise to continuing deterioration (Taneda *et al.* 1987; St Louis *et al.* 1998). On the other hand, patients with cerebellar haematomas larger than 3–4 cm in size may retain a nearly normal level of consciousness (drowsy, disorientated, or both) and subsequently survive without operation (Bogousslavsky *et al.* 1984; Gerritsen van der Hoop *et al.* 1988).

A second contentious issue is that some neurosurgeons argue that it is not direct compression of the brainstem, but obstructive hydrocephalus that is the main problem, and that ventriculostomy is a sufficient measure to prevent a fatal outcome (Shenkin & Zavala 1982). Such an approach may be justified in some patients, with progressive obtundation and hydrocephalus without clinical signs of brainstem compression. Against the adoption of ventricular shunting as a panacea for cerebellar haematomas is the rapid disappearance of pupillary, corneal and oculocephalic reflexes, something not seen with acute hydrocephalus from other causes (van Gijn *et al.* 1985), and also the frequent failure of ventricular shunting to improve the level of consciousness (Mathew *et al.* 1995).

Surgical evacuation of cerebellar haematomas can be life-saving, often with surprisingly few neurological sequelae. Sound indications for evacuation are the combination of a depressed level of consciousness with signs of progressive brainstem compression (unless all brainstem reflexes have been lost for more than a few hours, in which case a fatal outcome is unavoidable), or haematoma greater than 3–4 cm in diameter. If the patient has a depressed level of consciousness and hydrocephalus, without signs of brainstem compression and with a haematoma less than 3 cm, ventriculostomy can be carried out as an initial (and perhaps only) procedure.

As with supratentorial haemorrhage, some patients with cerebellar haemorrhage have been successfully treated by stereotactic aspiration, with or without instillation of fibrinolytic drugs (Niizuma & Suzuki 1987). Any advantage of these techniques over the conventional approach with suboccipital craniotomy remains to be proved.

Pontine haemorrhages

Pontine haemorrhages are not as invariably fatal as when the diagnosis could only be made at post-mortem, but the case fatality is still about 60% (Kushner & Bressman 1985; Masiyama *et al.* 1985) (section 8.8.2) (Fig. 12.3). The management of these patients is usually conservative, but some case reports have documented successful stereotactic aspiration (Beatty & Zervas 1973; Bosch & Beute 1985; Niizuma

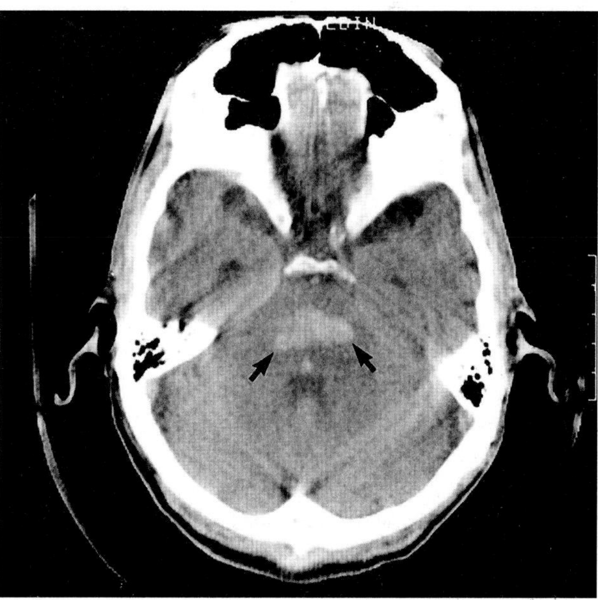

Fig. 12.3 CT brain scan, showing a pontine haematoma (arrows) in a patient who walked, unsteadily, into (and out of) the out-patient clinic.

& Suzuki 1987). The natural history may or may not have been influenced by these interventions, and surgical failures in similar cases are likely to receive rather less medical publicity.

References

Please note that all references taken from *The Cochrane Library* are given a current date as this database is updated on a quarterly basis. Please refer to the current *Cochrane Library* article for the latest review. The same applies to the *British Medical Journal* 'Clinical Evidence' series which is updated every six months.

Adams, R.E. & Diringer, M.N. (1998) Response to external ventricular drainage in spontaneous intracerebral hemorrhage with hydrocephalus. *Neurology* **50**, 519–523.

Arakawa, S., Saku, Y., Ibayashi, S., Nagao, T. & Fujishima, M. (1998) Blood pressure control and recurrence of hypertensive brain hemorrhage. *Stroke* **29**, 1806–1809.

Auer, L.M., Deinsberger, W., Niederkorn, K. *et al.* (1989) Endoscopic surgery versus medical treatment for spontaneous intracerebral hematoma: a randomized study. *Journal of Neurosurgery* **70**, 530–535.

Batjer, H.H., Reisch, J.S., Allen, B.C., Plaizier, L.J. & Su, C.J. (1990) Failure of surgery to improve outcome in hypertensive putaminal hemorrhage: a prospective randomized trial. *Archives of Neurology* **47**, 1103–1106.

Bayer, A.J., Pathy, M.S. & Newcombe, R. (1987) Double-blind randomised trial of intravenous glycerol in acute stroke. *Lancet* **i**, 405–408.

Beatty, R.M. & Zervas, N.T. (1973) Stereotactic aspiration of a brain stem hematoma. *Neurosurgery* **13**, 204–207.

Becker, K.J., Baxter, A.B., Bybee, H.M., Tirschwell, D.L. & Abouelsaad, T. (1999) Extravasation of radiographic contrast is an independent predictor of death in primary intracerebral hemorrhage. *Stroke* **30**, 2025–2032.

Bell, B.A., Smith, M.A., Kean, D.M., McGhee, C.N. *et al.* (1987) Brain water measured by magnetic resonance imaging: correlation with direct estimation and changes after mannitol and dexamethasone. *Lancet* **1**, 66–69.

Boeer, A., Voth, E., Henze, T. & Prange, H.W. (1991) Early heparin therapy in patients with spontaneous intracerebral haemorrhage. *Journal of Neurology, Neurosurgery and Psychiatry* **54**, 466–467.

Bogousslavsky, J., Regli, F. & Jeanrenaud, X. (1984) Benign outcome in unoperated large cerebellar haemorrhage: report of 2 cases. *Acta Neurochirurgica (Wien)* **73**, 59–65.

Bosch, D.A. & Beute, G.N. (1985) Successful stereotaxic evacuation of an acute pontomedullary hematoma: case report. *Journal of Neurosurgery* **62**, 153–156.

Brillman, J. (1979) Acute hydrocephalus and death one month after nonsurgical treatment for acute cerebellar hemorrhage: case report. *Journal of Neurosurgery* **50**, 374–376.

Brisman, M.H., Bederson, J.B., Sen, C.N., Germano, I.M., Moore, F. & Post, K.D. (1996) Intracerebral hemorrhage occurring remote from the craniotomy site. *Neurosurgery* **39**, 1114–1121.

Broderick, J.P, Brott, T., Tomsick, T., Tew, J., Duldner, J. & Huster, G. (1994) Management of intracerebral hemorrhage in a large metropolitan population. *Neurosurgery* **34**, 882–887.

Broderick, J.P., Adams, H.P. Jr, Barsan, W. *et al.* (1999) Guidelines for the management of spontaneous intracerebral hemorrhage: a statement for healthcare professionals from a special writing group of the Stroke Council, American Heart Association. *Stroke* **30**, 905–915.

Butler, A.C. & Tait, R.C. (1998) Management of oral anticoagulant-induced intracranial haemorrhage. *Blood Reviews* **12**, 35–44.

Collins, R., Scrimgeour, A., Yusuf, S. & Peto, R. (1988) Reduction in fatal pulmonary embolism and venous thrombosis by perioperative administration of subcutaneous heparin: overview of results of randomized trials in general, orthopedic, and urologic surgery. *New England Journal of Medicine* **318**, 1162–1173.

Darby, J.M., Yonas, H., Marion, D.W. & Latchaw, R.E. (1988) Local 'inverse steal' induced by hyperventilation in head injury. *Neurosurgery* **23**, 84–88.

Daverat, P., Castel, J.P., Dartigues, J.F. & Orgogozo, J.M. (1991) Death and functional outcome after spontaneous intracerebral hemorrhage: a prospective study of 166 cases using multivariate analysis. *Stroke* **22**, 1–6.

Dickmann, U., Voth, E., Schicha, H., Henze, T., Prange, H. & Emrich, D. (1988) Heparin therapy, deep-vein thrombosis and pulmonary embolism after intracerebral hemorrhage. *Klinische Wochenschrift* **66**, 1182–1183.

Diringer, M.N., Edwards, D.F. & Zazulia, A.R. (1998) Hydrocephalus: a previously unrecognized predictor of poor outcome from supratentorial intracerebral hemorrhage. *Stroke* **29**, 1352–1357.

Dunne, J.W., Chakera, T. & Kermode, S. (1987) Cerebellar haemorrhage: diagnosis and treatment: a study of 75 consecutive cases. *Quarterly Journal of Medicine* **64**, 739–754.

Eleff, S.M., Borel, C., Bell, W.R. & Long, D.M. (1990) Acute management of intracranial hemorrhage in patients receiving thrombolytic therapy: case reports. *Neurosurgery* **26**, 867–869.

Fisher, C.M., Picard, E.H., Polak, A., Dalal, P. & Ojemann, R. (1965) Acute hypertensive cerebellar hemorrhage. *Journal of Nervous and Mental Disease* **140**, 38–57.

Fogelholm, R., Nuutila, M. & Vuorela, A.L. (1992) Primary intracerebral haemorrhage in the Jyvaskyla region, central Finland, 1985–89: incidence, case fatality rate, and functional outcome. *Journal of Neurology, Neurosurgery and Psychiatry* **55**, 546–552.

Fogelholm, R., Avikainen, S. & Murros, K. (1997) Prognostic value and determinants of first-day mean arterial pressure in spontaneous supratentorial intracerebral hemorrhage. *Stroke* **28**, 1396–1400.

Franke, C.L., de Jonge, J., van Swieten, J.C., Op de Coul, A.A.W. & van Gijn, J. (1990) Intracerebral hematomas during anticoagulant treatment. *Stroke* **21**, 726–730.

Franke, C.L., van Swieten, J.C., Algra, A. & van Gijn, J. (1992) Prognostic factors in patients with intracerebral haematoma. *Journal of Neurology, Neurosurgery and Psychiatry* **55**, 653–657.

Fredriksson, K., Norrving, B. & Stromblad, L.G. (1992) Emergency reversal of anticoagulation after intracerebral hemorrhage. *Stroke* **23**, 972–977.

Gerritsen van der Hoop, R., Vermeulen, M. & van Gijn, J. (1988) Cerebellar hemorrhage: diagnosis and treatment. *Surgical Neurology* **29**, 6–10.

van Gijn, J., Hijdra, A., Wijdicks, E.F.M., Vermeulen, M. & van Crevel, H. (1985) Acute hydrocephalus after aneurysmal subarachnoid hemorrhage. *Journal of Neurosurgery* **63**, 355–362.

Gujjar, A.R., Deibert, E., Manno, E.M., Duff, S. & Diringer, M.N. (1998) Mechanical ventilation for ischemic stroke and intracerebral hemorrhage: indications, timing, and outcome. *Neurology* **51**, 447–451.

Hårdemark, H.G., Wesslén, N. & Persson, H. (1999) Influence of clinical factors, CT findings and early management on outcome in supratentorial intracerebral hemorrhage. *Cerebrovascular Diseases* **9**, 10–21.

Hirano, T., Read, S.J., Abbott, D.F. *et al.* (1999) No evidence of hypoxic tissue on ^{18}F-fluoromisonidazole PET after intracerebral hemorrhage. *Neurology* **53**, 2179–2182.

Izumihara, A., Ishihara, T., Iwamoto, N., Yamashita, K. & Ito, H. (1999) Postoperative outcome of 37 patients with lobar intracerebral hemorrhage related to cerebral amyloid angiopathy. *Stroke* **30**, 29–33.

Juvela, S. (1995) Risk factors for impaired outcome after spontaneous intracerebral hemorrhage. *Archives of Neurology* **52**, 1193–1200.

Juvela, S., Heiskanen, O., Poranen, A. *et al.* (1989) The treatment of spontaneous intracerebral hemorrhage: a prospective randomized trial of surgical and conservative treatment. *Journal of Neurosurgery* **70**, 755–758.

Kase, C.S., Robinson, R.K., Stein, R.W. *et al.* (1985) Anticoagulant-related intracerebral hemorrhage. *Neurology* **35**, 943–948.

Kaufman, H.H. (1993) Treatment of deep spontaneous intracerebral hematomas: a review. *Stroke* **24**, I101–I106.

Keir, S.L., Lewis, S.C., Wardlaw, J.M., Sandercock, P.A. on behalf of IST and CAST collaborative groups (2000) Effect of aspirin or heparin given to patients with hemorrhagic stroke. *Stroke* **31**, 314 (abstract).

Kobayashi, S., Sato, A., Kageyama, Y., Nakamura, H., Watanabe, Y. & Yamaura, A. (1994) Treatment of hypertensive cerebellar hemorrhage: surgical or conservative management? *Neurosurgery* **34**, 246–250.

Kushner, M.J. & Bressman, S.B. (1985) The clinical manifestations of pontine hemorrhage. *Neurology* **35**, 637–643.

Leker, R.R. & Abramsky, O. (1998) Early anticoagulation in patients with prosthetic heart valves and intracerebral hematoma. *Neurology* **50**, 1489–1491.

Lisk, D.R., Pasteur, W., Rhoades, H., Putnam, R.D. & Grotta, J.C. (1994) Early presentation of hemispheric intracerebral hemorrhage: prediction of outcome and guidelines for treatment allocation. *Neurology* **44**, 133–139.

Lui, T.N., Fairholm, D.J., Shu, T.F., Chang, C.N., Lee, S.T. & Chen, H.R. (1985) Surgical treatment of spontaneous cerebellar hemorrhage. *Surgical*

Neurology **23**, 555–558.

McKissock, W., Richardson, A. & Walsh, L. (1959) Primary intracerebral haematoma: results of surgical treatment in 244 consecutive cases. *Lancet* **ii**, 683–686.

McKissock, W., Richardson, A. & Taylor, J. (1961) Primary intracerebral haemorrhage: a controlled trial of surgical and conservative treatment in 180 unselected cases. *Lancet* **ii**, 221–226.

Mahaffey, K.W., Granger, C.B., Sloan, M.A. *et al.* (1999) Neurosurgical evacuation of intracranial hemorrhage after thrombolytic therapy for acute myocardial infarction: experience from the GUSTO-I Trial. *American Heart Journal* **138**, 493–499.

Masiyama, S., Niizuma, H. & Suzuki, J. (1985) Pontine haemorrhage: a clinical analysis of 26 cases. *Journal of Neurology, Neurosurgery and Psychiatry* **48**, 658–662.

Mathew, P., Teasdale, G., Bannan, A. & Oluoch-Olunya, D. (1995) Neurosurgical management of cerebellar haematoma and infarct. *Journal of Neurology, Neurosurgery and Psychiatry* **59**, 287–292.

Matsumoto, K. & Hondo, H. (1984) CT-guided stereotaxic evacuation of hypertensive intracerebral hematomas. *Journal of Neurosurgery* **61**, 440–448.

Mendelow, A.D. (1993) Mechanisms of ischemic brain damage with intracerebral hemorrhage. *Stroke* **24** (Suppl. I), 115–117.

Miller, D.W., Barnett, G.H., Kormos, D.W. & Steiner, C.P. (1993) Stereotactically guided thrombolysis of deep cerebral hemorrhage: preliminary results. *Cleveland Clinic Journal of Medicine* **60**, 321–324.

Mitsuno, T., Kanaya, H., Shirakata, S., Ohsawa, K. & Ishikawa, Y. (1966) Surgical treatment of hypertensive intracerebral hemorrhage. *Journal of Neurosurgery* **24**, 70–76.

Mohadjer, M., Braus, D.F., Myers, A., Scheremet, R. & Krauss, J.K. (1992) CT-stereotactic fibrinolysis of spontaneous intracerebral hematomas. *Neurosurgical Review* **15**, 105–110.

Morgenstern, L.B., Frankowski, R.F., Shedden, P., Pasteur, W. & Grotta, J.C. (1998) Surgical treatment for intracerebral hemorrhage (STICH): a single-center, randomized clinical trial. *Neurology* **51**, 1359–1363.

Muizelaar, J.P., Lutz, H.A. & Becker, D.P. (1984) Effect of mannitol on ICP and CBF and correlation with pressure autoregulation in severely head-injured patients. *Journal of Neurosurgery* **61**, 700–706.

Muizelaar, J.P., Marmarou, A., Ward, J.D. *et al.* (1991) Adverse effects of prolonged hyperventilation in patients with severe head injury: a randomized clinical trial. *Journal of Neurosurgery* **75**, 731–739.

Nieuwkamp, D.J., de Gans, K., Rinkel, G.J.E. & Algra, A. (2000) Treatment and outcome of severe intraventricular extension in patients with subarachnoid or intracerebral hemorrhage: a systematic review of the literature. *Journal of Neurology* **247**, 117–121.

Niizuma, H. & Suzuki, J. (1987) Computed tomography-guided stereotactic aspiration of posterior fossa hematomas: a supine lateral retromastoid approach. *Neurosurgery* **21**, 422–427.

Niizuma, H., Shimizu, Y., Yonemitsu, T., Nakasato, N. & Suzuki, J. (1989) Results of stereotactic aspiration in 175 cases of putaminal hemorrhage. *Neurosurgery* **24**, 814–819.

Ogata, J., Imakita, M., Yutani, C., Miyamoto, S. & Kikuchi, H. (1988) Primary brainstem death: a clinico-pathological study. *Journal of Neurology, Neurosurgery and Psychiatry* **51**, 646–650.

Ott, K.H., Kase, C.S., Ojemann, R.G. & Mohr, J.P. (1974) Cerebellar hemorrhage: diagnosis and treatment: a review of 56 cases. *Archives of Neurology* **31**, 160–167.

Patrono, C., Ciabattoni, G., Patrignani, P. *et al.* (1985) Clinical pharmacology of platelet cyclooxygenase inhibition. *Circulation* **72**, 1177–1184.

Portenoy, R.K., Lipton, R.B., Berger, A.R., Lesser, M.L. & Lantos, G. (1987) Intracerebral haemorrhage: a model for the prediction of outcome. *Journal of Neurology, Neurosurgery and Psychiatry* **50**, 976–979.

Poungvarin, N., Bhoopat, W., Viriyavejakul, A. *et al.* (1987) Effects of dexamethasone in primary supratentorial intracerebral hemorrhage. *New England Journal of Medicine* **316**, 1229–1233.

Prasad, K. & Shrivastava, A. (2000) Surgery for primary supratentorial intracerebral haemorrhage. In: *The Cochrane Library*. Oxford: Update Software.

Ramas, R., Salem, B.I., De Pawlikowski, M.P., Goordes, C., Eisenberg, S. & Leidenfrost, R. (1996) The efficacy of pneumatic compression stockings in the prevention of pulmonary embolism after cardiac surgery. *Chest* **109**, 82–85.

Rohde, V., Schaller, C. & Hassler, W.E. (1995) Intraventricular recombinant tissue plasminogen activator for lysis of intraventricular haemorrhage. *Journal of Neurology, Neurosurgery and Psychiatry* **58**, 447–451.

Ropper, A.H. (1986) Lateral displacement of the brain and level of consciousness in patients with an acute hemispheral mass. *New England Journal of Medicine* **314**, 953–958.

Ropper, A.H. (1993) Treatment of intracranial hypertension. In: *Neurological and Neurosurgical Intensive Care* (ed. A.H. Ropper) 3rd edn, pp. 29–52. Raven Press, New York.

Ropper, A.H. & King, R.B. (1984) Intracranial pressure monitoring in comatose patients with cerebral hemorrhage. *Archives of Neurology* **41**, 725–728.

Sandercock, P., Collins, R., Counsell, C. *et al.* (1997) The International Stroke Trial (IST): a randomised trial of aspirin, subcutaneous heparin, both, or neither among 19,435 patients with acute ischaemic stroke. *Lancet* **349**, 1569–1581.

Shenkin, H.A. & Zavala, H. (1982) Cerebellar strokes: mortality, surgical indications, and results of ventricular drainage. *Lancet* **ii**, 429–431.

Sloan, M.A., Price, T.R., Petito, C.K. *et al.* (1995) Clinical features and pathogenesis of intracerebral hemorrhage after rt-PA and heparin therapy for acute myocardial infarction: the Thrombolysis in Myocardial Infarction (TIMI) II pilot and randomized clinical trial combined experience. *Neurology* **45**, 649–658.

St Louis, E.K., Wijdicks, E.F.M. & Li, H.Z. (1998) Predicting neurologic deterioration in patients with cerebellar hematomas. *Neurology* **51**, 1364–1369.

Taneda, M., Hayakawa, T. & Mogami, H. (1987) Primary cerebellar hemorrhage: quadrigeminal cistern obliteration on CT scans as a predictor of outcome. *Journal of Neurosurgery* **67**, 545–552.

Tellez, H. & Bauer, R.B. (1973) Dexamethasone as treatment in cerebrovascular disease, 1: a controlled study in intracerebral hemorrhage. *Stroke* **4**, 541–546.

Terayama, Y., Tanahashi, N., Fukuuchi, Y. & Gotoh, F. (1997) Prognostic value of admission blood pressure in patients with intracerebral hemorrhage: Keio Cooperative Stroke Study. *Stroke* **28**, 1185–1188.

Tuhrim, S., Dambrosia, J.M., Price, T.R. *et al.* (1988) Prediction of intracerebral hemorrhage survival. *Annals of Neurology* **24**, 258–263.

Tuhrim, S., Dambrosia, J.M., Price, T.R. *et al.* (1991) Intracerebral hemorrhage: external validation and extension of a model for prediction of 30-day survival. *Annals of Neurology* **29**, 658–663.

Waga, S., Shimosaka, S. & Sakakura, M. (1983) Intracerebral hemorrhage remote from the site of the initial neurosurgical procedure. *Neurosurgery* **13**, 662–665.

Wells, P.S., Lensing, A.W.A. & Hirsh, J. (1994) Graduated compression stockings in the prevention of postoperative venous thromboembolism: a meta-analysis. *Archives of Internal Medicine* **154**, 67–72.

Wijdicks, E.F.M., Schievink, W.I., Brown, R.D. & Mullany, C.J. (1998) The dilemma of discontinuation of anticoagulation therapy for patients with intracranial hemorrhage and mechanical heart valves. *Neurosurgery* **42**, 769–773.

Young, W.B., Lee, K.P., Pessin, M.S., Kwan, E.S., Rand, W.M. & Caplan, L.R. (1990) Prognostic significance of ventricular blood in supratentorial hemorrhage: a volumetric study. *Neurology* **40**, 616–619.

Yu, Y.L., Kumana, C.R., Lauder, I.J. *et al.* (1992) Treatment of acute cerebral hemorrhage with intravenous glycerol: a double-blind, placebo-controlled, randomized trial. *Stroke* **23**, 967–971.

Zuccarello, M., Brott, T., Derex, L. *et al.* (1999) Early surgical treatment for supratentorial intracerebral hemorrhage: a randomized feasibility study. *Stroke* **30**, 1833–1839.

CHAPTER THIRTEEN

Specific treatment of aneurysmal subarachnoid haemorrhage

13.1 General principles

The essence of managing patients with aneurysmal subarachnoid haemorrhage (SAH) is deceptively simple: make the diagnosis, locate the aneurysm and occlude it. And yet, on average, 50% of the patients still die (at least in figures from population-based studies), 50% of the survivors remain severely disabled, and even for functionally independent patients their quality of life is often impaired (Hijdra *et al.* 1987a; Hop *et al.* 1997; Olafsson *et al.* 1997; Hop *et al.* 1998). This disappointing overall outcome is partly explained by very early deaths: approximately 15% of patients die within hours of the onset (section 13.2.3). The main problem, however, is that many complications beset the course of the disease: re-bleeding, delayed cerebral ischaemia, hydrocephalus and a variety of systemic disorders. Tragically, treatment of one complication may produce another. Because distinguishing the different causes of secondary deterioration has many pitfalls, precise observations and definitions are essential for the management of individual patients, as well as for scientific studies directed at improving the outcome in the future (van Crevel 1980).

Despite the need for a precise distinction between different complications, a systematic survey of 184 consecutive articles about SAH published in nine neurosurgical and neurological journals between 1985 and 1992 was rather disappointing (van Gijn *et al.* 1994). Specific outcome events, i.e. re-bleeding, ischaemia and hydrocephalus, were sufficiently defined in only 31% of the articles, incompletely in 22%, and not at all in 47%. The proportion of acceptable definitions did not depend on the type of complication or the year of publication, but there was a relation with the type of journal. The four exclusively neurosurgical journals provided adequate definitions for any of the three outcome events in only 20% (of 209 instances), whereas the five mainly neurological journals published fewer articles on the subject (74 instances), but more often with precise criteria (65%). Research groups in different institutions may not always agree on the precise criteria for the complications of SAH, but the very least one can ask from authors is an attempt at formulating their criteria. The definitions we propose for distinguishing the different complications after SAH will be discussed in the separate sections about the management of each specific complication, but it should be emphasized at the outset that repeat computed tomography (CT) has a vital role to play.

Articles reporting the frequency of specific complications of subarachnoid haemorrhage are only worth reading if an adequate definition of those complications is given.

Occlusion of the ruptured aneurysm by the neurosurgeon or the interventional radiologist is the main aim of treatment in almost every patient with aneurysmal SAH, but the contribution of the neurologist to the management can be considerable. Firstly, continuous observation is the basis of management in these patients, before as well as after interventions to occlude the aneurysm. The neurologist is trained in assessing subtle changes in the neurological condition, and—not being tied up in the operating theatre—can be quickly on the spot to investigate any changes that the nursing staff have detected. Secondly, important systemic complications may occur after aneurysmal haemorrhage, and the neurologist is in an ideal position to investigate these and, if necessary, to liaise quickly with general physicians, anaesthetists and other specialists.

It is only in close collaboration with neurosurgeons and radiologists, however, that the neurologist can adequately fulfil this role (Fig. 13.1). Ideally, the investigation and treatment of patients with aneurysmal SAH should be planned by at least a day-to-day mutual consultation amongst specialists in these disciplines; the management plan can be jointly modified, depending on changes in the neurological condition. At any rate, patients should certainly not be cared for in general medical or neurological wards that have no immediate access to both neurosurgical expertise and modern neuroradiological facilities. The threshold for admission to an intensive-care unit should be low, because close observation cannot be guaranteed on general neurology wards. The need for expert referral applies even to so-called 'poor-grade patients' (section 13.2.1): these may be the very patients who need urgent intervention because of haematoma, hydrocephalus, or hypovolaemia, for example (Wijdicks 1995). In this chapter, we shall first discuss the general outcome and then follow the clinical course of a patient with SAH, especially the prevention and management of the possible complications.

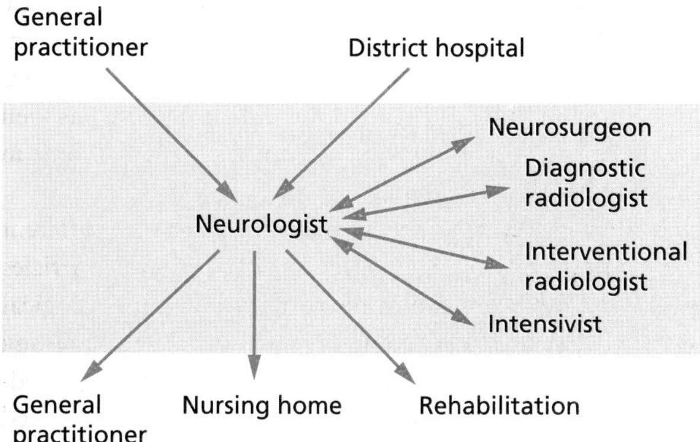

Fig. 13.1 The neurologist as case manager of patients with subarachnoid haemorrhage. The green box includes the relevant services required to manage acute subarachnoid haemorrhage, usually found in a neurology and neurosurgery centre.

13.2 Prognosis

Meaningful interpretation of patient outcome in any reported series requires an accurate description of the state of the patient on admission, the most relevant features of which will be discussed below, and on the length of time the patient has already survived the bleed (Alvord *et al.* 1972). The state of patients reported in hospital series will, in turn, depend heavily on the selection criteria for admission (Maurice-Williams & Marsh 1985). To begin with, a source of bias in any hospital-based series is that it cannot include the patients who died (approximately 15%) before they could be admitted (Crawford & Sarner 1965; Phillips *et al.* 1980; Ljunggren *et al.* 1985; Inagawa *et al.* 1995; Schievink *et al.* 1995). What is more, the average outcome will be much poorer in centres admitting patients regardless of their clinical condition than in, for example, a neurosurgical centre in which the policy is to operate on all patients within the first 3 days, with the result that moribund patients will usually be referred elsewhere, often as much by preselection on the part of the referring physicians as by discouragement from the centre in question (Fig. 9.1). For the same reason, reports dealing only with operated patients are meaningless, almost by definition. Even comprehensive series reflecting the overall management of patients with SAH cannot serve as a basis for comparison, unless one can be reasonably certain that the entire community has been included (Phillips *et al.* 1980; Ostbye *et al.* 1997).

13.2.1 'Grading' patients with aneurysmal subarachnoid haemorrhage

The neurological condition of the patient on admission, particularly the level of consciousness, is the most important clinical determinant of the eventual outcome (Hijdra *et al.* 1988). Several grading systems have been developed for this initial assessment, in most cases consisting of approximately five categories of severity, in hierarchical order. No single system has gained world-wide acceptance, but the Hunt and Hess system is still undeservedly popular (Hunt & Hess 1968). So was the Botterell scale in the 1960s and 1970s, both in the original version (Botterell *et al.* 1956) and in Nishioka's modification (Nishioka 1966). The constituent features of these grading systems are not only the level of consciousness, but also headache, neck stiffness and focal neurological deficit. Unfortunately, these more or less traditional systems are neither valid nor reliable.

Validity refers to whether a particular 'instrument' actually measures what it is supposed to measure—in this case prognosis. Headache and neck stiffness are very poor predictors of outcome in their own right, unless applied to patients from the pre-CT era and cerebrospinal fluid spectrophotometry, when the series must have included non-aneurysmal haemorrhage, and even patients with an innocuous but sudden headache followed by a traumatic lumbar puncture (section 5.6.3). Moreover, these grading scales attribute equal weight to the presence of impaired level of consciousness, focal deficit, or both, the actual grade depending on the severity. Finally, both of these features are classified in vague terms.

The reliability of a scale refers to its reproducibility, particularly with different observers. In view of the overlapping and equivocal terminology, it is not surprising that a formal study of observer variability demonstrated formidable inconsistencies when the same patients were graded by different physicians on either the Hunt and Hess scale, or on the Nishioka–Botterell scale (Lindsay *et al.* 1982). Up to four different grades were selected for the same patient! A similar inconsistency between observers was found with regard to the four clinical features on which the two scales are based (Lindsay *et al.* 1983).

Clearly, there is a need for a better grading system, which contains only relevant features for predicting prognosis (level of consciousness and the presence or absence of a focal deficit) and which defines and combines these in an unambiguous fashion. Classification into a few levels of the sum score of the Glasgow Coma Scale (GCS) (Table 3.5), which consists of eye-opening, motor response and verbal response, proved more reliable than any of the previous systems used to classify the degree of wakefulness (Teasdale & Jennett 1974; Lindsay *et al.* 1983). The Glasgow Coma Scale predicts outcome more accurately, even in compressed form, with five classes, than the time-honoured Hunt and Hess scale (Oshiro *et al.* 1997). The different elements of the Glasgow Coma Scale do not have the same prognostic value; for example, a patient being disoriented rather than alert has stronger implications for outcome than losing a point on the dimensions 'best motor response' or 'eye opening' (Hirai *et al.* 1996). A study aimed at selecting prognostically relevant cut-off points in the Glasgow Coma Scale proposed the following five grades: I (GCS score 15); II (GCS scores 11–14); III (GCS scores 8–10); IV (GCS scores 4–7); and V (GCS score 3) (Takagi *et al.* 1999).

A committee of the World Federation of Neurological Surgeons (WFNS) has proposed a new grading scale of five levels, essentially based on the GCS, with focal deficit making up one extra level for patients with a GCS score of 14 or 13 (Table 13.1). In other words, the WFNS Scale takes account of the fact that a focal neurological deficit in patients with SAH rarely occurs with a normal level of consciousness, and assumes that the presence or absence of such a deficit does not add much to the prognosis in patients with a GCS score of 12 or less (Drake *et al.* 1988). No formal studies of the validity and reliability of the WFNS Scale have yet been undertaken, but at least its core is made up by the GCS, which is extremely valid as a predictor of outcome (Oshiro *et al.* 1997). The reliability of the GCS is also good, although some have found that this only applies to experienced observers (Teasdale & Jennett 1974; Rowley & Fielding 1991).

It is often tacitly assumed that the initial clinical condition is related only to the impact of the first haemorrhage. This is incorrect, as some complications can occur within hours of the original rupture: early re-bleeding, cardiopulmonary dysfunction or acute hydrocephalus. Especially the presence of acute hydrocephalus may be sadly overlooked if the telltale history of increasing drowsiness in the first few hours after the bleed is not properly interpreted (section 13.3.2). Not surprisingly, the patients' worst clinical grade before the aneurysm is clipped or coiled is a better predictor of outcome than their condition on admission, or the best clinical grade (Chiang *et al.* 2000). However, we wish to emphasize that no grading scale, whatever its merits, should ever be used as the only guide to management. A patient without any deficit at all may, perhaps rightly, be regarded as a candidate for early surgical or endovascular intervention, but conversely a patient 'in a bad grade' should not be left alone to recover or die, or be aggressively treated according to a standard protocol (Bailes *et al.* 1990). Instead, the patient should be thoroughly investigated and receive specific treatments according to the problems that are identified.

Table 13.1 Grading system for the initial classification of patients with subarachnoid haemorrhage, according to the World Federation of Neurological Surgeons (WFNS) Scale (Drake *et al.* 1988).

WFNS grade	Glasgow Coma Scale	Focal deficit
I	15	Absent
II	14–13	Absent
III	14–13	Present
IV	12–7	Present or absent
V	6–3	Present or absent

'Grading' patients with subarachnoid haemorrhage is a misguided attempt to create a uniform baseline measure of overall condition. The patient's clinical state should be recorded in descriptive, not in codified terms: level of consciousness (Glasgow Coma Scale) and any focal neurological deficits. Specific causes of early neurological deficit should be identified: intracranial haematoma, acute hydrocephalus, or cardiorespiratory complications.

13.2.2 Methods of outcome assessment

Most studies attempt not only to report case fatality, but also to define morbidity. Before the 1980s, surviving patients were usually categorized as 'good', 'fair' or 'poor', but with widely varying definitions of each. Fortunately, the Glasgow Outcome Scale (Table 13.2) is now widely used (van Gijn *et al.* 1994). This scale was originally devised for assessing patients with head injury, but its general terminology allows its use as a measure of outcome for any serious brain disease. The World Federation of Neurological Surgeons has recommended its future use in patients with subarachnoid haemorrhage (Drake *et al.* 1988). It is a simple hybrid of a disability and a handicap scale, very similar to the modified Rankin scale (sometimes called the Oxford Handicap Scale) that is often used in assessing outcome after ischaemic stroke (section 17.6.3). There is little variation between observers who use the Glasgow Outcome Scale (Maas *et al.* 1983). The main difference from the modified Rankin Scale is that the Glasgow Outcome Scale does not allow any distinction within the stratum of patients who have some impairment but are independent, i.e. between those who do or do not need some help every day. Whether this is a disadvantage in terms of sensitivity in comparisons between groups has not been studied.

Table 13.2 The Glasgow Outcome Scale (from Jennett & Bond 1975).

Grade	Description	Definition
1	Good recovery	Patient can lead an independent life, with or without minimal neurological deficit
2	Moderately disabled	Patient has neurological or intellectual impairment, but is independent
3	Severely disabled	Patient conscious, but totally dependent on others to get through daily activities
4	Vegetative survival	
5	Dead	

At the very least, any study of the outcome after subarachnoid haemorrhage should report the case fatality (at about 1 month) and the morbidity (at about 6 months) by means of the Glasgow Outcome Scale or the (modified) Rankin scale.

13.2.3 Case fatality

Only studies up to the mid-1960s can illustrate the results of conservative treatment alone. However, it should be kept in mind that at that time, not only the methods of treatment but also the methods of diagnosis differed from current practice, and that the series necessarily included varieties of non-aneurysmal haemorrhage that CT scanning would now exclude. With this qualification, Pakarinen's population-based study from Finland can be regarded as the standard of management results before the era of aneurysm surgery; the total case fatality was 62%, with most deaths occurring in the first 6 weeks (Pakarinen 1967).

Death outside hospital occurs in approximately 15% of patients (Crawford & Sarner 1965; Phillips *et al.* 1980; Ljunggren *et al.* 1985; Inagawa *et al.* 1995; Schievink *et al.* 1995). This proportion is unlikely to have changed over the years; it may be impossible to change it ever, because the damage of the initial bleed cannot be undone (Hijdra & van Gijn 1982). Of those patients who do reach hospital alive, a further 10–12% die within 24 h of the first bleed (Locksley 1966; Hijdra & van Gijn 1982; Broderick *et al.* 1994). In one of these series, serial CT scanning identified re-bleeding in 50% (16 of 31) of the patients who died within the first day of admission (Hijdra & van Gijn 1982); even that high proportion is perhaps an underestimate, because re-bleeding occurs relatively often within the first few hours—that is, before the first CT scan is done (Inagawa *et al.* 1987).

Bearing in mind that some 25% of patients die within 24 h of the onset of symptoms, outside or just inside hospital, and that these deaths are almost unavoidable, it is the subsequent case fatality and morbidity that is the realistic target for our medical and surgical interventions. In a large hospital series (not a population series) reported in the 1980s, 35% of those surviving the first day died within the subsequent 3 months, with approximately equal proportions of the total being contributed by poor condition from the initial haemorrhage, re-bleeding and delayed cerebral ischaemia (Hijdra *et al.* 1987a). To assess whether the case fatality has improved after the introduction of modern management strategies such as the operating microscope, liberal administration of fluids, avoidance of antihypertensive drugs, and nimodipine for prevention of delayed cerebral ischaemia, Hop *et al.* (1997) studied the outcome in all 21 population-based studies from 1960 through the mid-1990s. Case fatality ranged between 32% and 67%, with only one exception. Nearly all deaths occurred within the first 3 weeks. The case fatality decreased by 0.5% per year over the study period (95% confidence interval (CI), −0.1% to 1.2%). This decline was steeper after adjustment for age and sex (0.9% per year; 95% CI, 0.7%–2.6%). Projection of this trend into the future indicates that, whatever new developments in the management of patients with SAH may arise, the effect on the *overall* death rate is likely to remain modest.

For patients who survive SAH and do not have their ruptured aneurysm occluded, the risk of re-bleeding remains a substantial 3.5% per year (section 13.11.2).

13.2.4 Factors related to outcome

Outcome (defined as the proportion of patients dead or dependent after 3–6 months) after subarachnoid haemorrhage (SAH) depends on a large variety of factors, and it may be helpful to interpret these in the light of three general principles. The first is that many of the prognostic factors are interrelated. For that reason, univariate analysis may be misleading, since a single factor may not be a determinant in itself but merely a marker of a confounding factor, that is, a 'true' (i.e. independent) prognostic factor. For example, people who carry matches in their pockets are at high risk of lung cancer, but not because of the matches! The cigarettes are the confounding factor. In the same way, finding that outcome after craniotomy for SAH is best in centres with a large volume of aneurysm operations may reflect not just surgical skill (Solomon *et al.* 1996). The alternative explanation is referral bias: large centres recruit patients from a wide area, and patients in good condition will be relatively more likely to reach the 'centre of excellence'. Another example is that middle cerebral artery aneurysms have been associated with a poor outcome in univariate analysis (Kassell *et al.* 1990; Rinne *et al.* 1996). This is probably explained not by the site of the aneurysm *per se,* but by the associated haematomas, as the prognostic value disappears when the clinical condition and the amount of extravasated blood are introduced into the model (Kassell *et al.* 1990).

The second principle that should be kept in mind when prognostic factors after SAH are interpreted is that the main cause of poor outcome in patients who reach hospital alive is secondary deterioration, especially from re-bleeding and delayed ischaemia (Enblad & Persson 1997; Linn *et al.* 2000). Of these two complications, only delayed ischaemia is associated with some of the baseline factors that also determine outcome in general (Hijdra *et al.* 1988). Re-bleeding, in contrast, although a major and sometimes the dominant contributor to poor outcome, even in centres aiming at early surgery (Roos *et al.* 1997; Vermeij *et al.* 1998), occurs more or less at random in all types of patients, regardless of their clinical and radiological characteristics at baseline (Hijdra *et al.* 1988).

The third principle—partly related to the previous one—in understanding prognostic factors after SAH is that their predictive power is relatively weak. Patients in poor clinical condition, predicted to do badly, may sometimes still do well (Le Roux *et al.* 1996); the same is true of aged patients (Fridriksson *et al.* 1995; Stachniak *et al.* 1996). On the other hand, the unpredictability of re-bleeding requires considerable caution in predicting a good outcome in patients who are in perfect clinical condition, apart from their headache.

The three baseline variables most closely related to poor outcome are the level of consciousness, age and the amount of subarachnoid blood on the CT scan (Table 13.3).

Conscious level

The largest body of information is derived from the multicentre American Cooperative Study, which included 3521 patients (Kassell *et al.* 1990). Nevertheless, in that study the level of consciousness on admission was not strictly defined (four categories), whereas most other studies are based on the Glasgow Coma Scale. The predictive value for overall outcome of the Glasgow Coma Scale, even in a compressed form (five classes), is better than that of the traditional, largely intuition-based Hunt and Hess scale (Oshiro *et al.* 1997) (section 13.2.1). Not all elements of the Glasgow Coma scale have the same prognostic value; for example, being disoriented rather than alert has far graver implications for outcome than losing a point on the dimensions 'best motor response' or 'eye opening' (Hirai *et al.* 1996). The level of consciousness on admission is related to loss of consciousness at the time of aneurysm rupture, which is the strongest predictor for delayed ischaemia (Hop *et al.* 1999).

The amount of blood in the subarachnoid space

The amount of subarachnoid blood in the American study was estimated from the maximal thickness of the clot (Fisher *et al.* 1980), against a sum score for each of 10 cisterns in the European study of prognostic factors; only the latter method has been subjected to an interobserver study, with satisfactory results (Hijdra *et al.* 1990). Of course, the amount of blood may merely reflect the damage that occurred at the time of the haemorrhage, as is the case for the level of consciousness, and the prognostic importance of the blood load by no means implies that removal of subarachnoid blood will improve outcome.

Age

Not surprisingly, increasing age was an adverse factor in several studies (Table 13.3). In a separate study dedicated to aneurysmal haemorrhage in patients over 65 years of age, case fatality resulted mostly from intracranial complications, whereas the proportion of medical complications was not markedly different from that in younger patients (Muizelaar *et al.* 1988).

The other prognostic factors in Table 13.3 have been included only if their association with poor outcome was

Table 13.3 Factors with prognostic value for poor outcome (death or severe disability) after subarachnoid haemorrhage; the first three factors are the most powerful predictors.

Prognostic factor	Identified in multivariate analysis	Identified only in univariate analysis
Decreased level of consciousness on admission*	Hijdra *et al.* 1988 Kassell *et al.* 1990a	
Increasing age	Kassell *et al.* 1990a Lanzino *et al.* 1996	
Large amount of blood on CT scan*	Hijdra *et al.* 1990 Kassell *et al.* 1990a	
High blood pressure on admission	Kassell *et al.* 1990a Simpson *et al.* 1991	Toftdahl *et al.* 1995
Pre-existing medical condition	Kassell *et al.* 1990a	
Use of anticoagulants	Rinkel *et al.* 1997	
Intravenous drug abuse	Simpson *et al.* 1991	
Associated intracranial haematoma	Hauerberg *et al.* 1994	
Aneurysm in posterior circulation*	Kassell *et al.* 1990a	Schievink *et al.* 1995b
Level of creatinine kinase BB in cerebrospinal fluid	(Coplin *et al.* 1999)	

*For definitions and further discussion, see text.

confirmed at least once by multivariate modelling. Familial aneurysmal SAH does not seem to have an adverse effect on outcome (Ronkainen *et al.* 1999).

Delays in admission frequently occur in patients with SAH, if only because the condition is too uncommon to always be recognized quickly by the average primary-care physician (Adams *et al.* 1980; Kassell *et al.* 1985). Several hospital-based studies have proposed the notion that delay is associated with a worse outcome and, consequently, that earlier referral would substantially improve outcome (Mayer *et al.* 1996; Jakobsson *et al.* 1996; Neil-Dwyer & Lang 1997). But it remains to be proved that the episodes of secondary deterioration that usually prompted the delayed referral would not have occurred in hospital; an observational study estimated that the gains of earlier admission would have been very modest indeed (Linn *et al.* 2000).

The main adverse factors for outcome after subarachnoid haemorrhage are level of consciousness, amount of blood in the subarachnoid space and increasing age.

13.3 Indications for immediate operation

13.3.1 Intracranial haematomas

Intraparenchymal haematomas occur in up to 30% of patients with ruptured aneurysms (van Gijn & van Dongen 1982). Not surprisingly, the average outcome is worse than in patients with purely subarachnoid blood (Hauerberg *et al.* 1994). When a large haematoma is the most likely cause of gradual deterioration in the level of consciousness within the first few days (Fig. 13.2), its immediate evacuation should be seriously considered (with simultaneous clipping of the aneurysm, if it can be identified)—often with the aneurysm having been demonstrated only by magnetic resonance (MR) angiography or CT angiography (section 9.4.3). There has been an impression that surgical treatment is not only life-saving in patients with impending transtentorial herniation, particularly with temporal haematomas, but that it may even result in independent survival (Brandt *et al.* 1987). Fortunately, this notion has been backed up by a randomized controlled trial, albeit a small one, in which 11 of 15 patients in the operated group survived, against three of 15 in the conservatively treated group (relative risk 0.27; 95% confidence interval, 0.09 to 0.74) (Heiskanen *et al.* 1988).

If patients with large intraparenchymal or subdural haematomas, likely to be caused by a ruptured aneurysm, become increasingly drowsy in the first few hours after subarachnoid haemorrhage, they are candidates for immediate surgical evacuation of the haematoma, preferably preceded by CT angiography, but not necessarily by catheter angiography, to display the relevant aneurysm.

An acute subdural haematoma, which is usually associated with recurrent aneurysmal rupture (section 8.10), may be

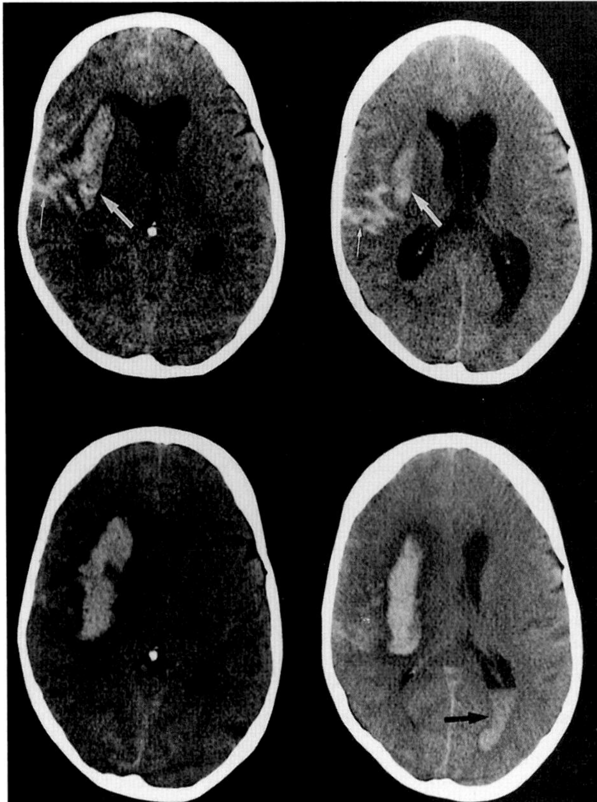

Fig. 13.2 'Enlarging haematoma'. *Top:* CT brain scan on the day of subarachnoid haemorrhage from a ruptured aneurysm of the right middle cerebral artery, in a 51-year-old man receiving anticoagulant medication for myocardial infarction with mitral valve insufficiency. There is a haematoma in the right Sylvian fissure (thin arrow) and in the subinsular cortex (thick arrow); at the time of the scan, anticoagulation had already been reversed by infusion of a concentrate of coagulation factors. *Bottom:* CT brain scan 5 days after the haemorrhage, showing a marked increase of the space-occupying effect, with compression of the right lateral ventricle and the third ventricle. The increased mass effect results not only from a newly formed rim of oedema around the haematoma (short arrow), but also from an increase in size of the haematoma itself. There had been no new neurological signs or other clinical features indicating re-bleeding. The newly formed collection of blood in the posterior horn of the left lateral ventricle (long arrow) is often seen in the absence of re-bleeding (sedimentation effect).

equally life-threatening; evacuation is also called for in these cases (O'Sullivan *et al.* 1994).

13.3.2 Symptomatic hydrocephalus

Gradual obtundation within 24 h of haemorrhage, sometimes accompanied by slow pupillary responses to light and downward deviation of the eyes, is fairly characteristic of acute hydrocephalus (van Gijn *et al.* 1985; Rinkel *et al.* 1990). If the diagnosis is confirmed by CT, early ventricular drainage may be required, although some patients do improve spontaneously in the first 24 h. The management priorities of acute hydrocephalus are discussed more fully below in the section on secondary deterioration (section 13.9.2).

13.3.3 Early death without realistic options for surgical intervention

Not all patients who arrive moribund can be saved. In a consecutive series of 31 patients who died on the first day, nine had a potentially treatable supratentorial haematoma, but 16 had primary dysfunction of the brainstem from massive intraventricular haemorrhage on CT, including distension of the fourth ventricle with blood (in eight cases this occurred together with an intracerebral haematoma). Surgical evacuation of a 'packed' intraventricular haemorrhage is pointless (Shimoda *et al.* 1999). In the six remaining patients, neither a supratentorial haematoma nor intraventricular haemorrhage could explain the progressive dysfunction of the brainstem and the fatal outcome, the CT scan showing no abnormality other than subarachnoid blood (Hijdra & van Gijn 1982). The most likely explanation is a prolonged period of global cerebral ischaemia at the time of haemorrhage, as a result of the pressure in the cerebrospinal fluid spaces being elevated to the level of that in the arteries, perhaps only for a few minutes. Such a potentially lethal arrest of the circulation to the brain is indeed suggested by post-mortem evidence, by the recording of intracranial pressure, and by transcranial Doppler sonography at the time of recurrent aneurysmal haemorrhage (Smith 1963; Grote & Hassler 1988).

Ventricular fibrillation may occur, but its frequency at the onset of SAH is unknown. There is a single report of 26 patients who received out-of-hospital cardiopulmonary resuscitation (and of whom one-third had a good outcome), but it inevitably lacked details about the precise nature of the cardiorespiratory disturbance (Shapiro 1996). Ventricular fibrillation is probably a relatively rare cause of sudden death in hospitalized patients with ruptured aneurysm (section 13.10.2). The only prospective hospital study of this problem reported 43 consecutive episodes of cardiorespiratory complications in patients with aneurysmal haemorrhage (mostly days or weeks after the initial haemorrhage). Thirty-seven episodes consisted of primary respiratory arrest, in one case followed within minutes by ventricular fibrillation. Only two patients had ventricular fibrillation at onset, and in four patients the course of events was uncertain because they died suddenly, without vital signs having been recorded (Hijdra *et al.* 1984).

13.4 General care

13.4.1 Blood pressure

Management of hypertension is a difficult issue in patients

with subarachnoid haemorrhage (SAH), especially if the pressure rises above about 200/110 mmHg. Following intracranial haemorrhage, the range between the upper and lower limits of the autoregulation of cerebral blood flow becomes narrower, which makes the perfusion of brain more dependent on arterial blood pressure (Kaneko *et al.* 1983) (section 11.1.3). Consequently, aggressive treatment of surges of blood pressure entails a definite risk of ischaemia in brain areas with no autoregulation. The rationalistic approach is therefore to advise against treating hypertension following aneurysmal rupture (Calhoun & Oparil 1990). The empirical evidence from clinical trials is sparse, but tends to support the avoidance of antihypertensive drugs. In the American Cooperative Study, conducted between 1963 and 1970, 1005 patients with ruptured aneurysms were randomized between four treatment modalities; one arm consisted of drug-induced lowering of the blood pressure, another of bed rest alone (the other two arms were surgical: carotid ligation and intracranial surgery). In the intention-to-treat analysis, antihypertensive drugs failed to reduce either case fatality or the rate of re-bleeding within the first 6 months after the initial event; on-treatment analysis suggested that induced hypotension did decrease the rate of re-bleeding in comparison with bed rest, but not the case fatality (Torner *et al.* 1981b). However, it should be kept in mind that the diagnosis of re-bleeding was made in the pre-CT era and was therefore probably inaccurate (section 13.7.1). The same caveat applies to the finding from the same study that the rate of re-bleeding was not dependent on the degree of blood pressure reduction (Nibbelink *et al.* 1981). An observational study from the 1980s, in which all events had been documented by serial CT scanning, compared patients in whom hypertension had been newly treated with normotensive controls; the rate of re-bleeding was lower but the rate of cerebral infarction was higher than in untreated patients, despite the blood pressures still being, on average, higher than in the controls (Wijdicks *et al.* 1990). This suggests that hypertension after SAH is a compensatory phenomenon, at least to some extent, and one that should not be interfered with. In keeping with this, a further observational study from the same centre (Rotterdam) suggested that the combined strategy of avoiding antihypertensive medication and increasing fluid intake may decrease the risk of cerebral infarction (Hasan *et al.* 1989a).

It seems best to only use antihypertensive therapy (other than any drugs the patients were on already) in patients with extreme elevations of blood pressure as well as evidence of rapidly progressive end-organ deterioration, diagnosed from either clinical signs (e.g. new retinopathy, heart failure, etc.) or laboratory evidence (e.g. signs of left-ventricular failure on chest X-ray, proteinuria or oliguria with a rapid rise of plasma creatinine levels). Effective treatments are:

- diazoxide (50–150 mg by intravenous bolus, repeated after 5–10 min, or 15–30 mg/min by intravenous infusion, up to 600 mg);
- labetalol hydrochloride (20–80 mg by intravenous bolus every 10 min, or 2 mg/min by intravenous infusion, up to 300 mg) (Calhoun & Oparil 1990; Gifford *et al.* 1991). Labetalol, however, may be ineffective in patients previously treated with betablockers and is contraindicated in heart failure and asthma;
- nitroprusside (intravenously) has also been advocated in hypertensive crises, but is probably not a first-line drug in this situation because animal studies have shown that it increases intracranial pressure (Candia *et al.* 1978).

It is reasonable to aim for a 25% decrease in mean arterial pressure below the initial baseline. For monitoring the blood pressure in these situations, an arterial line is almost mandatory. In practice, however, there is rarely any need for antihypertensive therapy. In many patients, surges of high blood pressure can be attenuated by adequate pain management or sedation, for example when the patient is resisting the ventilator.

Hypertension in the acute phase of subarachnoid haemorrhage can be left untreated unless there are signs of end-organ damage by high blood pressure. Existing antihypertensive drugs can be continued.

13.4.2 Fluids and electrolytes

Fluid management in subarachnoid haemorrhage is important to prevent a reduction in plasma volume, which may contribute to the development of cerebral ischaemia (section 13.8). Nevertheless, the arguments for a liberal (some might say aggressive) regimen of fluid administration are indirect. In approximately one-third of patients, their plasma volume decreases by more than 10% between the second and tenth day after the haemorrhage; this is significantly associated with a negative sodium balance. In other words, there is loss of sodium as well as of water, or 'cerebral salt wasting' (Wijdicks *et al.* 1985a; Hasan *et al.* 1990). Moreover, fluid restriction in patients with hyponatraemia is associated with an increased risk of cerebral ischaemia (Wijdicks *et al.* 1985b). Fluid restriction was applied in the past because hyponatraemia was erroneously attributed to water retention, via inappropriate secretion of antidiuretic hormone. Two non-randomized studies with historical controls suggest that a daily intake of at least 3 L of saline (against 1.5–2.0 L in the past) is associated with a lower rate of delayed cerebral ischaemia and a better overall outcome (Hasan *et al.* 1989a; Vermeij *et al.* 1998). The interpretation of these two studies is difficult not only because of their observational nature, but also because the liberal administration of saline in the second period was confounded by avoidance of antihypertensive drugs. Two randomized studies of hypervolaemia have been published. One included only 30 patients (Rosenwasser *et al.* 1983). Treatment allocation was not blinded (personal information obtained from the authors), and outcome was not assessed beyond the time of operation (days 7–10); at that time, the rate of delayed ischaemia had been reduced by two-thirds (67%; 95% CI, 1%–89%). In the second trial, 82 patients were randomized between normovolaemia and hypervolaemia (monitored by means of cardiac filling pressures); 20% in each group had an episode of secondary deterioration interpreted as delayed cerebral ischaemia, and blood volume and cerebral blood flow measurements were also similar in the two groups (Lennihan *et al.* 2000).

Despite the incomplete evidence, it seems reasonable to prevent hypovolaemia. We favour giving 2.5–3.5 L/day of normal saline, unless contraindicated by signs of impending cardiac failure (see below). The amount of intravenous saline should be reduced if the patient is also receiving nutritional solution via the enteral route; most commercially prepared enteral solutions deliver 1–2 cal/mL (4–8 J/mL). Nevertheless, it appears that many patients need a daily fluid intake of 4–6 L (sometimes as much as 10 L) to balance the production of urine plus estimated insensible losses (via perspiration and expired air). In patients with fever, from whatever cause (section 13.4.3), fluid intake should be gradually increased. Fluid requirements may be guided by recording the central venous pressure (the directly measured value should be above 8 mmHg) or pulmonary wedge pressure (to be kept above 7 mmHg), but frequent calculation of fluid balance (four times per day until approximately day 10) is the main way of estimating how much fluid should be given. There is a good indication for measuring central venous pressure, via a catheter in the subclavian or internal jugular vein, in patients who develop hyponatraemia or a negative fluid balance; pulmonary artery balloon catheters are used in patients with a history of cardiopulmonary disease.

A high fluid intake is essential in patients with aneurysmal subarachnoid haemorrhage, to compensate for 'cerebral salt wasting' and to prevent hypovolaemia, because this predisposes to cerebral ischaemia. The daily minimum is 2.5–3.5 L of normal saline, by the oral or intravenous route; more may be needed to balance the volume of urine, or with fever.

13.4.3 Analgesics and general nursing care

As long as the aneurysm has not been occluded, the patient should be kept on complete bed rest, traditionally flat and in dimmed light, on the assumption that any form of excitement increases the risk of re-bleeding. Patients in whom a good angiographic study has not shown an aneurysm can usually be allowed to sit up as soon as the headache subsides, but with an aneurysmal pattern of haemorrhage on the CT scan it is wise to keep them under the close supervision of the nursing staff until the repeat angiogram has been done (section 9.4.6). Continuous assessment of the level of consciousness is essential. This should preferably be recorded by means of the Glasgow Coma Scale (section 3.3.2), although it must be remembered that with inexperienced observers errors of more than one point can occur (Teasdale & Jennett 1974; Rowley & Fielding 1991). Any change in the level of consciousness may signify early cerebral ischaemia, rebleeding, enlargement of the ventricles, or a systemic medical complication. The nurses should be familiar with the peak times of occurrence of re-bleeding and cerebral ischaemia, and they should be able to detect the early signs of delirium, which is seldom caused by subarachnoid haemorrhage (SAH) *per se* but more often by the combined effects of isolation, sleep deprivation, narcotic drugs and alcohol withdrawal.

Headache can sometimes be managed with mild analgesics such as paracetamol, with or without dextropropoxyphene; salicylates should be avoided until the aneurysm has been occluded, because of their inhibitory effect on haemostasis. However, usually the pain is so severe that codeine needs to be added, and this will not mask neurological signs. Sometimes, pain can be alleviated with anxiolytic drugs such as midazolam. Even a synthetic opiate such as piritramide may be needed to obtain relief. As a last resort, severe headache can be treated with morphine given intravenously in small increments of 1–2 mg; many patients benefit from the euphoriant effect. A potential adverse effect of morphine is hypotension, because it is a potent vasodilator. The blood pressure should be checked frequently until the pain has subsided. Constipation is a common disadvantage of morphine, as well as of codeine.

Coughing and straining must be rigorously prevented because of the attendant overshoots in arterial blood pressure. Stool softeners should be prescribed routinely. Enemas are contraindicated because they markedly increase intra-abdominal pressure and secondarily intracranial pressure. A urinary catheter is almost always needed, except in men who are alert and have perfect bladder control. Proper control of fluid balance requires the volume of urine to be precisely measured; condom devices leak or slip off too often to be of any use in these critically ill patients. Intermittent catheterization may substantially decrease the risk of urinary infections, but the procedure is too stressful for patients with SAH (and requires more time from the nursing staff than most hospital budgets allow).

Headache is a typical and distressing problem in patients with subarachnoid haemorrhage. In those with a decreased level of consciousness, it may manifest as restlessness. The 'analgesic staircase' consists of frequent doses (every 3–4 h) of paracetamol 500 mg orally; add codeine 20 mg orally; piritramide 20 mg subcutaneously; morphine 2 mg intravenously, with 1–2 mg increments.

If they are pulling at equipment, confused patients should be restrained by means of girdles and Velcro wristbands that can be attached to the side of the bed. Of course, specific causes of confusion should be excluded, such as pain, hypoxia, alcohol withdrawal, infection or a blocked urinary catheter. Self-extubation is a potentially life-threatening event, and sedation, restraint, or proximity of nursing personnel do not necessarily decrease the risk (Coppolo & May 1990).

A reliable intravenous route should be maintained for emergency administration of plasma expanders or anticonvulsants. Oral administration of antacids is said to be sufficient to protect against stress-induced gastric bleeding; H_2-receptor antagonists or proton-pump inhibitors are expensive and should be considered only in mechanically ventilated patients, or in patients with a previous history of peptic ulcers.

The body temperature should be frequently measured, up to four times per day, depending on the interval after SAH, and the level of consciousness. In the first few days, mild fever (up to 38.5 °C) often results from the inflammatory reaction in the subarachnoid space; in that case, the pulse rate is characteristically normal (Rousseaux *et al.* 1980). Infection should be suspected if the temperature exceeds 38.5 °C, if the pulse rate is elevated as well, or if the patient has vomited.

Deep venous thrombosis (DVT) is not as common after SAH as ischaemic stroke, presumably because the patients are restless, mostly younger and—most importantly—have no paralysed leg. In a large and prospective series, DVT was diagnosed clinically in only 4% (Vermeulen *et al.* 1984a). In general, DVT can be prevented by subcutaneous low-dose heparin or heparinoids (section 15.13), but the obvious concern is that anticoagulation will not be confined to the venous system and that the risk of aneurysmal re-bleeding will be increased. No systematic studies have disproved this concern, but many physicians prefer to err on the side of caution and do not prophylactically institute treatment with heparin or its low-molecular analogues. Graduated compression stockings are of confirmed benefit in preventing DVT in patients undergoing general surgical, neurosurgical or orthopaedic procedures (Wells *et al.* 1994; Nurmohamed *et al.* 1996; Agnelli *et al.* 1998), and are also the preferred form of thrombosis prevention in patients with SAH before aneurysm occlusion, a piece of advice admittedly lacking support from a clinical trial in this specific situation. Because these stockings must be individually fitted to be efficacious, some favour pneumatic devices that apply intermittent venous compression to the leg. A study specifically performed in patients with SAH, but with non-randomized controls, suggested DVT could be successfully prevented in this way (Black *et al.* 1986). A snag is that the pneumatic stockings can only be successfully employed if backed up by a repair service that keeps them running (Clarke Pearson *et al.* 1984). The devices are well tolerated by patients and can be managed easily by the nursing staff. It has been argued that impedance plethysmography or duplex Doppler sonography should be performed to exclude clinically occult thrombosis before any kind of compression is applied to the calves, but no systematic studies have addressed the question of whether the danger of dislodging emboli to the lungs is imaginary or not.

The prophylactic use of antiepileptic medication is controversial. Seizures in the first few weeks after aneurysmal rupture occur in about 10% of patients and may be easily confused with re-bleeding (Rose & Sarner 1965; Hart *et al.* 1981; Hasan *et al.* 1993; Pinto *et al.* 1996). The majority occur soon after the initial haemorrhage. Predictive factors for epileptic seizures have not been consistently identified. Intracranial haematoma and intracranial surgery probably increase the risk, but a randomized trial of anticonvulsants after supratentorial craniotomy for benign lesions (not only aneurysms) failed to show benefit in terms of seizure rate or case fatality, although the confidence intervals were wide (Foy *et al.* 1992). Currently, we adhere to the principle *in dubio abstine,* because the possible disadvantage of a serious drug reaction may well outweigh the benefits. If phenytoin is given, absorption by the oral route is severely impaired when patients receive continuous nasogastric tube feeding (Bauer 1982). Absorption will improve if the continuous feeding is stopped 2 h before the dose is given, the suspension or crushed tablets are flushed down the nasogastric tube with 60 mL of water, and two additional hours are allowed to elapse before feeding is resumed; but larger than usual doses will still be required.

Our recommendations for the general management of patients with SAH are summarized in Table 13.4. Before discussing the diagnosis and prevention of all the possible complications, we shall address the *prevention* of the two most common ones: re-bleeding and cerebral ischaemia.

13.5 Prevention of re-bleeding

13.5.1 Risk of re-bleeding

In the first few hours after admission for the initial haemorrhage, up to 15% of patients experience a sudden episode of clinical deterioration that suggests re-bleeding (Kassell & Torner 1983; Hijdra *et al.* 1987b; Fujii *et al.* 1996). As such sudden episodes often occur before the first CT scan, or even before admission to hospital, a definite diagnosis is difficult, and the true frequency of re-bleeding on the first day is invariably underestimated. A study from Japan, in which 150 patients were investigated after an amazingly short delay of 6 h or less from symptom onset, found that of the 33 patients who eventually re-bled, 29 did so on the first day, and 23 within the first 6 h of symptom onset (Inagawa *et al.* 1987). In patients who survive the first day, the risk of re-bleeding

Table 13.4 Recommendations for nursing and general management of patients with subarachnoid haemorrhage.

Nursing
Continuous observation (Glasgow Coma Scale, temperature, ECG monitoring, pupils, any focal neurological deficits)

Nutrition
—*Oral route:*
Only with intact cough and swallowing reflexes (section 15.17)
Keep stools soft by adequate fluid intake and by restriction of milk content; if necessary add laxatives
—*Nasogastric tube:* deflate endotracheal cuff (if present) on insertion
Confirm proper placement by X-ray
Begin with small test feeds of 5% dextrose
Prevent aspiration by feeding in sitting position and by checking gastric residue every hour
Tablets should be crushed and flushed down (phenytoin levels will not be adequate in conventional doses)
—*Total parenteral nutrition should only be used as a last resort*

Blood pressure
Do not treat hypertension unless there is clinical or laboratory evidence of progressive end organ damage

Fluids and electrolytes
Intravenous line mandatory
Give at least 3 L/day (normal saline, 0.9%)
Insert an indwelling urinary catheter if there is incontinence
Compensate for a negative fluid balance and for fever
Monitoring of electrolytes (and leukocyte count), at least every other day

Pain
Start with paracetamol and/or dextropropoxyphene; avoid aspirin
Midazolam can be used if pain is accompanied by anxiety (5 mg bolus)
For severe pain, use codeine or, as a last resort, morphine

Prevention of deep venous thrombosis and pulmonary embolism
Apply compression stockings or intermittent compression by pneumatic devices

is more or less evenly distributed over the next 4 weeks, although there may be a second peak early in the third week (Hijdra *et al.* 1987b). Given that the proportion of patients who eventually re-bled amounted to 32% in a consecutive series of patients not treated with antifibrinolytic agents, but in whom one-third of the patients had undergone aneurysm clipping around day 12, the risk of re-bleeding without medical or surgical intervention in the 4 weeks after the first day must be about 35–40% (Hijdra *et al.* 1987b). A more precise estimate is difficult to obtain, because currently patients in good condition often undergo operation or endovascular occlusion much sooner, within 3 days. In previous studies, before the advent of CT, the occurrence of re-bleeding was probably overestimated (Vermeulen *et al.* 1984b). Between 4 weeks and 6 months after the haemorrhage, the risk of re-bleeding gradually decreases, from the initial level of 1–2% per day to a constant level of about 3% per year (section 13.11.2).

The risk of re-bleeding after rupture of an intracranial aneurysm, without medical or surgical intervention is: in all patients, about 20% on the first day; and in survivors of the first day, about 40% in the first month. Therefore the cumulative risk for all patients in the first month is about 50%.

The case fatality of re-bleeding is high, around 50%, compared with the 35% overall case fatality within 3 months for patients who survive the first day (Hijdra *et al.* 1987b) (section 13.2.3). Together with its frequency, this means that re-bleeding is still the main cause of a poor outcome, even in centres aiming at early occlusion of the aneurysm (Roos *et al.* 1997; Vermeij *et al.* 1998). Unfortunately, there are few prognostic factors that predict an increased risk of re-bleeding. Some studies suggest that re-bleeding occurs more often in patients with a decreased level of consciousness (Torner *et al.* 1981a; Aoyagi & Hayakawa 1984). This could not be confirmed in a study in which the diagnosis of re-bleeding was rigorous, based on serial CT scanning (Hijdra *et al.* 1987b). A single post-mortem study suggested that the risk of re-bleeding increases with the size of the aneurysm (Inagawa & Hirano 1990). On the other hand, this does not apply to true giant aneurysms (Khurana *et al.* 1998). Even if the difference between certain subgroups is substantial, therapeutic measures for the prevention of re-bleeding should not be restricted to only high-risk groups because of the prevention paradox (Rose 1992); treatment would then be denied to most patients eventually going on to suffer the event in question, in this case re-bleeding (section 18.5.2).

Re-bleeding of a ruptured aneurysm cannot be predicted reliably.

13.5.2 Operation and its timing

A classical study from the Atkinson Morley's Hospital in London was the first to establish in a randomized controlled trial that operation (at that time mainly carotid ligation) was preferable to conservative management for patients who had recovered from the immediate effects of rupture of an aneurysm—in that series, aneurysms of the posterior communicating artery (McKissock *et al.* 1960). A subsequent study of aneurysms of the anterior communicating artery complex showed no difference between surgical and conservative treatment, but nevertheless surgical treatment of intracranial aneurysms became more and more the standard treatment, without further controlled trials being done (McKissock *et al.* 1965). In those days, the aneurysm was usually clipped after at least 12 days had elapsed. The second week was notorious for its ischaemic complications, even without operation, and attempts at very early intervention were disappointing.

Improvements in anaesthetic technique, and especially the introduction of the operating microscope, have radically changed this policy of delayed surgery. Nowadays, many neurosurgeons clip aneurysms early, i.e. within 3 days of the initial bleed. The main rationale for early surgery is, of course, optimal prevention of re-bleeding. Some also believe that ischaemia might be prevented by early operation, because the clots that surround blood vessels in the subarachnoid space can be washed away and no longer contribute their putative effect in the development of vasospasm (Mizukami *et al.* 1982). However, a clinical trial of intraoperative thrombolysis with recombinant tissue plasminogen activator (rt-PA) failed to show any convincing benefit (Findlay *et al.* 1995), and in an uncontrolled and small study there was no difference in outcome according to the dose of rt-PA that was used (Öhman *et al.* 1991). Another theoretical advantage of early aneurysm clipping is that if cerebral ischaemia does develop, there is an opportunity for hypertensive and hypervolaemic treatment without the danger of re-bleeding.

The theoretical advantages of early surgery have not yet been proven by any systematic studies, which is an uncomfortable thought. A remarkable study was done in Finland and, to date, it is the only randomized controlled trial of the timing of operation. The 216 enrolled patients were allocated to surgery within 3 days, after 7 days, or in the intermediate period (Öhman & Heiskanen 1989). The outcome tended to be better after early than intermediate or late surgery, but as the difference was not statistically significant, a disadvantage of early surgery could not be excluded. The same result—no difference in outcome after early or late operation—emerged from observational studies: a multicentre study from North America (Kassell *et al.* 1990), and a single-institution review in Cambridge, England (Whitfield *et al.* 1996). The US study found the worst outcome in patients who underwent surgery between day 7 and 10 after the initial haemorrhage. This disadvantageous period for performing the operation, in the second week after subarachnoid haemorrhage, coincides with the peak time of cerebral ischaemia (Hijdra *et al.* 1986) and of cerebral vasospasm (Weir *et al.* 1978), both phenomena being most common from day 4 to day 12.

Although early aneurysm operation in patients in good clinical condition is now the usual practice, this policy is vulnerable to challenge and reversal, because it has not been supported by any randomized controlled trial.

In addition to the introduction of the operating microscope, the neurosurgical technique has also undergone considerable evolution in other ways as well. Although this is not a textbook of the technical details of operative treatment, it is useful for physicians to know something about these developments (Table 13.5). A most unusual complication of operative treatment of aneurysms is a delayed-type hypersensitivity against the metal alloy, which may necessitate removal of the clip (Ross *et al.* 1998).

13.5.3 Antifibrinolytic drugs

Because re-bleeding is such an important cause of death and disability, and as it is thought to originate from dissolution of the clot at the site of the ruptured aneurysm, prevention by drug treatment is a logical aim. The clot dissolution probably results from fibrinolytic activity in the cerebrospinal fluid after subarachnoid haemorrhage (SAH). Because antifibrinolytic agents reduce fibrinolytic activity and cross the blood–brain barrier rapidly after SAH, antifibrinolytic therapy was suggested as a means of reducing the occurrence of re-bleeds and improving the outcome (Fodstad *et al.* 1981). The two most commonly used drugs are tranexamic acid (TEA; usual dose 1 g intravenously or 1.5 g orally, four to six times daily), or epsilon-aminocaproic acid (EACA; 3–4.5 g/3 h intravenously or orally). Both agents are structurally similar to

Table 13.5 Special neurosurgical techniques used in obliteration of aneurysms.

Vessel reconstruction, with fusiform aneurysms or giant aneurysms
Permanent occlusion of parent vessel (Anson *et al.* 1996; Drake & Peerless 1997)
Temporary occlusion of parent vessel (Ogilvy *et al.* 1996; Piepgras *et al.* 1998)
'Trapping', without revascularization (Drake & Peerless 1997)
Aneurysmorrhaphy and thrombectomy (Sinson *et al.* 1996; Anson *et al.* 1996)
Excision of aneurysm, with end-to-end anastomosis (Chang *et al.* 1986; Anson *et al.* 1996).
Excision of aneurysm, with large-artery bypass (Tulleken and Verdaasdonk, 1995; Tulleken *et al.* 1998)
Combination with endovascular techniques
Intraoperative angiography, to verify clip placement (Derdeyn *et al.* 1997)
Clipping, followed by endovascular coiling (Forsting *et al.* 1996)
Special clips
Clips with different shapes and physical properties (Ooka *et al.* 1997)
Titanium clips, which cause no artifacts on magnetic resonance imaging (Lawton *et al.* 1996)
Special approaches to basilar artery aneurysms
Transpetrous approach (Friedman *et al.* 1997; Lawton *et al.* 1997)

lysine and so block the lysine sites by which the plasminogen molecules bind to complementary sites on fibrin. In this way, these drugs prevent fibrinolysis in general and lysis of the clot around the recently ruptured aneurysm in particular. It is assumed that it takes 36 h to achieve complete inhibition of fibrinolysis in the cerebrospinal fluid.

In 1967, Gibbs and O'Gorman published the first report on antifibrinolytic treatment in patients with SAH (Gibbs & O'Gorman 1967). Since then, over 30 studies on antifibrinolytic therapy in aneurysmal SAH have been published (Roos *et al.* 2000a). Unfortunately, most are uncontrolled and only a minority of the controlled studies are randomized. Moreover, the results of some of the individual randomized studies contradict each other. The randomized studies have been reviewed as part of the Cochrane Collaboration (Roos *et al.* 2000a).

Eight trials met the predefined inclusion criteria, including 937 patients of whom 476 were randomized to receive antifibrinolytic drugs; 364 received placebo treatment (in five trials) and 97 patients received open control treatment. By far the largest study was the Dutch–Scottish trial reported in 1984 (Vermeulen *et al.* 1984a). In only one study, with 39 patients, EACA was used (Girvin 1973); in all others, TEA was the experimental drug. Only two studies recorded not just case fatality, but also dependency, and only these two could therefore be used in the main analysis, of 'poor outcome'. In that analysis, antifibrinolytic treatment did not provide any evidence of benefit (odds ratio [OR] 1.05; 95% CI, 0.76–1.46) (Fig. 13.3). The outcome measure 'death from any cause' was reported in all eight included studies, and again this comparison provided no evidence of any benefit of antifibrinolytic treatment (OR 0.96; 95% CI, 0.72–1.26).

On the other hand, the analysis of specific event rates did show striking differences. The risk of *re-bleeding* was significantly reduced by antifibrinolytic therapy (OR 0.59; 95% CI, 0.42–0.81). This was also true in the analysis of just the five double-blind and placebo-controlled studies (OR 0.50; 95% CI, 0.34–0.73), as well as in the sensitivity analysis of the two studies with re-bleeds confirmed by CT scan or post-mortem (OR 0.35; 95% CI, 0.22–0.57). In contrast, in the four trials which reported *cerebral ischaemia* rates, antifibrinolytic treatment increased the risk (OR 2.03; 95% CI, 1.40–2.94). Again, this was consistent in the analysis of the two placebo-controlled trials among these four (OR 1.97; 95% CI, 1.33–2.92), and in the sensitivity analysis on the two trials in which cerebral ischaemia was confirmed by CT scan or post-mortem (OR 1.82; 95% CI, 1.15–2.90). *Hydrocephalus* was reported in four trials; antifibrinolytic treatment had no overall effect (OR 1.05; 95% CI, 0.71–1.56).

Antifibrinolytic drugs prevent re-bleeding after aneurysmal rupture, but because they increase the risk of cerebral ischaemia there is no useful effect on overall outcome.

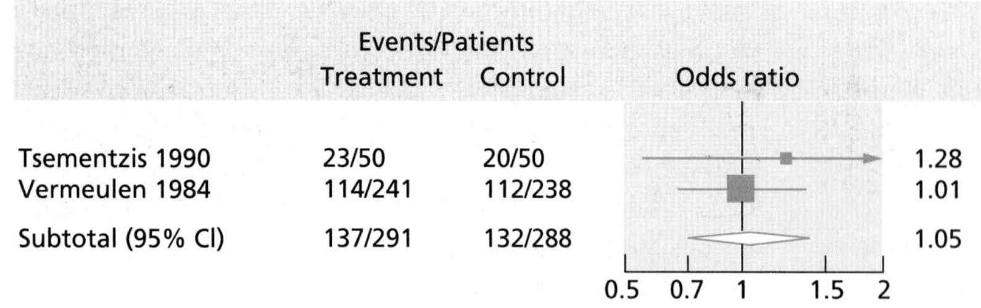

Events/Patients
Treatment
Control
Odds ratio
Tsementzis 1990
23/50
20/50
1.28
Vermeulen 1984
114/241
112/238
1.01
Subtotal (95% CI)
137/291
132/288
1.05
0.5
0.7
1
1.5
2

Fig. 13.3 The results of a systematic review of two placebo controlled randomized trials that examined the effect of antifibrinolytic agents for patients with subarachnoid haemorrhage, in terms of odd ratios for death or dependence. The horizontal error bars indicate the 95% confidence intervals. An odds ratio of greater than 1.0 indicates that more patients were dead or disabled in the group treated with antifibrinolytic agents (with permission from Roos *et al.* 2000a).

In brief, antifibrinolytic drugs work, but they do not help. This does not necessarily mean the end of the story, if measures could be found to prevent the attendant ischaemia. How antifibrinolytic treatment precipitates cerebral ischaemia is still unclear. Possible explanations include increased blood viscosity, the development of microthrombi, delayed clearance of blood clots around the arteries at the base of the brain, and the development of hydrocephalus through delayed resorption of blood. In the Dutch–Scottish trial of TEA, it was after day 6 that the rate of cerebral infarction in patients on the active drug started to exceed that in the placebo group, raising the possibility that a shorter period of treatment might still inhibit re-bleeding yet avoid the ischaemic complications (Vermeulen *et al.* 1984a). Disappointingly, however, a pilot study in which TEA was given for only 4 days produced the reverse of the desired result: the rate of re-bleeding was as high as one would expect in untreated patients, and cerebral ischaemia was as frequent as in previous patients on long-term treatment (Wijdicks *et al.* 1989).

In the meantime, several measures have emerged that are effective in the prevention of ischaemic complications: maintenance of an adequate intake of water and sodium; avoidance of antihypertensive treatment; calcium antagonists; and, if necessary, plasma volume expansion (section 13.6). It is theoretically possible that antifibrinolytic drugs might prevent re-bleeds and yet improve overall outcome if they were combined with these measures to prevent cerebral ischaemia. A preliminary study in which antifibrinolytic drugs and calcium antagonists were combined showed promising results (Beck *et al.* 1988). A new clinical trial has recently been completed in the Netherlands, in which all 492 patients were maximally protected against ischaemia by means of calcium antagonists and hypervolemia, and 229 were randomized to additional treatment with tranexamic acid (Roos 2000b). Tranexamic acid again significantly reduced the rate of re-bleeding, from 33% in the control group to 19% with active treatment (relative risk reduction, 0.58; 95% CI, 0.42–0.80). However, the overall outcome was no different between the two groups, mainly because of cerebral ischaemia. This complication occurred relatively less often in patients with a normal level of consciousness on admission, with a trend towards improvement of overall outcome by tranexamic acid. Unfortunately, even if the result of this post-hoc subgroup analysis is true, it is unlikely to be of any practical use, since nowadays alert patients tend to undergo surgery or coil placement early, despite the lack of evidence (section 13.5.2).

13.5.4 Endovascular occlusion

Until the 1990s, endovascular treatment of aneurysms was restricted to patients in whom the aneurysm was unsuitable for clipping because of its size or location (especially in the posterior circulation), or in whom operation was contraindicated. The technique consisted initially of balloon occlusion, but a more novel development is to pack the aneurysm with coils, first of a pushable kind and more recently with a system for controlled detachment (Guglielmi *et al.* 1992) (Fig. 13.4). Ideally, after coiling, the remaining aneurysmal lumen becomes occluded by a process of reactive thrombosis; post-mortem studies have shown, however, that endothelialization of the aneurysm orifice after placement of coils is the

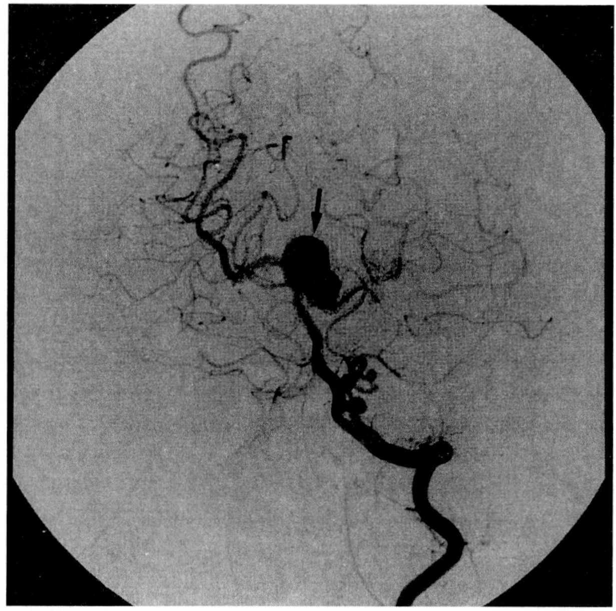

(a)

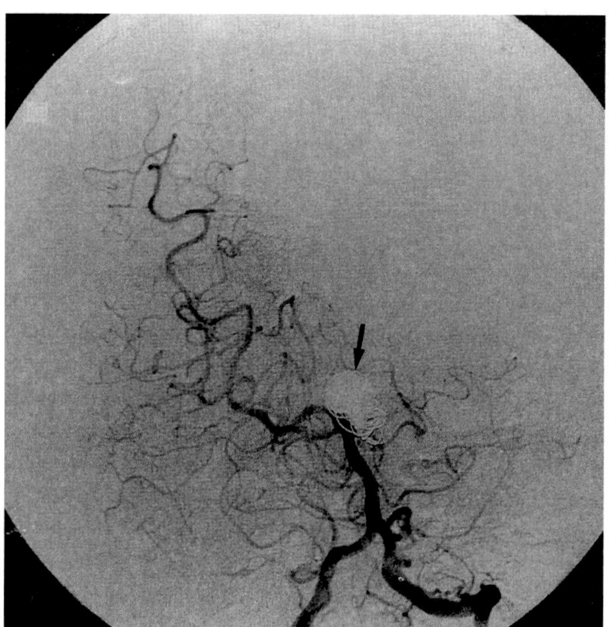

(b)

Fig. 13.4 (a) Catheter angiogram showing an aneurysm (arrow) at the tip of the basilar artery. (b) A repeat angiogram after occlusion of the aneurysm with detachable coils (arrow), through an endovascular approach.

exception rather than the rule (Stiver *et al.* 1998; Bavinzski *et al.* 1999a). In large aneurysms, the process of intra-aneurysm clot organization seems to be delayed and incomplete; tiny open spaces between the coils and an incomplete membranous covering in the region of the neck are frequently encountered (Molyneux *et al.* 1995; Bavinzski *et al.* 1999a).

The technique is much less invasive than surgical treatment, but is not without its hazards. Firstly, the aneurysm may rupture during the procedure, a complication much more difficult to control than during surgical exploration (McDougall *et al.* 1998). Secondly, if the process of reactive thrombosis extends to the parent vessel, infarction of brain tissue may occur. Of course, in patients with ruptured aneurysms, ischaemic complications may occur even without any intervention at all, but the rate may be as high as 38% in patients treated within 3 days, against 22% in patients treated surgically (Gruber *et al.* 1998a). For that reason, most interventional radiologists institute heparin after the procedure, at least for a few days. Finally, one or more coils may become dislodged and herniate or embolize into the parent vessel, which again may lead to ischaemic brain damage (Spetzger *et al.* 1997). The risk of this complication is greater with wide-necked aneurysms; special coils that can expand in three dimensions are being devised to minimize this danger (Malek *et al.* 1999). With detachable coils, the overall rate of ischaemic complications is of the order of 8–9%, and that of re-bleeding 2–3%(Brilstra *et al.* 1999).

Recent years have seen an increasing trend towards detachable coils being used for the treatment of aneurysms that are easily amenable to surgical treatment. Numerous observational studies have published complication rates, occlusion rates and short-term follow-up results. These were summarized, up to March 1997, in a systematic review of 48 eligible studies including 1383 patients (Brilstra *et al.* 1999). Permanent complications of the procedure occurred in 3.7% of 1256 patients in whom this was recorded (95% CI, 2.7%–4.9%); complete occlusion of the aneurysm was achieved in 400 of 744 aneurysms when this information was available (54%; 95% CI, 50%–57%), and of the 569 patients who were followed up, 90% were independent. Of course, this pooled series was biased towards large aneurysms and aneurysms of the posterior circulation, but weighted regression analysis did not demonstrate a relationship between the outcome and aneurysm size, aneurysm neck size, aneurysm location, the aneurysm being ruptured or unruptured, the initial condition of patients (which must reflect a rather homogeneous sample of alert patients), or any other baseline variable (Brilstra *et al.* 1999). Results not markedly different from this compilation have been reported in a few later series (Nichols *et al.* 1997; Raymond & Roy 1997; Raymond *et al.* 1997; Debrun *et al.* 1998; Eskridge & Song 1998; Kuether *et al.* 1998; Bavinzski *et al.* 1999b; Gruber *et al.* 1999a; Murayama *et al.* 1999). Coiling is an especially attractive option in patients with multiple aneurysms (Solander *et al.* 1999) and in patients with sickle cell anaemia (McQuaker *et al.* 1999). Dissecting aneurysms have also been treated by coiling, especially in the posterior fossa (Yamaura *et al.* 1999).

However, non-randomized comparisons between endovascular and surgical treatment are quite inappropriate, if only because there are so many differences in study design, patients, and aneurysms. Moreover, re-rupture of aneurysms may occur even months after apparently successful coiling, and the long-term re-bleeding rates after endovascular coiling still need to be established (Manabe *et al.* 1998; Byrne *et al.* 1999). A first report from a single centre (Oxford, UK), in which more than 300 patients had been followed up after aneurysm embolization for a median period of almost 2 years, reported re-bleeding rates of 0.8% in the first year, 0.6% in the second year and 2.4% in the third year, with no re-bleeding subsequently (Byrne *et al.* 1999). On the other hand, it should not be assumed that surgical treatment is always definitive: in a retrospective review of postoperative angiograms in a series of 66 patients with ruptured aneurysms and 12 additional aneurysms, all treated by surgical clipping, 8% of the patients had aneurysms with a residual lumen, or aneurysms that were previously undetected (Macdonald *et al.* 1993).

For many patients with giant aneurysms, endovascular treatment is the only option, although the difficulties are still considerable (Malisch *et al.* 1997). In some patients with giant aneurysms, coiling is combined with surgical treatment, before or after the operation (Civit *et al.* 1996; Malisch *et al.* 1997; Thielen *et al.* 1997; Hacein-Bey *et al.* 1998; Cockroft *et al.* 2000). In others, vascular reconstruction with balloons is attempted before coiling (Levy & Ku 1997; Levy 1997) or with stenting (Higashida *et al.* 1997; Sekhon *et al.* 1998; Lanzino *et al.* 1999a).

Randomized controlled trials are urgently needed in patients with aneurysms in whom it is uncertain whether surgical clipping or endovascular coiling should be the preferred treatment. A first such study, although small (109 patients), found no difference in outcome at 3 months between the surgical group and the endovascular group (Vanninen *et al.* 1999). Fortunately, some larger studies are now under way. An international study coordinated from Oxford had randomized more than 1000 patients at the time of writing, and is still actively recruiting (http://users.ox.ac.uk/~isat/). Since the safety and efficacy of coiling compared with clipping is not known, the most efficient way to evaluate the new technology is to offer it only within the context of a randomized trial. Enthusiasts for coiling may find it difficult to accept this stricture, but it is all too easy for such new technologies to creep into routine clinical practice without proper evaluation; innovation is not necessarily the same as progress.

13.6 Prevention of delayed cerebral ischaemia

13.6.1 Pathogenesis and risk factors

Unlike stroke occurring as a result of disease of the extracranial or intracranial arteries, cerebral ischaemia or infarction after subarachnoid haemorrhage (SAH) is not confined to the territory of a single cerebral artery or one of its branches (Hijdra *et al.* 1986) (Figs 13.5 & 13.6). Vasospasm is often implicated, because its peak frequency from day 5 to day 14 coincides with that of delayed ischaemia (Weir *et al.* 1978), and also because it is often generalized, in keeping with the multifocal or diffuse nature of the clinical manifestations and of the ischaemic lesions found on CT and at post-mortem (Heros *et al.* 1983; Kistler *et al.* 1983). None the less, there are strong objections to the widespread use of the term

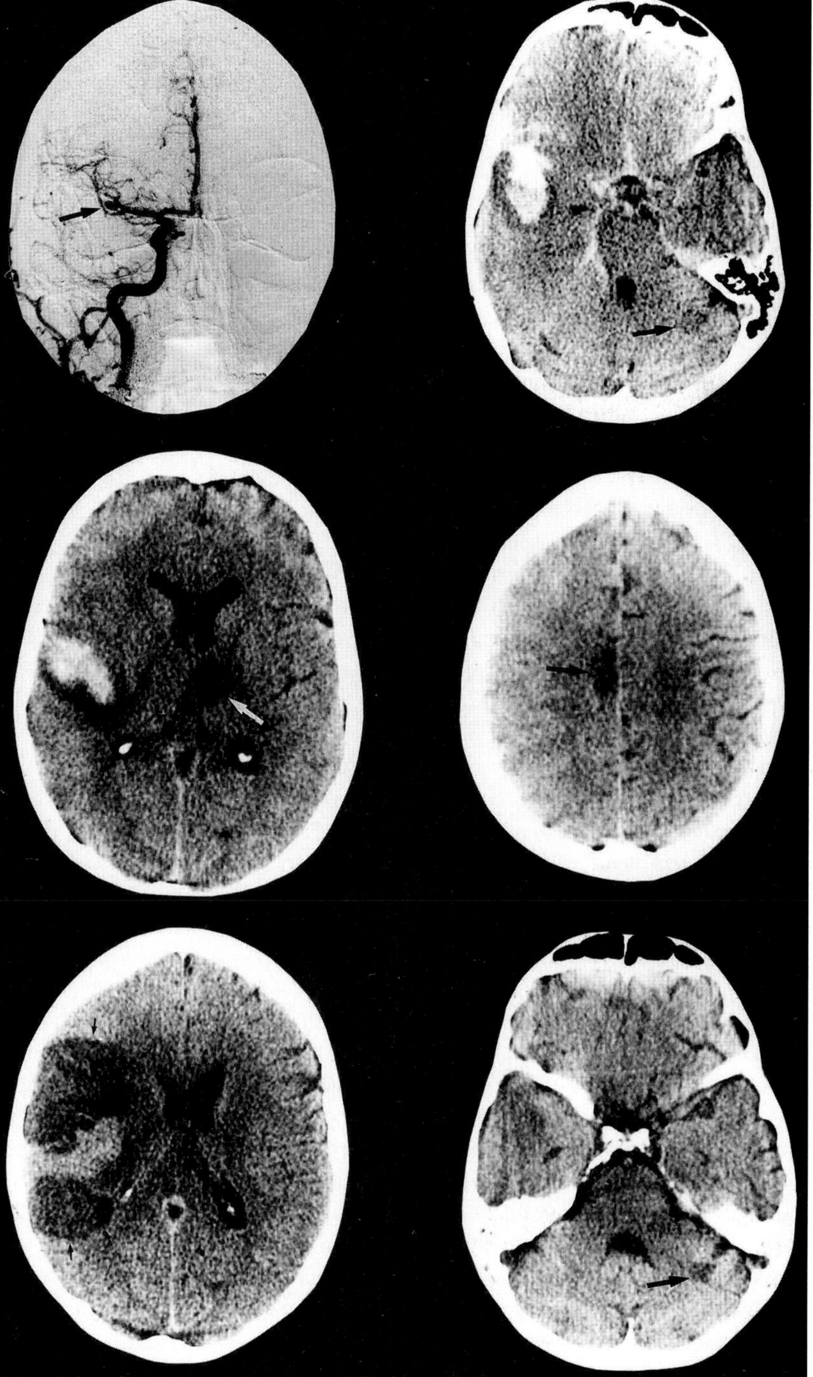

Fig. 13.5 Delayed cerebral ischaemia after subarachnoid haemorrhage, with scattered lesions. Cerebral catheter angiography and CT brain scans of a 43-year-old woman with subarachnoid haemorrhage. Angiography on the day of the haemorrhage (upper row, left) showed an aneurysm of the right middle cerebral artery (arrow), consistent with the CT scan on admission (not shown). On the second day, after a gradual decline in the level of consciousness, a repeat CT scan (upper row, right) showed unchanged blood in the basal cisterns and an unchanged intracranial haematoma at the site of the aneurysm, but also a newly developed focal hypodensity in the left cerebellar hemisphere (arrow). On the fifth day after the haemorrhage, she developed hemiparesis on the left, with a further decline in the level of consciousness. The CT now showed infarcts in the left thalamus (middle row, left: white arrow), and in the distal territory of the right anterior cerebral artery (middle row, right: black arrow). Ten days after the haemorrhage, the haematoma had resolved, leaving a large area of ischaemia (bottom row, left: arrows). One month after the haemorrhage, the left cerebellar infarct is still clearly visible (bottom row, right: arrow) (with permission from Hop *et al.* 1996).

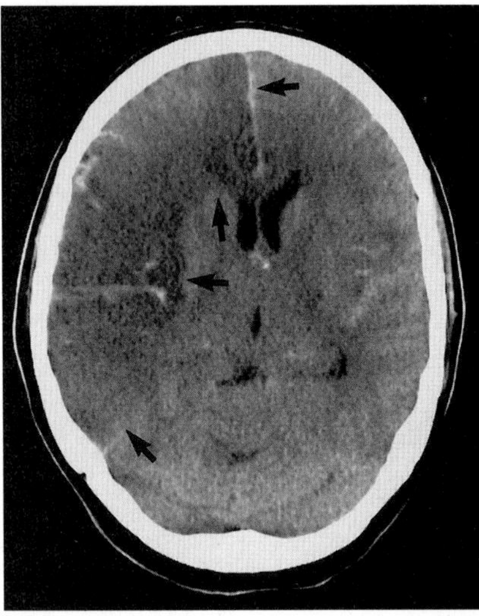
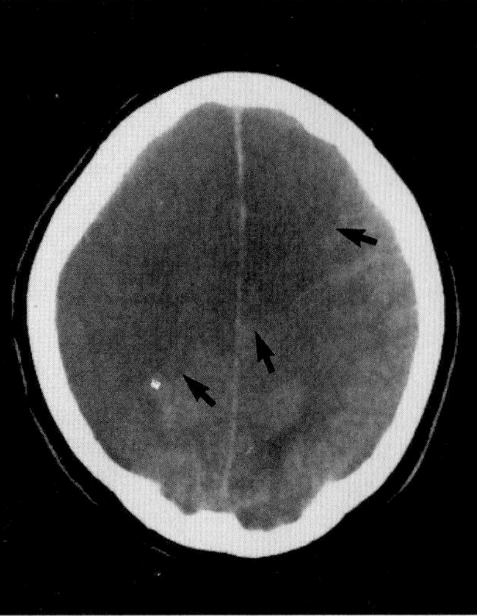

Fig. 13.6 Diffuse ischaemia in the right hemisphere and in the frontal lobe of the left hemisphere (arrows), in a 47-year-old woman with a ruptured aneurysm of the anterior communicating artery; she was not admitted until 1 week after the onset of acute headache, when her level of consciousness started to deteriorate. Within 2 days of admission, she became brain dead.

'vasospasm' as a synonym for delayed cerebral ischaemia—not so much out of fastidiousness on our part, but because the exchange of one term for the other impedes understanding and, even worse, progress. There are at least five reasons why vasospasm is not synonymous with delayed cerebral ischaemia:

• firstly, arterial narrowing does not necessarily signify contraction of smooth muscle in the arterial wall, but may represent necrosis and secondary oedema in the wall (Conway & McDonald 1972; Hughes & Schianchi 1978; Smith *et al.* 1983; Findlay *et al.* 1989). Intimal proliferation is another possibility—a process shown to underlie restenosis in coronary arteries after balloon angioplasty (Post *et al.* 1994);

• secondly, arterial narrowing can be asymptomatic, even if severe (Millikan 1975; Fisher *et al.* 1977);

• thirdly, the interpretation of angiographic appearances relating to the severity or even the presence of arterial narrowing is subject to considerable variation between observers (Eskesen *et al.* 1987);

• fourthly, treatment with nimodipine is very effective in preventing delayed cerebral ischaemia (see below), but it does not significantly affect the frequency of arterial narrowing (Pickard *et al.* 1989);

• finally, vasospasm is only one of the factors involved in the pathogenesis of cerebral infarction in patients with ruptured aneurysms (Table 13.6).

Many of the predictive factors for delayed cerebral ischaemia listed in Table 13.6 are interrelated, or depend on intermediate factors; these interactions are complex and poorly understood. They include the development of hyponatraemia and hypovolaemia (section 13.10.1). An often-quoted study postulated a close relationship between the location of subarachnoid blood and the 'thickness' of the clot, on the one hand, and the occurrence of vasospasm and delayed cerebral ischaemia, on the other, but these observations were based on only 41 patients (Kistler *et al.* 1983). Moreover, the method of assessing local amounts of subarachnoid blood (called the Fisher scale, after the last author), is associated with wide interobserver variation (Svensson *et al.* 1996). Although there is little doubt that the overall amount of subarachnoid blood, as seen on CT scan, is a powerful predictor of delayed cerebral ischaemia, larger series have failed to show any relationship between the anatomical distribution or even the side of infarction and the site of the extravasated blood in the subarachnoid space (Hijdra *et al.* 1986; Brouwers *et al.* 1992). Another awkward fact, often conveniently overlooked, is that delayed cerebral ischaemia is rare after SAH from arteriovenous malformations, despite arterial narrowing in some cases (Maeda *et al.* 1997), and that it does not occur at all in non-aneurysmal perimesencephalic SAH, even after matching for the amount of extravasated blood

Table 13.6 Factors associated with delayed cerebral ischaemia after subarachnoid haemorrhage.

Arterial narrowing (Kistler *et al.* 1983)
But also:
Loss of consciousness >1 h at onset (Brouwers *et al.* 1992; Hop *et al.* 1999)
Amount of subarachnoid blood on early CT scanning (Hijdra *et al.* 1988; Öhman *et al.* 1991; Brouwers *et al.* 1992)
Acute hydrocephalus (van Gijn *et al.* 1985; Hasan *et al.* 1991b; Fujii *et al.* 1997)
Hyponatraemia and hypovolaemia (Wijdicks *et al.* 1985a; Wijdicks *et al.* 1985b; Hasan *et al.* 1990)
Treatment with antihypertensive drugs (Wijdicks *et al.* 1990)
Treatment with antifibrinolytic drugs (Vermeulen *et al.* 1984a)
Previous cigarette smoking? (Lasner *et al.* 1997)
Detection of emboli on transcranial Doppler monitoring, after surgical clipping (Giller *et al.* 1998)

(Rinkel *et al.* 1991). It is not too far-fetched to speculate that damage to the wall of an artery, or a generalized perfusion deficit at the time of bleeding, or both, are necessary determinants of delayed cerebral ischaemia.

> *Cerebral ischaemia after subarachnoid haemorrhage occurs only if the source is a ruptured aneurysm; whether or not it develops is strongly related to the total amount of subarachnoid blood, but much less to the distribution of the extravasated blood.*

The search for substances that might act as mediators for arterial narrowing in the development of delayed cerebral ischaemia has been intensified after the recognition of several new candidate molecules. Firstly, nitrous oxide is an important regulatory molecule by which endothelial cells regulate vascular tone through the layer of smooth-muscle cells. Secondly, similar roles have been attributed to endothelin and protein C kinase (Sobey & Faraci 1998). Other intermediate factors that have been implicated are coagulation factors (Fujii *et al.* 1997; Peltonen *et al.* 1997; Ikeda *et al.* 1997), cytokines (Gaetani *et al.* 1998) and adhesion molecules (Polin *et al.* 1998a), but the results of these studies are inconsistent and often contradictory.

In summary, any causal relationship between the amount of extravasated blood and the development of delayed cerebral ischaemia is not sufficiently explained by the production of putative toxic substances released from clots around the large arteries at the base of the brain. As loss of consciousness at the time of the haemorrhage is an important and independent predictive factor for delayed cerebral ischaemia (Brouwers *et al.* 1992), it is conceivable that global ischaemia during this brief period, along with a massive increase in intracranial pressure, may sensitize neurones to marginal perfusion associated with later complications, such as diffuse vasospasm or hypovolaemia.

Practical measures that may help to prevent ischaemia are avoidance of antihypertensive drugs, an adequate intake of fluid and sodium, although the benefit of such regimens is supported by indirect evidence only (Rosenwasser *et al.* 1983; Hasan *et al.* 1989a; Vermeij *et al.* 1998) (section 13.4.2). Of possible drug treatments, randomized controlled trials so far support only routine administration of calcium antagonists (section 13.6.2). Other theoretically attractive pharmacological interventions remain largely unproven so far: maintaining plasma volume by means of fludrocortisone acetate or albumin, neuroprotection via hydroxyl radical scavengers, and—after aneurysm occlusion—prophylaxis with antithrombotic drugs such as aspirin.

13.6.2 Calcium antagonists

Calcium entry blocking drugs have been used because they inhibit the contractile properties of smooth-muscle cells, particularly those in cerebral arteries, and also because they may to some extent protect neurones against the deleterious effect of calcium influx after ischaemic damage (Greenberg 1987) (section 11.1.4). A Cochrane Review has assessed the clinical trials that addressed the question of whether calcium antagonists improve outcome in patients with aneurysmal subarachnoid haemorrhage (SAH) (Feigin *et al.* 2000). The Cochrane Stroke Review Group's search strategy, plus hand searching and personal contacts with trialists and pharmaceutical companies marketing calcium antagonists, identified 11 completed, unconfounded, truly randomized controlled trials comparing any calcium antagonist with control within 10 days of SAH onset. In the 11 trials, 2804 patients with subarachnoid haemorrhage had been randomized (1376 in the treatment and 1428 in the control group). The drugs analysed were: nimodipine (eight trials, 1574 patients), nicardipine (two trials, 954 patients), and AT-877 (fasudil; one trial, 276 patients). In 92% of the patients, aneurysms were confirmed by angiography or post-mortem.

Overall, calcium antagonists significantly reduced the risk of a poor outcome (relative risk (RR) 0.82; 95% CI, 0.72–0.93); the absolute risk reduction was 5.1%, and the corresponding number of patients needed to treat to prevent a single poor outcome event was 20. For oral nimodipine alone, the RR was 0.69 (95% CI, 0.58–0.84). The RR of death on treatment with calcium antagonists was 0.94 (95% CI, 0.80–1.10), that of ischaemic neurological deficits 0.67 (95% CI, 0.59–0.76), and that of CT-documented cerebral infarction was 0.80 (95% CI, 0.71–0.89). Calcium antagonists reduced the proportion of patients with poor outcome and ischaemic neurological deficits after aneurysmal SAH, but the risk reduction for overall case fatality alone was not statistically significant. The results for 'poor outcome' were statistically robust, but depended mainly on trials with oral nimodipine, and especially on a single large trial (Pickard *et al.* 1989); the evidence for nicardipine and AT-877 was inconclusive. The intermediate factors through which nimodipine exerts its beneficial effect after aneurysmal SAH remain uncertain. Interestingly, several studies with nimodipine found there was no difference between treated patients and controls with regard to the frequency of arterial narrowing on a repeat angiogram (Philippon *et al.* 1986; Petruk *et al.* 1988; Pickard *et al.* 1989). Therefore, at least with this particular calcium antagonist, the protective effect on neurones seems to be more important than any amelioration of vasospasm. An uncontrolled study, in which nimodipine was stopped after 2 weeks if there had been no signs of ischaemia up to that time, found no deleterious effects (Toyota 1999).

The practical implications are that the regimen in the dominant nimodipine trial (60 mg orally every 4 h, continued for 3 weeks) is currently regarded as the standard treatment in patients with aneurysmal subarachnoid haemorrhage. If the patient is unable to swallow, the tablets should be crushed and washed down a nasogastric tube with normal saline.

And yet almost all the evidence about efficacy and dosage of nimodipine hinges on this single, large clinical trial (Pickard *et al.* 1989). Given the uncertain effect on overall case fatality, and the possibility that the results of the meta-analysis might be affected by unpublished negative trials, the benefits of nimodipine cannot be regarded as being beyond all reasonable doubt.

Oral nimodipine probably reduces the risk of a poor outcome after subarachnoid haemorrhage by about one-third.

Low blood pressure may complicate administration of nimodipine, not only with the intravenous route but also when the drug is given orally (Feigin *et al.* 2000). If no blood loss has occurred or any other cause for hypotension is found, the dose of nimodipine should be halved (to 60 mg t.d.s.), and subsequently discontinued if the blood pressure does not come back to initial levels.

13.6.3 Increasing plasma volume

Because of its mineralocorticoid activity (reabsorption of sodium in the distal tubules of the kidney), fludrocortisone might, in theory, prevent a negative sodium balance, hypovolaemia and so ischaemic complications (Wijdicks *et al.* 1988a). A randomized study in which 91 patients were entered soon after admission showed that fludrocortisone acetate significantly reduced natriuresis in the first 6 days after the haemorrhage. Reductions in the plasma volume depletion and of ischaemic complications were not statistically significant, but such beneficial effects may have been masked because patients in the control group were often treated with plasma expanders after they had developed clinical signs of ischaemia (Hasan *et al.* 1989b). These results were confirmed by a smaller trial in 30 patients (Mori *et al.* 1999). The available evidence is insufficiently conclusive to warrant routine administration of fludrocortisone to all patients with subarachnoid haemorrhage.

A small randomized trial of 5% albumin (2-hourly, until central venous pressures of 5–8 mmHg were reached), resulted in an even sodium balance in the experimental group of 19 patients after aneurysm operation, against an average sodium loss in 24 randomized controls in whom central venous pressure was kept below 5 mmHg; there was no difference in blood volume, while the number of patients was too small to allow conclusions about prevention of ischaemia (Mayer *et al.* 1998).

13.6.4 Free radical scavengers

Tirilazad mesylate, a 21-aminosteroid free radical scavenger, has so far failed to show consistent improvement of outcome in four randomized controlled trials, with a total of more than 3500 patients (Kassell *et al.* 1996; Haley *et al.* 1997; Lanzino & Kassell 1999; Lanzino *et al.* 1999b). The only beneficial effect on the overall outcome was seen in a single subgroup of a single trial, i.e. those treated with 6 mg/kg/day (two other groups received 0.2 mg/kg/day or 2 mg/kg/day) (Kassell *et al.* 1996). Unfortunately, this possible benefit could not be reproduced in the corresponding subgroup in a parallel trial (Haley *et al.* 1997), nor in two further trials with an even higher dose (15 mg/kg/day) in women (Lanzino & Kassell 1999; Lanzino *et al.* 1999b); the sex distinction was made because in the first two trials women did not seem to respond as well as men. Delayed cerebral ischaemia was reduced in only one of the four trials—but in the one that failed to show an effect on overall outcome (Lanzino *et al.* 1999b), and not in the other three. A paper reporting that patients receiving the study drug in a small subgroup in New Zealand had less fatigue and better neuropsychological performance than controls suggests desperation rather than conviction among the investigators and the sponsoring company (Ogden *et al.* 1998). A formal overview of the complete clinical evidence is not yet available, but the case for the drug seems weak, for any dose and in either sex.

A single trial with another hydroxyl radical scavenger, *N'*-propylenedinicotinamide (nicaraven) in 162 patients, showed a decreased rate of delayed cerebral ischaemia but no reduction in the rate of poor outcomes at 3 months after subarachnoid haemorrhage (SAH) (Asano *et al.* 1996). Curiously enough, the reverse was found in a trial of 286 patients with ebselen, a seleno-organic compound with antioxidant activity through a glutathione peroxidase-like action: improved outcome at 3 months after SAH, but without any reduction in the frequency of delayed ischaemia (Saito *et al.* 1998).

13.6.5 Aspirin and other antiplatelet agents

Several studies have found that blood platelets are activated from day 3 after subarachnoid haemorrhage (SAH). This is mostly inferred from increased levels of thromboxane B_2, the stable metabolite of thromboxane A_2, which promotes platelet aggregation and vasoconstriction (Vinge *et al.* 1988; Juvela *et al.* 1990; Ohkuma *et al.* 1991) (section 11.1.3). The practical question is whether interventions aimed at counteracting platelet activation are therapeutically useful. A retrospective analysis of 242 patients who had survived the first 4 days after SAH suggested that patients who had used salicylates before their haemorrhage (by history and urine screening) had significantly less delayed cerebral ischaemia, with or without permanent deficits (relative risk, 0.40; 95% CI, 0.18–0.93) (Juvela 1995). The first clinical trial was carried out as early as 1982, and failed to show benefit from aspirin (Mendelow *et al.* 1982); however, the number of patients was small (53), unoperated patients were also included, and all were treated with tranexamic acid, which increases the risk of ischaemia (section 13.5.3) This therapeutic option warrants a prospective and randomized study of salicylates or other antiplatelet drugs as a preventive measure against delayed cerebral ischaemia—preferably after clipping or coiling the aneurysm, to avoid re-bleeding being precipitated by the antiplatelet and so antihaemostatic action. A pilot study of aspirin after early operation in 50 patients has shown that this treatment is feasible and probably safe (Hop *et al.*, unpublished observations).

Four antiplatelet drugs other than aspirin have been tested in separate trials of patients with SAH:

- dipyridamole (100 mg/day orally or 10 mg/day intravenously), in 320 patients (Shaw *et al.* 1985);
- the thromboxane A_2 synthetase inhibitor nizofenone (10 mg/day intravenously), in 77 patients (Saito *et al.* 1983);
- the thromboxane A_2 synthetase inhibitor Cataclot (ozagrel sodium, 1 µg/kg/min intravenously), in 24 patients (Tokiyoshi *et al.* 1991);
- the experimental antiplatelet agent OKY-46, 160 mg or 800 mg orally, in 256 patients (Suzuki *et al.* 1989).

Ischaemic neurological deficits were reduced in one study (Suzuki *et al.* 1989), but not in the other study that assessed this outcome event (Tokiyoshi *et al.* 1991). In a systematic overview of these four trials, and the two aspirin trials mentioned in the preceding paragraph, poor outcome was not significantly different between patients treated with antiplatelet agents and controls (Raupp *et al.*, unpublished review).

13.7 Management of re-bleeding

13.7.1 Diagnosis

Loss of consciousness was the cardinal feature of re-bleeding in a prospective series of 39 patients with a CT-proven re-bleed: of the 36 patients who were awake at the time, 35 lost consciousness, preceded by headache in one-third; in the remaining patient, a sudden increase in headache was the only symptom (Hijdra *et al.* 1987b). In the same study, only serial CT scanning uncovered re-bleeding in two of the three remaining patients, in whom the level of consciousness was already minimal; in other words, no 'silent re-bleeding' was found in awake patients. In patients with a first episode of subarachnoid haemorrhage (SAH), loss of consciousness is less common, occurring in slightly less than 50% (Vermeulen *et al.* 1984a). This difference in the proportion with unconsciousness at onset confirms that re-bleeding has a more severe impact on the brain than the first bleed (Fig. 13.7), which also follows from the higher case fatality (50%). In fatal episodes of re-bleeding, most patients immediately lose their brainstem reflexes at the same time as consciousness, but without initial apnoea (Hijdra *et al.* 1987b).

Re-bleeding is not the only cause of a sudden deterioration of consciousness in a patient with a ruptured aneurysm. Other complications underlie about one-third of all episodes of sudden deterioration (Table 13.7). The frequency of re-bleeding is overestimated to an even greater degree if the mode of onset is not precisely known (Maurice-Williams 1982). Once the respiratory and circulatory state of the patient has sufficiently stabilized, it is mandatory to confirm the diagnosis of re-bleeding by repeat brain CT, which may show successive layers of fresh blood in the brain substance or the ventricular system, each layer corresponding to an episode of clinical deterioration (Vermeulen *et al.* 1984b). Lumbar puncture, apart from its dangers, is unreliable for the diagnosis of re-bleeding (Vermeulen *et al.* 1983).

13.7.2 To resuscitate or not?

The question of whether patients with a re-bleed should be resuscitated and artificially ventilated if respiratory arrest occurs is not academic. In the series of 39 patients with a CT-confirmed re-bleed mentioned earlier, 14 had initial respiratory abnormalities that called for assisted ventilation. Spontaneous respiration returned within an hour in eight of these 14 patients, and in three more between one and 24 hours (Hijdra *et al.* 1984). In a study of episodes of respiratory arrest in which first bleeds were also included, the answer to the question of whether the patient would or would not regain spontaneous respiration could not be predicted from the anatomical site of haemorrhage on CT, the initial presence or absence of brainstem reflexes, or the type of respiratory disorder (Hijdra *et al.* 1984). Many patients with initial apnoea who were successfully resuscitated later died from subsequent complications—but the message to be remembered is that survival without brain damage is possible, even after respiratory arrest. That is another important reason why patients with a recently ruptured aneurysm should be under close and continuous observation. After resuscitation, it will usually become clear within a matter of hours whether the patient will indeed survive the episode, or whether dysfunction of the brainstem will persist. There are no good grounds to fear that the intervention will only result in prolongation of a vegetative state. Furthermore, in those patients who progress to brain death from a devastating re-bleed, usually with massive hydrocephalus and large intraventricular clots, the resuscitation procedure has at least allowed organ donation to be considered, with benefits to others.

Table 13.7 Specific causes of sudden deterioration in patients with aneurysmal subarachnoid haemorrhage (from Vermeulen *et al.* 1984b).

Re-bleeding (two-thirds) (section 13.7)
Epileptic seizure (section 13.4.3)
Delayed cerebral ischaemia, with atypical, sudden onset (section 13.8)
Ventricular fibrillation (section 13.10.2)

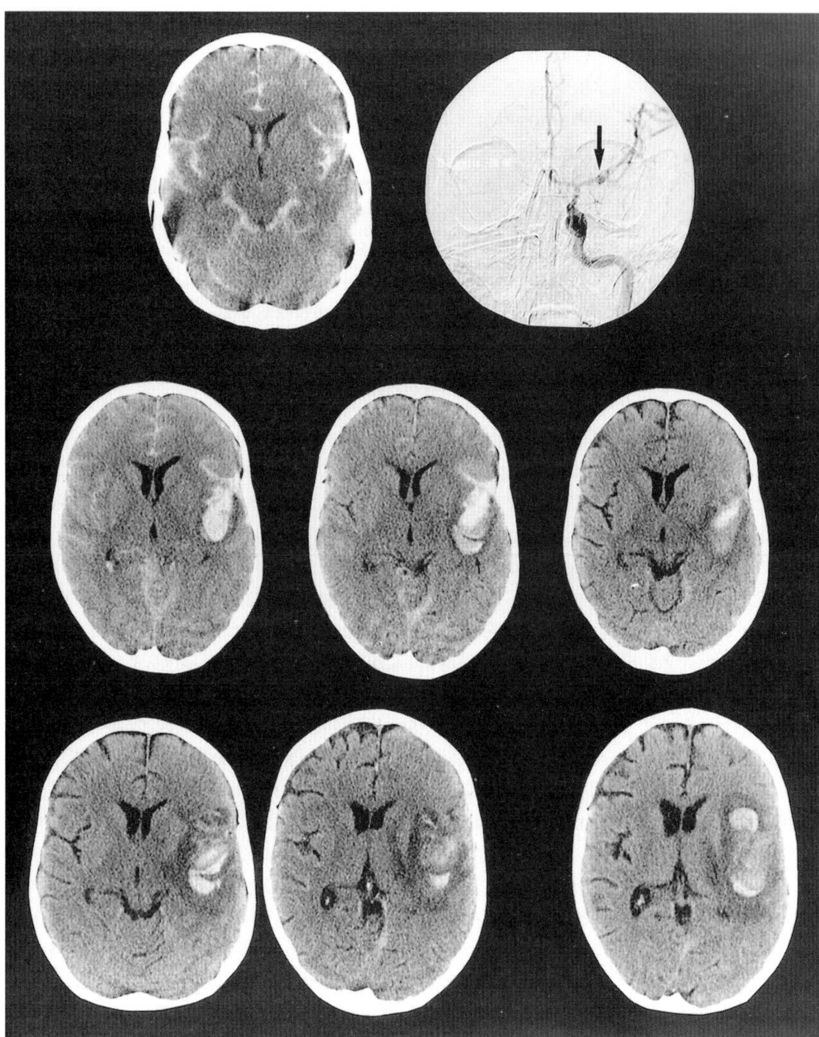

Fig. 13.7 Serial CT brain scans with multiple episodes of re-bleeding. *Top, left:* diffuse haemorrhage throughout all the subarachnoid spaces, in a 45-year-old man (day 0). *Middle row, left:* CT scan showing a haematoma in the left Sylvian fissure, after a sudden episode of clinical deterioration (day 1). *Top, right:* angiogram, made on day 3, after substantial improvement in the level of consciousness; aneurysm of the left middle cerebral artery (arrow). *Middle row, centre:* CT scan after angiography (day 3), following a second episode of sudden deterioration. There is a new compartment of blood at the posterior end of the previous haematoma (arrow). *Middle row, right:* resorption of the haematoma (day 12). *Bottom row, left and centre:* CT scan showing fresh blood, after a third episode of clinical deterioration (day 15). *Bottom, right:* CT scan showing fresh haematoma at site of aneurysm, following a fourth episode, with a sudden decrease in the level of consciousness (day 24). Eventually, the patient successfully underwent surgery on day 53.

Sudden apnoea in a patient with subarachnoid haemorrhage usually signifies re-bleeding. With full resuscitative measures, spontaneous respiration will rapidly return in approximately 50% of the cases, followed within hours by return of consciousness and of brainstem reflexes if these were lost at the same time. If spontaneous respiration does not return, then organ donation should be considered.

13.7.3 Emergency clipping or coiling of the aneurysm

A large haematoma that causes brain shift without gross intraventricular haemorrhage is an infrequent finding after re-bleeding, occurring in around 10% (Hijdra *et al.* 1987b). In these rare cases, evacuation of the haematoma may be indicated (section 13.3.1). A more common reason for neurosurgical intervention after re-bleeding is the concern that amongst the survivors, 50–75% have a further re-bleed (Inagawa *et al.* 1987; Hijdra *et al.* 1987b). This implies that emergency clipping or coiling of the aneurysm should be seriously considered in patients who regain consciousness after re-bleeding. Of course, the risk of the operation is increased after a re-bleed, but the risks of a wait-and-see policy at that stage seem even more intimidating. The management of re-bleeding is summarized in Table 13.8.

13.8 Management of cerebral ischaemia

13.8.1 Diagnosis

The clinical manifestations of delayed cerebral ischaemia evolve gradually, over several hours, and usually between days 4 and 12 after the haemorrhage. In a quarter of the patients, ischaemia causes hemispheric focal deficits; in another quarter, a decrease in the level of consciousness; and in the remaining half of the patients, these two features develop at the same time (Hijdra *et al.* 1986). The diagnosis

Table 13.8 Management of re-bleeding.

In case of respiratory arrest, resuscitate and ventilate; within hours, either spontaneous respiration will return or all other brainstem functions will be lost
Repeat CT brain scan
Consider emergency clipping or coiling of the aneurysm after recovery, as the majority will re-bleed again, with a high case fatality; any intracranial haematoma can be removed at the same time

of cerebral ischaemia should be based not only on this clinical picture, but also on the results of a repeat CT brain scan (Fig. 13.5). The scan serves to exclude other intracranial causes of subacute deterioration such as oedema surrounding an intracranial haematoma, dilatation of the ventricular system, or unsuspected re-bleeding (Table 13.9). Positive evidence of ischaemia is shown by CT in about 80% of patients after exclusion of these other causes, at least after a few days (Hijdra *et al.* 1986). Magnetic resonance imaging is probably more sensitive in detecting early changes in the water content of the brain parenchyma, but the acquisition time needed to obtain good images is often too long for ill and restless patients. Single photon emission computed tomography (SPECT) scanning may be helpful, but hypoperfusion may also result from oedema around a resolving haematoma or, if it occurs in the basal parts of the brain, from hydrocephalus (Davis *et al.* 1990; Hasan *et al.* 1991a). Transcranial Doppler sonography may suggest impending cerebral ischaemia by means of the increased blood flow velocity from arterial narrowing in the middle cerebral artery or in the posterior circulation, but there is considerable overlap with patients who do not develop ischaemia (Sloan *et al.* 1989, 1994). One reason is that narrowing in distal branches of the middle cerebral artery often escapes detection (Okada *et al.* 1999). A recent study specified that only velocities below 120 cm/s or above 200 cm/s were reasonably accurate in excluding or predicting delayed ischaemia, respectively, but almost 60% of patients were in the intermediate range (Vora *et al.* 1999). Even then, demonstration of arterial narrowing does not prove in itself that clinical deterioration has been caused by ischaemia. Furthermore, factors such as intracranial pressure, arterial blood pressure and respiration may all influence the velocity waveform.

Table 13.9 Causes of subacute clinical deterioration after subarachnoid haemorrhage.

Oedema surrounding intracranial haematoma (section 13.3.1)
Cerebral ischaemia (section 13.8.1)
Hydrocephalus (section 13.9.1)
Unsuspected re-bleeding (section 13.7.1)
Systemic complications (section 13.10)
Hyponatraemia
Disturbance of heart rhythm
Neurogenic pulmonary oedema
Hypotension
Infection

13.8.2 Induced hypertension and volume expansion

Since the 1960s, induced hypertension has been used to combat ischaemic deficits in patients with subarachnoid haemorrhage (SAH) (Farhat & Schneider 1967). Later, induced hypertension was often combined with volume expansion. Particularly remarkable was the case of a 50-year-old woman with a ruptured middle cerebral artery aneurysm who developed aphasia and a right-sided hemiparesis postoperatively. Her deficits cleared when she was treated with noradrenaline and blood transfusion, which raised her blood pressure from 120/70 to 180/110 mmHg. Numerous attempts during the next few days to allow the blood pressure to fall into the normal range were always met by worsening of her neurological condition. This treatment regimen was also successful in five of six other patients (Kosnik & Hunt 1976). The effect of induced hypertension and volume expansion was later assessed in a larger series of patients with progressive neurological deterioration and angiographically confirmed 'vasospasm' (Kassell *et al.* 1982). The authors were able to reverse the deficits in 47 of 58 cases, and permanently in 43. In 16 patients who responded to this treatment, the neurological deficits recurred when the blood pressure transiently dropped, but again resolved when the pressure increased. Similar results have been obtained in two other series, although both reported the degree of improvement in rather vague terms (Awad *et al.* 1987; Miller *et al.* 1995). The most plausible explanation for these phenomena is a defect of cerebral autoregulation that makes the perfusion of the brain passively dependent on the systemic blood pressure.

The risks of deliberately increasing the arterial pressure and plasma volume include re-bleeding of an untreated aneurysm, increased cerebral oedema, or haemorrhagic transformation in areas of infarction (Amin-Hanjani *et al.* 1999), myocardial infarction and congestive heart failure. If cardiac failure is refractory to maximum pressor and inotropic infusions, an intra-aortic balloon pump may bridge the critical period (Apostolides *et al.* 1996). At any rate, the circulatory system should be closely monitored with an arterial line and either a central venous or pulmonary artery catheter. These monitoring procedures carry their own risks: infection, pneumothorax, haemothorax, ventricular dysrhythmias and pulmonary infarction (Rosenwasser *et al.* 1995). Some have found that the development of neurological deficits was more closely related to the pulmonary capillary wedge pressure than to the blood pressure, or to a measure of cardiac output (Finn *et al.* 1986). A currently recommended regimen, although it is not supported by rigorously controlled trials, is to start with plasma volume expansion with hetastarch or another colloid solution (Table 13.10). Administration of albumin 5% does not increase plasma volume (Mayer *et al.* 1998). The aim is to raise the central venous filling pressure to approximately 8–12 mmHg, or the pulmonary capillary wedge pressure to about 14–18 mmHg. If no clinical improvement is obtained with these measures, one might consider raising the blood pressure with dopamine or dobutamine to a level of 20–40 mmHg above pretreatment values (Biller *et al.* 1988). These procedures should only be carried out in an intensive-care unit with facilities for specialized care and close monitoring.

13.8.3 Translumenal angioplasty

A few centres have reported on the endovascular approach in the treatment of 'symptomatic vasospasm' (Higashida *et al.* 1989; Newell *et al.* 1989; Nichols *et al.* 1994; Firlik *et al.* 1997; Bejjani *et al.* 1998; Eskridge *et al.* 1998). These reports document sustained improvement in more than half the cases, but the series were uncontrolled and evidently there must be publication bias. Others have reported results only for arteries, and not for patients (Elliott *et al.* 1998; Eskridge *et al.* 1999). Re-bleeding may be precipitated by this procedure, even after the aneurysm has been clipped (Newell *et al.* 1989; Linskey *et al.* 1991). A post-mortem study in two patients showed that the procedure had resulted in stretching and disruption of a degenerate muscular layer, as well as of proliferated collagen tissue (Honma *et al.* 1995). Hyperperfusion injury has also been reported (Schoser *et al.* 1997). In view of the risks, the high costs and the lack of randomized controlled trials, translumenal angioplasty should presently be regarded as a strictly experimental procedure.

Table 13.10 Management of cerebral ischaemia.

Immediately administer 500 mL of plasma expander
Insert subclavian vein catheter or pulmonary arterial balloon catheter; maintain central venous pressure between 8 and 12 mmHg, or pulmonary wedge pressure between 14 and 18 mmHg
Keep arterial pressure 20–40 mmHg above baseline values
Maintain fluid intake with at least 3 L of normal saline (0.9%) per 24 h
Correct hyponatraemia, if severe (Table 13.12)

The same applies to uncontrolled reports of improvement of ischaemic deficits after intra-arterial infusion of papaverine, following superselective catheterization (Kaku *et al.* 1992; Elliott *et al.* 1998; Fandino *et al.* 1998); moreover, not all of these impressions are positive (Polin *et al.* 1998b).

13.8.4 Pharmacological intervention

Calcitonin gene-related peptide (CGRP) is a potent vasodilator in the carotid vascular bed, but a randomized, multicentre, single-blind clinical trial in 62 patients failed to bear out any benefit in terms of overall outcome: the relative risk of a poor outcome in CGRP-treated patients was 0.88 (95% CI, 0.60–1.28) (Anon. 1992). Cyclosporin A also failed to produce improvement in nine patients (Manno *et al.* 1997).

13.9 Management of acute hydrocephalus

13.9.1 Diagnosis

In several series of patients admitted within 3 days of subarachnoid haemorrhage who were not selected for aneurysm surgery, the frequency of acute hydrocephalus (defined as a bicaudate index above the 95th percentile for age; Fig. 13.8) was consistently around 20% (van Gijn *et al.* 1985; Milhorat 1987; Hasan *et al.* 1991b). Of those, only 10–28% had a normal level of consciousness, but approximately one-third of them deteriorated in the next few days (Hasan *et al.* 1989c).

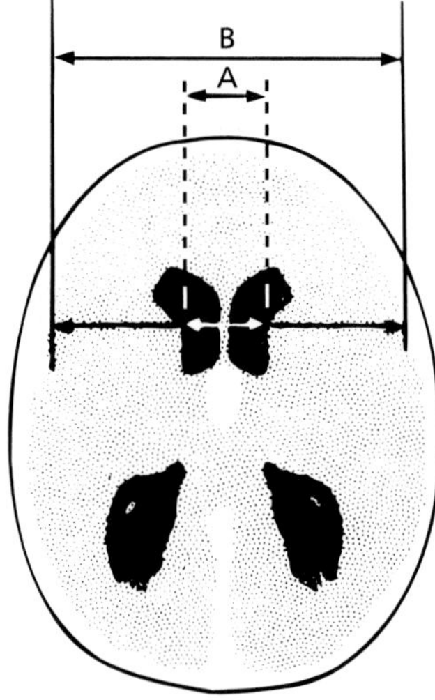

Fig. 13.8 Diagram showing the bicaudate index (A/B), a simple and linear method for measuring the size of the ventricular system. A is the width of the frontal horns between the parallel walls of the caudate nuclei, at the level of the foramina of Monro, B the diameter of the brain at the same level. The 95th percentile for the bicaudate index is 0.16 at age 30 years or under, 0.18 at 50 years, 0.19 at 60 years, 0.21 at 80 years, and 0.25 at 100 years (with permission from van Gijn *et al.* 1985).

The classical presentation of acute hydrocephalus is that of a patient who is alert immediately after the initial haemorrhage, but who in the next few hours becomes increasingly drowsy, to the point that the patient only moans and localizes to pain. However, only 50% of all patients with acute hydrocephalus present in this way (van Gijn *et al.* 1985). In the other 50%, consciousness is impaired from the onset, or the course is unknown because the patient was alone at the time of haemorrhage. If the patient is admitted very early and secondary deterioration occurs because of hydrocephalus, serial brain CTs may show that the level of consciousness correlates more or less inversely with the width of the lateral ventricles (Rinkel *et al.* 1990) (Fig. 13.9). When different patients are compared within one series, however, the relationship between the level of consciousness and the degree of ventricular dilatation is rather erratic (van Gijn *et al.* 1985; Hasan *et al.* 1989c). Ocular signs do not always accompany obtundation as a result of acute hydrocephalus; they help to corroborate the diagnosis, but not to exclude it. In a prospective study in which 30 of 34 patients with acute hydroceph-

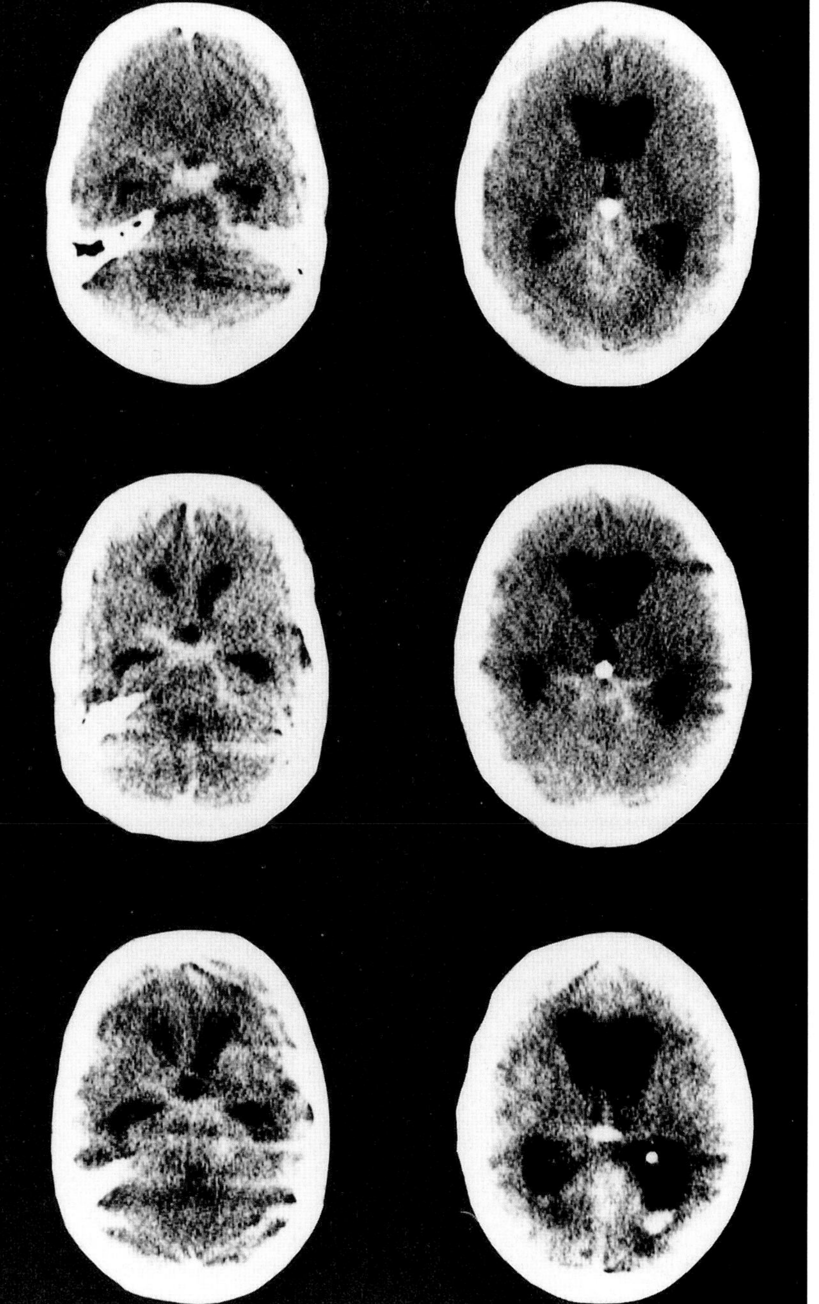

(a)

Fig. 13.9 (a) Non-contrast CT brain scans in a patient with subarachnoid haemorrhage—incidentally, this was not from a ruptured aneurysm, but from an unidentified source, presumably a ruptured vein (section 9.1.2), in the perimesencephalic cisterns. In this case, the site at which the cerebrospinal fluid is obstructed is not so much the ventricular system itself but the tentorial hiatus, through which the outflow from the fourth ventricle has to pass in order to reach the arachnoid villi at the convexity of the brain. *Left:* slices at the level of the basal cisterns. *Right:* slices at the level of the pineal gland. Upper row (4 h after the ictus): haemorrhage in the basal cisterns, with most of the blood located in the interpeduncular fossa and the left ambiens cistern; relative size of lateral ventricles (ratio between actual and normal value of bicaudate index (Fig. 13.8) for age) = 1.4. *Middle row* (9 h after the ictus): amount of blood in the basal cistern unchanged; relative size of lateral ventricles 1.4. *Bottom row* (28 h after the ictus): some sedimentation of blood in the posterior horns; relative size of lateral ventricles 1.8. (b) CT scan 5 weeks after the haemorrhage, and 4 weeks after insertion of a ventricular catheter; relative size of lateral ventricles 1.2. (c) Serial measurements of the relative size of the lateral and third ventricles, and total scores on the Glasgow Coma Scale (with permission from Rinkel *et al.* 1990). (*continued* p. 542)

(b)

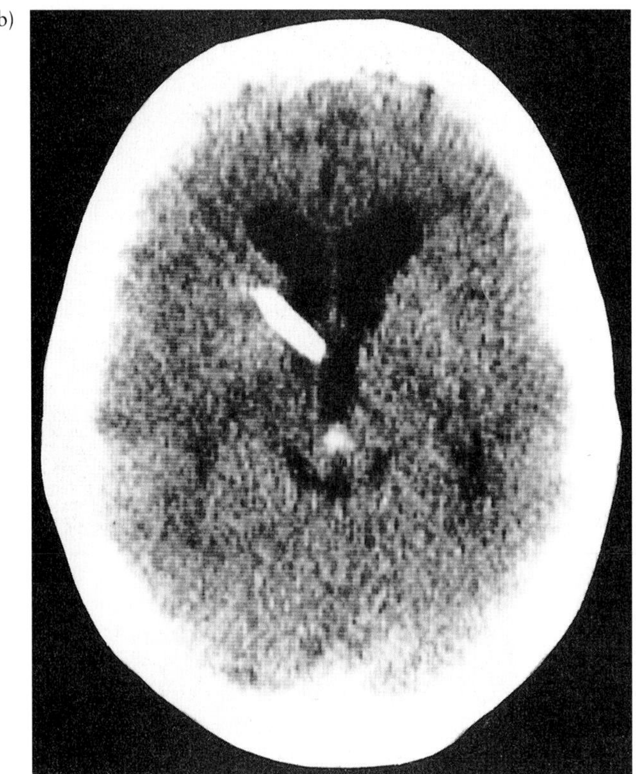

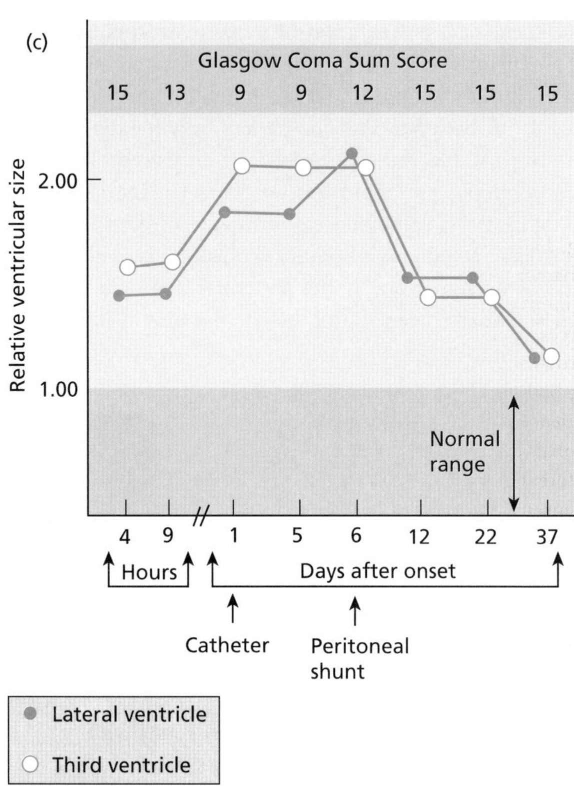

Fig. 13.9 (*continued*)

alus had an impaired level of consciousness, nine of these 30 had small, non-reactive pupils, and four of the nine also showed persistent downward deviation of the eyes, with otherwise intact brainstem reflexes (van Gijn *et al.* 1985). These eye signs reflect dilatation of the proximal part of the aqueduct, which causes dysfunction of the pretectal area (Swash 1974). All nine patients with non-reactive pupils had a relative ventricular size of more than 1.20 and were in coma—i.e. they did not open their eyes, did not obey commands and did not utter words.

Repeat CT scanning is required to diagnose or exclude hydrocephalus in a patient with subarachnoid haemorrhage who deteriorates within hours or days of the initial event, with or without eye signs of hydrocephalus (small, unreactive pupils and downward deviation of gaze). Patients with intraventricular blood or with extensive haemorrhage in the perimesencephalic cisterns are predisposed to developing acute hydrocephalus.

Intraventricular blood was found to be associated with acute hydrocephalus in all studies that addressed this question (Fig. 13.10), at least if there was enough to suggest direct intraventricular haemorrhage rather than just sedimentation in the posterior horns, which reflects diffusion of red blood cells throughout the cerebrospinal fluid spaces (van Gijn *et al.* 1985; Graff-Radford *et al.* 1989; Hasan *et al.* 1991b; Mehta *et al.* 1996). On the other hand, not all patients with acute hydrocephalus have intraventricular blood (the proportions varied between 35 and 65% in these studies), and it is an erroneous notion that acute hydrocephalus is, by definition, the result of intraventricular obstruction. In some patients, it is probable that clots obstructing the tentorial hiatus are partly or wholly responsible (Fig. 13.9) (Hasan & Tanghe 1992; Rinkel *et al.* 1992).

13.9.2 Possible interventions (Table 13.11)

Wait-and-see policy

Applying a wait-and-see policy for 24 h is eminently justified in patients with dilated ventricles who are alert, because only about one-third of them will become symptomatic in the next few days (Hasan *et al.* 1989c). Postponing interventions for a day can be rewarding, even if the level of consciousness is decreased. The reason is that spontaneous improvement within this period has been documented in approximately 50% of the patients (seven of 13) with acute hydrocephalus who were only drowsy, and also in almost 50% of the patients (19 of 43) who had a Glasgow Coma Score of 12/14 or worse but no massive intraventricular haemorrhage (Hasan *et al.* 1989c). On the other hand, it is not always easy to make a definitive decision on the need for surgical

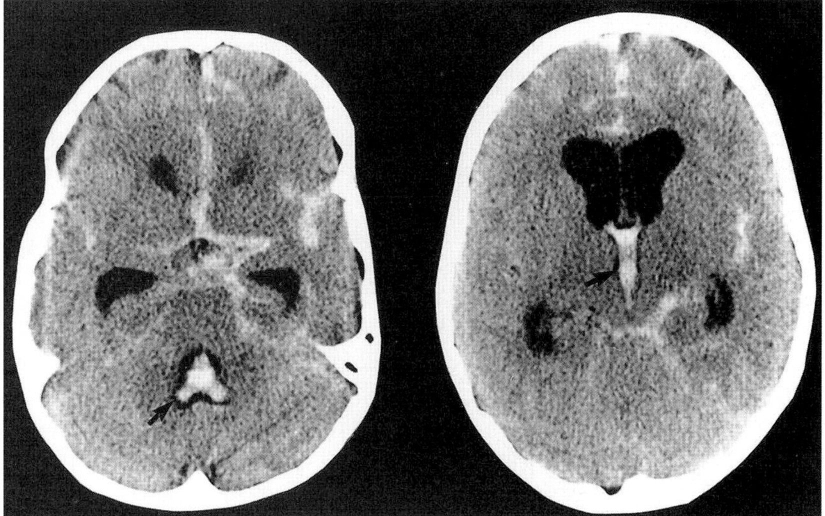

Fig. 13.10 Acute hydrocephalus after subarachnoid haemorrhage, as a result of intraventricular obstruction of cerebrospinal fluid flow: the fourth (left: arrow) and third (right: arrow) ventricles are both filled with blood (day 0); the patient was a 24-year-old woman, who probably had an earlier episode 7 days before (not investigated). The site of the aneurysm was not identified, due to her poor condition.

Table 13.11 Management of acute hydrocephalus.

Consider the diagnosis if conscious level gradually deteriorates, particularly on the first day after the bleed
Repeat the CT brain scan and compare the bicaudate index with that on any previous scan
Spontaneous improvement occurs within 24 h in 50% of the patients (except those with massive intraventricular haemorrhage); take action if patient further deteriorates or fails to improve within 24 h
Lumbar punctures are reasonably safe if there is no brain shift, and effective in about 50% of the patients who have no intraventricular obstruction
External drainage of the ventricles is very effective in restoring the level of consciousness, but carries a high risk of re-bleeding (consider emergency clipping or coiling of the aneurysm at the same time), and of infection (this may to some degree be prevented by prophylactic antibiotics or subcutaneous tunnelling)

measures even after a day has elapsed, because patients may temporarily improve to some extent, but then reach a plateau phase or again deteriorate; such fluctuations were encountered in about one-third of the cases (Hasan *et al.* 1989c). Any further deterioration in the level of consciousness warrants active intervention.

Lumbar puncture

Lumbar puncture was suggested as a therapeutic measure a long time ago, but formal studies are scarce (Kolluri & Sengupta 1984). In a prospective but uncontrolled study, Hasan *et al.* treated 17 patients in this way. They had acute hydrocephalus with neither a haematoma nor gross intraventricular haemorrhage, i.e. less than complete filling of the third or fourth ventricle (Hasan *et al.* 1991b). Between one and seven spinal taps per patient were performed in the first 10 days, the number depending on the rate of improvement; each time, a maximum of 20 mL of cerebrospinal fluid was removed, the aim being to achieve a closing pressure of 15 cmH_2O. Five of the 17 patients had a decreased level of consciousness on admission, and in these patients the lumbar punctures were started immediately; in 11 of the remaining 12 patients, deterioration occurred a few days after admission, and the last patient had a fluctuating level of consciousness. Of the 17 patients, 12 showed initial improvement, and of these, six fully recovered, two showed incomplete improvement but fully recovered after insertion of an internal shunt, and the four others died of other complications several days after the lumbar punctures had been started. Of the five remaining patients in whom lumbar puncture had no effect, two recovered after an internal shunt and three died of other complications. The rate of re-bleeding (two of the 17 patients) was similar to what might have been expected, but of course the numbers were small (Hasan *et al.* 1991b). Until randomized controlled trials are available—and we think these are still needed and ethically justifiable—the tentative conclusion is that lumbar puncture seems a safe and reasonably effective way of treating those forms of acute hydrocephalus that are not obviously caused by intraventricular obstruction.

In patients deteriorating from acute hydrocephalus after subarachnoid haemorrhage, it is worth trying lumbar punctures if spontaneous improvement does not occur within 24 h, and if the probable site of obstruction is in the subarachnoid space, not in the ventricular system.

External ventricular drainage

External drainage of the cerebral ventricles by a catheter inserted through a burr hole is, in many centres, the most common method of treating acute hydrocephalus. Internal drainage, to the right atrium or the peritoneal cavity, is rarely considered in the first few days, because the blood in the cerebrospinal fluid will almost inevitably block the shunt. After insertion of an external catheter, the improvement is usually rapid and sometimes dramatic (van Gijn *et al.* 1985; Hasan *et al.* 1989c). Unfortunately other problems tend to intervene soon, particularly re-bleeding and ventriculitis.

Re-bleeding after insertion of an external drain occurs significantly more often than in patients with acute hydrocephalus who do not undergo shunt treatment or in patients without hydrocephalus (Raimondi & Torres 1973; Papo *et al.* 1984; van Gijn *et al.* 1985; Hasan *et al.* 1989c; Paré *et al.* 1992; Kawai *et al.* 1997). This complication did not occur in only one published series (Mehta *et al.* 1996). None of these studies had a randomized design for assessing the effect of shunt insertion, and it is conceivable that the development of acute hydrocephalus is associated with a more severely disrupted aneurysm that is more prone to re-bleeding as part of its natural history. But it seems plausible that the increased risk of aneurysmal re-bleeding in patients undergoing ventricular drainage results from a rise in aneurysmal transmural pressure, since intracranial pressure is rapidly lowered by ventricular drainage. It has been suggested that an excess of re-bleeding can be prevented by keeping the pressure of the cerebrospinal fluid between 15 and 25 mmHg (Pickard 1984). Disappointingly, this has not been borne out by subsequent experience (Hasan *et al.* 1989c). Milhorat advocated capitalizing on the expected improvement after external drainage by performing early aneurysm surgery at the same time (Milhorat 1987). His results sound impressive: of 42 patients with acute hydrocephalus, 35 underwent external drainage and 29 survived. This is clearly another area in which a randomized controlled trial is needed.

Ventriculitis is a frequent complication after external drainage, especially if drainage is continued for more than 3 days. Of 31 patients treated with external drainage, 17 had died after 3 months, and infection contributed to the death of five (Hasan *et al.* 1989c). The use of prophylactic antibiotics or a long subcutaneous tunnel has been advocated, but these measures have not been subjected to a controlled study.

13.10 Management of systemic complications

Neurologists and neurosurgeons are regularly confronted by non-neurological complications in patients with aneurysmal subarachnoid haemorrhage—complications that require intensive therapeutic intervention (Gruber *et al.* 1999b). Forty per cent had at least one life-threatening complication in a series of 451 patients enrolled in a clinical trial of nicardipine (Solenski *et al.* 1995), and a similar proportion of medical complications (37%) accounts for deaths (Gruber *et al.* 1998b). Hyponatraemia is the most common of these, but several other systemic disorders may cause secondary neurological deterioration. Clinical detection of these metabolic derangements requires a high index of suspicion.

13.10.1 Hyponatraemia

Hyponatraemia, with or without intravascular volume change, is the most common electrolyte disturbance following aneurysmal rupture. The frequency depends on the chosen cut-off point; if defined as a sodium level of 134 mmol/L or less on at least two consecutive days, it occurs in about one-third of patients (Hasan *et al.* 1989a). It develops most commonly between the second and tenth day (Wijdicks *et al.* 1985a).

The clinical manifestations of hyponatraemia include an impaired level of consciousness, asterixis, hemiparesis, seizures and coma (Arieff *et al.* 1976). These usually do not occur until the plasma sodium is less than 125 mmol/L, but irritability, restlessness and confusion can result from a rapid decline of sodium, particularly if the downward trend continues over a few days. Sodium levels below 100 mmol/L almost always give rise to seizures, and rarely ventricular tachycardia or fibrillation (Arieff 1986). But the most dreaded complication of hyponatraemia is the precipitation of delayed cerebral ischaemia, through associated hypovolaemia.

In general, the causes of hyponatraemia depend on the patient's volume status. In most but not all cases, the total body sodium has remained constant, but the water content of the extracellular volume is at fault; therefore hyponatraemia can be best classified according to the extracellular volume status. After the syndrome of inappropriate secretion of antidiuretic hormone (SIADH) was first described in the 1950s (Bartter & Schwarz 1967), hyponatraemia in subarachnoid haemorrhage (SAH) has often been incorrectly attributed to this syndrome (Doczi *et al.* 1981). In SIADH, there is a continuing secretion of ADH that is not appropriate to changes in plasma volume and osmolality. The extracellular volume increases, and due to the expansion of the intravascular component of this volume, a *dilutional hyponatraemia* ensues. Natriuresis takes place, because the volume expansion increases the glomerular filtration rate and inhibits the secretion of aldosterone. Balance studies have shown that the degree of natriuresis is relatively small and approximately equals intake. The high concentration of urinary sodium in SIADH can be simply explained by the fact that the sodium intake must be excreted in a small volume of urine.

In contrast, hyponatraemia after SAH results from excessive natriuresis, or *cerebral salt wasting* (Harrigan 1996). A prospective study of 21 patients demonstrated that the plasma volume decreased in most patients who developed hyponatraemia, and that this was preceded by a negative sodium balance in all instances (Wijdicks *et al.* 1985a). Plasma volume considerably decreased, even in some patients with normal sodium levels, usually as a result of excessive natriuresis. Serum vasopressin levels were increased or normal on admission, but had decreased by the time hyponatraemia occurred. It is clear that the volume status in these patients is extremely important.

A possible contributing factor in the development of hyponatraemia may be hydrocephalus, particularly enlargement of the third ventricle (van Gijn *et al.* 1985; Wijdicks *et al.* 1988b). This relationship is independent of the amount of cisternal blood or the location of the ruptured aneurysm, but is partly dependent on the amount of intraventricular blood. Mechanical pressure on the hypothalamus can perhaps disturb sodium and water homeostasis. Three substances have been identified as being related to natriuresis and possibly act as intermediary factors: a digoxin-like substance (Wijdicks *et al.* 1987), atrial natriuretic factor (Diringer *et al.* 1988; Rosenfeld *et al.* 1989; Wijdicks *et al.* 1991; Wijdicks *et al.* 1997), and brain natriuretic peptide (Berendes *et al.* 1997; Wijdicks *et al.* 1997; Tomida *et al.* 1998).

Correction of hyponatraemia in SAH is truly a problem of correcting volume depletion (Table 13.12). Acute symptomatic hyponatraemia is rare, and requires urgent treatment with hypertonic saline (1.8% or even 3%). On the other hand, over-rapid infusion of sodium may precipitate myelinolysis in the pons and the white matter of the cerebral hemispheres. A retrospective survey suggests that the maximal rate of correction should be by 12 mmol/L per day (Sterns *et al.* 1986), but others maintain that more rapid correction is safe as long as the plasma sodium level does not exceed 126 mmol/L during the first 24 h (Ayus *et al.* 1987). A mild degree of hyponatraemia (125–134 mmol/L) is usually well tolerated and self-limiting, and need not be treated. Hyponatraemia in patients with evidence of a negative fluid balance, or excessive natriuresis, is corrected with saline (0.9%; sodium concentration, 150 mmol/L) or with a mixture of glucose and saline.

Table 13.12 Management of hyponatraemia.

Almost invariably caused by sodium *depletion*, not by sodium dilution (syndrome of inappropriate secretion of antidiuretic hormone)
Associated hypovolaemia increases risk of delayed cerebral ischaemia
Give isotonic saline (with or without plasma expander) or a mixture of glucose and saline; no free water
If necessary, add fludrocortisone acetate, 400 mg/day in two doses, orally or intravenously
Keep central venous pressure between 8 and 12 mmHg, or pulmonary capillary wedge pressure between 14 and 18 mmHg

Hyponatraemia after subarachnoid haemorrhage usually reflects cerebral salt wasting (sodium depletion) and not secretion of antidiuretic hormone (sodium dilution). Because hyponatraemia may lead to hypovolaemia, it should be vigorously treated to prevent cerebral ischaemia.

13.10.2 Disorders of heart rhythm

Aneurysmal rupture is commonly associated with cardiac dysrhythmias and electrocardiographic (ECG) abnormalities. This is one of the reasons why patients with subarachnoid haemorrhage (SAH) may be initially misdiagnosed as acute myocardial infarction and admitted to coronary care units. Cardiogenic shock may occur, usually in combination with pulmonary oedema (section 13.10.3). A popular explanation is sustained sympathetic stimulation, sometimes resulting in structural damage to the myocardium, which is often evident on echocardiograms (Pollick *et al.* 1988; Mayer *et al.* 1999). The histological features of myocardial damage are contraction bands, focal myocardial necrosis and subendocardial ischaemia. A more unconventional theory is the existence of an arrhythmogenic centre in the insular cortex (Svigelj *et al.* 1994).

The most common ECG abnormalities in SAH (Fig. 13.11) are S–T segment and T segment changes, prominent U waves, Q–T prolongation and sinus dysrhythmias (Marion *et al.* 1986; Stober *et al.* 1988; Brouwers *et al.* 1989). Life-threatening dysrhythmias such as ventricular fibrillation or *torsade de pointes* may be seen on 24-h monitoring, but are extremely rare (Carruth & Silverman 1980; Hijdra *et al.* 1984; Andreoli *et al.* 1987). A striking finding in a large series of patients investigated by serial ECGs was that every patient had at least one abnormal ECG (Brouwers *et al.* 1989). Virtually all ECG abnormalities changed to other abnormalities, in no consistent order, and then disappeared, during an observation period of 10 days. Some patients had ECG changes that closely resembled those in acute myocardial infarction; these spontaneously disappeared the following day without any change in the neurological or cardiac condition. Potentially dangerous dysrhythmias or actual death from cardiac failure did not occur in this limited series. By contrast, others found runs of ventricular tachycardia in 20% of those monitored, and prolonged Q–T intervals in 60% (Estanol Vidal *et al.* 1979). Prolonged Q–T intervals often represent delayed ventricular repolarization, and predispose to ventricular dysrhythmias. The prognostic value of these ECG changes is unclear, but in patients with SAH they are more important as indicators of severe intracranial

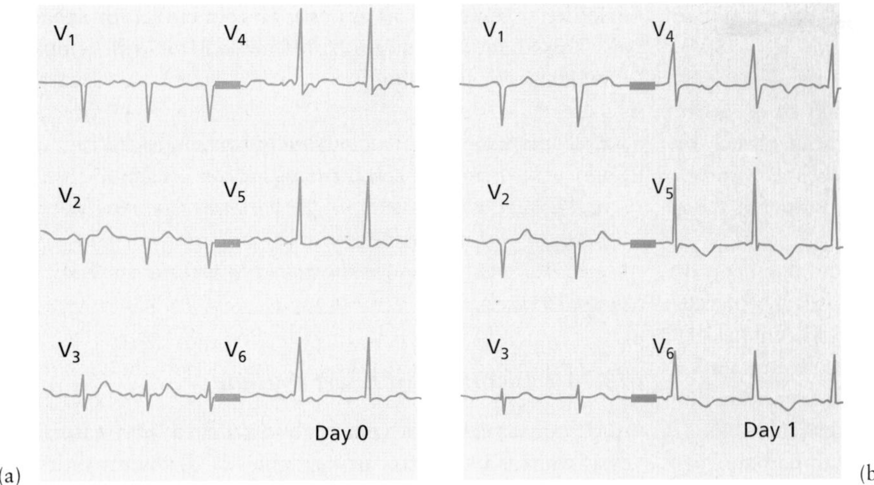

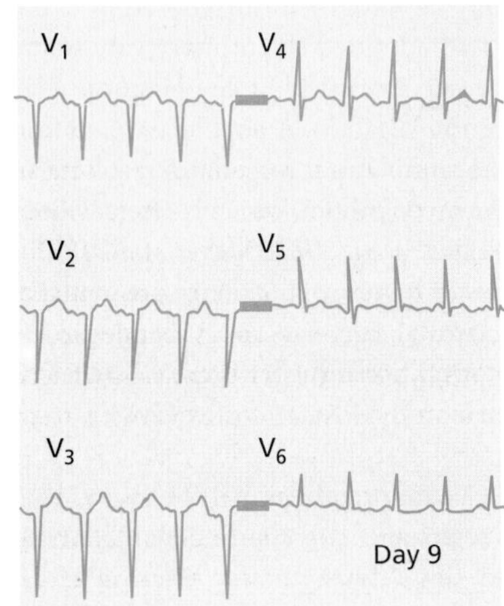

Fig. 13.11 Electrocardiographic (ECG) abnormalities in a 74-year-old woman with subarachnoid haemorrhage. (a) Day 0: ischaemic S–T segment, prominent U wave and prolonged Q–T_c interval. (b) Day 1: sinus bradycardia, ischaemic S–T segment, ischaemic T wave, prolonged Q–T_c interval and signs of left ventricular hypertrophy. (c) Day 9: sinus tachycardia, transient pathological Q wave and ischaemic S–T segment.

disease than as predictors of potentially serious cardiac complications (Brouwers *et al.* 1989; Manninen *et al.* 1995).

Abnormalities of heart rhythm after subarachnoid haemorrhage represent 'smoke' rather than 'fire', and rarely need to be treated.

Generally, severe ventricular dysrhythmias are of short duration. Betablockade has been proposed as a preventive treatment aimed at lowering the sympathetic tone. In patients with head injury, a double-blind, randomized study found that betablockers reduced catecholamine-induced cardiac necrosis, but not in-hospital case fatality (Cruickshank *et al.* 1987). In patients with SAH, routine administration of betablockers is not warranted until there is evidence of improved overall outcome; the net benefits may be disappointing, because betablockers also lower blood pressure. Randomized controlled trials of cardioprotective agents in SAH are scarce, but are less pressing than those aimed at the neurological complications.

13.10.3 Neurogenic pulmonary oedema

Neurogenic pulmonary oedema is a dramatic and dangerous complication (Wijdicks *et al.* 1998). After subarachnoid haemorrhage (SAH), it usually has an extremely rapid onset, within hours, although a delayed course has been reported (Fisher & Aboul Nasr 1979). What triggers pulmonary oedema is unclear. Elevated intracranial pressure can lead to a massive sympathetic discharge mediated by the anterior hypothalamus. Systemic hypertension often co-exists, but pulmonary oedema may present or even worsen during the lowering of systemic or pulmonary pressures. It has also been suggested that increased sympathetic activity leads to generalized vasoconstriction, including the pulmonary vasculature, and that direct damage to endothelial cells may result in increased permeability (Theodore & Robin 1976).

Fortunately, pulmonary oedema is not common, occurring in less than 10% of patients with SAH. It is related to the severity of aneurysmal haemorrhage, and is rarely seen in patients with a normal level of consciousness (Weir 1978).

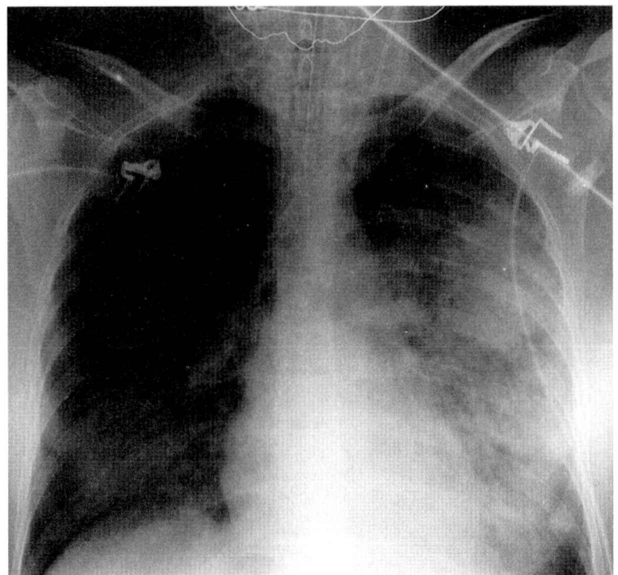

Fig. 13.12 Chest X-ray showing neurogenic pulmonary oedema (same patient as in Fig. 13.10).

The typical clinical picture consists of unexpected dyspnoea, cyanosis and production of pink and frothy sputum. Many patients are pale, sweat excessively and are hypertensive. A chest X-ray usually demonstrates impressive pulmonary oedema (Fig. 13.12), which may disappear in a matter of hours following positive end-expiratory pressure ventilation (Wauchob *et al.* 1984). Diuretics are often used as standard therapy, and it has been claimed that labetalol or chlorpromazine are also beneficial (Wohns *et al.* 1985; Harrier 1988). A problem is that liberal administration of fluids is beneficial for brain perfusion, but may delay recovery of pulmonary oedema and hence impair brain oxygenation; while positive end-expiratory pressure ventilation increases intracranial pressure.

Neurogenic pulmonary oedema may be complicated by reversible decompensation of the left ventricle, clinically manifested by sudden hypotension following initially elevated blood pressure, transient lactic acidosis, mild elevation of the creatine kinase muscle–brain (MB) fraction and varied ECG changes during the first day, followed by widespread and persistent T-wave inversion (Mayer *et al.* 1994; Parr *et al.* 1996). In these cases of pulmonary oedema with secondary cardiac injury, treatment with pressor agents may be indicated.

13.11 Late complications

13.11.1 Vitreous haemorrhages

Preretinal haemorrhages associated with subarachnoid haemorrhage (SAH) may break into the vitreous cavity (Terson's syndrome) (section 5.6.1). They may also occur with other disorders associated with an abrupt rise in intracranial pressure, such as head injury (Medele *et al.* 1998). In a prospective study of 99 patients with SAH, any intraocular haemorrhage was found in 17% of patients, and vitreous haemorrhages in 7%; the rates were three times as high in patients who had lost consciousness at some stage (Pfausler *et al.* 1996; Frizzell *et al.* 1997). These haemorrhages occur in one or both eyes, usually at the time of SAH onset, but sometimes several days later, and then mostly in association with re-bleeding or sometimes angiography. It may, however, take days or weeks before the patient is sufficiently alert to complain about blurred vision. In most cases, the vitreous haemorrhage clears spontaneously in a matter of weeks to months. In patients with bilateral, severe haemorrhages, vitrectomy may be required to improve vision during the period of neurological recovery (Weingeist *et al.* 1986; Huber *et al.* 1988; Kuhn *et al.* 1998).

13.11.2 Late re-bleeding

When the ruptured aneurysm is left untreated, the rate of re-bleeding, after the first 6 months have passed, is about 3% per year during the first decade (Winn *et al.* 1977). This situation is now increasingly unusual. In patients with a successfully occluded aneurysm, the most important question is about the risk of bleeding from any associated unruptured aneurysms as well as aneurysms formed *de novo*, or from regrowth of the aneurysm that caused the first bleed. A study in 220 successfully operated patients in Japan, followed up for an average of 10 years, found that the risk of re-bleeding was far from negligible: calculated according to the Kaplan–Meier method, the cumulative recurrence rate of subarachnoid haemorrhage (SAH) was 2.2% at 10 years and 9.0% at 20 years after the original treatment (Tsutsumi *et al.* 1998). This result, so far unconfirmed, substantially exceeds the risk in the general population: assuming an annual incidence of SAH of six per 100 000, which is the closest estimate for European countries other than Finland (Linn *et al.* 1996), the cumulative rate in the general population would be only around 0.06% after 10 years, and 0.12% after 20 years.

13.11.3 Late hydrocephalus

Even 2–3 weeks after the initial haemorrhage, some patients with mild and untreated hydrocephalus at onset may still deteriorate and require shunting; others may newly develop hydrocephalus. Together, these two groups amounted to about one-fifth of all surviving patients in the two neurosurgical series which addressed this problem (Vale *et al.* 1997; Gruber *et al.* 1999c). Within the first 3 days, symptomatic hydrocephalus ('acute hydrocephalus') is found in an approximately similar proportion of 20% (section 13.9.1). Half of the patients with acute hydrocephalus spontaneously improve (Hasan *et al.* 1989c), but an equal proportion develop symptomatic hydrocephalus after day 5 (Vermeij *et al.* 1994). Early dilatation of the ventricles and intraventricular haemorrhage are the most powerful risk factors (Tapaninaho *et al.* 1993; Vermeij *et al.* 1994). Additional and independent predictors for late hydrocephalus are the sum score of cisternal blood on initial CT, and long-term treatment with tranexamic acid (Vermeij *et al.* 1994). The frequency of chronic hydrocephalus is no lower after endovascular treatment, compared with surgical clipping (Gruber *et al.* 1999c). If fenestration of the lamina terminalis is performed, as part of the microsurgical procedure for aneurysm repair, late hydrocephalus is a rare event (Tomasello *et al.* 1999). Occasionally, hydrocephalus develops after a latent period of more than 4 weeks, after the patient has been discharged home.

13.12 Management of unruptured aneurysms

Most aneurysms never rupture. On the assumption that up to 5% of the population eventually develop at least one aneurysm in their lifetime (section 9.1.1), and that the annual incidence of aneurysmal subarachnoid haemorrhage is approximately six per 100 000, which corresponds with a lifetime risk of 0.5%, only about one in 10 cerebral aneurysms ever ruptures. In individual patients, the following questions arise: does this particular patient have a higher than average risk of harbouring an aneurysm? Given the characteristics of the patient and the aneurysm, is the risk of rupture higher or lower than average? What are the risks of occluding an unruptured aneurysm? On the basis of what is known so far, should incidental aneurysms be treated? And finally, can we identify specific groups of people at high risk, in whom systematic screening for aneurysms is warranted?

13.12.1 Prevalence of unruptured aneurysms

In a systematic review addressing the prevalence of intracranial aneurysms in patients studied for reasons other than subarachnoid haemorrhage, 23 studies were identified, totalling 56 304 patients; 6685 (12%) of these patients were from 15 angiography studies (Rinkel *et al.* 1998). In retrospective post-mortem studies, the prevalence was lowest, at 0.4% (95% CI, 0.4%–0.5%), in prospective post-mortem studies it was 3.6% (95% CI, 3.1%–4.1%), in retrospective angiography studies 3.7% (95% CI, 3.0%–4.4%), and in prospective angiography studies 6.0% (95% CI, 5.3%–6.8%). The angiography studies were somewhat biased towards overestimation, because in around 15% the indication was a planned operation for a suspected pituitary tumour, polycystic kidney disease, or familial subarachnoid haemorrhage—conditions in which the frequency of aneurysms is higher than average. For adults without specific risk factors for aneurysms, the prevalence was 2.3% (95% CI, 1.7%–3.1%), and it tended to increase with age. In the general population, the prevalence of *known* aneurysms in Olmsted County, Minnesota, was estimated at 0.83% (Menghini *et al.* 1998), which implies that even in that highly investigated region only one out of four aneurysms is detected.

The prevalence of aneurysms is greater than average in a number of specific conditions (section 9.1.1). Relatively common among these is familial subarachnoid haemorrhage, defined as two or more first-degree relatives being affected; it accounts for 7–20% of episodes of subarachnoid haemorrhage (Schievink 1997). The mean age at the time of haemorrhage in patients with the familial form is some 7 years lower than in those with the sporadic form, although part of the difference may be explained by detection bias; also, middle cerebral artery aneurysms occur more often in patients with familial disease (Bromberg *et al.* 1995a). Observations differ on whether the risk of a poor outcome after subarachnoid haemorrhage is relatively greater in familial cases or not (Bromberg *et al.* 1995b; Ronkainen *et al.* 1999). In such families, the frequency of aneurysms on investigation of other first-degree relatives is 8–10% (Ronkainen *et al.* 1994; Ronkainen *et al.* 1997; Raaymakers *et al.* 1998a). A single study (so far) found that the presence of an aneurysm in these families was associated with elevated levels of lipoprotein(a) (Phillips *et al.* 1997).

Autosomal dominant polycystic kidney disease (ADPKD) is classically associated with intracranial aneurysms, although these occur in only a minority of patients (Chauveau *et al.* 1994; Pirson & Chauveau 1995). Angiographic screening of ADKPD patients in two different studies yielded aneurysms in eight of 56 patients with a family history of subarachnoid haemorrhage (14%; 95% CI, 6%–26%), and in five of 115 without such family history (4%; 95% CI, 1%–10%)(Chapman *et al.* 1992; Huston *et al.* 1993). Follow-up of 10 ADKPD patients with aneurysms showed no growth or new aneurysms, during an average period of 3 years (Huston *et al.* 1996). Aneurysms of this type that rupture are found more often in males, at a relatively young age, and predominantly on the middle cerebral artery; there is no correlation with arterial hypertension (Lozano & Leblanc 1992).

A special category of unruptured aneurysms is in patients who are symptomatic, but through clinical manifestations other than subarachnoid haemorrhage, with acute symptoms (ischaemia, headache, seizure, or cranial neuropathy) or chronic symptoms attributed to mass effect: headache, visual loss, pyramidal tract dysfunction, or facial pain (Raps *et al.* 1993).

13.12.2 Risk of rupture

It is difficult to find unbiased reports of patients with unruptured aneurysms, from which to determine the risk of aneurysmal rupture. Series reported from surgical centres are inevitably incomplete, in that some—if not most—patients undergo prophylactic surgical treatment; therefore, it is not inconceivable that patients elected for treatment have a risk of rupture that is different from the residual group. Even in series reported by 'ultraconservative' neurologists, patients may have removed themselves by seeking a surgical option elsewhere. Another potential source of bias is the indication for performing angiography. Even after exclusion of subarachnoid haemorrhage (SAH), this was often related to other kinds of vascular disease, associated with risk factors that also operate for subarachnoid haemorrhage. Magnetic resonance angiography is so recent a development that follow-up studies of unbiased cohorts are not yet available.

A systematic review of studies up to 1998 identified nine, including 3709 patients, that addressed the risk of aneurysm rupture (Rinkel *et al.* 1998). The overall risk of rupture was 1.9% per annum (95% CI, 1.5%–2.4%). Aneurysms were significantly more likely to rupture in women than in men (relative risk (RR), 2.1; 95% CI, 1.1%–3.9%), and the risk of rupture increased with age: in patients aged 60–79 years, the relative risk of rupture was 1.7 (95% CI, 0.7–4.0) compared with those aged 40–59 years. But the risk of rupture was even more dependent on the characteristics of the aneurysm than on those of the patient. Symptomatic aneurysms (RR 8.3; 95% CI, 4.0–17), posterior circulation aneurysms (RR 4.1; 95% CI, 1.5–11) and large (>10 mm diameter) aneurysms (RR 5.5; 95% CI, 3.3–9.4) were relatively more likely to rupture. The absolute risk of rupture for aneurysms with a diameter of 10 mm or less was 0.7% per annum. Additional aneurysms (i.e. in addition to the one that had already ruptured) were more prone to bleeding, but the difference was not statistically significant.

Subsequent to this overview, a multicentre retrospective study (coordinated by the Mayo Clinic) was published, in which 1449 patients with 1937 intracranial aneurysms greater than 2 mm in diameter were followed up for an average period of 8.3 years (Wiebers *et al.* 1998); half the patients had no history of SAH from a different aneurysm, while the other half had a history of SAH from an aneurysm that had been successfully repaired. In the first group, the cumulative rate of rupture of aneurysms that were less than 10 mm in diameter at diagnosis was less than 0.05% per year; in the second group, the rate was approximately 11 times as high (0.5% per year). Again, the size and location of the aneurysm were independent predictors of rupture: the relative risk was 11.6 for aneurysms greater than 10 mm, 13.7 for posterior circulation aneurysms, and 8.0 for posterior communicating artery aneurysms.

The striking difference in the absolute risk of rupture for incidental aneurysms smaller than 10 mm between the study by Rinkel *et al.* (0.7% per annum) and the large international study by Wiebers *et al.* (0.05% per annum) cannot be explained, because it is impossible to extract from each data set the sources of bias alluded to above. An identifiable factor that may have led to underestimation in the international study is the inclusion criterion of a complete set of angiograms being available (films of patients who died in the meantime may have been removed from the hospital records). A prospective study from the same international group is still in progress, and may resolve some of the controversies.

Estimates for the annual risk of bleeding from an (as yet) unruptured aneurysm so far suffer from biases of various kinds. Therefore, they vary a great deal—between one in 20 and one in 200. The risk is relatively great for aneurysms larger than 10 mm (including most symptomatic aneurysms) and for posterior circulation aneurysms.

The importance of aneurysm size for the risk of rupture is a paradox that puzzles many physicians and surgeons, because most ruptured aneurysms encountered in clinical practice are smaller than 10 mm, or even 5 mm (Jane *et al.* 1985; Juvela *et al.* 1993). Some neurosurgeons advocate prophylactic operation on small aneurysms for that reason (Rosenorn & Eskesen 1993). The most likely explanation is that the vast majority of aneurysms are of small size, and that even a minute fraction of those rupturing will still outnumber a large proportion of the smaller group of larger aneurysms that rupture (in the same way that most children with Down's syndrome are born to young mothers, even though the risk increases with age). The corollary of this notion is the 'prevention paradox' (Rose 1992): screening the population for people at highest risk (large aneurysms) will do little to change the burden of the disease (i.e. ruptured aneurysms), because most patients who actually suffer subarachnoid haemorrhage have small aneurysms (section 18.5.2).

13.12.3 Complications of treatment

A systematic review of the complications of surgery for unruptured aneurysms included 61 studies that involved 2460 patients, reported between 1966 and 1996 (Raaymakers *et al.* 1998b). Somewhat more than half (57%) of the patients were women, and the mean age was 50 years; the total number of unruptured aneurysms was at least 2568 (27% > 25 mm, 30% located on the posterior circulation). Case fatality was 2.6% (95% CI, 2.0%–3.3%). Permanent morbidity occurred in 10.9% (95% CI, 9.6%–12.2%) of patients. Postoperative mortality and morbidity were significantly lower in more recent years for non-giant aneurysms and aneurysms with an anterior location. In the international study of unruptured aneurysms, not yet included in this overview, the overall rate of surgery-related mortality and permanent morbidity (persisting until 1 year) for 1172 unruptured aneurysms was similar, at 13.6% or 13.1%, depending on whether the patient had or had not previously undergone surgery after bleeding from another aneurysm (Wiebers *et al.* 1998). Age independently predicted surgical outcome.

A recent cooperative study suggested that endovascular treatment for unruptured aneurysms (255 patients) was associated with less death and dependency than surgical treatment (2357 patients), after adjustment for known prognostic factors; nevertheless, selection bias for other factors may have influenced the results, and a randomized trial is needed (Johnston *et al.* 1999a).

13.12.4 When to operate on incidental aneurysms?

Whenever a cerebral aneurysm is a surprise finding on an angiographic study performed for another purpose, the practical dilemma arises of whether the operative risk associated with preventive clipping or coiling of the aneurysm is outweighed by the morbidity from eventual rupture of untreated aneurysms. 'Intuition' fails in balancing the short-term risks against the long-term risks, although it was found some years ago that many neurosurgeons had adopted an approach of either 'never operate', or 'always operate' (van Crevel *et al.* 1986). In the United States, opinion in favour of active treatment seems to predominate (at least, it did a decade ago), since almost one-quarter of medical costs for aneurysm surgery could be attributed to unruptured aneurysms (Wiebers *et al.* 1992). It is especially in such situations that the technique of decision analysis is helpful. The five most important factors can be estimated: the annual risk of rupture, given the characteristics of the aneurysm (section 13.12.2); the case fatality and morbidity after rupture; the risk of surgery (for the aneurysm in question and for the neurosurgeon in question; section 13.12.3); the life expectancy (not necessarily actuarial; it makes sense to adjust the life expectancy according to 'biological age'); and lastly, the disutility of being handicapped, which is generally perceived as a greater disadvantage—even per year—in the immediate than in the more distant future (van Crevel *et al.* 1986). In addition, a family history of subarachnoid haemorrhage probably increases the risk of rupture (section 13.12.1).

Incidentally discovered aneurysms of 10–25 mm in diameter are associated with an annual risk of rupture that has been estimated at as low as 1% (Wiebers *et al.* 1998), or as high as 10% (Rinkel *et al.* 1998), or in between (Auger & Wiebers 1991); sensitivity analyses should take account of this range. A recent modelling study came down at 10 mm as the cut-off point above which operation was cost-effective (Johnston *et al.* 1999b).

An unruptured aneurysm is not an inevitable 'time bomb', because only one in 10 ever ruptures. Whether operation or coiling is warranted depends on the patient's age, the size of the aneurysm (above 10 mm the risk of bleeding is relatively great), the family history, and the risk of intervention. The eventual decision is also influenced by the patient's own perception of risk.

In patients with unruptured aneurysms, control of conventional risk factors for vascular disease (smoking, blood pressure, oral contraceptives, high alcohol intake, obesity) seems sensible, even more than for the population in general.

13.12.5 Who should be screened?

In families with two or more first-degree relatives affected by subarachnoid haemorrhage, the initiative for screening is often taken by the remaining relatives. The efficiency of screening in the families is relatively high, with a yield of 8–10% in the first-degree relatives of rupture cases (Ronkainen *et al.* 1994; Ronkainen *et al.* 1997; Raaymakers *et al.* 1998a). Also, the risk of rupture in untreated aneurysms may be greater than in sporadic cases. But a theoretical modelling exercise predicted that screening in families with two or more affected members will not reduce mortality and morbidity in first-degree relatives unless the expected frequency of aneurysms is considerably greater than 10% (Crawley *et al.* 1999). Not surprisingly, this applies *a fortiori* to screening of the general population (Yoshimoto & Wakai 1999). Even if there is no scientific evidence in favour of screening such families, the level of anxiety and distress is often the decisive factor in justifying investigations and prophylactic treatment in relatives who demand this. But a negative result of screening raises questions about diagnostic accuracy (section 9.4.3 on computed tomographic angiography and 9.4.4 on magnetic resonance angiography). Also, at present there is absolutely no evidence to answer the question of how frequently screening should be repeated—if at all. A 5-year interval is arbitrarily adopted by many physicians caring for members of affected families, but of course counselling involves more than periodically filling out an X-ray request form.

It is a completely different situation when physicians take the initiative for screening. Such medical action, which transforms healthy people into potential patients, requires very persuasive evidence about the benefits for individual relatives, and about the cost-effectiveness of the programme in comparison with other measures to improve health in the general population. A potential target is first-degree relatives of patients with 'sporadic' aneurysmal subarachnoid haemorrhage (SAH) (Mathieu *et al.* 1997). Studies suggesting an increased risk for such family members often suffer from one or more problems: incomplete ascertainment of all living relatives; failure to distinguish different degrees of kinship; and no allowance for expected prevalence (De Braekeleer *et al.* 1996; Mathieu *et al.* 1997). A study in which these disadvantages were avoided found an odds ratio for first-degree relatives against second-degree relatives of 6.5 for definite or probable episodes of SAH (95% CI, 2.0–21); if possible episodes were also included, the odds ratio dropped to 2.8 (95% CI, 1.4–5.7). The frequency of SAH in second-degree relatives was of the same order of magnitude as for the general population (Bromberg *et al.* 1995c). In a Finnish study, the relative risk for relatives with only a single affected member was 1.8, but with a wide confidence interval (95% CI, 0.7–4.8) (Ronkainen *et al.* 1998). The increased risk for first-degree relatives was not statistically significant in a case–control study in China, of 149 incident patients with SAH and 298 external controls matched for age and sex (Wang *et al.* 1995), but problems with that study are that the criteria for the diagnosis of SAH through an interview were unspecified, medical records were not obtained for verification, although this is indispensable (Bromberg *et al.* 1996), and the fate of almost 10% of the first-degree relatives was unknown.

These results prompted a study of screening amongst first-degree relatives of patients with 'sporadic' aneurysmal SAH in the Netherlands (Raaymakers *et al.* 1999a). Starting from 160 index SAH patients, 626 first-degree relatives (parents, siblings or children) were screened by means of magnetic resonance angiography; conventional catheter angiography was performed in positive cases. Aneurysms were found in 25 relatives (4.0%; 95%, CI, 2.6%–5.8%) (Raaymakers *et al.* 1999b); this is about twice the estimated prevalence in the general population (section 13.12.1), and half the prevalence in families with two or more affected members (Ronkainen *et al.* 1994; Ronkainen *et al.* 1997; Raaymakers *et al.* 1998a). Eighteen relatives underwent surgery, which resulted in a decrease in functional health in 11 (disabling in one). There was no parallel control group, but on the basis of a decision-analytical model it was estimated that operation resulted in a gain in life expectancy of 2.5 years for each of these 18 persons (equalling 0.9 months for each of the 626 'screenees'), at the expense of 19 years of decreased functional health per person (6.6 months per 'screenee'). The number of relatives needed to screen for preventing one episode of SAH was 149 (298 to prevent a fatal episode) (Raaymakers *et al.* 1999a). A Canadian group studied 19 second-generation siblings in four families with an affected mother and child, and calculated that catheter angiography was justified in such situations if life expectancy exceeded 32 years (Leblanc *et al.* 1994).

In general, the modest gain in life expectancy and the substantial risk of postoperative sequelae do not at present seem to warrant physician-driven screening programmes. Perhaps this conclusion should be revised if in the future endovascular treatment proves safer as well as effective (Johnson *et al.* 2000).

Screening for unruptured aneurysms is defensible in families with two or more first-degree relatives affected by subarachnoid haemorrhage (especially with mother–child pairs and with high levels of anxiety), or if there is a single affected relative in families with autosomal dominant polycystic kidney disease. Screening should be discouraged in relatives of patients with 'sporadic' aneurysmal subarachnoid haemorrhage.

References

Please note that all references taken from *The Cochrane Library* are given a current date as this database is updated on a quarterly basis. Please refer to the current *Cochrane Library* article for the latest review. The same applies to the *British Medical Journal* 'Clinical Evidence' series which is updated every six months.

Adams, H.P. Jr, Jergenson, D.D., Kassell, N.F. & Sahs, A.L. (1980) Pitfalls in the recognition of subarachnoid hemorrhage. *Journal of the American Medical Association* **244**, 794–796.

Agnelli, G., Piovella, F., Buoncristiani, P. *et al.* (1998) Enoxaparin plus compression stockings compared with compression stockings alone in the prevention of venous thromboembolism after elective neurosurgery. *New England Journal of Medicine* **339**, 80–85.

Alvord, E.C., Loeser, J.D., Bailey, W.L. & Copass, M.K. (1972) Subarachnoid hemorrhage due to ruptured aneurysms: a simple method of estimating prognosis. *Archives of Neurology* **27**, 273–284.

Amin-Hanjani, S., Schwartz, R.B., Sathi, S. & Stieg, P.E. (1999) Hypertensive encephalopathy as a complication of hyperdynamic therapy for vasospasm: report of two cases. *Neurosurgery* **44**, 1113–1116.

Andreoli, A., di Pasquale, G., Pinelli, G., Grazi, P., Tognetti, F. & Testa, C. (1987) Subarachnoid hemorrhage: frequency and severity of cardiac arrhythmias. A survey of 70 cases studied in the acute phase. *Stroke* **18**, 558–564.

Anon. (1992) Protease inhibitors for delayed cerebral ischemia after subarachnoid haemorrhage? *Lancet* **339**, 1199–1200.

Anson, J.A., Lawton, M.T. & Spetzler, R.F. (1996) Characteristics and surgical treatment of dolichoectatic and fusiform aneurysms. *Journal of Neurosurgery* **84**, 185–193.

Aoyagi, N. & Hayakawa, I. (1984) Analysis of 223 ruptured intracranial aneurysms with special reference to rerupture. *Surgical Neurology* **21**, 445–452.

Apostolides, P.J., Greene, K.A., Zabramski, J.M., Fitzgerald, J.W. & Spetzler, R.F. (1996) Intra-aortic balloon pump counterpulsation in the management of concomitant cerebral vasospasm and cardiac failure after subarachnoid hemorrhage: Technical case report. *Neurosurgery* **38**, 1056–1059.

Arieff, A.I. (1986) Hyponatremia, convulsions, respiratory arrest, and permanent brain damage after elective surgery in healthy women. *New England Journal of Medicine* **314**, 1529–1535.

Arieff, A.I., Llach, F. & Massry, S.G. (1976) Neurological manifestations and morbidity of hyponatremia: correlation with brain water and electrolytes. *Medicine (Baltimore)* **55**, 121–129.

Asano, T., Takakura, K., Sano, K. *et al.* (1996) Effects of a hydroxyl radical scavenger on delayed ischemic neurological deficits following aneurysmal subarachnoid hemorrhage: results of a multicenter, placebo-controlled double-blind trial. *Journal of Neurosurgery* **84**, 792–803.

Auger, R.G. & Wiebers, D.O. (1991) Management of unruptured intracranial aneurysms: a decision analysis. *Journal of Stroke and Cerebrovascular Disease* **1**, 174–181.

Awad, I.A., Carter, L.P., Spetzler, R.F., Medina, M. & Williams, F.C. Jr (1987) Clinical vasospasm after subarachnoid hemorrhage: response to hypervolemic hemodilution and arterial hypertension. *Stroke* **18**, 365–372.

Ayus, J.C., Krothapalli, R.K. & Arieff, A.I. (1987) Treatment of symptomatic hyponatremia and its relation to brain damage: a prospective study. *New England Journal of Medicine* **317**, 1190–1195.

Bailes, J.E., Spetzler, R.F., Hadley, M.N. & Baldwin, H.Z. (1990) Management morbidity and mortality of poor-grade aneurysm patients. *Journal of Neurosurgery* **72**, 559–566.

Bartter, F.C. & Schwarz, W.B. (1967) The syndrome of inappropriate secretion of antidiuretic hormone. *American Journal of Medicine* **42**, 790–806.

Bauer, L.A. (1982) Interference of oral phenytoin absorption by continuous nasogastric feedings. *Neurology* **32**, 570–572.

Bavinzski, G., Talazoglu, V., Killer, M. *et al.* (1999a) Gross and microscopic histopathological findings in aneurysms of the human brain treated with Guglielmi detachable coils. *Journal of Neurosurgery* **91**, 284–293.

Bavinzski, G., Killer, M., Gruber, A., Reinprecht, A., Gross, C.E. & Richling, B. (1999b) Treatment of basilar artery bifurcation aneurysms by using Guglielmi detachable coils: a 6-year experience. *Journal of Neurosurgery* **90**, 843–852.

Beck, D.W., Adams, H.P. Jr, Flamm, E.S., Godersky, J.C. & Loftus, C.M.

(1988) Combination of aminocaproic acid and nicardipine in treatment of aneurysmal subarachnoid hemorrhage. *Stroke* **19**, 63–67.

Bejjani, G.K., Bank, W.O., Olan, W.J. & Sekhar, L.N. (1998) The efficacy and safety of angioplasty for cerebral vasospasm after subarachnoid hemorrhage. *Neurosurgery* **42**, 979–986.

Berendes, E., Walter, M., Cullen, P. *et al.* (1997) Secretion of brain natriuretic peptide in patients with aneurysmal subarachnoid haemorrhage. *Lancet* **349**, 245–249.

Biller, J., Godersky, J.C. & Adams, H.P. Jr (1988) Management of aneurysmal subarachnoid hemorrhage. *Stroke* **19**, 1300–1305.

Black, P.M., Crowell, R.M. & Abbott, W.M. (1986) External pneumatic calf compression reduces deep venous thrombosis in patients with ruptured intracranial aneurysms. *Neurosurgery* **18**, 25–28.

Botterell, E.H., Lougheed, W.M., Scott, J.W. & Vandewater, S.L. (1956) Hypothermia, and interruption of carotid, or carotid and vertebral circulation, in the surgical management of intracranial aneurysms. *Journal of Neurosurgery* **13**, 1–42.

Brandt, L., Sonesson, B., Ljunggren, B. & Såveland, H. (1987) Ruptured middle cerebral artery aneurysm with intracerebral hemorrhage in younger patients appearing moribund: emergency operation? *Neurosurgery* **20**, 925–929.

Brilstra, E.H., Rinkel, G.J.E., van der Graaf, Y., van Rooij, W.J.J. & Algra, A. (1999) Treatment of intracranial aneurysms by embolization with coils: a systematic review. *Stroke* **30**, 470–476.

Broderick, J.P., Brott, T.G., Duldner, J.E., Tomsick, T. & Leach, A. (1994) Initial and recurrent bleeding are the major causes of death following subarachnoid hemorrhage. *Stroke* **25**, 1342–1347.

Bromberg, J.E.C., Rinkel, G.J.E., Algra, A. *et al.* (1995a) Familial subarachnoid hemorrhage: distinctive features and patterns of inheritance. *Annals of Neurology* **38**, 929–934.

Bromberg, J.E.C., Rinkel, G.J.E., Algra, A., Limburg, M. & van Gijn, J. (1995b) Outcome in familial subarachnoid hemorrhage. *Stroke* **26**, 961–963.

Bromberg, J.E.C., Rinkel, G.J.E., Algra, A. *et al.* (1995c) Subarachnoid haemorrhage in first and second degree relatives of patients with subarachnoid haemorrhage. *British Medical Journal* **311**, 288–289.

Bromberg, J.E.C., Rinkel, G.J.E., Algra, A., Greebe, P., Beldman, T. & van Gijn, J. (1996) Validation of family history in subarachnoid hemorrhage. *Stroke* **27**, 630–632.

Brouwers, P.J.A.M., Wijdicks, E.F.M., Hasan, D. *et al.* (1989) Serial electrocardiographic recording in aneurysmal subarachnoid hemorrhage. *Stroke* **20**, 1162–1167.

Brouwers, P.J.A.M., Wijdicks, E.F.M. & van Gijn, J. (1992) Infarction after aneurysm rupture does not depend on distribution or clearance rate of blood. *Stroke* **23**, 374–379.

Byrne, J.V., Sohn, N.J. & Molyneux, A.J. (1999) Five-year experience in using coil embolization for ruptured intracranial aneurysms: outcomes and incidence of late rebleeding. *Journal of Neurosurgery* **90**, 656–663.

Calhoun, D.A. & Oparil, S. (1990) Treatment of hypertensive crisis. *New England Journal of Medicine* **323**, 1177–1183.

Candia, G.J., Heros, R.C., Lavyne, M.H., Zervas, N.T. & Nelson, C.N. (1978) Effect of intravenous sodium nitroprusside on cerebral blood flow and intracranial pressure. *Neurosurgery* **3**, 50–53.

Carruth, J.E. & Silverman, M.E. (1980) *Torsade de pointe* atypical ventricular tachycardia complicating subarachnoid hemorrhage. *Chest* **78**, 886–888.

Chang, H.S., Fukushima, T., Miyazaki, S. & Tamagawa, T. (1986) Fusiform posterior cerebral artery aneurysm treated with excision and end-to-end anastomosis: case report. *Journal of Neurosurgery* **64**, 501–504.

Chapman, A.B., Rubinstein, D., Hughes, R. *et al.* (1992) Intracranial aneurysms in autosomal dominant polycystic kidney disease. *New England Journal of Medicine* **327**, 916–920.

Chauveau, D., Pirson, Y., Verellen Dumoulin, C., Macnicol, A., Gonzalo, A. & Grunfeld, J.P. (1994) Intracranial aneurysms in autosomal dominant polycystic kidney disease. *Kidney International* **45**, 1140–1146.

Chiang, V.L.S., Claus, E.B. & Awad, I.A. (2000) Toward more rational prediction of outcome in patients with high-grade subarachnoid hemorrhage. *Neurosurgery* **46**, 28–35.

Civit, T., Auque, J., Marchal, J.C., Bracard, S., Picard, L. & Hepner, H. (1996) Aneurysm clipping after endovascular treatment with coils: a report of eight patients. *Neurosurgery* **38**, 955–960.

Clarke Pearson, D.L., Synan, I.S., Hinshaw, W.M., Coleman, R.E. & Creasman, W.T. (1984) Prevention of postoperative venous thromboembolism by external pneumatic calf compression in patients with gynecologic malignancy. *Obstetrics and Gynecology* **63**, 92–98.

Cockroft, K.M., Marks, M.P. & Steinberg, G.K. (2000) Planned direct dual-modality treatment of complex broad-necked intracranial aneurysms: four technical case reports. *Neurosurgery* **46**, 226–230.

Conway, L.W. & McDonald, L.W. (1972) Structural changes of the intradural arteries following subarachnoid hemorrhage. *Journal of Neurosurgery* **37**, 715–723.

Coplin, W.M., Longstreth, W.T. Jr, Lam, A.M. *et al.* (1999) Cerebrospinal fluid creatine kinase-BB isoenzyme activity and outcome after subarachnoid hemorrhage. *Archives of Neurology* **56**, 1348–1352.

Coppolo, D.P. & May, J.J. (1990) Self-extubations: a 12-month experience. *Chest* **98**, 165–169.

Crawford, M.D. & Sarner, M. (1965) Ruptured intracranial aneurysm: a community study. *Lancet* **ii**, 1254–1257.

Crawley, F., Clifton, A. & Brown, M.M. (1999) Should we screen for familial intracranial aneurysm? *Stroke* **30**, 312–316.

van Crevel, H. (1980) Pitfalls in the diagnosis of rebleeding from intracranial aneurysm. *Clinical Neurology and Neurosurgery* **82**, 1–9.

van Crevel, H., Habbema, J.D. & Braakman, R. (1986) Decision analysis of the management of incidental intracranial saccular aneurysms. *Neurology* **36**, 1335–1339.

Cruickshank, J.M., Neil-Dwyer, G., Degaute, J.P. *et al.* (1987) Reduction of stress/catecholamine-induced cardiac necrosis by beta 1-selective blockade. *Lancet* **2**, 585–589.

Davis, S., Andrews, J., Lichtenstein, M. *et al.* (1990) A single-photon emission computed tomography study of hypoperfusion after subarachnoid hemorrhage. *Stroke* **21**, 252–259.

De Braekeleer, M., Pérusse, L., Cantin, L., Bouchard, J.M. & Mathieu, J. (1996) A study of inbreeding and kinship in intracranial aneurysms in the Saguenay Lac-Saint-Jean region (Quebec, Canada). *Annals of Human Genetics* **60**, 99–104.

Debrun, G.M., Aletich, V.A., Kehrli, P., Misra, M., Ausman, J.I. & Charbel, F. (1998) Selection of cerebral aneurysms for treatment using Guglielmi detachable coils: the preliminary University of Illinois at Chicago experience. *Neurosurgery* **43**, 1281–1295.

Derdeyn, C.P., Moran, C.J., Cross, D.T. III, Sherburn, E.W. & Dacey, R.G. Jr (1997) Intracranial aneurysm: anatomic factors that predict the usefulness of intraoperative angiography. *Radiology* **205**, 335–339.

Diringer, M., Ladenson, P.W., Stern, B.J., Schleimer, J. & Hanley, D.F. (1988) Plasma atrial natriuretic factor and subarachnoid hemorrhage. *Stroke* **19**, 1119–1124.

Doczi, T., Bende, J., Huszka, E. & Kiss, J. (1981) Syndrome of inappropriate secretion of antidiuretic hormone after subarachnoid hemorrhage. *Neurosurgery* **9**, 394–397.

Drake, C.G. & Peerless, S.J. (1997) Giant fusiform intracranial aneurysms: review of 120 patients treated surgically from 1965 to 1992. *Journal of Neurosurgery* **87**, 141–162.

Drake, C.G., Hunt, W.E., Sano, K. *et al.* (1988) Report of World Federation of Neurological Surgeons Committee on a universal subarachnoid hemorrhage grading scale. *Journal of Neurosurgery* **68**, 985–986.

Elliott, J.P., Newell, D.W., Lam, D.J. *et al.* (1998) Comparison of balloon angioplasty and papaverine infusion for the treatment of vasospasm following aneurysmal subarachnoid hemorrhage. *Journal of Neurosurgery* **88**, 277–284.

Enblad, P. & Persson, L. (1997) Impact on clinical outcome of secondary brain insults during the neurointensive care of patients with subarachnoid haemorrhage: a pilot study. *Journal of Neurology, Neurosurgery and Psychiatry* **62**, 512–516.

Eskesen, V., Karle, A., Kruse, A., Kruse Larsen, C., Praestholm, J. & Schmidt, K. (1987) Observer variability in assessment of angiographic vasospasm after aneurysmal subarachnoid haemorrhage. *Acta Neurochirurgica (Wien)* **87**, 54–57.

Eskridge, J.M. & Song, J.K. (1998) Endovascular embolization of 150 basilar tip aneurysms with Guglielmi detachable coils: results of the Food and Drug Administration multicenter clinical trial. *Journal of Neurosurgery* **89**, 81–86.

Eskridge, J.M., McAuliffe, W., Song, J.K. *et al.* (1998) Balloon angioplasty for the treatment of vasospasm: results of first 50 cases. *Neurosurgery* **42**, 510–516.

Eskridge, J.M., Song, J.K., Elliot, J.P., Newell, D.W., Grady, M.S. & Winn, H.R. (1999) Balloon angioplasty of the A_1 segment of the anterior cerebral artery narrowed by vasospasm. *Journal of Neurosurgery* **91**, 153–156.

Estanol Vidal, B., Badui Dergal, E., Cesarman, E. *et al.* (1979) Cardiac arrhythmias associated with subarachnoid hemorrhage: prospective study. *Neurosurgery* **5**, 675–680.

Fandino, J., Kaku, Y., Schuknecht, B., Valavanis, A. & Yonekawa, Y. (1998) Improvement of cerebral oxygenation patterns and metabolic validation of super-selective intraarterial infusion of papaverine for the treatment of cerebral vasospasm. *Journal of Neurosurgery* **89**, 93–100.

Farhat, S.M. & Schneider, R.C. (1967) Observations on the effect of systemic blood pressure on intracranial circulation in patients with cerebrovascular insufficiency. *Journal of Neurosurgery* **27**, 441–445.

Feigin, V.L., Rinkel, G.J.E., Algra, A., Vermeulen, M. & van Gijn, J. (2000) Calcium antagonists for aneurysmal subarachnoid haemorrhage (Cochrane Review). In: *The Cochrane Library*. Oxford: Software Update.

Findlay, J.M., Weir, B.K., Kanamaru, K. & Espinosa, F. (1989) Arterial wall changes in cerebral vasospasm. *Neurosurgery* **25**, 736–745.

Findlay, J.M., Kassell, N.F., Weir, B.K.A. *et al.* (1995) A randomized trial of intraoperative, intracisternal tissue plasminogen activator for the prevention of vasospasm. *Neurosurgery* **37**, 168–178.

Finn, S.S., Stephensen, S.A., Miller, C.A., Drobnich, L. & Hunt, W.E. (1986) Observations on the perioperative management of aneurysmal subarachnoid hemorrhage. *Journal of Neurosurgery* **65**, 48–62.

Firlik, A.D., Kaufmann, A.M., Jungreis, C.A. & Yonas, H. (1997) Effect of transluminal angioplasty on cerebral blood flow in the management of symptomatic vasospasm following aneurysmal subarachnoid hemorrhage. *Journal of Neurosurgery* **86**, 830–839.

Fisher, A. & Aboul Nasr, H.T. (1979) Delayed nonfatal pulmonary edema following subarachnoid hemorrhage: case report. *Journal of Neurosurgery* **51**, 856–859.

Fisher, C.M., Roberson, G.H. & Ojemann, R.G. (1977) Cerebral vasospasm with ruptured saccular aneurysm: the clinical manifestations. *Neurosurgery* **1**, 245–248.

Fisher, C.M., Kistler, J.P. & Davis, J.M. (1980) Relation of cerebral vasospasm to subarachnoid hemorrhage visualized by computerized tomographic scanning. *Neurosurgery* **6**, 1–9.

Fodstad, H., Pilbrant, A., Schannong, M. & Strömberg, S. (1981) Determination of tranexamic acid and fibrin/fibrinogen degradation products in cerebrospinal fluid after aneurysmal subarachnoid haemorrhage. *Acta Neurochirurgica (Wien)* **58**, 1–13.

Forsting, M., Albert, F.K., Jansen, O. *et al.* (1996) Coil placement after clipping—endovascular treatment of incompletely clipped cerebral aneurysms: report of two cases. *Journal of Neurosurgery* **85**, 966–969.

Foy, P.M., Chadwick, D.W., Rajgopalan, N., Johnson, A.L. & Shaw, M.D. (1992) Do prophylactic anticonvulsant drugs alter the pattern of seizures after craniotomy? *Journal of Neurology, Neurosurgery and Psychiatry* **55**, 753–757.

Fridriksson, S.M., Hillman, J., Säveland, H. & Brandt, L. (1995) Intracranial aneurysm surgery in the 8th and 9th decades of life: impact on population-based management outcome. *Neurosurgery* **37**, 627–631.

Friedman, R.A., Pensak, M.L., Tauber, M., Tew, J.M. Jr & Van Loveren, H.R. (1997) Anterior petrosectomy approach to infraclinoidal basilar artery aneurysms: the emerging role of the neuro-otologist in multidisciplinary management of basilar artery aneurysms. *Laryngoscope* **107**, 977–983.

Frizzell, R.T., Kuhn, F., Morris, R., Quinn, C. & Fisher, W.S. III (1997) Screening for ocular hemorrhages in patients with ruptured cerebral aneurysms: a prospective study of 99 patients. *Neurosurgery* **41**, 529–533.

Fujii, Y., Takeuchi, S., Sasaki, O., Minakawa, T., Koike, T. & Tanaka, R. (1996) Ultra-early rebleeding in spontaneous subarachnoid hemorrhage. *Journal of Neurosurgery* **84**, 35–42.

Fujii, Y., Takeuchi, S., Sasaki, O., Minakawa, T., Koike, T. & Tanaka, R. (1997) Serial changes of hemostasis in aneurysmal subarachnoid hemorrhage, with special reference to delayed ischemic neurological deficits. *Journal of Neurosurgery* **86**, 594–602.

Gaetani, P., Tartara, F., Pignatti, P., Tancioni, F., Baena, R.R.Y. & De Benedetti, F. (1998) Cisternal CSF levels of cytokines after subarachnoid hemorrhage. *Neurological Research* **20**, 337–342.

Gibbs, J.R. & O'Gorman, P. (1967) Fibrinolysis in subarachnoid haemorrhage. *Postgraduate Medical Journal* **43**, 779–784.

Gifford, R.W. Jr (1991) Management of hypertensive crises. *Journal of the American Medical Association* **266**, 829–835.

van Gijn, J. & van Dongen, K.J. (1982) The time course of aneurysmal haemorrhage on computed tomograms. *Neuroradiology* **23**, 153–156.

van Gijn, J., Hijdra, A., Wijdicks, E.F.M., Vermeulen, M. & van Crevel, H. (1985) Acute hydrocephalus after aneurysmal subarachnoid hemorrhage. *Journal of Neurosurgery* **63**, 355–362.

van Gijn, J., Bromberg, J.E., Lindsay, K.W., Hasan, D. & Vermeulen, M. (1994) Definition of initial grading, specific events, and overall outcome in patients with aneurysmal subarachnoid hemorrhage: a survey. *Stroke* **25**, 1623–1627.

Giller, C.A., Giller, A.M. & Landreneau, F. (1998) Detection of emboli after surgery for intracerebral aneurysms. *Neurosurgery* **42**, 490–493.

Girvin, J.P. (1973) The use of antifibrinolytic agents in the preoperative treatment of ruptured intracranial aneurysms. *Transactions of the American Neurological Association* **98**, 150–152.

Graff-Radford, N.R., Torner, J., Adams, H.P. Jr & Kassell, N.F. (1989) Factors associated with hydrocephalus after subarachnoid hemorrhage: a report of the Cooperative Aneurysm Study. *Archives of Neurology* **46**, 744–752.

Greenberg, D.A. (1987) Calcium channels and calcium channel antagonists. *Annals of Neurology* **21**, 317–330.

Grote, E. & Hassler, W. (1988) The critical first minutes after subarachnoid hemorrhage. *Neurosurgery* **22**, 654–661.

Gruber, A., Ungersböck, K., Reinprecht, A. *et al.* (1998a) Evaluation of cerebral vasospasm after early surgical and endovascular treatment of ruptured intracranial aneurysms. *Neurosurgery* **42**, 258–267.

Gruber, A., Reinprecht, A., Görzer, H. *et al.* (1998b) Pulmonary function and radiographic abnormalities related to neurological outcome after aneurysmal subarachnoid hemorrhage. *Journal of Neurosurgery* **88**, 28–37.

Gruber, A., Killer, M., Bavinzski, G. & Richling, B. (1999a) Clinical and angiographic results of endosaccular coiling treatment of giant and very large intracranial aneurysms: a 7-year, single-center experience. *Neurosurgery* **45**, 793–803.

Gruber, A., Reinprecht, A., Illievich, U.M. *et al.* (1999b) Extracerebral organ dysfunction and neurologic outcome after aneurysmal subarachnoid hemorrhage. *Critical Care Medicine* **27**, 505–514.

Gruber, A., Reinprecht, A., Bavinzski, G., Czech, T. & Richling, B. (1999c) Chronic shunt-dependent hydrocephalus after early surgical and early endovascular treatment of ruptured intracranial aneurysms. *Neurosurgery* **44**, 503–509.

Guglielmi, G., Vinuela, F., Duckwiler, G. *et al.* (1992) Endovascular treatment of posterior circulation aneurysms by electrothrombosis using electrically detachable coils. *Journal of Neurosurgery* **77**, 515–524.

Hacein-Bey, L., Connolly, E.S. Jr, Mayer, S.A., Young, W.L., Pile-Spellman, J. & Solomon, R.A. (1998) Complex intracranial aneurysms: combined operative and endovascular approaches. *Neurosurgery* **43**, 1304–1312.

Haley, E.C. Jr, Kassell, N.F., Apperson-Hansen, C., Maile, M.H. & Alves, W.M. (1997) A randomized, double-blind, vehicle-controlled trial of tirilazad mesylate in patients with aneurysmal subarachnoid hemorrhage: a cooperative study in North America. *Journal of Neurosurgery* **86**, 467–474.

Harrier, H.D. (1988) Use of labetalol in trauma. *Critical Care Medicine* **16**, 1159–1160.

Harrigan, M.R. (1996) Cerebral salt wasting syndrome: a review. *Neurosurgery* **38**, 152–160.

Hart, R.G., Byer, J.A., Slaughter, J.R., Hewett, J.E. & Easton, J.D. (1981) Occurrence and implications of seizures in subarachnoid hemorrhage due to ruptured intracranial aneurysms. *Neurosurgery* **8**, 417–421.

Hasan, D. & Tanghe, H.L. (1992) Distribution of cisternal blood in patients with acute hydrocephalus after subarachnoid hemorrhage. *Annals of Neurology* **31**, 374–378.

Hasan, D., Vermeulen, M., Wijdicks, E.F.M., Hijdra, A. & van Gijn, J. (1989a) Effect of fluid intake and antihypertensive treatment on cerebral ischemia after subarachnoid hemorrhage. *Stroke* **20**, 1511–1515.

Hasan, D., Lindsay, K.W., Wijdicks, E.F.M. *et al.* (1989b) Effect of fludrocortisone acetate in patients with subarachnoid hemorrhage. *Stroke* **20**, 1156–1161.

Hasan, D., Vermeulen, M., Wijdicks, E.F.M., Hijdra, A. & van Gijn, J. (1989c) Management problems in acute hydrocephalus after subarachnoid hemorrhage. *Stroke* **20**, 747–753.

Hasan, D., Wijdicks, E.F.M. & Vermeulen, M. (1990) Hyponatremia is associated with cerebral ischemia in patients with aneurysmal subarachnoid hemorrhage. *Annals of Neurology* **27**, 106–108.

Hasan, D., van Peski, J., Loeve, I., Krenning, E.P. & Vermeulen, M. (1991a) Single photon emission computed tomography in patients with acute hydrocephalus or with cerebral ischaemia after subarachnoid haemorrhage.

Journal of Neurology, Neurosurgery and Psychiatry **54**, 490–493.

Hasan, D., Lindsay, K.W. & Vermeulen, M. (1991b) Treatment of acute hydrocephalus after subarachnoid hemorrhage with serial lumbar puncture. *Stroke* **22**, 190–194.

Hasan, D., Schonck, R.S., Avezaat, C.J., Tanghe, H.L., van Gijn, J. & van der Lugt, P.J. (1993) Epileptic seizures after subarachnoid hemorrhage. *Annals of Neurology* **33**, 286–291.

Hauerberg, J., Eskesen, V. & Rosenorn, J. (1994) The prognostic significance of intracerebral haematoma as shown on CT scanning after aneurysmal subarachnoid haemorrhage. *British Journal of Neurosurgery* **8**, 333–339.

Heiskanen, O., Poranen, A., Kuurne, T., Valtonen, S. & Kaste, M. (1988) Acute surgery for intracerebral haematomas caused by rupture of an intracranial arterial aneurysm: a prospective randomized study. *Acta Neurochirurgica (Wien)* **90**, 81–83.

Heros, R.C., Zervas, N.T. & Varsos, V. (1983) Cerebral vasospasm after subarachnoid hemorrhage: an update. *Annals of Neurology* **14**, 599–608.

Higashida, R.T., Halbach, V.V., Cahan, L.D. *et al.* (1989) Transluminal angioplasty for treatment of intracranial arterial vasospasm. *Journal of Neurosurgery* **71**, 648–653.

Higashida, R.T., Smith, W., Gress, D., Urwin, R. *et al.* (1997) Intravascular stent and endovascular coil placement for a ruptured fusiform aneurysm of the basilar artery: case report and review of the literature. *Journal of Neurosurgery* **87**, 944–949.

Hijdra, A. & van Gijn, J. (1982) Early death from rupture of an intracranial aneurysm. *Journal of Neurosurgery* **57**, 765–768.

Hijdra, A., Vermeulen, M., van Gijn, J. & van Crevel, H. (1984) Respiratory arrest in subarachnoid hemorrhage. *Neurology* **34**, 1501–1503.

Hijdra, A., van Gijn, J., Stefanko, S. *et al.* (1986) Delayed cerebral ischemia after aneurysmal subarachnoid hemorrhage: clinicoanatomic correlations. *Neurology* **36**, 329–333.

Hijdra, A., Braakman, R., van Gijn, J., Vermeulen, M. & van Crevel, H. (1987a) Aneurysmal subarachnoid hemorrhage: complications and outcome in a hospital population. *Stroke* **18**, 1061–1067.

Hijdra, A., Vermeulen, M., van Gijn, J. & van Crevel, H. (1987b) Rerupture of intracranial aneurysms: a clinicoanatomic study. *Journal of Neurosurgery* **67**, 29–33.

Hijdra, A., van Gijn, J., Nagelkerke, N.J., Vermeulen, M. & van Crevel, H. (1988) Prediction of delayed cerebral ischemia, rebleeding, and outcome after aneurysmal subarachnoid hemorrhage. *Stroke* **19**, 1250–1256.

Hijdra, A., Brouwers, P.J., Vermeulen, M. & van Gijn, J. (1990) Grading the amount of blood on computed tomograms after subarachnoid hemorrhage. *Stroke* **21**, 1156–1161.

Hirai, S., Ono, J. & Yamaura, A. (1996) Clinical grading and outcome after early surgery in aneurysmal subarachnoid hemorrhage. *Neurosurgery* **39**, 441–446.

Honma, Y., Fujiwara, T., Irie, K., Ohkawa, M. & Nagao, S. (1995) Morphological changes in human cerebral arteries after percutaneous transluminal angioplasty for vasospasm caused by subarachnoid hemorrhage. *Neurosurgery* **36**, 1073–1081.

Hop, J.W., Rinkel, G.J.E., Algra, A. & van Gijn, J. (1997) Case-fatality rates and functional outcome after subarachnoid hemorrhage: a systematic review. *Stroke* **28**, 660–664.

Hop, J.W., Rinkel, G.J.E., Algra, A. & van Gijn, J. (1998) Quality of life in patients and partners after aneurysmal subarachnoid hemorrhage. *Stroke* **29**, 798–804.

Hop, J.W., Rinkel, G.J.E., Algra, A. & van Gijn, J. (1999) Initial loss of consciousness and risk of delayed cerebral ischemia after aneurysmal subarachnoid hemorrhage. *Stroke* **30**, 2268–2271.

Huber, A., Klöti, R. & Landolt, E. (1988) Terson's syndrome. *Neuro-ophthalmology* **8**, 223–233.

Hughes, J.T. & Schianchi, P.M. (1978) Cerebral artery spasm: a histological study at necropsy of the blood vessels in cases of subarachnoid hemorrhage. *Journal of Neurosurgery* **48**, 515–525.

Hunt, W.E. & Hess, R.M. (1968) Surgical risk as related to time of intervention in the repair of intracranial aneurysms. *Journal of Neurosurgery* **28**, 14–20.

Huston, J. III, Torres, V.E., Sulivan, P.P., Offord, K.P. & Wiebers, D.O. (1993) Value of magnetic resonance angiography for the detection of intracranial aneurysms in autosomal dominant polycystic kidney disease. *Journal of the American Society of Nephrology* **3**, 1871–1877.

Huston, J. III, Torres, V.E., Wiebers, D.O. & Schievink, W.I. (1996) Follow-up of intracranial aneurysms in autosomal dominant polycystic kidney disease by magnetic resonance angiography. *Journal of the American Society of Nephrology* **7**, 2135–2141.

Ikeda, K., Asakura, H., Futami, K. & Yamashita, J. (1997) Coagulative and fibrinolytic activation in cerebrospinal fluid and plasma after subarachnoid hemorrhage. *Neurosurgery* **41**, 344–349.

Inagawa, T. & Hirano, A. (1990) Ruptured intracranial aneurysms: an autopsy study of 133 patients. *Surgical Neurology* **33**, 117–123.

Inagawa, T., Kamiya, K., Ogasawara, H. & Yano, T. (1987) Rebleeding of ruptured intracranial aneurysms in the acute stage. *Surgical Neurology* **28**, 93–99.

Inagawa, T., Tokuda, Y., Ohbayashi, N., Takaya, M. & Moritake, K. (1995) Study of aneurysmal subarachnoid hemorrhage in Izumo City, Japan. *Stroke* **26**, 761–766.

Jakobsson, K.E., Saveland, H., Hillman, J. *et al.* (1996) Warning leak and management outcome in aneurysmal subarachnoid hemorrhage. *Journal of Neurosurgery* **85**, 995–999.

Jane, J.A., Kassell, N.F., Torner, J.C. & Winn, H.R. (1985) The natural history of aneurysms and arteriovenous malformations. *Journal of Neurosurgery* **62**, 321–323.

Jennett, B. & Bond, M. (1975) Assessment of outcome after severe brain damage: a practical scale. *Lancet* **i**, 480–484.

Johnston, S.C., Dudley, R.A., Gress, D.R. & Ono, L. (1999a) Surgical and endovascular treatment of unruptured cerebral aneurysms at University hospitals. *Neurology* **52**, 1799–1805.

Johnston, S.C., Gress, D.R. & Kahn, J.G. (1999b) Which unruptured cerebral aneurysms should be treated? A cost-utility analysis. *Neurology* **52**, 1806–1815.

Johnston, S.C., Wilson, C.B., Halbach, V.V. *et al.* (2000) Endovascular and surgical treatment of unruptured cerebral aneurysms: comparison of risks. *Annals of Neurology* **48**, 11–19.

Juvela, S. (1995) Aspirin and delayed cerebral ischemia after aneurysmal subarachnoid hemorrhage. *Journal of Neurosurgery* **82**, 945–952.

Juvela, S., Kaste, M. & Hillbom, M. (1990) Platelet thromboxane release after subarachnoid hemorrhage and surgery. *Stroke* **21**, 566–571.

Juvela, S., Porras, M. & Heiskanen, O. (1993) Natural history of unruptured intracranial aneurysms: a long-term follow-up study. *Journal of Neurosurgery* **79**, 174–182.

Kaku, Y., Yonekawa, Y., Tsukahara, T. & Kazekawa, K. (1992) Superselective intra-arterial infusion of papaverine for the treatment of cerebral vasospasm after subarachnoid hemorrhage. *Journal of Neurosurgery* **77**, 842–847.

Kaneko, T., Sawada, T. & Niimi, T. (1983) Lower limit of blood pressure in treatment of acute hypertensive intracranial hemorrhage (AHCH). *Journal of Cerebral Blood Flow and Metabolism* **3** (Suppl. 1), S51–S52.

Kassell, N.F. & Torner, J.C. (1983) Aneurysmal rebleeding: a preliminary report from the Cooperative Aneurysm Study. *Neurosurgery* **13**, 479–481.

Kassell, N.F., Peerless, S.J., Durward, Q.J., Beck, D.W., Drake, C.G. & Adams, H.P. Jr (1982) Treatment of ischemic deficits from vasospasm with intravascular volume expansion and induced arterial hypertension. *Neurosurgery* **11**, 337–343.

Kassell, N.F., Kongable, G.L., Torner, J.C., Adams, H.P. Jr & Mazuz, H. (1985) Delay in referral of patients with ruptured aneurysms to neurosurgical attention. *Stroke* **16**, 587–590.

Kassell, N.F., Torner, J.C., Haley, E.C. Jr, Jane, J.A., Adams, H.P. Jr & Kongable, G.L. (1990) The International Cooperative Study on the Timing of Aneurysm Surgery, 1: overall management results. *Journal of Neurosurgery* **73**, 18–36.

Kassell, N.F., Haley, E.C. Jr, Apperson-Hansen, C. *et al.* (1996) Randomized, double-blind, vehicle-controlled trial of tirilazad mesylate in patients with aneurysmal subarachnoid hemorrhage: a cooperative study in Europe, Australia, and New Zealand. *Journal of Neurosurgery* **84**, 221–228.

Kawai, K., Nagashima, H., Narita, K. *et al.* (1997) Efficacy and risk of ventricular drainage in cases of grade V subarachnoid hemorrhage. *Neurological Research* **19**, 649–653.

Khurana, V.G., Piepgras, D.G. & Whisnant, J.P. (1998) Ruptured giant intracranial aneurysms, 1: a study of rebleeding. *Journal of Neurosurgery* **88**, 425–429.

Kistler, J.P., Crowell, R.M., Davis, K.R. *et al.* (1983) The relation of cerebral vasospasm to the extent and location of subarachnoid blood visualized by CT scan: a prospective study. *Neurology* **33**, 424–436.

Kolluri, V.R. & Sengupta, R.P. (1984) Symptomatic hydrocephalus following aneurysmal subarachnoid hemorrhage. *Surgical Neurology* **21**, 402–404.

Kosnik, E.J. & Hunt, W.E. (1976) Postoperative hypertension in the management of patients with intracranial arterial aneurysms. *Journal of Neurosurgery* **45**, 148–154.

Kuether, T.A., Nesbit, G.M. & Barnwell, S.L. (1998) Clinical and angiographic outcomes, with treatment data, for patients with cerebral aneurysms treated with Guglielmi detachable coils: a single-center experience. *Neurosurgery* **43**, 1016–1023.

Kuhn, F., Morris, R., Witherspoon, C.D. & Mester, V. (1998) Terson syndrome: results of vitrectomy and the significance of vitreous hemorrhage in patients with subarachnoid hemorrhage. *Ophthalmology* **105**, 472–477.

Lanzino, G. & Kassell, N.F. (1999) Double-blind, randomized, vehicle-controlled study of high-dose tirilazad mesylate in women with aneurysmal subarachnoid hemorrhage, 2: a cooperative study in North America. *Journal of Neurosurgery* **90**, 1018–1024.

Lanzino, G., Kassell, N.F., Germanson, T.P. *et al.* (1996) Age and outcome after aneurysmal subarachnoid hemorrhage: why do older patients fare worse? *Journal of Neurosurgery* **85**, 410–418.

Lanzino, G., Wakhloo, A.K., Fessler, R.D., Hartney, M.L., Guterman, L.R. & Hopkins, L.N. (1999a) Efficacy and current limitations of intravascular stents for intracranial internal carotid, vertebral, and basilar artery aneurysms. *Journal of Neurosurgery* **91**, 538–546.

Lanzino, G., Kassell, N.F., Dorsch, N.W.C. *et al.* (1999b) Double-blind, randomized, vehicle-controlled study of high-dose tirilazad mesylate in women with aneurysmal subarachnoid hemorrhage, 1: a cooperative study in Europe, Australia, New Zealand, and South Africa. *Journal of Neurosurgery* **90**, 1011–1017.

Lasner, T.M., Weil, R.J., Riina, H.A. *et al.* (1997) Cigarette smoking-induced increase in the risk of symptomatic vasospasm after aneurysmal subarachnoid hemorrhage. *Journal of Neurosurgery* **87**, 381–384.

Lawton, M.T., Heiserman, J.E., Prendergast, V.C., Zabramski, J.M. & Spetzler, R.F. (1996) Titanium aneurysm clips, 3: clinical application in 16 patients with subarachnoid hemorrhage. *Neurosurgery* **38**, 1170–1175.

Lawton, M.T., Daspit, C.P. & Spetzler, R.F. (1997) Technical aspects and recent trends in the management of large and giant midbasilar artery aneurysms. *Neurosurgery* **41**, 513–520.

Leblanc, R., Worsley, K.J., Melanson, D. & Tampieri, D. (1994) Angiographic screening and elective surgery of familial cerebral aneurysms: a decision analysis. *Neurosurgery* **35**, 9–18.

Le Roux, P.D., Elliott, J.P., Newell, D.W., Grady, M.S. & Winn, H.R. (1996) Predicting outcome in poor-grade patients with subarachnoid hemorrhage: a retrospective review of 159 aggressively managed cases. *Journal of Neurosurgery* **85**, 39–49.

Lennihan, L., Mayer, S.A., Fink, M.E. *et al.* (2000) Effect of hypervolemic therapy on cerebral blood flow after subarachnoid hemorrhage: a randomized controlled trial. *Stroke* **31**, 383–391.

Levy, D.I. (1997) Embolization of wide-necked anterior communicating artery aneurysm: technical note. *Neurosurgery* **41**, 979–982.

Levy, D.I. & Ku, A. (1997) Balloon-assisted coil placement in wide-necked aneurysms: technical note. *Journal of Neurosurgery* **86**, 724–727.

Lindsay, K.W., Teasdale, G., Knill Jones, R.P. & Murray, L. (1982) Observer variability in grading patients with subarachnoid hemorrhage. *Journal of Neurosurgery* **56**, 628–633.

Lindsay, K.W., Teasdale, G.M. & Knill Jones, R.P. (1983) Observer variability in assessing the clinical features of subarachnoid hemorrhage. *Journal of Neurosurgery* **58**, 57–62.

Linn, F.H.H., Rinkel, G.J.E., Algra, A. & van Gijn, J. (1996) Incidence of subarachnoid hemorrhage—role of region, year, and rate of computed tomography: a meta-analysis. *Stroke* **27**, 625–629.

Linn, F.H.H., Rinkel, G.J.E., Algra, A. & van Gijn, J. (2000) The notion of 'warning leaks' in subarachnoid haemorrhage: are such patients in fact admitted with a rebleed? *Journal of Neurology, Neurosurgery and Psychiatry* **68**, 332–336.

Linskey, M.E., Horton, J.A., Rao, G.R. & Yonas, H. (1991) Fatal rupture of the intracranial carotid artery during transluminal angioplasty for vasospasm induced by subarachnoid hemorrhage: case report. *Journal of Neurosurgery* **74**, 985–990.

Ljunggren, B., Saveland, H., Brandt, L. & Zygmunt, S. (1985) Early operation and overall outcome in aneurysmal subarachnoid hemorrhage. *Journal of Neurosurgery* **62**, 547–551.

Locksley, H.B. (1966) Report of the Cooperative Study on intracranial aneurysms and subarachnoid hemorrhage: Section V, part II. Natural history of subarachnoid hemorrhage, intracranial aneurysms, and arteriovenous malformations. *Journal of Neurosurgery* **25**, 321–368.

Lozano, A.M. & Leblanc, R. (1992) Cerebral aneurysms and polycystic kidney disease: a critical review. *Canadian Journal of Neurological Sciences* **19**, 222–227.

Maas, A.I., Braakman, R., Schouten, H.J., Minderhoud, J.M. & van Zomeren, A.H. (1983) Agreement between physicians on assessment of outcome following severe head injury. *Journal of Neurosurgery* **58**, 321–325.

Macdonald, R.L., Wallace, M.C. & Kestle, J.R. (1993) Role of angiography following aneurysm surgery. *Journal of Neurosurgery* **79**, 826–832.

McDougall, C.G., Halbach, V.V., Dowd, C.F., Higashida, R.T., Larsen, D.W. & Hieshima, G.B. (1998) Causes and management of aneurysmal hemorrhage occurring during embolization with Guglielmi detachable coils. *Journal of Neurosurgery* **89**, 87–92.

McKissock, W., Richardson, A. & Walsh, L. (1960) 'Posterior-communicating aneurysms': a controlled trial of conservative and surgical treatment of ruptured aneurysms of the internal carotid artery at or near the point of origin of the posterior communicating artery. *Lancet* **i**, 1203–1206.

McKissock, W., Richardson, A. & Walsh, L. (1965) Anterior communicating aneurysms: a trial of conservative and surgical treatment. *Lancet* **i**, 873–876.

McQuaker, I.G., Jaspan, T., McConachie, N.S. & Dolan, G. (1999) Coil embolization of cerebral aneurysms in patients with sickling disorders. *British Journal of Haematology* **106**, 388–390.

Maeda, K., Kurita, H., Nakamura, T. *et al.* (1997) Occurrence of severe vasospasm following intraventricular hemorrhage from an arteriovenous malformation: report of two cases. *Journal of Neurosurgery* **87**, 436–439.

Malek, A.M., Higashida, R.T., Phatouros, C.C., Dowd, C.F. & Halbach, V.V. (1999) Treatment of an intracranial aneurysm using a new three-dimensional-shape Guglielmi detachable coil: technical case report. *Neurosurgery* **44**, 1142–1144.

Malisch, T.W., Guglielmi, G., Vinuela, F. *et al.* (1997) Intracranial aneurysms treated with the Guglielmi detachable coil: midterm clinical results in a consecutive series of 100 patients. *Journal of Neurosurgery* **87**, 176–183.

Manabe, H., Fujita, S., Hatayama, T., Suzuki, S. & Yagihashi, S. (1998) Rerupture of coil-embolized aneurysm during long-term observation: case report. *Journal of Neurosurgery* **88**, 1096–1098.

Manninen, P.H., Ayra, B., Gelb, A.W. & Pelz, D. (1995) Association between electrocardiographic abnormalities and intracranial blood in patients following acute subarachnoid hemorrhage. *Journal of Neurosurgical Anesthesiology* **7**, 12–16.

Manno, E.M., Gress, D.R., Ogilvy, C.S., Stone, C.M. & Zervas, N.T. (1997) The safety and efficacy of cyclosporine A in the prevention of vasospasm in patients with Fisher grade 3 subarachnoid hemorrhages: a pilot study. *Neurosurgery* **40**, 289–293.

Marion, D.W., Segal, R. & Thompson, M.E. (1986) Subarachnoid hemorrhage and the heart. *Neurosurgery* **18**, 101–106.

Mathieu, J., Hébert, G., Pérusse, L. *et al.* (1997) Familial intracranial aneurysms: recurrence risk and accidental aggregation study. *Canadian Journal of Neurological Sciences* **24**, 326–331.

Maurice-Williams, R.S. (1982) Ruptured intracranial aneurysms: has the incidence of early rebleeding been over-estimated? *Journal of Neurology, Neurosurgery and Psychiatry* **45**, 774–779.

Maurice-Williams, R.S. & Marsh, H. (1985) Ruptured intracranial aneurysms: the overall effect of treatment and the influence of patient selection and data presentation on the reported outcome. *Journal of Neurology, Neurosurgery and Psychiatry* **48**, 1208–1212.

Mayer, P.L., Awad, I.A., Todor, R. *et al.* (1996) Misdiagnosis of symptomatic cerebral aneurysm: prevalence and correlation with outcome at four institutions. *Stroke* **27**, 1558–1563.

Mayer, S.A., Fink, M.E., Homma, S. *et al.* (1994) Cardiac injury associated with neurogenic pulmonary edema following subarachnoid hemorrhage. *Neurology* **44**, 815–820.

Mayer, S.A., Solomon, R.A., Fink, M.E. *et al.* (1998) Effect of 5% albumin solution on sodium balance and blood volume after subarachnoid hemorrhage. *Neurosurgery* **42**, 759–767.

Mayer, S.A., Lin, J., Homma, S. *et al.* (1999) Myocardial injury and left ventricular performance after subarachnoid hemorrhage. *Stroke* **30**, 780–786.

Medele, R.J., Stummer, W., Mueller, A.J., Steiger, H.J. & Reulen, H.J. (1998) Terson's syndrome in subarachnoid hemorrhage and severe brain injury accompanied by acutely raised intracranial pressure. *Journal of Neurosurgery* **88**, 851–854.

Mehta, V., Holness, R.O., Connolly, K., Walling, S. & Hall, R. (1996) Acute hydrocephalus following aneurysmal subarachnoid hemorrhage. *Canadian Journal of Neurological Sciences* **23**, 40–45.

Mendelow, A.D., Stockdill, G., Steers, A.J., Hayes, J. & Gillingham, F.J. (1982) Double-blind trial of aspirin in patient receiving tranexamic acid for subarachnoid hemorrhage. *Acta Neurochirurgica (Wien)* **62**, 195–202.

Menghini, V.V., Brown, R.D. Jr, Sicks, J.D., O'Fallon, W.M. & Wiebers, D.O. (1998) Incidence and prevalence of intracranial aneurysms and hemorrhage in Olmsted County, Minnesota, 1965–95. *Neurology* **51**, 405–411.

Milhorat, T.H. (1987) Acute hydrocephalus after aneurysmal subarachnoid hemorrhage. *Neurosurgery* **20**, 15–20.

Miller, J.A., Dacey, R.G. Jr & Diringer, M.N. (1995) Safety of hypertensive hypervolemic therapy with phenylephrine in the treatment of delayed ischemic deficits after subarachnoid hemorrhage. *Stroke* **26**, 2260–2266.

Millikan, C.H. (1975) Cerebral vasospasm and ruptured intracranial aneurysm. *Archives of Neurology* **32**, 433–449.

Mizukami, M., Kawase, T., Usami, T. & Tazawa, T. (1982) Prevention of vasospasm by early operation with removal of subarachnoid blood. *Neurosurgery* **10**, 301–307.

Molyneux, A.J., Ellison, D.W., Morris, J. & Byrne, J.V. (1995) Histological findings in giant aneurysms treated with Guglielmi detachable coils: report of two cases with autopsy correlation. *Journal of Neurosurgery* **83**, 129–132.

Mori, T., Katayama, Y., Kawamata, T. & Hirayama, T. (1999) Improved efficiency of hypervolemic therapy with inhibition of natriuresis by fludrocortisone in patients with aneurysmal subarachnoid hemorrhage. *Journal of Neurosurgery* **91**, 947–952.

Muizelaar, J.P., Vermeulen, M., van Crevel, H. *et al.* (1988) Outcome of aneurysmal subarachnoid hemorrhage in patients 66 years of age and older. *Clinical Neurology and Neurosurgery* **90**, 203–207.

Murayama, Y., Viñuela, F., Duckwiler, G.R., Gobin, Y.P. & Guglielmi, G. (1999) Embolization of incidental cerebral aneurysms by using the Guglielmi detachable coil system. *Journal of Neurosurgery* **90**, 207–214.

Neil-Dwyer, G. & Lang, D. (1997) 'Brain attack'—aneurysmal subarachnoid haemorrhage: death due to delayed diagnosis. *Journal of the Royal College of Physicians of London* **31**, 49–52.

Newell, D.W., Eskridge, J.M., Mayberg, M.R., Grady, M.S. & Winn, H.R. (1989) Angioplasty for the treatment of symptomatic vasospasm following subarachnoid hemorrhage. *Journal of Neurosurgery* **71**, 654–660.

Nibbelink, D.W., Torner, J.C. & Henderson, W.G. (1981) Randomised treatment study: drug-induced hypotension. In: *Aneurysmal Subarachnoid Haemorrhage. Report of the Cooperative Study* (eds A.L. Sahs, D.W. Nibbelink & J.C. Torner), pp. 77–106. Urban & Schwarzenberg, Baltimore.

Nichols, D.A., Meyer, F.B., Piepgras, D.G. & Smith, P.L. (1994) Endovascular treatment of intracranial aneurysms. *Mayo Clinic Proceedings* **69**, 272–285.

Nichols, D.A., Brown, R.D. Jr, Thielen, K.R., Meyer, F.B., Atkinson, J.L. & Piepgras, D.G. (1997) Endovascular treatment of ruptured posterior circulation aneurysms using electrolytically detachable coils. *Journal of Neurosurgery* **87**, 374–380.

Nishioka, H. (1966) Report on the cooperative study of intracranial aneurysms and subarachnoid hemorrhage. Section VII, I. Evaluation of the conservative management of ruptured intracranial aneurysms. *Journal of Neurosurgery* **25**, 574–592.

Nurmohamed, M.T., van Riel, A.M., Henkens, C.M. *et al.* (1996) Low molecular weight heparin and compression stockings in the prevention of venous thromboembolism in neurosurgery. *Thrombosis and Haemostasis* **75**, 233–238.

Ogden, J.A., Mee, E.W. & Utley, T. (1998) Too little, too late: does tirilazad mesylate reduce fatigue after subarachnoid hemorrhage? *Neurosurgery* **43**, 782–787.

Ogilvy, C.S., Carter, B.S., Kaplan, S., Rich, C. & Crowell, R.M. (1996) Temporary vessel occlusion for aneurysm surgery: risk factors for stroke in patients protected by induced hypothermia and hypertension and intravenous mannitol administration. *Journal of Neurosurgery* **84**, 785–791.

Ohkuma, H., Suzuki, S., Kimura, M. & Sobata, E. (1991) Role of platelet function in symptomatic cerebral vasospasm following aneurysmal subarachnoid hemorrhage. *Stroke* **22**, 854–859.

Öhman, J. & Heiskanen, O. (1989) Timing of operation for ruptured supratentorial aneurysms: a prospective randomized study. *Journal of Neurosurgery* **70**, 55–60.

Öhman, J., Servo, A. & Heiskanen, O. (1991) Risks factors for cerebral infarction in good-grade patients after aneurysmal subarachnoid hemorrhage and surgery: a prospective study. *Journal of Neurosurgery* **74**, 14–20.

Okada, Y., Shima, T., Nishida, M. *et al.* (1999) Comparison of transcranial Doppler investigation of aneurysmal vasospasm with digital subtraction angiographic and clinical findings. *Neurosurgery* **45**, 443–449.

Olafsson, E., Hauser, W.A. & Gudmundsson, G. (1997) A population-based study of prognosis of ruptured cerebral aneurysm: mortality and recurrence of subarachnoid hemorrhage. *Neurology* **48**, 1191–1195.

Ooka, K., Shibuya, M. & Suzuki, Y. (1997) A comparative study of intracranial aneurysm clips: closing and opening forces and physical endurance. *Neurosurgery* **40**, 318–323.

Oshiro, E.M., Walter, K.A., Piantadosi, S., Witham, T.F. & Tamargo, R.J. (1997) A new subarachnoid hemorrhage grading system based on the Glasgow Coma Scale: a comparison with the Hunt and Hess and World Federation of Neurological Surgeons Scales in a clinical series. *Neurosurgery* **41**, 140–147.

Ostbye, T., Levy, A.R. & Mayo, N.E. (1997) Hospitalization and case-fatality rates for subarachnoid hemorrhage in Canada from 1982 through 1991: the Canadian Collaborative Study Group of Stroke Hospitalizations. *Stroke* **28**, 793–798.

O'Sullivan, M.G., Dorward, N., Whittle, I.R., Steers, A.J. & Miller, J.D. (1994) Management and long-term outcome following subarachnoid haemorrhage and intracranial aneurysm surgery in elderly patients: an audit of 199 consecutive cases. *British Journal of Neurosurgery* **8**, 23–30.

Pakarinen, S. (1967) Incidence, aetiology and prognosis of primary subarachnoid haemorrhage. *Acta Neurologica Scandinavica* **43** (Suppl. 29), 1–128.

Papo, I., Bodosi, M., Merei, T.F. & Luongo, A. (1984) L'hydrocephalie apres hemorragie sous-arachnoidienne [hydrocephalus following subarachnoid hemorrhage]. *Neurochirurgie* **30**, 159–164.

Paré, L., Delfino, R. & Leblanc, R. (1992) The relationship of ventricular drainage to aneurysmal rebleeding. *Journal of Neurosurgery* **76**, 422–427.

Parr, M.J., Finfer, S.R. & Morgan, M.K. (1996) Reversible cardiogenic shock complicating subarachnoid haemorrhage. *British Medical Journal* **313**, 681–683.

Peltonen, S., Juvela, S., Kaste, M. & Lassila, R. (1997) Hemostasis and fibrinolysis activation after subarachnoid hemorrhage. *Journal of Neurosurgery* **87**, 207–214.

Petruk, K.C., West, M., Mohr, G. *et al.* (1988) Nimodipine treatment in poor-grade aneurysm patients: results of a multicenter double-blind placebo-controlled trial. *Journal of Neurosurgery* **68**, 505–517.

Pfausler, B., Belcl, R., Metzler, R., Mohsenipour, I. & Schmutzhard, E. (1996) Terson's syndrome in spontaneous subarachnoid hemorrhage: a prospective study in 60 consecutive patients. *Journal of Neurosurgery* **85**, 392–394.

Philippon, J., Grob, R., Dagreou, F., Guggiari, M., Rivierez, M. & Viars, P. (1986) Prevention of vasospasm in subarachnoid haemorrhage: a controlled study with nimodipine. *Acta Neurochirurgica (Wien)* **82**, 110–114.

Phillips, J., Roberts, G., Bolger, C. *et al.* (1997) Lipoprotein(a): a potential biological marker for unruptured intracranial aneurysms. *Neurosurgery* **40**, 1112–1115.

Phillips, L.H., Whisnant, J.P., O'Fallon, W.M. & Sundt, T.M. (1980) The unchanging pattern of subarachnoid hemorrhage in a community. *Neurology* **30**, 1034–1040.

Pickard, J.D. (1984) Early posthaemorrhagic hydrocephalus. *British Medical Journal* **289**, 569–570.

Pickard, J.D., Murray, G.D., Illingworth, R. *et al.* (1989) Effect of oral nimodipine on cerebral infarction and outcome after subarachnoid haemorrhage: British aneurysm nimodipine trial. *British Medical Journal* **298**, 636–642.

Piepgras, D.G., Khurana, V.G. & Whisnant, J.P. (1998) Ruptured giant intracranial aneurysms, 2: a retrospective analysis of timing and outcome of surgical treatment. *Journal of Neurosurgery* **88**, 430–435.

Pinto, A.N., Canhao, P. & Ferro, J.M. (1996) Seizures at the onset of subarachnoid haemorrhage. *Journal of Neurology* **243**, 161–164.

Pirson, Y. & Chauveau, D. (1995) ADPKD-associated intracranial aneurysm: new insights and unanswered questions. *Contributions to Nephrology* **115**, 53–58.

Polin, R.S., Bavbek, M., Shaffrey, M.E. *et al.* (1998a) Detection of soluble E-selectin, ICAM-1, VCAM-1, and L-selectin in the cerebrospinal fluid of patients after subarachnoid hemorrhage. *Journal of Neurosurgery* **89**, 559–567.

Polin, R.S., Hansen, C.A., German, P., Chadduck, J.B. & Kassell, N.F. (1998b) Intra-arterially administered papaverine for the treatment of symptomatic cerebral vasospasm. *Neurosurgery* **42**, 1256–1264.

Pollick, C., Cujec, B., Parker, S. & Tator, C. (1988) Left ventricular wall motion abnormalities in subarachnoid hemorrhage: an echocardiographic study. *Journal of the American College of Cardiology* **12**, 600–605.

Post, M.J., Borst, C. & Kuntz, R.E. (1994) The relative importance of arterial remodeling compared with intimal hyperplasia in lumen renarrowing after balloon angioplasty: a study in the normal rabbit and the hypercholesterolemic Yucatan micropig. *Circulation* **89**, 2816–2821.

Raaymakers, T.W.M., Rinkel, G.J.E. & Ramos, L.M.P. (1998a) Initial and follow-up screening for aneurysms in families with familial subarachnoid hemorrhage. *Neurology* **51**, 1125–1130.

Raaymakers, T.W.M., Rinkel, G.J.E., Limburg, M. & Algra, A. (1998b) Mortality and morbidity of surgery for unruptured intracranial aneurysms: a meta-analysis. *Stroke* **29**, 1531–1538.

Raaymakers, T.W.M., Rinkel, G.J.E., van Gijn, J. *et al.* (1999a) Risks and benefits of screening for intracranial aneurysms in first-degree relatives of patients with sporadic subarachnoid hemorrhage. *New England Journal of Medicine* **341**, 1344–1350.

Raaymakers, T.W.M. & the MARS Study Group (1999b) Aneurysms in relatives of patients with subarachnoid hemorrhage: frequency and risk factors. *Neurology* **53**, 982–988.

Raimondi, A.J. & Torres, H. (1973) Acute hydrocephalus as a complication of subarachnoid hemorrhage. *Surgical Neurology* **1**, 23–26.

Raps, E.C., Rogers, J.D., Galetta, S.L. *et al.* (1993) The clinical spectrum of unruptured intracranial aneurysms. *Archives of Neurology* **50**, 265–268.

Raymond, J. & Roy, D. (1997) Safety and efficacy of endovascular treatment of acutely ruptured aneurysms. *Neurosurgery* **41**, 1235–1245.

Raymond, J., Roy, D., Bojanowski, M., Moumdjian, R. & L'Espérance, G. (1997) Endovascular treatment of acutely ruptured and unruptured aneurysms of the basilar bifurcation. *Journal of Neurosurgery* **86**, 211–219.

Rinkel, G.J.E., Wijdicks, E.F.M., Ramos, L.M.P. & van Gijn, J. (1990) Progression of acute hydrocephalus in subarachnoid haemorrhage: a case report documented by serial CT scanning. *Journal of Neurology, Neurosurgery and Psychiatry* **53**, 354–355.

Rinkel, G.J.E., Wijdicks, E.F.M., Vermeulen, M., Hasan, D., Brouwers, P.J.A.M. & van Gijn, J. (1991) The clinical course of perimesencephalic nonaneurysmal subarachnoid hemorrhage. *Annals of Neurology* **29**, 463–468.

Rinkel, G.J.E., Wijdicks, E.F.M., Vermeulen, M., Tans, J.T.J., Hasan, D. & van Gijn, J. (1992) Acute hydrocephalus in nonaneurysmal perimesencephalic hemorrhage: evidence of CSF block at the tentorial hiatus. *Neurology* **42**, 1805–1807.

Rinkel, G.J.E., Djibuti, M., Algra, A. & van Gijn, J. (1998) Prevalence and risk of rupture of intracranial aneurysms: a systematic review. *Stroke* **29**, 251–256.

Rinne, J., Hernesniemi, J., Niskanen, M. & Vapalahti, M. (1996) Analysis of 561 patients with 690 middle cerebral artery aneurysms: anatomic and clinical features as correlated to management outcome. *Neurosurgery* **38**, 2–11.

Ronkainen, A., Hernesniemi, J., Ryynanen, M., Puranen, M. & Kuivaniemi, H. (1994) A ten percent prevalence of asymptomatic familial intracranial aneurysms: preliminary report on 110 magnetic resonance angiography studies in members of 21 Finnish familial intracranial aneurysm families. *Neurosurgery* **35**, 208–212.

Ronkainen, A., Hernesniemi, J., Puranen, M. *et al.* (1997) Familial intracranial aneurysms. *Lancet* **349**, 380–384.

Ronkainen, A., Miettinen, H., Karkola, K. *et al.* (1998) Risk of harboring an unruptured intracranial aneurysm. *Stroke* **29**, 359–362.

Ronkainen, A., Niskanen, M., Piironen, R. & Hernesniemi, J. (1999) Familial subarachnoid hemorrhage: outcome study. *Stroke* **30**, 1099–1102.

Roos, Y.B.W.E.M., Beenen, L.F., Groen, R.J., Albrecht, K.W. & Vermeulen, M. (1997) Timing of surgery in patients with aneurysmal subarachnoid haemorrhage: rebleeding is still the major cause of poor outcome in neurosurgical units that aim at early surgery. *Journal of Neurology, Neurosurgery and Psychiatry* **63**, 490–493.

Roos, Y.B.W.E.M., Rinkel, G.J.E., Vermeulen, M., Algra, A. & van Gijn, J. (2000a) Antifibrinolytic treatment in aneurysmal subarachnoid haemorrhage. *The Cochrane Library Issue* **1**, 2000.

Roos, Y.B.W.E.M., for the STAR Study Group (2000b) Antifibrinolytic treatment in subarachnoid hemorrhage: a randomized placebo-controlled trial. *Neurology* **54**, 77–82.

Rose, F.C. & Sarner, M. (1965) Epilepsy after ruptured intracranial aneurysm. *British Medical Journal* **1**, 18–21.

Rose, G. (1992) *The Strategy of Preventive Medicine*. Oxford Medical Publications, Oxford.

Rosenfeld, J.V., Barnett, G.H., Sila, C.A., Little, J.R., Bravo, E.L. & Beck, G.J. (1989) The effect of subarachnoid hemorrhage on blood and CSF atrial natriuretic factor. *Journal of Neurosurgery* **71**, 32–37.

Rosenorn, J. & Eskesen, V. (1993) Does a safe size-limit exist for unruptured intracranial aneurysms? *Acta Neurochirurgica (Wien)* **121**, 113–118.

Rosenwasser, R.H., Delgado, T.E., Buchheit, W.A. & Freed, M.H. (1983) Control of hypertension and prophylaxis against vasospasm in cases of subarachnoid hemorrhage: a preliminary report. *Neurosurgery* **12**, 658–661.

Rosenwasser, R.H., Jallo, J.I., Getch, C.C. & Liebman, K.E. (1995) Complications of Swan–Ganz catheterization for hemodynamic monitoring in patients with subarachnoid hemorrhage. *Neurosurgery* **37**, 872–875.

Ross, I.B., Warrington, R.J. & Halliday, W.C. (1998) Cell-mediated allergy to a cerebral aneurysm clip: case report. *Neurosurgery* **43**, 1209–1211.

Rousseaux, P., Scherpereel, R., Bernard, M.H., Graftieaux, J.P. & Guyot, J.F. (1980) Fever and cerebral vasospasm in intracranial aneurysms. *Surgical Neurology* **14**, 459–465.

Rowley, G. & Fielding, K. (1991) Reliability and accuracy of the Glasgow Coma Scale with experienced and inexperienced users. *Lancet* **337**, 535–538.

Saito, I., Asano, T., Ochiai, C., Takakura, K., Tamura, A. & Sano, K. (1983) A double-blind clinical evaluation of the effect of nizofenone (Y-9179) on delayed ischemic neurological deficits following aneurysmal rupture. *Neurological Research* **5**, 29–47.

Saito, I., Asano, T., Sano, K. *et al.* (1998) Neuroprotective effect of an antioxidant, ebselen, in patients with delayed neurological deficits after aneurysmal subarachnoid hemorrhage. *Neurosurgery* **42**, 269–277.

Schievink, W.I. (1997) Genetics of intracranial aneurysms. *Neurosurgery* **40**, 651–662.

Schievink, W.I., Wijdicks, E.F.M., Parisi, J.E., Piepgras, D.G. & Whisnant, J.P. (1995) Sudden death from aneurysmal subarachnoid hemorrhage. *Neurology* **45**, 871–874.

Schoser, B.G., Heesen, C., Eckert, B. & Thie, A. (1997) Cerebral hyperperfusion injury after percutaneous transluminal angioplasty of extracranial arteries. *Journal of Neurology* **244**, 101–104.

Sekhon, L.H.S., Morgan, M.K., Sorby, W. & Grinnell, V. (1998) Combined endovascular stent implantation and endosaccular coil placement for the treatment of a wide-necked vertebral artery aneurysm: technical case report. *Neurosurgery* **43**, 380–383.

Shapiro, S. (1996) Management of subarachnoid hemorrhage patients who presented with respiratory arrest resuscitated with bystander CPR. *Stroke* **27**, 1780–1782.

Shaw, M.D., Foy, P.M., Conway, M. *et al.* (1985) Dipyridamole and postoperative ischemic deficits in aneurysmal subarachnoid hemorrhage. *Journal of Neurosurgery* **63**, 699–703.

Shimoda, M., Oda, S., Shibata, M., Tominaga, J., Kittaka, M. & Tsugane, R. (1999) Results of early surgical evacuation of packed intraventricular hemorrhage from aneurysm rupture in patients with poor-grade subarachnoid hemorrhage. *Journal of Neurosurgery* **91**, 408–414.

Sinson, G., Philips, M.F. & Flamm, E.S. (1996) Intraoperative endovascular surgery for cerebral aneurysms. *Journal of Neurosurgery* **84**, 63–70.

Sloan, M.A., Haley, E.C. Jr, Kassell, N.F. *et al.* (1989) Sensitivity and specificity of transcranial Doppler ultrasonography in the diagnosis of vasospasm following subarachnoid hemorrhage. *Neurology* **39**, 1514–1518.

Sloan, M.A., Burch, C.M., Wozniak, M.A. *et al.* (1994) Transcranial Doppler detection of vertebrobasilar vasospasm following subarachnoid hemorrhage. *Stroke* **25**, 2187–2197.

Smith, B. (1963) Cerebral pathology in subarachnoid haemorrhage. *Journal of Neurology, Neurosurgery and Psychiatry* **26**, 67–70.

Smith, R.R., Clower, B.R., Peeler, D.F. Jr & Yoshioka, J. (1983) The angiopathy of subarachnoid hemorrhage: angiographic and morphologic correlates. *Stroke* **14**, 240–245.

Sobey, C.G. & Faraci, F.M. (1998) Subarachnoid haemorrhage: what happens to the cerebral arteries? *Clinical and Experimental Pharmacology and Physiology* **25**, 867–876.

Solander, S., Ulhoa, A., Viñuela, F. *et al.* (1999) Endovascular treatment of multiple intracranial aneurysms by using Guglielmi detachable coils. *Journal of Neurosurgery* **90**, 857–864.

Solenski, N.J., Haley, E.C. Jr, Kassell, N.F., *et al.* (1995) Medical complications of aneurysmal subarachnoid hemorrhage: a report of the Multicenter Cooperative Aneurysm Study. *Critical Care Medicine* **23**, 1007–1017.

Solomon, R.A., Mayer, S.A. & Tarmey, J.J. (1996) Relationship between the volume of craniotomies for cerebral aneurysm performed at New York State hospitals and in-hospital mortality. *Stroke* **27**, 13–17.

Spetzger, U., Reul, J., Thron, A., Warnke, J.P. & Gilsbach, J.M. (1997) Microsurgical embolectomy and removal of a migrated coil from the middle cerebral artery. *Cerebrovascular Diseases* 7, 226–231.

Stachniak, J.B., Layon, A.J., Day, A.L. & Gallagher, T.J. (1996) Craniotomy for intracranial aneurysm and subarachnoid hemorrhage: is course, cost, or outcome affected by age? *Stroke* 27, 276–281.

Sterns, R.H., Riggs, J.E. & Schochet, S.S. Jr (1986) Osmotic demyelination syndrome following correction of hyponatremia. *New England Journal of Medicine* **314**, 1535–1542.

Stiver, S.I., Porter, P.J., Willinsky, R.A. & Wallace, C. (1998) Acute human histopathology of an intracranial aneurysm treated using Guglielmi detachable coils: case report and review of the literature. *Neurosurgery* **43**, 1203–1207.

Stober, T., Anstatt, T., Sen, S., Schimrigk, K. & Jager, H. (1988) Cardiac arrhythmias in subarachnoid haemorrhage. *Acta Neurochirurgica (Wien)* **93**, 37–44.

Suzuki, S., Sano, K., Handa, H. *et al.* (1989) Clinical study of OKY-046, a thromboxane synthetase inhibitor, in prevention of cerebral vasospasms and delayed cerebral ischaemic symptoms after subarachnoid haemorrhage due to aneurysmal rupture: a randomized double-blind study. *Neurological Research* **11**, 79–88.

Svensson, E., Starmark, J.E., Ekholm, S., Von Essen, C. & Johansson, A. (1996) Analysis of interobserver disagreement in the assessment of subarachnoid blood and acute hydrocephalus on CT scans. *Neurological Research* **18**, 487–494.

Svigelj, V., Grad, A., Tekavcic, I. & Kiauta, T. (1994) Cardiac arrhythmia associated with reversible damage to insula in a patient with subarachnoid hemorrhage. *Stroke* **25**, 1053–1055.

Swash, M. (1974) Periaqueductal dysfunction (the Sylvian aqueduct syndrome): a sign of hydrocephalus? *Journal of Neurology, Neurosurgery and Psychiatry* **37**, 21–26.

Takagi, K., Tamura, A., Nakagomi, T. *et al.* (1999) How should a subarachnoid hemorrhage grading scale be determined? A combinatorial approach based solely on the Glasgow Coma Scale. *Journal of Neurosurgery* **90**, 680–687.

Tapaninaho, A., Hernesniemi, J., Vapalahti, M. *et al.* (1993) Shunt-dependent hydrocephalus after subarachnoid haemorrhage and aneurysm surgery: timing of surgery is not a risk factor. *Acta Neurochirurgica (Wien)* **123**, 118–124.

Teasdale, G. & Jennett, B. (1974) Assessment of coma and impaired consciousness: a practical scale. *Lancet* **ii**, 81–84.

Theodore, J. & Robin, E.D. (1976) Speculations on neurogenic pulmonary edema (NPE). *American Review of Respiratory Disease* **113**, 405–411.

Thielen, K.R., Nichols, D.A., Fulgham, J.R. & Piepgras, D.G. (1997) Endovascular treatment of cerebral aneurysms following incomplete clipping. *Journal of Neurosurgery* **87**, 184–189.

Tokiyoshi, K., Ohnishi, T. & Nii, Y. (1991) Efficacy and toxicity of thromboxane synthetase inhibitor for cerebral vasospasm after subarachnoid hemorrhage. *Surgical Neurology* **36**, 112–118.

Tomasello, F., D'Avella, D. & De Divitiis, O. (1999) Does lamina terminalis fenestration reduce the incidence of chronic hydrocephalus after subarachnoid hemorrhage? *Neurosurgery* **45**, 827–831.

Tomida, M., Muraki, M., Uemura, K. & Yamasaki, K. (1998) Plasma concentrations of brain natriuretic peptide in patients with subarachnoid hemorrhage. *Stroke* **29**, 1584–1587.

Torner, J.C., Kassell, N.F., Wallace, R.B. & Adams, H.P. Jr (1981a) Preoperative prognostic factors for rebleeding and survival in aneurysm patients receiving antifibrinolytic therapy: report of the Cooperative Aneurysm Study. *Neurosurgery* **9**, 506–513.

Torner, J.C., Nibbelink, D.W. & Burmeister, L.F. (1981b) Statistical comparisons of end results of a randomised treatment study. In: *Aneurysmal Subarachnoid Hemorrhage. Report of the Cooperative Study* (eds A.L. Sahs, D.W. Nibbelink & J.C. Torner), pp. 249–275. Urban & Schwarzenberg, Baltimore.

Toyota, B.D. (1999) The efficacy of an abbreviated course of nimodipine in patients with good-grade aneurysmal subarachnoid hemorrhage. *Journal of Neurosurgery* **90**, 203–206.

Tsutsumi, K., Ueki, K., Usui, M., Kwak, S. & Kirino, T. (1998) Risk of recurrent subarachnoid hemorrhage after complete obliteration of cerebral aneurysms. *Stroke* **29**, 2511–2513.

Tulleken, C.A.F. & Verdaasdonk, R.M. (1995) First clinical experience with Excimer assisted high flow bypass surgery of the brain. *Acta Neurochirurgica (Wien)* **134**, 66–70.

Tulleken, C.A.F., van der Zwan, A., Van Rooij, W.J. & Ramos, L.M.P. (1998) High-flow bypass using nonocclusive excimer laser-assisted end-to-side anastomosis of the external carotid artery to the P_1 segment of the posterior cerebral artery via the sylvian route: technical note. *Journal of Neurosurgery* **88**, 925–927.

Vale, F.L., Bradley, E.L. & Fisher, W.S. III (1997) The relationship of subarachnoid hemorrhage and the need for postoperative shunting. *Journal of Neurosurgery* **86**, 462–466.

Vanninen, R., Koivisto, T., Saari, T., Hernesniemi, J. & Vapalahti, M. (1999) Ruptured intracranial aneurysms—acute endovascular treatment with electrolytically detachable coils: a prospective randomized study. *Radiology* **211**, 325–336.

Vermeij, F.H., Hasan, D., Vermeulen, M., Tanghe, H.L. & van Gijn, J. (1994) Predictive factors for deterioration from hydrocephalus after subarachnoid hemorrhage. *Neurology* **44**, 1851–1855.

Vermeij, F.H., Hasan, D., Bijvoet, H.W.C. & Avezaat, C.J.J. (1998) Impact of medical treatment on the outcome of patients after aneurysmal subarachnoid hemorrhage. *Stroke* **29**, 924–930.

Vermeulen, M., van Gijn, J. & Blijenberg, B.G. (1983) Spectrophotometric analysis of CSF after subarachnoid hemorrhage: limitations in the diagnosis of rebleeding. *Neurology* **33**, 112–115.

Vermeulen, M., Lindsay, K.W., Murray, G.D. *et al.* (1984a) Antifibrinolytic treatment in subarachnoid hemorrhage. *New England Journal of Medicine* **311**, 432–437.

Vermeulen, M., van Gijn, J., Hijdra, A. & van Crevel, H. (1984b) Causes of acute deterioration in patients with a ruptured intracranial aneurysm: a prospective study with serial CT scanning. *Journal of Neurosurgery* **60**, 935–939.

Vinge, E., Brandt, L., Ljunggren, B. & Andersson, K.E. (1988) Thromboxane B_2 levels in serum during continuous administration of nimodipine to patients with aneurysmal subarachnoid hemorrhage. *Stroke* **19**, 644–647.

Vora, Y.Y., Suarez-Almazor, M., Steinke, D.E., Martin, M.L. & Findlay, J.M. (1999) Role of transcranial Doppler monitoring in the diagnosis of cerebral vasospasm after subarachnoid hemorrhage. *Neurosurgery* **44**, 1237–1247.

Wang, P.S., Longstreth, W.T. Jr & Koepsell, T.D. (1995) Subarachnoid hemorrhage and family history: a population-based case-control study. *Archives of Neurology* **52**, 202–204.

Wauchob, T.D., Brooks, R.J. & Harrison, K.M. (1984) Neurogenic pulmonary oedema. *Anaesthesia* **39**, 529–534.

Weingeist, T.A., Goldman, E.J., Folk, J.C., Packer, A.J. & Ossoinig, K.C. (1986) Terson's syndrome: clinicopathologic correlations. *Ophthalmology* **93**, 1435–1442.

Weir, B.K. (1978) Pulmonary edema following fatal aneurysm rupture. *Journal of Neurosurgery* **49**, 502–507.

Weir, B., Grace, M., Hansen, J. & Rothberg, C. (1978) Time course of vasospasm in man. *Journal of Neurosurgery* **48**, 173–178.

Wells, P.S., Lensing, A.W.A. & Hirsh, J. (1994) Graduated compression stockings in the prevention of postoperative venous thromboembolism: a meta-analysis. *Archives of Internal Medicine* **154**, 67–72.

Whitfield, P.C., Moss, H., O'Hare, D., Smielewski, P., Pickard, J.D. & Kirkpatrick, P.J. (1996) An audit of aneurysmal subarachnoid haemorrhage: earlier resuscitation and surgery reduces inpatient stay and deaths from rebleeding. *Journal of Neurology, Neurosurgery and Psychiatry* **60**, 301–306.

Wiebers, D.O., Torner, J.C. & Meissner, I. (1992) Impact of unruptured intracranial aneurysms on public health in the United States. *Stroke* **23**, 1416–1419.

Wiebers, D., Whisnant, J., Forbes, G. *et al.* (1998) Unruptured intracranial aneurysms: risk of rupture and risks of surgical intervention. *New England Journal of Medicine* **339**, 1725–1733.

Wijdicks, E.F.M. (1995) Worst-case scenario: management in poor-grade aneurysmal subarachnoid hemorrhage. *Cerebrovascular Diseases* **5**, 163–169.

Wijdicks, E.F.M., Vermeulen, M., ten Haaf, J.A., Hijdra, A., Bakker, W.H. & van Gijn, J. (1985a) Volume depletion and natriuresis in patients with a ruptured intracranial aneurysm. *Annals of Neurology* **18**, 211–216.

Wijdicks, E.F.M., Vermeulen, M., Hijdra, A. & van Gijn, J. (1985b) Hyponatremia and cerebral infarction in patients with ruptured intracranial aneurysms: is fluid restriction harmful? *Annals of Neurology* **17**, 137–140.

Wijdicks, E.F.M., Vermeulen, M., van Brummelen, P., den Boer, N.C. & van Gijn, J. (1987) Digoxin-like immunoreactive substance in patients with aneurysmal subarachnoid haemorrhage. *British Medical Journal* **294**, 729–732.

Wijdicks, E.F.M., Vermeulen, M., van Brummelen, P. & van Gijn, J. (1988a) The effect of fludrocortisone acetate on plasma Volume and natriuresis in patients with aneurysmal subarachnoid hemorrhage. *Clinical Neurology and Neurosurgery* **90**, 209–214.

Wijdicks, E.F.M., van Dongen, K.J., van Gijn, J., Hijdra, A. & Vermeulen, M. (1988b) Enlargement of the third ventricle and hyponatraemia in aneurysmal subarachnoid haemorrhage. *Journal of Neurology, Neurosurgery and Psychiatry* **51**, 516–520.

Wijdicks, E.F.M., Hasan, D., Lindsay, K.W. *et al.* (1989) Short-term tranexamic acid treatment in aneurysmal subarachnoid hemorrhage. *Stroke* **20**, 1674–1679.

Wijdicks, E.F.M., Vermeulen, M., Murray, G.D., Hijdra, A. & van Gijn, J. (1990) The effects of treating hypertension following aneurysmal subarachnoid hemorrhage. *Clinical Neurology and Neurosurgery* **92**, 111–117.

Wijdicks, E.F.M., Ropper, A.H., Hunnicutt, E.J., Richardson, G.S. & Nathanson, J.A. (1991) Atrial natriuretic factor and salt wasting after aneurysmal subarachnoid hemorrhage. *Stroke* **22**, 1519–1524.

Wijdicks, E.F.M., Schievink, W.I. & Burnett, J.C. Jr (1997) Natriuretic peptide system and endothelin in aneurysmal subarachnoid hemorrhage. *Journal of Neurosurgery* **87**, 275–280.

Wijdicks, E.F.M., Kokmen, E. & O'Brien, P.C. (1998) Measurement of impaired consciousness in the neurological intensive care unit: a new test. *Journal of Neurology, Neurosurgery and Psychiatry* **64**, 117–119.

Winn, H.R., Richardson, A.E. & Jane, J.A. (1977) The long-term prognosis in untreated cerebral aneurysms, 1: the incidence of late hemorrhage in cerebral aneurysm: a 10-year evaluation of 364 patients. *Annals of Neurology* **1**, 358–370.

Wohns, R.N., Tamas, L., Pierce, K.R. & Howe, J.F. (1985) Chlorpromazine treatment for neurogenic pulmonary edema. *Critical Care Medicine* **13**, 210–211.

Yamaura, I., Tani, E., Yokota, M. *et al.* (1999) Endovascular treatment of ruptured dissecting aneurysms aimed at occlusion of the dissected site by using Guglielmi detachable coils. *Journal of Neurosurgery* **90**, 853–856.

Yoshimoto, Y. & Wakai, S. (1999) Cost-effectiveness analysis of screening for asymptomatic, unruptured intracranial aneurysms: a mathematical model. *Stroke* 30, 1621–1627.

CHAPTER FOURTEEN

Specific treatment of intracranial vascular malformations

14.1 Introduction

This chapter will deal mostly with arteriovenous malformations (AVMs) in the strict sense of the term, and only briefly with cavernous angiomas and dural arteriovenous fistulae. Venous angiomas and telangiectasias rarely, if ever, require any therapeutic intervention (sections 8.2.6 and 8.2.7). A general point to be made about the management of AVMs in the brain is that there is no hurry. Even if the malformation has presented with haemorrhage, the risk of early re-bleeding is low. It is extremely unusual for recurrent haemorrhage to supervene whilst the attendant physicians and surgeons are still in the process of balancing the risks and benefits of the various treatment options.

Recurrent haemorrhage from arteriovenous malformations may occur, but the interval is commonly counted in months or years, not in days or weeks as with ruptured aneurysms. This leaves time for ample consultation between neurologists, neurosurgeons and neuroradiologists on whether intervention is feasible and desirable.

The delay is necessary not just for thinking. If a haemorrhage has been the presenting feature and has resulted in neurological deficits, one needs to take the degree of recovery into consideration; at the very least, a few weeks are required for the eventual disability to be estimated with any confidence. These considerations also imply that if a first angiogram has not shown the expected AVM, it is safe to wait 4–6 weeks before repeating the study, in case the AVM has been compressed by the mass effect of the haematoma (Willinsky *et al.* 1993; Halpin *et al.* 1994; Hino *et al.* 1998).

14.1.1 Heterogeneity of arteriovenous malformations

An important point is that no two patients with arteriovenous malformations are alike or have the same prognosis, which makes it difficult to outline a general management strategy—much more so than for ruptured aneurysms at the base of the brain, for example. First of all, the clinical manifestations are diverse: not only haemorrhage or epilepsy, but also progressive neurological deterioration, benign intracranial hypertension and migrainous headaches, to name the most common presentations (section 14.1.2). The most important determinants of the therapeutic management are the size and location of the malformation, along with the type of venous drainage. For example, a small and superficial AVM in one occipital lobe is much more easily accessible to surgical treatment than an anomaly involving almost an entire hemisphere, with feeders from all major arteries and with extensive drainage into the deep venous system. For these reasons, Spetzler and Martin (1986) have proposed a grading system for AVMs that takes account of these three key features. This grading bears mainly on the feasibility of surgical treatment, and not so much on the risk of haemorrhage (Figs 14.1–14.3) (Table 14.1). Of course, it is more useful to describe the three features separately than to rely on the sum score alone; in the process of summation important information gets lost.

A cautionary note is appropriate about the dangers of making too facile a distinction between 'eloquent' and so-called 'silent' areas of the brain. Operating in specialized areas of the cerebral cortex may result in easily recognizable deficits such as hemiparesis, aphasia or a visual field defect, but this does not imply that less specialized areas of the brain are functionally unimportant. Surgical excision of, say, the right temporal lobe will not result in impairments that are obvious when the patient is making a brief visit to a hospital clinic. But a conversation with the patient's life partner will drastically cure any previous belief on the part of the surgeon that 'silent' areas of the brain can be excised without any consequences for the patient's mood or personality. To illustrate this point with a comparison: if the function of the intact brain is symbolized by a beautiful painting, lesions in

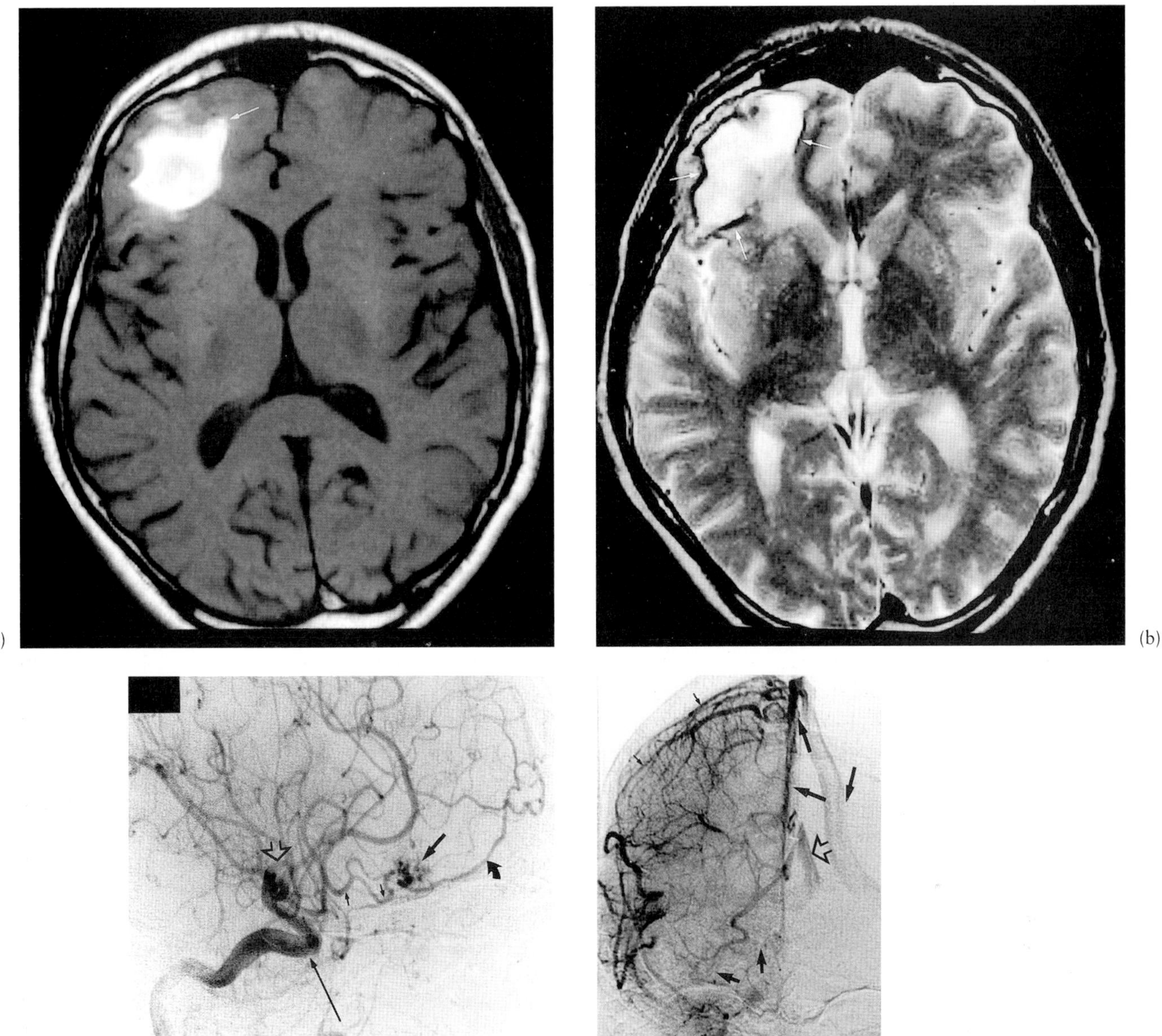

Fig. 14.1 Small arteriovenous malformation (AVM) (<3 cm), in a 59-year-old man. (a) T1-weighted axial magnetic resonance (MR) scan showing a haematoma in the right frontal lobe (arrow). (b) T2-weighted MR scan, showing a rim of haemosiderin (low signal) around the haematoma (arrow). (c) Right carotid angiogram, arterial phase, oblique lateral view: small AVM in frontal lobe (thick solid arrow), fed by a branch of the anterior cerebral artery (short thin arrows). An early draining vein is visible (curved arrow). The middle cerebral artery (viewed mainly end on because of the projection – open arrow) and internal carotid artery (long thin arrow) are also seen. (d) Right carotid angiogram, venous phase, antero-posterior view: drainage via veins on the cortical surface (short arrows). Note the veins draining the AVM (short thick arrows) have virtually emptied as they fill earlier than the normal cortical veins (short thin arrows). The superior sagittal sinus (thick solid arrows), straight sinus (open arrow) and normal cortical veins (short thin arrows) are also shown.

'eloquent' brain areas can be compared with holes or blots in the picture, whereas lesions in 'silent' areas correspond with darkening of the varnish and fading of the colours. The fallacy of the notion that some areas of the brain are unimportant is perpetuated by the preoperative application of 'functional' imaging techniques, such as functional magnetic resonance imaging (MRI) (Latchaw *et al.* 1995; Maldjian *et al.* 1996; Schlosser *et al.* 1997) or positron emission tomography (Leblanc *et al.* 1995). Only elementary functions show up on such studies, whereas complex mental processes—no less important—are diluted through the interaction between different parts of the brain. Attempts to

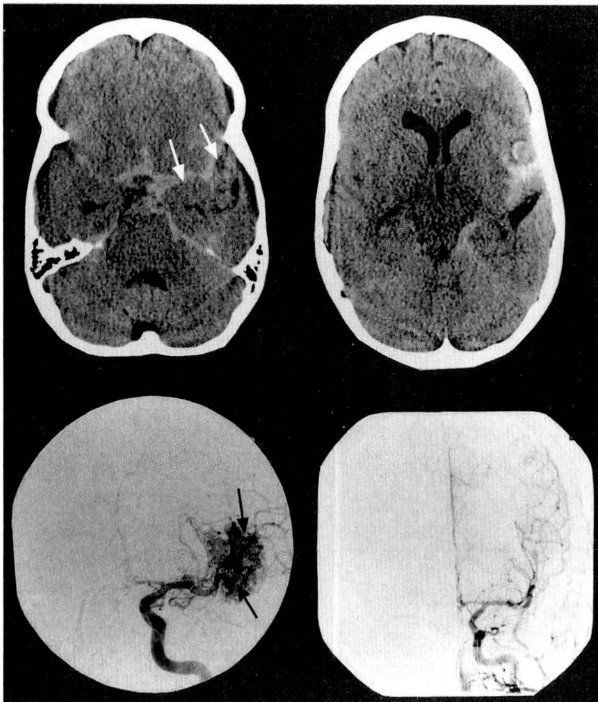

Fig. 14.2 Medium-sized arteriovenous malformation (AVM) (3–6 cm), in a 31-year-old woman. Top: CT brain scan, showing subarachnoid haemorrhage, predominantly in the left Sylvian fissure (arrows). Bottom, left: left carotid angiogram, antero-posterior view, shows AVM in the left temporal lobe (arrows) supplied by branches of the left middle cerebral artery. Bottom, right: repeat angiogram after excision of the AVM.

distinguish 'highly eloquent' and 'less eloquent' areas suffer from the same overemphasis of single brain functions over general functions (Schaller *et al.* 1998).

> *The term 'silent area of the brain' should be interpreted as an area with a general rather than a specific function (such as language or movements), not as an area that is redundant.*

14.1.2 Clinical presentations other than haemorrhage

Intracranial haemorrhage is the initial manifestation of arteriovenous malformations (AVMs) in at least 50% of cases, although the exact proportion depends to some extent on whether the series has been collected in a neurological or neurosurgical centre (Lobato *et al.* 1992; Brown *et al.* 1996; Kupersmith *et al.* 1996). The other clinical features are similar in children and adults, except that in neonates high-volume intracranial shunts may cause congestive heart failure or hydrocephalus (Hayashi *et al.* 1996; Kelly *et al.* 1978).

> *Clinical presentations of arteriovenous malformations are haemorrhage (50%), epilepsy (35%), progressive ischaemia (10%), benign intracranial hypertension, migrainous headaches, and cranial nerve dysfunction (all rare).*

Epilepsy, usually with partial seizures, is the initial manifestation in about one-third of cases, and progressive neurological deterioration in about 10%. Insidiously developing neurological deficits can be focal or more general, in the form of problems with memory or cognition (Jaillard *et al.* 1999); in both cases, the explanation is that shunting through a low-resistance AVM results in underperfusion of the surrounding normal brain tissue, a phenomenon known as vascular 'steal' (Brown *et al.* 1988; Leblanc & Little 1990; Sheth & Bodensteiner 1995). An argument against this explanation may be that in patients with an AVM and focal deficits, the blood flow velocity in feeding arteries, as measured with transcranial Doppler techniques, is no higher than in other patients with AVMs (Mast *et al.* 1995). The pathophysiological events resulting from AVMs must be more complex than can be explained by blood velocity alone. The syndrome of benign intracranial hypertension, with headache or visual symptoms, may result if the malformation drains into the superior sagittal sinus, which leads to increased cerebro-

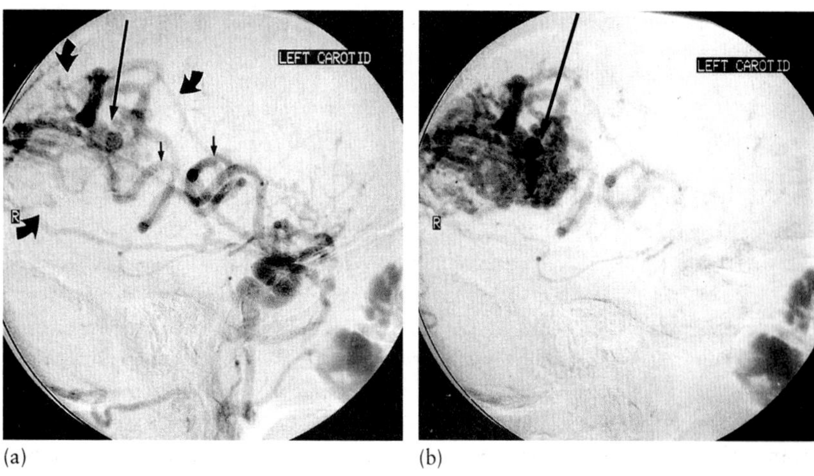

Fig. 14.3 (a) Cerebral angiogram (left common carotid injection, lateral projection) of a large parieto-occipital arteriovenous malformation (AVM) (> 6 cm), fed by dilated branches of the middle cerebral artery (short arrows). The nidus is beginning to fill (long arrow). The full extent is indicated by the curved arrows. (b) Film from later in the sequence showing the nidus more clearly.

Table 14.1 Grading system for arteriovenous malformations, according to Spetzler and Martin (1986)

Graded feature	Points assigned
Size of arteriovenous malformation	
Small (< 3 cm)	1
Medium (3–6 cm)	2
Large (> 6 cm)	3
Location	
Non-eloquent area	0
Eloquent area	1
Pattern of venous drainage	
Superficial only	0
Deep (any part)	1

Grade = [size] + [eloquence] + [venous drainage], i.e. [1, 2 or 3] = [0 or 1] + [0 or 1].

spinal fluid pressure (Chimowitz *et al.* 1990; Verm & Lee 1997).

Migrainous headaches may, in a tiny minority of migraineurs, be associated with AVMs in the occipital region (Bruyn 1984; Haas 1991). There is little to distinguish these patients from ordinary migraineurs except the hemianopic deficit is always on the same side, and the hemianopia may follow rather than precede the headache. However, in view of the dilemmas with regard to invasive treatment of AVMs, it is far from certain that a patient with migraine benefits from the knowledge that there is an underlying AVM. Another disadvantage of ordering imaging studies in all migraineurs with stereotyped attacks is the cost, discomfort and risk of the negative investigations in the vast majority.

An exceptional manifestation of AVMs is cranial nerve dysfunction, such as hemifacial spasm, through pressure by a dilated draining vein (Konan *et al.* 1999); trigeminal neuralgia has occurred in this way after partial embolization of an AVM (Mineura *et al.* 1998).

14.1.3 Can the natural history be improved upon?

Even if the presentation and the future risks of patients with AVMs were less heterogeneous, balancing the pros and cons of the available treatment options would be difficult, for several reasons. Occasionally, AVMs may even disappear spontaneously (Fig. 14.4).

Firstly, the natural history of AVMs in general is known only vaguely, because most series have been retrospectively collected, usually with a limited period of follow-up, and because easily operable lesions are almost never included, causing a bias towards AVMs that are large, deep, or located in 'eloquent' areas of the brain. Notwithstanding these shortcomings, a reasonable overall estimate is an annual risk of bleeding of 2–4% (Jane *et al.* 1985; Aminoff 1987; Heros & Tu 1987; Brown *et al.* 1988; Ondra *et al.* 1990). Depending on the characteristics of the AVM, however, the annual risk can be as low as 1%, or as high as 18% (Pollock *et al.* 1996a; Mast *et al.* 1997). Several studies have addressed the difference between baseline characteristics of AVMs presenting with haemorrhage and AVMs with other clinical manifestations (mainly epilepsy), and a single study prospectively followed two such groups for an average period of 10 months (Mast *et al.* 1997). Risk factors for haemorrhage identified by more than one study, and therefore not likely to represent a chance finding, are:

- history of a previous haemorrhage (Pollock *et al.* 1996a; Mast *et al.* 1997);
- deep venous drainage (Miyasaka *et al.* 1992; Turjman *et al.* 1995; Mast *et al.* 1997; Duong *et al.* 1998; Langer *et al.* 1998);
- the presence of a single draining vein (Miyasaka *et al.* 1992; Pollock *et al.* 1996a);
- the presence of intranidal aneurysms (Brown *et al.* 1988; Turjman *et al.* 1995; Redekop *et al.* 1998).

Such associated aneurysms may also bleed during or after treatment of the AVM (Thompson *et al.* 1998). Patient characteristics such as age, sex, or a history of hypertension have not been consistently identified as determinants of the risk of rupture. Spontaneous obliteration of AVMs does occur, but is a rare phenomenon (Wakai *et al.* 1983; Ezura & Kagawa 1992; Guazzo & Xuereb 1994; Abdulrauf *et al.* 1999) (Fig. 14.4).

The case fatality for a first bleed is around 10%, ranging between 0% and 25% in different studies (Iansek *et al.* 1983; Brown *et al.* 1988; Ondra *et al.* 1990; Neil-Dwyer & Lang 1997; Hartmann *et al.* 1998). This proportion is much lower than for ruptured aneurysms, in which approximately 50% of first episodes are fatal in hospital series (section 13.2.3).

The average risk of haemorrhage from an arteriovenous malformation is 2–4% per annum. Unfavourable factors (with higher risk) are a previous haemorrhage, an associated saccular aneurysm, and venous drainage via the deep venous system or via a single vein.

A second problem is that the benefits and risks of any treatment can only be measured over many years, particularly if the lesion has not been completely obliterated and if the unwanted effects of treatment do not emerge until years later, as with radiosurgery. Nevertheless, decision analyses have been attempted, especially with a view to surgical treatment (Iansek *et al.* 1983; Aminoff 1987). A third factor that is difficult to quantify in decision analyses is the patient's psychological attitude to living with an unoperated lesion in the brain that may unexpectedly bleed. Some patients show

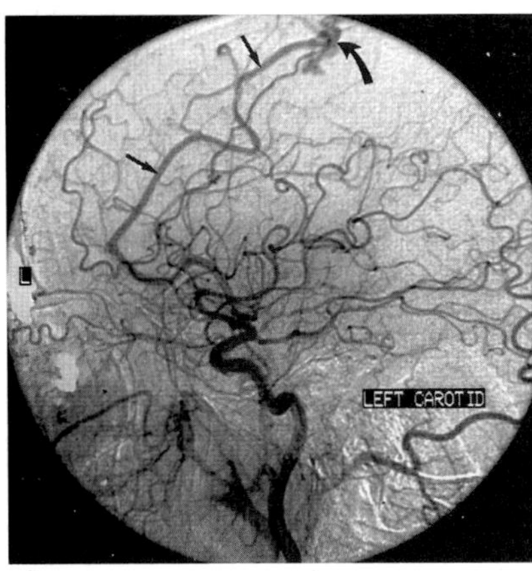

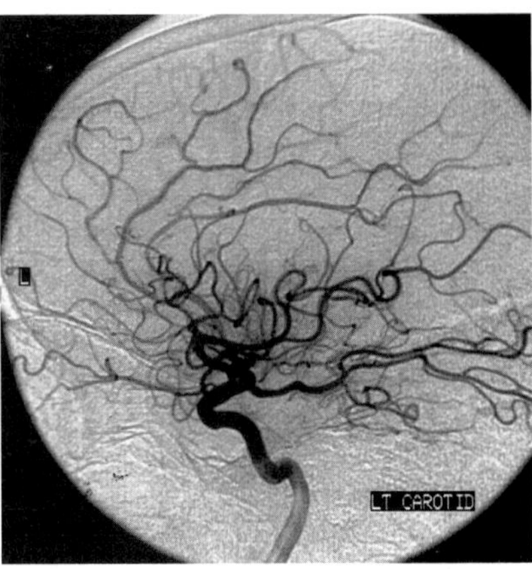

Fig. 14.4 A 51-year-old man presented with epilepsy. His cerebral angiogram (left-hand panel) revealed a small left parasagittal arteriovenous malformation (AVM) (curved arrows) fed by a single, dilated callosomarginal branch (straight arrow) of the left anterior cerebral artery, and draining into a dilated vein. Two months later, at attempted glue embolization, the AVM had vanished (right-hand panel).

admirable sang-froid in coping with this knowledge, but in other cases the patient's life may turn out to be so dominated by the perceived danger that he or she insists on intervention even when the balance of risks would seem to argue against such a course of action. Finally, the balance between benefits and risks for any form of treatment (surgical excision, endovascular embolization, or radiosurgery) has never been assessed in randomized controlled trials. Despite the heterogeneity of lesions, such trials, necessarily in the form of a multicentre effort, are the only possible way of therapeutic advancement in this area, unless in the improbable circumstance that some form of intervention is completely harmless.

Randomized controlled trials of treatment in patients with arteriovenous malformations are difficult because the lesions are rare and heterogeneous—but this does not absolve the neurological and neurosurgical community from the moral obligation to start organizing them.

The available options for treatment are: medical management; surgical excision; endovascular embolization; radiosurgery; and some combination of these treatment modalities.

14.2 Medical management

In any patients with an arteriovenous malformation (AVM), antithrombotic drugs should probably be avoided, including aspirin and other non-steroidal anti-inflammatory drugs that interfere with cyclo-oxygenase and thereby with platelet aggregation. Hypertension, if present, should be controlled. In patients with symptomatic epilepsy, anticonvulsants are usually indicated. At present there is no evidence in favour of anticonvulsant treatment in patients with AVMs who have never had seizures, even in those with neurological sequelae after a haemorrhage.

Pregnant patients with unoperated AVMs should be managed in the same way as other patients, at least until childbirth (Horton *et al.* 1990; Finnerty *et al.* 1999). It is controversial whether any anticonvulsant medication should be changed to a supposedly 'safe' drug such as carbamazepine, firstly because there are no adequately controlled studies, and secondly because organogenesis is often completed by the time a woman discovers she is pregnant (Donaldson 1989). During delivery, the risk of rupture with bearing down and its attendant overshoots of arterial blood pressure is generally thought to be high enough to justify an elective Caesarean section at 38 weeks' gestation (Donaldson 1989). Again, we should emphasize that such actions are based not on controlled trials but on 'clinical intuition', with all its pitfalls. In fact, evidence from observational studies does not suggest any difference in outcome for mother or child between vaginal delivery and Caesarean section (Dias & Sekhar 1990).

14.3 Surgical excision

Excision of an arteriovenous malformation (AVM) is the most definitive treatment, and therefore this approach is preferred if the operation is technically feasible and if the risks of neurological sequelae seem acceptable. Deep-seated lesions in the thalamus or basal ganglia can also be resected, but with higher risk (Tew *et al.* 1995). Ligation of feeding arteries alone is now considered out of date, because invariably new feeding vessels will emerge, being subject to the draining forces resulting from the low resistance of dilated veins that can be accessed without a capillary network; in the few cases in which this does not occur, the brain tissue in the involved area may become irreversibly ischaemic.

Details of operative technique can be found elsewhere (Stein *et al.* 1998). Here, only the general principles will be outlined. A superselective catheter angiogram is essential for accurate localization during the operation—particularly of the superficial veins, which can usually be recognized on the angiogram by their shape. From here, the feeding arteries at the margin of the malformation are uncovered by microdissection, although these are often hidden in the depths of the sulci. Often, there is a well-defined layer of glial tissue between the AVM and normal brain, in which plane the dissection can be found. Small arteries are occluded by cautery, bipolar cautery having the great advantage that the vessel does not stick to the forceps, with the danger of bleeding when the forceps are retracted. Metallic clips are used for larger feeding arteries, but care is necessary to ensure feeders supplying both brain tissue and the AVM are left alone, and that only the branches to the malformation itself are ligated. In this fashion, surgeons slowly work their way around the malformation, a meticulous process that takes hours and sometimes even the greater part of a day. During this process, it is often possible to decrease the size of draining veins by gentle cauterization. The deepest part of the AVM is often found near the ventricular system, with numerous small arteries that are frequently related to the anterior or posterior choroidal arteries, or both, and that have subependymal draining veins. Some surgeons prefer to use hypotension in this phase of the operation. One large draining vein, superficial or deep, should be left intact until the very end of the procedure, to prevent congestion in neighbouring brain structures. The probability of complete removal may be increased by intraoperative angiography or computer-assisted image guidance (Munshi *et al.* 1999; Pelak *et al.* 1999).

After the operation, close monitoring is needed for the first 24 h, in view of the danger of haemorrhage or brain swelling. These complications are most common in AVMs 4 cm or more in diameter (Morgan *et al.* 1999), particularly if preoperative single photon emission computed tomography scanning has shown hypoperfusion of the parenchyma distal to the AVM nidus, and in AVMs arising directly off proximal cerebral arteries or, conversely, in a distal or border-zone location (Awad *et al.* 1994; Kato *et al.* 1997). Haemorrhages within days of surgical treatment may arise not only in the field of operation, e.g. from small remaining portions of the AVM, but also from small vessels at some distance from the lesion; in either case, the vascular bed cannot withstand the pressure of the large volume of blood that has been redirected—the so-called 'breakthrough' phenomenon (Spetzler *et al.* 1978; Young *et al.* 1996). Brain swelling may also result from a redistribution of blood flow, or more specifically from occlusion of venous outflow (al Rodhan *et al.* 1993).

Ischaemic deficits after surgical treatment of AVMs are especially likely if the arterial supply is through the lenticulostriate vessels (Morgan *et al.* 1997). Clinical improvement is still possible in the long term, by adaptive phenomena or because not all the damage to neurones has been irreversible (Heros *et al.* 1990). Even in carefully selected patients, the overall rate of serious permanent morbidity is about 8% (Heros *et al.* 1990).

The risk of postoperative seizures can perhaps be decreased by prophylactic anticonvulsants if the patient is not already receiving them; the benefits are estimated to exceed the risks, although no evidence from randomized controlled trials is available; but at any rate the drugs should be slowly withdrawn after a few months if no fits have occurred.

Recurrent haemorrhage may occur even after apparently complete resection of an AVM (Gabriel *et al.* 1996; Kader *et al.* 1996; Pellettieri *et al.* 1997). A possible explanation is regrowth of abnormal vessels through the action of angiogenetic factors, especially in children (Kader *et al.* 1996); others postulate the existence of 'hidden compartments'—portions of the malformation that were already there but only filled with blood after resection of the main part (Pellettieri *et al.* 1997).

In patients with small AVMs for which radiosurgical treatment is also possible, analysis of the balance of risks seems to favour resection as the most efficacious procedure in most cases, and also as the most cost-effective (Porter *et al.* 1997; Schaller & Schramm 1997; Giller *et al.* 1998; Chang & Nihei 1999).

14.4 Endovascular embolization

The development of microcatheters has allowed the delivery of foreign material into arteriovenous malformations (AVMs), with the aim of occluding the anomalous vessels and thereby reducing the risk of subsequent haemorrhage and other complications (Luessenhop & Presper 1984). The substances that were used initially consisted of particulate matter, such as ceramic pellets, silastic pellets, gelfoam and isopropyl alcohol fragments. At present, rapidly polymerizing liquid glues are often preferred, such as bucrylate (Vinuela *et al.* 1983) or cellulose acetate polymer (Tokunaga *et al.* 1999). With time, it has become clear that total obliteration of the AVM by means of embolization can be achieved in only 5% (Frizzel & Fisher 1995). In many centres, the procedure is therefore used mainly as an adjunct to operation or radiosurgery, especially with deep AVMs; preoperative embolization can often successfully decrease the size of the malformation to such a degree that subsequent intervention is probably safer and more complete than it would have been otherwise (Stein & Wolpert 1980; Luessenhop & Rosa 1984; Fournier *et al.* 1991; Deruty *et al.* 1995; Lawton *et al.* 1995; Wallace *et al.* 1995; Lundqvist *et al.* 1996; Debrun *et al.* 1997). Not only are the technical difficulties of the operation reduced, but also the postoperative haemodynamic consequences are more gradual, which decreases the risk of the breakthrough phenomenon mentioned above. The annual risk of haemorrhage in partially occluded AVMs does not seem unexpectedly high, at 3% per annum in a single series (Gobin *et al.* 1996). Some surgeons inject embolic material into cannulated blood vessels at the time of operation, but the course of the material is more difficult to control under these circumstances than when the vascular bed downstream from the catheter can be visualized with soluble contrast (Deruty *et al.* 1985).

Complications of endovascular embolization in the immediate phase include:

• cerebral infarction by inadvertent obliteration of an artery to normal brain;
• haemorrhage associated with manipulation of the catheter, or with distension of the microballoon—but this is a rare phenomenon even before injection of embolic material;
• haemorrhage as a result of haemodynamic changes due to vessel occlusion, leading to rupture of a feeding artery, a draining vein, or dilated capillaries (Kvam *et al.* 1980; Luessenhop & Presper 1984; Vinuela *et al.* 1986); and
• pulmonary infarction after passage of the embolic material through the malformation.

Rarely, delayed haemorrhage occurs, which may be explained by toxic effects of bucrylate on the vessel wall, with angionecrosis and extravasation of bucrylate (Deruty *et al.* 1985; Vinters *et al.* 1986). Although serious complications of embolization are few and far between in the series reported by the world experts cited above, these results cannot necessarily be generalized. In a series of 53 consecutive patients treated in the 1980s in the Netherlands by a dedicated neuroradiologist to whom patients were referred from all over the country, five patients died and 17 had permanent deficits, four of whom were no longer able to lead an independent life (Tjan & de Jonge, unpublished observations). Techniques to make the procedure more efficient as well as safe include intra-arterial blood pressure monitoring (Sorimachi *et al.* 1995), transvenous pressure monitoring (Murayama *et al.* 1996), estimation of flow patterns by means of non-soluble contrast material (Wakhloo *et al.* 1998) or colour-coded transcranial ultrasound (Klötzsch *et al.* 1995), and induction of temporary asystole and hypotension by an intravenous bolus of adenosine (Pile-Spellman *et al.* 1999).

14.5 Radiosurgery

Focused radiation is an increasingly important option in the management of arteriovenous malformations (AVMs) that are considered to be inaccessible to surgical treatment—i.e. lesions in the deep regions of a cerebral hemisphere, in the brainstem, or in important primary projection areas, such as for language or for motor control of the dominant hand. With these techniques, highly collimated quantities of high-energy radiation are directed from many different angles at the lesion, resulting in a steep dosage gradient between the target and the normal brain tissue surrounding it. Lesions of more than 3.5 cm in size are not suitable for radiosurgical treatment, because the dose to normal tissues would be excessive. The rationale for this treatment is that radiation damages and eventually occludes the blood vessels constituting the AVM (Ogilvy 1990). This takes place in the long term, after months or years. In the meantime there is still a risk of haemorrhage, but probably no higher than without intervention (Friedman *et al.* 1996; Pollock *et al.* 1996b). The tissue changes consist of damage to endothelial cells, deposition of collagen in the subendothelial region and proliferation of the muscle layer (Schneider *et al.* 1997; Szeifert *et al.* 1997). These alterations occur more extensively in arteries than veins, particularly in small arteries. Magnetic resonance (MR) imaging and MR angiography reflect these changes, showing a decreasing calibre in the feeding vessels and AVM nidus volumes from an early stage, 3 months after radiosurgery (Guo *et al.* 1995, 1996; Morikawa *et al.* 1996). The brain around the nidus often shows hyperintense changes on T2-weighted images (Morikawa *et al.* 1996). MR imaging correctly identifies the stage of complete obliteration and probably obviates the need for repeat catheter angiography (Guo *et al.* 1996; Pollock *et al.* 1996c). Contrast enhancement on CT or MRI may still be visible after the stage of obliteration; in many cases this phenomenon disappears over the next few years, but not in all (Yamamoto *et al.* 1995a; Kihlström *et al.* 1997).

Two different techniques have been developed: the 'gamma knife' and the linear accelerator, on the one hand, delivering photons; and the proton beam technique, on the other (Heros & Korosue 1990). Both methods use a stereotactic device for the delivery of radiation and require an extensive infrastructure of particle physics expertise that restricts their application to only a few centres in the world. Not surprisingly, radiosurgery is sometimes used in combination with surgical resection (Steinberg *et al.* 1996; Firlik *et al.* 1998), endovascular treatment (Gobin *et al.* 1996; Lundqvist *et al.* 1996), or both (Smith *et al.* 1997).

The *gamma knife*, developed by the Swedish neurosurgeon Leksell, is a system that uses a cobalt source for generating highly collimated gamma rays that converge at a focal point in the brain. A summary of the results in three groups of patients treated with the gamma knife has shown that between 79 and 84% of the patients had complete angiographic obliteration of the AVM after 2 years (Lindquist & Steiner 1988). An important determinant of success is the ratio between the size of the lesion and the minimum dose of radiation, up to an optimum of 25 Gy (Flickinger *et al.* 1996; Karlsson *et al.* 1997a, 1999). Treatment failures can mostly be explained by errors in targeting (Ellis *et al.* 1998; Gallina *et al.* 1998). In these cases, a second procedure is warranted (Pollock *et al.* 1996d; Karlsson *et al.* 1998). The obliteration rate reported by the Mayo Clinic group was 75% (Yamamoto *et al.* 1995b), and the rate reported by the Pittsburgh group was 90% (Flickinger *et al.* 1996). The latter group identified the following factors as predictors of successful obliteration, apart from the minimum dose: small AVM volume, number of draining veins, young patient age, and hemispheric AVM location (Pollock *et al.* 1998). A group in Komaki (Japan) confirmed that the success rate is relatively high in children (Tanaka *et al.* 1996). In children with epilepsy as the presenting symptom, seizure control after radiosurgery is generally good (Gerszten *et al.* 1996). Complications of gamma-knife treatment (radiation necrosis) are equally dependent on dose and on location (Flickinger *et al.* 1997; Karlsson *et al.* 1997b); this is a serious consideration, especially in AVMs of the brainstem (Karlsson *et al.* 1996). Long-term complications include progressive neurological deficit from an expanding, encapsulated haematoma (Kurita *et al.* 1996) or a cyst (Yamamoto *et al.* 1996; Yamamoto *et al.* 1998); such cysts may also be asymptomatic (Kihlström *et al.* 1997). Gamma-knife treatment has also been implicated in diffuse leukoaraiosis (Yamamoto *et al.* 1997a) and middle cerebral artery stenosis (Yamamoto *et al.* 1997b), but the proof for any causal association is rather weak.

Three groups using a related technique with a *linear accelerator*, which delivers radiation to a defined volume of tissue, have reported similar results, with complete arteriovenous malformation obliteration after 2 years in between 70% and 80% (Betti *et al.* 1989; Colombo *et al.* 1989; Pica *et al.* 1996). The rate of symptomatic radiation necrosis with either the gamma knife or the linear accelerator was of the order of 3%. It should be kept in mind that, as a rule, these two techniques were applied only in patients with AVMs measuring less than 3.5 cm in diameter. Neuropsychological testing, up to 1 year after treatment, produced no evidence for a deleterious effect on intellect, but of course could not exclude more delayed problems (Wenz *et al.* 1998).

The other method, the *proton beam* technique, uses the so-called Bragg peak of the proton beam generated at the Harvard University cyclotron (Kjellberg *et al.* 1983a). The proton beam is designed to reach its peak in a defined volume of tissue. The reported rate of complete obliteration was only of the order of 22%, but this series was associated with a less than 2% risk of serious complications and involved a high proportion of larger lesions and low doses of radiation (Kjellberg *et al.* 1983b; Heros & Korosue 1990). Unfortunately, the risk of haemorrhage from any AVM is not reduced, or may even be increased, until complete obliteration has been achieved (Ogilvy 1990). For smaller lesions measuring less than 3.5 cm in diameter, a group in Stanford used helium-ion Bragg-peak radiation and found an obliteration rate of 39% after 1 year, 84% after 2 years and 97% after 3 years (Steinberg *et al.* 1990). Even 70% of the larger lesions were no longer detectable on angiography after 3 years. On the other hand, the risk of disabling neurological complications as a result of treatment was 9%. With larger AVMs, the chance of obliteration decreases and the risk of complications increases, as higher doses are needed (Miyawaki *et al.* 1999). Little is known at present about possible adverse effects in the long term, particularly tumour formation.

In summary, if any intervention at all is needed, the technique of focused radiation is not much safer and is probably less effective than surgical resection, certainly in the short term. This approach should be reserved for AVMs that are completely inaccessible to surgery or embolization, i.e. small and deep lesions, fed by small blood vessels.

The techniques for removal of arteriovenous malformations have not been properly compared with the natural history, or with each other. Provisionally, it seems that open surgery is best for superficial arteriovenous malformations; endovascular embolization is preferable for deep and large (> 3.5 cm) lesions, often in combination with open surgery; and radiosurgery is reserved for small, deep arteriovenous malformations.

14.6 Treatment of cavernous angiomas

The complete lack of randomized controlled clinical trials is even worse with cavernomas than with deep haemorrhages from degenerative small vessel disease. Some surgeons advocate surgical removal of most, if not all, symptomatic cavernomas in the cerebral hemispheres (excluding the basal ganglia) and in the cerebellum, especially those that have bled (Ojemann *et al.* 1993). Others even include deep cavernomas, through stereotactic methods (Esposito *et al.* 1994), or cavernomas in the brainstem, if they are superficially located or if there are recurrent symptoms (Fahlbusch *et al.* 1990; Zimmerman *et al.* 1991). Although we admire the technical skills that are displayed in these operations, we deplore the disregard of the natural history of the lesions, which is often quite favourable (section 8.2.5). It has been claimed that intractable epilepsy associated with cortical cavernomas can be greatly improved by operation if the seizure history is under 1 year and if there is good concordance with electrophysiological studies, but again there is no evidence from controlled studies (Cohen *et al.* 1995; Casazza *et al.* 1996).

14.7 Treatment of dural arteriovenous fistulae

The natural history of these lesions may be favourable, especially if they present other than with haemorrhage (section 8.2.8). Despite this, different surgical techniques have been applied, depending on the location of the fistula and the type of venous drainage (Lucas *et al.* 1997). The risk of haemorrhage is greatest if drainage is via leptomeningeal vessels (Cognard *et al.* 1995); in that situation, ligation of the draining vessels is the preferred treatment (Collice *et al.* 1996). Other possible treatments are transvenous embolization (Urtasun *et al.* 1996; Roy & Raymond 1997), radiosurgery (Link *et al.* 1996), arterial embolization, especially if there is an unbearable audible bruit (Link *et al.* 1996), and occlusion of a part of the superior sagittal sinus (Lucas *et al.* 1996).

References

Please note that all references taken from *The Cochrane Library* are given a current date as this database is updated on a quarterly basis. Please refer to the current *Cochrane Library* article for the latest review. The same applies to the *British Medical Journal* 'Clinical Evidence' series which is updated every six months.

Abdulrauf, S.I., Malik, G.M. & Awad, I.A. (1999) Spontaneous angiographic obliteration of cerebral arteriovenous malformations. *Neurosurgery* **44**, 280–287.

al Rodhan, N.R., Sundt, T.M. Jr, Piepgras, D.G., Nichols, D.A., Rufenacht, D. & Stevens, L.N. (1993) Occlusive hyperemia: a theory for the hemodynamic complications following resection of intracerebral arteriovenous malformations. *Journal of Neurosurgery* **78**, 167–175.

Aminoff, M.J. (1987) Treatment of unruptured cerebral arteriovenous malformations. *Neurology* **37**, 815–819.

Awad, I.A., Magdinec, M. & Schubert, A. (1994) Intracranial hypertension after resection of cerebral arteriovenous malformations: predisposing factors and management strategy. *Stroke* **25**, 611–620.

Betti, O.O., Munari, C. & Rosler, R. (1989) Stereotactic radiosurgery with the linear accelerator: treatment of arteriovenous malformations. *Neurosurgery* **24**, 311–321.

Brown, R.D. Jr, Wiebers, D.O., Forbes, G. *et al.* (1988) The natural history of unruptured intracranial arteriovenous malformations. *Journal of Neurosurgery* **68**, 352–357.

Brown, R.D. Jr, Wiebers, D.O., Torner, J.C. & O'Fallon, W.M. (1996) Frequency of intracranial hemorrhage as a presenting symptom and subtype analysis: a population-based study of intracranial vascular malformations in Olmsted County, Minnesota. *Journal of Neurosurgery* **85**, 29–32.

Bruyn, G.W. (1984) Intracranial arteriovenous malformation and migraine. *Cephalalgia* **4**, 191–207.

Casazza, M., Broggi, G., Franzini, A. *et al.* (1996) Supratentorial cavernous angiomas and epileptic seizures: preoperative course and postoperative outcome. *Neurosurgery* **39**, 26–32.

Chang, H.S. & Nihei, H. (1999) Theoretical comparison of surgery and radiosurgery in cerebral arteriovenous malformations. *Journal of Neurosurgery* **90**, 709–719.

Chimowitz, M.I., Little, J.R., Awad, I.A., Sila, C.A., Kosmorsky, G. & Furlan, A.J. (1990) Intracranial hypertension associated with unruptured cerebral arteriovenous malformations. *Annals of Neurology* **27**, 474–479.

Cognard, C., Gobin, Y.P., Pierot, L. *et al.* (1995) Cerebral dural arteriovenous fistulas: clinical and angiographic correlation, with a revised classification of venous drainage. *Radiology* **194**, 671–680.

Cohen, D.S., Zubay, G.P. & Goodman, R.R. (1995) Seizure outcome after lesionectomy for cavernous malformations. *Journal of Neurosurgery* **83**, 237–242.

Collice, M., D'Aliberti, G., Talamonti, G. *et al.* (1996) Surgical interruption of leptomeningeal drainage as treatment for intracranial dural arteriovenous fistulas without dural sinus drainage. *Journal of Neurosurgery* **84**, 810–817.

Colombo, F., Benedetti, A., Pozza, F., Marchetti, C. & Chierego, G. (1989) Linear accelerator radiosurgery of cerebral arteriovenous malformations. *Neurosurgery* **24**, 833–840.

Debrun, G.M., Aletich, V., Ausman, J.I., Charbel, F. & Dujovny, M. (1997) Embolization of the nidus of brain arteriovenous malformations with *n*-butyl cyanoacrylate. *Neurosurgery* **40**, 112–120.

Deruty, R., Lapras, C., Pierluca, P. *et al.* (1985) Embolisation peropératoire des malformations arterio-veineuses cérébrales par le butyl-cyanoacrylate (18 cas) [peroperative embolization of cerebral arteriovenous malformations with butylcyanoacrylate (18 cases)]. *Neurochirurgie* **31**, 21–29.

Deruty, R., Pelissou-Guyotat, I., Amat, D. *et al.* (1995) Multidisciplinary treatment of cerebral arteriovenous malformations. *Neurological Research* **17**, 169–177.

Dias, M.S. & Sekhar, L.N. (1990) Intracranial hemorrhage from aneurysms and arteriovenous malformations during pregnancy and the puerperium. *Neurosurgery* **27**, 855–865.

Donaldson, J.O. (1989) *The Neurology of Pregnancy,* 2nd edn. Saunders, London.

Duong, D.H., Young, W.L., Vang, M.C. *et al.* (1998) Feeding artery pressure and venous drainage pattern are primary determinants of hemorrhage from cerebral arteriovenous malformations. *Stroke* **29**, 1167–1176.

Ellis, T.L., Friedman, W.A., Bova, F.J., Kubilis, P.S. & Buatti, J.M. (1998) Analysis of treatment failure after radiosurgery for arteriovenous malformations. *Journal of Neurosurgery* **89**, 104–110.

Esposito, V., Oppido, P.A., Delfini, R. & Cantore, G. (1994) A simple method for stereotactic microsurgical excision of small, deep-seated cavernous angiomas. *Neurosurgery* **34**, 515–518.

Ezura, M. & Kagawa, S. (1992) Spontaneous disappearance of a huge cerebral arteriovenous malformation: case report. *Neurosurgery* **30**, 595–599.

Fahlbusch, R., Strauss, C., Huk, W., Rockelein, G., Kompf, D. & Ruprecht, K.W. (1990) Surgical removal of pontomesencephalic cavernous hemangiomas. *Neurosurgery* **26**, 449–456.

Finnerty, J.J., Chisholm, C.A., Chapple, H., Login, I.S. & Pinkerton, J.V. (1999) Cerebral arteriovenous malformation in pregnancy: presentation and neurologic, obstetric, and ethical significance. *American Journal of Obstetrics and Gynecology* **181**, 296–301.

Firlik, A.D., Levy, E.I., Kondziolka, D. & Yonas, H. (1998) Staged volume radiosurgery followed by microsurgical resection, a novel treatment for giant cerebral arteriovenous malformations: technical case report. *Neurosurgery* **43**, 1223–1227.

Flickinger, J.C., Pollock, B.E., Kondziolka, D. & Lunsford, L.D. (1996) A dose–response analysis of arteriovenous malformation obliteration after radiosurgery. *International Journal of Radiation Oncology, Biology, Physics* **36**, 873–879.

Flickinger, J.C., Kondziolka, D., Pollock, B.E., Maitz, A.H. & Lunsford, L.D. (1997) Complications from arteriovenous malformation radiosurgery: multivariate analysis and risk modeling. *International Journal of Radiation Oncology, Biology, Physics* **38**, 485–490.

Fournier, D., TerBrugge, K.G., Willinsky, R.A., Lasjaunias, P. & Montanera, W. (1991) Endovascular treatment of intracerebral arteriovenous malformations: experience in 49 cases. *Journal of Neurosurgery* **75**, 228–233.

Friedman, W.A., Blatt, D.L., Bova, F.J., Buatti, J.M., Mendenhall, W.M. & Kubilis, P.S. (1996) The risk of hemorrhage after radiosurgery for arteriovenous malformations. *Journal of Neurosurgery* **84**, 912–919.

Frizzel, R.T. & Fisher, W.S. III (1995) Cure, morbidity, and mortality associated with embolization of brain arteriovenous malformations: a review of 1246 patients in 32 series over a 35-year period. *Neurosurgery* **37**, 1031–1039.

Gabriel, E.M., Sampson, J.H. & Wilkins, R.H. (1996) Recurrence of a cerebral arteriovenous malformation after surgical excision. *Journal of Neurosurgery* **84**, 879–882.

Gallina, P., Merienne, L., Meder, J.F., Schlienger, M., Lefkopoulos, D. & Merland, J.L. (1998) Failure in radiosurgery treatment of cerebral arteriovenous malformations. *Neurosurgery* **42**, 996–1002.

Gerszten, P.C., Adelson, P.D., Kondziolka, D., Flickinger, J.C. & Lunsford, L.D. (1996) Seizure outcome in children treated for arteriovenous malformations using gamma knife radiosurgery. *Pediatric Neurosurgery* **24**, 139–144.

Giller, C.A., Giller, A.M. & Landreneau, F. (1998) Detection of emboli after surgery for intracerebral aneurysms. *Neurosurgery* **42**, 490–493.

Gobin, Y.P., Laurent, A., Merienne, L. *et al.* (1996) Treatment of brain arteriovenous malformations by embolization and radiosurgery. *Journal of Neurosurgery* **85**, 19–28.

Guazzo, E.P. & Xuereb, J.H. (1994) Spontaneous thrombosis of an arteriovenous malformation. *Journal of Neurology, Neurosurgery and Psychiatry* **57**, 1410–1412.

Guo, W.Y., Pan, D.H.C., Liu, R.S. *et al.* (1995) Early irradiation effects observed on magnetic resonance imaging and angiography, and positron emission tomography for arteriovenous malformations treated by gamma knife radiosurgery. *Stereotactic and Functional Neurosurgery* **64** (Suppl. 1), 258–269.

Guo, W.Y., Pan, H.C., Chung, W.Y., Wang, L.W. & Teng, M.M.H. (1996) Do we need conventional angiography? The role of magnetic resonance imaging in verifying obliteration of arteriovenous malformations after gamma knife surgery. *Stereotactic and Functional Neurosurgery* **66**, 71–84.

Haas, D.C. (1991) Arteriovenous malformations and migraine: case reports and an analysis of the relationship. *Headache* **31**, 509–513.

Halpin, S.F., Britton, J.A., Byrne, J.V., Clifton, A., Hart, G. & Moore, A. (1994) Prospective evaluation of cerebral angiography and computed tomography in cerebral haematoma. *Journal of Neurology, Neurosurgery and Psychiatry* **57**, 1180–1186.

Hartmann, A., Mast, H., Mohr, J.P. *et al.* (1998) Morbidity of intracranial hemorrhage in patients with cerebral arteriovenous malformation. *Stroke* **29**, 931–934.

Hayashi, T., Ichiyama, T., Nishikawa, M. *et al.* (1996) A case of a large neonatal arteriovenous malformation with heart failure: color Doppler sonography, MRI and MR angiography as early non-invasive diagnostic procedures. *Brain and Development* **18**, 236–238.

Heros, R.C. & Korosue, K. (1990) Radiation treatment of cerebral arteriovenous malformations. *New England Journal of Medicine* **323**, 127–129.

Heros, R.C. & Tu, Y.K. (1987) Is surgical therapy needed for unruptured arteriovenous malformations? *Neurology* **37**, 279–286.

Heros, R.C., Korosue, K. & Diebold, P.M. (1990) Surgical excision of cerebral arteriovenous malformations: late results. *Neurosurgery* **26**, 570–577.

Hino, A., Fujimoto, M., Yamaki, T., Iwamoto, Y. & Katsumori, T. (1998) Value of repeat angiography in patients with spontaneous subcortical hemorrhage. *Stroke* **29**, 2517–2521.

Horton, J.C., Chambers, W.A., Lyons, S.L., Adams, R.D. & Kjellberg, R.N. (1990) Pregnancy and the risk of hemorrhage from cerebral arteriovenous malformations. *Neurosurgery* **27**, 867–871.

Iansek, R., Elstein, A.S. & Balla, J.I. (1983) Application of decision analysis to management of cerebral arteriovenous malformation. *Lancet* **i**, 1132–1135.

Jaillard, A.S., Peres, B. & Hommel, M. (1999) Neuropsychological features of dementia due to dural arteriovenous malformation. *Cerebrovascular Diseases* **9**, 91–97.

Jane, J.A., Kassell, N.F., Torner, J.C. & Winn, H.R. (1985) The natural history of aneurysms and arteriovenous malformations. *Journal of Neurosurgery* **62**, 321–323.

Kader, A., Goodrich, J.T., Sonstein, W.J., Stein, B.M., Carmel, P.W. & Michelsen, W.J. (1996) Recurrent cerebral arteriovenous malformations after negative postoperative angiograms. *Journal of Neurosurgery* **85**, 14–18.

Karlsson, B., Lax, I., Soderman, M., Kihlström, L. & Lindquist, C. (1996) Prediction of results following gamma knife surgery for brain stem and other centrally located arteriovenous malformations: relation to natural course. *Stereotactic and Functional Neurosurgery* **66**, 260–268.

Karlsson, B., Lindquist, C. & Steiner, L. (1997a) Prediction of obliteration after gamma knife surgery for cerebral arteriovenous malformations. *Neurosurgery* **40**, 425–430.

Karlsson, B., Lax, I. & Söderman, M. (1997b) Factors influencing the risk for complications following gamma knife radiosurgery of cerebral arteriovenous malformations. *Radiotherapy and Oncology* **43**, 275–280.

Karlsson, B., Kihlström, L., Lindquist, C. & Steiner, L. (1998) Gamma knife surgery for previously irradiated arteriovenous malformations. *Neurosurgery* **42**, 1–5.

Karlsson, B., Lax, I. & Söderman, M. (1999) Can the probability for obliteration after radiosurgery for arteriovenous malformations be accurately predicted? *International Journal of Radiation Oncology, Biology, Physics* **43**, 313–319.

Kato, Y., Sano, H., Nonomura, K. *et al.* (1997) Normal perfusion pressure breakthrough syndrome in giant arteriovenous malformations. *Neurological Research* **19**, 117–123.

Kelly, J.J., Mellinger, J.F. & Sundt, T.M. (1978) Intracranial arteriovenous malformations in childhood. *Annals of Neurology* **3**, 338–343.

Kihlström, L., Guo, W.Y., Karlsson, B., Lindquist, C. & Lindqvist, M. (1997) Magnetic resonance imaging of obliterated arteriovenous malformations up to 23 years after radiosurgery. *Journal of Neurosurgery* **86**, 589–593.

Kjellberg, R.N., Hanamura, T., Davis, K.R., Lyons, S.L. & Adams, R.D. (1983a) Bragg-peak proton-beam therapy for arteriovenous malformations of the brain. *New England Journal of Medicine* **309**, 269–274.

Kjellberg, R.N., Davis, K.R., Lyons, S., Butler, W. & Adams, R.D. (1983b) Bragg peak proton beam therapy for arteriovenous malformation of the brain. *Clinical Neurosurgery* **31**, 248–290.

Klötzsch, C., Henkes, H., Nahser, H.C., Kühne, D. & Berlit, P. (1995) Transcranial color-coded duplex sonography in cerebral arteriovenous malformations. *Stroke* **26**, 2298–2301.

Konan, A.V., Roy, D. & Raymond, J. (1999) Endovascular treatment of hemifacial spasm associated with a cerebral arteriovenous malformation using transvenous embolization: case report. *Neurosurgery* **44**, 663–666.

Kupersmith, M.J., Vargas, M.E., Yashar, A. *et al.* (1996) Occipital arteriovenous malformations: visual disturbances and presentation. *Neurology* **46**, 953–957.

Kurita, H., Sasaki, T., Kawamoto, S. *et al.* (1996) Chronic encapsulated expanding hematoma in association with gamma knife stereotactic radiosurgery for a cerebral arteriovenous malformation. *Journal of Neurosurgery* **84**, 874–878.

Kvam, D.A., Michelsen, W.J. & Quest, D.O. (1980) Intracerebral hemorrhage as a complication of artificial embolization. *Neurosurgery* **7**, 491–494.

Langer, D.J., Lasner, T.M., Hurst, R.W., Flamm, E.S., Zager, E.L. & King, J.T. Jr (1998) Hypertension, small size, and deep venous drainage are associated with risk of hemorrhagic presentation of cerebral arteriovenous malformations. *Neurosurgery* **42**, 481–486.

Latchaw, R.E., Hu, X.P., Ugurbil, K., Hall, W.A., Madison, M.T. & Heros, R.C. (1995) Functional magnetic resonance imaging as a management tool for cerebral arteriovenous malformations. *Neurosurgery* **37**, 619–625.

Lawton, M.T., Hamilton, M.G. & Spetzler, R.F. (1995) Multimodality treatment of deep arteriovenous malformations: thalamus, basal ganglia, and brain stem. *Neurosurgery* **37**, 29–36.

Leblanc, R. & Little, J.R. (1990) Hemodynamics of arteriovenous malformations. *Clinical Neurosurgery* **36**, 299–317.

Leblanc, R., Meyer, E., Zatorre, R., Tampieri, D. & Evans, A. (1995) Functional PET scanning in the preoperative assessment of cerebral arteriovenous malformations. *Stereotactic and Functional Neurosurgery* **65**, 60–64.

Lindquist, C. & Steiner, L. (1988) Stereotactic radiosurgical treatment of arteriovenous malformations. In: *Modern Stereotactic Neurosurgery* (ed. L.D. Lunsford), pp. 491–505. Martinus Nyhoff, Boston.

Link, M.J., Coffey, R.J., Nichols, D.A. & Gorman, D.A. (1996) The role of radiosurgery and particulate embolization in the treatment of dural arteriovenous fistulas. *Journal of Neurosurgery* **84**, 804–809.

Lobato, R.D., Rivas, J.J., Gomez, P.A., Cabrera, A., Sarabia, R. & Lamas, E. (1992) Comparison of the clinical presentation of symptomatic arteriovenous malformations (angiographically visualized) and occult vascular malformations. *Neurosurgery* **31**, 391–396.

Lucas, C.P., De Oliveira, E., Tedeschi, H. *et al.* (1996) Sinus skeletonization, a treatment for dural arteriovenous malformations of the tentorial apex: report of two cases. *Journal of Neurosurgery* **84**, 514–517.

Lucas, C.P., Zabramski, J.M., Spetzler, R.F. & Jacobowitz, R. (1997) Treatment for intracranial dural arteriovenous malformations: a meta-analysis from the English language literature. *Neurosurgery* **40**, 1119–1130.

Luessenhop, A.J. & Presper, J.H. (1984) Surgical embolization of cerebral arteriovenous malformations through internal carotid and vertebral arteries: long term results. *Journal of Neurosurgery* **60**, 14–22.

Luessenhop, A.J. & Rosa, L. (1984) Cerebral arteriovenous malformations: indications for and results of surgery, and the role of intravascular techniques. *Journal of Neurosurgery* **60**, 14–22.

Lundqvist, C., Wikholm, G. & Svendsen, P. (1996) Embolization of cerebral arteriovenous malformations, 2: aspects of complications and late outcome. *Neurosurgery* **39**, 460–467.

Maldjian, J., Atlas, S.W., Howard, R.S. II *et al.* (1996) Functional magnetic resonance imaging of regional brain activity in patients with intracerebral arteriovenous malformations before surgical or endovascular therapy. *Journal of Neurosurgery* **84**, 477–483.

Mast, H., Mohr, J.P., Osipov, A. *et al.* (1995) 'Steal' is an unestablished mechanism for the clinical presentation of cerebral arteriovenous malformations. *Stroke* **26**, 1215–1220.

Mast, H., Young, W.L., Koennecke, H.C. *et al.* (1997) Risk of spontaneous haemorrhage after diagnosis of cerebral arteriovenous malformation. *Lancet* **350**, 1065–1068.

Mineura, K., Sasajima, H., Itoh, Y., Kowada, M., Tomura, N. & Goto, K. (1998) Development of a huge varix following endovascular embolization for cerebellar arteriovenous malformation: a case report. *Acta Radiologica* **39**, 189–192.

Miyasaka, Y., Yada, K., Ohwada, T., Kitahara, T., Kurata, A. & Irikura, K. (1992) An analysis of the venous drainage system as a factor in hemorrhage from arteriovenous malformations. *Journal of Neurosurgery* **76**, 239–243.

Miyawaki, L., Dowd, C., Wara, W. *et al.* (1999) Five year results of LINAC radiosurgery for arteriovenous malformations: outcome for large AVMs. *International Journal of Radiation Oncology, Biology, Physics* **44**, 1089–1106.

Morgan, M.K., Drummond, K.J., Grinnell, V. & Sorby, W. (1997) Surgery for cerebral arteriovenous malformation: risks related to lenticulostriate arterial supply. *Journal of Neurosurgery* **86**, 801–805.

Morgan, M.K., Sekhon, L.H.S., Finfer, S. & Grinnell, V. (1999) Delayed neurological deterioration following resection of arteriovenous malformations of the brain. *Journal of Neurosurgery* **90**, 695–701.

Morikawa, M., Numaguchi, Y., Rigamonti, D. *et al.* (1996) Radiosurgery for cerebral arteriovenous malformations: assessment of early phase magnetic resonance imaging and significance of gadolinium-DTPA enhancement. *International Journal of Radiation Oncology, Biology, Physics* **34**, 663–675.

Munshi, I., Macdonald, R.L. & Weir, B.K.A. (1999) Intraoperative angiography of brain arteriovenous malformations. *Neurosurgery* **45**, 491–497.

Murayama, Y., Usami, S., Hata, Y. *et al.* (1996) Transvenous hemodynamic assessment of arteriovenous malformations and fistulas: preliminary clinical experience in Doppler guidewire monitoring of embolotherapy. *Stroke* **27**, 1358–1364.

Neil-Dwyer, G. & Lang, D. (1997) 'Brain attack'—aneurysmal subarachnoid haemorrhage: death due to delayed diagnosis. *Journal of the Royal College of Physicians of London* **31**, 49–52.

Ogilvy, C.S. (1990) Radiation therapy for arteriovenous malformations: a review. *Neurosurgery* **26**, 725–735.

Ojemann, R.G., Crowell, R.M. & Ogilvy, C.S. (1993) Management of cranial and spinal cavernous angiomas. *Clinical Neurosurgery* **40**, 98–123.

Ondra, S.L., Troupp, H., George, E.D. & Schwab, K. (1990) The natural history of symptomatic arteriovenous malformations of the brain: a 24-year follow-up assessment. *Journal of Neurosurgery* **73**, 387–391.

Pelak, V.S., Galetta, S.L., Grossman, R.I., Townsend, J.J. & Volpe, N.J. (1999) Evidence for preganglionic pupillary involvement in superficial siderosis. *Neurology* **53**, 1130–1132.

Pellettieri, L., Svendsen, G., Wikholm, G. & Carlsson, C.A. (1997) Hidden compartments in AVMs: a new concept. *Acta Radiologica* **38**, 2–7.

Pica, A., Ayzac, L., Sentenac, I. *et al.* (1996) Stereotactic radiosurgery for arteriovenous malformations of the brain using a standard linear accelerator: the Lyon experience. *Radiotherapy and Oncology* **40**, 51–54.

Pile-Spellman, J., Young, W.L., Joshi, S. *et al.* (1999) Adenosine-induced cardiac pause for endovascular embolization of cerebral arteriovenous malformations: technical case report. *Neurosurgery* **44**, 881–886.

Pollock, B.E., Flickinger, J.C., Lunsford, L.D., Bissonette, D.J. & Kondziolka, D. (1996a) Factors that predict the bleeding risk of cerebral arteriovenous malformations. *Stroke* **27**, 1–6.

Pollock, B.E., Flickinger, J.C., Lunsford, L.D., Bissonette, D.J. & Kondziolka, D. (1996b) Hemorrhage risk after stereotactic radiosurgery of cerebral arteriovenous malformations. *Neurosurgery* **38**, 652–659.

Pollock, B.E., Kondziolka, D., Flickinger, J.C., Patel, A.K., Bissonette, D.J. & Lunsford, L.D. (1996c) Magnetic resonance imaging: an accurate method to evaluate arteriovenous malformations after stereotactic radiosurgery. *Journal of Neurosurgery* **85**, 1044–1049.

Pollock, B.E., Kondziolka, D., Lunsford, L.D., Bissonette, D. & Flickinger, J.C. (1996d) Repeat stereotactic radiosurgery of arteriovenous malformations: factors associated with incomplete obliteration. *Neurosurgery* **38**, 318–323.

Pollock, B.E., Flickinger, J.C., Lunsford, L.D., Maitz, A. & Kondziolka, D. (1998) Factors associated with successful arteriovenous malformation radiosurgery. *Neurosurgery* **42**, 1239–1244.

Porter, P.J., Shin, A.Y., Detsky, A.S., Lefaive, L. & Wallace, M.C. (1997) Surgery versus stereotactic radiosurgery for small, operable cerebral arteriovenous malformations: a clinical and cost comparison. *Neurosurgery* **41**, 757–764.

Redekop, G., Terbrugge, K., Montanera, W. & Willinsky, R. (1998) Arterial aneurysms associated with cerebral arteriovenous malformations: classification, incidence, and risk of hemorrhage. *Journal of Neurosurgery* **89**, 539–546.

Roy, D. & Raymond, J. (1997) The role of transvenous embolization in the treatment of intracranial dural arteriovenous fistulas. *Neurosurgery* **40**, 1133–1141.

Schaller, C. & Schramm, J. (1997) Microsurgical results for small arteriovenous malformations accessible for radiosurgical or embolization treatment. *Neurosurgery* **40**, 664–672.

Schaller, C., Schramm, J. & Haun, D. (1998) Significance of factors contributing to surgical complications and to late outcome after elective surgery of cerebral arteriovenous malformations. *Journal of Neurology, Neurosurgery and Psychiatry* **65**, 547–554.

Schlosser, M.J., McCarthy, G., Fulbright, R.K., Gore, J.C. & Awad, I.A. (1997) Cerebral vascular malformations adjacent to sensorimotor and visual cortex: functional magnetic resonance imaging studies before and after therapeutic intervention. *Stroke* **28**, 1130–1137.

Schneider, B.F., Eberhard, D.A. & Steiner, L.E. (1997) Histopathology of arteriovenous malformations after gamma knife radiosurgery. *Journal of Neurosurgery* **87**, 352–357.

Sheth, R.D. & Bodensteiner, J.B. (1995) Progressive neurologic impairment from an arteriovenous malformation vascular steal. *Pediatric Neurology* **13**, 352–354.

Smith, K.A., Shetter, A., Speiser, B. & Spetzler, R.F. (1997) Angiographic follow-up in 37 patients after radiosurgery for cerebral arteriovenous malformations as part of a multimodality treatment approach. *Stereotactic and Functional Neurosurgery* **69**, 136–142.

Sorimachi, T., Takeuchi, S., Koike, T., Minakawa, T., Abe, H. & Tanaka, R. (1995) Blood pressure monitoring in feeding arteries of cerebral arteriovenous malformations during embolization: a preventive role in hemodynamic complications. *Neurosurgery* **37**, 1041–1047.

Spetzler, R.F. & Martin, N.A. (1986) A proposed grading system for arteriovenous malformations. *Journal of Neurosurgery* **65**, 476–483.

Spetzler, R.F., Wilson, C.B., Weinstein, P., Mehdorn, M., Townsend, J. & Telles, D. (1978) Normal perfusion pressure breakthrough phenomenon. *Clinical Neurosurgery* **25**, 651–672.

Stein, B.M. & Wolpert, S.M. (1980) Arteriovenous malformations of the brain, 2: current concepts and treatment. *Archives of Neurology* **37**, 69–75.

Stein, B.M., Pile-Spellman, J. & Isaacson, S.R. (1998) Vascular malformations of the brain and dura. In: *Stroke—Pathophysiology, Diagnosis, and Management* (eds H.J.M. Barnett, J.P. Mohr, B.M. Stein & F.M. Yatsu), 3rd edn, pp. 1309–1347. Churchill Livingstone, New York.

Steinberg, G.K., Fabrikant, J.I., Marks, M.P. *et al.* (1990) Stereotactic heavy-charged-particle Bragg-peak radiation for intracranial arteriovenous malformations. *New England Journal of Medicine* **323**, 96–101.

Steinberg, G.K., Chang, S.D., Levy, R.P., Marks, M.P., Frankel, K. & Marcellus, M. (1996) Surgical resection of large incompletely treated intracranial arteriovenous malformations following stereotactic radiosurgery. *Journal of Neurosurgery* **84**, 920–928.

Szeifert, G.T., Kemeny, A.A., Timperley, W.R. & Forster, D.M.C. (1997) The potential role of myofibroblasts in the obliteration of arteriovenous malformations after radiosurgery. *Neurosurgery* **40**, 61–65.

Tanaka, T., Kobayashi, T., Kida, Y., Oyama, H. & Niwa, M. (1996) Comparison between adult and pediatric arteriovenous malformations treated by gamma knife radiosurgery. *Stereotactic and Functional Neurosurgery* **66**, 288–295.

Tew, J.M. Jr, Lewis, A.I. & Reichert, K.W. (1995) Management strategies and surgical techniques for deep-seated supratentorial arteriovenous malformations. *Neurosurgery* **36**, 1065–1072.

Thompson, R.C., Steinberg, G.K., Levy, R.P. & Marks, M.P. (1998) The management of patients with arteriovenous malformations and associated intracranial aneurysms. *Neurosurgery* **43**, 202–211.

Tokunaga, K., Kinugasa, K., Kawada, S. *et al.* (1999) Embolization of cerebral arteriovenous malformations with cellulose acetate polymer: a clinical, radiological, and histological study. *Neurosurgery* **44**, 981–989.

Turjman, F., Massoud, T.F., Vinuela, F., Sayre, J.W., Guglielmi, G. & Duckwiler, G. (1995) Correlation of the angioarchitectural features of cerebral arteriovenous malformations with clinical presentation of hemorrhage. *Neurosurgery* **37**, 856–860.

Urtasun, F., Biondi, A., Casaco, A. *et al.* (1996) Cerebral dural arteriovenous fistulas: percutaneous transvenous embolization. *Radiology* **199**, 209–217.

Verm, A. & Lee, A.G. (1997) Bilateral optic disk edema with macular exudates as the manifesting sign of a cerebral arteriovenous malformation. *American Journal of Ophthalmology* **123**, 422–424.

Vinters, H.V., Lundie, M.J. & Kaufmann, J.C. (1986) Long-term pathological follow-up of cerebral arteriovenous malformations treated by embolization with bucrylate. *New England Journal of Medicine* **314**, 477–483.

Vinuela, F.V., Debrun, G.M., Fox, A.J., Girvin, J.P. & Peerless, S.J. (1983) Dominant-hemisphere arteriovenous malformations: therapeutic embolization with isobutyl-2-cyanoacrylate. *American Journal of Neuroradiology* **4**, 959–966.

Vinuela, F., Fox, A.J., Pelz, D. & Debrun, G. (1986) Angiographic follow-up of large cerebral AVMs incompletely embolized with isobutyl-2-cyanoacrylate. *American Journal of Neuroradiology* **7**, 919–925.

Wakai, S., Chen, C.H., Wu, K.Y. & Chiu, C.W. (1983) Spontaneous regression of a cerebral arteriovenous malformation: report of a case and review of the literature. *Archives of Neurology* **40**, 377–380.

Wakhloo, A.K., Lieber, B.B., Rudin, S., Fronckowiak, M.D., Mericle, R.A. & Hopkins, L.N. (1998) A novel approach to flow quantification in brain arteriovenous malformations prior to enbucrilate embolization: use of insoluble contrast (Ethiodol droplet) angiography. *Journal of Neurosurgery* **89**, 395–404.

Wallace, R.C., Flom, R.A., Khayata, M.H. *et al.* (1995) The safety and effectiveness of brain arteriovenous malformation embolization using acrylic and particles: the experiences of a single institution. *Neurosurgery* **37**, 606–615.

Wenz, F., Steinvorth, S., Wildermuth, S. *et al.* (1998) Assessment of neuropsychological changes in patients with arteriovenous malformation (AVM) after radiosurgery. *International Journal of Radiation Oncology, Biology, Physics* **42**, 995–999.

Willinsky, R.A., Fitzgerald, M., Terbrugge, K., Montanera, W. & Wallace, M. (1993) Delayed angiography in the investigation of intracerebral hematomas caused by small arteriovenous malformations. *Neuroradiology* **35**, 307–311.

Yamamoto, M., Jimbo, M., Ide, M., Lindquist, C. & Steiner, L. (1995a) Gamma knife radiosurgery in cerebral arteriovenous malformations: post-obliteration nidus changes observed on neurodiagnostic imaging. *Stereotactic and Functional Neurosurgery* **64** (Suppl. 1), 126–133.

Yamamoto, M., Coffey, R.J., Nichols, D.A. & Shaw, E.G. (1995b) Interim report on the radiosurgical treatment of cerebral arteriovenous malformations: the influence of size, dose, time, and technical factors on obliteration rate. *Journal of Neurosurgery* **83**, 832–837.

Yamamoto, M., Jimbo, M., Hara, M., Saito, I. & Mori, K. (1996) Gamma knife radiosurgery for arteriovenous malformations: long-term follow-up results focusing on complications occurring more than 5 years after irradiation. *Neurosurgery* **38**, 906–914.

Yamamoto, M., Ban, S., Ide, M. & Jimbo, M. (1997a) A diffuse white matter ischemic lesion appearing 7 years after stereotactic radiosurgery for cerebral arteriovenous malformations: case report. *Neurosurgery* **41**, 1405–1409.

Yamamoto, M., Ide, M., Jimbo, M. & Ono, Y. (1997b) Middle cerebral artery stenosis caused by relatively low-dose irradiation with stereotactic radiosurgery for cerebral arteriovenous malformations: case report. *Neurosurgery* **41**, 474–477.

Yamamoto, M., Ide, M., Jimbo, M., Hamazaki, M. & Ban, S. (1998) Late cyst convolution after gamma knife radiosurgery for cerebral arteriovenous malformations. *Stereotactic and Functional Neurosurgery* **70**, 166–178.

Young, W.L., Kader, A., Ornstein, E. *et al.* (1996) Cerebral hyperemia after arteriovenous malformation resection is related to 'breakthrough' complications but not to feeding artery pressure. *Neurosurgery* **38**, 1085–1093.

Zimmerman, R.S., Spetzler, R.F., Lee, K.S., Zabramski, J.M. & Hargraves, R.W. (1991) Cavernous malformations of the brain stem. *Journal of Neurosurgery* **75**, 32–39.

CHAPTER FIFTEEN

What are this person's problems? A problem-based approach to the general management of stroke

15.1 Introduction

The patient's general management, as distinct from the specific treatment of their stroke (Chapters 11–14), is primarily aimed at identifying and solving existing problems, as well as anticipating and preventing potential problems, at different stages of their illness. This chapter will cover the common problems which occur in patients who have had a stroke. Each section is loosely structured as follows:

• *General description of each problem,* which includes a definition, its frequency, causes and clinical significance, and prognosis.

• *Assessment,* including methods of detection, simple clinical assessments and measures which may be appropriate for use in goal setting, audit or research.

• *Prognosis and treatment,* including what is known about recovery and those interventions which may hasten it.

Unfortunately, relatively little research has focused on these aspects of stroke. Few post-stroke problems have been systematically identified in community-based incidence studies (section 17.2.1) so their frequency in unselected populations is unknown. More importantly, there are few large randomized controlled trials or systematic reviews to guide our management. This is partly because there are major methodological difficulties in performing randomized controlled trials and systematic reviews to evaluate non-pharmacological interventions (Table 15.1). Therefore, the content of this chapter will reflect more our own clinical experience rather than high-quality evidence which, at present, is limited. Many of the topics are not specific to stroke medicine but might be included in any textbook of internal medicine or surgery. We have not attempted to provide comprehensive reviews, but instead have concentrated on those aspects of assessment and management which are particularly relevant to stroke patients.

Table 15.1 Problems in performing randomized controlled trials and systematic reviews of physical therapy interventions.

Lack of theoretical model or rationale founded on basic science for many interventions
Ethical problems of performing randomized controlled trials due to therapists' certainty about the effectiveness of their own therapy in individual patients
Difficulty in getting patients, and therapists, to accept the possibility of 'no treatment'
Strong patient preferences based on their belief in the benefits and acceptability of therapy
Difficulty in blinding patients to treatment allocation
Difficulty in designing convincing placebo treatments, or establishing appropriate 'controls'
Difficulties in defining a therapy (in terms of type, dose, frequency, timing and duration) which has to be tailored to the individual patient. This leads to difficulties in applying the results in practice
Failure to identify key components or interactions between components of intervention
Moderate treatment effects mean that large numbers of patients need to be randomized
The need to randomize large numbers of patients may necessitate multicentre trials but these raise difficulties in standardizing and monitoring treatment
Therapy is very labour intensive and therefore expensive, so that bodies which fund research may not be willing to fund the therapy
Difficulties agreeing suitable measures of outcome which are sensitive both to the things which therapists expect to influence, and those which are relevant to the patient and family
In unblinded trials, patient loyalty to a therapist may bias their responses to subjective outcome scales
Heterogeneity of reported outcome measures which hinders systematic review of trials
Problems due to complex interactions with other therapies given simultaneously

15.2 Airway, breathing and circulation

Inadequate airway, breathing or circulation are life-threatening. Urgent resuscitative measures must be taken. Even if not an immediate threat to survival, it seems sensible to optimize the delivery of oxygen and glucose to the brain to minimize brain damage and so achieve the best possible outcome for the patient (section 11.1.3).

15.2.1 Maintenance of a clear airway

Patients with a decreased level of consciousness, impaired bulbar function or who have aspirated may have an obstructed or partially obstructed airway. Central cyanosis, noisy airflow with grunting, snoring or gurgling, an irregular breathing pattern and indrawing of the suprasternal area and intercostal muscles may all indicate an obstructed airway. It is important that apnoeic spells due to an obstructed airway are not mistakenly attributed to periodic respiration (e.g. Cheyne–Stokes) (section 15.2.2). If an obstructed airway is suspected, the oropharynx should be cleared of any foreign matter with a sweep of a gloved finger, the patient's jaw pulled forward, and the neck extended to stop the tongue falling back to obstruct the airway (Fig. 15.1). Positioning the patient in the coma (i.e. recovery) position (Fig. 15.2) may be enough to keep the airway clear, although in some situations an oropharyngeal or nasopharyngeal airway, or even endotracheal intubation, may be required.

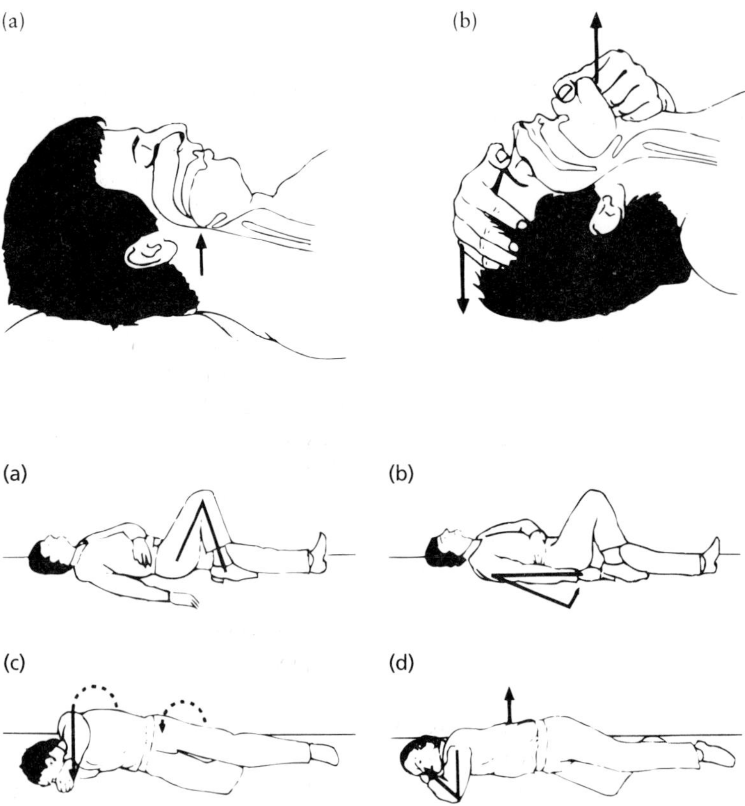

Fig. 15.1 It is essential to maintain a patent airway in a patient with a decreased level of consciousness. (a) In a comatose patient with their head in a resting or flexed position the tongue falls backwards to obstruct the hypopharnyx (arrow) and the epiglottis obstructs the larnyx. (b) Tilting the head back by lifting the chin stretches the anterior neck structures which opens the airway.

Fig. 15.2 If the patient has a decreased level of consciousness and is not maintaining their airway (but does not require resuscitation) one can help maintain an open airway by putting the patient in the recovery position. (a) Flex the patient's leg closest to you. (b) Put their hand closest to you under their buttock. (c) Gently roll the patient towards you. (d) Tilt their head backwards and put their upper hand under their lower cheek to prevent the patient rolling onto their face. Their head should be kept low to encourage secretions to drain away.

Do not mistakenly attribute apnoeic spells due to intermittent airway obstruction to periodic or Cheyne–Stokes respiration.

15.2.2 Inadequate breathing

Strokes may weaken the intercostal muscles and the diaphragm, leading to reduced ventilation, poor cough, and perhaps an increased risk of pneumonia (Houston *et al.* 1995). They may directly, or more often indirectly, impair the function of the respiratory centre in the medulla which results in various disordered patterns of breathing (Fig. 15.3) whilst the patient is awake, but much more commonly during sleep (Bassetti *et al.* 1997).

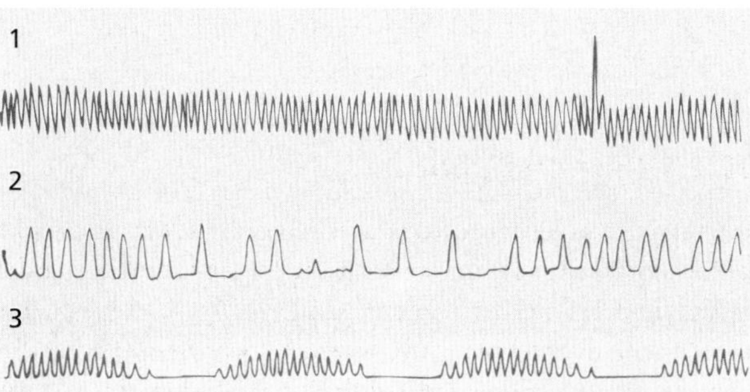

Fig. 15.3 Diagram showing abnormal patterns of breathing which may occur after a stroke: 1, hyperventilation 2, irregular 3, Cheyne–Stokes (with permission from Rout *et al.* 1971).

Abnormal patterns of breathing

The abnormal patterns of breathing associated with stroke include obstructive and central sleep apnoea, periodic respiration (Cheynes–Stokes), hyperventilation ('forced respiration'), irregular (ataxic) breathing, apneustic (held in expiration) breathing and, ultimately, complete apnoea (North & Jennett 1974; Bassetti & Aldrich 1999).

Sleep apnoea has been identified in up to 69% of hospital-admitted patients, depending on the definitions and detection methods used. It is usually 'obstructive' although may occasionally be 'central' and is probably the commonest abnormality (Askenasy & Goldhammer 1988; Wessendorf *et al.* 2000). It has been associated with greater age, body mass index, stroke severity, and diabetes (Bassetti & Aldrich 1999). The clinical significance of this potentially treatable phenomenon is still uncertain. It is plausible that the resulting hypoxia or rise in blood pressure might be associated with poorer outcomes, or increased risk of recurrence.

Periodic respiration (Cheyne–Stokes), where there are regular alternating phases of hyperventilation and hypoventilation, is well recognized. Other neurological functions, e.g.

wakefulness, often vary in phase with the cycle. Periodic respiration, although originally described in left-ventricular failure, has been observed in normal wakeful and sleeping subjects, patients with central sleep apnoea and those with acute and chronic neurological damage (Cheyne 1818; Sprecht & Fruhmann 1972; North & Jennett 1974; Webb 1974; O'Sullivan *et al.* 1984). In 121 (12%) of 991 patients hospitalized with acute stroke, periodic respiration was recorded in the medical notes, but this is likely to be an underestimate because the patients were not continuously monitored (Turney *et al.* 1984). Another study of 39 conscious patients with ischaemic stroke demonstrated periodic respiration in four (10%) whilst awake, and in 11 (28%) during sleep using non-invasive monitoring techniques (Bassetti *et al.* 1997). The mechanisms of periodic respiration are still debated but it probably reflects a change in the sensitivity of the brainstem respiratory centre to the arterial pressure of carbon dioxide ($Paco_2$) and slowed central circulation, with a resultant delay in the feedback loop controlling respiration (Brown & Plum 1961; Karp *et al.* 1961). Whilst periodic respiration may, in an unconscious or drowsy patient, be associated with a poor chance of survival, it is seen quite frequently in patients who are alert and who subsequently make a reasonable recovery (Rout *et al.* 1971; Nachtmann *et al.* 1995).

Periodic respiration (Cheyne–Stokes) does not necessarily imply a hopeless prognosis.

Associated with these abnormalities of breathing pattern one can observe changes in blood gas tension, pH and middle cerebral artery blood velocities, all of which might exacerbate cerebral ischaemia, but their relevance has not been researched adequately (Rout *et al.* 1971; Askenasy & Goldhammer 1988; Wardlaw 1993; Nachtmann *et al.* 1995).

Co-existing cardiopulmonary disease (e.g. chronic obstructive pulmonary disease, pneumonia) is probably a more frequent cause of inadequate ventilation than the abnormal breathing patterns due to the stroke itself. Its detection depends on a thorough initial assessment including an adequate history, physical examination and some simple investigations, e.g. electrocardiogram (section 10.3.2).

Assessment

The adequacy of ventilation should be assessed clinically by checking for central cyanosis and examining the chest and, where there is doubt, by measuring the arterial blood gases. We increasingly use pulse oximetry to assess and monitor our patients. Finger probes are more accurate than those on the ear, and it probably does not matter whether the probe is placed on the paretic or non-paretic hand (Jensen *et al.* 1998; Roffe *et al.* 1999).

Treatment

If the patient is hypoxic, the inspired oxygen concentration should be increased, but with care if the patient has chronic lung disease and a tendency to hypercapnoea, in which case 24% oxygen should be used initially with careful monitoring of the patient's respiration, neurological function (section 15.5), and arterial blood gases. There are currently no data to support the *routine* administration of increased concentrations of oxygen to patients who are not hypoxic, nor the use of continuous positive airways pressure (CPAP) in patients with obstructive sleep apnoea which is identified after an acute stroke (Ronning & Guldvog 1999). Treatment for any co-existing lung or cardiac disease should be given. Although sitting the patient up may help to improve oxygenation, this has not been a consistent finding in all studies (Pang *et al.* 1988; Elizabeth *et al.* 1993; Misra *et al.* 1997; Rowat *et al.* 1998). If the patient is sat out of bed, it is important that they are well supported in an upright position and not slumped in the chair, the latter position worsens ventilation. Sitting may also reduce the intracranial pressure, but may cause other problems (section 15.11).

Tracheal intubation and mechanical ventilation are sometimes useful, either to maintain ventilation or reduce intracranial pressure (section 11.8.4), however, practice varies greatly between centres and there is little reliable evidence to guide such treatment decisions (Gujjar *et al.* 1998; Bushnell *et al.* 1999). Often, such aggressive management is considered inappropriate because of the patient's low probability of regaining a good quality of life (section 10.4). Sedative drugs, given to promote sleep, to facilitate imaging or to control seizures, may precipitate periodic respiration or respiratory failure and should generally be avoided although interestingly there is a suggestion that some, e.g. benzodiazepines, may potentially be neuroprotective (section 11.6). Although theophylline has been used successfully to reverse periodic respiration, the indications for its use are unclear (Nachtmann *et al.* 1995).

If the patient is nursed in a sitting position, it is best if they are well supported and upright in a chair rather than slumped in bed or a chair, the latter position makes breathing more difficult.

15.2.3 Poor circulation

Both severe brainstem dysfunction and massive subarachnoid haemorrhage can cause major circulatory problems such as neurogenic pulmonary oedema, cardiac dysrhythmias and erratic blood pressure with severe hyper- or hypotension (section 13.10). More frequently, circulatory failure, with or without hypotension or hypoxia related to pulmonary oedema, is due to co-existent heart disease (e.g. congestive cardiac failure, myocardial infarction, atrial fibrillation), hypovolaemia (e.g. dehydration, bleeding), or severe infection.

Cardiac dysrhythmias

Cardiac dysrhythmias are quite common after an acute stroke, although they rarely cause major problems (Reinstein *et al.* 1972; Lavy *et al.* 1974; Norris *et al.* 1978; Britton *et al.* 1979; Mikolich *et al.* 1981; Rem *et al.* 1985). The most clinically important, in terms of frequency and effect on management, is atrial fibrillation which occurs in about 17% of patients with stroke, 18% of those with ischaemic stroke and 11% of those with primary intracerebral haemorrhage (Sandercock *et al.* 1992). In the majority of cases, atrial fibrillation precedes the stroke and in some it is presumably the cause of the stroke (section 6.5). Of course, a small proportion of ischaemic strokes (5% in the Oxfordshire Community Stroke Project) occur in the context of a recent (within 6 weeks) myocardial infarction (section 7.10) (Sandercock *et al.* 1989). *Routine* monitoring of the patient's cardiac rhythm is probably not necessary unless there is a clinical problem (e.g. palpitations, syncope, unexplained breathlessness or recent myocardial infarction). Ambulatory recording of the electrocardiogram can be useful to establish whether patients have paroxysmal atrial fibrillation which will influence decisions about anticoagulation for secondary prevention (section 16.5).

Cardiac dysrhythmias are quite common after an acute stroke, but seldom seem to be a problem unless they are due not to the stroke itself but to a recent myocardial infarction.

Myocardial injury

It is important to identify the presence and likely cause of any circulatory failure, by clinical assessment of the cardiovascular system backed up with relevant investigations (e.g. cardiac enzymes, electrocardiogram (ECG) or echocardiography). ST-segment depression on 24-h ECG monitoring occurred in 15 (37%) of 40 acute stroke patients in one study although it is unclear whether this was due to myocardial ischaemia and whether this finding has any predictive value with respect to outcome (Raicevic *et al.* 1998). Raised plasma creatine kinase (CK) levels are not found uncommonly but the interpretation may be difficult where the patient has fallen, been injured, lain on a hard floor or had a generalized seizure which may all increase the CK level. Measurement of more cardiac specific isoenzymes (i.e. muscle–brain (MB) fraction) may only partially resolve the difficulties and the value of cardiac troponins as an indicator of myocardial damage has not yet been established in acute stroke (Norris *et al.* 1979; James *et al.* 2000). Transient rises in cardiac enzymes have been attributed to focal regions of myocardial necrosis (i.e. myocytolysis) which have been identified at post-mortem, but their clinical importance is uncertain (Dimant & Grob 1977; Norris *et al.* 1979). One population-based study suggested that about 1% of strokes occurred in the context of a recent (<28 days) myocardial infarction (Mooe *et al.* 1999). Patients with circulatory failure, atrial fibrillation and recent myocardial infarction have a poor prognosis for survival and functional recovery after stroke (Sandercock *et al.* 1992; Mooe *et al.* 1999). Active treatment of these problems is likely to improve the patients' outcome but a detailed account is beyond the scope of this book.

Gastrointestinal haemorrhage

Although so-called 'stress ulceration' with associated bleeding is well described in critically ill patients, including those with head injury, little has been written about gastrointestinal haemorrhage after stroke (Gottlieb *et al.* 1986; Metz *et al.* 1993). Early studies showed very high rates of gastrointestinal haemorrhage varying from 10% (Messina *et al.* 1979) to 19% (Kitimura & Ito 1976) but the patients in these series were not representative of the generality of even those strokes admitted to hospital. Wijdicks *et al.* (1994) reported a frequency of only 0.1% in patients admitted to the Mayo Clinic, but relied on routinely coded data and so may well have underestimated the real frequency. In one of our hospitals, 18 (3%) of 607 patients admitted with a stroke had a documented upper gastrointestinal bleed, 50% of which were associated with systemic hypotension (systolic blood pressure <100 mmHg) or a fall of at least 2 g/dL in haemoglobin concentration (Davenport *et al.* 1996a). Bleeds were more common in elderly patients and those with severe strokes and, perhaps for this reason, few patients were thoroughly investigated to establish the source of bleeding. Kitimura and Ito (1976) performed routine endoscopic gastroscopy in 177 Japanese acute stroke patients, 75 with intracerebral haemorrhage, 54 with ischaemic stroke and 48 with subarachnoid haemorrhage. Thirty-three (19%) had haematemesis or malaena and 64 (36%) had evidence of bleeding on endoscopy. Ten (6%) of the 177 had an acute ulcer, 19 (11%) had erosions, and 63 (36%) had petechiae on endoscopy. These endoscopic changes and gastrointestinal haemorrhage were most frequent in haemorrhagic strokes, those with decreased conscious level and were associated, not surprisingly, with an increased mortality. In our study, 10 (56%) of the 18 patients with gastrointestinal haemorrhage died and only five of the eight survivors were eventually discharged to their own home (Davenport *et al.* 1996a). Clearly, hypotension and anaemia might both exacerbate cerebral ischaemia and worsen the neurological outcome. Although there is little evidence to support routine prophylaxis with acid-suppressing or mucosal protecting drugs after stroke, one should obviously be aware of these patients' bleeding potential when prescribing antithrombotic and anti-inflammatory medication (Koch *et al.* 1996). We try to avoid using non-steroidal anti-inflammatory drugs unless there is a strong indication.

15.3 Reduced level of consciousness

About 15% of stroke patients in the Oxfordshire Community Stroke Project had a reduced level of consciousness (Table 15.2) during the first few days after the stroke, whilst 420 (42%) of 991 patients admitted to the Mayo Clinic were recorded as having a reduced level of consciousness (Turney *et al.* 1984). Clearly, the higher proportion in the hospital-based study is likely to have been due to referral bias, i.e. severe strokes were over-represented. The causes of drowsiness or unconsciousness in stroke patients are not entirely clear (Plum & Posner 1980). It may arise from direct (e.g. haemorrhage or infarction), or more commonly indirect damage (from raised intracranial pressure) to the brainstem. However, we not infrequently see patients with large ischaemic, apparently unilateral hemispheric strokes who become drowsy within hours of onset, before one would expect enough oedema to have developed to raise intracranial pressure markedly and with little or no apparent mass effect on brain imaging (Melo *et al.* 1992). Indeed, in one study, only a minority of patients whose conscious level deteriorated after a large hemispheric ischaemic stroke had globally raised intracranial pressure on invasive monitoring (Frank 1995). It has been argued that differences in pressure between brain compartments may be more important. Level of consciousness is an important indicator of the severity of the stroke and a valuable prognostic variable (section 10.2.7). The patient's level of consciousness is frequently used to guide the need for intervention, and those who are drowsy or unconscious are at greater risk of developing secondary complications, for example, aspiration or pressure sores.

Assessment

The most commonly used measure of level of consciousness is the Glasgow Coma Scale (GCS) (Table 3.5), which reliably documents the patient's spontaneous actions as well as those in response to verbal and painful stimuli (Wijdicks *et al.* 1998). Although useful, this scale, which was originally designed for patients with head injury, has a number of problems when applied to stroke. The most important is that many patients with stroke are dysphasic and therefore have a reduced score on the verbal response scale. Thus, a patient may have a reduced total score on the GCS but a normal level of consciousness. In such cases it is reasonable to ignore the verbal score (Prasad & Menon 1998). Inexperienced users may apply the motor scale to the affected arm in a patient with a hemiparesis and obtain a reduced motor response rather than the 'best' response. The GCS communicates most information if the component scores are recorded separately. The Reaction Level Scale, a unidimensional scale, although less widely used than the GCS, is an alternative tool for monitoring level of consciousness and may be more sensitive to

Table 15.2 The frequency of various clinical features amongst 675 patients with a first-ever-in-a-lifetime stroke at their initial assessment by a study neurologist (from the Oxfordshire Community Stroke Project, unpublished data).

Clinical feature	Number (%)	Not assessable (%)
Glasgow Coma Scale (motor < 6)	86 (13)	15 (2)
Glasgow Coma Scale (eyes < 4)	98 (15)	16 (2)
Glasgow Coma Scale (eyes + motor < 10)	111 (16)	16 (2)
High blood pressure (systolic > 160 mmHg)	311 (46)	19 (3)
Very high blood pressure (systolic > 200 mmHg)	90 (13)	19 (3)
High blood pressure (diastolic > 100 mmHg)	131 (19)	22 (3)
Very high blood pressure (diastolic > 120 mmHg)	23 (3)	22 (3)
Epileptic seizures within 24 h	14 (2)	0 (0)
Facial weakness	256 (38)	40 (6)
Arm or hand weakness	344 (51)	32 (5)
Leg weakness	307 (45)	34 (5)
Unilateral weakness of at least two of face, arm and leg	331 (49)	0 (0)
Sensory loss (proprioception)	101 (15)	168 (25)
Sensory loss (spinothalamic)	196 (29)	140 (21)
Homonymous visual field defect	113 (18)	134 (20)
Gaze palsy	50 (7)	36 (5)
Mental test score < 8/10 (Hodkinson 1972)	85 (13)	135 (20)
Visuospatial dysfunction	81 (12)	179 (27)
Dysphasia	122 (19)	111 (16)
Dysarthria	135 (20)	127 (19)

mild reductions in conscious level, and be more easily interpreted in aphasic patients (Starmark *et al.* 1988; Johnstone *et al.* 1993).

Patients who have a reduced level of consciousness are at greater risk of developing complications (Table 15.3), so expert nursing care is needed to minimize these risks. Also, a falling level of consciousness may alert one to an important and potentially reversible condition (Table 15.4). Therefore, patients with severe strokes, and in whom active treatment would be considered, should be monitored with the GCS for the first few days, especially where staff change frequently, to avoid delays in initiating investigation and treatment of any worsening condition. We usually decrease the frequency of monitoring, e.g. hourly, two, three or six hourly, over the first few days after the stroke. The rate at which the frequency of monitoring is reduced will depend on the team's judgement about the likelihood of deterioration and the appropriateness and urgency of any intervention aimed at reversing the deterioration. Also, the availability of nursing staff to perform the measurements and the patient's need for unbroken sleep have to be taken into account. Therefore, one might monitor a patient's GCS hourly during the first 2 days after a cerebellar haematoma (in whom decompressive surgery would be considered) but only six hourly in a patient who is stable 2 days after a mild ischaemic stroke. The investigation and treatment of patients with a falling level of consciousness are similar to those with other indicators of worsening and are discussed in section 15.5. The specific treatment of patients with raised intracranial pressure is discussed in section 11.8.

Table 15.3 Common complications in patients with a depressed level of consciousness after stroke.

Complication	Section
Urinary incontinence	15.14
Faecal incontinence or constipation	15.15
Airway obstruction	15.2.1
Fever and infection	15.12
Aspiration	15.17
Dehydration	15.18.1
Malnutrition	15.19.1
Pressure sores	15.16

Table 15.4 Remediable causes of a reduced level of consciousness after stroke.

Causes	Section
General	
Hypoxia	15.2.2
Hypotension	15.2.3
Severe infection	15.12
Electrolyte imbalance	15.18.2
Drugs, e.g. benzodiazepines, opiate analgesics	
Neurological	
Epileptic seizures	15.8
Raised intracranial pressure	11.8, 12.2.2
Obstructive hydrocephalus (e.g. in cerebellar haematoma)	12.2.6
Cerebral ischaemia after subarachnoid haemorrhage	13.8

15.4 Severe stroke vs. apparently severe stroke

It is important to be aware that severe concurrent illness or stroke complications may make a stroke appear much worse than it really is (Table 15.5). The clinical features indicating a severe stroke (e.g. reduced level of consciousness) and poor prognosis may be due to the complicating illness. For example, a patient with a pure motor stroke (lacunar syndrome) (section 4.3.2) and a severe chest or urinary infection may be drowsy or confused. It is then difficult to differentiate this clinical picture from that due to a major middle cere-

Table 15.5 Causes of apparently severe strokes.

Non-neurological	
Infection	Respiratory Urinary Septicaemia
Metabolic	Dehydration Electrolyte disturbance Hypoglycaemia
Drugs	Major and minor tranquillizers Baclofen Lithium toxicity Anticonvulsant toxicity Antiemetics
Hypoxia	Pulmonary embolism Chronic pulmonary disease Pulmonary oedema
Hypercapnoea	Chronic pulmonary disease
Others	Limb or bowel ischaemia in patients with a cardiac or aortic arch source of embolism
Neurological	
Obstructive hydrocephalus in patients with stroke in the posterior fossa, or subarachnoid haemorrhage	
Epileptic seizures, including complex partial seizures	

bral artery territory infarction (total anterior circulation infarction). Of course, an infection is more easily treated than a large volume of necrotic brain, so with appropriate therapy the prognosis of the two patients will be quite different. A thorough general examination will identify signs such as fever, confusion and agitation, increased respiratory rate, tender abdomen or purulent urine, and usually indicate any relevant co-existing disorder. Simple investigations such as a white blood cell count, erythrocyte sedimentation rate, urea and electrolytes, urine microscopy and culture, chest X-ray, ECG and blood cultures are useful, not only to identify the cause of the stroke (sections 6.7.1 and 6.7.2), but also to alert one to serious co-existing non-stroke disease. Seizures that have occurred since stroke onset make the assessment of stroke severity particularly difficult so that treatment may be needed to prevent further seizures (section 15.8). It is important not to overlook the possibility that any decreased conscious level is due to sedative drugs.The treatment of apparently severe strokes will depend on the specific problem identified or suspected.

A 70-year-old man was found unconscious at home and admitted to hospital. In the receiving unit he had a partial seizure affecting his right side with secondary generalization. Subsequent neurological examination revealed a reduced conscious level (Glasgow Coma Scale: eye 2, motor 4, verbal 1), deviated gaze and a flaccid paralysis of the right side. Brain CT scan on the day of admission was normal. A diagnosis of a severe ischaemic stroke was made and the decision not to resuscitate was recorded in the notes. He was given intravenous fluids but no anticonvulsants. He was later reviewed by the stroke physician who having found occasional twitching movements of the right hand, reversed the decision not to resuscitate and started anticonvulsants with an initial loading dose. The patient improved and 4 days later was discharged from hospital without residual neurological deficits. Therefore, do not 'write off' people with apparently severe strokes and recent seizures.

15.5 Worsening after a stroke

Although stroke onset is usually abrupt, the patient's neurological condition may worsen hours, days or, rarely, weeks after the initial assessment. Patients may exhibit a reducing level of consciousness, worsening of existing neurological deficits, or new deficits indicating dysfunction in another part of the brain. A large number of terms including 'stroke-in-evolution', 'stroke-in-progression' and 'progressing stroke' have been applied to this situation, which probably reflects the considerable level of interest in the problem and uncertainty as to its causes (Gautier 1985; Asplund 1992; Castillo 1999). After all, here is a situation where one might be able to intervene to prevent a major stroke. Unfortunately, definitions vary and the literature, as well as clinicians, are confused. Clearly, if we accept that the neurological deficit commonly increases over minutes or hours, then the earlier in the course of the stroke we first see the patient, the more likely we are to observe subsequent worsening. Indeed, it is likely that, as we attempt to introduce acute treatments for stroke, we will become much more aware of the 'normal' worsening over the first few hours and days after stroke onset. We will probably see patients earlier in the development of their stroke and monitor them more closely because they will be in clinical trials, or given a specific treatment for acute stroke. Not surprisingly therefore, estimates of the frequency of worsening in the first day or two have varied considerably but have been reported in up to 40% of hospital-admitted patients (Davalos *et al.* 1997).

The factors underlying the progression of neurological deficits in the first day or two after stroke onset are unclear. For example, what causes the progression of deficits in some patients with lacunar infarction? (Nakamura *et al.* 1999). It has been suggested that worsening in the first day or two is more likely to be due to a neurological mechanism than due to a systemic complication of the stroke. Early worsening is likely to reflect complex interactions between biochemical and haemodynamic factors which are known to be important in the development of ischaemic stroke (sections 11.1.3 and 11.1.4). A history of diabetes, coronary disease, low and high arterial blood pressure, early computed tomography (CT) signs of infarction, evidence of siphon or middle cerebral artery occlusion, and various biochemical parameters including serum glucose and glutamate have all been associated with a greater risk of early worsening (Castillo 1999). Greater age, initial stroke severity and the presence of cerebral oedema on scanning have been associated with late deterioration (Castillo 1999).

Worsening has a number of recognized causes, some reversible, so it is important to detect and treat them early. The literature has tended to emphasize the neurological causes (Table 15.6) but it is important not to miss the non-neurological ones which are more treatable. There is, not surprisingly, considerable overlap with the causes of 'apparently severe stroke' (Table 15.5). The outcome of patients whose neurological condition worsens after initial presentation is predictably poorer than that of patients who remain stable or improve rapidly.

Assessment

To ensure that clinical worsening is identified as early as possible, i.e. when the potential for reversal is usually greatest, it is important to monitor the patient's condition. Regular measurements such as those in Table 15.7 will usually alert one to any problem. However, experienced nursing staff who have regular close contact with the patient may detect a problem at an early stage before it becomes obvious to other

Table 15.6 Causes of worsening after stroke.

Neurological
Progression/completion of the stroke
Extension/early recurrence (section 16.1)
Haemorrhagic transformation of an infarct (section 5.4)
Development of oedema around the infarct or haemorrhage* (section 11.1.5)
Obstructive hydrocephalus in patients with stroke in the posterior fossa, or after subarachnoid haemorrhage* (sections 12.2.6 and 13.9.2)
Epileptic seizures* (section 15.8)
Delayed ischaemia* (in subarachnoid haemorrhage; sections 13.6 and 13.8)
Incorrect diagnosis
Cerebral tumour (section 3.4.4)
Cerebral abscess* (section 3.4.6)
Encephalitis* (section 3.4.6)
Chronic subdural haematoma* (section 3.4.4)
Subdural empyema* (section 3.4.6)
*Non-neurological**
See Table 15.5

*Remediable causes of worsening.

Table 15.7 Parameters to monitor and detect worsening.

Conscious level, i.e. Glasgow Coma Scale (sections 3.3.2 and 15.3)
Pupillary responses (section 3.3.6)
Eye movements (section 3.3.6)
Limb movements (section 3.3.4)
Temperature (section 15.12)
Pulse rate (section 15.2.3)
Blood pressure (section 15.7)
Respiratory rate (sections 15.2.2 and 15.12)
Pulse oximetry (section 15.2.2)
Fluid balance (section 15.18.1)

members of the team. Family members, who often spend long periods with ill patients, may also detect subtle but important changes in the patient's condition. It is important that the physician caring for the patient encourages free communication so this sort of information is made known to those directing the patient's care.

Although there is a long list of the causes of worsening, it is important to consider first those that are most readily reversible (Table 15.6). The majority can be diagnosed by a clinical assessment supplemented by simple laboratory investigations. An urgent repeat CT brain scan is advisable in some situations, for example deterioration in conscious level in a patient with a posterior fossa stroke or subarachnoid haemorrhage who may be developing obstructive hydrocephalus, which may be amenable to neurosurgical intervention. The detection of haemorrhagic transformation of infarction in a patient receiving antithrombotic drugs may influence the decision to continue the medication or not, although there is no available evidence concerning the best policy in this situation (sections 5.4, 11.3.2 and 11.4.2). A CT brain scan that shows that the deterioration was due to an early recurrent ischaemic stroke, especially one in a different arterial territory to the initial stroke, may encourage one to investigate further for a proximal arterial or cardiac source of embolism.

Treatment

Clearly, any treatment will depend on the reason for the worsening (see relevant sections) but it should be emphasized that at present there is little evidence from randomized controlled trials to support the use of treatments such as anticoagulants, thrombolysis, neuroprotection, haemodilution and manipulation of blood pressure (Chapter 11). A small trial which randomized 98 patients to either routine care or intensive physiological monitoring showed that the more intensively monitored patients received more intensive treatment (e.g. supplementary oxygen) and deteriorated less frequently (Davis *et al.* 1999). This preliminary finding, which needs to be confirmed in larger studies, could have important implications for the management of patients with acute stroke (section 17.4.2).

A 65-year-old woman had an acute ischaemic stroke affecting her cerebellum and brainstem. This occurred on a background of a previous occipital ischaemic stroke, impaired renal function and hypertension. After a stormy early course requiring drainage of obstructive hydrocephalus and ventilation on the intensive care unit, she made good progress. She could sit independently, help with washing herself and dressing, and could take a soft diet and fluids safely. She had diplopia, poor balance and complained of vertigo and vomiting which was exacerbated by movement. She was started on regular oral metoclopramide with some relief of these symptoms. She was transferred to a separate rehabilitation ward on a Friday afternoon. Over the weekend she deteriorated. Her speech became very unclear, her swallowing unsafe and she was unable to sit. Infection, metabolic abnormalities and recurrent hydrocephalus were excluded and a repeat MR scan showed no new stroke lesion although this seemed the most likely explanation. The family were advised that the prognosis for a good recovery was poor. The speech therapist, assessing the patient prior to insertion of a percutaneous endoscopic gastrostomy, remarked that the patient's tongue movements were like those of a patient with Parkinson's disease—the penny dropped! The drug chart was reviewed, the metoclopramide was withdrawn and the patient returned to her previous functional state over the next week. She was eventually discharged home, walking and requiring minimal help with everyday activities.

15.6 Co-existing medical problems

Co-existing medical problems are common in stroke patients because they are usually elderly and have associated vascular disease (Table 15.8). Although we have already mentioned the importance of cardiorespiratory diseases in the immediate management of the patient (section 15.2), these and other conditions can be important for many other reasons, not least that they may require treatment in their own right. Severe non-stroke illness can make a mild stroke *appear* severe and thus lead to an inaccurate prognosis and possibly inappropriate treatment (section 15.4). Co-existent cardiorespiratory (e.g. angina, cardiac failure, chronic obstructive pulmonary disease), musculoskeletal (e.g. arthritis, back pain, amputation) and psychiatric (e.g. depression, anxiety) often compound stroke-related disability. So, for example, after several months' rehabilitation, one might have taught a patient with a severe hemiparesis to walk again, but if they also have chronic obstructive pulmonary disease the added effort of walking with a hemiplegic gait over that with a normal gait may mean the patient cannot walk any useful distance. It is important to be aware of the limitations on rehabilitation imposed by pre-existing disease before spending months trying to make a patient walk. It may be more realistic to teach the patient to be independent in a wheelchair. Even if one cannot estimate the impact of non-stroke disease on recovery, knowledge of its existence may explain why a patient is not achieving their rehabilitation goals (section 10.3.4).

Although most patients who survive a stroke improve over weeks or months, many of the co-existing problems, which contribute to disability, progress. Thus, a patient may reach their optimal functional recovery some months after a stroke and then deteriorate due to progression of a co-morbid condition. If this kind of deterioration can be anticipated, it may allow for a more flexible package of care to cope with such fluctuations. There can be few things more dispiriting than to strive to discharge a patient into one form of accommodation and then hear that within a few months their condition has deteriorated to such an extent that the accommodation is no longer suitable. This can shatter the morale of the patient and their carer.

Table 15.8 Frequency of co-existing pathology amongst 675 patients with a first-ever-in-a-lifetime stroke (from the Oxfordshire Community Stroke Project, unpublished data).

	n	(%)
Previous angina	106	(16)
Previous myocardial infarction	112	(17)
Cardiac failure	52	(8)
Intermittent claudication	112	(17)
Diabetes mellitus	63	(9)
Previous epileptic seizures	19	(3)
Previous malignancy	74	(11)
Dependent before stroke (Rankin > 2)	103	(15)

No data were available on respiratory or musculoskeletal problems.

Functional deterioration months after a stroke is unlikely to be due to the initial stroke and much more likely to be caused by a recurrent stroke or the progression of some co-morbid condition such as angina, arthritis or intermittent claudication.

Assessment

A thorough history and examination at the time of admission, perhaps with reassessment when the patient is more active, should identify the main co-existing medical problems. An assessment of the patient's pre-stroke functional status (i.e. what could they do and not do?) is invaluable, not only in predicting outcome (section 10.2.7), but also for identifying co-existing problems. Unfortunately, this is often not recorded in medical records unless specifically prompted (Davenport *et al.* 1995; Rudd *et al.* 1999). One approach might be to estimate routinely a pre-stroke Barthel Index (see Table 17.19) since this covers most of the important activities of daily living (ADL). This sort of ADL checklist is also useful in making a prognosis and in setting rehabilitation goals since, depending on the cause and duration, the pre-stroke functional impairment will determine the best achievable post-stroke functional status. If a patient has, as a result of arthritis, been immobile for 10 years before the stroke, it is ridiculous to try to get the patient to walk after the stroke. Unfortunately, this is often attempted simply because nobody has obtained an accurate picture of the patient's pre-stroke function. This is more likely to happen where the patient has difficulties with communication and no carer is available.

An assessment of the patient's pre-stroke function may also be very important in making decisions within the first few hours after the stroke. Although it may be impossible for anyone to judge a person's quality of life, other than that person themselves, one may deduce something from the patient's function. This may be important where, for example, one is considering antibiotics for a severe infection, or neurosurgery for acute obstructive hydrocephalus in a patient with a cerebellar stroke. It may not be appropriate to submit a previously very disabled or demented patient, who will almost certainly have a poor long-term outcome, to uncomfortable procedures (section 10.4).

Treatment

Clearly, one should aim to minimize the effect of co-morbidity by giving as effective treatments as possible. Where it is not possible to influence the disease directly, it is important to take account of co-morbidity in one's overall approach to the patient. One's intermediate and long-term goals also have to take this into account (section 10.3.3).

15.7 High and low blood pressure after stroke

15.7.1 High blood pressure

High blood pressure is often noted on admission to hospital after a stroke but it then usually falls spontaneously over the next few days (Bath & Bath 1997). Although the raised blood pressure may, in part, reflect the physical and mental stress of hospital admission, or the 'white coat' effect, some of the rise seems to be due to the acute stroke itself (Harper *et al.* 1994b). Raised blood pressure detected during the initial assessment may also indicate chronic hypertension since about 50% of stroke patients are hypertensive before the onset (i.e. at least two readings of > 160/90 mmHg; Sandercock *et al.* 1989). These patients will tend to have higher blood pressures than those without previous hypertension and are more likely to show evidence of end-organ damage, e.g. hypertensive retinopathy, impaired renal function and left-ventricular hypertrophy. Blood pressure in the acute phase is generally higher in patients with intracerebral haemorrhage than ischaemic stroke (Allen 1983; Carlberg *et al.* 1991; Harper *et al.* 1994a).

Assessment

There is considerable variation in the methods used and the frequency of monitoring blood pressure after acute stroke. Traditionally, the blood pressure has been measured in the standard way with a sphygmomanometer and an appropriately sized cuff kept at the level of the patient's heart. However, increasingly, automated non-invasive systems are used which allow more frequent monitoring (even when nursing staff are few) and thus earlier intervention. In the intensive care unit, intra-arterial monitoring is frequently used although this can very occasionally cause peripheral ischaemia. More intensive monitoring is often accompanied by more manipulation of blood pressure, the value of which is currently unclear (see below).

There is no consistent difference between the blood pressure measured in the weak arm and unaffected arm, although there is often a difference between arms which is unrelated to the side of the stroke and probably reflects occlusive vascular disease affecting one arm (Panayiotou *et al.* 1993). Therefore, the blood pressure should be checked in both arms on at least one occasion and monitored consistently in the arm giving the highest reading to avoid a spurious label of labile blood pressure. If the blood pressure is raised on admission it should be monitored to establish whether or not it falls spontaneously. If the blood pressure is high it is important to look for evidence of end-organ damage including hypertensive retinopathy; left-ventricular hypertrophy on clinical assessment, ECG or echocardiography; and renal dysfunction with proteinuria or renal failure. The presence of end-organ damage suggests that the high blood pressure is not simply a response to the acute stroke.

Treatment

There is considerable uncertainty about the relative risks and benefits of lowering the blood pressure in the acute phase of stroke. Treatment may theoretically reduce the likelihood of re-bleeding in intracerebral and subarachnoid haemorrhage and of brain oedema and haemorrhagic transformation in cerebral infarction. However, lowering the blood pressure may reduce cerebral perfusion where cerebral autoregulation is impaired and thus further increase ischaemic damage (Bath & Bath 1997; Potter 1999) (section 11.9). Intravenous calcium channel blockers which, apart from their potential neuroprotective action, also lower arterial blood pressure have been associated with worse outcomes in several randomized controlled trials (RCTs) (Horn *et al.* 2000) (section 11.9). Small trials have not established how blood pressure should be manipulated in the acute phase of stroke and large trials are required to determine how and when we should do so (Bath & Bath 1997; Blood Pressure in Acute Stroke Collaboration 2000).

Until randomized trials are available to answer this question directly, we offer the following advice. If the blood pressure remains elevated (i.e. > 160/90 mmHg) for a couple of weeks, or where there is evidence of end-organ damage, we would give the patient general advice (i.e. salt restriction, weight loss and moderation of alcohol intake) and start an antihypertensive drug, accepting that this timing is arbitrary. The issues of when to start antihypertensive treatment and the choice of agent, for the purposes of secondary prevention, are addressed in section 16.3.1. Our management is similar whatever the pathological type of stroke. Where the patient is already on antihypertensive treatment, it seems reasonable to continue it as long as the patient can swallow the tablets safely and has not become hypovolaemic, which may increase its effect and lead to marked and potentially damaging hypotension. If the blood pressure is very high (i.e. > 220/> 120 mmHg) there may be evidence of organ damage which prompts earlier initiation of blood pressure lowering drugs (Table 15.9). The aim of therapy should be a moderate reduction in blood pressure over a day or so, not minutes. An oral betablocker (in the absence of contraindications) is a reasonable first choice but some authorities advise intravenous nitroprusside or labetalol, with very careful intra-

Table 15.9 Circumstances in which we would consider lowering the blood pressure immediately after an acute stroke.

Papilloedema or retinal haemorrhages and exudates indicating severe hypertensive retinopathy
Marked renal failure with microscopic haematuria and proteinuria
Left-ventricular failure established on clinical features and supported by evidence from the chest x-ray and/or echocardiogram
Features of hypertensive encephalopathy, e.g. seizures, reduced conscious level
Aortic dissection

Note: even these features may be misleading in acute stroke because left-heart failure may frequently be related to co-existent ischaemic heart disease, and seizures and drowsiness may occur due to the stroke itself.

arterial monitoring of blood pressure for resistant cases (Phillips 1994). Nitroprusside has the advantage of a very short half-life so that turning off the infusion quickly reverses the hypotensive effect.

Do not lower the blood pressure in the first few days after a stroke unless there is evidence of accelerated hypertension or end-organ damage.

15.7.2 Low blood pressure

It is difficult to define low blood pressure since, although one could set an arbitrary lower value for the systolic or mean blood pressure, clinically significant hypotension is that which leads to dysfunction of one or more organs. The level at which this occurs will depend on the patients' age, their normal blood pressure, the state of their arterial tree and whether autoregulation is intact or impaired. There is good evidence that autoregulation in the brain is impaired after stroke so that even if a patient has the same blood pressure after stroke as before, cerebral perfusion might be reduced. Unfortunately, judgements about the optimal level of blood pressure after acute stroke are very difficult in routine practice since we have no easy and reliable techniques for assessing organ perfusion. Of course, when blood pressure is very low, patients may show signs of 'shock' (e.g. cold extremities, low urine output, worsening renal function, mental confusion, lactic acidosis) and actions to improve organ perfusion are required. In the International Stroke Trial, low blood pressure after acute stroke was associated with poor outcome even having adjusted for stroke severity (Signorini *et al.* 1999). However, the low blood pressure might not be the cause of the poor outcome but rather the consequence of important co-morbidity (e.g. heart failure, atrial fibrillation) or complications (e.g. dehydration, pulmonary embolism).

Assessment

The monitoring of blood pressure after stroke has been discussed in section 15.7.1. The assessment of the clinical importance of hypotension should include a clinical examination and some simple investigations (e.g. blood urea, arterial blood gases) to identify the features of 'shock' mentioned already. Having established that the patient has low blood pressure which is associated with under-perfusion of tissues, it is then important to establish the cause. Is the patient hypovolaemic, due to dehydration (section 15.18.1) or blood loss (section 15.2.3)? Has the patient had a pulmonary embolus (section 15.13), are they in heart failure (section 15.2.3) or are they septic (section 15.12)? Is the patient on drugs which could lower blood pressure excessively? These questions can normally be answered following a thorough clinical examination, review of the drug and fluid balance charts, and some simple investigations including haemoglobin and haematocrit, neutrophil count, C-reactive protein, urine and blood cultures, cardiac enzymes, an ECG and chest X-ray. Occasionally, further investigation with, for example, an isotope lung scan, an echocardiogram or measurement of right-atrial or pulmonary wedge pressures is required to sort out the cause.

Treatment

This will obviously depend on the cause of the low blood pressure. In our experience, hypovolaemia is the most frequent problem and patients usually improve with intravenous fluids. Obviously, it is important to exclude cardiac failure before giving fluids in this way.

15.8 Epileptic seizures

15.8.1 Early seizures

About 5% of patients have an epileptic seizure within the first week or two of their stroke (so-called onset seizures), the majority occurring within 24 h (Kilpatrick *et al.* 1990; Giroud *et al.* 1994; So *et al.* 1996; Reith *et al.* 1997; Burn *et al.* 1998). Inevitably, estimates of the frequency of onset seizures vary because of differences in case selection, diagnostic criteria, lack of witnesses and methods of follow-up (Pohlmann-Eden *et al.* 1996). The majority of onset seizures are partial although often with secondary generalization (Kilpatrick *et al.* 1990; Reith *et al.* 1997) (section 3.4.2) (Table 15.2). Onset seizures are more common in severe strokes, those due to haemorrhage and those involving the cerebral cortex (Kilpatrick *et al.* 1990; Giroud *et al.* 1994; So *et al.* 1996; Reith *et al.* 1997; Burn *et al.* 1998).

15.8.2 Later seizures

In population-based cohorts, which are relatively unaffected by hospital referral bias, the risk of having a first seizure, excluding onset seizures, is between 3% and 5% in the first year after a stroke and about 1–2%/year thereafter (So *et al.* 1996; Burn *et al.* 1998) (Fig. 15.4). This represents a greatly increased relative risk of seizure (perhaps 20-fold) compared with stroke-free individuals of similar age. Patients with onset seizures, haemorrhagic strokes and infarcts involving the cerebral cortex have the highest overall risk of seizures (Kilpatrick *et al.* 1992; Burn *et al.* 1998). Seizures may recur in about 50% of the patients, but are rarely troublesome if accurately diagnosed and appropriately treated. Patients who become functionally independent and who have not yet had a seizure are at very low risk of post-stroke seizures. The *theoretical* future risk of seizures is not great enough to prevent the patient driving (Burn *et al.* 1998).

The risk of having an epileptic seizure after a first-ever-in-a-lifetime stroke is, on average, about 5% in the first year and 1–2% per year thereafter. However, the risk is higher in patients with haemorrhagic stroke, large ischaemic strokes involving the cortex and lower in patients with lacunar and posterior circulation strokes.

Assessment

The diagnosis of seizures should, as usual, be based on a detailed description of the attack from the patient, and if possible a witness, and may very occasionally be confirmed by electroencephalography (EEG) during a seizure. If patients have seizures in the first few days after the stroke, and especially if they are partial, they should be investigated. Non-stroke lesions complicated by post-seizure impairments (e.g. Todd's paresis) may mimic strokes (section 3.4.2). Because the neurological deficits and conscious level may be temporarily much worse immediately after a seizure, 'onset seizures' can make the assessment of stroke severity unreliable (section 15.4). We have also seen occasional patients who have had non-convulsive status epilepticus, a diagnosis which can only be confirmed by EEG, who may, for example, be severely dysphasic, and who have improved dramatically with anticonvulsant treatment. Also, seizures should not automatically be attributed to the stroke since many other causes may be present coincidentally, or as a consequence of the stroke (Table 15.10): appropriate investigations should be performed to exclude these. Finally, seizures may mimic recurrent stroke if associated with worsening of the original focal deficit; this is particularly confusing if any seizures have been unwitnessed and the patient presents with worsening of their earlier stroke (section 15.5).

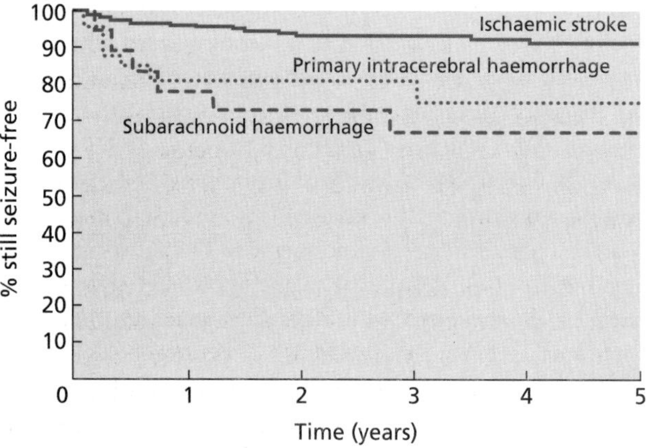

Fig. 15.4 A Kaplan–Meier plot showing the proportion of patients remaining seizure free at increasing intervals after a first-ever-in-a-lifetime stroke. Separate plots are shown for patients with ischaemic stroke ($n = 545$), primary intracerebral haemorrhage ($n = 66$) and subarachnoid haemorrhage ($n = 33$). Adapted from Burn *et al.* (1998).

Treatment

Any precipitating cause should be treated. Status epilepticus, although rare, should be managed in the normal way (Lowenstein & Alldredge 1998). There is no evidence to support the routine use of prophylactic anticonvulsants in stroke

Table 15.10 Causes of epileptic seizures after 'stroke'.

General
Alcohol withdrawal
Anticonvulsant withdrawal
Hypoglycaemia (section 15.18.4)
Hyperglycaemia, especially non-ketotic hyperglycaemia (section 15.18.3)
Hyper/hyponatraemia (sections 15.18.1 and 15.18.2)
Hypocalcaemia or hypomagnesaemia
Drugs:
- Baclofen given for spasticity
- Antibiotics for infections, e.g. ciprofloxacin
- Antidepressants given for emotionalism or depression
- Phenothiazines given for agitation or hiccups
- Antiarrhythmics for associated atrial fibrillation

Neurological
Due to the primary stroke lesion
Haemorrhagic transformation of infarction (section 5.4)
Underlying pathology:
- Arteriovenous malformation (section 8.2.4)
- Intracranial venous thrombosis (section 5.5.2)
- Mitochondrial cytopathy (section 7.19)
- Hypertensive encephalopathy (section 3.4.5)

Wrong diagnosis (section 3.4)
Herpes simplex encephalitis
Cerebral abscess
Cerebral tumour
Subdural empyema

patients (including those with subarachnoid haemorrhage (section 13.4.3) who have not yet had a seizure but who are thought to be at high risk. Usually, an isolated seizure does not require anticonvulsants since the risk of further seizures is only about 50% over the next few years. However, if seizures recur, or if the patient wishes to minimize the risk of recurrence because of its implications for driving, employment or leisure activities, treatment after the first seizure may be warranted. We are not aware of any studies which have compared the efficacy of different anticonvulsants in preventing seizures after stroke. Indeed, there is little evidence to suggest that any one of the most commonly used first-line drugs (i.e. phenytoin, sodium valproate and carbamazepine) is more effective than any other in preventing partial or generalized seizures in adults. Each drug has its pros and cons. The direct costs of phenytoin are lower than the others but adverse effects are probably more frequent. The relatively close relationship between drug levels and toxic effects for phenytoin may make the differentiation of toxic effects from other causes of neurological worsening after stroke easier. Some clinicians believe that carbamazepine is the logical choice in stroke patients in whom seizures are usually partial, with or without secondary generalization. We could not come to a consensus on which we should recommend as first choice for treating seizures after stroke. Patients who have had a seizure should be advised not to drive (for a period which varies depending on national regulations), and to inform the necessary authorities. However, many stroke patients who have seizures are too disabled to drive anyway (section 15.32.2).

15.9 Headache, nausea and vomiting

Headache is quite a common symptom after stroke and may provide clues to the pathological type of stroke (e.g. haemorrhagic) and its cause (e.g. giant cell arteritis) (sections 3.3.10 and 6.6.6). It is often associated with nausea or vomiting, most commonly in haemorrhagic and vertebrobasilar strokes (Canhao *et al.* 1997). Nausea or vomiting without headache is often secondary to vertigo. These symptoms, which can be severe initially, usually improve within a few days. Having established that there is no sinister underlying cause, most patients simply require reassurance that the pain will improve, adequate analgesia and/or antiemetics. However, these drugs may have adverse effects (see case history in section 15.5). Persistent vertigo which may be positional and associated with nausea or vomiting can be a particularly troublesome symptom, most commonly after vertebrobasilar strokes. It may not respond to antiemetics, indeed some authorities believe that these may inhibit tolerance developing. The place of so-called vestibular rehabilitation in such cases is unclear.

Table 15.11 Some of the drugs used to treat hiccups (most have important adverse effects) (from Launois *et al.* 1993).

Chlorpromazine
Haloperidol
Metoclopramide
Sodium valproate
Phenytoin
Carbamazepine
Nifedipine
Amitriptyline
Baclofen

15.10 Hiccups

Hiccups are due to involuntary diaphragmatic contractions with closure of the glottis. The precise cause is unclear. They may be persistent and troublesome in patients with strokes affecting the medulla. If they persist, other causes should be considered (e.g. uraemia, diaphragmatic irritation). Numerous folk cures, e.g. sudden frights, and drugs (Table 15.11) have been suggested as effective treatments. Drugs may occasionally be worth trying where hiccups are persistent and distressing to the patient but most have significant adverse effects. The management of hiccups has been thoroughly reviewed elsewhere (Launois *et al.* 1993; Friedman 1996).

15.11 Immobility and poor positioning

Immobility is a major consequence of impaired conscious level; severe motor deficits including weakness, ataxia and apraxia; and less commonly of sensory (i.e. proprioceptive) and visuospatial deficits. Immobility makes the patient vulnerable to a number of complications such as infections (section 15.12), deep venous thrombosis (DVT) and pulmonary embolism (section 15.13), pressure sores (section 15.16), contractures (section 15.20) falls and resulting injuries (section 15.26). Immobile patients are unable to position themselves to maintain comfort, facilitate activities such as drinking and passing urine, or to relieve pressure over bony prominences. They are in the ignominious situation of always having to ask others to position them.

There has been little formal research of positioning after stroke. For example, after a stroke should the patient be nursed sitting or lying, and if lying, on which side? There is some evidence regarding the optimum positioning of mechanically ventilated patients. Nursing semirecumbent has been shown to be associated with a lower risk of pneumonia (Drakulovic *et al.* 1999). In the self-ventilating stroke patient the optimal position(s) are unclear but decisions should take into account the following physiological factors:

• *Maintenance of a clear airway.* In unconscious patients correct positioning is vital to maintain a clear airway and so reduce the risk of aspiration (section 15.2.1).
• *Oxygenation.* Position may influence the patient's ability to breath, ventilate their lungs and oxygenate their blood (section 15.2.2).
• *Cerebral perfusion.* Patients who are hypovolaemic may have reduced systemic blood pressure when sitting which may reduce cerebral perfusion and possibly increase cerebral ischaemia. However, if intracranial pressure falls further on sitting, cerebral perfusion pressure may increase.
• *Cerebral oedema.* Intracranial pressure is highly dependent on posture, being higher in supine patients and lower when sitting (Feldman *et al.* 1992). The relationships between oxygenation, cerebral perfusion, intracranial pressure and cerebral blood flow are so complex that it is difficult to predict the optimum position for nursing an individual patient (Fig. 15.5). Whether our own anecdotal observation that some patients with severe strokes are more alert when sitting up than when lying is explained by reduced intracranial pressure, reduced cerebral oedema, improved oxygenation, and/or increased sensory or social stimulation is not at all clear.

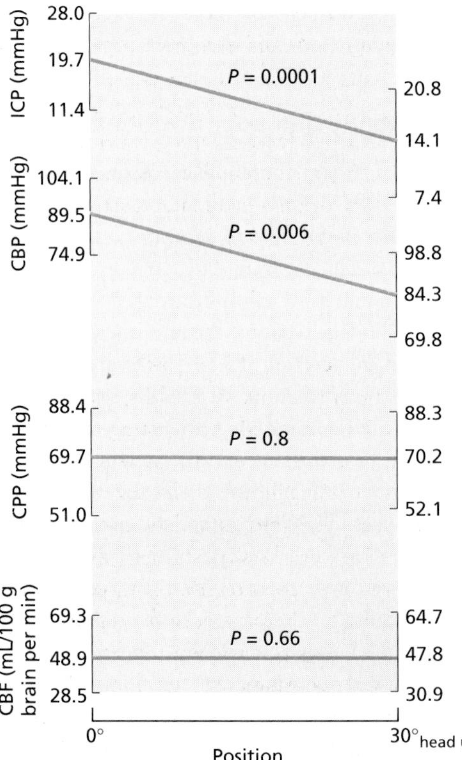

Fig. 15.5 Graph showing the interrelationships between intracranial pressure (ICP), carotid blood pressure (CBP), cerebral perfusion pressure (CPP) and cerebral blood flow (CBF) with changes in posture in patients with head injury (data from Feldman *et al.* 1992).

• *Tone.* The position of a patient influences the tone in their trunk and limbs. Positioning of the patient is used by physiotherapists and nurses to promote higher or lower tone, whichever seems most appropriate for that particular patient. Spasticity and the tendency to develop contractures may be reduced by careful positioning to reduce tone (section 15.20), whilst patients who have low tone in their truncal muscles may benefit from positioning which promotes increased tone and leads to better truncal control. The positioning charts which are so often strategically placed by the patient's bed to guide nursing care give the impression that we know what we are doing (see Fig. 15.14). However, although there is some agreement about the optimum positioning of patients with hemiplegia (e.g. fingers extended, spine straight), there are many areas of uncertainty (e.g. optimum position of the head, foot and unaffected limbs) (Carr & Kenney 1992). There is clearly a need for further research into this area although this will be hampered by difficulties in prescribing specific positioning regimens, in ensuring compliance, and in reliably assessing outcomes (section 15.20).
• *Swallowing.* Easier and safer if the patient is sitting up with their neck flexed (section 15.17).
• *Pressure area care.* For immobile patients who cannot shift their own weight, their position must be changed frequently enough to avoid developing ischaemia of the skin and subcutaneous tissues over bony prominences at weight bearing points (section 15.16).
• *Limb oedema.* The ankles and the paralysed arm of immobile hemiparetic patients frequently become oedematous and painful. This may increase muscle tone and further reduce function (section 15.25).
• *Stimulation.* It is difficult for patients to see what is going on around them when lying flat. This lack of sensory and social stimulation and contact with daily events will encourage sleep and may lead to boredom, reduced morale and sometimes confusion.

The team should assess (and regularly reassess) each patient and decide which of these potential problems are most important. For example, is the patient hypoxic or dysphagic or at particular risk of pressure sores? Depending on this assessment, a positioning regimen which sets out what are thought to be the best positions, and the frequency of repositioning, should be prescribed and re-evaluated.

15.12 Fever and infection

Fever is quite common after stroke although its frequency obviously depends on the population of stroke patients studied, the definitions used, the method, timing and duration of monitoring. All published studies have been of hospital-referred patients, most have defined fever as an axillary or rectal temperature of >37.5°C, and have monitored temperature up to two hourly for 2–7 days. Patients with fever during the first few days after stroke have a worse outcome than those without (Jorgensen *et al.* 1999; Hajat *et al.* 2000; Wang *et al.* 2000). It is unclear whether this adverse prognosis is simply because it is a marker of a severe stroke (i.e. due to loss of central temperature control or resorption of subarachnoid blood); an indicator of an infective complication (e.g. pneumonia or urinary infection); or increases cerebral damage. The last is an attractive, although unproven concept, since it is consistent with research in animal models which has shown that hyperthermia increases and hypothermia decreases ischaemic cerebral damage (Busto *et al.* 1987, 1989; Chen *et al.* 1991; Moyer *et al.* 1992). Table 15.12 lists some of the potential causes of fever after stroke, of which infections are probably the most common (Przelomski *et al.* 1986). Fever and infection may predate the stroke onset, and may actually cause or at least precipitate the stroke (sections 6.3.3, 6.6.7 and 7.11).

Chest infections. Immobile stroke patients are prone to infections, the most common sites being the chest and urinary tract (Dromerick & Reding 1994; Kalra *et al.* 1995; Davenport *et al.* 1996b; Langhorne *et al.* 2000). Chest infections are much more common in the acute stage than later, occurring in about 20% of patients within the first month or two. Chest infections may be due to aspiration, failure to clear secretions, the patient's immobility or reduced chest wall movement on the hemiparetic side. In one post-mortem study, pneumonia was usually bilateral and where it was unilateral there was no relationship with the side of the hemiparesis (Mulley 1981). However, others have found more clinical signs of pneumonia on the side of the hemiparesis (Kaldor & Berlin 1981). Chest infections may be minimized by careful positioning of the patient, physiotherapy and suction to avoid the accumulation of secretions, and care to avoid aspiration (section 15.17).

Table 15.12 Causes of fever after a stroke.

Causes	Section
Infective/inflammatory complications of the stroke	
Urinary infection	15.14
Pneumonia	15.12.1
Deep venous thrombosis	15.13
Pulmonary embolism	15.13
Pressure sores	15.16
Infected intravenous access site	
Vascular problems, e.g. infarction of myocardium, bowel or limb	
Inflammatory causes of the stroke itself	
Infective endocarditis	6.5, 8.2.11
Arteritis	7.3
Co-incidental conditions	
Upper respiratory tract infection	
Drug allergy	

Urinary infections. A prospective study has shown that about a quarter of hospitalized stroke patients develop a urinary infection within the first 2 months and this remains common over the subsequent months (Davenport *et al.* 1996b; Langhorne *et al.* 2000). Urinary infections can be avoided by maintaining adequate hydration and thus urine output, and by avoiding unnecessary bladder catheterization (section 15.14).

Infections are an important cause of mortality and morbidity after stroke and often interrupt rehabilitation (Bounds *et al.* 1981).

There is little evidence to support the use of prophylactic antibiotics to reduce the overall risk of infections after stroke. Ensuring the patient receives adequate nutrition may be important because malnutrition leads to immuneparesis (section 15.19).

Assessment

The patient's temperature should be monitored at least six hourly during the first few days after the stroke and thereafter if there are any other signs of infection, or functional deterioration. However, fever may not accompany infection, especially in elderly and immunocompromised patients. Any functional deterioration or failure to attain a rehabilitation goal should prompt a search for occult infection. Obviously, the cause of fever should be identified using clinical assessment supplemented with appropriate investigations (e.g. blood neutrophil count, C-reactive protein, cultures of urine, sputum or blood, chest X-ray).

Treatment

The treatment of fever will depend on the cause (Table 15.12). We quite often start a broad-spectrum antibiotic, once specimens for microbiological testing have been taken, since delays in treating infections may impede patients' progress. Appropriate antibiotics and supportive treatment (e.g. physiotherapy, oxygen) should be given in established infection. Also, it seems reasonable, whatever the cause of the fever, to use a fan and prescribe antipyretic medication such as paracetamol or aspirin since fever may worsen outcome (see above). Even if such interventions appear to be without risk, one must remember that they take up a nurse's time which might be spent to greater effect in some other activity. The widespread practice of treating fever in the absence of infection, as well as experimental attempts to induce hypothermia after stroke, are not supported by robust evidence from randomized trials (Correia *et al.* 2000).

Any functional deterioration or failure to attain a rehabilitation goal should prompt a search for occult infection.

15.13 Venous thromboembolism

Deep venous thrombosis (DVT) is common in patients with a recent stroke, particularly those with severe weakness of the leg and who are immobile. Studies using radio-labelled fibrinogen to identify thromboses, including those which are not clinically obvious, showed that about 50% of hemiplegic patients have DVT (Cope *et al.* 1973; Warlow *et al.* 1976; Gubitz *et al.* 2000). Studies using less sensitive screening techniques such as Doppler ultrasound and plethysmography suggest a lower frequency of perhaps 5–15%, although the types of patients included and the duration and timing of follow-up inevitably influence these estimates (Desmukh *et al.* 1991; Oczkowski *et al.* 1992). Clinically apparent DVT confirmed on investigation is even less common, occurring in less than 5%, but DVTs may not be symptomatic, or recognized, and still lead on to important complications (Kalra *et al.* 1995; Davenport *et al.* 1996b). Pulmonary embolism (PE) has been identified as an important cause of preventable death after stroke (Bounds *et al.* 1981). However, clinically evident PE has been variably estimated to affect only 1–16% of patients in prospective trials (McCarthy & Turner 1986; Gubitz *et al.* 2000) and 3–40% in observational studies (Langhorne *et al.* 2000). Fifty per cent of patients who die following an acute stroke showed evidence of PE at post-mortem, but it is difficult to judge how much these contributed to the patients' death (Warlow *et al.* 1976). After some of these studies were published, management has changed to include earlier mobilization, more aggressive hydration and antithrombotic drugs (sections 11.3 and 11.4) which may reduce the frequency of thrombosis. It is therefore difficult to judge how important DVT and PE are in determining the outcome after stroke in current practice.

Assessment

DVT should be suspected if a patient's leg becomes swollen, hot or painful or if the patient develops a fever. Unfortunately, the clinical diagnosis of DVT can be difficult because many paretic legs become swollen due to the effects of gravity and lack of movement. If a paretic leg swells whilst a patient is still being nursed in bed, DVT is a likely cause, but where a patient is sitting out or mobilizing the clinical diagnosis of DVT is much less certain. Non-stroke patients who develop a DVT will often complain of discomfort or swelling, but stroke patients who have communication difficulties, sensory loss or neglect may not complain, so that clinical detection will depend on the vigilance of members of the multidisciplinary team.

Where the patient develops clinical evidence of a DVT or pulmonary embolism, confirmatory investigations must be carried out if treatment with anticoagulants is being considered. We would normally use Doppler ultrasound in the first instance to confirm the diagnosis since this is non-invasive, widely available and reasonably sensitive (>90%) and specific (>90%) in detecting at least above-the-knee DVT in symptomatic patients (Tapson 1998). However, it is operator dependent and if there is doubt about the result, or if one wishes to exclude thrombosis in the calf veins, venography should be performed (Weinmann & Salzman 1994). The value of screening asymptomatic patients for DVT has not been established. In considering such a policy one has to remember that the sensitivity and specificity of non-invasive tests such as D-dimers, Doppler ultrasound, plethysmography and magnetic resonance imaging (MRI) is lower in patients who do not have symptoms of DVT than in those with symptoms, and more 'positives' will be 'false-positives' (Wells *et al.* 1995; Becker *et al.* 1996; Harvey *et al.* 1996; Davidson 1998). A ventilation/perfusion isotope lung scan may be helpful in determining the likelihood that respiratory symptoms are due to pulmonary embolism.

The clinical diagnosis of deep venous thrombosis in stroke patients is particularly difficult because, on the one hand, a swollen leg may be due to paralysis and dependancy whilst, on the other hand, a patient may not complain about pain and swelling because of language and perceptual problems.

Prevention

Manoeuvres which may reduce the risk of DVT and pulmonary embolism include the following:

Early mobilization of the patient and avoidance of prolonged bed rest, although the effectiveness of this regimen after stroke has never been tested in RCTs.

Routine use of *full-length graduated compression stockings*. Systematic reviews of RCTs of graduated compression stockings in patients undergoing *surgery* have shown 62–68% relative reduction in the odds of developing DVT (Wells *et al.* 1994; Agu *et al.* 1999; Lees & Amarigiri 2000; P. Roderick, personal communication). Most of these RCTs tested full-length stockings or did not specify the length. The data, from a few small RCTs, are insufficient to determine whether below-knee stockings are effective. The combination of graduated compression stockings and heparin (at least in perioperative patients) appears to be more effective than heparin alone (Agu *et al.* 1999). There have been very few RCTs testing graduated compression stockings in medical patients.

In stroke, unlike surgery, stockings cannot be applied before the onset of the insult (i.e. the surgery itself), so DVTs may develop before stockings can be applied, and patients may be immobile for weeks and have prolonged leg paralysis. Moreover, compression stockings have potential hazards: they occasionally cause acute limb ischaemia, particularly in those with diabetes, peripheral neuropathy or peripheral vascular disease (Fig. 15.6); they are uncomfortable and unpopular with patients and nurses; and considerable nursing resources are consumed in their application and monitoring. They are expensive in some countries and have to be replaced regularly. Only one small RCT evaluating compression stockings in acute stroke has been completed but was inconclusive (Chiodo Grandi *et al.* 2000; Muir *et al.* 2000). Thus it is not surprising that a recent survey of over 3000 UK physicians found no consensus on their value; 46% thought stockings were useful, 26% that they were useless and 28% were uncertain of their value in prevention of post-stroke DVT (Ebrahim & Redfern 1999). This variation must be unacceptable if stockings are effective (since perhaps as many as 50% of patients are currently denied them) or ineffective (since perhaps 50% of patients are subjected to discomfort and somebody must bear the costs). We currently use them in patients we judge to be at particularly high risk of DVT (e.g. patients with severe leg weakness, thrombophilia, cancer or previous venous thromboembolism) but avoid their use in patients with diabetes or symptoms or signs of peripheral vascular disease (Scottish Intercollegiate Guidelines Network 2000). If used, stockings should be fitted in accordance with the manufacturer's instructions and removed daily to check for problems with the skin. Ideally, we would enter patients into a large RCT to establish the effectiveness (or not) of compression stockings in prevention of DVT and PE after stroke (http://www.dcn.ed.ac.uk/CLOTS).

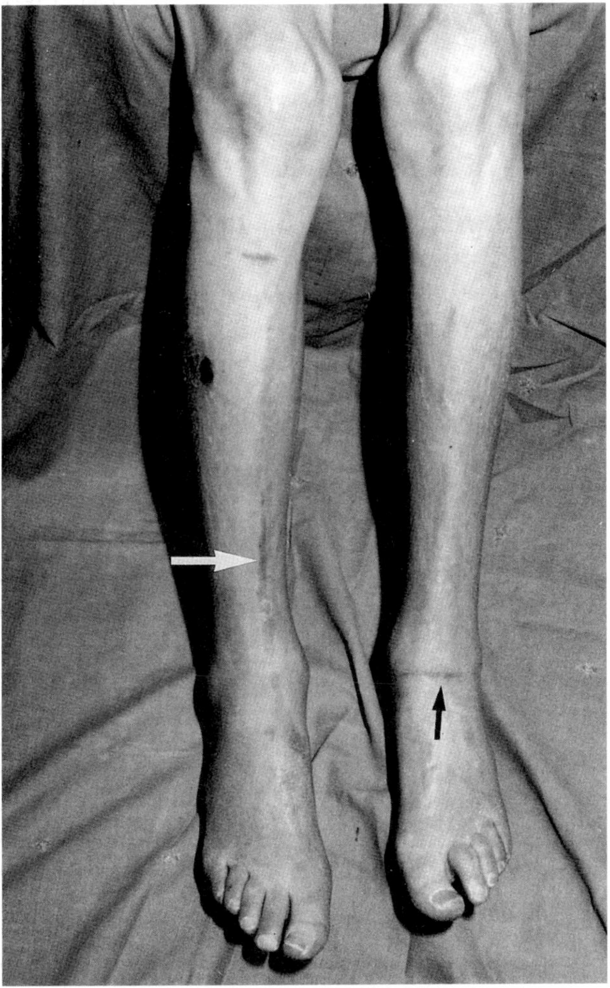

Fig. 15.6 Photograph showing a patient with peripheral vascular disease and diabetes mellitus who was fitted with graduated compression stockings. Note the necrotic skin over the anterior border of the tibia (white arrow) and where the stockings were creased at the ankle (black arrow). There were also necrotic areas over both heels which failed to heal and led to a right above-knee amputation following an unsuccessful revascularization procedure.

Aspirin, started within 48 h of a presumed ischaemic stroke, reduces the relative risk of PE by about 30% and improves the patients' long-term outcome (section 11.3.2). We start aspirin routinely (first dose 300 mg and 75 mg per day thereafter) as soon as we have excluded intracranial haemorrhage or other contraindications.

Heparin has been shown to reduce the risk of DVT in patients with ischaemic stroke, but this benefit is offset by a greater risk of haemorrhagic complications so that routine use of heparin does not improve outcome (section 11.4.2). We reserve heparin (5000 units of subcutaneous unfractionated heparin twice per day) for patients we judge to be at particularly high risk of DVT and PE and low risk of haemorrhagic complications, accepting that these judgements are based on inadequate evidence. Such patients might include those with an ischaemic stroke with leg weakness and immobility, and cancer, thrombophilia or previous venous thromboembolism (Scottish Intercollegiate Guidelines Network 2000) (section 11.4.3).

Other methods of prophylaxis, e.g. external pneumatic compression and functional electrical stimulation, have been suggested but not evaluated adequately (Prasad *et al.* 1982; Desmukh *et al.* 1991; Chiodo Grandi *et al.* 2000).

Hydration/fluids may influence the risk of venous thromboembolism. A systematic review of RCTs testing haemodilution in stroke indicated that it probably reduces the risk of DVT and PE (odds ratio 0.54, 95% confidence interval 0.30–0.99) (Asplund *et al.* 2000). It is unclear whether this is a specific effect of haemodilution or a non-specific effect of improved hydration. We give intravenous crystalloid to most of our patients with acute stroke and immobility, in part because these patients are often unable to take adequate fluids orally (sections 15.17 and 15.18.1).

Treatment

If a patient with a confirmed ischaemic stroke has a proven

DVT or pulmonary embolism, standard or low-molecular-weight heparin (either given subcutaneously or intravenously) should be given. We generally treat patients with anticoagulants even if the thrombus is restricted to the calf veins although this will also depend on the presence of any relative contraindications to treatment. An alternative strategy of repeating the Doppler ultrasound to identify those patients with propagation of the thrombus in the popliteal or femoral veins, and then treating only them is probably reasonable. Low-molecular-weight heparin has practical advantages: dosing is based on the patient's weight, and not regular monitoring of coagulation tests; injections are less frequent; and the subcutaneous route allows the patient to mobilize and thus attend therapy sessions. Low molecular weight heparin is at least as effective as standard heparin in prevention of pulmonary embolism and perhaps safer with respect to haemorrhagic complications, although a lower haemorrhagic complication rate has not been established in stroke patients (van den Belt *et al.* 2000) (section 11.4.6). We would normally continue heparin for a few days whilst starting oral anticoagulants which we continue for three to six months, depending on the patient's mobility (Castro *et al.* 2000; Hutten & Prins 2000). We do not believe that intracranial haemorrhage is an absolute contraindication to anticoagulation since, if a patient has a life-threatening pulmonary embolus, the risk of anticoagulation may be worth taking. We have occasionally anticoagulated patients with a large thrombus in the femoral vein, or a pulmonary embolus, with adjusted dose intravenous heparin within one week of an intracerebral haemorrhage without obvious ill effects. There are few studies which help us make this difficult decision but anticoagulation may be less hazardous than one might expect (Dickmann *et al.* 1988; Boeer *et al.* 1991; Feigin *et al.* 2000) (sections 11.4.4 and 12.2.3). In a small number of patients, insertion of a caval filter or even thrombolysis may need to be considered but these interventions have not been evaluated in RCTs in stroke patients. This is likely to remain the case.

15.14 Urinary incontinence and retention

Between one-and two-thirds of patients admitted to hospital are incontinent of urine in the first few days after an acute stroke (Brocklehurst *et al.* 1985; Borrie *et al.* 1986; Barer 1989a; Benbow *et al.* 1991; Nakayama *et al.* 1997). Urinary incontinence is more common in older patients, those with severe strokes, other disabling conditions and diabetes (Nakayama *et al.* 1997). Urinary incontinence may be caused by the stroke itself, but perhaps 20% of patients have been incontinent before the stroke (Borrie *et al.* 1986; Benbow *et al.* 1991). Although detrusor instability is the most common single cause of urinary incontinence after the first four weeks, many other factors may contribute in the acute stage (Table 15.13). Urinary incontinence is an important cause of distress to patients and carers, increases the risk of pressure sores, often interferes with rehabilitation (e.g. by interrupting physiotherapy sessions or increasing spasticity, section 15.20) and influences the patient's requirements for ongoing nursing care (Brittain *et al.* 2000).

Assessment

To identify patients with urinary incontinence one simply has to ask the carer or nursing staff. These are the people most aware of urinary problems since they have to deal with the consequences. It is important to ask, since many people consider incontinence an inevitable consequence of stroke and thus not worthy of mention. Routine use of a measure such as the Barthel Index to monitor patients' progress on the Stroke Unit should identify all patients with urinary incontinence (section 10.3.7) (see Table 17.19). It is often useful, but frequently overlooked, to ask the patients themselves what they think is causing their incontinence. This may, for instance, help distinguish true incontinence from accidental spillage of urine from a urinal which results from the patient's poor manual dexterity (Fig. 15.7). More detailed information, including urinary volumes, frequency and times of voiding, which can be collated with a micturition chart, may be useful in identifying the causes of incontinence (e.g. diuretics, communication difficulties) and in formulating a management plan.

Where the cause of urinary incontinence is unclear, and if it persists for more than a few days, the patient should be investigated. Urine microscopy and culture should identify infection. Measurement of postmicturition bladder volumes (by bladder ultrasound or catheterization) may be useful in assessing bladder sensation, contractility and outflow. We

Table 15.13 Factors which may contribute to urinary incontinence.

Reduced conscious level
Immobility (cannot get to the toilet in time)
Communication problems (cannot ask to go to the toilet)
Impaired upper limb function (cannot manipulate clothes or the urinal)
Dyspraxias
Loss of inhibition of bladder contraction (detrusor instability so cannot wait to go)
Urinary infection (often without other symptoms)
Urinary overflow due to outflow obstruction (e.g. prostatism)
Faecal impaction
Excess urinary flow due to high fluid intake, diuretics and poorly controlled diabetes
Too few carers/nurses (cannot attend to patients in time)
Importance of maintaining continence underestimated by carers/nurses

(a)

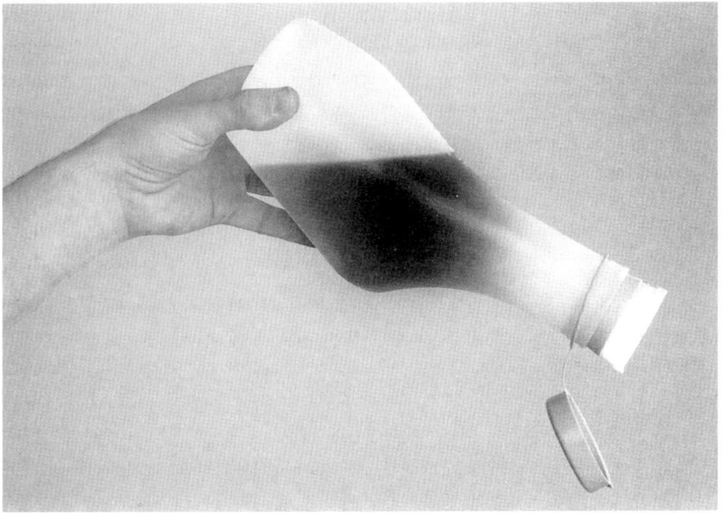

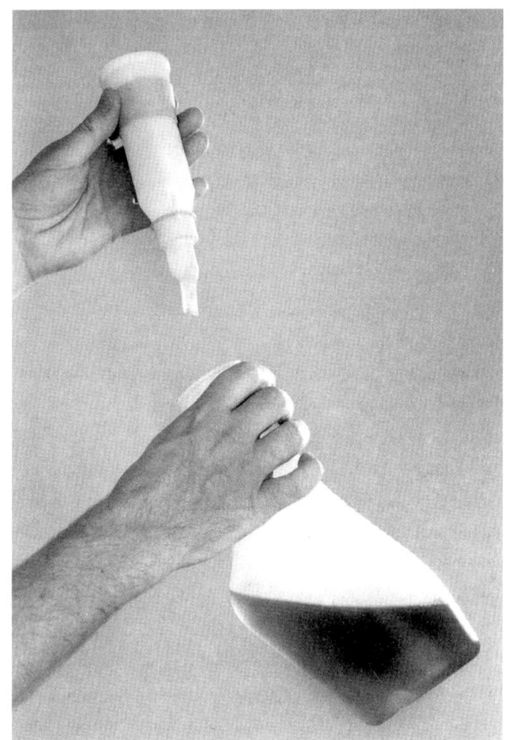

(b)

Fig. 15.7 Some patients have difficulty manipulating a urinal which leads to spills and, effectively, incontinence: (a) this urinal can be inverted without leaking; (b) a simple one-way valve inserted in the neck of the urinal prevents the contents spilling.

reserve formal urodynamic studies, which can identify detrusor hyper- and hyporeflexia and bladder outflow problems, for the few patients with unexplained, troublesome incontinence which persists for weeks after the stroke.

Prognosis

Urinary incontinence is an important predictor of poor survival and functional outcome (section 10.2.7). It reflects prestroke function as well as stroke severity. In one study, 60% of those incontinent on admission (excluding those with occasional accidents only) were dead at 6 months, 14% remained fully incontinent, 10% had occasional accidents and 16% were continent (Nakayama *et al.* 1997). In other words, in survivors, urinary incontinence often resolves spontaneously over the first week or two (Brocklehurst *et al.* 1985; Wade & Langton Hewer 1985; Borrie *et al.* 1986). The patients with persisting problems were often incontinent before their stroke, or immobile or confused (Borrie *et al.* 1986).

Treatment

If a patient is incontinent, but able to understand, then a careful explanation of the cause and likely prognosis should be given. Carers often benefit from such information too. Because urgency of micturition is such a common cause of incontinence in stroke patients, simple steps such as regular toileting, offering dysphasic patients some means to alert the nurses to their needs, improving their mobility, or providing a commode by the bed, can all be effective (Gelber *et al.* 1993). Obviously, one should strive to treat the underlying cause (e.g. infection, outflow obstruction) and where possible remove exacerbating factors (e.g. excessive fluids, uncontrolled hyperglycaemia or diuretics). Having excluded easily treatable causes, we first employ 'bladder retraining' where patients are prompted to void regularly (Gelber *et al.* 1993; Eustice *et al.* 2000; Roe *et al.* 2000). If this does not achieve continence, we use a bedside ultrasound machine to exclude a postmicturition residual of 100 mL or more and then introduce an anticholinergic drug (e.g. oxybutinin) assuming there are no contraindications, e.g. closed angle glaucoma (Azam *et al.* 2000). One must obviously be alert to the possible adverse effects of these drugs (Table 15.14). This approach achieves reasonable results with relatively few patients requiring formal urodynamic studies (Chan 1997; Khorsandi *et al.* 1998).

An *indwelling catheter* should be avoided if at all possible because this makes resolution of urinary incontinence impossible to detect, and may lead to a number of complications (Table 15.15). Intermittent catheterization facilitates detection of the resolution of incontinence but it is unclear whether complication rates are lower than with continuous use, and it is certainly more labour intensive. Other aids and appliances may be useful (Table 15.16) in avoiding unnecessary

Table 15.14 Drugs used to inhibit bladder contractility and their adverse effects.

Anticholinergic drugs
Flavoxate hydrochloride
Oxybutynin hydrochloride
Tolterodine tartrate
Propiverine hydrochloride
Propantheline bromide
Tricyclic antidepressants
Imipramine
Amitriptyline
Nortriptyline
Common adverse effects
Dry mouth
Blurred vision
Nausea/vomiting
Constipation/diarrhoea
Confusion in the elderly
Retention where there is bladder neck obstruction
Precipitation of acute glaucoma

catheterization. However, when patients are at high risk of pressure sores (section 15.16), and other means have failed to keep them dry, or if accurate monitoring of fluid balance is required for some reason, an indwelling catheter may be the best option. Catheterization may also be required to relieve urinary retention (see below) until any cause or precipitating factor can be removed, e.g. enlarged prostate, urinary infection, severe constipation, anticholinergic drugs.

Occasionally, if urinary incontinence is a bar to discharge into the community, long-term catheterization with a silastic catheter may be the preferred option. This issue should be discussed with the patient and, where appropriate, their carer. Continence advisors, nurses with specialist training in the management of incontinence and access to information, aids and appliances, can often help other professionals, patients and their carers. The choice of continence aids is huge but there are few rigorous studies to establish which are most cost-effective, and acceptable to patients and carers (Shirran and Brazzelli 2000). In many parts of the UK, laundry services run by health authorities or social services provide invaluable assistance to families having to cope with incontinence.

An indwelling catheter should be avoided if possible because this makes resolution of urinary incontinence impossible to detect and may lead to a number of complications.

Table 15.15 Problems (and solutions) with indwelling urinary catheters (from Belfield 1989).

Problem	Solution
Pain on insertion	Explain to the patient what is going to happen Use plenty of anaesthetic gel and allow time for it to work
Paraphimosis	Ensure foreskin is not left retracted after insertion
Poor self-esteem	Explain why catheter is needed, how it works and how long it will be in place Provide a discreet drainage bag
Immobility because of drainage bag	Use well-supported leg bag for mobile patients
Leakage	Use appropriate size of catheter Inhibit any involuntary bladder contraction which causes bypassing with an antimuscarinic drug (e.g. Table 15.14) Change catheter if blocked
Blockage	Ensure adequate urine flow Remove encrusted catheter
Infection	Avoid unnecessary catheterization since no proven method of preventing infection
Catheter falls out due to urethral dilatation or pelvic floor laxity	Ensure balloon inflated to correct volume or use larger volume balloon
Catheter rejection due to bladder contraction	Avoid large volume balloon Inhibit with antimuscarinic drug (Table 15.14)
Catheter pulled out by patient	Manage without a catheter to avoid further trauma
Pain on catheter removal	Avoid routine changes Explain procedure to patient Allow adequate time for balloon deflation
Failure of balloon deflation	Introduce ureteric catheter stylet along inflation channel

Urinary retention

Urinary retention, which may be acute or chronic, is quite common in stroke patients, more so in men. The main cause is pre-existing bladder outflow obstruction which may be precipitated by constipation, immobility, and drugs such as tricyclic antidepressants which have antimuscarinic effects. Urinary retention may present with dribbling incontinence, agitation or confusion and is easily missed in patients with a reduced conscious level, communication difficulties or other

Table 15.16 Aids and appliances which may be useful in patients with urinary incontinence (from Smith 1989).

Absorbent pads and pants
These vary in the volume of urine they can absorb, their shape, and the method of holding them in position.

Urinals
Useful for men who are immobile or have urgency which gives them insufficient time to reach the toilet. They can be fitted with a non-spill valve for patients who have poor manual dexterity (Fig. 15.7) or fluid absorbing granules to reduce spillage.

Bedside commode
Useful where urgency is associated with poor mobility so the patient has insufficient time to get to the toilet (Fig. 15.26b).

Penile sheath
Often viewed as an alternative to an indwelling catheter in men without bladder outflow obstruction, but they easily fall off and are therefore unsuitable for agitated or confused patients. Other problems include skin erosions due to urinary stasis or the adhesive strip, and twisting of the sheath and penile retraction during voiding which causes leakage.

cognitive problems. It is important to palpate the patient's abdomen on admission and, later, if urinary problems or agitation develop, to exclude a distended bladder. A urethral catheter provides prompt relief but in men with benign prostatic hypertophy, alpha-blocking drugs (e.g. prazosin) or finasteride (which inhibits the metabolism of testosterone to dihydrotestosterone in the prostate) may enable one to remove the catheter without recurrence of retention. Surgeons and anaesthetists are often unwilling to consider transurethral resection of an enlarged prostate until several months have passed. We are not aware of any evidence to indicate how long we should delay. Recent technologies such as prostatic stents, or so-called 'continent' catheters, may provide more acceptable and safer alternatives.

It is important to palpate the patient's abdomen on admission and, later, if urinary problems or agitation develop, to exclude a distended bladder.

15.15 Faecal incontinence and constipation

Constipation is common after stroke and may lead to faecal smearing or incontinence. Immobility, poor fluid and food intake, and constipating analgesics are common causative factors. Estimates of the frequency in stroke patients admitted to hospital vary between 25% and 40% (Brocklehurst *et al.* 1985; Nakayama *et al.* 1997). Faecal incontinence has been associated with increasing age, diabetes, other disabling conditions, stroke severity and size of brain lesion (Nakayama *et al.* 1997).

Assessment

The frequency of bowel movements should be monitored. Simple monitoring will detect constipation and diarrhoea and may help establish the pattern of any faecal incontinence. Abdominal and rectal examination will usually identify faecal impaction and indicate whether the constipated stool is hard or soft. Occasionally, it may be useful to culture the stool or to X-ray the abdomen to exclude infection or high faecal impaction, respectively, if the patient has faecal incontinence associated with diarrhoea. More detailed investigation is usually not required unless there are persistent unexplained problems.

Prognosis

In one study of 935 patients, 63% of those with faecal incontinence on hospital admission (excluding those with occasional accidents only) were dead at 6 months, 27% remained fully incontinent, 6% had occasional accidents and 20% were continent (Nakayama *et al.* 1997). Achieving continence of faeces is often a crucial step in discharging a patient home since incontinence is so practically and socially difficult to cope with, and is invariably a cause of considerable strain for the carer.

Faecal incontinence which is not associated with severe cognitive problems is almost always remediable by dealing with constipation or diarrhoea.

Treatment

Avoidance of constipation by ensuring an adequate intake of fluid and fibre is the best approach, but laxatives, suppositories and, occasionally, enemas are sometimes required. We find that stimulating laxatives (e.g. senna) are generally more effective than osmotic ones (e.g. lactulose) in elderly patients although the choice will also be influenced by whether the stool is hard or soft. It is important to remember that laxatives may cause incontinence in immobile patients. Where patients are unable to toilet themselves, and a carer is not constantly available, it may be necessary to induce constipation, with for example codeine phosphate, and then relieve this with regular enemas to coincide with visits from a carer.

15.16 Pressure sores

Pressure sores occur when local pressure on skin and subcutaneous tissues exceeds the capillary opening pressure for long enough to cause ischaemia. In addition, friction may cause blistering and tears in the skin. Pressure sores usually occur over weight-bearing bony prominences (Fig. 15.8). Sores occur in patients who are immobile and unable to redistribute their own weight when lying or sitting. The

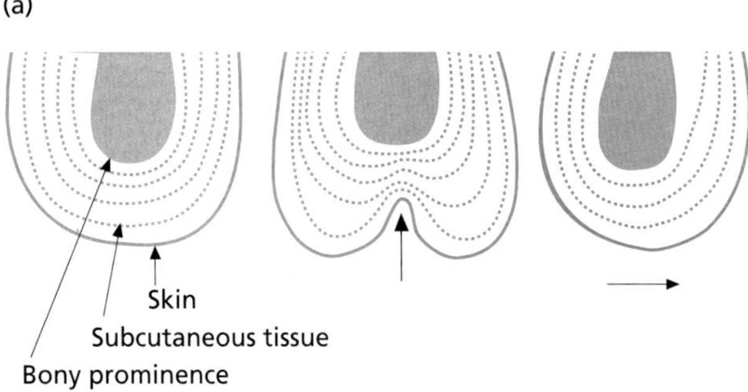

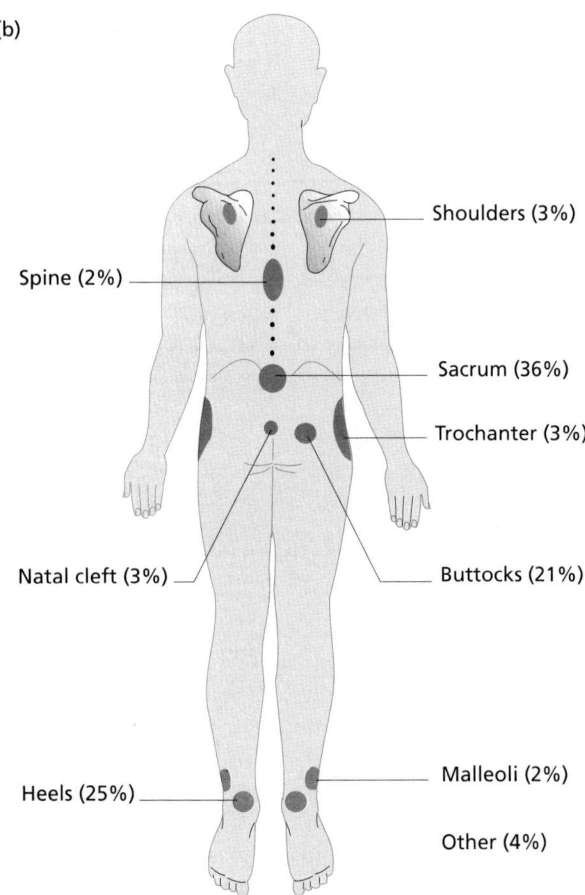

Fig. 15.8 Showing (a) the distortions of tissues over a bony prominence due to compression or shear which may lead to pressure sores and (b) the anatomical distribution of established pressure sores based on data from a cross-sectional survey in the UK of pressure sores in patients being nursed on the Pegasus Airwave System. Patients with cerebrovascular disease were the largest group in this sample but only comprised 14.1% of patients overall (from St Clair 1992).

reported frequency of pressure sores in hospitalized stroke patients is about 3%, but this is bound to vary depending on the population studied and the diagnostic criteria (Kalra *et al.* 1995). Also, one might expect the frequency to be less in the sorts of institutions which are prepared to publish their results. Pressure sores are more common in patients who are malnourished, infected, incontinent or have serious underlying disease (Berlowitz & Wilking 1989). They cause pain, increase spasticity, slow the recovery process, and may be fatal. They prolong length of stay in hospital, often require intensive treatment and can therefore be extremely expensive to health services (Cullum *et al.* 1995, 2000). They can and should be prevented, although they may develop in the interval between the onset of the stroke and admission to hospital.

Assessment

Immobile patients should be examined regularly (sometimes several times in a day) to identify early signs of pressure damage, i.e. skin redness. It is important that patients who are at particular risk of developing pressure sores are identified as early as possible so that preventive measures can be taken. The Waterlow Scale (Table 15.17) is one of many clinical scoring systems developed to indicate an individual patient's risk of pressure sores. Most scales include some measure of mobility, continence, cognitive function and nutritional status and none, based on less than ideal evaluations, is clearly superior to the others (Barratt 1988; Cullum *et al.* 1995).

> *Each patient's risk of pressure sores should be assessed and documented and actions, appropriate to the level of risk, should be taken to prevent pressures sores developing. Pressure sores can be prevented by good nursing.*

The clinician should be alert to behaviour which, in patients with communication and cognitive problems, may indicate a painful pressure area. Such patients may repeatedly move themselves out of a desired position. For example, patients, colloquially known as 'thrusters', with a painful sacrum may force themselves out of chairs by extending their bodies at the waist. This may become a major problem for nursing staff. If patients develop pressure sores it is useful to have some objective measure of their severity so that healing or lack of healing can be monitored. Photographs incorporating a centimetre scale are a convenient and reliable method to demonstrate change, but where this facility is not available, tracing the limits of the sore or simply measuring it in several planes is useful (Allman *et al.* 1987). Several grading scales have been developed for use in research but because they are less objective than say a photograph their inter-observer reliability is inferior (Shea 1975). Patients who are at risk of sores, or who have established pressure sores, should be investigated to exclude malnutrition, hypoalbuminaemia, anaemia and infection (in the pressure sore or elsewhere), all of which can slow healing (Allman *et al.* 1987).

Table 15.17 The Waterlow Scale to assess the risk of pressure sores.

Build/weight	Skin	Continence	Mobility	Sex/age	Appetite
Average 0	Healthy 0	Complete 0	Fully mobile 0	Male 1	Average 0
Above average 2	Tissue paper 1	Occasionally incontinent 1	Restricted/difficult 1	Female 2	Poor 1
Below average 3	Dry 1	Catheter/incontinent of faeces 2	Restless/fidgety 2	14–49 1	Anorexic 2
	Oedematous 1	Doubly incontinent 3	Apathetic 3	50–64 2	
	Clammy 1		Inert/ in traction 4	65–75 3	
	Discoloured 2			75–80 4	
	Broken 3			81+ 5	

A total score of 10 indicates a patient is at risk of pressures sores, one of 15 indicates a high risk and a score of 20 a very high risk. In addition to the basic scale in which the scores for each of the six domains (i.e. weight, skin, continence, mobility, age/sex and appetite) are summed, additional points are added for special risk factors: poor nutrition (8 points); sensory deprivation including stroke (5 points); high-dose anti-inflammatory drugs, steroids (3 points); smoking > 10/day (1 point); orthopaedic surgery or fracture below waist (3 points).

Prevention

The most important measure in preventing sores is to relieve the pressure on the tissues for long enough, and at frequent enough intervals, to allow the tissues to receive an adequate blood supply. This can usually be achieved by regular turning of patients (one or two hourly depending on the assessment of risk) but this takes up a lot of skilled nursing resources. Although the introduction of a variety of special mattresses and cushions (Table 15.18) may reduce the need for regular turning, most patients still need to be turned. Some beds are designed to turn the patient automatically (e.g. the net suspension bed).

Pressure-relieving mattresses and cushions can be divided into 'passive' and 'active' systems (Table 15.18). The 'passive' systems distribute the patient's weight through a larger area and make it easier for patients to reposition themselves (Kemp *et al.* 1993; Hofman *et al.* 1994). High specification foam mattresses are more effective in preventing pressure sores than standard foam mattresses (Cullum *et al.* 2000). 'Active' systems (Fig. 15.9b) usually work by inflating and deflating air cells to relieve pressure on each point at regular intervals, and are more effective than the 'passive' systems in intensive care patients (Cullum *et al.* 2000). However, they are expensive and can make certain nursing tasks more difficult, e.g. positioning a patient to reduce the risk of contractures, to help breathing and to facilitate swallowing, because they offer a less firm base. Local treatments (e.g. creams, lotions) are sometimes applied to unbroken areas of skin to prevent pressure sores developing. Their effectiveness has not yet been demonstrated (Clark 2000).

The ultimate choice of preventative method will depend on an assessment of the individual patient's risk of pressure sore, the availability of nurses, the patient's other needs, e.g. positioning, and available resources. Further research is required to identify the most cost-effective strategy for preventing pressure sores (Cullum *et al.* 1995, 2000). Studies will have to take into account patients' absolute risk of developing sores, the reduction in risk with each intervention and the cost of the intervention, as well as the cost of treating any pressure sores which develop. However, we believe that, whatever technology is employed, adequate numbers of skilled

Table 15.18 Specialized mattresses and cushions.

Passive systems

Sheepskin fleeces and bootees which reduce skin shear and moisture. The natural fleeces are better than man-made ones. They are rendered ineffective by poor cleaning and being covered by sheets

Padded mattresses containing polyester fibres, e.g. Spenco

Polystyrene bead system

Foam mattresses (e.g. Vaperm) vary in their pressure-relieving properties

Gel pads can be used under heels and sacrum

Roho cushions are effective but very expensive (Fig. 15.9a)

Active systems

Ripple mattresses and airwave systems provide alternating pressure; the larger the cells the better but they tend to break down and leak

Low air loss systems (e.g. Mediscus) providing constant low pressure; although effective, tend to be noisy, expensive and complex, needing regular maintenance and training (Fig. 15.9b)

Flotation beds, and deep water beds, are difficult to nurse patients on, are very heavy and some patients get motion sickness. Dry flotation providing constant low pressure produced by glass microspheres blown by air. Air can be turned off when the patient needs to be repositioned. Effective but bulky and expensive

Mechanical beds turn the patient, e.g. net suspension bed. Effectiveness uncertain, patients may not like being suspended (on view). Useful to turn patients who are in pain

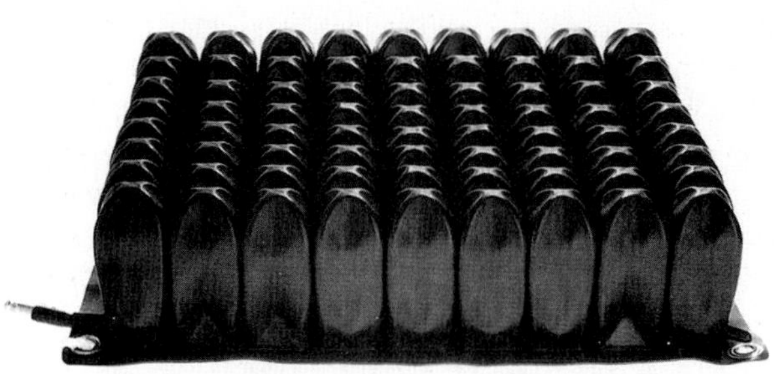

(a)

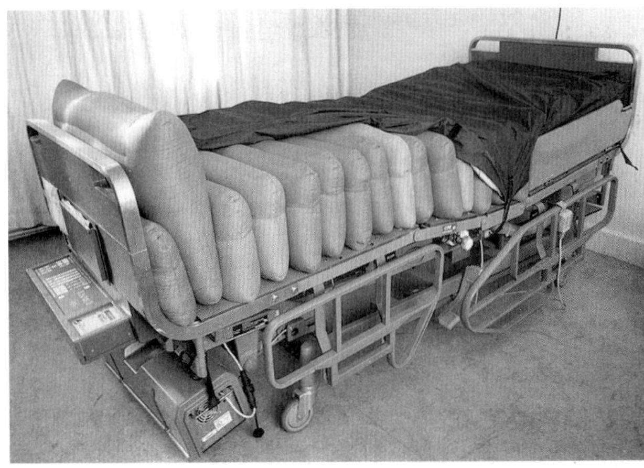

(b)

Fig. 15.9 Pressure-relieving cushion and bed. (a) Roho cushion; (b) low air loss bed.

nursing staff will still be essential if pressure sores are to be prevented.

Treatment

For patients with established pressure sores, the relief of pressure probably remains the most important factor in promoting healing. 'Active' pressure-relieving systems are more effective than 'passive' ones in treatment of established pressure sores (Cullum *et al.* 2000). In addition, it is important to optimize the patient's general condition by providing a good diet with adequate protein intake and by treating concurrent illness aggressively (e.g. infections, cardiac failure). This may need intensive nursing input in frail, elderly, anorexic patients who are drowsy or have swallowing problems. The pain associated with pressures sores may increase tone and lead to contractures which may hinder rehabilitation (Allman *et al.* 1987; Hofman *et al.* 1994). The discomfort may affect the patient's morale and further worsen their outcome. Adequate analgesia should be given to patients and opiates may sometimes be required, especially before renewal of dressings. Antibiotics may be required if there is local or systemic infection (spreading cellulitis, osteomyelitis). Debridement to remove necrotic tissue, and skin grafting to achieve skin coverage, may sometimes be necessary. A bewildering variety of local dressings and treatments (e.g. vitamin C, zinc, ultrasound, electrical stimulation, ultraviolet light) which aim to promote healing and reduce infection are available. Some small RCTs evaluating these have been reported, but need to be systematically reviewed and it is likely that larger studies evaluating the most promising interventions will be required (Bradley *et al.* 2000; Flemming & Cullum 2000a,b).

15.17 Swallowing problems

Up to 50% of conscious patients admitted to hospital with an acute stroke may have an unsafe swallow on bedside testing (Gordon *et al.* 1987; Barer 1989b; Smithard *et al.* 1996; Mann *et al.* 1999). However, estimates of the frequency of swallowing difficulties vary because of differences in definitions, timing and methods of detecting dysphagia and in selecting patients for study. Swallowing difficulties have been associated with a high case fatality and poor functional outcome and certainly put patients at risk of aspiration, pneumonia, dehydration and malnutrition (Smithard *et al.* 1996; Mann *et al.* 1999). However, much of the excess mortality and morbidity is probably due to the severity of the stroke itself rather than the swallowing difficulties.

15.17.1 Mechanisms of dysphagia

The following mechanisms of dysphagia after stroke have been identified with videofluoroscopy (Veis & Logemann 1985; Mann *et al.* 1999):

- poor oral control (oral preparatory phase) and delayed triggering of the swallow leads most often to aspiration before the swallow, i.e. liquid trickles over the back of the tongue before the swallow starts. In addition, patients with weakness or incoordination of the face or tongue often have difficulty keeping fluids in their mouth, and in chewing and manipulation of the food to produce a well-formed food bolus;
- failure of laryngeal adduction which leads to aspiration during the swallow itself;
- reduced pharyngeal 'peristalsis', or cricopharyngeal dysfunction, may allow food to collect in the pharynx and spill over, past the vocal cords and into the trachea. Thus, aspiration occurs after the swallow.

Poor oral control and a delayed triggering of the swallow are the most common mechanisms causing dysphagia after stroke but more than one abnormality can usually be identified.

15.17.2 Detection of dysphagia

Despite their frequency, and the serious consequences of failing to detect them, swallowing problems are often not sought systematically in patients admitted to hospital with an acute stroke (Davenport *et al.* 1995; Rudd *et al.* 1999). There is also no agreement about the best method of screening for dysphagia. Although videofluoroscopy (Fig. 15.10) is usually considered the 'gold-standard', it has a number of limitations, including its impracticality in the acute phase of stroke (Table 15.19). Because of the limitations of videofluoroscopy, a number of clinical tests which can be performed at the bedside to screen patients have been developed (Kidd *et al.* 1993; Smithard *et al.* 1998). Unfortunately, none of them detects all the patients who aspirate, which may be important since silent aspirators may be at greatest risk of complications (Holas *et al.* 1994). Typically, a clinical assessment might identify 50–80% of those with aspiration on videofluoroscopy (Smithard *et al.* 1998). Clinicians often use the gag reflex to indicate swallowing safety but this has been shown to be both inaccurate and unreliable (kappa = 0.3) (Ellul & Barer 1993; Smithard *et al.* 1998). It is unclear whether dysphagia identified on a bedside swallowing assessment, or videofluoroscopic findings, are better predictors of those who will develop complications such as pneumonia (Smithard *et al.* 1996; Mann *et al.* 1999). Some workers have emphasized that the integrity of patients' laryngeal cough reflex may be a more important determinant of the risk of pneumonia than their ability to swallow (Addington *et al.* 1999). The place of other techniques such as pulse oximetry to detect oxygen desaturation, and nasal endoscopy to visualize the pharynx and larynx, during swallowing is unclear. Until further studies have demonstrated which method of assessment most reliably detects clinically

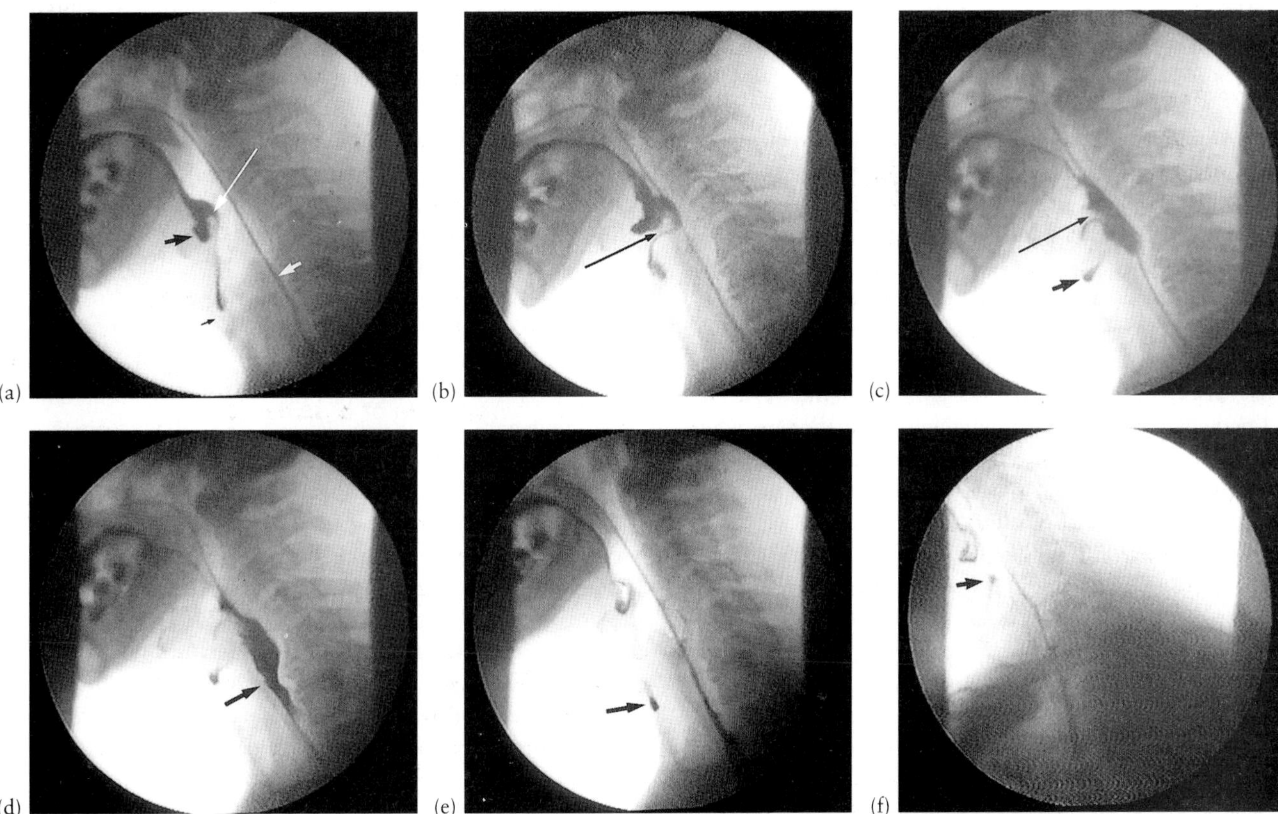

Fig. 15.10 A series of six frames taken from a videofluoroscopy examination in a stroke patient with swallowing difficulties. We have shown only the lateral views. (a) The food bolus containing radiodense material has been propelled into the pharynx by the tongue and has filled the vallecular space (large black arrow). Food is spilling over from the vallecular space, past the epiglottis (long white arrow) and is heading for the vocal cords (small black arrow). Note the nasogastric tube (short white arrow). The pharyngeal swallow has not yet been triggered. (b) The pharyngeal swallow has triggered (at last) with elevation and inversion of the epiglottis (arrow). (c) The epiglottis is fully inverted (long arrow). No further laryngeal penetration has occurred, indicating effective (but rather belated) laryngeal closure. However, some of the food bolus has passed the vocal cords (short arrow). (d) The food bolus is passing through the cricopharyngeal sphincter (arrow). (e) The swallow is complete but part of the food bolus remains below the vocal cords (arrow). The patient has not coughed indicating that sensation is impaired, i.e. this patient has silent aspiration. (f) The patient has been asked to cough and this voluntary cough is effective in clearing the aspirated food back into the pharynx (arrow) (videofluoroscopy provided by Diane Fraser).

Table 15.19 Limitations of videofluoroscopy.

Lack of general availability, especially in the acute situation
Lack of evidence that aspiration detected by this method is clinically important since studies have shown that normal people aspirate under some circumstances
Patients are tested under unfamiliar and artificial conditions which may influence their swallowing performance and limit the generalizability of the results
Exposure of patients to radiation
Use of radiological contrast which may cause lung damage if inhaled

important swallowing problems, i.e. those that worsen the outcome or require treatment to improve outcome, we suggest the following approach to screening for dysphagia.

The gag reflex is not a useful indicator of a stroke patient's swallowing ability.

Firstly, identify those patients who are *likely* to have problems swallowing, e.g. those with severe hemispheric, brainstem or bilateral strokes or impaired consciousness. Table 15.20 lists those features which individually, or more particularly in combination, should alert one to a high risk of swallowing difficulty.

Secondly, for patients without these features, or where access to a speech and language therapist with an interest in swallowing difficulties is limited, a doctor or nurse can usefully assess swallowing. Ask the patient to swallow a total of perhaps 50 mL of water, initially in 5 mL aliquots, whilst sitting supported in the upright position, with neck flexed (which keeps the airway closed) and the head tilted to the unaffected side (which avoids the water slipping down the neglected side of the oropharynx). Suction equipment should be available. The volume and speed of delivery of the water can be controlled using a teaspoon, or drinking straw as a pipette (Fig. 15.11). Patients may, if simply handed a cup to drink from, attempt to drink the whole quantity and aspirate large volumes. After each swallow, wait for an involuntary cough and ask the patient to speak. A cough or a change in the patient's voice (i.e. wet voice) may indicate aspiration. One should be particularly careful in assessing patients with existing respiratory disease who may be compromised by even minor degrees of aspiration.

Table 15.20 Features that indicate a likelihood of swallowing problems, derived from several studies (Kidd *et al.* 1993; Scottish Intercollegiate Guidelines Network 1997; Smithard *et al.* 1998).

Decreased level of consciousness (including confusion)
Poor sitting balance
Bilateral strokes
Older age
Abnormal tongue or palatal movement
Weak or absent voluntary cough
Moist or bubbling voice
Evidence of chest infection
Reduced pharyngeal sensation

Finally, if swallowing difficulties are likely, or are demonstrated on simple bedside testing, put the patient on 'nil by mouth' and hydrate them via an alternative route until a more detailed assessment can be made (section 15.18.1). To maintain the patient's comfort, their mouth should be kept moist and clean with regular mouth care.

Prognosis

Most patients with swallowing difficulties immediately after their stroke either die, or improve, so dysphagia which persists in patients who survive for more than a week or two is relatively uncommon. In one study, only one patient out of 357 had dysphagia 6 months after stroke onset (Barer 1989b). Interestingly, many patients who are eating a normal diet have persisting abnormalities, including aspiration on videofluoroscopy, for several months after the stroke but their significance is unclear (Smithard *et al.* 1997; Mann *et al.* 1999).

Treatment

An ongoing assessment of the patient's swallowing abilities by a speech and language therapist is valuable in guiding their fluid and feeding regimen, so that patients are not unnecessarily deprived of nutrition or put at risk of aspiration. Speech and language therapists may not be any more accurate in detecting the presence of a swallowing problem than nurses or doctors, but they do provide a more detailed assessment and potential solutions. Their assessment includes feeding the patient: in various positions (e.g. leaning to one side or the other); with different food textures (e.g. liquid, thickened fluids, purée or solids); with increasing bolus size; with different methods of delivery; and with different verbal cues or instructions (Smithard *et al.* 1998). Videofluoroscopy can be useful in patients with persisting swallowing difficulties; if the cause of the dysphagia is uncertain; where percutaneous endoscopic gastrostomy (PEG) is being considered (section 15.19); or where silent aspiration is suspected in patients with repeated chest infections.

Based on their swallowing assessment, which may or may not include videofluoroscopy, speech and language therapists may be able to teach the patient and carers methods of compensating for their problems until recovery occurs (Scottish Intercollegiate Guidelines Network 1997). Simple interventions which might allow a patient to swallow safely include the following:

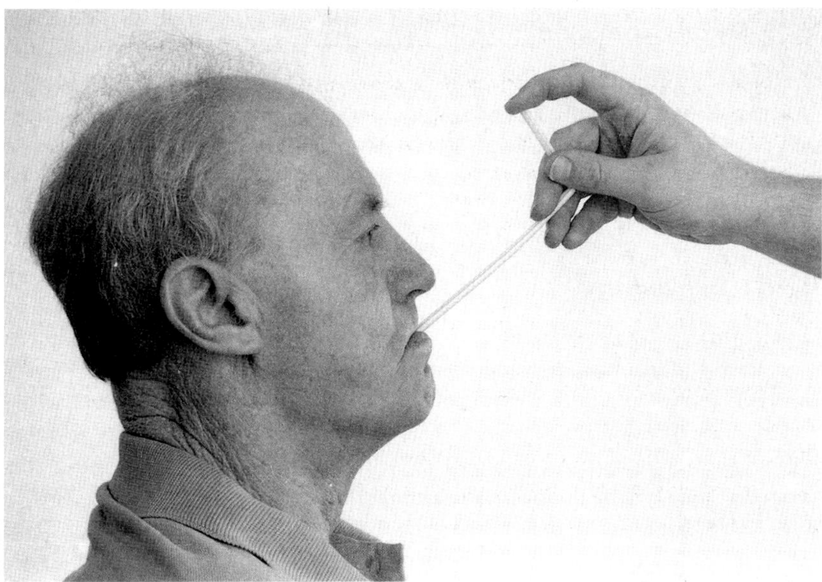

Fig. 15.11 One can control the volume of liquid a patient receives during a swallowing assessment with a drinking straw used as a pipette.

- ensure the patient is appropriately positioned, e.g. not slumped, semirecumbent to their hemiplegic side;
- teach the patient manoeuvres such as the 'chin tuck' or 'head turn' which make aspiration less likely;
- tailor the consistency of fluids and food to the patient's swallowing abilities. For instance, thickened fluids are usually more easily swallowed than water because they move less rapidly through the oropharynx and so give more time for the initiation of the swallow. Ideally a range of diets of specified consistency should be available. It is important that those responsible for distributing meals and refreshments, including well meaning relatives, are aware of patients' individual requirements;
- choose an appropriate type of drinking vessel. If the patient has not got a severe facial weakness and can suck, a drinking straw is often helpful. Beakers with spouts tend to encourage the patient to drink with an extended neck which opens the airway and encourages aspiration (Fig. 15.12).

These interventions, which involve swallowing food and fluids, are often termed 'direct' strategies, whilst exercises which do not actually involve swallowing anything and which aim to improve motor control are referred to as 'indirect' strategies. Unfortunately, there has been little formal evaluation of either strategy and there is no reliable evidence to suggest that therapy speeds the return of a normal swallow (Bath *et al.* 2000).

All those involved in giving a patient food or fluids, including their relatives, must be made aware of the patient's swallowing difficulties and what the patient can, and can't, swallow safely. Staff training and effective communication are essential.

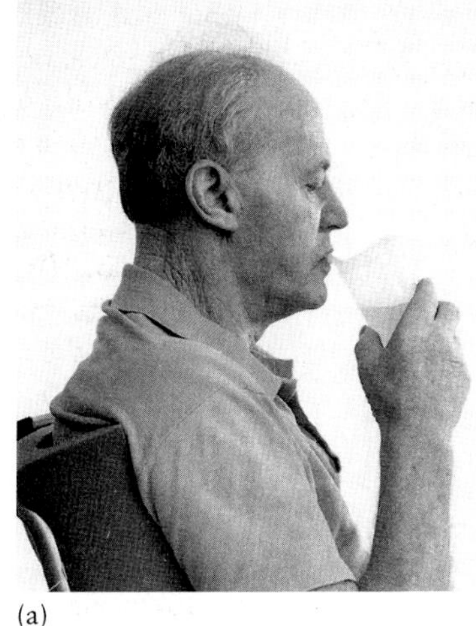

(a)

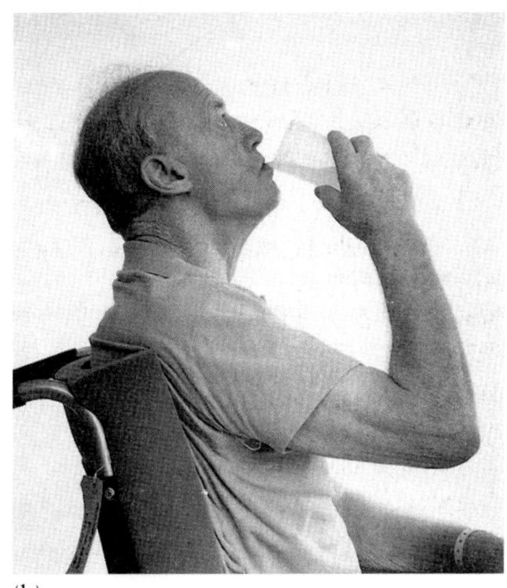

(b)

Fig. 15.12 Although beakers with a spout may prevent spills they have unfortunate associations with childhood which can make them unpopular with some patients. Also, they encourage patients to extend their neck when drinking which may lead to aspiration. The way *not* to do it: (a) bring the spout to the lips; (b) throw back the head, *open* the airway and inhale!

15.18 Metabolic disturbances

Metabolic disturbances, which may occasionally mimic stroke (sections 3.4.5 and 7.16), occur commonly in patients with severe strokes (Berkovic *et al.* 1984). They are important because they may cause 'worsening' (section 15.5), but are often easily reversed.

15.18.1 Dehydration

Patients with stroke are vulnerable to dehydration because:

• swallowing difficulties are common after acute stroke (section 15.17);

• immobility often means patients are dependent on others to provide them with drinks (section 15.11). They may even have been lying on the floor for several hours before being found;

• they may have communication problems (section 15.30) so they cannot ask for drinks;

• they may have visual neglect (section 15.28) so may not see the jug of water beside them;

• they are often elderly and therefore may have reduced sensitivity to thirst (O'Neill & McLean 1992); and

• they may have a fever, chest infection (section 15.12), hyperglycaemia (section 15.18.3) or be taking diuretics all of which increase their fluid losses.

Assessment

Clinical signs (Table 15.21) are helpful in identifying dehydration, but are not so reliable in older patients (Gross *et al.* 1992). Tachycardia, poor peripheral perfusion and a low jugular venous pressure are useful in severe cases but it is often impractical to test for orthostatic hypotension. Investigations, including the haematocrit, urea and electrolytes are probably more reliable than the bedside assessment. Where a patient is unwell with hypotension or renal failure, cannulation of a central vein to measure the right-atrial pressure directly, and to monitor fluid replacement, may occasionally be valuable. In hospital, charting of patients' fluid intake and output can be helpful but fluid charts are often inaccurate, not least because it is difficult, although not impossible, to monitor output when patients are incontinent (section 15.14). Hypernatraemia is usually due to water depletion without concomitant sodium depletion and often occurs if patients do not drink adequate amounts. It is only diagnosed by measuring the serum sodium since it is difficult to detect clinically. Very occasionally, hypernatraemia indicates a diabetic hyperosmolar state.

Table 15.21 Clinical indicators of dehydration.

General signs
Thirst
Reduced skin turgor
Dry mucous membranes
Sunken eyes
Cardiovascular
Cool peripheries
Collapsed peripheral veins
Postural hypotension
Low jugular venous pulse or central venous pressure
Low urine output
Investigations
Raised haemoglobin concentration
Raised haematocrit
Raised serum sodium (evidence of water depletion)
Raised urea (out of proportion to the serum creatinine)

Prevention and treatment

Patients who are unable or unwilling to take adequate oral fluids to prevent or reverse dehydration should be given fluid replacement by another route, i.e. intravenously, subcutaneously or by nasogastric tube. There is very little evidence to suggest that any one route is better than another (Challiner *et al.* 1994) (Table 15.22). Parenteral fluid replacement should be guided by regular monitoring of urea and electrolytes since patients' requirements for fluids are unpredictable (depending on urinary and insensible losses) and overhydration can occur (O'Neill *et al.* 1992). If patients are willing and able to take fluids orally they should be given adequate access to fluids (i.e. the cup and jug should be placed within their reach and not on the side of any neglect) and, importantly, regular encouragement to drink. Where the patient is hypernatraemic, adequate isotonic fluid replacement will usually normalize the serum sodium.

Always ensure that patients, or at least those who can swallow safely, have ready access to fluids.

15.18.2 Hyponatraemia

Hyponatraemia is uncommon after ischaemic stroke and primary intracerebral haemorrhage, compared with subarachnoid haemorrhage (section 13.4.2). One study suggested that hyponatraemia was more common in patients with haemorrhagic than ischaemic stroke, but this remains to be confirmed (Kusuda *et al.* 1989). It may be due to excess salt loss due to, for example, diuretics, or it may be dilutional (reflecting inappropriate secretion of antidiuretic hormone) in response to the brain injury or medical complications (O'Neill *et al.* 1992). Dilution is the conventional explanation for hyponatraemia after ischaemic stroke or intracerebral haemorrhage, but after subarachnoid haemorrhage,

Table 15.22 Advantages and disadvantages of different methods of hydrating patients who are unable to swallow.

Intravenous:	*Advantages* Can give large volumes rapidly in hypovolaemia Can give intravenous drugs or irritative solutions via cannula *Disadvantages* Can overload patient if not properly supervised Requires skilled person to insert cannula (so administration may be interrupted if cannula needs replacing) Infection at site of cannula can be serious Cannulae are expensive and should be replaced regularly
Subcutaneous:	*Advantages* Can be started by relatively unskilled staff (which may reduce interruptions) Needle can be placed where patient cannot reach it and so lessen likelihood of removal Unlikely to administer large volumes rapidly and therefore fluid overload less likely Butterfly cannulae are relatively inexpensive *Disadvantages* May be associated with local oedema, redness or even abscess Absorption can be unpredictable Unable to give large volumes rapidly to reverse hypovolaemia and severe dehyration Cannot use cannulae for drug administration or irritative solutions
Nasogastric:	*Advantages* More 'physiological' and volume overload unlikely Can feed the patient via tube as well as just hydrating them Can give oral medications via tube Does not necessarily require expensive giving sets or sterile fluids *Disadvantages* May increase risk of aspiration Frequently pulled out by restless patients and thus fluid administration interrupted Probably less acceptable to patients and relatives Radiation exposure if X-rays used to check position

hyponatraemia has been attributed to excessive renal salt loss (section 13.10.1). It is unclear how often this so-called 'cerebral salt wasting' occurs in other types of stroke. Joynt *et al.* (1981) demonstrated higher levels of antidiuretic hormone in stroke patients than controls but none of their patients had hyponatraemia. Hyponatraemia may occasionally cause patients to deteriorate neurologically, so it is important to detect since it is usually reversible.

Assessment

We measure urea and electrolytes in all stroke patients as part of the baseline assessment, and we monitor them regularly where the baseline assessment indicates an abnormality, in patients with severe stroke, and those with swallowing problems. A low serum sodium should prompt a search for the cause. This will include a review of the medication, a clinical assessment of hydration (Table 15.21) and fluid balance and, depending on the circumstances, some investigations, e.g. blood sugar, creatinine, plasma and urine osmolality and urinary sodium concentration, plasma antidiuretic hormone level (where available) and perhaps a chest X-ray to identify a cause of inappropriate secretion of antidiuretic hormone.

Treatment

The treatment of hyponatraemia will obviously depend on the cause, e.g. stopping diuretics, fluid restriction in dilutional hyponatraemia and cautious administration of intravenous isotonic saline where salt wasting is confirmed (sections 13.4.2 and 13.10.1). It is usually recommended that hyponatraemia is corrected slowly, over days rather than hours, to reduce the risk of central pontine myelinolysis (Burcar *et al.* 1977; Harris *et al.* 1993).

15.18.3 Hyperglycaemia

Hyperglycaemia (defined as a random plasma glucose of > 8.0 mmol/L, or 140 mg/dL, or a fasting level of > 6.7 mmol/L, or 120 mg/dL) has been estimated to occur in 20–43% of patients with acute stroke (Scott *et al.* 1998). Of these, about 25% are known to have diabetes mellitus already and another quarter have a raised HbA_{1c} which suggests that they had raised blood glucose for some period before the stroke, referred to as 'latent diabetes' (van Kooten *et al.* 1993). However, about one-half of the patients with hyperglycaemia have a normal HbA_{1c} suggesting that the hyperglycaemia was very recent and may be due to the stroke itself. Whether the hyperglycaemia is due to release of catecholamines and corticosteroids as part of the stress response is controversial (Scott *et al.* 1998).

Hyperglycaemia, like fever (section 15.12), after a stroke is associated with increased case fatality and poor functional outcome (Scott *et al.* 1998). This could be explained by more severe strokes producing a greater stress response and, thus, hyperglycaemia so that hyperglycaemia is simply a marker of severe stroke. However, some studies have demonstrated that hyperglycaemia is associated with a poor outcome having adjusted for stroke severity and other baseline prognostic factors (Weir *et al.* 1997; Bruno *et al.* 1999). This finding, along with some (but not all) animal work showing that hyperglycaemia can exacerbate ischaemic neuronal damage, has led many to hypothesize a causal relationship between hyperglycaemia and poor outcome. It is also likely that some of the excess morbidity and mortality associated with hyperglycaemia results from the micro- and macrovascular complications of known or latent diabetes.

Assessment

A random blood glucose should be measured in all patients with stroke. In those with hyperglycaemia, a fasting blood glucose and an HbA_{1c} will help distinguish latent diabetes from hyperglycaemia due to the stroke itself. A glucose tolerance test after the acute stage of the illness (i.e. when the patient is medically stable) may be helpful in sorting out which patients have diabetes or impaired glucose tolerance and which simply have hyperglycaemia related to the acute stroke. Patients with established diabetes and latent diabetes should be assessed to exclude vascular (both micro and macro) and neurological complications.

Treatment

The DIGAMI study, an RCT in diabetic patients with acute myocardial infarction, showed that tight control of blood glucose in the acute and recovery phases of their illness improved survival (Malmberg *et al.* 1995). This, along with a theoretical rationale (see above), has encouraged stroke physicians to plan large RCTs to evaluate a similar approach in patients with acute stroke. One small RCT has shown that glucose potassium insulin (GKI) infusions can be used with reasonable safety to control hyperglycaemia in acute stroke but larger studies are needed to demonstrate whether such an intervention improves patients' outcomes (Scott *et al.* 1999). Until trials are available in which we can enter our patients, we aim to keep blood sugars less than 11 mmol/L (200 mg/dL) in the first few days after an acute stroke. This will keep the patient free from thirst and avoid excessive diuresis which may cause dehydration. Whether more aggressive control of blood sugar is sensible will depend on any benefits, and the risks of hypoglycaemia, which will almost certainly depend on the intensity of monitoring available. Thus, GKI infusions may be safe in an intensive care unit, but not in a poorly staffed general ward.

15.18.4 Hypoglycaemia

Hypoglycaemia may mimic stroke or transient ischaemic attack (sections 3.4.5 and 7.16), but also occurs after stroke because patients' food intake and any requirement for hypoglycaemic agents may be less. Since hypoglycaemia may, if severe or undetected, cause worsening of the neurological deficit, the blood sugar should be monitored particularly carefully in diabetic patients on hypoglycaemic medication.

15.19 Nutrition

15.19.1 Malnutrition

Malnutrition is a common and often unrecognized problem in patients admitted to hospital, especially the elderly (Sullivan *et al.* 1999). Inevitably, the reported frequency of malnutrition after stroke has varied depending on patient selection, the definitions of malnutrition and the method and timing of assessments. Table 15.23 shows the various estimates of the frequency of malnutrition on admission to hospital after an acute stroke. It is not clear which factors are associated with malnutrition on admission, but the non-stroke literature suggests that malnutrition would be more frequent in older patients, those living in institutions and poor social circumstances, and those with prior cognitive impairment, physical disability or gastrointestinal disease. Several studies have shown that stroke patients' nutritional status may worsen during hospital admission (Axelsson *et al.* 1988; Unosson *et al.* 1994; Davalos *et al.* 1996; Smithard *et al.* 1996; Gariballa *et al.* 1998b). Stroke, like any acute illness, may lead to a negative energy balance and greater nutritional demands but stroke patients may be less able to meet these. Patients often have swallowing difficulties (section 15.17) and even those who can swallow may have a poor appetite because of intercurrent illness, depression, apathy, or medication and may eat slowly because of facial weakness, lack of dentures or poor arm function.

Poor nutrition has been associated with reduced muscle strength, reduced resistance to infection and impaired wound healing (although not specifically in stroke patients). Among patients with stroke, muscle weakness, infections and pressure sores are common and account for many deaths and much morbidity (Langhorne *et al.* 2000). Malnutrition has been associated with increased case fatality, poorer functional outcomes, increased frequency of infections and longer lengths of stay but it is unclear whether these associations are independent of stroke severity, or causal (Davalos *et al.* 1996; Gariballa *et al.* 1998b).

15.19.2 Obesity

Although under-nutrition is a concern, obesity can also be a problem during recovery from stroke. Where patients have restricted mobility, especially where they rely on others for help with transfers, obesity can be a crucial factor in how long they remain in hospital and how much support they require. It is also a problem in the long term in achieving adequate control of vascular risk factors such as hypertension (section 16.3.5) and diabetes. Patients quite often gain weight after stroke, presumably because of decreased energy expenditure and excessive calorie intake.

Table 15.23 Estimates of the frequency of malnutrition in various studies.

Study	No. at baseline	Type of patients	*n* (%) with low albumin	*n* (%) classified as malnourished and criteria	Factors associated with malnutrition on admission
Axelsson *et al.* 1988	100	Acute admissions	23 (23%)	16 (16%) > 2 low values†	Increased age* Females* Prior peptic ulcer* Atrial fibrillation**
Unosson *et al.* 1994	50	Acute admissions	31 (62%) < 36 g/L	4 (8%) > 2 low values†	n/a
Davalos *et al.* 1996	104	Acute admissions	8 (8%)	17 (16%) either low albumin or TSF/MAMC	n/a
Gariballa *et al.* 1998	201	All acute admissions	38 (19%) < 35 g/L	n/a	n/a
Choi-Kwon *et al.* 1998	88	Acute admitted females only (highly selected)		30 (34%) > 2 low values†	Haemorrhagic stroke
Finestrone *et al.* 1995	49	Rehabilitation only	n/a	Mild 7 (14%) Moderate 9 (19%) Severe 8 (16%) > 1 low level‡	Dysphagia* Diabetes** Previous stroke**

MAMC, midarm muscle circumference; n/a, not available from report; TSF, triceps skinfold thickness.

Derived from univariate* and multivariate** analyses.

† Low levels on a variable list of measures usually including anthropometry and blood tests but ‡ applying different normal ranges.

Assessment

In routine clinical practice there are practical difficulties in assessing stroke patients' nutritional status. A dietary and weight history may not be available because of patients' communication problems and an alternative source of this information may not be available if, as is common, the patient lives alone. Simple assessments of weight and height to estimate the body mass index (BMI) pose problems in immobile stroke patients. Specialized equipment, of limited availability, such as weighing beds or hoists and scales which accommodate wheelchairs, may be required and height may have to be estimated from the patient's demi-span or heel-knee length. Laboratory parameters such as haemoglobin, serum protein, albumin and transferrin may not necessarily reflect nutritional status. More complex anthropometric measures, vitamin estimations, antigen skin testing and bioelectric impedance are used in research but are not widely available. An awareness of the possibility of malnutrition is a key factor in identifying malnourished patients. A simple end-of-the-bed assessment reliably identifies most stroke patients with a low BMI and abnormal anthropometry (Mead *et al.* 1998). Estimation of the BMI, serial weights to identify weight loss, and monitoring of dietary intake should be used to screen patients on admission and monitor them whilst on the Stroke Unit. Simple laboratory tests including a serum albumin may be worth monitoring where there is clinical evidence of poor or worsening nutrition.

15.19.3 Prevention and treatment of malnutrition

General approach

It is useful to involve the speech and language therapist and dietician in the assessment and care of patients who have swallowing problems, or in whom nutritional intake may be inadequate for other reasons, e.g. confusion. Patients often eat very slowly after stroke and need supervision to ensure safe swallowing. Simple measures such as providing appetizing food of an appropriate consistency (section 15.17), placing the patient's meal in their intact visual field, and ensuring that the patient has well-fitting dentures should not be overlooked. Staff shortages may mean that patients receive insufficient food which will eventually cause malnutrition, or have food forced into them hurriedly by unthinking staff, which is very demeaning and adversely affects morale. Where trained staff are unable to cope, the patient's family or even volunteers can be easily trained to help with feeding.

Nutritional supplements

It is unclear how we should best support patients' nutritional status during the period when their oral intake is inadequate. A systematic review of all of the 30 available RCTs, including 2062 patients, suggested that oral or enteral (i.e. via a feeding tube) nutritional supplementation applied to diverse patient groups (and not specifically those with stroke) improved measures of nutrition and significantly reduced the odds of death (odds reduction, 34%; 95%CI, 9–52%) (Potter *et al.* 1998). However, when only more rigorous studies were included in the analysis, the effect on death was not statistically significant (odds reduction, 19%; 95%CI, 50% increase to 56% reduction). Although oral supplements after stroke may improve nutrition, their impact on survival and function is unclear (Gariballa *et al.* 1998a). Where swallowing is impaired it is unclear how long to wait before starting feeding and what is the best route (Bath *et al.* 2000). Whilst the patient cannot swallow adequate food their nutritional status will inevitably deteriorate unless supported. If tube feeding was well tolerated and carried no hazard then one would lose nothing by starting it early. Unfortunately, this is not the case although perceptions of patient tolerance and hazard vary; some clinicians prefer to introduce tube feeding very soon after the stroke, others delay for days and sometimes weeks.

Nasogastric and percutaneous endoscopic gastrostomy tubes

Nasogastric (NG) and percutaneous endoscopic gastrostomy (PEG) tubes are often inserted to allow fluid and food to be given to patients but they are not without their problems (Table 15.24). Patients find feeding via NG tube uncomfortable, feeding is often interrupted by repeated tube removal by the patient, and complications occur although no reliable estimates of complication rates have been published. By restraining the patient (e.g. tying hands to cot sides, use of mittens, or an American Football helmet!) (Fig. 15.13) one can probably improve the continuity of NG feeding but such restraints are considered unethical in some societies. A systematic review of studies reporting the complication rates associated with PEG feeding estimated the risk of death related to the procedure itself at 0.3% and the risk of major complications at 10% (Wollman *et al.* 1995). Several reports of the complication rates of PEG insertion, specifically amongst stroke patients, have been published (Wanklyn *et al.* 1995a; Norton *et al.* 1996; James *et al.* 1998; Skelly *et al.* 1999; Wijdicks & McMahon 1999). These included a total of 310 patients of whom about 8% died within a week or two of the procedure (it is impossible to know what proportion were due to the procedure itself) and 25% died during the hospital admission. The rates of various complications among these 310 patients, during variable follow-up periods, were: aspiration pneumonia 19%, tube blockage/breakage or removal 11%, wound infection 8%, gastrointestinal haemorrhage 0.6% (one fatal) and fatal gut perforation 0.3%.

Table 15.24 Advantages and disadvantages of nasogastric (NG) and percutaneous endoscopic gastrostomy (PEG) feeding.

	Advantages	Disadvantages
NG tube	Widely available Cheap	Often pulled out Unsightly Uncomfortable May lead to aspiration Nasal irritation/ulcer Interference with swallow
PEG	Rarely displaced Cosmetically acceptable Long-term use practical	Limited availability Expensive Aspiration when sedated Wound infections Bleeding Peritonitis

There have been only three small randomized comparisons of NG and PEG tube feeding (Baeten & Hoefnagels 1992; Park *et al.* 1992; Bath *et al.* 2000) and only one, involving only 30 patients, specifically in acute stroke (Norton *et al.* 1996). These suggest that PEG feeding is associated with more effective nutritional support, with less interruption of feeding, but they were too small to indicate reliably whether patients' outcomes were improved. Thus the relative merits of the two types of tube are uncertain, at least in the first month of so after the stroke. There is little doubt that a PEG tube is a better option if feeding is to be prolonged. Also, in practice, there may be no alternative to a PEG tube if feeding is required and NG feeding has been unsuccessful.

A survey of almost 3000 physicians who manage stroke in the UK demonstrated wide variation in the use of oral supplements and in the timing and method of feeding in dysphagic stroke patients (Ebrahim & Redfern 1999). Such variation reflects the lack of clear evidence to guide practice. A large multicentre randomized trial (the FOOD trial) is currently trying to establish the role of routine oral supplementation of hospital diet and the optimum timing and type of tube feeding after a stroke (http://www.dcn.ed.ac.uk/food).

15.19.4 Treatment of obesity

Patients who are obese, in particular if this causes problems with mobility or control of diabetes or blood pressure, should be encouraged to lose weight and be offered dietary advice.

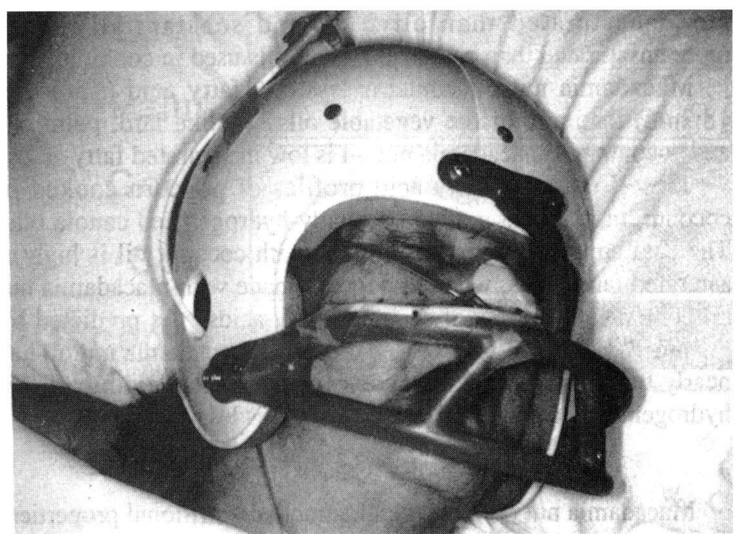

Fig. 15.13 Use of an American Football helmet to prevent the patient pulling out a nasogastric feeding tube (with permission from Levine & Morris 1995).

15.19.5 Other considerations

It is important to remember that eating plays an important role in our social lives and is a source of pleasure. Eating with other people during the recovery phase of stroke encourages communication and social interaction. Patients who are concerned by their appearance after a stroke (e.g. due to facial weakness) may gain confidence from this opportunity to socialize. On the other hand, dribbling or ending up with the food on the table or floor may distress the patient and inhibit social interaction. Advice from the occupational therapist regarding equipment to allow the patient to eat independently should be sought to maximize the positive, and minimize the negative, aspects of eating in a communal setting (section 15.32.6).

15.20 Spasticity and contractures

Spasticity has been defined as a motor disorder characterized by velocity dependent increase in muscle tone with exaggerated tendon reflexes. It is usually accompanied by muscle weakness and clumsiness and sometimes by flexor or extensor spasms. Immediately after a stroke the muscular tone in the limbs and trunk may be lower, the same as, or higher than normal (Gray *et al.* 1990). The reasons for this variation are unclear. Although tone may be lower than normal in the acute phase, in most patients who do not recover it tends to increase over the first few weeks (Brown *et al.* 1993). In patients with a hemiparesis, the tone in the arm is usually greater in the flexors than extensors, whilst in the leg it is greater in the extensors than the flexors. This explains the typical hemiplegic posture (i.e. elbow, wrist and fingers flexed and arm adducted and internally rotated whilst the leg is extended at the hip and knee and the foot is plantar flexed and inverted). Tone in the truncal muscles may also be abnormally high or low. Tone may increase in any muscle group so much that it restricts the active movement which the residual muscle strength can produce. Imbalance in muscle tone can eventually result in shortening of muscles and permanent deformity and so restrict the full range of movement, i.e. contractures. Closely allied to spasticity are 'associated reactions' which are involuntary movements of the affected side (most typically flexion of the arm) elicited by a variety of stimuli including the use of unaffected limbs (e.g. self-propelling a wheelchair; yawning or coughing) and the upright posture (Mulley 1982; Cornall 1991). Associated reactions become more obvious with increases in tone. Associated reactions may be misinterpreted as voluntary movements by family and ill-informed staff who should be educated about their significance to prevent them becoming unduly optimistic about the patient's motor recovery. Spasticity and contractures may cause pain, deformity, disability and, if severe, secondary complications such as pressure sores at points of contact between soft tissues (e.g. on the inner aspect of the knees in a patient with contractures of the adductors of the thighs).

Associated reactions may be misinterpreted as voluntary movements by family and ill-informed staff who should be educated about their significance to prevent them becoming unduly optimistic about the patient's motor recovery.

Assessment

Tone and spasticity. Physicians are trained to assess the tone in a limb by asking the patient to relax (which is almost guaranteed to have the opposite effect) and then moving the limb through its range of movement at each joint at different speeds and noting the resistance to these movements. Unfortunately, many physicians do not appreciate how much tone is influenced by factors such as the patient's position, anxiety, fatigue, pain and medication. Tone may change from minute to minute. This makes it difficult to assess objectively with good inter-observer reliability. Physiotherapists, who spend far more time handling patients than physicians, are more aware of changes in tone and try to take advantage of them in their therapy. Formal measurement of tone can be attempted using clinical scales (e.g. the modified Ashworth scale, Table 15.25) or techniques such as electrogoniometry or quantitative neurophysiology. Unfortunately, the last two are not widely available or practical in routine clinical practice. The inter-observer reliability of the clinical scales is generally good for assessing tone in the arm and around the knee but poor for assessing tone around the ankle (Gregson *et al.* 2000). In any case, when assessing the effectiveness of treatment in an individual patient, or in a group of patients in RCTs, it may be better to measure the patients' function (e.g. walking speed or dressing), or the achievement of a specific goal (to allow the palm of the hand to be accessed to maintain hygiene) than to rely on measurement of tone itself. Indeed, the management of abnormal tone, like all other aspects of rehabilitation, should be directed at achieving realistic, relevant and measurable goals (section 10.3.3).

Contractures are easier to assess than spasticity because, by definition, the deformity is fixed. Thus, one can objectively measure the range of movement around a joint and repeat the measure to determine whether or not an intervention has improved the range. However, occasionally an apparent contracture responds to injection of botulinum toxin (see below) indicating that the shortening is due to muscle contraction rather than permanent shortening of muscles or tendons.

Prevention and treatment

In rehabilitation our aim is to modulate changes in tone to the patient's advantage. For instance, to increase tone in a flaccid leg to provide the patient with a more secure base on which to walk, or reduce tone in the arm to facilitate more active movement. We use several complementary approaches to prevent the development of unwanted patterns of tone and to alleviate existing problems due to spasticity and contractures. Some are applicable to any patient whilst others are only required to deal with exceptional problems.

Avoidance of exacerbating factors. Pain, urinary retention, severe constipation, skin irritation, pressure sores, anxiety and any other unpleasant stimulus may cause an unwanted increase in tone. These factors must be avoided or alleviated.

Positioning and seating. Poor positioning, especially in immobile patients, can lead to detrimental changes in tone. For example, long periods spent lying supine will increase extensor spasms, presumably by facilitation of basic reflexes. Unfortunately, there appears to be quite a lot of uncertainty about the optimum positions for patients with hemiplegia and there are also practical difficulties in keeping patients in the required position, i.e. the patients tend to move (Carr & Kenney 1992). The positioning charts which can be found on most Stroke Units (Fig. 15.14) can only be used as a general guide. Finding the optimum position for a patient is often a matter of trial and error and relies on the experience of the therapists and nurses. Appropriate seating which can be tailored to the individual patient is essential (Fig. 15.15). Ideally, patients should be seated in a balanced, symmetrical and stable position which they find comfortable and which enables them to function, e.g. eat, drink, etc.

Passive movements and physiotherapy. It is important that muscles are not allowed to remain in a relaxed and shortened position for long periods. For example, if the arm is left in a flexed posture at the elbow, or the foot plantar flexed in bed, this can lead to permanent shortening and contractures. Patients' limbs should be moved passively to stretch the muscles and maintain the range of movement, even in the very acute stages. However, it is important that carers are taught to do this without causing damage to vulnerable structures such as the shoulder (section 15.24). Also, handling methods, during transfers for example, can influence tone, at least in the short term (Brown *et al.* 1993). Physiotherapists have an important role in teaching nurses and informal carers the correct positioning and handling techniques to minimize risk of injury (to patient and handler) and unwanted spasticity.

Patients with a hemiparesis may attempt to 'overuse' their sound side to achieve mobility but, as a consequence, the tone may increase in the affected side. Using the unaffected leg to self-propel a wheelchair is said to lead to increased spasticity in the affected arm and leg (Ashburn & Lynch 1988; Cornall 1991). The impact of any changes in tone associated with such activities on functional recovery has not been established. The aim of many of the facilitation and inhibition techniques used by therapists is to use basic reflexes and postural changes in tone to promote function.

Table 15.25 The modified Ashworth scale for the clinical assessment of muscle tone (from Ashworth 1964).

0	No increase in muscle tone
1	Slight increase in muscle tone, manifested by a catch and release, or by minimal resistance at the end of the range of motion when the affected part(s) is moved in flexion or extension
1+	Slight increase in muscle tone, manifested by a catch, followed by minimal resistance throughout the remainder (less than half) of the range of movement
2	More marked increase in muscle tone through most of the range of movement but affected parts easily moved
3	Considerable increase in muscle tone, passive movement difficult
4	Affected parts rigid in flexion or extension

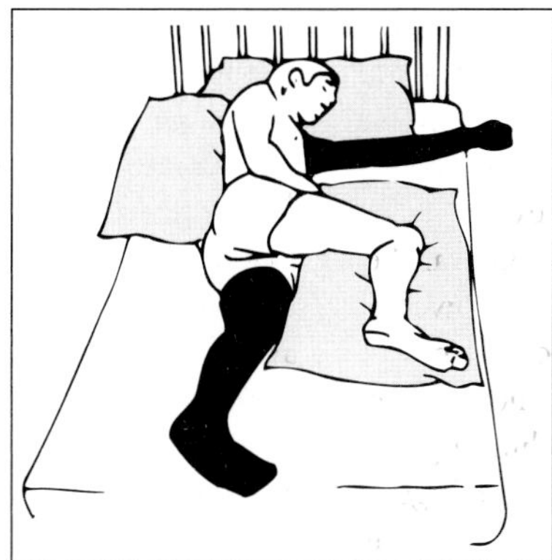

Lying on affected side
No backrest. 1 or 2 pillows for head.
Affected shoulder pulled well forward.
Place good leg forward on a pillow.
Pillow placed behind back.

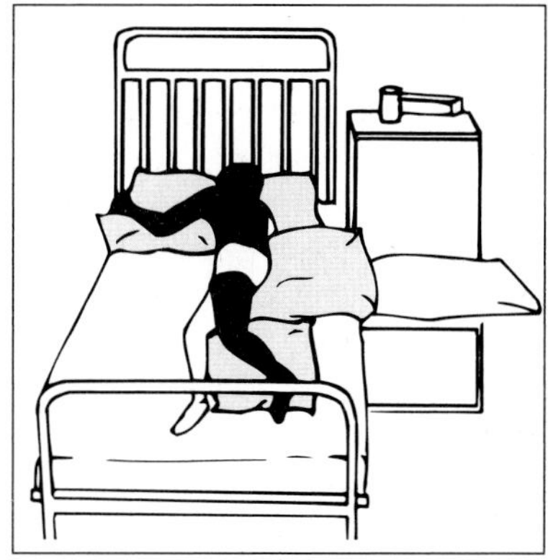

Lying on unaffected side
No backrest. 1 or 2 pillows for head.
Affected shoulder forward with arm on pillow.
Place affected leg backward on a pillow.
Pillow placed behind back.

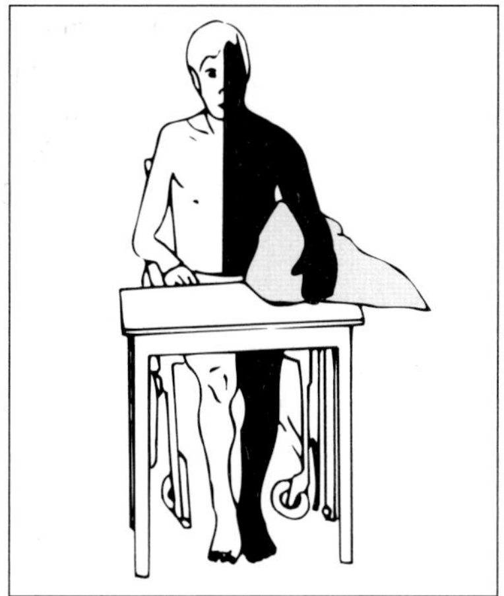

Sitting up
Sitting well back and in centre of chair.
Affected arm placed well forward on table or pillow.
Feet flat on floor.
Knees directly above the floor.

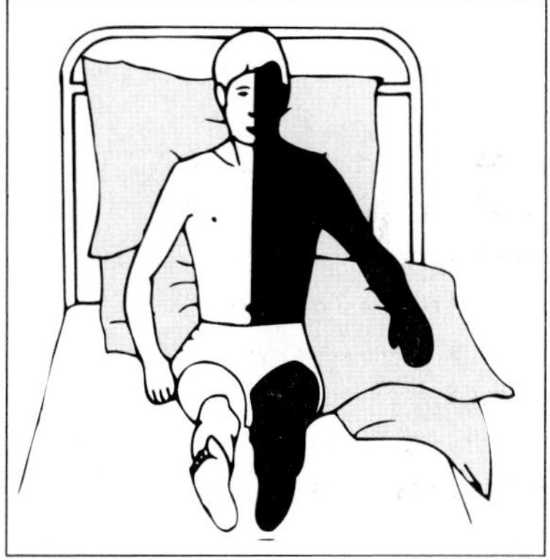

Sitting in bed
Sitting in bed is not desirable.
Affected arm placed on pillow.
Legs are straight.
Sitting upright and well supported.

Fig. 15.14 The typical chart used to guide the positioning of a stroke patient with hemiplegia (affected side in black).

These techniques, although widely accepted and used by therapists, have not been evaluated adequately in randomized controlled trials (section 15.21). Various physical techniques including the application of cold, of heat, splinting and electrical stimulation can, at least for a short time, reduce spasticity (Brown *et al.* 1993; Barnes 1998). This may relieve discomfort, allow improved hygiene, and plaster casts or splints to be applied. Whether these physical techniques have direct longer term benefits is unclear (Barnes 1998).

Splinting and casting. Occasionally these techniques may be necessary to prevent or treat contractures. Progressive splinting and application of casts can improve range of movement but the optimum duration and best methods are unclear. Also, badly fitted casts and splints can cause pain, pressure sores and tendon damage which may exacerbate rather than relieve spasticity and contractures.

Oral antispastic drugs. Where spasticity is not adequately controlled by physical techniques, or where the patient is suffering from painful muscle spasms, certain drugs have been advocated. These include baclofen, dantrolene, tizanidine and diazepam which reduce tone by altering neurotransmitter function or ion fluxes centrally, in the spinal cord or in muscles. Although some small RCTs have shown benefits in patients with established spasticity due to a variety of causes, it is difficult to know how applicable their results are to patients with stroke, especially in the acute phase (Gracies *et al.* 1997b; Shakespeare *et al.* 2000; Taricco *et al.* 2000). In our experience they rarely make much difference in stroke patients and they have a number of adverse effects (Table 15.26). We would normally use baclofen for a trial period in patients who our physiotherapists feel might benefit. Adverse effects are much more common in older patients but can be

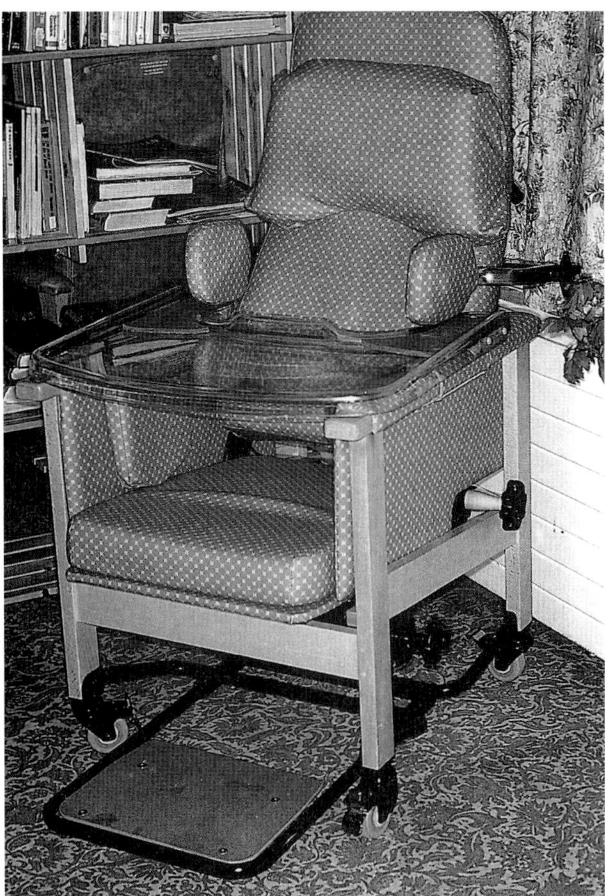

Fig. 15.15 A chair which can be tailored to the individual needs of the patient. This model can be raised, or lowered, the back rest and seat can be adjusted, arms can be altered and extra supports can be inserted.

minimized by starting with low doses and increasing the dose slowly until the desired effect is achieved, or adverse effects necessitate withdrawal.

Local and regional treatments. Injection of botulinum toxin directly into muscles can reduce troublesome spasticity. For example, it has been used to obtain better access to the palm of a hand affected by flexor deformity to allow cleaning and treatment of infected skin (Bhakta *et al.* 1996). Its effectiveness in reducing spasticity is supported by the results of several small RCTs although its impact on patients' disability is less well established (Burbaud *et al.* 1996; Simpson 1997; Bhakta *et al.* 2000; Intercollegiate Working Party for Stroke 2000). It appears to be safe, at least in the short term, but because its effects wear off over several months, repeated injections may be required and treatment costs can be very high. Sometimes, a single injection can allow simpler measures to be introduced which avoids the need for further injections. Very occasionally, and usually where simple measures (see above) have been inadequate, spasticity can be so troublesome as to warrant more invasive procedures. These include:

- local nerve blocks using injection of ethanol or phenol. Although occasionally useful to solve specifc problems, this technique can lead to unwanted muscle weakness and painful dysaesthesias (Gracies *et al.* 1997a);
- intrathecal infusion of baclofen using implantable pumps (Gracies *et al.* 1997b);
- surgical procedures such as anterior and posterior rhizotomy and more recently lesioning of the dorsal root entry zone (so called DREZ-otomy) (Barnes 1998); and
- tendon lengthening and transfers which can, for example, help to reduce equino-varus deformity (Barnes 1998).

Anecdotally, the prevalence of severe contractures appears to have declined dramatically over the last 30 years which is probably a result of improvements in the standards of general care. We now virtually never have to resort to the more invasive procedures described here.

15.21 Limb weakness, poor truncal control and unsteady gait

These three aspects of the patient's condition are impossible to separate and will therefore be discussed together. Weakness of an arm, leg or both, sometimes with unilateral facial weakness, is probably the most common and widely recognized impairment related to stroke. However, there are often associated but less obvious problems with the axial muscles which impair truncal control and walking.

Facial weakness, which affects about 40% of patients (Table 15.2), apart from its cosmetic effects, may contribute to dysarthria (section 15.30.2) and cause problems with the oral preparatory phase of swallowing (section 15.17). Weakness of the upper limb, which affects about 50% of patients (Table 15.2), along with changes in tone, is associated with the development of a painful shoulder (section 15.24) and swelling of the hand (section 15.25). Poor hand and arm function is a major cause of dependency in activities of daily living. Weakness of the leg, which affects about 45% of patients (Table 15.2), may be severe enough to immobilize the patient and thus predispose to the complications of immobility (section 15.11). Leg weakness, making it difficult to stand, transfer or walk independently, is one of the most important factors prolonging hospital stay in stroke patients. In patients with hemiparesis, which affects about 55% of patients, the arm is usually weaker than the leg (Table 15.2).

Assessment

Physiotherapists generally feel (and rightly so in our opinion) that physicians place too much emphasis on the assessment of muscle power and not enough on the associated abnormalities of tone, truncal control and patterns of movement which account for many of the functional consequences of stroke. In assessing a patient with stroke, it may be more useful to observe the range and control of voluntary move-

Table 15.26 Adverse effects of antispasticity drugs.

Adverse effect	Baclofen	Diazepam	Dantrolene	Tizanidine
Sedation/central nervous system depression	++	+++	+	+
Confusion	+	+		
Hypotonia/weakness	+	+	++	+
Unsteadiness/ataxia	+	++	+	+
Exacerbation of epileptic seizures	++			
Psychosis/hallucinations	++		+	
Insomnia	+			+
Headache	+	+		
Urinary retention	+	+	+	
Dry mouth			++	
Hypotension	+	+		+
Nausea/vomiting	+	+		+
Diarrhoea/constipation	+	+	+	+
Abnormal liver function	+	+	+++	+
Hyperglycaemia	+			
Visual disturbance	+	+		
Skin rashes	+	+	+	
Pericarditis/pleural effusions			+	
Blood dyscrasia		+		
Withdrawal symptoms	+	++		
Drug interactions	++	+	+	

+, reported occasionally; ++, quite frequent; +++, potentially fatal.

ments of the limbs than assessing muscle power. For instance, does the patient have only coarse movement around the hip or shoulder, or have they retained movement at the more distal joints? In stroke patients, distal movements are usually more severely impaired than proximal ones. The assessment of motor function and truncal control has already been described (section 3.3.4).

Recovery from a hemiplegic stroke has been likened to early infant development, in that the recovery of truncal control follows the same general pattern as that of a growing child. Head control returns first, followed by rolling over, sitting balance and then standing balance, and lastly the patient can walk with increasing steadiness and speed (see Fig. 10.14). After a stroke it is useful to know where the patient is on this 'developmental ladder' when assessing prognosis and setting goals for rehabilitation. It is important to assess truncal control and gait since truncal ataxia can occur without limb incoordination in patients with midline cerebellar lesions. It is not unknown for patients to undergo full gastrointestinal and metabolic investigation to elucidate the cause of vomiting before their truncal ataxia is noted and a cerebellar stroke diagnosed. It also seems absurd that, although immobility is the main reason for a stroke patient needing to stay in hospital for rehabilitation, mobility and balance are often not assessed properly by doctors admitting stroke patients (Davenport *et al.* 1995). Having stressed the importance of testing truncal control and gait, it is important that in doing so neither the patient nor the doctor are put at risk of injury. Poor handling and lifting technique may dislocate a patient's flaccid shoulder (section 15.24), result in a fracture from a fall (section 15.26) and may even injure the doctor's back! Physiotherapists should ideally provide appropriate training to *all* staff, and informal carers, who are involved in handling patients.

The severity of weakness of individual muscle groups is often graded with the Medical Research Council (MRC) Scale (Table 15.27). This was originally designed to assess motor weakness arising from injuries to single peripheral nerves, not stroke. Unfortunately, although the MRC scale has good inter-observer reliability if applied rigorously (Gregson *et al.* 2000), it is often misused and the optional expansion to include extra grades (e.g. 4^+, 5^-) makes it even less reliable in the routine recording of motor weakness. The Motricity Index, a modification of the MRC Scale (Table 15.27), for use in patients with stroke, allows the observer to grade the severity of the hemiparesis rather than each separate muscle group (Demeurisse *et al.* 1980). This can be useful in charting patients' progress for research purposes but is of limited value in routine clinical practice because it is difficult to remember the weights applied to individual movements and it requires a small block to assess grip strength. There are several other tools available for objectively measuring and recording motor function (Table 15.28).

Table 15.27 The MRC Scale of Weakness and the Motricity Index which was developed from the MRC Scale for use in stroke patients (Medical Research Council 1982).

MRC scale		
0	No contraction	
1	Flicker or trace of contraction	
2	Active movement with gravity eliminated	
3	Active movement against gravity	
4	Active movement against resistance	
5	Full strength	
The motricity index		
Arm	Pinch grip	—
	Elbow flexion (from 90°)	—
	Shoulder abduction (from chest)	—
	Total arm score	—
Leg	Ankle dorsi-flexion (from plantar flexed)	—
	Knee extension (from 90°)	—
	Hip flexion	—
	Total leg score	—
Scoring system for pinch grip		
0	Pinch grip, no movement	
11	Beginnings of prehension	
19	Grips block (not against gravity)	
22	Grips block against gravity	
26	Against pull but weak	
33	Normal	
Scoring system for movements other than pinch grip		
0	No movement	
9	Palpable contraction only	
14	Movement but not against gravity/limited range	
19	Movement against gravity/full range	
25	Weaker than other side	
33	Normal	

Table 15.28 Measurements of motor function (from Wade 1992a,b).

Impairments
MRC Scale (Table 15.27)
Motricity index (Table 15.27)
Trunk control test
Motor club assessment
Rivermead motor assessment
Dynamometry

Disability
Upper limb
- Nine-hole peg test
- Frenchay arm test/battery
- Action research arm test

Truncal control/mobility
- Standing balance
- Functional ambulation category
- Timed 10-m walk
- Truncal control
- Rivermead mobility index (Table 15.44)
- Subsection of Office of Population Censuses and Surveys (OPCS) scale (Martin *et al.* 1988)

Treatment

Spontaneous recovery of motor function is highly variable. The more severe the initial impairment, the less likely is full recovery. Duncan *et al.* (1992) showed that motor and sensory function 5 days after stroke onset explained 74% of the variance in motor function at 6 months with the Fugl-Meyer scale. The pattern of recovery of motor function parallels that of other stroke-related deficits, with the most rapid recovery occurring in the first few weeks and then the pace of improvement slows over subsequent months (section 10.2.5). In patients with hemiparesis it is generally thought that motor function in the leg improves more than that in the arm, although this has been questioned (Duncan *et al.* 1994). Also, unless the patient has some return of grip within one month of the stroke, useful return of function is unlikely, although not impossible (Sunderland *et al.* 1989).

Physiotherapy is the main therapeutic option in hemiparesis although techniques vary. The two broad approaches most commonly employed are the 'facilitation and inhibition' technique and the 'functional' approach. The facilitation and inhibition technique is based on the premise that posture and sensory stimuli can modify basic reflex patterns which emerge after cerebral damage. If one observes a hemiplegic patient one might notice that the erect posture exaggerates the typical hemiplegic posture. Similarly, turning the head towards the affected side decreases the flexor tone in the arm, whilst turning the head away from the affected arm increases the tone. Several workers have developed different treatments based on facilitation and inhibition, the best known being those of Bobath (1978) and Brunnstrom (1970). Although these techniques differ, certain features have been identified as common to all (Table 15.29). They all aim to achieve as normal a posture and pattern of movement on the affected side as possible. On the other hand, the functional approach simply aims, through training and strengthening of the unaffected side, to compensate for the impairment to achieve maximum function. For example, patients may be encouraged to transfer and walk as soon as possible after the stroke. Supporters of the facilitation and inhibition approach claim that although the functional approach might achieve earlier independence, it results in more abnormal patterns of tone and movement which in the long term may lead to contractures and loss of function. Vigorous activity involving the unaffected side may increase the tone in the affected limbs during the activity. This does not seem to occur with all activities (e.g. pedaling) and any long-term effects on tone

Table 15.29 Common features of facilitation/inhibition-based therapy (from Flanagan 1967).

Recognition of the intimate relationship between sensation and movement
Recognition of the importance of basic reflex activity
Use of sensory input and different postures to facilitate or inhibit reflex activity and movement
Motor relearning based on repetition of activity and frequency of stimulation
Treatment of the body as an integrated unit rather than focusing on one part
Close personal interaction between the therapist and patient

are unclear (Brown & Kautz 1998). We believe there is a place for both approaches in clinical practice. Quite often, where a patient has not achieved useful independent mobility despite a prolonged period of physiotherapy (with the facilitation and inhibition approach), we switch to a functional approach to maximize the patient's autonomy. For example, we will train patients to transfer independently and self-propel a wheelchair even though this may be associated with, at least in the short term, unwanted changes in tone.

Although physiotherapists appreciate the complex nature of the motor problems in hemiparesis, including the subtle problems which affect the contralateral limbs, this focus on the motor impairments may distract attention from the associated sensory, cognitive and visuospatial problems which may often be more important in limiting the patient's functional recovery.

There has been very little formal evaluation of the physiotherapy techniques. Although several small RCTs have been reported, no definite conclusions about the relative merits of different approaches can be drawn (Stern *et al.* 1970; Dickstein *et al.* 1986; Jongbloed *et al.* 1989; Wagenaar *et al.* 1990; Pollock *et al.* 2000). In any case, comparisons of different techniques may have limited relevance to current clinical practice as many therapists adopt an eclectic approach, using selected aspects of each technique where appropriate for individual patients. There are, therefore, some important questions about physiotherapy after stroke which need to be addressed in properly designed RCTs:

- when should physiotherapy start?
- how long should it continue?
- what is the optimum intensity of physiotherapy?
- which specific therapeutic interventions are the *most* effective?
- is therapy provided by relatively unskilled therapists as effective as that provided by skilled therapists?
- which patients gain most from physiotherapy and can we prospectively identify them?

The results of small RCTs support the hypothesis that physiotherapy, especially that focused on achieving particular tasks, improves function even when started late after the stroke (Wade *et al.* 1992; Dean & Shepherd 1997; Kwakkel *et al.* 1999a, b). The trials generally indicate that therapy has a greater impact on specific motor impairments than the resulting disability. This may be because the resulting disabilities are the consequence of sensory and cognitive as well as motor problems. The size of any treatment effect is probably influenced by the intensity of treatment (Langhorne *et al.* 1996; Kwakkel *et al.* 1997; Feys *et al.* 1998). However, many older, sicker patients may not be able to tolerate intensive regimes which indicates the need for research to identify the optimum physiotherapy regime for particular subgroups of patients (Lincoln *et al.* 1999). Given the methodological difficulties in systematically reviewing and performing RCTs of physiotherapy techniques (and those of other therapists), this is a daunting challenge (Table 15.1).

Other interventions

A large number of physical techniques have been developed with the aim of improving motor function or gait. Some have been evaluated in small RCTs which have included highly selected patients and focused more on impairment than disability as outcome measures. None are supported by enough evidence to recommend their routine use. These techniques have included:

- electromyographic (EMG) biofeedback (Schleenbaker and Mainous 1993; Moreland & Thomson 1994; Glanz *et al.* 1995; Moreland *et al.* 1998). Other types of biofeedback, including visual and auditory feedback may help patients achieve better sitting or standing balance, for example (Sackley & Lincoln 1997; Wong *et al.* 1997);
- functional electrical stimulation, which may act as an orthosis, e.g. when applied it can reduce foot drop to facilitate gait, it probably increases muscle strength, but it is unclear whether it improves functional outcome and many patients find it uncomfortable (Glanz *et al.* 1996; Burridge *et al.* 1997; Chae *et al.* 1998; Powell *et al.* 1999);
- acupuncture (Gosman-Hedstrom *et al.* 1998) and transcutaneous electrical nerve stimulation (TENS) (Tekeoolu *et al.* 1998);
- treadmill gait retraining with or without bodyweight support (Visintin *et al.* 1998);
- forced use where the unaffected arm is immobilized for a major part of the day and during physiotherapy sessions (van der Lee *et al.* 1999); and
- drugs to enhance motor recovery (Walker-Batson *et al.* 1995).

Complementary approaches

In this section we have dealt with interventions that aim to decrease disability by improving impairments. The complementary strategy involving the appropriate provision of mobility aids, e.g. walking sticks, splints and wheelchairs is dealt with elsewhere (section 15.32.1).

15.22 Sensory impairments

It is impossible to assess sensation adequately because of reduced conscious level, confusion or communication problems in about a one-fifth of patients with acute stroke, but about one-third of the remainder have impairment of at least one sensory modality (Table 15.2). Sensory problems are more easily identified in patients with right rather than left hemisphere stroke, probably because of the communication difficulties associated with left hemisphere strokes. Severe sensory loss may be as disabling as paralysis, especially when it affects proprioception. Loss of pain and temperature sensation in a limb, or sensory loss with neglect, may put a patient at risk of injury from hot water, etc. Disordered sensation with numbness or paraesthesia, even without functional difficulties may, if persistent, be as distressing to some patients as central post-stroke pain (section 15.23). We have discussed some of the difficulties in assessing sensory function earlier (section 3.3.5).

Patients often complain bitterly about what appears to the doctor to be a minor change in sensation. Do not underestimate the effect which facial numbness, or tingling in a hand, can have on the morale of a patient.

Little is known specifically about the recovery of sensation after stroke, although it probably follows the pattern of recovery seen in most other impairments (section 10.2.5). Sensory symptoms may worsen during intercurrent illness (e.g. infections) leading to concerns about recurrent stroke. Under these circumstance it is important to give appropriate explanation and reassurance to the patient and any carer. Although patients may be given sensory stimulation as part of their therapy little is known about the effect this or any other intervention has on sensation (Yekutiel & Guttman 1993). Where patients have lost temperature or pain sensation in a limb, especially if there is associated neglect, it is important to counsel them about commonsense strategies to avoid injury to the limb.

15.23 Pain

Pain is a common complaint amongst stroke patients. Langhorne *et al.* (2000) reported that 34% of 311 patients required analgesia for pain (excluding shoulder pain) during hospital admission after an acute stroke. There are many potential causes, some of which are coincidental and others of which are in some way due to the stroke (Table 15.30). Usually, the cause becomes obvious after one has asked the patient about the distribution, nature and onset of the pain and has examined the relevant area. However, some pains (e.g. due to spasticity, axial arthritis and central post-stroke pain) may be difficult for patients to describe and localize. Diagnosis, and assessment of analgesic requirements, are particularly difficult in patients with communication and cognitive problems (Kehayia *et al.* 1997).

Table 15.30 Causes of pain after stroke.

Headache due to vascular pathology (sections 3.3.10 and 15.9)
Painful shoulder (section 15.24)
Deep venous thrombosis and pulmonary embolism (section 15.13)
Pressure sores (section 15.16)
Limb spasticity (section 15.20)
Fractures (section 15.26)
Arterial occlusion with ischaemia of limb, bowel or myocardium
Co-existing arthritis exacerbated by immobility or therapy
Instrumentation, e.g. catheter, intravenous cannulae, nasogastric tube
Central *post-stroke* pain (thalamic pain/Dejerine–Roussy syndrome) (section 15.23)

The treatment of pain depends on the likely cause. Simple analgesics (e.g. paracetamol) along with some reassurance that the pain does not indicate any serious problem may be all that is needed. Other interventions such as local application of heat or cold, and use of transcutaneous electrical nerve stimulation (TENS) or acupuncture, may relieve symptoms with a low risk of adverse effects. Pain due to spasticity should initially be treated by alleviating exacerbating factors and by carefully positioning the patient (section 15.20). Antispasticity drugs are occasionally required, seldom work and have significant adverse effects (Table 15.26). Musculoskeletal pain can be treated with simple analgesics and, if these are ineffective and there are no contraindications, a non-steroidal anti-inflammatory drug. If a joint becomes acutely painful it may be necessary to rest it and investigate to exclude more serious causes, e.g. septic arthritis, fracture, or gout exacerbated by diuretics or aspirin. We find it useful to discuss the patient's pain at the multidisciplinary team meeting where one can establish the pattern, severity and control of pain in different settings, e.g. on the ward, at night, during therapy sessions. This can provide important clues to its cause and the best approach to treatment.

Central post-stroke pain (CPSP) is variably described as a superficial burning, lacerating or pricking sensation often exacerbated by factors including touch, movement, cold and anxiety (Bowsher 1996). It usually affects one-half of the body but may be more localized, affecting a quadrant, one limb or the face. Andersen *et al.* (1995b) reported that 16 (8%) of a group of 207 hospital-admitted stroke patients, who had survived 6 months and could communicate, had

CPSP and in 10 (5%) the pain was severe. This estimate is certainly higher than we would expect in our clinical practice. A less common, but related, problem is one of post-stroke pruritus (Kimyai-Asadi *et al.* 1999). Central post-stroke pain is usually associated with some abnormality of pin prick or temperature sensation and may be associated with autonomic changes, for example sweating or cold. It may start immediately after the stroke but more frequently after a delay of weeks or months (Bowsher 1996). Although the term 'thalamic pain' is commonly used synonymously with CPSP, this is misleading since the pain occurs in patients with stroke lesions affecting any part of the sensory pathways (Bowsher *et al.* 1998).

Central post-stroke pain is often resistant to therapy. Avoidance of those factors which exacerbate the symptoms is an important first step. Tricyclic antidepressants (e.g. nortryptiline) may alleviate the symptoms and also lift any associated depression (Leijon & Boivie 1989). A small dose should be used initially and be increased slowly until adequate symptom control is achieved or adverse effects become troublesome. If tricyclic antidepressants are ineffective, addition of gabapentin is probably a reasonable second-line treatment. A range of alternative drugs including other anticonvulsants (e.g. carbamazepine, phenytoin, valproate, clonazepam), antiarrhythmics (e.g. mexiletine), anaesthetics (e.g. ketamine), opiates and intrathecal baclofen have been advocated but none have been adequately evaluated in placebo-controlled randomized trials (Schott 1995; Wiffen *et al.* 2000). Analgesics of any kind are typically unhelpful, opiates included. Physical methods such as acupuncture and TENS are worth trying since they may occasionally provide relief and are at least fairly safe without any lasting adverse effects. Psychological interventions may help but have not been formally evaluated. More invasive and destructive techniques such as stereotactic mesencephalic tractotomy, or deep-brain stimulation, are occasionally used in severe cases which are resistant to other treatment modalities, but are not necessarily effective (Schott 1995).

15.24 Painful shoulder

Shoulder pain is a common problem after stroke. Wanklyn *et al.* (1996) reported that 63% of patients had shoulder pain in the first 6 months after hospital discharge, and in the Auckland community-based stroke register, about one-fifth of patients developed painful shoulders, usually within the first week and on the hemiparetic side (Ratnasabathy *et al.* 2000).

Although many factors (Table 15.31) have been associated with painful shoulder, their role in its development is unclear (Roy 1988; Van Langenberghe *et al.* 1988). A small propor-

Table 15.31 Factors associated with painful shoulder after stroke.

Associated features
Shoulder pain before the stroke
Low tone allowing glenohumeral subluxation/malalignment (Fig. 15.16)
Spasticity (section 15.20)
Severe weakness of the arm (section 15.21)
Sensory loss (section 15.22)
Neglect (section 15.28)
Visual field deficits (section 15.27.1)
Neurological mechanisms
Reflex sympathetic dystrophy (shoulder–hand syndrome)
Central post-stroke pain (section 15.23)
Brachial plexus injury
Orthopaedic problems
Adhesive capsulitis (frozen shoulder)
Rotator cuff tears due to improper handling or positioning
Acromioclavicular arthritis
Glenohumeral arthritis
Subdeltoid tendinitis

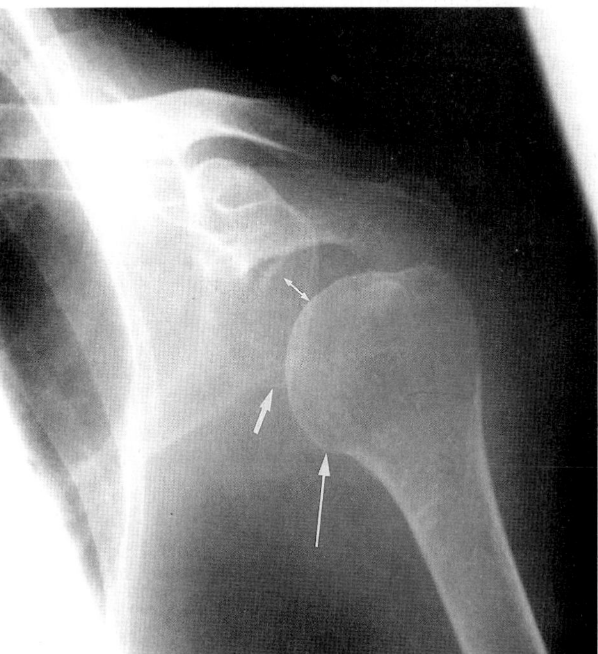

Fig. 15.16 X-ray of shoulder showing glenohumeral subluxation, a common finding in stroke patients, but does it matter? Note the widened joint space (double-headed arrow) and the increased distance between the lower border of the glenoid cavity (short arrow) and the lower border of the humeral head (long arrow) (photograph provided by Dr Allan Stephenson).

Table 15.32 Features of reflex sympathetic dystrophy.

Pain and tenderness on abduction, flexion and external rotation of the arm at the shoulder
Pain and swelling over the carpal bones
Swelling of metacarpophalangeal and proximal interphalangeal joints
Changes in temperature, colour and dryness of the skin on the hand
Loss of dorsal hand skin creases, and nail changes
Osteoporosis

Note: there is probably considerable overlap between reflex sympathetic dystrophy and the cold arms described by Wanklyn *et al.* (1995b) (section 15.25).

tion of patients who complain of a painful shoulder after a stroke have the other clinical features which comprise the syndrome of reflex sympathetic dystrophy or shoulder–hand syndrome (Table 15.32). It is unclear whether this represents a distinct entity or simply the severe end of a spectrum. Our ignorance of the causes and prognosis of shoulder pain is in part due to major problems of definition and the lack of well-validated and reliable assessment tools. Although our understanding of the epidemiology and causes of painful shoulder is incomplete, no-one involved in stroke rehabilitation can doubt its importance. It causes patients great discomfort, it may seriously affect morale, and can inhibit recovery. In some patients it persists for months, even years.

Table 15.33 General measures which may reduce the frequency of painful shoulder after stroke.

Instruct *all* staff and carers to:

Support the flaccid arm to reduce subluxation
Teach patients not to allow the affected arm to hang unsupported when sitting or standing. Whilst sitting they might use one of several arm supports which attach to the chair or wheelchair. All are more effective than a pillow which spends most of the time on the floor. Shoulder/arm orthoses may, depending on their design, prevent subluxation but have not been shown to reduce the frequency of painful shoulder (Fig. 15.17).

Avoid pulling on the affected arm when handling the patient
Staff and carers should be trained in methods of handling and lifting patients to avoid traction injuries.

Avoid any activity which causes shoulder discomfort
Therapy sessions sometimes do more harm than good.

Maintain range of passive shoulder movements

Prevention and treatment

Treatment of an established painful shoulder is often ineffective so that any measures to prevent its development are important. It is probably useful to introduce policies on the Stroke Unit which have been identified as being associated with a lower frequency of the problem in non-randomized studies (Table 15.33). It may also be useful to identify individuals who are at particularly high risk (based on the fac-

(a)
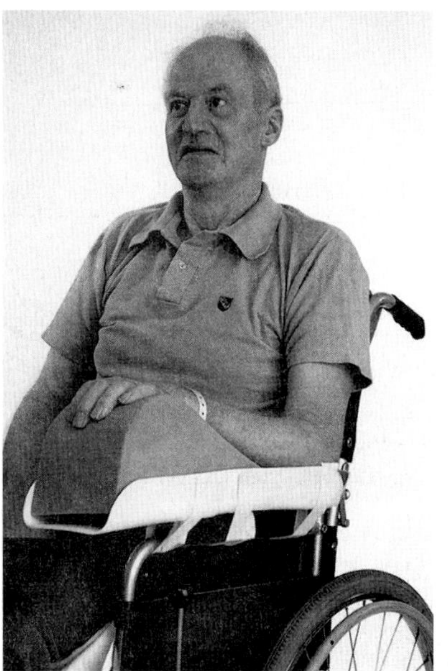
(b)
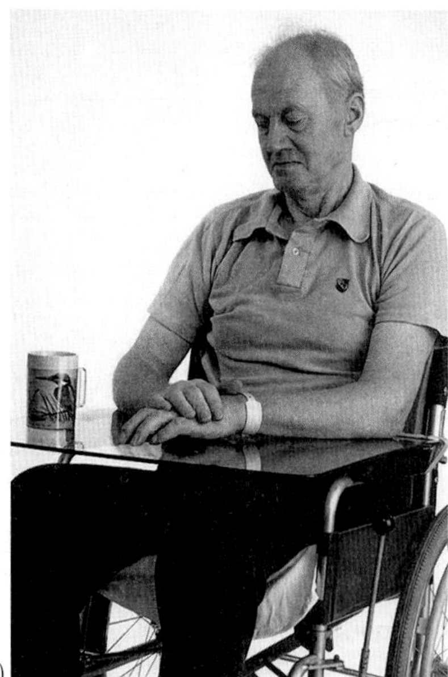
(c)
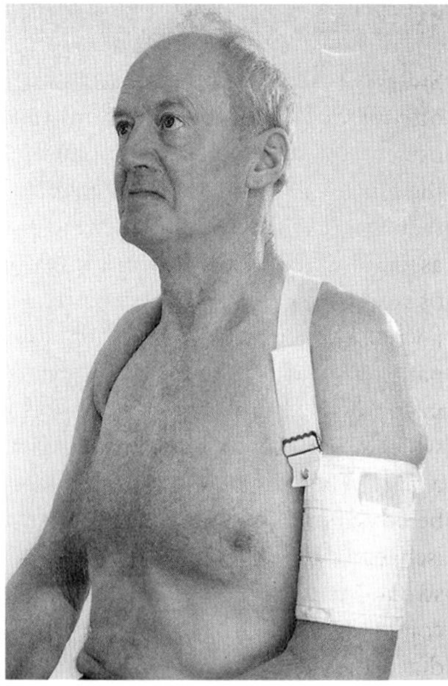

Fig. 15.17 By supporting the weight of the arm, glenohumeral subluxation can be reduced. This may be achieved when the patient is sitting using an arm support (a) which attaches to the chair or wheelchair or, alternatively, a perspex tray (b) which, because it is transparent, allows the patient to check on the position of their feet. Both are better than pillows which invariably end up on the floor. Several designs of sling (c) are available to reduce subluxation when patients are upright.

tors in Table 15.31) and make all staff aware of the potential problem. More specific interventions including slings and cuffs to support the flaccid arm (Fig. 15.17) (Brooke *et al.* 1991), and functional electrical stimulation (Linn *et al.* 1999; Price & Pandyan 2000), may reduce subluxation but their effect on the frequency of painful shoulder and arm function is unproven. Many therapists worry that the use of slings and cuffs will inhibit recovery of the arm because the arm is held in a position which promotes spasticity.

When a patient complains of shoulder pain it is important to exclude glenohumeral dislocation, fracture or specific shoulder syndromes. For example, painful arc (supraspinatus tendinitis) may respond better to specific measures (e.g. local steroid injection) although even the evidence supporting treatments for these specific syndromes is poor (Green *et al.* 1998, 2000). In established painful shoulder many treatments have been suggested, some have been evaluated in small RCTs, but further studies are needed to define the best treatments (Table 15.34) (Inaba & Piorkowski 1972; Braus *et al.* 1994). Some interventions are probably harmless (e.g. application of cold, heat, strapping, TENS) and if they produce even short-term relief they are worth trying (Leandri *et al.* 1990; Partridge *et al.* 1990; Ancliffe 1992). Others have potentially important adverse effects and costs (e.g. steroid injections) and therefore need to be evaluated further before being adopted into routine clinical practice (Dekker *et al.* 1997).

Shoulder pain after stroke is common, ill understood, difficult to prevent and none of the suggested treatments are supported by reliable evidence.

Table 15.34 Treatments used for painful shoulders.

Physiotherapy
Positioning and mobilization
Exercises (Partridge *et al.* 1990)
Heat or cold (Partridge *et al.* 1990)

Support
Strapping (Ancliffe 1992)
Shoulder/arm orthoses (Fig. 15.17)
Bobath sling
Rood support
Arm supports for bed or chairs
Lapboard (Fig. 15.17)
Forearm support
Wheelchair outrigger (Fig. 15.17)

Medication
Systemic:
- Analgesics
- Non-steroidal anti-inflammatory drugs
- Corticosteroids (Braus *et al.* 1994)
- Antispastic drugs (Table 15.26)
- Phenoxybenzamine
- Antidepressants

Local:
- Corticosteroid injection of shoulder (Dekker *et al.* 1997)
- Local anaesthetic
- Stellate ganglion block

Other physical
Ultrasound (Inaba & Piorkowski 1972)
Acupuncture
Biofeedback
Transcutaneous electrical nerve stimulation (TENS) (Leandri *et al.* 1990)

Surgery
Sympathectomy
Humeral head suspension
Relief of contractures

15.25 Swollen and cold limbs

Swelling with pitting oedema, and sometimes pain, quite often occurs in the paralysed or neglected hand, arm or leg, usually within the first few weeks. The swelling may limit the movement of the affected part and the pain not only further restricts movement but also exacerbates spasticity and associated reactions (section 15.20). Some patients complain of coldness of the limb, more often of the arm than the leg (Wanklyn *et al.* 1995b). Swelling often occurs in the legs of patients who sit for prolonged periods (section 15.13) and in a paralysed arm. Gravity and lack of muscle contraction, which reduce venous and lymphatic return, presumably play a part. There are a number of other causes which need to be considered (Table 15.35). People with fractures or acute ischaemia of the limb usually complain of severe pain, but stroke patients with sensory loss, visuospatial dysfunction or communication difficulties may not, which can lead to these diagnoses being overlooked.

Table 15.35 Causes of swollen limb after stroke.

Gravity in a dependent limb
Lack of muscle contraction
Deep venous thrombosis (section 15.13)
Compression of veins or lymphatics by tumour, etc.
Cardiac failure
Hypoalbuminaemia (section 15.19)
Occult injury (section 15.26)
Acute ischaemia
Reflex sympathetic dystrophy (section 15.24) (Table 15.32)

Assessment

The other causes of a swollen limb should be excluded by clinical examination and appropriate investigation before attributing the swelling simply to immobility or dependency.

Investigation is not usually necessary but Doppler ultrasound or venography to exclude deep venous thrombosis of the leg (section 15.13), simple X-ray of a swollen wrist or ankle to exclude a fracture, and a serum albumin may be useful. One can monitor the effect of any intervention by simply measuring the circumference of the limb although plethysmography has been used in research studies.

Treatment

The treatment obviously depends on the cause. Where the swelling appears to be due to immobility we try the following:

- elevation of the affected limb when at rest;
- encourage active movement (but this may be impossible with severe weakness but is important if neglect is the main cause);
- graduated compression stocking on the leg (full length or below-knee depending on extent of swelling) or a bandage on the arm, although the latter may worsen swelling of the hand; and
- intermittent compression of the limb although this was shown to be ineffective in reducing arm swelling in a randomized trial (Roper *et al.* 1999).

In addition, where the limb is painful, simple analgesia may ameliorate the secondary effects of pain on tone which lead to spasticity and contractures. Diuretics should be avoided unless there is evidence of heart failure, since immobile stroke patients have a tendency to become dehydrated (section 15.18.1) and incontinent (section 15.14).

15.26 Falls and fractures

Falls are common after stroke. Between 25 and 39% of patients have been reported as falling during in-patient rehabilitation, the higher figure coming from a prospective study in a unit dealing mainly with elderly patients (Dromerick & Reding 1994; Nyberg & Gustafson 1995; Langhorne *et al.* 2000). Falls are also frequent amongst stroke patients who are dependent in activities of daily living (ADL) following discharge from hospital. In one study, 79% of such patients fell in the first 6 months at home and the majority fell more than once (Forster & Young 1995). Many factors contribute to this tendency to fall, some are listed in Table 15.36. Some of these, and others (male sex, dependency in ADL, urinary incontinence, postural instability, bilateral motor impairment, bilateral brain lesion or leukoaraiosis on brain imaging, visuospatial neglect and use of diuretics, sedatives or antidepressants) have been incorporated in a risk assessment scale (Nyberg & Gustafson 1997). This needs to be simplified and validated in an independent cohort (section 10.2.7) before it is employed in routine practice.

A small proportion of falls occurring in hospital (<5%), or in the first few months at home (about 1%), result in serious injury, most often fracture of the hip, pelvis or wrist, but other injuries (e.g. head and soft tissue), fear and loss of confidence are very common consequences (Forster & Young 1995; Nyberg & Gustafson 1995). Stroke patients are two to four times more likely to suffer a fracture than unaffected individuals, and over 80% are secondary to falls (Ramnemark *et al.* 1998). Most hip fractures affect the hemiparetic side, probably because the patients tend to fall to that side, but the osteoporosis which develops on the side of the weakness may be a contributory factor (Ramnemark *et al.* 1999).

Table 15.36 Factors likely to contribute to falls after stroke.

The patient
Muscle weakness (especially of quadriceps) (section 15.21)
Sensory loss (especially visual impairments) (sections 15.22 and 15.27)
Impaired balance, righting reflexes and ataxia (section 15.21)
Confusion (section 15.29)
Visuospatial neglect, e.g. denial of hemiparesis (section 15.28)
Deformity, e.g. plantar flexion causing toe catching (section 15.20)
Epileptic seizures (section 15.8)
Postural hypotension due to drugs or dehydration (sections 15.2.3 and 15.18.1)
The environment
Inappropriate footwear, e.g. slippers
Slippery floors, deep pile carpets and loose rugs
Excess furniture
Poorly positioned rails and inappropriate aids
Lack of supervision
Fire doors (these may close automatically and hit slow-moving stroke patients)
Drugs: Sedatives and hypnotics
Hypotensive drugs
Antispastic drugs (Table 15.26)
Anticonvulsants

Stroke patients with communication problems, sensory loss or neglect may not report injury or pain so it is important to look for signs of fracture, i.e. deformity, swelling, bruising, on admission and after any accident. One should have a low threshold for X-raying suspected fractures.

Prevention and treatment

One could avoid falls, and thus fractures, by keeping the patient in bed, clearly not a solution during rehabilitation. The risk of falls and injuries may be minimized by the physiotherapist, nursing staff and carer working closely together to ensure that patients are mobilizing with adequate supervision and support. It is also useful to identify patients who are at particular risk of falling (see above). Withdrawal of unnecessary diuretics, and psychotropic drugs, and avoidance of any relevant environmental causes should help reduce the risk of falls (Hanlon *et al.* 1996) (Table 15.36). There is evidence, although not specifically in stroke patients, that attention to risk factors and exercise programmes can reduce the risk of falls (Campbell *et al.* 1999; Gillespie *et al.* 2000) and the use of hip protectors can reduce the risk of hip fracture in individuals prone to falls (Parker *et al.* 2000). Drugs such as Vitamin D or bisphosphonates might prevent osteoporosis of the affected limb and thus reduce the risk of fractures but large studies are required to establish whether the routine use of such interventions is worthwhile (Sato *et al.* 1997).

15.27 Visual problems

Stroke patients often have pre-existing visual problems due to refractive errors, cataracts, glaucoma, diabetic retinopathy and senile macular degeneration (Lotery *et al.* 2000). Although it is beyond the scope of this book to deal with their specific management, it is important that the clinician is aware of them, and their causes, because they may have an important influence on the patient's function.

Simple measures such as ensuring that a patient's glasses are clean, available and on their nose are obvious but easily overlooked.

15.27.1 Visual field defects

About 20% of stroke patients have a demonstrable field defect (Turney *et al.* 1984) (Table 15.2). However, a similar proportion are not assessable because of reduced conscious level or communication difficulties. The frequency in hospital patients will obviously depend on patient selection and the methods used to detect defects. Apart from their value in localizing the stroke lesion (section 3.3.6), visual field defects have some predictive value. A homonymous visual field defect in association with motor and cognitive deficits is usually due to a large stroke lesion and is associated with a relatively poor prognosis (section 4.3.4). Some patients who are mobile but unaware of their field loss may be at greater risk of injury. Many patients with field defects find reading and watching television difficult, although some of their difficulty may be due to associated problems with cognition and concentration. Homonymous field defects have important implications for patients who wish to drive (and sometimes for unfortunate pedestrians and cyclists!) (section 15.32.2). Some of the difficulties in detecting field defects in stroke patients have already been discussed in section 3.3.6.

There have been very few studies of the recovery of visual field defects after stroke. Gray *et al.* (1989) found that only 14 (17%) of 81 patients with an acute hemispheric stroke and complete homonymous hemianopia (more than half of the hemifield was lost) had normal visual fields 1 month after their stroke. Most of any recovery occurred within the first 10 days. Thirteen (72%) patients with only an incomplete hemianopia initially (less than half of the hemifield was lost) recovered over the same period. This study supports our clinical impression that usually, although there are exceptions, visual field defects persist unless they resolve early.

Usually, although there are exceptions, visual field defects persist unless they resolve early.

No treatment is known to enhance the recovery of visual field defects. Therefore, interventions which aim to reduce the resulting disability and handicap are most important. It seems sensible to avoid putting patients with a homonymous field defect in a bed next to the wall so they cannot see anything going on around them. One can imagine that this 'sensory deprivation' might be bad for morale. It may be possible to teach the patient to compensate for a field defect by strategies such as head turning. Hemianopia, even without associated neglect, makes reading difficult. Loss of the right visual field means that the patient has to track the words into a blind field, especially where they have no macular sparing. Loss of the left visual field makes it difficult to find the start of each line and patients lose their place easily. This can sometimes be helped by putting a ruler under each line and their hand or a bright coloured object at the left-hand margin, and to train them to look at this before starting a new line. Large print makes reading easier. Some patients with a right homonymous hemianopia find they can read more easily upside down because they can scan from right to left. Fresnel's lenses, which shift images in the hemianopic field into the intact one, were evaluated in one small randomized trial where they improved visual perception but not activities of daily living (Rossi *et al.* 1990). Patients with field defects spend a lot of money on new glasses within a few months of their stroke because they mistakenly believe that the problem is with their eyes. It is therefore important that the nature of the problem is explained to the patient and any carer and that new glasses are only prescribed where there is an uncorrected refractive error.

Patients often attribute their poor vision after a stroke to inadequate glasses. Explain to patients the nature and cause of their visual problems so they do not waste their money on inappropriate new glasses.

15.27.2 Disordered eye movements, diplopia and oscillopsia

Strokes may lead to conjugate gaze palsies so the patient is unable to look in a particular direction(s), or has diplopia due to dysconjugate eye movements (section 3.3.6). Conjugate gaze palsies were present in about 8% of 675 stroke patients at presentation in the Oxfordshire Community Stroke Project (Table 15.2) but are more common in hospital-based series, presumably because lacunar and minor cortical strokes are under-represented (Turney *et al.* 1984; Stone *et al.* 1993). The pattern of abnormal eye movements after stroke helps to localize the stroke lesion and the presence of a conjugate gaze palsy in a supratentorial stroke is associated with a poor outcome (Table 10.6).

Conjugate gaze palsies rarely cause disability or handicap. Double vision, which may result from dysconjugate eye movements, and oscillopsia associated with nystagmus, are much more troublesome, sometimes exacerbating gait problems and making reading, watching television and driving difficult. The practical difficulties in assessing eye movements after stroke have been discussed earlier (section 3.3.6).

The most effective way of relieving patients of double vision in the early stages is a patch over one eye (it probably does not matter which, although alternation is traditionally recommended). Diplopia often resolves in a few weeks of the stroke but if it remains a problem it can be helped by using glasses fitted with prism lenses. However, prisms are of no use where diplopia is associated with a variable degree of divergence. Of course, patients should be warned not to spend a lot of money on new glasses until they have reached a stable state. Oscillopsia rarely seems to persist which is fortunate since there are no effective remedies.

15.27.3 Visual hallucinations

Occasionally, patients report vivid visual hallucinations after strokes (section 3.3.6). However, more often they occur as part of an acute confusional state (section 15.29.1) and resolve, but if persistent it may be worth considering investigations to exclude epileptic seizures, particularly if the hallucinations are stereotyped and localized to a hemianopic field. Visual hallucinations, sometimes associated with confusion, are frequently seen after administering neuroprotective drugs (section 11.6), so if these drugs are shown to improve the outcome of stroke this problem may become much more common. Usually, patients simply require explanation and reassurance, although if hallucinations are associated with marked agitation a major tranquilliser may be needed.

15.28 Visuospatial dysfunction

Visuospatial dysfunction includes visual and sensory neglect, visual and sensory inattention or extinction, constructional dyspraxias and agnosias. Unfortunately, the nomenclature is complex and confused by the use of different terms for the same phenomena (Table 3.10).

The frequency of visuospatial dysfunction amongst stroke patients varies widely in the published literature because of patient selection, the timing of assessments and the use of different definitions and assessments (Bowen *et al.* 1999). Visual neglect has been reported in 33–85% of patients with right-hemisphere strokes and 0–47% of those with left-hemisphere strokes (Stone *et al.* 1993).

Assessment

More sensitive tests will naturally increase the apparent frequency of the problem. Stone *et al.* (1993) reported a high frequency of visuospatial dysfunction amongst 171 consecutive admissions to two hospitals in London, examined within two or three days of an acute hemispheric stroke using the Behavioural Inattention Test (Table 15.37). This contains various tests which aim to assess both sensory neglect (patient's perception of incoming stimuli) and motor neglect (the patient's willingness to explore external space) (Table 15.38). The frequency of visuopatial dysfunction in dominant hemisphere stroke may be underestimated because of the practical difficulties in assessing patients with a paralysed dominant hand or problems with language (section 3.3.3). With unstructured and non-standardized testing (usually including bilateral simultaneous stimulation for sensory and visual inattention, clock drawing and simple figure copying) we identified only 16% of assessable patients (25% were not assessable because of reduced level of consciousness, language problems or paralysis) in the Oxfordshire Community Stroke Project as having visuospatial dysfunction (Table 15.2). Testing visuospatial function is one of the most difficult aspects of the examination and therefore frequently omitted in routine practice (Davenport *et al.* 1995; Rudd *et al.* 1999). It is not surprising that the inter-observer reliability of unstructured testing is relatively poor (kappa = 0.4) (Table 3.20). We have already described some simple bedside assessments which are useful in detecting impairments of functional importance as well as in helping to localize the stroke lesion (Table 3.11).

Prognosis

Visuospatial problems are major causes of disability and handicap, impede functional recovery and have been associated, although not invariably so (Pedersen *et al.* 1997), with a poor outcome (Denes *et al.* 1982; Kinsella & Ford 1985) (Table 10.3). There have been few studies of the recovery of visuospatial function, but these suggest, as with most other stroke-related impairments, that recovery is most rapid in the first week or two and then slows (Cassidy *et al.* 1999; Ferro *et al.* 1999) (section 10.2.5). Between 10 and 20% of

Table 15.37 Frequency of visuospatial problems amongst hospitalized patients within three days of a hemispheric first stroke (Stone *et al.* 1993).

	Per cent of assessable patients with phenomena		Per cent not assessable	
	Right hemisphere ($n = 69$)	Left hemisphere ($n = 102$)	Right hemisphere ($n = 69$)	Left hemisphere ($n = 102$)
Visual neglect	82	65	11	27
Hemi-inattention	70	49	9	15
Tactile extinction	65	35	25	58
Allaesthesia	57	11	15	55
Visual extinction	23	2	13	21
Anosognosia	28	5	13	45
Anosodiaphoria	27	2	13	48
Non-belonging	36	29	20	53
Gaze paresis	29	25	0	3
Visual field defect	36	46	11	9

Note: The differences in frequency between left and right were statistically significant for all but non-belonging, gaze paresis and visual field defects. The relatively high frequency of these phenomena in this series (cf. Table 15.2) probably reflects the severity of the strokes in this hospital-referred series and the sensitivity of the test battery used.

patients with visual neglect in the acute stage have persisting problems 3 months later and recovery after this time is usually slow and incomplete (Stone *et al.* 1992). However, this study used a sensitive instrument to detect even mild cases so that in routine clinical practice, where only more marked impairments are detected, the prognosis may be worse. Stone *et al.* (1992) also showed that if visual neglect was severe and associated with anosognosia it was less likely to resolve.

Table 15.38 Components of the Behavioural Inattention Test (from Wilson *et al.* 1987).

Full version	Modified version
Line crossing	Pointing to objects in ward
Letter cancellation	Food on the plate
Star cancellation (Fig. 3.9)	Reading a menu
Figure and shape drawing	Reading a newspaper article
Line bisection	Star cancellation (Fig. 3.9)
Line cancellation	Picture scanning
Representational drawing	Coin selection
Telephone dialling	Figure copying
Menu reading	
Article reading	
Telling and setting time	
Coin sorting	
Address and sentence copying	
Map navigation	
Card sorting	

Treatment

Visuospatial dysfunction has a major impact on rehabilitation. For instance, it is difficult to persuade patients with anosognosia or denial to become involved in therapy. There have been very few randomized controlled trials (RCTs) of interventions aimed at improving visuospatial function after stroke and they have all suffered from the difficulties outlined previously (Table 15.1). Several small RCTs have shown an effect of specific interventions for neglect on performance on test batteries but less impact on activities of daily living (Robertson 1993; Ferro *et al.* 1999). In other words, any benefit of therapy appears to benefit performance on selected tasks but not usually on general visuospatial abilities.

Currently, therefore we have to adopt strategies which do not necessarily influence the severity of the underlying impairment but may reduce the resulting disability and handicap and help carers to cope. Carers are often bemused, frustrated or angered by the behavioural consequences of visuospatial dysfunction and it is very important to spend time explaining the unusual nature of the deficit. If this is not done, then carers may wrongly conclude that the patient is dementing, wilfully obstructive or even deliberately ignoring them.

Patients with unilateral neglect are often positioned so they have their intact side facing a wall to encourage them to respond to stimuli on the affected side. However, since there is little evidence that this strategy influences outcome, we generally aim to position the patient in the middle of the ward so they receive stimulation from both sides on the basis that their morale might suffer if they are not stimulated

(Loverro & Reding 1988). In our experience, patients with unilateral neglect and hemiparesis can be taught to walk, but often this is of limited functional use because they are so prone to falls. Unless supervised when walking, the patient's attention may become drawn to the unaffected side, which appears to inhibit activity on the affected side which leads to the fall. It can be difficult to persuade a patient who is unaware of their hemiparesis that they should only try to walk when supervised and that unsupervised walking carries a risk of falls and fractures (section 15.26). Patients with neglect are at risk in other situations, for example in the kitchen, because they are unaware of dangers to their affected side so that measures have to be taken to reduce this risk, for example use of a microwave rather than a conventional cooker.

Carers are often bemused, frustrated and angered by the behavioural consequences of visuospatial dysfunction and it is very important to spend time explaining the unusual nature of the deficit.

15.29 Cognitive dysfunction

The majority of patients with stroke are elderly and so pre-existing dementia is common. Its frequency has been estimated at 6–16% depending on the stroke population studied, the definitions and methods of ascertainment used (Gustafson *et al.* 1991; Henon *et al.* 1999). In clinical practice, as well as formal studies, it is important to gather information from the family about the patients' pre-stroke cognitive state, especially where patients have communication problems. The Informant Questionnaire on Cognitive Decline in the Elderly (IQCODE) is a well-validated assessment of previous cognitive status which makes use of information from the patient and their family (Jorm *et al.* 1991). Without this information it is impossible to distinguish pre-stroke dementia from acute confusional states, and dementia secondary to the stroke. These will have different potential for improvement.

15.29.1 Acute confusional states

In prospective hospital-based studies, the frequency of acute delirium, defined according to the criteria of the Diagnostic and Statistical Manual of Mental Disorders (DSM), version IIIR or IV is 24–48% (Gustafson *et al.* 1991; Henon *et al.* 1999). A similar range of frequencies has been found for disorientation in time, place or person within the first week or two among stroke patients admitted to hospital (Desmond *et al.* 1994; Pederson *et al.* 1998). Many risk factors for developing an acute confusional state after stroke have been identified but the most consistent are increasing age, pre-stroke dementia, and greater stroke severity. The frequency of acute confusional states amongst unselected stroke patients (i.e. including those not admitted to hospital) is likely to be lower than in the published hospital-based series given the association with stroke severity. Although acute confusional states after stroke may be a direct consequence of the cerebral dysfunction, or non-cerebral complications (Table 15.39), abnormal function of the hypothalamic–pituitary–adrenal axis has been associated with acute confusion (Mitchell 1997). Confusion with disorientation, poor memory and disruptive behaviour are distressing to other patients and carers and severely hamper rehabilitation. Patients with acute confusional states are more likely to have longer hospital stays, are less likely to be discharged home, and they have worse physical and cognitive outcomes (Gustafson *et al.* 1991; Henon *et al.* 1999).

Assessment

Cognitive impairments are often overlooked in elderly patients admitted to hospital (Arden *et al.* 1993). Unstructured assessments have been shown to have poor inter-observer reliability (kappa = 0.2–0.4) (Table 3.20). Therefore, it is important to include one of the large number of assess-

Table 15.39 Causes of cognitive dysfunction after stroke.

Coincidental (pre-existing)
Alzheimer's disease and other dementing illnesses

Directly caused by stroke
Large hemispheric lesions
Strategically located lesions, e.g. thalamus (section 3.3.3)
Vascular dementia (section 5.7.1)
Amyloid angiopathy (section 8.2.2)
Giant cell arteritis (section 7.3)*
Primary angiitis of the central nervous system (section 7.3)*
Infective endocarditis (sections 6.5 and 8.2.11)*

Complications of the stroke
Infections (section 15.12)*
Hypoxia, hypotension, etc. (section 15.2)*
Metabolic abnormalities (section 15.18)*
Depression (section 15.31.1)*
Hydrocephalus (section 12.2.6)*
Epileptic seizures (section 15.8)*
Urinary retention (section 15.14)*
Alcohol and drug withdrawal*
Drugs (e.g. neuroleptics, anticholinergic, antispastic, sedatives, antidepressants, diuretics)*

Conditions mimicking stroke (section 3.4)
Herpes encephalitis (section 3.4.6)
Chronic subdural haematoma (section 3.4.4)
Cerebral abscess or subdural empyema (section 3.4.6)
Cerebral tumour (section 3.4.4)
Creutzfeldt–Jakob disease (section 3.4.6)

*Potentially reversible causes.

ment tools available, e.g. the ten-item Hodkinson Abbreviated Mental Test (Table 15.40) or the longer Mini Mental State Examination (Table 15.41), in the routine assessment of patients on admission to the Stroke Unit. Having such a measure at baseline allows subsequent changes to be identified and the causes sought. Where patients are unable to communicate one usually has to rely on the family, and the team's observation of the patient's behaviour and learning capacity.

Treatment

Treatment should focus on any potentially reversible underlying cause such as infection, electrolyte imbalance or hypoxia (Table 15.39). Confused patients require closer observation to reduce the risk of falls, and inappropriate removal of oxygen masks, intravenous cannulae, nasogastric tubes and urinary catheters. The balance of risk and benefit must be carefully weighed in each patient before one resorts to other measures such as mattresses on the floor (which may reduce injury but increase disorientation and make nursing more hazardous), physical restraints (which some regard as unethical and may cause injury) and psychotropic drugs (which have many adverse effects including confusion, hypotension, dehydration and involuntary movements).

15.29.2 Post-stroke dementia

Some patients, who had no recognized cognitive problems before their stroke, develop cognitive deficits which persist after the acute illness, or develop over the following months. In the Framingham study, nine (12%) of 74 patients who had normal scores on their Mini Mental State Examination (MMSE) before their stroke scored less than 24 on the MMSE 6 months after the stroke (Kase *et al.* 1998). In several hospital-based studies which relied on retrospective diagnosis of pre-stroke dementia, the estimates of the frequency of new dementia in the first year after stroke were about 15% although rates of over 30% have been reported (Inzitari *et al.* 1998). Although cognitive dysfunction, in common with most other post-stroke impairments, during the first few months after stroke may subsequently improve (Desmond *et al.* 1996), one longitudinal study has shown that, among patients without significant cognitive impairment on hospital discharge, there was a 29% risk of dementia (according to DSM IIIR criteria) in the subsequent year (Treves *et al.* 1997). This suggests that stroke might trigger a progressive process in some patients. Predictably, older age and indicators of greater stroke severity have been found consistently to be associated with post-stroke dementia whilst other factors such as being female, previous stroke, primary intracerebral haemorrhage and atrial fibrillation and other cardiovascular problems have been identified in individual studies (Inzitari *et al.* 1998; Barba *et al.* 2000). Post-stroke dementia is associated with a worse long-term survival and worse functional outcomes (Tatemichi *et al.* 1994; Desmond *et al.* 1998).

Table 15.40 Hodkinson Abbreviated Mental Test (from Hodkinson 1972).

Patient's age
Time (estimated to nearest hour)
Mr John Brown, 42 West Street, Gateshead (should be repeated to ensure that the patient has heard it correctly and then recalled at end of test)
Name of hospital/place
Current year
Recognition of two people (e.g. doctor, nurse)
Patient's date of birth
Dates of World War I*
Present monarch†
Count down from 20 to 1

Patient scores one point for each correct response.

* It may now be more appropriate to ask for dates of World War II.
† Clearly in some countries it would be more relevant to ask who the president is.

Assessment

It is important to reassess patients' cognitive function, even months or years after the stroke, especially where a deterioration in cognition or functional status has been noted by the patient or carer. Simple bedside assessments such as the Mini Mental State Examination (Table 15.41) and CAMCOG (the cognitive and self-contained part of the Cambridge Examination for Mental Disorders of the Elderly (CAMDEX)) (De Koning *et al.* 1998) are usually adequate for this purpose but one has to be aware that such measures tend to emphasize language dysfunction and are less sensitive in identifying, for example, visuospatial problems (section 15.28). More detailed neuropsychological assessments (e.g. Raven's Progressive Matrices, Raven 1965) which depend less on intact language function may be required to give a true indication of the patient's degree of cognitive deficit.

Prevention and treatment

Unfortunately, post-stroke dementia is rarely reversible but it may possibly be prevented and progression slowed by treating vascular risk factors, antithrombotic drugs and other means (sections 16.3 and 16.4). Many drugs are widely used in the treatment of vascular dementia (e.g. piracetam, oxypentifylline, naftidrofuryl oxalate, codergocrine mesylate) though there is little evidence of their benefit. Donepezil and rivastigmine appear to improve cognitive function in patients with mild and moderate dementia due to Alzheimer's disease

Table 15.41 Mini Mental State Examination (adapted from Folstein *et al.* 1975).

Section	Questions	Max. points
1. Orientation	(a) Can you tell me today's (date)/(month)/(year)? Which (day of the week) is it today? Can you also tell me which (season) it is?	5
	(b) What city/town are we in? What is the (county)/(country)? What (building) are we in and on what (floor)?	5
2. Registration	I should like to test your memory (name 3 common objects, e.g. 'ball, car, man') Can you repeat the words I said? (*score 1 point for each word*) (repeat up to 6 trials until all three are remembered) (record number of trials needed here:)	3
3. Attention and calculation	(a) From 100 keep subtracting 7 and give each answer: stop after 5 answers (93_86_79_72_65_) *Alternatively* (b) Spell the word 'WORLD' backwards (D_L_R_O_W)	5
4. Recall	What were the three words I asked you to say earlier? (*skip this test if all three objects were not remembered during registration test*)	3
5. Language Naming Repeating	Name these objects (show a watch) (show a pencil) Repeat the following: 'no ifs, ands or buts'	2 1
6. Reading and writing	Show card or write 'CLOSE YOUR EYES' Read this sentence and do what it says	1
	Now can you write a short sentence for me?	1
7. Three stage command	Present paper Take this paper in your left (or right) hand, fold it in half, and put it on the floor	3
8 Construction	Will you copy this drawing please? (intersecting pentagons)	1
Total score		**30**

but their effectiveness in vascular dementia is not established. Of course, one should seek to exclude any factors which may cause acute confusion (section 15.29.1) and reversible causes of dementia (e.g. severe depression, hypothyroidism) (Kimura *et al.* 2000). In planning patients' rehabilitation, placement and longer-term care it is important to know whether the patient's cognitive state will improve over months, is stable or worsening. Unfortunately, only regular reassessment over a prolonged period can do this. If patients are disorientated or have memory problems the 'carry over' between therapy sessions is often poor, leading to slow progress with rehabilitation. Our current practice, which aims to make best use of scarce resources, is to try to identify patients with irreversible severe cognitive dysfunction as early as possible and, taking account of this, get on with planning long-term placement and a suitable package of care. Ideally, where cognitive dysfunction limits the patients' involvement in rehabilitation one should be able to arrange suitable supportive care for a period, after which a further assessment of their ability to benefit from rehabilitation could be made. Alas, the inflexibility of most stroke services currently makes this approach difficult (section 17.5.4).

Look systematically for pre- and post-stroke cognitive problems at an early stage in order to take account of them in the planning of rehabilitation, placement and long-term care.

15.30 Communication difficulties

The most common problems with communication after stroke are aphasia and dysarthria, which may occur separately but frequently co-exist. Aphasia is almost invariably associated with dysgraphia and sometimes dyslexia. Patients occasionally talk very quietly after a stroke, which sometimes appears to be due to difficulties in co-ordinating speech and breathing. Other abnormalities include aprosody (loss of emotional content of speech) which occurs with non-dominant hemisphere lesions.

15.30.1 Aphasia

Estimates of the frequency of aphasia have inevitably depended on the population and screening methods used. In the Oxfordshire Community Stroke Project, 19% of 564 assessable patients were thought to be dysphasic at first assessment (Table 15.2) whilst in the hospital-based Copenhagen Stroke Study 38% of 881 conscious patients were judged dysphasic according to the Scandinavian Stroke Scale (Pederson *et al.* 1995).

Assessment

A thorough assessment of patients' communication abilities is not only important to localize and classify the stroke lesion (section 3.3.3) but also to:

• find a way for the patient to express his or her feelings, make their needs known to the carers and so avoid unnecessary distress caused by, for example, urinary incontinence (section 15.14);

• find out how much the patient is capable of understanding so that one can tailor information-giving to their level of understanding. Also, therapists need to find a way of asking the patient to follow quite complex instructions, although many therapists are masters of non-verbal communication;

• assess the patient's prognosis and set appropriate rehabilitation goals; and

• protect the patient from losing control of their affairs. We have seen lawyers, oblivious to patients' severe aphasia and dyslexia, explaining complex documents and asking for (and obtaining) patients' signatures. The hazards of such apparent 'comprehension and consent' are self evident but often not considered by physicians. It is important that the family and lawyer are made aware of patients' level of comprehension.

Although communication problems may be obvious, it is not always easy, as we have already discussed, to distinguish aphasia from dysarthria (section 3.3.3). Table 3.9 outlines a simple assessment of language function. It is important not to overlook pre-existing impairments such as deafness, ill-fitting dentures and poor vision which can all adversely affect a patient's ability to communicate. Before testing comprehension the patient must be wearing their hearing aid which should be turned on and functioning properly.

It is quite common for language function to vary with factors such as fatigue, anxiety and intercurrent illness. If patients' communication deteriorates under these circumstance it is important to explain that they have not had a recurrent stroke. Different members of the rehabilitation team may judge the severity of an individual patient's problems differently. In our experience, nurses often overestimate the patient's ability to understand language in part because, in dealing with the patient, they use a lot of non-verbal cueing which is of course of immense value.

More formal testing of language function with one of the standardized instruments (e.g. Western Aphasia Test, Aachen Aphasia Score, Porch Index of Communication Ability, Boston Diagnostic Aphasia Examination) is sometimes useful where there is doubt about the diagnosis, or in research projects, but these are usually administered by a speech and language therapist. The Frenchay Aphasia Screening Test (FAST) has been developed for use in routine clinical practice by non-experts and has reasonable reliability and validity (Enderby *et al.* 1986, 1987; O'Neill *et al.* 1990).

Having established that the patient has a communication problem, one should ensure that all the simple measures to optimize a patient's ability to communicate are taken, e.g. correct false teeth, hearing aid and spectacles are being used. These simple things are easily overlooked but can make a great difference to the patient.

Prognosis

Aphasia is a frequent cause of long-term disability and handicap. The pattern of recovery and its dependence on initial severity is illustrated by data from the Copenhagen Stroke Study (Fig. 15.18). Most recovery usually occurs within the first few weeks and, not surprisingly, those with mild aphasia at stroke onset have a better outcome (Ferro *et al.* 1999).

Treatment

There is considerable controversy about the effectiveness of speech and language therapy in aphasia. The results of the randomized controlled trials (RCTs) have been disappointing, mainly because of methodological weaknesses, as outlined in Table 15.1 (Whurr *et al.* 1992; Ferro *et al.* 1999; Greener *et al.* 2000a). However, other criticisms include the failure to describe the interventions, use of weak or low-intensity interventions, inappropriate control therapies, unblinded assessments of outcome and large numbers of patients lost to follow-up or not complying with treatment. Although some studies have shown that intensive treatment may be effective (Hagen 1973; Wertz *et al.* 1986), others have shown no clear evidence of benefit from less intensive treatment (Lincoln *et al.* 1984). Several small RCTs have shown that, at least for selected patients, similar outcomes can be achieved from the input of volunteers working with guidance from a speech and language therapist vs. regular therapy from trained therapists (Meikle *et al.* 1979; David *et al.* 1982; Wertz *et al.* 1986; Hartman & Landau 1987;

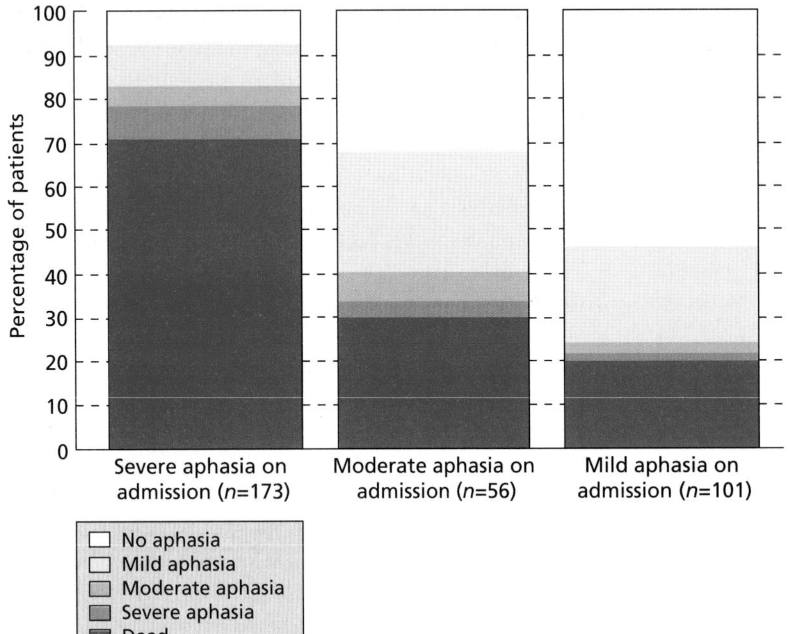

Fig. 15.18 The relationship between aphasia on hospital admission and outcome at six months in the Copenhagen Stroke Study. Of 881 assessable patients on admission, 173 had severe aphasia (i.e. could only say 'yes' and 'no' or less), 56 moderate aphasia (i.e. better than severe but could speak in sentences) and 101 mild aphasia (i.e. limited vocabulary). Fifty-six (17%) aphasia patients were not followed up at six months (with permission from Pederson *et al.* 1995).

Marshall *et al.* 1989). One meta-analysis, of both randomized and non-randomized studies of the effectiveness of therapy on language, concluded that therapy, whether introduced early or late, definitely enhanced spontaneous recovery (Roby 1998). This meta-analysis also concluded that greater intensity of treatment produced larger effects. However, another systematic review, but one which included only randomized trials, was far more cautious in its conclusions, suggesting that there was insufficient evidence of benefit (Greener *et al.* 1998). Both reviewers agree, however, that more methodologically robust RCTs are required to identify specific reproducible interventions which are effective in increasing the rate of recovery of aphasia and in decreasing the residual impairment, disability and handicap (Greener *et al.* 2000a).

There is some evidence that drugs might improve language function or enhance the effects of language therapy (Small 1994; Greener *et al.* 2000b). The most intensively studied is piracetam although evidence of its ability to potentiate the effect of speech therapy comes from small RCTs or posthoc subgroup analyses of larger ones (Huber 1999; Orgogozo 1999). We believe there is currently too little evidence to recommend the use of piracetam or other drugs outside RCTs.

Even though there is doubt about the effect that speech therapy has on aphasia, few clinicians, patients or families doubt the value of involving a speech and language therapist in a patient's care. Therapists can assess the patient's communication problems, make a precise diagnosis and explain this to other members of the team and, most importantly, to the patient and carer. They can offer advice about the likely prognosis based on their findings. They can also devise strategies to allow the patient and the family to cope with the communication handicap, perhaps by achieving communication in other ways, e.g. gesture, word/picture charts. It may be appropriate to refer some patients to stroke clubs, which in the UK specialize in supporting aphasic patients and their families. Thus, therapists may or may not be able to influence recovery of language function measured by specific tests, but they can certainly help improve communication, in its broadest sense, and reduce the distress associated with communication difficulties after stroke.

15.30.2 Dysarthria

Dysarthria affected 20% of 648 assessable patients in the Oxfordshire Community Stroke Project but only 6% in the Copenhagen Stroke Study (Pederson *et al.* 1995). It usually improves spontaneously and rarely causes major long-term problems. This is fortunate since, although speech and language therapists give patients exercises aimed at improving the clarity of speech, there has been little formal evaluation of these techniques (Sellars *et al.* 2000). In patients with dysarthria and intact language and cognitive functions, communication aids such as pen and paper, letter and picture charts, and electronic communicators may be helpful.

15.31 Psychological problems

15.31.1 Low mood and anxiety

Patients who have had a stroke have more psychological symptoms than age- and sex-matched controls (House *et al.*

1991; Burvill *et al.* 1995a,b; Beekman *et al.* 1998). Depressive symptoms, anxiety and non-specific psychological distress are particularly common.

Depression has been reported in as few as 11% and as many as 61% of stroke survivors (Robinson & Szetela 1981; House *et al.* 1991). This variation is due to differences in the definitions of depression used, methods of detection, the interval between stroke onset and assessment, and selection of patients (House 1987). Community-based studies have produced more consistent results: the frequency of major depression one month after stroke was estimated to be 11% and 25% in studies from Oxford and Umea, respectively; a study from Perth, Australia estimated the frequency at 4 months after stroke as 15% (House *et al.* 1991; Astrom *et al.* 1993; Burvill *et al.* 1995a).

The frequency of anxiety disorders has also varied considerably. Generalized anxiety disorders occur in 25–30% of hospital-admitted patients (Dennis *et al.* 2000) but are far less frequent in community-based samples, occurring in less than 5%. Interestingly, agorophobia was the most frequent anxiety disorder identified in the community-based studies (House *et al.* 1991; Burvill *et al.* 1995b).

A history of previous depression, stroke severity, poor physical function and low social activity are the risk factors most consistently associated with depression after stroke (Dennis *et al.* 2000; Singh *et al.* 2000). Although the literature has been dominated by many small studies relating the lesion location with post-stroke depression, two systematic reviews conclude that there is little or no evidence of such a relationship (Singh *et al.* 1998; Carson *et al.* 2000). Of course, depression is a frequent consequence of other non-neurological diseases and therefore depression after stroke may be a non-specific reaction to illness rather than due to the brain lesion itself. The aetiology of mood disorders after stroke is bound to be multifactorial and 'post-stroke depression' is probably not a discrete disease entity.

Symptoms of anxiety are far less obviously associated with stroke severity and poor outcome but are probably more common in women (Dennis *et al.* 2000). The high frequency of such symptoms is not surprising since a stroke, even a minor one, represents a considerable threat to most patients. Patients are likely to be frightened of dying, being left disabled or having another stroke. Their role in the family and their livelihood may be threatened. Some of these threats are amplified by the patient's and their family's lack of knowledge concerning stroke, which adds to their uncertainty. Patients very often have symptoms of both anxiety and depression.

Assessment

After a stroke it may be particularly difficult to diagnose depression, especially if the patient cannot communicate. A sad expression due to facial weakness, crying due to emotionalism (section 15.31.2) or frustration, apathy in right hemisphere lesions, and the loss of the normal modulation in tone when speaking (aprosody), may all lead to a mistaken impression of depression. However, one still needs to be aware of the possibility of depression in all patients who have had a stroke. Lack of progress with rehabilitation, a change in personality or mood, loss of weight or a poor sleep pattern may all indicate the onset of a depressive illness. If there is doubt, then a trial of an antidepressant may be justified, although it is sometimes helpful to obtain a formal psychiatric assessment first.

Several relatively short and simple questionnaires have been developed to detect depression and anxiety and some have been used in patients with stroke (Table 15.42). Unfortunately, response rates in patients with communication and other cognitive difficulties are often low and none of the instruments has sufficient sensitivity and specificity to be recommended as a screening tool in clinical practice (Shinar *et al.* 1986; House *et al.* 1989a; O'Rourke *et al.* 1998). They are more useful in research, although a structured psychiatric interview, e.g. the Present State Examination (PSE), Schedule for Affective Disorders and Schizophrenia (SADS) is recognized as the 'gold-standard' for making an accurate psychiatric diagnosis.

Prognosis

The prognosis of depression after stroke varies considerably between studies. Hospital-based studies provide a rather pessimistic view. On the other hand, community-based studies have estimated that perhaps 60% of patients who are depressed at one or four months after a stroke will have recovered at one year (Astrom *et al.* 1993; Burvill *et al.* 1995a). House *et al.* (1991), followed up 78 patients and identified only two who had major depression which persisted throughout the first year after their stroke. Patients who remain depressed at one year may be resistant to treatment (Astrom *et al.* 1993).

Prevention

It may be possible to reduce the psychological morbidity, in particular anxiety, by spending time with the patient and carer explaining the nature, prognosis and consequences of stroke although the effectiveness of such information-giving on emotional outcome has not been established (Friedland & McColl 1987; Mant *et al.* 1998; Rodgers *et al.* 1999; Knapp *et al.* 2000). It is important that patients and carers are aware that although the symptoms of stroke come on quickly, improvement occurs over weeks or months; they should be neither surprised nor disappointed that their recovery does not occur 'at a stroke' (section 10.2.5). Also, in our experience many patients have an overly pessimistic view of the risk of dying or having a recurrent stroke. Some realistic

Table 15.42 Self-report questionnaires which have been used to identify psychological problems after stroke (where data are available we have included estimates of sensitivity and specificity for diagnosing psychiatric disorder defined by psychiatric interview 'gold-standard').

Scale (and study)	Features of scale	Typical response rates (method of delivery)	Diagnosis	Sensitivity (%)	Specificity (%)
General Health Questionnaire	Several versions 12–60 item				
O'Rourke *et al.* 1998*	30 item, cut-off 9/10	92% (interview)	DSM IV depression	85	64
Johnson *et al.* 1995*	28 item, cut-off 5/6	—	DSM III depression	78	81
Beck Depression Inventory	21 item				
House *et al.* 1989a	Cut-off 9/10	77–88% (self-report)	DSM III depression	92	75
Hospital Anxiety and Depression Questionnaire	14 item				
Johnson *et al.* 1995*	Cut-off 5/6	—	DSM III depression	61	50
O'Rourke *et al.* 1998*	Cut-off 6/7	76% (self-report)	DSM IV depression	80	79
Centre for Epidemiologic Studies depression scale	20 item				
Shinar *et al.* 1986	Cut-off 15/16	—	DSM III depression	73	100
Agrell & Dehlin 1989	Cut-off 20	—	Informal clinical	56	91
Wakefield Depression Inventory	12 item	—	—	—	—
Geriatric depression scale	30 item				
Agrell & Dehlin 1989	Cut-off 10	—	Informal clinical	88	64
Johnson *et al.* 1995*	Cut-off 10/11	—	DSM III depression	84	66
Zung depression scale	20 item				
Agrell & Dehlin 1989	Cut-off 45	—	Informal clinical	76	96
Visual analogue mood scale					
House *et al.* 1989a	10-cm horizontal line	49%	—	—	—

*Some authors have published sensitivities and specificities for several cut-off points.

DSM, Diagnostic and Statistical Manual of Mental Disorders.

information about the risks may provide reassurance (sections 16.1 and 17.5.5). Patients are likely to need more than one opportunity to talk so that all the staff caring for the patient and their family should be able to address the issues in a consistent manner. The role of 'counselling' and stroke family support workers is unclear but such interventions are appreciated and some trials have demonstrated improved psychological outcomes for patients (Mant *et al.* 1999; Knapp *et al.* 2000) (section 17.5.3). Cognitive behaviour therapy which aims to teach patients and their carers how to identify and solve problems may improve psychological outcomes but this approach needs further rigorous evaluation, particularly since the necessary resources are seldom available to deliver it (House *et al.* 1999).

It is important that patients and carers are aware that although the symptoms of stroke come on quickly, improvement occurs over weeks or months; they should be neither surprised nor disappointed that their recovery does not occur 'at a stroke'.

Treatment

In patients with a depressive illness after stroke, antidepressants appear to improve mood although it is unclear whether this translates into better physical and social outcomes (Lipsey *et al.* 1984; Andersen *et al.* 1994; Dam *et al.* 1996; Wiart *et al.* 2000). It is wise to start with a small dose initially and then gradually increase to minimize adverse effects, but it is important not to use sub-therapeutic doses in the mistaken belief that depression after a stroke is somehow more drug sensitive. Improvements in mood attributable to antidepressants are usually delayed at least 2 weeks after treatment is started. There is no clear evidence that any one drug is more effective than another in this setting, although the frequency and type of adverse effects associated with each group of antidepressants often determines the choice (Song *et al.* 1993; Lauritzen *et al.* 1994). In elderly patients with a past history of depression who have previously relapsed when treatment has stopped, one should probably continue treatment indefinitely to prevent a relapse which could have serious functional consequences. Even where there is some doubt about the diagnosis of depression after stroke, perhaps because of communication difficulties, a trial of antidepressants may be worthwhile. Some drugs which are started after a stroke (e.g. betablockers to treat newly discovered hypertension) can themselves cause depression so it is important to review the drug chart before starting antidepressants. Cognitive behaviour therapy may help depression after stroke but is usually less available and more labour intensive (Hibbard *et al.* 1990). Electroconvulsive therapy may occasionally be required and has been used without complications after stroke (Murray *et al.* 1986).

Start with a small dose of antidepressant and gradually increase it to minimize adverse effects. It is important not to use sub-therapeutic doses in the mistaken belief that depression after a stroke is somehow more drug sensitive.

15.31.2 Emotionalism

About one-fifth of patients have difficulty controlling the expression of emotion in the year following a stroke (House *et al.* 1989b; Andersen *et al.* 1995a). This problem has been described using a variety of overlapping terms including emotionalism, pathological emotionalism, emotional lability, emotional incontinence, pathological crying/laughing and pseudobulbar affect. The patient abruptly starts to weep, or less commonly to laugh uncontrollably, sometimes with no obvious precipitant. More often, episodes are triggered by a kind word (e.g. how are you feeling?) or a thought with emotional overtones (e.g. thinking of grandchildren), but the emotional response is out of proportion to the degree of 'internal sadness' (or mirth). Usually, the episodes are short lived but may occur frequently enough to disrupt completely a conversation, therapy session or social event. Such outbursts cause considerable distress to the patient and their carer and may be a major obstacle to rehabilitation and social integration. Although classically described as a characteristic of pseudobulbar palsy (e.g. with bilateral strokes), emotionalism often occurs after a single, unilateral stroke. It is most common early on although may not be noticed in the first few days because of everything else that is going on. Usually, episodes of emotionalism become less severe and less frequent with time (House *et al.* 1989b). Patients with emotionalism have more severe strokes, more psychological symptoms, and tend to have worse cognitive function than unaffected patients so it is important not to overlook these additional sources of distress (House *et al.* 1989b; Andersen *et al.* 1995a; Calvert *et al.* 1998).

Assessment

Emotionalism should be suspected if the patient is more tearful, or cries more easily, than before the stroke. Ask the patient, carer or staff whether the crying is of sudden onset and whether the patient can control it. Patients may describe similar problems controlling laughter, but this is much less common. Having established that crying is a problem, one needs to assess whether this is solely due to emotionalism or whether it reflects frustration or depression. Crying which always occurs when the patient is trying, with difficulty, to perform a task (e.g. an aphasic patient trying to speak) suggests that the emotional outburst is due to frustration, although this does not mean there are no other psychological problems as well. One needs to talk to the patient, the carers and staff to assess whether or not the patient is depressed (section 15.31.1). It can be useful to ask the patient to keep a diary to document the frequency and severity of emotional outbursts, especially if one is planning to start treatment.

Treatment

Patients and carers are often confused and distressed by emotionalism. Therefore, it is important to explain that the problem is due to the stroke, that it is relatively common, that it does not represent the degree of distress it suggests, and that it usually becomes less severe with time. Do not walk away when the patient bursts into tears, but take the opportunity to explain the nature of the problem to them. If it is a persistent problem, and is either causing major distress to the patient and family, or disrupting therapy sessions, antidepressants can be effective, rather paradoxically because the problem is primarily one of psychomotor response rather than mood. Symptoms are usually improved within the first few days of initiating the treatment, unlike the symptoms of depression which rarely respond in less than 2 weeks. Small doses are often effective. It is best to start with 25 mg of amitryptyline in the first instance, taken at bedtime (Schiffer *et al.* 1985; Robinson *et al.* 1993). If the symptoms are not better in a week, increase the dose slowly until the patient responds or begins to have dose-related adverse effects. If the patient does not respond, citolapram or fluoxetine can be tried since the former has been shown to be effective in a randomized controlled trial and there are anecdotal reports of success of fluoxetine where a tricyclic has been ineffective (Sloan *et al.* 1992; Andersen *et al.* 1993).

Emotionalism after stroke can occur with single or multiple lesions in more-or-less any part of the brain. It is usually triggered by some sort of emotion (such as seeing grandchildren), but the response is completely out of proportion to the stimulus.

15.31.3 Boredom

Patients who remain in hospital for a long period of rehabilitation often complain of boredom, not surprisingly because much of their time is spent doing nothing (Lincoln *et al.* 1989). Boredom is a particular problem during weekends and evenings when the patients are not receiving therapy, or at least not receiving it from the therapists. It may also be a problem for patients after discharge home if they are housebound, socially isolated and unable to resume their normal leisure or work activities. Boredom leads to reduced motivation, low morale and can ultimately affect the patient's recovery. The team should remain alert to the problem and ask patients about it. There are a number of ways to alleviate boredom in hospitalized patients, which include the following:

- be as flexible as possible about visiting hours to maximize social contact with family and friends;
- provide patients with a variety of leisure activities on the unit. Some units even employ leisure activity coordinators;
- encourage families to take patients out of the hospital wherever this is practical, e.g. walks in the grounds, trips to the pub, trips home for a meal;
- introduce volunteers on the unit to work with the patients and develop group activities at weekends;
- encourage patients to keep their own timetable so they can plan their free time; and
- provide individual televisions with remote controls and headphones, videos and even computer games.

These interventions may be integrated with the rehabilitation programme and incorporated in goal setting, and so benefit the patient in other ways. Unfortunately, even in specialized Stroke Units, patients spend far too much of their time staring into space (Lincoln *et al.* 1996). For patients at home there are often clubs, day centres and voluntary organizations which can help to get them out of the house, meet other people, and involved in leisure activities.

15.31.4 Fatigue

Many of our patients, and others reported in the literature, complain of fatigue in the weeks and months after a stroke. Inglis *et al.* (1999) reported a frequency of 68%, twice that of age- and sex-matched stroke-free controls. Fatigue is often severe enough to limit involvement in rehabilitation and delay return to normal everyday activities. It has been measured in stroke patients using the fatigue impact scale, a self report questionairre (Fisk *et al.* 1994). It does not appear associated with stroke severity and our impression is that it may affect patients who seem to have made a full physical recovery. It often resolves spontaneously after a few months. Although fatigue may be a symptom of depression, it certainly occurs in patients without mood problems (Inglis *et al.* 1999). We normally look for obvious causes, such as depression or medications, e.g. betablockers, but in the majority no cause is identified. None the less, simple acknowledgement by the stroke team that fatigue is a recognized problem after stroke, and that it resolves, may be helpful to patients.

15.32 Dependency in activities of daily living

In previous sections we have discussed many of the impairments which result from stroke. In this section we will concentrate on the resulting disabilities, and the measures which can be taken to limit them. Their frequency in stroke survivors is shown in Table 15.43. Interventions aimed at reducing physical, cognitive and emotional impairments may all improve activities of daily living (ADL) function. However, there is increasing evidence from randomized controlled trials (RCTs) that occupational therapy, including training and practice, the introduction of aids and appliances, and alterations to the patients' environment, can also reduce dependency in ADL, and handicap (e.g. Langhorne *et al.* 1999; Walker *et al.* 1999; Gilbertson *et al.* 2000). With a few exceptions, these trials have not reported the effects of therapy on individual items of ADL (Drummond & Walker 1994b; Walker *et al.* 1994).

15.32.1 Mobility

Sections 15.11 and 15.21 addressed the immediate problems of immobility and the interventions described were those aimed at preventing complications and reducing the impairment. This section will deal with the disability and handicap as a consequence of reduced mobility. Many patients have mobility problems one year after their stroke (Table 15.43). Although the neurological consequences of the stroke account for the majority of these problems, other pathologies, in particular arthritis and hip fractures, add to the burden of walking disability (Collen & Wade 1991).

Table 15.43 Frequency of dependency in activities of daily living (based on the Barthel Index, see Table 17.19) amongst 246 consecutive patients surviving 1 year after their first-ever-in-a-lifetime stroke in the Oxfordshire Community Stroke Project (unpublished data).

Function	Dependent (%)	Independent (%)
Bowel function	23 (9)	223 (91)
Grooming	26 (11)	220 (89)
Toileting	30 (12)	216 (88)
Transfers	33 (13)	213 (87)
Walking inside	36 (15)	210 (85)
Bladder function	41 (17)	205 (83)
Feeding	44 (18)	202 (82)
Dressing	53 (22)	193 (78)
Stairs	64 (26)	182 (74)
Walking outside	76 (31)	171 (69)
Bathing	80 (33)	166 (67)

It is notable that there is a hierachy with stairs, walking outside and bathing being the most difficult tasks, whilst continence of bowels, grooming and toileting are attained by most patients.

Assessment

Simple history taking is surprisingly informative. Self-reported ability to turn over in bed, sit up, transfer (i.e. bed to chair, and sitting to standing), walk (and use of walking aids, furniture) and climb stairs (up, down or both, with or without rails) give a fairly clear picture of the patient's residual problems. It is useful to know whether the patient can (and does) walk outside, their range, and whether physical or verbal support from another person is needed. It is also important to establish the reason for any problem, i.e. is it due to painful joints or feet, breathlessness, angina, intermittent claudication, loss of confidence, environmental factors such as high steps, lack of handrails, or even the neighbour's aggressive dog? It is useful to observe the patient and the carer carrying out the various manoeuvres in their own home since environmental factors so often determine the level of handicap associated with impaired mobility. Several scales are available for measuring mobility, e.g. Rivermead Mobility Index (Wade 1992b) (Table 15.44). The timed 10-m walk is particularly useful because it is simple, objective, requires no more equipment than a watch with a second hand, and age-related normative data are available, i.e. < 60 years 10 s; 60–69 years 12.5 s; > 70 years 16.6 s (Wade *et al.* 1987).

Treatment

Where the patient has residual problems, a physiotherapist or occupational therapist can improve mobility (Wade *et al.* 1992). Patients' mobility quite often deteriorates, after a period of stability, in the months or years after a stroke. This may be attributed to further strokes, progression of co-existing pathology (e.g. arthritis) or attenuation of the benefits of regular physiotherapy. It is important that whoever is responsible for monitoring the patient's progress, most often the general (family) practitioner, is alert to this and refers the patient back to the physiotherapist. Although not backed up by RCTs, we have little doubt as to the value of so called 'top up' physiotherapy in patients such as this, although its effectiveness will inevitably depend on the cause of any deterioration. Therapy in the patient's own home may be more helpful than in a hospital out-patient department since the therapist can then address the real, everyday problems that the patient is experiencing. For example, patients can be taught to climb their *own* stairs and to overcome the particular problems associated with the layout of their *own* home. Two RCTs, which compared the effectiveness of home vs. hospital-based physiotherapy, showed that improvement in ADL function was slightly greater in those treated at home, but other outcomes were no different (Gladman *et al.* 1995). Although the therapist may be able to reduce the patient's degree of impairment, even when intervention starts very late after a stroke, the therapist's main tool at this point is the provision of mobility aids (Tables 15.45 and 15.46). When one prescribes an aid for patients, it is important to provide them and any carers with training in its use, and to ensure that it is maintained in good order (Intercollegiate Working Party for Stroke, 2000) (Figs 15.19–15.25). Many patients do not use the aids provided which is both a waste of resources and an indication of the lack of value of that aid. It is important to follow-up patients who have been given aids to ensure they

Table 15.44 Rivermead Mobility Index (from Collen *et al.* 1991).

1. *Turning over in bed*
   Do you turn over from your back to your side without help?
2. *Lying from sitting*
   From lying in bed, do you get up to sit on the edge of the bed on your own?
3. *Sitting balance*
   Do you sit on the edge of the bed without holding on for 10 s?
4. *Sitting to standing*
   Do you stand up (from any chair) in less than 15 s, and stand there for 15 s (using hands, and with an aid if necessary)?
5. *Standing unsupported*
   Observe standing for 10 s without any aid or support.
6. *Transfer*
   Do you manage to move, e.g. from bed to chair and back without any help?
7. *Walking inside, with an aid if needed*
   Do you walk 10 m, with an aid or furniture if necessary, but with no stand-by help?
8. *Stairs*
   Do you manage a flight of stairs without help?
9. *Walking outside (even ground)*
   Do you walk around outside, on pavements without help?
10. *Walking inside (with no aid)*
    Do you walk 10 m inside with no caliper, splint, aid or use of furniture, and no stand-by help?
11. *Picking off floor*
    If you drop something on the floor, do you manage to walk 5 m, pick it up and then walk back?
12. *Walking outside (uneven ground)*
    Do you walk over uneven ground (grass, gravel, dirt, snow, ice, etc.) without help?
13. *Bathing*
    Do you get in and out of a bath or shower unsupervised and wash yourself?
14. *Up and down four steps*
    Do you manage to go up and down four steps with no rail and without help, but using an aid if necessary?
15. *Running*
    Do you run 10 m without limping in 4 s (fast walk is acceptable)?

Note: only question 5 depends on direct observation. The index forms a hierarchy so that one does not have to ask all the questions. However, the authors point out that by asking all the questions, and finding out why patients cannot manage certain actions, useful information is obtained to guide management.

Table 15.45 Walking aids (from Mulley 1991).

Shoes
Should be comfortable, supportive and have non-slip soles
Occasionally, a smooth sole facilitates a smooth swing phase in patients with foot drop when walking on carpets

Walking sticks
May improve standing stability and walking speed but must be tailored to the patient (i.e. length, handle shape, weight and appearance) (Tyson & Ashburn 1994; Lu *et al.* 1997). A long stick can be used to encourage patients to put weight through their affected leg (Fig. 15.19d)
Replace worn rubber ferrule (i.e. rubber bit on end of stick)
Should be held in the unaffected hand in patients with hemiparesis but this means the patient's functioning hand is no longer available for other tasks
Other uses include extending the patient's reach and 'self-defence'

Tripods and quadrapods
Provide a broader base of support than a walking stick
Their weight may cause associated reactions (section 15.20) and may worsen the quality of gait (Tyson & Ashburn 1994)
Not useful on uneven ground

Walking frames (Fig. 15.19)
Available in many sizes and shapes with or without wheels
Useful where balance is poor, especially if the patient tends to lean backwards
Often give patients confidence
Needs good upper limb function and, of course, prevents patient from using hands or carrying things; many patients attach a basket or use a wheeled trolley to overcome this problem
Patients often try to pull up on their frame to rise from a chair, which can cause them to fall
Frames may trip up patients and be difficult to manoeuvre with lots of furniture and thick carpets
Cannot be used on stairs, therefore patients may require several frames, one on each level
Beware bent frames, protruding screws, loose hand grips and worn ferrules
Other uses, drying underclothes

Ankle–foot orthosis or brace (Fig. 15.20)
Usually of thermoplastic construction and tailored to the individual
Occasionally useful in spastic foot drop to improve gait pattern (Tyson *et al.* 1998), but does not improve spasticity (Beckerman *et al.* 1996) and may actually exacerbate the problem
Beware in patients with oedema and tendency to leg ulcers

Knee brace
Occasionally required to prevent hyperextension of the knee

Functional electrical stimulation
An experimental treatment which has been used to correct foot drop after stroke (section 15.21)

Hand rails
Short grab-rails can be useful to provide support, especially at thresholds and doorways
Full-length rails on staircases are invaluable to those with poor balance, confidence or vision
Advice on positioning hand rails should be obtained from an occupational therapist; poorly placed hand rails can cause accidents or may not be used

fit the patient's needs and are actually being used, and to retrieve any unused equipment.

If one prescribes an aid, one should teach the patient or carer how to use it, ensure that it solves the problem, ensure that it is maintained in good working order, and provide follow-up to ensure its continued use or appropriate removal.

Patients who are unable to walk outside, or who can walk only short distances, or who have difficulty using their own or public transport, may be helped by putting them in contact with any local transport schemes. For example, in the UK special financial allowances are available to help with the added cost of being immobile, specially adapted taxis can be provided and some shopping centres provide electric wheelchairs. In the last few years there has been a major campaign

Table 15.46 Other aids to mobility.

Chairs (Fig. 15.21)
Higher seats (but not so high as to cause the feet to dangle) without too much backward angle, and firm arm rests (of the correct height, shape and length) facilitate transfers
It is easier to stand from a chair if the patient can pull his/her heels under it
Chairs should be tailored to the individual's requirements, but existing chairs may be raised or lowered
Chairs on castors can be dangerous

Ejector chairs (Fig. 15.22)
The seat or chair may be sprung to provide an initial lift to allow the patient to rise
These must be tailored to the individual's weight to avoid the patient being catapulted across the room
Electric chairs which slowly bring the patient to a semi-erect position are occasionally useful but are expensive, bulky and require training to use properly

Beds
A firm mattress at the correct height will facilitate transfers from a bed
Blocks or leg extensions can be used to modify an existing bed
A grab-rail attached to the bed frame or floor can facilitate independent transfers (Fig. 15.23a)
It may be impossible to attach aids to a divan-style bed
Mechanical devices which help the patient to sit in bed can occasionally be helpful (Fig. 15.23b)

Wheelchairs
An invaluable means to improve mobility
Many hundreds of designs including self-propelled, carer-propelled and electric chairs
Need to be tailored to individual's requirements
Must be kept in good working order (Fig. 15.24)

Ramps
Useful to those in wheelchairs and their carers
Many designs available for different situations

Lifts
Many types, including:
Domestic stair-lifts (Fig. 15.25) for those who cannot manage stairs
Through-the-floor lifts for accessing upper floors in wheelchairs
Short-rise lifts for accessing vehicles in wheelchairs or where there is insufficient space for a ramp
Lifts are expensive and may require structural alterations to accommodate them

to improve access to public places for patients with disabilities.

15.32.2 Driving

Many people who have had a stroke never return to driving (Legh-Smith *et al.* 1986; Fisk *et al.* 1997). There are several reasons: severe residual motor, sensory, visual or cognitive impairments are the most common. In many countries the authorities place restrictions on driving after stroke, and particularly if the stroke is complicated by epileptic seizures (section 15.8). The variation in regulations probably reflects the dearth of relevant research in this area. Special, and usually more stringent regulations, sometimes apply to those who drive commercial vehicles and taxis.

In our experience, patients are often not asked by their doctors whether they drive so that many continue to drive and put lives at risk in contravention of their local regulations (Davenport *et al.* 1995; Fisk *et al.* 1997). It is the doctor's responsibility to ask patients whether or not they drive so they can be given the relevant information. Failure to do so might have serious consequences, although it is unclear whether patients who have had a stroke and return to driving are at greater risk of road traffic accidents (Haselkorn *et al.* 1998).

There appears to be little agreement about the optimal method of assessing a disabled patient's fitness to drive. Informal judgements are often made by patients or their family doctors (Fisk *et al.* 1997). Bedside testing of neurological impairments including cognitive function, assessments in driving simulators, and road tests have all been advocated. One might start with a bedside assessment to demonstrate any physical, and probably more importantly visual, visuospatial and cognitive impairments, which would make safe driving very unlikely (Nouri *et al.* 1987; Mazer *et al.* 1998). Patients who pass on the bedside testing could then be assessed on a driving simulator or an 'off-road' test which would identify those who are clearly unsafe to drive (Nouri & Tinson 1988; Fox *et al.* 1998). The remainder could then be given a road test in a dual-control car with an appropriately trained instructor. This stepwise approach should minimize the risk of injury to the patient, instructor and other road users. Many countries provide specialist centres for the assessment of disabled drivers. These centres not only assess driving skills, but also provide advice on the available vehicle adaptations which allow patients with severe physical disability to drive.

15.32.3 Toileting

The problems of urinary and faecal incontinence have been discussed in sections 15.14 and 15.15, respectively. In the Oxfordshire Community Stroke Project, 12% of surviving patients were still dependent in toileting one year after their first stroke (Table 15.43). Dependency may be due to an inability to transfer independently, walk, or dress and undress. For the cognitively intact patient, this is an embarrassing disability which severely damages their self-esteem.

An assessment by an occupational therapist should define the severity and cause of the problem. The patient's ability

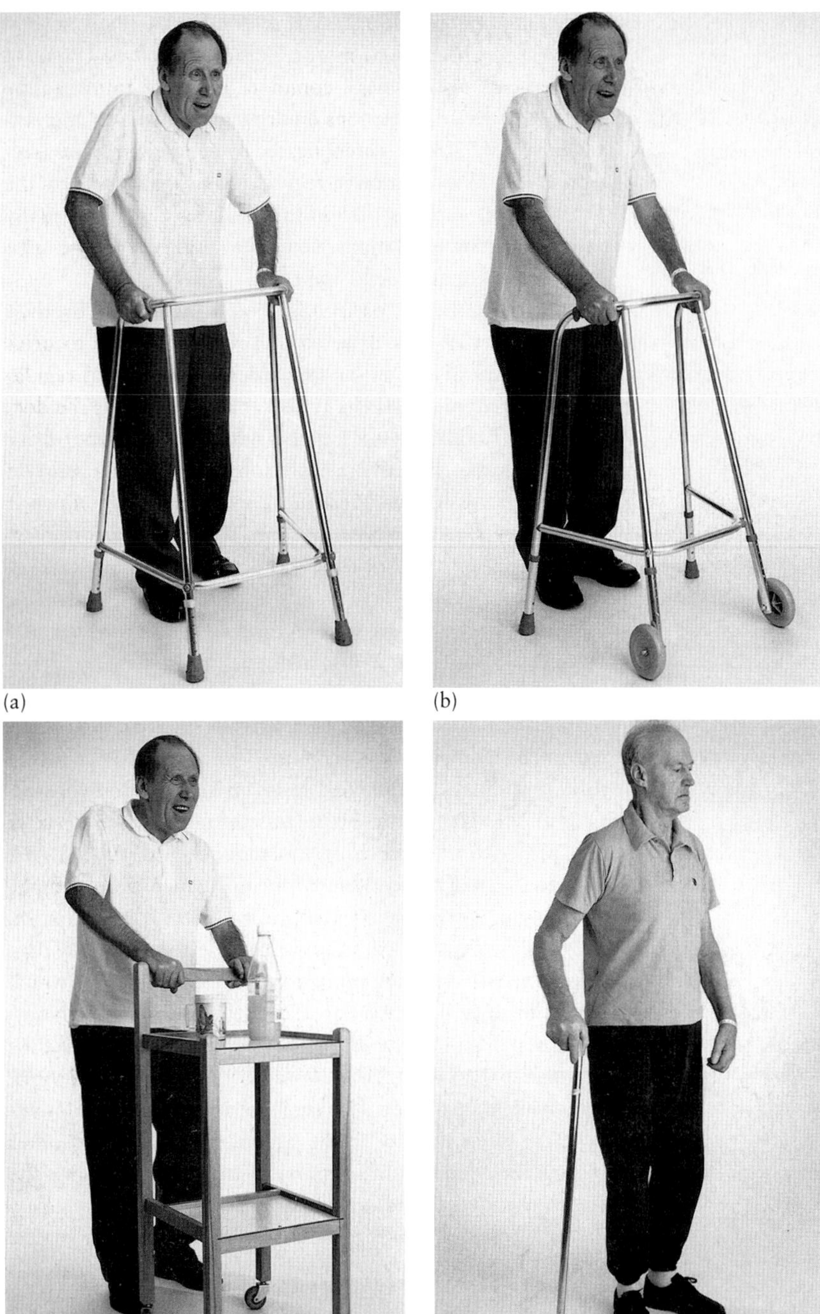

(a) (b) (c) (d)

Fig. 15.19 Walking aids. (a) A typical lightweight walking frame of adjustable height which may be useful if a patient has poor balance but reasonable arm and hand function. (b) A walking frame with wheels which may be better than (a) in patients who tend to fall backwards or who have Parkinson's disease. (c) A tea trolley which will provide the patient with support as well as allow them to take things from place to place. (d) A long walking stick held in the unaffected hand can be used to encourage the patient to put more of their weight through their affected leg.

to toilet themselves is very dependent on the environment so that a home assessment may be particularly useful. Simple factors such as the width of the door to the toilet or bathroom, the position and height of the toilet, and the position of the toilet roll holder can make a crucial difference to whether or not the patient can use the toilet independently.

Therapy aimed at improving performance in mobility, transfers and dressing will all facilitate independence in toileting. Table 15.47, p. 636 lists some common problems and some simple solutions, and Fig. 15.26, p. 637 shows some simple toilet aids.

15.32.4 Washing and bathing

About 11% and 33%, respectively, of patients one year after a first-ever-in-a-lifetime stroke are dependent in washing

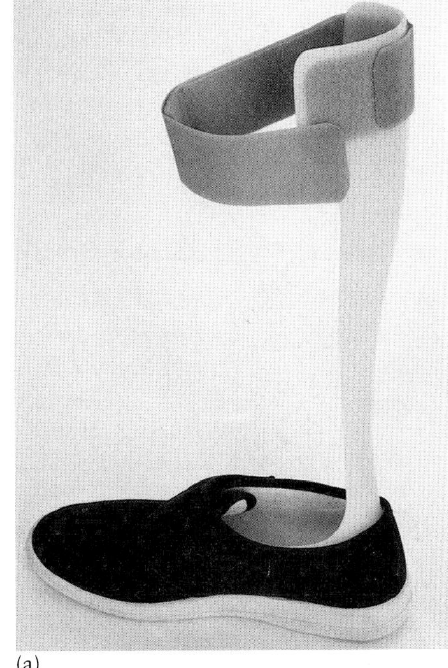

(a)

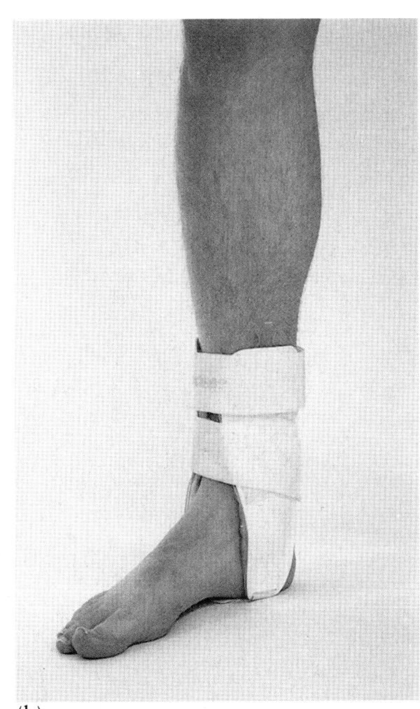

(b)

Fig. 15.20 Ankle supports. (a) A thermoplastic ankle–foot orthosis: the famous AFO splint. Although this is very useful in patients with foot drop secondary to lower motor neurone lesions, in stroke patients it can sometimes increase the tendency to plantar flexion by stimulating the sole of the foot. (b) A lateral ankle support may be useful in patients who have a tendency to invert their foot when walking.

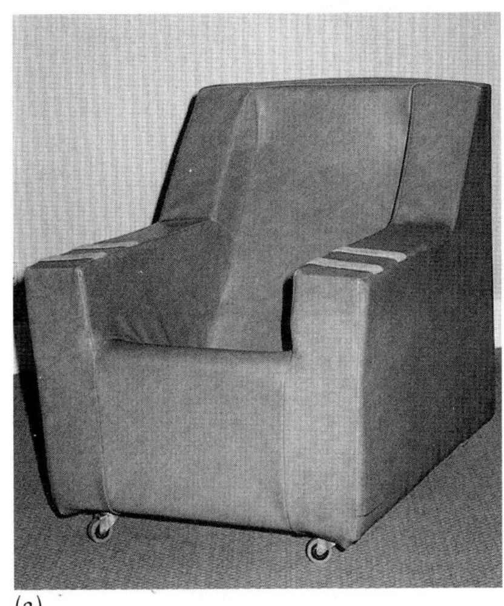

(a)

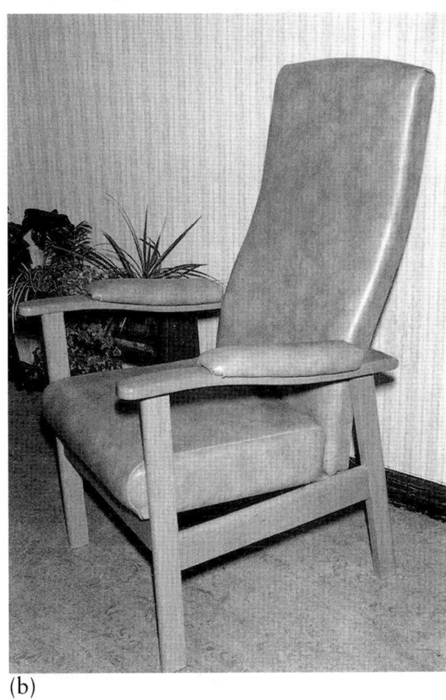

(b)

Fig. 15.21 Choosing an appropriate chair for a stroke patient who has difficulties getting from sitting to standing. (a) A bad chair to ensure the user never escapes! The seat is low and slopes backwards, the arms are soft and offer little resistance to allow the person to push up on them, the base is solid so they cannot pull their legs under them, and this chair is on castors so that if they eventually do manage to stand the chair slides away and causes them to fall backwards. Note the Velcro pads on the arms to allow a tray to be fixed across the user's escape route. (b) A good chair to facilitate easy transfers. This chair is of reasonable height, is upright, has firm but padded arms and allows the patient to pull their legs underneath them which makes it easier to get their weight over their feet. This chair does not have wings which may provide support for the head when sleeping but can stop interaction with other people sitting to either side.

and bathing (Table 15.43). Motor, sensory, visuospatial and cognitive impairments contribute most to these disabilities. Although poor arm function makes washing and grooming more difficult, most patients can perform these tasks with their unaffected arm, but patients with visuospatial and cognitive deficits, even when arm function seems quite good, may be unable to wash and groom themselves independently. Independence in bathing obviously requires some independence in mobility and transfers. Other disabling conditions in the elderly (e.g. painful arthritis) often contribute to the problems. A skilled assessment by an occupational therapist, preferably in the patient's own home, will delineate the problems. This assessment ensures there is adequate access to the bathroom (e.g. for a wheelchair). The size and layout of the bathroom will determine which aids can be used.

Therapy aimed at improving those impairments, especially motor impairments, which are contributing to the disability in bathing and washing may be of some help but, again, at

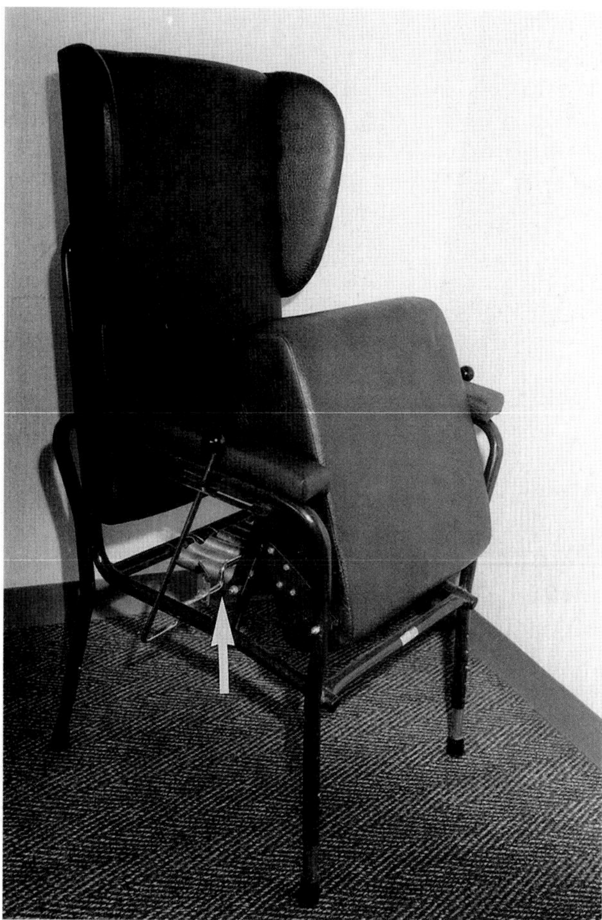

Fig. 15.22 An ejector chair. The number of springs (arrow) can be altered depending on the weight of the user. Some patients find that this type of chair pushes them off balance.

this stage the provision of aids to allow the patient to compensate for their impairments is more effective. There are a wide range of aids and adaptations to overcome most problems with bathing (Fig. 15.27 and Table 15.48, p. 637). Of course, in many countries patients prefer to take showers rather than a bath which generally reduces the difficulty. One general point is that a patient who has trouble bathing should ensure that somebody else is in the house and that the bathroom door is left unlocked, so that if they fall or are unable to get out of the bath somebody can easily reach them.

Patients who have difficulties bathing independently should not be left in their house alone whilst bathing. Some form of alarm or even a cordless or mobile telephone will increase safety.

Some bathroom adaptations are expensive and cause considerable disruption to the patient's home. It is important that a proper assessment is done to avoid unnecessary building work and to ensure that any modifications really are likely to help the patient and/or carer. For some patients who live alone, or where aids and adaptations are not appropriate, it may be necessary to recommend either a simple strip wash or to introduce a nurse, care assistant or family member to help with bathing and so allow the patient to remain in their own home.

15.32.5 Dressing

About 22% of surviving patients needed help from another person to dress one year after their first-ever-in-a-lifetime stroke in the Oxfordshire Community Stroke Project (Table 15.43). Dependency in dressing is usually due to a combination of arm weakness or incoordination, inability to stand independently to pull up lower garments, cognitive and visuospatial problems (Walker & Lincoln 1991). A painful shoulder makes dressing even more difficult (section 15.24). A detailed assessment by an occupational therapist should elucidate the causes and define the degree of disability.

Occupational therapists spend a considerable proportion of their time training patients to dress themselves. If the disability is due simply to a motor deficit, then 'dressing practice' where the patient is taught to compensate for their impairments, is often successful (Walker *et al.* 1994). If the patient has cognitive or visuospatial problems, or other non-stroke problems (e.g. arthritis), the benefit of this type of therapy is less obvious. There has been little formal evaluation of dressing therapy.

Advice on the best type of clothes can allow patients to become independent, i.e. avoidance of tight clothes with small buttons or zips, and of shoes with laces. Oval buttons are easier to manipulate than round ones (Huck & Bonhotal 1997). Velcro fastenings have revolutionized dressing for patients with only one functioning hand, being easier to use and preferred by patients (Huck & Bonhotal 1997). Some of the common problems and possible solutions are shown in Table 15.49 and Fig. 15.28, p. 638. If patients still cannot dress themselves, then care assistants or a member of the family will be needed to help.

15.32.6 Feeding

One year after a first-ever-in-a-lifetime stroke, about 18% of surviving patients in the Oxfordshire Community Stroke Project needed some help from another person to feed (Table 15.43). Dependency in feeding is one of the most demeaning problems because of its associations with infancy. Impaired function of the arm and hand is the most common cause, although problems with sitting balance, facial weakness, visuospatial and sensory function may be important as well. A small number of patients may have residual problems swallowing (section 15.17). Most problems can be identified simply by talking to the patient and/or carer, but often it is

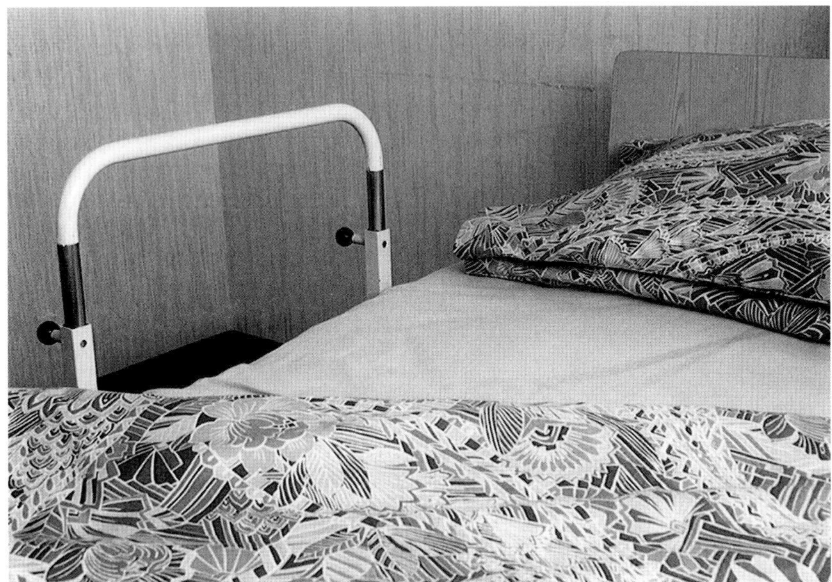
(a)

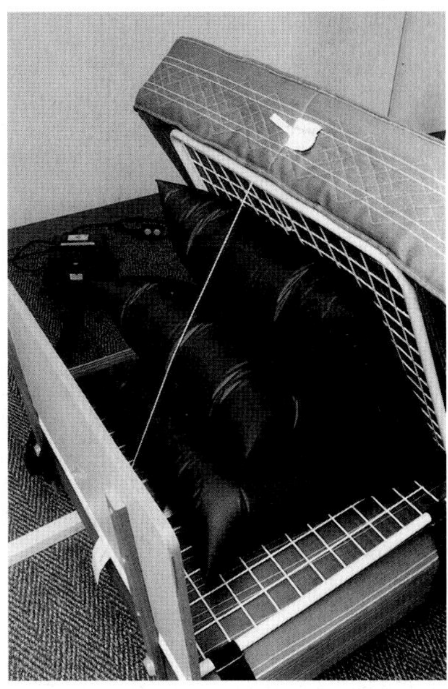
(b)

Fig. 15.23 Aids to getting out of bed. Although many people can get out of a bed independently during a therapy session when they are 'warmed up', they may need aids to get out in the middle of the night or first thing in the morning. (a) A grab-rail attached to the bed can facilitate transfers from lying to standing and may therefore prevent incontinence at night. The height of this model can be adjusted to suit the individual. (b) A pneumatic mattress elevator can be helpful in getting patients from lying to sitting.

useful for a trained observer, usually an occupational therapist, to assess the patient.

Intensive therapy may improve arm function (section 15.21), but late after stroke, the provision and training in the use of feeding aids is probably more effective. Sometimes very simple problems, which require very simple solutions, are overlooked. For instance, it is important that any dentures are in good working order and in the mouth rather than a glass of water on the bedside table, that the patient is sitting at a table on a chair of appropriate height, and that the knife is sharp. Furthermore, the type of food may make the difference between patients being able to feed themselves, or not. A hemiplegic patient may be independent eating sandwiches but dependent for eating a steak. Some of the more common feeding problems, and the aids which can help, are shown in Table 15.50 and Fig. 15.29, p. 639.

15.32.7 Preparing food

Many patients are unable to prepare food for themselves or their family because of a wide variety of post-stroke impairments. Cognitive and visuospatial problems may put patients, and others living in the same building, in danger from lacerations, burns, fires, gas poisoning, explosions and flooding. Again, problems are easily identified by talking to, or observing, the patient in the kitchen. An occupational therapist may be able to teach patients alternative methods of performing certain tasks and for many with physical rather than cognitive problems there is a large variety of kitchen aids available to help with specific difficulties (Table 15.51, p. 640). Patients with cognitive problems may be helped by things such as electric kettles which turn themselves off, and gas stoves which automatically ignite, but for those with severe cognitive problems it may be necessary to ban them from the kitchen or to remove cookers, etc.

Where patients cannot prepare food for themselves, it is obviously important to ensure delivery of prepared meals to their homes, or to provide a care assistant who can prepare meals. Often, relatives and social services provide these services.

15.33 Social difficulties

We have discussed how stroke-related impairments result in disability or dependency in activities of daily living. However, there is more to life than just these basic activities. Environmental factors become extremely important in determining the effect of the stroke on a person's role in society and their handicap. This section will address some of the social factors which are often of greatest concern to patients and their carers.

15.33.1 Accommodation

About 50% of the patients who survive a stroke are dependent in activities of daily living (ADL) (Table 15.43). Some patients with complex or worsening disability may not, if admitted to hospital, be able to return to their own home.

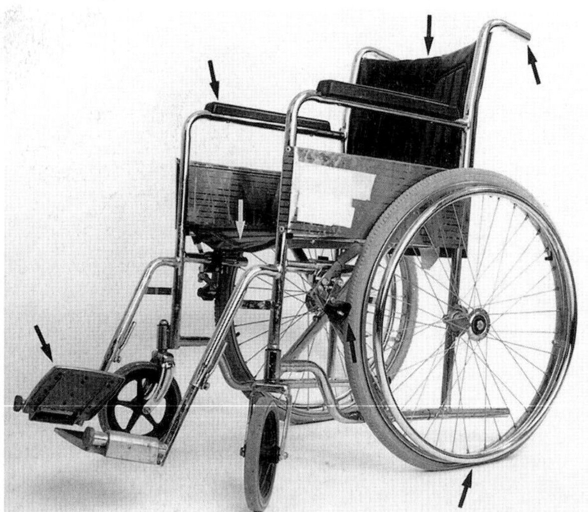

Fig. 15.24 Things to look for when examining a wheelchair. This wheelchair has many hazardous and uncomfortable features. Note the white sticky tape covering the name of the hospital on the side of this wheelchair, which wished, very reasonably, to remain anonymous. 1, Check that the tyres are properly inflated (arrow). Flat tyres make the wheelchair hard work to propel and the brakes inoperative. 2, Check the brakes work (arrow). 3, Check that the sides and arms (arrow) are removable to facilitate transfers onto toilets, into cars, etc. 4, Check that the foot plates are not fixed (arrow) or flapping about. Both may cause injury. The foot plates should fold neatly and securely out of the way when not in use. 5, Check that the arms (arrow) are properly padded to avoid discomfort and compression neuropathy of the ulnar nerve. 6, Check that the back (arrow) and seat (arrow) are not sagging and that the appropriate cushion is being used to reduce the risk of pressure sores. 7, Check that the grips on the handles are in good order (arrow).

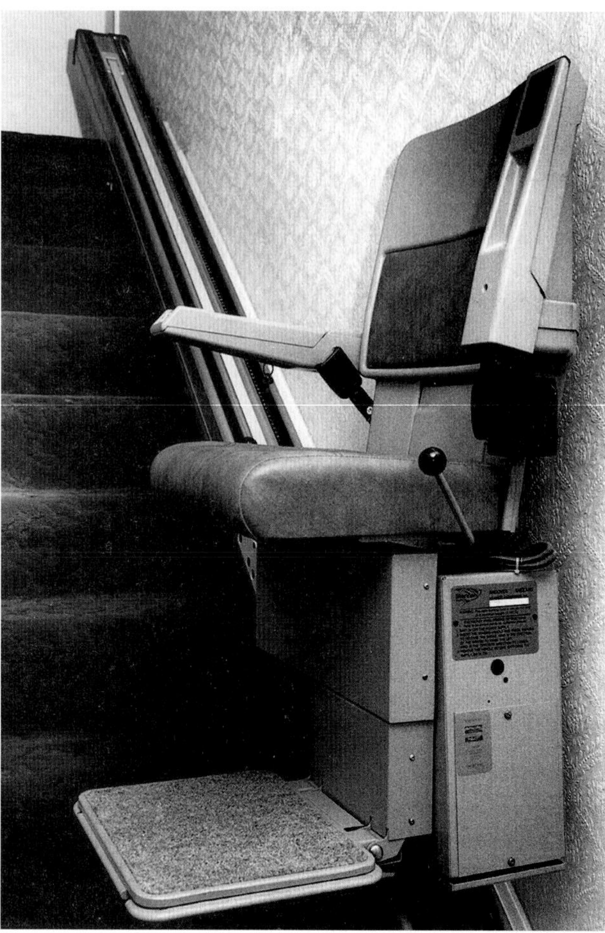

Fig. 15.25 A typical stair-lift for domestic use. The armrests fold out of the way to facilitate transfers. The foot rest and seat fold up when not in use. The controls are on the armrests.

In the Oxfordshire Community Stroke Project, 643 (95%) of 675 people were living at home before their first-ever-in-a-lifetime stroke. At one year, 418 (89%) of the 467 survivors were able to live at home. Thus, the proportion of patients in institutions had not increased greatly, but many of the 32 patients who had lived in an institution before their stroke had died. Patients' ability to return home depends on the answers to the following questions, amongst others:

- is the disability likely to improve or worsen with time?
- will aids and adaptations reduce dependency?
- what does the patient's accommodation comprise?
- what level of informal support is available, e.g. family?
- what level of community support is available, e.g. community nursing, home helps?

Any assessment has to identify the needs of the patient to determine whether those needs can be practically provided in the patient's current accommodation, or whether alternative or modified accommodation will be needed. This may involve one or more visits home with the patient and any carer to establish exactly what the practical problems are. If a short visit is not enough, then home visits for a few days

Table 15.47 Toileting problems and solutions.

Cannot get to toilet because of mobility or access problems	
Solutions:	Urinal (Fig. 15.7)
	Commode, many designs to suit individual needs (Fig. 15.26)
	Chemical toilet, useful where regular emptying of a commode is not possible
Cannot transfer on and off the toilet, or poor balance making manipulation of clothes difficult	
Solutions:	Grab-rails
	Toilet frame (Fig. 15.26)
	Raised or adjustable toilet seat (Fig. 15.26)
Cannot clean myself	
Solutions:	Toilet paper holder on the unaffected side which can be used with one hand
	Large aperture toilet seat
	Self-cleaning toilet, like a bidet and toilet in one

(a) 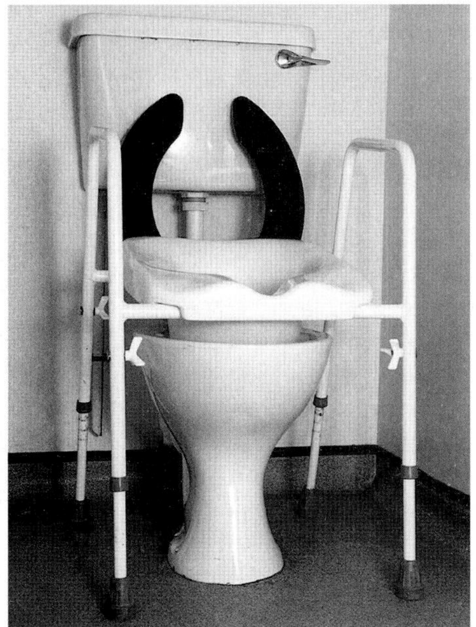 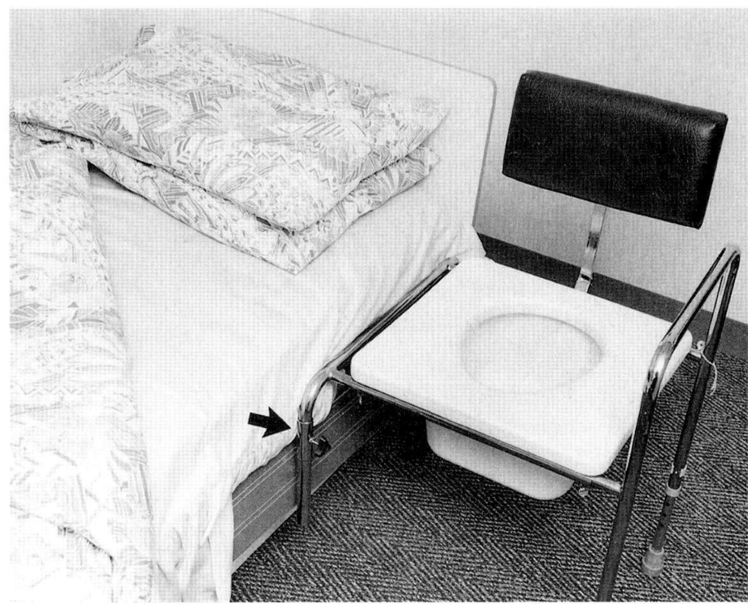 (b)

Fig. 15.26 Simple toilet aids. (a) A raised toilet seat with a frame. (b) A commode. This one attaches securely to the bed (arrow) for use at night.

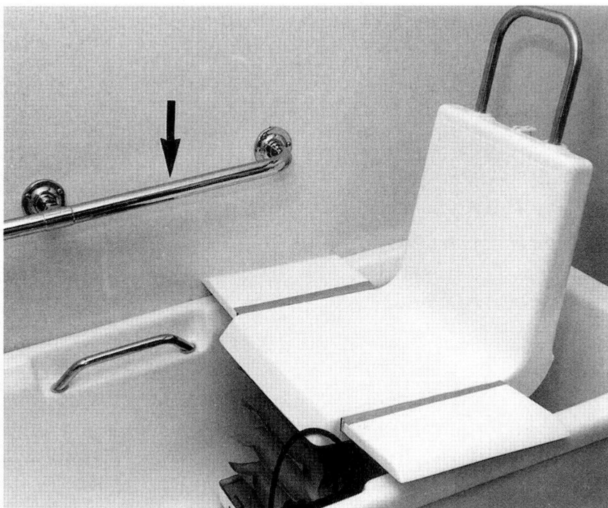

Fig. 15.27 A pneumatic bath aid to lower patients into and to lift them out of a bath. However, the humble bath rail (arrow) with some other simple aids is very commonly all that is needed to allow the person to use a bath independently.

Table 15.48 Problems with grooming or bathing/showering and solutions.

Cannot brush my dentures with one hand

Solutions: Half fill sink with water, attach brush with a suction pad to the sink and brush dentures with functioning hand

Cannot get into, and even more important, out of the bath

Solutions:
- Grab-rails appropriately mounted around bath
- Non-slip bath mat
- Bath stool
- Bath board
- Inflatable or hydraulic bath seats which can lower patients into or raise them out of the bath (Fig. 15.27)
- Hoists
- Replace bath with shower

and nights can be useful to predict how the patient and carer will cope in the longer term. The layout of the home is obviously important. Are there steps up to the front door which make access difficult? Are the toilet and bathroom upstairs? Is the house cluttered with furniture? Are the carpets deep pile which may cause difficulty for a patient with a foot drop? Some Stroke Units have predischarge apartments in the hospital which allow the team and the patient to assess under supervision how well the patient copes. This may not be the same as discharge into the community, however.

The timing of accommodation assessment is difficult because it often takes a considerable time to find alternative accommodation, or to make major structural changes to the patient's current home. Thus, if one is going to avoid unnecessary delays in hospital, one has to make a decision before the patient has achieved their optimal functional status. Considerable judgement is required to 'best guess' the patient's final functional level and to identify their accommodation needs well in advance of hospital discharge.

After a thorough assessment, the patient and their family, with help from the team, need to decide where they wish to live, taking into account all the practical issues including any financial constraints. After all, given unlimited funds, it is

Table 15.49 Problems with dressing and solutions (Fig. 15.28).

Cannot manage zips or buttons	
Solutions:	Button hook or toggle button hook allows patient to fasten buttons with one hand
	Replace round buttons with oval ones
	Hook to pull up zip
	Replace zips and buttons with Velcro
Cannot get shoes on or tie shoe laces	
Solutions:	Long-handled shoe horn
	Replace shoe laces with elastic ones or Velcro straps
	Shoe ties
Cannot reach or pull up clothes	
Solutions:	Dressing hook or even a walking stick
	Reaching aid

almost always possible to maintain even the most severely disabled patient at home. The final decision is often a result of negotiation between the patient, carer and team members. For instance, patients with visuospatial or cognitive problems may not appreciate the likely problems which will face their carers after discharge. For these sorts of reasons it is not always possible to fulfil the wishes of both patient and carer.

Options for alternative accommodation, and the availability of support in the community, vary from place to place, country to country, and from time to time. However, in general, one needs a range of accommodation offering a variety of levels of support and supervision to meet the needs of individual patients.

15.33.2 Employment

About one-third of patients who have a stroke are of employment age. In Oxfordshire, 76 (24%) of 318 men and 39 (11%) of 357 women were in paid employment before their stroke. Of these, 68 (59%) returned to work at some stage, the majority within 6 months of the stroke. Obviously, the nature of previous employment, residual impairments and disabilities, the patient's own wishes, and the attitudes and policies of employers will determine whether return to employment is feasible. It is also likely that the local arrangements for paying sickness benefit will influence whether patients return to work, and the timing of their return (Saeki *et al.* 1995). Of course, many patients who are approaching retirement age may not want to return to work anyway.

Assessment of the patient's ability to return to work is often left to the patient and family, but involvement of members of the team (i.e. occupational therapist, speech and language therapist, physiotherapist and social worker) can be very useful to help explore the possible work options. Some employers have occupational health departments which can provide further specialist advice on specific regulations covering return to work, and on any alterations to the working environment or job itself which would facilitate this.

It is important that patients and their families are counselled about the patient's limitations. Many patients and families are under the misconception that patients should rest after a stroke and that physical activity will bring on another stroke (Wellwood *et al.* 1994). This misconception may have made them rule out, inappropriately, the possibility of return to work.

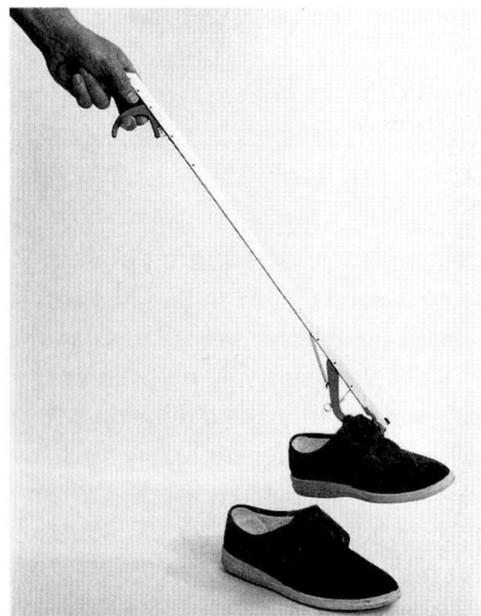
(a)

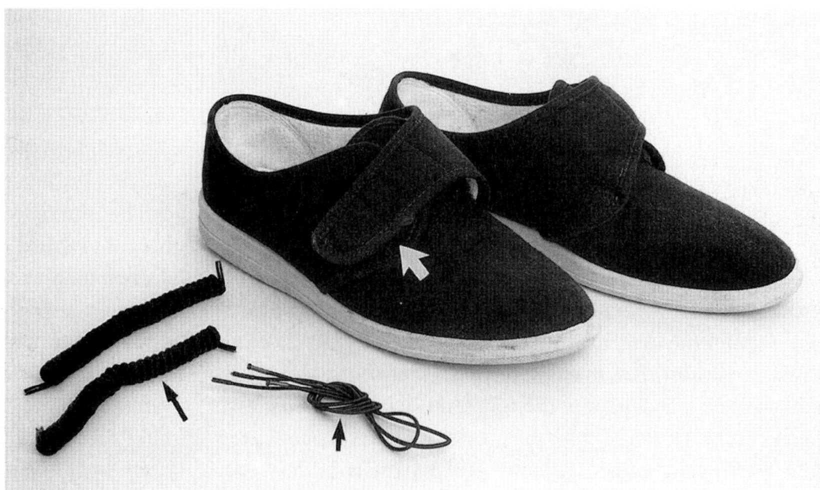
(b)

Fig. 15.28 Simple dressing aids. (a) A reaching aid. (b) Elastic laces (short black arrow), spiral laces which one simply pulls tight (long black arrow) and Velcro fasteners (white arrow) are invaluable dressing aids for those with only one functioning hand or poor manual dexterity.

Table 15.50 Feeding problems and solutions (Fig. 15.29).

Cannot cut up food because of poor arm function	
Solutions:	If moderate hand weakness, a large-handled sharp knife may be enough
	Alternatively, a combination knife and spoon or fork may help, but warn the patient to be careful not to cut their mouth
Cannot hold bowl or plate still when cutting or spooning	
Solution:	A non-slip mat or tray, or containers with suction pads
Cannot push peas onto fork or spoon	
Solution:	Provide a dish with a raised side or rim
Dribbling due to facial weakness	
Solutions:	A mug with a spout, or a straw may help. Straws are available with a non-return valve if the patient cannot suck using a conventional one because of facial weakness, but has an intact swallow

Many patients and their carers are under the misconception that exercise, hard work or stress will bring on another stroke. They should be counselled to dispel these myths.

Patients may require specific occupational therapy to improve physical skills required for particular jobs, and/or retraining to change employment. Patients often complain of marked fatigue (section 15.31.4) so that a return to part-time work, at least initially, is often more successful than the patient struggling to cope with full-time work. Patients often find that although they can perform the physical aspects of their work, their concentration may be impaired. In many countries, special schemes are available to provide employment for disabled people.

15.33.3 Leisure

Two-thirds of stroke patients are retired from employment. For them, resumption of a leisure activity is more relevant than work. Restriction in leisure activities may be the result of physical or cognitive impairments but may also be caused by psychological factors and even fear that an activity may bring on a further stroke. Many disabled stroke patients are unable to continue with their normal leisure activities and do not take up new ones which are within their abilities (Sjogren 1982; Drummond 1990). Reduction in leisure activities will exacerbate social isolation, lower mood and adversely affect relationships with carers (Sjogren 1982; Feibel & Springer 1982). The level of social activities, including leisure, can be measured using the Frenchay Activities Index but the Nottingham Leisure Questionnaire has been developed specifically for this purpose (Holbrook & Skilbeck 1983; Schuling *et al.* 1993; Drummond & Walker 1994a).

Counselling the patient and their carers about the value of maintaining leisure activities and social contacts may be useful, and can have dramatic consequences (Fig. 15.30), along with practical help in achieving them. Although therapy specifically directed at improving participation in leisure activities, or using leisure goals to improve activities of

(a)

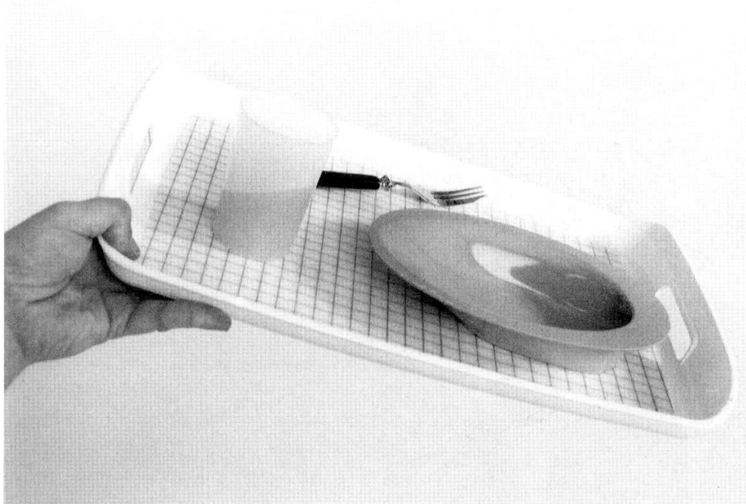

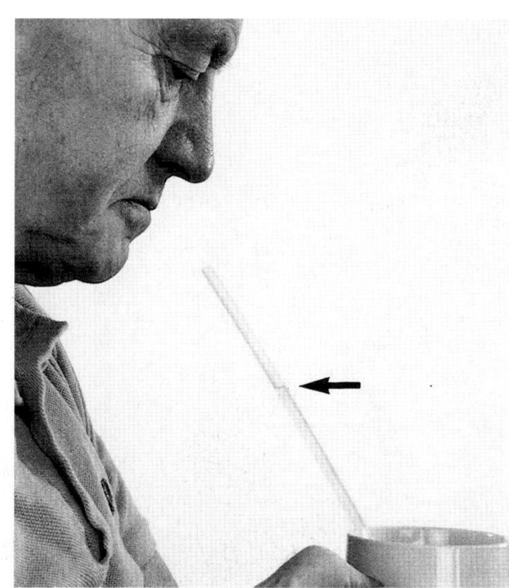

(b)

Fig. 15.29 Simple feeding aids. (a) A combination fork and knife, and a plate with a high side or plate guard may facilitate eating one handed. The non-slip tray also helps by fixing the plate and also reduces the risk of spills. (b) This drinking straw has a one-way valve so that when the user stops sucking the fluid does not fall back into the beaker (arrow). This may be useful in patients with facial weakness and poor lip closure but who have a normal swallow.

Table 15.51 Problems with food preparation and solutions.

Problem	Solution
Cannot open cans with one functional hand	Wall-mounted (electric) tin opener
Cannot open bottles with one functional hand	A bottle or jar stabilizer to fix the bottles to work surface
Cannot cut up or peel ingredients with one functional hand	A plate or board with spikes on which to impale the item to be cut

daily living function, was shown to be effective in small randomized controlled trials, a large trial (TOTAL) has failed to confirm this effect (Jongbloed & Morgan 1991; Drummond & Walker 1994b; J. Gladman, personal communication).

Air travel

We are frequently asked by patients and their families whether the patient can travel on a commercial flight after a stroke. We are not aware of any research into the safety, or otherwise, of flying after stroke. Prolonged immobility

(a)

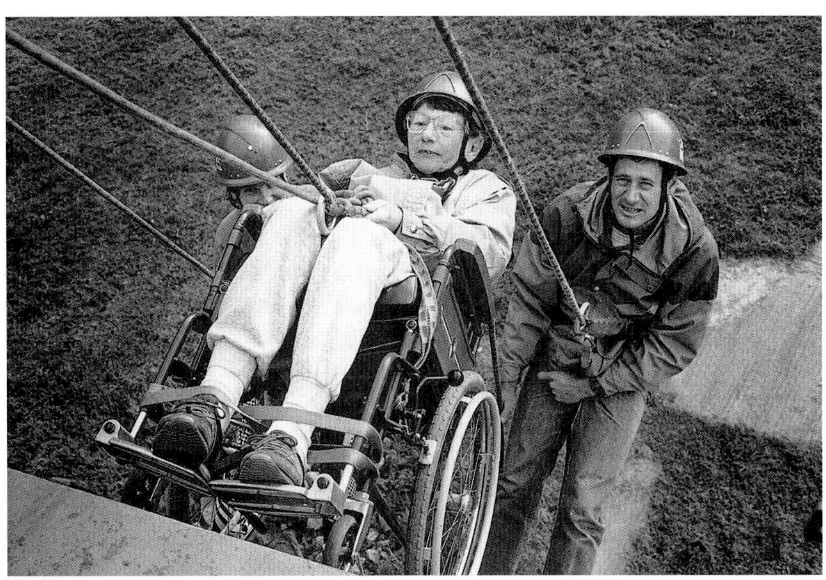

(b)

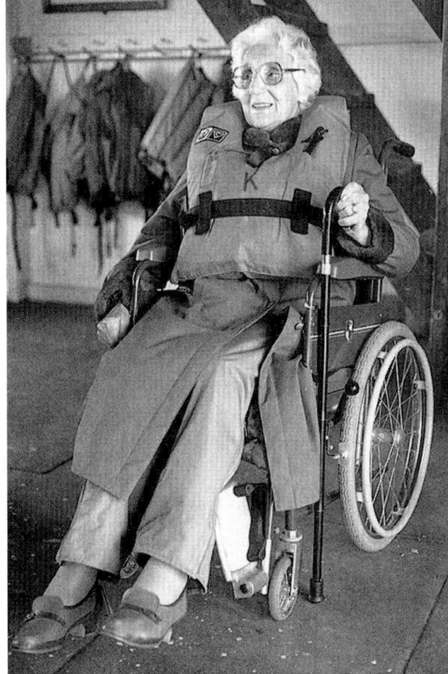

(c)

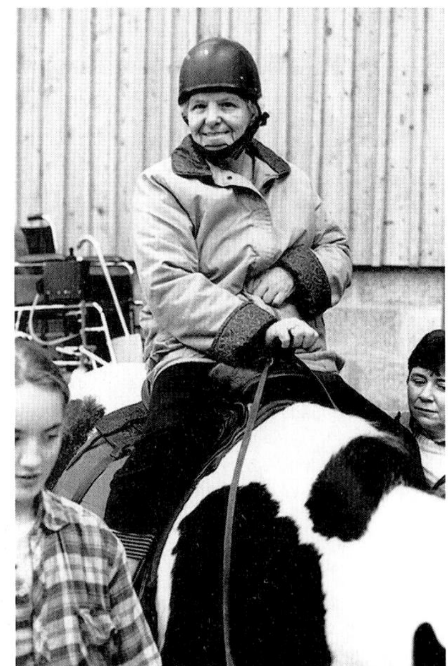

Fig. 15.30 Leisure activities for patients with mobility problems after stroke. (a) Abseiling in a wheelchair; (b) preparing for canoeing; (c) horse riding (photographs taken by Renzo Mazzolini for the Chest Heart and Stroke Association, Scotland).

on longhaul flights with the attendent risk of venous thromboembolism, and the effect of altitude (most commercial aeroplanes are pressurized to a level equivalent to an altitude of about 7000 feet) on the brain, are two issues which need to be considered. In giving advice one also needs to take into account the importance of the flight (e.g. is it to get home or simply part of a holiday?); the interval from the stroke since this will in part determine the risk of recurrent stroke; the ability of the patient to manage everyday activities, such as toileting and feeding on an aeroplane; the availability of an accompanying carer; and the attitude of the airline and the provider of the patient's travel insurance. Many patients who have a stroke whilst on holiday are repatriated by air within a week or two without apparent ill effects.

15.33.4 Sex

Although many stroke patients are elderly, they were often sexually active before their stroke. After stroke, libido, coital frequency and satisfaction are reduced among both patients and their partners (Angeleri *et al.* 1993; Korpelainen *et al.* 1999). This reduction in activity is due to both physical and psychosocial factors, the latter probably being of greater importance (Table 15.52). Reduced sexual activity may contribute to a worsening emotional relationship with a partner.

A patient and their partner may believe that reduced satisfaction with their sexual relationship is an inevitable consequence of stroke. Although we often feel embarrassed about talking to people about these aspects of their lives, it is important that sexual problems are addressed. Physical difficulties related to the patient's impairments can often be overcome with a little commonsense and a realization that intercourse, with vaginal penetration, is not an absolute requirement. The psychological problems contributing to sexual dysfunction are often the most difficult to sort out. Sometimes patients and their partners simply need to be reassured that sexual activity, like any other physical activity, will not precipitate another stroke. Verbal information may usefully be supplemented by leaflets, supplied by charities and patient organizations, which include advice for patients and carers (Duddle 1993).

Table 15.52 Causes of reduced sexual activity and satisfaction after a stroke.

Psychosocial factors
Loss of interest
Fear of impotence
Fear of bringing on another stroke
Emotional changes may adversely affect the relationship
Inability to discuss problems

Physical factors
Physical disability may make sexual intercourse difficult or impossible, e.g. indwelling catheter, contractures
Impotence and reduced libido due to:
- Drugs (e.g. thiazide diuretics, betablockers, tricyclic antidepressants)
- Co-morbidity (e.g. diabetes, peripheral vascular disease)

We encourage patients to resume sexual activity as soon as they wish to after a stroke. One exception might be a patient with a recent rupture of a saccular aneurysm which has not for some reason been clipped or coiled. One might imagine that the increase in blood pressure associated with orgasm could cause a re-bleed. Unfortunately, strokes can put tremendous strains on a relationship which are more difficult to manage. Where sexual dysfunction is due to medication (Table 15.52), withdrawal and substitution with an alternative drug may be effective. In men with impotence, sildenafil (Viagra) may be useful although experience of its use after stroke is limited and the manufacturers recommend caution in this situation. Many patients with stroke will be taking nitrates for ischaemic heart disease which precludes the concurrent use of sildenafil. Referral to a sexual dysfunction clinic, or for marital guidance, may be useful if problems persist after attending to the simple and obvious.

15.33.5 Finance

Stroke may place a considerable financial burden on patients and their families. Employment, and therefore income, may be affected (Holbrook 1982). Disability, and the aids and adaptations needed to overcome it, may also be costly. Even when the patient is still in hospital, carers may have difficulty meeting the costs of transport to visit the patient. This is important because the patient's morale may suffer if regular visiting is not possible and this may adversely affect outcome. Of course, in some unenlightened health systems, the patient or family may have to pay directly for their health care and financial constraints may even prevent patients from receiving the necessary treatment.

The professionals involved must be alert to the financial problems which affect patients and be ready to offer help as required. In the UK, and other countries, where the level of government support for home care is dependent on the patient's personal finances, a financial assessment may be necessary for planning care. In the UK, social workers are responsible for these assessments although other agencies may become involved.

Depending on assessment of the patient's and carer's needs, and sometimes a financial assessment, patients or carers may be eligible for financial benefits from government, charitable and other sources (e.g. superannuation schemes, insurance policies, etc.).

15.34 Carers

Looking after a patient with disability places considerable physical and emotional strains on the carer (Han & Haley 1999). Carers worry about the patients' needs and their ability to fulfil them. Caring may well limit the carer's employment and leisure activities and lead to social isolation and loneliness. Carers of disabled stroke patients are more often anxious, depressed, have more physical symptoms and are more dissatisfied with their jobs and social life than controls of similar age and sex (Han & Haley 1999). The extent of these difficulties appears to be related to the patient's level of dependency, mood, behaviour and cognitive function (Dennis *et al.* 1998; Han & Haley 1999). However, the magnitude of the burden of caregiving, as perceived by the carer, may relate to their own physical and emotional state as much as that of the patient (Scholte op Reimer *et al.* 1998). The impact that a stroke has on the family changes over time. Periods which are likely to cause carers particular stress and when extra support may be needed are:

- immediately after the stroke when the carer has to come to terms with what is potentially a life-threatening event and one which may have a major effect on the patient's and potential carer's future life together;
- during a prolonged period of in-patient care. Visiting may be difficult because of travelling and also because the patient's behaviour may put emotional pressure on the carer;
- around the period of hospital discharge. Suddenly the patient who has been looked after by a team of highly skilled professionals appears, at least to the carer, to be only the carer's responsibility; and
- during the weeks and months following hospital discharge when professional support dwindles (sometimes inappropriately and abruptly), friends stop calling, and the carer becomes physically and emotionally exhausted.

Holbrook (1982) made some helpful observations of the stages which families typically go through in adjusting to the change in their lives (Table 15.53). Although these do not apply to all carers, it is useful to be aware of them in managing patients and their families.

Although the physical aspects of caring for a person with a disabling stroke are hard, it is often the patient's psychological and resulting behavioural problems which cause most distress to carers (Brocklehurst *et al.* 1981). Carers may note a change in personality, the patient may become short-tempered and irritable, depressed or apathetic (Angeleri *et al.* 1993). Such changes may lead to a deterioration in their relationship which may be compounded by a cessation or disturbance of their sexual relationship (section 15.33.4).

Carers often have feelings of guilt which add to their distress. They worry that they contributed to the stroke, perhaps by giving the patient the wrong diet or because of some petty incident which the carer feels they should have avoided. They feel guilty about not visiting enough or for not having the patient home soon enough. After hospital discharge they feel guilty about wanting to carry on with their own lives. They often worry that the patient will fall, have another stroke or even die unless they are in constant attendance. These fears, apart from adding to the distress of carers, may also cause the carers to become overprotective towards the patient, which may prejudice the patient's outcome.

Table 15.53 Stages of adjustment amongst families of patients with a stroke (from Holbrook 1982).

Stage 1:	Crisis	Shock Confusion High anxiety
Stage 2:	Treatment stage	High expectation of recovery Denial that disability is permanent Periods of grieving Fears for the future Job Mobility Lifestyle About coping
Stage 3:	Realization of disability	Anger Feelings of rejection Despair Frustration Depression
Stage 4:	Adjustment	

Assessment

It is important that all those involved in managing a stroke patient are aware of the burden that caring for a disabled patient places on the family and other carers. The carer should be invited to discuss *their* problems. This is usually best done when the patient is absent since carers often feel uncomfortable or guilty when talking about *their* own problems if the patient is present. Indeed, carers often need a lot of encouragement to discuss their problems at all. However, they should be encouraged to do so not only for their own sake, but also for the patient's. If they are not coping this will adversely affect the patient.

It is important to assess the carer's physical and mental ability to go on providing the necessary care. If the patient is in hospital, it is often useful to get the carer to help with the patient's nursing care and attend their therapy sessions. This gives the carer an indication of what caring may involve, it can help the carer and team members identify and hopefully resolve problems before discharge, and it provides a valuable opportunity to 'train' the carer. Pre-discharge visits home for a day or weekend fulfil similar functions. Carers may need physical or simply psychological support.

Prevention and treatment

Physical support is usually limited whilst the patient is in hospital, although some carers may need help with finances (section 15.33.5) and visiting. However, physical support is likely to become more important after the patient is discharged home. Examples include:

- providing help with housework to give the carer more time for providing personal care;
- providing a care assistant or district nurse to help with the patient's personal care;
- providing a laundry service if the patient has persisting urinary or faecal incontinence;
- arranging for the patient to attend a day hospital or day centre or arranging 'patient sitting' services to allow the carer to go shopping, have their hair done, or attend some social function; and
- arranging regular respite admissions to a hospital or nursing home to allow the carer to go on holiday, or simply to give them a well-earned rest.

Such services may be expensive but they probably prevent or delay the need for long-term institutional care which may be even more expensive.

Psychological support. Carers often need help coming to terms with the changes in the person who has had a stroke. They have many questions and sources of concern (Table 15.54). Support is needed whilst the patient is in hospital and thereafter. It may take a variety of forms:

Table 15.54 Common questions asked by carers.

Acutely
What is a stroke?
Will they die?
Will they be disabled?
Why did this happen?
Was it my fault?
Will it happen again?

After hospital discharge
How long will they keep improving for?
Will their speech get better?
Why are they not the person I knew before?
Can I leave them alone to go out?
Can they exercise, will it bring on another stroke?
Will I always feel so tired?
Where can I get help with money?
Where can I get help with bathing?
Can I have a rest or holiday, i.e. respite?

- an informal talk with the consultant, nurse, therapist or social worker. These are valuable opportunities for carers to ask questions;
- a carers' group where they can ask team members questions, share experiences and provide mutual support (Mykyta *et al.* 1976; Holbrook 1982);
- formal sessions with a counsellor which may help them come to terms with their problems.

The setting in which support is given needs to be tailored to the individual since, for example, not everybody wants to attend a group. The need for these sorts of services may not be apparent whilst patients are in hospital, or when they attend an out-patient department. Also, for patients who are not admitted after their stroke, or who remain in hospital for just a few days, the opportunities for the patient and their carer to ask questions and obtain advice are often limited. One approach is to provide a dedicated stroke family support worker who can identify the physical and emotional needs of patients and their families and try to meet them using all available resources. In many places this role is already, at least partially, carried out by social workers and other members of the team, but there are often difficulties in bridging the gap between hospital and community care Although such support is valued by its recipients, its impact on patient and carer outcomes are unclear (section 17.5.3).

Giving information (section 17.5.5). Carers may know little about stroke, its causes and consequences and have often received misleading information from families and friends (Wellwood *et al.* 1994). Carers, like patients, vary in the amount, type and format of information they want about stroke. Information giving therefore needs to be tailored to the individual. Leaflets, audio or video tapes may usefully reinforce verbal transfer of information but more formal evaluation of their relative effectiveness is required (Lomer & McLellan 1987). Education programmes appear to increase carers' knowledge and satisfaction with information received but not necessarily their emotional outcome (Mant *et al.* 1998; Rodgers *et al.* 1999; Knapp *et al.* 2000). It is important that patients and carers are given consistent information and advice to avoid confusion. Good communication between potential providers of information is therefore vital.

References

Please note that all references taken from *The Cochrane Library* are given a current date as this database is updated on a quarterly basis. Please refer to the current *Cochrane Library* article for the latest review. The same applies to the *British Medical Journal* 'Clinical Evidence' series which is updated every six months.

Addington, W.R., Stephens, R.E. & Gilliland, K.A. (1999) Assessing the laryngeal cough reflex and the risk of developing pneumonia after stroke. An interhospital comparison. *Stroke* 30, 1203–1207.

Agrell, B. & Dehlin, O. (1989) Comparison of six depression rating scales in geriatric stroke patients. *Stroke* 20, 1190–1194.

Agu, O., Hamilton, G. & Baker, D. (1999) Graduated compression stockings in prevention of venous thromboembolism. *British Journal of Surgery* **86**, 992–1004.

Allen, C.M.C. (1983) Clinical diagnosis of the acute stroke syndrome. *Quarterly Journal of Medicine* **208**, 515–523.

Allman, R.M., Walker, J.M., Hart, M.K., Lapsade, C.A., Noel, L.B. & Smith, C.R. (1987) Air fluidised beds or conventional therapy for pressure sores. *Annals of Internal Medicine* **107**, 641–648.

Ancliffe, J. (1992) Strapping the shoulder in patients following cerebrovascular accident (CVA): a pilot study. *Australian Journal of Physiotherapy* **38**, 837–839.

Andersen, G., Vestergaard, K. & Riis, J.O. (1993) Citalopram for post-stroke pathological crying. *Lancet* **342**, 837–839.

Andersen, G., Vestergaard, K. & Lauritzen, L. (1994) Effective treatment of post stroke depression with the selective serotonin reuptake inhibitor citalopram. *Stroke* **25**, 1099–1104.

Andersen, G., Vestergaard, K. & Ingeman-Nielsen, M. (1995a) Post-stroke pathological crying: frequency and correlation to depression. *European Journal of Neurology* **2**, 45–50.

Andersen, G., Vestergaard, K., Ingeman-Nielsen, M. & Jensen, T.S. (1995b) Incidence of central post-stroke pain. *Pain* **61**, 187–193.

Angeleri, F., Angeleri, V.A., Foschi, N., Giaquinto, S. & Nolfe, G. (1993) The influence of depression, social activity and family stress on functional outcome after stroke. *Stroke* **24**, 1478–1483.

Arden, M., Mayou, R., Feldman, E. & Hawton, K. (1993) Cognitive impairment in the elderly medically ill: how often is it missed? *International Journal of Geriatric Psychiatry* **8**, 929–937.

Ashburn, A. & Lynch, M. (1988) Disadvantages of the early use of wheelchairs in the treatment of hemiplegia. *Clinical Rehabilitation* **2**, 327–331.

Ashworth, B. (1964) Preliminary trial of carisoprodol in multiple sclerosis. *Practitioner* **192**, 540–542.

Askenasy, J.J. & Goldhammer, I. (1988) Sleep apnea as a feature of bulbar stroke. *Stroke* **19**, 637–639.

Asplund, K. (1992) Any progress on progressing stroke? *Cerebrovascular Diseases* **2**, 317–319.

Asplund, K., Israelsson, K. & Schampi, I. (2000) Haemodilution for acute ischaemic stroke (Cochrane Review). In: *The Cochrane Library.* Oxford: Update Software.

Astrom, M., Adolfsson, R. & Asplund, K. (1993) Major depression in stroke patients. A 3 year longitudinal study. *Stroke* **24**, 976–982.

Axelsson, K., Asplund, K., Norberg, A. & Alafuzoff, I. (1988) Nutritional status in patients with acute stroke. *Acta Medica Scandinavica* **224**, 217–224.

Azam, U., Collin, P.G., Radley, S.C., Richmond, D.H. & Chapple, C.R. (2000) Anticholinergic drugs for urinary incontinence in adults (Protocol for a Cochrane Review). In: *The Cochrane Library.* Oxford: Update Software.

Baeten, C. & Hoefnagels, J. (1992) Feeding via nasogastric tube or percutaneous endoscopic gastrostomy: a comparison. *Scandinavian Journal of Gastroenterology* **27** (Suppl. 194), 95–98.

Barba, R., Martínez-Espinosa, S., Rodríguez-García, E., Pondal, M., Vivancos, J. & Del Ser, T. (2000) Poststroke dementia: clinical features and risk factors. *Stroke* **31**, 1494–1501.

Barer, D.H. (1989a) Continence after stroke: useful predictor or goal of therapy? *Age and Ageing* **18**, 183–191.

Barer, D.H. (1989b) The natural history and functional consequences of dysphagia after hemispheric stroke. *Journal of Neurology, Neurosurgery and Psychiatry* **52**, 236–241.

Barnes, M.P. (1998) Management of spasticity. *Age and Ageing* **27**, 239–245.

Barratt, E. (1988) A review of risk assessment methods. *Care-Science and Practice* **6**, 49–52.

Bassetti, C. & Aldrich, M.S. (1999) Sleep apnoea in acute cerebrovascular diseases: final report on 128 patients. *Sleep* **22**, 217–222.

Bassetti, C., Aldrich, M.S. & Quint, D. (1997) Sleep-disordered breathing in patients with acute supra- and intratentorial strokes. A prospective study of 39 patients. *Stroke* **28**, 1765–1772.

Bath, F.J. & Bath, P.M.W. (1997) What is the correct management of blood pressure in acute stroke? The blood pressure in acute stroke collaboration. *Cerebrovascular Diseases* **7**, 205–213.

Bath, P.M.W., Bath, F.J. & Smithard, D.G. (2000) Interventions for dysphagia in acute stroke (Cochrane Review). In: *The Cochrane Library.* Oxford: Update Software.

Becker, D., Philbrick, J., Bachhuber, T. & Humphries, J. (1996) D-dimer testing and acute venous thromboembolism. *Archives of Internal Medicine* **156**, 939–946.

Beckerman, H., Becher, J., Lankhorst, G.J., Verbeek, A.L.M. & Vogelaar, T.W. (1996) The efficacy of thermocoagulation of the tibial nerve and a polypropylene ankle-foot orthosis on spasticity of the leg in stroke patients: results of a randomized clinical trial. *Clinical Rehabilitation* **10**, 112–120.

Beekman, A.T.F., Penninx, B.W.J.H., Deeg, D.J.H. *et al.* (1998) Depression in survivors of stroke: a community-based study of prevalence, risk factors and consequences. *Social Psychiatry and Psychiatric Epidemiology* **33**, 463–470.

Belfield, P.W. (1989) Urinary catheters. In: *Everyday Aids and Appliances* (ed. G.P. Mulley), pp. 55–59. BMJ Publishers, London.

van den Belt, A.G.M., Prins, M.H., Lensing, A.W.A. *et al.* (2000) Fixed dose subcutaneous low molecular weight heparins versus adjusted dose unfractionated heparin for venous thromboembolism (Cochrane Review). In: *The Cochrane Library.* Oxford: Update Software.

Benbow, S., Sangster, G. & Barer, D. (1991) Incontinence after stroke. *Lancet* **338**, 1602–1603.

Berkovic, S.F., Bladin, P. & Darby, D.G. (1984) Metabolic disorders presenting as stroke. *Medical Journal of Australia* **140**, 421–424.

Berlowitz, D.R. & Wilking, S.V. (1989) Risk factors for pressure sores. A comparison of cross-sectional and cohort-derived data. *Journal of the American Geriatrics Society* **37**, 1043–1050.

Bhakta, B., Cozens, J.A., Chamberlain, M.A. & Bamford, J.M. (1996) Use of botulinum toxin in stroke patients with severe upper limb spasticity. *Journal of Neurology, Neurosurgery and Psychiatry* **61**, 30–35.

Bhakta, B., Cozens, J.A., Chamberlain, M.A. & Bamford, J.M. (2000) The impact of botulinum type A on disability and carer burden due to arm spasticity after stroke: a randomized double blind placebo controlled trial. *Journal of Neurology, Neurosurgery and Psychiatry* **69**, 217–221.

Blood Pressure in Acute Stroke Collaboration (BASC) (2000) Interventions for deliberately altering blood pressure in acute stroke (Cochrane Review). In: *The Cochrane Library.* Oxford: Update Software.

Bobath, B. (1978) *Adult Hemiplegia Evaluation and Treatment*, 2nd edn. Heinemann, London.

Boeer, A., Voth, E. & Prange, H.W. (1991) Early heparin therapy in patients with spontaneous intracerebral haemorrhage. *Journal of Neurology, Neurosurgery and Psychiatry* **54**, 466–467.

Borrie, M.J., Campbell, A., Caradoc-Davies, T.H. & Spears, G.F.S. (1986) Urinary incontinence after stroke: a prospective study. *Age and Ageing* **15**, 177–181.

Bounds, J.V., Wiebers, D.O., Whisnant, J.P. & Okazaki, H. (1981) Mechanisms and timing of deaths from cerebral infarction. *Stroke* **12**, 474–477.

Bowen, A., McKenna, K. & Tallis, R.C. (1999) Reasons for variability in the reported rate of occurrence of unilateral spatial neglect after stroke. *Stroke* **30**, 1196–1202.

Bowsher, D. (1996) Central pain: clinical and physiological characteristics. *Journal of Neurology, Neurosurgery and Psychiatry* **61**, 62–69.

Bowsher, D., Leijon, G. & Thoumas, K.A. (1998) Central post stroke pain: correlation of MRI with clinical pain characteristics and sensory abnormalities. *Neurology* **51**, 1352–1358.

Bradley, M., Nelson, E.A., Petticrew, M., Cullum, N. & Sheldon, T. (2000) Dressings for pressure sores (Protocol for a Cochrane Review). In: *The Cochrane Library.* Oxford: Update Software.

Braus, D.F., Krauss, J.K. & Strobel, J. (1994) The shoulder hand syndrome after stroke: a prospective clinical trial. *Annals of Neurology* **36**, 728–733.

Brittain, K.R., Perry, S.I., Shaw, C. *et al.* (2000) Prevalence and impact of urinary symptoms among community-dwelling stroke survivors. *Stroke* **31**, 886–891.

Britton, M., De Faire, U., Helmers, C., Miah, K., Ryding, C. & Wester, P.O. (1979) Arrhythmias in patients with acute cerebrovascular disease. *Acta Medica Scandinavica* **205**, 425–428.

Brocklehurst, J.C., Morris, P., Andrews, K., Richards, B. & Laycock, P. (1981) Social effects of stroke. *Social Science and Medicine* **15A**, 35–39.

Brocklehurst, J.C., Andrews, K., Richards, B. & Laycock, P.J. (1985) Incidence and correlates of incontinence in stroke patients. *Journal of the American Geriatrics Society* **33**, 540–542.

Brooke, M.M., de Lateur, B.J., Diana-Rigby, G.C. & Questad, K.A. (1991) Shoulder subluxation in hemiplegia: effects of three different supports. *Archives of Physical Medicine and Rehabilitation* **72**, 583–586.

Brown, D.A. & Kautz, S.A. (1998) Increased workload enhances force output during pedaling exercise in persons with post-stroke hemiplegia. *Stroke* **29**, 598–606.

Brown, H.W. & Plum, F. (1961) The neurologic basis of Cheyne–Stokes respiration. *American Journal of Medicine* **30**, 849–860.

Brown, R.A., Holdsworth, L., Leslie, G.C., Mutch, W.J. & Part, N.J. (1993) The effects of time after stroke and selected therapeutic techniques on quadriceps muscle tone in stroke patients. *Physiotherapy Theory and Practice* **9**, 131–142.

Brunnstrom, S. (1970) *Movement Therapy in Hemiplegia.* Harper & Row, New York.

Bruno, A., Biller, J., Adams, H.P. *et al.* (1999) Acute blood glucose level and outcome from ischemic stroke. *Neurology* **52**, 280–284.

Burbaud, P., Wiart, L., Dubos, J.L. *et al.* (1996) A randomized, double blind, placebo controlled trial of botulinum toxin in the treatment of spastic foot in hemiparetic patients. *Journal of Neurology, Neurosurgery and Psychiatry* **61**, 265–269.

Burcar, P.J., Notenberg, M.D. & Yarnell, P.R. (1977) Hyponatraemia and central pontine myelinolysis. *Neurology* **27**, 223–226.

Burn, J., Dennis, M., Bamford, J., Sandercock, P., Wade, D. & Warlow, C. (1998) Epileptic seizures after a first-ever stroke: the Oxfordshire Community Stroke Project. *British Medical Journal* **315**, 1582–1587.

Burridge, J.H., Taylor, P.N., Hagan, S.A., Wood, D.E. & Swain, I.D. (1997) The effects of common peroneal stimulation on the effort and speed of walking: a randomized controlled trial with chronic hemiplegic patients. *Clinical Rehabilitation* **11**, 201–210.

Burvill, P.W., Johnson, G.A., Jamrozik, K.D., Anderson, C.S., Stewart-Wynne, E.G. & Chakera, T.M.H. (1995a) Prevalence of depression after stroke: the Perth Community Stroke Study. *British Journal of Psychiatry* **166**, 320–327.

Burvill, P.W., Johnson, G.A., Jamrozik, K.D., Anderson, C.S., Stewart-Wynne, E.G. & Chakera, T.M.H. (1995b) Anxiety disorders after stroke: results from the Perth Community Stroke Study. *British Journal of Psychiatry* **166**, 328–332.

Bushnell, C.D., Phillips-Bute, B.G., Laskowitz, D.T., Lynch, J.R., Chilukuri, V. & Borel, C.O. (1999) Survival and outcome after endotracheal intubation for acute stroke. *Neurology* **52**, 1374–1381.

Busto, R., Dietrich, W.D., Globus, M.Y.T., Valdes, I., Scheinberg, P. & Ginsberg, M.D. (1987) Small differences in intra-ischemic brain temperature critically determine the extent of ischemic neuronal injury. *Journal of Cerebral Blood Flow and Metabolism* **7**, 729–738.

Busto, R., Dietrich, D., Globus, M.Y.T. & Ginsberg, M.D. (1989) The importance of brain temperature in cerebral ischaemic injury. *Stroke* **20**, 1113–1114.

Calvert, T., Knapp, P. & House, A. (1998) Psychological associations with emotionalism after stroke. *Journal of Neurology, Neurosurgery and Psychiatry* **65**, 928–929.

Campbell, A.J., Robertson, M.C., Gardner, M.M., Norton, R.N. & Buchner, D.M. (1999) Falls prevention over 2 years: a randomized controlled trial in women 80 years and older. *Age and Ageing* **28**, 513–518.

Canhao, P., Melo, T.P., Salgado, A.V. *et al.* (1997) Nausea and vomiting in acute ischemic stroke. *Cerebrovascular Diseases* **7**, 220–225.

Carlberg, B., Asplund, K. & Hagg, E. (1991) Course of blood pressure in different subsets of patients after acute stroke. *Cerebrovascular Diseases* **1**, 281–287.

Carr, E.K. & Kenney, F.D. (1992) Positioning of the stroke patient: a review of the literature. *International Journal of Nursing Studies* **29**, 355–369.

Carson, A.J., MacHale, S., Allen, K. *et al.* (2000) Depression after stroke is not associated with lesion location: a systematic review. *Lancet* **356**, 122–126.

Cassidy, T.P., Bruce, D.W., Lewis, S. & Gray, C.S. (1999) The association of visual field defecits and visuo-spatial neglect in acute right-hemisphere stroke patients. *Age and Ageing* **28**, 257–260.

Castillo, J. (1999) Deteriorating stroke: diagnostic criteria, predictors, mechanisms and treatment. *Cerebrovascular Diseases* **9** (Suppl. 3), 1–8.

Castro, A.A., Clark, O.A.C., Atallah, A.N. & Burihan, E. (2000) Duration of initial heparin treatment for deep-vein thrombosis (Protocol for a Cochrane Review). In: *The Cochrane Library.* Oxford: Update Software.

Chae, J., Bethoux, F., Bohine, T., Dobos, L., Davis, T. & Friedl, A. (1998) Neuromuscular stimulation for upper extremity motor and functional recovery in acute hemiplegia. *Stroke* **29**, 975–979.

Challiner, Y.C., Jarrett, D., Hayward, M.J., Al-Jubouri, M.A. & Julious, S.A. (1994) A comparison of intravenous and subcutaneous hydration in elderly acute stroke patients. *Postgraduate Medical Journal* **70**, 195–197.

Chan, H. (1997) Bladder management in acute care of stroke patients: a quality improvement project. *Journal of Neuroscience Nursing* **29**, 187–190.

Chen, H., Chopp, M. & Welch, K.M.A. (1991) Effect of mild hyperthermia on the ischaemic infarct volume after middle cerebral artery occlusion in the rat. *Neurology* **41**, 1133–1135.

Cheyne, J. (1818) A case of apoplexy in which the fleshy part of the heart was converted to fat. *Dublin Hospital Report* **2**, 216.

Chiodo Grandi, F., Miccio, M., Salvi, R., Antonutti, L. & Mazzone, C. (2000) Physical means for preventing deep vein thrombosis in stroke (Protocol for a Cochrane Review). In: *The Cochrane Library.* Oxford: Update Software.

Choi-Kwon, S., Yang, Y.H., Kim, E.K., Jeon, M.Y. & Kim, J.S. (1998) Nutritional status in acute stroke: undernutrition versus overnutrition in different stroke subtypes. *Acta Neurologica Scandinavica* **98**, 187–192.

Clark, M. (2000) Dressings and topical agents for the prevention of pressure sores (Protocol for a Cochrane Review). In: *The Cochrane Library.* Oxford: Update Software.

Collen, F.M. & Wade, D.T. (1991) Residual mobility problems after stroke. *International Disability Studies* **13**, 12–15.

Collen, F.M., Wade, D.T., Robb, G.F. & Bradshaw, C.M. (1991) The Rivermead Mobility Index: a further development of the Rivermead Motor Assessment. *International Disability Studies* **13**, 50–54.

Cope, C., Tyrone, M.R. & Skversky, N.J. (1973) Phlebographic analysis of the incidence of thrombosis in hemiplegia. *Radiology* **109**, 581–584.

Cornall, C. (1991) Self propelling wheelchairs: the effect on spasticity in hemiplegic patients. *Physiotherapy Theory and Practice* **7**, 13–21.

Correia, M., Silva, M. & Veloso, M. (2000) Cooling therapy for acute stroke (Cochrane Review). In: *The Cochrane Library.* Oxford: Update Software.

Cullum, N., Deeks, J., Fletcher, A. *et al.* (1995) The prevention and treatment of pressure sores. *Effective Health Care* **2**, 1–16.

Cullum, N., Deeks, J.J., Sheldon, T.A., Song, F. & Fletcher, A.W. (2000) Beds, mattresses and cushions for preventing and treating pressure sores. (Cochrane Review). In: *The Cochrane Library.* Oxford: Update Software.

Dam, M., Tonin, P., De Boni, A. *et al.* (1996) Effects of fluoxetine and maprotiline on functional recovery in post-stroke hemiplegic patients undergoing rehabilitation therapy. *Stroke* **27**, 1211–1214.

Davalos, A., Ricart, W., Gonzalez-Huix, F. *et al.* (1996) Effect of malnutrition after acute stroke on clinical outcome. *Stroke* **27**, 1028–1032.

Davalos, A., Castillo, J., Pumar, J.M. & Noya, M. (1997) Body temperature and fibrinogen are related to early neurological deterioration in acute ischemic stroke. *Cerebrovascular Diseases* **7**, 64–69.

Davenport, R.J., Dennis, M.S. & Warlow, C.P. (1995) Improving the recording of the clinical assessment of stroke patients using a clerking proforma. *Age and Ageing* **24**, 43–48.

Davenport, R.J., Dennis, M.S. & Warlow, C.P. (1996a) Gastrointestinal haemorrhage following acute stroke. *Stroke* **27**, 421–424.

Davenport, R.J., Dennis, M.S., Wellwood, I. & Warlow, C.P. (1996b) Complications following acute stroke. *Stroke* **27**, 415–420.

David, R., Enderby, P. & Bainton, D. (1982) Treatment of acquired aphasia: speech therapists and volunteers compared. *Journal of Neurology, Neurosurgery and Psychiatry* **45**, 957–961.

Davidson, B.L. (1998) What are the most reliable detection methods for deep vein thrombosis and pulmonary embolism to be used as endpoints in trials of venous thromboprophylaxis? *Haemostasis* **28** (Suppl. 3), 113–119.

Davis, M., Hollymann, C., McGiven, M., Chambers, I., Egbuji, J. & Barer, D. (1999) Physiological monitoring in acute stroke. *Age and Ageing* **28** (Suppl. 1), 45.

De Koning, I., van Kooten, F., Dippel, D.W.J. *et al.* (1998) The CAMCOG: a useful screening instrument for dementia in stroke patients. *Stroke* **29**, 2080–2086.

Dean, C.M. & Shepherd, R.B. (1997) Task related training improves performance in seated reaching tasks after stroke. A randomized controlled trial. *Stroke* **28**, 722–728.

Dekker, J.H.M., Wagenaar, R.C., Lankhorst, G.J. & de Jong, B.A. (1997) The painful hemiplegic shoulder. Effects of intra-articular triamcinalone acetonide. *American Journal of Physical Medicine and Rehabilitation* **76**, 43–48.

Demeurisse, G., Demol, O. & Robaye, E. (1980) Motor evaluation in vascular hemiplegia. *European Neurology* **19**, 382–389.

Denes, G., Semenza, C., Stoppa, E. & Lis, A. (1982) Unilateral spatial neglect and recovery from hemiplegia: a follow-up study. *Brain* **105**, 543–552.

Dennis, M., O'Rourke, S., Lewis, S., Sharpe, M. & Warlow, C. (1998) A quantitative study of the emotional outcome of people caring for stroke survivors. *Stroke* **29**, 1867–1872.

Dennis, M., O'Rourke, S., Lewis, S., Sharpe, M. & Warlow, C. (2000) Emotional outcomes after stroke: factors associated with poor outcome. *Journal of Neurology, Neurosurgery and Psychiatry* **68**, 47–52.

Desmond, D.W., Tetemichi, T.K., Figueroa, M., Gropen, T.I. & Stern, Y. (1994) Disorientation following stroke: frequency, course, and clinical correlates. *Journal of Neurology* **241**, 585–591.

Desmond, D.W., Moroney, J.T., Sano, M. & Stern, Y. (1996) Recovery of cognitive function after stroke. *Stroke* **27**, 1798–1803.

Desmond, D.W., Moroney, J.T., Bagiella, E., Sano, M. & Stern, Y. (1998) Dementia as a predictor of adverse outcomes following stroke. An evaluation of diagnostic methods. *Stroke* **29**, 69–74.

Desmukh, M., Bisignani, M., Landau, P. & Orchard, T.J. (1991) Deep vein thrombosis in rehabilitating stroke patients. Incidence, risk factors and prophylaxis. *American Journal of Physical Medicine and Rehabilitation* **70**, 313–316.

Dickmann, U., Voth, E., Schicha, H., Henze, T., Prange, H. & Emrich, D. (1988) Heparin therapy, deep vein thrombosis and pulmonary embolism after intracerebral haemorrhage. *Klinische Wochenschrift* **66**, 1182–1183.

Dickstein, R., Hocherman, S., Pillar, T. & Shaham, R. (1986) Stroke rehabilitation. Three exercise therapy approaches. *Physical Therapy* **66**, 1233–1238.

Dimant, J. & Grob, D. (1977) Electrocardiographic changes and myocardial damage in patients with acute cerebrovascular accidents. *Stroke* **8**, 448–455.

Drakulovic, M.B., Torres, A., Bauer, T.T., Nicolas, J.M., Hogue, S. & Ferrer, M. (1999) Supine body position as a risk factor for nosocomial pneumonia in mechanically ventilated patients: a randomized trial. *Lancet* **354**, 1851–1858.

Dromerick, A.E.R. & Reding, M. (1994) Medical and neurological complications during in-patient stroke rehabilitation. *Stroke* **25**, 358–361.

Drummond, A. (1990) Leisure activity after stroke. *International Disability Studies* **12**, 157–160.

Drummond, A.E.R. & Walker, M.F. (1994a) The Nottingham Leisure Questionnaire for stroke patients. *British Journal of Occupational Therapy* **57**, 414–418.

Drummond, A. & Walker, M.F. (1994b) A randomized controlled trial of leisure therapy after stroke. *Clinical Rehabilitation* **9**, 283–290.

Duddle, M. (1993) Sex after stroke illness. In: *Stroke Association Leaflet S16*. Stroke Association, London.

Duncan, P.W., Goldstein, L.B., Matchar, D., Divin, G.W. & Feussner, J. (1992) Measurement of motor recovery after stroke. Outcome assessment and sample size requirements. *Stroke* **23**, 1084–1089.

Duncan, P.W., Goldstein, L.B., Horner, R.D., Landsman, P.B., Samsa, G.P. & Matchar, D.B. (1994) Similar motor recovery of upper and lower extremities after stroke. *Stroke* **25**, 1181–1188.

Ebrahim, S. & Redfern, J. (1999) *Stroke Care—A matter of chance. A National Survey of Stroke Services.* The Stroke Association, London.

Elizabeth, J., Singarayar, J., Ellul, J., Barer, D. & Lye, M. (1993) Arterial oxygen saturation and posture in acute stroke. *Age and Ageing* **22**, 269–272.

Ellul, J. & Barer, D. (1993) Detection and management of dysphagia in patients with acute stroke. *Age and Ageing* **22** (Suppl. 2), 17 (Abstract).

Enderby, P.M., Wood, V.A., Wade, D.T. & Langton Hewer, R. (1986) The Frenchay Aphasia Screening Test: a short, simple test for aphasia appropriate for non-specialists. *International Rehabilitation Medicine* 8, 166–170.

Enderby, P.M., Wood, V.A. & Wade, D.T. (1987) *Frenchay Aphasia Screening Test Manual.* NFER-Nelson, Windsor.

Eustice, S., Paterson, J. & Roe, B. (2000) Prompted voiding for the management of urinary incontinence in adults (Protocol for a Cochrane Review). In: *The Cochrane Library.* Oxford: Update Software.

Feibel, J.H. & Springer, C.J. (1982) Depression and failure to resume social activities after stroke. *Archives of Physical Medicine and Rehabilitation* **63**, 276–278.

Feigin, V.L., Rinkel, G.J.E., Algra, A. & van Gijn, J. (2000) Standard heparin, heparinoids, or low-molecular weight heparin for primary intracerebral haemorrhage (Protocol for a Cochrane Review). In: *The Cochrane Library.* Oxford: Update Software.

Feldman, Z., Kanter, M.J., Robertson, C.S. *et al.* (1992) Effect of head elevation on intracranial pressure, cerebral perfusion pressure, and cerebral blood flow in head-injured patients. *Journal of Neurosurgery* **76**, 207–211.

Ferro, J.M., Mariano, G. & Madureira, S. (1999) Recovery from aphasia and neglect. *Cerebrovascular Diseases* **9** (Suppl. 5), 6–22.

Feys, H.M., De Weerdt, W.J., Selz, B.E. *et al.* (1998) Effect of a therapeutic intervention for the hemiplegic upper limb in the acute phase after stroke. A single blind, randomized, controlled multicentre trial. *Stroke* **29**, 785–792.

Finestone, H.M., Greene-Finestone, L.S., Wilson, E.S. & Teasell, R.W. (1995) Malnutrition in stroke patients on the rehabilitation service and at follow-up: prevalence and predictors. *Archives of Physical Medicine and Rehabilitation* **76**, 310–316.

Fisk, G.D., Owsley, C. & Pulley, L.V. (1997) Driving after stroke: driving exposure, advice, and evaluations. *Archives of Physical Medicine and Rehabilitation* **78**, 1338–1345.

Fisk, J.D., Ritvo, P.G., Ross, L., Haase, D.A., Marrie, T.J. & Schlech, W.F. (1994) Measuring the functional impact of fatigue: initial validation of the fatigue impact scale. *Clinical Infectious Diseases* **18** (Suppl. 5), 79–83.

Flanagan, E.M. (1967) Methods for facilitation and inhibition of motor activity. *American Journal of Physical Medicine* **46**, 1006–1011.

Flemming, K. & Cullum, N. (2000a) Therapeutic ultrasound for pressure sores (Protocol for a Cochrane Review). In: *The Cochrane Library.* Oxford: Update Software.

Flemming, K. & Cullum, N. (2000b) Electrical stimulation for pressure sores (Protocol for a Cochrane Review). In: *The Cochrane Library.* Oxford: Update Software.

Folstein, M.F., Folstein, S.E. & McHugh, P.R. (1975) Mini-Mental State: a practical method for grading cognitive state of patients for clinicians. *Journal of Psychiatric Research* **12**, 189–198.

Forster, A. & Young, J. (1995) Incidence and consequences of falls due to stroke: a systematic inquiry. *British Medical Journal* **311**, 83–86.

Fox, G.K., Bowden, S.C. & Smith, D.S. (1998) On-road assessment of driving competence after brain impairment: review of current practice and recommendations for a standardized examination. *Archives of Physical Medicine and Rehabilitation* **79**, 1288–1296.

Frank, J.I. (1995) Large hemispheric infarction, deterioration, and intracranial pressure. *Neurology* **45**, 1286–1290.

Friedland, J. & McColl, M.-A. (1987) Social support and psychological dysfunction after stroke: buffering effects in a community sample. *Archives of Physical Medicine and Rehabilitation* **68**, 475–480.

Friedman, N.L. (1996) Hiccups: a treatment review. *Pharmacotherapy* **16**, 986–995.

Gariballa, S.E., Parker, S.G. & Castleden, C.M. (1998a) A randomized controlled trial of nutritional supplementation after stroke. *Age and Ageing* **27** (Suppl 1), 66. (Abstract).

Gariballa, S.E., Parker, S.G., Taub, N. & Castleden, C.M. (1998b) Influence of nutritional status on clinical outcome after acute stroke. *American Journal of Clinical Nutrition* **68**, 275–281.

Gautier, J.C. (1985) Stroke in progression. *Stroke* **16**, 729–733.

Gelber, D.A., Good, D.C., Laven, L.J. & Verhulst, S.J. (1993) Causes of urinary incontinence after acute hemispheric stroke. *Stroke* **24**, 378–382.

Gilbertson, L., Langhorne, P., Walker, A. & Allen, A. (2000) Domiciliary occupational therapy for stroke patients discharged home from hospital: a randomized controlled trial. *British Medical Journal* **320**, 603–606.

Gillespie, L.D., Gillespie, W.J., Cumming, R., Lamb, S.E. & Rowe, B.H. (2000) Interventions for preventing falls in the elderly (Cochrane Review). In: *The Cochrane Library.* Oxford: Update Software.

Giroud, M., Gras, P., Fayolle, H., Andre, N., Soichot, P. & Dumas, R. (1994) Early seizures after acute stroke: a study of 1,640 cases. *Epilepsia* **35**, 959–964.

Gladman, J., Forster, A. & Young, J. (1995) Hospital- and home-based rehabilitation after discharge from hospital for stroke patients: analysis of two trials. *Age and Ageing* **24**, 49–53.

Glanz, M., Klawansky, S., Stason, W. *et al.* (1995) Biofeedback therapy in post-stroke rehabilitation: a meta-analysis of the randomized controlled trials. *Archives of Physical Medicine and Rehabilitation* **76**, 508–515.

Glanz, M., Klawansky, S., Stason, W., Berkey, C. & Chalmers, T.C. (1996) Functional electrical stimulation in post-stroke rehabilitation: a meta-analysis of the randomized controlled trials. *Archives of Physical Medicine and Rehabilitation* **77**, 549–553.

Gordon, C., Langton Hewer, R. & Wade, D.T. (1987) Dysphagia in acute stroke. *British Medical Journal* **295**, 411–414.

Gosman-Hedstrom, G., Claesson, L., Klingenstierna, U. *et al.* (1998) Effects of acupuncture treatment on daily life activities and quality of life. A controlled, prospective, and randomized study of acute stroke patients. *Stroke* **29**, 2100–2108.

Gottlieb, J.E., Menashe, P.I. & Cruz, E. (1986) Gastrointestinal complications in critically ill patients: the intensivists overview. *American Journal of Gastroenterology* **81**, 227–238.

Gracies, J.M., Elovic, E., McGuire, J. & Simpson, D.M. (1997a) Traditional pharmacological treatments for spasticity. Part I: Local treatments. *Muscle and Nerve* **6** (Suppl.), S61–S91.

Gracies, J.M., Nance, P., Elovic, E., McGuire, J. & Simpson, D.M. (1997b) Traditional pharmacological treatments for spasticity. Part II: General and regional treatments. *Muscle and Nerve* **6** (Suppl.), S92–S120.

Gray, C.S., French, J.M., Bates, D., Cartlidge, N.E.F., Venables, G.S. & James, O.F.W. (1989) Recovery of visual fields in acute stroke: homonymous hemianopia associated with adverse prognosis. *Age and Ageing* **18**, 419–421.

Gray, C.S., French, J.M., Bates, D., Cartlidge, N.E.F., James, O.F.W. & Venables, G. (1990) Motor recovery following acute stroke. *Age and Ageing* **19**, 179–184.

Green, S., Buchbinder, R., Glazier, R. & Forbes, A. (1998) Systematic review of randomized controlled trials of interventions for painful shoulder: selection criteria, outcome assessment, and efficacy. *British Medical Journal* **316**, 354–360.

Green, S., Buchbinder, R., Glazier, R. & Forbes, A. (2000) Interventions for shoulder pain (Cochrane Review). In: *The Cochrane Library*. Oxford: Update Software.

Greener, J., Enderby, P., Whurr, R. & Grant, A. (1998) Treatment for aphasia following stroke; evidence for effectiveness. *International Journal of Language and Communiction Disorders* **33**, 158–161.

Greener, J., Enderby, P. & Whurr, R. (2000a) Speech and language therapy for aphasia following stroke (Protocol for a Cochrane Review). In: *The Cochrane Library*. Oxford: Update Software.

Greener, J., Enderby, P. & Whurr, R. (2000b) Pharmacological treatment for aphasia following stroke (Protocol for a Cochrane Review). In: *The Cochrane Library*. Oxford: Update Software.

Gregson, J.M., Leathley, M.J., Moore, P.A., Smith, T.L., Sharma, A.K. & Watkins, C.L. (2000) An assessment of the reliability of the modified Ashworth scale for measuring muscle tone and the Medical Research Council scale for measuring muscle power in post-stroke patients. *Age and Ageing* **29**, 223–228.

Gross, C.R., Lindquist, R.D., Wooley, A.C., Granier, R., Allard, K. & Webster, B. (1992) Clinical indicators of dehydration severity in elderly patients. *Journal of Emergency Medicine* **10**, 267–274.

Gubitz, G., Counsell, C., Sandercock, P. & Signorini, D. (2000) Anticoagulants for acute ischaemic stroke (Cochrane Review). In: *The Cochrane Library*. Oxford: Update Software.

Gujjar, A.R., Deibert, E., Manno, E.M., Duff, S. & Diringer, M.N. (1998) Mechanical ventilation for ischemic stroke and intracerebral hemorrhage. Indications, timing, and outcome. *Neurology* **51**, 447–451.

Gustafson, Y., Olsson, T., Eriksson, S., Asplund, K. & Bucht, G. (1991) Acute confusional states (Delirium) in stroke patients. *Cerebrovascular Diseases* **1**, 257–264.

Hagen, C. (1973) Communication abilities in hemiplegia: effect of speech therapy. *Archives of Physical Medicine and Rehabilitation* **54**, 454–463.

Hajat, C., Hajat, S. & Sharma, P. (2000) Effects of post-stroke pyrexia on stroke outcome. A meta-analysis of studies in patients. *Stroke* **31**, 410–414.

Han, B. & Haley, W.E. (1999) Family caregiving for patients with stroke. Review and analysis. *Stroke* **30**, 1478–1485.

Hanlon, J.T., Cutson, T. & Ruby, C.M. (1996) Drug-related falls in the older adult. *Topics in Geriatric Rehabilitation* **11**, 38–54.

Harper, G., Castleden, C.M. & Potter, J.F. (1994a) Factors affecting changes in blood pressure after stroke. *Stroke* **25**, 1726–1729.

Harper, G., Fotherby, M.D., Panayiotou, B., Castelden, C.M. & Potter, J.F. (1994b) The changes in blood pressure after acute stroke: abolishing the 'white-coat effect' with 24-h ambulatory monitoring. *Journal of Internal Medicine* **235**, 343–346.

Harris, C.P., Townsend, J.J. & Baringer, S.R. (1993) Symptomatic hyponatraemia: can myelinolysis be prevented by treatment? *Journal of Neurology, Neurosurgery and Psychiatry* **56**, 626–632.

Hartman, J. & Landau, W.M. (1987) Comparison of formal language therapy with supportive counselling for aphasia due to acute vascular accident. *Archives of Neurology* **44**, 646–649.

Harvey, R.L., Roth, E.J., Yarnold, P.R., Durham, J.R. & Green, D. (1996) Deep vein thrombosis in stroke. The use of plasma D-dimer level as a screening test in the rehabilitation setting. *Stroke* **27**, 1516–1520.

Haselkorn, J.K., Mueller, B.A. & Rivara, F.A. (1998) Characteristics of drivers and driving record after traumatic and nontraumatic brain injury. *Archives of Physical Medicine and Rehabilitation* **79**, 738–742.

Henon, H., Lebert, F., Durieu, I. *et al.* (1999) Confusional state in stroke. Relation to preexisting dementia, patient characteristics, and outcome. *Stroke* **30**, 773–779.

Hibbard, M.R., Grober, S.E., Gordon, W.A., Aletta, E.G. & Freeman, A. (1990) Cognitive therapy and the treatment of post-stroke depression. *Topics in Geriatric Rehabilitation* **5** (3), 43–55.

Hodkinson, H.M. (1972) Evaluation of a mental test score for assessment of mental impairment in the elderly. *Age and Ageing* **1**, 233–238.

Hofman, A., Geelkerkern, R.H., Willie, J., Hamming, J.J., Herman, J. & Breslau, P.J. (1994) Pressure sores and pressure decreasing mattresses: controlled clinical trial. *Lancet* **343**, 568–571.

Holas, M.A., DePippo, K.L. & Reding, M.J. (1994) Aspiration and relative risk of medical complications following stroke. *Archives of Neurology* **51**, 1051–1053.

Holbrook, M. (1982) Stroke: social and emotional outcome. *Journal of the Royal College of Physicians of London* **116**, 100–104.

Holbrook, M. & Skilbeck, C.E. (1983) An activities index for use with stroke patients. *Age and Ageing* **12**, 166–170.

Horn, J. & Limburg, M. (2000) Calcium antagonists for acute ischemic stroke (Cochrane Review). In: *The Cochrane Library*. Oxford: Update Software.

House, A. (1987) Mood disorders after stroke: a review of the evidence. *International Journal of Geriatric Psychiatry* **2**, 211–221.

House, A., Dennis, M., Hawton, K. & Warlow, C. (1989a) Methods of identifying mood disorders in stroke patients: experience in the Oxfordshire Community Stroke Project. *Age and Ageing* **18**, 371–379.

House, A., Dennis, M., Molyneux, A., Warlow, C. & Hawton, K. (1989b) Emotionalism after stroke. *British Medical Journal* **298**, 991–994.

House, A., Dennis, M., Mogridge, L., Warlow, C., Hawton, K. & Jones, L. (1991) Mood disorders in the year after first stroke. *British Journal of Psychiatry* **158**, 83–92.

House, A., Knapp, P., Dempster, C. *et al.* (1999) *Does problem solving therapy improve psychological outcome after stroke?* NHS R&D Programme (Final report), University of Leeds.

Houston, J.G., Morris, A.D., Grosset, D.G., Lees, K.R., McMillan, N. & Bone, I. (1995) Ultrasonic evaluation of movement of the diaphragm after acute cerebral infarction. *Journal of Neurology, Neurosurgery and Psychiatry* **58**, 738–741.

Huber, W. (1999) The role of piracetam in the treatment of acute and chronic aphasia. *Pharmacopsychiatry* **32** (Suppl.), 38–43.

Huck, J. & Bonhotal, B.H. (1997) Fastener systems on apparel for hemiplegic stroke victims. *Applied Ergonomics* **28**, 277–282.

Hutten, B.A. & Prins, M.H. (2000) Duration of oral anticoagulant treatment for symptomatic venous thromboembolism (Protocol for a Cochrane Review). In: *The Cochrane Library*. Oxford: Update Software.

Inaba, M. & Piorkowski, M. (1972) Ultrasound in treatment of painful shoulders in patients with hemiplegia. *Physical Therapy* **52**, 737–741.

Inglis, J.L., Eskes, G.A. & Phillips, S.J. (1999) Fatigue after stroke. *Archives of Physical Medicine and Rehabilitation* **80**, 173–178.

Intercollegiate Working Party for Stroke (2000) *National Clinical Guidelines for Stroke*. Royal College of Physicians, London.

Inzitari, D., Di Carlo, A., Pracucci, G. *et al.* (1998) Incidence and determinants of post-stroke dementia as defined by an informant interview method in a hospital-based stroke registry. *Stroke* **29**, 2087–2093.

James, A., Kapur, K. & Hawthrone, A.B. (1998) Long-term outcome of percutaneous endoscopic gastrostomy feeding in patients with dysphagic stroke. *Age and Ageing* **27**, 671–676.

James, P., Ellis, C.J., Whitlock, R.M.L., McNeil, A.R., Henley, J. & Anderson, N.E. (2000) Relation between troponin T concentration and mortality in patients presenting with an acute stroke: observational study. *British Medical Journal* **320**, 1502–1504.

Jensen, L.A., Onyskiw, J.E. & Prasad, N.G.N. (1998) Meta-analysis of arterial oxygen saturation monitoring by pulse oximetry in adults. *Heart and Lung* **27**, 387–408.

Johnstone, A.J., Lohlun, J.C., Miller, J.D. *et al.* (1993) A comparison of the Glasgow Coma Scale and the Swedish Reaction Level Scale. *Brain Injury* **7**, 501–506.

Jongbloed, L. & Morgan, D. (1991) An investigation of involvement in leisure activities after a stroke. *American Journal of Occupational Therapy* **45**, 420–427.

Jongbloed, L., Stacey, S. & Brighton, C. (1989) Stroke rehabilitation: sensorimotor integrative treatment versus functional treatment. *American Journal of Occupational Therapy* **43**, 391–397.

Jorgensen, H.S., Reith, J., Nakayama, H., Kammersgaard, L.P., Raaschou, H.O. & Olsen, T.S. (1999) What determines good recovery in patients with the most severe strokes? The Copenhagen Stroke Study. *Stroke* **30**, 2008–2012.

Jorm, A.F., Scott, R., Cullen, J.S. & MacKinnon, A.J. (1991) Performance of the informant questionnaire on cognitive decline in the elderly (IQCODE) as a screening test for dementia. *Psychological Medicine* **21**, 785–790.

Joynt, R.J., Feibel, J.H. & Sladek, C.M. (1981) Antidiuretic hormone levels in stroke patients. *Annals of Neurology* **9**, 182–184.

Kaldor, A. & Berlin, I. (1981) Pneumonia, stroke, and laterality. *Lancet* **1**, 843.

Kalra, L., Yu, G., Wilson, K. & Roots, P. (1995) Medical complications during stroke rehabilitation. *Stroke* **26**, 990–994.

Karp, H.R., Sieker, H.O. & Heyman, A. (1961) Cerebral circulation and function in Cheyne–Stokes respiration. *American Journal of Medicine* **30**, 861–870.

Kase, C.S., Wolf, P.A., Kelly-Hayes, M., Kannel, W.B., BeiSeries, A. & D'Agostino, R.B. (1998) Intellectual decline after stroke. The Framingham Study. *Stroke* **29**, 805–812.

Kehayia, E., Korner-Bitensky, N., Singer, F. *et al.* (1997) Differences in pain medication use in stroke patients with and without aphasia. *Stroke* **28**, 1867–1870.

Kemp, M.G., Kopanke, D., Tordecilla, L. *et al.* (1993) The role of surfaces and patients attributes in preventing pressure ulcers in elderly patients. *Research in Nursing and Health* **16**, 89–96.

Khorsandi, M., Ginsberg, P.C. & Harkaway, R.C. (1998) Reassessing the role of urodynamics after cerebrovascular accident. Males versus females. *Urologia Internationalis* **61**, 142–146.

Kidd, D., Lawson, J., Nesbitt, R. & MacMahon, J. (1993) Aspiration in acute stroke: a clinical study with videofluroscopy. *Quarterly Journal of Medicine* **86**, 825–829.

Kilpatrick, C.J., Davis, S.M., Hopper, J.L. & Rossiter, S.C. (1992) Early seizures after acute stroke. Risk of late seizures. *Archives of Neurology* **49**, 509–511.

Kilpatrick, D.J., Davis, S.M., Tress, B.M., Rossiter, S.C., Hopper, J.L. & Vandendriesen, M.L. (1990) Epileptic seizures in acute stroke. *Archives of Neurology* **47**, 157–160.

Kimura, M., Robinson, R.G. & Kosier, J.T. (2000) Treatment of cognitive impairment after poststroke depression. A double-blind treatment trial. *Stroke* **31**, 1482–1486.

Kimyai-Asadi, A., Nousari, H.C., Kimyai-Asadi, T. & Milani, F. (1999) Post-stroke pruritus. *Stroke* **30**, 692–693.

Kinsella, G. & Ford, B. (1985) Hemi-inattention and the recovery patterns of stroke patients. *International Rehabilitation Medicine* **7**, 102–106.

Kitimura, T. & Ito, K. (1976) Acute gastric changes in patients with acute stroke. Part I: With reference to gastroendoscopic findings. *Stroke* **7**, 460–466.

Knapp, P., Young, J., House, A. & Forster, A. (2000) Non-drug strategies to resolve psycho-social difficulties after stroke. *Age and Ageing* **29**, 23–30.

Koch, M., Dezi, A., Ferrario, F. & Capurso, L. (1996) Prevention of non-steroidal anti-inflammatory drug-induced gastrointestinal mucosal injury. A meta-analysis of randomized controlled clinical trials. *Archives of Internal Medicine* **156**, 2321–2332.

van Kooten, F., Hoogerbrugge, N., Naarding, P. & Koudstaal, P.J. (1993) Hyperglycaemia in the acute phase of stroke is not caused by stress. *Stroke* **24**, 1129–1132.

Korpelainen, J.T., Nieminen, P. & Myllyla, V.V. (1999) Sexual functioning among stroke patients and their spouses. *Stroke* **30**, 715–719.

Kusuda, K., Saku, Y., Sadoshima, S., Kozo, I. & Fujishima, M. (1989) Disturbances of fluid and electrolyte balance in patients with acute stroke. *Nippon Ronen Igakkai Zasshi* **26**, 223–227.

Kwakkel, G., Wagenaar, R.C., Koelman, T.W., Lankhorst, G.J. & Koetsier, J.C. (1997) Effects of intensity of rehabilitation after stroke. A research synthesis. *Stroke* **28**, 1550–1556.

Kwakkel, G., Kollen, B.J. & Wagenaar, R.C. (1999a) Therapy impact on functional recovery in stroke rehabilitation. *Physiotherapy* **85**, 377–391.

Kwakkel, G., Wagenaar, R.C., Twisk, J.W.R., Lankhorst, G.J. & Koetsier, J.C. (1999b) Intensity of leg and arm training after primary middle-cerebral-artery stroke: a randomized trial. *Lancet* **354**, 191–196.

Langhorne, P. & Legg, L. on behalf of the Outpatient Therapy Trialists (1999) Therapy for stroke patients living at home. *Lancet* **354**, 1730–1731.

Langhorne, P., Wagenaar, R. & Partridge, C. (1996) Physiotherapy after stroke: more is better? *Physiotherapy Research International* **1**, 75–88.

Langhorne, P., Stott, D.J., Robertson, L. *et al.* (2000). Medical complications in hospitalised stroke patients: a multicentre study. *Stroke* **31**, 1223–1229.

Launois, S., Bizec, J.L., Whitelaw, W.A., Cabane, J. & Derenne, J.P. (1993) Hiccups in adults: an overview. *European Respiratory Journal* **6**, 563–575.

Lauritzen, L., Bjerg Bendsen, B., Vilmar, T., Bjerg Bendsen, E., Lunde, M. & Bech, P. (1994) Post-stroke depression: combined treatment with imipramine or desipramine and mianserin. A controlled clinical study. *Psychopharmacology* **114**, 119–122.

Lavy, S., Yaar, I. & Melamed, E. (1974) The effect of acute stroke on cardiac functions in an intensive care stroke unit. *Stroke* **5**, 775–780.

Leandri, M., Parodi, C.I., Corrieri, N. & Rigardo, S. (1990) Comparison of TENS treatments in hemiplegic shoulder pain. *Scandinavian Journal of Rehabilitation Medicine* **22**, 69–71.

van der Lee, J.H., Wagenaar, R.C., Lankhorst, G.J., Vogelaar, T.W., Deville, W.L. & Bouter, L.M. (1999) Forced use of the upper extremity in chronic stroke patients: results from a single-blind randomized clinical trial. *Stroke* **30**, 2369–2375.

Lees, T.A. & Amarigiri, S.V. (2000) Elastic compression stockings for prevention of deep vein thrombosis (Protocol for a Cochrane Review). In: *The Cochrane Library.* Oxford: Update Software.

Legh-Smith, J., Wade, D.T. & Langton Hewer, R. (1986) Driving after a stroke. *Journal of the Royal Society of Medicine* **79**, 200–203.

Leijon, G. & Boivie, J. (1989) Central post-stroke pain—a controlled trial of amitriptyline and carbamazepine. *Pain* **36**, 27–36.

Levine, J.A. & Morris, J.C. (1995) The use of a football helmet to secure a nasogastric tube. *Nutrition* **11**, 285.

Lincoln, N.B., Mulley, G.P., Jones, A.C., McGuirk, E., Lendrem, W. & Mitchell, R.A. (1984) Effectiveness of speech therapy for aphasic stroke patients. A randomized controlled trial. *Lancet* **1** (8388), 1197–1200.

Lincoln, N.B., Gamlen, R. & Thomason, H. (1989) Behavioural mapping of patients on a stroke unit. *International Disability Studies* **11**, 149–154.

Lincoln, N.B., Willis, D., Philips, S.A., Juby, L.C. & Berman, P. (1996) Comparison of rehabilitation practice on hospital wards for stroke patients. *Stroke* **27**, 18–23.

Lincoln, N.B., Parry, R.H. & Vass, C.D. (1999) Randomized, controlled trial to evaluate increased intensity of physiotherapy treatment of arm function after stroke. *Stroke* **30**, 573–579.

Linn, S.L., Granat, M.H. & Lees, K.R. (1999) Prevention of shoulder subluxation after stroke with electrical stimulation. *Stroke* **30**, 963–968.

Lipsey, J.R., Robinson, R.G., Pearlson, G.D., Rao, K. & Price, T.R. (1984) Nortriptyline treatment of post-stroke depression: a double-blind study. *Lancet* **1** (8372), 297–300.

Lomer, M. & McLellan, D.L. (1987) Informing hospital patients and their relatives about stroke. *Clinical Rehabilitation* **1**, 33–37.

Lotery, A., Wiggam, M.I., Jackson, A.J. *et al.* (2000) Correctable visual impairment in stroke rehabilitation patients. *Age and Ageing* **29**, 221–222.

Loverro, J. & Reding, M. (1988) Bed orientation and rehabilitation outcome for patients with stroke and hemianopsia or visual neglect. *Journal of Neurological Rehabilitation* **147**, 150.

Lowenstein, D.H. & Alldredge, B.K. (1998) Status epilepticus. *New England Journal of Medicine* **338**, 970–976.

Lu, C.L., Yu, B., Basford, J.R., Johnson, M.E. & An, K.N. (1997) Influences of cane length on the stability of stroke patients. *Journal of Rehabilitation Research and Development* **34**, 97–100.

McCarthy, S.T. & Turner, J. (1986) Low-dose subcutaneous heparin in the prevention of deep vein thrombosis and pulmonary emboli following acute stroke. *Age and Ageing* **15**, 85–88.

Malmberg, K., Ryden, L., Efendic, S. *et al.* (1995) Randomized trial of insulin glucose infusion followed by subcutaneous insulin treatment in diabetic patients with acute myocardial infarction (DIGAMI Study): effects on mortality at 1 year. *Journal of the American College of Cardiology* **26**, 57–65.

Mann, G., Dip, P.G., Hankey, G.J. & Cameron, D. (1999) Swallowing function after stroke. Prognosis and prognostic factors at 6 months. *Stroke* **30**, 744–748.

Mant, J., Carter, J., Wade, D.T. & Winner, S. (1998) The impact of an information pack on patients with stroke and their carers: a randomized controlled trial. *Clinical Rehabilitation* **12**, 465–476.

Mant, J., Carter, J., Wade, D.T. & Winner, S. (1999) Randomized controlled trial of a Stroke Family Support Organiser. *Cerebrovascular Diseases* **9**

(Suppl. 1), 123.

Marshall, R.C., Wertz, R.T., Weiss, D.G. *et al.* (1989) Home treatment for aphasic patients by trained non-professionals. *Journal of Speech and Hearing Disorders* **54**, 462–470.

Martin, J., Meltzer, H. & Elliot, D. (1988) *The Prevalence of Disability Among Adults*. Office of Population Censuses and Surveys, HMSO, London.

Mazer, B.L., Korner-Bitensky, N.A. & Sofer, S. (1998) Predicting ability to drive after stroke. *Archives of Physical Medicine and Rehabilitation* **79**, 743–750.

Mead, G.E., Donaldson, L., North, P. & Dennis, M.S. (1998) An informal assessment of nutritional status in acute stroke for use in an international multicentre trial of feeding regimens. *International Journal of Clinical Practice* **52**, 316–318.

Medical Research Council (1982) *Aids to the Examination of the Peripheral Nervous System*, pp. 1–60. Castle Press, Grimsby.

Meikle, M., Wechsler, E., Tupper, A.-M. *et al.* (1979) Comparative trial of volunteer and professional treatments of dysphasia after stroke. *British Medical Journal* **2**, 87–89.

Melo, T.P., de Mendonca, A., Crespo, M., Carvalho, M. & Ferro, J.M. (1992) An emergency room-based study of stroke coma. *Cerebrovascular Diseases* **2**, 93–101.

Messina, C., Di Rosa, A.E. & Leggiadro, N. (1979) Gastro-intestinal hemorrhage in stroke. *Acta Neurologica* **1**, 474–482.

Metz, C.A., Livinston, D.H., Smith, J.S., Larson, G.M. & Wilson, T.H. (1993) Impact of multiple risk factors and ranitidine prophylaxis on the development of stress-related upper gastrointestinal bleeding: a prospective, multicentre, double-blind, randomized trial. The Ranitidine Head Injury Study Group. *Critical Care Medicine* **21**, 1844–1849.

Mikolich, J.R., Jacobs, W.C. & Fletcher, G.F. (1981) Cardiac arrhythmias in patients with acute cerebrovascular accidents. *Journal of the American Medical Association* **246**, 1314–1317.

Misra, M., Dujovny, M., Alp, S. *et al.* (1997) Changes in cerebral oxygen saturation with change in posture: a preliminary report. *Journal of Stroke and Cerebrovascular Diseases* **6**, 337–340.

Mitchell, A.J. (1997) Clinical implications of post-stroke Hypothalamic-Pituitary Adrenal Axis Dysfunction: a critical literature review. *Journal of Stroke and Cerebrovascular Diseases* **6**, 377–388.

Mooe, T., Olofsson, B.O., Stegmayr, B. & Eriksson, P. (1999) Ischemic stroke. Impact of a recent myocardial infarction. *Stroke* **30**, 997–1001.

Moreland, J.D. & Thomson, M.A. (1994) Efficacy of electromyographic biofeedback compared with conventional physical therapy for upper-extremity function in patients following stroke: a research overview and meta-analysis. *Physical Therapy* **74**, 534–547.

Moreland, J.D., Thomson, M.A. & Fuoco, A.R. (1998) Electromyographic biofeedback to improve lower extremity function after stroke: a meta-analysis. *Archives of Physical Medicine and Rehabilitation* **79**, 134–140.

Moyer, D.J., Welsh, F.A. & Zager, E.L. (1992) Spontaneous cerebral hypothermia diminishes focal infarction in rat brain. *Stroke* **23**, 1812–1816.

Muir, K.W., Watt, A., Baxter, G., Grosset, D.G. & Lee, K.R. (2000) Randomized trial of graded compression stockings for prevention of deep-vein thrombosis after acute stroke. *Quarterly Journal of Medicine* **93**, 359–364.

Mulley, G.P. (1981) Pneumonia, stroke and laterality. *Lancet* **1** (8228), 1051 (letter).

Mulley, G. (1982) Associated reactions in the hemiplegic arm. *Scandinavian Journal of Rehabilitation Medicine* **14**, 117–120.

Mulley, G. (1991) Walking frames. In: *More Everyday Aids and Appliances* (ed. G. Mulley), pp. 174–181. BMJ Publishing, London.

Murray, G.B., Shea, V. & Conn, D.K. (1986) Electroconvulsive therapy for post stroke depression. *Journal of Clinical Psychiatry* **47**, 258–260.

Mykyta, L.J., Bowling, J.H., Nelson, D.A. & Lloyd, E.J. (1976) Caring for relatives of stroke patients. *Age and Ageing* **5**, 87–90.

Nachtmann, A., Siebler, M., Rose, G., Sitzer, M. & Steinmetz, H. (1995) Cheyne–Stokes respiration in ischemic stroke. *Neurology* **45**, 820–821.

Nakamura, K., Saku, Y., Ibayashi, S. & Fujishima, M. (1999) Progressive motor deficits in lacunar infarction. *Neurology* **52**, 29–33.

Nakayama, H., Jorgensen, H.S., Pedersen, P.M., Raaschou, H.O. & Olsen, T.S. (1997) Prevalence and risk factors of incontinence after stroke. The Copenhagen Stroke Study. *Stroke* **28**, 58–62.

Norris, J.W., Groggatt, G.M. & Hachinski, V.C. (1978) Cardiac arrhythmias in acute stroke. *Stroke* **9**, 392–396.

Norris, J.W., Hachinski, V.C., Myers, M.G., Callow, J., Wong, T. & Moore, R.W. (1979) Serum cardiac enzymes in stroke. *Stroke* **10**, 548–553.

North, J.B. & Jennett, S. (1974) Abnormal breathing patterns associated with acute brain damage. *Archives of Neurology* **31**, 338–344.

Norton, B., Homer-Ward, M., Donnelly, M.T., Long, R.G. & Holmes, G.K.T. (1996) A randomized prospective comparison of percutaneous endoscopic gastrostomy and nasogastric tube feeding after acute dysphagic stroke. *British Medical Journal* **312**, 13–16.

Nouri, F.M. & Tinson, D.J. (1988) A comparison of a driving simulator and a road test in the assessment of driving ability after a stroke. *Clinical Rehabilitation* **2**, 99–104.

Nouri, F.M., Tinson, D.J. & Lincoln, N.B. (1987) Cognitive ability and driving after stroke. *International Disability Studies* **9**, 110–115.

Nyberg, L. & Gustafson, Y. (1995) Patient falls in stroke rehabilitation. A challenge to rehabilitation strategies. *Stroke* **26**, 838–842.

Nyberg, L. & Gustafson, Y. (1997) Fall prediction index for patients in stroke rehabilitation. *Stroke* **28**, 716–721.

Oczkowski, W.J., Ginsberg, J.S., Shin, A. & Panju, A. (1992) Venous thromboembolism in patients undergoing rehabilitation for stroke. *Archives of Physical Medicine and Rehabilitation* **73**, 712–716.

O'Neill, P.A. & McLean, K.A. (1992) Water homeostasis and ageing. *Medical Laboratory Science* **49**, 291–298.

O'Neill, P.A., Cheadle, B., Wyatt, R., McGuffog, J. & Fullerton, K.J. (1990) The value of the Frenchay Aphasia Screening Test for dysphasia: better than the clinician? *Clinical Rehabilitation* **4**, 123–128.

O'Neill, P.A., Davies, I., Fullerton, K.J. & Bennett, D. (1992) Fluid balance in elderly patients following acute stroke. *Age and Ageing* **21**, 280–285.

Orgogozo (1999) Piracetam in the treatment of acute stroke. *Pharmacopsychiatry* **32** (Suppl. 1), 25–32.

O'Rourke, S., McHale, S., Slattery, J. & Dennis, M. (1998) Detecting psychiatric morbidity after stroke: a comparison of the General Health Questionnaire and the Hospital Anxiety and Depression Scale. *Stroke* **29**, 980–985.

O'Sullivan, C.E., Issa, F.G., Berthon-Jones, M. & Saunders, N.A. (1984) Pathophysiology of sleep apnea. In: *Sleep and Breathing* (eds N.A. Saunders & C.E. Sullivan), pp. 299–363. Marcel Dekker Inc., New York/Basel.

Panayiotou, B.N., Harper, G.D., Fotherby, M.D., Potter, J.F. & Castleden, C.M. (1993) Interarm blood pressure difference in acute hemiplegia. *Journal of the American Geriatrics Society* **41**, 422–423.

Pang, P.A., Yeung, V.T.F. & Zang, Y.G. (1988) Do postural changes affect gas exchange in acute hemiplegia? *British Journal of Clinical Practice* **42**, 501–502.

Park, R.H., Allison, M.C., Lang, J. *et al.* (1992) Randomized comparison of percutaneous endoscopic gastrostomy and nasogastric tube feeding in patients with persisting neurological dysphagia. *British Medical Journal* **304**, 1406–1409.

Parker, M.J., Gillespie, L.D. & Gillespie, W.J. (2000) Hip protectors for preventing hip fractures in the elderly (Cochrane Review). In: *The Cochrane Library*. Oxford: Update Software.

Partridge, C.J., Edwards, S.M., Mee, R. & Van Langenberghe, H.V.K. (1990) Hemiplegic shoulder pain: a study of two methods of physiotherapy treatment. *Clinical Rehabilitation* **4**, 43–49.

Pedersen, P.M., Jorgensen, H.S., Nakayama, H., Raaschou, H.O. & Olsen, T.S. (1995) Aphasia in acute stroke: incidence, determinants, and recovery. *Annals of Neurology* **38**, 659–666.

Pedersen, P.M., Jorgensen, H.S., Nakayama, H., Raaschou, H.O. & Olsen, T.S. (1997) Hemineglect in acute stroke—incidence and prognostic implications. The Copenhagen Stroke Study. *American Journal of Physical Medicine and Rehabilitation* **76**, 122–127.

Pedersen, P.M., Jorgensen, H.S., Nakayama, H., Raaschou, H.O. & Olsen, T.S. (1998) Impaired orientation in acute stroke: frequency, determinants, and time-course of recovery. *Cerebrovascular Diseases* **8**, 90–96.

Phillips, S.J. (1994) Pathophysiology and management of hypertension in acute ischemic stroke. *Hypertension* **23**, 131–136.

Plum, F. & Posner, J.B. (1980) Supratentorial lesions causing coma. In: *The Diagnosis of Stupor and Coma* (eds F. Plum & F.H. McDowell), pp. 134–136. FA Davis Company, Philadelphia.

Pohlmann-Eden, B., Hoch, D.B., Cochius, J.I. & Hennerici, M.G. (1996) Stroke and epilepsy: Critical review of the literature. *Cerebrovascular Diseases* **6**, 332–338.

Pollock, A., Langhorne, P. & Baer, G. (2000) Physiotherapy for the recovery of postural control and lower limb function following stroke (Protocol for a Cochrane Review). In: *The Cochrane Library*. Oxford: Update Software.

Potter, J.F. (1999) What should we do about blood pressure and stroke? *Quar-*

terly Journal of Medicine **92**, 63–66.

Potter, J.N., Langhorne, P. & Roberts, M. (1998) Routine protein energy supplementation in adults: systematic review. *British Medical Journal* **317**, 495–501.

Powell, J., Pandyan, A.D., Granat, M., Cameron, M. & Stott, D.J. (1999) Electrical stimulation of wrist extensors in post-stroke hemiplegia. *Stroke* **30**, 1384–1389.

Prasad, B.K., Banarjee, A.K. & Howard, H. (1982) Incidence of deep vein thrombosis and the effect of pneumatic compression of the calf in elderly hemiplegics. *Age and Ageing* **11**, 42–44.

Prasad, K. & Menon, G.R. (1998) Comparison of the three strategies of verbal scoring of the Glasgow Coma Scale in patients with stroke. *Cerebrovascular Diseases* **8**, 79–85.

Price, C.I.M. & Pandyan, A.D. (2000) Electrical stimulation for preventing and treating post-stroke shoulder pain (Protocol for a Cochrane Review). In: *The Cochrane Library.* Oxford: Update Software.

Przelomski, M.M., Roth, R.M., Gleckman, R.A. & Marcus, E.M. (1986) Fever in the wake of a stroke. *Neurology* **36**, 427–429.

Raicevic, R., Jovicic, A., Tavcioski, D., Dordevic, D. & Krgovic, M. (1998) Clinical predictors of cardiac complications in patients with acute ischemic brain disease. *Vojnosanitetski Pregled* **55**, 3–14.

Ramnemark, A., Nyberg, L., Borssen, B., Olsson, T. & Gustafson, Y. (1998) Fractures after stroke. *Osteoporosis International* **8**, 92–95.

Ramnemark, A., Nyberg, R.P.T., Lorentzon, R., Olsson, T. & Gustafson, Y. (1999) Hemiosteoporosis after severe stroke, independent of changes in body composition and weight. *Stroke* **30**, 755–760.

Ratnasabathy, Y., Broad, J.B., Baskett, J.J., Marshall, J. & Bonita, R. (2000) Shoulder pain in people with a stroke: a population based study. *Cerebrovascular Diseases* **10** (Suppl. 2), 11 (Abstract).

Raven, J.C. (1965) *Guide to Using the Coloured Progressive Matices.* HK Lewis & Co., London.

Reinstein, L., Gracey, J.G., Kline, J.A. & Van Buskirk, C. (1972) Cardiac monitoring in the acute stroke patient. *Archives of Physical Medicine and Rehabilitation* **53**, 311–314.

Reith, J., Jorgensen, H.S., Nakayama, H., Raaschou, H.O. & Olsen, T.S. (1997) Seizures in acute stroke: predictors and prognostic significance. The Copenhagen Stroke Study. *Stroke* **28**, 1585–1589.

Rem, J.A., Hachinski, V.C., Boughner, D.R. & Barnett, H.J.M. (1985) Value of cardiac monitoring and echocardiography in TIA and stroke patients. *Stroke* **16**, 950–956.

Robertson, I.H. (1993) Cognitive rehabilitation in neurologic disease. *Current Opinion in Neurology* **6**, 756–760.

Robinson, R.G. & Szetela, B. (1981) Mood change following left hemisphere brain injury. *Annals of Neurology* **40**, 195–202.

Robinson, R.G., Parikh, R.M., Lipsey, J.R., Starkstein, S.E. & Price, T.R. (1993) Pathological laughing and crying following stroke: validation of a measurement scale and a double-blind treatment study. *American Journal of Psychiatry* **150**, 286–293.

Roby, R.R. (1998) A meta-analysis of clinical outcomes in the treatment of aphasia. *Journal of Speech and Hearing Research* **41**, 172–187.

Rodgers, H., Atkinson, C., Bond, S., Suddes, M., Dobson, R. & Curless, R. (1999) Randomized controlled trial of a comprehensive stroke education programme for patients and caregivers. *Stroke* **30**, 2585–2591.

Roe, B., Williams, K. & Palmer, M. (2000) Bladder training for urinary incontinence (Cochrane Review). In: *The Cochrane Library.* Oxford: Update Software.

Roffe, C., Sills, S. & Crome, P. (1999) Should the pulse oximeter be attached to the affected or non-affected limb in patients with acute stroke? *Cerebrovascular Diseases* **9** (Suppl. 1), 86 (Abstract).

Ronning, O.M. & Guldvog, B. (1999) Should stroke victims routinely receive supplemental oxygen? A quasi randomized trial. *Stroke* **30**, 2033–2037.

Roper, T.A., Redford, S. & Tallis, R.C. (1999) Intermittent compression for the treatment of the oedematous hand in hemiplegic stroke: a randomized controlled trial. *Age and Ageing* **28**, 9–13.

Rossi, P.W., Kheyfets, S. & Reding, M.J. (1990) Fresnel prisms improve visual perception in stroke patients with homonymous hemianopia or unilateral visual neglect. *Neurology* **40**, 1597–1599.

Rout, M.W., Lane, D.J. & Wollner, L. (1971) Prognosis in acute cerebrovascular accidents in relation to respiratory pattern and blood gas tensions. *British Medical Journal* **3**, 7–9.

Rowat, A., Wardlaw, J.M., Dennis, M. *et al.* (1998) How does altering the posture of stroke patients affect their arterial oxygen saturation and blood pressure? *Cerebrovasacular Diseases* **8**, 29.

Roy, C.W. (1988) Shoulder pain in hemiplegia: a literature review. *Clinical Rehabilitation* **2**, 35–44.

Rudd, A.G., Irwin, P., Rutledge, Z. *et al.* (1999) The National Sentinel Audit for stroke: a tool for raising standards of care. *Journal of the Royal College of Physicians of London* **33**, 460–464.

Sackley, C.M. & Lincoln, N.B. (1997) Single blind randomized controlled trial of visual feedback after stroke: effects on stance symmetry and function. *Disability and Rehabilitation* **19**, 536–546.

Saeki, S., Ogata, H., Okubo, T., Takahashi, K. & Hoshuyama, T. (1995) Return to work after stroke. A follow-up study. *Stroke* **26**, 399–401.

Sandercock, P.A.G., Warlow, C.P., Jones, L.N. & Starkey, I.R. (1989) Predisposing factors for cerebral infarction: the Oxfordshire Community Stroke Project. *British Medical Journal* **298**, 75–80.

Sandercock, P.A.G., Bamford, J., Dennis, M. *et al.* (1992) Atrial fibrillation and stroke: prevalence in different types of stroke and influence on early and long term prognosis (Oxfordshire Community Stroke Project). *British Medical Journal* **305**, 1460–1465.

Sato, Y., Maruoka, H. & Oizumi, K. (1997) Amelioration of hemiplegia-associated osteopenia more than 4 years after stroke by 1 alpha-hydroxyvitamin D3 and calcium supplementation. *Stroke* **28**, 736–739.

Schiffer, R.B., Herndon, R.M. & Rudick, R.A. (1985) Treatment of pathologic laughing and weeping with amitriptyline. *New England Journal of Medicine* **312**, 1480–1482.

Schleenbaker, R.E. & Mainous, A.G.I. (1993) Electromyographic biofeedback for the neuromuscular re-education in the hemiplegic stroke patient: a meta analysis. *Archives of Physical Medicine and Rehabilitation* **74**, 1301–1304.

Scholte op Reimer, W.J.M., de Haan, R.J., Rijnders, P.T., Limburg, M. & van den Bos, G.A.M. (1998) The burden of caregiving in partners of long-term stroke survivors. *Stroke* **29**, 1605–1611.

Schott (1995) From thalamic syndrome to central post-stroke pain. *Journal of Neurology, Neurosurgery and Psychiatry* **61**, 560–564.

Schuling, J., de Haan, R., Limburg, M. & Groenier, K.H. (1993) The Frenchay Activities Index. Assessment of functional status in stroke patients. *Stroke* **24**, 1173–1177.

Scott, J.F., Gray, C.S., O'Connell, J.E. & Alberti, K.G.M.M. (1998) Glucose and insulin therapy in acute stroke; why delay further? *Quarterly Journal of Medicine* **91**, 511–515.

Scott, J.F., Robinson, G.M., French, J.M., O'Connell, J.E., Alberti, K.G.M.M. & Gray, C.S. (1999) Glucose Potassium Insulin Infusions in the treatment of acute stroke patients with mild to moderate hyperglycaemia. The Glucose Insulin in Stroke trial (GIST). *Stroke* **30**, 793–799.

Scottish Intercollegiate Guidelines Network (SIGN) (1997) Management of patients with stroke. III: Identification and management of dysphagia. SIGN, Edinburgh (www.show.scot.nhs.uk/sign/home.htm).

Scottish Intercollegiate Guidelines Network (SIGN) (2000) Prophylaxis of venous thromboembolism. SIGN, Edinburgh. (www.show.scot.nhs.uk/sign/home.htm).

Sellars, C., Hughes, T. & Langhorne, P. (2000) Speech and language therapy for dysarthria due to non-progressive brain damage. (Protocol for a Cochrane Review). In: *The Cochrane Library.* Oxford: Update Software.

Shakespeare, D.T., Young, C.A. & Boggild, M. (2000) Anti-spasticity agents for multiple sclerosis (Protocol for a Cochrane Review). In: *The Cochrane Library.* Oxford: Update Software.

Shea, J.D. (1975) Pressure sores: classification and management. *Clinical Orthopaedics* **112**, 89–100.

Shinar, D., Gross, C.R., Price, T.R., Banko, M., Bolduc, P.L. & Robinson, R.G. (1986) Screening for depression in stroke patients: the reliability and validity of the center for epidemiologic studies depression scale. *Stroke* **17**, 241–245.

Shirran, E. & Brazzelli, M. (2000) Absorbent products for the containment of urinary and/or faecal incontinence (Protocol for a Cochrane Review). In: *The Cochrane Library.* Oxford: Update Software.

Signorini, D.F., Sandercock, P.A.G., Warlow, C.P., for the, I.S.T. & Collaborative Group. (1999) Systolic blood pressure on randomisation and outcome in the International Stroke Trial. *Cerebrovascular Diseases* **9** (Suppl. 1), 34.

Simpson, D.M. (1997) Clinical trials of botulinum toxin in the treatment of spasticity. *Muscle and Nerve* **6** (Suppl.), S169–S175.

Singh, A., Herrmann, N. & Black, S.E. (1998) The importance of lesion location in post-stroke depression: a critical review. *Canadian Journal of Psy-*

chiatry **43**, 921–927.

Singh, A., Black, S.E., Herrmann, N. *et al.* (2000) Functional and neuro-anatomic correlations in post stroke depression. The Sunnybrook Stroke Study. *Stroke* **31**, 637–644.

Sjogren, K. (1982) Leisure after stroke. *International Rehabilitation Medicine* **4**, 80–87.

Skelly, R., Terry, H., Millar, E. & Cohen, D. (1999) Outcomes of percutaneous endoscopic gastrostomy feeding. *Age and Ageing* **28**, 416.

Sloan, R.L., Brown, K.W. & Pentland, B. (1992) Fluoxetine as a treatment for emotional lability after brain injury. *Brain Injury* **6**, 315–319.

Small, S.L. (1994) Pharmacotherapy of aphasia. A critical review. *Stroke* **25**, 1282–1289.

Smith, N. (1989) Aids for urinary incontinence. In: *Everyday Aids and Appliances* (ed. G.P. Mulley), pp. 50–54. BMJ Publishers, London.

Smithard, D.G., O'Neill, P.A., Park, C. *et al.* (1996) Complications and outcome after acute stroke. Does dysphagia matter? *Stroke* **27**, 1200–1204.

Smithard, D.G., O'Neill, P.A., England, R.E. *et al.* (1997) The natural history of dysphagia following a stroke. *Dysphagia* **12**, 188–193.

Smithard, D.G., O'Neill, P.A., Park, C. *et al.* (1998) Can bedside assessment reliably exclude aspiration following acute stroke? *Age and Ageing* **27**, 99–106.

So, E.L., Annegers, J.F., Hauser, W.A., O'Brien, P.C. & Whisnant, J.P. (1996) Population-based study of seizure disorders after cerebral infarction. *Neurology* **46**, 350–355.

Song, F., Freemantle, N., Sheldon, T.A. *et al.* (1993) Selective serotonin reuptake inhibitors: meta-analysis of efficacy and acceptability. *British Medical Journal* **306**, 683–687.

Sprecht, H. & Fruhmann, G. (1972) Incidence of periodic breathing in 2000 subjects without pulmonary or neurological disease. *Bulletin de Physiopathologie Respiratoire* **8**, 1075–1083.

St Clair, M. (1992) Survey of the uses of the Pegasus Airwave System in the United Kingdom. *Journal of Tissue Viability* **2**, 9–16.

Starmark, J.E., Stalhammar, S. & Holmgren, E. (1988) The reaction level scale (RLS85): manual and guidelines. *Acta Neurochirurgica* **91**, 12–20.

Stern, P.H., McDowell, F., Miller, J.M. & Robinson, M. (1970) Effects of facilitation exercise techniques in stroke rehabilitation. *Archives of Physical Medicine and Rehabilitation* **50**, 526–531.

Stone, S.P., Patel, P., Greenwood, R.J.˙ & Halligan, P.W. (1992) Measuring visual neglect in acute stroke and predicting its recovery: the visual neglect recovery index. *Journal of Neurology, Neurosurgery and Psychiatry* **55**, 431–436.

Stone, S.P., Halligan, P.W. & Greenwood, R.J. (1993) The incidence of neglect phenomena and related disorders in patients with an acute right or left hemisphere stroke. *Age and Ageing* **22**, 46–52.

Sullivan, D.H., Sun, S. & Walls, R.C. (1999) Protein-energy undernutrition among elderly hospitalized patients: a prospective study. *Journal of the American Medical Association* **281**, 2013–2019.

Sunderland, A., Tinson, D., Bradley, L. & Langton Hewer, R. (1989) Arm function after stroke. An evaluation of grip strength as a measure of recovery and a prognostic indicator. *Journal of Neurology, Neurosurgery and Psychiatry* **52**, 1267–1272.

Tapson, V.F. (1998) The diagnostic and therapeutic approach to acute venous thromboembolism. *Proceedings of the Royal College of Physicians of Edinburgh* **28**, 173–186.

Taricco, M., Telaro, E., Adone, R. & Pagliacci, C. (2000) Pharmacological interventions for spasticity following spinal cord injury (Protocol for a Cochrane Review). In: *The Cochrane Library.* Oxford: Update Software.

Tatemichi, T.K., Paik, M., Bagiella, E., Desmond, D.W., Pirro, M. & Hanzawa, L.K. (1994) Dementia after stroke is a predictor of long term survival. *Stroke* **25**, 1915–1919.

Tekeoolu, Y., Adak, B. & Goksoy, T. (1998) Effect of transcutaneous electrical nerve stimulation (TENS) on Barthel Activities of Daily Living (ADL) index score following stroke. *Clinical Rehabilitation* **12**, 277–280.

Treves, T.A., Aronovich, B.D., Bormstein, N.M. & Korczyn, A.D. (1997) Risk of dementia after a first-ever ischemic stroke: a 3 year longitudinal study. *Cerebrovascular Diseases* **7**, 48–52.

Turney, T.M., Garraway, W.M. & Whisnant, J.P. (1984) The natural history of hemispheric and brainstem infarction in Rochester, Minnesota. *Stroke* **15**, 790–794.

Tyson, S.F. & Ashburn, A. (1994) The influence of walking aids on hemiplegic gait. *Physiotherapy Theory and Practice* **10**, 77–86.

Tyson, S., Thornton, H. & Downes, A. (1998) The effect of a hinged ankle-foot orthosis on hemiplegic gait: four single case studies. *Physiotherapy Theory and Practice* **14**, 75–85.

Unosson, M., Ek, A.C., Bjurulf, P., von Schenck, H. & Larsson, J. (1994) Feeding dependence and nutritional status after acute stroke. *Stroke* **25**, 366–371.

Van Langenberghe, H.V.K., Partridge, C.J., Edwards, M.S. & Mee, R. (1988) Shoulder pain in hemiplegia—a literature review. *Physiotherapy Theory and Practice* **4**, 155–162.

Veis, S.L. & Logemann, J.A. (1985) Swallowing disorders in persons with cerebrovascular accident. *Archives of Physical Medicine and Rehabilitation* **66**, 372–375.

Visintin, M., Barbeau, H., Korner-Bitensky, N. & Mayo, N.E. (1998) A new approach to retrain gait in stroke patients through body weight support and treadmill stimulation. *Stroke* **29**, 1122–1128.

Wade, D.T. (1992a) Measures of motor impairment. In: *Measurement in Neurological Rehabilitation,* pp. 147–165. Oxford Medical Publications, Oxford.

Wade, D.T. (1992b) Measures of focal disability. In: *Measurement in Neurological Rehabilitation,* pp. 166–174. Oxford Medical Publications, Oxford.

Wade, D.T. & Langton Hewer, R. (1985) Outlook after an acute stroke: urinary incontinence and loss of consciousness compared in 532 patients. *Quarterly Journal of Medicine* **56**, 601–608.

Wade, D., Wood, V., Heller, A. *et al.* (1987) Walking after stroke; measurement and recovery over the first three months. *Scandinavian Journal of Rehabilitation Medicine* **9**, 25–30.

Wade, D.T., Collen, F.M., Robb, G.F. & Warlow, C.P. (1992) Physiotherapy intervention late after stroke and mobility. *British Medical Journal* **304**, 609–613.

Wagenaar, R.C., Meijer, O.G., van Wieringen, P.C.W. *et al.* (1990) The functional recovery of stroke: a comparison between neuro-developmental treatment and the Brunnstrom method. *Scandinavian Journal of Rehabilitation Medicine* **22**, 1–8.

Walker, M.F. & Lincoln, N.B. (1991) Factors influencing dressing performance after stroke. *Journal of Neurology, Neurosurgery and Psychiatry* **54**, 699–701.

Walker, M.F., Drummond, A. & Lincoln, N.B. (1994) Dressing after stroke. *Clinical Rehabilitation* **8**, 86 (Abstract).

Walker, M.F., Gladman, J.R.F., Lincoln, N.B., Siemonsma, P. & Whitely, T. (1999) Occupational therapy for stroke patients not admitted to hospital: a randomized controlled trial. *Lancet* **354**, 278–280.

Walker-Batson, D., Smith, P., Curtis, S., Unwin, H. & Greenlee, R. (1995) Amphetamine paired with physical therapy accelerates motor recovery after stroke. Further evidence. *Stroke* **26**, 2254–2259.

Wang, Y., Lim, L.L.V., Levi, C., Heller, R.F., Fisher, J. & Maths, B. (2000) Influence of admission body temperature on stroke mortality. *Stroke* **31**, 404–409.

Wanklyn, P., Cox, N. & Belfield, P. (1995a) Outcome in patients who require a gastrostomy after stroke. *Age and Ageing* **24**, 510–514.

Wanklyn, P., Forster, A., Young, J. & Mulley, G. (1995b) Prevalence and associated features of the cold hemiplegic arm. *Stroke* **26**, 1867–1870.

Wanklyn, P., Forster, A. & Young, J. (1996) Hemiplegic shoulder pain (HSP): natural history and investigation of associated features. *Disability and Rehabilitation* **18**, 497–501.

Wardlaw, J.M. (1993) Cheyne–Stokes respiration in patients with acute ischaemic stroke: observations on middle cerebral artery blood velocity changes using transcranial doppler ultrasound. *Cerebrovascular Diseases* **3**, 377–380.

Warlow, C., Ogston, D. & Douglas, A.S. (1976) Deep venous thrombosis of the legs after strokes. Part 1. Incidence and predisposing factors. *British Medical Journal* **1**, 1178–1181.

Webb, P. (1974) Periodic breathing during sleep. *Journal of Applied Physiology* **37**, 899–903.

Weinmann, E.E. & Salzman, E.W. (1994) Deep vein thrombosis (review). *New England Journal of Medicine* **331**, 1630–1641.

Weir, C.J., Murray, G.D., Dyker, A.G. & Lees, K.R. (1997) Is hyperglycaemia an independent predictor of poor outcome after acute stroke? Results of a long-term follow-up study. *British Medical Journal* **314**, 1303–1306.

Wells, P.S., Lensing, A.W.A. & Hirsh, J. (1994) Graduated compression stockings in the prevention of postoperative venous thromboembolism: a meta analysis. *Archives of Internal Medicine* **154**, 67–72.

Wells, P.S., Lensing, A.W.A., Davidson, B.L., Prins, M.H. & Hirsh, J. (1995) Accuracy of ultrasound for the diagnosis of deep venous thrombosis in asymptomatic patients after orthopoedic surgery. A meta-analysis. *Annals of Internal Medicine* **122**, 47–53.

Wellwood, I., Dennis, M.S. & Warlow, C.P. (1994) Perceptions and knowledge of stroke among surviving patients with stroke and their carers. *Age and Ageing* **23**, 293–298.

Wertz, R.T., Weiss, D.G., Aten, J.L. *et al.* (1986) Comparison of clinic, home and deferred language treatment for aphasia. A veterans administration cooperative study. *Archives of Neurology* **43**, 653–657.

Wessendorf, T.E., Teschler, H., Wang, Y.-M., Konietzko, N. & Thilmann, A.F. (2000) Sleep-disordered breathing among patients with first-ever stroke. *Journal of Neurology* **247**, 41–47.

Whurr, R., Perlman Lorch, M. & Nye, C. (1992) A meta-analysis of studies carried out between 1946 and 1988 concerned with the efficacy of speech and language therapy treatment for aphasic patients. *European Journal of Disorders of Communication* **27**, 1–17.

Wiart, L., Petit, H., Joseph, P.A., Mazaux, J.M. & Barat, M. (2000) Fluoxetine in early poststroke depression. A double-blind placebo-controlled study. *Stroke* **31**, 1829–1832.

Wiffen, P., McQuay, H., Carroll, D., Jadad, A. & Moore, A. (2000) Anticonvulsant drugs for acute and chronic pain. In: *The Cochrane Library.* Oxford: Update Software.

Wijdicks, E.F.M. & McMahon, M.M. (1999) Percutaneous endoscopic gastrostomy after actue stroke: complications and outcome. *Cerebrovascular Diseases* **9**, 109–111.

Wijdicks, E.F.M., Fulgham, J.R. & Batts, K.P. (1994) Gastrointestinal bleeding in stroke. *Stroke* **25**, 2146–2148.

Wijdicks, E.F.M., Kokmen, E. & O'Brien, P. (1998) Measurement of impaired consciousness in the neurological intensive care unit: a new test. *Journal of Neurology, Neurosurgery and Psychiatry* **64**, 117–119.

Wilson, B., Cockburn, J. & Halligan, P. (1987) *Behavioural Inattention Test.* Thames Valley Test Company, Titchfield, Hants.

Wollman, B., D'Agostino, H.B., Walus-Wigle, J.R., Easter, D.W. & Beale, A. (1995) Radiologic, endoscopic and surgical gastrostomy: an institutional evaluation and a meta-analysis of the literature. *Radiology* **197**, 699–704.

Wong, A.M., Lee, M.Y., Kuo, J.K. & Tang, F.T. (1997) The development and clinical evaluation of a standing biofeedback trainer. *Journal of Rehabilitation Research and Development* **34**, 322–327.

Yekutiel, M. & Guttman, E. (1993) A controlled trial of the retraining of the sensory function of the hand in stroke patients. *Journal of Neurology, Neurosurgery and Psychiatry* **56**, 241–244.

CHAPTER SIXTEEN

Preventing recurrent stroke and other serious vascular events

16.1 Prognosis and prediction of future vascular events

The prognosis for early death and disability after stroke has been discussed in section 10.2. This section describes the long-term prognosis of patients with transient ischaemic attacks (TIAs) and stroke for important future vascular events, particularly those such as recurrent stroke, that might be prevented by appropriate treatment strategies. As highlighted in section 10.2, much of the information we have about the prognosis of these patients comes from following large cohorts of patients over time. But, because the prognosis of each individual patient may vary considerably from the prognosis of all patients *en masse* (because of the different underlying causes of the TIA/stroke and different co-morbidities, etc.—see below), it is important that the prognostic data from cohort studies are interpreted in their proper context. This section is therefore structured to help apply the results of cohort studies to individual patients to answer the question 'What is the risk of another important vascular event for *this* patient?' and thereby to be able to identify the appropriate goals and treatments for *this* patient.

16.1.1 Prognosis after transient ischaemic attack and mild ischaemic stroke

Patients with TIA and mild ischaemic stroke are not only *qualitatively* similar in terms of age, sex and prevalence of co-existent vascular diseases and risk factors, but they also share a similar prognosis for future stroke and death and will therefore be considered together (Wiebers *et al.* 1982; Dennis *et al.* 1989; Koudstaal *et al.* 1992b) (section 3.2.3).

Cohorts of patients with TIA and mild ischaemic stroke

The prognosis of patients with TIA and mild ischaemic stroke, as a group, varies considerably amongst different studies due to differences in study methodology and casemix (Hankey *et al.* 1993a) (Table 16.1). Before the results of the different studies can be accepted and validly compared, they should ideally meet most, if not all, of the criteria listed in Table 10.1. The few prognostic studies which are comparable indicate that the prognosis of hospital-referred TIA patients is better than that of community-based patients (Dennis *et al.* 1990; Hankey *et al.* 1991; Dutch TIA Trial Study Group 1993; Hankey & Warlow 1994). This is mainly because hospital series tend not to include patients in whom a very early stroke occurred (at home) before they had time to reach hospital, and because older patients (who have a worse prognosis because of a greater frequency of adverse prognostic factors) are less likely to be referred to hospital (Hankey *et al.* 1993a). Even so, TIA patients as a group, whether hospital- or community-based, have an increased absolute risk of stroke and other serious vascular events compared with age- and sex-matched controls (Howard *et al.* 1994) (Table 16.2). This is because patients with symptomatic cerebrovascular disease almost always have co-existent symptomatic or asymptomatic vascular disease elsewhere, such as in the coronary, peripheral and renal arteries (section 6.3.1).

The risk of stroke is highest soon after the TIA. In the *first* year, the absolute risk of stroke is about 12% in community studies and 7% in hospital series (Fig. 16.1 and Table 16.2). The relative risk is about 12 times that of people of the same age and sex who have not had a TIA (Dennis *et al.* 1990). This higher early risk of stroke reflects not just iatrogenic post-angiographic and post-carotid endarterectomy strokes in some patients, but presumably the presence of unstable and 'active' arterial embolic sources, such as an unstable atherosclerotic plaque which has released a small embolus which is soon followed by a larger one, before the endothelium heals (Whisnant & Wiebers 1987; Dennis *et al.* 1990; Hankey *et al.* 1991; European Carotid Surgery Trialists' Collaborative Group 1998) (section 6.3.2).

After transient ischaemic attack and ischaemic stroke the risk of recurrent stroke is highest within the first few weeks and months: about 10% in the first year, and then about 5% per year.

Table 16.2 lists the approximate average annual risk and relative risk (compared with people of the same age and sex who have not had a TIA) of each of the important outcome events over the first 5 years after a TIA (Hankey & Warlow 1994). Heart disease is the most common cause of death; about 40% of deaths after TIA are due to heart disease, 25% to stroke, 5% to other vascular diseases such as ruptured aortic aneurysm, and 30% to non-vascular disorders (Hankey & Warlow 1994). However, the relative frequency of stroke, coronary events and non-vascular events changes with time after TIA and first-ever-in-a-lifetime stroke; during the first year after a TIA or stroke, most vascular events are strokes, and after that the number of coronary events and non-vascular events (e.g. cancer) exceeds the number

Table 16.1 Methodological explanations which might account for the different prognosis of cohorts of patients with transient ischaemic attack and mild ischaemic stroke in different studies (from Sackett *et al.* 1991).

Study nature (e.g. prospective or retrospective)
Referral patterns
Small sample size and hence imprecision
Case selection
Diagnostic criteria
Time delay between the last transient ischaemic attack and entry into the study
Pathogenesis of transient ischaemic attack
Prevalence and level of important prognostic factors
Treatments
Adequacy of follow-up
Outcome criteria
Methods of survival analysis

Table 16.2 Comparison of absolute average annual risk and relative risk of important outcome events after transient ischaemic attack and stroke in hospital-referred and community samples followed at the same time using the same methods (from Dennis *et al.* 1993; Hankey & Warlow 1994; Burn *et al.* 1994).

	Absolute annual risk (%)		
	Hospital-referred	Community	Relative risk
After transient ischaemic attack			
Death	5	8	1.4
Stroke			
0–1 year	7	12	12
0–5 years	4	7	7
Myocardial infarction	3	3	Unknown
Stroke, myocardial infarction or vascular death	6	9	Unknown
Stroke, myocardial infarction or death	8	10	Unknown
After stroke			
Death			
0–30 days		20 (PICH 50%, IS 10%)	Unknown
30 days–1 year		10	3
0–1 year		30	8
30 days–5 years		9	2
Recurrent stroke			
0–1 year		10–16	15
1–5 years		4	Unknown
0–5 years		4–8	9

IS, ischaemic stroke; PICH, primary intracerebral haemorrhage.

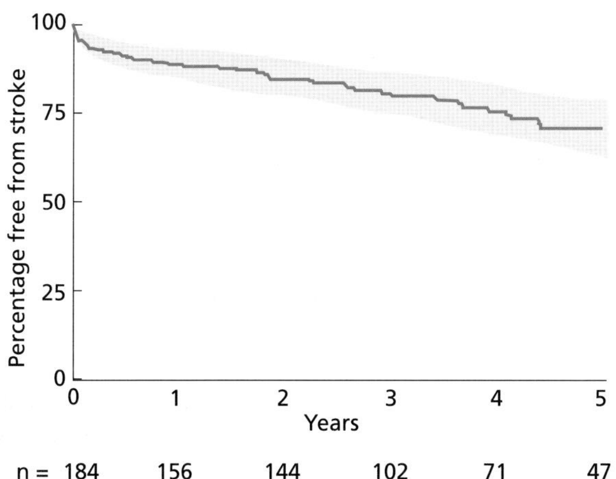

Fig. 16.1 Kaplan–Meier plot showing survival free of stroke in 184 transient ischaemic attack patients in the Oxfordshire Community Stroke Project. The shading indicates 95% confidence intervals. The numbers along the *x*-axis indicate the number of people still at risk of stroke at the beginning of each year of follow-up (with permission from Dennis *et al.* 1990).

of strokes (Dennis *et al.* 1993; Hankey & Warlow 1994; Hankey *et al.* 2000a).

Data on the site, nature and severity of stroke after TIA are limited but it seems that most strokes are ischaemic, about two-thirds are major disabling strokes, about one-half to two-thirds occur in the same vascular territory as the presenting TIA (particularly carotid territory events), and about 20% of the latter (i.e. strokes in the same vascular territory) are lacunar infarcts (Dennis *et al.* 1990; Hankey *et al.* 1991; Cillessen *et al.* 1993). In the Dutch TIA trial, patients with TIA or non-disabling ischaemic stroke due to large vessel disease were more likely to experience a recurrent ischaemic stroke of the same type during follow-up than patients with small vessel disease. The most plausible reason is that some patients in whom small vessel disease was the cause of the index event had pre-existing large vessel disease that became symptomatic later (Kappelle *et al.* 1995.

After transient ischaemic attacks and ischaemic stroke it is important to recognize the importance of non-stroke vascular events such as myocardial infarction; indeed, coronary heart disease is a more likely cause of death than stroke in the long term.

Individual TIA patients

Although TIA patients as a *group* have an increased risk of stroke and other serious vascular events, the prognosis of TIA patients as *individuals* is extremely variable; some have a benign prognosis and others a poor prognosis. This is because of differences in 'casemix', i.e. differences in the causes of TIAs amongst different patients and also differences in the presence and level of important prognostic factors (Hankey *et al.* 1993a; Landi *et al.* 1993). A good example of different prognoses for TIA patients with presumed different causes comes from the Dutch TIA trial: although TIA patients with 'atypical' symptoms (episodes of cerebral or visual dysfunction that were not fully compatible with the internationally accepted criteria for a TIA) were found to have a similar overall risk of major vascular events as patients with 'typical' symptoms, they had a lower risk of stroke and a higher risk of major cardiac events, suggesting that 'atypical' TIAs may have been due to heart disease, perhaps a cardiac dysrhythmia (Koudstaal *et al.* 1992a). On the other hand, the nature of the symptomatic vascular disease did not seem to be relevant to the prognosis: patients with TIA and mild ischaemic stroke who were thought to have intracranial small vessel disease on the basis of their clinical features and computed tomography (CT) scan of the brain at baseline had an identical annual stroke rate of 3.6% as those with presumed large vessel disease (Kappelle *et al.* 1995).

Table 16.3 lists the important independent adverse prognostic factors for stroke, coronary events and the composite outcome event of stroke, myocardial infarction and vascular death (whichever occurred first) that have been identified in each of two large studies (Hankey *et al.* 1992, 1993b; Dutch TIA Trial Study Group 1993; Pop *et al.* 1994; van Latum *et al.* 1995). The combined outcome event of stroke, myocardial infarction or vascular death is used because the underlying arterial pathology is similar (mostly atherosclerosis); the underlying pathology is likely to respond to the same treatment (e.g. antithrombotic drugs); and combining the outcome events generates the biggest number and with that comes greater statistical power and therefore certainty about what the exact risks are, and what the treatment effect really is.

Table 16.3 Important independent predictors of major vascular events in transient ischaemic attack (TIA) patients (from Hankey *et al.* 1992; Dutch TIA Trial Study Group 1993; Pop *et al.* 1994). These studies aimed to investigate the relationship between each of several potential prognostic variables and the occurrence of stroke in TIA patients. Multiple regression analysis was used to examine the independent effect of each of the variables on the subsequent risk of stroke by taking into account and adjusting for the effect of the other variables.

Stroke
Large number of TIAs in the 3 months before presentation
Increasing age
Peripheral vascular disease
TIA of the brain (compared with the eye)
Coronary event
Increasing age
Male sex
Ischaemic heart disease (angina pectoris, anterior myocardial infarction or T-wave inversion on electrocardiogram)
Stroke, myocardial infarction or vascular death
Increasing age
Peripheral vascular disease
Large number of TIAs in the 3 months before presentation
Male sex
TIAs of the brain (compared with the eye)
Left-ventricular hypertrophy on the electrocardiogram

Other studies have identified other factors such as blurred vision (as opposed to blackened vision), and impaired cerebrovascular reserve as potential markers of an increased risk of recurrent stroke and other vascular events (Evans *et al.* 1994; Streifler *et al.* 1995; Donders *et al.* 1996; Yamauchi *et al.* 1996). The long-term follow-up and analysis of the large cohorts of medically treated patients with TIA and non-disabling ischaemic stroke in the European Carotid Surgery Trial and the North American Symptomatic Carotid Endarterectomy Trial, have provided more reliable data about prognostic factors as will be discussed later (section 16.8.8) (Eliasziw *et al.* 1995; Paddock-Eliasziw *et al.* 1996; Rothwell & Warlow 1999b, 2000b, c; Rothwell *et al.* 2000).

Based on the presence and power of the significant prognostic factors in one of these studies (Hankey *et al.* 1993b), prediction models (equations) of both the relative risk and absolute risk of stroke (Table 16.4), coronary events (Table 16.5) and of all serious vascular events (Table 16.6) have been developed. The serious vascular events model is available for use at http://www.dcn.ed.ac.uk/model/predict.htm. The aim of these prediction models is to enable clinicians to stratify TIA (and stroke) patients according to their risk of subsequent vascular events, and use this information to target specific effective medical and surgical treatments to the appropriate patients. For example, it is not appropriate (or cost-effective) for patients at very low risk of subsequent events to be prescribed costly medications (e.g. clopidogrel) or referred for potentially risky operations (e.g. carotid endarterectomy), whereas both interventions may be appropriate for higher risk patients. Prediction models should be used with caution, however. They need to be externally valid and robust (Hier & Edelstein 1991). The models in Tables 16.4–16.6 have been applied to two independent cohorts of TIA patients to test their external validity and are fairly reliable predictors of outcome, particularly for patients predicted to be at low risk. However, these prediction models, and those derived from the Dutch TIA trial, are not sufficiently reliable and valid to apply with confidence in individual patients; we need more reliable predictors of recurrence risk (Dippel & Koudstaal 1997a). Furthermore, prediction

Table 16.4 Prediction equation for survival free of stroke in a patient with transient ischaemic attacks (TIAs).

Age in years minus 60	multiplied by	4.5
Female	subtract	36
TIA of the eye (amaurosis fugax) only	subtract	72
Carotid as well as vertebrobasilar TIAs	add	53
Number of TIAs in the last 3 months (n)	add	$1.6 \times (n-1)$
Peripheral vascular disease	add	76
Left-ventricular hypertrophy (ECG)	add	68
Residual neurological signs	add	74
	Total score =	y
Divide y by 100 and exponentiate ($e^{y/100}$) =	x	
Probability of survival free of stroke:	at 1 year = 0.96^x	
	at 5 years = 0.88^x	

Example: A 65-year-old woman with five episodes of amaurosis fugax in the last 3 months and ECG shows left-ventricular hypertrophy

		Cumulative score
65 – 60 years = 5	multiplied by 4.5	22.5
Female	subtract 36	–13.5
TIA of the eye (amaurosis fugax) only	subtract 72	–85.5
Five TIAs in the last 3 months	add $1.6 \times (5-1)$	–79.1
Left-ventricular hypertrophy (ECG)	add 68	–11.1
	Total score =	–11.1
Divide –11.1 by 100 and exponentiate ($e^{-0.111}$)	$= 1/(e^{-0.111})$	
	= 1/1.117	
	= 0.895	
Probability of survival free of stroke:	at 1 year = $0.96^{0.895}$ = 0.96 or 96%	
	at 5 years = $0.88^{0.895}$ = 0.89 or 89%	

Table 16.5 Prediction equation for survival free of a coronary event in a patient with transient ischaemic attacks (TIAs).

Age in years minus 60	multiplied by	8.1
Female	subtract	102
TIA of the eye (amaurosis fugax) only	subtract	44
Number of TIAs in the last 3 months (n)	add	$0.97 \times (n-1)$
Carotid as well as vertebrobasilar TIAs	add	107
Peripheral vascular disease	add	59
Residual neurological signs	add	48
Left-ventricular hypertrophy (ECG)	add	33
Ischaemic heart disease	add	87
	Total score =	y
Divide y by 100 and exponentiate ($e^{y/100}$) =	x	
Probability of survival free of a coronary event:	at 1 year = 0.99^x	
	at 5 years = 0.92^x	

Example: A 70-year-old woman with one TIA of the brain in the last 3 months and a history of angina

		Cumulative score
70 – 60 years = 10	multiplied by 8.1	81
Female	subtract 102	–21
Ischaemic heart disease	add 87	66
	Total score =	66
Divide 66 by 100 and exponentiate ($e^{0.66}$) =	1.93	
Probability of survival free of a coronary event:	at 1 year = $0.99^{1.93}$ = 0.98 or 98%	
	at 5 years = $0.92^{1.93}$ = 0.85 or 85%	

Age in years minus 60	multiplied by	6
Female	subtract	68
TIA of the eye (amaurosis fugax) only	subtract	56
Number of TIAs in the last 3 months (n)	add	$1.5 \times (n-1)$
Carotid as well as vertebrobasilar TIAs	add	71
Peripheral vascular disease	add	84
Residual neurological signs	add	66
Left-ventricular hypertrophy (ECG)	add	54
	Total score =	y

Divide y by 100 and exponentiate ($e^{y/100}$) = x

Probability of survival free of stroke, myocardial infarction or vascular death:

at 1 year = 0.95^x

at 5 years = 0.79^x

Example: A 65-year-old woman with five episodes of amaurosis fugax only in last 3 months and ECG shows left ventricular hypertrophy

		Cumulative score
65 – 60 years = 5	multiplied by 6	30
Female	subtract 68	–38
TIA of the eye (amaurosis fugax) only	subtract 56	–94
Five TIAs in the last 3 months	add $(1.5 \times [5-1])$	–88
Left-ventricular hypertrophy (ECG)	add 54	–34
	Total score =	–34

Divide –34 by 100 and exponentiate ($e^{-0.34}$) $= 1/(e^{0.34})$

$= 1/1.4$

$= 0.7$

Probability of survival free of stroke, myocardial infarction or vascular death:

at 1 year = $0.95^{0.7} = 0.96$ or 96%

at 5 years = $0.79^{0.7} = 0.85$ or 85%

Table 16.6 Prediction equation for survival free of stroke, myocardial infarction or vascular death in a patient with transient ischaemic attacks (TIAs). (For interactive use see http://www.dcn.ed.ac.uk/model/predict.htm)

models should not lead to overemphasis on the need to identify and treat *only* high-risk patients because most strokes, and other vascular outcome events, occur in patients who are predicted to be at lower risk (in the same way that most strokes occur in people with 'normal' blood pressure, who are considered to be at low risk) (section 18.5.2).

16.1.2 Prognosis after stroke (ischaemic and haemorrhagic stroke combined)

Most of the data about the prognosis after stroke come from studies that have examined 'all stroke', not particular stroke types such as ischaemic stroke or even mild ischaemic stroke compared with primary intracerebral haemorrhage (PICH). These data are useful for clinicians who, for whatever reason, are not able to classify strokes into pathological types.

Cohorts of stroke patients

Community studies indicate that about 20% of all patients with a first-ever stroke die within 1 month (section 10.2.3). After the first month, the average annual risk of death falls appreciably to about 9%/year over the next few years (Fig. 10.2) (Table 16.2). Although some studies have shown a greater risk of dying over the first 5 years after stroke (i.e. >9%/year), the poorer survival may have been, in part, because these studies included patients with recurrent strokes (and not just first-ever-in-a-lifetime strokes) in their inception cohort (Schmidt *et al.* 1988; Kojima *et al.* 1990). However, there is in fact remarkably little information about differences in case fatality amongst patients with first-ever-in-a-lifetime and recurrent stroke (section 10.2.3). Amongst the 80% or so of stroke patients who survive the first 30 days after stroke, the relative risk of dying is about twice the risk of people in the general population (Dennis *et al.* 1993; Hankey *et al.* 2000a) (Fig. 10.2). This excess risk of death persists for several years, probably because stroke patients have co-existent vascular risk factors and diseases such as hypertension and coronary heart disease (Sacco *et al.* 1982).

It is not always easy to distinguish a recurrent stroke from other causes of worsening in the first week or so after a stroke (section 15.5). Bearing this in mind, it seems that the risk of recurrent stroke is greatest early after the first

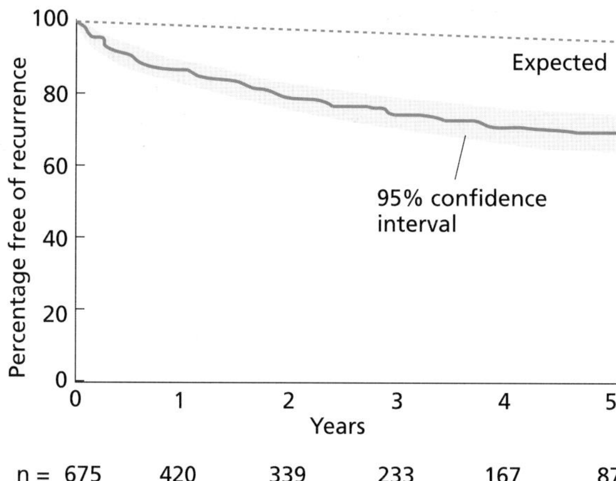

Fig. 16.2 Kaplan–Meier plot showing the probability that, given survival, first-ever-in-a-lifetime stroke patients will remain free from recurrent stroke, compared with the expected probability of people in the same general population remaining free from a first-ever-in-a-lifetime stroke (derived from Oxfordshire Community Stroke Project incidence data 1981–86). The shading indicates 95% confidence intervals. The numbers along the x-axis indicate the number of people still at risk of recurrent stroke at the beginning of each year of follow-up (with permission from Burn *et al.* 1994).

stroke: about 2–3% of survivors of first-ever-in-a-lifetime stroke have a recurrent stroke within the first 30 days, about 9% in the first 6 months and 10–16% within 1 year, which is about 15 times greater than the risk in the general population of the same age and sex (Matsumoto *et al.* 1973; Viitanen *et al.* 1988; Terent 1989; Broderick *et al.* 1992; Burn *et al.* 1994; Lauria *et al.* 1995; Easton 1997; Sandercock & Tangkanakul 1997; Hankey *et al.* 1998) (Fig. 16.2 and Table 16.2). After the first year, the average annual risk of recurrent stroke for the next 4 years falls to about 5% (and about 40% of these recurrences are not of functional significance to the patient) (Marquardsen 1969; Matsumoto *et al.* 1973; Sacco *et al.* 1982; Sage & van Uitert 1983; Dombovy *et al.* 1987; Meissner *et al.* 1988; Schmidt *et al.* 1988; Viitanen *et al.* 1988; Terent 1989; Broderick *et al.* 1992; Burn *et al.* 1994; Hankey *et al.* 1998). This risk is very similar to that of TIA patients and is about nine times the risk of stroke in the general population of the same age and sex (Burn *et al.* 1994) (Table 16.2). The pathological type of recurrent stroke is the same as the index stroke in the vast majority of cases (Yamamoto & Bogousslavsky 1997; Hankey *et al.* 1998). Although the decision to treat with secondary prevention measures, and for how long, is based on the absolute risk of recurrent stroke for a patient rather than the relative risk (section 16.2), and the results of clinical trials, these data emphasize that effective prevention measures should be started as soon as possible and continued for at least a few years, if not longer.

The risk of recurrent stroke is highest early after a first-ever-in-a-lifetime stroke, demanding early intervention with appropriate and effective secondary prevention strategies.

As with TIA patients, the prognosis of individual stroke patients is extremely variable: some patients die immediately, some die later, some survive and are left with a permanent disability and some recover completely. Factors that increase the risk of a first-ever-in-a-lifetime stroke may not necessarily be so important in predicting a recurrent stroke. Unfortunately, the data we have on the long-term follow-up of community-based stroke patients are limited and so the results of statistical analyses of prognostic variables are not robust and are hence inconsistent. An increased risk of recurrent stroke has been associated with advanced age (Hankey *et al.* 1998); male gender (Jorgensen *et al.* 1997); a history of TIA (Jorgensen *et al.* 1997) or diabetes mellitus (Hier *et al.* 1991; Hankey *et al.* 1998); haemorrhagic stroke (Hankey *et al.* 1998); high blood pressure (Hier *et al.* 1991; Alter *et al.* 1994; Lai *et al.* 1994; Jorgensen *et al.* 1997); low blood pressure (Irie *et al.* 1993); valvular heart disease and congestive heart failure (Broderick *et al.* 1992); atrial fibrillation (Lai *et al.* 1994, Jorgensen *et al.* 1997); and an abnormal initial CT brain scan. A lower risk of recurrent stroke has been associated with a low diastolic blood pressure, no history of stroke, no history of diabetes and an infarct of unknown cause (Hier *et al.* 1991).

16.1.3 Prognosis after ischaemic stroke

Cohorts of ischaemic stroke patients

The overall case fatality of patients with first-ever-in-a-lifetime ischaemic stroke is about 7% at 7 days, 10–15% at 30 days, 20% at 6 months, 25–30% at 1 year, and 50–55% at 5 years (Petty *et al.* 1998) (Fig. 10.3). Young adults (< 45 years of age) have a better prognosis with a lower overall case fatality of about 2% at 30 days and a low risk of subsequent fatal events (Abraham *et al.* 1971; Marshall 1982; Lanzino *et al.* 1991; Ferro & Crespo 1994); a long-term follow-up of 296 young adults with ischaemic stroke over a mean of 6 years reported an annual mortality from vascular death of 1.7% (Kappelle *et al.* 1994).

The overall risk of recurrent stroke after a first-ever-in-a-lifetime ischaemic stroke is about 2% at 7 days, 4% at 30 days, 12% at 1 year, and 30% at 5 years (Bamford *et al.* 1987, 1990, 1991; Hier *et al.* 1991; Burn *et al.* 1994; Sacco *et al.* 1994; Petty *et al.* 1998).

Individual ischaemic stroke patients

Amongst patients with ischaemic stroke, the reported significant independent predictors of recurrent stroke are increasing age (Sacco *et al.* 1982; Petty *et al.* 1998); diabetes mellitus (Sacco *et al.* 1982; Hier *et al.* 1991; Petty *et al.* 1998); hypertension (Hier *et al.* 1991; Sacco *et al.* 1994); valvular heart disease (Broderick *et al.* 1992); congestive heart failure (Sacco *et al.* 1982; Viitanen *et al.* 1988; Broderick *et al.* 1992); and myocardial infarction or other ischaemic heart disease (Sacco *et al.* 1982). In the Oxfordshire Community Stroke Project, the 1-year rates of recurrent stroke also varied amongst the four clinical subtypes of ischaemic stroke: total anterior circulation infarction (TACI) 6%, lacunar infarction (LACI) 9%, partial anterior circulation infarction (PACI) 17% and posterior circulation infarction (POCI) 20% (Bamford *et al.* 1991). Furthermore, there were three different patterns of recurrence (Fig. 16.3); patients with PACI had a high early recurrence rate (suggesting an active source of recurrent embolism), patients with POCI had a moderately high early recurrence rate with further episodes throughout the first year, and those with LACI had a low and fairly constant recurrence rate, supporting the notion that LACIs occur as a result of occlusion of a single perforating artery and are not usually due to an active single source of recurrent embolism (Bamford *et al.* 1987, 1991; Sacco *et al.* 1989; Mead *et al.* 2000). There is some evidence that at least half of recurrent infarcts in patients after LACIs are lacunar again, also supporting the hypothesis that LACIs are usually caused by a general disorder of intracranial small vessels (Boiten & Lodder 1993; Salgado *et al.* 1996; Samuelsson *et al.* 1996; Yamamoto & Bogousslavsky 1997, 1998). However, not all recurrences are lacunar infarcts and, indeed, other studies have found that recurrent LACIs account for no more than about 25% of recurrences (which is similar to the proportion of patients with first-ever-in-a-lifetime ischaemic stroke who are found to have a LACI) (Gandolfo *et al.* 1986; Sacco *et al.* 1991; Clavier *et al.* 1994; Kappelle *et al.* 1995).

Although atrial fibrillation (AF) is a risk factor for first ischaemic stroke (Whisnant *et al.* 1996), it has not been identified as a significant independent predictor of stroke recurrence in community-based studies (Broderick *et al.* 1992; Sandercock *et al.* 1992; Sacco *et al.* 1994). This may be because AF is associated with a high case fatality and, among survivors, AF is recognized and treated appropriately with cardioversion or anticoagulation.

The risk of recurrent stroke is highest early after first-ever-in-a-lifetime stroke, demanding early intervention with appropriate and effective secondary prevention strategies.

16.1.4 Prognosis after primary intracerebral haemorrhage

Cohorts of primary intracerebral haemorrhage patients

There have been many studies of the prognosis of PICH, but most have been retrospective hospital-based studies of selected patients, some before the era of CT scanning, or prospective hospital-based studies with short follow-up. Such hospital-based studies may be biased by omitting patients with milder strokes who do not require admission, severely

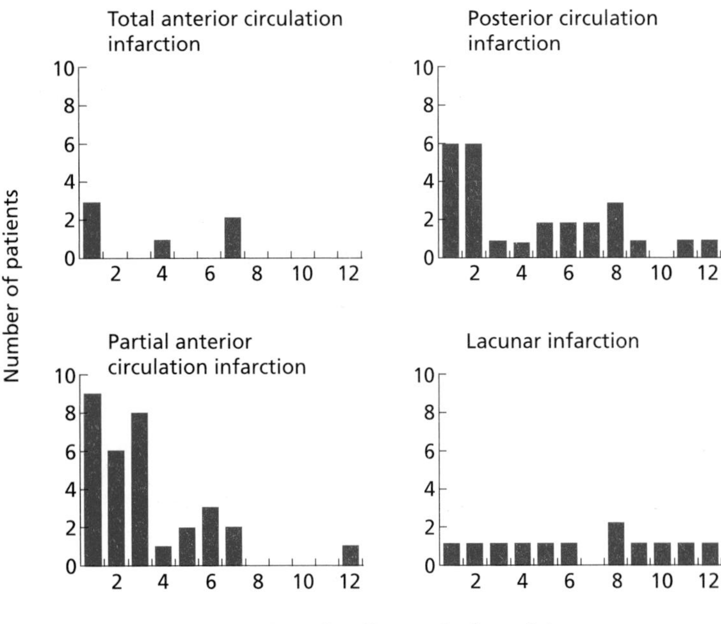

Fig. 16.3 The timing of recurrent stroke in different subtypes of ischaemic stroke. These histograms show the number of patients who experienced a first recurrent stroke at different time intervals (months) after an initial first-ever-in-a-lifetime ischaemic stroke of each clinical subtype. These data come from the Oxfordshire Community Stroke Project (with permission from Bamford *et al.* 1991).

ill patients who die before they can be admitted, and elderly patients who remain in nursing homes. A few community-based studies have provided information on PICH, but most were undertaken before the era of freely available CT scans, or only reported relatively short follow-up, and they were all small. Therefore, although much is now known about the long-term risk of death, disability and subsequent vascular events in patients with ischaemic stroke, there have been very few community-based studies of the long-term follow-up of patients with CT brain scan evidence of PICH. A population study in the Jyvaskyla region, Central Finland, of 158 patients with CT- or autopsy-confirmed PICH, all of whom were followed up for a median of 32 months, found that the 30-day case fatality was 50%, but after the first month the probability of survival did not differ from an age- and sex-matched normal population (Fogelholm *et al.* 1992). In the Oxfordshire Community Stroke Project (OCSP), which registered 66 patients with PICH, the 30-day case fatality was also about half (52%) (Bamford *et al.* 1990; Counsell *et al.* 1995a). However, the long-term case fatality was worse than in Finland; all surviving patients were followed for up to 6 years and the average death rate for those surviving 30 days was 8%/year for the first 5 years, which is similar to that for patients with ischaemic stroke (section 16.1.3). The main causes of 'late' deaths (> 30 days) were non-stroke vascular disease such as myocardial infarction (55%) and the complications of immobility due to the initial or a recurrent stroke (45%).

The long-term risk of death or of recurrent stroke after primary intracerebral haemorrhage is not precisely known because there have been no large community-based studies.

The risk of recurrent stroke following PICH is poorly documented in many studies due to varying duration and intensity of follow-up. In the OCSP, each patient was carefully assessed for recurrent stroke, but the numbers were very small. Amongst those surviving 30 days, the annual risk of recurrent stroke was about 7% and of death and/or recurrent stroke about 11% (Counsell *et al.* 1995a) (Fig. 16.4). These rates are similar to those following ischaemic stroke (section 16.1.3). At least 25% of the recurrences were definite haemorrhages, and in those patients there was a high chance of underlying cerebral amyloid angiopathy (section 8.2.2). The population study in the Jyvaskyla region, Central Finland, found that amongst patients who had survived 10 days or more, six (4%) had a recurrent PICH (diagnosed by CT or autopsy) and another five had a recurrent ischaemic or non-defined acute stroke at some time between 36 and 1210 days after the initial bleed (Fogelholm *et al.* 1992).

Of course, the risk of recurrence is influenced by the aetiology of the initial intracerebral haemorrhage. Haemorrhages due to arteriovenous malformations and cerebral amyloid angiopathy (which are commonly lobar haemorrhages) more often recur (Neau *et al.* 1997). Patients with hypertensive haemorrhages also have an increased risk of re-bleeding, often in a different site, if their blood pressure is not well controlled over a sustained period (Lee *et al.* 1990; Passero *et al.* 1995; Arakawa *et al.* 1998; Gonzales-Duarte *et al.* 1998; Bae *et al.* 1999).

Individual primary intracerebral haemorrhage patients

There have not been any prospective community-based follow-up studies of patients with PICH which have recorded sufficient numbers of recurrent strokes to have the statistical power to identify reliably any predictive factors. If it were possible to reliably predict those at low risk of recurrent haemorrhage, it may then be possible to reliably identify subgroups of patients who would benefit from aspirin to prevent fatal *cardio*vascular disease or recurrent *ischaemic*

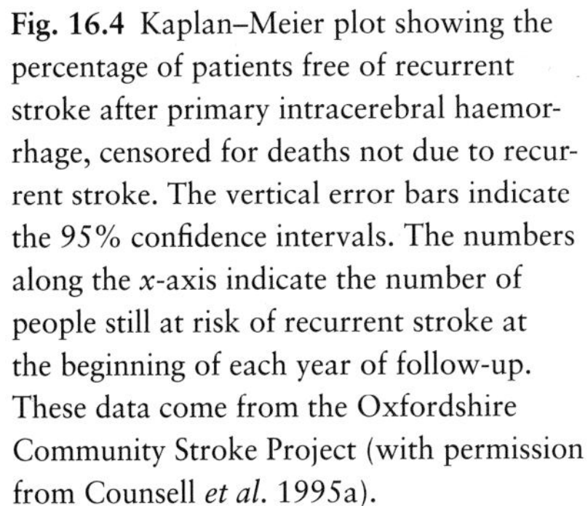

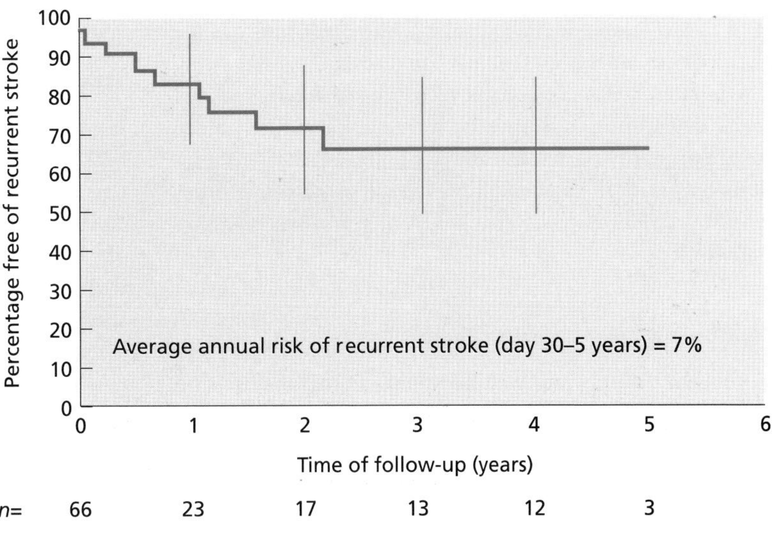

Fig. 16.4 Kaplan–Meier plot showing the percentage of patients free of recurrent stroke after primary intracerebral haemorrhage, censored for deaths not due to recurrent stroke. The vertical error bars indicate the 95% confidence intervals. The numbers along the x-axis indicate the number of people still at risk of recurrent stroke at the beginning of each year of follow-up. These data come from the Oxfordshire Community Stroke Project (with permission from Counsell *et al.* 1995a).

stroke. However, at the moment aspirin is not recommended in the acute aftermath of a PICH because of an unproven fear of exacerbating any recurrent intracerebral bleeding that may occur (unless the patient is at greater risk of an ischaemic event) (section 16.4.3). A recently published cohort study of 71 hospital-referred patients with lobar intracerebral haemorrhage identified a 2-year cumulative rate of recurrent haemorrhagic stroke of 21%, and the apolipoprotein E genotype (E2 and E4 alleles) was associated with an increased risk of recurrence (O'Donnell *et al.* 2000). This finding awaits confirmation.

16.2 General approach to preventing recurrent stroke and other serious vascular events

'Mass' vs. 'high-risk' strategy

There are two approaches to stroke prevention: the 'mass' and the 'high-risk' strategy. The mass strategy involves making small changes to every member of the general stroke-free population (such as a reduction by a few millimetres of mercury of diastolic blood pressure), which has the effect of reducing the mean blood pressure of the entire population (section 18.6). Such changes are achieved by alterations in lifestyle or in the environment. The high-risk strategy is to seek out individuals with high levels of risk, such as those labelled as having hypertension, and then to give them medical or surgical treatments to reduce that risk (section 18.5). It seems at first counter-intuitive, but it is none the less true, that the mass strategy is likely to have as great an impact on stroke incidence as all the medical activity entailed in the high-risk strategy (Rose 1992). This is not to belittle the efforts of doctors, but merely to point out that their efforts must be supported by wider, population-based efforts.

Primary prevention is in the hands of primary health care doctors, governmental public health departments and politicians. Politicians have a much greater influence than doctors over the measures which are central to the success of primary stroke prevention (i.e. the measures which could improve the health of the entire population: a ban on tobacco advertising, a reduction in the salt content of processed foods, reduced social deprivation and poverty, to name but a few). Since we are primarily physicians and not politicians, this chapter deals only with the *secondary* prevention of stroke; in other words, preventing stroke after a TIA or a first-ever-in-a-lifetime stroke.

Patients at greatest absolute risk benefit most

Throughout the chapter we will emphasize that the decision whether or not to apply a preventive measure should be based mostly on the likely *absolute* benefit (e.g. avoid 50 events per 1000 patients treated) rather than on the *relative* reduction in risk. An impressive 50% relative risk reduction will yield an absolute benefit of only 10 per 1000 patients treated when applied to patients at low risk of the event (e.g. 2% in controls reduced to 1% in the treated group) (Table 16.7). Section 11.2.1. and Table 11.2 explain the meaning of the terms relative and absolute benefit.

The decision to treat a patient depends more on the absolute benefit of treatment than the relative reduction of risk provided by the treatment. Patients at very low absolute risk of recurrent stroke (e.g. 1%) are still at low absolute risk, even if the treatment reduces their risk by 50% (i.e. to 0.5%); the 0.5% absolute reduction in risk of recurrent stroke (or absolute benefit) means 200 patients have to be treated to prevent one having a stroke (i.e. 100/0.5).

Preventing other types of vascular events and 'vascular dementia'

Patients with stroke and TIA are not just at high risk of stroke, but also of myocardial infarction, lower limb ischaemia and death from vascular disease. Stroke physicians therefore need to pay attention to the heart and peripheral vascular tree both in their clinical examination and also when deciding on treatments for secondary prevention. 'Vascular dementia' is a very heterogeneous condition, but some stroke and TIA patients do become demented from vascular disease of the brain, although the factors which predict vascular dementia after stroke are not well characterized (Foster & Hickenbottom 1999) (section 15.29.2). However, if the frequency of vascular dementia after stroke can be reduced, that would be important. A number of current trials of interventions which primarily aim to prevent recurrent stroke (such as blood pressure reduction, cholesterol reduction, homocysteine lowering and aspirin), are seeking to determine whether the intervention also reduces the frequency and severity of cognitive impairment due to cerebrovascular disease (see relevant section on each of the specific interventions).

Treat any specific underlying cause

It goes without saying that if a treatable cause for the cerebral ischaemia has been identified, such as arteritis or infective endocarditis, then specific treatment should be given (section 16.7). However, this is likely to apply to less than 5% of unselected patients (Chapter 7). Of course, patients with stroke often have other vascular disorders which require specific treatment or preventive action in their own right; the assessment and treatment of angina, heart failure, cardiac dysrhythmias, valvular heart disease, abdominal aortic aneurysm and peripheral vascular disease may not directly reduce the risk of further stroke, but should at least improve quality of life and reduce the risk of other serious vascular events.

General strategies for all patients and specific strategies for patients after cerebral ischaemia

Strategies for secondary stroke prevention are, broadly, divided into two. Firstly, those which apply to all patients with cerebrovascular disease, irrespective of whether ischaemic or haemorrhagic (chiefly risk factor modification) (section 16.3) and secondly, those which apply only to patients with ischaemic stroke or TIA in whom appropriately timed brain CT or magnetic resonance (MR) imaging has ruled out intracranial haemorrhage: antiplatelet drugs (section 16.4); anticoagulants (section 16.5); angiotensin-converting enzyme inhibitors (section 16.6); treatment of various specific underlying causes (section 16.7); and vascular surgical procedures (sections 16.8–16.13).

16.3 Risk factor control for patients with transient ischaemic attack, ischaemic stroke and primary intracerebral haemorrhage

This section deals with the interventions which are applicable to all patients with acute cerebrovascular events irrespective of pathological type; for example, long-term blood pressure reduction applies to patients with hypertension whether the event was ischaemic or haemorrhagic. Smoking cessation is important for any patient with symptomatic vascular disease (even if cessation may not definitely reduce the risk of recurrent stroke). Recommendations by guideline groups from Europe and North America are broadly similar, but differ in some important details; in any event any guidelines should always be adapted to meet local circumstances (Scottish Intercollegiate Guidelines Network 1999; Wolf *et al.* 1999, Wade 2000).

16.3.1 Blood pressure reduction

Raised blood pressure is the most important treatable and causal risk factor for stroke (section 6.3.3). This relationship is much stronger than had previously been realized. Two things have clarified the relationship: systematic reviews of the observational epidemiological studies and the realization that random error in the measurement of the baseline blood pressure must be corrected for (MacMahon *et al.* 1990; Collins & MacMahon 1994). The technical term for this error is the 'regression–dilution bias' and its importance (and how to correct for it) are explained in detail elsewhere (MacMahon *et al.* 1990; MacMahon & Rodgers 1994a). A systematic review, correcting for this error, showed that for each 7.5 mmHg rise in usual diastolic blood pressure there is a *doubling* in the risk of stroke (Collins & MacMahon 1994; MacMahon & Rodgers 1994a) (Fig. 6.9). There is rather more limited evidence about the relationship between usual diastolic blood pressure and the risk of subsequent recurrent stroke amongst survivors of stroke (MacMahon & Rodgers 1994a). However, data from two independent sources, the UK-TIA Aspirin Trial and the Anti-Thrombotic Trialists' Collaboration strongly suggest that, after correction for the regression–dilution bias, there is a strong linear relationship between usual blood pressure and risk of stroke amongst survivors of minor ischaemic stroke and TIA (Rodgers *et al.* 1996) (Fig. 16.5). These observational data highlight the high absolute risk (section 16.1.1) of stroke in such patients and that blood pressure reduction *might* lead to worthwhile absolute reduction in the risk of recurrent stroke even amongst individuals whose blood pressure is apparently 'normal', or only modestly elevated (MacMahon & Rodgers 1994a, PROGRESS Management Committee 1996) (Fig. 16.6).

Evidence from randomized trials in primary stroke prevention

Antihypertensive drugs for primary stroke prevention amongst patients with moderate to severe hypertension have been evaluated in trials which have recruited almost 50 000 individuals (MacMahon & Rodgers 1994a). Conventional antihypertensive drugs reduced the risk of stroke by about 38%, and most of the benefit becomes apparent within a year

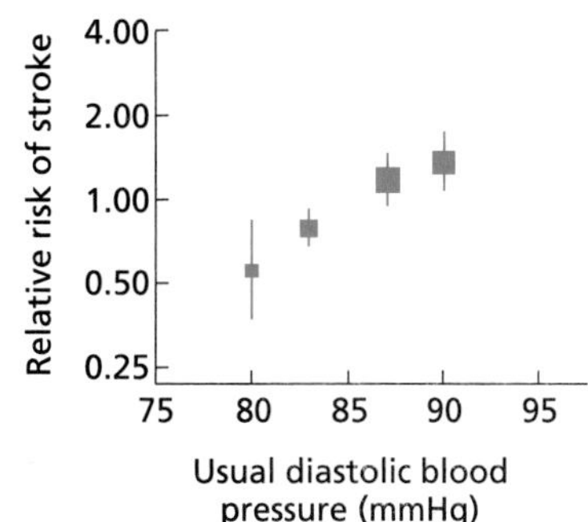

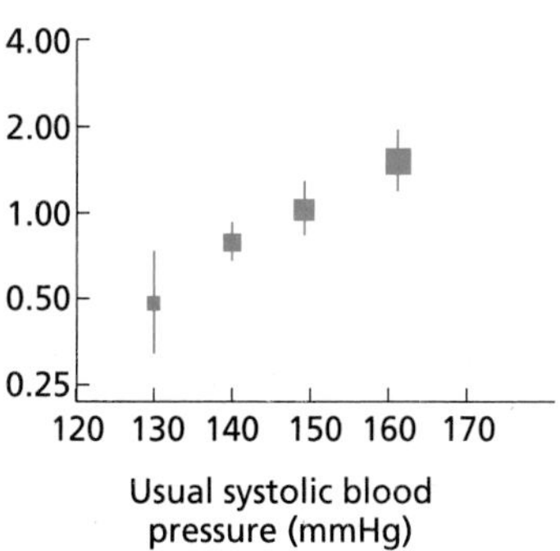

Fig. 16.5 Relative risk of stroke by approximate usual systolic and diastolic blood pressure amongst 2435 patients with a history of transient ischaemic attack or minor stroke. Solid squares represent stroke risk in each category relative to the risk in the whole study population. The sizes of the squares are proportional to the number of events in each category of usual blood pressure. The vertical lines indicate the 95% confidence intervals (with permission from PROGRESS Management Committee 1996).

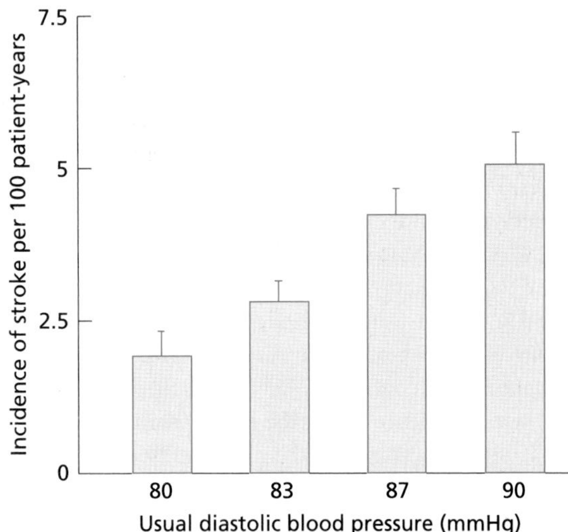

Fig. 16.6 Absolute risk of stroke by approximate usual diastolic blood pressure amongst 2201 patients with a history of transient ischaemic attack or minor stroke. The vertical error bars indicate 1 SD (with permission from S. MacMahon, personal communication 1996).

or two of starting treatment (Collins & MacMahon 1994; MacMahon & Rodgers 1994a,b) (Figs 16.7 and 16.8).

Limited evidence on secondary stroke prevention

There have been only two small trials, with a total of 549 patients, evaluating the effect of antihypertensive drugs amongst stroke survivors (i.e. of secondary stroke prevention). Patients were included in these trials some weeks after their stroke. A systematic review of the data from these two trials showed that treatment was similarly associated with a 38% reduction in the risk of (recurrent) stroke, but the confidence interval was wide and included both the possibility that blood pressure reduction more than halved the risk of stroke or gave almost no benefit at all (Fig. 16.7). The addition of data from two other trials evaluating betablockers (not primarily designed to reduce blood pressure), the Treatment of Early Stroke Trial (TEST) study and the betablocker component of the Dutch TIA Trial, increased the amount of data available. Putting these four studies together, with a total of 2742 patients, the relative reduction in the risk of stroke was 19%, which was not statistically significant (MacMahon & Rodgers 1994a,b; PROGRESS Management Committee 1996) (Fig. 16.9). Since then, a large placebo-controlled trial in China of blood pressure reduction with the diuretic indapamide in 5665 stroke survivors (some of whom were 'normotensive') has published a preliminary report suggesting that the treatment achieved a reduction of 2 mmHg in diastolic blood pressure over 2 years which was associated with a 29% relative reduction in stroke risk (PATS Collaborating Group 1995). A meta-analysis, including the preliminary PATS trial results, yielded similar estimates, but since the PATS study dominated the overall results, the authors concluded that firm conclusions were not possible until the PROGRESS trial results were available (INDANA Project Collaborators 1997). It was also not possible to determine whether the benefit depended on the level of baseline blood pressure.

The absolute benefits of blood pressure reduction might well be substantial amongst individuals with a history of stroke or TIA, in whom the risk of stroke is about 10% in the first year after the event and about 5%/year thereafter (section 16.1.1). The difference in absolute risk and absolute risk difference is illustrated well in the lower part of Fig. 16.7; in primary prevention, antihypertensive drugs reduced the risk of stroke from 3.2% to 2.0%, an absolute risk reduction of 1.2% (i.e. treat 83 to prevent one stroke), whereas in secondary prevention, the difference was 27.3% vs. 18.8% = 8.5% (i.e. treat 12 to prevent one stroke). But, whilst blood pressure reduction in hypertensive patients may confer a similar relative reduction in primary and secondary stroke incidence, the true size of the benefit for secondary prevention is somewhat uncertain and the benefits could be much smaller (MacMahon & Rodgers 1994b, PROGRESS Management Committee 1996). The results of PROGRESS are expected in 2001 (PROGRESS Management Committee 1999).

Individuals with recent stroke or transient ischaemic attack have a much higher absolute risk of stroke than most individuals in the general population. Because of this, even those transient ischaemic attack or stroke patients with relatively 'normal' blood pressure may benefit substantially from blood pressure reduction after stroke. It seems likely that benefits from blood pressure reduction will be determined more by the patient's general characteristics and mix of risk factors for vascular disease than solely by their absolute level of blood pressure. Which individuals with 'normal blood pressure' and 'mild elevations' of blood pressure benefit most from blood pressure reduction after stroke will be determined by trials currently in progress.

In general, the decision on whether or not to use antihypertensive drugs in a given individual who has not had a TIA or stroke should therefore be based, not on their level of blood pressure, but rather on that individual's absolute risk of a serious vascular event, cardiac as well as cerebral. In general, patients with a blood pressure of 150–170 mmHg systolic, or 90–100 mmHg diastolic, or both, should be given treatment to lower blood pressure if the risk of a major vascular event

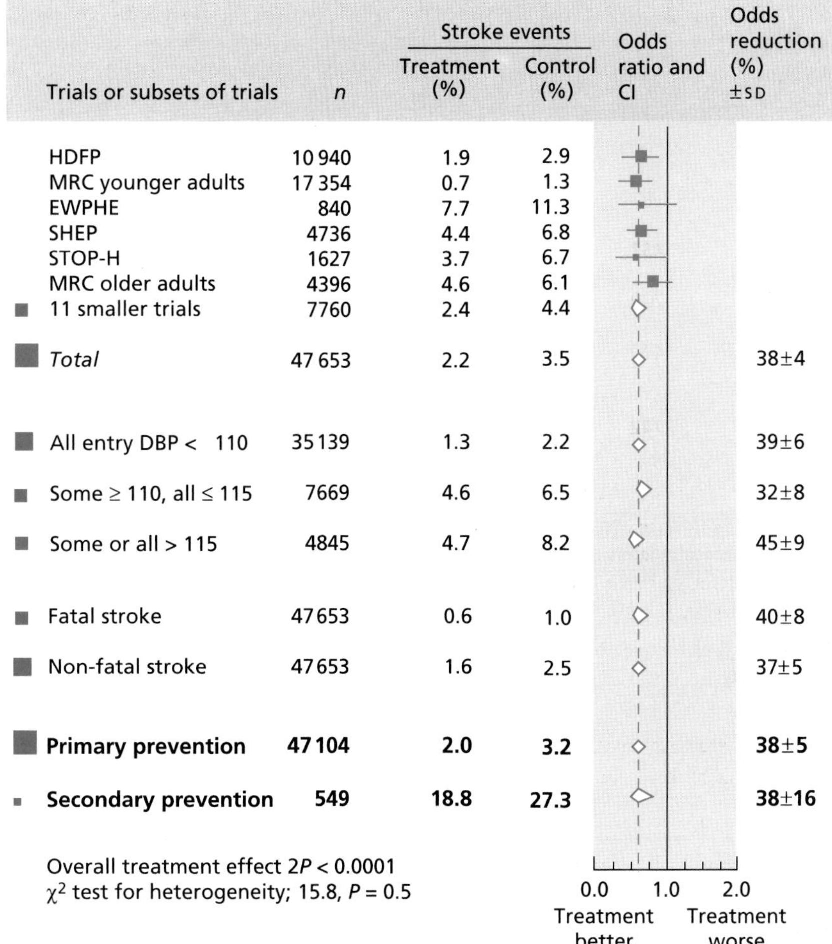

Trials or subsets of trials | n | Stroke events: Treatment (%) | Control (%) | Odds ratio and CI | Odds reduction (%) ±SD
HDFP | 10 940 | 1.9 | 2.9
MRC younger adults | 17 354 | 0.7 | 1.3
EWPHE | 840 | 7.7 | 11.3
SHEP | 4736 | 4.4 | 6.8
STOP-H | 1627 | 3.7 | 6.7
MRC older adults | 4396 | 4.6 | 6.1
11 smaller trials | 7760 | 2.4 | 4.4
Total | 47 653 | 2.2 | 3.5 | 38±4
All entry DBP < 110 | 35139 | 1.3 | 2.2 | 39±6
Some ≥ 110, all ≤ 115 | 7669 | 4.6 | 6.5 | 32±8
Some or all > 115 | 4845 | 4.7 | 8.2 | 45±9
Fatal stroke | 47653 | 0.6 | 1.0 | 40±8
Non-fatal stroke | 47653 | 1.6 | 2.5 | 37±5
Primary prevention | 47 104 | 2.0 | 3.2 | 38±5
Secondary prevention | 549 | 18.8 | 27.3 | 38±16
Overall treatment effect 2P < 0.0001
χ2 test for heterogeneity; 15.8, P = 0.5
0.0
1.0
2.0
Treatment better
Treatment worse

Fig. 16.7 Overview of the results from 17 randomized trials of antihypertensive therapy on stroke risk. The ratio of odds of stroke in the treatment group compared with the control group is plotted for each trial (black square: area proportional to number of strokes), along with the 99% confidence interval (horizontal line). A dark green square to the left of the solid vertical line suggests benefit but this benefit is significant at the level of $2P < 0.01$ only if the entire confidence interval is to the left of the solid vertical line. Overviews of several trial results (and 95% confidence interval) are represented by open diamonds (with permission from MacMahon & Rodgers 1994a).

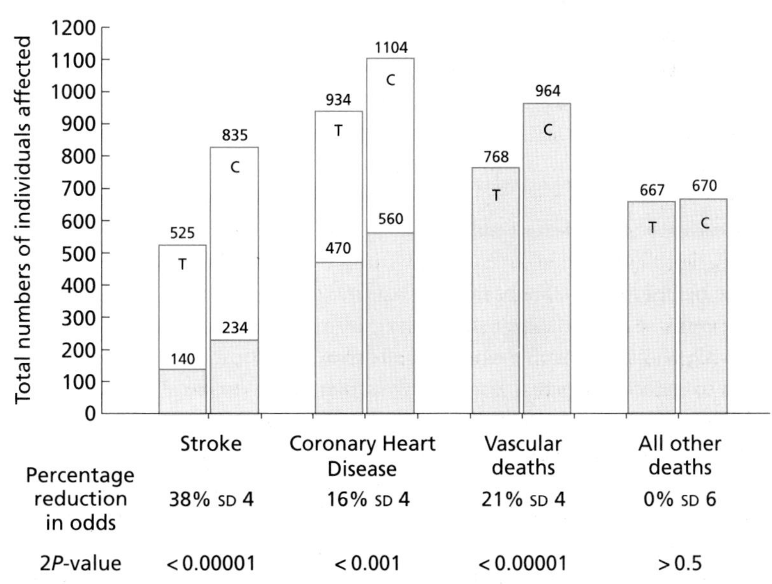

Fig. 16.8 Absolute benefit of antihypertensive drug treatment over five years. Overview of the results of 17 randomized trials of blood pressure lowering including a total of 47 667 individuals in whom there was a mean diastolic blood pressure difference between treated patients and controls, during follow-up, of 5–6 mmHg. Fatal events are represented by green shaded columns. C, control; T, treatment (with permission from Collins & MacMahon 1994).

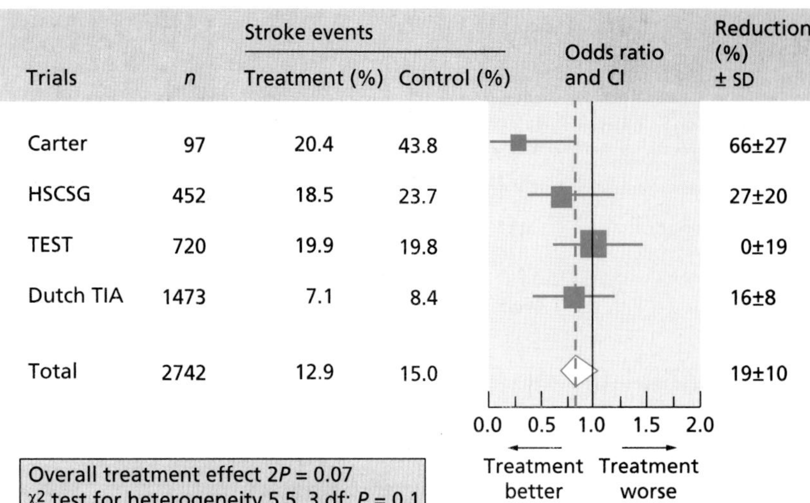

Trials
n
Stroke events
Treatment (%)
Control (%)
Odds ratio and CI
Reduction (%) ± SD
Carter 97 20.4 43.8 66±27
HSCSG 452 18.5 23.7 27±20
TEST 720 19.9 19.8 0±19
Dutch TIA 1473 7.1 8.4 16±8
Total 2742 12.9 15.0 19±10
0.0 0.5 1.0 1.5 2.0
Treatment better
Treatment worse
Overall treatment effect 2P = 0.07
χ2 test for heterogeneity 5.5, 3 df; P = 0.1

Fig. 16.9 The results of a systematic review of four randomized trials to estimate the reduction in stroke risk with blood pressure reduction in stroke and transient ischaemic attack patients with (and without) hypertension. The ratio of odds of stroke in the treatment group compared with the control group is plotted for each trial (black square: area proportional to number of strokes), along with the 99% confidence interval (horizontal line). A dark green square to the left of the solid vertical line suggests benefit, but this benefit is significant at the level of $2P < 0.01$ only if the entire confidence interval is to the left of the solid vertical line. An overview of all of the trial results (and 95% confidence interval) is represented by an open diamond (with permission from PROGRESS Management Committee 1996).

Table 16.7 Relative and absolute reduction in risk achievable if diastolic blood pressure is reduced by 5–6 mmHg.

	60-year-old woman with initial diastolic blood pressure of 100 mmHg and no other risk factors for vascular disease	70-year-old man with initial diastolic blood pressure of 95 mmHg and multiple risk factors for vascular disease
Absolute risk of serious vascular event in next 10 years (%) (i.e. of stroke, myocardial infarction or vascular death):		
Without treatment	10	50
With treatment	7	33
Absolute reduction in risk (per 1000 patients)	30 (i.e. 10% down to 7%)	170 (i.e. 50% down to 33%)
Relative reduction in risk	One-third	One-third
Need to treat this number of similar individuals to avoid one serious vascular event within the next 10 years*	33	6

*This is the 'number-needed-to-treat' (modified from Jackson *et al.* 1993).

in the next 10 years is more than 20% (Jackson et al. 1993). The results of clinical trials indicate that, at this level of absolute risk, about 150 people would require treatment for 2 or 3 years to reduce the annual number of vascular events by one. Since the absolute risk of stroke rises with age, and since antihypertensive drugs are effective in older people, elderly hypertensive patients stand to gain as much (or even more) from blood pressure reduction as younger patients (Table 16.7), although they are also at higher risk of adverse events from the treatment (MacMahon & Rodgers 1994a,b; Mulrow et al. 2000).

Who to treat: implications for practice

Direct trial evidence is not strong and does not support routine long-term use of drugs to lower blood pressure in 'hypertensive' or 'normotensive' stroke and TIA patients. None the less, because almost all stroke and TIA survivors have a risk of further vascular events of at least 20% over the next 10 years, then one should at least consider blood pressure reduction in all hyperensive survivors. Until the results of current trials in stroke and TIA survivors are available (see below), we use antihypertensive drugs only in patients at highest risk, and remain uncertain about how to treat lower risk individuals (and how best to define 'high' and 'low' risk). In particular, we will need to have a clearer idea whether the *relative* benefits of treatment vary with the level of *absolute* risk defined at baseline. This explains our caution in extrapolating too far from the available blood pressure lowering trial data in primary prevention, to help us to decide how to manage stroke and TIA survivors.

Who to treat: implications for research

There are substantial uncertainties about the wisdom of blood pressure reduction in patients after stroke, mainly because of concerns that this may precipitate a further stroke. Whether this risk applies to the generality of stroke and TIA survivors or just to a particular subset (e.g. those with severe carotid or vertebral artery stenosis) is not known. In the light of these uncertainties, a large trial evaluating the balance of risk and benefits of blood pressure reduction in a wide variety of TIA and stroke survivors is now under way—the Protection Against Recurrent Stroke Study (PROGRESS) trial (PROGRESS Management Committee 1996). The principal eligibility criterion was that the responsible physician was substantially uncertain about whether or not to give antihypertensive drugs. Therefore, patients with a blood pressure which would conventionally be considered 'normal', and patients with only moderate elevations of blood pressure, were included. Some individuals were even included with quite high levels of blood pressure in whom the clinicians were uncertain about the value of treatment for some reason. Some 6100 patients were randomized between a regimen consisting of the angiotensin-converting enzyme inhibitor perindopril combined with the diuretic indapamide, or perindopril alone, versus placebo controls (PROGRESS Management Committee 1999). The results of the study are expected in 2001.

When to start antihypertensive treatment after an acute stroke

There are enormous variations in clinical practice. Some clinicians prefer to start treatment for hypertension almost immediately, within hours of stroke onset, whereas others prefer to delay treatment by at least 1 or 2 weeks (Lindley *et al.* 1995a,b). Our own practice is equally variable since there is no good evidence to guide us. As a practical point, blood pressure tends to fall spontaneously without treatment over the first 2 weeks after stroke onset, and so provided there is no evidence that the patient has accelerated hypertension it may be best to defer any treatment decision for 1 or 2 weeks (sections 11.9 and 15.7.2). If a patient already on an antihypertensive drug is admitted with a stroke, should one stop or continue it? Again, there is no good evidence. We take note of the admission blood pressure, and if it is high and the patient can swallow, we will continue, otherwise we will often stop treatment. Sometimes, however, patients whose blood pressure has fallen to apparently normal levels by the time of hospital discharge are found to have raised blood pressures at their post-discharge clinic visit. This may be a spurious elevation of blood pressure due to the 'white coat' effect (i.e. the stress of seeing a doctor), but the rise does highlight the need to check the blood pressure amongst stroke survivors on more than one occasion after discharge from hospital.

It is unclear when raised blood pressure should be lowered immediately after acute stroke. Unless the patient has accelerated hypertension, we tend to wait for 1 or 2 weeks.

Which antihypertensive drug?

Systematic reviews have shown that diuretics and betablockers should be the first-line agents in the treatment of stroke-free people with hypertension and in the elderly, since they both have proven benefits in reducing morbidity and mortality (Psaty *et al.* 1997; Mulrow *et al.* 2000; Mulrow & Jackson 2000). A calcium antagonist, nitrendipine, has been compared with placebo for primary stroke prevention in elderly patients with systolic hypertension and is effective, but has not been compared with conventional drugs (Staessen *et al.* 1997). Although calcium channel blockers and angiotensin-converting enzyme inhibitors reduce blood pressure in hypertensive patients, they are a great deal more expensive and the clinical trials do not show greater reductions in the risk of stroke or cardiovascular events than conventional agents. Furthermore, there is evidence that the short-acting non-dihydropyridine calcium channel blockers may cause harm (Psaty *et al.* 1997; Cutler 1999; Hansson *et al.* 1999a; Mulrow & Jackson 2000). Overall indications of tolerability and quality of life are more favourable for diuretics and betablockers than for the newer drugs (Mulrow & Jackson 2000).

Ferner and Neil (1995) calculated, using data from the Medical Research Council (MRC) trial of treatment of mild hypertension, that to treat 800 patients with bendrofluazide for 1 year in order to prevent one vascular event would cost £1400 per event prevented. If the efficacy is similar, treating the same number of hypertensive patients with angiotensin-converting enzyme inhibitors would cost approximately £100 000 per vascular event prevented (see also Table 11.3) (Ferner & Neil 1995).

There are no completed trials comparing newer agents with standard antihypertensive drugs post stroke, but the choice will be informed by three ongoing trials. The PROGRESS trial is comparing perindopril with perindopril plus the diuretic indapamide with placebo (PROGRESS Management Committee 1996, 1999). A study in 4000 stroke survivors will compare the effects of the angiotensin antagonist eprosartan with the calcium antagonist nitrendipine on 'death from any cause or hospitalization from cardiovascular or cerebrovascular events' (Schrader 2000). A smaller, open trial in 500 hypertensive stroke patients, will compare the effects of a calcium antagonist with an angiotensin-converting enzyme inhibitor with no antihypertensive treatment on stroke recurrence (Fujishima 1999). The blood pressure reductions achieved in the Heart Outcomes Prevention Evaluation (HOPE) trial were small (the differences in systolic and diastolic blood pressure between treated and control groups at 2 years were 3 mmHg and 2 mmHg, respectively), but the data provide additional confirmation that angiotensin-converting enzyme inhibitors can reduce the risk of vascular events as well as lowering blood pressure (Heart Outcomes Prevention Evaluation (HOPE) Study Investigators 2000a–c) (section 16.6).

In the absence of specific contraindications, low-dose diuretics or low-dose betablockers should be used for first-line treatment to prevent recurrent stroke, although their use is supported only by indirect evidence from the randomized trials in primary stroke prevention.

Reduce blood pressure after stroke by dietary salt reduction or potassium supplementation

Analysis of the observational data relating salt intake to blood pressure, and of the randomized trials of different interventions to reduce salt intake, has shown that a reduction in dietary salt has substantial promise as an effective means of blood pressure control (Frost *et al.* 1991; Law *et al.* 1991a,b) (section 6.3.3). This holds true both for whole populations and for individuals. A relatively simple modification of the diet (not adding salt at the table, avoiding salty foods) can lead to a reduction in salt intake of up to 100 mmol/day. This degree of salt reduction in a 20–29-year-old on the fifth centile of the blood pressure distribution is likely to lead to a 1 mmHg fall in diastolic blood pressure. By contrast, the same reduction in dietary salt intake in a patient aged 60–69 years on the 95th centile is likely to lead to a 7 mmHg fall in diastolic blood pressure, comparable to the reduction which can be achieved with diuretics or betablockers. It therefore seems reasonable to advise older hypertensive stroke survivors to reduce their dietary salt intake. This can be achieved without major discomfort and, in the patients most likely to benefit (i.e. elderly hypertensive stroke survivors), is likely to lead both to a worthwhile reduction in diastolic blood pressure and to minimize the need for drug therapy with all the attendant adverse effects.

The value of universal dietary salt restriction as a means of preventing stroke in the general population has been challenged (Alderman *et al.* 1998; Graudal *et al.* 1998). However, the weight of evidence still suggests it is a valuable option for blood pressure reduction in individuals with hypertension (Mulrow & Jackson 2000).

Potassium supplementation appears to be an effective alternative for blood pressure reduction, particularly in people who are unable to reduce their intake of sodium (Whelton *et al.* 1997).

Reducing dietary salt intake reduces blood pressure, particularly in older people with high blood pressure.

Effect of blood pressure reduction on vascular dementia

A *post hoc* subgroup analysis of the Systolic Hypertension in Europe (Syst-Eur) trial suggested that treatment of systolic hypertension might reduce the frequency of vascular dementia in older patients (Forette *et al.* 1998). However, the number of cases with dementia of any cause was very small: 21 (0.8%) among those allocated treatment treated vs. 11 (0.4%) among controls. In the only comparable previous study, dementia was also infrequent, but slightly less frequent in the treated group (1.6% vs. 1.9%) (SHEP Cooperative Research Group 1991). These data suggest that, in stroke-free individuals at low absolute risk of vascular dementia, antihypertensive drugs might reduce the relative risk by about a quarter, with an absolute benefit of about three per 1000. In stroke and TIA survivors, in whom the risk of vascular dementia is likely to be higher, the absolute benefits might be greater. However, until the PROGRESS and SCOPE trials have been completed (they are prospectively assessing cognitive function in all patients), the 'jury is still out' on whether blood pressure reduction prevents vascular dementia (Clarfield & Paltiel 1999; Hansson *et al.* 1999b).

16.3.2 Cholesterol reduction

Observational epidemiology: cholesterol, coronary heart disease and stroke

A systematic review of the relationship between baseline cholesterol and the risk of subsequent coronary heart disease, corrected for regression–dilution bias, has shown that the association is strong (and much stronger than that directly inferred from individual prospective studies) (Law *et al.* 1994a,b) (section 6.3.3). From these observational cohort studies (which included about 500 000 men and 18 000 coronary heart disease events) it is estimated that a long-term reduction in plasma cholesterol of 0.6 mmol/L (about 10%), which can be achieved by modest dietary change, lowers the relative risk of ischaemic heart disease by about 50% at age 40 years, falling to 20% at age 70 years. There is no clear relationship between plasma cholesterol and total stroke, but evidence is beginning to emerge of a weak positive association between cholesterol level and the risk of ischaemic stroke and a weak negative association with haemorrhagic stroke (Fig. 6.11). The excess risk of haemorrhagic stroke only appeared amongst individuals with baseline cholesterol concentrations below about 5 mmol/L (relative risk 1.9, 95% confidence interval (CI), 1.4–2.5). In other words, reducing cholesterol might somewhat reduce ischaemic stroke and slightly increase haemorrhagic stroke (Iso *et al.* 1989; Law *et al.* 1994a,b; Prospective Studies Collaboration 1995; Eastern Stroke and Coronary Heart Disease Collaborative Research Group 1998).

Effect of cholesterol reduction on coronary heart disease and death

In patients with and without symptomatic coronary artery disease, cholesterol reduction with drugs reduces the risk of *cardiac* morbidity and mortality and also reduces the number of patients requiring cardiac interventions (e.g. surgical coronary revascularization) (Probstfield 2000). People with a history of coronary heart disease have a higher risk of events than those without, and so the absolute benefits are greater in secondary prevention than in primary prevention (Probstfield 2000). The randomized controlled trials (based on 45 000 people and 4000 ischaemic heart disease events) also showed that the full effect of reduction in risk is achieved within 5 years (Law *et al.* 1994a,b). There has been considerable debate whether or not cholesterol reduction reduces death from all causes, and whether the reduction in death from coronary heart disease is offset by an increase in death from cancer, suicide and other non-vascular causes. However, a careful and systematic review of all the observational data and the relevant randomized controlled trials did not support this concern (Iso *et al.* 1989; Law *et al.* 1994a,b; Probstfield 2000).

At least one further study is under way. The British Heart Foundation/Medical Research Council (BHF/MRC) Heart Protection Study has recruited about 18 000 patients at high risk of serious vascular events (because of a history of past myocardial infarction, stroke, TIA or other vascular disease). Patients have been randomized between cholesterol reduction with simvastatin and control and are then to be followed for at least 5 years, and follow-up continues. This study will have sufficient power to detect worthwhile reductions in death from all causes as well as in fatal and non-fatal coronary events (Keech *et al.* 1994; Collins & Peto 1999).

Effect of cholesterol reduction on stroke

A systematic review of the randomized controlled trials in the primary and secondary prevention of stroke and coronary heart disease showed that cholesterol reduction with non-statin drugs did not appear to affect the risk of fatal or non-fatal stroke (Table 16.8) (Di Mascio *et al.* 2000). However, statin drugs were associated with larger reductions in cholesterol and a 23% relative reduction in fatal or non-fatal stroke, but the confidence interval was wide (95% CI for reduction in odds of stroke, 13–33%). The effects of cholesterol reduction on fatal stroke and on haemorrhagic stroke remain unclear. Existing trial data cannot exclude the possibility that statins increase the risk of haemorrhagic stroke (Plehn *et al.* 1999; White *et al.* 2000).

Table 16.8 Effects of cholesterol reduction stroke; evidence from all available randomized trials (from Di Mascio *et al.* 2000).

	Trials	Total cholesterol reduction, % (SD)	Number of stroke events included in this analysis	Odds reduction (%)	(95% CI)
Clinical setting					
Primary prevention	9	15 (6)	273	4	(–21–24)
Secondary prevention	25	18 (7)	1071	20	(9–29)*
Treatment					
Statin drugs	16	22 (4)	846	23	(13–33)*
Other drugs	12	13 (6)	439	–4	(–28–15)
Other interventions	5	14 (4)	69	28	(–17–66)
Total cholesterol reduction (%)					
< 10	8	9 (1)	427	–4	(–28–15)
10–20	13	15 (3)	670	23	(10–34)*
> 20	12	24 (4)	257	25	(4–41)*

SD, standard deviation. Negative numbers indicate that treatment increases the odds of stroke (i.e. is harmful). Confidence intervals with only positive numbers (*) indicate a statistically significant reduction in the odds of stroke (at the $P < 0.05$ level at least).

The BHF/MRC Heart Protection Study will include about 6000 patients with a past history of stroke or TIA and there should be sufficient stroke outcome events to provide reliable estimates of the effects on 'total stroke' (i.e. whether any increase in haemorrhagic stroke is offset by a greater reduction in ischaemic stroke) (Keech *et al.* 1994; Collins & Peto 1999). It will also provide useful evidence on the effects of statins in older patients. A second trial, the Stroke Prevention by Aggressive Reduction in Cholesterol Levels (SPARCL), has recently started; it is comparing atorvastatin with placebo in 4200 patients with minor stroke or TIA and primary assessment of outcome is the effect on total stroke (http://www.neuro.wustl.edu/stroke/trials/). It is plausible that cholesterol reduction may prevent vascular dementia as well as ischaemic stroke. This hypothesis is being tested in the pravastatin in the prevention of cerebrovascular disease and its consequences in the elderly (PROSPER) study (Gaw *et al.* 1999).

Effect of cholesterol reduction on carotid and vertebral atheroma

There have been several trials evaluating the effect of cholesterol-lowering drugs (chiefly statins and fibrates) on the progression of carotid atheroma, and it appears that the treatment may slow or arrest progression. Individually, none of the trials have followed patients for long enough to know reliably whether this reduces either the risk of stroke, or avoids the need for vascular surgical procedures on the carotid or vertebral arteries (Mack *et al.* 1993; Adams *et al.* 1995; Crouse *et al.* 1995; Hodis *et al.* 1996; Mercuri *et al.* 1996; MacMahon *et al.* 1998). A systematic review of these trials to examine the effects of cholesterol reduction on the progression of carotid atheroma would be helpful.

Who to treat: dietary advice to reduce fat intake for all

Blood lipid levels should either be measured within 48 h of stroke onset or at 3 months after the stroke, if a reliable reading is required to guide treatment (Butterworth *et al.* 1997). As with blood pressure, there is no threshold level of cholesterol below which the risk of coronary events does not fall so, in general, 'the lower the cholesterol the better'. It therefore seems prudent to advise all survivors of ischaemic stroke (almost all of whom have a cholesterol higher than 3 mmol/L) to reduce their dietary intake of saturated fat. Moderate dietary change, which can reduce plasma cholesterol by 0.6 mmol/L, can lead to a worthwhile reduction in the risk of coronary events (Law *et al.* 1994a,b). Patients are more likely to achieve cholesterol reduction by diet if they have been told their cholesterol level, or at least have been informed that it is high (Elton *et al.* 1994). Individualized dietary advice can reduce blood cholesterol by 5.3% (Tang *et al.* 1998).

The rationale for suggesting dietary cholesterol reduction in survivors of ischaemic stroke and TIA is simply that their *cerebro*vascular event immediately identifies them as being at higher risk of all vascular events, including coronary events, than normal people (section 16.1). The presence of symptomatic vascular disease (i.e. the stroke) shifts the relationship between cholesterol and coronary heart disease to the left. So that, for a given level of cholesterol, the risk of a coronary event is substantially higher (Fig. 16.10). This is confirmed by the lipid research clinic programme data (Fig. 16.11) showing the difference in risk of future coronary

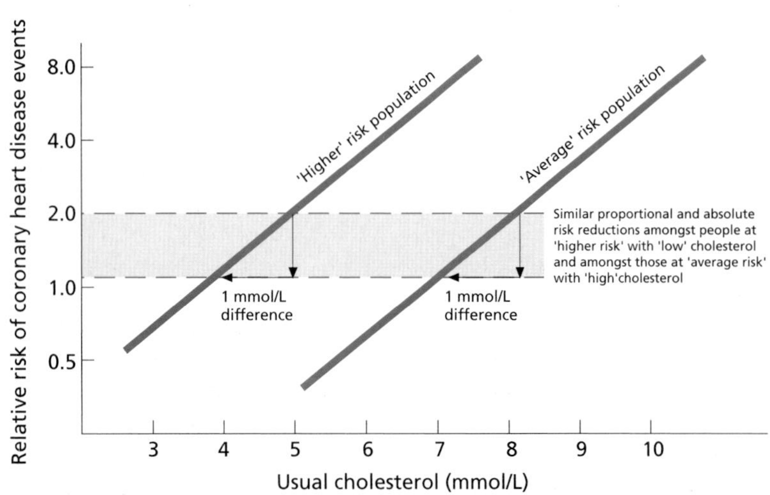

Fig. 16.10 Relative risk of coronary heart disease (CHD) at various levels of plasma cholesterol. The right-hand regression line indicates the relationship between usual cholesterol and CHD in an 'average-risk population' (generally individuals who are free of vascular disease at baseline). The left-hand regression line (higher risk population) represents the relationship between CHD and cholesterol amongst individuals at higher risk, usually because of the presence of symptomatic vascular disease at baseline. In both categories of patients a similar reduction in cholesterol (1.0 mmol) leads to an approximate halving of the risk of CHD. However, in high-risk populations, a cholesterol level of 5.0 mmol/L is associated with a four-fold higher risk of CHD than a similar cholesterol level in the average risk population (J. Armitage, personal communication 1996).

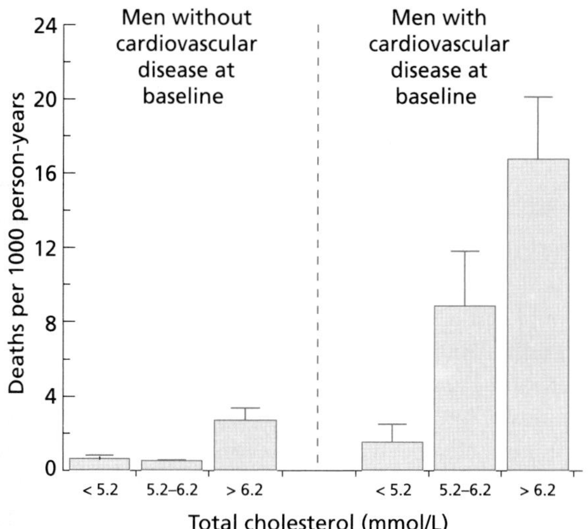

Fig. 16.11 Lipid Research Clinics Programme Prevention Study: this figure further illustrates the difference between high- and low-risk populations. Amongst a high-risk population (men with symptomatic cardiovascular disease (CVD) at baseline) a given level of cholesterol is associated with a substantially higher risk of future death from coronary heart disease than in a low-risk population (men without symptomatic CVD at baseline) (with permission from Pekkanen *et al.* 1990).

events in individuals with and without symptomatic cardiovascular disease at baseline, in relation to their plasma cholesterol levels (Pekkanen *et al.* 1990).

Thus, the decision to reduce cholesterol is based not just on the level of cholesterol, but on the presence of other clinical predictors of outcome such as the presence of symptomatic cerebrovascular or coronary artery disease. Given everyone should consider reducing their cholesterol by diet, it seems reasonable to tell people their cholesterol level and give simple dietary advice. Dieticians in different hospitals have different criteria (i.e. different levels of cholesterol) for accepting referrals for dietary intervention. Many different organizations produce appropriate leaflets advising on suitable dietary change. The Scottish Intercollegiate Guidelines Network (2000) has published useful guidelines on lipid management (also available at http://www.show.nhs.uk/sign/clinical.htm).

It seems prudent to advise all survivors of stroke to reduce their dietary intake of saturated fat. Moderate dietary change can lead to a worthwhile reduction in the risk of coronary events.

Cholesterol reduction with statins

The results of available trials suggest that any patient with a history of ischaemic stroke or TIA *and* coronary heart disease and a cholesterol level greater than 5.0 mmol/L (or low-density lipoprotein (LDL) cholesterol > 3 mmol/L) is likely to benefit from cholesterol reduction with a statin (Consensus Conference on Lipid Lowering to Prevent Vascular Events 1999; Probstfield 2000). We would not recommend *routine* use of statins in TIA and stroke patients until the results from the MRC/BHF Heart Protection Study are available; in the interim, useful guidelines on the assessment and management of hyperlipidaemia are published in *Clinical Evidence* (Godlee *et al.* 2000) and by the Scottish Intercollegiate Guidelines Network (2000).

Cholesterol reduction by dietary means is advisable in all patients with recent stroke or transient ischaemic attack. This should reduce the risk of coronary events. Which patients benefit the most from cholesterol reduction with drugs will be determined by current trials, but present evidence suggests that statins are indicated in transient ischaemic attack and ischaemic stroke patients with a history of myocardial infarction or angina.

Agent/dose/adverse effects/cost

Pravastatin has been licensed by the US Food and Drug Aministration for stroke prevention in patients with coronary heart disease and average levels of cholesterol (< 6.2 mmol/L) and simvastatin has been approved for treatment of patients with coronary heart disease and high levels of cholesterol (5.8–8.0 mmol/L) (Gorelick & Mazzone 1999). The natural statins lovastatin, pravastatin and simvastatin are fermentation-derived and have a similar structure, whereas the newer synthetic statins (atorvastatin, cerivastatin and fluvastatin) have very different structures; it is not clear which is the best agent for the prevention of vascular events or stroke (Furberg 1999).

The reduction in cholesterol level with statins is dose related, but the optimum dose for the prevention of vascular events is unclear. Adverse effects are uncommon, and dose related: increases in liver transaminases occur in about 0.5%; slight rises in muscle enzyme level in about 5–10%; muscle pain associated with marked increases in muscle enzymes > 10 times the normal range is rare (< 0.1%) and reversible; increases in cerebral haemorrhage, cancer and non-vascular deaths have all been suggested, but not confirmed (Sudlow & Baigent 2000a; Probstfield 2000). The rarer adverse events with statins and other cholesterol-reducing agents have been reviewed in detail elsewhere (Knopp 1999).

Though effective and relatively safe, statins are expensive. Whilst the costs per life year gained for people with an annual risk of coronary events of more than 3% are high, and lie between £6000 and £11 000, this is comparable to other interventions in secondary prevention (Pickin & McCabe 1999). However, the total cost to health service providers will be large. In a typical general practice population of 10 000 patients, 353 patients with coronary artery disease might require treatment, at a total annual cost of £176 000 to £214 000 (Pickin & McCabe 1999). If every person aged 45–74 in the UK with clinical evidence of coronary heart disease were treated with a statin for 5 years, about 22 000 deaths and major clinical events would be avoided, at a cost £228 million (Davey Smith & Ebrahim 1999).

16.3.3 Smoking cessation

Smoking and the risk of stroke

In 1995, smoking caused three million deaths and it is forecast that, by the year 2025, smoking could cause perhaps 10 million deaths per year worldwide (Peto 1994). Long-term follow-up studies, started in the 1950s, have shown that the association between smoking and deaths from cancer and vascular diseases is far stronger than had previously been thought. The old statement, based partly on the first 20 years of the Study of British Doctors, that 'at least a quarter' of all regular cigarette smokers would be killed by the habit now needs revision. In fact, the proportion is about 50% (Peto 1994). Smoking is clearly a risk factor for ischaemic stroke (section 6.3.3) and for subarachnoid haemorrhage (section 9.1.1); its effect on the risk of primary intracerebral haemorrhage is less clear (Shinton & Beevers 1989; Donnan *et al.* 1993, Hankey 1999b). Passive smoking is also a risk factor for stroke (Bonita *et al.* 1999) (section 6.3.3).

Benefits of stopping

There have been no satisfactory controlled trials randomizing people between 'continue smoking' and 'stop smoking', but the adverse health effects of smoking are so clearly established that all who use tobacco in any form (cigarettes, pipe, cigars or chewing tobacco) should be advised to stop; the risks of stroke are likely to decline within 2–5 years of stopping (Peto 1994; Nicholas & Kottke 2000).

Table 16.9 Effectiveness of different forms of nicotine replacement therapy (NRT) in achieving smoking cessation (quitting) (modified from Silagy *et al.*1999).

	Proportion quitting		
	Treated (%)	Control (%)	Odds ratio (95% CI)
Gum	19	12	1.6 (1.5–1.8)
Patches	14	8	1.8 (1.6–2.0)
Nasal spray	24	12	2.3 (1.6–3.2)
Inhaler	17	9	2.0 (1.4–3.0)
All NRT trials	16	10	1.7 (1.6–1.8)

Note: an odds ratio of 1.7 indicates that nicotine replacement therapy increased the odds of quitting 1.7-fold (or by 70%), or if 16 smokers are given nicotine replacement therapy, one will quit.

Best methods to aid smoking cessation

There is now clear evidence that simple advice from a physician and nicotine replacement therapy (NRT) are both effective (and cost-effective) aids to smoking cessation (Silagy & Ketteridge 2000; Silagy *et al.* 2000) (Table 16.9). A formal review of the randomized controlled trials evaluating different forms of NRT showed that all of the commercially available forms (nicotine gum, transdermal patch, and in some countries, the nicotine nasal spray, nicotine inhaler and nicotine sublingual tablets) are effective as part of a strategy to promote smoking cessation. They increase quit rates approximately 1.5–2-fold regardless of the setting (Silagy *et al.* 2000). For patients who are particularly nicotine dependent, the 4 mg gum is significantly more effective than the lower dose. In less highly dependent smokers, the different preparations are comparable in their efficacy, but nicotine patches offer greater convenience and minimal need for instruction; nicotine patches appear safe in people with coronary artery disease (Ness & Lonn 2000). Inhalers and nasal sprays are useful in patients with particularly severe nicotine craving.

Training the physicians who give advice on smoking cessation improves their effectiveness (Thorogood 2000). Encouraging smoking partners of patients also to quit smoking may help the patient to abstain and will also reduce the patient's exposure to environmental tobacco smoke; both of these effects are likely to beneficial.

Smoking cessation, aided by nicotine replacement therapy if necessary, is advisable for all smokers whether they have had a stroke or not.

16.3.4 Reduction in alcohol intake

High levels of alcohol consumption are associated with high blood pressure, and are also a risk factor for stroke and vascular dementia in a number of observational studies (Hillbom *et al.* 1999) (section 6.3.3). However, some studies have suggested that people who abstain completely from alcohol have a somewhat higher risk of cardiovascular events (possibly including stroke) than individuals who drink a modest to a moderate amount of alcohol regularly (Hillbom *et al.* 1999) (section 6.3.3). Reducing heavy alcohol intake is therefore advisable, since it is likely to reduce blood pressure, although whether this will reduce the risk of stroke or vascular dementia is not known; complete abstinence, however, may not be a good idea (Hillbom *et al.* 1999; Mulrow & Jackson 2000).

16.3.5 Healthy diet and weight reduction

Observational epidemiological studies show, with reasonable consistency, that a diet rich in fresh fruit and vegetables is associated with a lower risk of stroke (Ness & Powles 1999) (section 6.3.3). The average westerner must make several changes to achieve a healthier diet: reduce the total fat content of the diet to no more than 30% of calorie intake; switch from saturated animal fat to unsaturated vegetable fats; increase the intake of vegetables and fresh fruit and dietary fibre; and reduce the consumption of low-residue processed foods. Such a diet is also likely to reduce blood pressure slightly (Mulrow & Jackson 2000). The role of a healthy diet and/or increased vitamin C and fish consumption in the primary prevention of stroke and vascular disease remains unclear, but a diet rich in these nutrients has the potential to be protective (Khaw & Woodhouse 1995; Morris *et al.* 1995, Ness & Powles 1999, Ness 2000; Mulrow & Jackson 2000).

Randomized trials of different dietary interventions after myocardial infarction (advising patients to eat a more Mediterranean diet: more oily fish, more fruit and vegetables, bread, pasta and olive oil) may result in substantial survival benefit (Ness & Lonn 2000). It therefore seems reasonable to inform stroke survivors with a history of ischaemic heart disease about the components of a healthy diet. Weight reduction with or without restriction of sodium intake is a safe and effective way of reducing blood pressure in hypertensive older people (Whelton *et al.* 1998; Brand *et al.* 2000; Mulrow & Jackson 2000).

16.3.6 Vitamins, antioxidants and fish oil

Folic acid

A raised plasma homocysteine is a risk factor for stroke and vascular disease (Perry 1999; Hankey & Eikelboom 1999) (section 6.3.3). Increasing folate intake with dietary supplements of 0.5–5 mg folic acid (with about 0.5 mg vitamin B_{12}) can lower plasma homocysteine levels by one-quarter to one-third (Homocysteine Lowering Trialists' Collaboration 1998). The effects of folic acid supplements in the secondary prevention of vascular events after stroke are being studied in two current trials; at present there is no indication for routine folate supplementation after stroke (Hankey 1999a; Hankey & Eikelboom 1999; Toole 1999). Further details of the Vitamins in Stroke Prevention (VISP) and VITAmins TO Prevent Stroke (VITATOPS) trials are available at http://www.neuro.wustl.edu/stroke/trials/index.htm and http://www.health.wa.gov.au/VITATOPS/ respectively.

Antioxidants

Laboratory evidence suggests that oxidative modification of LDL cholesterol may be an important stage in the formation and rupture of atherosclerotic plaques (Witzum 1994). The few observational studies of intake of antioxidants and stroke risk suggest that low antioxidant levels (chiefly beta-carotene and vitamin C) are associated with an increased risk of stroke (Manson *et al.* 1993; Keli *et al.* 1996; Neve 1996; Daviglus *et al.* 1997; Ness & Powles 1999) (section 6.3.3). This suggested that administering antioxidant compounds, by protecting cholesterol from oxidation, may reduce the risk of ischaemic stroke. A number of dietary constituents have antioxidant properties, such as certain minerals (e.g. selenium, copper, zinc, manganese), vitamins (C, E), provitamins (beta-carotene) and flavonoids. But the trials to date have not provided evidence of benefit. The trials of beta-carotene supplements in either primary or secondary prevention of vascular events did not provide evidence of benefit and there was some evidence of harm overall (Ness & Powles 1999; Ness 2000; Ness & Lonn 2000). Vitamin E supplements were not effective after myocardial infarction (GISSI-Prevenzione Investigators 1999). In the second part of the HOPE trial, patients were given vitamin E or placebo. After up to 4.5 years of use, vitamin E had not reduced the incidence of myocardial infarction, stroke or cardiovascular deaths, thus confirming previous studies. However, this part of the study is to continue with the aim of assessing the impact of prolonged vitamin E treatment on prevention of cancers as well as of vascular disease (Heart Outcomes Prevention Evaluation (HOPE) Study Investigators 2000a). The effects of a cocktail of antioxidant vitamins in stroke prevention are being evaluated in the ongoing MRC/BHF Heart Protection Study (Keech *et al.* 1994; Collins & Peto 1999). The Women's Health Initiative (WHI) and the Women's Antioxidant and Cardiovascular Study (WACS) are also assessing the effects of antioxidants on vascular events (see http://www.cardiosource.com and Manson *et al.* (1995)). At present, there is no indication to use antioxidant supplements routinely for secondary prevention after stroke.

Fish oil

Fish oil supplements might reduce the risk of vascular disease and lower blood pressure slightly, but the available evidence is insufficient to support their routine use for primary or secondary stroke prevention (Hooper *et al.* 2000; Mulrow & Jackson 2000). In patients with previous myocardial infarction, a dietary supplement of *n*-3 polyunsaturated fats (a component of fish oil) was associated with a reduction in death from cardiovascular causes, with no apparent effect on fatal or non-fatal stroke (GISSI-Prevenzione Investigators 1999).

16.3.7 Management of diabetes mellitus and glucose intolerance

Diabetes mellitus and glucose intolerance are important risk factors for ischaemic stroke (Tuomilehto & Rastenye 1999) (section 6.3.3). The randomized trials have shown that more intensive treatment of hyperglycaemia results in fewer microvascular complications of diabetes (retinopathy and renal damage) but not necessarily fewer macrovascular complications (i.e. stroke and myocardial infarction). None the less, early detection of diabetes and glucose intolerance, followed by careful control of glycaemia and attention to vascular risk factors are very likely to improve long-term outcome (Tuomilehto & Rastenye 1999; Sigal 2000). The management of hyperglycaemia and diabetes mellitus in the acute phase of stroke is discussed in section 15.18.3.

16.3.8 Exercise

Observational studies show reasonably consistently that physical activity is associated with a lower risk of stroke, independent of other factors (Evenson *et al.* 1999; Wannamethee & Shaper 1999) (section 6.3.3). A systematic review of rather questionable quality, of largely non-randomized evidence, estimated that exercise programmes for people aged 45 and over might be both effective in primary stroke prevention and also cost-effective (Nicholl *et al.* 1994). Cardiac rehabilitation programmes (of which exercise is just a part) reduce the frequency of major cardiac events after myocardial infarction. Aerobic exercise reduces blood pressure, but the effects of exercise programmes alone after myocardial infarction or stroke on the occurrence of further vascular events are unknown (Mulrow & Jackson 2000; Ness & Lonn 2000). After a stroke, patients should be encouraged to return to normal physical activities, but the levels of physical activity likely to reduce the risk of further vascular events may not be achievable. However, exercise may bring other benefits; in the elderly, structured exercise programmes may reduce the risk of falls (Campbell *et al.* 1998; Gillespie *et al.* 2000).

16.4 Antiplatelet drugs

Patients with a history of symptomatic vascular disease (i.e. myocardial infarction, ischaemic stroke, transient ischaemic attack (TIA), angina, intermittent claudication, etc.) are at particular risk of vascular death or of further cardiac or cerebrovascular events. Platelets are involved in the pathophysiology, not just of acute thrombosis occurring in arteries and veins, but possibly also in the process of atherogenesis in arterial walls (section 6.3.2). Antiplatelet drugs should, in theory, therefore reduce the risk of recurrent vascular events.

16.4.1 Evidence

Measures of outcome

Antiplatelet drugs may prevent not just ischaemic stroke, but also myocardial infarction and deaths from other forms of vascular disease involving thrombosis. The most appropriate analysis of efficacy is therefore based on the composite outcome of 'stroke, myocardial infarction or vascular death' (whichever occurs first). This composite outcome will be referred to as 'vascular events': it also includes haemorrhagic stroke and any deaths from bleeding, so it also provides a convenient summation of benefit (any reductions in ischaemic events) plus risk (any increases in haemorrhages). Because the number of events is greater, the composite also provides more statistical power, and therefore precision, in estimating treatment effect than any of the individual components. However, if the number of outcome events is sufficient, it is not unreasonable to at least explore treatment effects on individual outcomes, such as stroke or coronary events. There is increasing interest in whether aspirin might reduce the risk of progressive cognitive impairment and vascular dementia in high-risk subjects, through a variety of intermediate factors (Williams *et al.* 2000).

Data available

A systematic review by the Antiplatelet Trialists' Collaboration (APT) of the trials available in 1994 provided clear evidence of the benefits of antiplatelet drugs (Antiplatelet Trialists' Collaboration 1994). The review group is now broadened to include trials of anticoagulants, so it was renamed the Antithrombotic Trialists Collaboration (ATT). The analyses were updated to include all the antiplatelet trials available by 1997 (Antithrombotic Trialists' Collaboration 2000): 198 trials (140 000 patients) comparing antiplatelet drug(s) with control; 10 trials (6500 patients) directly comparing different daily doses of aspirin; 27 trials (34 000 patients) comparing another single antiplatelet drug with aspirin alone and 43 trials (37 000 patients) comparing aspirin plus another antiplatelet drug with aspirin alone.

Effects in people at high risk

For these analyses, 'high risk' was defined by the presence—at the time of randomization in the trial—of some form of symptomatic vascular disease such as myocardial infarction, angina, stroke, TIA or intermittent claudication. Among patients with acute ischaemic stroke, immediate

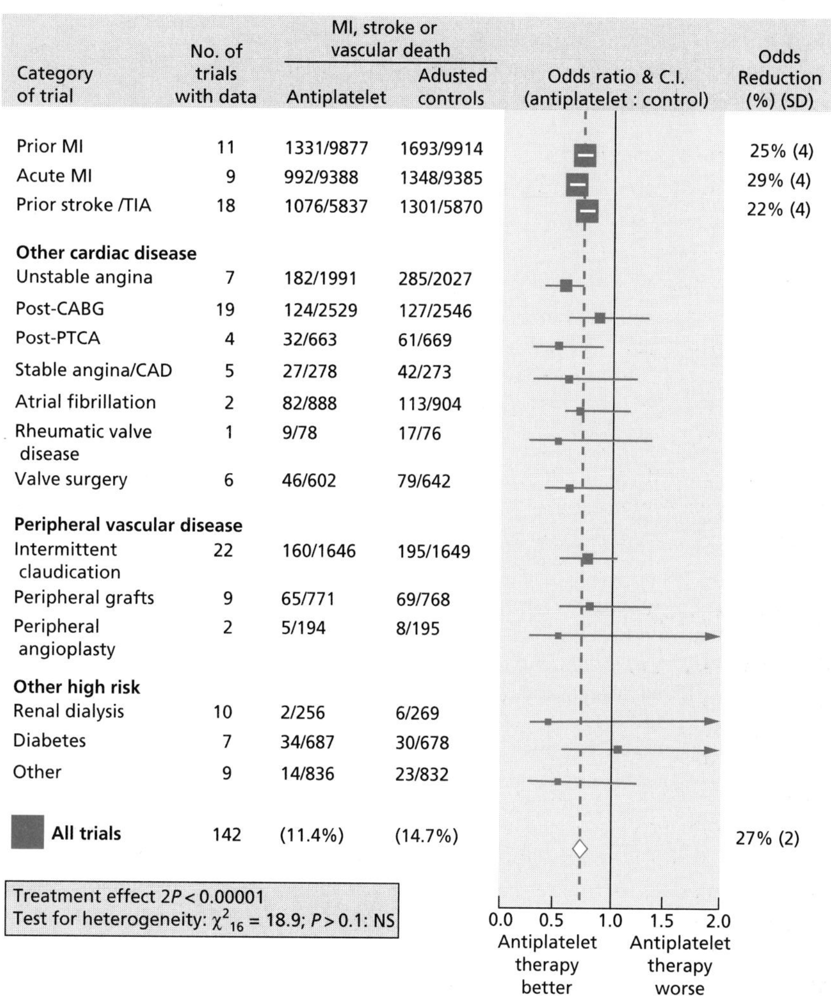

Category of trial
No. of trials with data
MI, stroke or vascular death
Antiplatelet
Adusted controls
Odds ratio & C.I. (antiplatelet : control)
Odds Reduction (%) (SD)
Prior MI 11 1331/9877 1693/9914 25% (4)
Acute MI 9 992/9388 1348/9385 29% (4)
Prior stroke /TIA 18 1076/5837 1301/5870 22% (4)
Other cardiac disease
Unstable angina 7 182/1991 285/2027
Post-CABG 19 124/2529 127/2546
Post-PTCA 4 32/663 61/669
Stable angina/CAD 5 27/278 42/273
Atrial fibrillation 2 82/888 113/904
Rheumatic valve disease 1 9/78 17/76
Valve surgery 6 46/602 79/642
Peripheral vascular disease
Intermittent claudication 22 160/1646 195/1649
Peripheral grafts 9 65/771 69/768
Peripheral angioplasty 2 5/194 8/195
Other high risk
Renal dialysis 10 2/256 6/269
Diabetes 7 34/687 30/678
Other 9 14/836 23/832
All trials 142 (11.4%) (14.7%) 27% (2)
Treatment effect 2P < 0.00001
Test for heterogeneity: χ²16 = 18.9; P > 0.1: NS
0.0 0.5 1.0 1.5 2.0
Antiplatelet therapy better
Antiplatelet therapy worse

Fig. 16.12 Proportional effects of antiplatelet therapy on serious vascular events in 142 trials of antiplatelet therapy vs. control in patients subdivided by type of trial. CABG, coronary artery bypass grafting; CAD, coronary artery disease; MI, myocardial infarction; PTCA, percutaneous transluminal coronary angioplasty. In most trials, patients were allocated roughly evenly between treatment groups, but in some more were deliberately allocated to active treatment; to allow direct comparisons between percentages having an event in each treatment group, in this figure and elsewhere, adjusted totals have been calculated after converting any unevenly randomized trials to even ones by counting control patients more than once. Statistical calculations are, however, based on actual numbers from individual trials. The ratio of the odds of an event in the treatment group compared with that in the control group is plotted for each trial (dark green square: area proportional to amount of statistical information contributed by trial) along with its 99% confidence interval (horizontal line). Stratified overview of the result of all trials (and 95% confidence interval) is represented by an open diamond, indicating odds ratio of 0.73 (SD 0.02) or, equivalently, an odds reduction of 27% (SD 2) (with permission from the Antiplatelet Trialists' Collaboration 1994). An updated version of this figure that includes the results of the Antithrombotic Trialists' Collaboration 2000 analyses will be available at http://www.dcn.ed.ac.uk/spgm.

antiplatelet therapy reduced the odds of a vascular event by 11%, corresponding to the avoidance of about 12 vascular events for every 1000 patients treated for about 1 month (section 11.3.2). In the 1994 APT analyses, for all other categories of high-risk patients, antiplatelet drugs reduced the odds of a serious vascular event by about one-quarter and this proportional reduction was remarkably consistent across different categories of high-risk patients (Fig. 16.12). The studies evaluating antiplatelet drugs in patients with a history of past stroke or TIA suggested they reduced the risk of vascular events from about 22% to about 18%, equivalent to the avoidance of 37 serious vascular events per 1000 patients treated over about 3 years (Fig. 16.13). In other words, about 27 of these high-risk individuals need to receive antiplatelet drugs for 3 years to avoid one serious vascular event. The similar absolute benefits for antiplatelet drugs amongst patients who are at risk for other reasons are also shown in Fig. 16.13. The final results of the ATT 2000 analyses were broadly similar. A link to the publication reporting the results will be available on the website associated with this book (http://www.dcn.ed.ac.uk/spgm).

Antiplatelet drugs are antihaemostatic and so, not surprisingly, associated with a small but definite excess of haemorrhagic strokes. In the overview of the long-term trials, haemorrhagic strokes occurred in 0.2% of controls and 0.3% of treated patients, i.e. an excess of about one per 1000 patients treated over an average of 2.5 years (Antiplatelet Trialists' Collaboration 1994). However, this small but definite hazard is enormously outweighed by the reduction of recurrent ischaemic stroke, both in the acute phase of stroke, and in long-term secondary prevention. The balance of risk and benefit is therefore favourable for most individuals at high vascular risk as a result of a TIA or an ischaemic stroke (section 16.4.2).

There are limited data from the trials comparing antiplatelet drugs with control for primary and secondary stroke pre-

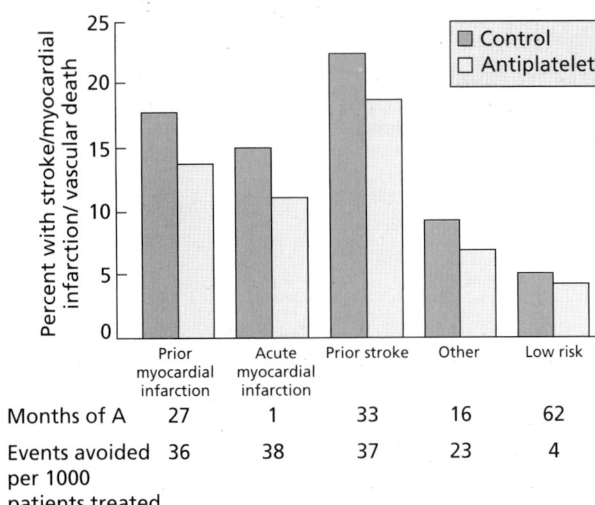

Fig. 16.13 Absolute effects of antiplatelet therapy (145 trials) on serious vascular events (myocardial infarction, stroke or vascular death) in four high-risk categories of patient (secondary prevention) and in low-risk people (primary prevention). Adjusted totals calculated after converting any unevenly randomized trials to even ones by counting control patients more than once. Statistical significance (2*P*) based on stratified analyses of original, unadjusted numbers in each trial. Months of A, means of scheduled antiplatelet therapy duration. No trial lasted under 1 month (with permission from Antiplatelet Trialists' Collaboration 1994). An updated version of this figure that includes the results of the Antithrombotic Trialists' Collaboration 2000 analyses will be available at http://www.dcn.ed.ac.uk/spgm.

vention in patients with atrial fibrillation. The numbers of events in the trials were small, so the confidence intervals were wide, but the point estimate for the benefit was similar to that seen in patients without atrial fibrillation: the relative reduction in risk of stroke was 24% (95% CI, 7–39%) and of vascular events was 19% (95% CI, 1–34%) (Atrial Fibrillation Investigators 1999; Hart *et al.* 1999; Benavente *et al.* 2000). These analyses did not identify any subgroup of patient which was particularly responsive (or unresponsive) to aspirin. In primary prevention, about 10 strokes would be avoided yearly for every 1000 patients treated with aspirin and about 24 per year in secondary prevention (Hart *et al.* 1999, Benavente *et al.* 2000). The evidence from the trials which compared warfarin with aspirin is discussed in section 16.5.1.

Likewise, the effects of aspirin on preventing early recurrence during the acute phase of stroke, are similar in patients with and without atrial fibrillation. The International Stroke Trial (IST) and the Chinese Acute Stroke Trial (CAST) included 4500 patients with acute ischaemic stroke who were in atrial fibrillation at the time of randomization. In these patients, the risk of recurrent stroke in hospital within the first 2–4 weeks was 2.9% in the controls and 2.0% in patients allocated aspirin. The one-third reduction in the odds of recurrent ischaemic stroke with aspirin was again no different to that seen in patients without atrial fibrillation (Chen *et al.* 2000).

The rather sparse data on the choice of antithrombotic regimen in patients in whom atrial fibrillation is associated with various other cardiac disorders, such as valvular heart disease, cardiomyopathy, etc. have recently been published and summarized in guidelines (Salen *et al.* 1998; Stein *et al.* 1998; Scottish Intercollegiate Guidelines Network 1999, also available at: http://www.show.scot.nhs.uk/sign/clinical.htm).

Cardiac lesions other than atrial fibrillation

Data are available from 14 trials comparing antiplatelet drugs with controls in about 5000 patients with a cardiac lesion associated with a high embolic risk. About half of these patients had been randomized in trials where the presence of atrial fibrillation was a primary eligibility criterion, and the remainder had either valvular heart disease or prosthetic heart valves. The one-quarter relative reduction in vascular events with antiplatelet drugs was not significantly different from that observed in other high-risk groups (Antithrombotic Trialists' Collaboration 2000). The rather poor quality evidence comparing the effects of antiplatelet drugs with anticoagulants and other antithrombotic agents in this heterogeneous group has been reviewed in a number of consensus and guideline documents (Salen *et al.* 1998; Stein *et al.* 1998; Scottish Intercollegiate Guidelines Network 1999, also available at http://www.show.scot.nhs.uk/sign/clinical.htm) (section 16.5.1).

Effects in people at low risk

Individuals who are asymptomatic, free of vascular risk factors and with no history of previous symptomatic vascular disease, are at extremely low vascular risk. Three trials examined the effects of aspirin in 29 000 people (almost all physicians). None had a history of prior vascular events, but some had vascular risk factors, so their average annual risk of a serious vascular event was 1% or less. The four per 1000 reduction in vascular events over an average of 5 years was not statistically or clinically significant (Antiplatelet Trialists' Collaboration 1994).

Two trials have examined the effects of aspirin in people who have not had a symptomatic vascular event but who did have identifiable vascular risk factors. The Hypertension Optimal Treatment (HOT) trial aimed to evaluate the effects of aspirin in people at slightly higher than average risk of vascular disease as a result of hypertension. In this study, 18 790 hypertensive people were randomly allocated to 75 mg aspirin daily or open control in a factorial design with various interventions to lower blood pressure to different target levels (Hansson *et al.* 1998). The risk of stroke in this population was very low—just 1.6% in the controls over 3.8 years, or 0.4%/year. Although low-dose aspirin reduced the annual risk of vascular events from 10.5 to 8.9 per 1000 patient years, the absolute risk reduction was small (0.16%), so 625 hypertensive individuals would need to be treated for 1 year to prevent a single vascular event. There was no apparent effect on total stroke, fatal stroke or fatal haemorrhagic stroke, but there was a significant excess of non-fatal haemorrhages with aspirin, chiefly gastrointestinal, but again the absolute risk was low, and the excess was less than 0.5%/year (1.4% aspirin vs. 0.7% control over 3.8 years).

The thrombosis prevention trial evaluated low-intensity oral anticoagulation (target international normalized ratio (INR) 1.5), 75 mg aspirin daily, both or neither in the primary prevention of ischaemic heart disease (IHD) in a two-by-two factorial design (Meade *et al.* 1998). About 5500 men aged between 45 years and 69 years without prior stroke or myocardial infarction, but with a high risk of IHD, as defined by a risk score, were included. Compared with control, aspirin reduced 'all IHD' by 20%, almost entirely due to a 32% relative reduction in non-fatal events; the absolute reduction in 'all IHD' due to aspirin was 2.3 per 1000 person years. The 0.7% reduction in non-fatal ischaemic stroke was offset by a similar-sized increase in haemorrhagic or fatal stroke, so that overall, there was no difference in total stroke (2.9% aspirin, 3.0% control).

At least two other studies are ongoing. The Women's Health Study is examining the effects of aspirin in a randomized trial involving 40 000 apparently healthy postmenopausal women and results are expected soon (Buring & Hennekens 1992). The Aspirin in Asymptomatic Atherosclerosis (AAA) trial is examining the effects of aspirin in avoiding vascular events in 3000 patients with asymptomatic peripheral vascular disease (G. Fowkes, personal communication).

A recent meta-analysis of all of the clinical trials in low-risk individuals did not show evidence of a reduction in total strokes with aspirin, so we would not recommend it (Hart *et al.* 2000a; Sudlow & Baigent 2000b).

Effects on vascular dementia

Thromboxane biosynthesis is increased in stroke patients who develop vascular dementia, though it is not clear what part this plays in pathogenesis (van Kooten *et al.* 1999). Aspirin both inhibits thromboxane biosynthesis and prevents recurrent strokes, so might be expected to reduce either the frequency or severity of vascular dementia. A systematic review of aspirin in the prevention of vascular dementia identified only one inconclusive trial (Williams *et al.* 2000). However, a small substudy from the thrombosis prevention trial reported that patients allocated antithrombotic therapy had greater verbal fluency and mental flexibility (Richards *et al.* 1997). A planned substudy in the AAA trial will also examine the effects of aspirin on the occurrence of cognitive decline and frank dementia (G. Fowkes, personal communication).

16.4.2 Who to treat

Patients with transient ischaemic attack or ischaemic stroke

Almost all patients with TIA or ischaemic stroke have a sufficiently high risk of further vascular events to justify the use of long-term antiplatelet drugs (section 16.1.1). The relative reductions in the risk of vascular events were identical in patients presenting with TIAs and with completed ischaemic stroke (Antiplatelet Trialists' Collaboration 1994; Antithrombotic Trialists' Collaboration 2000). In high-risk individuals the proportional reductions in vascular events were approximately similar in males and females, diabetics and non-diabetics, older patients and younger patients, and in patients with and without hypertension (Antiplatelet Trialists' Collaboration 1994).

> *In general, we would treat most patients with symptomatic vascular disease—including ischaemic stroke and transient ischaemic attack—with antiplatelet drugs because all these patients are at sufficiently high risk of serious vascular events to justify the inconvenience, cost and small risks of treatment.*

Patients with transient ischaemic attack or ischaemic stroke and atrial fibrillation unsuitable for anticoagulation

Most patients with atrial fibrillation and a history of ischaemic stroke or TIA have a sufficiently high risk to justify the use of oral anticoagulants (section 16.5). However, for patients with contraindications to warfarin, aspirin is a safe though less effective alternative. Restoration of (and maintenance of) sinus rhythm as a further means of avoiding the need for anticoagulation is discussed in section 16.7.1.

Cardiac lesions other than atrial fibrillation.

Some patients with a potential cardiac source of embolism other than atrial fibrillation may benefit from antiplatelet drugs. The list is extensive and includes: mitral valve prolapse, isolated aortic stenosis, mitral annulus calcification, cardiac failure, patent foramen ovale and bioprosthetic heart valve (Scottish Intercollegiate Guidelines Network 1999, also available at http://www.show.scot.nhs.uk/sign/clinical.htm). For patients with any of these conditions, if there is a history of systemic embolism (or TIA or ischaemic stroke), or if atrial fibrillation is present, anticoagulants may be preferable to antiplatelet drugs (sections 16.5.2 and 16.7.2). However, if oral anticoagulants are contraindicated, or the risk of embolism is low, then antiplatelet drugs are likely to be beneficial. The risk of recurrent vascular events in most individuals with mitral valve prolapse and TIA or stroke who are in sinus rhythm is very low, so antiplatelet drugs are probably adequate (Orencia *et al.* 1995).

We would seldom use antiplatelet drugs in a TIA or ischaemic stroke patient under the age of 40 years with only one of these asymptomatic cardiac abnormalities and no evidence of atrial fibrillation or symptomatic vascular disease in the heart, legs or brain. In older patients, aged over 40 years with such cardiac lesions, we would be more likely to use antiplatelet drugs, particularly if there was also evidence of symptomatic vascular disease.

If we were faced with a woman aged 40, with a transient focal neurological disturbance (which was probably migrainous but might possibly have been thromboembolic), no vascular risk factors, and uncomplicated mitral valve prolapse on echocardiography, we would probably give aspirin empirically. If the attack recurred, we would be more inclined to use aspirin. We would all be very reluctant to use anticoagulants.

Asymptomatic carotid stenosis

There is some debate about whether patients with asymptomatic carotid stenosis have a sufficiently high risk of stroke to justify antiplatelet drugs. A recent small trial did not provide clear evidence of benefit (Cote *et al.* 1995). Since many individuals with asymptomatic stenosis have symptomatic coronary or peripheral vascular disease (and such patients clearly benefit from antiplatelet therapy), the decision about whether or not to use antiplatelet drugs should be governed not so much by the presence or absence of a stenosis, but whether or not the patient has *symptomatic* vascular disease. The role of aspirin in asymptomatic peripheral vascular disease is being examined in the Aspirin in Asymptomatic Atherosclerosis (AAA) trial (G. Fowkes, personal communication).

Patients without symptomatic vascular disease, but with vascular risk factors

Since the unselective use of aspirin in individuals without evidence of cardio- or cerebrovascular disease might damage large numbers of previously healthy individuals, we do not recommend routine aspirin use in these patients.

16.4.3 Who not to treat

It seems illogical to treat somebody with an acute primary intracerebral or subarachnoid haemorrhage (SAH) (at least before any aneurysm is clipped) with an antihaemostatic drug like aspirin. On the other hand, if a patient has an ischaemic stroke and the brain imaging shows haemorrhagic transformation, we would perhaps not start aspirin immediately, but would certainly wish to ensure the patient was discharged on aspirin for long-term secondary prevention. Patients with a history of recent gastrointestinal bleeding (haematemesis or malaena), or with symptoms suggestive of active peptic ulceration, should probably not receive antiplatelet drugs. Those with a definite allergy to aspirin should obviously avoid it. Those with neutropenia should avoid ticlopidine (and probably clopidogrel as well). However, some patients with primary intracerebral haemorrhage or SAH may have a clear indication for aspirin, such as a recent myocardial infarction or unstable angina; in patients with haemorrhagic stroke, long-term aspirin is probably safe after the acute stage, but we cannot be sure for lack of appropriate evidence. After SAH, and clipping of the responsible aneurysm, aspirin is also probably safe.

16.4.4 Agent/dose

Direct and indirect comparisons

The relative efficacy of different antiplatelet agents may be compared in two different ways. *Indirect comparisons* compare the effects of drug X vs. control in disease A, with the effects of drug Y vs. control in disease A, or related disease B. This has obvious limitations, since the drugs X and Y are being compared in somewhat different types of patients. *Direct randomized comparisons*, where patients are randomized in a single trial to receive either drug X or drug Y avoid the bias inherent in indirect comparisons, but are likely to have limited statistical power (Antiplatelet Trialists' Collaboration 1994).

Aspirin ... and what is the right dose?

In the APT and ATT reviews, aspirin was the most extensively tested drug, accounting for about two-thirds of the data. There is proof beyond all reasonable doubt that aspirin is effective; it reduced the odds of a vascular event by about a quarter. The indirect comparisons of the different aspirin dose categories (< 75 mg daily, 75–150 mg daily, 160–325 mg daily and 500–1500 mg daily) did not show any significant heterogeneity of treatment effect (Fig. 16.14). However, in the three trials which compared less than 75 mg daily with control (total 3600 patients), the benefit appeared somewhat smaller and was not statistically significant (odds reduction 13%; 95% CI, 9% increase to 30% reduction). In the direct randomized comparisons there was no clear evidence that any one aspirin dose was more effective than another (Antithrombotic Trialists' Collaboration 2000). However, the confidence intervals were wide, so one cannot exclude clinically important differences between low-dose aspirin (below 75 mg daily) and higher doses (Antithrombotic Trialists' Collaboration 2000). A meta-regression analysis of a smaller set of trials did not provide evidence that the reduction in stroke with aspirin was related to dose in the range 50–1500 mg/day (Johnson *et al.* 1999). Since the ATT review was completed, the Aspirin after Carotid Endarterectomy (ACE) trial has reported its results. The trial compared 3 months' treatment with aspirin at one of four different doses (81 mg, 325 mg, 650 mg and 1300 mg daily) in about 2900 patients undergoing carotid endarterectomy. In this rather specialized setting the odds of serious vascular events over 3 months was 27% (95% CI, 3–45%) lower in patients allocated either of the two lower doses (Taylor *et al.* 1999).

Our preferred dose of aspirin for long-term secondary prevention is 75 mg daily.

Thienopyridines (ticlopidine and clopidogrel) compared with controls

Ticlopidine inhibits the binding of adenosine diphosphate (ADP) to its receptor on platelets, thereby inhibiting ADP-dependent activation of the glycoprotein IIb/IIIa complex, the major receptor for fibrinogen on the platelet surface and the final common pathway of platelet activation (McTavish *et al.* 1990). Clopidogrel is a new thienopyridine derivative, chemically related to ticlopidine. It also inhibits platelet activation by selectively and irreversibly blocking the binding of ADP to its receptor on platelets.

Forty-five trials comparing ticlopidine with control, including 7600 patients, have been completed. Ticlopidine reduced the odds of a serious vascular event by 31% (95% CI, 18–42%) (Antithrombotic Trialists' Collaboration 2000). Ticlopidine alone is an effective antiplatelet drug, and although there were no trials comparing clopidogrel with a control (such trials would rightly have been regarded as

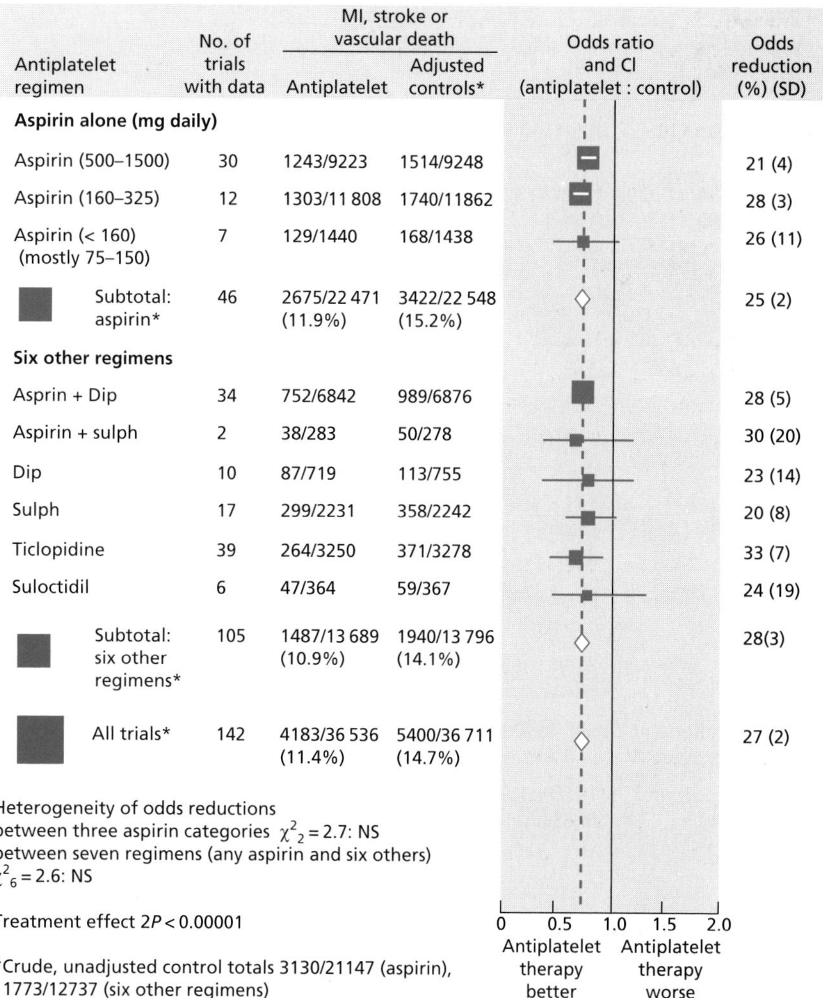

Antiplatelet regimen
No. of trials with data
MI, stroke or vascular death
Antiplatelet
Adjusted controls*
Odds ratio and CI (antiplatelet : control)
Odds reduction (%) (SD)
Aspirin alone (mg daily)
Aspirin (500–1500) 30 1243/9223 1514/9248 21 (4)
Aspirin (160–325) 12 1303/11 808 1740/11862 28 (3)
Aspirin (< 160) (mostly 75–150) 7 129/1440 168/1438 26 (11)
Subtotal: aspirin* 46 2675/22 471 (11.9%) 3422/22 548 (15.2%) 25 (2)
Six other regimens
Asprin + Dip 34 752/6842 989/6876 28 (5)
Aspirin + sulph 2 38/283 50/278 30 (20)
Dip 10 87/719 113/755 23 (14)
Sulph 17 299/2231 358/2242 20 (8)
Ticlopidine 39 264/3250 371/3278 33 (7)
Suloctidil 6 47/364 59/367 24 (19)
Subtotal: six other regimens* 105 1487/13 689 (10.9%) 1940/13 796 (14.1%) 28(3)
All trials* 142 4183/36 536 (11.4%) 5400/36 711 (14.7%) 27 (2)
Heterogeneity of odds reductions
between three aspirin categories $\chi^2_2 = 2.7$: NS
between seven regimens (any aspirin and six others)
$\chi^2_6 = 2.6$: NS
Treatment effect $2P < 0.00001$
0 0.5 1.0 1.5 2.0
Antiplatelet therapy better
Antiplatelet therapy worse
*Crude, unadjusted control totals 3130/21147 (aspirin), 1773/12737 (six other regimens)
NB: some trials contributed to more than one comparison

Fig. 16.14 Indirect comparisons of proportional effects on serious vascular events of different antiplatelet regimens in 142 trials in high-risk patients. The ratio of odds of myocardial infarction (MI), stroke or vascular death in the treatment group compared with the control group is plotted for each trial (dark green square: area proportional to the number of strokes), along with 99% confidence interval (horizontal line). The presence of a green square to the left of the solid vertical line suggests benefit, but this benefit is significant at the level of $2P < 0.01$ only if the entire confidence interval is to the left of the solid vertical line. An overview of all of the trial results (and 95% confidence interval) is represented by an open diamond, beside which is given the overall relative reduction in risk of MI, stroke and vascular death. Dip, dipyridamole; Sulph, sulphinpyrazone (with permission from the Antiplatelet Trialists' Collaboration 1994). An updated version of this figure, that includes the results of the Antithrombotic Trialists' Collaboration 2000 analyses, will be available at http://www.dcn.ed.ac.uk/spgm.

unethical), the data are consistent with the hypothesis that both drugs are effective (Hankey *et al.* 2000b).

Thienopyridines (ticlopidine and clopidogrel) compared with aspirin

Since both drugs are chemically related thienopyridines, with similar effects on platelets, a systematic review of the trials comparing them with aspirin is appropriate (Hankey *et al.* 2000b,c). Four trials involving a total of 22 656 high vascular risk patients were included. The trials were of high quality. Aspirin was compared with ticlopidine in three trials (3471 patients) and with clopidogrel in one trial (19 185 patients) (CAPRIE Steering Committee 1996). Allocation to a thienopyridine was associated with a marginal, yet just statistically significant, 9% reduction in the odds of a serious vascular event (95% CI, 2–16%), corresponding to the avoidance of about 11 serious vascular events per 1000 patients treated for about 2 years (Fig. 16.15a). There was also a 12% reduction in the odds of stroke (95% CI, 2–21%) (Fig. 16.15b). The absolute reduction in stroke was small; about seven strokes avoided per 1000 patients treated for 2 years.

In the subset of patients who were entered in the trials with a TIA or ischaemic stroke, the proportional reductions in vascular events and stroke were similar to those for all types of patients combined. However, since these patients are at particularly high risk of stroke, allocation to a thienopyri-

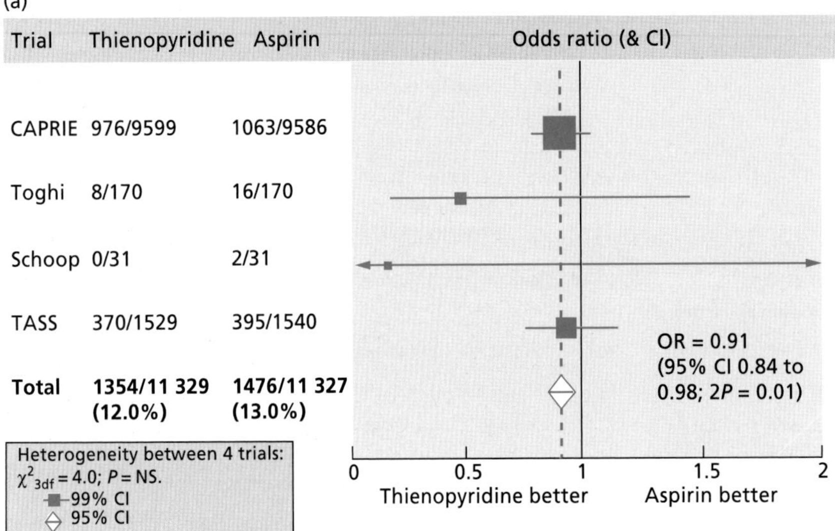

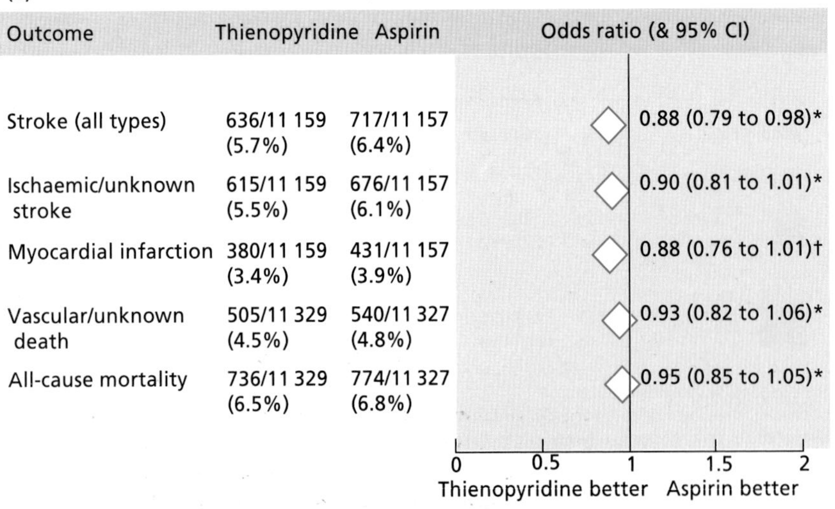

Fig. 16.15 Systematic review of randomized trials comparing thienopyridines with aspirin. (a) Effects on the primary outcome (stroke, myocardial infarction or vascular death). Each trial is represented by a solid dark green square proportional in size to the number of outcome events and a horizontal line representing the 99% confidence interval. The open diamond represents the overall result of the meta-analysis. TASS, Ticlopidine Aspirin Stroke Study; CAPRIE, Clopidogrel vs. aspirin in Patients at Risk of Ischaemic Events. (b) Effects on secondary outcomes. More detailed data available on version published in the Cochrane Library (Hankey *et al.* 2000b). (With permission from Hankey *et al.* 2000b.)

dine was associated with a somewhat larger absolute reduction in stroke (10.4% vs. 12.0%); corresponding to 16 (95% CI, 3–28) strokes avoided per 1000 patients treated for 2 years. A limited amount of additional information on the relative effects of ticlopidine and aspirin will come from the ongoing African-American Stroke Prevention Study (AASPS) (Gorelick *et al.* 1998).

If the overall point estimate is indeed the true effect (i.e. a 9% odds reduction with thienopyridines) then, compared with aspirin, the thienopyridines reduce the rate of serious vascular events at about 2 years from 13.0% to 12.0% in high vascular risk patients. This is an absolute risk reduction of 1.0% over about 2 years, meaning that about 100 high-risk patients need to be treated with a thienopyridine for about 2 years to prevent or delay one vascular event (or 200 patients to prevent one event per year). The *Drug and Therapeutics Bulletin*, an independent UK publication which reviews new treatments concluded 'clopidogrel appears to offer little or no advantage over aspirin' (Anon. 1999a). The standard dose of clopidogrel is 75 mg daily.

Adding ticlopidine or clopidogrel to aspirin

In patients undergoing cardiac stent procedures, ticlopidine may add benefit compared with aspirin alone, but these conclusions are based on one small trial of 30 days or less duration with only about 1100 patients (Antithrombotic Trialists' Collaboration 2000). Much more reliable data will be available from the the Chinese Acute Myocardial Infarction trial, which will randomize 30 000 patients within 24 h of acute myocardial infarction to: aspirin 162 mg, or aspirin 162 mg plus clopidogrel 75 mg, in a two-by-two factorial design with metoprolol. This study started in 1999; it is not clear whether comparable large-scale studies will be undertaken in patients at high risk of stroke.

Dipyridamole compared with control

Dipyridamole was originally introduced in 1959 as a vasodilator for the treatment of patients with angina. In 1965, its antiplatelet properties were discovered, and by 1969 the first randomized controlled trial of its use in stroke prevention was reported. The 15 trials (over 5700 patients) available by 1997 comparing dipyridamole alone with control did not provide clear evidence of benefit; the 16% reduction in the odds of vascular events was only marginally significant (95% CI, 3–28%) (Antithrombotic Trialists' Collaboration 2000). Dipyridamole alone therefore may not be an effective antiplatelet agent.

Adding dipyridamole to aspirin

Much interest has focused on whether dipyridamole adds useful antithrombotic effect to aspirin alone. The data available in 1994 did not resolve this question (Antiplatelet Trialists' Collaboration 1994). The second European Stroke Prevention Study (ESPS-2) was therefore designed to try and answer this dilemma once and for all (Diener *et al.* 1996). It compared 50 mg daily of enteric-coated aspirin with control and 400 mg daily of slow-release dipyridamole with control in a two-by-two factorial design. The study included over 6000 patients with ischaemic stroke. On its own, the ESPS-2 appeared to show that the combination had a small but definite advantage over aspirin alone (Diener *et al.* 1996). However, in the meta-analysis of all trials, confidence intervals around the estimate of treatment effect on vascular events were wide and included the possibility of no difference at all between the combination and aspirin alone (Wilterdink & Easton 1999) (Fig. 16.16). However, the 23% reduction in non-fatal strokes was significant. Expressed differently, the confidence interval around the observed small difference between aspirin and aspirin plus dipyridamole was wide and included the possibility of substantial extra benefit or slight disadvantage in terms of serious vascular events. In 1998, the combination of aspirin with dipyridamole was licensed for stroke prevention.

Clinicians and statisticians have taken differing views about how best to interpret these data; some prefer to focus on the results of ESPS-2 alone, whereas others prefer to take a broader view and look at the totality of the evidence. To resolve the debate, the European/Australian Stroke Prevention in Reversible Ischaemia (ESPRIT) trial is comparing aspirin (30–325 mg daily) with aspirin plus 200 mg slow-

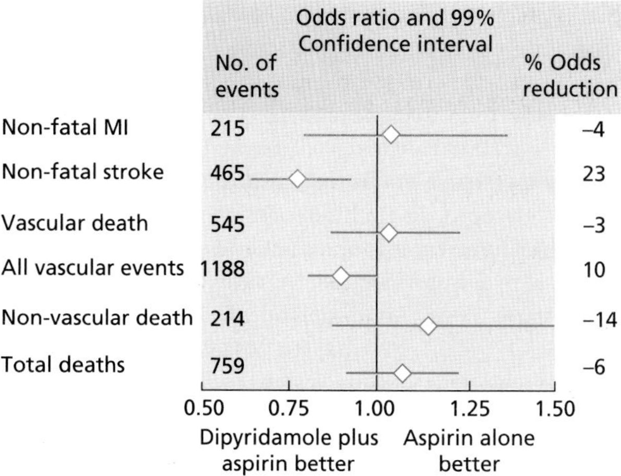

Fig. 16.16 Systematic review of the trials comparing aspirin plus dipyridamole with aspirin alone. Proportional effects on different vascular events. Each outcome is represented by a diamond with its 99% confidence interval shown as a horizontal line. MI, myocardial infarction. (With permission from Wilterdink & Easton 1999.)

release dipyridamole twice daily with oral anticoagulant (INR 2–3), in 4200 patients with TIA and ischaemic stroke. It will provide additional evidence on this question (De Schryver & Algra 2000; http://home.wxs.nl/~esprit/).

Dipyridamole alone is not effective, and until the ESPRIT trial is completed there will be continuing dispute about how much benefit there is from adding dipyridamole to aspirin (Wilterdink & Easton 1999); the available evidence falls short of 'proof beyond all reasonable doubt' that the combination is better than aspirin alone in preventing 'vascular events'. The data are, however, suggestive though not conclusive, that the combination may convey greater protection against stroke than aspirin alone. Because of the cost and extra adverse effects, we would not use the combination as first-line therapy, but would consider adding dipyridamole if recurrent ischaemic events occurred on aspirin alone.

Other antiplatelet drugs

A number of other drugs with a variety of antiplatelet actions have been tested. The evidence from the randomized trials comparing sulphinpyrazone, suloctidil, indobufen or triflusal with controls is not sufficient to support their routine use for the secondary prevention of vascular events (Antithrombotic Trialists' Collaboration 2000) (Fig. 16.14). Two trials are underway, each comparing aspirin with triflusal, but both are small and unlikely to provide reliable evidence (Culebras 1998; Matias-Guiu 1999).

New agents: platelet glycoprotein IIb/IIIa receptor blockers and antagonists

This is a rapidly evolving area of medical research and practice. A number of new antithrombotic agents are undergoing clinical development and several have been licensed, chiefly for use in acute coronary ischaemia and in patients undergoing coronary revascularization. A systematic review of the 15 trials (29 000 patients) available in 1997 provided proof beyond reasonable doubt that, in this cardiological setting, platelet glycoprotein IIb/IIIa receptor blockers and antagonists given intravenously and combined with aspirin reduced the odds of serious vascular events by one-fifth compared with aspirin alone (Antithrombotic Trialists' Collaboration 2000).

Many questions remain: Is this class of agent safe and effective when given long term for stroke prevention? What is the best agent (and its optimum dose)? Will readministration provoke a major allergic reaction? (Vorchheimer *et al.* 1999). Furthermore, these agents have to be given parenterally and are also associated with a significant bleeding risk. An effective and safe oral preparation for long-term use to prevent stroke is yet to be identified, but this remains a promising area of research (Patrono *et al.* 1998).

At least one trial in stroke patients began in 1999; the Blockade of the gpIIb/IIIa Receptor to Avoid Vascular Occlusion (BRAVO) trial is comparing the oral agent lotrafiban with placebo in patients with TIA, stroke, myocardial infarction or unstable angina, who are taking aspirin, to assess its effects on serious vascular events (http://www.neuro.wustl.edu/stroke/trials).

Although glycoprotein IIb/IIIa agents clearly have a place in the management of patients with acute coronary syndromes and after coronary stenting, we are guarded in our expectations of their likely benefits in stroke prevention.

16.4.5 Adverse effects and cost

Adverse effects of aspirin and how to minimize them (reduce the dose!)

Any aspirin dose between 75 mg and 1500 mg daily is likely to be effective. The commonest adverse effects of aspirin (nausea, dyspepsia and constipation) are dose related, and therefore lower dose regimens (75–325 mg daily) are likely to cause fewer adverse effects and to be associated with better compliance (UK-TIA Study Group 1991; Patrono *et al.* 1998). It is not clear whether the bleeding risks associated with aspirin are dose related.

The evidence from trials comparing doses of less than 75 mg daily with control is less robust than for higher doses, but for patients unable to tolerate higher doses, doses as low as 30 mg aspirin daily may still have useful antithrombotic effects (Dutch TIA Trial Study Group 1991; van Gijn 1999). For patients who develop adverse effects on 300 mg daily, the dose may therefore be progressively reduced to 30 mg daily (Dutch TIA Trial Study Group 1991; SALT Collaborative Group 1991).

For patients who experience adverse effects even on low doses, various alternative preparations of aspirin are now available: buffered, enteric-coated and modified-release aspirin. These newer formulations may reduce dyspepsia (and hence improve compliance), but there is no good evidence that changing to these preparations will necessarily reduce the risk of bleeding (Kelly *et al.* 1996; Anon. 1997).

Adverse effects of dipyridamole

Headaches (which tend to reduce with prolonged use), diarrhoea and other gastrointestinal upsets are well-known adverse effects of dipyridamole that may limit its tolerability and hence reduce compliance (Diener *et al.* 1996).

Adverse effects of ticlopidine and clopidogrel

Compared with aspirin 325 mg, thienopyridines produced a significant reduction in the odds of gastrointestinal haemorrhage and other upper gastrointestinal upset, but a significant increase in the odds of skin rash and of diarrhoea. Allocation to ticlopidine, but not clopidogrel, was associated with a significant 1.7-fold increase in the odds of neutropenia (95% CI, 1.5–4.8-fold relative increase); the frequency was 2.3% with ticlopidine vs. 0.8% on control (Hankey *et al.* 2000b). Ticlopidine-associated neutropenia is usually reversible. Rare but more serious reactions have also been reported: irreversible agranulocytosis, pancytopenia, aplastic anaemia, thrombotic thrombocytopenic purpura, atypical microangiopathy and toxic erythroderma (Shear & Appel 1995; Gill *et al.* 1997; Alba *et al.* 1998; Bennett *et al.* 1998, 2000; Steinhubl *et al.* 1999).

Cost

Aspirin is inexpensive; a few tens of pounds (or dollars) per year, depending on formulation. The cost in the year 2000 of treating 100 patients for 2 years with clopidogrel, at about US$800/patient/year, totals about $160 000 to prevent one vascular event (Hankey *et al.* 2000b). As this is likely to exceed the average cost of the vascular event prevented, it seems prudent, at this stage at least, to infer that thienopyridines should not replace aspirin as the first-choice antiplatelet agent for all high vascular risk patients.

These health care costs would have to be compared with other effective but expensive interventions (Tables 18.2 and 18.3). Any economic evaluation of the relative merits of different forms of health care that might be applied for stroke prevention in patients at risk of recurrent stroke would need to consider the relative cost-effectiveness of carotid endarterectomy and lipid-lowering therapy if one is taking a broader view. An even broader view might consider the question of whether spending large sums of money on clopidogrel (and thereby avoiding more strokes) might divert money away from other more effective forms of health care for stroke patients (such as stroke units).

The estimates of the benefits of dipyridamole have been submitted to formal economic analyses. If the economic analysis is based on the ESPS-2 estimate of treatment effect, the combination would prevent more strokes than aspirin alone and this would cost, from the perspective of the UK National Health Service, about £5500 per stroke avoided over 5 years. If the economic model was adjusted to take the perspective of society as a whole, and looking over a patient's anticipated lifetime, the use of the combination might plausibly be associated with net cost saving (Chambers *et al.* 1998). However, the Antithrombotic Trialists' (ATT) estimates of effect are far less optimistic (and include the possibility of net disadvantage) and therefore any economic analyses, based on the ATT estimates, would be much less favourable.

16.4.6 How long should treatment continue?

Most of the trials evaluating aspirin in high-risk patients lasted just 2 or 3 years (Antiplatelet Trialists' Collaboration 1994). The benefits of continuing aspirin beyond this period have therefore not been evaluated formally. There was clear evidence of benefit for up to 2 years' treatment with probable additive benefit between years two and three. Although there is no firm evidence from trials to support this, it seems highly likely that individuals who are at continuing high risk because of past stroke or TIA should probably continue aspirin lifelong, provided there are no adverse effects.

> *Aspirin 75 mg daily is effective, safe and inexpensive. It is the antiplatelet drug of first choice for most patients with a history of recent transient ischaemic attack or ischaemic stroke and should be continued for life.*

16.4.7 What to do with aspirin 'failures' and aspirin intolerance

Aspirin 'failures' (i.e. further vascular events on aspirin)

Firstly, no treatment is 100% effective, so inevitably many patients will have further events while on aspirin. In one sense, therefore, one such event is not a 'failure'. However, if a patient continues to have vascular events while on aspirin, it is worth checking: Is the patient really taking the tablets (and if not, why not)? Is the clinical diagnosis correct (are the attacks perhaps not vascular in origin at all)? If vascular, is the cause likely to be atherothromboembolism and are vascular risk factors being managed optimally? Have other treatable causes been excluded or treated (e.g. severe symptomatic carotid stenosis)? If all these have been checked, some clinicians then increase the dose of aspirin, but there is no evidence to support increasing the dose above 75–150 mg aspirin daily. Clopidogrel or ticlopidine are effective alternatives to aspirin (and clopidogrel is less likely to cause neutropenia, thrombotic thrombocytopenic purpura and diarrhoea than ticlopidine). However, one must accept that 'continuing attacks despite aspirin' was not an eligibility criterion for the trials of ticlopidine and clopidogrel, so the benefits of these agents in aspirin 'failures' are not clearly established. Adding dipyridamole may add benefit, but the size of the extra benefit is controversial; again, the trials were not of aspirin 'failures' who might well be more resistant to antiplatelet drugs (for whatever reason) and so 'fail' not just on aspirin but on other antiplatelet drugs as well.

At present, there is no evidence that, for patients in sinus rhythm, oral anticoagulants alone, or in combination with aspirin, offer any definite net advantage over aspirin alone, and they can do harm. We would, however, use heparin, then warfarin, in patients who are having very frequent TIAs on aspirin (section 16.5.2).

Aspirin intolerance

Many patients who are apparently intolerant of aspirin may be able to tolerate it, just by reducing the dose. For those whose symptoms are not alleviated by reducing the dose, changing the formulation may help (e.g. to enteric coating). There is no strong evidence to support the routine use of prostaglandin analogues such as misoprostol, H_2 antagonists or proton pump inhibitors to reduce the gastrointestinal toxicity of aspirin and other non-steroidal anti-inflammatory drugs (Rostom *et al.* 2000). Although clopidogrel has a role for patients who are intolerant, or allergic to, aspirin, one must accept the caveat that there is no direct evidence of the relative effectiveness of thienopyridines compared with aspirin in these patients, because they were excluded from the randomized trials.

Patients (and their doctors) often become quite worried if they have had a stroke or TIA and turn out to be completely intolerant of even very low-dose aspirin or other antiplatelet drugs. It is worth remembering that, for such patients, the benefits of antiplatelet agents are only moderate and that blood pressure reduction, smoking cessation and modification of cholesterol levels may produce benefits which are at least as big as, if not bigger than, the effects of antiplatelet therapy. Furthermore, if the results of the HOPE trial are confirmed, angiotensin-converting enzyme inhibitors are likely to add substantial extra benefit (section 16.6).

The writing of a prescription for aspirin in patients with transient ischaemic attacks or minor strokes is still, all too often, the end of the search for potential ways of reducing stroke risk; it should be just the beginning!

16.5 Anticoagulants

Emboli arising in the heart, extracranial arteries or elsewhere often contain fibrin. Inhibitors of the coagulation cascade prevent conversion of fibrinogen to fibrin, so anticoagulants should reduce the thromboembolic complications of occlusive arterial disease. These drugs first became available for clinical use in the 1950s and have been extensively used in patients with stroke and TIA ever since, despite the lack of reliable trial evidence. The therapeutic question can be reduced to: 'for which categories of patients do the benefits of anticoagulants (prevention of ischaemic events) outweigh the risks (increased risk of haemorrhagic events)?'

16.5.1 Evidence

Primary stroke prevention in survivors of myocardial infarction

A systematic review of the trials comparing long-term full-dose oral anticoagulants with a control in survivors of myocardial infarction suggested that treatment reduced the risk of stroke and vascular death (Antman *et al.* 1992; Vaitkus *et al.* 1992; Aspect Research Group 1994). However, the relevant comparison is now with aspirin, not with a control. Low fixed-dose warfarin (1 mg or 3 mg daily) was no better than 160 mg aspirin daily (Coumadin Aspirin Reinfarction Study (CARS) Investigators 1997). For the majority of survivors of uncomplicated myocardial infarction, antiplatelet drugs are the preferred option for long-term prevention of further vascular events because of their lower bleeding risk, complexity and cost (Cairns 1994; Scottish Intercollegiate Guidelines Network 1999). In selected individuals with above average risk of further events, for example those with persistent atrial fibrillation, long-term oral anticoagulants may be justifiable (Scottish Intercollegiate Guidelines Network 1999).

The available evidence is not conclusive and at least one further trial is under way to clarify the optimum intensity of anticoagulation, the benefits of combination therapy with aspirin, and the selection of patients most likely to benefit from anticoagulants. Anticoagulants in the Secondary Prevention of Events in Coronary Thrombosis (ASPECT-II) will compare the efficacy and safety of three regimens of long-term antithrombotic treatment in 8700 patients with acute cardiac ischaemic syndromes: adjusted full-intensity oral anticoagulation (target range 3.0–4.0 INR), low-dose aspirin, or combined therapy of low-dose aspirin and adjusted low-intensity oral anticoagulation (target range INR: 2.0–2.5) (Van *et al.* 1997).

Prevention of stroke in survivors of ischaemic stroke or transient ischaemic attack without atrial fibrillation: secondary stroke prevention

A systematic review of the few, methodologically poor, trials of oral anticoagulants vs. control for the long-term secondary prevention of stroke in patients who have had a TIA or ischaemic stroke but were *not* in atrial fibrillation suggested that: anticoagulants increased the risk of fatal intracranial haemorrhage; the balance of risk and benefit from anticoagulants was unclear; and that anticoagulants could not be recommended for routine practice (Liu *et al.* 2000). Further methodologically sound studies are clearly required.

The largest trial comparing anticoagulants with aspirin is the Stroke Prevention in Recurrent Ischaemia Trial (SPIRIT)

(Algra *et al.* 1997). It compared, in a single-blind trial, the efficacy and safety of 30 mg aspirin daily with oral anticoagulation (INR 3.0–4.5), in 1316 patients with TIA or minor ischaemic stroke. The primary measure of outcome was the composite event 'death from all vascular causes, non-fatal stroke, non-fatal myocardial infarction or non-fatal major bleeding complication'. The trial was stopped at the first interim analysis, when the mean duration of follow-up was 14 months. There was an excess of the primary outcome event in the anticoagulated group: 12.4% vs. 5.4% in the aspirin group (hazard ratio, 2.3; 95% CI, 1.6–3.5). This adverse effect was due to an excess of major bleeding complications with anticoagulants: 53 (27 intracranial, 17 fatal), compared with six on aspirin (3 intracranial, 1 fatal). The bleeding risk increased by a factor of 1.43 (95% CI, 0.96–2.13) for each 0.5 unit increase of the achieved INR. The authors concluded that in such patients, anticoagulation with an INR range of 3.0–4.5 was not safe. The presence of leukoaraiosis on the pre-treatment brain scan and age over 65 increased the risk of anticoagulant-related haemorrhage. The risk of intracranial haemorrhage appears to be higher in patients with strokes of arterial origin compared with patients in atrial fibrillation (Gorter 1999).

The Stroke Prevention with Warfarin or Aspirin Trial (SWAT) randomized 178 patients with 'small stroke' or TIA to warfarin (INR 2–3), warfarin plus 80 mg aspirin daily, or aspirin 1300 mg daily. Only 30 non-TIA outcome events were recorded, so the trial was too small for any reliable conclusions (Stewart *et al.* 1998).

The efficacy of lower intensity anticoagulation regimens therefore remains to be determined. Three trials are now under way (WARSS, ESPRIT and WAIAS) and a fourth is planned (ARCH). The Warfarin Aspirin Recurrent Stroke Study (WARSS) is comparing warfarin (INR 1.4–2.8) with aspirin 325 mg daily in a double-blind placebo-controlled trial (Sacco *et al.* 1997). The WARSS primary outcome is death or symptomatic ischaemic stroke recurrence. Recruitment of the planned sample size of 1920 patients with ischaemic stroke is completed and follow-up continues.

The ESPRIT trial plans to recruit 4500 patients with TIA or minor ischaemic stroke who will be allocated to aspirin (30–325 mg daily), aspirin plus dipyridamole (200 mg slow-release twice daily), or oral anticoagulants (INR 2–3) (Algra 2000; http://home.wxs.nl/~esprit/).

The Warfarin vs. Aspirin for Intracranial Artery Stenosis study (WAIAS) will compare warfarin (INR 2–3) with 1300 mg aspirin daily in 800 patients with TIA or ischaemic stroke due to intracranial artery stenosis greater than 50% (http://www.neuro.wustl.edu/stroke/trials).

The Aortic Arch-related Cerebral Hazard (ARCH) trial is planning to recruit 800 patients with brain infarction of unknown cause and atheromatous plaques thicker than 4 mm in the aortic arch, between warfarin (INR 2–3), aspirin 300 mg daily, and aspirin plus clopidogrel 75 mg daily (P. Amarenco, personal communication).

In ischaemic stroke and transient ischaemic attack patients who are in sinus rhythm, 'high-intensity' oral anticoagulation (INR 3.0–4.5) is associated with a definite net hazard, chiefly due to the increased risk of intracranial haemorrhage, and should be avoided. It is not clear whether 'low to moderate intensity' anticoagulation (INR 1.4–3.0) offers any advantage over aspirin, but the ongoing trials (WARSS, ESPRIT, ARCH and WAIAS) comparing the two should provide useful information. For now, in most patients, aspirin is the first-line antithrombotic agent of choice. We would encourage clinicians to randomize eligible patients in the ongoing trials, so that we may have more reliable evidence in this area.

Primary stroke prevention in patients with atrial fibrillation

A systematic review of the five studies comparing 'moderate-intensity' oral anticoagulants (INR 2–3) with control for the primary prevention of stroke in patients in atrial fibrillation showed that anticoagulation reduced the risk of 'all stroke' by 61% (95% CI, 41–74%) and of 'fatal or disabling stroke' by 53% (95% CI, 20–72%) (Fig. 16.17). For primary prevention in patients with atrial fibrillation who have an average annual stroke risk of 4%, for every 1000 treated with oral anticoagulants, about 25 strokes and 12 disabling strokes would be avoided per year (Atrial Fibrillation Investigators 1994; Hart *et al.* 1999; Benavente *et al.* 2000). There is some evidence to suggest that in such patients, anticoagulants may have a greater protective effect against cardioembolic strokes, whereas aspirin has greater effects against atherothrombotic strokes (Hart *et al.* 2000b).

Several trials have compared oral anticoagulation of varying intensity with aspirin (Atrial Fibrillation Investigators 1994; Hart *et al.* 1999). The Second Stroke Prevention in Atrial Fibrillation Trial (SPAF-II) compared warfarin (INR 2–4.5) with aspirin 325 mg daily. Event rates in both treatment groups were low and the trial did not show that anticoagulants were clearly superior. Furthermore, in older patients, the reduction in ischaemic stroke with warfarin was offset by an increase in intracranial haemorrhage, perhaps related to the rather high intensity of the anticoagulant regimen (Stroke Prevention in Atrial Fibrillation Investigators 1994). A study in the Netherlands, which used screening in primary care to identify patients, also found low event rates (about 2%/year) and no difference between moderate-intensity oral anticoagulants (INR 2.5–3.5), low-intensity oral anticoagulants (INR 1.1–1.6) and aspirin 150 mg daily (Hellemans *et al.* 1999). The second Copenhagen Atrial Fibrillation, Aspirin and Anticoagulation Study (AFASAK-II) stopped prematurely in the light of other trial evidence, but again did not provide any evidence of a difference between oral anticoagulants (INR 2–3) and aspirin 300 mg daily (Gullov *et al.* 1998). A systematic review of these trials of low-intensity regimens is clearly needed!

Several trials have compared adjusted 'moderate-intensity' oral anticoagulants with 'fixed minidose' regimens with or without aspirin in primary stroke prevention. In the third Stroke Prevention in Atrial Fibrillation Trial (SPAF-III), 'low-intensity' anticoagulants with a fixed-dose warfarin regimen (INR 1.2–1.5) combined with aspirin 325 mg daily turned out to be significantly less effective than adjusted-dose anticoagulants (INR 2–3) (SPAF-III Writing Committee 1996). Two further studies then stopped prematurely in the light of the SPAF-III results. The AFASAK-II trial results were consistent with SPAF-III; minidose warfarin, with or without aspirin, was less effective than adjusted dose (Gullov *et al.* 1998). Similarly, a study in Italy comparing adjusted-dose with fixed minidose warfarin, though inconclusive when terminated, was consistent with SPAF-III (Pengo *et al.* 1998). A systematic review of these data would be helpful, but it does not appear at present that fixed minidose regimens are effective in primary stroke prevention for patients in atrial fibrillation.

Secondary prevention of stroke in survivors of ischaemic stroke or transient ischaemic attack in atrial fibrillation

The average annual risk of stroke among controls in the largest secondary prevention trial, the European Atrial Fibrillation Trial (EAFT), was 12% compared with just over 4% amongst controls in the primary prevention trials (Figs 16.18 and 16.19). In the EAFT, anticoagulants reduced the risk of stroke by two-thirds, from 12% to 4%/year. The annual risk of stroke, myocardial infarction, systemic embolism or vascular death was reduced by about 50%, from 17% in controls to 8% in anticoagulant-allocated patients (European Atrial Fibrillation Trial Study Group 1993; Atrial Fibrillation Investigators 1994; Koudstaal 2000a).

Only three trials have directly compared anticoagulants with antiplatelet drugs in secondary stroke prevention. In the EAFT, anticoagulation within the range of INR 2–3 appeared to be more effective than aspirin (European Atrial Fibrillation Trial Study Group 1993). The risk of major bleeding complications was low, both on anticoagulation (2.8%/year) and on aspirin (0.9%/year) and, as it happened, no intra-

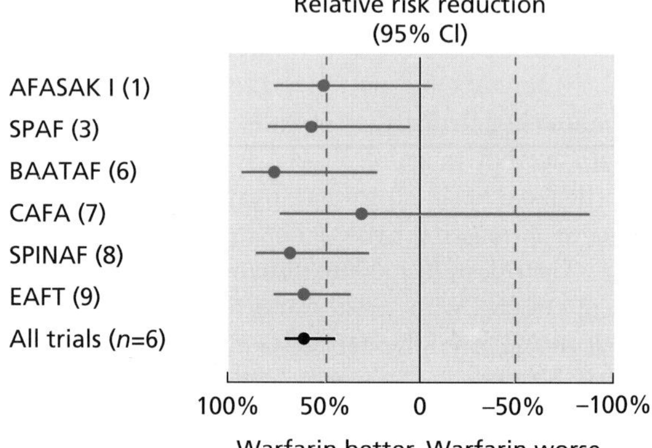

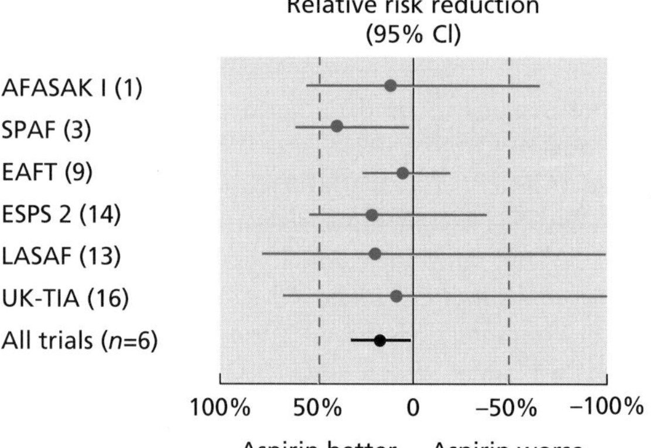

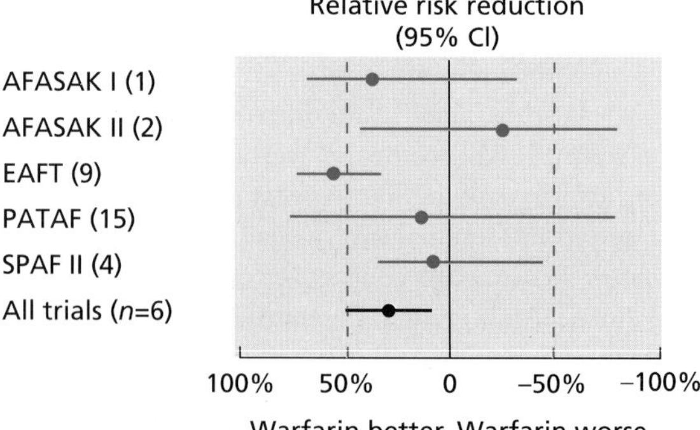

Fig. 16.17 Effects on all stroke (ischaemic and haemorrhagic) of antithrombotic drugs for patients with atrial fibrillation. (a) Adjusted-dose warfarin compared with placebo (six randomized trials). (b) Aspirin compared with placebo (six randomized trials). (c) Adjusted-dose warfarin compared with aspirin (five randomized trials). Horizontal lines are 95% confidence intervals around the point estimates. AFASAK, Copenhagen Atrial Fibrillation, Aspirin and Anticoagulation Study; BAATAF, Boston Area Anticoagulation Trial for Atrial Fibrillation; CAFA, Canadian Atrial Fibrillation Anticoagulation Study; EAFT, European Atrial Fibrillation Trial; ESPS-II, European Stroke Prevention Study 2; LASAF, Low-Dose Aspirin, Stroke and Atrial Fibrillation Pilot Study; PATAF, Prevention of Arterial Thromboembolism in Atrial Fibrillation; SPAF, Stroke Prevention in Atrial Fibrillation Study; SPINAF, Stroke Prevention in Non-rheumatic Atrial Fibrillation; UK-TIA, United Kingdom TIA Aspirin Study (with permission from Hart *et al.* 1999).

cranial bleeds were identified. Forty-six patients in the Veterans Administration Stroke Prevention in Atrial Fibrillation (VA-SPINAF) study had a history of prior stroke or TIA at the time of randomization. A third small trial compared adjusted-dose warfarin with the antiplatelet agent, indobufen, but again, adjusted-dose warfarin was associated with a non-significantly lower stroke rate (Morocutti *et al.* 1997). Compared with aspirin, if 1000 patients are treated with anticoagulants for 1 year, about 90 serious vascular events (mostly strokes) are avoided; about 11 ischaemic stroke or TIA survivors need to be treated with anticoagulants to prevent one vascular event per year (stroke, myocardial infarction, systemic embolism or vascular death) (Koudstaal 2000b,c).

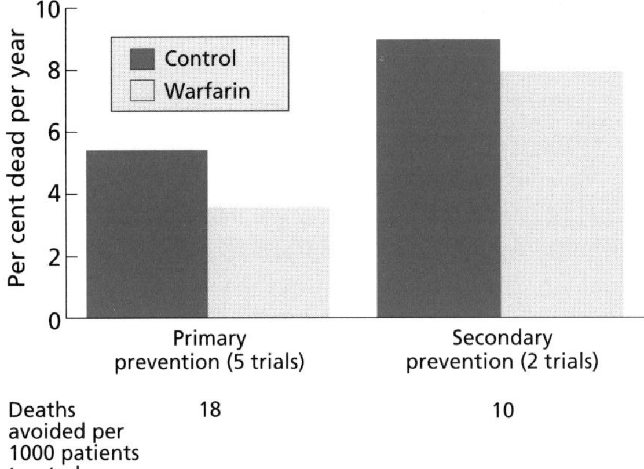

Fig. 16.18 The absolute effects, in terms of death from all causes, of anticoagulants in patients with atrial fibrillation based on a systematic review of five trials compared with the effect in two secondary prevention trials (data from European Atrial Fibrillation Trial Study Group 1993; Atrial Fibrillation Trial Investigators 1994).

A small trial in Japan compared moderate-intensity oral anticoagulants (INR 2.2–3.5) with low-intensity anticoagulants (INR 1.5–2.1) in stroke or TIA patients with atrial fibrillation. It was stopped prematurely after 112 patients had been randomized, because of a high risk of bleeding in the higher intensity group (Minematsu *et al.* 1999).

Moderate-intensity anticoagulants (INR 2–3) appear to be effective and safe for secondary prevention in patients with atrial fibrillation and a recent ischaemic stroke or TIA, and are more effective than aspirin alone. Fixed minidose regimens, either alone or in combination with aspirin, have not been adequately evaluated for secondary prevention. Their lack of effect in the primary prevention trials suggests that further randomized trials, to identify the lowest effective anticoagulant intensity for secondary prevention of stroke in survivors of ischaemic stroke or TIA with atrial fibrillation, would be worthwhile.

16.5.2 Who to treat

Some of the same factors that increase the risk of haemorrhage *with* treatment also increase the risk of stroke *without* treatment, particularly hypertension (Atrial Fibrillation Investigators 1994; van Latum *et al.* 1995). Many other factors have been identified which alone, or in combination with other factors, identify those patients with stroke (or TIA) and atrial fibrillation who are at highest risk of stroke without treatment (and therefore have the most to gain) (Atrial Fibrillation Investigators 1994; Di Pasquale *et al.* 1995; van Latum *et al.* 1995; Hart *et al.* 1999) (Fig. 16.19 and Table 16.10).

Survivors of ischaemic stroke or transient ischaemic attack in atrial fibrillation

For long-term secondary prevention after TIA or ischaemic

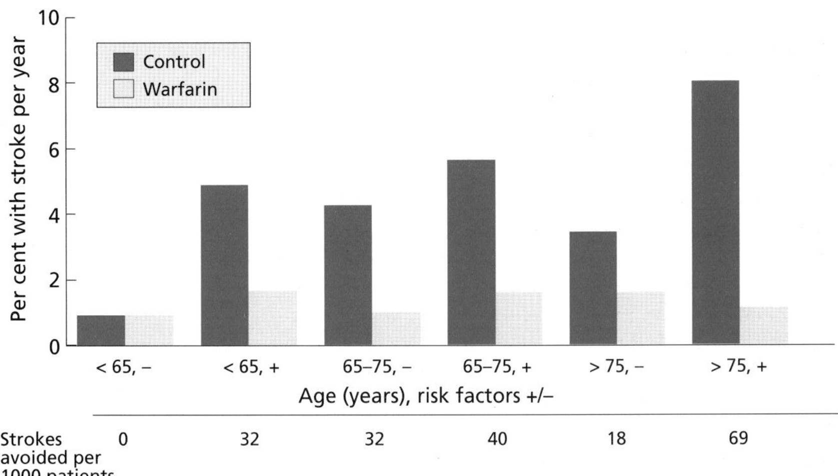

Fig. 16.19 The absolute effects, in terms of stroke prevention, of anticoagulants in primary prevention of stroke in patients with atrial fibrillation based on a systematic review of five trials: absolute risk of stroke in relation to age and presence (+) or absence (–) of risk factors (data from the Atrial Fibrillation Investigators 1994).

stroke in patients in atrial fibrillation we would routinely attempt to use moderate-intensity oral anticoagulants (INR 2–3) rather than antiplatelet drugs. However, survivors of non-disabling ischaemic stroke (i.e. independent in activities of daily living) and TIA patients are a fairly heterogeneous group, and certain factors may make clinicans reluctant to prescribe long-term anticoagulants; for example, a history of uncontrolled hypertension, recent gastrointestinal bleeding, alcoholic liver disease, confusion or dementia, tendency to falls, difficulties with access to an anticoagulant clinic, or the presence of extensive leukoaraiosis on CT scanning. These factors either increase the likelihood of over-anticoagulation or intracranial bleeding (or both) (Hart *et al.* 1995; Levine *et al.* 1998). In patients with prior stroke or TIA, echocardiographic findings are unlikely to influence any decision whether or not to use anticoagulants (Sudlow *et al.* 1998).

Patients with atrial fibrillation, no history of stroke or transient ischaemic attack, but at high risk of vascular events: primary stroke prevention

In patients with atrial fibrillation but no history of stroke or TIA, routine echocardiography is not likely to influence decisions about anticoagulation (unless the patient is younger than 75 years, has no clinical risk factors for stroke and no contraindications to anticoagulants) (Sudlow *et al.* 1998). Patients at high risk (defined by the clinical factors outlined in Table 16.10), that is an annual stroke risk of over 3%, should be considered for anticoagulation with warfarin at a target INR of 2.5 (range 2.0–3.0). The balance of risks and benefits of warfarin should be assessed and discussed with the patient, and reassessed annually (Scottish Intercollegiate Guidelines Network 1999, also available at http://www.show.scot.nhs.uk/sign/clinical.htm).

Translating the evidence into clinical practice

It is difficult to translate these research findings on the benefits of anticoagulants into clinical practice. People with atrial fibrillation in the general population are likely to be less compliant with, and less carefully monitored than, patients within the trials; this may reduce the benefits and increase the risks (Green *et al.* 1997). It is also likely that, when applied to the generality of patients with ischaemic stroke and TIA, the benefits of anticoagulants are less extreme than suggested by the trials.

The use of different risk stratification methods will result in different proportions of patients being offered anticoagulants (section 6.5). A study applied the SPAF-I criteria, the Atrial Fibrillation Investigators (AFI) pooled analysis and the SPAF-III criteria to a community sample of atrial fibrillation patients; the criteria suggested that 61%, 49% and 41%, respectively, were at high enough risk to gain net benefit from anticoagulants (Sudlow *et al.* 1998). Furthermore, the quality of national and local guideline documents on the use of anticoagulants in atrial fibrillation can vary; a survey of UK documents revealed considerable variation in whether anticoagulant treatment was recommended (range 13–100%) (Thomson *et al.* 1998). The way doctors interact with patients is also important. Giving information to patients about the risks and benefits of anticoagulants led to a low uptake of anticoagulants (Howitt & Armstrong 1999).

There will therefore need to be major changes in health service provision to match the increased need for anticoagu-

Table 16.10 Annual risk of stroke on no treatment, aspirin or warfarin in high-, moderate- and low-risk patients with non-valvular atrial fibrillation (Scottish Intercollegiate Guidelines Network 1999).

Risk group	Untreated	Aspirin	Warfarin	NNT*
Very high				
Previous ischaemic stroke or transient ischaemic attack	12%	10%	5%	13
High				
Age over 65 and one other risk factor:	5–8%	4–6%	2–3%	22–47
Hypertension				
Diabetes mellitus				
Heart failure				
Left-ventricular dysfunction				
Moderate				
Age over 65, no other risk factors	3–5%	2–4%	1–2%	47–83
Age under 65, other risk factors				
Low				
Age under 65, no other risk factors	1.2%	1%	*c.* 0.5%	200

*Number-needed-to-treat with warfarin *instead of aspirin* for 1 year to prevent one stroke.

lant therapy and to ensure that it is delivered consistently, effectively and safely (Sudlow *et al.* 1995). Better means of ensuring that patients make well-informed decisions are also needed.

Anticoagulants are indicated for many patients with recent transient ischaemic attack or ischaemic stroke who are in atrial fibrillation, provided there are no contraindications. It is important to assess the risk of anticoagulation for each individual patient and to provide a safe and accessible anticoagulant service.

Anticoagulants for patients with repeated transient ischaemic attacks or ischaemic strokes despite optimum antiplatelet drug therapy

In our experience, this situation is relatively uncommon. The first step should be to verify again that the attacks are truly ischaemic in nature and do not represent structural brain disease, epilepsy, migraine, psychogenic disorder, etc. (section 3.1). If the diagnosis is correct, these admittedly rare patients are often very worried, as are their doctors. Of course, those with carotid ischaemic events and severe symptomatic carotid stenosis should be considered for endarterectomy, but sometimes this is not possible or practical (section 16.8), and very occasionally the attacks continue after what appears to be a technically adequate operation. Two or 3 months of moderate-intensity oral anticoagulants (INR 2–3) may reduce the frequency and severity of the TIAs, which is comforting to the patient and reduces anxiety all round. We generally do this in the full knowledge that this treatment may not reduce the risk of stroke or vascular death; it is purely given for symptom control. It is often possible to withdraw the anticoagulants gradually and replace them with aspirin. In such cases, the unstable atheromatous plaque that was causing the frequent attacks (we presume) has perhaps 'healed' and become covered with endothelium (section 6.3.2).

16.5.3 Who not to treat

In general, the main contraindication to oral anticoagulation is a high risk of bleeding. However, many of the conditions which increase the risk of bleeding also increase the risk of thromboembolism.

CT or MR brain scan not available

We always obtain a brain CT (or MR) scan to exclude intracranial haemorrhage, because anticoagulation of patients with intracranial bleeding is presumably unwise, at least in the short term, if not in the long term. We would want the imaging (especially if it was a CT, performed within the first few days of the stroke to maximize the chances of finding intracranial haemorrhage (section 5.3.4). It is not clear whether or not the presence of haemorrhagic transformation of a cerebral infarct is an absolute contraindication to the use of anticoagulants. If we felt the patient had a clear indication for immediate anticoagulation, we would not delay if the scan showed a minor degree of haemorrhagic transformation (i.e. a few cortical petechae). On the other hand, if there was confluent haemorrhage or a parenchymatous haematoma, we would prefer to wait a week or two at least.

Patients with atrial fibrillation at low risk of stroke

For low-risk individuals, with an annual stroke risk below 3%, the risks of oral anticoagulants are generally not justifiable. For such patients, aspirin is a safe and effective alternative to anticoagulants (Scottish Intercollegiate Guidelines Network 1999, also available at: http://www.show.scot.nhs.uk/sign/clinical.htm) (section 16.4.2).

Infective endocarditis

Patients with active endocarditis should not be treated with oral anticoagulants because of their high risk of intracerebral haemorrhage (Hart *et al.* 1995).

Other relative contraindications

These have all been mentioned previously but bear repeating (section 11.4.4) (Tables 11.5 and 11.7). The risk of bleeding complications from long-term anticoagulants is likely to be higher in patients: who are older, have a history of previous gastrointestinal bleeding, uncontrolled hypertension, alcoholic liver disease, or are unable to attend for regular blood tests for monitoring (Levine *et al.* 1998). It is often difficult to judge whether or not a patient will be compliant with treatment, but clearly a history of poor compliance with some previous medication is at least an indicator. The presence of leukoaraiosis on CT scanning was a predictor of intracranial haemorrhage in the SPIRIT trial, and it is therefore potentially a relative contraindication to anticoagulants (Gorter 1999).

16.5.4 Agent/dose/adverse effects

If oral anticoagulants are to be used for long-term secondary prevention, a baseline full blood count, platelet count, INR and liver function tests should be done—and the results known—before treatment is started.

On the rare occasions when there is an urgent need for immediate anticoagulation, heparin can be given, since oral anticoagulants take several days to become effective. Intravenous unfractionated heparin is monitored by measuring the activated partial thromboplastin time (APTT). Reagents for this test vary and must be standardized by the local laboratory, so dosing schedules must be determined by local guidelines. In some hospitals, fixed-dose low molecular weight heparin regimens are used in preference to intravenous unfractionated heparin. We advise you to follow local practice guidelines.

Should patients be given heparin before starting oral anticoagulants in non-urgent situations?

After taking the first few doses of oral anticoagulants without concomitant heparin, patients may develop a transient pro-coagulant state. In patients with protein S or protein C deficiency, this may be severe enough to cause warfarin-induced skin necrosis (Miura *et al.* 1996). Patients with the antiphospholipid syndrome may also have low levels of protein S and protein C, and therefore be at risk of warfarin-induced skin necrosis (C. Ludlam, personal communication). For patients without any evidence of protein S or protein C deficiency who do not have antiphospholipid syndrome, the risks of a clinically important pro-coagulant state developing are more theoretical than real. In general, therefore, in non-urgent situations, we start oral anticoagulants *without* heparin but would seek advice from a local haematologist if we felt there was a high risk of a transient pro-coagulant state.

Convenient warfarin dosing schedules are given in Table 16.11. A low-dose induction regimen was found to have advantages over this standard regimen for patients aged over 75 (Gedge *et al.* 2000). Commonly used drugs which interact with warfarin are given in Table 16.12. Patients should be followed up regularly. The frequency of follow-up will be determined by local facilities and by how far the patient lives from the hospital. Follow-up by the local general (family) practitioner may be feasible.

Table 16.11 A schedule for dosage and monitoring of full-dose warfarin therapy (from the Scottish Intercollegiate Guidelines Network 1999).

Day	INR (9–11 AM)	Warfarin dose (mg) given at 5–7 PM
1	< 1.4	10
2	< 1.8	10
	1.8	1
	> 1.8	0.5
3	<2.0	10
	2.0–2.1	5
	2.2–2.3	4.5
	2.4–2.5	4
	2.6–2.7	3.5
	2.8–2.9	3
	3.0–3.1	2.5
	3.2–3.3	2
	3.4	1.5
	3.5	1
	3.6–4.0	0.5
	> 4.0	0
Predicted maintenance dose		
4	< 4	> 8
	1.4	8
	1.5	7.5
	1.6–1.7	7
	1.8	6.5
	1.9	6
	2.0–2.1	5.5
	2.2–2.3	5
	2.4–2.6	4.5
	2.7–3.0	4
	3.1–3.5	3.5
	3.6–4.0	3
	4.1–4.5	Miss out next day dose then give 2 mg
	4.5	Miss out 2 days' doses then give 1 mg

Note: Measurement of International Normalized Ratio (INR) levels in patients receiving heparin during the initiation of oral anticoagulants. It is advisable to check both the activated partial thromboplastin time (APTT) and the INR. The APTT should be within or below the therapeutic range (1.5–2.5 times control). If the APTT is above this range, the heparin effect on INR should be neutralized by adding protamine (0.4 mg/mL plasma) to the sample.

Dose and target international normalized ratio (INR)

It is now clear, and not surprising, that bleeding risk is closely related to the intensity of oral anticoagulation (Levine *et al.* 1998). The target INR varies according to the indication for anticoagulation and is given in Table 16.13 (Scottish Intercollegiate Guidelines Network 1999, also available at http://www.show.scot.nhs.uk/sign/clinical.htm). The trials of anticoagulation in patients with atrial fibrillation evaluated oral anticoagulants aiming for an INR of 1.5–4.5 (Hart *et al.* 1999). Non-randomized evidence from the EAFT suggested that an INR above 5.0 was associated with an unacceptably high risk of haemorrhage, and an INR below 2.0 carried a high risk of recurrent stroke because of inadequate treatment (European Atrial Fibrillation Trial Study Group 1995). The recommended target INR for patients with atrial fibrillation is therefore 2.5, but a range of 2.0–3.0 is acceptable (Scottish Intercollegiate Guidelines Network 1999).

Long-term subcutaneous heparin therapy

A small trial compared 'usual therapy' with 'usual therapy' plus

Table 16.12 Drugs which interact with oral anticoagulants (adapted from the Scottish Intercollegiate Guidelines Network 1999).

Avoid			Sulphonamides
Aspirin	Except where combination specifically indicated	Thyroid	Carbimazole
			Thiouracils
Analgesics	Co-proxamol		Thyroxine
	Ketorolac (postoperative)	Non-steroidal anti-inflammatory	Diflunisal
Antifungals	Miconazole	Gout	Allopurinol
Diabetes	Glucagon		Sulphinpyrazone
Non-steroidal anti-inflammatory	Azopropazone	Others	Aminoglutethimide
	Phenylbutazone		Barbiturates
Others	Enteral feeds containing vitamin K		Cyclosporin
			Mercaptopurine
			Oral contraceptives
Adjust dose			
Ulcer healing	Cimetidine	***Monitor International Normalized Ratio***	
	Omeprazole	Gastrointestinal motility	Cisapride
Antiarrhythmics	Amiodarone	Antiarrythmics	Quinidine
	Propafenone		Cholestyramine
Lipid-lowering antiepileptics	Fibrates		Statins
	Carbamazepine	Antidepressants	Serotonin uptake antagonists
	Phenobarbitone	Antibiotics/antifungals	Check product data sheet, if not listed under 'adjust dose'
	Phenytoin		
	Primidone	Diabetes	Tolbutamide
Alcohol dependency	Disulfiram	Non-steroidal anti-inflammatory	Check product data sheet, if not listed under 'avoid' or 'adjust dose'
Antibiotics/antifungals	Aztreonam		
	Cephamandole		
	Chloramphenicol	Others	Anabolic steroids
	Ciprofloxacin		Corticosteroids
	Co-trimoxazole		Hormone antagonists
	Erythromycin		Ifosfamide
	Griseofulvin		Influenza vaccine
	Metronidazole		Rawachol
	Ofloxacin		Sucralfate
	Rifampicin		

once daily subcutaneous unfractionated heparin (12 500 IU) in 1095 patients with TIA and minor stroke (Nerni Serneri *et al.* 1999). The trial results were somewhat confounded, because there was a higher use of antiplatelet drugs in the control group. However, there was no significant difference in the proportion of patients with stroke or death (10.9% among patients allocated heparin vs. 11.7% among controls). The hazards of heparin are discussed in section 11.4.6.

Mesoglycan

Mesoglycan is a novel antithrombotic drug consisting of dermatan sulphate and heparin sulphate. It has been compared with aspirin in 1398 patients with recent ischaemic stroke. There were no clear differences in major outcome events between the two groups (Forconi *et al.* 1995). The agent is worthy of further study, but cannot be recommended for routine use at present.

Adding aspirin to anticoagulants

A systematic review of the six trials comparing oral anticoagulants with oral anticoagulants plus aspirin, included 3874 patients with cardio- and cerebrovascular disease and found that the addition of aspirin approximately doubled the risk of intracranial haemorrhage (Hart & Benavente 1999). For most categories of patients, and especially those at high risk of bleeding with anticoagulants, the combination should be avoided. However, in some categories of patients at particularly high risk of thromboembolism (e.g. mechanical prosthetic valves), the greater antithrombotic benefit of the combination may outweigh the extra bleeding risk (Loewen *et al.* 1998).

When to stop anticoagulants?

Most of the trials have tested only a few years of anticoagulants, and it is not yet known whether the balance of risk

Table 16.13 Target International Normalized Ratio (INR) for different indications (adapted from Scottish Intercollegiate Guidelines Network 1999).

Indication	Target (desired range) of INR
Prophylaxis of central venous catheter thrombosis	Minidose warfarin (1 mg/day) with no INR monitoring
Prophylaxis of venous thromboembolism in high-risk patients	2.5 (2.0–3.0)
Treatment of venous thromboembolism	
Prophylaxis of cardiac thromboembolism	
Atrial fibrillation	
Heart valve disease, heart failure, cardiomyopathy	
Bioprosthetic heart valves	
Acute myocardial infarction (selected patients)	
Mechanical heart valves	
First generation (e.g. Starr–Edwards, Bjork–Shiley)	3.5 (3.0–4.0)
Second generation (e.g. St Jude, Medtronic, Monostrut)	3.0 (2.0–3.0)

For fuller list see: Scottish Intercollegiate Guidelines Network 1999 (http://www.show.scot.nhs.uk/sign/clinical.htm).

and benefit alters with prolonged therapy, particularly as the patient passes the age of 70 years. However, the risk of bleeding does appear to increase with increasing duration of treatment (Levine *et al.* 1998).

If a patient has a serious haemorrhage, not due to over-anticoagulation, then the reason for giving anticoagulants should be reviewed, and the risk of thromboembolism reassessed. Since occult pathological lesions in the gastrointestinal tract and genitourinary system often present with bleeding, investigation of such patients (even if apparently over-anticoagulated) is usually justified (Levine *et al.* 1998).

Further research is clearly required to determine the optimum duration of treatment. If we considered that a patient remained at high risk (whatever their age), no bleeding events had occurred, and no factors which might increase the risk of bleeding had developed (e.g. falling or dementia), most of us would keep the patient on anticoagulants.

16.6 Angiotensin-converting enzyme inhibitors

16.6.1 Rationale

The findings of the Heart Outcomes Prevention Evaluation (HOPE) study suggest that the benefits of inhibition of the angiotensin-converting enzyme, with ramipril, are greater than might be expected from the small reduction in blood pressure it produced (Heart Outcomes Prevention Evaluation Study Investigators 2000a–c). The study also showed that the drug has vasculoprotective and renoprotective properties in diabetics. These data have generated hypotheses that activation of the renin–angiotensin system is an independent risk factor for cardiovascular disease and that angiotensin-converting enzyme inhibitors might have protective effects on the arterial wall.

16.6.2 Evidence

The HOPE study involved 267 centres from 19 countries in North America, South America and Europe and included 9297 patients with any evidence of coronary artery disease, stroke or peripheral vascular disease. Patients were randomly assigned to ramipril 10 mg daily or placebo. It included 3577 patients with diabetes mellitus (Heart Outcomes Prevention Evaluation Study Investigators 2000a–c). The primary outcome was a composite of myocardial infarction, stroke or death from cardiovascular causes. Secondary outcomes were revascularization, congestive heart failure, unstable angina or diabetic complications. The mean age of patients was 66 years, 27% were women, 90% had evidence of coronary artery disease and 38% had diabetes. Follow-up was for 4–6 years. In March 1999, the trial was terminated early on the recommendation of the trial's data and safety monitoring board. At this time, 13.9% of patients given ramipril had reached the primary outcome compared with 17.5% of patients given placebo (relative risk 0.78; 95% CI 0.70–0.86, $P < 0.000002$). These results correspond to a relative risk reduction of 25% for cardiovascular death, of 20% for myocardial infarction, and of 32% for stroke (Yusuf *et al.* 2000). Of the secondary outcomes, the ramipril group had a 15% relative risk reduction in revascularization and a 17% reduction in diabetic complications. Furthermore, subgroup analysis showed that these reductions were very similar for patients with normal cardiac function, for patients with or without hypertension, for patients with or without coronary artery disease, and for patients with diabetes.

16.6.3 Implications for clinical practice

The implications of this trial for clinical practice are potentially enormous if a large proportion of stroke patients are to be treated with angiotensin-converting enzyme inhibitors. If 50% of high-risk people in developed countries and 25% of people in developing countries with vascular disease were to take angiotensin-converting enzyme inhibitors, 400 000 deaths and 600 000 non-fatal cardiovascular events could be prevented every year, but at enormous cost (Heart Outcomes Prevention Evaluation Study Investigators 2000a,b,c). The choice of antihypertensive agent after stroke will be further informed by the results of the PROGRESS trial and other studies currently under way (section 16.3.1).

16.7 Treatment of specific underlying causes

16.7.1 Cardioversion of atrial fibrillation to sinus rhythm

There is limited agreement amongst cardiologists on the comparative merits of cardioversion by electric shock, cardioversion by drugs, and long-term oral anticoagulants; a consensus statement highlighted the need for further trials (Anon. 1999b). A decision analysis suggested that long-term antiarrhythmic drugs such as amiodarone may be preferable to anticoagulants in primary prevention; no calculations were provided for secondary prevention (Middlekauff *et al.* 1995). The selection of patients for cardioversion may be guided by the results of transoesophageal echocardiography (Kinch & Davidoff 1995; Di Pasquale *et al.* 1995).

We now quite often discuss whether or not to try and convert patients with atrial fibrillation and a recent TIA or ischaemic stroke to sinus rhythm with our local cardiological colleagues. Further trials to evaluate the best policy in this area are clearly needed.

16.7.2 Other cardiac lesions

For patients who have cardiac disorders with a high risk of embolism (e.g. rheumatic atrial fibrillation, mechanical prosthetic heart valves), the criteria for selecting which patients should be anticoagulated—and at what intensity—are reasonably clear (Stein *et al.* 1998; Scottish Intercollegiate Guidelines Network 1999, also available at http://www.show.scot.nhs.uk/sign/clinical.htm) (Table 16.13). The management of stroke in patients with prosthetic mechanical valves already on anticoagulants was discussed in sections 6.5 and 11.4.

The criteria to select which of the patients with structural lesions—such as patent foramen ovale, atrial septum aneurysm, mitral valve prolapse, mitral annular calcification, aortic sclerosis and left-ventricular aneurysms—should have surgical correction are not clear (Salen *et al.* 1998). In the treatment of these conditions which have the *potential* to be a source of embolism, but are associated with lower risks of thromboembolism, the choice of antithrombotic regimen is also problematic and recommendations by experts vary (Salen *et al.* 1998; Stein *et al.* 1998; Scottish Intercollegiate Guidelines Network 1999).

The management of ischaemic stroke and other thromboembolic events amongst pregnant patients with prosthetic heart valves is highly controversial and has been discussed in detail elsewhere (Greaves 1993; Sbarouni & Oakley 1994; Ginsberg and Hirsh 1998; Chan *et al.* 2000). Briefly, thromboprophylaxis of women with mechanical heart valves during pregnancy is best achieved with oral anticoagulants; however, this increases the risk of fetal abnormalities. Substituting oral anticoagulants with heparin between 6 and 12 weeks reduces the risk of fetal defects, but with an increased risk of thromboembolic complications. The use of low-dose heparin is definitely inadequate; the use of adjusted-dose heparin warrants aggressive monitoring and appropriate dose adjustment (Chan *et al.* 2000).

16.7.3 Dissection of the carotid and vertebral arteries

Thrombus may form at sites of intimal damage, and embolize to the brain, causing further infarction and a progressive stroke syndrome (section 7.2.1). If the dissection can be confirmed by ultrasound, MR angiography or catheter angiography, the difficult decision about whether or not to give anticoagulants or aspirin to prevent recurrent stroke often arises, and has been discussed earlier (section 11.4.2).

16.7.4 Antiphospholipid syndrome

This acquired disorder of the clotting system (section 7.3), which predisposes to thrombosis, may be treated with antiplatelet or anticoagulant drugs. There are few randomized trials. A small trial in 80 pregnant women with antiphospholipid syndrome and a history of recurrent miscarriage showed that heparin plus aspirin yielded a higher rate of live births than aspirin alone (Rai *et al.* 1997). A nonrandomized retrospective study suggested that warfarin was associated with a lower frequency of vascular events than aspirin, but the difference in vascular event rates between warfarin-treated patients and controls may have been related more to patient selection than to the treatment itself (Khamashta *et al.* 1995; Greaves 1999). The relative effects of anticoagulants and antiplatelet drugs on major vascular events needs to be evaluated by a larger scale randomized trial.

If you consider that clinical features suggest that antiphospholipid antibodies are contributing to stroke risk, it is probably reasonable to use antiplatelet drugs in the first instance, and then oral anticoagulants if the patient has a further thrombotic or embolic event (Scottish Intercollegiate Guidelines Network 1999, also available at http://www.show.scot.nhs.uk/sign/clinical.htm).

16.7.5 Homocysteinaemia

Observational epidemiological studies and case–control studies have suggested that a moderate increase in plasma homocysteine is a risk factor for premature vascular disease and stroke (sections 6.3.3 and 7.20). Treatment of young patients who have high levels of homocysteine with high-dose oral folate has been reported to yield some benefit in terms of neurological function, but whether this leads to a reduction in the risk of serious vascular events is not known. The place of routine folate supplementation is discussed in section 16.3.6.

16.7.6 Migraine

Migraine may be a modest independent risk factor for stroke, but the proportion of all strokes attributable to migraine must be extremely small. The risk of stroke in an individual migraineur is so low that prophylactic treatment purely to prevent migrainous stroke cannot be justified (section 7.8). Patients who have frequent severe migraine and other vascular risk factors should of course have their vascular risk factors dealt with conventionally; those who have *symptomatic* vascular disease should be on aspirin anyway. In the US Physicians's Study, patients allocated to aspirin had a 20% lower relative risk of recurrent migraine than those allocated placebo (Buring *et al.* 1990).

16.7.7 Hyperviscosity

Stroke is a rare complication of the hyperviscosity syndrome (section 7.9). Management should be guided by the treatment of the underlying disorder (i.e. by the type and severity of the underlying pathology, e.g. myeloma), and not by the stroke.

16.7.8 Oral contraceptives and hormone replacement therapy

Young women who have a stroke of any pathological type whilst on oral contraceptives should probably stop them (section 7.13.1). A substantial proportion of these women have other vascular risk factors (usually smoking, but other factors may be present as well, such as hypertension) and these require attention in their own right. Alternative forms of contraception should be offered.

A small proportion of postmenopausal women on hormone replacement therapy (HRT) have a stroke (section 7.13.2). For them, the question then arises 'should the treatment be stopped or continued?' Observational epidemiological data suggest that, amongst women free of vascular disease when they start treatment, HRT is more likely to prevent coronary heart disease events than cause cancer of the breast or uterine cavity and there may also be a small reduction in the risk of limb bone fractures. There are several ongoing randomized trials of HRT in primary and secondary prevention of vascular disease. The most relevant of these is the Women's Estrogen for Stroke Trial (WEST) study which is comparing, in postmenopausal women with recent stroke or TIA, HRT with control, to see whether there is a net reduction in the risk of stroke and other serious vascular events in such high-risk individuals (Horwitz & Brass 1994).

The ESPRIT-UK trial is evaluating oestrogen in the secondary prevention of reinfarction in female survivors of myocardial infarction; the trial protocol is not published, but for details of this trial and of the two large trials of hormone replacement in primary prevention of vascular disease (Women's Health Initiative (WHI) (Buring & Hennekens 1992) and Women's International Study of Long Duration Oestrogen after Menopause (WISDOM)); see http://www.cardiosource.com. Pending the results of these trials in primary and secondary prevention, guidance for an individual woman having a stroke whilst on HRT must be based on guesswork rather than facts. Women will be influenced in their decision whether to stop or continue HRT after their stroke by the severity of the symptoms which led to the initiation of HRT; those who had had severe menopausal symptoms may wish to continue and those with mild or no symptoms (e.g. they were taking HRT for prophylaxis of osteoporosis) may wish to stop.

The role of hormone replacement therapy in postmenopausal women for primary and secondary stroke prevention is the subject of current research; firm guidelines cannot be given at present but there is no overwhelming reason for women who have a stroke to stop their hormonal treatment.

16.7.9 Infections

Less than 1% of all strokes are due to unusual infections, but if rare treatable conditions such as Lyme disease, human immunodeficiency virus (HIV) or syphilis are diagnosed clinically and confirmed serologically, then specific treatment is required (section 7.11).

16.7.10 Sickle cell disease

Repeated blood transfusion can—in the short term—prevent stroke in children with sickle cell disease and stroke (section 7.9); and appears to be effective in preventing both a first stroke and recurrent stroke (Adams *et al.* 1998). However, the trials to date have been small, the treatment is expensive and intrusive and can lead to long-term iron overload: long-term trials evaluating long-term complications are needed.

16.8 Endarterectomy for symptomatic carotid stenosis

16.8.1 Introduction

Soon after the introduction of cerebral angiography, and the rediscovery that atherothrombotic stenosis at the origin of the internal carotid artery (ICA) could cause ischaemic stroke (which had actually been suggested many decades earlier, section 2.5), surgeons began to devise methods to remove or bypass the arterial lesion (Thompson 1996). After early surgical attempts in China and Argentina, the first successful endarterectomy was done by DeBakey in 1953, but not reported until more than 20 years later (Chao *et al.* 1938; Carrea *et al.* 1955; DeBakey 1975). However, it was really the report of Felix Eastcott's successful carotid reconstruction in a patient with frequent 'low-flow' TIAs at St Mary's Hospital in London that gave the impetus to what was to become, in North America at least, an epidemic of carotid endarterectomies for asymptomatic as well as symptomatic stenosis (Eastcott *et al.* 1954; Pokras & Dyken 1988). ICA occlusion generally came to be regarded as inoperable and surgical attempts to correct carotid coils, kinks and fibromuscular dysplasia are not supported by any good evidence.

Innumerable surgical case series have been published. Although they provide some idea of the risk of surgery and how it might be minimized, they cannot demonstrate any certain benefit because most economized by foregoing the luxury of any control group at all and the rest used only non-randomized controls. The two early randomized trials were inconclusive (Fields *et al.* 1970; Shaw *et al.* 1984). Not surprisingly, in view of the lack of reliable data, there were soon huge variations in surgery rates between countries, and even within the same country (UK-TIA Study Group 1983; Warlow 1984). Under these highly unsatisfactory circumstances, physcians began to question publicly the utility of carotid endarterectomy, inappropriate use of surgery was documented, and the number of operations—perhaps as a consequence—began to fall (Barnett *et al.* 1984; Warlow 1984; Pokras & Dyken 1988; Winslow *et al.* 1988; Tu *et al.* 1998). Eventually, in the early 1980s, these pressures persuaded surgeons and physicians to mount randomized trials large enough to be conclusive, and the first results in patients with *symptomatic* stenosis began to appear in the early 1990s (European Carotid Surgery Trialists' Collaborative Group 1991; Mayberg *et al.* 1991; North American Symptomatic Carotid Endarterectomy Trial Collaborators 1991). Surgery clearly did prevent stroke in patients with recently symptomatic severe ICA stenosis, but at a price: the risk of stroke as a consequence of surgery, the risk of other complications of surgery, the cost of surgery, and the risk and cost of the investigations to select suitable patients (section 6.7.5). By then carotid endarterectomy was rapidly becoming one of the most studied surgical procedures ever and the stage was set for clinical guidelines supported by something other than whim, the beginnings of economic analyses (section 16.8.6), an estimate of the public health impact of surgery (section 18.4.1), and comparisons of risk between institutions and even individual surgeons (section 16.8.7). Not surprisingly, surgery rates have started rising again. However, there is concern in North America that much of this rise is to do with operating on *asymptomatic* stenosis which may well not be appropriate, and on patients with non-specific symptoms which is definitely inappropriate (Cebul *et al.* 1998; Tu *et al.* 1998) (section 16.9). Paradoxically, there is also concern at unmet needs, at least in the UK (Ferris *et al.* 1998). Nowadays, the challenge is to decide which individuals should be offered surgery: not 'does surgery work?' because—on average—it clearly does, but 'for whom is surgery most appropriate?' (sections 16.8.7–16.8.9).

16.8.2 The carotid endarterectomy operation

The carotid bifurcation is exposed, gently mobilized, and slings placed around the internal, external and common carotid arteries (Fig. 16.20). During this exposure, embolic material may be inadvertently dislodged from the arterial lumen, and nerves which lie close to the artery can be damaged (section 16.8.4). After applying clamps to these three arteries, away from any atheromatous plaque, the bifurcation is opened through a longitudinal incision, the entire stenotic lesion cored out, the distal intimal margin secured, the arteriotomy closed, and the clamps released to restore blood flow to the brain. Most patients should already be on antiplatelet drugs before surgery and these should be continued afterwards because the patients are still at high risk of ischaemic stroke in the territory of other arteries, and of coronary events (section 16.1). In addition, most surgeons heparinize patients during the procedure itself. Controlling systemic blood pressure before, during and after surgery is crucial to avoid hypotension, which will make any cerebral ischaemia worse, and hypertension which may cause cerebral oedema or even intracerebral haemorrhage (section 16.8.3). Operative damage to the nerve to the carotid sinus, or changes in the carotid sinus itself, may make control of postoperative blood pressure more of a problem, but in the long term has

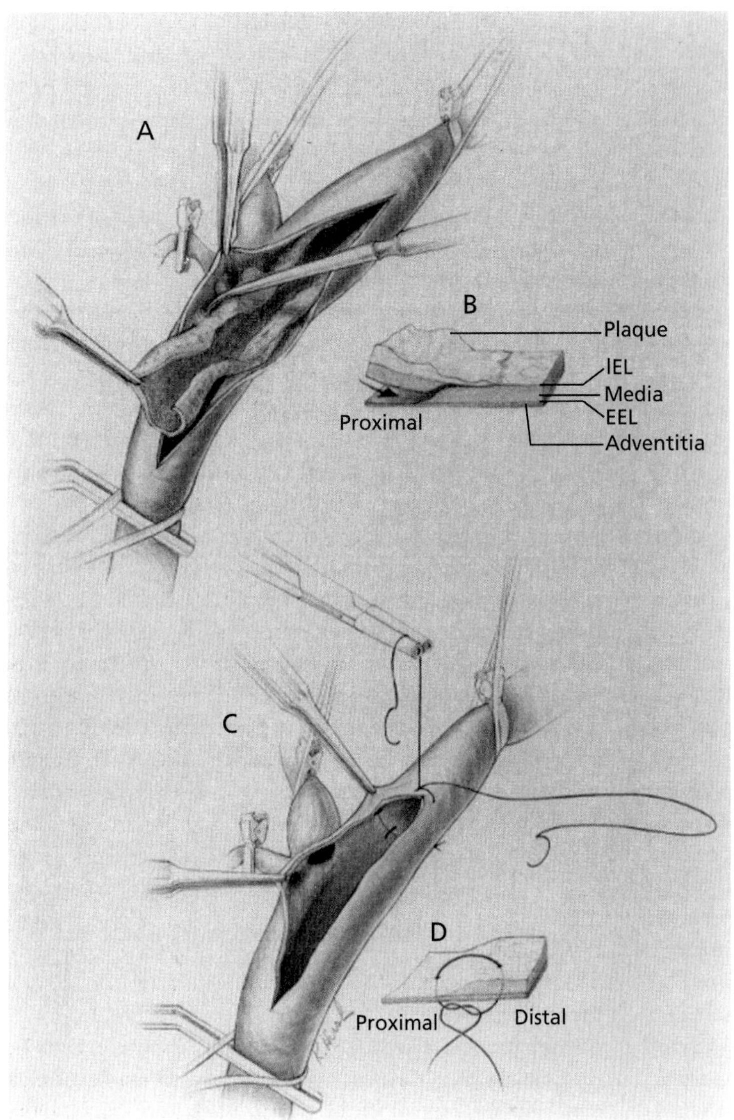

Fig. 16.20 Illustration of a standard carotid endarterectomy. At A the atherothrombotic plaque is being cored out, the plane of dissection usually being between the media and external elastic lamina (EEL) at B. At C the artery is being closed with particular attention to tacking down the distal intimal flap at D. IEL, internal elastic lamina. (With permission from Zarins & Gewertz 1987.)

little if any effect (Eliasziw *et al.* 1998). This then is the operation at its simplest, and for nearly 50 years surgeons have been attempting to make it safer by using various modifications on the basic technique, which has remained essentially unchanged, although a few surgeons prefer eversion endarterectomy rather than the standard procedure (Loftus & Quest 1987; Darling *et al.* 1996; Cao *et al.* 1998).

Cerebral protection (shunting)

In theory, it should be possible to prevent low cerebral blood flow during carotid clamping, and so perhaps an ischaemic stroke, by inserting a temporary intralumenal shunt from the common carotid artery (CCA) to the ICA distal to the operation site. Some surgeons routinely shunt for this reason, and to allow more time to teach trainees, but there are problems:

- insertion may be difficult, particularly with small-calibre arteries, and the shunt can dissect the arterial wall or dislodge atherothrombotic material which embolizes to the brain;
- clot may form in the shunt and embolize, or even occlude the shunt completely;
- the shunt may be obstructed by kinking, or if the end abuts against the arterial wall;
- the shunt can transmit emboli from thrombus in the CCA damaged during shunt insertion;
- the shunt itself may make the operation technically more difficult, and longer, and the more extensive surgical exposure required may increase the chance of nerve damage, postoperative haematoma and infection.

A compromise is to selectively shunt only patients *likely* to develop, or who actually are experiencing, cerebral ischaemia as a result of low flow. But who exactly are they? There have been enormous but inconclusive efforts to identify the patients who need shunting (Ferguson 1986; Ojemann & Heros 1986; Naylor *et al.* 1992). Some believe that a shunt should be used if there is contralateral ICA occlusion, or if the patient has had a recent ischaemic stroke. Others shunt patients who have a low ICA 'stump' pressure (measured distal to the ICA clamp), perhaps indicating poor collateral blood flow to the ipsilateral cerebral hemisphere. Collateralization itself can possibly be predicted preoperatively with transcranial Doppler techniques (Schneider *et al.* 1988). Intraoperative monitoring of the electroencephalogram, sensory evoked potentials, regional cerebral blood flow, middle cerebral artery blood flow and emboli detection with transcranial Doppler, jugular venous oxygen saturation, cerebrovascular haemoglobin oxygen saturation with near-infrared spectroscopy, and the neurological state of the patient if operated under regional anaesthesia, may provide early warning of cerebral ischaemia. But, all this may be too late for a quickly inserted shunt, or abandoned operation, to ameliorate the consequences of cerebral ischaemia which may not even be reversible at all if actually due to embolism from the operation site rather than low flow.

The risk of stroke as a consequence of carotid endarterectomy is so low that to have a 90% probability of detecting the effect of an intervention that further reduces this risk by as much as 50%—say from 6% to 3%—requires at least 1000 patients in each of two arms of a randomized trial comparing the intervention with control. The same problem of power and sample size applies to non-randomized comparisons although these are far less reliable because of their many potential biases.

Unfortunately, it is almost impossible to demonstrate reliably that any particular policy reduces perioperative stroke risk, because it is already so small that very large numbers of patients are required to avoid random error (Schroeder 1990; Halsey 1992). Even putting what randomized evidence there is about shunting together in a meta-analysis is inconclusive (Counsell *et al.* 2000a). Furthermore, it is difficult to distinguish the rather small number of preventable (by shunting) strokes due to low flow from the larger number of unpreventable (by shunting) strokes due to embolism (section 16.8.3). As a result, there is no standard policy for either operative monitoring or the use of shunts, and surgeons rely on their own experience, commonsense, and whatever technique of monitoring they have available and are comfortable with.

There is no standard method to predict reliably which patients will have an ischaemic stroke during carotid clamping. It is therefore difficult to select patients who should be protected by a shunt during carotid endarterectomy, which is why there is so much variation in practice.

Restenosis and patch angioplasty

After carotid endarterectomy the long-term risk of ischaemic stroke ipsilateral to the operated artery is so low that recurrent stenosis cannot be of any great clinical concern, in the sense of causing stroke (section 16.8.5). If stenosis does recur then a second endarterectomy is more difficult and risky, and angioplasty or stenting may be preferable, although there is no randomized evidence for either procedure in symptomatic or asymptomatic restenosis (Yadav *et al.* 1996). In fact, the reported rate of restenosis varies enormously depending on whether the study was prospective or retrospective, the completeness and length of follow-up, the sensitivity and specificity of the imaging method used, and the definition of restenosis (Frericks *et al.* 1998). Sometimes, a restenosis is not a restenosis at all but a residual stenosis from a technically inadequate carotid endarterectomy. Certainly, recurrent atherothrombotic stenosis can occur, but usually not for some years, whilst early restenosis (within a year or so) is more likely to be due to neointimal hyperplasia (Hunter *et al.* 1987). On balance, therefore, there is no point in repeated clinical or ultrasonographic follow-up just to detect asymptomatic restenosis, but if a restenosis becomes symptomatic then a repeat carotid endarterectomy is probably reasonable.

Many surgeons routinely use a patch of autologous vein, or synthetic material, to close the artery, enlarge the lumen and so—they hope—reduce the risk of restenosis and, more importantly, of stroke. Meta-analysis of the few randomized trials, many of which were of low quality, suggested a possible reduction in restenosis and fewer perioperative arterial occlusions but, not surprisingly, there were so few strokes that any effect on their risk was very uncertain (Counsell *et al.* 1998, 2000b). Patching increases the surgery time, there are two suture lines rather than one and there are complications, albeit rarely: the centre of a vein patch can become necrotic and rupture to cause a life-threatening neck haematoma, perhaps less often if the vein is harvested from the thigh than the ankle; aneurysmal bulging and dilatation of the carotid bifurcation; and synthetic grafts can become infected. Also, it may be impossible to find enough leg vein left over after any earlier coronary artery surgery, and removing what vein there is can cause local haematoma, infection, ulceration and discomfort. Further randomized trials are clearly required but the stroke rates are now so low, or should be, that very large numbers will be required to show that patching reduces not just restenosis, but what really matters—stroke.

General vs. regional anaesthesia

Surgery is more often performed under general than regional anaesthesia. Both types have their strong supporters and detractors. With general anaesthesia, the patient lies perfectly still and there is good control over the cardiovascular system, but there is probably a higher risk of coronary and pulmonary complications. With regional anaesthesia, there is a much lower shunt rate because it is immediately obvious when a shunt is needed to restore blood flow distal to the carotid clamps, elaborate intraoperative monitoring is unnecessary, and hospital stay may be shorter. On the other hand, some patients will not tolerate the procedure and a quick change to general anaesthesia may be required. What little evidence there is favours regional anaesthesia (Tangkanakul *et al.* 2000). Only a large definitive trial will confirm what might turn out to be a substantially lower operative stroke risk and this has been started in the UK (http://www.dcn.ed.ac.uk/gala).

Early technical failure

Just occasionally the carotid artery occludes immediately, or a few days after surgery, as a result of thrombosis, dissection or excessive kinking at the operation site. This does not necessarily cause stroke if the collateral supply to the brain is sufficient. Both thrombosis and dissection are thought to be largely due to poor operative technique, particularly if the distal intimal flap has been left unsecured or there is a ridge of arterial tissue due to faulty suturing. Residual disease is another cause of thrombosis. Therefore, before closing the skin, some surgeons check the endarterectomy site with conventional ultrasonography, angiography, angioscopy or intravascular ultrasound and, if necessary, reopen the artery to improve the anatomical result. Whether this has much effect on surgical or later stroke risk is unknown.

16.8.3 Perioperative stroke

The most feared complication of carotid endarterectomy is stroke, the very thing the operation is designed to prevent (Naylor & Ruckley 1996; Ferguson *et al.* 1999) (Table 16.14). The reported risk ranges from an implausibly low 1% or less, to an unacceptably high of 20% or more. This variation may be explained by differences in: the definition of stroke; whether all or only some strokes are included; the accuracy of stroke diagnosis; the completeness of the clinical details; whether the study was retrospective or prospective; whether the diagnosis of stroke was based on patient observation or just medical record review; variation in casemix, surgical and anaesthetic skills; whether the rate is per patient or per operated artery; chance and random variation; and publication bias (Campbell 1993; Rothwell *et al.* 1996b). No more than 20% of perioperative strokes are likely to be fatal, being mostly either total or partial anterior circulation

Table 16.14 Complications of carotid endarterectomy.

Ischaemic stroke or transient ischaemic attack (almost always ipsilateral to the operated artery) due to:
Embolism from the operation site during surgery
Embolism from the operation site after surgery
Carotid dissection
Perioperative internal carotid artery occlusion
Low cerebral blood flow during surgery
Perioperative systemic hypotension

Haemorrhagic stroke (almost always ipsilateral to the operated artery) due to:
Perioperative hypertension
Postendarterectomy cerebral hyperperfusion
Antithrombotic drugs

Death due to:
Stroke
Myocardial infarction
Pulmonary embolism
Rupture of arterial operation site

Cardiovascular and respiratory complications:
Myocardial infarction
Angina
Hypotension/hypertension
Cardiac arrhythmia
Cardiac failure
Chest infection

Local complications:
Cranial and peripheral nerve injury (recurrent and superior laryngeal, vagal, hypoglossal, marginal mandibular branch of facial, spinal accessory, greater auricular, transverse cervical nerves)
Wound infection
Neck haematoma
Aneurysmal dilatation at operation site
Patch disruption and haemorrhage
Malignant tumour in the scar
Chyle fistula

Others:
Deep venous thrombosis and pulmonary embolism
Transhemispheric cerebral oedema
Headache
Focal epileptic seizures
Facial (parotid) pain
Pain at vein donor site after vein patch angioplasty

infarcts with 30-day case fatalities of about 40% and 5%, respectively (Table 10.2). Therefore, reports of less than four times as many non-fatal as fatal strokes are almost certainly undercounting mild strokes, a tendency which may well be due to surgeons reporting their own results without the 'help' of any neurologists (Rothwell & Warlow 1995). Despite the obvious implications for service planning, it has been all but impossible to sort out whether there really is a systematic difference in risk between surgeons. This is largely due to the problems of adjusting for casemix, as well as chance effects due to the inevitably rather small numbers operated on by each surgeon (Rothwell *et al.* 1999a). One might anticipate that 'practice makes perfect' and there is at least some casemix-adjusted evidence that high-volume surgeons have lower operative risks than low-volume surgeons (Kucey *et al.* 1998). But, whatever anyone claims, and even though the size of any stroke risk depends on the study quoted, there is no doubt that there is a risk of stroke and death, realistically somewhere between 3% and 10%, depending on various factors (section 16.8.7).

There are several causes for perioperative stroke but these are difficult to identify when it occurs during general anaesthesia, or even afterwards. In an emergency situation on a surgical ward, it may be impossible to get one or more of a neurologist, brain CT scan, carotid ultrasound and angiogram quickly enough to allow any useful corrective action (see below). Clinical details are often so poorly recorded that, in retrospect, it can be impossible to establish a cause. Also, despite attempts to do so, it is difficult to be sure whether *any* stroke, let alone a perioperative stroke, is due to embolism or low flow (Steed *et al.* 1982; Krul *et al.* 1989; Riles *et al.* 1994; Spencer 1997) (section 6.6.5).

Embolism from the operation site

This is probably the most common cause of stroke *during* surgery. Atherothrombotic debris may be released whilst the carotid bifurcation is being mobilized, as the carotid clamps are applied, when any shunt is inserted, and when the clamps are removed. Indeed, air bubbles or particulate emboli during surgery are very commonly detected by transcranial Doppler ultrasound, although most seem to be of little clinical consequence (Gaunt *et al.* 1993; Jansen *et al.* 1994a). *Postoperative* ischaemic stroke is usually due to embolism from residual but disrupted atheromatous plaque; thrombus forming on the endarterectomized surface or on suture lines, or more probably on a loose distal intimal flap where the lesion has been carelessly snapped off; thrombus complicating damaged arterial wall as a result of the clamps; and thrombus complicating arterial dissection starting at a loose intimal flap of the ICA or as a result of shunt damage to the arterial wall. A high rate of postoperative microembolic signals on transcranial Doppler monitoring may predict ischaemic stroke, but the numbers of strokes is very small so it is difficult to be sure (Levi *et al.* 1997).

Stroke complicating carotid endarterectomy is most commonly due to embolism from the operation site during or soon after surgery. Ischaemic stroke due to interruption of carotid blood flow during surgery is less common and intracerebral haemorrhage is very rare.

Acute internal carotid artery occlusion

This is caused by occlusive thrombosis or dissection, usually a result of technical failure during surgery (see above). It may not cause stroke if the collateral blood supply is adequate.

Low-flow ischaemic stroke

Clearly, temporary reduction in ICA blood flow during carotid clamping may cause ipsilateral ischaemic stroke if the collateral supply from the contralateral ICA and vertebrobasilar system, through the circle of Willis, is inadequate, particularly if there is already maximal cerebral vasodilatation (i.e. cerebrovascular reserve is exhausted). Rarely, systemic hypotension may cause ischaemic stroke and low-flow infarction contralateral to surgery, but probably only if the contralateral ICA is occluded.

Haemorrhagic stroke and cerebral hyperperfusion

Intracranial haemorrhage is most unusual. It can occur during surgery or up to about 1 week later, almost always ipsilateral to the operated artery. It may be due to the increase in perfusion pressure and cerebral blood flow that occurs after removal of a severe ICA stenosis, particularly if cerebral autoregulation is defective as a consequence of a recent cerebral infarct (Ouriel *et al.* 1999). Antithrombotic drugs and uncontrolled hypertension may also play a part (Solomon *et al.* 1986; Hafner *et al.* 1987; Piepgras *et al.* 1988; Jansen *et al.* 1994b).

Interestingly, transient cerebral hyperperfusion, ipsilateral but sometimes bilateral, lasting some days is quite common after carotid endarterectomy, particularly if the lesion is severely stenosing and cerebrovascular reserve is already poor with impaired autoregulation. This may be the cause of the occasional case of ipsilateral transhemispheric cerebral oedema, intracerebral haemorrhage, focal epileptic seizures and headache which can all occur a few days after surgery. Clearly this syndrome is different from ischaemic stroke due to low flow or embolism, and is distinguished by the slower onset, as well as by brain and arterial imaging (Andrews *et al.* 1987; Schroeder *et al.* 1987; Naylor *et al.* 1993b; Chambers *et al.* 1994; Breen *et al.* 1996). To complicate matters, a very similar clinical syndrome has been described as a result of cerebral vasoconstriction (Lopez-Valdes *et al.* 1997).

Management of perioperative stroke

Unless the operation was under regional anaesthesia, or cerebral ischaemia has not already been suspected by intraoperative monitoring, the first clue that a patient has had an intraoperative stroke is usually delay or failure to awaken from general anaesthesia. It is then vital to determine, within minutes if possible, whether the cause is thrombosis at the operation site, because this is amenable to correction. If transcranial Doppler monitoring has been used during the operation, a change in the middle cerebral artery velocity signal may have suggested a problem at the endarterectomy site (any confusion with intracerebral haemorrhage distorting the Doppler signal is most unlikely). Ideally, a rapid bedside duplex scan should be done and the neck immediately reopened if ICA occlusion is suspected, even taking the very low risk that there is actually an intracerebral haemorrhage. Passage of a Fogarty catheter, restoration of flow, and correction of any technical fault which caused the thrombosis can, in some circumstances, be followed by complete neurological recovery. The later after operation a stroke occurs the less likely that return to theatre is either practical or effective, but how late is too late is a guess.

If the operated ICA is still patent, then the next question is whether the stroke is due to intracerebral haemorrhage. A brain CT scan is therefore needed and further management is the same as for spontaneous stroke (Chapter 10).

16.8.4 Other complications

Carotid endarterectomy is associated with a wide variety of potential complications (Naylor & Ruckley 1996) (Table 16.14).

Death is reported in about 1–2% of patients and is generally due to stroke, myocardial infarction or some other complication of the frequently associated coronary heart disease or, rarely, to pulmonary embolism (Rothwell *et al.* 1996a). Higher rates can be found in 'administrative data sets' which may be a more realistic reflection of routine practice than large randomized trials, but any comparisons are confounded by variation in casemix, particularly the proportion of patients with asymptomatic stenosis who have a lower case fatality (Rothwell *et al.* 1996b; Wennberg *et al.* 1998).

Cardiovascular and respiratory complications. Myocardial infarction during, or in the early days after surgery, occurs in 1–2% of patients, more often if there is symptomatic coronary heart disease, and particularly if myocardial infarction has occurred in the previous few months or if the patient has unstable angina. Perioperative myocardial infarction can be painless so clues to the diagnosis are unexplained hypotension, tachycardia and dysrhythmias. Congestive cardiac failure, angina and cardiac dysrhythmias are also occasional concerns (Riles *et al.* 1979; North American Symptomatic Carotid Endarterectomy Trial Collaborators 1991; Urbinati *et al.* 1994; Paciaroni *et al.* 1999). Postoperative hypertension and hypotension may be a problem, perhaps due to operative interference with the carotid baroreceptors, but it is transient. Postoperative chest infection occurs in less than 1%.

Cranial and peripheral nerve injuries as a result of traction, pressure or transection occur in up to 20% of cases, the frequency partly depending on how hard one looks (Fig. 16.21). However, these injuries are not necessarily symptomatic, and are seldom of any long-term consequence. Damage to the recurrent and superior laryngeal branches of the vagus nerve, or more probably the vagus itself, causes change of voice quality, hoarseness, difficulty coughing and sometimes dyspnoea on exertion due to vocal cord paralysis. If a simultaneous or staged bilateral carotid endarterectomy is done, and causes bilateral vocal cord paralysis, then airway obstruction can occur. Hypoglossal nerve injury causes ipsilateral weakness of the tongue which can lead to temporary or even permanent dysarthria, difficulty with mastication or dysphagia. Again, bilateral damage causes much more serious speech and swallowing problems, and sometimes even upper airway obstruction. Damage to the marginal mandibular branch of the facial nerve causes rather trivial weakness at the corner of the mouth. Spinal accessory nerve injury is rare and causes pain and stiffness in the shoulder and neck, along with weakness of the sternomastoid and trapezius muscles. A high incision can cut the greater auricular nerve to cause numbness over the ear lobe and angle of the jaw, which may persist and be irritating for the patient. Damage to the transverse cervical nerves is almost inevitable and causes numbness around the scar area which is seldom a problem. Clearly, permanent disability from a nerve injury can be as bad as a mild stroke and needs to be taken into account when considering the risks and benefits of surgery (Gutrecht & Jones 1988; Maniglia & Han 1991; Sweeney & Wilbourn 1992).

> *Permanent disability from surgical injury to a nerve in the neck is very rare but can be as bad or worse than many operative strokes, and must be taken into account when assessing the risk of surgery.*

Therefore, if a patient has symptoms referable to *both* severely stenosed carotid arteries, requiring bilateral carotid endarterectomy, it is probably safer to do the operations a few weeks apart rather than under the same anaesthetic, mostly because of the dangers of bilateral hypoglossal or vagal nerve damage.

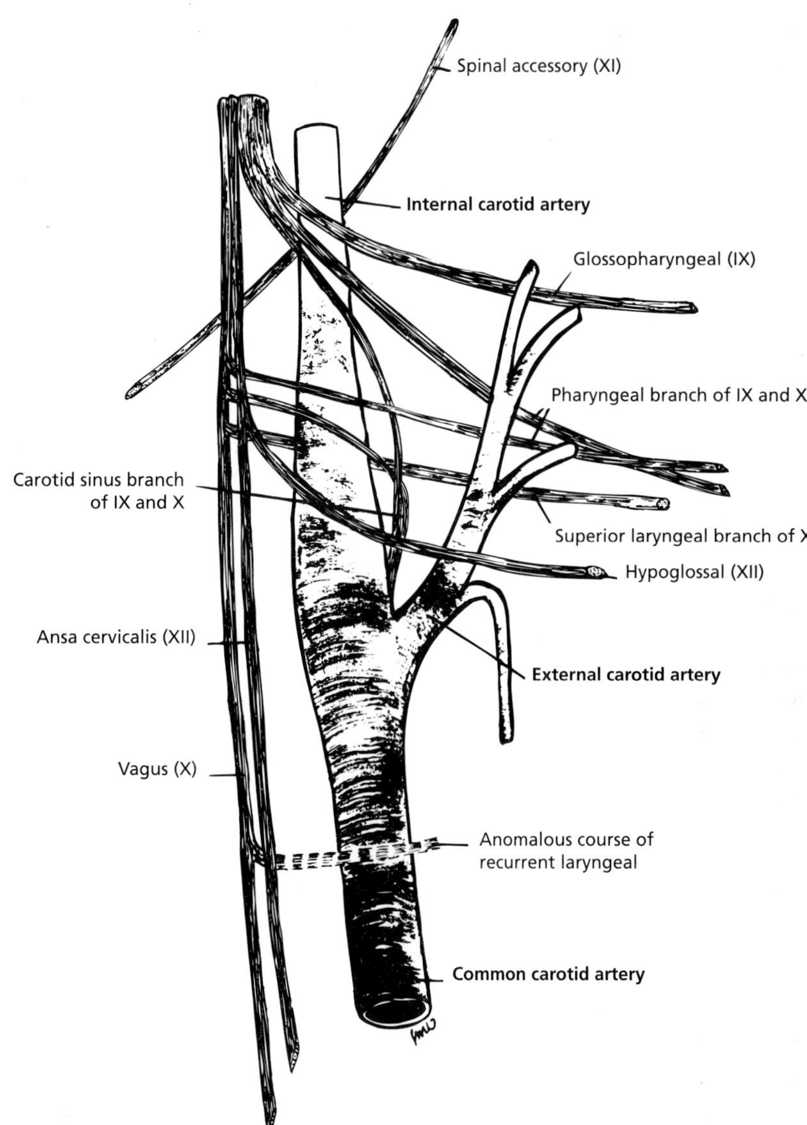

Fig. 16.21 Diagram of the nerves in the neck which may be damaged during carotid endarterectomy (adapted with permission from Schroeder & Levi 1999).

Before a staged second carotid endarterectomy it is always wise to inspect the tongue and vocal cords to ensure there has been no subclinical unilateral nerve damage from the first operation because, if so, the second operation should be postponed.

Local wound complications include: infection; haematoma or, rarely, major haemorrhage, due to leakage or rupture of the arteriotomy or patch which can be life threatening if it causes tracheal compression; aneurysm formation weeks or years later; and malignant tumour in the scar—all are rare (Graver & Mulcare 1986; Martin-Negrier *et al.* 1996). Although surgeons often notice the haemostatic defect caused by preoperative aspirin, this probably does not increase the rate of reoperation for bleeding (Lindblad *et al.* 1993). Very rarely the thoracic duct can be damaged and cause a chyle fistula.

Headache ipsilateral to the operation may occur and is perhaps related to transient cerebral hyperperfusion (section 16.8.3), uncontrolled hypertension or something akin to cluster headache due to subtle damage to the sympathetic plexus around the carotid artery (De Marinis *et al.* 1991; Ille *et al.* 1995). Very rarely, *focal epileptic seizures* occur as well as headache (Youkey *et al.* 1984). Of course, seizures may occasionally complicate perioperative stroke, just like any other stroke (sections 6.6.6 and 15.8).

Facial pain ipsilateral to surgery and related to eating is most unusual and may in some way be due to disturbed innervation of the parotid gland (Truax 1989).

16.8.5 Evidence of benefit

As a result of the large randomized controlled trials, it is now quite clear that endarterectomy of recently symptomatic *severe* carotid stenosis almost completely abolishes the high risk of ischaemic stroke ipsilateral to the operated artery over the subsequent 2 or 3 years. Moreover, this effect is durable over at least 8 years (European Carotid Surgery Trialists' Collaborative Group 1991, 1998; North American Symptomatic Carotid Endarterectomy Trial Collaborators 1991; Mayberg *et al.* 1991; Barnett *et al.* 1998). Indeed, the ipsilateral stroke risk becomes so low that presumably both embolic and low-flow strokes are being prevented (Fig. 16.22b). Because so few strokes in these patients are anything other than ipsilateral and ischaemic (Fig. 16.22c), and taking account of the early risk of surgical death or stroke (Fig. 16.22a), the balance of surgical risk and long-term benefit is—on average—in favour of surgery combined with best medical treatment compared with best medical treatment alone (i.e. treatment of hypertension, stopping smoking, antithrombotic drugs, etc.) (Fig. 16.22d).

On average, there is clearly an advantage to surgery when the symptomatic stenosis exceeds 80% diameter reduction of the arterial lumen using the European Carotid Surgery Trial (ECST) method, which is about the same as 70% using the North American Symptomatic Carotid Endarterectomy Trial (NASCET) method (section 6.7.4). The risk of surgery is much the same at all degrees of stenosis and so, because the unoperated risk of stroke in patients with less than 60% (ECST) stenosis is so low, the risk of surgery is not worthwhile for them (Fig. 16.22). Presumably, most of these patients have had TIAs, and some will have strokes in the future, due not just to embolism from the mildly diseased carotid bifurcation but to undiscovered (by imaging) atherothrombosis elsewhere, or cardiac sources of embolism, or to intracranial small vessel disease. For patients with between 60% and 80% (ECST) stenosis there is still some uncertainty left because there may be a few patients at high enough risk of stroke who would gain from surgery, if only we knew who they were (section 16.8.8).

The high risk of stroke with unoperated severe stenosis rapidly attenuates in the first 2 years after presentation, and within 3 years it is the same as in patients with mild stenosis (Fig. 16.23). This can also be inferred from inspection of the survival curves of unoperated and operated patients which become parallel after about 2 years (Fig. 16.24). Where the curves cross at about 6 months, the risk of stroke is equal

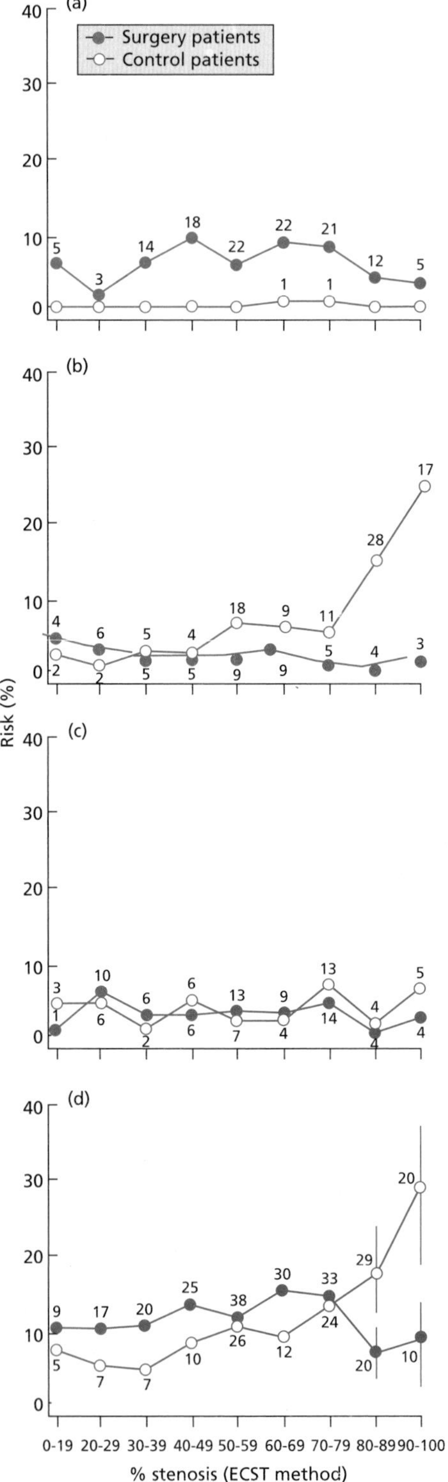

Fig. 16.22 Risk (%) of outcome events at 3 years in the surgery vs. no surgery control group by severity of carotid diameter stenosis in the European Carotid Surgery Trial (ECST). (a) The surgical risk: actual risk of stroke lasting more than 7 days and all deaths within 30 days of trial surgery. (b) The surgical benefit: predicted risk of ipsilateral ischaemic stroke lasting more than 7 days. (c) The noise: predicted risk of all other strokes lasting more than 7 days. (d) The net benefit by combining the surgical risk, the surgical benefit and the noise: predicted risk of any stroke lasting more than 7 days and the actual risk of a stroke lasting more than 7 days or death as a result of surgery (with permission from European Carotid Surgery Trialists' Collaborative Group 1998). The numbers at each point indicate the number of patients with an event. The vertical lines are 95% confidence intervals.

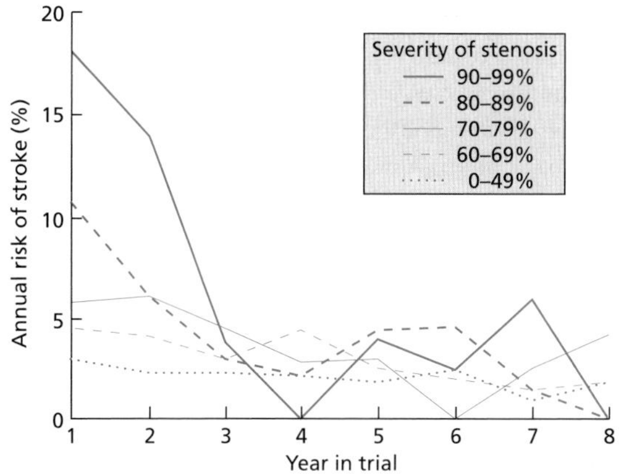

Fig. 16.23 Risk (%) of any stroke lasting more than 7 days (first or subsequent) in the no-surgery patients in the European Carotid Surgery Trial by severity of carotid diameter stenosis and in each of the 8 years following randomization (with permission from European Carotid Surgery Trialists' Collaborative Group 1998).

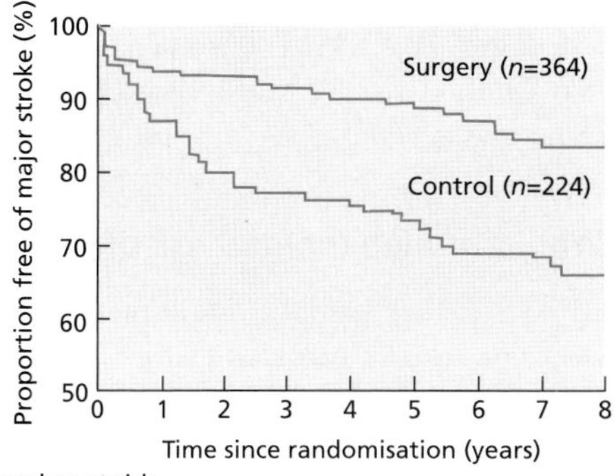

Fig. 16.24 Kaplan–Meier survival curves to show survival free of stroke lasting more than 7 days (non-stroke deaths occurring more than 30 days after surgery are censored) in the surgery and no-surgery control patients with 80–99% diameter stenosis of the symptomatic carotid artery in the European Carotid Surgery Trial (with permission from European Carotid Surgery Trialists' Collaborative Group 1998).

in surgical and non-surgical patients but, because the surgical strokes have occurred earlier and may have caused persisting disability, the surgery group is not advantaged until 6 months after this point when the two groups have a similar number of 'stroke–disability' years.

After successful surgery for recently symptomatic severe carotid stenosis, the high risk of ischaemic stroke ipsilateral to the operated artery is almost completely removed. For patients with recently symptomatic mild and moderate stenosis the unoperated risk of stroke is not high enough to make the immediate risk of surgery worthwhile.

Because the risk of stroke in moderate stenosis patients remains low for several years (Fig. 16.23), there is no point in duplex follow-up in case the stenosis becomes more severe. No doubt severe stenosis does sometimes develop but, unless there are further symptoms, the stenosis by this time is essentially asymptomatic and carries such a low risk of stroke that there is no overall advantage for surgery (section 16.9). It is preferable to ask the patient to return if there are any further cerebrovascular symptoms and, if the stenosis is *then* 80% (ECST) or more, it is reasonable to recommend carotid endarterectomy.

Cognitive performance

Carotid endarterectomy may not merely reduce stroke risk, but may also improve cognitive performance, perhaps by increasing cerebral blood flow or by reducing the frequency of subclinical emboli which declines after surgery (Markus *et al.* 1995; van Zuilen *et al.* 1995). On the other hand, subtle cognitive difficulties short of an obvious stroke may complicate the procedure itself. Unfortunately, studies addressing this issue have been beset with such methodological difficulties that no conclusions can be drawn (Lunn *et al.* 1999). Indeed, it is difficult to imagine that this balance of cognitive benefit and risk will ever be resolved because further randomized trials will probably never be done, at least not in symptomatic stenosis patients.

Cerebral reactivity

It is conceivable that patients with impaired cerebral reactivity and raised oxygen extraction fraction are at particular risk of stroke without surgery, and that this impairment can be corrected by carotid endarterectomy, but the studies have been too small to be sure (Schroeder 1988; Naylor *et al.* 1993a; Yonas *et al.* 1993; Hartl *et al.* 1994; Yamauchi *et al.* 1996; Visser *et al.* 1997). Also, we do not know what proportion of strokes in patients with recently symptomatic severe carotid stenosis are actually due to impaired cerebral reactivity, either as a direct result of low flow or perhaps indirectly as a result of an inadequate collateral circulation to compensate for acute arterial occlusion if it should occur. Nor do we know whether the risk of surgery is higher in these patients and so whether on balance carotid endarterectomy will indeed reduce stroke risk any more than in those without impaired reactivity. Finally, there are a great variety of techniques for measuring cerebrovascular reactivity which do not necessarily correlate with each other (section 6.7.9).

16.8.6 Selection of patients for carotid endarterectomy

Patients find carotid endarterectomy not only inconvenient

and frightening, but there are a number of usually trivial and temporary problems such as nerve palsies, and there is always some risk of stroke and even of death. To these must be added the risk of any preceding catheter angiography unless non-invasive imaging alone is adequate to display the relevant parts of the cerebral circulation (section 6.7.4). On average, patients even with severe stenosis are unlikely to gain more than a year or two of stroke-free life (European Carotid Surgery Trialists' Collaborative Group 1998). Clearly, therefore, several essential conditions must be fulfilled before recommending surgery (Table 16.15). After all, we are not dealing with a simple, cheap, safe and widely available treatment such as aspirin.

If the combined angiographic and surgical risk of stroke is, say, 10% in routine clinical practice rather than the more optimistic estimates of some surgeons, if the unoperated risk of stroke is 20% after 2 years which is on average the case for severe stenosis, and if successful surgery reduces this risk of stroke to zero which is not far from the truth, then doing 10 operations would cause one stroke and avoid two. The net gain would be one stroke avoided. If one only considers disabling strokes, comprising about half the total number, then the 'number-needed-to-treat' doubles to a rather daunting 20. Clearly, to reduce this number of patients that have to be operated on to prevent one having a stroke, and therefore to maximize cost-effectiveness, we need to know more exactly who is at highest risk of surgical stroke, and who will survive to be at highest risk of ipsilateral ischaemic stroke if surgery is not done. It is therefore essential that safe surgery is offered to those patients who have most to gain (i.e. those at highest risk of ipsilateral ischaemic stroke without surgery) and who are most likely to survive for a number of years to enjoy that gain. Ideally we must focus surgery on the small number of patients who *will* have a stroke without it, not on the larger number of patients who *might* have a stroke, because in the latter group there will be a lot of unnecessary operations. After all, even with more than 90% stenosis, seven out of 10 patients will *not* have a stroke in 3 years (Fig. 16.22b). Furthermore, surgery is not cheap. Excluding the cost of working up the very large number of TIA and stroke patients to find the 5% or so suitable for surgery, the charges in 1985 were US$4000 and $6000 in a private and university hospital, respectively; the cost in Sweden in 1991 was estimated at US$11 602; and in Canada in 1996 it was about $7000 (Green & McNamara 1987; Asplund *et al.* 1993; Smurawska *et al.* 1998).

Table 16.15 Conditions to be fulfilled before recommending patients for carotid endarterectomy.

A patient with one or more carotid distribution* transient ischaemic attacks or non-disabling ischaemic strokes in the previous few months and who has, therefore, everything or almost everything to lose from a major hemisphere stroke. Vascular risk factors should be under control (section 16.3) and most patients should be taking antiplatelet drugs (section 16.4).

Duplex sonography shows severe carotid bifurcation disease of the symptomatic artery (likely to be at least 70% stenosis by European Carotid Surgery Trial measurement on catheter angiography).

The patient is prepared to consider and accept the early risk and inconvenience of surgery for long-term benefit.

The patient is fit for surgery: no recent myocardial infarction; angina controlled; no cardiac failure; hypertension controlled; reasonable lung function; and biologically not too aged.

If catheter angiography is still being used, the institution has an experienced neuroradiology team with a low complication rate, preferably kept under prospective and independent audit.

The institution has an experienced surgical and anaesthetic team with a low surgical complication rate, preferably kept under prospective and independent audit.

*For distinction between carotid and vertebrobasilar distribution attacks, see Table 4.4.

16.8.7 Who is at high (or low) risk of surgery?

Perioperative stroke risk (and the risk of the few non-stroke deaths which are usually cardiac in origin) is presumably related to the skill of the surgeon; the skill of the anaesthetist; aspects of the surgical technique; patient age and sex; co-existing pathology, such as coronary heart disease; the state of the brain and any ischaemic damage; and the state of the arterial supply to the brain.

Surgeon and surgical factors. Although surgical and anaesthetic skill must be important, the risk of surgery is not necessarily related to the number of operations done by each surgeon. In any event, the risk is difficult to quantify accurately, particularly when the risk of surgical stroke is so low and when most surgeons operate on a relatively small number of patients every year (Rothwell *et al.* 1999a). A surgeon doing as many operations as one per week might not expect to have more than five stroke complications in 2 years, i.e. 5%, but with a 95% confidence interval of about 2–11%. In the next 2 years his or her complication rate might, just by chance alone, be as good as 2% or as bad as 11%. Variation in surgical technique—the use of shunts, patches, etc.—is mostly of uncertain benefit with respect to perioperative stroke risk (section 16.8.2).

Patient factors. Very few serious attempts have been made to sort out which patient-related factors affect perioperative stroke risk, and then which factors are independent from each other so they can be used in combination to predict surgical risk in individuals (Sundt *et al.* 1975; McCrory *et al.* 1993; Goldstein *et al.* 1994; Riles *et al.* 1994; Golledge *et al.* 1996; Kucey *et al.* 1998; Ferguson *et al.* 1999). Risk factors almost certainly include increasing age, female sex, hypertension, peripheral vascular disease, ischaemia of the brain rather than the eye, contralateral internal carotid occlusion, and stenosis of the ipsilateral external carotid artery and carotid siphon (Rothwell *et al.* 1997). Operating on the left carotid artery being more risky than on the right clearly needs confirmation and, if true, might be to do with the easier detection of verbal than non-verbal cognitive deficits, or with the surgical feeling that it is more difficult operating on the left side (Barnett *et al.* 1998; Kucey *et al.* 1998; Ferguson *et al.* 1999). The *independent* surgical risk factors for patients in the ECST were female sex, hypertension and peripheral vascular disease, but the predictive model derived from these patients must be validated in a completely independent data set (Table 16.16).

It is said that surgery very soon after stroke is more risky than waiting for a few weeks, but the evidence is very weak (Pritz 1997). It makes sense to operate as soon as possible, bearing in mind the high risk of stroke early after presentation, provided the patient's neurological state is reasonably stable. Whether *emergency* surgery is sensible, particularly for patients with a very recent stroke, is controversial and even the enthusiasts recommend randomized trials into which we hope they will enter their own patients (Eckstein *et al.* 1999).

Recent myocardial infarction, or unstable angina, are both thought to increase the risk of perioperative cardiac complications. When any coronary artery bypass should be done is discussed in section 16.8.11.

Perioperative stroke risk depends not just on the skill of the surgeon and anaesthetist, but also on various patient-related factors such as age, female sex, peripheral vascular disease, contralateral internal carotid artery occlusion and hypertension.

Audit and monitoring of surgical results. It is completely impossible to compare surgical morbidity between surgeons or institutions, or in the same place at different times, or before and after the introduction of a particular change in the technique, without adjusting adequately for casemix—in other words, for the patient's inherent surgical risk. In addition, large enough numbers have to be collected to avoid random error (Rothwell *et al.* 1999a). This level of sophistication has never been achieved, and nor probably have adequate methods of routine data collection to support it, in normal clinical practice. It is clearly important, however, to have some idea of the risk of surgery in one's own hospital (*and* of any preceding catheter angiography, section 6.7.4) in the sort of patients that are usually operated on. Risks reported in the literature are irrelevant because they are not generalizable to one's own institution.

Table 16.16 Models to predict ipsilateral ischaemic stroke (the medical model) and surgical stroke or death (the surgical model) derived from the European Carotid Surgery Trial (Rothwell *et al.* 1999).

Prognostic variable	Hazard ratio	(95% CI)	*P*	Risk points	Predictive points
Medical model					
Cerebral vs. ocular events	2.45	(1.09–3.71)	0.02	1	1
Plaque surface irregularity	2.09	(1.21–3.62)	0.008	1	1
Any events within the last 2 months	1.82	(1.02–3.18)	0.04	1	1
Carotid stenosis (per 10% stenosis)	1.30	(1.10–1.40)	0.001	0–2	0–2
Surgical model					
Female sex	2.05	(1.29–3.24)	0.002	1	−0.5
Peripheral vascular disease	2.48	(1.51–4.13)	0.0004	1	−0.5
Systolic BP > 180 mmHg	2.21	(1.29–3.79)	0.004	1	−0.5

Medical model: a Cox's proportional hazards model for ipsilateral carotid territory major ischaemic stroke (i.e. fatal or lasting longer than 7 days) on medical treatment derived from the 857 patients with 0–69% stenosis randomized to no-surgery in the European Carotid Surgery Trial.

Surgical model: a multiple logistic regression model for any major stroke (i.e. fatal or lasting longer than 7 days) or death from other causes within 30 days of carotid endarterectomy derived from the 1203 patients with 0–69% stenosis randomized to surgery in the European Carotid Surgery Trial.

In the risk factor model, which should be applied to the 70–99% stenosis group, surgical predictive points are subtracted (i.e. become negative) and their weighting is reduced by 50%.

Valid comparison of surgical stroke risk between different surgeons or institutions, or in the same place at different times, is impossible without both adjustment for casemix and many hundreds of patients in each comparison group. Such a worthy ideal has never been, and may never be, achieved.

16.8.8 Who will survive to be at high (or low) risk of ipsilateral ischaemic stroke without surgery?

Not *all* patients with even extremely severe symptomatic stenosis go on to have an ipsilateral ischaemic stroke, far from it. In the ECST, although about 30% with 90–99% stenosis had a stroke in 3 years, 70% did not and these 70% could only have been harmed by surgery, never helped (Fig. 16.22b). Both the ECST and NASCET have shown very clearly the importance of increasing severity of carotid stenosis ipsilateral to the cerebral or ocular symptoms in the prediction of ischaemic stroke in the same arterial distribution, although if the ICA 'collapses' distal to an extreme stenosis the risk may be less (Morgenstern *et al.* 1997; Rothwell *et al.* 2000b) (Fig. 16.22b). *Angiographically* demonstrated 'ulceration' or 'irregularity' increases the stroke risk even more, but it is unclear whether this can be translated to the appearances on ultrasound (Eliasziw *et al.* 1994; Rothwell *et al.* 2000a). A prognostic model, as yet not completely validated, suggests that two additional independent variables have predictive importance: having any cerebrovascular events in the previous 2 months and having brain rather than ocular events (Table 16.16). Although it would be nice to refine this model with, for example, measurements of cerebral reactivity and emboli load on transcranial Doppler, these techniques were not used in the large trial from which the model was derived, and much more work needs to be done in this 'physiological' area where so far the numbers are very small (Molloy & Markus 1999) (section 6.7.9).

The risk of ischaemic stroke ipsilateral to symptomatic carotid stenosis increases as the stenosis becomes more severe, particularly when it is more than about 80% (ECST method) of the vessel diameter. On the other hand, the risk of perioperative stroke is largely independent of the amount of stenosis. Therefore, on average, the more severe the stenosis, the more a patient has to gain from successful carotid endarterectomy. In practice, the risk of surgery is unacceptable if the stenosis is less than about 70–80% (ECST), but the exact break-even point must depend on other factors which predict stroke without surgery, such as ischaemia in the brain rather than the eye.

To complicate matters further one also must avoid offering surgery to patients unlikely to survive long enough to enjoy any benefit of stroke prevention and so for whom the immediate surgical risks would not be worthwhile. These include the very elderly and patients with advanced cancer. It would also seem sensible to avoid surgery in patients with severe symptomatic cardiac disease who are likely to die a cardiac death within a year or two.

16.8.9 Balancing competing risks: early hazard vs. late benefit

Ideally, one would like to know for an individual patient their unoperated risk of ipsilateral ischaemic stroke over the next few years, their risk of carotid endarterectomy, and their chance of surviving long enough to make the risk of surgery worthwhile in the sense of enjoying a stroke-free life. One must also remember that the risk of stroke declines with time after a TIA or stroke (Fig. 16.23). If the diagnosis is delayed by several months, then the risk of surgery may no longer be justifiable; exactly how many months delay is allowable in this situation is uncertain and one can but recommend that patients be investigated quickly and efficiently to minimize the problem.

In recently symptomatic severe carotid stenosis, the risk of stroke is highest within the first weeks or months of the most recent cerebrovascular event. It follows, therefore, that the benefit of surgery is maximized if it is done reasonably quickly after patients present to medical attention.

At present, we do not know precisely what these risks are for *individuals* but we do have an approximate idea what they may be in *groups of individuals*. By adding risk points from the 'medical' model predicting stroke without surgery, and subtracting the risk points from the 'surgical' model predicting the risk of surgery, we can come up with a score which may be clinically useful (Table 16.16). In the 16% or so of patients in the ECST, with recently symptomatic and severe carotid stenosis and a score above 3.5, there was an advantage to surgery but with a lower score there was no clear advantage and even net harm (Fig. 16.25). Clearly this kind of approach must be validated in other data sets before it can be widely recommended. But if successful, it will reduce the 'numbers-needed-to-treat' for one patient to avoid a stroke from 10 to about three, i.e. only two out of every three operations will be unnecessary, rather than nine out of 10 (Rothwell *et al.* 1999b).

Gaining truly informed consent is not a problem just confined to randomized controlled trials, but a reality of everyday clinical practice. Deciding who should have surgery is difficult enough, but then explaining the various competing risks to a worried patient and how taking an early risk might prevent later stroke is much more difficult. Quoting a

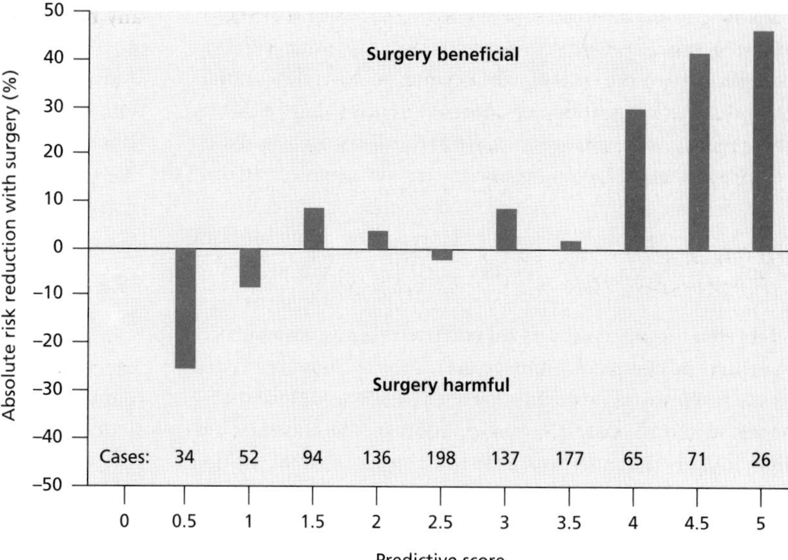

Fig. 16.25 The reduction in 5-year predicted absolute risk of ipsilateral carotid ischaemic stroke lasting more than 7 days, and any surgical death or stroke lasting more than 7 days, in the surgery group compared with the no-surgery group in patients with more than 70% symptomatic carotid stenosis in the European Carotid Surgery Trial, divided into strata by their predictive score (with permission from Rothwell *et al.* 1999b).

relative risk reduction of 50% (i.e. from 20% to 10% stroke risk) is more likely to lead to operative consent than either quoting the equivalent absolute risk reduction of 10%, or the statement that 'operating on 10 patients like you will prevent one having a stroke'. One cannot assume that an apparently rational clinical decision will reflect what a patient wants to have done, particularly after one has explained that surgery will not improve any neurological impairment that may already be present from an earlier stroke.

16.8.10 Management of patients with other potential causes of stroke as well as carotid stenosis

An occasional patient with a lacunar ischaemic stroke or TIA may have ipsilateral severe carotid stenosis (section 6.4). The question then arises whether the stenosis is 'symptomatic' (i.e. a small deep lacunar infarct has, unusually, been caused by artery-to-artery embolism or low flow) or 'asymptomatic' (i.e. the stenosis is a coincidental bystander and the infarct was really due to intracranial small vessel disease). Unfortunately, but not surprisingly, the number of such patients in the randomized trials is so small that it is not really certain what the effect of surgery is (Boiten *et al.* 1996; Inzitari *et al.* 2000a). The observational studies mostly show that severe stenosis is about equally rare in the symptomatic and contralateral carotid arteries, which rather supports the notion of the stenosis being coincidental, but the numbers are too small to be sure (Mead *et al.* 2000). Under the circumstances, we suspect that most people would recommend surgery, particularly if the stenosis is *very* severe (> 90%), because even if the artery was in truth asymptomatic at least with this degree of stenosis there is some evidence that the risk of ipsilateral ischaemic stroke is high enough to justify the risk of surgery (section 16.9.2). The same arguments probably apply if there is also a major co-existing source of embolism from the heart (such as non-rheumatic atrial fibrillation), in which case the patient may reasonably be offered surgery as well as anticoagulation (section 16.5.2).

16.8.11 Carotid endarterectomy before, during or after coronary artery surgery?

If patients with recently symptomatic carotid stenosis also have *symptomatic* coronary heart disease requiring surgery, it is profoundly unclear whether coronary bypass should be done before the carotid endarterectomy (and risk a stroke during the procedure), after the carotid endarterectomy (and risk cardiac complications during carotid endarterectomy) or simultaneously under the same general anaesthetic (and risk both stroke and cardiac complications all at once) (Graor & Hertzer 1988; Akins 1995; Davenport *et al.* 1995). The apparently high risk of the last option may well be unacceptable, although a small quasi-randomized trial suggests otherwise (Hertzer *et al.* 1989; Borger *et al.* 1999). Which option to choose must depend on the individual patient and close collaboration between neurologist, cardiologist and surgeon; there is no clear guidance from randomized trials.

It is uncertain whether carotid endarterectomy should precede, follow or be combined with coronary artery bypass surgery in patients who have both cerebrovascular and cardiac symptoms severe enough to require surgery.

Whatever one believes about the excess risk of stroke during cardiac or any other surgery in patients with *asymp-*

tomatic carotid stenosis (section 7.18), the risk of stroke is still very low. Not all these strokes, or any other cerebral complications, are necessarily related to low flow rather than other complications of coronary surgery. Furthermore, there is no good evidence that the carotid stenosis should be removed at any stage unless one rejects the argument against operating on asymptomatic carotid stenosis in general (section 16.9). Although carotid angioplasty with or without stenting is increasingly recommended before coronary surgery, there is even less evidence to support the apparent logic of this practice than there is for endarterectomy; either procedure may be completely unnecessary. Proper trials are needed and not more and more uninformative non-randomized case series. After all, despite some opinion to the contrary, the human body does not just consist of a series of tubes waiting to be stented (Waigand *et al.* 1998).

16.9 Endarterectomy for asymptomatic carotid stenosis

As far as one can tell, less than 20% of ischaemic stroke patients have had any preceding transient ischaemic attacks (TIAs), even when the stroke is likely to have been due to the embolic or low-flow consequences of severe carotid stenosis, i.e. total and partial anterior circulation infarcts (Table 6.1). A large proportion of strokes are unheralded by TIAs and, until the moment of stroke, any stenosis was 'asymptomatic'. If these asymptomatic stenoses could be detected before the stroke, then might not unheralded (by TIA) stroke be preventable by carotid endarterectomy, particularly as surgery is beneficial in patients whose stenosis has revealed itself by becoming 'symptomatic' (section 16.8)?

It is not difficult to identify asymptomatic carotid stenosis and to quantify its extent by duplex sonography in several categories of patient:

- during screening programmes of apparently healthy people when a carotid bruit is heard and/or carotid ultrasound is being used routinely;
- as a result of hearing a carotid bruit or doing an ultrasound examination during the course of working up patients with non-cerebral symptoms, particularly if they are presenting with vascular disease below the neck (angina, claudication, etc.) or non-focal neurological symptoms;
- when bilateral carotid imaging is done in patients with unilateral carotid symptoms (i.e. the patient is symptomatic but one carotid artery is asymptomatic);
- when patients are being worked up for major surgery below the neck and a carotid bruit is heard or an ultrasound reveals carotid stenosis;
- one might also argue that any carotid stenosis is 'asymptomatic' in a patient with a lacunar TIA or ischaemic stroke (section 6.8.2), or in a fibrillating ischaemic stroke or TIA patient (section 6.8.3), even if the cerebral ischaemia was in the distribution of the stenosed artery.

However asymptomatic carotid stenosis comes to attention, four questions arise: What is the risk of operating on it? What is the risk (of stroke) if the stenosis is left unoperated? Does surgery reduce the risk of stroke? What is the balance of immediate surgical risk vs. long-term benefit?

16.9.1 Risk of carotid endarterectomy for asymptomatic carotid stenosis

There are a large number of case series with very different reported surgical stroke risks for the same reasons as in symptomatic carotid stenosis (section 16.8.3). Although the risk is about half that for symptomatic carotid stenosis (Rothwell *et al.* 1996b), there is still *some* risk. Indeed, the risk may not necessarily be very low in, for example, patients with angina whose carotid stenosis was discovered during preparation for coronary artery surgery, or in patients who have already had an endarterectomy on one side and are at risk of bilateral vagal or hypoglossal nerve palsies if both sides are operated on (section 16.8.4). As for symptomatic stenosis, the risk of surgery cannot be generalized from the literature to one's own institution, a risk that should be known locally. In competent hands, the risk of stroke and/or death within 30 days of surgery is probably under 5%.

16.9.2 Prognosis of asymptomatic carotid stenosis

There have not been many prospective studies of large num-

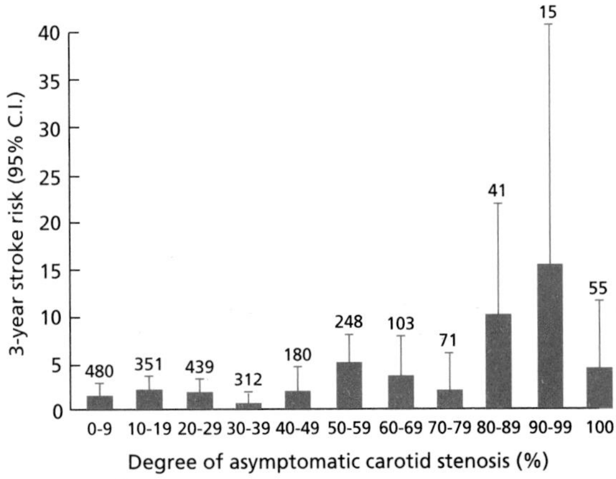

Fig. 16.26 Kaplan–Meier 3-year estimates (with 95% confidence intervals) of the risk of stroke lasting more than 7 days in the distribution of the asymptomatic carotid artery in patients in the European Carotid Surgery Trial by deciles of diameter carotid stenosis. The numbers above each error bar refer to the numbers of patients in each stenosis group (with permission from European Carotid Surgery Trialists' Collaborative Group 1995).

bers of patients in which all or most of them escaped a carotid endarterectomy at some stage during follow-up, and which used actuarial analysis stratified by degree of stenosis at study entry. In particular, one needs to know the risk of ischaemic stroke ipsilateral to the asymptomatic stenosis since, by analogy with symptomatic stenosis, endarterectomy is unlikely to reduce the risk of any other type of stroke. In fact, it seems that the absolute risk of stroke is surprisingly low, considerably lower than in symptomatic stenosis: for *severe* asymptomatic stenosis, i.e. a stenosis of at least 70% of the arterial lumen, the annual risk of stroke is perhaps 3%/year, and of ipsilateral ischaemic stroke about 2%/year (Table 18.10b). With extreme (> 90%) stenosis, there is some evidence that the risk of ipsilateral ischaemic stroke becomes rather more, but this information is based on very small numbers and some of those strokes are lacunar or cardio-embolic, and so are unlikely to be prevented by carotid endarterectomy (Fig. 16.26) (Inzitari *et al.* 2000b). Perhaps even severely stenosed arteries are relatively 'safe' unless either the atherothrombotic plaque becomes unstable and emboli are released, or a fall in systemic blood pressure causes focal cerebral ischaemia. Interestingly, asymptomatic stenosis is less likely than symptomatic stenosis to be associated with transcranial Doppler-detected emboli (Markus *et al.* 1995). Over and above the severity of stenosis, other factors associated with a higher risk of stroke may include hypertension, coronary heart disease, a high frequency of transcranial Doppler-detected emboli, impaired cerebral reactivity, the nature of the stenotic plaque on imaging and the rate of plaque progression, but much larger numbers are needed to sort all this out (Dippel *et al.* 1997b; Mackey *et al.* 1997).

The available studies also emphasize that the risk of coronary as well as cerebrovascular events increases with the severity of asymptomatic carotid stenosis. Therefore, a patient at risk of stroke is quite likely to die a cardiac death, possibly before enough time has passed to allow the benefit (if any) of carotid endarterectomy to occur (Chimowitz *et al.* 1994).

16.9.3 Surgical benefit

By extrapolating from the trials in symptomatic carotid stenosis (section 16.8.5), one would expect endarterectomy of severe asymptomatic stenosis to reduce the risk of ischaemic stroke ipsilateral to the operation. And indeed it does, by about 50% in one meta-analysis and 30% in another (Benavente *et al.* 1998; Chambers *et al.* 2000) (Fig. 16.27). However, the confidence intervals around these estimates are quite large and more information will emerge from at least one ongoing trial (Chaturvedi & Halliday 1998). For now, one has to realize that even though the relative risk reduction seems impressive, the *absolute* risk reduction is hardly worthwhile given the low risk of stroke in unoperated patients; about 50 patients have to have surgery to prevent one having a stroke in the next 3 years, double that number if only disabling strokes are counted. Far too many patients have to be operated on unnecessarily. This is hardly cost-effective medicine unless it turns out that over several years the low annual unoperated risk of stroke continues and so the cumulative risk becomes much higher than the early surgical risk. However, one has to bear in mind that the patient may die a cardiac death before any stroke occurs (see above).

16.9.4 Balance of surgical risk and benefit

Given the surgical risk (which to some extent must depend

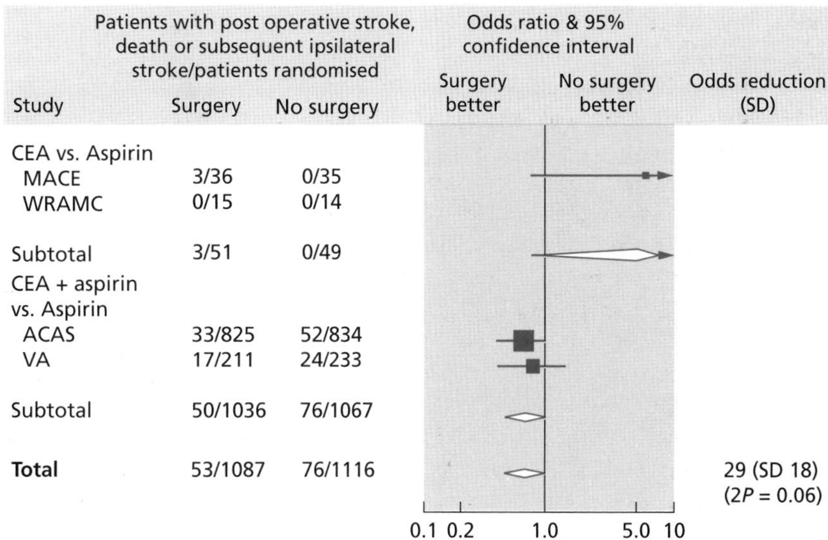

Patients with post operative stroke, death or subsequent ipsilateral stroke/patients randomised
Odds ratio & 95% confidence interval
Study
Surgery
No surgery
Surgery better
No surgery better
Odds reduction (SD)
CEA vs. Aspirin
MACE 3/36 0/35
WRAMC 0/15 0/14
Subtotal 3/51 0/49
CEA + aspirin vs. Aspirin
ACAS 33/825 52/834
VA 17/211 24/233
Subtotal 50/1036 76/1067
Total 53/1087 76/1116
29 (SD 18) (2P = 0.06)
0.1 0.2 1.0 5.0 10

Fig. 16.27 A Cochrane review meta-analysis of carotid endarterectomy vs. medical management in patients with asymptomatic and fairly severe carotid stenosis. The outcome is surgical stroke and death, and subsequent ipsilateral stroke. Each randomized trial is represented by a horizontal line reflecting the 95% confidence interval and a dark green square representing the point estimate of the relative reduction in odds of a poor outcome (in favour of surgery to the left of the 1.0 odds ratio line of no effect). The diamonds are pooled risk ratios with 95% confidence intervals. CEA, carotid endarterectomy (with permission from Chambers *et al.* 2000).

on the type of patient under consideration as well as surgical skill), the added risk of any preceding catheter angiography unless non-invasive vascular imaging is deemed sufficiently accurate, and what appears to be a remarkably low risk of stroke in unoperated patients (even when they have major surgery below the neck), there is clearly no reason to recommend *routine* carotid endarterectomy for asymptomatic stenosis. It follows that deliberately screening apparently healthy people for carotid stenosis is also most unwise (section 18.5.5). What is needed is a prognostic model to pick out those very few patients whose asymptomatic stenosis is particularly likely to cause stroke, and then operate only on them. For now, however, patients with extreme stenosis who may possibly have a higher unoperated ipsilateral ischaemic stroke risk than the average 2%/year of severe stenosis patients in general, and the very rare patient with an unbearable self-audible bruit due to the stenosis, might be surgical candidates.

Although carotid endarterectomy may even halve the risk of stroke in patients with asymptomatic severe stenosis, the absolute unoperated risk of stroke is usually so low in these patients that surgery is hardly ever worthwhile.

16.10 Carotid angioplasty and stenting

If endarterectomy of a recently symptomatic severe carotid stenosis more-or-less abolishes the risk of ipsilateral ischaemic stroke, then clearly, percutaneous transluminal balloon

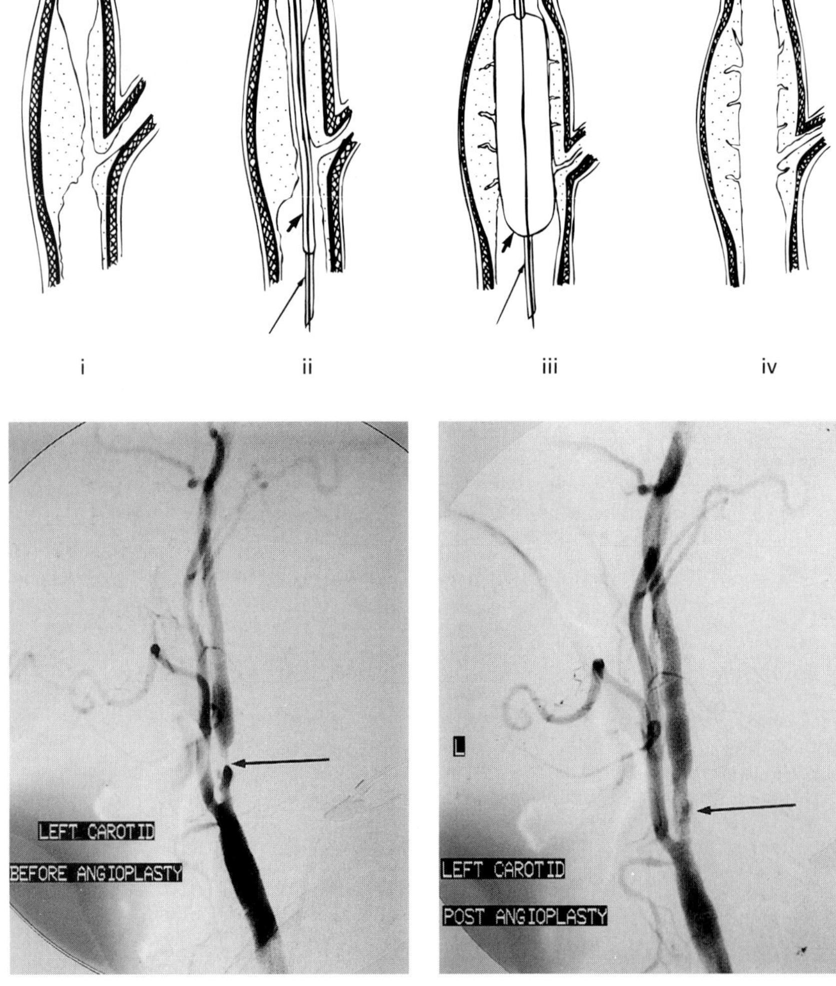

Fig. 16.28 Percutaneous transluminal balloon angioplasty of the carotid artery. (a) Diagram to show the principle of angioplasty: (i) the carotid bifurcation with a large atherothrombotic stenosis; (ii) the guidewire (small short arrow) with the (deflated—short arrow) balloon catheter (long arrows) is passed across the stenosis; (iii) the balloon is inflated (in some systems the guidewire may be withdrawn prior to inflation, in others it is left in) and the plaque is pushed outwards, so stretching the arterial wall and cracking the plaque; (iv) after the balloon is deflated and removed, the lumen has been widened, the arterial wall remains stretched and the plaque remains. (b) Carotid angiogram to show stenosis: (i) before (arrow) and (ii) after (arrow) angioplasty; the tight stenosis has been converted to a more normal (looking) lumen.

angioplasty, with or without stenting to maintain arterial patency, may do so as well (Mathur *et al.* 1998) (Fig. 16.28). However, major concerns are:

- the angioplasty balloon may dislodge atherothrombotic debris which then embolizes to the brain or eye;
- the procedure may cause arterial wall dissection at the time or afterwards;
- thrombus may form on the stretched and so damaged plaque, and then embolize;
- the angioplasty balloon may obstruct carotid blood flow for long enough to cause low-flow ischaemic stroke;
- dilatation of the balloon may cause bradycardia or hypotension due to carotid sinus stimulation;
- overdistension of the arterial wall may cause aneurysm formation and even arterial rupture;
- the stent may erode through the arterial wall;
- the stent may fracture;
- angioplasty may precipitate vasospasm;
- and stenosis may recur and be followed by stroke, so that the durability of any stroke prevention is compromised.

Of course, angioplasty is less unpleasant and less invasive than carotid endarterectomy, and generally more convenient and quicker. Being done under local anaesthetic, there may be less problem with perioperative hypertension although cerebral haemorrhage and hyperperfusion have been reported (McCabe *et al.* 1999; Qureshi *et al.* 1999). It is unlikely to cause nerve injuries, wound infection, venous thromboembolism or myocardial infarction (if the last occurs, the intra-arterial access allows immediate coronary revascularization), and hospital stay may be shorter. At present, however, it is not clear just how risky the procedure is because not very many patient series have been reported and anyway non-randomized case series are no way to compare the procedure with carotid surgery. The one reasonably large randomized trial so far available suggests that the procedural stroke complication rate is similar to carotid endarterectomy (albeit with wide confidence intervals) and that there are few strokes in the long term (with even wider confidence intervals) (CAVATAS Investigators 2000). Clearly much larger trials are needed, and are being done, to establish both the safety and durability of angioplasty and stenting compared with surgery, hopefully before we are engulfed by an epidemic of ineffective procedures (Crawley & Brown 2000a).

If the benefits do turn out to be greater than the risks, angioplasty, with or without stenting, may be applicable not just to patients presently eligible for carotid endarterectomy but also to those who are unfit for surgery—or at least for a general anaesthetic—because of coronary heart disease or other problems, for stenoses too distal for direct surgery, and for other causes of arterial stenosis such as irradiation and fibromuscular dysplasia.

At present, there is no evidence to support the routine use of carotid angioplasty, with or without stenting, outside well-conducted randomized trials.

16.11 Extra-to-intracranial bypass surgery

About 10% of patients with minor carotid ischaemic events have occlusion of the internal carotid artery (ICA), or stenosis of the ICA well distal to the bifurcation, or middle cerebral artery (MCA) occlusion or stenosis. All these lesions are inoperable, or out of reach of the vascular surgeon, if not of the angioplasty enthusiast's balloon. These lesions can all be bypassed by anastomosing a branch of the external carotid artery (usually the superficial temporal) via a skull burr hole to a cortical branch of the MCA. This 'surgical collateral' was reckoned to improve the blood supply in the distal MCA bed and so reduce the risk of stroke, and to reduce the severity of any stroke that did occur. However, there are several reasons why the procedure might not work (Latchaw *et al.* 1979; Hankey & Warlow 1991; Karnik *et al.* 1992; Klijn *et al.* 1997; Powers *et al.* 2000):

- the artery feeding the anastomosis can take months to dilate into an effective collateral channel;
- many patients have good collateral flow already from orbital collaterals or via the circle of Willis;
- not all strokes distal to ICA/MCA occlusion or inaccessible stenosis are due to low flow (section 6.2.3);
- the risk of stroke in patients with ICA occlusion is not that high compared with severe and recently symptomatic ICA stenosis (less than 10%/year) and, anyway, not all of these strokes are ipsilateral to the occlusion;
- neither resting cerebral blood flow nor cerebral reactivity are necessarily depressed in these patients;
- the risk of surgery may outweigh the benefit, if any.

The risk–benefit relationship has been evaluated in only one randomized trial and this failed to show any benefit from routine surgery (EC–IC Bypass Study Group 1985). However, it has been argued that patients with impaired cerebrovascular reactivity, or with maximal oxygen extraction, were not identified and perhaps it is *these* patients who *might* be benefited by surgery (Warlow 1986). But to show whether stroke is prevented, and not just that pathophysiology is improved, would require another randomized trial in this specific subgroup, not a series of anecdotes, however persuasive (Karnik *et al.* 1992).

At present routine extra-to-intracranial bypass surgery cannot be recommended.

16.12 Surgery and angioplasty for vertebrobasilar ischaemia

There is no good evidence (i.e. there are no large randomized trials) (Crawley & Brown 2000b) that surgery improves the prognosis for patients with vertebrobasilar ischaemia. There is, however, no shortage of ingenious, if technically demanding, techniques which are far from risk free (Diaz *et al.* 1984; Harward *et al.* 1984; Thevenet & Ruotolo 1984; Hopkins *et al.* 1987; Spetzler *et al.* 1987; Terada *et al.* 1996; Malek *et al.* 1999):

- endarterectomy of severe carotid stenosis to improve collateral blood flow, via the circle of Willis, to the basilar artery distal to severe vertebral or basilar artery stenosis or occlusion;
- resection and anastomosis, resection and reimplantation, bypass or endarterectomy of proximal vertebral artery stenosis;
- release of the vertebral artery from compressive fibrous bands or osteophytes;
- various extra-to-intracranial procedures to bypass vertebral artery stenosis or occlusion;
- angioplasty of the vertebral and basilar arteries.

Subclavian (and innominate) steal, although commonly detected with ultrasonography, very rarely causes neurological symptoms and does not seem to lead on to ischaemic stroke (section 6.7.6). However, incapacitatingly frequent vertebrobasilar TIAs in the presence of demonstrated unilateral or bilateral retrograde vertebral artery flow distal to severe subclavian or innominate disease may sometimes be relieved by endarterectomy or angioplasty of the subclavian artery; carotid-to-subclavian or femoral-to-subclavian bypass; transposition of the subclavian artery to the common carotid artery (CCA); transposition of the vertebral artery to the CCA; and axillary-to-axillary artery bypass grafting. All these procedures carry a risk and it is not clear which is the most sensible. Irrespective of the neurological situation, some kind of vascular surgical procedure may be needed if the hand and arm become ischaemic distal to subclavian or innominate artery disease

16.13 Other surgical procedures

Aortic arch atheroma is now increasingly diagnosed by transoesophageal echocardiography in patients with TIAs or ischaemic stroke, but so far there are no surgical, or indeed medical, treatment options over and above controlling vascular risk factors (section 16.3) and antiplatelet drugs (section 16.4). One trial has been started, the ARCH trial (section 16.5.1).

Innominate or proximal common carotid artery stenosis or occlusion is quite often seen on angiograms in symptomatic patients but, unless very severe, does not influence the decision about endarterectomy for any internal carotid artery stenosis. Although it is possible to bypass such lesions it is highly doubtful whether this reduces the risk of stroke unless, perhaps, several major neck vessels are involved and the patient has low-flow cerebral or ocular symptoms (section 6.6.5). This very rare situation can be due to atheroma, Takayasu's disease or aortic dissection. Clearly, close consultation between physicians and vascular surgeons is needed to sort out, on an individual patient basis, what to do for the best.

Coronary artery bypass surgery (or angioplasty) may of course be indicated for patients presenting with cerebrovascular events who also happen to have cardiac symptoms. But, in addition, because asymptomatic coronary artery disease is so often associated with symptomatic cerebrovascular disease (section 6.7.10), would coronary intervention also be worthwhile even if there were no cardiac symptoms or signs? Given the high risk of cardiac events which might be reduced in the long term (section 16.1), this is a perfectly reasonable question, but one which could only be answered by a randomized controlled trial, perhaps first in patients who are thought to be at particularly high risk of coronary events on the basis of clinical features, or non-invasive cardiac investigation.

References

Please note that all references taken from *The Cochrane Library* are given a current date as this database is updated on a quarterly basis. Please refer to the current *Cochrane Library* article for the latest review. The same applies to the *British Medical Journal* 'Clinical Evidence' series which is updated every six months.

Abraham, J., Shetty, G. & Jose, C.J. (1971) Strokes in the young. *Stroke* **2**, 258–267.

Adams, H.P., Byington, R.P., Hoen, H., Dempsey, R. & Furberg, C.D. (1995) Effect of cholesterol lowering medications on progression of mild atherosclerotic lesions of the carotid arteries and on the risk of stroke. *Cerebrovascular Diseases* **5**, 171–177.

Adams, R.J., McKie, V., Hsu, L. *et al.* (1998) Prevention of a first stroke by transfusions in children with sickle cell anaemia and abnormal results on trancranial doppler sonography. *New England Journal of Medicine* **339**, 5–11.

Akins, C.W. (1995) The case for concomitant carotid and coronary artery surgery. *British Heart Journal* **74**, 97–98.

Alba, P.M., Baez, J.M., Paz, A. *et al.* (1998) Atypical microangiopathy in a patient treated with ticlopidine. *Haematologica* **83**, 380–381.

Alderman, M.H., Cohen, H. & Madhavan, S. (1998) Dietary intake and mortality: the National Health and Nutrition Examination Survey (NHANES I). *Lancet* **351**, 781–785.

Algra, A. (2000) Anticoagulants versus aspirin and the combination of aspirin and dipyridamole versus aspirin only in patients with transient ischaemic attacks or non-disabling stroke. ESPRIT (European/Australian Stroke Prevention in Reversible Cerebral Ischaemia Trial). *Stroke* **31**, 557.

Algra, A., Franke, C.L., Koehler, P.J.J. *et al.* (1997) A randomized trial of anticoagulants versus aspirin after cerebral ischemia of presumed arterial origin. *Annals of Neurology* **42**, 857–865.

Alter, M., Friday, G., Lai, S.M., O'Connell, J. & Sobel, E. (1994) Hypertension and risk of stroke recurrence. *Stroke* **25**, 1605–1610.

Andrews, B.T., Levy, M.L., Dillon, W. & Weinstein, P.R. (1987) Unilateral normal perfusion pressure breakthrough after carotid endarterectomy: case report. *Neurosurgery* **21**, 568–571.

Anon. (1997) Which prophylactic aspirin? *Drug and Therapeutics Bulletin* **35** (1), 7–8.

Anon. (1999a) Clopidogrel and ticlopidine—improvements on aspirin? *Drug and Therapeutics Bulletin* **37** (8), 59–61.

Anon. (1999b) Atrial fibrillation in hospital and general practice: the Sir James Mackenzie consensus conference. *Proceedings of the Royal College of Physicians of Edinburgh* **29**, 2–3.

Antiplatelet Trialists' Collaboration (1994) Collaborative overview of randomised trials of antiplatelet therapy. I. Prevention of death, myocardial infarction, and stroke by prolonged antiplatelet therapy in various categories of patients. *British Medical Journal* **308**, 81–106.

Antithrombotic Trialists' Collaboration (2000) Collaborative overview of randomised trials of antithrombotic therapy—1: prevention of death, myocardial infarction and stroke by various antiplatelet regimens in 269 trials among 210 107 patients of high risk of cardiovacsular disease. *British Medical Journal* (submitted).

Antman, E.M., Lau, J., Kupelnick, B., Mosteller, F. & Chalmers, T.C. (1992) A comparison of results of meta-analyses of randomised control trials and recommendations of clinical experts. Treatments for myocardial infarction. *Journal of the American Medical Association* **268** (2), 240–248.

Arakawa, S., Saku, Y., Ibayashi, S., Nagao, T. & Fujishima, M. (1998) Blood pressure control and recurrence of hypertensive brain hemorrhage. *Stroke* **29**, 1806–1809.

Aspect Research Group (1994) Effect of long term oral anticoagulant treatment on mortality and cardiovascular morbidity after myocardial infarction. *Lancet* **343**, 499–503.

Asplund, K., Marke, L.-A., Terent, A., Gustafsson, C. & Wester, P.O. (1993) Costs and gains in stroke prevention: European perspective. *Cerebrovascular Diseases* **3**, 34–42.

Atrial Fibrillation Investigators (1994) Risk factors for stroke and efficacy of antithrombotic therapy in atrial fibrillation. Analysis of pooled data from five randomised controlled trials. *Archives of Internal Medicine* **154**, 1449–1457.

Atrial Fibrillation Investigators (1999) Efficacy of aspirin in patients with atrial fibrillation. Analysis of pooled data from three randomised controlled trials. *Archives of Internal Medicine* **157**, 1237–1240.

Bae, H.-G., Jeong, D.-S., Doh, J.-W., Lee, K.-S. & Yun, I.-G. (1999) Recurrence of bleeding in patients with hypertensive intracerebral hemorrhage. *Cerebrovascular Diseases* **9**, 102–108.

Bamford, J., Sandercock, P., Jones, L. & Warlow, C. (1987) The natural history of lacunar infarction: the Oxfordshire Community Stroke Project. *Stroke* **18**, 545–551.

Bamford, J., Sandercock, P., Dennis, M., Burn, J. & Warlow, C. (1990) A prospective study of acute cerebrovascular disease in the community: the Oxfordshire Community Stroke Project—1981–86. Incidence, case fatality rates and overall outcome at one year of cerebral infarction, primary intracerebral haemorrhage and subarachnoid haemorrhage. *Journal of Neurology, Neurosurgery and Psychiatry* **53**, 16–22.

Bamford, J., Sandercock, P., Dennis, M., Burn, J. & Warlow, C. (1991) Classification and natural history of clinically identifiable subtypes of cerebral infarction. *Lancet* **337**, 1521–1526.

Barnett, H.J.M. & Meldrum, H. (1994) Status of carotid endarterectomy. *Current Opinion in Neurology* **7**, 54–59.

Barnett, H.J.M, Taylor, D.W., Eliasziw, M. *et al.* for the North American Symptomatic Carotid Endarterectomy Trial Collaborators (1998) Benefit of carotid endarterectomy in patients with symptomatic moderate or severe stenosis. *New England Journal of Medicine* **339**, 1415–1425.

Benavente, O., Moher, D. & Pham, B. (1998) Carotid endarterectomy for asymptomatic carotid stenosis: a meta-analysis. *British Medical Journal* **317**, 1477–1480.

Benavente, O., Hart, R., Koudstaal, P., Laupacis, A. & Mcbride, R. (2000) Oral anticoagulants for preventing stroke in patients with non-valvular atrial fibrillation and no history of stroke or transient ischaemic attack. In: *The Cochrane Library*. Oxford: Update Software.

Bennett, C.L., Weiberg, P.D., Rozenber-Ben-Dror, K. *et al.* (1998) Thrombotic thrombocytopaenic purpura associated with ticlopidine: a review of 60 cases. *Annals of Internal Medicine* **128**, 541–544.

Bennett, C.L., Connors, J.M., Carwile, J.M. *et al.* (2000) Thrombotic thrombocytopaenic purpura associated with clopidogrel. *New England Journal of Medicine* **342**, 1773–1777.

Boiten, J. & Lodder, J. (1993) Prognosis for survival, handicap and recurrence of stroke in lacunar and superficial infarction. *Cerebrovascular Diseases* **3**, 221–226.

Boiten, J., Rothwell, P.M., Slattery, J. & Warlow, C.P. for the European Carotid Surgery Trialists' Collaborative Group (1996) Lacunar stroke in the European Carotid Surgery Trial: risk factors, distribution of carotid stenosis, effect of surgery and type of recurrent stroke. *Cerebrovascular Diseases* **6**, 281–287.

Bonita, R., Duncan, J., Truelson, T., Jackson, R. & Beaglehole, R. (1999) Passive smoking as well as active smoking increases the risk of stroke. *Tobacco Control* **8**, 156–160.

Borger, M.A., Fremes, S.E., Weisel, R.D. *et al.* (1999) Coronary bypass and carotid endartertomy: a combined approach increase risk? A meta-analysis. *Annals of Thoracic Surgery* **68**, 14–21.

Brand, M.B., Mulrow, C.D., Chiquette, E. *et al.* (2000) Dieting to reduce body weight for controlling hypertension in adults. In: *The Cochrane Library*. Oxford: Update Software.

Breen, J.C., Caplan, L.R., Dewitt, L.D., Belkin, M., Mackey, W.C. & O'Donnell, T.P. (1996) Brain oedema after carotid surgery. *Neurology* **46**, 175–181.

Broderick, J.P., Phillips, S.J., O'Fallon, W.M., Frey, R.L. & Whisnant, J.P. (1992) Relationship of cardiac disease to stroke occurrence, recurrence, and mortality. *Stroke* **23**, 1250–1256.

Buring, J.E., Peto, R. & Hennekens, C.H. (1990) Low-dose aspirin for migraine prophylaxis. *Journal of the American Medical Association* **264**, 1711–1713.

Buring, J. & Hennekens, C. for the Women's Health Study Research Group (1992) Women's Health Study: study design. *Journal of Myocardial Ischemia* **4**, 27–29.

Burn, J., Dennis, M., Bamford, J., Sandercock, P., Wade, D. & Warlow, C. (1994) Long-term risk of recurrent stroke after a first-ever stroke. The Oxfordshire Community Stroke Project. *Stroke* **25**, 333–337.

Butterworth, R., Marshall, W. & Bath, P. (1997) Changes in serum lipid measurements following acute ischaemic stroke. *Cerebrovascular Diseases* **7**, 10–13.

Cairns, J.A. (1994) Oral anticoagulants or aspirin after myocardial infarction? *Lancet* **343**, 497–498.

Campbell, A.J., Robertson, M., Garner, M.M., Norton, R.N., Tilyard, M. & Buchner, D. (1998) Randomised controlled trial of a general practice programme home based exercise to prevent falls in elderly women. *British Medical Journal* **315**, 1065–1069.

Campbell, W.B. (1993) Can reported carotid surgical results be misleading?. In: *Surgery for Stroke* (eds R.M. Greenhalgh & L.H. Hollier), pp. 331–337. WB Saunders, London.

Cao, P., Giordano, G., De Rango, P. *et al.* and Collaborators of the EVEREST Study Group (1998) A randomised study on eversion versus standard carotid endarterectomy: study design and preliminary results: the Everest Trial. *Journal of Vascular Surgery* **27**, 595–605.

CAPRIE Steering Committee (1996) A randomised, blinded, trial of clopidogrel versus aspirin in patients at risk of ischaemic events (CAPRIE). *Lancet* **348**, 1329–39.

Carrea, R., Molins, M. & Murphy, G. (1955) Surgical treatment of spontaneous thrombosis of the internal carotid artery in the neck. Carotid-carotideal anastomosis. Report of a case. *Acta Neurologica Latin America* **1**, 71–78.

CAVATAS Investigators (2000) Carotid and vertebral artery transluminal angioplasty study (CAVATAS): results in patients with carotid artery stenosis randomised between surgery and angioplasty. *Lancet* (submitted).

Cebul, R.D., Snow, R.J., Pine, R., Hertzer, N.R. & Norris, D.G. (1998) Indications, outcomes, and provider volumes for carotid endarterectomy. *Journal of the American Medical Association* **279**, 1282–1287.

Chambers, B.R., Smidt, V. & Koh, P. (1994) Hyperfusion post-endarterectomy. *Cerebrovascular Diseases* **4**, 32–37.

Chambers, B.R., You, R.X. & Donnan, G.A. (2000) Carotid endarterectomy for asymptomatic stenosis. In: *The Cochrane Library*. Oxford: Update Software.

Chambers, M., Forbes, C., Gladman, J. & Hutton, J. (1998) Cost-effectiveness of antiplatelet therapy in preventing recurrent stroke: duration of follow-up, cost perspective and background risk. *Cerebrovascular Diseases* **8** (Suppl. 4), 50.

Chan, W.S., Anand, S. & Ginsberg, J.S. (2000) Anticoagulation of pregnant women with mechanical heart valves. A systematic review of the literature. *Archives of Internal Medicine* **160**, 191–196.

Chao, W.H., Kwan, S.T., Lyman, R.S. & Loucks, H.H. (1938) Thrombosis of the left internal carotid artery. *Archives of Surgery* **37**, 100–111.

Chaturvedi, S. & Halliday, A. (1998) Is another clinical trial warranted regarding endarterectomy for asymptomatic carotid stenosis? *Cerebrovascular Diseases* **8**, 210–213.

Chen, Z.M., Sandercock, P., Pan, H.C. *et al.* on behalf of the CAST and IST Collaborative Groups (2000) Indications for early aspirin use in acute ischaemic stroke. A combined analysis of 40 000 randomized patients from the Chinese Acute Stroke Trial and the International Stroke Trial. *Stroke* **31**, 1240–1249.

Chimowitz, M.I., Weiss, D.G., Cohen, S.L., Starling, M.R., Hobson, R.W. & the Veterans Affairs Cooperative Study Group 167 (1994) Cardiac prognosis of patients with carotid stenosis and no history of coronary artery disease. *Stroke* **25**, 759–765.

Cillessen, J.P.M., Kappelle, L.J., van Swieten, J.C., Algra, A. & van Gijn, J. (1993) Dose cerebral infarction after a previous warning occur in the same vascular territory? *Stroke* **24**, 351–354.

Clarfield, A.M. & Paltiel, O. (1999) Commentary. *ACP Journal Club* **130**, 57.

Clavier, I., Hommel, M., Besson, G., Noelle, B. & Perret, J.E.F. (1994) Long-term prognosis of symptomatic lacunar infarcts. *Stroke* **25**, 2005–2009.

Collins, R. & MacMahon, S. (1994) Blood pressure, antihypertensive drug treatment and the risks of stroke and of coronary heart disease. *British Medical Bulletin* **50** (2), 272–298.

Collins, R. & Peto, R. (1999) MRC/BHF Heart Protection Study. *Stroke* **30**, 1304.

Consensus Conference on Lipid Lowering to Prevent Vascular Events (1999) Final consensus statement. *Journal of the Royal College of Physicians of Edinburgh* **29** (2), 2–4.

Cote, R., Batista, M., Abramowicz, M., Langlois, Y., Bourque, F. & Mackey, A. (1995) Lack of effect of aspirin in patients with carotid bruits and substantial carotid narrowing. The asymptomatic cervical study group. *Annals of Internal Medicine* **123**, 720–722.

Coumadin Aspirin Reinfarction Study (CARS) Investigators (1997) Randomised double-blind trial of fixed low-dose warfarin with aspirin after myocardial infarction. *Lancet* **350**, 389–396.

Counsell, C.E., Salinas, R., Naylor, R. & Warlow, C.P. (1997) A systematic review of the randomised trials of carotid patch angioplasty in carotid endarterectomy. *European Journal of Vascular and Endovascular Surgery* **13**, 345–354.

Counsell, C., Naylor, R. & Warlow, C. (1998) Regarding 'Prospective randomized trials of carotid endarterectomy with primary closure and patch reconstruction: the problem is power'. *Journal of Vascular Surgery* **27**, 386–387.

Counsell, C., Salinas, R., Naylor, R. & Warlow, C.P. (2000a) Routine or selective carotid artery shunting during carotid endarterectomy and the difference methods of monitoring in selective shunting. In: *The Cochrane Library*. Oxford: Update Software.

Counsell, C., Salinas, R., Warlow, C. & Naylor, R. (2000b) Patch angioplasty versus primary closure for carotid endarterectomy. In: *The Cochrane Library*. Oxford: Update Software.

Crawley, F. & Brown, M.M. (2000a) Percutaneous transluminal angioplasty and stenting for carotid artery stenosis. In: *The Cochrane Library*. Oxford: Update Software.

Crawley, F. & Brown, M.M. (2000b) Percutaneous transluminal angioplasty and stenting for vertebral artery stenosis. In: *The Cochrane Library*. Oxford: Update Software.

Crouse, J.R., Byington, R.P., Bond, M.G. *et al.* (1995) Pravastatin, lipids and atherosclerosis in the carotid arteries (PLAC-II). *American Journal of Cardiology* **75**, 455–459.

Culebras, A. (1998) Triflusal versus Aspirin for Prevention Infarction Randomised Stroke Sudy (TAPIRSS). *Stroke* **29**, 553.

Cutler, J. (1999) Which drug for treatment of hypertension? *Lancet* **353**, 604–605.

Darling, R.C., Paty, P.S.K., Shah, D.M., Chang, B.B. & Leather, R.P. (1996) Eversion endarterectomy of the internal carotid artery: technique and results in 449 procedures. *Surgery* **120**, 635–639.

Davenport, R.J., Starkey, I.R., Ruckley, C.V., Dennis, M., Sandercock, P.A.G. & Warlow, C.P. (1995) A difficult case: how should a patient presenting with unstable angina and a recent stroke be managed? *British Medical Journal* **310**, 1449–1452.

Davey Smith, G. & Ebrahim, S. (1999) Cholesterol lowering. *Lancet* **353**, 1097.

Daviglus, M.L., Orencia, A.J., Dyer, A.R. *et al.* (1997) Dietary vitamin C, beta-carotene and 30-year risk of stroke: results from the Western Electric Study. *Neuroepidemiology* **16**, 69–77.

De Marinis, M., Zaccaria, A., Faraglia, V., Fiorani, P., Maira, G. & Agnoli, A. (1991) Post-endarterectomy headache and the role of the oculosympathetic system. *Journal of Neurology, Neurosurgery and Psychiatry* **54**, 314–317.

De Schryver, E. & Algra, A. (2000) Dipyridamole plus aspirin versus aspirin for preventing stroke. In: *The Cochrane Library*. Oxford: Update Software.

DeBakey, M.E. (1975) Successful carotid endarterectomy for cerebrovascular insufficiency. Nineteen-year follow-up. *Journal of the American Medical Association* **233**, 1083–1085.

Dennis, M.S., Bamford, J.M., Sandercock, P.A.G. & Warlow, C.P. (1989) A comparison of risk factors and prognosis for transient ischaemic attacks and minor ischaemic strokes. The Oxfordshire Community Stroke Project. *Stroke* **20**, 1494–1499.

Dennis, M., Bamford, J., Sandercock, P. & Warlow, C. (1990) Prognosis of transient ischaemic attacks in the Oxfordshire Community Stroke Project. *Stroke* **21**, 848–853.

Dennis, M.S., Burn, J.P.S., Sandercock, P.A.G., Bamford, J.M., Wade, D.T. & Warlow, C.P. (1993) Long-term survival after first-ever stroke: the Oxfordshire Community Stroke Project. *Stroke* **24**, 796–800.

Di Mascio, R., Marchioli, R. & Tognoni, G. (2000) Cholesterol reduction and stroke occurrence: an overview of randomized clinical trials. *Cerebrovascular Diseases* **10**, 85–92.

Di Pasquale, G., Urbinatti, S. & Pinelli, G. (1995) New echocardiographic markers of embolic risk in atrial fibrillation. *Cerebrovascular Diseases* **5**, 315–322.

Diaz, F.G., Ausman, J.I., de los Reyes, R.A. *et al.* (1984) Surgical reconstruction of the proximal vertebral artery. *Journal of Neurosurgery* **61**, 874–881.

Diener, H.C., Cunha, L., Forbes, C., Sivenius, J., Smets, P. & Lowenthal, A. (1996) European Stroke Prevention Study. 2. Dipyridamole and acetylsalicylic acid in the secondary prevention of stroke. *Journal of Neurological Sciences* **143**, 1–13.

Dippel, D.W.J. & Koudstaal, P.J. on behalf of the Dutch TIA Trial Study Group (1997a) We need stronger predictors of major vascular events in patients with a recent transient ischaemic attack or nondisabling stroke. *Stroke* **28**, 774–776.

Dippel, D.W.J., Koudstaal, P.J., van Urk, H. *et al.* on behalf of the European Carotid Surgery Trialists' Collaborative Group (1997b) After successful endarterectomy for symptomatic carotid stenosis, should any contralateral but asymptomatic carotid stenosis be operated on as well? *Cerebrovascular Diseases* **7**, 34–42.

Dombovy, M., Basford, J., Whisnant, J. & Bergstrahl, E. (1987) Disability and use of rehabilitation services following stroke in Rochester, Minnesota, 1975–79. *Stroke* **18**, 830–836.

Donders, R.C.J.M., Kappelle, L.J., Algra, A. *et al.* (1996) Subtypes of transient monocular blindness and subsequent risk of vascular complications. *Cerebrovascular Diseases* **6**, 241–247.

Donnan, G.A., You, R., Thrift, A. & Mcneil, J.J. (1993) Smoking as a risk factor for stroke. *Cerebrovascular Diseases* **3**, 129–138.

Dutch TIA Trial Study Group (1991) A comparison of two doses of aspirin (30 mg versus 283 mg a day) in patients after a transient ischaemic attack or minor ischaemic stroke. *New England Journal of Medicine* **325** (18), 1261–1266.

Dutch TIA Trial Study Group (1993) Predictors of major vascular events in patients with a transient ischaemic attack of non-disabling stroke. *Stroke* **24**, 527–531.

Eastcott, H.H.G., Pickering, G.W. & Rob, C.G. (1954) Reconstruction of internal carotid artery in a patient with intermittent attacks of hemiplegia. *Lancet* **ii**, 994–996.

Eastern Stroke and Coronary Heart Disease Collaborative Research Group (1998) Blood pressure, cholesterol and stroke in Eastern Asia. *Lancet* **352**, 1801–1807.

Easton, J.D. (1997) Epidemiology of stroke recurrence. *Cerebrovascular Diseases* **7** (Suppl. 1), 2–4.

EC–IC Bypass Study Group (1985) Failure of extracranial–intracranial arterial bypass to reduce the risk of ischaemic stroke: results of an international randomised trial. *New England Journal of Medicine* **313**, 1191–1200.

Eckstein, H., Schumacher, H., Klemm, K. *et al.* (1999) Emergency carotid endarterectomy. *Cerebrovascular Diseases* 9, 270–281.

Eliasziw, M., Streifler, J.Y., Fox, A.J., Hachinski, V.C., Ferguson, G.G. & Barnett, H.J.M. for the North American Symptomatic Carotid Endarterectomy Trial (1994) Significance of plaque ulceration in symptomatic patients with high-grade carotid stenosis. *Stroke* 25, 304–308.

Eliasziw, M., Streifler, J.Y., Spence, J.D., Fox, A.J., Hachinski, V.C. & Barnett, H.J.M. for the North American Symptomatic Carotid Endarterectomy Trial (NASCET) Group (1995) Prognosis for patients following a transient ischaemic attack with and without a cerebral infarction on brain CT. *Neurology* 45, 428–431.

Eliasziw, M., Spence, J.D. & Barnett, H.J.M for the North American Symptomatic Carotid Endarterectomy Trial (1998) Carotid endarterectomy does not affect long term blood pressure: observations from the NASCET. *Cerebrovascular Diseases* 8, 20–24.

Elton, P.J., Ryman, A., Hammer, M. & Page, F. (1994) Randomised controlled trial in northern England of the effect of a person knowing their own serum cholesterol concentration. *Journal of Epidemiology and Community Health* 48, 22–25.

European Atrial Fibrillation Trial Study Group (1993) Secondary prevention in nonrheumatic trial fibrillation after transient ischaemic attack or minor stroke. *Lancet* 342, 1255–1262.

European Atrial Fibrillation Trial Study Group (1995) Optimal oral anticoagulant therapy in patients with nonrheumatic atrial fibrillation and recent cerebral ischaemia. *New England Journal of Medicine* 333 (1), 5–10.

European Carotid Surgery Trialists' Collaborative Group (1991) MRC European Carotid Surgery Trial: interim results for symptomatic patients with severe (70–99%) or with mild (0–29%) carotid stenosis. *Lancet* 337, 1235–1243.

European Carotid Surgery Trialists' Collaborative Group (1995) Risk of stroke in the distribution of an asymptomatic carotid artery. *Lancet* 345, 209–212.

European Carotid Surgery Trialists' Collaborative Group (1998) Randomised trial of endarterectomy for recently symptomatic carotid stenosis: final results of the MRC European Carotid Surgery Trial (ECST). *Lancet* 351, 1379–1387.

Evans, B.A., Sicks, J.D. & Whisnant, J.P. (1994) Factors affecting survival and occurrence of stroke in patients with transient ischaemic attacks. *Mayo Clinic Proceedings* 69, 416–421.

Evenson, K.R., Rosamond, W., Cai, J. *et al.* (1999) Physical activity and ischaemic stroke risk. *Stroke* 30, 1333–1339.

Ferguson, G.G. (1986) Carotid endarterectomy. To shunt or not to shunt? *Archives of Neurology* 43, 615–618.

Ferguson, G.G., Eliasziw, M., Barr, H.W.K. *et al.* for the North American Symptomatic Carotid Endarterectomy Trial (NASCET) Collaborators (1999) The North American Symptomatic Carotid Endarterectomy Trial: surgical results in 1415 patients. *Stroke* 30, 1751–1758.

Ferner, R.E. & Neil, H.A.W. (1995) A suitable case for treatment. *Lancet* 345, 1051.

Ferris, G., Roderick, P., Smithies, A. *et al.* (1998) An epidemiological needs assessment of carotid endarterectomy in an English health region. Is the need being met? *British Medical Journal* 317, 447–451.

Ferro, J.M. & Crespo, M. (1994) Prognosis after transient ischaemic attack and ischaemic stroke in young adults. *Stroke* 25, 1611–1616.

Fields, W.S., Maslenikov, V., Meyer, J.S., Hass, W.K., Remington, R.D. & Macdonald, M. (1970) Joint study of extracranial arterial occlusion. V. Progress report of prognosis following surgery or nonsurgical treatment for transient cerebral ischaemic attacks and cervical carotid artery lesions. *Journal of the American Medical Association* 211, 1993–2003.

Fogelholm, R., Nuutila, M. & Vuorela, A.L. (1992) Primary intracerebral haemorrhage in the Jyvaskyla region, Central Finland, 1985–89: incidence, case fatality rate, and functional outcome. *Journal of Neurology, Neurosurgery and Psychiatry* 55, 546–552.

Forconi, S., Battistini, N., Guerrini, M. & Passero, S.G. (1995) A randomised, ASA-controlled trial of mesoglycan in secondary prevention after cerebral ischaemic events. *Cerebrovascular Diseases* 5, 334–341.

Forette, F., Seux, M.L., Staessen, J.A., Thijs, L., Birkenhager, W.H. & Babarskiene, M.R. (1998) Prevention of dementia in randomised double-blind placebo-controlled Systolic Hypertension in Europe (Syst-Eur) trial. *Lancet* 352, 1347–1351.

Foster, N.L. & Hickenbottom, S. (1999) When do strokes cause dementia? *Archives of Neurology* 56, 778–779.

Frericks, H., Kievit, J., van Baalen, J.M. & van Bockel, J.H. (1998) Carotid recurrent stenosis and risk of ipsilateral stroke: a systematic review of the literature. *Stroke* 29, 244–250.

Frost, C.D., Law, M.R. & Wald, N.J. (1991) II Analysis of observational data within populations. *British Medical Journal* 302, 815–819.

Fujishima, M. (1999) Stroke hypertension and recurrence in Kyushu (SHARK). *Stroke* 30, 1304.

Furberg, C. (1999) Natural statins and stroke risk. *Circulation* 99, 185–188.

Gandolfo, C., Moretti, C., Dall Agata, D. *et al.* (1986) Long-term prognosis of patients with lacunar syndromes. *Acta Neurologica Scandinavica* 74, 224–229.

Gaunt, M.E., Naylor, A.R., Sayers, R.D., Ratliff, D.A. & Bell, P.R.F. (1993) Sources of air embolisation during carotid surgery: the role of transcranial Doppler ultrasonography. *British Journal of Surgery* 80, 1121.

Gaw, A., Shepherd, J., Blauw, G. & Murphy, M. (1999) Pravastatin in the prevention of cerebrovascular disease and its consequences in the elderly—the PROSPER design. *Stroke* 30, 251.

Gedge, J., Orme, S., Hampton, K., Channer, K. & Hendra, T. (2000) A comparison of a low-dose warfarin reduction regimen with the modified Fennerty regimen in elderly inpatients. *Age and Ageing* 29, 31–34.

van Gijn, J. (1999) Low doses of aspirin in stroke prevention. *Lancet* 353, 2172–2173.

Gill, S., Majumdar, S., Brown, N.E. & Armstrong, P.W. (1997) Ticlopidine-associated pancytopaenia; implications of an acetylsalicylic acid alternative. *Canadian Journal of Cardiology* 13, 909–913.

Gillespie, L.D., Gillespie, W.J., Cumming, R., Lamb, S.E. & Rowe, B.H. (2000) Interventions for preventing falls in the elderly. In: *The Cochrane Library*. Oxford: Update Software.

Ginsberg, J. & Hirsh, J. (1998) Use of antithrombotic agents during pregnancy. *Chest* 114, 524S–530S.

GISSI-Prevenzione Investigators (1999) Dietary supplementation with n-3 polyunsaturated fatty acids and vitamin E after myocardial infarction: results of the GISSI-Prevenzione trial. *Lancet* 354, 447–455.

Godlee, F., Goldmann, D., Donald, A. & Barton, S. (eds) (2000) *Clinical Evidence*. BMJ Publishing Group, London.

Goldstein, L.B., McCrory, D.C., Landsman, P.B. *et al.* (1994) Multicenter review of preoperative risk factors for carotid endarterectomy in patients with ipsilateral symptoms. *Stroke* 25, 1116–1121.

Golledge, J., Cuming, R., Beattie, D.K., Davies, A.H. & Greenhalgh, R.M. (1996) Influence of patient-related variables on the outcome of carotid endarterectomy. *Journal of Vascular Surgery* 24, 120–126.

Gonzales-Duarte, A., Canu, C., Ruiz-Sandoval, J. & Barinagarrementeria, F. (1998) Recurrent primary intracerebral haemorrhage. *Stroke* 29, 1802–1805.

Gorelick, P. & Mazzone, T. (1999) Plasma lipids and stroke. *Journal of Cardiovascular Risk* 6, 217–221.

Gorelick, P., Leurgans, S., Richardson, D. *et al.* (1998) The African American Antiplatelet Stroke Study. *Journal of Stroke and Cerebrovascular Diseases* 7, 426–434.

Gorter, J.W. for the Stroke Prevention in Reversible Ishaemia (SPIRIT) and European Atrial Fibrillation (EAFT) Study Groups (1999) Major bleeding during anticoagulation after cerebral ischaemia: patterns and risk factors. *Neurology* 53, 1319–1327.

Graor, R.A. & Hertzer, N.R. (1988) Management of coexistent carotid artery and coronary artery disease. *Stroke* 19, 1441–1443.

Graudal, N.A., Galloe, A.M. & Garred, P. (1998) Effects of sodium restriction on blood pressure, renin, aldosterone, catecholamines, cholesterols, and triglyceride: a meta-analysis. *Journal of the American Medical Association* 279, 1383–1391.

Graver, L.M. & Mulcare, R.J. (1986) Pseudoaneurysm after carotid endarterectomy. *Journal of Cardiovascular Surgery* 27, 294–297.

Greaves, M. (1993) Anticoagulants in pregnancy. *Pharmacology and Therapeutics* 59, 311–327.

Greaves, M. (1999) Antiphospholipid antibodies and thrombosis. *Lancet* 353, 1348–1353.

Green, C.J., Hadorn, D. & Kazanjian, A. (1997) Anticoagulation in chronic non-valvular atrial fibrillation: critical appraisal and meta-analysis. *Canadian Journal of Cardiology* 13, 811–815.

Green, R.M. & McNamara, J. (1987) Optimal resources for carotid endarterectomy. *Surgery* 102, 743–748.

Gullov, A.L., Koefoed, B.G., Petersen, P. *et al.* (1998) Fixed minidose warfarin and aspirin alone and in combination vs adjusted-dose warfarin for stroke prevention in atrial fibrillation: Second Copenhagen Atrial Fibrillation, Aspirin, and Anticoagulation Study. *Archives of Internal Medicine* **158**, 513–521.

Gutrecht, J.A. & Jones, H.R. (1988) Bilateral hypoglossal nerve injury after bilateral carotid endarterectomy. *Stroke* **19**, 261–262.

Hafner, D.H., Smith, R.B., King, O.W. *et al.* (1987) Massive intracerebral haemorrhage following carotid endarterectomy. *Archives of Surgery* **122**, 305–307.

Halsey, J.H. for the International Transcranial Doppler Collaborators (1992) Risk and benefits of shunting in carotid endarterectomy. *Stroke* **23**, 1583–1587.

Hankey, G.J. (1999a) VITAmins TO Prevent Stroke (VITATOPS). *Stroke* **30**, 1305.

Hankey, G.J. (1999b) Smoking and risk of stroke. *Journal of Cardiovascular Risk* **6**, 207–211.

Hankey, G.J. & Eikelboom, J. (1999) Homocysteine and vascular disease. *Lancet* **354**, 407–413.

Hankey, G.J. & Warlow, C.P. (1991) Prognosis of symptomatic carotid artery occlusion. An overview. *Cerebrovascular Diseases* **1**, 245–256.

Hankey, G.J. & Warlow, C.P. (1994) *Transient Ischaemic Attacks of the Brain and Eye*. W.B. Saunders, London.

Hankey, G.J., Slattery, J.M. & Warlow, C.P. (1991) The prognosis of hospital-referred transient ischaemic attacks. *Journal of Neurology, Neurosurgery and Psychiatry* **54**, 793–802.

Hankey, G.J., Slattery, J.M. & Warlow, C.P. (1992) Transient ischaemic attacks: which patients are at high (and low) risk of serious vascular events? *Journal of Neurology, Neurosurgery and Psychiatry* **55**, 640–652.

Hankey, G.J., Dennis, M.S., Slattery, J.M. & Warlow, C.P. (1993a) Why is the outcome of transient ischaemic attacks different in different groups of patients? *British Medical Journal* **306**, 1107–1111.

Hankey, G.J., Slattery, J.M. & Warlow, C.P. (1993b) Can the long term outcome of individual patients with transient ischaemic attacks be predicted accurately? *Journal of Neurology, Neurosurgery and Psychiatry* **56**, 752–759.

Hankey, G.J., Jamrozik, K., Broadhurst, R.J. *et al.* (1998) Long-term risk of first recurrent stroke in the Perth Community Stroke Study. *Stroke* **29**, 2491–2500.

Hankey, G.J., Jamrozik, K., Broadhurst, R.J. *et al.* (2000a) Five year survival after first-ever stroke and related prognostic factors in the Perth Community Stroke Study. *Stroke* **31** (in press).

Hankey, G.J., Sudlow, C. & Dunbabin, D. (2000b) Thienopyridine derivatives (ticlopidine, clopidogrel) versus aspirin for prevention of stroke and other serious vascular events in high vascular risk patients. In: *The Cochrane Library*. Oxford: Update Software.

Hankey, G.J., Sudlow, C.M. & Dunbabin, D.W. (2000c) Thienopyridines or aspirin to prevent stroke and other serious events in patients at high risk of vascular disease? A systematic review of the evidence from randomized trials. *Stroke* **31**, 1779–1784.

Hansson, L., Zanchetti, A., Carruthers, S.G. *et al.* (1998) Effects of intensive blood-pressure lowering and low-dose aspirin in patients with hypertension: principal results of the Hypertension Optimal Treatment (HOT) randomised trial. HOT Study Group. *Lancet* **351**, 1755–1762.

Hansson, L., Lindholm, L., Niskanen, L. *et al.* (1999a) Effect of angiotensin-converting enzyme inhibition compared with conventional therapy on cardiovascular morbidity and mortality in hypertension: the Captopril Prevention Project (CAPP) randomised trial. *Lancet* **353**, 611–616.

Hansson, L., Lithell, H. Skoog, I. *et al.* (1999b) Study on Cognition and Prognisis in the Elderly (SCOPE). *Blood Pressure* **8**, 177–183.

Hart, R.G. & Benavente, O. (1999) Increased risk of intracranial hemorrhage when aspirin is added to warfarin: a meta-analysis. *Stroke* **30**, 258.

Hart, R.G., Boop, B.S. & Anderson, D.C. (1995) Oral anticoagulants and intracranial haemorrhage. Facts and hypotheses. *Stroke* **26**, 1471–1477.

Hart, R.G., Benavente, O., Mcbride, R. & Pearce, L.A. (1999) Antithrombotic therapy to prevent stroke in patients with atrial fibrillation: a meta-analysis. *Archives of Internal Medicine* **131**, 492–501.

Hart, R.G., Halperin, J.L., McBride, R., Benavente, O., Man-Son-Hing, M. & Kronmal, R. (2000a) Aspirin for primary prevention of stroke and other major vascular events. Meta-analyses and hypotheses. *Archives of Neurology* **57**, 326–332.

Hart, R.G., Pearce, L.A., Miller, V.T. *et al.* (2000b) Cardioembolic vs. non cardioembolic strokes in atrial fibrillation: frequency and effect of antithrombotic agents in the Stroke Prevention in Atrial Fibrillation studies. *Cerebrovascular Diseases* **10**, 39–43.

Hartl, W.H., Janssen, I. & Furst, H. (1994) Effect of carotid endarterectomy on patterns of cerebrovascular reactivity in patients with unilateral carotid artery stenosis. *Stroke* **25**, 1952–1957.

Harward, T.R.S., Wickbom, I.G., Otis, S.M., Bernstein, E.F. & Dilley, R.B. (1984) Posterior communicating artery visualization in predicting results of carotid endarterectomy for vertebrobasilar insufficiency. *American Journal of Surgery* **148**, 43–48.

Heart Outcomes Prevention Evaluation Study Investigators (2000a) Vitamin E supplementation and cardiovascular events in high-risk patients. *New England Journal of Medicine* **342**, 154–160.

Heart Outcomes Prevention Evaluation Study Investigators (2000b) Effects of an agiotensin-converting enzyme inhibitor, ramipiril, on cardiovascular events in high-risk patients. *New England Journal of Medicine* **342**, 145–153.

Heart Outcomes Prevention Evaluation Study Investigators (2000c) Effects of ramipiril on cardiovascular and microvascular outcomes in people with diabetes mellitus: results of the HOPE study and MICRO-HOPE substudy. *Lancet* **355**, 253–259.

Hebert, P.R., Gaziano, JM. & Hennekens, C.H. (1995) An overview of trials in cholesterol lowering and risk of stroke. *Archives of Internal Medicine* **155**, 50–55.

Hebert, P.R., Gaziano, J.M., Chan, K.S. & Hennekens, C.H. (1997) Cholesterol lowering with statin drugs, risk of stroke and total mortality: an overview of randomized trials. *Journal of the American Medical Association* **278** (4), 313–321.

Hellemans, B., Langenberg, M., Lodder, J. *et al.* (1999) Primary prevention of arterial thromboembolism in non-rheumatic atrial fibrillation in primary care: randomised controlled trial comparing two intensities of coumadin with aspirin. *British Medical Journal* **319**, 958–964.

Hertzer, N.R., Loop, F.D., Beven, E.G., O'Hara, P.J. & Krajewski, L.P. (1989) Surgical staging for simultaneous coronary and carotid disease: a study including prospective randomisation. *Journal of Vascular Surgery* **9**, 455–463.

Hier, D.B. & Edelstein, G. (1991) Deriving clinical prediction rules from stroke outcome research. *Stroke* **22**, 1431–1436.

Hier, D.B., Foulkes, M.A., Swiontoniowski, M. *et al.* (1991) Stroke recurrence within 2 years after ischaemic infarction. *Stroke* **22**, 155–161.

Hillbom, M., Juvela, S. & Numminen, H. (1999) Alcohol intake and risk of stroke. *Journal of Cardiovascular Risk* **6**, 223–228.

Hodis, H.N., Mack, W.J., Labree, L. *et al.* (1996) Reduction in carotid arterial wall thickness using lovastatin and dietary therapy: a randomized controlled clinical trial. *Annals of Internal Medicine* **124**, 548–556.

Homocysteine Lowering Trialists' Collaboration (1998) Lowering blood homocysteine with folic acid based supplements: meta-analysis of randomised trials. *British Medical Journal* **316**, 894–898.

Hooper, L., Capps, N., Clements, G. *et al.* (2000) Food or supplements rich in omega-3 fatty acids for prevention of cardiovascular disease in patients with ischaemic heart disease. In: *The Cochrane Library*. Oxford: Update Software.

Hopkins, L.N., Martin, N.A., Hadley, M.N., Spetzler, R.F., Budny, J. & Carter, L.P. (1987) Vertebrobasilar insufficiency. Part 2: microsurgical treatment of intracranial vertebrobasilar disease. *Journal of Neurosurgery* **66**, 662–674.

Horwitz, R.I. & Brass, L.M. (1994) Women's Estrogen for Stroke Trial (WEST). *Stroke* **25**, 545 (Abstract).

Howard, G., Evans, G.W., Crouse, J.R. *et al.* (1994) A prospective reevaluation of transient ischaemic attacks as a risk factor for death and fatal or nonfatal cardiovascular events. *Stroke* **25**, 342–345.

Howitt, A. & Armstrong, D. (1999) Implementing evidence-based medicine in general practice audit and qualitative study of antithrombotic treatment for atrial fibrillation. *British Medical Journal* **318**, 1324–1327.

Hunter, G.C., Palmaz, J.C., Hayashi, H.H., Raviola, C.A., Vogt, P.J. & Guernsey, J.M. (1987) The aetiology of symptoms in patients with recurrent carotid stenosis. *Archives of Surgery* **122**, 311–315.

Ille, O., Woimant, F., Pruna, A., Corabianu, O., Idatte, J.M. & Haguenau, M. (1995) Hypertensive encephalopathy after bilateral carotid endarterectomy. *Stroke* **26**, 488–491.

INDANA (Individual Data Analysis of Antihypertensive Intervention Trials)

Project Collaborators (1997) Effect of antihypertensive treatment in patients having already suffered a stroke. *Stroke* **28**, 2557–2562.

Inzitari, D., Eliasziw, M., Sharpe, B.L., Fox, A.J. & Barnett, H.J.M. for the North American Symptomatic Carotid Endarterectomy Trial Group (2000a) Risk factors and outcome of patients with carotid artery stenosis presenting with lacunar stroke. *Neurology* **54**, 660–666.

Inzitari, D., Eliasziw, M., Gates, P., Sharpe, B.L., Chan, R.K.T., Meldrum, H.E. & barnett, H.J.M. for the North American Symptomatic Carotid Endarterectomy Trial Group (2000b) The causes and risk of stroke in patients with asymptomatic internal-carotid-artery stenosis. *New England Journal of Medicine* **342**, 1693–1700.

Irie, K., Yamaguchi, T., Minematsu, K. & Omae, T. (1993) The J-curve phenomenon in stroke recurrence. *Stroke* **24**, 1844–1849.

Iso, H., Jacobs, D.R., Wentworth, D., Neaton, J.D. & Cohen, J.D. (1989) Serum cholesterol levels and six year mortality from stroke in 350 977 men screened for the multiple risk factor intervention trial. *New England Journal of Medicine* **320**, 904–910.

Jackson, R., Barham, P., Bills, J. *et al.* (1993) Management of raised blood pressure in New Zealand: a discussion document. *British Medical Journal* **307**, 107–110.

Jansen, C., Ramos, L.M.P., van Heesewijk, J.P.M., Moll, F.L., van Gijn, J. & Ackerstaff, R.G.A. (1994a) Impact of microembolism and hemodynamic changes in the brain during carotid endarterectomy. *Stroke* **25**, 992–997.

Jansen, C., Sprengers, A.M., Moll, F.L. *et al.* (1994b) Prediction of intracerebral haemorrhage after carotid endarterectomy by clinical criteria and intraoperative transcranial Doppler monitoring. *European Journal of Vascular Surgery* **8**, 303–308.

Johnson, E.S., Lanes, S.F., Wentworth, C.E. *et al.* (1999) A metaregression analysis of the dose–response effect of aspirin on stroke. *Archives of Internal Medicine* **159**, 1248–1253.

Jorgensen, H.S., Nakayama, H., Reith, J., Raaschou, H.O. & Olsen, T.S. (1997) Stroke recurrence: predictors, severity, and prognosis. The Copenhagen Stroke Study. *Neurology* **48**, 891–895.

Kappelle, L.J., Adams, H.P. Jr, Heffner, M.L., Torner, J.C., Gomez, F. & Biller, J. (1994) Prognosis of young adults with ischaemic stroke. *Stroke* **25**, 1360–1365.

Kappelle, L.J., van Latum, J.C., van Swieten, J.C., Algra, A., Koudstaal, P.J. & van Gijn, J. for the Dutch TIA Trial Study Group (1995) Recurrent stroke after transient ischaemic attack or minor ischaemic stroke: does the distinction between small and large vessel disease remain true to type? *Journal of Neurology, Neurosurgery and Psychiatry* **59**, 127–131.

Karnik, R., Valentin, A., Ammerer, H.-P., Donath, P. & Slany, J. (1992) Evaluation of vasomotor reactivity by transcranial Doppler and acetazolamide test before and after extracranial–intracranial bypass in patients with internal carotid artery occlusion. *Stroke* **23**, 812–817.

Keech, A., Collins, R., Macmahon, S. *et al.* (1994) Three year follow up of the Oxford Cholesterol Study: assessment of the efficacy and safety in simvastatin in preparation for a large mortality study. *European Heart Journal* **15**, 255–269.

Keli, S.O., Hertog, M.G.L., Feskens, E.J.M. & Kromhout, D. (1996) Dietary flavonoids, antioxidant vitamins, and incidence of stroke. *Archives of Internal Medicine* **156**, 637–642.

Kelly, J., Kaufman, D., Jurgelon, J. *et al.* (1996) Risk of aspirin-associated major upper gastrointestinal bleeding with enteric or coated product. *Lancet* **348**, 1413–1416.

Khamashta, M.A., Cuadrado, M.J., Mujic, F., Taub, N.A., Hunt, B.J. & Hughes, G.R.V. (1995) The management of thrombosis in the antiphospholipid-antibody syndrome. *New England Journal of Medicine* **332** (15), 993–997.

Khaw, K.T. & Woodhouse, P. (1995) Interrelation of vitamin C, infection, haemostatic factors and cardiovascular disease. *British Medical Journal* **310**, 1559–1563.

Kinch, J.W. & Davidoff, R. (1995) Prevention of embolic events after cardioversion of atrial fibrillation. Current and evolving strategies. *Archives of Internal Medicine* **155**, 1353–1360.

Klijn, C.J.M., Kappelle, L.J., Tulleken, C.A.F. & van Gijn, J. (1997) Symptomatic carotid artery occlusion. A reappraisal of haemodynamic factors. *Stroke* **28**, 2084–2093.

Knopp, R.H. (1999) Drug treatment of lipid disorders. *New England Journal of Medicine* **341**, 498–511.

Kojima, S., Omura, T., Wakamatsu, W. *et al.* (1990) Prognosis and disability of stroke patients after 5 years in Akita, Japan. *Stroke* **21**, 72–77.

van Kooten, F., Ciabattoni, G., Koudstaal, P.J., Grobbee, D., Kluft, C. & Patrono, C. (1999) Increased thromboxane biosynthesis is associated with poststroke dementia. *Stroke* **30**, 1542–1547.

Koudstaal, P. (2000a) Anticoagulants for preventing stroke in patients with nonrheumatic atrial fibrillation and a history of stroke or transient ischemic attacks. In: *The Cochrane Library*. Oxford: Update Software.

Koudstaal, P. (2000b) Anticoagulants versus antiplatelet therapy for preventing stroke in patients with nonrheumatic atrial fibrillation and a history of stroke or transient ischemic attacks. In: *The Cochrane Library*. Oxford: Update Software.

Koudstaal, P (2000c) Antiplatelet therapy for preventing stroke in patients with nonrheumatic atrial fibrillation and a history of stroke or transient ischemic attacks. In: *The Cochrane Library*. Oxford: Update Software.

Koudstaal, P.J., van Gijn, J., Frenken C.W.G.M. *et al.* for the Dutch Transient Ischaemic Attack Group (1992a) TIA, RIND, minor stroke: a continuum, or different subgroups? *Journal of Neurology, Neurosurgery and Psychiatry* **55**, 95–97.

Koudstaal, P.J., Algra, A., Pop, G.A.M., Kappelle, L.J., van Latum, J.C. & van Gijn, J. for the Dutch TIA Study Group (1992b) Risk of cardiac events in atypical transient ischaemic attack or minor stroke. *Lancet* **340**, 630–633.

Krul, J.M.J., van Gijn, J., Ackerstaff, R.G.A., Eikelboom, B.C., Theodorides, T. & Vermeulen, F.E.E. (1989) Site and pathogenesis of infarcts associated with carotid endarterectomy. *Stroke* **20**, 324–328.

Kucey, D.S., Bowyer, B., Iron, K., Austin, P., Anderson, G. & Tu, J.V. (1998) Determinants of outcome after carotid endarterectomy. *Journal of Vascular Surgery* **28**, 1051–1058.

Lai, S.M., Alter, M., Friday, G. & Sobel, E. (1994) A multifactorial analysis of risk factors for recurrence of ischaemic stroke. *Stroke* **25**, 958–962.

Landi, G., Motto, C., Cella, E. *et al.* (1993) Pathogenetic and prognostic features of lacunar transient ischaemic attack syndromes. *Journal of Neurology, Neurosurgery and Psychiatry* **56**, 1265–1270.

Latchaw, R.E., Ausman, J.I. & Lee, M.C. (1979) Superficial temporal–middle cerebral artery bypass. A detailed analysis of multiple pre- and postoperative angiograms in 40 consecutive patients. *Journal of Neurosurgery* **51**, 455–465.

van Latum, J.C., Koudstaal, P.J., Venables, G.S., van Gijn, J., Kappelle, L.J. & Algra, A. for the European Atrial Fibrillation Trial (EAFT) Study Group (1995) Predictors of major vascular events in patients with a transient ischaemic attack or minor ischaemic stroke and with nonrheumatic atrial fibrillation. *Stroke* **16**, 801–806.

Lauria, G., Gentile, M., Fassetta, G. *et al.* (1995) Incidence and prognosis of stroke in the Belluno Province, Italy: first year results of a community-based study. *Stroke* **26**, 1787–1793.

Law, M.R., Frost, C.D. & Wald, N.J. (1991a) III Analysis of data from trials of salt reduction. *British Medical Journal* **302**, 819–824.

Law, M.R., Frost, C.D. & Wald, N.J. (1991b) I Analysis of observational data among populations. By how much does dietary salt reduction lower blood pressure? *British Medical Journal* **302**, 811–815.

Law, M.R., Thomson, S.G. & Wald, N.J. (1994a) Assessing possible hazards of reducing serum cholesterol. *British Medical Journal* **308**, 373–379.

Law, M.R., Wald, N.J., Wu, T., Hackshaw, A. & Bailey, A. (1994b) Systematic underestimation of association between serum cholesterol concentration and ischaemic heart disease in observational studies: data from the BUPA study. *British Medical Journal* **308**, 363–379.

Lee, K.S., Bae, H.G. & Yun, I.G. (1990) Recurrent intracerebral haemorrhage due to hypertension. *Neurosurgery* **26**, 586–590.

Levi, C.R., O'Malley, H.M., Fell, G. *et al.* (1997) Transcranial Doppler detected cerebral microembolism following carotid endarterectomy. High microembolic signal loads predict postoperative cerebral ischaemia. *Brain* **120**, 621–629.

Levine, M., Raskob, G., Landefeld, S. & Kearon, C. (1998) Haemorrhagic complications of anticoagulant treatment. *Chest* **114**, 511S–523S.

Lindblad, B., Persson, N.H., Takolander, R. & Bergqvist, D. (1993) Does low-dose acetylsalicylic acid prevent stroke after carotid surgery? A double-blind, placebo-controlled randomised trial. *Stroke* **24**, 1125–1128.

Lindley, R.I., Amayo, E.O., Marshall, J., Sandercock, P., Dennis, M. & Warlow, C. (1995a) Hospital services for patients with acute stroke in the United Kingdom. The Stroke Association Survey of Consultant Opinion. *Age and Ageing* **24**, 525–532.

Lindley, R.I., Amayo, E.O., Marshall, J., Sandercock, P. & Warlow, C. (1995b)

Acute stroke treatment in UK hospitals: the Stroke Association Survey of Consultant Opinion. *Journal of the Royal College of Physicians* **29**, 479–484.

Liu, M., Counsell, C. & Sandercock, P. (2000) Anticoagulants for preventing recurrence following ischaemic stroke or transient ischaemic attack. In: *The Cochrane Library*. Oxford: Update Software.

Loewen, P., Sunderji, R. & Gin, K. (1998) The efficacy and safety of combination warfarin and ASA therapy—a systematic review of the literature and update of guidelines. *Canadian Journal of Cardiology* **14** (5), 717–726.

Loftus, C.M. & Quest, D.O. (1987) Technical controversies in carotid artery surgery. *Neurosurgery* **20**, 490–495.

Lopez-Valdes, E., Chang, H.M., Pessin, M.S. & Caplan, L.R. (1997) Cerebral vasoconstriction after carotid surgery. *Neurology* **49**, 303–304.

Lunn, S., Crawley, F., Harrison, M.J.G., Brown, M.M. & Newman, S.P. (1999) Impact of carotid endarterectomy upon cognitive functioning. A systematic review of the literature. *Cerebrovascular Diseases* **9**, 74–81.

McCabe, D.J.H., Brown, M.M. & Clifton, A. (1999) Fatal cerebral reperfusion haemorrhage after carotid stenting. *Stroke* **30**, 2483–2486.

McCrory, D.C., Goldstein, L.B., Samsa, G.P. *et al.* (1993) Predicting complications of carotid endarterectomy. *Stroke* **24**, 1285–1291.

Mack, W.J., Selzer, R.H., Hodis, H.N. *et al.* (1993) One year reduction and longitudinal analysis of carotid intima-media thickness associated with colestipol/niacin therapy. *Stroke* **24**, 1779–1783.

Mackey, A.E., Abrahamowicz, M., Langlois, Y. *et al.* and the Asymptomatic Cervical Bruit Study Group (1997) Outcome of asymptomatic patients with carotid disease. *Neurology* **48**, 896–903.

MacMahon, S. & Rodgers, A. (1994a) The epidemiological association between blood pressure and stroke: implications for primary and secondary prevention. *Hypertension Research* **17** (Suppl. I), S23–S32.

MacMahon, S. & Rodgers, A. (1994b) Blood pressure, antihypertensive treatment and stroke risk. *Journal of Hypertension* **12** (Suppl. 10), S5–S14.

MacMahon, S., Peto, R., Cutler, J. *et al.* (1990) Blood pressure, stroke and coronary heart disease. Part 1—prolonged differences in blood pressure: prospective observational studies corrected for the regression dilution bias. *Lancet* **335**, 765–774.

MacMahon, S., Sharpe, N., Gamble, G. *et al.* (1998) Effects of lowering average of below-average cholesterol levels on the progression of carotid atherosclerosis: results of the LIPID Atherosclerosis Substudy. LIPID Trial Research Group. *Circulation* **97**, 1784–1790.

McTavish, D., Faulds, G. & Goa, K.L. (1990) Ticlopidine: an updated review of its pharmacology and therapeutic use in platelet-dependent disorders. *Drugs* **40**, 238–259.

Malek, A.M., Higashida, R.T., Phatouros, C.C. *et al.* (1999) Treatment of posterior circulation ischaemia with extracranial percutaneous balloon angioplasty and stent placement. *Stroke* **30**, 2073–2085.

Maniglia, A.J. & Han, D.P. (1991) Cranial nerve injuries following carotid endarterectomy: an analysis of 336 procedures. *Head and Neck* **13**, 121–124.

Manson, J.E., Stampfer, M.J., Willett, W.C., Colditz, G.A., Speitzer, F.E. & Hennekens, C.H. (1993) Antioxidant vitamin consumption and incidence of stroke in women. *Circulation* **87**, 678 (Abstract).

Manson, J.E., Gaziano, J.M., Spelsberg, A. *et al.* (1995) A secondary prevention trial of antioxidant vitamins and cardiovascular disease in women: rationale, design, and methods. *Annals of Epidemiology* **5**, 261–269.

Markus, H.S., Thomson, N.D. & Brown, M.M. (1995) Asymptomatic cerebral embolic signals in symptomatic and asymptomatic carotid artery disease. *Brain* **118**, 1005–1011.

Marquardsen, J. (1969) The natural history of acute cerebrovascular disease: a retrospective study of 769 patients. *Acta Neurologica Scandinavica* **45** (Suppl. 38), 11–155.

Marshall, J. (1982) The cause and prognosis of strokes in people under 50 years. *Journal of Neurological Sciences* **53**, 473–488.

Martin-Negrier, M.-L., Belleannee, G., Vital, C. & Orgogozo, J.-M. (1996) Primitive malignant fibrous histiocytoma of the neck with carotid occlusion and multiple cerebral ischaemic lesions. *Stroke* **27**, 536–537.

Mathur, A., Roubin, G.S., Iyer, S.S. *et al.* (1998) Predictors of stroke complicating carotid artery stenting. *Circulation* **97**, 1239–1245.

Matias-Guiu, J. (1999) Triflusal versus acetylsalicylic acid in secondary prevention of cerebral infarction (TACIP). *Stroke* **30**, 1305.

Matsumoto, N., Whisnant, J.P., Kurland, L.T. & Okazaki, H. (1973) Natural history of stroke in Rochester, Minnesota 1955–1969: an extension of a previous study 1945–1954. *Stroke* **4**, 20–29.

Mayberg, M.R., Wilson, E., Yatsu, F. *et al.* for the Veterans Affairs Cooperative Studies Programe 309 Trialist Group (1991) Carotid endarterectomy and prevention of cerebral ischaemia in symptomatic carotid stenosis. *Journal of the American Medical Association* **266**, 3289–3294.

Mead, G.E., Lewis, S.C., Wardlaw, J.M., Dennis, M.S. & Warlow, C.P. (2000) Severe ipsilateral carotid stenosis in lacunar ischaemic stroke: an innocent bystander? *Journal of Neurology, Neurosurgery and Psychiatry* (submitted).

Meade, T.W., Brennan, P.J., Wilkes, H.C. & Zuhrie, S.R. (1998) Thrombosis prevention trial: randomised trial of low-intensity oral anticoagulation with warfarin and low-dose aspirin in the primary prevention of ischaemic heart disease in men at increased risk. *Lancet* **351**, 233–241.

Meissner, I., Whisnant, J.P. & Garraway, W.M. (1988) Hypertension management and stroke recurrrence in a community (Rochester, Minnesota, 1950–1979). *Stroke* **19**, 459–463.

Mercuri, M., Bond, M.G., Sirtori, C.R. *et al.* (1996) Pravastatin reduces carotid intima-media thickness progression in an asymptomatic hypercholesterolemic mediterranean population: the Carotid Atherosclerosis Italian Ultrasound Study. *American Journal of Medicine* **101**, 627–634.

Middlekauff, H.R., Stevenson, W.G. & Gornbein, J.A. (1995) Antiarrhythmic prophylaxis versus warfarin anticoagulation to prevention thromboembolic events among patients with atrial fibrillation. *Archives of Internal Medicine* **155**, 913–920.

Minematsu, K., Yasaka, M. & Yamaguchi, T. for Japanese NV-AF Study Group (1999) Optimal intensity for secondary prevention of stroke in patients with non-valvular atrial fibrillation: a prospective, randomised multicentre trial. *Stroke* **30**, 241.

Miura, Y., Ardenghy, M., Ramaastry, S., Korach, R. & Hochberg, J. (1996) Coumadin necrosis of the skin: report of four patients. *Annals of Plastic Surgery* **37**, 332–337.

Molloy, J. & Markus, H.S. (1999) Asymptomatic embolization predicts stroke and TIA risk in patients with carotid artery stenosis. *Stroke* **30**, 1440–1443.

Morgenstern, L.B., Fox, A.J., Sharpe, B.L., Eliasziw, M., Barnett, H.J.M. & Grotta, J.C for the North American Symptomatic Carotid Endarterectomy Trial (NASCET) Group. (1997) The risks and benefits of carotid endarterectomy in patients with near occlusion of the carotid artery. *Neurology* **48**, 911–915.

Morocutti, C., Amabile, G., Fattapposta, F. *et al.* (1997) Indobufen versus warfarin in the secondary prevention of major vascular events in nonrheumatic atrial fibrillation. *Stroke* **28**, 1015–1021.

Morris, M.C., Mandson, J.E., Rosner, B., Buring, J.E., Willett, W.C. & Hennekens, C.H. (1995) Fish consumption and cardiovascular disease in the Physicians' Health Study. A prospective study. *American Journal of Epidemiology* **14** (2), 166–175.

Mulrow, C. & Jackson, R. (2000) Treating primary hypertension. In: *Clinical Evidence* (eds F. Godlee, D. Goldmann, A. Donald & S. Barton), pp. 61–63. BMJ Publishing Group, London.

Mulrow, C., Lau, J., Cornell, J. & Brand, M. (2000) Pharmacotherapy for hypertension in the elderly. In: *The Cochrane Library*. Oxford: Update Software.

Naylor, A.R. & Ruckley, C.V. (1996) Complications after carotid surgery. In: *Complications in Arterial Surgery. A Practical Approach to Management* (ed. B. Campbell), pp. 73–88. Butterworth-Heinemann, Oxford.

Naylor, A.R., Bell, P.R.F. & Ruckley, C.V. (1992) Monitoring and cerebral protection during carotid endarterectomy. *British Journal of Surgery* **79**, 735–741.

Naylor, A.R., Merrick, M.V., Sandercock, P.A.G. *et al.* (1993a) Serial imaging of the carotid bifurcation and cerebrovascular reserve after carotid endarterectomy. *British Journal of Surgery* **80**, 1278–1282.

Naylor, A.R., Whyman, M.R., Wildsmith, J.A.W. *et al.* (1993b) Factors influencing the hyperaemic response after carotid endarterectomy. *British Journal of Surgery* **80**, 1523–1527.

Neau, J.P., Ingrand, P., Couderq, C. *et al.* (1997) Recurrent intracerebral hemorrhage. *Neurology* **49**, 106–113.

Nerni Serneri, G.G., Gensini, M., Carnovali, G. *et al.* (1999) Low-dose heparin in stroke prevention; preliminary efficacy analysis. *Cerebrovascular Diseases* **9** (Suppl. 1), 67.

Ness, A. (2000) Dietary interventions. In: *Clinical Evidence* (eds F. Godlee, D. Goldmann, A. Donald & S. Barton), pp. 520–522. BMJ Publishing Group, London.

Ness, A. & Lonn, E. (2000) Dietary interventions, antioxidant vitamins, cardiac rehabilitation including exercise, smoking cessation. In: *Clinical Evidence* (eds F. Godlee, D. Goldmann, A. Donald & S. Barton), pp. 91–99. BMJ Publishing Group, London.

Ness, A. & Powles, J. (1999) The role of diet, fruit and vegetables and antioxidants in the aetiology of stroke. *Journal of Cardiovascular Risk* **6**, 229–234.

Nicholas, J. & Kottke, T. (2000) Smoking cessation. In: *Clinical Evidence* (eds F. Godlee, D. Goldmann, A. Donald & S. Barton), pp. 54–54. BMJ Publishing Group, London.

Nicholl, J.P., Coleman, P. & Brazier, J.E. (1994) Health and healthcare costs and benefits of exercise. *Pharmacoeconomics* **5** (2), 109–122.

North American Symptomatic Carotid Endarterectomy Trial Collaborators (1991) Beneficial effect of carotid endarterectomy in symptomatic patients with high-grade carotid stenosis. *New England Journal of Medicine* **325**, 445–453.

O'Donnell, H.C., Rosand, J., Knudsen, K. *et al.* (2000) Apolipoprotein E genotype and the risk of recurrent lobar intracerebral haemorrhage. *New England Journal of Medicine* **342**, 240–245.

Ojemann, R.G. & Heros, R.C. (1986) Carotid endarterectomy. To shunt or not to shunt? *Archives of Neurology* **43**, 617–618.

Orencia, A.J., Petty, G.W., Khandheria, B.K. *et al.* (1995) Risk of stroke with mitral valve prolapse in population-based cohort study. *Stroke* **26**, 7–13.

Ouriel, K., Shortell, C.K., Illig, K.A., Greenberg, R.K. & Green, R.M. (1999) Intracerebral haemorrhage after carotid endarterectomy: incidence, contribution to neurologic morbidity, and predictive factors. *Journal of Vascular Surgery* **29**, 82–89.

Paciaroni, M., Eliasziw, M., Kappelle, L.J., Finan, J.W., Ferguson, G.G. & Barnett, H.J.M. for the North American Symptomatic Carotid Endarterectomy Trial (NASCET) Collaborators (1999) Medical complications associated with carotid endarterectomy. *Stroke* **30**, 1759–1763.

Paddock-Eliasziw, L.M., Eliasziw, M., Barr, H.W.K. & Barnett, H.J.M. for the North American Symptomatic Carotid Endarterectomy Trial Group (1996) Long-term prognosis and the effect of carotid endarterectomy in patients with recurrent ipsilateral ischaemic events. *Neurology* **47**, 1158–1162.

Passero, S., Burgalassi, L., D'Andrea, P. & Battistini, N. (1995) Recurrence of bleeding in patients with primary intracerebral haemorrhage. *Stroke* **26**, 1189–1192.

Patrono, C., Coller, B., Dalen, J. *et al.* (1998) Platelet-active drugs. The relationship between dose, effectiveness, and side effects. *Chest* **114**, 470S–488S.

PATS Collaborating Group (1995) Epidemiology survey. Post-stroke antihypertensive treatment study: a preliminary result. *Chinese Medical Journal* **108** (9), 710–717.

Pekkanen, J., Linn, S., Heiss, G. *et al.* (1990) Ten year mortality from cardiovascular disease in relation to cholesterol level among men with and without preexisting cardiovascular disease. *New England Journal of Medicine* **322**, 1700–1707.

Pengo, V., Zasso, A., Barbero, F. *et al.* (1998) Effectiveness of fixed minidose warfarin in the prevention of thromboembolism and vascular death in nonrheumatic atrial fibrillation. *American Journal of Cardiology* **82**, 433–437.

Perry, I. (1999) Homocysteine and risk of stroke. *Journal of Cardiovascular Risk* **6**, 235–240.

Peto, R. (1994) Smoking and death: the past 40 years and the next 40. *British Medical Journal* **309**, 937–939.

Petty, G.W., Brown, R.D. Jr, Whisnant, J.P., Sicks, J.D., O'Fallon, W.M. & Wiebers, D.O. (1998) Survival and recurrence after first cerebral infarction. A population-based study in Rochester, Minnesota, 1975 through 1989. *Neurology* **50**, 208–216.

Pickin, D. & McCabe, C. (1999) Lipid lowering in the United Kingdom National Health Service: effectiveness and cost-economic view. *Proceedings of the Royal College of Physicians of Edinburgh* **29**, 31–40.

Piepgras, D.G., Morgan, M.K., Sundt, T.M., Yanagihara, T. & Mussman, L.M. (1988) Intracerebral haemorrhage after carotid endarterectomy. *Journal of Neurosurgery* **68**, 532–536.

Plehn, J.F., Davis, B., Sacks, F. *et al.* (1999) Reduction of stroke after myocardial infarction with pravastatin. *Circulation* **99**, 216–223.

Pokras, R. & Dyken, M.L. (1988) Dramatic changes in the performance of endarterectomy for diseases of the extracranial arteries of the head. *Stroke* **19**, 1289–1290.

Pop, G.A.M., Koudstaal, P.J., Meeder, H.J., Algra, A., van Latum, J.C. & van Gijn, J. for the Dutch TIA Trial Study Group (1994) Predictive value of clinical history and electrocardiogram in patients with transient ischaemic attack or minor ischaemic stroke for subsequent cardiac and cerebral ischaemic events. *Archives of Neurology* **51**, 333–341.

Porta, M., Munari, L.M., Belloni, G., Moschini, L. & Bonaldi, G. (1991) Percutaneous angioplasty of atherosclerotic carotid arteries. *Cerebrovascular Diseases* **1**, 265–272.

Powers, W.J., Derdeyn, C.P., Fritsch, S.M. *et al.* (2000) Benign prognosis of never-symptomatic carotid occlusion. *Neurology* **54**, 878–882.

Pritz, M.B. (1997) Timing of carotid endarterectomy after stroke. *Stroke* **28**, 2563–2567.

Probstfield, J. (2000) Cholesterol lowering drugs. In: *Clinical Evidence* (eds F. Godlee, D. Goldmann, A. Donald & S. Barton), pp. 63–65, 88–90. BMJ Publishing Group, London.

PROGRESS Management Committee (1996) Blood pressure lowering for the secondary prevention of stroke: rationale and design of PROGRESS. *Journal of Hypertension* **14**, S41–S46.

PROGRESS Management Committee (1999) Perindopril Protection Against Recurrent Stroke Study: characteristics of study population at baseline. *Journal of Hypertension* **17**, 1647–1655.

Prospective Studies Collaboration (1995) Cholesterol, diastolic blood pressure, and stroke: 13 000 strokes in 450 000 people in 45 prospective cohorts. *Lancet* **346**, 1647–1653.

Psaty, B.M., Smith, N.L., Siscovick, D.S. *et al.* (1997) Health outcomes associated with antihypertensive therapies used as first-line agents: a systematic review and meta-analysis. *Journal of the American Medical Association* **277** (9), 739–745.

Qureshi, A.I., Luft, A.R., Sharma, M. *et al.* (1999) Frequency and determinants of postprocedural haemodynamic instability after carotid angioplasty and stenting. *Stroke* **30**, 2086–2093.

Rai, R., Cohen, H., Dave, M. & Regan, L. (1997) Randomised controlled trial of aspirin plus heparin in pregnant women with recurrent miscarriage associated with phospholipid antibodies (or antiphospholipid antibodies). *British Medical Journal* **314**, 253–257.

Richards, M., Meade, T.W., Peart, S., Brennan, P.J. & Mann, A.H. (1997) Is there any evidence for a protective effect of antithrombotic medication on cognitive function in men at risk of cardiovascular disease? Some preliminary findings. *Journal of Neurology, Neurosurgery and Psychiatry* **62**, 269–272.

Riles, T.S., Kopelman, I. & Imparato, A.M. (1979) Myocardial infarction following carotid endarterectomy. A review of 683 operations. *Surgery* **85**, 249–252.

Riles, T.S., Imparato, A.M., Jacobowitz, G.R. *et al.* (1994) The cause of perioperative stroke after carotid endarterectomy. *Journal of Vascular Surgery* **19**, 206–216.

Rodgers, A., MacMahon, S., Gamble, G., Slattery, J., Sandercock, P. & Warlow, C. (1996) Blood pressure is an important predictor of future stroke risk in individuals with cerebrovascular disease. *British Medical Journal* **313**, 147.

Rose, G. (1992) *The Strategy of Preventive Medicine*. Oxford University Press, Oxford.

Rostom, A., Welch, V., Wells, G. *et al.* (2000) Prostaglandin analogues, H_2-receptor antagonists and proton pump inhibitors for the prevention of chronic NSAID induced upper gastrointestinal toxicity in adults. In: *The Cochrane Library*. Oxford: Update Software.

Rothwell, P.M. & Warlow, C.P. (1995) Is self-audit reliable? *Lancet* **346**, 1623.

Rothwell, P.M. & Warlow, C.P. on behalf of the European Carotid Surgery Trialists' Collaborative Group (1999a) Interpretation of operative risks of individual surgeons. *Lancet* **353**, 1325.

Rothwell, P.M. & Warlow, C.P. on behalf of the European Carotid Surgery Trialists' Collaborative Group (1999b) Prediction of benefit from carotid endarterectomy in individual patients: a risk modelling study. *Lancet* **353**, 2105–2110.

Rothwell, P.M., Slattery, J. & Warlow, C.P. (1996a) A systematic comparison of the risk of stroke and death due to carotid endarterectomy for symptomatic and asymptomatic stenosis. *Stroke* **27**, 266–269.

Rothwell, P.M., Slattery, J. & Warlow, C.P. (1996b) A systematic review of the risk of stroke and death due to carotid endarterectomy. *Stroke* **27**, 260–265.

Rothwell, P.M., Slattery, J. & Warlow, C.P. (1997) Clinical and angiographic predictors of stroke and death from carotid endarterectomy: systematic review. *British Medical Journal* **315**, 1571–1577.

Rothwell, P.M., Gibson, R. & Warlow, C.P. on behalf of the European Carotid Surgery Trialists' Collaborative Group (2000a) Interrelation between plaque surface morphology and degree of stenosis on carotid angiograms and the risk of ischaemic stroke in patients with symptomatic carotid stenosis. *Stroke* **31**, 615–621.

Rothwell, P.M. & Warlow, C.P. on behalf of the European Carotid Surgery Trialists' Collaborative Group (2000b) Low risk of ischaemic stroke in patients with reduced internal carotid artery lumen diameter distal to severe symptomatic carotid stenosis. *Stroke* **31**, 622–630.

Sacco, R.L., Wolf, P.A., Kannel, W.B. & McNamara, P.M. (1982) Survival and recurrence following stroke: the Framingham study. *Stroke* **13**, 290–295.

Sacco, R.L., Foulkes, M.A., Mohr, J.P., Wolf, P.A., Hier, D.B. & Price, T.R. (1989) Determinants of early recurrence of cerebral infarction: the Stroke Data Bank. *Stroke* **20**, 983–989.

Sacco, S.E., Whisnant, J.P., Broderick, J.P., Phillips, S.J. & O'Fallon, W.M. (1991) Epidemiological characteristics of lacunar infarcts in a population. *Stroke* **22**, 1236–1241.

Sacco, R.L., Shi, T., Zamanillo, M.C. & Zargman, D.E. (1994) Predictors of mortality and recurrence after hospitalised cerebral infarction in an urban community: the North Manhattan Stroke Study. *Neurology* **44**, 626–634.

Sacco, R.L, Pullicino, P., Karanjia, P. *et al.* (1997) The feasibility of a collaborative double-blind study using an anticoagulant. *Cerebrovascular Diseases* **7**, 100–112.

Sackett, D.L., Haynes, R.B., Guyatt, G.H. & Tugwell, P. (1991) Making a prognosis. In: *Clinical Epidemiology. A Basic Science for Clinical Medicine*, 2nd edn, pp. 173–185. Little, Brown, Boston.

Sage, J.I. & van Uitert, R.L. (1983) Risk of recurrent stroke with atrial fibrillation: differences between rheumatic and atherosclerotic heart disease. *Stroke* **14**, 537–540.

Salen, D., Levine, H., Pauker, S., Eckman, M. & Daudelin, D. (1998) Antithrombotic therapy in valvular heart disease. *Chest* **114**, 590S–601S.

Salgado, A.V., Ferro, J.M. & Gouveira-Oliveira, A. (1996) Long-term prognosis of first-ever lacunar strokes. A hospital-based study. *Stroke* **27**, 661–666.

SALT Collaborative Group (1991) Swedish Aspirin Low-dose Trial (SALT) of 75 mg aspirin as secondary prophylaxis after cerebrovascular ischaemic events. *Lancet* **338** (8779), 1345–1349.

Samuelsson, M., Lindell, D. & Norrving, B. (1996) Presumed pathogenetic mechanisms of recurrent stroke after lacunar infarction. *Cerebrovascular Diseases* **6**, 128–136.

Sandercock, P. & Tangkanakul, C. (1997) Very early prevention of stroke recurrence. *Cerebrovascular Diseases* 7 (Suppl. 1), 10–15.

Sandercock, P., Bamford, J., Dennis, M. *et al.* (1992) Atrial fibrillation and stroke: prevalence in different types of stroke and influence on early and long term prognosis (Oxfordshire Community Stroke Project). *British Medical Journal* **305**, 1460–1465.

Sbarouni, E. & Oakley, C.M. (1994) Outcome of pregnancy in women with valve prostheses. *British Heart Journal* **71**, 196–201.

Schmidt, E.V., Smirnov, V.E. & Ryabova, V.S. (1988) Results of the seven year prospective study of stroke patients. *Stroke* **19**, 942–949.

Schneider, P.A., Ringelstein, B., Rossman, M.E. *et al.* (1988) Importance of cerebral collateral pathways during carotid endarterectomy. *Stroke* **19**, 1328–1334.

Schrader, J. (2000) Acute candesartan cilexitil evaluation in stroke survivors. *Stroke* **31**, 557.

Schroeder, T. (1988) Hemodynamic significance of internal carotid artery disease. *Acta Neurologica Scandinavica* 77, 353–72.

Schroeder, T. (1990) How to predict which patient with carotid atherosclerosis is 'high risk'. *Acta Chirurgica Scandinavica Supplement* **555**, 209–222.

Schroeder, T.V. & Levi, N. (1999) What steps can I take to minimise inadvertent cranial nerve injury. In: *Carotid Artery Surgery: a Problem Based Approach* (eds A.R. Naylor & W.C. Mackey). Saunders, London.

Schroeder, T., Sillesen, H., Sorensen, O. & Engell, H.C. (1987) Cerebral hyperfusion following carotid endarterectomy. *Journal of Neurosurgery* **66**, 824–829.

Scottish Intercollegiate Guidelines Network (1999) *Antithrombotic Therapy*. Edinburgh: Royal College of Physicians of Edinburgh. (http://www.show.scot.nhs.uk/sign/home.htm).

Scottish Intercollegiate Guidelines Network (2000) *Lipids and the Primary Prevention of Coronary Heart Disease*. Edinburgh: Royal College of Physicians of Edinburgh (http://www.show.scot.nhs.uk/sign/home.htm).

Shaw, D.A., Venables, G.S., Cartlidge, N.E.F., Bates, D. & Dickinson, P.H. (1984) Carotid endarterectomy in patients with transient cerebral ischaemia. *Journal of Neurological Sciences* **64**, 45–53.

Shear, N.H. & Appel, C. (1995) Prevention of ischemic stroke. *New England Journal of Medicine* **333**, 460.

SHEP Cooperative Research Group (1991) Prevention of stroke by antihypertensive drug treatment in older persons with isolated systolic hypertension. Final results of the Systolic Hypertension in the Elderly Program (SHEP). *Journal of the American Medical Association* **265**, 3255–3264.

Shinton, R. & Beevers, G. (1989) Meta-analysis of relation between cigarette smoking and stroke. *British Medical Journal* **298**, 789–794.

Sigal, R. (2000) Cardiovascular disease in diabetes mellitus. In: *Clinical Evidence* (eds F. Godlee, D. Goldmann, A. Donald & S. Barton), pp. 258–267. BMJ Publishing Group, London.

Silagy, C. & Ketteridge, S. (2000) Physician advice for smoking cessation. In: *The Cochrane Library*. Oxford: Update Software.

Silagy, C., Mant, D., Fowler, G. & Lancaster, T. (2000) Nicotine replacement therapy for smoking cessation. In: *The Cochrane Library*. Oxford: Update Software.

Smurawska, L.T., Bowyer, B., Rowed, D., Maggisano, R., Oh, P. & Norris, J.W. (1998) Changing practice and costs of carotid endarterectomy in Toronto, Canada. *Stroke* **29**, 2014–2017.

Solomon, R.A., Loftus, C.M., Quest, D.O. & Correll, J.W. (1986) Incidence and etiology of intracerebral haemorrhage following carotid endarterectomy. *Journal of Neurosurgery* **64**, 29–34.

SPAF-III Writing Committee for the Stroke Prevention in Atrial Fibrillation Investigators (1996) Adjusted-dose warfarin versus low intensity fixed-dose warfarin plus aspirin for high risk patients with atrial fibrillation: Stroke Prevention in Atrial Fibrillation III randomised clinical trial. *Lancet* **348**, 633–638.

Spencer, M.P. (1997) Transcranial Doppler monitoring and causes of stroke from carotid endarterectomy. *Stroke* **28**, 685–691.

Spetzler, R.F., Hadley, M.N., Martin, N.A., Hopkins, L.N., Carter, L.P. & Budny, J. (1987) Vertebrobasilar insufficiency. Part 1: microsurgical treatment of extracranial vertebrobsilar disease. *Journal of Neurosurgery* **66**, 648–661.

Staessen, J.A., Fagard, R., Thijs, L., Celis, H., Arabidze, G.G. & Birkenheger, W..H. (1997) Randomised double-blind comparison of placebo and active treatment for older patients with isolated systolic hypertension. *Lancet* **350**, 757–764.

Steed, D.L., Peitzman, A.B., Grundy, B.L. & Webster, M.W. (1982) Causes of stroke in carotid endarterectomy. *Surgery* **92**, 634–639.

Stein, P.D., Alpert, J.S., Dalen, J., Horstkotte, D. & Turpie, A.G.G. (1998) Antithrombotic therapy in patients with mechanical and biological prosthetic valves. *Chest* **114**, 602S–610S.

Steinberg, D. (1995) Clinical trials of antioxidants in atherosclerosis: are we doing the right thing? *Lancet* **346**, 36–38.

Steinhubl, S.R., Tan, W.A., Foody, J.M. & Topol, E.J. for the EPISTENT Investigators (1999) Incidence and time course of thrombolytic thrombocytopaenia purpura due to ticlopidine following coronary stenting. *Journal of the American Medical Association* **281**, 806–810.

Stewart, B., Shuaib, A. & Veloso, F. for the SWAT Investigators (1998) Stroke Prevention with Warfarin or Aspirin Trial (SWAT). *Stroke* **29**, 304.

Streifler, J.Y., Eliasziw, M., Benavente, O.R. *et al.* for the North American Symptomatic Carotid Endarterectomy Trial (1995) The risk of stroke in patients with first-ever retinal vs hemispheric transient ischaemic attacks and high-grade carotid stenosis. *Archives of Neurology* **52**, 246–249.

Stroke Prevention in Atrial Fibrillation Investigators (1994) Warfarin versus aspirin for prevention of thrombo embolism in atrial fibrillation: Stroke Prevention in Atrial Fibrillation II Study. *Lancet* **343**, 687–691.

Sudlow, C. & Baigent, C. (2000a) Secondary prevention. Cholesterol reduction. In: *Clinical Evidence* (eds F. Godlee, D. Goldmann, A. Donald & S. Barton), pp. 121–122. BMJ Publishing Group, London.

Sudlow, C. & Baigent, C. (2000b) Primary prevention. Antithrombotic treatment. In: *Clinical Evidence* (eds F. Godlee, D. Goldmann, A. Donald & S.

Barton), pp. 65–66. BMJ Publishing Group, London.

Sudlow, C.M., Rodgers, H., Kenny, R.A. & Thomson, R.G. (1995) Service provision and use of anticoagulants in atrial fibrillation. *British Medical Journal* **311**, 558–561.

Sudlow, C.M., Thomson, R., Thwaites, B., Rodgers, H. & Kenny, R.A. (1998) Prevalence of atrial fibrillation and elegibility for anticoagulants in the community. *Lancet* **352**, 1167–1171.

Sundt, T.M., Sandok, B.A. & Whisnant, J.P. (1975) Carotid endarterectomy. Complications and preoperative assessment of risk. *Mayo Clinic Proceedings* **50**, 301–306.

Sweeney, P.J. & Wilbourn, A.J. (1992) Spinal accessory (11th) nerve palsy following carotid endarterectomy. *Neurology* **42**, 674–675.

Tang, J.L., Armitage, J., Lancaster, T., Silagy, C., Fowler, G. & Neil, H. (1998) Systematic review of dietary interventions to lower cholesterol in free-living subjects. *British Medical Journal* **316**, 1213–1220.

Tangkanakul, C., Counsell, C. & Warlow, C. (2000) Local versus general anaesthesia for carotid endarterectomy. In: *The Cochrane Library*. Oxford: Update Software.

Taylor, D.W., Barnett, H.J.M., Haynes, R.B. *et al.* (1999) Low-dose and high-dose acetylsalicylic acid for patients undergoing carotid endarterectomy: a randomised controlled trial. *Lancet* **353**, 2179–2184.

Terada, T., Higashida, R.T., Halbach, V.V. *et al.* (1996) Transluminal angioplasty for arteriosclerotic disease of the distal vertebral and basilar arteries. *Journal of Neurology, Neurosurgery and Psychiatry* **60**, 377–381.

Terent, A. (1989) Survival after stroke and TIA during the 1970s and 1980s. *Stroke* **20**, 1320–1326.

Thevenet, A. & Ruotolo, C. (1984) Surgical repair of vertebral artery stenoses. *Journal of Cardiovascular Surgery* **25**, 101–110.

Thompson, J.E. (1996) The evolution of surgery for the treatment and prevention of stroke. The Willis Lecture. *Stroke* **27**, 1427–1434.

Thomson, R., McElroy, H. & Sudlow, M. (1998) Guidelines on anticoagulant treatment in atrial fibrillation in Great Britain: variation in content and implications for treatment. *British Medical Journal* **316**, 509–513.

Thorogood, M. (2000) Changing behaviour. In: *Clinical Evidence* (eds F. Godlee, D. Goldmann, A. Donald & S. Barton), pp. 16–29. BMJ Publishing Group, London.

Toole, J. (1999) Vitamin Intervention for Stroke Prevention (VISP). *Stroke* **30**, 1305.

Tu, J.V., Hannan, E.L., Anderson, G.M. *et al.* (1998) The fall and rise of carotid endarterectomy in the United States and Canada. *New England Journal of Medicine* **339**, 1441–1447.

Tuomilehto, J. & Rastenye, D. (1999) Diabetes and glucose intolerance as risk factors for stroke. *Journal of Cardiovascular Risk* **6**, 241–249.

Turpie, A.G.G., Gent, M., Laupacis, A., Latour, Y., Gunnstensen, J. & Basile, F. (1993) A comparison of aspirin with placebo in patients treated with warfarin after heart valve replacement. *New England Journal of Medicine* **329**, 524–529.

UK-TIA Study Group (1983) Variation in the use of angiography and carotid endarterectomy by neurologists in the UK-TIA aspirin trial. *British Medical Journal* **286**, 514–517.

UK-TIA Study Group (1991) The United Kingdom Transient Ischaemic Attack (UK-TIA) aspirin trial: final results. *Journal of Neurology, Neurosurgery and Psychiatry* **54**, 1044–1054.

Urbinati, S., di Pasquale, G., Andreoli, A. *et al.* (1994) Preoperative noninvasive coronary risk stratification in candidates for carotid endarterectomy. *Stroke* **25**, 2022–2027.

Vaitkus, P.T., Berlin, J.A., Schwartz, J.S. & Barnathan, E.S. (1992) Stroke complicating acute myocardial infarction. A meta-analysis of risk modification by anticoagulation and thrombolytic therapy. *Archives of Internal Medicine* **152**, 2020–2024.

Van, E.R.F., Grobbee, D.E., Deckers, J.W., Bak, A.A.A., Verheugt, F.W.A. & Jonker, J.J.C. (1997) Antitrombotische behandeling na een acute ischemische hartziekte: acetylsalicylzuur en (of) orale anticoagulantia? [Antithrombotic treatment for an acute myocardial infarction: aspirin and (or) oral anticoagulants?] Aspect-II, een nieuw onderzoek. *Nederlands Tijdschrift Voor Geneeskunde* **141**, 2129–2131.

Viitanen, M., Eriksson, S. & Asplund, K. (1988) Risk of recurrent stroke, myocardial infarction and epilepsy during long term follow up after stroke. *European Neurology* **28**, 227–231.

Visser, G.H., van Huffelen, A.C., Wieneke, G.H. & Eikelboom, B.C. (1997) Bilateral increase in CO_2 reactivity after unilateral carotid endarterectomy. *Stroke* **28**, 899–905.

Vorchheimer, D.A., Badimon, J.J. & Fuster, V. (1999) Platelet glycoprotein IIb/IIIa receptor antagonists in cardiovascular disease. *Journal of the American Medical Association* **281**, 1407–1414.

Wade, D.T. and the Intercollegiate Working Party (2000) *National Clinical Guidelines for Stroke*. London: Royal College of Physicians (http://www.rcplondon.ac.uk).

Waigand, J., Gross, C.M., Uhlich, F. *et al.* (1998) Elective stenting of carotid artery stenosis in patients with severe coronary artery disease. *European Heart Journal* **19**, 1365–1370.

Wannamethee, S.G. & Shaper, A. (1999) Physical activity and the prevention of stroke. *Journal of Cardiovascular Risk* **6**, 213–216.

Warlow, C.P. (1984) Carotid endarterectomy: does it work? *Stroke* **15**, 1068–1076.

Warlow, C.P. (1986) Extracranial to intracranial bypass and the prevention of stroke. *Journal of Neurology* **233**, 129–130.

Wennberg, D.E., Lucas, F.L., Birkmeyer, J.D., Bredenberg, C.E. & Fisher, E.S. (1998) Variation in carotid endarterectomy mortality in the Medicare population: trial hospitals, volume, and patient characteristics. *Journal of the American Medical Association* **279**, 1278–1281.

Whelton, P.K, He, J., Cutler, J.A., Brancati, F.L., Appel, L..J., Follmann, D. & Klag, M.J. (1997) Effects of oral potassium on blood pressure: meta-analysis of randomized controlled clinical trials. *Journal of the American Medical Association* **277**, 1624–1632.

Whelton, P.K., Appel, L.J., Espeland, M.A., Applegate, W.B., Ettinger, W.H. Jr & Kostis, J.B. (1998) Sodium reduction and weight loss in the treatment of hypertension in older persons: a randomized controlled trial of nonpharmacologic interventions in the elderly (TONE). *Journal of the American Medical Association* **279**, 839–846.

Whisnant, J.P. & Wiebers, D.O. (1987) Clinical epidemiology of transient cerebral ischaemic attacks (TIA) in the anterior and posterior cerebral circulation. In: *Occlusive Cerebrovascular Disease, Diagnosis and Surgical Management* (ed. T.M. Sundt Jr), pp. 60–65. W.B. Saunders, Philadelphia.

Whisnant, J.P., Wiebers, D.O., O'Fallon, W.M., Sicks, J.D. & Frye, R.L. (1996) A population-based model of risk factors for ischemic stroke: Rochester, Minnesota. *Neurology* **47**, 1420–1428.

White, H.D., Simes, J., Anderson, N.E. *et al.* (2000) Pravastatin therapy and risk of stroke. *New England Journal of Medicine* **343**, 317–326.

Wiebers, D.O., Whisnant, J.P. & O'Fallon, W.M. (1982) Reversible ischaemic neurological deficit (RIND) in a community: Rochester, Minnesota, 1955–1974. *Neurology* **32**, 459–465.

Williams, P.S., Spector, A., Orrell, M. & Rands, G. (2000) Aspirin for vascular dementia. In: *The Cochrane Library*. Oxford: Update Software.

Wilterdink, J. & Easton, D. (1999) Dipyridamole plus aspirin in cerebrovascular disease. *Archives of Neurology* **56**, 1087–1092.

Winslow, C.M., Solomon, D.H., Chassin, M.R., Kosecoff, J., Merrick, N.J. & Brook, R.H. (1988) The appropriateness of carotid endarterectomy. *New England Journal of Medicine* **318**, 721–727.

Witzum, J.L. (1994) The oxidation hypothesis of atherosclerosis. *Lancet* **344**, 793–795.

Wolf, P.A., Clagett, G.P., Easton, J.D. *et al.* (1999) Preventing ischemic stroke in patients with prior stroke and transient ischemic attack: a statement for healthcare professionals from the Stroke Council of the American Heart Association. *Stroke* **30**, 1991–1994.

Yadav, J.S., Roubin, G.S., King, P., Iyer, S. & Vitek, J. (1996) Angioplasty and stenting for restenosis after carotid endarterectomy. Initial experience. *Stroke* **27**, 2075–2079.

Yamamoto, H. & Bogousslavsky, J. (1997) Pathophysiological patterns of stroke recurrence. *Cerebrovascular Diseases* **7** (Suppl. 1), 5–9.

Yamamoto, H. & Bogousslavsky, J. (1998) Mechanisms of second and further strokes. *Journal of Neurology, Neurosurgery and Psychiatry* **64**, 771–776.

Yamauchi, H., Fukuyama, H., Nagahama, Y. *et al.* (1996) Evidence of misery perfusion and risk of recurrent stroke in major cerebral arterial occlusive diseases from PET. *Journal of Neurology, Neurosurgery and Psychiatry* **61**, 18–25.

Yonas, H., Smith, H.A., Durham, S.R., Pentheny, S.L. & Johnson, D.W. (1993) Increased stroke risk predicted by compromised cerebral blood flow reactivity. *Journal of Neurosurgery* **79**, 483–489.

Youkey, J.R., Clagett, G.P., Jaffin, J.H., Parisi, J.E. & Rich, N.M. (1984) Focal motor seizures complicating carotid endarterectomy. *Archives of Surgery* **119**, 1080–1084.

Zarins, C.K. & Gewertz, B.L. (eds) (1987) *Atlas of Vascular Surgery*. Churchill Livingstone, New York.

van Zuilen, E.V., Moll, F.L., Vermeulen, F.E.E., Mauser, H.W., van Gijn, J. & Ackerstaff, R.G.A. (1995) Detection of cerebral microemboli by means of transcranial Doppler monitoring before and after carotid endarterectomy. *Stroke* **26**, 210–213.

CHAPTER SEVENTEEN

The organization of stroke services

17.1 Introduction

The burden

Stroke is the third most common cause of death in most developed countries, after coronary heart disease and cancer, and accounts for millions of deaths in the rest of the world (Murray & Lopez 1997). It accounts for 12% of deaths in England and Wales (Secretary of State for Health 1992) and is one of the most important causes of severe disability (Martin *et al.* 1988). In Scotland, about 7% of hospital-bed days are accounted for by stroke patients, who represent 2% of hospital discharges. Stroke accounts for 6% of hospital costs and 4.6% of National Health Service costs in Scotland (Isard & Forbes 1992). Studies from some countries (e.g. Sweden, US, Canada and Netherlands) suggest that the financial burden may be greater than in the UK, possibly because of greater expenditure on health services (Persson *et al.* 1990; Smurawska *et al.* 1994; Taylor *et al.* 1996; Evers *et al.* 1997; Caro *et al.* 2000). Many stroke patients have pre-existing illnesses, so that even before the stroke they place a substantial burden on health services. However, even taking this into account, stroke causes an increased use of health services, and thus direct costs (Leibson *et al.* 1996). Although the direct hospital costs are important early after a stroke, it is the costs relating to the long-term care of disabled survivors that dominate the lifetime costs (Bergman *et al.* 1995; Taylor *et al.* 1996). The financial burden on our society as a whole is likely to be huge, but is extremely difficult to estimate because it is borne by patients' families (e.g. lost income) and, in many countries, by social services. Approximately one-third of people who have a stroke are of working age, so that we also have to consider its indirect costs such as the impact on national productivity (section 15.33.2). Even if the incidence is falling (section 18.2.2), the burden of stroke is likely to remain very substantial for the foreseeable future because of the increasing numbers of elderly people at risk.

Governments, and in particular those responsible for providing health care, have become increasingly aware of the impact that stroke has on the health of the population and the cost to the community. In the UK, relatively little attention was paid to stroke until the publication of the King's Fund Consensus Conference (1988) on the treatment of stroke. This highlighted the many deficiencies in the services provided for stroke patients, concluding that 'services were often haphazard and poorly tailored to the patient's needs'. In England, stroke has moved up the political agenda, and was identified as one of the five key areas for improving the health of the nation in the 1990s (Secretary of State for Health 1992). There has been a similar and continuing emphasis on stroke in many other countries. These changes have led to a tremendous surge of interest in stroke in general, and in stroke services in particular. Over the last few years, an increasing amount of research has been carried out to determine the best and most cost-effective ways of providing care for stroke patients. This chapter will cover the organization of services for people who have had a stroke. Inevitably, the discussion will reflect the UK—and to some extent the Australian and Dutch—models of care, but we hope it will have some relevance for services elsewhere.

Aims of stroke services

The overall aim of stroke services is to deliver the care

Table 17.1 The components for the management of patients with transient ischaemic attack and stroke.

Prompt and accurate diagnosis (Chapter 3)
Specific acute medical and surgical treatment (Chapters 11, 12, 13 and 14)
Assessment of patients' problems (section 10.3.2)
General care, including interventions to resolve problems (includes many aspects of rehabilitation) (Chapter 15)
Terminal care for patients who are unlikely to survive (section 10.4)
Hospital discharge and placement (section 17.5.3)
Continuing or long-term care for severely disabled patients (section 17.4)
Follow-up to detect and manage late-onset problems (section 17.5.4)
Secondary prevention of further vascular events (Chapter 16)

required by patients and their families in the most efficient, effective, equitable and humane manner possible. Services may not necessarily be stroke-specific, but may be part of those for internal medicine, care of the elderly, neurology, rehabilitation and continuing care. It is good organization which is probably the most important factor in determining service effectiveness. When considering exactly how stroke services should best be organized, it is useful to consider the main components of caring for patients with stroke and transient ischaemic attack (TIA) (Table 17.1). Stroke services should also provide information and support to the patients and their families. In addition, given the lack of evidence for many of our interventions, services should facilitate research and education. We have not included primary prevention amongst the components of care, although this is potentially the most effective method of reducing stroke-related death, disability and handicap (Chapter 18). Primary stroke prevention has so much in common with the prevention of other vascular diseases that it would seem to make more sense to link these preventive services together, especially as their success depends more on political and social change than on health services.

A comprehensive stroke service has to provide the facilities and expertise to fulfil all of the functions outlined in Table 17.1. The manner in which the service is best provided will depend on local history, geography, needs, resources, people and politics. Any stroke service must therefore be tailored to the local conditions to achieve maximum effectiveness. For this reason, it is difficult to be dogmatic about exactly how services should be organized. However, in this chapter we will attempt to provide general guidance and to elucidate the principles that should be of use to the clinician, public health physician, or health service manager (administrator) in planning a service. In planning or reviewing stroke services, it is useful to start by trying to answer several questions:

- what are the needs of the population to be served by the stroke service?
- assuming that resources are limited, to what extent can the needs of the population realistically be met?
- what are the *current* resources, people and facilities committed to the management of patients with TIAs and stroke?
- what is the evidence for the cost-effectiveness of the components of both the existing and planned stroke service?
- what are the major gaps in the present provision of services (i.e. unmet needs and failure to provide effective interventions)?
- what resources, people and facilities will be needed to meet the needs of the population?
- how should these resources best be organized?
- how can performance of the stroke services be monitored?

Local stroke services must be tailored to local conditions; there is no perfect blueprint that can be applied everywhere.

17.2 Determining the needs of the population

If the aim of the service is to provide care for all those in the population who require it, not just those who can afford to pay for it, then the first factor to consider is the incidence of stroke and transient ischaemic attack in that population. This information should be the basis of a 'needs assessment' which those responsible for ensuring adequate health-care provision must develop. This is fundamental to determining *how much* stroke service should be provided.

17.2.1 Incidence of acute stroke and transient ischaemic attack

Despite the huge burden that cerebrovascular disease places on communities throughout the world, there are less reliable data on its burden than one might expect. Although a large number of 'incidence' studies have appeared in the literature over the past 30 years, the majority have had methodological weaknesses that make their results, at least in part, unreliable. The criteria for an 'ideal' study of the incidence of stroke and transient ischaemic attack (TIA) are listed in Table 17.2. The age-specific incidence provided by some more-or-less 'ideal' studies are given in Table 17.3, all of which were based on white populations because no reasonably up-to-date and reliable information is available in other populations.

There are quite good data on the incidence of stroke in many white populations, except in the Americas, some data on Oriental populations, and no reliable data at all for other parts of Asia or the whole of sub-Saharan Africa.

Table 17.2 Criteria for an 'ideal' stroke and transient ischaemic attack (TIA) incidence study (adapted from Malmgren *et al.* 1987 and Sudlow & Warlow 1996).

A large, stable well-defined study population; the number and sex of the people in the population should be available in at least 10-year age intervals during the study. This usually requires a recent census.

Complete ascertainment of all patients with either stroke or TIA occurring in that population, whether referred to hospital or not. This requires multiple overlapping methods to detect cases, including contacting primary health teams, review of hospital admissions and death certificates.

Accurate assessment of the cross-boundary flows in both directions.

First-ever-in-a-lifetime strokes and TIAs should be distinguished from recurrent strokes and TIAs.

Prospective assessment of all suspected cases so that standard diagnostic criteria (WHO definition) can be applied rigorously soon after the patient presents for medical attention (so-called 'hot pursuit').

Studies should register patients with 'TIAs' as well as strokes to ensure that mild strokes, which may be misclassified as TIAs by referring doctors in routine clinical practice, are not under-represented.

Use of brain imaging to determine the pathological type of stroke. This should be performed early enough after stroke onset to reliably distinguish ischaemic and haemorrhagic stroke.

Case ascertainment over whole years to avoid bias due to any seasonal fluctuations in incidence.

Standard methods of data presentation—i.e. not more than 5 years' data averaged together, incidence for men and women presented separately, incidence in those over 85 years old if possible, incidence presented as mid-decade age bands (e.g. 55–64 years) but 5-year bands available; 95% confidence intervals should be given for incidence.

Possible approaches to assessing need

Because of the dearth of reliable incidence data (i.e. the number of first-ever-in-a-lifetime cases of stroke occurring in the population over a defined time period), those planning stroke services may decide to base their estimates of need on routinely collected mortality data (i.e. the number of deaths attributed to stroke in the population over a defined time period). They should, however, be aware of the potential problems of adopting this policy.

Mortality statistics depend on the collation of data from death certificates. They are thus dependent on the accuracy of death certification, which even in countries with quite high post-mortem rates such as the UK and US is known to be poor (section 18.2.1). The accuracy of mortality statistics also depends on the accuracy of the population denominators used and thus on the reliability and timing of the most recent census. Furthermore, mortality statistics only include the deaths attributed to stroke (and not the number of stroke episodes), and are not in themselves of much value in estimating the need for health services. Although they are bound to reflect, at least indirectly, the incidence of stroke in the population, the case fatality may differ from place to place, and so there will not be a uniform relationship between stroke mortality and incidence. There is some evidence that case fatality is falling, whilst incidence is not (section 18.2.1).

Hospital admission or discharge statistics are an alternative source of information which may reflect the incidence of stroke. Out-patient attendances are seldom recorded. Again, inaccuracies in diagnostic codes may limit their usefulness (Leibson *et al.* 1994; Davenport *et al.* 1996b). Also, data may be distorted by double counting, which frequently occurs when patients are transferred from an acute centre to a rehabilitation or continuing care facility. A study in Norway found that stroke incidence estimated from hospital discharge data was much higher than that derived from a population-based stroke register (Ellekjaer *et al.* 1999). The major problem is that these data, even if accurate, only include those patients who are admitted to the hospital with a stroke. They are therefore a better measure of the hospital service that is currently provided than of the population's needs. The relationship between stroke incidence and hospitalization can only be known with certainty where a reliable stroke incidence study has been performed to determine the proportion of stroke patients who attend hospital. Where hospital admission rates have been determined, they vary considerably between places—55% to over 95% in developed countries, whilst there is no information from Asia and Africa (Bamford *et al.* 1986; Asplund *et al.* 1995). There is also no information about changes in admission rates with time. The hospital admission rate, or even the attendance at an out-patient clinic, depends on several factors that are independent of population need:

- the quality and availability of primary health-care facilities;
- the quality and availability of hospital facilities;
- the population's expectations—do people expect to be hospitalized after a stroke, or does the culture allow for care in the community?;
- the availability of support services, which may be informal (i.e. the extended family) or formal (i.e. community services);
- the relative cost to the patient and the patient's family of home vs. hospital care; and
- the value of hospital admission as perceived by doctors.

17.2.2 Stroke prevalence

Another measure of the frequency of stroke that some suggest is useful in planning services is stroke prevalence—i.e. the number of people who have ever had a stroke living in the population at any one point in time. They argue that the

Table 17.3 Annual age-specific incidence of stroke per 100 000 population in the 1980s and 1990s (adapted from Sudlow & Warlow 1997).

	Age (years)					
Place and mid-year of study	0–44	45–54	55–64	65–74	75–84	≥85
Australia, Perth (1989) Anderson *et al.* (1993a,b)	17	98	207	511	1679	2369
Denmark, Frederiksberg (1989) Jorgensen *et al.* (1992)	4	104	306	712	1298	1599
France, Dijon (1987) Giroud *et al.* (1989a,b)	10	62	119	410	979	1641
Germany, Erlangen (1995) Kolominsky-Rabas *et al.* (1998)	16	105	196	508	1226	2117
Greece, Arcadia (1994) Vemmos *et al.* (1999)	14	82	218	568	1220	2661
Italy, Aosta (1989) D'Alessandro *et al.* (1992)	13	82	255	707	1607	3237
Italy, Belluno (1993) Lauria *et al.* (1995)	10	114	242	720	1317	3413
Italy, Umbria (1988) Ricci *et al.*)1991)	5	115	280	541	1458	2180
New Zealand, Auckland (1991) Bonita *et al.* (1993)	18*	82	253	647	1267	1967
Norway, Innherred (1995) Ellekjaer *et al.* (1997)	12†	40	217	741	1820	3039
Poland, Warsaw‡ (1991) Czlonkowska *et al.* (1994)	14	76	268	408	901§	1355¶
Russia, Novosibirsk (1992) Feigin *et al.* (1995)	28	246	496	1060	1554	1513
Sweden, Soderhamn (1990) Terent (1988)	12	67	313	976	2056	2995
UK, London (1996) Stewart *et al.* (1999)	21	87	221	516	891	1892
UK, Oxfordshire (1984) Bamford *et al.* (1988)	9	57	291	690	1428	2009
UK, Teesside (1996) Thomson *et al.* (1999)	11	89	297	611	1247	2099
US, Rochester (1988) Broderick *et al.* (1989)	9	62	269	642	1272	2111

* Age group 15–44 years.
† Age group 15–44 years.
‡ Subarachnoid haemorrhage excluded.
§ Age group 75–79 years.
¶ Age group ≥80 years.

prevalence of stroke is more important than the incidence in determining the needs for long-term support services in the community. However, we would argue that the greater the time that elapses after an acute stroke or transient ischaemic attack (TIA), the less important disease-specific services become. If one is interested in determining the need for long-term support services, it is more useful to estimate the prevalence of disability due to *all* causes, rather than just that related to stroke. Furthermore, patients with stroke are often elderly and suffer from other disabling conditions (e.g. arthritis, dementia), so that it is almost impossible to tease out which disability is attributable to stroke rather than these other causes. In addition, stroke prevalence can never reflect the true burden of stroke, because the patients who die soon after a stroke are not represented. There are also a number of important methodological difficulties associated with measuring the prevalence of stroke and TIA, not least the need to make accurate diagnoses sometimes years after the actual event and to survey thousands of people. As a quicker alternative, one can estimate the prevalence of stroke from its

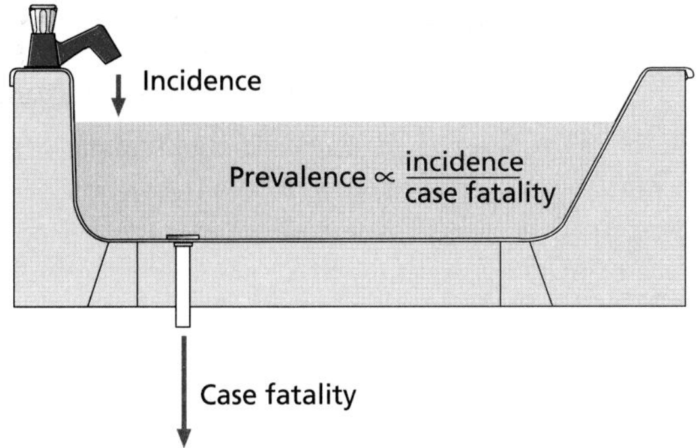

Fig. 17.1 A bath with water running in (representing incident cases), the water level (representing prevalence) and water going down the plug hole (representing deaths in prevalent cases). The prevalence is directly proportional to the incidence and inversely proportional to the case fatality amongst prevalent cases, although the mathematical relationship is quite complex.

incidence and case fatality using the 'bath principle' (Fig. 17.1). Where this has been done for a predominantly white population in New Zealand, the prevalence was estimated to be 833 per 100 000 population (991 in men, 706 in women) aged 15 years and older (Bonita *et al.* 1997b). Of the prevalent cases, around 55% had not made a complete recovery from their stroke, and 21% needed help with self-care activities.

Stroke prevalence is difficult to measure directly, and is not particularly useful.

17.2.3 A practical approach to needs assessment

The vast majority of health service planners are not fortunate enough to have had a recent, methodologically sound, stroke incidence study performed in the population they serve. Rather than carrying out their own incidence study, which is time-consuming and expensive (but technically not that difficult), we recommend the following approach for determining local needs, which uses both local data and information from incidence studies from other areas. If one looks at the estimates of incidence from the most reliable studies (i.e. those fulfilling most of the criteria of an 'ideal' study), it is surprising how little variation there is in the incidence of stroke (given the limits of the studies' precision) (Table 17.3). However, it is important to point out that these are based mainly on white populations, and the incidence may vary in different ethnic groups. For instance, in both New York and London, the incidence of stroke is significantly higher in blacks than in whites (Sacco *et al.* 1998; Stewart *et al.* 1999). Also, the incidence of stroke amongst people of Pacific origin is higher than in those of European origin (Bonita *et al.* 1997a). However, the incidence of stroke amongst ethnic groups may not be the same as the incidence in the same ethnic group living in the original population from which they came.

One should start with the age-specific and sex-specific stroke incidence in the population that is closest to the local one in terms of geography, ethnic composition and culture. These rates can then be applied to the local population numbers to obtain an age-specific and sex-standardized incidence rate (Table 17.4). A comparison of routinely collected data from the area in which the stroke incidence study was performed with similar data from one's own vicinity may give further evidence of the relevance of the incidence data. The cause-specific mortality rates are likely to be the most reliable and easily obtained. A large difference compared with one's own area should alert one to potential differences in stroke incidence, although this may be related to the accuracy of death certification, or different case fatalities. One can then judge whether the incidence locally is likely to be greater or less than that in the available incidence study.

An alternative approach might be to use local hospital admission or discharge data and to adjust them to take account of the likely proportion of stroke patients admitted.

Table 17.4 A step-by-step guide to estimating approximately the number of strokes in a local population of interest.

Step 1	Obtain the most accurate census data for the population of interest for each sex and age category.
Step 2	Identify the 'ideal' incidence study that is likely to have been done in a similar population to the one of interest (e.g. geography, race).
Step 3	Multiply each age-specific and sex-specific incidence rate by the number of people of that age and sex in the population of interest—e.g. if the incidence in men 65–74 years old is 690 per 100 000 and there are 11 000 men in this age band in the population of interest, one would expect about 76 men (i.e. (690 × 11 000)/100 000) between 65 and 74 years of age to suffer a stroke each year in the population of interest.
Step 4	Sum the numbers of patients of each sex in each age band expected to have stroke, to obtain the total number expected in the population.
Step 5	Consider making an adjustment for any marked differences in, for example, the cause-specific mortality between the population of interest and the population in which the incidence study was done.
Step 6	If one is interested in transient ischaemic attacks, then their incidence is usually about 20% that of stroke (Dennis *et al.* 1989).
Step 7	The number of recurrent strokes is of the order of 30% of first-ever-in-a-lifetime strokes, so that to estimate the total number of strokes likely to occur in the population of interest, the number of incident strokes should be inflated by 30%.

This will be more reliable for stroke than for transient ischaemic attacks (TIAs). One could estimate this proportion by surveying the local primary health teams and asking them to report the proportion of patients with acute stroke whom they refer to hospital. This may be reliable enough if they report that they refer virtually all cases (as in Sweden), but if the proportion is smaller, their estimate may be misleading (Asplund *et al.* 1995). Also, hospital discharge data may be inaccurate for a number of reasons (Leibson *et al.* 1994; Davenport *et al.* 1996b):

- inaccuracy of routine clinical diagnosis, especially of TIAs;
- lack of computed tomography (CT) brain scans to confirm the stroke diagnosis and exclude other diagnoses;
- delay in CT scanning, so that ischaemic and haemorrhagic strokes are not reliably distinguished;
- use of vague terms, e.g. 'acute hemiparesis', 'cerebrovascular disease' in medical records and discharge summaries from which routine codes may be derived;
- coding errors;
- failure to distinguish acute stroke admissions from those due to complications of an earlier stroke; and
- failure to code strokes occurring in hospital, or in the context of another diagnosis.

Table 17.5 gives the likelihood that a patient allocated one of the cerebrovascular codes on discharge from one of five Scottish hospitals would have actually had an acute stroke. Ellekjaer *et al.* (1999) in Norway also identified that certain

Table 17.5 The proportion of patients who were allocated a cerebrovascular code (ICD 9 or 10) on discharge from (or having died in) one of five Scottish hospitals and who actually had had an acute stroke. The positive predictive values associated with these codes are higher if only emergency admissions are considered. Of course, diagnostic accuracy and coding procedures vary between institutions, so that these data are not easily applied to other settings. In this study, we did not identify patients who had actually had a stroke but who received a non-stroke code (data provided by N. Weir and the Scottish Stroke Outcomes Group).

	Positive predictive value: all admissions		Positive predictive value: emergency admissions only	
Code	*n*	%	*n*	%
Subarachnoid haemorrhage				
430.9	99	85	77	88
160	83	88	67	93
Intracranial haemorrhage				
431.9	78	91	65	94
161	255	87	226	92
Non-traumatic intracranial haemorrhage				
432.9	4	75	4	75
162	26	58	24	63
Stenosis/occlusion of a precerebral artery				
433	80	1	7	0
Ischaemic stroke				
434	210	83	170	86
163	684	93	614	95
Transient ischaemic attack				
435	155	5	141	6
Stroke, unspecified				
436.9	710	78	598	82
164	1204	87	1071	88
Cerebrovascular disease, unspecified				
437	110	25	78	31
167	319	28	222	31
Cerebrovascular disease sequelae				
438	4	0	0	0

diagnostic codes were more likely to identify true strokes than others. Therefore, if one plans to use hospital discharge data, one would be wise to be selective in one's choice of discharge codes.

The crude incidence of stroke tells one how common the problem is, but in itself is not sufficient to determine the health service needs of the population. Before one can plan a service, one needs to have estimates of the following:

Age-and sex-specific incidence. Younger patients require different facilities from older ones, e.g. retraining for employment. Older women more often live alone, and may require more formal support in the community. Table 17.3 shows the age-specific incidence from those studies that were identified in a systematic review as having used satisfactory or near 'ideal' methodology (Sudlow & Warlow 1996, 1997). There does not appear to be a consistent difference in the incidence between the sexes in these studies, women having a slightly higher incidence at young ages (where numbers are small) and at very old ages.

Type-specific incidence (that is transient ischaemic attack, ischaemic stroke, primary intracerebral haemorrhage and subarachnoid haemorrhage). These data may be useful in more detailed planning of the population's needs. Patients with transient ischaemic attack and minor ischaemic stroke require prompt diagnosis, investigation and initiation and supervision of secondary prevention but not prolonged inpatient care (if at all), rehabilitation, or community support services. Patients with subarachnoid haemorrhage usually require emergency hospitalization and neurosurgical facilities (Chapter 13). Haemorrhagic strokes have a higher early case fatality, so although they may require more care in the very early stages the longer term burden of severe disability may be less than for patients with ischaemic stroke (Table 10.2). The estimates of the relative frequency of the pathological type of stroke are remarkably similar in most of the published incidence studies, which come from predominantly white populations (Fig. 17.2). Although the proportion of patients who are haemorrhagic is probably higher in Oriental populations, it is difficult to be certain, because there are no recent more or less 'ideal' studies from non-white populations. The proportion of strokes due to subarachnoid haemorrhage and primary intracerebral haemorrhage is greater in the young than the old.

The prognosis of stroke and its subtypes. From the type-specific incidence and case fatality, one can estimate the likely requirements for assessment and diagnostic services, acute care, rehabilitation and terminal care services, long-term care, community support and secondary prevention. The prognosis of stroke and its subtypes has been discussed elsewhere (sections 10.2 and 16.1). Information on stroke severity and co-morbidity would be invaluable, since these will be major determinants of patients' health service use. However, such data are unlikely to be routinely available unless a stroke register has been kept.

Changes over time. When one is planning a stroke service, one has to take account of any changes that may occur in the future, because one's service will need to alter to take these into account. Trends in stroke mortality and incidence are discussed later (section 18.2), and there is some evidence that the incidence, and maybe even the severity, of stroke is falling in many Western populations. Apart from the changing incidence, one also has to take into account changing demographics. In most developed countries, older people account for an increasing proportion of the population. Therefore, in a disease such as stroke in which the incidence is much higher in older people (Table 17.3), the total number of strokes will

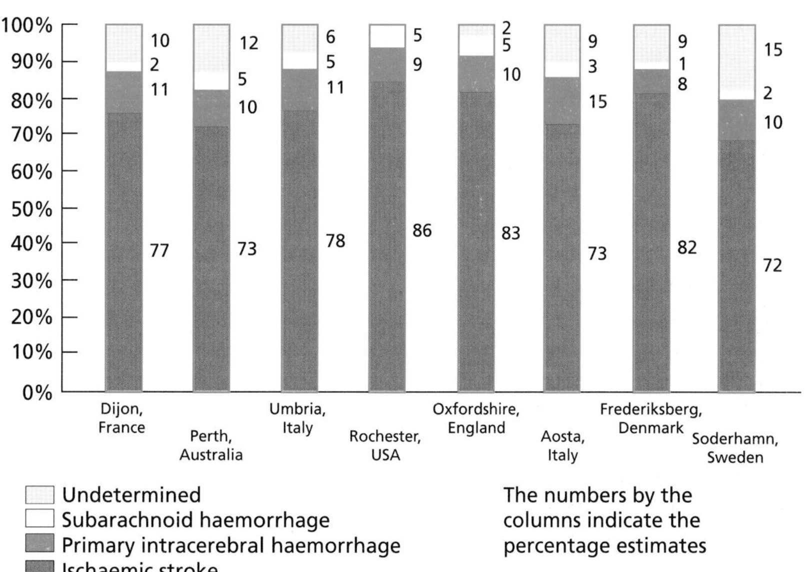

Fig. 17.2 Histogram showing the proportions of patients aged between 45 and 84 years with a first-ever-in-a-lifetime stroke due to ischaemia, primary intracerebral haemorrhage, subarachnoid haemorrhage and uncertain, in more-or-less 'ideal' incidence studies. Only studies with a computed tomography (CT) scan rate of more than 70%, and including patients with subarachnoid haemorrhage, are covered. The study from Rochester did not have an 'uncertain' category, because the small proportion of patients who did not have a CT scan or post-mortem were counted as having ischaemic strokes (Sudlow & Warlow 1997).

increase unless offset by a falling incidence. However, one has to remember that case fatality is higher in older patients (Fig. 10.9) and in those with prior disability, and therefore fewer of these older stroke patients will survive to require long-term care. Malmgren *et al.* (1989) calculated that over 30 years the number of new strokes occurring each year in the UK might increase, but there would be fewer *newly* disabled survivors. This type of forecast is potentially useful in determining the services one plans for the future. If there are going to be more acute strokes, one will need to plan for more acute services, but if fewer survive the acute stage, rehabilitation and long-term care facilities may not need to expand to the same degree. Changes in clinical practice are likely to force rapid alterations in the shape of clinical services for stroke. For example, if a highly cost-effective acute treatment for ischaemic stroke was identified (e.g. thrombolysis), but could only be given in hospital, this would markedly increase the hospitalization rate in those countries in which a sizeable proportion of strokes are currently managed at home (section 11.5). Conversely, if rehabilitation at home is more cost-effective than in hospital, this would require a transfer of hospital-based resources into the community (section 17.5.3). The changes in management of stroke have, until now, been small and gradual, but with recent increases in research efforts, major changes are more likely and the needs of the population could alter rapidly and unpredictably. People's expectations of health care, often driven by media reports of medical successes and failures, may also force changes in services that go beyond the evidence of effectiveness.

17.2.4 Assuming that resources are limited, to what extent will the needs of the population be met?

Having obtained an estimate of one's local age-specific, sex-specific and type-specific incidence and outcome of stroke and transient ischaemic attack, one is still a long way from determining the needs of the population. After all, this estimate does not indicate the actual resources these people will require, and of course at some stage somebody has to make a political decision about how completely the population's needs are to be met. Inevitably, where there are limited resources for health services, choices have to be made about allocating resources between areas (e.g. should one build a new hospital or a new school?). Having been given limited resources, however, it is important that those planning stroke services should use them in as an efficient a manner as possible and should prioritize (i.e. ration) to make sure that sufficient funds are available for whatever are perceived to be the most important aspects of the service. These decisions are usually taken by politicians but, because they depend on information about the effectiveness of components of the stroke services, it is vital for the politicians to receive sound medical advice.

17.3 Planning a stroke service

Having established the aims of the service, the needs of the population and the degree to which one expects to fulfil these, one can then plan the development of services. Usually, one starts with the existing services, even if these are inadequate and chaotic. It is then useful to consider the following questions prior to making any changes:

- what are the current resources committed to the management of patients with transient ischaemic attacks and stroke?
- what are the major gaps (i.e. unmet needs and failure to provide cost-effective interventions) in the present provision of services?

One needs to establish the strengths and weaknesses of the current services in order to identify the most important areas for improvement. Priority should be given to providing patients with basic care (e.g. nursing to provide for basic needs) and to delivering those interventions that are of proven effectiveness.

Although information regarding current services may already be available, it is likely that in addition to routinely collected data, it will be useful to carry out a survey to determine the following:

- how many and what sort of patients are currently being managed (i.e. demographic and clinical data)?
- where are they being managed (i.e. in the hospital or community, in neurology, internal medicine or geriatric medicine)?
- by whom are they being managed (i.e. general or family practitioner, neurologist, general physician)?
- how are they being managed (i.e. the process of care)?
- what resources are currently being used?

A community-based register that identified all patients in the population who had a stroke or TIA would be an ideal but expensive and impractical way of answering these questions. A hospital-based stroke register is a practical alternative that can help to answer most of the questions, although clearly it cannot provide detailed information about patients who are not referred to hospital. A register is an invaluable tool for monitoring the performance of services as well as planning them (section 17.6).

Set up a hospital-based stroke register to get some idea of the current state of the local stroke service—however fragmented and chaotic it is.

The simplest, quickest and most practical approach is to carry out a survey of the current services against certain standards. Those working within a service are often fully aware of its deficiencies, and their knowledge should not be ignored. However, this approach will only work where there is a willingness to acknowledge deficiencies and to change practice. This approach can identify areas of strength and weakness, and may determine which area to concentrate on first (e.g. Scottish Stroke Services Audit 1999).

An honest, objective appraisal of services against some agreed standards by those involved in providing them, perhaps facilitated by an independent observer, may be the best stimulus for service development.

The immediate priorities for improving a service will also depend on how easily or cheaply particular problems can be solved. For instance, poor standards of medical assessment may be improved by the introduction of a protocol and education for junior medical staff with little implication for resources, whilst the provision of an occupational therapy department where one is lacking has major resource implications.

What is the evidence for the cost-effectiveness of components of the stroke service? (Section 17.7)

Stroke services should first concentrate on providing basic care for the patients and their families and then aim to give priority to those aspects of care that are generally accepted as being, or have been proven to be, effective. Evidence from randomized trials and formal statistical overviews of groups of trials provide the most reliable unbiased evidence. The Stroke Review Group of the Cochrane Collaboration is an excellent source of this type of information, providing an increasing number of systematic reviews (Counsell *et al.* 1995) (section 11.2.1) (website http://www.dcn.ed.ac.uk/csrg). It is important that those who are responsible for planning services should be aware of all the available evidence concerning the effectiveness of interventions and the methods of delivering these interventions to the appropriate patients. If there are data concerning the cost of interventions and various other aspects of the service, this may allow healthcare planners to make more informed choices about which services should be provided.

The best and quickest way to access information on the effectiveness of interventions in stroke is the regularly updated electronic database provided by the Cochrane Collaboration. However, it is important to remember that any lack of evidence of benefit is not equivalent to evidence of lack of benefit. Often evidence of benefit is lacking because of the methodological difficulties in reliably evaluating interventions.

17.4 Where should stroke patients be managed?

17.4.1 Caring for stroke patients in the community

Why admit stroke patients to hospital?

The vast majority of patients who have a stroke have it in the community and not in hospital. Many of them require help from medical and social services. Community-based incidence studies have shown wide variations in hospital admission rates, varying from 55% in Oxfordshire, UK in the 1980s to about 95% in Sweden and Germany in the 1990s (Bamford *et al.* 1986; Asplund *et al.* 1995; Kolominsky-Rabas *et al.* 1998). The main reason for admission to hospital in the UK in the 1980s was for nursing care rather than diagnosis and treatment (Bamford *et al.* 1986). The higher rates in other studies may reflect differences in social factors—in particular, the support available in the community, housing and the wishes and expectations of the patients and their families. However, in the last decade the need to use CT scanning to establish whether a stroke is ischaemic or haemorrhagic has become accepted, and the potential for early intervention is increasingly being recognized (Adams *et al.* 1994; European Ad Hoc Consensus Group 1996; Scottish Intercollegiate Guidelines Network (SIGN) 1997; http://www.show.scot.nhs.uk/sign/home.htm) (Chapter 11). Thus, referral to hospital for assessment, even if only on an outpatient basis, is probably becoming more common.

Is care in the community safe, effective and less costly than hospital-based care?

It is interesting that in the UK, which already has a lower hospital admission rate for stroke than most other developed countries, there have been moves to admit even fewer patients to hospital (Wade 1992). This is probably based on two assumptions: that care in the community is at least as effective as care in hospital and may be cheaper; and that patients and families prefer to be cared for at home. The adoption of a policy of non-admission for stroke patients carries the considerable risk that 'community care' may become synonymous with 'inadequate care'. This concern is fuelled by data from a community-based stroke register in the UK, which showed that non-admitted patients were less often investigated and assessed in accordance with accepted guidelines, and rarely received rehabilitation (Rodgers *et al.* 1999). It is far easier, and cheaper, to overlook the needs of patients when they are at home rather than in hospital, and it is far harder to monitor what is going on.

Do not move the care of stroke patients into the community until there is reliable evidence that this is at least as cost-effective as hospital-based care, and that it is preferred by patients and their families.

The data from randomized studies comparing the effectiveness and cost of a policy of avoiding admission by providing care at home with a conventional policy of admitting most patients to hospital are sparse, and do not indicate that either model is superior (Langhorne *et al.* 2000a). Indeed, in one randomized controlled trial that compared hospital care with avoidance of hospital for 'appropriate' patients with acute stroke, almost a third of those allocated to care in the community had to be admitted for a variety of reasons (Evans *et al.* 2000). This confirms the earlier finding from a large non-randomized study that preventing admission is not always feasible (Wade *et al.* 1985). Of course, changes in the acute treatment of stroke may make the results of such studies irrelevant. Also, we have little information concerning patients' and families' preferences. Therefore, it would be unwise to introduce a major shift in the pattern of where patients are managed before more evidence about cost-effectiveness is available.

How feasible is community-based care?

Certainly, many of the components of care shown in Table 17.1 can very reasonably be provided without admission to hospital. We will discuss here how each of these can be provided in the community.

Diagnosis and assessment. The clinical diagnosis and initial assessment of stroke, including simple blood tests and an electrocardiogram, do not in themselves require referral to hospital. Assuming a reasonable level of knowledge and competence, all this could be done by a primary care physician in the patient's own home. CT brain scanning is an out-patient procedure, and although a relatively small proportion of patients will need a CT scan to confirm the diagnosis of stroke, the majority will need one to plan further treatment—in particular, secondary prevention (section 5.3.3). However, one will probably need to liaise with the radiology department to restructure the service to ensure that CT scans are performed soon after stroke onset so as to allow reliable differentiation between haemorrhage and infarction (section 5.3.4) and early initiation of antithrombotic treatment (sections 11.4, 11.5, 16.4 and 16.5). Other investigations (e.g. chest X-ray, duplex sonography, echocardiography) can also be performed as out-patient procedures. But all this does rely on an efficient means of transporting patients—some of whom may be disabled—to and from hospital, and once they get there on having an efficient and streamlined system to access the results and care for the patients. So called 'one-stop' out-patient neurovascular clinics can provide such facilities.

Transient events, transient ischaemic attacks (TIAs) and episodes that may be confused with them (Table 3.14) are less reliably diagnosed than strokes and more often require input from a specialist, especially when the diagnosis is crucial to future decision-making—for example, in distinguishing between carotid and posterior circulation TIAs in a patient with severe carotid stenosis (Table 4.4). The large range of final diagnoses in patients referred to the Oxfordshire Community Stroke Project with 'probable TIAs' by general (family) practitioners is shown in Table 3.19 (section 3.6).

Although the clinical diagnosis of stroke may be quite straightforward a day or two after the onset, it is increasingly apparent, as we encourage earlier referral to hospital, that diagnosis is more difficult in the hyper-acute phase (section 3.2.3). Doctors working in the community will of course see patients even earlier, and probably have less experience and training in neurological diagnosis than those in hospital. Moreover, even if the correct diagnosis has been made, the assessment guiding the further management needs to be both thorough and accurate (section 10.3.2). There is evidence from audits of case-notes that hospital-admitted patients often have incomplete and inaccurate assessments (Davenport *et al.* 1995; Rudd *et al.* 1999). Evidence from our own and other studies of assessments in primary care indicate that these are often superficial and even less complete (Rodgers *et al.* 1999). Of course, there is as yet little evidence that improving the completeness of assessment significantly alters outcome—but equally, no evidence exists that sloppy assessment is as effective as a good assessment. Also, one must not overlook the possibility that a thorough assessment of the patient's and carer's problems and needs has advantages beyond those measured by crude clinical outcome (e.g. patient's perception of self-value, etc.).

Acute treatment. In some societies, the high hospital admission rates may in part reflect the belief amongst both physicians and the public that specific acute therapy is effective, or that close monitoring and manipulation of physiological parameters (e.g. blood pressure, blood glucose) lead to better outcomes. Certainly in Italy, where the admission rate is probably about 85%, acute treatments such as glycerol are much more in vogue than in the UK (Ricci *et al.* 1991; D'Alessandro *et al.* 1992) (section 11.2.4). In some places, early initiation of aspirin treatment after acute ischaemic stroke (section 11.3.3) and the current evidence regarding the impact of thrombolytic therapy (section 11.5.2) in a highly selected subgroup of patients with ischaemic stroke, may not be seen as adequate justification for referring all patients to hospital in the acute stage. However, if more effective or widely applicable acute treatments are found, then this may have a profound effect on where stroke patients are managed. For example, if a treatment has to be preceded by brain CT or another hospital-based procedure, or if it is given by intravenous infusion, more stroke patients will have to be admitted to hospital. Also, it seems likely that hospital admission will normally be required for entry into the randomized trials that are needed to test the effectiveness of novel therapies. Of course, if the treatment could be administered in the community and haemorrhage did not have to be excluded by brain CT prior to drug administration, the hospital admission rate might actually fall, since a proportion of patients might improve to such an extent that they did not require admission.

General care may be provided either in hospital or in the community, although most patients with a severe stroke will need admission to hospital unless considerably more extensive support services are available in the community than currently. The data available from both randomized and non-randomized trials suggests that only a proportion of hospital admissions can be avoided by providing a rapid-response service in the community to support patients in their own home, and the overall use of hospital facilities may not be reduced (Wade *et al.* 1985; Langhorne *et al.* 2000a; Kalra *et al.* 2000). However, there are insufficient data for definite conclusions to be drawn about the feasibility and cost-effectiveness of such an approach.

Rehabilitation. It is possible to rehabilitate patients in hospital, in their own homes, or in hospital-based facilities such as day hospitals. In hospital, patients spend relatively little time with physical therapists, although in stroke units, where the nurses adopt a more 'therapeutic role', patients spend a greater proportion of their time in therapeutic activities (Lincoln *et al.* 1996; Indredavik *et al.* 1999a). Patients' limited contact with therapists and the large proportion of their time in which they are engaged in non-therapeutic activities indicate that rehabilitation could be provided to patients living at home. Unfortunately, although the patients and families may prefer this option, practical difficulties in providing and coordinating enough care for patients in the community often prevent early discharge. These include the practical problems (e.g. transport, time) of several different people visiting the patient at home and coordination of a geographically dispersed team. Multidisciplinary stroke teams which aim to allow patients to be discharged earlier from hospital, and which can provide ongoing rehabilitation and care for patients at home, have been set up and evaluated in randomized trials. The pooled results of the trials in which community care was coordinated suggest that the length of the initial hospital stay can be reduced, whilst patient and carer outcomes are equivalent or slightly better than in conventional hospital-based care (Rudd *et al.* 1997; Rodgers *et al.* 1997; Widen Holmqvist *et al.* 1998; Anderson *et al.* 2000b; Early Supported Discharge Trialists 2000; Mayo *et al.* 2000). Economic analyses of these trials, which took account of the costs of community care, suggest that a shorter length of stay could be achieved with fewer resources (McNamee *et al.* 1998; Beech *et al.* 1999; Anderson *et al.* 2000a). One trial that evaluated early discharge, but crucially did not provide a coordinated multidisciplinary team in the community, achieved shorter lengths of hospital stay but at the expense of inferior patient outcomes (Ronning & Guldvog 1998). Of course, the results of these small single-centre trials may not necessarily apply to different health-care and social environments, but if the results of the several ongoing trials produce consistent results, this will demonstrate that early supported discharge is a cost-effective approach that is widely applicable (Early Supported Discharge Trialists 2000).

The effectiveness of domiciliary physiotherapy and of physiotherapy provided in a day hospital have been compared in randomized trials (Young & Forster 1992; Gladman *et al.* 1993; Gladman & Lincoln 1994). A combined analysis of these demonstrated only small differences in outcome in patients treated in different settings (Gladman *et al.* 1995). The relative costs of providing care in these settings varied between the studies, with day hospital treatment costing more (Gladman *et al.* 1994) or less (Young & Forster 1993) than domiciliary physiotherapy. The evidence from a systematic review of randomized trials in frail elderly patients (not just those with stroke) suggests that day hospital care, compared with no organized service, prevents deterioration in activities of daily living (Forster *et al.* 2000a). This finding might be expected to apply at least to frail elderly stroke patients.

Continuing care and maintenance, almost by definition, is provided in the community, although certain aspects may be hospital-based—e.g. day hospital, respite care, etc. The emphasis on long-term institutional care varies from country to country.

Secondary prevention. There is little doubt that most of this aspect of stroke care can be very effectively managed in the community. However, there are now several effective options for the secondary prevention of stroke (Chapter 16), and some (e.g. anticoagulation and carotid surgery) need detailed assessment prior to implementation. Patients with TIAs and mild stroke can usually be managed mainly as out-patients or day patients. By providing rapid and easy access to a specialist opinion for out-patients, it may be possible to avoid unnecessary hospital admission, which will save resources. Some centres are able to offer a one-visit assessment during which patients can be assessed clinically, with all the non-invasive investigations (e.g. blood tests, electrocardiography (ECG), carotid duplex ultrasound, chest X-ray and brain CT) being performed to allow the clinician to plan secondary prevention. It makes no sense to admit patients as the only way of obtaining rapid access to investigatory facilities. After all, the common investigations, except for catheter angiography, can all be routinely performed on an out-patient basis. Hopefully, in the next few years non-invasive arterial imaging with ultrasound and magnetic resonance will completely replace the more invasive and hazardous techniques (section 6.7.5). Those responsible for organizing stroke services should ensure that patients have rapid access to investigations on an out-patient or day case basis and so avoid unnecessary admissions to hospital, and that there is an efficient system to process the patients, get the results of investigations back to the physician, and then translate them into advice for the patient (Gubitz *et al.* 1999).

The risk of stroke after a TIA, or of recurrent stroke after a first stroke, is much higher in the early period and tails off later (section 16.1.1). Thus, one has most to gain from starting secondary prevention as early as possible. Also, since the accurate diagnosis of TIAs depends on a good history, it makes sense to assess the patients as soon after the event as possible.

In many centres, so-called 'one-stop' neurovascular, TIA, or stroke clinics have been set up, which are characterized by:

- providing rapid access to a specialist opinion regarding TIAs, minor strokes and episodes that may mimic them;
- streamlined access to the necessary investigations (which requires close liaison with the radiology department);
- close links with surgeons who can offer carotid endarterectomy.

These clinics should minimize unnecessary hospital admission and delays in accessing specialist opinion, investigations and treatment. However, such clinics attract patients with a wide range of neurological conditions (Table 17.6), so the clinician must have neurological training, or at least easy access to sound neurological advice (Martin *et al.* 1997; Karunaratne *et al.* 1999).

'One-stop' neurovascular clinics should provide rapid clinical assessment of patients who may have had a transient ischaemic attack or minor stroke, with streamlined and cost-effective investigations and early intervention to reduce the risk of a serious vascular event.

Coordination of care by a multidisciplinary team. There is now evidence that care in a dedicated stroke unit, which is coordinated by a specialist with an interested multidisciplinary team, is more effective than care provided in general wards (Stroke Unit Trialists' Collaboration 1997, 2000). It therefore seems likely that specialist care would be superior to non-specialist care delivered in the community. It is even conceivable that care in the community could be coordinated by a specialist multidisciplinary team, but this would need to be evaluated properly. However, there may be considerable practical difficulties in attempting to deliver intensive packages of care in the community and any evaluation must address the possibility that community care may be effective in one setting but not another, depending on local factors that hamper or facilitate this model of care—e.g. how dispersed a population is, public transport, etc. Table 17.7 summarizes our recommendations for the development of community-based stroke services.

Table 17.6 Some of the non-cerebrovascular problems referred to one of our neurovascular clinics by general practitioners in Edinburgh over the last 5 years. There were, of course, countless patients with transient symptoms in whom no definite diagnosis was made.

General medical problems
Cardiac syncope: dysrhythmias, aortic stenosis
Cough syncope
Postural hypotension
Hyperventilation
Sleep apnoea
Hypoglycaemia

Neurological problems
Migraine (both with and without headache)
Epilepsy
Transient global amnesia
Glioma
Meningioma
Cerebral metastases
Subdural haematoma
Lymphocytic meningitis
Peripheral neuropathy
Compression mononeuropathy
Guillain–Barré syndrome
Cervical myelopathy
Brachial neuritis
Herpes zoster neuropathy
Bell's palsy
Syringobulbia
Myasthenia gravis
Multiple sclerosis
Motor neurone disease

Psychiatric problems
Somatization disorder

Ophthalmic problems
Retinal vein occlusion
Glaucoma

Table 17.7 Summary of recommendations for the development of community-based stroke services.

No major changes to the balance between community and hospital care be introduced unless there is good evidence that one model of care is superior. This situation may change if effective acute treatments for stroke are identified.

The assessment of stroke patients in the community should be improved by:
Introducing assessment guidelines and more education for primary care physicians;
Offering rapid and easy access to a 'one stop' out-patient assessment by a specialist;
Developing multidisciplinary teams in the community, or encouraging those based in hospitals to develop outreach services.

Coordination be improved so that those working in the community and hospital work together to develop guidelines to help decide which patients are best managed at home and which should be admitted to hospital. Specialists in hospital should be available to offer advice (perhaps by telephone) on individual patients.

Further research is carried out to determine the relative effectiveness of care in the community vs. that in hospital.

17.4.2 Hospital-based care

The type of stroke services that hospitals provide varies considerably from place to place. To some extent, this reflects differences in local conditions and needs, but it also reflects the lack of evidence that one particular model of care is any better than another. The results of a systematic review are therefore important, because they provide good evidence that hospital-based stroke services should be *organized* (Stroke Unit Trialists' Collaboration 1997, 2000). This review examined all the randomized controlled trials that compared the outcome for stroke patients cared for in a specialist stroke unit with those cared for in general medical wards: patients managed in stroke units were less likely to die, need long-term institutional care, or be dependent on others for everyday activities up to 12 months after stroke (Fig. 17.3) (Table 17.8). The results of individual trials suggest that stroke units may also improve the patients' quality of life, and that improvements in outcome persist for several years (Juby *et al.* 1996; Indredavik *et al.* 1998, 1999a).

Whatever else, stroke services should be organized by people who are both knowledgeable and enthusiastic.

The trials included in the meta-analysis were testing much more heterogeneous interventions than is usual in drug trials, where the intervention is defined in terms of the chemical, the dose and the timing. Because of this heterogeneity of input—but not of the results—it is difficult to generalize from the stroke unit overview, and some important questions are left when applying the results to everyday clinical practice.

Stroke patients managed in a stroke unit are less likely to have a poor outcome than those managed in a general medical ward.

What is a stroke unit?

Most of the Stroke Unit Trialists did not describe their units in detail, but many of the units had some features in common (Table 17.9). Most of the trials were of geographically defined stroke units. Beyond this, it is not possible to determine whether the effectiveness of the units is due to the total package of care or to particular components of care. Some of the individual components could be evaluated in randomized trials (e.g. guidelines for prevention of deep venous thrombosis, intensive physiotherapy, etc.), and trials can be reviewed systematically to provide reliable data, but some of the less well-defined components and the possible synergy between them will make this difficult. For example, better communication between health professionals, stroke patients and their carers, which is so often inadequate and a major source of dissatisfaction in non-specialized wards, may in part explain the success of stroke units, but this would be difficult, if not impossible, to prove (Wellwood *et al.* 1995a; O'Mahony *et al.* 1997). The term 'stroke unit' means different things to different people. So it is important to define the terms we use before proceeding (Table 17.10).

Stroke intensive care units

In some centres, particularly those in North America and Germany, there has been a vogue for admitting patients with severe strokes to areas with facilities for intensive moni-

Study name	Events/patients: Stroke unit	Events/patients: Medical ward	Odds ratio & 95% CI (Stroke unit better / Stroke unit worse)	Odds reduction (SD)
Akershus	101/271	113/279		
Dover	61/116	66/117		
Edinburgh	66/155	78/156		
Goteborg-Ostra	49/215	43/202		
Helsinki	36/121	46/122		
Illinois	22/56	17/35		
Kuopio	22/50	23/45		
Montreal	57/65	52/65		
New York	15/42	17/40		
Newcastle	18/34	21/33		
Nottingham	62/176	53/139		
Orpington 1993	33/124	52/121		
Orpington 1995	18/36	30/37		
Perth	6/29	14/30		
Svendborg	18/31	20/34		
Tampere	43/98	42/113		
Trondheim	41/110	61/110		
Umea	51/110	105/183		
Uppsala	40/60	35/52		
Total (95%CI)	759/1899	888/1913		23% (6) (2*P* <0.001)

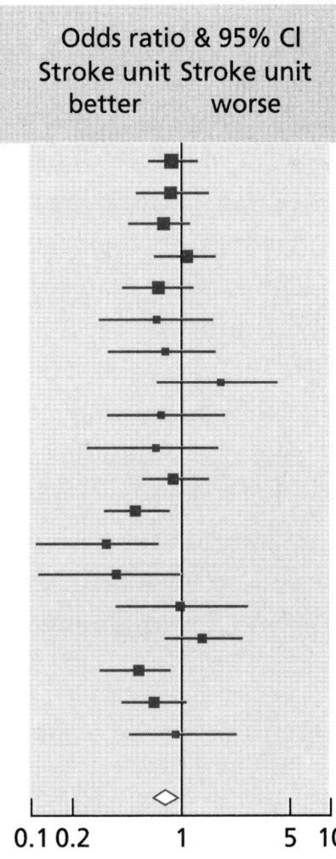

Fig. 17.3 The results of a systematic review of randomized trials testing the effectiveness of stroke unit care compared with a general medical ward. The result of each individual trial, expressed as the odds ratio, is represented by a solid square with a horizontal line indicating the 95% confidence interval. The solid square size is proportional to the amount of information in the trial. An odds ratio to the left of the vertical line indicates that the odds of the outcome (in this case events refer to death or living in an institution between 6 and 12 months after randomization) is less with stroke unit care than care in general wards. The estimate based on an overview of all the trials is represented by an open diamond (with permission from the Stroke Unit Trialists' Collaboration 2000).

Table 17.8 The relative and absolute benefits of stroke units compared with less organized systems of care. This table shows the proportion (%) of patients with various outcomes at the end of scheduled follow up (median 1 year) in the randomized trials of stroke unit care vs. conventional care. The absolute risk reduction equates to the percentage of outcomes achieved (+) or avoided (–), and the number of outcomes for every 1000 patients cared for in a stroke unit assuming the absolute risk of an outcome in the population is similar to that in the trials.

	Stroke unit (%)	Conventional care (%)	Odds ratio (95% CI)	Absolute risk reduction (%) (95% CI)	Approximate no. of outcomes/ 1000 admitted
Home (independent)	44	38	1.33 (1.15, 1.54)	6 (2, 9)	60
Home (dependent)	16	16	1.04 (0.72, 1.50)	0 (–2, 2)	0
Institution	18	21	0.84 (0.71, 0.99)	–3 (–6, –1)	30
Dead	22	25	0.83 (0.71, 0.97)	–3 (–6, 0)	30
Dead/institution	40	46	0.77 (0.68, 0.88)	–6 (–9, –3)	60
Dead/dependent	56	62	0.75 (0.65, 0.87)	–6 (–9, –3)	60

These figures are approximate. They are based on data from the Stroke Unit Trialists' Collaboration 2000 and unpublished data relating to subgroups of trials that reported particular outcomes.

Table 17.9 Core features of stroke units included in a systematic review of randomized trials (Stroke Unit Trialists' Collaboration 1997).

Care co-ordinated by a multidisciplinary team
Team meets to discuss patients at least weekly
Nurses have expertise in rehabilitation
Team consists of professionals interested and specializing in stroke
Regular in-service training for staff is provided
Involvement of carers in patient care

toring of many physiological functions (cardiac, respiratory and neurological). Interventions are introduced to correct these abnormalities (e.g. raised intracranial pressure, systemic hypertension, etc.), in the belief that this will improve outcome (Hacke *et al.* 1994). There have been several non-randomized studies of stroke intensive care units, but there is no good evidence that these improve patient outcome, and due to their high staffing levels and expensive equipment, they inevitably require extra resources (Kennedy *et al.* 1970; Drake *et al.* 1973; Pitner & Mance 1973). Also, there is little evidence from randomized trials that the various individual interventions employed are effective. Stroke intensive care units may help, but there is no evidence one way or the other; so we need randomized trials to evaluate them. Of course, if an effective treatment is developed that requires intensive care, then that would be different.

Acute stroke units, or stroke rehabilitation units, or both?

About 50% of the trials in the meta-analysis were of acute stroke units, whilst the rest were primarily of stroke rehabilitation units. Admitting all acute stroke patients directly into a unit makes the introduction of assessment protocols easier, allows expertise to be focused, and will certainly facilitate the very large randomized trials of acute treatments that are needed to identify effective treatments (Bath *et al.* 1996). Also, admission of patients directly to an acute stroke unit facilitates a policy of aggressive early mobilization (section 15.11), hydration (section 15.18.1), control of temperature (section 15.12), avoidance of hypoxia (section 15.2.2) and large changes in blood pressure (section 15.7). Although there are no reliable data from randomized trials demonstrating that any one of these interventions improves outcomes, they are supported by a reasonable theoretical rationale and some observational data (Davis *et al.* 1999; Indredavik *et al.* 1999b; Langhorne 1999). Alternatively, this might all be achieved by setting up a stroke assessment area on an acute general medical ward, which would need some organizational changes but might not necessarily require extra resources. One randomized trial has compared an acute stroke unit that did not provide ongoing rehabilitation with non-specialist care, and this failed to demonstrate improvements in survival or functional status—although other potential benefits (e.g. training, research, communication) were not sought (Ilmavirta *et al.* 1994). Perhaps the most successful model is the comprehensive stroke unit, which admits patients acutely and then provides at least a few weeks of rehabilitation. Such a model, which is widespread in Norway and Sweden, is supported by several trials included in the systematic review and data from a national stroke register in Sweden (Stegmayr *et al.* 1999). However, although we believe that rehabilitation should start on the day of the stroke, some patients are more appropriately cared for in an acute ward than in one in which the emphasis is just on rehabilitation. For example, very sick stroke patients might

Table 17.10 Definitions relating to stroke units.

Stroke service	The overall organization for delivering care to individuals with transient ischaemic attacks and strokes. A stroke service may (and probably should) include a stroke unit, but is more than just a stroke unit
Acute stroke assessment area	Where stroke patients are admitted directly to be assessed and cared for acutely
Stroke rehabilitation unit	A unit in which the emphasis is on rehabilitation rather than acute care. Patients are not admitted with acute stroke directly from the community to stroke rehabilitation units
Acute stroke unit	A unit to which patients are admitted directly and may also remain for a variable time to be rehabilitated, i.e. combining an acute stroke assessment area with a stroke rehabilitation unit. This is distinct from a stroke intensive care unit, and is sometimes referred to as a *comprehensive stroke unit*
Stroke intensive care unit	A unit to which patients are admitted directly for only a short period to be closely monitored in a 'high-tech' environment, similar to that in a coronary care unit
Stroke unit	A rather vague term that refers to those units included in the systematic overview which all had at their heart a multidisciplinary team, but in which the balance between acute care and rehabilitation varied and was often unclear (Stroke Unit Trialists' Collaboration 2000)

require care that would disrupt a rehabilitation unit, at a time when they are unlikely to benefit from a rehabilitation environment. We believe that the best model is one in which patients are admitted into an acute stroke assessment area and then move to a stroke rehabilitation unit as soon as they are medically stable and can participate in rehabilitation and benefit from that environment. Ideally, the acute assessment area and rehabilitation units would be closely integrated (perhaps with an acute stroke bay actually on the rehabilitation unit), sharing staff and methods of working. Models that separate acute assessment and rehabilitation areas may disorientate some patients (and their families), and can compromise continuity of care.

Stroke-specific unit or not?

The meta-analysis included trials of organized care within stroke-specific units, neurology wards and geriatric rehabilitation units compared with in acute general wards. Some studies directly compared a stroke rehabilitation unit with geriatric rehabilitation units. However, there are insufficient data to decide whether stroke-specific units are better or not. In smaller hospitals, there may be too few patients with acute stroke to make stroke-specific services viable. Stroke-specific services certainly allow more specialization amongst the team members, which enhances the educational and research potential of the service. Training of junior doctors and other staff, which might suffer if all the stroke patients are managed by a single team, can be protected and probably improved by organizing rotation of staff through the unit. Moreover, stroke specialists are more likely to be enthusiastic about teaching students and staff about strokes than generalists, or those with another specialist interest.

Geographically defined unit or not?

The meta-analysis predominantly included trials of geographically defined stroke units, but it did include one trial of a stroke team that cared for patients scattered in different wards of the hospital (Wood-Dauphinee *et al.* 1984). This study, and another more recent one, provide little evidence that a stroke team working on general wards can achieve outcomes as good those of a team working on a stroke unit (Evans *et al.* 2000). The most important advantage of having the patients in one location is that the nursing staff can play a greater role in the rehabilitation process. Inevitably, when patients are scattered, it is more difficult to incorporate the nurses, who have such an essential role to play in the team (section 10.3.6). Also, stroke patients managed in acute general areas have to compete for nursing time with patients who may be perceived to have more urgent needs (e.g. chest pain). Stroke patients may, for example, need regular toileting to maintain continence and thus dignity. These aspects of care are very important, but can be seen as less urgent, and when nursing resources are stretched they may not be a priority. A geographically defined stroke unit removes this competition for nursing time, and allows the nurses to take on a new role—not just as carers, but also as facilitators of patients' independence—and to continue therapy (directed by specialist therapists) throughout the 24-h period. Some argue that having stroke patients together in one area may adversely affect the morale of patients and staff. We have not found this a particular problem, although it depends on the mix of individual patients and therefore varies with time. A good physical environment, positive attitudes amongst the staff, and attempts to relieve the boredom of hospital (section 15.31.3) can all avoid poor morale amongst patients and their families. Poor morale amongst staff can be avoided by ensuring adequate staffing for the given workload, as well as in-service education.

> *The main advantage of caring for stroke patients in one place is that the nurses can play a major role in the rehabilitation process.*

Which patients gain most from stroke unit care?

The trials included in the meta-analysis usually selected patients before randomization. Stratification of patients within the meta-analysis by stroke severity showed that patients with mild, moderate and severe strokes are all likely to benefit from stroke unit care (Stroke Unit Trialists' Collaboration 1997, 2000). However, most units adopted a system of triage based on the patient's likely needs, and many excluded patients with non-disabling stroke or those with little hope of survival. Data from non-randomized, and thus potentially biased, comparisons of outcomes following admission to a stroke unit or general care support the notion that stroke unit care benefits unselected stroke patients (Jorgensen *et al.* 1999; Stegmayr *et al.* 1999).

Patients with severe strokes and a reduced conscious level who are unlikely to survive are probably better managed on an acute ward or unit until they either die or improve to a level at which they can actively take part in rehabilitation. These patients obviously need skilled nursing, which can be provided on an acute ward, with input from the stroke team (e.g. advice on positioning and swallowing safety), to prevent complications such as pressure sores, aspiration pneumonia and shoulder injuries.

Patients with severe stroke who survive the first few weeks but show few signs of any functional improvement pose a particular problem. We believe that such patients are best managed on an acute ward until they can be transferred to a facility to provide long-term nursing care. Often, the type of problem they have—e.g. a high risk of pressure sores (section 15.16), or a need for nasogastric or gastrostomy feeding (section 15.19)—makes placement in a nursing home difficult unless staff have appropriate expertise and training. Occasionally, such patients may unexpectedly improve to the extent that they may benefit from more active input from the multidisciplinary stroke team. Nursing staff should ideally be trained to reassess patients regularly and to make appropriate referrals for further rehabilitation.

Should the stroke service be restricted to patients of a particular age?

In the meta-analysis of trials, there was little evidence that patients of particular ages gained more or less from care in a stroke unit (Stroke Unit Trialists' Collaboration 1997, 2000). Although we think that *needs* rather than *age* should dictate where and by whom patients are managed, local conditions will often dictate whether an 'age-related service' is the best option. For example, where an age-related geriatric service (e.g. one that admits any patient who is over 75 years old, whatever the problem) provides effective stroke rehabilitation, there may be a case for adding a new service for younger stroke patients rather than dismantling the current service. Professionals and patients' families are often concerned that younger patients' morale will suffer if they are treated in a ward with mainly older patients. Further research into patient attitudes is needed to clarify this question.

How long should patients remain in the unit?

Some units—particularly those that admit patients acutely—define maximum lengths of stay, but often transfer patients on to 'slower-stream' rehabilitation facilities (Indredavik *et al.* 1991). It seems to us that the only reason to define a maximum length of stay is to remove 'bed blockers' and allow admission of new cases. If the unit is of sufficient size for the population's needs, works flexibly and is efficient in discharging patients, then a defined maximum length of stay should not be needed. If one does insist on a maximum length of stay, one must ensure that the facilities and staff exist elsewhere to deliver appropriate continuing care and that patients are not left to languish on an acute medical ward. One might argue that patients who are no longer improving, but are having to wait for placement in the community or an institution, should not be kept in a stroke unit. However, for some individuals the unit may offer the best environment to maintain any functional improvement already gained. Also, to move them to another part of the hospital to await their placement may not be optimal for a patient and their family who may have built up close relationships with the stroke unit staff. Moves under these situations should only be considered where beds are limited and patients who are judged likely to gain more from the unit environment are waiting to be admitted.

How large should a stroke unit be?

Age-specific and sex-specific stroke incidence data and details of the hospital catchment population, along with hospital activity data, should allow an estimate of the number of patients who are likely to require admission to hospital each year (section 17.2.3). Unfortunately, there may be variations due simply to chance or the season of the year. Although consistent seasonal differences in the incidence of stroke have not been demonstrated in community-based studies, at least in temperate regions, an excess of hospital admissions and stroke deaths during the winter has been found (Kelly Hayes *et al.* 1995; Rothwell *et al.* 1996). Of course, this apparent winter excess in hospital-based and mortality studies may simply reflect referral bias and a higher case fatality during cold weather. Whatever the explanation for any seasonal variation, it does cause difficulties when planning stroke services. Prior to the development of a stroke unit, a survey in one of our own medical units, which admits between 200 and 250 stroke patients each year, demonstrated that the number of stroke in-patients on any one day varied between nine and 35 over a year. Therefore, whatever organization one sets up to manage these patients, it must be flexible enough to cope with large fluctuations in their numbers. To ensure the best use of beds, the unit—whether for acute assessment, rehabilitation, or both—should be able to accommodate different proportions of men and women, as the proportions are bound to fluctuate. One problem of a geographically defined stroke unit is the inevitable limit on the number of beds. However, this problem may be overcome by ensuring that the stroke unit is part of a larger area, into which it can expand with demand and then contract again. The patients we cannot immediately accommodate in our stroke rehabilitation unit are cared for on the acute medical wards, although the stroke team still coordinates their care. Ideally, the excess patients would be in a rehabilitation area rather than in an acute general ward, so that they would not have to compete for nursing time with acutely ill patients. Such arrangements also mean that, at times, non-stroke patients are cared for in the stroke unit. Where large fluctuations in demand exist, it is also important that the team should be able to draw on extra resources to manage the larger number of patients. Inevitably, there are times when resources are not adequate to meet all the needs of the patients, and it is then important for the team to support its members in the difficult task of prioritizing—or in other words rationing—care.

A survey in one of our own medical units, which admits between 200 and 250 stroke patients each year, demonstrated that the number of stroke in-patients on any one day varied between nine and 35 over a year. Therefore, stroke services must be flexible enough to cope with large fluctuations in the numbers and types of patients referred.

Who should run the stroke unit?

The units included in the review were run by geriatricians, neurologists, general (internal) physicians and rehabilitationists. Indirect comparisons of the benefits of units run by different specialist groups did not show any significant differences (Stroke Unit Trialists' Collaboration 1997, 2000). One randomized trial showed that within a stroke unit, elderly patients who were allocated care by a geriatric team with access to day hospital after discharge had better functional outcomes than those for whom care was provided by neurologists without access to a day hospital (Hui *et al.* 1995). However, this was primarily a trial evaluating day hospital care. We believe that whoever is responsible should have the necessary knowledge, training and above all enthusiasm to take on the task. The most appropriate professional group will vary from place to place. For example, in the Netherlands, practically all stroke patients are managed by neurologists, whilst in the UK the majority are managed, at least initially, by general physicians and geriatricians (Ebrahim & Redfern 1999). British neurologists may have the knowledge and training to diagnose and investigate stroke patients, but unfortunately most do not have the time (because of their limited numbers and other responsibilities), access to beds, or training in rehabilitation to run a stroke service without help from other specialists. In the UK, geriatricians are often in the best position to take a leading role, although most would need extra training in neurology and the active participation of their local neurologist—who can very usefully contribute to diagnosis and management of patients, especially those with unusual causes of stroke, as well as patients with 'funny turns' and the many and varied neurological problems that arise in in-patient and out-patient stroke care (Table 17.6). An increasing number of hospitals are appointing specialist stroke physicians to coordinate stroke services.

Overcoming resistance to change

Although there is now good evidence for the effectiveness of stroke units, the development of such units is often resisted by those who perceive them as a threat. Fears that setting up a stroke unit might divert resources from other areas can be countered by pointing out that stroke units generally make more efficient use of existing staff and beds, and so may eventually even increase the resources available to other specialities. Some physicians worry that a specialized stroke team will de-skill their junior medical, nursing and paramedical staff and reduce their access to patients for teaching, but this can be overcome by rotating staff and students through the unit. Opposition may be reduced by adopting an evolutionary approach to developing the service. For example, one might introduce a stroke assessment protocol before trying to set up an acute assessment area, or a stroke team working on the general medical wards before trying to set up a geographically defined stroke unit. Where resistance persists, one can try to influence the local organizations that fund health care (i.e. health authorities and general or family practitioners in the UK; health insurers in other countries) to exert pressure for change, since they are generally keen to fund services for which there is scientific evidence of efficacy (curiously, neither coronary care units nor regional oncology services have been nearly as well evaluated as stroke units, and yet their utility is said to be 'obvious' and they are widely encouraged). It is important to be flexible in the model of stroke service that is adopted, since its structure must be tailored to local needs, resources, geography, people and politics (Table 17.11).

Table 17.11 Summary of recommendations for the organization of in-patient stroke care.

A stroke unit is an important component of a coordinated stroke service, but additional facilities are needed to provide a comprehensive service
Although admitting stroke patients to a defined geographical area has several important advantages, it does not necessarily require more resources
The most obvious factors that contribute to the effectiveness of stroke units are their organization and the involvement of a multidisciplinary team, the members of which are knowledgeable and enthusiastic about stroke
One needs a system of clinical triage to identify the patients most likely to benefit from a stroke rehabilitation unit
Ward-based rehabilitation units facilitate the fuller involvement of the nursing staff and carers in the rehabilitation process
A coordinated stroke service facilitates research and education for the professionals involved, the patients and their carers
A stroke service consisting of a stroke unit (i.e. a ward) must develop a system for dealing with fluctuations in demand
An organized stroke service may reduce the overall cost of caring for stroke patients in hospital
Rotate staff and students to facilitate training and education
Stroke services should be tailored to local conditions

17.5 Integration of services

Inevitably, the majority of stroke patients require both community-based and hospital-based resources at some stage of their illness. It is therefore important to consider how these can be integrated to ensure that patients are appropriately placed at each stage of their illness and that transfers between each part of the service are as seamless as possible. Figure 17.4 illustrates how the components of a stroke service might fit together.

17.5.1 Transfers from community to hospital

Patients are admitted to hospital after an acute stroke for a variety of reasons (Bamford *et al.* 1986). In countries with well-organized primary health-care systems, patients are often assessed by their general (family) practitioner prior to admission. This allows for some patients to remain at home if they do not require immediate hospitalization, but it can cause delays in admission. Delays in admission not only preclude very early thrombolytic treatment of ischaemic stroke (section 11.5), but may lead to other problems. A patient who is very dependent may be left at home for a few days 'to see how they will do' and so either avoid admission, or allow the patient to die at home. This delay, although sometimes justified, may put the patient at risk of

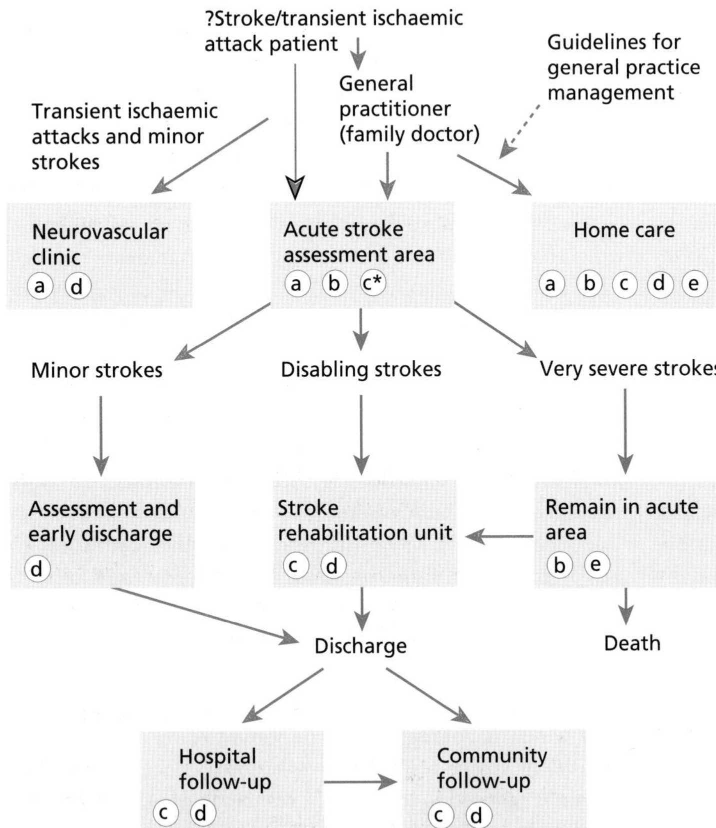

Fig. 17.4 A diagram illustrating the components, functions and interrelationships of a hospital-based stroke service that is integrated with community services: (a) diagnosis, (b) acute care, (c) rehabilitation, (d) secondary prevention, (e) terminal care. *We believe that elements of the rehabilitation process are important even on the day of the stroke onset.

unnecessary complications of immobility and mishandling. If the carers are given inadequate support, even for a few days, this may prejudice their attitudes later to accepting responsibility for caring after discharge from hospital. Thus, an attempt to avoid hospital admission can sometimes prolong any admission and even lead to long-term institutionalization. To avoid these problems, one needs to develop joint guidelines between the primary and secondary health-care systems concerning which patients should be managed at home, which patients should be referred immediately for admission, and which might be referred to an out-patient clinic.

It seems likely that medical treatments for acute stroke will be more effective if given very early after symptom onset; for example, thrombolysis within 3 h of symptom onset appears safer and perhaps more effective than that given later (section 11.5.2). Currently, in most health-care systems, there are delays in admitting patients to hospital (Chaturvedi *et al.* 1998; Wester *et al.* 1999). Factors associated with greater delays include: ischaemic rather than haemorrhagic stroke, gradual onset of symptoms, mild symptoms, living alone, delays in contacting medical services, attendance at a primary care facility, and failure to use ambulance transportation (Wester *et al.* 1999). These are likely to vary between health-care systems. Alberts *et al.* (1992) demonstrated that by informing the public, training primary care physicians and paramedics, and improving organization, the delay in hospital admission can be reduced significantly. Of course, the diurnal variation in stroke onset influences early access to medical therapy. About 25% of patients with ischaemic stroke, and rather fewer of those with primary intracerebral haemorrhage, wake from sleep with symptoms of stroke. Most strokes become apparent between 6 AM and 12 PM, when medical services are perhaps most able to deliver acute treatment (Wroe *et al.* 1992). Unfortunately, the inevitable delay between stroke onset during sleep and the patient waking to notice the symptoms for the first time may reduce the effectiveness of any acute treatment.

17.5.2 Integration of hospital-based services

Many places will have the necessary facilities and skills to provide an excellent hospital-based service to patients with stroke. More often, the problem lies with the organization and integration of these facilities. For example, where patients are admitted to acute general neurological or medical wards but have to be referred to a separate institution for rehabilitation, needless delays can result. In such circumstances, one will read in the case-notes 'waiting for rehabilitation'—when, of course, rehabilitation should have started on the day of the stroke (section 10.3). Thus, one needs to organize services so that the patient's needs are matched by the care provided at all stages of his or her illness.

Delivering acute medical treatments

Even when patients arrive at the hospital within a few hours of stroke onset, there are often unnecessary delays in assessing the patients clinically, obtaining a CT or magnetic resonance (MR) scan and actually administering the treatment (Wester *et al.* 1999). One needs to ensure that patients with symptoms of stroke who may be candidates for acute medical treatment do not wait to be assessed by an admitting physician in the Accident and Emergency Department (Johnston *et al.* 1999). Patients who might benefit from acute treatment should be identified early, either by paramedical staff in the ambulances or by triage nurses in the emergency room, using simple algorithms, so they can be fast-tracked through the admission system (http://www.dcn.ed.ac.uk/spgm). One needs to establish, in collaboration with the radiology service, a system for obtaining urgent brain imaging at any time, as well as the means to move the patient rapidly to a place at which treatment can be administered promptly and safely. One approach has been to establish so-called 'acute stroke teams' or 'brain attack teams' that can be activated by paramedics or triage nurses (National Institute of Neurological Disorders and Stroke rt-PA Stroke Study Group 1997).

Neurosurgical facilities

These facilities should be readily available, because urgent neurosurgery can occasionally be life-saving and produce a good functional outcome (Chapters 12 and 13). Inevitably, many smaller hospitals do not have these facilities. However, for the 1–2% of stroke patients who are at risk of deteriorating rapidly with a surgically remediable complication (e.g. acute hydrocephalus), a management plan should be available. This should include a policy to ensure the early identification and safe transfer of suitable patients to a neurosurgical centre.

The hazards of transfer

Where patients have to be transferred between institutions (and teams) to receive the appropriate care, there is a real danger that continuity of care will suffer. A consistent approach to patients and their families may not be achieved without excellent communication between the professionals involved. Patients' medical records should follow them through the system, and ideally at least one health professional should be involved in a patient's care from admission to discharge, and perhaps even beyond.

17.5.3 Transfers from hospital to community

One of the main areas of concern to patients, and more particularly to carers, is the organization (or rather the lack of organization) of the hospital discharge (Pound *et al.* 1994;

Wellwood *et al.* 1995a). One can well understand their concern. One day patients are being cared for in hospital by a team of professionals, and the next day they are at home and the responsibility of the carers. A number of things can reduce the stress related to the transition from hospital to home:

• providing adequate information (section 17.5.5) and training the carers whilst the patient is in hospital. This might include inviting the carers along to therapy sessions and involving them in the patient's care on the unit;

• predischarge home visits with the patient and one or more members of the team to ensure that the home environment is tailored to the patient's needs. Also, informal visits home, initially for a day and then graduating to overnight and weekend stays, allow the patient and carer to gain confidence, identify potential problems, and help maintain morale (section 15.31);

• predischarge case conferences (section 10.3.7) to allow the patient and carer to meet with the hospital-based team and any professionals who are to be involved in their care in the community;

• clear guidelines about who to contact in the event of problems. General (family) practitioners, or one of their team, are the ideal points of contact, but they can only fulfil this role if adequately briefed before the patient's discharge. It follows that detailed records of the patient's problems, and the plans for support in the community, must be relayed to those expected to monitor the home situation.

In some circumstances, it may be appropriate to further break down the boundary between hospital and home by organizing for the patient to attend a day hospital or outpatient department regularly to be reviewed medically, or to receive further physical therapy. This can then be withdrawn gradually, depending on the patient's and carer's needs.

In parts of the UK, specialist workers have been introduced (with a variety of titles, including 'stroke family support worker') to help support patients and their carers in the community. They contact the patient and their family early in the hospital admission, when they can spend time educating them about stroke and answering any questions. They are then available to help them over the period of the discharge and for as long as they need support. They are in an ideal position to identify any problems or unmet needs and to develop customized solutions. They may do this by taking action themselves or by making appropriate referrals to other agencies. Although randomized trials of such interventions have not demonstrated major effects on patients' physical outcomes, these workers are valued by patients and their carers and may improve the psychological outcome (Forster & Young 1996; Dennis *et al.* 1997c; Dowswell *et al.* 1997; Mant *et al.* 1999; Knapp *et al.* 2000; Mant *et al.* 2000).

17.5.4 Follow-up and maintenance

Some patients and their carers develop problems that become apparent after discharge from hospital, but only after several weeks or months (Table 17.12). It is important to have a system in place to detect these problems before they cause irreversible breakdown of the social situation. Hospital follow-up may be useful, but problems of this type may not be detected in a brief visit to a clinic, and patients and their carers may not be forthcoming or even admit to anything being wrong in response to a specific enquiry. A member of the primary care team, or a stroke family support worker, who can visit the patient in the home is in a far better position to deal with this situation (section 17.5.3). A small proportion of patients make little progress in the first few months after the stroke (perhaps due to intercurrent illness) and are discharged to a supported environment, but then unexpectedly begin to improve. Ideally, such patients should be identified and should re-enter a rehabilitation programme, but few services are sufficiently well organized or adequately resourced to offer this.

Although there is little evidence for the effectiveness of *continuing* rehabilitation after stroke, our experience suggests that some patients do require therapy to promote continued recovery or to maintain the progress gained in hospital. There is uncertainty about the most effective method of delivering continuing therapy—e.g. domiciliary vs. day hospital (section 17.4.1).

Although secondary prevention should be started as soon after the stroke as possible, for the reasons outlined in Chap-

Table 17.12 Common problems that arise late after a stroke, often when the patient is no longer in hospital.

Patient
Deteriorating function due to:
Overprotective carer
Progressing co-morbidities
Lack of continuing physical therapy?
Depression or anxiety, even agoraphobia (section 15.31)
Social isolation financial difficulties (section 15.33.5)
Sexual dysfunction (section 15.33.4)
Undetected rise in blood pressure
Central post-stroke pain (section 15.23)
Carer (section 15.34)
Physical ill health due to the strain of caring
Depression or anxiety
Poor relationship with patient because of personality change
Social isolation because unable to get out to meet people
Financial difficulties

Table 17.13 A stroke follow-up checklist.

Review	
Impairments	Weakness, balance, speech, etc.
Disabilities	What can you do for yourself?
	Do you need help with any everyday activities?
	Ask specifically about 'activities of daily living' functions
Aids and adaptations	Do you need any aids?
	Have they been delivered yet?
	Are you using them?
	Are they in good working order?
Support services	Are they happening?
	Are they appropriate and adequate?
Have any new problems arisen since last seen (Table 17.12)?	
Is there anything you can't do, but want to do?	
Are you back to work?	
Are you driving a car?	
How is your carer (if any) coping?	
Is everything being done to prevent a recurrent vascular event?	
Check the blood pressure, cholesterol and glucose (if diabetic)	
Enquire about smoking, diet and exercise	
Check compliance with medication	

ter 16, the interventions (e.g. modification of blood pressure, cholesterol, control of diabetes, and antiplatelet drugs) need to be continued and monitored. This can be done in a hospital-based clinic, but would be managed better and more conveniently (for the patient) in the primary health-care sector, since many of these interventions will be lifelong. A follow-up checklist should ensure that late problems are not overlooked (Table 17.13).

Secondary prevention, which will be lifelong, can be provided in a hospital-based clinic, but is managed more conveniently (for the patient) in the primary health-care sector.

17.5.5 Information for patients and carers

Studies of the attitudes of patients and their carers to medical services in general, and stroke services in particular, have demonstrated that one of the greatest sources of dissatisfaction is with communication (Pound *et al.* 1994; Wellwood *et al.* 1995a). Patients and carers may receive very little information about the nature of stroke, its cause, management and likely prognosis (Wellwood *et al.* 1994). Even where information is provided, it may be in a form that is difficult to understand or retain.

Patients' and carers' perceptions of the stroke service are likely to depend not just on the degree of recovery, but also on the quality of communication. Although it is easy to show that many patients receive little information, one must also remember that for some it may be enough. We have shown that some patients do not want a lot of information, preferring to trust in the professionals' judgement (Wellwood *et al.* 1994). This will undoubtedly vary from place to place, and may change over time. It is therefore important to tailor the provision of information to the individual's needs and wishes. This information should probably be provided using a number of different media, including:

- a notice-board on the unit (Fig. 17.5);
- an information pack containing appropriate leaflets;
- audio and video tapes;
- individual interviews with patients and carers by members of the team; and
- patient and carer groups.

However, there is probably no substitute for one of the team sitting down with the patient and family on one or more occasions to explain the situation and answer any specific questions. This can then be backed up with written material. One approach, which has been used in other areas (e.g. oncology), is to record the interview and give the recording to the patient or family so that they can review what has been said as they wish (Scott *et al.* 2000). This might overcome the problem of patients and families only taking in a small proportion of the information given to them. Randomized trials of educational programmes for patients and carers suggest that they improve recipients' knowledge and satisfaction with the information received, but do not significantly improve their physical or psychological status (Forster *et al.* 2000b; Knapp *et al.* 2000). Like all other areas of stroke care, a service needs to establish a system ensuring that input—in this case the provision of information—is tailored to the individual needs of patients and carers (Table 17.14).

17.6 Monitoring and evaluating stroke services

We believe that the most reliable way of determining the relative effectiveness of interventions is an appropriately designed randomized trial, or a meta-analysis if more than one trial is available (section 11.2.1). Unfortunately, this is not a very practical option in the evaluation of a local stroke service rather than stroke services in general (Table 17.15), so we have to rely on less robust methodologies.

Non-randomized comparisons of the process of care, or of patient and carer outcomes achieved by services—in different places at the same time or in the same place over time—are the only practical methods of evaluation. If one is setting up a new service in a hospital, the process, or outcomes, can be compared with those in a nearby hospital without a new service. Alternatively, one could measure the process and

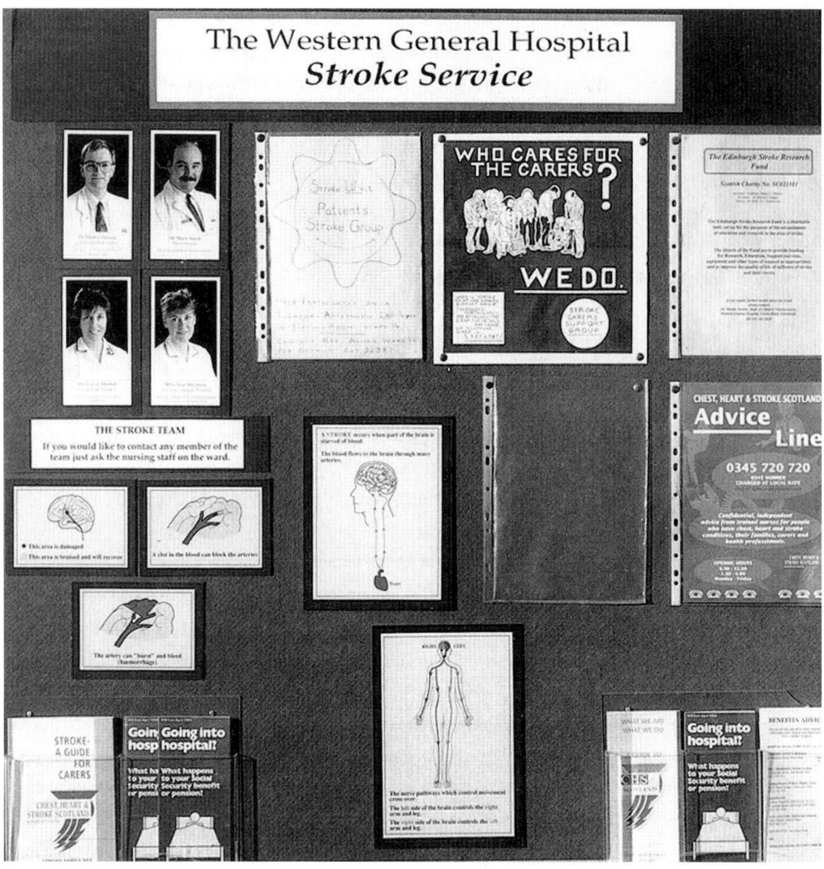

Fig. 17.5 A notice-board at the entrance to a stroke unit. Typically it introduces the members of the stroke team, indicating how they might be contacted. It presents, in simple terms, what a stroke is and how it might affect the patient. We also include useful pamphlets and information relating to patient and carer groups.

Table 17.14 Tips on improving communication with carers of hospitalized stroke patients.

Provide a notice-board at the entrance to the unit introducing staff and informing relatives about how to contact members of the team
Hold ward rounds during visiting times
Hold a regular 'open access' clinic where carers can meet the consultant
Invite carers to participate in patient care
Invite carers to therapy sessions
Set up a carers' group
Document the content of any discussions with relatives in the notes and report these at team meetings to ensure consistency
Arrange predischarge case conferences or family meetings
Back up verbal communication with written or audio material

outcomes achieved by the existing service and then measure whether these are improved after the new service has been established (i.e. a before-and-after study). However, such evaluations can be misleading. They may be able to demonstrate improvements (or worsening), or differences in the process or outcome of care, but they cannot provide reliable data to indicate that any changes are actually due to the

Table 17.15 Reasons why it is not practical to perform a randomized controlled trial to evaluate a new stroke unit.

Some would argue that given the strong evidence for the effectiveness of organized stroke care it is ethically unacceptable to randomize patients to disorganized care.
In a single institution, it may be impossible to isolate the treatment and control groups. Thus, there may be contamination of the control group that will reduce the power of the study to demonstrate significant differences in outcomes. Where one is comparing services in several institutions, it may become difficult to distinguish the effects of the services from the effects of factors unique to the institutions themselves (e.g. admission policy).
In a single institution, it is often impractical to randomize sufficient patients to provide a statistically robust result.
Although the benefits of a service may be measured in terms of crude outcomes—e.g. death—more subtle but valuable benefits such as patient satisfaction are less easily measured.
Randomized trials need resources—e.g. randomization services, maintenance of at least two parallel services, blinded outcome assessments, data collection, storage and analysis—all of which make them relatively unattractive to purchasers of health care. For example, in a recently completed trial of a stroke family support worker, the trial cost as much as the intervention itself (Dennis *et al.* 1997c).

new service (section 17.6.3). There may be systematic differences in the patients treated by services in different hospitals, or in the same hospital over time. For example, in one of our own hospitals, the development of a new stroke service was accompanied by closure of the accident and emergency department, which may have accounted for fewer patients with severe stroke being admitted. We observed a marked fall in case fatality and length of stay, but was this due to our new stroke service (Davenport *et al.* 1996a)? Almost certainly not. Other changes might influence the results of any evaluation. For example, new legislation concerning care in the community accompanied the setting up of our unit. Could this account for our reduced length of stay? Probably not.

Clearly, one cannot rely on such non-randomized evaluations to influence practice elsewhere, but they may fulfil important *local* functions. One could reasonably argue that, as long as the new service is not much more expensive to run, it does not matter whether any improvements observed can be attributed directly to that service. Obviously, if the new service was very costly, one would want reassurance that the improvements had not occurred spontaneously. Also, if a non-randomized evaluation demonstrates either no improvement or even a worse outcome, it is difficult to know how to respond. Were the changes due to the new service, in which case it ought to be modified, or were they due to some unforeseen confounding factor?

There are several other methodological problems, which can affect randomized as well as non-randomized comparisons, and which need to be considered:

- small numbers of patients, so that any change observed may be accounted for by the play of chance;
- missing a moderate but real change because too few patients were studied; and
- observer bias in assessing the process or outcome. Often, the observers have an interest in the result of the evaluation, which may influence their judgements.

What aspects of a service can we measure? A stroke service may include some components for which there is little doubt of their effectiveness, but many others of uncertain benefit. When assessing performance, it is therefore most important to monitor how well the service delivers those components whose effectiveness is established (e.g. aspirin for secondary prevention; section 16.4). The simplest way to monitor the service is to measure the amount of work being carried out. Unfortunately, politicians and those who fund health care place too much emphasis on the volume rather than quality of service. The number of cases managed by a service tells one very little about the quality of care given to those patients.

In assessing the quality of care (or 'clinical audit', as it tends to be called) one should consider three aspects of the service (Donabedian 1988): the structure, or facilities available; the process of care; and the outcomes for those treated.

17.6.1 Structure

From all that has been said above, it should be fairly obvious that a stroke service needs certain essential facilities to provide all the components necessary to care for patients with strokes and transient ischaemic attacks. This makes the setting of standards and the measurement of performance for structure relatively straightforward. Some basic standards for structure might include:

- an identified individual who is responsible for the organization of services;
- a multidisciplinary team (section 10.3.5);
- immediate access to acute hospital beds;
- prompt out-patient assessment by a specialist for patients who do not need admission to hospital (i.e. a 'one-stop' neurovascular out-patient clinic; section 17.4.1);
- prompt access to CT scanning for in-patients and out-patients (section 17.4.1);
- prompt access to non-invasive vascular imaging, carotid angiography and surgery if necessary (section 16.8);
- a stroke unit (section 17.4.2); and
- continuing care facilities, both community-based and institutional.

However, care has to be taken in defining these standards. For example, what does 'prompt access' mean, what is a specialist, what does a stroke unit consist of? One could very quickly fulfil a requirement for a stroke unit by simply relabelling a general medical ward, but of course one is unlikely to accrue the undoubted benefits of stroke unit care (section 17.4.2). There is also an inevitable overlap with measures of process and outcome when defining the quality of these elements. For example, the multidisciplinary team will only be effective if it meets regularly, the non-invasive vascular imaging must be accurate (section 6.7.5), and the carotid angiography and surgery must be delivered at low risk (section 16.8).

17.6.2 Process

Although some aspects of the process of care are easily monitored, e.g. waiting times for appointments, those relating to clinical care are much more difficult. It may be relatively easy to define a standard (for example, patients with transient ischaemic attacks and ischaemic strokes should be given aspirin to reduce the risk of further vascular events, unless there are contraindications), but for other procedures for which there is less scientific justification, it is more difficult. The lack of scientific justification can, and frequently is, overcome by using the combined views of recognized experts, i.e. a consensus. Thus, it is possible, by one means or another, to produce standards to which we may aspire even when there is limited evidence on which to base clinical practice (section 17.6.4). However, as we have already stressed, the care an individual receives should be based on a thorough assessment and tailored to the individual's particular condition and needs (section 10.3.2). So, for example, one might set the standard that all patients should have a thorough assessment of their visuospatial function on admission because any abnormality may have important effects on their function and prognosis. However, detailed testing of visuospatial function cannot be carried out in unconscious patients, or in those who are unable to communicate or use their dominant hand. Thus, what appears to be a fairly straightforward standard cannot be applied sensibly to every patient. To overcome this difficulty, one has to develop standards with criteria attached where lower standards may be acceptable. The National Sentinel Audit of Stroke (Rudd *et al.* 1999) addressed this problem by having a 'no but ...' clause attached to each standard (Fig. 17.6). This is essential for the process of care to be compared in different groups of patients—so that, for example, if there is a higher proportion of unconscious patients in one group (i.e. a difference in casemix), the process with regard to assessing visuospatial function will not necessarily be worse.

Monitoring the process of care by case-note review raises a number of important methodological problems that must be addressed if one's assessment is to be useful and valid.

Another difficulty with measuring the process of care is that, by directly observing the care, one is likely to alter its delivery (the so-called Hawthorne effect). For example, if junior—or senior, for that matter—doctors are observed when performing an assessment, they are likely to take extra care with the assessment. Also, such an approach is likely to be very costly if performed on all stroke admissions. The alternative is to audit the records of care, but this immediately raises the question of the validity of the medical record—i.e. whether the records reflect the actual care provided. However, most people would agree that good records probably do reflect good care given, and that this is a reasonable method of measuring the process of care. The other methodological problems involved in audits of case-notes are summarized in Table 17.16.

Although one may be measuring the performance against some 'ideal' standard, one is likely to want to compare the performance in the same service over time, or to compare performances between services. To do this meaningfully, one has to have a valid and reliable measure of performance, one needs to audit enough cases to produce statistically robust results, and one must be able to take into account differences in casemix between services or changes over time. The *Stroke Audit Package* published by the Royal College of Physicians (1994) was developed to overcome these methodological problems and enable valid comparisons to be made (Gompertz *et al.* 1994; Hancock *et al.* 1997). This package only addressed a limited number of the more medical aspects of care, and the Royal College of Physicians therefore also developed the National Sentinel Audit, which also addressed other important aspects of care delivered by different members of the multidisciplinary team (Rudd *et al.* 1999).

17.6.3 Outcome

The term 'outcome' causes confusion due to variation in usage. Clinicians use the term to refer to the clinical outcome of the patient or carer. Outcomes therefore include survival,

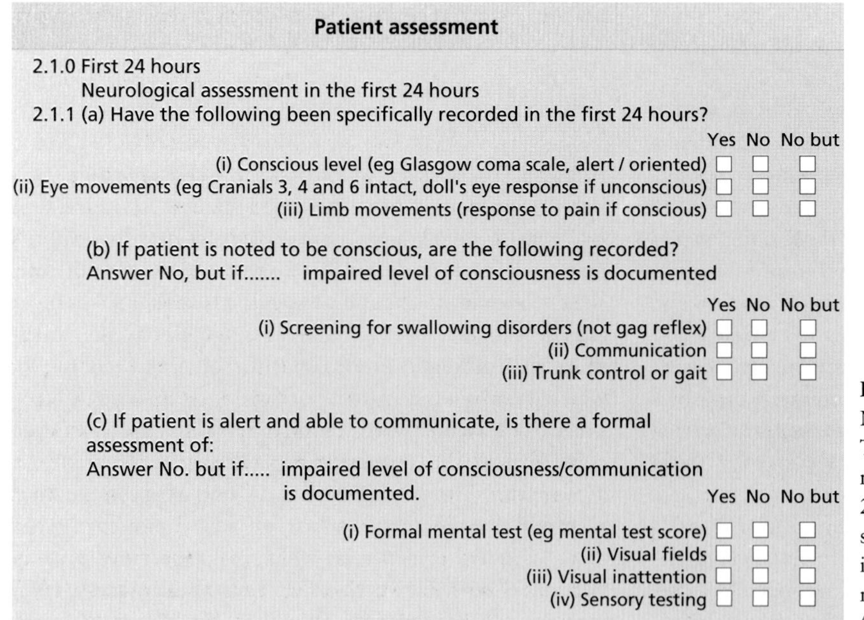

Patient assessment

2.1.0 First 24 hours

Neurological assessment in the first 24 hours

2.1.1 (a) Have the following been specifically recorded in the first 24 hours?

	Yes	No	No but
(i) Conscious level (eg Glasgow coma scale, alert / oriented)	☐	☐	☐
(ii) Eye movements (eg Cranials 3, 4 and 6 intact, doll's eye response if unconscious)	☐	☐	☐
(iii) Limb movements (response to pain if conscious)	☐	☐	☐

(b) If patient is noted to be conscious, are the following recorded?
Answer No, but if....... impaired level of consciousness is documented

	Yes	No	No but
(i) Screening for swallowing disorders (not gag reflex)	☐	☐	☐
(ii) Communication	☐	☐	☐
(iii) Trunk control or gait	☐	☐	☐

(c) If patient is alert and able to communicate, is there a formal assessment of:
Answer No. but if..... impaired level of consciousness/communication is documented.

	Yes	No	No but
(i) Formal mental test (eg mental test score)	☐	☐	☐
(ii) Visual fields	☐	☐	☐
(iii) Visual inattention	☐	☐	☐
(iv) Sensory testing	☐	☐	☐

Fig. 17.6 One of the sections from the National Sentinel Audit of Stroke (1998). This one relates to the recording of the neurological examination. The interval (e.g. 24 h) since admission at which these data should be recorded, and the circumstances in which it is acceptable for the information not to be recorded, are given in each section (Rudd *et al.* 1999).

Table 17.16 Important methodological issues in the audit of case-notes.

Patient selection bias	The case-notes audited should be a representative sample of all those treated—thus it might be a consecutive series or a random sample
Case-note retrieval bias	Poor-quality case-notes or those of dead patients may be more difficult to retrieve, which might bias the audit in a favourable direction. A high rate of retrieval is an important step in reducing bias (Vickers & Pollock 1993)
Lack of precision	A sufficiently large number of case-notes should be audited to provide a precise estimate of performance and to allow precise comparisons to be made with other centres, or with audits performed at different times in the same centre
Observer bias	Auditors may have an interest in the result of the audit, which may influence their assessment of performance; blinded, or at least impartial, observers should be employed if possible
Poor interobserver reliability of measure	If the measure of performance is not reliable, then it will be more difficult to demonstrate real differences between centres. Also, if there is a consistent difference in the way an audit measure is applied by different auditors, this may produce invalid comparisons
Differences in casemix	A standard that is applicable to one patient may not apply to another. It is important that standards should be adjusted for differences in casemix

functional status, complications, or less easily defined concepts such as quality of life. Others, particularly those with a management background, use the term 'outcome' to refer to any result of an intervention, e.g. reduced waiting times or readmission rates. Certain aspects, such as patient satisfaction with care, are variably referred to as either indicators of process or as an outcome. In this section, we use 'outcome' to refer to the *clinical* outcome of patients (i.e. physical, functional, cognitive, emotional, etc.).

Since the main aim of stroke services is to optimize the outcome for patients and carers, the measurement of outcome is obviously the most relevant criterion by which to judge the performance of a service. Unfortunately, the use of outcomes to reflect the quality of care is the most challenging area of stroke audit (Gompertz *et al.* 1995; Dennis 2000). The difficulties in using outcome data to reflect the quality of care have been extensively studied (Goldstein & Spiegelhalter 1996; Davies & Crombie 1997; Thomas & Hofer 1998). Until these can be overcome, those involved in providing and monitoring health services must be extremely careful not to misinterpret outcome data. The observed outcome in a group of patients treated by a particular service will be determined by four factors:

- the quality and effectiveness of the care provided;
- the method of measurement of outcome (e.g. who is measuring it, and how?);
- chance (or random error); and
- casemix (or prognostic factors).

The quality and effectiveness of the care provided

This is the aspect we hope outcomes will reflect. However, it is important to remember that most interventions have only small or moderate-sized effects, which may be difficult to detect even in large randomized trials. Even a wildly implausible 50% relative reduction in the death rate from 30% to 15% after the opening of a stroke unit, for instance, would require a sample of 200 patients both before and after its introduction to eliminate the effects of chance, let alone bias of various sorts. The systematic review suggests that the impact of stroke unit care is far less than this (Stroke Unit Trialists' Collaboration 2000) (section 17.4.2) (Table 18.1c).

The method of measurement of outcome

Many attempts to monitor the quality of service by measuring patient outcomes have relied on mortality data, presumably because they are often routinely available, objective and may indicate where there are major problems. Unfortunately, mortality is unlikely to be influenced by many components of care (discharge planning being one obvious example). Some outcome measures that may better reflect the quality of care are shown in Table 17.17. They measure outcome at different levels of disease—pathology, impairment, disability, handicap and quality of life (section 10.1). It is important that they should have acceptable validity (i.e. that they measure what they are intended to measure) and reliability (i.e. that they are reproducible in different settings and when used by different people). A number of different types of scale have been developed and used to measure outcome after stroke. The choice of scale will depend on the question being asked, but there are a number of features that one should look for in choosing an outcome measure (Table 17.18) (van Gijn & Warlow 1992). One can loosely categorize the measures of outcome after stroke under the following headings.

Stroke scales. So-called 'stroke scales' (e.g. the Scandinavian Stroke Scale, Canadian Stroke Scale, National Institutes of Health Stroke Scale) were largely developed to describe the severity of acute stroke and to monitor changes in the patient's condition (Scandinavian Stroke Study Group 1985; Cote *et al.* 1986, 1989; Brott *et al.* 1989). Most concentrate

Table 17.17 Aspects of outcome that may be relevant in assessing stroke services, and some tools for measuring these outcomes.

Outcome	Promising measurement tools
Survival	Case fatality during a defined time period, e.g. at 30 days or 6 months after stroke onset
Complications	Proportion of patients developing pressure sores or fractures; there are difficulties in defining these and reliably recording them. Paradoxically, better services may identify more and record them more often (Davenport *et al.* 1996c)
Residual impairments	Probably not very useful, and not easily collected after hospital discharge
Mobility	10-m walking speed
Arm function	Nine-hole peg test
Psychological outcome	Hospital anxiety and depression scale General health questionnaire (Table 15.42) Many of the most disabled patients will not be capable of responding to measures of psychological outcome
Disability	Barthel Index (Table 17.19) Functional Independence Measure (FIM) Three simple questions (Fig. 17.7) Office of Population Censuses and Surveys disability scale (Martin *et al.* 1988) Oxford Handicap Scale (also known as the Modified Rankin Scale) (Table 17.21)—should be measured at defined point after the stroke, e.g. 6 months. Easily collected after hospital discharge
Handicap	London Handicap Scale (Harwood *et al.* 1994)—a difficult area with no well-tested measures. The Oxford Handicap Scale does not really address handicap in isolation
Patient or carer satisfaction	Hospsat and Homesat (Pound *et al.* 1994)—is this an outcome or process measure?
General health or health-related quality of life	Nottingham Health Profile Short Form 36 EuroQol—Potentially interesting because it could allow comparisons with other disease states. However, many stroke patients cannot complete the questionnaires because of cognitive problems

on the type and severity of the neurological impairments, although some (e.g. Mathew's Scale) also include a disability element (Mathew *et al.* 1972). They have been criticized for lacking relevance for patients, being complex and therefore impractical, and for summing 'apples and pears' (van Gijn & Warlow 1992). They rely on a clinical examination, and therefore cannot be used other than in a 'face-to-face' situation. We do not think they are useful in evaluating stroke services. They might be used as a measure of casemix, and even for describing short-term changes early after acute stroke, when measuring disability, handicap, or quality of life is both difficult and inappropriate.

> *'Far better an approximate answer to the right question, which is often vague, than an exact answer to the wrong question, which can always be made precise' (Tukey 1962).*

Functional scales include measures of disability or dependence in activities of daily living (ADL), such as the Barthel Index (Table 17.19), the Nottingham ADL Scale and the Functional Independence Measure (FIM) (Mahoney & Barthel 1965; Ebrahim *et al.* 1985; State University of New York at Buffalo 1993). Under this heading one could also include the so-called extended ADL scales (EADL), which identify whether patients are participating in more complex activities such as shopping, leisure, or work. The latter type of scale includes the Frenchay Activities Index and the Nottingham Extended ADL Scale (Holbrook & Skilbeck 1983; Nouri & Lincoln 1987; Schuling *et al.* 1993). These appear to measure relevant aspects of outcome, although some demonstrate ceiling effects (e.g. the Barthel Index) and may not pick up problems in particular areas, e.g. communication (Wellwood *et al.* 1995b). They are in general 'ordinal scales', so that care must be taken in choosing the appropriate statistical method to describe or compare groups of patients (Table 17.20). One disability scale, the Office of Population Censuses and Surveys (OPCS) disability instrument, could be considered an 'interval' scale, and it appears to cover most aspects of disability (Martin *et al.* 1988). However, it is probably too com-

Table 17.18 Important features of scales for the measurement of outcome after stoke.

Validity
The scale should measure that aspect of outcome it purports to measure. Different types of validity include: criterion validity, when the measure is related to an accepted 'gold-standard'; construct validity, where the measure is related to existing measures of similar aspects of outcome; content (or face) validity, which relies on expert agreement that the measure is a reasonable reflection of what it is supposed to be measuring. There are considerable difficulties in demonstrating the validity of a particular measure (Lyden & Lau 1991)

Reliability
This refers to the reproducibility of a measurement, most commonly between observers (inter-observer reliability) and over time (intra-observer or test–retest reliability)

Relevance
The scale should measure some aspect of outcome that is relevant to the patient or carer as well as to the doctor. Thus, the size of a cerebral infarct on a CT brain scan is of little relevance, whilst patients' ability to look after themselves is very important to the patient and carer

Practicality
Scales vary in their complexity and the time taken to complete an assessment. Studies of long-term outcome involving hundreds of patients need very simple measures which can be completed by postal or telephone questionnaire, whilst smaller studies in hospital can afford to use more complex measures

Sensitivity
It is important that a scale can distinguish patients who have different outcomes or can detect important changes in a particular patient. Usually, more sensitive scales are more complex and unfortunately less reliable

Communicability
It is useful if the measure means something to other health professions or even patients. It is more useful to know that a patient feels 'fine' than to be told that their score on a particular stroke scale was 23 out of 100, for example

plex for routine use in large studies (McPherson *et al.* 1993; Wellwood *et al.* 1995b). Some of these scales are simple enough to incorporate into a postal or telephone questionnaire, and may therefore be used in large studies of long-term outcome (Shinar *et al.* 1987).

Handicap is difficult to define and therefore difficult to measure, but is undoubtedly of relevance to stroke patients and their carers. The Oxford Handicap Scale (Table 17.21), which is a modification of the Rankin Scale, sounds from its name as if it measures handicap, but it probably measures a combination of symptoms, dependency and change in lifestyle (Rankin 1957; Bamford *et al.* 1989). However, it has been widely used, is relevant and simple enough to be used reliably over the telephone, and is therefore useful in large studies (Candelize *et al.* 1994). The London Handicap Scale is a promising measure of handicap after stroke, but it requires further evaluation (Harwood *et al.* 1994; Jenkinson *et al.* 2000).

Quality of life, like handicap, is difficult to define and thus measure. A large number of generic measures (otherwise known as multidimensional measures) have been developed that attempt to measure outcomes in relation to various aspects, including physical function, psychological function, pain and social function. They include the Short Form 36, Nottingham Health Profile, EuroQol, and the Sickness Impact Profile (Bergner *et al.* 1981; Hunt *et al.* 1985; Ebrahim *et al.* 1986; EuroQol Group 1990; Brazier *et al.* 1992; Ware & Sherbourne 1992; De Haan *et al.* 1993; Dorman *et al.* 1997a,b; Buck *et al.* 2000). Most provide a profile of outcome rather than an overall measure, and group comparisons are therefore complex. However, the EuroQol provides a single measure of 'utility', and researchers have made some headway in deriving summary scores for other measures. Because they are generic, i.e. can be used across many different health states, they do offer health economists and colleagues the opportunity to compare the utility of different health outcomes in different diseases. Some are long and complex (e.g. the Sickness Impact Profile) and are not suited to large-scale studies in which face-to-face administration is not practical. Also, they rely on patients' views of their health status, which limits their use in patients with severe communication and cognitive difficulties. It is unclear how valid the carers' responses on behalf of the patient are to these questionnaires (Dorman *et al.* 1997c).

Like motherhood, quality of life is much admired, difficult to define and even more difficult to measure.

Three simple questions. We have used 'three simple questions' to categorize patients into those with poor, fair and good outcomes after stroke (Fig. 17.7) (Dennis *et al.* 1997a,b). This approach to the measurement of outcome after stroke appears to be reasonably valid and reliable, and is certainly practical when the outcome of very large numbers of patients needs to be measured (International Stroke Trial Collaborative Group 1997). Further work is required to establish the optimal wording of the simple questions and to test them in different languages and settings.

Patient satisfaction. Many health-care systems are being influenced by market forces and the idea that patients are consumers. This has placed increasing importance on the satisfaction of our 'clients' with their health care. Many health service managers regard patient satisfaction as being an important outcome, although some would consider satisfaction to be a measure of process. Pound *et al.* (1994) have developed measures of patient and carer satisfaction with hospital and home care. However, these measures need to

Item	Score		Categories
Bowels	0	0	Incontinent or needs enemas
	5	1	Occasional incontinence (< once per week)
	10	2	Continent
Bladder	0	0	Incontinent/unable to manage catheter
	5	1	Occasional accident (< once per day)
	10	2	Continent
Grooming	0	0	Needs help with shaving, washing, hair or teeth
	5	1	Independent
Toilet use	0	0	Dependent
	5	1	Needs some help
	10	2	Independent on, off, dressing and cleaning
Feeding	0	0	Dependent
	5	1	Needs some help (e.g. with cutting, spreading)
	10	2	Independent if food provided within reach
Transfer (e.g. bed to chair)	0	0	Unable and no sitting balance
	5	1	Needs major help
	10	2	Needs minor help
	15	3	Independent
Mobility	0	0	Unable
	5	1	Wheelchair independent indoors
	10	2	Walks with help or supervision
	15	3	Independent (but may use aid)
Dressing	0	0	Dependent
	5	1	Needs some help
	10	2	Independent, including fasteners
Stairs	0	0	Unable
	5	1	Needs some help or supervision
	10	2	Independent up and down
Bathing	0	0	Dependent
	5	1	Independent in bath or shower
Total	100	20	

Table 17.19 Barthel Index, showing two alternative scoring systems (from Mahoney & Barthel 1965).

be evaluated further in different settings before they can be recommended for general use. Patient and carer satisfaction appears to reflect the process of care and the patients' outcomes. As one would expect, those with poorer physical outcomes and depression are likely to report less satisfaction with care (Pound *et al.* 1999). However, patients—and particularly women and the elderly—appear to have low expectations and are often satisfied with what professionals would regard as poor treatment (Wellwood *et al.* 1995a; Pound *et al.* 1999).

When should we measure outcome? Outcomes some months after the stroke are probably most relevant to patients, but are more difficult and expensive to measure than at an earlier stage. Many services monitor the patient's functional status at the time of hospital discharge, and this information is easily and cheaply collected. However, because patients usually improve for several months after a stroke, the longer they stay in hospital the better their outcome at discharge. Thus, such measures are easily manipulated and impossible to interpret. It is more relevant to measure the outcome at

Table 17.20 Types of measurement scales and their properties (adapted from Wade 1992a).

	Nominal scale	Ordinal scale	Interval scale	Ratio scale
Features	Categories for classification with no order	Rank order but non-uniform intervals	Uniform intervals but no zero	Uniform intervals with zero
General example	Rainy, snowy and windy	Hot, warm, cool and cold	Degrees centigrade	Degrees Kelvin
Stroke example	Total anterior circulation infarct, lacunar infarct	Oxford Handicap Scale	OPCS disability measure	Timed 10-m walk
Use of numbers	Descriptive only	Just to put in order	Indicate order or difference	Indicate order, difference or absolute value
Group description	Frequencies Proportions Mode	Median Range (interquartile)	Mean (Variance)	Mean (Variance) Coefficient of variation
Group comparison	Chi-square Odds ratio	Mann–Whitney Wilcoxon	*t*-test Analysis of variance	*t*-test Analysis of variance

OPCS, Office of Population Censuses and Survey.

Table 17.21 The Oxford Handicap Scale (also known as the modified Rankin scale). The dotted line shows how the scale can be dichotomized to distinguish between patients who are independent in everyday activities and those who are not. The three simple questions (Fig. 17.7) aim to dichotomize patients in a similar way.

Grade	Description
0	No symptoms
1	Minor symptoms that do not interfere with lifestyle
2	Minor handicap. Symptoms that lead to some restriction in lifestyle, but do not interfere with the patients' ability to look after themselves
······	······
3	Moderate handicap. Symptoms that significantly restrict lifestyle and prevent totally independent existence
4	Moderately severe handicap. Symptoms that clearly prevent independent existence, although the patient does not need constant care and attention
5	Severe handicap. Totally dependent, requiring constant attention day and night

a fixed interval from the stroke, but after discharge this will inevitably be more time-consuming and expensive. However, some of the simpler measures can be completed by telephone or postal questionnaire (Shinar *et al.* 1987; Candelise *et al.* 1994; Lindley *et al.* 1994). Some measures (e.g. EuroQol), which seem ideally suited for use as postal questionnaires, include visual analogue scales, which appear to be particularly unreliable in stroke patients (Price *et al.* 1999).

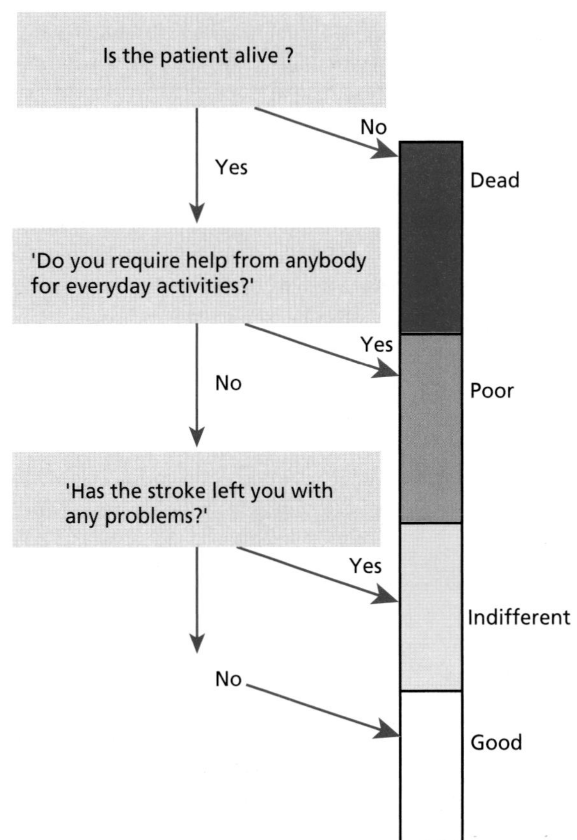

Fig. 17.7 'Three simple questions' that can be used to place stroke patients into four different outcome categories (from Lindley *et al.* 1994).

How to score dead patients? Because many patients die after stroke, outcome measurements can only be applied to the survivors. If these measures are averaged, and groups of patients compared, then there may be a serious problem of interpretation if there are more survivors in one group than in the other. Some workers attempt to get round this by giving the worst score to the dead patients and then including them in the analysis but, depending on the scale used, this is not necessarily valid. One solution is to measure the proportion of patients who are 'dead or disabled/handicapped', but this may sacrifice sensitivity. However, in studies including large numbers, such dichotomized outcomes may be adequate (Peto 1980).

Chance (or random error)

With small numbers, the imprecision of the estimate of performance may prevent useful comparisons being made. Thus, it is important to measure outcomes in a large, representative sample of patients or carers. This has implications for the type of measure of outcome used, since it must be simple and practical to administer to large numbers, exactly as in large, simple randomized trials. A consequence of the need to have adequate numbers of patients in order to obtain precise estimates of outcome is that it may take several years for a hospital to accumulate enough data to provide such a precise estimate—for example, of its case fatality. Thus, there is likely to be a considerable delay between a change in the quality of care and any statistically significant change in measured outcomes. Figure 17.8 shows the case fatality before and after the introduction of an organized stroke service, and illustrates that even with several hundred patients, the 95% confidence interval around the estimates of case fatality are surprisingly wide, even before taking into account any effect of casemix adjustment (see below). We suggest that power calculations should be performed (as for randomized trials) before instigating any audit to demonstrate changes in the outcomes following modification of a service.

When planning an audit, estimate the likely number of cases that will need to be included in order to identify a difference reliably (i.e. do a power calculation).

Although the evidence that institutions with greater throughput have better outcomes is conflicting (e.g. for carotid endarterectomy), one argument for stipulating a minimum patient volume per year is to ensure that measures of performance can be reasonably precise. If one's local surgeon performed 50 operations in the previous year, with only two deaths or perioperative strokes, this is a very acceptable 4% complication rate. However, the 95% confidence interval extends up to a very unacceptable 14%. It is therefore very difficult to know with any certainty whether one's local surgeon has results that make carotid endarterectomy worthwhile.

If the outcomes are measured in a relatively small number of patients or carers, bad outcomes may reflect bad luck rather than bad care, while conversely, good outcomes may reflect good luck rather than good care.

Casemix

The most important determinant of outcome is probably not the *quality* or *effectiveness* of care, but the type of patient treated. The patient's age, pre-stroke status and the severity of the stroke are bound to have an overwhelming effect on the outcome, and may obscure any real effect that our treatments may have. That is why large randomized trials are required to demonstrate modest treatment effects. This casemix can vary considerably in different services and in the same service over time, which means that raw outcome data simply cannot be used to reflect the quality or effectiveness of care; they have to be adjusted for differences in casemix. Unfortunately, this assumes that we know how to adjust for casemix in stroke, which is not the case. Good casemix descriptors include those factors that are highly pre-

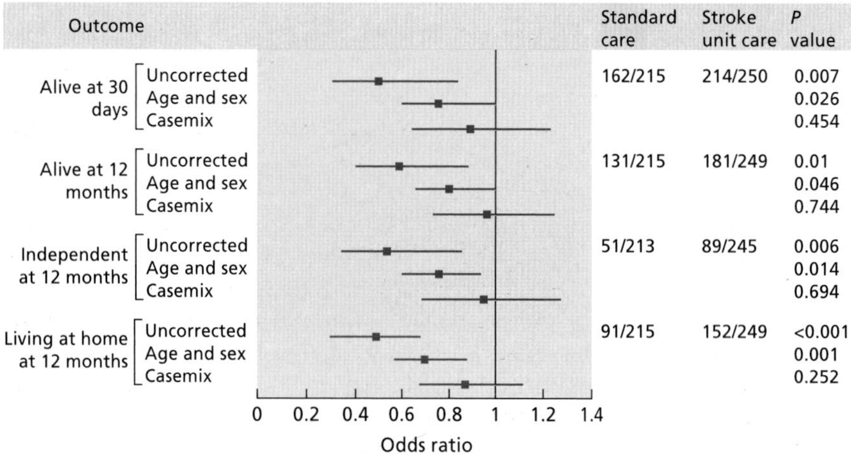

Fig. 17.8 The odds ratios (95% confidence intervals indicated by horizontal lines) comparing outcome before ($n = 216$) and after ($n = 252$) a change in the organization from standard to stroke unit care in one of our institutions: data for four outcomes, before and after adjustment for differences in age and sex only, and then other casemix variables (Table 10.7). Odds ratios to the left of the vertical line indicate a better outcome in the stroke unit.

dictive of outcome. But as we have already seen, our ability to predict outcome after stroke, even in terms of survival, is relatively poor (section 10.2.7). Also, we can only correct for those prognostic factors that we can identify and measure reliably. After all, we rely on randomized controlled trials to provide evidence of the effectiveness of interventions simply because randomization ensures that the different treatment groups are balanced for recognized, unrecognized and unmeasurable prognostic factors and that the treatment allocation is not biased. In the report comparing outcomes after stroke in Scottish hospitals, the only prognostic factors that were routinely collected, and could therefore be adjusted for, were age, sex and social deprivation (Clinical Outcomes Working Group 1999). If more powerful predictive factors such as those identified in the Oxfordshire Community Stroke Project (Table 10.7) are taken into account, most of the variation between hospitals with respect to case fatality disappears and can be accounted for by chance alone (Weir & the Scottish Stroke Outcomes Group 1999). Unfortunately, these variables are not routinely available to allow such adjustment. If variations in outcome remain, it is impossible to know whether they are due to failure to completely adjust for casemix or some aspect of the care given (Wolfe *et al.* 1999). In accounting for random variation, one must also take into account the imprecision of any statistical model used, which will depend on the size of the cohort from which the model was derived. The problems of adjusting for casemix are even greater if one considers other relevant outcomes such as quality of life, where we know almost nothing about the factors that predict this. Before we use outcomes to reflect the effectiveness and quality of care, and to alter services as a consequence of these, we have to develop reliable methods of interpreting them. It will be interesting to see whether this will ever be possible.

Crude measures of patient outcome do not necessarily reflect the quality or effectiveness of the care provided. Even adjusting for casemix may not solve this problem.

Measuring the 'efficiency' of a service. Rather than attempting to interpret measures of outcome at a particular interval after the stroke, the change in the patient's condition can be used as an 'outcome'. For example, some research groups have used the functional independence measure (FIM) to assess patients on admission to and discharge from a treatment programme. Other measures, such as the Barthel Index, could be used in the same way. Any change in the FIM might be considered, at least in part, to be a measure of the effectiveness of the treatment programme, although most of the improvement may actually be spontaneous. The change in FIM can be divided by some measure of the amount of treatment provided, e.g. length of stay, to give an idea of 'efficiency'. In some ways, this approach is similar to that described above, since one could consider the FIM on admission to be a casemix descriptor. Unfortunately, differences in casemix such as age, severity and location of the brain lesion and other medical problems, as well as the interval since the stroke, are likely to influence the rate of change in the FIM. To interpret the change in the FIM as a reflection of effectiveness or efficiency would therefore still require a measure of casemix (Alexander 1994). Another problem is that measures such as the FIM are not 'interval' scales (Table 17.20). A change of 10 points at one end of the scale is therefore not equivalent to a 10-point change at the other. This makes changes in score difficult to interpret.

17.6.4 A practical approach

Given the limitations of using structure, process or outcome measurement (see 17.6.3), it is probably best not to rely on any one method, but to use a combination of methods. This has the advantage of reflecting most aspects of the service. Also, if one relies on only a small number of performance indicators, it can have a number of adverse effects on health services. Effort and resources may be directed at improving one service or one aspect of a service, to the detriment of other areas (this has been called 'measure fixation').

Clinicians and managers whose income or reputations depend on the indicators may alter their practice (e.g. refuse to treat sicker patients) or manipulate data to enhance their apparent performance (i.e. gaming). For instance, by altering the coding of any factors used to adjust for casemix (e.g. stroke severity), one can increase the expected mortality for one's patients and thus improve one's apparent performance (i.e. the observed/expected mortality ratio). The best example of such gaming was documented following the publication of institution-specific and surgeon-specific death rates for cardiac surgery in New York (Green & Wintfeld 1995). The reported proportion of patients with co-morbidities, such as renal failure and chronic obstructive pulmonary disease, which were used to adjust outcomes for casemix, increased several-fold over 2 years. It is highly unlikely that the type of patient had changed. The surgeons were simply *reporting* more co-morbidity.

We suggest the following approach to assessing the quality of stroke services, although this will inevitably change as our understanding improves:

• perform a structural audit to ensure that services include access to the facilities shown in Table 17.22;

• assess the process of care by performing a regular audit of a representative sample of case-notes using a well-tested and reliable audit instrument that will allow comparisons to be made with other units, or in the same unit over time, e.g. the National Sentinel Audit of Stroke (Rudd *et al.* 1999). The results of such an audit should identify where the problems lie (Crombie & Davies 1998). Also, by setting challenging targets one could use this approach to drive forward improvements in services;

Table 17.22 Facilities needed for a comprehensive stroke service.

Primary care physicians (e.g. general practitioners, family doctors)
Immediate access to acute hospital beds (ideally in a dedicated acute stroke unit)
Access to a 'one-stop' neurovascular out-patient clinic within a few days
Immediate access to diagnostic imaging, e.g. brain CT, duplex sonography
Easy access to vascular surgery and other specialties which have occasional input (Table 10.11)
Stroke rehabilitation unit with multidisciplinary team
Ability to perform predischarge home assessments
Facilities to continue therapy after hospital discharge in various settings, e.g. out-patients, day hospital, patient's home
Facilities to follow patients up medically
Outreach multidisciplinary team or a community team which can link with hospital-based team
Resources to provide personal care to dependent patients living in the community
Long-term institutional care for patients with severe disability who cannot be managed at home

• collect any outcome data that purchasers or commissioners of the stroke service require—but these should be kept simple, to minimize the cost and because they are likely to be easier to interpret. However, any interpretation will require more complex data about the patients whom the service treats. The casemix and outcome data together could form the basis for a minimum data set. Our suggestions as to what this might include are outlined in Table 17.23, and include those variables that we have found useful in predicting outcomes after stroke (section 10.2.7). These items include some demographic data, which are usually collected routinely (e.g. age, marital status) and which are likely to relate to outcome—the latter probably having an influence on place of residence, since having a potential carer may increase the likelihood of returning home. Pre-stroke function, which will also reflect co-morbidity, is bound to relate closely to functional outcome, and pre-stroke dependence is known to increase the risk of death. One could suggest a wide range of different indicators of stroke severity, such as conscious level, urinary incontinence, severity of motor weakness, or the proportion of patients with total anterior circulation syndromes (section 4.3.4). Poor outcomes may at best reflect poor care, but do not—unlike audits of process—identify the areas in which the service needs to be improved;

• monitor the frequency of complications after stroke. Although this is unlikely to provide any quantitative information about the quality of care, the data might be used to identify problems. For example, a high or rising proportion of patients with pressure sores may indicate inadequate numbers of nurses or poor-quality nursing care. Unfortunately,

Table 17.23 Minimum data set for stroke. This reflects known factors that influence the outcome after stroke (Tables 10.3 and 10.7) and also data that may be routinely available to health service workers.

Casemix data
Age
Sex
Marital status, or living alone before the stroke
Pre-stroke function, i.e. was the patient independent in activities of daily living?
Stroke severity:
Conscious level (normal or reduced?)
Can they talk?
Is the patient orientated in time, place and person?
Severity of weakness (can they lift an affected limb against gravity? can they walk independently?)
Urinary incontinence during first 7 days after the stroke
Process
Number of physicians responsible for stroke care. A lower number suggests more specialization
Proportion of patients discussed by a multidisciplinary team
Proportion of patients managed on a stroke unit
Proportion of patients having CT or magnetic resonance scans
Proportion of patients with ischaemic stroke on aspirin at discharge
Proportion of patients with ischaemic stroke and atrial fibrillation on anticoagulants at discharge
*Outcomes**
Survival to 30 days
Independence/dependence in activities of daily living at 6 months
Complications, e.g. pressure sores
Place of residence at 6 months

*Note: there is little point routinely collecting other outcomes, even if they are as relevant to patients and their carers, since we know even less about the factors that predict them and cannot therefore make any adjustments for casemix.

there are considerable problems in defining complications and in providing reliable diagnostic criteria to allow monitoring (Kalra *et al.* 1995; Davenport *et al.* 1996c; Langhorne *et al.* 2000b). Pressure sores and fractures are probably the most reliably monitored complications, but both are uncommon. A system of critical incident recording might focus on these and other problems and provide a simple indicator that the service may be performing poorly;

• provide an environment in which the identification of problems is encouraged and not penalized. One suspects that informal judgements that 'there may be a problem with quality' made by those working within a service, or using a service, would be as sensitive a method of identifying major problems as any of those discussed above. This approach will only be effective if those working within a service are objective and honest and if the system does not punish health-care workers, but encourages everyone constantly to provide better services;

• develop a system to provide an external and independent review of services by professionals from another centre. This can usefully identify problems that need to be addressed.

It is essential that politicians and health service managers should understand the difficulties in interpreting measures of process and outcome, and their limitations. They must not make important decisions about the distribution of resources on the basis of simplistic analyses of these crude types of data. However, large discrepancies in the apparent performance of different stroke services should trigger a detailed enquiry to look into the possible explanation. Also, it is important not to use the results of a non-randomized evaluation of a local stroke service to guide service development elsewhere.

Stroke guidelines

In recent years, huge numbers of guidelines have been written to indicate how to manage stroke patients. These are intended to describe best practice in the most common clinical situations, and do not necessarily indicate how every individual patient should be treated. They provide useful standards against which at least the process of care can be monitored. In the past, guidelines have been based on incomplete and thus potentially biased and misleading assessments of the evidence for the effectiveness of interventions. However, the methodology for guideline development is becoming increasingly rigorous, with recommendations being based on systematic reviews of the literature. Standards exist against which one can assess the quality of a clinical guideline (Scottish Intercollegiate Guidelines Network (SIGN) 1999; http://www.show.scot.nhs.uk/sign/home.htm). If guidelines are to improve clinical practice, it is important for them to be effectively implemented. Several factors have been identified (Table 17.24) that are associated with a greater chance of improving practice in accordance with guidelines (Bero *et al.* 1998).

When one has to decide whether to implement clinical guidelines, it is important to assess the methodological rigour with which they were developed. Failure to do so could lead to the adoption of ineffective or even harmful practices.

Integrated care pathways (for an example, see http://www.dcn.ed.ac.uk/spgm)

Clearly, a multifaceted approach must be taken to ensure that stroke patients are managed in line with guidelines unless there is a valid reason to deviate from the guidelines in an individual patient. One approach that is increasingly used in stroke units is the integrated care pathway, which often facilitates local activities that are very likely to increase adherence to guidelines (Table 17.24). The development of integrated care pathways usually requires local scrutiny of available guidelines and discussion of how patients should be managed, and introducing them involves local educational sessions. They usually incorporate patient-specific reminders, i.e. guidance on how to manage common problems. They are often a focus of local audits, which measure the degree of compliance with the pathways and the reasons for any deviations, and feed these back to the staff in the unit. Although there is no robust evidence from large randomized trials that integrated care pathways lead to better patient outcomes, they may improve documentation (Moloney *et al.* 1999; Sulch *et al.* 2000).

Table 17.24 Factors associated with a greater chance of improving practice in accordance with guidelines (adapted from Bero *et al.* 1998).

Consistently effective interventions

Educational outreach visits (for prescribing in North America)

Patient-specific reminders (manual or computerized)

Multifaceted interventions (a combination that includes two or more of the following: audit and feedback, reminders, local consensus processes, or marketing)

Interactive educational meetings (participation of health-care providers in workshops that include discussion or practice)

Interventions of variable effectiveness

Audit and feedback (or any summary of clinical performance)

The use of local opinion leaders (practitioners identified by their colleagues as influential)

Local consensus processes (inclusion of participating practitioners in discussions to ensure they agree that the chosen clinical problem is important and the approach to managing the problem is appropriate)

Patient-mediated interventions (any intervention aimed at changing the performance of health-care providers for which specific information was sought from or given to patients)

Interventions that have little or no effect

Educational materials (distribution of recommendations for clinical care, including clinical practice guidelines, audio-visual materials, and electronic publications)

Educational meetings (such as lectures)

17.7 Cost-effectiveness of stroke services

Because of its frequency in most populations, the resulting severe disability and the need for prolonged institutional care, stroke places a very considerable financial burden on most societies (section 17.1). Therefore, when planning stroke services it is important not only to aim for maximum effectiveness, in terms of achieving the best possible outcomes for the patients and their families, but also to do this as efficiently as possible. As we have seen, there is little reliable information about the effectiveness of many interventions, but there is even less about the relative costs of treatment. One can use several different types of economic analysis to relate the effect of treatment and its associated costs (Table 17.25). Ideally, data regarding both the effectiveness and the costs of treatment will come from the same study, but such data are rarely available. More often, we have to use data from a variety of sources. Also, any conclusions from economic analyses are likely to be very sensitive to the assumptions made and to whether both direct and indirect costs are estimated.

Hospital costs account for the majority of the costs associated with acute stroke, at least in countries with sophisticated health-care systems (Terent *et al.* 1994). Figure 17.9 shows the relative size of the components of the cost of hospital care for acute stroke patients in one of our institutions. It appears that at least in the British model of care, and probably in other models as well, most of the direct hospital costs are accounted for by nursing salaries and hospital overheads, with relatively little being spent on investigation or specific treatments (Bowen & Yaste 1994; Smurawska *et al.* 1994; Dennis *et al.* 1995). Even in the United States, where patients stay in an acute hospital for only a few days, assessment, investigations and treatment account for less than half of the costs, and the length of stay is the most important predictor of hospital costs (Diringer *et al.* 1999). Thus, the cost to the health service of managing a patient with stroke is highly dependent on the length of hospital stay—assuming that the intensity of nursing input remains constant (Holloway *et al.* 1996).

Where most of the cost of stroke care in hospital is accounted for by nursing services and overheads, it does not make sense to waste time arguing about even quite large changes in the cost of investigations and treatments.

Attempts to restrict or rationalize the use of investigations or drug therapies can only have a marginal effect on the overall hospital costs. Several non-randomized studies from the United States have shown that the introduction of care pathways for stroke patients can reduce hospital costs (or charges), mainly by reducing length of stay (Odderson & McKenna 1993; Bowen & Yaste 1994; Wentworth & Atkinson 1996; Mamoli *et al.* 1999). A policy of accelerated discharge is likely to reduce the per capita costs considerably, although—depending on funding arrangements—this is likely be transferred onto another budget, e.g. community care and families. In fact, the limited evidence available from randomized trials suggests that early supported discharge schemes are marginally cheaper overall than more prolonged hospital-based rehabilitation (section 17.5.3). Interventions that promote more rapid or complete recovery may be very cost-effective, as long as they are not themselves very expensive. The evidence from the systematic review of stroke unit trials suggests that patients not only more often survive, but

Table 17.25 Some terms used in health economics (Robinson 1993a,b,c; Drummond *et al.* 1996).

Types of economic analysis

Cost minimization refers to situations in which the health outcomes are similar in different treatment groups and the analysis aims to identify which group is associated with lower costs, i.e. what the most efficient way of achieving a particular goal is

Cost-effectiveness aims to relate improvement in health outcome using natural units (e.g. life-years gained, recurrent strokes avoided) to the cost of achieving those outcomes

Cost-utility analyses relate improvement in health outcome expressed in terms of non-financial value of the gain in health outcome (e.g. quality-adjusted life-years, healthy-years equivalents)

Cost-benefit analyses simply relate the overall cost in financial terms of competing strategies. For example, the benefits from a treatment are expressed in the reduction in expenditure that would result. Thus, one might relate the cost of preventing a recurrent stroke to the costs of treating the strokes that would occur if prevention was not attempted

Types of direct cost

Health service costs. These include staff time, medical supplies, hotel services, use of capital equipment (including depreciation, interest paid) and overheads, e.g. heating, lighting. Some costs are fixed (i.e. independent of activity), whilst others are variable (e.g. dependent on number of patients treated)

Costs borne by patients and relatives, e.g. transport to visit, cost of home care

Costs borne by other agencies and society generally, e.g. social services providing home care or nursing-home care

Types of indirect cost

Loss of income for patient or family members

Loss of production for society

'Cost' of psychological distress or pain suffered. These costs are impossible to put a financial value on, except in the law courts

Other terms

Discounting puts greater value on costs or savings now compared with the same costs or savings that might accrue in the future

Marginal costs refer to the extra costs incurred in providing more service. The cost per extra operation may be quite different from the average cost per operation overall

Charges that may be levied by an organization providing health care, which may include profit or which may be subsidizing another service, are distinct from costs

Sensitivity analyses are used to take account of uncertainty about the costs and effectiveness of treatments. The components of the evaluation are varied to examine any effect on the conclusion of the economic analysis. One can vary one variable at a time, or several

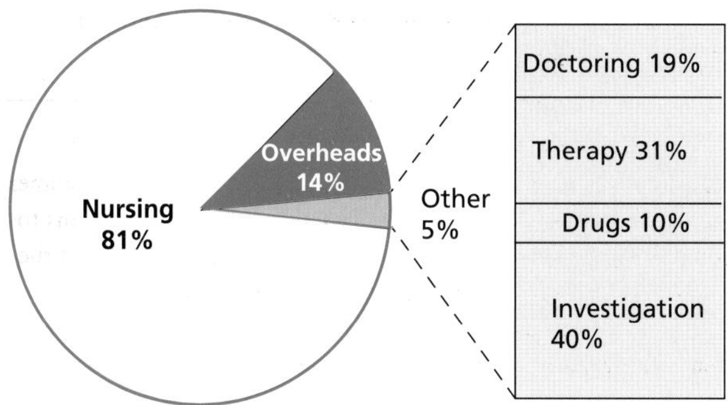

Fig. 17.9 The proportion of direct hospital costs attributable to different aspects of care provided in Edinburgh, Scotland. These data relate to a period before stroke services were organized. The development of a stroke team and unit may have altered the proportions, although probably not by very much (from Dennis *et al.* 1995).

also have a better functional outcome (Stroke Unit Trialists' Collaboration 1997, 2000). An analysis of the cost-effectiveness of stroke unit care suggested that better patient outcomes could be achieved with at worst moderate increases in costs (and at best small decreases in cost), and that stroke unit care was more cost-effective than that in general medical settings (Major & Walker 1998). Thus, it seems likely that by providing better-coordinated stroke care in units, the cost of managing a patient with stroke in hospital can be reduced. Of course, what we do not know is whether, for example, by doubling the amount of therapy that patients receive we might increase the rate of recovery and thus shorten the length of hospital admission, so that the increased therapy would pay for itself.

A practical approach to monitoring the cost-effectiveness of a stroke service might include collecting data about the total length of stay in hospital (i.e. in both the acute and rehabilitation units), since this appears to be—at least in the UK—a reasonable reflection of direct hospital costs (Dennis *et al.* 1995). However, note would have to be taken of any major changes in nursing costs or those related to investigations and treatment. The length of stay needs to be interpreted in the light of data about the destination on discharge and the patient's functional status. It is easy to reduce the length of stay by discharging patients into nursing homes instead of to their own homes, and by discharging more severely dependent patients into the community, but this adds to the costs (financial, physical and emotional) to the family and social services. Except for billing purposes, setting up systems for collecting detailed data about exactly what investigations, drugs and therapy patients receive would be time-consuming and expensive, and would probably provide little extra information about the overall cost of care. Reducing the length of stay by just one day would probably pay for all of the average patients' investigations and drugs.

An organized stroke service may be cheaper than a disorganized one, and it could release resources for other areas.

References

Please note that all references taken from *The Cochrane Library* are given a current date as this database is updated on a quarterly basis. Please refer to the current *Cochrane Library* article for the latest review. The same applies to the *British Medical Journal* 'Clinical Evidence' series which is updated every six months.

Adams, H.P., Brott, T.G., Crowell, R.M. *et al.* (1994) Guidelines for the management of patients with acute ischaemic stroke: a statement for healthcare professionals from a special writing group of the Stroke Council, American Heart Association. *Stroke* **25**, 1901–1914.

Alberts, M.J., Perry, A., Dawson, D.V. & Bertels, C. (1992) Effects of public and professional education on reducing the delay in presentation and referral of stroke patients. *Stroke* **23**, 352–356.

Alexander, M.P. (1994) Stroke rehabilitation outcome: a potential use of predictive variables to establish levels of care. *Stroke* **25**, 128–134.

Anderson, C.S., Jamrozik, K.D., Burvill, P.W., Chakera, T.M., Johnson, G.A. & Stewart-Wynne, E.G. (1993a) Ascertaining the true incidence of stroke: experience from the Perth Community Stroke Study, 1989–90. *Medical Journal of Australia* **158**, 80–84.

Anderson, C.S., Jamrozik, K.D., Burvill, P.W., Chakera, T.M., Johnson, G.A. & Stewart-Wynne, E.G. (1993b) Determining the incidence of different subtypes of stroke: results from the Perth Community Stroke Study. 1989–90. *Medical Journal of Australia* **158**, 85–89.

Anderson, C., Mhurcha, C.N., Rubenach, S., Clark, M., Spencer, C. & Winsor, A. (2000a) Home or hospital for stroke rehabilitation? Results of a randomized controlled trial. II: Cost minimization analysis at 6 months. *Stroke* **31**, 1032–1037.

Anderson, C., Rubenach, S., Mhurcha, C.N., Clark, M., Spencer, C. & WInsor, A. (2000b) Home or hospital for stroke rehabilitation? Results of a randomized controlled trial. I: Health outcomes at 6 months. *Stroke* **31**, 1024–1031.

Asplund, K., Bonita, R., Kuulasmaa, K. *et al.* (1995) Multinational comparisons of stroke epidemiology: evaluation of case ascertainment in the WHO MONICA Stroke Study. *Stroke* **26**, 355–360.

Bamford, J., Sandercock, P., Warlow, C. & Gray, M. (1986) Why are patients with acute stroke admitted to hospital? *British Medical Journal* **292**, 1369–1372.

Bamford, J., Sandercock, P., Dennis, M. *et al.* (1988) A prospective study of acute cerebrovascular disease in the community: the Oxfordshire Community Stroke Project 1981–86, 1: methodology, demography and incident cases of first-ever stroke. *Journal of Neurology, Neurosurgery and Psychiatry* **51**, 1373–1380.

Bamford, J.L., Sandercock, P.A.G., Warlow, C.P. & Slattery, J. (1989) Interobserver agreement for the assessment of handicap in stroke patients [letter]. *Stroke* **20**, 828.

Bath, P.M.W., Soo, J., Butterworth, R.J. & Kerr, J.E. (1996) Do acute stroke units improve care? *Cerebrovascular Diseases* **6**, 346–349.

Beech, R., Rudd, A.G., Tilling, K. & Wolfe, C.D.A. (1999) Economic consequences of early inpatient discharge to community-based rehabilitation for stroke in an inner-London teaching hospital. *Stroke* **30**, 729–735.

Bergman, L., van de Meulen, J.H.P., Limburg, M. & Habbema, D.F. (1995) Costs of medical care after first-ever stroke in the Netherlands. *Stroke* **26**, 1830–1836.

Bergner, M., Bobbitt, R.A., Carter, W.B. & Gilson, B.S. (1981) The Sickness Impact Profile: development and final revision of a health status measure. *Medical Care* **19**, 787–805.

Bero, L.A., Grilli, R., Grimshaw, J.M. *et al.* (1998) Closing the gap between research and practice: an overview of systematic reviews of interventions to promote the implementation of research findings. *British Medical Journal* **317**, 465–468.

Bonita, R., Broad, J.B. & Beaglehole, R. (1993) Changes in stroke incidence and case-fatality in Auckland, New Zealand, 1981–91. *Lancet* **342**, 1470–1473.

Bonita, R., Broad, J.B. & Beaglehole, R. (1997a) Ethnic differences in stroke incidence and case fatality in Auckland, New Zealand. *Stroke* **28**, 758–761.

Bonita, R., Solomon, N. & Broad, J.B. (1997b) Prevalence of stroke and stroke-related disability: estimates from the Auckland Stroke Studies. *Stroke* **28**, 1898–1902.

Bowen, J. & Yaste, C. (1994) Effect of a stroke protocol on hospital costs of stroke patients. *Neurology* **44**, 1961–1964.

Brazier, J.E., Harper, R., Jones, N.M.B. *et al.* (1992) Validating the SF-36 health survey questionnaire: new outcome measure for primary care. *British Medical Journal* **305**, 160–164.

Broderick, J.P., Phillips, S.J., Whisnant, J.P., O'Fallon, W.M. & Bergstrahl, E.J. (1989) Incidence rates of stroke in the eighties: the end of the decline in stroke? *Stroke* **20**, 577–582.

Brott, T., Adams, H.P., Olinger, C.P. *et al.* (1989) Measurements of acute cerebral infarction: a clinical examination scale. *Stroke* **20**, 864–870.

Buck, D., Jacoby, A., Massey, A. & Ford, G. (2000) Evaluation of measures used to assess quality of life after stroke. *Stroke* **31**, 2004–2010.

Candelise, L., Pinardi, G., Aritzu, E. & Musicco, M. (1994) Telephone interview for stroke outcome assessment. *Cerebrovascular Diseases* **4**, 341–343.

Caro, J.J., Huybrechts, K.F. & Duchesne, I. for the Stroke Economic Analysis Group (2000) Management patterns and costs of acute ischemic stroke. An international study. *Stroke* **31**, 582–590.

Chaturvedi, S., Bertasio, B. & Femino, L. (1998) Emergency physician attitudes toward thrombolytic therapy in acute stroke. *Health Services Research* **7**, 442–445.

Clinical Outcomes Working Group (1999) *Clinical Outcome Indicators.* Scottish Executive Health Dept., Edinburgh.

Cote, R., Hachinski, V.C., Shurvell, B.L., Norris, J.W. & Wolfson, C. (1986) The Canadian Neurological Scale: a preliminary study in acute stroke. *Stroke* **17**, 731–737.

Cote, R., Battista, R.N.N., Wolfson, C., Boucher, J., Adam, J. & Hachinski, V. (1989) The Canadian Neurological Scale: validation and reliability assessment. *Neurology* **39**, 638–643.

Counsell, C., Warlow, C., Sandercock, P., Fraser, H. & van Gijn, J. (1995) The Cochrane Collaboration Stroke Review Group: meeting the need for systematic reviews in stroke care. *Stroke* **26**, 498–502.

Crombie, I.K. & Davies, H.T.A. (1998) Beyond health outcomes: the advantages of measuring process. *Journal of Evaluation in Clinical Practice* **4**, 31–38.

Czlonkowska, A., Ryglewicz, D., Weissbein, T., Baranska-Gieruszczak, M. & Hier, D.B. (1994) A prospective community-based study of stroke in Warsaw, Poland. *Stroke* **25**, 547–551.

D'Alessandro, G., Di Giovanni, G., Roveyaz, L. *et al.* (1992) Incidence and prognosis of stroke in the Valle d'Aosta, Italy: first-year results of a community-based study. *Stroke* **23**, 1712–1715.

Davenport, R.J., Dennis, M.S. & Warlow, C.P. (1995) Improving the recording of the clinical assessment of stroke patients using a clerking proforma. *Age and Ageing* **24**, 43–48.

Davenport, R.J., Dennis, M.S. & Warlow, C.P. (1996a) Effect of correcting outcome data for case mix: an example from stroke medicine. *British Medical Journal* **1996** (312), 1503–1505.

Davenport, R.J., Dennis, M.S. & Warlow, C.P. (1996b) The accuracy of Scottish Morbidity Record (SMR1) data for identifying hospitalised stroke patients. *Health Bulletin* **54**, 402–405.

Davenport, R.J., Dennis, M.S., Wellwood, I. & Warlow, C.P. (1996c) Complications following acute stroke. *Stroke* **27**, 415–420.

Davies, H.T.A. & Crombie, I.K. (1997) Interpreting health outcomes. *Journal of Evaluation in Clinical Practice* **3**, 187–199.

Davis, M., Hollymann, C., McGiven, M., Chambers, I., Egbuji, J. & Barer, D. (1999) Physiological monitoring in acute stroke. *Age and Ageing* **28** (Suppl. 1), P45.

De Haan, R., Horn, J., Limburg, M., Van Der Meulen, J. & Bossuyt, P. (1993) A comparison of five stroke scales with measures of disability, handicap, and quality of life. *Stroke* **24**, 1178–1181.

Dennis, M. (2000) Stroke services: the good, the bad, and the .... *Journal of the Royal College of Physicians of London* **34**, 92–96.

Dennis, M., Bamford, J., Sandercock, P. & Warlow, C.P. (1989) Incidence of transient ischaemic attacks in Oxfordshire, England. *Stroke* **20**, 333–339.

Dennis, M., Wellwood, I., McGregor, K., Dent, J. & Forbes, J. (1995) What are the major components of the cost of caring for stroke patients in hospital in the UK? [abstract]. *Cerebrovascular Diseases* **5**, 243.

Dennis, M.S., Wellwood, I., O'Rourke, S., MacHale, S. & Warlow, C.P. (1997a) How reliable are simple questions in assessing outcome after stroke? *Cerebrovascular Diseases* **7**, 19–21.

Dennis, M.S., Wellwood, I. & Warlow, C.P. (1997b) Are simple questions a valid measure of outcome after stroke? *Cerebrovascular Diseases* **7**, 22–27.

Dennis, M., O'Rourke, S., Slattery, J., Staniforth, T. & Warlow, C. (1997c) Evaluation of a stroke family care worker: results of a randomised controlled trial. *British Medical Journal* **314**, 1071–1076.

Diringer, M.N., Edwards, D.F. & Mattson, D.T. (1999) Predictors of acute hospital costs for treatment of ischemic stroke in an academic center. *Stroke* **30**, 724–728.

Donabedian, A. (1988) The quality of care: how can it be assessed? *Journal of the American Medical Association* **260**, 19–26.

Dorman, P.J., Slattery, J., Farrell, F., Dennis, M., Sandercock, P.A.G. & the United Kingdom collaborators in the International Stroke Trial (1997a) A randomised comparison of the EuroQol and short-Form 36 after stroke. *British Medical Journal* **315**, 461.

Dorman, P.J., Waddell, F., Slattery, J., Dennis, M. & Sandercock, P. (1997b) Is the EuroQol a valid measure of health-related quality of life after stroke? *Stroke* **28**, 1876–1882.

Dorman, P.J., Waddell, F., Slattery, J., Dennis, M. & Sandercock, P. (1997c) Are proxy assessments of health status after stroke with the EuroQol questionnaires feasible, accurate and unbiased? *Stroke* **28**, 1883–1887.

Dowswell, G., Lawler, J., Young, J., Forster, A. & Hearn, J. (1997) A qualitative study of specialist nurse support for stroke patients and care-givers at home. *Clinical Rehabilitation* **11**, 293–301.

Drake, W.E., Hamilton, M.J., Carlsson, M., Kand, F. & Blumenkrantz, J. (1973) Acute stroke management and patient outcome: the value of neurovascular care units (NCU). *Stroke* **4**, 933–945.

Drummond, M.F. & Jefferson, T.O., on behalf of the BMJ Economic Evaluation Working Party (1996) Guidelines for authors and peer reviewers of economic submissions to the BMJ. *British Medical Journal* **313**, 275–283.

Early Supported Discharge Trialists (2000) Services for reducing duration of hospital care for acute stroke patients. In: *The Cochrane Library*. Oxford: Update Software.

Ebrahim, S. & Redfern, J. (1999) *Stroke Care: a Matter of Chance—a National Survey of Stroke Services.* The Stroke Association, London.

Ebrahim, S.B., Nouri, F. & Barer, D. (1985) Measuring disability after a stroke. *Journal of Epidemiology and Community Health* **39**, 86–89.

Ebrahim, S.B., Barer, D. & Nouri, F. (1986) Use of the Nottingham Health Profile with patients after a stroke. *Journal of Epidemiology and Community Health* **40**, 166–169.

Ellekjaer, H., Holmen, J., Indredavik, B. & Terent, A. (1997) Epidemiology of stroke in Innherred, Norway, 1994–96: incidence and 30 day case-fatality rate. *Stroke* **28**, 2180–2184.

Ellekjaer, H., Holmen, J., Kruger, O. & Terent, A. (1999) Identification of incident stroke in Norway: hospital discharge data compared with a population-based stroke register. *Stroke* **30**, 56–60.

European Ad Hoc Consensus Group (1996) European strategies for early intervention in stroke. *Cerebrovascular Diseases* **6**, 315–324.

EuroQol Group (1990) EuroQol: a new facility for the measurement of health-related quality of life. *Health Policy* **16**, 199–208.

Evans, A., Perez, I., Melbourn, A., Steadman, J. & Kalra, L. (2000) Alternative strategies in stroke: a randomized controlled trial of three strategies of stroke management and rehabilitation. *Cerebrovascular Diseases* **10** (Suppl. 2), 60.

Evers, S.M.A.A., Engel, G.L. & Ament, A.J.H.A. (1997) Cost of stroke in the Netherlands from a societal perspective. *Stroke* **28**, 1375–1381.

Feigin, V.L., Wiebers, D.O., Nikitin, Y.P., O'Fallon, W.M. & Whisnant, J.P. (1995) Stroke epidemiology in Novosibirsk, Russia: a population-based study. *Mayo Clinic Proceedings* **70**, 847–852.

Forster, A. & Young, J. (1996) Specialist nurse support for patients with stroke in the community: a randomised controlled trial. *British Medical Journal* **312**, 1642–1646.

Forster, A., Young, J., Langhorne, P. for the Day Hospital Group (2000a) Medical day hospital care for the elderly versus alternative forms of care. In: *The Cochrane Library*. Oxford: Update Software.

Forster, A., Young, J., Smith, J., Knapp, P., House, A. & Knight, J. (2000b) Information provision for stroke patients and their caregivers (protocol for a Cochrane Review). In: *The Cochrane Library.* Oxford: Update Software.

van Gijn, J. & Warlow, C.P. (1992) Down with stroke scales. *Cerebrovascular Diseases* **2**, 239–247.

Giroud, M., Gras, P., Chadan, N. *et al.* (1991a) Cerebral haemorrhage in a French prospective population study. *Journal of Neurology, Neurosurgery and Psychiatry* **54**, 595–598.

Giroud, M., Milan, C., Beuriat, P. *et al.* (1991b) Incidence and survival rates during a two-year period of intracerebral and subarachnoid haemorrhages, cortical infarcts, lacunes and transient ischaemic attacks: the stroke registry of Dijon, 1985–89. *International Journal of Epidemiology* **20**, 892–899.

Gladman, J.R.F. & Lincoln, N.B. (1994) Follow-up of a controlled trial of domiciliary stroke rehabilitation (DOMINO Study). *Age and Ageing* **23**, 9–13.

Gladman, J.R.F., Lincoln, N.B. & Barer, D.H. (1993) A randomised controlled trial of domiciliary and hospital-based rehabilitation for stroke patients after discharge from hospital. *Journal of Neurology, Neurosurgery and Psychiatry* **56**, 960–966.

Gladman, J.R.F., Whynes, D. & Lincoln, N. (1994) Cost comparison of domiciliary and hospital-based stroke rehabilitation (DOMINO Study Group). *Age and Ageing* **23**, 241–245.

Gladman, J.R.F., Forster, A. & Young, J. (1995) Hospital- and home-based rehabilitation after discharge from hospital for stroke patients: analysis of two trials. *Age and Ageing* **24**, 49–53.

Goldstein, H. & Spiegelhalter, D.J. (1996) League tables and their limitations: statistical issues in comparisons of institutional performance. *Journal of the Royal Statistical Society* **159**, 385–443.

Gompertz, P., Dennis, M., Hopkins, A. & Ebrahim, S. (1994) Development and reliability of the Royal College of Physicians Stroke Audit Form. *Age and Ageing* **22**, 378–383.

Gompertz, P., Pound, P., Briffa, J. & Ebrahim, S. (1995) How useful are non-random comparisons of outcomes and quality of care in purchasing hospital stroke services. *Age and Ageing* **24**, 137–141.

Green, J. & Wintfeld, N. (1995) Report cards on cardiac surgeons: assessing New York State's Approach. *New England Journal of Medicine* **332**, 1229–1232.

Gubitz, G., Phillips, S. & Dwyer, V. (1999) What is the cost of admitting patients with transient ischaemic attacks to hospital? *Cerebrovascular Diseases* **9**, 210–214.

Hacke, W., Schwab, S. & De Georgia, M. (1994) Intensive care of acute ischemic stroke. *Cerebrovascular Diseases* **4**, 385–392.

Hancock, R.J.Y., Oddy, M., Saweirs, W.M. & Court, B. (1997) The RCP stroke audit package in practice. *Journal of the Royal College of Physicians of London* **31**, 74–78.

Harwood, R.H., Gompertz, P. & Ebrahim, S. (1994) Handicap one year after a stroke: validity of a new scale. *Journal of Neurology, Neurosurgery and Psychiatry* **57**, 825–829.

Holbrook, M. & Skilbeck, C.E. (1983) An activities index for use with stroke patients. *Age and Ageing* **12**, 166–170.

Holloway, R.G., Witter, D.M., Lawton, K.B., Lipscomb, J. & Samsa G. (1996) Inpatient costs of specific cerebrovascular events at five academic medical centers. *Neurology* **46**, 854–860.

Hui, E., Lum, C.M., Woo, J., Or, K.H. & Kay, R.L. (1995) Outcomes of elderly stroke patients: day hospital versus conventional medical management. *Stroke* **26**, 1616–1619.

Hunt, S., McEwan, J. & McKenna, S. (1985) Measuring health status: a new tool for clinicians and epidemiologists. *Journal of the Royal College of General Practitioners* **35**, 185–188.

Ilmavirta, M., Frey, H., Erila, T. & Fogelholm, R. (1994) *Stroke outcome and outcome of brain infarction. A prospective randomised study comparing outcomes of patients with acute brain infarction treated in a stroke unit and in an ordinary neurological ward.* Academic dissertation, Vol. 410 (Series A), University of Tampere Faculty of Medicine, Tampere.

Indredavik, B., Bakke, F., Solberg, R., Rokseth, R., Haaheim, L.L. & Holme, I. (1991) Benefit of a stroke unit: a randomized controlled trial. *Stroke* **22**, 1026–1031.

Indredavik, B., Bakke, F., Slordahl, S.A., Rokseth, R. & Haheim, L.L. (1998) Stroke unit treatment improves long-term quality of life: a randomized controlled trial. *Stroke* **29**, 895–899.

Indredavik, B., Bakke, F., Slordahl, S.A., Rokseth, R. & Haheim, L.L. (1999a) Stroke unit treatment: 10 year follow up. *Stroke* **30**, 1524–1527.

Indredavik, B., Bakke, F., Slordahl, S.A., Rokseth, R. & Haheim, L.L. (1999b) Treatment in a combined acute and rehabilitation stroke unit: which aspects are most important? *Stroke* **30**, 917–923.

International Stroke Trial Collaborative Group (1997) The International Stroke Trial (IST): a randomised trial of aspirin, subcutaneous heparin, both, or neither among 19 345 patients with acute ischaemic stroke. *Lancet* **349**, 1569–1582.

Isard, P.A. & Forbes, J.F. (1992) The cost of stroke to the National Health Service in Scotland. *Cerebrovascular Diseases* **2**, 47–50.

Jenkinson, C., Mant, J., Carter, J., Wade, D. & Winner, S. (2000) The London Handicap Scale: a re-evaluation of its validity using a standard scoring and simple summation. *Journal of Neurology, Neurosurgery and Psychiatry* **68**, 365–367.

Johnston, F., Wardlaw, J., Dennis, M.S. *et al.* (1999) Delays in stroke referrals. *Lancet* **354**, 47–48.

Jorgensen, H.S., Plesner, A.M., Hubbe, P. & Larsen, K. (1992) Marked increase of stroke incidence in men between 1972 and 1990 in Frederiksberg, Denmark. *Stroke* **23**, 1701–1704.

Jorgensen, H.S., Kammersgaard, L.P., Nakayama, H. *et al.* (1999) Treatment and rehabilitation on a stroke unit improves 5-year survival: a community-based study. *Stroke* **30**, 930–933.

Juby, L.C., Lincoln, N.B., Berman, P. for the Stroke Unit Evaluation Study Group (1996) The effect of a stroke unit rehabilitation unit on functional and psychological outcome: a randomised controlled trial. *Cerebrovascular Diseases* **6**, 106–110.

Kalra, L., Yu, G., Wilson, K. & Roots, P. (1995) Medical complications during stroke rehabilitation. *Stroke* **26**, 990–994.

Karunaratne, P.M., Norris, C.A. & Syme, P.D. (1999) Analysis of six months' referrals to a 'one-stop' neurovascular clinic in a district general hospital: implications for purchasers of a stroke service. *Health Bulletin* **57**, 17–26.

Kelly-Hayes, M., Wolf, P.A., Kase, C.S., Brand, F.N., McGuirk, J.M. & D'Agostino, R.B. (1995) Temporal patterns of stroke onset: the Framingham study. *Stroke* **26**, 1343–1347.

Kennedy, F.B., Pozen, T.J., Gabelman, E.H., Tuthill, J.E. & Zaentz, S.D. (1970) Stroke intensive care: an appraisal. *American Health Journal* **80**, 188–196.

King's Fund Consensus Conference (1988) Treatment of stroke. *British Medical Journal* **297**, 126–128.

Knapp, P., Young, J., House, A. & Forster, A. (2000) Non-drug strategies to resolve psycho-social difficulties after stroke. *Age and Ageing* **29**, 23–30.

Kolominsky-Rabas, P.L., Sarti, C., Heuschmann, P.U. *et al.* (1998) A prospective community-based study of stroke in Germany—the Erlangen Stroke Project (ESPro): incidence and case fatality at 1, 3, and 12 months. *Stroke* **29**, 2501–2506.

Langhorne, P. (1999) Measures to improve recovery in the acute phase of stroke. *Cerebrovascular Diseases* **9** (Suppl. 5), 2–5.

Langhorne, P., Dennis, M.S. & collaborators (2000a) Services for preventing hospital admission of acute stroke patients. In: *The Cochrane Library.* Oxford: Update Software.

Langhorne, P., Stott, D.J., Robertson, L. *et al.* (2000b) Medical complications in hospitalised stroke patients: a multicentre study. *Stroke* **31**, 1223–1229.

Leibson, C.L., Naessens, J.M., Brown, R.D. & Whisnant, J.P. (1994) Accuracy of hospital discharge abstracts for identifying stroke. *Stroke* **25**, 2348–2355.

Leibson, C.L., Hu, T., Brown, R.D., Hass, S.L., O'Fallon, W.M. & Whisnant, J.P. (1996) Utilization of acute care services in the year before and after first stroke: a population-based study. *Neurology* **46**, 861–869.

Lincoln, N.B., Willis, D., Philips, S.A., Juby, L.C. & Berman, P. (1996) Comparison of rehabilitation practice on hospital wards for stroke patients. *Stroke* **27**, 18–23.

Lindley, R.I., Waddell, F., Livingstone, M. *et al.* (1994) Can simple questions assess outcome after stroke? *Cerebrovascular Diseases* **4**, 314–324.

Lyden, P.D. & Lau, G.T. (1991) A critical appraisal for stroke evaluation and rating scales. *Stroke* **22**, 1345–1352.

McNamee, P., Christensen, J., Soutter, J. *et al.* (1998) Cost analysis of early supported hospital discharge for stroke. *Age and Ageing* **27**, 345–351.

McPherson, K., Sloan, R., Hunter, J. & Dowell, C. (1993) Validation studies of the OPCS scale: more useful than the Barthel Index? *Clinical Rehabilitation* **7**, 105–112.

Mahoney, F. & Barthel, D. (1965) Functional evaluation: the Barthel Index. *Maryland State Medical Journal* **14**, 61–65.

Major, K. & Walker, A. (1998) Economics of stroke unit care. In: *Stroke Units: an Evidence-Based Approach* (eds P. Langhorne & M. Dennis), pp. 56–65. BMJ Books, London.

Malmgren, R., Warlow, C., Bamford, J. & Sandercock, P. (1987) Geographical and secular trends in stroke incidence. *Lancet* ii, 1196–1200.

Malmgren, R., Bamford, J., Warlow, C., Sandercock, P. & Slattery, J. (1989) Projecting the number of patients with first-ever strokes and patients newly handicapped by stroke in England and Wales. *British Medical Journal* **298**, 656–660.

Mamoli, A., Censori, B., Casto, L., Sileo, C., Cesana, B. & Camerlingo, M. (1999) An analysis of the costs of ischemic stroke in an Italian stroke unit. *Neurology* **53**, 112–116.

Mant, J., Carter, J., Wade, D.T. & Winner, S. (1999) Randomised controlled trial of a Stroke Family Support Organiser. *Cerebrovascular Diseases* **9** (Suppl. 1), 123.

Mant, J., Langhorne, P., Dennis, M. & Winner, S. (2000) Stroke liaison workers for stroke survivors and their carers. In: *The Cochrane Library*. Oxford: Update Software.

Martin, J., Meltzer, H. & Elliot, D. (1988) *The Prevalence of Disability Among Adults*. Office of Population Censuses and Surveys. HMSO, London.

Martin, P.J., Young, G., Enevoldson, T.P. & Humphrey, P.R.D. (1997) Overdiagnosis of TIA and minor stroke: experience at a regional neurovascular clinic. *Quarterly Journal of Medicine* **90**, 759–763.

Mathew, N.T., Rivera, V.M., Meyer, J.S., Charney, J.Z. & Hartmann, A. (1972) Double-blind evaluation of glycerol therapy in acute cerebral infarction. *Lancet* ii, 1327–1329.

Mayo, N.E., Wood Dauphinee, S., Côte, R. *et al.* (2000) There's no place like home. An evaluation of early supported discharge for stroke. *Stroke* **31**, 1016–1023.

Moloney, A., Critchelow, B. & Jones, K. (1999) A multi-disciplinary care pathway in stroke: does it improve care? *Age and Ageing* **28** (Suppl. 1), 42–43.

Murray, C.J.L. & Lopez, A.D. (1997) Mortality by cause for eight regions of the world: Global Burden of Disease Study. *Lancet* **349**, 1269–1276.

National Institute of Neurological Disorders and Stroke (NINDS) rt-PA Stroke Study Group (1997) A systems approach to the immediate evaluation and management of hyperacute stroke: experience at eight centers and implications for community practice and patient care. *Stroke* **28**, 1530–1540.

Nouri, F.M. & Lincoln, N.B. (1987) An extended activities of daily living scale for stroke patients. *Clinical Rehabilitation* **1**, 301–305.

Odderson, I.R. & McKenna, B.S. (1993) A model for management of patients with stroke during the acute phase: outcome and economic implications. *Stroke* **24**, 1823–1827.

O'Mahony, P.G., Rodgers, H., Thompson, R., Dobson, R. & James, O.F.W. (1997) Satisfaction with information and advice received by stroke patients. *Clinical Rehabilitation* **11**, 68–72.

Persson, U., Silverberg, R., Lindgren, B. *et al.* (1990) Direct costs of stroke for a Swedish population. *International Journal of Technology Assessment in Health Care* **6**, 125–137.

Peto, R. (1980) Monitoring cancer patients in clinical trials need not be precise. In: *Cancer: Assessment and Monitoring* (eds T. Symington, A.E. Williams & J.G. McVie), pp. 377–381. Churchill Livingstone, Edinburgh.

Pitner, S.E. & Mance, C.J. (1973) An evaluation of stroke intensive care: results of a municipal hospital. *Stroke* **4**, 737–741.

Pound, P., Gompertz, P. & Ebrahim, S. (1994) Patients' satisfaction with stroke services. *Clinical Rehabilitation* **8**, 7–17.

Pound, P., Tilling, K., Rudd, A.G. & Wolfe, C.D.A. (1999) Does patient satisfaction reflect differences in care received after stroke? *Stroke* **30**, 49–55.

Price, C.I.M., Curless, R.H. & Rodgers, H. (1999) Can stroke patients use visual analogue scales? *Stroke* **30**, 1357–1361.

Rankin, J. (1957) Cerebral vascular accidents in people over the age of 60, 2: prognosis. *Scottish Medical Journal* **2**, 200–215.

Ricci, S., Celani, M.G., La Rosa, F. *et al.* (1991) SEPIVAC: a community-based study of stroke incidence in Umbria, Italy. *Journal of Neurology, Neurosurgery and Psychiatry* **54**, 695–698.

Robinson, R. (1993a) Economic evaluation and health care: what does it mean? *British Medical Journal* **307**, 670–673.

Robinson, R. (1993b) Economic evaluation and health care: costs and cost-minimisation analysis. *British Medical Journal* **307**, 670–673.

Robinson, R. (1993c) Economic evaluation and health care: cost-effectiveness analysis. *British Medical Journal* **307**, 793–795.

Rodgers, H., Soutter, J., Kaiser, W. *et al.* (1997) Early supported hospital discharge following acute stroke: pilot study results. *Clinical Rehabilitation* **11**, 280–287.

Rodgers, H., Thomson, R.G., Gani, A. *et al.* (1999) *Teesside Stroke Register Final Report. II. Service utilization final report for NHS R&D Programme, University of Newcastle.*

Ronning, O.M. & Guldvog, B. (1998) Outcome of subacute stroke rehabilitation: a randomized controlled trial. *Stroke* **29**, 779–784.

Rothwell, P.M., Wroe, S.J., Slattery, J. & Warlow, C.P. (1996) Is stroke incidence related to season or temperature? *Lancet* **347**, 934–936.

Royal College of Physicians Research Unit & UK Stroke Audit Group (1994) *Stroke Audit Package*. Royal College of Physicians, London.

Rudd, A.G., Wolfe, C.D., Tilling, K. & Beech, R. (1997) Randomised controlled trial to evaluate early discharge scheme for patients with stroke. *British Medical Journal* **315**, 1039–1044.

Rudd, A.G., Irwin, P., Rutledge, Z. *et al.* (1999) The National Sentinel Audit for stroke: a tool for raising standards of care. *Journal of the Royal College of Physicians of London* **33**, 460–464.

Sacco, R.L., Boden-Albala, B., Gan, R., Chen, X., Kargman, D.E. & Shea, S. (1998) Stroke incidence among white, black, and Hispanic residents of an urban community: the North Manhattan stroke study. *American Journal of Epidemiology* **147**, 259–268.

Scandinavian Stroke Study Group (1985) Multicenter trial of hemodilution in ischemic stroke: background and study protocol. *Stroke* **16**, 885–890.

Schuling, J., De Haan, R., Limburg, M. & Groenier, K.H. (1993) The Frenchay Activities Index: assessment of functional status in stroke patients. *Stroke* **24**, 1173–1177.

Scott, J.T., Entwistle, V.A., Sowden, A.J. & Watt, I. (2000) Provision of recordings or summaries of consultations to people with cancer. In: *The Cochrane Library*. Oxford: Update Software.

Scottish Intercollegiate Guidelines Network (SIGN) (1997) *The Management of Patients with Stroke, 1: Assessment, Investigation, Immediate Management and Secondary Prevention*. SIGN, Edinburgh.

Scottish Intercollegiate Guidelines Network (SIGN) (1999) *An Introduction to SIGN Methodology for the Development of Evidence-Based Clinical Guidelines*. SIGN, Edinburgh.

Scottish Stroke Services Audit (1999) *Report on an Audit of the Organisation of Services for Stroke Patients, 1997–98*. Royal College of Physicians and Surgeons of Glasgow, Glasgow.

Secretary of State for Health (1992) *The Health of the Nation*. HMSO, London.

Shinar, D., Gross, C.R., Bronstein, K.S. *et al.* (1987) Reliability of the activities of daily living scale and its use in telephone interview. *Archives of Physical Medicine and Rehabilitation* **68**, 723–728.

Smurawska, L.T., Alexandrov, A.V., Bladin, C.F. & Norris, J.W. (1994) Cost of acute stroke care in Toronto, Canada. *Stroke* **25**, 1628–1631.

State University of New York at Buffalo (1993) *Guide for Use of the Uniform Data Set for Medical Rehabilitation (Adult FIM)*, Version 4.0. State University of New York at Buffalo, Buffalo, NY.

Stegmayr, B., Asplund, K., Hulter-Asberg, K. *et al.* (1999) Stroke units in their natural habitat: can results of randomized trials be reproduced in routine clinical practice? *Stroke* **30**, 709–714.

Stewart, J.A., Dundas, R., Howard, R.S., Rudd, A.G. & Wolfe, C.D.A. (1999) Ethnic differences in incidence of stroke: prospective study with stroke register. *British Medical Journal* **318**, 967–971.

Stroke Unit Trialists' Collaboration (1997) Collaborative systematic review of the randomised trials of organised inpatient (stroke unit) care after stroke. *British Medical Journal* **314**, 1151–1159.

Stroke Unit Trialists' Collaboration (2000) Organised inpatient (stroke unit) care for stroke. In: *The Cochrane Library*. Oxford: Update Software.

Sudlow, C.L.M. & Warlow, C.P. (1996) Comparing stroke incidence worldwide: what makes studies comparable? *Stroke* **27**, 550–558.

Sudlow, C.L.M. & Warlow, C.P. (1997) Comparable studies of the incidence of stroke and its pathological types: results from an international collaboration. *Stroke* **28**, 491–499.

Sulch, D., Peraz, I., Melbourn, A. & Kalra, L. (2000) Randomized controlled trial of integrated (managed) care pathway for stroke rehabilitation. *Stroke* **31**, 1929–1934.

Taylor, T.N., Davis, P.H., Torner, J.C., Holmes, J., Meyer, J.W. & Jacobson, M.F. (1996) Lifetime cost of stroke in the United States. *Stroke* **27**, 1459–1466.

Terent, A. (1988) Increasing incidence of stroke amongst Swedish women. *Stroke* **19**, 598–603.

Terent, A., Marke, L.A., Asplund, K., Norrving, B., Jonsson, E. & Wester, P.-O. (1994) Costs of stroke in Sweden: a National perspective. *Stroke* **25**, 2363–2369.

Thomas, J.W. & Hofer, T.P. (1998) Research evidence on the validity of risk-adjusted mortality rate as a measure of hospital quality of care. *Medical Care Research and Review* **55**, 371–404.

Thomson, R.G., Rodgers, H., Gani, A. *et al.* (1999) *Teesside Stroke Register Final Report. I. Epidemiology final report for NHS R&D Programme, University of Newcastle.*

Tukey, J.W. (1962) The future of data analysis. *Annals of Mathematical Statistics* **33**, 1–67.

Vemmos, K.N., Bots, M.L., Tsibouris, P.K. *et al.* (1999) Stroke incidence and case fatality in southern Greece: the Arcadia Stroke Registry. *Stroke* **30**, 363–370.

Vickers, N. & Pollock, A. (1993) Incompleteness and retrieval of case note in a case note audit of colorectal cancer. *Quality in Health Care* **2**, 170–174.

Wade, D.T. (1992) *Epidemiologically Based Needs Assessment, Report 3: Stroke.* NHS Management Executive, London.

Wade, D.T., Langton-Hewer, R., Skilbeck, C.E., Bainton, D. & Burns-Cox, C. (1985) Controlled trial of a home-care service for acute stroke patients. *Lancet* **i**, 323–326.

Ware, J.E. & Sherbourne, C.D. (1992) The MOS 36-item short form health survey (SF-36), 1: conceptual framework and item selection. *Medical Care* **30**, 473–483.

Weir, N. & the Scottish Stroke Outcomes Group (1999) Stroke league tables: are they likely to reflect differences in quality? *Cerebrovascular Diseases* **9** (Suppl. 1), 115.

Wellwood, I., Dennis, M.S. & Warlow, C.P. (1994) Perceptions and knowledge of stroke among surviving patients with stroke and their carers. *Age and Ageing* **23**, 293–298.

Wellwood, I., Dennis, M. & Warlow, C. (1995a) Patients' and carers' satisfaction with acute stroke management. *Age and Ageing* **24**, 519–524.

Wellwood, I., Dennis, M.S. & Warlow, C.P. (1995b) A comparison of the Barthel Index and the OPCS disability instrument used to measure outcome after acute stroke. *Age and Ageing* **24**, 54–57.

Wentworth, D.A. & Atkinson, R.P. (1996) Implementation of an acute stroke program decreases hospitalization costs and length of stay. *Stroke* **27**, 1040–1043.

Wester, P., Radberg, J., Lundgren, B., Peltonen, M. for the Seek-Medical-Attention-in-Time Study Group (1999) Factors associated with delayed admission to hospital and in-hospital delays in acute stroke and TIA: a prospective, multicentre study. *Stroke* **30**, 40–48.

Widen Holmqvist, L., von Koch, L., Kostulas, V. *et al.* (1998) A randomized controlled trial of rehabilitation at home after stroke in southwest Stockholm. *Stroke* **29**, 591–597.

Wolfe, C.D.A., Tilling, K., Beech, R., Rudd, A.G. for the European BIOMED Study of Stroke Care Group (1999) Variations in case fatality and dependency from stroke in Western and Central Europe. *Stroke* **30**, 350–356.

Wood-Dauphinee, S., Shapiro, S., Bass, E. *et al.* (1984) A randomized trial of team care following stroke. *Stroke* **15** (5), 864–872.

Wroe, S.J., Sandercock, P., Bamford, J., Dennis, M., Slattery, J. & Warlow, C. (1992) Diurnal variation in incidence of stroke: Oxfordshire Community Stroke Project. *British Medical Journal* **304**, 155–157.

Young, J.B. & Forster, A. (1992) The Bradford community stroke trial: results at six months. *British Medical Journal* **304**, 1085–1089.

Young, J.B. & Forster, A. (1993) Day hospital and home physiotherapy for stroke patients: a comparative cost-effectiveness study. *Journal of the Royal College of Physicians of London* **27** (3), 252–257.

CHAPTER EIGHTEEN

Reducing the burden of stroke and improving the public health

18.1 Introduction

The huge burden of stroke on patients, their families and friends, and society is constantly and appropriately being emphasized (Warlow 1998a). Stroke is the third most common cause of death worldwide after coronary heart disease and all cancers put together, causing about 4.4 million deaths in 1990 (Murray & Lopez 1997). It is the most common life-threatening neurological condition and stroke disability is the most important single cause of severe disability in people living in their own homes in the UK (Martin *et al.* 1988). In Scotland, stroke consumes almost 5% of the entire National Health Service budget (Isard & Forbes 1992). In descending order of interest to most clinicians but, as we shall see, not in order of likely impact on the public health, there are four complementary strategies to reduce stroke burden (Fig. 18.1):

- treating first-ever-in-a-lifetime and recurrent acute strokes to reduce case fatality and maximize independence and quality of life in the survivors (section 18.3);
- reducing the risk of stroke after transient ischaemic attack (TIA), and of recurrent stroke after a first-ever-in-a-lifetime stroke (secondary prevention) (section 18.4);
- seeking out and treating people at particularly high risk of stroke to reduce their risk (the 'high-risk' strategy for primary prevention) (section 18.5);
- reducing the average level of causative risk factors in the whole population (the 'mass' strategy for primary prevention) (section 18.6).

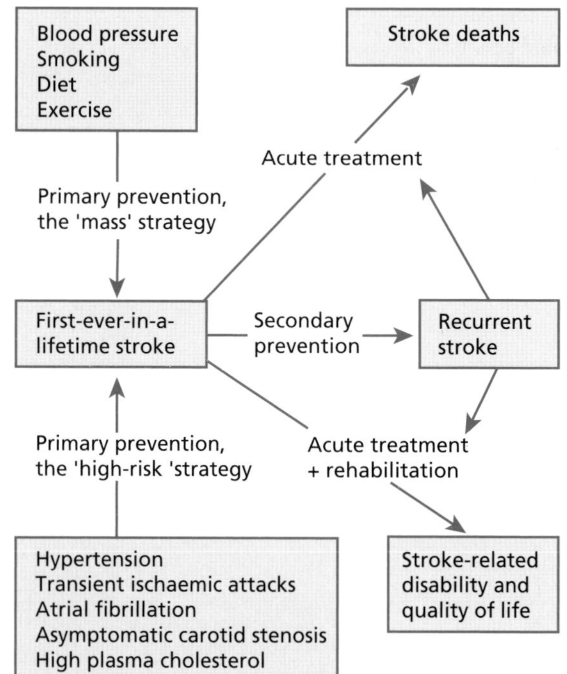

Fig. 18.1 Strategies for reducing the burden of stroke.

However, we must first consider how the burden of stroke can be monitored routinely over time so that goals to reduce it can be set, and then worked towards by implementing the four strategies. Secondly, we must compare their effectiveness, practicability and cost where we can.

Stroke is the third most common cause of death worldwide, the most common life-threatening neurological condition, and the most important single cause of severe disability in people living in their own homes.

18.2 Changes in the burden of stroke with time

At present, mortality statistics are the only *routinely* available method for monitoring the burden of stroke with time. But, even this method is woefully inaccurate in almost all developing countries, and leaves much to be desired even in developed countries. No country in the world has a routine method of monitoring stroke *incidence* because this is so difficult to measure at one point in time, let alone at several (section 18.2.2). Hospital discharge rates are unreliable: admitted patients generally have more severe strokes, the proportion of strokes admitted is mostly unknown and could change unpredictably and unmeasurably with time as a result of bed availability, new treatments, and variation in admission policy (Giroud *et al.* 1997) (section 17.2.1). Moreover, many routine coding systems double-count patients as they move from one service to another within the same hospital. Nor is there a routine method for monitoring stroke case fatality and outcome in survivors, and certainly not for monitoring the cost of stroke. Stroke prevalence depends on both incidence and case fatality. Therefore, any change would be impossible to interpret without also measuring one of its two components. In any event, prevalence is tedious and time consuming to measure; it is probably inaccurate because distant and mild strokes are forgotten and the evidence for any past stroke may not be very good. Different screening methods can yield very different estimates in the same population and we have no idea if the answers to screening questions are affected by cultural factors, or at different time periods in the same culture (Di Carlo *et al.* 1999) (section 17.2.2). Therefore, unless community-based incidence studies can be repeated, or sustained over time with rigorous standardization of their methods, which has seldom been achieved, the only realistic way to assess the success of strategies for reducing stroke burden is by monitoring stroke mortality (section 18.7). So, how reliable are routine stroke mortality statistics, what do they mean, and is stroke mortality changing?

18.2.1 Time trends in stroke mortality

There is no doubt there have been substantial changes in stroke mortality in both men and women at all ages, over the past few decades (Bonita & Beaglehole 1993). In most Western countries and Japan, rates have fallen by up to 7% per year in parallel with falling (but not so fast) mortality for coronary heart disease (Fig. 18.2). However, in some countries, particularly in Eastern Europe, both stroke and coronary heart disease mortality have been rising from an already high level, while in the United States stroke mortality has levelled off (Gillum & Sempos 1997; Massing *et al.* 1998). What explains these changing rates? Is stroke incidence changing, the most common assumption, or are there other plausible explanations?

Changes in death certification practice

The decline in stroke mortality has been so consistent in so many countries that it is unlikely to be entirely due to a systematic change in how death certificates have been completed and then coded. However, there are many ambiguous situations where coding practices may vary. For example, when a patient who remains bedridden after a stroke and dies of pneumonia 6 months later, the underlying cause of death may be coded either as pneumonia, with stroke not

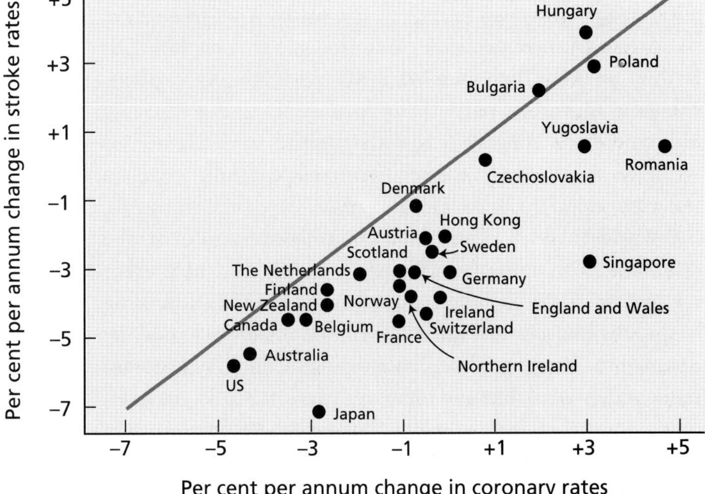

Fig. 18.2 A comparison of the annual percentage decline of age-standardized mortality due to stroke, and to coronary heart disease, in men aged 40–69 years between 1970 and 1985 in 27 countries with reasonably reliable data (with permission from Bonita *et al.* 1990).

even mentioned on the death certificate, or as stroke. The documented inaccuracy of death certification of stroke, particularly in the elderly where most strokes occur, is of concern, even though this may be improving at least when stroke patients are admitted to hospitals with CT scanning facilities (Corwin *et al.* 1982; Hasuo *et al.* 1989; Iso *et al.* 1990). In times past, sudden death may have been certified as due to stroke but, as we now know, only subarachnoid haemorrhage causes death within minutes of symptom onset (section 5.6.1). Sudden death is far more likely to be caused by some complication of coronary heart disease, particularly a dysrhythmia (Phillips *et al.* 1977; Thomas *et al.* 1988). Recognizing and then avoiding this artifact may explain some of the decline in stroke mortality, particularly in Japan in the early postwar years (Netsky & Miyaji 1976). However, this artifact is unlikely to be the explanation for the later fall in stroke mortality in Japan, as well as in western European and North American countries.

Errors in age standardization

Older populations have a higher stroke mortality than younger populations. Therefore, if mortality is measured in age-band strata that are too wide, any change in the distribution of the age of people within various substrata of a single stratum could lead to apparent rather than real changes in stroke mortality. After all, even across a mere 10-year age difference, stroke mortality can more than double (Bonita & Beaglehole 1993). This problem is particularly pertinent in the oldest age stratum with an open upper end (e.g. 80 years plus), because this stratum might contain people of very different ages and the proportion of people at these different ages may change with time.

Changes in diagnostic accuracy

The clinical diagnosis of stroke vs. not-stroke as a cause of death should be reasonably secure in countries with good health care even though post-mortem rates to confirm the diagnosis have declined precipitously (Lanska 1993). It is thus unlikely that inaccurate diagnosis wholly explains changing mortality, particularly in patients under 75 years old where the diagnosis is rather easier and, rightly or wrongly, more likely to be attempted carefully than in the very elderly. Of course, for *epidemiological* purposes, the World Health Organization clinical definition of stroke (Hatano 1976) must be adhered to rigidly and at present we can see no compelling reason for any modification using brain imaging. A definition based on imaging would be doomed to change with time as imaging technology becomes more widely available, and improves (section 3.2.3). In developing countries, and indeed in cultures where post-mortem is culturally unacceptable, the technique of 'verbal autopsy' may be better than nothing but there is no standard methodology. It requires questioning of all relevant family, carers, witnesses, medical and other staff as soon after death as possible, as well as local validation against some reasonable 'gold-standard', which has seldom been achieved (Chandramohan *et al.* 1994; Kaufman *et al.* 1997).

Competing causes of death

It has been argued that stroke mortality is declining because those likely to die of stroke are now dying earlier of coronary heart disease, or some other non-stroke cause. Actually, this is unlikely because, in countries where stroke mortality is falling, coronary heart disease and overall mortality are also falling (Fig. 18.2). In fact, because myocardial infarction and ischaemic stroke share the same risk factors, and so the same sort of people have both, it is conceivable that more effective treatment after acute myocardial infarction, and so longer survival, might leave *more* people at high risk of stroke and so *increase* stroke mortality (Bonneux *et al.* 1997).

Changes in the mixture of stroke types

Certain types of stroke are far more likely to cause death than others. For example, the 30-day case fatality after lacunar infarction is less than 5%, whereas after total anterior circulation infarction it is about 40% (Table 10.2). If, therefore, the proportion of strokes due to lacunar infarction is increasing, and the proportion due to total anterior circulation infarction is decreasing, then stroke mortality would fall even if overall stroke incidence remained constant. This kind of detail of stroke type is simply not available or accurate in routine mortality statistics, and even in incidence studies it is difficult to achieve (section 17.2.1).

Changes in case fatality

There is evidence that patients are surviving longer after stroke (Immonen-Raiha *et al.* 1997; Peltonen *et al.* 1998). This might have the effect of reducing stroke mortality (but not incidence) because patients remaining alive longer would be more likely to die of an intercedent non-stroke event, such as myocardial infarction, than of the stroke itself. Improved survival could be due to:

- a change in the relative proportion of various stroke types for which there is no evidence one way or the other (e.g. a higher proportion of lacunar strokes, see above);
- improvements in drug treatment of acute stroke, which is unlikely because until recently none have been effective (section 11.2.3);
- improvements in nursing care which is plausible but unproven;
- the introduction of Stroke Units, but this is only a recent and as yet far from widespread development (section 17.4.2); or

• strokes may have been getting milder.

Of course, another, quite likely, explanation is simply that milder strokes are now more often *identified*, because patient expectations are rising and we are all becoming diagnostically more competent and increasingly helped by more sensitive brain imaging. Naturally, stroke survival then 'improves'. Also, perhaps what were once called transient ischaemic attacks are now called strokes, a tendency that would again apparently improve stroke survival.

In summary therefore, there are several more-or-less plausible reasons for changes in stroke mortality which are nothing to do with changes in incidence. A fall (or rise) in stroke mortality does not necessarily mean that there has been a fall (or rise) in incidence. Unfortunately, stroke incidence is tedious and expensive to measure at one point in time (section 17.2.1), and even more so at several points in time (section 18.2.2), and nowhere is this routine practice. Indeed, it might be more cost-effective to improve on all the possible biases and inaccuracies of routinely collected mortality statistics and then use them as an (imperfect) surrogate for stroke incidence. However, there will be continuing concern about their accuracy, particularly between different countries, and also even within one country at different times. At present, it is very uncertain that stroke mortality can be safely extrapolated to stroke incidence, particularly when it seems as though changes in mortality have been much more dramatic than changes in incidence (section 18.2.2).

Stroke mortality is falling in many countries, but it is unclear whether this is due to a fall in stroke incidence, lower case fatality, or some artifact of the collection and analysis of routine mortality data.

18.2.2 Time trends in stroke incidence

Measuring stroke incidence accurately is not technically difficult but requires more resources than are available in routine clinical and public health practice, and it is time consuming (Sudlow & Warlow 1996). As a consequence, not many stroke incidence studies meet an ideal standard, or even a more-or-less ideal standard, when set against explicit methodological criteria; those that do come only from developed countries (section 17.2.1). Very few have been repeated, or continued for long enough, to provide reliable time trend information. The best known comes from Rochester, Minnesota, USA, where stroke incidence fell remarkably in the 1960s and 1970s, but then stabilized and slightly increased (Brown *et al.* 1996). Elsewhere the situation is confused. Although incidence has fallen in Hisayama, Japan, Novosibirsk, Russia, Finland, and Perth, Australia (Ueda *et al.* 1981; Feigin *et al.* 1995; Tuomilehto *et al.* 1996; Jamrozik *et al.* 1999), it has not in Auckland, New Zealand, Dijon, France or Shanghai, China (Bonita *et al.* 1993; Hong *et al.* 1994; Lemesle *et al.* 1999). It has actually risen in Soderhamn, Sweden and Frederiksberg, Denmark (Terent 1988; Jorgensen *et al.* 1992). For other parts of the world there is simply no reliable information. Very few time trend studies have divided strokes into their different pathological types. Indeed, not only are the numbers of intracerebral haemorrhages much smaller than ischaemic strokes so that estimates of frequency are imprecise, but brain computed tomography to differentiate between them has either not been practicable in community-based incidence studies (which are essential for measuring stroke incidence), or has only become widely available relatively recently. Although the numbers are again small, the incidence of aneurysmal subarachnoid haemorrhage has probably not changed in reality, but has been markedly over-estimated in the past (Linn *et al.* 1996). Community-based stroke incidence studies can also, with very few extra resources, keep track of survival and dependency in survivors as potential indicators of the quality of stroke care, if both casemix and chance are allowed for (section 17.6.3).

In the few places where it has been measured reasonably reliably, stroke incidence seems to have declined, stayed the same, or increased. However, it has been very difficult to use consistent methods and to obtain large enough sample sizes for precise estimates. In truth, it is not very clear what incidence rates are doing.

It is distinctly odd that stroke mortality has fallen so much in places like Sweden and New Zealand where stroke incidence has not (Bonita *et al.* 1993; Peltonen *et al.* 1998). In Auckland, it seems stroke severity has declined but maybe the medical services became better at recognizing mild strokes. However, in Perth, Australia, case fatality has not changed (Jamrozic *et al.* 1999). As well as the problems with mortality statistics (section 18.2.1), another possibility for this incidence/mortality disparity, is the imprecision of most incidence studies and the play of chance. Not only do these studies have to be sustained over time, or repeated at two different times, without any change in their methods (case-finding, definitions, etc.), but, most importantly, they have to be big enough to minimize the effect of chance and so provide precise incidence estimates (Asplund *et al.* 1995; WHO MONICA Project 1997). For example, to have a 90% probability of reliably demonstrating a 1% per annum decline in incidence over 10 years requires a population of one million people to be surveyed twice (about 2000 first-ever-in-a-lifetime strokes in the first year, and 1800 in the tenth). This size has not so far been achieved. Finally, if hospital admission rates have risen for mild strokes, then incidence studies which relied on most stroke patients being admitted to hospital would incorrectly conclude that strokes are getting milder. Certainly, overall hospital admission rates have changed with time, for example increasing from 79% to 88% in Perth, Australia (Jamrozic *et al.* 1999).

18.2.3 Why is stroke incidence changing, if it really is?

If we do not really know whether stroke incidence is changing, then it is perhaps premature to ask *why* it is changing. However, many people have assumed, rightly or wrongly, that because stroke mortality is declining in many countries, stroke incidence *must* be declining and have then attempted to provide explanations. A further assumption is often made that this decline is to do with the medical treatment of causative risk factors, particularly hypertension (Whisnant 1984). However, calculations have shown that the drug treatment of hypertension cannot possibly explain more than 25% of the decline in stroke mortality, although this may not necessarily reflect incidence (Bonita 1994). Nor can the identification and treatment of TIAs have had much impact on stroke incidence, largely because only a small proportion of strokes are preceded by TIAs (Warlow 1998b) (section 18.4.1). A general decline in the prevalence and level of causative risk factors in the population, such as high blood pressure, has been suggested. Indeed, there is some evidence for this impacting on stroke mortality but not, curiously, on stroke incidence, and there is some evidence for an impact on coronary heart disease as well (Tuomilehto *et al.* 1991; Vartiainen *et al.* 1994, 1995; Hu *et al.* 2000). It is conceivable that reduction of the salt content of preserved food as a consequence of refrigeration *might* have lowered the average population blood pressure, but we cannot be sure. On the other hand, there is a lot of salt in modern processed food.

Therefore, although stroke mortality has almost certainly declined in most developed countries, it is not at all clear that this reflects declining stroke incidence. It could be that incidence is not changing at all. Of course, because most populations are ageing, the *number* of stroke patients will certainly increase even if the incidence does not. However, the number of *newly* dependent stroke survivors will not necessarily increase as much because elderly dependent people are more likely to die early as a consequence of stroke than young independent people (Malmgren *et al.* 1989).

Rather than attempt to look backwards to explain, with difficulty, any change in stroke burden which may or may not have occurred, it is surely more productive to look forwards and consider the four strategies which *might* reduce stroke burden in the future, whether such strategies could be implemented, and how the effects, if any, could be better monitored from now on. There are still far more questions than answers in this last area, and it is hardly surprising that, at present, no goals based on stroke incidence, severity or outcome are being set, at least not by the UK Government. There are only mortality goals, despite the well-appreciated but much glossed-over imperfections of routinely collected mortality statistics.

18.3 Likely effect of acute stroke treatment on stroke burden in the population

Enormous efforts are being devoted to developing and testing promising new treatments for acute stroke and at long last there has been some progress for ischaemic stroke (Chapter 11). Also, reorganizing haphazard stroke care into Stroke Units is not just an effective strategy to reduce case fatality and dependency, but greatly facilitates randomized trials of new treatments (section 17.4.2).

But what impact might the present treatment of acute stroke be having on the overall burden of stroke? Clearly, it will have no effect on stroke incidence, except that some patients otherwise destined to have a stroke might only have a TIA if they are successfully treated within a few hours of onset. Unfortunately, any impact on stroke mortality will be small. For example, if thrombolysis really did reduce case fatality and could be given to as many as 10% of all ischaemic stroke patients, and not just the 1% or so apparently being achieved in the United States, then overall stroke mortality would be reduced by a mere 0.5% (Table 18.1a). Although aspirin is far less effective than thrombolysis, it can be given to almost all ischaemic stroke patients and therefore could reduce mortality by more, but still by only about 1.5% (Table 18.1b). Stroke Units might reduce overall mortality by 3% (Table 18.1c). Of course, if the national mortality statistics are exaggerated, and many people coded as dying of stroke are in fact dying of something else (section 18.2.1), then the relative (proportional), but still not the absolute, reduction in stroke mortality attributable to acute stroke treatment would be higher. None the less, in the near future, any measurable decline in stroke mortality is most unlikely to be due to the treatment of acute stroke.

The treatment of acute stroke has surprisingly little impact on stroke mortality in the population because either the effect of treatment is weak (like aspirin) or it can only be applied to a small proportion of patients (like thrombolysis).

This rather gloomy message for the public health is because patients die before treatment can be started; treatment is far from completely effective; treatment may be contraindicated in various types of patients, and has risks; and treatment may only work if given within a few hours of stroke onset. Of course, treatment should reduce dependency as well as case fatality but the proportional impact on overall stroke burden is, not surprisingly, very similar (Table 18.2). In fact, stroke dependency cannot easily be monitored over time. It clearly has to be assessed at a fixed time after stroke onset, but so often the patient has gone home so this may be impractical; there are many possible instruments available (section 17.6.3); and there may well be trans-cultural differences in

Table 18.1 The estimated effect of treatment for acute stroke on stroke mortality in England and Wales.

(a) *Thrombolysis with recombinant tissue plasminogen activator (rt-PA) within 3 h of stroke onset*
About 130 000 patients per annum have a first-ever-in-a-lifetime (Bamford *et al.* 1988) or recurrent stroke (Jamrozic *et al.* 1999) of whom about 104 000 (80%) are ischaemic strokes. About 20% die in the first few months (Dennis *et al.* 1993). If rt-PA could be given to as many as 10% of the ischaemic stroke patients (10 400), and if that reduced case fatality by even as much as 3% as suggested by the most widely cited trial which may well be over-optimistic in comparison with the Cochrane review (Wardlaw *et al.* 2000), from 20% to 17% (National Institute of Neurological Disorders and Stroke rt-PA Stroke Study Group 1995) (2080 to1768 dead), then 312 deaths would be avoided or postponed. This is a relative risk reduction of 15%.

However, stroke mortality in England and Wales is 68 000 deaths per annum (Secretary of State for Health 1992).

Therefore, the proportion of stroke mortality avoided or postponed by treatment with rt-PA would be:

$(312/68\,000) \times 100 = \approx 0.5\%$

(b) *Aspirin within 48 h of stroke onset*
About 130 000 patients per annum have a first-ever-in-a-lifetime (Bamford *et al.* 1988) or recurrent stroke (Jamrozic *et al.* 1999) of whom about 104 000 (80%) are ischaemic strokes. About 20% die in the first few months (Dennis *et al.* 1993). If aspirin could be given to all the ischaemic stroke patients, and if that reduced case fatality by 1% (International Stroke Trial Collaborative Group 1997) from 20% to 19% (20 800 to 19 760), then 1040 deaths would be avoided or postponed. This is a relative risk reduction of 5%.

However, stroke mortality in England and Wales is 68 000 deaths per annum (Secretary of State for Health 1992).

Therefore, the proportion of stroke mortality avoided or postponed by treatment with aspirin would be:

$(1040/68\,000) \times 100 = \approx 1.5\%$

(c) *Stroke Units*
About 130 000 patients per annum have a first-ever-in-a-lifetime (Bamford *et al.* 1988) or recurrent stroke (Jamrozic *et al.* 1999) of whom about 104 000 (80%) are ischaemic strokes. About 20% die in the first few months (Dennis *et al.* 1993). If say 70% of all stroke patients (91 000) were admitted to hospital and cared for in a Stroke Unit rather than a general medical ward, and if that reduced case fatality by 2.4%, from 20% to 17.6% (Stroke Unit Trialists' Collaboration 2000) (18 200 to 16 000 dead), then 2200 deaths would be avoided or postponed. This is a relative risk reduction of 12%.

However, stroke mortality in England and Wales is 68 000 deaths per annum (Secretary of State for Health 1992).

Therefore, the proportion of stroke mortality avoided or postponed by treatment in a Stroke Unit would be:

$(2200/68\,000) \times 100 = \approx 3\%$

---

what 'dependency' means. Therefore, it is probably impractical to use dependency as a goal in reducing stroke burden.

18.4 Likely effect and cost of long-term treatment of transient ischaemic attack patients and ischaemic stroke survivors on stroke occurrence: secondary stroke prevention

18.4.1 Effect

Transient ischaemic attack (TIA) patients are at high risk of stroke (section 16.1.1). Of course, TIAs are, in a sense, ischaemic strokes which have recovered in 24 h and so treating TIAs is really secondary stroke prevention. About 25% of TIA patients will have a stroke in 5 years and as many or more a serious cardiac event. Much the same risks apply to ischaemic stroke survivors (section 16.1.3). For many of these individual patients, treatments such as aspirin, which reduces stroke risk by about one-quarter (section 16.4.1), or carotid endarterectomy which reduces stroke risk in suitable patients by about one-half (section 16.8.5), are clearly reasonable. But, what impact will these and other effective treatments for individual TIA, or surviving stroke patients, have at the population level? Very little. Lowering the blood pressure and plasma cholesterol, stopping smoking, antiplatelet drugs for those in sinus rhythm and anticoagulation for those in atrial fibrillation, and carotid endarterectomy will each individually knock off only a few percentage points from stroke incidence and recurrence (Warlow 1998b) (Table 18.3). In combination they might be additive, but we don't know. The reasons for this disappointingly small effect on stroke risk are:

- only about 15% of strokes are preceded by TIAs (see Table 6.1);
- of these TIAs, only about 50% come to medical attention (Dennis *et al.* 1989);
- strokes can occur, or recur, so quickly after presentation that treatment cannot be started in time (section 16.1.1);
- treatment is always much less than 100% effective (Table 18.3);
- there are risks of treatment (Chapter 16); and
- not all patients comply with treatment.

Also, although most patients are eligible for aspirin (section 16.4.2), and many patients for blood pressure control (section 16.3.1), the same cannot be said for carotid endarterectomy which is only indicated in recently symptomatic patients who are fit for surgery and who have severe carotid stenosis—perhaps about 8% of all hospital-referred TIA cases (Hankey *et al.* 1991).

So, we are frustrated by the prevention paradox (section 18.5.2). Although treatment for a relatively small number of high-risk (e.g. TIA) patients will be reasonably effective for many (but not all) in terms of reduced stroke risk, it will have little impact on stroke incidence in the population because

Table 18.2 The estimated effect of treatments for acute stroke on death and dependency in a population of 1 million people of whom about 2400 have a first-ever-in-a-lifetime stroke or recurrent stroke in one year (from Hankey & Warlow 1999).

Intervention	Death or dependency (%)		Relative risk reduction (%)	Absolute risk reduction (%)	Number of deaths/dependents avoided per 1000 patients treated	Number of patients needed to treat to avoid one death or dependency	Target population (% of all 2400 strokes)	Number (%) of deaths/dependents avoided in population of 1 million with 2400 strokes
	Control	Intervention						
Thrombolysis	62.7	56.4	10	6.3	63	16	240 (10)	15 (1.2)
Aspirin	47.0	45.8	3	1.2	12	83	1900 (80)	23 (1.8)
Stroke Unit	62.0	56.4	9	5.6	56	18	1920 (80)	107 (8.3)

Table 18.3 Secondary prevention of stroke: an estimate of the effectiveness and cost of various long-term interventions to reduce the risk of stroke in 12 000 transient ischaemic attack (TIA) patients and stroke survivors in a population of 1 million people (from Hankey & Warlow 1999).

Strategy/ intervention	Stroke risk per year (%)		Relative risk reduction (%)	Absolute risk reduction (%)	Number of strokes avoided per 1000 treated per year	No. of TIA/stroke patients needed to treat to avoid one stroke per year	Target population (% of all prevalent TIA and stroke survivors)	Number of strokes avoided per year among target population	% of all 2400 strokes avoided each year in population of 1 million	Approximate cost per stroke avoided (Australian $)
	Control	Intervention								
Blood pressure lowering drugs	7.0	4.8	28	2.2	22	45	6000 (50)	132	5.5	$1350 (diuretic) $18 000 (ACE inhibitor)
Smoking cessation	7.0	4.7	33	2.3	23	43	3600 (30)	84	3.5	$0 (voluntary) $ < 19 600 (patches for all)
Cholesterol lowering drugs	7.0	5.3	24	1.7	17	59	4800 (40)	81	3.4	$41 000
Antiplatelet drugs							8000 (75% of 10 650 TIA/ ischaemic strokes)			
Aspirin*	7.0	6.0	13	1.0	10	100		80	3.3	$2000
Clopidogrel	7.0	5.4	10	1.6	16	62 (166†)		128 (48†)	5.3 (2.0†)	$74 400
Aspirin + dipyridamole	7.0	5.1	15	1.9	19	53 (111†)		152 (72†)	6.3 (3.0†)	$18 500
Anticoagulants	12.0	4.0	67	8.0	80	12	2130 (20% of 10 650 TIA/ ischaemic strokes) but only up to 1065 (50%) realistically	85	3.5	> $1200
Carotid endarterectomy	8.8	5.0	44	3.8	38	26	850 (8% of 10 650 TIA/ ischaemic strokes)	32	1.3	$182 000

* Relative risk reduction based on only the aspirin vs. control trials in transient ischaemic attack and mild ischaemic stroke patients, not on all antiplatelet drugs vs. control in all high vascular risk patients. † Over and above the effect of aspirin alone.

most strokes occur in patients who have not had a TIA and who are at a lower risk of stroke. Of course, the same treatments are also appropriate after mild first-ever-in-a-lifetime ischaemic stroke and will therefore reduce the risk of recurrent stroke, but this will have no effect on stroke incidence (i.e. the frequency of first-ever-in-a-lifetime stroke). On the other hand, control of vascular risk factors and antithrombotic drugs will usefully reduce the risk of coronary events.

Prevention of stroke after transient ischaemic attacks is an example of the 'high-risk' prevention strategy and will have little effect on stroke incidence, even though the individual transient ischaemic attack patient may have much to gain.

18.4.2 Cost

Any estimates of cost will inevitably have considerable uncertainty around them, but the ranking and relative costs in Table 18.3 are probably reasonably robust even though they do not include the cost of adverse effects and treatment monitoring (Hankey & Warlow 1999). Aspirin, anticoagulants, diuretics and stopping smoking (with will-power rather than nicotine patches), are all affordable and cost much less than a stroke. Angiotensin converting enzyme inhibitors, dipyridamole, statins and clopidogrel are far more expensive and it is clearly crucial to sort out just how effective they are and do more sophisticated economic analyses before widespread prescribing. Carotid endarterectomy is very expensive per stroke avoided which is another reason, as well as its risk, to restrict it to patients who are at *particularly* high risk (section 16.8.9).

18.5 Likely effect of the 'high-risk' strategy for primary stroke prevention

18.5.1 Screening and case-finding for asymptomatic individuals at high risk of stroke

For years it has been axiomatic that we should seek out people who are at the highest risk of a disorder, and then intervene to reduce their individual risks. But, these days there is concern about just what this strategy can achieve in terms of reduced disease burden, at what cost, and to balance any benefits against the potential adverse effects of labelling and treating people as 'patients' when they had previously regarded themselves as perfectly well. Well-intentioned attempts have been made to identify and treat people with severe hypertension to reduce their risk of stroke, people with high plasma cholesterol to reduce their risk of coronary events, people who drink alcohol heavily, people who are obese, people who smoke, and so on. This strategy requires major efforts, particularly in primary care, to identify the 'cases' by systematic screening of everyone in the community (or on a family practice register); or by identifying just high-risk patients with a self-administered questionnaire; or by opportunistic 'case-finding' (for example, by measuring the blood pressure of all adults attending a doctor or nurse for whatever reason) (Holmen *et al.* 1991; Hutchison *et al.* 1998). This activity in itself requires considerable resources. But these pale into insignificance when set against the resources required to actually treat all those at high risk of stroke, i.e. the people who are now deemed to be patients, with behavioural modification or with drugs for years, perhaps for the rest of their lives (Langham *et al.* 1996; Wonderling *et al.* 1996). Moreover, there is increasing evidence that, for many reasons, compliance with treatment in 'real life' is considerably less than in randomized controlled trials, and efforts at health promotion have transient effects, so the overall effectiveness of any treatment is attenuated (Andrade *et al.* 1995; Cupples & McKnight 1999). One must also always remember that it is unethical to identify an individual as high-risk and then be unable to reduce that risk through lack of resources; the individual has gained nothing and may even have lost something by being labelled as 'sick' (Rose 1991). However, despite many potential barriers to the implementation of stroke prevention strategies (Table 18.4), attempts at risk factor control are now quite widespread, at least in people who, in a sense, have shown that they are at the highest risk of all by actually having a stroke (Kalra *et al.* 1998).

Naturally, the 'high-risk' strategy becomes harder to sustain as one attempts to identify and treat not just those at the very highest risk of stroke (e.g. people with a diastolic blood pressure >120 mmHg), but also the many more at somewhat lower risk but who are still clearly *at risk* (e.g. people with a diastolic blood pressure of 110–120 mmHg, all other risk factors being equal) (Fig. 18.3). Also, to make matters worse, the lower the risk of stroke in a group of people (e.g. with moderate rather than severe hypertension), the greater the number who have to be detected and treated to prevent one of them having a stroke. In other words, the less cost-effective treatment becomes (section 18.5.2) (see Tables 11.2 and 18.5). Indeed, it becomes extraordinarily expensive to prevent one stroke if, for example, middle-aged patients with moderate hypertension are treated with even quite inexpensive drugs (Asplund *et al.* 1993).

The 'high-risk' strategy for stroke prevention requires the identification and treatment of people at particularly high-risk of stroke; hypertensives, smokers, diabetics, and those in atrial fibrillation or with severe carotid stenosis.

In places such as North Karelia in Finland, Wales, Japan and China, non-randomized evaluation of the 'high-risk' strategy has sometimes, but not always, shown a reduction in vascular events (Vartiainen *et al.* 1994; Iso *et al.* 1998; Tudor-Smith *et al.* 1998; ; Fang *et al.* 1999). But this is very weak

Table 18.4 Some barriers to the implementation of stroke prevention.

Patients
Lack of knowledge and motivation, so leading to low attendance for blood pressure screening, reporting transient ischaemic attack symptoms, etc.
Poor access to care due to financial or social disadvantage
Cultural factors ('I never see the doctor', etc.)
Interventions may have obvious adverse effects
The cost to the patient if no third-party payer
Intuitive discounting of any stroke in the distant future

Doctors
Lack of knowledge and skills
Lack of time
Lack of training
Lack of incentives, including financial
No positive feedback (prevented strokes are never seen, only the failures of prevention)
Lack of prestige for prevention services
Trained to be reactive rather than proactive philosophy
Failure to delegate to nurses, dieticians, etc.

Health care settings
Other priorities (e.g. acute stroke care)
Lack of resources and systems for preventive care
Lack of status for prevention
Lack of policies, standards and guidelines
Poor communication between primary and secondary care (i.e. no shared-care programmes)

Politicians
Competing demands for fixed and limited resources (e.g. cancer services)
Lack of information from experts
Any political benefits are too long-term to influence re-election prospects

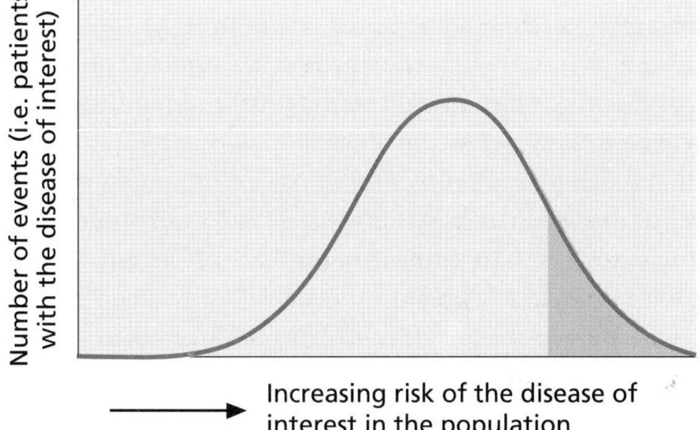

Fig. 18.3 Most cases of a disease occur in people at moderate risk, rather few (shaded) occur in people at the very highest risk in the right-hand tail of a normal distribution.

evidence based on potentially biased observational data. In contrast, any benefit has been disappointingly small in the context of well-organized randomized trials. Indeed, it has proved exceptionally difficult to demonstrate that the 'high-risk' strategy reduces all cause mortality, or coronary and stroke events at all. Perhaps this is because:

- the required sample size is all but impossible to achieve, even with meta-analysis;
- the populations treated were not at high enough risk to have any serious chance of showing any benefit over and above any risks from the interventions;
- the trials were too short-term;
- the patients simply did not have enough incentive to keep up the interventions; or
- randomized trials involving large communities in primary prevention strategies impose too many constraints to be generalizable to real clinical life.

None the less, it is an uncomfortable possibility that the non-randomized comparisons were, as is so often the case, biased and that the 'high-risk' strategy itself is flawed. If so, any more 'health promotion' strategies aimed at essentially asymptomatic, albeit high vascular risk, individuals should be more thoroughly justified and certainly not detract from national fiscal and legislative policies that underpin the 'mass' prevention strategy (McCormick & Skrabanek 1988; Ebrahim & Davey Smith 1997) (section 18.6). After all, when intervention is planned in an apparently healthy population rather than in symptomatic individuals, it is even more important that we are absolutely sure that our efforts are 'effective, affordable, acceptable, humane, accessible and equitable' (Ebrahim & Harwood 1999).

18.5.2 Relative (proportional) vs. absolute risk reduction and the prevention paradox

The higher an individual's risk of the disease to be prevented, and provided the same proportional reduction in risk is achievable from treatment at all levels of baseline risk (see below), then the more he or she has to gain from prevention, and the more cost-effective the intervention becomes (Field *et al.* 1995). In other words, given a constant proportional risk reduction, individuals at highest absolute risk without treatment gain the most from treatment, and the fewer need to be treated to prevent one having a poor outcome (Jackson *et al.* 1993) (Table 18.5). However, the assumption that the *proportional* risk reduction is similar at all levels of baseline risk has seldom been tested. Indeed, to do so requires quite sophisticated modelling of individual patient data at baseline in large randomized trials and meta-analyses to estimate the risk of a poor outcome in each individual, then to place them into strata of risk at the time treatment was started, and then doing a subgroup analysis of treatment effect within

Table 18.5 The number-needed-to-treat to prevent one patient having a poor outcome depends on the baseline absolute risk of the disorder to be prevented as well as on the proportional reduction in risk achieved by treatment.

(a) The effect of increasing baseline risk of stroke (as age and blood pressure increase) on the number of men who need to be treated each year (over the next decade) to prevent one of them having a stroke, assuming a 39% relative, i.e. proportional, risk reduction by treatment at all levels of baseline risk (Kawachi & Purdie 1989)

	Diastolic blood pressure (mmHg)		
Age (years)	90	100	110
30	4292	3217	2423
40	1746	1315	997
50	1059	654	398
60	540	403	281

(b) The effect of increasing baseline risk of coronary death (as age increases, and given the higher risk in men than women) on the number of people who need to be screened and then, if plasma cholesterol > 6.5 mmol/L, treated to prevent one of them dying a coronary death in the next 5 years, assuming a 20% relative, i.e. proportional, risk reduction by treatment at all levels of baseline risk (Khaw & Rose 1989)

Age (years)	Men	Women
25–34	21 067	137 320
35–44	2463	23 244
45–54	586	2224
55–64	231	450

each stratum. For example, there is some unconfirmed evidence that aspirin is less effective at high baseline levels of long-term vascular risk (Rothwell 1995) although the effect is similar in patients with various prior diseases (myocardial infarction, stroke, etc.) and risk factors (hypertensive vs. not, etc.) (Antiplatelet Trialists' Collaboration 1994). Blood pressure lowering has a similar proportional effect at different levels of baseline blood pressure, but people with the same blood pressure can have very different risks depending on the presence of other risk factors (Collins & MacMahon 1994) (section 16.3.1). The assumption of similar proportional risk reductions is clearly *not* true when there is a high risk of treatment at all levels of baseline risk of the disease to be prevented, and yet the treatment benefit is confined to those at the highest risk. For example, the risk of carotid endarterectomy is not worth taking in patients at low risk of stroke where the net proportional risk reduction conferred by surgery is low or even negative. On the other hand, even though the surgical risk is the same, the net benefit is clearly favourable in patients at high baseline risk of stroke, i.e. those with recently symptomatic severe carotid stenosis with additional poor prognostic factors (Rothwell *et al.* 1999) (section 16.8.9). It is conceivable that thrombolytic treatment in acute ischaemic stroke is more effective in mild than severe strokes (Wardlaw *et al.* 1999). Therefore, it is very important that reliable and robust models are developed to estimate individual risk of a poor outcome at baseline, validated in several independent data sets, and then applied to the individual patient data in randomized trials and meta-analyses so that treatment vs. no-treatment can be directly compared within strata of baseline risk. With this approach, the conventional distinction between primary and secondary prevention will become increasingly blurred because there may well be asymptomatic people with an extremely high risk of a first stroke (e.g. elderly man in rheumatic atrial fibrillation with cardiac failure) but symptomatic patients with perhaps a TIA, but with a rather low risk of stroke (e.g. young woman with one episode of amaurosis fugax 6 months ago, a normal heart and no vascular risk factors).

An unfortunate paradox is that the more one refines the 'high-risk' strategy to make it cost-effective (i.e. by focusing preventive efforts on those individuals at highest risk and so reducing the number who need to be treated to prevent one having a stroke), the smaller becomes the proportion of *all* events prevented. What is best for the individual is not necessarily best for society (Rose 1992). This is because most events occur *not* in those at highest risk (because their numbers are small), but in those at moderate risk (because their numbers are very much greater) even though their absolute risk is less than in individuals at highest risk (Whelton 1994) (Fig. 18.3) (Table 18.6). It is said that one-third of all strokes arise from about 20% of the population identified on the basis of a combination of various risk factors (D'Agostino *et al.* 1994). However, it would be enormously expensive to find and treat them all successfully and we would still be failing to prevent the other two-thirds of strokes. It has been further claimed that as many as 80% of all strokes arise in the 20% predicted to be at highest risk, although such precision seems most unlikely to be borne out in practice and the predictive model has not been validated (Coppola *et al.* 1995).

All this risk assessment does of course require doctors to fairly accurately define the absolute risk of stroke in an individual based on a *combination* of risk factors, not just on the level of one (such as blood pressure), and not by guesswork. This is already happening for the risk of coronary events (Grover *et al.* 1995a,b; Wilson *et al.* 1998; Jackson 2000). If a risk is above some pre-specified cut-off level, then intervention is deemed sensible. However, the cut-off point selected must itself depend on the cost and risk of the intervention, as well as the expected benefit in reducing the absolute risk of stroke over a specified period of time (Robson *et al.* 2000). But to do all this, we need well validated and reliable risk tables or equations, most likely programmed into a handheld or desk-top computer. These are becoming available for

Table 18.6 Examples to show that only a small proportion of events occur in people at the highest risk of those events, and that most events occur in people at moderate risk.

(a) Systolic blood pressure and the risk of stroke in men aged 40–49 years. The prevalence of various levels of blood pressure and the incidence and expected number of cases of stroke arising in each blood pressure stratum over 24 years, using Framingham Study data (from Table 2.3 in Ebrahim & Harwood 1999)

Systolic blood pressure (mmHg)	Prevalence (%)	Stroke incidence per 100/24 years	Expected number of strokes calculated from 2nd and 3rd columns (cumulative %)
< 120	16	1.7	27 (5)
120–139	43	3.6	155 (32)
140–159	29	5.6	162 (60)
160–179	8	12.8	102 (78)
180 +	4	31.8	127 (100)
Total			573 (100)

i.e. 78% of strokes occur in people with a systolic blood pressure less than 180 mmHg, and over half of all strokes (60%) in people with levels of less than 160 mmHg

(b) The estimated number and proportion of serious vascular events (stroke, myocardial infarction and vascular death) within 5 years of a transient ischaemic attack or mild ischaemic stroke stratified by the baseline level of risk (from Hankey *et al.* 1993; using UK-TIA Aspirin Trial patients)

Predicted risk of serious vascular events within 5 years (%)	Number of patients in each predicted risk stratum	Predicted number (and cumulative %) of serious vascular events arising in stratum
0–10	236	17 (5)
11–20	509	86 (28)
21–30	389	92 (52)
31–40	220	61 (69)
41–50	117	49 (82)
51–60	73	24 (88)
61–70	42	16 (92)
71–80	30	14 (96)
81–90	24	10 (99)
91–100	13	4 (100)
Total	1653	373 (100)

i.e. only 68 out of 373 (18%) events arise in patients at greater than 50% risk of a serious vascular event

(*continued p. 774*)

estimating the risk of coronary events, notwithstanding the difficulty in deciding which risk estimator to use because the results are not necessarily the same and concerns that a risk model derived from one population does not necessarily 'fit' another population (Menotti *et al.* 2000; Ramachandran *et al.* 2000). It is obviously important to 'set' the sensitivity and specificity of the predictive instrument appropriately (Ramsay *et al.* 1996; Durrington *et al.* 1999; Haq *et al.* 1999; Baker *et al.* 2000). The Framingham model for stroke (and coronary) risk prediction is available on http://www.hbroussais.fr/scientific/fram.eng.html where an individual's risk factors can be entered and a probability of stroke emerges. However, confidence intervals are not provided and the model has not yet been properly validated in an independent data set.

But, inevitably, the 'high-risk' strategy which concentrates on the right-hand end of the normal distribution (i.e. the deviants) misses out the large middle portion (i.e. the normals) from which most strokes will arise, the prevention paradox which has been repeatedly emphasized (Rose 1992) (Fig. 18.3).

Because most strokes arise in people at moderate risk of stroke, concentrating preventive measures only on those at highest risk will have rather little effect on stroke incidence.

18.5.3 Blood pressure lowering and primary stroke prevention

In the context of hypertension, drug treatment reduces an

Table 18.6 (*continued*)

(c) The number and proportion of ipsilateral ischaemic strokes lasting more than 7 days estimated to arise over about 6 years in carotid transient ischaemic attack patients without carotid surgery, stratified by extent of symptomatic carotid stenosis (measured by the European Carotid Surgery Trial method; section 6.7.5)

Symptomatic carotid stenosis (%)	Number of patients in each stenosis stratum*	% risk of stroke ipsilateral to the symptomatic carotid artery†	Number (and cumulative %) of all strokes calculated from 2nd and 3rd columns
0–19	84	6.5	5 (22)
20–29	27	5.1	1 (26)
30–39	22	6.5	2 (35)
40–49	4	6.6	0 (35)
50–59	18	10.8	2 (43)
60–69	17	10.2	2 (52)
70–79	18	8.8	2 (61)
80–89	15	21.4	3 (74)
90–99	9	31.7	3 (87)
Occluded	15	20	3 (100)
Total	229	11.2	23 (100)

i.e. about 50% of strokes occur in patients with less than 70% stenosis, and only about one-quarter of the strokes arise in patients with severe carotid stenosis (80–99%), the range in which carotid endarterectomy is beneficial (section 16.8.5)

* Unpublished data from Hankey *et al.* (1991): a hospital-referred cohort of 229 TIA patients fit enough to be considered for carotid angiography with a view to carotid endarterectomy and studied before the availability of non-invasive carotid tests to screen out from angiography those patients without severe carotid stenosis.
† From the European Carotid Surgery Trial, no-surgery patients, over about 6 years (European Carotid Surgery Trialists' Collaborative Group 1998).

individual's stroke risk by about 38% within a few years (Collins & MacMahon 1994) (section 16.3.1). This sounds, and is, impressive. But if, somehow, treatment were to be given to *all* those people with a systolic blood pressure of 160 mmHg or more, irrespective of their absolute risk of stroke (which would be impossible to achieve in practice, maybe undesirable in the very elderly, as well as costly) then stroke incidence would still be reduced by only 15% (Table 18.7). But, given the lack of effort on the part of some doctors who only see their failures (the strokes) and are never rewarded by their successes (the patients who remain stroke free), the lack of compliance on the part of many patients who felt well until the treatment made them feel unwell, and that it is clearly not cost-effective to treat every 'hypertensive' irrespective of their baseline risk of stroke, the actual effect of blood pressure lowering on stroke incidence will be far less in practice.

18.5.4 Atrial fibrillation and primary stroke prevention

About 20% of patients with first-ever-in-a-lifetime stroke are in atrial fibrillation at or before presentation (Sandercock *et al.* 1992). Therefore, the treatment of fibrillating people could not possibly prevent more than 20% of all strokes. In fact, the likely proportion prevented would be more like 4% if anticoagulation could be delivered to even as many as 50% of all the fibrillating people under the age of 80 years, notwithstanding the considerable logistical problems and the evidence that at present these patients are either untreated or undertreated for various reasons which are difficult to discern (Hart *et al.* 1996; Anderson *et al.* 1998; Mead *et al.* 1999) (section 16.5.1) (Table 18.8). Because aspirin can be given to more fibrillating people than warfarin, where the difficulties and risks of treatment may be unacceptably high, this might also reduce overall stroke incidence by 3% even though it is relatively less effective than warfarin. Aspirin may even reduce overall stroke incidence by about 4% if it were given to fibrillators in all age groups and not just to those under the age of 80 years (Table 18.8). Of course, the more that anticoagulants are focused on those who wish to take them, and who are most likely to have a stroke and the least likely to bleed, the fewer patients have to undergo the rigours of treatment unnecessarily and the less it will cost to prevent one stroke, and to gain one Quality Adjusted Life Year (Atrial Fibrillation Investigators 1994; Howitt & Armstrong 1999; Lip 1999) (Table 18.9). But, the proportion of all incident strokes prevented would be less because of the prevention paradox (section 18.5.2).

Table 18.7 The estimated effect of treating hypertension (defined as systolic blood pressure > 160 mmHg) and so reducing the risk of stroke by 38% (Collins & MacMahon 1994), on stroke incidence, using the population data from Framingham in Table 18.6a.

Systolic blood pressure (mmHg)	Prevalence before treatment (%)	Expected number of strokes before treatment	Expected number of strokes after treatment
Not treated			
< 120	16	27	27
120–139	43	155	155
140–159	29	162	162
Treated			
160–179	8	102	63
180 +	4	127	79
Total		573	486

i.e. a proportional (relative) reduction of (573 − 486)/573 × 100 = 15% in stroke numbers (and in stroke incidence)

Table 18.8 The estimated effect that the antithrombotic treatment of atrial fibrillation might have on stroke incidence.

(a) The prevalence (per 100 population) of patients with atrial fibrillation (AF) by age in various community-based studies, both sexes combined

Reference	Age (years) 50–59	60–69	70–79	80 +
Ostrander *et al.* (1965) Michigan, USA	0.5	1.3	4.1	2.9
Rose *et al.* (1978) Male London civil servants	0.4	N/A	N/A	N/A
Evans (1985) South Tyneside, England	N/A	N/A	3.2	8.0
Hill *et al.* (1987) British General Practice	N/A	N/A	3.0	5.6
Wolf *et al.* (1991) Framingham, USA	0.5	1.8	4.8	8.8
Langenberg *et al.* (1996) Dutch General Practice	N/A	2.8	6.6	10.0
Furberg *et al.* (1994) USA	N/A	N/A	5.8	7.3
Overall approximation*	0.5	2.0	5.0	8.0

(b) The estimated number of strokes likely to occur in Scotland, with and without anticoagulation or aspirin, in patients in AF in 1 year

Age (years)	Number of people in Scotland†	Prevalence of AF/100 population‡	Number of people with AF (from columns 2 and 3)	No treatment§	Anticoagulation¶ (and number of strokes prevented)	Aspirin** (and number of strokes prevented)
50–59	556 956	0.5	2785	111	43 (68)	84 (27)
60–69	515 593	2.0	10 312	412	161 (251)	313 (99)
70–79	345 859	5.0	17 293	692	270 (422)	526 (166)
80 +	168 247	8.0	13 460	538	210 (328)	409 (129)
Total 50 +	1 586 655	2.8	43 850	1753	684 (1069)	1332 (421)

(*continued p. 776*)

Table 18.8 *(continued)*

(c) Calculation of the impact of treatment on stroke incidence

About 30 000 people in Scotland under the age of 80 years are in AF (many would not use anticoagulation over that age because of the risks) (Table 18.8b)
Perhaps 50%, i.e. 15 000 might have no contraindications and be suitable and willing for anticoagulation with warfarin
Of these, about 4% will have a stroke per annum, i.e. 600 (section 16.5.1)
This could be reduced by 61% with warfarin, i.e. to about 234 (section 16.5.1)
Therefore: 600 – 234 = 366 strokes avoided or postponed

In Scotland, there are about 10 000 first-ever-in-a-lifetime strokes per annum (National Medical Advisory Committee 1993)
Therefore: warfarin might reduce stroke incidence by about 366 × 100/10 000 = 4%

Or, if aspirin were given to all 30 000 fibrillating people under the age of 80 years, strokes could be reduced by 24%, i.e. from about 1200 to 912 (section 16.4.1)
Therefore: aspirin might reduce stroke incidence by about 288 × 100/10 000 = 3%

If aspirin were to be given to the 44 000 patients at *all* ages, then the percentage reduction in stroke incidence would be about 4%

* Formal analysis not possible because the studies did not all provide numerators and denominators.
† Official Scottish Population Statistics for 1990, General Registrar for Scotland.
‡ From Table 18.8a.
§ Assuming risk of first-ever-in-a-lifetime stroke of about 4%/year at all ages, and that most fibrillation is 'non-rheumatic' (section 16.5.1).
¶ Relative risk reduction of 61% (section 16.5.1).
** Relative risk reduction of 24% (section 16.4.1).

N/A, not available.

Table 18.9 Results of a decision analysis comparing warfarin with aspirin among people with non-rheumatic atrial fibrillation at three levels of baseline risk (Gage *et al.* 1995).

		Quality adjusted life years gained by treatment			
Risk level	Annual stroke risk (%)	Warfarin treatment	Aspirin treatment	No treatment	Extra cost per QALY, warfarin vs. aspirin
High	5 +	6.51	6.27	6.01	Cheaper
Medium	2.6–4.5	6.60	6.46	6.23	$8000
Low	< 1.6	6.70	6.69	6.51	$370 000

18.5.5 Endarterectomy for asymptomatic carotid stenosis and primary stroke prevention

Although carotid endarterectomy reduces the relative risk of stroke ipsilateral to 'severe' asymptomatic carotid stenosis by between one-third and one-half, the cost-effectiveness is highly questionable; about 50 patients must be operated on to prevent one having a stroke in 3 years (section 16.9.3). None the less, some advocate screening for asymptomatic carotid stenosis and then offering surgery to those fit for surgery (perhaps under the age of 80 years). Not only would this be hugely expensive (about 60 000 carotid endarterectomies would be needed in Scotland to clear the prevalent backlog of 'cases', a country with only about 30 vascular surgeons), but even if surgery was done on *all* those aged 50–79 years, stroke incidence would only be reduced by about 6% in the next year, and maybe by a similar amount in each subsequent year if the unoperated risk of stroke remains constant (Table 18.10). As the years go by, *new* cases of severe stenosis would appear and could be operated on but that would require regular re-screening and the effect on stroke incidence is unclear. Moreover, because the prevalence of asymptomatic stenosis is so low, and no screening test is perfect, screening is likely to identify far more false-positive than true-positive stenoses which could actually lead to more harm than good if inappropriate surgery followed (Lee *et al.* 1997; Whitty *et al.* 1998). It is therefore incumbent on any remaining proponents of screening for asymptomatic carotid stenosis to prove their point in a randomized trial. Until then, screening should be strongly discouraged.

Table 18.10 The estimated effect that endarterectomy for asymptomatic carotid stenosis might have on stroke incidence.

(a) Prevalence of carotid stenosis (about 50–99%) in various studies* by age, males and females combined

	Age (years)			
Reference	50–59	60–69	70–79	80+
Ricci *et al.* (1991) Italy	1/138 (0.7%)	1/101 (1%)	9/60 (15%)	4/21 (19%)
O'Leary *et al.* (1992) USA	N/A	N/A	73/1458 (5%)	28/322 (7%)
Prati *et al.* (1992) Italy	1/236 (0.4%)	8/194 (4%)	13/139 (9%)	5/47 (11%)
Willeit & Kiechl (1993) Austria	6/228 (3%)	22/232 (10%)	25/206 (12%)	N/A
Total	8/602 (1.3%)	31/527 (5.9%)	120/1863 (6.4%)	37/390 (9.5%)

(b) Some studies† reporting the risk of stroke in the distribution of an asymptomatic carotid stenosis

	Number of patients	Mean age (years)	Per cent stenosis‡	Approximate risk of ipsilateral stroke (%)
Meissner *et al.* (1987)	292	67	80+	2.1/year
Norris *et al.* (1991)	177	64	75–99	2.5/year
Hobson *et al.* (1993)	233	65	50–99	9.4 in 4 years
European Carotid Surgery Trialists' Collaborative Group (1995)	127	64	70–99	5.7 in 3 years
Asymptomatic Carotid Atherosclerosis Study Group (1995)	834	67	60–99	11.0 in 5 years

(*continued p. 778*)

18.5.6 Lowering plasma cholesterol and primary stroke prevention

Although increasing plasma cholesterol does not seem to be a risk factor for stroke in observational studies (section 6.3.3), there is persuasive evidence from randomized trials that lowering it does reduce the risk of stroke, non-fatal rather more than fatal, in patients at high risk of coronary events (section 16.3.2). Just how this might translate into reduced stroke incidence is difficult to work out, at least until it is clearer what the long-term stroke risk is in populations at high risk of coronary events, and what level of coronary risk is deemed sufficient to justify the considerable present expense of statin drugs.

18.5.7 Other interventions

At present there are no definitely effective and routine treatments for a raised plasma fibrinogen and trials are in progress to assess the impact of plasma homocysteine lowering (sections 6.3.3 and 16.3.6). Therefore, no calculations have been done to examine the impact of these treatments on stroke incidence. Presumably, amongst all the many benefits of quitting smoking, reduction in stroke incidence is one. Long-term aspirin has nothing to offer apparently healthy middle-aged people because their risk of stroke, and other serious vascular events, is so low. Indeed, the risk of serious intra- and extracranial haemorrhage with aspirin may actually be higher than the risk of stroke. Any risk at all of such adverse events may be unacceptable to people without symptoms (Sudlow & Baigent 1999) (section 16.4.1).

In summary, therefore, identifying and treating patients at particularly high risk of stroke will prevent strokes and benefit some, but by no means all, of those individual patients. However, because most strokes do not occur in those at highest risk, and in many of those at highest risk treatment itself is impracticable or too risky or too expensive to be justified, the 'high-risk' prevention strategy will not have a major impact on stroke incidence. Furthermore, it would be unfortunate if pursuing just the 'high-risk' strategy not only had little effect on stroke incidence, but also distracted us from those at moderate risk who might then believe it was safe to smoke and indulge in other 'unhealthy' activities, because it is from the large number of these moderate risk people that most strokes emerge (Kinlay & Heller 1990).

Table 18.10 (*continued*)

(c) Estimate of the number of strokes avoided or postponed if all patients in Scotland with asymptomatic and 'severe' carotid stenosis were operated on

Age (years)	Population of Scotland§	Per cent with asymptomatic 50–99% carotid stenosis¶	Number with asymptomatic 50–99% carotid stenosis from columns 2 and 3	Number with strokes ipsilateral to asymptomatic carotid stenosis per annum		
				No surgery**	Surgery††	Strokes avoided
50–59	556 956	1.3	7240	145	72	73
60–69	515 593	5.9	30 420	608	304	304
70–79	345 859	6.4	22 135	443	222	221
80 +	168 247	9.5	15 983	320	160	160
Total	1 586 655	—	75 778	1516	758	758

(d) Proportion of first-ever-in-a-lifetime strokes which might be prevented by a policy of screening for asymptomatic carotid stenosis and offering surgery to all those under the age of 80 years

Number of people in Scotland between the ages of 50 and 80 years (above this age surgery not usually recommended) (Table 18.10c): 1 418 408

Number of people with approximately 50–99% asymptomatic carotid stenosis (Table 18.10c): 59 795

Assuming a 2% per annum risk of stroke in the asymptomatic carotid stenosis distribution (Table 18.10b and c), then the number of people with such a stroke each year would be 1196

Assuming a 50% relative reduction in stroke risk with carotid endarterectomy (Table 18.10c), then the number of strokes avoided per annum would be: 1196 × 50/100 = 598

In Scotland about 10 000 first-ever-in-a-lifetime strokes per annum‡‡

Therefore: surgery would avoid about 598 × 100/10 000 of all first strokes in the next year, i.e. about 6%§§

* Studies selected were reasonably large, gave age bands in decades, recorded carotid diameter stenosis at about 50–99% by age, and were population based.

† The selected studies were reasonably large ($n > 100$), mostly prospective, the carotid stenosis was 'severe' and usually unoperated unless it became symptomatic.

‡ Stenosis measured in various different ways.

§ Official Scottish Population Statistics for 1990, General Registrar for Scotland.

¶ From Table 18.10a.

** About 2% per annum, from Table 18.10b.

†† Assuming a 50% relative risk reduction in stroke (section 16.9.3).

‡‡ National Medical Advisory Committee (1993).

§§ It is not possible to calculate the annual figure because the incidence of the development of severe asymptomatic carotid stenosis is unknown.

N/A, not available.

18.6 Likely effect of the 'mass' strategy for primary stroke prevention

In recent years epidemiologists have begun to calculate what the effect might be of not just truncating the right-hand tail of the risk distribution (Fig. 18.3) by treating the high-risk individuals (the 'high-risk' prevention strategy), but of shifting the entire distribution slightly to the left (the 'mass' prevention strategy) (Fig. 18.4). This would not only reduce the mean value of a continuously varying risk factor (such as blood pressure or plasma cholesterol level) but also the number of patients at particularly high risk who are labelled as 'diseased' and so requiring treatment (Table 18.11). But what matters just as much if not more, is not the few events prevented by reducing the small number of high-risk individuals, but the greater number of events avoided in the much larger number of people at moderate risk. As an example, reducing the population mean systolic blood pressure by a mere 1–2% should reduce the incidence of stroke by about 10% (Table 18.12). This sort of reduction in blood pressure

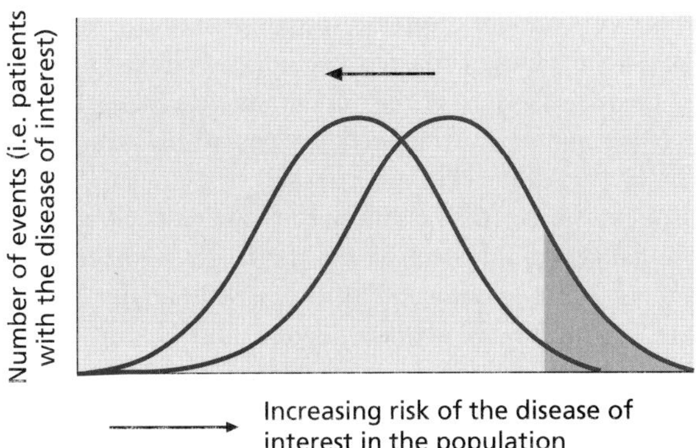

Fig.18.4 The 'mass' strategy of disease prevention involves a small left shift in the risk distribution.

might be achievable by a 'mass' public health strategy, usually involving relatively risk-free lifestyle changes, aimed at the *whole* population where everyone reduces their risk by just a little bit: a slightly lower blood pressure in everyone as well as fewer 'hypertensives', and likewise fewer cigarettes smoked by all smokers as well as more quitters, somewhat more exercise all round as well as more marathon runners, a little less alcohol for all drinkers as well as fewer alcoholics, a touch of weight reduction for all as well as fewer morbidly obese, facilitation of regular exercise by children and adults by discouraging car use and provision of sports grounds and safe cycling facilities, and so on. Also, reducing the prevalence of smoking by a mere 1% could have a surprising impact on stroke burden and cost (Lightwood & Glantz 1997) However, because each individual has very little to gain from this approach, the interventions must be perceived as desirable, fashionable, and enjoyable (cycle tracks, sports fields for sports and not buildings, smoke-free public places, healthy inexpensive non-fattening food, etc.).

The 'mass' strategy for stroke prevention requires, among other things, a small downward shift in the mean population blood pressure by a few millimetres of mercury. This should have a surprisingly large impact on stroke incidence although each individual will gain very little.

Fortunately, an individual's blood pressure is not entirely a matter of genetics, we know this if only because that average blood pressure is lower in the summer than winter (Khaw 1994). Therefore, it may be possible to lower the mean population blood pressure by several millimetres of

Table 18.11 The estimated effect of reducing the mean level of a risk factor in the population on the prevalence of abnormally high values (i.e. of 'disease') (from Rose & Day 1990).

		Predicted fall in prevalence of high values (%)	
Risk factor	Reduction in mean value	From	To
Systolic blood pressure	5 mmHg	15	11
Body weight	1 kg	6	4
Alcohol intake	15 mL/week*	17	15

*Given in mL because equivalence of units of alcohol varies somewhat between countries.

Table 18.12 The estimated effect on stroke incidence of a downward shift in the population mean systolic blood pressure by 1–2% using population data from Framingham (Table 18.7) (from Ebrahim & Harwood 1999).

Systolic blood pressure (mmHg)	Prevalence before intervention (%)	Prevalence after intervention (%)	Expected number of strokes before intervention	Expected number of strokes after intervention
< 120	16	18	27	31
120–139	43	43	155	155
140–159	29	29	162	162
160–179	8	8	102	102
180 +	4	2	127	64
Total			573	514

i.e. a proportional reduction of (573–514)/573 × 100 = 10% in stroke numbers (and incidence) mercury by any one of several non-pharmacological interventions although it has been remarkably difficult to prove this (Cutler 1991; Law *et al.* 1991; Arroll & Beaglehole 1993; Alderman 1994; Whelton *et al.* 1997; Kassirer & Angell 1998; Ebrahim & Davey Smith 1998; Pratt 1999) (sections 6.3.3 and 16.3.1):

• a reduction in salt intake by a tolerable 3 g/day by means of a public health campaign and insistence on labelling the salt content of processed and other foods with a gradual reduction in the permitted concentration, admittedly a hotly debated issue;
• perhaps potassium supplementation of the diet;
• reduced heavy alcohol consumption by safe drinking campaigns;
• stress reduction;
• a general emphasis on weight control by promoting regular exercise and calorie labelling of foods.

Regular exercise and weight control will also reduce the prevalence of diabetes and high plasma cholesterol (Scottish Intercollegiate Guidelines Network 1996; http://www.show.scot.nhs.uk/sign/home.htm). All these interventions depend on education, reduction in poverty, peer pressure, role models, advertising, the media and political action and very little, if at all, on action at the individual doctor level. Moreover, the political will must come not just from the Department of Health but also from the Departments of Finance, Education, Housing, Social Security, Agriculture, Transport and the Environment. In other words, from across the whole of Government. This point is so often missed by commentators who claim that any improvement (or deterioration) in 'health' is inevitably just to do with the Department of Health. These interventions are no more invasive or prescriptive than providing a clean water supply or mass immunization, both of which are clearly in the domain of public health services. But, naturally, one has to accept the prevention paradox, that a strategy that brings large benefits to the community offers very little to each participating individual who is mostly at low risk of stroke (Rose 1981).

This 'mass' strategy cannot be evaluated by a randomized controlled trial, not because the outcome is unmeasurable or because the sample size would have to be too big or it would take too long to demonstrate an effect, but because the strategy requires everybody to be 'treated' and it would simply be impracticable to apply the 'treatment' to a random 50% of the population. The effectiveness has to be taken on trust. But, because it is simple, probably inexpensive and, in theory, makes sense, it would surely be worth pursuing. Of course, because moving the distribution of a risk factor to the left may increase the number of individuals at very low risk of the disease in question, one would need to be reasonably confident that these same individuals would not be systematically disadvantaged in some way:

• if mean population blood pressure was lowered, would the larger number of patients with 'low' blood pressure be put at risk of some unexpected disorder, perhaps, for example, depression or fatigue (Barrett-Connor & Palinkas 1994)?
• if the mean weight of the population was reduced, would the larger number of 'thin' people be put at risk in some way, hypothermia in the elderly perhaps?
• if the mean cigarette consumption was reduced what possible danger could there be for the larger numbers of ex-smokers and non-smokers? And what about the effect on society from loss of taxation income and jobs in cigarette factories?
• would the increased number of non-drinkers really have a higher mortality, particularly from coronary heart disease (section 6.3.3)?
• does very low cholesterol concentration really cause haemorrhagic stroke, or even suicide, if not cancer (section 6.3.3)?
• would increased exercise cause too many injuries, particularly in the osteoporotic elderly, and so attenuate or even reverse the cardiovascular advantages?

Because being simple goes against the grain of societies which believe in a quick technological or mystical fix for illness, or which may crave short-term results in the marketplace, and in societies which exalt the individual over the community, the 'mass' prevention strategy may be very difficult to implement. However, the argument in favour of this strategy for not just stroke prevention, but for health promotion and the prevention of disease in general, is persuasive, if not compelling (Rose 1992).

18.7 Goals, strategies and measuring success (or failure)

Setting targets or goals in any human endeavour is surely reasonable provided they are not so easily achieved that no effort is required, or so difficult that demoralization sets in. This certainly applies to stroke rehabilitation (section 10.3.3) and could be applied to reducing the burden of stroke in the whole community. The difficulty is deciding which target to select. It has to be at the level of the whole community, or a random sample of it, to avoid selection bias; it has to be simple so that it is measurable in very large numbers of people at reasonable cost; it has to be robust so that it can be measured reliably at various points in time; it must be valid and so measure something meaningful; and it almost certainly has to be measurable in routine practice to ensure complete coverage for the foreseeable future. At present, the *only* measure which comes anywhere near fulfilling these criteria is stroke mortality, despite its imperfections (section 18.2.1). Anything else is impracticable (Dennis & Warlow 1991). However, one can reasonably hope, and even expect, that an intervention which reduces stroke incidence and disability would also have *some* impact on stroke mortality, although this impact could well be attenuated by the fact that not all types of stroke are fatal, mortality statistics are inaccurate, and so on. One fear is that in our efforts to improve the accuracy of death certification and coding we might cause an artifactual decline in stroke mortality simply by appropriately moving some patients to another more plausible category of cause of death. After all, there must be something wrong with the mortality data if one year after stroke about 30% of the patients are dead (i.e. 39 000 out of 130 000 first and recurrent strokes in England and Wales in a year) (section 10.2.3), and yet stroke is recorded as the cause of death in about 68 000 patients a year (Secretary of State for Health 1992).

At present, mortality statistics are, despite their imperfections, the only routinely available method to measure the success or failure of stroke prevention programmes.

In the meantime it is surely important to develop some routine method of measuring stroke incidence, as well as of outcome and survival, at the level of the whole community, not just in hospitalized patients. This must be practicable, and inexpensive, which will take time to achieve. At the very least, one might think that routine measurement of stroke outcome is required to inform health-care decisions, for how else can one system or provider of care be compared with another? But maybe even this is too fraught with difficulties to be useful, and measuring process of care is probably more meaningful (section 17.6.3).

As to which stroke prevention strategy to choose, it seems sensible to pursue all of them whilst accepting that each one on its own will not have a dramatic effect (Table 18.13). It would be impossible to deny an effective treatment to an individual if the benefits outweighed the risks, and the cost was acceptable, either to the individual or to a third-party payer. It would be inconceivable not to continue to search for and evaluate treatments for acute stroke. And it would be unforgivable to ignore the theoretical attractions of the 'mass' strategy for stroke prevention.

Finally, almost any strategy for stroke prevention must be intimately linked with almost any strategy for the prevention of coronary heart disease and peripheral vascular disease, because they are largely caused by the same underlying degenerative vascular disorders. So, stroke prevention should not be considered in isolation, but as part of a general strategy for the prevention of all forms of vascular disease, including stroke.

Table 18.13 Summary of the estimated effect of various interventions on stroke incidence, and of the number of people who need to be treated to prevent one having a stroke in 1 year.

Intervention	% reduction in stroke incidence	Number needed to be treated to prevent one stroke in 1 year
Treat systolic blood pressure ≥ 160 mmHg	15 (Table 18.7)	Hundreds, depending on age (Table 18.5)
Reduce population mean systolic blood pressure by 1–2%	10 (Table 18.12)	Thousands
Endarterectomy for asymptomatic severe carotid stenosis	6* (Table 18.10d)	100 (Table 18.10c)
Treatment of hypertension in transient ischaemic attack patients	6 (Table 18.3)	45 (Table 18.3)
Aspirin for atrial fibrillation, all ages	4 (Table 18.8c)	104 (Table 18.8c)
Anticoagulation for atrial fibrillation, age < 80 years	4 (Table 18.8c)	41 (Table 18.8c)
Aspirin for atrial fibrillation, age < 80 years	3 (Table 18.8c)	104 (Table 18.8c)
Aspirin for transient ischaemic attacks	3 (Table 18.3)	100 (Table 18.3)
Endarterectomy for recently symptomatic severe carotid stenosis	1 (Table 18.3)	26 (Table 18.3)

* This figure would decline with time because it can be calculated only for the first year after surgery for all prevalent cases of asymptomatic carotid stenosis; how many *new* cases which might appear thereafter is unknown.

Stroke prevention must not be seen in isolation, but as part of a programme to prevent the clinical manifestations of all forms of degenerative vascular disease.

References

Please note that all references taken from *The Cochrane Library* are given a current date as this database is updated on a quarterly basis. Please refer to the current *Cochrane Library* article for the latest review. The same applies to the *British Medical Journal* 'Clinical Evidence' series which is updated every six months.

Alderman, M.H. (1994) Non-pharmacological treatment of hypertension. *Lancet* **344**, 307–311.

Anderson, D.C., Koller, R.L., Asinger, R.W., Bundlie, S.R. & Pearce, L.A. (1998) Atrial fibrillation and stroke: epidemiology, pathophysiology, and management. *Neurologist* **4**, 235–258.

Andrade, S.E., Walker, A.M., Gottlieb, L.K., *et al.* (1995) Discontinuation of antihyperlipidemic drugs – do rates reported in clinical trials reflect rates in primary care settings? *New England Journal of Medicine* **332**, 1125–1131.

Antiplatelet Trialists' Collaboration (1994) Collaborative overview of randomised trials of antiplatelet therapy I: Prevention of death, myocardial infarction, and stroke by prolonged antiplatelet therapy in various categories of patients. *British Medical Journal* **308**, 81–106.

Arroll, B. & Beaglehole, R. (1993) Exercise for hypertension. *Lancet* **341**, 1248–1249.

Asplund, K., Marke, L., Terent, A., Gustafsson, C. & Wester, P.O. (1993) Costs and gains in stroke prevention: European perspective. *Cerebrovascular Diseases* **3** (Suppl. 1), 34–42.

Asplund, K., Bonita, R., Kuulasmaa, K. *et al.* (1995) Multinational comparisons of stroke epidemiology. Evaluation of case ascertainment in the WHO MONICA Stroke Study. *Stroke* **26**, 355–360.

Asymptomatic Carotid Atherosclerosis Group (1995) Carotid endarterectomy for patients with asymptomatic internal carotid artery stenosis. *Journal of the American Medical Association* **273**, 1421–1428.

Atrial Fibrillation Investigators (1994) Risk factors for stroke and efficacy of antithrombotic therapy in atrial fibrillation. Analysis of pooled data from five randomised controlled trials. *Archives of Internal Medicine* **154**, 1449–1457.

Baker, S., Priest, P. & Jackson, R. (2000) Using thresholds based on risk of cardiovascular disease to target treatment for hypertension: modelling events averted and number treated. *British Medical Journal* **320**, 680–685.

Bamford, J., Sandercock, P., Dennis, M. *et al.* (1988) A prospective study of acute cerebrovascular disease in the community: the Oxfordshire Community Stroke Project 1981–86. I. Methodology, demography and incident cases of first-ever stroke. *Journal of Neurology, Neurosurgery and Psychiatry* **51**, 1373–1389.

Barrett-Connor, E. & Palinkas, L.A. (1994) Low blood pressure and depression in older men: a population based study. *British Medical Journal* **308**, 446–449.

Bonita, R. (1994) Epidemiological studies and the prevention of stroke. *Cerebrovascular Diseases* **4** (Suppl. 1), 2–10.

Bonita, R. & Beaglehole, R. (1993) Explaining stroke mortality trends. *Lancet* **341**, 1510–1511.

Bonita, R., Stewart, A. & Beaglehole, R. (1990) International trends in stroke mortality: 1970–85. *Stroke* **21**, 989–992.

Bonita, R., Broad, J.B. & Beaglehole, R. (1993) Changes in stroke incidence and case-fatality in Auckland, New Zealand 1981–91. *Lancet* **342**, 1470–1473.

Bonneux, L., Looman, C.W.N., Barendregt, J.J. & Van der Maas, P.J. (1997) Regression analysis of recent changes in cardiovascular morbidity and mortality in The Netherlands. *British Medical Journal* **314**, 789–792.

Brown, R.D., Whisnant, J.P., Sicks, J.D., O'Fallon, W.M. & Wiebers, D.O. (1996) Stroke incidence, prevalence, and survival. Secular trends in Rochester, Minnesota, through 1989. *Stroke* **27**, 373–380.

Chandramohan, D., Maude, G.H., Rodrigues, L.C. & Hayes, R.J. (1994) Verbal autopsies for adult deaths: issues in their development and validation. *International Journal of Epidemiology* **23**, 213–222.

Collins, R. & MacMahon, S. (1994) Blood pressure, antihypertensive drug treatment and the risks of stroke and of coronary heart disease. *British Medical Bulletin* **50**, 272–298.

Coppola, W.G.T., Whincup, P.H., Papacosta, O., Walker, M. & Ebrahim, S. (1995) Scoring system to identify men at high risk of stroke: a strategy for general practice. *British Journal of General Practice* **45**, 185–189.

Corwin, L.E., Wolf, P.A., Kannel, W.B. & McNamara, P.M. (1982) Accuracy of death certification of stroke: the Framingham study. *Stroke* **13**, 818–821.

Cupples, M.E. & McKnight, A. (1999) Five year follow up of patients at high cardiovascular risk who took part in randomised controlled trial of health promotion. *British Medical Journal* **319**, 687–688.

Cutler, J.A. (1991) Randomised clinical trials of weight reduction in nonhypertensive persons. *Annals of Epidemiology* **1**, 363–370.

D'Agostino, R.B., Wolf, P.A., Belanger, A.J. & Kannel, W.B. (1994) Stroke risk profile: adjustment for antihypertensive medication. The Framingham Study. *Stroke* **25**, 40–43.

Dennis, M. & Warlow, C. (1991) Strategy for stroke. *British Medical Journal* **303**, 636–638.

Dennis, M.S., Bamford, J., Sandercock, P. & Warlow, C.P. (1989) Incidence of transient ischaemic attacks in Oxfordshire, England. *Stroke* **20**, 333–339.

Dennis, M.S., Burn, J.P.S., Sandercock, P.A., Bamford, J.M., Wade, D.T. & Warlow, C.P. (1993) Long-term survival after first-ever stroke: the Oxfordshire Community Stroke Project. *Stroke* **24**, 796–800.

Di Carlo, A., Candelise, L., Gandolfo, C. *et al.* (1999) Influence of different screening procedures on the stroke prevalence estimates: The Italian Longitudinal Study on Aging. *Cerebrovascular Diseases* **9**, 231–237.

Durrington, P.N., Prais, H., Bhatnagar, D. *et al.* (1999) Indications for cholesterol-lowering medication: comparison of risk-assessment methods. *Lancet* **353**, 278–281.

Ebrahim, S. & Davey Smith, G. (1997) Systematic review of randomised controlled trials of multiple risk factor interventions for preventing coronary heart disease. *British Medical Journal* **314**, 1666–1674.

Ebrahim, S. & Davey Smith, G. (1998) Lowering blood pressure: a systematic review of sustained effects of non-pharmacological interventions. *Journal of Public Health Medicine* **20**, 441–448.

Ebrahim, S. & Harwood, R. (1999) *Stroke: Epidemiology, Evidence and Clinical Practice*. Oxford University Press, Oxford.

European Carotid Surgery Trialists' Collaborative Group (1995) Risk of stroke in the distribution of an asymptomatic carotid artery. *Lancet* **345**, 209–212.

European Carotid Surgery Trialists' Collaborative Group (1998) Randomised trial of endarterectomy for recently symptomatic carotid stenosis: final results of the MRC European Carotid Surgery Trial (ECST). *Lancet* **351**, 1379–1387.

Evans, G.J. (1985) *Risk factors for stroke in the elderly*. MD Thesis, University of Cambridge.

Fang, X.-H., Kronmal, R.A., Li, S.-C. *et al.* (1999) Prevention of stroke in Urban China. A community-based intervention trial. *Stroke* **30**, 495–501.

Feigin, V.L., Wiebers, D.O., Whisnant, J.P. & O'Fallon, M. (1995) Stroke incidence and 30-day case-fatality rates in Novosibirsk, Russia, 1982 through 1992. *Stroke* **26**, 924–929.

Field, K., Thorogood, M., Silagy, C., Normand, C., O'Neill, C. & Muir, J. (1995) Strategies for reducing coronary risk factors in primary care: which is most cost effective? *British Medical Journal* **310**, 1109–1112.

Furberg, C.D., Psaty, B.M., Manolio, T.A., Gardin, J.M., Smith, V.E. & Rautaharju, P.M. (1994) Prevalence of atrial fibrillation in elderly subjects (the Cardiovascular Health Study). *American Journal of Cardiology* **74**, 236–241.

Gage, B.F., Cardinalli, A.B., Albers, G.W. & Owens, D.K. (1995) Cost effectiveness of warfarin and aspirin for prophylaxis of stroke in patients with nonvalvular atrial fibrillation. *Journal of the American Medical Association* **274**, 1839–1845.

Gillum, R.F. & Sempos, C.T. (1997) The end of the long-term decline in stroke mortality in the United States? *Stroke* **28**, 1527–1529.

Giroud, M., Lemesle, M., Quantin, C. *et al.* (1997) A hospital-based and a population-based stroke registry yield different results: the experience in Dijon, France. *Neuroepidemiology* **16**, 15–21.

Grover, S.A., Coupal, L. & Hu, X.-P. (1995a) Identifying adults at increased risk of coronary disease. How well do the current cholesterol guidelines work? *Journal of the American Medical Association* **274**, 801–806.

Grover, S.A., Lowensteyn, I., Esrey, K.L., Steinert, Y., Joseph, L. & Abrahamowicz, M. (1995b) Do doctors accurately assess coronary risk in their patients? Preliminary results of the coronary health assessment study. *Brit-*

ish Medical Journal 310, 975–978.

Hankey, G.J. & Warlow, C.P. (1999) The treatment and secondary prevention of stroke: evidence, costs and effects on individuals and populations. *Lancet* **354**, 1457–1463.

Hankey, G.J., Slattery, J.M. & Warlow, C.P. (1991) The prognosis of hospital-referred transient ischaemic attacks. *Journal of Neurology, Neurosurgery and Psychiatry* **54**, 793–802.

Hankey, G.J., Slattery, J.M. & Warlow, C.P. (1993) Can the long term outcome of individual patients with transient ischaemic attacks be predicted accurately? *Journal of Neurology, Neurosurgery and Psychiatry* **56**, 752–759.

Haq, I.U., Ramsay, L.E., Jackson, P.R. & Wallis, E.J. (1999) Prediction of coronary risk for primary prevention of coronary heart disease: a comparison of methods. *Quarterly Journal of Medicine* **92**, 379–385.

Hart, R.G., Talbert, R.L., Kadri, K. & Amato, M. (1996) Warfarin for prevention of stroke: a practical, clinical review. *Neurologist* **2**, 319–341.

Hasuo, Y., Ueda, K., Kiyohara, Y. *et al.* (1989) Accuracy of diagnosis on death certificates for underlying causes of death in a long-term autopsy-based population study in Hisayama, Japan; with special reference to cardiovascular diseases. *Journal of Clinical Epidemiology* **42**, 577–584.

Hatano, S. (1976) Experience from a multicentre stroke register: a pre-liminary report. *Bulletin of the World Health Organisation* **54**, 541–553.

Hill, J.D., Mottram, E.M. & Killeen, P.D. (1987) Study of the prevalence of atrial fibrillation in general practice patients over 65 years of age. *Journal of the Royal College of General Practitioners* **37**, 172–173.

Hobson, R.W., Weiss, D.G., Fields, W.S. *et al.* (1993) Efficacy of carotid endarterectomy for asymptomatic carotid stenosis. *New England Journal of Medicine* **328**, 221–227.

Holmen, J., Forsen, L., Hjort, P.F., Midthjell, K., Waaler, H.T. & Bjorndal, A. (1991) Detecting hypertension: screening versus case finding in Norway. *British Medical Journal* **302**, 219–222.

Hong, Y., Bots, M.L., Pan, X., Hofman, A., Grobbee, D.E. & Chen, H. (1994) Stroke incidence and mortality in rural and urban Shanghai from 1984 through 1991. Findings from a community-based registry. *Stroke* **25**, 1165–1169.

Howitt, A. & Armstrong, D. (1999) Implementing evidence based medicine in general practice: audit and qualitative study of antithrombotic treatment for atrial fibrillation. *British Medical Journal* **18**, 1324–1327.

Hu, F.B., Stampfer, M.J., Manson, J.E. *et al.* (2000) Trends in the incidence of coronary heart disease and changes in diet and lifestyle in women. *New England Journal of Medicine* **343**, 530–537.

Hutchison, B., Birch, S., Evans, C.E. *et al.* (1998) Screening for hypercholesterolaemia in primary care: randomised controlled trial of postal questionnaire appraising risk of coronary heart disease. *British Medical Journal* **316**, 1208–1213.

Immonen-Raiha, P., Mahonen, M., Tuomilehto, J. *et al.* (1997) Trends in case-fatality of stroke in Finland during 1983–92. *Stroke* **28**, 2493–2499.

International Stroke Trial Collaborative Group (1997) The International Stroke Trial (IST): a randomised trial of aspirin, subcutaneous heparin, both, or neither among 19,435 patients with acute ischaemic stroke. *Lancet* **349**, 1569–1581.

Isard, P.A. & Forbes, J.F. (1992) The cost of stroke to the National Health Service in Scotland. *Cerebrovascular Diseases* **2**, 47–50.

Iso, H., Jacobs, D.R. & Goldman, L. (1990) Accuracy of death certificate diagnosis of intracranial haemorrhage and nonhaemorrhagic stroke. *American Journal of Epidemiology* **132**, 993–998.

Iso, H., Shimamoto, T., Naito, Y., Sato, S. *et al.* (1998) Effects of a long-term hypertension control program on stroke incidence and prevalence in a rural community in northeastern Japan. *Stroke* **29**, 1510–1518.

Jackson, R. (2000) Updated New Zealand cardiovascular disease risk-benefit prediction guide. *British Medical Journal* **320**, 709–710.

Jackson, R., Barham, P., Bills, J. *et al.* (1993) Management of raised blood pressure in New Zealand: a discussion document. *British Medical Journal* **307**, 107–110.

Jamrozik, K., Broadhurst, R.J., Lai, N., Hankey, G.J., Burvill, P.W. & Anderson, C.S. (1999) Trends in the incidence, severity, and short-term outcome of stroke in Perth, Western Australia. *Stroke* **30**, 2105–2111.

Jorgensen, H.S., Plesner, A.-M., Hubbe, P. & Larsen, K. (1992) Marked increase of stroke incidence in men between 1972 and 1990 in Frederiksberg, Denmark. *Stroke* **23**, 1701–1704.

Kalra, L., Perez, I. & Melbourn, A. (1998) Stroke risk management: changes in mainstream practice. *Stroke* **29**, 53–57.

Kassirer, J.P. & Angell, M. (1998) Losing weight: an ill-fated New Year's resolution. *New England Journal of Medicine* **338**, 52–54.

Kaufman, J.S., Asuzu, M.C., Rotimi, C.N., Johnson, O.O., Owoaje, E.E. & Cooper, R.S. (1997) The absence of adult mortality data for sub-Saharan Africa: a practical solution. *Bulletin of the World Health Organization* **75**, 389–395.

Kawachi, I. & Purdie, G. (1989) The benefits and risks of treating mild to moderate hypertension. *New Zealand Medical Journal* **102**, 377–379.

Khaw, K.-T. (1994) Genetics and environment: Geoffrey Rose revisited. *Lancet* **343**, 838–839.

Khaw, K.-T. & Rose, G. (1989) Cholesterol screening programmes: how much potential benefit? *British Medical Journal* **299**, 606–607.

Kinlay, S. & Heller, R.F. (1990) Effectiveness and hazards of case finding for a high cholesterol concentration. *British Medical Journal* **300**, 1545–1547.

Langenberg, M., Hellemons, B.S.P., van Ree, J.W. *et al.* (1996) Atrial fibrillation in elderly patients: prevalence and comorbidity in general practice. *British Medical Journal* **313**, 1534.

Langham, S., Thorogood, M., Normand, C., Muir, J., Jones, L. & Fowler, G. (1996) Costs and cost effectiveness of health checks conducted by nurses in primary care: the Oxcheck study. *British Medical Journal* **312**, 1265–1268.

Lanska, D.J. (1993) Decline in autopsies for deaths attributed to cerebrovascular disease. *Stroke* **24**, 71–75.

Law, M.R., Frost, C.D. & Wald, N.J. (1991) By how much does dietary salt reduction lower blood pressure? III Analysis of data from trials of salt reduction. *British Medical Journal* **302**, 819–824.

Lee, T.T., Solomon, N.A., Heidenreich, P.A., Oehlert, J. & Garber, A.M. (1997) Cost-effectiveness of screening for carotid stenosis in asymptomatic persons. *Annals of Internal Medicine* **126**, 337–346.

Lemesle, M., Milan, C., Faivre, J., Moreau, T., Giroud, M. & Dumas, R. (1999) Incidence trends of ischaemic stroke and transient ischaemic attacks in a well-defined French population from 1985 through 1994. *Stroke* **30**, 371–377.

Lightwood, J.M. & Glantz, S.A. (1997) Short-term economic and health benefits of smoking cessation: myocardial infarction and stroke. *Circulation* **96**, 1089–1096.

Linn, F.H.H., Rinkel, G.J.E., Algra, A. & van Gijn, J. (1996) Incidence of subarachnoid haemorrhage. Role of region, year, and rate of computed tomography: a meta-analysis. *Stroke* **27**, 625–629.

Lip, G.Y.H. (1999) Thromboprophylaxis for atrial fibrillation. *Lancet* **353**, 4–6.

McCormick, J. & Skrabanek, P. (1988) Coronary heart disease is not preventable by population interventions. *Lancet* **2**, 839–841.

Malmgren, R., Bamford, J., Warlow, C., Sandercock, P. & Slattery, J. (1989) Projecting the number of patients with first-ever strokes and patients newly handicapped by stroke in England and Wales. *British Medical Journal* **298**, 656–660.

Martin, J., Meltzer, H. & Elliot, D. (1988) OPCS surveys of disability in Great Britain Report 1. In: *The Prevalence of Disability Among Adults.* Office of Population Censuses and Surveys, HMSO, London.

Massing, M.W., Rywik, S.L., Jasinski, B., Manolio, T.A., Williams, O.D. & Tyroler, H.A. (1998) Opposing national stroke mortality trends in Poland and for African Americans and Whites in the United States. 1968–94. *Stroke* **29**, 1366–1372.

Mead, G.E., Wardlaw, J.M., Lewis, S.C., McDowall, M. & Dennis, M.S. (1999) The influence of randomised trials on the use of anticoagulants for atrial fibrillation. *Age and Ageing* **28**, 441–446.

Meissner, I., Wiebers, D.O., Whisnant, J.P. & O'Fallon, W.M. (1987) The natural history of asymptomatic carotid artery occlusive lesions. *Journal of the American Medical Association* **258**, 2704–2707.

Menotti, A., Puddu, P.E. & Lanti, M. (2000) Comparison of the Framingham risk function-based coronary chart with risk function from an Italian population study. *European Heart Journal* **21**, 365–370.

Murray, C.J.L. & Lopez, A.D. (1997) Mortality by cause for eight regions of the world: Global Burden of Disease Study. *Lancet* **349**, 1269–1276.

National Institute of Neurological Disorders, Stroke rt-PA Stroke Study Group (1995) Tissue plasminogen activator for acute ischaemic stroke. *New England Journal of Medicine* **333**, 1581–1587.

National Medical Advisory Committee (1993) *The Management of Patients with Stroke.* HMSO, Edinburgh.

Netsky, M.G. & Miyaji, T. (1976) Prevalence of cerebral haemorrhage and thrombosis in Japan: study of the major causes of death. *Journal of Chronic Disorders* **29**, 711–721.

Norris, J.W., Zhu, C.Z., Bornstein, N.M. & Chambers, B.R. (1991) Vascular risks of asymptomatic carotid stenosis. *Stroke* **22**, 1485–1490.

O'Leary, D.H., Anderson, K.M., Wolf, P.A., Evans, J.C. & Poehlman, H.W. (1992) Cholesterol and carotid atherosclerosis in older persons: the Framingham Study. *Annals of Epidemiology* **2**, 147–153.

Ostrander, L.D., Brandt, R.L., Kjelsberg, M.O. & Epstein, F.H. (1965) Electrocardiographic findings among the adult population of a total natural community, Tecumseh, Michigan. *Circulation* **31**, 888–898.

Peltonen, M., Stegmayr, B. & Asplund, K. (1998) Time trends in long-term survival after stroke: the Northern Sweden Multinational Monitoring of Trends and Determinants in Cardiovascular Disease (MONICA) study. 1985–94. *Stroke* **29**, 1358–1365.

Phillips, L.H., Whisnant, J.P. & Reagan, T.J. (1977) Sudden death from stroke. *Stroke* **8**, 392–395.

Prati, P., Vanuzzo, D., Casaroli, M., *et al.* (1992) Prevalence and determinants of carotid atherosclerosis in a general population. *Stroke* **23**, 1705–1711.

Pratt, M. (1999) Benefits of lifestyle activity vs. structured exercise. *Journal of the American Medical Association* **281**, 375–376.

Ramachandran, S., French, J.M., Vanderpump, M.P.J., Croft, P. & Neary, R.H. (2000) Using the Framingham model to predict heart disease in the United Kingdom: retrospective study. *British Medical Journal* **320**, 676–677.

Ramsay, L.E., Haq, I.U., Jackson, P.R., Yeo, W.W., Pickin, D.M. & Payne, J.N. (1996) Targeting lipid-lowering drug therapy for primary prevention of coronary disease: an updated Sheffield table. *Lancet* **348**, 387–388.

Ricci, S., Flamini, F.O., Celani, M.G. *et al.* (1991) Prevalence of internal carotid-artery stenosis in subjects older than 49 years: a population study. *Cerebrovascular Diseases* **1**, 16–19.

Robson, J., Boomla, K., Hart, B. & Feder, G. (2000) Estimating cardiovascular risk for primary prevention: outstanding questions for primary care. *British Medical Journal* **320**, 702–704.

Rose, G. (1981) Strategy of prevention: lessons from cardiovascular disease. *British Medical Journal* **282**, 1847–1851.

Rose, G. (1991) Ancel Keys lecture. *Circulation* **84**, 1405–1409.

Rose, G. (1992) *The Strategy of Preventive Medicine.* Oxford University Press, Oxford.

Rose, G. & Day, S. (1990) The population mean predicts the number of deviant individuals. *British Medical Journal* **301**, 1031–1034.

Rose, G., Baxter, P.J., Reid, D.D. & McCartney, P. (1978) Prevalence and prognosis of electrocardiographic findings in middle-aged men. *British Heart Journal* **40**, 636–643.

Rothwell, P.M. (1995) Can overall results of clinical trials be applied to all patients? *Lancet* **345**, 1616–1619.

Rothwell, P.M. & Warlow, C.P. on behalf of the European Carotid Surgery Trialists' Collaborative Group (1999) Prediction of benefit from carotid endarterectomy in individual patients: a risk-modelling study. *Lancet* **353**, 2105–2110.

Sandercock, P.A.G., Bamford, J., Dennis, M.S. *et al.* (1992) Atrial Fibrillation and stroke: prevalence in different types of stroke and influence on early and long term prognosis (Oxfordshire Community Stroke Project). *British Medical Journal* **305**, 1460–1465.

Scottish Intercollegiate Guidelines Network (1996) *Obesity in Scotland. Integrating Prevention with Weight Management.* Royal College of Physicians, Edinburgh.

Secretary of State for Health (1992) *The Health of the Nation.* HMSO, London.

Stroke Unit Trialists' Collaboration (2000) Organised inpatient (stroke unit) care for stroke. In: *The Cochrane Library*. Oxford: Update Software.

Sudlow, C. & Baigent, C. (1999) Antithrombotic treatment. In: *Clinical Evidence*, p. 532. BMJ Publishing Group, London.

Sudlow, C.L.M. & Warlow, C.P. (1996) Comparing stroke incidence worldwide. What makes studies comparable? *Stroke* **27**, 550–558.

Terent, A. (1988) Increasing incidence of stroke among Swedish women. *Stroke* **19**, 598–603.

Thomas, A.C., Knapman, P.A., Krikler, D.M. & Davies, M.J. (1988) Community study of the causes of 'natural' sudden death. *British Medical Journal* **297**, 1453–1456.

Tudor-Smith, C., Nutbeam, D., Moore, L. & Catford, J. (1998) Effects of the Heartbeat Wales programme over five years on behavioural risks for cardiovascular disease: quasi-experimental comparison of results from Wales and a matched reference area. *British Medical Journal* **316**, 818–822.

Tuomilehto, J., Bonita, R., Stewart, A., Nissinen, A. & Salonen, J.T. (1991) Hypertension, cigarette smoking, and the decline in stroke incidence in Eastern Finland. *Stroke* **22**, 7–11.

Tuomilehto, J., Rastenyte, D., Sivenius, J. *et al.* (1996) Ten-year trends in stroke incidence and mortality in the FINMONICA Stroke Study. *Stroke* **27**, 825–832.

Ueda, K., Omae, T., Hirota, Y. *et al.* (1981) Decreasing trend in incidence and mortality from stroke in Hisayama residents, Japan. *Stroke* **12**, 154–160.

Vartiainen, E., Puska, P., Pekkanen, J., Tuomilehto, J. & Jousilahti, P. (1994) Changes in risk factors explain changes in mortality from ischaemic heart disease in Finland. *British Medical Journal* **309**, 23–27.

Vartiainen, E., Sarti, C., Tuomilehto, J. & Kuulasmaa, K. (1995) Do changes in cardiovascular risk factors explain changes in mortality from stroke in Finland? *British Medical Journal* **310**, 901–904.

Wardlaw, J.M., Dorman, P.J., Candelise, L., Signorini, D.F. (1999) The influence of baseline prognostic variables on outcome after thrombolysis. *Journal of Neurology* **246**, 1059–1062.

Wardlaw, J.M., del Zoppo, G. & Yamaguchi, T. (2000) Thrombolysis for acute ischaemic stroke. In: *The Cochrane Library.* Oxford: Update Software.

Warlow, C.P. (1998a) Epidemiology of stroke. *Lancet* **352** (Suppl. 3), SIII1–4.

Warlow, C.P. (1998b) Can neurologists influence stroke incidence and do they? *Journal of the Royal College of Physicians of London* **32**, 466–472.

Whelton, P.K. (1994) Epidemiology of hypertension. *Lancet* **344**, 101–106.

Whelton, P.K., He, J., Cutler, J.A. *et al.* (1997) Effects of oral potassium on blood pressure. Meta-analysis of randomised controlled clinical trials. *Journal of the American Medical Association* **277**, 1624–1632.

Whisnant, J.P. (1984) The decline of stroke. *Stroke* **15**, 160–168.

Whitty, C.J.M., Sudlow, C.L.M. & Warlow, C.P. (1998) Investigating individual subjects and screening populations for asymptomatic carotid stenosis can be harmful. *Journal of Neurology, Neurosurgery and Psychiatry* **64**, 619–623.

WHO MONICA Project prepared by Thorvaldsen, P., Kuulasmaa, K., Rajakangas, A.-M., Rastenyte, D., Sarti, C. & Wilhelmsen, L. (1997) Stroke trends in the WHO MONICA Project. *Stroke* **28**, 500–506.

Willeit, J. & Kiechl, S. (1993) Prevalence and risk factors of asymptomatic extracranial carotid artery atherosclerosis. A population-based study. *Arteriosclerosis and Thrombosis* **13**, 661–668.

Wilson, P.W., D'Agostino, R.B., Levy, D., Belanger, A.M., Silbershatz, H. & Kannel, W.B. (1998) Prediction of coronary heart disease using risk factor categories. *Circulation* **97**, 1837–1847.

Wolf, P.A., Abbott, R.D. & Kannel, W.B. (1991) Atrial fibrillation as an independent risk factor for stroke: the Framingham Study. *Stroke* **22**, 983–988.

Wonderling, D., McDermott, C., Buxton, M. *et al.* (1996) Costs and cost effectiveness of cardiovascular screening and intervention: the British family heart study. *British Medical Journal* **312**, 1269–1273.

Index

Note: page numbers in *italics* refer to figures, those in **bold** refer to tables.

UNIVERSITY of WOLVERHAMPTON

PATHOPHYSIOLOGY

CONCEPTS OF ALTERED HEALTH STATES

12/04

UNIVERSITY OF WOLVERHAMPTON ENTERPRISE LTD.

Harrison Learning Centre
Wolverhampton Campus
University of Wolverhampton
St Peter's Square
Wolverhampton WV1 1RH
Wolverhampton (01902) 322305

ONE WEEK LOAN

16 MAY 2006
29 SEP 2006
-8 NOV 2007
24 SEP 2010

Telephone Renewals: 01902 321333
Please RETURN this item on or before the last date shown above.
Fines will be charged if items are returned late.
See tariff of fines displayed at the Counter. (L2)

WITHDRAWN

Study Guide to Accompany Porth's

Pathophysiology

Concepts of Altered Health States, Seventh Edition

Aug 2004 • 416 pages • Softbound • ISBN: 0-7817-5097-0

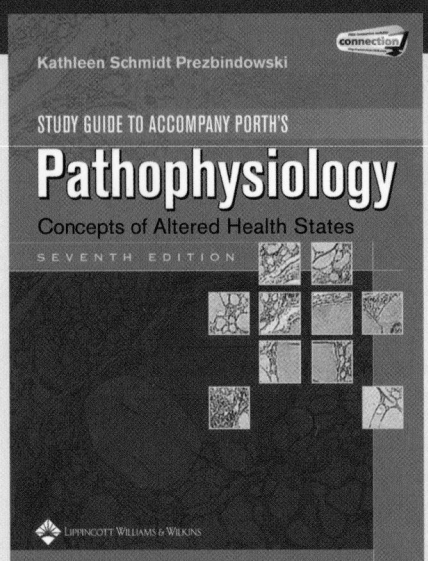

Study Guide to Accompany
Pathophysiology: Concepts of Altered Health States
Seventh Edition
Kathleen Schmidt Prezbindowski, PhD, MSN

Understanding and integrating the complex concepts governing pathophysiology can be challenging. This concise learning tool lets you review, chapter-by-chapter, all the vital material addressed by one of the most successful educational resources in the field: **Porth's Pathophysiology: Concepts of Altered Health States, Seventh Edition.**

Meet the challenges of important exams and clinical practice with confidence!

- Reader-friendly format mirrors the layout of the textbook, assuring thorough coverage and easy cross-referencing.
- Review questions related to each chapter subsection allow ample opportunities to reinforce your understanding and enhance your critical thinking skills.
- A range of learning tools—including short-answer, matching, fill-in, multiple choice, and labeling exercises—test your comprehension and prepare you for any exam.
- Answer key with rationales at the end of the guide explains the how and why behind correct responses—a great way to assess your strengths and identify areas in need of further review.

Make this knowledge-builder your new study partner!

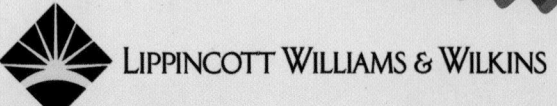

Order Online at LWW.com/nursing or call 1-800-399-3110

PATHOPHYSIOLOGY

CONCEPTS OF ALTERED HEALTH STATES

Seventh Edition

Carol Mattson Porth, RN, MSN, PhD (Physiology)

Professor Emeritus, School of Nursing
University of Wisconsin—Milwaukee
Milwaukee, Wisconsin

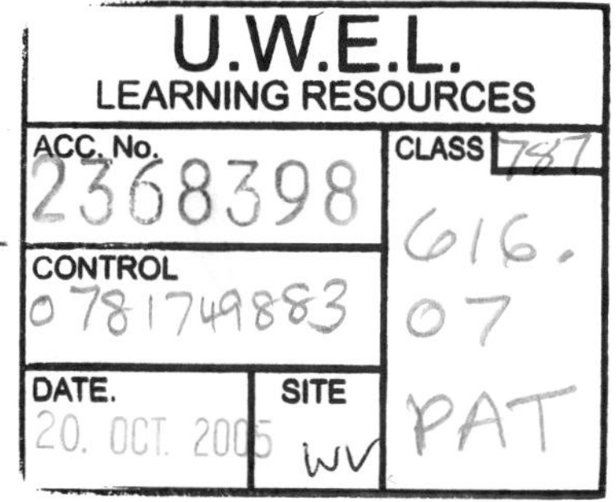

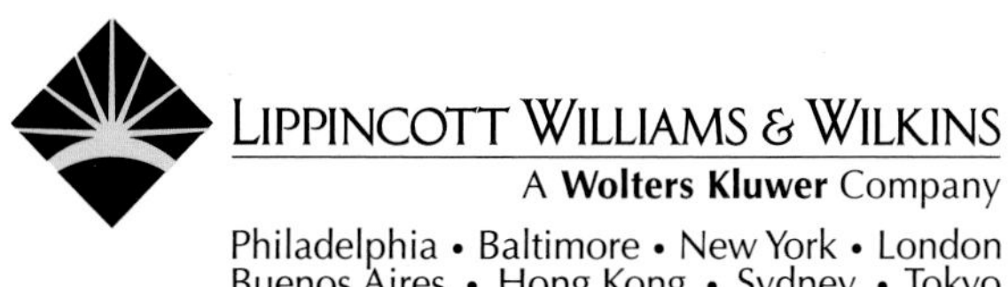

Philadelphia • Baltimore • New York • London
Buenos Aires • Hong Kong • Sydney • Tokyo

Senior Acquisitions Editor: Margaret Zuccarini
Managing Editor: Helen Kogut
Editorial Assistant: Carol DeVault
Senior Production Editor: Sandra Cherrey Scheinin
Director of Nursing Production: Helen Ewan
Managing Editor/Production: Erika Kors
Art Director: Carolyn O'Brien
Design Coordinator: Brett MacNaughton
Cover Designer: Melissa Walter
Interior Designer: Melissa Olson
Senior Manufacturing Manager: William Alberti
Indexer: Coughlin Indexing Services, Inc.
Compositor: Circle Graphics
Printer: R.R. Donnelley–Willard

7th Edition

Copyright © 2005 by Lippincott Williams & Wilkins.
Copyright © 2002 by Lippincott Williams & Wilkins. Copyright © 1998 by Lippincott-Raven Publishers. Copyright © 1994 by J.B. Lippincott Company. All rights reserved. This book is protected by copyright. No part of it may be reproduced, stored in a retrieval system, or transmitted, in any form or by any means—electronic, mechanical, photocopy, recording, or otherwise—without prior written permission of the publisher, except for brief quotations embodied in critical articles and reviews and testing and evaluation materials provided by publisher to instructors whose schools have adopted its accompanying textbook. Printed in the United States of America. For information write Lippincott Williams & Wilkins, 530 Walnut Street, Philadelphia PA 19106.

Materials appearing in this book prepared by individuals as part of their official duties as U.S. Government employees are not covered by the above-mentioned copyright.

9 8 7 6 5 4 3 2

Library of Congress Cataloging-in-Publication Data

Porth, Carol.
Pathophysiology : concepts of altered health states / Carol Mattson Porth.—7th ed.
p. ; cm.
Includes bibliographical references and index.
ISBN 0-7817-4988-3 (alk. paper)
1. Physiology, Pathological. 2. Nursing. I. Title.
[DNLM: 1. Disease—Nurses' Instruction. 2. Pathology—Nurses' Instruction. 3. Physiology—Nurses' Instruction. QZ 4 P851p 2005]
RB113.P67 2005
616.07—dc22

2004005807

U.W.E.

Care has been taken to confirm the accuracy of the information presented and to describe generally accepted practices. However, the authors, editors, and publisher are not responsible for errors or omissions or for any consequences from application of the information in this book and make no warranty, express or implied, with respect to the content of the publication.

The authors, editors, and publisher have exerted every effort to ensure that drug selection and dosage set forth in this text are in accordance with the current recommendations and practice at the time of publication. However, in view of ongoing research, changes in government regulations, and the constant flow of information relating to drug therapy and drug reactions, the reader is urged to check the package insert for each drug for any change in indications and dosage and for added warnings and precautions. This is particularly important when the recommended agent is a new or infrequently employed drug.

Some drugs and medical devices presented in this publication have Food and Drug Administration (FDA) clearance for limited use in restricted research settings. It is the responsibility of the health care provider to ascertain the FDA status of each drug or device planned for use in his or her clinical practice.

LWW.com

Learning without thought is labor lost.

—Confucius

This book is dedicated to the students, past and present, for whom this book was written.

Consultants

Edward W. Carroll, BS, MS, PhD
Clinical Assistant Professor
Department of Biological Sciences
Marquette University
Milwaukee, Wisconsin

Kathryn J. Gaspard, PhD
Clinical Associate Professor
College of Nursing
University of Wisconsin—Milwaukee
Milwaukee, Wisconsin

Glenn Matfin, BSc (Hons), MB ChB, DGM, MRCP(UK), MFPM, FACE, FACP
Senior Director
Global Clinical Research
Novartis Pharmaceuticals
East Hanover, New Jersey

Contributors

Diane S. Book, MD
Assistant Professor of Neurology
Medical College of Wisconsin
Milwaukee, Wisconsin

Edward W. Carroll, BS, MS, PhD
Clinical Assistant Professor
Department of Biomedical Sciences
Marquette University
Milwaukee, Wisconsin

Robin Curtis, PhD
Professor, Retired
Department of Cellular Biology, Neurobiology, and Anatomy
Medical College of Wisconsin
Milwaukee, Wisconsin

Elizabeth C. Devine, BSN, MSN, PhD, FAAN
Professor
College of Nursing
University of Wisconsin
Milwaukee, Wisconsin

W. Michael Dunne, Jr., PhD
Professor of Pathology & Immunology
Washington University School of Medicine
St. Louis, Missouri

Susan A. Fontana, RN, PhD, APRN, BC
Family Nurse Practitioner
Associate Professor, College of Nursing
University of Wisconsin—Milwaukee
Milwaukee, Wisconsin

Kathryn J. Gaspard, PhD
Clinical Associate Professor
College of Nursing
University of Wisconsin—Milwaukee
Milwaukee, Wisconsin

Kathleen E. Gunta, RN, MSN, ONC
Clinical Nurse Specialist
St. Luke's Medical Center
Milwaukee, Wisconsin

Safak Guven, MD, FACE, FACP
Assistant Professor
Clinical Director, Obesity/Metabolic Syndrome Clinic
Medical College of Wisconsin
Milwaukee, Wisconsin

Georgianne H. Heymann, RN, BSN
Science Editor
Milwaukee, Wisconsin

Marilyn King Hightower, RN, MSN
Lecturer, Clinical Instructor in Pediatrics
Louise Herrington School of Nursing
Baylor University
Dallas, Texas

Mary Kay Jiricka, RN, MSN, APN-BC
Clinical Nurse Specialist
St. Luke's Medical Center
Milwaukee, Wisconsin

Julie Kuenzi, RN, MSN, CDE, BC-ADM
Clinical Nurse Specialist
Diabetes Care Center Coordinator
Froedtert Hospital
Milwaukee, Wisconsin

Mary Pat Kunert, RN, BSN, PhD
Associate Professor
College of Nursing
University of Wisconsin—Milwaukee
Milwaukee, Wisconsin

Judy Wright Lott, RNC, DSN, NNP, FAAN
Dean & Professor of Nursing
Louise Herrington School of Nursing
Baylor University
Dallas, Texas

Glenn Matfin, BSc (Hons), MB ChB, DGM, MRCP(UK), MFPM, FACE, FACP
Senior Director
Global Clinical Research
Novartis Pharmaceuticals
East Hanover, New Jersey

Patricia McCowen Mehring, RNC, MSN, WHNP
Nurse Practitioner
Medical College of Wisconsin
Milwaukee, Wisconsin

Janice Kuiper Pikna, RN, MSN, CS
Clinical Nurse Specialist—Gerontology
Senior Health Program
Froedtert Hospital
Milwaukee, Wisconsin

Sandra Kawczynski Pasch, RN, MS, MA
Assistant Professor
Columbia College of Nursing
Milwaukee, Wisconsin

Joan Pleuss, RD, MS, CDE, CD
Program Manager/Bionutrition Core
General Clinical Research Center
Medical College of Wisconsin
Milwaukee, Wisconsin

Debra Bancroft Rizzo, RN, MSN, FNP-C
Rheumatology Nurse Practitioner
Rheumatic Disease Center
Milwaukee, Wisconsin

Gladys Simandl, RN, PhD
Professor
Columbia College of Nursing
Milwaukee, Wisconsin

Cynthia V. Sommer, PhD, MT(ASCP)
Associate Professor Emeritus
Department of Biological Sciences
University of Wisconsin—Milwaukee
Milwaukee, Wisconsin

Kathleen A. Sweeney, RN, MS, CNS, ACRN
Women's Statewide Outreach Coordinator
Medical College of Wisconsin
Wisconsin HIV Primary Care Support Network
Milwaukee, Wisconsin

Kerry Twite, RN, MSN, AOCN
Clinical Nurse Specialist—Oncology
St. Luke's Medical Center
Milwaukee, Wisconsin

Jill M. White Winters, RN, PhD
Associate Professor
College of Nursing
Marquette University
Milwaukee, Wisconsin

Reviewers

Pattie Clark, RN, MSN
Associate Professor of Nursing
Abraham Baldwin College
Tifton, Georgia

Brenda Lohri-Posey, RN, EdD
Assistant Dean for Learning, Nursing, and Program Coordination
Belmont Technical College
University of Phoenix Online
Phoenix, Arizona

Nancy E. Lynch, RN, BSN
Nursing Instructor
College of New Caledonia
British Columbia, Canada

Bernadette Madara, EdD, APRN
Associate Professor
Southern Connecticut State University
New Haven, Connecticut

James J. McPherson, PhD
Associate Professor, Director of Graduate Studies, Interim Chair
Occupational Therapy Program
Gannon University
Erie, Pennsylvania

Denise D. Wilson, PhD, APN, FNP, ANP
Associate Professor and Graduate Program Director
Mennonite College of Nursing at Illinois State University
Normal, Illinois

Preface

The preparation of this edition has been both challenging and humbling. Challenging to incorporate the myriad of new information; humbling to realize that despite advances in science and technology, illness and disease continue to occur and take their toll in terms of the physiologic as well as the social, psychological, and economic well-being of individuals, their families and communities, and the world.

As the others before it, the seventh edition has been carefully critiqued, reorganized, updated, and revised. Careful attention has been given to the incorporation of the most recent advances from the fields of genetics and molecular biology. This edition maintains many of the features of the previous edition including the introductory chapter on health and disease, the chapter on sleep and sleep disorders, and the chapter on neurobiology of thought and mood disorders, which has been enlarged to include a discussion of the physiology of hallucinations and delusions. In addition, the content on inflammation and wound healing has been pulled out and presented as a separate chapter. Other additions include a section on bioterrorism and the threat of global infectious diseases that appears in the chapter on mechanisms of infectious diseases and a discussion of the metabolic syndrome that appears in the chapter on diabetes.

The integration of full color into the design and illustrations has continued. Over a hundred of the illustrations that appear in this edition are new or have been extensively modified. The illustrations have been carefully chosen to support the concepts that are presented in the text, while maintaining a balance between line drawings of anatomic structures and pathophysiologic processes, flow charts, and photographic illustrations of disease states. This offers not only visual appeal but also enhances conceptual learning, linking text content to illustration content. This edition also retains the list of suffixes and prefixes, the table of normal laboratory values, the glossary, and the list of Internet addresses that were in the sixth edition. Objectives continue to appear at the beginning of each major section in a chapter, and summary statements appear at the end. The key concept boxes have been retained at the end of each chapter. They are intended to help the reader retain and use text information by providing a mechanism to incorporate the information into a larger conceptual unit as opposed to merely memorizing a string of related and unrelated facts. Review exercises are a new to this edition. They appear at the end of each chapter and assist the reader in using the conceptual approach to solving problems related to chapter content.

Despite the extensive changes and revision, every attempt has been made to present content in a manner that is logical, understandable, and inspires reader interest. The content has been arranged so that concepts build on one another. Words are defined as content is presented. Concepts from physiology, biochemistry, physics, and other sciences are reviewed as deemed appropriate. A conceptual model that integrates the developmental and preventative aspects of health has been used. Selection of content was based on common health problems, including the special needs of children and elderly persons. Although intended as a course textbook, it also is designed to serve as a reference book that students can take with them and use in their practice once the course is finished. The book was written with undergraduate students in mind, but is also appropriate for graduate students in nurse practitioner and clinical nurse specialist programs and for students in other health care disciplines.

And finally, as a nurse-physiologist, my major emphasis with each revision has been to relate normal body functioning to the physiologic changes that participate in disease production and occur as a result of disease, as well as the body's remarkable ability to compensate for these changes. The beauty of physiology is that it integrates all of the aspects of the individual cells and organs of the human body into a total functional whole that can be used to explain both the physical and psychological aspects of altered health. Indeed, it has been my philosophy to share the beauty of the human body and to emphasize that in disease as in health, there is more "going right" in the body than is "going wrong." This book is an extension of my career and, as such, of my philosophy. It is my hope that readers will learn to appreciate the marvelous potential of the body, incorporating it into their own philosophy and ultimately sharing it with their clients.

Carol Mattson Porth

To the Reader

This book was written with the intent of making the subject of pathophysiology an exciting exploration that relates normal body functioning to the physiologic changes that occur as a result of disease, as well as the body's remarkable ability to compensate for these changes. Indeed, it is these changes that represent the signs and symptoms of disease.

Using a book such as this can be simplified by taking the time to find what is in the book and how to locate information when it is needed. The *table of contents* at the beginning of the book provides an overall view of the organization and content of the book. It also provides clues as to the relationships among areas of content. For example, the location of the chapter on neoplasia within the unit on cell function and growth indicates that neoplasms are products of altered cell growth. The *index,* which appears at the end of the book, can be viewed as a road map for locating content. It can be used to quickly locate related content in different chapters of the book or to answer questions that come up in other courses.

Organization

The book is organized into units and chapters. The *units* identify broad areas of content, such as alterations in the circulatory system. Many of the units have a chapter that contains essential information about the structures being discussed in the unit. These chapters provide the foundation for understanding the pathophysiology content presented in the subsequent chapters. The *chapters* focus on specific areas of content, such as heart failure and circulatory shock. The *chapter outline* that appears at the beginning of each chapter provides an overall view of the chapter content and organization. *Icons* identify specific content related to infants and children, pregnant women, and older adults.

Reading and Learning Aids

In an ever-expanding world of information you will not be able to read, let alone remember, everything that is in this book, or in any book, for that matter. With this in mind, we have developed a number of special features that will help you focus on and master the essential content for your current as well as future needs.

The *objectives* that appear at the beginning of each major area of content provide a focus for your study. After you have finished each of these areas of content, you may want to go back and make sure that you have met each of the objectives.

It is essential for any professional to use and understand the vocabulary of his or her profession. Throughout the text, you will encounter terms in italics. This is a signal that a word and the ideas associated with it are important to learn. In addition, two aids are provided to help you expand your vocabulary and improve your comprehension of what you are reading: the glossary and the list of prefixes and suffixes.

The *glossary* contains concise definitions of frequently encountered terms. If you are unsure of the meaning of a term you encounter in your reading, check the glossary in the back of the book before proceeding.

The *list of prefixes and suffixes* is a tool to help you derive the meaning of words you may be unfamiliar with and increase your vocabulary. Many disciplines establish a vocabulary by affixing one or more letters to the beginning or end of a word or base to form a derivative word. Prefixes are added to the beginning of a word or base, and suffixes are added to the end. If you know the meanings of common prefixes and suffixes, you can usually derive the meaning of a word, even if you have never encountered it before. A list of prefixes and suffixes can be found on the inside back covers.

Boxes

Boxes are used throughout the text to summarize and highlight key information. You will encounter two types of boxes: Key Concept Boxes and Summary Boxes.

One of the ways to approach learning is to focus on the major ideas or concepts rather than trying to memorize a list of related and unrelated bits of information. As you have probably already discovered, it is impossible to memorize everything that is in a particular section or chapter of the book. Not only does your brain have a difficult time trying to figure out where to store all the different bits of information, your brain doesn't know how to retrieve the information when you need it. Most important of all, memorized lists of content can seldom, if ever, be applied directly to an actual clinical situation. The *Key Concept Boxes* guide you in identifying the major ideas or concepts that form the foundation for truly understanding the major areas of content. When you understand the concepts in the Key Concept boxes, you will have a framework for remembering and using the facts given in the text.

THE INFLAMMATORY RESPONSE

- Inflammation represents the response of body tissue to immune reactions, injury, or ischemic damage.
- The classic response to inflammation includes redness, swelling, heat, pain or discomfort, and loss of function.
- The manifestations of an acute inflammatory response can be attributed to the immediate vascular changes that occur (vasodilation and increased capillary permeability), the influx of inflammatory cells such as neutrophils, and, in some cases, the widespread effects of inflammatory mediators, which produce fever and other systemic signs and symptoms.
- The manifestations of chronic inflammation are due to infiltration with macrophages, lymphocytes, and fibroblasts, leading to persistent inflammation, fibroblast proliferation, and scar formation.

The *Summary Boxes* at the end of each section provide a review and a reinforcement of the main content that has been covered. Use the summaries to assure that you have covered and understand what you have read.

In summary, heart failure occurs when the heart fails to pump sufficient blood to meet the metabolic needs of body tissues. The physiology of heart failure reflects an interplay between a decrease in cardiac output that accompanies impaired function of the failing heart and the compensatory mechanisms designed to preserve the cardiac reserve. Adaptive mechanisms include the Frank-Starling mechanism, sympathetic nervous system activation, the renin-angiotensin-aldosterone mechanism, natriuretic peptides, the endothelins, and myocardial hypertrophy and remodeling. In the failing heart, early decreases in cardiac function may go unnoticed because these compensatory mechanisms maintain the cardiac output. This is called *compensated heart failure.* Unfortunately, the mechanisms were not intended for long-term use, and in severe and prolonged decompensated heart failure, the compensatory mechanisms no longer are effective, and instead contribute to the progression of cardiac heart failure.

Heart failure may be described as high-output or low-output failure, systolic or diastolic failure, and right-sided or left-sided failure. With high-output failure, the function of the heart may be supranormal but inadequate because of excessive metabolic needs, and low-output failure is caused by disorders that impair the pumping ability of the heart. With systolic dysfunction, there is impaired ejection of blood from the heart during systole; with diastolic dysfunction, there is impaired filling of the heart during diastole. Right-sided failure is characterized by congestion in the peripheral circulation, and left-sided failure by congestion in the pulmonary circulation.

The manifestations of heart failure include edema, nocturia, fatigue and impaired exercise tolerance, cyanosis, signs of increased sympathetic nervous system activity, and impaired gastrointestinal function and malnutrition. In right-sided failure, there is dependent edema of the lower parts of the body, engorgement of the liver, and ascites. In left-sided failure, shortness of breath and chronic, nonproductive cough are common.

The diagnostic methods in heart failure are directed toward establishing the cause and extent of the disorder. Treatment is directed toward correcting the cause whenever possible, improving cardiac function, maintaining the fluid volume within a compensatory level, and developing an activity pattern consistent with individual limitations in cardiac reserve. Among the medications used in the treatment of heart failure are diuretics, digoxin, ACE inhibitors, and β-blockers.

Acute pulmonary edema is a life-threatening condition in which the accumulation of fluid in the interstitium of the lung and alveoli interferes with lung expansion and gas exchange. It is characterized by extreme breathlessness, rales, frothy sputum, cyanosis, and signs of hypoxemia. In cardiogenic shock, there is failure to eject blood from the heart, hypotension, inadequate cardiac output, and impaired perfusion of peripheral tissues. Mechanical support devices, including the intraaortic balloon pump (for acute failure) and the VAD, sustain life in persons with severe heart failure. Heart transplantation remains the treatment of choice for many persons with end-stage heart failure.

Tables and Charts

Tables and charts are designed to present complex information in a format that makes it more meaningful and easier to remember. Tables have two or more columns, and are often used for the purpose of comparing or contrasting information. Charts have one column and are used to summarize information.

TABLE 34-4 Causes and Manifestations of Respiratory Acidosis

Causes	Manifestations
Depression of Respiratory Center Drug overdose Head injury **Lung Disease** Bronchial asthma Emphysema Chronic bronchitis Pneumonia Pulmonary edema Respiratory distress syndrome **Airway Obstruction, Disorders of Chest Wall and Respiratory Muscles** Paralysis of respiratory muscles Chest injuries Kyphoscoliosis Extreme obesity Treatment with paralytic drugs **Breathing Air With High CO_2 Content**	**Blood pH, CO_2, HCO_3^-** pH decreased PCO_2 (primary) increased HCO_3^- (compensatory) increased **Neural Function** Dilation of cerebral vessels and depression of neural function Headache Weakness Behavior changes Confusion Depression Paranoia Hallucinations Tremors Paralysis Stupor and coma **Skin** Skin warm and flushed **Signs of Compensation** Acid urine

CHART 31-1

*Causes of Respiratory Failure**

Impaired Ventilation

Upper airway obstruction
- Infection (*e.g.,* epiglottitis)
- Foreign body
- Laryngospasm
- Tumors

Weakness or paralysis of respiratory muscles
- Brain injury
- Drug overdose
- Guillain-Barré syndrome
- Muscular dystrophy
- Spinal cord injury

Chest wall injury

Impaired Matching of Ventilation and Perfusion

Chronic obstructive pulmonary disease
Restrictive lung disease
Severe pneumonia
Atelectasis

Impaired Diffusion

Pulmonary edema
Acute respiratory distress syndrome

*This list is not intended to be inclusive.

Illustrations

The full-color illustrations will help you to build your own mental image of the content that is being presented. Each drawing has been developed to fully support and build upon the ideas in the text. Some illustrations are used to help you picture the complex interactions of the multiple phenomena that are involved in the development of a particular disease; others can help you to visualize normal function or understand the mechanisms whereby the disease processes exert their effects. In addition, photographs of pathologic processes and lesions provide a realistic view of selected pathologic processes and lesions.

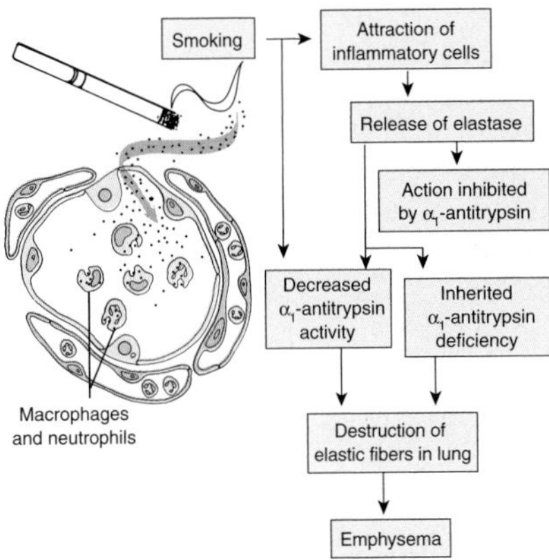

FIGURE 31-10 Smoking and protease–antiprotease mechanisms of emphysema. Smoking inhibits antielastase and favors the recruitment of leukocytes and release of elastase, with elastic tissue destruction in the lung and development of emphysema.

Material for Review

An important feature has been built into the text to help you verify your understanding of the material presented. After you have finished reading and studying the chapter, work on answering the *review exercises* at the end of the chapter. They are designed to help you integrate and synthesize material. If you are unable to answer a question, reread the relevant section in the chapter.

REVIEW EXERCISES

A 12-year-old boy with sickle cell disease presents in the emergency room with severe chest pain. His mother reports that he was doing well until he came down with a respiratory tract infection. She also says he insisted on playing basketball with the other boys in the neighborhood even though he was not feeling well.

A. What is the most likely cause of pain in this boy?

B. Infections and aerobic exercise that increase the levels of deoxygenated hemoglobin produce sickling in persons who are homozygous for the sickle cell gene and have sickle cell disease, but not in persons who are heterozygous and have sickle cell trait. Explain.

C. People with sickle disease experience anemia but not iron deficiency. Explain.

Appendices

Your book contains two appendices. Appendix A, "Laboratory Values," provides rapid access to normal values for many laboratory tests, as well as a description of the prefixes, symbols, and factors (*e.g.*, micro, μ, 10^{-6}) used for describing these values. Knowledge of normal values can help you to put abnormal values in context. Appendix B, "Weblinks," is provided to help you in obtaining additional information on topics that are of interest to you. The websites in Appendix B will also help you to keep abreast of new information that is constantly evolving. For your convenience, these weblinks are also found on the book's Connection site.

We hope that this guide has given you a clear picture of how to use this book. Good luck and enjoy the journey!

Acknowledgments

As in past editions, many persons participated in the creation of this work. The contributing authors deserve a special mention, for they worked long hours preparing the content for the seventh edition of *Pathophysiology: Concepts of Altered Health States,* I would also like to acknowledge Dr. Edward W. Carroll, Dr. Kathryn Gaspard, and Dr. Glenn Matfin for their consultation and help.

Several other persons deserve special recognition. Georgianne Heymann assisted in editing the manuscript. As with previous editions, she provided not only excellent editorial assistance, but also encouragement and support when the tasks associated with manuscript preparation became most frustrating. Brett MacNaughton deserves recognition for his work in coordinating the development and revision of illustrations in the book. I would also like to acknowledge the contributions of other authors who have shared their illustrations and photos.

I would also like to recognize the efforts of the editorial and production staff at Lippincott Williams & Wilkins that were directed by Margaret Zuccarini, Senior Acquisitions Editor. I particularly want to thank Carol DeVault who served as Editorial Assistant; Helen Kogut, who served as Managing Editor; and Sandra Cherrey Scheinin for her dedication as Production Editor.

Past and present students in my classes also deserve a special salute, for they are the inspiration upon which this book is founded. They have provided the questions, suggestions, and contact with the "real world" of patient care that have directed the organization and selection of content for the book.

And last, but not least, I would like to acknowledge my family, my friends, and my colleagues for their patience, their understanding, and their encouragement throughout the entire process.

Contents

UNIT III

Integrative Body Functions 185

UNIT VII

Respiratory Function *631*

CHAPTER 29

Control of Respiratory Function 633

CHAPTER 30

Respiratory Tract Infections, Neoplasms, and Childhood Disorders 659

CHAPTER 31

Disorders of Ventilation and Gas Exchange 689

UNIT VIII

Renal Function and Fluids and Electrolytes *725*

CHAPTER 32

Control of Renal Function 727

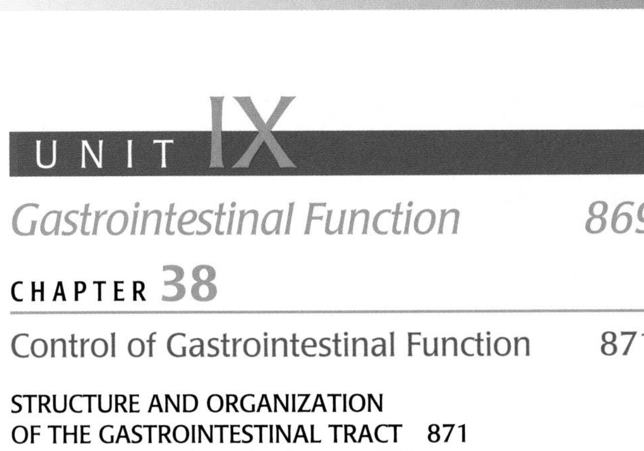

UNIT IX Gastrointestinal Function 869

CHAPTER 38

Control of Gastrointestinal Function 871

CHAPTER 39

Disorders of Gastrointestinal Function 885

CHAPTER 40

Disorders of Hepatobiliary and Exocrine Pancreas Function 917

UNIT X Endocrine Function 949

CHAPTER 41

Mechanisms of Endocrine Control 951

Glenn Matfin, Julie A. Kuenzi, and Safak Guven

CHAPTER 42

Disorders of Endocrine Control of Growth and Metabolism 961

Glenn Matfin, Julie A. Kuenzi, and Safak Guven

UNIT I

Concepts of Health and Disease

Early peoples were considered long-lived if they reached 30 years of age—that is, if they survived infancy. For many centuries, infant mortality was so great that large families became the tradition; many children in a family ensured that at least some would survive. Life expectancy has increased over the centuries, and today an individual in a developed country can expect to live about 71 to 79 years. Although life expectancy has increased radically since ancient times, human longevity has remained fundamentally unchanged.

The quest to solve the mystery of human longevity, which appears to be genetically programmed, began with Gregor Mendel (1822–1884), an Augustinian monk. Mendel laid the foundation of modern genetics with the pea experiments he performed in a monastery garden. Today, geneticists search for the determinant, or determinants, of the human life span. Up to this time, scientists have failed to identify an aging gene that would account for a limited life span. However, they have found that cells have a finite reproductive capacity. As they age, genes are increasingly unable to perform their functions. The cells become poorer and poorer at making the substances they need for their own special tasks or even for their own maintenance. Free radicals, mutation in a cell's DNA, and the process of programmed cell death are some of the factors that work together to affect a cell's functioning.

CHAPTER

1

Concepts of Health and Disease

Georgianne H. Heymann
Carol M. Porth

The concepts of what constituted health and disease at the beginning of the last century were far different from those of this century. In most of the industrialized nations of the world, people now are living longer and enjoying a healthier lifestyle. Much of this has been made possible by recent advances in science and technology. There has been an increased knowledge of immune mechanisms; the discovery of antibiotics to cure infections; and the development of vaccines to prevent disease, chemotherapy to attack cancers, and drugs to control the manifestations of mental illness.

The introduction of the birth control pill and improved prenatal care have led to decreased birth rates and declines in infant and child mortality. The benefits of science and technology also have increased the survival of infants born prematurely and of children with previously untreatable illnesses, such as immunodeficiency states and leukemia. There also has been an increase in the survival of very seriously ill and critically injured persons of all age groups. Consequently, there has been an increase in longevity, a shift in the age distribution of the population, and an increase in age-related diseases. Coronary heart disease, stroke, and cancer have now replaced pneumonia, tuberculosis, and diarrhea and enteritis—the leading causes of death in the 1900s.

This chapter, which is intended to serve as an introduction to the book, is organized into four sections: health and society, historical perspectives on health and disease, perspectives on health and disease in individuals, and perspectives on health and disease in populations. The chapter is intended to provide the reader with the ability to view within a larger framework the historical aspects of health and disease and the relationship of health and disease to individuals and populations, and to introduce the reader to terms, such as *etiology* and *pathogenesis*, that are used throughout this text.

Health and Society

Everyone who is born holds dual citizenship in the kingdom of the well and in the kingdom of the sick. Although we all prefer to use only the good passport, sooner or later each of us is obligated, at least for a spell, to identify ourselves as citizens of that other place.[1]

After completing this section of the chapter, you should be able to meet the following objectives:

- Describe the concepts used to establish belief systems within a community and the effects on its health care practices
- Identify a disease believed to be generated by specific emotions and the characteristics ascribed to it
- Explain how mythologizing disease can be detrimental to individuals in a society

There is a long history that documents the concern of humans for their own health and well-being and that of their community. It is not always evident what particular beliefs were held by early humans concerning health and disease. Still, there is evidence that whenever humans have formed social groups, some individuals have taken the role of the healer, responsible for the health of the community by preventing disease and curing the sick.

In prehistoric times, people believed that angry gods or evil spirits caused ill health and disease. To cure the sick, the gods had to be pacified or the evil spirits driven from the body. In time, this task became the job of the healers, or tribal priests. They tried to pacify the gods or drive out the evil spirits using magic charms, spells, and incantations. There also is evidence of surgical treatment. Trephining involved the use of a stone instrument to cut a hole in the skull of the sick person. It is believed that this was done to release spirits responsible for illness. Prehistoric healers probably also discovered that many plants can be used as drugs.

The community as a whole also was involved in securing the health of its members. It was the community that often functioned to take care of those considered ill or disabled. The earliest evidence of this comes from an Old Stone Age cave site, Riparo del Romio, in southern Italy. There the remains of an adolescent dwarf were found. Despite his severe condition, which must have greatly limited his ability to contribute to either hunting or gathering, the young man survived to the age of 17 years. He must have been supported throughout his life by the rest of the community, which had incorporated compassion for its members into its belief system.[2] Communities such as this probably existed throughout prehistory; separated from each other and without any formal routes of communication, they relied on herbal medicines and group activity to maintain health.

Throughout history, peoples and cultures have developed their health practices based on their belief systems. Many traditions construed sickness and health primarily in the context of an understanding of the relations of human beings to the planets, stars, mountains, rivers, spirits, and ancestors, gods and demons, the heavens and underworld. Some traditions, such as those reflected in Chinese and Indian cultures, although concerned with a cosmic scope, do not pay great attention to the supernatural.

Over time, modern Western thinking has shed its adherence to all such elements. Originating with the Greek tradition—which dismissed supernatural powers, although not environmental influences—and further shaped by the flourishing anatomic and physiologic programs of the Renaissance, the Western tradition was created based on the belief that everything that needed to be known essentially could be discovered by probing more deeply and ever more minutely into the flesh, its systems, tissues, cells, and DNA.[3] Through Western political and economic domination, these health beliefs now have powerful influence worldwide.

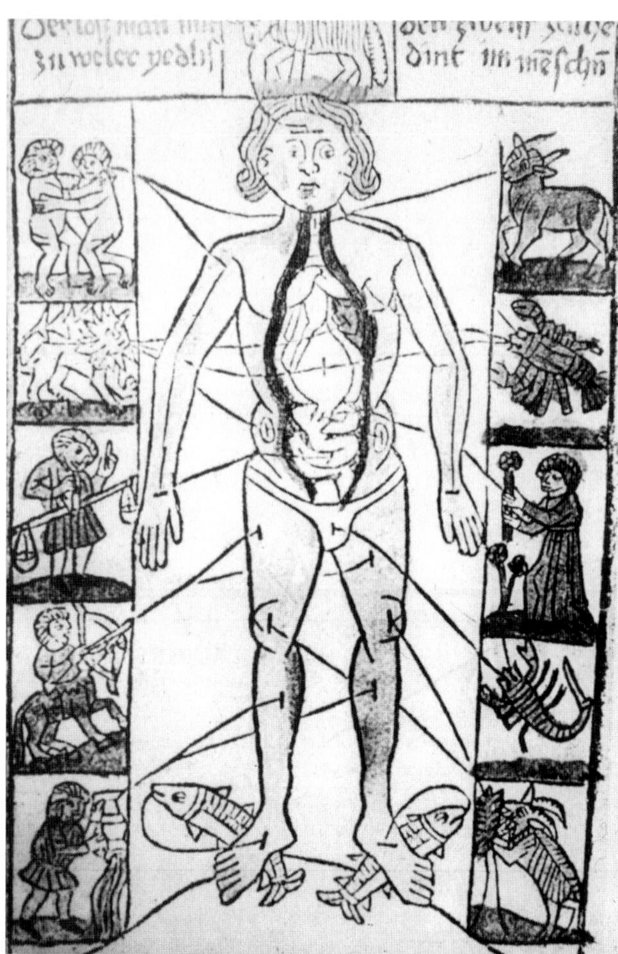

Influences of zodiac signs on the human body. (Courtesy of the National Library of Medicine)

Every society has its own ideas and beliefs about life, death, and disease. It is these perceptions that shape the concept of health in a society. Although some customs and beliefs tend to safeguard human communities from disease, others invite and provoke disease outbreaks.

The beliefs that people have concerning health and disease can change the destiny of nations. The conquering of the Aztec empire may be one example. Historians have speculated how Hernando Cortez, starting off with fewer than 600 men, could conquer the Aztec empire, whose subjects numbered millions. Historian William H. McNeill suggests a sequence of events that may explain how a tiny handful of men could subjugate a nation of millions.

Although the Aztecs first thought the mounted, gunpowered Spaniards were gods, experience soon showed otherwise. Armed clashes revealed the limitations of horseflesh and of primitive guns, and the Aztecs were able to drive Cortez and his men from their city. Unbeknownst to the Aztecs, the Spaniards had a more devastating weapon than any firearm: smallpox. An epidemic of smallpox broke out among the Aztecs after their skirmishes with the Spaniards. Because the population lacked inherited or acquired immunity, the results were catastrophic. It is presumed that a quarter to a third of the population died from the initial onslaught.

Even more devastating were the psychological implications of the disease: it killed only American Indians and left Spaniards unharmed. A way of life built around the old Indian gods could not survive such a demonstration of the superior power of the God the Spaniards worshipped. It is not hard to imagine then that the Indians accepted Christianity and submitted meekly to Spanish control.[4] Although we live in an age of science, science has not eliminated fantasies about health; the stigmas of sickness and the moral meanings that they carry continue. Whereas people in previous centuries wove stories around leprosy, plague, and tuberculosis to create fear and guilt, the modern age has created similar taboos and mythologies about cancer and acquired immunodeficiency syndrome (AIDS).

The myth of tuberculosis (TB) was that a person who suffered from it was of a melancholy, superior character—sensitive, creative, a being apart. Melancholy, or sadness, made one "interesting" or romantic. The general perception of TB as "romantic" was not just a literary device. It was a way of thinking that insinuated itself into the sensibilities and made it possible to ignore the social conditions, such as overcrowding and poor sanitation and nutrition, that helped breed tuberculosis.

The infusion of beliefs into public awareness often is surreptitious. Just as tuberculosis often had been regarded sentimentally, as an enhancement of identity, cancer was regarded with irrational revulsion, as a diminution of the self.[1] Current accounts of the psychological aspects of cancer often cite old authorities, starting with the Greek physician Galen, who observed that "melancholy women" are more likely to get breast cancer than "sanguine women."

Grief and anxiety were cited as causes of cancer, as well as personal losses. Public figures such as Napoleon, Ulysses S. Grant, Robert A. Taft, and Hubert Humphrey have all had their cancers diagnosed as the reaction to political defeat and the end to their political ambitions. Although distress can affect immunologic responsiveness, there is no scientific evidence to support the view that specific emotions, or emotions in general, can produce specific diseases—or that cancer is the result of a "cancer personality," described as emotionally withdrawn, lacking self-confidence, and depressive.

These disease mythologies contribute to the stigmatizing of certain illnesses and, by extension, of those who are ill. The beliefs about health and disease have the power to trap or empower people. They may inhibit people from seeking early treatment, diminish personal responsibility for practicing healthful behaviors, or encourage fear and social isolation. Conversely, they also can be the impetus for compassion to those who are ill, for commitment to improving one's own health, and for support of efforts to improve the health status of others.

In summary, what constitutes health and disease changes over time. Prehistoric times were marked by beliefs that angry gods or evil spirits caused ill health and disease. To cure the sick, the gods had to be pacified or the evil spirits driven from the body. Tribal healers, or priests, emerged to accomplish this task. Prehistoric healers used a myriad of treatments, including magic charms, spells, and incantations; surgical treatment; and plant medicines.

Throughout history, the concept of health in a society has been shaped by its beliefs about life, death, and disease. Some beliefs and customs, such as exhibiting compassion for disabled community members, tend to safeguard human communities and increase the quality of life for all community members. Others invite and provoke disease outbreaks, such as myths about the causes of disease.

Even though science and technology have advanced the understanding and treatment of disease, misconceptions and fantasies about disease still arise. In previous centuries, diseases such as leprosy, plague, and tuberculosis were fodder for taboos and mythologies; today, it is cancer and AIDS. The psychological effects of disease mythologies can be positive or negative. At their worst, they can stigmatize and isolate those who are ill; at their best, they can educate the community and improve the health of its members.

Health and Disease: A Historical Perspective

After completing this section of the chapter, you should be able to meet the following objectives:

- Describe the contributions of the early Greek, Italian, and English scholars to the understanding of anatomy, physiology, and pathology
- State two important advances of the nineteenth century that helped to pave the way for prevention of disease
- State three significant advances of the twentieth century that have revolutionized diagnosis and treatment of disease
- Propose developments that will both hamper and contribute to the promotion of health and the elimination of disease in the twenty-first century

It has been said that those who do not know history are condemned to repeat it. There are many contributors to the understanding of how the body is constructed and how it works, and what disease is and how it can be treated, which in turn leads to an understanding of what health is and how can it be maintained.

Much of what we take for granted in terms of treating the diseases that afflict humankind has had its origin in the past. Although they are seemingly small contributions in terms of today's scientific advances, it is the knowledge produced by the great thinkers of the past that has made possible the many things we now take for granted.

THE INFLUENCE OF EARLY SCHOLARS

Knowledge of anatomy, physiology, and pathology as we now know it began to emerge with the ancient Greeks. They were the first to recognize the distinction between internal and external causes of illness.

To Hippocrates and his followers, we owe the foundations of the clinical principles and the ethics that grew into modern medical science. Hippocrates (460–377 BC) was a blend of scientist and artist. He believed that disease occurred when the four humors—blood from the heart, yellow bile from the liver, black bile from the spleen, and phlegm from the brain—became out of balance. These humors were said to govern character as well as health, producing phlegmatic, sanguine, choleric, and melancholic personalities. This belief paralleled the even older Chinese tradition, which was founded on the complementary principles of yin (female principle) and yang (male), whose correct proportions were essential for health. Hippocrates is identified with an approach to health that dictated plenty of healthy exercise, rest in illness, and a moderate, sober diet.

It was Aristotle (384–322 BC) who, through his dissection of small animals and description of their internal anatomy, laid the foundations for the later scrutiny of the human body. For Aristotle, the heart was the most important organ. He believed it to be the center of the blood system as well as the center of the emotions. However, Aristotle's main contributions were made to science in general.

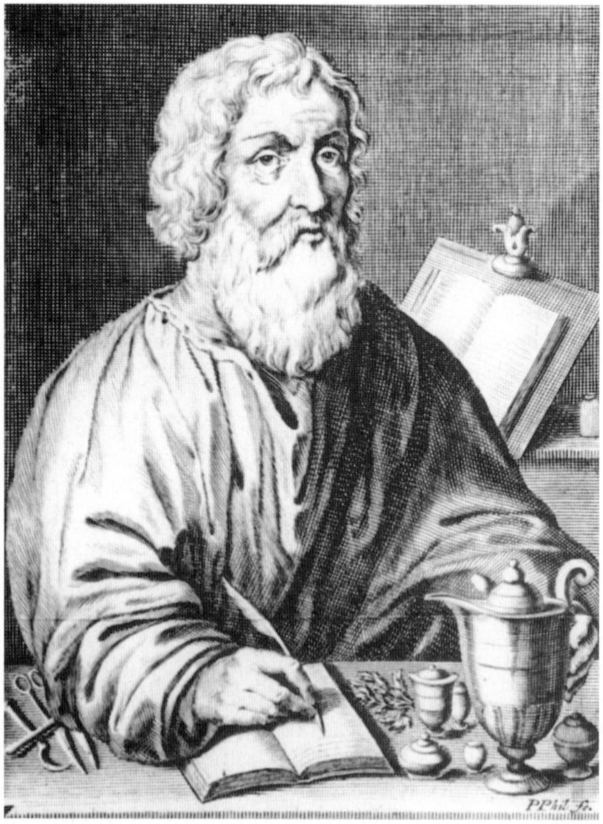

Hippocrates: A blend of scientist and scholar. (Courtesy of the National Library of Medicine)

The person who took the next major step was Galen (AD 129–199), a physician to the emperors and gladiators of ancient Rome. Galen expanded on the Hippocratic doctrines and introduced experimentation into the study of healing. His work came to be regarded as the encyclopedia of anatomy and physiology. He demoted the heart—in his view, the liver was primary for venous blood, whereas the seat of all thought was the brain. He described the arteries and veins and even revealed the working of the nervous system by severing a pig's spinal cord at different points and demonstrating that corresponding parts of the body became paralyzed. According to Galen, the body carried three kinds of blood that contained spirits charged by various organs: the veins carried "natural spirit" from the liver; the arteries, "vital spirit" from the lungs; the nerves, "animal spirit" from the brain. The heart merely warmed the blood. After Galen's death, however, anatomic research ceased, and his work was considered infallible for almost 1400 years.

As the great medical schools of universities reformed the teaching of anatomy in the early 1500s and integrated it into medical studies, it became apparent to anatomists that Galen's data—taken from dogs, pigs, and apes—often were riddled with error. It was only with the work of Andreas Vesalius (1514–1564) that Galen's ideas truly were challenged.

Vesalius, professor of anatomy and surgery at Padua, Italy, dedicated a lifetime to the study of the human body. Vesalius carried out some unprecedentedly scrupulous dissections and used the latest in artistic techniques and printing for the more than 200 woodcuts in his *De Humani Corporis Fabrica* ("On the Fabric [Structure] of the Human Body"). He showed not only what bodily parts looked like but also how they worked. The book, published in 1543, set a new standard for the understanding of human anatomy. With this work, Vesalius became a leading figure in the revolt against Galen's teachings.

One of the most historically significant discoveries was made by William Harvey (1578–1657), an English physician and physiologist. He established that the blood circulates in a closed system impelled mechanically by a "pumplike" heart. He also measured the amount of blood in the circulatory system in any given unit of time—one of the first applications of quantitative methods in biology. Harvey's work, published in *On the Motion of the Heart and Blood in Animals* (1628), provided a foundation of physiologic principles that led to an understanding of blood pressure and set the stage for innovative techniques such as cardiac catheterization.

With the refinement of the microscope by the Dutch lens maker Anton van Leeuwenhoek (1632–1723), the stage was set for the era of cellular biology. Another early user of the microscope, English scientist Robert Hooke (1635–1703), published his *Micrographia* in 1665 in which

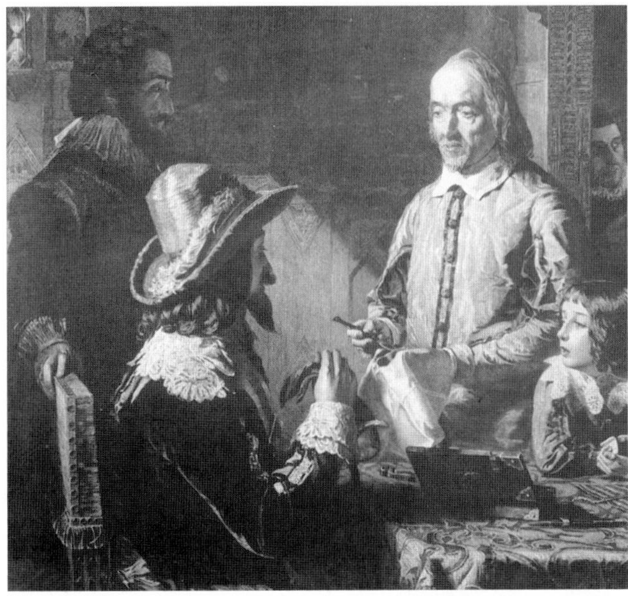

William Harvey's most eminent patient, King Charles I, and the future King Charles II look on as Harvey displays a dissected deer heart. (Courtesy of the National Library of Medicine)

he formally described the plant cells in cork and presented his theories of light and combustion and his studies of insect anatomy. His book presented the great potential of the microscope for biologic investigation. In it, he inaugurated the modern biologic usage of the word *cell*. A century later, German-born botanist Mathias Schleiden (1804–1881) and physiologist Theodor Schwann (1810–1882) observed that animal tissues also were composed of cells.

Although Harvey contributed greatly to the understanding of anatomy and physiology, he was not interested in the chemistry of life. It was not until French chemist Antoine Lavoisier (1743–1794), who was schooled as a lawyer but devoted to scientific pursuits, overturned 100-year-old theories of chemistry and established the basis of modern chemistry that new paths to examine body processes, such as metabolism, opened up. His restructured chemistry also gave scientists, including Louis Pasteur, the tools to develop organic chemistry.

In 1796, Edward Jenner (1749–1823) conducted the first vaccination by injecting the fluid from a dairymaid's cowpox lesion into a young boy's arm. The vaccination by this English country doctor successfully protected the child from smallpox. Jenner's discovery led to the development of vaccines to prevent many other diseases as well. Jenner's classic experiment was the first officially recorded vaccination.

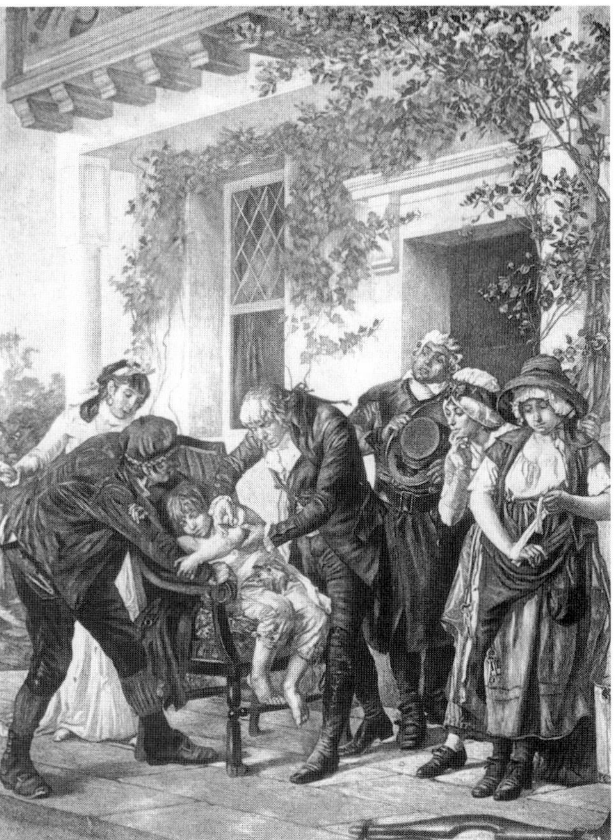

Painting by Georges-Gaston Mélingue (1894). The first vaccination. Here Dr. Jenner introduces cowpox taken from dairymaid Sarah Nelmes (*right*) and introduces it into two incisions on the arm of James Phipps, a healthy 8-year-old boy. The boy developed cowpox, but not smallpox, when Jenner introduced the organism into his arm 48 days later. (Courtesy of the National Library of Medicine)

THE NINETEENTH CENTURY

The nineteenth century was a time of spectacular leaps forward in the understanding of infectious diseases. For many centuries, rival epidemiologic theories associated disease and epidemics like cholera with poisonous fumes given off from dung heaps and decaying matter (poisons in the air, exuded from rotting animal and vegetable material, the soil, and standing water) or with contagion (person-to-person contact).

In 1865, English surgeon Joseph Lister (1827–1912) concluded that microbes caused wound infections. He began to use carbolic acid on wounds to kill microbes and reduce infection after surgery. However, Lister was not alone in identifying hazards in the immediate environment as detrimental to health. English nurse Florence Nightingale (1820–1910) was a leading proponent of sanitation and hygiene as weapons against disease. It was at the English base at Scutari during the Crimean War (1854–1856) that Nightingale waged her battle. Arriving at the army hospital with a party of 38 nurses, Nightingale found nearly 2000 wounded and sick inhabiting foul, rat-infested wards. The war raged on, deluging the hospital with wounded as Nightingale not only organized the nursing care of the wounded but also provided meals, supplied bedding, and saw to the laundry. Within 6 months, she had brought about a transformation and slashed the death rate from approximately 40% to 2%.[3]

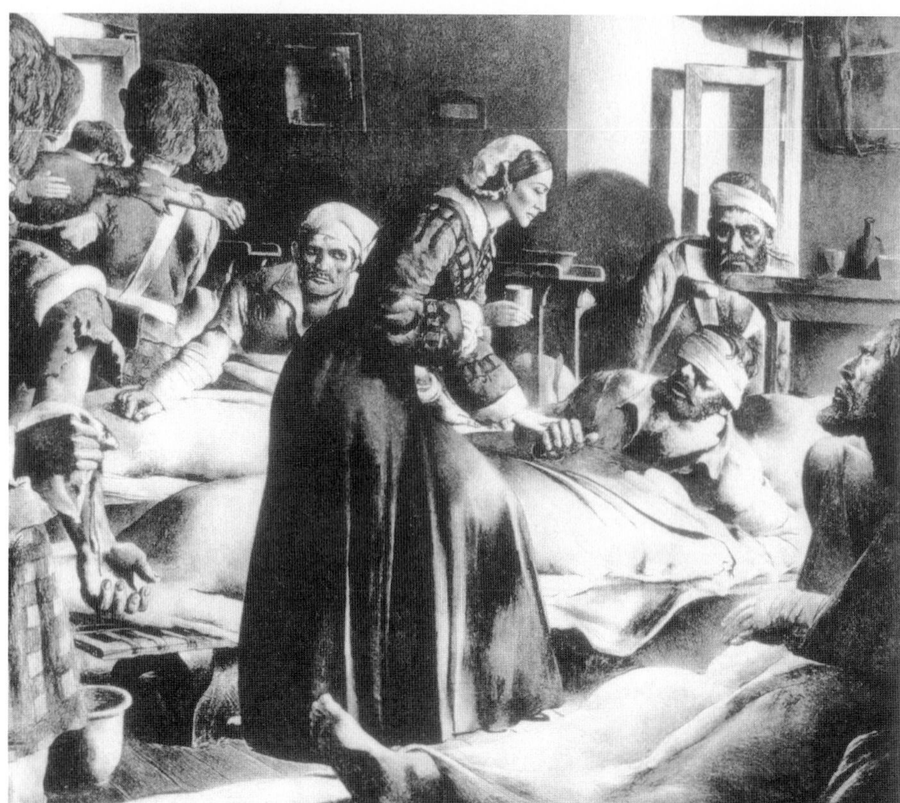

Florence Nightingale caring for wounded at Scutari, Turkey, during the Crimean War. (Courtesy of the National Library of Medicine)

From the 1860s, the rise of bacteriology, associated especially with chemist and microbiologist Louis Pasteur in France and bacteriologist Robert Koch in Germany, established the role of microorganismal pathogens. Almost for the first time in medicine, bacteriology led directly to dramatic new cures.

The technique of pasteurization is named after Louis Pasteur (1822–1895). He introduced the method in 1865 to prevent the souring of wine. Pasteur's studies of fermentation convinced him that it depended on the presence of microscopic forms of life, with each fermenting medium serving as a unique food for a specific microorganism. He developed techniques for culturing microbes in liquid broths. Through his work, he was able to dispel the disease theory that predominated in the mid-nineteenth century, attributing fevers to "miasmas," or fumes, and laid the foundation for the germ theory of disease.

The anthrax bacillus, discovered by Robert Koch (1843–1910), was the first microorganism identified as a cause of illness. Koch's trailblazing work also included identifying the organism responsible for tuberculosis and the discovery of a tuberculosis skin-testing material.

In 1895, German physicist Wilhelm Röntgen (1845–1923) discovered X rays. For the first time without a catastrophic event, the most hidden parts of a human body were revealed. Even though he understood that it was a significant discovery, Röntgen did not initially recognize the amazing diagnostic potential of the process he had discovered.

THE TWENTIETH CENTURY

The twentieth century was a period of revolutionary industry in the science and politics of health. Concerns about the care of infants and children and the spread of infectious disease became prevailing themes in public and political arenas alike. It was during this time that private duty and public health nursing emerged as the means of delivering health care to people in their homes and in their communities. Social service agencies like the Henry Street Settlement in New York, founded by Lillian Wald, sent nurses into tenements to care for the sick.[5] The placement of nurses in schools began in New York City in 1902 at the urging of Wald, who offered to supply a Henry Street nurse for 1 month without charge.[5] Efforts to broaden the delivery of health care from the city to rural areas also were initiated during the early 1900s. The American Red Cross, which was reorganized and granted a new charter by Congress in 1905, established a nursing service for the rural poor that eventually expanded to serve the small town poor as well.[5]

Scientific discoveries and innovations abounded in the twentieth century. In the early 1900s, German bacteriologist Paul Ehrlich (1854–1915) theorized that certain substances could act as "magic bullets," attacking disease-causing microbes but leaving the rest of the body undamaged. In 1910, he introduced his discovery: using the arsenic compound Salvarsan, he had found an effective weapon against syphilis. Through his work, Ehrlich launched the science of chemotherapy.

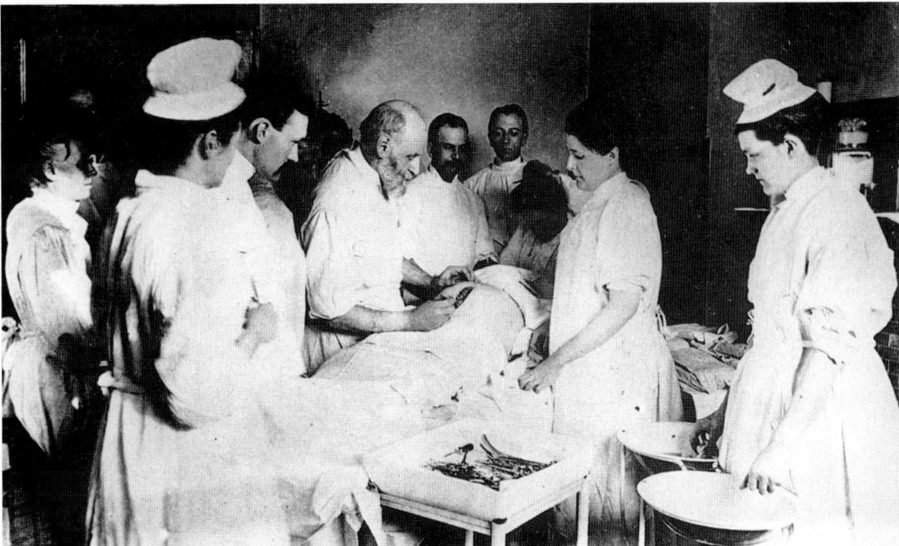

The operating room. With the advent of anesthesia, knowledge of how microbes cause disease, and availability of incandescent lighting in the operating room, surgery became an option for treating disease. Rubber gloves had not yet been invented and the surgical team worked with bare hands to perform surgery. (Hahnemann Hospital, Chicago, IL. Courtesy Bette Clemons, Phoenix, AZ)

The first antibiotic was discovered in 1928 by English bacteriologist Sir Alexander Fleming (1881–1955). As he studied the relationship between bacteria and the mold *Penicillium,* he discovered its ability to kill staphylococci. However, it was not until the 1940s that later researchers, who were searching for substances produced by one microorganism that might kill other microorganisms, produced penicillin as a clinically useful antibiotic.

By the 1930s, innovative researchers had produced a cornucopia of new drugs that could be used to treat many of the most common illnesses that left their victims either severely disabled or dead. The medical community now had at its disposal medications such as digoxin to treat heart failure; sulfa drugs, which produced near-miraculous cures for infections such as scarlet fever; and insulin to treat diabetes.

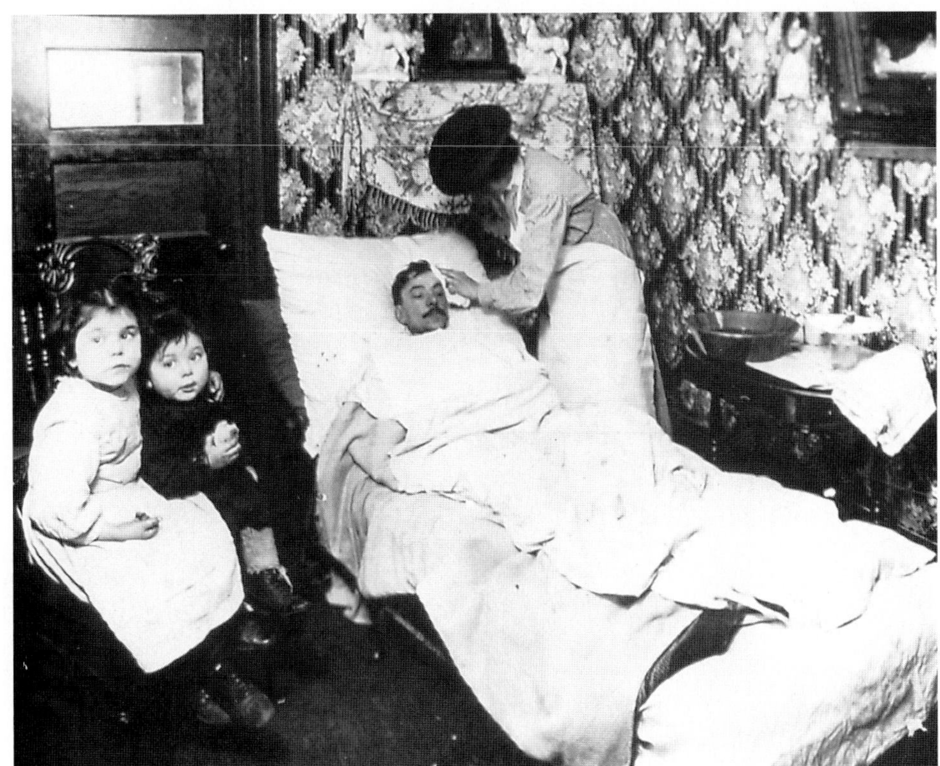

At the turn of the century, social service agencies like Henry Street Settlement in New York sent nurses into tenements to care for the sick. (Schorr T.M., Kennedy S.M. [1999]. *100 years of American nursing* [p. 12]. Philadelphia: Lippincott Williams & Wilkins)

With the discovery of insulin, a once-fatal disease known from antiquity no longer carried a death sentence. Working together, Canadian physician Sir Frederick Banting (1891–1941) and physiologist Charles Best (1899–1978) isolated insulin from the pancreas of a dog in 1921. The extract, when given to diabetic dogs, restored their health. In January 1922, they successfully treated a young boy dying of diabetes with their pancreatic extracts. Although still incurable, it became possible to live with diabetes.

One disease that remained not only incurable but untreatable through much of the twentieth century was tuberculosis. With no cure or preventive vaccine forthcoming, efforts at the turn of the century were dedicated to controlling the spread of tuberculosis. It was then that an alliance between organized medicine and the public resulted in the formation of voluntary local organizations to battle the disease. These organizations focused on education to counteract the fear of tuberculosis; at the same time, they warned against the disease. In 1904, the local organizations joined together to form a national organization, the National Association for the Study and Prevention of Tuberculosis. In 1918, the name was changed to the National Tuberculosis Association, which was renamed the American Lung Association in 1973.[6]

The national and local tuberculosis associations played a vital role in educating the public by running campaigns urging people to have skin tests and chest x-rays as a means of diagnosing tuberculosis. Once tuberculosis was diagnosed, an individual was likely to be sent to a sanatorium or tuberculosis hospital. There, good nourishment, fresh air, and bed rest were prescribed in the belief that if the body's natural defenses were strengthened, they would be able to overcome the tuberculosis bacillus. For almost half a century, this would be the prevailing treatment. It was not until 1945, with the introduction of chemotherapy, that streptomycin was used to treat tuberculosis.

Outbreaks of poliomyelitis, which had increased in the early decades of the 1900s, served as the impetus for the work of American microbiologist Jonas Salk (1914–1995). At its peak, the virus was claiming 50,000 victims annually in the United States.[3] Test trials of Salk's vaccine with inactivated virus began in 1953, and it proved to prevent the development of polio. By 1955, the massive testing was complete, and the vaccine was quickly put into wide use.

Surgical techniques also flourished during this time. A single technical innovation was responsible for opening up the last surgical frontier—the heart. Up to this time, the heart had been out of bounds; surgeons did not have the means to take over the function of the heart for long enough to get inside and operate.[7] American surgeon John Gibbon (1903–1973) addressed this problem when he developed the heart-lung machine. Dramatic advances followed its successful use in 1953—probably none more so than the first successful heart transplantation performed in 1967 by South African surgeon Christiaan Barnard (1922–2001).

For centuries, the inheritance of traits had been explained in religious or philosophical terms. Although English naturalist Charles Darwin's (1809–1882) work dispelled long-held beliefs about inherited traits, it was Austrian bo-

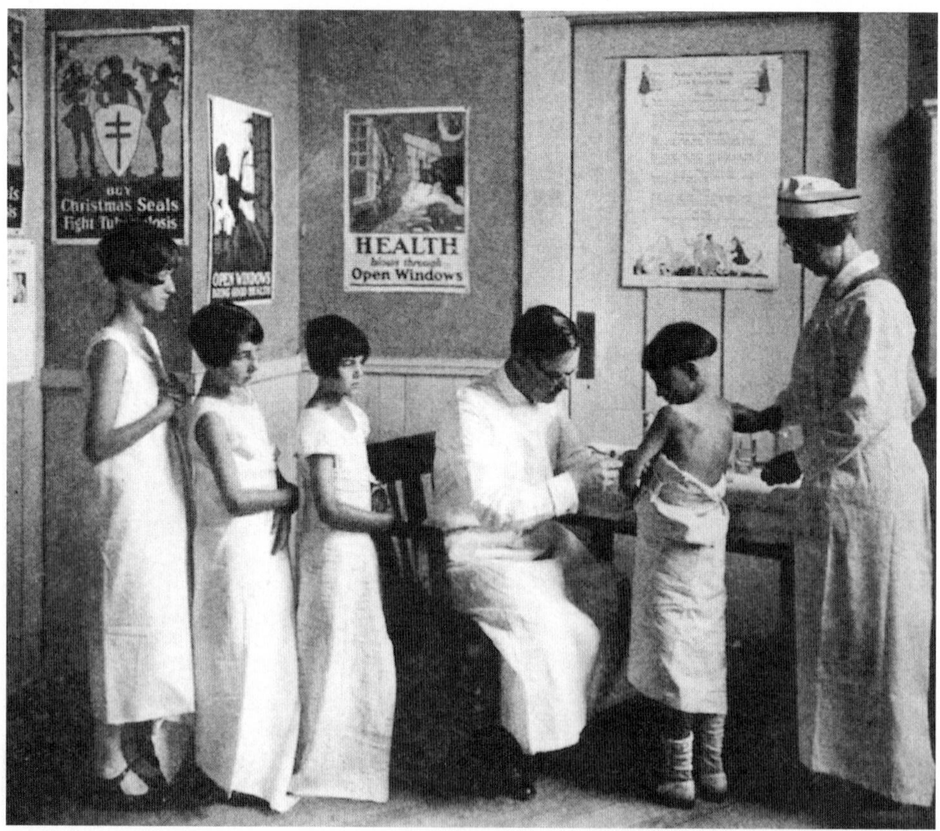

A tuberculosis skin testing clinic. (Schorr T.M., Kennedy S.M. [1999]. *100 years of American nursing* [p. 49]. Philadelphia: Lippincott Williams & Wilkins)

of the disease process include the etiology, pathogenesis, morphologic changes, clinical manifestations, diagnosis, and clinical course.

Etiology

The causes of disease are known as *etiologic factors.* Among the recognized etiologic agents are biologic agents (*e.g.*, bacteria, viruses), physical forces (*e.g.*, trauma, burns, radiation), chemical agents (*e.g.*, poisons, alcohol), and nutritional excesses or deficits. At the molecular level, it is important to distinguish between sick molecules and molecules that cause disease.[13] This is true of diseases such as cystic fibrosis, sickle cell anemia, and familial hypercholesterolemia, in which genetic abnormality of a single amino acid, transporter molecule, or receptor protein produces widespread effects on health.

Most disease-causing agents are nonspecific, and many different agents can cause disease of a single organ. For example, lung disease can result from trauma, infection, exposure to physical and chemical agents, or neoplasia. With severe lung involvement, each of these agents has the potential to cause respiratory failure. On the other hand, a single agent or traumatic event can lead to disease of a number of organs or systems. For example, severe circulatory shock can cause multiorgan failure.

Although a disease agent can affect more than a single organ, and a number of disease agents can affect the same organ, most disease states do not have a single cause. Instead, most diseases are multifactorial in origin. This is particularly true of diseases such as cancer, heart disease, and diabetes. The multiple factors that predispose to a particular disease often are referred to as *risk factors.*

One way to view the factors that cause disease is to group them into categories according to whether they were present at birth or acquired later in life. *Congenital conditions* are defects that are present at birth, although they may not be evident until later in life. Congenital malformation may be caused by genetic influences, environmental factors (*e.g.*, viral infections in the mother, maternal drug use, irradiation, or intrauterine crowding), or a combination of genetic and environmental factors. Not all genetic disorders are evident at birth. Many genetic disorders, such as familial hypercholesterolemia and polycystic kidney disease, take years to develop. *Acquired defects* are those that are caused by events that occur after birth. These include injury, exposure to infectious agents, inadequate nutrition, lack of oxygen, inappropriate immune responses, and neoplasia. Many diseases are thought to be the result of a genetic predisposition and an environmental event or events that serve as a trigger to initiate disease development.

Pathogenesis

Pathogenesis is the sequence of cellular and tissue events that take place from the time of initial contact with an etiologic agent until the ultimate expression of a disease. Etiology describes what sets the disease process in motion, and pathogenesis, how the disease process evolves. Although the two terms often are used interchangeably, their meanings are quite different. For example, atherosclerosis often is cited as the cause or etiology of coronary heart disease. In reality, the progression from fatty streak to the occlusive vessel lesion seen in persons with coronary heart disease represents the pathogenesis of the disorder. The true etiology of atherosclerosis remains largely uncertain.

Morphology

Morphology refers to the fundamental structure or form of cells or tissues. *Morphologic changes* are concerned with both the gross anatomic and microscopic changes that are characteristic of a disease. *Histology* deals with the study of the cells and extracellular matrix of body tissues. The most common method used in the study of tissues is the preparation of histologic sections that can be studied with the aid of a microscope. Because tissues and organs usually are too thick to be examined under a microscope, they must be sectioned to obtain thin, translucent sections. Histologic sections play an important role in the diagnosis of many types of cancer. A *lesion* represents a pathologic or traumatic discontinuity of a body organ or tissue. Descriptions of lesion size and characteristics often can be obtained through the use of radiographs, ultrasonography, and other imaging methods. Lesions also may be sampled by biopsy and the tissue samples subjected to histologic study.

Clinical Manifestations

Disease can be manifest in a number of ways. Sometimes, the condition produces manifestations, such as fever, that make it evident that the person is sick. Other diseases are silent at the onset and are detected during examination for other purposes or after the disease is far advanced.

Signs and *symptoms* are terms used to describe the structural and functional changes that accompany a disease. A *symptom* is a subjective complaint that is noted by the person with a disorder, whereas a *sign* is a manifestation that is noted by an observer. Pain, difficulty in breathing, and dizziness are symptoms of a disease. An elevated temperature, a swollen extremity, and changes in pupil size are objective signs that can be observed by someone other than the person with the disease. Signs and symptoms may be related to the primary disorder, or they may represent the body's attempt to compensate for the altered function caused by the pathologic condition. Many pathologic states are not observed directly—one cannot see a sick heart or a failing kidney. Instead, what can be observed is the body's attempt to compensate for changes in function brought about by the disease, such as the tachycardia that accompanies blood loss or the increased respiratory rate that occurs with pneumonia.

It is important to recognize that a single sign or symptom may be associated with a number of different disease states. For example, an elevated temperature can indicate the presence of an infection, heat stroke, brain tumor, or any number of other disorders. A differential diagnosis that describes the origin of a disorder usually requires information regarding a number of signs and symptoms. For example, the presence of fever, a reddened sore throat, and positive throat culture describe a "strep throat" infection. A *syndrome* is a compilation of signs and symptoms (*e.g.*, chronic fatigue syndrome) that are characteristic of a specific disease state. *Complications* are possible adverse ex-

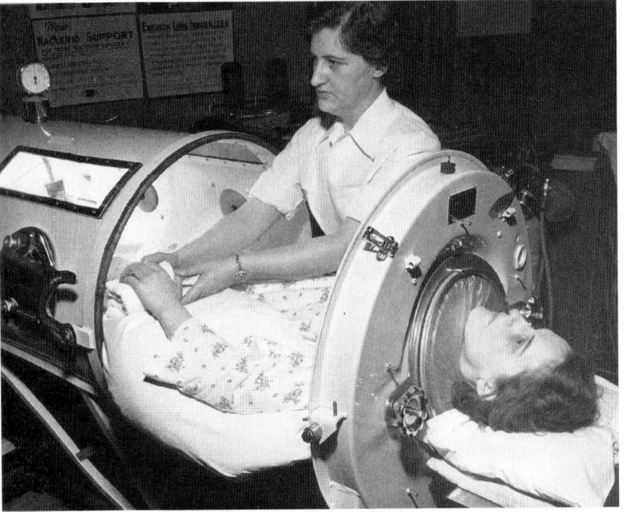

The "iron lung," which used negative pressure to draw air into the lungs, was used to provide ventilatory support for persons with "bulbar polio." (Schorr T.M., Kennedy S.M. [1999]. *100 years of American nursing* [p. 91]. Philadelphia: Lippincott Williams & Wilkins)

tanist Gregor Mendel's (1822–1884) revolutionary theories on the segregation of traits, largely ignored until 1902, that laid the groundwork for establishing the chromosome as the structural unit of heredity. Many other scientists and researchers contributed to the storehouse of genetic knowledge. With the work by American geneticist James Watson (1928–) and British biophysicists Francis Crick (1916–) and Maurice Wilkins (1916–) in the early 1950s, which established the double-helical structure of DNA, the way to investigating and understanding our genetic heritage was opened.

It is difficult, if not impossible, to single out all the landmark events of the twentieth century that contributed to the health of humankind. Among the other notable achievements are the development of kidney dialysis, oral contraceptives, transplant surgery, the computed axial tomography (CAT) scanner, and coronary angioplasty.

Not all of the important advances in modern medicine are as dramatic as open-heart surgery. Often, they are the result of dogged work by many people and yield results only after a number of years, and then they frequently go unheralded. For example, vaccination programs, control of infectious diseases through improvements in sanitation of water and waste disposal, safer and healthier foods free from microbial contamination, identification of health risks from behaviors such as smoking, and improved prenatal care all have saved many lives in the twentieth century.

THE TWENTY-FIRST CENTURY

The twenty-first century reveals new horizons, but also new problems. In greater numbers than ever, goods and people travel the world. There is unprecedented physical mobility—travel and migration from villages to cities and country to country—and interconnectedness. However, the benefits of physical mobility and interconnectedness are accompanied by risks. Diseases such as AIDS remind us that nothing is regional, local, or limited in its reach: contagious illness has a worldwide arena.

The challenges of maintaining health and well-being in this global community are increasingly apparent. The inadvertent introduction of pathogens poses an unrelenting threat to public health, as does the deliberate use of microorganisms as weapons (see Chapter 18 for a discussion of bioterrorism and emerging global infectious diseases). In February 2003, the viral respiratory illness named *severe acute respiratory syndrome* (SARS) by the World Health Organization was first recognized in China.[8] In the next few months, the illness swept through parts of Asia and spread to more than two dozen countries in North America, South America, and Europe. The disease was characterized by rapid onset and variable severity, ranging from mild illness to death. The prevention of SARS was a particular challenge because preventive interventions (*e.g.*, vaccines and antibiotics) were unavailable. Containment became a global collaboration, with public health authorities utilizing isolation and quarantine to focus delivery of health care to people who were ill and to protect healthy people from getting sick. During the February to July outbreak, more than 8000 people worldwide became infected, and more than 900 died.

Commerce also is an integral part of the growing world community, bringing goods and services once unobtainable into the global marketplace. Expanded international trade also provides the vehicle for the unwitting introduction or transmission of disease. One such instance occurred in the spring of 2003 in the United States.[9] A multistate outbreak of human monkeypox, first identified in the Democratic Republic of the Congo in 1970, was traced by investigators to pet prairie dogs. The prairie dogs became infected when they were housed or transported along with infected Gambian giant rats, dormice, and rope squirrels that were part of a shipment of small mammals from Ghana. Spread of nonindigenous zoonotic pathogens to indigenous susceptible animal populations can be rapid and deadly. With such outbreaks lurks an additional danger—the potential for interspecies exchange, including between humans and animals such as pets.

The widespread distribution of infected and potentially infected animals allowed epizootic spread of monkeypox through several states before effective interventions could be put into place. One of the challenges to the world health community will be to study the role of international travel and commerce in the emergence of infectious diseases through the dissemination of pathogens and their vectors throughout the world and then to develop long-term strategies of surveillance and intervention with the ultimate goal of curtailing their occurrence.

In 1976, the World Health Organization (WHO) actually succeeded in eliminating smallpox from the face of the earth.[10] This triumph gave substance to the idea that other infections, like measles, also might disappear if sufficient efforts were directed at worldwide campaigns to isolate and cure them. However, new infectious diseases, such as Lyme disease and Legionnaire's disease, and new forms of old diseases, such as resistant strains of tuberculosis and malaria, have emerged and are readily spread worldwide. The powerful interventions used to fight these infections have had the unexpected effect of accelerating their biologic evolution and making them impervious to one after another form of chemical attack.

Pathogens also can be introduced into the food chain and travel worldwide. The discovery that beef from cattle infected with bovine spongiform encephalopathy (BSE) may be the source of Creutzfeldt-Jakob disease led many countries to ban beef products from the United Kingdom when BSE was found to be prevalent in English herds. The introduction of such pathogens can be the result of ignorance, carelessness, or greed. Tobacco is a product that serves as a pathogen. In a quest for ever-increasing profits, the tobacco industry created a demand for its product by artificially raising the nicotine content of cigarettes so as to increase their addictive potential. This was done with the knowledge of the health risks of tobacco products, thanks to experiments conducted by the tobacco companies' own medical scientists, but kept secret.

If there is a blueprint for future advances, it is in the genes. The twenty-first century is destined to be dominated by advances in genetics. With the mapping of the human genome comes hope of cure for some of the most dreaded crippling and fatal diseases. The mapping of the human genome also has posed new ethical dilemmas, for with it comes the potential to predict the future health of persons based on their genes. It soon may be possible to differentiate between persons who will develop certain debilitating diseases and those who will not.

Although advances in science and technology will continue to provide new treatments for many diseases, it has become apparent that there are more impressive rewards to be had by preventing diseases from becoming established in the first place. Ultimately, maintaining health is more resource conservative and cost effective than relying on the treatment of disease. Many decades ago, we learned that even though the "magic bullets" such as antibiotics had the ability to cure what was once considered incurable, much of our freedom from communicable disease is due to clean water, efficient sanitation, and good nutrition. We have become increasingly aware of the importance of preventive measures against noninfectious conditions, especially cancer and coronary heart disease. There is no better way to prevent disease and maintain health than by leading a healthy life, and increasingly, it will be the individual who is responsible for ensuring a healthy passage through life.

In summary, Greek scholars were responsible for establishing the fundamentals of anatomy, physiology, and pathology that served as the earliest knowledge base for understanding health and disease. It was Hippocrates (460–377 BC) and his followers who laid the foundations of the clinical principles and ethics that grew into modern science. Although his belief that disease occurred when the four humors—blood, yellow and black bile, and phlegm—became out of balance was disproved, his approach to health that dictated plenty of healthy exercise, rest in illness, and a moderate, sober diet remains valid. Galen (AD 129–199) took the next major step, expanding on Hippocratic doctrines and introducing experimentation into the study of healing. His work, gleaned through his role as physician to the emperors and gladiators of Rome and animal dissections, came to be regarded as the encyclopedia of anatomy and physiology and was considered infallible for almost 1400 years.

Significant challenges to long-held beliefs began with the work of Andreas Vesalius (1514–1564), professor of anatomy and surgery at Padua, Italy. His published work, *On the Fabric [Structure] of the Human Body,* showing how the parts of the body looked and worked, set a new standard for the understanding of human anatomy. Other significant early contributions were made by scholars such as William Harvey (1578–1657), the English physician and physiologist, who in his book, *On the Motion of the Heart and Blood in Animals,* provided a physiologic framework for the circulation of blood; Anton van Leeuwenhoek (1632–1723), the Dutch lens maker who refined the microscope and set the stage for the era of cellular biology; and Edward Jenner (1749–1823), the English country physician who conducted the first successful vaccination.

The nineteenth century was a time of major discoveries that paved the way for understanding infectious diseases. Significant contributions were made by such scientists as Joseph Lister, the English surgeon who concluded that microbes caused wound infections; German bacteriologist Robert Koch, who discovered the anthrax bacillus, thus identifying for the first time a microorganism and the illness it caused; and French chemist and microbiologist Louis Pasteur, who developed the technique of pasteurization. Perhaps the most notable technical innovation of the century was the discovery of X rays by German physicist Wilhelm Röntgen.

The scientific undertakings and discoveries of the twentieth century were revolutionary. In 1910, Paul Ehrlich introduced chemotherapy, and in 1928, Sir Alexander Fleming discovered the first antibiotic as he studied the relationship between bacteria and the mold *Penicillium.* Diseases that had once been fatal or crippling were managed or prevented by new advances, such as the discovery of insulin by Sir Frederick Banting and Charles Best in 1922 and the development of the polio vaccine by Jonas Salk in 1953. Technical innovations set the stage for new surgical techniques. The creation of the heart-lung machine by American surgeon John Gibbon paved the way for coronary bypass surgery and the first successful heart transplantation in 1967, which was performed by Christiaan Barnard, a South African surgeon. Other important advances included kidney dialysis, oral contraceptives, the CAT scanner, and coronary angioplasty. Public health programs also were responsible for greatly affecting the health of populations, such as those dedicated to increasing vaccination, improving sanitation of water and waste disposal, and identifying health risks.

Knowledge about the influence of heredity on health and disease originated with Charles Darwin's (1809–1882) evolutionary theories about inherited traits and with Gregor Mendel's (1822–1884) theories on the segregation of traits, which laid the groundwork for establishing the chromosome as the structural unit of heredity. In the early 1950s, geneticist James Watson of the United States and British biophysicists Francis Crick and Maurice Wilkins presented their findings on the double-helical structure of DNA.

The twenty-first century is predicted to be a time of great advances in the field of genetics, already evidenced by the substantial mapping of the human genome that has taken place. Scientists look to genetic research to provide advances that not only will predict who may develop disease but also will provide new treatments for those diseases. However promising future advances may appear, it is readily apparent that prevention is an equally important tool in maintaining health.

Perspectives on Health and Disease in Individuals

After completing this section of the chapter, you should be able to meet the following objectives:

- State the World Health Organization definition of health
- Describe the function of adaptation as it relates to health and disease
- State a definition of pathophysiology
- Characterize the disease process in terms of etiology, pathogenesis, morphology, clinical manifestations, and prognosis
- Explain the meanings of reliability, validity, sensitivity, specificity, and predictive value as they relate to observations and tests used in the diagnosis of disease

What constitutes health and disease often is difficult to determine because of the way different people view the topic. What is defined as health is determined by many factors, including heredity, age and sex, cultural and ethnic differences, as well as individual, group, and governmental expectations.

HEALTH

The World Health Organization (WHO) in 1948 defined health as a "state of complete physical, mental, and social well-being and not merely the absence of disease and infirmity."[10] Although ideal for many people, this was an unrealistic goal. At the World Health Assembly in 1977, representatives of the member governments of WHO agreed that their goal was to have all citizens of the world reach a level of health by the year 2000 that allows them to live a socially and economically productive life.[10] The U.S. Department of Health and Human Services in *Healthy People 2010* described the determinants of health as an interaction between an individual's biology and behavior, physical and social environments, government policies and interventions, and access to quality health care.[11]

HEALTH AND DISEASE AS STATES OF ADAPTATION

The ability of the body to adapt both physically and psychologically to the many stresses that occur in both health and disease is affected by a number of factors, including age, health status, psychosocial resources, and the rapidity with which the need to adapt occurs (see Chapter 9). Generally speaking, adaptation affects the whole person. When adapting to stresses that are threats to health, the body uses those behaviors that are the most efficient and effective. It does not use long-term mechanisms when short-term adaptation is sufficient. The increase in heart rate that accompanies a febrile illness is a temporary response designed to deliver additional oxygen to tissues during the short period that the elevated temperature increases metabolic needs. On the other hand, hypertrophy of the left ventricle is a long-term adaptive response that occurs in persons with chronic hypertension.

Adaptation is further affected by the availability of adaptive responses and the ability of the body to select the most appropriate response. The ability to adapt is dependent on the availability of adaptive responses—the greater number of available responses, the more effective the capacity to adapt. Adaptive capacity is decreased with extremes of age and with disease conditions that limit the availability of adaptive responses. The immaturity of the infant impairs the ability to adapt, as does the decline in functional reserve that occurs in the elderly. For example, infants have difficulty concentrating urine because of the immaturity of their renal tubular structures and therefore are less able than an older child or adult to cope with decreased water intake or exaggerated water losses. Similarly, persons with preexisting heart disease are less able to adapt to health problems that require recruitment of cardiovascular responses. Adaptation also is less effective when changes in health status occur suddenly rather than gradually. For instance, it is possible to lose a liter of blood through chronic gastrointestinal bleeding without developing signs of shock. On the other hand, a sudden hemorrhage that causes the loss of an equal amount of blood is apt to produce hypotension and circulatory shock. Even in advanced disease states, the body retains much of its adaptive capacity and is able to maintain the internal environment within relatively normal limits.

DISEASE

The term *pathophysiology,* which is the focus of this book, may be defined as the physiology of altered health. The term combines the words *pathology* and *physiology.* Pathology (from the Greek *pathos,* meaning "disease") deals with the study of the structural and functional changes in cells, tissues, and organs of the body that cause or are caused by disease. Physiology deals with the functions of the human body. Thus, pathophysiology deals not only with the cellular and organ changes that occur with disease but also with the effects that these changes have on total body function. Pathophysiology also focuses on the mechanisms of the underlying disease and provides the background for preventive as well as therapeutic health care measures and practices.

A disease has been defined as any deviation from or interruption of the normal structure or function of a part, organ, or system of the body that is manifested by a characteristic set of symptoms or signs; the etiology, pathology, and prognosis may be known or unknown.[12] The aspects

tensions of a disease or outcomes from treatment. *Sequelae* are lesions or impairments that follow or are caused by a disease.

Diagnosis

A *diagnosis* is the designation as to the nature or cause of a health problem (*e.g.,* bacterial pneumonia or hemorrhagic stroke). The diagnostic process usually requires a careful history and physical examination. The history is used to obtain a person's account of his or her symptoms, their progression, and the factors that contribute to a diagnosis. The physical examination is done to observe for signs of altered body structure or function.

The development of a diagnosis involves weighing competing possibilities and selecting the most likely one from among the conditions that might be responsible for the person's clinical presentation. The clinical probability of a given disease in a person of a given age, sex, race, lifestyle, and locality often is influential in arriving at a presumptive diagnosis. Laboratory tests, radiologic studies, CT scans, and other tests often are used to confirm a diagnosis.

Normality. An important factor when interpreting diagnostic test results is the determination of whether they are normal or abnormal. Is a blood count above normal, within the normal range, or below normal? Normality usually determines whether further tests are needed or if interventions are necessary. What is termed a *normal* value for a laboratory test is established statistically from test results obtained from a selected sample of people. The normal values refer to the 95% distribution (mean plus or minus two standard deviations [mean ± 2 SD]) of test results for the reference population.[14] Thus, the normal levels for serum sodium (135 to 145 mEq/L) represent the mean serum level for the reference population ± 2 SD. The normal values for some laboratory tests are adjusted for sex or age. For example, the normal hemoglobin range for women is 12.0 to 16.0 g/dL and for men, 14.0 to 17.4 g/dL.[15] Serum creatinine level often is adjusted for age in the elderly (see Chapter 36), and normal values for serum phosphate differ between adults and children.

Reliability, Validity, Sensitivity, Specificity, and Predictive Value. The quality of data on which a diagnosis is based may be judged for its reliability, validity, sensitivity, specificity, and predictive value.[16,17] *Reliability* refers to the extent to which an observation, if repeated, gives the same result. A poorly calibrated blood pressure machine may give inconsistent measurements of blood pressure, particularly of pressures in either the high or low range. Reliability also depends on the persons making the measurements. For example, blood pressure measurements may vary from one observer to another because of the technique that is used (*e.g.,* different observers may deflate the cuff at a different rate, thus obtaining different values), the way the numbers on the manometer are read, or differences in hearing acuity. *Validity* refers to the extent to which a measurement tool measures what it is intended to measure. This often is assessed by comparing a measurement method with the best possible method of measure that is available. For example, the validity of blood pressure measurements obtained by a sphygmomanometer might be compared with those obtained by intraarterial measurements.

Measures of sensitivity and specificity are concerned with determining how well the test or observation identifies people with the disease and people without the disease. *Sensitivity* refers to the proportion of people with a disease who are positive for that disease on a given test or observation (called a *true-positive* result). *Specificity* refers to the proportion of people without the disease who are negative on a given test or observation (called a *true-negative* result). A test that is 95% specific correctly identifies 95 of 100 normal people. The other 5% are *false-positive* results. A false-positive test result, particularly for conditions such as human immunodeficiency virus (HIV) infection, can be unduly stressful for the person being tested (see Chapter 22). In the case of HIV testing, a positive result on the initial antibody test is followed up with a more sensitive test. On the other hand, *false-negative* test results in conditions such as cancer can delay diagnosis and jeopardize the outcome of treatment.

Predictive value is the extent to which an observation or test result is able to predict the presence of a given disease or condition. A *positive predictive value* refers to the proportion of true-positive results that occurs in a given population. In a group of women found to have "suspect breast nodules" in a cancer-screening program, the proportion later determined to have breast cancer would constitute the positive predictive value. A *negative predictive value* refers to the true-negative observations in a population. In a screening test for breast cancer, the negative predictive value represents the proportion of women without suspect nodules who do not have breast cancer. Although predictive values rely in part on sensitivity and specificity, they depend more heavily on the prevalence of the condition in the population. Despite unchanging sensitivity and specificity, the positive predictive value of an observation rises with prevalence, whereas the negative predictive value falls.

Clinical Course

The clinical course describes the evolution of a disease. A disease can have an acute, subacute, or chronic course. An *acute disorder* is one that is relatively severe, but self-limiting. *Chronic disease* implies a continuous, long-term process. A chronic disease can run a continuous course, or it can present with exacerbations (aggravation of symptoms and severity of the disease) and remissions (a period during which there is a lessening of severity and a decrease in symptoms). *Subacute disease* is intermediate or between acute and chronic: it is not as severe as an acute disease and not as prolonged as a chronic disease.

The spectrum of disease severity for infectious diseases such as hepatitis B can range from preclinical to persistent chronic infection. During the *preclinical stage,* the disease is not clinically evident but is destined to progress to clinical disease. As with hepatitis B, it is possible to transmit the virus during the preclinical stage. *Subclinical disease* is not clinically apparent and is not destined to become clinically apparent. It is diagnosed with antibody or culture tests. Most cases of tuberculosis are not clinically apparent, and evidence of their presence is established by skin tests.

Clinical disease is manifested by signs and symptoms. A persistent chronic infectious disease persists for years, sometimes for life. *Carrier status* refers to an individual who harbors an organism but is not infected, as evidenced by antibody response or clinical manifestations. This person still can infect others. Carrier status may be of limited duration, or it may be chronic, lasting for months or years.

In summary, health is determined by many factors, including genetics, age and sex, and cultural and ethnic differences. The WHO defines health as a "state of complete physical, mental, and social well-being and not merely the absence of disease and infirmity."

The ability of the body to adapt to changes that occur in both health and disease is affected by such factors as age, health status, and psychosocial resources. Adaptation is further affected by the availability and number of adaptive responses. Extreme age and disease conditions, such as when changes occur suddenly rather than gradually, also affect the capacity to adapt.

The term *pathophysiology* may be defined as the physiology of altered health. A *disease* has been defined as any deviation from or interruption of the normal structure or function of any part, organ, or system of the body that is manifested by a characteristic set of symptoms or signs and whose etiology, pathology, and prognosis may be known or unknown. The causes of disease are known as *etiologic factors.* Recognized etiologic agents include biologic agents (bacteria, viruses), physical forces (trauma, burns, radiation), chemical agents (poisons, alcohol), and nutritional excesses or deficits. *Pathogenesis* describes how the disease process evolves. *Morphology* refers to the structure or form of cells or tissues; *morphologic changes* are changes in structure or form that are characteristic of a disease.

Disease can manifest itself through signs and symptoms. A symptom is a subjective complaint, such as pain or dizziness; a sign is an observable manifestation, such as an elevated temperature or a reddened sore throat. A syndrome is a compilation of signs and symptoms that are characteristic of a specific disease state.

The clinical course of a disease describes its evolution. It can be acute (relatively severe, but self-limiting), chronic (continuous or episodic, but taking place over a long period), or subacute (not as severe as acute or as prolonged as chronic). Within the disease spectrum, a disease can be designated preclinical, or not clinically evident; subclinical, not clinically apparent and not destined to become clinically apparent; or clinical, characterized by signs and symptoms.

Perspectives on Health and Disease in Populations

After completing this section of the chapter, you should be able to meet the following objectives:

- Define the term *epidemiology*
- Compare the meaning of the terms *incidence* and *prevalence* as they relate to measures of disease frequency
- Compare the sources of information and limitations of mortality and morbidity statistics
- Characterize the natural history of a disease
- Differentiate primary, secondary, and tertiary levels of prevention
- Propose ways in which practice guidelines can be used to improve health care

The health of individuals is closely linked to the health of the community and to the population it encompasses. The ability to traverse continents in a matter of hours has opened the world to issues of populations at a global level. Diseases that once were confined to local areas of the world now pose a threat to populations throughout the world.

As we move through the twenty-first century, we are continually reminded that the health care system and the services it delivers are targeted to particular populations. Managed care systems are focused on a population-based approach to planning, delivering, providing, and evaluating health care. The focus of health care also has begun to emerge as a partnership in which individuals are asked to assume greater responsibility for their own health.

EPIDEMIOLOGY AND PATTERNS OF DISEASE

Epidemiology is the study of disease in populations. It was initially developed to explain the spread of infectious diseases during epidemics and has emerged as a science to study risk factors for multifactorial diseases, such as heart disease and cancer. Epidemiology looks for patterns, such as age, race, dietary habits, lifestyle, or geographic location of persons affected with a particular disorder. In contrast to biomedical researchers, who seek to elucidate the mechanisms of disease production, epidemiologists are more concerned with whether something happens than how it happens.[18] For example, the epidemiologist is more concerned with whether smoking itself is related to cardiovascular disease and whether the risk for heart disease decreases when smoking ceases. On the other hand, the biomedical researcher is more concerned about the causative agent in cigarette smoke and the pathway by which it contributes to heart disease.

Much of our knowledge about disease comes from epidemiologic studies. Epidemiologic methods are used to determine how a disease is spread, how to control it, how to prevent it, and how to eliminate it. Epidemiologic methods also are used to study the natural history of disease, to evaluate new preventative and treatment strategies, to explore the impact of different patterns of health care delivery, and to predict future health care needs. As such, epidemiologic studies serve as a basis for clinical decision making, allocation of health care dollars, and development of policies related to public health issues.

Prevalence and Incidence

Measures of disease frequency are an important aspect of epidemiology. They establish a means for predicting what diseases are present in a population and provide an indication of the rate at which they are increasing or decreasing. A *disease case* can be either an existing case or the number of new episodes of a particular illness that is diagnosed within a given period. *Incidence* is the number of new cases arising in a population during a specified time. It is determined by dividing the number of new cases of a disease by the population at risk for development of the disease during the same period. *Prevalence* is the number of people in a population who have a particular disease at a given point in time or period. It is determined by dividing the existing number of cases by the population at risk for development of the disorder during the same period. Incidence and prevalence rates always are reported as proportions (*e.g.*, cases per 100 or cases per 100,000).

Morbidity and Mortality

Morbidity and mortality statistics provide information about the functional effects (morbidity) and death-producing (mortality) characteristics of a disease. These statistics are useful in terms of anticipating health care needs, planning of public education programs, directing health research efforts, and allocating health care dollars.

Mortality or death statistics provide information about the trends in the health of a population. In most countries, people are legally required to record certain facts such as age, sex, and cause of death on a death certificate. Internationally agreed classification procedures (the International Classification of Diseases by the WHO) are used for coding the cause of death, and the data are expressed as death rates.[10] Crude mortality rates (*i.e.*, number of deaths in a given period) do not account for age, sex, race, socioeconomic status, and other factors. For this reason, mortality often is expressed as death rates for a specific population, such as the infant mortality rate. Mortality also can be described in terms of the leading causes of death according to age, sex, race, and ethnicity. Among all persons 65 years of age and older, the five leading causes of death in the United States are heart disease, cancer, stroke, chronic obstructive lung disease, and pneumonia and influenza[9] (Fig. 1-1). In 1997, for example, diabetes was the third leading cause of death among American Indians 65 years of age and older, the fourth leading cause of death among older Hispanic and black persons, and the sixth leading cause of death among older white persons and Asian Americans.[11]

Morbidity describes the effects an illness has on a person's life. Many diseases, such as arthritis, have low death rates but have a significant impact on a person's life. Morbidity is concerned not only with the occurrence or incidence of a disease but also with persistence and the long-term consequences of the disease.

DETERMINATION OF RISK FACTORS

Conditions suspected of contributing to the development of a disease are called *risk factors*. They may be inherent to the person (high blood pressure or overweight) or external (smoking or drinking alcohol). There are different types of studies used to determine risk factors, including cross-sectional studies, case-control studies, and cohort studies. *Cross-sectional studies* use the simultaneous collection of information necessary for classification of exposure and outcome status. They can be used to compare the prevalence of a disease in those with the factor (or exposure) with the prevalence of a disease in those who are unexposed to the factor, such as the prevalence of coronary heart disease in smokers and nonsmokers. *Case-control studies* are designed to compare persons known to have the outcome of interest (*cases*) and those known not to have

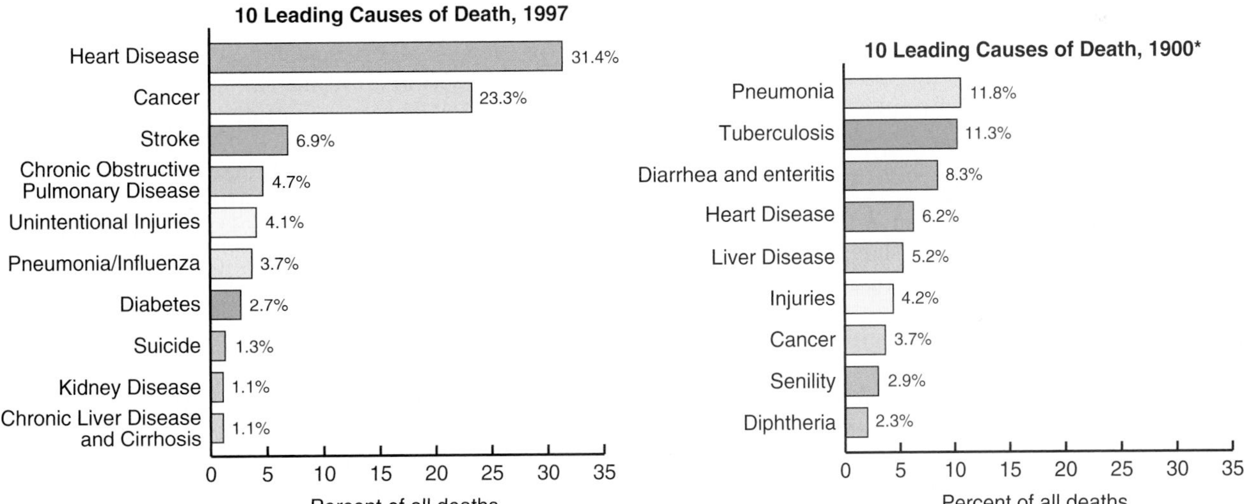

FIGURE 1-1 The 10 leading causes of death as a percentage of deaths in the United States, 1900 and 1997. (U.S. Department of Health and Human Services. [2000]. *Healthy people 2010.* Centers for Disease Control and Prevention, National Center for Health Statistics, National Vital Statistics System. [Unpublished data, 1997.] Accessible at http://web.health.gov/healthypeople/)

the outcome of interest (*control*). Information on exposures or characteristics of interest is then collected from persons in both groups. For example, the characteristics of maternal alcohol consumption in infants born with fetal alcohol syndrome (cases) can be compared with those in infants born without the syndrome (control). A *cohort* is a group of persons who were born at approximately the same time or share some characteristics of interest. Persons enrolled in a cohort study (also called a *longitudinal study*) are followed over a period to observe some health outcome. A cohort may consist of a single group of persons chosen because they have or have not been exposed to suspected risk factors; two groups specifically selected because one has been exposed and the other has not; or a single exposed group in which the results are compared with the general population. The Framingham Study, which examined the characteristics of people who would later experience coronary heart disease, and the Nurses' Health Study, which initially explored the relationship between oral contraceptives and breast cancer, are two well-known cohort studies.

The Framingham Study

One of the best-known examples of a cohort study is the Framingham Study, which was carried out in Framingham, Massachusetts.[19] Framingham was selected because of the size of the population, the relative ease with which the people could be contacted, and the stability of the population in terms of moving into and out of the area. This longitudinal study, which began in 1950, was set up by the U.S. Public Health Service to study the characteristics of people who would later develop coronary heart disease. The study consisted of 5000 persons, aged 30 to 59 years, selected at random and followed for an initial period of 20 years, during which time it was predicted that 1500 of them would develop coronary heart disease. The advantage of such a study is that it can study a number of risk factors at the same time and determine the relative importance of each. Another advantage is that the risk factors can be related later to other diseases such as stroke. Chart 1-1 describes some of the significant milestones from the Framingham Study.

CHART 1-1

Framingham Study: Significant Milestones

- 1960—Cigarette smoking found to increase risk of heart disease
- 1961—Cholesterol level, blood pressure, and electrocardiogram abnormalities found to increase risk of heart disease
- 1967—Physical activity found to reduce risk of heart disease and obesity to increase risk of heart disease
- 1970—High blood pressure found to increase risk of stroke
- 1976—Menopause found to increase risk of heart disease
- 1977—Effects of triglycerides and low-density lipoprotein (LDL) and high-density lipoprotein (HDL) cholesterol noted
- 1978—Psychosocial factors found to affect heart disease
- 1986—First report on dementia
- 1988—High levels of HDL cholesterol found to reduce risk of death
- 1994—Enlarged left ventricle shown to increase risk of stroke
- 1996—Progression from hypertension to heart failure described
- 1997—Report of cumulative effects of smoking and high cholesterol on the risk of atherosclerosis

(Abstracted from Framingham Heart Study. [2001]. Research milestones. [On-line.] Available: http://rover.nhlbi.nih.gov/about/framingham/timeline.htm.)

The Nurses' Health Study

A second well-known cohort study is the Nurses' Health Study, which was developed by Harvard University and Brigham and Women's Hospital. The study began in 1976 with a cohort of 121,700 female nurses, 30 to 55 years of age, living in the United States.[20] Initially designed to explore the relationship between oral contraceptives and breast cancer, nurses in the study have provided answers to detailed questions about their menstrual cycle, smoking habits, diet, weight and waist measurements, activity patterns, health problems, and medication use. They have collected urine and blood samples and even provided researchers with their toenail clippings.[21] In selecting the cohort, it was reasoned that nurses would be well organized, accurate, and observant in their responses and that physiologically they would be no different from other groups of women. It also was anticipated that their childbearing, eating, and smoking patterns would be similar to those of other working women.

The Nurses' Health Study has yielded over 250 published papers on subjects as diverse as body mass index, weight change, and risk for adult-onset asthma in women[22]; smoking cessation and time course to decreased risk for coronary heart disease in middle-aged women[23]; electric blanket use and breast cancer[24]; waist circumference, waist:hip ratio, and risk for breast cancer[25]; and aspirin and risk for colorectal cancer.[26] After 25 years, 90% of the nurses still respond promptly to the biennial questionnaire—a rate that far exceeds the average for other longitudinal studies.

NATURAL HISTORY

The *natural history* of disease refers to the progression and projected outcome of a disease without medical intervention. By studying the patterns of a disease over time in populations, epidemiologists can better understand its natural history. A knowledge of the natural history can be used to determine disease outcome, establish priorities for health care services, determine the effects of screening and early detection programs on disease outcome, and compare the results of new treatments with the expected outcome without treatment.

There are some diseases for which there are no effective treatment methods available, or the current treatment measures are effective only in certain people. In this case, the natural history of the disease can be used as a predictor of outcome. For example, the natural history of hepatitis C indicates that 80% of people who become infected with the virus fail to clear the virus and progress to chronic infection.[27] Information about the natural history of a disease and the availability of effective treatment methods provides directions for preventive measures. In the case of hepatitis C, careful screening of blood donations and education of intravenous drug abusers can be used to prevent transfer of the virus. At the same time, scientists are striving to develop a vaccine that will prevent infection in persons exposed to the virus. The development of vaccines to prevent the spread of infectious diseases such as polio and hepatitis B undoubtedly has been motivated by knowledge about the natural history of these diseases and the lack of effective intervention measures. With other diseases, such as breast cancer, early detection through use of breast self-examination and mammography increases the chances for a cure.

Prognosis refers to the probable outcome and prospect of recovery from a disease. It can be designated as chances for full recovery, possibility of complications, or anticipated survival time. Prognosis often is presented in relation to treatment options—that is, the expected outcomes or chances for survival with or without a certain type of treatment. The prognosis associated with a given type of treatment usually is presented along with the risk associated with the treatment.

LEVELS OF PREVENTION

Basically, leading a healthy life contributes to the prevention of disease. There are three fundamental types of prevention: primary prevention, secondary prevention, and tertiary prevention[28] (Chart 1-2). *Primary prevention* is directed at keeping disease from occurring by removing all risk factors. Immunizations are examples of primary prevention. *Secondary prevention* detects disease early when it is still asymptomatic and treatment measures can affect a cure. The use of a Papanicolaou (Pap) smear for early detection of cervical cancer is an example of secondary prevention. *Tertiary prevention* is directed at clinical interventions that prevent further deterioration or reduce the complications of a disease once it has been diagnosed. An example is the use of β-adrenergic drugs to reduce the risk for death in persons who have had a heart attack. Tertiary prevention measures also include measures to limit physical impairment and social consequences of an illness.

Primary prevention often is accomplished outside the health care system. Chlorination and fluoridation of water supplies and laws that mandate seat belt use are examples of community-wide primary prevention. There are fewer community-wide efforts directed at secondary prevention, and those that are available usually do not involve the entire community. Examples include breast self-examination education programs and blood pressure screening programs. Nevertheless, many health care clinics are becoming increasingly devoted to primary and secondary prevention through such activities as prenatal and well-child care, immunizations, lifestyle counseling, and screening for early disease detection or risk factors. There are many fewer tertiary prevention efforts outside the health care system.

CHART 1-2

Levels of Prevention

- Primary prevention: Actions aimed at prevention of disease
- Secondary prevention: Actions aimed at early detection and prompt treatment of disease
- Tertiary prevention: Treatment and rehabilitation measures aimed at preventing further progress of the disease

EVIDENCE-BASED PRACTICE AND PRACTICE GUIDELINES

Evidence-based practice and evidence-based practice guidelines have recently gained popularity with clinicians, public health practitioners, health care organizations, and the public as a means of improving the quality and efficiency of health care.[29,30] Their development has been prompted, at least in part, by the enormous amounts of published information about diagnostic and treatment measures for various disease conditions as well as demands for better and more cost-effective health care.

Evidence-based practice has been defined as "the conscientious, explicit, and judicious use of current best evidence in making decisions about the care of individual patients."[29] It is based on the integration of the individual expertise of the practitioner with the best external clinical evidence from systematic research.[29] The term *clinical expertise* implies the proficiency and judgment that individual clinicians gain through clinical experience and clinical practice. The best external clinical evidence relies on the identification of clinically relevant research, often from the basic sciences, but especially from patient-centered clinical studies that focus on the accuracy and precision of diagnostic tests and methods, the power of prognostic indicators, and the effectiveness and safety of therapeutic, rehabilitative, and preventive regimens.

Clinical practice guidelines are systematically developed statements intended to inform practitioners and clients in making decisions about health care for specific clinical circumstances.[31,32] They not only should review various outcomes but also must weigh various outcomes, both positive and negative, and make recommendations. Guidelines are different from systematic reviews. They can take the form of algorithms, which are step-by-step methods for solving a problem, written directives for care, or a combination thereof.

The development of evidence-based practice guidelines often uses methods such as meta-analysis to combine evidence from different studies to produce a more precise estimate of the accuracy of a diagnostic method or the effects of an intervention method.[33] It also requires review: by practitioners with expertise in clinical content, who can verify the completeness of the literature review and ensure clinical sensibility; by experts in guideline development who can examine the method by which the guideline was developed; and by potential users of the guideline.[31]

Once developed, practice guidelines must be continually reviewed and changed to keep pace with new research findings and with new diagnostic and treatment methods. For example, the Guidelines for the Prevention, Evaluation, and Treatment of High Blood Pressure (see Chapter 25), first developed in 1972 by the Joint National Committee, have been revised seven times, and the Guidelines for the Diagnosis and Management of Asthma (see Chapter 31), first developed in 1991 by the Expert Panel, have undergone three revisions.

Evidence-based practice guidelines, which are intended to direct client care, are also important in directing research into the best methods of diagnosing and treating specific health problems. This is because health care providers use the same criteria for diagnosing the extent and severity of a particular condition such as hypertension and because they use the same protocols for treatment.

In summary, the health of individuals is closely linked to the health of the community and to the population it encompasses. Epidemiology is the study of disease in populations. It looks for patterns such as age, race, and dietary habits of persons who are affected with a particular disorder to determine under what circumstances the particular disorder will occur. Using epidemiologic methods, researchers determine how a disease is spread, how to control it, how to prevent it, and how to eliminate it.

Epidemiologists use measures of disease frequency to predict what diseases are present in a population and as an indication of the rate at which they are increasing or decreasing. Incidence is the number of new cases arising in a population during a specified time. Prevalence is the number of people in a population who have a particular disease at a given point in time or period.

Morbidity and mortality provide epidemiologists with information about the functional effects and death-producing characteristics of a disease. Mortality or death statistics provide information about the trends in the health of a population. Morbidity describes the effects an illness has on a person's life. It is concerned with the incidence of disease as well as its persistence and long-term consequences.

Conditions suspected of contributing to the development of a disease are called *risk factors*. They may be inherent to a person (high blood pressure) or external (smoking). Studies used to determine risk factors include cross-sectional studies, case-control studies, and cohort studies. Cross-sectional studies use the simultaneous collection of information necessary for classification of exposure and outcome status. Case-control studies are designed to compare subjects who are known to have the outcome of interest (cases) with those who are known not to have the outcome of interest (control). Cohort studies involve groups of persons who were born at approximately the same time or share some characteristic of interest. The Framingham Study, which examined the characteristics of people in whom coronary heart disease would later develop, and the Nurses' Health Study, which initially explored the relationship between oral contraceptives and breast cancer, are two well-known cohort studies.

The natural history of disease refers to the progression and projected outcome of a disease without medical intervention. It can be used to determine disease outcome, establish priorities for health care services, provide direction for prevention and early detection programs, and compare treatment methods and their outcomes with untreated outcomes. *Prognosis* is the term used to designate the probable outcome and prospect of recovery from a disease.

The three fundamental types of prevention are primary prevention, secondary prevention, and tertiary prevention. Primary prevention, such as immunizations, is directed at removing risk factors so that disease does not occur. Secondary prevention, such as a Pap smear, detects disease when it still is asymptomatic and curable with treatment. Tertiary prevention, such as β-adrenergic drugs to reduce the risk for death in persons who have had a heart attack, focuses on clinical interventions that prevent further deterioration or reduce the complications of a disease.

Evidence-based practice and evidence-based practice guidelines are mechanisms that use the current best evidence to make decisions about the health care of individuals. They are based on the expertise of the individual practitioner integrated with the best clinical evidence from systematic review of credible research studies. Practice guidelines may take the form of algorithms, which are step-by-step methods for solving a problem, written directives, or a combination thereof.

References

1. Sontag S. (1990). *Illness as metaphor.* New York: Doubleday, Anchor Books.
2. James P., Thorpe N. (1995). *Ancient inventions.* New York: Random House, Ballantine Books.
3. Porter R. (1998). *The greatest benefit to mankind: A medical history of humanity.* New York: W.W. Norton & Company.
4. McNeill W.H. (1998). *Plagues and peoples.* New York: Doubleday, Anchor Books.
5. Schorr T.M., Kennedy M.S. (1999). *100 Years of American nursing.* Philadelphia: Lippincott Williams & Wilkins.
6. American Lung Association. (1982, March). From Koch to today. *American Lung Association Bulletin 68,* 2–3.
7. Le Fanu J. (2000). *The rise and fall of modern medicine.* New York: Carroll & Graf.
8. CDC. (2003). Update: Severe acute respiratory syndrome–worldwide and United States, 2003. *MMWR Morbidity and Mortality Weekly Report 52,* 664–665.
9. CDC. (2003). Multistate outbreak of monkeypox: Illinois, Indiana, and Wisconsin, 2003. *MMWR Morbidity and Mortality Weekly Report 52,* 537–540.
10. World Health Organization. (2001). About WHO: Definition of health; disease eradication/elimination goals. [On-line.] Available: http://www.int/aboutwho/en/history/htm. Accessed February 19, 2004.

11. U.S. Department of Health and Human Services. (2000). *Healthy people 2010.* National Health Information Center. [On-line.] Available: http://www.healthypeople./gov.
12. *Dorland's illustrated medical dictionary* (29th ed., p. 511). (2000). Philadelphia: W.B. Saunders.
13. Waldenstrom J. (1989). Sick molecules and our concepts of illness. *Journal of Internal Medicine 225,* 221–227.
14. Brigden M.L., Heathcote J.C. (2000). Problems with interpreting laboratory tests. *Postgraduate Medicine 107*(7), 145–162.
15. Fischbach F. (2004). *A manual of laboratory and diagnostic tests* (6th ed., p. 74). Philadelphia: Lippincott Williams & Wilkins.
16. Bickley L. (2003). *Bates' guide to physical assessment and history taking* (7th ed., pp. 783–802). Philadelphia: Lippincott Williams & Wilkins.
17. Dawson-Saunders B., Trapp R.G. (1990). Evaluating diagnostic procedures. In Dawson-Saunders B., Trapp R.G. (Eds.), *Basic and clinical biostatistics* (pp. 229–244). Norwalk, CT: Appleton & Lange.
18. Vetter N., Mathews I. (1999). *Epidemiology and public health maintenance.* Edinburgh: Churchill Livingstone.
19. Framingham Heart Study. (2001). *Framingham Heart Study: Design, rationale, objectives, and research milestones.* [On-line.] Available: http://www.nhlbi.nih.gov/about/framingham/design.htm. Accessed February 19, 2004.
20. Channing Laboratory. (2004). *Nurses health study.* [On-line]. Available: http://www.channing.harvard.edu/nhs/hist.html. Accessed February 19, 2004.
21. Garland M., Morris J.S., Stamfer M.J., et al. (1995). Prospective study of toenail selenium levels and cancer among women. *Journal of the National Cancer Institute 87,* 497–505.
22. Carmago C.A., Weiss S.T., Zhang S., et al. (1999). Prospective study of body mass index, weight gain, and risk of adult-onset asthma in women. *Archives of Internal Medicine 159,* 2582–2588.
23. Kawachi I., Colditz G.A., Stamfer M.J., et al. (1994). Smoking cessation and time course of decreased risks of coronary heart disease in middle-aged women. *Archives of Internal Medicine 154,* 169–175.
24. Laden F., Neas L.M., Tolbert P.E., et al. (2000). Electric blanket use and breast cancer in the Nurses' Health Study. *American Journal of Epidemiology 152,* 41–49.
25. Huang Z., Willett W.C., Colditz G.A., et al. (1999). Waist circumference, waist:hip ratio, and risk of breast cancer in the Nurses' Health Study. *American Journal of Epidemiology 150,* 1316–1324.
26. Giovannucci E., Egan K.M., Hunter D.J., et al. (1995). Aspirin and the risk of colorectal cancer in women. *New England Journal of Medicine 333,* 609–614.
27. Liang J., Reherman B., Seeff L.B., et al. (2000). Pathogenesis, natural history, treatment, and prevention of hepatitis C. *Annals of Internal Medicine 132,* 296–305.
28. Stanhope M., Lancaster J. (2000). *Community and public health nursing* (5th ed., p. 43). St. Louis: Mosby.
29. Sackett D.L. (1996). Evidence based medicine: What it is and what it isn't. *British Medical Journal 312,* 71–72.
30. Youngblut J.M., Brooten D. (2001). Evidence-based practice: Why is it important. *AACN Clinical Issues 12,* 468–475.
31. Shekelle P.G., Woolff S.H., Eccles M., et al. (1999). Developing guidelines. *British Medical Journal 318,* 593–596.
32. Natsch S, van der Meer J.W.M. (2003). The role of clinical guidelines, policies, and stewardship. *Journal of Hospital Infection 53,* 172–176.
33. Acton G.J. (2001). Meta-analysis: A tool for evidence-based practice. *AACN Clinical Issues 12,* 539–545.

CHAPTER

2

Concepts of Altered Health in Children

Judy Wright Lott

Children are not miniature adults. Physical and psychological maturation and development strongly influence the type of illnesses children experience and their responses to these illnesses. Although many signs and symptoms are the same in persons of all ages, some diseases and complications are more likely to occur in the child. This chapter provides an overview of the developmental stages of childhood and the related health care needs of children. Specific diseases are presented throughout other sections of the book.

At the beginning of the 20th century, a child in the United States had little chance of reaching adulthood: the infant mortality rate was 200 deaths per 1000 live births.[1] Infectious diseases were rampant, and children, with their immature and inexperienced immune systems and their frequent exposure to other infected children, were especially vulnerable. With the introduction of antimicrobial agents, infectious disease control, and nutritional and technologic advances, infant mortality decreased dramatically. Although infant mortality has declined over past decades, the record low of 6.9 infant deaths per 1000 live births in 2000 placed the United States only 28th in relation to other industrialized nations.[2,3] Also of great concern is the difference in mortality rates for white and nonwhite infants. Infant death rates among African Americans, Native Americans, Alaska Natives, and Hispanics/Latinos in 2000 were all above the national average of 6.9 deaths per 1000 live births. The greatest disparity exists for African Americans, whose infant death rate (14.1 per 1000 in 2000) is nearly 2.5 times that of white infants (5.7 per 1000 in 2000). Recent data indicate that the racial disparities between white and African-American infant mortality rates are increasing.[1–4]

One of the more perplexing causes of infant mortality is the incidence of preterm birth among women of all races and classes. Despite continued, gradual declines in the overall infant mortality rate during the latter part of the 20th century, the incidence of premature births continues as a challenge to reducing the racial disparities as well as the overall incidence. Prematurity and consequent low birth weight is the leading cause of death in African-American infants. For white infants, the leading cause of death is congenital anomalies.[1–3] Sudden infant death syndrome (SIDS) is the third leading cause of overall infant mortality among all races in the United States, accounting for approximately 9% of infant deaths.[4]

Congenital anomalies (birth defects) account for the most infant deaths, causing approximately one in five infant deaths overall. Efforts to decrease mortality rates are aimed at improving access to prenatal care and understanding the underlying causes of neonatal (*i.e.,* infants younger than 28 days of age) mortality, congenital anomalies, and preterm delivery, which are still poorly understood despite continuing research. Many of the major causes of death during the post-neonatal period (*i.e.,* age 28 days to 1 year)—SIDS, death from infectious diseases (*e.g.*, pneumonia, influenza), and accidents—may be preventable through health promotion efforts such as routine infant care instruction, immunizations, and teaching of parenting skills.

Growth and Development

After completing this section of the chapter, you should be able to meet the following objectives:

- ✦ Characterize the use of percentiles to describe growth and development during infancy and childhood
- ✦ Describe the major events that occur during prenatal development from fertilization to birth
- ✦ Define the terms *low birth weight, small for gestational age,* and *large for gestational age*
- ✦ Identify reasons for abnormal intrauterine growth
- ✦ Describe assessment methods for determination of gestational age

The phrase *growth and development* describes a process whereby a fertilized ovum becomes an adult person. *Physical growth* describes changes in the body as a whole or in its individual parts. *Development,* on the other hand, embraces other aspects of differentiation, such as changes in body function and psychosocial behaviors.

Physical growth occurs in a cephalocaudal (head-to-toe) direction. Relative body proportions change over the life span. In early fetal development, the head is the largest part of the body, but proportional size changes as the individual grows (Fig. 2-1).

The average newborn weighs approximately 3000 to 4000 g and is 50 to 53 cm long. The first year is a period of rapid growth demonstrated by lengthening of the trunk and deposition of subcutaneous fat.[5] After the first year until onset of puberty, the legs grow more rapidly than any other part of the body.

The onset of puberty is marked by significant alterations in body proportions because of the effects of the pubertal growth spurt. The feet and hands are the first to grow. Because the trunk grows faster than the legs, at adolescence a large portion of the increase in height is a result of trunk growth. The brain also undergoes a period of rapid growth. At birth, the brain is 25% of adult size; at 1 year, it is 50% of adult size; and at 5 years, it is 90% of adult size. The size of the head reflects brain growth.[6] Linear growth is a result of skeletal growth. After maturation of the skeleton is complete, linear growth is complete. By 2 years of age, the length is 50% of the adult height. Beginning with the third year, the growth rate is 5 to 6 cm for the next 9 years. A growth spurt during adolescence is necessary for adult height to be reached. Males add approximately 20 cm and females 16 cm to height during this time. Weight is rapidly increased after birth. Generally by 6 months of age, the birth weight is doubled; by 1 year of age it is tripled. The average weight increase is 2 to 2.75 kg per year until the adolescent growth spurt begins.[7]

Growth and development encompass a complex interaction between genetic and environmental influences. The experience of each child is unique, and the patterns of growth and development may be profoundly different for individual children within the context of what is considered *normal.* Because of the wide variability, these norms often can be expressed only in statistical terms.

Evaluation of growth and development requires comparison of an individual's growth and development to a standard. Statistics are calculations derived from measurements that are used to describe the sample measured or to make predictions about the rest of the population represented by the sample. Because all individuals grow and develop at different rates, the standard must somehow take this individual variation into account. The standard typically is derived from measurements made on a sample of individuals deemed representative of the total population. When multiple measurements of biologic variables such as height, weight, head circumference, and blood pressure are made, most values fall around the center or middle of all the values. Plotting the data on a graph yields a bell-shaped curve, which depicts the normal distribution of these continuously variable values (Fig. 2-2).

The mean and standard deviation are common statistics used in describing the characteristics of a population. The mean represents the average of the measurements; it is the sum of the values divided by the number of values. A normal bell-shaped curve is symmetric, with the mean falling in the center of the curve and with one half of the values falling on either side of the mean. The standard de-

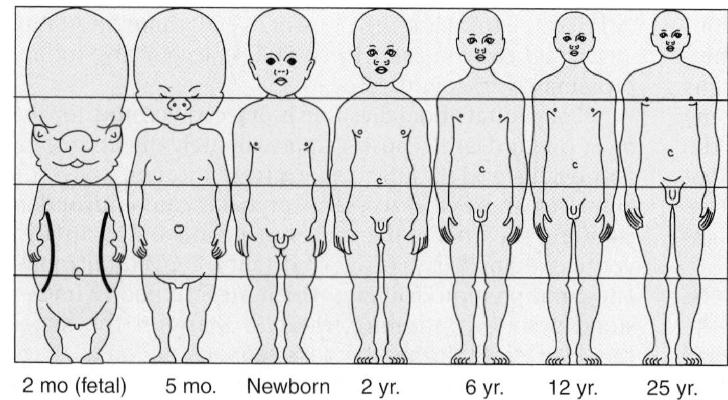

FIGURE 2-1 Changes in body proportions from the 2nd fetal month to adulthood. (Robbins W.J., Brody S., Hogan A.G., et al. [1928]. *Growth.* New Haven: Yale University Press. By permission of publisher)

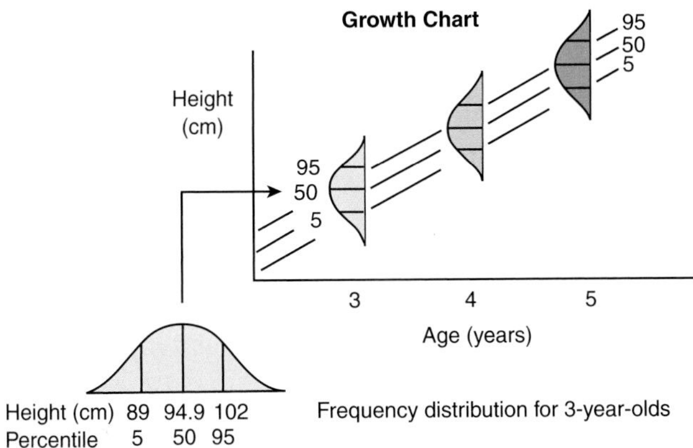

FIGURE 2-2 Relationship between percentile lines on the growth curve and frequency distributions of height at different ages. (Behrman R.E., Kliegman R.M., Jenson H.B. [2000]. *Nelson textbook of pediatrics* [16th ed., pp. 23–65]. Philadelphia: W.B. Saunders)

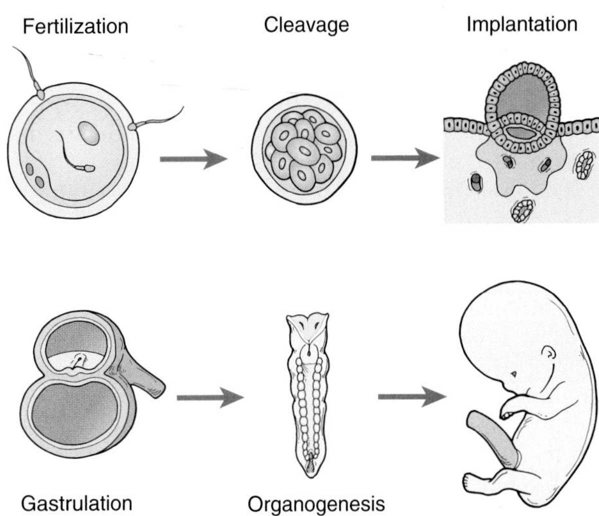

FIGURE 2-3 Milestones in development.

viation determines how far a value varies or deviates from the mean. The points 1 standard deviation above and below the mean include 68% of all values, 2 standard deviations 95% of all values, and 3 standard deviations 99.7% of all values.[5] If a child's height is within 1 standard deviation of the mean, he or she is as tall as 68% of children in the population. If a child's height is greater than 3 standard deviations, he or she is taller than 99.7% of children in the population.

The bell-shaped curve can also be marked by percentiles, which are useful for comparison of an individual's values with other values. When quantitative data are arranged in ascending and descending order, a middle value, called the *median,* can be described with one half (50%) of the values falling on either side. The values can be further divided into percentiles. A percentile is a number that indicates the percentage of values for the population that are equal to or below the number. Percentiles are used most often to compare an individual's value with a set of norms. They are used extensively to develop and interpret physical growth charts and measurements of ability and intelligence.

PRENATAL GROWTH AND DEVELOPMENT

Human development is considered to begin with fertilization, the union of sperm and ovum resulting in a zygote (Fig. 2-3). The process begins with the intermingling of a haploid number of paternal (23,X or Y) and maternal (23,X) chromosomes in the ampulla of the oviduct that fuse to form a zygote. Within 24 hours, the unicellular organism becomes a two-cell organism and, within 72 hours, it is a 16-cell organism called a *morula.* This series of mitotic divisions is called *cleavage.* During cleavage, the rapidly developing cell mass travels down the oviduct to the uterus by a series of peristaltic movements. The morula enters the uterus approximately 3 days after fertilization. On the fourth day, the morula is separated into two parts by fluid from the uterus. The outer layer gives rise to the placenta (trophoblast), and the inner layer gives rise to the embryo (embryoblast). The structure is now called a *blastocyst.* By the sixth day, the blastocyst attaches to the endometrium. This is the beginning of *implantation,* and it is completed during the second week of development.[8]

Prenatal development is divided into two main periods. The first, or embryonic, period begins during the second week and continues through the eighth week after fertilization.[6,8] During the embryonic period, the main organ systems are developed, and many function at a minimal level (see Chapter 7). The second, or fetal, period begins during the ninth week. During the fetal period, the growth and differentiation of the body and organ systems occur.

Embryonic Development

Human development progresses through three phases.[6] During the first stage of embryonic development, growth occurs through an increase in cell numbers and the elaboration of cell products. The second stage of development is one of morphogenesis (development of form), which

PRENATAL DEVELOPMENT

- The prenatal period, which begins with implantation of the blastocyst, is divided into two periods: the embryonic period and the fetal period.
- The embryonic period spans the second through the eighth weeks of gestation. This period is marked by the formation of the germ layers, early tissue differentiation, and development of the major organs and systems of the body.
- The fetal period extends from the ninth week to birth. Development during the fetal period is largely concerned with rapid growth and differentiation of tissues, organs, and body systems.

includes mass cell movement. During this stage, the movement of cells allows them to interact with each other in the formation of tissues and organs. The third stage is the stage of differentiation or maturation of physiologic processes. Completion of differentiation results in organs that are capable of performing specialized functions.

With the onset of embryonic development, which begins during the second week of gestation, the trophoblast continues its rapid proliferation and differentiation, and the embryoblast evolves into a bilaminar embryonic disk. This flattened, circular plate of cells gives rise to all three germ layers of the embryo (*i.e.,* ectoderm, mesoderm, endoderm). The third week is a period of rapid development, noted for the conversion of the bilaminar embryonic disk into a trilaminar embryonic disk through a process called *gastrulation*[6,8] (see Fig. 2-3). The ectoderm differentiates into the epidermis and nervous system, and the endoderm gives rise to the epithelial linings of the respiratory passages, digestive tract, and glandular cells of organs such as the liver and pancreas. The mesoderm becomes smooth muscle tissue, connective tissue, blood vessels, blood cells, bone marrow, skeletal tissue, striated muscle tissue, and reproductive and excretory organs.

The notochord, which is the primitive axis about which the axial skeleton forms, is also formed during the third week (see Chapter 49). The neurologic system begins its development during this period. *Neurulation,* a process that involves formation of the neural plate, neural folds, and their closure, is completed by the fourth week. Disturbances during this period can result in brain and spinal defects such as spina bifida. The cardiovascular system is the first functional organ system to develop. The primitive heart, which beats and circulates blood, develops during this period (see Chapter 26).

By the fourth week, the neural tube is formed. The embryo begins to curve and fold into a characteristic C-shaped structure. The limb buds are visible, as are the otic pits (*i.e.,* primordia of the internal ears) and the lens placodes (primordia of the lens of the eyes). The fifth week is notable for the rapid growth of the head secondary to brain growth.

During the sixth week, the upper limbs are formed by fusion of the swellings around the branchial groove. In the seventh week, there is the beginning of the digits, and the intestines enter the umbilical cord (umbilical herniation). By the eighth week, the embryo is human-like in appearance—eyes are open, and eyelids and ear auricles are easily identified.

Fetal Development

The fetal period extends from the ninth week to birth.[6,8] During the 9th to 12th weeks, fetal head growth slows, whereas body length growth is greatly accelerated. By the 11th week, the intestines in the proximal portion of the cord have returned to the abdomen. The primary ossification centers are present in the skull and long bones, and maturation of the fetal external genitalia is established by the 12th week. During the fetal period, the liver is the major site of red blood cell formation (*i.e.,* erythropoiesis); at 12 weeks, this activity has decreased, and erythropoiesis begins in the spleen. Urine begins to form during the 9th to 12th weeks and is excreted into the amniotic fluid.[8]

The 13th through 16th weeks are notable for ossification of the skeleton, scalp hair patterning, and differentiation of the ovaries in female fetuses. By the 17th through 20th week, growth has slowed. The fetal skin is covered with a fine hair called *lanugo* and a white, cheeselike material called *vernix caseosa.* Eyebrows and head hair are visible. In male fetuses, the testes begin to descend, and in female fetuses, the uterus is formed. Brown fat also forms during this period. Brown fat is a specialized type of adipose tissue that produces heat by oxidizing fatty acids. Brown fat is similar to white fat but has larger and more numerous mitochondria, which provide its brown color. Brown fat is found near the heart and blood vessels that supply the brain and kidneys and is thought to play a role in maintaining the temperature of these organs during exposure to environmental changes that occur after birth.

During the 21st through 25th weeks, significant fetal weight gain occurs. The type II alveolar cells of the lung begin to secrete surfactant (see Chapter 29). The pulmonary system becomes more mature and able to support respiration during the 26th through 29th weeks. Breathing movements are present as a result of central nervous system (CNS) maturation. At this age, a fetus can survive if born prematurely and given intensive care. There also is an increasing amount of subcutaneous fat, with white fat making up 3.5% of body weight.[6]

The 30th through 34th weeks are significant for an increasing amount of white fat (8% of body weight), which gives the fetal limbs an almost chubby appearance.[6] During the 35th week, grasp and the pupillary light reflex are present. If a normal-weight fetus is born during this period, it is premature by "date" as opposed to premature by "weight."[6]

Expected time of birth is 266 days, or 38 weeks after fertilization, or 40 weeks after the last menstrual period (LMP).[6] At this time, the neurologic, cardiovascular, and pulmonary systems are developed enough for the infant to make the transition to extrauterine life. The survival of the newborn depends on this adaptation after the placenta is removed.

Fetal Growth and Weight Gain. Development during the fetal period is primarily concerned with rapid growth and differentiation of tissues, organs, and systems. Fetal weight gain is linear from 20 weeks' gestation through 38 weeks' gestation. In the last half of pregnancy, the fetus gains 85% of birth weight. After 38 weeks' gestation, the rate of growth declines, probably related to the constraint of uterine size and decreased placental function. After birth, weight gain again increases, similar to intrauterine rates. Birth weight can be affected by a variety of factors, including maternal nutrition, genetic factors, chronic maternal diseases, placental abnormalities, sex, socioeconomic factors; multiple births, chromosomal abnormalities, and infectious diseases.

BIRTH WEIGHT AND GESTATIONAL AGE

At birth, the average weight of the full-term newborn is 3000 to 4000 g. Before 1961, infants weighing less than 2500 g were classified as premature. In 1961, owing to the recognition that factors other than gestational age affect birth weight, infants weighing less than 2500 g were classified as low birth weight (LBW). Lubchenco and Battaglia established standards for birth weight, gestational age, and intrauterine growth in the United States in the 1960s[9,10] (Fig. 2-4). With these standards, gestational age can be assessed, and normal and abnormal growth can be identified. The Colorado Growth Curve places newborns into percentiles.[9] The 10th through 90th percentiles of intrauterine growth encompass 80% of births.[11] Growth is considered abnormal when a newborn falls above or below the 90th and 10th percentiles, respectively.

An infant is considered term when born between the beginning of the 38th week and completion of the 41st week. An infant is considered premature when born before the end of the 37th week and post-mature when born after the end of the 41st week. The lowest mortality rates occur among newborns with weights between 3000 and 4000 g with gestational ages of 38 to 42 weeks.[12–14]

Abnormal Intrauterine Growth

Growth of the fetus in the uterus depends on a multitude of intrinsic and extrinsic factors. Optimal fetal growth depends on efficient placental function, adequate provision of energy and growth substrates, appropriate hormonal environment, and adequate room in the uterus. Birth weight variability in a population is primarily determined by maternal heredity, intrinsic fetal growth potential, and environmental factors. Abnormal growth, which can occur at any time during fetal development, can have immediate and long-term consequences for the infant.

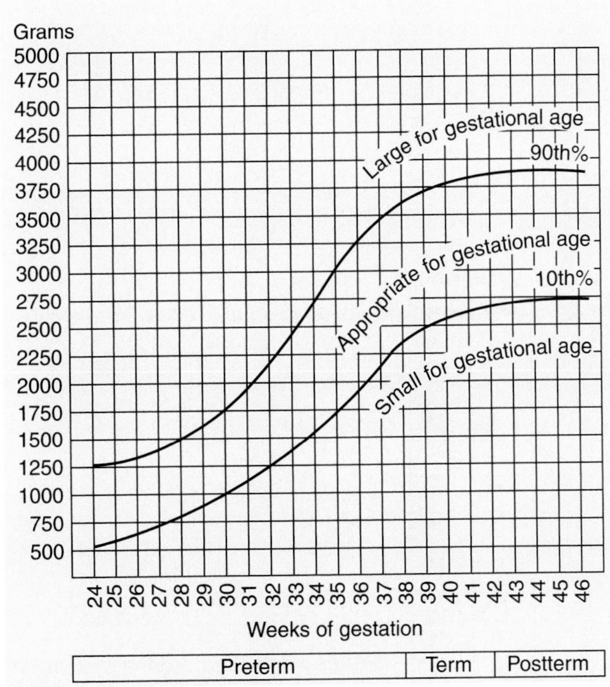

FIGURE 2-4 Classification of newborns by birth weight and gestational age. (Redrawn from Battaglia F.C., Lubchenco L.O. [1967]. A practical classification of newborn infants by weight and gestational age. *Journal of Pediatrics* 71, 159)

Small for Gestational Age. *Small for gestational age* (SGA) is a term that denotes fetal undergrowth. SGA is defined as birth weight less than 2 standard deviations below the mean for gestational age, or below the 10th percentile. It often is used interchangeably with *intrauterine growth retardation* (IUGR). Worldwide, between 30% and 40% of infants born at weights less than 2500 g are SGA. Mortality rates of severely affected SGA infants are five to six times those of normally grown infants of comparable gestational age.

Fetal growth retardation can occur at any time during fetal development. Depending on the time of insult, the infant can have symmetric or proportional growth retardation or asymmetric or disproportional growth retardation. Impaired growth that occurs early in pregnancy during the hyperplastic phase of growth results in symmetric growth retardation. Because mitosis is affected, organs and tissues are smaller as a result of overall decreased cell number. Head circumference, length, and weight usually are represented within similar percentile grids, although the head may be smaller, as in microcephaly.[15] This is irreversible postnatally. Causes of proportional IUGR include chromosomal abnormalities, congenital infections, and exposure to environmental toxins.

Impaired growth that occurs later in pregnancy during the hypertrophic phase of growth results in asymmetric growth retardation.[12–14] Infants with IUGR due to intrauterine malnutrition often have weight reduction out of proportion to length or head circumference but are spared impairment of head and brain growth.[7] Tissues and organs are small because of decreased cell size, not decreased cell numbers. Postnatally, the impairment may be partially corrected with good nutrition.

Maternal, placental, and environmental factors affect fetal growth. Because of the effects on the placenta (it also is undergrown), the risk for perinatal complications is higher. These include birth asphyxia, hyperglycemia, polycythemia, meconium (*i.e.*, dark green, mucilaginous newborn stool) aspiration, and hypothermia. The long-term effects of growth retardation depend on the timing and severity of the insult. Many of these infants have developmental disabilities on follow-up examination, especially if the growth retardation is symmetric. They may remain small, especially if the insult occurred early. If the insult occurred later because of placental insufficiency or uterine restraint, with good nutrition catch-up growth can occur, and the infant may attain appropriate growth.

Large for Gestational Age. *Large for gestational age* (LGA) is a term that denotes fetal overgrowth. The definition of LGA is birth weight greater than 2 standard deviations above the mean for gestation, or above the 90th percentile. The excessive growth may result from a genetic predisposition or may be stimulated by abnormal conditions in utero. Infants of diabetic mothers may be LGA, especially if the diabetes was poorly controlled during pregnancy. Maternal hyperglycemia exposes the fetus to increased levels of glucose, which stimulates fetal secretion of insulin. Insulin increases fat deposition, and the result is a macrosomic (large body size) infant. Infants with macrosomia have enlarged viscera and are large and plump because of an increase in body fat. Complications when an infant is LGA include birth asphyxia and trauma due to mechanical difficulties during the birth process, hypoglycemia, and polycythemia.[12]

Assessment Methods

Gestational age assessment can be divided into two categories: prenatal assessment and postnatal assessment. *Prenatal assessment* of gestational age most commonly includes careful menstrual history, physical milestones during pregnancy (*e.g.*, uterine size, detection of fetal heart rate and movements), and prenatal tests for maturity (*e.g.*, ultrasound, amniotic fluid studies). Nägele's rule uses the first day of the LMP to calculate the day of labor by adding 7 days to the LMP and counting back 3 months.[12] This method may be inaccurate if the mother is not a good historian or has a history of irregular menses, which interferes with identification of a normal cycle.

Postnatal assessment of gestational age is done by examination of external physical and neuromuscular characteristics alone or in combination. Assessment of gestational age should be a part of every initial newborn examination. Accurate assessment of gestational age facilitates risk assessment and identification of abnormalities and allows for earlier interventions. Dubowitz or Ballard developed the most common methods used in nurseries today. The Dubowitz method is comprehensive and includes 21 criteria using external physical (11) and neuromuscular (10) signs.[16] The estimate of gestational age is best done within 12 hours of birth and is accurate within 1 week. The method is less accurate for infants born at less than 30 weeks' gestational age. The Ballard method is an abbreviated Dubowitz method that includes 12 criteria, using 6 external physical and 6 neuromuscular signs (Fig. 2-5). The New Ballard Score (NBS) was updated and modified to include newborns at gestational ages of 20 to 44 weeks and is the most commonly used method. If performed within 12 hours post-birth by an experienced examiner, it is accurate to within 1 week.[11]

In summary, growth and development begin with union of ovum and sperm and are ongoing throughout a child's life to adulthood. Abnormalities during this process can have profound effects on the infant. Prenatal development is com-

Neuromuscular Maturity

	-1	0	1	2	3	4	5
Posture							
Square Window (wrist)	>90°	90°	60°	45°	30°	0°	
Arm Recoil		180°	140°-180°	110° 140°	90-110°	<90°	
Popliteal Angle	180°	160°	140°	120°	100°	90°	<90°
Scarf Sign							
Heel to Ear							

Physical Maturity

Skin	sticky friable transparent	gelatinous red, translucent	smooth pink, visible veins	superficial peeling &/or rash. few veins	cracking pale areas rare veins	parchment deep cracking no vessels	leathery cracked wrinkled
Lanugo	none	sparse	abundant	thinning	bald areas	mostly bald	
Plantar Surface	heel-toe 40-50 mm: -1 <40 mm: -2	>50mm no crease	faint red marks	anterior transverse crease only	creases ant. 2/3	creases over entire sole	
Breast	imperceptible	barely perceptible	flat areola no bud	stippled areola 1-2mm bud	raised areola 3-4mm bud	full areola 5-10mm bud	
Eye/Ear	lids fused loosely:-1 tightly:-2	lids open pinna flat stays folded	sl. curved pinna; soft; slow recoil	well-curved pinna; soft but :eady recoil	formed &firm instant recoil	thick cartilage ear stiff	
Genitals male	scrotum flat, smooth	scrotum empty faint rugae	testes in upper canal rare rugae	testes descending few rugae	testes down good rugae	testes pendulous deep rugae	
Genitals female	clitoris prominent labia flat	prominent clitoris small labia minora	prominent clitoris enlarging minora	majora & minora equally prominent	majora large minora small	majora cover clitoris & minora	

Maturity Rating

score	weeks
-10	20
-5	22
0	24
5	26
10	28
15	30
20	32
25	34
30	36
35	38
40	40
45	42
50	44

FIGURE 2-5 Ballard scoring system for determining gestational age in weeks. (Bickley L.S. [2003]. Bates' guide to physical examination and history taking [p. 737]. Philadelphia: Lippincott Williams & Wilkins)

posed of two periods—the embryonic period and the fetal period. During these periods, the zygote becomes the newborn with the organ maturity to make the adjustments necessary for extrauterine life. Infants born before this process is completed are called *premature* and can have major problems with extrauterine adjustments. Postnatal growth is rapid and ongoing and proceeds in an orderly and predictable manner.

Infancy

After completing this section of the chapter, you should be able to meet the following objectives:

- Describe the use of the Apgar score in evaluating infant well-being at birth
- List three injuries that can occur during the birth process
- Describe physical growth and organ development during the first year of life
- Explain how the common health care needs of the premature infant differ from the health care needs of the term newborn or infant
- Differentiate between organic and nonorganic failure to thrive syndrome

Infancy is defined as that time from birth to approximately 18 months of age, the first 4 weeks of which are designated as the newborn or neonatal period. This is a period of rapid physical growth and maturation. The infant begins life as a relatively helpless organism and, through a process of progressive development, gains the skills to interact and cope with the environment. The infant begins life with a number of primitive reflexes and little body control. By 18 months, a child is able to run, grasp and manipulate objects, feed himself or herself, play with toys, and communicate with others.

GROWTH AND DEVELOPMENT

Physical growth is rapid during infancy. After birth, there is a period of relative starvation as the infant adjusts to enteral feeding. Typically, infants lose approximately 5% to 10% of their birth weight, but within days, they begin to gain weight, and by 2 weeks, they are back to birth weight. Average birth weight for a term newborn is 3000 to 4000 g, and this weight usually is doubled by 6 months and tripled by approximately 1 year after birth.

The median height at birth is 49.9 cm for girls and 50.5 cm for boys. During the first 6 months, height increases by 2.5 cm per month. By 1 year, the increase in length is 50% of the birth length. This increase is primarily in trunk growth. Median head circumference at birth is 34.5 cm for girls and 34.8 cm for boys. The skull bones of newborn infants are incomplete and are connected by bands of connective tissue called sutures. At the junction of the sutures are wider spaces of unossified membranous tissue called fontanels. The larger anterior fontanel is palpable until about 18 months to 2 years of age; the smaller ones are replaced by bone by the end of the first year. The fontanels allow the infant's head to be compressed slightly during birth and allow rapid brain growth. Premature closure of any suture in the skull is called craniostenosis or craniosynostosis. The clinical consequences of premature closure depends on which suture is affected. The closed suture prevents growth from occurring in the affected area, but growth continues in the unaffected sutures, resulting in an abnormally shaped head.

The rapid increase in head circumference during the first year, is a good indicator of brain growth. Head circumference increases by 1.5 cm per month the first 6 months and 0.5 cm per month the second 6 months. Chest circumference at birth is smaller than head circumference. By 1 year, the head and chest are approximately equal in circumference; after 1 year, chest circumference exceeds head circumference.[7] After birth, most organ systems continue to grow and mature in an orderly fashion. Variations in growth and development are responsible for the differences in body proportions. For example, during the fetal period, the head is the predominant part because of the rapidly growing brain, whereas during infancy, the trunk predominates, and in childhood, the legs predominate. The patterns of growth are cephalocaudal, proximodistal, and mass (size) to specific.

INFANCY

- Infancy, which is the time from birth to 18 months of age, is a period of rapid physical growth and maturation.
- From an average birth weight of 3000 to 4000 g in the full-term infant and a median height of 49.9 cm for girls and 50.5 cm for boys, the infant manages to triple its weight and increase its length by 50% at 1 year of age.
- Developmentally, the infant begins life with a number of primitive reflexes and little body control. By 18 months, a child is able to run, grasp and manipulate objects, feed himself/herself, play with toys, and communicate with others.
- Basic trust, the first of Erikson's psychosocial stages, develops as infants learn that basic needs are met regularly.
- At the age of 18 months or the end of the infancy period, the emergence of symbolic thought causes a reorganization of behaviors with implications for the many developmental domains that lie ahead as the child moves to the early childhood stage of development.

Organ Systems

Organ systems must continue to grow and mature after delivery. Many are at a minimal level of functioning at birth. This often places the infant at risk for health problems.

Respiratory System. Onset of respiration must begin at birth for survival. By the late fetal period, the lungs are capable of respiration because the alveolar capillary membrane is sufficiently thin to allow for gas exchange.

Characteristically, mature alveoli do not form until after birth. Before birth, the primordial alveoli appear as small ridges on the walls of the respiratory bronchioles and terminal saccules. After birth, the primordial alveoli enlarge as the lungs expand, but the most important increase in the size of the lungs results from an increase in the number of alveoli and growth of the airways. Infants are obligatory nose breathers until 3 to 4 months of age; any upper airway obstruction may cause respiratory distress.[7] The trachea is small and close to the bronchi, and the bronchi's branching structures enable infectious agents to be easily transmitted throughout the lungs. The softness of the supporting cartilage in the trachea, along with its small diameter, places the infant at risk for airway obstruction. The auditory (eustachian) tube is short and straight and closely communicates with the ear, putting the infant at risk for middle ear infections (see Chapter 55).

Cardiovascular System. Birth initiates major changes in the cardiovascular system when the circulation of fetal blood through the placenta ceases and the infant's lungs expand and begin to function. The fetal shunts that allowed the blood to bypass the lungs (foramen ovale, ductus arteriosus) and the liver (ductus venous) close and cease to function. At birth, the size of the heart is large in relation to the chest cavity. The size and weight of the heart double the first year. Initially, the right ventricle is more muscular than the left ventricle, but this reverses in infancy. The heart rate gradually slows, and systolic blood pressure rises.

Hematopoietic System. The hematopoietic system is responsible for the production of blood cells. The hematopoietic system is composed of pluripotent stem cells that differentiate to form the red blood cells (RBCs), white blood cells (WBCs), and platelets through a process called hematopoiesis. New blood cells are constantly being generated to replace older blood cells that are broken down. A balance between new blood cell production and blood cell breakdown is necessary for normal circulating volume. As red blood cells are broken down, one of the major byproducts of the breakdown of hemoglobin is bilirubin (see Chapter 16). The lipid-soluble form of bilirubin, which is called *unconjugated bilirubin* or *indirect reacting bilirubin,* combines with plasma proteins for transport in the blood and interstitial fluids. Unconjugated bilirubin is removed from the blood by the liver and conjugated to form a water-soluble form of bilirubin. Conjugated (direct-acting) bilirubin is excreted from the liver cells into the biliary system and then into the intestinal tract. Normally, about two thirds of the unconjugated bilirubin produced by a term newborn can be effectively cleared by the liver. However, the relative immaturity of the newborn liver and the shortened life span of the fetal red blood cells may predispose the term newborn to hyperbilirubinemia and yellowish pigmentation of the skin, known as *jaundice* (Fig. 2-6). With the establishment of sufficient enteral nutrition, regular bowel elimination, and normal fluid volume, the liver is usually able to clear the excess bilirubin. The presence of jaundice with elevation of either indirect or direct bilirubin that is present at birth, appears within the first 24 hours of life, or is persistent indicates a pathophysiologic cause and should be investigated.

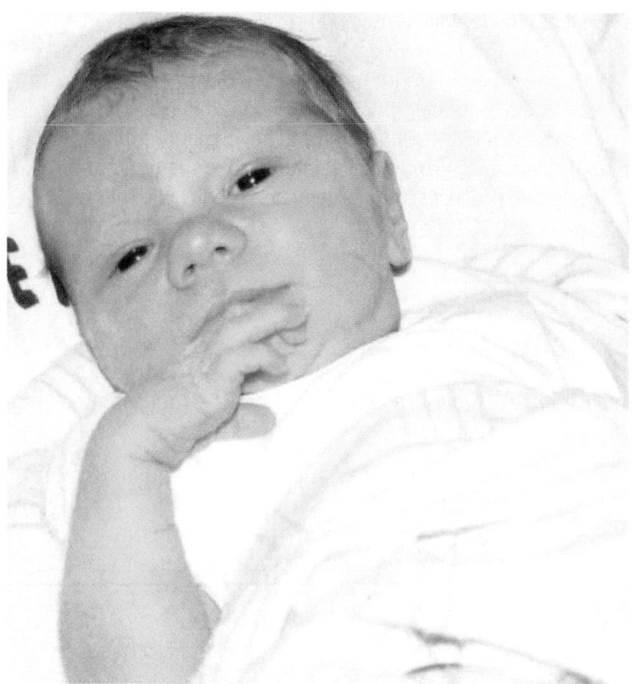

FIGURE 2-6 Photo of a newborn infant with jaundice.

Gastrointestinal System. The infant's gastrointestinal system is immature, and most digestive processes are poorly functioning until approximately 3 months of age. Solid food may pass incompletely digested and be evident in the stool. The newborn's first stool is called *meconium* and is composed of amniotic fluid, intestinal secretions, shed mucosal cells, and sometimes blood from ingested maternal blood or minor bleeding of intestinal tract vessels. Passage of meconium should occur within the first 24 to 48 hours in healthy term newborns but may be delayed for up to 7 days in preterm newborns or in newborns who do not receive enteral nutrition owing to illness.

At birth, sucking may be poor and require several days to become effective. The tongue thrust reflex is present and aids in sucking, but it disappears at approximately 6 months of age. Stomach capacity increases rapidly in the first months, but because of the limited capacity and rapid emptying, infants require frequent feeding.[7] The infant's genitourinary system is functionally immature at birth. There is difficulty in concentrating urine, and the ability to adjust to a restricted fluid intake is limited. The small bladder capacity causes frequent voiding.

Nervous System. The nervous system undergoes rapid maturation and growth during the infancy period. In contrast to other systems that grow rapidly after birth, the nervous system grows proportionately more rapidly before birth. The most rapid period of fetal brain growth is between 15 and 20 weeks of gestation, at which time there is a significant increase in neurons. A second increase occurs between 30 weeks' gestation and 1 year of age. At birth, the average brain weighs approximately 325 g. By 1 year of age, the weight has tripled, and the brain weighs approximately 1000 g.[7] Head circumference, one of the best indicators of brain growth, increases six times as much during the first year as it does during the second year of life.

At birth, the nervous system is incompletely integrated but sufficiently developed to sustain extrauterine life. Most of the neurologic reflexes are primitive reflexes. Normal newborn reflexes, which include the Moro (startle), rooting (sucking), and stepping (placing) reflexes, can be used to evaluate the newborn and infant's developing central nervous system.

The maturation of the nervous system includes an increase in the size of neurons, size and number of glial cells, and number of interneuron connections and branching of axons and dendrites. As this maturation progresses, the level of infant functioning increases from simple to complex and from primitive reflexes to purposeful movement. Cortical control of motor functions is closely associated with myelination of nerve fibers. Myelination of the various nerve tracts progresses rapidly after birth and follows a cephalocaudal and proximodistal direction sequence, beginning with myelination of the spinal cord and cranial nerves and followed by the brain stem and corticospinal tracts.[7] In general, sensory pathways become myelinated before motor pathways. The acquisition of fine and gross motor skills depends on this myelination and maturation.

The first year of life also is filled with psychosocial developmental milestones for the infant. Basic needs must be met before the infant can accomplish these developmental tasks. Erikson described the development of a sense of trust as the task of the first stage.[17] If trust is not acquired, the infant becomes mistrustful of others and frustrated with his or her inability to control the surrounding environment.

COMMON HEALTH PROBLEMS

The birth process is a critical event. Prenatal influences, birth trauma, and prematurity have an immediate impact on survival and health. The common health problems in this section have been divided into three subsections: health problems of the newborn, special needs of the premature infant, and health problems of the infant.

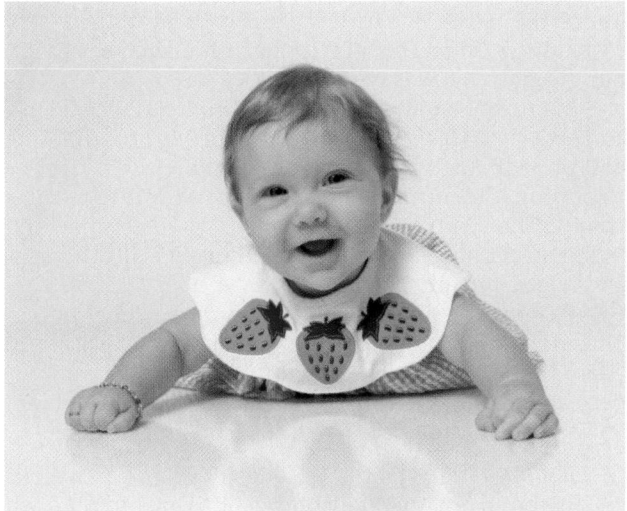

Health Problems of the Newborn

The most profound physiologic change required of the newborn is the transition from intrauterine to extrauterine existence. Onset of respiration must begin at birth for survival. The first breath expands the alveoli and initiates gas exchange. The infant's respiratory rate initially is rapid and primarily abdominal, but with maturation, the respiratory rate gradually slows. Birth also initiates major changes in the cardiovascular system. The fetal shunts, the foramen ovale and ductus arteriosus, begin to close, and the circulation of blood changes from a serial to a parallel circuit. (See Chapter 26 for further discussion.)

In addition to establishing respiration, heat regulation is another response critical to the infant's survival. At birth, the newborn's temperature is about 0.5°C higher than the mother's temperature. The temperature gradient causes vasodilation; thus, heat is lost rapidly, especially in a cold delivery room. The newborn's large surface area and lack of subcutaneous fat predisposes to excessive heat loss. Marked heat loss and the consequent lowering of body temperature can cause an otherwise healthy newborn to develop respiratory distress.

Distress at Birth and the Apgar Score. The Apgar score, devised by Dr. Virginia Apgar, is a scoring system that evaluates infant well-being at birth.[15] The system addresses five categories (*i.e.,* heart rate, respiratory effort, muscle tone, reflex irritability, and color) with a total score ranging from 0 to 10, depending on the degree to which these functions are presented (Table 2-1). Evaluations are performed at 1 minute and 5 minutes after delivery. A score of 0 to 3 is indicative of severe distress, 4 to 6 of moderate distress, and 7 to 10 of mild to no distress. Most infants score 6 to 7 at 1 minute and 8 to 9 at 5 minutes. If the score is 7 or less, the evaluation should be repeated every 5 minutes until a score of 7 or greater is obtained. An abnormal score at 5 minutes is more predictive of problems with survival and neurologic outcome than at 1 minute.[12]

Birth Injuries. Injuries sustained during the birth process are responsible for a significant amount of neonatal mortality and morbidity. In 2000, birth injuries ranked as the eighth leading cause of infant death in the United States. Predisposing factors for birth injuries include macrosomia, prematurity, cephalopelvic disproportion, and dystocia (*i.e.,* abnormal labor or childbirth).[12,18]

Cranial Injuries. The contour of the head of the newborn often reflects the effects of the delivery presentation. In vertex (head-first) deliveries, the head is usually flattened at the forehead, with the apex rising and forming a plane at the end of the parietal bones and the posterior skull or occiput dropping abruptly. By 1 to 2 days of age, the head has taken on a more oval shape. Such head molding does not occur in babies born by breech presentation or by cesarian section.

Caput succedaneum is a localized area of scalp edema caused by sustained pressure of the presenting part against

TABLE 2-1 Apgar Score Assessment

Criterion	Score* 0	1	2
Heart rate	Absent	<100	>100
Respiratory effort	Absent	Weak, irregular	Crying
Muscle tone	Limp	Some flexion	Well flexed
Reflex irritability	No response	Grimace	Cry, gag
Color	Pale	Cyanotic	Pink
Total	0	5	10

* The Apgar score should be assigned at 1 minute and 5 minutes after birth, using a timer. Each criterion is assessed and assigned a 0, 1, or 2. The total score is the assigned Apgar score. If resuscitation is required beyond the 5 minutes, additional Apgar scores also may be assigned as a method to document the response of the newborn to the resuscitation.

the cervix. An accumulation of serum or blood forms above the periosteum from the high pressure caused by the obstruction. The caput succedaneum may extend across suture lines and have overlying petechiae, purpura, or ecchymosis. No treatment is needed, and it usually resolves over the first week of life.[12,18]

Cephalohematoma is a subperiosteal collection of blood from ruptured blood vessels. The margins are sharply delineated and do not cross suture lines. It usually is unilateral, but it may be bilateral, and it usually occurs over the parietal area. The swelling may not be apparent for 24 to 48 hours because subperiosteal bleeding is slow. The overlying skin is not discolored. An underlying skull fracture may be present. Treatment is not needed unless the cephalohematoma is large and results in severe blood loss or significant hyperbilirubinemia. Skull fracture and intracranial hemorrhage are associated complications. An uncomplicated cephalohematoma usually resolves within 2 weeks to 3 months.[11,15]

Fractures. Skull fractures are uncommon because the infant's compressible skull is able to mold to fit the contours of the birth canal. However, fractures can occur and more often follow a forceps delivery or severe contraction of the pelvis associated with prolonged, difficult labor. Skull fractures may be linear or depressed. Uncomplicated linear fractures often are asymptomatic and do not require treatment. Depressed skull fractures are observable by the palpable indentation of the infant's head. They require surgical intervention if there is compression of underlying brain tissue. A simple linear fracture usually heals within several months.[12,18]

The clavicle is the bone most frequently fractured during the birth process. It is more common in LGA infants and occurs when delivery of the shoulders is difficult in vertex (*i.e.,* head) or breech presentations. The infant may or may not demonstrate restricted motion of the upper extremity, but passive motion elicits pain. There may be discoloration or deformity and, on palpation, crepitus (*i.e.,* a crackling sound from bones rubbing together), and irregularity may be found. Treatment consists of immobilizing the affected arm and shoulder and providing pain relief.[12,18]

Peripheral Nerve Injuries. The brachial plexuses are situated above the clavicles in the anterolateral bases of the neck. They are composed of the ventral rami of the fifth cervical nerves through the first thoracic nerves. During vertex deliveries, excessive lateral traction of the head and neck away from the shoulders may cause a stretch injury to the brachial plexus on that side. In a breech presentation, excessive lateral traction on the trunk before delivery of the head may tear the lower roots of the cervical cord. If the breech presentation includes delivery with the arms overhead, an injury to the fifth and sixth cervical roots may result. When injury to the brachial plexus occurs, it causes paralysis of the upper extremity. The paralysis often is incomplete.[12,18,19]

Brachial plexus injuries include three types: Erb-Duchenne paralysis (*i.e.,* upper arm), Klumpke's paralysis (*i.e.,* lower arm), and paralysis of the entire arm. Risk factors include an LGA infant and a difficult, traumatic delivery. Erb-Duchenne paralysis occurs with injury to the fifth and sixth cervical roots. It is the most common type of brachial plexus injury and manifests with variable degrees of paralysis of the shoulder and arm. The position of the affected arm is adducted and internally rotated, with extension at the elbow, pronation of the forearm, and flexion of the wrist. When the infant is lifted, the affected extremity is limp. The Moro reflex is impaired or absent, but the grasp reflex is present.

Klumpke's paralysis results from injury to the seventh and eighth cervical and first thoracic nerve roots. It is rare and presents with paralysis of the hand. The infant has wrist drop, the fingers are relaxed, and the grasp reflex is absent. The Moro reflex is impaired, with the upper extremity extending and abducting normally while the wrist and fingers remain flaccid.[12,18,19]

Treatment of brachial plexus injuries includes immobilization, appropriate positioning, and an exercise program. Most infants recover in 3 to 6 months. If paralysis persists beyond this time, surgical repair (neuroplasty, end-to-end anastomosis, nerve grafting) may be done.[19]

Congenital Malformations. Congenital malformations are anatomic or structural abnormalities present at birth (see Chapter 7). They are a major cause of morbidity and mortality in children. In 2000, congenital anomalies accounted for 20.5% of infant deaths, including 22% of neonatal deaths and 17.3% of infant deaths beyond the neonatal period.[3,4] Anomalies of the cardiovascular system and CNS account for most deaths due to congenital anomalies.[3] Some stages of embryonic development are more at risk than others for development of congenital malformations after teratogen exposure. The causes of congenital malformations may be classified as genetic, environmental, or multifactorial.

Health Problems of the Premature Infant

Infants born before 37 weeks' gestation are considered premature. They often fall into the LBW category, defined as birth weight less than 2500 g. LBW and prematurity often go hand in hand. Most infants weighing less than 2500 g, and almost all weighing less than 1500 g, are premature. Mortality and morbidity are increased in the premature population and are inversely proportional to the length of gestation. The shorter the time of gestation, the greater is the risk for death or disability. The immaturity of the organ systems interferes with the successful transition to extrauterine life, predisposing this population to complications. Included in this group are those premature infants who have grown abnormally during their shortened gestation (*i.e.,* LGA or SGA). Abnormal growth places an added stress on their transition to extrauterine life.

Despite the advances in obstetric management since the late 1960s, the rate of premature delivery has not significantly changed. The incidence of preterm births (<37 weeks' gestation) has gradually increased since the mid-1980s from 9.5% to 11.6%. The cause of this increase is not known. African Americans are two to three times more likely to have a preterm delivery; almost one of every five African-American births is premature.[20] In the United States, LBW is responsible for two thirds of neonatal deaths despite an increase in the survival rate of the LBW infant. Contributing risk factors for prematurity also are associated with LBW. Risk factors associated with prematurity and LBW include maternal age (*i.e.,* younger than 16, older than 35 years), race (*i.e.,* African American more than white), socioeconomic status, marital status (*i.e.,* single more than married), smoking, substance abuse, malnutrition, poor or no prenatal care, medical risks predating pregnancy, and medical risks in current pregnancy.[12,21]

The premature infant is poorly equipped to withstand the rigors of extrauterine transition. The organ systems are immature and may not be able to sustain life. The respiratory system may not be able to support gas exchange; the skin may be thin and gelatinous and easily damaged; the immune system is compromised and may not effectively fight infection; and the lack of subcutaneous fat puts the infant at risk for temperature instability. Complications of prematurity include respiratory distress syndrome, pulmonary hemorrhage, transient tachypnea, congenital pneumonia, pulmonary air leaks, bronchopulmonary dysplasia, recurrent apnea, glucose instability, hypocalcemia, hyperbilirubinemia, anemia, intraventricular hemorrhage, necrotizing enterocolitis, circulatory instability, hypothermia, bacterial or viral infection, retinopathy of prematurity, and disseminated intravascular coagulopathies.

Respiratory Problems. The *respiratory distress syndrome* (RDS), frequently referred to as *hyaline membrane disease,* is the most common complication of prematurity. In the United States, RDS develops in approximately 10% to 15% of newborns weighing less than 2500 g and 60% of infants born at 29 weeks' gestation. The incidence of RDS is lower in African-American than in white infants and in female than in male infants.

The primary cause of RDS is the lack of surfactant in the lungs (see respiratory distress syndrome, Chapter 30). Surfactant is produced by type II alveolar cells in the lungs. It is a combination of several phospholipids that lowers the alveolar surface tension and facilitates lung expansion (see Chapters 29). At 24 weeks' gestation, there are small amounts of surfactant and few terminal air sacs (*i.e.,* primitive alveoli) with underdeveloped pulmonary vascularity. If an infant is born at this time, there is little chance of survival. By 26 to 28 weeks' gestation, there usually is sufficient surfactant and lung development to permit survival.

The availability of exogenous surfactant replacement therapy has improved the outcome of RDS and has been recognized as the main factor responsible for the 6.2% decrease in the infant mortality rate in the United States from 1989 to 1990. However, because the survival rate of the sickest infants has improved and because their management is more complex, the incidence of other complications has increased. These include air leak syndromes, bronchopulmonary dysplasia, and intracranial hemorrhage.[12,21]

Apnea and *periodic breathing* are other common respiratory problems in premature infants. Because the respiratory center in the medulla oblongata is underdeveloped in the premature infant, the ability for sustained ventilatory drive often is impaired. *Apnea* is defined as cessation of breathing; it is characterized by failure to breathe for 20 seconds or more and often is accompanied by bradycardia or cyanosis. Among infants weighing less than 1.5 kg, 50% require intervention for significant apneic spells.[12,21] Although apnea may be caused by an underlying disease process such as infection, this is not apnea of prematurity and should not be treated as such.

Periodic breathing commonly occurs in those infants weighing less than 1.8 kg. It is an intermittent failure to breathe for periods lasting less than 10 to 15 seconds. Management of apnea and periodic breathing includes use of medications or ventilatory support until the CNS is developed and able to sustain adequate ventilatory drive.[12,21]

Intraventricular Hemorrhage. Intraventricular hemorrhage (IVH) is a common problem almost exclusive to premature infants. It ranks second only to RDS as a major cause of death in the premature infant. In infants born after less than 35 weeks' gestation or weighing less than 1400 g, the incidence is 40% to 50%, with the most immature at the highest risk for IVH. The hemorrhage often occurs in a subependymal germinal matrix layer (Fig. 2-7). This is a periventricular structure located between the caudate nucleus and the thalamus at the level of or slightly posterior to the foramen of Monro. The germinal matrix is

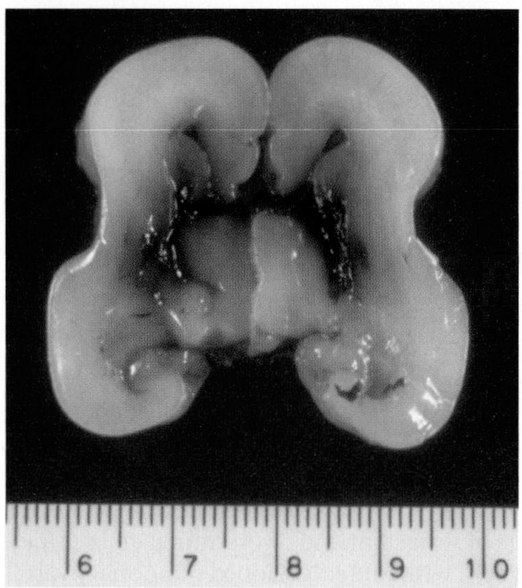

FIGURE 2-7 Intraventricular hemorrhage in a premature infant. (From Rubin E., Farber J.L. [1999]. *Pathophysiology* [3rd ed.] Philadelphia: Lippincott-Raven)

an early developmental structure that contains a fragile vascular area that is poorly supported by connective tissue. By term, this structure is gone.

Risk factors for IVH include pneumothorax, hypotension, acidosis, coagulopathy, respiratory distress syndrome, and volume expansion. The proposed mechanisms for IVH include a hypoxic-ischemic insult resulting in cerebral hyperperfusion of the germinal matrix area that causes vessel rupture. Another proposed mechanism is disruption of vascular integrity in the germinal matrix caused by hypotension. Four grades of hemorrhage have been identified.[12,18] Most hemorrhages resolve, but the more severe hemorrhages may obstruct the flow of cerebrospinal fluid, causing a progressive hydrocephalus (Table 2-2).

Necrotizing Enterocolitis. Necrotizing enterocolitis (NEC) is an acquired gastrointestinal disease process that is a major problem in preterm infants. The incidence is 1% to 5% of admissions to the neonatal intensive care unit. Although approximately 90% of infants affected are preterm infants weighing less than 1500 g, 10% of infants affected are term infants. The mortality rate varies from 20% to 40%.

The exact cause of NEC is unknown, but it is thought to be multifactorial. Risk factors for NEC include birth asphyxia, umbilical artery catheterization, patent ductus arteriosus, polycythemia, enteral feeding, and medications such as indomethacin, vitamin E, and xanthines.[22] There is agreement that the process begins with diminished perfusion of the intestinal wall, which results in ischemia and hypoxia that leads to necrosis and gangrene. Although bacterial infection plays a role in the disease, it is not thought to be the initiating event. Milk feeding has been implicated. Approximately 93% of infants in whom NEC develops have been fed enterally.[23] Human milk and commercial formulas serve as substrates for bacterial growth in the gut.

The ileum is most commonly affected, followed by the ascending colon, cecum, transverse colon, and rectosigmoid. The necrosis of the intestine may be superficial, affecting only the mucosa or submucosa, or it may extend through the entire intestinal wall. Perforation can occur and lead to peritonitis.[22,24] The manifestations of NEC are variable, but the usual presentation includes abdominal distention, gastric aspirates, bilious stools, lethargy, apnea, and hypoperfusion. The infant often appears septic. Laboratory examination may reveal leukocytosis or leukopenia, neutropenia, thrombocytopenia, glucose instability, electrolyte imbalance, metabolic acidosis, hypoxia, hypercapnia, and disseminated intravascular coagulation. Blood cultures are positive for only approximately 30% of these patients. Microorganisms reported in NEC include *Escherichia coli, Clostridium difficile, Clostridium perfringens,* and *Klebsiella, Enterobacter, Pseudomonas,* and *Salmonella* species.[22]

Clinical diagnosis is primarily radiographic. The radiographic hallmark of NEC is pneumatosis intestinalis or intramural air. Pneumoperitoneum is indicative of intestinal perforation. A large, stationary, distended loop of in-

TABLE 2-2 Classification of Periventricular/Intraventricular Hemorrhage

Grade	Location of Hemorrhage and Radiologic Appearance
Mild (grade I)	Subependymal region, germinal matrix
Moderate (grade II)	Subependymal hemorrhage with minimal filling (10%–40%) of lateral ventricles with no or little ventricular enlargement
Severe (grade III)	Subependymal hemorrhage with significant filling of lateral ventricles (>50%) with significant ventricular enlargement
Periventricular hemorrhagic infarction	Intraparenchymal venous hemorrhage

(From Fanaroff A.A., Martin R.J. [1997]. The central nervous system: Intracranial hemorrhage. In *Neonatal-perinatal medicine: Diseases of the fetus and infant* [6th ed., pp. 891–893]. Philadelphia: W.B. Saunders and Volpe J.J. [1995]. Intracranial hemorrhage: Germinal matrix hemorrhage of the premature infant. In *Neurology of the newborn* [3rd ed., pp. 403–463]. Philadelphia: W.B. Saunders.)

testine on repeated radiographs may indicate gangrene, and a gasless abdomen may indicate peritonitis.[22]

Treatment includes cessation of feedings, stomach decompression, broad-spectrum antibiotic coverage, and supportive treatment. Intestinal perforation requires surgical intervention. Intestinal resection of dead intestine with a diverting ostomy is the procedure of choice.[22]

Infection and Sepsis. Infants are at increased risk for infection due to the immaturity and relative inexperience of their immune system. Preterm infants are at even higher risk because the majority of maternal antibodies are transferred during the latter weeks of gestation. In addition, preterm infants often require invasive treatments that further increase their susceptibility to microbial invasion. Maternal risk factors that increase the likelihood of infection in the preterm infant include inadequate prenatal care, poor nutrition, low socioeconomic status, prolonged rupture of membranes, maternal fever, foul-smelling amniotic fluid, or presence of a urinary tract infection. Neonatal factors associated with the development of infection include antenatal or intrapartal asphyxia, congenital abnormalities, male sex, multiple gestations, concurrent neonatal diseases, invasive diagnostic or therapeutic procedures, iatrogenic complications, and administration of medications that alter normal microbial flora.

Newborns are at risk for infection by bacterial, viral, fungal, or protozoal microorganisms; the most common form is bacterial sepsis or bloodstream infection. Bacterial sepsis is characterized by signs of systemic infection in the presence of bacteria in the bloodstream. The incidence of bacterial sepsis in the newborn is about 1 to 8 newborns per every 1000 live births and 160 to 300 per 1000 newborns less than 1500 g (very low birth weight [VLBW]).[25,26] Almost 30% of babies admitted to neonatal intensive care units may have positive blood cultures. Because of the severe consequences of untreated bacterial sepsis and the association of infection as the cause of preterm labor, preterm babies often are treated for sepsis despite the absence of a confirmatory positive blood culture. Incidence of infection can vary by geographic region, nursery, and time of year. Mortality of neonatal bacterial sepsis is about 25% despite the use of potent antibacterial agents and supportive care.[26,27] Sepsis from group B beta-hemolytic streptococcus carries a higher mortality rate.[28]

Microorganisms. The microorganisms responsible for newborn infection have changed over the past decades. Because there are significant regional variations, it is necessary to know the specific microorganisms and antibacterial agent susceptibilities in specific institutions, as well as the general predominant bacterial patterns. In this way, early therapy can be selected for the most likely bacteria when sepsis is suspected. Early diagnosis and treatment of the bacterial sepsis provides better outcomes. Group B streptococcus and *E. coli* account for 70% to 80% of positive blood cultures in the neonatal population.[26] Other bacteria, such as *Listeria monocytogenes,* enterococci, and gram-negative enteric bacilli (other than *E. coli*), occur less commonly but must be considered.

Group B beta-hemolytic streptococcus (GBS) is the most common bacteria causing early-onset bacterial sepsis in newborns, especially preterm newborns. Streptococci are gram-positive diplococcal bacteria that exist in pairs or chains during replication. GBS can be found in cultures of body fluids, blood, urine, cerebrospinal fluid (CSF), or other bodily secretions of infected newborns. Early-onset GBS disease typically presents with respiratory distress, hypotension, and other signs characteristic of sepsis. Signs of neurologic involvement are more common in late-onset infection.

Administration of antimicrobial agents to mothers during the intrapartal period or to newborns immediately postpartum has been shown to reduce the risk for early-onset group B streptococcal infection. The Centers for Disease Control (CDC), in collaboration with the American College of Obstetricians and Gynecologists and the American Academy of Pediatrics, developed guidelines for prevention of neonatal GBS disease in 1996.[25,29,30] These guidelines recommended the use of either a risk-based approach or a screening-based approach. The risk-based approach resulted in a 40% reduction, and the screening-based approach resulted in an 80% reduction in the occurrence of neonatal GBS disease.[29,30] Subsequent studies show there has been a 65% reduction of GBS disease in areas where surveillance data were collected.[25] GBS disease continues to be a threat to the newborn owing to the high mortality and morbidity of the disease and the increased survival of smaller and more preterm newborns with a higher risk for GBS disease.

Patterns of Bacterial Sepsis. Bacterial sepsis occurs in two distinct patterns, early onset and late onset, that differ in clinical presentation, epidemiology, pathogenesis, and prognosis. *Early-onset infection* is a severe, rapidly progressive, multiorgan system illness that occurs within the first few days of life. Pneumonia is common in early-onset infection. There may be a history of obstetrical complications, such as prolonged rupture of membranes, prolonged second stage of labor, or leaking membranes. The microorganisms causing early-onset infection are those that are usually found in the mother's genital tract and include streptococci, *L. monocytogenes,* and *E. coli.* Mortality of early-onset infection, reported as 5% to 50%, is high.

Late-onset infection occurs after post-birth day 5. It has a slower progression than early-onset infection and usually has a focal site. Meningitis is seen more often with late-onset infection than with early-onset infection. In addition to those microorganisms responsible for early-onset infection, *Staphylococcus aureus, Staphylococcus epidermidis,* and other enterobacteria as well as pseudomonads are common in late-onset infections. The mortality rate for late-onset infection is about 2% to 6%.[26]

Manifestations of Bacterial Sepsis. The manifestations of bacterial infection in the newborn result from two sources: the effects of the bacterial invasion of the microorganism and the response of the newborn's immune system to the invasion. Bacteria release endotoxins and other vasoactive substances, causing central vasodilation, peripheral vasoconstriction, and systemic hypovolemia. The immune response to the endotoxins leads to hemodynamic, metabolic, respiratory, central nervous system, gastrointestinal, and dermatologic changes.

The signs of bacterial sepsis in a newborn, which can occur in all body systems, are generally nonspecific and are not easily distinguished from other causes. Therefore, it is important to have a high index of suspicion for sepsis in the newborn, especially the preterm newborn. The observation that there has been a subtle change in a baby's general condition, often marked by the nursing assessment that the baby "is not doing right," may be the first indication of infection. However, as the septicemia progresses, the signs become more severe and more specific.

Optimal prognosis depends on early diagnosis and implementation of appropriate therapy; thus, frequent and careful assessment and evaluation of the baby's physical condition can have a significant impact on outcome. Table 2-3 outlines the assessment for indicators of infection in the newborn and infant.

Health Problems of the Infant

Infants are prone to numerous health problems during the first year of life, which may become serious if not recognized and treated appropriately. Many of them may be precipitated by the relative immaturity of the organ systems. Infants are prone to nutritional disturbances, feeding difficulties, problems with food allergies, gastroesophageal reflux, and colic. Injuries, the major cause of death during infancy, are caused by events such as aspiration of foreign objects, suffocation, motor vehicle accidents, falls, poisoning, burns, and drowning. Childhood diseases may be a problem if the infant is not adequately immunized.

Issues Related to Nutrition. Good nutrition is important during infancy because of rapid growth. Human milk or commercial infant formulas form the basis for the early nutritional needs of the newborn and young infant. The American Academy of Pediatrics recommends breastfeeding for the first 12 months of life. Human milk from a well-nourished mother is easily digested, provides sufficient nutrients and calories for normal growth and development, and has the added benefit of offering some immune protection. Fluoride is recommended for breastfed infants and those receiving formula made with water containing less than 0.3 ppm of fluoride. Dietary or supplemental iron is added at approximately 6 months of age, when the fetal iron stores are depleted.

Mothers who do not choose to breast-feed their child or who are unable to breast-feed may choose from a variety of commercial formulas designed to closely match the nutrition of human milk. Several companies produce infant formulas that contain the essential nutrients for infants. Although there are some minor differences, most infant formulas are similar, regardless of which company produces the formula.

Some infants may experience difficulties in consuming mother's milk or infant formulas that are based on cow's milk because of lactase deficiency. Lactase is an enzyme that breaks down lactose, the carbohydrate found in human milk and cow's milk. Some infant formulas contain carbohydrates other than lactose. These formulas are made from soybeans. Other feeding intolerances also may occur. Treatment of any milk or formula intolerance depends on identification of the specific offender and elimination of it from the diet. Newborns and infants frequently exhibit "spitting up" or regurgitation of formula, despite the absence of a formula intolerance. In general, cow's milk–based formulas are preferable to soy-based formulas, and changing to a soy-based formula should be undertaken only when there is a proven case of intolerance. It is important that all claims of formula intolerance be thoroughly investigated before an infant is changed to a soy-based formula. Education of the parents about the signs and symptoms of intolerance and reassurance that spitting up formula is normal may be all that is required. An infant that is gaining weight, appears alert and well nourished, has adequate stools, and demonstrates normal hunger is unlikely to have a formula intolerance.

One area of infant nutrition that is still the subject of much controversy is the introduction of solid foods. There is great variation in advice regarding when to start solid foods and what solid foods to introduce. In general, human milk or iron-fortified infant formulas should supply most infant nutrition during the first year of life. However, solid foods usually are introduced beginning at 6 months. When solid foods are being introduced, they should be considered as supplemental to the total nutrition and not as the main component of nutrition. Solid foods should be introduced only by spoon-feeding. The addition of cereal to formula in a bottle or in "infant feeders" is not recommended. It has never been shown that early introduction of solid foods causes the infant to sleep longer at night.

Bland infant cereals, such as rice cereal, usually are introduced first. Slow progression to the addition of individual vegetables, fruits, and, finally, meats occurs as the infant learns to chew and swallow food. Infants also become able to drink from a cup rather than a bottle during this time. The addition of desserts is not recommended because these add calories without adding substantial nutrition.

Sometime between 9 and 12 months, the infant's intake of solid foods and formula increases, and the infant can be weaned from the breast or bottle. Much anxiety can accompany weaning, so it should be done gradually. Mothers may need reassurance that their infant is progressing normally at that time.

Irritable Infant Syndrome or Colic. Colic is usually defined as paroxysmal abdominal pain or cramping in an infant and usually is manifested by loud crying, drawing up of the legs to the abdomen, and extreme irritability. Episodes of colic may last from several minutes to several hours a day. During this time, most efforts to soothe the infant or relieve the distress are unsuccessful. Colic is most common in infants younger than 3 months of age but can persist up to 9 months of age.

Caring for an infant with colic can be frustrating. There is no single etiologic factor that causes colic; therefore, the treatment of colic is not precise. Many nonmedical techniques and pharmacologic preparations such

TABLE 2-3 Assessment of Infection in the Newborn

Evaluation	Data
Are there maternal risk factors?	Premature labor <37 weeks' gestation
	Group B streptococcal colonization
	Premature rupture of membranes (>18 hours delivery)
	Inadequate prenatal care
	Low socioeconomic status
	Poor nutrition
	Substance abuse
	Maternal infection or fever
Are there intrapartal risk factors?	Perinatal complications
	Foul-smelling amniotic fluid
	Maternal fever
Are there neonatal risk factors?	Prematurity <37 weeks' gestation
	Congenital anomalies
	Perinatal asphyxia
	Male sex
	Multiple birth
	Concurrent neonatal disease
Are there environmental risk factors?	Invasive diagnostic or therapeutic procedures
	Antimicrobial agent administration
	Nursery environment
Are there general signs of infection?	Poor feeding
	Irritability
	Lethargy
	Temperature instability
Are there skin signs of infection?	Petechiae
	Pustules
	Edema
	Jaundice
	Sclerema
Are there respiratory signs of infection?	Nasal flaring
	Expiratory grunting
	Intercostal retractions
	Tachypnea
	Apnea
Are there cardiovascular signs of infection?	Tachycardia
	Bradycardia
	Hypotension
	Cyanosis
	Decreased perfusion
	Hepatosplenomegaly
Are there gastrointestinal signs of infection?	Emesis or residuals from feeding
	Abdominal distention
	Bloody stools
	Diarrhea
Are there central nervous system signs of infection?	Hypotonia
	Hypertonia
	Poor spontaneous movement
	Seizures
Is the complete blood count abnormal?	Granulocytopenia
	Neutropenia
	Increased ratio of immature neutrophils
	Döhle bodies
	Toxic granules in cells
	Thrombocytopenia
	Anemia

as antispasmodics, sedatives, and antiflatulents have been tried. Nonpharmacologic interventions should be attempted before administration of drugs. Support of the parents is probably the single most important factor in the treatment of colic. Many times, the mother (or primary care provider) may be afraid to state just how frustrated she is with her inability to console the infant. An open discussion of this frustration can help the mothers or care providers recognize that their feelings of frustration are normal; frequently, this gives them the added support needed to deal with their infant.

Failure to Thrive. *Failure to thrive* is a term that refers to inadequate growth of the child due to the inability to obtain or use essential nutrients. Failure to thrive may be organic or nonorganic. Organic failure to thrive is the result of a physiologic cause that prevents the infant from obtaining or using nutrients appropriately. An example of organic failure to thrive is inadequate growth of an infant with deficient energy reserve because of a congenital defect that makes sucking and feeding difficult. Nonorganic failure to thrive is the result of psychological factors that prevent adequate intake of nutrition. An example of nonorganic failure to thrive is inadequate weight gain due to inadequate intake of nutrients because of parental neglect.

Diagnosis of the type of failure to thrive depends on careful examination and history of the infant and follow-up evaluations. An individual infant's growth can be compared with the standards for normal growth and development. Cases of organic failure to thrive usually are easier to diagnose than cases of nonorganic failure to thrive. Diagnosis of nonorganic failure to thrive requires extensive investigation of history, family situation, relationship of the care provider to the infant, and evaluation of feeding practices. The nonorganic basis should be considered early in every case of failure to thrive.

Therapy for failure to thrive depends on the cause. Because long-term nutritional deficiencies can result in impaired physical and intellectual growth, provision of optimal nutrition is essential. Methods to increase nutritional intake by adjusting caloric density of the formula or by parenteral nutrition may be required in cases of organic failure to thrive.

Sudden Infant Death Syndrome (SIDS). Defined as the sudden death of an infant younger than 1 year of age that remains unexplained after autopsy, investigation of the death scene, and review of the history, SIDS is the third leading cause of overall infant mortality among all races in the United States, accounting for approximately 10% of infant deaths.[4] SIDS is the leading cause of infant death in the United States during the postneonatal period, between 1 and 12 months of age. Approximately 7000 infants die of SIDS each year.[23,31,32] The specific cause of SIDS is not known. Factors associated with an increased prevalence of SIDS include prone sleeping position, African-American or Native-American race, prematurity, LBW, young maternal age, lack of prenatal care or inadequate prenatal care, smoking or substance use during pregnancy, and exposure to environmental cigarette smoke.[4]

The prone sleeping position is a significant risk factor in SIDS. The frequency of SIDS is more than threefold greater when infants sleep on their stomachs compared with sleeping on their backs.[4] Population-based education programs to decrease the practice of having infants sleep on their stomachs have resulted in a substantial decrease in SIDS.

The exact cause of SIDS is unknown. Theories focus on brain stem abnormality, which prevents effective cardiorespiratory control. Features of SIDS include prolonged sleep apnea, increased frequency of brief inspiratory pauses, excessive periodic breathing, and impaired response to increased carbon dioxide or decreased oxygen. A diagnosis of SIDS can be made only if an autopsy is performed to exclude other causes of death. Differentiation of child abuse from SIDS is an important consideration, and each case of SIDS must be subjected to careful examination.

Support of the family of an infant who dies of SIDS is crucial. Parents frequently feel guilty or inadequate as parents. The fact that there must be close scrutiny to differentiate a SIDS death from a death by child abuse adds to the guilt and disappointment felt by the family. After a diagnosis of SIDS is made, it is important that the parents and other family members receive information about SIDS. Health care providers need to be fully aware of resources available to families with a SIDS death. The siblings of the child who died should not be overlooked. Children also need information and support to get through the grief process. Children may blame themselves for the death or fear that they, too, may die of SIDS. Too many times they are not given information because the adults are trying to protect them.

Injuries. Injuries are the major cause of death in infants 6 to 12 months of age. Aspiration of foreign objects, suffocation, falls, poisonings, drowning, burns, and other bodily damage may occur because of the infant's increasing ability to investigate the environment. Childproofing the environment can be an important precaution to prevent injuries. No home or environment can be completely childproofed, but close supervision of the child by a competent care provider is essential to prevent injury.

Motor vehicle accidents are responsible for a significant number of infant deaths. After 1 year of age, motor vehicle accidents become the number one cause of accidental death. Most states require that infants be placed in an approved infant safety restraint while riding in a vehicle. The middle of the back seat is considered the safest place for the infant to ride. Many hospitals do not discharge an infant unless there is a safety restraint system in the car. If a family cannot afford a restraint system, programs are available that donate or loan the family a restraint. Health care providers must be involved in educating the public about the dangers of carrying infants in vehicles without taking proper precautions to protect them.

Infectious Diseases. One of the most dramatic improvements in infant health has been related to widespread immunization of infants and children to the major communicable childhood diseases, including diphtheria, pertussis, tetanus, polio, measles, mumps, rubella, hepatitis, and *Haemophilus influenzae* type B infection. Immunizations to these infectious diseases have greatly reduced morbidity and mortality in infants and young children. These immunizations are given at standard times as part of health promotion in infants and children. However, immunization programs have not completely eradicated these diseases, but have only lowered their prevalence. Immunization programs are effective only if all children receive the immunizations. Although most immunizations can be received through local health departments at no or low cost, many infants or young children do not routinely receive immunizations or do not receive the full regimen of immunizations. Methods to improve compliance and access to immunizations are needed. Immunization recommendations are subject to change as research leads to development of improved vaccines or more understanding of the microorganisms.

In summary, infancy is defined as that period from birth to 18 months of age. During this time, growth and development are ongoing. The relative immaturity of many of the organ systems places the infant at risk for a variety of illnesses. Birth initiates many changes in the organ systems as a means of adjusting to postnatal life. The birth process is a critical event, and maladjustments and injuries during the birth process are a major cause of death or disability. Premature delivery is a significant health problem in the United States. The premature infant is at risk for numerous health problems because of the interruption of intrauterine growth and immaturity of organ systems.

Early Childhood

After completing this section of the chapter, you should be able to meet the following objectives:

- Define *early childhood*
- Describe the growth and development of early childhood
- Discuss the common health problems of early childhood

Early childhood is considered the period of 18 months through 5 years of age. During this time, the child passes through the stages of toddler (*i.e.,* 18 months to 3 years) and preschooler (*i.e.,* 3 to 5 years). There are many changes as the child moves from infancy through the toddler and preschool years. The major achievements are the development and refinement of locomotion and language, which take place as children progress from dependence to independence.[12,21]

GROWTH AND DEVELOPMENT

Early childhood is a period of continued physical growth and maturation. Compared with infancy, physical growth is not as dramatic. Weight gain during the toddler stage is 1.8 to 2.7 kg per year (an average of 2.3 kg per year). At 2 years, the average weight is 12 kg, and by 2.5 years, the birth weight has quadrupled. By the preschool years, growth slows considerably. The average weight gain is approximately 2.3 kg per year, and almost all organ systems have reached full maturity. At 3 years, the average weight is 14.5 kg, and by 6 years, it has increased to 21 kg. During early childhood, height increases an average 7.5 cm per year and comes primarily through an increase in leg length. At 2 years of age, the average height is 86.6 cm, and by 6 years, it has reached 116 cm. In the first 2 years of life, head circumference increases by 2.5 cm per year. After 2 years of age, head circumference growth slows, and by 5 years, the average increase in head circumference is 1.25 cm per year.[7]

EARLY CHILDHOOD

- Early childhood, which encompasses the period from 18 months through 5 years of age, is a period of continued growth and development.
- During this time, the child passes through the stages of toddler (*i.e.,* 18 months to 3 years) and preschooler (*i.e.,* 3 years through 5 years).
- The major achievements are the development and refinement of locomotion and language, which take place as children progress from dependence to independence.
- During early childhood, the child begins to develop independence. The toddler must acquire a sense of autonomy while overcoming a sense of doubt and shame. The preschooler must acquire a sense of initiative and develop a conscience.
- Learning is ongoing and progressive and includes interactions with others, appropriate social behavior, and sex role functions.

The maturation of organ systems is ongoing during early childhood. The respiratory system continues its growth and maturation, but because of the relative immaturity of the airway structures, otitis media and respiratory infections are common. The barrel-shaped chest that is characteristic of infancy has begun to change to a more adult shape. The respiratory rate of infancy has slowed and averages 20 to 30 breaths/minute. Respirations remain abdominal until 7 years of age.[7]

Neural growth remains rapid during early childhood. Growth is primarily hypertrophic. The brain is 90% of adult size by 2 years of age. The cephalocaudal, proximodistal principle is followed as myelinization of the cortex, brain stem, and spinal cord is completed. The spinal cord is completely myelinated by 2 years of age. At that time, control of anal and urethral sphincters and the motor skills of locomotion can be achieved and mastered. The continuing maturation of the neuromuscular system is increasingly evident as complex gross and fine motor skills are acquired throughout early childhood.

Growth and maturation in the musculoskeletal system continue with ossification of the skeletal system, growth of the legs, and changes in muscle and fat proportions. Legs grow faster than the trunk in early childhood; after the first year of life, approximately two thirds of the increase in

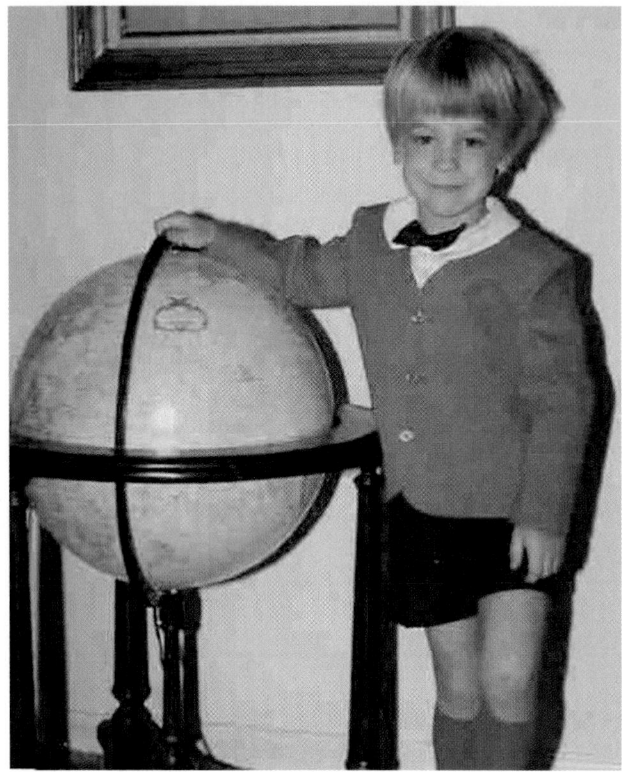

height is leg growth. Muscle growth is balanced by a corresponding decrease in adipose tissue accumulation.

During early childhood, many important psychosocial tasks are mastered by the child. Independence begins to develop, and the child is on the way to becoming a social being in control of the environment. Development and refinement of gross and fine motor abilities allow involvement with a potentially infinite number of tasks and activities. Learning is ongoing and progressive and includes interactions with others, appropriate social behavior, and sex role functions. Erikson described the tasks that must be accomplished in early childhood. The toddler must acquire a sense of autonomy while overcoming a sense of doubt and shame. The preschooler must acquire a sense of initiative and develop a conscience.[17]

COMMON HEALTH PROBLEMS

The early childhood years can pose significant health risks to the growing and maturing child. Injuries are the leading cause of death in children between the ages of 1 and 4 years; only adolescents experience more injuries. Locomotion, together with a lack of awareness of danger, places toddlers and preschoolers at special risk for injuries. Motor vehicle accidents are responsible for almost 50% of all accidental deaths in this group. Many of the injuries and deaths can be prevented by appropriate seat belts and restraints in car seats. Other major causes of injuries include drowning, burns, poisoning, falls, aspiration and suffocation, and bodily damage.[7]

Infectious diseases can be a problem for children during early childhood because of their susceptibility. This also may be the time when children first enter day care, which increases their exposure to other children and infectious diseases. The major disorders include the communicable childhood diseases (*e.g.,* common cold, influenza, varicella [chicken pox], and gastrointestinal tract infections).[6]

Child maltreatment is an increasing problem in the United States. Although the numbers vary according to the methods and definitions used, the best estimates indicate that approximately 1.4 million children in the United States undergo some form of abuse.[33] Child maltreatment includes physical and emotional neglect, physical abuse, and sexual abuse. Neglect is the most common type of maltreatment and can take the form of deprivation of basic necessities or failure to meet the child's emotional needs. It is often attributed to poor parenting skills. Physical abuse is the deliberate infliction of injury. The cause is probably multifactorial, with predisposing factors that include the parent, child, and environment. Sexual abuse is on the rise and includes a spectrum of types. The typical abuser is male. Children often do not report the abuse because they are afraid of not being believed.[7,33]

In summary, early childhood is defined as the period from 18 months to 5 years of age—the toddler and preschool years. Growth and development continue but are not as dramatic as during the prenatal and infancy periods. Early childhood is a time when most organ systems reach maturity and the child becomes an independent, mobile being. There continue to be significant health risks during this period, especially from infectious diseases and injuries. Injuries are the leading cause of death during this period. Child abuse is rapidly increasing as a major health problem.

Early School Years to Late Childhood

After completing this section of the chapter, you should be able to meet the following objectives:

- Define *early school years*
- Characterize the growth and development that occurs during the early school years
- Discuss the common health problems of the early school years

In this text, early school years or late childhood is defined as the period in which a child begins school through the beginning of adolescence. These 6 years involve a great deal of change; when one recollects "childhood," these are the years most often remembered. The experiences of this period have a profound effect on the physical, cognitive, and psychosocial development of the child and contribute greatly to the adult that the child will become.

GROWTH AND DEVELOPMENT

Although physical growth is steady throughout the early school years, it is slower than in the previous periods and the adolescent period to follow. During late childhood,

MIDDLE CHILDHOOD

- The middle childhood years (6 to 12 years) are those during which the child begins school through the beginning of adolescence.
- Growth during this period averages 3 to 3.5 kg and 6 cm per year, and occurs in approximately three to four bursts per year that last for approximately 8 weeks.
- Muscular strength, coordination, and stamina increase progressively, as does the ability to perform complex movements such as shooting basketballs, playing the piano, and dancing.
- During this stage, the child develops the cognitive skills that are needed to consider several factors simultaneously and to evaluate oneself and perceive others' evaluations.

children typically gain approximately 3 to 3.5 kg and grow an average of 6 cm per year.[5] The average 6-year-old child is 116 cm tall and weighs approximately 21 kg. By 12 years of age, the same child may weigh 40 kg and be 150 cm tall. There is only a slight difference in the body sizes of boys and girls during this period, with boys being only slightly taller and heavier than girls.[7]

During late childhood, a child's legs grow longer, posture improves, and his or her center of gravity descends to a lower point. These changes make children more graceful and help them to be successful at climbing, bike riding, roller skating, and other physical activities. Body fat distribution decreases and, in combination with the lengthening skeleton, gives the child a thinner appearance. As body fat decreases, lean muscle mass increases. By 12 years of age, boys and girls have doubled their body strength and physical capabilities. Although muscular strength increases, the muscles are still relatively immature, and injury from overstrenuous activities, such as difficult sports, can occur. With the gains in length, the head circumference decreases in relation to height, waist circumference decreases in relation to height, and leg length increases in relation to height.

Facial proportions change as the face grows faster in relation to the rest of the cranium. The brain and skull grow very little during late childhood. Primary teeth are lost and replaced by permanent teeth. When the permanent teeth first appear, they may appear to be too big for the mouth and face. This is a temporary imbalance that is alleviated as the face grows. Caloric requirements usually are lower compared with previous periods and with the adolescent period to follow. Cardiac growth is slow. Heart rate and respiratory rates continue to decrease, and blood pressure gradually rises. Growth of the eye continues, and the normal farsightedness of the preschool child is gradually converted to 20/20 vision by approximately 11 to 12 years. Frequent vision assessment is recommended during late childhood as part of normal routine health screenings.[7]

Bone ossification and mineralization continues. Bones cannot resist muscle pressure and pull as well as mature bones. Precautions should be taken to prevent alterations in bone structure, such as providing properly fitting shoes and adequate desks to prevent poor posture. Children should be checked routinely and often for scoliosis (see Chapter 58) during this period.

Toward the end of late childhood, the physical differences between the two sexes become apparent. Females usually enter pubescence approximately 2 years before males, resulting in noticeable differences in height, weight, and development of secondary sex characteristics. There is much individual variation among children of the same sex. These differences can be extremely difficult for children to cope with.

Entry into the school setting has a major impact on the psychosocial development of the child at this age. The child begins to develop relationships with other children, forming groups. Peers become more important as the child moves out of the security of the family and into the bigger world. Usually during this period, children begin to form closer bonds with individual "best friends." However, the best-friend relationships may frequently change. The personality of the child begins to appear. Although the personality is still developing, the basic temperament and approach to life become apparent. Although changes in personality occur with maturity, the basic elements may not change. The major task of this stage, as identified by Erikson, is the development of industry or accomplishment.[17] Failure to meet this task results in a sense of inferiority or incompetence, which can impede further progress.

COMMON HEALTH PROBLEMS

Because of the high level of immune system competence in late childhood, these children have an immunologic advantage over earlier years. Respiratory infections are the leading cause of illness at this time, followed by gastrointestinal disorders. The chief cause of mortality is accidents, primarily motor vehicle accidents. Immunization against the major communicable diseases of childhood has greatly improved the health of children in their early childhood years.

Health promotion includes appropriate dental care. The incidence of dental caries has decreased since the addition of fluoride to most water systems in the United States. There is a high incidence of dental caries during late childhood that is related to inadequate dental care and a high amount of dietary sugar. Children at the early part of this stage may not be as effective in brushing their teeth and may require adult assistance, but they may be reluctant to allow parental help.

Infections with bacterial and fungal agents are a common problem in childhood. These infections commonly occur as respiratory, gastrointestinal, or skin diseases. Infections of the skin occur more frequently in this age group than in any other age group, probably related to increased exposure to skin lesions. Other acute or chronic health problems may surface for the first time. Asthma,

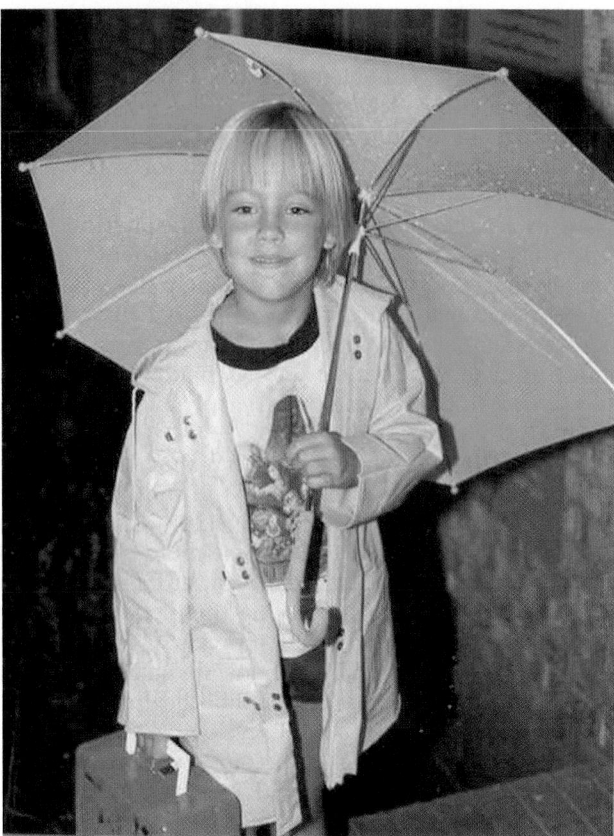

caused by allergic reactions, frequently manifests for the first time during the early school years. Epilepsy also may be first diagnosed during this period. Many childhood cancers also may appear. Developmental disabilities or specific learning disabilities may become apparent as the child enters school.

In summary, early school years to late childhood is defined as that period from beginning school through adolescence. During these 6 years, growth is steady but much slower than in the previous periods. Entry into school begins the formation of relationships with peers and has a major impact on psychological development. This is a wonderful period of relatively good health secondary to an immunologic advantage, but respiratory disease poses a leading cause of illness, and motor vehicle accidents are the major cause of death. Several chronic health problems, such as asthma, epilepsy, and childhood cancers, may surface during this time.

Adolescence

After completing this section of the chapter, you should be able to meet the following objectives:

- Define what is meant by the period known as *adolescence*
- Characterize the physical and psychosocial changes that occur during adolescence
- Cite the developmental tasks that adolescents need to fulfill
- Describe common concerns of parents regarding their adolescent child
- Discuss how the changes that occur during adolescence can influence the health care needs of the adolescent

Adolescence is a transitional period between childhood and adulthood. Significant physical, social, psychological, and cognitive changes occur during adolescence. The changes of adolescence do not occur on a strict timeline; instead, they occur at different times according to a unique internal calendar. For definition's sake, adolescence is considered to begin with the development of secondary sex characteristics, around 11 or 12 years of age, and to end with the completion of somatic growth from approximately 18 to 20 years of age. Girls usually begin and end adolescence earlier than boys. The adolescent period is conveniently referred to as the *teenaged years,* from 13 through 19 years of age.

Several "tasks" that adolescents need to fulfill have been identified. These tasks include achieving independence from parents, adopting peer codes and making personal lifestyle choices, forming or revising individual body image and coming to terms with one's body image if it is not "perfect," and establishing sexual, ego, vocational, and moral identities.

GROWTH AND DEVELOPMENT

Adolescence is influenced by CNS-mediated hormonal activity. Physical growth occurs simultaneously with sexual maturation. Adolescents typically experience gains of 20% to 25% in linear growth. An adolescent growth spurt lasting approximately 24 to 36 months accounts for most of this somatic growth. The age at onset, duration, and extent of the growth varies between males and females and among individuals. In females, the growth spurt usually begins around 10 to 14 years of age. It begins earlier in females than in males and ends earlier, with less dramatic changes in weight and height. Females usually gain approximately 5 to 20 cm in height and 7 to 25 kg in weight. Most females have completed their growth spurt by 16 or

ADOLESCENT PERIOD

- The adolescent period, which extends from 13 through 19 years of age, is a time of rapid changes in body size and shape, and physical, psychological, and social functioning.
- Adolescence is a time when hormones and sexual maturation interact with social structures in fostering the transition from childhood to adulthood.
- The development tasks of adolescence include achieving independence from parents, adopting peer codes and making personal lifestyle choices, forming or revising individual body image, and coming to terms with one's body image.

17 years of age. Males begin their growth spurt later, but it usually is more pronounced, with an increase in height of 10 to 30 cm and an increase in weight of 7 to 30 kg. Males may continue to gain in height until 18 to 20 years of age. Increases in height are possible until approximately 25 years of age.[34]

The changes in physical body size have a characteristic pattern. Growth in arms, legs, hands, feet, and neck is followed by increases in hip and chest size and several months later by increases in shoulder width and depth and trunk length. The period of these rapid and dramatic changes may be difficult for the adolescent and parents. Shoe size may change several times over several months. Although brain size is not significantly increased during adolescence, the size and shape of the skull and facial bones change, making the features of the face appear to be out of proportion until full adult growth is attained.[6,34] Muscle mass and strength also increase during adolescence. Sometimes, there may be a discrepancy between the growth of bone and muscle mass, creating a temporary dysfunction with slower or less smooth movements resulting from the mismatch of bone and muscle. Body proportions undergo typical changes during adolescence. In males, the thorax becomes broader, and the pelvis remains narrow. In females, the opposite occurs: the thorax remains narrow, and the pelvis widens.

Organ systems also undergo changes in function, and some have changes in structure. The heart increases in size as the result of increased muscle cell size. Heart rate decreases to normal adult rates, whereas blood pressure increases rapidly to adult rates. Circulating blood volume and hemoglobin concentration increase. Males demonstrate greater changes in blood volume and higher hemoglobin concentrations because of the influence of testosterone and the relatively higher muscle mass.

Skin becomes thicker, and additional hair growth occurs in both sexes. Sebaceous and sweat gland activity increases. Plugged sebaceous glands frequently result in acne (see Chapter 61). Increased sweat gland activity results in perspiration and body odor. The eyes undergo changes that may contribute to increased myopia. Auditory acuity peaks in adolescence and begins to decline after approximately 13 years of age.

Voice changes are of significant importance during adolescence for both sexes; however, the change is more pronounced in males. The voice change results from the growth of the larynx. There is more growth of the larynx in males than in females. The paranasal sinuses reach adult proportions, which increases the resonance of the voice, adding to the adult sound of the voice.[6,34]

Changes in the endocrine system are of great importance in the initiation and continuation of the adolescent growth spurt. The hormones involved include growth hormone (GH), thyroid hormones, adrenal hormones, insulin, and the gonadotropic hormones. GH regulates growth in childhood but is essentially replaced by sex hormones as the primary impetus for growth during adolescence. The exact role of GH in the adolescent growth spurt is unclear. Thyroid hormone, a significant hormone in the regulation of metabolism during childhood, continues to be important during adolescence. The relation of thyroid hormone to the other hormones and its role in the adolescent growth spurt is unclear. The thyroid gland becomes larger during adolescence, and it is believed that production of thyroid hormones is increased during this period. Insulin is necessary for appropriate growth at all stages, including adolescence. Insulin must be present for GH to be effective. The pancreatic islets of Langerhans increase in size during adolescence.[6,34]

The anterior pituitary gland produces the gonadotropic hormones, follicle-stimulating hormone, and luteinizing hormone. These hormones influence target organs to secrete sex hormones. The ovaries respond by secreting estrogens and progesterone, and the testes respond by producing androgens, resulting in the maturation of the primary sex characteristics and the appearance of secondary sex characteristics. Primary sex characteristics are those involved in reproductive function (*i.e.,* internal and external genitalia). The secondary sex characteristics are the physical signs that signal the presence of sexual maturity but are not directly involved in reproduction (*i.e.,* pubic and axillary hair). Androgens initiate the beginning of the growth spurt. Sex hormones, including androgens, also conclude height growth by causing bone maturity, epiphyseal closure of bones, and discontinuation of skeletal growth.

The dramatic and extensive physical changes that occur during the transition from child to adult are matched only by the psychosocial changes that occur during the adolescent period. It is not possible to develop one guide that adequately describes and explains the tremendous changes that occur during adolescence because the experience is unique for each adolescent. There are, fortunately, some commonalities within the process that can be used to facilitate understanding of these changes. The transition from child to adult is not a smooth, continuous, or uniform process. There are frequent periods of rapid change, followed by brief plateaus. These periods can change with little or no warning, which makes living with an adolescent difficult at times.

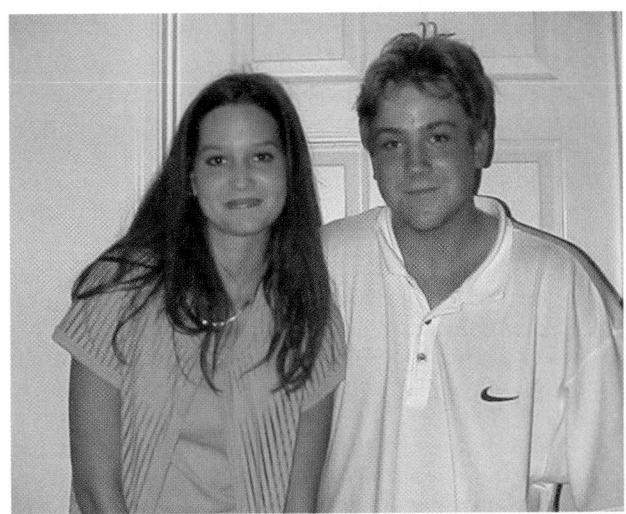

One thing that persons who deal with adolescents must remember: no matter how rocky the transition from child to adult, adolescence is not a permanent disability! Eighty percent of adolescents go through adolescence with little or no lasting difficulties. Health care professionals who care for adolescents may need to offer support to worried parents that the difficulties their adolescent is experiencing, and that the entire family is experiencing as a result, may be normal. The adolescent also may need reassurance that his or her feelings are not abnormal.[6,34]

Common concerns of adolescents include conflicts with parents, conflicts with siblings, concerns about school, and concerns about peers and peer relationships. Personal identity is an overwhelming concern expressed by adolescents. Common health problems experienced by adolescents include headache, stomachache, and insomnia. These disorders may be psychosomatic in origin. Adolescents also may exhibit situational anxiety and mild depression. The health care worker may need to refer adolescents for specialized counseling or medical care if any of the health care concerns are exaggerated.

Parents of adolescents also may have concerns about their child during the adolescent period. Common concerns related to the adolescent's behavior include rebelliousness, wasting time, risk-taking behaviors, mood swings, drug experimentation, school problems, psychosomatic complaints, and sexual activity.[34] Adolescence is a period of transition from childhood to adulthood and is often filled with conflicts as the adolescent attempts to take on an adult role. Open communication between the adolescent and family can help make the transition less stressful; however, communication between parents and adolescents is more difficult.

COMMON HEALTH PROBLEMS

Adolescence is considered to be a relatively healthy period; however, significant morbidity and mortality do occur. Health promotion is of extreme importance during the adolescent period. There are fewer actual physical health problems during this period, but there is a greater risk for morbidity and mortality from other causes, such as accidents, homicide, or suicide.

Several factors contribute to the risk for injury during adolescence. The adolescent often is unable to recognize potentially dangerous situations, possibly because of a discrepancy between physical maturity and cognitive and emotional development. Certain behavioral and developmental characteristics of the adolescent exaggerate this problem. Adolescents typically feel the need to challenge parental or other authority. They also have a strong desire to "fit in" with the peer group. Adolescents exhibit a type of magical thinking and have a need to experiment with potentially dangerous situations or behaviors. They believe that bad things will not happen to them, despite engaging in risky behaviors.

More than 80% of deaths during adolescence are attributed to injuries. Leading causes of nonintentional injuries are automobile accidents (number 1), motorcycle accidents, and drowning (number 2). Other accidental injuries include those from falls, striking objects, firearm mishaps (number 3), and sports. Accidental injuries kill more adolescents every year than all other causes of death combined, with males accounting for four of five injury victims. Automobile accidents account for 50% of all deaths of adolescents from ages 16 through 19 years.[6,34] Drowning, which is more common in males than females, decreases in prevalence after 18 years of age. Most drownings occur on weekends from May through August, are associated with alcohol use, and occur in fresh water rather than in the ocean. Firearm injuries are the third leading cause of nonintentional mortality in adolescents. Firearm accidents occur much more frequently in males between the ages of 15 and 24 years than in males of any other age.[6] Many of these accidents occur in the adolescent's home while cleaning or playing with the gun.

Other nonintentional causes of death include poisoning, skateboard injuries, all-terrain vehicle accidents, and participation in sports. However, most sports injuries are not fatal. Approximately one third to one half of all injuries occur in school. Falls are the most common cause of injury in high schools, with contusions, abrasions, swelling, sprains, strains, and dislocations being the most common injuries.[2,26] Cancer is the fourth leading cause of death in adolescents, but it is the leading cause of death from nonviolent sources. There is an increased incidence of certain types of cancer during adolescence, including lymphomas, Hodgkin's disease, and bone and genital tumors. Leukemia is the leading cause of cancer mortality in persons between the ages of 15 and 24 years.[34]

Adolescents also are subject to intentional injuries, such as homicide and suicide. Suicide rates have risen dramatically for adolescents since the 1950s, to approximately 13 to 14 per 100,000. Most of the increase can be attributed to the greater number of suicides committed by white males. It also is thought that the rate of adolescent suicide may be higher than what is reported because of underreporting on death certificates. Almost 60% of suicides involve firearms.[34]

The increasing prevalence of sexual activity among adolescents has created unique health problems. These include adolescent pregnancy, sexually transmitted diseases, and human immunodeficiency virus (HIV) transmission. Associated problems include substance abuse, such as alcohol, tobacco, inhalants, and other illicit drugs. Health care providers must not neglect discussing sexual activity with the adolescent. Nonjudgmental, open, factual communication is essential for dealing with an adolescent's sexual practices. Discussion of sexual activity frequently is difficult for the adolescent and the adolescent's family. If a relationship exists between the adolescent and the health care provider, this may provide a valuable forum for the adolescent to get accurate information about safe sex, including contraception and avoidance of high-risk behaviors for acquiring sexually transmitted diseases or acquired immunodeficiency syndrome (AIDS).[34]

Substance abuse among adolescents increased rapidly in the 1960s and 1970s but has declined since that time. However, substance abuse still is prevalent in the adolescent age group. Health care workers must be knowledgeable about the symptoms of drug abuse, the consequences of drug abuse, and the appropriate management of adolescents with substance abuse problems. Substance abuse among adolescents includes the use of tobacco products, cigarettes, and "smokeless" tobacco (*e.g.*, snuff, chewing tobacco). Other substances include alcohol, marijuana, stimulants, inhalants, cocaine, hallucinogens, tranquilizers, and sedatives. Adolescents are at high risk for succumbing to the peer pressure to participate in substance abuse. They have a strong desire to fit in and be accepted by their peer group. It is difficult for them to "just say no." Magical thinking leads adolescents to believe that they will not get "hooked" or that the bad consequences will not happen to them. Adolescents and the rest of society are constantly bombarded with the glamorous side of substance use. Television shows, movies, and magazine advertisements are filled with beautiful, healthy, successful, happy, and popular persons who are smoking cigarettes or drinking beer or other alcoholic beverages. Adolescents are trying to achieve the lifestyle depicted in those ads, and it takes tremendous willpower to resist that temptation. It is important that adolescents be provided with "the rest of the story" through education and constant communication.[6,34]

Pregnancy has become a major problem of the teen years. Approximately 1 million adolescents in the United States become pregnant annually.[2] Four of every 10 teenage females become pregnant before reaching 20 years of age. One fifth of all pregnancies occur within the first month after beginning sexual activity; one half occur within the first 6 months of sexual activity. Of the slightly more than 1 million pregnant adolescents, 47% delivered, 40% had therapeutic abortions, and 13% had spontaneous abortions.[6]

Adolescent pregnancy carries significant risks to the mother and to the fetus or newborn. The topic of adolescent pregnancy involves issues related to physical and biologic maturity of the adolescent, growth requirements of the adolescent and fetus, and unique prenatal care requirements of the pregnant adolescent. Emotional responses and psychological issues regarding relationships of the adolescent in her family and with the father of the baby, as well as how the pregnancy will affect the adolescent's future, must be considered.

In summary, adolescence is a transitional period between childhood and adulthood. It begins with development of secondary sex characteristics (11 to 12 years) and ends with cessation of somatic growth (18 to 20 years). This is the period of a major growth spurt, which is more pronounced in males. The endocrine system is of great importance with its numerous hormonal changes and their initiation and continuation of the growth spurt. Psychosocial changes are equally dramatic during this period and often place tremendous pressure on relationships between adults and the adolescent. Adolescence is a relatively healthy period, but significant morbidity and mortality exist as a result of accidents, homicide, and suicide. The increasing prevalence of sexual activity and substance abuse places the adolescent at risk for HIV infection; alcohol, tobacco, and other drug abuse; and adolescent pregnancy.

REVIEW EXERCISES

The vital signs of a full-term 1-day-old newborn are as follows: temperature, 101.4°F (axillary); pulse, 188 beats/minute; respirations, 70 breaths/minute; blood pressure, 56/36 mm Hg.

A. What laboratory test or tests should be performed?

B. What information could be obtained from review of the maternal record that may be helpful in establishing a differential diagnosis for this infant?

C. What other clinical signs should be assessed?

A preterm newborn, approximately 30 weeks' gestation, is admitted to the newborn intensive care unit. The baby exhibits respiratory distress, including tachypnea, retractions, and expiratory grunting.

A. Identify the two most common causes for respiratory distress in this baby.

B. Explain the etiology of the two causes identified.

An adolescent male is seen in the health clinic for a routine sports examination. The nurse practitioner notes that the adolescent has a mild to moderate case of facial acne. The nurse practitioner discusses the causes, prevention, and treatment of acne with the young man.

A. What physiologic changes contribute to the development of acne in adolescents?

B. What other physical changes also occur during adolescence?

C. What are common health problems in adolescents?

References

1. U.S. Department of Health and Human Services. (2000). *Healthy children 2000.* Washington, DC: Author.
2. Anderson, R.N. (2002). Deaths: Leading causes for 2000. *National Vital Statistics Reports 50*(16).
3. Centers for Disease Control and Prevention, National Center for Health Statistics. (2000). *Health, United States, 2000.*
4. Pastore G., Guala A., Zaffaroni M. (2003). Back to sleep: Risk factors for SIDS as targets for public health campaigns. *Journal of Pediatrics 142*(4), 453–454.
5. Needlman R.D. (2000). Growth and development. In Behrman R.E., Kliegman R.M., Jenson H.B. (Eds.), *Nelson textbook of pediatrics* (16th ed., pp. 23–65). Philadelphia: W.B. Saunders.
6. Moore K.L., Persaud T.V.N., Chabner D.E.B. (2003) *The developing human: Clinically oriented embryology* (7th ed.). Philadelphia: W.B. Saunders.
7. Zitelli B.J., Davis H.J. (2002). *Atlas of pediatric physical diagnosis* (4th ed.). St. Louis: Mosby–Year Book.
8. O'Brien P. (2003). *Langman's medical embryology* (9th ed.). Philadelphia: Lippincott Williams & Wilkins.
9. Lubchenco L.O., Hansman C., Dressler M., et al. (1963). Intrauterine growth as estimated from liveborn birthweight data at 24 to 42 weeks of gestation. *Pediatrics 32,* 793–800.
10. Battaglia F.C., Lubchenco L.O. (1967). A practical classification of newborn infants by weight and gestational age. *Journal of Pediatrics 71,* 748–758.

11. Ballard J.L., Khoury J.C., Wedig K., et al. (1991). New Ballard score, expanded to include extremely premature infants. *Journal of Pediatrics 119,* 417–423.
12. Sansoucie D.A., Calvaliere T.A. (2003). Newborn and infant assessment. In Kenner C., Lott J.W. (Eds.), *Comprehensive neonatal nursing: A physiologic perspective* (pp. 308–347). Philadelphia: W.B. Saunders.
13. Harmon J. (2003). High-risk pregnancy. In Kenner C., Lott J.W. (Eds.), *Comprehensive neonatal nursing: A physiologic perspective* (pp. 173–196). Philadelphia: W.B. Saunders.
14. Barnes F.L. (2000). The effects of the early uterine environment on the subsequent development of embryo and fetus [Review]. *Theriogenology 53*(2):649–658.
15. Apgar V. (1953). A proposal for a new method of evaluation of the newborn infant. *Current Research in Anesthesia and Analgesia 32,* 260.
16. Dubowitz L.M., Dubowitz V., Goldberg C. (1970). Clinical assessment of gestational age in the newborn infant. *Journal of Pediatrics 77,* 1–10.
17. Erikson E. (1963). *Childhood and society.* New York: W.W. Norton.
18. Blackburn S.T. (2003). Assessment and management of neurologic dysfunction. In Kenner C., Lott J.W. (Eds.), *Comprehensive neonatal nursing: A physiologic perspective* (pp. 624–660). Philadelphia: W.B. Saunders.
19. Stoll B.J., Kliegman R.M. (2000). The fetus and the neonatal infant. In Behrman R.E., Kliegman R.M., Jenson H.B. (Eds.), *Nelson textbook of pediatrics* (16th ed., pp. 487–492). Philadelphia: W.B. Saunders.
20. Brandt I., Sticker E.J., Lentze M.J. (2003) Catch-up growth of head circumference of very low birth weight, small for gestational age preterm infants and mental development to adulthood. *Journal of Pediatrics 142*(5), 463–470.
21. Cifuentes J., Segars A.H., Ross M., Carlo W. (2003). Assessment and management of respiratory dysfunction. In Kenner C., Lott J.W. (Eds.), *Comprehensive neonatal nursing: A physiologic perspective* (pp. 348–362). Philadelphia: W.B. Saunders.
22. Thigpen J., Kenner, C. (2003). Assessment and management of gastrointestinal dysfunction. In Kenner C., Lott J.W. (Eds.), *Comprehensive neonatal nursing: A physiologic perspective* (pp. 448–485). Philadelphia: W.B. Saunders.
23. Beckwith J.B. Defining the sudden infant death syndrome [Review]. (2003). *Archives of Pediatric and Adolescent Medicine 157*(3), 286–290.
24. Wyckoff M.M., McGrath J.M., Griffin T., Malan J. (2003). Nutrition: Physiologic basis of metabolism and management of enteral and parenteral nutrition. In Kenner C., Lott J.W. (Eds.), *Comprehensive neonatal nursing: A physiologic perspective* (pp 425–447). Philadelphia: W.B. Saunders.
25. Baltimore S., Huie S., Meek J., et al. (2001). Early-onset neonatal sepsis in the era of group B Streptococcal prevention. *Pediatrics 108*(5), 1094–1098.
26. Klein J., Remington J.S. (2001). Current concepts of infections of the fetus and newborn infant. In: Remington J.S., Klein J.O. (Eds.), *Infectious disease in the fetus and newborn infant* (5th ed., pp. 1–23). Philadelphia: W.B. Saunders.
27. Batra S., Kumar R., Seema K.A., Ray G. (2000). Alterations in antioxidant status during neonatal sepsis. *Annals of Tropical Paediatrics 20,* 27–33.
28. Edwards M., Baker C. (2001). Group B streptococcal infections. In Remington J.S., Klein J.O. (Eds.), *Infectious disease in the fetus and newborn infant* (5th ed., pp. 1091–1156). Philadelphia: W.B. Saunders.
29. Rosenstein N.E., Sucuchat A., for the Neonatal Group B Study Group (1997). Opportunities for prevention of perinatal group B streptococcal disease: a multi-state analysis. *Obstetrics and Gynecology 90,* 901–906.
30. Moore M.R., Schrag S.J., Schuchat A. (2001). Effects of intrapartum antimicrobial prophylaxis for prevention of group-B-streptococcal disease on the incidence and ecology of early-onset neonatal sepsis. *Lancet Infectious Diseases 3*(4), 201–213.
31. Hunt C. (2000). Sudden infant death syndrome. In Behrman R.E., Kliegman R.M., Jenson H.B. (Eds.), *Nelson textbook of pediatrics* (16th ed., pp. 2139–2143). Philadelphia: W.B. Saunders.
32. Hunt C.E., Lesko S.M., Vezina R.M., et al. (2003). Infant sleep position and associated health outcomes. *Archives of Pediatric and Adolescent Medicine 157*(5), 469–474.
33. Leventhal J.M. (2003). The field of child maltreatment enters its fifth decade. *Child Abuse and Neglect, 27*(1), 1–4.
34. Lopez R.I., Kelly K. (2002). The teen health book: A parents' guide to adolescent health and well-being (pp. 3–37, 561–575). New York: W.W. Norton.

CHAPTER

3

Concepts of Altered Health in Older Adults

Janice Kuiper Pikna

For age is opportunity no less than youth, itself, though in another dress. And as the evening twilight fades away the sky is filled with stars, invisible by day.

—Henry Wadsworth Longfellow

Aging is a natural, lifelong process that brings with it unique biopsychosocial changes. These changes create special health care needs for the older adult population that merit consideration. Because the prediction for the future is a continuous increase in the older adult population, there is a need to focus on the special health care needs of this group. *Gerontology* is the discipline that studies aging and the aged from biologic, psychological, and sociologic perspectives. It explores the dynamic processes of complex physical changes, adjustments in psychological functioning, and alterations in social identities. Through a holistic approach, health care providers specializing in gerontology seek to assist older adults in maximizing their functional abilities while attempting to prevent and minimize illness and disability.

An important first distinction is that aging and disease are not synonymous. Unfortunately, a common assumption is that growing older is inevitably accompanied by illness, disability, and overall decline in function. The fact is that the aging body can accomplish most, if not all, of the functions of its youth; the difference is that they may take longer, require greater motivation, and be less precise. But as in youth, maintenance of physiologic function occurs through continued use.

The Elderly and Theories of Aging

After completing this section of the chapter, you should be able to meet the following objectives:

- State a definition for *young-old, middle-old,* and *old-old,* and characterize the changing trend in the elderly population
- State a philosophy of aging that incorporates the positive aspects of the aging process
- Compare the focus of programmed change and stochastic theories of aging

WHO ARE THE ELDERLY?

The older adult population is typically defined in chronologic terms and includes individuals 65 years of age and older. This age was chosen somewhat arbitrarily, and historically it is linked to the Social Security Act of 1935. With this Act, the first national pension system in the United States, which designated 65 years as the pensionable age, was developed. Since then, the expression *old age* has been understood to apply to anyone older than 65 years. Because there is considerable heterogeneity among this group, older adults often are subgrouped into young-old (65 to 74 years), middle-old (75 to 84 years), and old-old (85+ years) to reflect more accurately the changes in function that occur. Age parameters, however, are somewhat irrelevant because chronologic age is a poor predictor of biologic function. However, chronologic age does help to quantify the number of individuals in a group and allows predictions to be made for the future.

In the year 2000, 12.4% of the total United States population (34.4 million) was 65 years of age or older. The proportion of older adults declined for the first time in the 1990s, due partly to the relatively low number of births in the late 1920s and early 1930s. This trend is not expected to continue, however, as the "baby boomers" (born from 1946 to 1964) reach age 65, beginning in the year 2011. During the 1990s, the most rapid growth of the elderly population occurred in the oldest age groups. Those 85 years and older increased by 38%, whereas the 75- to 84-year-olds increased by 23% and the 65- to 74-year-old group increased by less than 2%. The entire population of older adults is expected to grow to over 70 million by the year 2030 (Fig. 3-1). Average life expectancy has increased as a result of overall advances in health care technology, improved nutrition, and improved sanitation. Women who are now 65 years of age can expect to live an additional 19.2 years (84.2 years of age), and men an additional 16 years (81 years old).[1,2]

Aging can be thought of somewhat as a women's issue because women tend to outlive men. In the year 2000, there was a sex ratio of 143 women for every 100 men older than 65 years in the United States. This ratio increases to as high as 243 women for every 100 men in the 85 years and older age group. Marital status also changes with advancing age. In 2000, almost half of all older women living in the community were widows, and there were four times as many widows as there were widowers.[1,2]

Although about 4 million older adults were in the workforce in 2000 (*i.e.*, working or actively seeking work), most were retired.[1] Retirement represents a significant role change for older adults. Attitudes and adjustment to retirement are influenced by preretirement lifestyles and values. Individuals with leisure pursuits during their work life seem to adjust better to retirement than those whose lives were dominated by work. For many of today's cohort of older adults, the work ethic of the Great Depression remains profoundly ingrained as the central purpose in life. When work is gone, a significant loss is felt, and something must be substituted in its place. Because leisure has not always been a highly valued activity, older adults may have difficulty learning to engage in meaningful leisure pursuits.

Loss of productive work is just one of many losses that can accompany the aging process. Loss of a spouse is a highly significant life event that commonly has negative implications for the survivor. Experts cite an increased mortality among recently bereaved older adults (especially men), an increased incidence of depression, psychological distress, loneliness, and higher rates of chronic illness. Loss of physical health and loss of independence are other changes that can affect the psychosocial aspects of aging, as can relocation, loss of friends and relatives, and changes in the family structure.

Poverty is common among the elderly population. In 2001, 10% of those 65 years of age and older lived below the poverty line, and another 6.5% were classified as "near poor" (income between the poverty level and 125% of this level). Poverty rates vary among elderly subgroups, with 21.9% of elderly African Americans at poverty level in 1999, 21.8% of elderly Hispanics, and 8.9% of elderly Caucasians. The main sources of income for older persons in 1998 were Social Security (90% of older persons), income from assets (59%), public and private pensions (41.6%), and earnings (22%).[1]

Contrary to popular belief, most older adults live in community settings. Most live in some type of family setting, with a spouse, their children, or other relatives, and approximately 30% live alone. Only 4.5% of all individuals 65 years of age and older reside in long-term care facil-

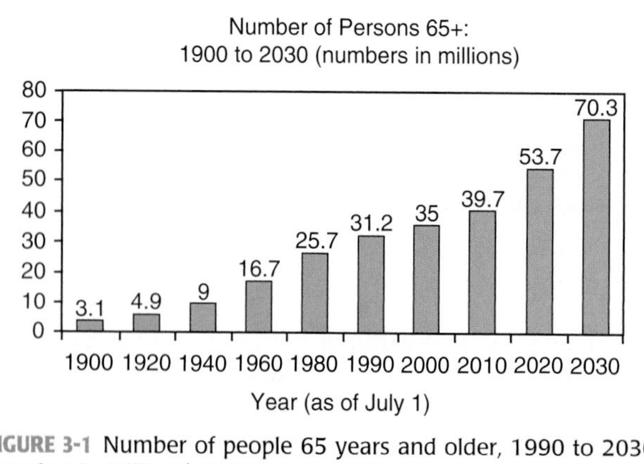

FIGURE 3-1 Number of people 65 years and older, 1990 to 2030 (number in millions). *Note: increments in years are uneven. Based on U.S. Bureau of Census.* (From: *A profile of older Americans: 2002.* U.S. Department of Health and Human Services: Administration on Aging).

THE ELDERLY

- The older population, which is subgrouped into the young-old (65 to 74 years), the middle-old (75 to 84 years), and the old-old (85+ years), has increased dramatically during the past century and is expected to continue to grow as the result of overall advances in health care technology, improved nutrition, and improved sanitation.
- As the result of increased years, many older adults are confronted with retirement, changes in lifestyle, loss of significant others, and a decline in physical functioning.
- Although aging brings with it a unique set of biophysiologic changes, it is not synonymous with disease and disability. Most older adults can perform most or all of the activities they performed in earlier years, although they often take longer and require greater motivation.

ities or nursing homes. However, this number increases to 18.2% for persons 85 years of age or older.[1]

Older adults are the largest consumers of health care. In 1997, more than half of the population (54.5%) reported having one or more disabilities. One third had at least one severe disability, and approximately one sixth (14%) had difficulties with activities of daily living (ADL). Almost half of all adult hospital beds are filled with patients 65 years of age and older.[2]

THEORIES OF AGING

The lifestyle changes that occur with aging have been described in various developmental theories. Probably the most widely known is Erikson's eight stages of development. According to this theory, the first seven developmental stages span the period from childbirth through middle adulthood. The eighth stage, in older adulthood, focuses on "ego integrity versus despair." Ego integrity is the acceptance of one's life in relation to humanity and one's place in history. Lack of ego integrity leads to despair, signified by nonacceptance of one's lifestyle and a fear of death. Despair may be manifested as apathy, depression, or decreased life satisfaction.[3,4]

The stages of physical change that occur as part of the aging process are less well articulated. Several theories attempt to explain the biology of aging through a variety of scientific observations at the molecular, cellular, organ, and system levels. No one theory explains all of the aging processes, but each holds some clues. In reality, it is reasonable to suppose that there are multiple influences that affect the aging process. The various theories of aging can be categorized as either programmed change theories or stochastic theories. *Developmental-genetic theories* propose that the changes that occur with aging are genetically programmed, whereas *stochastic theories* maintain that the changes result from an accumulation of random events or damage from environmental agents or influences.[5] It is accepted now that the process of aging and longevity is multifaceted, with both genetics and environmental factors playing a role. In animal studies, genetics accounted for less that 35% of the effects of aging, whereas environmental influences accounted for more than 65% of the effects.[6]

The developmental-genetic theory resides with genetic influences that determine physical condition, occurrence of disease, age of death, cause of death, and other factors contributing to longevity.[5,7] At the cellular level, Hayflick and Moorhead observed more than 35 years ago that cultured human fibroblasts have a limited ability to replicate (approximately 50 population doublings) and then die.[8] Before achieving this maximum, they slow their rate of division and manifest identifiable and predictable morphologic changes characteristic of senescent cells. Another explanation of cellular aging resides with an enzyme called *telomerase* that is believed to govern chromosomal aging through its action on telomeres, the outermost extremities of the chromosome arms. With each cell division, a small segment of telomeric deoxyribonucleic acid (DNA) is lost, unless a cell has a constant supply of telomerase. In the absence of telomerase, the telomeres shorten, resulting in senescence-associated gene expression and inhibition of cell replication. It is thought that in certain cells, such as cancer cells, telomerase maintains telomere length, thereby enhancing cell replication. Currently, there is interest in developing telomerase therapy that could be used to initiate cell death in selected targets such as cancer cells and preventing cell senescence in other cell types, such as the chondrocytes in joints, the retinal epithelial cells in the eye, and the lymphocytes in the immune system.[5,9]

The stochastic theories propose that aging is caused by random damage to vital cell molecules.[5] The damage eventually accumulates to a level sufficient to result in the physiologic decline associated with aging. The most prominent example of the stochastic theory is the somatic mutation theory of aging, which states that the longevity and function of cells in various tissues of the body are determined by the double-stranded DNA molecule and its specific repair enzymes. DNA undergoes continuous change in response both to exogenous agents and intrinsic processes. It has been suggested that aging results from conditions that produce mutations in DNA or deficits in DNA repair mechanisms. The oxidative free radical theory is a stochastic idea in which aging is thought to result partially from oxidative metabolism and the effects of free radical damage (see Chapter 5). The major byproducts of oxidative metabolism include superoxides that react with DNA, ribonucleic acid, proteins, and lipids, leading to cellular damage and aging. Another damage theory, the wear and tear theory, proposes that accumulated damage to vital parts of the cell leads to aging and death. Cellular DNA is cited as an example. If repair to damaged DNA is incomplete or defective, as is thought to occur with aging, declines in cellular function might occur.[5,7]

Although these theories help to explain some of the biologic phenomena of aging, many questions remain. It seems likely that the human genome project will begin to explain some of the questions regarding the genetics of aging, but many questions need to be answered regarding the effects of environmental influences on aging.

In summary, aging is a natural, lifelong process that brings with it unique biopsychosocial changes. Aging is not synonymous with disease or ill health. The aging body can accomplish most or all of the functions of its youth, although they may take longer, require greater motivation, and be less precise.

The older adult population is typically defined in chronologic terms as individuals 65 years of age and older and can be further defined as young-old (65 to 74 years), middle-old (75 to 84 years), and old-old (85+ years). The number of older persons has increased and is expected to continue to grow in the future, with an anticipated 70 million Americans older than age 65 by the year 2030.

There are two main types of theories used to explain the biologic changes that occur with aging: programmed change theories, which propose that aging changes are genetically programmed, and stochastic theories, which maintain that aging changes result from an accumulation of random events or damage from environmental hazards.

Physiologic Changes of Aging

After completing this section of the chapter, you should be able to meet the following objectives:

- Describe common skin changes that occur with aging
- Explain how muscle changes that occur with aging affect high-speed performance and endurance
- Describe the process of bone loss that occurs with aging
- State the common changes in blood pressure regulation that occur with aging
- List the changes in respiratory function that occur with aging
- Relate aging changes in neural function to the overall function of the body
- Briefly discuss the effects of aging on vision, hearing, taste, and smell
- Describe three changes that occur in the gastrointestinal tract with aging
- State the significance of decreased lean body mass on interpretation of the glomerular filtration rate using serum creatinine levels

The physiologic changes seen in the elderly reflect not only the aging process but also the effects of years of exposure to environmental agents, such as sunlight and cigarette smoke, and disease processes such as diabetes mellitus. Overall, there is a general decline in the structure and function of the body with advancing age. The decline results in a decreased reserve capacity of the various organ systems that consequently produce reduced homeostatic capabilities, making the older adult more vulnerable to stressors such as illness, trauma, surgery, medications, and environmental changes.

Research to identify true age-related changes as opposed to disease states is difficult. Studies using cross-sectional methodologies are the easiest to perform; however, mortality can confound the results. Although longitudinal studies tend to be more precise, they require years to perform and may not be able to account for numerous variables that enter into the aging equation, such as environment, occupation, and diet. However, it is important to differentiate, as much as possible, those changes that occur in the body as a result of aging from those that occur because of disease. This distinction allows for more accurate diagnosis and treatment of disease conditions and helps to avoid inappropriate labeling of aging changes.

Regardless of the difficulty in defining normal aging as it relates to the various organ systems, there is a pattern of gradual loss that occurs. Many of these losses begin in early adulthood, but because of the large physiologic reserve of most organ systems, the decrement does not become functionally significant until the loss reaches a certain level. Some changes, such as those that affect the skin and posture, are more visible, whereas others, such as those affecting the kidney, may go unnoticed until the person is challenged with situations such as metabolizing and eliminating medications.

SKIN

Changes in the skin more obviously reflect the aging process than do changes in other organ systems (see Chapter 61). Aging can impinge on the primary functions of the skin: protection from the environment, temperature regulation, fluid and electrolyte balance, sensory function, and excretion of metabolic wastes. Exposure to sunlight and harsh weather accelerates aging of the skin.

With aging, the skin becomes wrinkled and dry and develops uneven pigmentation. The thickness of the dermis, or middle layer of skin, decreases by approximately 20%, which gives the skin an overall thin and transparent quality. This is especially true for areas exposed to sunlight. Dermal collagen fibers rearrange and degenerate, resulting in decreased skin strength and elasticity. Cellularity and vascularity of the dermis decrease with advancing age and can cause vascular fragility, leading to senile purpura (*i.e.,* skin hemorrhages) and slow skin healing. Delayed wound healing may be influenced by other factors such as poor nutrition and circulation and by changes in immune function.[10,11] The function of the sebaceous glands diminishes with age and leads to a decrease in sebum secretion. The decrease in size, number, and activity of the eccrine sweat glands causes a decrease in their capacity to produce sweat.[10,11]

Fingernails and toenails become dull, brittle, and thick, mostly as a result of decreased vascularity of the nail beds. Age-related changes in hair occur as well. Owing to a decline in melanin production by the hair follicle, approximately one half of the population older than 50 years of age has at least 50% gray hair, regardless of sex or original hair color. Changes in hair growth and distribution also are seen.[10,11] Hair on the scalp, axillae, and pubis becomes more sparse, and the hairs of the ears and nostrils coarsen. Skin disorders are common among the older adult population and can include skin cancers, keratoses (*i.e.,* warty lesions), xerosis (*i.e.,* excessive dryness), dermatitis, and pruritus (*i.e.,* generalized itching).

STATURE AND MUSCULOSKELETAL FUNCTION

Aging is accompanied by a progressive decline in height, especially among older women. This decline in height is attributed mainly to compression of the spinal column. Body composition changes as well. The amount of fat increases, and lean body mass and total body water decrease with advancing age.

With aging, there is a reduction in muscle size and strength that is related to a loss of muscle fibers and a reduction in the size of the existing fibers. Although the decline in strength that occurs with aging cannot be halted, its progress can be slowed with exercise. There is a decline in high-speed performance and reaction time because of a decrease in type II muscle fibers.[12,13] Impairments in the nervous system also can cause movements to slow. However, type I muscle fibers, which offer endurance, are thought to remain consistent with age (see Chapter 12).

Numerous studies have reported a loss of bone mass with aging, regardless of sex, race, or body size. With aging, the process of bone formation (*i.e.*, renewal) is slowed in relation to bone resorption (*i.e.*, breakdown), resulting in a loss of bone mass and weakened bone structure. This is especially true for postmenopausal women. By 65 years of age, most women have lost two thirds of their skeletal mass owing to a decrease in estrogen production.[13] Skeletal bone loss is not a uniform process. At approximately 30 years of age, bone loss begins, predominantly in the trabecular bone (*i.e.*, fine network of bony struts and braces in the medullary cavity) of the heads of the femora and radii and in the vertebral bodies.[13,14] By 80 years of age, women have lost nearly 43% of their trabecular bone, and men have lost 27%. This process becomes pathologic (*i.e.*, osteoporosis) when it significantly increases the predisposition to fracture and associated complications (see Chapter 58).

The prevalence of joint disease is increased among the elderly. By age 65 years, 80% of the population has some articular disease. Osteoarthritis is so common among elderly persons that it is often incorrectly assumed to be a normal age-related change rather than a disease. The synovial joints ultimately are affected by osteoarthritis, most commonly the joints of the hands, feet, knees, hips, and shoulders. It is characterized by cartilage loss and new bone formation, accounting for a distortion in articulation, limited range of motion, and joint instability (see Chapter 59). Age is the single greatest risk factor for development of osteoarthritis, in part because of the mechanical impact on joints over time, but it also is related to injury, altered physical condition of the articular cartilage, obesity (*e.g.*, knee), congenital deformity (*e.g.*, hip), crystal deposition in articular cartilage (*e.g.*, knee), and heredity. Pain, immobility, and joint inflammation often ensue. Treatment is aimed at minimizing risk factors, weight loss if indicated, exercise to increase muscle strength, and pain relief measures.

CARDIOVASCULAR FUNCTION

Cardiovascular disease remains the leading cause of morbidity and mortality in older adults. It often is difficult to separate true age-related changes in the cardiovascular system from disease processes. The aorta and arteries tend to become stiffer and less distensible with age, the heart becomes less responsive to the catecholamines, the maximal exercise heart rate declines, and there is a decreased rate of diastolic relaxation.[15]

Although approximately 40% of older adults have hypertension, the disorder is not considered a normal age-related process.[16] The relationship between blood pressure and risk for cardiovascular disease is continuous, consistent, and independent of other risk factors. It has been shown that the higher the blood pressure, the greater the chance of heart attack, heart failure, stroke, and kidney disease. In persons older than 50 years, systolic blood pressure (SBP) greater than 140 mm Hg is a more important risk factor than a rise in diastolic blood pressure (DBP). The risk for developing cardiovascular disease beginning at 115/75 mm Hg doubles with each increment of 20/10 mmHg. Individuals who are normotensive at age 55 have a 90% lifetime risk for developing hypertension. There is now a push to intervene when individuals are prehypertensive (*i.e.*, SBP of 120 to 139 mm Hg or DBP of 80 to 89 mm Hg) with lifestyle modification strategies to prevent hypertension. There is also a move to treat hypertension aggressively in order to minimize negative outcomes.[16] With advancing age, the elevation in blood pressure is generally more pronounced for the SBP than for the DBP, probably as a result of increased aortic stiffness. In the older adult, compensatory cardiovascular mechanisms often are delayed or insufficient, so that a drop in blood pressure due to position change or consumption of a meal is common.[17,18] Orthostatic hypotension, or a significant drop in systolic blood pressure on assumption of the upright position, is more common among elderly persons (see Chapter 25). Even in the absence of orthostatic hypotension, older adults respond to postural stress with diminished changes in heart rate and diastolic pressure. This altered response to orthostatic stress is thought to result from changes in autonomic nervous system function, inadequate functioning of the circulatory system, or both.[19]

Senescent cardiac muscle typically displays a decreased response to β-adrenergic stimulation and circulating catecholamines, and there is increased diastolic stiffness of the ventricles that impedes filling, probably because of a slower rate of diastolic relaxation. Although early diastolic filling decreases by approximately 50% between 20 and 80 years of age, filling volumes are maintained, most likely as a result of an enhanced atrial contraction and its contribution to ventricular filling. The afterload (*i.e.*, opposition to left ventricular ejection) rises steadily with age as the ascending aorta becomes more rigid and the resistance in peripheral arterial vessels increases. Although the overall size of the heart does not increase, the thickness of the left ventricular wall may increase with age, in part responding to the increased afterload that develops because of blood vessel changes.[15] The resting heart rate remains unchanged or decreases only slightly with age; however, the maximum heart rate that can be achieved during maximal exercise is decreased.

Despite aging changes and cardiovascular disease, overall cardiovascular function at rest in most healthy elderly persons is considered adequate to meet the body's needs. Cardiac output is essentially maintained in healthy older adults (men more than women) during exercise despite the decreased heart rate response, apparently because of a greater stroke volume resulting from increased end-diastolic volume (*i.e.*, Frank-Starling mechanism) during exercise.[17,20]

RESPIRATORY FUNCTION

As lung function changes with age, it often is difficult to differentiate the effects of age from those of environmental and disease factors. Maximal oxygen consumption (VO_2 max), a measure used to determine overall cardiopulmonary function, declines with age. Numerous studies have indicated that VO_2 max can improve significantly with exercise and that the VO_2 max of older adult master athletes can meet and exceed that of their younger counterparts.

A progressive loss of elastic recoil in the lung is caused by changes in the amount of elastin and composition of collagen fibers. Calcification of the soft tissues of the chest wall causes increased stiffness and thus increases the workload of the respiratory muscles. There is a loss of alveolar structure that decreases the surface area of gas exchange. Although the total lung capacity remains constant, the consequences of these changes result in an increased residual lung volume, increased functional reserve capacity, and a decline in vital capacity. There is a linear decrease in arterial oxygen tension (PO_2) of approximately 20 mm Hg from 20 to 70 years of age. This is thought to result primarily from the ventilation-perfusion mismatching of the aging lung.[21]

NEUROLOGIC FUNCTION

Changes at the structural, chemical, and functional levels of the nervous system occur with normal aging, but overall, they do not interfere with day-to-day routines unless specific neurologic diseases come into play. The weight of the brain decreases with age, and there is a loss of neurons in the brain and spinal cord. Neuron loss is most pronounced in the cerebral cortex, especially in the superior temporal area. Additional changes take place in the neurons and supporting cells. Atrophy of the neuronal dendrites results in impaired synaptic connections, diminished electrochemical reactions, and neural dysfunction. Synaptic transmissions also are affected by changes in the chemical neurotransmitters dopamine, acetylcholine, and serotonin. As a result, many neural processes slow. Lipofuscin deposits (*i.e.*, yellow, insoluble intracellular material) are found in greater amounts in the aged brain.[22,23]

Sensorimotor changes show a decline in motor strength, slowed reaction time, diminished reflexes (especially in the ankles), and proprioception changes. These changes can cause the balance problems and slow, more deliberate movements that are frequently seen in older individuals.[24]

Even though changes in the brain are associated with aging, overall cognitive abilities remain intact. Although language skills and attention are not altered with advanced age, performance and constructional task abilities can decline, as can short-term memory and immediate recall. A change in personality or significant cognitive deficits is considered unusual with normal aging, and if either occurs, evaluation is in order. Dementia or depression can frequently be the cause.

SPECIAL SENSES

Sensory changes with aging can greatly affect the older adult's level of functioning and quality of life. Vision and hearing impairments due to disease states, for example, can interfere with communication and may lead to social isolation and depression.

Vision

There is a general decline in visual acuity with age, and nearly all individuals older than 55 years of age require vision correction for reading or distance. The decline occurs as a result of a smaller pupil diameter, loss of refractive power of the lens, and an increase in the scattering of light. The most common visual problem among older adults is presbyopia, or difficulty focusing on near objects. It is caused mainly by decreased elasticity of the lens and atrophy of the ciliary muscle (see Chapter 54).

Glare and abrupt changes in light pose particular problems for older adults. Both are reasons that the elderly frequently give up night driving; they also increase their risk for falls and injury. Color discrimination changes also take place with aging. In particular, older adults have more difficulty identifying blues and greens. This is thought to be related to problems associated with filtering short wavelengths of light (*i.e.*, violet, blue, green) through a yellowed, opaque lens. Corneal sensitivity also may diminish with age, so that older adults may be less aware of injury or infection.[25,26]

Ophthalmologic diseases and disorders are common in the elderly. Cataracts, glaucoma, and macular degeneration are seen frequently and can greatly impair vision and function. Low-vision aids, such as special magnifiers and high-intensity lighting that mimics sunlight, can assist in optimizing vision in otherwise uncorrectable ophthalmologic problems.

Hearing

Hearing loss is common among older adults, and some degree of impairment is almost inevitable with advancing age. It has been reported that 30% of independent individuals older than 65 years and about half of those older than 85 years have a hearing impairment.[27–29]

Presbycusis, or the hearing loss of old age, is characterized by a gradual, progressive onset of bilateral and symmetric sensorineural hearing loss of high-frequency tones (see Chapter 55). The hearing deficit often has both a peripheral and a central component. Speech discrimination, or the ability to distinguish among words that are near-homonyms or distinguish words spoken by several different speakers, often is impaired.[27] Accelerated speech and shouting can increase distortion and further compound the problem. When speaking to hearing-impaired older adults, it is helpful to face them directly so that they can observe lip movements and facial expressions. Speech should be slow and direct. Loudness can be irritating. Rephrasing misunderstood messages also can improve understanding of the spoken word. Hearing aids can be effective for various levels of hearing loss and may greatly improve the ability to hear and communicate. However, the usefulness of a hearing aid may be limited if the hearing deficit is multifactorial, with both a central and a peripheral component. In one study of hearing in the elderly, it was suggested that speech audiometry is a good indicator of real hearing difficulties faced by older adults and may be more valuable than pure-tone audiometry. Hearing deficits with age are not always limited to an increased detection threshold; both include other aspects of hearing, such as sound, comprehension of speech, and noise discrimination, as noted earlier.[28]

Cerumen (*i.e.,* ear wax) impaction in the external auditory canal also is commonly seen in older adults and can impair hearing. The cerumen glands, which are modified apocrine sweat glands, atrophy and produce drier cerumen. This may be partially responsible for more frequent cerumen impactions in the older adult population.[27]

Taste and Smell

Olfaction, or the sense of smell, declines with aging possibly as a result of generalized atrophy of the olfactory bulbs and a moderate loss of olfactory neurons. Smell is a protective mechanism, and persons who cannot smell may be at risk for exposure to environmental hazards. For example, people who cannot smell smoke would be at particular risk if a fire broke out.

The sense of taste decreases with aging, but it is believed to be less affected than olfaction. Because taste and smell are necessary for the enjoyment of food flavor, older adults may not enjoy eating as much as in their youth. Drugs and disease also may affect taste. Alterations in taste and smell, along with other factors such as eating alone, decreased ability to purchase and prepare food, and the high cost of some foods, may account for poor nutritional intake in some older adults. Conversely, the lack of sensory feedback may lead the person to eat more and gain weight. A decline in taste is more pronounced among older adults with Alzheimer's disease, presumably because of the neuropathologic changes in the brain.[30]

IMMUNE FUNCTION

An overall decline in immune system capabilities with aging can pose an increased risk for some infections (see Chapter 19). Involution of the thymus gland is complete by approximately 45 to 50 years of age, and although the total number of T cells remains unchanged, there are changes in the function of helper T cells that alter the cellular immune response of older adults. There also is evidence of an increase in various autoantibodies (*e.g.,* rheumatoid factor) as a person ages, increasing the risk for autoimmune disorders. Older adults are more susceptible to urinary tract infections, respiratory tract infections, wound infections, and nosocomial infections. The mortality rate from influenza and bronchopneumonia is increased for the older adult population. Local organ factors and coincident diseases probably play a bigger role in the acquisition of these infections than age-related changes in immunity.[31]

Early detection of infections is more difficult in older adults because the typical symptoms, such as fever and elevated white blood cell count, often are absent.[32] A change in mental status or decline in function often is the only presenting sign. It has been reported that frank delirium occurs in 50% of older adults with infections. Thus, infections in elderly persons may be far advanced at the time of diagnosis.

GASTROINTESTINAL FUNCTION

The gastrointestinal tract shows less age-associated change in function than many other organ systems. Although tooth loss is common, and approximately 40% to 50% of the older adult population is edentulous, it is not considered part of the normal aging process. Poor dental hygiene with associated caries and periodontal disease is the main reason for the loss. *Edentia,* or toothlessness, can lead to dietary changes and can be associated with malnutrition. Use of dentures can enhance mastication; however, taste sensation is inhibited. Because of improved dental technology and the fluoridated water supply, more persons are able to keep their teeth into their later years. *Xerostomia,* or dry mouth, also is common, but it is not universal among older adults and typically occurs as a result of decreased salivary secretions. Other causes of dry mouth can include medications, such as anticholinergics and tranquilizers, radiation therapy, and obstructive nasal diseases that induce mouth breathing.

Soergel and colleagues (1964) coined the term *presbyesophagus* to denote changes in esophageal function, such as decreased motility and inadequate relaxation of the lower esophageal sphincter, that occur with aging.[33] However, in studies that controlled for disease states such as diabetes mellitus and neuropathies, no increase in abnormal motility was observed. In general, the physiologic function of the esophagus appears to remain intact with advancing age.

Atrophy of the gastric mucosa and a decrease in gastric secretions can occur in older adults. Achlorhydria (*i.e.,* decrease in hydrochloric acid secretion) occurs, probably as a result of a loss of parietal cells. Although not universal, achlorhydria is more prevalent among older adults and can cause impaired gastric absorption of substances requiring an acid environment.

Atrophic gastritis and decreased secretion of intrinsic factor are more common with aging and result in a malabsorption of vitamin B_{12}. Because vitamin B_{12} is necessary for the maturation of red blood cells, a deficiency can lead to a type of macrocytic anemia called *pernicious anemia.* Vitamin B_{12} deficiency also can cause neurologic abnormalities such as peripheral neuropathy, ataxia, and even dementia. Treatment consists of regular periodic vitamin B_{12} replacement therapy through injection because the oral form is not absorbed owing to a lack of intrinsic factor.[34]

The small intestine shows some age-related morphologic changes, such as mucosal atrophy; however, absorption of most nutrients and other functions appear to remain intact. Absorption of calcium, however, decreases with aging and may reflect decreased intestinal absorption along with other factors, such as reduced intake of vitamin D, decreased formation of vitamin D_3 by the skin because of reduced sun exposure, and decreased activation of vitamin D_3 by the liver and kidney.

Diverticula of the colon are common among older adults, with more than 50% of individuals older than 80 years having diverticular disease. The high incidence appears to result mainly from a low-fiber diet. Constipation, or infrequent passage of hard stool, is another frequently occurring phenomenon. It often is attributed to immobility and decreased physical activity, a low-fiber diet, decreased fluid intake, and medications; malignancies and other disease states also can be responsible. Complications of constipation can include fecal impaction or obstruction, megacolon, rectal prolapse, hemorrhoids, and laxative abuse.

RENAL FUNCTION

Although age-related anatomic and physiologic changes occur, the aging kidney remains capable of maintaining fluid and electrolyte balance remarkably well. Aging changes result in a decreased reserve capacity, which may alter the kidney's ability to maintain homeostasis in the face of illnesses or stressors. Overall, there is a general decline in kidney mass with aging, predominantly in the renal cortex. The number of functional glomeruli decreases by 30% to 50%, with an increased percentage of sclerotic or abnormal glomeruli.[35]

Numerous cross-sectional and longitudinal studies have documented a steady, age-related decline in total renal blood flow of approximately 10% per decade after 20 years of age, so that the renal blood flow of an 80-year-old person averages approximately 300 mL/minute, compared with 600 mL/minute in a younger adult. The major decline in blood flow occurs in the cortical area of the kidney, causing a progressive, age-related decrease in the glomerular filtration rate (GFR). Serum creatinine, a byproduct of muscle metabolism, often is used as a measure of GFR. The decline in GFR that occurs with aging is not accompanied by an equivalent increase in serum creatinine levels because the production of creatinine is reduced as muscle mass declines with age.[36] Serum creatinine levels often are used as an index of kidney function when prescribing and calculating drug doses for medications that are eliminated through the kidneys; this has important implications for older adults. If not carefully addressed, improper drug dosing can lead to an excess accumulation of circulating drugs and result in toxicity. A formula that adjusts for age-related changes in serum creatinine for individuals 40 through 80 years of age is available (see Chapter 36).

Renal tubular function declines with advancing age, and the ability to concentrate and dilute urine in response to fluid and electrolyte impairments is diminished. The aging kidney's ability to conserve sodium in response to sodium depletion is impaired and can result in hyponatremia. A decreased ability to concentrate urine, an age-related decrease in responsiveness to antidiuretic hormone, and an impaired thirst mechanism may account for the older adult's greater predisposition to dehydration during periods of stress and illness. Older adults also are more prone to hyperkalemia and hypokalemia when stressed than are younger individuals. An elevated serum potassium may result from a decreased GFR, lower renin and aldosterone levels, and changes in tubular function. Low potassium levels, on the other hand, are more commonly caused by gastrointestinal disorders or diuretic use. Neither is the result of aging.[36]

GENITOURINARY FUNCTION

Changes in the bladder occur with the aging process, resulting in a possible decline in function. Overall, the smooth muscle and supportive elastic tissue are replaced with fibrous connective tissue. This can cause incomplete bladder emptying and a diminished force of urine stream. Bladder capacity also decreases with age, whereas the frequency of urination increases. As elastic tissue and muscles weaken, stress incontinence becomes more prevalent.

In aging women, atrophy of perineal structures can cause the urethral meatus to recede along the vaginal wall. Atrophy of other pelvic organs occurs in the aging woman because of diminished estrogen production after menopause: vaginal secretions diminish; the vaginal lining is thinner, drier, less elastic, and more easily traumatized; and normal flora are altered. These changes can result in vaginal infections, pruritus, and painful intercourse.[37]

In aging men, benign prostatic hyperplasia (BPH) is very common. The incidence progressively increases to approximately 80% of men by 80 years of age. The condition often is asymptomatic until approximately 50 years of age. Thereafter, the incidence and severity of symptoms increase with age. BPH can cause obstructive symptoms such as urinary hesitancy, diminished force of stream, retention, and postvoid dribbling; it also can cause irritative symptoms such as frequency, nocturia, urgency, and even urge incontinence[38] (see Chapter 45).

Sexual activity remains possible into late life for men and women. In general, the duration and intensity of the sexual response cycle is diminished in both sexes. Penile erection takes longer to develop because of changes in neural innervation and vascular supply. Women take longer to experience the physiologic changes of vaginal expansion and lubrication during the excitement phase. Social factors affecting sexual behavior include the desire to remain sexually active, access to a sexually functioning partner, and availability of a conducive environment.[39,40]

In summary, there is a general decline in the structure and function of the body with advancing age, resulting in a decreased reserve capacity of the various organ systems, including the integumentary, musculoskeletal, cardiorespiratory, nervous, sensory, immune, gastrointestinal, and genitourinary systems. This results in a reduction of homeostatic capabilities, making the older adult more vulnerable to stressors such as illness, trauma, surgery, medication administration, and environmental changes.

Functional Problems of Aging

After completing this section of the chapter, you should be able to meet the following objectives:

- Compare information obtained from functional assessment with that obtained from a physical examination used to arrive at a medical diagnosis

- ✦ Cite the differences between chronic and transient urinary incontinence
- ✦ State four risk factors for falls in older individuals
- ✦ List five symptoms of depression in older adults
- ✦ Name a tool that can be used for assessing cognitive function
- ✦ State the difference between delirium and dementia

Although aging is not synonymous with disease, the aging process does lend itself to an increased incidence of illness. As chronologic age increases, so does the probability of having multiple chronic diseases. It has been estimated that 86% of older adults have at least one chronic condition, and most actually have more than one. The extent of these problems is described in Table 3-1. Older adults are more likely to experience a decline in overall health and function because of the increased incidence of chronic illness that occurs with advancing age. Because aging also brings with it a decreased ability to maintain homeostasis, illnesses often manifest in an atypical manner. For example, myocardial infarction may occur without chest pain or other presenting symptoms. Sepsis without fever is common, and pneumonia may present with acute confusion but lack the prodromal symptom of cough.

In addition to chronic illnesses, older adults suffer disproportionately from functional disabilities, or the inability to perform the necessary activities of daily living (ADL). It is most likely that the decrements in health that can accompany the aging process are responsible for these functional disabilities. Among the more common functional problems of the older adult are urinary incontinence, instability and falls, sensory impairment, depression, dementia, and delirium.

FUNCTIONAL ASSESSMENT

Evaluation of the older adult's functional abilities is a key component in gerontologic health care. Medical diagnoses alone are incomplete without an assessment of function. Two older adults with similar medical diagnoses of arthritis, hypertension, and osteoporosis, for example, can be at opposite ends of the spectrum of functional abilities.

TABLE 3-1 Common Health Problems in the Elderly

Health Problems	Percentage With Problems
Arthritis	49
Hypertension	36
Hearing impairment	30
Heart disease	27
Orthopedic impairments	18
Cataracts	17
Sinusitis	12
Diabetes	10

(Data from American Association of Retired Persons. [2000]. *A profile of older Americans*. www.aarp.org)

Assessing functional status can be done in many different ways, using a variety of methods. Measures of function should attempt systematically and objectively to evaluate the level at which an individual is functioning in a variety of areas, including biologic, psychological, and social health.

Selection of a screening tool to measure function depends on the purpose of data collection, the individual or target population to be assessed, availability and applicability of the instruments, reliability and validity of the screening tools, and the setting or environment. An issue that arises when assessing function is the question of capability versus performance. For example, an older adult may be able to bathe without supervision; however, the long-term care facility where the person resides may discourage it for safety reasons. Among the more commonly used assessment tools are those that measure the ability to perform ADL and the patient's cognitive function.

When evaluating levels of function, determination of the older adult's ability to perform ADL and instrumental ADL (IADL) should be included. Activities of daily living are basic self-care tasks, such as bathing, dressing, grooming, ambulating, transferring (*e.g.*, from a chair to bed), feeding, and communicating. Instrumental activities of daily living are more complex tasks that are necessary to function in society, such as writing, reading, cooking, cleaning, shopping, laundering, climbing stairs, using the telephone, managing money, managing medications, and using transportation. The IADL tasks indirectly examine cognitive abilities as well because they require a certain level of cognitive skills to complete.

Several tools are available for measuring functional status. One of the more commonly used tools is the Index of Activities of Daily Living. Developed by Katz in 1963 and revised in 1970, it summarizes performance in six functions: bathing, dressing, toileting, transferring, continence, and feeding. It is used as an assessment tool to determine the need for care and the appropriateness of treatment and as a teaching aid in rehabilitation settings. Through questioning and observation, the rater forms a mental picture of the older adult's functional status as it existed during a 2-week period preceding the evaluation, using the most dependent degree of performance.[41,42] Numerous studies using the Katz Index tool show significant validity and reliability. The advantage of the tool is that it is easy to administer and provides a "snapshot" of the older adult's level of physical functioning. The disadvantage is that it does not include IADL categories that are of equal importance, especially for older adults living in the community.

URINARY INCONTINENCE

Urinary incontinence, or involuntary loss of urine, plagues more than 30% of community-living individuals older than 60 years of age, 50% of hospitalized older adults, and 60% of residents in long-term care facilities. These estimates may be low because individuals often fail to report symptoms of urinary incontinence, perhaps owing to the attached social stigma. Health care professionals often neglect to elicit such information as well.

Incontinence is an expensive problem. A conservative estimate of cost for direct care of adults with incontinence is more than $15 billion annually.[43] Urinary incontinence can have deleterious consequences, such as social isolation and embarrassment, depression and dependency, skin rashes and pressure sores, and financial hardship. Although urinary incontinence is a common disorder, it is not considered a normal aspect of aging. Studies reveal that 60% to 70% of community-dwelling older adults with urinary incontinence can be successfully treated and even cured.

Changes in the micturition cycle that accompany the aging process make the older adult prone to urinary incontinence. Decreases in bladder capacity, in bladder and sphincter tone, and in the ability to inhibit detrusor (*i.e.,* bladder muscle) contractions, combined with the nervous system's increased variability to interpret bladder signals, can cause incontinence (see Chapter 37). Impaired mobility and a slower reaction time also can aggravate incontinence.

The causes of incontinence can be divided into two categories: transient and chronic. Of particular importance is the role of pharmaceuticals as a cause of transient urinary incontinence. Numerous medications, such as long-acting sedatives and hypnotics, psychotropics, and diuretics, can induce incontinence. Treatment of transient urinary incontinence is aimed at ameliorating or relieving the cause on the assumption that the incontinence will resolve.

Chronic, or established, urinary incontinence occurs as a failure of the bladder to store urine or a failure to empty urine. Failure to store urine can occur as a result of detrusor muscle overactivity with inappropriate bladder contractions (*i.e.,* urge incontinence). There is an inability to delay voiding after the sensation of bladder fullness is perceived. Urge incontinence is typically characterized by large-volume leakage episodes occurring at various times of day. Urethral incompetence (*i.e.,* stress incontinence) also causes a bladder storage problem. The bladder pressure overcomes the resistance of the urethra and results in urine leakage. Stress incontinence causes an involuntary loss of small amounts of urine with activities that increase intraabdominal pressure, such as coughing, sneezing, laughing, or exercising.[43–45]

Failure of the bladder to empty urine can occur because of detrusor hyper-reflexia, resulting in urine retention and overflow incontinence. Also called *neurogenic incontinence,* this type of incontinence can be seen with neurologic damage from conditions such as diabetes mellitus and spinal cord injury. Outlet obstruction, as with prostate enlargement and urethral stricture, also can cause urinary retention with overflow incontinence. Functional incontinence, or urine leakage due to toileting problems, occurs because cognitive, physical, or environmental barriers impair appropriate use of the toilet.[44,45]

After a specific diagnosis of urinary incontinence is established, treatment is aimed at correcting or ameliorating the problem. Probably the most effective interventions for older adults with incontinence are behavioral techniques. These strategies involve educating the individual and providing reinforcement for effort and progress. Techniques include bladder training, timed voiding or habit training, prompted voiding, pelvic floor muscle (*i.e.,* Kegel) exercises, and dietary modifications. Biofeedback, a training technique to teach pelvic floor muscle exercises, uses computerized instruments to relay information to individuals about their physiologic functions. Biofeedback can be helpful when used in conjunction with other behavioral treatment techniques. Use of pads or other absorbent products should be seen as a temporary help measure and not as a cure. Numerous types of products are available to meet many different consumer needs.

Pharmacologic intervention may be helpful for some individuals. Estrogen replacement therapy in postmenopausal women, for example, was thought to help relieve stress incontinence. However, it is no longer recommended as a treatment approach, in light of newer information about the cardiovascular side effects and increased cancer risks that estrogen can pose. Drugs with anticholinergic and bladder smooth muscle relaxant properties (*e.g.,* oxybutynin, tolterodine) may help with urge incontinence. These medications are not without side effects, however, and their use must be carefully weighed against the possible benefits.

Surgical intervention may help to relieve urinary incontinence symptoms in appropriate patients. Bladder neck suspension may assist with stress incontinence unrelieved by other interventions, and prostatectomy is appropriate for men with overflow incontinence due to enlarged prostate. However, older adults may have medical conditions that preclude surgery. Other treatments include intermittent self-catheterization for some types of overflow incontinence.

INSTABILITY AND FALLS

Unstable gait and falls are a common source of concern for the older adult population. The literature reveals that 30% of community-dwelling individuals older than 65 years of age and 50% of nursing home residents fall each year. Most falls do not result in serious injury, but the potential for serious complications and even death is real. Accidents are the seventh leading cause of death among older adults, with falls ranking first in this category. Hip fractures are one of the most feared complications from a fall. More than 340,000 individuals fracture a hip each year; most of these are elderly women. Significant morbidity occurs as a result of a hip fracture. The literature varies, but as many as 50% of older adults who sustain a hip fracture are reported to require nursing home care for at least 1 year, and up to 20% die in the year after a hip fracture. Other bones frequently fractured by older adults who fall are the humerus, wrist, and pelvis. These bones bear the brunt of osteoporotic changes and, as a result, are more vulnerable to injury. Soft tissue injuries such as sprains and strains also can result from falls.[46–48]

An individual's activity may be restricted because of fear on the individual's or caregiver's part about possible falling. These anxieties may lead to unnecessary restrictions in independence and mobility and commonly are mentioned as a reason for institutionalization.

Although some falls have a single, obvious cause, such as a slip on a wet or icy surface, most are the result of several factors. Risk factors that predispose to falling include a combination of age-related biopsychosocial changes, chronic illnesses, and situational and environmental hazards. Gait and stability require the integration of information from the special senses, the nervous system, and the musculoskeletal system. Changes in gait and posture that occur in healthy aged individuals also contribute to the problem of falls. The older person's stride shortens; the elbows, trunk, and knees become more flexed; toe and heel lift decrease while walking; and sway while standing increases. Muscle strength and postural control of balance decrease, proprioception input diminishes, and righting reflexes slow. All these factors predispose the older adult to the possibility of falling.[49]

Because the central nervous system integrates sensory input and sends signals to the effector components of the musculoskeletal system, any alteration in neural function can predispose to falls. For this reason, falls have been associated with strokes, Parkinson's disease, and normal-pressure hydrocephalus. Similarly, diseases or disabilities that affect the musculoskeletal system, such as arthritis, muscle weakness, or foot deformities, are associated with an increase in the incidence of falls. Age- and disease-related alterations in vision and hearing impair sensory input and can contribute to falls. Vestibular system alterations such as benign positional vertigo or Ménière's disease cause balance problems that can result in falls. Cognitive impairments such as dementia have been associated with an increased risk for falling, most likely because of impaired judgment and problem-solving abilities.

Input from the cardiovascular and respiratory systems influences function and ambulation. Cardiovascular diseases, especially postural hypotension, can cause recurrent falls, solely or in association with the previously mentioned factors. The dramatic drop in blood pressure on rising that is seen in postural hypotension can cause falls because of syncope and dizziness.

Medications are an important and potentially correctable cause of instability and falls. Centrally acting medications, such as sedatives and hypnotics, have been associated with an increase in the risk for falling and injury. Diuretics can cause volume depletion, electrolyte disturbances, and fatigue, predisposing to falls. Antihypertensive drugs can cause fatigue, orthostatic hypotension, and impaired alertness, contributing to the risk for falls.

Environmental hazards play a significant role in falling. More than 70% of falls occur in the home and often involve objects that are tripped over, such as cords, scatter rugs, and small items left on the floor. Poor lighting, ill-fitting shoes, surfaces with glare, and improper use of ambulatory devices such as canes or walkers also contribute to the problem.[47,48] Table 3-2 summarizes the possible causes of falls.

Preventing falls is the key to controlling the potential complications that can result. Because multiple factors usually contribute to falling, the aim of the clinical evaluation is to identify risk factors that can be modified. Assessment

TABLE 3-2 Risk Factors for Falls

Category of Risk Factors	Examples
Accidents and environmental hazards	Slips, trips Clutter, cords, throw rugs
Age-related functional changes	Decreased muscle strength, slowed reaction time, decreased proprioception, impaired righting reflexes, increased postural sway, altered gait, impaired visual and hearing function
Cardiovascular disorders	Aortic stenosis, cardiac dysrhythmias, autonomic nervous system dysfunction, hypovolemia, orthostatic hypotension, carotid sinus syncope, vertebrobasilar insufficiency
Gastrointestinal disorders	Diarrhea, postprandial syncope, vasovagal response
Genitourinary disorders	Urinary incontinence, urinary urgency/frequency, nocturia
Medication use	Alcohol, antihypertensives, cardiac medications, diuretics, narcotics, oral hypoglycemic agents, psychotropic medications, drug–drug interactions, polypharmacy
Metabolic disorders	Anemia, dehydration, electrolyte imbalance, hypothyroidism
Musculoskeletal disorders	Osteoarthritis, rheumatoid arthritis, myopathy
Neurologic disorders	Balance/gait disorders, cerebellar dysfunction, stroke with residual effects, cervical spondylosis, central nervous system lesions, delirium, dementia, normal-pressure hydrocephalus, peripheral neuropathy, Parkinson's disease, seizure disorders, transient ischemic attack
Prolonged bed rest	Hypovolemia, muscle weakness from disuse and deconditioning
Respiratory disorders	Hypoxia, pneumonia
Sensory impairments	Decreased visual acuity, cataract, glaucoma, macular degeneration, hearing impairment, vestibular disorders

of sensory, neurologic, and musculoskeletal systems; direct observation of gait and balance; and a careful medication inventory can help identify possible causes. Dizziness, either transient due to a self-limiting illness or recurring, is a risk factor for falls. In one study, 24% of persons older than 72 years of age reported at least once-monthly episodes of dizziness.[50] Dizziness was associated with several conditions, including cardiovascular disorders, sensory impairment, balance disturbances, and psychological conditions. The number of medications the person took also was associated with episodes of dizziness.[50]

Preventive measures can include a variety of interventions, such as surgery for cataracts or cerumen removal for hearing impairment related to excessive earwax accumulation. Other interventions may include podiatric care, discontinuation or alteration of the medication regimen, exercise programs, physical therapy, and appropriate adaptive devices. The home also should be assessed by an appropriate health care professional (*e.g.,* occupational therapist) and recommendations made regarding modifications to promote safety. Simple changes such as removing scatter rugs, improving the lighting, and installing grab bars in the bathtub can help prevent falling. These interventions can maximize the older adult's independence and prevent the morbidity and mortality that can occur as a result of a fall.

SENSORY IMPAIRMENT

Although sensory impairments are not imminently life threatening, their impact on health can be substantial. Hearing impairment is associated with decreased quality of life, depression, isolation, and dementia. Visual impairment is related to increased risk for falls, hip fractures, physical disability, and depression. Nursing home residents with visual impairment are more likely to require assistance with ADLs and can be at risk for falls and hip fractures. Visual impairment also appears to increase mortality.[27,51,52]

Sensory impairment results not only from deficits in peripheral sensory structures but also from the central processing of sensory information. The older person's difficulty in processing multisensory information is seen most strikingly when there is a rapid fluctuation in the nature of the information that is received from the environment.[27]

It has been reported that a lack of sensory information can predispose to psychological symptoms. Charles Bonnet syndrome is an organic disorder occurring in the elderly that is characterized by complex visual hallucinations. It is associated with ocular disease and, strictly speaking, is seen in older adults with preserved intellectual functions.[53] In one study, 10% of persons (mean age, 75 years) with severe visual disability experienced visual hallucinations.[54] These persons retained insight into the problem and needed only reassurance that their hallucinations did not represent mental illness. Both auditory and visual impairment can have important psychological effects in association with dementia. Delusions have been associated with hearing impairment. In one study that used a case-control method, elderly persons with late-life psychosis with paranoid symptomatology were four times more likely to have hearing impairments compared with control subjects.[55]

DEPRESSION

Depression is a significant health problem that affects the older adult population. Estimates of depression in older adults vary widely; however, there is a consensus that the size of the problem is underestimated owing to misdiagnosis and mistreatment. Approximately 15% of community-dwelling older adults are thought to have depressive symptoms. The estimate drops to approximately 3% when diagnosis is restricted to major depression. Depressive symptoms are seen in approximately 15% to 25% of nursing home residents.[56]

The term *depression* is used to describe a symptom, syndrome, or disease. As listed in the American Psychiatric Association's 1994 *Diagnostic and Statistical Manual of Mental Disorders* (DSM-IVR), the criteria for the diagnosis and treatment of major depression include at least five of the following symptoms during the same 2-week period, with at least one of the symptoms being depressed mood or anhedonia (*i.e.,* loss of interest or pleasure): depressed or irritable mood; loss of interest or pleasure in usual activities; appetite and weight changes; sleep disturbance; psychomotor agitation or retardation; fatigue and loss of energy; feelings of worthlessness, self-reproach, or excessive guilt; diminished ability to think or concentrate; and suicidal ideation, plan, or attempt.[57]

Depressive symptomatology can be incorrectly attributed to the aging process, making recognition and diagnosis difficult. Depressed mood, the signature symptom of depression, may be less prominent in the older adult, and more somatic complaints and increased anxiety are reported, confusing the diagnosis. Symptoms of cognitive impairment can be seen in the depressed older adult. Because it can be misdiagnosed as dementia, a thorough medical evaluation is in order. Unlike true dementia, pseudodementia of depression usually improves with treatment for depression. Although they are similar in clinical presentation, there are some subtle distinctions between the two conditions (Table 3-3). Physical illnesses can complicate the diagnosis as well. Depression can be a symptom of a medical condition, such as pancreatic cancer, hypothyroidism or hyperthyroidism, pneumonia and other infections, congestive heart failure, dementia, and stroke.[56,58] Medications such as sedatives, hypnotics, steroids, antihypertensives, and analgesics also can induce a depressive state. Numerous confounding social problems, such as bereavement, loss of job or income, and loss of social support, can obscure or complicate the diagnosis.[58,59]

The course of depression in older adults is similar to that in younger persons. As many as 40% experience recurrences. Suicide rates are highest among the elderly population. There is a linear increase in suicide with age, most notably among white men older than 60 years of age. Although the exact reasons are unclear, it may be caused by the emotional alienation that can accompany the aging process, combined with complex biopsychosocial losses.[58–60]

Because diagnosis of depression can be difficult, use of a screening tool may help to measure affective functioning objectively. The *Geriatric Depression Scale,* an instrument of known reliability and validity, was developed to

TABLE 3-3 Characteristics That Distinguish Dementia From Pseudodementia of Depression

Dementia	Pseudodementia of Depression
Insidious onset	Rapid onset
Symptoms present for long duration	Symptoms present for relatively short time
Inaccurate in answering orientation questions; attempts to cover up inaccuracies	May show lack of interest in answering questions; frequent "don't know" or "don't care" response
May try to conceal deficits	May tend to emphasize deficits; highlight disabilities
Consistently performs poorly on tasks of similar difficulty	May display marked variability in performing tasks of similar difficulty
Mood and behavior tend to be labile	Mood consistently depressed; may have superimposed agitation or anxiety
May have neurologic symptoms of dysphasia, apraxia, or agnosia	Neurologic symptoms not present

measure depression specifically in the noninstitutionalized older adult population. The 30-item dichotomous scale elicits information on topics relevant to symptoms of depression among older adults, such as memory loss and anxiety.[61] Many other screening tools, each with its own advantages and disadvantages, exist to evaluate the older adult's level of psychological functioning, in its entirety or as specific, separate components of function.

Treatment goals for older adults with depression are to decrease the symptoms of depression, improve the quality of life, reduce the risk for recurrences, improve health status, decrease health care costs, and decrease mortality. Pharmacotherapy (*i.e.*, use of antidepressants) is an effective treatment approach for the depressed older adult. The selection of a particular medication depends on a variety of factors, such as a prior positive or negative response, history of first-degree relatives responding to medication, concurrent medical illnesses that may interfere with medication use, concomitant use of nonpsychotropic medications that may alter the metabolism or increase the side-effect profile, likelihood of adherence, patient preference, and cost.

Selective serotonin reuptake inhibitors (SSRIs), a class of antidepressants (*e.g.*, sertraline, paroxetine, escitalopram), provide high specificity by blocking or slowing serotonin reuptake without the antagonism of neurotransmitter receptors or direct cardiac effects. Because of this, they are an attractive first choice for pharmacotherapy. Dosing is usually once per day, creating ease of administration. They also are less lethal in overdose than other types of antidepressants, such as the tricyclics, an important consideration because of the high suicide rate among older adults. The anticholinergic and cardiovascular side effects that can be problematic with tricyclic antidepressants (*e.g.*, nortriptyline, desipramine, amitriptyline) are minimal with SSRIs. Regardless of the classification, psychotropic medications should be given in low doses initially and gradually titrated according to response and side effects. Response to antidepressants usually requires 4 to 6 weeks at therapeutic dose levels. For a single episode of major depression, drug therapy usually should continue for a minimum of 6 months to 1 year, and 2 to 5 years for recurrent depression, to prevent relapse.[56,58,59]

Electroconvulsive therapy (ECT) may be the treatment of choice for older adults with severe, pharmacologically resistant major depressive episodes. Studies indicate that individuals older than 60 years of age are the largest group of patients who receive ECT. Despite the negative publicity that has been associated with ECT, the evidence for its efficacy in the treatment of depression is strong. Unfortunately, relapse after ECT is common, and alternative treatment strategies, including maintenance ECT or maintenance antidepressants after ECT, are being used.[62]

"Talking therapy," such as supportive counseling or psychotherapy, is considered to be an important part of the treatment regimen, alone or in combination with pharmacotherapy or ECT. Alterations in life roles, lack of social support, and chronic medical illnesses are just a few examples of life event changes that may require psychosocial support and new coping skills. Counseling in the older adult population requires special considerations. Individuals with significant vision, hearing, or cognitive impairments may require special approaches. Many elderly persons do not see themselves as depressed and reject referrals to mental health professionals. Special efforts are needed to engage these individuals in treatment. Family therapy can be beneficial as a way to help the family understand more about depression and its complexities and as an important source of support for the older adult. Although depression can impose great risks for older adults, it is thought to be the most treatable psychiatric disorder in late life and therefore warrants aggressive case finding and intervention.

DEMENTIA

Dementia is a complex and devastating problem that is a major cause of disability in the older adult population. Although the actual prevalence of dementia is unknown, estimates range from 2.5% to 24.6% of those older than 65 years of age, with the number increasing with advanced age. In long-term care facilities, up to 70% of residents have cognitive impairments.[63,64]

Although there can be a decline in intellectual function with aging, dementia, sometimes called *senility,* is not a normal aging process. Dementia is a syndrome of acquired, persistent impairment in several domains of intellectual function, including memory, language, visuospatial ability, and cognition (*i.e.,* abstraction, calculation, judgment, and problem solving). Mood disturbances and changes in personality and behavior often accompany the intellectual deterioration.[57]

Dementia can result from a wide variety of conditions, including degenerative, vascular, neoplastic, demyelinating, infectious, inflammatory, toxic, metabolic, and psychiatric disorders. Up to 70% of older adults with dementia (5 million Americans) are thought to have Alzheimer's disease, a chronic, progressive neurologic disorder of unknown cause.[63] Multi-infarct dementia is the second most common disorder, with 10% to 20% of dementias attributed to this vascular disorder in which multiple emboli disseminate throughout the brain, causing infarctions.[57,65,67]

Much work is being done in the diagnosis and treatment of dementia, in particular of Alzheimer's disease. Amyloid plaques and neurofibrillary tangles are the hallmarks of the disease pathology. Recent research has identified enzymes called secretases, which are believed to play a role in the formation of the amyloid plaques. Studies are also investigating abnormal tau proteins that form the tangles involved in Alzheimer's disease. One of the more recent genetic findings was the discovery of apolipoprotein E alleles (apoE2, apoE3, and apoE4) on chromosome 19. Apolipoprotein E is a normal protein that helps transport blood cholesterol. It is thought that apoE2 is protective against Alzheimer's disease, apoE3 (the most common apoE allele found in the general population) plays a neutral role, and apoE4 increases the risk for developing late-onset Alzheimer's disease. The precise mechanism in not yet known.[65,66,68] Although advancements in research continue, as yet there are no specific diagnostic tests to determine the presence of Alzheimer's disease, and the diagnosis is made by excluding other possible causes of the dementia symptoms.

A commonly used measure of cognitive function is the Mini-Mental State Examination (MMSE) developed by Folstein and colleagues in 1975.[69] This tool provides a brief, objective measure of cognitive functioning and has been widely used. The MMSE, which can be administered in 5 to 10 minutes, consists of a variety of questions that cover memory, orientation, attention, and constructional abilities. The test has been studied and found to fulfill its original goal of providing a brief screening tool that quantifies cognitive impairments and documents cognitive changes over time. However, it has been cautioned that this examination should not be used by itself as a diagnostic tool to identify dementia.

Several medications have become available over the past decade to help halt further cognitive decline in Alzheimer's disease. Emphasis has been on increasing cholinergic synaptic transmission in areas of the brain that are concerned with memory and cognition. Drugs that inhibit the breakdown of acetylcholine at the synaptic cleft have been developed and have been shown to be effective in slowing the progression of the disease in some persons. At present, four drugs—tacrine, donepezil, rivastigmine, and galantamine—are available in the therapeutic category of cognitive-enhancing agents, although tacrine is no longer marketed in the United States. All four medications are acetylcholinesterase inhibitors whose action elevates acetylcholine concentrations in the cerebral cortex by slowing degradation of acetylcholine released by still-intact neurons. The magnitude of the cognitive-enhancing effects of tacrine, the first-released drug in this category, have been modest and associated with significant side effects that generally preclude its use. Donepezil has been shown to be a more potent, specific inhibitor of acetylcholinesterase with minimal side effects.[70] The newer agents, rivastigmine and galantamine, are thought to be more selective in the binding and inactivation of acetylcholinesterase; however, adverse reactions, especially gastrointestinal symptoms, can impede therapeutic dosing. Although there still is no cure for dementia, cholinesterase inhibitors are considered efficacious as antidementia drugs on the basis of improvements seen on standardized cognitive tests, as well as slower decline in loss of function due to the disease process. Evidence suggest that the cognitive-enhancing drugs are also beneficial in individuals with vascular dementia.[71] Antiglutamatergic treatment is currently under investigation for use in moderate-to-severe Alzheimer's disease. This novel neurochemical approach assumes that overstimulation of the *N*-methyl-D-aspartate (NMDA) receptor by glutamate is implicated in neurodegenerative disorders. Memantine, an NMDA antagonist, shows promising results—subjects showed less decline in both cognitive and functional abilities while on the drug. Memantine has recently been approved by the U.S. Food and Drug Administration (FDA) for general use.[72]

Among the neuroprotective drugs that are proposed to delay the onset or progression of Alzheimer's disease are extracts of *Ginkgo biloba,* vitamin E, nonsteroidal anti-inflammatory drugs (NSAIDs), and calcium channel blockers. Extracts of *Ginkgo biloba,* derived from the leaf of a subtropical tree, are available in health food stores. The compounds, which supposedly have antioxidant, neurotrophic, and anti-inflammatory properties, are promoted as a remedy for memory problems in persons with Alzheimer's disease.[73] A metaanalysis of five studies that examined the efficacy of the compound on cognition concluded that *Ginkgo biloba* extract improves cognition slightly.[74] The pathology of Alzheimer's disease may involve oxidative stress and the accumulation of free radicals, leading to neuronal degeneration in the brain. Vitamin E, a fat-soluble vitamin, interacts with cell membranes, traps free radicals, and may interrupt chain reactions that damage cells.[75] In the past, estrogen was felt to have neuroprotective effects for postmenopausal women. More recently, however, multicenter randomized placebo-controlled trials failed to show any improvement associated with the use of estrogen in women who already have Alzheimer's disease.[76] As a result, current evidence does not support the use of estrogen in the treatment of Alzheimer's disease. [77] The NSAIDs are thought to decrease the inflammatory response to inflammatory mediators released from injured or degenerating nerve cells. Calcium channel blockers prevent calcium influx, which is proposed to cause neuronal death due to release of intracellular enzymes. Use of *Ginkgo biloba,* NSAIDs, and calcium channel blockers for Alzheimer's disease is generally not advised; however, most clinicians do advocate the use of vitamin E.

The term mild cognitive impairment (MCI) has been used to denote cognitive impairment with aging that does not meet criteria for dementia and that is not attributed to any known medical condition. Studies suggest, however, that most of those diagnosed with MCI will go on to develop Alzheimer's disease. Treatment approaches are aimed at slowing declining over time and generally include both pharmacologic and behavioral approaches.

Management of older adults with Alzheimer's disease and other dementias usually involves assuming increasing responsibility for and supplying increasing care to individuals as the illness renders them incapable. Impaired judgment and cognition can prevent the older adult from making reasonable decisions and choices and eventually threatens their overall well-being. Family members often assume the monumental task of caring for older adults with dementia until the burden becomes too great, at which time many older adults may be relocated to long-term care facilities.

Some specific behavioral problems commonly are seen in older adults with dementia, including agitation, depression, hallucinations, aggressiveness, and wandering. It may be necessary to use low doses of pharmacologic agents such as neuroleptics, antidepressants, and anxiolytics. Nonpharmacologic interventions can help control behavioral problems and may preclude the need for medications. Ensuring that the individual's physical needs, such as hygiene, bowel and bladder elimination, safety, and nutrition, are met can help prevent catastrophic reactions. Providing a consistent routine in familiar surroundings also helps to alleviate stress. Matching the cognitive needs of the older adult by avoiding understimulation and overstimulation assists in preventing behavior problems.

The work of Hall has shown positive results in the care of older adults with Alzheimer's disease.[77] Hall's conceptual model, progressively lowered stress threshold (PLST), proposes that the demented individual's ability to tolerate any type of stress progressively declines as the disease advances. Interventions for the older adult with dementia therefore center on eliminating and avoiding stressors as a way to prevent dysfunctional behaviors. These stressors include fatigue, change of routine, excessive demands, overwhelming stimuli, and physical stressors. Hall's work with the PLST model has shown that individuals tend to awaken less at night, use less sedatives and hypnotics, eat better, socialize more, function at a higher level, and experience fewer episodes of anxiety, agitation, and other dysfunctional behaviors. Further work has shown that family caregivers trained using the PLST model improved their abilities to provide care to loved ones with dementia and lowered their own stress levels.[78]

DELIRIUM

It is important to differentiate dementia from delirium, also referred to as *acute confusional state*. The demented older adult is far more likely to become delirious. The onset of delirium in the demented individual may be mistaken as an exacerbation of the dementia and consequently not treated.[79,80]

Delirium is an acute disorder developing over a period of hours to days and is seen frequently in hospitalized elderly patients. Prevalence rates range from 14% to 56% of hospitalized older adults and up to 90% of older adults admitted to psychiatric hospitals. Delirium is defined by the DSM-IVR as an organic mental syndrome featuring a global cognitive impairment, disturbances of attention, reduced level of consciousness, increased or decreased psychomotor activity, and a disorganized sleep–wake cycle. The severity of the symptoms tends to fluctuate unpredictably but often is more pronounced at night.[57]

Delirium can be a presenting feature of a physical illness and may be seen with disorders such as myocardial infarction, pneumonia and other infections, cancer, and hypothyroidism. Patients with drug toxicities may present with delirium. Malnutrition, use of physical restraints, and iatrogenic events also can precipitate delirium.

The exact reason that delirium occurs is unclear. It is speculated that the decreased central nervous system capacity in older adults may precipitate delirium. Other possible contributing factors include vision and hearing impairments, psychological stress, and diseases of other organ systems. Delirium has a high mortality rate, ranging between 20% and 40%. Agitation, disorientation, and fearfulness—the key symptoms of delirium—place the individual at high risk for injuries such as a fracture from a fall.[79,80]

Diagnosis of delirium involves recognition of the syndrome and identification of its causes. Management involves treatment of the underlying disease condition and symptomatic relief through supportive therapy, including good nutrition and hydration, rest, comfort measures, and emotional support. Prevention of delirium is the overall goal; avoidance of the devastating and life-threatening acute confusional state is the key to successful management and treatment.[81]

In summary, health care for older adults requires unique considerations, taking into account age-related physiologic changes and specific disease states common in this population. Although aging is not synonymous with disease, the aging process does lend itself to an increased incidence of illness. The overall goal is to assist the older adult in maximizing independence and functional capabilities and minimizing disabilities that can result from various acute and chronic illnesses.

The evaluation of the older adult's functional abilities is a key component in gerontologic health care. Medical diagnoses alone are incomplete without an assessment of function. When evaluating levels of function, determination of the older adult's ability to perform ADL and IADL should be included.

Among the functional disorders that are common in the older population are urinary incontinence, instability and falls, sensory impairment, depression, dementia, and delirium. The older adult is especially prone to urinary incontinence because of changes in the micturition cycle that accompany the aging process. Behavioral techniques can be an effective way to treat incontinence problems in the older adult population. Falls are a common source of concern for the older adult population. Although most falls do not result in serious injury, the potential for serious complications and even death is real. Most falls are the result of several risk factors, including age-related biopsychosocial changes, chronic illness, and situational and environmental hazards. Both hearing and visual impairment, which are common in elderly persons, contribute to communication problems, depression, and social isolation. Depression is a significant but treatable health problem that often is misdiagnosed and mistreated in the older adult population. Dementia is a syndrome of acquired, persistent impairment in several domains of intellectual function, including memory, language, visuospatial ability, and cognition (*i.e.*, abstraction, calculation, judgment, and problem solving). Although there can be a slight decline in intellectual function with aging, dementia is not a normal aging process. Delirium is an acute confusional disorder developing over a period of hours to days and often is seen as a presenting feature of a physical illness or drug toxicity.

Drug Therapy in the Older Adult

After completing this section of the chapter, you should be able to meet the following objectives:

- Characterize drug therapy in the older adult population
- List five factors that contribute to adverse drug reactions in the elderly
- Cite cautions to be used in prescribing medications for elderly persons

Drug therapy in the older adult population is a complex phenomenon influenced by numerous biopsychosocial factors. The elderly population is the largest group of consumers of prescription and over-the-counter drugs. Although the older population comprises only 12.4% of the U.S. population, they consume one third of all prescription drugs and 50% of all over-the-counter medications.[82] The incidence of adverse drug reactions in the elderly is two to three times that found in young adults. This is considered to be a conservative estimate because drug reactions are less well recognized in older adults and reactions often can mimic symptoms of specific disease states.

Errors in the administration of medications and compliance are common among the older adult population, estimated by several authorities to be between 25% and 50% for community-dwelling elderly persons. Reasons for this high volume of errors are numerous. Poor manual dexterity, failing eyesight, lack of understanding about the treatment regimen, attitudes and beliefs about medication use, mistrust of health care providers, and forgetfulness or confusion are but a few factors that can affect the adherence to medication regimens. The role of the health care provider also can contribute to improper medication use. There can be a tendency to treat symptoms with drugs rather than fully investigate the cause of those symptoms. To compound matters, accurate diagnosis of specific disease states can be difficult because older adults tend to underreport symptoms and because presenting symptoms are often atypical.[82,83]

Age-related physiologic changes also account for adverse effects of medications. In general, the absorption of orally ingested drugs remains essentially unchanged with age, even though the gastric pH is known to rise and gastric emptying time can be delayed. Changes in drug distribution, however, are clinically significant. Because lean body mass and total body water decrease with advancing age, water-soluble drugs such as digoxin and propranolol tend to have a smaller volume of distribution, resulting in higher plasma concentrations for a given dose and increased likelihood of a toxic reaction. Conversely, fat-soluble drugs such as diazepam are more widely distributed and accumulate in fatty tissue owing to an increase in adipose tissue with aging. This can cause a delay in elimination and accumulation of the drug over time (*i.e.*, prolonged half-life) with multiple doses of the same drug. Drug metabolism through the liver is thought to be altered owing to the decrease in hepatic blood flow seen in the older adult. Renal excretion controls the elimination of drugs from the body, and because kidney function declines with age, the rate of drug excretion decreases. This can result in an increased half-life of drugs and is why estimates of creatinine clearance are recommended to determine drug dosing.[84,85]

Drug use for older adults warrants a cautious approach. "Start low and go slow" is the adage governing drug prescribing in geriatric pharmacology. Older adults often can achieve therapeutic results on small doses of medications. If necessary, dosing can then be titrated slowly according to response.

Further complicating matters is the issue of polypharmacy in older adults, who often have multiple disorders that may require multiple drug therapies. Polypharmacy increases the risk for drug interactions and adverse drug reactions and decreases compliance. Drugs and disease states also can interact, causing adverse effects. For example, psychotropic drugs administered to older adults with dementia may cause a worsening of confusion; β-blocking agents administered to an individual with chronic obstructive pulmonary disease may induce bronchoconstriction; and nonsteroidal anti-inflammatory medications given to an older adult with hypertension can raise blood pressure further.

The use of certain types of medications carries a high risk for older adults and should be avoided if possible. In general, long-acting drugs or drugs with prolonged half-lives can be problematic. Many sedatives and hypnotics fit into this category, and drugs such as diazepam and flurazepam should be avoided. Other classes of drugs, such as antidepressants and anxiolytics, may provide the necessary symptomatic relief and may be more appropriate for older adults than sedatives and hypnotics. Use of these agents warrants caution, however, with consideration for the unique pharmacokinetic changes that accompany aging. Drugs that possess anticholinergic properties should also be used with caution. Anticholinergics are used for a variety of conditions; however, side effects such as dry mouth and eyes, blurred vision, and constipation are common. These drugs can also cause more serious side effects, such as confusion, urinary retention, and orthostatic hypotension.

Agents that enter the central nervous system, including narcotics and alcohol, can cause a variety of problems, most notably delirium. These problems most likely occur as a result of a decreased central nervous system reserve capacity.[85,86]

Because of the serious implications of medication use in the elderly, strategies need to be used to enhance therapeutic effects and prevent harm. Careful evaluation of the need for the medication by the health care provider is the first step. Once decided, analysis of the individual's current medication regimen and disease states is necessary to prevent drug–drug interactions, drug–disease interactions, and adverse responses. Dosing should be at the low end, and frequency of drug administration should be kept to a minimum to simplify the routine and enhance compliance. Timing the dose to a specific activity of daily living (*e.g.*, "take with breakfast") can also improve compliance, as can special packaging devices such as pill boxes and blister packs. The cost of medications is another important factor for older adults on reduced, fixed incomes. Choosing less expensive products of equal efficacy can increase compliance. The importance of educating the individual about the medication cannot be overemphasized. Health care professionals need to provide verbal and written information on the principles of medication use and on the specific medications being used. This facilitates active, involved participation by the older adult and enhances the individual's ability to make informed decisions.

In summary, drug therapy in the older adult population is a complex phenomenon influenced by numerous biopsychosocial factors. Alterations in pharmacokinetics occur with advancing age and increase the likelihood of toxic reactions. "Start low and go slow" is the adage governing geriatric pharmacology. Centrally acting drugs and drugs with long half-lives should be avoided when possible. Drug–drug interactions, drug–disease interactions, and adverse reactions increase in the elderly population. Educating the older adult about drug use is an important factor in ensuring compliance and accurate medication administration.

REVIEW EXERCISES

It is said that the aging body can accomplish most, if not all, of the functions of its youth; the difference is that they may take longer, require greater motivation, and be less precise.

A. Explain how this concept might contribute to falls in elderly persons.

Nocturia or the need to urinate during the night is a common problem of the elderly.

A. Explain the rationale for this complaint.

Errors and adverse drug reactions are a continual threat for the elderly.

A. Explain common causes of inappropriate medication use in the elderly.

References

1. U.S Census Bureau. The 65 years and older population (2000). [On-line.] Available: www.census.gov/population/www/socdemo/age.html#older.
2. American Association of Retired Persons (2002). A profile of older Americans. [On-line.] Available: www/aarp.org/.
3. Erikson E. (1963). *Childhood and society*. New York: W.W. Norton.
4. Erikson E.H., Erikson J.M., Kivirck H.Q. (1986). *Vital involvement in old age*. New York: W.W. Norton.
5. Troen B.R. (2003). The biology of aging. *Mount Sinai Journal of Medicine 70,* 3–22.
6. Finch C.E., Tanzi R.E. (1997). Genetics of aging. *Science 278,* 407–412.
7. Slagboom P.E., Bastiann T.H., Beekman M., et al. (2000). Genetics of human aging. *Annals of the New York Academy of Science 908,* 50–61.
8. Hayflick L, Moorehead P.S. (1965). The limited in vitro lifetime of human diploid cell strains. *Experimental Cell Research 37,* 614–636.
9. Fossell M. (1998). Telomerase and the aging cell. *Journal of the American Medical Association 279,* 1732–1735.
10. Timiras M.L. (2003). The skin. In Timiras P. (Ed.), *Physiological basis of aging and geriatrics* (3rd ed., pp. 397–404). Boca Raton, FL: CRC Press.
11. Smith E.S., Fleischer AB Jr., Feldman S.R. (2001). Demographics of aging and skin disease. *Clinics in geriatric medicine 17,* 631–641.
12. Taaffe D.R., Marcus R. (2000). Musculoskeletal health and the older adult. *Journal of Rehabilitation Research and Development 37,* 245–254.
13. Timiras P.S. (2003). The skeleton, joints, and skeletal and cardiac muscles In Timiras P.S. (Ed.), *Physiological basis of aging and geriatrics* (3rd ed., pp. 375–395). Boca Raton, FL: CRC Press.
14. Loeser R.F., Delbono O. (2003). Aging of the muscles and joints. In Hazzard W.R., Blass J.P., Halter J.B., et al. (Eds.), *Principles of geriatric medicine and gerontology* (5th ed., pp. 905–918). New York: McGraw-Hill.
15. Lakatta E.G. (1999). Cardiovascular aging research. *Journal of the American Gerontological Society 47,* 613–625.
16. Joint National Committee. (2003). *The seventh report of Joint National Committee on Prevention, Detection, Evaluation, and Treatment of High Blood Pressure*. NIH publication no. 03-5233. Bethesda, MD: National Institutes of Health.
17. Taffet G.E., Lakatta E. (2003). Aging of the cardiovascular system. In Hazzard W.R., Blass J.P., Halter J.B., et al. (Eds.), *Principles of geriatric medicine and gerontology* (5th ed., pp. 403–421). New York: McGraw-Hill.
18. Smith N.L., Psaty B.M., Rutan G.H., et al. (2003). The association between time since last meal and blood pressure in older adults: The cardiovascular health study. *Journal of the American Geriatrics Society 51,* 824–828.
19. Lakatta E.G. (2000). Cardiovascular aging in health. *Clinical Geriatric Medicine 16,* 419–444.
20. Schwartz R.S., Kohrt W.M. (2003). Exercise in elderly people: Physiologic and functional effects. In Hazzard W.R., Blass J.P., Halter J.B. et al. (Eds.), *Principles of geriatric medicine and gerontology* (5th ed., pp. 931–946). New York: McGraw-Hill.
21. Timiras P.S. (2003). The pulmonary respiration, hematopoiesis and erythrocytes. In Timiras P.S. (Ed.), *Physiological basis of aging and geriatrics* (3rd ed., pp. 319–336). Boca Raton, FL: CRC Press.
22. Timiras P.S. (2003). Aging of the nervous system: Structural and biochemical changes. In Timiras P.S. (Ed.), *Physiological basis of aging and geriatrics* (3rd ed., pp. 99–117). Boca Raton, FL: CRC Press.

23. Timiras P.S. (2003). The nervous system: Functional changes. In Timieas P.S. (Ed.), *Physiological basis of aging and geriatrics* (3rd ed., pp. 119–140). Boca Raton, FL: CRC Press.
24. Odenheimer G.L. (1998). Geriatric neurology. *Neurology Clinics 16,* 561–567.
25. Schneck M.E., Haegerstrom-Portnoy G. (2003). Practical assessment of vision in the elderly. *Ophthalmology Clinics of North America 16,* 269–287.
26. Meisani E., Brown C., Emerle H. (2003). Sensory systems: Normal aging, disorder, and treatment of vision and hearing in humans. In Timiras P.S. (Ed.), *Physiological basis of aging and geriatrics* (3rd ed., pp.141–165). Boca Raton, FL: CRC Press.
27. Nusbaum N.J. (1999). Aging and sensory senescence. *Southern Medical Journal 92,* 267–275.
28. Martini A., Mazzoli M., Rosignoli M., et al. (2001). Hearing in the elderly: A population study. *Audiology 40,* 285–293.
29. Mills J.A. (2003). Age-related changes in the auditory system. In Hazzard W.R., Blass J.P., Halter J.B., et al. (Eds.), *Principles of geriatric medicine and gerontology* (5th ed., pp. 1239–1251). New York: McGraw-Hill.
30. Finkelstein J.A., Schiffman S.S. (1999). Workshop on taste and smell in the elderly: An overview. *Physiology and behavior 66,* 173–176.
31. Ginaldi L., Strennberg H. (2003). The immune system. In Timiras P.S. (Ed.), *Physiological basis of aging and geriatrics* (3rd ed., pp. 265–283). Boca Raton, FL: CRC Press.
32. Mouton C.P., Pierce B., Espino D.V. (2001). Common infections in older adults. *American Family Practitioner 63,* 257–268.
33. Soergel K.H., Zboralske F.E., Amberg J.R. (1964). Presbyesophagus: Esophageal motility in nonagenarians. *Journal of Clinical Investigation 43,* 1472–1476.
34. Hall K.E. (2003). Effects of aging on the gastrointestinal function. In Hazzard W.R., Blass J.P., Halter J.B., et al. (Eds.), *Principles of geriatric medicine and gerontology* (5th ed., pp. 593–600). New York: McGraw-Hill.
35. Lindeman R.D. (1998). Renal and electrolyte disorders. In Duthie E.H. Jr., Katz P.R. (Eds.), *Practice in geriatrics* (3rd ed., pp. 546–561). Philadelphia: W.B. Saunders.
36. Wiggins J. (2003). Changes in renal function. In Hazzard W.R., Blass J.P., Halter J.B., et al. (Eds.), *Principles of geriatric medicine and gerontology* (5th ed., pp. 543–549). New York: McGraw-Hill.
37. Smith M. (1998). Gynecological disorders. In Duthie E.H. Jr., Katz P.R. (Eds.), *Practice in geriatrics* (3rd ed., pp. 524–534). Philadelphia: W.B. Saunders.
38. DuBeau C. (2003). Benign prostate disorders. In Hazzard W.R., Blass J.P., Halter J.B., et al. (Eds.), *Principles of geriatric medicine and gerontology* (5th ed., pp. 1303–1310). New York: McGraw-Hill.
39. Weidner W., Altwein J., Hauck E., et al. (2001). Sexuality of the elderly. *Urologia Internationalis 66,* 181–184.
40. Kingsberg S. (2002). The impact of aging on sexual function in women and their partners. *Archives of Sexual Behavior 31,* 431–437.
41. Katz S., Ford A.B., Jackson B.A., Jaffee M.W. (1963). Studies of illness in the aged: The index of ADL. *Journal of the American Medical Association 185,* 914–919.
42. Katz S., Downs T.D., Cash H.R., Grotz R.C. (1970). Progress in development of the Index of ADL. *Gerontologist 10,* 20–30.
43. Fantl J.A., Neuman D.F., Colling J., et al. (1996). *Urinary incontinence in adults: Acute and chronic management.* Clinical practice guideline no. 2, 1996 update. Publication no. 96–06. Rockville, MD: Agency for Health Care Policy and Research.
44. Yee S., Phanumus D., Fields S.D. (2000). Urinary incontinence: A primary care guide to managing acute and chronic symptoms in older adults. *Geriatrics 55*(11), 65–71.
45. Wymann J.F. (2003). Treatment of urinary incontinence in men and older women. In Newman D.K., Palmer M.H. (Eds.), *The state of the science on urinary incontinence. American Journal of Nursing Supplement 3,* 26–35.
46. King M.B. (2003). Falls. In Hazzard W.R., Blass J.P., Halter J.B., et al. (Eds.), *Principles of geriatric medicine and gerontology* (5th ed., pp. 1517–1529). New York: McGraw-Hill.
47. Fuller G.F. (2000). Falls in the elderly. *American Family Practitioner 61,* 2159–2168, 2173–2174.
48. Marks R., Allegrante J., MacKenzie C, Lane J. (2003). Hip fractures among the elderly: Causes, consequences and control. *Ageing Research Reviews 2,* 57–93.
49. Hausdorff J.M., Edelberg H.K., Cudkowicz M.E., et al. (1997). The relationship between gait and falls. *Journal of the American Geriatric Society 45,* 1406.
50. Tennetti M.E., Williams C.S., Gill T.M. (2000). Dizziness among older adults: A possible geriatric syndrome. *Annals of Internal Medicine 132,* 337–344.
51. Keller B.K., Morton J.L., Thomas V.S., Potter J.F. (1999). The effect of visual and hearing impairment on functional status. *Journal of the American Gerontological Society 47,* 1319–1325.
52. Reuben D.B., Mui S., Damesyn M., et al. (1999). The prognostic value of sensory impairment in older persons. *Journal of the American Gerontological Society 47,* 930–935.
53. Mojica T.R., Baily P.P. (2000). Hallucinations in the vision-impaired elderly: The Charles Bonnet Syndrome. *Nurse Practitioner 25*(8), 74–76.
54. Teunisse R.J., Cruysberg J.R., Hoefnagels W.H., et al. (1996). Visual hallucinations in psychologically normal people: Charles Bonnet's syndrome. *Lancet 347,* 794–797.
55. Almedia O.P., Howard R.J., Levy R. (1995). Psychotic states arising in late life (late paraphrenia): The role of risk factors. *British Journal of Psychiatry 166,* 215–228.
56. NIH Consensus Development Panel. (1995). Diagnosis and treatment of depression in late life. *Journal of the American Medical Association 268,* 1018–1024.
57. American Psychiatric Association. (1994). *Diagnostic and statistical manual of mental disorders* (4th ed., rev.). Washington, DC: Author.
58. Pollock B.G., Reynolds C.F. 3rd (2000). Depression late in life. *Harvard Mental Health Letter 17*(3), 3–5.
59. Depression Guideline Panel. (1993). *Depression in primary care: Treatment of major depression* (Vol. 2). Clinical practice guideline no. 5, 1993. Publication no. 93-0551. Rockville, MD: Agency for Health Care Policy and Research.
60. Bharucha A.J., Satlin A. (1997). Late life suicide: A review. *Harvard Review of Psychiatry 5*(2), 55–65.
61. Yesavage J.A., Brink T.L., Rose T.L., et al. (1983). Development and validation of a geriatric depression scale: A preliminary report. *Journal of Psychiatric Research 17,* 37–49.
62. Kelly K.G., Zisselman M. (2000). Update on electroconvulsive therapy (ECT) in older adults. *Journal of the American Geriatric Society 48,* 560–566.
63. Clark C.M., Karlawish J.H.T. (2003). Alzheimer's disease: Current concepts and emerging diagnostic and therapeutic strategies. *Annals of Internal Medicine 138,* 400–410.
64. Karlawish J.H.T., Clark C.M. (2003). Diagnostic evaluation of elderly patients with mild memory problems. *Annals of Internal Medicine 138,* 411–419.
65. Portfolio for progress: The aging mind: Alzheimer's disease and normal aging (2003). National Institutes on Aging. [On-line.] Available: http://www.nia.nih.gov/health/pubs/portfolio/html/mind.htm.
66. Garand L., Hall G.R. (2000). The biological basis of behavioral symptoms in dementia. *Issues in Mental Health Nursing 21,* 91–107.

67. Loeb C., Meyer J.S. (2000). Criteria for diagnosis of vascular dementia. *Archives of Neurology* 67, 615–618.
68. Beck C., Cody M., Souder E., et al. (2000). Dementia diagnostic guidelines: Methodologies, results, implementation costs. *Journal of the American Geriatric Society 48,* 1195–1203.
69. Folstein M.F., Folstein B.E., McHugh P.R. (1975). "Mini-Mental State": A practical method for grading the cognitive state of patients for the clinician. *Journal of Psychiatric Research 12,* 189–198.
70. Feldman H., Gauthier S., Hecker J., et al. (2003). Efficacy of donepezil on maintenance of activities of daily loving in patients with moderate to severe Alzheimer's disease and the effect on caregiver burden. *Journal of the American Geriatrics Society 51,* 737–744.
71. Pratt R.D., Perdomo C.A. (2002). Donepezil-treated patients with probable vascular dementia demonstrate cognitive benefits. *Annals of the New York Academy of Sciences 977,* 513–522.
72. Reisberg B., Doody R., Stoffler A., et al. (2003). Memantine in moderate-to-severe Alzheimer's disease. *New England Journal of Medicine 348,* 1333–1341.
73. LeBars P.L., Katz M.M., Berman N., et al. (1997). A placebo-controlled, double-blind, randomized trial of *Ginkgo biloba* for dementia. *Journal of the American Medical Association 278,* 1327–1332.
74. Oken B.S., Storzbach D.M., Kaye J.A. (1998). The efficacy of *Ginkgo biloba* on cognitive function in Alzheimer's disease. *Archives of Neurology 55,* 1409–1415.
75. Sono M., Ernesto M.S., Thomas R.G., et al. (1997). A controlled trial of selegiline, alpha-tocopherol, or both as treatment for Alzheimer's disease. *New England Journal of Medicine 336,* 1216–1222.
76. Writing Group for the Women's Health Initiative Investigators (2002). Risks and benefits of estrogen plus progestin in healthy postmenopausal women. *Journal of the American Medical Association 288,* 321–333.
77. Hall G.R., LaBudakis D. (1999). A behavioral approach to Alzheimer's disease. The progressively lowered stress threshold model. *Advanced Nurse Practitioner 7*(7), 39–41, 81.
78. Stolley J.M., Reed D., Buckwalter K.C. (2002). Caregiver appraisal and intervention based on the progressively lowered stress threshold model. *American Journal of Alzheimer's Disease and Other Dementias 17,* 110–120.
79. O'Keefe S.T. (1999). Delirium in the elderly. *Age and Aging 28*(Suppl. 2): 5–8.
80. Wakefield B.J. (2002). Risk for acute confusion in hospital admissions. *Clinical Nursing Research 11,* 153–172.
81. Inouye S.K., Bogarous S.T., Charpentier P.A., et al. (1999). A multicomponent intervention to prevent delirium in hospitalized older patients. *New England Journal of Medicine 340,* 669–676.
82. William C.M. (2002). Using medications appropriately in older adults. *American Family Physician 66,* 1917–1924.
83. Aparasu R.R., Mort J.R. (2000). Inappropriate prescribing for the elderly: Peers criteria-based review. *Annals of Pharmacology 34,* 338–346.
84. Timiras M.L., Luxenberg J. (2003). Pharmacology and drug management in the elderly. In Timiras P. (Ed.), *Physiological basis of aging and geriatrics* (3rd ed., pp. 407–414). Boca Raton, FL: CRC Press.
85. Beyth R.J., Shorr R.I. (2002). Principles of drug therapy in older patients: Rational drug prescribing. *Clinics in Geriatric Medicine 18,* 577–592.
86. Katzung B.G. (2001). Special aspects of geriatric pharmacology. In Katzung B.G. (Ed.), *Basic and Clinical Pharmacology* (8th ed., pp. 1036–1044). New York: Lange Medical Books/ McGraw-Hill.

UNIT II

Cell Function and Growth

With its elegant structure and astonishing range of functions, the living cell is an object of wonder. It is the basic unit of all living organisms. There are more than 300 trillion cells in the human body, and every second of every day, more than 10 million die and are replaced.

In 1665, these impressive structures were named. While examining a thin slice of cork, Robert Hooke (1635–1703), an English scientist and pioneer microscopist, noted that it was made up of tiny boxlike units. The units reminded him of the small enclosures in which monks lived, and he named the microscopic spaces "cells," from the Latin word cells, meaning "small enclosures."

Although Hooke, as well as other scientists, intently studied microscopic life, few guessed the significance of the cells. That would be delayed until microscopes were advanced enough to yield more detailed information. It was with the work of Anton van Leeuwenhoek (1632–1723), a Dutch biologist and microscopist, that the mysteries and importance of the cell were revealed. He ground a single lens to such perfection that he was able to produce a microscope with great resolving power—one that was capable of magnifying a specimen from approximately 50 to 300 times in diameter. Van Leeuwenhoek's work, which included constructing an aquatic microscope that he used to study red blood cells and their flow through the body, was responsible for helping scientists investigate human tissue in ways that once they only dreamed of.

CHAPTER

4

Cell and Tissue Characteristics

Edward W. Carroll

In most organisms, the *cell* is the smallest functional unit that can retain the characteristics necessary for life. Cells are organized into larger functional units called *tissues* based on their embryonic origin. These tissues combine to form the various body structures and organs. Although the cells of different tissues and organs vary in structure and function, certain characteristics are common to all cells. Cells are remarkably similar in their ability to exchange materials with their immediate environment, obtaining energy from organic nutrients, synthesizing complex molecules, and replicating themselves. Because most disease processes are initiated at the cellular level, an understanding of cell function is crucial to understanding the disease process. Some diseases affect the cells of a single organ, others affect the cells of a particular tissue type, and still others affect the cells of the entire organism. This chapter discusses the structural and functional components of the cell, integration of cell function and growth, movement of molecules such as ions across the cell membrane and membrane potentials, and tissue types.

Functional Components of the Cell

After you have completed this section of the chapter, you should be able to meet the following objectives:

- ✦ List the major components of the cell protoplasm
- ✦ State why the nucleus is called the "control center" of the cell

- ✦ Explain the relationships among DNA, genes, and chromosomes
- ✦ Name the three types of RNA and describe their role in protein synthesis
- ✦ List the cellular organelles and state their functions
- ✦ State four functions of the cell membrane

Although diverse in their organization, all eukaryotic cells have in common structures that perform unique functions. When seen under a light microscope, three major components of the cell become evident: the nucleus, the cytoplasm, and the cell membrane (Fig. 4-1).

PROTOPLASM

Biologists call the internal matrix of the cell *protoplasm.* Protoplasm is composed of water, proteins, lipids, carbohydrates, and electrolytes. Two distinct regions of protoplasm exist in the cell: the *cytoplasm,* which lies outside the nucleus, and the *karyoplasm* or *nucleoplasm,* which lies inside the nucleus.

Water makes up 70% to 85% of the cell's protoplasm. The second most abundant constituents (10% to 20%) of protoplasm are the cell proteins, which form cell structures and the enzymes necessary for cellular reactions. Proteins can be bound to other compounds to form nucleoproteins, glycoproteins, and lipoproteins. Lipids comprise 2% to 3% of most cells. The most important lipids are the phospholipids and cholesterol, which are mainly insoluble in water; they combine with proteins to form the cell membrane and the membranous barriers that separate different cell compartments. Some cells also contain large quantities of triglycerides. In the fat cells, triglycerides can compose up to 95% of the total cell mass. This fat represents stored energy, which can be mobilized and used wherever it is needed in the body. Only a few carbohydrates are found in the cell, and these serve primarily as a rapid source of energy. Potassium, magnesium, phosphate, sulfate, and bicarbonate are the major intracellular electrolytes. Small quantities of sodium, chloride, and calcium ions are also present in the cell. These electrolytes help in the generation and transmission of electrochemical impulses in nerve and muscle cells. Intracellular electrolytes participate in reactions that are necessary for the cell's metabolism.

THE NUCLEUS

The nucleus of the cell appears as a rounded or elongated structure situated near the center of the cell (see Fig. 4-1). The nucleus, which is enclosed by the nuclear envelope (membrane), contains genetic material known as chromatin and a distinct region called the *nucleolus.* All eukaryotic cells

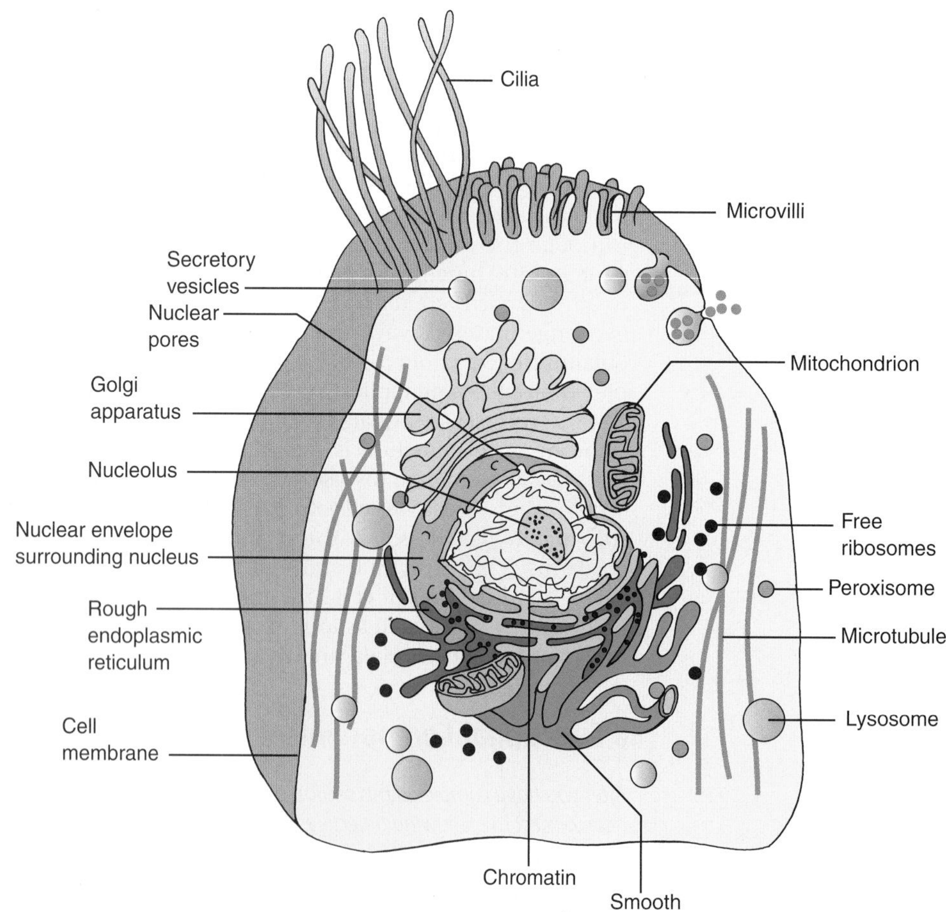

FIGURE 4-1 Composite cell designed to show in one cell all of the various components of the nucleus and cytoplasm.

THE FUNCTIONAL ORGANIZATION OF THE CELL

- Cells are the smallest functional unit of the body. They contain structures that are strikingly similar to those needed to maintain total body function.
- The nucleus is the control center for the cell. It also contains most of the hereditary material.
- The organelles, which are analogous to the organs of the body, are contained in the cytoplasm. They include the mitochondria, which supply the energy needs of the cell; the ribosomes, which synthesize proteins and other materials needed for cell function; and the lysosomes and proteosomes, which function as the cell's digestive system.
- The cell membrane encloses the cell and provides for intracellular and intercellular communication, transport of materials into and out of the cell, and maintenance of the electrical activities that power cell function.

have at least one nucleus (prokaryotic cells, such as bacteria, lack a nucleus and nuclear membrane). Some cells contain more than one nucleus; osteoclasts (a type of bone cell) typically contain 12 or more. The platelet-producing cell, the megakaryocyte, has only one nucleus but usually contains 16 times the normal chromatin amount.

The nucleus is the control center for the cell. It contains deoxyribonucleic acid (DNA) that is essential to the cell because its genes contain the information necessary for the synthesis of proteins that the cell must produce to stay alive. These proteins include structural proteins and enzymes used to synthesize other substances, including carbohydrates and lipids. Genes also represent the individual units of inheritance that transmit information from one generation to another. The nucleus is also the site of ribonucleic acid (RNA) synthesis. Three types of RNA exist in the cell: messenger RNA (mRNA), which copies and carries the DNA instructions for protein synthesis to the cytoplasm; ribosomal RNA (rRNA), which moves to the cytoplasm, where it becomes the site of protein synthesis; and transfer RNA (tRNA), which also moves into the cytoplasm, where it transports amino acids to the elongating protein being synthesized (see Chapter 6).

Chromatin is the term used to describe the complex structure of DNA and DNA-associated proteins dispersed in the nuclear matrix. Two extremely long, double-stranded helical chains containing variable sequences of four nitrogenous bases comprise each DNA molecule. These bases form the genetic code. Each double-stranded DNA molecule periodically coils around basic proteins called *histones,* forming regularly spaced spherical structures called *nucleosomes* that resemble beads on a string (Fig. 4-2). This string of beads further winds into filaments that make up the structure of chromatin. Additional coiling produces structures known as *chromosomes,* which are visible during cell division.

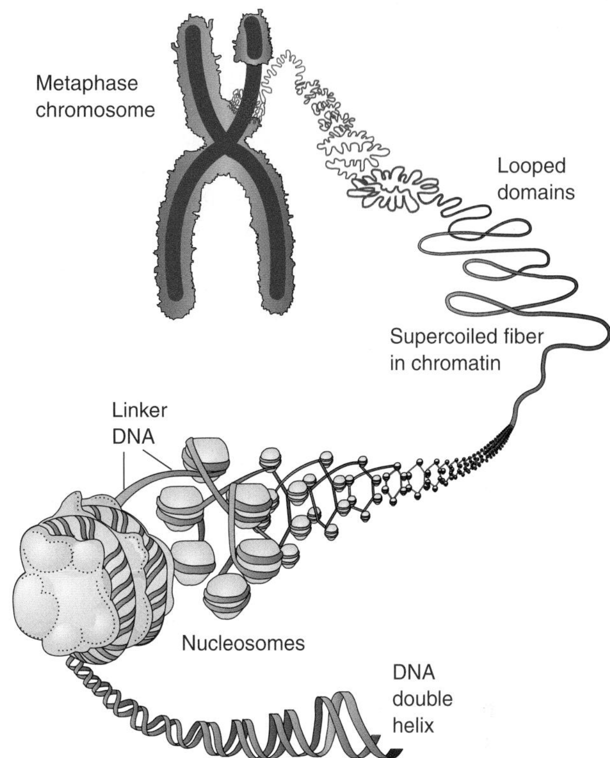

FIGURE 4-2 Increasing orders of DNA compaction in chromatin and mitotic chromosomes. (From Cormack D.H. [1993]. *Essential histology.* Philadelphia: J.B. Lippincott)

Although each DNA molecule contains many genetic instructions, it also contains additional material. Stretches of meaningless DNA can lie between one gene and the next and sometimes reside within the gene sequence itself. The amino acid sequences of the gene interpreted are the *exon,* whereas *introns* are the interspersed, meaningless portions. In cells that are about to divide, the DNA must be replicated before mitosis or cell division occurs. Replication generates two complementary DNA strands, such that each daughter cell receives an identical set of genes.

Chromosome condensation occurs during mitosis, a process rendering the chromosomes visible under the microscope; at other times during the cell cycle, they are not observable. In the mature or nondividing cell, chromatin may exist in a less active, condensed form called *heterochromatin* or a transcriptionally more active form called *euchromatin.* Because heterochromatic regions of the nucleus stain more intensely than regions consisting of euchromatin, nuclear staining can be a guide to cell activity. A nucleus containing primarily euchromatin stains less intense.

The nucleus also contains the darkly stained round body called the *nucleolus.* Although nucleoli were first described in 1781, their function was unknown until the early 1960s: it was determined that transcription of RNA occurs exclusively in the nucleolus. Nucleoli are structures composed of regions from five different chromosomes, each with a part of the genetic code needed for the synthesis of rRNA. Euchromatic nuclei and prominent nucleoli are characteristic of cells that are actively synthesizing proteins.

Surrounding the nucleus is a doubled membrane called the *nuclear envelope* or *nuclear membrane.* The nuclear membrane contains many structurally complex circular pores where the two membranes fuse to form a gap filled with a thin protein diaphragm. Evidence suggests that many classes of molecules, including fluids, electrolytes, RNA, some proteins, and perhaps some hormones, can move in both directions through the nuclear pores. Nuclear pores apparently regulate the exchange of molecules between the cytoplasm and the nucleus.

THE CYTOPLASM AND ITS ORGANELLES

The cytoplasm surrounds the nucleus, and it is in the cytoplasm that the work of the cell takes place. Cytoplasm is essentially a colloidal solution that contains water, electrolytes, suspended proteins, neutral fats, and glycogen molecules. Although they do not contribute to the cell's function, pigments may also accumulate in the cytoplasm. Some pigments, such as melanin, which gives skin its color, are normal constituents of the cell. Bilirubin is a normal major pigment of bile; however, excess accumulation of bilirubin within cells is abnormal. This is evidenced clinically by a yellowish discoloration of the skin and sclera, a condition called *jaundice.*

Embedded in the cytoplasm are various *organelles,* which function as the organs of the cell. These organelles include the ribosomes, endoplasmic reticulum (ER), Golgi complex, mitochondria, lysosomes, microtubules, filaments, peroxisomes, and centrioles.

Ribosomes

The ribosomes serve as sites of protein synthesis in the cell. They are small particles of nucleoproteins (rRNA and proteins) that can be found attached to the wall of the ER or as free ribosomes (Fig. 4-3). Scattered in the cytoplasm individually or joined by strands of mRNA are the functional units called *polyribosomes.* Free ribosomes are involved in the synthesis of proteins, mainly enzymes that aid in the control of cell function.

Endoplasmic Reticulum

The ER is an extensive system of paired membranes and flat vesicles that connects various parts of the inner cell (see Fig. 4-3). Between the paired ER membranes is a fluid-filled space called the *matrix.* The matrix connects the space between the two membranes of the double-layered nuclear membrane, the cell membrane, and various cytoplasmic organelles. It functions as a tubular communication system transporting various substances from one part of the cell to another. A large surface area and multiple enzyme systems attached to the ER membranes also provide the machinery for a major share of the metabolic functions of the cell.

Two forms of ER exist in cells: rough and smooth. Rough ER is studded with ribosomes attached to specific binding sites on the membrane. Ribosomes, with their accompanying strand of mRNA, synthesize proteins. Proteins produced by the rough ER are usually destined for incorporation into cell membranes and lysosomal enzymes

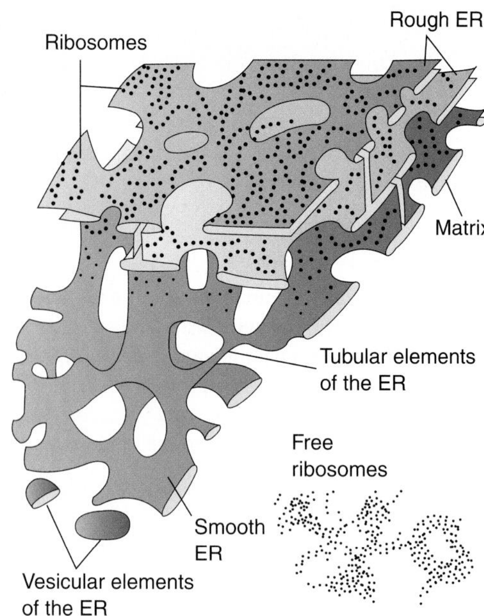

FIGURE 4-3 Three-dimensional view of the rough endoplasmic reticulum (ER) with its attached ribosomal RNA and the smooth endoplasmic reticulum.

or for exportation from the cell. The rough ER segregates these proteins from other components of the cytoplasm and modifies their structure for a specific function. For example, the synthesis of both digestive enzymes by pancreatic acinar cells and plasma proteins by liver cells takes place in the rough ER. All cells require a rough ER for the synthesis of lysosomal enzymes.

The smooth ER is free of ribosomes and is continuous with the rough ER. It does not participate in protein synthesis; instead, its enzymes are involved in the synthesis of lipid molecules, regulation of intracellular calcium, and metabolism and detoxification of certain hormones and drugs. It is the site of lipid, lipoprotein, and steroid hormone synthesis. The sarcoplasmic reticulum of skeletal and cardiac muscle cells is a form of smooth ER. Calcium ions needed for muscle contraction are stored and released from cisternae of the sarcoplasmic reticulum. Smooth ER of the liver is involved in glycogen storage and metabolism of lipid-soluble drugs.

Golgi Complex

The Golgi apparatus, sometimes called the *Golgi complex,* consists of stacks of thin, flattened vesicles or sacs. These Golgi bodies are found near the nucleus and function in association with the ER. By way of transfer vesicles, the Golgi complex receives the small membrane-covered materials produced in the ER. Many cells synthesize proteins that are larger than the active product. As an example, the Golgi complex of the beta cells of the pancreas cuts apart proinsulin, the inactive form of insulin, into the smaller active form. The Golgi complex modifies these substances and packages them into secretory granules or vesicles. These secretory vesicles contain enzymes destined for export from the cell. After appropriate signals, secretory vesicles move out of the Golgi complex into the cytoplasm, fuse to the inner side of the plasma membrane, and release their contents into the extracellular fluid. Figure 4-4 is a diagram of the synthesis and movement of a hormone through the rough ER and Golgi complex. In addition, the Golgi may produce large carbohydrate molecules that combine with proteins produced by the rough ER to form glycoproteins.

Lysosomes and Peroxisomes

Physiologists often view lysosomes as the digestive system of the cell. These small, membrane-enclosed sacs contain powerful hydrolytic enzymes. These enzymes can break down and recycle worn-out cell parts. They also break down foreign substances such as bacteria taken into the cell. All of the lysosomal enzymes are acid hydrolases, which means that they require an acid environment. The lysosomes provide this environment by maintaining a pH of approximately 5 in their interior. The pH of the cytoplasm, which is approximately 7.2, serves to protect other cellular structures from this acidity. Like many other organelles, lysosomes have a unique surrounding membrane that can be pinched off to form vesicles that transport materials throughout the cytoplasm.

Synthesis of lysosomal enzymes occurs in the rough ER. After transport to and uptake by the Golgi apparatus, the Golgi biochemically modifies and packages these materials as lysosomes. Unlike other organelles, the sizes and functions of lysosomes vary considerably. This diversity is determined by the type of enzyme packaged in the lysosome by the Golgi complex. *Primary lysosomes* contain hydrolytic enzymes that have not yet entered the digestive process. They become *secondary lysosomes* after activation of their enzymes has occurred and the chemical degradation process has begun. Primary lysosomes can form secondary lysosomes in one of two ways: heterophagy or autophagy (Fig. 4-5). *Heterophagocytosis* refers to the uptake of material from outside the cell. An infolding of the cell membrane takes external materials into the cell to form a surrounding phagocytic vesicle or *phagosome*. Primary lysosomes then fuse with phagosomes to form secondary lysosomes. Heterophagocytosis is most common in phagocytic white blood cells such as neutrophils and macrophages. *Autophagocytosis* involves the removal of damaged cellular organelles, such as mitochondria or ER, which the lysosomes must remove if the cell's normal function is to continue. Autophagocytosis is most pronounced in cells undergoing atrophy.

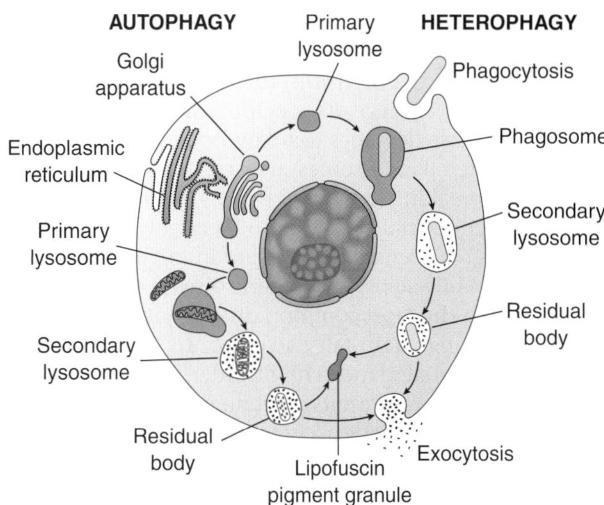

FIGURE 4-5 The process of autophagy and heterophagy, showing the primary and secondary lysosomes, residual bodies, extrusion of residual body contents from the cell, and lipofuscin-containing residual bodies.

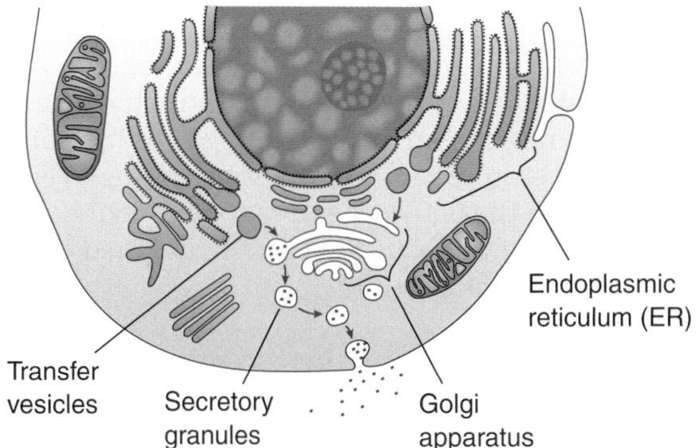

FIGURE 4-4 Hormone synthesis and secretion. In hormone secretion, the hormone is synthesized by the ribosomes attached to the rough endoplasmic reticulum. It moves from the rough ER to the Golgi complex, where it is stored in the form of secretory granules. These leave the Golgi complex and are stored within the cytoplasm until released from the cell in response to an appropriate signal.

Although enzymes in the secondary lysosomes can break down most proteins, carbohydrates, and lipids to their basic constituents, some materials remain undigested. These undigested materials may remain in the cytoplasm as *residual bodies* or are extruded from the cell by exocytosis. In some long-lived cells, such as neurons and heart muscle cells, large quantities of residual bodies accumulate as lipofuscin granules or age pigment. Other indigestible pigments, such as inhaled carbon particles and tattoo pigments, also accumulate and may persist in residual bodies for decades.

Lysosomes play an important role in the normal metabolism of certain substances in the body. In some inherited diseases known as *lysosomal storage diseases,* a specific lysosomal enzyme is absent or inactive, in which case the digestion of certain cellular substances (*e.g.,* glucocerebrosides, gangliosides, sphingomyelin) does not occur. As a result, these substances accumulate in the cell. In Tay-Sachs disease, an autosomal recessive disorder, hexosaminidase A, which is the lysosomal enzyme needed for degrading the GM_2 ganglioside found in nerve cell membranes, is deficient. Although GM_2 ganglioside accumulates in many tissues, such as the heart, liver, and spleen, its accumulation in the nervous system and retina of the eye causes the most damage (see Chapter 7).

Smaller than lysosomes, spherical membrane-bound organelles called *peroxisomes* contain a special enzyme that degrades peroxides (*e.g.,* hydrogen peroxide). Peroxisomes function in the control of free radicals (see Chapter 5). Unless degraded, these highly unstable chemical compounds would otherwise damage other cytoplasmic molecules. For example, catalase degrades toxic hydrogen peroxide molecules to water. Peroxisomes also contain the enzymes needed for breaking down very-long-chain fatty acids, which mitochondrial enzymes ineffectively degrade. In liver cells, peroxisomal enzymes are involved in the formation of the bile acids. In a genetic disease called *adrenoleukodystrophy,* the most common disorder of peroxisomes, a buildup of long-chain fatty acids occurs in the nervous system and adrenal gland. The disorder, which is rapidly progressive and fatal, results in dementia and adrenal insufficiency because of the accumulation of the fatty acids.

Proteasomes

Three major cellular mechanisms are involved in the breakdown of proteins (*proteolysis*). One of these is by the previously mentioned endosomal-lysosomal degradation. Another cytoplasmic degradation mechanism is the *caspase pathway* that that is involved in apoptotic cell death (see Chapter 5). The third method of *proteolysis* occurs within an organelle called the *proteasome.* Proteasomes are quite large (approximately 2000 kd) and are thought to be present in the nucleus and the cytoplasm. This organelle recognizes misformed and misfolded proteins that are destined for degradation, including transcription factors and the cyclins that are important in controlling the cell cycle. It has been suggested that as many as one third of the newly formed polypeptide chains are selected for proteasome degradation due to quality control mechanisms within the cell.

Mitochondria

The mitochondria are literally the "power plants" of the cell because they transform organic compounds into energy that is easily accessible to the cell. Mitochondria do not make energy, but they extract it from organic compounds. Mitochondria contain the enzymes needed for capturing most of the energy in foodstuffs and converting it into cellular energy. Generally, this multistep process is called *cellular respiration* because it requires oxygen. Cells store most of this energy as high-energy phosphate bonds found in compounds such as adenosine triphosphate (ATP), which powers the various cellular activities. Energy that is not used or stored is dissipated as heat used to maintain body temperature.

Mitochondria are found close to the site of energy consumption in the cell (*e.g.,* near the myofibrils in muscle cells). The number of mitochondria in a given cell type varies by the type of activity the cell performs and the energy needed to undertake this activity. For example, a dramatic increase in mitochondria occurs in skeletal muscle repeatedly stimulated to contract.

Mitochondria are composed of two membranes: an outer membrane that encloses the periphery of the mitochondrion and an inner membrane, which forms shelf-like projections, called *cristae* (Fig. 4-6). The outer and inner membranes form two spaces. An outer space is found between the two membranes. Deep to the outer space, the inner or *matrix space* contains an amorphous matrix. The outer mitochondrial membrane is involved in lipid synthesis and fatty acid metabolism, whereas the inner membrane contains the respiratory chain enzymes and transport proteins needed for the synthesis of ATP.

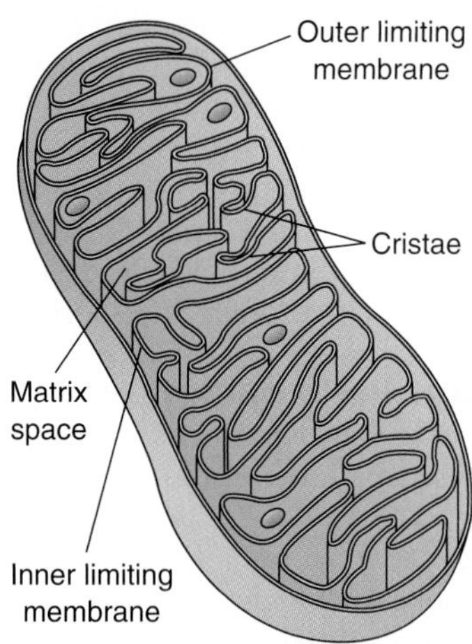

FIGURE 4-6 Mitochondrion. The inner membrane forms transverse folds called cristae, where the enzymes needed for the final step in adenosine triphosphate (ATP) production (*i.e.,* oxidative phosphorylation) are located.

Mitochondria contain their own DNA and ribosomes and are self-replicating. The DNA is found in the mitochondrial matrix and is distinct from the chromosomal DNA found in the nucleus. Mitochondrial DNA, known as the "other human genome," is a double-stranded, circular molecule that encodes the ribosomal RNA (rRNA) and transfer RNA (tRNA) required for intramitochrondial synthesis of proteins needed for the energy-generating function of the mitochondria. Although mitochondrial DNA directs the synthesis of 13 of the proteins required for mitochondrial function, the DNA of the nucleus encodes the structural proteins of the mitochondria and other proteins needed to carry out cellular respiration.

Mitochondrial DNA is inherited matrilineally (*i.e.,* from the mother), thus providing a basis for familial lineage studies. Mutations have been found in each of the mitochondrial genes, and an understanding of the role of mitochondrial DNA in certain diseases is beginning to emerge. Most tissues in the body depend to some extent on oxidative metabolism and can therefore be affected by mitochondrial DNA mutations.

THE CYTOSKELETON

Besides its organelles, the cytoplasm contains a network of microtubules, microfilaments, intermediate filaments, and thick filaments (Fig. 4-7). Because they control cell shape and movement, these structures are a major component of the structural elements called the *cytoskeleton.*

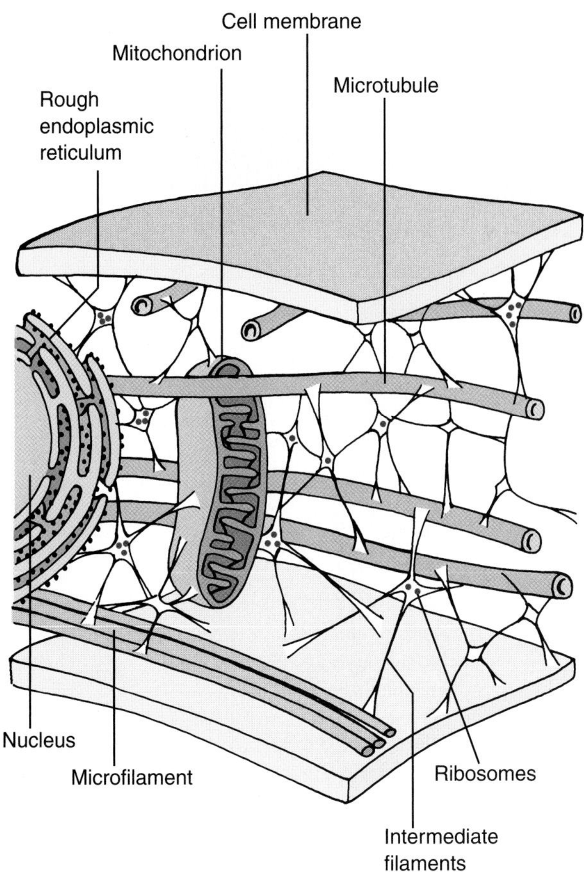

FIGURE 4-7 Microtubes and microfilaments of the cell. The microfilaments associate with the inner surface of the cell and aid in cell motility. The microtubules form the cytoskeleton and maintain the position of the organelles.

Microtubules

The microtubules are slender tubular structures composed of globular proteins called *tubulin*. Microtubules function in many ways, including development and maintenance of cell form. They participate in intracellular transport mechanisms, including axoplasmic transport in neurons and melanin dispersion in pigment cells of the skin. Other functions include formation of the basic structure for several complex cytoplasmic organelles, including the centrioles, basal bodies, cilia, and flagella. Abnormalities of the cytoskeleton may contribute to alterations in cell mobility and function. For example, proper functioning of the microtubules is essential for various stages of leukocyte (white blood cell) migration. In certain disease conditions, such as diabetes mellitus, alterations in leukocyte mobility and migration may interfere with the chemotaxis and phagocytosis of the inflammatory response and predispose toward the development of bacterial infection.

Cells can rapidly assemble and disassemble microtubules according to specific needs. The action of the plant alkaloid colchicine halts the assembly of microtubules. This compound stops cell mitosis by interfering with formation of the mitotic spindle. Colchicine is often used for cytogenetic (chromosome) studies. It is also used as a drug for treating gout. The drug's ability to reduce the inflammatory reaction associated with this condition may stem from its ability to interfere with microtubular function of white blood cells and their migration into the area.

Cilia and Flagella. Cilia and flagella are hairlike processes extending from the cell membrane that are capable of sweeping and flailing movements, which can move surrounding fluids or move the cell through fluid media (Fig. 4-8). Both contain identically organized cores of microtubules that consist of two microtubules surrounded at the periphery by clusters of paired microtubules. Each cilium and flagellum is anchored to a basal body that is responsible for the formation of the microtubular core. Cilia are found on the apical (luminal) surfaces of many epithelial linings, including the nasal sinuses or passages such as the upper respiratory system. Removal of mucus from the respiratory passages is highly dependent on proper function of the cilia. Flagella form the tail-like structures that provide motility for sperm.

Genetic defects can result in improper microtubule formation and, as a result, the cilia may be nonfunctional. One of these disorders, the *immobile cilia syndrome,* impairs sperm motility, causing male sterility while also immobilizing the cilia of the respiratory tract, thus interfering with clearance of inhaled bacteria, leading to a chronic lung disease called *bronchiectasis*.

Centrioles and Basal Bodies. Centrioles and basal bodies are structurally identical organelles composed of an array of highly organized microtubules. Internally, centrioles and basal bodies have an amorphous central core surrounded by clusters formed of triplet sets of microtubules. In dividing cells, the two cylindrical centrioles form the mitotic spindle that aids in the separation and movement of the chromosomes. Basal bodies are more numerous than centrioles and are found near the cell membrane in association with cilia and flagella. They are responsible for the formation of the highly organized core of microtubules found in cilia and flagella. The internal microtubular arrangement of centrioles and basal bodies is different from that found in cilia and flagella.

Microfilaments

Microfilaments are thin, threadlike cytoplasmic structures. Three classes of microfilaments exist: thin microfilaments, which are equivalent to the thin actin filaments in muscle; intermediate filaments, which are a heterogeneous group of filaments with diameter sizes between the thick and thin filaments; and thick myosin filaments, which are present in muscle cells but may also exist temporarily in other cells.

Muscle contraction depends on the interaction between the thin actin filaments and thick myosin filaments. Microfilaments are present in the superficial zone of the cytoplasm in most cells. Contractile activities involving the microfilaments and associated thick myosin filaments contribute to movement of the cytoplasm and cell membrane during endocytosis and exocytosis. Microfilaments

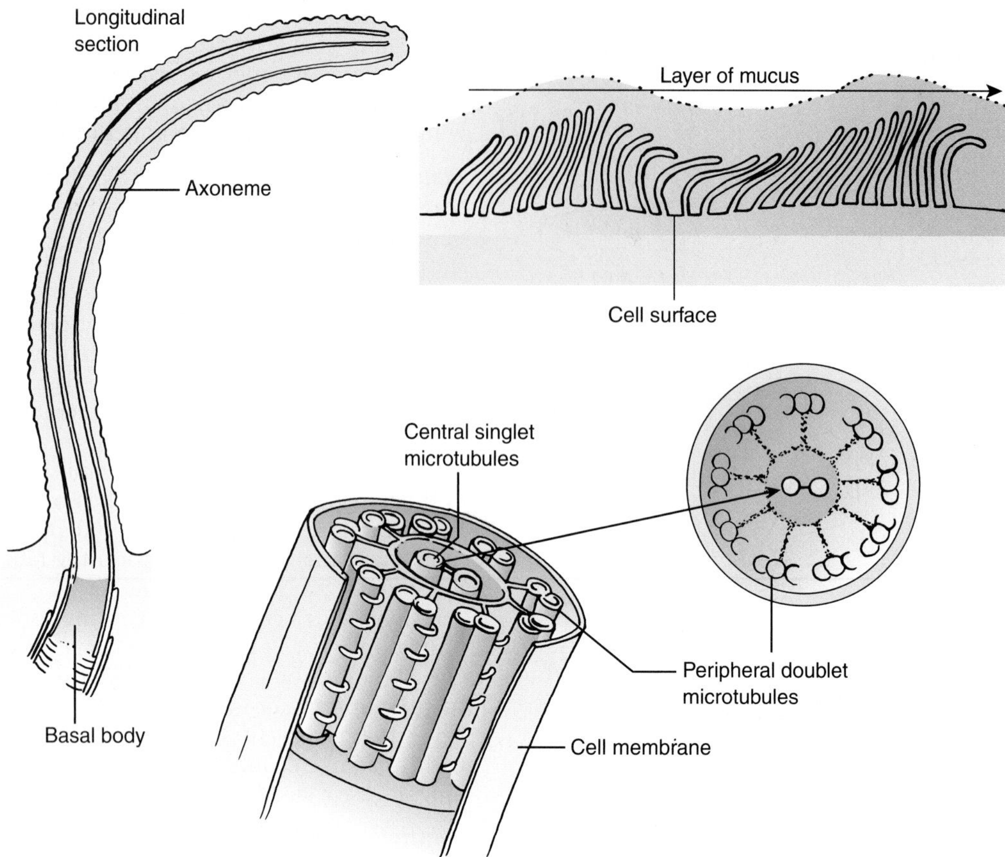

FIGURE 4-8 Structure of cilium. (Adapted from Cormack D. H. [1993]. *Essential histology* [p. 79]. Philadelphia: J.B. Lippincott)

are also present in the microvilli of the intestine. The intermediate filaments assist in supporting and maintaining the asymmetric shape of cells. Examples of intermediate filaments are the keratin filaments that are found anchored to the cell membrane of epidermal keratinocytes of the skin and the glial filaments that are found in astrocytes and other glial cells of the nervous system. The *neurofibrillary tangle* found in the brain in Alzheimer's disease contains microtubule-associated proteins and neurofilaments, evidence of a disrupted neuronal cytoskeleton.

THE CELL MEMBRANE

The cell is enclosed in a thin membrane that separates the intracellular contents from the extracellular environment. To differentiate it from the other cell membranes, such as the mitochondrial or nuclear membranes, the cell membrane is often called the *plasma membrane*. In many respects, the plasma membrane is one of the most important parts of the cell. It acts as a semipermeable structure that separates the intracellular and extracellular environments. It provides receptors for hormones and other biologically active substances, participates in the electrical events that occur in nerve and muscle cells, and aids in the regulation of cell growth and proliferation. The cell membrane may play an important role in the behavior of cancer cells (discussed in Chapter 8).

The cell membrane consists of an organized arrangement of lipids, carbohydrates, and proteins (Fig. 4-9). A main structural component of the membrane is its lipid bilayer. It is a bimolecular layer that consists primarily of phospholipids, with glycolipids and cholesterol. Lipids form a bilayer structure that is essentially impermeable to all but lipid-soluble substances. Approximately 75% of the lipids are phospholipids, each with a hydrophilic (water-soluble) head and a hydrophobic (water-insoluble) tail. Phospholipid molecules, along with the glycolipids, are aligned such that their hydrophilic heads face outward on each side of the membrane and their hydrophobic tails project toward the middle of the membrane. The hydrophilic heads retain water and help cells stick to each other. At normal body temperature, the viscosity of the lipid component of the membrane is equivalent to that of olive oil. The presence of cholesterol stiffens the membrane.

Although the lipid bilayer provides the basic structure of the cell membrane, proteins carry out most of the specific functions. Some proteins, called *transmembrane proteins*, pass directly through the membrane and communicate with the intracellular and extracellular environments. *Integral proteins*

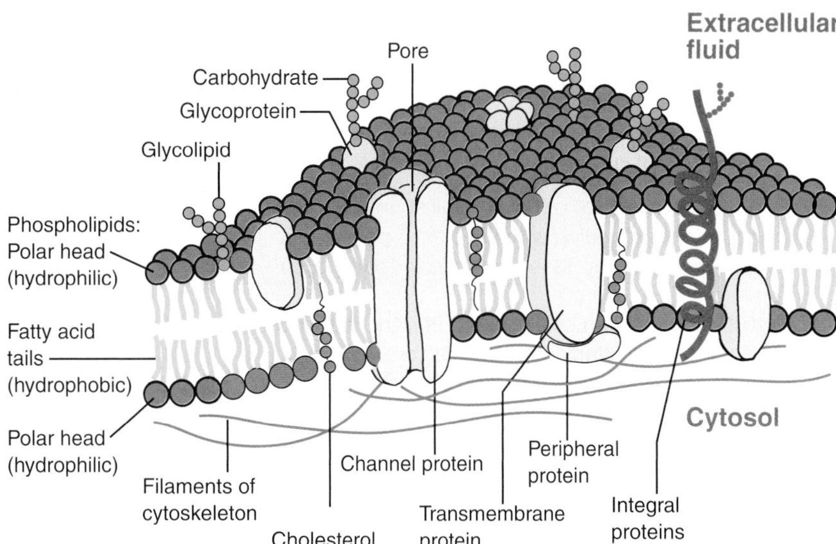

FIGURE 4-9 The structure of the cell membrane showing the hydrophilic (polar) heads and the hydrophobic (fatty acid) tails and the position of the integral and peripheral proteins in relation to the interior and exterior of the cell.

are transmembrane proteins tightly bound to lipids in the bilayer and are essentially part of the membrane. A second type of protein, the *peripheral proteins,* are bound to one or the other side of the membrane and do not pass into the lipid bilayer. Removal of peripheral proteins from the membrane surface usually causes damage to the membrane.

The manner in which proteins are associated with the cell membrane often determines their function. Thus, peripheral proteins are associated with functions involving the inner or outer side of the membrane where they are found. Peripheral proteins usually serve as receptors or are involved in intracellular signaling systems. By contrast, only the transmembrane proteins can function on both sides of the membrane or transport molecules across it.

Many integral transmembrane proteins form the ion channels found on the cell surface. These channel proteins have a complex morphology and are selective with respect to the substances they transmit. Mutations in these channel proteins, often called *channelopathies,* are responsible for a host of genetic disorders. For example, in *cystic fibrosis,* the primary defect resides in an abnormal chloride channel, which results in increased sodium and water reabsorption that causes respiratory tract secretions to thicken and occlude the airways (see Chapter 31).

A fuzzy-looking layer surrounds the cell surface called the *cell coat,* or *glycocalyx.* The structure of the glycocalyx consists of long, complex carbohydrate chains attached to protein molecules that penetrate the outside portion of the membrane (*i.e.,* glycoproteins); outward-facing membrane lipids (*i.e.,* glycolipids); and carbohydrate-binding proteins called *lectins.* The cell coat participates in cell-to-cell recognition and adhesion. It contains tissue transplant antigens that label cells as self or nonself. The cell coat of a red blood cell contains the ABO blood group antigens. An intimate relationship exists between the cell membrane and the cell coat. If the cell coat is enzymatically removed, the cell remains viable and can generate a new cell coat, but damage to the cell membrane usually results in cell death.

In summary, the cell is a remarkably autonomous structure that functions strikingly similarly to that of the total organism. In most cells, a single nucleus controls cell function and is the mastermind of the cell. It contains DNA, which provides the information necessary for the synthesis of the various proteins that the cell must produce to stay alive and to transmit information from one generation to another.

The cytoplasm contains the cell's organelles and the enzymes necessary for glycolysis. Ribosomes serve as sites for protein synthesis in the cell. The ER functions as a tubular communication system that transports substances from one part of the cell to another and as the site of protein (rough ER), carbohydrate, and lipid (smooth ER) synthesis. Golgi bodies modify materials synthesized in the ER and package them into secretory granules for transport within the cell or for export from the cell. Lysosomes, which are viewed as the digestive system of the cell, contain hydrolytic enzymes that digest worn-out cell parts and foreign materials. They are membranous structures formed in the Golgi complex from hydrolytic enzymes synthesized in the rough ER. Another organelle, the proteosome, digests misformed and misfolded proteins. The mitochondria serve as power plants for the cell because they transform food energy into ATP, to power cell activities. Mitochondria contain their own extrachromosomal DNA, important in the synthesis of mitochondrial RNAs and proteins used in oxidative metabolism. Microtubules are slender, stiff, tubular structures that influence cell shape, provide a means of moving organelles through the cytoplasm, and affect movement of the cilia and of chromosomes during cell division. Several types of threadlike filaments, including actin and myosin filaments, participate in muscle contraction.

The plasma membrane is a lipid bilayer that surrounds the cell and separates it from its surrounding external environment. A fuzzy-looking layer, the cell coat or glycocalyx, surrounds the cell surface; it contains tissue antigens and participates in cell-to-cell recognition and adhesion.

Integration of Cell Function and Replication

After you have completed this section of the chapter, you should be able to meet the following objectives:

- Trace the pathway for cell communication, beginning at the receptor and ending with effector response, and explain why the process is often referred to as *signal transduction*
- Describe the function of G proteins in signal transduction
- List three classifications of growth factors
- Relate the function of ATP to cell metabolism
- Differentiate anabolism and catabolism
- Compare the processes involved in aerobic and anaerobic metabolism
- Describe the five phases of the cell cycle

CELL COMMUNICATION

Cells in multicellular organisms need to communicate with one another to coordinate their function and control their growth. The human body has several means of transmitting information between cells. These mechanisms include direct communication between adjacent cells through gap junctions, autocrine and paracrine signaling, and endocrine or synaptic signaling. *Autocrine signaling* occurs when a cell releases a chemical into the extracellular fluid that affects its own activity (Fig. 4-10). With *paracrine signaling,* enzymes rapidly metabolize the chemical mediators and therefore act mainly on nearby cells. *Endocrine signaling* relies on hormones carried in the bloodstream to cells throughout the body. *Synaptic signaling* occurs in the nervous system, where neurotransmitters act only on adjacent nerve cells through special contact areas called *synapses*. In some parts of the body, the same chemical messenger can function as a neurotransmitter, a paracrine mediator, and a hormone secreted by neurons into the bloodstream.

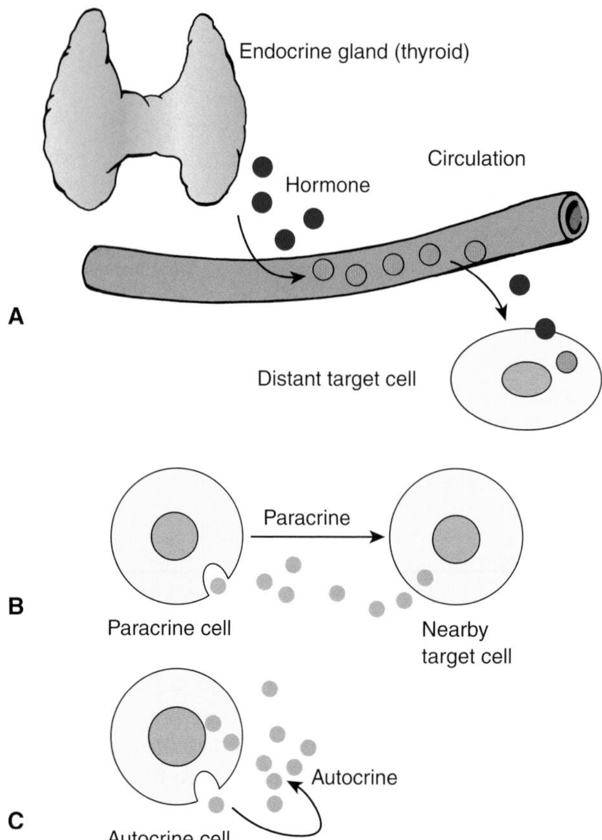

FIGURE 4-10 Examples of endocrine (**A**), paracrine (**B**), and autocrine (**C**) secretions.

CELL RECEPTORS

Signaling systems consist of receptors that reside either in the cell membrane (surface receptors) or within the cells (intracellular receptors). Receptors are activated by a variety of extracellular signals or *first messengers,* including neurotransmitters, protein hormones and growth factors, steroids, and other chemical messengers. Some lipid-soluble chemical messengers move through the membrane and bind to cytoplasmic or nuclear receptors to exert their physiologic effects. Signaling systems also include transducers and effectors that are involved in conversion of the signal into a physiologic response. The pathway may include additional intracellular mechanisms, called *second messengers*. Many molecules involved in signal transduction are proteins. A unique property of proteins that allows them to function in this way is their ability to change their shape or conformation, thereby changing their function and consequently the functions of the cell. Proteins often accomplish these conformational changes through enzymes called *protein kinases* that catalyze the phosphorylation of amino acids in the protein structure.

Cell Surface Receptors

Each cell type in the body contains a distinctive set of surface receptors that enable it to respond to a complementary set of signaling molecules in a specific, preprogrammed

> **CELL COMMUNICATION**
>
> - Cells communicate with each other and with the internal and external environments by a number of mechanisms, including electrical and chemical signaling systems that control electrical potentials, the overall function of a cell, and gene activity needed for cell division and cell replication.
> - Chemical messengers exert their effects by binding to cell membrane proteins or receptors that convert the chemical signal into signals within the cell, in a process called *signal transduction.*
> - Cells can regulate their responses to chemical messengers by increasing or decreasing the number of active receptors on their surface.

way. These proteins are not static components of the cell membrane; they increase or decrease in number according to the needs of the cell. When excess chemical messengers are present, the number of active receptors decreases in a process called *down-regulation;* when there is a deficiency of the messenger, the number of active receptors increases through *up-regulation.* Three known classes of cell surface receptor proteins exist: G-protein linked, ion-channel linked, and enzyme linked.

G-Protein–Linked Receptors. With more than 1000 members, G-protein–linked receptors are the largest family of cell surface receptors. Although many intercellular messengers exist, they usually rely on the intermediary activity of a separate class of membrane-bound regulatory proteins to convert external signals (first messengers) into internal signals (second messengers). Because these regulatory proteins bind to guanine nucleotides such as guanine diphosphate (GDP) and guanine triphosphate (GTP), they are called *G proteins.* G-protein–linked receptors mediate cellular responses for numerous types of first messengers, including proteins, small peptides, amino acids, and fatty acids derivatives such as the prostaglandins.

All G-protein–linked signal transduction systems rely on a series of orchestrated biochemical events (Fig. 4-11). They all have a receptor component, which functions as a signal discriminator by recognizing a specific first messenger, and they all undergo conformational changes with receptor binding that activate the G protein. The activated G protein, in turn, acts as a transducer, passing the message on to other membrane-bound intermediates called *effectors.* Often, the effector is an enzyme that converts an inactive precursor molecule into a second messenger, which diffuses into the cytoplasm and carries the signal beyond the cell membrane. A common second messenger is cyclic adenosine monophosphate (cAMP). It is activated by the enzyme *adenyl cyclase,* which generates cAMP by transferring phosphate groups from ATP to other proteins. This transfer changes the form and function of these proteins. Such changes eventually produce the cell response to the first messenger, whether it is a secretion, muscle contraction or relaxation, or a change in cell metabolism. Sometimes, it is the opening or closing of ion channels in the cell membrane.

Although there are differences among the G-protein–linked receptors, all share a number of features. All are found on the cytoplasmic side of the cell membrane, and all incorporate the *GTPase cycle,* which functions as the on–off switch for G-protein activity. GTPase is an enzyme that converts GTP with its three phosphate groups to GDP with its two phosphate groups. In the inactive state, G proteins contain tightly bound GDP. When a receptor coupled to a G protein is activated, the G protein releases the GDP and binds GTP. This causes the G protein to dissociate from the receptor and activate the effector. During the process of signal transduction, GTPase converts bound GTP to GDP, thereby returning the G protein to its resting state and switching the signal off. Certain bacterial toxins can bind to the G proteins, causing inhibition or stimulation of its signal function. One such toxin, the toxin of *Vibrio cholerae,* binds and activates the stimulatory G protein linked to the cAMP system that controls the secretion of fluid into the intestine. In response to the cholera toxin, these cells overproduce fluid, leading to severe diarrhea and life-threatening depletion of extracellular fluid volume.

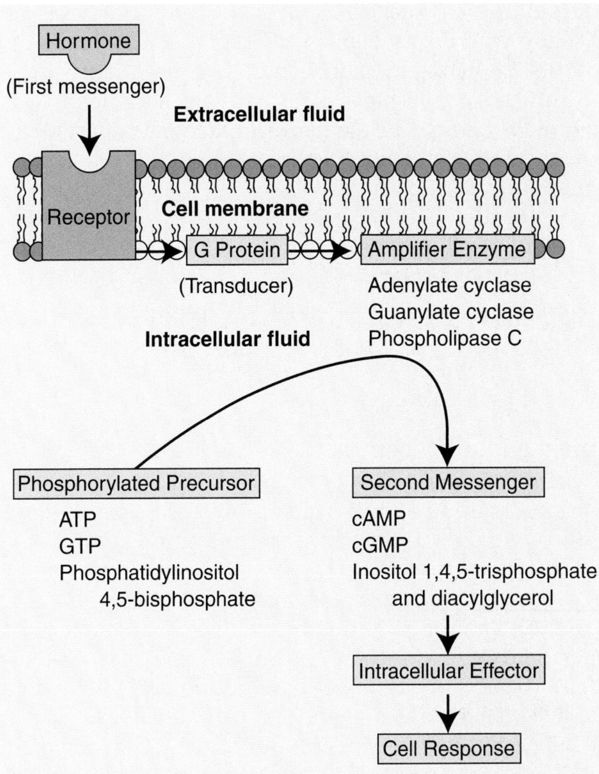

FIGURE 4-11 Signal transduction pattern common to several second messenger systems. A protein or peptide hormone is the first messenger to a membrane receptor, stimulating or inhibiting a membrane-bound enzyme by means of a G protein. The amplifier enzyme catalyzes the production of a second messenger from a phosphorylated precursor. The second messenger then activates an internal effector, which leads to the cell response. (Redrawn from Rhoades R.A., Tanner G.A. [1996]. *Medical physiology.* Boston: Little, Brown)

Ion-Channel–Linked Receptors. Ion-channel–linked receptors are involved in the rapid synaptic signaling between electrically excitable cells. A few neurotransmitters mediate this type of signaling by transiently opening or closing ion channels formed by integral proteins in the cell membrane. This type of signaling is involved in the transmission of impulses in nerve and muscle cells.

Enzyme-Linked Receptors. Many hormones, growth factors, and cytokines signal their target cells by binding to a class of receptors that activate an intracellular domain with enzyme (tyrosine kinase) activity. The enzyme catalyzes the phosphorylation of tyrosine residues in the receptor and target proteins, thereby transferring an external message to the cell interior. Enzyme-linked receptors mediate cellular responses such as calcium influx, increased sodium–potassium exchange, and stimulation of glucose and amino acid uptake. Insulin acts by binding to a surface receptor with tyrosine kinase activity (see Chapter 43).

The signaling cascades generated by the activation of tyrosine kinase receptors are also involved in the function of growth factors. As their name implies, many growth factors are important messengers in signaling cell replacement and cell growth. Most of the growth factors belong to one of three groups: factors that foster the multiplication and development of various cell types (*e.g.*, growth factor and epidermal growth factor); cytokines, which are important in the regulation of the immune system (see Chapter 19); and colony-stimulating factors, which regulate the proliferation and maturation of white and red blood cells (see Chapter 14).

Intracellular Receptors

Some messengers, such as thyroid hormone and steroid hormones, do not bind to membrane receptors but move directly across the lipid layer of the cell membrane and are carried to the cell nucleus, where they influence DNA activity. Many of these hormones bind to a cytoplasmic receptor, and together they are carried to the nucleus. In the nucleus, the receptor–hormone complex binds to DNA, thereby increasing transcription of messenger RNA (mRNA). The mRNAs are translated in the ribosomes, with the production of increased amounts of proteins that alter cell function.

THE CELL CYCLE AND CELL DIVISION

The life of a cell is called the *cell cycle.* It is usually divided into five phases or gaps: G_0, G_1, S, G_2, and M. Some cells may not have a G_1 phase, and others may not have a G_2 stage. However, all cells must grow, replicate their genetic material if they are to divide, and undergo the process of mitosis if they are to replicate. G_0 is the stage during which the cell may leave the cell cycle and either remain in a state of inactivity or reenter the cell cycle at another time. G_1 is the stage during which the cell is starting to prepare for mitosis through DNA and protein synthesis and an increase in organelle and cytoskeletal elements. The S phase is the synthesis phase, during which DNA replication occurs and the centrioles are beginning to replicate. G_2 is the premitotic phase and is similar to G_1 as for RNA and protein synthesis. The M phase is the phase during which cell mitosis occurs. Nondividing cells, such as mature nerve cells and cells not preparing for mitosis, are said to be in the G_0 phase of the cell cycle (Fig. 4-12).

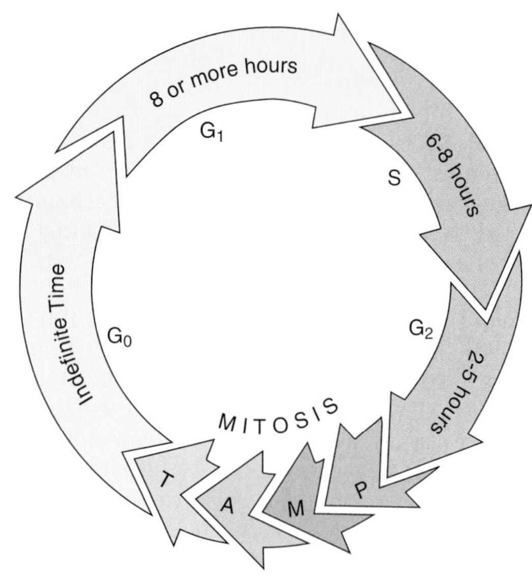

FIGURE 4-12 Cell cycle. G_0, nondividing cell; G_1, cell growth; S, DNA replication; G_2, protein synthesis; M, mitosis, which lasts for 1 to 3 hours and is followed by cytokinesis or cell division. (teleophase [T], anaphase [A], mitosis [M], prophase [P])

Cell Division

Cell division, or *mitosis,* which was first described in 1875, is the process during which a parent cell divides and each daughter cell receives a chromosomal karyotype identical to the parent cell. Cell division gives the body a means of replacing cells that have a limited life span, such as skin and blood cells; increasing tissue mass during periods of growth; and providing for tissue repair and wound healing. Despite the early cytologic description of the four stages of mitosis, it was not until the early 1950s that the importance of the cell cycle was realized.

Mitosis, which is a dynamic and continuous process, usually lasts from 1 to 1½ hours. It is divided into four stages: prophase, metaphase, anaphase, and telophase (Fig. 4-13). The phase during which the cell is not undergoing division is called *interphase.* During *prophase,* the chromosomes become visible because of increased coiling of the DNA, the two centrioles replicate, and a pair moves to each side of the cell. Simultaneously, the microtubules of the mitotic spindle appear between the two pairs of centrioles. Later in prophase, the nuclear envelope and nucleolus disappear. *Metaphase* involves the organization of the chromosome pairs in the midline of the cell and the formation of a mitotic spindle composed of the microtubules. *Anaphase* is the period during which separation of the chromosome pairs occurs, with the microtubules pulling one member of each pair of 46 chromosomes toward the opposite cell pole. Cell division, or *cytokinesis,* is completed after *telophase,* the stage during which the mitotic spindle vanishes and a new nuclear

THE CELL CYCLE AND CELL DIVISION

- The cell cycle, which represents the life of a cell, is divided into two main phases: the synthesis or S phase, during which DNA is replicated and the M phase, during which mitosis occurs.
- Extra gaps are inserted to allow for growth and protein– G_1 to prepare for the S phase and G_2 to prepare for the M phase.
- A third gap, G_0, provides a time for cells to leave the cell cycle.

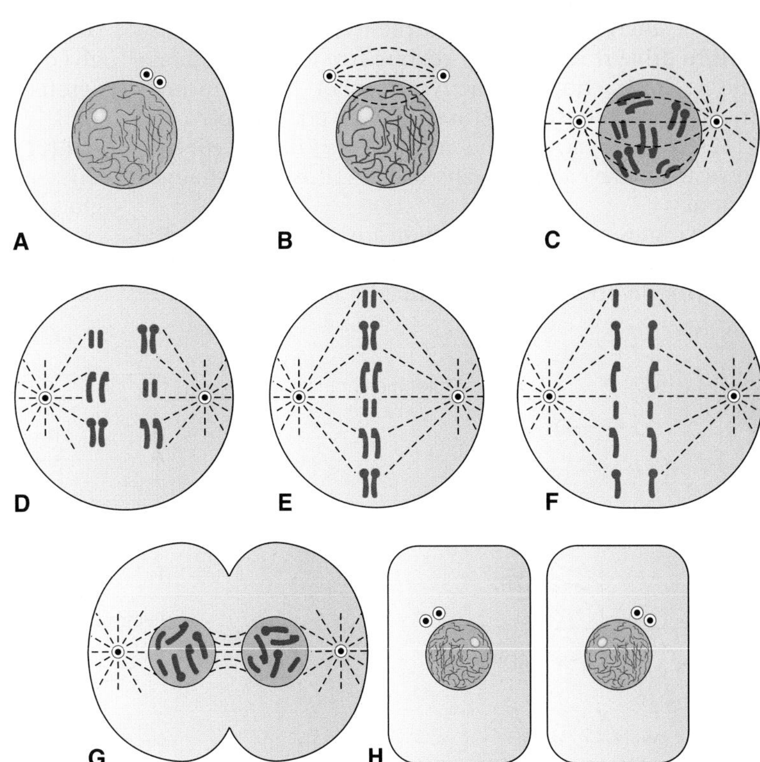

FIGURE 4-13 Cell mitosis. **A** and **H** represent the nondividing cell; **B, C,** and **D** represent prophase; **E** and **F** represent anaphase; and **G** represents telophase.

membrane develops and encloses each complete set of chromosomes.

Cell division is controlled by changes in the intracellular concentrations and activity of three major groups of intracellular proteins: (1) cyclins, (2) cyclin-dependent kinases, and (3) the anaphase-promoting complex. The central components of the cell cycle control system are the cyclin-dependent kinases, whose activity depends on association with the regulatory units called *cyclins*. Oscillations in the activity of the various cyclin-dependent kinases lead to initiation of the different phases of the cell cycle. For example, activation of the S-phase cyclin-dependent kinases initiates the S phase of the cell cycle, whereas activation of the M-phase cyclin-dependent kinases triggers mitosis. The anaphase-promoting complex is responsible for the breakdown of the M cyclins and other regulators of mitosis.

Cell division is also controlled by several external factors, including the presence of cytokines, various growth factors, or even adhesion factors when the cell is associated with other cells in a tissue. In addition, the cell cycle is regulated by several checkpoints that determine whether DNA replication has occurred with a high degree of fidelity. Two of the better understood are the DNA damage and the spindle formation checkpoints. If these biochemical checkpoints are not faithfully met, the cell may default to programmed cell death or apoptosis.

CELL METABOLISM AND ENERGY SOURCES

Energy is the ability to do work. Cells use oxygen and the breakdown products of the foods we eat to produce the energy needed for muscle contraction, transport of ions and molecules, and the synthesis of enzymes, hormones, and other macromolecules. *Energy metabolism* refers to the processes by which fats, proteins, and carbohydrates from the foods we eat are converted into energy or complex energy sources in the cell. Catabolism and anabolism are the two phases of metabolism. *Catabolism* consists of breaking down stored nutrients and body tissues to produce energy. *Anabolism* is a constructive process in which more complex molecules are formed from simpler ones.

The special carrier for cellular energy is ATP. ATP molecules consist of adenosine, a nitrogenous base; ribose, a five-carbon sugar; and three phosphate groups (see Fig. 4-14). The phosphate groups are attached by two high-energy bonds. Large amounts of free energy are released when ATP is hydrolyzed to form adenosine diphosphate (ADP), an adenosine molecule that contains two phosphate groups.

High-energy bonds
Adenine
Ribose
Phosphates
Adenosine

FIGURE 4-14 Structure of the adenosine triphosphate (ATP) molecule.

The free energy liberated from the hydrolysis of ATP is used to drive reactions that require free energy, such as muscle contraction and active transport mechanisms. Energy from foodstuffs is used to convert ADP back to ATP. ATP is often called the *energy currency* of the cell; energy can be "saved" or "spent" using ATP as an exchange currency.

Two sites of energy production are present in the cell: the *anaerobic* (*i.e.*, without oxygen) glycolytic pathway, occurring in the cytoplasm, and the *aerobic* (*i.e.*, with oxygen) pathways in the mitochondria. The anaerobic glycolytic pathway serves as an important prelude to the aerobic pathways.

Anaerobic Metabolism

Glycolysis is the process by which energy is liberated from glucose (Fig. 4-15). It is an important energy provider for cells that lack mitochondria, the cell organelle in which aerobic metabolism occurs. This process also provides energy in situations when delivery of oxygen to the cell is

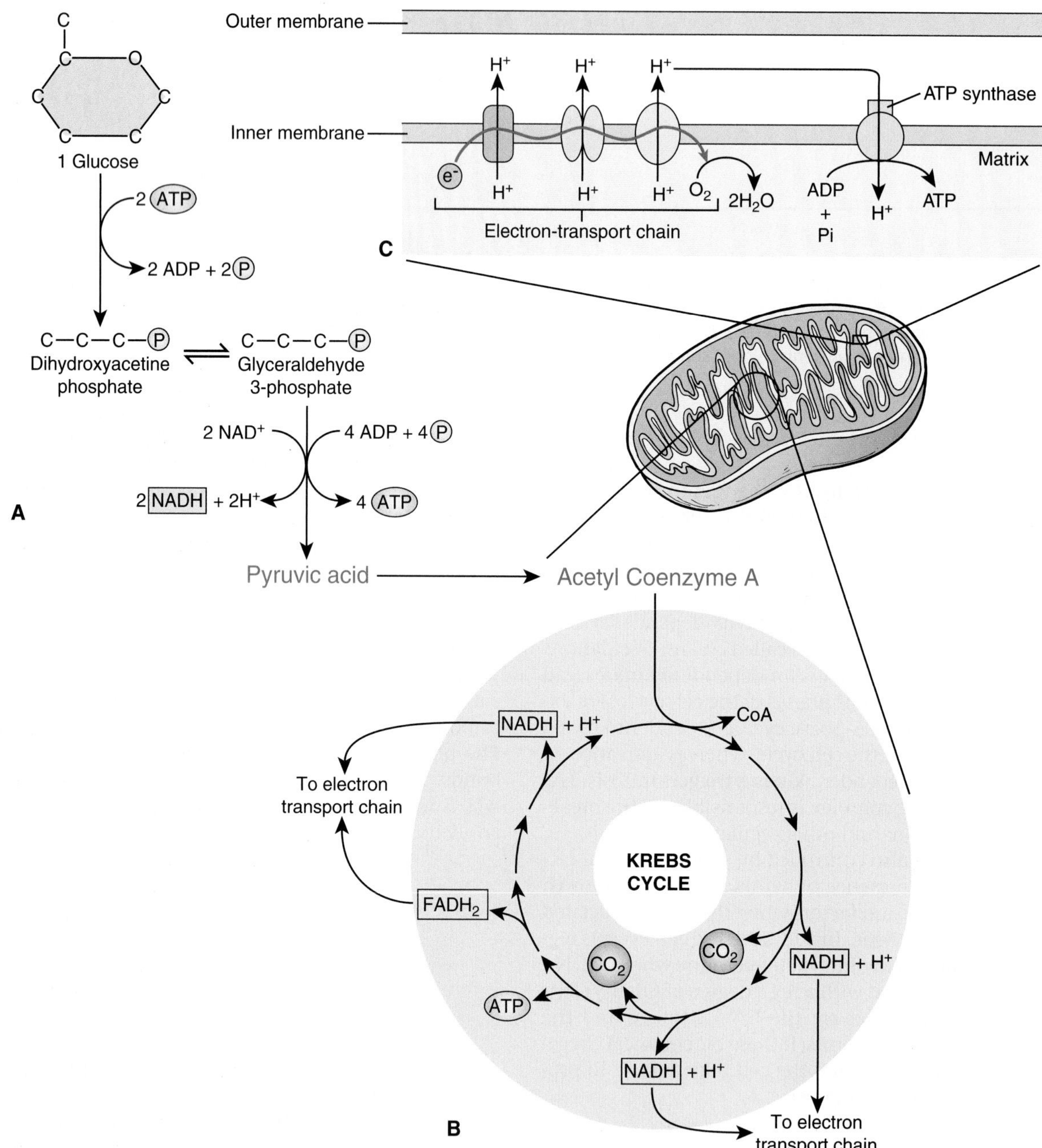

FIGURE 4-15 Simplified version of (**A**) the glycolytic or anaerobic pathway that occurs in the cytoplasm, (**B**) the mitochondrial citric acid or aerobic pathway, and (**C**) the electron transport chain, in which the hydrogen (H^+) ions and electrons (e^-) from NADH+ H^+ complexes generated in the glycolytic and citric acid pathways are converted to ATP and water in the presence of oxygen (O_2).

delayed or impaired. Glycolysis involves a sequence of reactions that converts glucose to pyruvate, with the concomitant production of ATP from ADP. The net gain of energy from the glycolysis of one molecule of glucose is two ATP molecules. Although comparatively inefficient as to energy yield, the glycolytic pathway is important during periods of decreased oxygen delivery, as occurs in skeletal muscle during the first few minutes of exercise.

Glycolysis requires the presence of nicotinamide-adenine dinucleotide (NAD^+), a hydrogen (H^+) carrier. Important end products of glycolysis are pyruvate and NADH + H^+. When oxygen is present, pyruvate moves into the aerobic mitochondrial pathway, and the NADH + H^+ delivers the H^+ and its electron to the oxidative electron transport system (to be discussed). Transfer of hydrogen from NADH to the electron transport system allows the glycolytic process to continue by facilitating the regeneration of NAD^+. Under anaerobic conditions, such as cardiac arrest or circulatory shock, pyruvate is converted to lactic acid, which diffuses out of the cells into the extracellular fluid. Conversion of pyruvate to lactic acid is reversible, and after the oxygen supply has been restored, lactic acid is reconverted back to pyruvate and used directly for energy or to synthesize glucose.

Much of the reconversion of lactic acid occurs in the liver, but a small amount can occur in other tissues. The liver removes lactic acid from the bloodstream and converts it to glucose in a process called *gluconeogenesis*. This glucose is released into the bloodstream to be used again by the muscles or by the central nervous system. This recycling of lactic acid is called the *Cori cycle*. Heart muscle is also efficient in converting lactic acid to pyruvic acid and then using the pyruvic acid for fuel. Pyruvic acid is a particularly important source of fuel for the heart during heavy exercise when the skeletal muscles are producing large amounts of lactic acid and releasing it into the bloodstream.

Aerobic Metabolism

Aerobic metabolism occurs in the cell's mitochondria and involves the citric acid cycle and oxidative phosphorylation. It is here that hydrogen and carbon molecules from the fats, proteins, and carbohydrates in our diet are broken down and combined with molecular oxygen to form carbon dioxide and water as energy is released. Unlike lactic acid, which is an end product of anaerobic metabolism, carbon dioxide and water are generally harmless and easily eliminated from the body. In a 24-hour period, oxidative metabolism produces 300 to 500 mL of water.

The citric acid cycle, sometimes called the *tricarboxylic acid* or *Krebs cycle,* provides the final common pathway for the metabolism of nutrients (see Fig. 4-15). In the citric acid cycle, an activated two-carbon molecule of acetyl coenzyme A (acetyl-CoA) condenses with a four-carbon molecule of oxaloacetic acid and moves through a series of enzyme-mediated steps. This process produces hydrogen and carbon dioxide. As hydrogen is generated, it combines with one of two special carriers, NAD^+ or flavin adenine dinucleotide ($FADH^+$), for transfer to the electron transport system. The carbon dioxide is converted to bicarbonate or carried to the lungs and exhaled. In the citric acid cycle, each of the two pyruvate molecules formed in the cytoplasm from one molecule of glucose yields another molecule of ATP along with two molecules of carbon dioxide and eight hydrogen atoms. These hydrogen atoms are transferred to the electron transport system on the inner mitochondrial membrane for oxidation. Besides pyruvate from the glycolysis of glucose, products of amino acid and fatty acid degradation enter the citric acid cycle and contribute to the generation of ATP.

Oxidative metabolism, which supplies 90% of the body's energy needs, is the process by which hydrogen generated during the citric acid cycle combines with oxygen to form ATP and water. It is accomplished by a series of enzymatically catalyzed reactions that split each hydrogen atom into a H^+ ion and an electron. During the process of ionization, the electrons removed from the hydrogen atoms enter an electron transport system found on the inner membrane of the mitochondrion (Fig. 4-15). This electron transport chain consists of electron acceptors that can be reversibly reduced or oxidized by accepting or giving up electrons. Among the members of the electron transport system are several proteins, including a set of iron-containing molecules called *cytochromes*. Each electron is shuttled from one acceptor to another until it reaches the end of the chain, where its final two electrons are used to reduce elemental oxygen, which combines with the hydrogen ions to form water. As the electrons move along the electron transport chain, large amounts of energy are released. This energy is used to convert ADP to ATP. Because the formation of ATP involves the addition of a high-energy phosphate bond to ADP, the process is sometimes called *oxidative phosphorylation*. Cyanide poisoning kills by binding to the enzymes needed for a final step in the oxidative phosphorylation sequence.

In summary, cells communicate with each other by means of chemical messenger systems. In some tissues, chemical messengers move from cell to cell through gap junctions without entering the extracellular fluid. Other types of chemical messengers bind to receptors on or near the cell surface. Three classes of cell surface receptor proteins are: G-protein linked, ion-channel linked, and enzyme linked. G-protein–linked receptors rely on a class of molecules called *G proteins* that function as an on–off switch to convert external signals (first messengers) into internal signals (second messengers). Ion-linked signaling is mediated by neurotransmitters that transiently open or close ion channels formed by integral proteins in the cell membrane. Enzyme-linked receptors interact with certain peptide hormones, such as insulin and growth factors, and directly initiate the activity of the intracellular protein–tyrosine kinase enzyme.

The life of a cell is called the cell cycle. It is usually divided into five phases: G_0, or the resting phase; G_1, during which the cell begins to prepare for division through DNA and protein synthesis; the S or synthetic phase, during which DNA replication occurs; G_2, which is the premitotic phase and is similar to G_1 regarding RNA and protein synthesis; and the M phase, during which cell division occurs. Cell division, or mitosis, is the process during which a parent cell divides into two daughter cells, with each receiving an identical pair of chromosomes. The process of mitosis is dynamic and continuous and is divided into four stages: prophase, metaphase, anaphase, and telophase.

Metabolism is the process by which the carbohydrates, fats, and proteins we eat are broken down and subsequently converted into the energy needed for cell function. Energy is converted to ATP, the energy currency of the cell. Two sites of energy conversion are present in cells: the mitochondria and the cytoplasmic matrix. The most efficient of these pathways is the aerobic citric acid pathway in the mitochondria. This pathway requires oxygen and produces carbon dioxide and water as end products. The glycolytic pathway within the cytoplasm involves the breakdown of glucose to form ATP. This pathway can function without oxygen by producing lactic acid.

Movement Across the Cell Membrane and Membrane Potentials

After you have completed this section of the chapter, you should be able to meet the following objectives:

- Discuss the mechanisms of membrane transport associated with diffusion, osmosis, endocytosis, and exocytosis and compare with active transport mechanisms
- Describe the function of ion channels
- Describe the basis for membrane potentials
- Explain the relationship between membrane permeability and membrane potential

The cell membrane serves as a barrier that controls which substances enter and leave the cell. This barrier function allows materials that are essential for cell function to enter the cell, while excluding those that are harmful. It is responsible for differences in the composition of intracellular and extracellular fluids.

MOVEMENT OF SUBSTANCES ACROSS THE CELL MEMBRANE

Movement through the cell membrane occurs in essentially two ways: passively, without an expenditure of energy, or actively, using energy-consuming processes. The cell membrane can also engulf a particle, forming a membrane-coated vesicle; this membrane-coated vesicle is moved into the cell by *endocytosis* or out of the cell by *exocytosis*.

Passive Movement

Passive movement of particles or ions across the cell membrane is directly influenced by chemical or electrical gradients and does not require an expenditure of energy. A difference in the number of particles on either side of the membrane creates a chemical gradient, and a difference in charged particle or ions creates an electrical gradient. Chemical and electrical gradients are often linked and are called *electrochemical gradients*.

Diffusion. Diffusion refers to the process by which molecules and other particles in a solution become widely dispersed and reach a uniform concentration because of energy created by their spontaneous kinetic movements (Fig. 4-16). Electrolytes and other substances move from an area of higher to an area of lower concentration. With

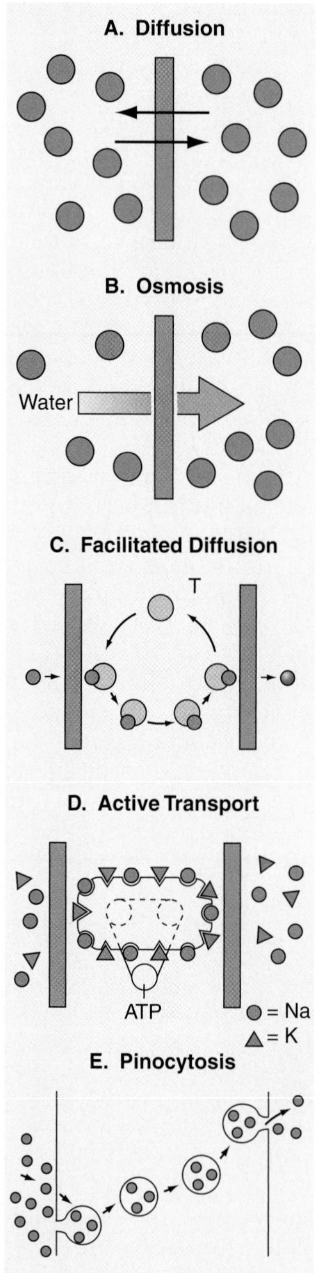

FIGURE 4-16 Mechanisms of membrane transport. (**A**) Diffusion, in which particles move to become equally distributed across the membrane. (**B**) The osmotically active particles regulate the flow of water. (**C**) Facilitated diffusion uses a carrier system. (**D**) In active transport, selected molecules are transported across the membrane using the energy-driven ATP pump. (**E**) The membrane forms a vesicle that engulfs the particle and transports it across the membrane, where it is released. This is called *pinocytosis.*

ions, diffusion is affected by energy supplied by their electrical charge. Lipid-soluble molecules, such as oxygen, carbon dioxide, alcohol, and fatty acids, become dissolved in the lipid matrix of the cell membrane and diffuse through the membrane in the same manner that diffusion occurs in water. Other substances diffuse through minute pores of the cell membrane. The rate of movement depends on how many particles are available for diffusion and the velocity of the kinetic movement of the particles. The number of openings in the cell membrane through which the particles can move also determines transfer rates. Temperature changes the motion of the particles; the greater the temperature, the greater is the thermal motion of the molecules. Thus, diffusion increases in proportion to the increased temperature.

Osmosis. Most cell membranes are semipermeable in that they are permeable to water but not all solute particles. Water moves through a semipermeable membrane along a concentration gradient, moving from an area of higher to one of lower concentration (see Fig. 4-16). This process is called *osmosis,* and the pressure that water generates as it moves through the membrane is called *osmotic pressure.*

Osmosis is regulated by the concentration of nondiffusible particles on either side of a semipermeable membrane. When there is a difference in the concentration of particles, water moves from the side with the lower concentration of particles and higher concentration of water to the side with the higher concentration of particles and lower concentration of water. The movement of water continues until the concentration of particles on both sides of the membrane is equally diluted or until the hydrostatic (osmotic) pressure created by the movement of water opposes its flow.

Facilitated Diffusion. Facilitated diffusion occurs through a transport protein that is not linked to metabolic energy (see Fig. 4-16). Some substances, such as glucose, cannot pass unassisted through the cell membrane because they are not lipid soluble or are too large to pass through the membrane's pores. These substances, combined with special transport proteins at the membrane's outer surface, are carried across the membrane attached to the transporter and then released. In facilitated diffusion, a substance can move only from an area of higher concentration to one of lower concentration. The rate at which a substance moves across the membrane because of facilitated diffusion depends on the difference in concentration between the two sides of the membrane. Also important are the availability of transport proteins and the rapidity with which they can bind and release the substance being transported. It is thought that insulin, which facilitates the movement of glucose into cells, acts by increasing the availability of glucose transporters in the cell membrane.

Active Transport and Cotransport

Active transport mechanisms involve the expenditure of energy. The process of diffusion describes particle movement from an area of higher concentration to one of lower concentration, resulting in an equal distribution across the cell membrane. Sometimes, however, different concentrations of a substance are needed in the intracellular and extracellular fluids. For example, the intracellular functioning of the cell requires a much higher concentration of potassium than is present in the extracellular fluid while maintaining a much lower concentration of sodium than in the extracellular fluid. In these situations, energy is required to pump the ions "uphill" or against their concentration gradient. When cells use energy to move ions against an electrical or chemical gradient, the process is called *active transport.*

The active transport system studied in the greatest detail is the sodium–potassium (Na^+/K^+) ATPase pump (see Fig. 4-16). This pump moves sodium from inside the cell to the extracellular region, where its concentration is approximately 14 times greater than inside; the pump also returns potassium to the inside, where its concentration is approximately 35 times greater than it is outside the cell. Energy used to pump sodium out of the cell and potassium into the cell is obtained by splitting and releasing energy from the high-energy phosphate bond in ATP by the enzyme ATPase. Were it not for the activity of the sodium–potassium pump, the osmotically active sodium particles would accumulate in the cell, causing cellular swelling because of an accompanying influx of water (see Chapter 5).

Two types of active transport systems exist: primary active transport and secondary active transport. In *primary active transport,* the source of energy (*e.g.,* ATP) is used directly in the transport of a substance. *Secondary active transport* mechanisms harness the energy derived from the primary active transport of one substance, usually sodium ions, for the cotransport of a second substance. For example, when sodium ions are actively transported out of a cell by primary active transport, a large concentration gradient develops (*i.e.,* high concentration on the outside and low on the inside). This concentration gradient represents a large storehouse of energy because sodium ions are always attempting to diffuse into the cell. Similar to facilitated diffusion, secondary transport mechanisms use membrane transport proteins. These proteins have two binding sites, one for sodium ions and the other for the substance undergoing secondary transport. Secondary transport systems are classified into two groups: *cotransport* or *symport* systems, in which the sodium ion and solute are transported in the same direction, and *countertransport* or *antiport* systems, in which sodium ions and the solute are transported in the opposite direction (Fig. 4-17). An example of cotransport occurs in the intestine, where the absorption of glucose and amino acids is coupled with sodium transport.

Endocytosis and Exocytosis

Endocytosis is the process by which cells engulf materials from their surroundings. It includes pinocytosis and phagocytosis. *Pinocytosis* involves the ingestion of small solid or fluid particles. The particles are engulfed into small, membrane-surrounded vesicles for movement into the cytoplasm. The process of pinocytosis is important in the transport of proteins and strong solutions of electrolytes (see Fig. 4-16).

Phagocytosis literally means *cell eating* and can be compared with pinocytosis, which means *cell drinking.* It

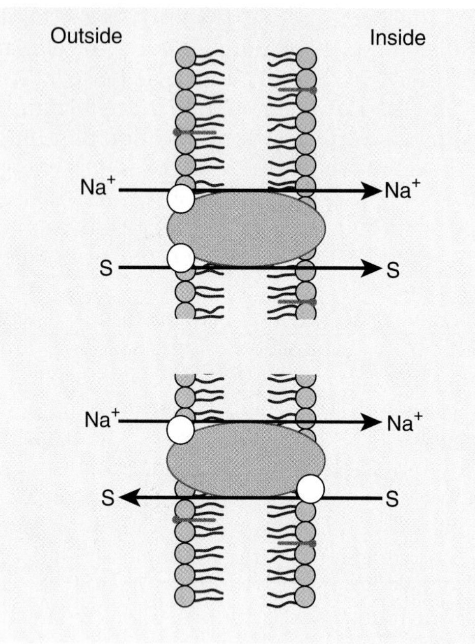

FIGURE 4-17 Secondary active transport systems. Symport or cotransport (*top*) carries the transported solute (**s**) in the same direction as the Na^+ ion. Antiport or counter-transport carries the solute and Na^+ in the opposite direction. (Rhoades R.A., Tanner G.A. [1996]. *Medical physiology.* Boston: Little, Brown)

involves the engulfment and subsequent killing or degradation of microorganisms and other particulate matter. During phagocytosis, a particle contacts the cell surface and is surrounded on all sides by the cell membrane, forming a phagocytic vesicle or phagosome. Once formed, the phagosome breaks away from the cell membrane and moves into the cytoplasm, where it eventually fuses with a lysosome, allowing the ingested material to be degraded by lysosomal enzymes. Certain cells, such as macrophages and polymorphonuclear leukocytes (neutrophils), are adept at engulfing and disposing of invading organisms, damaged cells, and unneeded extracellular constituents (see Chapter 20).

Receptor-mediated endocytosis involves the binding of substances such as low-density lipoproteins to a receptor on the cell surface. Binding of a ligand (*i.e.,* a substance with a high affinity for a receptor) to its receptor normally causes widely distributed receptors to accumulate in clathrin-coated pits. An aggregation of special proteins on the cytoplasmic side of the pit causes the coated pit to invaginate and pinch off, forming a clathrin-coated vesicle that carries the ligand and its receptor into the cell.

Exocytosis is the mechanism for the secretion of intracellular substances into the extracellular spaces. It is the reverse of endocytosis in that a secretory granule fuses to the inner side of the cell membrane, and an opening occurs in the cell membrane. This opening allows the contents of the granule to be released into the extracellular fluid. Exocytosis is important in removing cellular debris and releasing substances, such as hormones, synthesized in the cell.

During endocytosis, portions of the cell membrane become an endocytotic vesicle. During exocytosis, the vesicular membrane is incorporated into the plasma membrane. In this way, cell membranes can be conserved and reused.

Ion Channels

The electrical charge on small ions such as Na^+ and K^+ makes it difficult for these ions to move across the lipid layer of the cell membrane. However, rapid movement of these ions is required for many types of cell functions, such as nerve activity. This is accomplished by facilitated diffusion through selective ion channels. Ion channels are integral proteins that span the width of the cell membrane and are normally composed of several polypeptides or protein subunits that form a gating system. Specific stimuli cause the protein subunits to undergo conformational changes to form an open channel or gate through which the ions can move (Fig. 4-18). In this way, ions do not need to cross the lipid-soluble portion of the membrane but can remain in the aqueous solution that fills the ion channel. Ion channels are highly selective; some channels allow only for passage of sodium ions, and others are selective for potassium, calcium, or chloride ions. Specific interactions between the ions and the sides of the channel can produce an extremely rapid rate of ion movement. For example, ion channels can become negatively charged, promoting the rapid movement of positively charged ions.

The plasma membrane contains two basic groups of ion channels: leakage channels and gated channels. Leakage channels are open even in the unstimulated state, whereas gated channels open and close in response to specific stimuli. Three types of gated channels are present in the plasma membrane: *voltage-gated channels,* which have electrically operated gates that open when the membrane potential changes beyond a certain point; *ligand-gated channels,* which have chemically operated gates that respond to specific receptor-bound ligands, such as the neurotransmitter acetylcholine; and *mechanically gated channels,* which open or close in response to such mechanical stimulations as vibrations, tissue stretching, and pressure.

RESTING MEMBRANE POTENTIALS

Electrical potentials exist across the membranes of most cells in the body. Because these potentials occur at the level of the cell membrane, they are called *membrane potentials.* In excitable tissues, such as nerve or muscle cells, changes in the membrane potential are necessary for generation and conduction of nerve impulses and muscle contraction. In other types of cells, such as glandular cells, changes in the membrane potential contribute to hormone secretion and other functions.

Electrical Potentials

Electrical potential, measured in volts (V), describes the ability of separated electrical charges of opposite polarity (+ and –) to do work. The potential difference is the difference between the separated charges. The terms *potential dif-*

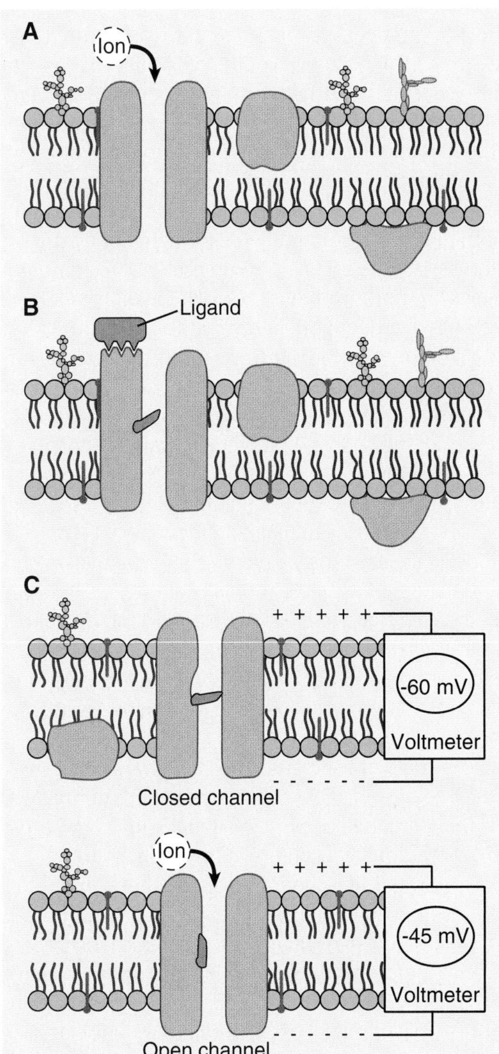

FIGURE 4-18 Ion channels. (**A**) Nongated ion channel remains open, permitting free movement of ions across the membrane. (**B**) Ligand-gated channel is controlled by ligand binding to the receptor. (**C**) Voltage-gated channel is controlled by a change in membrane potential. (Rhoades R.A., Tanner G.A. [1996]. *Medical physiology.* Boston: Little, Brown)

ference and *voltage* are synonymous. Voltage is always measured with respect to two points in a system. For example, the voltage in a car battery (6 or 12 V) is the potential difference between the two battery terminals. Because the total amount of charge that can be separated by a biologic membrane is small, the potential differences are small and are measured in *millivolts* (1/1000 of a volt). Potential differences across the cell membrane can be measured by inserting a very fine electrode into the cell and another into the extracellular fluid surrounding the cell and connecting the two electrodes to a voltmeter (Fig. 4-19). The movement of charge between two points is called *current.* It occurs when a potential difference has been established and a connection is made such that the charged particles can move between the two points.

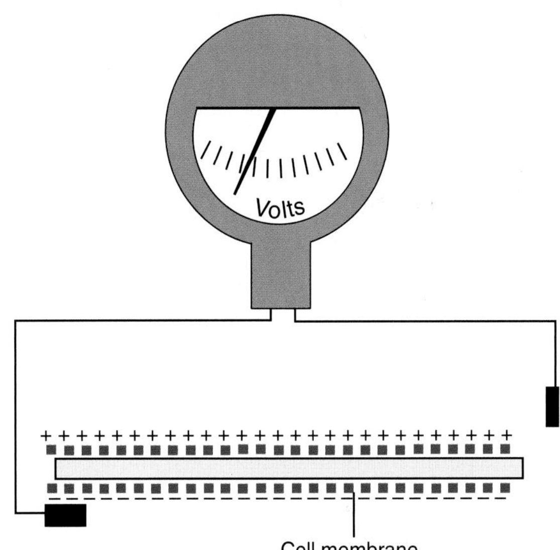

FIGURE 4-19 Alignment of charge along the cell membrane. The electrical potential is negative on the inside of the cell membrane in relation to the outside.

Extracellular and intracellular fluids are electrolyte solutions containing approximately 150 to 160 mmol/L of positively charged ions and an equal concentration of negatively charged ions. These are the current-carrying ions responsible for generating and conducting membrane potentials. Usually, a small excess of positively charged ions exists at the outer surface of the cell membrane. This is represented as positive charges on the outside of the membrane and is balanced by an equal number of negative charges on the inside of the membrane. Because of the extreme thinness of the cell membrane, the accumulation of these ions at the surfaces of the membrane contributes to the establishment of a *resting membrane potential. Action potentials* (discussed in Chapter 49) represent abrupt and pulselike changes in the membrane potential that are propagated along a nerve or muscle fiber. They occur when the membrane potential reaches a threshold level, increasing membrane permeability and allowing charged ions such as sodium to move across the cell membrane.

Diffusion Potentials

A diffusion potential describes the voltage generated by ions that diffuse across the membrane. Two conditions are necessary for a membrane potential to occur by diffusion: the membrane must be selectively permeable, allowing a single type of ion to diffuse through membrane pores, and the concentration of the diffusible ion must be greater on one side of the membrane than on the other. In the resting or unexcited state, when the membrane is highly permeable to potassium, the concentration of potassium ions inside the cell is approximately 35 times greater than outside. Because of the large concentration gradient existing across the cell membrane, potassium ions tend to diffuse outward. As they do so, they carry their positive charges with them, and the inside becomes negative in relation to the outside. This new potential difference repels further outward movement of the positively charged potassium ions. The same phenomenon occurs during an action potential, when the membrane is highly permeable to sodium. Sodium ions move inside the cell, creating a membrane potential of the opposite polarity. An *equilibrium potential* is one in which no net movement of ions occurs because the diffusion and electrical forces are exactly balanced (see accompanying box). For potassium, this represents the *resting membrane potential.*

Variations in Membrane Potentials

The resting membrane potential and membrane excitability can be altered by changes in ion concentration or membrane permeability. For example, calcium ions decrease membrane permeability to sodium ions, and vice versa. If insufficient calcium ions are available, as in severe hypocalcemia, the permeability to sodium increases. As a result, membrane excitability increases—sometimes causing spontaneous muscle movements (tetany) to occur. Local anesthetic agents (*e.g.,* procaine, cocaine) act directly on neural membranes to decrease their permeability to sodium.

CLINICAL APPLICATION

The Nernst Equation for Calculating an Equilibrium Potential

The following equation, known as the *Nernst equation,* can be used to calculate the equilibrium potential (electromotive force [EMF] in millivolts [mV] of a univalent ion at body temperature of 37°C).

$$\text{EMF (mV)} = -61 \times \log_{10} (\text{ion concentration inside/ion concentration outside})$$

For example, if the concentration of an ion inside the membrane is 100 mmol/L and the concentration outside the membrane is 10 mmol/L, the EMF (mV) for that ion would be $-61 \times \log_{10}$ (100/10 [$\log_{10}$ of 10 is 1]). Therefore, it would take 61 mV of charge inside the membrane to balance the diffusion potential created by the concentration difference across the membrane for the ion.

The EMF for potassium ions using a normal estimated intracellular concentration of 140 mmol/L and a normal extracellular concentration of 4 mmol/L is –94 mV:

$$-94 \text{ mV} = -61 \times \log_{10} (140 \text{ mmol inside}/4 \text{ mmol outside})$$

This value assumes the membrane is permeable only to potassium. This value approximates the –70 to –90 mV *resting membrane potential* for nerve fibers measured in laboratory studies.

When a membrane is permeable to several different ions, the diffusion potential reflects the sum of the equilibrium potentials for each of the ions.

In summary, movement of materials across the cell's membrane is essential for survival of the cell. Diffusion is a process by which substances such as ions move from areas of greater concentration to areas of lesser concentration to attempt uniform distribution. Osmosis refers to the diffusion of water molecules through a semipermeable membrane along a concentration gradient. In facilitated diffusion, molecules that cannot normally pass through the cell's membranes can do so with the assistance of a carrier molecule. Diffusion of water molecules by osmosis or ions by facilitated diffusion does not require an expenditure of energy by the cell and is therefore passive in nature. Another type of transport, called *active transport,* requires the cell to expend energy in moving ions against a concentration gradient. Two types of active transport exist, primary and secondary; both require carrier proteins. The Na^+/K^+ ATPase pump is the best-known type of active transport. It is estimated that up to one third of the energy expenditure of the cell is used to maintain the Na^+/K^+ ATPase pump.

Endocytosis is a process by which cells engulf materials from the surrounding medium. Small particles are ingested by a process called *pinocytosis* and larger particles by *phagocytosis.* Some particles require bonding with a ligand, and the process is called *receptor-mediated endocytosis.* Exocytosis involves the removal of large particles from the cell and is essentially the reverse of endocytosis.

Ion channels are integral transmembrane proteins that span the width of the cell membrane and are normally composed of polypeptide or protein subunits that form a gating system. Many ions can diffuse through the cell membrane only if conformational changes occur in the membrane proteins that comprise the ion channel. Two basic groups of ion channels exist: leakage channels and gated channels.

Electrical potentials (negative on the inside and positive on the outside) exist across the membranes of most cells in the body. These electrical potentials result from the selective permeability of the cell membrane to Na^+ and K^+; the presence of nondiffusible anions inside the cell membrane; and the activity of the sodium–potassium membrane pump, which extrudes Na^+ from inside the membrane and returns K^+ to the inside. An equilibrium or diffusion potential is one in which no net movement of ions occurs because the diffusion and electrical forces are exactly balanced.

Body Tissues

After you have completed this section of the chapter, you should be able to meet the following objectives:

- Explain the process of cell differentiation in terms of development of organ systems in the embryo and the continued regeneration of tissues in postnatal life
- Explain the function of stem cells
- Describe the characteristics of the four different tissue types
- Explain the function of intercellular adhesions and junctions
- Characterize the composition and functions of the extracellular components of tissue

In the preceding sections, we discussed the individual cell, its metabolic processes, and mechanisms of communication and replication. Although cells are similar, their structure and function vary according to the special needs of the body. For example, muscle cells perform different functions from skin cells or nerve cells. Groups of cells that are closely associated in structure and have common or similar functions are called *tissues*. Four categories of tissue exist: (1) epithelium, (2) connective (supportive) tissue, (3) muscle, and (4) nerve. These tissues do not exist in isolated units, but in association with each other and in variable proportions, forming different structures and organs. This section provides a brief overview of the cells in each of these four tissue types, the structures that hold these cells together, and the extracellular matrix in which they live.

CELL DIFFERENTIATION

After conception, the fertilized ovum undergoes a series of divisions, ultimately forming approximately 200 different cell types. The formation of different types of cells and the disposition of these cells into tissue types is called *cell differentiation,* a process controlled by a system that switches genes on and off. Embryonic cells must become different to develop into all of the various organ systems, and they must remain different after the signal that initiated cell diversification has disappeared. The process of cell differentiation is controlled by cell memory, which is maintained through regulatory proteins contained in the individual members of a particular cell type. Cell differentiation also involves the sequential activation of multiple genes and their protein products. This means that after differentiation has occurred, the tissue type does not revert to an earlier stage of differentiation. The process of cell differentiation normally moves forward, producing cells that are more specialized than their predecessors. Usually, highly differentiated cell types, such as skeletal muscle and nervous tissue, lose their ability to undergo cell division.

Although most cells differentiate into specialized cell types, many tissues contain a few *stem cells* that apparently are only partially differentiated. These stem cells are still capable of cell division and serve as a reserve source for specialized cells throughout the life of the organism. They are the major source of cells that make regeneration possible in some tissues. Stem cells have varying abilities to differentiate. Some tissues, such as skeletal muscle tissue, lack sufficient numbers of undifferentiated cells and have limited regenerative capacity. Stem cells of the hematopoietic (blood) system have the greatest potential for differentiation. These cells can potentially reconstitute the entire blood-producing and immune systems. They are the major ingredient in bone marrow transplants. Other stem cells, such as those that replenish the mucosal surface of the gastrointestinal tract, are less general but can still differentiate. Cancer cells are thought to originate from undifferentiated stem cells (see Chapter 8).

EMBRYONIC ORIGIN OF TISSUE TYPES

All of the approximately 200 different types of body cells can be classified into four basic or primary tissue types: epithelial, connective, muscle, and nervous (Table 4-1). These basic tissue types are often described by their embryonic origin. The embryo is essentially a three-layered tubular structure (Fig. 4-20). The outer layer of the tube is called the *ectoderm;* the middle layer, the *mesoderm;* and the inner layer, the *endoderm.* All of the adult body tissues originate from these three cellular layers. Epithelium has its origin in all three embryonic layers, connective tissue and muscle develop mainly from the mesoderm, and nervous tissue develops from the ectoderm.

EPITHELIAL TISSUE

Origin and Characteristics

Epithelial tissue forms sheets that cover the body's outer surface, line the internal surfaces, and form the glandular tissue. Underneath all types of epithelial tissue is an extracellular matrix, called the *basement membrane.* A basement membrane consists of the basal lamina and an underlying reticular layer. The terms *basal lamina* and *basement membrane* are often used interchangeably. Epithelial cells have strong intracellular protein filaments (*i.e.,* cytoskeleton) that are important in transmitting mechanical stresses from one cell to another. Cells of epithelial tissue are tightly bound together by specialized junctions. These specialized junctions enable these cells to form barriers to the movement of water, solutes, and cells from one body compartment to the next. Epithelial tissue is avascular (*i.e.,* without blood vessels) and must therefore receive oxygen and nutrients from the capillaries of the connective tissue on which the epithelial tissue rests (Fig. 4-21). Epithelial tissues contain neural receptors (*i.e.,* pressure, thermal, and pain) that serve to sample the internal and external environments. To survive, epithelial tissue must be kept moist. Even the seemingly dry skin epithelium is kept moist by a nonvitalized, waterproof layer of superficial skin cells called *keratin,* which prevents evaporation of moisture from the deeper living cells.

Epithelia are derived from all three embryonic layers. Most epithelia of the skin, mouth, nose, and anus are derived from the ectoderm. Linings of the respiratory tract, the gastrointestinal tract, and the glands of the digestive tract are of endodermal origin. The endothelial lining of blood vessels originates from the mesoderm. Many types of epithelial tissue retain the ability to differentiate and undergo rapid proliferation for replacing injured tissue.

Types of Epithelial Cells

Epithelial tissues are classified according to the shape of the cells and the number of layers that are present: *simple, stratified,* and *pseudostratified.* The terms *squamous* (thin and flat), *cuboidal* (cube shaped), and *columnar* (resembling a column) refer to the cells' shape (Fig. 4-22).

Simple Epithelium. *Simple epithelium* contains a single layer of cells, all of which rest on the basement membrane.

TABLE 4-1 Classification of Tissue Types

Tissue Type	Location
Epithelial Tissue	
Covering and lining of body surfaces	
Simple epithelium	
Squamous	Lining of blood vessels, body cavities, alveoli of lungs
Cuboidal	Collecting tubules of kidney; covering of ovaries
Columnar	Lining of intestine and gallbladder
Stratified epithelium	
Squamous keratinized	Skin
Squamous nonkeratinized	Mucous membranes of mouth, esophagus, and vagina
Cuboidal	Ducts of sweat glands
Columnar	Large ducts of salivary and mammary glands; also found in conjunctiva
Transitional	Bladder, ureters, renal pelvis
Pseudostratified	Tracheal and respiratory passages
Glandular	
Endocrine	Pituitary gland, thyroid gland, adrenal, and other glands
Exocrine	Sweat glands and glands in gastrointestinal tract
Neuroepithelium	Olfactory mucosa, retina, tongue
Reproductive epithelium	Seminiferous tubules of testis; cortical portion of ovary
Connective Tissue	
Embryonic connective tissue	
Mesenchymal	Embryonic mesoderm
Mucous	Umbilical cord (Wharton's jelly)
Adult connective tissue	
Loose or areolar	Subcutaneous areas
Dense regular	Tendons and ligaments
Dense irregular	Dermis of skin
Adipose	Fat pads, subcutaneous layers
Reticular	Framework of lymphoid organs, bone marrow, liver
Specialized connective tissue	
Bone	Long bones, flat bones
Cartilage	Tracheal rings, external ear, articular surfaces
Hematopoietic	Blood cells, myeloid tissue (bone marrow)
Muscle Tissue	
Skeletal	Skeletal muscles
Cardiac	Heart muscles
Smooth	Gastrointestinal tract, blood vessels, bronchi, bladder, and others
Nervous Tissue	
Neurons	Central and peripheral neurons and nerve fibers
Supporting cells	Glial and ependymal cells in central nervous system; Schwann and satellite cells in peripheral nervous system

Simple squamous epithelium is adapted for filtration; it is found lining the blood vessels, lymph nodes, and alveoli of the lungs. The single layer of squamous epithelium lining the heart and blood vessels is known as the *endothelium.* A similar type of layer, called the *mesothelium,* forms the serous membranes that line the pleural, pericardial, and peritoneal cavities and cover the organs of these cavities. A *simple cuboidal epithelium* is found on the surface of the ovary and in the thyroid. *Simple columnar epithelium* lines the intestine. One form of a simple columnar epithelium has hairlike projections called *cilia,* often with specialized mucus-secreting cells called *goblet cells.* This form of simple columnar epithelium lines the airways of the respiratory tract.

Stratified and Pseudostratified Epithelium. *Stratified epithelium* contains more than one layer of cells, with only the deepest layer resting on the basement membrane. It is designed to protect the body surface. *Stratified squamous keratinized* epithelium makes up the epidermis of the skin. *Keratin* is a tough, fibrous protein existing as filaments in the outer cells of skin. A stratified squamous keratinized epithelium is made up of many layers. The layers closest to the underlying tissues are cuboidal or columnar. The cells become more irregular and thinner as they move closer to the surface. Surface cells become totally filled with keratin and die, are sloughed off, and then are replaced by the deeper cells. A stratified squamous nonkeratinized epithelium is found on moist surfaces such as the

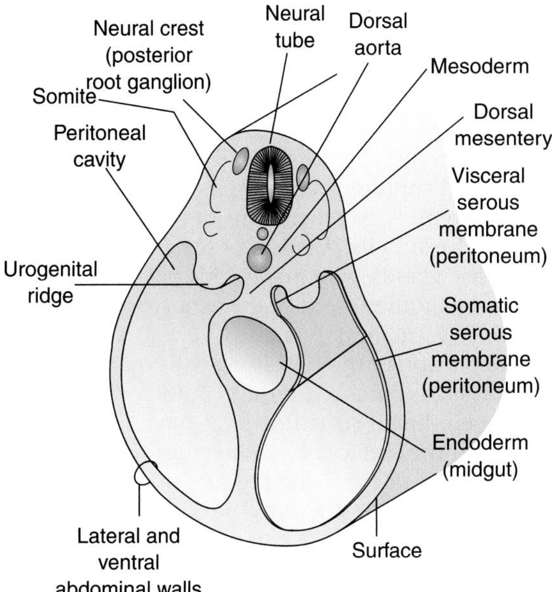

FIGURE 4-20 Cross section of a human embryo illustrating the development of the somatic and visceral structures.

ORGANIZATION OF CELLS INTO TISSUES

- Cells with a similar embryonic origin or function are often organized into larger functional units called *tissues,* and these tissues in turn associate with other, dissimilar tissues to form the various organs of the body.
- Connective tissue is the most abundant tissue of the body. It is found in a variety of forms, ranging from solid bone to blood cells that circulate in the vascular system.
- Epithelial tissue forms sheets that cover the body's outer surface, lines internal surfaces, and forms glandular tissue. It is supported by a basement membrane, is avascular, and must receive nourishment from capillaries in supporting connective tissues.
- Muscle tissue contains actin and myosin filaments that allow it to contract and provide locomotion and movement of skeletal structures (skeletal muscle), pumping of blood through the heart (cardiac muscle), and contraction of blood vessels and visceral organs (smooth muscle).
- Nervous tissue provides the means for controlling body function and for sensing and moving about in the external environment. It consists of two major types of cells: the neurons, which function in communication, and the neuroglial cells, which support the neurons.

mouth and tongue. Stratified cuboidal and columnar epithelia are found in the ducts of salivary glands and the larger ducts of the mammary glands. In smokers, the normal columnar ciliated epithelial cells of the trachea and bronchi are often replaced with stratified squamous epithelium cells that are better able to withstand the irritating effects of cigarette smoke.

Pseudostratified epithelium is a type of epithelium in which all of the cells are in contact with the underlying intercellular matrix, but some do not extend to the surface. A pseudostratified ciliated columnar epithelium with goblet cells forms the lining of most of the upper respiratory tract. All of the tall cells reaching the surface of this type of epithelium are either ciliated cells or mucus-producing goblet cells. The basal cells that do not reach the surface serve as stem cells for ciliated and goblet cells. *Transitional epithelium* is a stratified epithelium characterized by cells that can change shape and become thinner when the tissue is stretched. Such tissue can be stretched without pulling the superficial cells apart. Transitional epithelium is well adapted for the lining of organs that are constantly changing their volume, such as the urinary bladder.

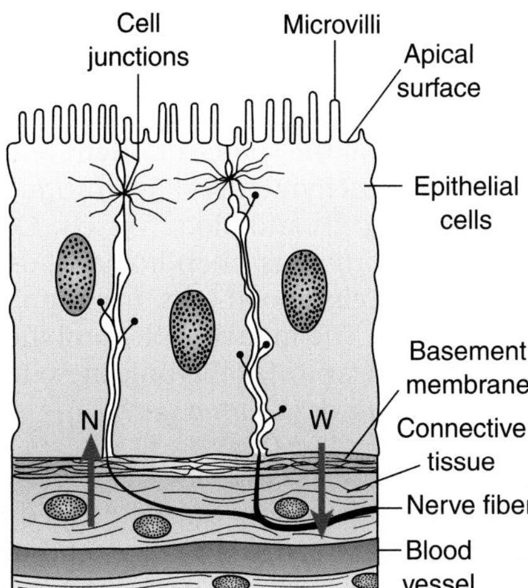

FIGURE 4-21 Typical arrangement of epithelial cells in relation to underlying tissues and blood supply. Epithelial tissue has no blood supply of its own but relies on the blood vessels in the underlying connective tissue for nutrition (**N**) and elimination of wastes (**W**).

Glandular Epithelium. *Glandular epithelial tissue* is formed by cells specialized to produce a fluid secretion. This process is usually accompanied by the intracellular synthesis of macromolecules. The chemical nature of these macromolecules is variable. The macromolecules typically are stored in the cells in small, membrane-bound vesicles called *secretory granules.* For example, glandular epithelia can synthesize, store, and secrete proteins (*e.g.,* insulin), lipids (*e.g.,* adrenocortical hormones, secretions of the sebaceous glands), and complexes of carbohydrates and proteins (*e.g.,* saliva). Less common are secretions such as those produced by the sweat glands, which require minimal synthetic activity.

All glandular cells arise from surface epithelia by means of cell proliferation and invasion of the underlying connective tissue, and all release their contents or secretions into the extracellular compartment. *Exocrine glands,* such as the sweat glands and lactating mammary glands, retain their

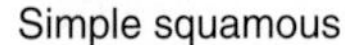

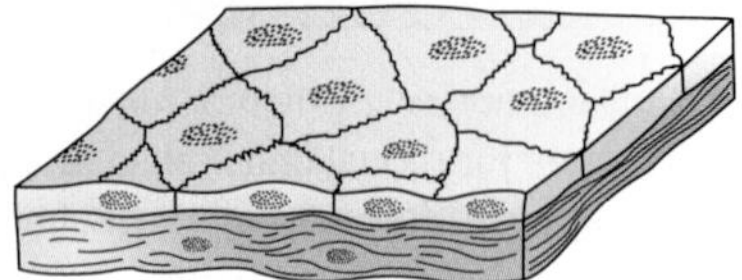

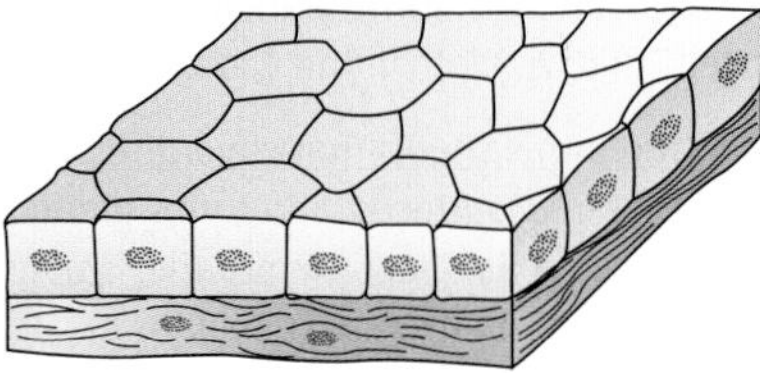

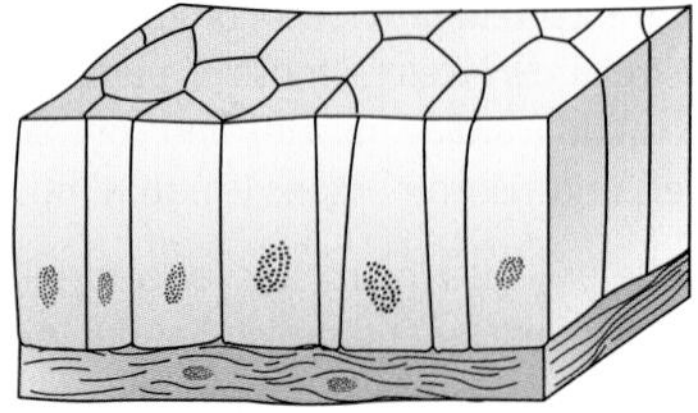

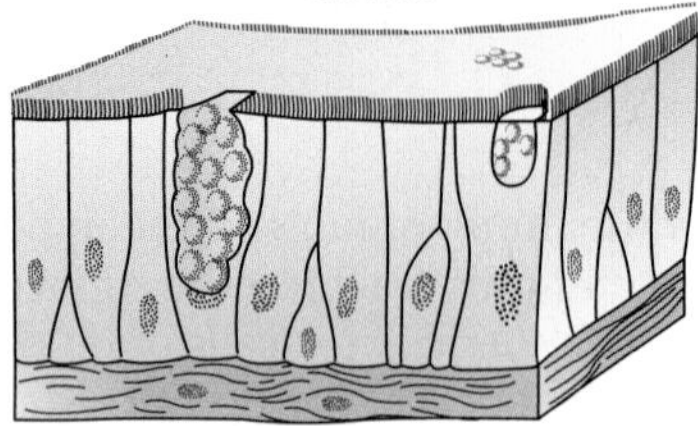

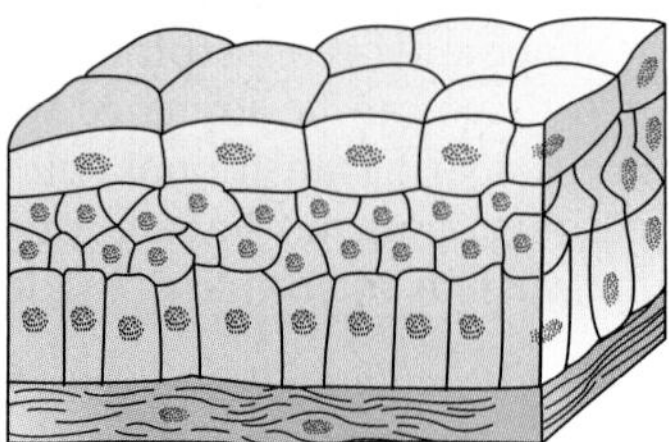

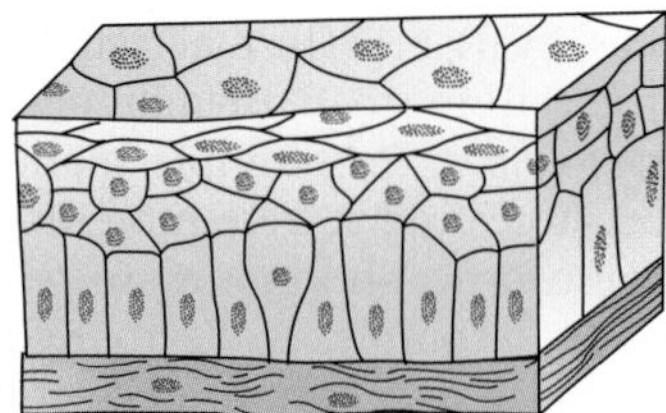

FIGURE 4-22 Representation of the various epithelial tissue types.

connection with the surface epithelium from which they originated. This connection takes the form of epithelium-lined tubular ducts through which the secretions pass to reach the surface. Exocrine glands are often classified according to the way secretory products are released by their cells. In *holocrine*-type cells (*e.g.,* sebaceous glands), the glandular cell ruptures, releasing its entire contents into the duct system. New generations of cells are replaced by mitosis of basal cells. *Merocrine-* or *eccrine*-type glands (*e.g.,* salivary glands, exocrine glands of the pancreas) release their glandular products by exocytosis. In apocrine secretions (*e.g.,* mammary glands, certain sweat glands), the apical portion of the cell, along with small portions of the cytoplasm, is pinched off the glandular cells. *Endocrine glands* are epithelial structures that have had their connection with the surface obliterated during development. These glands are ductless and produce secretions (*i.e.,* hormones) that move directly into the bloodstream.

CONNECTIVE OR SUPPORTIVE TISSUE

Origin and Characteristics

Connective tissue (or supportive tissue) is the most abundant tissue in the body. As its name suggests, it connects and binds or supports the various tissues. The capsules that surround organs of the body are composed of connective tissue. Bone, adipose tissue, and cartilage are specialized types of connective tissue that function to support the soft tissues of the body and store fat. Connective tissue is unique in that its cells produce the extracellular matrix that supports and holds tissues together. Connective tissue has a role in tissue nutrition. The proximity of the extracellular matrix to blood vessels allows it to function as an exchange medium through which nutrients and metabolic wastes pass.

Most connective tissue is derived from the embryonic mesoderm, but some is derived from the neural crest, a derivative of the ectoderm. During embryonic development, mesodermal cells migrate from their site of origin and then surround and penetrate the developing organ. These cells are called *mesenchymal cells,* and the tissue they form is called *mesenchyme.* Tissues derived from embryonic mesenchymal cells include bone, cartilage, and adipose (fat) cells. Besides providing the source or origin of most connective tissues, mesenchyme develops into other structures, such as blood cells and blood vessels. Connective tissue cells include fibroblasts, chondroblasts, osteoblasts, hematopoietic stem cells, blood cells, macrophages, mast cells, and adipocytes. The matrix of the umbilical cord is composed of a second type of embryonic mesoderm called *mucous connective tissue* or *Wharton's jelly.*

Types of Connective Tissue

Adult connective tissue proper can be divided into four types: loose or areolar, reticular, adipose, and dense connective tissue. Dense connective tissue is further subdivided into irregular and regular connective tissue. Specialized connective tissues, such as blood and blood-forming tissues, are discussed in Chapter 14; cartilage and bone are discussed in Chapter 56.

Loose Connective and Adipose Tissue. Loose connective tissue, also known as *areolar tissue,* is soft and pliable. Although it is more cellular than dense connective tissue, it contains large amounts of intercellular substance (Fig. 4-23). It fills spaces between muscle sheaths and forms a layer that encases blood and lymphatic vessels. Areolar connective tissue supports the epithelial tissues and provides the means by which these tissues are nourished. In an organ containing functioning epithelial tissue and supporting connective tissue, the term *parenchymal tissue* is used to describe the functioning epithelium as opposed to the connective tissue framework or stroma.

Cells of loose connective tissue include fibroblasts, mast cells, adipose or fat cells, macrophages, plasma cells, and leukocytes. Loose connective tissue cells secrete substances that form the extracellular matrix that supports and connects body cells. Fibroblasts are the most abundant of these cells. They are responsible for the synthesis of the fibrous and gel-like substance that fills the intercellular spaces of the body and for the production of collagen, elastic, and reticular fibers.

The *basal lamina* is a special type of intercellular matrix that is present where connective tissue contacts the tissue it supports. It is visible only with an electron microscope and is produced by the epithelial cells. In many locations, reticular fibers, produced by the connective tissue cells, are associated with the basal lamina. Together, the basal lamina and the reticular layer form the basement membrane seen by light microscopy. A basement membrane is found along the interface between connective tissue and muscle fibers, on Schwann cells of the peripheral nervous system, on the basal surface of endothelial cells, and on fat cells. These basement membranes bond cells to the underlying or surrounding connective tissues, serve as selective filters for particles that pass between connective tissue and other cells, and contribute to cell regeneration and repair.

Adipose tissue is a special form of connective tissue in which adipocytes predominate. Adipocytes do not generate an extracellular matrix but maintain a large intracellular space. These cells store large quantities of triglycerides and are the largest repository of energy in the body. Adipose tissue helps fill spaces between tissues and helps to keep organs in place. The subcutaneous layers of fat help to shape the body. Because fat is a poor conductor of heat, adipose tissue serves as thermal insulation for the body. Adipose tissue exists in two forms. Unilocular (white) adipose tissue is composed of cells in which the fat is contained in a single, large droplet in the cytoplasm. Multilocular (brown) adipose tissue is composed of cells that contain multiple droplets of fat and numerous mitochondria. These two types of fat are discussed in Chapter 11.

Reticular Connective Tissue. *Reticular tissue* is characterized by a network of reticular fibers associated with reticular cells. These reticular cells are believed to retain

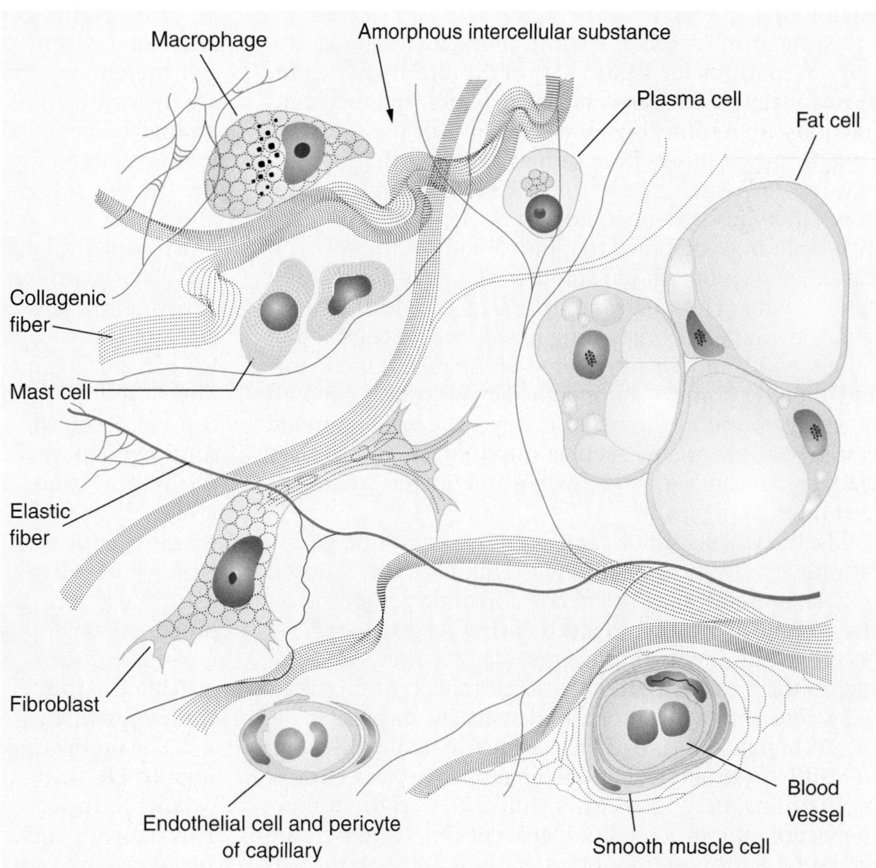

FIGURE 4-23 Diagrammatic representation of cells that may be seen in loose connective tissue. The cells lie in the extracellular matrix that is bathed in tissue fluid that originates in capillaries. (From Cormack D.H. [1987]. *Ham's histology* [9th ed.]. Philadelphia: J.B. Lippincott)

multipotential capabilities similar to undifferentiated mesenchymal cells. Reticular tissues comprise the framework of the liver, bone marrow, and lymphoid tissues such as the spleen.

Dense Connective Tissue. Dense connective tissue exists in two forms: dense irregular and dense regular. Dense irregular connective tissue consists of the same components found in loose connective tissue, but exhibiting a predominance of collagen fibers and fewer cells. This type of tissue can be found in the dermis of the skin (*i.e.,* reticular layer), the fibrous capsules of many organs, and the fibrous sheaths of cartilage (*i.e.,* perichondrium) and bone (*i.e.,* periosteum). It also forms the fascia that invests muscles and organs. Dense regular connective tissues are rich in collagen fibers and form the tendons and aponeuroses that join muscles to bone or other muscles and the ligaments that join bones to bone. Tendons and ligaments are white fibers because of an abundance of collagen. Ligaments such as the ligamenta flava of the vertebral column and the true vocal folds are called *yellow fibers* because of the abundance of elastic fibers.

MUSCLE TISSUE

Three types of muscle tissues exist: *skeletal, cardiac,* and *smooth.* Skeletal and cardiac muscles are striated muscles. The actin and myosin filaments are arranged in large parallel arrays in bundles, giving the muscle fibers a striped or striated appearance when they are viewed through a microscope.

Skeletal muscle is the most abundant tissue in the body, accounting for 40% to 45% of the total body weight. Most skeletal muscles are attached to bones, and their contractions are responsible for movements of the skeleton. Skeletal muscle differs from cardiac and smooth muscle in that it is enervated by the somatic rather than the autonomic nervous system. Cardiac muscle, comprising the myocardium, is designed to pump blood continuously. It has inherent properties of automaticity, rhythmicity, and conductivity. The pumping action of the heart is controlled by impulses originating in the cardiac conduction system and is modified by blood-borne neural mediators and impulses from the autonomic nervous system. Smooth muscle is found in the iris of the eye, the walls of blood vessels, hollow organs such as the stomach and urinary bladder, and hollow tubes, such as the ureters, that connect internal organs.

Neither skeletal nor cardiac muscle can undergo the mitotic activity needed to replace injured cells. Smooth muscle, however, may proliferate and undergo mitotic activity. Some increases in smooth muscle are physiologic, as occurs in the uterus during pregnancy. Other increases, such as the increase in smooth muscle that occurs in the arteries of persons with chronic hypertension, are pathologic.

Although the three types of muscle tissue differ significantly in structure, contractile properties, and control mechanisms, they have many similarities. In the following section, the structural properties of skeletal muscle are presented as the prototype of striated muscle tissue. Smooth muscle and the ways in which it differs from skeletal muscle are also discussed. Cardiac muscle is described in Chapter 23.

Skeletal Muscle

Skeletal muscle tissue is packaged into skeletal muscles that attach to and cover the body skeleton. Each skeletal muscle is a discrete organ made up of hundreds or thousands of muscle fibers. At the periphery of skeletal muscle fibers, randomly scattered satellite cells are found. They represent a source of undifferentiated myoblast cells that may be involved in the limited regeneration capabilities of skeletal muscle. Although muscle fibers predominate, substantial amounts of connective tissue, blood vessels, and nerve fibers are also present.

Organization and Structure. In an intact muscle, the individual muscle fibers are held together by several different layers of connective tissue. Skeletal muscles such as the biceps brachii are surrounded by a dense, irregular connective tissue covering called the *epimysium* (Fig. 4-24). Each muscle is subdivided into smaller bundles called *fascicles,* which are surrounded by a connective tissue covering called the *perimysium.* The number of fascicles and their size vary among muscles. Fascicles consist of many elongated structures called *muscle fibers,* each of which is surrounded by connective tissue called the *endomysium.* Skeletal muscles are syncytial or multinucleated structures, meaning there are no true cell boundaries within a skeletal muscle fiber.

The cytoplasm of the muscle fiber (*i.e.,* sarcoplasm) is contained within the sarcolemma, which represents the cell membrane. Embedded throughout the sarcoplasm are the contractile elements actin and myosin, which are arranged in parallel bundles (*i.e.,* myofibrils). The thin, lighter-staining myofilaments are composed of actin, and the thicker, darker-staining myofilaments are composed of myosin. Each myofibril consists of regularly repeating units along the length of the myofibril; each of these units is called a *sarcomere* (see Fig. 4-24). Sarcomeres are the structural and functional units of cardiac and skeletal muscle. A sarcomere extends from one Z line to another Z line. Within the sarcomere are alternating light and dark bands. The central portion of the sarcomere contains the dark band (A band) containing mainly myosin filaments, with some overlap with actin filaments. Straddling the Z band, the lighter I band contains only actin filaments; therefore, it takes two sarcomeres to complete an I band. An H zone is found in the middle of the A band and represents the region where only myosin filaments are found. In the center of the H zone is a thin, dark band, the M band or line, produced by linkages between the myosin filaments. Z bands consist of short elements that interconnect and provide the thin actin filaments from two adjoining sarcomeres with an anchoring point.

The *sarcoplasmic reticulum,* which is comparable to the smooth ER, is composed of longitudinal tubules that run parallel to the muscle fiber and surround each myofibril. This network ends in enlarged, saclike regions called the *lateral sacs* or *terminal cisternae.* These sacs store calcium to

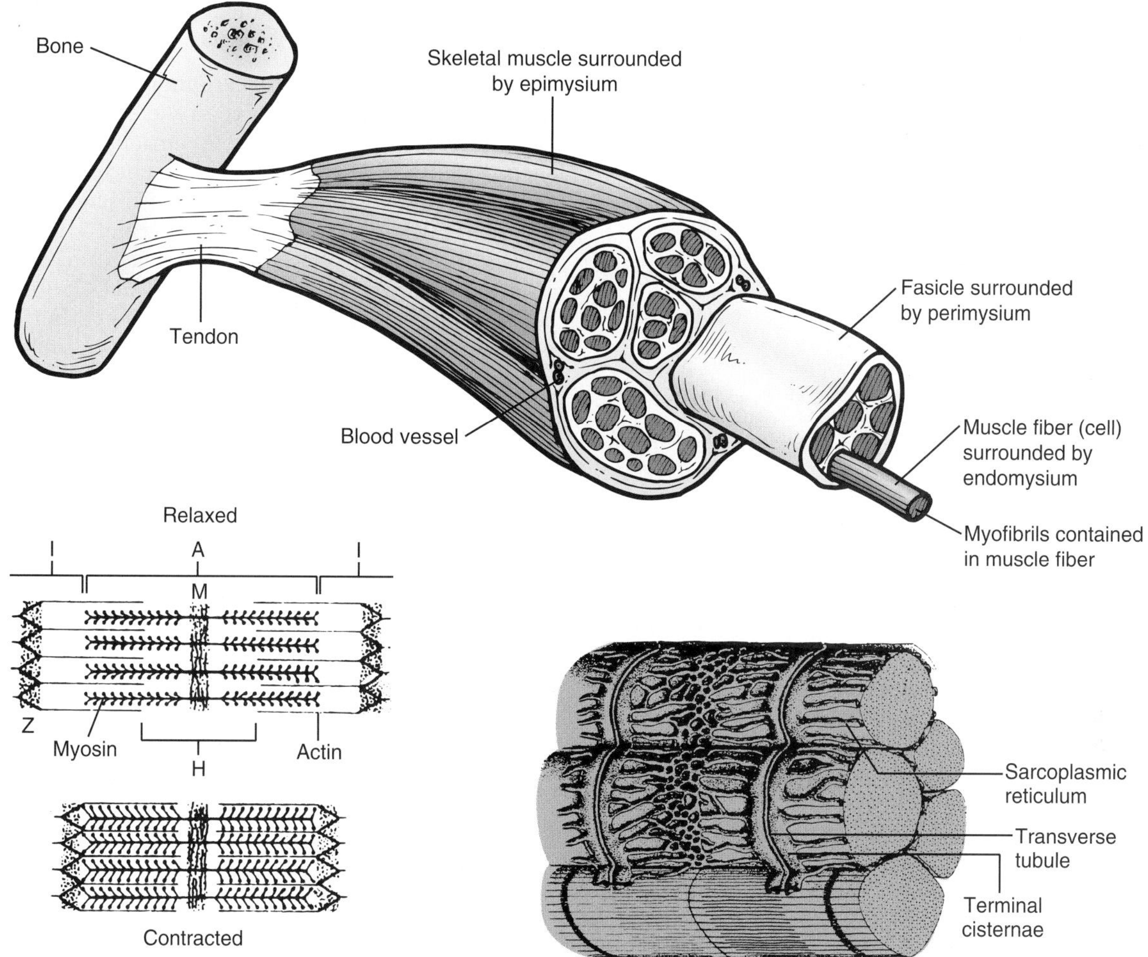

FIGURE 4-24 Connective tissue components of a skeletal muscle. The structure of the myofibril and the relationship between actin and myosin myofilaments are also shown.

be released during muscle contraction. A binding protein called *calsequestrin* found in the terminal cisternae enables a high concentration of calcium ions to be sequestered in the cisternae. Concentration levels of calcium ions in the cisternae are 10,000 times higher than in the sarcoplasm.

A second system of tubules consists of the *transverse* or *T tubules,* which are extensions of the plasma membrane and run perpendicular to the muscle fiber. The hollow portion or lumen of the transverse tubule is continuous with the extracellular fluid compartment. Action potentials, which are rapidly conducted over the surface of the muscle fiber, are in turn propagated by the T tubules and into the sarcoplasmic reticulum. As the action potential moves through the lateral sacs, the sacs release calcium, initiating muscle contraction. The membrane of the sarcoplasmic reticulum also has an active transport mechanism for pumping calcium ions back into the reticulum. This prevents interactions between calcium ions and the actin and myosin myofilaments after cessation of a muscle contraction.

Skeletal Muscle Contraction. During muscle contraction, the thick myosin and thin actin filaments slide over each other, causing shortening of the muscle fiber, although the length of the individual thick and thin filaments remains unchanged. The structures that produce the sliding of the filaments are the myosin heads that form cross-bridges with the thin actin filaments (Fig. 4-25). When activated by ATP, the cross-bridges swivel in a fixed arc, much like the oars of a boat, as they become attached to the actin filament. During contraction, each cross-bridge undergoes its own cycle of movement, forming a bridge attachment and releasing it, and moving to another site where the same sequence of movement occurs. This pulls the thin and thick filaments past each other.

Myosin is the chief constituent of the thick filament. It consists of a thin tail, which provides the structural backbone for the filament, and a globular head. Each globular head contains a binding site able to bind to a complementary site on the actin molecule. Besides the binding site for actin, each myosin head has a separate active site that catalyzes the breakdown of ATP to provide the energy needed to activate the myosin head so that it can form a cross-bridge with actin. After contraction, myosin also binds ATP, thus breaking the linkage between actin and myosin.

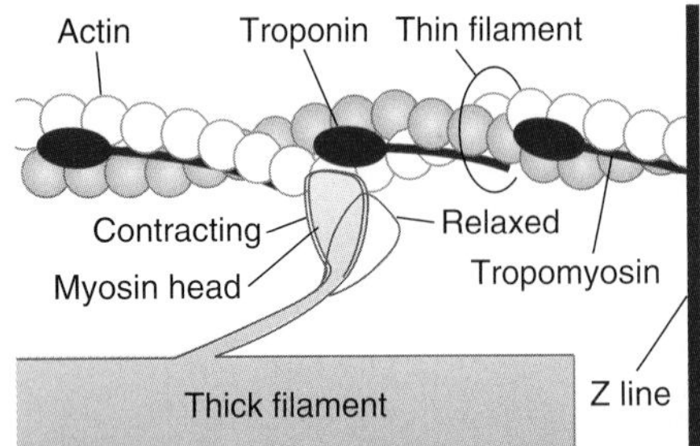

FIGURE 4-25 Molecular structure of the thin actin filament and the thicker myosin filament of striated muscle. The thin filament is a double-stranded helix of actin molecules with tropomyosin and troponin molecules lying along the grooves of the actin strands. During muscle contraction, the ATP-activated heads of the thick myosin filament swivel into position, much like the oars on a boat, form a cross-bridge with a reactive site on tropomyosin, and then pull the actin filament forward. During muscle relaxation, the troponin molecules cover the reactive sites on tropomyosin.

Myosin molecules are bundled together side by side in the thick filaments such that one half have their heads toward one end of the filament and their tails toward the other end; the other half are arranged in the opposite manner. The thin filaments are composed mainly of actin, a globular protein lined up in two rows that coil around each other to form a long helical strand. Associated with each actin filament are two regulatory proteins, tropomyosin and troponin (see Fig. 4-25). *Tropomyosin,* which lies in grooves of the actin strand, provides the site for attachment of the globular heads of the myosin filament. In the noncontracted state, *troponin* covers the tropomyosin-binding sites and prevents formation of cross-bridges between the actin and myosin. During an action potential, calcium ions released from the sarcoplasmic reticulum diffuse to the adjacent myofibrils, where they bind to troponin. Binding of calcium to troponin uncovers the tropomyosin-binding sites such that the myosin heads can attach and form cross-bridges. Energy from ATP is used to break the actin and myosin cross-bridges, stopping the muscle contraction. After breaking of the linkage between actin and myosin, the concentration of calcium around the myofibrils decreases as calcium is actively transported into the sarcoplasmic reticulum by a membrane pump that uses energy derived from ATP.

The basis of rigor mortis can be explained by the binding of actin and myosin. As the muscle begins to degenerate after death, the sarcoplasmic cisternae release their calcium ions, which enable the myosin heads to combine with their sites on the actin molecule. As ATP supplies diminish, no energy source is available to start the normal interaction between actin and myosin, and the muscle is in a state of rigor until further degeneration destroys the cross-bridges between actin and myosin.

Smooth Muscle

Smooth muscle is often called *involuntary muscle* because its activity arises spontaneously or through activity of the autonomic nervous system. Smooth muscle contractions are slower and more sustained than skeletal or cardiac muscle contractions.

Organization and Structure. Smooth muscle cells are spindle shaped and smaller than skeletal muscle fibers. Each smooth muscle cell has one centrally positioned nucleus. Z bands or M lines are not present in smooth muscle fibers, and the cross-striations are absent because the bundles of filaments are not parallel but crisscross obliquely through the cell. Instead, the actin filaments are attached to structures called *dense bodies.* Some dense bodies are attached to the cell membrane; others are dispersed in the cell and linked together by structural proteins (Fig. 4-26).

The lack of Z lines and of regular overlapping of the contractile elements provides a greater range of tension development. This is important in hollow organs that undergo changes in volume, with consequent changes in the length of the smooth muscle fibers in their walls. Even with the distention of a hollow organ, the smooth muscle fiber retains some ability to develop tension, whereas such distention would stretch skeletal muscle beyond the area where the thick and thin filaments overlap.

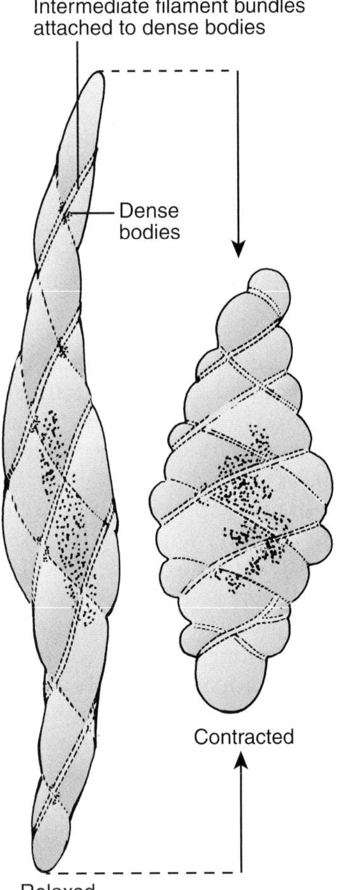

FIGURE 4-26 Structure of smooth muscle showing the dense bodies. In smooth muscle, the force of contraction is transmitted to the cell membrane by bundles of intermediate fibers. (Cormack D.H. [1993]. *Essential histology* [p. 229]. Philadelphia: J.B. Lippincott).

Smooth muscle is usually arranged in sheets or bundles. In hollow organs, such as the intestines, the bundles are organized into the two-layered muscularis externa consisting of an outer, longitudinal layer and an inner, circular layer. A thinner muscularis mucosa often lies between the muscularis externa and the endothelium. In blood vessels, the bundles are arranged circularly or helically around the vessel wall.

Smooth Muscle Contraction. As with cardiac and skeletal muscle, smooth muscle contraction is initiated by an increase in intracellular calcium. However, smooth muscle differs from skeletal muscle in the way its cross-bridges are formed. The sarcoplasmic reticulum of smooth muscle is less developed than in skeletal muscle, and no transverse tubules are present. Smooth muscle relies on the entrance of extracellular calcium and its release from the sarcoplasmic reticulum for muscle contraction. This dependence on movement of extracellular calcium across the cell membrane during muscle contraction is the basis for the action of calcium-blocking drugs used in treatment of cardiovascular disease.

Smooth muscle also lacks the calcium-binding regulatory protein, troponin, which is found in skeletal and cardiac muscle. Instead, it relies on another calcium-binding protein called *calmodulin*. The calcium–calmodulin complex binds to and activates the myosin-containing thick filaments, which interact with actin.

Types of Smooth Muscle. Smooth muscle may be divided into two broad categories according to the mode of activation: multiunit and single-unit smooth muscle. In *multiunit* smooth muscle, each unit operates almost independently of the others and is often enervated by a single nerve, such as occurs in skeletal muscle. It has little or no inherent activity and depends on the autonomic nervous system for its activation. This type of smooth muscle is found in the iris, in the walls of the vas deferens, and attached to hairs in the skin. The fibers in *single-unit* smooth muscle are in close contact with each other and can contract spontaneously without nerve or hormonal stimulation. Normally, most muscle fibers contract synchronously, hence the term *single-unit* smooth muscle. Some single-unit smooth muscle, such as that found in the gastrointestinal tract, is self-excitable. This is usually associated with a basic slow-wave rhythm transmitted from cell to cell by nexus (*i.e.*, gap junctions) formed by the fusion of adjacent cell membranes. The cause of this slow wave is unknown. The intensity of contraction increases with the frequency of the action potential. Certain hormones, other agents, and local factors can modify smooth muscle activity by depolarizing or hyperpolarizing the membrane. Smooth muscle cells found in the uterus and small-diameter blood vessels are also single-unit smooth muscle.

NERVE TISSUE

Nerve tissue is distributed throughout the body as an integrated communication system. Anatomically, the nervous system is divided into the central nervous system (CNS), which consists of the brain and spinal cord, and the peripheral nervous system (PNS), composed of nerve fibers and ganglia that exist outside the CNS. Nerve cells develop from the embryonic ectoderm. Nerve cells are highly differentiated and therefore incapable of regeneration in postnatal life. Embryonic development of the nervous system and the structure and functions of the nervous system are discussed more fully in Chapter 50.

Structurally, nerve tissue consists of two cell types: nerve cells or neurons and glial or supporting cells. Most nerve cells consist of three parts: the soma or cell body, dendrites, and axon. The cytoplasm-filled dendrites, which are multiple, elongated processes, receive and carry stimuli from the environment, from sensory epithelial cells, and from other neurons to the cell. The axon, which is a single cytoplasm-filled process, is specialized for generating and conducting nerve impulses away from the cell body to other nerve cells, muscle cells, and glandular cells.

Neurons can be classified as afferent and efferent neurons according to their function. Afferent or sensory neurons carry information toward the CNS; they are involved in the reception of sensory information from the external environment and from within the body. Efferent or motor neurons carry information away from the CNS; they are needed for control of muscle fibers and endocrine and exocrine glands.

Communication between neurons and effector organs, such as muscle cells, occurs at specialized structures called *synapses*. At the synapse, chemical messengers (*i.e.*, neurotransmitters) alter the membrane potential to conduct impulses from one nerve to another or from a neuron to an effector cell. In addition, electrical synapses exist in which nerve cells are linked through gap junctions that permit the passage of ions from one cell to another.

Neuroglia (*glia* means "glue") are the cells that support neurons, form myelin, and have trophic and phagocytic functions. Four types of neuroglia are found in the CNS: astrocytes, oligodendrocytes, microglia, and ependymal cells. Astrocytes are the most abundant of the neuroglia. They have many long processes that surround blood vessels in the CNS. They provide structural support for the neurons, and their extensions form a sealed barrier that protects the CNS. The oligodendrocytes provide myelination of neuronal processes in the CNS. The microglia are phagocytic cells that represent the mononuclear phagocytic system in the nervous system. Ependymal cells line the cavities of the brain and spinal cord and are in contact with the cerebrospinal fluid. In the PNS, supporting cells consist of the Schwann and satellite cells. The Schwann cells provide myelination of the axons and dendrites, and the satellite cells enclose and protect the dorsal root ganglia and autonomic ganglion cells.

EXTRACELLULAR TISSUE COMPONENTS

The discussion thus far has focused on the cellular components of the different tissue types. Within tissues, cells are held together by cell junctions; the space between cells is filled with an extracellular matrix; and adhesion molecules form intercellular contacts.

Cell Junctions and Cell-to-Cell Adhesions

Cell junctions occur at many points in cell-to-cell contact, but they are particularly plentiful and important in epithelial tissue. Four basic types of intercellular junctions are observed: tight junctions, adhering junctions, gap junctions, and hemidesmosomes (Fig. 4-27). Often, the cells in epithelial tissue are joined by all four types of junctions.

Tight Junctions. *Continuous tight* or occluding junctions (*i.e.,* zona occludens), which are found only in epithelial tissue, seal the surface membranes of adjacent cells together. This type of intercellular junction prevents materials such as macromolecules present in the intestinal contents from entering the intercellular space.

Adhering Junctions. *Adhering junctions* represent a site of strong adhesion between cells. The primary role of adhering junctions may be that of preventing cell separation. Adhering junctions are not restricted to epithelial tissue; they provide adherence between adjacent cardiac muscle cells as well. Adhering junctions are found as continuous, beltlike adhesive junctions (*i.e.,* zonula adherens), or scattered, spotlike adhesive junctions called *desmosomes* (*i.e.,* macula adherens). A special feature of the adhesion belt junction is that it provides a site for anchorage of microfilaments to the cell membrane. In epithelial desmosomes, bundles of keratin-containing intermediate filaments (*i.e.,* tonofilaments) are anchored to the junction on the cytoplasmic area of the cell membrane. A primary disease of desmosomes is pemphigus. This disease is caused by a buildup of antibodies to the proteins of the desmosomes. Persons affected have skin and mucous membrane blistering.

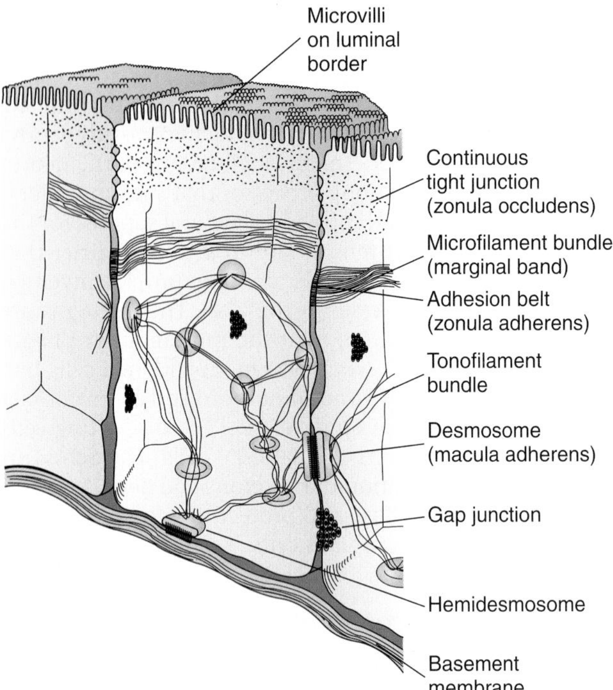

FIGURE 4-27 The chief types of intercellular junctions found in epithelial tissue. (From Cormack D.H. [1993]. *Essential histology.* Philadelphia: J.B. Lippincott)

Gap Junctions. *Gap junctions,* or *nexus junctions,* involve the close adherence of adjoining cell membranes with the formation of channels that link the cytoplasm of the two cells. Gap junctions are not unique to epithelial tissue; they play an essential role in many types of cell-to-cell communication. Because they are low-resistance channels, gap junctions are important in cell-to-cell conduction of electrical signals (*e.g.,* between cells in sheets of smooth muscle or between adjacent cardiac muscle cells, where they function as electrical synapses). These multiple communication channels also enable ions and small molecules to pass directly from one cell to another. Gap junctions are associated with a variety of diseases, among which are inner ear deafness, cardiac arrhythmias, and Charcot-Marie-Tooth disease (the most common inherited peripheral neuropathy).

Hemidesmosomes. Hemidesmosomes are another type of junction. They are found at the base of epithelial cells and help attach the epithelial cell to the underlying connective tissue. They resemble half a desmosome, hence their name.

Extracellular Matrix

Tissues are not made up solely of cells. A large part of their volume is made up of an extracellular matrix. This matrix is composed of a variety of proteins and polysaccharides (*i.e.,* a molecule made up of many sugars). These proteins and polysaccharides are secreted locally and are organized into a supporting meshwork in close association with the cells that produced them. The amount and composition of the matrix vary with the different tissues and their function. In bone, for example, the matrix is more plentiful than the cells that surround it; in the brain, the cells are much more abundant, and the matrix is only a minor constituent.

Two main classes of extracellular macromolecules make up the extracellular matrix. The first is composed of polysaccharide chains of a class called *glycosaminoglycans* (GAGs), which are usually found linked to protein as proteoglycans. The second type consists of the fibrous proteins (*i.e.,* collagen and elastin) and the fibrous adhesive proteins (*i.e.,* fibronectin and laminin) that are found in the basement membrane. Members of each of these two classes of extracellular macromolecules come in a variety of shapes and sizes.

The proteoglycan and GAG molecules in connective tissue form a highly hydrated, gel-like substance, or tissue gel, in which the fibrous proteins are embedded. The polysaccharide gel resists compressive forces, the collagen fibers strengthen and help organize the matrix, the rubber-like elastin adds resilience, and the adhesive proteins help cells attach to the appropriate part of the matrix. Polysaccharides in the tissue gel are highly hydrophilic, and they form gels even at low concentrations. They also accumulate a negative charge that attracts cations such as sodium, which are osmotically active, causing large amounts of water to be sucked into the matrix. This creates a swelling pressure, or turgor, that enables the matrix to withstand extensive compressive forces. This is in contrast to collagen, which resists stretching forces. For example, the cartilage matrix that lines the knee joint can support pressures of hundreds of atmospheres by this mechanism.

Glycosaminoglycan and proteoglycan molecules in connective tissue usually constitute less than 10% by weight of fibrous tissue. Because they form a hydrated gel, the molecules fill most of the extracellular space, providing mechanical support to the tissues while ensuring rapid diffusion of water and electrolytes and the migration of cells. One GAG, hyaluronan or hyaluronic acid, is thought to play an important role as a space-filler during embryonic development. It creates a cell-free space into which cells subsequently migrate. When cell migration and organ development are complete, the excess hyaluronan is degraded by the enzyme hyaluronidase. Hyaluronan is also important in directing the cell replacement that occurs during wound repair (see Chapter 20).

Three types of fibers are found in the extracellular space: collagen, elastin, and reticular fibers. *Collagen* is the most common protein in the body. It is a tough white fiber that serves as the structural framework for skin, ligaments, tendons, and many other structures. *Elastin* acts like a rubber band; it can be stretched and then returns to its original form. Elastin fibers are abundant in structures subjected to frequent stretching, such as the aorta and some ligaments. *Reticular fibers* are extremely thin fibers that create a flexible network in organs subjected to changes in form or volume, such as the spleen, liver, uterus, or intestinal muscle layer.

Adhesion Molecules

Important classes of extracellular macromolecules are the adhesion molecules. The two major classes of adhesion molecules that provide and maintain intercellular contacts are calcium ion–dependent and calcium ion–independent adhesion molecules. The calcium-dependent adhesion molecules include the *cadherins* and some *selectins,* whereas the calcium-independent adhesion molecules include the integrins, the magnesium ion–dependent selectins, and the immunoglobulin superfamily (*neural cell adhesion molecules* [NCAMs] and *intercellular adhesion molecules* [ICAMs]).

Cadherins. Cadherins link parts of the internal cytoskeleton (actin and structures called catenins) with extracellular cadherins of an adjacent cell. This type of linkage is called *homophilic,* meaning that molecules on one cell bind to other molecules of the same type on adjacent cells (Fig. 4-28). More than 40 different types of cadherins are known, and they are found in such intercellular junctions as the zonula and macula adherens.

Selectins. Selectins bind carbohydrates present on the ligands of an adjacent cell in a *heterophilic* type of interaction (see Fig. 4-28). In heterophilic interactions, the molecules on one cell bind to molecules of a different type on adjacent cells. Selectins are found on activated endothelial cells of blood vessels, on leukocytes, and on platelets. They, together with integrins and immunoglobulins (Ig), participate in leukocyte movement through the endothelial lining of blood vessels during inflammation.

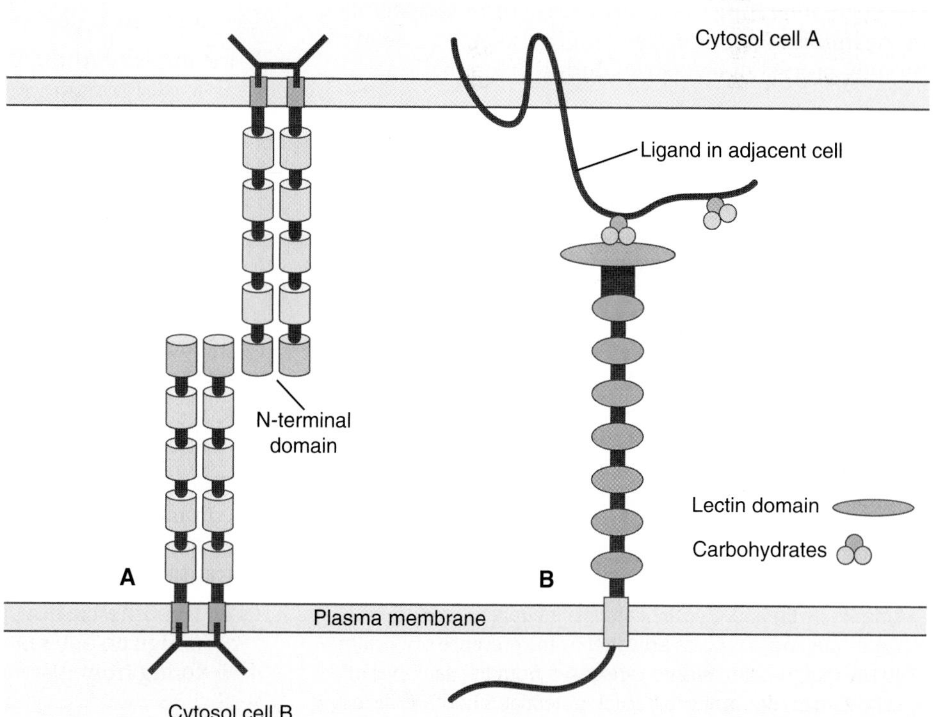

FIGURE 4-28 Homophilic and heterophilic cell adhesions. Examples of a homophilic intercellular adhesion between two identical cadherin dimer molecules joined at the N-terminal domain (**A**) and a heterophilic binding of the lectin domain of an integrin with the carbohydrate portions of a ligand (**B**). (Courtesy Edward W. Carroll.)

Integrins. Integrins usually assist in attaching epithelial cells to the underlying basement membrane. Unlike other cell adhesion molecules, they are heterodimers consisting of alpha and beta subunits. Extracellularly, they are attached to fibronectin and laminin, the two major components of the basement membrane. Like the cadherins, their intracellular portion is linked to actin (see Fig. 4-28).

One group of integrins is associated with hemidesmosomes, whereas others are associated with the surface of white blood cells, macrophages, and platelets. Integrins usually have a weak affinity for their ligands unless they are associated with cellular focal contacts and hemidesmosomes. This allows some movement between cells except where a firm attachment is required to attach epithelial cells to the underlying connective tissue.

Certain integrins play an important role in allowing white blood cells to pass through the vessel wall, a process called *transmigration*. Persons affected with leukocyte adhesion deficiency are unable to synthesize appropriate integrin molecules. As a result, they experience repeated bacterial infections because their white blood cells are not able to transmigrate through vessel walls.

Immunoglobulin Superfamily. NCAMs belong to a super family of immunoglobulins that includes several related types. All types are calcium ion independent but, unlike other adhesion molecules, may participate in homophilic or heterophilic interactions. Heterophilic attachments are to other members of the superfamily such as ICAMs and vascular cell adhesion molecules (VCAMS). During early development of the central nervous system, cells at the roof of neural tube express high levels of NCAMs on their cell surface and are unable to move because of intercellular adhesions. Future neural crest cells lose their NCAMs and begin migrating to various areas of the body. Members of the immunoglobulin superfamily also play a role in the homing process of leukocytes during inflammation.

In summary, body cells are organized into four basic tissue types: epithelial, connective, muscle, and nervous. The epithelium covers and lines the body surfaces and forms the functional components of glandular structures. Epithelial tissue is classified into three types according to the shape of the cells and the number of layers that are present: simple, stratified, and pseudostratified. The cells in epithelial tissue are held together by four types of intercellular junctions: tight, adhering, gap, and hemidesmosomes. Connective tissue supports and connects body structures; it forms the bones and skeletal system, the joint structures, the blood cells, and the intercellular substances. Adult connective tissue can be divided into four types: loose or areolar, reticular, adipose, and dense (regular and irregular).

Muscle tissue is a specialized tissue designed for contractility. Three types of muscle tissue exist: skeletal, cardiac, and smooth. Actin and myosin filaments interact to produce muscle shortening, a process activated by the presence of calcium. In skeletal muscle, calcium is released from the sarcoplasmic reticulum in response to an action potential. Smooth muscle is often called *involuntary muscle* because it contracts spontaneously or through activity of the autonomic nervous system. It differs from skeletal muscle in that its sarcoplasmic reticulum is less defined and it depends on the entry of extracellular calcium ions for muscle contraction.

Nervous tissue is designed for communication purposes and includes the neurons, the supporting neural structures, and the ependymal cells that line the ventricles of the brain and the spinal canal.

The extracellular matrix is made up of a variety of proteins and polysaccharides. These proteins and polysaccharides are secreted locally and are organized into a supporting meshwork in close association with the cells that produced them. The amount and composition of matrix vary with the different tissues and their function. Extracellular fibers include collagen fibers, which compose tendons and ligaments; elastic fibers, found in large arteries and some ligaments; and thin reticular fibers, which are plentiful in organs that are subject to a change in volume (*e.g.,* spleen and liver).

Cell adhesion molecules are an important set of macromolecule having a variety of structures and functions. These functions include leukocyte migration into extracellular tissue and integral structural components of several cell-to-cell junctions, such as desmosomes. Other adhesion molecules are involved in attaching epithelial cells to the underlying connective tissue by way of hemidesmosomes.

REVIEW EXERCISES

Tattoos consist of pigments that have been injected into the skin.

A. Explain what happens to the dye once it is injected and why it does not eventually wash away.

Insulin is synthesized in the beta cells of the pancreas as a prohormone and then is secreted as an active hormone.

A. Using your knowledge of the function of DNA, the RNAs, the endoplasmic reticulum, and the Golgi complex, propose a pathway for the synthesis of insulin.

Persons who drink sufficient amounts of alcohol display rapid changes in central nervous system function, including both motor and behavioral changes, and the odor of alcohol can be detected on their breath.

A. Use the concepts related to lipid bilayer structure of the cell membrane to explain this observation.

The absorption of glucose from the intestine involves a cotransport mechanism in which the active primary transport of sodium is used to provide for the secondary transport of glucose.

A. Hypothesize how this information might be used to design an oral rehydration solution for someone suffering from diarrhea.

Bibliography

Alberts B., Johnson A., Lewis J., et al. (2002). *Molecular biology of the cell* (4th ed., pp. 129–188, 583–614, 771–792, 852–870, 1065–1126). New York: Garland Science.

Ashcroft F.M. (2000). *Ion channels and disease* (pp. 67–96, 95–133, 211–229). San Diego: Academic Press.

Baserga R. (1999). Introduction to the cell cycle. In Stein G.S., Baserga R., Giordano A., Denhardt D.T. (Eds.). *The molecular basis of cell cycle and growth control* (pp. 1–14). New York: Wiley-Liss.

Goldberg A.L., Elledge S.J., Harper J.W. (2001). The cellular chamber of doom. *Scientific American* 68–73.

Guyton A.C., Hall J.E. (2000). *Textbook of medical physiology* (10th ed., p. 85). Philadelphia: W. B. Saunders.

Joachim F. (1998). How the ribosome works. *American Scientist* *86*(5), 428–439.

Kerr J.B. (1999). *Atlas of functional histology* (pp. 1–24, 25–37, 81–106). London: Mosby.

Kierszenbaum A.L. (2003). *Histology and cell biology: An introduction to pathology* (pp. 65–68; 91). St. Louis: Mosby.

Kimball Biology Pages. (2000, May 21). The cell cycle. [On-line]. Available at: http://www.ultranet.com/~jkimball/BiologyPages/C/CellCycle.html. Accessed July 24, 2000.

Kumar V., Cotran R.S., Robbins S.L. (2003). *Robbins' basic pathology* (7th ed., pp. 221–225, 464–465, 838–839, 841–843). Philadelphia: W. B. Saunders.

Mathews C.K., van Holde K.E., Ahern K.G. (2000). *Biochemistry* (3rd ed., pp. 446–482). San Francisco: Benjamin/Cummings.

Moore K.L., Persaud T.V.N. (2003). *The developing human: Clinically oriented embryology* (7th ed., pp. 15–42). Philadelphia: W. B. Saunders.

Nelson D.L., Cox M.M. (2000). *Lehninger's principles of biochemistry* (3rd ed., pp. 567–597). New York: Worth Publishers.

Thiry M., Goessens G. (1996). Historical overview. In *Molecular biology intelligence unit: The nucleolus during the cell cycle.* (pp. 1–11). Georgetown, TX: R. G. Landes Co.

Tortora G.J., Grabowski S.R. (2003). *Principles of anatomy and physiology* (10th ed., pp. 59–102, 273–307, 385–418). New York: John Wiley & Sons.

United Mitochondrial Disease Foundation. (2001). *Mitochondrial disease: Basis of disease.* [On-line]. Available at http://www.umdf.org/mitodisease. Accessed June 20, 2001.

Wallace D.C. (1997). Mitochondrial DNA in aging and disease. *Scientific American 277*(2), 40–47.

CHAPTER

5

Cellular Adaptation, Injury, and Death

When confronted with stresses that endanger its normal structure and function, the cell undergoes adaptive changes that permit survival and maintenance of function. It is only when the stress is overwhelming or adaptation is ineffective that cell injury and death occur. This chapter focuses on cellular adaptation, injury, and death.

Cellular Adaptation

After you have completed this section of the chapter, you should be able to meet the following objectives:

- ✦ Cite the general purpose of changes in cell structure and function that occur as the result of normal adaptive processes
- ✦ Describe cell changes that occur with atrophy, hypertrophy, hyperplasia, metaplasia, and dysplasia and state general conditions under which the changes occur
- ✦ Cite three sources of intracellular accumulations
- ✦ Compare the pathogenesis and effects of dystrophic and metastatic calcifications

Cells adapt to changes in the internal environment, just as the total organism adapts to changes in the external environment. Cells may adapt by undergoing changes in size, number, and type. These changes, occurring singly or in combination, may lead to atrophy, hypertrophy, hyperplasia, metaplasia, and dysplasia (Fig. 5-1). Adaptive cellular responses also include intracellular accumulations and storage of products in abnormal amounts.[1,2]

Numerous molecular mechanisms mediate cellular adaptation, including factors produced by other cells or by the cells themselves. These mechanisms depend largely on signals transmitted by chemical messengers that exert their effects by altering gene function. In general, the genes expressed in all cells fall into two categories: "housekeeping" genes that are necessary for normal function of a cell, and genes that determine the differentiating characteristics of a particular cell type. In many adaptive cellular responses, the expression of the differentiation genes is altered, whereas that of the housekeeping genes remains unaffected. Thus, a cell is able to change size or form without compromising its normal function. Once the stimulus for adaptation is removed, the effect on expression of the differentiating genes is removed, and the cell resumes its previous state of specialized function. Whether adaptive cellular changes are normal or abnormal depends on whether the response was mediated by an appropriate stimulus. Normal adaptive responses occur in response to need and an appropriate stimulus. After the need has been removed, the adaptive response ceases.

ATROPHY

When confronted with a decrease in work demands or adverse environmental conditions, most cells are able to revert to a smaller size and a lower and more efficient level

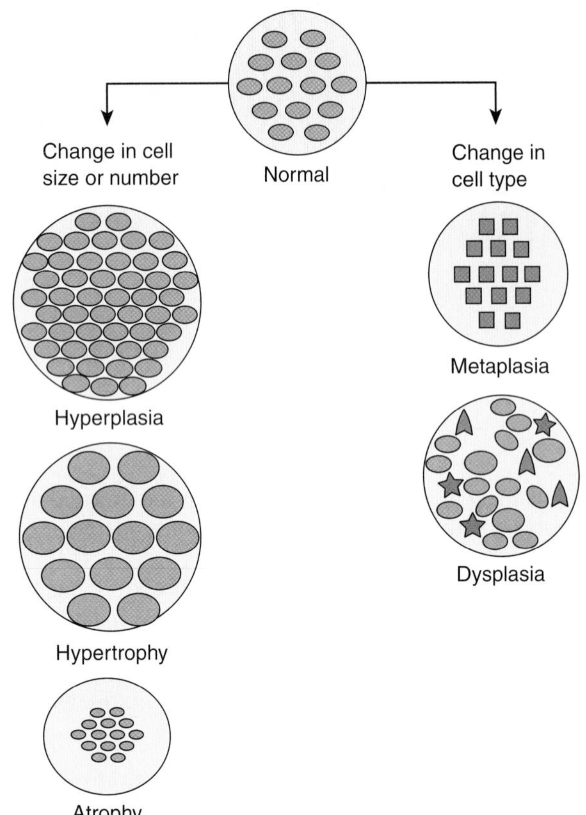

FIGURE 5-1 Adaptive tissue (*large circles*) and cell responses involving a change in number (hyperplasia), cell size (hypertrophy and atrophy), cell type (metaplasia), or size, shape, and organization (dysplasia).

of functioning that is compatible with survival. This decrease in cell size is called *atrophy*. Cell size, particularly in muscle tissue, is related to workload. As the workload of a cell declines, oxygen consumption and protein synthesis decrease. Cells that are atrophied reduce their oxygen consumption and other cellular functions by decreasing the number and size of their organelles and other structures. There are fewer mitochondria, myofilaments, and endoplasmic reticulum structures. When a sufficient number of cells are involved, the entire tissue or muscle atrophies.

The general causes of atrophy can be grouped into five categories: (1) disuse, (2) denervation, (3) loss of endocrine stimulation, (4) inadequate nutrition, and (5) ischemia or decreased blood flow. Disuse atrophy occurs when there is a reduction in skeletal muscle use. An extreme example of disuse atrophy is seen in the muscles of extremities that have been encased in plaster casts. Because atrophy is adaptive and reversible, muscle size is restored after the cast is removed and muscle use is resumed. Denervation atrophy is a form of disuse atrophy that occurs in the muscles of paralyzed limbs. Lack of endocrine stimulation produces a form of disuse atrophy. In women, the loss of estrogen stimulation during menopause results in atrophic changes in the reproductive organs. With malnutrition and decreased blood flow, cells decrease their size and energy requirements as a means of survival.

CELLULAR ADAPTATIONS

- Cells are able to adapt to increased work demands or threats to survival by changing their size (atrophy and hypertrophy), number (hyperplasia), and form (metaplasia).
- Normal cellular adaptation occurs in response to an appropriate stimulus and ceases once the need for adaptation has ceased.

HYPERTROPHY

Hypertrophy represents an increase in cell size and with it an increase in the amount of functioning tissue mass. It results from an increased workload imposed on an organ or body part and is commonly seen in cardiac and skeletal muscle tissue, which cannot adapt to an increase in workload through mitotic division and formation of more cells. Hypertrophy involves an increase in the functional components of the cell that allows it to achieve equilibrium between demand and functional capacity. For example, as muscle cells hypertrophy, additional actin and myosin filaments, cell enzymes, and adenosine triphosphate (ATP) are synthesized.

Hypertrophy may occur as the result of normal physiologic or abnormal pathologic conditions. The increase in muscle mass associated with exercise is an example of physiologic hypertrophy. Pathologic hypertrophy occurs as the result of disease conditions and may be adaptive or compensatory. Examples of adaptive hypertrophy are the thickening of the urinary bladder from long-continued obstruction of urinary outflow and the myocardial hypertrophy that results from valvular heart disease or hypertension. Compensatory hypertrophy is the enlargement of a remaining organ or tissue after a portion has been surgically removed or rendered inactive. For instance, if one kidney is removed, the remaining kidney enlarges to compensate for the loss.

The precise signal for hypertrophy is unknown. It may be related to ATP depletion, mechanical forces such as stretching of the muscle fibers, activation of cell degradation products, or hormonal factors.[1] Whatever the mechanism, a limit is eventually reached beyond which further enlargement of the tissue mass is no longer able to compensate for the increased work demands. The limiting factors for continued hypertrophy might be related to limitations in blood flow. In hypertension, for example, the increased workload required to pump blood against an elevated arterial pressure results in a progressive increase in left ventricular muscle mass and need for coronary blood flow (Fig. 5-2).

There has been recent interest in the signaling pathways that control the arrangement of contractile elements in myocardial hypertrophy. Research suggests that certain signal molecules can alter gene expression, controlling the size and assembly of the contractile proteins in hypertrophied myocardial cells. For example, the hypertrophied

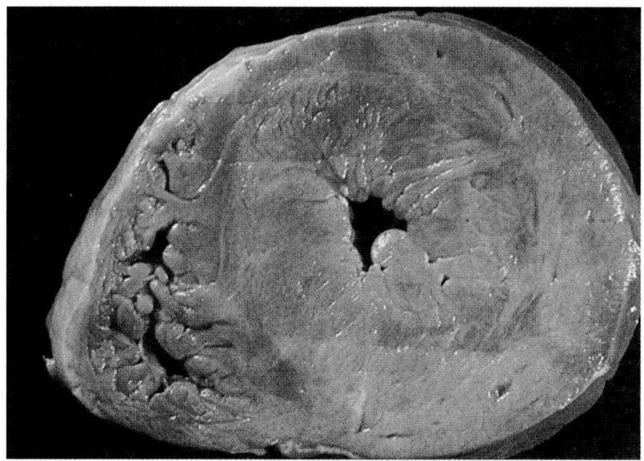

FIGURE 5-2 Myocardial hypertrophy. Cross-section of the heart in a patient with long-standing hypertension. (From Rubin E., Farber J.L. [1999]. *Pathology* [3rd ed., p. 9]. Philadelphia: Lippincott-Raven)

myocardial cells of well-trained athletes have proportional increases in width and length. This is in contrast to the hypertrophy that develops in dilated cardiomyopathy, in which the hypertrophied cells have a relatively greater increase in length than width. In pressure overload, as occurs with hypertension, the hypertrophied cells have greater width than length.[3] It is anticipated that further elucidation of the signal pathways that determine the adaptive and nonadaptive features of cardiac hypertrophy will lead to new targets for treatment.

HYPERPLASIA

Hyperplasia refers to an increase in the number of cells in an organ or tissue. It occurs in tissues with cells that are capable of mitotic division, such as the epidermis, intestinal epithelium, and glandular tissue. Nerve, skeletal, and cardiac muscle cells do not divide and therefore have no capacity for hyperplastic growth. There is evidence that hyperplasia involves activation of genes controlling cell proliferation and the presence of intracellular messengers that control cell replication and growth. As with other normal adaptive cellular responses, hyperplasia is a controlled process that occurs in response to an appropriate stimulus and ceases after the stimulus has been removed.

The stimuli that induce hyperplasia may be physiologic or nonphysiologic. There are two common types of physiologic hyperplasia: hormonal and compensatory. Breast and uterine enlargement during pregnancy are examples of a physiologic hyperplasia that results from estrogen stimulation. The regeneration of the liver that occurs after partial hepatectomy (*i.e.,* partial removal of the liver) is an example of compensatory hyperplasia. Hyperplasia is also an important response of connective tissue in wound healing, during which proliferating fibroblasts and blood vessels contribute to wound repair. Although hypertrophy and hyperplasia are two distinct processes, they may occur together and are often triggered by the same mechanism.[1] For example, the pregnant uterus undergoes both hypertrophy and hyperplasia as the result of estrogen stimulation.

Most forms of nonphysiologic hyperplasia are due to excessive hormonal stimulation or the effects of growth factors on target tissues.[2] Excessive estrogen production can cause endometrial hyperplasia and abnormal menstrual bleeding (see Chapter 47). Benign prostatic hyperplasia, which is a common disorder of men older than 50 years of age, is thought to be related to the action of androgens (see Chapter 45). Skin warts are an example of hyperplasia caused by growth factors produced by certain viruses, such as the papillomaviruses.

METAPLASIA

Metaplasia represents a reversible change in which one adult cell type (epithelial or mesenchymal) is replaced by another adult cell type. Metaplasia is thought to involve the reprogramming of undifferentiated stem cells that are present in the tissue undergoing the metaplastic changes.

Metaplasia usually occurs in response to chronic irritation and inflammation and allows for substitution of cells that are better able to survive under circumstances in which a more fragile cell type might succumb. However, the conversion of cell types never oversteps the boundaries of the primary groups of tissue (*e.g.,* one type of epithelial cell may be converted to another type of epithelial cell, but not to a connective tissue cell). An example of metaplasia is the adaptive substitution of stratified squamous epithelial cells for the ciliated columnar epithelial cells in the trachea and large airways of a habitual cigarette smoker. Although the squamous epithelium is better able to survive in these situations, the protective function that the ciliated epithelium provides for the respiratory tract is lost. Also, continued exposure to the influences that cause metaplasia may predispose to cancerous transformation of the metaplastic epithelium.

DYSPLASIA

Dysplasia is characterized by deranged cell growth of a specific tissue that results in cells that vary in size, shape, and organization. Minor degrees of dysplasia are associated with chronic irritation or inflammation. The pattern is most frequently encountered in areas of metaplastic squamous epithelium of the respiratory tract and uterine cervix. Although dysplasia is abnormal, it is adaptive in that it is potentially reversible after the irritating cause has been removed. Dysplasia is strongly implicated as a precursor of cancer. In cancers of the respiratory tract and the uterine cervix, dysplastic changes have been found adjacent to the foci of cancerous transformation. Through the use of the Papanicolaou (Pap) test, it has been documented that cancer of the uterine cervix develops in a series of incremental epithelial changes ranging from severe dysplasia to invasive cancer. However, dysplasia is an adaptive process and as such does not necessarily lead to cancer. In many cases, the dysplastic cells revert to their former structure and function.

INTRACELLULAR ACCUMULATIONS

Intracellular accumulations represent the buildup of substances that cells cannot immediately use or dispose of. The substances may accumulate in the cytoplasm (frequently in the lysosomes) or in the nucleus. In some cases, the accumulation may be an abnormal substance that the cell has produced, and in other cases, the cell may be storing exogenous materials or products of pathologic processes occurring elsewhere in the body. These substances can be grouped into three categories: (1) normal body substances, such as lipids, proteins, carbohydrates, melanin, and bilirubin, that are present in abnormally large amounts; (2) abnormal endogenous products, such as those resulting from inborn errors of metabolism; and (3) exogenous products, such as environmental agents and pigments that cannot be broken down by the cell.[2] These substances may accumulate transiently or permanently, and they may be harmless or, in some cases, toxic.

The accumulation of normal cellular constituents occurs when a substance is produced at a rate that exceeds its metabolism or removal. An example of this type of process is fatty changes in the liver due to intracellular accumulation of triglycerides. Liver cells normally contain some fat, which is either oxidized and used for energy or converted to triglycerides. This fat is derived from free fatty acids released from adipose tissue. Abnormal accumulation occurs when the delivery of free fatty acids to the liver is increased, as in starvation and diabetes mellitus, or when the intrahepatic metabolism of lipids is disturbed, as in alcoholism.

Intracellular accumulation can result from genetic disorders that disrupt the metabolism of selected substances. A normal enzyme may be replaced with an abnormal one, resulting in the formation of a substance that cannot be used or eliminated from the cell, or an enzyme may be missing, so that an intermediate product accumulates in the cell. For example, there are at least 10 genetic disorders that affect glycogen metabolism, most of which lead to the accumulation of intracellular glycogen stores. In the most common form of this disorder, von Gierke's disease, large amounts of glycogen accumulate in the liver and kidneys because of a deficiency of the enzyme glucose-6-phosphatase. Without this enzyme, glycogen cannot be broken down to form glucose. The disorder leads not only to an accumulation of glycogen but also to a reduction in blood glucose levels. In Tay-Sachs disease, another genetic disorder, abnormal lipids accumulate in the brain and other tissues, causing motor and mental deterioration beginning at approximately 6 months of age, followed by death at 2 to 3 years of age. In a similar manner, other enzyme defects lead to the accumulation of other substances.

Pigments are colored substances that may accumulate in cells. They can be endogenous (*i.e.,* arising from within the body) or exogenous (*i.e.,* arising from outside the body). Icterus, also called *jaundice,* is characterized by a yellow discoloration of tissue due to the retention of bilirubin, an endogenous bile pigment. This condition may result from increased bilirubin production from red blood cell destruction, obstruction of bile passage into the intestine, or toxic diseases that affect the liver's ability to remove bilirubin from the blood. Lipofuscin is a yellow-brown pigment that results from the accumulation of the indigestible residues produced during normal turnover of cell structures (Fig. 5-3). The accumulation of lipofuscin increases with age and is sometimes referred to as the *wear-and-tear pigment.* It is more common in heart, nerve, and liver cells than other tissues and is seen more often in conditions associated with atrophy of an organ.

One of the most common exogenous pigments is carbon in the form of coal dust. In coal miners or persons exposed to heavily polluted environments, the accumulation of carbon dust blackens the lung tissue and may cause serious lung disease. The formation of a blue lead line along the margins of the gum is one of the diagnostic features of lead poisoning. Tattoos are the result of insoluble pigments introduced into the skin, where they are engulfed by macrophages and persist for a lifetime.

The significance of intracellular accumulations depends on the cause and severity of the condition. Many accumulations, such as lipofuscin and mild fatty change, have no effect on cell function. Some conditions, such as the hyperbilirubinemia that causes jaundice, are reversible. Other disorders, such as glycogen storage diseases, produce accumulations that result in organ dysfunction and other alterations in physiologic function.

PATHOLOGIC CALCIFICATIONS

Pathologic calcification involves the abnormal tissue deposition of calcium salts, together with smaller amounts of iron, magnesium, and other minerals. It is known as *dystrophic calcification* when it occurs in dead or dying tissue and as *metastatic calcification* when it occurs in normal tissue.

Dystrophic Calcification

Dystrophic calcification represents the macroscopic deposition of calcium salts in injured tissue. It is often visible to the naked eye as deposits that range from gritty sandlike grains to firm, hard, rock material. The pathogenesis of

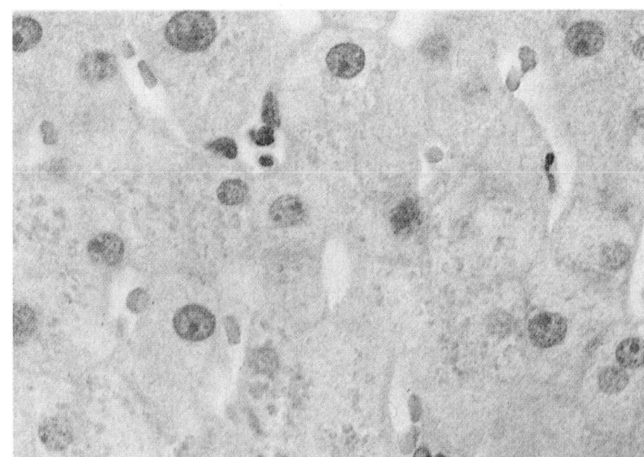

FIGURE 5-3 Accumulation of intracellular lipofuscin. A photomicrograph of the liver of an 80-year-old man shows golden cytoplasmic granules, which represent lysosomal storage of lipofuscin. (From Rubin E., Farber J.L. [1999]. *Pathology* [3rd ed., p. 13]. Philadelphia: Lippincott-Raven)

dystrophic calcification involves the intracellular or extracellular formation of crystalline calcium phosphate. The components of the calcium deposits are derived from the bodies of dead or dying cells as well as from the circulation and interstitial fluid.

Dystrophic calcification is commonly seen in atheromatous lesions of advanced atherosclerosis, areas of injury in the aorta and large blood vessels, and damaged heart valves. Although the presence of calcification may only indicate the presence of previous cell injury, as in healed tuberculosis lesions, it is also a frequent cause of organ dysfunction. For example, calcification of the aortic valve is a frequent cause of aortic stenosis in elderly people (Fig. 5-4).

Metastatic Calcification

In contrast to dystrophic calcification, which occurs in injured tissues, metastatic calcification occurs in normal tissues as the result of increased serum calcium levels (hypercalcemia). Almost any condition that increases the serum calcium level can lead to calcification in inappropriate sites, such as the lung, renal tubules, and blood vessels. The major causes of hypercalcemia are hyperparathyroidism, either primary or secondary to phosphate retention in renal failure; increased mobilization of calcium from bone, as in Paget disease, cancer with metastatic bone lesions, or immobilization; and vitamin D intoxication.

In summary, cells adapt to changes in their environment and in their work demands by changing their size, number, and characteristics. These adaptive changes are consistent with the needs of the cell and occur in response to an appropriate stimulus. The changes are usually reversed after the stimulus has been withdrawn.

When confronted with a decrease in work demands or adverse environmental conditions, cells atrophy or reduce their size and revert to a lower and more efficient level of functioning. Hypertrophy results from an increase in work demands and is characterized by an increase in tissue size brought about by an increase in cell size and functional components in the cell. An increase in the number of cells in an organ or tissue that is still capable of mitotic division is called hyperplasia. Metaplasia occurs in response to chronic irritation and represents the substitution of cells of a type that are better able to survive under circumstances in which a more fragile cell type might succumb. Dysplasia is characterized by deranged cell growth of a specific tissue that results in cells that vary in size, shape, and appearance. It is a precursor of cancer.

Under some circumstances, cells may accumulate abnormal amounts of various substances. If the accumulation reflects a correctable systemic disorder, such as the hyperbilirubinemia that causes jaundice, the accumulation is reversible. If the disorder cannot be corrected, as often occurs in many inborn errors of metabolism, the cells become overloaded, causing cell injury and death.

Pathologic calcification involves the abnormal tissue deposition of calcium salts. Dystrophic calcification occurs in dead or dying tissue. Although the presence of dystrophic calcification may only indicate the presence of previous cell injury, it is also a frequent cause of organ dysfunction (*e.g.,* when it affects the heart valves). Metastatic calcification occurs in normal tissues as the result of elevated serum calcium levels. Almost any condition that increases the serum calcium level can lead to calcification in inappropriate sites such as the lung, renal tubules, and blood vessels.

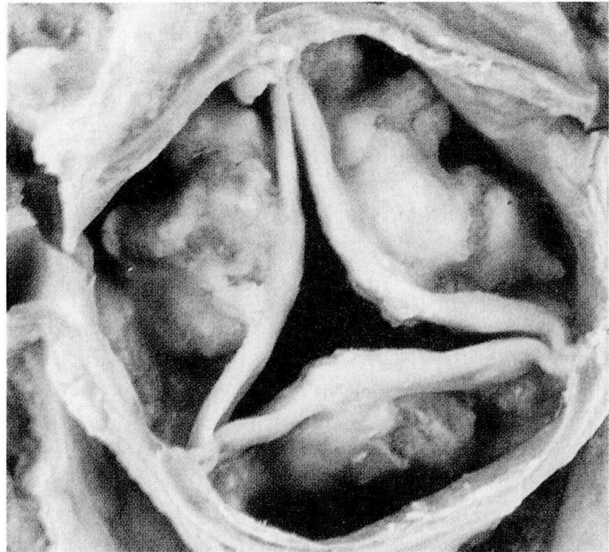

FIGURE 5-4 Calcific aortic stenosis. Large deposits of calcium salts are evident in the cusps and free margins of the thickened aortic valve as viewed from above. (From Rubin E., Farber J.L. [1999]. *Pathology* [3rd ed., p. 28]. Philadelphia: Lippincott-Raven)

Cell Injury and Death

After you have completed this section of the chapter, you should be able to meet the following objectives:

- Describe the mechanisms whereby physical agents such as blunt trauma, electrical forces, and extremes of temperature produce cell injury
- Differentiate between the effects of ionizing and nonionizing radiation in terms of their ability to cause cell injury
- Explain how the injurious effects of biologic agents differ from those produced by physical and chemical agents
- State the mechanisms and manifestations of cell injury associated with lead poisoning
- State how nutritional imbalances contribute to cell injury
- Describe three types of reversible cell changes that can occur with cell injury
- Define *free radical* and relate free radical formation to cell injury and death
- Describe cell changes that occur with ischemic and hypoxic cell injury
- Relate the effects of impaired calcium homeostasis to cell injury and death
- Differentiate cell death associated with necrosis and apoptosis
- Cite the reasons for the changes that occur with the wet and dry forms of gangrene

Cells can be injured in many ways. The extent to which any injurious agent can cause cell injury and death depends in large measure on the intensity and duration of the injury and the type of cell that is involved. Cell injury is usually reversible up to a certain point, after which irreversible cell injury and death occur. Whether a specific stress causes irreversible or reversible cell injury depends on the severity of the insult and on variables such as blood supply, nutritional status, and regenerative capacity. Cell injury and death are ongoing processes, and in the healthy state, they are balanced by cell renewal.

CAUSES OF CELL INJURY

Cell damage can occur in many ways. For purposes of discussion, the ways by which cells are injured have been grouped into five categories: (1) injury from physical agents, (2) radiation injury, (3) chemical injury, (4) injury from biologic agents, and (5) injury from nutritional imbalances.

Injury From Physical Agents

Physical agents responsible for cell and tissue injury include mechanical forces, extremes of temperature, and electrical forces. They are common causes of injuries due to environmental exposure, occupational and transportation accidents, and physical violence and assault.

Mechanical Forces. Injury or trauma due to mechanical forces occurs as the result of body impact with another object. The body or the mass can be in motion, or as sometimes happens, both can be in motion at the time of impact. These types of injuries split and tear tissue, fracture bones, injure blood vessels, and disrupt blood flow.

Extremes of Temperature. Extremes of heat and cold cause damage to the cell, its organelles, and its enzyme systems. Exposure to low-intensity heat (43° to 46°C), such as occurs with partial-thickness burns and severe heat stroke, causes cell injury by inducing vascular injury, accelerating cell metabolism, inactivating temperature-sensitive enzymes, and disrupting the cell membrane. With more intense heat, coagulation of blood vessels and tissue proteins occurs. Exposure to cold increases blood viscosity and induces vasoconstriction by direct action on blood vessels and through reflex activity of the sympathetic nervous system. The resultant decrease in blood flow may lead to hypoxic tissue injury, depending on the degree and duration of cold exposure. Injury from freezing probably results from a combination of ice crystal formation and vasoconstriction. The decreased blood flow leads to capillary stasis and arteriolar and capillary thrombosis. Edema results from increased capillary permeability.

Electrical Injuries. Electrical injuries can affect the body through extensive tissue injury and disruption of neural and cardiac impulses. The effect of electricity on the body is mainly determined by its voltage, the type of current (*i.e.,* direct or alternating), its amperage, the resistance of the intervening tissue, the pathway of the current, and the duration of exposure.[4]

Lightning and high-voltage wires that carry several thousand volts produce the most severe damage.[2] Alternating current (AC) is usually more dangerous than direct current (DC) because it causes violent muscle contractions, preventing the person from releasing the electrical source and sometimes resulting in fractures and dislocations. In electrical injuries, the body acts as a conductor of the electrical current. The current enters the body from an electrical source, such as an exposed wire, and passes through the body and exits to another conductor, such as the moisture on the ground or a piece of metal the person is holding. The pathway that a current takes is critical because the electrical energy disrupts impulses in excitable tissues. Current flow through the brain may interrupt impulses from respiratory centers in the brain stem, and current flow through the chest may cause fatal cardiac arrhythmias.

The resistance to the flow of current in electrical circuits transforms electrical energy into heat. This is why the elements in electrical heating devices are made of highly resistive metals. Much of the tissue damage produced by electrical injuries is caused by heat production in tissues that have the highest electrical resistance. Resistance to electrical current varies from the greatest to the least in bone, fat, tendons, skin, muscles, blood, and nerves. The most severe tissue injury usually occurs at the skin sites where the current enters and leaves the body. After electricity has penetrated the skin, it passes rapidly through the body along the lines of least resistance—through body fluids and nerves. Degeneration of vessel walls may occur, and thrombi may form as current flows along the blood vessels. This can cause extensive muscle and deep tissue injury. Thick, dry skin is more resistant to the flow of electricity than thin, wet skin. It is generally believed that the greater the skin resistance, the greater is the amount of local skin burn, and the less the resistance, the greater are the deep and systemic effects.

Radiation Injury

Electromagnetic radiation comprises a wide spectrum of wave-propagated energy, ranging from ionizing gamma rays to radiofrequency waves (Fig. 5-5). A photon is a par-

CELL INJURY

- Cells can be damaged in a number of ways, including physical trauma, extremes of temperature, electrical injury, exposure to damaging chemicals, radiation damage, injury from biologic agents, and nutritional factors.
- Most injurious agents exert their damaging effects through uncontrolled free radical production, impaired oxygen delivery or utilization, or the destructive effects of uncontrolled intracellular calcium release.
- Cell injury can be reversible, allowing the cell to recover, or it can be irreversible, causing cell death and necrosis.
- In contrast to necrosis, which results from tissue injury, apoptosis is a normal physiologic process designed to remove injured or worn-out cells.

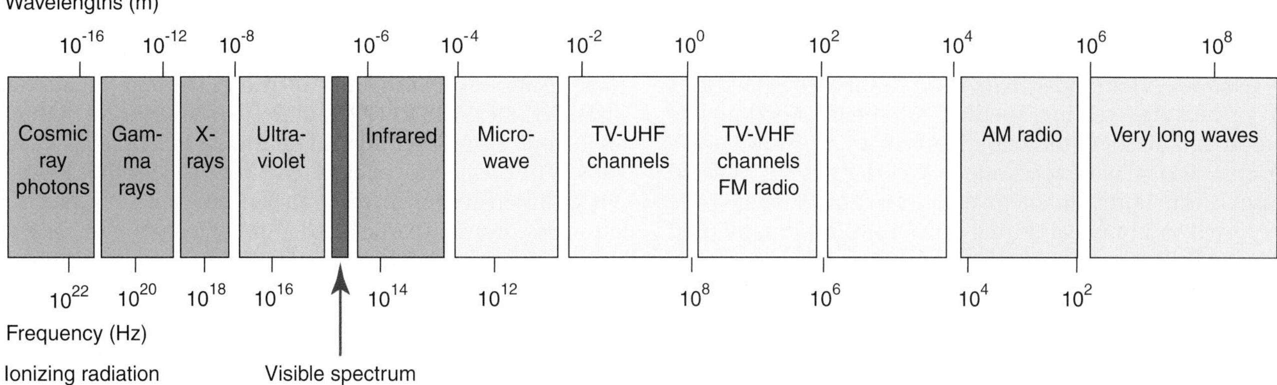

FIGURE 5-5 Spectrum of electromagnetic radiation.

ticle of radiation energy. Radiation energy above the ultraviolet (UV) range is called *ionizing radiation* because the photons have enough energy to knock electrons off atoms and molecules. *Nonionizing radiation* refers to radiation energy at frequencies below that of visible light. *UV radiation* represents the portion of the spectrum of electromagnetic radiation just above the visible range. It contains increasingly energetic rays that are powerful enough to disrupt intracellular bonds and cause sunburn.

Ionizing Radiation. Ionizing radiation affects cells by causing ionization of molecules and atoms in the cell, by directly hitting the target molecules in the cell, or by producing free radicals that interact with critical cell components.[1,2,5] It can immediately kill cells, interrupt cell replication, or cause a variety of genetic mutations, which may or may not be lethal. Most radiation injury is caused by localized irradiation that is used in treatment of cancer (see Chapter 8). Except for unusual circumstances such as the use of high-dose irradiation that precedes bone marrow transplantation, exposure to whole-body irradiation is rare.

The injurious effects of ionizing radiation vary with the dose, dose rate (a single dose can cause greater injury than divided or fractionated doses), and the differential sensitivity of the exposed tissue to radiation injury. Because of the effect on DNA synthesis and interference with mitosis, rapidly dividing cells of the bone marrow and intestine are much more vulnerable to radiation injury than tissues such as bone and skeletal muscle. Over time, occupational and accidental exposure to ionizing radiation can result in increased risk for the development of various types of cancers, including skin cancers, leukemia, osteogenic sarcomas, and lung cancer.

Many of the clinical manifestations of radiation injury result from acute cell injury, dose-dependent changes in the blood vessels that supply the irradiated tissues, and fibrotic tissue replacement. The cell's initial response to radiation injury involves swelling, disruption of the mitochondria and other organelles, alterations in the cell membrane, and marked changes in the nucleus. The endothelial cells in blood vessels are particularly sensitive to irradiation. During the immediate postirradiation period, only vessel dilation takes place (*e.g.,* the initial erythema of the skin after radiation therapy). Later or with higher levels of radiation, destructive changes occur in small blood vessels such as the capillaries and venules. Acute reversible necrosis is represented by such disorders as radiation cystitis, dermatitis, and diarrhea from enteritis. More persistent damage can be attributed to acute necrosis of tissue cells that are not capable of regeneration and chronic ischemia. Chronic effects of radiation damage are characterized by fibrosis and scarring of tissues and organs in the irradiated area (*e.g.,* interstitial fibrosis of the heart and lungs after irradiation of the chest). Because the radiation delivered in radiation therapy inevitably travels through the skin, radiation dermatitis is common. There may be necrosis of the skin, impaired wound healing, and chronic radiation dermatitis.

Ultraviolet Radiation. Ultraviolet radiation causes sunburn and increases the risk for skin cancers (see Chapter 61). The degree of risk depends on the type of UV rays, the intensity of exposure, and the amount of protective melanin pigment in the skin. Skin damage induced by UV radiation is thought to be caused by reactive oxygen species and by damage to melanin-producing processes in the skin. UV radiation also damages DNA, resulting in the formation of pyrimidine dimers (*i.e.,* the insertion of two identical pyrimidine bases into replicating DNA instead of one). Other forms of DNA damage include the production of single-stranded breaks and formation of DNA–protein cross-links. Normally, errors that occur during DNA replication are repaired by enzymes that remove the faulty section of DNA and repair the damage. The importance of the DNA repair process in protecting against UV radiation injury is evidenced by the vulnerability of persons who lack the enzymes needed to repair UV-induced DNA damage. In a genetic disorder called *xeroderma pigmentosum,* an enzyme needed to repair sunlight-induced DNA damage is lacking. This autosomal recessive disorder is characterized by extreme photosensitivity and a 2000-fold increased risk for skin cancer in sun-exposed skin.[2]

Nonionizing Radiation. Nonionizing radiation includes infrared light, ultrasound, microwaves, and laser energy. Unlike ionizing radiation, which can directly break chemical bonds, nonionizing radiation exerts its effects by causing vibration and rotation of atoms and molecules. All of this vibrational and rotational energy is eventually converted to thermal energy. Low-frequency nonionizing radiation is used widely in radar, television, industrial operations (*e.g.*, heating, welding, melting of metals, processing of wood and plastic), household appliances (*e.g.*, microwave ovens), and medical applications (*e.g.*, diathermy). Isolated cases of skin burns and thermal injury to deeper tissues have occurred in industrial settings and from improperly used household microwave ovens. Injury from these sources is mainly thermal and, because of the deep penetration of the infrared or microwave rays, tends to involve dermal and subcutaneous tissue injury.

Chemical Injury

Chemicals capable of damaging cells are everywhere around us. Air and water pollution contain chemicals capable of tissue injury, as does tobacco smoke and some processed or preserved foods. Some of the most damaging chemicals exist in our environment, including gases such as carbon monoxide, insecticides, and trace metals such as lead.

Chemical agents can injure the cell membrane and other cell structures, block enzymatic pathways, coagulate cell proteins, and disrupt the osmotic and ionic balance of the cell. Corrosive substances such as strong acids and bases destroy cells as the substances come into contact with the body. Other chemicals may injure cells in the process of metabolism or elimination. Carbon tetrachloride (CCl_4), for example, causes little damage until it is metabolized by liver enzymes to a highly reactive free radical ($CCl_3^{\bullet}$). Carbon tetrachloride is extremely toxic to liver cells.

Drugs. Many drugs—alcohol, prescription drugs, over-the-counter drugs, and street drugs—are capable of directly or indirectly damaging tissues. Ethyl alcohol can harm the gastric mucosa, liver (see Chapter 40), developing fetus (see Chapter 7), and other organs. Antineoplastic (anticancer) and immunosuppressant drugs can directly injure cells. Other drugs produce metabolic end products that are toxic to cells. Acetaminophen, a commonly used over-the-counter analgesic drug, is detoxified in the liver, where small amounts of the drug are converted to a highly toxic metabolite. This metabolite is detoxified by a metabolic pathway that uses a substance (*i.e.*, glutathione) normally present in the liver. When large amounts of the drug are ingested, this pathway becomes overwhelmed, and toxic metabolites accumulate, causing massive liver necrosis.

Lead Toxicity. Lead is a particularly toxic metal. Small amounts accumulate to reach toxic levels. There are innumerable sources of lead in the environment, including flaking paint, lead-contaminated dust and soil, lead-contaminated root vegetables, lead water pipes or soldered joints, pottery glazes, and newsprint. Adults often encounter lead through occupational exposure. Lead and other metal smelters, miners, welders, storage battery workers, and pottery makers are particularly at risk.[1,6] Children are exposed to lead through ingestion of peeling lead paint, by breathing dust from lead paint (*e.g.*, during remodeling), or from playing in contaminated soil. There has been a substantial decline in blood lead levels of the entire population since the removal of lead from gasoline and from soldered food cans.[7] However, high lead blood levels continue to be a problem, particularly among children. In the Third National Health and Nutrition Examination Survey (NHANES III, 1988 to 1991), blood lead levels were highest in 1- to 2-year-old children and lowest in 12- to 19-year-olds.[7] The prevalence of elevated blood lead levels is higher for children living in more urbanized areas. By race or ethnicity, non-Hispanic black children residing in central cities with a population of 1 million or more have the highest proportion of elevated blood lead levels. A high percentage of Mexican-American children living in the most urbanized areas also had elevated lead levels.[8]

Lead is absorbed through the gastrointestinal tract or the lungs into the blood. A deficiency in calcium, iron, or zinc increases lead absorption. In children, most lead is absorbed through the lungs. Although children may have the same or a lower intake of lead, the absorption in infants and children is greater; thus, they are more vulnerable to lead toxicity.[2] Lead crosses the placenta, exposing the fetus to levels of lead that are comparable with those of the mother. Lead is stored in bone and eliminated by the kidneys. Approximately 85% of absorbed lead is stored in bone (and teeth of young children), 5% to 10% remains in the blood, and the remainder accumulates in soft tissue deposits. Although the half-life of lead is hours to days, bone deposits serve as a repository from which blood levels are maintained. In a sense, bone protects other tissues, but the slow turnover maintains blood levels for months to years.

The toxicity of lead is related to its multiple biochemical effects.[2] It has the ability to inactivate enzymes, compete with calcium for incorporation into bone, and interfere with nerve transmission and brain development. The major targets of lead toxicity are the red blood cells, the gastrointestinal tract, the kidneys, and the nervous system.

Anemia is a cardinal sign of lead toxicity. Lead competes with the enzymes required for hemoglobin synthesis and with the membrane-associated enzymes that prevent hemolysis of red blood cells. The resulting red cells are microscopic and hypochromic, resembling those seen in iron-deficiency anemia. The life span of the red cell is also decreased. The gastrointestinal tract is the main source of symptoms in the adult. This is characterized by "lead colic," a severe and poorly localized form of acute abdominal pain. A lead line formed by precipitated lead sulfite may appear along the gingival margins. The lead line is seldom seen in children. The kidneys are the major route for excretion of lead. Lead can cause diffuse kidney damage, eventually leading to renal failure. Even without overt signs of kidney damage, lead toxicity leads to hypertension.

In the nervous system, lead toxicity is characterized by demyelination of cerebral and cerebellar white matter and death of cortical cells. When this occurs in early childhood, it can affect neurobehavioral development and result in lower IQ levels and poorer classroom performance.[9] Peripheral demyelinating neuropathy may occur in adults. The most serious manifestation of lead poisoning is acute encephalopathy. It is manifested by persistent vomiting, ataxia, seizures, papilledema, impaired consciousness, and coma. Acute encephalopathy may manifest suddenly, or it may be preceded by other signs of lead toxicity such as behavioral changes or abdominal complaints.

Because of the long-term neurobehavioral and cognitive deficits that occur in children with even moderately elevated lead levels, the Centers for Disease Control and Prevention and the American Academy of Pediatrics have issued recommendations for childhood lead screening.[10–12] A safe blood level of lead is still uncertain. At one time, 25 μg/dL was considered safe. Surveys have shown abnormally low IQs in children with levels as low as 10 to 15 μg/dL; in 1991, the safe level was lowered to 10 μg/dL.[13] Recent research suggests that even levels below 10 μg/dL are associated with declines in children's IQ at 3 to 5 years of age.[14]

Screening for lead toxicity involves use of capillary blood obtained from a finger stick to measure free erythrocyte protoporphyrin (EP). Elevated levels of EP result from the inhibition by lead of the enzymes required for heme synthesis in red blood cells. The EP test is useful in detecting high lead levels but usually does not detect levels below 20 to 25 μg/dL. Thus, capillary screening test values greater than 10 μg/dL should be confirmed with those from a venous blood sample. This test also reflects the effects of iron deficiency, a condition that increases lead absorption.[13]

Because the symptoms of lead toxicity usually are vague, diagnosis is often delayed. Anemia may provide the first clues to the disorder. Laboratory tests are necessary to establish a diagnosis. Measurement of lead levels in venous blood is usually used. Treatment involves removal of the lead source and, in cases of severe toxicity, administration of a chelating agent. Asymptomatic children with blood levels of 45 to 69 μg/dL usually are treated. A public health team should evaluate the source of lead because meticulous removal is needed.

Injury From Biologic Agents

Biologic agents differ from other injurious agents in that they are able to replicate and can continue to produce their injurious effects. These agents range from submicroscopic viruses to the larger parasites. Biologic agents injure cells by diverse mechanisms. Viruses enter the cell and become incorporated into its DNA synthetic machinery. Certain bacteria elaborate exotoxins that interfere with cellular production of ATP. Other bacteria, such as the gram-negative bacilli, release endotoxins that cause cell injury and increased capillary permeability.

Injury From Nutritional Imbalances

Nutritional excesses and nutritional deficiencies predispose cells to injury. Obesity and diets high in saturated fats are thought to predispose persons to atherosclerosis. The body requires more than 60 organic and inorganic substances in amounts ranging from micrograms to grams. These nutrients include minerals, vitamins, certain fatty acids, and specific amino acids. Dietary deficiencies can occur in the form of starvation, in which there is a deficiency of all nutrients and vitamins, or because of a selective deficiency of a single nutrient or vitamin. Iron-deficiency anemia, scurvy, beriberi, and pellagra are examples of injury caused by the lack of specific vitamins or minerals. The protein and calorie deficiencies that occur with starvation cause widespread tissue damage.

MECHANISMS OF CELL INJURY

The mechanisms by which injurious agents cause cell injury and death are complex. Some agents, such as heat, produce direct cell injury; other factors, such as genetic derangements, produce their effects indirectly through metabolic disturbances and altered immune responses. There seem to be at least three major mechanisms whereby most injurious agents exert their effects: free radical formation, hypoxia and ATP depletion, and disruption of intracellular calcium homeostasis.

Free Radical Injury

Many injurious agents exert their damaging effects through a reactive chemical species called a *free radical*.[1,2,15–17] Free radical injury is rapidly emerging as a final common pathway for tissue damage by many injurious agents.

In most atoms, the outer electron orbits are filled with paired electrons moving in opposite directions to balance their spins. A free radical is a highly reactive chemical species arising from an atom that has a single unpaired electron in an outer orbit (Fig. 5-6). In this state, the radical is highly unstable and can enter into reactions with cellular constituents, particularly key molecules in cell membranes and nucleic acids. Moreover, free radicals can establish chain reactions, sometimes thousands of events long, as the molecules they react with in turn form free radicals. Chain reactions may branch, causing even greater damage. Uncontrolled free radical production causes damage to cell membranes, cross-linking of cell proteins, inactivation of enzyme systems, or damage to the nucleic acids that make up DNA.

Free radical formation is a byproduct of many normal cellular reactions in the body, including energy generation, breakdown of lipids and proteins, and inflammatory processes. For example, free radical generation is the main mechanism for killing microbes by phagocytic white blood cells. Molecular oxygen (O_2), with its two unpaired outer electrons, is the main source of free radicals. During the course of normal cellular respiration, molecular oxygen is sequentially reduced in the mitochondria by the addition of four electrons to produce water. During the process, small amounts of partially reduced intermediate species are converted to free radicals. These reactive species include the superoxide radicals (one electron), hydrogen peroxide (two electrons), and the hydroxyl radical (three electrons). Transition metals, such as copper and iron, which can accept or donate free electrons during intracellular reactions, are also a source of free radicals. Nitric oxide (NO), an important mediator that is normally synthesized by a variety of cell types, can act as a free radical or be converted into a highly reactive nitrite species.

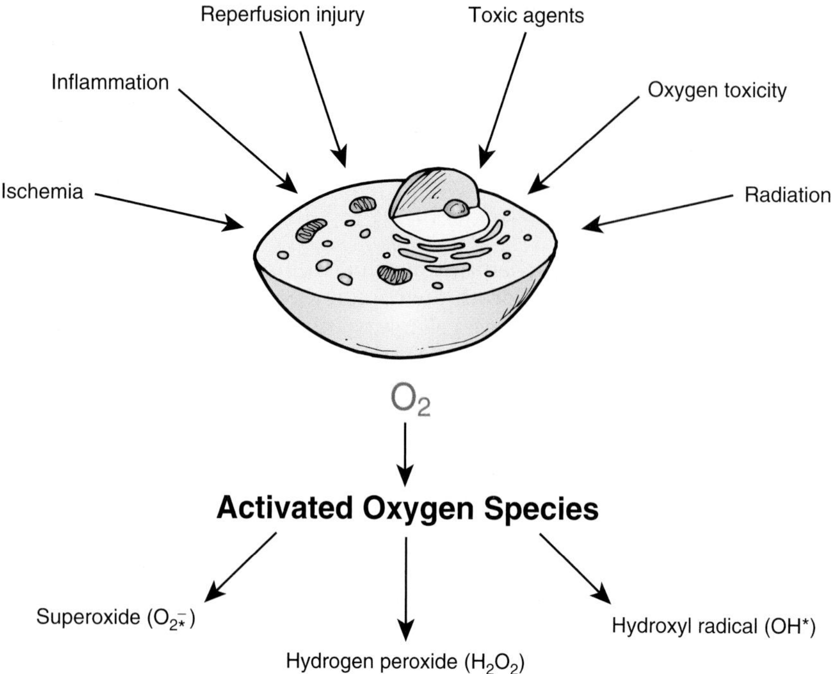

FIGURE 5-6 Generation of free radicals.

Although the effects of these reactive species are wide-ranging, three types of effects are particularly important in cell injury: lipid peroxidation, oxidative modification of proteins, and DNA effects (Fig. 5-7). Destruction of the phospholipids in cell membranes, including the outer plasma membrane and those of the intracellular organelles, results in loss of membrane integrity. Free radical attack on cell proteins, particularly those of critical enzymes, can interrupt vital processes throughout the cell. DNA is an important target of the hydroxyl free radical. Damage can involve single-stranded breaks in DNA, modification of base pairs, and cross-links between strands. In most cases, various DNA repair pathways can repair the damage. However, if the damage is extensive, the cell dies. The effects of free radical–mediated DNA changes have also been implicated in aging and malignant transformation of cells.

Damage to vital cell proteins, including enzymes

DNA damage

Lipid peroxidation and injury to cell membranes

FIGURE 5-7 Mechanisms of free radical cell damage.

Under normal conditions, most cells have chemical mechanisms that protect them from the injurious effects of free radicals. These mechanisms commonly break down when the cell is deprived of oxygen or exposed to certain chemical agents, radiation, or other injurious agents. Free radical formation is a particular threat to tissues in which the blood flow has been interrupted and then restored. During the period of interrupted flow, the intracellular mechanisms that control free radicals are inactivated or damaged. When blood flow is restored, the cell is suddenly confronted with an excess of free radicals that it cannot control.

Scientists continue to investigate the use of free radical scavengers to protect against cell injury during periods when protective cellular mechanisms are impaired. Defenses against free radicals include vitamins E and C.[17,18] Vitamin E is the major lipid-soluble antioxidant present in all cellular membranes. Vitamin C is an important water-soluble cytosolic chain-breaking antioxidant; it acts directly with superoxide and singlet oxygen radicals. β-carotene, a pigment found in most plants, reacts with singlet oxygen and can also function as an antioxidant.[19]

Hypoxic Cell Injury

Hypoxia deprives the cell of oxygen and interrupts oxidative metabolism and the generation of ATP. The actual time necessary to produce irreversible cell damage depends on the degree of oxygen deprivation and the metabolic needs of the cell. Well-differentiated cells, such as those in the heart, brain, and kidneys, require large amounts of oxygen to provide energy for their special functions. Brain cells, for example, begin to undergo permanent damage after 4 to 6 minutes of oxygen deprivation. A thin margin can exist between the time involved in reversible and irreversible cell damage. One study found that the epithelial cells of the proximal tubule of the kidney in the rat could survive 20 but not 30 minutes of ischemia.[20]

Hypoxia can result from an inadequate amount of oxygen in the air, respiratory disease, ischemia (*i.e.,* decreased blood flow due to circulatory disorders), anemia, edema, or inability of the cells to use oxygen. Ischemia is characterized by impaired oxygen delivery and impaired removal of metabolic end products such as lactic acid. In contrast to pure hypoxia, which affects the oxygen content of the blood and affects all of the cells in the body, ischemia commonly affects blood flow through small numbers of blood vessels and produces local tissue injury. In cases of edema, the distance for diffusion of oxygen may become a limiting factor. In hypermetabolic states, the cells may require more oxygen than can be supplied by normal respiratory function and oxygen transport. Hypoxia also serves as the ultimate cause of cell death in other injuries. For example, toxins from certain microorganisms can interfere with cellular use of oxygen, and a physical agent such as cold can cause severe vasoconstriction and impair blood flow.

Hypoxia literally causes a power failure in the cell, with widespread effects on the cell's functional and structural components. As oxygen tension in the cell falls, oxidative metabolism ceases, and the cell reverts to anaerobic metabolism, using its limited glycogen stores in an attempt to maintain vital cell functions. Cellular pH falls as lactic acid accumulates in the cell. This reduction in pH can have profound effects on intracellular structures. The nuclear chromatin clumps and myelin figures, which derive from destructive changes in cell membranes and intracellular structures, are seen in the cytoplasm and extracellular spaces.

One of the earliest effects of reduced ATP is acute cellular swelling caused by failure of the energy-dependent sodium/potassium (Na^+/K^+)-ATPase membrane pump, which extrudes sodium from and returns potassium to the cell. With impaired function of this pump, intracellular potassium levels decrease, and sodium and water accumulate in the cell. The movement of fluid and ions into the cell is associated with dilation of the endoplasmic reticulum, increased membrane permeability, and decreased mitochondrial function.[2] To this point, the cellular changes due to ischemia are reversible if oxygenation is restored. If the oxygen supply is not restored, however, there is a continued loss of essential enzymes, proteins, and ribonucleic acid through the hyperpermeable membrane of the cell. Injury to the lysosomal membranes results in leakage of destructive lysosomal enzymes into the cytoplasm and enzymatic digestion of cell components. Leakage of intracellular enzymes through the permeable cell membrane into the extracellular fluid is used as an important clinical indicator of cell injury and death. These enzymes enter the blood and can be measured by laboratory tests.

Impaired Calcium Homeostasis

Calcium functions as a messenger for the release of many intracellular enzymes. Normally, intracellular calcium levels are kept extremely low compared with extracellular levels. These low intracellular levels are maintained by energy-dependent membrane-associated calcium/magnesium (Ca^{2+}/Mg^{2+})-ATPase exchange systems.[2] Ischemia and certain toxins lead to an increase in cytosolic calcium because of increased influx across the cell membrane and the release of calcium stored in the mitochondria and endoplasmic reticulum. The increased calcium level activates a number of enzymes with potentially damaging effects. The enzymes include the phospholipases responsible for damaging the cell membrane, proteases that damage the cytoskeleton and membrane proteins, ATPases that break down ATP and hasten its depletion, and endonucleases that fragment chromatin. Although it is known that injured cells accumulate calcium, it is unknown whether this is the ultimate cause of irreversible cell injury.

REVERSIBLE CELL INJURY AND CELL DEATH

The mechanisms of cell injury can produce sublethal and reversible cellular damage or lead to irreversible injury with cell destruction or death (Fig. 5-8). Cell destruction and removal can involve one of two mechanisms: apoptosis,

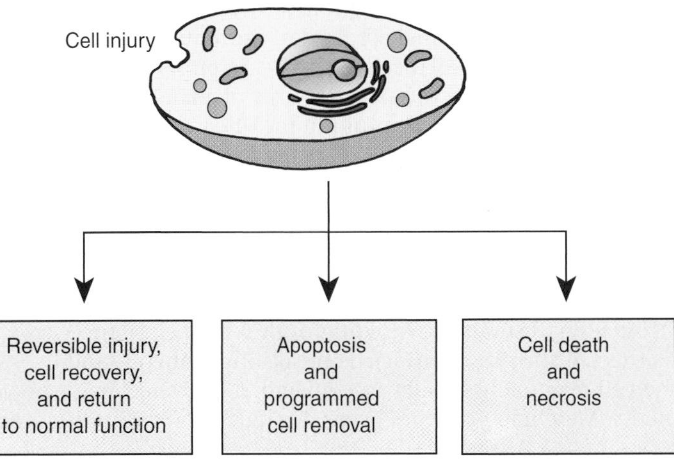

FIGURE 5-8 Outcomes of cell injury: reversible cell injury, apoptosis and programmed cell removal, cell death and necrosis.

which is designed to remove injured or worn-out cells, or cell death and necrosis, which occurs in irreversibly damaged cells.

Reversible Cell Injury

Reversible cell injury, although impairing cell function, does not result in cell death. Two patterns of reversible cell injury can be observed under the microscope: cellular swelling and fatty change. Cellular swelling occurs with impairment of the energy-dependent Na^+/K^+-ATPase membrane pump, usually as the result of hypoxic cell injury.

Fatty changes are linked to intracellular accumulation of fat. When fatty changes occur, small vacuoles of fat disperse throughout the cytoplasm. The process is usually more ominous than cellular swelling, and although it is reversible, it usually indicates severe injury. These fatty changes may occur because normal cells are presented with an increased fat load or because injured cells are unable to metabolize the fat properly. In obese persons, fatty infiltrates often occur within and between the cells of the liver and heart because of an increased fat load. Pathways for fat metabolism may be impaired during cell injury, and fat may accumulate in the cell as production exceeds use and export. The liver, where most fats are synthesized and metabolized, is particularly susceptible to fatty change, but fatty changes may also occur in the kidney, the heart, and other organs.

Programmed Cell Death

In each cell line, the control of cell number is regulated by a balance of cell proliferation and cell death. Cell death can involve apoptosis or necrosis. Apoptotic cell death involves controlled cell destruction and is involved in normal cell deletion and renewal. For example, blood cells that undergo constant renewal from progenitor cells in the bone marrow are removed by apoptotic cell death.

Apoptosis, from Greek *apo* for "apart" and *ptosis* for "fallen," means *fallen apart.* Apoptotic cell death, which is equated with cell suicide, eliminates cells that are worn out, have been produced in excess, have developed improperly, or have genetic damage. In normal cell turnover, this process provides the space needed for cell replacement. The process, which was first described in 1972, has become one of the most vigorously investigated processes in biology.[21] Apoptosis is thought to be involved in several physiologic and pathologic processes. Current research is focusing on the control mechanisms of apoptosis in an attempt to understand the pathogenesis of many disease states, such as cancer and autoimmune disease.

Apoptotic cell death is characterized by controlled autodigestion of cell components. Cells appear to initiate their own death through the activation of endogenous enzymes. This results in cell shrinkage brought about by disruption of the cytoskeleton, condensation of the cytoplasmic organelles, disruption and clumping of nuclear DNA, and a distinctive wrinkling of the cell membrane.[2] As the cell shrinks, the nucleus breaks into spheres, and the cell eventually divides into membrane-covered fragments. Membrane changes occur during the process, signaling surrounding phagocytic cells to engulf the apoptotic cell parts and complete the degradation process (Fig. 5-9).

Apoptosis is thought to be responsible for several normal physiologic processes, including programmed destruction of cells during embryonic development, hormone-dependent involution of tissues, death of immune cells, cell death by cytotoxic T cells, and cell death in proliferating cell populations. During embryogenesis, in the development of a number of organs such as the heart, which begins as a single pulsating tube and is gradually modified to become a four-chambered pump, apoptotic cell death allows for the next stage of organ development. It also separates the webbed fingers and toes of the developing embryo (Fig. 5-10). Apoptotic cell death occurs in the hormone-dependent involution of endometrial cells during the menstrual cycle and in the regression of breast tissue after weaning from breast-feeding. The control of immune cell numbers and destruction of autoreactive T cells in the thymus have been credited to apoptosis. Cytotoxic T cells and natural killer cells are thought to destroy target cells by inducing apoptotic cell death.

Apoptosis appears to be linked to several pathologic processes. For example, suppression of apoptosis may be a determinant in the growth of cancers. Apoptosis is also thought to be involved in the cell death associated with certain viral infections, such as hepatitis B and C, and in cell death caused by a variety of injurious agents, such as mild thermal injury and radiation injury. Apoptosis may also be involved in neurodegenerative disorders such as Alzheimer's disease, Parkinson's disease, and amyotrophic lateral sclerosis (ALS). The loss of cells in these disorders does not induce inflammation; although the initiating event is unknown, apoptosis appears to be the mechanism of cell death.[22]

Several mechanisms appear to be involved in initiating cell death by apoptosis. As in the case of endometrial changes that occur during the menstrual cycle, the process

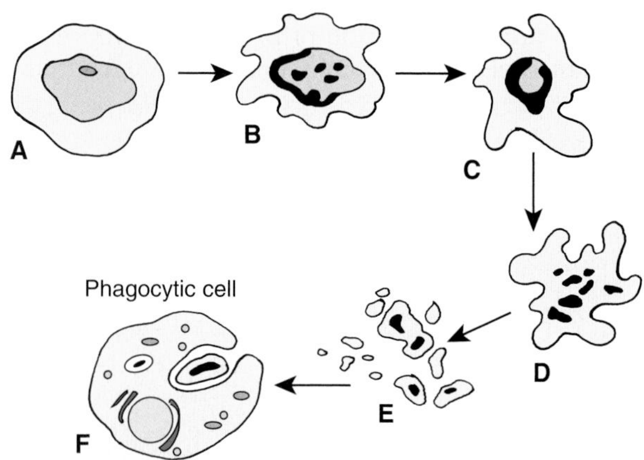

FIGURE 5-9 Apoptotic cell removal: **(A)** shrinking of the cell structures, **(B** and **C)** condensation and fragmentation of the nuclear chromatin, **(D** and **E)** separation of nuclear fragments and cytoplasmic organelles into apoptotic bodies, and **(F)** engulfment of apoptotic fragments by phagocytic cell.

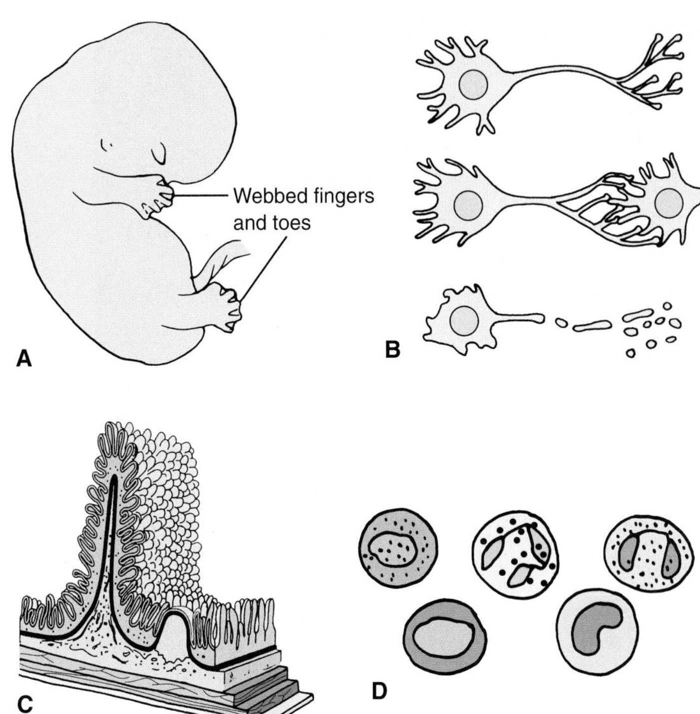

FIGURE 5-10 Examples of apoptosis: (**A**) separation of webbed fingers and toes in embryo, (**B**) development of neural-appropriate connections, (**C**) removal of cells from intestinal villa, and (**D**) removal of senescent blood cells.

can be triggered by the addition or withdrawal of hormones. In hepatitis B and C, the virus seems to sensitize the hepatocytes to apoptosis.[23] Certain oncogenes and suppressor genes involved in the development of cancer seem to play an active role in stimulation or suppression of apoptosis. Injured cells may induce apoptotic cell death through increased cytoplasmic calcium, which leads to activation of nuclear enzymes that break down DNA. In some instances, gene transcription and protein synthesis, the events that produce new cells, may be the initiating factors. In other cases, cell surface signaling or receptor activation appears to be the influencing force.

Necrosis

Necrosis refers to cell death in an organ or tissue that is still part of a living person.[24] Necrosis differs from apoptosis in that it involves unregulated enzymatic digestion of cell components, loss of cell membrane integrity with uncontrolled release of the products of cell death into the intracellular space, and initiation of the inflammatory response.[25] In contrast to apoptosis, which functions in removing cells so that new cells can replace them, necrosis often interferes with cell replacement and tissue regeneration.

With necrotic cell death, there are marked changes in the appearance of the cytoplasmic contents and the nucleus. These changes often are not visible, even under the microscope, for hours after cell death. The dissolution of the necrotic cell or tissue can follow several paths. The cell can undergo liquefaction (*i.e.,* liquefaction necrosis); it can be transformed to a gray, firm mass (*i.e.,* coagulation necrosis); or it can be converted to a cheesy material by infiltration of fatlike substances (*i.e.,* caseous necrosis). *Liquefaction necrosis* occurs when some of the cells die but their catalytic enzymes are not destroyed. An example of liquefaction necrosis is the softening of the center of an abscess with discharge of its contents. During *coagulation necrosis,* acidosis develops and denatures the enzymatic and structural proteins of the cell. This type of necrosis is characteristic of hypoxic injury and is seen in infarcted areas. *Infarction* (*i.e.,* tissue death) occurs when an artery supplying an organ or part of the body becomes occluded and no other source of blood supply exists. As a rule, the infarct's shape is conical and corresponds to the distribution of the artery and its branches. An artery may be occluded by an embolus, a thrombus, disease of the arterial wall, or pressure from outside the vessel.

Caseous necrosis is a distinctive form of coagulation necrosis in which the dead cells persist indefinitely as soft, cheeselike debris.[1] It is most commonly found in the center of tuberculosis granulomas, or tubercles, and is thought to result from immune mechanisms (see Chapter 20).

Gangrene. The term *gangrene* is applied when a considerable mass of tissue undergoes necrosis. Gangrene may be classified as dry or moist. In dry gangrene, the part becomes dry and shrinks, the skin wrinkles, and its color changes to dark brown or black. The spread of dry gangrene is slow, and its symptoms are not as marked as those of wet gangrene. The irritation caused by the dead tissue produces a line of inflammatory reaction (*i.e.,* line of demarcation) between the dead tissue of the gangrenous area and the healthy tissue (Fig. 5-11). Dry gangrene

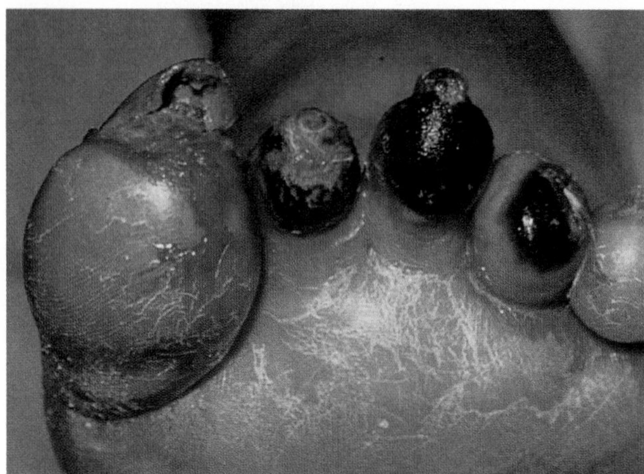

FIGURE 5-11 Gangrenous toes. (Biomedical Communications Group, Southern Illinois University School of Medicine, Springfield, IL)

usually results from interference with arterial blood supply to a part without interference with venous return and is a form of coagulation necrosis.

In moist or wet gangrene, the area is cold, swollen, and pulseless. The skin is moist, black, and under tension. Blebs form on the surface, liquefaction occurs, and a foul odor is caused by bacterial action. There is no line of demarcation between the normal and diseased tissues, and the spread of tissue damage is rapid. Systemic symptoms are usually severe, and death may occur unless the condition can be arrested. Moist or wet gangrene primarily results from interference with venous return from the part. Bacterial invasion plays an important role in the development of wet gangrene and is responsible for many of its prominent symptoms. Dry gangrene is confined almost exclusively to the extremities, whereas moist gangrene may affect the internal organs or the extremities. If bacteria invade the necrotic tissue, dry gangrene may be converted to wet gangrene.

Gas gangrene is a special type of gangrene that results from infection of devitalized tissues by one of several *Clostridium* bacteria, most commonly *Clostridium perfringens*. These anaerobic and spore-forming organisms are widespread in nature, particularly in soil; gas gangrene is prone to occur in trauma and compound fractures in which dirt and debris are embedded. Some species have been isolated in the stomach, gallbladder, intestine, vagina, and skin of healthy persons. The bacteria produce toxins that dissolve cell membranes, causing death of muscle cells, massive spreading edema, hemolysis of red blood cells, hemolytic anemia, hemoglobinuria, and renal failure.[25] Characteristic of this disorder are the bubbles of hydrogen sulfide gas that form in the muscle. Gas gangrene is a serious and potentially fatal disease. Antibiotics are used to treat the infection, and surgical methods are used to remove the infected tissue. Amputation may be required to prevent spreading infection involving a limb. Hyperbaric oxygen therapy has been used, but clinical data supporting its efficacy have not been rigorously assessed.

In summary, cell injury can be caused by a number of agents, including physical agents, chemicals, biologic agents, and nutritional factors. Among the physical agents that generate cell injury are mechanical forces that produce tissue trauma, extremes of temperature, electricity, radiation, and nutritional disorders. Chemical agents can cause cell injury through several mechanisms: they can block enzymatic pathways, cause coagulation of tissues, or disrupt the osmotic or ionic balance of the cell. Biologic agents differ from other injurious agents in that they are able to replicate and continue to produce injury. Among the nutritional factors that contribute to cell injury are excesses and deficiencies of nutrients, vitamins, and minerals.

Injurious agents exert their effects largely through generation of free radicals, production of cell hypoxia, or unregulated intracellular calcium levels. Partially reduced oxygen species called *free radicals* are important mediators of cell injury in many pathologic conditions. They are an important cause of cell injury in hypoxia and after exposure to radiation and certain chemical agents. Lack of oxygen underlies the pathogenesis of cell injury in hypoxia and ischemia. Hypoxia can result from inadequate oxygen in the air, cardiorespiratory disease, anemia, or the inability of the cells to use oxygen. Increased intracellular calcium activates a number of enzymes with potentially damaging effects.

Injurious agents may produce sublethal and reversible cellular damage or may lead to irreversible cell injury and death. Cell death can involve two mechanisms: apoptosis and necrosis. Apoptosis involves controlled cell destruction and is the means by which the body removes and replaces cells that have been produced in excess, developed improperly, have genetic damage, or are worn out. Necrosis refers to cell death that is characterized by cell swelling, rupture of the cell membrane, and inflammation.

REVIEW EXERCISES

A 30-year-old man sustained a fracture of his leg 2 months ago. The leg had been encased in a cast, which was just removed. The patient is amazed at the degree to which the muscles in his leg have shrunk.

A. Would you consider the changes in the patient's muscles to be a normal adaptive response? Explain.

B. Will these changes have an immediate or long-term effect on the function of the leg?

C. What type of measures can be taken to restore full function to the leg?

A 45-year-old woman has been receiving radiation therapy for breast cancer.

A. Explain the effects of ionizing radiation in eradicating the tumor cells.

B. Why is the radiation treatment given in small divided or fractionated doses, rather than as a single large dose?

C. Part way through the treatment schedule, the woman notices that her skin over the irradiated area has become reddened and irritated. What is the reason for this?

People who have had a heart attack may experience additional damage once blood flow has been restored, a phenomenon referred to *reperfusion injury*.

A. What is the proposed mechanism underlying reperfusion injury?

B. What factors might influence this mechanism?

Every day, blood cells in our body become senescent and die without producing signs of inflammation, and yet, massive injury or destruction of tissue, such as occurs with a heart attack, produces significant signs of inflammation.

A. Explain.

References

1. Rubin E., Farber J.L. (Eds.). (1999). *Pathology* (3rd ed., pp. 6–13, 87–103, 329–330, 338–341). Philadelphia: Lippincott-Raven.
2. Kumar V., Cotran R.S., Robbins S.L., Collins T. (2003). *Robbins basic pathology* (7th ed., pp. 3–31, 275–290). Philadelphia: W. B. Saunders.
3. Hunter J.J., Chien K.R. (1999). Signaling pathways in cardiac hypertrophy and failure. *New England Journal of Medicine 341*(17), 1276–1283.
4. Anastassios C., Koumbourlis M.D. (2002). Electrical injuries. *Critical Care Medicine 30*(Suppl), S424–S430.
5. Hahn S.M., Glatstein E. (2001). Radiation injury. In Braunwald E., Fauci A., Kasper D.L., et al. (Eds.). *Harrison's principles of internal medicine* (15th ed., pp. 2585–2590). New York: McGraw Hill.
6. Landrigan P.J., Todd A.C. (1994). Lead poisoning. *Western Journal of Medicine 161,* 153–156.
7. Brody D.J., Pirkle J.L, Kramer R.A. (1994). Blood lead levels in the US population: Phase I of the Third National Health and Nutrition Examination Survey (NHANES III, 1988–1991). *Journal of the American Medical Association 272*(4), 277–283.
8. Pirkle J.L., Brody D.J., Gunter E.W. (1994). The decline in blood lead levels in the United States: The National Health and Nutrition Examination Surveys (NHANES). *Journal of the American Medical Association 272*(4), 284–291.
9. Markowitz M. (2004). Lead poisoning. In Behrman R.E., Kliegman R.M., Jenson H.B. (Eds.). *Nelson textbook of pediatrics* (17th ed., pp. 2358–2362). Philadelphia: W. B. Saunders.
10. Ellis M.R., Kane K.Y. (2000). Lightening the lead load in children. *American Family Physician* 62, 545–554, 559–560.
11. Centers for Disease Control and Prevention. (1997). *Screening young children for lead poisoning: Guidance for state and local health officials.* Atlanta: Centers for Disease Control and Prevention, National Center for Environmental Health, U.S. Department of Health and Human Services, Public Health Service.
12. American Academy of Pediatrics Committee on Environmental Health. (1998). Screening for elevated blood levels. *Pediatrics 101,* 1072–1078.
13. Centers for Disease Control. (1991). *Preventing lead poisoning in young children: A statement by the Centers for Disease Control.* Atlanta: U.S. Department of Health and Human Services, Public Health Service.
14. Canfield R.L., Henderson C.R. Jr., Cory-Slechta D.A., et al. (2003). Intellectual impairment in children with blood lead concentrations below 10 µg per deciliter. *New England Journal of Medicine 348,* 1517–1526.
15. McCord J.M. (2000). The evolution of free radicals and oxidative stress. *American Journal of Medicine 108,* 652–659.
16. Kerr M.E., Bender C.M., Monti E.J. (1996). An introduction to oxygen free radicals. *Heart and Lung 25,* 200–209.
17. Chyanyu C.L., Jackson R.M. (2002). Reactive species mechanisms of cellular hypoxia-reoxygenation injury. *American Journal of Physiology: Cell Physiology 282,* C227–C241.
18. Machlin L.J., Bendich A. (1987). Free radical tissue damage: Protective role of antioxidant nutrients. *FASEB Journal 1*(6), 441–445.
19. Fang Y., Yang S., Wu G. (2002). Free radicals, antioxidants, and nutrition. *Nutrition 18,* 872–879.
20. Vogt M.T., Farber E. (1968). On the molecular pathology of ischemic renal cell death: Reversible and irreversible cellular and mitochondrial metabolic alterations. *American Journal of Pathology 53,* 1–26.
21. Skikumar P., Dong Z., Mikhailov V., et al. (1999). Apoptosis: Definitions, mechanisms, and relevance to disease. *American Journal of Medicine 107,* 490–505.
22. Thompson C.B. (1995). Apoptosis in the pathogenesis and treatment of disease. *Science 267,* 1456–1462.
23. Rust C., Gores G.J. (2000). Apoptosis and liver disease. *American Journal of Medicine 108,* 568–575.
24. Proskuryakov S.Y., Konoplyannikov A.G., Gabai V.L. (2003). Necrosis: A specific form of programmed cell death. *Experimental Cell Research 283,* 1–16.
25. Kasper D.L., Zaleznik D.F. (2001). Gas gangrene, antibiotic-associated colitis, and other clostridial infections. In Braunwald E., Fauci A., Kasper D.L. et al. (Eds.). *Harrison's principles of internal medicine* (15th ed., pp. 922–927). New York: McGraw Hill.

CHAPTER

6

Genetic Control of Cell Function and Inheritance

Edward W. Carroll

Our genetic information is stored in the structure of *deoxyribonucleic acid* (DNA). DNA is an extremely stable macromolecule found in the nucleus of each cell. The gene is the unit of heredity passed from generation to generation. Because of the stable structure of DNA, the genetic information can survive the many processes of reduction division, in which the gametes (*i.e.,* ovum and sperm) are formed, and the fertilization process. This stability is also maintained throughout the many mitotic cell divisions involved in the formation of a new organism from the single-celled fertilized ovum called the *zygote.*

The term *gene* is used to describe a part of the DNA molecule that contains the information needed to code for the many types of proteins and enzymes needed for the day-to-day function of the cells in the body. For example, genes control the type and quantity of hormones that a cell produces, the antigens and receptors that are present on the cell membrane, and the synthesis of enzymes needed for metabolism. Of the over 30,000 estimated genes that humans possess, more than 12,000 have been identified and mapped to a particular chromosome. With few exceptions, each gene provides the instructions for the synthesis of a single protein. This chapter includes discussions of genetic regulation of cell function, chromosomal structure, patterns of inheritance, and gene technology.

Genetic Control of Cell Function

After completing this section of the chapter, you should be able to meet the following objectives:

- ✦ Describe the structure of a gene
- ✦ Explain the mechanisms by which genes control cell function and another generation
- ✦ Describe the concepts of induction and repression as they apply to gene function
- ✦ Describe the pathogenesis of gene mutation
- ✦ Explain how gene expressivity and penetrance determine the effects of a mutant gene that codes for the production of an essential enzyme

The genetic information needed for protein synthesis is encoded in the DNA contained in the cell nucleus. A second type of nucleic acid, *ribonucleic acid* (RNA), is involved in the actual synthesis of cellular enzymes and proteins. Cells contain several types of RNA: messenger RNA, transfer RNA, and ribosomal RNA. *Messenger RNA* (mRNA) contains the transcribed instructions for protein synthesis obtained from the DNA molecule and carries them into the cytoplasm. Transcription is followed by translation, the synthesis of proteins according to the instructions carried by mRNA. *Ribosomal RNA* (rRNA) provides the machinery needed for protein synthesis. *Transfer RNA* (tRNA) reads the instructions and delivers the appropriate amino acids to the ribosome, where they are incorporated into the protein being synthesized. The mechanism for genetic control of cell function is illustrated in Figure 6-1. The nuclei of all the cells in an organism contain the same accumulation of genes derived from the gametes of the two parents. This means that liver cells contain the same genetic information as skin and muscle cells. For this to be true, the molecular code must be duplicated before each succeeding cell division, or mitosis. In theory, although this has not yet been achieved in humans, any of the highly differentiated cells of an organism could be used to produce a complete, genetically identical organism, or *clone*. Each particular cell type in a tissue uses only part of the information stored in the genetic code. Although information required for the development and differentiation of the other cell types is still present, it is repressed.

Besides nuclear DNA, part of the DNA of a cell resides in the mitochondria. Mitochondrial DNA is inherited from the mother by her offspring (*i.e.*, matrilineal inheritance). Several genetic disorders are attributed to defects in mitochondrial DNA. Leber's hereditary optic neuropathy was the first human disease attributed to mutation in mitochondrial DNA.

FUNCTION OF DNA IN CONTROLLING CELL FUNCTION

- The information needed for the control of cell structure and function is embedded in the genetic information encoded in the stable DNA molecule.
- Although every cell in the body contains the same genetic information, each cell type uses only a portion of the information, depending on its structure and function.
- The production of the proteins that control cell function is accomplished by (1) the transcription of the DNA code for assembly of the protein onto messenger RNA, (2) the translation of the code from messenger RNA and assembly of the protein by ribosomal RNA in the cytoplasm, and (3) the delivery of the amino acids needed for protein synthesis to ribosomal RNA by transfer RNA.

GENE STRUCTURE

The structure that stores the genetic information in the nucleus is a long, double-stranded, helical molecule of DNA. DNA is composed of *nucleotides*, which consist of phosphoric acid, a five-carbon sugar called *deoxyribose*, and one of four nitrogenous bases. These nitrogenous bases carry the genetic information and are divided into two groups: the *purine bases*, adenine and guanine, which have two nitrogen ring structures, and the *pyrimidine bases*, thymine and cytosine, which have one ring. The backbone of DNA consists of alternating groups of sugar and phosphoric acid; the paired bases project inward from the sides of the sugar molecule. DNA resembles a spiral staircase, with the paired bases representing the steps (Fig. 6-2). A precise complementary pairing of purine and pyrimidine bases occurs in the double-stranded DNA molecule. Adenine is paired with thymine, and guanine is paired with cytosine. Each nucleotide in a pair is on one strand of the DNA molecule, with the bases on opposite DNA strands bound together by hydrogen bonds that are extremely stable under normal conditions. Enzymes called *DNA helicases* separate the two strands so that the genetic information can be duplicated or transcribed.

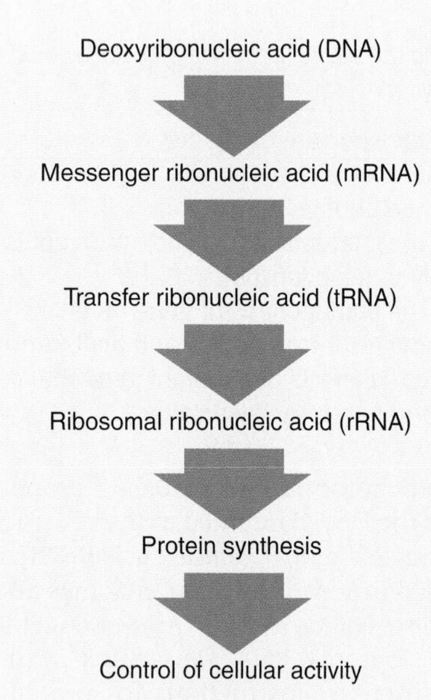

FIGURE 6-1 DNA-directed control of cellular activity through synthesis of cellular proteins. Messenger RNA carries the transcribed message, which directs protein synthesis, from the nucleus to the cytoplasm. Transfer RNA selects the appropriate amino acids and carries them to ribosomal RNA where assembly of the proteins takes place.

Several hundred to almost 1 million base pairs can represent a gene; the size is proportional to the protein product it encodes. Of the two DNA strands, only one is used in transcribing the information for the cell's polypeptide-building machinery. The genetic information of one strand is meaningful and is used as a template for transcription; the complementary code of the other strand does not make sense and is ignored. Both strands, however, are involved in DNA duplication. Before cell division, the two strands of the helix separate, and a complementary molecule is duplicated next to each original strand. Two strands become four strands. During cell division, the newly duplicated double-stranded molecules are separated and placed in each daughter cell by the mechanics of mitosis. As a result, each of the daughter cells again contains the meaningful strand and the complementary strand joined together as a double helix. In 1958, Meselson and Stahl characterized this replication of DNA as *semiconservative* as opposed to conservative (Fig. 6-3).

The DNA molecule is combined with several types of protein and small amounts of RNA into a complex known as *chromatin*. Chromatin is the readily stainable portion of

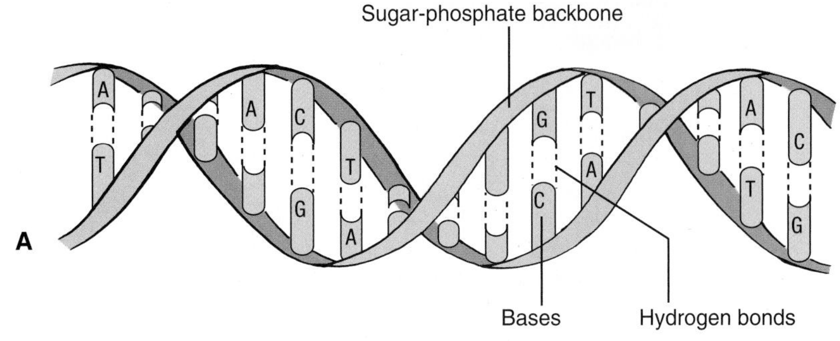

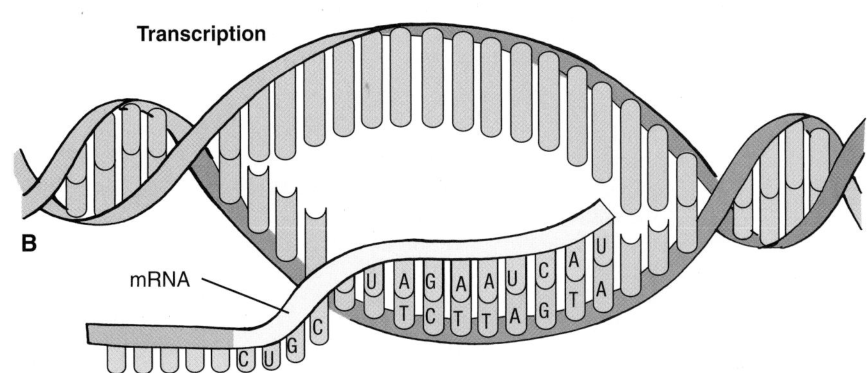

FIGURE 6-2 The DNA double helix and transcription of messenger RNA (mRNA). The top panel (**A**) shows the sequence of four bases (adenine [A], cytosine [C], guanine [G], and thymine [T]), which determines the specificity of genetic information. The bases face inward from the sugar-phosphate backbone and form pairs (*dashed lines*) with complementary bases on the opposing strand. In the bottom panel (**B**), transcription creates a complementary mRNA copy from one of the DNA strands in the double helix.

the cell nucleus. Some DNA proteins form binding sites for repressor molecules and hormones that regulate genetic transcription; others may block genetic transcription by preventing access of nucleotides to the surface of the DNA molecule. A specific group of proteins called *histones* is thought to control the folding of the DNA strands.

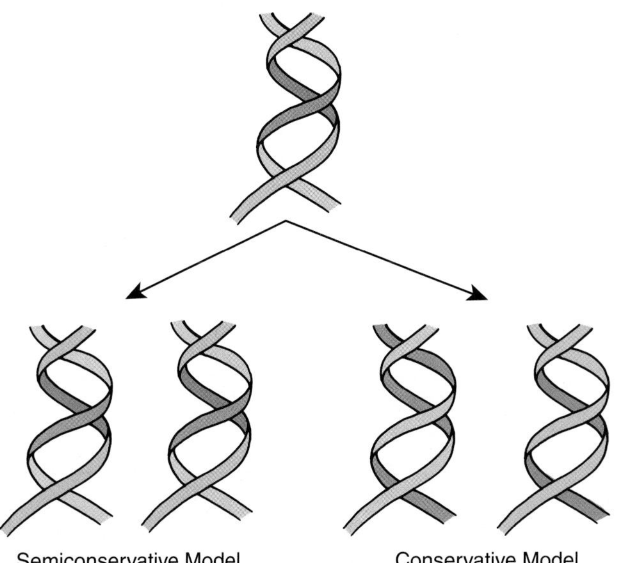

FIGURE 6-3 Semiconservative vs conservative models of DNA replication as proposed by Meselson and Stahl in 1958. In semiconservative DNA replication, the two original strands of DNA unwind and a complementary strand is formed along each original strand.

GENETIC CODE

The four bases—guanine, adenine, cytosine, and thymine (uracil is substituted for thymine in RNA)—make up the alphabet of the genetic code. A sequence of three of these bases forms the fundamental triplet code used in transmitting the genetic information needed for protein synthesis. This triplet code is called a *codon* (Table 6-1). An example is the nucleotide sequence GCU (guanine, cytosine, and uracil), which is the triplet RNA code for the amino acid alanine. The genetic code is a universal language used by most living cells (*i.e.,* the code for the amino acid tryptophan is the same in a bacterium, a plant, and a human being). *Stop codes,* which signal the end of a protein molecule, are also present. Mathematically, the four bases can be arranged in 64 different combinations. Sixty-one of the triplets correspond to particular amino acids, and three are stop signals. Only 20 amino acids are used in protein synthesis in humans. Several triplets code for the same amino acid; therefore, the genetic code is said to be *redundant* or *degenerate.* For example, AUG is a part of the initiation or start signal and the codon for the amino acid methionine. Codons that specify the same amino acid are called *synonyms.* Synonyms usually have the same first two bases but differ in the third base.

PROTEIN SYNTHESIS

Although DNA determines the type of biochemical product that the cell synthesizes, the transmission and decoding of information needed for protein synthesis are carried out by RNA, the formation of which is directed by DNA. The general structure of RNA differs from DNA in three

TABLE 6-1 Triplet Codes for Amino Acids

Amino Acid	RNA Codons					
Alanine	GCU	GCC	GCA	GCG		
Arginine	CGU	CGC	CGA	CGG	AGA	AGG
Asparagine	AAU	AAC				
Aspartic acid	GAU	GAC				
Cysteine	UGU	UGC				
Glutamic acid	GAA	GAG				
Glutamine	CAA	CAG				
Glycine	GGU	GGC	GGA	GGG		
Histidine	CAU	CAC				
Isoleucine	AUU	AUC	AUA			
Leucine	CUU	CUC	CUA	CUG	UUA	UUG
Lysine	AAA	AAG				
Methionine	AUG					
Phenylalanine	UUU	UUC				
Proline	CCU	CCC	CCA	CCG		
Serine	UCU	UCC	UCA	UCG	AGC	AGU
Threonine	ACU	ACC	ACA	ACG		
Tryptophan	UGG					
Tyrosine	UAU	UAC				
Valine	GUU	GUC	GUA	GUG		
Start (CI)	AUG					
Stop (CT)	UAA	UAG	UGA			

respects: RNA is a single-stranded rather than a double-stranded molecule; the sugar in each nucleotide of RNA is ribose instead of deoxyribose; and the pyrimidine base thymine in DNA is replaced by uracil in RNA. Three types of RNA are known: mRNA, tRNA, and rRNA. All three types are synthesized in the nucleus by RNA polymerase enzymes that take directions from DNA. Because the ribose sugars found in RNA are more susceptible to degradation than the sugars in DNA, the types of RNA molecules in the cytoplasm can be altered rapidly in response to extracellular signals.

Messenger RNA

Messenger RNA is the template for protein synthesis. It is a long molecule containing several hundred to several thousand nucleotides. Each group of three nucleotides forms a codon that is exactly complementary to the triplet of nucleotides of the DNA molecule. Messenger RNA is formed by a process called *transcription*. In this process, the weak hydrogen bonds of the DNA are broken so that free RNA nucleotides can pair with their exposed DNA counterparts on the meaningful strand of the DNA molecule (see Fig. 6-2). As with the base pairing of the DNA strands, complementary RNA bases pair with the DNA bases. In RNA, uracil replaces thymine and pairs with adenine.

During transcription, a specialized nuclear enzyme, called *RNA polymerase*, recognizes the beginning or start sequence of a gene. The RNA polymerase attaches to the double-stranded DNA and proceeds to copy the meaningful strand into a single strand of RNA as it travels along the length of the gene. On reaching the stop signal, the enzyme leaves the gene and releases the RNA strand. The RNA strand is then processed. Processing involves the addition of certain nucleic acids at the ends of the RNA strand and cutting and splicing of certain internal sequences. Splicing often involves the removal of stretches of RNA (Fig. 6-4). Because of the splicing process, the final mRNA sequence is different from the original DNA template. RNA sequences that are retained are called *exons*, and those excised are called *introns*. The functions of the in-

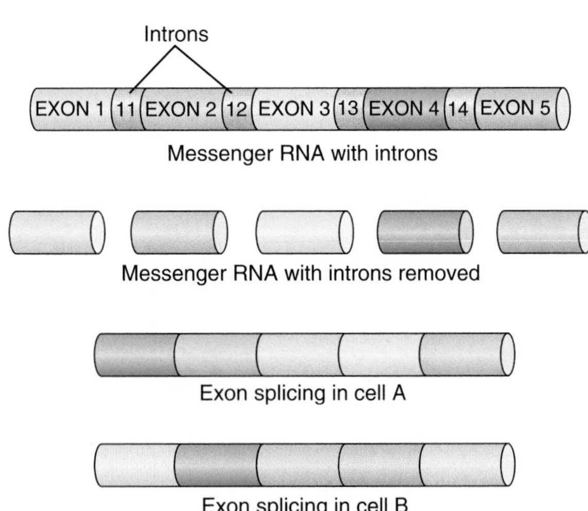

FIGURE 6-4 In different cells, an RNA strand may eventually produce different proteins depending on the sequencing of exons during gene splicing. This variation allows a gene to code for more than one protein. (Courtesy of Edward W. Carroll)

trons are unknown. They are thought to be involved in the activation or deactivation of genes during various stages of development.

Splicing permits a cell to produce a variety of mRNA molecules from a single gene. By varying the splicing segments of the initial mRNA, different mRNA molecules are formed. For example, in a muscle cell, the original tropomyosin mRNA is spliced in as many as 10 different ways, yielding distinctly different protein products. This permits different proteins to be expressed from a single gene and reduces how much DNA must be contained in the genome.

Transfer RNA

The clover-shaped tRNA molecule contains only 80 nucleotides, making it the smallest RNA molecule. Its function is to deliver the activated form of amino acids to protein molecules in the ribosomes. At least 20 different types of tRNA are known, each of which recognizes and binds to only one type of amino acid. Each tRNA molecule has two recognition sites: the first is complementary for the mRNA codon, the second for the amino acid itself. Each type of tRNA carries its own specific amino acid to the ribosomes, where protein synthesis is taking place; there it recognizes the appropriate codon on the mRNA and delivers the amino acid to the newly forming protein molecule.

Ribosomal RNA

The ribosome is the physical structure in the cytoplasm where protein synthesis takes place. Ribosomal RNA forms 60% of the ribosome; the remainder of the ribosome is composed of the structural proteins and enzymes needed for protein synthesis. As with the other types of RNA, rRNA is synthesized in the nucleus. Unlike other RNAs, ribosomal RNA is produced in a specialized nuclear structure called the *nucleolus*. The formed rRNA combines with ribosomal proteins in the nucleus to produce the ribosome, which is then transported into the cytoplasm. On reaching the cytoplasm, most ribosomes become attached to the endoplasmic reticulum and begin the task of protein synthesis.

Proteins are made from a standard set of amino acids, which are joined end to end to form the long polypeptide chains of protein molecules. Each polypeptide chain may have as many as 100 to more than 300 amino acids in it. The process of protein synthesis is called *translation* because the genetic code is translated into the production language needed for protein assembly. Besides rRNA, translation requires the coordinated actions of mRNA and tRNA (Fig. 6-5). Each of the 20 different tRNA molecules transports its specific amino acid to the ribosome for incorporation into the developing protein molecule. Messenger RNA provides the information needed for placing the amino acids in their proper order for each specific type of protein. During protein synthesis, mRNA contacts and passes through the ribosome, which "reads" the directions for protein synthesis in much the same way that a tape is read as it passes through a tape player. As mRNA passes through the ribosome, tRNA delivers the appropriate amino acids for attachment to the growing polypeptide chain. The long mRNA molecule usually travels through and directs protein synthesis in more than one ribosome at a

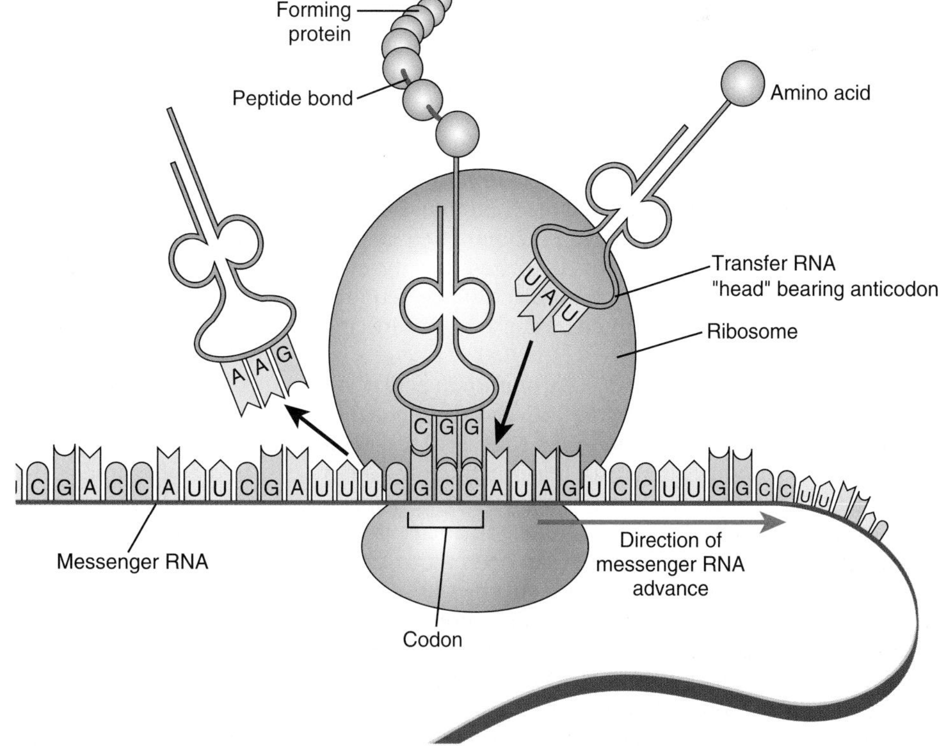

FIGURE 6-5 Protein synthesis. A messenger RNA strand is moving through a small ribosomal RNA subunit in the cytoplasm. Transfer RNA transports amino acids to the mRNA strand and recognizes the RNA codon calling for the amino acid by base pairing (through its anticodon). The ribosome then adds the amino acid to the growing polypeptide chain. The ribosome moves along the mRNA strand and is read sequently. As each amino acid is bound to the next by a peptide bond, its tRNA is released.

time. After the first ribosome reads the first part of the mRNA, it moves on to read a second and a third. As a result, ribosomes that are actively involved in protein synthesis are often found in clusters called *polyribosomes.*

REGULATION OF GENE EXPRESSION

Although all cells contain the same genes, not all genes are active all of the time, nor are the same genes active in all cell types. On the contrary, only a small, select group of genes is active in directing protein synthesis in the cell, and this group varies from one cell type to another. For the differentiation process of cells to occur in the various organs and tissues of the body, protein synthesis in some cells must be different from that in others. To adapt to an ever-changing environment, certain cells may need to produce varying amounts and types of proteins. Certain enzymes, such as carbonic anhydrase, are synthesized by all cells for the fundamental metabolic processes on which life depends.

The degree to which a gene or particular group of genes is active is called *gene expression.* A phenomenon termed *induction* is an important process by which gene expression is increased. Except in early embryonic development, induction is promoted by some external influence. *Gene repression* is a process by which a regulatory gene acts to reduce or prevent gene expression. Some genes are normally dormant but can be activated by inducer substances; other genes are naturally active and can be inhibited by repressor substances. Genetic mechanisms for the control of protein synthesis are better understood in microorganisms than in humans. It can be assumed, however, that the same general principles apply.

The mechanism that has been most extensively studied is the one by which the synthesis of particular proteins can be turned on and off. For example, in the bacterium *Escherichia coli* grown in a nutrient medium containing the disaccharide lactose, the enzyme galactosidase can be isolated. The galactosidase catalyzes the splitting of lactose into a molecule of glucose and a molecule of galactose. This is necessary if lactose is to be metabolized by *E. coli.* However, if the *E. coli* is grown in a medium that does not contain lactose, very little of the enzyme is produced. From these and other studies, it is theorized that the synthesis of a particular protein, such as galactosidase, requires a series of reactions, each of which is catalyzed by a specific enzyme.

At least two types of genes control protein synthesis: *structural genes* that specify the amino acid sequence of a polypeptide chain and *regulator genes* that serve a regulatory function without stipulating the structure of protein molecules. The regulation of protein synthesis is controlled by a sequence of genes, called an *operon,* on adjacent sites on the same chromosome (Fig. 6-6). An operon consists of a set of structural genes that code for enzymes used in the synthesis of a particular product and a promoter site that binds RNA polymerase and initiates transcription of the structural genes. The function of the operon is further regulated by activator and repressor operators, which induce or repress the function of the promoter. Activator and repressor sites commonly monitor levels of the synthesized product and regulate the activity of the operon through a negative feedback mechanism. Whenever product levels decrease, the function of the operon is activated, and when levels increase, its function is repressed. Regulatory genes found elsewhere in the genetic complex can exert control over an operon through activator or repressor substances. Not all genes are subject to induction and repression.

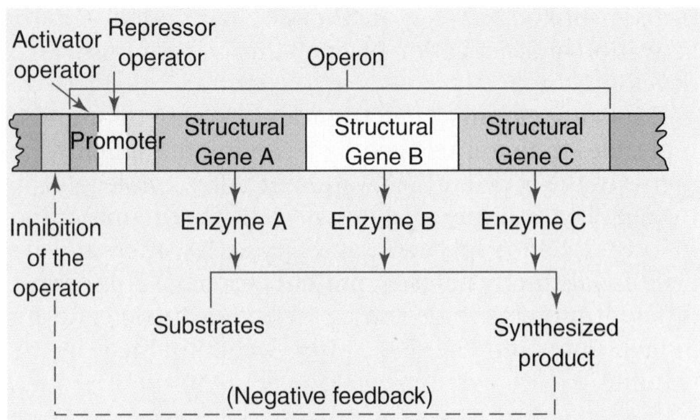

FIGURE 6-6 Function of the operon to control biosynthesis. The synthesized product exerts negative feedback to inhibit function of the operon, in this way automatically controlling the concentration of the product itself. (Guyton A., Hall J.E. [2000]. *Textbook of medical physiology* [10th ed., p. 31]. Philadelphia: W.B. Saunders)

GENE MUTATIONS

Rarely, accidental errors in duplication of DNA occur. These errors are called *mutations.* Mutations result from the substitution of one base pair for another, the loss or addition of one or more base pairs, or rearrangements of base pairs. Many of these mutations occur spontaneously; others occur because of environmental agents, chemicals, and radiation. Mutations may arise in somatic cells or in germ cells. Only those DNA changes that occur in germ cells can be inherited. A somatic mutation affects a cell line that differentiates into one or more of the many tissues of the body and is not transmissible to the next generation. Somatic mutations that do not have an impact on the health or functioning of a person are called *polymorphisms.* Occasionally, a person is born with one brown eye and one blue eye because of a somatic mutation. The change or loss of gene information is just as likely to affect the fundamental processes of cell function or organ differentiation. Such somatic mutations in the early embryonic period can result in embryonic death or congenital malformations.

Somatic mutations are important causes of cancer and other tumors in which cell differentiation and growth get out of control. Each year, hundreds of thousands of random changes occur in the DNA molecule because of environmental events or metabolic accidents. Fortunately, less than 1 in 1000 base pair changes result in serious mutations. Most of these defects are corrected by DNA repair mechanisms. Several mechanisms exist, and each depends on specific enzymes such as DNA repair nucleases. Fishermen, farmers, and others who are excessively exposed to the ultraviolet radiation of sunlight have an increased risk for development of skin cancer because of potential radiation damage to the genetic structure of the skin-forming cells.

In summary, genes are the fundamental unit of information storage in the cell. They determine the types of proteins and enzymes made by the cell and therefore control inheritance and day-to-day cell function. Genes store information in a stable macromolecule called *DNA.* Genes transmit information contained in the DNA molecule as a triplet code. The genetic code is determined by the arrangement of the nitrogenous bases of the four nucleotides (*i.e.,* adenine, guanine, thymine [or uracil in RNA], and cytosine). The transfer of stored information into production of cell products is accomplished through a second type of macromolecule called *RNA.* Messenger RNA transcribes the instructions for product synthesis from the DNA molecule and carries it into the cell's cytoplasm, where ribosomal RNA uses the information to direct product synthesis. Transfer RNA acts as a carrier system for delivering the appropriate amino acids to the ribosomes, where the synthesis of cell products occurs. Although all cells contain the same genes, only a small, select group of genes is active in a given cell type. In all cells, some genetic information is repressed, whereas other information is expressed. Gene mutations represent accidental errors in duplication, rearrangement, or deletion of parts of the genetic code. Fortunately, most mutations are corrected by DNA repair mechanisms in the cell.

Chromosomes

After completing this section of the chapter, you should be able to meet the following objectives:

- Define the terms *autosomes, chromatin, meiosis,* and *mitosis*
- List the steps in constructing a karyotype using cytogenetic studies
- Explain the significance of the Barr body

Most genetic information of a cell is organized, stored, and retrieved in small intracellular structures called *chromosomes.* Although the chromosomes are visible only in dividing cells, they retain their integrity between cell divisions. The chromosomes are arranged in pairs; one member of the pair is inherited from the father, the other from the mother. Each species has a characteristic number of chromosomes. In a particular species of an ant, the females have a single pair of chromosomes, whereas the males have only one chromosome; 630 pairs of chromosomes are present in certain ferns. In humans, 46 single or 23 pairs of chromosomes are present. Of the 23 pairs of human chromosomes, 22 are called *autosomes* and are alike in both males and females. Each of the 22 pairs of autosomes has the same appearance in all individuals, and each has been given a numeric designation for classification purposes (Fig. 6-7).

The sex chromosomes make up the 23rd pair of chromosomes. Two sex chromosomes determine the sex of a

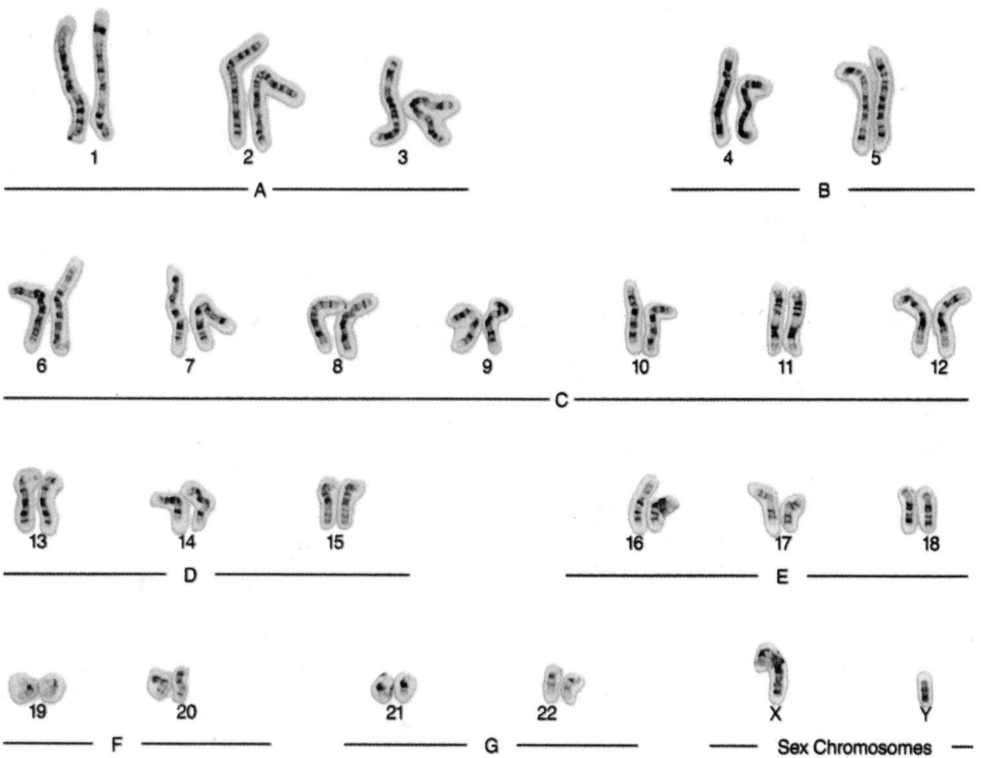

FIGURE 6-7 Karyotype of normal human body. (Courtesy of the Prenatal Diagnostic and Imaging Center, Sacramento, CA. Frederick W. Hansen, MD, Medical Director)

CHROMOSOME STRUCTURE

- The DNA that stores genetic material is organized into 23 pairs of chromosomes. There are 22 pairs of autosomes, which are alike for males and females, and one pair of sex chromosomes, with XX pairing in females and XY pairing in males.
- Cell division involves the duplication of the chromosomes. Duplication of chromosomes in somatic cell lines involves mitosis, in which each daughter cell receives a pair of 23 chromosomes. Meiosis is limited to replicating germ cells and results in formation of a single set of 23 chromosomes.

person. All males have an X and Y chromosome (*i.e.,* an X chromosome from the mother and a Y chromosome from the father); all females have two X chromosomes (*i.e.,* one from each parent). The much smaller Y chromosome contains the *male-specific region* (MSY) that determines sex. This region constitutes more than 90 percent of the length of the Y chromosome.

Only one X chromosome in the female is active in controlling the expression of genetic traits; however, both X chromosomes are activated during gametogenesis. In the female, the active X chromosome is invisible, but the inactive X chromosome can be demonstrated with appropriate nuclear staining. Inactivation is thought to involve the addition of a methyl group to the X chromosome. This inactive chromatin mass is seen as the *Barr body* in epithelial cells or as the drumstick body in the chromatin of neutrophils. The genetic sex of a child can be determined by microscopic study of cell or tissue samples. The total number of X chromosomes is equal to the number of Barr bodies plus one (*i.e.,* an inactive plus an active X chromosome). For example, the cells of a normal female have one Barr body and therefore a total of two X chromosomes. A normal male has no Barr bodies. Males with Klinefelter's syndrome (one Y, an inactive X, and an active X chromosome) exhibit one Barr body. In the female, whether the X chromosome derived from the mother or that derived from the father is active is determined within a few days after conception; the selection is random for each postmitotic cell line. This is called the *Lyon principle,* after Mary Lyon, the British geneticist who described it.

CELL DIVISION

Two types of cell division occur in humans and many other animals: mitosis and meiosis. *Meiosis* is limited to replicating germ cells and takes place only once in a cell line. It results in the formation of gametes or reproductive cells (*i.e.,* ovum and sperm), each of which has only a single set of 23 chromosomes. Meiosis is typically divided into two distinct phases, meiotic divisions I and II. Similar to mitosis, cells about to undergo the first meiotic division replicate their DNA during interphase. During metaphase I, homologous chromosomes pair up, forming a synapsis or tetrad (two chromatids per chromosome). They are sometimes called *bivalents.* The X and Y chromosomes are not homologs and do not form bivalents. While in metaphase I, an interchange of chromatid segments can occur. This process is called *crossing over* (Fig. 6-8). Crossing over allows for new combinations of genes, increasing genetic variability. After telophase I, each of the two daughter cells contains one member of each homologous pair of chromosomes and a sex chromosome (23 double-stranded chromosomes). No DNA synthesis occurs before meiotic division II. During anaphase II, the 23 double-stranded chromosomes (two chromatids) of each of the two daughter cells from meiosis I divide at their centromeres. Each subsequent daughter cell receives 23 single-stranded chromatids. Thus, a total of four daughter cells are formed by a meiotic division of one cell (Fig. 6-9).

Meiosis, occurring only in the gamete-producing cells found in either testes or ovaries, has a different outcome in males and females. In males, meiosis (spermatogenesis) results in four viable daughter cells called *spermatids* that differentiate into sperm cells. In females, gamete formation or oogenesis is quite different. After the first meiotic division of a primary oocyte, a secondary oocyte and another structure called a *polar body* are formed. This small polar body contains little cytoplasm, but it may undergo a second meiotic division, resulting in two polar bodies (Fig. 6-10). The secondary oocyte undergoes its second meiotic division, producing one mature oocyte and another polar body. Four viable sperm cells are produced during spermatogenesis, but only one ovum from oogenesis.

CHROMOSOME STRUCTURE

Cytogenetics is the study of the structure and numeric characteristics of the cell's chromosomes. Chromosome studies can be done on any tissue or cell that grows and divides in culture. Lymphocytes from venous blood are frequently used for this purpose. After the cells have been cultured, a drug called *colchicine* is used to arrest mitosis in metaphase. A chromosome spread is prepared by fixing

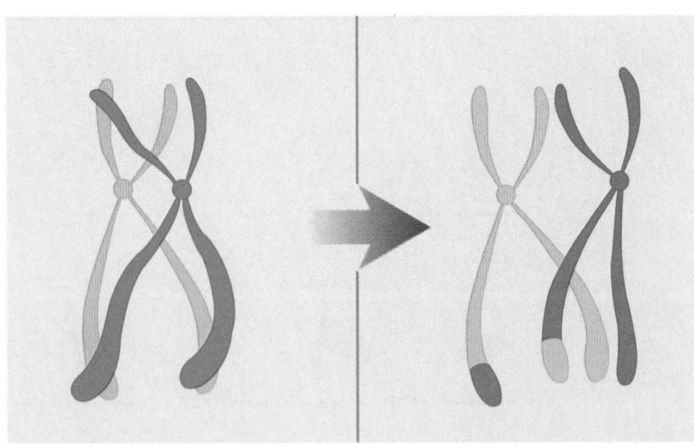

FIGURE 6-8 Crossing over of DNA at the time of meiosis.

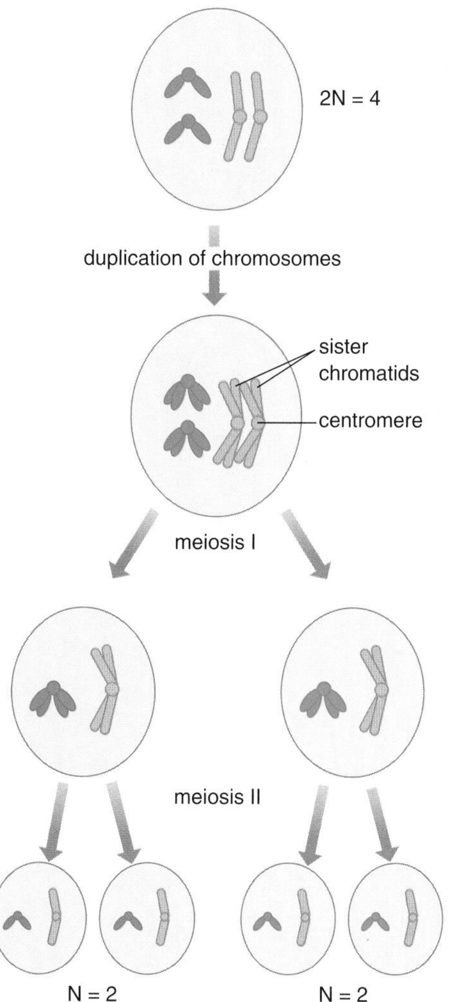

FIGURE 6-9 Separation of chromosomes at the time of meiosis.

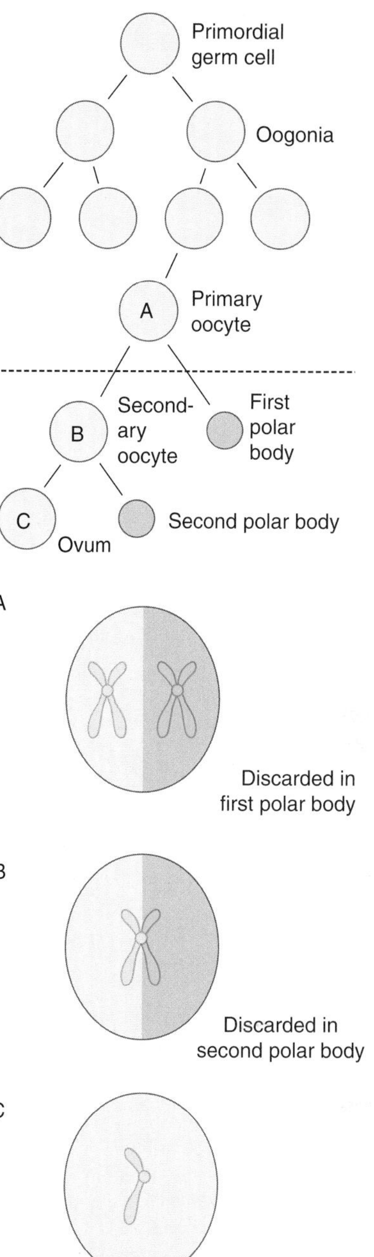

FIGURE 6-10 Essential stages of meiosis in a female, with discarding of the first and second polar bodies and formation of the ovum with the haploid number of chromosomes. The *dotted line* indicates reduction division. (Adapted from Cormack D.H. [1993]. *Essential histology.* Philadelphia: J.B. Lippincott)

and spreading the chromosomes on a slide. Subsequently, appropriate staining techniques show the chromosomal banding patterns so that they can be identified. The chromosomes are photographed, and the photomicrograph of each chromosome is cut out and arranged in pairs according to a standard classification system (see Fig. 6-7). The completed picture is called a *karyotype,* and the procedure for preparing the picture is called *karyotyping.* A uniform system of chromosome classification was originally formulated at the 1971 Paris Chromosome Conference and was later revised to describe the chromosomes as seen in more elongated prophase and prometaphase preparations.

In the metaphase spread, each chromosome takes the form of chromatids to form an "X" or "wishbone" pattern. Human chromosomes are divided into three types according to the position of the centromere (Fig. 6-11). If the centromere is in the center and the arms are of approximately the same length, the chromosome is said to be *metacentric;* if it is not centered and the arms are of clearly different lengths, it is *submetacentric;* and if it is near one end, it is *acrocentric.* The short arm of the chromosome is designated as "p" for "petite," and the long arm is designated as "q" for no other reason than it is the next letter of the alphabet. The arms of the chromosome are indicated by the chromosome number followed by the p or q designation (*e.g.,* 15p). Chromosomes 13, 14, 15, 21, and 22 have small masses of chromatin called *satellites* attached to their short arms by narrow stalks. At the ends of each chromosome are special DNA sequences called *telomeres.* Telomeres allow the end of the DNA molecule to be replicated completely.

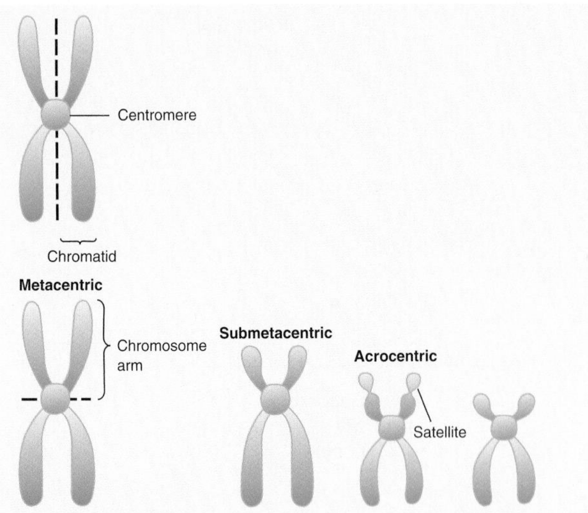

FIGURE 6-11 Three basic shapes and the component parts of human metaphase chromosomes. The relative size of the satellite on the acrocentric is exaggerated for visibility. (Adapted from Cormack D.H. [1993]. *Essential histology*. Philadelphia: J.B. Lippincott)

The banding patterns of a chromosome are used in describing the position of a gene on the chromosome. Each arm of a chromosome is divided into regions, which are numbered from the centromere outward (*e.g.,* 1,2). The regions are further divided into bands, which are also numbered (Fig. 6-12). These numbers are used in designating the position of a gene on a chromosome. For example, Xp22 refers to band 2, region 2 of the short arm (p) of the X chromosome.

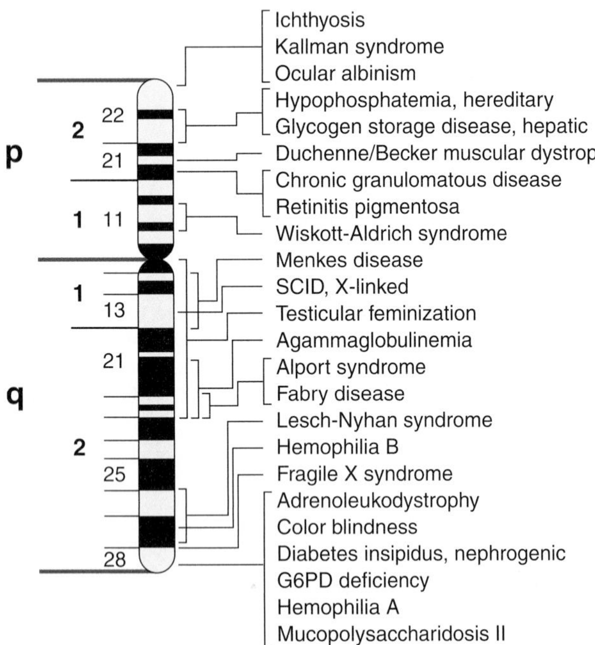

FIGURE 6-12 The localization of representative inherited diseases on the X chromosome. Notice the nomenclature of arms (P,Q), regions (1,2), bands (*e.g.,* 11,22). (Rubin E., Farber J.L. [1999]. *Pathology* [3rd ed., p. 260]. Philadelphia: Lippincott-Raven)

In summary, the genetic information in a cell is organized, stored, and retrieved as small cellular structures called *chromosomes.* Forty-six chromosomes arranged in 23 pairs are present in the human being. Twenty-two of these pairs are autosomes. The 23rd pair is the sex chromosomes, which determine the sex of a person. Two types of cell division occur, meiosis and mitosis. Meiosis is limited to replicating germ cells and results in the formation of gametes or reproductive cells (ovum and sperm), each of which has only a single set of 23 chromosomes. Mitotic division occurs in somatic cells and results in the formation of 23 pairs of chromosomes. A karyotype is a photograph of a person's chromosomes. It is prepared by special laboratory techniques in which body cells are cultured, fixed, and then stained to display identifiable banding patterns. A photomicrograph is then made. Often, the individual chromosomes are cut out and regrouped according to chromosome number.

Patterns of Inheritance

After completing this section of the chapter, you should be able to meet the following objectives:

- ✦ Construct a hypothetical pedigree for a recessive and dominant trait according to Mendel's law
- ✦ Contrast genotype and phenotype
- ✦ Define the terms *allele, locus, expressivity,* and *penetrance*

The characteristics inherited from a person's parents are inscribed in gene pairs found along the length of the chromosomes. Alternate forms of the same gene are possible (*i.e.,* one inherited from the mother and the other from the father), and each may produce a different aspect of a trait.

DEFINITIONS

Genetics has its own set of definitions. The *genotype* of a person is the genetic information stored in the base sequence triplet code. The *phenotype* refers to the recognizable traits, physical or biochemical, associated with a specific genotype. Often, the genotype is not evident by available detection methods. More than one genotype may have the same phenotype. Some brown-eyed persons are carriers of the code for blue eyes, and other brown-eyed persons are not. Phenotypically, these two types of brown-eyed persons are the same, but genotypically, they are different.

When it comes to a genetic disorder, not all persons with a mutant gene are affected to the same extent. *Expressivity* refers to the manner in which the gene is expressed in the phenotype, which can range from mild to severe. *Penetrance* represents the ability of a gene to express its function. Seventy-five percent penetrance means that 75% of persons of a particular genotype present with a recog-

TRANSMISSION OF GENETIC INFORMATION

- The transmission of information from one generation to the next is vested in genetic material transferred from each parent at the time of conception.
- Alleles are the alternate forms of a gene (one from each parent), and the locus is the position that they occupy on the chromosome.
- The genotype of a person represents the sum total of the genetic information in the cells and the phenotype the physical manifestations of that information.
- Penetrance is the percentage in a population with a particular genotype in which that genotype is phenotypically manifested, whereas expressivity is the manner in which the gene is expressed.
- Mendelian, or single-gene, patterns of inheritance include autosomal dominant and recessive traits that are transmitted from parents to their offspring in a predictable manner. Polygenic inheritance, which involves multiple genes, and multifactorial inheritance, which involves multiple genes as well as environmental factors, are less predictable.

nizable phenotype. Syndactyly and blue sclera are genetic mutations that often do not exhibit 100% penetrance.

The position of a gene on a chromosome is called its *locus,* and alternate forms of a gene at the same locus are called *alleles.* When only one pair of genes is involved in the transmission of information, the term *single-gene trait* is used. Single-gene traits follow the mendelian laws of inheritance (to be discussed).

Polygenic inheritance involves multiple genes at different loci, with each gene exerting a small additive effect in determining a trait. Most human traits are determined by multiple pairs of genes, many with alternate codes, accounting for some dissimilar forms that occur with certain genetic disorders. Polygenic traits are predictable, but with less reliability than single-gene traits. *Multifactorial* inheritance is similar to polygenic inheritance in that multiple alleles at different loci affect the outcome; the difference is that multifactorial inheritance includes environmental effects on the genes.

Many other gene–gene interactions are known. These include *epistasis,* in which one gene masks the phenotypic effects of another nonallelic gene; *multiple alleles,* in which more than one allele affects the same trait (*e.g.,* ABO blood types); *complementary genes,* in which each gene is mutually dependent on the other; and *collaborative genes,* in which two different genes influencing the same trait interact to produce a phenotype that neither gene alone could produce.

GENETIC IMPRINTING

Besides autosomal and sex-linked genes and mitochondrial inheritance, it was found that certain genes exhibit a "parent of origin" type of transmission in which the parental genomes do not always contribute equally in the development of an individual (Fig. 6-13). The transmission of this phenomenon was given the name *genomic imprinting* by Helen Crouse in 1960. Although rare, it is estimated that approximately 100 genes exhibit genomic, or genetic, imprinting. Evidence suggests that a genetic conflict occurs in

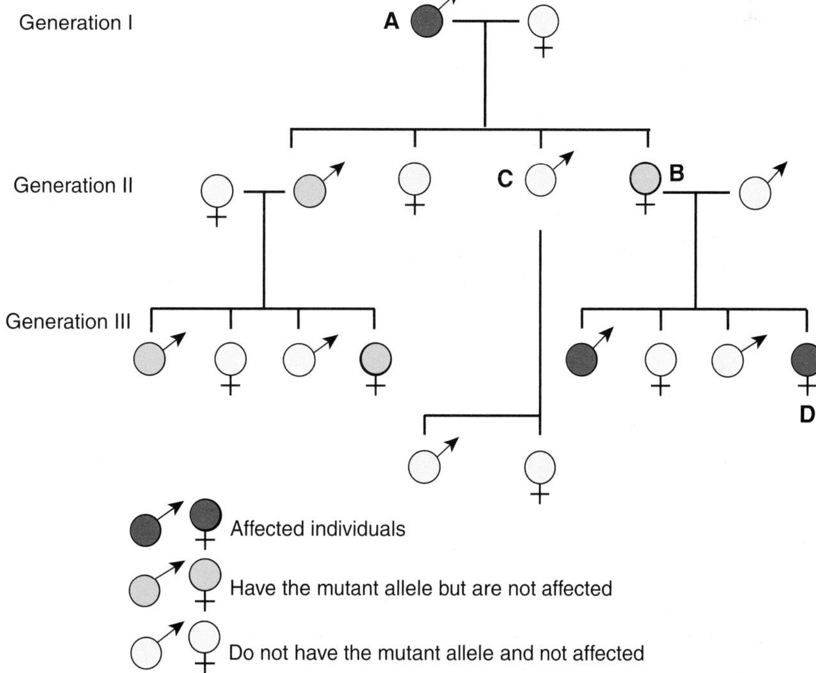

FIGURE 6-13 Pedigree of genetic imprinting. In generation I, male **A** has inherited a mutant allele from his affected mother (not shown); the gene is "turned off" during spermatogenesis, and therefore none of his offspring (generation II) will express the mutant allele, regardless if they are carriers. However, the gene will be "turned on" again during oogenesis in any of his daughters (**B**) who inherit the allele. All offspring (generation III) who inherit the mutant allele will be affected. All offspring of normal children (**C**) will produce normal offspring. Children of female **D** will all express the mutation if they inherit the allele.

the developing embryo: the male genome attempts to establish larger offspring, whereas the female prefers smaller offspring to conserve her energy for the current and subsequent pregnancies.

It was the pathologic analysis of ovarian teratomas (tumors made up of various cell types derived from an undifferentiated germ cell) and hydatidiform moles (gestational tumors made up of trophoblastic tissue) that yielded the first evidence of genetic imprinting. All ovarian teratomas were found to have a 46,XX karyotype. The results of detailed chromosomal polymorphism analysis confirmed that these tumors developed without the paternally derived genome. Conversely, analysis of hydatidiform moles suggested that they were tumors of paternal origin.

A well-known example of genomic imprinting is the transmission of the mutations in Prader-Willi and Angelman's syndromes. Both syndromes exhibit mental retardation as a common feature. It was also found that both disorders had the same deletion in chromosome 15. When the deletion is inherited from the mother, the infant presents with Angelman's ("happy puppet") syndrome; when the same deletion is inherited from the father, Prader-Willi syndrome results.

A related chromosomal disorder is *uniparental disomy*. This occurs when two chromosomes of the same number are inherited from one parent. Normally, this is not a problem except in cases in which a chromosome has been imprinted by a parent. If an allele is inactivated by imprinting, the offspring will have only one working copy of the chromosome, resulting in possible problems.

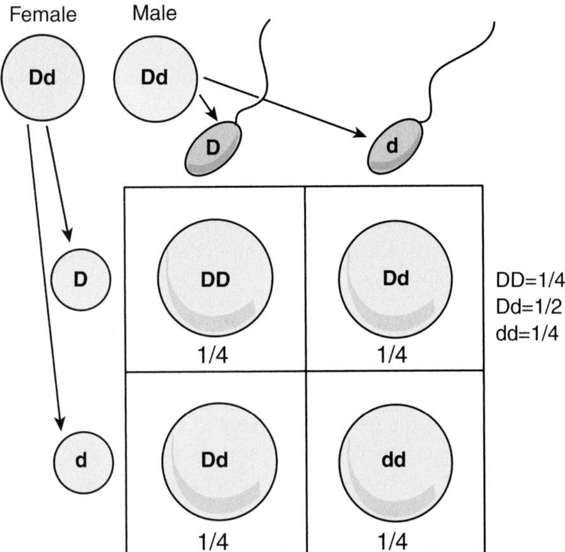

FIGURE 6-14 The Punnett square showing all possible combinations for transmission of a single gene trait (dimpled cheeks). The example shown is when both parents are heterozygous (dD) for the trait. The alleles carried by the mother are on the left and those carried by the father are on the top. The D allele is dominant and the d allele is recessive. The DD and Dd offspring have dimples and the dd offspring does not.

MENDEL'S LAW

A main feature of inheritance is predictability: given certain conditions, the likelihood of the occurrence or recurrence of a specific trait is remarkably predictable. The units of inheritance are the genes, and the pattern of single-gene expression can often be predicted using Mendel's laws of genetic transmission. Techniques and discoveries since Gregor Mendel's original work was published in 1865 have led to some modification of his original laws.

Mendel discovered the basic pattern of inheritance by conducting carefully planned experiments with simple garden peas. Experimenting with several phenotypic traits in peas, Mendel proposed that inherited traits are transmitted from parents to offspring by means of independently inherited factors—now known as genes—and that these factors are transmitted as recessive and dominant traits. Mendel labeled dominant factors (his round peas) "A" and recessive factors (his wrinkled peas) "a." Geneticists continue to use capital letters to designate dominant traits and lowercase letters to identify recessive traits. The possible combinations that can occur with transmission of single-gene dominant and recessive traits can be described by constructing a figure called a *Punnett square* using capital and lowercase letters (Fig. 6-14).

The observable traits of single-gene inheritance are inherited by the offspring from the parents. During maturation, the primordial germ cells (*i.e.,* sperm and ovum) of both parents undergo meiosis, or reduction division, in which the number of chromosomes is divided in half (from 46 to 23). At this time, the two alleles from a gene locus separate so that each germ cell receives only one allele from each pair (*i.e.,* Mendel's first law). According to Mendel's second law, the alleles from the different gene loci segregate independently and recombine randomly in the zygote. Persons in whom the two alleles of a given pair are the same (AA or aa) are called *homozygotes. Heterozygotes* have different alleles (Aa) at a gene locus. A *recessive trait* is one expressed only in a homozygous pairing; a *dominant trait* is one expressed in either a homozygous or a heterozygous pairing. All persons with a dominant allele (depending on the penetrance of the genes) manifest that trait. A *carrier* is a person who is heterozygous for a recessive trait and does not manifest the trait. For example, the genes for blond hair are recessive, and those for brown hair are dominant. Therefore, only persons with a genotype having two alleles for blond hair would be blond; persons with either one or two brown alleles would have dark hair.

PEDIGREE

A pedigree is a graphic method for portraying a family history of an inherited trait. It is constructed from a carefully obtained family history and is useful for tracing the pattern of inheritance for a particular trait.

In summary, inheritance represents the likelihood of the occurrence or recurrence of a specific genetic trait. The genotype refers to information stored in the genetic code of a person, whereas the phenotype represents the recognizable traits, physical and biochemical, associated with the genotype. Expressivity refers to the expression of a gene in the phenotype, and penetrance is the ability of a gene to express its function. The point on the DNA molecule that controls the inheritance of a particular trait is called a *gene locus.* Alternate forms of a gene at a gene locus are called *alleles.* The alleles at a gene locus may carry recessive or dominant traits. A recessive trait is one expressed only when two copies (homozygous) of the recessive allele are present. Dominant traits are expressed with either homozygous or heterozygous pairing of the alleles. A pedigree is a graphic method for portraying a family history of an inherited trait.

Gene Technology

After completing this section of the chapter, you should be able to meet the following objectives:

- Define genomic mapping
- Briefly describe the methods used in linkage studies, dosage studies, and hybridization studies

GENOMIC MAPPING

The genome is the gene complement of an organism. Genomic mapping is the assignment of genes to specific chromosomes or parts of the chromosome. The Human Genome Project, which started in 1990 and was completed in 2003, was an international project to identify and localize the over 30,000 estimated genes in the human genome. This was a phenomenal undertaking because approximately 3 million base pairs are present in the human genome. The results of the project are expected to reveal the chemical basis for as many as 4000 genetic diseases, provide information needed for developing screening and diagnostic tests for genetic disorders, and become the basis for new treatment methods for these disorders.

Two types of genomic maps exist: genetic maps and physical maps. Genetic maps are like highway maps. They use linkage studies (*e.g.,* dosage, hybridization) to estimate the distances between chromosomal landmarks (*i.e.,* gene markers). Physical maps are similar to a surveyor's map. They measure the actual physical distance between chromosomal elements in biochemical units, the smallest being the nucleotide base.

Genetic maps and physical maps have been refined over the decades. The earliest mapping efforts localized genes on the X chromosome. The initial assignment of a gene to a particular chromosome was made in 1911 for the color blindness gene inherited from the mother (*i.e.,* following the X-linked pattern of inheritance). In 1968, the specific location of the Duffy blood group on the long arm of chromosome 1 was determined. The locations of more than 12,000 expressed human genes have been mapped to a specific chromosome, and most of them to a specific region on the chromosome. However, genetic mapping is continuing so rapidly that these numbers are constantly being updated. Documentation of gene assignments to specific human chromosomes is updated almost daily in the *Online Mendelian Inheritance in Man* (http://www.ncbi.nlm.nih.gov/Omim), an encyclopedia of expressed gene loci. Many methods have been used for developing genetic maps. The most important ones are family linkage studies, gene dosage methods, and hybridization studies. Often, the specific assignment of a gene is made using information from several mapping techniques.

Most of the genome mapping has been accomplished by a method called *transcript mapping.* The two-part process begins with isolating mRNAs immediately after they are transcribed. Next, the complementary DNA molecule is prepared. Although transcript mapping may provide knowledge of the gene sequence, it does not automatically mean that the function of the genetic material has been determined.

> **GENE MAPPING**
>
> - Gene mapping involves the assignment of a gene to a specific chromosome or part of a chromosome.
> - Linked genes are found on the same chromosome; the degree of linkage of two genes is based on their physical distance from each other on the chromosome.
> - Somatic cell hybridization allows geneticists to study which chromosomes contain the coding for various enzymes.
> - In situ hybridization uses specific sequences of DNA or RNA to locate genes that do not express themselves in cell culture.

Linkage Studies

Mendel's laws were often insufficient to explain the transmission of several well-known traits such as color blindness and hemophilia A. In some families, it was noted that these two conditions were transmitted together. In 1937, Bell and Haldane concluded that somehow the two mutations were coupled or "linked." Detailed analyses of other familial conditions have concluded that several exceptions to Mendel's laws exist.

Linkage studies assume that genes occur in a linear array along the chromosomes. During meiosis, the paired chromosomes of the diploid germ cell exchange genetic material because of the crossing-over phenomenon (see Fig. 6-9). This exchange usually involves more than one gene; large blocks of genes (representing large portions of the chromosome) are usually exchanged. Although the point at which the block separates from another occurs randomly, the closer together two genes are on the same chromosome, the greater the chance that they will be passed on together to the offspring. When two inherited traits occur together at a rate greater than would occur by chance alone, they are said to be *linked.*

Several methods take advantage of the crossing over and recombination of genes to map a particular gene. In one method, any gene that is already assigned to a chromosome can be used as a marker to assign other linked genes. For example, it was found that an extra long chromosome 1 and the Duffy blood group were inherited as a dominant trait, placing the position of the blood group gene close to the extra material on chromosome 1. Color blindness has been linked to classic hemophilia A (*i.e.,* lack of factor VIII) in some pedigrees; hemophilia A has been linked to glucose-6-phosphate dehydrogenase deficiency in others; and color blindness has been linked to glucose-6-phosphate dehydrogenase deficiency in still others. Because the gene for color blindness is found on the X chromosome, all three genes must be found in a small section of the X chromosome. Linkage analysis can be used clinically to identify affected persons in a family with a known genetic defect. Males, because they have one X and one Y chromosome, are said to be *hemizygous* for sex-linked traits. Females can be homozygous (normal or mutant) or heterozygous for sex-linked traits. Heterozygous females are known as *carriers* for X-linked defects.

One autosomal recessive disorder that has been successfully diagnosed prenatally by linkage studies using amniocentesis is congenital adrenal hyperplasia (due to 21-hydroxylase deficiency), which is linked to an immune response gene (human leukocyte antigen [HLA] type). Postnatal linkage studies have been used in diagnosing hemochromatosis, which is closely linked to another HLA type. Persons with this disorder are unable to metabolize iron, and it accumulates in the liver and other organs. It cannot be diagnosed by conventional means until irreversible damage has been done. Given a family history of the disorder, HLA typing can determine whether the gene is present, and if it is present, dietary restriction of iron intake may be used to prevent organ damage.

Dosage Studies

Dosage studies involve measuring enzyme activity. Autosomal genes are normally arranged in pairs, and normally both are expressed. If both alleles are present and both are expressed, the activity of the enzyme should be 100%. If one member of the gene pair is missing, only 50% of the enzyme activity is present, reflecting the activity of the remaining normal allele.

Hybridization Studies

A recent biologic discovery revealed that two somatic cells from different species, when grown together in the same culture, occasionally fuse to form a new hybrid cell. Two types of hybridization methods are used in genomic studies: somatic cell hybridization and in situ hybridization.

Somatic cell hybridization involves the fusion of human somatic cells with those of a different species (typically, the mouse) to yield a cell containing the chromosomes of both species. Because these hybrid cells are unstable, they begin to lose chromosomes of both species during subsequent cell divisions. This makes it possible to obtain cells with different partial combinations of human chromosomes. By studying the enzymes that these cells produce, detecting that an enzyme is produced is possible only when a certain chromosome is present; the coding for that enzyme must be located on that chromosome.

In situ hybridization involves the use of specific sequences of DNA or RNA to locate genes that do not express themselves in cell culture. DNA and RNA can be chemically tagged with radioactive or fluorescent markers. These chemically tagged DNA or RNA sequences are used as probes to detect gene location. The probe is added to a chromosome spread after the DNA strands have been separated. If the probe matches the complementary DNA of a chromosome segment, it hybridizes and remains at the precise location (therefore the term *in situ*) on a chromosome. Radioactive or fluorescent markers are used to find the location of the probe.

RECOMBINANT DNA TECHNOLOGY

During the past several decades, genetic engineering has provided the methods for manipulating nucleic acids and recombining genes (recombinant DNA) into hybrid molecules that can be inserted into unicellular organisms and reproduced many times over. Each hybrid molecule produces a genetically identical population, called a *clone,* that reflects its common ancestor.

Gene isolation and cloning techniques rely on the fact that the genes of all organisms, from bacteria through mammals, are based on similar molecular organization. Gene cloning requires cutting a DNA molecule apart, modifying and reassembling its fragments, and producing copies of the modified DNA, its mRNA, and its gene product. The DNA molecule is cut apart by using a bacterial enzyme, called a *restriction enzyme,* that binds to DNA wherever a particular short sequence of base pairs is found and cleaves the molecule at a specific nucleotide site. In this way, a long DNA molecule can be broken down into smaller, discrete fragments with the intent that one fragment contains the gene of interest. More than 100 restriction enzymes are commercially available that cut DNA at different recognition sites.

The selected gene fragment is replicated through insertion into a unicellular organism, such as a bacterium. To do this, a cloning vector such as a bacterial virus or a small DNA circle that is found in most bacteria, called a *plasmid,* is used. Viral and plasmid vectors replicate autonomously in the host bacterial cell. During gene cloning, a bacterial vector and the DNA fragment are mixed and joined by a special enzyme called a *DNA ligase.* The recombinant vectors formed are then introduced into a suitable culture of bacteria, and the bacteria are allowed to replicate and express the recombinant vector gene. Sometimes, mRNA taken from a tissue that expresses a high level of the gene is used to produce a complementary DNA molecule that can be used in the cloning process. Because the fragments of the entire DNA molecule are used in the cloning process, additional steps are taken to identify and separate the clone that contains the gene of interest.

As for biologic research and technology, cloning makes it possible to identify the DNA sequence in a gene and produce the protein product encoded by a gene. The specific nucleotide sequence of a cloned DNA fragment can often be identified by analyzing the amino acid sequence and mRNA codons of its protein product. Short sequences of base pairs can be synthesized, radioactively labeled, and subsequently used to identify their complementary sequence. In this way, identifying normal and abnormal gene structures is possible. Proteins that formerly were available only in small amounts can now be made in large quantities once their respective genes have been isolated. For example, genes encoding for an insulin and growth hormone have been cloned to produce these hormones for pharmacologic use.

GENE THERAPY

Although quite different from inserting genetic material into a unicellular organism such as bacteria, techniques are available for inserting genes into the genome of intact multicellular plants and animals. Promising delivery vehicles for these genes are the adenoviruses. These viruses are ideal vehicles because their DNA does not become integrated into the host genome; however, repeated inoculations are often needed because the body's immune system usually targets cells expressing adenovirus proteins. Sterically stable liposomes also show promise as DNA delivery mechanisms. This type of therapy is one of the more promising methods for the treatment of genetic disorders, certain cancers, cystic fibrosis, and many infectious diseases. Two main approaches are used in gene therapy: transferred genes can replace defective genes, or they can selectively inhibit deleterious genes. Cloned DNA sequences or ribosomes are usually the compounds used in gene therapy. However, the introduction of the cloned gene into the multicellular organism can influence only the few cells that get the gene. An answer to this problem would be the insertion of the gene into a sperm or ovum; after fertilization, the gene would be replicated in all of the differentiating cell types. Even so, techniques for cell insertion are limited. Not only are moral and ethical issues involved, but also these techniques cannot direct the inserted DNA to attach to a particular chromosome or supplant an existing gene by knocking it out of its place.

DNA FINGERPRINTING

The technique of DNA fingerprinting is based in part on those techniques used in recombinant DNA technology and those originally used in medical genetics to detect slight variations in the genomes of different individuals. Using restrictive endonucleases, DNA is cleaved at specific regions. The DNA fragments are separated according to size by electrophoresis (*i.e.*, Southern blot) and transferred to a nylon membrane. The fragments are then broken apart and subsequently annealed with a series of radioactive probes specific for regions in each fragment. An autoradiograph reveals the DNA fragments on the membrane. When used in forensic pathology, this procedure is undertaken on specimens from the suspect and the forensic specimen. Banding patterns are then analyzed to see if they match. With conventional methods of analysis of blood and serum enzymes, a 1 in 100 to 1000 chance exists that the two specimens match because of chance. With DNA fingerprinting, these odds are 1 in 100,000 to 1 million.

In summary, the genome is the gene complement of an organism. Genomic mapping is a method used to assign genes to particular chromosomes or parts of a chromosome. The most important ones used are family linkage studies, gene dosage methods, and hybridization studies. Often the specific assignment of a gene is determined by using information from several mapping techniques. Linkage studies assign a chromosome location to genes based on their close association with other genes of known location. Recombinant DNA studies involve the extraction of specific types of messenger RNA used in synthesis of complementary DNA strands. The complementary DNA strands, labeled with a radioisotope, bind with the genes for which they are complementary and are used as gene probes. Now underway is an international project to identify and localize the over 30,000 estimated genes in the human genome. Genetic engineering has provided the methods for manipulating nucleic acids and recombining genes (recombinant DNA) into hybrid molecules that can be inserted into unicellular organisms and reproduced many times over. As a result, proteins that formerly were available only in small amounts can now be made in large quantities once their respective genes have been isolated. DNA fingerprinting, which relies on recombinant DNA technologies and those of genetic mapping, is often used in forensic investigations.

REVIEW EXERCISES

Cystic fibrosis is a disorder of a cell membrane chloride channel that causes the exocrine glands of the body to produce abnormally thick mucus, with the resultant development of chronic obstructive lung disease, pancreatitis, and infertility in men.

A. Explain how a single mutant gene can produce such devastating effects.

B. The disease is transmitted as a single-gene recessive trait. Describe the inheritance of the disorder using Figure 6-15.

Adult polycystic kidney disease is transmitted as an autosomal dominant trait.

A. Explain the parent-to-child transmission of this disorder.

B. Although the disease is transmitted as an autosomal dominant trait, some people who inherit the gene may develop symptoms early in life. Others may develop it later in life, and still others may never develop significant symptoms of the disease during their lifetime. Explain.

Human insulin, prepared by recombinant DNA technology, is now available for treatment of diabetes mellitus.

A. Explain the techniques used for the production of a human hormone using this technology.

Bibliography

Alberts B., Johnson A., Lewis J., Raff M., et al. (2002). *Molecular biology of the cell* (4th ed., pp. 191–468, 386–387). New York: Garland Science.

Aparicio S. A. J. R. (2000). How to count human genes. *Nature Genetics 25*(2), 129–130. [On-line]. Available: http://www.nature.com. Accessed July 13, 2000.

Carlson B. M. (1999). *Human embryology and developmental biology* (2nd ed., pp. 2–23, 128–145). St. Louis: Mosby.

Ewing B., Green P. (2000). Analysis of expressed sequence tags indicates 35,000 human genes. *Nature Genetics 25*(2) 232–234. [On-line]. Available: http://www.nature.com. Accessed July 13, 2000.

Guyton A. C., Hall J. E. (2000). *Textbook of medical physiology* (10th ed., pp. 24–37). Philadelphia: W. B. Saunders.

Hattori M., Fujyama A., Taylor H., et al. (2000). The DNA sequence of human chromosome 21. *Nature 405,* 311–319. [On-line]. Available: http://www.nature.com. Accessed July 13, 2000.

Hawley R. S., Mori C. A. (1999). *The human genome: A user's guide.* San Diego: Harcourt Academic Press.

Human Genome Project. (2000). *Columbia encyclopedia* (6th ed.). [On-line]. Available: http://www.bartleby.com/65/hu/_HumanG.html. Accessed October 22, 2000.

The International RH Mapping Consortium. (2000). *A new gene map of the human genome.* [On-line]. Available: http://www.ncbi.nlm.nih.gov/genemap99. Accessed July 13, 2000.

Jain H. K. (1999). *Genetics: Principles, concepts and implications.* Enfield, NH: Science Publishers.

Jegalian K., Lahn B. T. (2001). Why the Y is so weird. *Scientific American* February, 56–61.

Kierszenbaum A. L. (2003). *Histology and cell biology: An introduction to pathology* (pp. 87–88). St. Louis: Mosby.

Liang F., Holt I., Pertea G., et al. (2000). Gene index analysis of the human genome estimates approximately 120,000 genes. *Nature Genetics 25* (2) 239–240. [On-line]. Available: http://www.nature.com. Accessed July 13, 2000.

Marieb E. N. (2001). *Human anatomy and physiology.* (5th ed., pp. 1159–1160). San Francisco: Addison Wesley.

Moore K. L., Persaud T. V. N. (1998). *The developing human: Clinically orientated embryology.* (6th ed., pp. 17–46). Philadelphia: W. B. Saunders.

Ostrer H. (1998). *Non-mendelian genetics in humans.* New York: Oxford University Press.

Sadler R. W. (2003). *Langman's medical embryology* (9th ed., pp. 3–30). Philadelphia: Lippincott Williams & Wilkins.

Sapienza C. (1990). Parenteral imprinting of genes. *Scientific American 263*(4), 52–60.

Skaletsky H., Kuroda-Kawaguchi T., Minx P., Cordom H., et. al. (2003). *The male-specific region of the Y chromosome is a mosaic of discrete sequence classes.* Nature 423(6942), 825–837. [On-line.] Available: http://gateway1.ovid.com:80/ovidweb.cgi. Accessed August 1, 2003.

Snustad D. P., Simmons J. M. (Eds.). (2000). *Principles of genetics* (2nd ed., pp. 3–21, 52–71, 91–115, 665–669). New York: John Wiley & Sons.

Steinberg D. (2002). *Embryonic germ cells show gene imprinting.* [On-line.] Available: http://www.the-scientist.com/yr2001/sep/research_020902.html. Accessed July 22, 2003.

Wilson J. F. (2001). *Gene therapy, stem cells: Prime for vision restoration.* [On-line.] Available: http://www.the-scientist.com/yr2001/sep/research1_010917.html. Accessed July 22, 2003.

CHAPTER

7

Genetic and Congenital Disorders

Genetic and congenital defects are important at all levels of health care because they affect all age groups and can involve almost any of the body tissues and organs. Congenital defects, sometimes called *birth defects,* develop during prenatal life and are present at birth, although some, such as cardiac abnormalities, may not become apparent until some years later. The term congenital does not imply or exclude genetic disorders, which are usually hereditary in origin.

Birth defects, which affect more than 150,000 infants each year, are the leading cause of infant death.[1] Birth defects may be caused by genetic factors (*i.e.,* single-gene or multifactorial inheritance or chromosomal aberrations), or they may be caused by environmental factors that occurred during embryonic or fetal development (*i.e.,* maternal disease, infections, or drugs taken during pregnancy). In rare cases, congenital defects may be the result of intrauterine factors such as fetal crowding, positioning, or entanglement of fetal parts with the amnion. This chapter provides an overview of genetic and congenital disorders and is divided into three parts: (1) genetic and chromosomal disorders, (2) disorders caused by environmental agents, and (3) diagnosis and counseling.

Genetic and Chromosomal Disorders

After you have completed this section of the chapter, you should be able to meet the following objectives:

- Define the terms *congenital, allele, gene locus, gene mutation, genotype, phenotype, homozygous, heterozygous, polymorphism, gene penetrance,* and *gene expression*
- Describe three types of single-gene disorders
- Differentiate between mitochondrial and nuclear genes
- Contrast disorders due to multifactorial inheritance with those caused by single-gene inheritance
- Describe two chromosomal abnormalities that demonstrate aneuploidy
- Describe three patterns of chromosomal breakage and rearrangement
- Relate maternal age and occurrence of Down syndrome

Genetic disorders can be described as a discrete event that affects gene expression in a group of cells related to each other by gene linkage. Most genetic disorders are caused by an alteration in DNA sequences that alter the synthesis of a single-gene product. However, some genetic disorders are caused by chromosome rearrangements that result in deletion or duplication of a group of closely linked genes or by mistakes during mitosis or meiosis that result in an abnormal number of chromosomes.[2]

The genes on each chromosome are arranged in pairs and in strict order, with each gene occupying a specific location or *locus.* The two members of a gene pair, one inherited from the mother and the other from the father, are called *alleles*. If the members of a gene pair are identical (*i.e.*, code the exact same gene product), the person is *homozygous*, and if the two members are different, the person is *heterozygous*. The genetic composition of a person is called a *genotype*, whereas the *phenotype* is the observable expression of a genotype in terms of morphologic, biochemical, or molecular traits. If the trait is expressed in the heterozygote (one member of the gene pair codes for the trait), it is said to be *dominant;* if it is expressed only in the homozygote (both members of the gene pair code for the trait), it is *recessive*.

Although gene expression usually follows a dominant or recessive pattern, it is possible for both alleles (members) of a gene pair to be fully expressed in the heterozygote, a condition called *codominance*. Many genes have only one normal version, which geneticists call the *wild-type* allele. Other genes have more than one normal allele (alternate forms) at the same locus. This is called *polymorphism*. Blood group inheritance (*e.g.*, AO, BO, AB) is an example of codominance and polymorphism.

A gene *mutation* is a biochemical event such as nucleotide change, deletion, or insertion that produces a new allele. A single mutant gene may be expressed in many different parts of the body. Marfan's syndrome is a defect in connective tissue that has widespread effects involving skeletal, eye, and cardiovascular structures. In other single-gene disorders, the same defect can be caused by mutations at several different loci. Childhood deafness can result from at least 16 different types of autosomal recessive mutations.

Genetic disorders involve a permanent change (or mutation) in the genome. A genetic disorder can involve a single-gene trait, multifactorial inheritance, or a chromosome disorder.

SINGLE-GENE DISORDERS

Single-gene disorders are caused by a single defective or mutant gene. The defective gene may be present on an autosome or the X chromosome, and it may affect only one member of an autosomal gene pair (matched with a normal gene) or both members of the pair. Single-gene defects follow the mendelian patterns of inheritance (see Chapter 6) and are often called *mendelian disorders*. At last count, there were more than 8000 single-gene disorders, many of which have been mapped to a specific chromosome.[3]

Single-gene disorders are characterized by their patterns of transmission, which usually are obtained through a family genetic history. The patterns of inheritance depend on whether the phenotype is dominant or recessive and on whether the gene is located on an autosomal or sex chromosome. Disorders of autosomal inheritance include autosomal dominant and autosomal recessive traits. Among the approximate 8000 single-gene disorders, more than half are autosomal dominant. Autosomal recessive phenotypes are less common, accounting for approximately one third of single-gene disorders.[4] Currently, all sex-linked genetic disorders are thought to be X linked, and most are recessive. The only mutations affecting the Y-linked genes are involved in spermatogenesis and male fertility and hence are not transmitted. A few additional genes with homologs on the X chromosome have been mapped to the Y chromosome, but to date, no disorders resulting from mutations in these genes have been described.

Virtually all single-gene disorders lead to formation of an abnormal protein or decreased production of a gene product. The defect can result in defective or decreased amounts of an enzyme, defects in receptor proteins and their function, alterations in nonenzyme proteins, or mutations resulting in unusual reactions to drugs. Table 7-1 lists some of the common single-gene disorders and their manifestations.

GENETIC AND CHROMOSOMAL DISORDERS

- Genetic disorders are inherited as autosomal dominant disorders, in which each child has a 50% chance of inheriting the disorder, and as autosomal recessive disorders, in which each child has a 25% chance of being affected, a 50% chance of being a carrier, and a 25% chance of being unaffected.
- Sex-linked disorders almost always are associated with the X chromosome and are predominantly recessive.
- Chromosomal disorders reflect events that occur at the time of meiosis and result from defective movement of an entire chromosome or from breakage of a chromosome with loss or translocation of genetic material.

Autosomal Dominant Disorders

In autosomal dominant disorders, a single mutant allele from an affected parent is transmitted to an offspring regardless of sex. The affected parent has a 50% chance of transmitting the disorder to each offspring (Fig. 7-1). The unaffected relatives of the parent or unaffected siblings of the offspring do not transmit the disorder. In many conditions, the age of onset is delayed, and the signs and symptoms of the disorder do not appear until later in life, as in Huntington's chorea (see Chapter 53).

Autosomal dominant disorders also may manifest as a new mutation. Whether the mutation is passed on to the next generation depends on the affected person's reproductive capacity. Many new autosomal dominant mutations are accompanied by reduced reproductive capacity; therefore, the defect is not perpetuated in future generations. If an autosomal defect is accompanied by a total inability to reproduce, essentially all new cases of the disorder will be due to new mutations. If the defect does not affect reproductive capacity, it is more likely to be inherited.

Although there is a 50% chance of inheriting a dominant genetic disorder from an affected parent, there can be wide variation in gene penetration and expression. When a person inherits a dominant mutant gene but fails to express it, the trait is described as having *reduced penetrance*. Penetrance is expressed in mathematical terms: a 50%

TABLE 7-1 Some Disorders of Mendelian or Single-Gene Inheritance and Their Significance

Disorder	Significance
Autosomal Dominant	
Achondroplasia	Short-limb dwarfism
Adult polycystic kidney disease	Kidney failure
Huntington's chorea	Neurodegenerative disorder
Familial hypercholesterolemia	Premature atherosclerosis
Marfan's syndrome	Connective tissue disorder with abnormalities in skeletal, ocular, cardiovascular systems
Neurofibromatosis (NF)	Neurogenic tumors: fibromatous skin tumors, pigmented skin lesions, and ocular nodules in NF-1; bilateral acoustic neuromas in NF-2
Osteogenesis imperfecta	Molecular defects of collagen
Spherocytosis	Disorder of red blood cells
von Willebrand's disease	Bleeding disorder
Autosomal Recessive	
Color blindness	Color blindness
Cystic fibrosis	Disorder of membrane transport of chloride ions in exocrine glands causing lung and pancreatic disease
Glycogen storage diseases	Excess accumulation of glycogen in the liver and hypoglycemia (von Gierke's disease); glycogen accumulation in striated muscle in myopathic forms
Oculocutaneous albinism	Hypopigmentation of skin, hair, eyes as result of inability to synthesize melanin
Phenylketonuria (PKU)	Lack of phenylalanine hydroxylase with hyperphenylalaninemia and impaired brain development
Sickle cell disease	Red blood cell defect
Tay-Sachs disease	Deficiency of hexosaminidase A; severe mental and physical deterioration beginning in infancy
X-Linked Recessive	
Bruton-type hypogammaglobulinemia	Immunodeficiency
Hemophilia A	Bleeding disorder
Duchenne dystrophy	Muscular dystrophy
Fragile X syndrome	Mental retardation

penetrance indicates that a person who inherits the defective gene has a 50% chance of expressing the disorder. The person who has a mutant gene but does not express it is an important exception to the rule that unaffected persons do not transmit an autosomal dominant trait. These persons can transmit the gene to their descendants and so produce a skipped generation. Autosomal dominant disorders also can display *variable expressivity,* meaning that they can be expressed differently among individuals. Polydactyly or supernumerary digits, for example, may be expressed in the fingers or the toes.

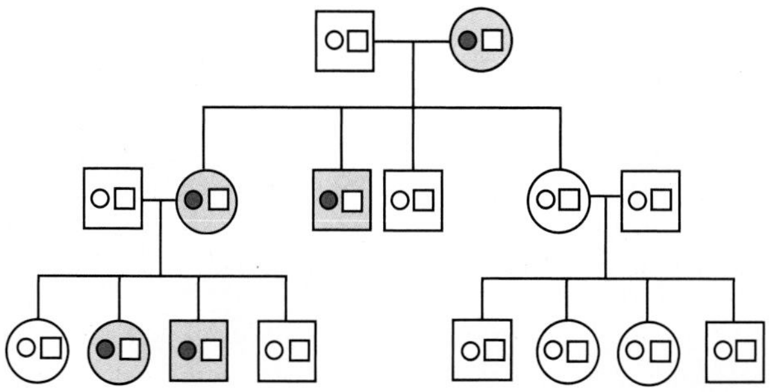

FIGURE 7-1 Simple pedigree for inheritance of an autosomal dominant trait. The small, colored circle represents the mutant gene. An affected parent with an autosomal dominant trait has a 50% chance of passing the mutant gene on to each child regardless of sex.

The gene products of autosomal dominant disorders usually are regulatory proteins involved in rate-limiting components of complex metabolic pathways or key components of structural proteins such as collagen.[5,6] Two disorders of autosomal inheritance, Marfan's syndrome and neurofibromatosis (NF), are described in this chapter.

Marfan's Syndrome. Marfan's syndrome is an autosomal dominant connective tissue disorder. The basic biochemical abnormality in Marfan's syndrome affects *fibrillin I,* a major component of microfibrils found in the extracellular matrix. [6] These microfibrils form the scaffolding for the deposition of elastin and are considered integral components of elastic fibers. Fibrillin I is encoded by the FBNI gene, which maps to chromosome 15q21. More than 100 mutations in the FBNI gene have been found, making genetic diagnosis unfeasible. The prevalence of Marfan's syndrome is estimated to be 2 to 3 per 10,000. Approximately 75% are familial, and the remainder are sporadic, arising from new mutations in the germ cells of parents.[6]

Skeletal, ocular, and cardiovascular structures are affected by the connective tissue changes that occur in Marfan's syndrome. There is a wide range of variation in the expression of the disorder. Persons may have abnormalities of one or all three types of structures. The skeletal deformities, which are the most obvious features of the disorder, include a long, thin body with exceptionally long extremities and long, tapering fingers, sometimes called *arachnodactyly* or *spider fingers* (Fig. 7-2); hyperextensible joints; and a variety of spinal deformities, including kyphoscoliosis. Chest deformity, pectus excavatum (*i.e.,* deeply depressed sternum), or pigeon chest deformity, often is present. The most common eye disorder is bilateral dislocation of the lens due to weakness of the suspensory ligaments. Myopia and predisposition to retinal detachment also are common, the result of increased optic globe length due to altered connective tissue support of ocular structures. However, the most life-threatening aspects of the disorder are the cardiovascular defects, which include mitral valve prolapse, progressive dilation of the aortic valve ring, and weakness of the wall of the aorta and other arteries. Dissection and rupture of the aorta often lead to premature death. The average age of death in persons with Marfan's syndrome is 30 to 40 years.[5]

Neurofibromatosis. Neurofibromatosis is a condition involving neurogenic tumors that arise from Schwann cells and other elements of the peripheral nervous system.[5,6] There are at least two genetically and clinically distinct forms of the disorder: type 1 NF (NF-1), also known as *von Recklinghausen disease,* and type 2 NF (NF-2), previously called acoustic NF. Both of these disorders result from a genetic defect in a protein that regulates cell growth. The gene for NF-1 has been mapped to chromosome 17, and the gene for NF-2 has been mapped to chromosome 22.

NF-1 is a relatively common disorder with a frequency of 1 in 3500.[5] Approximately 50% of cases have a family history of autosomal dominant transmission, and the remaining 50% appear to represent a new mutation. In more than 90% of persons with NF-1, cutaneous and subcutaneous neurofibromas develop in late childhood or adolescence. The cutaneous neurofibromas, which vary in number from a few to many hundreds, manifest as soft, pedunculated lesions that project from the skin. They are the most common type of lesion, often are not apparent until puberty, and are present in greatest density over the trunk (Fig. 7-3). The subcutaneous lesions grow just below the skin; they are firm and round and may be painful. Plexiform neurofibromas involve the larger peripheral nerves. They tend to form large tumors that cause severe disfigurement of the face or an extremity. Pigmented nodules of the iris (Lisch nodules), which are specific for NF-1, usually are present after 6 years of age. They do not present any clinical problem but are useful in establishing a diagnosis.

A second major component of NF-1 is the presence of large (usually ≥15 mm in diameter), flat cutaneous pigmentations, known as *café-au-lait spots.* They are usually a uniform light brown in whites and darker brown in African Americans, with sharply demarcated edges.

Although small single lesions may be found in normal children, larger lesions or six or more spots larger than 1.5 cm in diameter suggest NF-1. The skin pigmentations become more evident with age as the melanosomes in the epidermal cells accumulate melanin.

In addition to neurofibromatoses, persons with NF-1 have a variety of other associated lesions, the most common being skeletal lesions such as scoliosis and erosive bone defects. Persons with NF-1 also are at increased risk for development of other nervous system tumors such as meningiomas, optic gliomas, and pheochromocytomas.

NF-2 is characterized by tumors of the acoustic nerve. Most often, the disorder is asymptomatic through the first 15 years of life. The most frequent symptoms are headaches, hearing loss, and tinnitus (*i.e.,* ringing in the ears). There may be associated intracranial and spinal meningiomas. The condition is made worse by pregnancy, and oral contraceptives may increase the growth and symptoms of tumors. Persons with the disorder should be warned that severe disorientation may occur during diving or swimming underwater, and drowning may result. Surgery may be indicated for debulking or removal of the tumors.

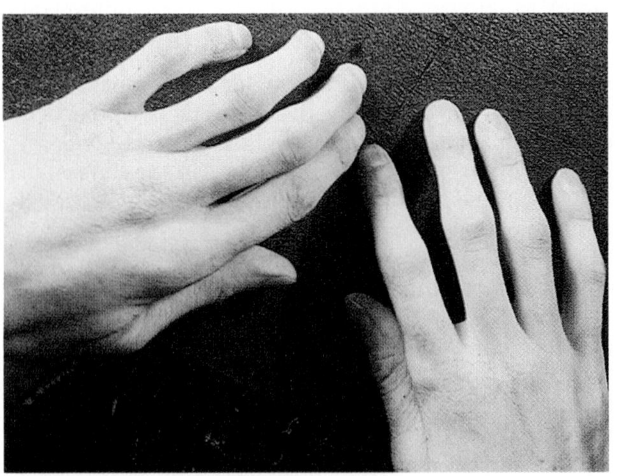

FIGURE 7-2 Long, slender fingers (arachnodactyly) in a patient with Marfan's syndrome. (Rubin E., Farber J.L. [1999]. *Pathology* [3rd ed., p. 242]. Philadelphia: Lippincott-Raven)

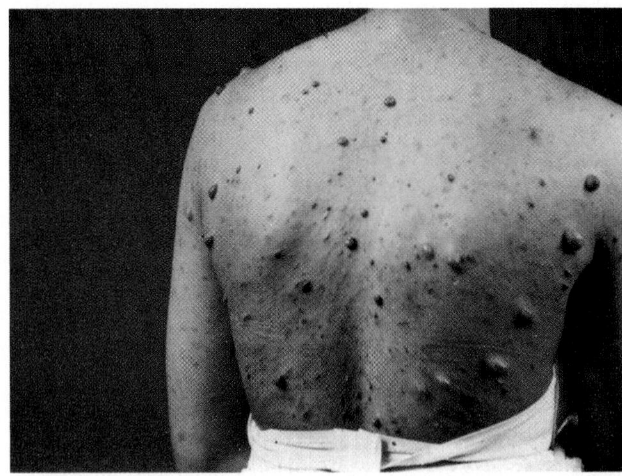

FIGURE 7-3 Neurofibromatosis on the back. (Reed and Carnick Pharmaceuticals) (Sauer G.C., Hall J.C. [1996]. *Manual of skin diseases.* Philadelphia: Lippincott-Raven)

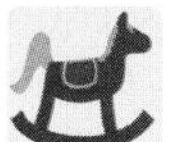

Autosomal Recessive Disorders

Autosomal recessive disorders are manifested only when both members of the gene pair are affected. In this case, both parents may be unaffected but are carriers of the defective gene. Autosomal recessive disorders affect both sexes. The occurrence risk in each pregnancy is one in four for an affected child, two in four for a carrier child, and one in four for a normal (noncarrier, unaffected) homozygous child (Fig. 7-4).

With autosomal recessive disorders, the age of onset is frequently early in life; the symptomatology tends to be more uniform than with autosomal dominant disorders; and the disorders are characteristically caused by deficiencies in enzymes rather than abnormalities in structural proteins. In the case of a heterozygous carrier, the presence of a mutant gene usually does not produce symptoms because equal amounts of normal and defective enzymes are synthesized. The "margin of safety" ensures that cells with half their usual amount of enzyme function normally. By contrast, the inactivation of both alleles in a homozygote results in complete loss of enzyme activity. Autosomal recessive disorders include almost all inborn errors of metabolism. Enzyme disorders that impair catabolic pathways result in an accumulation of dietary substances (*e.g.*, phenylketonuria) or cellular constituents (*e.g.*, lysosomal storage diseases). Other disorders result from a defect in the enzyme-mediated synthesis of an essential protein (*e.g.*, the cystic fibrosis transmembrane conductance regulator in cystic fibrosis [Chapter 31]). Two examples of autosomal recessive disorders that are not covered elsewhere in this book are phenylketonuria and Tay-Sachs disease.

Phenylketonuria. Phenylketonuria (PKU) is a rare metabolic disorder caused by a deficiency of the liver enzyme phenylalanine hydroxylase. As a result of this deficiency, toxic levels of the amino acid phenylalanine accumulate in the blood and other tissues. The disorder, which affects approximately 1 in every 15,000 infants in the United States, is usually inherited as a recessive trait and is manifested only in the homozygote.[7] If untreated, the disorder results in mental retardation, microcephaly, delayed speech, and other signs of impaired neurologic development.

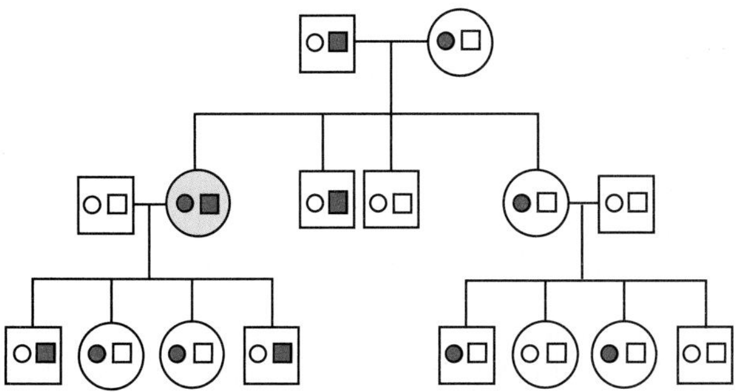

FIGURE 7-4 Simple pedigree for inheritance of an autosomal recessive trait. The small, colored circle and square represent a mutant gene. When both parents are carriers of a mutant gene, there is a 25% chance of having an affected child, a 50% chance of a carrier child, and a 25% chance of a nonaffected or noncarrier child, regardless of sex. All children (100%) of an affected parent are carriers.

Because the symptoms of untreated PKU develop gradually and would often go undetected until irreversible mental retardation had occurred, newborn infants are routinely screened for abnormal levels of serum phenylalanine. It is important that blood samples for PKU screening be obtained at least 12 hours after birth to ensure accuracy.[8] It also is possible to identify carriers of the trait by subjecting them to a phenylalanine test, in which a large dose of phenylalanine is administered orally and the rate at which it disappears from the bloodstream is measured.

In 2000, the National Institutes of Health (NIH) released a consensus statement on the screening and management of PKU.[7] This statement emphasized the need for a nationwide approach to newborn screening that includes appropriate specimen collection; specimen tracking; laboratory analysis; data collection and analysis; locating and notifying families with abnormal results; diagnosis; treatment; and long-term management, including psychological, nursing and social services, nutritional therapy, and genetic and family counseling.[9]

Infants with the disorder are treated with a special diet that restricts phenylalanine intake. The results of dietary therapy of children with PKU have been impressive. The diet can prevent mental retardation as well as other neurodegenerative effects of untreated PKU. However, dietary treatment must be started early in neonatal life to prevent brain damage. Infants with elevated phenylalanine levels (>10 mg/dL) should begin treatment by 7 to 10 days of age, indicating the need for early diagnosis. Evidence suggests that high levels of phenylalanine, even during the first 2 weeks of life, can affect the structural development of the visual system, although visual deficits are usually mild.[9]

The NIH consensus panel recommends that dietary control of phenylalanine levels is necessary throughout the lifetime of a person with PKU. The panel recommends that infants with PKU should have phenylalanine levels measured weekly during the first year of life; twice monthly from 1 to 12 years of age; and monthly after 12 years of age.[7] Women with PKU who wish to have children require careful attention to their diet, both before conception and during pregnancy, as a means of controlling their phenylalanine levels.[7]

Tay-Sachs Disease. Tay-Sachs disease is a variant of a class of lysosomal storage diseases, known as *gangliosidoses,* in which substances (gangliosides) found in the membranes of nervous tissue are deposited in neurons of the central nervous system and retina because of a failure of lysosomal degradation.[5,6] The disease is particularly prevalent among eastern European (Ashkenazi) Jews. Infants with Tay-Sachs disease appear normal at birth but begin to manifest progressive weakness, muscle flaccidity, and decreased attentiveness at approximately 6 to 10 months of age. This is followed by rapid deterioration of motor and mental function, often with development of generalized seizures. Retinal involvement leads to visual impairment and eventual blindness. Death usually occurs before 4 years of age. Although there is no cure for the disease, analysis of the blood serum for a deficiency of the lysosomal enzyme, hexosaminidase A, which is deficient in Tay-Sachs disease, allows for accurate identification of the genetic carriers for the disease.

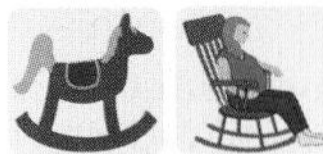

X-Linked Disorders

Sex-linked disorders are almost always associated with the X, or female, chromosome, and the inheritance pattern is predominantly recessive. Because of a normal paired gene, female heterozygotes rarely experience the effects of a defective gene. The common pattern of inheritance is one in which an unaffected mother carries one normal and one mutant allele on the X chromosome. This means that she has a 50% chance of transmitting the defective gene to her sons, and her daughters have a 50% chance of being carriers of the mutant gene (Fig. 7-5). When the affected son procreates, he transmits the defective gene to all of his daughters, who become carriers of the mutant gene. Because the genes of the Y chromosome are unaffected, the affected male does not transmit the defect to any of his sons, and they will not be carriers or transmit the disorder to their children. X-linked recessive disorders include the fragile X syndrome, glucose-6-phosphate dehydrogenase deficiency (see Chapter 16), hemophilia A (see Chapter 15), and X-linked agammaglobulinemia (see Chapter 21).

Fragile X Syndrome. Fragile X syndrome is an X-linked disorder associated with a fragile site on the X chromosome where the chromatin fails to condense during mitosis. As with other X-linked disorders, fragile X syndrome affects males more often than females. The disorder, which affects approximately 1 in 1000 male infants, is the second most common cause of mental retardation, after Down syndrome.[2,10]

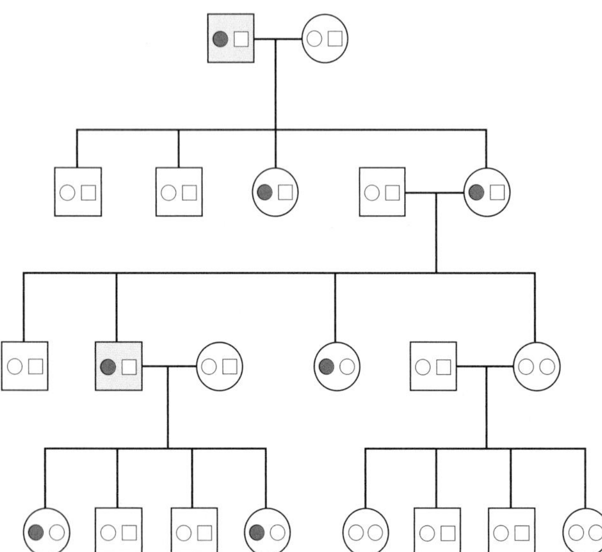

FIGURE 7-5 Simple pedigree for inheritance of an X-linked recessive trait. X-linked recessive traits are expressed phenotypically in the male offspring. The *small colored circle* represents the X chromosome with the defective gene and the *larger colored square* the affected male. The affected male passes the mutant gene to all of his daughters, who become carriers of the trait and have a 50% chance of passing the gene to their sons and their daughters, who have a 50% chance of being carriers of the gene.

Affected males are mentally retarded and share a common physical phenotype that includes a long face with large mandible and large, everted ears. Hyperextensible joints, a high-arched palate, and mitral valve prolapse, which is observed in some cases, mimic a connective tissue disorder. Some physical abnormalities may be subtle or absent. The most distinctive feature, which is present in 90% of prepubertal males, is macro-orchidism or large testes.[2,10]

In 1991, the fragile X syndrome was mapped to a small area between bands Xq27 and Xq28 on the X chromosome, now designated FMR-1 (fragile X, mental retardation 1) site.[2,10] The mechanism by which the normal FMR-1 gene is converted to an altered, or mutant, gene capable of producing the disorder involves an increase in the length of the gene. A small region of the gene that contains the CCG triplet code undergoes repeated duplication, resulting in a longer gene. The longer gene is susceptible to methylation, a chemical process that results in inactivation of the gene. When the number of repeats is small (<200), the person often has few or no manifestations of the disorder, compared with those evidenced in persons with a larger number of repeats.

In fragile X families, the probability of being affected with the disorder is related to the position in the pedigree. Later generations are more likely to be affected than earlier generations. For example, brothers of transmitting males are at a 9% risk for mental retardation, whereas grandsons of transmitting males are at a 40% risk.[2,6] The increase in occurrence of the disorder in successive generations is referred to as *genetic anticipation*.[2] In the case of the fragile X syndrome, genetic anticipation is caused by the progressive expansion of the CCG triplet repeat.[11]

Approximately 20% of males who have been shown to carry the fragile X mutation are clinically and cytogenetically normal. Because male carriers transmit the trait through all their daughters (who are phenotypically normal) to affected grandchildren, they are called *transmitting males*. Approximately 50% of female carriers are affected (mentally retarded), a proportion that is higher than with other X-linked disorders.[5]

Mitochondrial Gene Disorders

The mitochondria generate energy for cellular processes through oxidative phosphorylation and the generation of adenosine triphosphate (ATP). These cellular structures contain their own DNA, which is distinct from the DNA contained in the cell nucleus (see Chapter 4). Mitochondrial DNA, which is packaged in a double-stranded circular chromosome located inside the mitochondria, is often referred to as the "other human genome."[12,13] Mitochondrial DNA is subject to mutations at a higher rate than nuclear DNA and has no repair mechanisms. It is inherited maternally and does not recombine; thus, mothers transmit mitochondrial genes to all their offspring—male and female. However, daughters transmit the DNA further to their offspring, but sons do not.

The mitochondrial DNA contains 37 genes. The genes encode two types of ribosomal RNA, 22 types of transfer RNA, and 13 polypeptides that are subunits of enzymes that participate in oxidative phosphorylation.[4] Another 74 polypeptides that participate in oxidative phosphorylation are encoded by the nuclear genome. Consequently, disorders of mitochondrial function can result from mutations in either mitochondrial or nuclear DNA. Oxidative phosphorylation is central to three of the major functions of the mitochondria: (1) production of energy for the cell, (2) generation of reactive oxygen species as a result of oxidative phosphorylation, and (3) generation of signals that initiate apoptosis.[4] The mitochondrial myopathies are often associated with the so-called ragged red fibers, a histologic phenotype resulting from the degeneration of muscle fibers and the proliferation of abnormal muscle mitochondria.[4]

The understanding of the role of mitochondrial DNA has evolved since 1988, when the first mutation of mitochondrial DNA was discovered.[12] Since that time, more than 100 different disease-related rearrangements and point mutations have been identified.[4] The range of these diseases is diverse, although neuromuscular disorders predominate. Table 7-2 describes representative examples of disorders due to mutations in mitochondrial DNA.

MULTIFACTORIAL INHERITANCE DISORDERS

Multifactorial inheritance disorders are caused by multiple genes and, in many cases, environmental factors. The exact number of genes contributing to multifactorial traits is not known, and these traits do not follow a clear-cut pattern of inheritance, as do single-gene disorders. Multifactorial inheritance has been described as a threshold phenomenon in which the factors contributing to the trait might be compared with water filling a glass.[13] Using this analogy, one might say that expression of the disorder occurs when the glass overflows. Disorders of multifactorial inheritance can be expressed during fetal life and can be present at birth, or they may be expressed later in life. Congenital disorders that are thought to arise through multifactorial inheritance include cleft lip or palate, clubfoot, congenital dislocation of the hip, congenital heart disease, pyloric stenosis, and urinary tract malformation. Environmental factors are thought to play a greater role in disorders of multifactorial inheritance that develop in adult life, such as coronary artery disease, diabetes mellitus, hypertension, cancer, and common psychiatric disorders such as manic-depressive psychoses and schizophrenia.

Although multifactorial traits cannot be predicted with the same degree of accuracy as the mendelian single-gene mutations, characteristic patterns exist. First, multifactorial congenital malformations tend to involve a single organ or tissue derived from the same embryonic developmental field. Second, the risk for recurrence in future pregnancies is for the same or a similar defect. This means that parents of a child with a cleft palate defect are at increased risk for having another child with a cleft palate, but not with spina bifida. Third, the increased risk (compared with the general population) among first-degree relatives of the affected person is 2% to 7%, and among second-degree relatives, it is approximately one half that amount.[6] The risk increases with increasing incidence of the defect among relatives. This means that the risk is greatly increased when a second child with the defect is born to a couple. The risk also increases with severity of the disorder and when the defect occurs in the sex not usually affected by the disorder.

CHROMOSOMAL DISORDERS

Chromosomal disorders form a major category of genetic disease, accounting for a large proportion of reproductive wastage (early gestational abortions), congenital malformations, and mental retardation. Specific chromosomal

TABLE 7-2 Some Disorders of Organ Systems Associated With Mitochondrial DNA Mutations

Disorder	Manifestations
Leigh disease	Proximal muscle weakness, sensory neuropathy, developmental delay, ataxia, seizures, dementia, and visual impairment due to retinal pigment degeneration
Myoclonic epilepsy with ragged red fibers	Myoclonic seizures, cerebellar ataxia, mitochondrial myopathy (muscle weakness, fatigue)
Leber's hereditary optic neuropathy	Painless, subacute, bilateral visual loss, with central blind spots (scotomas) and abnormal color vision
MELAS	*M*itochondrial *E*ncephalomyopathy (cerebral structural changes), *L*actic *A*cidosis, and *S*trokelike syndrome, seizures, and other clinical and laboratory abnormalities. May manifest only as diabetes mellitus
MERRF	*M*yoclonic *E*pilepsy, *R*agged *R*ed *F*ibers in muscle, ataxia, sensorineural deafness
Deafness	Progressive sensorineural deafness, often associated with aminoglycoside antibiotics
Chronic progressive external ophthalmoplegia	Progressive weakness of the extraocular muscles
Kearns-Sayre syndrome	Progressive weakness of the extraocular muscles of early onset with heart block, retinal pigmentation

abnormalities can be linked to more than 60 identifiable syndromes that are present in 0.7% of all live births, 2% of all pregnancies in women older than 35 years of age, and 50% of all first-term abortions.[4]

During cell division (*i.e.,* mitosis) in nongerm cells, the chromosomes replicate so that each cell receives a full diploid number. In germ cells, a different form of division (*i.e.,* meiosis) takes place. During meiosis, the double sets of 22 autosomes and the 2 sex chromosomes (normal diploid number) are reduced to single sets (haploid number) in each gamete. At the time of conception, the haploid number in the ovum and that in the sperm join and restore the diploid number of chromosomes. Chromosomal defects usually develop because of defective movement during meiosis or because of breakage of a chromosome with loss or translocation of genetic material.

Chromosome abnormalities are commonly described according to the shorthand description of the karyotype. In this system, the total number of chromosomes is given first, followed by the sex chromosome complement, and then the description of any abnormality. For example, a male with trisomy 21 is designated 47,XY, +21.

Alterations in Chromosome Duplication

Mosaicism is the presence in one individual of two or more cell lines characterized by distinctive karyotypes. This defect results from an accident during chromosomal duplication. Sometimes, mosaicism consists of an abnormal karyotype and a normal one, in which case the physical deformities caused by the abnormal cell line usually are less severe.

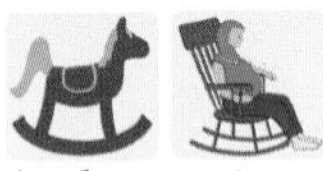

Alterations in Chromosome Number

A change in chromosome number is called *aneuploidy.* Among the causes of aneuploidy is failure of the chromosomes to separate during oogenesis or spermatogenesis. This can occur in the autosomes or the sex chromosomes and is called *nondisjunction.* Nondisjunction gives rise to germ cells that have an even number of chromosomes (22 or 24). The products of conception formed from this even number of chromosomes have an uneven number of chromosomes, 45 or 47. *Monosomy* refers to the presence of only one member of a chromosome pair. The defects associated with monosomy of the autosomes are severe and usually cause abortion. Monosomy of the X chromosome (45,X), or Turner's syndrome, causes less severe defects. *Polysomy,* or the presence of more than two chromosomes to a set, occurs when a germ cell containing more than 23 chromosomes is involved in conception. This defect has been described for the autosomes and the sex chromosomes. Trisomies of chromosomes 8, 13, 18, and 21 are the more common forms of polysomy of the autosomes. There are several forms of polysomy of the sex chromosomes in which extra X or Y chromosomes are present.

Down Syndrome. First described in 1866 by John Langon Down, trisomy 21, or Down syndrome, causes a combination of birth defects including some degree of mental retardation, characteristic facial features, and other health problems. According to the National Down Syndrome Association, it is the most common chromosomal disorder, occurring approximately once in every 800 to 1000 births. Currently, there are approximately 350,000 people in the United States with Down syndrome.[14]

Approximately 95% of cases of Down syndrome are caused by nondisjunction or an error in cell division during meiosis, resulting in a trisomy of chromosome 21. Most of the remaining cases are due to a translocation in which part of chromosome 21 breaks off and attaches to another chromosome (usually chromosome 14). Although there still are only 46 chromosomes in the cell, the presence of the extra part of chromosome 21 causes the features of Down syndrome (to be discussed).

The risk for having a child with Down syndrome increases with maternal age—it is 1/1300 at 25 years of age, 1/365 at 35 years, and 1/30 at 45 years of age.[15] The reason for the correlation between maternal age and nondisjunction is unknown but is thought to reflect some aspect of aging of the oocyte. Although males continue to produce sperm throughout their reproductive life, females are born with all the oocytes they ever will have. These oocytes may change as a result of the aging process. With increasing age, there is a greater chance of a woman having been exposed to damaging environmental agents, such as drugs, chemicals, and radiation. Unlike trisomy 21, Down syndrome due to a chromosome (21;14) translocation shows no relation to maternal age but has a relatively high recurrence risk in families when a parent, particularly the mother, is a carrier.

The physical features of a child with Down syndrome are distinctive, and therefore the condition usually is apparent at birth. These features include a small and rather square head. There is upward slanting of the eyes; small, low-set, and malformed ears; a fat pad at the back of the neck; an open mouth; and a large, protruding tongue (Fig. 7-6). The child's hands usually are short and stubby,

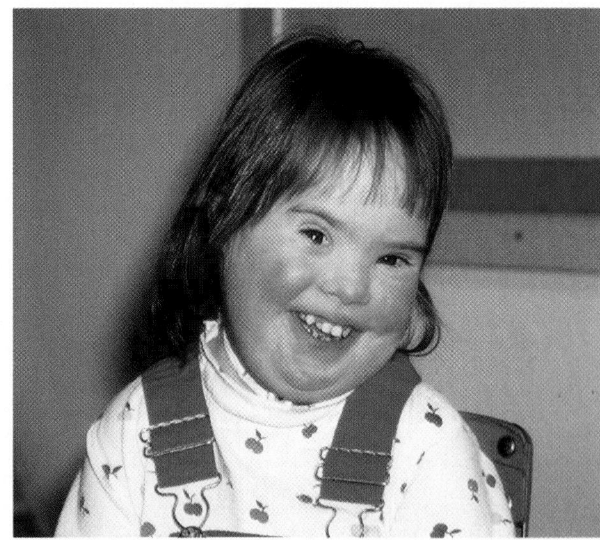

FIGURE 7-6 A child with Down syndrome. (Courtesy of March of Dimes Birth Defects Foundation, White Plains, NY)

with fingers that curl inward, and there usually is only a single palmar (*i.e.,* simian) crease. Hypotonia and joint laxity also are present in infants and young children. There often are accompanying congenital heart defects and an increased risk for gastrointestinal malformations. Approximately 1% of persons with trisomy 21 Down syndrome have mosaicism (*i.e.,* cell populations with the normal chromosome number and trisomy 21); these persons may be less severely affected. Of particular concern is the much greater risk for development of acute leukemia among children with Down syndrome—10 to 20 times greater than that of other children.[5] With increased life expectancy due to improved health care, it has been found that there also is an increased risk for Alzheimer's disease among older persons with Down syndrome.

Several prenatal screening tests can be done to determine the risk for having a child with Down syndrome. The most commonly used test is the triple screen—α-fetoprotein (AFP), human chorionic gonadotropin (HCG), and unconjugated estriol. The results of these tests, which usually are done between 15 and 20 weeks of gestation, together with the woman's age often are used to determine the probability of a pregnant woman having a child with Down syndrome. These tests are able to detect accurately only approximately 60% of fetuses with Down syndrome. Some women are given false-positive readings, and some are given false-negative readings. In 1992, fetal nuchal (back of neck) translucency, as measured by ultrasonography in the first trimester, was proposed as another screening measure; the nucha was found to be thicker in fetuses with Down syndrome.[16] This test, which must be done by a highly trained professional, continues to be investigated as a screening method. The only way to determine accurately the presence of Down syndrome in the fetus is through chromosome analysis using chorionic villus sampling, amniocentesis, or percutaneous umbilical blood sampling.

Turner's Syndrome. Turner's syndrome is the result of complete or partial X-chromosome monosomy in a phenotypic female, associated with characteristic clinical features, the most consistent being short stature and ovarian dysgenesis. The disorder affects approximately 1 of every 2500 live births, and it has been estimated that more than 99% of fetuses are spontaneously aborted in the first trimester.[4,16,17] Unlike Down syndrome, the disorder does not appear to be associated with advanced parental age.

Turner's syndrome is characterized cytogenetically by a monosomy of the X chromosome, the presence of an abnormal X chromosome, or a mosaicism of a 45,X cell line with another cell line (*e.g.,* 45,X/46,XX, 45,X). Pure 45,X monosomy is the most common karyotype and is associated with the most abnormal phenotype.

Characteristically, the female with Turner's syndrome is short in stature, but her body proportions are normal (Fig 7-7). She does not menstruate and shows no signs of secondary sex characteristics. Variations in the syndrome range from essentially none to webbing of the neck with redundant skin folds and low hairline, nonpitting lymphedema of the hands and feet, and congenital heart defects, particularly coarctation of the aorta. There also may be abnormalities in kidney development (*i.e.,* abnormal location, abnormal vascular supply, or double collecting system), changes in nail growth, high-arched palate, short fourth metacarpal, and strabismus. When a mosaic cell line is present, the manifestations associated with the chromosomal defect tend to be less severe.

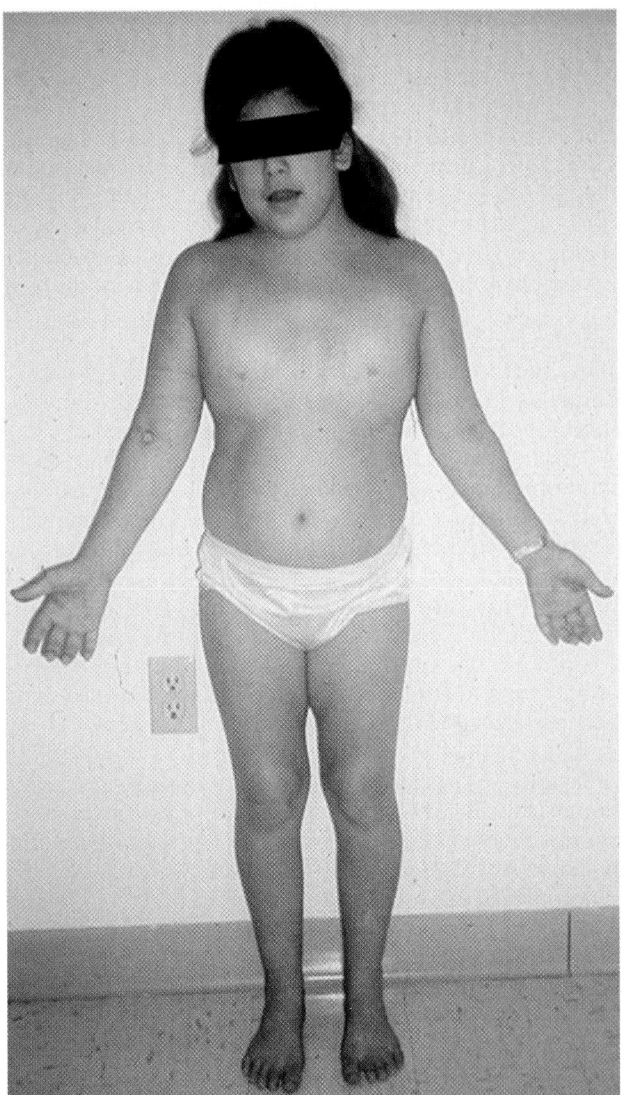

FIGURE 7-7 Turner syndrome. Short stature, stocky build, crest chest, lack of breast development, and cubitus valgus are evident in this 13-year-old girl. (Shulman D., Beru B. [2000]. *Atlas of clinical endocrinology: Neuroendocrinology and pituitary disease.* Philadelphia: Current Medicine Inc)

Treatment of Turner's syndrome begins during childhood. Growth hormone therapy is now standard treatment and can result in a gain of 6 to 10 cm in final height. Estrogen therapy, which is instituted around the normal age of puberty, is used to promote development and maintenance of secondary sexual characteristics.[16–19]

The diagnosis of Turner's syndrome often is delayed until late childhood or early adolescence in girls who do not present with the classic features of the syndrome.[17]

Early diagnosis is an important aspect of treatment of Turner's syndrome. It allows for counseling about the phenotypic characteristics of the disorder; screening for cardiac, renal, thyroid, and other abnormalities; provision of emotional support for the girl and her family; and planning for growth hormone therapy and estrogen replacement therapy.[20] Because of the potential for delay in diagnosis, it has been recommended that girls with unexplained short stature (height below the fifth percentile), webbed neck, peripheral lymphedema, coarctation of the aorta, or delayed puberty have chromosome studies done. In addition, chromosome analysis should be considered for girls who remain above the fifth percentile but have two or more features of Turner's syndrome, including high palate, nail deformities, short fourth metacarpal, and strabismus.[18]

There is also concern for adult women with Turner's syndrome. Until recently, females with Turner's syndrome received intensive medical care during childhood but were discharged from specialty clinics after induction of puberty and attainment of final height. It is now known that women with Turner's disease have increased morbidity due to cardiovascular disease and gastrointestinal, renal, and other endocrine disorders.[19] Adults with Turner's syndrome continue to have reduced bone mass, and this has been associated with increased risk for fractures.

Klinefelter's Syndrome. Klinefelter's syndrome is a condition of testicular dysgenesis accompanied by the presence of one or more extra X chromosomes in excess of the normal male XY complement.[4] Most males with Klinefelter's syndrome have one extra X chromosome (47,XXY). In rare cases, there may be more than one extra X chromosome (48,XXXY). The presence of the extra X chromosome in the 47,XXY male results from nondisjunction during meiotic division in one of the parents. The additional X chromosome (or chromosomes) is of maternal origin in approximately two thirds of cases and of paternal origin in the remaining one third.[5] The cause of the nondisjunction is unknown. Advanced maternal age increases the risk, but only slightly.

Based on studies conducted in the 1970s, including one sponsored by the National Institutes of Health and Human Development that checked the chromosomes of more than 40,000 infants, it has been estimated that the 47,XXY syndrome is one of the most common genetic abnormalities known, occurring as frequently as 1 in 500 to 1 in 1000 male births.[21] Although the presence of the extra chromosome is fairly common, the syndrome, with its accompanying signs and symptoms that may result from the extra chromosome, is uncommon. Many men live their lives without being aware that they have an additional chromosome. For this reason, it has been suggested that the term *Klinefelter's syndrome* be replaced with *47,XXY male*.[22]

Klinefelter's syndrome is characterized by enlarged breasts, sparse facial and body hair, small testes, and the inability to produce sperm.[21] Regardless of the number of X chromosomes present, the male phenotype is retained. The condition often goes undetected at birth. The infant usually has normal male genitalia, with a small penis and small, firm testicles. At puberty, the intrinsically abnormal testes do not respond to stimulation from the gonadotropins and undergo degeneration. This leads to a tall stature with abnormal body proportions in which the lower part of the body is longer than the upper part. Later in life, the body build may become heavy, with a female distribution of subcutaneous fat and variable degrees of breast enlargement. There may be deficient secondary male sex characteristics, such as a voice that remains feminine in pitch and sparse beard and pubic hair. There may be sexual dysfunction along with the complete infertility that occurs owing to the inability to produce sperm. Regular administration of testosterone, beginning at puberty, can promote more normal growth and development of secondary sexual characteristics. Although the intellect usually is normal, most 47,XXY males have some degree of language impairment. They often learn to talk later than do other children and often have trouble with learning to read and write.

Alterations in Chromosome Structure

Aberrations in chromosome structure occur when there is a break in one or more of the chromosomes followed by rearrangement or deletion of the chromosome parts. Among the factors believed to cause chromosome breakage are exposure to radiation sources, such as x-rays; influence of certain chemicals; extreme changes in the cellular environment; and viral infections.

Several patterns of chromosome breakage and rearrangement can occur (Fig. 7-8). There can be a *deletion* of the broken portion of the chromosome. When one chromosome is involved, the broken parts may be *inverted*. *Isochromosome formation* occurs when the centromere, or central portion, of the chromosome separates horizontally instead of vertically. *Ring formation* results when deletion is followed by uniting of the chromatids to form a ring. *Translocation* occurs when there are simultaneous breaks in two chromosomes from different pairs, with exchange of chromosome parts. With a balanced reciprocal translocation, no genetic information is lost; therefore, persons with translocations usually are normal. However, these persons are translocation carriers and may have normal and abnormal children.

A special form of translocation called a *centric fusion* or *Robertsonian translocation* involves two acrocentric chromosomes in which the centromere is near the end (see Fig. 7-8). Typically, the break occurs near the centromere affecting the short arm in one chromosome and the long arm in the other. Transfer of the chromosome fragments leads to one long and one extremely short chromosome. The short fragments commonly are lost. In this case, the person has only 45 chromosomes, but the amount of genetic material that is lost is so small that it often goes unnoticed. Difficulty, however, arises during meiosis, with gametes receiving either no chromosome or the translocated chromosome.

A rare form of Down syndrome can occur in the offspring of persons in whom there has been a translocation involving the long arm of chromosome 21q and the long arm of one of the acrocentric chromosomes (most often 14 or 22). The translocation adds to the normal long arm of chromosome 21; therefore, the person with this type of

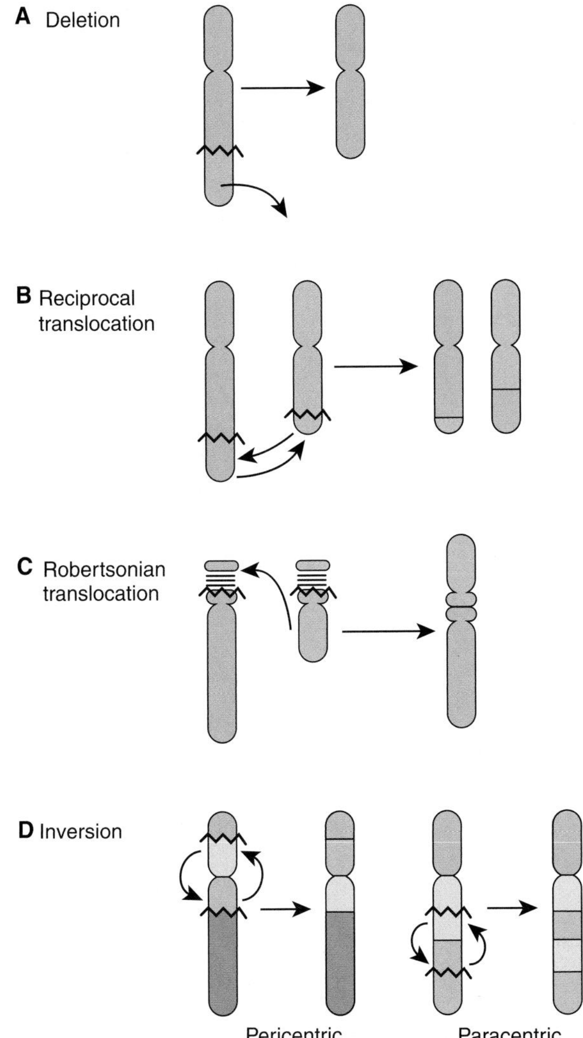

FIGURE 7-8 Structural abnormalities in the human chromosome. (**A**) Deletion of part of a chromosome leads to loss of genetic material and shortening of the chromosome; (**B**) A reciprocal translocation involves two nonhomologous chromosomes, with exchange of the acentric segment. (**C**) Robertsonian translocation in which two nonhomologous acrocentric chromosomes break near their centromeres, after which the long arms fuse to form one large metacentric chromosome; (**D**) Inversion, which requires two breaks in a single chromosome with inversion to the opposite side of the centromere (pericentric, or paracentric if the breaks are on the same arm). (Adapted from Rubin E., Farber J.L. [1999]. *Pathology* [3rd ed., p. 225]. Philadelphia: Lippincott-Raven)

Down syndrome has 46 chromosomes, but essentially a trisomy of 21q.[4–6]

The manifestations of aberrations in chromosome structure depend to a great extent on the amount of genetic material that is lost. Many cells sustaining unrestored breaks are eliminated within the next few mitoses because of deficiencies that may in themselves be fatal. This is beneficial because it prevents the damaged cells from becoming a permanent part of the organism or, if it occurs in the gametes, from giving rise to grossly defective zygotes. Some altered chromosomes, such as those that occur with translocations, are passed on to the next generation.

In summary, genetic disorders can affect a single gene (mendelian inheritance) or several genes (polygenic inheritance). Single-gene disorders may be present on an autosome or on the X chromosome, and they may be expressed as a dominant or recessive trait. In autosomal dominant disorders, a single mutant allele from an affected parent is transmitted to an offspring regardless of sex. The affected parent has a 50% chance of transmitting the disorder to each offspring. Autosomal recessive disorders are manifested only when both members of the gene pair are affected. Usually, both parents are unaffected but are carriers of the defective gene. Their chances of having an affected child are one in four; of having a carrier child, two in four; and of having a noncarrier unaffected child, one in four. Sex-linked disorders, which are associated with the X chromosome, are those in which an unaffected mother carries one normal and one mutant allele on the X chromosome. She has a 50% chance of transmitting the defective gene to her sons, and her daughters have a 50% chance of being carriers of the mutant gene. Because of a normal paired gene, female heterozygotes rarely experience the effects of a defective gene. Multifactorial inheritance disorders are caused by multiple genes and, in many cases, environmental factors.

The mitochondria contain their own DNA, which is distinct from nuclear DNA. This DNA, which is inherited maternally, is subject to mutations at a higher rate than nuclear DNA and has no repair mechanisms. Disorders of mitochondrial genes interfere with production of cellular energy, lead to the production of energy-reactive oxygen species, or disrupt the generation of signals that initiate apoptosis. The range of mitochondrial gene disorders is diverse, with neuromuscular disorders predominating.

Chromosomal disorders result from a change in chromosome number or structure. A change in chromosome number is called *aneuploidy. Monosomy* involves the presence of only one member of a chromosome pair; it is seen in Turner's syndrome, in which there is monosomy of the X chromosome. *Polysomy* refers to the presence of more than two chromosomes in a set. Klinefelter's syndrome involves polysomy of the X chromosome. Trisomy 21 (*i.e.,* Down syndrome) is the most common form of chromosome disorder. Alterations in chromosome structure involve deletion or addition of genetic material, which may involve a translocation of genetic material from one chromosome pair to another.

Disorders Due to Environmental Influences

After you have completed this section of the chapter, you should be able to meet the following objectives:

- Cite the most susceptible period of intrauterine life for development of defects due to environmental agents

- ✦ State the cautions that should be observed when considering use of drugs during pregnancy
- ✦ Describe the effects of alcohol and cocaine abuse on fetal development and birth outcomes
- ✦ List four infectious agents that cause congenital defects

The developing embryo is subject to many nongenetic influences. After conception, development is influenced by the environmental factors that the embryo shares with the mother. The physiologic status of the mother—her hormone balance, her general state of health, her nutritional status, and the drugs she takes—undoubtedly influences the development of the unborn child. For example, diabetes mellitus is associated with increased risk for congenital anomalies. Smoking is associated with lower than normal neonatal weight. Alcohol, in the context of chronic alcoholism, is known to cause fetal abnormalities. Some agents cause early abortion. Measles and other infectious agents cause congenital malformations. Other agents, such as radiation, can cause chromosomal and genetic defects and produce developmental disorders.

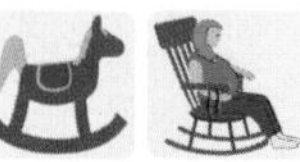

PERIOD OF VULNERABILITY

The embryo's development is most easily disturbed during the period when differentiation and development of the organs are taking place. This time interval, which is often referred to as the period of *organogenesis,* extends from day 15 to day 60 after conception. Environmental influences during the first 2 weeks after fertilization may interfere with implantation and result in abortion or early resorption of the products of conception. Each organ has a critical period during which it is highly susceptible to environmental derangements (Fig. 7-9). Often, the effect is expressed at the biochemical level just before the organ begins to develop. The same agent may affect different organ systems that are developing at the same time.

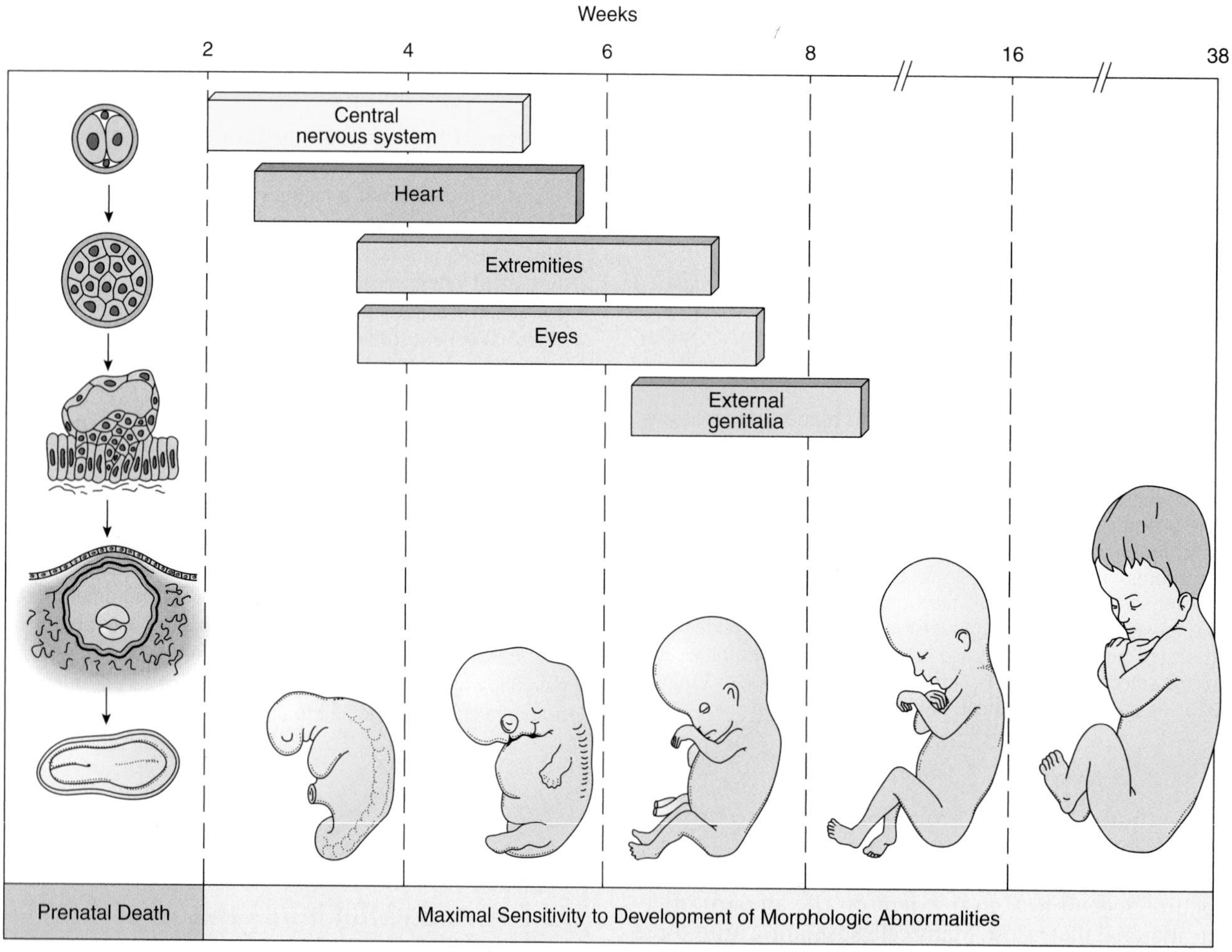

Weeks: 2, 4, 6, 8, 16, 38

Central nervous system | Heart | Extremities | Eyes | External genitalia

Prenatal Death | Maximal Sensitivity to Development of Morphologic Abnormalities

FIGURE 7-9 Sensitivity of specific organs to teratogenic agents at critical periods in embryogenesis. Exposure of adverse influences in the preimplantation and early postimplantation stages of development (*far left*) leads to prenatal death. Periods of maximal sensitivity to teratogens (*horizontal red bars*) vary for different organ systems but overall are limited to the first 8 weeks of pregnancy. (Rubin E., Farber J.L. [1999]. *Pathology* [3rd ed., p. 216]. Philadelphia: Lippincott-Raven)

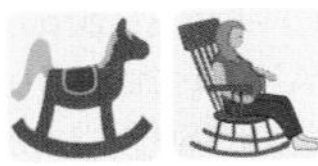

TERATOGENIC AGENTS

A teratogenic agent is an environmental agent that produces abnormalities during embryonic or fetal development. It is important to remember that, in this case, the environment is that of the embryo and fetus. Maternal disease or altered metabolic state also can affect the environment of the embryo or fetus. For discussion purposes, teratogenic agents have been divided into three groups: radiation, drugs and chemical substances, and infectious agents. Chart 7-1 lists commonly identified agents in each of these groups. Theoretically, environmental agents can cause birth defects in three ways: by direct exposure of the pregnant woman and the embryo or fetus to the agent; through exposure of the soon-to-be-pregnant woman with an agent that has a slow clearance rate such that a teratogenic dose is retained during early pregnancy; or as a result of mutagenic effects of an environmental agent that occur before pregnancy, causing permanent damage to a woman's (or a man's) reproductive cells.

Radiation

Heavy doses of ionizing radiation have been shown to cause microcephaly, skeletal malformations, and mental retardation. There is no evidence that diagnostic levels of radiation cause congenital abnormalities. Because the question of safety remains, however, many agencies require that the day of a woman's last menstrual period be noted on all radiologic requisitions. Other institutions may require a pregnancy test before any extensive diagnostic x-ray studies are performed. Radiation is teratogenic and mutagenic, and there is the possibility of effecting inheritable changes in genetic materials. Administration of therapeutic doses of radioactive iodine (^{131}I) during the 13th week of gestation, the time when the fetal thyroid is beginning to concentrate iodine, has been shown to interfere with thyroid development.

CHART 7-1

*Teratogenic Agents**

Radiation

Drugs and Chemical Substances

Alcohol
Anticoagulants
  Warfarin
Anticonvulsants
Cancer drugs
  Aminopterin
  Methotrexate
  6-Mercaptopurine
Isotretinoin (Accutane)
Propylthiouracil
Tetracycline
Thalidomide

Infectious Agents

Viruses
  Cytomegalovirus
  Herpes simplex virus
  Measles (rubella)
  Mumps
  Varicella-zoster virus (chickenpox)
Nonviral factors
  Syphilis
  Toxoplasmosis

* Not inclusive.

Chemicals and Drugs

Environmental chemicals and drugs can cross the placenta and cause damage to the developing embryo and fetus. It has been estimated that only 2% to 3% of developmental defects have a known drug or environmental origin. Some of the best-documented environmental teratogens are the organic mercurials, which cause neurologic deficits and blindness. Sources of exposure to mercury include contaminated food (fish) and water.[23] The precise mechanism by which chemicals and drugs exert their teratogenic effects is largely unknown. They may produce cytotoxic (cell-killing), antimetabolic, or growth-inhibiting properties. Often their effects depend on the time of exposure (in terms of embryonic and fetal development) and extent of exposure (dosage).

Drugs top the list of chemical teratogens, probably because they are regularly used at elevated doses. Most drugs can cross the placenta and expose the fetus to both the pharmacologic and teratogenic effects. Factors that affect placental drug transfer and drug effects on the fetus include the rate at which the drug crosses the placenta, the duration of exposure, and the stage of placental and fetal development at the time of exposure.[24] Lipid-soluble drugs tend to cross the placenta more readily and enter the fetal circulation. The molecular weight of a drug also influences the rate of transfer and the amount of drug transferred across the placenta. Drugs with a molecular weight of less than 500 can cross the placenta easily, depending on lipid solubility and degree of ionization; those with a molecular weight of 500 to 1000 cross the placenta with more difficulty; and those with molecular weights of more than 1000 cross very poorly.[24]

A number of drugs are suspected of being teratogens, but only a few have been identified with certainty.[25] Perhaps the best known of these drugs is thalidomide, which has been shown to give rise to a full range of malformations, including phocomelia (*i.e.*, short, flipper-like appendages) of all four extremities. Other drugs known to cause fetal abnormalities are the antimetabolites that are used in the treatment of cancer, the anticoagulant drug warfarin, several of the anticonvulsant drugs, ethyl alcohol, and cocaine. Some drugs affect a single developing structure; for example, propylthiouracil can impair thyroid development, and tetracycline can interfere with the mineralization phase of tooth development. More recently, vitamin A and its derivatives (the retinoids) have been targeted for concern because of their teratogenic potential. Concern over the teratogenic effects of vitamin A derivatives became evident with the introduction of the acne drug isotretinoin (Accutane). Fetal abnormalities such as cleft palate, heart defects, retinal and optic nerve abnormalities, and central nervous system malformations were observed in women ingesting therapeutic doses of the drug during the first trimester of pregnancy.[26] There also is concern about the teratogenic effects when a woman consumes high doses of vitamin A, such as those contained in some dietary supplements or vitamin pills. It is currently recommended that doses greater than 10,000 IU should be avoided.[27]

In 1983, the U.S. Food and Drug Administration established a system for classifying drugs according to probable risks to the fetus. According to this system, drugs are put into five categories: A, B, C, D, and X. Drugs in category A are the least dangerous, and categories B, C, and D are increasingly more dangerous. Those in category X are contraindicated during pregnancy because of proven teratogenicity.[28] The law does not require classification of drugs that were in use before 1983.

Because many drugs are suspected of causing fetal abnormalities, and even those that were once thought to be safe are now being viewed critically, it is recommended that women in their childbearing years avoid unnecessary use of drugs. This pertains to nonpregnant women as well as pregnant women because many developmental defects occur early in pregnancy. As happened with thalidomide, the damage to the embryo may occur before pregnancy is suspected or confirmed. Two drugs of particular importance are alcohol and cocaine.

Fetal Alcohol Syndrome. The term *fetal alcohol syndrome* (FAS) refers to a constellation of physical, behavioral, and cognitive abnormalities resulting from maternal alcohol consumption. It has been reported that 1 in 1000 infants born in the United States manifests some characteristics of the syndrome.[29] Alcohol, which is lipid soluble and has a molecular weight between 600 and 1000, passes freely across the placental barrier; concentrations of alcohol in the fetus are at least as high as in the mother. Unlike other teratogens, the harmful effects of alcohol are not restricted to the sensitive period of early gestation, but extend throughout pregnancy.

Alcohol has widely variable effects on fetal development, ranging from minor abnormalities to FAS. Criteria for defining FAS were standardized by the Fetal Alcohol Study Group of the Research Society on Alcoholism in 1980,[30] and modifications were proposed in 1989.[31] The proposed criteria are prenatal or postnatal growth retardation (*i.e.,* weight or length below the 10th percentile); central nervous system involvement, including neurologic abnormalities, developmental delays, behavioral dysfunction, intellectual impairment, and skull and brain malformation; and a characteristic face with short palpebral fissures (*i.e.,* eye openings), a thin upper lip, and an elongated, flattened midface and philtrum (*i.e.,* the groove in the middle of the upper lip). The facial features of FAS may not be as apparent in the newborn but become more prominent as the infant develops (Fig. 7-10). As the children grow into adulthood, the facial features become more subtle, making diagnosis of FAS in older individuals more difficult.[32] Each of these defects can vary in severity, probably reflecting the timing of alcohol consumption in terms of the period of fetal development, amount of alcohol consumed, and hereditary and environmental influences. Because of problems with terminology and the diagnostic criteria, the Institute of Medicine in 1996 proposed the terms *alcohol-related neurodevelopmental disorder* (ARND) and *alcohol-related birth defects* (ARBD) to describe conditions in which there is a history of maternal alcohol consumption.[33] This new terminology uses pathophysiologic diagnostic categories to describe the conditions resulting

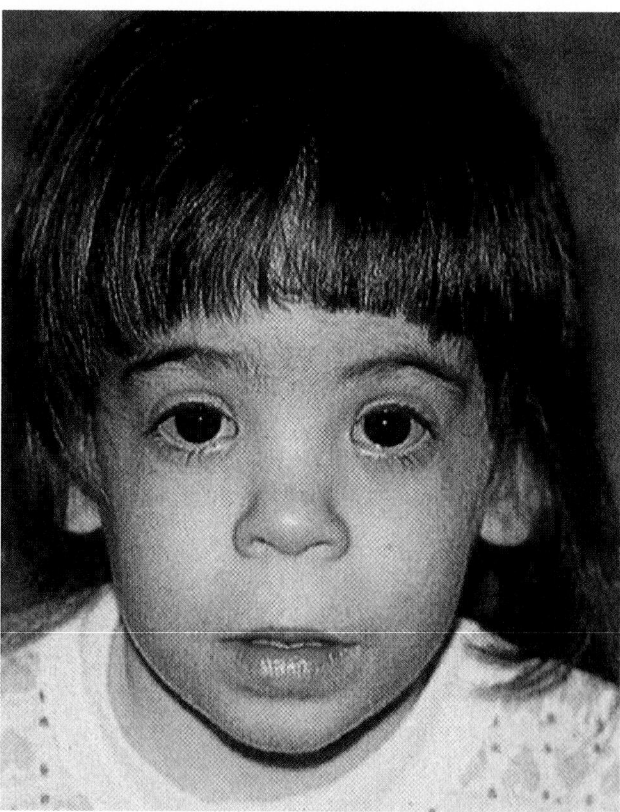

FIGURE 7-10 Child with fetal alcohol syndrome. (Goldman B., Schnell J., Spencer P. [2002] *Atlas of clinical neurology.* Philadelphia: Current Medicine Inc)

TERATOGENIC AGENTS

- Teratogenic agents such as radiation, chemicals, and drugs, and infectious organisms are agents that produce abnormalities in the developing embryo.
- The stage of development of the embryo determines the susceptibility to teratogens. The period during which the embryo is most susceptible to teratogenic agents is the time during which rapid differentiation and development of body organs and tissues are taking place, usually from days 15 to 60 postconception.

from confirmed alcohol exposure. For example, facial abnormalities, growth retardation, and central nervous system abnormalities would be classified as FAS; central nervous system and cognitive abnormalities would be classified as ARND; and birth defects would be ARBD.[33,34]

The mechanisms whereby alcohol exerts its teratogenic effects are unclear. Evidence suggests that the effects of alcohol observed in children with FAS are related to the timing of alcohol consumption and peak alcohol dose.

The amount of alcohol that can be safely consumed during pregnancy also is unknown. Animal studies suggest that the fetotoxic effects of alcohol are dose dependent rather than threshold dependent. Studies suggest that even three drinks per day may be associated with a lower IQ at 4 years of age.[35] However, it may be that the time during which alcohol is consumed is equally important. Even small amounts of alcohol consumed during critical periods of fetal development may be teratogenic. For example, if alcohol is consumed during the period of organogenesis, a variety of skeletal and organ defects may result. When alcohol is consumed later in gestation, when the brain is undergoing rapid development, there may be behavioral and cognitive disorders in the absence of physical abnormalities. Chronic alcohol consumption throughout pregnancy may result in a variety of effects, ranging from physical abnormalities to growth retardation and compromised central nervous system functioning. Evidence suggests that short-lived high concentrations of alcohol such as those that occur with binge drinking may be particularly significant, with abnormalities being unique to the period of exposure. The recommendation of both the U.S. Surgeon General and the Academy of Pediatrics is that women abstain completely from alcohol during pregnancy.[34,36]

Cocaine Babies. Of concern is the increasing use of cocaine by pregnant women. In 1992, approximately 45,000 women in this country used cocaine during their pregnancy.[37] Determining the exposure of infants to maternal cocaine use often is difficult. In utero exposure often is ascertained by testing maternal urine for cocaine and its metabolites and by interviewing the mother. Urine testing provides evidence only of recent cocaine use, and information from an interview may be inaccurate. Urine testing of infants provides evidence only of recent exposure to cocaine.

Among the effects of cocaine use during pregnancy is a decrease in uteroplacental blood flow, maternal hypertension, stimulation of uterine contractions, and fetal vasoconstriction. The decrease in uteroplacental blood flow is associated with an increase in preterm births, intrauterine growth retardation, microcephaly, and neurologic abnormalities.[38,39] Furthermore, there appears to be a dose-related relationship between increasing levels of chronic cocaine abuse and impaired fetal growth and neurologic function.[38,39] Maternal hypertension may increase the risk for abruptio placentae, particularly if it is accompanied by a decrease in uteroplacental blood flow.[39] Fetal vasoconstriction has been suggested as the cause of fetal anomalies, particularly limb reduction defects and urogenital tract defects such as hydronephrosis, hypospadias, and undescended testicles, as well as ambiguous genitalia.[40,41] Exposure of the fetus to cocaine also may lead to destructive lesions of the brain, including cerebral infarction and intracranial hemorrhage. Sudden infant death syndrome (SIDS) also has been more common in infants of mothers who have used cocaine during their pregnancy.[42]

Although the immediate effects of maternal cocaine use on infant behavior are being reported, the long-term effects are largely unknown. Unfortunately, cocaine addiction often affects the behavior of the pregnant woman to the extent that the need to procure larger amounts of the drug overwhelms all other considerations of maternal and fetal well-being; other factors such as malnutrition, use of other drugs and teratogens, and lack of prenatal care also may contribute to fetal disorders.

Folic Acid Deficiency. Although most birth defects are related to exposure to a teratogenic agent, deficiencies of nutrients and vitamins also may be a factor. Folic acid deficiency has been implicated in the development of neural tube defects (*e.g.,* anencephaly, spina bifida, encephalocele). Studies have shown a reduction in neural tube defects when folic acid was taken before conception and continued during the first trimester of pregnancy.[43,44] The Public Health Service recommends that all women of childbearing age should take 400 (micrograms) μg of folic acid daily. It has been suggested that this recommendation may help to prevent as many as 50% of neural tube defects.[45] The Institute of Medicine Panel for Folate and Other B Vitamins and Choline has recently revised the Recommended Dietary Allowance for pregnant women to 600 μg.[46] These recommendations are particularly important for women who have previously had an affected pregnancy, for couples with a close relative with the disorder, and for women with diabetes mellitus and those on anticonvulsant drugs who are at increased risk for having infants with birth defects.

Since 1998, all enriched cereal grain products in the United States have been fortified with folic acid. To achieve an adequate intake of folic acid, pregnant women should couple a diet that contains folate-rich foods (*e.g.,* orange juice, dark green leafy vegetables, and legumes) with sources of synthetic folic acid, such as fortified food products.[46]

Infectious Agents

Many microorganisms cross the placenta and enter the fetal circulation, often producing multiple malformations. The acronym TORCH stands for *t*oxoplasmosis, *o*ther, *r*ubella (*i.e.,* German measles), *c*ytomegalovirus, and *h*erpes, which are the agents most frequently implicated in fetal anomalies.[4] Other infections include varicella-zoster virus infection, listeriosis, leptospirosis, Epstein-Barr virus infection, tuberculosis, and syphilis. The TORCH screening test examines the infant's serum for the presence of antibodies to these agents. These infections tend to cause similar clinical manifestations, including microcephaly, hydrocephalus, defects of the eye, and hearing problems.

Toxoplasmosis is a protozoal infection caused by *Toxoplasma gondii*. The infection can be contracted by eating raw or inadequately cooked meat or food that has come in contact with infected meat.[47] The domestic cat can carry the organism, excreting the protozoa in its feces. It has been suggested that pregnant women should avoid contact with excrement from the family cat. The introduction of the rubella vaccine in the United States has virtually eliminated congenital rubella. The epidemiology of cytomegalovirus infection is largely unknown. Some infants are severely affected at birth, and others, although having evidence of the infection, have no symptoms. In some symptom-free infants, brain damage becomes evident over a span of several years. There also is evidence that some infants contract the infection during the first year of life, and in some of them, the infection leads to retardation a year or two later. Herpes simplex type 2 infection is considered to be a genital infection and usually is transmitted through sexual contact. The infant acquires this infection in utero or in passage through the birth canal.

In summary, a teratogenic agent is one that produces abnormalities during embryonic or fetal life. It is during the early part of pregnancy (15 to 60 days after conception) that environmental agents are most apt to produce their deleterious effects on the developing embryo. A number of environmental agents can be damaging to the unborn child, including radiation, drugs and chemicals, and infectious agents. FAS is a risk in infants of women who regularly consume alcohol during pregnancy. Of recent concern is the use of cocaine by pregnant women. Because many drugs have the potential for causing fetal abnormalities, often at an early stage of pregnancy, it is recommended that women of childbearing age avoid unnecessary use of drugs. It also has been shown that folic acid deficiency can contribute to neural tube defects. The acronym TORCH stands for *t*oxoplasmosis, *o*ther, *r*ubella, *c*ytomegalovirus, and *h*erpes, which are the infectious agents most frequently implicated in fetal anomalies.

Diagnosis and Counseling

After you have completed this section of the chapter, you should be able to meet the following objectives:

- Describe the process of genetic assessment
- Cite the rationale for prenatal diagnosis
- Describe methods used in arriving at a prenatal diagnosis, including ultrasonography, amniocentesis, chorionic villus sampling, percutaneous umbilical fetal blood sampling, and laboratory methods to determine the biochemical and genetic makeup of the fetus

The birth of a defective child is a traumatic event in any parent's life. Usually two issues must be resolved. The first deals with the immediate and future care of the affected child, and the second with the possibility of future children in the family having a similar defect. Genetic assessment and counseling can help to determine whether the defect was inherited and the risk for recurrence. Prenatal diagnosis provides a means of determining whether the unborn child has certain types of abnormalities.

GENETIC ASSESSMENT

Effective genetic counseling involves accurate diagnosis and communication of the findings and risks for recurrence to the parents and other family members who need such information. Counseling may be provided after the birth of an affected child, or it may be offered to persons at risk for having defective children (*i.e.,* siblings of persons with birth defects). A team of trained counselors can help the family to understand the problem and can support their decisions about having more children.

Assessment of genetic risk and prognosis usually is directed by a clinical geneticist, often with the aid of laboratory and clinical specialists. A detailed family history (*i.e.,* pedigree), a pregnancy history, and detailed accounts of the birth process and postnatal health and development are included. A careful physical examination of the affected child and often of the parents and siblings usually is needed. Laboratory tests, including chromosomal analysis and biochemical studies, often precedes a definitive diagnosis.

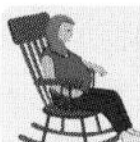

PRENATAL DIAGNOSIS

Prenatal diagnosis should begin with measures to identify pregnancies in which there is a recognizable risk for a diagnosable fetal disorder.[4,48] The use of a questionnaire to elicit genetic information is recommended by the American College of Obstetricians and Gynecologists before prenatal diagnosis is undertaken.[48]

The purpose of prenatal diagnosis is not just to detect fetal abnormalities. Rather, it has the following objectives: to provide parents with information needed to make an informed choice about having a child with an abnormality; to provide reassurance and reduce anxiety among high-risk groups; and to allow parents at risk for having a child with a specific defect, who might otherwise forgo having a child, to begin pregnancy with the assurance that knowledge about the presence or absence of the disorder in the fetus can be confirmed by testing. Prenatal screening cannot be used to rule out all possible fetal abnormalities. It is limited to determining whether the fetus has (or probably has) designated conditions indicated by late maternal age, family history, or well-defined risk factors.[4]

Among the methods used for fetal diagnosis are maternal blood screening, ultrasonography, amniocentesis, chorionic villus sampling, and percutaneous umbilical fetal blood sampling.[4] Termination of pregnancy is indicated only in a small number of cases; in the rest, the fetus is normal, and the procedure provides reassurance for the parents. Prenatal diagnosis can also provide the information needed for prescribing prenatal treatment for the fetus. For example, if congenital adrenal hyperplasia is diagnosed, the mother can be treated with adrenal cortical hormones to prevent masculinization of a female fetus.

Maternal Serum Markers

Maternal blood testing began in the early 1980s with the test for AFP. AFP is a major fetal plasma protein and has a structure similar to the albumin that is found in postnatal life. AFP is made initially by the yolk sac and later by the liver. It peaks at approximately 12 to 14 weeks in the fetus and falls thereafter. AFP is found in the amniotic fluid at approximately 1/100 the concentration found in fetal serum. AFP reaches the maternal bloodstream and can be measured by laboratory methods. The normal maternal serum AFP level rises from 13 weeks and peaks at 32 weeks of gestation. In pregnancies where the fetus has a neural tube defect (*i.e.,* anencephaly and open spina bifida) or certain other malformations such as an anterior abdominal wall defect, maternal and amniotic levels of AFP are elevated because open neural tube and ventral wall defects are associated with exposed fetal membrane and blood vessel surfaces that increase the AFP in the amniotic fluid and maternal blood. Screening of maternal blood samples usually is done between weeks 16 and 18 of gestation.[4,48]

Although neural tube defects have been associated with elevated levels of AFP, decreased levels have been associated with Down syndrome. The single maternal serum marker that yields the highest detection rate for Down syndrome is an elevated level of HCG. The combined use of three maternal serum markers, decreased AFP and unconjugated estriol and elevated HCG, between 16 and 20 weeks of pregnancy has been shown to detect as many as 60% of Down syndrome pregnancies.[4,48] The use of ultrasound to verify fetal age can reduce the number of false-positive tests with this screening method.

Ultrasound

Ultrasound is a noninvasive diagnostic method that uses reflections of high-frequency sound waves to visualize soft tissue structures. Since its introduction in 1958, it has been used during pregnancy to determine number of fetuses, fetal size, fetal position, amount of amniotic fluid that is present, and placental location. It also is possible to assess fetal movement, breathing movements, and heart pattern. Improved resolution and real-time units have enhanced the ability of ultrasound scanners to detect congenital anomalies. With this more sophisticated equipment, it is possible to obtain information such as measurements of hourly urine output in a high-risk fetus. Ultrasound makes possible the in utero diagnosis of hydrocephalus, spina bifida, facial defects, congenital heart defects, congenital diaphragmatic hernias, disorders of the gastrointestinal tract, and skeletal anomalies. Cardiovascular abnormalities are the most commonly missed malformation. A four-chamber view of the fetal heart improves the detection of cardiac malformations. Intrauterine diagnosis of congenital abnormalities permits planning of surgical correction shortly after birth, preterm delivery for early correction, selection of cesarean section to reduce fetal injury, and, in some cases, intrauterine therapy. When a congenital abnormality is suspected, a diagnosis made using ultrasound usually can be obtained by weeks 16 to 18 of gestation.

Amniocentesis

Amniocentesis involves the withdrawal of a sample of amniotic fluid from the pregnant uterus by means of a needle inserted through the abdominal wall (Fig. 7-11).

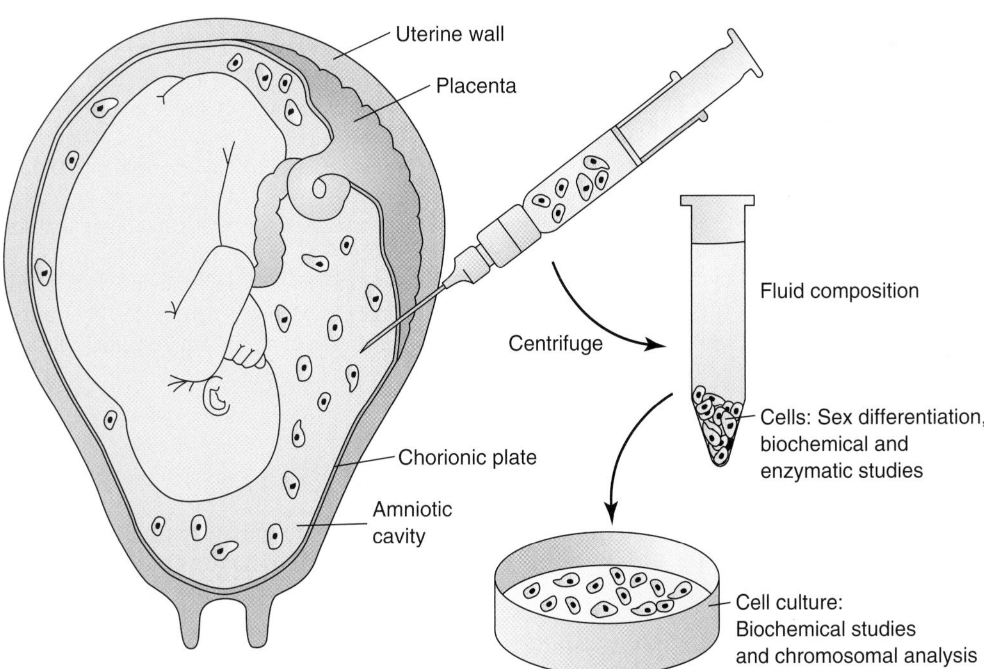

FIGURE 7-11 Amniocentesis. A needle is inserted into the uterus through the abdominal wall, and a sample of amniotic fluid is withdrawn for chromosomal and biochemical studies. (Department of Health, Education, and Welfare. [1977]. *What are the facts about genetic disease?* Washington, DC: DHEW)

The procedure is useful in women older than 35 years of age, who have an increased risk for giving birth to an infant with Down syndrome; in parents who have another child with chromosomal abnormalities; and in situations in which a parent is known to be a carrier of an inherited disease. Ultrasound is used to gain additional information and to guide the placement of the amniocentesis needle. The amniotic fluid and cells that have been shed by the fetus are studied. Usually, a determination of fetal status can be made by the 16th to 17th week of pregnancy.[48–50] For chromosomal analysis, the fetal cells are grown in culture, and the result is available in 10 to 14 days. The amniotic fluid also can be tested using various biochemical tests.[4]

Early amniocentesis (before 15 weeks) can be done. However, its safety has not been established. The volume of fluid removed in relation to total amniotic fluid is greater, which may produce fetal loss or have an effect on fetal lung function.

Chorionic Villus Sampling

Sampling of the chorionic villi usually is done after 10 weeks of gestation.[49,50] Doing the test before that time is not recommended because of the danger of limb reduction defects in the fetus. The chorionic villi are the site of exchange of nutrients between the maternal blood and the embryo—the chorionic sac encloses the early amniotic sac and fetus, and the villi are the primitive blood vessels that develop into the placenta. The sampling procedure usually is performed using a transabdominal approach. The tissue that is obtained can be used for fetal chromosome studies, DNA analysis, and biochemical studies. The fetal tissue does not have to be cultured, and fetal chromosome analysis can be made available in 24 hours. DNA analysis and biochemical tests can be completed in 1 to 2 weeks.[50]

Percutaneous Umbilical Blood Sampling

Percutaneous fetal blood sampling involves the transcutaneous insertion of a needle through the uterine wall and into the umbilical artery. It is performed under ultrasound guidance and can be done any time after 16 weeks of gestation. It is used for prenatal diagnosis of hemoglobinopathies, coagulation disorders, metabolic and cytogenic disorders, and immunodeficiencies. Fetal infections such as rubella and toxoplasmosis can be detected through measurement of immunoglobulin M antibodies or direct blood cultures. Results from cytogenic studies usually are available within 48 to 72 hours. Because the procedure carries a greater risk for pregnancy loss than amniocentesis, it usually is reserved for situations in which rapid cytogenic analysis is needed or in which diagnostic information cannot be obtained by other methods.

Fetal Biopsy

Fetal biopsy is done with a fetoscope under ultrasound guidance. It is used to detect certain genetic skin defects that cannot be diagnosed with DNA analysis. It also may be done to obtain muscle tissue for use in diagnosis of Duchenne muscular dystrophy.

Cytogenic and Biochemical Analyses

Amniocentesis and chorionic villus sampling yield cells that can be used for cytogenetic and DNA analyses. Biochemical analyses can be used to detect abnormal levels of AFP and abnormal biochemical products in the maternal blood and in specimens of amniotic fluid and fetal blood.

Cytogenetic studies are used for fetal karyotyping to determine the chromosomal makeup of the fetus. They are done to detect abnormalities of chromosome number and structure. Karyotyping also reveals the sex of the fetus. This may be useful when an inherited defect is known to affect only one sex.

Analysis of DNA is done on cells extracted from the amniotic fluid, chorionic villus sampling, or fetal blood from percutaneous umbilical sampling to detect genetic defects such as inborn errors of metabolism. The defect may be established through direct demonstration of the molecular defect or through methods that break the DNA into fragments so that the fragments may be studied to determine the presence of an abnormal gene. Direct demonstration of the molecular defect is done by growing the amniotic fluid cells in culture and measuring the enzymes that the cultured cells produce. Many of the enzymes are expressed in the chorionic villi; this permits earlier prenatal diagnosis because the cells do not need to be subjected to prior culture. DNA studies are used to detect genetic defects that cause inborn errors of metabolism, such as Tay-Sachs disease, glycogen storage diseases, and familial hypercholesterolemia. Prenatal diagnoses are possible for more than 70 inborn errors of metabolism.

In summary, genetic and prenatal diagnosis and counseling are done in an effort to determine the risk for having a child with a genetic or chromosomal disorder. They often involve a detailed family history (*i.e.,* pedigree), examination of any affected and other family members, and laboratory studies including chromosomal analysis and biochemical studies. They usually are done by a genetic counselor and a specially prepared team of health care professionals. Ultrasound and amniocentesis can be used to screen for congenital defects. Ultrasound is used for determination of fetal size and position and for the presence of structural anomalies. Amniocentesis and chorionic villus sampling are used to obtain specimens for cytogenetic and biochemical studies. They are used in the prenatal diagnosis of more than 70 genetic disorders.

REVIEW EXERCISES

A 23-year-old woman with sickle cell anemia and her husband want to have a child but worry that their child will be born with the disease.

A. What is the mother's genotype in terms of the sickle cell gene? Is she heterozygous or homozygous?

B. If the father is found to not have the sickle cell gene, what is the probability of their child having the disease or being a carrier of the disease?

C. If both the mother and father are found to be heterozygous (carriers) of the sickle cell gene, what are the chances that their child would have sickle cell disease or be a carrier of the trait?

A couple has a child who was born with a congenital heart defect.

A. Would you consider the defect to be the result of a single gene or a polygenic trait?

B. Would these parents be at greater risk for having another child with a heart defect, or would they be at equal risk for having a child with a defect in another organ system, such as a cleft palate?

A 26-year-old woman is planning to become pregnant.

A. What information would you give her regarding the effects of medications and drugs on the fetus? What stage of fetal development is associated with greatest risk?

B. What is the rationale for ensuring that she has an adequate intake of folic acid before conception and during pregnancy?

C. She and her husband have an indoor cat. What precautions should she use in caring for the cat?

References

1. March of Dimes Birth Defects Foundation. (2003). Birth defects information. [On-line]. Available: http://www.modimes.org.
2. Barsch G. (2002). Genetic diseases. In McPhee S. J., Linappa V. R., Ganong W. F., et al. (Eds.). *Pathology of disease* (4th ed., pp. 2–27). New York: McGraw-Hill.
3. Online Mendelian Inheritance in Man (OMIN™). (2003). Baltimore, MD: McKusick-Nathans Institute of Genetic Medicine, Johns Hopkins University; and Bethesda, MD: National Center for Biotechnology Information, National Library of Medicine. [On-line]. Available: http://www.ncbi.nlm.nih.gov/omim.
4. Nussbaum R. L., McInnes R. R., Willard H. F. (2001). *Thompson and Thompson genetics in medicine* (6th ed., pp. 51–78, 135, 159, 173–176, 244–249, 359–388). Philadelphia: W. B. Saunders.
5. Rubin E., Farber J. E. (Eds.). (1999). *Pathology* (3rd ed., pp. 123–157). Philadelphia: Lippincott-Raven.
6. Maitra A., Kumar V. (2003). Genetic and pediatric diseases. In Cotran R. S., Collins T., Robbins S. L. (Eds.). (2003). *Robbins basic pathology* (7th ed., pp. 211–263). Philadelphia: W. B. Saunders.
7. National Institute of Health Consensus Statement. (2000). Phenylketonuria (PKU): Screening and management. [On-line]. Available: http://consensus.nih.gov.
8. Koch R. K. (1999). Issues in newborn screening for phenylketonuria. *American Family Physician 60,* 1462–1466.
9. Hellekson K. L. (2001). Practice guidelines: NIH consensus statement on phenylketonuria. *American Family Physician 63,* 1430–1432.
10. National Institute of Child Health and Human Development. (2000). Facts about fragile X syndrome. [On-line]. Available: http://www.nichd.nih.gov/publications/pubs/Fragilex.htm.
11. Warren S. T. (1997). Trinucleotide repetition and fragile X syndrome. *Hospital Practice 31*(4), 73–85, 90–98.
12. Johns D. R. (1995). Mitochondrial DNA and disease. *New England Journal of Medicine 333,* 638–644.
13. Haslam R. H. A. (2000). Mitochondrial encephalomyopathies. In Behrman R. E., Kliegman R. M., Jenson H. B. (Eds.). *Nelson textbook of pediatrics* (16th ed., pp. 1845–1847). Philadelphia: W. B. Saunders.
14. Riccardi V. M. (1977). *The genetic approach to human disease* (p. 92). New York: Oxford University Press.
15. March of Dimes. (2003). Down syndrome. [On-line]. Available: http://www.modimes.org/HealthLibrary2/FactSheets/Down_syndrome.htm.
16. Newberger D. S. (2000). Down syndrome: Prenatal risk assessment and diagnosis. *American Family Physician 62,* 825–832, 837–838.
17. Wald N. J., Watt H. C., Hacshaw A. K. (1999). Integrated screening for Down's syndrome based on tests performed during the first and second trimester. *New England Journal of Medicine 341,* 461–467.
18. Rosenfeld R. G. (2000). Turner's syndrome: A growing concern. *Pediatrics 137,* 443–444.
19. Saenger P. (1996). Turner's syndrome. *New England Journal of Medicine 335,* 1749–1754.
20. Elsheikh M., Dunger D. B., Conway G. S., et al. (2002). Turner's syndrome in adulthood. *Endocrine Reviews 21,* 120–140.
21. Savendahl L., Davenport M. (2000). Delayed diagnoses of Turner's syndrome: Proposed guidelines for change. *Journal of Pediatrics 137,* 455–459.
22. National Institute of Child Health and Human Development. (2000). A guide for XXY males and their family. [On-line]. Available: http://www.nichd.nih.gov/publications/pubs/klinefelter.htm.
23. Steurerwald U., Weibe P., Jorgensen P. J., et al. (2000). Maternal seafood diet, methylmercury exposure, and neonatal neurologic function. *Journal of Pediatrics 136,* 599–605.
24. Katzung B. D. (1998). *Basic and clinical pharmacology* (7th ed., pp. 979–988). Stamford, CT: Appleton & Lange.
25. Koren G., Pstuszak A., Ito S. (1998). Drugs in pregnancy. *New England Journal of Medicine 338,* 1128–1137.
26. Ross S. A., McCaffery P. J., Drager U. C., et al. (2000). Retinoids in embryonal development. *Physiological Reviews 80,* 1021–1055.
27. Oakley G. P., Erickson J. D. (1995). Vitamin A and birth defects. *New England Journal of Medicine 333,* 1414–1415.
28. U.S. Food and Drug Administration. (2000). Pregnancy categories. [On-line]. Available: http://www.fda.gov.
29. March of Dimes. (1999). Leading categories of birth defects. [On-line]. Available: http://www.modimes.org/HealthLibrary2/InfantHealthStatistics/bdtable.htm.
30. Rosett H. L. (1980). A clinical perspective of the fetal alcohol syndrome. *Alcoholism, Clinical and Experimental Research 4,* 162–164.
31. Sokol R. J., Clarren S. K. (1980). Guidelines for use of terminology describing the impact of prenatal alcohol on the offspring. *Alcoholism, Clinical and Experimental Research 13,* 587–589.
32. Lewis D. D., Woods S. E. (1994). Fetal alcohol syndrome. *American Family Physician 50,* 1025–1032.
33. Stratton K., Howe C., Battaglia F. (Eds.). (1996). *Fetal alcohol syndrome: Diagnosis, epidemiology, prevention and treatment* (pp. 4–21). Washington, DC: National Academy Press.
34. American Academy of Pediatrics (2000). Fetal alcohol syndrome and alcohol-related neurodevelopmental disorders. *Pediatrics 106,* 358–361.
35. Ernhart C. B., Bowden D. M., Astley S. J. (1987). Alcohol teratogenicity in the human: A detailed assessment of specificity,

critical period, and threshold. *American Journal of Obstetrics and Gynecology 156,* 33–39.
36. Surgeon General's advisory on alcohol and pregnancy. (1981). *FDA Drug Bulletin 2,* 10.
37. March of Dimes. (2000). Cocaine use during pregnancy. [Online]. Available: http://www.modimes.org/HealthLibrary2/FactSheets/Cocaine_use_during_pregnancy.htm.
38. Volpe J. J. (1972). Effect of cocaine use on the fetus. *New England Journal of Medicine 327,* 399–407.
39. Chiriboga C. A., Brust C. M., Bateman D., et al. (1999). Dose-response effect of fetal cocaine exposure on newborn neurologic function. *Pediatrics 103,* 79–85.
40. MacGregor S. N., Keith L. G., Chasnoff I. J., et al. (1987). Cocaine use during pregnancy: Adverse outcome. *American Journal of Obstetrics and Gynecology 157,* 686–690.
41. Chasnoff I. J., Chisum G. M., Kaplan W. E. (1988). Maternal cocaine use and genitourinary malformations. *Teratology 37,* 201–204.
42. Riley J. B., Brodsky N. L., Porat R. (1988). Risk of SIDS in infants with in utero cocaine exposure: A prospective study [Abstract]. *Pediatric Research 23,* 454A.
43. Committee on Genetics. (1993). Folic acid for the prevention of neural tube defects. *Pediatrics 92,* 493–494.
44. Centers for Disease Control and Prevention. (1992). Recommendations for use of folic acid to reduce the number of cases of spina bifida and other neural tube defects. *Morbidity and Mortality Weekly Report 41,* 1–8.
45. Scholl T. O., Johnson W. G. (2000). Folic acid: Influence on outcome of pregnancy. *American Journal of Clinical Nutrition 71* (Suppl.), 1295S–1303S.
46. Bailey L. B. (2000). New standard for dietary folate intake in pregnant women. *American Journal of Clinical Nutrition 71* (Suppl.), 1304S–1307S.
47. Jones J., Lopez A., Wilson M. (2003). Congenital toxoplasmosis. *American Family Physician 67,* 2131–2138.
48. D'Alton M. E., DeCherney A. H. (1993). Prenatal diagnosis. *New England Journal of Medicine 328,* 114–120.
49. American College of Obstetricians and Gynecologists. (1987). *Antenatal diagnosis of genetic disorders* (pp. 1–8). Technical bulletin no. 108. Washington, DC: Author.
50. Wilson R. D. (2000). Amniocentesis and chorionic villus sampling. *Current Opinion in Obstetrics and Gynecology 12,* 81–86.

CHAPTER

8

Neoplasia

Kerry Twite

Cancer is the second leading cause of death in the United States. The disease affects all age groups, causing more death in children 1 to 14 years of age than any other disease. According to estimates of the American Cancer Society, 1.3 million new cases of cancer were diagnosed in the United States in 2003, and 556,500 people died of the disease.[1] Trends in cancer survival demonstrate that relative 5-year survival rates have improved since the early 1960s. Approximately 62% of people who develop cancer each year will be alive 5 years later.[1] Although the mortality rate has decreased, the number of cancer deaths has increased due to the aging and expanding population.

Cancer is not a single disease. Cancer can originate in almost any organ, with the prostate being the most common site in men and the breast in women (Fig. 8-1). The ability of cancer to be cured varies considerably and depends on the type of cancer and the extent of the disease at the time of diagnosis. Cancers such as acute lymphocytic leukemia, Hodgkin's disease, testicular cancer, and osteosarcoma, which only a few decades ago had poor prognoses, are today cured in many cases. However, lung cancer, which is the leading cause of death in men and women in the United States, is resistant to therapy, and although some progress has been made in its treatment, mortality rates remain high.

This chapter is divided into six sections: concepts of cell differentiation and growth, characteristics of benign and malignant neoplasms, etiology of cancer, clinical manifestations, diagnosis and treatment, and childhood cancers. Hematologic malignancies (lymphomas and leukemias) are presented in Chapter 17.

Ten Leading Cancer Types for the Estimated New Cancer Cases and Deaths, by Sex, US. 2003*

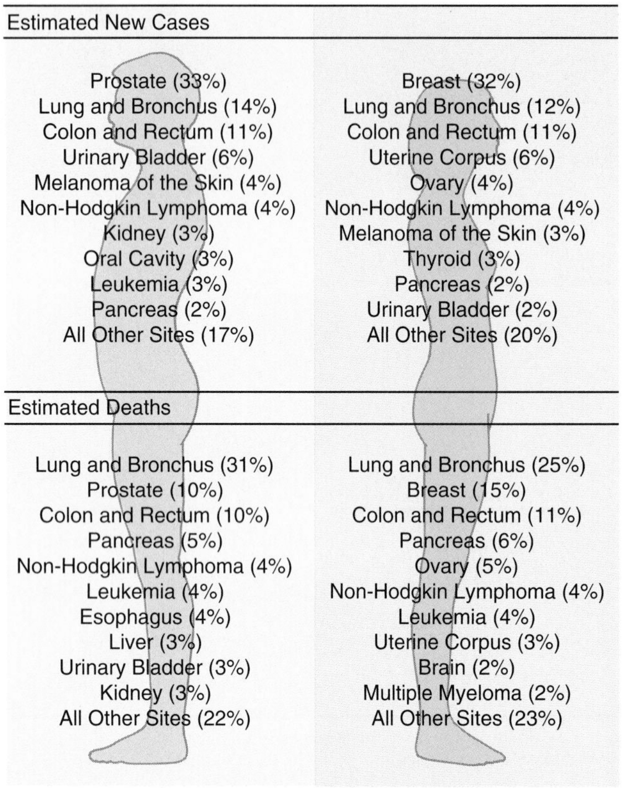

Estimated New Cases	
Prostate (33%)	Breast (32%)
Lung and Bronchus (14%)	Lung and Bronchus (12%)
Colon and Rectum (11%)	Colon and Rectum (11%)
Urinary Bladder (6%)	Uterine Corpus (6%)
Melanoma of the Skin (4%)	Ovary (4%)
Non-Hodgkin Lymphoma (4%)	Non-Hodgkin Lymphoma (4%)
Kidney (3%)	Melanoma of the Skin (3%)
Oral Cavity (3%)	Thyroid (3%)
Leukemia (3%)	Pancreas (2%)
Pancreas (2%)	Urinary Bladder (2%)
All Other Sites (17%)	All Other Sites (20%)
Estimated Deaths	
Lung and Bronchus (31%)	Lung and Bronchus (25%)
Prostate (10%)	Breast (15%)
Colon and Rectum (10%)	Colon and Rectum (11%)
Pancreas (5%)	Pancreas (6%)
Non-Hodgkin Lymphoma (4%)	Ovary (5%)
Leukemia (4%)	Non-Hodgkin Lymphoma (4%)
Esophagus (4%)	Leukemia (4%)
Liver (3%)	Uterine Corpus (3%)
Urinary Bladder (3%)	Brain (2%)
Kidney (3%)	Multiple Myeloma (2%)
All Other Sites (22%)	All Other Sites (23%)

*Excludes basal and squamous cell skin cancers and in situ carcinomas except urinary bladder.
Note: Percentages may not total 100 percent due to rounding.

FIGURE 8-1 Cancer incidence and mortality by site and sex. (Adapted from Jemel, A. et al. [2003]. Cancer statistics, 2003. *CA: A Cancer Journal for Clinicians 53*, 9.)

Concepts of Cell Differentiation and Growth

After completing this section of the chapter, you should be able to meet the following objectives:

- Define *neoplasm* and explain how neoplastic growth differs from the normal adaptive changes seen in atrophy, hypertrophy, and hyperplasia
- Distinguish between cell proliferation and differentiation
- Describe the five phases of the cell cycle
- Explain the function of cyclins, cyclin-dependent kinases, and cyclin-dependent kinase inhibitors in terms of regulating the cell cycle
- Characterize the properties of stem cells

Cancer is a disorder of altered cell differentiation and growth. The resulting process is called *neoplasia,* meaning "new growth," and the new growth is called a *neoplasm.* Unlike changes in tissue growth that occur with hypertrophy and hyperplasia, the growth of a neoplasm is uncoordinated and relatively autonomous in that it lacks normal regulatory controls over cell growth and division. Neoplasms tend to increase in size and continue to grow after the stimulus that evoked the change has ceased or the needs of the organism have been met.

Tissue renewal and repair involve two components: cell proliferation and differentiation. *Proliferation,* or the process of cell division, is an inherent adaptive mechanism for replacing body cells when old cells die or additional cells are needed. *Differentiation* is the process of specialization whereby new cells acquire the structure and function of the cells they replace. *Apoptosis,* which is discussed in Chapter 5, is a form of programmed cell death designed to eliminate senescent cells or unwanted cells. In adult tissues, the size of a population of cells is determined by the rates of cell proliferation, differentiation, and death by apoptosis.[2]

THE CELL CYCLE

The cell cycle is the interval between each cell division. During the cell cycle, genetic information is duplicated, and the duplicated chromosomes are appropriately aligned for distribution between two genetically identical daughter cells. In addition, checkpoints or pauses in the cell cycle provide opportunities for monitoring the accuracy of deoxyribonucleic acid (DNA) replication. These checkpoints allow for any defects to be edited and repaired, thereby ensuring that each daughter cell receives a full complement of genetic information, identical to that of the parent cell.[2,3]

The cell cycle is divided into four distinct phases referred to as G_1, S, G_2, and M (Fig. 8-2). G_1 (*gap 1*), is the postmitotic phase during which DNA synthesis ceases while ribonucleic acid (RNA) and protein synthesis and cell growth take place. During the *S phase,* DNA synthesis occurs, giving rise to two separate sets of chromosomes, one for each daughter cell. G_2 (*gap 2*) is the premitotic phase and is similar to G_1 in that DNA synthesis ceases while RNA and protein synthesis continues.[4] The *M phase* is the phase of cellular division or mitosis. Continually dividing cells, such as the stratified squamous epithelium of the skin, continuously cycle from one mitosis to the next mitosis. Cells

CELL PROLIFERATION AND GROWTH

- Tissue growth and repair involve cell proliferation and differentiation.
- Cell proliferation is the process whereby tissues acquire new or replacement cells through cell division.
- Cell differentiation is the orderly process in which proliferating cells are transformed into different and more specialized types. It determines the microscopic characteristics of the cell, how the cell functions, and how long it will live.
- Cells that are fully differentiated are no longer capable of cell division.

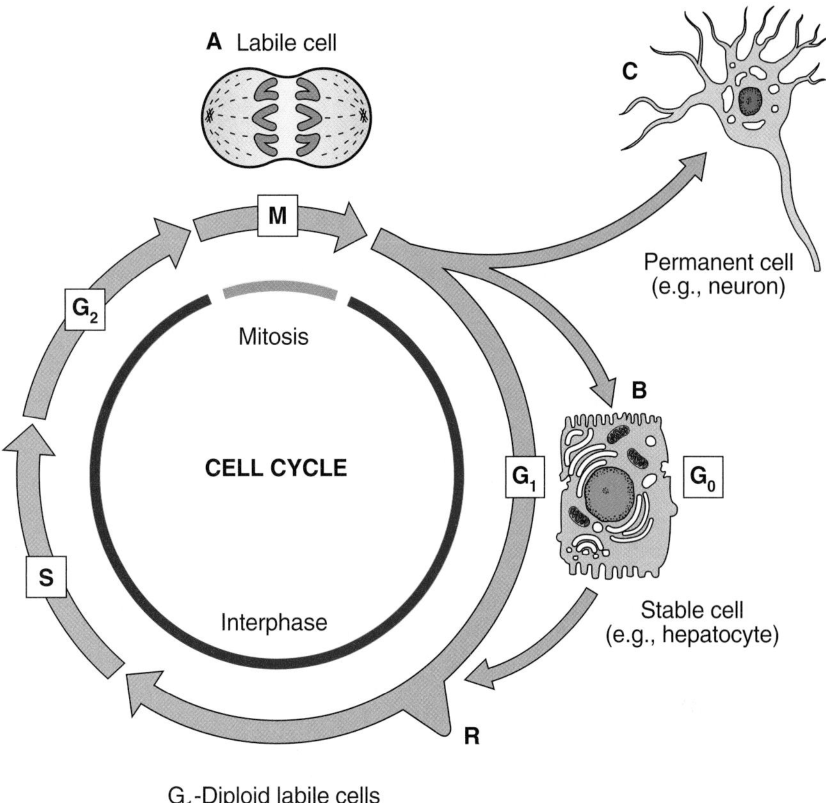

FIGURE 8-2 The cell cycle. (**A**) Labile cells (*e.g.*, intestinal crypt cells) undergo continuous replication and the interval between two consecutive mitoses is designated the cell cycle. After division, the cells enter a gap (G_1) during which DNA synthesis ceases and RNA and protein synthesis takes place as the cell develops its own specialized type of function. Cells that continue in the cell cycle pass the restriction point (R), which commits them to a new round of cell division and continuation to the synthesis (S) phase during which all the chromosomes are replicated. The S phase is followed by the short gap (G_2) during which DNA synthesis ceases and protein synthesis continues. The M phase is the period of mitosis. After each cycle, one daughter cell will become committed to differentiation and the other will continue cycling. (**B**) Some cell types, such as hepatocytes, are stable. After cell mitosis, the cells take up their specialized functions (G_0) and do not reenter the cell cycle unless stimulated by the loss of other cells. (**C**) Permanent cells (neurons) become terminally differentiated after mitosis and cannot reenter the cell cycle. (Rubin E., Farber J.L. [1999]. *Pathology* (3rd ed., p. 85). Philadelphia: Lippincott-Raven)

that are not actively dividing are quiescent and reside in G_0, or the resting phase of the cell cycle. These quiescent cells reenter the cell cycle in response to extracellular nutrients, growth factors, hormones, and other signals such as blood loss or tissue injury that signal for cell renewal.[5] Nondividing permanent cells, such as neurons, exit the cell cycle and are unable to undergo further cell division.

The duration of the phases of the cell cycle vary depending on the cell type, frequency with which the cells divide, and host characteristics such as the presence of appropriate growth factors. Very rapidly dividing cells can complete the cell cycle in less than 8 hours, whereas others can take longer than 1 year. Most of this variability occurs in the G_0 and G_1 phases. The duration of the S phase (10 to 20 hours), the G_2 phase (2 to 10 hours), and the M phase (0.5 to 1 hour) appears to be relatively constant.

A family of proteins called *cyclins* controls entry and progression of cells through the cell cycle. Cyclins act by complexing with (and thereby activating) proteins called cyclin-dependent kinases (CDKs). Kinases are enzymes that phosphorylate proteins. The CDKs phosphorylate specific target proteins and are expressed continuously during the cell cycle but in an inactive form; whereas the cyclins are synthesized during specific phases of the cell cycle and then rapidly degraded once their task is completed. Different combinations of cyclins and CDKs are associated with each of the stages of the cell cycle. For example, cyclin B and CDK1 control the transition from G_2 to M. As the cell moves into G_2, cyclin B is synthesized and binds to CDK1. The cyclin B–CDK1 complex then directs the event leading to mitosis, including DNA replication and assembly of the mitotic spindle. Although each phase of the cell cycle is monitored carefully, the transition from G_2 to M is believed to be one of the most important checkpoints in the cell cycle clock. In addition to the synthesis and degradation of the cyclins, the cyclin–CDK complexes are regulated by the binding of CDK inhibitors. The CDK inhibitors are particularly important in regulating cell cycle checkpoints during which mistakes in DNA replication are repaired. Recent understanding of the cyclins, CDKs, and CDK inhibitors has prompted exciting research into the development of new approaches in cancer treatment.[6]

CELL PROLIFERATION

Cell proliferation is the process by which cells divide and reproduce. In normal tissue, cell proliferation is regulated so that the number of cells actively dividing is equivalent to the number dying or being shed. In humans, there are two major categories of cells: gametes and somatic cells. The *gametes* (ovum and sperm) are *haploid,* having only one set of chromosomes from one parent and are designed specifically for sexual fusion. After fusion, a *diploid* cell containing both sets of chromosomes is formed. This cell is the *somatic cell* that goes on to form the rest of the body.

In terms of cell proliferation, the 200 or more cell types of the body can be divided into three large groups: the well-differentiated neurons and cells of skeletal and cardiac muscle that are unable to divide and reproduce; the parent, or progenitor cells, that continue to divide and reproduce, such as blood cells, skin cells, and liver cells; and the undifferentiated stem cells that can be triggered to enter the cell cycle and produce large numbers of progenitor cells when the need arises. The rates of reproduction of these cells vary greatly. White blood cells and cells that line the gastrointestinal tract live several days and must be replaced constantly. In most tissues, the rate of cell reproduction is greatly increased when tissue is injured or lost. Bleeding, for example, stimulates the rapid reproduction of the blood-forming cells of the bone marrow. In some types of tissue, the genetic program for cell replication normally is suppressed, but can be reactivated under certain conditions. The liver, for example, has extensive regenerative capabilities under certain conditions.

CELL DIFFERENTIATION

Cell differentiation is the process whereby proliferating cells are transformed into different and more specialized cell types. This process results in a fully differentiated, adult cell that has achieved its specific set of structural, functional, and life expectancy characteristics. For example, a red blood cell is programmed to develop into a concave disk that functions as a vehicle for oxygen transport and lives approximately 120 days.

All of the different cell types of the body originate from a single cell—the fertilized ovum. As the embryonic cells increase in number, they engage in an orderly process of differentiation that is necessary for the development of all the various organs of the body. The process of differentiation is regulated by a combination of internal processes involving the expression of specific genes and external stimuli provided by neighboring cells, exposure to substances in the maternal circulation, and a variety of growth factors, nutrients, oxygen, and ions.[6]

What makes the cells of one organ different from those of another organ is the type of genes that are expressed. Although all cells have the same complement of genes, only a small number of these genes are expressed in postnatal life. When cells, such as those of the developing embryo, differentiate and give rise to committed cells of a particular tissue type, the appropriate genes are maintained in an active state while the remainder are inactive. Normally, the rate of cell reproduction and the process of cell differentiation are precisely controlled in prenatal and postnatal life so that both of these mechanisms cease once the appropriate numbers and types of cells are formed.

The process of differentiation occurs in orderly steps; with each progressive step, increased specialization is exchanged for a loss of ability to develop different cell characteristics and different cell lines. The more highly specialized a cell becomes, the more likely it is to lose its ability to undergo mitosis. Neurons, which are the most highly specialized cells in the body, lose their ability to divide and reproduce once development of the nervous system is complete. More importantly, there are no reserve or parent cells to direct their replacement. However, appropriate numbers of these cell types are generated in the embryo such that loss of a certain percentage of cells does not affect the total cell population. Although these cells cannot divide and are not replaced if lost, they exist in sufficient numbers to carry out their specific functions. In other, less specialized tissues, such as the skin and mucosal lining of the gastrointestinal tract, cell renewal continues throughout life.

Even in the continuously renewing cell populations, highly specialized cells are similarly unable to divide. However, progenitor cells of the same lineage that have not yet differentiated to the extent that they have lost their ability to divide are able to provide an alternative mechanism for cell replacement. These cells are sufficiently "committed" that their daughter cells are restricted to producing a single type of cell, but they are not well enough differentiated to preclude the potential for active proliferation. As a result, these parent or progenitor cells are able to provide large numbers of replacement cells.

Another type of cell, called a *stem cell,* remains incompletely differentiated throughout life. Stem cells are reserve cells that remain quiescent until there is a need for cell replenishment, in which case they divide, producing other stem cells and cells that can carry out the functions of the differentiated cell (Fig. 8-3). When a stem cell divides, one daughter cell retains the stem cell characteristics, and the other daughter cell becomes a progenitor cell that proceeds through an irreversible process that leads to terminal differentiation. The progeny of each progenitor cell continues along the same genetic program, with the differentiating cells undergoing multiple mitotic divisions in the process of becoming a mature cell type and with each generation of cells becoming more specialized. In this way, a single stem cell can give rise to the many cells needed for normal tissue repair or blood cell production. When the dividing cells become fully differentiated, they no longer are capable of mitosis. In the immune system, for example, appropriately stimulated B lymphocytes be-

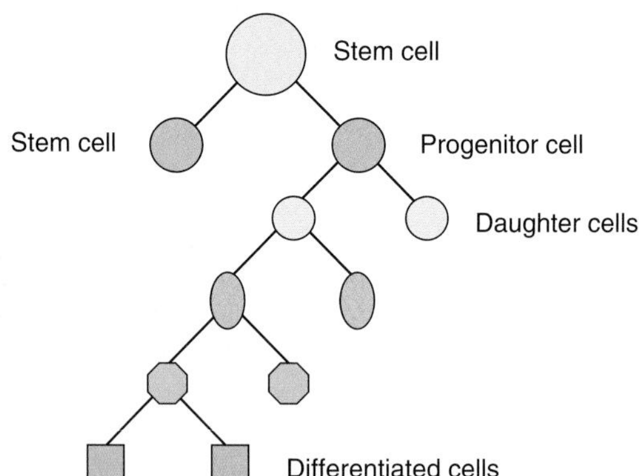

FIGURE 8-3 Mechanism of stem cell–mediated cell replacement. Division of a stem cell with an unlimited potential for proliferation results in one daughter cell, which retains the characteristics of a stem cell, and a second daughter cell, which differentiates into a progenitor or parent cell, with a limited potential for differentiation and proliferation. As the daughter cells of the progenitor cell proliferate, they become more differentiated, until reaching the stage where they are fully differentiated and no longer able to divide.

come progressively more differentiated as they undergo successive mitotic divisions, until they become mature plasma cells that no longer can divide but are capable of releasing large amounts of membrane-bound antibody.

There are several types of stem cells, some of which include the muscle satellite cell, the epidermal stem cell, the spermatogonium, and the basal cell of the olfactory epithelium. These stem cells are unipotent in that they give rise only to one type of differentiated cell. Oligopotent stem cells can produce a small number of cells, and pluripotent stem cells, such as those involved in hematopoiesis, give rise to numerous cell types.[5] Stem cells are the primary cellular component responsible for bone marrow replenishing blood cell progenitors in transplantation (discussed later).

In summary, the term *neoplasm* refers to an abnormal mass of tissue in which the growth exceeds and is uncoordinated with that of the normal tissues. Unlike normal cellular adaptive processes such as hypertrophy and hyperplasia, neoplasms do not obey the laws of normal cell growth. They serve no useful purpose, they do not occur in response to an appropriate stimulus, and they continue to grow at the expense of the host.

The process of cell growth and division is called the *cell cycle.* It is divided into four phases: G_1, the postmitotic phase, during which DNA synthesis ceases while RNA and protein synthesis and cell growth take place; S, the phase during which DNA synthesis occurs, giving rise to two separate sets of chromosomes; G_2, the premitotic phase, during which RNA and protein synthesis continues; and M, the phase of cell mitosis or cell division. The G_0 phase is a resting or quiescent phase in which nondividing cells reside. The entry into and the progression through the various stages of the cell cycle are controlled by cyclins, cyclin-dependent kinases, and cyclin-dependent kinase inhibitors.

Cell proliferation is the process whereby cells divide and bear offspring; it normally is regulated so that the number of cells that are actively dividing is equal to the number dying or being shed. Cell differentiation is the process whereby cells are transformed into different and more specialized cell types as they proliferate. It determines the structure, function, and life span of a cell. There are three types of cells: well-differentiated cells that are no longer able to divide, progenitor or parent cells that continue to divide and bear offspring, and undifferentiated stem cells that can be recruited to become progenitor cells when the need arises. As a cell line becomes more differentiated, it becomes more highly specialized in its function and less able to divide.

Characteristics of Benign and Malignant Neoplasms

After completing this section of the chapter, you should be able to meet the following objectives:

- Cite the method used for naming benign and malignant neoplasms
- State at least five ways in which benign and malignant neoplasms differ
- Relate the properties of cell differentiation to the development of a cancer cell line and the behavior of the tumor
- Trace the pathway for hematologic spread of a metastatic cancer cell
- Use the concepts of growth fraction and doubling time to explain the growth of cancerous tissue

Body organs are composed of two types of tissue: parenchymal tissue and stromal or supporting tissue. The *parenchymal tissue cells* represent the functional components of an organ. The parenchymal cells of a tumor determine its behavior and are the component for which a tumor is named. The *supporting tissue* includes the extracellular matrix and connective tissue that surround the parenchymal cells. It contains the blood vessels that provide nourishment and support for the parenchymal cells.

TERMINOLOGY

By definition, a *tumor* is a swelling that can be caused by a number of conditions, including inflammation and trauma. Although they are not synonymous, the terms *tumor* and *neoplasm* often are used interchangeably. Neoplasms usually are classified as benign or malignant. Neoplasms that contain well-differentiated cells that are clustered together in a single mass are considered to be *benign.* These tumors usually do not cause death unless their location or size interferes with vital functions. In contrast, malignant neoplasms are less well differentiated and have the ability to break loose, enter the circulatory or lymphatic systems, and form secondary malignant tumors at other sites. *Malignant neoplasms* usually cause suffering and death if untreated or uncontrolled.

Tumors usually are named by adding the suffix *-oma* to the parenchymal tissue type from which the growth originated.[7] Thus, a benign tumor of glandular epithelial tissue is called an *adenoma,* and a benign tumor of bone tissue is called an *osteoma.* The term *carcinoma* is used to designate a malignant tumor of epithelial tissue origin. In the case of a malignant tumor of glandular epithelial tissue, the term *adenocarcinoma* is used. Malignant tumors of mesenchymal origin are called *sarcomas* (*e.g.,* osteosarcoma). *Papillomas* are benign microscopic or macroscopic finger-like projections that grow on any surface. A *polyp* is growth that projects from a mucosal surface, such as the intestine. Although the term usually implies a benign neoplasm, some malignant tumors also appear as polyps.[2,7] Adenomatous polyps are considered precursors to adenocarcinomas of the colon. *Cancer in situ* refers to marked neoplasic changes in cells that are found localized to the tissue of origin, that is, a preinvasive neoplasm. *Oncology* is the study of tumors and their treatment. Table 8-1 lists the names of selected benign and malignant tumors according to tissue types.

Benign and malignant neoplasms usually are differentiated by their (1) cell characteristics, (2) rate of growth, (3) manner of growth, (4) capacity to metastasize and spread to other parts of the body, and (5) potential for causing death. The characteristics of benign and malignant neoplasms are summarized in Table 8-2.

TABLE 8-1 Names of Selected Benign and Malignant Tumors According to Tissue Types

Tissue Type	Benign Tumors	Malignant Tumors
Epithelial		
Surface	Papilloma	Squamous cell carcinoma
Glandular	Adenoma	Adenocarcinoma
Connective		
Fibrous	Fibroma	Fibrosarcoma
Adipose	Lipoma	Liposarcoma
Cartilage	Chondroma	Chondrosarcoma
Bone	Osteoma	Osteosarcoma
Blood vessels	Hemangioma	Hemangiosarcoma
Lymph vessels	Lymphangioma	Lymphangiosarcoma
Lymph tissue		Lymphosarcoma
Muscle		
Smooth	Leiomyoma	Leiomyosarcoma
Striated	Rhabdomyoma	Rhabdomyosarcoma
Neural Tissue		
Nerve cell	Neuroma	Neuroblastoma
Glial tissue	Glioma (benign)	Glioblastoma, astrocytoma, medulloblastoma, oligodendroglioma
Nerve sheaths	Neurilemmoma	Neurilemmal sarcoma
Meninges	Meningioma	Meningeal sarcoma
Hematologic		
Granulocytic		Myelocytic leukemia
Erythrocytic		Erythrocytic leukemia
Plasma cells		Multiple myeloma
Lymphocytic		Lymphocytic leukemia or lymphoma
Monocytic		Monocytic leukemia
Endothelial Tissue		
Blood vessels	Hemangioma	Hemangiosarcoma
Lymph vessels	Lymphangioma	Lymphangiosarcoma
Endothelial lining		Ewing's sarcoma

BENIGN NEOPLASMS

Benign tumors are characterized by a slow, progressive rate of growth that may come to a standstill or regress, an expansive manner of growth, and inability to metastasize to distant sites. Benign tumors are composed of well-differentiated cells that resemble the cells of the tissue of origin. For example, the cells of a uterine leiomyoma resemble uterine smooth muscle cells. For unknown reasons, benign tumors seem to have lost the ability to suppress the genetic program for cell replication but retain the program for normal cell differentiation. Benign tumors grow by expansion and are usually enclosed in a fibrous capsule (Fig. 8-4). This is in sharp contrast to malignant neoplasms, which grow by infiltrating the surrounding tissue. The capsule is responsible for a sharp line of demarcation between the benign tumor and the adjacent tissues, a factor that facilitates surgical removal. The formation of the capsule is thought to represent the reaction of the surrounding tissues to the tumor.

BENIGN AND MALIGNANT NEOPLASMS

- A tumor is a new growth or neoplasm.
- Benign neoplasms are well-differentiated tumors that resemble the tissues of origin but have lost the ability to control cell proliferation. They grow by expansion, are enclosed in a fibrous capsule, and do not cause death unless their location is such that it interrupts vital body functions.
- Malignant neoplasms are less well-differentiated tumors that have lost the ability to control both cell proliferation and differentiation. They grow in a crablike manner to invade surrounding tissues, have cells that break loose and travel to distant sites to form metastases, and inevitably cause suffering and death unless their growth can be controlled through treatment.

Benign tumors do not usually undergo degenerative changes as readily as malignant tumors, and they usually do not cause death unless they interfere with vital functions because of their location. For instance, a benign tumor growing in the cranial cavity can eventually cause death by compressing brain structures. Benign tumors also can cause disturbances in the function of adjacent or distant structures by producing pressure on tissues, blood vessels, or nerves. Some benign tumors are also known for

TABLE 8-2 Characteristics of Benign and Malignant Neoplasms

Characteristics	Benign	Malignant
Cell characteristics	Well-differentiated cells that resemble cells in the tissue of origin	Cells are undifferentiated, with anaplasia and atypical structure that often bears little resemblance to cells in the tissue of origin
Rate of growth	Usually progressive and slow; may come to a standstill or regress	Variable and depends on level of differentiation; the more anaplastic the cells, the more rapid the rate of growth
Mode of growth	Grows by expansion without invading the surrounding tissues; usually encapsulated	Grows by invasion, sending out processes that infiltrate the surrounding tissues
Metastasis	Does not spread by metastasis	Gains access to blood and lymph channels to metastasize to other areas of the body

their ability to cause alterations in body function through abnormal elaboration of hormones.

MALIGNANT NEOPLASMS

Malignant neoplasms tend to grow rapidly, spread widely, and have the potential to kill regardless of their original location. Because of their rapid rate of growth, malignant tumors tend to compress blood vessels and outgrow their blood supply, causing ischemia and tissue necrosis; rob normal tissues of essential nutrients; and liberate enzymes and toxins that destroy tumor tissue and normal tissue.

There are two categories of malignant neoplasms—solid tumors and hematologic cancers. Solid tumors initially are confined to a specific tissue or organ. As the growth of a solid tumor progresses, cells are shed from the original tumor mass and travel through the blood and lymph system to produce metastasis in distant sites. Hematologic cancers involve the blood-forming cells that naturally migrate to the blood and lymph systems, thereby making them disseminated diseases from the beginning.

Cancer in situ is a localized preinvasive lesion. Depending on its location, this type of lesion usually can be removed surgically or treated so that the chances of recurrence are small. For example, cancer in situ of the cervix is essentially 100% curable.

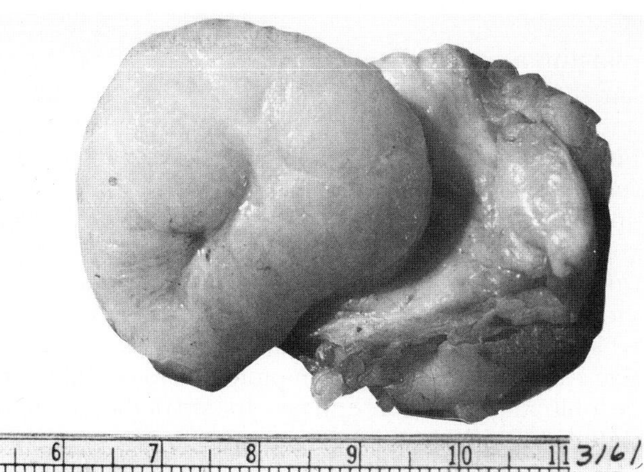

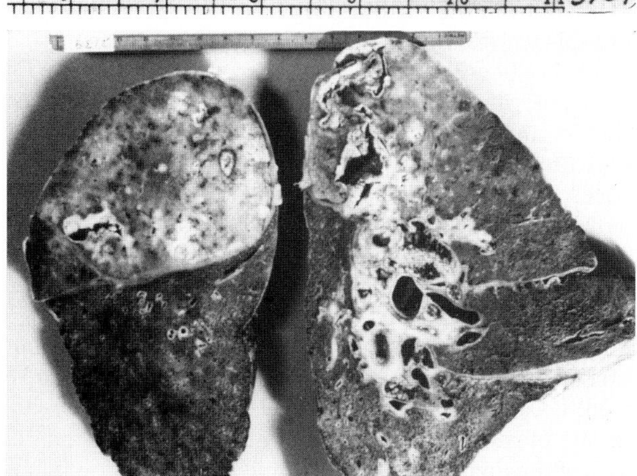

FIGURE 8-4 Photographs of a benign encapsulated fibroadenoma of the breast (**top**) and a bronchogenic carcinoma of the lung (**bottom**). The fibroadenoma has sharply defined edges, but the bronchogenic carcinoma is diffuse and infiltrates the surrounding tissues.

Cancer Cell Characteristics

Cancer cells, unlike normal cells, fail to undergo normal cell proliferation and differentiation. It is thought that cancer cells develop from mutations that occur during the differentiation process. When the mutation occurs early in the process, the resulting tumor is poorly differentiated and highly malignant; when it occurs later in the process, the tumor is more fully differentiated and less malignant (Fig. 8-5).

The term *anaplasia* is used to describe the lack of cell differentiation in cancerous tissue. Undifferentiated cancer cells display marked variations in size and shape. Their nuclei are variable in size and bizarre in shape, the chromatin is coarse and clumped, and the nucleoli are often exceedingly large. In descending the scale of differentiation, enzymes and specialized pathways of metabolism are lost, and cells undergo functional simplification.[2] Highly anaplastic cancer cells, whatever their tissue of origin, begin to resemble each other more than they do their tissue of origin. For example, when examined under the microscope, anaplastic cancerous tissue that originates in the liver does not have the appearance of normal liver tissue. Some cancers display only slight anaplasia, and others display marked anaplasia. The cytologic-histologic grading of tumors is based on the degree of differentiation and the number of proliferating cells.[8] The closer the tumor cells resemble comparable normal cells, both morphologically

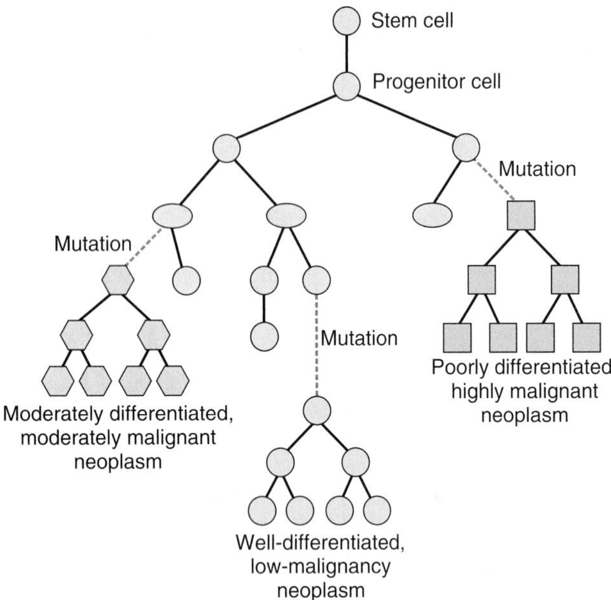

FIGURE 8-5 Mutation of a cell line. Generally, mutations that occur early in the differentiation process result in poorly differentiated neoplasms and those that appear late in the differentiation process result in relatively well-differentiated neoplasms.

and functionally, the lower the grade. Accordingly, grade I neoplasms are well differentiated, and grade IV are poorly differentiated and display marked anaplasia.

Because cancer cells lack differentiation, they do not function properly, nor do they die according to the time frame of normal cells. In some types of leukemia, for example, the lymphocytes do not follow the normal developmental process. They do not differentiate fully, acquire the ability to destroy bacteria, or die on schedule. Instead, these long-lived, defective cells continue to grow, crowding the normal developing blood cells and thereby affecting the development of other cell lineages such as the erythrocytes, platelets, and other white blood cells. This results in reduced numbers of mature, effectively functioning cells, producing immature white blood cells that cannot effectively fight infection, a decreased pool of erythrocytes that cannot effectively transport oxygen to tissues, and a diminished number of platelets that cannot participate in the blood clotting process.

Alterations in cell differentiation also are accompanied by changes in cell characteristics and cell function that distinguish cancer cells from their fully differentiated normal counterparts. These changes include alterations in contact inhibition, loss of cohesiveness and adhesion, impaired cell-to-cell communication, expression of altered tissue antigens, and elaboration of degradative enzymes that enable invasion and metastatic spread.

Contact inhibition is the cessation of growth after a cell comes in contact with another cell. Contact inhibition usually switches off cell growth by blocking the synthesis of DNA, RNA, and protein. In wound healing, contact inhibition causes fibrous tissue growth to cease at the point where the edges of the wound come together. Cancer cells, however, tend to grow rampantly without regard for adjacent tissue. The reduced tendency of cancer cells to stick together (*i.e., cohesiveness* and *adhesiveness*) permits shedding of the tumor's surface cells; these cells appear in the surrounding body fluids or secretions and often can be detected using the cytologic examination. Impaired cell-to-cell communication may interfere with formation of intercellular connections and responsiveness to membrane-derived signals.

Cancer cells also express a number of cell surface molecules or antigens that are immunologically identified as foreign. These *tissue antigens* are coded by the genes of a cell. Many transformed cancer cells revert to earlier stages of gene expression and produce antigens that are immunologically distinct from the antigens that are expressed by cells of the well-differentiated tissue from which the cancer originated. Some cancers express fetal antigens that are not produced by comparable cells in the adult. Tumor antigens may be clinically useful as markers to indicate the presence, recurrence, or progressive growth of a cancer. Response to treatment can be evaluated based on an increase or decrease in tumor antigens.

Cancers may also engage in the abnormal production of substances that affect body function. For example, nonendrocrine tumors may assume hormone synthesis, or cancer cells may produce procoagulant materials that affect blood clotting mechanisms.

Invasion and Metastasis

Cancer spreads by direct invasion and extension, seeding of cancer cells in body cavities, and metastatic spread through the blood or lymph pathways. Unlike benign tumors, which grow by expansion and usually are surrounded by a capsule, malignant tumors grow by extensive infiltration and invasion of the surrounding tissues. The word *cancer* is derived from the Latin word meaning *crablike* because cancerous growth spreads by sending crablike projections into the surrounding tissues. Most cancers synthesize and secrete enzymes that break down proteins and contribute to the infiltration, invasion, and penetration of the surrounding tissues. The lack of a sharp line of demarcation separating them from the surrounding tissue makes the complete surgical removal of malignant tumors more difficult than removal of benign tumors.

The *seeding* of cancer cells into body cavities occurs when a tumor erodes and sheds cells into these spaces. Most often, the peritoneal cavity is involved, but other spaces such as the pleural cavity, pericardial cavity, and joint spaces may be involved. Seeding into the peritoneal cavity is particularly common with ovarian cancers.

The term *metastasis* is used to describe the development of a secondary tumor in a location distant from the primary tumor. Metastatic tumors retain many of the characteristics of the primary tumor from which they were derived. Because of this, it usually is possible to determine the site of the primary tumor from the cellular characteristics of the metastatic tumor. Some tumors tend to metastasize early in their developmental course, whereas others do not metastasize until later. Occasionally, a metastatic tumor will be found far advanced before the primary tumor becomes clinically detectable. Malignant tumors of the kidney, for example, may go completely undetected and be asymptomatic even when a metastatic lesion is found in the lung.

Metastasis occurs by way of the lymph channels (*i.e.*, lymphatic spread) and the blood vessels (*i.e.*, hematogenic spread).[2,8] Lymphatic spread is more typical of carcinomas and hematogenic spread of sarcomas. In many types of cancer, the first evidence of disseminated disease is the presence of tumor cells in the lymph nodes that drain the tumor area. When metastasis occurs by way of the lymphatic channels, the tumor cells lodge first in the regional lymph nodes that received drainage from the tumor site. Once in the lymph node, the cells may die because of the lack of a proper environment, grow into a discernible mass, or remain dormant for unknown reasons. Because the lymphatic channels empty into the venous system, cancer cells that survive may eventually break loose and gain access to the circulatory system. In patients with breast cancer, lymphatic spread and, therefore, extent of disease may be determined by performing a sentinel lymph node biopsy, which is done by injecting a radioactive tracer and blue dye into the tumor to determine the first lymph node in the route of lymph drainage from the cancer. Once the sentinel lymph node is identified, it is examined to determine the presence or absence of cancer cells.

With hematologic spread, the blood-borne cancer cells typically follow the venous flow that drains the site of the neoplasm. Before entering the general circulation, venous blood from the gastrointestinal tract, pancreas, and spleen is routed through the portal vein to the liver. The liver is therefore a common site for metastatic spread of cancers that originate in these organs. Although the site of hematologic spread usually is related to vascular drainage of the primary tumor, some tumors metastasize to distant and unrelated sites. One explanation is that cells of different tumors tend to metastasize to specific target organs that provide substances such as cytokines or growth factors that are needed for their survival.[2] For example, transferrin, a growth-promoting substance isolated from lung tissue, has been found to stimulate the growth of extremely malignant cells that typically metastasize to the lungs. Other organs that are preferential sites for metastasis contain their own specific sets of cytokines.

The selective nature of hematologic spread indicates that metastasis is a finely orchestrated, multistep process, and only a small, select clone of cancer cells has the right combination of gene products to perform all of the steps needed for establishment of a secondary tumor (Fig. 8-6). It has been estimated that fewer than 1 in 10,000 tumor cells that leave a primary tumor survives to start a secondary tumor.[9] To metastasize, a cancer cell must be able to break loose from the primary tumor, invade the surrounding extracellular matrix, gain access to a blood vessel, survive its passage in the bloodstream, emerge from the bloodstream at a favorable location, invade the surrounding tissue, and begin to grow.

Considerable evidence suggests that cancer cells capable of metastasis secrete enzymes that break down the surrounding extracellular matrix, allowing them to move through the degraded matrix and gain access to a blood vessel. Once in the circulation, the tumor cells are vulnerable to destruction by host immune cells. Some tumor cells gain protection from the antitumor host cells by aggregating and adhering to circulating blood components, particularly platelets, to form tumor emboli. Tumor cells that survive their travel in the circulation must be able to halt their passage by adhering to the vessel wall. Tumor cells express various cell surface attachment factors such as laminin receptors that facilitate their anchoring to the capillary basement membrane. After attachment, the tumor cells secrete proteolytic enzymes such as type IV collagenase that degrade the basement membrane and facilitate the migration of the tumor cells through the capillary wall into the interstitial area, where they subsequently establish growth of a secondary tumor.

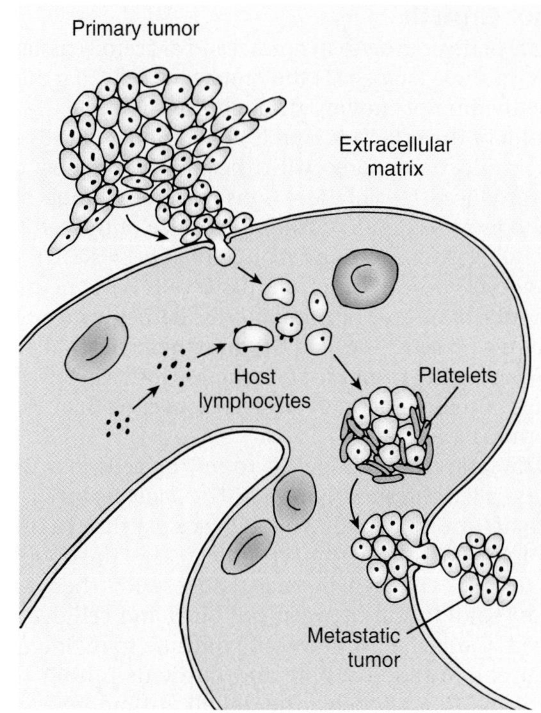

FIGURE 8-6 The pathogenesis of metastasis. (Adapted from Kumar V., Cotran R.S., Robbins S.L. [1992]. *Basic pathology* [7th ed., p. 196]. Philadelphia: W.B. Saunders)

Once in the target tissue, the process of tumor development depends on the establishment of blood vessels and specific growth factors that promote proliferation of the tumor cells. Tumor cells secrete tumor-associated angiogenic factors, which enables the development of new blood vessels in the tumor, a process termed *angiogenesis*.[8] The presence of stimulatory or inhibitory growth factors correlates with the site-specific pattern of metastasis. For example, a potent growth-stimulating factor has been isolated from lung tissue, and stromal cells in bone have been shown to produce a factor that stimulates growth of prostatic cancer cells.[8]

Tumor Growth

The rate of tissue growth in normal and cancerous tissue depends on three factors: (1) the number of cells that are actively dividing or moving through the cell cycle, (2) the duration of the cell cycle, and (3) the number of cells that are being lost compared with the number of new cells being produced. One of the reasons cancerous tumors often seem to grow so rapidly relates to the size of the cell pool that is actively engaged in cycling. It has been shown that the cell cycle time of cancerous tissue cells is not necessarily shorter than that of normal cells. Rather, cancer cells do not die on schedule, and the growth factors that allow cells to enter the G_0 phase are lacking. Thus, a greater percentage of cells are actively engaged in cycling than occurs in normal tissue.

The ratio of dividing cells to resting cells in a tissue mass is called the *growth fraction*. The *doubling time* is the length of time it takes for the total mass of cells in a tumor to double. As the growth fraction increases, the doubling time decreases. When normal tissues reach their adult size, an equilibrium between cell birth and cell death is reached. Cancer cells, however, continue to divide until limitations in blood supply and nutrients inhibit their growth. As this happens, the doubling time for cancer cells decreases. If tumor growth is plotted against time on a semilogarithmic scale, the initial growth rate is exponential and then tends to decrease or flatten out over time. This characterization of tumor growth is called the *Gompertzian model*.[10]

A tumor usually is undetectable until it has doubled 30 times and contains more than 1 billion (10^9) cells. At this point, it is approximately 1 cm in size (Fig. 8-7). After 35 doublings, the mass contains more than 1 trillion (10^{12}) cells, which is a sufficient number to kill the host.

In summary, neoplasms may be either benign or malignant. Benign and malignant tumors differ in terms of cell characteristics, manner of growth, rate of growth, potential for metastasis, ability to produce generalized effects, tendency to cause tissue destruction, and capacity to cause death. The growth of a benign tumor is restricted to the site of origin, and the tumor usually does not cause death unless it interferes with vital functions. Malignant neoplasms grow wildly and without organization, spread to distant parts of the body, and cause death unless their growth is inhibited or stopped by treatment. There are two types of cancer: solid tumors and hematologic tumors. Solid tumors initially are confined to a specific organ or tissue, whereas hematologic cancers are disseminated from the onset.

Cancer is a disorder of cell proliferation and differentiation. Cancer cells often are poorly differentiated compared with normal cells. They have abnormal karyotypes, display abnormal cell membrane antigens and characteristics, and produce abnormal biochemical products. All cancers result from nonlethal genetic changes that transform a normal cell into a cancer cell. The spread of cancer occurs through three pathways: direct invasion and extension, seeding of cancer cells in body cavities, and metastatic spread through vascular or lymphatic pathways. Only a proportionately small clone of cancer cells is capable of metastasis. To metastasize, a cancer cell must be able to break loose from the primary tumor, invade the surrounding extracellular matrix, gain access to a blood vessel, survive its passage in the bloodstream, emerge from the bloodstream at a favorable location, invade the surrounding tissue, and begin to grow. The rate of growth of cancerous tissue depends on the ratio of dividing to resting cells (growth fraction) and the time it takes for the total cells in the tumor to double (doubling time). A tumor is usually undetectable until it has doubled 30 times and contains more than a billion cells.

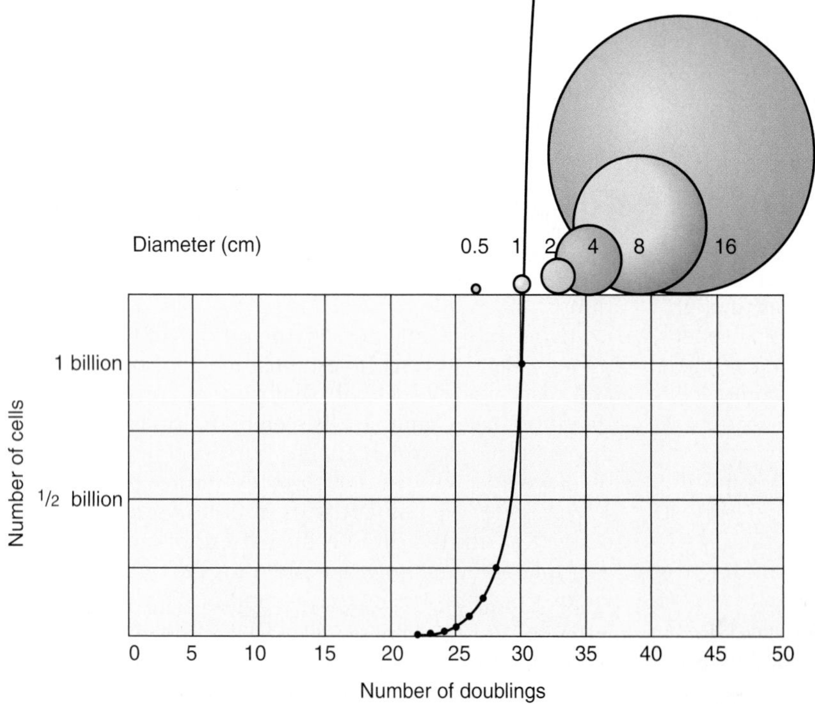

FIGURE 8-7 Growth curve of a hypothetical tumor on arithmetic coordinates. Notice the number of doubling times before the tumor reaches an appreciable size. (Adapted from Collins V.P., et al. [1956]. Observations of growth rates of human tumors. *Am J Roent Rad Ther Nuclear Med 76,* 988.)

Etiology of Cancer

After completing this section of the chapter, you should be able to meet the following objectives:

- Describe the role of proto-oncogenes, tumor suppressor genes, apoptosis genes, and genes that control signal pathways in the development of a cancer cell line
- State the importance of angiogenesis in cancer growth and metastasis
- Explain how host factors such as heredity, levels of endogenous hormones, and immune system function increase the risk for development of selected cancers
- Relate the effects of environmental factors such as chemical carcinogens, radiation, and oncogenic viruses to the risk for cancer development
- Briefly describe the steps in the transformation of normal cells to cancer cells by carcinogens

The cause of cancer can be viewed from two perspectives: a molecular origin within cells and an external origin in which factors such as age, heredity, and environmental agents influence its inception and growth. Together, both mechanisms contribute to a multidimensional web of causation by which cancers develop and progress over time.

MOLECULAR BASIS OF CANCER

The molecular pathogenesis of cancer is thought to have origin in genetic damage or mutation (oncogenesis) and the resultant changes in cell physiology that transform a normally functioning cell into a cancer cell.

Oncogenesis

The term *oncogenesis* refers to the genetic mechanism whereby normal cells are transformed into cancer cells. Three kinds of genes control cell growth and replication: *proto-oncogenes, tumor suppressor genes,* and genes that control programmed cell death or *apoptosis.*[2] In addition to these three classes of genes, a fourth category of genes, those that regulate repair of damaged DNA, is also implicated in the process of oncogenesis (Fig. 8-8). The DNA repair genes affect cell proliferation and survival indirectly through their ability to repair nonlethal damage in other genes including proto-oncogenes, tumor suppressor genes, and the genes that control apoptosis.[2] These genes have been implicated as the principal targets of genetic damage occurring during the development of a cancer cells.[11] Such genetic damage may be caused by the action of chemicals, radiation, or viruses, or it may be inherited in the germ line. Significantly, it appears that the acquisition of a single gene mutation is not sufficient to transform normal cells into cancer cells. Instead, cancerous transformation appears to require the activation of many independently mutated genes.

Genes that promote autonomous cell growth in cancer cells are called oncogenes. They are derived from mutations in proto-oncogenes and are characterized by the ability to promote cell growth in the absence of normal growth-promoting signals. A key feature of oncogene activity is that a single altered copy of a gene regulating any of the steps in this process leads to unregulated cell growth. Selected oncogenes have been associated with numerous cancer types. For example, the human epidermal growth factor receptor-2 (*HER-2/neu*) gene is amplified in up to 30% of breast cancers and indicates a tumor that is aggressive with a poor prognosis.[12] One of the newer cancer drugs is trastuzumab (Herceptin), a monoclonal antibody

ONCOGENESIS

- Normal cell growth is controlled by growth-promoting proto-oncogenes and growth-suppressing anti-oncogenes. Normally, cell growth is genetically controlled so that potentially malignant cells are targeted for elimination by tumor-suppressing genes.
- Oncogenesis is a genetic process whereby normal cells are transformed into cancer cells. It involves mutations in the normal growth-regulating genes.
- The transformation of normal cells into cancer cells is multifactorial, involving the inheritance of cancer susceptibility genes and environmental factors such as chemicals, radiation, and viruses.

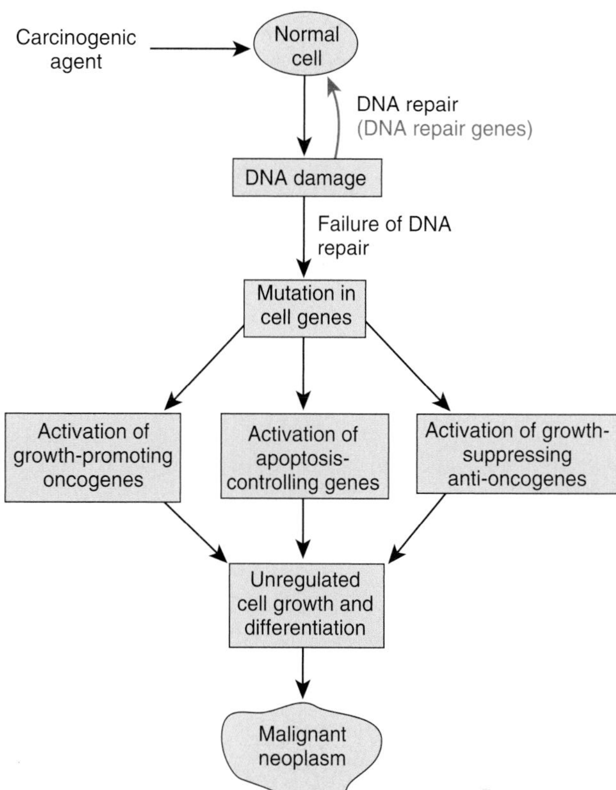

FIGURE 8-8 Flowchart depicting the stages in the development of a malignant neoplasm resulting from exposure to an oncogenic agent that produces DNA damage. When DNA repair genes are present (*red arrow*) the DNA is repaired and gene mutation does not occur.

that selectively binds to the HER-2, inhibiting the proliferation of tumor cells that overexpress the HER-2.

Tumor suppressor genes, or antioncogenes, inhibit the proliferation of cells in a tumor. When this type of gene is inactivated, a genetic signal that normally inhibits proliferation is removed, thereby causing unregulated growth to begin. Numerous tumor suppressor genes have been identified and linked to inherited and sporadic cancers.[2] Of particular interest in this group is the *TP53* gene. Located on the short arm of chromosome 17, it codes for the p53 protein, which functions as a suppressor of tumor growth. Mutations in the *TP53* gene have been implicated in the development of lung, breast, and colon cancer—the three leading causes of cancer death.[2] The *TP53* gene also appears to initiate apoptosis in radiation and chemotherapy damaged tumor cells. Thus, tumors that retain normal *TP53* function are more likely to respond to such therapy than tumors that carry a defective *TP53* gene.[2]

A relatively common pathway by which cancer cells gain autonomous growth is by mutations in genes that control signaling pathways. These signaling pathways couple growth factors receptors to their nuclear targets. Under normal conditions, cell proliferation involves the binding of a growth factor to its receptor on the cell membrane, activation of the growth factor receptor on the inner surface of the cell membrane, the transfer of the signal across the cytosol to the nucleus through signal-transducing proteins that function as second messengers, induction and activation of regulatory factors that initiate DNA transcription, and the entry of the cell into the cell cycle (Fig. 8-9). Many of the proteins involved in the signaling pathways that control the action of growth factors exert their effects through enzymes called *kinases* that phosphorylate proteins. In some types of cancer, such as chronic myeloid leukemia, mutation in a proto-oncogene controlling tyrosine kinase activity occurs, causing unregulated cell growth and proliferation.

Even with all the genetic abnormalities described earlier, tumors cannot enlarge unless angiogenesis occurs and supplies them with the blood vessels necessary for survival. Angiogenesis is required not only for continued tumor growth but also for metastasis. The molecular basis for the angiogenic switch is unknown, but it appears to involve increased production of angiogenic factors or loss of angiogenic inhibitors. The normal *TP53* gene appears to inhibit angiogenesis by inducing the synthesis of an antiangiogenic molecule called *thrombospondin-1*.[2] With mutational inactivation of both *TP53* alleles (as occurs in many cancers), the levels of thrombospondin-1 drop precipitously, tilting the balance in favor of angiogenic factors. Angiogenesis is also influenced by hypoxia and release of proteases that are involved in regulating the balance between angiogenic and antiangiogenic factors. Because of the crucial role of angiogenic factors in tumor growth, much interest is focused on the development of antiangiogenesis therapy.

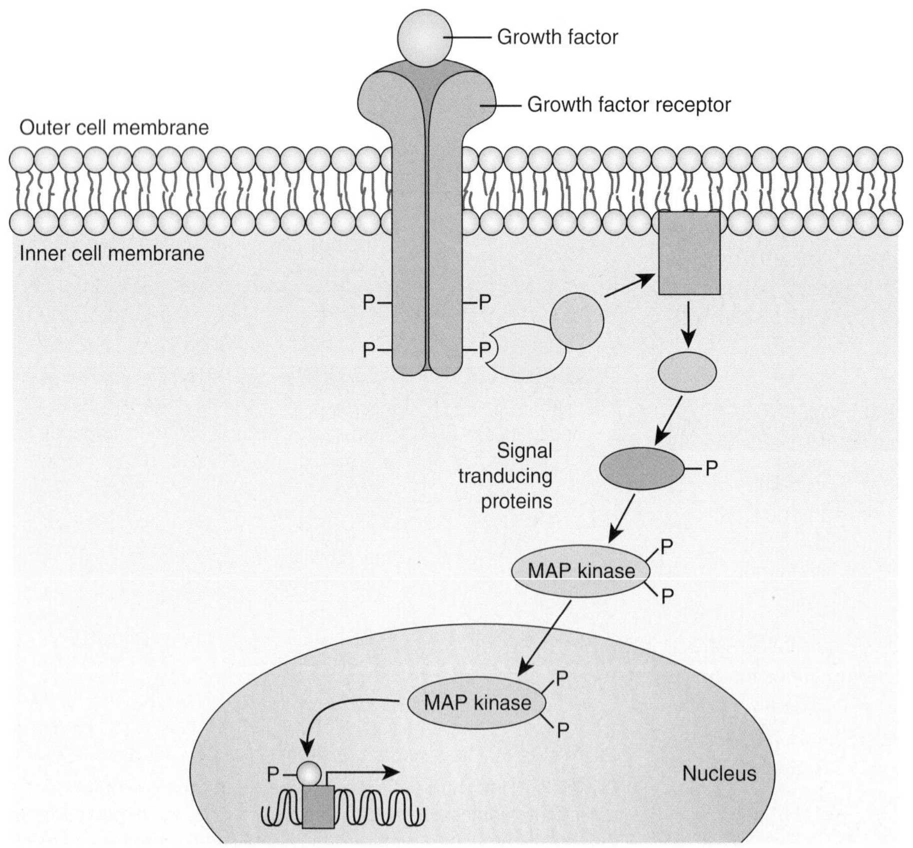

FIGURE 8-9 Pathway for genes regulating cell growth and replication. Stimulation of a normal cell by a growth factor results in activation of the growth factor receptor and signaling proteins that transmit the growth-promoting signal to the nucleus, where it modulates gene transcription and progression through the cell cycle. Many of these signaling proteins exert their effects through enzymes called *kinases* that phosphorylate proteins.

Cancer Cell Transformation

The transformation of normal cells into cancer cells by carcinogenic agents is a multistep process that can be divided into three stages: initiation, promotion, and progression (Fig. 8-10). *Initiation* involves the exposure of cells to appropriate doses of a carcinogenic agent that makes them susceptible to malignant transformation. The carcinogenic agents can be chemical, physical, or biologic, and they produce irreversible changes in the genome of a previously normal cell. Because the effects of initiating agents are irreversible, multiple divided doses may achieve the same effects as single exposures of the same comparable dose or small amounts of highly carcinogenic substances. The most susceptible cells for mutagenic alterations in the genome are the cells that are actively synthesizing DNA.[13]

Promotion involves the induction of unregulated accelerated growth in already initiated cells by various chemicals and growth factors. Promotion is reversible if the promoter substance is removed. Cells that have been irreversibly initiated may be promoted even after long latency periods. The latency period varies with the type of agent, the dosage, and the characteristics of the target cells. Many chemical carcinogens are called *complete carcinogens* because they can initiate and promote neoplastic transformation. *Progression* is the process whereby tumor cells acquire malignant phenotypic changes that promote invasiveness, metastatic competence, autonomous growth tendencies, and increased karyotypic instability.[14]

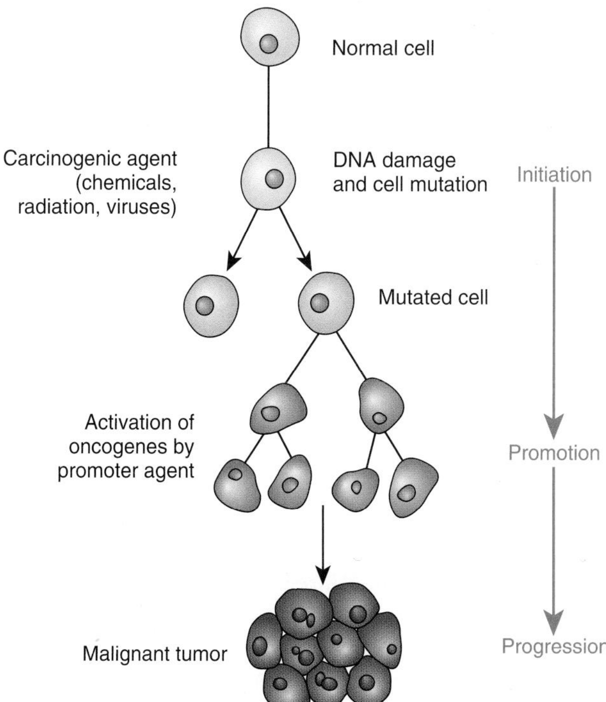

FIGURE 8-10 The process of initiation, promotion, and progression in the clonal evolution of malignant tumors. Initiation involves the exposure of cells to appropriate doses of a carcinogenic agent; promotion, the unregulated and accelerated growth of the mutated cells; and progression, the acquisition of malignant characteristics by the tumor cells.

HOST AND ENVIRONMENTAL FACTORS

Because cancer is not a single disease, it is reasonable to assume that it does not have a single cause. More likely, cancer occurs because of interactions among multiple risk factors or repeated exposure to a single carcinogenic (cancer-producing) agent. Among the risk factors that have been linked to cancer are heredity, hormonal factors, immunologic mechanisms, and environmental agents such as chemicals, radiation, and cancer-causing viruses.

Heredity

A hereditary predisposition to approximately 50 types of cancer has been observed in families. Breast cancer, for example, occurs more frequently in women whose grandmothers, mothers, aunts, and sisters also have experienced a breast malignancy. The genetic predisposition for development of cancer has been documented for a number of cancerous and precancerous lesions that follow mendelian inheritance patterns. Cancer is found in approximately 10% of persons having one affected first-degree relative, in approximately 15% of persons having two affected family members, and in 30% of persons having three affected family members. The risk increases to approximately 50% in women 65 years of age who have multiple family members with breast cancer. Two oncogenes, called *BRCA-1* (breast carcinoma 1) and *BRCA-2* (breast carcinoma 2), have been implicated in a genetic susceptibility to breast cancer.[2] Individuals carrying a *BRCA* mutation have a lifetime risk (if they live to the age of 85 years) of 80% for developing breast cancer. The lifetime risk for developing ovarian cancer is 10% to 20% for *BRCA-2* mutations and 40% to 60% for *BRCA-1* mutations. These oncogenes have also been associated with an increased risk for prostate, pancreatic, colon, and other cancers.[15]

Several cancers exhibit an autosomal dominant inheritance pattern. In approximately 40% of cases, retinoblastoma is inherited as an autosomal dominant trait; the remaining cases are nonhereditary. The penetrance of the genetic trait is high; in carriers of the dominant retinoblastoma gene, the penetrance for this gene is 95% for at least one tumor, and the affected person may be unilaterally or bilaterally affected.[16] Familial adenomatous polyposis of the colon also follows an autosomal dominant inheritance pattern. In people who inherit this gene, hundreds of adenomatous polyps may develop, some of which inevitably become malignant.[2]

Hormones

Hormones have received considerable research attention with respect to cancer of the breast, ovary, and endometrium in women and of the prostate and testis in men. Although the link between hormones and the development of cancer is unclear, it has been suggested that it may reside with the ability of hormones to drive the cell division of a malignant phenotype. Neoplasms of tissues that are responsive to hormones are responsible for 35% of all newly diagnosed tumors in men and 40% of all newly diagnosed tumors in women in the United States.[17] Because of the evidence that endogenous hormones affect the risk for these cancers, concern exists regarding the effects on cancer risk if the same or closely related hormones are administered for therapeutic purposes.

Immunologic Mechanisms

There is growing evidence for the immune system's participation in resistance against the progression and spread of cancer. The central concept, known as the immune surveillance hypothesis, which was first proposed by Paul Ehrlich in 1909, postulates that the immune system plays a central role in resistance against the development of tumors.[18] In addition to cancer–host interactions as a mechanism of cancer development, immunologic mechanisms provide a means for the detection, classification, and prognostic evaluation of cancers and as a potential method of treatment. *Immunotherapy* (discussed later in this chapter) is a cancer treatment modality designed to heighten the patient's general immune responses so as to increase tumor cell destruction.

It has been suggested that the development of cancer might be associated with impairment or decline in the surveillance capacity of the immune system. For example, increases in cancer incidence have been observed in people with immunodeficiency diseases and in those with organ transplants who are receiving immunosuppressant drugs. The incidence of cancer also is increased in the elderly, in whom there is a known decrease in immune activity. The association of Kaposi's sarcoma with acquired immunodeficiency syndrome (AIDS) further emphasizes the role of the immune system in preventing malignant cell proliferation.

It has been shown that most tumor cells have molecular configurations that can be specifically recognized by immune T cells or by antibodies and hence are termed *tumor antigens*. The most relevant tumor antigens fall into two categories: unique tumor-specific antigens found only on tumor cells, and tumor-associated antigens found on tumor cells and on normal cells. Quantitative and qualitative differences permit the use of these tumor-associated antigens to distinguish cancer cells from normal cells.[19]

Virtually all of the components of the immune system have the potential for eradicating cancer cells, including T lymphocytes, B lymphocytes and antibodies, macrophages, and natural killer (NK) cells (see Chapter 19). The T-cell response is undoubtedly one of the most important host responses for controlling the growth of antigenic tumor cells; it is responsible for direct killing of tumor cells and for activation of other components of the immune system. The T-cell immunity to cancer cells reflects the function of two subsets of T cells: the $CD4^+$ helper T cells and $CD8^+$ cytotoxic T cells. The finding of tumor-reactive antibodies in the serum of people with cancer supports the role of the B cell as a member of the immune surveillance team. Antibodies can destroy cancer cells through complement-mediated mechanisms or through antibody-dependent cellular cytotoxicity, in which the antibody binds the cancer cell to another effector cell, such as the NK cell, that does the actual killing of the cancer cell. NK cells do not require antigen recognition and can lyse a wide variety of target cells. The cytotoxic activity of NK cells can be augmented by the cytokines, interleukin-2 (IL-2), and interferon, and its activity can be amplified by immune T-cell responses.[20] Macrophages are important in tumor immunity as antigen-presenting cells to initiate the immune response and as potential effector cells to participate in tumor cell lysis.

Chemical Carcinogens

A carcinogen is an agent capable of causing cancer. The role of environmental agents in causation of cancer was first noted in 1775 by Sir Percivall Pott, who related the high incidence of scrotal cancer in chimneysweeps to their exposure to coal soot.[7] In 1915, a group of Japanese investigators conducted the first experiments in which a chemical agent was used to produce cancer.[7] These investigators found that a cancerous growth developed when they painted a rabbit's ear with coal tar. Coal tar has since been found to contain potent polycyclic aromatic hydrocarbons. Since then, many carcinogenic agents have been identified (Chart 8-1).

More than 6 million chemicals have been identified. It is estimated that less than 1000 of these have been extensively examined for their carcinogenic potential.[21] Some have been found to cause cancers in animals, and others are known to cause cancers in humans. These agents include both natural (*e.g.*, aflatoxin B_1) and artificial products (*e.g.*, vinyl chloride).

CHART 8-1

Chemical and Environmental Agents Known to be Carcinogenic in Humans

Polycyclic Hydrocarbons

Soots, tars, and oils
Cigarette smoke

Industrial Agents

Aniline and azo dyes
Arsenic compounds
Asbestos
β-Naphthylamine
Benzene
Benzo[*a*]pyrene
Carbon tetrachloride
Insecticides, fungicides
Nickel and chromium compounds
Polychlorinated biphenyls
Vinyl chloride

Food and Drugs

Smoked foods
Nitrosamines
Aflatoxin B_1
Diethylstilbestrol
Anticancer drugs (*e.g.*, alkylating agents, cyclophosphamide, chlorambucil, nitrosourea)

Chemical carcinogens can be divided into two groups: direct-reacting agents, which do not require activation in the body to become carcinogenic; and indirect-reacting agents, called *procarcinogens or initiators,* which become active only after metabolic conversion. Direct- and indirect-acting initiators form highly reactive species (*i.e.,* electrophiles and free radicals) that bind with the nucleophilic residues on DNA, RNA, or cellular proteins. The action of these reactive species tends to cause cell mutation or alteration in synthesis of cell enzymes and structural proteins in a manner that alters cell replication and interferes with cell regulatory controls. The carcinogenicity of some chemicals is augmented by agents called *promoters* that, by themselves, have little or no cancer-causing ability. It is believed that promoters exert their effect by changing the expression of genetic material in a cell, increasing DNA synthesis, enhancing gene amplification (*i.e.,* number of gene copies that are made), and altering intercellular communication.

The exposure to many chemical carcinogens is associated with lifestyle risk factors, such as smoking, dietary factors, and alcohol consumption. Cigarette smoke contains both procarcinogens and promoters. It is directly associated with lung and laryngeal cancer and has been linked with cancers of the mouth, nasal cavities, pharynx, esophagus, pancreas, liver, kidney, uterus, cervix, and bladder and myeloid leukemias.[22] Chewing tobacco or tobacco products increases the risk for cancers of the oral cavity and esophagus. It has been estimated that 30% of all cancer deaths and 87% of lung cancer deaths in the United States are related to tobacco.[22] Not only is the smoker at risk, but others passively exposed to cigarette smoke are also at risk. Environmental tobacco smoke has been classified as a group A carcinogen based on the U.S. Environmental Protection Agency's system of carcinogen classification. Each year, about 3000 nonsmoking adults die of lung cancer as a result of environmental tobacco smoke.[22]

There is strong evidence that certain elements in the diet contain chemicals that contribute to cancer risk. Most known dietary carcinogens either occur naturally in plants or are produced during food preparation.[23] Afloxin is a naturally occurring agent produced by a mold that grows in improperly stored grains or nuts. Benzo[*a*]pyrene and other polycyclic hydrocarbons are converted to carcinogens when foods are fried in fat that has been reused multiple times. Among the most potent of the procarcinogens are the polycyclic aromatic hydrocarbons. The polycyclic aromatic hydrocarbons are of particular interest because they are produced from animal fat in the process of charcoal-broiling meats and are present in smoked meats and fish. They also are produced in the combustion of tobacco and are present in cigarette smoke. Nitrosamines, which are powerful carcinogens, are formed in foods that are smoked, salted, cured, or pickled using nitrites or nitrates as preservatives.[23] Formation of these nitrosamines may be inhibited by the presence of antioxidants such as vitamin C found in fruits and vegetables. Cancer of the colon has been associated with high dietary intake of fat and red meat and a low intake of dietary fiber. A high-fat diet is thought to be carcinogenic because it increases the flow of primary bile acids that are converted to secondary bile acids in the presence of anaerobic bacteria in the colon, producing carcinogens or promoters. Recent studies have identified obesity and lowered physical activity, in addition to a high-fat diet, with an increased risk for colon cancer.[23]

Alcohol modifies the metabolism of carcinogens in the liver and esophagus.[7] It is believed to influence the transport of carcinogens, increasing the contact between an externally induced carcinogen and the stem cells that line the upper oral cavity, larynx, and esophagus. The carcinogenic effect of cigarette smoke can be enhanced by concomitant consumption of alcohol; persons who smoke and drink considerable amounts of alcohol are at increased risk for development of cancer of the oral cavity, larynx, and esophagus.

The effects of carcinogenic agents usually are dose dependent—the larger the dose or the longer the duration of exposure, the greater the risk that cancer will develop. Some chemical carcinogens may act in concert with other carcinogenic influences, such as viruses or radiation, to induce neoplasia. There usually is a time delay ranging from 5 to 30 years from the time of chemical carcinogen exposure to the development of overt cancer. This is unfortunate because many people may have been exposed to the agent and its carcinogenic effects before the association is recognized. This occurred, for example, with the use of diethylstilbestrol, which was widely used in the United States from the mid-1940s to 1970 to prevent miscarriages. It was not until the late 1960s, however, that many cases of vaginal adenosis and adenocarcinoma in young women were found to be the result of their exposure in utero to diethylstilbestrol.[24]

Radiation

The effects of *ionizing radiation* in carcinogenesis have been well documented in atomic bomb survivors, in patients diagnostically exposed, and in industrial workers, scientists, and physicians who were exposed during employment. Malignant epitheliomas of the skin and leukemia were significantly elevated in these populations. Between 1950 and 1970, the death rate from leukemia alone in the most heavily exposed population groups of the atomic bomb survivors in Hiroshima and Nagasaki was 147 per 100,000 persons, 30 times the expected rate.[25]

The type of cancer that developed depended on the dose of radiation, the sex of the person, and the age at which exposure occurred. For instance, approximately 25 to 30 years after total-body or trunk irradiation, there were increased incidences of leukemia and cancers of the breast, lung, stomach, thyroid, salivary gland, gastrointestinal system, and lymphoid tissues. The length of time between exposure and the onset of cancer is related to the age of the individual. For example, children exposed to ionizing radiation in utero have an increased risk for developing leukemias and childhood tumors, particularly 2 to 3 years after birth. This latency period for leukemia extends to 5 to 10 years if the child was exposed after birth and to 20 years for certain solid tumors.[26] As another example, the latency period for the development of thyroid cancer in infants and small children who received radiation to the head and neck to decrease the size of the tonsils or thymus was as long as 35 years after exposure.

The association between sunlight and the development of skin cancer (see Chapter 61) has been reported for more than 100 years. *Ultraviolet radiation* emits relatively low-energy rays that do not deeply penetrate the skin. The evidence supporting the role of ultraviolet radiation in the cause of skin cancer includes skin cancer that develops primarily on the areas of skin more frequently exposed to sunlight (*e.g.*, the head and neck, arms, hands, and legs), a higher incidence in light-complexioned individuals who lack the ultraviolet-filtering skin pigment melanin, and the fact that the intensity of ultraviolet exposure is directly related to the incidence of skin cancer, as evidenced by higher rates occurring in Australia and the American Southwest.[26] There also are studies suggesting that intense, episodic exposure to sunlight, particularly during childhood, is more important in the development of melanoma than prolonged low-intensity exposure. As with other carcinogens, the effects of ultraviolet radiation usually are additive, and there usually is a long delay between the time of exposure and the time that cancer can be detected.

Oncogenic Viruses

An oncogenic virus is one that can induce cancer. It has been suspected for some time that viruses play an important role in the development of certain forms of cancer, particularly leukemia and lymphoma. Ellermann in 1908 and Rous in 1911 were the first to describe the transmissibility of avian leukemia and sarcoma, respectively.[27] Interest in the field of viral oncology, particularly in human populations, has burgeoned with the discovery of reverse transcriptase, the development of recombinant DNA technology, and more recently with the discovery of oncogenes and tumor suppressor genes.

Viruses, which are small particles containing genetic (DNA or RNA) material, enter a host cell and become incorporated into its chromosomal DNA or take control of the cell's machinery for the purpose of producing viral proteins. A large number of DNA and RNA viruses (*i.e.*, retroviruses) have been shown to be oncogenic in animals. However, only a few viruses have been linked to cancer in humans.

Four DNA viruses have been implicated in human cancers: the human papillomavirus (HPV), Epstein-Barr virus (EBV), hepatitis B virus (HBV), and human herpesvirus-8 (HHV-8).[2] HHV-8, which causes Kaposi's sarcoma in persons with AIDS, is discussed in Chapter 22. There are more than 60 genetically different types of HPV. Some types (*i.e.*, types 1, 2, 4, 7) have been shown to cause benign squamous papillomas (*i.e.*, warts). HPVs also have been implicated in squamous cell carcinoma of the cervix and anogenital region. HPV types 16 and 18 are found in approximately 75% to 100% of squamous cell carcinomas of the cervix and presumed precursors (*i.e.*, severe cervical dysplasia and carcinoma in situ).[2]

EBV is a member of the herpesvirus family. It has been implicated in the pathogenesis of four human cancers: Burkitt's lymphoma, nasopharyngeal cancer, B-cell lymphomas in immunosuppressed individuals such as those with AIDS, and some cases of Hodgkin's lymphoma. Burkitt's lymphoma, a tumor of B lymphocytes, is endemic in parts of East Africa and occurs sporadically in other areas worldwide. In persons with normal immune function, the EBV-driven B-cell proliferation is readily controlled, and the person becomes asymptomatic or experiences a self-limited episode of infectious mononucleosis (see Chapter 17). In regions of the world where Burkitt's lymphoma is endemic, concurrent malaria or other infections cause impaired immune function, allowing sustained B-lymphocyte proliferation. The incidence of nasopharyngeal cancer is high in some areas of China, particularly southern China, and in the Cantonese population in Singapore. An increased risk for B-cell lymphomas is seen in individuals with drug-suppressed immune systems, for examples, individuals with transplanted organs.

HBV is the etiologic agent in the development of hepatitis B, cirrhosis, and hepatocellular carcinoma. There is a significant correlation between elevated rates of hepatocellular carcinoma worldwide and the prevalence of HBV carriers. The precise mechanism by which HBV induces hepatocellular cancer has not been determined, although it has been suggested that it may be the result of prolonged HBV-induced liver damage and regeneration. Other etiologic factors also may contribute to the development of liver cancer, including ingestion of aflatoxin and infection with the hepatitis C virus (HCV).

Although there are a number of retroviruses (RNA viruses) that cause cancer in animals, human T-cell leukemia virus-1 (HTLV-1) is the only known retrovirus to cause cancer in humans. HTLV-1 is associated with a form of T-cell leukemia that is endemic in certain parts of Japan and some areas of the Caribbean and Africa, and is found sporadically elsewhere, including the United States and Europe.[2] Similar to the AIDS virus, HTLV-1 is attracted to the $CD4^+$ T cells, and this subset of T cells is therefore the major target for cancerous transformation. The virus requires transmission of infected T cells by way of sexual intercourse, infected blood, or breast milk.

In summary, the cause of cancer can be viewed from two perspectives: a molecular origin within cells and an external origin in which factors such as age, heredity, and environmental agents influence its inception and growth. The molecular pathogenesis of cancer is thought to have its origin in genetic damage or mutation (oncogenesis) and changes in cell physiology that transform a normally functioning cell into a cancer cell. There are four kinds of genes that control cell growth and replication: growth-promoting regulatory genes (proto-oncogenes), growth-inhibiting regulatory genes (tumor suppressor genes), genes that control programmed cell death (apoptosis genes), and genes that regulate the repair of damaged DNA.

Because cancer is not a single disease, it is likely that multiple factors interact at the genetic level to transform normal cells into cancer cells. Such genetic damage may be interactions between multiple risk factors or repeated exposure to a single carcinogenic (cancer-producing) agent. Among the risk factors that have been linked to cancer are heredity, hormonal factors, immunologic mechanisms, and environmental agents such as chemicals, radiation, and cancer-causing viruses.

Clinical Manifestations

After completing this section of the chapter, you should be able to meet the following objectives:

- Describe the many possible ways by which cancer acts to disrupt organ function
- Characterize the mechanisms involved in the fatigue, tissue wasting, loss of appetite, and pain experienced by cancer patients
- Define the term *paraneoplastic syndrome* and explain its pathogenesis and manifestations

There probably is no single body function left unaffected by the presence of cancer. Because tumor cells replace normally functioning parenchymal tissue, the initial manifestations of cancer usually reflect the primary site of involvement. For example, cancer of the lung initially produces impairment of respiratory function; as the tumor grows and metastasizes, other body structures become affected. Cancer also produces generalized manifestations such as fatigue, anorexia and involuntary weight loss, anemia, and other symptoms unrelated to the tumor site. Many of these manifestations are compounded by the side effects of methods used to treat the disease.

TISSUE INTEGRITY

Cancer disrupts tissue integrity. As cancers grow, they compress and erode blood vessels, causing ulceration and necrosis along with frank bleeding and sometimes hemorrhage. One of the early warning signals of colorectal cancer is blood in the stool. Cancer cells also may produce enzymes and metabolic toxins that are destructive to the surrounding tissues. Usually, tissue damaged by cancerous growth does not heal normally. Instead, the damaged area persists and often continues to grow; a sore that does not heal is another warning signal of cancer. Cancer has no regard for normal anatomic boundaries; as it grows, it invades and compresses adjacent structures. Abdominal cancer, for example, may compress the viscera and cause bowel obstruction. Cancer may also obstruct lymph flow and penetrate serous cavities, causing pleural effusion or ascites.

In its late stages, cancer often causes pain (see Chapter 50). Pain is probably one of the most dreaded aspects of cancer, and pain management is one of the major treatment concerns for persons with incurable cancers.

CANCER CACHEXIA

Many cancers are associated with weight loss and wasting of body fat and muscle tissue, accompanied by profound weakness, anorexia, and anemia. This wasting syndrome is often referred to as the *cancer anorexia-cachexia syndrome.*[2,28,29] It is a common manifestation of most solid tumors with the exception of breast cancer. It has been estimated that 80% of persons with upper gastrointestinal cancer and 60% of persons with lung cancer have already experienced substantial weight loss at the time of diagnosis.[28] It is more common in children and elderly persons and becomes more pronounced as the disease progresses. The condition contributes to disease outcome and survival time. Persons with cancer cachexia also respond less well to chemotherapy and experience increased toxicity.

The cause of cancer anorexia-cachexia syndrome is probably multifactorial, resulting from tumor- or host-derived factors that cause anorexia directly by acting on satiety centers in the hypothalamus or indirectly by injuring tissues that subsequently release anorexigenic substances. Although anorexia, reduced food intake, and abnormalities of taste are common in people with cancer and often are accentuated by treatment methods, the extent of weight loss and protein wasting cannot be explained in terms of diminished food intake alone. There also is a disparity between the size of the tumor and the severity of cachexia, which supports the existence of other mediators in the development of cachexia.

Several cytokines have been proposed as mediators of the cachectic response, including tumor necrosis factor-α (TNF-α), interleukin (IL)-1 and IL-6, and interferon-γ.[28,29] High serum levels of these cytokines have been observed in some (but not all) persons with cancer, and their levels appear to correlate with progress of the tumors. TNF-α, secreted primarily from macrophages in response to tumor cell growth or gram-negative bacterial infections, was the first identified cytokine associated with cachexia and wasting. It causes anorexia by suppressing satiety centers and by suppressing the synthesis of lipoprotein lipase, an enzyme that facilitates the release of fatty acids from lipoproteins so that they can be used by tissues. It also induces a number of inflammatory responses, activates the coagulation system, suppresses bone marrow stem cell division, and acts on hepatocytes to increase the synthesis of specific serum proteins in response to inflammatory stimuli. IL-1 and IL-6 share many of the features of TNF-α in terms of the ability to initiate cachexia.[28]

In addition to loss of appetite and decreased nutrient intake, malignant disease appears to be associated with a hypermetabolic state and altered nutrient metabolism. Most solid tumors produce large amounts of lactate, which is converted back to glucose in the liver. The production of glucose (gluconeogenesis) from lactate uses adenosine triphosphate (ATP) and is very energy inefficient. A 40% increase in hepatic glucose production has been reported in persons with cancer cachexia, which may also be a consequence of meeting the tumor's metabolic needs.[28] Abnormalities in fat and protein metabolism have also been reported. During starvation in persons without cancer, ketones derived from fat replace the glucose normally used by the brain, leading to decreased gluconeogenesis from amino acids with conservation of muscle mass. In patients with cancer cachexia, amino acids are not spared, and there is depletion of lean body mass, a condition thought to contribute to a decrease in survival time.

PARANEOPLASTIC SYNDROMES

In addition to signs and symptoms at the sites of primary and metastatic disease, cancer can produce manifestations in sites that are not directly affected by the disease. Such manifestations are collectively referred to as *paraneoplastic syndromes*.[2,30,31] Some of these manifestations are caused by the elaboration of hormones by cancer cells, and others result from the production of circulating factors that produce hematopoietic, neurologic, and dermatologic syndromes (Table 8-3). These syndromes are most commonly associated with lung, breast, and hematologic malignancies.[2]

A variety of peptide hormones are produced by both benign and malignant tumors. The biochemical pathways for the synthesis and release of peptide hormones (*e.g.*, antidiuretic [ADH], adrenocorticotropin [ACTH], and parathyroid [PTH] hormones) are present in most cells. Thus, the three most common endocrine syndromes associated with cancer are the syndrome of inappropriate ADH secretion (see Chapter 33), Cushing's syndrome due to ectopic ACTH production (see Chapter 42), and hypercalcemia[2,31,32] (see Chapter 33). Hypercalcemia of malignancy does not appear to be related to PTH but to a PTH-related protein, which shares several biologic actions with PTH. Hypercalcemia also can be caused by osteolytic processes induced by cancer such as multiple myeloma or bony metastases from other cancers.

Some paraneoplastic syndromes are associated with the production of circulating mediators that produce hematologic complications. For example, a variety of cancers may produce procoagulation factors that contribute to an increased risk for venous thrombosis and nonbacterial thrombotic endocarditis. Sometimes, unexplained thrombotic events are the first indication of an undiagnosed malignancy. The precise relationship between coagulation disorders and cancer is still unknown. Several malignancies, such as mucin-producing adenocarcinomas, release thromboplastic materials that may activate the clotting system.

The symptomatic paraneoplastic neurologic disorders are relatively rare with the exception of the Lambert-Eaton myasthenic syndrome, which affects about 3% of persons with small cell lung cancer; and myasthenia gravis, which affects about 15% of people with thymoma.[33] The Lambert-Eaton syndrome, or reverse myasthenia gravis, is seen almost exclusively in small cell lung cancer. It produces muscle weakness in the limbs rather than the initial bulbar and ocular muscle weakness seen in myasthenia gravis. The origin of paraneoplastic neurologic disorders is thought to be immune mediated. The altered immune response is initiated by the production of onconeural antigens (*e.g.*, antigens normally expressed in the nervous system) by the cancer cells. The immune system, in turn, recognizes the onconeural antigens as foreign and mounts an immune response. In many cases, the immune attack controls the growth of the cancer. The antibodies and cytotoxic T cells are not sufficient to cause neurologic disease unless they cross the blood–brain barrier and react with neurons expressing the onconeural antigen.[33]

Among the paraneoplastic dermatologic disorders is a disorder called *acanthosis nigricans*. It is characterized by the pigmented hyperkeratosis, consisting of symmetric verrucous and papillary lesions that occur in skin flexures, particularly the axillary and perineal areas.[31] The lesions are usually symmetric and may be accompanied by pruritus. The condition is usually associated with visceral adenocarcinomas, particularly of the stomach.

The paraneoplastic syndromes may be the earliest indication that a person has cancer, and should be regarded as such. They may also represent significant clinical problems, may be potentially lethal in persons with cancer, and may mimic metastatic disease and confound treatment.[2] Diagnostic methods focus both on identifying the cause of the disorder and on locating the malignancy responsible for the disorder. Techniques for precise identification of minute amounts of polypeptides may allow for early diagnosis of curable malignancies in asymptomatic individuals.[31] The treatment of paraneoplastic syndromes involves concurrent treatment of the underlying cancer and suppression of the mediator causing the syndrome.

TABLE 8-3 Common Paraneoplastic Syndromes

Type of Syndrome	Associated Tumor Type	Proposed Mechanism
Endocrinologic		
Syndrome of inappropriate ADH	Small cell lung cancer, others	Production and release of ADH by tumor
Cushing's syndrome	Small cell lung cancer, bronchial carcinoid cancers	Production and release of ACTH by tumor
Hypercalcemia	Squamous cell cancers of lung, head, neck, ovary	Production and release of polypeptide factor with close relationship to PTH
Hematologic		
Venous thrombosis	Pancreatic, lung, other cancers	Production of procoagulation factors.
Nonbacterial thrombolytic endocarditis	Advanced cancers	
Neurologic		
Eaton-Lambert syndrome	Small cell lung cancer	Autoimmune production of antibodies to motor end-plate structures
Myasthenia gravis	Thymoma	
Dermatologic		
Acanthosis nigricans	Gastric carcinoma	Possibly caused by production of growth factors (epidermal) by tumor cells

ADH, antidiuretic hormone; ACTH, adrenocorticotropic hormone; PTH, parathyroid hormone.

In summary, although the clinical manifestations vary with the type of cancer and the organ that is involved, there are some general manifestations related to the effects of tumor growth. Cancer compresses blood vessels, obstructs lymph flow, disrupts tissue integrity, invades serous cavities, and compresses visceral organs. It also produces chemical mediators, such as TNF, that produce weight loss and tissue wasting. Paraneoplastic syndromes arise from the ability of neoplasms to elaborate hormones and other chemical messengers to produce endocrine, hematopoietic, neurologic, and dermatologic syndromes.

Diagnosis and Treatment

After completing this section of the chapter, you should be able to meet the following objectives:

- ✦ Describe methods used in detection and diagnosis of cancer, including the Papanicolaou smear, tissue biopsy, and tumor markers
- ✦ Compare methods used in grading and staging cancers
- ✦ Explain the mechanism by which radiation exerts its beneficial effects in the treatment of cancer
- ✦ Describe the adverse effects of radiation therapy
- ✦ Compare the action of cell cycle–specific and cell cycle–independent chemotherapeutic drugs
- ✦ Describe the three mechanisms whereby biotherapy exerts its effects
- ✦ Describe three examples of targeted therapy used in the treatment of cancer

DIAGNOSTIC METHODS

The methods used in the diagnosis and staging of cancer are determined largely by the location and type of cancer suspected. A number of diagnostic procedures are used in the diagnosis of cancer, including x-ray studies, endoscopic examinations, urine and stool tests, blood tests for tumor markers, bone marrow aspirations, ultrasound imaging, magnetic resonance imaging (MRI), computed tomography (CT) scan, and positron-emission tomography (PET) scan.

The Papanicolaou Test

The Papanicolaou (Pap) test is a cytologic method that is used for detecting cancer cells. It consists of a microscopic examination of a properly prepared slide by a cytotechnologist or pathologist for the purpose of detecting the presence of abnormal cells. The usefulness of the Pap test relies on the fact that the cancer cells lack the cohesive properties and intercellular junctions that are characteristic of normal tissue; without these characteristics, cancer cells tend to exfoliate and become mixed with secretions surrounding the tumor growth. Although the Pap test is widely used as a screening test for cervical cancer (see Chapter 47), it can be performed on other body secretions, including nipple drainage, pleural or peritoneal fluid, and gastric washings.

Biopsy

Tissue biopsy is the removal of a tissue specimen for microscopic study. Biopsies are obtained in a number of ways, including needle aspiration (*i.e.,* fine, percutaneous, or core needle); endoscopic methods, such as bronchoscopy or cystoscopy, which involve the passage of an endoscope through an orifice and into the involved structure; or laparoscopic methods. In some instances, a surgical incision is made from which biopsy specimens are obtained. Excisional biopsies are those in which the entire tumor is removed. The tumors usually are small, solid, palpable masses. If the tumor is too large to be completely removed, a wedge of tissue from the mass can be excised for examination. Tissue diagnosis is of critical importance in designing the treatment plan should cancer cells be found.

Tumor Markers

Tumor markers are antigens that are expressed on the surface of tumor cells or substances released from normal cells in response to the presence of tumor.[2,34] Some substances, such as hormones and enzymes, are produced normally by the tissue involved but become overexpressed as a result of cancer. Other tumor markers, such as oncofetal protein, are produced during fetal development and are induced to reappear later in life as a result of benign and malignant neoplasms. Tumor markers are used for screening, diagnosis, establishing prognosis, monitoring treatment, and detecting recurrent disease.

As diagnostic tools, tumor markers have limitations. The value of a marker depends on its sensitivity, specificity, proportionality, and feasibility.[34] Sensitivity implies that the marker is apparent early in the development of the tumor and has few false-negative results. Specificity indicates that the marker is specific for the specific cancer and is not elevated in other disease conditions (*i.e.,* has few false-positive results). Proportionality means that the level of marker accurately reflects the growth of the tumor, such that higher levels reflect a larger growth. Feasibility implies that the methods are readily available and easy to use and that the cost is not prohibitive. Nearly all markers can be elevated in benign conditions, and most are not elevated in the early stages of malignancy. Hence, tumor markers have limited value as screening tests. Extremely elevated levels of a tumor marker can indicate a poor prognosis or the need for more aggressive treatment. Perhaps the greatest value of tumor markers is in monitoring therapy in people with widespread cancer. Nearly all markers show an association with the clinical course of the disease. The levels of most markers decrease with successful treatment and increase with recurrence or spread of the tumor.

The markers that have been most useful in clinical practice have been human chorionic gonadotropin (hCG), CA 125, prostate-specific antigen (PSA), alpha-fetoprotein (AFP), and carcinoembryonic antigen (CEA). HCG is a hormone normally produced by the placenta. It is used as a marker for diagnosing, prescribing treatment, and following the disease course in persons with high-risk gestational trophoblastic tumors. PSA is used as a marker in prostate cancer, and CA 125 is used as a marker in ovarian cancer.

Some cancers express fetal antigens, which are differentiation antigens normally present only during embryonal development.[2] The two that have proved most useful as tumor markers are AFP and CEA. AFP is synthesized by the fetal liver, yolk sac, and gastrointestinal tract and is the major serum protein in the fetus. Elevated levels are encountered in people with primary liver cancers and have also been observed in some testicular, ovarian, pancreatic, and stomach cancers. CEA normally is produced by embryonic tissue in the gut, pancreas, and liver and is elaborated by a number of different cancers. Depending on the serum level adopted for significant elevation, CEA is elevated in approximately 60% to 90% of colorectal carcinomas, 50% to 80% of pancreatic cancers, and 25% to 50% of gastric and breast tumors.[2] As with most other tumor markers, elevated levels of CEA and AFP are found in other, noncancerous conditions, and elevated levels of both depend on tumor size so that neither is useful as an early test for cancer.

CHART 8-2

TNM Classification System

T (tumor)

Tx	Tumor cannot be adequately assessed
T0	No evidence of primary tumor
Tis	Carcinoma in situ
T1–4	Progressive increase in tumor size or involvement

N (nodes)

Nx	Regional lymph nodes cannot be assessed
N0	No evidence of regional node metastasis
N1–3	Increasing involvement of regional lymph nodes

M (metastasis)

Mx	Not assessed
M0	No distant metastasis
M1	Distant metastasis present, specify sites

Staging and Grading of Tumors

The two basic methods for classifying cancers are *grading* according to the histologic or cellular characteristics of the tumor and *staging* according to the clinical spread of the disease. Both methods are used to determine the course of the disease and aid in selecting an appropriate treatment or management plan. Grading of tumors involves the microscopic examination of cancer cells to determine their level of differentiation and the number of mitoses. Cancers are classified as grades I, II, III, and IV with increasing anaplasia or lack of differentiation. Staging of cancers uses methods to determine the extent and spread of the disease. Surgery may be used to determine tumor size and lymph node involvement.

The clinical staging of cancer is intended to group patients according to the extent of their disease. It is useful in determining the choice of treatment for individual patients, estimating prognosis, and comparing the results of different treatment regimens. The TNM system of the American Joint Committee on Cancer (AJCC) is used by most cancer facilities.[35] This system, which is briefly described in Chart 8-2, classifies the disease into stages using three tumor components: *T* stands for the size and local spread of the primary tumor, *N* refers to the involvement of the regional lymph nodes, and *M* describes the extent of the metastatic involvement. The time of staging is indicated as clinical-diagnostic staging (cTNM); postsurgical resection-pathologic staging (pTNM); surgical-evaluative staging (sTNM); retreatment staging (rTNM); and autopsy staging (aTNM).[35]

CANCER TREATMENT

The goals of cancer treatment methods fall into three categories: curative, control, and palliative. The most common modalities are surgery, radiation, chemotherapy, hormonal therapy, and biotherapy. The treatment of cancer involves the use of a carefully planned program that combines the benefits of multiple treatment modalities and the expertise of an interdisciplinary team of specialists including medical, surgical, and radiation oncologists; clinical nurse specialists; nurse practitioners; pharmacists; and a variety of ancillary personnel.

Surgery

It is estimated that 90% of all patients with cancer will undergo a surgical procedure during the course of their management.[36] Surgery is often thought of as the first line of treatment for solid tumors. Surgery is used for diagnosis, staging of cancer, tumor removal, and palliation (*i.e.,* relief of symptoms) when a cure cannot be achieved. The type of surgery to be used is determined by the extent of the disease, the location and structures involved, the tumor growth rate and invasiveness, the surgical risk to the patient, and the quality of life the patient will experience after the surgery. If the tumor is small and has well-defined margins, the entire tumor often can be removed. If, however, the tumor is large or involves vital tissues, surgical removal may be difficult if not impossible.

Surgery provides several approaches for cancer treatment. For example, it can be the primary, curative treatment for cancers that are locally or regionally contained, have not metastasized, or have not invaded major organs. It also is used as a component of adjuvant therapy when used in combination with chemotherapy or radiation therapy in other types of cancers. Surgical techniques also may be used to control oncologic emergencies such as gastrointestinal hemorrhages. Another approach includes utilizing surgical techniques for cancer prophylaxis in families that have a high genetically confirmed risk for developing cancer. For instance, a total colectomy may be suggested for an individual with familial adenomatous polyposis coli because of the increased risk for developing cancer by age 40.

Surgical techniques have expanded to include cryosurgery, chemosurgery, laser surgery, and laparoscopic surgery. *Cryosurgery* involves the instillation of liquid nitrogen into the tumor through a probe. It is used in treating cancers of the liver and prostate. *Chemosurgery* is used in skin cancers. It involves the use of a corrosive paste in combination with multiple frozen sections to ensure complete removal of the tumor. *Laser surgery* uses a laser beam to resect a tumor. It has been used effectively in retinal and vocal cord surgery. *Laparoscopic surgery* involves the performance of abdominal surgery through two small incisions—one for viewing within the cavity and the other for insertion of the instruments to perform the surgery.

Cooperative efforts among cancer centers throughout the world have helped to standardize and improve surgical procedures, determine which cancers benefit from surgical intervention, and establish in what order surgical and other treatment modalities should be used. Increased emphasis also has been placed on the development of surgical techniques that preserve body image and form without compromising essential function. Nerve-sparing prostatectomy and limb-salvage surgery for soft tissue tumors preserve functional abilities while permitting complete removal of the tumor.[37]

Radiation Therapy

More than 60% of patients with cancer receive radiation therapy, alone or in combination with other forms of treatment.[38] The goal of radiation therapy is to achieve local-regional control of the cancerous growth without permanently damaging the surrounding normal tissue. Radiation can be used alone as a primary method of therapy, in combination with other forms of therapy, or as a palliative measure.

Radiation is well established as a primary therapy for squamous cell carcinomas of the head and neck, primary nervous system malignancies, some localized lymphomas, some germ cell tumors, and cervical, pancreatic, and prostate cancers.[39] When radiation is used as the primary treatment for cure, the duration of treatment usually is longer and the dose is higher than in palliative treatment modalities. In patients with acute lymphocytic leukemia in which the primary treatment is chemotherapy, radiation is used to treat sanctuary sites such as the central nervous system because it has been found to enhance the ability of chemotherapy to cross the blood–brain barrier. Radiation therapy also is used as an adjuvant treatment with surgery (administered presurgically or postsurgically), chemotherapy, or both chemotherapy and surgery.[39]

Radiation therapy is also used as a palliative treatment to reduce symptoms in approximately 50% of patients with advanced cancer. It is effective in reducing the pain associated with bone metastasis and, in some cases, improves mobility. Radiation also is used to treat several oncologic emergencies such as superior vena cava syndrome, spinal cord compression, bronchial obstruction, and hemorrhage.[40]

Mechanisms of Action. Ionizing radiation is radiation that is capable of ejecting one or more electrons from an atom. It affects cells by direct ionization of molecules or, more commonly, by indirect ionization.

Indirect ionization produced by x-rays and gamma rays causes cellular damage when these rays are absorbed into tissue and give up their energy by producing fast-moving electrons. These electrons interact with free or loosely bonded electrons of the absorber cells and subsequently produce free radicals that interact with critical cell components[41] (see Chapter 5). Radiation can immediately kill cells, delay or halt cell cycle progression, or, at dose levels commonly used in radiation therapy, cause damage in the nucleus that result in cell death after replication. Cell damage may be sublethal, in which case a single break in the strand of DNA can repair itself if there is time before the next radiation insult. Double-stranded breaks in DNA are generally believed to be the primary damage that leads to radiation death in cells. The consequence of unrepaired DNA is that cells may continue to function until they undergo cell mitosis, at which time the genetic damage from the irradiation may result in death of the cell.

The therapeutic effects of radiation therapy derive from the fact that the rapidly proliferating and poorly differentiated cells of a cancerous tumor are more likely to be injured than are the more slowly proliferating cells of normal tissue. To some extent, however, radiation is injurious to all rapidly proliferating cells, including those of the bone marrow and the mucosal lining of the gastrointestinal tract. In addition to its lethal effects, radiation also produces sublethal injury. Recovery from sublethal doses of radiation occurs in the interval between the first dose of radiation and subsequent doses. This is why large total doses of radiation can be tolerated when they are divided into multiple, smaller fractionated doses. Normal tissue usually is able to recover from radiation damage more readily than cancerous tissue.

Radiation, Sensitivity, and Responsiveness. The term *radiosensitivity* describes the inherent properties of a tumor that determine its responsiveness to radiation. It varies widely among the different types of cancers and is thought to vary as a function of their position in the cell cycle. Fast-growing cells, for example, that have cell cycle durations of 9 or 10 hours typically are more radiosensitive in mitosis (M) or late in the G_2 phase. More slowly growing cells that have longer S phases are more radioresistant.[41] Acute lymphocytic leukemia and lymphomas are highly radiosensitive cancers, but rhabdomyosarcomas and melanomas are much less so. The combination of selected cytotoxic drugs with radiation has demonstrated a radiosensitizing effect on tumor cells by altering the cell cycle distribution, increasing DNA damage, and decreasing DNA repair. Some radiosensitizers are hydroxyurea, 5-fluorouracil, paclitaxel, gemcitabine, cisplatin, etoposide, and camptothecin.[38]

The radiation dose that is chosen for treatment of a particular cancer is determined by factors such as the radiosensitivity of the tumor type, the size of the tumor, and, more importantly, the tolerance of the surrounding tissues. Dose-response curves, which express the extent of lethal tissue injury in relation to the dose of radiation, are determined by the number of cells that survive graded, fractional doses of radiation. With the use of more frequent fractionated doses, it is likely that the cancer cells will be dividing and in the vulnerable period of the cell cycle. This type of dose also allows time for normal tissues to repair the radiation damage. An important focus of research has been the search for drugs to reduce the biologic effects of radiation on normal tissue. These drugs, known as *radioprotectants,* would preferentially protect normal cells from the cytotoxic effects of radiation. One drug, amifostine, is approved to reduce the incidence of dryness of the mouth (*i.e.,* xerostomia) due to the effects of radiation on salivary gland function in patients undergoing radiation for head and neck cancers.[42]

Radiation responsiveness describes the manner in which a radiosensitive tumor responds to irradiation. One of the major determinants of radiation responsiveness is tumor oxygenation because oxygen is a rich source of free radicals that form and destroy essential cell components during irradiation. Many rapidly growing tumors outgrow their blood supply and become deprived of oxygen. The hypoxic cells of these tumors are more resistant to radiation than normal or well-oxygenated tumor cells. Methods of ensuring adequate oxygen delivery, such as adequate hemoglobin levels, are important. Concurrent administration of erythropoietin, a growth hormone for red blood cells, during radiation to increase hemoglobin concentrations above 13 g/dL has shown potential improvements in control and survival of patients with solid tumors, including cervical, bladder, and head and neck cancers.[42] Agents that increase the production of free radicals during radiation in a manner similar to oxygen are still under investigation.

Administration. Ionizing radiation exists in two distinct forms: electromagnetic and particulate. *Electromagnetic radiation* can be considered as a wave and a packet of energy (photon). It includes x-rays and gamma rays, both of which are similar in nature, but differ in the way they are made. X-rays are produced by electrical devices that accelerate electrons to high energy levels and abruptly stop them at a target. Gamma rays are emitted from the spontaneous decay of radioactive isotopes of elements such as cobalt and cesium. *Particulate radiation* consists of fast-moving, high-energy particles (*e.g.,* electrons, protons, alpha particles, neutrons, and heavy ions).[38] There has been limited clinical use of particulate radiation due to the complex and costly equipment used for its production.

Several types of equipment and sources can be used for administering radiation therapy. Radiation therapy can be delivered by either external beam radiation machines that have sources of radiation located some distance from the patient (sometimes called teletherapy) or by short-distance therapy (brachytherapy), in which a sealed radioactive source is placed close to or directly in the tumor site. Radioisotopes with a short half-life may be injected or given by mouth as a palliative or curative treatment for some cancers. Radiation delivery has to be carefully planned and controlled for absolute accuracy and optimum results.

External beam radiation is commonly delivered by a linear accelerator or a cobalt-60 machine. The linear accelerator is the preferred machine due to its versatility and precision of dose distribution as well as the speed with which treatment can be given. Linear accelerators produce ionizing radiation through a process in which electrons are accelerated at a very high rate, strike a target, and produce high-energy x-rays (photons). Photon energy generates a rectangular energy beam capable of penetrating deep within the tumor tissue. The linear accelerator can vary the level of radiation energy that is delivered so that different depths can be treated. The higher the level of radiation energy delivered by the radiation equipment, the greater the depth of penetration. Most linear accelerators also have electron beam capabilities. These high-energy electron beams are used for treating superficial structures, including lymph nodes and skin, while avoiding irradiation of deep-seated normal organs, such as the spinal cord. Various beam-modifying approaches are used to define and shape the beam size, thereby increasing the radiation damage to the tumor site while sparing the normal surrounding tissues. For example, a multileaf collimating system can be used to shape the treatment fields to conform to the tumor, by moving its 20 to 80 lead leaves or shields in front of the beam to customize the port through which the beam exits.[39] Three-dimensional (3-D) conformal therapy uses CT scans or MRIs to construct an image of the tumor. Intensity modulated radiation therapy (IMRT) uses computer imaging techniques to calculate the most efficient dosages and combinations of radiation treatments. This precise mapping of the tumor allows for the delivery of radiation beams that conform to the contours of the tumor, reducing the dose and therefore the toxicity to adjacent normal tissue.[15]

Cobalt-60 machines deliver gamma radiation equivalent to the photon energy produced by linear accelerators. Because the radiation source is a radioactive isotope undergoing constant decay, it needs to be replaced every 4 to 5 years to avoid lengthy treatment times. The cobalt-60 machines are still used widely in palliative situations and for targets close to the surface. Stereotactic radiosurgery is a method of destroying brain tumors and brain metastases by delivering a single large dose of radiation through stereotactically directed narrow beams. A gamma knife unit has been used most often for radiosurgery. It contains cobalt-60 sources that, when unshielded, emit multiple focused beams of gamma radiation.[38]

Brachytherapy involves the insertion of sealed radioactive sources into a body cavity (intracavitary) or directly into body tissues (interstitial). Radiation sources are sealed in applicators of almost any size or shape. Most commonly, they are packed into needles, beads, seeds, ribbons, or catheters, which are then implanted directly into the tumor. Remote afterloading machines make it possible to insert a radioactive material (*e.g.,* cesium-137, iridium-192) into a tumor area for a specific time and remove it while oncology personnel are outside the treatment room. This minimizes staff radiation exposure and decreases treatment times by allowing use of intermediate and high-dose radioactive sources.[43] Cancer of the cervix and uterus are often treated with these removable cesium or iridium insertions. Radioactive materials with a relatively short half-life, such as iodine-125 or palladium-103, are commonly encapsulated and used in permanent implants (*e.g.,* seed implants used to treat prostate cancer).

Unsealed internal radiation sources are injected intravenously or administered by mouth. Iodine-131, which is given by mouth, is used in the treatment of thyroid cancer. Strontium-89, administered intravenously, is given to control bone pain due to multiple skeletal metastases in patients with advanced breast, lung, or prostate cancer.[38]

Adverse Effects. Radiation cannot distinguish between malignant cells and the rapidly proliferating cells of normal tissue. During radiation treatment, injury to normal cells can produce adverse effects. Radiation effects are dose and fractionation dependent. Tissues, within the treatment fields, that are most frequently affected are the skin, the mucosal lining of the gastrointestinal tract, and the bone marrow. Anorexia, nausea, emesis, and diarrhea are common with abdominal and pelvic irradiation. These symptoms are usually controlled by medication and dietary measures. The primary systemic effect is fatigue. Most of these side effects are temporary and reversible.

Radiation can also cause bone marrow suppression, particularly when radiation is delivered to the bone marrow in skeletal sites. Subsequently, the complete blood count is affected, resulting in an initial decrease in the number of the leukocytes, followed by a decrease in thrombocytes (platelets) and, finally, red blood cells. This predisposes the individual to infection, bleeding, and anemia, respectively. Frequent blood counts are used during radiation therapy to monitor bone marrow function.

External beam radiation must first penetrate the skin; depending on the total dose and type of radiation used, skin reactions may develop. With moderate doses of radiation to the skin, the hair falls out spontaneously or when being combed, after the 10th to the 14th day; with larger doses, erythema develops (much like a sunburn) and may turn brown; and, at higher doses, patches of dry or moist desquamation may develop. Fortunately, epithelialization takes place after the treatments have been stopped. Mucositis, desquamation of the oral and pharyngeal mucous membranes, which sometimes may be severe, may occur as a predictable side effect in people receiving head and neck irradiation. Pain and difficulty eating and drinking can negatively affect the individual's nutritional status. Pelvic radiation can cause impotence or erectile dysfunction in men and vaginal irritation, dryness, discharge, dyspareunia, and as a late effect, vaginal stenosis in women.[44]

Chemotherapy

Cancer chemotherapy has evolved as one of the major systemic treatment modalities. Unlike surgery and radiation, cancer chemotherapy is a systemic treatment that enables drugs to reach the site of the tumor as well as distant sites. More than 50 different chemotherapeutic drugs are used alone or in various combinations.[45] Chemotherapeutic drugs may be the primary form of treatment, or they may be used as part of a multimodal treatment plan. Chemotherapy is the primary treatment for most hematologic and some solid tumors, including choriocarcinoma, testicular cancer, acute and chronic leukemia, Burkitt's lymphoma, Hodgkin's disease, and multiple myeloma.

Cancer chemotherapeutic drugs exert their effects through several mechanisms. At the cellular level, they exert their lethal action by targeting processes that prevent cell growth and replication. These mechanisms include disrupting production of essential enzymes; inhibiting DNA, RNA, and protein synthesis; and preventing cell mitosis.[6,45,46]

For most chemotherapy drugs, the relationship between tumor cell survival and drug dose is exponential, with the number of cells surviving being proportional to drug dose, and the number of cells at risk for exposure being proportional to the destructive action of the drug. Chemotherapeutic drugs are most effective in treating tumors that have a high growth fraction because of their ability to kill rapidly dividing cells. Exponential killing implies that a proportion or percentage of tumor cells are killed, rather than an absolute number (Fig. 8-11). This proportion is a constant percentage of the total number of cells. For this reason, multiple courses of treatment are needed if the tumor is to be eradicated.[46]

Cancer chemotherapy drugs may be classified as either cell cycle specific or cell cycle nonspecific. Drugs are cell cycle specific if they exert their action during a specific phase of the cell cycle. For example, methotrexate, an antimetabolite, acts by interfering with DNA synthesis and thereby interrupts the S phase of the cell cycle. Drugs that are cell cycle nonspecific affect cancer cells throughout all phases of the cell cycle. The alkylating agents are cell cycle nonspecific and act by disrupting DNA when the cells are in the resting state as well as when they are dividing. The site of action of chemotherapeutic drugs varies. Chemotherapy drugs that have similar structures and effects on cell func-

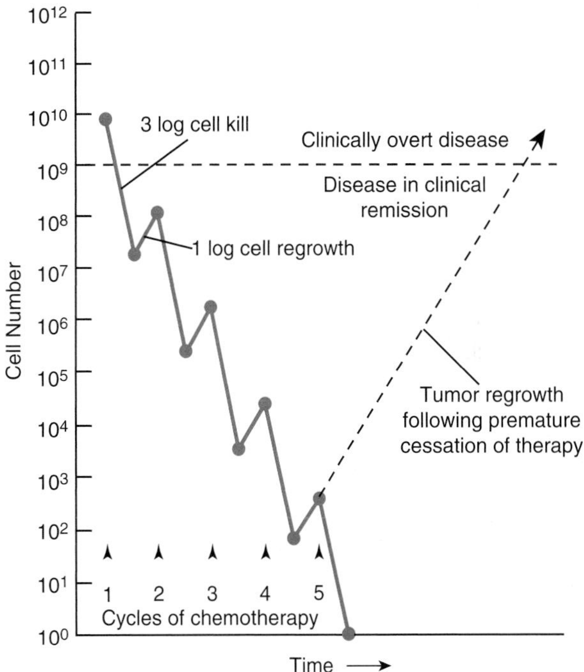

FIGURE 8-11 Relationship between tumor cell survival and administration of chemotherapy. The exponential relationship between drug dose and tumor cell survival dictates that a constant proportion, not number, of tumor cells are killed with each treatment cycle. In this example, each cycle of drug administration results in 99.9% (3 log) of cell kill, and 1 log of cell regrowth occurs between cycles. The *broken line* indicates what would occur if the last cycle of therapy were omitted: despite complete clinical remission of disease, the tumor ultimately would recur. (From Cooper M.R., Cooper M.R. [2001]. Basis for current major therapies for cancer: Systemic therapy. In Lenhard R.E., Osteen R.T., Gansler T. [Eds.], *The American Cancer Society's clinical oncology* [pp. 181]. Atlanta: American Cancer Society)

tion usually are grouped together, and these drugs usually have similar side-effect profiles. Because chemotherapy drugs differ in their mechanisms of action, cell cycle–specific and cell cycle–nonspecific agents are often combined to treat cancer.

Chemotherapy drugs are also classified according to their mechanism of action. The major classification of chemotherapy drugs are covalent DNA-binding drugs (alkylating agents), antimetabolites, antitumor antibiotics, microtubule-targeting drugs (mitotic inhibitors), DNA topoisomerase inhibitors, and enzymes. Alkylating agents share the same dose-related toxicity of myelesuppression. These drugs demonstrate a steep dose-response curve, making them ideal for the dose-intense preparative regimens needed for bone marrow transplantation. Antimetabolites, because of their S-phase specificity, have been shown to be more effective when given as a prolonged infusion. Efforts to minimize the toxicity profile of the antitumor antibiotics have resulted in the development of analog compounds (*e.g.,* idarubicin, epirubicin). Liposome technology has been used with two antitumor antibiotics (*e.g.,* doxorubicin and daunorubicin) to develop chemotherapy drugs that are encapsulated by coated liposomes. These drugs (*e.g.,* doxorubicin [Doxil] and daunorubicin [DaunoXome]) have been found to distribute more chemotherapy to the desired site with fewer side effects.[47]

The taxanes (*e.g.,* paclitaxel, docetaxel) and the vinca alkaloids (vincristine, vinblastine, vinorelbine) are drugs affecting the microtubule structures required for formation of the mitotic spindle. Although each group affects the microtubule, their mechanism of action differs. The side effect profile of the taxanes includes peripheral neuropathy and an increased incidence of hypersensitivity reactions.

The DNA-topoisomerase inhibitors are a relatively new class of chemotherapy agents, incorporating the older epipodophyllotoxins (etoposide and teniposide), with the new group of topoisomerase II inhibitors (topotecan, irinotecan).[45] These drugs are plant derivatives that inhibit the action of enzymes essential to the control, maintenance, and modification of the structure and function of DNA.

Combination chemotherapy has been found to be more effective than treatment with a single drug. Combination chemotherapy creates a more hostile environment for tumor cell growth through higher drug concentrations and prevents the development of resistant clones of cancer cells. With this method, several drugs with different mechanisms of action, metabolic pathways, times of onset of action and recovery, side effects, and onset of side effects are used. Drugs used in combination must be individually effective against the tumor and may be synergistic with each other. The regimens for combination therapy often are referred to by acronyms. Two well-known combinations are MOPP (Mustargen [nitrogen mustard], Oncovin [vincristine], prednisone, and procarbazine), used in the treatment of Hodgkin's disease, and AC-T (doxorubicin [adriamycin], cyclophosphamide, and paclitaxel [Taxol]), used in the treatment of breast cancer. Routes of administration and dosage schedules are carefully designed to ensure optimal delivery of the active forms of the drugs to a tumor during the sensitive phase of the cell cycle.

Many of these cancer chemotherapy drugs are administered intravenously. Venous access devices (VADs) often are used for people with poor venous access and those who require frequent or continuous intravenous therapy. The VAD can be used for home administration of chemotherapy drugs, blood sampling, and administration of blood components. These systems access the venous circulation either through an externalized catheter or an implanted catheter with access ports. In some cases, the drugs are administered by continuous infusion using an ambulatory infusion pump that allows the person to remain at home and maintain his or her activities.[45] Newer drugs (*e.g.,* capecitabine) have been formulated for the oral route. Although adherence to a dosing schedule and reimbursement for oral drugs are a challenge, these drugs provide a more convenient administration form for the patient.

Adverse Effects. Chemotherapy is administered on a dose-response basis (*i.e.,* the more drug administered, the greater the number of cancer cells killed). Chemotherapeutic drugs affect the neoplastic cells and the rapidly proliferating cells of normal tissue. The nadir (*i.e.,* lowest point) is the point of maximal toxicity for a given adverse effect of a drug and is stated in the time it takes to reach that point. The nadir for leukopenia with thiotepa, for example, occurs 14 days after initiation of treatment. Because many toxic effects of chemotherapeutic drugs persist for some time after the drug is discontinued, the nadir times and recovery rates are useful guides in evaluating the effects of cancer therapy. Some side effects appear immediately or after a few days (acute), some within a few weeks (intermediate), and others months to years after chemotherapy administration (long-term).

Most chemotherapeutic drugs suppress bone marrow function and formation of blood cells, leading to anemia, neutropenia, and thrombocytopenia. With neutropenia, there is risk for developing serious infections, whereas thrombocytopenia increases the risk for bleeding. The availability of hematopoietic growth factors (*e.g.,* granulocyte colony-stimulating factor [G-CSF]; erythropoietin, which stimulates red blood production; and IL-11, which stimulates platelet production) has shortened the period of myelosuppression, thereby reducing the need for hospitalizations due to infection and decreasing the need for blood products.[45]

Anorexia, nausea, and vomiting are common problems associated with cancer chemotherapy. The severity of the vomiting is related to the emetic potential of the particular drug. These symptoms can occur within minutes or hours of drug administration and are thought to be due to stimulation of the chemoreceptor trigger zone in the medulla that stimulates vomiting (see Chapter 39). The chemoreceptor trigger zone responds to levels of chemicals circulating in the blood. The acute symptoms usually subside within 24 to 48 hours and often can be relieved by antiemetics. The pharmacologic approaches to prevent chemotherapy-induced nausea and vomiting have greatly improved over several decades. The development of serotonin (5-HT_3) receptor antagonists (*e.g.,* ondansetron, granisetron, dolasetron, palonosetron) has facilitated the use of highly emetic chemotherapy drugs by more effectively reducing the nausea and vomiting induced by these drugs.[48] These antiemetics are effective when given by both the oral and intravenous routes. Aprepitant, a selective high-affinity antagonist of substance P/neuokinin-1 receptors, has recently been approved for use in treatment of nausea and vomiting that is associated with cancer chemotherapy.[48] The drug, which is given orally, has been shown to inhibit both the acute and chronic phases of chemotherapy-induced nausea and vomiting.

Diarrhea is another problem associated with cancer chemotherapy. Chemotherapy can cause temporary lactose intolerance or an increase in gastric motility. Pharmacologic and dietary interventions are helpful in reducing the severity of diarrhea. For example, Lomotil and Imodium are frequently prescribed, and patients should be advised to eat small, frequent, and low-residue meals; to refrain from eating spicy or greasy foods; to avoid extreme temperatures in foods or beverages; and to use nutritional supplements when necessary.[49] Some drugs cause stomatitis and damage to the rapidly proliferating cells of the gastrointestinal tract's mucosal lining. Despite advances in early detection and assessment, prevention and management of stomatitis continue to be problematic. Research is ongoing in an effort to resolve these troublesome side effects.

Fatigue is one of the most prevalent problems experienced by patients with cancer and is estimated to occur in 96% of individuals receiving chemotherapy (see Chapter 12). The cause is multifactorial. Hair loss results from impaired proliferation of the hair follicles and is a side effect of a number of cancer drugs; it usually is temporary, and the hair tends to regrow when treatment is stopped. The rapidly proliferating structures of the reproductive system are particularly sensitive to the action of cancer drugs. Women may experience changes in menstrual flow or have amenorrhea. Men may have a decreased sperm count (*i.e.*, oligospermia) or absence of sperm (*i.e.*, azoospermia). Many chemotherapeutic agents also may have teratogenic or mutagenic effects leading to fetal abnormalities.[50]

Chemotherapy drugs are toxic to all cells. The mutagenic, carcinogenic, and teratogenic potential of these drugs has been strongly supported by both animal and human studies. Because of these potential risks, special care is required when handling or administering the drugs. Drugs, drug containers, and administration equipment require special disposal as hazardous waste. Several organizations, including the Occupational Safety and Health Administration (OSHA), the Oncology Nursing Society (ONS), and the American Society of Hospital Pharmacists (ASHP), have developed special guidelines for the safe handling and disposal of antineoplastic drugs as well as for accidental spills and exposure.[50–52]

Epidemiologic studies have shown an increased risk for second malignancies such as acute nonlymphocytic leukemia after long-term use of alkylating agents[53,54] and semustine[55] for treatment of various forms of cancer. These second malignancies are thought to result from direct cellular changes produced by the drug or from suppression of the immune response.

Hormonal Therapy

Hormonal therapy consists of administration of drugs designed to negatively alter the hormonal environment of cancer cells negatively. It is used for cancers that are responsive to or dependent on hormones for growth. The actions of hormones and antihormones depend on the presence of specific receptors in the tumor. Among the tumors that are known to be responsive to hormonal manipulation are those of the breast, prostate, and the endometrium. Other cancers, such as Kaposi's sarcoma and renal, liver, ovarian, and pancreatic cancer, are also responsive to hormonal manipulation, but to a lesser degree.[56] The theory behind the majority of hormone-based cancer treatments is to deprive the cancer cells of the hormonal signals that otherwise would stimulate them to divide.

The therapeutic options for altering the hormonal environment in the woman with breast cancer or the man with prostate cancer include surgical and pharmacologic measures.[56] Surgery involves the removal of the organ responsible for the hormone production that is stimulating the target tissue (*e.g.*, oophorectomy in women or orchiectomy in men). Pharmacologic methods focus largely on reducing circulating hormone levels or changing the hormone receptors so that they no longer respond to the hormone. Pharmacologic suppression of circulating hormone levels can be effected through pituitary desensitization as with the administration of androgens or through the administration of gonadotropin-releasing hormone (GnRH) analogs that act at the level of the hypothalamus to inhibit gonadotropin production and release. Another class of drugs, the aromatase inhibitors, is used to treat breast cancer; these drugs act by interrupting the biochemical processes that convert androstenedione, an adrenally generated androgen, to estradiol in the peripheral tissues. Hormone receptor function can be altered by the administration of pharmacologic doses of exogenous hormones that act by producing a decrease in hormone receptors or by antihormone drugs that complex with hormone receptors (antiestrogens [tamoxifen, fulvestrant] and antiandrogens [flutamide, bicalutamide, nilutamide]) that complex with hormone receptors, making them inaccessible to hormone stimulation. Initially, patients often respond favorably to hormonal treatments, but eventually the cancer becomes resistant to hormonal manipulation, and other approaches must be sought to control the disease.

Biotherapy

Biotherapy involves the use of immunotherapy and biologic response modifiers as a means of changing the person's own immune response to cancer.[57,58] The major mechanisms by which biotherapy exerts its effects are modification of host responses, direct destruction of cancer cells by suppressing tumor growth or killing the tumor cell, and modification of tumor cell biology.[57]

Immunotherapy. Immunotherapy techniques include active and passive, or adoptive immunotherapy. Active immunotherapy involves nonspecific techniques such as bacille Calmette-Guérin (BCG). BCG is an attenuated strain of the bacterium that causes bovine tuberculosis. It acts as a nonspecific stimulant of the immune system and is instilled into the bladder as a means of treating superficial bladder cancer. Passive or adoptive immunotherapy involves the transfer of cultured immune cells into a tumor-bearing host. Early research efforts with adoptive immunotherapy involved the transfer of sensitized NK cells or T lymphocytes, combined with cytokines to the tumor-bearing host, in an attempt to augment the host's immune response. However, randomized clinical trials demonstrated no benefit from the addition of the cellular component beyond the benefit from the cytokine alone. Further research has focused on using antigen-presenting dendritic cells as delivery vehicles for tumor antigens. Dendritic cells are efficient at activating not only $CD4^+$ helper cells and $CD8^+$ killer T cells but also B cells and innate effectors such as NK cells.[58]

Biologic Response Modifiers. Biologic response modifiers (BRMs) can be grouped into three types: cytokines, which include the interferons and interleukins; monoclonal antibodies; and hematopoietic growth factors. Some agents, such as interferons, have more than one biologic function, including antiviral, immunomodulatory, and antiproliferative actions. The *interferons* are endogenous polypeptides that are synthesized by a number of cells in response to a variety of cellular or viral stimuli. The three major types of interferons are: alpha (α), beta (β), and gamma (γ), each group differing in terms of their cell surface receptors.[58] The interferons appear to inhibit viral replication and also may be involved in inhibiting tumor protein synthesis and in prolonging the cell cycle and increasing the percentage of cells in the G_0 phase. Interferons stimulate NK cells and T-lymphocyte killer cells. Interferon-γ has been approved for the treatment of hairy cell leukemia, AIDS-related Kaposi's sarcoma, and chronic myelogenous leukemia, and as adjuvant therapy for patients at high risk for recurrent melanoma.[59] Interferon-α has been used to treat some solid tumors (*e.g.,* renal cell carcinoma, colorectal cancer, carcinoid tumors, ovarian cancer) and hematologic neoplasms (*e.g.,* B-cell and T-cell lymphomas, cutaneous T-cell lymphoma, and multiple myeloma).[59] Research now is focusing on combining interferons with other forms of cancer therapy and establishing optimal doses and treatment protocols.

The *interleukins* (ILs) are cytokines that provide communication between cells, by binding to receptor sites on the cell-surface membranes of the target cells. Of the 18 known interleukins (see Chapter 19), IL-2 has been the most widely studied. A recombinant human IL-2 (rIL-2 aldesleukin) has been approved by the U.S. Food and Drug Administration (FDA) and is currently being used for the treatment of metastatic renal cell carcinoma and metastatic melanoma.[60]

Monoclonal antibodies (MoAbs) are highly specific antibodies derived from cloned cells or hybridomas. Scientists were able to produce large quantities of these MoAbs that are specific for tumor cells. The four types of therapeutic MoAbs are grouped according to the origin of the antibody: murine (mouse), human, chimeric (mixed mouse and human), and humanized (murine transformed to humanized format so that it is not recognized as foreign). For an MoAb to be therapeutic as a cancer treatment modality, a specific target antigen should be present on cancer cells only. Therapeutic monoclonal antibodies can be unconjugated (*i.e.,* "naked"), conjugated, or combined with a toxin, chemotherapy drug, or radioisotope.[61] A number of unconjugated MoAbs are available, including alemtuzumab (Campath), a humanized MoAb that targets the CD52 antigen of human B cells, T cells, NK cells, and monocyte-macrophages; rituximab (Rituxan), an anti-CD20 chimeric MoAb; and trastuzumab (Herceptin), a humanized MoAb that binds to the HER-2 receptor.[61,62] Three conjugated monoclonal antibodies have FDA approval: gemtuzumab ozogamicin (Mylotarg), a humanized antibody combined with an antitumor antibiotic; ibritumomab tiuxetan (Zevalin), a murine MoAb combined with a radioisotope; and tositumomab, a murine anti-CD20 MoAb bonded to radioactive iodine-131.[61]

Hematopoietic growth factors are growth and maturation factors that include the colony-stimulating factors (CSFs). The CSFs are factors that control the production of neutrophils and monocytes-macrophages, erythrocytes, and thrombopoietin.

Targeted Therapy

Researchers have been working diligently to produce drugs that target the processes of cancer cells specifically, leaving normal cells unharmed.[63] The characteristics and capabilities of cancer cells have been used to establish a framework for the development of such targeted agents. The first targeted therapies were the monoclonal antibodies. Researchers now are designing new drugs that can disrupt the molecular signaling pathways. The protein tyrosine kinases are intrinsic components of the signaling pathways for growth factors involved in the proliferation of lymphocytes and other cell types. Imatinib mesylate (Gleevec) is a protein tyrosine kinase inhibitor indicated in the treatment of chronic myeloid leukemia.[64] Gefitinib (Iressa), another tyrosine kinase inhibitor, is approved for the treatment of small cell lung cancer.[65] Thalidomide is one example of an antiangiogenic agent, developed to interfere with tumor neovascularization.[66] Its use as an antiangiogenic agent was suggested when researchers considered that the characteristic phocomelia ("seal limbs") produced by its use during pregnancy may have resulted from toxicity to vessels in the fetal limb buds. Cancer vaccines attempt to harness the body's immune system antigen recognition to boost tumor response rates. A number of vaccines for melanoma and prostate cancer are in research development.[64]

Bone Marrow and Peripheral Blood Stem Cell Transplantation

Bone marrow transplantation (BMT) and peripheral blood stem cell transplantation (PBSCT) are two treatment approaches for individuals with leukemias, certain solid tumors, and other cancers previously thought to be incurable. Both BMT and PBSCT involve high-dose chemotherapy and radiation therapy that are either marrow ablative (for hematologic cancers) or marrow suppressive (for solid tumors), followed by hematopoietic rescue.[67] BMT utilizes stem cells obtained from bone marrow, whereas PBSCT obtains stem cells through apheresis of the peripheral blood. Transplantation techniques can identify the source of the marrow or peripheral stem cells as *allogeneic,* in which the recipient receives stem cells from another person whose human leukocyte antigen (HLA) matches; *syngeneic,* in which the donor is an identical twin; and *autologous,* in which the recipient's own bone marrow or stem cells are used.

Allogeneic transplantation is used primarily to treat leukemia, lymphomas, and aplastic anemia. Advances in transplant medicine, such as supportive measures that include platelet administration, graft-versus-host disease pretreatment and prophylaxis, and hematopoietic growth factors, have increased survival and outcomes for patients. Autologous transplants are used for certain hematologic malignancies such as Hodgkin's and non-Hodgkin's lymphomas, and for some solid tumors such as neuroblastoma and testicular cancer. The primary goal of auto-BMT is to administer high-dose chemotherapy for maximum tumoricidal effect while providing a hematologic rescue to decrease the potentially fatal hematologic side effects.[68]

PBSCT, an alternative to BMT, uses the patient's peripheral blood stem cells to repopulate the bone marrow after extensive high-dose chemotherapy. It is a treatment option when there may be bone marrow abnormalities such as metastases or hypocellularity. PBSCT has been found to be more advantageous than BMT for a number of reasons. Stem cells can be harvested by apheresis techniques, which are less invasive and do not require general anesthesia. PBSCT is an outpatient procedure that is easier and safer for the patient and approximately half the cost of BMT. The period of aplasia after high-dose chemotherapy is shorter, thereby reducing the risks associated with granulocytopenia, the number of transfusions required, and the intensive supportive care needed during BMT. Despite the apparent advantages this technique has to offer, some disadvantages exist. Fewer pluripotent stem cells are contained in the peripheral blood; therefore, chemotherapy and growth factors must be given to mobilize sufficient stem cells for harvest by leukapheresis. There also may be the risk for infusing malignant cells, although this risk is less than with auto-BMT. PBSCT is rapidly becoming the preferred hematopoietic transplantation. Although the indications for PBSCT and the outcomes are similar to those of BMT, formal research and studies indicate some differences in rationale and outcomes.[67] Research is being undertaken to investigate the efficacy of PBSCT in fetal therapy, sequential PBSCTs in patients with residual disease, treatments involving combinations of PBSCT and auto-BMT, and the use of growth factors for cell mobilization to improve the quantity of cells harvested at one pheresis session.[69]

In summary, the methods used in the diagnosis of cancer vary with the type of cancer and its location. Because many cancers are curable if diagnosed early, health care practices designed to promote early detection are important. These practices include breast self-examination in the female, testicular self-examination in the male, and consulting a physician when any of the early warning signals of cancer are present. Pap smears, tissue biopsies, and tumor markers are used to detect the presence of cancer cells and make a diagnosis. Histologic studies are done in the laboratory using cells or tissue specimens. There are two basic methods of classifying tumors: (1) grading according to the histologic or tissue characteristics, and (2) clinical staging according to spread of the disease. The TNM system for clinical staging of cancer uses tumor size, lymph node involvement, and presence of metastasis.

Treatment plans that use more than one type of therapy, often in combination, are providing cures for a number of cancers that a few decades ago had a poor prognosis, and are increasing the life expectancy in other types of cancer. Surgical procedures are more precise and less invasive, preserving organ function and resulting in better quality-of-life outcomes. Newer radiation equipment and novel radiation techniques permit greater and more controlled destruction of cancer cells while sparing normal tissues. Successes with biotherapy techniques offer hope that the body's own defenses can be used in fighting cancer. Hybridoma technology has forged the frontier of the "magic bullet," whereby therapy is targeted to specific tumor antigens. BMT and PBSCT allow for a greater tumoricidal effect while replenishing the pluripotent stem cells, thus repopulating the bone marrow and restoring immune function.

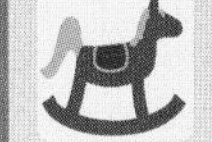

Childhood Cancers

After completing this section of the chapter, you should be able to meet the following objectives:

- Cite the early warning signs of cancer in children
- Discuss possible concerns of adult survivors of childhood cancer

In the United States, cancer is the leading cause of death in children 1 to 14 years of age.[1] The spectrum of cancers that affect children differs markedly from those that affect adults. Although most adult cancers are of epithelial cell origin (*e.g.,* lung cancer, breast cancer, colorectal cancers), childhood cancers usually involve the hematopoietic system, nervous system, or connective tissue. Leukemia accounts for 30% of the cases of childhood cancer and one third of the expected deaths.[22] Chart 8-3 lists the most common forms of solid childhood cancers.

As with adult cancers, there probably is no one cause of childhood cancer. However, many forms of childhood cancer repeat in families and may result from polygenic or single-gene inheritance, chromosomal aberrations (*e.g.,* translocations, deletions, insertions, inversions, duplications), exposure to mutagenic environmental agents, or a combination of these factors (see Chapter 7). If cancer develops in one child, the risk for cancer in siblings is approximately twice that of the general population, and if the disease develops in two children, the risk is even greater.

CHART 8-3

Common Solid Tumors of Childhood

Brain and nervous system tumors
- Medulloblastoma
- Glioma

Neuroblastoma
Wilms' tumor
Rhabdomyosarcoma and embryonal sarcoma
Retinoblastoma
Osteosarcoma
Ewing's sarcoma

Heritable forms of cancer tend to have an earlier age of onset, a higher frequency of multifocal lesions in a single organ, and bilateral involvement of paired organs or multiple primary tumors. The two-hit hypothesis has been used as one explanation of heritable cancers.[2] The first "hit" or mutation occurs prezygotically (*i.e.,* in germ cells before conception) and is present in the genetic material of all somatic cells. Cancer subsequently develops in one or several somatic cell lines that undergo a second mutation.

Children with heritable disorders are at increased risk for developing certain forms of cancer. For example, Down syndrome is associated with increased risk for leukemia; primary immunodeficiency disorders are associated with lymphoma, leukemia, and brain cancer; and xeroderma pigmentosum is associated with basal and squamous cell carcinoma and melanoma.

DIAGNOSIS AND TREATMENT

The early diagnosis of childhood cancers often is overlooked because the signs and symptoms often are similar to those of common childhood diseases and because cancer occurs less frequently in children than in adults.[70] Symptoms of prolonged fever, unexplained weight loss, and growing masses (especially in association with weight loss) should be viewed as warning signs of cancer in children. Diagnosis of childhood cancers involves many of the same methods that are used in adults. Accurate disease staging is especially beneficial in childhood cancers, in which the potential benefits of treatment must be carefully weighed against potential long-term effects.

The treatment of childhood cancers is complex, intensive, prolonged, and continuously evolving. Improved therapy and supportive care have led to progressive increases in survival. For children younger than 14 years of age, the 5-year survival rate between 1992 and 1998 for all cancer sites was 77%; for acute lymphocytic leukemia, 85%; for bone and joint cancer, 73%; for neuroblastoma, 69%; for brain and central nervous system, 70%; for Wilms' tumor, 90%; and for Hodgkin's disease, 94%.[1]

ADULT SURVIVORS OF CHILDHOOD CANCER

With improvement in treatment methods, the number of children who survive childhood cancer is continuing to increase. Almost 75% of childhood cancer survivors will be alive at 5 years, and the 10-year survival rate is approaching 70%.[71] Unfortunately, therapy may produce late sequelae, such as impaired growth, neurologic dysfunction, hormonal dysfunction, cardiomyopathy, pulmonary fibrosis, and risk for second malignancies. Although cures for large numbers of children have been possible only since the 1970s, much already is known about the potential for delayed effects.

Children reaching adulthood after cancer therapy may have reduced physical stature because of the therapy they received, particularly radiation, which retards the growth of normal tissues along with cancer tissue. The younger the age and the higher the radiation dose, the greater the deviation from normal growth. There also is concern that central nervous system radiation as a prophylactic measure in childhood leukemia has an effect on cognition and learning. Children younger than 6 years of age at the time of radiation and those receiving the highest radiation doses are most likely to have subsequent cognitive difficulties.

Delayed sexual maturation in both boys and girls can result from irradiation of the gonads. Delayed sexual maturation also is related to treatment of children with alkylating agents. Cranial irradiation may result in premature menarche in girls, with subsequent early closure of the epiphysis and a reduction in final growth achieved. Data related to fertility and health of the offspring of childhood cancer survivors is just becoming available.

Vital organs such as the heart and lungs may be affected by cancer treatment. Children who received anthracyclines (*i.e.,* doxorubicin or daunorubicin) may be at risk for developing cardiomyopathy and congestive heart failure. Pulmonary irradiation may cause lung dysfunction and restrictive lung disease. Drugs such as bleomycin, methotrexate, and bisulfan also can cause lung disease.

For survivors of childhood cancers, the risk for second cancers is reported to range from 3% to 12%. There is a special risk for second cancers in children with the retinoblastoma gene. Because of this risk, children who have been treated for cancer should be seen routinely for long-term follow-up.[72]

In summary, although most adult cancers are of epithelial cell origin, most childhood cancers usually involve the hematopoietic system, nervous system, or connective tissue. Heritable forms of cancer tend to have an earlier age of onset, a higher frequency of multifocal lesions in a single organ, and bilateral involvement of paired organs or multiple primary tumors. The early diagnosis of childhood cancers often is overlooked because the signs and symptoms mimic those of other childhood diseases. With improvement in treatment methods, the number of children who survive childhood cancer is continuing to increase. As these children approach adulthood, there is continued concern that the life-saving therapy they received during childhood may produce late effects, such as impaired growth, neurologic dysfunction, hormonal dysfunction, cardiomyopathy, pulmonary fibrosis, and risk for second malignancies.

REVIEW EXERCISES

A 30-year-old woman has experienced heavy menstrual bleeding and is told she has a uterine tumor called a *leiomyoma*. She is worried that this means she has cancer.

A. What is the difference between a leiomyoma and a leiomyosarcoma?

B. How would you go about explaining the difference to her?

The American Cancer Society recommends that all women have a yearly Pap test to screen for cervical cancer.

A. Use the characteristics of cancer cells to explain how this relatively simple test can be used as a screening method for cervical cancer.

A 48-year-old man presents at his health care clinic with complaints of leg weakness. He is a heavy smoker and has had a productive morning cough for years. Subsequent diagnostic tests reveal that he has small cell lung cancer with brain metastasis. His proposed plan of treatment includes chemotherapy and radiation therapy.

A. What is the probable cause of the leg weakness and is it related to his cancer?

B. Relate concepts of this man's smoking history to the development of lung cancer.

C. Explain the mechanism of cancer metastasis.

D. Explain the mechanisms whereby chemotherapy and irradiation destroy cancer cells.

References

1. Jemal A., Murray T., Samuels, A. et al. (2003). Cancer statistics, 2000. *CA: A Cancer Journal for Clinicians 53,* 5–26.
2. Kumar V., Cotran R.S., Robbins S.L. (Eds.) (2003). Neoplasia. In *Basic pathology* (7th ed., pp. 165–210). Philadelphia: W.B. Saunders.
3. Kasten M.B., Skopek S.X. (2001). Molecular basis of cancer: The cell cycle. In DeVita V.T. Jr., Hellman S., Rosenberg S.A. (Eds.), *Cancer: Principles and practice of oncology* (6th ed., pp. 91–108). Philadelphia: Lippincott Williams & Wilkins.
4. Martenez-Hernandez A. (2001). Repair, regeneration, and fibrosis. In Rubin E. (Ed.), *Essential pathology* (3rd ed., pp. 47–51). Philadelphia: Lippincott Williams & Wilkins.
5. Lee W.M.F., Dang C.V. (2000). Control of cell growth and differentiation. In Hoffman R., Benz E.K., Shattil S J., et al. (Eds.), *Hematology: Basic principles and practice* (3rd ed., pp. 57–71). New York: Churchill Livingstone.
6. Mitchel R.N., Cotran R.S. (2003). Tissue repair, cell regeneration, and fibrosis. In *Basic pathology* (7th ed., pp. 61–78). Philadelphia: W.B. Saunders.
7. Rubin E., Farber J.L. (1999). Neoplasia. In Rubin E., Hall J.E. *Pathology* (3rd ed., 155–211) Philadelphia: Lippincott-Raven.
8. Stetler W.G., Kliener D.E. (2001). Molecular biology of cancer: Invasion and metastasis. In DeVita V.T. Jr., Hellman S., Rosenberg S.A. (Eds.). *Cancer: Principles and practice of oncology* (6th ed., pp. 121–136). Philadelphia: Lippincott Williams & Wilkins.
9. Liotta L.A. (1992). Cancer cell invasion and metastasis. *Scientific American 266*(2), 54–63.
10. Yaeger T.E., Brady L.W. (2001). Basis for current major therapies in cancer. In Lenhard R.E., Osteen R.T., Gansler T. (Eds.), *The American Cancer Society's clinical oncology* (pp. 159–229). Atlanta: American Cancer Society.
11. Heath C.W., Fontham E.T. (2001). Cancer etiology. In Lenhard R.E., Osteen R.T., Gansler T. (Eds.), *American Cancer Society's clinical oncology* (9th ed., pp. 38–54). Atlanta: American Cancer Society.
12. Zhou B.P., Hung M.C. (2003). Dysregulation of cellular signaling by HER2/neu in breast cancer. *Seminars in Oncology 30*(5 Suppl. 16), 38–48.
13. Levine A.J. (1996). Tumor suppressor genes. In Pusztai L., Lewis C.E., Yap E. (Eds.), *Cell proliferation in cancer: Regulatory mechanisms of neoplastic cell growth* (pp. 86–104). Oxford: Oxford University Press.
14. Pusztai L., Cooper K. (1996). Introduction: Cell proliferation and carcinogenesis. In Pusztai L., Lewis C.E., Yap E. (Eds.), *Cell proliferation in cancer: Regulatory mechanisms of neoplastic cell growth* (pp. 3–24), Oxford: Oxford University Press.
15. Emory University. (2002). *Cancerquest.* [On-line]. Available: http://www.cancerquest.org. Retrieved December 14, 2003.
16. Knudson A.G. (1974). Heredity and human cancer. *American Journal of Pathology 77,* 77–84.
17. Cole P., Rodu B. (2001). Analytic epidemiology: Cancer causes. In DeVita V.T. Jr., Hellman S., Rosenberg S.A. (Eds.), *Cancer: Principles and practice of oncology* (6th ed., pp. 241–252). Philadelphia: Lippincott Williams & Wilkins.
18. Burnett F.M. (1967). Immunologic aspects of malignant disease. *Lancet 1,* 1171.
19. Beverley P. (1996). Tumor immunology. In Roitt I., Brostoff J., Male D. (Eds.), *Immunology* (4th ed., pp. 20.1–20.8). London: Mosby.
20. Greenberg P.D. (1997). Mechanisms of tumor immunology. In Roitt I., Brostoff J., Male D. (Eds.), *Medical immunology* (9th ed., pp. 631–639). Stamford, CT: Appleton & Lange.
21. Stellman J.M., Stellman S.D. (1996). Cancer and the workplace. *CA: A Cancer Journal for Clinicians 46,* 70–92.
22. American Cancer Society. (2003). *American Cancer Society facts and figures: 2003.* Atlanta, GA: Author.
23. Willett W.C. (2001). Cancer prevention: Diet and chemopreventive agents. In DeVita V.T. Jr., Hellman S., Rosenberg S.A. (Eds.), *Cancer: Principles and practice of oncology* (6th ed., pp. 561–614). Philadelphia: Lippincott Williams & Wilkins.
24. Poskanzer D.C., Herbst A. (1977). Epidemiology of vaginal adenosis and adenocarcinoma associated with exposure to stilbestrol in utero. *Cancer 39,* 1892–1895.
25. Jablon S., Kato H. (1972). Studies of the mortality of A-bomb survivors: 5. Radiation dose and mortality, 1950–1970. *Radiation Research 50,* 649–698.
26. Ruddon R.W. (Ed.) (1995). *Cancer biology* (pp. 3–60, 141–276). New York and Oxford: Oxford University Press.
27. Poeschla E.M., Wong-Staal F. (2001). Etiology of cancer: Viruses. In DeVita V.T. Jr., Hellman S., Rosenberg S.A. (Eds.), *Cancer: Principles and practice of oncology* (6th ed., pp. 149–178). Philadelphia: Lippincott Williams & Wilkins.
28. Imui A. (2002). Cancer anorexia-cachexia syndrome: Current issues in research and management. *CA: A Cancer Journal for Clinicians 52*(2), 72–91.
29. Rubin H. (2003). Cancer cachexia: Its correlations and causes. *Proceedings of the National Academy of Science 100*(9), 5384–5389.
30. Zumsteg M.M., Casperson D.S. (1998). Paraneoplastic syndromes in metastatic disease. *Seminars in Oncology Nursing 14*(3), 220–229.

31. Rosenthal P.E. (2001). Paraneoplastic and endocrine syndromes. In Lenhard R.E., Osteen R.T., Gansler T. (Eds.), *The American Cancer Society's clinical oncology* (pp. 721–732). Atlanta: American Cancer Society.
32. Shoback D., Funk J. (2001). Humoral manifestations of malignancy. In Greenspan F.S., Gardner D.G. (Eds.), *Basic and clinical endocrinology* (6th ed., 778–791). New York: McGraw-Hill.
33. Darnell R.B., Posner J.B. (2003). Paraneoplastic syndromes involving the nervous system. *New England Journal of Medicine 349*(16), 1543–1554.
34. Pfiefer J.D., Wick M.R. (2001). Pathologic evaluation of neoplastic diseases. In Lenhard R.E., Osteen R.T., Gansler T. (Eds.), *The American Cancer Society's clinical oncology* (pp. 123–147). Atlanta: American Cancer Society.
35. Green F.L., Page D.L., Fleming I.D. (2002). *AJCC cancer staging manual* (6th ed). New York: Springer-Verlag.
36. Rosenberg S.A. (2001). Cancer management: Principles of surgical oncology. In DeVita V.T. Jr., Hellman S., Rosenberg S.A. (Eds.), *Cancer: Principles and practice of oncology* (6th ed., pp. 253–264). Philadelphia: Lippincott Williams & Wilkins.
37. Bland K.B. (1997). Quality-of-life management for cancer patients. *CA: A Cancer Journal for Clinicians 47,* 194–197.
38. Dunne-Daly C.F. (1999). Principles of radiotherapy and radiobiology. *Seminars in Oncology Nursing 15*(4), 250–259.
39. Holden S.N., Rabinovitch R.A. (1999). Radiation therapy: An overview of fundamental concepts. *Highlights in Oncology Practice 17*(3), 48–53.
40. Hilderley L.J., Dow K.H. (1996). Radiation oncology. In McCorkle R., Grant M., Frank-Stromborg M., Baird S.B. (Eds.), *Cancer nursing: A comprehensive textbook* (2nd ed., pp. 331–358). Philadelphia: W.B. Saunders.
41. Hall E.J., Cox J.D. (1994). Physical and biologic basis of radiation therapy. In Cox J.D. (Ed.), *Moss' radiation oncology: Rationale, technique, results* (7th ed., pp. 3–66), St. Louis: Mosby.
42. Boelsen R., Jamar S. (2000). Advances in radiation oncology. *Oncology Nursing Updates 7*(3), 1–11.
43. Nicolaou N. (1999). Radiation therapy treatment planning and delivery. *Seminars in Oncology Nursing 15*(4), 260–269.
44. Kelly L.D. (1999). Nursing assessment and patient management. *Seminars in Oncology Nursing 15*(4), 282–291.
45. Miaskowski C., Viele C. (1999). Cancer chemotherapy. In *Oncology nursing assessment and clinical care* (pp. 83–106). St. Louis: Mosby.
46. Cooper M.R., Cooper M.R. (2001). Basis for current major therapies for cancer: Systemic therapy. In Lenhard R.E., Osteen R.T., Gansler T (Eds.), *The American Cancer Society's clinical oncology* (pp. 175–215). Atlanta: American Cancer Society.
47. Bogner J.R., Kronawitter U., Rolinski B., et al. (1994). Liposomal doxorubicin in the treatment of advanced AIDS-related Kaposi's sarcoma. *Journal of Acquired Immune Deficiency Syndrome 7,* 463–468.
48. Schnell F.M. (2003). Chemotherapy-induced nausea and vomiting: The importance of acute antiemetic control. *Oncologist 8,* 187–198.
49. Grant M., Ropka M.E. (1996). Alterations in nutrition. In McCorkle R., Grant M., Frank-Stromborg M., Baird S.B. (Eds.), *Cancer nursing: A comprehensive textbook* (2nd ed., pp. 919–943), Philadelphia: W.B. Saunders.
50. Oncology Nursing Society. (2002). *Cancer chemotherapy and biotherapy guidelines recommendations for practice.* Pittsburgh: Oncology Nursing Society.
51. U.S. Department of Labor, Office of Occupational Medicine, Occupational Safety and Health Administration (OSHA). (1986). *Work practice guidelines for personnel dealing with cytotoxic (antineoplastic) drugs.* Publication no. 8-1.1. Washington, DC: Author.
52. Polovich M., (2003). *Safe handling of hazardous drugs.* Pittsburgh: Oncology Nursing Society.
53. Pederson-Bjergaard J., Larson S.O. (1982). Incidence of acute nonlymphocytic leukemia, preleukemia and acute myeloproliferative syndrome up to 10 years after treatment of Hodgkin's disease. *New England Journal of Medicine 307,* 964–971.
54. Coltman C.A. Jr., Dixon D.O. (1982). Second malignancies complicating Hodgkin's disease: A Southwest Oncology Group 10 year followup. *Cancer Treatment Reports 66,* 1023–1033.
55. Boise J.D., Green M.H., Killen J.Y., et al. (1983). Leukemia, and preleukemia after adjuvant treatment of gastrointestinal cancer with semustine. *New England Journal of Medicine 309,* 1079–1084.
56. Hawkins R. (2002). Hormone therapy in cancer. *Oncology Nursing Updates 9*(3), 1–16.
57. DeMeyer E., Stein B.A. (1999). Biotherapy. In Miakowski C., Buchsel P. (Eds.), *Oncology nursing: Assessment and clinical care* (pp. 119–141). St. Louis: Mosby.
58. Reiger P.T. (2001). Biotherapy: An overview. In Reiger P.T. (Ed.), *Biotherapy: A comprehensive overview* (2nd ed., pp. 3–37) Sudbury, MA: Jones and Bartlett.
59. Kirkwood J.M. (2001). Interferons. In DeVita V.T. Jr., Hellman S., Rosenberg S.A. (Eds.), *Cancer: Principles and practice of oncology* (7th ed., pp. 461–471). Philadelphia: Lippincott Williams & Wilkins.
60. Mier J.W., Atkins M.B. (2001). Interleukin-2. In DeVita V.T. Jr., Hellman S., Rosenberg S.A. (Eds.), *Cancer: Principles and practice of oncology* (7th ed., pp. 471–478). Philadelphia: Lippincott Williams & Wilkins.
61. Schmidt K.V., Wood B.A. (2003). Trends in cancer therapy: Role of monoclonal antibodies. *Seminars in Oncology Nursing 19*(3), 169–179.
62. Von Mehren M., Adams G.P., Weiner L.M. (2003). Monoclonal antibody therapy for cancer. *Annual Review of Medicine 54,* 343–369.
63. Gemmill R., Idell C.S. (2003). Biological advances for new treatment approaches. *Seminars in Oncology Nursing 19*(3), 162–168.
64. Davey M.P. (2002). Imatinib mesylate. *Clinical Journal of Oncology Nursing 6*(2), 118–120.
65. Gale D.M. (2003). Molecular targets in cancer therapy. *Seminars in Oncology Nursing 19*(3), 193–205.
66. Waldman A.R. (2000). Thalidomide. *Clinical Journal of Oncology Nursing 4*(2), 99–100.
67. Buchsel P.C. Kapustay P.M. (2000). *Stem cell transplantation: A clinical textbook* (pp. 1.3–1.81, 2.3–2.23) Pittsburgh: Oncology Nursing Society.
68. Whedon M.B. (1995). Bone marrow transplantation nursing: Into the twenty-first century. In Buchsel P.C., Whedon M.B. (Eds.), *Bone marrow transplantation: Administrative and clinical strategies* (pp. 1–18). Boston: Jones and Bartlett.
69. Kessinger A. (2000). Reestablishing hematopoiesis with peripheral stem cells. In Armitage J.O., Antman K.H. (Eds.), *High-dose cancer therapy: Pharmacology, hematopoietins, stem cells* (3rd ed., pp. 273–282). Philadelphia: Lippincott Williams & Wilkins.
70. Behrman R.E., Kliegman R.M., Jensen H.B. (Eds.) (2004). *Nelson textbook of pediatrics* (17th ed., pp. 1679–1693). Philadelphia: W.B. Saunders.
71. Rowland J.H., Asis N., Tesauro G., et al. (2001). The changing face of cancer survivorship. *Seminar in Oncology Nursing 17*(4), 236–240.
72. Ward J.D. (2001). Pediatric cancer survivors. *Nurse Practitioner 26*(12), 18–37.

UNIT III

Integrative Body Functions

French physiologist Claude Bernard (1813–1878) was the first to theorize that, in a closely orchestrated process, the body strives to achieve and maintain a steady state. In the middle of the 19th century, Bernard proposed his concept of the *milieu intèrieur,* or the stable internal environment, regulated by a multitude of interacting control mechanisms geared to maintain the body's chemical and physical status. He proposed that internal secretions functioned as a part of the body's regulatory mechanism, maintaining a balance in response to a range of changing conditions imposed by the external environment.

Through his experiments, Bernard discovered a number of mechanisms that were dedicated to maintaining homeostasis. One of his discoveries was the process by which internal temperature is kept constant. He was able to show that the nervous system responds to internal cold by sending chemical messages to the blood vessels to constrict in order to conserve body heat. The product of his considerable work is the classic *Introduction to the Study of Experimental Medicine* (1865).

CHAPTER

9

Stress and Adaptation

Mary Pat Kunert

Stress has become an increasingly discussed topic in today's world. The concept is discussed extensively in the health care fields, and it is found as well in economics, political science, business, and education. At the level of the popular press, the term is exploited with messages about how stress can be prevented, managed, and even eliminated.

Whether stress is more prevalent today than it was in centuries past is uncertain. Certainly, the pressures that existed in the past were equally challenging, although of a different type. Social psychologists Richard Lazarus and Susan Folkman related that as early as the 14th century, the term was used to indicate hardship, straits, adversity, or affliction.[1] In the 17th century, *stress* and related terms appeared in the context of physical sciences: *load* was defined as an external force, *stress* as the ratio of internal force created by the load to the area over which the force acted, and *strain* as the deformation or distortion of the object.[1] These concepts are still used in engineering today.

The concepts of stress and strain survived, and throughout the 19th and early 20th centuries, stress and strain were thought to be the cause of "ill health" and "mental disease."[2] By the 20th century, stress had drawn considerable attention both as a health concern and as a research focus. In 1910, when Sir William Osler delivered his Lumleian Lectures on "Angina Pectoris," he described the relationship of stress and strain to angina pectoris.[3] Approximately 15 years later, Walter Cannon, well known for his work in physiology, began to use the word *stress* in relation to his laboratory experiments on the "fight-or-flight" response. It seems possible that the term emerged from his work with the homeostatic features of living organisms and their tendency to "bound back" and "resist disruption" when acted on by an "external force."[4] At about the same time, Hans Selye, who became known for his research and publications on stress, began using the term *stress* in a very special way to mean an orchestrated set of bodily responses to any form of noxious stimulus.[5]

The content in this chapter has been organized into three sections: homeostasis, the stress response and adaptation to stress, and disorders of the stress response.

Homeostasis

After completing this section of the chapter, you should be able to meet the following objectives:

- Cite Cannon's four features of homeostasis
- Describe the components of a control system, including the function of a negative feedback system

The concepts of stress and adaptation have their origin in the complexity of the human body and the interactions between the body cells and its many organ systems. These interactions require that a level of homeostasis or constancy be maintained during the many changes that occur in the internal and external environments. In effecting a state of constancy, homeostasis requires feedback control systems that regulate cellular function and integrate the function of the different body systems.

HOMEOSTASIS

- Homeostasis is the purposeful maintenance of a stable internal environment maintained by coordinated physiologic processes that oppose change.
- The physiologic control systems that oppose change operate by negative feedback mechanisms that are composed of a sensor that detects a change, an integrator/comparator that sums and compares incoming data with a set point, and an effector system that returns the sensed function to within the range of the set point.

CONSTANCY OF THE INTERNAL ENVIRONMENT

The environment in which body cells live is not the external environment that surrounds the organism, but rather the local fluid environment that surrounds each cell. Claude Bernard, a 19th century physiologist, was the first to describe clearly the central importance of a stable internal environment, which he termed the *milieu intèrieur.* Bernard recognized that body fluids surrounding the cells and the various organ systems provide the means for exchange between the external and the internal environments. It is from this internal environment that body cells receive their nourishment, and it is into this fluid that they secrete their wastes. Even the contents of the gastrointestinal tract and lungs do not become part of the internal environment until they have been absorbed into the extracellular fluid. A multicellular organism is able to survive only as long as the composition of the internal environment is compatible with the survival needs of the individual cells. For example, even a small change in the pH of the body fluids can disrupt the metabolic processes of individual cells.

The concept of a stable internal environment was supported by Walter B. Cannon, who proposed that this kind of stability, which he called *homeostasis,* was achieved through a system of carefully coordinated physiologic processes that oppose change.[6] Cannon pointed out that these processes were largely automatic and emphasized that homeostasis involves resistance to both internal and external disturbances.

In his book *Wisdom of the Body,* published in 1939, Cannon presented four tentative propositions to describe the general features of homeostasis.[6] With this set of propositions, Cannon emphasized that when a factor is known to shift homeostasis in one direction, it is reasonable to expect the existence of mechanisms that have the opposite effect. In the homeostatic regulation of blood sugar, for example, mechanisms that both raise and lower blood sugar would be expected to play a part. As long as the responding mechanism to the initiating disturbance can recover homeostasis, the integrity of the body and the status of normality are retained.

Constancy of the Internal Environment

1. Constancy in an open system, such as our bodies represent, requires mechanisms that act to maintain this constancy. Cannon based this proposition on insights into the ways by which steady states such as glucose concentrations, body temperature, and acid-base balance were regulated.
2. Steady-state conditions require that any tendency toward change automatically meets with factors that resist change. An increase in blood sugar results in thirst as the body attempts to dilute the concentration of sugar in the extracellular fluid.
3. The regulating system that determines the homeostatic state consists of a number of cooperating mechanisms acting simultaneously or successively. Blood sugar is regulated by insulin, glucagon, and other hormones that control its release from the liver or its uptake by the tissues.
4. Homeostasis does not occur by chance, but is the result of organized self-government.

(Cannon W.B. [1932]. *The wisdom of the body* (pp. 299–300). New York: W.W. Norton)

CONTROL SYSTEMS

The ability of the body to function and maintain homeostasis under conditions of change in the internal and external environment depends on the thousands of physiologic *control systems* that regulate body function. A homeostatic control system consists of a collection of interconnected components that function to keep a physical or chemical parameter of the body relatively constant. The body's control systems regulate cellular function, control life processes, and integrate functions of the different organ systems.

Of recent interest have been the neuroendocrine control systems that influence behavior. Biochemical messengers that exist in our brain serve to control nerve activity, regulate information flow, and, ultimately, influence behavior.[7] These control systems function in producing the emotional reactions to stressors. In persons with mental health disorders, they can interact in the production of symptoms associated with the disorder. The field of neuropharmacology has focused on the modulation of the endogenous messengers and signaling systems that control behavior in the treatment of mental disorders such as anxiety disorders, depression, and schizophrenia.

Feedback Systems

Most control systems in the body operate by *negative feedback mechanisms,* which function in a manner similar to the thermostat on a heating system. When the monitored function or value decreases below the set point of the system, the feedback mechanism causes the function or value to increase; and when the function or value is increased

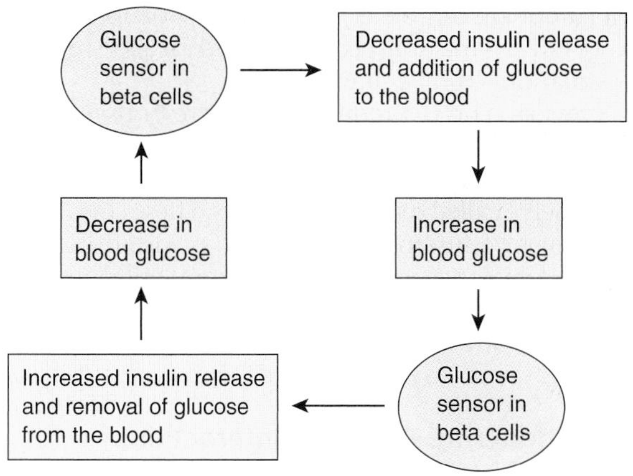

FIGURE 9-1 Illustration of negative feedback control mechanisms using blood glucose as an example.

above the set point, the feedback mechanism causes it to decrease (Fig. 9-1). For example, in the negative feedback mechanism that controls blood glucose levels, an increase in blood glucose stimulates an increase in insulin, which enhances the removal of glucose from the blood. When sufficient glucose has left the bloodstream to cause blood glucose levels to fall, insulin secretion is inhibited, and glucagon and other counterregulatory mechanisms stimulate the release of glucose from the liver, which causes the blood glucose to return to normal.

The reason most physiologic control systems function under negative rather than *positive feedback mechanisms* is that a positive feedback mechanism interjects instability rather than stability into a system. It produces a cycle in which the initiating stimulus produces more of the same. For example, in a positive feedback system, exposure to an increase in environmental temperature would invoke compensatory mechanisms designed to increase rather than decrease body temperature.

In summary, physiologic and psychological adaptation involves the ability to maintain the constancy of the internal environment (homeostasis) and behavior in the face of a wide range of changes in the internal and external environments. It involves negative feedback control systems that regulate cellular function, control life's processes, regulate behavior, and integrate the function of the different body systems.

Stress and Adaptation

After completing this section of the chapter, you should be able to meet the following objectives:

- State Selye's definition of stress
- Define *stressor*
- Cite two factors that influence the nature of the stress response
- Explain the interactions among components of the nervous system in mediating the stress response
- Describe the stress responses of the autonomic nervous system, the endocrine system, the immune system, and the musculoskeletal system
- Explain the purpose of adaptation
- List at least six factors that influence a person's adaptive capacity
- Relate experience and previous learning to the process of adaptation
- Contrast anatomic and physiologic reserve
- Propose a way by which social support may serve to buffer challenges to adaptation

The increased focus on health promotion has heightened interest in the roles of stress and biobehavioral stress responses in the development of disease.[8] Stress may contribute directly to the production or exacerbation of a disease, or it may contribute to the development of behaviors such as smoking, overeating, and drug abuse that increase the risk for disease.[9]

THE STRESS RESPONSE

In the early 1930s, the world-renowned endocrinologist Hans Selye was the first to describe a group of specific anatomic changes that occurred in rats that were exposed to a variety of different experimental stimuli. He came to an understanding that these changes were manifestations of the body's attempt to adapt to stimuli. Selye described *stress* as "a state manifested by a specific syndrome of the body developed in response to any stimuli that made an intense systemic demand on it."[10] As a young medical student, Selye noticed that patients with diverse disease conditions had many signs and symptoms in common. He observed that "whether a man suffers from a loss of blood, an infectious disease, or advanced cancer, he loses his appetite, his muscular strength, and his ambition to accomplish anything; usually the patient also loses weight and even his facial expression betrays that he is ill."[11] Selye referred to this as the "syndrome of just being sick."

In his early career as an experimental scientist, Selye noted that a triad of adrenal enlargement, thymic atrophy, and gastric ulcer appeared in rats he was using for his studies. These same three changes developed in response to many different or nonspecific experimental challenges. He assumed that the hypothalamic-pituitary-adrenal (HPA) axis played a pivotal role in the development of this response. To Selye, the response to stressors was a process that enabled the rats to resist the experimental challenge by using the function of the system best able to respond to it. He labeled the response the *general adaptation syndrome* (GAS): *general* because the effect was a general systemic reaction, *adaptive* because the response was in reaction to a stressor, and *syndrome* because the physical manifestations were coordinated and dependent on each other.[10]

According to Selye, the GAS involves three stages: the alarm stage, the resistance stage, and exhaustion stage. The *alarm stage* is characterized by a generalized stimulation of the sympathetic nervous system and the HPA axis, resulting in the release of catecholamines and cortisol. During the *resistance stage,* the body selects the most effective and economic channels of defense. During this stage, the increased cortisol levels present during the first stage drop because they are no longer needed. If the stressor is prolonged or overwhelms the ability of the body to defend itself, the *exhaustion stage* ensues, during which resources are depleted and signs of "wear and tear" or systemic damage appear.[12] Selye contended that many ailments, such as various emotional disturbances, mildly annoying headaches, insomnia, upset stomach, gastric and duodenal ulcers, certain types of rheumatic disorders, and cardiovascular and kidney diseases appear to be initiated or encouraged by the "body itself because of its faulty adaptive reactions to potentially injurious agents."[11]

The events or environmental agents responsible for initiating the stress response were called *stressors*. According to Selye, stressors could be endogenous, arising from within the body, or exogenous, arising from outside the body.[11] In explaining the stress response, Selye proposed that two factors determine the nature of the stress response: the properties of the stressor and the conditioning of the person being stressed. Selye indicated that not all stress was detrimental; hence, he coined the terms *eustress* and *distress*.[12] He suggested that mild, brief, and controllable periods of stress could be perceived as positive stimuli to emotional and intellectual growth and development. It is the severe, protracted, and uncontrolled situations of psychological and physical distress that are disruptive of health.[11] For example, the joy of becoming a new parent and the sorrow of losing a parent are completely different experiences, yet their stressor effect—the nonspecific demand for adjustment to a new situation—can be similar.

Stressors tend to produce different responses in different persons or in the same person at different times, indicating the influence of the adaptive capacity of the person, or what Selye called *conditioning factors*. These conditioning factors may be internal (*e.g.,* genetic predisposition, age, sex) or external (*e.g.,* exposure to environmental agents, life experiences, dietary factors, level of social support).[11] The relative risk for development of a stress-related pathologic process seems, at least in part, to depend on these factors.

Neuroendocrine–Immune Interactions

The manifestations of the stress response are strongly influenced by both the nervous and endocrine systems. The neuroendocrine systems integrate signals received along neurosensory pathways and from circulating mediators that are carried in the bloodstream. In addition, the immune system both affects and is affected by the stress response. Table 9-1 summarizes the action of hormones involved in the neuroendocrine responses to stress.

The stress response is meant to protect the person against acute threats to homeostasis and is normally time limited. Therefore, under normal circumstances, the neural responses and the hormones that are released during the response are not around long enough to cause damage to vital tissues. However, in situations in which the stress response is hyperactive or becomes habituated, the physiologic and behavioral changes (*e.g.,* immunosuppression, sympathetic system activation) induced by the response can themselves become a threat to homeostasis. If the stress response is

TABLE 9-1 Hormones Involved in the Neuroendocrine Response to Stress

Hormones Associated With the Stress Response	Source of the Hormone	Physiologic Effects
Catecholamines (norepinephrine, epinephrine)	Locus ceruleus, adrenal medulla	Produces a decrease in insulin release and an increase in glucagon release resulting in increased glycogenolysis, gluconeogenesis, lipolysis, proteolysis, and decreased glucose uptake by the peripheral tissues; an increase in heart rate, cardiac contractility, and vascular smooth muscle contraction; and relaxation of bronchial smooth muscle
Corticotropin-releasing factor (CRF)	Hypothalamus	Stimulates ACTH release from anterior pituitary and increased activity of neurons in locus ceruleus
Adrenocorticotropic hormone (ACTH)	Anterior pituitary	Stimulates the synthesis and release of cortisol
Glucocorticoid hormones (*e.g.,* cortisol)	Adrenal cortex	Potentiates the actions of epinephrine and glucagon; inhibits the release and/or actions of the reproductive hormones and thyroid-stimulating hormone; and produces a decrease in immune cells and inflammatory mediators
Mineralocorticoid hormones (*e.g.,* aldosterone)	Adrenal cortex	Increases sodium absorption by the kidney
Antidiuretic hormone (ADH, vasopressin)	Hypothalamus, posterior pituitary	Increases water absorption by the kidney; produces vasoconstriction of blood vessels; and stimulates the release of ACTH

hypoactive, the person may be more susceptible to diseases associated with overactivity of the immune response.[9]

Neuroendocrine Responses

The integration of the stress responses, which occurs at the level of the central nervous system (CNS), is complex and not completely understood. It relies on communication along neuronal pathways of the cerebral cortex, the limbic system, the thalamus, the hypothalamus, the pituitary gland, and the reticular activating system (RAS) (Fig. 9-2). The cerebral cortex is involved with vigilance, cognition, and focused attention, and the limbic system with emotional components (*e.g.*, fear, excitement, rage, anger) of the stress response. The thalamus functions as the relay center and is important in receiving, sorting out, and distributing sensory input. The hypothalamus coordinates the responses of the endocrine system and the autonomic nervous system (ANS). The RAS modulates mental alertness, ANS activity, and skeletal muscle tone, using input from other neural structures. The musculoskeletal tension that occurs during the stress response reflects the increased activity of the RAS and its influence on the reflex circuits that control muscle tone.

Locus Ceruleus. Central to the neural component of the neuroendocrine response to stress is an area of the brain stem called the locus ceruleus (LC).[13] The locus ceruleus is densely populated with neurons that produce norepinephrine (NE) and is thought to be the central integrating site for the ANS response to stressful stimuli (Fig. 9-3). The LC-NE system has afferent pathways to the hypothalamus, the limbic system, the hippocampus, and the cerebral cortex.

The LC-NE system confers an adaptive advantage during a stressful situation. The sympathetic nervous system manifestation of the stress reaction has been called the *fight-or-flight response*. This is the most rapid of the stress responses and represents the basic survival response of our primitive ancestors when confronted with the perils of the wilderness and its inhabitants. The increase in sympathetic activity in the brain increases attention and arousal and thus probably intensifies memory. The heart and respiratory rates increase, the hands and feet become moist, the pupils dilate, the mouth becomes dry, and the activity of the gastrointestinal tract decreases.

Corticotropin-releasing Factor. Corticotropin-releasing factor (CRF) is central to the endocrine component of the neuroendocrine response to stress (see Fig. 9-3). CRF is a small peptide hormone found in the hypothalamus and in extrahypothalamic structures, such as the limbic system and the brain stem. It is both an important endocrine regulator of pituitary and adrenal activity and a neurotransmitter involved in ANS activity, metabolism, and behavior.[9,14,15] Receptors for CRF are distributed throughout the brain as well as many peripheral sites. CRF from the hypothalamus induces the secretion of the adrenocorticotropic hormone (ACTH) from the anterior pituitary gland. ACTH, in turn, stimulates the adrenal gland to synthesize and secrete the glucocorticoid hormones (*e.g.*, cortisol).

The glucocorticoid hormones have a number of direct or indirect physiologic effects that mediate the stress response, enhance the action of other stress hormones, or suppress other components of the stress system. In this regard, cortisol acts both as a mediator of the stress response and an inhibitor of the stress response such that overactivation does not occur.[16] Cortisol maintains blood glucose levels by antagonizing the effects of insulin and enhances the effect of catecholamines on the cardiovascular system.

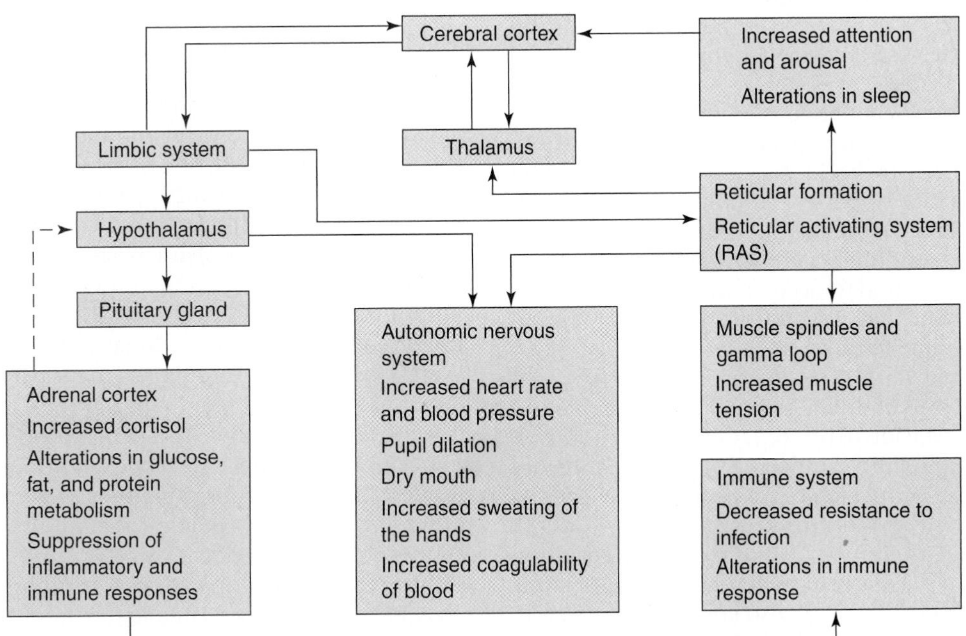

FIGURE 9-2 Stress pathways. The broken line represents negative feedback.

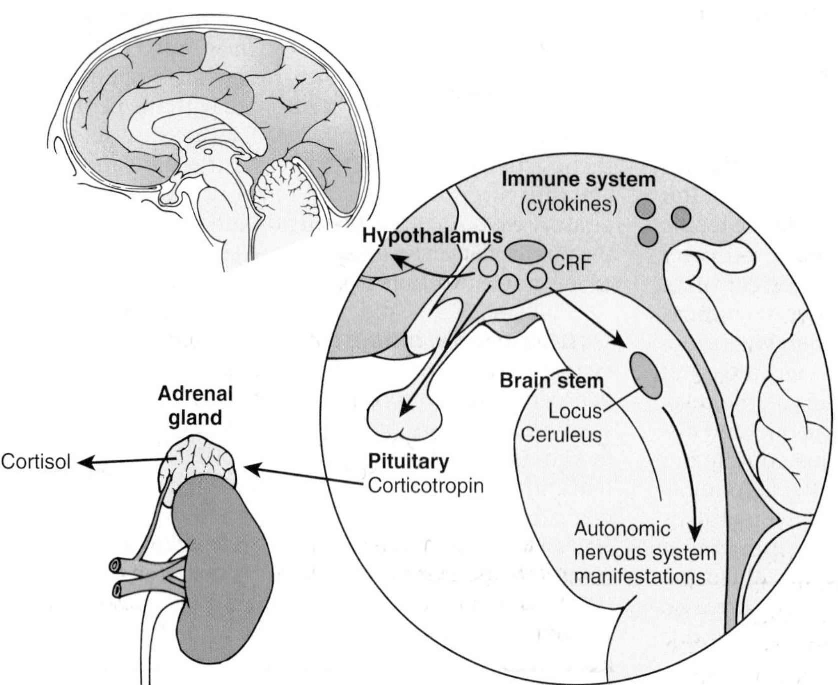

FIGURE 9-3 Neuroendocrine–immune system regulation of the stress response.

It also suppresses osteoblast activity, hematopoiesis, protein and collagen synthesis, and immune responses. All of these functions are meant to protect the organism against the effects of a stressor and to focus energy on regaining balance in the face of an acute challenge to homeostasis.

Other Hormones. A wide variety of other hormones, including growth hormones, thyroid hormone, and the reproductive hormones, also are responsive to stressful situations. Systems responsible for reproduction, growth, and immunity are directly linked to the stress system, and the hormonal effects of the stress response profoundly influence these systems.

Although growth hormone is initially elevated at the onset of stress, the prolonged presence of cortisol leads to suppression of growth hormone, somatomedin C, and other growth factors, exerting a chronically inhibitory effect on growth. In addition, CRF directly increases somatostatin, which in turn inhibits growth hormone secretion. Although the connection is speculative, the effects of stress on growth hormone may provide one of the vital links to understanding failure to thrive in children.

Stress-induced cortisol secretion also is associated with decreased levels of thyroid-stimulating hormone and inhibition of conversion of thyroxine (T_4) to the more biologically active triiodothyronine (T_3) in peripheral tissues (see Chapter 42). Both changes may serve as a means to conserve energy at times of stress.

Antidiuretic hormone (ADH) also is involved in the stress response, particularly in hypotensive stress or stress due to fluid volume loss. ADH, also known as *vasopressin,* increases water retention by the kidneys, produces vasoconstriction of blood vessels, and appears to synergize the capacity of CRF to increase the release of ACTH.

The reproductive hormones are inhibited by CRF at the hypophyseal level and by cortisol at the pituitary, gonadal, and target tissue levels.[11] Sepsis and severe trauma can induce anovulation and amenorrhea in women and decreased spermatogenesis and decreased levels of testosterone in men.

Immune Responses

The hallmark of the stress response, as first described by Selye, is the endocrine–immune interactions (*i.e.,* increased corticosteroid production and atrophy of the thymus) that are known to suppress the immune response. In concert, these two components of the stress system, through endocrine and neurotransmitter pathways, produce the physical and behavioral changes designed to adapt to acute stress. Much of the literature regarding stress and the immune response focuses on the causal role of stress in immune-related diseases. It has also been suggested that the reverse may occur; emotional and psychological manifestations of the stress response may be a reflection of alterations in the CNS resulting from the immune response (see Fig. 9-3). Immune cells such as monocytes and lymphocytes can penetrate the blood–brain barrier and take up residence in the brain, where they secrete cytokines and other inflammatory mediators that influence the stress response. In the case of cancer, this could mean that the subjective feelings of helplessness and hopelessness that have been repeatedly related to the onset and progression of cancers may arise secondary to the CNS effects of products released by immune cells during the early stage of the disease.[17]

The exact mechanism by which stress produces its effect on the immune response is unknown and probably varies from person to person, depending on genetic endowment and environmental factors. The most significant arguments for interaction between the neuroendocrine and immune systems derive from evidence that the immune and neuroendocrine systems share common signal pathways (*i.e.*, messenger molecules and receptors), that hormones and neuropeptides can alter the function of immune cells, and that the immune system and its mediators can modulate neuroendocrine function.[18] Receptors for a number of CNS-controlled hormones and neuromediators reportedly have been found on lymphocytes. Among these are receptors for glucocorticoids, insulin, testosterone, prolactin, catecholamines, estrogens, acetylcholine, and growth hormone, suggesting that these hormones influence lymphocyte function. For example, cortisol is known to suppress immune function, and pharmacologic doses of cortisol are used clinically to suppress the immune response. There is evidence that the immune system, in turn, influences neuroendocrine function.[19] It has been observed that the HPA axis is activated by cytokines such as interleukin-1, interleukin-6, and tumor necrosis factor that are released from immune cells (see Chapter 19).

A second possible route for neuroendocrine regulation of immune function is through the sympathetic nervous system and the release of catecholamines. The lymph nodes, thymus, and spleen are supplied with ANS nerve fibers. Centrally acting CRF activates the ANS through multisynaptic descending pathways, and circulating epinephrine acts synergistically with CRF and cortisol to inhibit the function of the immune system.

Not only is the quantity of immune expression changed because of stress, but also the quality of the response is changed. Stress hormones differentially stimulate the proliferation of subtypes of T lymphocyte helper cells. Because these helper T-cell subtypes secrete different cytokines, they stimulate different aspects of the immune response. One subtype tends to stimulate the cellular-mediated immune response, whereas a second type tends to activate B lymphocytes and humoral-mediated immune responses.[7]

Coping and Adaptation to Stress

The ability to adapt to a wide range of environments and stressors is not peculiar to humans. According to René Dubos (a microbiologist noted for his study of human responses to the total environment), "adaptability is found throughout life and is perhaps the one attribute that distinguishes most clearly the world of life from the world of inanimate matter."[20] Living organisms, no matter how primitive, do not submit passively to the impact of environmental forces. They attempt to respond adaptively, each in its own unique and most suitable manner. The higher the organism on the evolutionary scale, the larger its repertoire of adaptive mechanisms and its ability to select and limit aspects of the environment to which it responds. The most fully evolved mechanisms are the social responses through which individuals or groups modify their environments, their habits, or both to achieve a way of life that is best suited to their needs.

STRESS AND ADAPTATION

- Stress is a state manifested by symptoms that arise from the coordinated activation of the neuroendocrine and immune systems, which Selye called the general adaptation syndrome.
- The hormones and neurotransmitters (catecholamines and cortisol) that are released during the stress response function to alert the individual to a threat or challenge to homeostasis, to enhance cardiovascular and metabolic activity in order to manage the stressor, and to focus the energy of the body by suppressing the activity of other systems that are not immediately needed.
- Adaptation is the ability to respond to challenges of physical or psychological homeostasis and to return to a balanced state.
- The ability to adapt is influenced by previous learning, physiologic reserve, time, genetic endowment, age, health status and nutrition, sleep-wake cycles, and psychosocial factors.

Adaptation

Human beings, because of their highly developed nervous system and intellect, usually have alternative mechanisms for adapting and have the ability to control many aspects of their environment. Air conditioning and central heating limit the need to adapt to extreme changes in environmental temperature. The availability of antiseptic agents, immunizations, and antibiotics eliminates the need to respond to common infectious agents. At the same time, modern technology creates new challenges for adaptation and provides new sources of stress, such as increased noise, air pollution, exposure to harmful chemicals, and changes in biologic rhythms imposed by shift work and transcontinental air travel.

Of particular interest are the differences in the body's response to events that threaten the integrity of the body's physiologic environment and those that threaten the integrity of the person's psychosocial environment. Many of the body's responses to physiologic disturbances are controlled on a moment-by-moment basis by feedback mechanisms that limit their application and duration of action. For example, the baroreflex-mediated rise in heart rate that occurs when a person moves from the recumbent to the standing position is almost instantaneous and subsides within seconds. Furthermore, the response to physiologic disturbances that threaten the integrity of the internal environment is specific to the threat; the body usually does not raise the body temperature when an increase in heart rate is needed. In contrast, the response to psychological disturbances is not regulated with the same degree of specificity and feedback control; instead, the effect may be inappropriate and sustained.

Factors Affecting the Ability to Adapt

Adaptation implies that an individual has successfully created a new balance between the stressor and the ability to deal with it. The means used to attain this balance are called *coping strategies* or *coping mechanisms*. Coping mechanisms are the emotional and behavioral responses used to manage threats to our physiologic and psychological homeostasis. According to Lazarus, how we cope with stressful events depends on how we perceive and interpret the event.[21] Is the event perceived as a threat of harm or loss? And, is the event perceived as a challenge rather than a threat? Physiologic reserve, time, genetic endowment and age, health status, nutrition, sleep–wake cycles, hardiness, and psychosocial factors influence a person's appraisal of a stressor and the coping mechanisms used to adapt to the new situation (Fig. 9-4).

Physiologic and Anatomic Reserve. The trained athlete is able to increase cardiac output sixfold to sevenfold during exercise. The safety margin for adaptation of most body systems is considerably greater than that needed for normal activities. The red blood cells carry more oxygen than the tissues can use, the liver and fat cells store excess nutrients, and bone tissue stores calcium in excess of that needed for normal neuromuscular function. The ability of body systems to increase their function given the need to adapt is known as the *physiologic reserve*. Many of the body organs, such as the lungs, kidneys, and adrenals, are paired to provide anatomic reserve as well. Both organs are not needed to ensure the continued existence and maintenance of the internal environment. Many persons function normally with only one lung or one kidney. In kidney disease, for example, signs of renal failure do not occur until approximately 90% of the functioning nephrons have been destroyed.

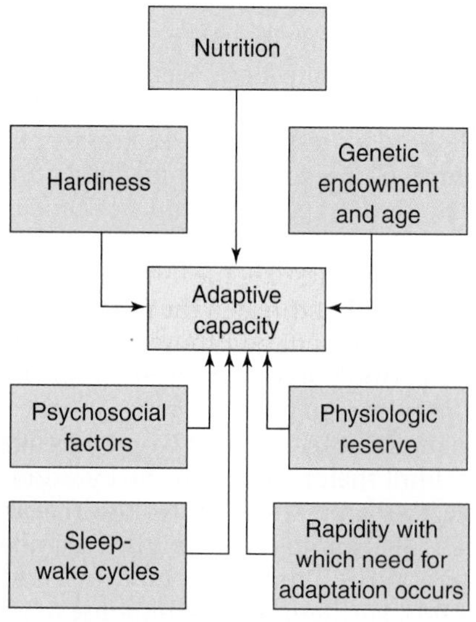

FIGURE 9-4 Factors affecting adaptation.

Time. Adaptation is most efficient when changes occur gradually rather than suddenly. It is possible, for instance, to lose a liter or more of blood through chronic gastrointestinal bleeding over a week without manifesting signs of shock. However, a sudden hemorrhage that causes rapid loss of an equal amount of blood is likely to cause hypotension and shock.

Genetic Endowment. Adaptation is further affected by the availability of adaptive responses and flexibility in selecting the most appropriate and economical response. The greater the number of available responses, the more effective is the capacity to adapt.

Genetic endowment can ensure that the systems that are essential to adaptation function adequately. Even a gene that has deleterious effects may prove adaptive in some environments. In Africa, the gene for sickle cell anemia persists in some populations because it provides some resistance to infection with the parasite that causes malaria.

Age. The capacity to adapt is decreased at the extremes of age. The ability to adapt is impaired by the immaturity of an infant, much as it is by the decline in functional reserve that occurs with age. For example, the infant has difficulty concentrating urine because of immature renal structures and therefore is less able than an adult to cope with decreased water intake or exaggerated water losses. A similar situation exists in the elderly owing to age-related changes in renal function.

Health Status. Physical and mental health status determines physiologic and psychological reserves and is a strong determinant of the ability to adapt. For example, persons with heart disease are less able to adjust to stresses that require the recruitment of cardiovascular responses. Severe emotional stress often produces disruption of physiologic function and limits the ability to make appropriate choices related to long-term adaptive needs. Those who have worked with acutely ill persons know that the will to live often has a profound influence on survival during life-threatening illnesses.

Nutrition. There are 50 to 60 essential nutrients, including minerals, lipids, certain fatty acids, vitamins, and specific amino acids. Deficiencies or excesses of any of these nutrients can alter a person's health status and impair the ability to adapt. The importance of nutrition to enzyme function, immune response, and wound healing is well known. On a worldwide basis, malnutrition may be one of the most common causes of immunodeficiency.

Among the problems associated with dietary excess are obesity and alcohol abuse. Obesity is a common problem. It predisposes to a number of health problems, including atherosclerosis and hypertension. Alcohol is commonly used in excess. It acutely affects brain function and, with long-term use, can seriously impair the function of the liver, brain, and other vital structures.

Sleep–Wake Cycles. Sleep is considered to be a restorative function in which energy is restored and tissues are regenerated.[22] Sleep occurs in a cyclic manner, alternating with periods of wakefulness and increased energy use. Biologic rhythms play an important role in adaptation to stress, development of illness, and response to medical treatment. Many rhythms, such as rest and activity, work and leisure, and eating and drinking, oscillate with a frequency similar to that of the 24-hour light–dark solar day. The term *circadian,* from the Latin *circa* (about) and *dies* (day), is used to describe these 24-hour diurnal rhythms.

Sleep disorders and alterations in the sleep–wake cycle have been shown to alter immune function, the normal circadian pattern of hormone secretion, and physical and psychological functioning.[23] The two most common manifestations of an alteration in the sleep–wake cycle are insomnia and sleep deprivation or increased somnolence. In some persons, stress may produce sleep disorders, and in others, sleep disorders may lead to stress. Acute stress and environmental disturbances, loss of a loved one, recovery from surgery, and pain are common causes of transient and short-term insomnia. Air travel and jet lag constitute additional causes of altered sleep–wake cycles, as does shift work. In persons with chronic insomnia, the bed often acquires many unpleasant secondary associations and becomes a place of stress and worry rather than a place of rest.[24]

Hardiness. Studies by social psychologists have focused on individuals' emotional reactions to stressful situations and their coping mechanisms to determine those characteristics that help some people remain healthy despite being challenged by high levels of stressors. For example, the concept of *hardiness* describes a personality characteristic that includes a sense of having control over the environment, a sense of having a purpose in life, and an ability to conceptualize stressors as a challenge rather than a threat.[25] Many studies by nurses and social psychologists suggest that hardiness is correlated with positive health outcomes.[25]

Psychosocial Factors. Several studies have related social factors and life events to illness. Scientific interest in the social environment as a cause of stress has gradually broadened to include the social environment as a resource that modulates the relation between stress and health. Presumably, persons who can mobilize strong supportive resources from within their social relationships are better able to withstand the negative effects of stress on their health. Studies suggest that social support has direct and indirect positive effects on health status and serves as a buffer or modifier of the physical and psychosocial effects of stress.[26]

Social networks contribute in a number of ways to a person's psychosocial and physical integrity. The configuration of significant others that constitutes this network functions to mobilize the resources of the person; these friends, colleagues, and family members share the person's tasks and provide monetary support, materials and tools, and guidance in improving problem-solving capabilities.[26] Persons with ample social networks are not as likely to experience many types of stress, such as being homeless or being lonely.[9] There is also evidence that persons who have social supports or social assets may live longer and have a lower incidence of somatic illness.[27]

Social support has been viewed in terms of the number of relationships a person has and the person's perception of these relationships.[28] Close relationships with others can involve positive effects as well as the potential for conflict and may, in some situations, leave the person less able to cope with life stressors.

In summary, the stress response involves the activation of several physiologic systems (sympathetic nervous system, the HPA axis, and the immune system) that work in a coordinated fashion to protect the body against damage from the intense demands made on it. Selye called this response the *general adaptation syndrome.* The stress response is divided into three stages: the *alarm stage,* with activation of the sympathetic nervous system and the HPA axis; the *resistance stage,* during which the body selects the most effective defenses; and the *exhaustion stage,* during which physiologic resources are depleted and signs of systemic damage appear.

The activation and control of the stress response are mediated by the combined efforts of the nervous and endocrine systems. The neuroendocrine systems integrate signals received along neurosensory pathways and from circulating mediators that are carried in the bloodstream. In addition, the immune system both affects and is affected by the stress response.

Adaptation is affected by a number of factors, including experience and previous learning, the rapidity with which the need to adapt occurs, genetic endowment and age, health status, nutrition, sleep–wake cycles, hardiness, and psychosocial factors.

Disorders of the Stress Response

After completing this section of the chapter, you should be able to meet the following objectives:

- Describe the physiologic and psychological effects of a chronic stress response
- Describe the three states characteristic of post-traumatic stress disorder
- List five nonpharmacologic methods of treating stress

For the most part, the stress response is meant to be acute and time limited. The time-limited nature of the process renders the accompanying catabolic and immunosuppressive effects advantageous. It is the chronicity of the response that is thought to be disruptive to physical and mental health.

Stressors can assume a number of patterns in relation to time. They may be classified as acute time-limited, chronic intermittent, or chronic sustained. An acute time-limited stressor is one that occurs over a short time and does not recur; a chronic intermittent stressor is one to which a person is chronically exposed. The frequency or chronicity of circumstances to which the body is asked to respond often determines the availability and efficiency of the stress responses. The response of the immune system, for example, is more rapid and efficient on second exposure to a pathogen than it is on first exposure, but chronic exposure to a stressor can fatigue the system and impair its effectiveness.

EFFECTS OF ACUTE STRESS

The reactions to acute stress are those associated with the ANS, the fight-or-flight response. The manifestations of the stress response—a pounding headache, cold and moist skin, a stiff neck—are all part of the acute stress response. Centrally, there is facilitation of neural pathways mediating arousal, alertness, vigilance, cognition, and focused attention as well as appropriate aggression. The acute stress response can result from either psychologically or physiologically threatening events. In situations of life-threatening trauma, these acute responses may be lifesaving in that they divert blood from less essential to more essential body functions. Increased alertness and cognitive functioning enables rapid processing of information and arrival at the most appropriate solution to the threatening situation.

However, for persons with limited coping abilities, either because of physical or mental health, the acute stress response may be detrimental. This is true of persons with preexisting heart disease in whom the overwhelming sympathetic behaviors associated with the stress response can lead to dysrhythmias. For people with other chronic health problems, such as headache disorder, acute stress may precipitate a reoccurrence. In healthy individuals, the acute stress response can redirect attention from behaviors that promote health, such as attention to proper meals and getting adequate sleep. For those with health problems, it can interrupt compliance with medication regimens and exercise programs. In some situations, the acute arousal state actually can be life threatening, physically immobilizing the person when movement would avert catastrophe (*e.g.*, moving out of the way of a speeding car).

EFFECTS OF CHRONIC STRESS

The stress response is designed to be an acute self-limited response in which activation of the ANS and the HPA axis is controlled in a negative feedback manner. As with all negative feedback systems, including the stress response system, pathophysiologic changes can occur. Function can be altered in several ways, including when a component of the system fails; when the neural and hormonal connections among the components of the system are dysfunctional; and when the original stimulus for the activation of the system is prolonged or of such magnitude that it overwhelms the ability of the system to respond appropriately. In these cases, the system may become overactive or underactive.

Chronicity and excessive activation of the stress response can result from chronic illnesses as well as contribute to the development of long-term health problems. Chronic activation of the stress response is an important public health issue from both a health and a cost perspective. The National Institute for Occupational Safety and Health declared stress a hazard of the workplace.[29] It is linked to a myriad of health disorders, such as diseases of the cardiovascular, gastrointestinal, immune, and neurologic systems, as well as depression, chronic alcoholism and drug abuse, eating disorders, accidents, and suicide.

Occurrence of the oral disease acute necrotizing gingivitis, in which the normal bacterial flora of the mouth become invasive, is known by dentists to be associated with acute stress, such as final examinations.[30] Similarly, herpes simplex type 1 infection (*i.e.*, cold sores) often develops during periods of inadequate rest, fever, ultraviolet radiation, and emotional upset. The resident herpesvirus is kept in check by body defenses, probably T lymphocytes, until a stressful event occurs that causes suppression of the immune system. Psychological stress is associated in a dose-response manner with an increased risk for development of the common cold, and this risk is attributable to increased rates of infection rather than frequency of symptoms after infection.[31]

In a study in which participants were infected with the influenza virus, those persons who reported the greatest amount of premorbid stress reported the most intense influenza symptoms and had a statistically greater production of interleukin-6, a cytokine that acts as a chemotactic agent for immune cells.[32] Elderly caregivers of a spouse with dementia had a significantly higher score for emotional distress and higher salivary cortisol than matched control subjects.[33] The higher stress was correlated with a decreased immune response to the influenza vaccine. The experience of stress also has been associated with delays in wound healing.[34]

POST-TRAUMATIC STRESS DISORDER

The post-traumatic stress disorder (PTSD) is an example of chronic activation of the stress response as a result of experiencing a potentially life-threatening event. It was formerly called *battle fatigue* or *shell shock* because it was first characterized in men and women returning from combat. Although war is still a significant cause of PTSD, other major catastrophic events, such as major weather-related disasters, airplane crashes, terrorist bombings, and rape or child abuse, also may result in the development of the disorder. The terrorist attack on the World Trade Center and Pentagon on September 11, 2001 represented an amalgam of interpersonal violence, loss, and threat to tens of thousands of people.[35] These events have influenced and will continue to influence the development of PTSD in a substantial number of people. On the basis of data obtained after the 1995 bombing of the Murrah Federal Building in Oklahoma City, it is predicted that PTSD will develop in approximately 35% of those who were directly exposed to the September 11 attacks.[36]

PTSD is characterized by a constellation of symptoms that are experienced as states of intrusion, avoidance, and hyperarousal. *Intrusion* refers to the occurrence of "flashbacks" during waking hours or nightmares in which the past traumatic event is relived, often in vivid and frightening detail. *Avoidance* refers to the emotional numbing that accompanies this disorder and disrupts important personal relationships. Because a person with PTSD has not been able to resolve the painful feelings associated with the trauma, depression is commonly a part of the clinical picture. Survivor guilt also may be a product of traumatic situations in which the person survived the disaster but loved ones did not. *Hyperarousal* refers to the presence of increased irritability, difficulty in concentration, an exaggerated startle reflex, and increased vigilance and concern over safety. In addition, memory problems, sleep disturbances, and excessive anxiety are commonly experienced by persons with PTSD.

To be given a diagnosis of PTSD, a person has to have been exposed to an extreme stress or a traumatic event and have symptoms that focus on intrusion, avoidance, and hyperarousal. The three types of symptoms must be present together for at least 1 month, and the disorder must have caused clinically significant distress or impairment in social, occupational, and other areas of functioning.[37]

Although the pathophysiology of PTSD is not completely understood, the revelation of physiologic changes related to the disorder has shed light on why some people recover from the disorder, whereas others do not. It has been hypothesized that the intrusive symptoms of PTSD may arise from exaggerated sympathetic nervous system activation in response to the traumatic event. Persons with chronic PTSD have been shown to have increased levels of norepinephrine and increased activity of α_2-adrenergic receptors.[35] The increase in catecholamines, in tandem with increased thyroid levels in persons with PTSD, is thought to explain some of the intrusive and somatic symptoms of the disorder.[35,38]

Recent neuroanatomic studies have identified alterations in two brain structures (the amygdala and hippocampus). Positron-emission tomography and functional magnetic resonance imaging (MRI) have shown increased reactivity of the amygdala and hippocampus and decreased reactivity of the anterior cingulate and orbitofrontal areas. These areas of the brain are involved in fear responses. The hippocampus also functions in memory processes. Differences in hippocampal function and memory processes suggest a neuroanatomic basis for the intrusive recollections and other cognitive problems that characterize PTSD.[35]

Importantly, the observed neuroanatomic changes in persons with PTSD do not uniformly resemble those seen with other types of stress.[39] For example, persons with PTSD demonstrate decreased cortisol levels, increased sensitivity of cortisol receptors, and an enhanced negative feedback inhibition of cortisol release with the dexamethasone suppression test. Dexamethasone is a synthetic glucocorticoid that mimics the effects of cortisol and directly inhibits the action of CRF and ACTH. This is in contrast to patients with major depression, who have a decreased sensitivity of glucocorticoid receptors, a high plasma level of cortisol, and a decreased dexamethasone suppression.[39] The hypersuppression of cortisol observed with the dexamethasone test suggests that persons with PTSD do not exhibit a classic stress response as described by Selye. Because this hypersuppression has not been described in other psychiatric disorders, it may serve as a relatively specific marker for PTSD.

Little is known about the risk factors that predispose people to the development of PTSD. It is important to note that less than half of all people who are exposed to a traumatic event develop PTSD. For example, only 15% to 30% of soldiers exposed to combat develop the disorder.[40] It also has been found that children exposed to violent events but who have strong family relationships rarely develop PTSD.[41] Statistics indicate there is a need for studies to determine risk factors for PTSD as a means of targeting individuals who may need intensive therapeutic measures after a life-threatening event. Research also is needed to determine the mechanisms by which the disorder develops so that it can be prevented, or if that is not possible, so that treatment methods can be created to decrease the devastating effects that this disorder has on affected individuals and their families.[38]

Health care professionals need to be aware that patients who present with symptoms of depression, anxiety, and alcohol or drug abuse may in fact be suffering from PTSD. The patient history should include questions concerning the occurrence of violence, major loss, or traumatic events in the person's life. Debriefing, or talking about the traumatic event at the time it happens, often is an effective therapeutic tool. Crisis teams are often among the first people to attend to the emotional needs of those caught in catastrophic events. Some people may need continued individual or group therapy. Often, concurrent pharmacotherapy with antidepressant and antianxiety agents is useful and helps the individual participate more fully in therapy.

Most importantly, the person with PTSD should not be made to feel responsible for the disorder or that it is evidence of a so-called character flaw. It is not uncommon for persons with this disorder to be told to "get over it" or "just get on with it, because others have." There is ample evidence to suggest that there is a biologic basis for the individual differences in responses to traumatic events, and these differences need to be taken into account.

TREATMENT AND RESEARCH OF STRESS DISORDERS

Treatment

The treatment of stress should be directed toward helping people avoid coping behaviors that impose a risk to their health and providing them with alternative stress-reducing strategies. Purposeful priority setting and problem solving can be used by persons who are overwhelmed by the number of life stresses to which they have been exposed. Other nonpharmacologic methods used for stress reduction are relaxation techniques, guided imagery, music therapy, massage, and biofeedback.

Relaxation. Practices for evoking the relaxation response are numerous. They are found in virtually every culture and are credited with producing a generalized decrease in sympathetic system activity and musculoskeletal tension. According to Herbert Benson, a physician who worked in developing the technique, four elements are integral to the various relaxation techniques: a repetitive mental device, a passive attitude, decreased mental tonus, and a quiet environment.[42] Benson developed a noncultural method that is commonly used for achieving relaxation (see accompanying box).

Progressive muscle relaxation, originally developed by Edmund Jacobson, who did extensive research on the muscle correlates of anxiety and tension, is another method of relieving tension. He observed that tension could be defined physiologically as the inappropriate contraction of muscle fibers. His procedure, which has been modified by a number of therapists, consists of systematic contraction and relaxation of major muscle groups.[43] As the person learns to relax, the various muscle groups are combined. Eventually, the person learns to relax individual muscle groups without first contracting them.

Imagery. Guided imagery is another technique that can be used to achieve relaxation. One method is scene visualization, in which the person is asked to sit back, close the eyes, and concentrate on a scene narrated by the therapist. Whenever possible, all five senses are involved: the person attempts to see, feel, hear, and taste aspects of the visual experience. Other types of imagery involve imagining the appearance of each of the major muscle groups and how they feel during tension and relaxation.

Music Therapy. Music therapy is used for both its physiologic and psychological effects. It involves listening to selected pieces of music as a means of ameliorating anxiety or stress, reducing pain, decreasing feelings of loneliness and isolation, buffering noise, and facilitating expression of emotion. Music is defined as having three components: rhythm, melody, and harmony.[44,45] Rhythm is the order in the movement of the music. Rhythm is the most dynamic aspect of music, and particular pieces of music often are selected because they harmonize with body rhythms such as heart rhythm, respiratory rhythm, or gait. The melody is created by the musical pitch and distance (or interval) between the musical tone. The melody contributes to the listener's emotional response to the music. The harmony results from the way pitches are blended together, with the combination of sounds described as consonant or dissonant by the listener. Music usually is selected based on a person's musical preference and past experiences with music. Depending on the setting, headphones may be used to screen out other distracting noises. Radio and television music is inappropriate for music therapy because of the inability to control the selection of pieces that are played, the interruptions that occur (*e.g.,* commercials and announcements), and the quality of the reception.

Massage Therapies. Massage is the manipulation of the soft tissues of the body to promote relaxation and relief of muscle tension. The technique that is used may involve a gentle stroking along the length of a muscle (effleurage), application of pressure across the width of a muscle (pétrissage), deep massage movements applied by a circular motion of the thumbs or fingertips (friction), squeezing across the width of a muscle (kneading), or use of light slaps or chopping actions (hacking).[46] Massage may be administered by practitioners who have received special training in its use or by less prepared persons such as parents of small children[47,48] or caregivers of confused elders.[49] It often is used as a means of physiologic relaxation and stress relief in critically ill patients.[50]

Biofeedback. Biofeedback is a technique in which an individual learns to control physiologic functioning. It involves electronic monitoring of one or more physiologic responses to stress with immediate feedback of the specific response to the person undergoing treatment. Several types of responses are used: electromyographic (EMG), electrothermal, and electrodermal (EDR).[51] The EMG response involves the measurement of electrical potentials from muscles, usually the forearm extensor or frontalis. This is used to gain control over the contraction of skeletal muscles that occurs with anxiety and tension. The electrodermal sensors monitor skin temperature in the fingers or toes. The sympathetic nervous system exerts significant control over blood flow in the distal parts of the body such as the digits of the hands and feet. Consequently, anxiety often is manifested by a decrease in skin temperature in the fingers and toes. EDR sensors measure conductivity of skin (usually the hands) in response to anxiety. Fearful and anxious people often have cold and clammy hands, which lead to a decrease in conductivity.

The Relaxation Response

- Sit quietly in a comfortable position.
- Deeply relax all your muscles, beginning at your feet and progressing up to your face.
- Breathe through your nose. Become aware of your breathing. As you breathe out, say the word "one" silently to yourself. Continue for 20 minutes. When you have finished, sit quietly for several minutes, first with your eyes closed and then with them open.
- Do not worry about whether you are successful in achieving a deep level of relaxation. Maintain a positive attitude and permit the relaxation to occur at its own rate. Expect distracting thoughts, ignore them, and continue repeating "one" as you breathe out.

(Modified from Benson H. [1977]. Systemic hypertension and the relaxation response. *New England Journal of Medicine* 296, 1152)

Research

Research in stress has focused on personal reports of the stress situation and the physiologic responses to stress. A number of interview guides and written instruments are available for measuring the personal responses to stress and coping in adults[52,53] and children.[54]

There are fewer methods available for measuring the physiologic responses to stress in humans because much of the research in the field of stress has been accomplished using animal models. There are some good reasons for this. First, the human experience of stress varies among individuals based on previous life experiences and availability of adaptive resources; therefore, it is difficult to find a stimulus that produces equivalent stress in all subjects in a study. Second, suitable methods for measuring the components of the stress response in humans are limited.

Some methods require invasive procedures, many demand expensive equipment, and all require investigator competency in their use.[55] In addition, many measurement methods, such as venipuncture, can introduce additional stress to the experimental condition.

Some of the current methods for studying the physiologic manifestations of the stress response include electrocardiographic recording of heart rate, blood pressure measurement, electrodermal measurement of skin resistance associated with sweating, and biochemical analyses of hormone levels.[55] Measurements of urinary and plasma catecholamines can be used as an index of ANS activation. Cortisol levels can be obtained from salivary samples. The effect of the stress response on the immune system can be studied through the use of blood tests to obtain immune cell (lymphocyte) counts and antibody levels.

Research that attempts to establish a link between the stress response and disease needs to be interpreted with caution owing to the influence that individual differences have on the way people respond to stress. Not everyone who experiences stressful life events develops a disease. The evidence for a link between the stress response system and the development of disease in susceptible persons is compelling but not conclusive. No study has established a direct cause-and-effect relationship between the stress response and disease occurrence. For example, depressive illness often is associated with an increase in both plasma cortisol and cerebrospinal fluid concentrations of CRF. The question that arises is whether this increased plasma cortisol is a cause or an effect of the depressive state. Although health care professionals continue to question the role of stressors and coping skills on the pathogenesis of disease states, we must resist the temptation to suggest that any disease is due to excessive stress or poor coping skills.

In summary, stress in itself is neither negative nor deleterious to health. The stress response is designed to be time limited and protective, but in situations of prolonged activation of the response because of overwhelming or chronic stressors, it could be damaging to health. PTSD is an example of chronic activation of the stress response as a result of experiencing a severe trauma. In this disorder, memory of the traumatic event seems to be enhanced. Flashbacks of the event are accompanied by intense activation of the neuroendocrine system.

Treatment of stress should be aimed at helping people avoid coping behaviors that can adversely affect their health and providing them with other ways to reduce stress. Nonpharmacologic methods used in the treatment of stress include relaxation techniques, guided imagery, music therapy, massage techniques, and biofeedback.

Research in stress has focused on personal reports of the stress situation and the physiologic responses to stress. A number of interview guides and written instruments are available for measuring the personal responses to acute and chronic stressors. Methods used for studying the physiologic manifestations of the stress response include electrocardiographic recording of heart rate, blood pressure measurement, electrodermal measurement of skin resistance associated with sweating, and biochemical analyses of hormone levels.

REVIEW EXERCISES

A 21-year-old college student notices that she frequently develops "cold sores" during stresses involved in final exam week.

A. What is the association between stress and the immune system?

B. One of her classmates suggests listening to music or trying relaxation exercises as a means of relieving stress. Explain how these interventions might work in relieving stress.

A 75-year-old woman with congestive heart failure complains that her condition gets worse when she worries and is under a lot of stress.

A. Relate the effects of stress on the neuroendocrine control of cardiovascular function and its possible relationship to a worsening of the woman's congestive heart failure.

B. She tells you that she dealt with much worse stresses when she was younger and never had any problems. How would you explain this?

A 30-year-old woman who was rescued from a collapsed building has been having nightmares recalling the event, excessive anxiety, and loss of appetite, and she is afraid to leave her home for fear something will happen.

A. Given her history and symptoms, what is a likely diagnosis?

B. How might she be treated?

References

1. Lazarus R. S., Folkman S. (1984). *Stress, appraisal, and coping.* New York: Springer.
2. Hinkle L. E. (1977). The concept of "stress" in the biological and social sciences. In Lipowskin Z. J., Lipsitt D. R., Whybrow P. C. (Eds.), *Psychosomatic medicine* (pp. 27–49). New York: Oxford University Press.
3. Osler W. (1910). The Lumleian lectures in angina pectoris. *Lancet 1,* 696–700, 839–844, 974–977.
4. Cannon W. B. (1935). Stresses and strains of homeostasis. *American Journal of Medical Science 189,* 1–5.
5. Selye H. (1946). The general adaptation syndrome and diseases of adaptation. *Journal of Clinical Endocrinology 6,* 117–124.
6. Cannon W. B. (1939). *The wisdom of the body* (pp. 299–300). New York: W. W. Norton.
7. Wilcox R. E., Gonzales R. A. (1995). Introduction to neurotransmitters, receptors, signal transduction, and second messengers. In Schatzberg A. F., Nemeroff C. B. (Eds.), *Textbook of psychopharmacology* (pp. 3–29). Washington, DC: American Psychiatric Press.
8. Elenkov I. J., Webster E. L., Torpy D. J., Chrousos G. P. (1999). Stress, corticotrophin-releasing hormone, glucocorticoids, and the immune/inflammatory response: Acute and chronic effects. *Annals of the New York Academy of Sciences 876,* 1–11.
9. Chrousos G. P. (1998). Stressors, stress, and neuroendocrine integration of the adaptive response. *Annals of the New York Academy of Sciences 851,* 311–335.
10. Selye H. (1976). *The stress of life* (rev. ed.). New York: McGraw-Hill.

11. Selye H. (1973). The evolution of the stress concept. *American Scientist 61,* 692–699.
12. Selye H. (1974). *Stress without distress* (p. 6). New York: New American Library.
13. Lopez J. F., Akil H., Watson S. J. (1999). Neural circuits mediating stress. *Biological Psychiatry 46,* 1461–1471.
14. Koob G. F. (1999). Corticotropin-releasing factor, norepinephrine, and stress. *Biological Psychiatry 46,* 1167–1180.
15. Lehnert H., Schulz C., Dieterich K. (1998). Physiological and neurochemical aspects of corticotrophin-releasing factor actions in the brain: The role of the locus ceruleus. *Neurochemical Research 23,* 1039–1052.
16. Sapolsky R. M., Romero L. M., Munck A. U. (2000). How do glucocorticoids influence stress responses? Integrating permissive, suppressive, stimulatory, and preparative actions. *Endocrine Reviews 21,* 55–89.
17. Dantzer R., Kelley K. W. (1989). Stress and immunity: An integrated view of relationships between the brain and immune system. *Life Sciences 44,* 1995–2008.
18. Falaschi P., Martocchia A., Proietti A., et al. (1994). Immune system and the hypothalamus-pituitary-adrenal axis. *Annals of the New York Academy of Sciences 741,* 223–231.
19. Woiciechowsky C., Schoning F., Lanksch W. R., et al. (1999). Mechanisms of brain mediated systemic anti-inflammatory syndrome causing immunodepression. *Journal of Molecular Medicine 77,* 769–780.
20. Dubos R. (1965). *Man adapting* (pp. 256, 258, 261, 264). New Haven: Yale University Press.
21. Lazarus R. (2000). Evolution of a model of stress, coping, and discrete emotions. In Rice V. H. (Ed.), *Handbook of stress, coping, and health* (pp. 195–222). Thousand Oaks, CA: Sage Publications.
22. Adams K., Oswold I. (1983). Protein synthesis, bodily renewal and sleep-wake cycle. *Clinical Science 65,* 561–567.
23. Gillin J. C., Byerley W. F. (1990). The diagnosis and management of insomnia. *New England Journal of Medicine 322,* 239–248.
24. Moldofsky H., Lue F. A., Davidson J. R., Gorezynski R. (1989). Effects of sleep deprivation on human immune functions. *FASEB Journal 3,* 1972–1977.
25. Ford-Gilboe M., Cohen J. A. (2000). Hardiness: A model of commitment, challenge, and control. In Rice V. H. (Ed.), *Handbook of stress, coping, and health* (pp. 425–436). Thousand Oaks, CA: Sage Publications.
26. Broadhead W. E., Kaplan B. H., James S. A., et al. (1983). The epidemiologic evidence for a relationship between social support and health. *American Journal of Epidemiology 117,* 521–537.
27. Greenblatt M., Becerra R. M., Serafetinides E. A. (1982). Social networks and mental health: An overview. *American Journal of Psychiatry 139,* 977–984.
28. Tilden V. P., Weinert C. (1987). Social support and the chronically ill individual. *Nursing Clinics of North America 33,* 613–620.
29. National Institute for Occupational Safety and Health. (1999). *Stress at work* (pp. 1–26). Publication no. 99-101, HE 20.7102:ST 8/4. Bethesda, MD: U.S. Department of Health and Human Services.
30. Dworkin S. F. (1969). Psychosomatic concepts and dentistry: Some perspectives. *Journal of Periodontology 40,* 647.
31. Cohen S., Tyrrell D. A. J., Smith A. P. (1991). Psychological stress and susceptibility to the common cold. *New England Journal of Medicine 325,* 606–612.
32. Cohen S., Doyle W. J., Skoner D. P. (1999). Psychological stress, cytokine production, and severity of upper respiratory illness. *Psychosomatic Medicine 61*(2), 175–180.
33. Vedhara K., Wilcock G. K., Lightman S. L., Shanks N. M. (1999). Chronic stress in elderly carers of dementia patients and antibody response to influenza vaccination. *Lancet 353,* 627–631.
34. Rozlog L. A., Kiecolt-Glaser J. K., Marucha P. T., et al. (1999). Stress and immunity: Implication for viral disease and wound healing. *Journal of Periodontology 70,* 786–792.
35. Yehuda R. (2002). Post-traumatic stress disorder. *New England Journal of Medicine 346,* 108–114.
36. North C. S., Nixon S. J., Shariat S., et al. (1999). Psychiatric disorders among survivors of the Oklahoma City bombing. *JAMA 282,* 755–762.
37. American Psychiatric Association. (1994). *Diagnostic and statistical manual of mental disorders* (4th ed., DSM-IV). Washington DC: American Psychiatric Association.
38. Yehuda R. (2000). Biology of posttraumatic stress disorder. *Journal of Clinical Psychiatry 61*(Suppl. 7), 14–21.
39. Yehuda R. (1998). Psychoneuroendocrinology of posttraumatic stress disorder. *Psychiatric Clinics of North America 21,* 359–379.
40. Sapolsky R. (1999). Stress and your shrinking brain (posttraumatic stress disorder's effect on the brain). *Discover 20*(3), 116.
41. McCloskey L. A. (2000). Posttraumatic stress in children exposed to family violence and single event trauma. *Journal of the American Academy of Child and Adolescent Psychiatry 39,* 108–115.
42. Benson H. (1977). Systemic hypertension and the relaxation response. *New England Journal of Medicine 296,* 1152–1154.
43. Jacobson E. (1958). *Progressive relaxation.* Chicago: University of Chicago Press.
44. Chlan L., Tracy M. F. (1999). Music therapy in critical care: Indications and guidelines for intervention. *Critical Care Nurse 19*(3), 35–41.
45. White J. M. (1999). Effects of relaxing music on cardiac autonomic balance and anxiety after acute myocardial infarction. *American Journal of Critical Care 8,* 220–230.
46. Vickers A., Zollman C. (1999). ABC of complementary therapies: Massage therapies. *British Medical Journal 319,* 1254–1257.
47. Rusy L. M., Weisman S. J. (2000). Complementary therapies for acute pediatric pain management. *Pediatric Clinics of North America 47,* 589–599.
48. Huhtala V., Lehtonen L., Heinonen R., Korvenranta H. (2000). Infant massage compared with crib vibrator in treatment of colicky infants. *Pediatrics 105*(6), E84.
49. Rowe M., Alfred D. (1999). The effectiveness of slow-stroke massage in diffusing agitated behaviors in individuals with Alzheimer's disease. *Journal of Gerontological Nursing 25*(6), 22–34.
50. Richards K. C. (1998). Effect of back massage and relaxation intervention on sleep in critically ill patients. *American Journal of Critical Care 7,* 288–299.
51. Fischer-Williams M., Nigl A. J., Sovine D. L. (1986). *A textbook of biological feedback.* New York: Human Sciences Press.
52. Wimbush F. B., Nelson M. L. (2000). Stress, psychosomatic illness, and health. In Rice V. H. (Ed.), *Handbook of stress, coping, and health* (pp. 143–194). Thousand Oaks, CA: Sage Publications.
53. Backer J. H., Bakas T., Bennett S. J., Pierce P. K. (2000). Coping with stress: Programs of nursing research. In Rice V. H. (Ed.), *Handbook of stress, coping, and health* (pp. 223–263). Thousand Oaks, CA: Sage Publications.
54. Ryan-Wenger N. A., Sharrer V. W., Wynd C. A. (2000). Stress, coping, and health in children. In Rice V. H. (Ed.), *Handbook of stress, coping, and health* (pp. 265–293). Thousand Oaks, CA: Sage Publications.
55. White J. M., Porth C. M. (2000). Physiological measurement of the stress response. In Rice V. H. (Ed.), *Handbook of stress, coping, and health* (pp. 69–94). Thousand Oaks, CA: Sage Publications.

CHAPTER

10

Alterations in Temperature Regulation

Mary Pat Kunert

Body temperature, at any given point in time, represents a balance between heat gain and heat loss. Body heat is generated in the core tissues of the body, transferred to the skin surface by the blood, and then released into the environment surrounding the body. Body temperature rises in fever as a result of cytokine-mediated changes in the hypothalamic temperature set point and in hyperthermia as a result of excessive heat production, inadequate heat dissipation, or a failure of thermoregulatory mechanisms. It falls during hypothermia caused by exposure to cold. This chapter is organized into three sections: regulation of body temperature, increased body temperature (fever and hyperthermia), and decreased body temperature (hypothermia).

Body Temperature Regulation

After completing this section of the chapter, you should be able to meet the following objectives:

- Differentiate between body core temperature and skin temperature and relate the differences to methods used for measuring body temperature
- Describe the mechanisms of heat production in the body
- Define the terms *conduction, radiation, convection,* and *evaporation,* and relate them to the mechanisms for heat loss from the body

Virtually all biochemical processes in the body are affected by changes in temperature. Metabolic processes speed up or slow down depending on whether body temperature is rising or falling. *Core body temperature* (*i.e.,* intracranial, intrathoracic, and intraabdominal) normally is maintained within a range of 36.0°C to 37.5°C (97.0°F to 99.5°F).[1–3] Within this range, there are individual differences and diurnal variations; internal core temperatures reach their highest point in late afternoon and evening and their lowest point in the early morning hours (Fig. 10-1).

Body temperature reflects the difference between heat production and heat loss and varies with exercise and extremes of environmental temperature. Properly protected, the body can function in environmental conditions that range from −50°C (−48°F) to +50°C (+122°F). Individual body cells, however, cannot tolerate such a wide range of temperatures—at −1°C (+32°F) ice crystals form, and at +45°C (+113°F), cell proteins coagulate.[4]

Most of the body's heat is produced by the deeper core tissues (*i.e.,* muscles and viscera), which are insulated from the environment and protected against heat loss by an outer shell of subcutaneous tissues and skin (Fig. 10-2). Because the shell lies between the core and the environment,

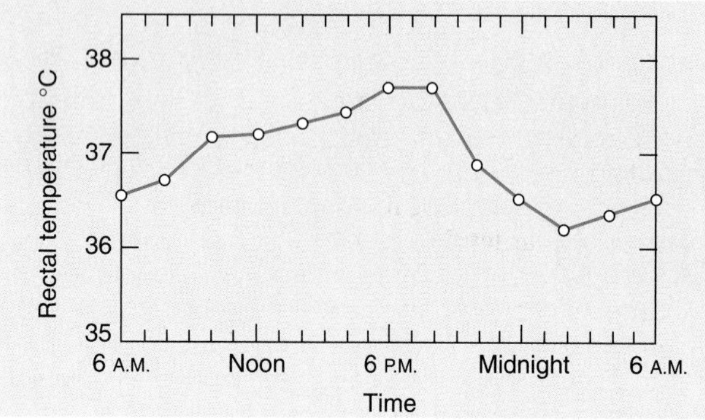

FIGURE 10-1 Normal diurnal variations in body temperature.

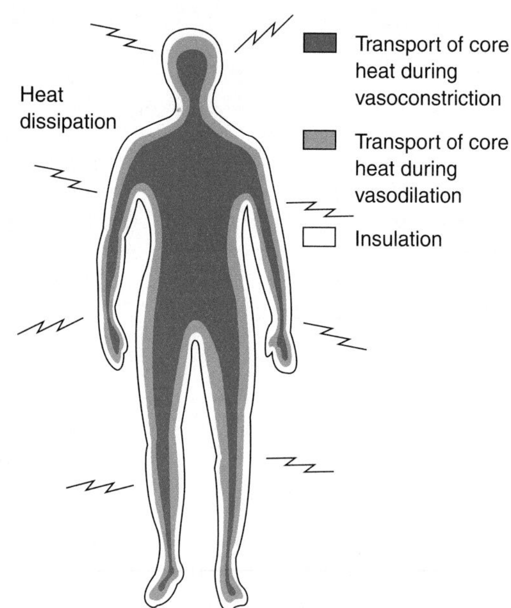

FIGURE 10-2 Control of heat loss. Body heat is produced in the deeper core tissues of the body, which is insulated by the subcutaneous tissues and skin to protect against heat loss. During vasodilatation, circulating blood transports heat to the skin surface, where it dissipates into the surrounding environment. Vasoconstriction decreases the transport of core heat to the skin surface, and vasodilatation increases transport.

all heat leaving the body core, with the exception of that lost through the respiratory tract, must pass through the outer shell.[2] The thickness of the shell depends on blood flow. In a warm environment, blood flow is increased, and the thickness of the outer shell is decreased, allowing for greater dissipation of heat. In a cold environment, blood flow to the skin and underlying tissues, including those of the limbs and more superficial muscles of the neck and trunk, constrict. This increases the thickness of the shell and helps to minimize the loss of core heat for the body. The subcutaneous fat layer contributes to the insulation value of the outer shell because of its thickness and because it conducts heat only about one third as effectively as other tissues.

Temperatures differ in various parts of the body, with core temperatures being higher than those at the skin surface. In general, the rectal temperature is used as a measure of core temperature. Rectal temperatures usually range from 37.3°C (99.2°F) to 37.6°C (99.6°F).[3] Core temperatures may also be obtained from the esophagus using a flexible thermometer, from a pulmonary artery catheter that is used for thermodilution measurement of cardiac output, or from a urinary catheter with a thermosensor that measures the temperature of urine in the bladder. Because of location, pulmonary artery and esophageal temperatures closely reflect the temperature of the heart and thoracic organs. This is the preferred measurement when body temperatures are changing rapidly and need to be followed reliably.[3]

THERMOREGULATION

- Core body temperature is a reflection of the balance between heat gain and heat loss by the body. Metabolic processes produce heat, which must be dissipated.
- The hypothalamus is the thermal control center for the body, receives information from peripheral and central thermoreceptors, and compares that information with its temperature set point.
- Heat loss occurs through transfer of body core heat to the surface through the circulation. Heat is lost from the skin through radiation, conduction, convection, and evaporation.
- An increase in core temperature is effected by vasoconstriction and shivering, a decrease in temperature by vasodilation, and sweating.

The oral temperature, taken sublingually, is usually 0.2°C (0.36°F) to 0.51°C (0.9°F) lower than the rectal temperature; however, it usually follows changes in core temperature closely. The axillary temperature also can be used as an estimate of core temperature. However, the parts of the axillary fossa must be pressed closely together for an extended period (5 to 10 minutes for a glass thermometer) because this method requires considerable heat to accumulate before the final temperature is reached.

Ear-based thermometry uses an infrared sensor to measure the flow of heat from the tympanic membrane and ear canal.[5] It has become popular in the pediatric setting because of its ease and speed of measurement, acceptability to parents and children, and cost savings in the personnel time that is required to take a child's temperature.[6] However, a debate continues regarding the accuracy of this method.[5,7] Several factors can alter the accuracy of ear-based thermometry: (1) the size of the probe cover must match the size of the ear canal; (2) the infrared reader must be directed at the tympanic membrane; and (3) the presence of any exudate (fluid or cerumen) in the ear canal or behind the tympanic membrane affects the accuracy of the reading.[7]

Core body temperature, rather than the surface temperature, is regulated by the *thermoregulatory center* in the hypothalamus. This center integrates input from cold and warm thermal receptors located throughout the body (and within the hypothalamus) and initiates output responses that conserve and generate body heat or increase its dissipation. The *thermostatic set point* of the thermoregulatory center is set so that the temperature of the body core is regulated within the normal range of 36.0° (97.0°F) to 37.5°C (99.5°F). When body temperature begins to rise above the set point, the hypothalamus signals the central and peripheral nervous systems to initiate heat-dissipating behaviors. Likewise, when the temperature falls below the set point, signals from the hypothalamus elicit physiologic behaviors that increase heat conservation and production. Core temperatures above 41°C (105.8°F) or below 34°C (93.2°F) usually mean that the body's ability to thermoregulate has been impaired (Fig. 10-3). Body responses that produce, conserve, and dissipate heat are described in Table 10-1.

In addition to physiologic thermoregulatory mechanisms, humans engage in voluntary behaviors to help regulate body temperature. These behaviors include the selection of proper clothing and regulation of environmental temperature through heating systems and air conditioning. Body positions that hold the extremities close to the body prevent heat loss and are commonly assumed in cold weather.

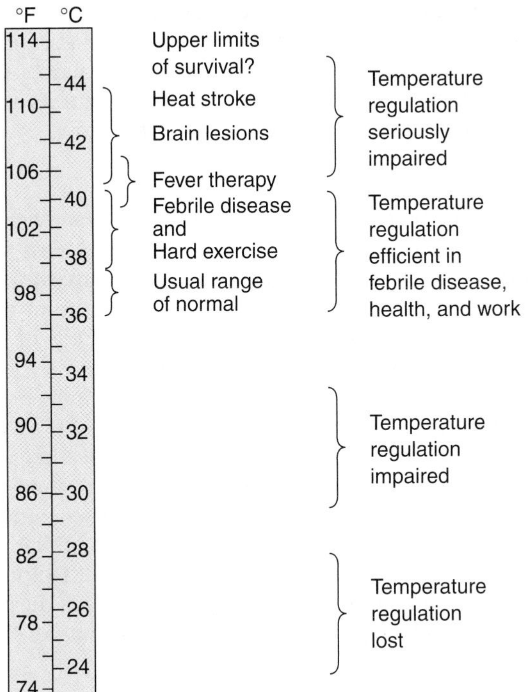

FIGURE 10-3 Body temperatures under different conditions. (Dubois, E. F. [1948]. *Fever and the regulation of body temperature.* Springfield, IL: Charles C. Thomas)

MECHANISMS OF HEAT PRODUCTION

Metabolism is the body's main source of heat production. There is a 0.56°C (1°F) increase in body temperature for every 7% increase in metabolism. The sympathetic neurotransmitters, epinephrine and norepinephrine, which are released when an increase in body temperature is needed, act at the cellular level to shift body metabolism to heat production rather than energy generation. This may be one of the reasons fever tends to produce feelings of weakness and fatigue. Thyroid hormone increases cellular metabolism, but this response usually requires several weeks to reach maximal effectiveness. The metabolic rate is typically 45% or more above normal in hyperthyroidism.[2]

Fine involuntary actions such as shivering and chattering of the teeth can produce a threefold to fivefold increase in body temperature. *Shivering* is initiated by impulses from the hypothalamus. The first muscle change that occurs with shivering is a general increase in muscle tone, followed by an oscillating rhythmic tremor involving the spinal-level reflex that controls muscle tone. Because no external work is performed, all the energy liberated by the metabolic processes from shivering is in the form of heat.[8]

Physical exertion increases body temperature. Muscles convert most of the energy in the fuels they consume into heat rather than mechanical work. With strenuous exercise, more than three fourths of the increased metabolism resulting from muscle activity appears as heat within the body, and the remainder appears as mechanical work.

MECHANISMS OF HEAT LOSS

Most of the body's heat losses occur at the skin surface as heat from the blood moves to the skin and from there into the surrounding environment. There are numerous arteriovenous (AV) shunts under the skin surface that allow blood to move directly from the arterial to the venous system[1] (Fig. 10-4). These AV shunts are much like the radiators in a heating system. When the shunts are open, body heat is freely dissipated to the skin and surrounding environment; when the shunts are closed, heat is retained in the body. The blood flow in the AV shunts is controlled almost exclusively by the sympathetic nervous system in response to changes in core temperature and environmental temperature. Contraction of the *pilomotor muscles* of the skin, which raises skin hairs and produces goose bumps, also aids in heat conservation by reducing the surface area available for heat loss.

Heat is lost from the body through radiation, conduction, and convection from the skin surface; through the evaporation of sweat and insensible perspiration; through the exhalation of air that has been warmed and humidified; and through heat lost in urine and feces. Of these mechanisms, only heat losses that occur at the skin surface are directly under hypothalamic control.

Conduction

Conduction is the direct transfer of heat from one molecule to another. Blood carries, or conducts, heat from the inner core of the body to the skin surface. Normally, only

TABLE 10-1 Heat Gain and Heat Loss Responses Used in Regulation of Body Temperature

Heat Gain		Heat Loss	
Body Response	Mechanism of Action	Body Response	Mechanism of Action
Vasoconstriction of the superficial blood vessels	Confines blood flow to the inner core of the body, with the skin and subcutaneous tissues acting as insulation to prevent loss of core heat	Dilatation of the superficial blood vessels	Delivers blood containing core heat to the periphery where it is dissipated through radiation, conduction, and convection
Contraction of the pilomotor muscles that surround the hairs on the skin	Reduces the heat loss surface of the skin	Sweating	Increases heat loss through evaporation
Assumption of the huddle position with the extremities held close to the body	Reduces the area for heat loss		
Shivering	Increases heat production by the muscles		
Increased production of epinephrine	Increases the heat production associated with metabolism		
Increased production of thyroid hormone	Is a long-term mechanism that increases metabolism and heat production		

a small amount of body heat is lost through conduction to a cooler surface. Cooling blankets or mattresses that are used for reducing fever rely on conduction of heat from the skin to the cool surface of the mattress. Heat also can be conducted in the opposite direction—from the external environment to the body surface. For instance, body temperature may rise slightly after a hot bath.

Water has a specific heat several times greater than air, so water absorbs far greater amounts of heat than air does. The loss of body heat can be excessive and life threatening in situations of cold water immersion or cold exposure in damp or wet clothing.

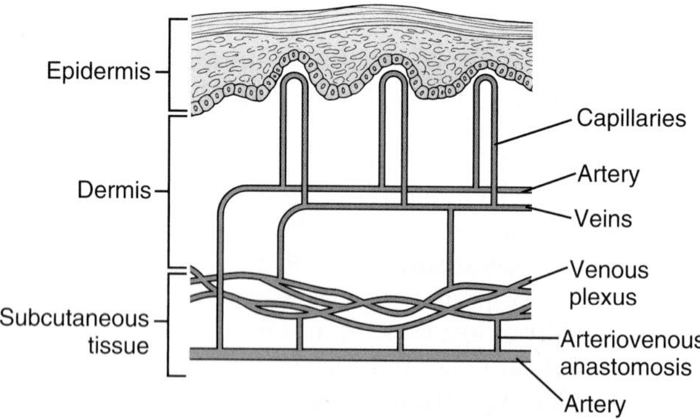

FIGURE 10-4 Skin circulation with arteriovenous shunts and venous plexus that participate in transfer of core heat to the skin. (Adapted from Guyton A., Hall J. E. [2002]. *Textbook of medical physiology* [10th ed., 823]. Philadelphia: W. B. Saunders with permission from Elsevier Science)

The conduction of heat to the body's surface is influenced by blood volume. In hot weather, the body compensates by increasing blood volume as a means of dissipating heat. Persons who are not acclimated to a hot environment can increase their total blood volume by 10% within 2 to 4 hours of heat exposure. A mild swelling of the ankles during hot weather (called heat edema) provides evidence of blood volume expansion. Exposure to cold produces a cold diuresis and a reduction in blood volume as a means of controlling the transfer of heat to the body's surface.

Radiation

Radiation is the transfer of heat through air or a vacuum. Heat from the sun is carried by radiation. Heat loss by radiation varies with the temperature of the environment. Environmental temperature must be less than that of the body for heat loss to occur. About 60% to 70% of body heat typically is dissipated by radiation.

Convection

Convection refers to heat transfer through the circulation of air currents. Normally, a layer of warm air tends to remain near the body's surface; convection causes continual removal of the warm layer and replacement with air from the surrounding environment. The windchill factor that often is included in the weather report combines the effect of convection due to wind with the still-air temperature.

Evaporation

Evaporation involves the use of body heat to convert water on the skin to water vapor. Water that diffuses through the skin independent of sweating is called *insensible perspira-*

tion. Insensible perspiration losses are greatest in a dry environment. Sweating occurs through the sweat glands and is controlled by the sympathetic nervous system. Unlike other sympathetically mediated functions, in which the catecholamines serve as neuromediators, sweating is mediated by acetylcholine. This means that anticholinergic drugs, such as atropine, can interfere with heat loss by interrupting sweating.

Evaporative heat losses involve insensible perspiration and sweating, with 0.58 calories being lost for each gram of water that is evaporated.[1] As long as body temperature is greater than the atmospheric temperature, heat is lost through radiation. However, when the temperature of the surrounding environment becomes greater than skin temperature, evaporation is the only way the body can rid itself of heat. Any condition that prevents evaporative heat losses causes the body temperature to rise.

In summary, body temperature is normally maintained within a range of 36.0°C to 37.4°C (97.0°F to 99.5°F). Most of the body's heat is produced by metabolic processes that occur within deeper core structures (*i.e.*, muscles and viscera) of the body. Heat loss occurs at the body's surface when heat from core structures is transported to the skin by the circulating blood. Heat is lost from the body through radiation, conduction, convection, and evaporation. The thermoregulatory center in the hypothalamus functions to modify heat production and heat losses as a means of regulating body temperature.

Increased Body Temperature

After completing this section of the chapter, you should be able to meet the following objectives:

- Characterize the physiology of fever
- Describe the four stages of fever
- Explain what is meant by intermittent, remittent, sustained, and relapsing fevers
- State the relation between body temperature and heart rate
- Differentiate between the physiologic mechanisms involved in fever and hyperthermia
- State the criteria for high-risk status of children 0 to 36 months of age
- State the definition of fever in elderly persons and cite possible mechanisms for altered febrile response in elderly persons
- Compare the characteristics of fevers caused by infectious agents and drug-related fevers
- Compare the mechanisms of malignant hyperthermia and neuroleptic malignant syndrome

Both fever and hyperthermia describe conditions in which body temperature is higher than the normal range. Fever is due to an upward displacement of the set point of the thermostatic center in the hypothalamus. This is in contrast to hyperthermia, in which the set point is unchanged, but the mechanisms that control body temperature are ineffective in maintaining body temperature within a normal range during situations when heat production outpaces the ability of the body to dissipate that heat.

FEVER

The literature on fever dates back to the writings of Hippocrates, which contain many descriptions of febrile-course diseases, such as typhoid fever.[9] However, it was not until the development of the thermometer that measurements of body temperature became possible. One of the first studies of body temperature was reported in 1868 by the German physician Carl Wunderlich. During a 20-year period, Wunderlich studied the body temperature of 25,000 patients with observations made twice daily with a foot-long thermometer held in the axilla for 20 minutes.[10] Wunderlich observed that the thermometer was a useful instrument for providing insight into the condition of the ill person. Today, temperature is one of the most frequent physiologic responses to be monitored during illness.

Mechanisms

Fever, or *pyrexia*, describes an elevation in body temperature that is caused by a cytokine-induced upward displacement of the set point of the hypothalamic thermoregulatory center. Fever is resolved or "broken" when the condition that caused the increase in the set point is removed. Fevers that are regulated by the hypothalamus usually do not rise above 41°C (105.8°F), suggesting a built-in thermostatic safety mechanism. Temperatures above that level are usually the result of superimposed activity, such as convulsions, hyperthermic states, or direct impairment of the temperature control center.

Pyrogens are exogenous or endogenous substances that produce fever. *Exogenous pyrogens* are derived from outside the body and include such substances as bacterial products, bacterial toxins, or whole microorganisms. Exogenous

FEVER

- Fever represents an increase in body temperature that results from a cytokine-induced increase in the set point of the thermostatic center in the hypothalamus.
- Fever is a nonspecific response that is mediated by endogenous pyrogens released from host cells in response to infectious or noninfectious disorders.
- The development of fever involves a prodrome, a chill during which the temperature rises until it reaches the new hypothalamic set point, a flush during which the skin vessels dilate and the temperature begins to fall, and a period of defervescence that is marked by sweating.
- Fever is resolved when the condition causing the increase in the set point of the thermostatic center in the hypothalamus is resolved.

pyrogens induce host cells to produce fever-producing mediators called *endogenous pyrogens.* Research has identified at least three chemical substances that act as endogenous pyrogens: interleukin-1, interleukin-6, and tumor necrosis factor.[11] These chemical mediators, also known as *cytokines,* are synthesized by a number of body cell types, including endothelial cells, epithelial cells, lymphocytes, fibroblasts, and monocytes. The endogenous pyrogens act to increase the set point of the hypothalamic thermoregulatory center. This effect is mediated through the local synthesis and release of prostaglandin E_2 (PGE_2). PGE_2, which is a metabolite of arachidonic acid (an intramembrane fatty acid), binds to receptors in the hypothalamus to induce changes in its set point through the second messenger cyclic adenosine monophosphate (cAMP).[12] In response to the increase in set point, the hypothalamus initiates shivering and vasoconstriction that increase the core body temperature to the new set point, and fever is established. In addition to their fever-producing actions, the endogenous pyrogens mediate a number of other responses. For example, interleukin-1 is an inflammatory mediator that produces other signs of inflammation, such as leukocytosis, anorexia, and malaise (see Chapter 20).

Many noninfectious disorders, such as myocardial infarction, pulmonary emboli, and neoplasms, produce fever. In these conditions, the injured or abnormal cells incite the production of endogenous pyrogen. For example, trauma and surgery can be associated with up to 3 days of fever. Some malignant cells, such as those of leukemia and Hodgkin's disease, secrete endogenous pyrogen.

A fever that has its origin in the central nervous system is sometimes referred to as a *neurogenic fever.* It usually is caused by damage to the hypothalamus due to central nervous system trauma, intracerebral bleeding, or an increase in intracranial pressure. Neurogenic fevers are characterized by a high temperature that is resistant to antipyretic therapy and is not associated with sweating.

Purpose

The purpose of fever is not completely understood. However, from a purely practical standpoint, fever is a valuable index to health status. For many, fever signals the presence of an infection and may legitimize the need for medical treatment. In ancient times, fever was thought to "cook" the poisons that caused the illness. With the availability of antipyretic drugs in the late 19th century, the belief that fever was useful began to wane, probably because most antipyretic drugs also had analgesic effects.

There is little research to support the belief that fever is harmful unless the temperature rises above 40°C (104°F). Animal studies have demonstrated a clear survival advantage in infected members with fever compared with animals that were unable to produce a fever. It has been shown that small elevations in temperature such as those that occur with fever enhance immune function. There is increased motility and activity of the white blood cells, stimulation of interferon production, and activation of T cells.[11,13] Many of the microbial agents that cause infection grow best at normal body temperatures, and their growth is inhibited by temperatures in the fever range. For example, the rhinoviruses responsible for the common cold are cultured best at 33°C (91.4°F), which is close to the temperature in the nasopharynx; temperature-sensitive mutants of the virus that cannot grow at temperatures above 37.5°C (99.5°F) produce fewer signs and symptoms.[14]

Patterns

The patterns of temperature change in persons with fever vary and may provide information about the nature of the causative agent.[15–17] These patterns can be described as intermittent, remittent, sustained, or relapsing (Fig. 10-5). An *intermittent fever* is one in which temperature returns to normal at least once every 24 hours. In a *remittent fever,* the temperature does not return to normal and varies a few degrees in either direction. In a *sustained* or *continuous fever,* the temperature remains above normal with minimal variations (usually less than 0.55°C or 1°F). A *recurrent* or *relapsing fever* is one in which there is one or more episodes of fever, each as long as several days, with one or more days of normal temperature between episodes.

Critical to the analysis of a fever pattern is the relation of heart rate to the level of temperature elevation. Normally, a 1°C rise in temperature produces a 15-beats/minute increase in heart rate (1°F, 10 beats/minute).[15] Most persons respond to an increase in temperature with an appropriate increase in heart rate. The observation that a rise in temperature is not accompanied by the anticipated change in heart rate can provide useful information about the cause of the fever. For example, a heart rate that is slower than would be anticipated can occur with Legionnaires' disease and drug fever, and a heart rate that is more rapid than anticipated can be symptomatic of hyperthyroidism and pulmonary emboli.

Manifestations

The physiologic behaviors that occur during the development of fever can be divided into four successive stages: a prodrome; a chill, during which the temperature rises; a flush; and defervescence (Fig. 10-6). During the *first* or *prodromal* period, there are nonspecific complaints such as mild headache and fatigue, general malaise, and fleeting aches and pains. During the *second stage* or *chill,* there is the uncomfortable sensation of being chilled and the onset of generalized shaking, although the temperature is rising. Vasoconstriction and piloerection usually precede the onset of shivering. At this point, the skin is pale and covered with goose flesh. There is a feeling of being cold and an urge to put on more clothing or covering and to curl up in a position that conserves body heat. When the shivering has caused the body temperature to reach the new set point of the temperature control center, the shivering ceases, and a sensation of warmth develops. At this point, the *third stage* or *flush* begins, during which cutaneous vasodilation occurs and the skin becomes warm and flushed. The *fourth,* or *defervescence,* stage of the febrile response is marked by the initiation of sweating. Not all persons proceed through the four stages of fever development. Sweating may be absent, and fever may develop gradually with no indication of a chill or shivering.

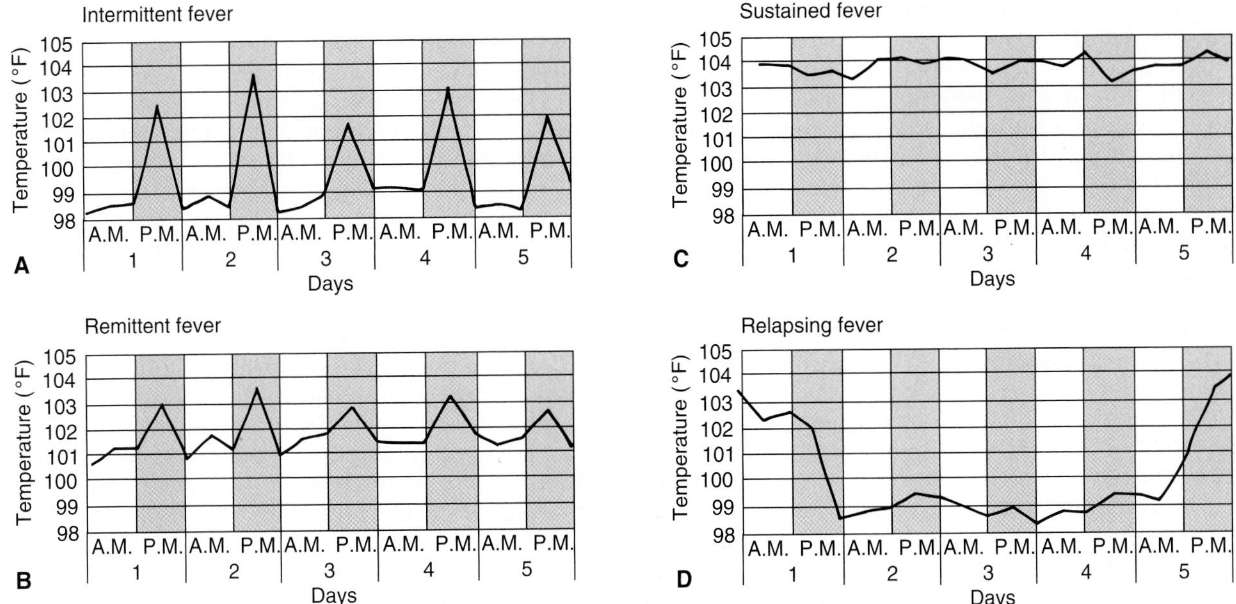

FIGURE 10-5 Schematic representation of fever patterns: (**A**) intermittent, (**B**) remittent, (**C**) sustained, and (**D**) recurrent or relapsing.

Common manifestations of fever are anorexia, myalgia, arthralgia, and fatigue. These discomforts are worse when the temperature rises rapidly or exceeds 39.5°C (103.1°F). Respiration is increased, and the heart rate usually is elevated. Dehydration occurs because of sweating and the increased vapor losses due to the rapid respiratory rate. The occurrence of chills commonly coincides with the introduction of pyrogen into the circulation. Many of the manifestations of fever are related to the increases in the metabolic rate, increases in oxygen demands, and use of body proteins as an energy source. During fever, the body switches from using glucose (an excellent medium for bacterial growth) to metabolism based on protein and fat breakdown.[18] With prolonged fever, there is an increased breakdown of endogenous fat stores. If fat breakdown is rapid, metabolic acidosis may result (see Chapter 34).

Headache is a common accompaniment of fever and is thought to result from the vasodilation of cerebral vessels occurring with fever. Delirium is possible when the temperature exceeds 40°C (104°F). In elderly persons, confusion

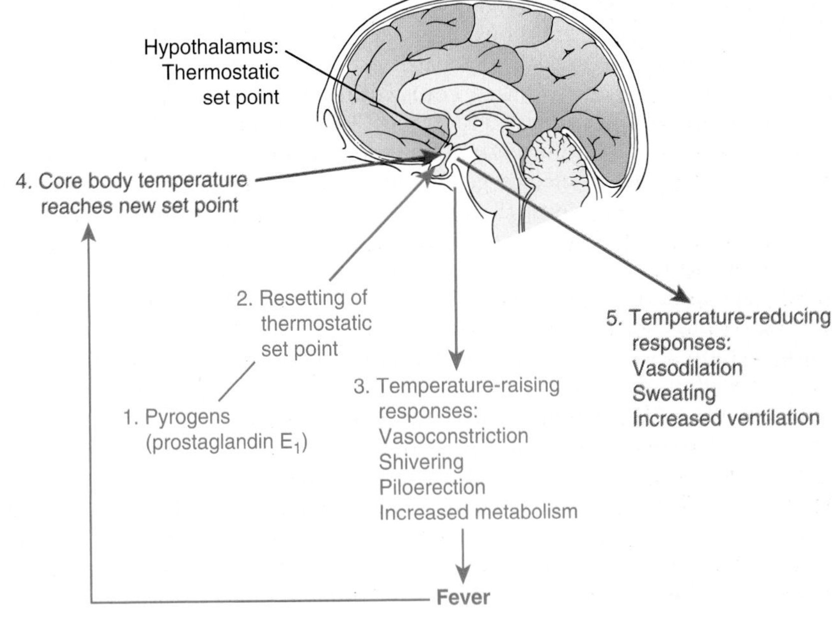

FIGURE 10-6 Mechanisms of fever. (1) Release of endogenous pyrogen from inflammatory cells, (2) resetting of hypothalamus thermostatic set point to a higher level (prodrome), (3) generation of hypothalamic-mediated responses that raise body temperature (chill), (4) development of fever with elevation of body to new thermostatic set point, and (5) production of temperature-lowering responses (flush and defervescence) and return of body temperature to a lower level.

and delirium may follow moderate elevations in temperature. Owing to increasingly poor oxygen uptake by the aging lung, pulmonary function may prove to be a limiting factor in the hypermetabolism that accompanies fever in older persons. Confusion, incoordination, and agitation commonly reflect cerebral hypoxemia. Febrile convulsions can occur in some children.[19] They usually occur with rapidly rising temperatures or at a threshold temperature that differs with each child.

The herpetic lesions, or fever blisters, that develop in some persons during fever are caused by a separate infection by the type 1 herpes simplex virus that established latency in the regional ganglia and is reactivated by a rise in body temperature.

Diagnosis and Treatment

Fever usually is a manifestation of a disease state, and as such, determining the cause of a fever is an important aspect of its treatment. For example, fevers from infectious diseases usually are treated with antibiotics, whereas other fevers, such as those resulting from a noninfectious inflammatory condition, may be treated symptomatically.

Sometimes, it is difficult to establish the cause of a fever. A prolonged fever for which the cause is difficult to ascertain is often referred to as *fever of unknown origin* (FUO). FUO is defined as a temperature elevation of 38.3°C (101°F) or higher that is present for 3 weeks or longer.[20] Among the causes of FUO are malignancies (*i.e.*, lymphomas, metastases to the liver and central nervous system); infections such as human immunodeficiency virus or tuberculosis, or abscessed infections; and drug fever. Malignancies, particularly non-Hodgkin's lymphoma, are important causes of FUO in elderly persons. Cirrhosis of the liver is another cause of FUO.

Recurrent or periodic fevers may occur in predictable intervals or without any discernible time pattern. They may be associated with no discernible cause, or they can be the presenting symptom of several serious illnesses and often precede the other symptoms of those diseases by weeks or months. The PFAPA syndrome, which is characterized by *p*eriodic *f*ever, *a*phthous (small ulcerative stomatitis), *p*haryngitis, and cervical *a*denopathy occurring every 21 to 28 days, is the most common cause of recurrent fevers in children younger than 5 years of age.[21] Other conditions in which recurrent fevers occur but do not follow a strictly periodic pattern include genetic disorders such as familial Mediterranean fever (FMF). FMF, an autosomal recessive disease, is characterized by early age of onset (<20 years), acute episodic peritonitis, and high fever with an average duration of less than 2 days. In some cases, pleuritis, pericarditis, and arthritis are present. The primary chronic complication is the presence of serum antibodies that can result in kidney or heart failure. This complication can be prevented by treatment with colchicine.[22]

Conditions that present with recurrent fevers occurring at irregular intervals include repeated viral or bacterial infections, parasitic and fungal infections, and some inflammatory conditions (*e.g.*, systemic juvenile arthritis and Crohn's disease). The clinical challenge is in the differential diagnosis of periodic or recurrent fever. The initial workup usually requires a thorough history and physical examination designed to rule out the more serious medical conditions that present initially with fever.

The methods of fever treatment focus on modifications of the external environment intended to increase heat transfer from the internal to the external environment, support of the hypermetabolic state that accompanies fever, protection of vulnerable body organs and systems, and treatment of the infection or condition causing the fever. Because fever is a disease symptom, its manifestation suggests the need for treatment of the primary cause.

Modification of the environment ensures that the environmental temperature facilitates heat transfer away from the body. Sponge baths with cool water or an alcohol solution can be used to increase evaporative heat losses. More profound cooling can be accomplished through the use of a cooling mattress, which facilitates the conduction of heat from the body into the coolant solution that circulates through the mattress. Care must be taken so that the cooling method does not produce vasoconstriction and shivering, which decrease heat loss and increase heat production.

Adequate fluids and sufficient amounts of simple carbohydrates are needed to support the hypermetabolic state and prevent the tissue breakdown that is characteristic of fever. Additional fluids are needed for sweating and to balance the insensible water losses from the lungs that accompany an increase in respiratory rate. Fluids also are needed to maintain an adequate vascular volume for heat transport to the skin surface.

Antipyretic drugs, such as aspirin and acetaminophen, often are used to alleviate the discomforts of fever and protect vulnerable organs, such as the brain, from extreme elevations in body temperature. These drugs act by resetting the hypothalamic temperature control center to a lower level, presumably by blocking the activity of cyclooxygenase, an enzyme that is required for the conversion of arachidonic acid to prostaglandin E_2.[23]

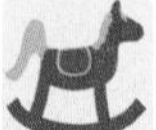

Fever in Children

The mechanisms for controlling temperature are not as well developed in infants as they are in older children and adults. In infants younger than 3 months, a mild elevation in temperature (*i.e.*, rectal temperature of 38°C [100.4°F]) can indicate serious infection that requires immediate medical attention.[24–26] Although infants with fever may not appear ill, this does not imply an absence of bacterial disease. Fever without a source occurs frequently in infants and children and is a common reason for visits to the clinic or emergency department.

Both minor and life-threatening infections are common in the infant to 3-year-old age group.[24,25] The most common causes of fever in children are minor or more serious infections of the respiratory system, urinary system, gastrointestinal tract, or central nervous system. Occult bacteremia and meningitis also occur in this age group and should be ruled out. The Agency for Health Care Policy and Research Expert Panel has developed clinical guidelines for use in the treatment of infants and children 0 to 36 months of age with fever without a source.[27] The guidelines define fever in this age group as an elevation in rectal temperature of at least 38°C (100.4°F). The guidelines also point out that fever may result from overbundling or a vaccine reaction. When overbundling is suspected, it is suggested that the infant be unbundled and the temperature retaken after 15 to 30 minutes.

Fever in infants and children can be classified as low risk or high risk, depending on the probability of the infection progressing to bacteremia or meningitis. Signs of toxicity include lethargy, poor feeding, hypoventilation, poor tissue oxygenation, and cyanosis. Infants can be considered low risk if they were delivered at term and sent home with their mother without complications and have been healthy with no previous hospitalizations or previous antimicrobial therapy. A white blood cell count and urinalysis are recommended as a means of confirming low-risk status. Blood and urine cultures, chest radiographs, and lumbar puncture usually are done in high-risk infants and children to determine the cause of fever.

The mean probability of serious bacterial infection in infants younger than 3 months of age is 8.6%; in children between 3 and 36 months of age, it is 4.5%.[25] Infants with fever who are considered to be low risk usually are managed on an outpatient basis provided that the parents or caregivers are deemed reliable. Older children with fever without a source also may be treated on an outpatient basis. Parents or caregivers require full instructions, preferably in writing, regarding assessment of the febrile child. They should be instructed to contact their health care provider should their child show signs suggesting sepsis. High-risk infants and infants who are younger than 28 days usually are hospitalized for evaluation of their fever and treatment. Parenteral antimicrobial therapy usually is initiated after samples for blood, urine, and spinal fluid cultures have been taken.

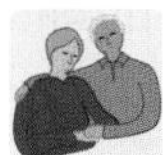

Fever in the Elderly

In the elderly, even slight elevations in temperature may indicate serious infection or disease. This is because elderly people often have a lower baseline temperature, and although they increase their temperature during an infection, it may fail to reach a level that is equated with significant fever.[28–30]

Normal body temperature and the circadian pattern of temperature variation often are altered in elderly people. Elderly persons are reported to have a lower basal temperature (36.4°C [97.6°F] in one study) than younger persons.[31] It has been recommended that the definition of fever in elderly persons be expanded to include an elevation of temperature of at least 1.1°C (2°F) above baseline values.[30]

It has been suggested that 20% to 30% of elders with serious infections present with an absent or blunted febrile response.[30] When fever is present in the elderly, it usually indicates the presence of serious infection, most often caused by bacteria. The absence of fever may delay diagnosis and initiation of antimicrobial treatment. Unexplained changes in functional capacity, worsening of mental status, weakness and fatigue, and weight loss are signs of infection in the elderly. They should be viewed as possible signs of infection and sepsis when fever is absent. The probable mechanisms for the blunted fever response include a disturbance in sensing of temperature by the thermoregulatory center in the hypothalamus, alterations in release of endogenous pyrogens, and failure to elicit responses such as vasoconstriction of skin vessels, increased heat production, and shivering that increase body temperature during a febrile response.

Another factor that may delay recognition of fever in the elderly is the method of temperature measurement. Oral temperature remains the most commonly used method for measuring temperature in the elderly. It has been suggested that rectal and tympanic membrane methods are more effective in detecting fever in elderly people. This is because conditions such as mouth breathing, tongue tremors, and agitation often make it difficult to obtain accurate oral temperatures in the elderly.

HYPERTHERMIA

Hyperthermia describes an increase in body temperature that occurs without a change in the set point of the hypothalamic thermoregulatory center. It occurs when the thermoregulatory mechanisms are overwhelmed by heat production, excessive environmental heat, or impaired dissipation of heat.[32] It includes (in order of increasing severity) heat cramps, heat exhaustion, and heatstroke. Malignant hyperthermia describes a rare genetic disorder of anesthetic-related hyperthermia. Fever and hyperthermia also may occur as the result of a drug reaction.

A number of factors predispose to hyperthermia. If muscle exertion is continued for long periods in warm weather, as often happens with athletes, military recruits, and laborers, excessive heat loads are generated.[32] Because adequate circulatory function is essential for heat dissipation, elderly persons and those with cardiovascular disease are at increased risk for hyperthermia. Drugs that increase muscle tone and metabolism or reduce heat loss (*e.g.*, diuretics, neuroleptics, drugs with anticholinergic action) can impair thermoregulation. Infants and small children who are left in a closed car for even short periods in hot weather are potential victims of hyperthermia.

HYPERTHERMIA

- Hyperthermia is a pathologic increase in core body temperature without a change in the hypothalamic set point. The thermoregulatory center is overwhelmed by either excess heat production, impaired heat loss, or excessive environmental heat.
- Malignant hyperthermia is an autosomal dominant disorder in which an abnormal release of intracellular stores of calcium causes uncontrolled skeletal muscle contractions, resulting in a rapid increase in core body temperature. This usually is in response to an anesthetic.

Additionally, several conditions are associated with a decreased ability to respond adequately to heat stress. For example, spinal cord injuries that transect the cord at T6 or above can seriously impair temperature regulation because the hypothalamus can no longer control skin blood flow or sweating.

The best approach to heat-related disorders is prevention, primarily by avoiding activity in hot environments, increasing fluid intake, and wearing climate- and activity-appropriate clothing. The ability to tolerate a hot environment depends on both temperature and humidity. A high relative humidity retards heat loss through sweating and evaporation and decreases the body's cooling ability. The *Heat Index* is the temperature that the body senses when both the temperature and humidity are combined. The Heat Index/Heat Disorder Table, produced by the National Weather Service, provides a useful guide for determining when to avoid outside activity (Table 10-2).

Heat Cramps

Heat cramps are slow, painful, skeletal muscle cramps and spasms, usually occurring in the muscles that are most heavily used and lasting for 1 to 3 minutes. Cramping results from salt depletion that occurs when fluid losses from heavy sweating are replaced by water alone. The muscles are tender, and the skin usually is moist. Body temperature may be normal or slightly elevated. There almost always is a history of vigorous activity preceding the onset of symptoms.

Treatment consists of drinking an oral saline solution (commercially prepared electrolyte solutions or 1 tsp of salt in 500 mL of water), stretching the affected muscles, and resting in a cool environment.[33] Because absorption is slow and unpredictable, salt tablets are not recommended. Salt tablets also can cause gastric irritation, vomiting, and cerebral edema. Strenuous physical activity should be avoided for several days while dietary sodium replacement is continued.

Heat Exhaustion

Heat exhaustion is related to a gradual loss of salt and water, usually after prolonged and heavy exertion in a hot environment. The symptoms include thirst, fatigue, nausea, oliguria, giddiness, and finally delirium. Gastrointestinal flulike symptoms are common. Hyperventilation in association with heat exhaustion may contribute to heat cramps and tetany by causing respiratory alkalosis (see Chapter 34). The skin is moist, the rectal temperature usually is higher than 37.8°C (100°F) but below 40°C (104°F), and the heart rate is elevated, usually by more than half again the normal resting rate. Signs of heat cramps may accompany heat exhaustion.

Like heat cramps, heat exhaustion is treated by rest in a cool environment, the provision of adequate hydration, and salt replacement. Intravenous fluids are administered when adequate oral intake cannot be achieved. If the individual has water-depleted heat exhaustion and is hypernatremic, rehydration needs to occur at a regulated rate to reduce the development of iatrogenic cerebral edema (see Chapter 33).[32]

Heatstroke

Heatstroke is a severe, life-threatening failure of thermoregulatory mechanisms resulting in an excessive rise in body temperature—a core temperature greater than 40°C (104°F), absence of sweating, and loss of consciousness. The risk for developing heatstroke in response to heat stress is increased in conditions (*i.e.,* alcoholism, obesity, diabetes mellitus, and chronic cardiac, renal or mental disease) and with drugs (*i.e.* alcohol, anticholinergics, β-blockers, or tricyclic antidepressants) that impair vasodilation and sweating.[34,35]

The pathophysiology of heatstroke is thought to result from the direct effect of heat on body cells and the release of cytokines (*e.g.,* interleukins, tumor necrosis factor, and interferon) from heat-stressed endothelial cells, leukocytes, and epithelial cells that protect against tissue injury. The net result is a combination of local and systemic inflammatory responses that may result in multiorgan dysfunction, encephalopathy, rhabdomyolysis, and acute renal failure.[34]

Heatstroke may be designated as *classic* or *nonexertional* when it arises as a consequence of exposure to high environmental temperatures or as *exertional* when it arises as a consequence of strenuous exercise.[33,34] The classic form of heatstroke is seen most commonly in elderly and disabled persons. An average of 1700 heatstroke-related deaths occur in the United States every year, with 80% of those deaths occurring in persons 50 years of age and older.[35] In elderly people, the problem often is one of impaired heat loss and failure of homeostatic mechanisms, such that body temperature rises with any increase in environmental temperature. Elderly persons with a decreased ability to perceive changes in environmental temperature or decreased mobility are at particular risk because they also may be unable to take appropriate measures such as

TABLE 10-2 Heat Index Values Associated With Possible Heat Disorders

Heat Index (Combination of Heat and Humidity Effects)	Possible Heat Disorder
80°F–90°F	Fatigue possible with prolonged exposure and physical activity
90°F–105°F	Sunstroke, heat cramps, and heat exhaustion possible
105°F–130°F	Sunstroke, heat cramps, and heat exhaustion likely, and heat stroke possible
130°F or greater	Heat stroke highly likely with continued exposure

Data from http://www.crh.noaa.gov/pub/heat.htm (U.S. National Weather Service).

removing clothing, moving to a cooler environment, and increasing fluid intake. This is particularly true of elderly persons who live alone in small and poorly ventilated housing units and who may be too confused or weak to complain or seek help at the onset of symptoms.

Exertional heatstroke occurs most often in summer and mainly affects athletes and laborers who are exposed to high temperature environments. Persons with exertional heatstroke often continue to perspire, a factor that often results in a delay in diagnosis. In addition, rhabdomyolysis and its complications (hyperkalemia, hyperphosphatemia, hypocalcemia, and myoglobinuria) contribute to the morbidity and mortality associated with the disorder.[33]

The symptoms of heatstroke include tachycardia, hyperventilation, dizziness, weakness, emotional lability, nausea and vomiting, confusion, delirium, blurred vision, convulsions, collapse, and coma. The skin is hot and usually dry, and the pulse is typically strong initially. The blood pressure may be elevated at first, but hypotension develops as the condition progresses. As vascular collapse occurs, the skin becomes cool. Associated abnormalities include electrocardiographic changes consistent with heart damage, blood coagulation disorders, potassium and sodium depletion, and signs of liver damage.

Early recognition and aggressive treatment of heatstroke is critical in order to reduce both the morbidity and mortality associated with the cellular injury due to direct heat and the effect of cytokine actions.[30,31] Treatment consists of rapidly reducing the core temperature. Care must be taken that the cooling methods used do not produce vasoconstriction or shivering and thereby decrease the cooling rate or induce heat production. Two general methods of cooling are used. One method involves submersion in cold water or application of ice packs, and the other involves spraying the body with tepid water while a fan is used to enhance heat dissipation through convection. Whatever method is used, it is important that the temperature of vital structures, such as the brain, heart, and liver, be reduced rapidly because tissue damage ensues when core temperatures rise above 43°C (109.4°F). Selective brain cooling has reportedly been achieved by fanning the face during hyperthermia.[3] Blood flows from the emissary venous pathways of the skin on the head through the bones of the skull to the brain. In hyperthermia, face fanning is thought to cool the venous blood that flows through these emissary veins and thereby produce brain cooling by enhancing heat exchange between the hot arterial blood and the surface-cooled venous blood in the intracranial venous spaces. Because reducing the body temperature may not modulate the inflammatory or coagulation responses elicited in response to heat stress, new pharmacologic interventions to inhibit or attenuate these responses are being investigated.[34]

Drug Fever

Drug fever has been defined as fever coinciding with the administration of a drug and disappearing after the drug has been discontinued.[36–38] Drugs can induce fever by several mechanisms. They can interfere with heat dissipation; they can alter temperature regulation by the hypothalamic centers; they can act as direct pyrogens; they can injure tissues directly; or they can induce an immune response.[39]

Exogenous thyroid hormone increases metabolic rate and can increase heat production and body temperature. Peripheral heat dissipation can be impaired by atropine, antihistamines, phenothiazines, and tricyclic antidepressants, which decrease sweating, or by sympathomimetic drugs, which produce peripheral vasoconstriction. Cimetidine, a histamine type 2 (H_2)-blocking drug that decreases gastric acid production, also blocks H_2 receptors in the hypothalamus and has been known to cause fever. Bleomycin (an anticancer drug), amphotericin B (an antifungal drug), and vaccines that contain bacterial and viral products all can act to induce the release of pyrogens. Intravenously administered drugs can lead to infusion-related phlebitis with production of cellular pyrogens that produce fever. Treatment with anticancer drugs can cause the release of endogenous pyrogen from the cancer cells that are destroyed.

The most common cause of drug fever is a *hypersensitivity reaction.* Hypersensitivity drug fevers develop after several weeks of exposure to the drug, cannot be explained in terms of the drug's pharmacologic action, are not related to drug dose, disappear when the drug is stopped, and reappear when the drug is readministered. The fever pattern is typically spiking in nature and exhibits a normal diurnal rhythm. Persons with drug fevers often experience other signs of hypersensitivity reactions, such as arthralgias, urticaria, myalgias, gastrointestinal discomfort, and rashes.

Temperatures of 38.8°C to 40.0°C (102°F to 104°F) are common in drug fever. The person may be unaware of the fever and appear to be well for the degree of fever that is present. The absence of an appropriate increase in heart rate for the degree of temperature elevation is an important clue to the diagnosis of drug fever. A fever often precedes other, more serious effects of a drug reaction; for this reason, the early recognition of drug fever is important. Drug fever should be suspected whenever the temperature elevation is unexpected and occurs despite improvement in the condition for which the drug was prescribed.

Malignant Hyperthermia

Malignant hyperthermia is an autosomal dominant metabolic disorder in which heat generated by uncontrolled skeletal muscle contraction can produce severe and potentially fatal hyperthermia. The muscle contraction is caused by an abnormal release of intracellular calcium from the mitochondria and sarcoplasmic reticulum (see Chapter 4).

In affected persons, an episode of malignant hyperthermia is triggered by exposure to certain stresses or general anesthetic agents. The syndrome most frequently is associated with the halogenated anesthetic agents and the depolarizing muscle relaxant succinylcholine.[40,41] There also are various nonoperative precipitating factors, including trauma, exercise, environmental heat stress, and infection. The condition is particularly dangerous in a young person who has a large muscle mass to generate heat.

During malignant hyperthermia, the body temperature can rise to as high as 43°C (109.4°F) at a rate of 1°C

(2°F) every 5 minutes. An initial sign of the disorder, when the condition occurs during anesthesia, is skeletal muscle rigidity. Cardiac arrhythmias and a hypermetabolic state follow in rapid sequence unless the triggering event is immediately discontinued. In addition to discontinuing the triggering agents, treatment includes measures to cool the body and the administration of dantrolene, a muscle relaxant drug that acts by blocking the release of calcium from the sarcoplasmic reticulum. There is no accurate screening test for the condition. A family history of malignant hyperthermia should be considered when general anesthesia is needed because there are anesthetic agents available that do not trigger the hyperthermic response.

Neuroleptic Malignant Syndrome

The neuroleptic malignant syndrome is associated with neuroleptic (psychotropic) medications and may occur in as many as 1% of persons taking such drugs. Some of the most commonly implicated drugs are haloperidol, chlorpromazine, thioridazine, and thiothixene. All of these drugs block dopamine receptors in the basal ganglia and hypothalamus. Hyperthermia is thought to result from alterations in the function of the hypothalamic thermoregulatory center caused by decreased dopamine levels or from uncontrolled muscle contraction like that occurring with anesthetic-induced malignant hyperthermia. Many of the neuroleptic drugs produce an increase in muscle contraction, suggesting that this mechanism may contribute to the neuroleptic malignant syndrome.

The syndrome usually has an explosive onset and is characterized by hyperthermia, muscle rigidity, alterations in consciousness, and autonomic nervous system dysfunction. The hyperthermia is accompanied by tachycardia (120 to 180 beats/minute), cardiac dysrhythmias, labile blood pressure (70/50 to 180/130 mm Hg), postural instability, dyspnea, and tachypnea (18 to 40 breaths/minute).[42] Permanent brain damage may result, and the mortality rate is nearly 30%.[43]

Treatment of neuroleptic malignant syndrome includes the immediate discontinuance of the neuroleptic drug, measures to decrease body temperature, and treatment of dysrhythmias and other complications of the disorder. Bromocriptine (a dopamine agonist) and dantrolene (a muscle relaxant) may be used as part of the treatment regimen.

In summary, fever and hyperthermia refer to an increase in body temperature outside the normal range. True fever is a disorder of thermoregulation in which there is an upward displacement of the set point for temperature control. In hyperthermia, the set point is unchanged, but the challenge to temperature regulation exceeds the thermoregulatory center's ability to control body temperature. Fever can be caused by a number of factors, including microorganisms, trauma, and drugs or chemicals, all of which incite the release of endogenous pyrogens. The reactions that occur during fever consist of four stages: a prodrome, a chill, a flush, and defervescence. A fever can follow an intermittent, remittent, sustained, or recurrent pattern. The manifestations of fever are largely related to dehydration and an increased metabolic rate. Even a low-grade fever in high-risk infants or in elderly persons can indicate serious infection.

The treatment of fever focuses on modifying the external environment as a means of increasing heat transfer to the external environment; supporting the hypermetabolic state that accompanies fever; protecting vulnerable body tissues; and treating the infection or condition causing the fever.

Hyperthermia, which varies in severity based on the degree of core temperature elevation and the severity of cardiovascular and nervous system involvement, includes heat cramps, heat exhaustion, and heatstroke. Among the factors that contribute to the development of hyperthermia are prolonged muscular exertion in a hot environment, disorders that compromise heat dissipation, and hypersensitivity drug reactions. Malignant hyperthermia is an autosomal dominant disorder that can produce a severe and potentially fatal increase in body temperature. The condition commonly is triggered by general anesthetic agents and muscle relaxants used during surgery. The neuroleptic malignant syndrome is associated with neuroleptic drug therapy and is thought to result from alterations in the function of the thermoregulatory center or from uncontrolled muscle contraction.

Decreased Body Temperature

After completing this section of the chapter, you should be able to meet the following objectives:

- Define *hypothermia*
- Compare the manifestations of mild, moderate, and severe hypothermia and relate them to changes in physiologic functioning that occur with decreased body temperature

HYPOTHERMIA

Hypothermia is defined as a core temperature (*i.e.,* rectal, esophageal, or tympanic) less than 35°C.[44] Core body temperatures in the range of 34°C to 35°C (93.2°F to 95°F) are considered mildly hypothermic; 30°C to 34°C (86°F to 93.2°F), moderately hypothermic; and less than 30°C (86°F), severely hypothermic.[44] In the United States from 1979 to 1998, an average of 700 deaths per year were attributable to hypothermia.[45]

HYPOTHERMIA

- Hypothermia is a pathologic decrease in core body temperature without a change in the hypothalamic set point.
- The compensatory physiologic responses meant to produce heat (shivering) and retain heat (vasoconstriction) are overwhelmed by unprotected exposure to cold environments.

Accidental hypothermia may be defined as a spontaneous decrease in core temperature, usually in a cold environment and associated with an acute problem but without a primary disorder of the temperature-regulating center. The term *submersion hypothermia* is used when cooling follows acute asphyxia, as occurs in drowning.[46] In children, the rapid cooling process, in addition to the diving reflex that triggers apnea and circulatory shunting to establish a heart–brain circulation, may account for the surprisingly high survival rate after submersion. The diving reflex is greatly diminished in adults. Children have been reported to survive 10 to 40 minutes of submersion asphyxia.[46,47] Controlled hypothermia may be used during certain types of surgeries to decrease brain metabolism.

Systemic hypothermia may result from exposure to prolonged cold (atmospheric or submersion). The condition may develop in otherwise healthy persons in the course of accidental exposure. Because water conducts heat more readily than air, body temperature drops rapidly when the body is submerged in cold water or when clothing becomes wet. In persons with altered homeostasis due to debility or disease, hypothermia may follow exposure to relatively small decreases in atmospheric temperature.

Many underlying conditions can contribute to the development of hypothermia.[48,49] Infants are at risk because of their high ratio of surface area to body mass. Elderly and inactive persons living in inadequately heated quarters are particularly vulnerable to hypothermia.[50] Malnutrition decreases the fuel available for heat generation, and loss of body fat decreases tissue insulation. Alcohol and sedative drugs dull mental awareness to cold and impair judgment to seek shelter or put on additional clothing.[49] Alcohol also inhibits shivering. Persons with cardiovascular disease, cerebrovascular disease, spinal cord injury, and hypothyroidism also are predisposed to hypothermia.

Manifestations

The signs and symptoms of hypothermia include poor coordination, stumbling, slurred speech, irrationality and poor judgment, amnesia, hallucinations, blueness and puffiness of the skin, dilation of the pupils, decreased respiratory rate, weak and irregular pulse, and stupor. With mild hypothermia, intense shivering generates heat, and sympathetic nervous system activity is raised to resist lowering of temperature. Vasoconstriction can be profound, heart rate is accelerated, and stroke volume is increased. Blood pressure increases slightly, and hyperventilation is common. Exposure to cold augments urinary flow (*i.e.,* cold diuresis) before there is any fall in temperature. Dehydration and increased hematocrit may develop within a few hours of even mild hypothermia, augmented by an extracellular-to-intracellular water shift.

With moderate hypothermia, shivering gradually decreases, and the muscles become rigid. Shivering usually ceases at 27°C (80.6°F). Heart rate and stroke volume are reduced, and blood pressure falls. The greatest effect of hypothermia is exerted through a decrease in the metabolic rate, which falls to 50% of normal at 28°C (82.4°F).[51] Associated with this decrease in metabolic rate is a decrease in oxygen consumption and carbon dioxide production. There is roughly a 6% decrease in oxygen consumption for every 1°C (2°F) decrease in temperature. A decrease in carbon dioxide production leads to a decrease in respiratory rate. Respirations decrease as temperatures drop below 32.2°C (90°F). Decreases in mentation, the cough reflex, and respiratory tract secretions may lead to difficulty in clearing secretions and aspiration. Consciousness usually is lost at 30°C (86°F).[51]

In terms of cardiovascular function, a gradual decline in heart rate and cardiac output occurs as hypothermia progresses. Blood pressure initially rises and then gradually falls. There is increased risk for dysrhythmia developing, probably from myocardial hypoxia and autonomic nervous system imbalance. Ventricular fibrillation is a major cause of death in hypothermia.

Carbohydrate metabolism and insulin activity are decreased, resulting in a hyperglycemia that is proportional to the level of cooling. A cold-induced loss of cell membrane integrity allows intravascular fluids to move into the skin, giving the skin a puffy appearance. Acid-base disorders occur with increased frequency at temperatures below 25°C (77°F) unless adequate ventilation is maintained. Extracellular sodium and potassium concentrations decrease, and chloride levels increase. There is a temporary loss of plasma from the circulation along with sludging of red blood cells and increased blood viscosity as the result of trapping in the small vessels and skin.

Diagnosis and Treatment

Oral temperatures are markedly inaccurate during hypothermia because of severe vasoconstriction and sluggish blood flow. Electronic thermometers with flexible probes are available for measuring rectal, bladder, and esophageal temperatures. However, rectal and bladder temperatures often lag behind fluctuations in core temperature, and esophageal temperatures may be elevated during inhalation of heated air.[52] Most clinical thermometers measure temperature only in the range of 35°C to 42°C (95°F to 107.6°F); a special thermometer that registers as low as 25°C (77°F) or an electrical thermistor probe is needed for monitoring temperatures in persons with hypothermia.

The treatment of hypothermia consists of rewarming, support of vital functions, and the prevention and treatment of complications.[53] There are three methods of rewarming: passive rewarming, active total rewarming, and active core rewarming. *Passive rewarming* is done by removing the person from the cold environment, covering with a blanket, supplying warm fluids (oral or intravenous), and allowing rewarming to occur at the person's own pace. *Active total rewarming* involves immersing the person in warm water or placing heating pads or hot water bottles on the surface of the body, including the extremities. Active core rewarming places a major emphasis on rewarming the trunk, leaving the extremities, containing the major metabolic mass, cold until the heart rewarms. *Active core rewarming* can be done by instilling warmed fluids into the gastrointestinal tract; by peritoneal dialysis; by extracorporeal blood warming, in which blood is removed from the body and passed through a heat exchanger and then returned to the body; or by inhalation of an oxygen mixture warmed to 42°C to 46°C (107.6°F to 114.8°F).

Persons with mild hypothermia usually respond well to passive rewarming in a warm bed. Persons with moderate or severe hypothermia do not have the thermoregulatory shivering mechanism and require active rewarming. During rewarming, the cold acidotic blood from the peripheral tissues is returned to the heart and central circulation. If this is done too rapidly or before cardiopulmonary function has been adequately reestablished, the hypothermic heart cannot respond to the increased metabolic demands of warm peripheral tissues.

In summary, hypothermia is a potentially life-threatening disorder in which the body's core temperature drops below 35°C (95°F). Accidental hypothermia can develop in otherwise healthy persons in the course of accidental exposure and in elderly or disabled persons with impaired perception of or response to cold. Alcoholism, cardiovascular disease, malnutrition, and hypothyroidism contribute to the risk for hypothermia. The greatest effect of hypothermia is a decrease in the metabolic rate, leading to a decrease in carbon dioxide production and respiratory rate. The signs and symptoms of hypothermia include poor coordination, stumbling, slurred speech, irrationality, poor judgment, amnesia, hallucinations, blueness and puffiness of the skin, dilation of the pupils, decreased respiratory rate, weak and irregular pulse, stupor, and coma. The treatment of moderate and severe hypothermia includes active rewarming.

REVIEW EXERCISES

A 3-year-old-child is seen in pediatric clinic with a temperature of 39°C (103°F) temperature. Her skin is warm and flushed, her pulse is 120 beats/minute, and her respirations are shallow and rapid at 32 breaths/minute. Her mother states that she has complained of a sore throat and has refused to drink or take medication to bring her temperature down.

A. Explain the physiologic mechanisms of fever generation.

B. Are the warm and flushed skin, rapid heart rate, and respirations consistent with this level of fever?

C. How might the refusal to take fluids contribute to temperature regulation in this child?

D. After receiving an appropriate dose of acetaminophen, the child begins to sweat, and the temperature drops to 37.2°C (99°F). Explain the physiologic mechanisms responsible for the drop in temperature.

A 25-year-old man was brought into the emergency room after having been found unconscious in a snow bank. The outdoor temperature at the time he was discovered was −10°F. His car, which was stalled a short distance away, contained liquor bottles suggesting he had been drinking. His temperature on admission was 28.9°C (84°F), his heart rate 40 beats/minute, and his respirations 8 breaths/minute and shallow. His skin is cold, his muscles rigid, and his digits blue.

A. What factors might have contributed to this man's state of hypothermia?

B. Is this man able to engage in physiologic behaviors to control loss of body heat (refer to Fig. 10-3)?

C. Given two methods that are available for taking this man's temperature (oral or rectal), which would be most accurate? Explain.

D. What precautions should be considered when deciding on a method for rewarming this man?

References

1. Guyton A. C., Hall J. E. (2000). *Textbook of medical physiology* (10th ed., pp. 822–833). Philadelphia: W. B. Saunders.
2. Wenger C. B. (2003). The regulation of body temperature. In Rhoades R. A., Tanner G. A. (Eds.), *Medical physiology* (2nd ed., pp. 527–550). Philadelphia: Lippincott Williams & Wilkins.
3. Gisolfi C. V., Mora F. (2000). *The hot brain: Survival, temperature, and the human body.* Cambridge, MA: MIT Press.
4. Vick R. (1984). *Contemporary medical physiology* (p. 886). Menlo Park, CA: Addison Wesley.
5. Erickson R. S. (1999). The continuing question of how best to measure body temperature. *Critical Care Medicine 27,* 2307–2314.
6. Beach P. S., McCormick D. P. (1991). Clinical applications of ear thermometry [Editorial]. *Clinical Pediatrics* (Suppl. 4), 3–4.
7. Knies R. B. (1998). Research applied to clinical practice: Temperature measurements in acute care. [On-line.] Available: http://www.ENW.org/Research-Thermometry.htm.
8. Jansky L. (1998). Shivering. In Blatteis C. M. (Ed.), *Physiology and pathophysiology of temperature regulation* (pp. 48–58). River Edge, NJ: World Scientific Publishing.
9. Atkins L. (1984). Fever: The old and new. *Journal of Infectious Diseases 149,* 339–348.
10. Stein M. T. (1991). Historical perspectives in fever and thermometry. *Clinical Pediatrics* (Suppl. 4), 5–7.
11. Mackowiak P. A. (1998). Concepts of fever. *Archives of Internal Medicine 158,* 1870–1881.
12. Dinarello, C. A., Gatti, S., Bartfai, T. (1999). Fever: Links with an ancient receptor. *Current Biology 9.* R147–R150.
13. Blatteis C. M. (1998). Fever. In Blatteis C. M. (Ed.), *Physiology and pathophysiology of temperature regulation* (pp. 178–192). River Edge, NJ: World Scientific Publishing.
14. Rodbard D. (1981). The role of regional temperature in the pathogenesis of disease. *New England Journal of Medicine 305,* 808–814.
15. McGee Z. A., Gorby G. L. (1987). The diagnostic value of fever patterns. *Hospital Practice 22*(10), 103–110.
16. Cunha B. A. (1984). Implications of fever in the critical care setting. *Heart and Lung 13,* 460–465.
17. Cunha B. A. (1996). The clinical significance of fever patterns. *Infectious Disease Clinics of North America 10,* 33–43.
18. Saper C. B., Breder C. D. (1994). The neurologic basis of fever. *New England Journal of Medicine 330,* 1880–1886.
19. Champi C., Gaffney-Yocum P. A. (1999). Managing febrile seizures in children. *Nurse Practitioner 24*(10), 28–30, 34–35.
20. Cunha B. A. (1996). Fever without source. *Infectious Disease Clinics of North America 10,* 111–127.
21. John C. C., Gillsdorf J. R (2002). Recurrent fever in children. *The Pediatric Infectious Disease Journal 21,* 1071–1077.

22. Drenth, J. P. H., Van Der Meer, J. W. M. (2001). Hereditary periodic fever. *New England Journal of Medicine 345*(24), 1748–1756.
23. Plaisance K. I., Mackowiak P. A. (2000). Antipyretic therapy: Physiologic rationale, diagnostic implications, and clinical consequences. *Archives of Internal Medicine 160,* 449–456.
24. Baker M. D. (1999). Evaluation and management of infants with fever. *Pediatric Clinics of North America 46,* 1061–1072.
25. Park J. W. (2000). Fever without source in children. *Postgraduate Medicine 107,* 259–266.
26. Luszczak M. (2001). Evaluation and management of infants and young children with fever. *American Family Physician 64,* 1219–1226.
27. Baraff L. J., Bass J. W., Fleisher G. R., et al. (1993). Practice guidelines for the management of infants and children 0 to 36 months of age with fever without source. Agency for Health Care Policy and Research. (Erratum appears in *Ann Emerg Med.* [1993]. *22*[9], 1490). *Annals of Emergency Medicine 22*(7), 1198–1210.
28. Castle S. C., Norman D. C., Yeh M., et al. (1991). Fever response in elderly nursing home residents: Are the older truly colder? *Journal of the American Geriatric Society 39*(9), 853–857.
29. Yoshikawa T. T., Norman D. C. (1996). Approach to fever and infections in the nursing home. *Journal of the American Geriatric Society 44,* 74–82.
30. Yoshikawa T. T., Norman, D. C. (1998). Fever in the elderly. *Infectious Medicine 15,* 704–706, 708.
31. Castle S. C., Yeh M., Toledo S., et al. (1993). Lowering the temperature criterion improves detection of infections in nursing home residents. *Aging Immunology and Infectious Disease 4,* 67–76.
32. Wexler, R. K. (2002). Evaluation and treatment of heat-related illnesses. *American Family Physician 65*(11): 2307–2314.
33. Bouchama A., Knochel, J. P. (2002). Heat stroke. *New England Journal of Medicine 346*(25), 1978–1988.
34. Hamdy, R. C. (2002). Heat Stroke. *Southern Medical Journal 95*(8): 791–792.
35. Ballester J. M., Harchelroad F. P. (1999). Hyperthermia: How to recognize and prevent heat-related illnesses. *Geriatrics 54*(7), 20–24.
36. Tabor P. A. (1986). Drug-induced fever. *Drug Intelligence and Clinical Pharmacy 20,* 413–420.
37. Mackowiak P. A., LeMaistre C. F. (1986). Drug fever: A critical appraisal of conventional concepts. *Annals of Internal Medicine 106,* 728–733.
38. Hofland S. L. (1985). Drug fever: Is your patient's fever drug-related? *Critical Care Nurse 5,* 29–34.
39. Johnson D. H., Cunha B. A. (1996). Drug fever. *Infectious Disease Clinics of North America 10,* 85–99.
40. Jurkat-Rott K., McCarthy T., Lehmann-Horn F. (2000). Genetics and pathogenesis of malignant hyperthermia. *Muscle and Nerve 23,* 4–17.
41. Denborough M. (1998). Malignant hyperthermia. *Lancet 352,* 1131–1136.
42. Parker W. A. (1987). Neuroleptic malignant syndrome. *Critical Care Nurse 7,* 40–46.
43. Goldwasser H. D., Hooper J. F. (1988). Neuroleptic malignant syndrome. *American Family Practice 38*(5), 211–216.
44. Mercer J. B. (1998). Hypothermia and cold injuries in man. In Blatteis C. M. (Ed.), *Physiology and pathophysiology of temperature regulation* (pp. 246–256). River Edge, NJ: World Scientific Publishing.
45. Centers for Disease Control and Prevention. (2003). Hypothermia-related deaths, Philadelphia—January 1996–December 2001, and United States, 1979–1999. *Morbidity and Mortality Weekly Reports 52*(5), 86–87.
46. Conn A. W. (1979). Near drowning and hypothermia. *Canadian Medical Association Journal 120,* 397–400.
47. Siebke H., Beivik H., Rod T. (1975). Survival after 40 minutes submersion with cerebral sequelae. *Lancet 1,* 1275–1277.
48. Biem J., Koehncke N., Classen D., Dosman J. (2003). Out of the cold: management of hypothermia and frostbite. *Canadian Medical Association Journal 168*(3), 305–311.
49. Moss J. F. (1988). The management of accidental severe hypothermia. *New York Journal of Medicine 88,* 411–413.
50. Ballester J. M., Harchelroad F. P. (1999). Hypothermia: An easy-to-miss, dangerous disorder in winter weather. *Geriatrics 54*(2), 51–57.
51. Wong K. C. (1983). Physiology and pharmacology of hypothermia. *Western Journal of Medicine 138,* 227–232.
52. Danzl D. F., Pozos R. S. (1994). Accidental hypothermia. *New England Journal of Medicine 331,* 1756–1760.
53. Hanania N. A., Zimmerman J. L. (1999). Accidental hypothermia. *Critical Care Clinics 15,* 235–249.

CHAPTER 11

Alterations in Nutritional Status

Joan Pleuss

"You are what you eat" is a familiar maxim. To a great extent, nutrition determines how a person looks, feels, and acts. The need for adequate nutrition begins at the time of conception and continues throughout life. Nutrition provided by food or supplements in the proper proportions enables the body to maintain life, to grow physically and intellectually, to heal and repair tissue, and to maintain the stamina necessary for well-being. This chapter addresses nutritional status, overnutrition and obesity, and undernutrition.

Nutritional Status

After completing this section of the chapter, you should be able to meet the following objectives:

- Define *nutritional status*
- Define *calorie* and state the number of calories derived from the oxidation of 1 g of protein, fat, or carbohydrate
- Explain the difference between anabolism and catabolism
- Relate the processes of glycogenolysis and gluconeogenesis to the regulation of blood glucose by the liver
- Define *basal metabolic rate* and cite factors that affect it
- State the purpose of the Recommended Dietary Allowance of calories, proteins, fats, carbohydrates, vitamins, and minerals
- Describe methods used for a nutritional assessment
- State the factors used in determining body mass index and explain its use in evaluating body weight in terms of undernutrition and overnutrition

Nutritional status describes the condition of the body related to the availability and use of nutrients. Nutrients are derived from the digestive tract through the ingestion of foods or, in some cases, through liquid feedings that are delivered directly into the gastrointestinal tract by a synthetic tube (*i.e.,* tube feedings). The exception occurs in persons with certain illnesses in which the digestive tract is bypassed and the nutrients are infused directly into the circulatory system. Once inside the body, nutrients are used for energy or as the building blocks for tissue growth and repair. When excess nutrients are available, they frequently are stored for future use. If the required nutrients are unavailable, the body adapts by conserving and using its nutrient stores.

ENERGY METABOLISM

Energy is measured in heat units called *calories.* A calorie, spelled with a small *c* and also called a *gram calorie,* is the amount of heat or energy required to raise the temperature of 1 g of water by 1°C. A *kilocalorie* (kcal), or *large calorie,* is the amount of energy needed to raise the temperature of 1 kg of water by 1°C.[1] Because a calorie is so small, kilocalories often are used in nutritional and physiologic studies. The oxidation of proteins provides 4 kcal/g; fats, 9 kcal/g; carbohydrates, 4 kcal/g; and alcohol, 7 kcal/g.

All body activities require energy, whether they involve an individual cell, a single organ, or the entire body. *Metabolism* is the organized process through which nutrients such as carbohydrates, fats, and proteins are broken down, transformed, or otherwise converted into cellular energy. The process of metabolism is unique in that it enables the continual release of energy, and it couples this energy with physiologic functioning. For example, the energy used for muscle contraction is derived largely from energy sources that are stored in muscle cells and then released as the muscle contracts. Because most of our energy sources come from the nutrients in the food that is eaten, the ability to store energy and control its release is important.

ENERGY METABOLISM

- All body activities require energy, whether they involve a single cell, a single organ, or the entire body.
- Energy, which is measured in kilocalories (kcal), is obtained from foods.
- Fats, which are a concentrated water-free energy source, contain 9 kcal/g. They are stored in fat cells as triglycerides, which are the main storage sites for energy.
- Carbohydrates are hydrated fuels, which supply 4 kcal/g. They are stored in limited quantities as glycogen and can be converted to fatty acids and stored in fat cells as triglycerides.
- Amino acids, which supply 4 kcal/g, are used in building body proteins. Amino acids in excess of those needed for protein synthesis are converted to fatty acids, ketones, or glucose and are stored or used as metabolic fuel.

Adipose Tissue

More than 90% of body energy is stored in the adipose tissues of the body. Adipocytes, or fat cells, occur singly or in small groups in loose connective tissue. In many parts of the body, they cushion body organs such as the kidneys. In addition to isolated groups of fat cells, entire regions of fat tissue are committed to fat storage. Collectively, fat cells constitute a large body organ that is metabolically active in the uptake, synthesis, storage, and mobilization of lipids, which are the main source of fuel storage for the body. Some tissues, such as liver cells, are able to store small amounts of lipids, but when these lipids accumulate, they begin to interfere with cell function. Adipose tissue not only serves as a storage site for body fuels but also provides insulation for the body, fills body crevices, and protects body organs.

Studies of adipocytes in the laboratory have shown that fully differentiated cells do not divide. However, such cells have a long life span, and anyone born with large numbers of adipocytes runs the risk of becoming obese. Some immature adipocytes capable of division are present in postnatal life; these cells respond to estrogen stimulation and are the potential source of additional fat cells during postnatal life.[1] Fat deposition results from proliferation of these existing immature adipocytes and can occur as a consequence of excessive caloric intake when a woman is breast-feeding or during estrogen stimulation around the time of puberty. An increase in fat cells also may occur during late adolescence and in middle-aged persons who already are overweight.

There are two types of adipose tissue: white fat and brown fat. *White fat,* which despite its name is cream colored or yellow, is the prevalent form of adipose tissue in postnatal life. It constitutes 10% to 20% of body weight in adult males and 15% to 25% in adult females. At body temperature, the lipid content of fat cells exists as an oil. It consists of triglycerides, which are made up of three molecules of fatty acids esterified to a glycerol molecule. Triglycerides, which contain no water, have the highest caloric content of all nutrients and are an efficient form of energy storage. Fat cells synthesize triglycerides from dietary fats and carbohydrates. Insulin is required for transport of glucose into fat cells. When calorie intake is restricted for any reason, fat cell triglycerides are broken down, and the resultant fatty acids and glycerol are released as energy sources.

Brown fat differs from white fat in terms of its thermogenic capacity or ability to produce heat. Brown fat, the site of diet-induced thermogenesis and nonshivering thermogenesis, is found primarily in early neonatal life in humans and in animals that hibernate. In humans, brown fat decreases with age but is still detectable in the sixth decade. This small amount of brown fat has a minimal effect on energy expenditure.

Anabolism and Catabolism

There are two phases of metabolism: anabolism and catabolism. *Anabolism* is the phase of metabolic storage and synthesis of cell constituents. Anabolism does not provide energy for the body; it requires energy. *Catabolism* involves the breakdown of complex molecules into substances that can be used in the production of energy. The chemical intermediates for anabolism and catabolism are called *metabolites (e.g.,* lactic acid is a metabolite formed when glucose is broken down in the absence of oxygen). Both anabolism and catabolism are catalyzed by enzyme systems located in body cells. A *substrate* is a substance on which an enzyme acts. Enzyme systems selectively transform fuel substrates into cellular energy and facilitate the use of energy in the process of assembling molecules to form energy substrates and storage forms of energy.

Because body energy cannot be stored as heat, the cellular oxidative processes that release energy are low-temperature reactions that convert food components to chemical energy that can be stored. The body transforms carbohydrates, fats, and proteins into the intermediary compound, *adenosine triphosphate* (ATP). ATP is called the *energy currency of the cell* because almost all body cells store and use ATP as their energy source (see Chapter 4). The metabolic events involved in ATP formation allow cellular energy to be stored, used, and replenished.

Glucose Metabolism

Glucose is a six-carbon molecule; it is an efficient fuel that, when metabolized in the presence of oxygen, breaks down to form carbon dioxide and water (Fig. 11-1). Although many tissues and organ systems are able to use other forms of fuel, such as fatty acids and ketones, the brain and nervous system rely almost exclusively on glucose as a fuel source. The nervous system can neither store nor synthesize glucose; instead, it relies on the minute-by-minute extraction of glucose from the blood to meet its energy needs. In the fed and early fasting state, the nervous system requires approximately 100 to 115 g of glucose per day to meet its metabolic needs.

The liver regulates the entry of glucose into the blood. Glucose ingested in the diet is transported from the gastrointestinal tract, through the portal vein, and to the liver before it gains access to the circulatory system (Fig. 11-2). The liver stores and synthesizes glucose. When blood sugar is increased, the liver removes glucose from the blood and stores it for future use. Conversely, the liver releases its glucose stores when blood sugar drops. In this way, the liver acts as a buffer system to regulate blood sugar levels. Blood sugar levels usually reflect the difference between the amount of glucose released into the circulation by the liver and the amount of glucose removed from the blood by body cells.

Excess glucose is stored in two forms. It can be converted to fatty acids and stored in fat cells as triglycerides, or it can be stored in the liver and skeletal muscle as glycogen (see Fig. 11-2). Small amounts of glycogen also are stored in the skin and in some of the glandular tissues.

Glycogenolysis. Glycogenolysis, or the breakdown of glycogen, is controlled by the action of two hormones: glucagon and epinephrine. Epinephrine is more effective in stimulating glycogen breakdown in muscle, whereas the liver is more responsive to glucagon. The synthesis and degradation of glycogen are important because they help maintain blood sugar levels during periods of fasting and strenuous exercise. Only the liver is able to release its glucose stores into the blood for use by other tissues, such as the brain and nervous system. Glycogen breaks down to form a phosphorylated glucose molecule, and in this form, it is too large to pass through the cell membrane. The liver, but not skeletal muscle, has the enzyme glucose-6-phosphatase, which is needed to remove the phosphate group and allow the glucose molecule to enter the bloodstream.

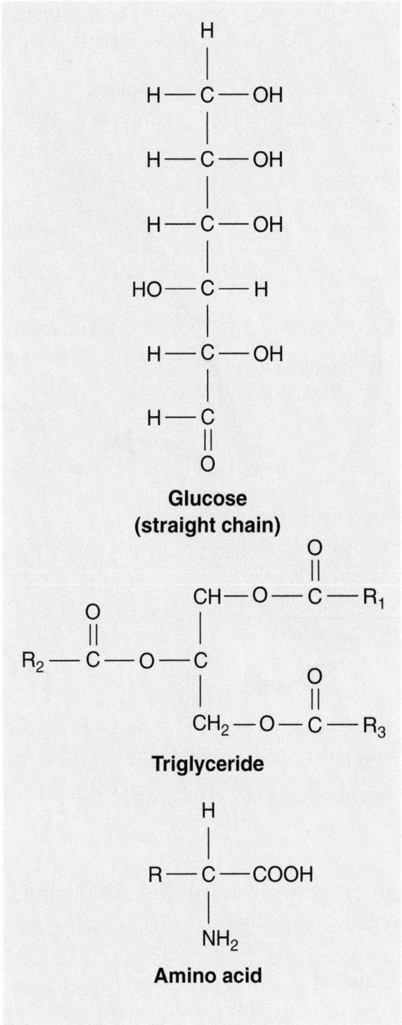

Glucose (straight chain)

Triglyceride

Amino acid

FIGURE 11-1 Glucose, triglyceride, and amino acid structure.

Gluconeogenesis. The synthesis of glucose is referred to as *gluconeogenesis,* or the building of glucose from new sources. The process of gluconeogenesis, most of which occurs in the liver, converts amino acids, lactate, and glycerol into glucose. Although many cells use fatty acids as a fuel source, they cannot be converted to glucose.

Glucose produced through the process of gluconeogenesis is either stored in the liver as glycogen or released into the general circulation. During periods of food deprivation or when the diet is low in carbohydrates, gluconeogenesis provides the glucose that is needed to meet the metabolic needs of the brain and other glucose-dependent tissues. Several hormones stimulate gluconeogenesis, including

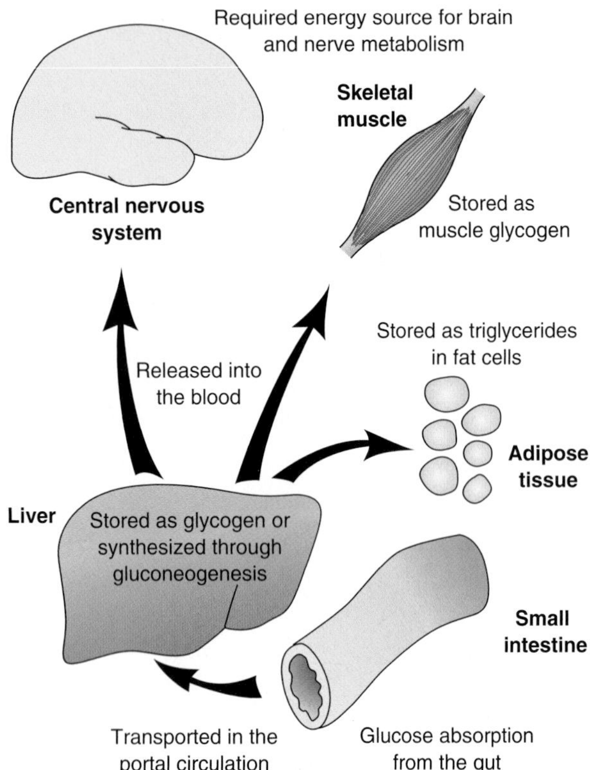

FIGURE 11-2 Regulation of blood glucose by the liver.

glucagon, glucocorticoid hormones from the adrenal cortex, and thyroid hormone.

Fat Metabolism

The average American diet provides approximately 33% of calories in the form of fats. In contrast to glucose, which yields only 4 kcal/g, each gram of fat yields 9 kcal. Another 30% to 50% of the carbohydrates consumed in the diet are converted to triglycerides for storage.

A triglyceride contains three fatty acids linked by a glycerol molecule (see Fig. 11-1). Fatty acids and triglycerides can be derived from dietary sources, they can be synthesized in the body, or they can be mobilized from fat depots. Excess carbohydrates are converted to triglycerides and transported to adipose cells for storage. One gram of anhydrous (water-free) fat stores more than six times as much energy as 1 hydrated gram of glycogen. One reason weight loss is greatest at the beginning of a fast or weight loss program is that this is when the body uses its water-containing glycogen stores. Later, when the body begins to use energy stored as triglycerides, water losses are decreased, and weight loss tends to plateau.

The mobilization of fatty acids for use in energy production is facilitated by the action of lipases (*i.e.*, enzymes) that break the triglycerides into three fatty acids and a glycerol molecule. The activation of lipases and subsequent mobilization of fatty acids is stimulated by epinephrine, glucocorticoid hormones, growth hormones, and glucagon. After triglycerides have been broken down, their fatty acids and glycerol enter the circulation and travel to the liver, where they are removed from the blood and used as a source of energy or converted to ketones.

The efficient burning of fatty acids requires a balance between carbohydrate and fat metabolism. The ratio of fatty acid and carbohydrate use is altered in situations that favor fat breakdown, such as diabetes mellitus and fasting. In these situations, the liver produces more ketones than it can use; this excess is released into the bloodstream. Ketones can be an important source of energy because even the brain adapts to the use of ketones during prolonged periods of starvation. A problem arises, however, when fat breakdown is accelerated and the production of ketones exceeds tissue use. Because ketones are organic acids, they cause ketoacidosis when they are present in excessive amounts.

Protein Metabolism

Approximately three fourths of body solids are proteins. Proteins are essential for the formation of all body structures, including genes, enzymes, contractile structures in muscle, matrix of bone, and hemoglobin of red blood cells.

Amino acids are the building blocks of proteins. Twenty amino acids are present in body proteins in significant quantities. Each amino acid has an acidic group (COOH) and an amino group (NH_2; see Fig. 11-1). Unlike glucose and fatty acids, there is only a limited facility for the storage of excess amino acids in the body. Most of the stored amino acids are contained in body proteins. Amino acids in excess of those needed for protein synthesis are converted to fatty acids, ketones, or glucose and are stored or used as metabolic fuel. Because fatty acids cannot be converted to glucose, the body must break down proteins and use the amino acids to generate glucose during periods when metabolic needs exceed food intake. The liver has the enzymes and mechanisms needed to deaminate and to convert the amino groups from the amino acid to urea. The breakdown or degradation of proteins and amino acids occurs primarily in the liver, which also is the site of gluconeogenesis.

ENERGY EXPENDITURE

The expenditure of body energy results from four mechanisms of heat production (*i.e.*, thermogenesis): basal metabolic rate or resting energy equivalent, diet-induced thermogenesis, exercise-induced thermogenesis, and thermogenesis in response to changes in environmental conditions. The amount of energy used varies with age, body size, rate of growth, and state of health.

Basal Metabolic Rate

The *basal metabolic rate* (BMR) refers to the chemical reactions occurring when the body is at rest. These reactions are necessary to provide energy for maintenance of normal body temperature, cardiovascular and respiratory function, muscle tone, and other essential activities of tissues and cells in the resting body. The resting metabolic rate constitutes 50% to 70% of body energy needs.[1] The BMR is measured using an instrument called a *metabolator* that measures the rate of oxygen use by a person. Oxygen consumption is measured under basal conditions: after a full night's sleep, after at least 12 hours without food, and while the person is awake and at rest in a warm and comfortable room. The BMR is then calculated in terms of calories per hour and normally averages approximately 65 to 70 calories per hour in an average 70-kg man.[1] Women in general have a 5% to 10% lower BMR than men because of their higher percentage of adipose tissue. Although much of the BMR is accounted for by essential activities of the central nervous system, kidneys, and other body organs, the variations in BMR among different individuals are related largely to skeletal muscle mass and body size. Under normal resting conditions, skeletal muscle accounts for 20% to 30% of the BMR.[1] For this reason, the BMR is commonly corrected for body size by expressing it as calories per hour per square meter of body surface area. Factors that affect the BMR are age, sex, physical state, and pregnancy. A progressive decline in the normal BMR occurs with aging[1] (Fig. 11-3). The BMR can be used to predict the calorie needs for maintenance of nutrition.

The *resting energy equivalent* (REE) is used for predicting energy expenditure. Several equations that determine REE have been published. Although the Harris-Benedict equation has been the most widely used, research indicates that the World Health Organization equation has better predicting value[2] (Table 11-1). Multiplying the REE by a factor of 1.2 usually adequately predicts the caloric needs for maintenance of nutrition during health. A factor of 1.5 usually provides the needed nutrients during repletion and during illnesses such as pneumonia, long bone fractures, cancer, peritonitis, and recovery from most types of surgery.

Diet- and Exercise-Induced Thermogenesis

Diet-induced thermogenesis, or thermic effect of food, describes the energy used by the body for the digestion, absorption, and assimilation of food after its ingestion. It is energy expended over and above the caloric value of the food and accounts for approximately 10% of the total calories expended. When food is eaten, the metabolic rate rises and then returns to normal within a few hours. The amount of energy expended for physical activity is determined by the type of activity performed, the length of participation, and the person's weight and physical fitness.

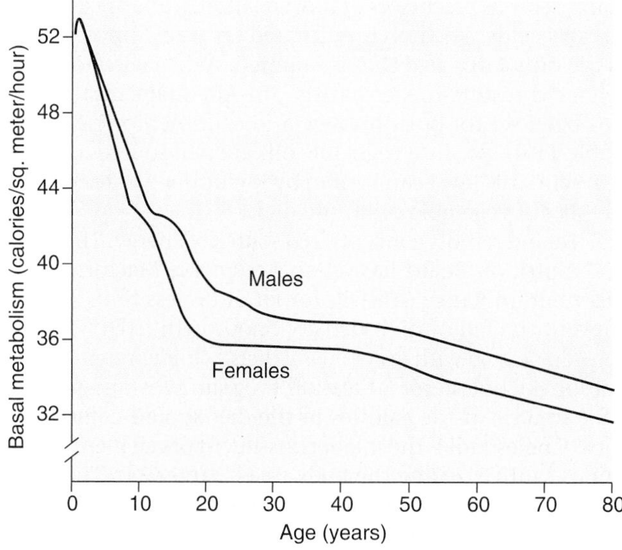

FIGURE 11-3 Normal basal metabolic rates at different ages for each sex. (Guyton A.C., Hall J.E. [1996]. *Medical physiology* [9th ed., p. 909]. Philadelphia: W.B. Saunders)

TABLE 11-1 Estimated Energy Requirements (EER) for Men and Women 30 Years of Age With a Body Mass Index of 18.5

Height (m [in])	PAL*	Weight (kg[lb])	EER†, men (kcal/d)	EER†, women (kcal/d)
1.50	Sedentary	41.6	1.848	1.625
(59)	Low active	(92)	2.009	1.803
	Active		2.215	2.025
	Very active		2.554	2.291
1.65	Sedentary	50.4	2.068	1.816
(65)	Low active	(111)	2.254	2.016
	Active		2.490	2.267
	Very active		2.880	2.567
1.80	Sedentary	59.9	2.301	2.015
(71)	Low active	(132)	2.513	2.239
	Active		2.782	2.519
	Very active		3.225	2.855

NOTE: For each year below 30 years of age, add 7 kcal/d for women and 10 kcal/d for men. For each year above 30 years of age, subtract 7 kcal/day for women and 10 kcal/d for men.

*PAL = total energy expenditure ÷ basal energy expenditure,
PA = 1.0 if PAL ≥1.0 <1.4 (sedentary)
PA = 1.12 if PAL ≥1.4 <1.6 (low activity)
PA = 1.27 if PAL ≥1.6 <1.9 (active)
PA = 1.45 if PAL ≥1.9 <2.5 (very active)

†EER derived from the following regression equations based on doubly labeled water data:
Adult man = 661.8 − 9.53 × age (y) × PA × (15.91 × wt [kg] + 539.6 × ht [m])
Adult woman = 354.1 − 6.91 × age (y) × PA × (9.36 × wt [kg] + 726 × ht [m]), where PA refers to coefficient for physical activity levels (PAL).

Adapted from Dietary reference intakes for energy carbohydrate, fiber, fat, fatty acids, cholesterol, protein, and amino acids (2002). This report may be accessed on-line via www.nap.edu. Copyright © 2002 by the National Academy of Sciences. All rights reserved.

RECOMMENDED DIETARY ALLOWANCES AND DIETARY REFERENCE INTAKES

The *Recommended Dietary Allowances* (RDAs) define the intakes that meet the nutrient needs of almost all healthy persons in a specific age and sex group.[3] The RDAs, which are periodically updated, have been published since 1941 by the National Academy of Sciences. The RDA is used in advising persons about the level of nutrient intake they need to decrease the risk of chronic disease.

The *Dietary Reference Intake* (DRI) includes a set of at least four nutrient-based reference values: the RDA, the Adequate Intake, the Estimated Average Requirement, and the Tolerable Upper Intake Level, each of which has specific uses.[4] The *Adequate Intake* (AI) is set when there is not enough scientific evidence to estimate an average requirement. The AI is derived from experimental or observational data that show a mean intake that appears to sustain a desired indicator of health. An *Estimated Average Requirement* is the intake that meets the estimated nutrient need of half of the persons in a specific group. This estimate is used as the basis for developing the RDA and is expected to be used by nutrition policy makers in the evaluation of the adequacy of a nutrient for a specific group and for planning how much of the nutrient the group should consume. The *Tolerable Upper Intake Level* is the maximum intake that is judged unlikely to pose a health risk in almost all healthy persons in a specified group. It refers to the total intakes from food, fortified food, and nutrient supplements. This value is not intended to be a recommended level of intake, and there is no established benefit for persons who consume nutrients at the RDA or AI levels.

The DRIs are regularly reviewed and updated by the Food and Nutrition Board of the Institute of Medicine and the National Academy of Sciences. The current recommended DRIs for selected vitamins and minerals that have been released between 1997 and 2001 are listed in Tables 11-2 and 11-3. In 2002, RDAs were established for dietary carbohydrate and protein. An AI was set for total fiber and linoleic and α-linolenic acids. The Food and Nutrition Board also established Acceptable Macronutrient Distribution Ranges (AMDR) as a percentage of energy intake for fat, carbohydrate, linoleic and α-linolenic acids, and protein[5] (Table 11-4).

Food and supplement labels use *Daily Values* (DVs), which are set by the U.S. Food and Drug Administration (FDA). However, the DVs are based on data that is older than the data used to determine the DRIs. Percent Daily Value (% DV) tells the consumer what percentage of the DV one serving of a food or supplement supplies.

Proteins, fats, carbohydrates, vitamins, and minerals each have their own function in providing the body with what it needs to maintain life and health. Recommended allowances have not been established for every nutrient; some are given as a safe and adequate intake, but others, such as carbohydrates and fats, are expressed as a percentage of the calorie intake.

NUTRITIONAL NEEDS

Calories

Energy requirements are greater during growth periods. Infants require approximately 115 kcal/kg at birth, 105 kcal/kg at 1 year, and 80 kcal/kg of body weight between 1 to 10 years of age. During adolescence, boys require 45 kcal/kg of body weight and girls require 38 kcal/kg of body weight. During pregnancy, a woman needs an extra 300 kcal/day above her usual requirement, and during the first 3 months of breast-feeding, she requires an additional 500 kcal.[3] Table 11-5 can be used to predict the caloric requirements of healthy adults.[5]

Proteins

Proteins are required for growth and maintenance of body tissues, enzymes and antibody formation, fluid and electrolyte balance, and nutrient transport. Proteins are composed of amino acids, nine of which are essential to the body. These are leucine, isoleucine, methionine, phenylalanine, threonine, tryptophan, valine, lysine, and histidine. The foods that provide these essential amino acids in adequate amounts are milk, eggs, meat, fish, and poultry. Dried peas and beans, nuts, seeds, and grains contain all the essential amino acids but in less than adequate proportions. These proteins need to be combined with each other or with complete proteins to meet the amino acid requirements for protein synthesis. Diets that are inadequate in protein can result in kwashiorkor. If calories and protein are inadequate, protein-calorie malnutrition occurs.

Unlike carbohydrates and fats, which are composed of hydrogen, carbon, and oxygen, proteins contain 16% nitrogen; therefore, nitrogen excretion is an indicator of protein intake. If the amount of nitrogen taken in by way of protein is equivalent to the nitrogen excreted, the person is said to be in nitrogen balance. A person is in positive nitrogen balance when the nitrogen consumed by way of protein is greater than the amount excreted. This occurs during growth, pregnancy, or healing after surgery or injury. A negative nitrogen balance often occurs with fever, illness, infection, trauma, or burns, when more nitrogen is excreted than is consumed. It represents a state of tissue breakdown.

Fats

Dietary fats are composed primarily of triglycerides (*i.e.*, a mixture of fatty acids and glycerol). The fatty acids are saturated (*i.e.*, no double bonds), monounsaturated (*i.e.*, one double bond), or polyunsaturated (*i.e.*, two or more double bonds). The saturated fatty acids elevate blood cholesterol, whereas the monounsaturated and polyunsaturated fats lower blood cholesterol. Saturated fats usually are from animal sources and remain solid at room temperature. With the exception of coconut and palm oils (which are saturated), unsaturated fats are found in plant oils and usually are liquid at room temperature. Dietary fats provide energy, function as carriers for the fat-soluble vitamins, serve as precursors of prostaglandins, and are a source of fatty acids. The polyunsaturated fatty acid linoleic acid is the only fatty acid that is required. A deficiency of linoleic acid results in dermatitis. An Adequate Intake (AI) has been set for both linoleic and α-linolenic acids[5] (see Table 11-4). Because vegetable oils are rich sources of linoleic acid, this level can be met by including two teaspoons per day of vegetable oil in the diet.

Fat is the most concentrated source of energy. The Food and Nutrition Board has set an Acceptable Macronutrient Distribution Range (AMDR) for fat of no less than 20% to prevent the fall of high-density lipoprotein (HDL) cholesterol associated with very-low-fat diets.[5] Guidelines from the National Cholesterol Education Program recommend that 25% to 35% of the calories in the diet should come from fats.[6] Cholesterol is the major constituent of cell membranes and is synthesized by the body (see Chapter 24). The daily dietary recommendation for cholesterol is less than 300 mg.

Carbohydrates

Dietary carbohydrates are composed of simple sugars, complex carbohydrates, and undigested carbohydrates

TABLE 11-2 Dietary Reference Intakes (DRIs): Recommended Intakes for Individuals, Vitamins Food and Nutrition Board, Institute of Medicine, National Academies

Life Stage Group	Vitamin A (µg/d)[a]	Vitamin C (mg/d)	Vitamin D (µg/d)[b,c]	Vitamin E (mg/d)[d]	Vitamin K (µg/d)	Thiamin (mg/d)	Riboflavin (mg/d)	Niacin (mg/d)[e]	Vitamin B_6 (mg/d)	Folate (µg/d)[f]	Vitamin B_{12} (µg/d)	Pantothenic Acid (mg/d)	Biotin (µg/d)	Choline[g] (mg/d)
Infants														
0–6 mo	400*	40*	5*	4*	2.0*	0.2*	0.3*	2*	0.1*	65*	0.4*	1.7*	5*	125*
7–12 mo	500*	50*	5*	5*	2.5*	0.3*	0.4*	4*	0.3*	80*	0.5*	1.8*	6*	150*
Children														
1–3 y	**300**	**15**	5*	**6**	30*	**0.5**	**0.5**	**6**	**0.5**	**150**	**0.9**	2*	8*	200*
4–8 y	**400**	**25**	5*	**7**	55*	**0.6**	**0.6**	**8**	**0.6**	**200**	**1.2**	3*	12*	250*
Males														
9–13 y	**600**	**45**	5*	**11**	60*	**0.9**	**0.9**	**12**	**1.0**	**300**	**1.8**	4*	20*	375*
14–18 y	**900**	**75**	5*	**15**	75*	**1.2**	**1.3**	**16**	**1.3**	**400**	**2.4**	5*	25*	550*
19–30 y	**900**	**90**	5*	**15**	120*	**1.2**	**1.3**	**16**	**1.3**	**400**	**2.4**	5*	30*	550*
31–50 y	**900**	**90**	5*	**15**	120*	**1.2**	**1.3**	**16**	**1.3**	**400**	**2.4**	5*	30*	550*
51–70 y	**900**	**90**	10*	**15**	120*	**1.2**	**1.3**	**16**	**1.7**	**400**	**2.4**[h]	5*	30*	550*
>70 y	**900**	**90**	15*	**15**	120*	**1.2**	**1.3**	**16**	**1.7**	**400**	**2.4**[h]	5*	30*	550*
Females														
9–13 y	**600**	**45**	5*	**11**	60*	**0.9**	**0.9**	**12**	**1.0**	**300**	**1.8**	4*	20*	375*
14–18 y	**700**	**65**	5*	**15**	75*	**1.0**	**1.0**	**14**	**1.2**	**400**[i]	**2.4**	5*	25*	400*
19–30 y	**700**	**75**	5*	**15**	90*	**1.1**	**1.1**	**14**	**1.3**	**400**[i]	**2.4**	5*	30*	425*
31–50 y	**700**	**75**	5*	**15**	90*	**1.1**	**1.1**	**14**	**1.3**	**400**[i]	**2.4**	5*	30*	425*
51–70 y	**700**	**75**	10*	**15**	90*	**1.1**	**1.1**	**14**	**1.5**	**400**	**2.4**[h]	5*	30*	425*
>70 y	**700**	**75**	15*	**15**	90*	**1.1**	**1.1**	**14**	**1.5**	**400**	**2.4**[h]	5*	30*	425*
Pregnancy														
≤18 y	**750**	**80**	5*	**15**	75*	**1.4**	**1.4**	**18**	**1.9**	**600**[j]	**2.6**	6*	30*	450*
19–30 y	**770**	**85**	5*	**15**	90*	**1.4**	**1.4**	**18**	**1.9**	**600**[j]	**2.6**	6*	30*	450*
31–50 y	**770**	**85**	5*	**15**	90*	**1.4**	**1.4**	**18**	**1.9**	**600**[j]	**2.6**	6*	30*	450*
Lactation														
≤18 y	**1,200**	**115**	5*	**19**	75*	**1.4**	**1.6**	**17**	**2.0**	**500**	**2.8**	7*	35*	550*
19–30 y	**1,300**	**120**	5*	**19**	90*	**1.4**	**1.6**	**17**	**2.0**	**500**	**2.8**	7*	35*	550*
31–50 y	**1,300**	**120**	5*	**19**	90*	**1.4**	**1.6**	**17**	**2.0**	**500**	**2.8**	7*	35*	550*

NOTE: This table (taken from the DRI reports, see www.nap.edu) presents Recommended Dietary Allowances (RDAs) in **bold type** and Adequate Intakes (AIs) in ordinary type followed by an asterisk (*) RDAs and AIs may both be used as goals for individual intake. RDAs are set to meet the needs of almost all (97 to 98 percent) individuals in a group. For healthy breastfed infants, the AI is the mean intake. The AI for other life stage and gender groups is believed to cover needs of all individuals in the group, but lack of data or uncertainty in the data prevent being able to specify with confidence the percentage of individuals covered by this intake.

[a] As retinol activity equivalents (RAEs). 1 RAE = 1 µg retinol, 12 µg β-carotene, 24 µg α-carotene, or 24 µg β-cryptoxanthin. The RAE for dietary provitamin A carotenoids is two-fold greater than retinol equivalents (RE), whereas the RAE for preformed vitamin A is the same as RE.

[b] Cholecalciferol. 1 µg cholecalciferol = 40 IU vitamin D.

[c] In the absence of adequate exposure to sunlight.

[d] As α-tocopherol. α-Tocopherol includes RRR-α-tocopherol, the only form of α-tocopherol that occurs naturally in foods, and the 2R-stereoisomeric forms of α-tocopherol (RRR-, RSR-, RRS-, and RSS-α-tocopherol) that occur in fortified foods and supplements. It does not include the 2S-stereoisomeric forms of α-tocopherol (SRR-, SSR-, SRS-, and SSS-α-tocopherol), also found in fortified foods and supplements.

[e] As niacin equivalents (NE). 1 mg of niacin = 60 mg of tryptophan, 0–6 months = preformed niacin (not NE).

[f] As dietary folate equivalents (DFE). 1 DFE = 1 µg food folate = 0.6 µg of folic acid from fortified food or as a supplement consumed with food = 0.5 µg of a supplement taken on an empty stomach.

[g] Although AIs have been set for choline, there are few data to assess whether a dietary supply of choline is needed at all stages of the life cycle, and it may be that the choline requirement can be met by endogenous synthesis at some of these stages.

[h] Because 10 to 30 percent of older people may malabsorb food-bound B_{12}, it is advisable for those older than 50 years to meet their RDA mainly by consuming foods fortified with B_{12} or a supplement containing B_{12}.

[i] In view of evidence linking folate intake with neural tube defects in the fetus, it is recommended that all women capable of becoming pregnant consume 400 µg from supplements or fortified foods in addition to intake of food folate from a varied diet.

[j] It is assumed that women will continue consuming 400 µg from supplements or fortified food until their pregnancy is confirmed and they enter prenatal care, which ordinarily occurs after the end of the periconceptional period—the critical time for formation of the neural tube.

Copyright 2001 by the National Academy of Sciences. All rights reserved.

TABLE 11-3 Dietary Reference Intakes (DRIs): Recommended Intakes for Individuals, Elements Food and Nutrition Board, Institute of Medicine, National Academies

Life Stage Group	Calcium (mg/d)	Chromium (μg/d)	Copper (μg/d)	Fluoride (mg/d)	Iodine (μg/d)	Iron (mg/d)	Magnesium (mg/d)	Manganese (mg/d)	Molybdenum (μg/d)	Phosphorus (mg/d)	Selenium (μg/d)	Zinc (mg/d)
Infants												
0–6 mo	210*	0.2*	200*	0.01*	110*	0.27*	30*	0.003*	2*	100*	15*	2*
7–12 mo	270*	5.5*	220*	0.5*	130*	**11**	75*	0.6*	3*	275*	20*	**3**
Children												
1–3 y	500*	11*	**340**	0.7*	**90**	**7**	**80**	1.2*	**17**	**460**	**20**	**3**
4–8 y	800*	15*	**440**	1*	**90**	**10**	**130**	1.5*	**22**	**500**	**30**	**5**
Males												
9–13 y	1,300*	25*	**700**	2*	**120**	**8**	**240**	1.9*	**34**	**1,250**	**40**	**8**
14–18 y	1,300*	35*	**890**	3*	**150**	**11**	**410**	2.2*	**43**	**1,250**	**55**	**11**
19–30 y	1,000*	35*	**900**	4*	**150**	**8**	**400**	2.3*	**45**	**700**	**55**	**11**
31–50 y	1,000*	35*	**900**	4*	**150**	**8**	**420**	2.3*	**45**	**700**	**55**	**11**
51–70 y	1,200*	30*	**900**	4*	**150**	**8**	**420**	2.3*	**45**	**700**	**55**	**11**
>70 y	1,200*	30*	**900**	4*	**150**	**8**	**420**	2.3*	**45**	**700**	**55**	**11**
Females												
9–13 y	1,300*	21*	**700**	2*	**120**	**8**	**240**	1.6*	**34**	**1,250**	**40**	**8**
14–18 y	1,300*	24*	**890**	3*	**150**	**15**	**360**	1.6*	**43**	**1,250**	**55**	**9**
19–30 y	1,000*	25*	**900**	3*	**150**	**18**	**310**	1.8*	**45**	**700**	**55**	**8**
31–50 y	1,000*	25*	**900**	3*	**150**	**18**	**320**	1.8*	**45**	**700**	**55**	**8**
51–70 y	1,200*	20*	**900**	3*	**150**	**8**	**320**	1.8*	**45**	**700**	**55**	**8**
>70 y	1,200*	20*	**900**	3*	**150**	**8**	**320**	1.8*	**45**	**700**	**55**	**8**
Pregnancy												
≤18 y	1,300*	29*	**1,000**	3*	**220**	**27**	**400**	2.0*	**50**	**1,250**	**60**	**12**
19–30 y	1,000*	30*	**1,000**	3*	**220**	**27**	**350**	2.0*	**50**	**700**	**60**	**11**
31–50 y	1,000*	30*	**1,000**	3*	**220**	**27**	**360**	2.0*	**50**	**700**	**60**	**11**
Lactation												
≤18 y	1,300*	44*	**1,300**	3*	**290**	**10**	**360**	2.6*	**50**	**1,250**	**70**	**13**
19–30 y	1,000*	45*	**1,300**	3*	**290**	**9**	**310**	2.6*	**50**	**700**	**70**	**12**
31–50 y	1,000*	45*	**1,300**	3*	**290**	**9**	**320**	2.6*	**50**	**700**	**70**	**12**

NOTE: This table presents Recommended Dietary Allowances (RDAs) in **bold type** and Adequate Intakes (AIs) in ordinary type followed by an asterisk (*). RDAs and AIs may both be used as goals for individual intake. RDAs are set to meet the needs of almost all (97 to 98 percent) individuals in a group. For healthy breastfed infants, the AI is the mean intake. The AI for other life stage and gender groups is believed to cover needs of all individuals in the group, but lack of data or uncertainty in the data prevent being able to specify with confidence the percentage of individuals covered by this intake.

SOURCES: Dietary Reference intakes for Calcium, Phosphorus, Magnesium, Vitamin D, and Fluoride (1997); Dietary Reference Intakes for Thiamin, Riboflavin, Niacin, Vitamin B_6, Folate, Vitamin B_{12}, Pantothenic Acid, Biotin, and Choline (1998); Dietary Reference Intakes for Vitamin C, Vitamin E, Selenium, and Carotenoids (2000); and Dietary Reference Intakes for Vitamin A, Vitamin K, Arsenic, Boron, Chromium, Copper, Iodine, Iron, Manganese, Molybdenum, Nickel, Silicon, Vanadium, and Zinc (2001). These reports may be accessed via www.nap.edu.

Copyright 2001 by The National Academies of Sciences. All rights reserved.

TABLE 11-4 Dietary Reference Intakes (DRIs): Recommended Intakes for Individuals, Macronutrients Food and Nutrition Board, Institute of Medicine, National Academies

Life Stage Group	Carbohydrate (g/d)	Total Fiber (g/d)	Fat (g/d)	Linoleic Acid (g/d)	α-Linolenic Acid (g/d)	Protein[a] (g/d)
Infants						
0–6 mo	60*	ND	31*	4.4*	0.5*	9.1*
7–12 mo	95*	ND	30*	4.6*	0.5*	**13.5**
Children						
1–3 y	**130**	19*	ND	7*	0.7*	**13**
4–8 y	**130**	25*	ND	10*	0.9*	**19**
Males						
9–13 y	**130**	31*	ND	12*	1.2*	**34**
14–18 y	**130**	38*	ND	16*	1.6*	**52**
19–30 y	**130**	38*	ND	17*	1.6*	**56**
31–50 y	**130**	38*	ND	17*	1.6*	**56**
51–70 y	**130**	30*	ND	14*	1.6*	**56**
>70 y	**130**	30*	ND	14*	1.6*	**56**
Females						
9–13 y	**130**	26*	ND	10*	1.0*	**34**
14–18 y	**130**	26*	ND	11*	1.1*	**46**
19–30 y	**130**	25*	ND	12*	1.1*	**46**
31–50 y	**130**	25*	ND	12*	1.1*	**46**
51–70 y	**130**	21*	ND	11*	1.1*	**46**
>70 y	**130**	21*	ND	11*	1.1*	**46**
Pregnancy						
14–18 y	**175**	28*	ND	13*	1.4*	**71**
19–30 y	**175**	28*	ND	13*	1.4*	**71**
31–50 y	**175**	28*	ND	13*	1.4*	**71**
Lactation						
14–18	**210**	29*	ND	13*	1.3*	**71**
19–30 y	**210**	29*	ND	13*	1.3*	**71**
31–50 y	**210**	29*	ND	13*	1.3*	**71**

NOTE: This table presents Recommended Dietary Allowances (RDAs) in **bold type** and Adequate Intakes (AIs) in ordinary type followed by an asterisk (*). RDAs and AIs may both be used as goals for individual intake. RDAs are set to meet the needs of almost all (97 to 98 percent) individuals in a group. For healthy breastfed infants, the AI is the mean intake. The AI for other life stage and gender groups is believed to cover needs of all individuals in the group but lack of data or uncertainty in the data prevent being able to specify with confidence the percentage of individuals covered by this intake.

[a]Based on 0.8g protein/kg body weight for reference body weight.

SOURCE: Dietary Reference Intakes for Energy, Carbohydrate, Fiber, Fat, Fatty Acids, Cholesterol, Protein, and Amino Acids (2002). This report may be accessed via www.nap.edu.

Copyright 2002 by the National Academy of Sciences. All rights reserved.

(*i.e.,* fiber). Because of their vitamin, mineral, and fiber content, it is recommended that the bulk of the carbohydrate content in the diet be in the complex form rather than as simple sugars that contain few nutrients. Sucrose (*i.e.,* table sugar) is implicated in the development of dental caries.

TABLE 11-5 Caloric Requirements Based on Body Weight and Activity Level

	Sedentary	Moderate	Active
Overweight	20–25 kcal/kg	30 kcal/kg	35 kcal/kg
Normal	30 kcal/kg	35 kcal/kg	40 kcal/kg
Underweight	30 kcal/kg	40 kcal/kg	45–50 kcal/kg

(Adapted from Goodhart R.S., Shils M.E. [1980]. *Modern nutrition in health and disease* [6th ed.]. Philadelphia: Lea and Febiger)

There is no specific dietary requirement for carbohydrates. All of the energy requirements of the body can be met by dietary fats and proteins. Although some tissues, such as the nervous system, require glucose as an energy source, this need can be met through the conversion of amino acids and the glycerol part of the triglyceride molecule to glucose. The fatty acids from triglycerides are converted to ketones and used for energy by other body tissues. A carbohydrate-deficient diet usually results in the loss of tissue proteins and the development of ketosis. Because protein and fat metabolism increases the production of osmotically active metabolic wastes that must be eliminated through the kidneys, there is danger of dehydration and electrolyte imbalances. The amount of carbohydrate needed to prevent tissue wasting and ketosis is 50 to 100 g/day. In practice, most of the daily energy requirement should be from carbohydrate. This is because protein is an expensive source of calories and because it is recommended that no more than 30% of the calories in the diet be derived from fat. The AMDR indicates that carbohydrate intake should be limited to no less than 45% of the calories in the diet to prevent high intakes of fat.[5]

Vitamins

Vitamins are a group of organic compounds that act as catalysts in various chemical reactions. A compound cannot be classified as a vitamin unless it is shown that a deficiency of it causes disease. Contrary to popular belief, vitamins do not provide energy directly. As catalysts, they are part of the enzyme systems required for the release of energy from protein, fat, and carbohydrates. Vitamins also are necessary for the formation of red blood cells, hormones, genetic materials, and the nervous system. They are essential for normal growth and development.

There are two types of vitamins: fat soluble and water soluble. The four fat-soluble vitamins are vitamins A, D, E, and K. The nine required water-soluble vitamins are thiamine, riboflavin, niacin, pyridoxine (vitamin B_6), pantothenic acid, vitamin B_{12}, folic acid, biotin, and vitamin C. Because the water-soluble vitamins are excreted in the urine, they are less likely to become toxic to the body, as compared with the fat-soluble vitamins that are stored in the body. Table 11-6 lists sources and functions of vitamins.

Minerals

Minerals serve many functions. They are involved in acid-base balance and in the maintenance of osmotic pressure in body compartments. Minerals are components of vitamins, hormones, and enzymes. They maintain normal hemoglobin levels, play a role in nervous system function, and are involved in muscle contraction and skeletal development and maintenance. Minerals that are present in relatively large amounts in the body are called *macrominerals.* These include calcium, phosphorus, sodium, chloride, potassium, magnesium, and sulfur. The remainder are classified as *trace minerals;* they include iron, manganese, copper, iodine, zinc, cobalt, fluorine, and selenium. Table 11-7 lists mineral sources and functions.

Fiber

Fiber, the portion of food that cannot be digested by the human intestinal tract, increases stool bulk and facilitates bowel movements. Soluble fiber, the type that produces a gel in the intestinal tract, binds with cholesterol and prevents it from being absorbed by the body. Soluble fiber also lowers blood glucose. More studies are needed to establish whether fiber prevents colon cancer and promotes weight loss. In 2002, the Food and Nutrition Board gave its first recommended intake for fiber. Men and women who are 50 years and younger should have 38 and 25 grams, respectively, of fiber daily, whereas those older than 50 years should have 30 and 21 grams, respectively, each day. The recommendation for children ranges from 19 to 31 grams, and for teenagers, it is similar to adults.[5]

NUTRITIONAL ASSESSMENT

The nutritional status can be assessed using the subjective global assessment (SGA). It includes weight status for the previous 6 months, dietary intake, gastrointestinal symptoms that impact food intake, and functional capacity and physical signs of fat loss and muscle wasting. Combined with objective measures such as albumin levels and body mass index, SGA will accurately identify malnourished individuals 90% of the time.[7]

Diet Assessment

A nutritional assessment includes an evaluation of the person's diet. This can be accomplished by recording the food consumed or by 24-hour recall and through the administration of a questionnaire or diet history. Each technique has its own shortcomings, such as the tendency to alter behavior when it is known that the behavior is being observed or reported.

Health Assessment

Health assessment, including a health history and physical examination, reveals weight changes, muscle wasting, fat stores, functional status, and nutritional status. Comparison of the person's current weight with previous weights identifies whether the person's weight is stable, changed drastically, or tends to fluctuate. For example, recent rapid weight loss can be a sign of cancer, a malfunctioning thyroid gland, or self-imposed starvation. A history of fluctuating weight could be associated with bulimia. Degradation of muscle, or muscle wasting, is a serious sign of malnutrition. Decreased ability to initiate or complete activities of daily living could result from a decrease in energy caused by a poor diet, a neurologic malfunction such as multiple sclerosis, or symptoms related to chronic obstructive pulmonary disease. Quality of the hair, absence of body hair, condition of gums, and skin lesions could signal poor nutritional status.

Anthropometric Measurements

Anthropometric measurements provide a means for assessing body composition, particularly fat stores and skeletal muscle mass. This is done by measuring height, weight, body circumferences, and thickness of various skinfolds. These measurements commonly are used to determine growth patterns in children and appropriateness of current weight in adults.

Body weight is the most frequently used method of assessing nutritional status; it should be used in combination with measurements of body height to establish whether a person is underweight or overweight.

An unintentional loss of 10% of body weight or more within the past 6 months usually is considered predictive of a poor clinical outcome, especially if weight loss is continuing.[8] The body mass index (BMI) uses height and weight to determine healthy weight (Table 11-8). It is calculated by dividing the weight in kilograms by the height in meters squared (BMI = weight [kg]/height [m^2]). A BMI between 18.5 and 25 has the lowest statistical health risk.[9] A BMI of

TABLE 11-6 Sources and Functions of Vitamins

Vitamin	Major Food Sources	Functions
Fat-Soluble Vitamins		
Vitamin A (retinol, provitamin, carotenoids)	Retinol: liver, butter, whole milk, cheese, egg yolks; provitamin A: carrots, green leafy vegetables, sweet potatoes, pumpkin, winter squash, apricots, cantaloupe, fortified margarine	Essential for normal retinal function; plays an essential role in cell growth and differentiation, particularly epithelial cells. Epidemiologic evidence suggests a role in preventing certain cancers
Vitamin D (calciferol)	Fortified dairy products, fortified margarine, fish oils, egg yolk	Increases intestinal absorption of calcium and promotes ossification of bones and teeth
Vitamin E (tocopherol)	Vegetable oil, margarine, shortening, green and leafy vegetables, wheat germ, whole-grain products, egg yolk, butter, liver	Functions as an antioxidant protecting vitamins A and C and fatty acids; prevents cell membrane injury
Water-Soluble Vitamins		
Vitamin C (ascorbic acid)	Broccoli, sweet and hot peppers, collards, brussel sprouts, kale, potatoes, spinach, tomatoes, citrus fruits, strawberries	Potent antioxidant involved in many oxidation–reduction reactions; required for synthesis of collagen; increases absorption of nonheme iron; is involved in wound healing and drug metabolism
Thiamin (vitamin B_1)	Pork, liver, meat, whole grains, fortified grain products, legumes, nuts	Coenzyme required for several important biochemical reactions in carbohydrate metabolism; thought to have an independent role in nerve conduction
Riboflavin (vitamin B_2)	Liver, milk, yogurt, cottage cheese, meat, fortified grain products	Coenzyme that participates in a variety of important oxidation–reduction reactions and an important component of a number of enzymes
Niacin (nicotinamide, nicotinic acid)	Liver, meat, poultry, fish, peanuts, fortified grain products	Essential component of the coenzymes nicotinamide adenine dinucleotide (NAD) and nicotinamide dinucleotide diphosphate (NADP), which are involved in many oxidative reduction reactions
Folacin (folic acid)	Liver, legumes, green leafy vegetables	Coenzyme in amino acid and nucleoprotein metabolism; promotes red cell formation
Vitamin B_6 (pyridoxine)	Meat, poultry, fish, shellfish, green and leafy vegetables, whole-grain products, legumes	A major coenzyme involved in the metabolism of amino acids; required for synthesis of heme
Vitamin B_{12}	Meat, poultry, fish, shellfish, eggs, dairy products	Coenzyme involved in nucleic acid synthesis; assists in development of red cells and maintenance of nerve function
Biotin	Kidney, liver, milk, egg yolks, most fresh vegetables	Coenzyme in fat synthesis, amino acid metabolism, and glycogen formation
Pantothenic acid	Liver, kidney, meats, milk, egg yolk, whole-grain products, legumes	Coenzyme involved in energy metabolism

(Data from *Vitamin facts*, National Dairy Council, and other sources)

less than 18.5 is classified as being underweight, and a BMI of 25 to 29.9 is considered overweight.[10] A BMI greater than 29.9 is diagnosed as obesity and is furthered classified into class I (BMI, 30.0–34.9), class II (BMI, 35.0–39.9), and class III or extreme obesity (BMI >40). Body weight reflects both lean body mass and adipose tissue and cannot be used as a method for describing body composition or the percentage of fat tissue present. Statistically, the best percentage of body fat for men is between 12% and 20%, and for women, it is between 20% and 30%.[10] During physical training, body fat usually decreases, and lean body mass increases.

Among the methods used to estimate body fat are skinfold thickness, body circumferences, hydrodensitometry, bioelectrical impedance, dual photon absorptiometry, computed tomography (CT), and magnetic resonance imaging (MRI). Measurements of *skinfold thickness* can provide a reasonable assessment of body fat, particularly if taken at multiple sites. They can provide information about the location of the fat and can be used, together with equations and tables, to estimate the percentage of lean body mass and fat tissue.[11,12] However, these measurements often are difficult to perform and subject to considerable variation

TABLE 11-7 Sources and Functions of Minerals

Mineral	Major Sources	Functions
Calcium	Milk and milk products, fish with bones, greens	Bone formation and maintenance; tooth formation, vitamin B absorption, blood clotting, nerve and muscle function
Chloride	Table salt, meats, milk, eggs	Regulates pH of stomach, acid-base balance, osmotic pressure of extracellular fluids
Cobalt	Organ meats, meats	Aids in maturation of red blood cells (as part of B_{12} molecule)
Copper	Cereals, nuts, legumes, liver, shellfish, grapes, meats	Catalyst for hemoglobin formation, formation of elastin and collagen, energy release (cytochrome oxidase and catalase), formation of melanin, formation of phospholipids for myelin sheath of nerves
Fluoride	Fluorinated water	Strengthens bones and teeth
Iodine	Iodized salt, fish (saltwater and anadromous)	Thyroid hormone synthesis and its function in maintenance of metabolic rate
Iron	Meats, heart, liver, clams, oysters, lima beans, spinach, dates, dried nuts, enriched and whole-grain cereals	Hemoglobin synthesis, cellular energy release (cytochrome pathway), killing bacteria (myeloperoxidase)
Magnesium	Milk, green vegetables, nuts, bread, cereals	Catalyst of many intracellular nerve impulses, retention of reactions, particularly those related to intracellular enzyme reactions; low magnesium levels produce an increase in irritability of the nervous system, vasodilatation, and cardiac dysrhythmias
Phosphorus	Meats, poultry, fish, milk and cheese, cereals, legumes, nuts	Bone formation and maintenance; essential component of nucleic acids and energy exchange forms such as adenosine triphosphate (ATP)
Potassium	Oranges, dried fruits, bananas, meats, potatoes, peanut butter, coffee	Maintenance of intracellular osmolality, acid-base balance, transmission of nerve impulses, catalyst in energy metabolism, formation of proteins, formation of glycogen
Sodium	Table salt, cured meats, meats, milk, olives	Maintenance of osmotic pressure of extracellular fluids, acid-base balance, neuromuscular function; absorption of glucose
Zinc	Whole-wheat cereals, eggs, legumes	Integral part of many enzymes, including carbonic anhydrase, which facilitates combination of carbon dioxide with water in red blood cells; component of lactate dehydrogenase, which is important in cellular metabolism; component of many peptidases; important in digestion of proteins in gastrointestinal tract

TABLE 11-8 Classification of Overweight and Obesity by BMI, Waist Circumference, and Associated Disease Risk*

			Disease Risk* Relative to Normal Weight and Waist Circumference	
	BMI (kg/m²)	Obesity Class	Men ≤102 cm (≤40 in) Women ≤88 cm (≤35 in)	Men >102 cm (>40 in) Women >88 cm (>35 in)
Underweight	<18.5		—	—
Normal†	18.5–24.9		—	—
Overweight	25.0–29.9		Increased	High
Obesity	30.0–34.9	I	High	Very high
	35.0–39.9	II	Very high	Very high
Extreme obesity	≥40	III	Extremely high	Extremely high

BMI, body mass index.
*Disease risk for type 2 diabetes, hypertension, and cardiovascular disease.
†Increased waist circumference also can be a marker for increased risk, even in persons of normal weight.
(Expert Panel. [1998]. Clinical guidelines on the identification, evaluation, and treatment of overweight and obesity in adults. National Institutes of Health. [On-line.] Available: http://nhlbi.nih.gov/guidelines/ob_gdlns.htm.

between observers, and they do not provide information about abdominal and intramuscular fat.

The measurement of *body circumferences* has received attention because excess visceral or intraabdominal fat is associated with increased risk for diabetes and cardiovascular disease.[13] Studies have also indicated that the subcutaneous fat at the abdomen is highly correlated with insulin resistance. A waist circumference greater than 40 inches in men and greater than 35 inches in women is considered high risk.[13] The remaining methods of determining body fat except for bioimpedance are expensive and not portable and are usually done in research settings. *Bioimpedance* is performed by attaching electrodes at the wrist and ankle that send a harmless current through the body. The flow of the current is affected by the amount of water in the body. Because fat-free tissue contains virtually all the water and the conducting electrolytes, measurements of the resistance (*i.e.*, impedance) to current flow can be used to estimate the percentage of body fat present.

Laboratory Studies

Various laboratory tests can aid in evaluating nutritional status. Some of the most commonly performed tests are serum albumin and prealbumin to assess the protein status, total lymphocyte count and delayed hypersensitivity reaction to assess cellular immunity, and creatinine–height index to assess skeletal muscle protein. Vitamin and mineral deficiencies can be determined by measurements of their levels in blood, saliva, and other body tissues or by measuring nutrient-specific chemical reactions. All of these tests are limited by confounding factors and therefore need to be evaluated along with other clinical data.

In summary, nutritional status describes the condition of the body related to the availability and use of nutrients. Nutrients provide the energy and materials necessary for performing the activities of daily living and for the growth and repair of body tissues. Metabolism is the organized process whereby nutrients such as carbohydrates, fats, and proteins are broken down, transformed, or otherwise converted to cellular energy. Glucose, fats, and amino acids from proteins serve as fuel sources for cellular metabolism. These fuel sources are ingested during meals and stored for future use. Glucose is stored as glycogen or converted to triglycerides in fat cells for storage. Fats are stored in adipose tissue as triglycerides. Amino acids are the building blocks of proteins, and most of the stored amino acids are contained in body proteins and as fuel sources for cellular metabolism. Energy is measured in heat units called *kilocalories.*

The expenditure of body energy results from heat production (*i.e.*, thermogenesis) associated with the BMR or basal energy equivalent, diet-induced thermogenesis, exercise-induced thermogenesis, and thermogenesis in response to changes in environmental conditions.

The body requires more than 40 nutrients on a daily basis. Nutritional status reflects the continued daily intake of nutrients over time and the deposition and use of these nutrients in the body. The DRI is the Daily Recommended Intake of essential nutrients considered to be adequate to meet the known nutritional needs of healthy persons. The DRI has 22 age and sex classifications and includes recommendations for calories, protein, fat, carbohydrates, vitamins, and minerals. The nutritional status of a person can be assessed by evaluation of dietary intake, anthropometric measurements, health assessment, and laboratory tests. Health assessment includes a health history and physical examination to determine weight changes, muscle wasting, fat stores, functional status, and nutritional status. Anthropometric measurements are used for assessing body composition; they include height and weight measurements and measurements to determine the composition of the body in relation to lean body mass and fat tissue (*e.g.*, skinfold thickness, body circumferences, hydrodensitometry, bioelectrical impedance, and CT scans).

Overnutrition and Obesity

After completing this section of the chapter, you should be able to meet the following objectives:

- Define and discuss the causes of obesity and health risks associated with obesity
- Differentiate upper and lower body obesity and their implications in terms of health risk
- Discuss the treatment of obesity in terms of diet, behavior modification, exercise, social support, and surgical methods

Obesity is defined as a condition characterized by excess body fat. Clinically, obesity and overweight have been defined in terms of the BMI. Historically, various world bodies have used different BMI cutoff points to define obesity. In 1997, the World Health Organization defined the various classifications of overweight (BMI ≥25) and obesity (BMI ≥30). This classification was subsequently adopted by the National Institutes of Health (NIH).[13] The use of a BMI cutoff of 25 as a measure of overweight raised some concern that the BMI in some men might be due to muscle rather than fat weight. However, it has been shown that a BMI cutoff of 25 can sensitively detect most overweight people and does not erroneously detect overlean people.[14]

Overweight and obesity have become national health problems, increasing the risk for hypertension, hyperlipidemia, type 2 diabetes, coronary heart disease, and other health problems. Sixty-four and one-half percent of the U.S. population is estimated to be overweight (BMI ≥25), and 30.5% of the population is obese (BMI ≥30).[15] There was no difference in prevalence among men of different racial and ethnic groups. However, black women had a significantly higher rate of overweight and obesity than did white women. Hispanic women fell between the two groups. The prevalence in overweight and obesity is alarming not only because of the number of people affected but also because the prevalence continues to increase from previous surveys. The prevalence of severe obesity is increasing at an even faster rate, with persons who self-reported a BMI of at least 40 having increased from 1 in 200 to 1 in 50; those with a

BMI of at least 50 from 1 in 2000 to 1 in 400; and those with a BMI of at least 30 from 1 in 10 to 1 in 5.[16]

CAUSES OF OBESITY

The excess body fat of obesity often significantly impairs health, and as a result, obesity is the second leading cause of preventable death in the United States.[17] This excess body fat is generated when the calories consumed exceed those expended through exercise and activity.[18] Although factors that lead to the development of obesity are not well understood, they are thought to involve the interaction of genotype and environmental factors, which include social, behavioral, and cultural, with the physiology, metabolism, and genetics of the individual.[19]

In studies of persons who were overweight, the metabolic factors contributing to overweight were a low energy expenditure rate; a high respiratory quotient (RQ), which indicates the carbohydrate-to-fat oxidation ratio; and a low level of spontaneous physical activity.[20] The average adjusted energy expenditure of overweight persons was 36.3 kcal/kg fat-free mass (FFM) but could range from 28 to 42 kcal/kg FFM. The RQ was likely to be high in those who gained weight, suggesting that the person was oxidizing more carbohydrate than fat.

Epidemiologic surveys indicate that the prevalence of overweight may also be related to social and economic conditions. The second (1976 through 1980) National Health and Nutrition Examination Survey (NHANES II) has shown that if American women are divided into two groups according to economic status, the prevalence of obesity is much higher among those in the poverty group.[21] In contrast, men above the poverty level had a higher prevalence of overweight than men below the poverty level.

Obesity is known to run in families, suggesting a hereditary component. The question that surrounds this observation is whether the disorder arises because of genetic endowment or environmental influences. Studies of twins and adopted children have provided evidence that heredity contributes to the disorder.[22] It is now believed that the heritability of the BMI is between 30% and 40%.[20]

Although genetic factors may explain some of the individual variations in terms of excess weight, environmental influences also must be taken into account. These influences include family dietary patterns, decreased level of activity because of labor-saving devices and time spent on the computer, reliance on the automobile for transportation, easy access to food, energy density of food, and super sizing of portions. The obese may be greatly influenced by the availability of food, the flavor of food, time of day, and other cues. The composition of the diet also may be a causal factor, and the percentage of dietary fat independent of total calorie intake may play a part in the development of obesity. Psychological factors include using food as a reward, comfort, or means of getting attention. Eating may be a way to cope with tension, anxiety, and mental fatigue. Some persons may overeat and use obesity as a means of avoiding emotionally threatening situations.

It has been suggested that the increased prevalence of obesity in the United States has resulted from increased caloric intake together with a sedentary lifestyle and energy-saving conveniences.[23] Even when a reasonable number of calories are consumed, fewer are expended because of inactivity. A low rate of energy expenditure may contribute to the prevalence of obesity in some families.

UPPER AND LOWER BODY OBESITY

Two types of obesity based on distribution of fat have been described: upper body and lower body obesity. *Upper body obesity* is also referred to as *central, abdominal,* or *male* obesity. Lower body obesity is known as *peripheral, gluteal-femoral,* or *female* obesity. The obesity type is determined by dividing the waist by the hip circumference. A waist-to-hip ratio greater than 1.0 in men and 0.8 in women indicates upper body obesity (Fig. 11-4). Research suggests that fat distribution may be a more important factor for morbidity and mortality than overweight or obesity.

The presence of excess fat in the abdomen out of proportion to total body fat is an independent predictor of risk factors and mortality. Waist circumference is positively correlated with abdominal fat content. Waist circumference of

OBESITY

- Obesity results from an imbalance between energy intake and energy consumption. Because fat is the main storage form of energy, obesity represents an excess of body fat.
- Overweight and obesity are determined by measurements of body mass index (BMI; weight [kg]/height [m^2]) and waist circumference. A BMI of 25 to 29.9 is considered overweight; a BMI of 30 or greater as obese; and a BMI greater than 40 as very or morbidly obese.
- Waist circumference is used to determine the distribution of body fat. Central, or abdominal, obesity is an independent predictor of morbidity and mortality associated with obesity.

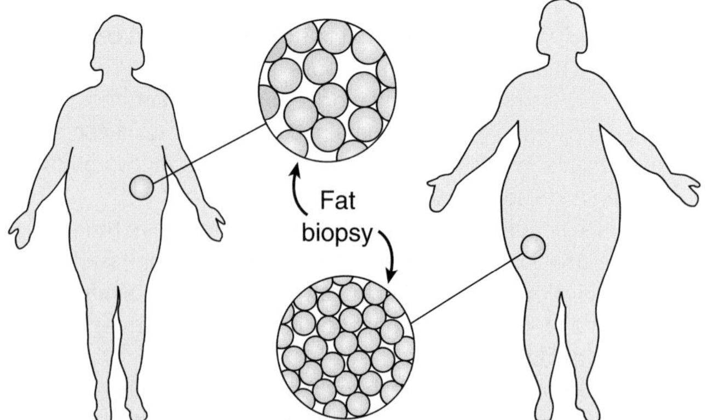

FIGURE 11-4 Distribution of body fat and size of fat cells in persons with upper and lower body obesity. (Courtesy of Ahmed Kissebah, M.D., Ph.D., Medical College of Wisconsin, Milwaukee)

35 inches or greater in women and 40 inches or greater in men has been associated with increased health risk[13] (see Table 11-8). Central obesity can be further differentiated into intraabdominal (viscera) fat and subcutaneous fat by the use of CT or MRI scans. However, intraabdominal fat usually is synonymous with central fat distribution. One of the characteristics of abdominal fat is that fatty acids released from the viscera go directly to the liver before entering the systemic circulation, having a potentially greater impact on hepatic function. Higher levels of circulating free fatty acids in obese persons, particularly those with upper body obesity, are thought to be associated with many of the adverse effects of obesity.[18]

In general, men have more intraabdominal fat and women more subcutaneous fat. As men age, the proportion of intraabdominal fat to subcutaneous fat increases. After menopause, women tend to acquire more central fat distribution. Increasing weight gain, alcohol, and low levels of activity are associated with upper body obesity. These changes place persons with upper body obesity at greater risk for ischemic heart disease, stroke, and death independent of total body fat. They also tend to exhibit hypertension, elevated levels of triglycerides and decreased levels of high-density lipoproteins, hyperinsulinemia and diabetes mellitus, breast and endometrial cancer, gallbladder disease, menstrual irregularities, and infertility. Visceral fat also is associated with abnormalities of metabolic and sex hormone levels.[24]

Weight loss causes a loss of visceral fat and has resulted in improvements in metabolic and hormonal abnormalities.[25,26] Although peripheral obesity is associated with varicose veins in the legs and mechanical problems, it does not increase the risk for heart disease.[27] In terms of weight reduction, some studies have shown that persons with upper body obesity are easier to treat than those with lower body obesity. Other studies have shown no difference in terms of success with weight reduction programs between the two types of obesity.

Weight cycling (the losing and gaining of weight) has been found to have little or no effect on metabolic variables, central obesity, or cardiovascular risk factors or future amount of weight loss.[28] More research is needed to determine its effect on dietary preference for fat, psychological adjustment, disordered eating, and mortality.[29,30] It is postulated that perhaps it is the underlying obesity and not the weight fluctuation that affects life expectancy.[31]

HEALTH RISKS ASSOCIATED WITH OBESITY

Obesity affects both psychosocial and physical well-being. In the United States as well as other countries, there are many negative stereotypes associated with obesity. People, especially women, are expected to be thin, and obesity may be seen as a sign of a lack of self-control. Obesity may negatively affect employment and educational opportunities as well as marital status. Obesity also may play a role in a person's treatment by health professionals.[32] Although nurses, physicians, and other health professionals are aware of the low success rate and difficulty in treating weight problems, they still may place the blame on the obese patient.[32]

In terms of health problems, obese persons are more likely to have high blood pressure, hyperlipidemia, cardiovascular disease, stroke, glucose intolerance, insulin resistance, type II diabetes, stroke, gallbladder disease, infertility, and cancer of the endometrium, prostate, colon, uterine, ovaries, kidney, gallbladder, and in postmenopausal women, breast.[20] The increased weight associated with obesity stresses the bones and joints, increasing the likelihood of arthritis. Other conditions associated with obesity include sleep apnea and pulmonary dysfunction, asthma, complications of pregnancy, menstrual irregularities, hirsutism, psychological distress, nonalcoholic steatohepatitis, carpal tunnel syndrome, venous insufficiency and deep vein thrombosis, and poor wound healing.[20] Because some drugs are lipophilic and exhibit increased distribution in fat tissue, the administration of these drugs, including some anesthetic agents, can be more dangerous in obese persons. If surgery is required, the obese person heals slower than a nonobese person of the same age.

Massive obesity, because of its close association with so many health problems, can be regarded as a disease in its own right.[33] It is the second leading cause of preventable death. In men who have never smoked, the risk for death increases from 1.06 at a BMI of 24.5 to 1.67 at a BMI higher than 26.[34] The waist-to-hip ratio is a less reliable predictor of mortality in women than BMI.

PREVENTION OF OBESITY

Emphasis is being placed on the prevention of obesity. It has been theorized that obesity is largely preventable because hereditary factors exert only a moderate effect. Some experts indicate that prevention should focus on young children, adolescents, and young adults,[35] while others would target the high-risk period from 25 to 35 years, menopause, and the year after successful weight loss.[36] A more active lifestyle together with a low-fat diet (<30% of calories) is seen as a strategy for prevention. Other strategies include the promotion of regular meals, avoidance of snacking, substituting water for calorie-containing beverages, decreased television viewing time, and increased activity.

TREATMENT OF OBESITY

The current recommendation is that treatment is indicated in all individuals who have a BMI of 30 or higher and those with a BMI of 25 to 29.9 or a high waist circumference plus two or more risk factors.[37] Treatment should focus on individualized lifestyle modification through a combination of a reduced-calorie diet, increased physical activity, and behavior therapy. Pharmacotherapy and surgery are available as an adjunct to lifestyle changes in individuals who meet specific criteria.

Before treatment begins, an assessment should be made of the degree of overweight and the overall risk status. The person should be assessed for the following risk factors: coronary heart disease and other atherosclerotic diseases, type 2 diabetes, sleep apnea, gynecologic abnormalities, osteoarthritis, gallstones, stress incontinence, cigarette smoking, hypertension, low-density lipoprotein cholesterol greater than 160 mg/dL, high-density lipoprotein cholesterol less than 35 mg/dL, impaired fasting glucose, family history of premature coronary heart disease, age 45 years or older in men or 55 years or older in women, physical inactivity, and high triglycerides.[38]

It also is advisable to determine the person's motivation to lose weight. Several factors can be evaluated to make this assessment. These include reasons and motivations for weight loss, previous history of weight loss attempts, social support, attitude toward physical activity, ability to participate in physical activity, time available for attempting intervention, understanding the causes of the obesity and its contribution to disease, and, finally, barriers the patient has for making changes.

The goals for weight loss are, at a minimum, prevention of further weight gain, but preferably reduction of current weight, and maintenance of a lowered body weight indefinitely. An algorithm has been designed for use in treating overweight and obesity. The initial goal in treatment is to lower body weight by 10% from baseline over a 6-month period with a 1- to 2-lb weight loss per week. Greater rates of weight loss do not achieve better long-term results.[38] This degree of weight loss requires a calorie reduction of 300 to 500 kcal/day in individuals with a BMI of 27 to 35. For those persons with a BMI greater than 35, the calorie intake needs to be reduced by 500 to 1000 kcal/day. After 6 months, the person should be given strategies for maintaining the new weight. Further weight loss can be considered after a period of weight maintenance. The person who is unable to achieve significant weight loss should be enrolled in a weight management program to prevent further weight gain.

Dietary Therapy

Dietary therapy should be individually prescribed based on the person's overweight status and risk profile. The diet should be a personalized plan that is 500 to 1000 kcal/day less than the current dietary intake. If the patient's risk status warrants it, the diet also should be decreased in saturated fat and contain 30% or less of total calories from fat. Reduction of dietary fat without a calorie deficit will not result in weight loss. Frequent contacts with a qualified dietetic professional help to achieve weight loss and then to maintain weight.

Physical Activity

Physical activity is important in the prevention of weight gain. In addition, it reduces cardiovascular and diabetes risk beyond that achieved by weight loss alone. Although physical activity is an important part of weight loss therapy, it does not lead to a significant weight loss. It may, however, help reduce body fat and prevent the decrease in muscle mass that often occurs with weight loss. Exercise should be started slowly with the duration and intensity increased independent of each other. The goal should be 30 minutes or more of moderate-intensity activity on most days of the week. The activity can be performed at one time or intermittently over the day.

Behavior Therapy

Techniques for changing behavior include self-monitoring of eating habits and physical activity, stress management, stimulus control, problem solving, contingency management, cognitive restructuring, social support, and relapse prevention.

Pharmacotherapy

Drugs approved by the FDA can be used as an adjunct to the aforementioned regimen in some patients with a BMI of 30 or more with no other risk factors or diseases and for patients with a BMI of 27 to 29.9 with concomitant risk factors or disease. The risk factors and diseases defined as warranting pharmacotherapy are coronary heart disease, type 2 diabetes, metabolic syndrome, gynecologic abnormalities, osteoarthritis, gallbladder disease, stress incontinence, and sleep apnea.[39]

Two FDA-approved prescription drugs are available for long-term weight loss therapy—sibutramine and orlistat. Sibutramine inhibits the reuptake of serotonin, norepinephrine, and dopamine. The drug produces weight loss by decreasing appetite.[40] Orlistat is a lipase inhibitor that works by decreasing fat absorption in the intestine. Both sibutramine and orlistat need careful monitoring for side effects. They also are contraindicated in certain patients.

Medication produces a 5% to 10% weight loss in clinical trials. This will provide medical benefit. Patients who do not lose a minimum of 4 pounds in the first 4 to 8 weeks of drug therapy should be considered nonresponders, and another antiobesity drug could be tried.[39] Even after weight loss has stopped, the medication can be continued as a part of a weight-maintenance program.

Over-the-counter (OTC) weight-loss products are not FDA regulated and should be used with a great deal of caution.

Weight Loss Surgery

The option of surgery is limited to persons with a BMI greater than 40; those with a BMI greater than 35 who have comorbid conditions and in whom efforts at medical therapy have failed; and those who have complications of extreme obesity. Vertical gastric banding and gastric bypass are two procedures that are used in subjects with acceptable operative risks. Persons who undergo surgical interventions also must continue in a program that provides guidance in nutrition and physical activity and behavioral and social support. These types of surgery have been shown to result in a reduction in BMI by 13.3 kg/m^2.[41]

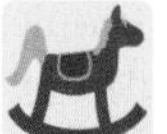

CHILDHOOD OBESITY

Obesity is the most prevalent nutritional disorder affecting the pediatric population in the United States. The findings from NHANES III, conducted between 1999 and 2000, indicated that 15% of children from ages 6 to 19 years were overweight.[42] This was a 4% increase from the previous NHANES study. Ten percent of children 2 to 5 years of age were overweight. The increase in prevalence was greater for those of African-American and Hispanic ethnicity. The definition for overweight for the NHANES III study was a BMI at or above the sex- and age-specific 95th percentile. Those who were between the 85th and 95th percentile were defined as at risk for overweight.

The major concern of childhood obesity is that obese children will grow up to become obese adults. Pediatricians are now beginning to see hypertension, dyslipidemia, and type 2 diabetes in obese children and adolescents. In North America, type 2 diabetes now accounts for half of all new diagnoses of diabetes (types 1 and 2) in some populations of adolescents.[43] In addition, there is a growing concern that childhood and adolescent obesity may be associated with negative psychosocial consequences such as low self-esteem and discrimination by adults and peers.[44]

Childhood obesity is determined by a combination of hereditary and environmental factors. It is associated with obese parents, higher socioeconomic status, increased parental education, small family size, and sedentary lifestyle.[45] Children with overweight parents are at highest risk; the risk in those with two overweight parents is much higher than that in children of families in which neither parent is obese. One of the trends leading to childhood obesity is the increase in inactivity. Increasing perceptions that neighborhoods are unsafe has resulted in less time spent outside playing and walking and more time spent indoors engaging in sedentary activities such as television viewing and computer usage. Television viewing is associated with consumption of calorie-dense snacks and decreased indoor activity. Studies have shown a 10% decrease in obesity risk for each hour per day of moderate-to-vigorous physical activity, whereas the risk increased by 12% for each hour per day of television viewing.[46] Obese children also may have a deficit in recognizing hunger sensations, stemming perhaps from parents who use food as gratification. The impact of fast food, increased portion size, energy density, sugar-sweetened soft drinks, and high glycemic index foods all are likely contributing to the increased weights in children and adolescents.

Because adolescent obesity is predictive of adult obesity, treatment of childhood obesity is desirable.[47] The goals of therapy in uncomplicated obesity are directed toward healthy eating and activity, not achievement of ideal body weight.[48] Families should be taught awareness of current eating habits, activity, and parenting behavior and how to modify them. In children with complications secondary to the obesity, the medial goal should be to improve that problem. Maintenance of baseline weight should be the initial step in weight control for all overweight children 2 years of age and older.[48] Children who have secondary complications of obesity will benefit from changes in eating and activity that will lead to weight loss of approximately 1 pound per month.[47] The weight loss interventions should include all family members and caregivers; begin early at a point when the family is ready for change; assist the family in learning to monitor eating and activity patterns and to make small and acceptable changes in these patterns; and teach the family to encourage and emphasize, not criticize.[48] They should include information about the medical complications of obesity, and they should be directed at permanent changes, not short-term diets or exercise programs aimed at rapid weight loss. Approaches can include a reduction of inactivity by limitation of television and computer and video games and by building activity into daily routine and on most days encouraging 30 minutes of unstructured outdoor play. Dietary goals are well-balanced, healthy meals with a healthy approach to eating using the Food Guide Pyramid as a model.[49] Specific strategies can include reduction of specific high-calorie foods or an appropriate balance of foods that are low, medium, and high calorie. Commercial diets are not recommended. Pharmacologic therapy and bariatric surgery should be reserved for children with complications and for severe obesity, respectively.[46]

In summary, obesity is defined as excess body fat resulting from consumption of calories in excess of those expended for exercise and activities. Heredity, socioeconomic, cultural, and environmental factors, psychological influences, and activity levels have been implicated as causative factors in the development of obesity. The health risks associated with obesity include hypertension and cardiovascular disease, hyperlipidemia, insulin resistance and type 2 diabetes mellitus, menstrual irregularities and infertility, cancer of the endometrium, breast, prostate, and colon, and gallbladder disease. There are two types of obesity—upper body and lower body obesity. Upper body obesity is associated with a higher incidence of complications. The treatment of obesity focuses on nutritionally adequate weight-loss diets, behavior modification, exercise, social support, and, in situations of marked obesity, surgical methods. Obesity is the most prevalent nutritional disorder affecting the pediatric population in the United States.

Undernutrition

After completing this section of the chapter, you should be able to meet the following objectives:

- List the major causes of malnutrition and starvation
- State the difference between protein-calorie starvation (*i.e.,* marasmus) and protein malnutrition (*i.e.,* kwashiorkor)
- Explain the effect of malnutrition on muscle mass, respiratory function, acid-base balance, wound healing, immune function, bone mineralization, the menstrual cycle, and testicular function
- State the causes of malnutrition in the hospitalized patient
- Compare the eating disorders and complications associated with anorexia nervosa, bulimia nervosa, and the binge-purge syndrome

Undernutrition ranges from the selective deficiency of a single nutrient to starvation in which there is deprivation of all ingested nutrients. Undernutrition can result from willful eating behaviors, as in anorexia nervosa and the binge-purge syndrome; lack of food availability; or health problems that impair food intake and decrease its absorption and use. Weight loss and malnutrition are common during illness, recovery from trauma, and hospitalization.

The prevalence of malnutrition in children is substantial. Globally, nearly 195 million children younger than 5 years of age are undernourished.[50] Malnutrition is most obvious in developing countries of the world, where the condition takes severe forms. Even in developed nations, malnutrition remains a problem. In 1992, it was estimated that 12 million American children consumed diets that were significantly below the recommended allowances of the National Academy of Sciences.[50]

MALNUTRITION AND STARVATION

Malnutrition and starvation are conditions in which a person does not receive or is unable to use an adequate amount of calories and nutrients for body function. Among the many causes of starvation, some are willful, such as the person with anorexia nervosa who does not consume enough food to maintain weight and health, and some are medical, such as persons with Crohn's disease who are unable to absorb their food. Most cases of food deprivation result in semistarvation with protein and calorie malnutrition.

In malnutrition and starvation, the amount of food consumed and absorbed is drastically reduced. It may be primary, resulting from inadequate food intake, or secondary to disease conditions that produce tissue wasting. Most of the literature on malnutrition and starvation has dealt with infants and children in underdeveloped countries. Malnutrition in this population commonly is divided into two distinct conditions: marasmus and kwashiorkor.

Marasmus represents a progressive loss of muscle mass and fat stores resulting from inadequate food intake that is equally deficient in calories and protein. The person appears emaciated, with sparse, dry, and dull hair and depressed heart rate, blood pressure, and body temperature. The child with marasmus has a wasted appearance, with stunted growth and loss of subcutaneous fat, but with relatively normal skin, hair, and liver function. *Kwashiorkor* is caused by protein deficiency. The term *kwashiorkor* comes from the African word meaning "the disease suffered by the displaced child" because the condition develops soon after a child is displaced from the breast after the arrival of a new infant and placed on a starchy gruel feeding. The child with kwashiorkor is characterized by edema, desquamating skin, discolored hair, enlarged abdomen, anorexia, and extreme apathy. There is less weight loss and wasting of skeletal muscles than in marasmus. Other manifestations include skin lesions, easily pluckable hair, enlarged liver and distended abdomen, cold extremities, and decreased cardiac output and tachycardia. *Marasmus-kwashiorkor* is an advanced protein-calorie deficit together with increased protein requirement or loss. This results in a rapid decrease in anthropometric measurements with obvious edema and wasting and loss of organ mass.

Protein-Calorie Malnutrition

Protein-calorie malnutrition represents a depletion of the body's lean tissues caused by starvation or a combination of starvation and catabolic stress. The lean tissues are the fat-free, metabolically active tissues of the body, namely, the skeletal muscles, viscera, and cells of the blood and immune system. They account for 35% to 50% of the total weight in the healthy young adult, with fat (20% to 30%), extracellular fluid (20%), and skeletal and connective tissues (10% to 15%).[51] Because the lean tissues are the largest body compartment, their rate of loss is the main determinant of total body weight in most cases of protein-calorie malnutrition.

Protein-calorie malnutrition is common in persons with trauma, sepsis, and serious illnesses such as cancer and acquired immunodeficiency syndrome. Approximately half of all persons with cancer experience tissue wasting in which the tumor induces metabolic changes leading to a loss of adipose tissue and muscle mass.[52] In healthy adults, body protein homeostasis is maintained by a cycle in which the net loss of protein in the postabsorptive state is matched by a net postprandial gain of protein.[53,54] In persons with severe injury or illness, net protein breakdown is accelerated and protein rebuilding disrupted. Consequently, these persons may lose up to 20% of body protein, much of which originates in skeletal muscle.[49] Protein mass is lost from the liver, gastrointestinal tract, kidneys, and heart. As protein is lost from the liver, hepatic synthesis of serum proteins decreases, and decreased levels of serum proteins are observed. There is a decrease in immune cells. Wound healing is poor, and the body is unable to fight off infection because of multiple immunologic malfunctions throughout the body. The gastrointestinal tract undergoes mucosal atrophy with loss of villi in the small intestine, resulting in malabsorption. The loss of protein from cardiac muscle leads to a decrease in myocardial contractility and cardiac output. The muscles used for breathing become weakened, and respiratory function becomes compromised as muscle proteins are used as a fuel source. A reduction in respiratory function has many implications, especially for persons with burns, trauma, infection, or chronic respiratory disease and for persons who are being mechanically ventilated because of respiratory failure.

In hospitalized patients, malnutrition increases morbidity and mortality rates, incidence of complications, and length of stay. Malnutrition may present at the time of admission or develop during hospitalization. The hospitalized patient often finds eating a healthful diet difficult and commonly has restrictions on food and water intake in preparation for tests and surgery. Pain, medications, special diets, and stress can decrease appetite. Even when the patient is well enough to eat, being alone in a room where unpleasant treatments may be given is not conducive to eating. Although hospitalized patients may appear to need fewer calories because they are on bed rest, their actual need for caloric intake may be higher because of other energy expenditures. For example, more calories are expended during fever, when the metabolic rate is increased. There also may be an increased need for protein to support tissue repair after trauma or surgery.

Diagnosis

No single diagnostic measure is sufficiently accurate to serve as a reliable test for malnutrition. Techniques of nutritional assessment include evaluation of dietary intake, anthropometric measurements, clinical examination, and laboratory tests. Evaluation of weight is particularly important. Body weight can be assessed in relation to height using the BMI. Evaluation of body composition can be performed by inspection or using anthropometic measurements such as skin-fold thickness. Serum albumin and prealbumin are used in the diagnosis of protein-calorie malnutrition. Albumin, which has historically been used as a determinant of nutrition status, has a relatively large body pool and a half-life of 20 days and is less sensitive to changes in nutrition than prealbumin, which has a shorter half-life and a relatively small body pool.[55]

Treatment

The treatment of severe protein-calorie malnutrition involves the use of measures to correct fluid and electrolyte abnormalities and replenish proteins, calories, and micronutrients.[56] Treatment is started with modest quantities of proteins and calories based on the person's actual weight. Concurrent administration of vitamins and minerals is needed. Either the enteral or parenteral route can be used. The treatment should be undertaken slowly to avoid complications. The administration of water and sodium with carbohydrates can overload a heart that has been weakened by malnutrition and result in congestive failure. Enteral feedings can result in malabsorptive symptoms due to abnormalities in the gastrointestinal tract. Refeeding edema is a benign dependent edema that results from renal retention of sodium and poor skin and blood vessel integrity. It is treated by elevation of the dependent area and modest sodium restrictions. Diuretics are ineffective and may aggravate electrolyte deficiencies.

EATING DISORDERS

Eating disorders affect an estimated 5 million Americans each year.[57] These illnesses, which include anorexia nervosa, bulimia nervosa, and binge-eating disorder and their variants, incorporate serious disturbances in eating, such as restriction of intake and binging, with an excessive concern over body shape or body weight. Eating disorders typically occur in adolescent girls and young women, although 5% to 15% of cases of anorexia nervosa and 40% of cases of binge-eating disorder occur in boys and men.[57] The mortality rate from anorexia nervosa, 0.56% per year, is more than 12 times the mortality rate among young women in the general population.[57]

Eating disorders are more prevalent in industrialized societies and occur in all socioeconomic and major ethnic groups. A combination of genetic, neurochemical, developmental, and sociocultural factors is thought to contribute to the development of the disorders.[58,59] The American Psychiatric Society's *Diagnostic and Statistical Manual of Mental Disorders, Text Revision* (DSM-IV-TR) has established criteria for the diagnosis of anorexia nervosa and bulimia nervosa.[60] Although these criteria allow clinicians to make a diagnosis in persons with a specific eating disorder, the symptoms often occur along a continuum between those of anorexia nervosa and bulimia nervosa. Preoccupation with weight and excessive self-evaluation of weight and shape are common to both disorders, and persons with eating disorders may demonstrate a mixture of both disorders.[60] The female athlete triad, which includes disordered eating, amenorrhea, and osteoporosis, does not meet the strict DSM-IV criteria for anorexia nervosa or bulimia nervosa, but shares many of the characteristics and therapeutic concerns of the two disorders (see Chapter 58). Persons with eating disorders may require concomitant evaluation for psychiatric illness because eating disorders often are accompanied by mood, anxiety, and personality disorders. Suicidal behavior may accompany anorexia nervosa and bulimia nervosa and should be ruled out.[57]

EATING DISORDERS

- Eating disorders are serious disturbances in eating, such as willful restriction of intake and binge eating, as well as excessive concern over body weight and shape.
- Anorexia nervosa is characterized by a refusal to maintain a minimally normal body weight (*e.g.,* at least 85% of minimal expected weight); an excessive concern over gaining weight and how the body is perceived in terms of size and shape; and amenorrhea (in girls and women after menarche).
- Bulimia nervosa is characterized by recurrent binge eating; inappropriate compensatory behaviors such as self-induced vomiting, fasting, or excessive exercise that follow the binge-eating episode; and extreme concern over body shape and weight.
- Binge eating consists of consuming unusually large quantities of food during a discrete period (*e.g.,* within any 2-hour period) along with lack of control over the binge-eating episode.
- Binge-eating disorders are characterized by eating behaviors such as eating rapidly, eating until becoming uncomfortably full, eating large amounts when not hungry, eating alone because of embarrassment, and disgust, depression, or guilt because of eating episodes.

Anorexia Nervosa

Anorexia nervosa was first described in the scientific literature more than 100 years ago by Sir William Gull.[61] The DSM-IV-TR diagnostic criteria for anorexia nervosa are (1) a refusal to maintain a minimally normal body weight for age and height (*e.g.,* at least 85% of minimal expected weight or BMI of at least 17.5); (2) an intense fear of gaining weight or becoming fat; (3) a disturbance in the way one's body size, weight, and shape are perceived; and (4) amenorrhea (in girls and women after menarche).[60] Anorexia nervosa is more prevalent among young women than men. The disorder typically begins in teenaged girls who are obese or perceive themselves as being obese. An interest in weight reduction becomes an obsession, with severely restricted caloric intake and frequently with excessive physical exercise. The term *anorexia,* meaning "loss of appetite," is a misnomer because hunger is felt, but in this case is denied.

Many organ systems are affected by the malnutrition that occurs in persons with anorexia nervosa. The severity of the abnormalities tends to be related to the degree of malnutrition and is reversed by refeeding. The most frequent complication of anorexia is amenorrhea and loss of secondary sex characteristics with decreased levels of estrogen, which can eventually lead to osteoporosis. Bone loss can occur in young women after as short a period of illness as 6 months.[57] Symptomatic compression fractures and kyphosis have been reported. Constipation, cold intolerance and failure to shiver in cold, bradycardia, hypotension, decreased heart size, electrocardiographic changes, blood and electrolyte abnormalities, and skin with lanugo (*i.e.,* increased amounts of fine hair) are common. Unexpected sudden deaths have been reported; the risk appears to increase as weight drops to less than 35% to 40% of ideal weight. It is believed that these deaths are caused by myocardial degeneration and heart failure rather than dysrhythmias.

The most exasperating aspect of the treatment of anorexia is the inability of the person with anorexia to recognize there is a problem. Because anorexia is a form of starvation, it can lead to death if left untreated. A multidisciplinary approach appears to be the most effective method of treating persons with the disorder.[62,63] The goals of treatment are eating and weight gain, resolution of issues with the family, healing of pain from the past, and efforts to work on psychological, relationship, and emotional issues.

Bulimia Nervosa and Binge Eating

Bulimia nervosa and binge eating are eating disorders that encompass an array of distinctive behaviors, feelings, and thoughts. Binge eating is characterized by the consumption of an unusually large quantity of food during a discrete time (*e.g.,* within any 2-hour period) along with lack of control over the binge-eating episode. A binge-eating/purging subtype of anorexia nervosa also exists.[60] Low body weight is the major factor that differentiates this subtype of anorexia nervosa from bulimia nervosa.

Bulimia Nervosa. Bulimia nervosa is 10 times more common in women than men; it usually begins between 13 and 20 years of age and affects up to 3% of young women.[64] The DSM-IV-TR criteria for bulimia nervosa are (1) recurrent binge eating (at least two times per week for 3 months); (2) inappropriate compensatory behaviors such as self-induced vomiting, abuse of laxatives or diuretics, fasting, or excessive exercise that follow the binge-eating episode; (3) self-evaluation that is unduly influenced by body shape and weight; and (4) a determination that the eating disorder does not occur exclusively during episodes of anorexia nervosa.[60] The diagnostic criteria for bulimia nervosa now include subtypes to distinguish patients who compensate by purging (*e.g.,* vomiting or abuse of laxatives or diuretics) and those who use nonpurging behaviors (*e.g.,* fasting or excessive exercise). The disorder may be associated with other psychiatric disorders, such as substance abuse.[57,64,65]

The complications of bulimia nervosa include those resulting from overeating, self-induced vomiting, and cathartic and diuretic abuse.[57,64–66] Among the complications of self-induced vomiting are dental disorders, parotitis, and fluid and electrolyte disorders. Dental abnormalities, such as sensitive teeth, increased dental caries, and periodontal disease, occur with frequent vomiting because the high acid content of the vomitus causes tooth enamel to dissolve. Esophagitis, dysphagia, and esophageal stricture are common. With frequent vomiting, there often is reflux of gastric contents into the lower esophagus because of relaxation of the lower esophageal sphincter. Vomiting may lead to aspiration pneumonia, especially in intoxicated or debilitated persons. Potassium, chloride, and hydrogen are lost in the vomitus, and frequent vomiting predisposes to metabolic acidosis with hypokalemia (see Chapter 34). An unexplained physical response to vomiting is the development of benign, painless parotid gland enlargement.

The weight of persons with bulimia nervosa may fluctuate, although not to the dangerously low levels seen in anorexia nervosa. Their thoughts and feelings range from fear of not being able to stop eating to a concern about gaining too much weight. They also experience feelings of sadness, anger, guilt, shame, and low self-esteem.

Treatment strategies include psychological and pharmacologic treatments. Unlike persons with anorexia nervosa, persons with bulimia nervosa or binge eating are upset by the behaviors practiced and the thoughts and feelings experienced, and they are more willing to accept help. Pharmacotherapeutic agents include the tricyclic antidepressants (*e.g.,* desipramine, imipramine), the selective serotonin reuptake inhibitors (*e.g.,* fluoxetine), and other antidepressant medications.[54]

Binge Eating. Binge eating is characterized by recurrent episodes of binge eating at least 2 days per week for 6 months and at least three of the following: (1) eating rapidly; (2) eating until becoming uncomfortably full; (3) eating large amounts when not hungry; (4) eating alone because of embarrassment; and (5) disgust, depression, or guilt because of eating episodes.[57,62,64] Most persons with binge-eating disorder are overweight, and in turn, obese persons have a higher prevalence of binge-eating disorder than the nonobese population.[66]

The primary goal of therapy for binge-eating disorders is to establish a regular, healthful eating pattern. Persons with binge-eating disorders who have been successfully treated for their eating disorder have reported that making meal plans, eating a balanced diet at three regular meals a day, avoiding high-sugar foods and other binge foods, recording food intake and binge-eating episodes, exercising regularly, finding alternative activities, and avoiding alcohol and drugs are helpful in maintaining their more healthful eating behaviors after treatment.

In summary, undernutrition can range from a selective deficiency of a single nutrient to starvation in which there is deprivation of all ingested nutrients. Malnutrition and starvation are among the most widespread causes of morbidity and mortality in the world. The body adapts to starvation through the use of fat stores and glucose synthesis to supply the energy needs of the central nervous system. Malnutrition is common during illness, recovery from trauma, and hospitalization. The effects of malnutrition and starvation on body function are widespread. They include loss of muscle mass, impaired wound healing, impaired immunologic function, decreased appetite, loss of calcium and phosphate from bone, anovulation and amenorrhea in women, and decreased testicular function in men.

Anorexia nervosa, bulimia nervosa, and binge eating are eating disorders that result in malnutrition. In anorexia nervosa, distorted attitudes about eating lead to serious weight loss and malnutrition. Bulimia nervosa is characterized by secretive episodes or binges of eating large quantities of easily consumed, high-calorie foods, followed by compensatory behaviors such as fasting, self-induced vomiting, or abuse of laxatives or diuretics. Binge-eating disorder is characterized by eating large quantities of food but is not accompanied by purging and other inappropriate compensatory behaviors seen in persons with bulimia nervosa.

REVIEW EXERCISES

A 25-year-old woman is 65 inches tall and weighs 300 pounds. She works as a receptionist in an office, brings her lunch to work with her, spends her evenings watching television, and gets very little exercise. She reports that she has been fat ever since she was a little girl, she has tried "every diet under the sun," and when she diets she loses some weight, but gains it all back again.

A. Calculate her BMI.

B. How would you classify her obesity?

C. What are her risk factors for obesity?

D. What would be one of the first steps in helping her develop a plan to lose weight?

A 16-year-old high school student is brought into the physician's office by her mother, who is worried because her daughter insists on dieting because she thinks she's too fat. The daughter is 67 inches tall and weighs 96 pounds. Her history reveals that she is a straight-A student, plays in the orchestra, and is on the track team. Although she had been having regular menstrual periods, she has not had a period in 4 months. She is given a tentative diagnosis of anorexia nervosa.

A. What are the diagnostic criteria for a diagnosis of anorexia nervosa?

B. What is the physiologic reason for her amenorrhea?

C. What are some of the physiologic manifestations associated with malnutrition and severe weight loss?

References

1. Guyton A.C., Hall J.E. (2000). *Textbook of medical physiology* (10th ed., pp. 815–821). Philadelphia: W.B. Saunders.
2. Garrel D.R., Jobin N., De Jonge L.H.M. (1996). Should we still use the Harris and Benedict equations? *Nutrition in Clinical Practice 11,* 99–103.
3. Subcommittee on the Tenth Edition of the RDAs. (1989). *Recommended dietary allowances* (10th ed.). Commission on Life Sciences-National Council. Washington, DC: National Academy Press.
4. Institute of Medicine. (2000). Introduction to dietary references intakes. In *Dietary reference intakes for vitamin C, vitamin E, selenium, and carotenoids.* Washington, DC: National Academy Press. [On-line.] Available: http://www.nap.edu/books/0309069351/html.
5. Trumbo P., Schlicker S., Yates A.A., et al. (2002). Dietary reference intakes for energy, carbohydrate, fiber, fat, fatty acids, cholesterol, protein, and amino acids. *Journal American Dietetic Association 102,* 1621–1630.
6. National Institutes of Health Expert Panel (2002). *Third report of the National Cholesterol Education Program (NCEP) Expert Panel on Detection, Evaluation, and Treatment of High Blood Cholesterol in Adults (Adult Treatment Panel III).* (NIH Publication No. 02–5215). Bethesda, MD: National Institutes of Health.
7. Carney D.E., Meguid M.M. (2002). Current concepts in nutritional assessment. *Archives Surgery 137,* 42–45.
8. Detsky A.S., Smalley P.S., Chang J. (1994). Is this patient malnourished? *Journal of the American Medical Association 271,* 54–58.
9. World Health Organization. (1989). *Measuring obesity: Classification and description of anthropometric data.* Copenhagen: World Health Organization.
10. Abernathy R.P., Black D.R. (1996). Healthy body weight: An alternative perspective. *American Journal of Clinical Nutrition 63*(Suppl.), 448S–451S.
11. Willett W.C., Dietz W.H., Colditz G.A. (1999). Guidelines to healthy weight. *New England Journal of Medicine 341,* 427–434.
12. Durnin J.V., deBrun H., Feunekas G.I. (1977). A comparison of skinfold method with extent of "overweight" and various weight-height relationships in assessment of obesity. *British Journal of Nutrition 77,* 3–7.
13. National Cholesterol Education Program Expert Panel on Detection, Evaluation, and Treatment of High Blood Cholesterol in Adults. (1998). *Clinical guidelines on the identification, evaluation, and treatment of overweight and obesity in adults.* NIH publication no. 98-4083. *Obesity Research* 6 (Suppl. 2), 51S–209S. Also available on-line: http://www.nhlbi.nih.gov/guidelines/ob_gdlns.htm.
14. Mokdad A.H., Serdula M.K., Dietz W.H., et al. (1999). The spread of the obesity epidemic in the United States, 1991–1998. *Journal of the American Medical Association 282,* 1519–1522.
15. Flegal K.M., Carroll, M.D., Ogden C.L., et al. (2002). Prevalence and trends in obesity among US adults, 1999–2000. *JAMA 288,* 1723–1727.
16. Sturm R. (2003). Increases in clinically severe obesity in the United States, 1986–2000. *Archives of Internal Medicine 163,* 2146–2148.
17. Allison D.B., Fontaine K.R., Manson J.E., et al. (1999). Annual deaths attributable to obesity in the United States. *JAMA 282,* 1530–1538.
18. Goran M.I. (2000). Energy metabolism and obesity. *Medical Clinics of North America 84,* 347–362.
19. Hill J.O., Wyatt H.R., Melanson E.L. (2000). Genetic and environmental contributions to obesity. *Medical Clinics of North America 84,* 333–346.
20. Pi-Sunyer F.X. (2002). The obesity epidemic: Pathophysiology and consequences of obesity. *Obesity Research 10*(Suppl 2), 972–104S.
21. McDowell A., Engel A., Massey J.T., et al. (1981). *Plan and operation of the National Health and Nutrition Examination Survey, 1976–1980.* Vital and Health Statistics Series 1(15), 1–144. Hyattsville, MD: National Center for Health Statistics.
22. Soreneson T.J., Holst C., Stunkard A.J., et al. (1992). Correlations of body mass index of adult adoptees and their biological

and adoptive relatives. *International Journal of Obesity and Related Metabolic Disorders 16,* 227–236.
23. Hill J.O., Melanson E.L. (1999). Overview of the determinants of overweight and obesity: Current evidence and research issues. *Medicine and Science in Sports and Exercise 31*(Suppl.), S515–S521.
24. Kissebah A.H., Krakower G.R. (1994). Regional adiposity and morbidity. *Physiological Reviews 74,* 761–811.
25. Fujoka S., Matsuzawa Y., Tounaja K., et al. (1991). Improvement of glucose and lipid metabolism associated with selective reduction of intra-abdominal fat in premenstrual women with visceral fat obesity. *International Journal of Obesity 15,* 853–859.
26. Pleuss J.A., Hoffman R.G., Sonnentag G.E., et al. (1993). Effects of abdominal fat on insulin and androgen levels. *Obesity Research 1* (Suppl. 1), 25F.
27. Ashwell M. (1994). Obesity in men and women. *International Journal of Obesity 18*(Suppl. 1), S1–S7.
28. Jeffery R.W. (1996). Does weight cycling present a health risk? *American Journal of Clinical Nutrition 63*(Suppl.), 452S–455S.
29. Muls E., Kempen K., Vansant G., et al. (1995). Is weight cycling detrimental to health? A review of the literature in humans. *International Journal of Obesity and Related Metabolic Disorders 19*(Suppl. 3), S46–S50.
30. Williamson D.F. (1996). "Weight cycling" and mortality: How do the epidemiologists explain the role of intentional weight loss? *Journal of the American College of Nutrition 15,* 6–13.
31. Garn S.M. (1996). Fractionating healthy weight. *American Journal of Clinical Nutrition 63*(Suppl.), 412S–414S.
32. Allison D.B., Saunders S.E. (2000). Obesity in North America: An overview. *Medical Clinics of North America 84,* 305–328.
33. Dwyer J. (1996). Policy and healthy weight. *American Journal of Nutrition 63*(Suppl. 3), 415S–418S.
34. Lee I., Manson J.E., Hennekens C.H., et al. (1993). Body weight and mortality: A 27-year follow-up of middle-aged men. *Journal of the American Medical Association 270,* 2823–2828.
35. Task Force on Prevention and Treatment of Obesity. (1994). Towards prevention of obesity: Research directives. *Obesity Research 2,* 571.
36. Wing R.R. (1995). Changing diet and exercise behaviors in individuals at risk for weight gain. *Obesity Research 3*(Suppl. 2), 277S–282S.
37. Pi-Sunyer F.X., Becker D.M., Bouchard C., et al. (1998). NHLBI Obesity Education Initiative Expert Panel on the Identification, Evaluation, and Treatment of Overweight and Obesity in Adults. *Obesity Research 6*(Suppl 2), 51S–209S.
38. U.S. Department of Health and Human Services (2000). *The practical guide: Identification, evaluation, and treatment of overweight and obesity in adults.* NIH Publication Number 00-4084. Rockville, MD: U.S. Department of Health and Human Service, National Institute of Health; National Heart, Lung, and Blood Institute; North American Association of the Study of Obesity.
39. Fujioka, K. (2002). Management of obesity as a chronic disease: Nonpharmacologic, pharmacologic, and surgical options. *Obesity Research 10,* 116S–123A.
40. Berke E.M., Morden N.E. (2000). Medical management of obesity. *American Family Physician 62,* 419–426.
41. Monteforte M.J., Turkelson C.M. (2000). Bariatric surgery for the morbid obese. *Obesity Surgery 10,* 391–401.
42. Ogden C.L., Flegal K.M., Carroll M.D., et al. (2002.). Prevalence and trends in overweight among US children and adolescents, 1999–2000. *JAMA 288,* 1728–1732.
43. Fagot-Campagna A., Pettitt D.J., Engelgau N.M., et al. (2000). Type 2 diabetes among North American children and adolescents: an epidemiologic review and a public health perspective. *Journal Pediatrics 136,* 664–672.
44. Hill J.O., Trowbridge F.L. (1998). Childhood obesity: Future directions and research priorities. *Pediatrics 101*(Suppl. 3), 570–574.
45. Birch L.L., Fisher J.O. (1998). Development of eating behaviors among children and adolescents. *Pediatrics 101*(Suppl. 3), 539–554.
46. Ebbeling C.B., Pawlak D.B., Ludwig D.S. (2002). Childhood obesity: public-health crisis, common sense cure. *Lancet 360,* 473–482.
47. Schonfeld-Warden N., Warden C.H. (1997). Childhood obesity. *Pediatric Clinics of North America 44,* 339–361.
48. Barlow S.E., Dietz W.H. (1998). Obesity evaluation and treatment: Expert Committee recommendations. *Pediatrics 102,* 1–11.
49. *The food guide pyramid.* U.S. Department of Agriculture, Center for Nutrition Policy and Promotion. [On-line]. Available: www.usda.gov/fcs/cnpp.htm.
50. Brown J.L., Pollitt E. (1996). Malnutrition, poverty, intellectual development. *Scientific American 274*(2), 38–43.
51. Hoffer I.J. (2001). Clinical nutrition. 1. Protein-energy malnutrition in the inpatient. *Canadian Medical Association Journal 165*(19), 1345–1349.
52. Tisdale M.J. (1999). Wasting in cancer. *Journal of Nutrition 129*(IS Suppl), 43S–46S.
53. Chiolero R., Revelly J., Tappy L. (1999). Energy metabolism in sepsis and injury. *Journal of Nutrition 129*(IS Suppl), 45S–51S.
54. Biolo G., Gabriele T., Cicchi B., et al. (1999). Metabolic response to injury and sepsis: Changes in protein metabolism. *Journal of Nutrition 129*(IS Suppl), 53S–57S.
55. Beck F.E., Rosenthal T.C. (2002). Prealbumin: A marker for nutritional evaluation. *American Family Physician 65*(8), 1575–1578.
56. Baron R.B. (2003). Nutrition. In Tierney L.M., McPhee S.J., Papadakis M.A. (Eds.), *Current diagnosis and treatment* (42nd ed., pp. 1212–1244). New York: Lange Medical Books/McGraw-Hill.
57. Becker A., Grinspoon S.K., Klibanski A., et al. (1999). Eating disorders. *New England Journal of Medicine 340,* 1092–1098.
58. Pritt S.D. (2003). Diagnosis of eating disorders in primary care. *American Family Physician 67,* 304–312.
59. Fairburn C.G., Harrison P.J. (2003). Eating disorders. *Lancet 361,* 407–416.
60. American Psychiatric Society. (2000). Practice guideline for treatment of patients with eating disorders (Revision). *American Journal of Psychiatry 157,* 1–38.
61. Gull W.W. (1868). Anorexia nervosa. *Transactions of the Clinical Society of London 7,* 22–27.
62. Kreipe R.E., Birndorf S.A. (2000). Eating disorders in adolescents and young adults. *Medical Clinics of North America 84,* 1027–1049.
63. Gordon A. (2001). Eating disorders: Anorexia nervosa. *Hospital Practice 36*(2), 36–38.
64. McGilley B.M., Pryor T.L. (1998). Assessment and treatment of bulimia nervosa. *American Family Physician 57*(6), 27–43.
65. Mehler P.S. (2003). Bulimia nervosa. *New England Journal of Medicine 349*(9), 875–881.
66. Schneider M. (2003). Bulimia nervosa and binge-eating disorders in adolescents. *Adolescent Medicine 14,* 119–131.

CHAPTER 12

Activity Tolerance and Fatigue

Mary Kay Jiricka

Health includes both physical and psychological components; it involves the ability to work, exercise, participate in leisure activities, and perform activities of daily living. To be able to perform these activities requires that the body have sufficient physiologic and psychological energy and stamina. When the body no longer can meet these energy demands, fatigue occurs. Fatigue may be acute, as in that resulting from increased physical activity, or it may be chronic. Conditions that impair health can affect a person's activity reserve and impose certain restrictions, such as bed rest and immobility, on the ability to perform work and other activities.

This chapter focuses on exercise and activity tolerance, activity intolerance and fatigue, and the physiologic and psychosocial responses to immobility and bed rest.

Exercise and Activity Tolerance

After completing this section of the chapter, you should be able to meet the following objectives:

- Describe the physiologic and psychological responses to exercise and work
- Define the term *maximal oxygen consumption* and state how it is measured
- Identify one physical method and two paper and pencil tools to assess work performance

Activity is defined as the process of energy expenditure for the purpose of accomplishing an effect. Humans interact with their environment in a cyclic pattern of periods of activity and rest, both of which have physical and psychological elements. Activity denotes the process of movement and expenditure of energy, whereas rest is characterized by inactivity and minimal energy expenditure. Movement and energy expenditure, as well as an overall conditioning of the body, when performed on a regular basis constitute a form of activity known as *exercise.*

EFFECTS OF EXERCISE AND ACTIVITY TOLERANCE

There is increasing interest in both the preventative and therapeutic effects of exercise. A regular program of exercise is recommended as a means of maintaining weight control and cardiovascular fitness.[1,2] The athletically fit person also has more reserves to call on when he or she becomes ill. Exercise also is becoming recognized as an integral part of the treatment regimen for many diseases. It

ACTIVITY TOLERANCE

- Activity is the process of purposeful energy expenditure. Exercise, a form of activity that results in overall conditioning of the body, can be aerobic or isometric.
- Exercise depends on the availability of energy substrates, cardiovascular fitness, muscle strength and flexibility, and motivation.
- The cardiovascular response to exercise includes increased heart rate, stroke volume, and mean arterial pressure. An increased percentage of cardiac output is distributed to working muscle.
- Pulmonary perfusion and pulmonary ventilation increase in response to exercise.
- Psychological effects of exercise include an increase in energy and in the ability to adapt to stress.

is recommended as a means of slowing, or even halting, the progression of atherosclerotic coronary artery disease; of lowering low-density lipoproteins (LDLs) and increasing high-density lipoproteins (HDLs) in persons with hyperlipidemia; of providing better regulation of blood glucose in persons with diabetes; and of improving activity tolerance in persons with cardiac and respiratory diseases.[3] Regular exercise also has psychological benefits. It can improve self-esteem, remedy depressive moods, and enhance quality of life.[1,2]

There are two main types of exercise: aerobic and isometric. *Aerobic,* or *endurance, exercise* involves the use of oxygen for transforming substrates such as glucose, fatty acids, and amino acids into energy. It involves a change in muscle length (contraction and elongation), such as during walking and running. During dynamic exercise that uses large muscle groups (*e.g.,* running), each person has a maximal oxygen uptake that cannot be exceeded, although it can be increased with appropriate training.[4] Aerobic exercise training results in muscles that use oxygen more efficiently such that the body can do more work with less cardiac and respiratory effort. The sustained type of muscle activity used during aerobic exercise does not promote significant muscle hypertrophy, even though the exercise may go on for hours.

During *isometric,* or *resistance, exercise* the muscles contract against an immovable force without changing length. Isometric exercise involves activities, such as weight lifting and high-resistance exercises, that improve overall muscle strength and tone and build muscle mass. The bulging biceps and chest muscle of professional weight lifters result from high-intensity resistance exercise. Here strength, not stamina, is important. Most exercise programs use a combination of aerobic and isometric activities.

Physical activity or exercise depends on four major components: cardiopulmonary fitness; muscle strength, flexibility, and endurance; availability of energy substrates to meet the increased energy demands imposed by increased physical activity; and motivation and mental endurance (Fig. 12-1).

Cardiopulmonary Responses

The cardiopulmonary responses to exercise include the circulatory functions of the heart and blood vessels and the gas exchange functions of the respiratory system. Collectively, they function to supply oxygen and energy substrates to the working muscle groups and to exchange oxygen and carbon dioxide with the atmosphere. Cardiopulmonary or aerobic exercise involves repetitive and rhythmic movements, uses large muscle groups, and results in the ability to perform vigorous exercise for an extended period. It also produces various physiologic responses and places a major stress on the cardiopulmonary system.[1]

The principal factor that determines how long and effectively a person will be able to exercise is the capacity of the heart, lungs, and circulation to deliver oxygen to the working muscles. The term *maximal oxygen consumption* ($\dot{V}O_2$ max) represents this principle. The $\dot{V}O_2$ max is determined by the rate at which oxygen is delivered to the working muscles, the oxygen-carrying capacity of blood, and the amount of oxygen extracted from the blood by the working muscles. It is measured as the volume of oxygen consumed, usually in liters or milliliters, per unit of time (*i.e.,* liters/minute). The $\dot{V}O_2$ max is an important determinant of the person's capacity to perform work and can increase up to 20-fold with strenuous exercise.[1,4]

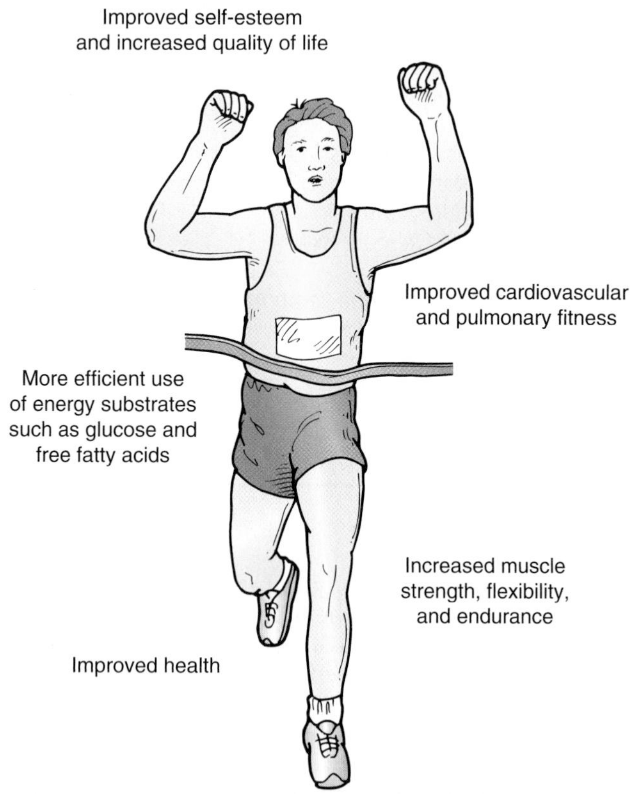
Improved self-esteem and increased quality of life
Improved cardiovascular and pulmonary fitness
More efficient use of energy substrates such as glucose and free fatty acids
Increased muscle strength, flexibility, and endurance
Improved health

FIGURE 12-1 Beneficial effects of physical activity and exercise.

The cardiovascular responses to exercise involve neural regulation (cardiovascular centers in the brain, with their autonomic output to the heart and blood vessels) in tandem with local control mechanisms that further regulate cardiac output, blood pressure, and local blood flow. The total neural activity is roughly proportional to muscle mass and its work intensity. Neural centers in the central nervous system (CNS) communicate with cardiovascular centers, reducing vagal tone and resetting the baroreceptors that control blood pressure. Local control is derived from release of metabolic end products such as lactic acid and from local vasoactive factors that dilate blood vessels. Local factors in the coronary vessels mediate coronary vasodilation, and increased sympathetic activity produces vasoconstriction of renal and gastrointestinal vessels, reducing blood flow to these organs.

During exercise, the cardiac output may increase from a resting level of 4 to 8 L/minute to as high as 15 L/minute for women and 22 L/minute for men. The increase in cardiac output that occurs during exercise is due to an increase in heart rate and stroke volume or the amount of blood that the heart pumps with each beat. The increase in heart rate is mediated through neural, hormonal, and intrinsic cardiovascular mechanisms. With anticipation of exercise, cardiovascular centers in the brain are stimulated to initiate sympathetic activity concomitant with inhibition of parasympathetic mechanisms. Stimulation of the sympathetic nervous system produces an increase in heart rate and cardiac contractility. At the start of exercise, the heart rate increases immediately and continues to increase until a plateau is reached. This plateau, or steady-state heart rate, is maintained until the exercise, or activity, is terminated. Release of epinephrine and norepinephrine from the adrenal glands helps to sustain the increased heart rate.[1,5] Also, contributing to the increased heart rate are mechanisms intrinsic to the heart. An increase in venous return stimulates right atrial stretch receptors that initiate an increase in heart rate, and an increase in ventricular filling stretches the myocardial fibers, resulting in a more forceful contraction and a more complete emptying of the ventricles with each beat through the *Frank-Starling mechanism*[1] (see Chapter 23).

Blood pressure also increases with exercise. With the onset of exercise, the systolic blood pressure increases because of the increase in cardiac output, while the diastolic pressure remains relatively unchanged because of vasodilatation and increased blood flow to the working muscles. The increased systolic pressure that occurs along with a nearly constant diastolic blood pressure produces an increase in pulse pressure and mean arterial pressure.[6] The increase in blood pressure is most pronounced when a medium muscle mass is working, such as the arms. This response results from the combination of a small (rather than large) dilated active muscle mass and a powerful central sympathetic drive.[4] Shoveling snow, which is a good example of exercise using primarily the arms, can substantially raise the systemic arterial pressure and increase the risk for heart attack and stroke in persons with coronary artery and cerebrovascular disease, respectively.

Exercise also causes an increase in blood flow that leads to increased shear stress on blood vessel walls. Enhanced shear stress results in several beneficial functions such as the production of vasodilators, antioxidants, and anticoagulants. This contributes to improved endothelial cell function, which results in vasodilation, inhibition of platelet activation, and increased fibrinolysis, thus leading to improved patency of the vasculature and maintenance of blood flow and vessel patency.[7] Adaptation to exercise also induces angiogenesis with an increased growth of vessels to support blood flow to the exercising muscle.[8] Because of the effects of exercise training on vascular function and angiogenesis, it has been proposed as a mechanism for improving blood flow and decreasing exercise-related leg pain (claudication) in persons with peripheral vascular disease.[9]

The role of the respiratory system during exercise is to increase the rate of oxygen and carbon dioxide exchange. This takes place through a series of physiologic responses. With the increase in cardiac output, a greater volume of blood under slightly increased pressure is delivered to the pulmonary vessels in the lungs. This results in the opening of more pulmonary capillary beds, producing better alveolar perfusion and a more efficient exchange of oxygen and carbon dioxide.[1,4] In addition to pulmonary perfusion being enhanced during exercise, pulmonary ventilation is increased. The respiratory rate and tidal volume increase, resulting in an increase in minute ventilation. This response is controlled by chemoreceptors—located in the medulla, the aorta, and the carotid arteries—that monitor blood gases and pH. During exercise, decreases in blood oxygen and pH and increases in carbon dioxide stimulate these receptors, producing an increase in both the rate and depth of respiration.[1]

Neuromuscular Responses

The integration of the neurologic and musculoskeletal systems is essential for body movement and participation in activity. To initiate and sustain increased activity, muscle strength, flexibility, and endurance are needed. *Muscle strength* is defined as the ability of muscle groups to produce force against resistance. *Flexibility* involves the range of movement of joints, and *muscle endurance* refers to the ability of the body or muscle groups to perform increased activity for an extended time.

Skeletal muscle consists of two distinct types of muscle fibers based on differences in their size, speed, contractile properties, endurance, and metabolic characteristics: red (dark) slow-twitch (type I) and white (light) fast-twitch (type II) muscle fibers.[1] Both heredity and activity influence the distribution of fast-twitch and slow-twitch fibers. Heredity appears to contribute to differences in muscle fiber composition, such that some people have considerably more fast-twitch than slow-twitch fibers, and others have more slow-twitch than fast-twitch fibers. This could determine to some extent the area of athletics for which a person is best suited.

The slow-twitch fibers, which are smaller than the fast-twitch fibers, tend to produce less overall force but are more energy efficient than fast-twitch fibers. They are better suited biochemically to perform lower-intensity work for prolonged periods of time. These fibers have a high oxidative capacity as a result of high concentrations of mitochondria and myoglobin. Slow-twitch fibers are highly fatigue resistant and ideally suited for prolonged aerobic exercise or activity. Slow-twitch fibers predominate in the large muscle groups such as the leg muscles; therefore, they play a major role in sustaining activity during prolonged exercise or endurance activities. Periods of sustained inactivity, such as prolonged immobility or bed rest, primarily affect slow-twitch fibers that quickly decondition.[1,10]

In contrast to slow-twitch fibers, fast-twitch fibers are larger and better suited for high-intensity work, but they fatigue more easily. These fibers have high myosin adenosine triphosphatase (ATPase) activity, few mitochondria, low myoglobin concentration, and high glycolytic capacity, resulting in dependence on anaerobic metabolism to supply adenosine triphosphate (ATP) for energy. Fast-twitch muscle fibers are most common in smaller muscle groups such as those found in the arms and eye. Fast-twitch fibers predominate during activities in which short bursts of intense energy are required, such as sprinting or weight lifting. Anabolic steroids enhance fast-twitch fiber activity.[1,10]

During aerobic activity, working muscles use oxygen 10 to 20 times faster than nonworking muscles. This increased oxygen demand is met by an increase in cardiac output and an increase in muscle blood flow. Skeletal muscles receive 85% to 95% of the cardiac output during aerobic activities and only 15% to 20% of the cardiac output at rest. The increased blood flow during aerobic activities is achieved through two mechanisms: dilation of blood vessels in the working muscles and constriction of blood vessels in the organs of low priority.[11]

Increased blood flow to working muscles is achieved by relaxation of the arterioles and the precapillary sphincters. Chemical changes such as decreased oxygen and pH and increased levels of potassium, adenosine, carbon dioxide, and phosphate contribute to the vasodilation during prolonged exercise and recovery from exercise.[11] Increased venous flow and, thus, return are enhanced by the alternate contraction and relaxation of working muscles.

Another mechanism that increases blood flow to the working muscles is the diversion of blood from the visceral organs.[4] The amount of blood diverted from the visceral organs is proportional to the level of exercise, and as exercise is increased, more blood is diverted to working muscles. This redistribution of blood flow results from selective vasoconstriction in organs, such as the kidneys and gastrointestinal structures, that are less active than the working muscles.[1,11]

Skeletal muscles hypertrophy and undergo other anatomic changes in response to exercise training. "Trained muscles" have an increased number of capillaries surrounding each muscle fiber that facilitates the delivery of oxygen to the working muscle cells during exercise. They are able to use oxygen more efficiently, probably because of enhanced enzymatic activity that increases oxidative capacity. The mitochondria appear to adapt by increasing the transport of oxygen and other substrates to the inner regions of the muscle fiber for more efficient use of oxygen.[1,11]

Metabolic and Thermal Responses

Unlike other tissues in the body, skeletal muscles switch between virtual inactivity when they are relaxed and using only minimal amounts of ATP to extremes of physical activity when they are using ATP at a rapid rate. However, the ATP inside muscle fibers is enough to power contraction for only a few seconds. If strenuous exercise is to continue for more than a few seconds, additional sources of ATP must be generated. The ATP that is used to power muscle contraction is obtained from three sources: creatine phosphate, glycogen, and fatty acids. Much like ATP, *creatine phosphate* (also known as *phosphocreatine*) contains high-energy phosphate bonds. It is unique to muscle fibers and is 8 to 10 times as abundant as ATP. Creatine is a small amino acid–like molecule that is both synthesized in the body and derived from foods. The enzyme creatine kinase (CK) catalyzes the transfer of the high-energy phosphate groups to creatine, forming creatine phosphate and ADP. When muscle contraction begins and ADP levels start to rise, CK catalyzes the transfer of a high-energy phosphate group back to ADP, thus forming new ATP molecules that can be used by the muscle for energy.

As the activity begins, especially aerobic activity, the body uses its energy sources in a characteristic pattern. The first sources for energy are stored ATP, creatine phosphate, and muscle glycogen. Short, intense periods of activity lasting 1 to 2 minutes exploit these energy sources through anaerobic metabolism. If the activity is to be performed for a period of 3 to 40 minutes, muscle glycogen and creatine phosphate are used to meet the energy requirements through both anaerobic and aerobic metabolism. For intense prolonged periods of activity, aerobic metabolism and the use of glucose, fatty acids, and amino acids become essential.[1]

To supply the energy needed for increased activity, a person must consume a balanced diet and have adequate hydration. General recommendations for a balanced diet include 55% complex carbohydrate sources, 30% fat sources (mainly polyunsaturated fats), and 15% protein (see Chapter 11). Although proteins are not used for energy sources during increased activity, they have an essential role in the building and rebuilding of tissues and organs. During increased activity and exercise, it is essential that an individual maintain adequate hydration. Increased activity can result in loss of fluids from the vascular compartment. If this is allowed to progress, the person may experience severe dehydration that may lead to vascular collapse. Before and during vigorous activity, a person should replenish body fluids with water and electrolyte solutions.[1]

Under normal resting conditions, the body is able to maintain its temperature within a set range. It does this by way of two mechanisms.[12] The first mechanism used by the body to regulate temperature is to change blood flow to the skin. When the blood vessels of the skin dilate, warm blood is shunted from the core tissues and organs to the skin surface, where heat is lost more easily to the surrounding environment (see Chapter 10). The second mechanism by which the body loses heat is through sweating, in which the evaporation of sweat from the skin surface contributes to the loss of body heat. Depending on training level and environmental conditions, the body may have difficulty regulating its temperature during vigorous exercise.[1,11] With sufficient training, the body adapts by increasing the rate of sweat production. As temperature regulation improves with training, the trained person begins to sweat sooner, often within 1 to 2 minutes of the start of exercise. Sweat production begins even before the core temperature rises, and a cooling effect is initiated soon after the start of exercise; the sweat produced is more dilute than that produced by a nontrained person. Sweat normally contains large amounts of sodium chloride; production of a dilute sweat allows evaporative cooling to take place while sodium chloride is conserved.[1]

During exercise, plasma proteins are shifted from the interstitial to the vascular compartment so that there is an increase in the amount of proteins in the blood. These proteins exert an osmotic force that draws fluid from the interstitial space into the vascular compartment. This contributes to an increase in vascular volume, which in turn is delivered to the working muscles and which also provides for more efficient heat dissipation.[1]

Gastrointestinal Function

The gastrointestinal system is affected by intense physical activity. During intense physical activity, blood flow is shunted away from the gastrointestinal tract toward the active skeletal muscles. As a result, gastrointestinal motility, secretory activity, and absorptive capacity are decreased. This can result in heartburn (reflux), vomiting, bloating, and stomach pain. It may also cause cramping, urge to defecate, and diarrhea. Although athletes may experience these symptoms, they are usually transient and do not have an effect on long-term health. In contrast to the effects of high-intensity exercise, repetitive low-intensity exercise may produce more long-term protective effects on the gastrointestinal tract. Evidence suggests that physical activity reduces the risk for colon cancer as well as diverticulosis, gastrointestinal hemorrhage, and inflammatory bowel disease.[13]

Hemostasis and Immune Function

Increased physical activity affects both hemostasis and the immune system. Increased epinephrine levels stimulate increased fibrinolytic (*i.e.*, breakdown of the fibrin strands in a blood clot) activity. Thus, regular strenuous exercise can result in increased fibrinolytic activity and a slowing of coagulation activity.[1]

The response of the immune system to exercise is varied and depends on frequency, intensity, and duration of the exercise. The immune system is stimulated by regular, moderate exercise and impaired with regular, repetitive, and intense exercise. A period of moderate-intensity exercise has been found to boost the immune system for several hours by producing an increase in circulating white blood cells, including neutrophils and lymphocytes. Of special note is the increased activity of natural killer (NK) cells. Chronic, intense, and exhaustive exercise produces different effects on the immune system. Elevation in body temperature, cytokine release, and increased levels of various stress-related hormones (*e.g.*, epinephrine, growth hormone, cortisol) may result in a temporary depression of the body's innate immune defenses. Strenuous exercise alters mucosal immunity of the upper respiratory tract. This may explain why elite athletes are susceptible to illness, especially upper respiratory tract infections. Strenuous exercise also lowers the production of the nonessential amino acid glutamine, which serves as an energy source for lymphocytes and macrophages.[1,14,15]

Psychological Responses

There is a mental component to the performance of increased activity and exercise. The mental aspect entails the motivation to initiate an activity, or exercise program, and the dedication to incorporate the regimen into one's lifestyle. Positive effects of regularly performed exercise include increased energy and motivation, positive self-image and self-esteem, decreased anxiety, and better management of stress.

Assessment of Activity Tolerance

The assessment of a person's ability to tolerate exercise and perform work can be conducted in several ways. It can be done by having the person report the perceived level of activity or level of fatigue on a pencil and paper test, or it can be measured by monitoring the person's response to exercise such as that performed using a treadmill or bicycle ergometer.

Pencil and Paper Tests. One subjective method involves the administration of a paper and pencil test in which participants describe their normal activities, their perceived level of activity tolerance, or their level of fatigue. An example of a paper and pencil test is the *Human Activity Profile* (HAP).[16] The HAP originally was developed to assess the quality of life for persons participating in a rehabilitation program for chronic obstructive pulmonary disease. After investigating numerous physiologic and psychological measures, it was noted that the most important aspect of quality of life was the amount of daily activity the person was able to perform. The HAP consists of 94 items that represent common activities that require known amounts of average energy expenditure. The person marks each item based on whether he or she is still able to perform the activity or has stopped performing the activity.

Another paper and pencil test is the *Fatigue Severity Scale*[17] (Chart 12-1). This tool consists of nine statements that describe symptoms of fatigue. Persons are instructed to choose a number from 1 to 7 that best indicates their agreement with each statement. The tool is brief, easy to administer, and easily interpreted. Paper and pencil tests provide an objective way to assess a person's activity tolerance.

Ergometry. *Ergometry* is a procedure for determining physical performance capacity. The ergometer is a specific tool that imposes a constant level of work. A specified workload, expressed in terms of watts or joules per second, is imposed while the person performs the task. During the performance of the work, the person's physiologic status is monitored, as is their subjective assessment of the work.[18]

Two examples of ergometers include the bicycle ergometer and the treadmill ergometer. A bicycle ergometer

CHART 12-1

*Fatigue Severity Scale**

1. My motivation is lower when I am fatigued.
2. Exercise brings on my fatigue.
3. I am easily fatigued.
4. Fatigue interferes with my physical functioning.
5. Fatigue causes frequent problems for me.
6. My fatigue prevents sustained physical functioning.
7. Fatigue interferes with carrying out certain duties and responsibilities.
8. Fatigue is among my three disabling symptoms.
9. Fatigue interferes with my work, family, or social life.

*Patients are instructed to choose a number from 1 to 7 that indicates their degree of agreement with each statement; 1 indicates strongly disagree, and 7 indicates strongly agree. (Krupp L.B., LaRocca N.G., Muire-Nash J., Steinberg A.D. [1989]. The Fatigue Severity Scale: Application to patients with multiple sclerosis and systemic lupus erythematosus. *Archives of Neurology 46,* 1122)

is a stationary bicycle that has a friction belt attached. The front wheel of the bicycle is rotated, and the braking force of the belt can be adjusted to alter the workload. A treadmill ergometer is used more frequently to assess workload performance, especially cardiac function. During treadmill testing, the person walks or runs on a moving belt. Changing the speed and incline of the treadmill alters the workload. This change usually is done in predetermined stages. During treadmill testing, the heart rate and electrocardiogram are monitored continuously, and the blood pressure is checked intermittently. Usually, the person being tested continues to exercise, completing successive stages of the test, until exhaustion intervenes or a predetermined or maximal heart rate is reached.[17]

Maximal heart rate is estimated by age. Tables of maximal heart rate by age are available, but as a general rule, the predicted maximal heart rate can be estimated by subtracting age from 220 (*e.g.,* the target heart rate for a 40-year-old person would be 180 beats/minute). The person may continue to exercise until the predicted maximum heart rate is achieved, or until 85% to 90% of the predicted maximal rate is reached.

Metabolic Equivalents. Metabolic equivalents (METs) are commonly used to express workload at various stages of work. One MET is equivalent to the energy expended in a resting position. METs are multiples of the basal metabolic rate, and as the type of activity performed (*e.g.,* walking, running) is changed, the MET requirement also changes. For example, walking at 4 miles per hour (mph), cycling at 11 mph, playing tennis (singles), or doing carpentry requires 5 to 6 METs. Running at 6 mph requires 10 METs, and running at 10 mph requires 17 METs. Physically trained persons are able to achieve workloads beyond 16 METs. Healthy sedentary persons seldom are able to exercise beyond 10 or 11 METs. In persons with coronary artery disease, workloads of 8 METs often produce angina.

During exercise stress testing, persons are asked to rate their subjective feelings of the exercise experience. A commonly used tool to measure the person's perception of the amount of work being performed is the Borg Rating of Perceived Exertion (RPE) Scale,[19] which is based on research that correlates heart rate to feelings of perceived exertion (Chart 12-2). The scale values range from 6 through 20. The numeric values on the RPE Scale increase linearly with workload, and the total scale reflects a 10-fold increase in heart rate. As the person is performing the exercise, he or she is asked to select a number that best corresponds to his or her feelings of exertion for the work being performed. The number chosen should be approximately 10 times the heart rate (*e.g.,* if the person rates the exercise experience as a 7, the heart rate should be 70 beats/minute). A newer category of scale with ratio properties has been developed. The numbers on this scale range from 0 to 10, with 0 representing nothing; 0.5, very, very weak; and 10, very, very strong. With this method, the expressions and the numbers they represent are placed in the correct position for a ratio scale. For example, because 1 represents very weak, 0.5 represents very, very weak or half that intensity.[20]

In summary, the response of the body to increased activity and exercise assumes that a healthy, normal person is performing the increased activity. In disease states, especially diseases of the cardiovascular, pulmonary, or musculoskeletal systems, the body's response to increased activity is compromised. The normal physiologic responses cannot be elicited. When a person experiences disease, activities of daily living and an exercise regimen must be adapted to the physiologic limitations.

The body reacts to the increased activity of exercise by a series of physiologic responses that increase its level of per-

CHART 12-2

The 15-Grade Scale for Rating of Perceived Exertion: the RPE Scale

6
7 Very, very light
8
9 Very light
10
11 Fairly light
12
13 Somewhat hard
14
15 Hard
16
17 Very hard
18
19 Very, very hard
20

Borg G.A.V. (1973). Perceived exertion: A note on "history" and methods. *Medicine and Science in Sports* 5, 90–93.

formance. Heart rate, cardiac output, and stroke volume increase to deliver more blood to working muscles. Minute ventilation and diffusion of oxygen and carbon dioxide increase to provide oxygen more efficiently to meet the rising metabolic demands. Local changes in the arterioles and capillaries contribute to enhanced perfusion of the working muscles. Over time and with training, temperature regulation is altered so that the body is able to perform activity without increasing its core temperature.

Activity tolerance is assessed by use of paper and pencil tests or with bicycle or treadmill ergometry. Persons are required to perform a prescribed amount of work. While performing this work, they are monitored for their cardiovascular response and their subjective feelings of exertion for the specified amount of work being performed.

Activity Tolerance and Fatigue

After completing this section of the chapter, you should be able to meet the following objectives:

- Differentiate acute from chronic fatigue
- List at least four health problems that are associated with chronic fatigue
- Define *chronic fatigue syndrome* and describe assessment findings, presenting symptoms, and laboratory values associated with the disorder
- Discuss treatment modalities for chronic fatigue syndrome

Activity intolerance can be viewed as not having sufficient physical or psychological energy reserve to endure or complete required or desired daily activities. Fatigue is the sensation that comes with having exhausted those energy reserves. It is a state that is experienced by everyone at some time in his or her life. Fatigue can be a normal physical response, as in the case of extreme exercise in healthy people, or it can be a symptom that is experienced by people with limited exercise reserve, such as people with cardiac or respiratory disease, anemia, or malnutrition, or those on certain types of drug therapy. Fatigue also may be related to lack of sleep or mental stress.

Like dyspnea and pain, fatigue is a subjective symptom. It often is described as a subjective feeling of tiredness that varies in terms of pleasantness, intensity, and duration and often is influenced by the time of day and a person's biorhythms.[21] Fatigue is different from the normal tiredness that people experience at the end of the day. Tiredness is relieved by a good night's sleep, whereas fatigue persists despite sufficient or adequate sleep. Although fatigue is one of the most common symptoms reported to health care professionals, it is one of the least understood of all health problems.

Fatigue may be described in terms of its underlying physiologic basis, by its origin or cause, or by its temporal patterns over time.[21] The physiologic basis of fatigue includes factors such as diaphragmatic, motor, or neurologic mechanisms. Diaphragmatic fatigue occurs in both acute and chronic respiratory conditions in which the force and duration of muscle work exceeds muscle energy stores. Neuromuscular fatigue involves the loss of maximal capacity to generate force during exercise.

MECHANISMS OF FATIGUE

The origin or cause of fatigue can be physiologic, psychological, pathologic, or of unknown cause (*e.g.*, chronic fatigue syndrome). Fatigue can be caused by environmental factors (*e.g.*, excessive noise, temperature extremes, changes in weather); drug-related incidents (*e.g.*, use of tranquilizers, alcohol, toxic chemical exposure); treatment-related causes (*e.g.*, chemotherapy, radiation therapy, surgery, anesthesia, diagnostic testing); physical exertion (*e.g.*, exercise); and psychological factors (*e.g.*, stress, monotony).

Clinically, fatigue can be defined or described by its temporal patterns over time, such as acute (*e.g.*, lasting less than 4 weeks) or chronic (*e.g.*, present for 50% of the day, or lasting 1 to 6 months or longer).[21] It is thought that both acute and chronic fatigue can exist in the same person, similar to acute and chronic pain.

ACUTE PHYSICAL FATIGUE

Acute fatigue has a rapid onset and is often defined as muscle fatigue associated with increased activity, or exercise, that is carried out to the point of exhaustion. It is relieved shortly after the activity ceases and serves as a protective mechanism. Physical conditioning can influence the onset of acute fatigue. People who engage in regular exercise compared with sedentary persons are able to perform an

ACTIVITY INTOLERANCE AND FATIGUE

- Activity intolerance is the inability of a person to complete activities because of insufficient psychological or physiologic energy.
- Fatigue may be due to situational stressors (environment, drug, therapies, physical or mental exertion) or developmental stressors (disease or emotional factors).
- Acute fatigue is muscle fatigue with a rapid onset and duration limited to the duration of the exercise. The time it takes to develop acute fatigue at any level of exercise depends on conditioning.
- Chronic fatigue has an insidious onset, a long duration unrelated to duration of activity, and intensity not related to the intensity of activity.
- Chronic fatigue syndrome (CFS) is characterized by disabling fatigue and many nonspecific symptoms, including cognitive impairments, sleep disturbances, and musculoskeletal pain. The etiology of CFS is unknown, but it is associated with several chronic diseases such as fibromyalgia, depression, and irritable bowel syndrome.

activity for longer periods before acute fatigue develops. They probably are able to do so because their muscles use oxygen and nutrients more efficiently, and their circulatory and respiratory systems are better able to deliver oxygen and nutrients to the exercising muscles.

Acute physical fatigue occurs more rapidly in deconditioned muscle. For example, acute fatigue often is seen in people who have been on bed rest because of a surgical procedure or in people who have had their activity curtailed because of chronic illness, such as heart or respiratory disease. In such cases, the acute fatigue often is out of proportion to the activity that is being performed (*e.g.,* dangling at the bedside, sitting in a chair for the first time). When resuming activity for the first time after a prolonged period of bed rest or inactivity, the person may experience tachycardia and hypotension. Unless these parameters are changed by medications such as β-adrenergic blocking drugs, heart rate and blood pressure become particularly sensitive indicators of activity tolerance or intolerance.

Another example of acute fatigue is that which occurs in people who require the use of assistive devices such as wheelchairs, walkers, or crutches. The upper arm muscles are less well adapted to prolonged exercise than the leg muscles. This is because arm muscles are primarily composed of type II muscle fibers. Type II muscle fibers, which are used when the body requires short bursts of energy, fatigue quickly. As a result, people who use wheelchairs or a pair of crutches may quickly experience fatigue until their arms become conditioned to the increased activity.

CHRONIC FATIGUE

Chronic fatigue differs from acute fatigue in terms of onset, intensity, perception, duration, and relief. In contrast to acute fatigue, chronic fatigue has an insidious onset, is typically perceived as being unusually intense relative to the amount of activity performed, lasts longer than 1 month, has a cumulative effect, and is not relieved by cessation of activity.[21] It is one of the more common problems experienced by people with chronic health problems (Table 12-1). In the primary care setting, 11% to 25% of patients present with chronic fatigue as their chief complaint. Of these, 20% to 45% will have a primary organic cause diagnosed for their fatigue, and 40% to 45% will have a primary psychiatric disorder diagnosed. The remainder will either meet the criteria for diagnosis of chronic fatigue syndrome (to be discussed) or will remain undiagnosed.

Although acute fatigue often serves a protective function, chronic fatigue does not. It limits the amount of activity that a person can perform and may interfere with employment, the performance of activities of daily living, and the quality of life in general. Although fatigue often is viewed as a symptom of anxiety and depression, it is important to recognize that these psychological manifes-

TABLE 12-1 Chronic Illnesses and Causes of Chronic Fatigue

Chronic Illness	Cause of Fatigue
Acquired immunodeficiency syndrome	Impaired immune function, anorexia, muscle weakness, and psychosocial factors associated with the disease
Anemia	Decreased oxygen-carrying capacity of blood
Arthritis	Pain and joint dysfunction lead to impaired mobility, loss of sleep, and emotional factors
Cancer	Presence of chemical products and catabolic processes associated with tumor growth; anorexia and difficulty eating; effects of chemotherapy and radiation therapy; and psychosocial factors such as depression, grieving, hopelessness, and fear
Cardiac disease	
Myocardial infarction	Death of myocardial tissue results in decreased cardiac output, poor tissue perfusion, and impaired delivery of oxygen and nutrients to vital organs
Congestive heart failure	Impaired pumping ability of the heart results in poor perfusion of muscle tissue and vital organs
Neurologic disorders	
Multiple sclerosis	Demyelinating disease of CNS characterized by slowing of nerve conduction, resulting in lower extremity weakness and fatigue
Myasthenia gravis	Disorder of postsynaptic acetylcholine receptors of the myoneural junction, resulting in muscle weakness and fatigue
Chronic lung disease	Increased work of breathing and impaired gas exchange
Chronic renal failure	Accumulation of metabolic wastes; fluid, electrolyte, and acid-base disorders; decreased red blood cell count and oxygen-carrying capacity due to impaired erythropoietin production
Metabolic disorders	
Hypothyroidism	Decrease in basal metabolic rate manifested by fatigue
Diabetes mellitus	Impaired cellular use of glucose by muscle cells
Obesity	Imbalance in nutritional intake and energy expenditure; increased workload due to excess weight
Steroid myopathy	Glucocorticosteroids interfere with protein and glycogen synthesis, which leads to muscle wasting

tations may be symptoms of the fatigue. For example, people with persistent fatigue due to a chronic illness may have to curtail their work schedules, decrease social activities, and limit their usual family responsibilities. These lifestyle changes may be the reasons for the depression rather than the depression being a cause of the fatigue.

Chronic fatigue occurs across a broad spectrum of disease states. It is a common complaint of persons with cancer, cardiac disease, end-stage renal disease, chronic lung disease, hepatitis C, arthritis, human immunodeficiency virus (HIV) and acquired immunodeficiency disease syndrome (AIDS), and neurologic disorders such as multiple sclerosis, postpolio syndrome, and Parkinson's disease.

Chronic fatigue is almost a universal phenomenon in persons with cancer, with prevalence rates ranging from 75% to 96%, depending on the form of treatment and stage of disease.[22–25] Cancer-related fatigue may be caused by the disease itself, or it may be caused by treatment. In fact, the majority of persons undergoing cancer chemotherapy or radiotherapy have reported significant fatigue during the course of treatment. Cancer-related fatigue involves a number of physiologic, sensory, affective, and cognitive dimensions.[26] There is often a sensation of feeling unusually tired with generalized weakness and a greater need for rest. There may also be a disturbing lack of motivation, anxiety, and sadness as well as an inability to concentrate or difficulty in thinking.

Several types of cancer-related factors may cause fatigue, the most prominent of which are factors that relate to energy imbalance. These include anemia, cachexia, stress, pain, infection, medications, and metabolic disorders.[26,27] The cytokine theory of cancer-related fatigue is just emerging. This theory is based, at least in part, on the observation that patients receiving agents such as interferon-α as part of their treatment plan experienced devastating fatigue that was dose limited. Interferon-α and other agents used to treat cancer also influence the release of other cytokines that are related to fatigue. Cancer cells and the immune system appear to produce or express a number of cytokines with the potential for manufacturing many of the factors that contribute to fatigue. One of these cytokines, tumor necrosis factor-α (TNF-α) is thought to interfere with appetite, produce weight loss, and cause depletion of the protein stores of skeletal muscle. As a result, muscle wasting occurs, and people have to expend more energy to perform simple activities such as sitting and standing.[27]

Management of Chronic Fatigue. Pathologic factors associated with fatigue include insomnia, anemia, psychological stress, and wasting or weakness.[21] Many of these conditions respond to appropriate treatment measures. Anemia, which is common among persons with HIV/AIDS, patients with end-stage renal disease, and cancer patients receiving chemotherapy, causes fatigue by interfering with the oxygen carrying capacity of the blood. It can often be treated with recombinant forms of erythropoietin (epoetin-alfa), an endogenous hormone normally produced by the kidney (see Chapter 16). Insomnia, which occurs for a number of reasons, including anxiety and depression, hot flashes, nocturia, and pain, is often amenable to nonpharmacologic and pharmacologic methods of treatment. Psychological disturbances, such as anxiety and depression, which are frequently associated with fatigue, can be treated with selected pharmacologic agents. Another cause of fatigue is loss of muscle mass, muscle strength, and endurance. This type of fatigue is common among persons with forced immobility, musculoskeletal disorders such as arthritis,[28] neuromuscular disorders such as multiple sclerosis, and wasting syndromes such as HIV/AIDS. Aerobic exercise has been shown to decrease this type of fatigue in AIDS[29] and multiple sclerosis patients.[30]

Chronic Fatigue Syndrome

Chronic fatigue syndrome (CFS) is a condition of disabling fatigue of at least 6 months' duration that is typically accompanied by an array of self-reported, nonspecific symptoms such as cognitive impairments, sleep disturbances, and musculoskeletal pain. CFS probably is not a new disease. Indeed, in the 19th century, the diagnosis of "neurasthenia" was a common diagnosis applied to a group of symptoms that are very similar to those found in CFS.[31,32] In the late 20th century and now into the 21st century, the disorder continues to be a relatively common problem. Because of differences in patients included in the diagnostic category of CFS, the prevalence data vary among studies. In general, approximately 10% to 20% of all patients in primary practice complained of fatigue of at least 6 months' duration. In community surveys, the prevalence of CFS is reported to be considerably lower (1% to 3%); however, this does not negate the importance of CFS as a major public health issue.[33]

Definition. Because the etiology of CFS is unknown, there are no biologic markers for the diagnosis of CFS, and there are no definitive treatments. Furthermore, the overlap of symptoms of CFS with other functional disorders such as fibromyalgia, multiple chemical sensitivities, depression, and irritable bowel syndrome, which also are characterized by fatigue, complicates the ability to define the syndrome with any degree of certainty.[34,35] In fact, CFS may describe a group of similar symptoms that develop with different pathophysiological disturbances.

Because of the need for diagnostic criteria, the case definition for CFS was established in 1988[36] by the Centers for Disease Control and Prevention (CDC) and revised through its International Chronic Fatigue Syndrome study group in 1994.[37] To be classified as CFS, the fatigue must be clinically evaluated, cause severe mental and physical exhaustion, and result in a significant reduction in the individual's premorbid activity level. In addition, there must be evidence of the concurrent occurrence of four of the following eight symptoms: sore throat, tender cervical or axillary lymph nodes, muscle pain, multijoint pain without swelling or redness, headaches, unrefreshing sleep, and postexertional malaise lasting more than 24 hours. The fatigue and concurrent symptoms must be of 6 months' duration or longer. Chart 12-3 outlines the criteria for diagnosis of CFS.[37]

Pathophysiology. Theories of the pathogenesis of CFS include infections, psychological disorders, a dysfunction in

CHART 12-3

Criteria for Diagnosis of Chronic Fatigue Syndrome

Clinically evaluated fatigue
- Fatigue of ≥6 months' duration (new or definite onset)
- Not relieved by rest
- Significant reduction in premorbid occupational, educational, social, or personal activities

Concurrent experience of at least four of the following symptoms:
- Impaired memory or concentration
- Sore throat
- Tender cervical or axillary lymph nodes
- Muscle pain
- Multijoint pain
- New headaches
- Unrefreshing sleep
- Postexertional malaise

Exclusionary diagnoses
- Any active medical condition that could explain the chronic fatigue
- Any previously diagnosed but incompletely resolved medical condition that could explain the chronic fatigue
- Any past or current diagnosis of a major depressive disorder, schizophrenia, delusional disorder, dementia, or anorexia or bulimia nervosa
- Alcohol or other substance abuse within 2 years of onset of chronic fatigue symptoms

(Developed from Fukuda K., Straus S.E., Hickie I., Sharpe M.C., Dobbins J.G., Komaroff A.L. [1994]. The chronic fatigue syndrome: A comprehensive approach to its definition and study. *Annals of Internal Medicine* 121, 953–959)

the hypothalamic-pituitary-adrenal axis, or an alteration in the autonomic nervous system.[38] Despite much research and the development of several theories, the pathophysiology of CFS remains elusive. Many people with CFS attribute the onset of their disease to an influenza-like infection. Thus, the link between infectious agents such as Epstein-Barr virus, human herpesvirus 6, enterovirus, human retrovirus, *Mycobacterium tuberculosis, Borrelia burgdorferi, Brucella,* and *Candida* species has been extensively studied.[32,35] To date, however, none of these agents has been conclusively linked in a cause-and-effect relationship with the development of CFS.

Psychological disorders often are associated with CFS, especially anxiety and depression, but this is difficult to evaluate. Persons with CFS are more likely than the general population to have experienced a psychological disorder such as major depression or panic disorder before the development of CFS; however, it also is true that a significant proportion of those persons with CFS have not had such episodes, either before or after the development of CFS.[31]

Several studies suggest that CFS may be due to a primary alteration in immune function. A number of immunologic abnormalities have been described in persons with CFS.[32,35] It is hypothesized that the immune system may overreact to an environmental agent (most likely an infectious agent) or internal stimuli and be unable to self-regulate after the infectious insult is over. Another possibility is that a viral infection may produce continued suppression of the immune system. Mononuclear cells from persons with CFS have been shown to have a decreased response to antigenic stimulation and proliferate at one half the normal rate. One of the most consistent immunologic findings is a low level of activity in NK cells.[39] It has been hypothesized that in a situation of prolonged immune activation, NK cells that find their way past the blood–brain barrier may damage brain cells and cause chronic neuroendocrine abnormalities and thus CFS.[39]

Diagnostic imaging studies have provided preliminary data suggesting that the CNS may be the final common pathway in the development of this disorder.[40] In brain imaging studies using magnetic resonance imaging (MRI) and positron-emission tomography (PET) scans, white matter abnormalities and hypoperfusion of the brain stem have been found in persons with CFS.[41,42] In other studies, abnormalities of the hypothalamic-pituitary-adrenal axis, such as attenuated activity of corticotropin-releasing hormone and changes in the circadian rhythm of cortisol secretion, have been documented. However, these findings remain unexplained.

Autonomic nervous system dysfunction also is thought to play a possible role in CFS. In a significant proportion of patients with CFS, there are abnormal responses to both parasympathetic and sympathetic laboratory challenges.[43] A statistically greater number of persons diagnosed with CFS have orthostatic hypotension and tachycardia with tilt table testing than do healthy control subjects.[31,43]

Manifestations. One of the most important findings in persons with CFS is the complaint of fatigue. Often, the symptom of fatigue is preceded by a cold or flulike illness. Frequently, the person describes the illness as recurring, with periods of exacerbations and remissions. With each subsequent episode of the illness, the fatigue increases.

Physical findings include low-grade fever. The fever is intermittent and occurs only when the illness recurs. Other findings include nonexudative pharyngitis, palpable and tender cervical lymph nodes, a mildly enlarged thyroid gland, wheezing, splenomegaly, myalgias, arthralgias, and heme-positive stool with subsequent negative sigmoidoscopies.

Psychological problems include impaired cognition, which the person describes as an inability to concentrate and perform previously mundane tasks. There are reports of mood and sleep disturbances, balance problems, visual disturbances, and various degrees of anxiety and depression.

Diagnosis and Treatment. The diagnosis of CFS is based on integration of the entire clinical picture of the person's symptoms, physical assessment findings, and the results of diagnostic tests. Laboratory tests are usually limited to blood counts and tests specific for the person's symptoms. Usually, the final diagnosis is based on the definition of CFS provided by the CDC[37] (see Chart 12-3).

Because there is no known cause of CFS, current treatment tends to remain symptomatic with a focus on management rather than cure.[41] It centers on education, emotional support, treatment of symptoms, and overall management of general health. Symptom management includes development of an exercise program that helps the person regain strength. Along with a structured activity program, persons should be encouraged to be as active as possible as they resume their activities of daily living.

A holistic approach to the treatment of CFS is essential. With proper treatment and support, most persons with CFS demonstrate improvement. However, relapses can occur. Persons diagnosed with CFS must continue to receive follow-up care and treatment on a regular basis. Local and national support groups are available for persons who experience CFS.

In summary, fatigue is a nonspecific, self-recognized state of physical and psychological exhaustion. It results in the person's not being able to perform routine activities and is not relieved with sleep or rest. Acute fatigue results from excessive use of the body or specific muscle groups and often is related to depletion of energy sources. Chronic fatigue often is associated with a specific disease or chronic illness and may be relieved when the effects of the disease are corrected. CFS is a complex illness that has physiologic and psychological manifestations. It is characterized by debilitating fatigue. Diagnosis often is made by a process of elimination, and treatment requires a holistic approach.

Bed Rest and Immobility

After completing this section of the chapter, you should be able to meet the following objectives:

- Describe the effects of gravity on the body
- Describe the effects of immobility and prolonged bed rest on the cardiovascular, pulmonary, renal, musculoskeletal, metabolic, and gastrointestinal body systems
- Discuss changes in fluid and electrolyte balance associated with immobility and prolonged bed rest
- Identify alterations in serum electrolyte and hematologic values that are related to immobility and prolonged bed rest
- Discuss changes in sensory perception that are consequences of immobility and prolonged bed rest
- Identify alterations in physical assessment findings that are related to the effects of immobility and prolonged bed rest
- Describe treatment interventions that counteract the negative effects of immobility and prolonged bed rest

Bed rest and immobility are the antithesis of exercise and mobility. They defy the active use of skeletal muscles, movement against gravity, conservation of body fluids, normal distribution of blood flow, and maintenance of cardiopulmonary reserves. Immobility may be dictated by an injury that requires stabilization to facilitate the healing process, or it may result from conditions that limit physical reserve. The effects of immobility can be restricted to a single extremity that is encased in a plaster cast; involve both legs, as in a person confined to a wheelchair; or involve the entire body, as in a person confined to bed rest. Bed rest and immobility are associated with various complications that include generalized weakness, orthostatic intolerance, atelectasis, pneumonia, pulmonary emboli, thrombophlebitis, muscle atrophy, osteoporosis, urinary retention, constipation, and impaired sensory perception[44–48] (Table 12-2). This section of the chapter describes the physiologic changes that occur with bed rest and immobility and the treatment interventions to counteract their effects.

Bed rest is one of the oldest and most commonly used methods of treatment for various medical conditions. Before the 1940s, bed rest was prescribed for 2 weeks after childbirth, 3 weeks after herniorrhaphy, and 4 to 6 weeks after myocardial infarction. It was believed that the complex biochemical and physical demands of physical activity diverted energy from the restorative and reparative processes of healing. Rest in bed was regarded as tantamount to optimal rest of the heart and entire body.

During World War II, the shortage of hospital beds and medical personnel forced early mobilization of many patients. As often happens with this kind of action, it soon was discovered that early mobilization lessened complications and improved patient outcome. The National Aeronautics and Space Administration (NASA) conducted research that described the damaging effects of prolonged inactivity and weightlessness. These studies indicate that weightlessness and the antigravity effects of bed rest produce similar responses.

ANTIGRAVITY EFFECTS OF BED REST

The supine position that often accompanies immobility and bed rest interferes with the effects of gravity. The force of gravity exerts beneficial effects on the body. As the body maintains a supine position, the absence of the force of gravity leads to many of the deconditioning effects associated with immobility and bed rest (Fig. 12-2).

While upright, the body compensates for the effects of gravity in a variety of ways. The skeletal muscles contract and exert pressure against veins and lymph vessels. This contraction counteracts the force of gravity that would cause blood and fluid to pool in the lower extremities. Blood is kept moving through the circulatory system. Bones remain stronger because longitudinal weight bearing keeps essential minerals, such as calcium, inside the structure of the bone.

PHYSIOLOGIC EFFECTS OF BED REST

Cardiovascular Responses

After a period of bed rest, the cardiovascular system exhibits changes that reflect the loss of gravitational and exercise stimuli. In effect, the cardiovascular system becomes

TABLE 12-2 Complications of Bed Rest and Immobility

System	Complication
Cardiovascular	Increased heart rate; decreased cardiac output and stroke volume contributing to decreased aerobic capacity; decreased size of the heart; decreased left ventricular end-diastolic volume; unchanged systolic-diastolic blood pressure; decreased fluid volume; orthostatic intolerance; venous thrombophlebitis
Pulmonary	Mechanical resistance to breathing; reduced cardiopulmonary functional capacity; relative hypoxemia; pneumonia
Musculoskeletal	Muscle atrophy and loss of strength and endurance; decreased strength of tendons and ligaments and their insertions on bone; decreased muscle oxidative capacity contributing to decreased aerobic capacity; osteoporosis (bone loss); contractures; immobilization hypercalcemia; osteoarthritis
Gastrointestinal	Loss of appetite; constipation
Genitourinary	Incontinence; renal calculi; urinary stasis and infection; electrolyte imbalance
Hematologic	Decreased total fluid volume; increased blood viscosity; thromboembolism
Metabolic and endocrine	Glucose intolerance; hyperglycemia; hyperinsulinemia; increased parathyroid hormone production
Skin	Pressure ulcers
Functional	Impaired ambulation and activity tolerance; impaired balance and coordination
Psychological	Sensory deprivation; altered sensory perception; confusion and disorientation; anxiety; depression; decreased intellectual capacity

Developed from information in Harper C.M., Lyles Y.M. (1988). Physiology and complications of bed rest. *Journal of the American Geriatric Society 36,* 1048.

deconditioned, resulting in an exaggeration of the hemodynamic changes normally seen with standing after brief bed rest. This deconditioning is manifest in three major alterations: postural hypotension, increased cardiac workload, and venous stasis with the potential for deep venous thrombosis.

BED REST AND IMMOBILITY

- The cardiovascular responses to bed rest include a redistribution of blood volume from the lower body to the central circulation, a deconditioning of the heart, and a reduction in total body water. Orthostatic intolerance may develop.
- Venous stasis due to bed rest encourages the development of deep vein thrombosis.
- Pulmonary changes due to bed rest include decreased tidal volume and functional residual capacity. Alveoli tend to collapse, resulting in areas of decreased pulmonary ventilation.
- Bed rest increases the risk for development of renal calculi and urinary tract infections.
- Muscle mass is reduced owing to disuse atrophy and bone mass is reduced because of an imbalance of activity between osteoclasts (bone resorption) and osteoblasts (bone generation).
- Pressure ulcers due to tissue ischemia may develop in areas in constant contact with the bed surface.
- Psychological effects of bed rest include anxiety and depression and decreased ability to concentrate and learn.

One of the most striking responses to assumption of the supine position during bed rest is the alteration of blood flow. In the supine position, approximately 500 mL of blood is redistributed from the lower extremities to the central circulation. Most of this blood is diverted to the lungs; a smaller portion is diverted to the arms and head. The increased fluid shifted to the head and thoracic cavity may result in the person experiencing headache, swelling of the nasal sinuses, nasal congestion, and puffiness of the eyelids.[49–54]

The increase in central blood volume results in an increase in stroke volume, which results in an increase in cardiac output. In the supine position, the normal cardiac output is 7 to 8 L/minute, compared with a cardiac output of 5 to 6 L/minute for a person in the standing position. Initially, the increase in stroke volume and cardiac output is accompanied by a slight decrease in heart rate and systemic vascular resistance and the maintenance of blood pressure. With extended periods of bed rest, there is an increase in venous compliance, which decreases venous return to the heart and thus compromises cardiac filling, resulting in an increase in heart rate and a decrease in stroke volume. With prolonged bed rest, heart rate can increase approximately 0.5 beat/minute each day.

The changes in cardiovascular function due to bed rest are often referred to as cardiovascular adaptation syndrome (CAS). Decreased cardiac output, along with decreased peripheral oxygen utilization, causes a decrease in maximal oxygen consumption ($\dot{V}O_2$ max). After days of bed rest, $\dot{V}O_2$ max 20 may decrease by as much as 27%. For persons with coronary artery disease, CAS may exaggerate the symptoms of angina.[53]

Bed rest also affects fluid balance. The increase in plasma volume in the central circulation stimulates baroreceptors. The stimulation of the baroreceptors results in

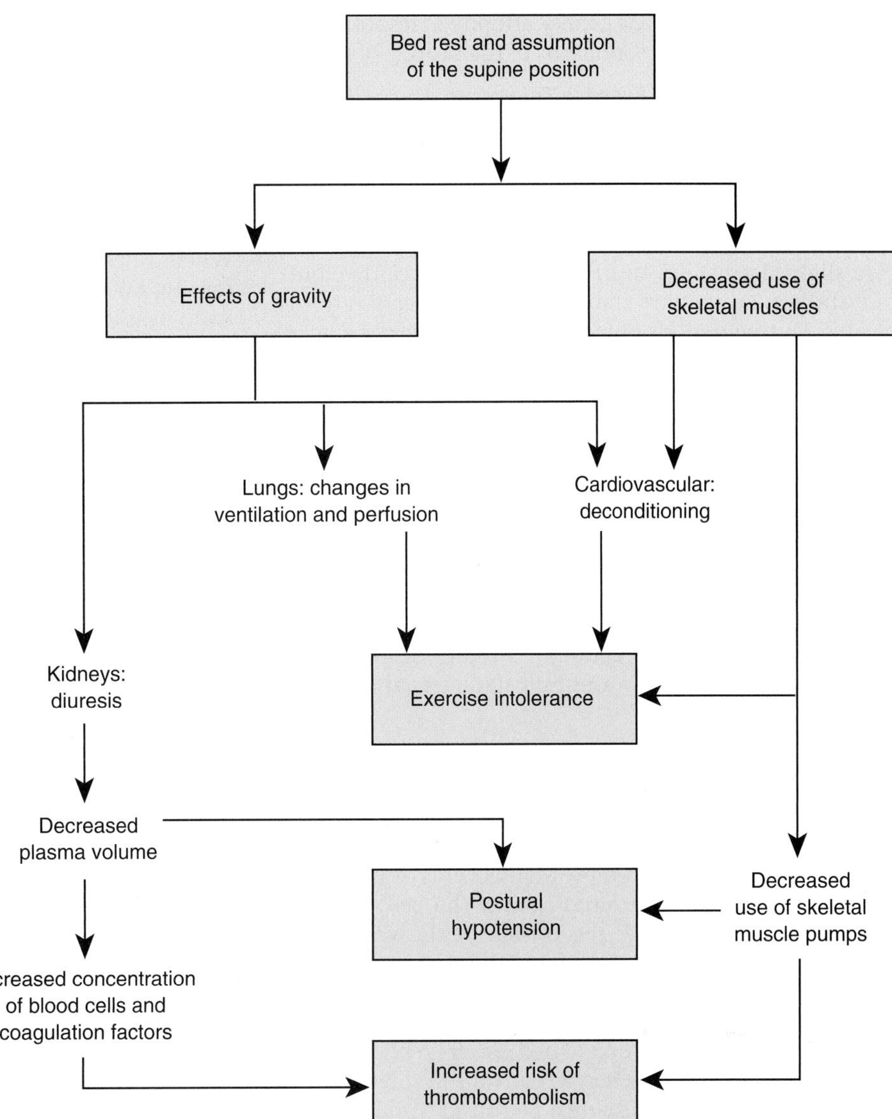

FIGURE 12-2 The effect of gravity and decreased use of the skeletal muscles during bed rest and assumption of the supine position on cardiovascular, respiratory, and renal function and their impact on exercise tolerance and the risk for complications such as thromboembolism and postural hypotension.

an inhibition of antidiuretic hormone and aldosterone, with a resultant water and sodium (*i.e.,* natriuresis) diuresis. In the supine position, diuresis begins on the first day with the shift of blood from the lower extremities to the thoracic cavity. The loss of water and sodium results in an increase in hematocrit, hemoglobin, and red cell mass owing to the loss of plasma volume.[45,46,50,54,55]

After approximately 4 days of bed rest, fluid losses reach an equilibrium. A possible explanation for this is that fluid is lost from the vascular compartment with a subsequent iso-osmotic shift of fluid from the extravascular space. Extravascular hydration is sacrificed to maintain adequate isotonic vascular volume. With a decrease in the extravascular volume and the reestablishment of intravascular volume, the osmoreceptors inhibit diuresis and natriuresis. Despite the reestablishment of intravascular volume, the extravascular spaces remain dehydrated.[45,46,50–53]

Orthostatic Hypotension. During bed rest, the forces of gravity and hydrostatic pressure are removed from the cardiovascular system. After 3 to 4 days of bed rest, resumption of the upright position results in orthostatic or postural intolerance. Standing after prolonged bed rest results in a decrease in central blood volume as blood is displaced to the lower extremities and dependent parts of the body. Decreases in stroke volume and cardiac output occur along with increases in heart rate and systemic vascular resistance. The signs and symptoms of postural intolerance include tachycardia, nausea, diaphoresis, and sometimes syncope or fainting.

It has been hypothesized that the underlying pathology for the bed rest–induced orthostatic intolerance is autonomic nervous system dysfunction. The reason for this is not completely understood because catecholamine levels and adrenergic receptor sensitivity do not change significantly with bed rest. Research suggests that an additional cardiovascular response is present that may contribute to orthostatic intolerance associated with bed rest. The decrease in stroke volume also may be caused by a reduction in left ventricular size and distensibility that occurs because of an apparent physiologic cardiac atrophy in response to a decrease in the loading conditions of the heart.[53,56]

Cardiac Workload and Exercise Tolerance. The major cardiovascular manifestation of deconditioning associated with bed rest is an increased workload on the heart. Initially, when a person assumes the supine position, venous return to the heart increases along with an increase in stroke volume and cardiac output, which is accompanied by a slight decrease in heart rate. Over time, cardiac output and stroke volume stabilize, whereas heart rate increases. During periods of tachycardia, the time the heart spends in diastole is decreased. With decreased time spent in diastole, the heart does not have sufficient time to fill with blood, and it has to work harder (expend more energy and use more oxygen) to perfuse vital organs and meet the metabolic demands of the body. This response is exaggerated when a person has to assume the upright position and begin activity after a prolonged period of bed rest. When a person begins submaximal exercise after prolonged bed rest, heart rate increases while stroke volume and cardiac output decrease. Between 5 and 10 weeks of reconditioning exercise is required for return of heart rate, stroke volume, and cardiac output parameters to their levels before bed rest.[49,51,53,57,58]

Venous Stasis. Venous stasis in the legs results from the lack of the skeletal muscle pump function that promotes venous return to the heart. The skeletal muscle pump function ceases after assumption of the supine position, and there is mechanical compression of veins from the position of the lower extremities against the bed. This increased pressure damages the intima of the vessel and causes platelets to adhere easily to the damaged vessel, encouraging clot formation.

The development of deep vein thrombosis (DVT) is the third major complication of bed rest. It is believed that three possible factors, Virchow's triad for thromboembolic disease, combine to predispose a person to thrombus formation. These factors are (a) a redistribution of circulating volume that leads to a decreased intravascular volume, which then contributes to increased blood viscosity and a hypercoagulable state; (b) venous stasis due to absence of the lower extremity muscle pumping effect; and (c) application of external pressure from the mattress against the veins.[53,59] However, most persons with DVT have other risk factors in addition to bed rest.[46] The development of DVT also predisposes to the development of pulmonary emboli. As persons begin to resume activity patterns, the risk that large thrombi may dislodge and work their way through the circulatory system and lodge in a pulmonary vessel increases.

Various theories have been advanced for the causes of the hypercoagulability and clot formation that occur with bed rest. One theory suggests that the development of dehydration with bed rest leads to an increased number of formed elements in the blood and contributes to increased blood viscosity. Increased viscosity contributes to clotting. Another theory points to the role of calcium. During bed rest, demineralization of bone occurs, and calcium and other minerals are released into the bloodstream. Calcium activates the conversion of prothrombin to thrombin, and thrombin becomes the activating enzyme that converts fibrinogen to fibrin. Fibrin then initiates the process of clot formation.[60]

Pulmonary Responses

Bed rest and assumption of the supine position produces changes in lung volumes and the mechanics of breathing. When a person is supine, the diaphragm moves upward, causing a decrease in the size of the thoracic compartment, and chest/lung expansion is limited because of the resistance of the bed. Lung expansion also is reduced by a decrease in lung compliance. In the supine position, normal tidal volume breathing is a function of the abdominal muscles, in contrast to breathing in the upright position, in which normal breathing is primarily a function of rib cage movement. Tidal volume and functional residual capacity are decreased, and the efficiency and effectiveness of ventilation are hindered. Regional changes in the ventilation-perfusion ratio in dependent areas of the lung occur when ventilation is decreased and perfusion is increased. This may result in arteriovenous shunting with a concomitant decrease in arterial oxygenation. Persons must work harder to breathe, and consequently they take fewer deep breaths. Alveoli tend to collapse, resulting in areas of atelectasis and a decrease in the surface for gas exchange. These changes in function contribute to respiratory complications associated with bed rest: atelectasis, accumulation of secretions, hypoxemia, and pulmonary emboli.[53]

Atelectasis is characterized by localized areas of lung collapse. It is caused by impaired mucociliary clearance of the airway, resulting in pooling of secretions. Also, poor fluid intake and dehydration may cause secretions to become thick and tenacious. Stasis of secretions provides an ideal medium for bacterial growth, especially pneumococcal, staphylococcal, and streptococcal organisms. To prevent the complication of pneumonia from developing, persons must perform coughing and deep-breathing exercises. However, with the combined need of overcoming resistance to chest and lung expansion and obstructed airways, more energy is required to breathe. More oxygen is used and more carbon dioxide is produced, causing the person to expend more energy to get less air.

Urinary Tract Responses

The kidneys are designed to function optimally with the body in the erect position (Fig. 12-3). The anatomy of the kidney is such that urine flows from the kidney pelvis by gravity, whereas the action of peristalsis moves urine through the ureters to the bladder. Prolonged bed rest affects the renal system by altering the composition of body fluids and predisposing to the development of kidney stones. In the supine position, urine is not readily drained from the renal pelvis. Bed rest also may predispose to urinary tract infections and urinary incontinence because of positional changes and difficulty in emptying the bladder.[52,53,58,61]

A major complication of prolonged bed rest is the increased risk for development of kidney stones. Prolonged bed rest causes muscle atrophy, protein breakdown, de-

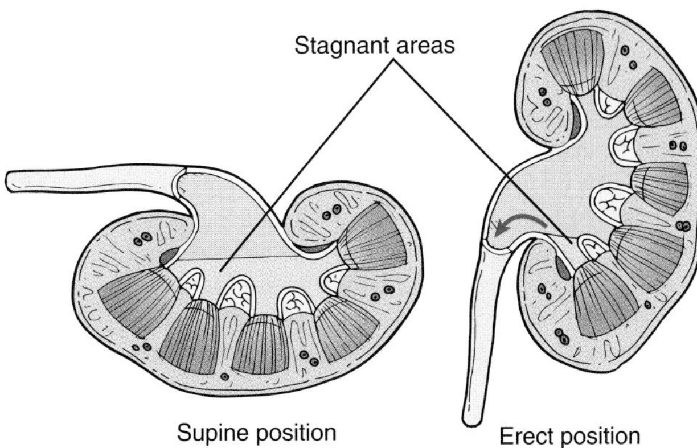

FIGURE 12-3 Effect of position on urine flow in the kidney.

mineralization of bone, and increased risk for development of calcium-containing kidney stones. The increased concentration of calcium salts (*i.e.,* calcium oxalate and calcium phosphate) in the urine resulting from demineralization of bone, along with urinary stasis, resulting from the supine position, favors crystallization of the stone-forming calcium salts. Moreover, urine levels of citrate, a prominent inhibitor of calcium stone formation, do not increase during bed rest.[52,53,58,60,61] Dehydration further increases the urinary concentration of stone-forming elements and risk for kidney stone formation. The pathogenesis and manifestations of kidney stones are discussed in Chapter 35.

Urinary tract infections and incontinence also may occur. The cause of incontinence is inadequate emptying of the bladder while the person is in the supine position. This position contributes to stagnation of urine in the bladder and may predispose the person to bladder and urinary tract infections.

Musculoskeletal Responses

Muscles are only as strong as they need to be to perform the work at hand. Disuse atrophy leads to loss of approximately one eighth of the muscle's strength with each week of disuse.[45,54,62] Weight loss occurs when normally healthy people are subjected to periods of prolonged bed rest. The weight loss occurs when people are placed on controlled diets, as well as when they are allowed to eat ad libitum.[62] The reduction in weight is associated with the loss of lean muscle mass and fat content. Immobilization also causes a reduction in force-generating capacity along with increased fatigability, primarily owing to a decrease in muscle mass and the cross-sectional area of muscle fiber.[54,63] The larger and the better trained the muscle, the faster the loss of muscle strength and the quicker the deconditioning occurs. The strength of fast-twitch (type II) fibers appears to decline at an accelerated rate compared with the decline in strength of slow-twitch (type I) fibers.[54] For example, leg muscles lose strength and mass more quickly than muscles of the arms in persons placed on prolonged bed rest.

In addition to loss of strength, muscles atrophy, change shape and appearance, and shorten when immobilized. There also is a decrease in the oxidative capacity of the muscle mitochondria. These changes affect individual muscle fibers and total muscle mass. Atrophy of muscles is reflected as an increase in urinary nitrogen excretion and a decrease in muscle weight. Because of the decreased oxidative capacity of the mitochondria, muscles fatigue more easily.[46,54,64]

Along with muscle, connective tissue undergoes changes when subjected to immobility or bed rest. Periarticular connective tissue, ligaments, tendons, and articular cartilage require motion to maintain health. Changes in structure and function of connective tissue become apparent 4 to 6 days after immobilization and remain even after normal activity has been resumed. It is believed that changes in the structure of collagen fibers contribute to the connective tissue changes associated with immobility.[53,54,64]

Muscle atrophy not only contributes to wasting and weakening of muscle tissue but also plays a role in the development of *contractures.* A contracture is the abnormal shortening of muscle tissue, rendering the muscle highly resistant to stretch. Muscles weaken and shorten with disuse. Contractures occur when muscles do not have the necessary strength to maintain their integrity (*i.e.,* their proper function and full range of motion). Contractures mainly develop over joints when there is an imbalance in the muscle strength of the antagonistic muscle groups. If allowed to progress, the contracture eventually involves the muscle groups, tendons, ligaments, and joint capsule. The joint becomes limited in its full use and range of motion. Proper body alignment decreases the risk for development of contractures.[46,60]

Another consequence of prolonged immobility and bed rest for the musculoskeletal system is the loss of bone mass and the development of osteoporosis. Bone is a dynamic tissue that undergoes continual deposition and replacement of minerals in response to the dual stimuli of weight bearing and muscle pull. According to Wolff's law, the density of bone is directly proportional to the stress placed upon it. When lack of stress is placed on bones, as occurs with bed rest or immobility, there is a greater amount of bone resorption than bone formation, resulting in a net loss of bone formation.[54] With immobility and bed rest, calcium loss from the bone begins almost immediately.

The maintenance of normal bone function depends on two types of cells: osteoblasts and osteoclasts (see Chapter 56). Osteoblasts function in building the osseous matrix of the bone, and osteoclasts function in the breakdown of the bone matrix. Through their opposing forces, the bone matrix is continually turned over, and new bone is generated. Osteoblasts depend on the stress of mobility and weight bearing to perform their function. During immobility and bed rest, the process of building new bone stops, but the osteoclast cells continue to perform their function. This results in structural changes in the bone. There also is an increase in the excretion of bone calcium and phosphorous. Despite the calcium loss from the bone, serum calcium remains normal because the excess calcium is excreted in the urine and feces.

Persons who experience disuse osteoporosis from prolonged immobility and bed rest develop soft, spongy bones.

The bones may easily compress and become deformed. Because of the lack of structural firmness, the bones may easily fracture. Persons with osteoporosis experience much pain when they begin weight-bearing activities. Despite the lack of calcium in the bone, a diet high in calcium will not enhance bone uptake of calcium. Unneeded calcium is added to the excess calcium that already is being excreted in the urine. This may precipitate the formation of calcium-containing renal stones. The best measure to prevent the occurrence of osteoporosis is to begin weight bearing as soon as possible.

Skin Responses

Except for the soles of the feet, the skin is not designed for weight bearing. However, during bed rest, the large surface area of the skin bears weight and is in constant contact with the surface of the bed. Constant pressure is transmitted to the skin, subcutaneous tissue, and muscle, especially to those tissues over bony prominences. This constant contact causes increased pressure and impairs normal capillary blood flow, which interferes with the exchange of nutrients and waste products. Tissue ischemia and necrosis may result and lead to the development of pressure ulcers. Also contributing to the development of pressure ulcers is moisture from skin that is in constant contact with bed linens, along with the forces of friction and shear that occur when the person is repositioned in bed.

Metabolic and Endocrine Responses

When a person is placed on bed rest, the basal metabolic rate drops in response to decreased energy requirements of the body. Anabolic processes are slowed, and catabolic processes become accelerated. Protein breakdown occurs and leads to a protein deficiency and a negative nitrogen balance.[47] Persons in a negative nitrogen balance experience nausea and anorexia, which contribute to the catabolic state. Carbohydrate intolerance has been noted to occur as early as the third day of immobility. Also, peripheral glucose uptake declines by 50% after 14 days of bed rest or immobility. The period of immobility correlates proportionally with the degree of carbohydrate intolerance. Glucose intolerance that often accompanies bed rest can be improved by implementing a regimen of isotonic exercises of the large muscle groups.[53]

The person on bed rest experiences an impaired responsiveness to the actions of insulin. During bed rest, it takes more insulin to maintain serum glucose. After 10 days of bed rest, there is a 100% increase in basal insulin concentration to maintain normal glucose control.[65,66] There also appears to be an induced insulin resistance that helps explain the negative nitrogen balance seen in patients who experience prolonged bed rest. The reason for this intolerance in not lack of insulin, but rather an increased resistance to the action of insulin that then results in a hyperglycemia and a hyperinsulinemia state.[53] Insulin also plays a role in regulating protein metabolism by inhibiting protein breakdown.

Possible reasons for the unresponsiveness of glucose to hyperinsulinemia include a change in the action of insulin because of the release of a substance that acts as an insulin inhibitor (this substance is believed to act at cell membrane–binding sites); a change in some aspect of the cellular membrane glucose transport system; or inhibition of the function of a second factor that has insulin-like activity. Research suggests that one or more factors are activated with physical exercise. These factors respond to the quantity of energy expenditure and are necessary for insulin, and possibly glucose, to function normally. In the absence of activity, the action of these factors may be suppressed. A final explanation for the unresponsiveness of glucose to hyperinsulinemia is a combination of the aforementioned causes.[65,66]

Another major hormonal change that occurs with prolonged periods of bed rest and immobility is an increase in the serum parathyroid hormone. The increased level is related to the hypercalcemia that occurs secondary to immobility. Triiodothyronine (T_3) blood levels are also elevated during periods of immobility.[53,67]

Persons who experience prolonged periods of bed rest have changes in the circadian release of various hormones. Normally, insulin and growth hormone peak twice a day. In people who experienced 30 days of bed rest, a single daily peak of these hormones occurred. Other hormonal changes include an afternoon peak of epinephrine rather than the normal early morning peak, and an early morning peak of aldosterone rather than the usual noonday peak that is seen in normally active persons.[68]

The immune system also is subject to physiologic changes associated with bed rest or immobility. Research demonstrates that after 4 weeks of bed rest, there is an increase in interleukin-1 production, which may play a role in the bone mineral loss that occurs during bed rest. Also seen is a decrease in interleukin-2 secretion, which may play a part in the infectious diseases that often occur during periods of bed rest.[69]

Gastrointestinal Responses

Gastrointestinal responses to bed rest vary. Loss of appetite, slowed rate of absorption, and distaste for food combine to contribute to nutritional hypoproteinemia. Passage of food through the gastrointestinal tract is slowed when the person is placed in the supine position. In a supine position, the velocity of peristaltic waves decreases by 60%. Also, the loss of plasma volume and dehydration can combine to exacerbate gastrointestinal problems. Thus, constipation and fecal impaction are frequent complications that occur when persons experience prolonged periods of immobility and bed rest. With inactivity, there is slowed movement of feces through the colon. The act of defecation requires the integration of the abdominal muscles, the diaphragm, and the levator ani. Muscle atrophy and loss of tone occur in the immobilized person and interfere with the normal act of defecation. Lack of privacy and the supine position may also compound problems with defecation.[45,47,53,60,61]

Sensory Responses

Immobility reduces the quality and quantity of sensory information available from kinesthetic, visual, auditory, and tactile sensation. It also reduces the person's ability to interact with the environment. Decreased kinesthetic stimulation occurs from both immobilization and assumption of the supine or recumbent position. Responses to decreased kinesthetic stimulation include an impaired functioning of thought processes and decreased sensory perception. Prolonged immobility and bed rest have been associated with a number of impaired sensory responses. Common occurrences include both visual and auditory hallucinations, vivid dreams, inefficient thought processes, loss of contact with reality, and alteration in tactile stimulation.

In addition to sensory deprivation related to prolonged bed rest and immobility, persons may experience a sensory monotony from the hospital environment. Repetitious and meaningless sounds from cardiac monitors, respirators, and hospital personnel, along with an environment that may be void of light and a normal day-night cycle, also contribute to impaired sensory perception.

PSYCHOSOCIAL RESPONSES

Immobility often sets the stage for changes in the person's response to illness. Persons adapt to prolonged bed rest and immobility through a series of physiologic responses and through changes in affect, perception, and cognition. Affective changes include increased anxiety, fear, depression, hostility, rapid mood changes, and alterations in normal sleep patterns. These changes in mood occur with hospitalized patients who are subjected to periods of prolonged bed rest and immobility and in persons in confinement, such as astronauts and prisoners. Research on immobilized or isolated persons has demonstrated that the motivation to learn decreases with periods of prolonged immobility, as does the ability to learn and retain new material and transfer newly learned material to a different situation. Persons are less able and less motivated to perform problem-solving activities; they are less able to concentrate and discriminate information.[68,70] These studies present major implications for the timing of patient education and the preparation of education materials.

Prolonged bed rest and immobility also contribute to the social isolation of the hospitalized person. Confined to a hospital bed, the person is unable to assume certain societal roles. The roles of spouse, parent, sibling, worker, and friend are altered either temporarily or permanently while the person is hospitalized. People may respond to this isolation by exhibiting various effective and ineffective coping behaviors, including increased anxiety, depression, restlessness, fear, and rapid mood changes.[70]

TIME COURSE OF PHYSIOLOGIC RESPONSES

The deconditioning responses to the inactivity of immobility and bed rest affect all body systems. One of the important factors to keep in mind is the rapidity with which the changes occur and the length of time required to overcome these effects. The body responds in a characteristic pattern to the effects of the supine position and bed rest (Table 12-3). During the first 3 days of bed rest, one of the first changes to occur is a massive diuresis. Accompanying the diuresis are increases in serum osmolality, hematocrit, venous compliance, and an increase of urinary sodium and chloride excretion. Fluid losses stabilize by approximately the fourth day. By days 4 to 7, there are changes in the hemolytic system. Fibrinogen and fibrinolytic activity

TABLE 12-3 Physiologic Changes During Bed Rest

0–3 Days	4–7 Days	8–14 Days	Over 15 Days
Increases in	**Increases in**	**Increases in**	**Increases in**
Urine volume	Urine creatinine, hydroxyproline, PO_4, N, and K excretion	Urine pyrophosphate	Peak hypercalciuria
Urine Na, Cl, Ca, and osmol excretion	Plasma globulin, phosphate, and glucose levels	Sweating sensitivity	Sensitivity to thermal threshold
Plasma osmolality	Blood fibrinogen	Exercise hyperthermia	Auditory threshold (secondary)
Hematocrit	Fibrinolytic activity and clotting time	Exercise maximal heart rate	
Venous compliance	Visual focal point		
	Hyperthermia of eye conjunctiva, dilation of retinal arteries and veins		
	Auditory threshold		
Decreases in	**Decreases in**	**Decreases in**	**Decreases in**
Total fluid intake	Near point of visual acuity	Red blood cell mass	Bone density
Extracellular and intracellular fluid	Orthostatic tolerance	Leukocyte phagocytosis	
Calf blood flow	Nitrogen balance	Tissue heat conductance	
Resting heart rate		Lean body mass	
Secretion of gastric acid			
Glucose tolerance			

(Greenleaf J.E. [1984]. Physiological responses to prolonged bed rest and fluid immersion in humans. *Journal of Applied Physiology: Respiratory, Environmental and Exercise Physiology* 57, 619–633)

increase, and clotting time is prolonged. The cardiovascular system responds with a decrease in cardiac output and stroke volume. The basal metabolic rate decreases, and glucose intolerance and a negative nitrogen balance begin to develop.[71]

Additional effects on the hemolytic system are observed on days 8 to 14. Red blood cell number is decreased, and the phagocytic ability of leukocytes is reduced. There is a decrease in lean body mass and, after 15 days of bed rest, osteoporosis and hypercalciuria occur. Aerobic power decreases, the cyclic excretion of some hormones is changed, and the person's thought patterns and sensory perception are altered.[71]

INTERVENTIONS

A holistic approach should be taken when caring for persons who are immobile or require prolonged periods of bed rest. Interventions and treatment should include actions that address the person's physical and psychosocial needs. The goals of care for the immobilized person include structuring a safe environment in which the person is not at risk for nosocomial complications, providing diversional activities to offset problems with sensory deprivation, and preventing complications of bed rest by implementing an interdisciplinary plan of care.

In summary, during the past 75 years, the use of bed rest has undergone a complete reversal as a standard of treatment for a variety of medical conditions. Over time, research findings have described the deleterious consequences of inactivity. All body systems are affected by complications of immobility and prolonged bed rest.

The responses to bed rest and immobility affect all body systems. One of the important factors is the rapidity with which the changes occur and the long time required to overcome the effects of prolonged bed rest and immobility. Adverse effects of prolonged immobility and bed rest include a decreased cardiac output, orthostatic intolerance, dehydration, and the potential for thrombophlebitis, pneumonia, formation of renal calculi, development of pressure ulcers, sensory deprivation, and impaired thought processes.

REVIEW EXERCISES

A 60-year-old man sustains an acute myocardial infarction (heart attack). He has been discharged from the hospital and is about to enter a phase II cardiac rehabilitation program. On his first day in the program, he is being examined for his tolerance to the exercise program.

A. One of tests that he is scheduled to undergo is the treadmill stress test. How will this test contribute to the evaluation of his ability to engage in an exercise test?

B. What other subjective tests might be used to determine his exercise tolerance?

A 40-year-old woman who is being treated with chemotherapy for breast cancer complains of excessive fatigue and activity intolerance. She claims she has so little energy she can hardly get up in the morning and has difficulty concentrating and doing such simple activities as going shopping.

A. What are some of the possible explanations for this woman's excessive fatigue?

B. What types of medical test might be done to identify possible causes of fatigue?

C. What types of treatment might be used to alleviate some of her symptoms?

A 23-year-old man, who has sustained multiple fractures and contusions in a motorcycle accident, is confined to bed rest in the supine position. He has been on bed rest for 2 days and has lost about 500 mL of extracellular fluid volume owing to diuresis.

A. Explain the physiologic rationale for the excessive diuresis.

B. Identify two complications of bed rest that might occur as the result of this loss of extracellular fluid volume.

C. Upon getting out of bed on the fourth day, he suddenly turns pale, has an increase in heart rate, and complains of dizziness. What has happened to this man?

References

1. McArdle W.D., Katch F.I., Katch V.I. (2001). *Exercise physiology: Energy, nutrition and human performance* (5th ed.). Baltimore: Lippincott Williams & Wilkins.
2. Jennings G.L.R. (1995). Mechanisms for reduction of cardiovascular risk by regular exercise. *Clinical and Experimental Pharmacology and Physiology 22,* 209–211.
3. Booth F.W., Gordon S.E., Carlson C.J., Hamilton M.T. (2000). Waging war on modern chronic diseases: Primary prevention through exercise biology. *Applied Journal of Physiology 88,* 774–787.
4. Martin B. (2003). Exercise physiology. In Rhoades R.A., Tanner G.A. (Eds.), *Medical physiology* (2nd ed., pp. 551–565). Philadelphia: Lippincott Williams & Wilkins.
5. Coote J.H., Bothams V.F. (2001). Cardiac vagal control before, during and after exercise. *Experimental Physiology 86*(6), 811–815.
6. Thompson P.D., Crouse S.F., Goodpaster B., et al. (2001). The acute versus the chronic response to exercise. *Medicine and Science in Sports and Exercise 33*(6 Suppl), S438–S445.
7. Sherman D.L. (2000). Exercise and endothelial function. *Coronary Artery Disease 11,* 117–122.
8. Gustafson T., Puntschart A., Kauser L., et al. (1999). Exercise-induced expression of angiogenesis-related transcription and growth factors in human skeletal muscle. *American Journal of Physiology 276,* H679–H685.
9. Stewart K.J., Hiatt W.R., Regensteiner J.G., Hirsch A.T. (2002). Exercise training for claudication. *New England Journal of Medicine 347,* 1941–1951.
10. Tonkonogi M., Sahlin K. (2002). Physical exercise and mitochondrial function in human skeletal muscle. *Exercise and Sport Sciences Reviews 30*(3), 129–137.

11. Buckwalter J.B., Clifford P.S. (2001). The paradox of sympathetic vasoconstriction in exercising skeletal muscle. *Exercise and Sport Sciences Reviews 29*(4), 159–163.
12. Kenney W.L., Johnson J.M. (1992). Control of skin blood flow during exercise. *Medicine and Science in Sports and Exercise 24,* 303–312.
13. Peters H.P., DeVries W.R. (2001). Potential benefits and hazards of physical activity and exercise on the gastrointestinal tract. *Gut 48,* 435–439.
14. MacKinnon L.T. (2000). Chronic exercise effects on immune function. *Medicine and Science in Sports and Exercise 32*(7 Suppl), S369–S376.
15. Rowbottom D.G., Green K.J. (2000). Acute exercise effects on the immune system. *Medicine and Science in Sports and Exercise 32*(7 Suppl), S396–S405.
16. Daughton D.M., Fix J.A. (1986). *Human Activity Profile (HAP) manual.* Lutz, FL: Psychological Assessment Resources, Inc.
17. Krupp L.B., LaRocca N.G., Muir-Nash J., Steinberg A.D. (1989). The Fatigue Severity Scale: Application to patients with multiple sclerosis and systemic lupus erythematosus. *Archives of Neurology 46,* 1121–1123.
18. Ulmer H.V. (1983). Work physiology: Environmental physiology. In Schmidt R.F., Thews G. (Eds.), *Human physiology* (pp. 548–564). New York: Springer-Verlag.
19. Borg G.A.V. (1973). Perceived exertion: A note on "history" and methods. *Medicine and Science in Sports and Exercise 5,* 90–93.
20. Borg G.A.V. (1982). Psychophysical bases of perceived exertion. *Medicine and Science in Sports and Exercise 14,* 377–381.
21. Piper B.F. (2003). Fatigue. In Carrieri-Kohlman V., Lindsey A.M., West C.W. (Eds.), *Pathophysiological phenomena in nursing: Human responses to illness* (pp. 209–234). Philadelphia: W.B. Saunders.
22. Curt C.A. (2000). The impact of fatigue on patients with cancer: overview of fatigue 1 and 2. *Oncologist 5* (Suppl 2), 9–12.
23. Hickok J.T., Morrow G.R., McDonald S., Bellig A.J. (1996). Frequency and correlates of fatigue in lung cancer patients receiving radiation therapy: Implications for management. *Journal of Pain and Symptom Management 11*(6), 370–377.
24. Woo B., Dibble S.L., Piper B.F., et al. (1998). Differences in treatment methods in women with breast cancer. *Oncology Nursing Forum 25*(5), 915–920.
25. Stone P., Hardy J., Broadley K., et al. (1999). Fatigue in advanced cancer. *European Journal of Cancer 34,* 1670–1676.
26. Gutstein H.B. (2001). The biologic basis of fatigue. *Cancer 6*(Suppl 6), 1678–1683.
27. Kurzrock R. (2001). The role of cytokines in cancer-related fatigue. *Cancer 6*(Suppl 6), 1684–1688.
28. Belza B. (1994). The impact of fatigue on exercise performance. *Arthritis Care and Research 7,* 176–180.
29. Smith B.A., Neidig J.L., Mitchell G.L., et al. (2001). Aerobic exercise: Effects on parameters related to fatigue, dyspnea, weight, and body composition in HIV-infected adults. *AIDS 15*(6), 693–701.
30. Ponichtera-Mulcare J.A. (1993). Exercise and multiple sclerosis. *Medicine and Science in Sports and Exercise 25,* 451–465.
31. Evengard B., Schacterle R.S., Komaroff L. (1999). Chronic fatigue syndrome: New insights and old ignorance. *Journal of Internal Medicine 256,* 455–469.
32. Evengdrd E., Klimas N. (2002). Chronic fatigue syndrome. *Drugs 62,* 2433–2446.
33. Lloyd A. (1998). Chronic fatigue syndrome: Shifting boundaries and attributions. *American Journal of Medicine 105*(3A), 7S–10S.
34. Demitrack M.A. (1998). Neuroendocrine aspects of chronic fatigue syndrome: A commentary. *American Journal of Medicine 105*(3A), 11S–14S.
35. Afari N., Buchwald D. (2003). Chronic fatigue syndrome: A review. *American Journal of Psychiatry 160,* 221–236.
36. Holmes G.P., Kaplan J.E., Gantz N.M., et al. (1988). Chronic fatigue syndrome: A working definition. *Annals of Internal Medicine 108,* 387–389.
37. Fukuda K., Straus S.E., Hickie I., et al. (1994). The chronic fatigue syndrome: A comprehensive approach to its definition and study. *Annals of Internal Medicine 121,* 953–959.
38. Demitrack M.A., Engleberg N.C. (1994). Chronic fatigue syndrome. *Current Therapy in Endocrinology and Metabolism 5,* 135–142.
39. Whiteside T.L., Friberg D. (1998). Natural killer cells and natural killer cell activity in chronic fatigue syndrome. *American Journal of Medicine 105*(3A), 27S–34S.
40. Craig T., Kakumanu S. (2002). Chronic fatigue syndrome: Evaluation and treatment. *American Family Physician 65,* 1083–1090.
41. Tirelli U., Chierichetti F., Tavio M., et al. (1998). Brain positron emission tomography (PET) in chronic fatigue syndrome: Preliminary data. *American Journal of Medicine 105*(3A), 54S–58S.
42. Lange G., Wang S., DeLuca J., Natelson B. (1998). Neuroimaging in chronic fatigue syndrome. *American Journal of Medicine 105*(3A), 50S–53S.
43. Pagani M., Lucini D. (1999). Chronic fatigue syndrome: A hypothesis focusing on the autonomic nervous system. *Clinical Science 96,* 117–125.
44. Harper C.M., Lyles Y.M. (1988). Physiology and complications of bed rest. *Journal of the American Geriatric Society 36,* 1047–1054.
45. Coletta E.M., Murphy J.B. (1992). The complications of immobility in the elderly stroke patient. *Journal of the American Board of Family Practice 5,* 389–397.
46. Dittmer D.K., Teasell, R. (1993). Complications of immobilization and bed rest. Part 1: Musculoskeletal and cardiovascular complications. *Canadian Family Physician 39,* 1428–1437.
47. Teasell R., Dittmer D.K. (1993). Complications of immobilization and bed rest. Part 2: Other complications. *Canadian Family Physician 39,* 1440–1446.
48. Convertino V.A., Bloomfield S.A., Greenleaf J.E. (1997). An overview of the issues: Physiological effects of bed rest and restricted physical activity. *Medicine and Science in Sports and Exercise 29*(2), 187–190.
49. Taylor H.L., Henschel A., Broek J., Keys A. (1949). Effects of bed rest on cardiovascular function and work performance. *Journal of Applied Physiology 11,* 223–239.
50. Dean E. (1993). Bedrest and deconditioning. *Neurology Report 17*(1), 6–9.
51. Convertino V.A. (1997). Cardiovascular consequences of bed rest: Effect on maximal oxygen uptake. *Medicine and Science in Sports and Exercise 29,* 191–197.
52. Faria S.H. (1998). Assessment of immobility hazards. *Home Care Provider 3,* 189–191.
53. Halar E.M., Bell K.R. (1998). *Immobility in rehabilitation medicine: Principles and practice* (3rd ed., pp. 1015–1034). Philadelphia: Lippincott-Raven Publishers.
54. Topp R., Ditmyer M.A., King K., et al. (2002). The effect of bed rest and potential of prehabilitation on patients in the intensive care unit. *AACN Clinical Issues 13*(2), 263–276.
55. Maloni J.A. (2000). Astronauts and pregnancy bed rest. *AWHONN Lifelines 6*(4), 318–323.
56. Levine B.D., Zuckerman J.H., Pawelczyk J.A. (1997). Cardiac atrophy after bed-rest deconditioning: A nonneural mechanism for orthostatic intolerance. *Circulation 96,* 517–525.
57. Saltin B., Blomquist G., Mitchell J.H., et al. (1968). Responses to exercise after bed rest and after training: A longitudinal study of adaptive changes in oxygen transport and body composition. *Circulation 38*(Suppl 7), 1–65.

58. Krasnoff J., Painter P. (1999). The physiological consequences of bed rest and inactivity. *Advances in Renal Replacement Therapy 6,* 124–132.
59. Slipman C.W., Lipetz J.S., Jackson H.B., Vresilovic E.J. (2000). Deep venous thrombosis and pulmonary embolism as a complication of bed rest and low back pain. *Archives of Physical Medicine and Rehabilitation 81,* 127–129.
60. Olson E.V., Thompson L.F., McCarthy J., et al. (1967). The hazards of immobility. *American Journal of Nursing 67,* 780–797.
61. Mobily P.R., Kelley L.S. (1991). Iatrogenesis in the elderly. *Journal of Gerontological Nursing 17*(9), 5–10.
62. Corcoran P.J. (1991). Use it or lose it: The hazards of bed rest and inactivity. *Western Journal of Medicine 154,* 536–538.
63. Ibebunjo C., Martyn J.A.J. (1999). Fiber atrophy, but not changes in acetylcholine receptor expression, contributes to the muscle dysfunction after immobilization. *Critical Care Medicine 27,* 275–285.
64. Hendricks T. (1995). The effects of immobilization on connective tissue. *Journal of Manual and Manipulative Therapy 3*(3), 98–103.
65. Dolkas C.B., Greenleaf J.E. (1977). Insulin and glucose responses during bed rest with isotonic and isometric exercise. *Journal of Applied Physiology 43,* 1033–1038.
66. Shangraw R.E., Stuart C.A., Prince M.J., et al. (1988). Insulin responsiveness of protein metabolism in vivo following bedrest in humans. *American Journal of Physiology 255,* E548–E558.
67. Schroth M., Dotsch J., Dorr H.G. (2001). Hypercalcemia and idiopathic hypoparathyroidism. *Journal of Clinical Pharmacy and Therapeutics 26,* 453–455.
68. Rubin M. (1988). The physiology of bed rest. *American Journal of Nursing 88,* 50–58.
69. Schmitt D.A., Schaffar L., Taylor G.R., et al. (1996). Use of bed rest and head-down tilt to simulate spaceflight-induced immune system changes. *Journal of Interferon and Cytokine Research 16,* 151–157.
70. Cunningham E. (1999) Coping with bed rest. *AWHONN Lifelines 5*(5), 50–55.
71. Greenleaf J.E., Kozlowski S. (1982). Physiological consequences of reduced physical activity during bed rest. In Terjung R.L. (Ed.), *Exercise and sport sciences reviews* (pp. 84–119). Syracuse, NY: American College of Sports Medicine.

CHAPTER

13

Sleep and Sleep Disorders

As humans, we spend approximately one third of our lives asleep. We all know what sleep feels like. Yet defining sleep, describing what happens when we sleep, and explaining why we sleep are more difficult. Of equal concern is an understanding of factors that interfere with sleep. For many people, the inability to engage in appropriate periods of normal, restful sleep seriously impairs their functioning. The content in this chapter is divided into three parts: (1) the neurobiology of sleep, (2) sleep disorders, and (3) sleep and sleep disorders in children and elderly persons.

Neurobiology of Sleep

After you have completed this section of the chapter, you should be able to meet the following objectives:

- Cite the major brain structures that are involved in sleep
- Describe the different stages of sleep in terms of the electroencephalogram tracing, eye movements, motor movements, heart rate, blood pressure, and cerebral activity
- Characterize the circadian rhythm as it relates to sleep and wakefulness
- Describe the possible role of melatonin in regulation of sleep

Sleep is part of what is called the *sleep–wake cycle.* In contrast to wakefulness, which is a time of mental activity and energy expenditure, sleep is a period of inactivity and restoration of mental and physical function. It has been suggested that sleep provides time for entering information that has been acquired during periods of wakefulness into memory and for reestablishing communication between various parts of the brain. Sleep also is a time when other body systems restore their energy and repair their tissues. Muscle activity and digestion decrease, and sympathetic nervous system activity is diminished. Many hormones, such as growth hormone, are produced in a cyclic manner correlating with the sleep–wake cycle, suggesting that growth and tissue repair may occur during sleep.

NEURAL STRUCTURES AND PATHWAYS

Anatomically, the sleep–wake cycle involves structures in the thalamus, associated areas of the cerebral cortex, and interneurons in the reticular formation of the midbrain, the pons, and the brain stem (Fig. 13-1). The reticular formation of the midbrain, pons, and brain stem monitors and modulates the activity of various circuits controlling wakefulness. The thalamus and the cerebral cortex function in

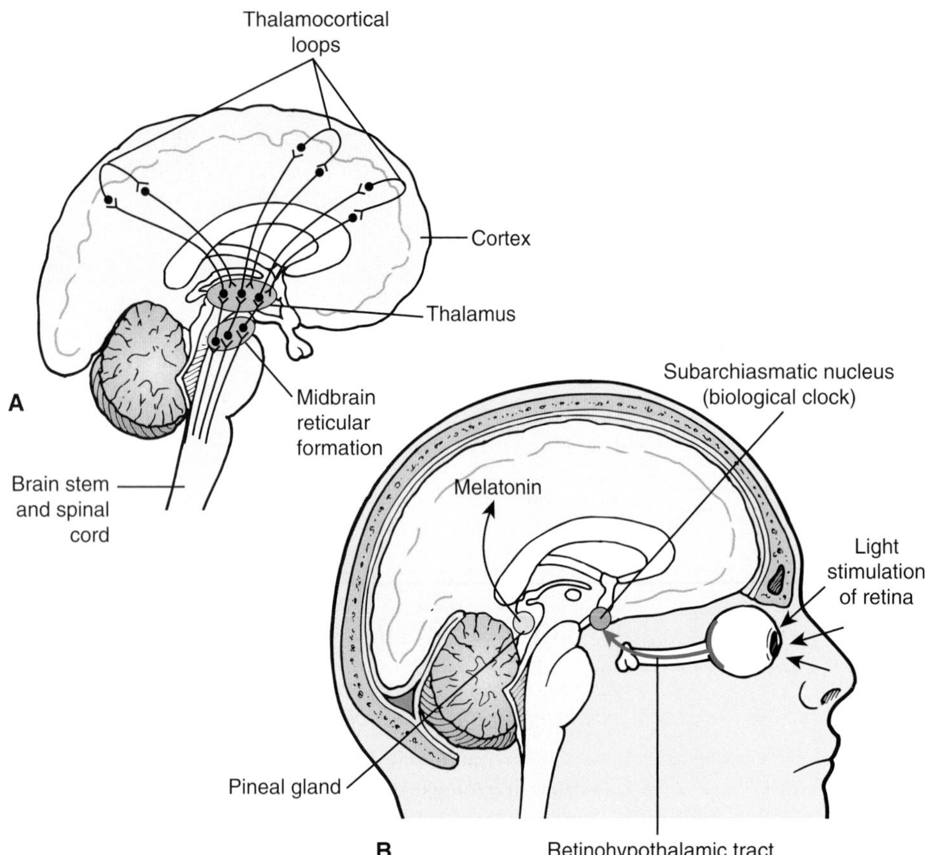

FIGURE 13-1 (**A**) Brain structures involved in sleep. (**B**) Location of the suprachiasmatic nucleus (biological clock) with input from the retina and its association with the pineal gland and melatonin production.

tandem, with all sensory information being relayed to the thalamus and from there to the cerebral cortex. For example, visual impulses from the retina go to the thalamus and are then relayed to the visual cortex. The pathways between each sensory area of the thalamus and the cortex form a two-way communication loop called the *thalamocortical loop*.[1] Communication between each sensory area of the thalamus and its companion area in the cortex is kept orderly by several neuronal control systems, including the midbrain reticular formation that controls the level of background activity so that external stimuli can be processed.

THE SLEEP–WAKE CYCLE

The sleep–wake cycle normally consists of a synchronous pattern of wakefulness and sleep. Wakefulness is a state of being aware of the environment—of receiving and responding to information arriving from all the senses, placing that information into memory, and recalling and integrating present experiences with previously stored memories. During wakefulness, both the thalamocortical loop and brain stem centers are active. A full repertoire of motor movements is made possible by corticospinal circuits that travel through the brain stem. Sleep represents a period of diminished consciousness from which a person can be aroused by sensory or other stimuli. It occurs in stages during which the brain remains active, but does not effectively process sensory information.

Brain Waves

Many of the advances in understanding the sleep–wake cycle have come about because of the ability to record brain waves through the use of the electroencephalogram (EEG). It was in 1928 that the German psychiatrist Hans

SLEEP–WAKE CYCLE

- The sleep–wake cycle normally consists of a synchronous pattern of wakefulness and sleep. Wakefulness is a state of being aware of the environment, receiving and responding to sensory input, recalling and integrating experiences into memory, and purposeful body movements.
- Sleep, which is a period of inactivity and restoration of mental and physical function, is characterized by alterations between non-REM and REM sleep.
- Non-REM sleep is a quiet type of sleep characterized by a relatively inactive, yet fully regulating brain, and fully movable body, whereas REM sleep is associated with rapid eye movements, loss of muscle movements, and vivid dreaming.

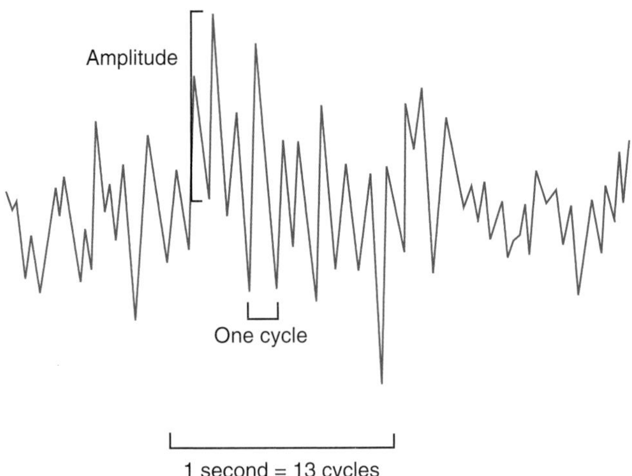

FIGURE 13-2 The amplitude and frequency characteristics of an EEG tracing.

Berger successfully recorded continuous electrical activity from the scalp of human subjects.[1] The source of the brain waves is the alternating excitatory and inhibitory nerve activity in postsynaptic neurons.[2] During the recording of an EEG, the postsynaptic potentials are averaged and filtered to improve the quality of the signal. As such, the EEG does not measure the activity of a single neuron, but rather the combined activity and "crosstalk" among many hundreds of neurons responding to a given stimulus.

The normal EEG consists of brain waves of various frequencies (measured in cycles per second, or hertz [Hz]) and amplitude (measured in microvolts [μV]; Fig. 13-2). Four types of EEG rhythms are used to describe brain activity during the sleep–wake cycle: alpha, beta, delta, and theta rhythms.[2,3] The *alpha* rhythm, which has a frequency of 7 to 13 Hz, occurs when a person is awake with eyes closed. When the eyes are open, the EEG becomes desynchronized and the dominant frequency changes to the low-amplitude *beta* rhythm with a frequency of 14 to 32 Hz. The increased frequency of the beta waves is thought to reflect a higher level of brain activity produced by firing of a large number of neurons and the low amplitude a lack of synchronization resulting from nerve activity occurring in many different brain sites at the same time. The *delta* (0.5 to 4 Hz) and *theta* (4 to 7 Hz) rhythms are observed during sleep. The low-frequency, higher-amplitude waves that occur during sleep indicate that fewer neurons are firing and that those that are active are more highly synchronized and less affected by sensory stimulation.

Sleep Stages

There are two types of sleep: rapid eye movement (REM) and non-REM sleep.[2,4] These two types of sleep alternate with each other and are characterized by differences in eye movements, muscle tone and body movements, heart rate and blood pressure, breathing patterns, brain wave activity, and dreaming (Table 13-1).

Non–Rapid Eye Movement Sleep. Non-REM sleep is a quiet type of sleep characterized by a relatively inactive, yet fully regulating brain, and fully movable body. The brain stem coordinates activity between the spinal cord and various reflexes, such as swallowing and chewing. Non-REM sleep normally is encountered when the person first becomes drowsy. It is divided into four stages that reflect an increasing depth of sleep (Fig. 13-3). *Stage 1* consists of low-voltage, mixed-frequency EEG activity. It occurs at sleep onset and is a brief (1 to 7 minutes) transitional stage between wakefulness and true sleep. During this stage, persons can be easily aroused simply by touching them, calling their name, or quietly closing a door. In addition to its role at sleep onset, stage 1 serves as a transitional stage for repeated sleep cycles throughout the night. A common sign of severely disrupted sleep is an increase or decrease in stage 1 sleep. *Stage 2,* which lasts approximately 10 to 25 minutes, is a deeper sleep during which EEG activity is interrupted by sleep spindles consisting of bursts of high-frequency (12 to 14 Hz) waves. *Stages 3 and 4* represent deep sleep and are dominated by high-voltage, low-frequency (1 to 3 Hz) waves. Stage 3 usually lasts only a few minutes and is transitional to stage 4, which lasts for approximately 20 to 40 minutes. During deep sleep, the muscles of the body relax, and posture is adjusted intermittently. The

TABLE 13-1 Electroencephalogram, Eye and Motor Movements, Vital Functions, and Cerebral Activity During Sleep

Sleep Stage	Electroencephalogram	Eye Movements	Motor Movements	Heart Rate, Blood Pressure, Respirations	Cerebral Activity
Stage 1	Low voltage, mixed frequency	Slow, rolling movements	Moderate activity	Slows	Decreases
Stage 2	Low voltage, 12- to 14-Hz spindles	Slow, rolling movements	Moderate activity	Slows	Decreases
Stages 3 and 4 (deep sleep)	Delta (1–3 Hz) waves (slow-wave sleep)	Slow, rolling movements	Moderate activity	Slows	Decreases
REM sleep	Low voltage, mixed frequency	Clusters of rapid eye movements	Suppressed with loss of muscle tone	Increases, variable	Increases

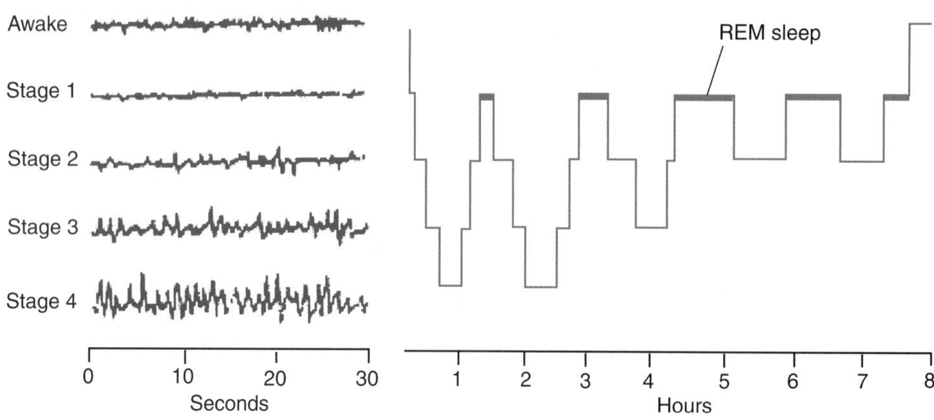

FIGURE 13-3 Brain waves during wakefulness and stages 1, 2, 3, and 4 sleep on the **left** and duration of wakefulness, REM, and non-REM sleep on the **right.** (Adapted from Kryger M. H., Roth T., Dement W. C. [Eds]. [1989]. *Principles and practices of sleep medicine.* Philadelphia: W. B. Saunders)

heart rate and blood pressure decrease, and gastrointestinal activity is slowed. An incrementally larger stimulus is required for arousal from slow-wave sleep.

REM Sleep. REM sleep is associated with rapid eye movements, loss of muscle movements, and vivid dreaming. It consists of low-voltage, high-frequency waves. External sensory input is inhibited, whereas internal sensory circuits such as those of the auditory and visual systems are aroused. During this time, the brain can replay previous memories but cannot acquire new sensory information (Fig. 13-4). At the same time, motor systems that control body movements are inhibited. There is a loss of muscle movement and muscle tone. The result is an extraordinary set of paradoxes, in which people see things in their dreams but cannot move. They imagine being engaged in activities such as running, flying, or dancing but are paralyzed.

There also are changes in autonomic nervous system–controlled functions during REM sleep: blood pressure, heart rate, and respirations increase and fluctuate, and

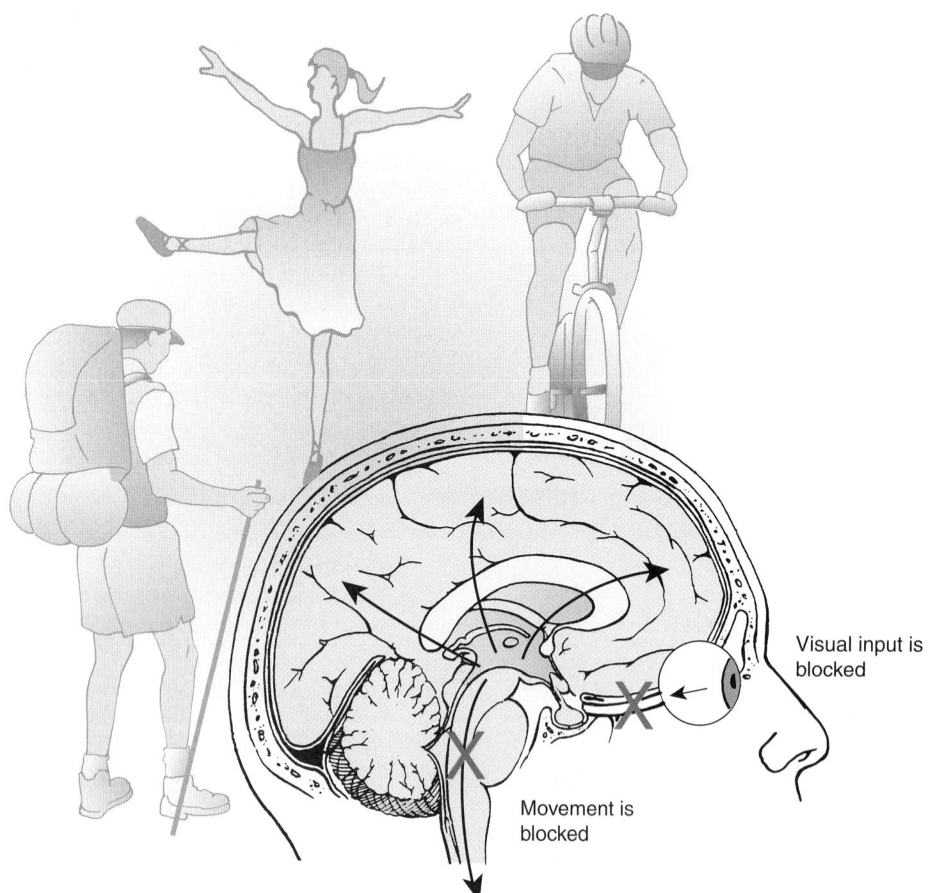

FIGURE 13-4 Dreaming during REM sleep when sensory and motor activity are blocked.

temperature regulation is lost. Cerebral blood flow and metabolic rate decrease. Sleep-related penile erection occurs during this stage of sleep.

It has been shown that adequate amounts of REM sleep are necessary for normal daytime functioning. Deprivation of REM sleep is associated with anxiety, irritability, inability to concentrate, and, if deprivation is severe enough, disturbed behavior.

Moving Between Sleep Stages. There is a rather predictable pattern of shifting between one non-REM stage and another during a typical night's sleep.[4] At sleep onset, there is a stepwise descent from lighter stage 1 sleep to deeper stage 4 sleep, followed by an abrupt ascent back toward stage 1. However, in place of stage 1, the first REM episode usually occurs. REM sleep is comparatively short (1 to 5 minutes) during the first sleep cycle, but gradually becomes longer across the night. Stages 3 and 4 occupy less time in the second and subsequent sleep cycles and disappear altogether in later cycles.

Breathing During Sleep

Breathing normally changes during sleep. Stages 1 and 2 of non-REM sleep are characterized by a cyclic waning and waxing of tidal volume and respiratory rate, which may include brief periods (5 to 15 seconds) of apnea. This pattern is called *periodic breathing*. Although the amount of periodic breathing that occurs during the first two stages of non-REM sleep differs among healthy persons, it is more common in persons older than 40 years of age.[5] After sleep has stabilized during stages 3 and 4 of non-REM sleep, breathing becomes more regular. Ventilation usually is 1 to 2 L/minute less than during quiet wakefulness; the PCO_2 levels are 2 to 8 mm Hg greater; the PO_2 levels are 5 to 10 mm Hg less; and the pH is 0.03 to 0.05 units less.[6] Involuntary respiratory control mechanisms, such as responses to hypercapnia, hypoxia, and lung inflation, are intact during non-REM sleep and critically important to maintaining ventilation.

During REM sleep, respirations become irregular, but not periodic, and may include short periods of apnea. Breathing during REM sleep has many features of the voluntary control that integrates breathing with acts such as walking, talking, and swallowing. However, their influence on breathing is diminished.

Dreaming

Dreams are recollections of mental activity that occurred during sleep. They occur during all stages of sleep but are more frequent during REM sleep. Approximately 80% of dreams occur during REM and sleep onset (stages 1 and 2).[7] Dreams that occur during REM sleep tend to be bizarre, with colorful, storybook-like detail.[1] Most nightmares occur during REM sleep. Dreams that occur during stages 1 and 2 of sleep tend to be shorter, have fewer associations, and lack the color and emotion of those that occur during REM sleep.

The purpose of dreaming is unclear. Evidence suggests that dreaming, like other physiologic functions, is important to learning and memory processing.[7] It has been suggested that dreaming may be the result of reprogramming of the central nervous system (*i.e.,* rearranging previous experiences) in preparation for the next day's conscious experiences.

CIRCADIAN RHYTHMS

Normally, sleep and wakefulness occur in a cyclic manner, integrated into the 24-hour light–dark solar day. The term *circadian,* from the Latin *circa* ("about") and *dies* ("day"), is used to describe these 24-hour diurnal rhythms. The function of the circadian time system is to provide a temporal organization for physiologic processes and behaviors as a means of promoting effective adaptation to the environment. At the behavioral level, this is expressed in regular cycles of sleep and waking and body functions such as temperature regulation and hormone secretion based on changes in the 24-hour light–dark solar day.

The daily rhythm of the sleep–wake cycle is part of a time-keeping system created by an internal pacemaker or clock.[8,9] Time isolation experiments, in which people were placed in an environment without time cues, showed that the cycle length of the human internal clock is in general from 23.5 to 26.5 hours.[8] Because the intrinsic cycle tends to be longer than 24 hours, a daily resetting of the circadian clock is necessary to synchronize with the environmental day. This process is called *entrainment* and normally is accomplished by exposure to the light–dark changes of the solar day.

The circadian clock appears to be controlled by a small group of hypothalamic cells, called the *suprachiasmatic nucleus* (SCN), located just above the optic chiasm and lateral to the third ventricle[8–10] (see Fig. 13-1). The SCN, which receives light–dark input from the retina, exhibits a rhythm of neuronal firing that is high during the day and low during the night. Although light serves as the primary stimulus for resetting the circadian clock, other stimuli, such as locomotion and activity, contribute to its regulation. The major projections from the SCN are to the anterior pituitary, with lesser ones to the basal forebrain and midline thalamus. Projections to the anterior pituitary provide for diurnal regulation of growth hormone and cortisol secretion; those to hypothalamic centers, for changes in metabolism and body temperature; and those to the brain stem reticular formation, for changes in autonomic nervous system–regulated functions such as heart rate and blood pressure (Fig. 13-5).

MELATONIN

Melatonin, a hormone produced by the pineal gland, is thought to help regulate the sleep–wake cycle and, possibly, circadian rhythm.[11–13] The pineal gland synthesizes and releases melatonin at night, a rhythm that is under the direct control of the SCN (see Fig. 13-1). Large numbers of melatonin receptors are present in the SCN, suggesting a feedback loop between the SCN and the pineal gland. Administration of melatonin produces phase-shifting changes in the circadian rhythm, similar to those caused by light. There has been recent interest in the use of melatonin in treatment of various sleep disorders, particularly those

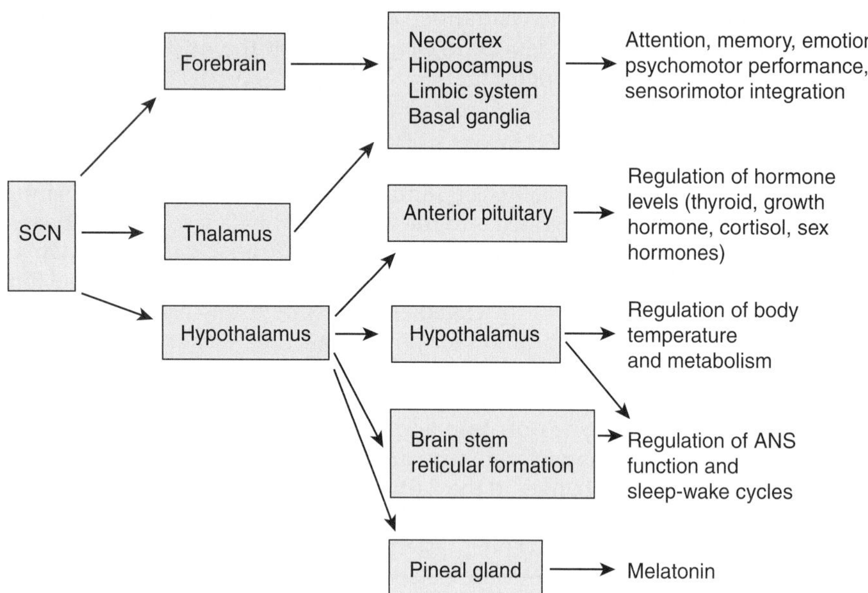

FIGURE 13-5 Projections from the suprachiasmatic nucleus (SCN) to the forebrain, thalamus, and hypothalamus.

related to a shift in the circadian rhythm. Although synthetic preparations are available without prescription in health food stores and pharmacies, their potency, purity, safety, and effectiveness cannot be ensured. There also is a lack of clinical trial evidence about appropriate dosage, adverse effects, drug interactions, and the effects of melatonin on various disease states.[12]

In summary, sleep is part of what is called the *sleep–wake cycle*. In contrast to wakefulness, which is a time of mental activity and energy expenditure, sleep is a period of inactivity and restoration of mental and physical function. There are two types of sleep: rapid eye movement (REM) and non-REM sleep. REM sleep is associated with rapid eye movements, loss of muscle movements, and vivid dreaming. External sensory input is inhibited, whereas internal sensory circuits such as those of the auditory and visual systems are aroused. Non-REM sleep is a quiet type of sleep characterized by a relatively inactive, yet fully regulating brain, and a fully movable body. It is divided into four stages that reflect an increasing depth of sleep. Stage 1 is a brief transitional stage that occurs at the onset of sleep, during which a person is easily aroused. Stage 2 is a deeper sleep, lasting approximately 10 to 25 minutes, during which EEG activity is interrupted by sleep spindles consisting of bursts of high-frequency waves. Stages 3 and 4 represent deep sleep, during which the muscles of the body relax, the heart rate and blood pressure decrease, and gastrointestinal activity is slowed.

Normally, sleep and wakefulness occur in a cyclic manner, called the *circadian rhythm,* that is integrated into the 24-hour light–dark solar day. The circadian clock is thought to be controlled by the SCN in the hypothalamus. The SCN, which receives light–dark input from the retina, exhibits a rhythm of neuronal firing that is high during the day and low during the night. Melatonin, a hormone produced by the pineal gland, is thought to help regulate the sleep–wake cycle.

Sleep Disorders

After you have completed this section of the chapter, you should be able to meet the following objectives:

- ✦ List the four categories of sleep disorders included in the International Classification of Sleep Disorders
- ✦ Describe the methods used in diagnosis of sleep disorders, including the sleep history, sleep diary, polysomnography, and wrist actigraphy
- ✦ Characterize the non–24-hour sleep–wake syndrome experienced by visually impaired individuals, sleep disorders associated with acute shifts in the sleep–wake cycle due to intercontinental travel and shift work, and advanced sleep phase and delayed sleep phase circadian rhythm sleep disorders
- ✦ Describe the causes, manifestations, diagnosis, and treatment of acute and chronic insomnia
- ✦ Differentiate periodic limb movement disorder and restless legs syndrome in terms of manifestations and treatment
- ✦ Explain the physiologic mechanisms, contributing factors, and manifestations of obstructive sleep apnea and describe the methods used in diagnosis and treatment of the disorder
- ✦ Define the term *parasomnias* and relate it to the manifestations of nightmare, sleep terrors, and sleep walking

In 1997, the American Sleep Disorders Association (ASDA) published a revision of the *International Classification of Sleep Disorders* (ICSD), which originally was developed in 1990.[14] The ICSD classifies sleep disorders into four categories: (1) dyssomnias, which are disorders of initiating and maintaining sleep and disorders of excessive sleepiness; (2) parasomnias, which are not responsible for disturbing the sleep–wake cycle but are undesirable phenomena that occur primarily during sleep; (3) sleep disorders associated with other medical or psychiatric disorders; and (4) proposed sleep disorders, such as pregnancy-induced sleep disruptions (Chart 13-1).

SLEEP DISORDERS

- Sleep disorders, which represent a disruption in the sleep–wake cycle, can be divided into four categories: dyssomnias; parasomnias; sleep disorders associated with mental, neurologic, or other medical conditions; and proposed sleep disorders.
- The dyssomnias, which are disorders that produce either excessive sleepiness or difficulty initiating or maintaining sleep, include circadian rhythm disorders, the various types of insomnia, narcolepsy, motor disorders that disrupt sleep, and sleep apnea.
- The parasomnias, which are undesirable physical phenomena that occur almost exclusively during sleep or are exaggerated by sleep, include nightmares, sleepwalking, and sleep terrors.

DIAGNOSTIC METHODS

The diagnosis of sleep disorders usually is based on adequate sleep history and physical examination. A sleep diary or sleep log often is helpful in describing sleep problems and arriving at a diagnosis.[15,16] In some cases, sleep laboratory studies may be needed to arrive at an accurate diagnosis.

Sleep History

A sleep history is fundamental to the process of identifying the nature of a sleep disorder.[16] The history should include the person's perception of the sleep problem, sleep schedule (*e.g.*, time of retiring and arising), problems with falling asleep and maintaining sleep, quality of sleep, daytime sleepiness and impact of the sleep disorder on daytime functioning, general emotional and physical problems, sleep hygiene (*e.g.*, eating and drinking before retiring), and sleep environment (*e.g.*, bed comfort, room temperature, noise, light). Because drugs such as over-the-counter medications, herbal preparations, and prescription medications can influence sleep, a careful drug history is important. It also is important to obtain information about the use of alcohol, caffeine, tobacco, and illegal substances.

Sleep Log/Diary

A sleep log/diary is a person's written account of his or her sleep experience. It usually is recommended that the diary be kept for at least 2 weeks. The diary should record the person's account of their bedtime, wakeup time, total sleep time, time of sleep onset, time needed to prepare for bed and to fall asleep, use of sleep medications, number of awakenings, subjective assessment of sleep quality, time out of bed in the morning, and daytime naps and symptoms. A number of sample forms are available to health care professionals for distribution to their clients.

CHART 13-1

International Classification of Sleep Disorders

Dyssomnias
Intrinsic sleep disorders
Extrinsic sleep disorders
Circadian rhythm sleep disorders

Parasomnias
Arousal disorders
Sleep–wake transition disorders
Parasomnias usually associated with REM sleep
Other parasomnias

Sleep Disorders Associated With Mental, Neurologic, or Other Medical Disorders
Associated with mental disorders
Associated with neurologic disorders
Associated with other medical disorders

Proposed Sleep Disorders

(From American Sleep Disorder Association. [1997]. *The international classification of sleep disorders: Revised.* Rochester, MN: Author.)

Polysomnography

A typical sleep study, or *polysomnography*, involves use of the EEG, electrooculogram (EOG), electromyogram (EMG), electrocardiogram (ECG), breathing movements, and pulse oximetry.[4] The EOG records eye movements. Because the eye is like a small battery with the retina negative to the cornea, an electrode placed on the skin near the eye records changes in voltage as the eye rotates in its socket. The EMG records the electrical activity from muscle movement. It is recorded from the surface of the skin. It typically is recorded from under the chin because muscles in this area of the body show very dramatic changes associated with the sleep cycle. The ECG is used to measure the heart rate and detect cardiac dysrhythmias. The pulse oximeter (ear or finger) measures arterial oxygen saturation.

The multiple sleep latency test (MSLT) is used to evaluate daytime sleepiness. This test usually is completed the morning after a diagnostic sleep study. An average adult requires 10 or more minutes to fall asleep. An MSLT result of less than 5 minutes is considered abnormal. Polysomnographic recordings are made during three to five naps spaced 2 hours apart during the day. Special attention is paid to how much time elapses from when the lights go out to the first evidence of sleep. This interval is called *sleep latency*.

Wrist actigraphy measures muscle motion and is used to obtain objective measurements of sleep duration and efficiency outside the sleep laboratory.[17] The actigraph is a compact device that is worn on the wrist and is used most often in conjunction with a sleep diary. Depending on the unit that is used, it can collect up to several weeks' worth of information.

DYSSOMNIAS

The dyssomnias are disorders that produce either excessive sleepiness or difficulty initiating or maintaining sleep. They represent the major cause of disturbed sleep or impaired wakefulness. They include the circadian rhythm disorders, the various types of insomnia, narcolepsy, motor disorders that disrupt sleep, and sleep apnea.

Circadian Rhythm Disorders

Sleep problems due to alterations in circadian rhythm tend to fall into three categories: non–24-hour sleep–wake syndrome (disorders of visual input and SCN function); acute shifts in the sleep–wake cycle (jet lag and shift work); and changes in sleep phase disorders (advanced and delayed sleep phase disorders).[9,18]

Non–24-Hour Sleep–Wake Syndrome. The non–24-hour sleep–wake syndrome consists of a lack of synchronization between the internal sleep–wake rhythm and the external 24-hour day. Most persons with the disorder are blind or have brain lesions that affect the SCN. Studies have shown that 70% or more of blind persons have chronic sleep–wake complaints.[18]

The non–24-hour syndrome often goes unrecognized. In sighted persons, a neurologic examination, including magnetic resonance imaging to detect possible SNC lesions, often is indicated. The disorder usually is unresponsive to sedative and stimulant medications. Some blind people seem to respond to a schedule of strict 24-hour cues.

Acute Shifts in the Sleep–Wake Cycle. The normal diurnal clock is set for a 24-hour day and resists changes in its pattern by as little as 1 to 2 hours per day. This means that there is a limited range of day lengths to which humans can synchronize. Imposed sleep–wake schedules of less than 23 hours or more than approximately 26 hours, such as those that occur with intercontinental jet travel and switches in the work shift, produce increasing sleep difficulties.

Time Zone Change (Jet Lag) Syndrome. Jet lag, a popular term for symptoms of sleep disturbances that occur with air travel that crosses several time zones, is caused by the sudden loss of synchrony between a traveler's intrinsic circadian clock and the local time of the flight's destination. The severity and duration of symptoms vary depending on the number of time zones crossed, direction of travel (eastward vs. westward), takeoff and arrival times, and age. Most people who cross three or four time zones experience some sleep disturbance, usually lasting 2 to 4 nights.

Circadian rhythms take longer to resynchronize to local time after eastward flights than westward flights, presumably because of the longer-than-24-hour intrinsic circadian period in most people.[18] Because the human time system seems to be less flexible in adjusting to sudden time changes after 35 years of age, age also affects adjustment to time zone changes.

Manifestations of jet lag syndrome include insomnia, daytime sleepiness, and decreased alertness and performance. Other symptoms, such as eye and nasal irritation, headache, abdominal distention, dependent edema, and intermittent dizziness, result from cabin conditions and usually remit sooner than symptoms of jet lag. Frequent travelers, such as airline personnel and business travelers, may develop chronic sleep disturbances accompanied by malaise, irritability, and performance impairment. Jet lag usually is milder in infrequent travelers but may reduce the enjoyment of a vacation or effectiveness of business transactions. Persons with preexisting sleep disorders such as sleep apnea often experience a worsening of symptoms with jet travel.

Management of jet lag focuses on efforts either to maintain the home time schedule or to adapt to the new time zone schedule. For persons crossing four or fewer time zones for only a few days, trying to maintain a schedule that is nearer to the home time schedule may be helpful, especially with westward travel. For longer stays, adapting to the new time schedule as quickly as possible is probably a better strategy. Use of artificial light may enhance the adjustment to the time shift. Getting outdoors and engaging in local social events enhances resynchronization by providing social cues and increasing exposure to the new light–dark environment.

Shift Work Sleep Disorder. The sleep disruption of night-shift work can be attributed to a clash between shift demands for wakefulness as part of the work environment and the sleep setting of the worker's intrinsic circadian clock. Shift work usually creates an environment in which some circadian clock-setting cues (*e.g.,* artificial light and rest–activity) are shifted, whereas others (*e.g.,* natural light–dark schedule, family and social routines) are not. This situation almost never allows for a complete shift of the circadian system. To complicate the situation, most night-shift workers revert to a nighttime sleeping schedule on days off. The effect of abruptly attempting to sleep at normal hours after working nights and sleeping days is biologically equivalent to a 6- to 10-hour eastbound jet flight.

Manifestations of sleep disorders of night-shift workers include shortened and interrupted daytime sleep after the night shift, somnolence and napping at work, sleepiness while commuting home, and insomnia on the nights off from work. Shift workers usually sleep less per scheduled sleep period than daytime workers and therefore are in a condition of chronic sleep deprivation.[18,19] Permanent night workers report averaging 6 hours of sleep on work days, approximately an hour less than evening and day workers.[18]

Arriving at a sleep schedule that is most supportive of the worker's intrinsic circadian rhythm often is difficult for night-shift workers. Beginning sleep at noon rather than earlier in the morning may produce a more normal sleep period in relation to shift onset but may exacerbate insomnia on nights off. Sleeping in absolute darkness during daytime by using blackout shades or eye masks may benefit the night worker's sleep.

Change in Sleep Phase Disorders. Change in sleep phase disorders include delayed sleep phase syndrome (DSPS) and advanced sleep phase syndrome (ASPS). The disorders may arise because of developmental changes in the sleep–wake cycle or because of poor sleep habits.

The main symptoms of *delayed sleep phase syndrome* are extreme difficulty falling asleep at a conventional hour of the night and awakening on time in the morning for school, work, or other responsibilities. Although most chronically sleep-deprived persons are sleepy in the late afternoon or evening, persons with DSPS report greatest alertness at these times of the day.[18]

The disorder is more common in adolescents and in persons older than 50 years of age.[18] In adults, there is evidence of association between some psychopathologic disorders and DSPS. Most cases are adolescents whose frustrated parents cannot wake them up in time for school and have trouble getting them to go to bed at night. Staying up late is fairly common among today's teenagers, who are strongly influenced by peer pressure, defiance of parental rules, and other pressures. It has been suggested that social pressure may contribute to, but may not be the only reason for, changes in a teenager's sleep pattern. Rather, puberty may be accompanied by a lengthening of the intrinsic circadian rhythm, with a corresponding increase in evening wakefulness, which in turn leads to later sleep onset and arising.

Diagnosis of DSPS usually can be made from information in a sleep history and confirmed with a 2-week sleep log or diary. The presence of concurrent psychopathologic disorders or chronic sedative or alcohol use should be considered.

There are no quick remedies for DSPS. In adolescents, commonsense remedies, such as setting earlier bedtimes and using multiple alarm clocks for waking up, have been used, but with minimal success. The use of bright light may be helpful in maintaining morning wakefulness. For some people, engagement in a regular morning exercise program, such as taking a daily 20- to 30-minute walk outdoors as soon as possible after arising each morning, may prove beneficial. In persons with psychopathologic disorders or sedative abuse, treatment of the underlying disorder is indicated.[18]

Advanced sleep phase syndrome basically is the mirror image of DSPS—early sleep onset and early arising. People with ASPS have trouble staying awake in the evening and have to curtail evening activities to avoid falling asleep. Unlike persons with depression, who awaken early with feelings of hopelessness and sadness, the person with ASPS obtains a normal amount of consolidated sleep and wakes up feeling refreshed.[18]

The pathophysiology of ASPS is presumed to be a partial defect in phase delay capability, with the possibility that persons with the disorder have an inherently fast circadian timing system. This disorder often is found in elderly people. Time isolation studies in middle-aged and older subjects suggest that the circadian timing system shortens with aging, usually beginning sometime in the sixth decade of life.[18]

Diagnosis of ASPS is based on history and information from a sleep log. Other pathologic causes, such as sleep apnea and depression, should be ruled out. The need for treatment depends on how disruptive a person perceives the problem to be. Current treatment methods, which focus largely on sleep schedule changes, are somewhat limited.

Insomnia

Insomnia probably is the most common of all sleep disorders. Every year, approximately 35% of the adult population has difficulty sleeping, and approximately half of these adults consider the problem serious.[15,20–22] Insomnia is more common in women and increases with age, psychological discomfort, and multiple health problems.

Insomnia represents a subjective problem of insufficient or nonrestorative sleep despite an adequate opportunity to sleep, thus differentiating insomnia from sleep deprivation. It includes difficulty falling asleep or maintaining sleep, waking up too early, or nonrefreshing sleep. Insomnia also involves daytime consequences such as tiredness, lack of energy, difficulty concentrating, and irritability.[15] Primary insomnia is sleep difficulty in which other causes of sleep disruption have been ruled out or treated.

Acute Insomnia. Acute insomnia is characterized by periods of sleep difficulty lasting between one night and a few weeks.[15] The primary consequences of acute insomnia are sleepiness, negative mood, and impairment of performance. The degree of impairment is related to the amount of sleep lost.

Acute insomnia often is caused by emotional and physical discomfort. Some common examples include an unfamiliar or nonconducive sleep environment, stress-related events, and sleep schedule problems. Probably one of the most common causes of acute insomnia is an unfamiliar sleep environment, such as that encountered when traveling. Factors that contribute to a nonconducive sleep environment include excessive noise, extremes of temperature, an uncomfortable sleep surface, or being forced to sleep in an uncomfortable position. Hospital intensive care units with their noise, intensive lighting, and frequent interruptions for monitoring vital signs and providing treatments are excellent examples of nonconducive sleep environments. Common stress-related causes of insomnia are expected occurrences such as being on call or stressful life events. Sleep schedule changes include jet lag and sleep disruption due to shift work.

Chronic Insomnia. Chronic insomnia refers to sleep difficulty of at least three nights per week for at least 1 month.[15] Persons with chronic insomnia frequently complain of fatigue; mood changes, such as irritability and depression; difficulty concentrating; and impaired performance.

Chronic insomnia often is related to medical or psychiatric disorders. Factors such as pain, immobility, and hormonal changes associated with pregnancy or menopause also can cause insomnia. Interrupted sleep can accompany other sleep disorders such as restless legs syndrome and sleep apnea. Many health problems worsen during the night. Heart failure, respiratory disease, and gastroesophageal reflux can cause frequent awakening during the night. Mood and anxiety disorders are the most frequent cause of insomnia in persons with psychiatric diagnoses.

A number of drugs can lead to poor-quality sleep. Drugs commonly related to insomnia are caffeine, nicotine, stimulating antidepressants, alcohol, and recreational drugs.[15,20,21] Approximately 10% to 15% of persons with insomnia have problems with chronic substance abuse, including alcohol.[21] Although alcohol initially may induce sleep, it often causes disrupted and fragmented sleep. Sleep also is disrupted in persons undergoing alcohol or sleep medication withdrawal.

Diagnosis and Treatment. The diagnosis of insomnia is aided by a sleep history. Questions should address both sleep and daytime functioning. If the person has a bed partner, it is important to ask if the person snores, has unusual movement during sleep, or is excessively drowsy during the day.[23] Because sleep needs vary from person to person, a 1- to 2-week sleep diary can be useful in diagnosing the sleep problem and in serving as a baseline for treatment effects.[15,16,20,23] Other factors that need to be explored are the use of drugs such as caffeine, tobacco, and alcohol as well as prescription and over-the-counter drugs that affect the sleep–wake cycle. Identification of physical and psychological factors that interfere with sleep also is important.

Treatment of insomnia includes education and counseling regarding better sleep habits (sleep hygiene), behavioral therapy aimed at changing maladaptive sleep habits, and the judicious use of pharmacologic interventions. The cause and duration of insomnia are particularly important in deciding on a treatment strategy. With transient insomnia, treatment stresses the development of good sleep hygiene and judicious short-term use of sedatives or hypnotics. Long-term and chronic insomnia require careful assessment to determine the cause of the disorder. Depending on the findings, treatment options include behavioral strategies such as relaxation therapy, sleep restriction therapy, stimulus control therapy, and cognitive therapy. Sedatives and hypnotics, which tend to become less effective with time and may cause dependence, are used with caution.

Sleep hygiene refers to a set of rules and information about personal and environmental activities that affect sleep.[15,16,20,21] These rules include establishing a regular wakeup time to help set the circadian clock and regularity of sleep onset; maintaining a practice of sleeping only as long as needed to feel refreshed; providing a quiet sleep environment that is neither too hot nor too cold; and avoiding the use of alcohol and caffeine (coffee, colas, tea, chocolate) before retiring for sleep. It is important that the bed and bedroom be identified with sleep and not with reading, watching television, or working. Persons who cannot fall asleep should be instructed to turn on the light and do something else outside the bed, preferably in another room.

Behavioral therapies include relaxation therapy, sleep restriction therapy, stimulus control therapy, and cognitive therapy.[16] Relaxation therapy is based on the premise that persons with insomnia tend to display high levels of physiologic, cognitive, and emotional arousal during both the day and the night.[15] Sleep restriction therapy consists of curtailing the amount of time spent in bed in an effort to increase the sleep efficiency (time asleep/time in bed). People with insomnia often increase their time in bed in the misguided belief that it will provide more opportunity to sleep. Stimulus control therapy focuses on reassociating the bed and bedroom with sleep rather than sleeplessness. Cognitive therapy involves the identification of dysfunctional beliefs and attitudes about sleep and replacing them with more adaptive substitutes.

Pharmacologic treatment usually is reserved for short-term management of insomnia—either as the sole treatment or as adjunctive therapy until the underlying problem can be addressed. The most common type of agents used to promote sleep are the benzodiazepine receptor agonists and a new class of nonbenzodiazepine hypnotics (zolpidem and zaleplon).[15,20,21,23] The nonbenzodiazepines are often preferred because of their rapid onset and shorter duration of action. Their use is generally limited to 7 to 10 days. Sedating antidepressants also may be prescribed, particularly when insomnia is due to depression. Antihistamines have sedative effects and may be used to induce sleep. The most commonly used agents are diphenhydramine and doxylamine. Most over-the-counter sleep medications include an antihistamine. Adverse effects of antihistamines include daytime sleepiness, cognitive impairments, and anticholinergic effects. Falls and fractures are more frequent in persons using hypnotic or other psychotherapeutic agents. The usefulness of melatonin in treating insomnia remains to be established.

Narcolepsy

Narcolepsy is a disorder of daytime sleep attacks, cataplexy (brief periods of muscle weakness), hypnagogic hallucinations occurring at the onset of sleep, and sleep paralysis.[24–26] Although the disorder is not progressive, it can be disabling and difficult to treat. Sixty to 80% of persons with narcolepsy have fallen asleep while driving, at work, or both.[24]

Daytime sleepiness is the most common initial symptom of narcolepsy. Sleepiness is most apparent in boring, sedentary situations and often is relieved by movement. Although the sleepiness that occurs with narcolepsy is similar to that experienced after sleep deprivation, it is different in that no amount of nighttime sleep produces full alertness. The periods of daytime sleep usually are brief, lasting 30 minutes or less, and often are accompanied by brief interruption of speech or irrelevant words, lapses in memory, and nonsensical activities. Cataplexy is characterized by brief periods of muscle weakness brought about by emotional reactions such as laughter, anger, or fear.

Some persons with narcolepsy have brief, intense, often frightening, dreamlike hallucinations (hypnagogic hallucinations) while dozing or falling asleep and brief periods of sleep paralysis.

The occurrence of REM sleep at sleep onset or within 10 to 15 minutes of sleep onset is the most characteristic and striking manifestation of the disorder. Periods of REM onset sleep are thought to indicate impaired sleep–wake regulation rather than increased need for REM sleep. The sleep paralysis, dreamlike hallucinations, and loss of muscle tone that occur during cataplexy are similar to behaviors that occur during REM sleep.

Narcolepsy affects men more often than women.[25] Onset is rare before 5 or after 50 years of age. The onset usually occurs during adolescence or during the early twenties. There is a second smaller peak of onset around 35 years of age.[24] The onset of symptoms often is insidious, with excessive daytime sleepiness preceding the onset of cataplexy. Sometimes it may have an abrupt onset attributed to head trauma, an infection, drug abuse, or pregnancy. Whether these events are causal or coincidental is unknown.

Although the cause of narcolepsy is unknown, there are indications that the disorder may have a genetic component. Persons with narcolepsy have been shown to have an unusually high rate of a specific human leukocyte antigen (HLA) subtype (HLA DQB1-0602).[25] Of persons with severe cataplexy, more than 85% to 95% have this HLA subtype. Most diseases associated with a specific HLA subtype have an autoimmune component. However, no autoimmune markers have been found to date. Recent research has suggested a link between a newly identified group of neurotransmitters called *hypocretins* and narcolepsy. The hypocretins (hypocretin 1 and hypocretin 2) are secreted by cells in the area of the hypothalamus that is related to wakefulness.[26] A mutation in the hypocretin 2 receptor was shown to cause canine narcolepsy.[27] Although the role of the hypocretin transmitter system in human narcolepsy is unclear, a small preliminary study has shown a lack of hypocretin 1 in the cerebrospinal fluid of 7 of 9 patients with the disorder.[28] Although these findings are preliminary, they suggest new avenues for research into the cause of narcolepsy.

Sleep laboratory studies most often are required for accurate diagnosis of narcolepsy. Both daytime and nighttime studies typically are done. Nighttime studies usually are performed after the person has been on a regular sleep schedule for 10 days or more to determine the presence and severity of sleep apnea, limb movement disorders, and nocturnal sleep disturbance. A daytime MSLT usually is done the next day. People with narcolepsy are observed to have a short period of sleep latency (2 to 4 minutes) during daytime studies, along with a rapid onset of REM sleep (usually within 10 minutes). A mean sleep latency of less than 5 minutes and two or more periods of sleep-onset REM during the repeated nap opportunities is considered diagnostic of narcolepsy.[24]

The treatment of narcolepsy focuses on the use of stimulant medications such as mazindol, methylphenidate, methamphetamine, and modafinil to counteract daytime sleepiness. Only modafinil, a nonamphetamine stimulant, has been studied and approved for use in treatment of narcolepsy. The mechanism of action of modafinil is unknown, although animal studies indicate the drug acts in areas of the brain involved in the sleep–wake cycle. Tricyclic antidepressants may be used to treat the cataleptic attacks. Nonpharmacologic treatment includes prevention of sleep deprivation, regular sleep and wake times, work in a stimulating environment, and avoidance of shift work. Scheduled short naps may be effective in reducing daytime sleepiness.

Motor Disorders of Sleep

A variety of spontaneous movements can occur during sleep. Some occur during normal sleep in all persons at some time. Others are not part of normal sleep patterns and can be disruptive of sleep. Among the abnormal motor disorders are periodic limb movement disorder (PLMD) and restless legs syndrome (RLS).

Limb movements can demonstrate characteristic rates and patterns during certain stages of sleep. Motoneuron depression is minimal during non-REM sleep and maximal during REM sleep. Many movement disorders occur during stage 2 non-REM sleep.

Periodic Limb Movement Disorder. Periodic limb movement disorder is characterized by episodes of repetitive movement of the large toe with flexion of the ankle, knee, and hip during sleep.[29] Both lower extremities are usually affected in an asymmetric manner. The condition occurs most frequently during light (stages 1 and 2 non-REM) sleep compared with deep (stages 3 and 4 non-REM) sleep and REM sleep. The disorder frequently accompanies RLS.

Periodic limb movement disorder, which occurs equally in men and women, is found in up to 11% of the population.[29] It rarely is diagnosed before 30 years of age and the prevalence increases with age. It may occur in as many as 20% of persons older than 65 years of age. The cause of PLMD is largely unknown. It has been observed that the movements mimic the Babinski reflex, suggesting removal of an excitatory influence over a subcortical inhibitory system allowing for facilitation of abnormal movements during sleep.[29] Diagnosis of PLMD is facilitated with use of EMG recordings from both tibialis anterior muscles. Four or more consecutive muscle contractions, each lasting 5 to 90 seconds (typically 20 to 40 seconds) and recurring at intervals of 5 to 90 seconds, is indicative of PLMD.

Restless Legs Syndrome. Restless legs syndrome is a neurologic disorder characterized by an irresistible urge to move the legs, usually because of a "creeping," "crawling," or uncomfortable sensation.[29–32] It usually is worse during periods of inactivity and often interferes with sleep. Occasionally, the condition occurs during the day after long periods of sitting. The prevalence of the condition peaks in middle age and reportedly occurs in 2% to 15% of the elderly population.[31] Although the prevalence increases with age, it has a variable age of onset and can occur in children.

The disorder, which is thought to have its origin in the central nervous system, can occur as a primary or secondary disorder. There is a high familial incidence of primary RLS, suggesting a genetic disorder. Secondary causes of RLS include iron deficiency, neurologic disorders such as spinal cord and peripheral nerve lesions, pregnancy, uremia, and medications. Although the neurologic basis of RLS has not been determined, it has been suggested that the disorder may involve disruption of descending inhibitory input to brain stem and spinal cord circuits. Based on classes of medications proved to be effective in treating the disorder, there is evidence for involvement of the dopaminergic, adrenergic, and opioid systems in the pathogenesis of the disorder.

Diagnosis of RLS is based on a history of (1) a compelling urge to move the legs, usually associated with paresthesias; (2) motor restlessness, as seen by activities such as pacing, tossing and turning in bed, or rubbing the legs; (3) symptoms that become worse at rest and are relieved by activity; and (4) symptoms that are worse in the evening or at night.[31] Laboratory tests to determine secondary causes of RLS usually are done. Because RLS may be a symptom of iron deficiency, serum ferritin and iron saturation should be assessed. This is important because iron deficiency is frequently present in the absence of anemia.[30] Sleep studies usually are not required because the condition can be diagnosed on the basis of history and clinical findings.

Treatment of RLS varies depending on the severity of symptoms. Dopaminergic agents are the first-line drugs for most persons with RLS. These include precursors of dopamine (carbidopa-levodopa), dopamine agonists (pergolide, pramipexole, ropinirole), and facilitating agents (selegiline). Benzodiazepines (*e.g.,* clonazepam, temazepam), opioids (*e.g.,* codeine, hydrocodone), and antiseizure agents (carbamazepine, gabapentin) are alternative agents. Although pharmacologic treatment is helpful for many persons with RLS, those with mild symptoms may not require medications. For many persons, deliberate manipulation of the muscles through ambulation, kicking movements, stretching, or massage may provide relief.[32] Good sleep habits are important. A high prevalence of iron deficiency has been found among persons with RLS, and treatment of the deficiency has been reported to improve or resolve symptoms.[30]

Obstructive Sleep Apnea

Sleep apnea is a serious, potentially life-threatening disorder characterized by brief periods of apnea or breathing cessation during sleep. There are two types of sleep apnea: obstructive and central. Obstructive apnea, which is caused by upper airway obstruction and characterized by snoring, disrupted sleep, and excessive daytime sleepiness, is the much more common type.[33] Central sleep apnea, which is caused by disorders affecting the respiratory center in the brain, is rare.

Apnea is defined as cessation of airflow through the nose and mouth for 10 seconds or longer. The apneic periods typically last for 15 to 120 seconds, and some persons may have as many as 500 apneic periods per night. An accompanying reduction in tidal volume due to a decrease in the depth and rate of respiration (called *hypopnea*) is associated with a decrease in arterial oxygen saturation. The average number of apnea-hypopnea periods per hour is called the *apnea-hypopnea index* (AHI).[34] An adult may experience up to five events an hour without symptoms. As the AHI increases, so does the severity of symptoms. An AHI of five or greater in combination with reports of excessive daytime sleepiness is indicative of sleep apnea.[35]

All skeletal muscles except the diaphragm undergo a decrease in tone during sleep. This loss of muscle tone is most pronounced during REM sleep. The loss of muscle tone in the upper airways predisposes to airway obstruction as the negative airway pressure produced by contraction of the diaphragm brings the vocal cords together, collapses the pharyngeal wall, and sucks the tongue back into the throat[36] (Fig. 13-6). Airway collapse is accentuated in persons with conditions that cause narrowing of the upper airway or weakness of the throat muscles.

Conditions that predispose to sleep apnea include male sex, increasing age, and obesity. Alcohol and other drugs that depress the central nervous system tend to increase the severity of obstructive episodes. It has been estimated that sleep apnea affects up to 4% of middle-aged men and 2% of middle-aged women.[5] Most persons who develop sleep apnea are obese. Large neck girth in both male and female snorers is highly predictive of sleep apnea.

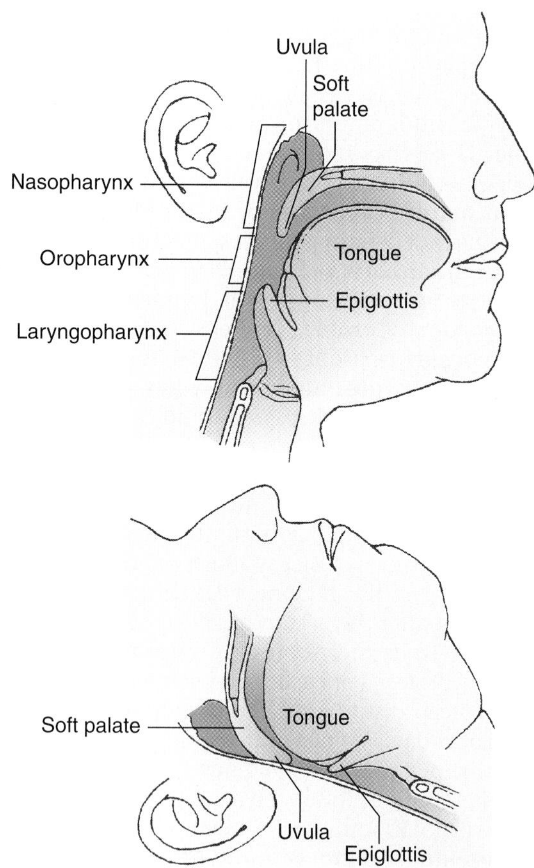

FIGURE 13-6 Principal mechanism of obstructive sleep apnea. When the person is awake (**top**), the airway is kept open by the activity of the pharyngeal musculature. During sleep (**bottom**), this activity is decreased, causing airway obstruction, most commonly in the area behind the uvula, soft palate, and posterior tongue.

Men with a neck circumference greater than 17 inches and women with a neck circumference greater than 16 inches are at higher risk for sleep apnea.[34] The pickwickian syndrome, named after the fat boy in Charles Dickens' *The Posthumous Papers of the Pickwick Club,* published in 1837, is characterized by obesity, hypersomnolence, periodic breathing, hypoxemia, and right-sided heart failure.[37]

Obstructive sleep apnea is characterized by loud snoring interrupted by periods of silence. Abnormal gross motor movements during sleep are common. In many cases, the snoring precedes by many years the onset of other signs of sleep apnea. Persons with sleep apnea often complain of persistent daytime sleepiness, morning headache, memory and judgment problems, irritability, difficulty concentrating, and depression. They also are more likely to fall asleep at inappropriate times and have higher rates of automobile and work-related accidents. Men may complain of impotence. In children, a decline in school performance may be the only indication of the problem.

Sleep apnea also is associated with sleep-related cardiac dysrhythmias and hypertension. Usually, bradycardia is observed, but ventricular tachycardia may occur in situations of severe hypoxemia. Frequent apneic periods may result in increased systemic and pulmonary blood pressures. The morning blood pressure has been shown to increase almost linearly with increasing apnea episodes. In severe cases, pulmonary hypertension, polycythemia, and cor pulmonale may develop. The signs and symptoms of sleep apnea are summarized in Chart 13-2.

Diagnosis and Treatment. Sleep apnea usually is suspected from a history of snoring, disturbed sleep, and daytime sleepiness. A definitive diagnosis is accomplished with sleep studies done in a sleep laboratory using polysomnography.[5,6,38] Currently, this procedure requires an overnight stay in a sleep laboratory. The procedure consists of EEG and EOG to determine the sleep stages; monitoring of the airflow; an ECG to detect arrhythmias; methods to measure ventilatory effort; and pulse oximetry to detect changes in oxygen saturation. An MSLT may be done to rule out narcolepsy in persons who exhibit excessive daytime sleepiness.

CHART 13-2

Signs and Symptoms of Sleep Apnea

- Noisy snoring
- Insomnia
- Abnormal movements during sleep
- Morning headaches
- Excessive daytime sleepiness
- Cognitive and personality changes
- Sexual impotence
- Systemic hypertension
- Pulmonary hypertension, cor pulmonale
- Polycythemia

Home evaluation using pulse oximetry and portable monitors may be used to screen for sleep apnea. This method is less expensive than laboratory sleep tests but often is less accurate.[34] Home evaluation is most useful in persons with severe sleep apnea, in whom the results clearly are positive.

The treatment of sleep apnea is determined by the severity of the condition. Behavioral measures may be the only treatment needed for persons with mild sleep apnea. These include weight loss, eliminating evening alcohol and sedatives, and proper bed positioning. Weight loss often is beneficial for persons with obstructive apnea. In many instances, the disordered breathing events are confined to the supine sleeping position, so that training the person to sleep in the lateral position may help to alleviate the problem.

Oral or dental appliances that displace the tongue forward and move the mandible to a more anterior and forward position may be an option for persons with mild to moderate sleep apnea. Persons who snore but do not have sleep apnea also may use these devices. They should be fitted by a dentist or orthodontist experienced in their use. Side effects of the devices include excessive salivation and temporomandibular joint discomfort.

The application of nasal continuous positive airway pressure (NCPAP) at night has proved helpful in treating obstructive sleep apnea. This method uses an occlusive nasal mask or a device that fits into the nares, an expiratory valve and tubing, and a blower system to generate positive pressure. The main difficulty with NCPAP is that many persons find it unacceptable. Common complaints include dryness of the mouth, claustrophobia, and noise.

Several surgical procedures have been used to correct airway obstruction, including nasal septoplasty (*i.e.,* repair of the nasal septum) and uvulopalatopharyngoplasty (*i.e.,* excision of excess soft tissue on the palate, uvula, and posterior pharyngeal wall). Both of these procedures have met with limited success. Severe cases of sleep apnea may require a tracheostomy (*i.e.,* surgical placement of a tube into the trachea for the purpose of maintaining an open airway). The tracheostomy tube remains occluded during the day and is opened during the night.

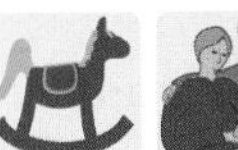
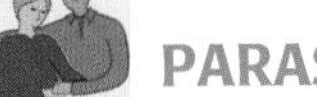

PARASOMNIAS

The parasomnias are undesirable physical phenomena that occur almost exclusively during sleep or are exaggerated by sleep.[39] They include nightmares, sleepwalking (somnambulism) and sleep terrors, teeth grinding, and bed-wetting (enuresis). Sleepwalking, sleep terrors, and bed-wetting often are seen in children and may be considered normal to some degree at a certain age. They are less common in adults and may be indicative of other pathologies. For example, sleepwalking and sleep terrors may occur in persons with poorly controlled cardiac insufficiency after myocardial infarction. In rare cases, sleepwalking and sleep terrors may be the first sign of a slowly evolving brain tumor. Finally, sleepwalking and sleep terrors may be triggered by disorders interacting with the sleep–wake cycle. Particularly in the elderly, health problems such as a febrile illness may enhance non-REM sleep nightmares, sleep terrors, and sleepwalking.

Nightmares

Nightmares are vivid and terrifying nocturnal episodes in which the dreamer is abruptly awakened from sleep. Usually, there is difficulty returning to sleep. Nightmares affect 20% to 39% of children between 5 and 12 years of age and 5% to 8% of adults.[40] Most nightmares occur during REM sleep. Most REM-altering disorders and medications that affect REM sleep affect dreaming.

Nightmares are a defining symptom of posttraumatic stress disorder (PTSD).[7] These nightmares occur after intensely frightening or highly emotional experiences and are associated with disturbed sleep and daytime hyperarousability. Persons with PTSD report awakening from dreams that involve reliving the trauma. The frequency of PTSD nightmares increases with the severity of trauma, and they can persist for long periods after the traumatic experience. It has been reported that 30% of veterans of the Vietnam War are affected by PTSD.[7] Among the civilian population, PTSD affects approximately 25% of persons who have experienced severe emotional and physical trauma or have had a severe medical illness.

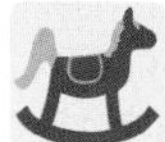
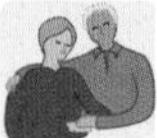

Sleepwalking and Sleep Terrors

Sleepwalking and sleep terrors usually occur during stages 3 and 4 of non-REM sleep. Because stages 3 and 4 are more prolonged during the first third of the night, sleepwalking and sleep terrors usually occur during this time. Sleep terrors are characterized by sudden, loud, terrified screaming and prominent autonomic nervous system activation (tachycardia, tachypnea, diaphoresis, and mydriasis). Sleepwalking is characterized by complex automatic behaviors, such as aimless wandering, furniture rearranging, urinating in closets, and going outdoors. During a typical episode, the sleepwalker appears dazed and relatively unresponsive to the communication efforts of others. On awakening, there may be a brief period of confusion or disorientation. The sleepwalker usually has no memory or only a vague awareness of what has happened.

Sleep terrors are more common in children and are discussed later in the chapter. In children, sleepwalking usually is a benign and self-limited disorder. In adults, sleepwalking occurs almost three times more often per year and persists for a longer period than in children. It often is associated with stress or major life events.[40] New-onset sleepwalking in older adults is uncommon and usually is a manifestation of another disorder such as delirium, drug toxicity, or seizure disorders.[40] Although rare, sleepwalking can occur during complex partial seizures.

Diagnosis and treatment of sleepwalking and sleep terrors depend on age. Because most children eventually outgrow the disorders, parents may need simply to be reassured and instructed in safety measures. Insufficient sleep may precipitate episodes of sleepwalking, so parents should make certain that the child goes to bed on time and gets enough sleep. In adults, a thorough medical, psychiatric, and sleep history should be done to eliminate other causes of the disorder. Because sleepwalking can be dangerous, it is important that the environment be safe. Dangerous objects should be removed, and bolts should be placed on doors and windows. No attempt should be made to interrupt the sleepwalking event because such efforts may be frightening.

Pharmacologic treatment includes the selective use of the benzodiazepines (particularly diazepam and clonazepam) or the tricyclic antidepressant imipramine.[40] In elderly persons, treatment focuses on reversing the underlying causes of delirium. Because medications are a frequent cause of delirium in the elderly, a complete drug history should be done with the intent of eliminating medications that might be causing the disorder.

In summary, the ICSD classifies sleep disorders into four categories: (1) dyssomnias, which are disorders of initiating and maintaining sleep and disorders of excessive sleepiness; (2) parasomnias, which are not responsible for disturbing the sleep–wake cycle but are undesirable phenomena that occur primarily during sleep; (3) sleep disorders associated with other medical and psychiatric disorders; and (4) proposed sleep disorders such as pregnancy-induced sleep disruptions.

The dyssomnias include circadian rhythm sleep disorders, insomnia, narcolepsy, disorders of leg movement, and sleep apnea. Sleep problems due to alterations in circadian rhythm tend to fall into three categories: non–24-hour sleep–wake syndrome (disorders of visual input and SCN function); acute shifts in the sleep–wake cycle (jet lag and shift work); and changes in sleep phase disorders (advanced and delayed sleep phase disorders). Insomnia represents a subjective problem of insufficient or nonrestorative sleep despite an adequate opportunity to sleep. It includes transient and chronic problems in falling asleep and maintaining sleep, waking up too early, or nonrefreshing sleep. Narcolepsy is a disorder of daytime sleep attacks, cataplexy, hallucinations occurring at the onset of sleep, and sleep paralysis. Among the abnormal motor disorders that occur during sleep are PLMD and RLS. PLMD is characterized by episodes of repetitive movement of the large toe with flexion of the ankle, knee, and hip during sleep, usually involving both legs. RLS is a neurologic disorder characterized by an irresistible urge to move the legs, usually owing to a "creeping," "crawling," or uncomfortable sensation. It usually is worse during periods of inactivity and often interferes with sleep. Obstructive sleep apnea is a serious, potentially life-threatening disorder characterized by brief periods of apnea or breathing cessation during sleep, loud snoring interrupted by periods of silence, and abnormal gross motor movements. It is accompanied by complaints of persistent daytime sleepiness, morning headache, memory and judgment problems, irritability, difficulty concentrating, and depression. Sleep apnea also is associated with sleep-related cardiac dysrhythmias and hypertension.

The parasomnias are undesirable physical phenomena that occur almost exclusively during sleep or are exaggerated by sleep. They include nightmares, sleepwalking and sleep terrors, teeth grinding, and bed-wetting (enuresis).

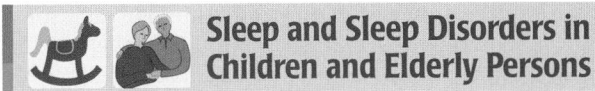

Sleep and Sleep Disorders in Children and Elderly Persons

After you have completed this section of the chapter, you should be able to meet the following objectives:

- Characterize normal sleep patterns of the infant and small child and relate to the development of sleep disorders
- Describe the normal changes in sleep stages that occur with aging and relate to sleep problems in the elderly

It has been said that "sleep is of the brain, by the brain, and for the brain."[1] Thus, sleep changes as the brain develops in the fetus and neonate, matures during adolescence and early adulthood, and begins to decline with aging.

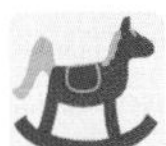

SLEEP DISORDERS IN CHILDREN

A child's circadian rhythms and sleep patterns are established early in life. There is evidence that many of the sleep patterns in the newborn are present at birth.[1] The first behavioral manifestations of sleep patterns occur between 28 to 30 weeks of gestation, when movement of the fetus is interrupted by periods of quiet. At 32 weeks, periods of quiescence begin to occur at regular intervals, suggesting the beginnings of a sleep–wake cycle.

An infant born at full term sleeps approximately 16 to 17 hours a day, half of which is spent in REM sleep. The other half of the infant's sleep resembles adult non-REM sleep.[1,41] Not only does the infant spend more time in REM sleep than adults, but also the behavioral manifestations of REM sleep are more exaggerated. This probably is because inhibitory systems in the infant's brain are relatively immature. Thus, an infant's sleep behavior includes a wide range of physical behaviors such as changes in facial expression, cooing sounds, and movement and stretching of the extremities.

Although infants have some capacity to concentrate sleep in one part of the day, this capacity must be developed in the weeks after birth. As development progresses, the infant is able to concentrate sleep during the night and remain awake for longer periods during the day. By 5 to 6 months, the infant may sleep through the night and may nap at predictable times during the day. As the cyclic structure of the sleep–wake cycle progresses, the amount of time spent in REM sleep decreases. By the time the child is 8 months of age, the duration of sleep has decreased to approximately 13 hours, and REM sleep occupies only approximately one third of that time. At 12 to 15 years of age, sleep has decreased to approximately 8 hours, with one fourth being spent in REM sleep.

Although complaints of sleep are common among adults, children usually do not complain about sleep problems, although their parents might. The usual concerns of parents include irregular sleep habits, insufficient or too much sleep, nightmares, sleep terrors, sleepwalking, and bed-wetting. Complaints of excessive daytime sleepiness or sleep attacks not accounted for by an inadequate amount of sleep may be due to a more serious health or sleep problem (*e.g.*, narcolepsy), in which case a careful sleep history, physical examination, and other diagnostic tests may be needed. Three of the more common sleep problems of children are discussed in this section of the chapter: sleep terrors, confusional arousals, and sleepwalking.

Sleep Terrors

Sleep terrors are marked by repeated episodes of awakening from sleep. They usually occur during the first half of sleep in the first interval of non-REM sleep.[41,42] The age of onset usually is between 4 and 12 years. The course is variable, usually occurring at intervals of days or weeks. The disorder gradually resolves in children and usually disappears during adolescence.

In a typical episode, the child sits up abruptly in bed, appears frightened, and demonstrates signs of extreme anxiety, including dilated pupils, excessive perspiration, rapid breathing, and tachycardia. Until the agitation and confusion subside, efforts to comfort or help the child are futile. There usually is no memory of the episode. Occasionally, the child recounts a sense of terror on being aroused during a night terror, but there is only fragmentary recall of dreamlike images. Treatment consists primarily of educating and reassuring the family. The child should be assisted in settling down without awakening. The child must be protected if he or she gets up and walks about during the episodes.

Confusional Arousals

Confusional arousals are common in infants and toddlers.[43] They usually occur during the first third of the night when the brain is partially asleep while remaining partially awake. During these events, children present with marked confusion, slow and inappropriate responses to questions, and nonpurposeful activities. They do express fear, terror, or panic. Children spontaneously return to sleep and have no recollection of the event in the morning. Recovery from sleep deprivation tends to increase the incidence of confusional arousals.

Sleepwalking

Sleepwalking involves repeated episodes of complex motor movements that lead to leaving the bed and walking without the child being conscious of the episode or remembering that it occurred. As with sleep terrors, it normally occurs in non-REM sleep stages 3 and 4 during the first half of the sleep period.

A sleepwalking episode typically lasts for a few minutes to half an hour, during which time the child sits up; makes purposeful movements such as picking at the bed coverings; then proceeds to semipurposeful movements such as getting out of bed, walking around, opening doors, dressing, or going to the bathroom. Often they end up in the parent's bedroom. Commonly, they are unresponsive to the efforts of others to communicate with them. Confusion and disorientation are typical of the events, and on awakening, there is no memory of the event. There may be manifestations of extreme autonomic nervous system activity such as tachycardia, rapid breathing, perspiration, and urination.

Approximately 10% to 15% of children have had isolated sleepwalking events.[40] It occurs more commonly in boys than in girls and is more frequent in children in whom there is a family history of sleepwalking. The onset usually is between 4 and 8 years of age, and it lasts several years. Usually symptoms resolve by the end of the teens or in the early 20s. The primary concern is injury during an episode. Children may bump into things, fall down stairs, or even leave their home during an episode. Therefore, gates should be placed across stairs and windows, and doors should be locked so the child cannot leave the house.

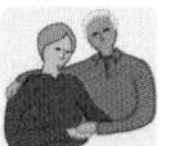

SLEEP DISORDERS IN ELDERLY PERSONS

Complaints of difficulty sleeping increase with aging. In a National Institute of Aging Study of more than 9000 persons aged 65 years and older, more than one half of the men and women reported at least one chronic sleep complaint.[44] The consequences of chronic sleep problems in elderly persons can be considerable. Left uncorrected, a sleep disorder affects the quality of life. Loss of sleep and use of sedating medications may lead to falls and accidents. Sleep-related disorders of breathing may have serious cardiovascular, pulmonary, and central nervous system effects.

A number of changes occur in the sleep–wake cycle as a person ages. Elderly persons have more fragmented sleep and shorter duration of stage 3 and 4 sleep. Although REM sleep tends to be preserved, the deepest stages of non-REM sleep frequently are reduced or nonexistent.[44–47] Compared with younger persons, elderly persons tend to achieve less total nighttime sleep. They often take longer to fall asleep, they awaken earlier, and they have more nighttime arousals. Environmental influences, particularly auditory stimuli, often are more disruptive in the elderly population. With an increase in nighttime wakefulness, there is an increase in daytime fatigue and daytime napping. An often overlooked cause of nocturnal awakenings in the elderly population is nocturia or need to urinate during the night.[45]

The causes of sleep disorders in the elderly include age-related changes in sleep architecture, secondary sleep disturbances, primary sleep disorders, lack of exercise, and poor sleep habits. Factors that predispose to secondary sleep disturbances include physical and mental illness, medication effects, and emotional stress. A variety of medical illnesses contribute to sleep disorders in the elderly, including arthritic pain, respiratory problems and cardiac disease, and neurologic disorders. Nightmares and nighttime fears are common in elderly persons with Parkinson's disease, particularly those who are receiving levodopa. Psychiatric illness, such as depression, is a common cause of disturbed sleep in this age group. Primary sleep disorders such as sleep apnea, RLS, and PLMD also increase in old age. Many medications have stimulating effects and interfere with sleep. These include some of the antidepressants, decongestants, bronchodilators, corticosteroids, and some antihypertensives. Alcohol use also may serve as a deterrent to sleep in the elderly. Sleep–wake problems may be compounded further by inappropriate interventions initiated by the older person, his or her family, or health care providers.

Sleep also is disturbed in disorders characterized by dementia. Episodes of nocturnal wandering, confusion, and delirium can occur despite normal daytime functioning. Persons with Alzheimer's disease often have increased periods of nighttime awakening and daytime napping.

Diagnosis of sleep disorders in elderly persons requires a comprehensive sleep history, inquiries about pain and anxiety or depression, review of current sleep hygiene practices, drug use history, spousal or bed partner reports, a comprehensive physical examination, and appropriate laboratory tests.[48,49] Treatment of a medical disorder and changes in medication regimens and timing of medication doses can improve sleep. Avoidance of alcohol and stimulants before bedtime and improving sleep hygiene are other measures that can be used to improve sleep. Although hypnotics can be used to treat transient insomnia, they often fail to provide long-term relief of chronic sleep disturbances.

In summary, circadian rhythms and sleep patterns are established early in life. In the newborn, REM sleep occurs at sleep onset, and periods of sleep and awakening are distributed throughout the day. As the cyclic structure of the sleep–wake cycle progresses, the amount of time spent in REM sleep decreases. By the time the child is 8 months of age, the duration of sleep has decreased to approximately 13 hours, and REM sleep occupies only approximately one third of that time. At 12 to 15 years of age, sleep has decreased to approximately 8 hours, with one fourth being spent in REM sleep. Although complaints of sleep are common among adults, children usually do not complain about sleep problems, although their parents might. The usual concerns of parents include irregular sleep habits, insufficient or too much sleep, nightmares, sleep terrors, sleepwalking, and bed-wetting.

Complaints of sleep disorders are common in elderly persons. The sleep–wake cycle changes with aging, resulting in more fragmented sleep, shorter duration of stage 3 and 4 sleep, and reduced REM sleep. The circadian rhythm of a typical sleep period also changes; elderly persons tend to go to bed earlier in the evening and awaken earlier in the morning. Elderly persons also have more health problems that interrupt sleep, they are apt to be on medications that interfere with sleep, and they are more likely to have sleep disorders such as insomnia, RLS, and sleep apnea. Left uncorrected, sleep disorders in the elderly affect their quality of life. Loss of sleep and use of sedating medications may lead to falls and accidents.

REVIEW EXERCISES

A frustrated mother complains that her teenage son stays up at night and then has trouble waking up and getting to school on time.

A. Is there a developmental explanation for these behaviors?

B. What suggestions would you make to the mother?

A 30-year-old woman presents with complaints of fatigue, irritability, and difficulty concentrating. She relates that for the past 3 months or more, she has had difficulty falling asleep and staying asleep despite remaining in bed and focusing on measures to help her sleep. She laughingly tells you that she has even tried counting sheep.

A. What type of diagnostic methods would prove useful in determining whether this woman's problem is related to insomnia?

B. If the woman is determined to suffer from insomnia, what type of treatments would be indicated?

A 50-year-old man presents with hypertension, daytime sleepiness and difficulty concentrating, and injuries sustained from an auto accident that occurred when he fell asleep at the wheel. He weighs 250 pounds, is 69 inches tall, and leads a sedentary lifestyle. He states that his wife has moved into the guest bedroom because his snoring disturbs her sleep.

A. What is the possible cause of this man's problems?

B. What diagnostic tests could be used to confirm the diagnosis?

C. What type of lifestyle changes and other treatments might be used?

References

1. Hobson J. A. (1989). *Sleep* (pp. 1–21, 74–78, 117–134, 121, 159–169). New York: Scientific American Library.
2. McCarley R. W. (1995). Sleep, dreams, and states of consciousness. In Conn P. M. (Ed.), *Neuroscience in medicine* (pp. 537–583). Philadelphia: J. B. Lippincott.
3. Carskadon M. A., Dement W. C. (2000). Normal human sleep. In Kryger M. H., Roth T., Dement W. C. (Eds.), *Principles and practices of sleep medicine* (3rd ed., pp. 15–25). Philadelphia: W. B. Saunders.
4. Carskadon M. A., Rechtschaffen A. (2000). Monitoring and staging human sleep. In Kryger M. H., Roth T., Dement W. C. (Eds.), *Principles and practices of sleep medicine* (3rd ed., pp. 1197–1230). Philadelphia: W. B. Saunders.
5. Strollo P. J., Rogers R. M. (1996). Obstructive sleep apnea. *New England Journal of Medicine 334,* 99–104.
6. Berry R. A. (1995). Sleep-related breathing disorders. In George R. B., Light R. W., Matthay M. A., Matthay R. A. (Eds.), *Chest medicine* (3rd ed., pp. 247–268). Baltimore: Williams & Wilkins.
7. Pagel J. F. (2000). Nightmares and disorders of dreaming. *American Family Physician 61,* 2037–2042, 2044.
8. Moore M. C., Czeisler C. A., Richardson G. S. (1983). Circadian timekeeping in health and disease. *New England Journal of Medicine 309,* 469–473.
9. Moore R. Y. (1997). Circadian rhythms: Basic neurobiology and clinical applications. *Annual Review of Medicine 48,* 253–266.
10. Richardson G., Tate B. (2000). Hormonal and pharmacological manipulation of the circadian clock: Recent developments and future strategies. *Sleep 23*(Suppl. 3), S77–S85.
11. Brzezinski A. (1997). Melatonin in humans. *New England Journal of Medicine 336,* 186–195.
12. Cupp M. J. (1997). Melatonin. *American Family Physician 56*(5), 1421–1488.
13. Ahrendt J. (2000). Melatonin, circadian rhythms, and sleep. *New England Journal of Medicine 343,* 1114–1115.
14. American Sleep Disorders Association. (1997). *The international classification of sleep disorders.* Rochester, MN: Author.
15. Members of National Heart, Lung, and Blood Institute Working Group on Insomnia. (1998). *Insomnia: Assessment and management in primary care.* NIH publication no. 98-4088. Bethesda, MD: National Institutes of Health.
16. Epstein D. R., Bootzin R. R. (2002). Insomnia. *Nursing Clinics of North America 37,* 611–631.
17. Ancoli-Israel S. (2000). Actigraphy. In Kryger M. H., Roth T., Dement W. C. (Eds.), *Principles and practices of sleep medicine* (3rd ed., pp. 1295–1301). Philadelphia: W. B. Saunders.
18. Wagner D. R. (1996). Disorders of the circadian sleep-wake cycle. *Neurologic Clinics 14,* 651–669.
19. Pilcher J. J., Lambert B. J., Huffcutt A. I. (2000). Differential effects of permanent and rotating shifts on self-report sleep length: A meta-analytic view. *Sleep 23,* 155–163.
20. Rajput V., Bromley S. M. (1999). Chronic insomnia: A practical review. *American Family Physician 60,* 1431–1442.
21. Meyer T. J. (1998). Evaluation and management of insomnia. *Hospital Practice 33*(12), 75–86.
22. Vgontzas A. N., Kales A. (1999). Sleep and its disorders. *Annual Review of Medicine 50,* 387–400.
23. Kupfer D. J., Reynold C. F. (1997). Management of insomnia. *New England Journal of Medicine 336,* 341–345.
24. Rogers A. E., Dreher H. M. (2002). Narcolepsy. *Nursing Clinics of North America 37,* 675–692.
25. Guilleminault C., Anagnos A. (2000). Narcolepsy. In Kryger M. H., Roth T., Dement W. C. (Eds.), *Principles and practices of sleep medicine* (3rd ed., pp. 676–686). Philadelphia: W. B. Saunders.
26. Krahn L. E., Black J. L., Silber M. H. (2001). Narcolepsy: A new understanding of irresistible sleep. *Mayo Clinic Proceedings 76,* 185–194.
27. Lin L., Faraco J., Li R. (1999). The sleep disorder canine narcolepsy is caused by a mutation in hypocretin (oxexin) receptor 2 gene. *Cell 98,* 365–376.
28. Nishino S., Ripley B., Overseem S., et al. (2000). Hypocretin (orexin) deficiency in human narcolepsy [Letter]. *Lancet 355,* 39–40.
29. Dyken M. E., Rodnitzky R. L. (1992). Periodic, aperiodic, and rhythmic limb movements and restless motor disorders of sleep. *Neurology 42*(Suppl. 6), 68–74.
30. Earley C. J. (2003). Restless legs syndrome. *New England Journal of Medicine 348,* 2103–2109.
31. National Center on Sleep Disorders Research. (2000). *Restless legs syndrome: Detection and management in primary care.* NIH publication no. 00-3788. Bethesda, MD: National Institutes of Health.
32. Paulson G. W. (2000). Restless legs syndrome: How to provide symptom relief with drug and nondrug therapies. *Geriatrics 55*(6), 35–48.
33. Guilleminault C., Stoohs R., Quera-Salva M. (1992). Sleep-related obstructive and nonobstructive apneas and neurologic disorders. *Neurology 42*(Suppl. 6), 53–60.
34. Members of the National Heart, Lung, and Blood Institute Working Group on Sleep Apnea. (1995). *Sleep apnea: Is your patient at risk?* NIH publication no. 95-3803. Bethesda, MD: National Institutes of Health.
35. Flemons W. W. (2002). Obstructive sleep apnea. *New England Journal of Medicine 347*(7), 498–504.

36. Victor L. D. (1999). Obstructive sleep apnea. *American Family Physician 60,* 2279–2286.
37. Burwell C. S., Robin E. D., Whaley R. D., et al. (1956). Extreme obesity associated with alveolar hypoventilation: A pickwickian syndrome. *American Journal of Medicine 21,* 811–818.
38. Ross S. D., Sheinhait I. A., Harrison K. J., et al. (2000). Systematic review and meta-analysis of the literature regarding the diagnosis of sleep apnea. *Sleep 23,* 519–533.
39. Schenck C. H., Mahowald M. W. (2000). Parasomnias. *Postgraduate Medicine 107*(3), 145–156.
40. Masand R., Popli A. P. (1995). Sleepwalking. *American Family Physician 51,* 649–653.
41. Ferber R. (1996). Childhood sleep disorders. *Neurologic Clinics 14,* 493–451.
42. Garcia J., Wills L. (2000). Sleep disorders in children and teens. *Postgraduate Medicine 107*(3), 161–178.
43. Ward T., Mason T. B. A. (2002). Sleep disorders in children. *Nursing Clinics of North America 37,* 693–706.
44. Foley D. J., Monjan A. A., Brown S. L., et al. (1995). Sleep complaints among elderly persons: An epidemiologic study of three communities. *Sleep 18,* 425–432.
45. Bliwise D. (2000). Normal aging. In Kryger M. H., Roth T., Dement W. C. (Eds.), *Principles and practices of sleep medicine* (3rd ed., pp. 26–42). Philadelphia: W. B. Saunders.
46. Neubauer D. N. (1999). Sleep problems in the elderly. *American Family Physician 59,* 2551–2559.
47. Ancoli-Israel S. (2000). Insomnia in the elderly: A review for the primary care practitioner. *Sleep 23*(Suppl. 1), S23–S29.
48. Foreman M. D., Wykle M. (1995). Nursing standard-of-practice protocol: Sleep disturbances in elderly patients. *Geriatric Nursing 16,* 238–243.
49. Vitello M. V. (1999). Effective treatments for age-related sleep disturbances. *Geriatrics 54*(11), 47–52.

UNIT IV

Hematopoietic Function

From ancient times, the importance of blood as a determinant of health was recognized. Its life-affecting powers are well described in the written treatises of Greek physician Galen (AD 130–200). Galen, who reigned as the foremost medical authority for nearly 1500 years, believed that an individual stayed healthy as long as four body fluids—blood, phlegm, yellow bile, and black bile—remained in the right proportion. He also believed that the four humors determined one's basic temperament. Whether an individual was sanguine, sluggish and dull, quick to anger, or melancholy was determined by the degree to which one or another of the humors predominated. The most desirable personality type was achieved when blood was thought to predominate, yielding a warm and cheerful person.

The workings of blood were traced by Galen from its creation, which he believed took place in the liver, throughout the body. He came to believe that disease manifested itself if any one of the fluids was in excess or deficient and was carried in the blood. The theory led to bloodletting—the drawing of blood from the vein of a sick person so the disease could flow out with the blood. For many centuries, bloodletting was the standard treatment for a myriad of ills.

CHAPTER

14

Hematopoietic System

Kathryn J. Gaspard

Blood consists of blood cells (*i.e.,* red blood cells, thrombocytes or platelets, and white blood cells) and the plasma in which the cells are suspended. Blood cells have a relatively short life span and must be continually replaced. The generation of blood cells takes place in the *hematopoietic* (from the Greek *haima* "blood" and *poiesis* "making") system. The hematopoietic system encompasses all of the blood cells and their precursors, the bone marrow where blood cells have their origin, and the lymphoid tissues where some blood cells circulate as they develop and mature.

Composition of Blood and Formation of Blood Cells

After completing this section of the chapter, you should be able to meet the following objectives:

- Describe the composition of plasma
- Name the formed elements of blood and cite their function and life span
- Trace the process of hematopoiesis from stem cell to mature blood cell

When blood is removed from the circulatory system, it clots. The clot contains the blood cells and fibrin strands formed from the conversion of the plasma protein fibrinogen. It is surrounded by a yellow liquid called *serum.* Blood that is kept from clotting by the addition of an anticoagulant (*e.g.,* heparin, citrate) and then centrifuged separates into layers (Fig. 14-1). The lower layer (approximately 42% to 47% of the whole-blood volume) contains the erythrocytes, or red blood cells, and is referred to as the *hematocrit.* The intermediate layer (approximately 1%) containing the leukocytes is white or gray and is called the *buffy layer.* Above the leukocytes is a thin layer of platelets that is not discernible to the naked eye. The translucent, yellowish fluid that forms on the top of the cells is the *plasma,* which comprises approximately 55% of the total volume.

PLASMA

The plasma component of blood carries the cells that transport gases, aid in body defenses, and prevent blood loss. It transports nutrients that are absorbed from the gastrointestinal tract to body cells and delivers the waste products from cellular metabolism to the kidney for elimination; it transports hormones and permits the exchange of chemical messengers; it facilitates the exchange of body heat; and it participates in electrolyte and acid-base balance and the osmotic regulation of body fluids. Plasma is 90% to 91% water by weight, 6.5% to 8% proteins by weight, and 2% other small molecular substances (Table 14-1).

PLASMA PROTEINS

The plasma proteins are the most abundant solutes in plasma. Most proteins are formed in the liver and serve a variety of functions. The major types are albumin, globulins, and fibrinogen. Albumin is the most abundant and makes up approximately 54% of the plasma proteins. It does not diffuse through the vascular endothelium and therefore contributes to plasma osmotic pressure and the maintenance of blood volume (see Chapter 33). Albumin also serves as a carrier for certain substances and acts as a blood buffer. The globulins comprise approximately 38% of plasma proteins. There are three types of globulins: the

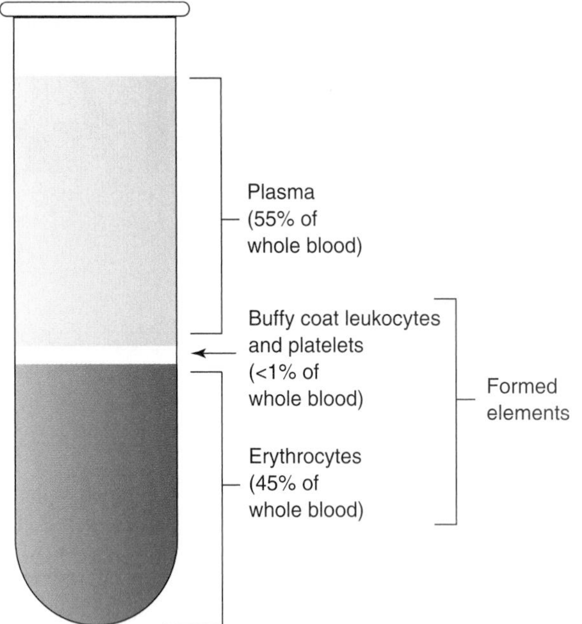

FIGURE 14-1 Layering of blood components in an anticoagulated and centrifuged blood sample.

alpha globulins that transport bilirubin and steroids, the beta globulins that transport iron and copper, and the gamma globulins that constitute the antibodies of the immune system. Fibrinogen makes up approximately 7% of the plasma proteins and is converted to fibrin in the clotting process. The remaining 1% of circulating proteins includes hormones, enzymes, complement, and carriers for lipids.

BLOOD CELLS

The blood cells include the erythrocytes or red blood cells, the leukocytes or white blood cells, and platelets (Table 14-2). The blood cells, or formed elements, are not all true cells, and most survive for only a few days in the circulation or tissues as a result of their function. They do not divide and thus must be continually renewed by the process of hematopoiesis in the bone marrow.

> **COMPOSITION OF THE BLOOD**
>
> - Blood is a liquid that fills the vascular compartment and serves to transport dissolved materials and blood cells throughout the body.
> - The most abundant of the blood cells, the erythrocytes or red blood cells, function in oxygen and carbon dioxide transport.
> - The leukocytes, or white blood cells, serve various roles in immunity and inflammation.
> - Platelets are small cell fragments that are involved in blood clotting.

Erythrocytes

The erythrocytes, or red blood cells, are the most numerous of the formed elements. They are small, biconcave disks with a large surface area and can easily deform in small capillaries. They contain the oxygen-carrying protein, hemoglobin, that functions in the transport of oxygen. The erythrocytes are derived from the myeloid or bone marrow stem cell and live approximately 120 days in the circulation (see Chapter 16).

Leukocytes

The leukocytes, or white blood cells, constitute only 1% of the total blood volume. They originate in the bone marrow and circulate throughout the lymphoid tissues of the body. There they function in the inflammatory and immune processes. They include the granulocytes, the lymphocytes, and the monocytes (Fig. 14-2).

Granulocytes. The granulocytes are all phagocytic cells and are identifiable because of their cytoplasmic granules. These white blood cells are spherical and have distinctive multilobar nuclei. The granulocytes are divided into three types (neutrophils, eosinophils, and basophils) according to the staining properties of the granules. Functionally, all granulocytes are phagocytes.

Neutrophils. The neutrophils, which constitute 55% to 65% of the total number of white blood cells, have granules that are neutral and hence do not stain with an acidic or a basic dye. Because these white cells have nuclei that are divided into three to five lobes, they are often called *polymorphonuclear leukocytes.*

The neutrophils are primarily responsible for maintaining normal host defenses against invading bacteria and fungi, cell remains, and a variety of foreign substances. The cytoplasm of mature neutrophils contains fine granules. These granules contain degrading enzymes that are used in destroying foreign substances and correspond to lysosomes found in other cells (see Chapter 4). Enzymes and oxidizing agents associated with these granules are capable of degrading a variety of natural and synthetic substances, including complex polysaccharides, proteins, and lipids. These enzymes are important in maintaining normal host defenses and in mediating inflammation.

The neutrophils have their origin in the myeloblasts that are found in the bone marrow (Fig. 14-3). The myeloblasts are the committed precursors of the granulocyte pathway and do not normally appear in the peripheral circulation. When they are present, it suggests a disorder of blood cell proliferation and differentiation. The myeloblasts differentiate into promyelocytes and then myelocytes. Usually, a cell is not called a *myelocyte* until it has at least 12 granules. The myelocytes mature to become metamyelocytes (Greek *meta,* "beyond"), at which point they lose their capacity for mitosis. Subsequent development of the neutrophil involves reduction in size, with transformation from an indented to an oval to a horseshoe-shaped nucleus (*i.e.,* band cell) and then to a mature cell with a

TABLE 14-1 Plasma Components

Plasma	Percentage of Plasma Volume	Description
Water	90–91	
Proteins	6.5–8	
Albumin		54% Plasma proteins
Globulins		38% Plasma proteins
Fibrinogen		7% Plasma proteins
Other substances	1–2	Hormones, enzymes, carbohydrates, fats, amino acids, gases, electrolytes, excretory products

segmented nucleus. These mature neutrophils are often referred to as *segs* because of their segmented nucleus. Development from stem cell to mature neutrophil takes approximately 2 weeks. It is at this point that the neutrophil enters the bloodstream.

After release from the marrow, the neutrophils spend only approximately 4 to 8 hours in the circulation before moving into the tissues. Their survival in the tissues lasts approximately 4 to 5 days. They die in the tissues in discharging their phagocytic function or they die of senescence. The pool of circulating neutrophils (*i.e.,* those that appear in the blood count) is in closely maintained equilibrium with a similar-sized pool of cells marginating along the walls of small blood vessels. These are the neutrophils that respond to chemotactic factors and migrate into the tissues toward the offending agent. Epinephrine, exercise, stress, and corticosteroid drug therapy can cause rapid increases in the circulating neutrophil count by shifting cells from the marginating to the circulating pool. Endotoxins or microbes have the opposite effect, producing a transient decrease in neutrophils by attracting neutrophils into the tissues.

Eosinophils. The cytoplasmic granules of the eosinophils stain red with the acidic dye eosin. These leukocytes constitute 1% to 3% of the total number of white blood cells and increase in number during allergic reactions and parasitic infections. In allergic reactions, it is thought that they release enzymes or chemical mediators that detoxify the agents associated with allergic reactions. In parasitic infections, the eosinophils use surface markers to attach themselves to the parasite and then release hydrolytic enzymes that kill it.

Basophils. The granules of the basophils stain blue with a basic dye. These cells constitute only approximately 0.3% to 0.5% of the white blood cells. The granules in the basophils contain heparin, an anticoagulant, and histamine, a vasodilator. The basophils share properties of mast cells and are thought to be involved in allergic and stress responses.

Lymphocytes. The lymphocytes constitute 20% to 30% of the white blood cell count. They originate in the bone marrow from lymphoid stem cells. They have no identifiable granules in the cytoplasm and are also called *agranulocytes*. The lymphocytes play an important role in the immune response. They move between blood and lymph tissue, where they may be stored for hours or years. Their function in the lymph nodes or spleen is to defend against

TABLE 14-2 Blood Cell Counts

Blood Cells	Number of Cells/μL	Percentage of White Blood Cells
Red blood cell count	$4.2–5.4 \times 10^6$, $3.6–5.0 \times 10^6$ *	
White blood cell count	$4.40–11.3 \times 10^3$	
Differential count		
Granulocytes		
Neutrophils		
Segs		47–63
Bands		0–4
Eosinophils		0–3
Basophils		0–2
Lymphocytes		24–40
Monocytes		4–9
Platelet count	$150–400 \times 10^3$	

*First value is for men and the second for women.

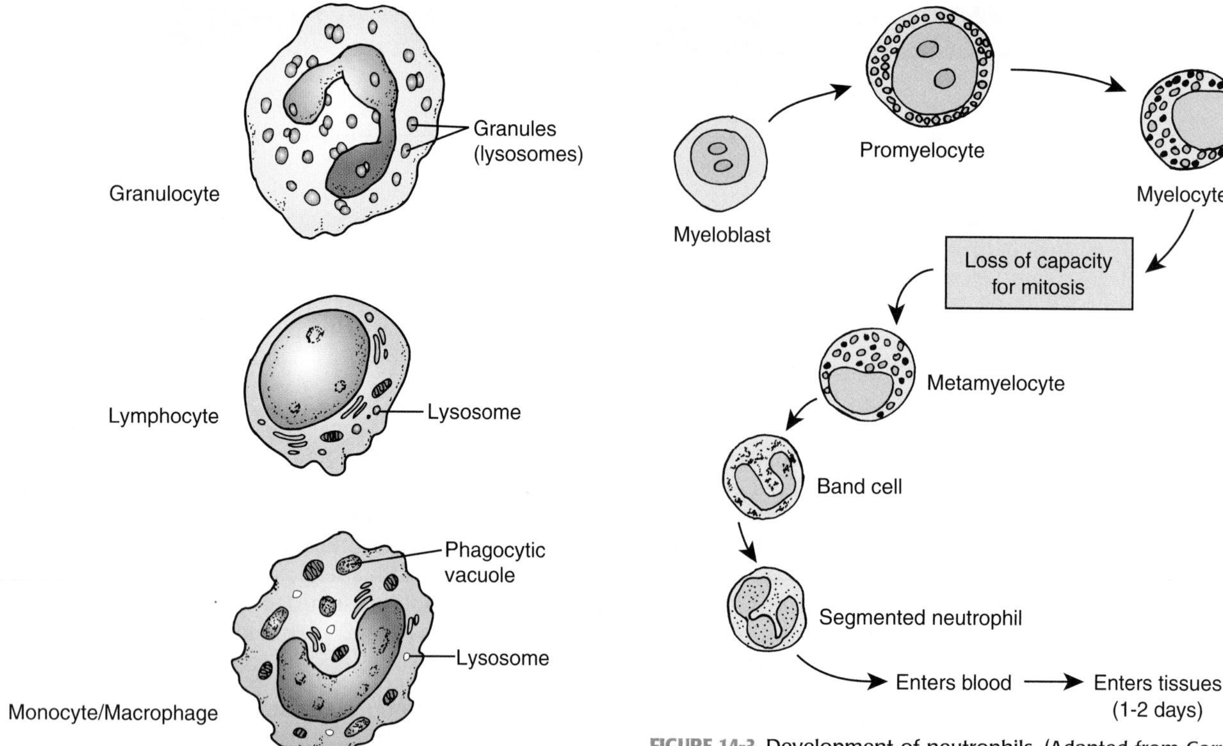

FIGURE 14-2 White blood cells.

FIGURE 14-3 Development of neutrophils. (Adapted from Cormack D. H. [1993]. *Ham's histology* [9th ed.]. Philadelphia: J. B. Lippincott)

microorganisms in the immune response (see Chapter 19). There are two types of lymphocytes: B lymphocytes and T lymphocytes. The B lymphocytes differentiate to form antibody-producing plasma cells and are involved in humoral-mediated immunity. The T lymphocytes activate other cells of the immune system and are involved in cell-mediated immunity.

Monocytes and Macrophages. Monocytes are the largest of the white blood cells and constitute approximately 3% to 8% of the total leukocyte count. The life span of the circulating monocyte is approximately 1 to 3 days, three to four times longer than that of the granulocytes. These cells survive for months to years in the tissues. The monocytes, which are phagocytic cells, are often referred to as *macrophages* when they enter the tissues. The monocytes engulf larger and greater quantities of foreign material than the neutrophils. These leukocytes play an important role in chronic inflammation and are also involved in the immune response by activating lymphocytes and by presenting antigen to T cells. When the monocyte leaves the vascular system and enters the tissues, it functions as a macrophage with specific activity. The macrophages are known as *histiocytes* in loose connective tissue, *microglial cells* in the brain, and *Kupffer cells* in the liver. Some macrophages function in the alveoli.

Granulomatous inflammation is a distinctive pattern of chronic inflammation in which the macrophages form a capsule around insoluble materials that cannot be digested. Foreign-body granulomas are incited by relatively inert foreign bodies, such as talc or surgical sutures. Immune granulomas are caused by insoluble particles that are capable of inciting a cell-mediated immune response. The tubercle that forms in primary tuberculosis infections is an example of an immune granuloma (see Chapter 30).

Thrombocytes

Thrombocytes, or platelets, are circulating cell fragments of the large megakaryocytes that are derived from the myeloid stem cell. They function to form a platelet plug to control bleeding after injury to a vessel wall (see Chapter 15). Their cytoplasmic granules release mediators required for hemostasis. Thrombocytes have no nucleus, cannot replicate, and, if not used, last approximately 8 to 9 days in the circulation before they are removed by the phagocytic cells of the spleen.

HEMATOPOIESIS

The generation of blood cells begins in the endothelial cells of the developing blood vessels during the fifth week of gestation and then continues in the liver and spleen. After birth, this function is gradually taken over by the bone marrow. The marrow is a network of connective tissue containing immature blood cells. At sites where the marrow is hematopoietically active, it produces so many erythrocytes that it is red, hence the name *red bone marrow*. Fat cells are also present in bone marrow, but they are in-

HEMATOPOIESIS

- Blood cells originate from pluripotent stem cells in the bone marrow.
- The proliferation, differentiation, and functional abilities of the various blood cells are controlled by hormone-like growth factors called *cytokines*.

active in terms of blood cell generation. Marrow made up predominantly of fat cells is called *yellow bone marrow*. During active skeletal growth, red marrow is gradually replaced by yellow marrow in most of the long bones. In adults, red marrow is largely restricted to the flat bones of the pelvis, ribs, and sternum. As a person ages, the cellularity of the marrow declines. When the demand for red cell replacement increases, as in hemolytic anemia, there can be resubstitution of red marrow for yellow marrow. Some hematopoiesis may also be generated in the spleen and the liver.

Blood Cell Precursors

The blood-forming population of bone marrow is made up of three types of cells: self-renewing stem cells, differentiated progenitor (parent) cells, and functional mature blood cells. All of the blood cell precursors of the erythrocyte (*i.e.,* red cell), myelocyte (*i.e.,* granulocyte or monocyte), lymphocyte (*i.e.,* T lymphocyte and B lymphocyte), and megakaryocyte (*i.e.,* platelet) series are derived from a small population of primitive cells called the *pluripotent stem cells* (Fig. 14-4). Their lifelong potential for proliferation and self-renewal makes them an indispensable and lifesaving source of reserve cells for the entire hematopoietic system. Several levels of differentiation lead to the development of committed unipotential cells, which are the progenitors for each of the blood cell types. These cells are referred to as *colony-forming units* or *burst-forming units*. These progenitor cells lose their capacity for self-renewal but retain the potential to differentiate in response to lineage-specific growth factors. They develop into the precursor cells that give rise to mature erythrocytes, myelocytes, megakaryocytes, or lymphocytes.

Disorders of hematopoietic stem cells include aplastic anemia and the leukemias. Today, potential cures for these

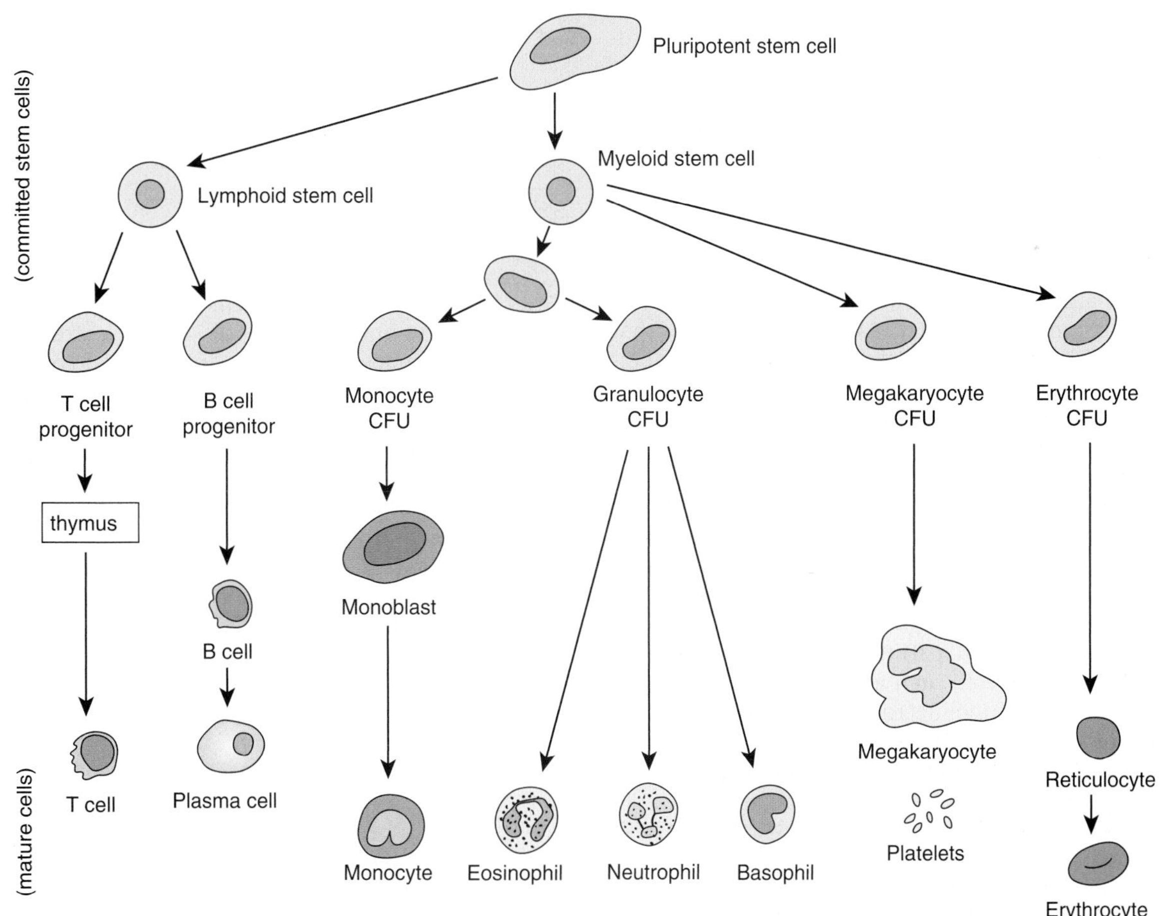

FIGURE 14-4 Major maturational stages of blood cells. CFU, colony forming units.

and many other disorders require hematopoietic stem cell transplantation. Stem cell transplants correct bone marrow failure, immune deficiencies, hematologic defects and malignancies, and inherited errors of metabolism. Sources of the stem cells include bone marrow, peripheral blood, and umbilical cord blood, all of which replenish the recipient with a normal population of pluripotent stem cells. Bone marrow and peripheral blood transplants may be derived from the patient (autologous) or from a histocompatible donor (allogeneic). Autologous transplants are often used to replenish stem cells after high-dose chemotherapy or irradiation. Peripheral blood stem cells are harvested from the blood after the administration of a cytokine growth factor that increases the quantity and migration of the cells from the bone marrow. Umbilical cord blood from HLA-matched donors is a transplant option for children and carries less risk for graft-versus-host disease. Methods of collecting, propagating, and preserving stem cells are still being investigated.

Regulation of Hematopoiesis

Under normal conditions, the numbers and total mass for each type of circulating blood cell remain relatively constant. The blood cells are produced in different numbers according to needs and regulatory factors. This regulation of blood cells is thought to be at least partially controlled by hormone-like growth factors called *cytokines*. The cytokines are a family of glycoproteins that stimulate the proliferation, differentiation, and functional activation of the various blood cell precursors in bone marrow. Many cytokines are produced by bone marrow stromal cells that include macrophages, endothelial cells, fibroblasts, and lymphocytes and act locally in the bone marrow by binding to cell surface receptors. Other cytokines are produced in the liver and kidney.

Some cytokines are colony-stimulating factors (CSFs) that were named for their ability to promote growth of blood cell colonies in culture. Major growth factors that act on committed progenitor cells include: erythropoietin (EPO), which stimulates red blood cell production; granulocyte-monocyte colony-stimulating factor (GM-CSF), which stimulates progenitors for granulocytes, monocytes, erythrocytes, and megakaryocytes; granulocyte colony-stimulating factor (G-CSF), which promotes the proliferation of neutrophils; macrophage colony-stimulating factor (M-CSF), which induces macrophage colonies, and thrombopoietin (TPO), which stimulates the differentiation of platelets. The CSFs act at different points in the proliferation and differentiation pathway, and their functions overlap. Other cytokines, such as the many interleukins, the interferons, and tumor necrosis factor, support the proliferation of stem cells and the development of lymphocytes and act synergistically to aid the multiple functions of the CSFs (see Chapter 19).

The genes for most hematopoietic growth factors have been cloned, and their recombinant proteins have been generated for use in a wide range of clinical problems. The clinically useful factors include EPO, TPO, G-CSF, and GM-CSF. They are used to treat bone marrow failure caused by chemotherapy or aplastic anemia, the anemia of kidney failure, hematopoietic neoplasms, infectious diseases such as acquired immunodeficiency syndrome (AIDS), congenital and myeloproliferative disorders, and some solid tumors. Growth factors are used to increase peripheral stem cells for transplantation and to accelerate cell proliferation after bone marrow engraftment. Many of these uses are still investigational.

In summary, blood is composed of plasma, plasma proteins, formed elements or blood cells, and substances such as hormones, enzymes, electrolytes, and byproducts of cellular waste. The blood cells consist of erythrocytes or red blood cells, leukocytes or white blood cells, and thrombocytes or platelets. Blood cells are generated from pluripotent stem cells located in the bone marrow. Blood cell production is regulated by chemical messengers called *cytokines* and *growth factors*.

Diagnostic Tests

After completing this section of the chapter, you should be able to meet the following objectives:

- Cite information gained from a complete blood count
- State the purpose of the erythrocyte sedimentation rate
- Describe the procedure used in bone marrow aspiration

Blood specimens can be obtained through skin puncture (capillary blood), venipuncture, arterial puncture, or bone marrow aspiration.

BLOOD COUNT

Tests of the hematologic system provide information regarding the number of blood cells and their structural and functional characteristics. A complete blood count (CBC) is a commonly performed screening test that determines the number of red blood cells, white blood cells, and platelets per unit of blood. The white cell differential count is the determination of the relative proportions (percentages) of individual white cell types. Measurement of hemoglobin, hematocrit, mean corpuscular volume (MCV), mean corpuscular hemoglobin concentration (MCHC), and mean cell hemoglobin (MCH) is usually included in the CBC. Inspection of the blood smear identifies morphologic abnormalities such as a change in size, shape, or color of cells. Specific tests of red blood cell function are found in Chapter 16 and of white blood cell function in Chapter 17.

ERYTHROCYTE SEDIMENTATION RATE

The erythrocyte sedimentation rate (ESR) is a screening test for monitoring the fluctuations in the clinical course of a disease. In anticoagulated blood, red blood cells aggregate and sediment to the bottom of a tube. The rate of fall of the aggregates is accelerated in the presence of fibrinogen and other plasma proteins that are often increased in inflammatory diseases. The ESR is the distance in millimeters that a red cell column travels in 1 hour. Normal values are 1 to 13 mm/hour for men and 1 to 20 mm/hour for women.

BONE MARROW ASPIRATION AND BIOPSY

Tests of bone marrow function are done on samples obtained using bone marrow aspiration or bone marrow biopsy. Bone marrow aspiration is performed with a special needle inserted into the bone marrow cavity, and a sample of marrow is withdrawn. Usually, the posterior iliac crest is used in all persons older than 12 to 18 months of age. Other sites include the anterior iliac crest, sternum, and spinous processes T10 through L4. The sternum is not commonly used in children because the cavity is too shallow and there is danger of mediastinal and cardiac perforation. Because aspiration disturbs the marrow architecture, this technique is used primarily to determine the type of cells present and their relative numbers. Stained smears of bone marrow aspirates are usually subjected to several studies: determination of the erythroid to myeloid cell count (*i.e.*, normal ratio is 1:3); differential cell count, search for abnormal cells, evaluation of iron stores in reticulum cells, and special stains and immunochemical studies.

Bone marrow biopsy is done with a special biopsy needle inserted into the posterior iliac crest. Biopsy removes an actual sample of bone marrow tissue and allows study of the architecture of the tissue. It is used to determine the marrow-to-fat ratio and the presence of fibrosis, plasma cells, granulomas, and cancer cells. The major hazard of these procedures is the slight risk for hemorrhage. This risk is increased in persons with a reduced platelet count.

In summary, diagnostic tests of the blood include the complete blood count, which is used to describe the number and characteristics of the erythrocytes, leukocytes, and platelets. The erythrocyte sedimentation rate is used to detect inflammation. Bone marrow aspiration is used to determine the function of the bone marrow in generating blood cells.

REVIEW EXERCISES

Many of the primary immunodeficiency disorders in which there is a defect in the development of immune cells of T or B lymphocyte origin can be cured with allogeneic stem cell transplantation from an unaffected donor.

A. Explain why stem cells are used rather than mature lymphocytes. You might want to refer to Figure 14-4.

B. Describe how the stem cells would go about the process of repopulating the bone marrow.

Bibliography

Alexander W. S. (1998). Cytokines in hematopoiesis. *International Reviews of Immunology 16,* 651–682.

Bonner H., Bagg A., Cossman J. (1999). The blood and lymphoid organs. In Rubin E., Farber J. L. (Eds.), *Pathology* (3rd ed., pp. 1066–1087). Philadelphia: Lippincott-Raven.

Davoren J. B. (2000). Blood disorders. In McPhee S. J., Lingappa V. R., Ganong W. F., Lange J. D. (Eds.), *Pathophysiology of disease* (3rd ed., pp. 98–123). New York: Lange Medical Books/McGraw-Hill.

Guyton A. C., Hall J. E. (2000). *Textbook of medical physiology* (10th ed.). Philadelphia: W. B. Saunders.

Hoffman R., Benz E. J., Shattil S. J., et al. (2000). *Hematology: Basic principles and practice* (3rd ed.). New York: Churchill Livingstone.

Jansen J., Thompson J. M., Dugan M. J., et al. (2002). Peripheral blood progenitor cell transplantation. *Therapeutic Apheresis 6*(1), 5–14.

Lovell-Badge R. (2001). The future for stem cell research. *Nature 414*(6859), 88–91.

Rocha V., Wagner J. E., Sobocinski K., et al. (2000). Graft-versus-host disease in children who have received a cord-blood or bone marrow transplant from an HLA-identical sibling. *New England Journal of Medicine 342,* 1846–1854.

Rubin R. N., Leopold L. (1998). *Hematologic pathophysiology*. Madison, CT: Fence Creek Publishing.

Stamatoyannopoulos G., Majerus P. W., Perlmutter R. M., Varmus H. (2001). *The molecular basis of blood diseases* (3rd ed.). Philadelphia: W. B. Saunders.

Wadlow R. C., Porter D. L. (2002). Umbilical cord blood transplant: Where do we stand? *Biology of Blood and Marrow Transplantation,* 637–647.

CHAPTER

15

Disorders of Hemostasis

Kathryn J. Gaspard

MECHANISMS OF HEMOSTASIS
- Vessel Spasm
- Formation of the Platelet Plug
- Blood Coagulation
- Clot Retraction
- Clot Dissolution

HYPERCOAGULABILITY STATES
- Increased Platelet Function
- Increased Clotting Activity
  - *Inherited Disorders*
  - *Acquired Disorders*

BLEEDING DISORDERS
- Platelet Defects
  - *Thrombocytopenia*
  - *Impaired Platelet Function*
- Coagulation Defects
  - *Impaired Synthesis of Coagulation Factors*
  - *Hereditary Disorders*
- Disseminated Intravascular Coagulation
- Vascular Disorders

The term *hemostasis* refers to the stoppage of blood flow. The normal process of hemostasis is regulated by a complex array of activators and inhibitors that maintain blood fluidity and prevent blood from leaving the vascular compartment. Hemostasis is normal when it seals a blood vessel to prevent blood loss and hemorrhage. It is abnormal when it causes inappropriate blood clotting or when clotting is insufficient to stop the flow of blood from the vascular compartment. Disorders of hemostasis fall into two main categories: the inappropriate formation of clots within the vascular system (*i.e.*, thrombosis) and the failure of blood to clot in response to an appropriate stimulus (*i.e.*, bleeding).

Mechanisms of Hemostasis

After completing this section of the chapter, you should be able to meet the following objectives:

- State the five stages of hemostasis
- Describe the formation of the platelet plug
- State the purpose of coagulation
- State the function of clot retraction
- Trace the process of fibrinolysis

Hemostasis is divided into five stages: (1) vessel spasm, (2) formation of the platelet plug, (3) blood coagulation or development of an insoluble fibrin clot, (4) clot retraction, and (5) clot dissolution (Fig. 15-1).

VESSEL SPASM

Vessel spasm is initiated by endothelial injury and caused by local and humoral mechanisms. A spasm constricts the vessel and reduces blood flow. It is a transient event that usually lasts less than 1 minute. Thromboxane A_2 (TXA_2), a prostaglandin released from the platelets and cells, and other mediators contribute to vasoconstriction. Prostacyclin, another prostaglandin released from the vessel endothelium, produces vasodilation and inhibits platelet aggregation.

FORMATION OF THE PLATELET PLUG

The platelet plug, the second line of defense, is initiated as platelets come in contact with the vessel wall. Tiny breaks in the vessel wall are often sealed with the platelet plug rather than a blood clot.

Platelets, also called *thrombocytes,* are large fragments from the cytoplasm of bone marrow cells called *megakaryocytes.*[1] They are enclosed in a membrane but have no nucleus and cannot reproduce. Although they lack a nucleus, they have many of the characteristics of a whole cell. They have mitochondria and enzyme systems capable of producing adenosine triphosphate (ATP) and adenosine diphosphate (ADP), and they have the enzymes needed for synthesis of prostaglandins, which are required for their function in hemostasis. The newly formed platelets that are released from the bone marrow spend up to 8 hours in the spleen before they are released into the blood.

The life span of a platelet is only 8 to 9 days. Platelet production is controlled by a protein called *thrombopoietin*

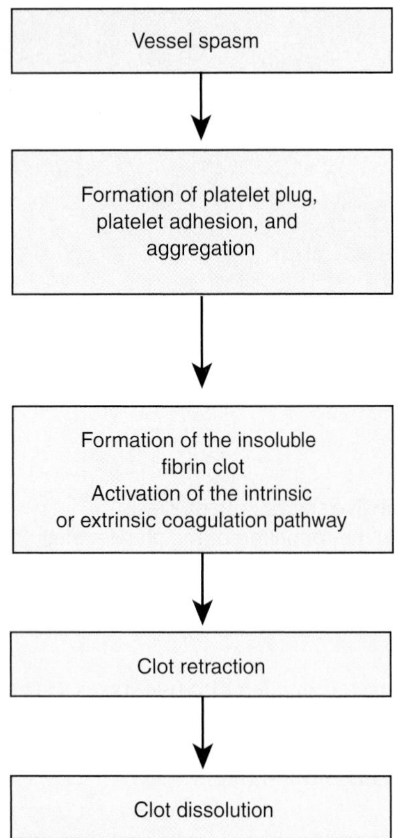

FIGURE 15-1 Steps in hemostasis.

that causes proliferation and maturation of megakaryocytes.[2] The sources of thrombopoietin include the liver, kidney, smooth muscle, and bone marrow. Its production and release are regulated by the number of platelets in the circulation.

Platelets contain two specific types of granules (α- and δ-granules) that release mediators for hemostasis. The α-granules express the P-selectin on their surface (see Chapter 4) and contain fibrinogen, fibronectin, factors V and VIII, platelet factor 4 (a heparin-binding chemokine), platelet-derived growth factor (PDGF), and transforming growth factor-α (TGF-α).[3] The release of growth factors causes vascular endothelial cells, smooth muscle cells, and fibroblasts to proliferate and grow. The δ-granules, or dense granules, contain ADP and ATP, ionized calcium, histamine, serotonin, and epinephrine.[3]

Platelet plug formation involves adhesion and aggregation of platelets (Fig. 15-2A). Platelets are attracted to a damaged vessel wall, become activated, and change from smooth disks to spiny spheres, exposing receptors on their surfaces. Platelet adhesion requires a protein molecule called *von Willebrand factor* (vWF). This factor is produced by the endothelial cells of blood vessels and circulates in the blood as a carrier protein for coagulation factor VIII. Adhesion to the vessel subendothelial layer occurs when the platelet receptor binds to vWF at the injury site, linking the platelet to exposed collagen fibers.

Platelet aggregation occurs soon after adhesion. It is mediated by the secretion of the contents of the platelet granules. The release of the dense body contents is particularly important because calcium is required for the coagulation component of hemostasis, and ADP is a mediator of platelet aggregation. ADP release also facilitates the release of ADP from other platelets, leading to amplification

HEMOSTASIS

- Hemostasis is the orderly, stepwise process for stopping bleeding that involves vasospasm, formation of a platelet plug, and the development of a fibrin clot.
- The blood clotting process requires the presence of platelets produced in the bone marrow, von Willebrand factor generated by the vessel endothelium, and clotting factors synthesized in the liver, using vitamin K.
- The final step of the process involves fibrinolysis or clot dissolution, which prevents excess clot formation.

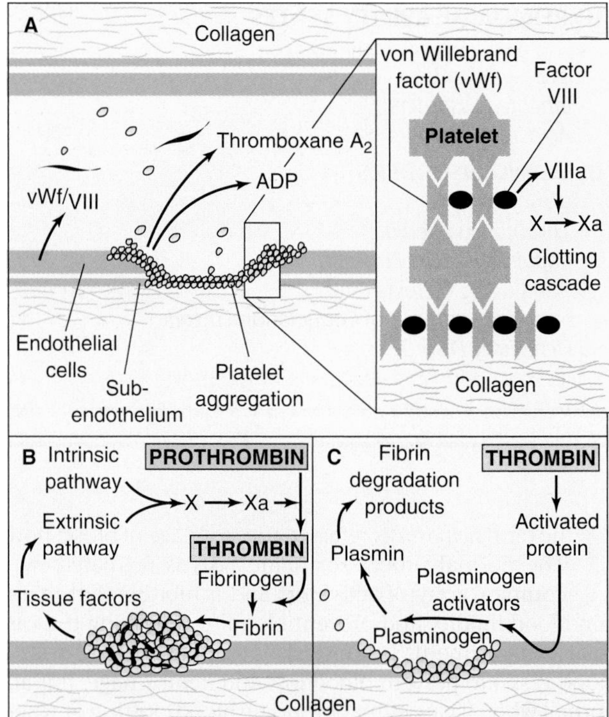

FIGURE 15-2 (**A**) The platelet plug occurs seconds after vessel injury. Von Willebrand's factor, released from the endothelial cells, binds to platelet receptors, causing *adhesion* of platelets to the exposed collagen. Platelet *aggregation* is induced by release of thromboxane A_2 and adenosine diphosphate. (**B**) Coagulation factors, activated on the platelet surface, lead to the formation of thrombin and fibrin, which stabilize the platelet plug. (**C**) Control of the coagulation process and clot dissolution are governed by thrombin and plasminogen activators. Thrombin activates protein C, which stimulates the release of plasminogen activators. The plasminogen activators in turn promote the formation of plasmin, which digests the fibrin strands.

of the aggregation process. Besides ADP, platelets also secrete the vasoconstrictor prostaglandin TXA_2, which is an important stimulus for platelet aggregation. The combined actions of ADP and TXA_2 lead to the buildup of the enlarging platelet aggregate, which becomes the primary hemostatic plug. Stabilization of the platelet plug occurs as the coagulation pathway is activated on the platelet surface and fibrinogen is converted to fibrin, thereby creating a fibrin meshwork that cements the platelets and other blood components together (see Fig. 15-2B). The primary aggregation and formation of the platelet plug is reversible up to the point at which the coagulation cascade has been activated and the platelets have been irreversibly fused together by the fibrin meshwork.

The platelet membrane plays an important role in platelet adhesion and the coagulation process. It has a coat of glycoproteins on its surface that control interactions with the vessel endothelium. Platelets normally avoid adherence to the endothelium but interact with injured areas of the vessel wall and the deeper exposed collagen.[1] Glycoprotein IIb/IIIa (GpIIb/IIIa) receptors on the platelet membrane bind fibrinogen and link platelets together. Drugs, which act as glycoprotein receptor agonists, have been developed for use in the treatment of acute myocardial infarction (see Chapter 26). Phospholipids, which are also present in the platelet membrane, provide critical binding sites for calcium and coagulation factors in the intrinsic coagulation pathway.

Defective platelet plug formation causes bleeding in persons who are deficient in platelet receptor sites or vWF. In addition to sealing vascular breaks, platelets play an almost continuous role in maintaining normal vascular integrity. They may supply growth factors for the endothelial cells and arterial smooth muscle cells. Persons with platelet deficiency have increased capillary permeability and sustain small skin hemorrhages from the slightest trauma or change in blood pressure.

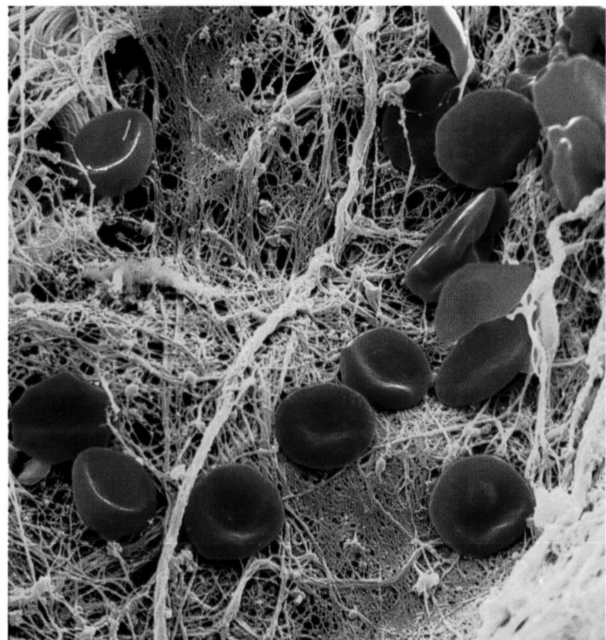

FIGURE 15-3 Scanning electron micrograph of a blood clot (×3600). The fibrous bridges that form a meshwork between red blood cells are fibrin fibers. (© Oliver Meckes, Science Source/Photo Researchers)

BLOOD COAGULATION

The coagulation cascade is the third component of the hemostatic process. It is a stepwise process resulting in the conversion of the soluble plasma protein, fibrinogen, into fibrin. The insoluble fibrin strands create a meshwork that cements platelets and other blood components together to form the clot (Fig. 15-3).

The coagulation process results from the activation of what has traditionally been designated the *intrinsic* or the *extrinsic* pathways (Fig. 15-4). The intrinsic pathway, which is a relatively slow process, begins in the blood itself. The extrinsic pathway, which is a much faster process, begins with trauma to the blood vessel or surrounding tissues and the release of tissue factor. The terminal steps in both pathways are the same: the activation of factor X and the conversion of prothrombin to thrombin. Thrombin then acts as an enzyme to convert fibrinogen to fibrin, the material that stabilizes a clot. Both pathways are needed for normal hemostasis, and many interrelations exist between them. Each system is activated when blood passes out of the vascular system. The intrinsic system is activated as blood comes in contact with collagen in the injured vessel wall; the extrinsic system is activated when blood is exposed to tissue extracts. Bleeding, when it occurs because of defects in the extrinsic system, usually is not as severe as that which results from defects in the intrinsic pathway.

The coagulation process is controlled by many substances that promote clotting (*i.e.*, procoagulation factors) or inhibit it (*i.e.*, anticoagulation factors). Each of the procoagulation or coagulation factors, identified by Roman numerals, performs a specific step in the coagulation process. The activation of one procoagulation factor or proenzyme is designed to activate the next factor in the sequence (*i.e.*, cascade effect). Because most of the inactive procoagulation factors are present in the blood at all times, the multistep process ensures that a massive episode of intravascular clotting does not occur by chance. It also means that abnormalities of the clotting process occur when one or more of the factors are deficient or when conditions lead to inappropriate activation of any of the steps.

Most of the coagulation factors are proteins synthesized in the liver. Vitamin K is necessary for the synthesis of factors VII, IX, X, prothrombin, and protein C. Calcium (factor IV) is required in all but the first two steps of the clotting process. The body usually has sufficient amounts of calcium for these reactions. Inactivation of the calcium ion prevents blood from clotting when it is removed from the body. The addition of citrate to blood stored for transfusion purposes prevents clotting by chelating ionic calcium. EDTA, another chelator, is often added to blood samples used for analysis in the clinical laboratory.

Blood coagulation is regulated by several natural anticoagulants. Antithrombin III inactivates coagulation factors and neutralizes thrombin, the last enzyme in the pathway

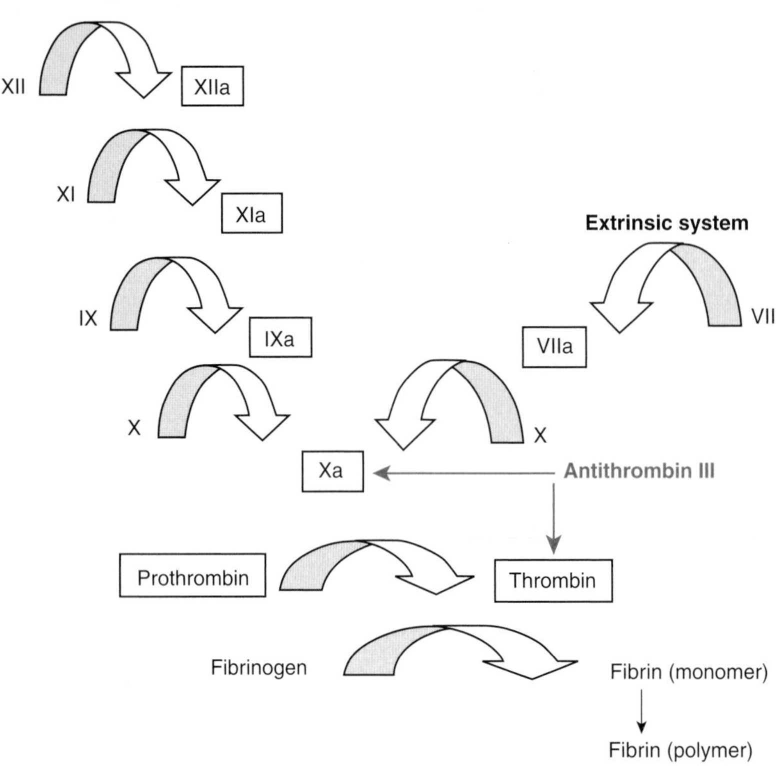

FIGURE 15-4 Intrinsic and extrinsic coagulation pathways. The terminal steps in both pathways are the same. Calcium, factors X and V, and platelet phospholipids combine to form prothrombin activator, which then converts prothrombin to thrombin. This interaction causes conversion of fibrinogen into the fibrin strands that create the insoluble blood clot.

for the conversion of fibrinogen to fibrin. When antithrombin III is complexed with naturally occurring heparin, its action is accelerated and provides protection against uncontrolled thrombus formation on the endothelial surface. Protein C, a plasma protein, acts as an anticoagulant by inactivating factors V and VIII. Protein S, another plasma protein, accelerates the action of protein C. Plasmin breaks down fibrin into fibrin degradation products that act as anticoagulants. It has been suggested that some of these natural anticoagulants may play a role in the bleeding that occurs with disseminated intravascular coagulation (DIC; discussed later).

The anticoagulant drugs warfarin and heparin are used to prevent thromboembolic disorders, such as deep vein thrombosis and pulmonary embolism. Warfarin acts by decreasing prothrombin and other procoagulation factors. It alters vitamin K such that it reduces its availability to participate in synthesis of the vitamin K–dependent coagulation factors in the liver. Warfarin is readily absorbed after oral administration. Its maximum effect takes 36 to 72 hours because of the varying half-lives of preformed clotting factors that remain in the circulation. Heparin is naturally formed and released in small amounts by mast cells in connective tissue surrounding capillaries. Pharmacologic preparations of heparin are extracted from animal tissues. Heparin binds to antithrombin III, causing a conformational change that increases the ability of antithrombin III to inactivate thrombin, factor Xa, and other clotting factors. By promoting the inactivation of clotting factors, heparin ultimately suppresses the formation of fibrin. Heparin is unable to cross the membranes of the gastrointestinal tract and must be given by injection, usually by intravenous infusion. A low-molecular-weight heparin has been developed that inhibits activation of factor X but has little effect on thrombin and other coagulation factors. The low-molecular-weight heparins are given by subcutaneous injection and require less frequent administration.

CLOT RETRACTION

Clot retraction normally occurs within 20 to 60 minutes after a clot has formed, contributing to hemostasis by squeezing serum from the clot and joining the edges of the broken vessel. Clot retraction requires large numbers of platelets. Therefore, failure of clot retraction is indicative of a low platelet count.

CLOT DISSOLUTION

The dissolution of a blood clot begins shortly after its formation; this allows blood flow to be reestablished and permanent tissue repair to take place (see Fig. 15-2C). The process by which a blood clot dissolves is called *fibrinolysis*. As with clot formation, clot dissolution requires a sequence of steps controlled by activators and inhibitors (Fig. 15-5).

Plasminogen, the proenzyme for the fibrinolytic process, normally is present in the blood in its inactive form.

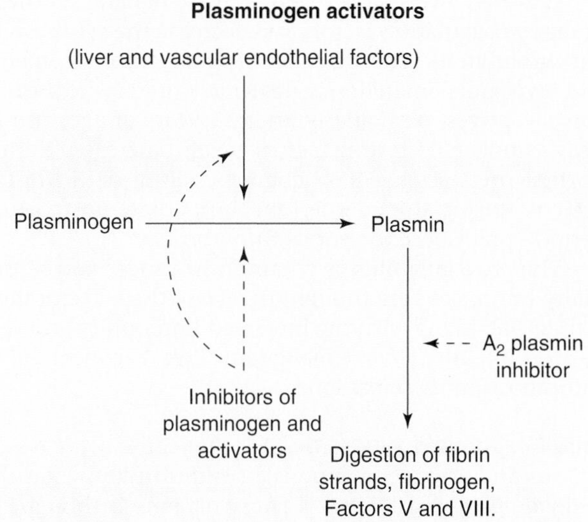

FIGURE 15-5 Fibrinolytic system and its modifiers. The *solid lines* indicate activation, and the *broken lines* indicate inactivation.

It is converted to its active form, plasmin, by plasminogen activators formed in the vascular endothelium, liver, and kidneys. The plasmin formed from plasminogen digests the fibrin strands of the clot and certain clotting factors, such as fibrinogen, factor V, factor VIII, prothrombin, and factor XII. Circulating plasmin is rapidly inactivated by α_2-plasmin inhibitor, which limits fibrinolysis to the local clot and prevents it from occurring in the entire circulation.

Two naturally occurring plasminogen activators are tissue-type plasminogen activator and urokinase-type plasminogen activator. The liver, plasma, and vascular endothelium are the major sources of physiologic activators. These activators are released in response to a number of stimuli, including vasoactive drugs, venous occlusion, elevated body temperature, and exercise. The activators are unstable and rapidly inactivated by inhibitors synthesized by the endothelium and the liver. For this reason, chronic liver disease may cause altered fibrinolytic activity. A major inhibitor, plasminogen activator inhibitor-1, in high concentrations has been associated with deep vein thrombosis, coronary artery disease, and myocardial infarction.[4]

In summary, hemostasis is designed to maintain the integrity of the vascular compartment. The process is divided into five phases: vessel spasm, which constricts the size of the vessel and reduces blood flow; platelet adherence and formation of the platelet plug; formation of the fibrin clot, which cements the platelet plug together; clot retraction, which pulls the edges of the injured vessel together; and clot dissolution, which involves the action of plasmin that dissolves the clot and allows blood flow to be reestablished and tissue healing to take place. Blood coagulation requires the stepwise activation of coagulation factors, carefully controlled by activators and inhibitors.

Hypercoagulability States

After completing this section of the chapter, you should be able to meet the following objectives:

- Compare normal and abnormal clotting
- State the causes and effects of increased platelet function
- State two conditions that contribute to increased clotting activity

There are two general forms of hypercoagulability states: conditions that create increased platelet function and conditions that cause accelerated activity of the coagulation system. Hypercoagulability represents hemostasis in an exaggerated form and predisposes to thrombosis. Arterial thrombi due to turbulence are composed of platelet aggregates, and venous thrombi due to stasis are largely composed of platelet aggregates and fibrin complexes that result from excess coagulation. Chart 15-1 summarizes conditions commonly associated with hypercoagulability states.

INCREASED PLATELET FUNCTION

Increased platelet function results in platelet adhesion, formation of platelet clots, and the disruption of blood flow. The causes of increased platelet function are disturbances in flow, endothelial damage, and increased sensitivity of platelets to factors that cause adhesiveness and aggregation. Atherosclerotic plaques disturb flow, cause endothelial damage, and promote platelet adherence. Platelets that adhere to the vessel wall release growth factors that cause proliferation of smooth muscle and thereby contribute to the development of atherosclerosis. Smoking, elevated levels of blood lipids and cholesterol, hemodynamic stress, diabetes mellitus, and immune mechanisms may cause vessel damage, platelet adherence, and, eventually, thrombosis. The term *thrombocytosis* is used to describe elevations in the platelet count above 1,000,000/mm^3. This occurs in some malignancies, in chronic inflammatory states, and after splenectomy. Myeloproliferative disorders

CHART 15-1

Conditions Associated With Hypercoagulability States

Increased Platelet Function

Atherosclerosis
Diabetes mellitus
Smoking
Elevated blood lipid and cholesterol levels
Increased platelet levels

Accelerated Activity of the Clotting System

Pregnancy and the puerperium
Use of oral contraceptives
Postsurgical state
Immobility
Congestive heart failure
Malignant diseases

HYPERCOAGULABILITY STATES

- Hypercoagulability states increase the risk of clot or thrombus formation in either the arterial or venous circulations.
- Arterial thrombi are associated with conditions that produce turbulent blood flow and platelet adherence.
- Venous thrombi are associated with conditions that cause stasis of blood flow with increased concentrations of coagulation factors.

such as polycythemia vera produce excess platelets that may predispose to thrombosis or, paradoxically, bleeding when the rapidly produced platelets are defective.

INCREASED CLOTTING ACTIVITY

Thrombus formation due to activation of the coagulation system can result from primary (genetic) or secondary (acquired) disorders affecting the coagulation components of the blood (*i.e.,* an increase in procoagulation factors or a decrease in anticoagulation factors).

Inherited Disorders

Of the inherited causes of hyperactivity, mutations in the factor V gene and prothrombin gene are the most common.[3] In persons with inherited defects in factor V, the mutant factor Va cannot be inactivated by protein C; as a result, an important antithrombotic counterregulatory mechanism is lost. Approximately 2% to 15% of the white population carries a specific factor V mutation (referred to as the Leiden mutation, because of the Dutch city where it was first discovered).[3] The defect predisposes to venous thrombosis; and among patients with recurrent deep vein thrombosis, the frequency of the mutation is even higher. Less common primary hypercoagulable states include inherited deficiencies of anticoagulants such as antithrombin III, protein C, and protein S.[3] Another hereditary defect results in high circulating levels of homocysteine and also predisposes to venous and arterial thrombosis by activating platelets and altering antithrombotic mechanisms.[3]

Acquired Disorders

Among the acquired or secondary factors that lead to increased coagulation and thrombosis are stasis due to prolonged bed rest or immobilization, myocardial infarction, cancer, hyperestrogenic states, and oral contraceptives. Smoking and obesity promote hypercoagulability for unknown reasons.

Stasis causes the accumulation of activated clotting factors and platelets and prevents their interactions with inhibitors. Slow and disturbed flow is a common cause of venous thrombosis in the immobilized or postsurgical patient. Heart failure also contributes to venous congestion and thrombosis. Hyperviscosity syndromes (polycythemia) and deformed red cells in sickle cell anemia increase the resistance to flow and cause small vessel stasis.

Elevated levels of estrogen increase hepatic synthesis of many coagulation factors and decrease the synthesis of antithrombin III.[5] The incidence of stroke, thromboemboli, and myocardial infarction is greater in women who use oral contraceptives, particularly after 35 years of age, and in heavy smokers.[5] Clotting factors are also increased during normal pregnancy. These changes, along with limited activity during the puerperium (immediate postpartum period), predispose to venous thrombosis.

Hypercoagulability is common in cancer and sepsis. Many tumor cells are thought to release tissue factor molecules that, along with the increased immobility and sepsis seen in patients with malignant disease, contribute to thrombosis in these patients.

Antiphospholipid Syndrome. Another cause of increased venous and arterial clotting is a condition known as the *antiphospholipid syndrome.*[6,7] The syndrome is thought to be an autoimmune hypercoagulability disorder characterized by antiphospholipid antibodies and at least one clinical manifestation, the most common being venous and arterial thrombosis and recurrent fetal loss. The disorder can manifest as a primary condition occurring in isolation with signs of hypercoagulability or as a secondary condition usually associated with systemic lupus erythematosus. The most common manifestation is thrombosis that may affect many organs. Venous thrombosis of the lower leg occurs in up to 55% of persons with the condition, and half of those develop pulmonary emboli. Arterial thrombosis in the brain affects 50% of individuals and is associated with transient ischemic attacks or strokes.[5]

Women with the disorder commonly have a history of recurrent pregnancy losses after the tenth week of gestation because of ischemia and thrombosis of the placental vessels. These women are at increased risk for giving birth to a premature infant because of pregnancy-associated hypertension and uteroplacental insufficiency.

In most persons with antiphospholipid syndrome, the thrombotic events occur as a single episode at one anatomic site. In some persons, recurrences may occur months or years later and mimic the initial event. Occasionally, someone may present with multiple vascular occlusions involving many organ systems. This rapid-onset condition is termed *catastrophic antiphospholipid syndrome* and is associated with high mortality.

The mechanisms for the syndrome are unknown; however, several potential pathways have been identified.[6,7] One is that the antibodies may directly interfere with regulation of the coagulation cascade, leading to hypercoagulability. Examples include inhibition of activated protein C and antithrombin pathways, inhibition of fibrinolysis, or upregulation of tissue factor activation. The second implicates activation of endothelial cells. Antibody binding to endothelial cells may cause secretion of cytokines that promote coagulation and platelet aggregation. Finally, it is likely that other factors may be required before clinical manifestations of the syndrome develop. This may include traumatic injury to the vascular bed, the generation of nonimmunologic procoagulation factors, or the presence of infection leading to cytokine production and endothelial cell activation.[6,7]

Treatment focuses on removal or reduction in factors that predispose to thrombosis, including advice to stop smoking and counseling against use of estrogen-containing oral contraceptives by women. The acute thrombotic event is treated with anticoagulants (heparin and warfarin) and immune suppression in refractory cases. Aspirin and anticoagulant drugs may be used to prevent future thrombosis.

In summary, hypercoagulability causes excessive clotting and contributes to thrombus formation. It results from conditions that create increased platelet function or that cause accelerated activity of the coagulation system. Increased platelet function usually results from disorders such as atherosclerosis that damage the vessel endothelium and disturb blood flow or from conditions such as smoking that cause increased sensitivity of platelets to factors that promote adhesiveness and aggregation. Factors that cause accelerated activity of the coagulation system include blood flow stasis, resulting in an accumulation of coagulation factors, and alterations in the components of the coagulation system (*i.e.*, an increase in procoagulation factors or a decrease in anticoagulation factors). The antiphospholipid syndrome is another cause of venous and arterial clotting and is manifest as a primary disorder or a secondary disorder associated with systemic lupus erythematosus. It is associated with antiphospholipid antibodies that promote thrombosis and that can affect many organs.

Bleeding Disorders

After completing this section of the chapter, you should be able to meet the following objectives:

- State the mechanisms of drug-induced thrombocytopenia and idiopathic thrombocytopenia and the differing features in terms of onset and resolution of the disorders
- Describe the manifestations of thrombocytopenia
- Describe the role of vitamin K in coagulation
- State three common defects of coagulation factors and the causes of each
- Differentiate between the mechanisms of bleeding in hemophilia A and von Willebrand disease
- Describe the physiologic basis of acute disseminated intravascular coagulation
- Describe the effect of vascular disorders on hemostasis

Bleeding disorders or impairment of blood coagulation can result from defects in any of the factors that contribute to hemostasis. Defects are associated with platelets, coagulation factors, and vascular integrity.

PLATELET DEFECTS

Bleeding can occur as a result of a decrease in the number of circulating platelets or impaired platelet function. The depletion of platelets must be relatively severe (10,000 to 20,000/mL, compared with the normal values of 150,000 to 400,000/mL) before hemorrhagic tendencies or spontaneous bleeding becomes evident. Bleeding that results from platelet deficiency commonly occurs in small vessels and is characterized by petechiae (*i.e.*, pinpoint purplish-red spots) and purpura (*i.e.*, purple areas of bruising) on the arms and thighs. Bleeding from mucous membranes of the nose, mouth, gastrointestinal tract, and vagina is characteristic. Bleeding of the intracranial vessels is a rare danger with severe platelet depletion.

BLEEDING DISORDERS

- Bleeding disorders are caused by defects associated with platelets, coagulation factors, and vessel integrity.
- Disorders of platelet plug formation include a decrease in platelet numbers due to inadequate platelet production (bone marrow dysfunction), excess platelet destruction (thrombocytopenia), abnormal platelet function (thrombocytopathia), or defects in von Willebrand factor.
- Impairment of the coagulation stage of hemostasis is caused by a deficiency in one or more of the clotting factors.
- Disorders of blood vessel integrity result from structurally weak vessels or vessel damage due to inflammation and immune mechanisms.

Thrombocytopenia

Thrombocytopenia is a decrease in the number of circulating platelets to a level less than 100,000/mL. It can result from a decrease in platelet production by the bone marrow, an increased pooling of platelets in the spleen, or decreased platelet survival due to immune destruction or nonimmune mechanisms. Massive blood or plasma transfusions may cause a dilutional thrombocytopenia because blood stored for more than 24 hours has no viable platelets.

Loss of bone marrow function in aplastic anemia (see Chapter 16) or replacement of bone marrow by malignant cells, such as occurs in leukemia, results in decreased production of platelets. Infection with human immunodeficiency virus (HIV) suppresses the production of megakaryocytes, the platelet precursors. Radiation therapy and drugs such as those used in the treatment of cancer may depress bone marrow function and reduce platelet production.

There may be normal production of platelets but excessive pooling of platelets in the spleen. The spleen normally sequesters approximately 30% to 40% of the platelets before release into the circulation. However, when the spleen is enlarged, as in *splenomegaly,* as many as 80% of the platelets can be sequestered in the spleen. Splenomegaly also occurs in cirrhosis with portal hypertension and in lymphomas.

Reduced platelet survival occurs by a variety of immune and nonimmune mechanisms. Platelet destruction may be caused by antiplatelet antibodies. The antibodies may be directed against the platelet self-antigens or against antigens on the platelets from blood transfusions or during pregnancy. The antibodies target the platelet membrane glycoproteins. Nonimmune destruction of platelets results from mechanical injury due to prosthetic heart valves or malignant hypertension that results in small vessel narrowing. In acute DIC or thrombotic thrombocytopenic purpura (TTP), excessive platelet consumption leads to a deficiency.

Drug-induced Thrombocytopenia. Some drugs, such as quinine, quinidine, and certain sulfa-containing antibiotics, may induce thrombocytopenia. These drugs act as haptens and induce an antigen–antibody response and formation of immune complexes that cause platelet destruction by complement-mediated lysis (see Chapter 19). In persons with drug-associated thrombocytopenia, there is a rapid fall in platelet count within 2 to 3 days of resuming a drug or 7 or more days (*i.e.,* the time needed to mount an immune response) after starting a drug for the first time. The platelet count rises rapidly after the drug is discontinued. The anticoagulant drug heparin has been increasingly implicated in thrombocytopenia and, paradoxically, in thrombosis. The complications typically occur 5 days after the start of therapy and result from heparin-dependent antiplatelet antibodies that cause aggregation of platelets and their removal from the circulation. The antibodies often bind to vessel walls, causing thrombosis and complications such as stroke and myocardial infarction. The newer low-molecular-weight heparin has been shown to be effective in reducing the incidence of heparin-induced complications compared with the older high-molecular-weight form of the drug.[8]

Idiopathic Thrombocytopenic Purpura. Idiopathic thrombocytopenic purpura (ITP), an autoimmune disorder, results in platelet antibody formation and excess destruction of platelets. The immunoglobulin G (IgG) antibody commonly binds to two identified membrane glycoproteins (GpIIb/IIIa and GpIb/IX) while in the circulation. The platelets, which are made more susceptible to phagocytosis because of the antibody, are destroyed in the spleen and the liver.

Half of the cases of ITP occur as an acute disorder in children, affecting both boys and girls.[9] The disorder occurs in young children and usually follows a viral infection. It is characterized by sudden onset of petechiae and purpura and is a self-limited disorder with no treatment. Most children recover in a few weeks. In contrast, ITP in adults is a chronic disorder with insidious onset and seldom follows an infection. It is a disease of young people, with a peak incidence between the ages of 18 and 40 years, and is seen twice as often in women as in men. Secondary forms of ITP may be associated with acquired immunodeficiency syndrome (AIDS), systemic lupus erythematosus, antiphospholipid syndrome, lymphoproliferative disorders, hepatitis C, and drugs such as heparin and quinidine. The condition may be discovered incidentally or as a result of bleeding, often into the skin (*i.e.,* purpura and petechiae) or oral mucosa. There is commonly a history of bruising, bleeding from gums, epistaxis (*i.e.,* nosebleeds), and abnormal menstrual bleeding in those with moderately reduced platelet counts. Half of the persons with ITP have platelet counts less than 10,000/mL and are at risk for internal bleeding. Because the spleen is the site of platelet destruction, splenic enlargement may occur.

Diagnosis usually is based on severe thrombocytopenia (platelet count <20,000/mL), and exclusion of other causes. Tests for the platelet-bound antibodies are available but lack specificity (*e.g.,* they react with platelet antibodies from other sources). Treatment includes the initial use of corticosteroid drugs, intravenous immune globulin, and splenectomy for those who relapse or do not respond to drugs.[9]

Thrombotic Thrombocytopenic Purpura. Thrombotic thrombocytopenic purpura is a combination of thrombocytopenia, hemolytic anemia, renal failure, fever, and neurologic abnormalities. It is a rare disorder occurring predominately in adult women. The onset is abrupt, and the outcome may be fatal. Widespread vascular occlusions consist of thrombi in arterioles and capillaries of many organs, including the heart, brain, and kidneys. Erythrocytes become fragmented as they circulate through the partly occluded vessels and cause the hemolytic anemia and jaundice. The clinical manifestations include purpura, petechiae, and vaginal bleeding and neurologic symptoms ranging from headache to seizures and altered consciousness. TTP is probably caused by widespread endothelial damage and activation of intravascular thrombosis. The disorder is similar to DIC but does not involve the clotting system. The inciting agent of TTP is unknown but may be viral in origin. Toxins produced by some strains of *Escherichia coli* (*e.g., E. coli* O157:H7) cause endothelial injury and are responsible for a similar condition, *hemolytic uremic syndrome* (see Chapter 39).

Treatment for TTP includes *plasmapheresis,* a procedure that involves removal of plasma from withdrawn blood and replacement with fresh-frozen plasma. The treatment is continued until remission occurs. With plasmapheresis treatment, there is a complete recovery in 80% to 90% of cases.

Impaired Platelet Function

Impaired platelet function (also called *thrombocytopathia*) may result from inherited disorders of adhesion (*e.g.,* von Willebrand disease) or acquired defects caused by drugs, disease, or extracorporeal circulation. Defective platelet function is also common in uremia, presumably because of unexcreted waste products. Cardiopulmonary bypass also causes platelet defects and destruction.

The use of aspirin and other nonsteroidal antiinflammatory drugs (NSAIDs) is the most common cause of impaired platelet function. Aspirin produces irreversible acetylation of platelet cyclooxygenase activity and consequently the synthesis of prostaglandin TXA_2, which is required for platelet aggregation. The effect of aspirin on platelet aggregation lasts for the life of the platelet—usually approximately 8 to 9 days. In contrast to the effects of aspirin, the inhibition of cyclooxygenase by other NSAIDs is reversible and lasts only for the duration of drug action.[10]

CHART 15-2

Drugs That May Predispose to Bleeding

Interference With Platelet Production or Function

Acetazolamide
Alcohol
Antimetabolite and anticancer drugs
Antibiotics such as penicillin and the cephalosporins
Aspirin and salicylates
Carbamazepine
Clofibrate
Colchicine
Dextran
Dipyridamole
Thiazide diuretics
Gold salts
Heparin
Nonsteroidal anti-inflammatory drugs
Quinine derivatives (quinidine and hydroxychloroquine)
Sulfinpyrazone
Sulfonamides

Interference With Coagulation Factors

Amiodarone
Anabolic steroids
Warfarin
Heparin

Decrease in Vitamin K Levels

Antibiotics
Clofibrate

Aspirin (81 mg daily) commonly is used to prevent formation of arterial thrombi and reduce the risk for heart attack and stroke. Chart 15-2 lists other drugs that impair platelet function.

COAGULATION DEFECTS

Blood coagulation defects can result from deficiencies or impairment of one or more of the clotting factors. Deficiencies can arise because of defective synthesis, inherited disease, or increased consumption of the clotting factors. Bleeding that results from clotting factor deficiency typically occurs after injury or trauma. Large bruises, hematomas, or prolonged bleeding into the gastrointestinal or urinary tracts or joints is common.

Impaired Synthesis of Coagulation Factors

Coagulation factors V, VII, IX, X, XI, and XII, prothrombin, and fibrinogen are synthesized in the liver. In liver disease, synthesis of these clotting factors is reduced, and bleeding may result. Of the coagulation factors synthesized in the liver, factors VII, IX, and X and prothrombin require the presence of vitamin K for normal activity. In vitamin K deficiency, the liver produces the clotting factor, but in an inactive form. Vitamin K is a fat-soluble vitamin that is continuously being synthesized by intestinal bacteria. This means that a deficiency in vitamin K is not likely to occur unless intestinal synthesis is interrupted or absorption of the vitamin is impaired. Vitamin K deficiency can occur in the newborn infant before the establishment of the intestinal flora; it can also occur as a result of treatment with broad-spectrum antibiotics that destroy intestinal flora. Because vitamin K is a fat-soluble vitamin, its absorption requires bile salts. Vitamin K deficiency may result from impaired fat absorption caused by liver or gallbladder disease.

Hereditary Disorders

Hereditary defects have been reported for each of the clotting factors, but most are rare diseases. The most common bleeding disorders involve the factor VIII–vWF complex. Factor VIII deficiency (hemophilia A) affects 1 in 5000 male live births, and von Willebrand disease may affect more than 1 in 1000.[11] Factor IX deficiency (*i.e.,* hemophilia B) occurs in approximately 1 in 30,000 persons and is genetically and clinically similar to hemophilia A.

Circulating factor VIII is part of a complex molecule, bound to vWF. Factor VIII coagulant protein is the functional portion produced by the liver and endothelial cells. vWF, synthesized by the endothelium and megakaryocytes, binds and stabilizes factor VIII in the circulation by preventing proteolysis. It is also required for platelet adhesion to the subendothelial layer.

Hemophilia A. Hemophilia A is an X-linked recessive disorder that primarily affects males. Although it is a hereditary disorder, there is no family history of the disorder in approximately 30% of newly diagnosed cases, suggesting that it has arisen as a new mutation in the factor VIII gene.[11] Approximately 90% of persons with hemophilia produce insufficient quantities of the factor, and 10% produce a defective form. The percentage of normal factor VIII activity in the circulation depends on the genetic defect and determines the severity of hemophilia (*i.e.,* 6% to 30% in mild hemophilia, 2% to 5% in moderate hemophilia, and 1% or less in severe forms of hemophilia). In mild or moderate forms of the disease, bleeding usually does not occur unless there is a local lesion or trauma such as surgery or dental procedures. The mild disorder may not be detected in childhood. In severe hemophilia, bleeding usually occurs in childhood (*e.g.,* it may be noticed at the time of circumcision) and is spontaneous and severe, often occurring several times a month.

Characteristically, bleeding occurs in soft tissues, the gastrointestinal tract, and the hip, knee, elbow, and ankle joints. Joint bleeding usually begins when a child begins to walk. Often, a target joint is prone to repeated bleeding. The bleeding causes inflammation of the synovium, with acute pain and swelling. Without proper treatment, chronic bleeding and inflammation cause joint fibrosis and contractures, resulting in major disability. Muscle hematomas may be present in 30% of episodes, and intracranial hemorrhage is an important cause of death.[12]

Factor VIII replacement therapy administered at home has reduced the typical musculoskeletal damage. It is initiated when bleeding occurs or as prophylaxis with repeated bleeding episodes. Highly purified factor VIII and factor IX concentrates prepared from human plasma are the usual replacement products for persons with severe hemophilia. Before blood was tested for infectious diseases, these products were prepared from multiple donor samples and carried a high risk for exposure to viruses for hepatitis and AIDS. Sixty to 70% of persons treated with the older plasma-derived products developed HIV or chronic hepatitis B or C, leading to complications such as Kaposi's sarcoma, non-Hodgkin's lymphoma, cirrhosis, or hepatocellular carcinoma.[11] Effective donor screening and the development of purification and viral-inactivation procedures now provide a safer product.

Factor VIII produced by recombinant DNA technology has been available since the early 1990s and does not have the potential for transmitting viral disease. It is costly, however, which prevents its widespread use. The development of inhibitory antibodies to recombinant factor VIII is still a major complication of treatment. Ten to fifteen percent of treated persons produce high titers of antibodies. The rate of antibody production for plasma-derived products is about the same. New preparations of recombinant factor VIII that contain no human or animal protein to incite antibody formation are now in clinical trials.[11] The newer recombinant products and continuous-infusion pumps may allow prevention rather than therapy for hemorrhage.

The cloning of the factor VIII gene and progress in gene delivery systems have led to the hope that hemophilia A may be cured by gene replacement therapy. Currently, clinical trials present encouraging data. Carrier detection and prenatal diagnosis can now be done by analysis of direct gene mutation or DNA linkage studies. Prenatal amniocentesis or chorionic villus sampling is used to predict complications and determine therapy. It may eventually be used to select patients for gene addition.

Von Willebrand Disease. Von Willebrand disease, which typically is diagnosed in adulthood, is the most common hereditary bleeding disorder. Transmitted as an autosomal trait, it is caused by a deficiency of or defect in vWF. This deficiency results in reduced platelet adhesion. There are many variants of the disease, and manifestations range from mild to severe. Because vWF carries factor VIII, its deficiency may also be accompanied by reduced levels of factor VIII and results in defective clot formation. Symptoms include bruising, excessive menstrual flow, and bleeding from the nose, mouth, and gastrointestinal tract. Many persons with the disorder are diagnosed when surgery or dental extraction results in prolonged bleeding. Most cases are mild and untreated. In severe cases, life-threatening gastrointestinal bleeding and joint hemorrhage may be similar to hemophilia.

Treatment of all forms of the disease includes factor VIII products that contain vWF. The disorder also responds to desmopressin acetate (DDAVP), a synthetic analog of the hormone vasopressin, which stimulates the endothelial cells to release vWF and plasminogen activator. DDAVP can also be used to treat mild hemophilia A and platelet dysfunction caused by uremia, heart bypass, and the effects of aspirin.[13]

DISSEMINATED INTRAVASCULAR COAGULATION

Disseminated intravascular coagulation is a paradox in the hemostatic sequence and is characterized by widespread coagulation and bleeding in the vascular compartment. It is not a primary disease but occurs as a complication of a wide variety of conditions. DIC begins with massive activation of the coagulation sequence as a result of unregulated generation of thrombin, resulting in systemic formation of fibrin. In addition, levels of all the major anticoagulants are reduced (Fig. 15-6). The microthrombi that result cause vessel occlusion and tissue ischemia. Multiple organ failure may ensue. Clot formation consumes all available coagulation proteins and platelets, and severe hemorrhage results.

The disorder can be initiated by activation of the intrinsic or extrinsic pathways. Activation through the extrinsic pathway occurs with liberation of tissue factors, as in obstetric complications, trauma, bacterial sepsis, and cancers. The intrinsic pathway may be activated through extensive endothelial damage caused by viruses, infections, immune mechanisms, stasis of blood, or temperature extremes. Common clinical conditions that may cause DIC include obstetrical disorders, massive trauma, shock, infections, and malignant disease. Chart 15-3 summarizes the conditions associated with DIC.

The factors involved in the conditions that cause DIC are often interrelated. In obstetrical complications, tissue factors released from necrotic placental or fetal tissue or amniotic fluid may enter the circulation, inciting the DIC. Hypoxia, shock, and acidosis that may coexist also contribute by causing endothelial injury. Gram-negative bacterial infections result in the release of endotoxins, which activate both the extrinsic pathway by release of tissue factor and the intrinsic pathway through endothelial damage. Endotoxins also inhibit the activity of protein C, an anticoagulant. Antigen–antibody complexes associated with infection can activate platelets through complement fragments.[14]

There is increasing evidence that the underlying cause of DIC is infection or inflammation and the cytokines liberated in the process are the pivotal mediators.[15] Cytokines and endotoxins activate the fibrinolytic system early in DIC. They later activate the coagulation system and inhibit fibrinolysis, causing a procoagulant state.[16]

Although coagulation and formation of microemboli characterize DIC, its acute manifestations usually are more directly related to the bleeding problems that occur. The bleeding may be present as petechiae, purpura, oozing from puncture sites, or severe hemorrhage. Uncontrolled postpartum bleeding may indicate DIC. Microemboli may obstruct blood vessels and cause tissue hypoxia and necrotic damage to organ structures, such as the kidneys, heart, lungs, and brain. As a result, common clinical signs may be due to renal, circulatory or respiratory failure, or convulsions and coma. A form of hemolytic anemia may develop as red cells are damaged as they pass through vessels partially blocked by thrombus.

The treatment of DIC is directed toward managing the primary disease, replacing clotting components, and pre-

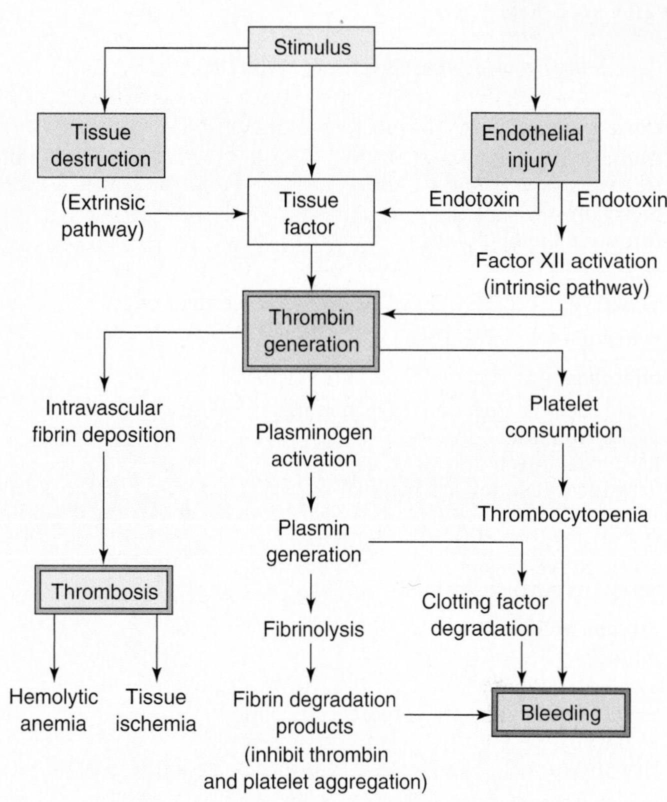

FIGURE 15-6 Pathophysiology of disseminated intravascular coagulation.

venting further activation of clotting mechanisms. Transfusions of fresh-frozen plasma, platelets, or fibrinogen-containing cryoprecipitate may correct the clotting factor deficiency. Heparin may be given to decrease blood coagulation, thereby interrupting the clotting process. Heparin therapy is controversial, however, and the risk for hemorrhage may limit its use to severe cases. It typically is given as a continuous intravenous infusion that can be interrupted promptly if bleeding is accentuated. Tissue factor pathway inhibitors, antithrombin, and protein C concentrates are being evaluated as potential therapies.[15]

VASCULAR DISORDERS

Bleeding from small blood vessels may result from vascular disorders. These disorders may occur because of structurally weak vessel walls or because of damage to vessels by inflammation or immune responses. Among the vascular disorders that cause bleeding are hemorrhagic telangiectasia, an uncommon autosomal dominant disorder characterized by thin-walled, dilated capillaries and arterioles; vitamin C deficiency (*i.e.*, scurvy), resulting in poor collagen synthesis and failure of the endothelial cells to be cemented together properly, which causes a fragile wall; Cushing's disease, causing protein wasting and loss of vessel tissue support because of excess cortisol; and senile purpura (*i.e.*, bruising in elderly persons) caused by the aging process. Vascular defects also occur in the course of DIC as a result of the presence of microthrombi and corticosteroid therapy.

Vascular disorders are characterized by easy bruising and the spontaneous appearance of petechiae and purpura of the skin and mucous membranes. In persons with bleeding disorders caused by vascular defects, the platelet count and results of other tests for coagulation factors are normal.

In summary, bleeding disorders or impairment of blood coagulation can result from defects in any of the factors that contribute to hemostasis: platelets, coagulation factors, or vascular integrity. The number of circulating platelets can be decreased (*i.e.*, thrombocytopenia), or platelet function can be impaired (*i.e.*, thrombocytopathia). Impairment of blood coagulation can result from deficiencies of one or more of the known clotting factors. Deficiencies can arise because of defective synthesis (*i.e.*, liver disease or vitamin K deficiency), inherited diseases (*i.e.*, hemophilia A or von Willebrand disease), or increased consumption of the clotting factors (DIC). Bleeding may also occur from structurally weak vessels that result from impaired synthesis of vessel wall components (*i.e.*, vitamin C deficiency, excessive cortisol levels as in Cushing's disease, or the aging process) or from damage by genetic mechanisms (*i.e.*, hemorrhagic telangiectasia) or the presence of microthrombi.

CHART 15-3

Conditions That Have Been Associated With DIC

Obstetric Conditions

Abruptio placentae
Dead fetus syndrome
Preeclampsia and eclampsia
Amniotic fluid embolism

Cancers

Metastatic cancer
Leukemia

Infections

Acute bacterial infections (*e.g.*, meningococcal meningitis)
Acute viral infections
Rickettsial infections (*e.g.*, Rocky Mountain spotted fever)
Parasitic infection (*e.g.*, malaria)

Shock

Septic shock
Severe hypovolemic shock

Trauma or Surgery

Burns
Massive trauma
Surgery involving extracorporeal circulation
Snake bite
Heatstroke

Hematologic Conditions

Blood transfusion reactions

REVIEW EXERCISES

A 55-year-old man has begun taking one 81-mg aspirin tablet daily on the recommendation of his physician. The physician told him that this would help to prevent heart attack and stroke.

A. What is the action of aspirin in terms of heart attack and stroke prevention?

The drug DDAVP increases the half-life of factor VIII and is sometimes used to treat bleeding in males with mild hemophilia A.

A. Explain.

A 29-year-old new mother, who delivered her baby 3 days ago, is admitted to the emergency department with chest pain and is diagnosed as having venous thrombosis with pulmonary emboli.

A. What factors would contribute to this woman's risk for developing thromboemboli?

B. She is admitted to the intensive care unit and started on low-molecular-weight heparin and warfarin. She is told that she will be discharged in 1 or 2 days and will remain on the heparin for 5 days and the warfarin for at least 3 months. Use Figure 15-4 to explain the action of heparin and warfarin. Why is heparin administered for 5 days during the initiation of warfarin?

C. Anticoagulation with the heparin and warfarin is not a definitive treatment for clot removal in pulmonary emboli, but a form of secondary prevention. Explain.

References

1. Guyton A. C., Hall J. E. (2000). *Textbook of medical physiology* (10th ed., pp. 419–429). Philadelphia: W. B. Saunders.
2. Kaushansky K. (1998). Thrombopoietin. *New England Journal of Medicine 339,* 746–754.
3. Mitchell R. N., Cotran R. (2003). Hemodynamic disorders, thrombosis, and shock. In Kumar V., Cotran R. S., Robbins S. L. *Basic pathology* (7th ed., pp.79–95). Philadelphia: W. B. Saunders.
4. Kohler H. P., Grant P. J. (2000). Plasminogen-activator inhibitor type 1 and coronary artery disease. *New England Journal of Medicine 342,* 1792–1801.
5. Chrousos G. P., Zoumakis E. N., Gravania A. (2001). The gonadal hormones and inhibitors. In Katzung B. G. (Ed.), *Basic and clinical pharmacology* (8th ed., p. 683–684). Norwalk, CT: Appleton & Lange.
6. Levine J. S., Branch D. W., Rausch J. (2002). The antiphospholipid syndrome. *New England Journal of Medicine 346*(10), 752–763.
7. Hanly J. C. (2003). Antiphospholipid syndrome: an overview. *Canadian Medical Association Journal 168*(13), 1675–1682.
8. Warkentin T. E., Chong B. H., Greinacher A. (1998). Heparin-induced thrombocytopenia: Towards consensus. *Thrombosis and Haemostasis 79,* 1–7.
9. Cines D. B., Blanchette V. S. (2002). Immune thrombocytopenic purpura. *New England Journal of Medicine 346,* 995–1008.
10. George J. N., Shattil S. J. (2000). Acquired disorders of platelet function. In Hoffman R., Benz E. J., Shattil S. J., et al. (Eds.), *Hematology* (3rd ed., p. 2176). New York: Churchill Livingstone.
11. Mannucci P. M., Tuddenham E. G. D. (2001). The hemophilias—from royal genes to gene therapy. *New England Journal of Medicine 344,* 1773–1779.
12. Klinge J., Ananyeva N. M., Hauser C., Saenko E. L. (2002). Hemophilia A—from basic science to clinical practice. *Seminars in Thrombosis and Hemostasis 28,* 309–322.
13. Mannucci P. M. (1997). Desmopressin (DDAVP) in the treatment of bleeding disorders: The first 20 years. *Blood 90,* 2515–2521.
14. Cotran R. S. (1999). Red cells and bleeding disorders. In Cotran R. S., Kumar V., Collins T. (Eds.) *Robbins pathologic basis of disease* (6th ed., p. 641). Philadelphia: W. B. Saunders.
15. Levi M., Jonge E., van der Poll T., ten Cate H. (2001). Advances in the understanding of the pathogenetic pathways of disseminated intravascular coagulation result in more insight in the clinical picture and better management strategies. *Seminars in Thrombosis and Hemostasis 27,* 569–575.
16. Van der Poll T., Jonge E., Levi M. (2001). Regulatory role of cytokines in disseminated intravascular coagulation. *Seminars in Thrombosis and Hemostasis 27,* 639–651.

CHAPTER

16

Red Blood Cell Disorders

Kathryn J. Gaspard

Although the lungs provide the means for gas exchange between the external and internal environments, it is the hemoglobin in the red blood cells that transports oxygen to the tissues. The red blood cells also function as carriers of carbon dioxide and participate in acid-base balance. The function of the red blood cells, in terms of oxygen transport, is discussed in Chapter 29, and acid-base balance is covered in Chapter 34. This chapter focuses on the red blood cell, anemia, and polycythemia.

The Red Blood Cell

After completing this section of the chapter, you should be able to meet the following objectives:

- Trace the development of a red blood cell from erythroblast to erythrocyte
- Discuss the function of iron in the formation of hemoglobin
- Describe the formation, transport, and elimination of bilirubin
- Explain the function of the enzyme glucose-6-phosphate dehydrogenase in the red blood cell
- State the meaning of the red blood cell count, percentage of reticulocytes, hemoglobin, hematocrit, mean corpuscular volume, and mean corpuscular hemoglobin concentration as it relates to the diagnosis of anemia

The mature red blood cell, the erythrocyte, is a nonnucleated, biconcave disk (Fig. 16-1). This shape increases the surface area available for diffusion of oxygen and allows the cell to change in volume and shape without rupturing its membrane. A complex cytoskeleton, which consists of an insoluble mesh of fibrous proteins attached to the inside of the cell membrane, provides this unique shape and flexibility. The biconcave form presents the plasma with a surface 20 to 30 times greater than if the red blood cell were an absolute sphere. The erythrocytes, 500 to 1000 times more numerous than other blood cells, are the most common type of blood cell.

The function of the red blood cell, facilitated by the hemoglobin molecule, is to transport oxygen to the tissues. Hemoglobin also binds some carbon dioxide and carries it from the tissues to the lungs. The hemoglobin molecule is composed of two pairs of structurally different polypeptide chains (Fig. 16-2). Each of the four polypeptide chains consists of a globin (protein) portion and heme unit, which surrounds an atom of iron that binds oxygen. Thus,

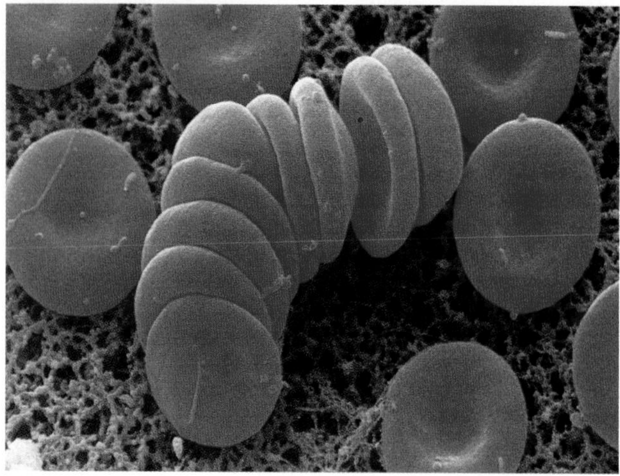

FIGURE 16-1 Scanning micrograph of normal red blood cells shows their normal concave appearance (× 3000). (© Andrew Syred, Science Photo Lab, Science Source/Photo Researchers)

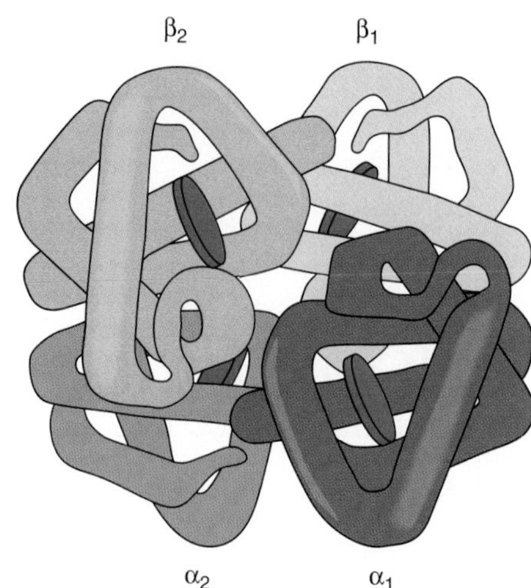

FIGURE 16-2 Structure of the hemoglobin molecule, showing the four subunits.

each molecule of hemoglobin can carry four molecules of oxygen. The production of each type of globin chain is controlled by individual structural genes with five different gene loci. Mutations, which can occur anywhere in these five loci, have resulted in more than 550 types of abnormal hemoglobin molecules.[1]

The two major types of normal hemoglobin are adult hemoglobin (HbA) and fetal hemoglobin (HbF). HbA consists of a pair of α chains and a pair of β chains. HbF is the predominant hemoglobin in the fetus from the third through the ninth month of gestation. It has a pair of γ chains substituted for the α chains. Because of this chain substitution, HbF has a high affinity for oxygen. This facilitates the transfer of oxygen across the placenta. HbF is replaced within 6 months of birth with HbA.

The rate at which hemoglobin is synthesized depends on the availability of iron for heme synthesis. A lack of iron results in relatively small amounts of hemoglobin in the red blood cells. The amount of iron in the body is approximately 35 to 50 mg/kg of body weight for males and less for females. Body iron is found in several compartments. Most iron (80%) is complexed to heme in hemoglobin, with small amounts found in the myoglobin of muscle, the cytochromes, and iron-containing enzymes. Approximately 20% is stored in the bone marrow, liver, spleen, and other organs. Iron in the hemoglobin compartment is recycled. When red blood cells age and are destroyed in the spleen, the iron from their hemoglobin is released into the circulation and returned to the bone marrow for incorporation into new cells or to the liver and other tissues for storage.

Dietary iron also helps to maintain body stores. Iron, principally derived from meat, is absorbed in the small intestine, especially the duodenum (Fig. 16-3). When body stores of iron are diminished or erythropoiesis is stimulated, absorption is increased. In iron overload, excretion of iron is accelerated. Normally, some iron is sequestered in the intestinal epithelial cells and is lost in the feces as these cells slough off. The iron that is absorbed enters the circulation, where it immediately combines with a beta globulin, *apotransferrin,* to form *transferrin,* which is then transported in the plasma. From the plasma, iron can be deposited in tissues such as the liver, where it is stored as *ferritin,* a protein–iron complex, which can easily return to the circulation. Serum ferritin levels, which can be measured in the laboratory, provide an index of body iron stores. Clinically, decreased ferritin levels usually indicate the need for prescription of iron supplements. Transferrin can also deliver iron to the developing red cell in bone marrow by binding to membrane receptors. The iron is taken up by the developing red cell, where it is used in heme synthesis.

RED BLOOD CELLS

- The function of red blood cells, facilitated by the iron-containing hemoglobin molecule, is to transport oxygen from the lungs to the tissues.
- The production of red blood cells, which is regulated by erythropoietin, occurs in the bone marrow and requires iron, vitamin B_{12}, and folate.
- The red blood cell, which has a life span of approximately 120 days, is broken down in the spleen; the degradation products such as iron and amino acids are recycled.
- The heme molecule, which is released from the red blood cell during the degradation process, is converted to bilirubin and transported to the liver, where it is removed and rendered water soluble for elimination in the bile.

RED CELL PRODUCTION

Erythropoiesis is the production of red blood cells. After birth, red cells are produced in the red bone marrow. Until age 5 years, almost all bones produce red cells to meet

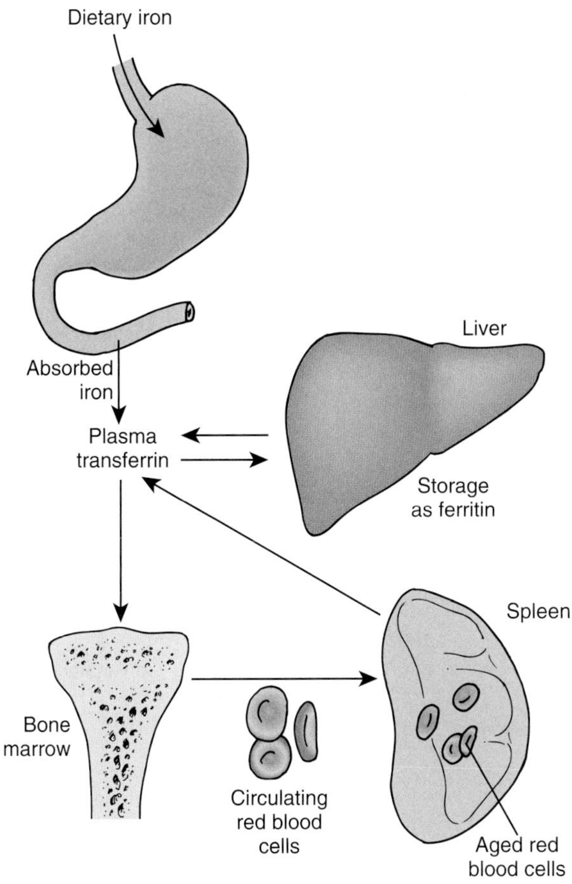

FIGURE 16-3 Iron cycle.

growth needs. After this period, bone marrow activity gradually declines. After 20 years of age, red cell production takes place mainly in the membranous bones of the vertebrae, sternum, ribs, and pelvis. With this reduction in activity, the red bone marrow is replaced with fatty yellow bone marrow.

The red cells are derived from precursor cells called erythroblasts, which are continuously being formed from the pluripotent stem cells in the bone marrow (Fig. 16-4). The red cell precursors move through a series of divisions, each producing a smaller cell as they continue to develop into mature red blood cells. Hemoglobin synthesis begins at the early erythroblast stage and continues until the cell becomes a mature erythrocyte. During its transformation from normoblast to reticulocyte, the red blood cell accumulates hemoglobin as the nucleus condenses and is finally lost. The period from stem cell to emergence of the reticulocyte in the circulation normally takes approximately 1 week. Maturation of reticulocyte to erythrocyte takes approximately 24 to 48 hours. During this process, the red cell loses its mitochondria and ribosomes, along with its ability to produce hemoglobin and engage in oxidative metabolism. Most maturing red cells enter the blood as reticulocytes. Approximately 1% of the body's total complement of red blood cells is generated from bone marrow each day, and the reticulocyte count therefore serves as an index of the erythropoietic activity of the bone marrow.

Erythropoiesis is governed for the most part by tissue oxygen needs. Any condition that causes a decrease in the amount of oxygen that is transported in the blood produces an increase in red cell production. The oxygen content of the blood does not act directly on the bone marrow to stimulate red blood cell production. Instead, the decreased

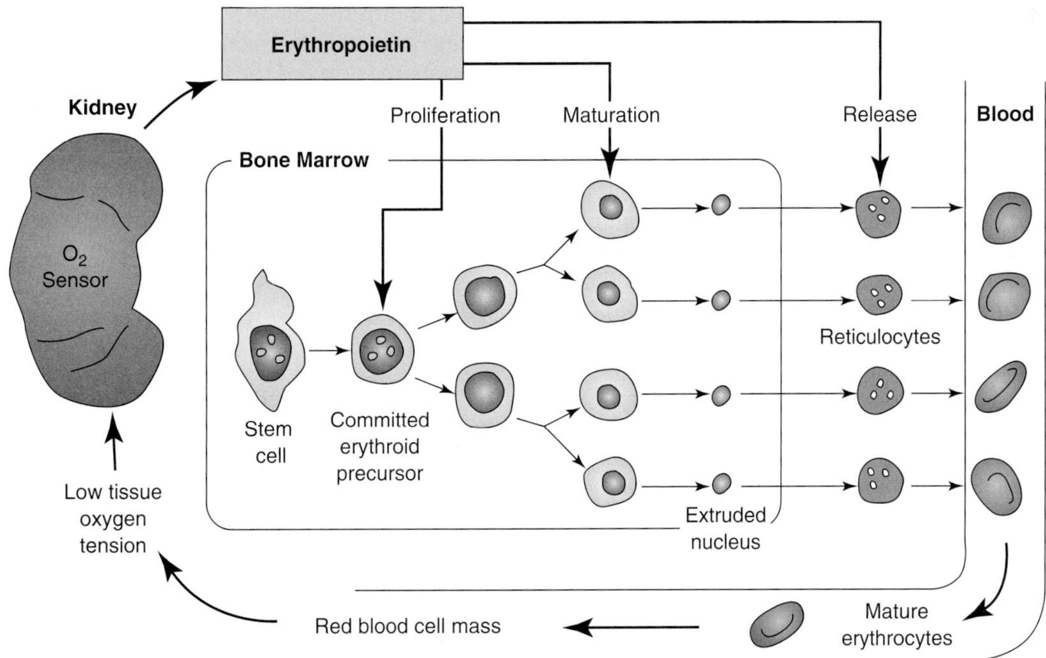

FIGURE 16-4 Red blood cell development.

oxygen content is sensed by the kidneys, which then produce a hormone called *erythropoietin.* Normally, the kidneys produce about 90% of erythropoietin, with the remaining 10% being released from the liver. In the absence of erythropoietin, as in kidney failure, hypoxia has little or no effect on red blood cell production. Erythropoietin takes several days to effect the release of red blood cells from the bone marrow, and only after 5 days or more does red blood cell production reach a maximum.

Erythropoietin acts in the bone marrow by binding to receptors on committed stem cells. It functions on many levels to promote hemoglobin synthesis, increase production of membrane proteins, and cause differentiation of erythroblasts. Human erythropoietin can be produced by recombinant DNA technology. It is used for the management of anemia in cases of chronic renal failure, for anemias induced by chemotherapy in persons with malignancies, and in the treatment of anemia in human immunodeficiency virus (HIV)–infected persons treated with zidovudine.

Because red blood cells are released into the blood as reticulocytes, the percentage of these cells is higher when there is a marked increase in red blood cell production. In some severe anemias, the reticulocytes may account for as much as 30% of the total red cell count. In some situations, red cell production is so accelerated that numerous erythroblasts appear in the blood.

RED CELL DESTRUCTION

Mature red blood cells have a life span of approximately 4 months, or 120 days. As the red blood cell ages, a number of changes occur. Metabolic activity in the cell decreases, enzyme activity declines, and adenosine triphosphate (ATP) decreases. Membrane lipids are reduced, causing the cell membrane to become more fragile. The cell ruptures as it travels through narrow places in the circulation and in the small trabecular spaces in the spleen. The rate of red cell destruction (1% per day) normally is equal to red cell production, but in conditions such as hemolytic anemia, the cell's life span may be shorter.

The destruction of red blood cells is accomplished by a group of large phagocytic cells found in the spleen, liver, bone marrow, and lymph nodes. These phagocytic cells recognize old and defective red cells and then ingest and destroy them in a series of enzymatic reactions. During these reactions, the amino acids from the globulin chains and iron from the heme units are salvaged and reused (Fig. 16-5). The bulk of the heme unit is converted to bilirubin, the pigment of bile, which is insoluble in plasma and attaches to the plasma proteins for transport. Bilirubin is removed from the blood by the liver and conjugated with glucuronide to render it water soluble so that it can be excreted in the bile. The plasma-insoluble form of bilirubin is referred to as *unconjugated bilirubin;* the water-soluble form is referred to as *conjugated bilirubin.* Serum levels of conjugated and unconjugated bilirubin can be measured in the laboratory and are reported as direct and indirect, respectively. If red cell destruction and consequent bilirubin production are excessive, unconjugated bilirubin accumulates in the blood. This results in a yellow discoloration of the skin, called *jaundice.*

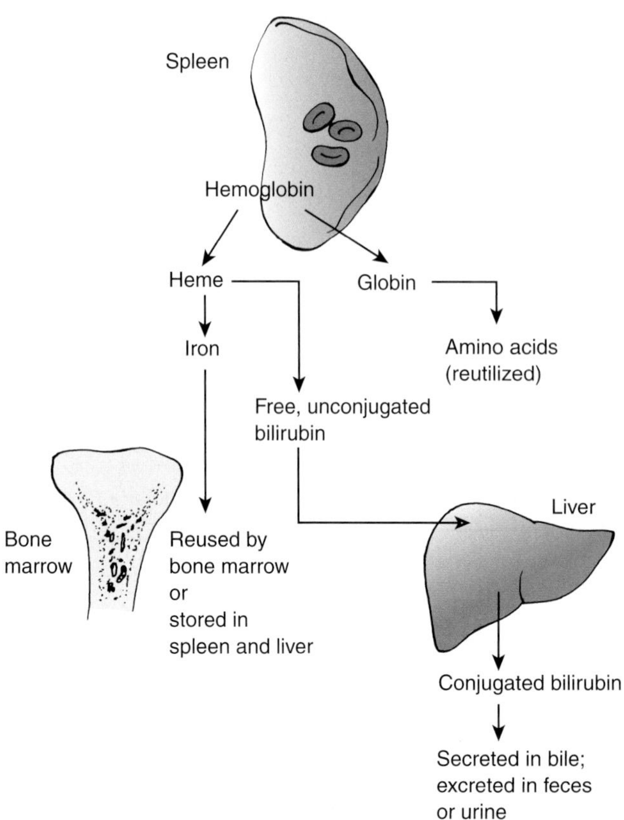

FIGURE 16-5 Destruction of red blood cells and fate of hemoglobin.

When red blood cell destruction takes place in the circulation, as in hemolytic anemia, the hemoglobin remains in the plasma. The plasma contains a hemoglobin-binding protein called *haptoglobin.* Other plasma proteins, such as albumin, can also bind hemoglobin. With extensive intravascular destruction of red blood cells, hemoglobin levels may exceed the hemoglobin-binding capacity of haptoglobin and other plasma proteins. When this happens, free hemoglobin appears in the blood (*i.e.,* hemoglobinemia) and is excreted in the urine (*i.e.,* hemoglobinuria). Because excessive red blood cell destruction can occur in hemolytic transfusion reactions, urine samples are tested for free hemoglobin after a transfusion reaction.

RED CELL METABOLISM AND HEMOGLOBIN OXIDATION

The red blood cell, which lacks mitochondria, relies on glucose and the glycolytic pathway for its metabolic needs (see Chapter 4). The enzyme-mediated anaerobic metabolism of glucose generates the ATP needed for normal membrane function and ion transport. The depletion of glucose or the functional deficiency of one of the glycolytic enzymes leads to the premature death of the red blood cell. An offshoot of the glycolytic pathway is the production of 2,3-diphosphoglycerate (2,3-DPG), which binds to the hemoglobin molecule and reduces the affinity of hemoglobin for oxygen. This facilitates the release of oxygen at the tissue level. An increase in the concentration of 2,3-DPG occurs in conditions of chronic hypoxia such as chronic lung disease, anemia, and high altitudes.

The oxidation of hemoglobin—the combining of hemoglobin with oxygen—can be interrupted by certain chemicals (*e.g.,* nitrates and sulfates) and drugs that oxidize hemoglobin to an inactive form. For example, the nitrite ion reacts with hemoglobin to produce *methemoglobin,* which has a low affinity for oxygen. Large doses of nitrites can result in high levels of methemoglobin, causing pseudocyanosis and tissue hypoxia. For example, sodium nitrate, which is used in curing meats, can produce methemoglobin when taken in large amounts. In nursing infants, the intestinal flora is capable of converting significant amounts of inorganic nitrate (*e.g.,* from well water) to nitrite. This inadvertent exposure to nitrates can cause serious toxic effects. A hereditary deficiency of glucose-6-phosphate dehydrogenase (G6PD; to be discussed) predisposes to oxidative denaturation of hemoglobin, with resultant red cell injury and lysis. Hemolysis occurs as the result of oxidative stress generated by either an infection or exposure to certain drugs.

LABORATORY TESTS

Red blood cells can be studied by means of a sample of blood (Table 16-1). In the laboratory, automated blood cell counters rapidly provide accurate measurements of red cell content and cell indices. The *red blood cell count* (RBC) measures the total number of red blood cells in 1 mm^3 of blood. The *percentage of reticulocytes* (normally approximately 1%) provides an index of the rate of red cell production. The *hemoglobin* (grams per 100 mL of blood) measures the hemoglobin content of the blood. The major components of blood are the red cell mass and plasma volume. The *hematocrit* measures the volume of red cell mass in 100 mL of plasma volume. To determine the hematocrit, a sample of blood is placed in a glass tube, which is then centrifuged to separate the cells and the plasma. The hematocrit may be deceptive because it varies with the quantity of extracellular fluid, rising with dehydration and falling with overexpansion of extracellular fluid volume.

Red cell indices are used to differentiate types of anemias by size or color of red cells. The *mean corpuscular volume* (MCV) reflects the volume or size of the red cells. The MCV falls in microcytic (small cell) anemia and rises in macrocytic (large cell) anemia. Some anemias are normocytic (*i.e.,* cells are of normal size or MCV). The *mean corpuscular hemoglobin concentration* (MCHC) is the concentration of hemoglobin in each cell. Hemoglobin accounts for the color of red blood cells. Anemias are described as *normochromic* (normal color or MCHC) or *hypochromic* (decreased color or MCHC). *Mean cell hemoglobin* (MCH) refers to the mass of the red cell and is less useful in classifying anemias.

A stained blood smear provides information about the size, color, and shape of red cells and the presence of immature or abnormal cells. If blood smear results are abnormal, examination of the bone marrow may be important. Marrow commonly is aspirated with a special needle from the posterior iliac crest or the sternum. The aspirate is stained and observed for number and maturity of cells and abnormal types.

In summary, the red blood cell provides the means for transporting oxygen from the lungs to the tissues. Red cells develop from stem cells in the bone marrow and are released as reticulocytes into the blood, where they become mature erythrocytes. Red blood cell production is regulated by the hormone erythropoietin, which is produced by the kidney in response to a decrease in oxygen levels. The life span of a red blood cell is approximately 120 days. Red cell destruction normally occurs in the spleen, liver, bone marrow, and lymph nodes. In the process of destruction, the heme portion of the hemoglobin molecule is converted to bilirubin. Bilirubin, which is insoluble in plasma, attaches to plasma proteins for transport in the blood. It is removed from the blood by the liver and conjugated to a water-soluble form so that it can be excreted in the bile.

The red blood cell, which lacks mitochondria, relies on glucose and the glycolytic pathway for its metabolic needs. The

TABLE 16-1 Standard Laboratory Values for Red Blood Cells

Test	Normal Values	Significance
Red blood cell count (RBC)		
Men	$4.2–5.4 \times 10^6/\mu L$	Number of red cells in the blood
Women	$3.6–5.0 \times 10^6/\mu L$	
Reticulocytes	1.0%–1.5% of total RBC	Rate of red cell production
Hemoglobin		
Men	14–16.5 g/dL	Hemoglobin content of the blood
Women	12–15 g/dL	
Hematocrit		
Men	40%–50%	Volume of cells in 100 mL of blood
Women	37%–47%	
Mean corpuscular volume	85–100 fL/red cell	Size of the red cell
Mean corpuscular hemoglobin concentration	31–35 g/dL	Concentration of hemoglobin in the red cell
Mean cell hemoglobin	27–34 pg/cell	Red cell mass

end product of the glycolytic pathway, 2,3-DPG, increases the release of oxygen to the tissues during conditions of hypoxia by reducing hemoglobin's affinity for oxygen.

In the laboratory, automated blood cell counters rapidly provide accurate measurements of red cell content and cell indices. A stained blood smear provides information about the size, color, and shape of red cells and the presence of immature or abnormal cells. If blood smear results are abnormal, examination of the bone marrow may be important.

Anemia

After completing this section of the chapter, you should be able to meet the following objectives:

- Describe the manifestations of anemia and their mechanisms
- Explain the difference between intravascular and extravascular hemolysis
- Compare the hemoglobinopathies associated with sickle cell anemia and thalassemia
- Explain the cause of sickling in sickle cell anemia
- Cite common causes of iron-deficiency anemia in infancy, adolescence, and adulthood
- Describe the relation between vitamin B_{12} deficiency and megaloblastic anemia
- List three causes of aplastic anemia
- Compare characteristics of the red blood cells in acute blood loss, hereditary spherocytosis, sickle cell anemia, iron-deficiency anemia, and aplastic anemia

Anemia is defined as an abnormally low number of circulating red blood cells or level of hemoglobin, or both, resulting in diminished oxygen-carrying capacity. Anemia usually results from excessive loss (*i.e.*, bleeding) or destruction (*i.e.*, hemolysis) of red blood cells or from deficient red blood cell production because of a lack of nutritional elements or bone marrow failure.

MANIFESTATIONS

Anemia is not a disease, but an indication of some disease process or alteration in body function. The manifestations of anemia can be grouped into three categories: (1) impaired oxygen transport with the resulting compensatory mechanisms, (2) reduction in red cell indices and hemoglobin levels, and (3) signs and symptoms associated with the pathologic process that is causing the anemia. The manifestations of anemia also depend on its severity, the rapidity of its development, and the person's age and health status. Because the body adapts to slowly developing anemia, the amount of red cell mass lost may reach 50% without the occurrence of signs and symptoms.[2] However, with rapid blood loss, circulatory shock and circulatory collapse may occur.

In anemia, the oxygen-carrying capacity of hemoglobin is reduced, causing tissue hypoxia. Tissue hypoxia can give rise to fatigue, weakness, dyspnea, and sometimes angina. Brain hypoxia results in headache, faintness, and dim vision. The redistribution of the blood from cutaneous tissues or a lack of hemoglobin causes pallor of the skin, mucous membranes, conjunctiva, and nail beds. Tachycardia and palpitations may occur as the body tries to compensate with an increase in cardiac output. A flow-type systolic murmur may result from changes in blood viscosity. Ventricular hypertrophy and high-output heart failure may develop in persons with severe anemia, particularly those with preexisting heart disease. Erythropoiesis is accelerated and may be manifested by diffuse bone pain and sternal tenderness. The production of 2,3-DPG is a compensatory mechanism that reduces the hemoglobin affinity for oxygen, as evidenced by a shift to the right in the oxygen–hemoglobin saturation curve; this causes more oxygen to be released to the tissues rather than remaining bound to hemoglobin. In addition to the common anemic manifestations, hemolytic anemias are accompanied by jaundice caused by increased blood levels of bilirubin. In aplastic anemia, petechiae and purpura (*i.e.*, red spots caused by small-vessel bleeding) are the result of reduced platelet function.

ANEMIA

- Anemia, which is a deficiency of red cells or hemoglobin, results from excessive loss (blood loss anemia), increased destruction (hemolytic anemia), or impaired production of red blood cells (iron-deficiency, megaloblastic, and aplastic anemias).
- Blood loss anemia is characterized by loss of iron-containing red blood cells from the body; hemolytic anemia involves destruction of red blood cells in the body with iron being retained in the body.
- Manifestations of anemia are caused by the decreased presence of hemoglobin in the blood (pallor), tissue hypoxia due to deficient oxygen transport (weakness and fatigue), and recruitment of compensatory mechanisms (tachycardia and palpitations) designed to increase oxygen delivery to the tissues.

BLOOD LOSS ANEMIA

With anemia caused by bleeding, iron and other components of the erythrocyte are lost from the body. Blood loss may be acute or chronic. Acute blood loss carries a risk for hypovolemia and shock (see Chapter 28). The red cells are normal in size and color. A fall in the red blood cell count, hematocrit, and hemoglobin are caused by hemodilution resulting from movement of fluid into the vascular compartment. The hypoxia that results from blood loss stimulates red cell production by the bone marrow. If the bleeding is controlled and sufficient iron stores are available, the red cell concentration returns to normal within 3 to 4 weeks. Chronic blood loss does not affect blood volume but instead leads to iron-deficiency anemia when iron stores are depleted. Because of compensatory mechanisms, patients are commonly asymptomatic until the hemoglobin level is less than 8 g/dL. The red cells that are produced have too little hemoglobin, giving rise to microcytic hypochromic anemia.

HEMOLYTIC ANEMIAS

Hemolytic anemia is characterized by the premature destruction of red cells, the retention in the body of iron and the other products of hemoglobin destruction, and an increase in erythropoiesis. Almost all types of hemolytic anemia are distinguished by normocytic and normochromic red cells. Because of the red blood cell's shortened life span, the bone marrow usually is hyperactive, resulting in an increase in the number of reticulocytes in the circulating blood. As with other types of anemia, the person experiences easy fatigability, dyspnea, and other signs and symptoms of impaired oxygen transport. The person may have mild jaundice due to the bilirubin in serum. In hemolytic anemia, red cell breakdown can occur in the vascular compartment, or it can result from phagocytosis by the reticuloendothelial system. Intravascular hemolysis occurs as a result of complement fixation in transfusion reactions, mechanical injury, or toxic factors. It is characterized by hemoglobinemia and hemoglobinuria. Extravascular hemolysis occurs when abnormal red cells are phagocytized in the spleen. A common example is sickle cell anemia.

The cause of hemolytic anemia can be intrinsic or extrinsic to the red blood cell. Intrinsic or inherited causes include defects of the red cell membrane, the various hemoglobinopathies, and inherited enzyme defects. Two main types of hemoglobinopathies can cause red cell hemolysis: the abnormal substitution of an amino acid in the hemoglobin molecule, as in sickle cell anemia, and the defective synthesis of one of the polypeptide chains that form the globin portion of hemoglobin, as in the thalassemias. Acquired forms of hemolytic anemia are caused by agents extrinsic to the red blood cell, such as drugs, bacterial and other toxins, antibodies, and physical trauma. Although all these factors can cause premature and accelerated destruction of red cells, they cannot all be treated in the same way. Some respond to splenectomy, others respond to treatment with corticosteroid hormones, and still others do not resolve until the primary disorder is corrected.

Inherited Disorders of the Red Cell Membrane

Hereditary spherocytosis, transmitted as an autosomal dominant trait, is the most common inherited disorder of the red cell membrane. The disorder is a deficiency of membrane proteins (*i.e.*, spectrin and ankyrin) that leads to the gradual loss of the membrane surface during the life span of the red blood cell, resulting in a tight sphere instead of a concave disk. Although the spherical cell retains its ability to transport oxygen, it is poorly deformable and susceptible to destruction as it passes through the venous sinuses of the splenic circulation. Clinical signs are variable but typically include mild anemia, jaundice, splenomegaly, and bilirubin gallstones. A life-threatening aplastic crisis may occur when a sudden disruption of red cell production (in most cases from a viral infection) causes a rapid drop in hematocrit and the hemoglobin level. The disorder usually is treated with splenectomy to reduce red cell destruction.

Sickle Cell Anemia

Sickle cell anemia results from a point mutation in the β chain of the hemoglobin molecule, with an abnormal substitution of a single amino acid, valine, for glutamic acid. Sickle hemoglobin (HbS) is transmitted by recessive inheritance and can manifest as sickle cell trait (*i.e.*, heterozygote with one HbS gene) or sickle cell disease (*i.e.*, homozygote with 2 HbS genes). In the heterozygote, only approximately 40% of the hemoglobin is HbS, but in the homozygote, 80% to 95% of the hemoglobin is HbS. Variations in proportions exist, and the concentration of HbS correlates with the risk for sickling.[3]

Sickle cell disease affects approximately 50,000 (0.1% to 0.2%) black Americans. Approximately 10% of black Americans carry the trait.[4] In parts of Africa, where malaria is endemic, the gene frequency approaches 30%, attributed to the slight protective effect against *Plasmodium falciparum* malaria.[3]

Pathophysiology. In the homozygote with sickle cell disease, the HbS becomes sickled when deoxygenated or at a low oxygen tension. The deoxygenated hemoglobin aggregates and polymerizes, creating a semisolid gel that changes the shape and deformability of the cell (Fig. 16-6). The sickled cell may return to normal shape with oxygenation in the lungs. However, after repeated episodes of deoxygenation, the cells remain permanently sickled.

There are two major consequences of red blood cell sickling: chronic hemolytic anemia and blood vessel occlusion. Premature destruction of the cells due to the rigid, nondeformable membrane causes hemolysis and a reduction in red cell numbers resulting in the anemia. Vessel occlusion with its consequent tissue hypoxia also contributes to the pathophysiology of sickle cell disease. The

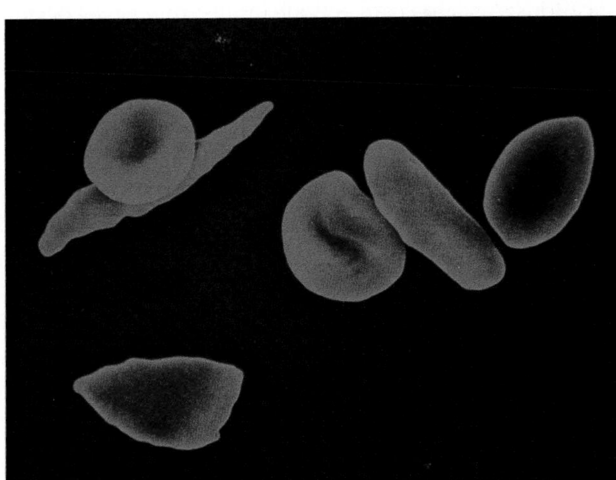

FIGURE 16-6 Photograph of a sickled cell and a normal red blood cell. (© Dr. Gopal Murti, Science Photo Library, Science Source/Photo Researchers)

sickled cells adhere to endothelial cells by surface antigens and cause endothelial activation with the liberation of activator substances that include interleukins, tumor necrosis factor, thrombin, and endotoxin.[3] These activators promote hypercoagulation, increased platelet activation, and thrombin generation resulting in thrombosis. Also, vasoconstrictor substances are released, and the release of nitric oxide, an important vasodilator, is impaired. These alterations further contribute to the vessel occlusion in sickle cell disease.

The person with sickle cell trait who has less HbS has little tendency to sickle except during severe hypoxia and is virtually asymptomatic. Fetal hemoglobin (HbF) inhibits the polymerization of HbS; therefore, most infants with sickle cell disease do not begin to experience the effects of the sickling until sometime after 4 to 6 months of age, when the HbF has been replaced by HbS.

Factors That Contribute to Sickling. The factors associated with sickling and vessel occlusion include cold, stress, physical exertion, infection, and illnesses that cause hypoxia, dehydration, or acidosis. The rate of HbS polymerization is affected by the concentration of hemoglobin in the cell. Dehydration increases the hemoglobin concentration and contributes to the polymerization and resulting sickling. Acidosis reduces the affinity of hemoglobin for oxygen, resulting in more deoxygenated hemoglobin and increased sickling. Even such trivial incidents as reduced oxygen tension induced by sleep may contribute to the sickling process.

Clinical Course. Sickle cell anemia is a chronic disorder resulting in anemia and in pain and organ failure due to vessel occlusion. Affected persons experience severe hemolytic anemia, chronic hyperbilirubinemia, and vasoocclusive crises. Hemolysis produces an anemia with hematocrit values ranging from 18% to 30%.[5] The hyperbilirubinemia that results from the breakdown products of hemoglobin often leads to jaundice and the production of pigment stones in the gallbladder.

Blood vessel occlusion causes most of the severe complications. An acute pain episode results from vessel occlusion and can occur suddenly in almost any part of the body. Common sites obstructed by sickled cells include the abdomen, chest, bones, and joints. Many areas may be affected simultaneously. Infarctions caused by sluggish blood flow may cause chronic damage to the liver, spleen, heart, kidneys, retina, and other organs. *Acute chest syndrome* is an atypical pneumonia resulting from pulmonary infarction. It is the second leading cause of hospitalization in persons with sickle cell disease and is characterized by pulmonary infiltrates, shortness of breath, fever, chest pain, and cough.[6] The syndrome can cause chronic respiratory insufficiency and is a leading cause of death in sickle cell disease. Children may experience growth retardation and susceptibility to osteomyelitis. Painful bone crises may be caused by marrow infarcts of the bones of the hands and feet and result in swelling of those extremities. Twenty-five percent of persons with sickle cell disease have neurologic complications related to vessel occlusion.[6] Stroke occurs in children 1 to 15 years of age and may recur in two thirds of those afflicted. Transient ischemic attack or cerebral hemorrhage may precede the stroke.

The spleen is especially susceptible to damage by sickle cell hemoglobin. Because of the spleen's sluggish blood flow and low oxygen tension, hemoglobin is deoxygenated and causes ischemia. Splenic injury begins as early as 3 to 6 months of age with intense congestion and is usually asymptomatic.[7] The congestion causes functional asplenia and predisposes the person to life-threatening infections by encapsulated organisms such as *Streptococcus pneumoniae, Haemophilus influenzae* type b, and *Klebsiella* species. Neonates and small children have not had time to create antibodies to these organisms and rely on the spleen for their removal. In the absence of specific antibody to the polysaccharide capsular antigens of these organisms, splenic activity is essential for removing these organisms when they enter the blood.

Diagnosis and Screening. Neonatal diagnosis of sickle cell disease is made on the basis of clinical findings and hemoglobin solubility results, which are confirmed by hemoglobin electrophoresis. Prenatal diagnosis is done by the analysis of fetal DNA obtained by amniocentesis.[3]

In the United States, screening programs have been implemented to detect newborns with sickle cell disease and other hemoglobinopathies. Cord blood or heel-stick samples are subjected to electrophoresis to separate the HbF from the small amount of HbA and HbS. Other hemoglobins may be detected and quantified by further laboratory evaluation. Many states mandate neonatal screening of all newborns, regardless of ethnic origin. Ideally, the effective screening program also includes expert genetic counseling and education about pregnancy options.

Management. There is no known cure for sickle cell anemia; treatment to reduce symptoms includes pain control, hydration, and management of complications. The person is advised to avoid situations that precipitate sickling episodes, such as infections, cold exposure, severe physical exertion, acidosis, and dehydration. Infections are aggressively treated, and blood transfusions may be warranted in a crisis or given chronically in severe disease.

Most children with sickle cell disease are at risk for fulminant septicemia and death during the first 3 years of life, when bacteremia from encapsulated organisms occurs commonly even in normal children. Prophylactic penicillin should be begun as early as 2 months of age and continued until at least 5 years of age.[8] Maintaining full immunization, including *H. influenzae* vaccine and hepatitis B vaccine, is recommended. The National Institutes of Health Committee on Management of Sickle Cell Disease also recommends administration of the 7-valent pneumococcal vaccine beginning at 2 to 6 months of age.[8] The 7-valent vaccine should be followed by immunization with the 23-valent pneumococcal vaccine at 24 months of age or later.

Hydroxyurea is a cytotoxic drug used to prevent complications of sickle cell disease. The drug allows synthesis of more HbF and less HbS, thereby decreasing sickling. Hydroxyurea reduces by 50% the pain episodes and pulmonary events in about 60% of the persons treated.[9] The others do not respond. Long-term effects on organ damage, growth and development, and risk for malignancies are unknown. Other therapies under investigation include drugs that affect globin gene expression; prevent polymerization, membrane damage, and cell dehydration; inhibit sickle cell adhesion to endothelial cells; and promote anticoagulation.[9] Nitric oxide (NO) appears to be a promising new drug. It regulates blood vessel tone, platelet activity, and endothelial cell adhesion—all factors that contribute to vessel occlusion. It has been shown that when NO concentrations, which are low in sickle cell disease, are increased through the use of supplemental oral arginine (a precursor of NO), pulmonary complications are reduced.[9]

Bone marrow or stem cell transplantation has the potential for cure in symptomatic children but carries the risk for graft-versus-host disease. The bone marrow transplant survival rate for HLA-identical sibling-donor transplants is about 93%. For those without family donors, transplants of unrelated-donor stem cells, cord blood, and mixed donor-host transplants offer possibilities of cure with about a 70% success rate.[9] Progress in gene therapy to treat sickle cell disease has been slow but promising and may be a future option.

Thalassemias

The thalassemias are a group of inherited disorders of hemoglobin synthesis due to absent or defective synthesis of the α or the β chains of adult hemoglobin. The β-thalassemias result from one of nearly 200 point mutations in the β-globin gene causing a defect in β-chain synthesis.[10] The α-thalassemias are caused by a gene deletion that results in defective α-chain synthesis. The defect is inherited as a mendelian trait, and a person may be heterozygous for the trait and have a mild form of the disease or be homozygous and have the severe form of the disease. Like sickle cell anemia, the thalassemias occur with high degree of frequency in certain populations. The β-thalassemias, sometimes called *Cooley's anemia* or *Mediterranean anemia,* are most common in the Mediterranean populations of southern Italy and Greece, and the α-thalassemias are most common among Asians. Both α- and β-thalassemias are common in Africans and black Americans.

Two factors contribute to the anemia that occurs in thalassemia: reduced hemoglobin synthesis and an imbalance in globin chain production. In α- and β-thalassemia, defective globin chain production leads to deficient hemoglobin production and the development of a hypochromic microcytic anemia. The unaffected type of chain continues to be synthesized, accumulates in the red cell, interferes with normal maturation, and triggers oxygen free radicals that contribute to red cell hemolysis and anemia. In β-thalassemia, the excess α chains are denatured to form precipitates (*i.e.,* Heinz bodies) in the bone marrow red cell precursors. These Heinz bodies impair DNA synthesis and cause damage to the red cell membrane. Severely affected red cell precursors are destroyed in the bone marrow, and those that escape intramedullary death are at increased risk for destruction in the spleen. In addition to the anemia, persons with moderate to severe forms of the disease suffer from coagulation abnormalities. Thrombotic events (stroke and pulmonary embolism) appear to be related to altered platelet function, endothelial activation, and an imbalance of procoagulants and anticoagulants.[10]

The β-Thalassemias. The clinical manifestations of β-thalassemias are based on the severity of the anemia. The presence of one normal gene in heterozygous persons (thalassemia minor) usually results in sufficient normal hemoglobin synthesis to prevent severe anemia. Persons who are homozygous for the trait (thalassemia major) have severe, transfusion-dependent anemia that is evident at 6 to 9 months of age. If transfusion therapy is not started early in life, severe growth retardation occurs in children with the disorder. Increased hematopoiesis, in response to erythropoietin, causes bone marrow expansion, impairs bone growth, and causes bone abnormalities. Bone marrow expansion leads to thinning of the cortical bone, with new bone formation evident on the maxilla and frontal bones of the face (*i.e.,* "chipmunk facies"). The long bones, ribs, and vertebrae may become vulnerable to fracture. Splenomegaly and hepatomegaly result from increased red cell destruction. Iron overload is a major complication of β-thalassemia. Excess iron stores, which accumulate from increased dietary absorption and repeated transfusions, are deposited in the myocardium, liver, and endocrine organs and induce organ damage. Cardiac and hepatic diseases are common causes of death from iron overload. Disorders of the pituitary, thyroid, and adrenal glands and the pancreas result in significant morbidity.[11]

Frequent transfusions (every 3 to 4 weeks) prevent most of the complications, and iron chelation therapy can reduce the iron overload and extend life expectancy.[11] Bone marrow transplantation is a potential cure for some patients, particularly younger persons with no complications of the disease or its treatment.[11] In the future, stem cell gene replacement may provide a cure for many with the disease.

The α-Thalassemias. Synthesis of the α-globin chains of hemoglobin is controlled by two pairs of genes; hence, α-thalassemia shows great variations in severity. Silent carriers who have a deletion of a single α-globin gene are asymptomatic, and those with deletion of two genes have mild hemolytic anemia. Deletion of three of the four α-chain genes leads to unstable aggregates of β chains called *hemoglobin H* (HbH). This disorder is the most important clinical form and is common in Asians. The β chains are more soluble than the α chains, and their accumulation is less toxic to the red cells; thus, senescent rather than precursor red cells are affected. Most persons with HbH have chronic moderate hemolytic anemia and may require transfusions in time of fever or illness or with certain medications.[11] The most severe form of α-thalassemia occurs in infants in whom all four α-globin genes are deleted. Such a defect results in a hemoglobin molecule (Hb Bart's) that is formed exclusively from the chains of HbF. Hb Bart's, which has an extremely high oxygen affinity, cannot release oxygen in the tissues. This disorder usually results in death in utero or shortly after birth. The few survivors are transfusion dependent and have other malformations.[11]

Inherited Enzyme Defects

The most common inherited enzyme defect that results in hemolytic anemia is a deficiency of G6PD. The gene that determines this enzyme is located on the X chromosome, and the defect is expressed only in males and homozygous females. There are more than 350 genetic variants of this disorder found in all populations. The African variant has been found in 15% of black Americans.[4] The disorder makes red cells more vulnerable to oxidants and causes direct oxidation of hemoglobin to methemoglobin and the denaturing of the hemoglobin molecule to form Heinz bodies, which are precipitated in the red blood cell. Hemolysis usually occurs as the damaged red blood cells move through the narrow vessels of the spleen, causing hemoglobinemia, hemoglobinuria, and jaundice. The hemolysis is short lived, occurring 2 to 3 days after the trigger event. In blacks, the defect is mildly expressed and is not associated with chronic hemolytic anemia unless triggered by oxidant drugs, acidosis, or infection.

The antimalarial drug primaquine, the sulfonamides, nitrofurantoin, aspirin, phenacetin, some chemotherapeutics, and other drugs cause hemolysis. Free radicals generated by phagocytes during infections also are possible triggers. A more severe deficiency of G6PD is found in people of Mediterranean descent (*e.g.*, Sardinians, Sephardic Jews, Arabs). In some of these persons, chronic hemolysis occurs in the absence of exposure to oxidants. The disorder can be diagnosed through the use of a G6PD assay or screening test.

Acquired Hemolytic Anemias

Several acquired factors exogenous to the red blood cell produce hemolysis by direct membrane destruction or by antibody-mediated lysis. Various drugs, chemicals, toxins, venoms, and infections such as malaria destroy red cell membranes. Hemolysis can also be caused by mechanical factors such as prosthetic heart valves, vasculitis, and severe burns. Obstructions in the microcirculation, as in disseminated intravascular coagulation, thrombotic thrombocytopenic purpura, and renal disease, may traumatize the red cells by producing turbulence and changing pressure gradients.

Many hemolytic anemias are immune mediated, caused by antibodies that destroy the red cell. Autoantibodies may be produced by a person in response to drugs and disease. Alloantibodies come from an exogenous source and are responsible for transfusion reactions and hemolytic disease of the newborn.

The autoantibodies that cause red cell destruction are of two types: warm-reacting antibodies of the immunoglobulin G (IgG) type, which are maximally active at 37°C, and cold-reacting antibodies of the immunoglobulin M (IgM) type, which are optimally active at or near 4°C. The warm-reacting antibodies cause no morphologic or metabolic alteration in the red cell. Instead, they react with antigens on the red cell membrane, causing destructive changes that lead to spherocytosis, with subsequent phagocytic destruction in the spleen or reticuloendothelial system. They lack specificity for the ABO antigens but may react with the Rh antigens. The hemolytic reactions associated with the warm-reacting antibodies occur with an incidence of approximately 10 per 1 million. The reactions have a rapid onset, and persons usually have mild jaundice and manifestations of anemia. There are varied causes; approximately 50% are idiopathic, and 50% are drug induced or are related to cancers of the lymphoproliferative system (*e.g.*, chronic lymphocytic leukemia, lymphoma), collagen diseases (*e.g.*, systemic lupus erythematosus), viral infections, and inflammatory disorders (*e.g.*, ulcerative colitis).[4] The antihypertensive drug α-methyldopa and the antiarrhythmic drug quinidine account for a small number of cases.[4] The drug-induced hemolysis is commonly benign.

The cold-reacting antibodies activate complement. Chronic hemolytic anemia caused by cold-reacting antibodies occurs with lymphoproliferative disorders and as an idiopathic disorder of unknown cause. The hemolytic process occurs in distal body parts, where the temperature may fall below 30°C. Vascular obstruction by red cells results in pallor, cyanosis of the body parts exposed to cold temperatures, and Raynaud's phenomenon (see Chapter 24). Hemolytic anemia caused by cold-reacting antibodies develops in only a few persons and is rarely severe.

Coombs' test, or the antiglobulin test, is used to diagnose immune hemolytic anemias. It detects the presence of antibody or complement on the surface of the red cell. The direct antiglobulin test (DAT) detects the antibody on red blood cells. In this test, red cells that have been washed free of serum are mixed with antihuman globulin reagent. The red cells agglutinate if the reagent binds to and bridges the antibody or complement on adjacent red cells. The DAT result is positive in cases of autoimmune hemolytic anemia, erythroblastosis fetalis (*i.e.*, Rh disease of the newborn), transfusion reactions, and drug-induced hemolysis. The indirect antiglobulin test detects antibody in the serum, and the result is positive for specific antibodies. It is used for antibody detection and crossmatching before transfusion.

ANEMIAS OF DEFICIENT RED CELL PRODUCTION

Anemia may result from the decreased production of erythrocytes by the bone marrow. A deficiency of nutrients for hemoglobin synthesis (iron) or DNA synthesis (cobalamin or folic acid) may reduce red cell production by the bone marrow. A deficiency of red cells also results when the marrow itself fails or is replaced by nonfunctional tissue.

Iron-Deficiency Anemia

Iron deficiency is a common worldwide cause of anemia affecting persons of all ages. The anemia results from dietary deficiency, loss of iron through bleeding, or increased demands. Because iron is a component of heme, a deficiency leads to decreased hemoglobin synthesis and consequent impairment of oxygen delivery.

Body iron is used repeatedly. When red cells become senescent and are broken down, their iron is released and reused in the production of new red cells. Despite this efficiency, small amounts of iron are lost in the feces and need to be replaced by dietary uptake. Iron balance is maintained by the absorption of 0.5 to 1.5 mg daily to replace the 1 mg lost in the feces. The average Western diet supplies this amount. The absorbed iron is more than sufficient to supply the needs of most individuals but may be barely adequate in women and infants and toddlers. Dietary deficiency of iron is not common in developed countries except in certain populations. Most iron is derived from meat, and when meat is not available, as for deprived populations, or is not a dietary constituent, as for vegetarians, iron deficiency may occur.

The usual reason for iron deficiency in adults is chronic blood loss because iron cannot be recycled to the pool. In men and postmenopausal women, blood loss may occur from gastrointestinal bleeding because of peptic ulcer, intestinal polyps, hemorrhoids, or cancer. Excessive aspirin intake may cause undetected gastrointestinal bleeding. In women, menstruation may account for an average of 1.5 mg of iron lost per day, causing a deficiency.[12] Although cessation of menstruation removes a major source of iron loss in the pregnant woman, iron requirements increase at this time, and deficiency is common. The expansion of the mother's blood volume requires approximately 500 mg of additional iron, and the growing fetus requires approximately 360 mg during pregnancy. In the postnatal period, lactation requires approximately 1.0 mg of iron daily.[12]

A child's growth places extra demands on the body. Blood volume increases, with a greater need for iron. Iron requirements are proportionally higher in infancy (3 to 24 months) than at any other age, although they are also increased in childhood and adolescence. In infancy, the two main causes of iron-deficiency anemia are low iron levels at birth because of maternal deficiency and a diet consisting mainly of cow's milk, which is low in absorbable iron. Adolescents are also susceptible to iron deficiency because of high requirements due to growth spurts, dietary deficiencies, and menstrual loss.[13]

Iron deficiency is characterized by low hemoglobin and hematocrit values, decreased iron stores, and low serum iron and ferritin levels. The red cells are decreased in number and are microcytic and hypochromic. Poikilocytosis (irregular shape) and anisocytosis (irregular size) are also present (Fig. 16-7). The laboratory values indicate reduced MCHC and MCV. Membrane changes may predispose to hemolysis, causing further loss of red cells.

The manifestations of iron-deficiency anemia are related to impaired oxygen transport and lack of hemoglobin. Depending on the severity of the anemia, fatigability, palpitations, dyspnea, angina, and tachycardia may occur. Epithelial atrophy is common and results in waxy pallor, brittle hair and nails, smooth tongue, sores in the corners of the mouth, and sometimes dysphagia and decreased acid secretion. A poorly understood symptom that sometimes is seen is pica, the bizarre compulsive eating of ice, dirt, or other abnormal substances. Iron deficiency in children may also result in neurologic manifestations such as developmental delay, stroke, and cranial nerve palsies.[14]

Prevention of iron deficiency is a primary concern in infants and children. Avoidance of cow's milk, iron supplementation at 4 to 6 months of age in breast-fed infants, and use of iron-fortified formulas and cereals is recommended for infants younger than 1 year of age.[15] In the second year, a diet rich in iron-containing foods and use of iron-fortified vitamins will help prevent iron deficiency. The treatment of iron-deficiency anemia in children and adults is directed toward controlling chronic blood loss, increasing dietary intake of iron, and administering supplemental iron. Ferrous sulfate, which is the usual oral replacement therapy, replenishes iron stores in several months. Parenteral iron (iron dextran) therapy may be used when oral forms are not tolerated or are ineffective. Because of the possibility of severe hypersensitivity reactions, an initial test dose should be administered before administration of the first therapeutic dose of the drug. It is recommended that the test dose be administered in an environment equipped for treatment of severe allergic or anaphylactic reactions. Iron dextran can be given intravenously or injected deep intramuscularly using the Z-track injection method in which the skin is pulled to one side before inserting the needle to prevent leakage into the tissues, with subsequent skin discoloration. In the future, gastric delivery systems may provide good therapy without side effects.

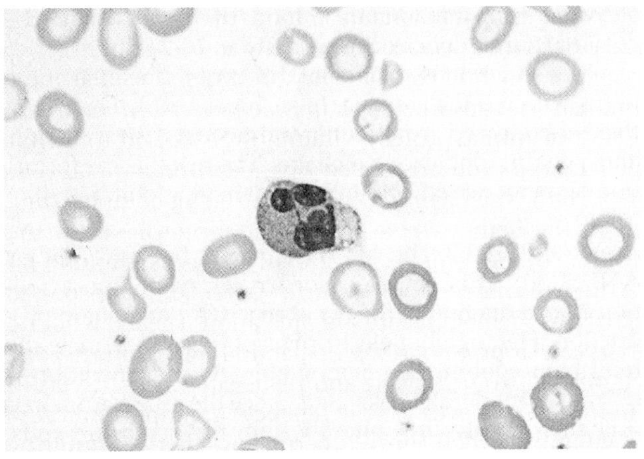

FIGURE 16-7 Iron deficiency anemia. A peripheral smear shows hypochromic and microcytic erythrocytes. Poikilocytosis (irregular shape) and anisocytosis (irregular size) are often observed. (Rubin E., Farber J. L. [1999]. *Pathology* [3rd ed., p. 1077]. Philadelphia: Lippincott-Raven)

Megaloblastic Anemias

Megaloblastic anemias are caused by abnormal nucleic acid synthesis that results in enlarged red cells (MCV > 100 fL) and deficient nuclear maturation. Cobalamin (vitamin B_{12}) and folic acid deficiencies are the most common megaloblastic anemias. Because megaloblastic anemias develop slowly, there are often few symptoms until the anemia is far advanced.

Cobalamin (Vitamin B_{12})–Deficiency Anemia. Vitamin B_{12} serves as a cofactor for two important reactions in humans. It is essential for the synthesis of DNA. When it is deficient, nuclear maturation and cell division, especially of the rapidly proliferating red cells, fail to occur. It is also involved in a reaction that prevents abnormal fatty acids from being incorporated into neuronal lipids. This abnormality may predispose to myelin breakdown and produce some of the neurologic complications of vitamin B_{12} deficiency.

Vitamin B_{12} is found in all foods of animal origin. Dietary deficiency is rare and usually found only in strict vegetarians who avoid all dairy products as well as meat and fish. It is absorbed by a unique process. After release from the animal protein, vitamin B_{12} is bound to intrinsic factor, a protein secreted by the gastric parietal cells (Fig. 16-8). The vitamin B_{12}–intrinsic factor complex travels to the ileum, where membrane receptors allow the binding of the complex to the epithelial cells. Vitamin B_{12} is then separated from intrinsic factor and transported across the membrane into the circulation. There it is bound to its carrier protein, transcobalamin II, which transports vitamin B_{12} to its storage and tissue sites. Any defects in this pathway may cause a deficiency. An important cause of vitamin B_{12} deficiency is pernicious anemia, resulting from a hereditary atrophic gastritis. As discussed in Chapter 39, immune-mediated chronic atrophic gastritis is a disorder that destroys the gastric mucosa, with loss of parietal cells and production of antibodies that interfere with the binding of vitamin B_{12} to intrinsic factor. Other causes of vitamin B_{12} deficiency anemia include gastrectomy, ileal resection, inflammation or neoplasms in the terminal ileum, and malabsorption syndromes in which vitamin B_{12} and other vitamin B compounds are poorly absorbed.

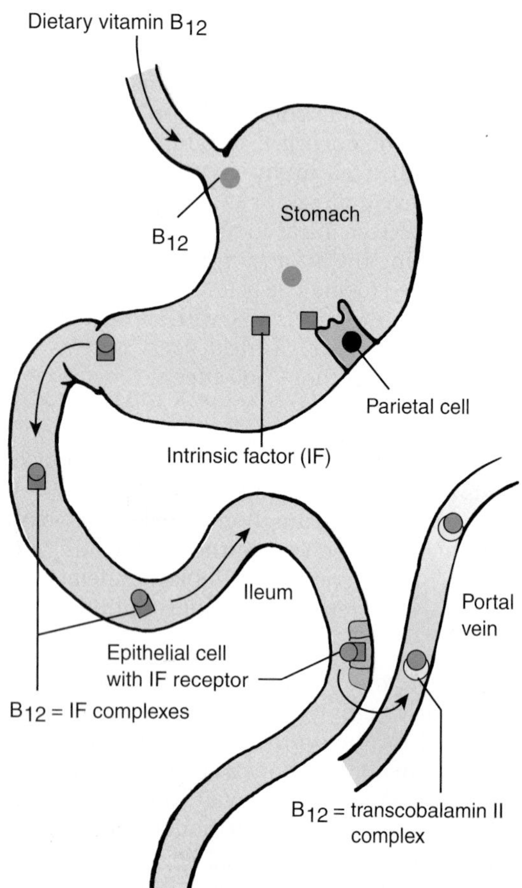

FIGURE 16-8 Absorption of vitamin B_{12}.

The hallmark of vitamin B_{12} deficiency is megaloblastic anemia. When vitamin B_{12} is deficient, the red cells that are produced are abnormally large because of excess ribonucleic acid production of hemoglobin and structural protein (Fig. 16-9). The cells have immature nuclei and show evidence of cellular destruction. They have flimsy membranes and are oval rather than biconcave. These oddly shaped cells have a short life span that can be measured in weeks rather than months. The MCV is elevated, and the MCHC is normal.

Neurologic changes that accompany the disorder are caused by deranged methylation of myelin protein. Demyelination of the dorsal and lateral columns of the spinal cord causes symmetric paresthesias of the feet and fingers, loss of vibratory and position sense, and eventual spastic ataxia. In more advanced cases, cerebral function may be altered. In some cases, dementia and other neuropsychiatric changes may precede hematologic changes.

Diagnosis of vitamin B_{12} deficiency is made by finding an abnormally low vitamin B_{12} serum level. The Schilling test, which measures the 24-hour urinary excretion of radiolabeled vitamin B_{12} administered orally, has been commonly used in the past to document decreased absorption of vitamin B_{12}. Currently, the diagnosis of pernicious anemia is usually made by the detection of parietal cell and intrinsic factor antibodies.[16] Lifelong treatment consisting of intramuscular injections of vitamin B_{12} reverses the anemia and improves the neurologic changes.

Folic Acid–Deficiency Anemia. Folic acid is also required for DNA synthesis and red cell maturation, and its deficiency produces the same type of megaloblastic red cell changes that occur in vitamin B_{12} deficiency anemia (*i.e.,* increased MCV and normal MCHC). Symptoms are also similar, but the neurologic manifestations are not present.

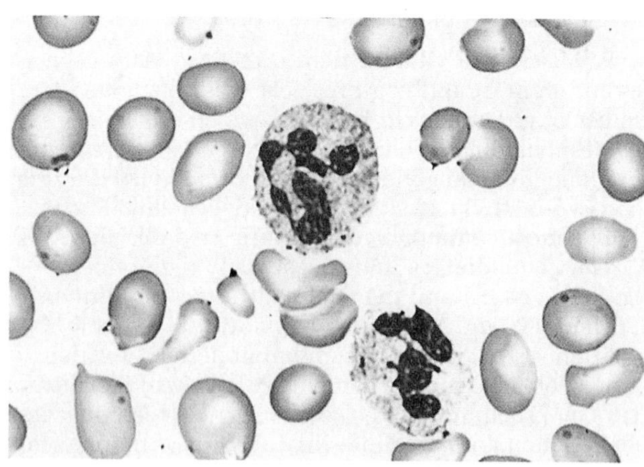

FIGURE 16-9 Peripheral blood smear of patient with vitamin B_{12} deficiency (pernicious anemia) that shows prominent megaloblastic anemia. The erythrocytes are large, often with oval shape, and are associated with poikilocytosis and teardrop shapes. The neutrophils are hypersegmented. (Rubin E., Farber J. L. [1999]. *Pathology* [3rd ed., p. 1076]. Philadelphia: Lippincott-Raven)

Folic acid is readily absorbed from the intestine. It is found in vegetables (particularly the green leafy types), fruits, cereals, and meats. Much of the vitamin, however, is lost in cooking. The most common causes of folic acid deficiency are malnutrition or dietary lack, especially in the elderly or in association with alcoholism. Total body stores of folic acid amount to 2000 to 5000 micrograms (μg), and 50 μg is required in the daily diet.[4] A dietary deficiency may result in anemia in a few months. Malabsorption of folic acid may be due to syndromes such as sprue or other intestinal disorders. Some drugs used to treat seizure disorders (*e.g.,* primidone, phenytoin, phenobarbital) and triamterene, a diuretic, predispose to a deficiency by interfering with folic acid absorption. In neoplastic disease, tumor cells compete for folate, and deficiency is common. Methotrexate, a folic acid analog used in the treatment of cancer, impairs the action of folic acid by blocking its conversion to the active form.

Because pregnancy increases the need for folic acid 5- to 10-fold, a deficiency commonly occurs. Poor dietary habits, anorexia, and nausea are other reasons for folic acid deficiency during pregnancy. Studies also show an association between folate deficiency and neural tube defects.[17] The U.S. Public Health Service recommends that all women of childbearing age should take 400 μg of folic acid daily. It is estimated that 50% of neural tube defects could thus be prevented.[18] The Institute of Medicine Panel on Folate and Other B Vitamins has revised the recommended daily allowance for pregnant women to 600 μg daily.[19] To ensure adequate folate consumption, the U.S. Food and Drug Administration mandated the addition of folate to cereal grain products effective January 1, 1998.

Aplastic Anemia

Aplastic anemia (*i.e.,* bone marrow depression) describes a primary condition of bone marrow stem cells that results in a reduction of all three hematopoietic cell lines—red blood cells, white blood cells, and platelets—with fatty replacement of bone marrow. Pure red cell aplasia, in which only the red cells are affected, rarely occurs.

Anemia results from the failure of the marrow to replace senescent red cells that are destroyed and leave the circulation, although the cells that remain are of normal size and color. At the same time, because the leukocytes, particularly the neutrophils, and the thrombocytes have a short life span, a deficiency of these cells usually is apparent before the anemia becomes severe.

The onset of aplastic anemia may be insidious, or it may strike with suddenness and great severity. It can occur at any age. The initial presenting symptoms include weakness, fatigability, and pallor caused by anemia. Petechiae (*i.e.,* small, punctate skin hemorrhages) and ecchymoses (*i.e.,* bruises) often occur on the skin, and bleeding from the nose, gums, vagina, or gastrointestinal tract may occur because of decreased platelet levels. The decrease in the number of neutrophils increases susceptibility to infection.

Among the causes of aplastic anemia is exposure to high doses of radiation, chemicals, and toxins that suppress hematopoiesis directly or through immune mechanisms. Chemotherapy and irradiation commonly result in bone marrow depression, which causes anemia, thrombocytopenia, and neutropenia. Identified toxic agents include benzene, the antibiotic chloramphenicol, and the alkylating agents and antimetabolites used in the treatment of cancer (see Chapter 8). Aplastic anemia caused by exposure to chemical agents may be an idiosyncratic reaction because it affects only certain susceptible persons. It typically occurs weeks after a drug is initiated. Such reactions often are severe and sometimes are irreversible and fatal. Aplastic anemia can develop in the course of many infections and has been reported most often as a complication of viral hepatitis, mononucleosis, and other viral illnesses, including acquired immunodeficiency syndrome (AIDS). In two thirds of cases, the cause is unknown, in which case it is called *idiopathic aplastic anemia.*

Therapy for aplastic anemia in young and severely affected patients includes stem cell replacement by bone marrow or peripheral blood transplantation. Histocompatible donors supply the stem cells to replace the patient's destroyed marrow cells. Graft-versus-host disease, rejection, and infections are major risks of the procedure, yet 70% or more survive.[20] For those who are not transplantation candidates, immunosuppressive therapy with lymphocyte immune globulin (*i.e.,* antithymocyte globulin) prevents suppression of proliferating stem cells, producing remission in up to 50% of patients.[20] Patients with aplastic anemia should avoid the offending agents and be treated with antibiotics for infection. Red cell transfusions to correct the anemia and platelets and corticosteroid therapy to minimize bleeding may also be required.

Chronic Disease Anemias

Anemia often occurs as a complication of chronic infections, inflammation, and cancer. Chronic diseases commonly associated with anemia include tuberculosis, AIDS, osteomyelitis, rheumatoid arthritis, systemic lupus erythematosus, and Hodgkin's disease. It is theorized that the short life span, deficient red cell production in response to erythropoietin, and low serum iron are caused by actions of macrophages and lymphocytes in response to cell injury. Macrophages sequester iron in the spleen and contribute to red cell destruction. The lymphocytes release cytokines (*e.g.,* interleukin-1 and interferon) that suppress the erythropoietin response, inhibit erythroid precursors, and reduce iron transport.[21] The moderate to severe anemia is similar to iron deficiency with microcytic, hypochromic red cells. The anemia may be reversed when the underlying disease is treated or with erythropoietin therapy.[21]

Chronic renal failure almost always results in a normocytic, normochromic anemia, primarily because of a deficiency of erythropoietin. Unidentified uremic toxins and retained nitrogen also interfere with the actions of erythropoietin and with red cell production and survival. Hemolysis and blood loss associated with hemodialysis and bleeding tendencies also contribute to the anemia of renal failure. In persons whose hematocrits are 30% to 35%, recombinant erythropoietin injected several times a week eliminates the need for transfusions.[21] Oral iron is sometimes required for a good response.

In summary, anemia is a condition of an abnormally low number of circulating red blood cells or hemoglobin level, or both. It is not a disease but rather a manifestation of a disease process or alteration in body function. Anemia can result from excessive blood loss, red cell destruction due to hemolysis, or deficient hemoglobin or red cell production. Blood loss anemia can be acute or chronic. With bleeding, iron and other components of the erythrocyte are lost from the body. Hemolytic anemia is characterized by the premature destruction of red cells, with retention in the body of iron and the other products of red cell destruction. Hemolytic anemia can be caused by defects in the red cell membrane, hemoglobinopathies (sickle cell anemia or thalassemia), or inherited enzyme defects (G6PD deficiency). Acquired forms of hemolytic anemia are caused by agents extrinsic to the red blood cell, such as drugs, bacterial and other toxins, antibodies, and physical trauma. Iron-deficiency anemia, which is characterized by decreased hemoglobin synthesis, can result from dietary deficiency, loss of iron through bleeding, or increased demands for red cell production. Vitamin B_{12} and folic acid deficiency impair red cell production by interfering with DNA synthesis. Aplastic anemia is caused by bone marrow suppression and usually results in a reduction of white blood cells and platelets as well as red blood cells.

The manifestations of anemia are those associated with impaired oxygen transport; alterations in red blood cell number, hemoglobin content, and cell structure; and the signs and symptoms of the underlying process causing the anemia.

Transfusion Therapy

After completing this section of the chapter, you should be able to meet the following objectives:

- ✦ Differentiate red cell antigens from antibodies in persons with type A, B, AB, or O blood
- ✦ Explain the determination of the Rh factor
- ✦ List the signs and symptoms of a blood transfusion reaction

Anemias of various causes are treated with transfusions of whole blood or red blood cells only when oxygen delivery to the tissues is compromised, as evidenced by measures of oxygen transport and use, hemoglobin, and hematocrit. Current recommendations suggest transfusion for patients with hemoglobin levels less than 7 to 8 g/dL, depending on age, illness, risk factors, and surgical procedures.[21] Acute massive blood loss usually is replaced with whole-blood transfusion. Most anemias, however, are treated with transfusions of red cell concentrates, which supply only the blood component that is deficient. Since the 1960s, devices that mechanically separate a unit of blood into its constituents provide red cell components, platelets, fresh-frozen plasma, cryoprecipitate, and clotting factor concentrates. In this way, a unit of blood can be used efficiently for several recipients to correct specific deficiencies.

Several red cell components that are used for transfusion are prepared and stored under specific conditions and have unique uses, as described in Table 16-2. These red cell components are derived principally from voluntary blood donors. In the future, red cell substitutes, such as hemoglobin solutions, may be used, particularly in the trauma setting.[22] The potential advantages are better storage, longer shelf life, and no risk for transfusion reaction.

The use of autologous donation and transfusion has been advocated since the early 1980s. Autologous transfusion refers to the procedure of receiving one's own blood—usually to replenish a surgical loss—thereby eliminating the risk for blood-borne disease or transfusion reaction. In 1992, a reported 8.5% of transfusions were autologous.[23] Autologous blood can be provided by several means: predeposit, hemodilution, and intraoperative salvage. A patient who is anticipating elective orthopedic, vascular, or open-heart surgery may predeposit blood (*i.e.,* have the blood collected up to 6 weeks in advance and stored) for later transfusion during the surgery. Hemodilution involves phlebotomy before surgery with transfusion of the patient's blood at the completion of surgery. The procedure requires the use of fluid infusions to maintain blood volume and is commonly used in open-heart surgery. Intraoperative blood salvage is the collection of blood shed from the operative site for reinfusion into the patient. Semiautomated devices are used to collect, anticoagulate, wash, and resuspend red cells for reinfusion during many procedures, including vascular, cardiac, and orthopedic surgery. Potential risks of autologous transfusion may include bacterial and other contamination, volume overload, and administrative errors.[22]

Before a red cell or whole-blood transfusion from a volunteer donor source can occur, a series of procedures are required to ensure a successful transfusion. Donor samples are first tested for blood-borne diseases, such as hepatitis B and hepatitis C, HIV types 1 and 2, human T cell lymphotropic viruses (HTLV-I and -II), and syphilis. Donor and recipient samples are typed to determine ABO and Rh groups and screened for unexpected red cell antibodies. The crossmatch is performed by incubating the donor cells with the recipient's serum and observing for agglutination. If none appears, the donor and recipient blood types are compatible.

ABO BLOOD GROUPS

ABO compatibility is essential for effective transfusion therapy and requires knowledge of ABO antigens and antibodies. There are four major ABO blood groups as determined by the presence or absence of two red cell antigens (A and B). Persons who have neither A nor B antigens are classified as having type O blood; those with A antigens are classified as having type A blood; those with B antigens, as having type B blood; and those with A and B antigens, as having type AB blood (Table 16-3). The ABO blood groups are genetically determined. The type O gene is apparently functionless in production of a red cell antigen. Each of the other genes is expressed by the presence of a

TABLE 16-2 Red Blood Cell Components Used in Transfusion Therapy

Component	Preparation	Use	Limitations
Whole blood	Drawn from donor Anticoagulant–preservative solutions added, usually citrate-phosphate-dextrose (CPDA-1) adenine; stored at 1°–6°C until expiration, up to 35 days	Replacement of blood volume and oxygen-carrying capacity lost in massive bleeding	Contains few viable platelets or granulocytes and is deficient in coagulation factors V and VIII; may cause hypervolemia, febrile and allergic reactions and infectious disease (*i.e.*, hepatitis and AIDS)
Red blood cells	Removal of two thirds of plasma by centrifugation; additive solution contains adenine and dextrose to extend shelf life up to 42 days and maintain ATP levels	Standard transfusion to increase oxygen-carrying capacity in chronic anemia and slow hemorrhage; reduce danger of hypervolemia	Contains no viable platelets or granulocytes; risk of reactions and infectious disease
Leukocyte-reduced red blood cells	Removal of 99% of leukocytes, platelets, and debris by centrifugation or filtration	Reduces risk of nonhemolytic febrile reactions in susceptible persons	Preparation may reduce red cell mass to 80%; 24-hr outdate and infectious disease risk
Washed red blood cells	Red cells are washed in normal saline solution and centrifuged several times to remove plasma and constituents.	Reduces risk of febrile and allergic reactions	Loss of red cell mass, 24-hr outdate, costly preparation, and infectious disease risk
Frozen red blood cells	Red cells are mixed with glycerol to prevent ice crystals from forming and rupturing the cell membrane; cells must be thawed, deglycerolized, and washed before transfusing.	Reduces risk of severe febrile reactions; preserves rare and autologous (self-donated) units for transfusion up to 10 yr	Costly and lengthy preparation; loss of red cell mass, 24-hr outdate, and infectious disease risk

ATP, adenosine triphosphate.
(Data from Vengelen-Tyler V. [Ed.] [1996]. *Technical manual.* [12th ed., pp. 135–142]. Bethesda, MD: American Association of Blood Banks)

strong antigen on the surface of the red cell. Six genotypes, or gene combinations, result in four phenotypes, or blood type expressions. ABO antibodies predictably develop in the serum of persons whose red cells lack the corresponding antigen. Persons with type A antigens on their red cells develop type B antibodies; persons with type B antigens develop type A antibodies in their serum; persons with type O blood develop type A and type B antibodies; and persons with type AB blood develop neither A nor B antibodies. The ABO antibodies usually are not present at birth but begin to develop at 3 to 6 months of age and reach maximum levels between the ages of 5 and 10 years.[24]

TABLE 16-3 ABO System for Blood Typing

Genotype	Red Cell Antigens	Blood Type	Serum Antibodies
OO	None	O	AB
AO	A	A	B
AA	A	A	B
BO	B	B	A
BB	B	B	A
AB	AB	AB	None

RH TYPES

The D antigen of the Rh system is also important in transfusion compatibility and is routinely tested. The Rh type is coded by three gene pairs: C, c; D, d; and E, e. Each allele, with the exception of d, codes for a specific antigen. The D antigen is the most immunogenic. Persons who express the D antigen are designated Rh positive, and those who do not express the D antigen are Rh negative. Unlike serum antibodies for the ABO blood types, which develop spontaneously after birth, Rh antibodies develop after exposure to one or more of the Rh antigens. More than 80% of Rh-negative persons develop the antibody to D antigen if they are exposed to Rh-positive blood.[25] Because it takes several weeks to produce antibodies, a reaction may be delayed and usually is mild. If subsequent transfusions of Rh-positive blood are given to a person who has become sensitized, the person may have a severe, immediate reaction.

BLOOD TRANSFUSION REACTIONS

The seriousness of blood transfusion reactions prompts the need for extreme caution when blood is administered. Because most transfusion reactions result from administrative errors or misidentification, care should be taken to correctly identify the recipient and the transfusion source. The recipient's vital signs should be monitored before and during the transfusion, and careful observation for signs of transfusion reaction is imperative. The most feared and lethal transfusion reaction is the destruction of donor red cells by reaction with antibody in the recipient's serum. This immediate hemolytic reaction usually is caused by ABO incompatibility. The signs and symptoms of such a reaction include sensation of heat along the vein where the blood is being infused, flushing of the face, urticaria, headache, pain in the lumbar area, chills, fever, constricting pain in the chest, cramping pain in the abdomen, nausea, vomiting, tachycardia, hypotension, and dyspnea. If any of these adverse effects occur, the transfusion should be stopped immediately. Access to a vein should be maintained because it may be necessary to infuse intravenous solutions to ensure diuresis, administer medications, and take blood samples. The blood must be saved for studies to determine the cause of the reaction.

Hemoglobin that is released from the hemolyzed donor cells is filtered in the glomeruli of the kidneys. Two possible complications of a blood transfusion reaction are oliguria and renal shutdown because of the adverse effects of the filtered hemoglobin on renal tubular flow. The urine should be examined for the presence of hemoglobin, urobilinogen, and red blood cells. Delayed hemolytic reactions may occur more than 10 days after transfusion and are caused by undetected antibodies in the recipient's serum. The reaction is accompanied by a fall in hematocrit and jaundice, but most recipients are asymptomatic.

A febrile reaction, the most common transfusion reaction, occurs in approximately 2% of transfusions. Recipient antibodies directed against the donor's white cells or platelets cause chills and fever. Antipyretics are used to treat this reaction. Future febrile reactions may be avoided by the use of leukocyte-reduced blood.

Allergic reactions are caused by patient antibodies against donor proteins, particularly immunoglobulin G. Urticaria and itching occur and can be relieved with antihistamines. Susceptible persons may be transfused with washed red cells to prevent reactions.

In summary, transfusion therapy provides the means for replacement of red blood cells and other blood components. Red blood cells contain surface antigens, and reciprocal antibodies are found in the serum. Four major ABO blood types are determined by the presence or absence of two red cell antigens: A and B. The D antigen determines the Rh-positive type; absence of the D antigen determines the Rh-negative type. ABO and Rh types must be determined in recipient and donor blood before transfusion to ensure compatibility.

Polycythemia

After completing this section of the chapter, you should be able to meet the following objectives:

- Define the term *polycythemia*
- Compare polycythemia vera and secondary polycythemia

Polycythemia is an abnormally high total red blood cell mass with a hematocrit greater than 50%. It is categorized as relative or absolute. In relative polycythemia, the hematocrit rises because of a loss of plasma volume without a corresponding decrease in red cells. This may occur with water deprivation, excess use of diuretics, or gastrointestinal losses. Relative polycythemia is corrected by increasing the vascular fluid volume.

Absolute polycythemia is a rise in hematocrit due to an increase in total red cell mass and is classified as primary or secondary. Primary polycythemia, or polycythemia vera, is a proliferative disease of the pluripotent cells of the bone marrow characterized by an absolute increase in total red blood cell mass accompanied by elevated white cell and platelet counts. It most commonly is seen in men between the ages of 40 and 60 years. In polycythemia vera, the manifestations are related to an increase in the red cell count, hemoglobin level, and hematocrit with increased blood volume and viscosity. Viscosity rises exponentially with the hematocrit and interferes with cardiac output and blood flow. Hypertension is common, and there may be complaints of headache, inability to concentrate, and some difficulty with hearing and vision because of decreased cerebral blood flow. Venous stasis gives rise to a plethoric appearance or dusky redness—even cyanosis—particularly of the lips, fingernails, and mucous membranes. Because of the increased concentration of blood cells, the person may experience itching and pain in the fingers or toes, and the hypermetabolism may induce night sweats and weight loss. Thromboembolism occurs in 15% to 60% of persons with polycythemia vera and contributes to death in 10% to 40% of the cases.[26] Hemorrhage, due to platelet abnormalities, occurs in 15% to 35% of cases and is also an important cause of death. The goal of treatment in primary polycythemia is to reduce blood viscosity. This can be done by withdrawing blood by means of periodic phlebotomy to reduce red cell volume. Control of platelet and white cell counts is accomplished by suppressing bone marrow function with chemotherapy.

Secondary polycythemia results from a physiologic increase in the level of erythropoietin, commonly as a compensatory response to hypoxia. Conditions causing hypoxia include living at high altitudes, chronic heart and lung disease, and smoking. The resultant release of erythropoietin by the kidney causes the increased formation of red blood cells in the bone marrow. Neoplasms that secrete erythropoietin may also cause a secondary polycythemia. Treatment of secondary polycythemia focuses on relieving hypoxia. For example, continuous low-flow oxygen therapy can be used to correct the severe hypoxia that occurs in some persons with chronic obstructive lung disease. This form of treatment is thought to relieve the pulmonary hypertension and polycythemia and to delay the onset of cor pulmonale.

In summary, polycythemia describes a condition in which the red blood cell mass is increased. It can present as a relative, primary, or secondary disorder. Relative polycythemia results from a loss of vascular fluid and is corrected by replacing the fluid. Primary polycythemia, or polycythemia vera, is a proliferative disease of the bone marrow with an absolute increase in total red blood cell mass accompanied by elevated white cell and platelet counts. Secondary polycythemia results from increased erythropoietin levels caused by hypoxic conditions such as chronic heart and lung disease. Many of the manifestations of polycythemia are related to increased blood volume and viscosity that lead to hypertension and stagnation of blood flow.

Age-Related Changes in Red Blood Cells

After completing this section of the chapter, you should be able to meet the following objectives:

- Cite the function of hemoglobin F in the neonate and describe the red blood cell changes that occur during the early neonatal period
- Cite the factors that predispose to hyperbilirubinemia in the infant
- Describe the pathogenesis of hemolytic disease of the newborn
- Compare conjugated and unconjugated bilirubin in terms of production of encephalopathy in the neonate
- Explain the action of phototherapy in the treatment of hyperbilirubinemia in the neonate
- State the changes in the red blood cells that occur with aging

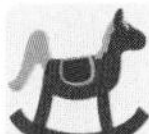

RED CELL CHANGES IN THE NEONATE

At birth, changes in the red blood cell indices reflect the transition to extrauterine life and the need to transport oxygen from the lungs (Table 16-4). Hemoglobin concentrations at birth are high, reflecting the high synthetic activity in utero to provide adequate oxygen delivery. Toward the end of the first postnatal week, hemoglobin concentration begins to decline, gradually falling to a minimum value at approximately age 2 months. The red cell count, hematocrit, and MCV likewise fall. The factors responsible for the decline include reduced red cell production and plasma dilution caused by increased blood volume with growth. Neonatal red cells also have a shorter life span of 50 to 70 days and are thought to be more fragile than those of older persons. During the early neonatal period, there is also a switch from HbF to HbA. The amount of HbF in term infants averages about 70% of the total hemoglobin and declines to trace amounts by 6 to 12 months of age.[27] The switch to HbA provides greater unloading of oxygen to the tissues because HbA has a lower affinity for oxygen compared with HbF. Infants who are small for gestational age or born to diabetic or smoking mothers or who experienced hypoxia in utero have higher total hemoglobin levels, higher HbF levels, and a delayed switch to HbA.

A physiologic anemia of the newborn develops at approximately 2 months of age. It seldom produces symptoms and cannot be altered by nutritional supplements. Anemia of prematurity, an exaggerated physiologic response in low-birth-weight infants, is thought to result from a poor erythropoietin response. The hemoglobin level rapidly declines after birth to a low of 7 to 10 g/dL at approximately 6 weeks of age. Signs and symptoms include apnea, poor weight gain, pallor, decreased activity, and tachycardia. In infants born before 33 weeks' gestation and those with hematocrits below 33%, the clinical features are more evident. One study suggests that the protein content

TABLE 16-4 Red Cell Values for Term Infants

Age	RBC × 10^6/μL Mean ± SD	Hb (g/dL) Mean ± SD	Hct (%) Mean ± SD	MCV (fL) Mean ± SD
Days				
1	5.14 ± 0.7	19.3 ± 2.2	61 ± 7.4	119 ± 9.4
4	5.00 ± 0.6	18.6 ± 2.1	57 ± 8.1	114 ± 7.5
7	4.86 ± 0.6	17.9 ± 2.5	56 ± 9.4	118 ± 11.2
Weeks				
1–2	4.80 ± 0.8	17.3 ± 2.3	54 ± 8.3	112 ± 19.0
3–4	4.00 ± 0.6	14.2 ± 2.1	43 ± 5.7	105 ± 7.5
8–9	3.40 ± 0.5	10.7 ± 0.9	31 ± 2.5	93 ± 12.0
11–12	3.70 ± 0.3	11.3 ± 0.9	33 ± 3.3	88 ± 7.9

Hb, hemoglobin; Hct, hematocrit; MCV, mean corpuscular volume.
(Adapted from Matoth Y., Zaizor R., Varsano I. [1971]. Postnatal changes in some red cell parameters. *Acta Paediatrica Scandinavica* 60, 317)

of breast milk may not be sufficient for hematopoiesis in the premature infant. Protein supplementation significantly increases the hemoglobin concentrations between the ages of 4 and 10 weeks.[28]

Anemia at birth, characterized by pallor, congestive heart failure, or shock, usually is caused by hemolytic disease of the newborn. Bleeding from the umbilical cord, internal hemorrhage, congenital hemolytic disease, and frequent blood sampling are other possible causes of anemia. The severity of symptoms and presence of coexisting disease may warrant red cell transfusion.

Hyperbilirubinemia in the Neonate

Hyperbilirubinemia, an increased level of serum bilirubin, is a common cause of jaundice in the neonate. A benign, self-limited condition, it most often is related to the developmental state of the neonate. Rarely, cases of hyperbilirubinemia are pathologic and may lead to kernicterus and serious brain damage.

In the first week of life, approximately 60% of term and 80% of preterm neonates are jaundiced.[29] This physiologic jaundice appears in term infants on the second or third day of life. Ordinarily, the indirect bilirubin in umbilical cord blood is 1 to 3 mg/dL and increases less than 5 mg/dL in 24 hours, giving rise to jaundice. The levels peak at 5 to 6 mg/dL between days 2 and 4 and decrease to less than 2 mg/dL by days 5 to 7.[29] The increase in bilirubin is related to the increased red cell breakdown and the inability of the immature liver to conjugate bilirubin. Premature infants exhibit a slower rise and longer duration in serum bilirubin levels, perhaps because of poor hepatic uptake and reduced albumin binding of bilirubin. Peak bilirubin levels of 8 to 12 mg/dL appear on days 5 to 7. Most neonatal jaundice resolves within 1 week and is untreated.

The cause of jaundice is determined on the basis of history and clinical and laboratory findings. Generally, a search for the cause should be made when (1) the jaundice appears in the first 24 to 36 hours after birth and lasts more than 10 to 14 days, (2) serum bilirubin rises at a rate greater than 5 mg/dL per 24 hours, (3) serum bilirubin is greater than 12 mg/dL in a full-term infant or 10 to 14 mg/dL in a preterm infant, or (4) the direct-reacting bilirubin is greater than 2 mg/dL at any time.[29] Many factors cause elevated bilirubin levels in the neonate, including breast-feeding, hemolytic disease of the newborn, hypoxia, infections, and acidosis. Bowel or biliary obstruction and liver disease are less common causes. Associated risk factors include prematurity, Asian ancestry, and maternal diabetes. Breast milk jaundice occurs in approximately 2% of breast-fed infants.[29] These neonates accumulate significant levels of unconjugated bilirubin 7 days after birth and reach maximum levels of 10 to 30 mg/dL in the third week of life. It is thought that the breast milk contains fatty acids that inhibit bilirubin conjugation in the neonatal liver. A factor in breast milk is also thought to increase the absorption of bilirubin in the duodenum. This type of jaundice disappears if breast-feeding is discontinued. Nursing can be resumed in 3 to 4 days without any hyperbilirubinemia ensuing.

Hyperbilirubinemia places the neonate at risk for the development of a neurologic syndrome called *kernicterus*. This condition is caused by the accumulation of unconjugated bilirubin in brain cells. Unconjugated bilirubin is lipid soluble, crosses the permeable blood–brain barrier of the neonate, and is deposited in cells of the basal ganglia, causing brain damage. Asphyxia and hyperosmolality may also contribute by damaging the blood–brain barrier and allowing bilirubin to cross and enter the cells. The level of unconjugated bilirubin and the duration of exposure that will be toxic to the infant are unknown. The less mature infant, however, is at greater risk for kernicterus.[29]

Symptoms may appear 2 to 5 days after birth in term infants or by day 7 in premature infants. Lethargy, poor feeding, and short-term behavioral changes may be evident in mildly affected infants. Severe manifestations include rigidity, tremors, ataxia, and hearing loss. Extreme cases cause seizures and death. Most survivors are seriously damaged and by 3 years of age exhibit involuntary muscle spasm, seizures, mental retardation, and deafness.

Hyperbilirubinemia in the neonate is treated with phototherapy or exchange transfusion. Phototherapy is more commonly used to treat jaundiced infants and reduce the risk for kernicterus. Exposure to fluorescent light in the blue range of the visible spectrum (420- to 470-nm wavelength) reduces bilirubin levels. Bilirubin in the skin absorbs the light energy and is converted to a structural isomer that is more water soluble and can be excreted in the stool and urine. Effective treatment depends on the area of skin exposed and the infant's ability to metabolize and excrete bilirubin. Frequent monitoring of bilirubin levels, body temperature, and hydration is critical to the infant's care. Exchange transfusion is considered when signs of kernicterus are evident or hyperbilirubinemia is sustained or rising and unresponsive to phototherapy.

Hemolytic Disease of the Newborn

Erythroblastosis fetalis, or hemolytic disease of the newborn, occurs in Rh-positive infants of Rh-negative mothers who have been sensitized. The mother can produce anti-Rh antibodies from pregnancies in which the infants are Rh positive or by blood transfusions of Rh-positive blood. The Rh-negative mother usually becomes sensitized during the first few days after delivery, when fetal Rh-positive red cells from the placental site are released into the maternal circulation. Because the antibodies take several weeks to develop, the first Rh-positive infant of an Rh-negative mother usually is not affected. Infants with Rh-negative blood have no antigens on their red cells to react with the maternal antibodies and are not affected.

After an Rh-negative mother has been sensitized, the Rh antibodies from her blood are transferred to subsequent infants through the placental circulation. These antibodies react with the red cell antigens of the Rh-positive infant, causing agglutination and hemolysis. This leads to severe anemia with compensatory hyperplasia and enlargement of the blood-forming organs, including the spleen and liver, in the fetus. Liver function may be impaired, with decreased production of albumin causing massive edema, called *hydrops fetalis*. If blood levels of unconjugated bilirubin are abnormally high because of red cell hemolysis, there is a danger of kernicterus developing in the infant, resulting in severe brain damage or death.

Several advances have served to decrease significantly the threat to infants born to Rh-negative mothers: prevention of sensitization, antenatal identification of the at-risk fetus, and intrauterine transfusion to the affected fetus. The injection of Rh immune globulin (*i.e.*, gamma-globulin–containing Rh antibody) prevents sensitization in Rh-negative mothers who have given birth to Rh-positive infants if administered at 28 weeks' gestation and within 72 hours of delivery, abortion, genetic amniocentesis, or fetal-maternal bleeding. After sensitization has developed, the immune globulin is of no value. Since 1968, the year Rh immune globulin was introduced, the incidence of sensitization of Rh-negative women has dropped dramatically. Early prenatal care and screening of maternal blood continue to be important in reducing immunization. Efforts to improve therapy are aimed at production of monoclonal anti-D, the Rh antibody.

In the past, approximately 20% of erythroblastotic fetuses died in utero. Fetal Rh phenotyping can now be performed to identify at-risk fetuses in the first trimester using fetal blood or amniotic cells.[30] Hemolysis in these fetuses can be treated by intrauterine transfusions of red cells through the umbilical cord. Exchange transfusions are administered after birth by removing and replacing the infant's blood volume with type O Rh-negative blood. The exchange transfusion removes most of the hemolyzed red cells and some of the total bilirubin, treating the anemia and hyperbilirubinemia.

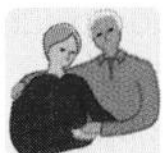

RED CELL CHANGES WITH AGING

Anemia is an increasingly common health problem in elderly people, affecting approximately 12% of persons aged 60 years and older.[31] Its prevalence is known to increase with age, with the highest prevalence occurring in men aged 85 years and older. Undiagnosed and untreated anemia can have severe consequences and is associated with increased risk for mortality, lower functional ability, self-care deficits, and depression. It can also cause neurologic and cognitive disorders and cardiovascular complications.

Hemoglobin levels decline after middle age. In studies of men older than 60 years of age, mean hemoglobin levels ranged from 15.3 to 12.4 g/dL, with the lowest levels found in the oldest persons. The decline is less in women, with mean levels ranging from 13.8 to 11.7 mg/dL.[32] In most asymptomatic elderly persons, lower hemoglobin levels result from iron deficiency and anemia of chronic disease. Anemia of chronic disease is associated with a number of conditions such as acute infections, chronic infections (tuberculosis), chronic inflammatory disorders (rheumatoid arthritis), malignancy, and protein-energy malnutrition.[31]

As with other body systems, the capacity for red cell production changes with aging. The location of bone cells involved in red cell production shifts toward the axial skeleton, and the number of progenitor cells declines from approximately 50% at age 65 years to approximately 30% at age 75 years. [32] Despite these changes, the elderly are able to maintain hemoglobin and hematocrit levels within a range that is similar to younger adults.[33] However, during a stress situation such as bleeding, the red blood cells of the elderly are not replaced as promptly as those of their younger counterparts. This inability to replace red blood cells closely correlates with the increased prevalence of anemia in the elderly.

Although the age-associated decline in the hematopoietic reserve in the elderly is not completely understood, several factors seem to play a role, including a reduction in hematopoietic progenitors, reduced production of hematopoietic growth factors, and reduced sensitivity of hematopoietic progenitors (*e.g.*, erythropoietin).[31,34] Inflammatory cytokines, which have been found to increase with age, may mediate this reduced sensitivity to erythropoietin.

The diagnosis of anemia in the elderly requires a complete physical examination, a complete blood count, and studies to rule out comorbid conditions such as malignancy, gastrointestinal conditions that cause bleeding, and pernicious anemia. The complete blood count should include a peripheral blood smear and a reticulocyte count and index. If the reticulocyte index is appropriately increased for the level of anemia, then blood loss or red cell destruction should be suspected. If the reticulocyte index is inappropriately low, then decreased red cell production is indicated.[34]

Treatment of anemia in the elderly should focus on the underlying cause and correction of the red cell deficit. An important aspect of anemia of chronic disease is the inability to use and mobilize iron effectively.[31] Orally administered iron is poorly used in older adults, despite normal iron absorption.[32] Although erythropoietin remains the treatment of choice for anemias associated with cancer and renal disease, its potential use in treating anemias associated with aging remains to be established.

In summary, hemoglobin concentrations at birth are high, reflecting the in utero need for oxygen delivery; toward the end of the first postnatal week, these levels begin to decline, gradually falling to a minimum value at approximately 2 months of age. During the early neonatal period, there is a shift from fetal to adult hemoglobin. Many infants have physiologic jaundice because of hyperbilirubinemia during the first week of life, probably related to increased red cell breakdown and the inability of the infant's liver to conjugate bilirubin. The term *kernicterus* describes elevated levels of lipid-soluble, unconjugated bilirubin, which can be toxic to brain cells. Depending on severity, it is treated with phototherapy, exchange transfusions, or both. Hemolytic disease of the newborn occurs in Rh-positive infants of Rh-negative mothers who have been sensitized. It involves hemolysis of infant red cells in response to maternal Rh antibodies that have crossed the placenta. Administration of Rh immune globulin to the mother within 72 hours of delivery of an Rh-positive infant, abortion, or amniocentesis prevents sensitization.

Anemia is an increasingly common health problem in the elderly, affecting approximately 12% of persons aged 60 years and older. As with many other tissue cells, the capacity for red cell replacement decreases with aging. Although most elderly persons are able to maintain their hemoglobin and hematocrit levels within a normal range, they are unable to replace their red cells as promptly as their younger counterparts during a stress situation such as bleeding. This inability to replace red blood cells closely correlates with the increased prevalence of anemia in elderly people, which is usually the result of bleeding, infection, malignancy, or chronic disease.

REVIEW EXERCISES

A 29-year-old woman complains of generalized fatigue. Her physical exam reveals a heart rate of 115 beats/minute, blood pressure of 115/75 mm Hg, and respiratory rate of 28 breaths/minute. Her skin and nail beds are pale. Her laboratory results include RBC $3.0 \times 10^6/\mu L$, hematocrit 30%, hemoglobin 9 g/dL, and a decrease in serum ferritin levels.

A. What disorder do you suspect this woman has?

B. What additional data would be helpful in determining the etiology of her condition?

C. Which of her signs reflect the body's attempt to compensate for the disorder?

D. What is the significance of the low ferritin level, and how could it be used to make decisions related to her treatment?

A 65-year-old woman is being seen in the clinic because of numbness in her lower legs and feet and difficulty walking. She has no other complaints. She takes a blood pressure pill, two calcium pills, and a multivitamin pill daily. Her laboratory results include RBC $3.0 \times 10^6/\mu L$, hematocrit 20%, hemoglobin 9 g/dL, and a markedly elevated MVC.

A. What type of anemia does she have?

B. What is the reason for her neurologic symptoms?

C. What type of treatment would be appropriate?

A 12-year-old boy with sickle cell disease presents in the emergency room with severe chest pain. His mother reports that he was doing well until he came down with a respiratory tract infection. She also says he insisted on playing basketball with the other boys in the neighborhood even though he was not feeling well.

A. What is the most likely cause of pain in this boy?

B. Infections and aerobic exercise that increase the levels of deoxygenated hemoglobin produce sickling in persons who are homozygous for the sickle cell gene and have sickle cell disease, but not in persons who are heterozygous and have sickle cell trait. Explain.

C. People with sickle disease experience anemia but not iron deficiency. Explain.

References

1. English E. (2003). Blood components, immunity, and hemostasis. In Rhoades R. A., Tanner R. A. *Medical physiology* (2nd ed., pp. 191–197), Philadelphia: Lippincott Williams & Wilkins.
2. Beck W. S. (1991). Erythropoiesis and introduction to the anemias. In Beck W. S. (Ed.), *Hematology* (5th ed., pp. 27, 29). Cambridge, MA: MIT Press.
3. Steinberg M. H., Rodgers, G. P. (2001). Pathophysiology of sickle cell disease: role of cellular and genetic modifiers. *Seminars in Hematology 38,* 299–306.
4. Bonner H., Bagg A., Cossman J. (1999). The blood and lymphoid organs. In Rubin E., Farber J. L. (Eds.), *Pathology* (3rd ed., pp. 1075–1085). Philadelphia: Lippincott-Raven.
5. Kumar V., Cotran R. S., Robbins S. L. (2003). *Robbins basic pathology* (7th ed., pp. 407–418). Philadelphia: W. B. Saunders.
6. Ballas S. K. (2001). Sickle cell disease. *Seminars in Hematology 38,* 307–314.
7. Lane P. (1996). Sickle cell disease. *Pediatric Clinics of North America 43,* 639–666.
8. National Institutes of Health. (2002). *The management of sickle cell disease.* NIH Publication No. 02-2117. [On-line.] Available at http://www.nhlbi.nih.gov/health/prof/blood/sickle/index.htm.
9. Vichinsky E. (2002). New therapies in sickle cell disease. *Lancet 360,* 629–631.
10. Rund D., Rachmilewitz E. (2001). Pathophysiology of alpha- and β-thalassemia: therapeutic implications. *Seminars in Hematology 38,* 343–349.
11. Lo L., Singer S. T. (2002). Thalassemia: current approach to an old disease. *Pediatric Clinics of North America 49,* 1165–1191.
12. Brittenham G. M. (2000). Disorders of iron metabolism: Iron deficiency and overload. In Hoffman R., Benz E. J., Shattil S. J., et al. (Eds.), *Hematology: Basic principles and practice* (3rd ed., pp. 405, 413). New York: Churchill Livingstone.
13. Glader B. (2004). Anemia of inadequate production. In Behrman R. E., Kliegman R. M., Jenson H. B. (Eds.), *Nelson textbook of pediatrics* (17th ed., pp. 1606–1607), Philadelphia: Saunders.
14. Yager J. Y., Hartfield D. S. (2002). Neurologic manifestations of iron deficiency in childhood. *Pediatric Neurology 27,* 85–92.
15. Kazal L. A. (2002). Prevention of iron deficiency in infants and toddlers. *American Family Physician 66,* 1217–1224.
16. Oh R., Brown D. L. (2003). Vitamin B_{12} deficiency. *American Family Physician 67,* 979–986.
17. Hoffbrand A. V., Herbert V. (1999). Nutritional anemias. *Seminars in Hematology 36*(Suppl. 7), 13–23.
18. Johnston M. V., Kinsman S. (2004). Congenital anomalies of the central nervous system. In Behrman R. E., Kliegman R. M., Jenson H. B. (Eds.), *Nelson textbook of pediatrics* (17th ed., pp. 1983–1984), Philadelphia: W. B. Saunders.
19. Bailey L. B. (2000). New standard for folate intake in pregnant women. *American Journal of Clinical Nutrition 71*(5 Suppl.), 1304S–1307S.
20. Young N. S., Maciejewski J. P. (2000). Aplastic anemias. In Hoffman R., Benz E. J., Shattil S. J., et al. (Eds.), *Hematology: Basic principles and practice* (3rd ed., pp. 316, 318). New York: Churchill Livingstone.
21. Hillman R. S., Ault K. A. (2002). *Hematology in clinical practice* (3rd ed., pp. 46, 12). New York: McGraw-Hill.
22. Goodnough L. T., Brecher M. E., Kanter M. H., AuBuchon J. P. (1999). Blood conservation. *New England Journal of Medicine 340,* 525–533.
23. Goodnough L. T., Brecher M. E., Kanter M. H., AuBuchon J. P. (1999). Blood transfusion. *New England Journal of Medicine 340,* 438–447.

24. Pittiglio D. H. (Ed.). (1983). *Modern blood banking and transfusion practices* (pp. 91–92). Philadelphia: F. A. Davis.
25. Vengelen-Tyler V. (Ed.). (1996). *Technical manual* (12th ed., pp. 135–142, 256). Bethesda, MD: American Association of Blood Banks.
26. Hocking W. G. (2002). Primary and secondary erythrocytosis. In Mazza J. J., *Manual of clinical hematology* (3rd ed., p. 80). Philadelphia: Lippincott Williams & Wilkins.
27. Ohls R. K., Christensen R. D. (2004). Development of the hematopoietic system. In Behrman R. E., Kliegman R. M., Jenson H. B. (Eds.), *Nelson textbook of pediatrics* (17th ed., pp. 1599–1604). Philadelphia: W. B. Saunders.
28. Brown M. S. (1988). Physiologic anemia of infancy: Nutritional factors and abnormal states. In Stockman J. A., Pochedly C. (Eds.), *Developmental and neonatal hematology* (pp. 252, 274). New York: Raven Press.
29. Stoll B. J., Kliegman R. M. (2004). Jaundice and hyperbilirubinemia in the newborn. In Behrman R. E., Kliegman R. M., Jenson H. B. (Eds.), *Nelson textbook of pediatrics* (17th ed., pp. 592–599). Philadelphia: W. B. Saunders.
30. Kramer K., Cohen H. J. (2000). Antenatal diagnosis of hematologic disorders. In Hoffman R., Benz E. J., Shattil S. J., et al. (Eds.), *Hematology: Basic principles and practice* (3rd ed., p. 2495). New York: Churchill Livingstone.
31. Williams W. J. (1995). Hematology in the aged. In Beutler E., Lichtman A., Coller B. S., Kipps T. J. (Eds.), *Williams' hematology* (5th ed., p. 73). New York: McGraw-Hill.
32. Balducci L. (2003). Epidemiology of anemia in the elderly: Information on diagnostic evaluation. *Journal of the American Geriatrics Society 51*(Suppl. 3), S2–S9.
33. Rothstein G. (2003). Disordered hematopoiesis and myelodysplasia in the elderly. *Journal of the American Geriatrics Society 51*(Suppl. 3), S22–S26.
34. Lipschitz D. (2003). Medical and functional consequences of anemia in the elderly. *Journal of the American Geriatrics Society 51* (Suppl. 3), S10–S13.

CHAPTER

17

Disorders of White Blood Cells and Lymphoid Tissues

Kerry Twite

The white blood cells and lymphoid tissue where these cells originate, mature, and function protect the body against invasion by foreign agents. Disorders of the white blood cells include a deficiency of leukocytes (leukopenia) and proliferative disorders. The proliferative disorders may be reactive, such as occurs with infection, or neoplastic, such as with the leukemias and lymphomas. This chapter focuses on leukopenia, infectious mononucleosis, malignant lymphomas, leukemias, and plasma cell dyscrasias (multiple myeloma).

Hematopoietic and Lymphoid Tissues

After completing this section of the chapter, you should be able to meet the following objectives:

- List the cells and tissues of the hematopoietic system
- Trace the development of the different blood cells from their origin in the pluripotent bone marrow stem cell to their circulation in the bloodstream

The hematopoietic system encompasses all the blood cells, their precursors, and their derivatives: the red blood cells, the thrombocytes or platelets, and the white blood cells. It includes the myeloid or bone marrow tissue in which the white blood cells are formed and the lymphoid tissues of the lymph nodes, thymus, and spleen, in which the white blood cells circulate and mature. The development of different cell lineages depends on cellular interactions and exposure to cytokines.

LEUKOCYTES (WHITE BLOOD CELLS)

The white blood cells include the granulocytes (*i.e.*, neutrophils, eosinophils, and basophils), the monocyte and macrophage lineage, and the lymphocytes. Granulocytes and monocytes are derived from the myeloid stem cell in the bone marrow and circulate in the blood. T lymphocytes (T cells) and B lymphocytes (B cells) originate in the bone marrow and migrate between the blood and the lymph (see Chapter 19). T lymphocytes mature in the thymus, and the B lymphocytes mature in the bone marrow—the mammalian equivalent of the avian bursa of Fabricius. The T lymphocytes differentiate to form helper T cells, which serve to orchestrate the immune response, and cytotoxic T cells, which provide for cell-mediated immune responses. The B lymphocytes differentiate to form immunoglobulin-producing plasma cells. Another population of lymphocytes includes the large granular lymphocytes, or *natural killer cells,* which do not share the specificity or characteristics of the T lymphocytes or the B lymphocytes, but have the ability to lyse target cells.[1]

HEMATOPOIESIS

- The white blood cells are formed from hematopoietic stem cells that differentiate into committed progenitor cells that in turn develop into the myelogenous and lymphocytic lineages needed for the formation of the different types of white blood cell.
- The growth and reproduction of the different stem cells is controlled by CSFs and other cytokines and chemical mediators.
- The life span of white blood cells is relatively short so that constant renewal is necessary to maintain normal blood levels. Any conditions that decrease the availability of stem cells or hematopoietic growth factors produce a decrease in white blood cells.

BONE MARROW AND HEMATOPOIESIS

The entire hematopoietic system, in all its complexity, arises from a small number of stem cells that differentiate to form blood cells and replenish bone marrow by a process of self-renewal. All the hematopoietic precursors, including the erythroid (red blood cell), myelocyte (granulocyte and monocyte), lymphocyte (T cell and B cell), and megakaryocyte (platelet) series, are derived from a small population of cells called the *pluripotent stem cells* (Chapter 14, Fig. 14-2). These cells are capable of providing *progenitor cells* (*i.e.,* parent cells) for lymphopoiesis and myelopoiesis, processes by which lymphoid and myeloid blood cells are made, respectively. Several levels of differentiation lead to the development of committed *unipotent cells,* which are the progenitors for each of the blood cell types. The progenitor cells lose their capacity for self-renewal but retain the potential to differentiate into erythrocytes, monocytes, megakaryocytes, or lymphocytes. This regulation of blood cells is thought to be at least partially controlled by protein messenger molecules, called *cytokines,* that regulate the function of other cells, in this case the blood cell precursors.[1]

The different committed stem cells, when grown in culture, produce colonies of specific types of blood cells. A committed stem cell that forms a specific type of blood cell is called a *colony-forming unit.* The *hematopoietic growth factors* are a family of glycoproteins that support hematopoietic colony formation (see Chapter 14). These growth factors can be categorized into three functional groups: those that are involved in the development of a specific cell lineage, those that affect the early multipotential progenitor cells, and those that indirectly regulate hematopoiesis by inducing the expression of growth factor genes in other cells.[2]

There are several lineage-specific growth factors: erythropoietin, granulocyte-macrophage colony-stimulating factor (GM-CSF), and monocyte-macrophage colony-stimulating factor (M-CSF). Although the hematopoietic growth factors act at different points in the proliferation and differentiation pathway, their functions overlap. Other cytokines, such as interleukin (IL)-1, IL-4, IL-6, and interferon, act synergistically to support the functions of the growth factors.[3]

Many of the hematopoietic growth factors have multiple functions and affect a variety of cell types. For example, GM-CSF stimulates the erythropoietic burst-forming units; stimulates the growth and function of granulocyte, macrophage, and eosinophil progenitor cells; and induces IL-1 gene expression in neutrophils and peripheral mononuclear leukocytes. Other growth factors, such as IL-3, act on the most immature marrow progenitor cells, thereby promoting the development of cells that can differentiate into a number of cell types. Stem cell factor (also called *c-kit ligand*) mediates the activation of stem cells and stimulates their differentiation into various cell lineages.[2]

The identification and characterization of the various cytokines and growth factors have led to their use in treating a wide range of diseases, including bone marrow failure, hematopoietic neoplasms, infectious diseases, and congenital and myeloproliferative disorders. Many of these uses are investigational.

LYMPHOID TISSUES

The body's lymphatic system, which consists of the lymphatic vessels, lymph nodes, spleen, and thymus, is made up of lymphoid tissue (see Chapter 19). Lymph is body fluid that originates as excess fluid from the capillaries. It is returned to the vascular compartment and the right side of the heart through lymphatic vessels.

The lymph nodes, which are situated along the lymphatic channels, filter the lymph before it is returned to the circulation (Fig. 17-1). Lymph enters a lymph node through afferent lymphatic channels, percolates through

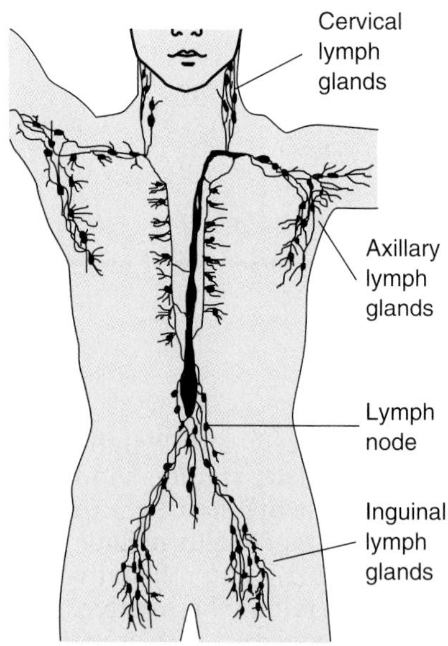

FIGURE 17-1 Location of a portion of the lymph nodes in the human body. (*What you need to know about Hodgkin's disease.* [1981]. Washington, DC: Department of Health and Human Services)

a labyrinthine system of minute channels lined with endothelial and phagocytic cells, and then emerges through efferent lymphatic vessels. A number of efferent vessels join to form collecting trunks. Each collecting trunk drains a definite area of the body. By filtering bacteria and other particulate matter, the lymph nodes serve as a secondary line of defense even when clinical disease is not present. In the event of malignant neoplasm development, cancer cells are filtered and retained by the lymph nodes for a period before being disseminated to other parts of the body. Because of their contribution to the development of the immune system, lymph nodes are relatively large at birth and progressively atrophy throughout life.

In summary, the hematopoietic system consists of a number of cells derived from the pluripotent stem cells originating in the bone marrow. These cells differentiate into committed cell lines that mature into red blood cells, platelets, and a variety of white blood cells. The lymphoid system consists of a network of lymphatic vessels, nodes, and tissues whose function is to drain lymph fluid from specific areas of the body and to filter particulate matter such as bacteria and cancer cells.

Nonneoplastic Disorders of White Blood Cells

After completing this section of the chapter, you should be able to meet the following objectives:

- Define the terms *leukopenia, neutropenia, granulocytopenia,* and *aplastic anemia*
- Cite two general causes of neutropenia
- Describe the mechanism of symptom production in neutropenia

The number of leukocytes, or white blood cells, in the peripheral circulation normally ranges from 5000 to 10,000/μL of blood. The term *leukopenia* describes an absolute decrease in white blood cell numbers. The disorder may affect any of the specific types of white blood cells, but most often it affects the neutrophils, which are the predominant type of granulocyte.

NEUTROPENIA (AGRANULOCYTOSIS)

Neutropenia refers specifically to a decrease in neutrophils. It commonly is defined as a circulating neutrophil count of less than 1500 cells/μL. Agranulocytosis, which denotes a severe neutropenia, is characterized by a circulating neutrophil count of less than 200 cells/μL.[4]

The reduction in granulocytes can occur because there is reduced or ineffective production of neutrophils or because there is excessive removal of neutrophils from the blood. The causes of neutropenia are summarized in Table 17-1.

Acquired Neutropenia

Granulopoiesis may be impaired as a result of a variety of bone marrow disorders, such as aplastic anemia or bone marrow depression due to cancer chemotherapy and irradiation, which interfere with the formation of all blood cells. Overgrowth of neoplastic cells in cases of nonmyelogenous leukemia and lymphoma also may suppress the function of neutrophil precursors. Infections by viruses or bacteria may drain neutrophils from the blood faster than they can be replaced, thereby depleting the neutrophil storage pool in the bone marrow.[4] Because of the neutrophil's short life span of approximately 1 day in the peripheral blood, neutropenia occurs rapidly when granulopoiesis is impaired. Under these conditions, neutropenia usually is accompanied by thrombocytopenia (*i.e.,* platelet deficiency).

TABLE 17-1 Causes of Neutropenia

Cause	Mechanism
Accelerated removal (*e.g.,* inflammation and infection)	Removal of neutrophils from the circulation exceeds production
Drug-induced granulocytopenia	
Defective production	
Cytotoxic drugs used in cancer therapy	Predictable damage to precursor cells, usually dose dependent
Phenothiazine, thiouracil, chloramphenicol, phenylbutazone, and others	Idiosyncratic depression of bone marrow function
Hydantoinates, primidone, and others	Intramedullary destruction of granulocytes
Immune destruction	Immunologic mechanisms with cytolysis or leukoagglutination
Aminopyrine and others	
Periodic or cyclic neutropenia (occurs during infancy and later)	Unknown
Neoplasms involving bone marrow (*e.g.,* leukemias and lymphomas)	Overgrowth of neoplastic cells, which crowd out granulopoietic precursors
Idiopathic neutropenia that occurs in the absence of other disease or provoking influence	Autoimmune reaction
Felty's syndrome	Intrasplenic destruction of neutrophils

In *aplastic anemia,* all of the myeloid stem cells are affected, resulting in anemia, thrombocytopenia, and agranulocytosis. Autoimmune disorders or idiosyncratic drug reactions may cause increased and premature destruction of neutrophils. In splenomegaly, neutrophils may be trapped in the spleen along with other blood cells. In Felty's syndrome, a variant of rheumatoid arthritis, there is increased destruction of neutrophils in the spleen.

Most cases of neutropenia are drug related. Chemotherapeutic drugs used in the treatment of cancer (*e.g.,* alkylating agents, antimetabolites) cause predictable dose-dependent suppression of bone marrow function. The term *idiosyncratic* is used to describe drug reactions that are different from the effects obtained in most persons and that cannot be explained in terms of allergy. A number of drugs, such as chloramphenicol (an antibiotic), phenothiazine tranquilizers, sulfonamides, propylthiouracil (used in the treatment of hyperthyroidism), and phenylbutazone (used in the treatment of arthritis), may cause idiosyncratic depression of bone marrow function. Some drugs, such as hydantoin derivatives and primidone (used in the treatment of seizure disorders), can cause intramedullary destruction of granulocytes and thereby impair production. Many idiosyncratic cases of drug-induced neutropenia are thought to be caused by immunologic mechanisms, with the drug or its metabolites acting as antigens (*i.e.,* haptens) to incite the production of antibodies reactive against the neutrophils. Neutrophils possess human leukocyte antigens (HLA) and other antigens specific to a given leukocyte line. Antibodies to these specific antigens have been identified in some cases of drug-induced neutropenia.[4]

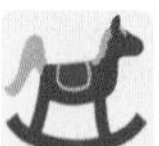

Congenital Neutropenia

A decreased production of granulocytes is a feature of a group of hereditary hematologic disorders, including cyclic neutropenia and Kostmann's syndrome. *Periodic* or *cyclic neutropenia* is an autosomal dominant disorder with variable expression that begins in infancy and persists for decades. It is characterized by periodic neutropenia that develops every 21 to 30 days and lasts approximately 3 to 6 days. Although the cause is undetermined, it is thought to result from impaired feedback regulation of granulocyte production and release. *Kostmann's syndrome,* which occurs sporadically or as an autosomal recessive disorder, causes severe neutropenia while preserving the erythroid and megakaryocyte cell lineages that result in red blood cell and platelet production. The total white blood cell count may be within normal limits, but the neutrophil count is less than 200/µL. Monocyte and eosinophil levels may be elevated. Treatment includes the administration of recombinant human granulocyte colony-stimulating factor (rhG-CSF).[5]

A transient neutropenia may occur in neonates whose mothers have hypertension. It usually lasts from 1 to 60 hours but can persist for 3 to 30 days. This type of neutropenia, which is associated with increased risk for nosocomial infection, is thought to result from transiently reduced neutrophil production.[4]

Clinical Course

The clinical features of neutropenia usually depend on the severity of neutropenia and the cause of the disorder. Because the neutrophil is essential to the cellular phase of inflammation, infections are common in persons with neutropenia, and extreme caution is needed to protect them from exposure to infectious organisms. Infections that may go unnoticed in a person with a normal neutrophil count could prove fatal in a person with neutropenia. These infections commonly are caused by organisms that normally colonize the skin, vagina, and gastrointestinal tract.

The signs and symptoms of neutropenia initially are those of bacterial or fungal infections. They include malaise, chills, and fever, followed by extreme weakness and fatigue. The white blood cell count often is reduced to 1000/µL and, in certain cases, may fall to 200 to 300/µL. The most frequent site of serious infection is the respiratory tract, a result of bacteria, fungi, and protozoa that frequently colonize the airways. Ulcerative necrotizing lesions of the mouth are common in neutropenia. Ulcerations of the skin, vagina, and gastrointestinal tract also may occur.[4]

Antibiotics are used to treat infections in those situations in which neutrophil destruction can be controlled or the neutropoietic function of the bone marrow can be recovered. Hematopoietic growth factors such as GM-CSF are being used more commonly to stimulate the maturation and differentiation of the granulocyte cell lineage. Treatment with these biologic response modifiers has reduced the period of neutropenia and the risk for development of potentially fatal septicemia.[4]

INFECTIOUS MONONUCLEOSIS

Infectious mononucleosis is a self-limiting lymphoproliferative disorder caused by the Epstein-Barr virus (EBV), a member of the herpesvirus family.[6,7] EBV is commonly present in all human populations. Infectious mononucleosis is most prevalent in adolescents and young adults in the upper socioeconomic classes in developed countries. This is probably because the disease, which is relatively asymptomatic when it occurs during childhood, confers complete immunity to the virus. In families from upper socioeconomic classes, exposure to the virus may be delayed until late adolescence or early adulthood. In such persons, mode of infection, size of the viral pool, and physiologic and immunologic condition of the host may determine whether the infection occurs.

Pathogenesis

Infectious mononucleosis is largely transmitted through oral contact with EBV-contaminated saliva. The virus initially penetrates the nasopharyngeal, oropharyngeal, and salivary epithelial cells. It then spreads to the underlying oropharyngeal lymphoid tissue and, more specifically, to B lymphocytes, all of which have receptors for EBV. Infection of the B cells may take one of two forms—it may kill the infected B cell, or it may become incorporated into its genome. A small number of infected B cells are killed and in the process release the virions. In most cells, however, the virus associates with the B-cell genome. The B cells that harbor the EBV genome proliferate in the circulation and produce the well-known *heterophil* antibodies that are used for the diagnosis of infectious mononucleosis.[7] A heterophil antibody is an immunoglobulin that reacts with antigens from another species, in this case, sheep red blood cells.

The normal immune response is important in controlling the proliferation of the EBV-infected B cells and cell-free virus. Most important in controlling the proliferation of EBV-infected B cells are the cytotoxic CD8$^+$ T cells and natural killer (NK) cells. The virus-specific T cells appear as large atypical lymphocytes that are characteristic of the infection.[7] In otherwise healthy persons, the humoral and cellular immune responses control viral shedding by limiting the number of infected B cells rather than eliminating them.

Although infectious B cells and free virions disappear from the blood following recovery from the disease, the virus remains in a few transformed B cells in the oropharyngeal region and is shed in the saliva. Once infected with the virus, persons remain asymptomatically infected for life, and a few intermittently shed EBV. Immunosuppressed persons shed the virus more frequently. A symptomatic shedding of EBV by healthy persons accounts for most of the spread of infectious mononucleosis, despite the fact that it is not a highly contagious disease.

Clinical Course

The onset of infectious mononucleosis usually is insidious. The incubation period lasts 4 to 8 weeks.[8] A prodromal period, which lasts for several days, follows and is characterized by malaise, anorexia, and chills. The prodromal period precedes the onset of fever, pharyngitis, and lymphadenopathy. Occasionally, the disorder comes on abruptly with a high fever. Most persons seek medical attention for severe pharyngitis, which usually is most severe on days 5 to 7 and persists for 7 to 14 days. Severe toxic pharyngotonsillitis may cause airway obstruction.

The lymph nodes are typically enlarged throughout the body, particularly in the cervical, axillary, and groin areas. Hepatitis and splenomegaly are common manifestations of the disease and are thought to be immune mediated. Hepatitis is characterized by hepatomegaly, nausea, anorexia, and jaundice. Although discomforting, it usually is a benign condition that resolves without causing permanent liver damage. The spleen may be enlarged two to three times its normal size, and rupture of the spleen is an infrequent complication. A rash that resembles rubella develops in 10% to 15% of cases.[7] In less than 1% of cases, mostly in the adult age group, complications of the central nervous system (CNS) develop. These complications include cranial nerve palsies, encephalitis, meningitis, transverse myelitis, and Guillain-Barré syndrome.

The peripheral blood usually shows an increase in the number of leukocytes, with a white blood cell count between 12,000 and 18,000/μL, 95% of which are lymphocytes.[7] The rise in white blood cells begins during the first week, continues during the second week of the infection, and then returns to normal around the fourth week. Although leukocytosis is common, leukopenia may be seen in some persons during the first 3 days of the illness. Atypical lymphocytes are common, constituting more than 20% of the total lymphocyte count. Heterophil antibodies usually appear during the second or third week and decline after the acute illness has subsided. They may, however, be detectable for up to 9 months after onset of the disease.

Most persons with infectious mononucleosis recover without incident. The acute phase of the illness usually lasts for 2 to 3 weeks, after which recovery occurs rapidly. Some degree of debility and lethargy may persist for 2 to 3 months. Treatment is primarily symptomatic and supportive. It includes bed rest and analgesics such as aspirin to relieve the fever, headache, and sore throat.[8]

In summary, neutropenia, a marked reduction in the number of circulating neutrophils, is one of the major disorders of the white blood cells. It can be acquired or congenital and can result from a combination of mechanisms. Severe neutropenia can occur as a complication of lymphoproliferative diseases, in which neoplastic cells crowd out neutrophil precursor cells, or of radiation therapy or treatment with cytotoxic drugs, which destroy neutrophil precursor cells. Neutropenia also may be encountered as an idiosyncratic reaction to various drugs. Because the neutrophil is essential to the cellular stage of inflammation, severe and often life-threatening infections are common in persons with neutropenia.

Infectious mononucleosis is a self-limited lymphoproliferative disorder caused by the B-lymphocytotropic EBV, a member of the herpesvirus family. The highest incidence of infectious mononucleosis is found in adolescents and young adults, and it is seen more frequently in the upper socioeconomic classes of developed countries. The virus is usually transmitted in the saliva. The disease is characterized by fever, generalized lymphadenopathy, sore throat, and the appearance in the blood of atypical lymphocytes and several antibodies, including the well-known heterophil antibodies that are used in the diagnosis of infectious mononucleosis. Most persons with infectious mononucleosis recover without incident. Treatment is largely symptomatic and supportive.

Neoplastic Disorders of Hematopoietic and Lymphoid Origin

After completing this section of the chapter, you should be able to meet the following objectives:

- Use the concepts regarding the central and peripheral lymphoid tissues to describe the site of origin of the malignant lymphomas, leukemias, and plasma cell dyscrasias
- Explain how changes in chromosomal structure and gene function can contribute to the development of malignant lymphomas, leukemias, and plasma cell dyscrasias
- Contrast and compare the signs and symptoms of Hodgkin's disease and non-Hodgkin's lymphoma
- Describe the treatment measures used in Hodgkin's disease and non-Hodgkin's lymphoma

- Use the predominant white blood cell type and classification of acute or chronic to describe the four general types of leukemia
- Explain the manifestations of leukemia in terms of altered cell differentiation
- Describe the following complications of acute leukemia and its treatment: leukostasis, tumor lysis syndrome, hyperuricemia, and blast crisis
- Relate the clonal expansion of immunoglobulin-producing plasma cells and accompanying destructive skeletal changes that occur with multiple myeloma in terms of manifestations and clinical course for the disorder

The neoplastic disorders of hematopoietic and lymphoid origin represent the most important of the white cell disorders. They include somewhat overlapping categories: the lymphomas (Hodgkin's disease and non-Hodgkin's lymphoma), the leukemias, and the plasma cell dyscrasias (multiple myeloma). The clinical features of these neoplasms are largely determined by their site of origin, the progenitor cell from which they originated, and the molecular events involved in their transformation into a malignant neoplasm. The leukemias, which arise from hematopoietic precursors in the bone marrow, can involve lymphocytes, granulocytes, and other blood cells. Because blood cells circulate throughout the body, these neoplasms are disseminated from the onset. The lymphomas originate in peripheral lymphoid structures such as the lymph nodes where B and T lymphocytes undergo further differentiation and proliferation as they interact with antigens. The plasma cell dyscrasias originate in the bone marrow where B cells differentiate into plasma cells.

MALIGNANT LYMPHOMAS

The lymphomas, Hodgkin's disease and non-Hodgkin's lymphoma, represent solid tumors derived from neoplastic lymphoid tissue cells (*i.e.,* lymphocytes or histiocytes) and their precursors or derivatives. The sixth most common cancer in the United States, the lymphomas are among the most studied human tumors and among the most curable.

Hodgkin's Disease

Hodgkin's disease is a specialized form of lymphoma that features the presence of an abnormal cell called a *Reed-Sternberg cell.*[9] In 2003, there were an estimated 7600 newly diagnosed cases and 1300 deaths from Hodgkin's disease.[10] Distribution of the disease is bimodal; the incidence rises sharply after 10 years of age, peaks in the early 20s, and then declines until 50 years of age. After 50 years of age, the incidence again increases steadily with age. The younger adult group consists equally of men and women, but after age 50 years, the incidence is higher among men.[11] The overall incidence of Hodgkin's disease has declined significantly since the late 1980s at a rate of 0.9% per year.[10]

The cause of Hodgkin's disease is unknown. There is a long-standing suspicion that the disease may begin as an inflammatory reaction to an infectious agent, possibly a virus. This belief is supported by epidemiologic data that include the clustering of the disease among family members and among students who have attended the same school. A suspected etiologic agent is EBV because a significant percentage of biopsy specimens have exhibited EBV DNA. In a number of studies that assessed the relationship between Hodgkin's disease and an infectious etiology, a threefold increased incidence of Hodgkin's disease was found in patients with a previous history of mononucleosis. Findings contradictory to the proposed viral hypothesis include an absence of occurrence in marital partners. There also seems to be an association between the presence of the disease and a deficient immune state. Although exposure to carcinogens or viruses, as well as genetic and immune mechanisms, have been proposed as causes, none have proved to be involved in the pathogenesis of Hodgkin's disease.

Manifestations. Hodgkin's disease is characterized by painless and progressive enlargement of a single node or group of nodes. It is believed to originate in one area of the lymphatic system, and if unchecked, it spreads throughout the lymphatic network. The initial lymph node involvement typically is above the level of the diaphragm. An exception is in elderly persons, in whom the subdiaphragmatic lymph nodes may be the first to be involved. Involvement of the liver, spleen, and bone marrow occurs after the disease becomes generalized.

The Reed-Sternberg cell, a distinctive tumor cell, is considered to be the true neoplastic element in Hodgkin's disease.[9,12] The classic Reed-Sternberg cell is a binucleated cell with mirror-image nuclei that contain clear chromatin and a large eosinophilic nucleolus in each lobe (Fig. 17-2). These malignant proliferating cells may invade almost any area of the body and may produce a wide variety of signs and symptoms. The spleen is involved in one third of the cases at the time of diagnosis.[12] A common finding in Hodgkin's disease is the presence of painless lymph node

MALIGNANT LYMPHOMAS

- The lymphoma represent malignancies that arise in the peripheral lymphoid tissues.
- Hodgkin's disease is a group of cancers characterized by Reed-Sternberg cells that begins as a malignancy in a single lymph node and then spreads to contiguous lymph nodes.
- Non-Hodgkin's lymphomas represent a group of heterogeneous lymphocytic cancers that are multicentric in origin and spread to various tissues throughout the body, including the bone marrow.
- Both types of lymphomas are characterized by manifestations related to uncontrolled lymph node and lymphoid tissue growth, bone marrow involvement, and constitutional symptoms (fever, fatigue, weight loss) related to the rapid growth of abnormal lymphoid cells and tissues.

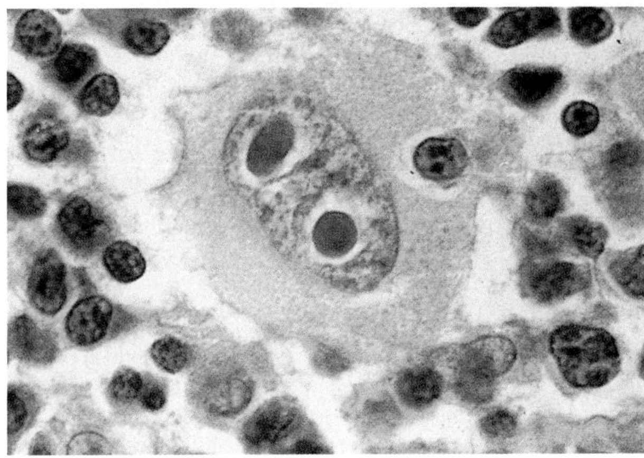

FIGURE 17-2 Classic Reed-Sternberg cell. Mirror-image nuclei contain large eosinophilic nucleoli. (Rubin E., Farber J.L. [1999]. *Pathology* [3rd ed., p. 1144]. Philadelphia: Lippincott-Raven)

enlargement, involving a single lymph node or groups of lymph nodes. The cervical and mediastinal nodes are involved most frequently. Less commonly, the axillary, inguinal, and retroperitoneal nodes are initially involved.[12] Additional symptoms that suggest Hodgkin's disease include fevers, chills, night sweats, and weight loss.

Persons with Hodgkin's disease are commonly designated as stage A if they lack constitutional symptoms and stage B if significant weight loss, fevers, pruritus, or night sweats are present. Approximately 40% of persons with Hodgkin's disease exhibit the stage B symptoms.[12] Other symptoms, such as fatigue and anemia, are indicative of disease spread. In the advanced stages of Hodgkin's disease, the liver, lungs, digestive tract, and, occasionally, CNS may be involved. As the disease progresses, the rapid proliferation of abnormal lymphocytes leads to an immunologic defect, particularly in cell-mediated responses, rendering the person more susceptible to viral, fungal, and protozoal infections. Anergy, or the failure to develop a positive response to skin tests, such as the tuberculin test, is common early in the course of the disease. An increased neutrophil count and mild anemia are often noted.

Diagnosis and Treatment. A definitive diagnosis of Hodgkin's disease requires that the Reed-Sternberg cell be present in a biopsy specimen of lymph node tissue.[12,13] Computed tomography (CT) scans of the chest and abdomen commonly are used to assess for involvement of mediastinal, abdominal, and pelvic lymph nodes.[14] A bipedal lymphangiogram may detect structural changes in the lymph nodes too small to visualize on CT scan. If with initial screenings the extent of lymph node involvement cannot be determined, positron-emission tomography (PET) may be helpful. A bilateral bone marrow biopsy should be performed in patients who are suspected of having disseminated disease.

The staging of Hodgkin's disease is of great clinical importance because the choice of treatment and the prognosis ultimately are related to the distribution of the disease. Staging is determined by the number of lymph nodes that are involved, whether the lymph nodes are on one or both sides of the diaphragm, and whether there is disseminated disease involving the bone marrow, liver, lung, or skin.

Irradiation and chemotherapy are used in treating the disease. Most people with localized disease are treated with radiation therapy. A combined approach using radiation and chemotherapy is used when the patient has adverse prognostic factors such as stage B symptoms, bulky masses, or disease involving nodes in the lower abdomen. As the accuracy of staging techniques, delivery of radiation, and curative efficacy of combination chemotherapy regimens have improved, the survival of people with Hodgkin's disease also has improved. With modern treatment methods, a 5-year cure rate of 85% can be achieved.[10]

Non-Hodgkin's Lymphomas

The non-Hodgkin's lymphomas (NHLs) are a heterogeneous group of solid tumors composed of neoplastic lymphoid cells. The heterogeneity reflects the potential for malignant transformation at any stage of B- and T-lymphocyte differentiation. Non-Hodgkin's occurs three times more frequently than Hodgkin's disease. In 2003, approximately 53,400 new cases of NHL were diagnosed in the United States, and approximately 23,400 deaths resulted from these disorders.[10] Non-Hodgkin's lymphomas are the sixth most common malignancy in both men and women. Since the early 1970s, the incidence rates for NHL have nearly doubled, then stabilized in the 1990s as a result of the decline in NHLs related to acquired immunodeficiency disease (AIDS).[10]

The etiology of most of the NHLs is unknown. A viral cause is suspected in at least some of the lymphomas. There is evidence of EBV infection in 95% of people with Burkitt's lymphoma, which is endemic to some parts of Africa.[9,12] A second virus, the human T-cell lymphoma virus (HTLV-1), which is endemic in the southwestern islands of Japan, has been associated with adult T-cell leukemia-lymphoma. Non-Hodgkin's lymphoma is also seen with increased frequency in persons infected with human immunodeficiency virus (HIV), in those who have received chronic immunosuppressive therapy after organ transplantation, and in individuals with acquired or congenital immunodeficiencies.[13,15] There is also a reported association between chronic *Helicobacter pylori* infection and low-grade, mucosa-associated lymphoid tissue (MALT) lymphoma of the stomach.[15] Other possible risk factors include occupational exposures to herbicides and chemical carcinogens.[10]

Pathogenesis. Non-Hodgkin's lymphomas result from the malignant transformation of normal lymphoid tissue at specific stages of differentiation. Lymphoid tissues can be divided into two major categories: central and peripheral lymphoid tissues (see Chapter 19). The peripheral lymphoid structures, which are the site of origin for the lymphomas, consist of the lymph nodes, spleen, and mucosa-associated lymphoid tissue of the gastrointestinal and respiratory tracts. The lymph nodes, which are located at strategic sites throughout the body, process antigens in lymph drained from most organs through afferent lymph nodes (see Chapter 19, Fig. 19-12). Lymph nodes have a capsule, a cortex, a medulla, and sinuses. The cortex is divided into the follicular and diffuse (paracortical) regions, and the medulla is separated into medullary cords and sinuses. The T lymphocytes are more abundant in the paracortex, and the B lymphocytes are more abundant in the follicles and germinal centers located in the outer cortex. The T lymphocytes proliferate on antigenic stimulation and migrate to the follicles, where they interact with B lymphocytes. These activated follicles become germinal centers, containing macrophages, follicular dendritic cells, and maturing T and B cells.

Non-Hodgkin's lymphomas can originate from malignant transformation of either the T or B cells during their differentiation in the peripheral lymphoid tissues.[9,12] Most (80% to 85%) are of B-cell origin, with the remainder being largely of T-cell origin. Although NHLs can develop in any of the lymphoid tissues, they most commonly originate in the lymph nodes and are classified as follicular, diffuse, or centrocytic.[13] Approximately 35% of NHLs in the United States and 22% in Europe are classified as follicular lymphomas.[16] Non-Hodgkin's lymphomas have the potential to spread to various lymphoid tissues throughout the body, especially the liver, spleen, and bone marrow.

The non-Hodgkin's lymphomas commonly are divided into three groups, depending on the grade of the tumor: low-grade lymphomas, which are predominantly B-cell tumors; intermediate-grade lymphomas, which include B-cell and some T-cell lymphomas; and high-grade lymphomas, which are largely immunoblastic (B-cell), lymphoblastic (T-cell), Burkitt's, and non-Burkitt's lymphomas.[12]

Manifestations. The manifestations of NHL depend on lymphoma type and the stage of the disease. For example, the small lymphocyte tumors are low-grade tumors that tend to progress slowly and are often asymptomatic for long periods. With or without treatment, the natural course of the disease may fluctuate over 5 to 10 or more years. Low-grade lymphomas eventually transform into more aggressive forms of lymphoma-leukemia and cause death of the patient. The diffuse large B-cell lymphomas, which account for about 50% of all NHLs, are particularly aggressive tumors.[9] They are diagnosed with significant symptoms, grow, metastasize rapidly, and are fatal if not treated. Because of their high growth fraction, these lymphomas tend to be radiosensitive and chemosensitive. Hence, with intensive combination chemotherapy, complete remission can be achieved in 60% to 80% of cases.[17]

The most frequently occurring clinical manifestation of NHL is painless, superficial lymphadenopathy. There may be noncontiguous nodal spread of the disease with involvement of the gastrointestinal tract, lung, liver, testes, and bone marrow. Frequently, there is increased susceptibility to bacterial, viral, and fungal infections associated with hypogammaglobulinemia and a poor humoral antibody response, rather than the impaired cellular immunity seen with Hodgkin's disease. Leukemic transformation with high peripheral lymphocytic counts occurs in a small percentage of persons with NHL.[9]

Diagnosis and Treatment. A lymph node biopsy is used to confirm the diagnosis of NHL and immunophenotyping to determine the lymphocyte lineage and clonality. Lymphomas can be grouped according to surface markers or phenotypic properties (*e.g.*, $CD20^+$).[14] Staging of the disease is important in selecting a treatment for persons with NHL. Bone marrow biopsy, blood studies, chest and abdominal CT scans, and nuclear medicine studies often are used to determine the stage of the disease. Cytologic examination of the cerebrospinal fluid may be positive in patients with aggressive NHL.

Treatment of NHL depends on the histologic type and stage of the disease. For early-stage disease, localized radiation may be used as a single treatment modality. However, because most people present with late-stage disease, combination chemotherapy, combined adjuvant radiation therapy, or both are recommended. Persons with lymphomas that carry a risk for CNS involvement usually receive CNS prophylaxis with high doses of chemotherapeutic agents that can cross the blood–brain barrier, intrathecal chemotherapy, or cranial irradiation. About 30% to 60% of patients do not achieve a complete response or relapse after standard-dose chemotherapy.[17]

Several monoclonal antibodies have recently become available for use in the treatment of NHL. Rituximab (Rituxan), which was the first to be approved by the U.S. Food and Drug Administration (FDA), recognizes and attaches to the CD20 antigen found on most B-cell lymphomas.[18,19] For aggressive lymphomas, the combination of chemotherapy and rituximab has shown dramatic response rates, indicating a synergistic effect. Because lymphoma cells tend to be very sensitive to radiation, newer forms of monoclonal antibodies have been developed that are similar to rituximab, but with radioactive molecules attached to them. The first to be approved by the FDA was ibritumomab tiuxetan (Zevalin), which is a monoclonal antibody conjugated with yttrium-90. It is being used for treatment in patients with follicular lymphomas who have relapsed after therapy. The second drug to be approved was tositumomab (Bexxar), which is an antibody conjugated to iodine-131. It is also being used in treatment of follicular lymphomas that have not responded to initial therapy.

Passive immunotherapy with anti–B-cell antibodies and radioimmunotherapy are significant advances in the therapeutic options for individuals with NHL.[18] Bone marrow and peripheral stem cell transplantation are potentially curative treatments for people with highly resistant forms of the disease.

The survival rates for lymphomas vary widely by cell type and stage of disease. At present, the overall 5-year survival rate for NHL is 55%.[10] Significant progress has been made with the introduction of monoclonal antibody–based therapy, but further studies are needed to prove that these new treatment options alter the natural history of the disease.

LEUKEMIAS

The leukemias are malignant neoplasms of cells originally derived from hematopoietic stem cells. They are characterized by diffuse replacement of bone marrow with unregulated, proliferating, immature neoplastic cells. In most cases, the leukemic cells spill out into the blood, where they are seen in large numbers. The term *leukemia* (*i.e.*, "white blood") was first used by Virchow to describe a reversal of the usual ratio of red blood cells to white blood cells. The leukemic cells may also infiltrate the liver, spleen, lymph nodes, and other tissues throughout the body, causing enlargement of these organs.

Approximately 30,600 new cases of leukemia were diagnosed in 2003, and approximately 21,900 persons died of the disease.[10] More children are stricken with leukemia than with any other form of cancer, and it is the leading cause of death in children between the ages of 1 and 14 years. Although leukemia commonly is thought of as a childhood disease, it strikes more adults than children. The overall trend in the 1990s has been a decrease in the incidence of leukemia in both men and women, with a slower decrease in deaths from leukemia.[10]

Classification

The leukemias commonly are classified according to their predominant cell type (*i.e.*, lymphocytic or myelogenous) and whether the condition is acute or chronic. Biphenotypic leukemias demonstrate characteristics of both lymphoid and myeloid lineages. A rudimentary classification system divides leukemia into four types: acute lymphocytic (lymphoblastic) leukemia (ALL), chronic lymphocytic leukemia (CLL), acute myelogenous (myeloblastic) leukemia (AML), and chronic myelogenous leukemia (CML). The *lymphocytic leukemias* involve immature lymphocytes and their progenitors that originate in the bone marrow but infiltrate the spleen, lymph nodes, CNS, and other tissues. The *myelogenous leukemias,* which involve the pluripotent myeloid stem cells in bone marrow, interfere with the maturation of all blood cells, including the granulocytes, erythrocytes, and thrombocytes.

Etiology and Molecular Biology

The causes of leukemia are largely unknown. The incidence of leukemia among persons who have been exposed to high levels of radiation is unusually high. The number of cases of leukemia reported in the most heavily exposed survivors of the atomic blasts at Hiroshima and Nagasaki during the 20-year period from 1950 to 1970 was nearly 30 times the expected rate.[20] An increased incidence of leukemia also is associated with exposure to benzene and the use of antitumor drugs (*i.e.*, mechlorethamine, procarbazine, cyclophosphamide, chloramphenicol, and the epipodophyllotoxins).[21] Leukemia may occur as a second cancer after aggressive chemotherapy for other cancers, such as Hodgkin's disease.[22] The existence of a genetic predisposition to develop acute leukemia is suggested by the increased leukemia incidence among a number of congenital disorders, including Down syndrome, von Reckinghausen's disease, and Fanconi's anemia. In individuals with Down syndrome, the incidence of acute leukemia is 10 times that of the general population.[23] Also, there are numerous reports of multiple cases of acute leukemia occurring within the same family. Some T-cell leukemias, hairy cell leukemia, and lymphoma are caused by retroviruses, HTLV-1 and HTLV-2.

The molecular biology of leukemia suggests that the event or events causing the disorders exert their effects through disruption or dysregulation of genes that normally regulate blood cell development, blood cell homeostasis, or both.[24] Cytogenetic studies have shown that recurrent chromosomal changes occur in over one half of all cases of leukemia.[25] Most commonly, these are structural changes classified as translocations, inversions, or deletions. It is the disruption or dysregulation of specific genes and gene products occurring at the site of these chromosome aberrations that contribute to the development of leukemia.[24] In many instances, these genes have also been found to be directly or indirectly involved in the normal development or maintenance of the hematopoietic system. Thus, it would appear that leukemia results, at least in part, from disruption in the activity of genes that normally regulate blood cell development. Currently, more than 500 recurring translocations have been described in hematologic malignancies.[25] One of the more studied is the reciprocal translocation from the long arm of chromosome 22 to the long arm of chromosome 9 that occurs in the Philadelphia (Ph) chromosome (discussed later). Almost all cases of CML and 22% to 25% of adult ALL are associated with the Ph chromosome karyotype. Advances in the understanding of the molecular biology of leukemia are beginning to provide a more complete understanding of the molecular complexity of leukemia for the purposes of diagnosis, classification, treatment, and monitoring of clinical outcomes.[24]

LEUKEMIAS

- Leukemias are malignant neoplasms arising from the transformation of a single blood cell line derived from hematopoietic stem cells.
- The leukemias are classified as acute and chronic lymphocytic (lymphocytes) or myelogenous (granulocytes, monocytes) leukemias according to their cell lineage.
- Because leukemic cells are immature and poorly differentiated, they proliferate rapidly and have a long life span, they do not function normally, they interfere with the maturation of normal blood cells, and they circulate in the bloodstream, cross the blood–brain barrier, and infiltrate many body organs.

Acute Leukemias

Acute leukemia is a cancer of the hematopoietic progenitor cells. It usually has a sudden and stormy onset with signs and symptoms related to depressed bone marrow function (Table 17-2). Acute lymphocytic leukemia (ALL) is the most common leukemia in childhood, constituting 80% to 85% of leukemia cases.[25] The peak incidence occurs between 2 and 4 years of age. Acute myelogenous leukemia (AML) is chiefly an adult disease; however, it is also seen in children and young adults. The incidence steadily increases

TABLE 17-2 Clinical Manifestations of Leukemia and Their Pathologic Basis*

Clinical Manifestations	Pathologic Basis
Bone marrow depression	
Malaise, easy fatigability	Anemia
Fever	Infection or increased metabolism by neoplastic cells
Bleeding	Decreased thrombocytes
Petechiae	
Ecchymosis	
Gingival bleeding	
Epistaxis	
Bone pain and tenderness upon palpation	Subperiosteal bone infiltration, bone marrow expansion, and bone resorption
Headache, nausea, vomiting, papilledema, cranial nerve palsies, seizures, coma	Leukemic infiltration of the central nervous system
Abdominal discomfort	Generalized lymphadenopathy, hepatomegaly, splenomegaly due to leukemic cell infiltration
Increased vulnerability to infections	Immaturity of the white cells and ineffective immune function
Hematologic abnormalities	Physical and metabolic encroachment of leukemia cells on red blood cell and thrombocyte precursors
Anemia	
Thrombocytopenia	
Hyperuricemia and other metabolic disorders	Abnormal proliferation and metabolism of leukemic cells

*Manifestations vary with the type of leukemia.

after middle age, with the median age of 60 to 65 years for adult AML.[25]

ALL encompasses a group of neoplasms composed of immature precursor B or T lymphocytes (Fig. 17-3). Most cases (about 85%) of ALL are of pre–B-cell origin.[9] The AMLs are an extremely heterogeneous group of disorders. Some arise from the pluripotent stem cells in which myeloblasts predominate, and others arise from the monocyte-granulocyte precursor, which is the cell of origin for myelomonocytic leukemia. Of all the leukemias, AML is most strongly linked with toxins and underlying congenital and hematologic disorders. It is the type of leukemia associated with Down syndrome.

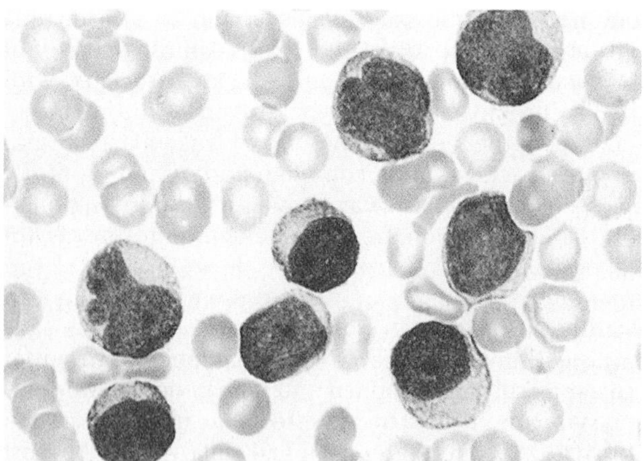

FIGURE 17-3 Acute lymphoblastic anemia (L2 ALL). The lymphoblasts in the peripheral blood contain irregular and indented nuclei with prominent nucleoli and a moderate amount of cytoplasm. (Rubin E., Farber J.L. [1999]. *Pathology* [3rd ed., p. 1129]. Philadelphia: Lippincott-Raven)

Manifestations. Although ALL and AML are distinct disorders, they typically present with similar clinical features. The warning signs and symptoms of acute leukemia are fatigue, pallor, weight loss, repeated infections, easy bruising, nosebleeds, and other types of hemorrhage. These features often appear suddenly in children.

Persons with acute leukemia usually present for medical evaluation within 3 months of the onset of symptoms. Both ALL and AML are characterized by fatigue resulting from anemia; low-grade fever, night sweats, and weight loss due to the rapid proliferation and hypermetabolism of the leukemic cells; bleeding because of a decreased platelet count; and bone pain and tenderness due to bone marrow expansion.[26] Infection results from neutropenia, with the risk for infection becoming high as the neutrophil count falls below 500 cells/μL. Generalized lymphadenopathy, splenomegaly, and hepatomegaly caused by infiltration of leukemic cells occur in all acute leukemias but are more common in ALL. In addition to the common manifestations of acute leukemia (*i.e.,* fatigue, weight loss, fever, easy bruising), infiltration of malignant cells in the skin, gums, and other soft tissues is particularly common in the monocytic form of AML. The leukemic cells may also cross the blood–brain barrier and establish sanctuary in the CNS. CNS involvement is more common in ALL than AML and is more common in children than adults. Signs and symptoms of CNS involvement include cranial nerve palsies, headache, nausea, vomiting, papilledema, and occasionally seizures and coma.

Leukostasis is a condition in which the circulating blast count is markedly elevated (usually 100,000 cells/μL). The high number of circulating leukemic blasts increases blood viscosity and predisposes to the development of leukoblastic emboli with obstruction of small vessels in the pulmonary and cerebral circulations. Occlusion of the pulmonary vessels leads to vessel rupture and infiltration of lung tissue, resulting in sudden shortness of breath and progressive dyspnea. Cerebral leukostasis leads to diffuse headache and lethargy, which can progress to confusion and coma. Once identified, leukostasis requires immediate and effective treatment to lower the blast count rapidly. Initial treatment employs apheresis to remove excess blast cells, followed by chemotherapy to stop leukemic cell production in the marrow.[26]

Hyperuricemia occurs as the result of increased proliferation or increased breakdown of purine nucleotides (*i.e.,* one of the compounds of nucleic acid) secondary to leukemic cell death that results from chemotherapy. It may increase before and during treatment. Prophylactic therapy with allopurinol, a drug that inhibits uric acid synthesis, is routinely administered to prevent renal complications secondary to uric acid crystallization in the urine.

Diagnosis and Staging. A definitive diagnosis of acute leukemia is based on blood and bone marrow studies; it requires the demonstration of leukemic cells in the peripheral blood, bone marrow, or extramedullary tissue. Laboratory findings reveal the presence of immature (blasts) white blood cells in the circulation and bone marrow, where they may constitute 60% to 100% of the cells. As these cells proliferate and begin to crowd the bone marrow, the development of other blood cell lines in the marrow is suppressed. Consequently, there is a loss of mature myeloid cells, such as erythrocytes, granulocytes, and platelets. Anemia is almost always present, and the platelet count is decreased. Bone marrow specimens are used to determine the molecular characteristics of the leukemia, the degree of bone marrow involvement, and the morphology and histology of the disease. Immunophenotyping is performed to determine the lineage subtype of the leukemic cells.[26]

In ALL, the staging always includes a lumbar puncture to assess CNS involvement. Imaging studies that include CT scans of the chest, abdomen, and pelvis may also be obtained to identify additional sites of disease.

Treatment. Treatment of ALL and AML consists of several phases and includes induction therapy, which is designed to elicit a remission; intensification therapy, which is used to produce a further reduction in leukemic cells after a remission is achieved; and maintenance therapy, which serves to maintain the remission. The goal of induction therapy is the production of a severe bone marrow response with destruction of leukemic progenitor cells followed by normal bone marrow recovery. The criteria for complete remission are (1) less than 5% blasts in the bone marrow, (2) normal peripheral blood counts, (3) absence of cytogenetic abnormalities, and (4) return to pre-illness performance status. The likelihood of achieving a remission depends on a number of factors, including age, type of leukemia, and stage of the disease at time of presentation. Of these factors, age is probably the most significant prognostic variable.

Treatment of ALL usually consists of four phases: induction therapy designed to elicit a remission; CNS prophylaxis; consolidation or intensification therapy; and maintenance therapy. Induction therapy incorporates a number of chemotherapeutic agents designed to achieve remission. CNS prophylaxis may be accomplished through the administration of intrathecal chemotherapy or cranial irradiation concurrent with systemic chemotherapy.[26] Because of its side effects, CNS irradiation is being used less frequently than in the past. The use of high-dose chemotherapy that crosses the blood–brain barrier may make separate CNS treatment unnecessary in the future. Although CNS involvement is a major problem in children, the incidence in adults at the time of diagnosis is less than 10%. Consolidation therapy consists of high doses of chemotherapy given to patients who have achieved remission with their induction therapy. Maintenance therapy usually is accomplished with lower doses of chemotherapy given over a long period of time (*e.g.,* 2 years) to patients after consolidation therapy. Although almost 80% of children are cured of ALL, only about 30% to 40% of adults achieve long-term disease-free survival.[27,28]

Massive necrosis of malignant cells can occur during the initial phase of treatment. This phenomenon, known as *tumor lysis syndrome,* can lead to life-threatening metabolic disorders, including hyperkalemia, hyperphosphatemia, hyperuricemia, hypomagnesemia, hypocalcemia, and acidosis, with the potential for causing acute renal failure. Aggressive prophylactic hydration with alkaline solutions and administration of allopurinol to reduce uric acid levels are given to counteract these effects.

As with ALL, treatment of AML consists of a number of phases. Treatment usually consists of induction therapy followed by intensive consolidation therapy. Induction therapy consists of intensive chemotherapy to effect aplasia of the bone marrow. During this period, supportive transfusion and antibiotic therapy often are needed. Gemtuzumab ozogamicin (Mylotarg) is another treatment option for patients with relapsed AML who are older than 60 years of age. It is a monoclonal antibody conjugated with chemotherapy that targets the CD33 antigen found on 90% of AML blast cells.[28] Response rates for standard chemotherapy treatment of AML approach 66%, with a 4-year disease-free survival rate of 30% to 40%.[26]

One type of AML, acute promyelocytic leukemia (APL), is treated differently than AML. About 90% of APL cases are a result of a chromosomal translocation (15:17) that blocks cellular differentiation and maturation at the level of the promyelocyte. Tretinoin, a vitamin A derivative, is a differentiating agent that, when combined with chemotherapy, induces the maturation of immature cancer cells into mature granulocytes. With the addition of tretinoin to standard chemotherapy, 90% to 95% of newly diagnosed patients with APL achieve a complete remission. For the 25% to 30% of APL patients who eventually relapse and require additional treatment, arsenic trioxide (Trisonox) is another option. Trisonox has been shown to inhibit growth, induce apoptosis, and promote differentiation in a variety of hematologic cancers.[28]

Bone marrow or stem cell transplantation may be considered for persons with ALL and AML who have failed to respond to other forms of therapy.[21,26] Because of the risk for complications, bone marrow transplantation is not usually recommended for patients older than 50 to 55 years of age.[21] Because the median age of patients with AML is approximately 65 years, most patients are not eligible for this type of treatment. For younger patients, the availability of acceptable HLA-matched donors is a limiting factor. The lack of suitable donors has prompted the use of the patient's (autologous) bone marrow or peripheral stem cells in transplantation. One of the potential disadvantages of this method is the potential contamination of the autologous graft with residual host leukemic cells.

Chronic Leukemias

In contrast to acute leukemias, chronic leukemias are malignancies involving the proliferation of well-differentiated myeloid and lymphoid cells. The two major types of chronic leukemia are chronic lymphocytic leukemia (CLL) and chronic myelogenous leukemia (CML). CLL is mainly a disorder of older persons; fewer than 10% of those who develop the disease are younger than 50 years of age. Men are affected twice as frequently as women. CML accounts for 15% of all leukemias in adults. It is predominantly a disorder of adults between the ages of 30 and 50 years, but it can affect children as well. The incidence is slightly higher in men than women.

Chronic lymphocytic leukemia is a lymphoproliferative disorder characterized by lymphocytosis, lymphadenopathy, and splenomegaly. Most cases (95%) result from the malignant transformation of relatively mature B lymphocytes that are immunologically incompetent (Fig. 17-4). The leukemic B cells fail to respond to antigenic stimulation; hence, persons with CLL have hypogammaglobulinemia. Infections remain a major cause of morbidity and mortality. Immunologic abnormalities, including autoimmune hemolytic anemia and immune-mediated thrombocytopenia, are also common, reflecting the abnormal immunoregulation inherent in the lymphocytic origin of the disorder.

Chronic myelogenous leukemia is a myeloproliferative disorder that results from the malignant transformation of a pluripotent hematopoietic stem cell. CML is associated with the presence of the Philadelphia (Ph) chromosome, representing a reciprocal translocation between the long arm of chromosome 22 and the long arm of chromosome 9[9,29,30] (Fig 17-5). The portion of the translocated long arm of chromosome 9 contains the *ABL* proto-oncogene that is the cellular homolog of the Abelson's murine leukemia virus. The *ABL* gene is received at a specific site on the long arm of chromosome 22, the *break point cluster region (BCR)*.[31] The resulting *BCR-ABL* fusion gene codes for the BCR-ABL fusion protein, which is a constitutively active cytoplasmic tyrosine kinase that can phosphorylate several substrates, resulting in cell growth and proliferation. It is generally believed that CML develops when a single pluripotential hematopoietic stem cell acquires a Ph chromosome carrying the *BCR-ABL* fusion gene. Because the tyrosine kinase generated by the *BCR-ABL* gene is constitutively active, the affected cells bypass the regulated signals that control normal cell growth and differentiation and instead undergo malignant transformation to become leukemic cells. The mechanism by which the Ph chromosome is first formed and the time required for progression to overt disease is unknown. It has been proposed that the close proximity of the *BCR* and *ABL* genes in the hematopoietic cells during interphase (see Chapter 4) may favor translocation between the two chromosomes.[31] In about 95% of persons with CML, the Ph chromosome can be identified in granulocytic, erythroid, and megakaryocytic precursors as well as B cells, and in some cases, T cells.[9] Although CML orig-

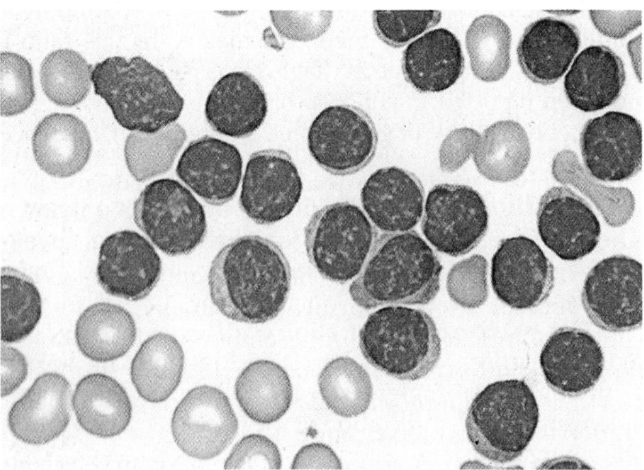

FIGURE 17-4 Chronic lymphocytic leukemia. A smear of peripheral blood shows numerous small-to-medium-sized lymphocytes. (Rubin E., Farber J.L. [1999]. *Pathology* [3rd ed., p. 1125]. Philadelphia: Lippincott-Raven)

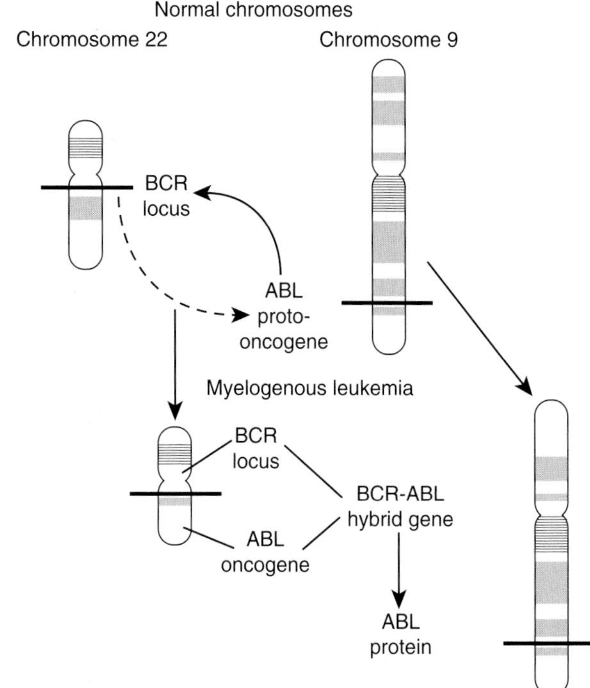

FIGURE 17-5 The Philadelphia (Ph) chromosome in which the breaks at the end of the long arms of chromosome 9 and 22 occur, allowing the ABL proto-oncogene on chromosome 9 to be translocated to breakpoint cluster region (BCR) on chromosome 22. The result is a shortened version of chromosome 22 with a new fusion gene coding for the BCR-ABL protein, which is presumably involved in the pathogenesis of chronic myelogenous leukemia.

inates in the pluripotent stem cells, granulocyte precursors remain the dominant leukemic cell type.

Manifestations. Both CLL and CML have a more insidious onset than acute leukemias and may be discovered during a routine medical examination by a blood count. The two types of chronic leukemias differ, however, in their manifestations and clinical course.

CLL typically follows a slow and indolent course. The clinical signs and symptoms are largely related to the progressive infiltration of neoplastic lymphocytes in the bone marrow and extramedullary tissue and to secondary immunologic defects. Often affected persons are asymptomatic at the time of diagnosis, and lymphocytosis is noted on a complete blood count obtained for another, unrelated disorder. Fatigue, reduced exercise tolerance, enlargement of superficial lymph nodes, or splenomegaly usually reflects a more advanced stage. As the disease progresses, lymph nodes gradually increase in size, and new nodes are involved, sometimes in unusual areas such as the scalp, orbit, pharynx, pleura, gastrointestinal tract, liver, prostate, and gonads. Severe fatigue, recurrent or persistent infections, pallor, edema, thrombophlebitis, and pain are also experienced. As the malignant cell population increases, the proportion of normal marrow precursors is reduced until only lymphocytes remain in the marrow.[30]

Typically, CML follows a triphasic course: (1) a chronic phase of variable length, (2) a short accelerated phase, and (3) a terminal blast crisis phase. The onset of the chronic phase is usually slow with nonspecific symptoms such as weakness and weight loss. The most characteristic laboratory finding at the time of presentation is leukocytosis with immature granulocyte cell types in the peripheral blood. Anemia and, eventually, thrombocytopenia develop. Anemia causes weakness, easy fatigability, and exertional dyspnea. Splenomegaly is often present at the time of diagnosis; hepatomegaly is less common; and lymphadenopathy is relatively uncommon. Although persons in the early chronic phase of CML generally are asymptomatic, without effective treatment most will enter the accelerated phase within 4 years.[30]

The accelerated phase is characterized by enlargement of the spleen and progressive symptoms. Splenomegaly often causes a feeling of abdominal fullness and discomfort. An increase in basophil count and more immature cells in the blood or bone marrow confirm transformation to the accelerated phase. During this phase, constitutional symptoms such as low-grade fever, night sweats, bone pain, and weight loss develop because of rapid proliferation and hypermetabolism of the leukemic cells. Bleeding and easy bruising may arise from dysfunctional platelets. Generally, the accelerated phase is short (6 to 12 months).[29]

The terminal blast crisis phase of CML represents evolution to acute leukemia and is characterized by an increasing number of myeloid precursors, especially blast cells. Constitutional symptoms become more pronounced during this period, and splenomegaly may increase significantly. Isolated infiltrates of leukemic cells can involve the skin, lymph nodes, bones, and CNS. With very high blast counts (100,000/μL), symptoms of leukostasis may occur. The prognosis for patients who are in the blast crisis phase is poor, with a median survival of 3 months.[30]

Diagnosis and Treatment. The diagnosis of chronic leukemia is based on blood and bone marrow studies. The treatment varies with the type of leukemic cell, the stage of the disease, other health problems, and the person's age.

Most early cases of CLL require no specific treatment. Reassurance that persons with the disorder can live a normal life for many years is important. Indications for chemotherapy or monoclonal antibodies include progressive fatigue, troublesome lymphadenopathy, anemia, thrombocytopenia, and a lymphocyte count of more than 150,000/mm^3. Initially, chemotherapy with alkylating agents (chlorambucil) and the antimetabolite fludarabine is used. Alemtuzumab (Campath) is indicated for the treatment of CLL in patients who have not responded to chemotherapy. This humanized monoclonal antibody is directed against the CD52 cell surface antigen present on lymphocyte cells of almost all patients with B-cell and T-cell CLL.[32] Complications such as autoimmune hemolytic anemia or thrombocytopenia may require treatment with corticosteroids or splenectomy.

In younger patients with aggressive disease, an allogeneic ablative or nonablative stem cell transplantation is a treatment option. In a nonablative type of transplantation, the goal is marrow suppression, destruction of leukemia cells by the donor's lymphocytes, known as "graft-versus-leukemia" effect, and marrow recovery with donor cells. The survival time for patients with CLL ranges from less than 2 years for aggressive forms of the disease to longer than 10 years for early-stage disease.[30]

The goals of treatment for CML include a hematologic response characterized by normalized blood counts; a cytogenetic response demonstrated by the reduction or elimination of the Ph chromosome from the bone marrow, and a molecular response confirmed by the elimination of the BCR-ABL fusion protein.[30] In the past, standard treatment included the use of single-agent chemotherapy (hydroxyurea) as well as interferon-alfa. In patients in the chronic phase, both agents normalized blood counts and reduced symptoms, but cytogenetic and molecular responses were rare. With its FDA approval in 2001, imatinib mesylate (Gleevec) has largely replaced hydroxyurea and interferon as standard therapy for CML.[30] Imatinib mesylate is a protein-tyrosine kinase inhibitor that selectively targets BCR-ABL–expressing leukemic cells for apoptosis.[33–35] The efficacy of imatinib mesylate has been demonstrated in hematologic, cytogenetic, and molecular response rates. Its side-effect profile and ease of administration (oral route) have dramatically changed the treatment of CML.[26]

Allogeneic bone marrow or stem cell transplantation offers a potential cure for CML. In most transplantation centers, full myoablative (destruction of bone marrow cells by irradiation or chemotherapy) transplantation is available to children and adults younger than 60 years of age who have sibling HLA-matched donors or molecular-matched unrelated donors. Nonmyoablative or "mini" transplantations are available to patients younger than 70 years of age who have sibling-matched or molecular-matched donors.

Cord blood transplantations have been performed successfully in small numbers of children and adults.

Allogeneic bone marrow transplantation cures CML by initial cytoreduction followed by long-term immunologic control mediated by the donor's immune system. This immunologic control, often referred to as *graft-versus-leukemia effect,* is provided as immune cells from the transplant donor destroy recurring leukemic cells in the transplant recipient. The recurrence of disease after allogeneic transplantation can often be reversed by infusion of T lymphocytes from the initial bone marrow donor. This procedure, called *donor lymphocyte infusion,* can lead to long-term remission in 60% to 70% of cases.[30] For persons with CML, the current median survival without transplantation is 3 to 4 years, with fewer than 50% of persons alive at 5 years.[23]

PLASMA CELL DYSCRASIAS

Plasma cell dyscrasias are characterized by expansion of a single clone of immunoglobulin-producing plasma cells and a resultant increase in serum levels of a single monoclonal immunoglobulin or its fragments. The plasma cell dyscrasias include multiple myeloma; localized plasmacytoma (solitary myeloma); lymphoplasmacytic lymphoma; primary or immunocyte amyloidosis due to excessive production of light chains; and monoclonal gammopathy of undetermined significance. *Monoclonal gammopathy of undetermined significance* (MGUS) is characterized by the presence of the M proteins in the serum without other findings of multiple myeloma. M proteins can be detected in the serum of 1% to 3% of healthy persons older than 50 years of age. MGUS is considered a premalignant condition.[36] Approximately 20% of persons with MGUS go on to develop a plasma cell dyscrasia (multiple myeloma, lymphoplasmacytic lymphoma, or amyloidosis) over a period of 10 to 15 years.

Multiple Myeloma

Multiple myeloma is by far the most frequent of the malignant plasma cell dyscrasias, accounting for 1% of all cancers and 10% of all hematologic malignancies in Caucasians and 20% in African Americans.[37] It occurs most frequently in persons older than 60 years of age with the median age of patients with multiple myeloma being 71 years. The occurrence of the disease tends to be more frequent in men than in women.

The cause of multiple myeloma is unknown. Risk factors are thought to include chronic immune stimulation, autoimmune disorders, exposure to ionizing radiation, and occupational exposure to pesticides or herbicides (*e.g.,* dioxin).[36] Multiple myeloma has been associated with exposure to Agent Orange during the Vietnam War. A number of viruses have been associated with the pathogenesis of myeloma. There is a 4.5-fold increase in the likelihood of developing myeloma for persons with HIV.[36] Hereditary and genetic factors may predispose to myeloma development. From family studies, researchers have identified 20 families in France where the risk for developing myeloma is as high as 5%.

Pathogenesis. Multiple myeloma is characterized by proliferation of malignant plasma cells in the bone marrow and osteolytic bone lesions throughout the skeletal system. As with other hematopoietic malignancies, it is now recognized that multiple myeloma is associated with chromosomal translocations, specifically those involving the immunoglobulin G (IgG) locus on chromosome 14. One fusion partner is a fibroblast growth factor receptor gene on chromosome 4, which is truncated to produce a constitutively active receptor. There is also a reported overexpression by myeloma cells of a gene, called the dickkopf 1 (*DKK1*) gene, which codes for a protein product that inhibits differentiation of osteoblast precursor cells, thereby contributing to the osteolytic lesions that occur with the disease.[38]

One of the characteristics of multiple myelomas is the unregulated production of a monoclonal antibody referred to as the *M protein* because it is detected as an M spike on protein electrophoresis. In most cases, the M protein is either IgG (60%) or IgA (20% to 25%).[39] In the remaining 15% to 20% of cases, the plasma cells produce only abnormal proteins, termed *Bence Jones proteins,* that consist of light chains of the immunoglobulin molecule. Because of their low molecular weight, the Bence Jones proteins are readily excreted in the urine. Persons with this form of the disease (light-chain disease) have Bence Jones proteins in their serum but lack the M component. However, up to 80% of myeloma cells produce both complete immunoglobulins as well as excess light chains; therefore, both M proteins and Bence Jones proteins are present. Many of the light chain proteins are directly toxic to renal tubular structures, which may lead to tubular destruction and, eventually, to renal failure.

Cytokines are important in the pathogenesis of the disorder. The multiple myeloma cell has a surface-membrane receptor for IL-6, which is known to be a growth factor for the disorder. Another important growth factor for the myeloma cell is IL-1, which has important osteoclast activity.[40] Other growth factors that are implicated in multiple myeloma include granulocyte-colony stimulating factor, interferon-alfa, and IL-10. Replacement of the bone marrow (and perhaps humoral suppression of myelopoiesis) leads initially to anemia and later to general bone marrow failure. The proliferation of neoplastic myeloma cells is supported by the cytokine IL-6 produced by fibroblasts and macrophages in the bone marrow stroma.

Manifestations. The main sites involved in multiple myeloma are the bones and bone marrow. In addition to the abnormal proliferation of marrow plasma cells, there is proliferation and activation of osteoclasts that leads to bone resorption and destruction (Fig. 17-6). This increased bone resorption predisposes the individual to pathologic fractures and hypercalcemia. Paraproteins secreted by the plasma cells may cause a hyperviscosity of body fluids and may break down into amyloid, a proteinaceous substance deposited between cells, causing heart failure and neuropathy. Although multiple myeloma is characterized by excessive production of monoclonal immunoglobulin, levels of normal immunoglobulins are usually depressed. This

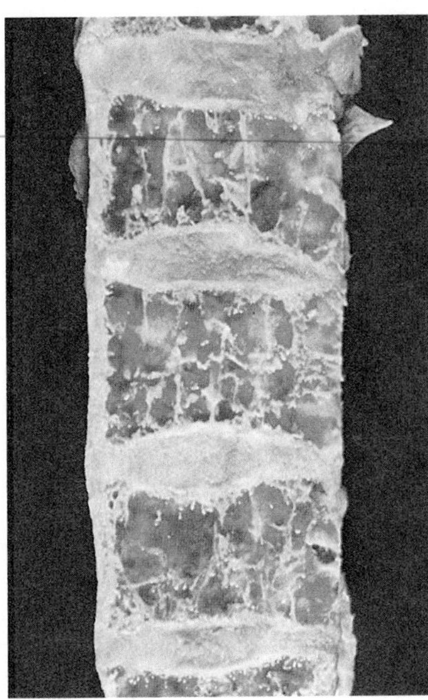

FIGURE 17-6 Multiple myeloma. Multiple lytic lesions of the vertebrae are present. (Rubin E., Farber J.L. [1999]. *Pathology* [3rd ed., p. 1148]. Philadelphia: Lippincott-Raven)

contributes to a general susceptibility to recurrent bacterial infections.

The malignant plasma cells also can form plasmacytomas (plasma cell tumors) in bone and soft tissue sites. The most common site of soft tissue plasmacytomas is the gastrointestinal tract. The development of plasmacytomas in bone tissue is associated with bone destruction and localized pain. Osteolytic lesions and compression fractures may be seen in the axial skeleton and proximal long bones. Occasionally, the lesions may affect the spinal column causing vertebral collapse and spinal cord compression.[36]

Bone pain is one of the first symptoms occurring in approximately three fourths of all individuals diagnosed with multiple myeloma. Bone destruction also impairs the production of erythrocytes and leukocytes and predisposes the patient to anemia and recurrent infections. Many patients experience weight loss and weakness. Renal insufficiency occurs in 50% of patients. Neurologic manifestations caused by neuropathy or spinal cord compression also may be present.

Diagnosis and Treatment. Diagnosis of multiple myeloma is based on clinical manifestations, blood tests, and bone marrow examination. The classic triad of bone marrow plasmacytosis (more than 10% plasma cells), lytic bone lesions, and either the serum M-protein spike or the presence of Bence Jones proteins in the urine is definitive for a diagnosis of multiple myeloma. Bone radiographs, skeletal survey, and magnetic resonance imaging (MRI) are important in establishing the presence of bone lesions. The Durie and Salmon staging system correlates clinical parameters with the burden of myeloma disease by examining the level of M and Bence Jones proteins for elevation, assessing for the presence and location of bone lesions, and evaluating the patient for hypercalcemia and anemia.[42]

For several decades, melphalan and prednisone have remained the cornerstone for treatment of multiple myeloma. The overall response rate for this regimen was about 50%. The addition of anthracyclines, alternate alkylating agents, and interferon has yielded minimal improvement in treatment outcomes. Although multiple myeloma is a radiosensitive disease, radiation therapy provides only supportive therapy or pain relief from lytic bone lesions and compression fractures. With conventional treatment, only 5% to 10% of patients achieve complete remission. Drug resistance develops rapidly.

Treatment with bisphosphonates (*e.g.,* pamidronate and zoledronic acid) has (1) reduced the incidence of skeletal events (pathologic fractures, spinal cord compression), (2) prevented hypercalcemia, (3) alleviated bone pain, and (4) improved the patient's quality of life. Anemia is a source of distress and fatigue. Erythropoietin therapy can be used to improve the anemia associated with myeloma and is well tolerated.

Recently, thalidomide, an agent with antiangiogenic properties, emerged as an active agent for relapsed and refractory multiple myeloma. As a single agent, thalidomide has been shown to induce response rates of 25% to 35% in persons whose myeloma was refractory to conventional therapies.[41] Thalidomide combined with dexamethasone pulsing has shown promising results (response rates of more than 75%) in previously treated and in newly diagnosed patients, and the combination of dexamethasone and thalidomide was added to the list of options for the primary treatment of advanced disease.[42,43] Because of its teratogenicity, the use of thalidomide in pregnant women is absolutely contraindicated.

High-dose chemotherapy with autologous stem cell transplantation is now considered appropriate front-line therapy for newly diagnosed multiple myeloma patients, younger than 70 years of age. Allogeneic transplantation offers prolonged disease-free outcomes and potential cure, but at a high cost of treatment-related mortality. Because of this, "mini transplants" providing nonmarrow ablative chemotherapy may be used to provide sufficient immune suppression to allow donor engraftment and subsequent graft-versus-tumor effect.

Clinical trials are underway investigating arsenic trioxide, a drug thought to exert its antimyeloma activity by inducing apoptosis and by inhibiting proliferation of drug-resistant myeloma cell lines and angiogenesis.[41,43] Bortezomib (Velcade), a reversible 26S proteasome inhibitor, was recently approved for treatment of progressive myeloma after previous treatment failures. Proteasomes are intracellular enzymes that degrade many proteins regulating the cell cycle, RNA transcription, apoptosis, cell adhesion, angiogenesis, and antigen presentation.[41,43]

Proteolysis by the 26S proteasome is fundamental to multiple signaling pathways within the cell, and disruption of this homeostatic pathway by bortezomib can lead to cell death and a delay in tumor growth.

In summary, the lymphomas (Hodgkin's disease and non-Hodgkin's lymphoma) represent malignant neoplasms of cells native to lymphoid tissue (*i.e.,* lymphocytes and histiocytes) that have their origin in the secondary lymphoid structures such as the lymph nodes and mucosa-associated lymphoid tissues. Hodgkin's disease is characterized by painless and progressive enlargement of a single node or group of nodes. It is believed to originate in one area of the lymphatic system and, if unchecked, spreads throughout the lymphatic network. The non-Hodgkin's lymphomas are a group of neoplastic disorders that originate in the lymphoid tissues, usually the lymph nodes. The non-Hodgkin's lymphomas are multicentric in origin and spread early to various lymphoid tissues throughout the body, especially the liver, spleen, and bone marrow.

The leukemias are malignant neoplasms of the hematopoietic stem cells that originate in the bone marrow. They are classified according to cell type (*i.e.,* lymphocytic or myelogenous) and whether the disease is acute or chronic. The lymphocytic leukemias involve immature lymphocytes and their progenitors that originate in the bone marrow but infiltrate the spleen, lymph nodes, CNS, and other tissues. The myelogenous leukemias involve the pluripotent myeloid stem cells in bone marrow and interfere with the maturation of all blood cells, including the granulocytes, erythrocytes, and thrombocytes.

The acute leukemias (*i.e.,* ALL, which primarily affects children, and AML, which primarily affects adults) have a sudden and stormy onset with symptoms of depressed bone marrow function (anemia, fatigue, bleeding, and infections); bone pain; and generalized lymphadenopathy, splenomegaly, and hepatomegaly. The chronic leukemias, which largely affect adults, have a more insidious onset. CLL often has the most favorable clinical course, with many persons living long enough to die of other, unrelated causes. The course of CML is slow and progressive, with transformation to a course resembling that of AML.

Multiple myeloma is a plasma cell dyscrasia characterized by expansion of a single clone of immunoglobulin-producing plasma cells and a resultant increase in serum levels of a single monoclonal immunoglobulin or its fragments. The main sites involved in multiple myeloma are the bones and bone marrow. In addition to the abnormal proliferation of marrow plasma cells, there is proliferation and activation of osteoclasts that leads to bone resorption and destruction and predisposes to increased risk for pathologic fractures and development of hypercalcemia. Paraproteins secreted by the plasma cells may cause a hyperviscosity of body fluids and may break down into amyloid, a proteinaceous substance deposited between cells, causing heart failure and neuropathy. Bone marrow involvement leads to increased risk for infection because of suppressed humoral and cell-mediated immunity and anemia due to impaired red cell production.

REVIEW EXERCISES

A mother brings her 4-year-old son into the pediatric clinic because of irritability, loss of appetite, low-grade fever, pallor, and complaints that his legs hurt. Blood tests reveal anemia, thrombocytopenia, and an elevated leukocyte count with atypical lymphocytes. A diagnosis of acute lymphocytic leukemia (ALL) is confirmed using bone marrow studies.

A. What is the origin of the anemia, thrombocytopenia, elevated leukocyte count, and atypical lymphocytes seen in this child?

B. Explain the pathophysiology underlying the child's fever, pallor, increased bleeding, and bone pain.

C. The parents are informed that treatment of ALL consists of aggressive chemotherapy with the purpose of achieving a remission. Explain the rationale for using chemotherapy to treat leukemia.

D. The parents are also told that the child will need intrathecal chemotherapy administered by a lumbar puncture. Why is this treatment necessary?

A 36-year-old man presents at his health care clinic with fever, night sweats, weight loss, and a feeling of fullness in his abdomen. Subsequent lymph node biopsy reveals a diagnosis of non-Hodgkin's lymphoma (NHL).

A. Although lymphomas can originate in any of the lymphoid tissues of the body, most originate in lymph nodes, and most (80% to 85%) are of B-cell origin. Hypothesize as to why B cells are more commonly affected than T cells.

B. The monoclonal antibody rituximab is often used in the treatment of NHL. Explain how this medication exerts its effect and why it is specific for B-cell lymphoma.

References

1. Guyton A.C., Hall J.E. (2000). *Textbook of medical physiology* (10th ed. pp. 392–401). Philadelphia: W.B. Saunders.
2. Metcalf D. (1999). Cellular hematopoiesis in the twentieth century. *Seminars in Hematology 36*(Suppl. 7), 5–12.
3. Alexander W.S. (1998). Cytokines in hematopoiesis. *International Reviews of Immunology 16,* 651–682.
4. Curnutte J.T., Coates T.D. (2000). Disorders of phagocyte function and number. In Hoffman R., Benz E.K., Shattil S.J., et al. (Eds.), *Hematology: Basic principles and practice* (3rd ed., pp. 720–762). New York: Churchill Livingstone.
5. Boxer L.A. (2004). Leukopenia. In Behrman R.E., Kliegman R.M., Jenson H.B. et al. (Eds.), *Textbook of pediatrics* (17th ed, pp. 717–723). Philadelphia: W.B. Saunders.
6. Sullivan J.L. (2000). Infectious mononucleosis and other Epstein-Barr virus-associated diseases. In Hoffman R., Benz E.K., Shattil S.J., et al. (Eds.), *Hematology: Basic principles and practice* (3rd ed., pp. 812–821). New York: Churchill Livingstone.
7. Samuelson J. (1999). *Infectious diseases.* In Cotran R.S., Kumar V., Collins T. (Eds.). In *Pathologic basis of disease* (6th ed., pp. 371–373). Philadelphia: W.B. Saunders.
8. Godshall S.E., Krichner J.T. (2000). Infectious mononucleosis: Complexities of a common syndrome. *Postgraduate Medicine 107,* 175–186.
9. Aster J. (2003). The hematopoietic and lymphoid systems. In Kumar V., Cotran R.S., Robbins S.L. (Eds.). *Robbins basic pathology* (7th ed., pp. 416–433). Philadelphia: W.B. Saunders.

10. American Cancer Society. (2003). *Cancer facts and figures 2003.* Atlanta: American Cancer Society.
11. Diehl V., Mauch P.M., Harris N.L. (2001). Hodgkin's disease. In DeVita V.T., Hellman S., Rosenberg S.A. (Eds.), *Cancer: Principles and practice of oncology* (6th ed., pp. 2339–2387). Philadelphia: Lippincott Williams & Wilkins.
12. Bonner H., Bagg A., Cossman J. (1999). The blood and lymphoid organs. In Rubin E., Farber J.L. *Pathology* (3rd ed. pp. 1117–1150). Philadelphia: Lippincott-Raven.
13. Cheson B.D. (2001). Hodgkin's disease and non-Hodgkin's lymphomas. In Lenbard R.E., Jr., Osteen R.T., Gansler T. (Eds.), *The American Cancer Society's clinical oncology* (pp. 497–516). Atlanta: American Cancer Society.
14. National Comprehensive Cancer Network. (2003). *NCCN clinical practice guidelines in oncology: Hodgkin's disease.* Jenkintown, PA: National Comprehensive Cancer Network.
15. Vose J.M., Chiu B.C-H, Cheson B.D., et al. (2002). Update on epidemiology and therapeutics in non-Hodgkin's lymphoma. *Hematology* 241–262.
16. Reiser M., Diehl V. (2002). Current treatment of follicular non-Hodgkin's lymphoma. *European Journal of Cancer 38,* 1167–1172.
17. Bilodeau, B.A., Fessele, K.L. (1998). Non-Hodgkin's lymphoma. *Seminars in Oncology Nursing 14*(4), 273–283.
18. Vose J.M. (2002). Immunotherapy for non-Hodgkin's lymphoma. *Clinical Oncology Updates 5*(4), 1–15.
19. McCune S.L., Gockerman J.P., Rizzieri D.A. (2001). Monoclonal antibody therapy in treatment of non-Hodgkin's lymphoma. *JAMA 286*(10), 1149–1152.
20. Jablon S., Kato H. (1972). Studies of the mortality of A-bomb survivors. *Radiation Research 50,* 649–698.
21. Scheinberg D.A., Maslak P., Weiss M. (2001). Acute leukemias. In DeVita V.T., Hellman S., Rosenberg S.A. (Eds.), *Cancer: Principles and practice of oncology* (6th ed., pp. 2404–2433). Philadelphia: Lippincott Williams & Wilkins.
22. Kaldor J.M., Day N.E., Clarke E.A., et al. (1990). Leukemia following Hodgkin's disease. *New England Journal of Medicine 322,* 1–6.
23. Miller K.B., Grodman H.M. (2001). Leukemia. In Lenbard R.E., Jr., Osteen R.T., Gansler T. *The American Cancer Society's clinical oncology* (pp. 527–551). Atlanta: American Cancer Society.
24. Bloomfield C.D., Caligiuri M.A. (2001). Biology of leukemias. In DeVita V.T., Hellman S., Rosenberg S.A. (Eds.), *Cancer: Principles and practice of oncology* (6th ed., pp. 2390–2402). Philadelphia: Lippincott Williams & Wilkins.
25. Wujcik D. (2003). Molecular biology of leukemia. *Seminars in Oncology Nursing 19*(2), 83–89.
26. Viele C.S. (2003). Diagnosis, treatment, and nursing care of acute leukemia. *Seminars in Oncology Nursing 19*(2), 98–108.
27. Faderi S., Jeha S., Kantajian H.M. (2003). The biology and therapy of adult acute lymphoblastic leukemia. *Cancer 98*(7), 1337–1354.
28. Stull D.M. (2003). Targeted therapies for the treatment of leukemia. *Seminars in Oncology Nursing 19*(2), 90–97.
29. Thijsen S.F.T., Schuurhuis G.J., van Oostveen J.W., Ossenkippele G.J. (1999). Chronic myeloid leukemia from basics to bedside. *Leukemia 13,* 1646–1674.
30. Breed C.D. (2003). Diagnosis, treatment, and nursing care of patients with chronic leukemia. *Seminars in Oncology Nursing 19*(2), 109–117.
31. Goldman J.M., Melo J.V. (2003). Chronic myeloid leukemia: Advances in biology and new approaches to treatment. *New England Journal of Medicine 349,* 1451–1464.
32. Vlahorvic G., Crawford J. (2003). Activation of tyrosine kinases in cancer. *Oncologist 8,* 531–538.
33. Kantarjian H., Sawyers C., Hochhaus A., et al. (International ST1571 CML Study Group). (2002). Hematologic and cytogenetic response to imatinib mesylate in chronic myelogenous leukemia. *New England Journal of Medicine 346*(9), 645–652.
34. Sorokin P. (2001). Campath-1H. *Clinical Journal of Oncology Nursing 5*(2), 65–66.
35. Zitella L. (2000). Tyrosine kinase inhibitors: A cure for chronic myeloid leukemia? *Clinical Journal of Oncology Nursing 4*(5), 227–229.
36. Zaidi A.A., Vesole D.H. (2001). Multiple myeloma: An old disease with new hope for the future. *CA: A Cancer Journal for Clinicians 51*(51), 273–285.
37. Rosenthal D.S., Schnipper L.E., McCaffrey R.P. et al. (2001). Multiple myeloma. In Lenbard R.E., Jr., Osteen R.T., Gansler T. *The American Cancer Society's clinical oncology* (pp. 516–525). Atlanta: American Cancer Society.
38. Triko G. (2000). Multiple myeloma and other plasma cell disorders. In Hoffman R., Benz E.K., Shattil S.J., et al. (Eds.), *Hematology: Basic principles and practice* (3rd ed., pp. 1398–1416). New York: Churchill Livingstone.
39. Glass D.A., Patel M.S., Karsenty G. (2003). A new insight into the formation of osteolytic lesions in multiple myeloma. *New England Journal of Medicine 349*(26), 2479–2481.
40. Bataille R., Harousseau J. (1997). Multiple myeloma. *New England Journal of Medicine 336,* 1657–1664.
41. Rajkumar S.V., Gertz M.A., Kyle R.A., Greiff P.R. (2002). Current therapy for multiple myeloma. *Mayo Clinic Proceedings 77,* 813–822.
42. National Comprehensive Cancer Network. (2003). *NCCN clinical practice guidelines in oncology: Multiple myeloma.* Jenkintown, PA: National Comprehensive Cancer Network.
43. Tariman J.D. (2003). Understanding novel therapeutic agents for multiple myeloma. *Clinical Journal of Oncology Nursing 7*(5), 521–528.

UNIT V

Infection, Inflammation, and Immunity

The quest to understand the mechanism of disease and ways to prevent it permeates humankind's history. Many civilizations contributed to the storehouse of knowledge. Among the early accomplishments of the Chinese are a number of practices they developed to prevent disease, one of which took the form of inoculation.

The deadly smallpox had been one of the world's most dreaded diseases. During the Middle Ages, epidemics were frequent; they swept across Asia and other parts of the world, leaving widespread death in their wake. In the 1400s, the Chinese created a technique to protect themselves during an epidemic. They collected the crusts of smallpox sores and allowed them to dry. The dried material was ground into powder and inhaled. The procedure was found to be hazardous, but it remains one of the first attempts at vaccination.

CHAPTER 18

Mechanisms of Infectious Disease

W. Michael Dunne, Jr.

All living creatures share two basic objectives in life: survival and reproduction. This doctrine applies equally to humans and to members of the microbial world, including bacteria, viruses, fungi, and protozoa. To satisfy these goals, organisms must extract from the environment essential nutrients for growth and proliferation; for countless microscopic organisms, that environment is the human body. Normally, the contact between humans and microorganisms is incidental and, in certain situations, may actually benefit both organisms. Under extraordinary circumstances, however, the invasion of the human body by microorganisms can produce harmful and potentially lethal consequences. The consequences of these invasions are collectively called *infectious diseases.*

Infectious Diseases

After completing this section of the chapter, you should be able to meet the following objectives:

- Define the terms *host, infectious disease, colonization, microflora, virulence, pathogen,* and *saprophyte*
- Describe host–microorganism interactions using the concepts of commensalism, mutualism, and parasitic relationships
- Describe the structural characteristics and mechanisms of reproduction for prions, viruses, bacteria, rickettsiae, and chlamydiae, fungi, and parasites
- Use the concepts of incidence, portal of entry, source of infection, symptomatology, disease course, site of infection, agent, and host characteristics to explain the mechanisms of infectious diseases

TERMINOLOGY

All scientific disciplines evolve with a distinct vocabulary, and the study of infectious diseases is no exception. The most appropriate way to approach this subject is with a brief discussion of the terminology used to characterize interactions between humans and microbes.

Any organism capable of supporting the nutritional and physical growth requirements of another is called a *host.* Throughout this chapter, the term host most often refers to humans supporting the growth of microorganisms. The term *infection* describes the presence and multiplication of a living organism on or within the host. Occasionally, infection and *colonization* are used interchangeably.

One common misconception should be dispelled right away: not all interactions between microorganisms and humans are detrimental. The internal and external exposed surfaces of the human body are normally and harmlessly inhabited by a multitude of bacteria, collectively referred to as the normal *microflora* (Table 18-1). Although the colonizing bacteria acquire nutritional needs and shelter, the host is not adversely affected by the relationship. An interaction such as this is called *commensalism,* and the colonizing microorganisms are sometimes referred to as *commensal flora.* The term *mutualism* is applied to an infection in which the microorganism and the host derive benefits from the interaction. For example, certain inhabitants of the human intestinal tract extract nutrients from the host and secrete essential vitamin byproducts of metabolism (*e.g.,* vitamin K), which are absorbed and used by the host. A *parasitic relationship* is one in which only the infecting organism benefits from the relationship. If the host sustains injury or pathologic damage in response to a parasitic infection, the process is called an infectious disease.

The severity of an infectious disease can range from mild to life threatening, depending on many variables, including the health of the host at the time of infection and the *virulence* (disease-producing potential) of the microorganism. A select group of microorganisms called *pathogens* are so virulent that they are rarely found in the absence of disease. Fortunately, there are few human pathogens in the microbial world. Most microorganisms are harmless *saprophytes* (*i.e.,* free-living organisms obtaining their growth from dead or decaying organic material from the environment). All microorganisms, even saprophytes and members of the normal flora, can be *opportunistic pathogens,* capable of producing an infectious disease when the health and immunity of the host have been severely weakened by illness, famine, or medical therapy.

AGENTS OF INFECTIOUS DISEASE

The agents of infectious disease include prions, viruses, bacteria, rickettsiae, and chlamydiae, fungi, and parasites.

TABLE 18-1 Location and Variety of Nonpathogenic Normal Human Microflora

Area	Sites	Bacteria	
		Gram-positive	Gram-negative
Upper respiratory tract	Mouth, nose Nasopharynx Throat	+++ (Aerobes and anaerobes)	+++ (Aerobes and anaerobes)
Lower respiratory tract	Larynx Trachea Lungs	0 0 0	0 0 0
External surfaces	Skin Outer ear Eyes	++++ (Aerobes and anaerobes) (Transient)	+ (Transient) 0
Upper gastrointestinal tract	Stomach Duodenum Esophagus Jejunum	+ (Transient) 0 0	+ (Transient) 0 0
Lower gastrointestinal tract	Ileum Colon	+++ (Predominantly anaerobes)	++++ (Predominantly anaerobes)
External genitourinary tract	Vagina Anterior urethra	++ 0	++ 0
Internal genitourinary tract	Cervix, ovaries Fallopian tubes Uterus, prostate Bladder, kidney Testes, epididymis	0 0 0 0 0	0 0 0 0 0
Body fluids	Blood, urine Spinal fluid Synovial fluid Peritoneal fluid	0 0 0 0	0 0 0 0

Key: 0, none; +, rare; ++, few; +++, moderate; ++++, many.

Prions

Can a protein alone cause a transmissible infectious disease? Until recently, microbiologists assumed that all infectious agents must possess a genetic master plan (a genome of either RNA or DNA) that codes for the production of the essential proteins and enzymes necessary for survival and reproduction. Prions, protein particles that lack any kind of a demonstrable genome, appear to be an exception to this rule because they are infectious and capable of duplication. A number of prion-associated diseases have been identified, the most famous of which include Creutzfeldt-Jakob disease and kuru in humans, and scrapie and bovine spongiform encephalopathy (BSE, or mad cow disease) in animals. The various prion-associated diseases produce very similar symptomatology and pathology in the host and are collectively called *transmissible neurodegenerative diseases.* All are characterized by a slowly progressive noninflammatory neuronal degeneration, leading to loss of coordination (ataxia), dementia, and death over a period of time ranging from months to years. In fact, recent studies indicate that prion proteins (called PrP^{SC}) are actually altered or mutated forms of a normal host protein called PrP^{C}. The mutated protein accumulates to a high concentration in neurons, leading to a toxic condition and cell death.

AGENTS OF INFECTIOUS DISEASE

- The agents of infectious disease represent a diversity of microorganisms that are not visible to the human eye.
- Microorganisms can be separated into eukaryotes (fungi and parasites), organisms containing a membrane-bound nucleus, and prokaryotes (bacteria), organisms in which the nucleus is not separated.
- Eukaryotes and prokaryotes are organisms because they contain all the enzymes required for their replication and possess all the biologic equipment necessary for exploiting metabolic energy.
- Viruses, which are the smallest pathogens, have no organized cellular structure, but consist of protein coat surrounding a nucleic acid core of DNA or RNA. Unlike eukaryotes and prokaryotes, viruses are incapable of replication outside of a living cell.
- Parasites (protozoa, helminths, and arthropods) are members of the animal kingdom that infect and cause disease in other animals, which then transmit them to humans.

Mycobacteria	Parasites	Mycoplasmas	Fungi	Chlamydia/Rickettsia	Spirochetes
+	+	+	+	0	+
0	(Protozoans)	0	(Yeast)	0	0
0	0	0	0	0	0
0	0	0	0	0	0
0	0	0	0	0	0
+	0	0	+	0	0
0	0	0	(Yeast)	0	0
0	0	0	0	0	0
+	0	0	0	0	0
(Transient)					
0	0	0	0	0	0
0					
+	+	0	+	0	+
0	(Protozoans)	0	(Yeast)		0
0	0	+	+	0	0
0	0	0	(Yeast)	0	0
0	0	0	0	0	0
0	0	0	0	0	0
0	0	0	0	0	0
0	0	0	0	0	0
0	0	0	0	0	0
0	0	0	0	0	0
0	0	0	0	0	0
0	0	0	0	0	0
0	0	0	0	0	0

Studies of the transmission of prion disease in animals clearly demonstrate that prions replicate, leading researchers to investigate how proteins can reproduce in the absence of genetic material. One theory postulates that the interaction between the normal PrP^{C} and the abnormal PrP^{SC} leads to a structural change in the normal protein, resulting in two PrP^{SC} molecules. PrP^{SC} then accumulates and spreads within the axons of the nerve cells, causing progressively greater damage of host neurons and the eventual incapacitation of the host. Because prions lack reproductive and metabolic functions, the currently available antibacterial and antiviral agents are useless.

Viruses

Viruses are the smallest obligate intracellular pathogens. They are incapable of replication outside of a living cell. They have no organized cellular structures but instead consist of a protein coat, or capsid, surrounding a nucleic acid core, or genome, of RNA or DNA—never both (Fig. 18-1). Some viruses are enclosed within a lipoprotein envelope derived from the cytoplasmic membrane of the parasitized host cell. Certain viruses are continuously shed from the infected cell surface enveloped in buds pinched from the cytoplasmic membrane. Enveloped viruses include members of the herpesvirus group and paramyxoviruses such as influenza and poxviruses.

Viruses must penetrate a susceptible living cell and use the biosynthetic machinery of the cell to produce viral progeny. The process of viral replication is shown in Figure 18-2. Not every viral agent causes lysis and death of the host cell during the course of replication. Some viruses enter the host cell and insert their genome into the host cell chromosome, where it remains in a latent, nonreplicating state for long periods without causing disease. Under the appropriate stimulation, the virus undergoes active replication and produces symptoms of disease months to years later. Members of the herpesvirus group and adenovirus are the best examples of latent viruses. Herpesviruses include the viral agents of chickenpox and zoster (shingles), genital herpes, cytomegalovirus infections, infectious mononucleosis, fever blisters, and Kaposi's sarcoma. In each of these, the resumption of the latent viral replication may produce symptoms of primary disease (*e.g.*, genital herpes) or cause an entirely different symptomatology (*e.g.*, shingles instead of chickenpox).

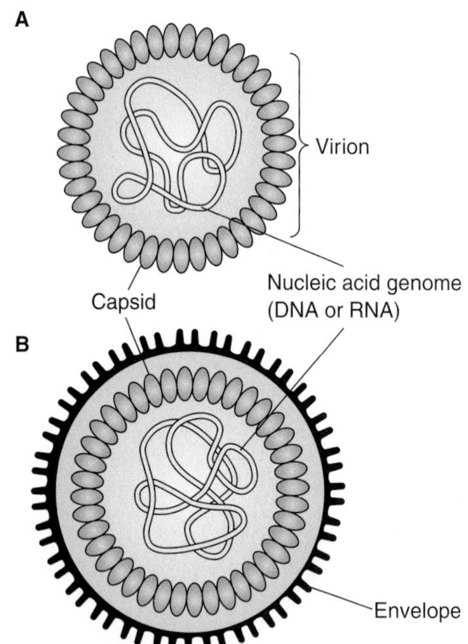

FIGURE 18-1 (**A**) The basic structure of a virus includes a protein coat surrounding an inner core of nucleic acid (DNA or RNA). (**B**) Some viruses may also be enclosed in a lipoprotein outer envelope.

Within the past two plus decades, members of the retrovirus group have received considerable attention after identification of the human immunodeficiency viruses (HIV) as the causative agent of acquired immunodeficiency syndrome (AIDS). The retroviruses have a unique mechanism of replication. After entry into the host cell, the viral RNA genome is first translated into DNA by a viral enzyme called *reverse transcriptase.* The viral DNA copy is integrated into the host chromosome and exists in a latent state similar to the herpesviruses. Reactivation and replication require a reversal of the entire process. Some retroviruses lyse the host cell during the process of replication. In the case of HIV, the infected cells regulate the immunologic defense system of the host, and their lysis leads to a permanent suppression of the immune response.

In addition to causing infectious diseases, certain viruses also have the ability to transform normal host cells into malignant cells during the replication cycle. This group of viruses is referred to as *oncogenic* and includes certain retroviruses and DNA viruses, such as the herpesviruses, adenoviruses, and papovaviruses.

The viruses of humans and animals have been categorized somewhat arbitrarily according to various characteristics. These include the type of viral genome (single-stranded or double-stranded DNA or RNA), the mechanism of replication (*e.g.*, retroviruses), the mode of transmission (*e.g.*, arthropod-borne viruses, enteroviruses), and the type of disease produced (*e.g.*, hepatitis A, B, C, D, and E viruses), just to name a few.

Bacteria

Bacteria are autonomously replicating unicellular organisms known as *prokaryotes* because they lack an organized nucleus. Compared with nucleated eukaryotic cells (see Chapter 4), the structure of the bacterial cell is small and relatively primitive (Fig. 18-3). Bacteria approximate the size of the eukaryotic mitochondria (about 1 mm in diameter) and may be the evolutionary ancestors of mitochondria.

Bacteria generally contain no organized intracellular organelles, and the genome consists of only a single chromosome of DNA. Many bacteria transiently harbor smaller extrachromosomal pieces of circular DNA called *plasmids.* Occasionally, plasmids contain genetic information that increases the virulence of the organism. Similar to eukaryotic cells, but unlike viruses, bacteria contain DNA and RNA.

The prokaryotic cell is organized into an internal compartment called the *cytoplasm,* which contains the reproductive and metabolic machinery of the cell (Fig. 18-4). The

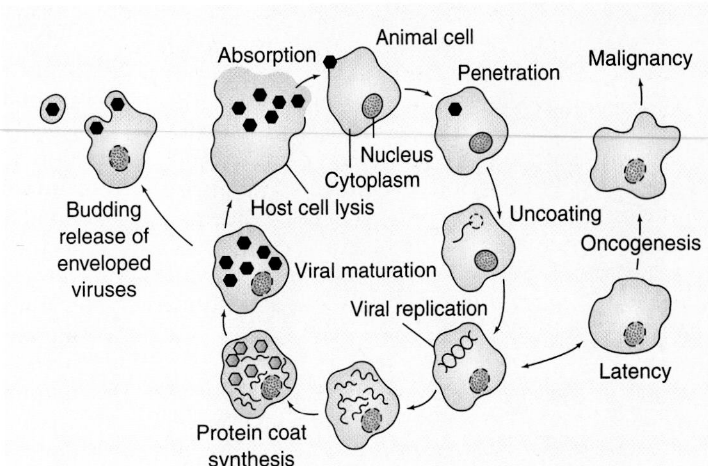

FIGURE 18-2 Schematic representation of the many possible consequences of viral infection of host cells, including cell lysis (poliovirus), continuous release of budding viral particles, or latency (herpesviruses) and oncogenesis (papovaviruses).

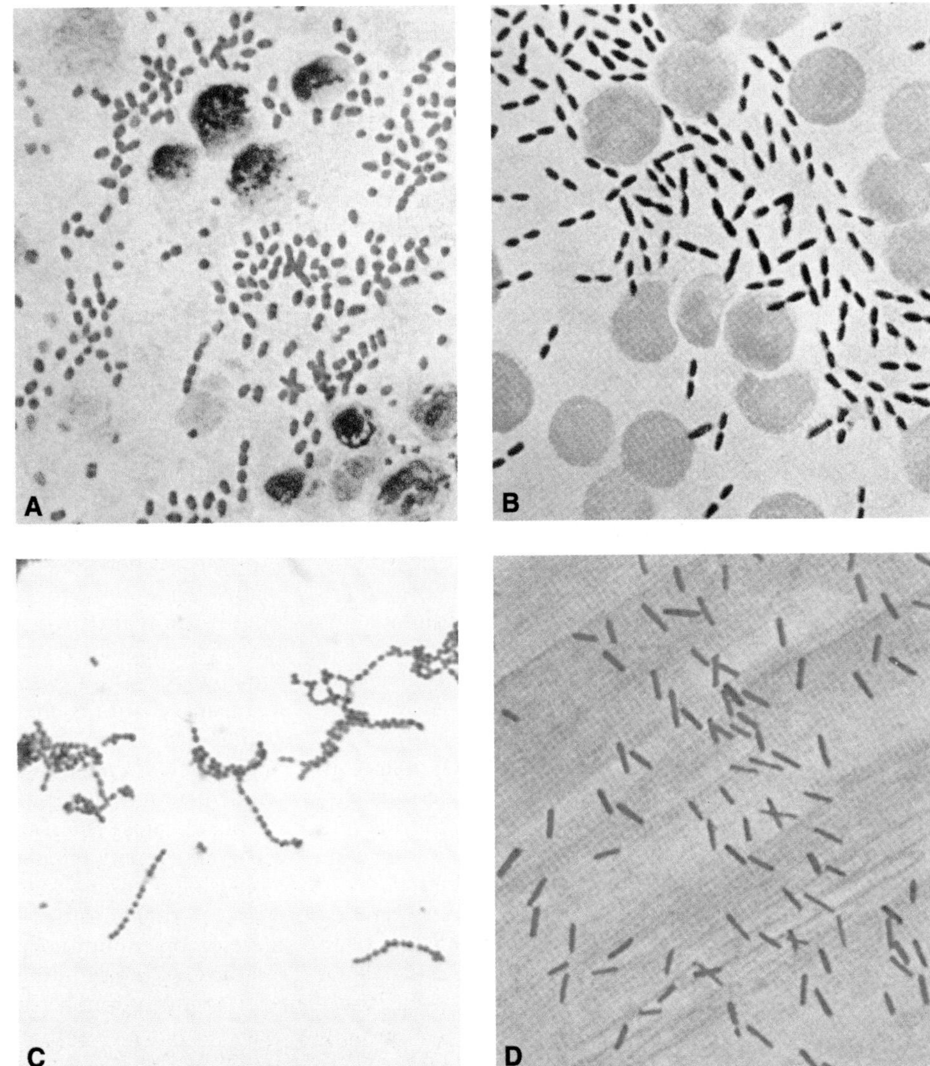

FIGURE 18-3 A sampling of microscopic morphology of bacteria demonstrating the variability of size and shape: (**A**) *Yersinia pestis;* (**B**) gram-positive diplococcus typical of *Streptococcus pneumoniae*; (**C**) *Streptococcus species* using Gram stain; (**D**) *Escherichia coli* using Gram stain. (Public Images Library, Centers for Disease Control and Prevention. Available: http://phil.cdc.gov/phil/detail.?id=2170)

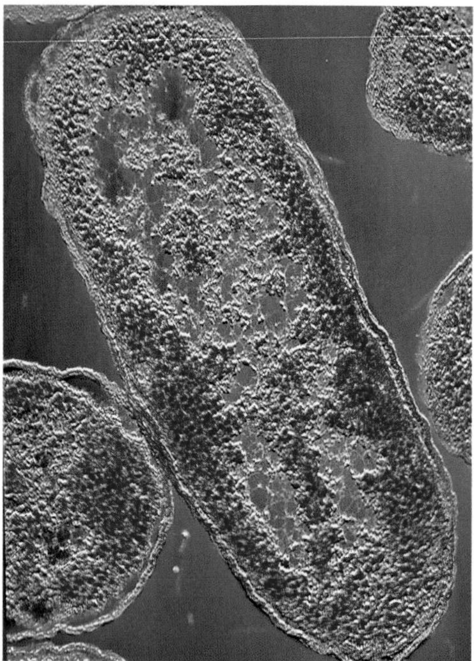

FIGURE 18-4 False-color transmission electron micrograph of the rod-shaped, gram-negative bacterium *Escherichia coli,* showing the simple prokaryotic cell structure including the cytoplasm, the cytoplasmic membrane, and the rigid cell wall. (© Science Source/Photo Researchers)

cytoplasm is surrounded by a flexible lipid membrane, called the *cytoplasmic membrane.* This in turn is enclosed within a rigid cell wall. The structure and synthesis of the cell wall determine the microscopic shape of the bacterium (*e.g.,* spherical [cocci], helical [spirilla], or elongated [bacilli]). Most bacteria produce a cell wall composed of a distinctive polymer known as *peptidoglycan.* This polymer is only produced by prokaryotes and is therefore an attractive target for antibacterial therapy. Several bacteria synthesize an extracellular capsule composed of protein or carbohydrate. The capsule protects the organism from environmental hazards such as the immunologic defenses of the host.

Certain bacteria are motile as the result of external whiplike appendages called *flagella.* The rotary action of the flagella transports the organism through a liquid environment like a propeller. Bacteria can also produce hairlike structures projecting from the cell surface called *pili* or *fimbriae,* which enable the organism to adhere to surfaces such as mucous membranes or other bacteria.

Most prokaryotes reproduce asexually by simple cellular division. The number of planes in which an organism divides can influence the microscopic morphology. For instance, when the cocci divide in chains, they are called streptococci; in pairs, diplococci; and in clusters, staphylococci. The growth rate of bacteria varies significantly among different species and depends greatly on physical growth conditions and the availability of nutrients. In the laboratory, a single bacterium placed in a suitable growth environment, such as an agar plate, reproduces to the extent that it forms a visible colony composed of millions of bacteria within a few hours. In nature, however, bacteria rarely exist as single cells floating in an aqueous environment. Rather, bacteria prefer to stick to and colonize environmental surfaces, producing highly structured communities called *biofilms.* Biofilms exist with a fair degree of organization and structure to permit access to available nutrients and elimination of metabolic waste. Within the biofilm, individual organisms use a primitive cellular communication in the form of chemical signaling to represent the state of the environment. These signals inform members of the community when sufficient nutrients are available for proliferation or when environmental conditions warrant dormancy or evacuation. Examples of biofilms abound in nature and are found on surfaces of marine environments and humans. One only has to disassemble a clogged sink drain to see a perfect example of a bacterial biofilm.

The physical appearance of a colony of bacteria grown on an agar plate can be quite distinctive for each species. Some produce pigments that give colonies a unique color. Some bacteria produce highly resistant spores when faced with an unfavorable environment. The spores can exist in a quiescent state almost indefinitely until suitable growth conditions are encountered. The spores germinate, and the organism resumes normal metabolism and replication.

Bacteria are extremely adaptable life forms. They inhabit almost every environmental extreme on earth, including humans. However, each individual bacterial species has a well-defined set of growth parameters, including nutrition, temperature, light, humidity, and atmosphere. Bacteria with extremely strict growth requirements are called *fastidious.* For example, *Neisseria gonorrhoeae,* the bacterium that causes gonorrhea, cannot live for extended periods outside the human body. Some bacteria require oxygen for growth and metabolism and are called *aerobes;* others cannot survive in an oxygen-containing environment and are called *anaerobes.* An organism capable of adapting its metabolism to aerobic or anaerobic conditions is called *facultatively anaerobic.*

In the laboratory, bacteria are generally classified according to the microscopic appearance and staining properties of the cell. Gram's stain, originally developed in 1884 by the Danish bacteriologist Christian Gram, is still the most widely used staining procedure. Bacteria are designated as *gram-positive* organisms if they are stained purple by a primary basic dye (usually crystal violet); those that are not stained by the crystal violet but are counterstained red by a second dye (safranin) are called *gram-negative* organisms. Staining characteristics and microscopic morphology are used in combination to describe bacteria. For example, *Streptococcus pyogenes,* the agent of scarlet fever and rheumatic fever, is a gram-positive streptococcal organism that is spherical, grows in chains, and stains purple by Gram's stain. *Legionella pneumophila,* the bacterium responsible for Legionnaire's disease, is a gram-negative rod.

Another means of classifying bacteria according to microscopic staining properties is called the *acid-fast stain.* Because of their unique cell membrane fatty acid content and composition, certain bacteria are resistant to the decolorization of a primary stain (either carbol fuchsin or a combination of auramine and rhodamine) when treated with a solution of acid alcohol. These organisms are termed *acid fast* and include a number of significant human pathogens, most notably *Mycobacterium tuberculosis* (the cause of tuberculosis) and other mycobacteria and a variety of filamentous bacteria, including several species of *Nocardia*—*N. asteroides* complex and *N. braziliensis*.

For purposes of taxonomy (*e.g.*, identification and classification), each member of the bacterial kingdom is categorized into a small group of biochemically and genetically related organisms called the *genus* and further subdivided into distinct individuals within the genus called *species*. The genus and species assignment of the organism is reflected in its name (*e.g.*, *Staphylococcus* [genus] *aureus* [species]).

Spirochetes. The spirochetes are an eccentric category of bacteria that are mentioned separately because of their unusual cellular morphology and distinctive mechanism of motility. Technically, the spirochetes are gram-negative rods but are unique in that the cell's shape is helical and the length of the organism is many times its width. A series of filaments are wound about the cell wall and extend the entire length of the cell. These filaments propel the organism through an aqueous environment in a corkscrew motion.

Spirochetes are anaerobic or facultatively anaerobic organisms and contain three genera: *Leptospira, Borrelia,* and *Treponema*. Each genus has saprophytic and pathogenic strains. The pathogenic leptospires infect a wide variety of wild and domestic animals. Infected animals shed the organisms into the environment through the urinary tract. Transmission to humans occurs by contact with infected animals or urine-contaminated surroundings. Leptospires gain access to the host directly through mucous membranes or breaks in the skin and can produce a severe and potentially fatal illness called *Weil's syndrome*. In contrast, the borreliae are transmitted from infected animals to humans through the bite of an arthropod vector such as lice or ticks. Included among the genus *Borrelia* are the agents of relapsing fever (*B. recurrentis*) and Lyme disease (*B. burgdorferi*). Pathogenic *Treponema* species require no intermediates and are spread from person to person by direct contact. The most important member of the genus is *Treponema pallidum,* the cause of syphilis.

Mycoplasmas. The mycoplasmas are unicellular prokaryotes capable of independent replication. These organisms are less than one third the size of bacteria and contain a small DNA genome approximately one half the size of the bacterial chromosome. The cell is composed of cytoplasm surrounded by a membrane, but unlike bacteria, the mycoplasmas do not produce a rigid peptidoglycan cell wall. As a consequence, the microscopic appearance of the cell is highly variable, ranging from coccoid forms to filaments, and the mycoplasmas are resistant to cell wall–inhibiting antibiotics such as penicillins and cephalosporins.

The mycoplasmas of humans are divided into three genera: *Mycoplasma, Ureaplasma,* and *Acholeplasma*. The first two of these require cholesterol from the environment to produce the cell membrane; the *Acholeplasma* do not. In the human host, mycoplasmas are commensals. However, a number of species are capable of producing serious diseases, including pneumonia (*Mycoplasma pneumoniae*), genital infections (*Mycoplasma hominis* and *Ureaplasma urealyticum*), and maternally transmitted respiratory infections to low-birth-weight infants (*U. urealyticum*).

Rickettsiae, Chlamydiae, Ehrlichieae, and *Coxiella*

This interesting group of organisms combines the characteristics of viral and bacterial agents to produce disease in humans. All are obligate intracellular pathogens like the viruses but produce a rigid peptidoglycan cell wall, reproduce asexually by cellular division, and contain RNA and DNA similar to the bacteria.

The rickettsiae depend on the host cell for essential vitamins and nutrients, but the chlamydiae appear to scavenge intermediates of energy metabolism such as adenosine triphosphate (ATP). The rickettsiae infect but do not produce disease in the cells of certain arthropods such as fleas, ticks, and lice. The organisms are accidentally transmitted to humans through the bite of the arthropod (*i.e.*, vector) and produce a number of potentially lethal diseases, including Rocky Mountain spotted fever and epidemic typhus.

The chlamydiae are slightly smaller than the rickettsiae but are structurally similar. Unlike the rickettsiae, chlamydiae are transmitted directly between susceptible vertebrates without an intermediate arthropod host. Transmission and replication of chlamydiae occur through a defined life cycle. The infectious form, called an *elementary body,* attaches to and enters the host cell, where it transforms into a larger reticulate body. The latter undergoes active replication into multiple elementary bodies, which are then shed into the extracellular environment to initiate another infectious cycle. Chlamydial diseases of humans include sexually transmitted genital infections (see Chapter 48); ocular infections and pneumonia of newborns (*Chlamydia trachomatis*); upper and lower respiratory tract infections in children, adolescents, and young adults (*Chlamydia pneumoniae*); and respiratory disease acquired from infected birds (*Chlamydia psittaci*).

Organisms classically referred to as ehrlichiae (including the reorganized genera *Ehrlichia, Anaplasma, Neorickettsia, Aegyptianella,* and *Wolbachia*) are also obligate intracellular organisms that resemble the rickettsiae in structure and produce a variety of veterinarian and human diseases, some of which have a tick vector. These organisms target host mononuclear and polymorphonuclear white blood cells for infection and, similar to the chlamydiae, multiply in the cytoplasm of infected leukocytes within vacuoles called *morulae*. Unlike the chlamydiae, however, the Ehrlichiae do not have a defined life cycle and are independent of the host cell for energy production. In the Far East, *Neorickettsia sennetsu* produces a disease in humans called sennetsu fever that resembles infectious mononucleosis. In the United States, the most frequent manifestation of ehrlichiae infection is human monocytotropic ehrlichiosis (HME), a disease caused by *ehrlichia chaffeensis* that is easily confused with Rocky Mountain spotted fever. *Anaplasma phagocytophilum* is the agent of human granulocytic ehrlichiosis (HGE) and is transmitted by the same tick vector as Lyme disease. The resulting illness is generally one of high fever, headache, and muscle pain, with gastrointestinal, central nervous system, or respiratory involvement. A rash is less likely to occur among patients with HGE.

The genus *Coxiella* contains only one species, *C. burnetii.* Like its rickettsial counterparts, it too is a gram-negative intracellular organism that infects a variety of animals, including cattle, sheep, and goats. In humans, *Coxiella* infection produces a disease called Q fever, characterized by a nonspecific febrile illness often accompanied by headache, chills, arthralgias, and mild pneumonia. The organism produces a highly resistant spore stage that is transmitted to humans when animal tissue is aerosolized (*e.g.,* as during meat processing) or by ingestion of contaminated milk.

Fungi

The fungi are free-living, eukaryotic saprophytes found in every habitat on earth. Some are members of the normal human microflora. Fortunately, few fungi are capable of causing diseases in humans, and most of these are incidental self-limited infections of skin and subcutaneous tissue. Serious fungal infections are rare and usually initiated through puncture wounds or inhalation. Despite their normally harmless nature, fungi can cause serious life-threatening opportunistic diseases when host defense capabilities have been disabled.

The fungi can be separated into two groups, yeasts and molds, based on rudimentary differences in their morphology (Fig. 18-5). The yeasts are single-celled organisms, approximately the size of red blood cells that reproduce by a budding process. The buds separate from the parent cell and mature into identical daughter cells. Molds produce long, hollow, branching filaments called *hyphae.* Some molds produce cross walls, which segregate the hyphae into compartments, and others do not. A limited number of fungi are capable of growing as yeasts at one temperature and as molds at another. These organisms are called *dimorphic fungi* and include a number of human pathogens such as the agents of blastomycosis, histoplasmosis, and coccidioidomycosis (San Joaquin fever).

The visual appearance of a fungal colony tends to reflect its cellular composition. Colonies of yeast are generally smooth with a waxy or creamy texture. Molds tend to produce cottony or powdery colonies composed of mats of hyphae collectively called a *mycelium.* The mycelium can penetrate the growth surface or project above the colony like the roots and branches of a tree. Yeasts and molds produce a rigid cell wall layer that is chemically unrelated to the peptidoglycan of bacteria and is therefore not susceptible to the effects of penicillin-like antibiotics.

Most fungi are capable of sexual or asexual reproduction. The former process involves the fusion of zygotes with the production of a recombinant zygospore. Asexual reproduction involves the formation of highly resistant spores called *conidia* or *sporangiospores,* which are borne by specialized structures that arise from the hyphae. Molds are identified in the laboratory by the characteristic microscopic appearance of the asexual fruiting structures and spores.

Just like the bacterial pathogens of humans, fungi can only produce disease in the human host if they can grow at the temperature of the infected body site. For example, a number of fungal pathogens called the *dermatophytes* are incapable of growing at core body temperature (37°C), and the infection is limited to the cooler cutaneous surfaces. Diseases caused by these organisms, including ringworm, athlete's foot, and jock itch, are collectively called *superficial mycoses. Systemic mycoses* are serious fungal infections of deep tissues and, by definition, are caused by organisms capable of growth at 37°C. Yeasts such as *Candida albicans* are commensal flora of the skin, mucous membranes, and gastrointestinal tract and are capable of growth at a wider range of temperatures. Intact immune mechanisms and competition for nutrients provided by the bacterial flora normally keep colonizing fungi in check. Alterations in either of these components by disease states or antibiotic therapy can upset the balance, permitting fungal overgrowth and setting the stage for opportunistic infections.

Parasites

In a strict sense, any organism that derives benefits from its biologic relationship with another organism is a parasite. In the study of clinical microbiology, however, the term *parasite* has evolved to designate members of the animal kingdom that infect and cause disease in other animals and includes protozoa, helminths, and arthropods.

The protozoa are unicellular animals with a complete complement of eukaryotic cellular machinery, including a well-defined nucleus and organelles. Reproduction may be sexual or asexual, and life cycles may be simple or complicated with several maturation stages requiring more than one host for completion. Most are saprophytes, but a few have adapted to the accommodations of the human environment and produce a variety of diseases, including malaria, amebic dysentery, and giardiasis. Protozoan infections can be passed directly from host to host such as through sexual contact, indirectly through contaminated water or food, or by way of an arthropod vector. Direct or indirect transmission results from the ingestion of highly resistant cysts or spores that are shed in the feces of an infected host. When the cysts reach the intestine, they mature into vegetative forms called *trophozoites,* which are capable of asexual reproduction or cyst formation. Most trophozoites are motile by means of flagella, cilia, or ameboid motion.

The helminths are a collection of wormlike parasites, which include the nematodes or roundworms, cestodes or tapeworms, and trematodes or flukes. The helminths reproduce sexually within the definitive host, and some require an intermediate host for the development and maturation of offspring. Humans can serve as the definitive or intermediate host and, in certain diseases such as trichinosis, as both. Transmission of helminth diseases occurs primarily through the ingestion of fertilized eggs (ova) or the penetration of infectious larval stages through the skin—directly or with the aid of an arthropod vector. Helminth infections can involve many organ systems and sites, including the liver and lung, urinary and intestinal tracts, circulatory and central nervous systems, and muscle. Although most helminth diseases have been eradicated from the United States, they are still a major health concern of developing nations.

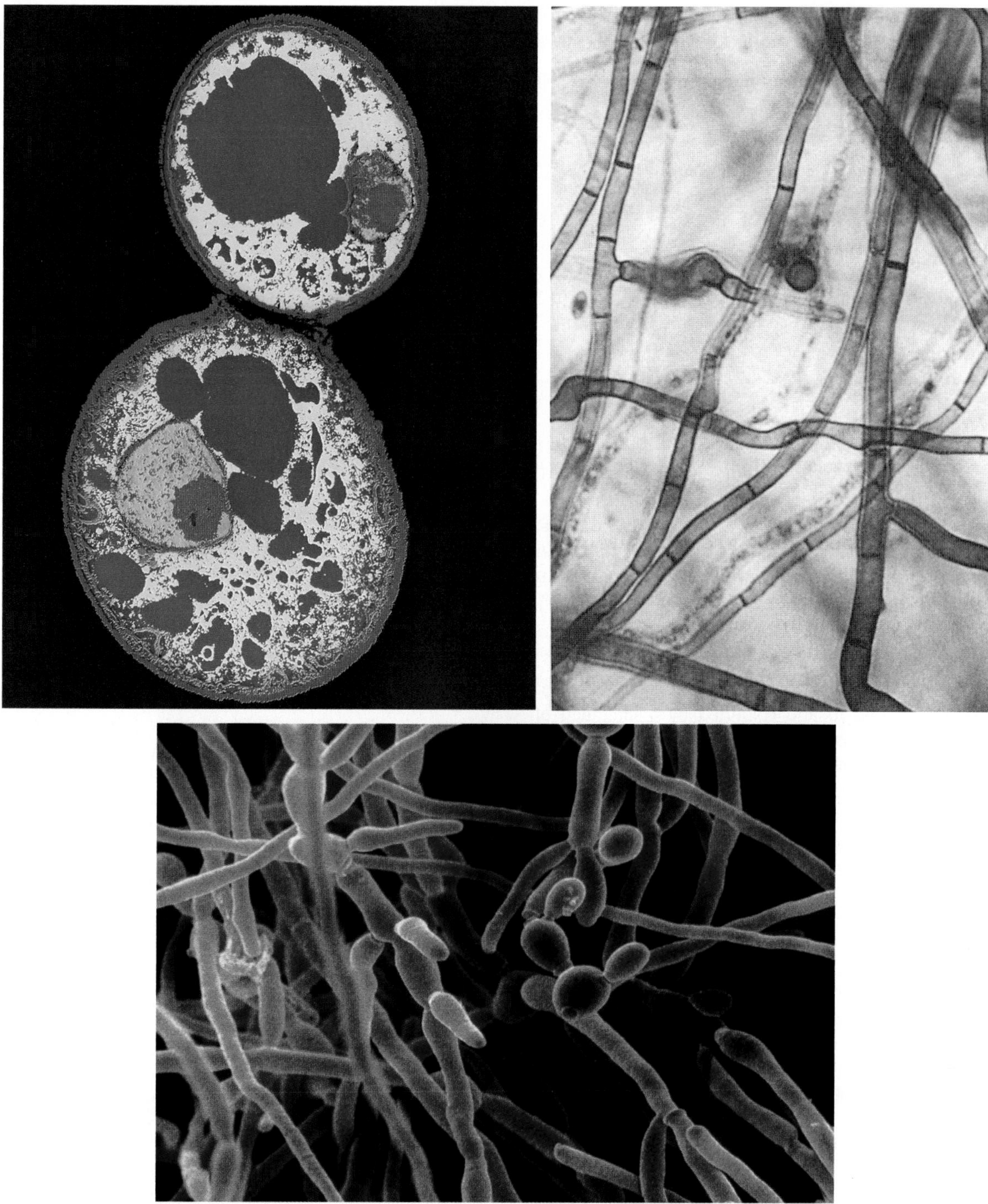

FIGURE 18-5 The microscopic morphology of fungal pathogens in humans. The yeasts are single-celled organisms that reproduce by the budding process (**upper left**). The molds (**right**) produce long branched or unbranched filaments called hyphae. *Candida albicans* (**lower left**) is a budding yeast that produces pseudohyphae both in culture and in tissues and exudates. (Upper left and lower left © Science Source/ Photo Researchers)

The parasitic arthropods of humans and animals include the vectors of infectious diseases (*e.g.*, ticks, mosquitoes, biting flies) and the ectoparasites. The ectoparasites infest external body surfaces and cause localized tissue damage or inflammation secondary to the bite or burrowing action of the arthropod. The most prominent human ectoparasites are mites (scabies), chiggers, lice (head, body, and pubic), and fleas. Transmission of ectoparasites occurs directly by contact with immature or mature forms of the arthropod or its eggs found on the infested host or the

TABLE 18-2 Comparison of Characteristics of Human Microbial Pathogens

Organism	Defined Nucleus	Genomic Material	Size*	Intracellular or Extracellular	Motility
Viruses	No	DNA or RNA	0.02–0.3	I	–
Bacteria	No	DNA	0.5–15	I/E	±
Mycoplasmas	No	DNA	0.2–0.3	E	–
Spirochetes	No	DNA	6–15	E	+
Rickettsiae	No	DNA	0.2–2	I	–
Chlamydiae	No	DNA	0.3–1	I	–
Yeasts	Yes	DNA	2–60	I/E	–
Molds	Yes	DNA	2–15 (hyphal width)	E	–
Protozoans	Yes	DNA	1–60	I/E	+
Helminths	Yes	DNA	2 mm–> 1 m	E	+

*Micrometers unless indicated.

host's clothing, bedding, or grooming articles such as combs and brushes. Many of the ectoparasites are vectors of other infectious diseases, including endemic typhus and bubonic plague (fleas) and epidemic typhus (lice). A summary of the salient characteristics of human microbial pathogens is presented in Table 18-2.

In summary, throughout life, humans are continuously and harmlessly exposed to and colonized by a multitude of microscopic organisms. This relationship is kept in check by the intact defense mechanisms of the host (*e.g.,* mucosal and cutaneous barriers, normal immune function) and the innocuous nature of most environmental microorganisms. Those factors that weaken the resistance of the host or increase the virulence of colonizing microorganisms can disturb the equilibrium of the relationship and cause disease. The degree to which the balance is shifted in favor of the microorganism determines the severity of illness.

There is an extreme diversity of prokaryotic and eukaryotic microorganisms capable of causing infectious diseases in humans. With the advent of immunosuppressive medical therapy and immunosuppressive diseases such as AIDS, the number and type of potential microbic pathogens, the so-called opportunistic pathogens, have increased dramatically. However, most infectious illnesses in humans continue to be caused by only a small fraction of the organisms that comprise the microscopic world.

Mechanisms of Infection

After completing this section of the chapter, you should be able to meet the following objectives:

- ✦ Differentiate between incidence and prevalence and among endemic, epidemic, and panepidemic
- ✦ Describe the stages of an infectious disease after the point at which the potential pathogen enters the body
- ✦ List the systemic manifestations of infectious disease
- ✦ Describe mechanisms and significance of antimicrobial and antiviral drug resistance
- ✦ Explain the actions of intravenous immunoglobulin and cytokines in the treatment of infectious illnesses

EPIDEMIOLOGY OF INFECTIOUS DISEASES

Epidemiology, in the context of this chapter, is the study of factors, events, and circumstances that influence the transmission of infectious diseases among humans. The ultimate goal of the epidemiologist is to devise strategies that interrupt or eliminate the spread of an infectious agent. To accomplish this, infectious diseases must be classified according to incidence, portal of entry, source, symptoms, disease course, site of infection, and virulence factors so that potential outbreaks may be predicted and averted or appropriately treated. Each of these categories is discussed in detail with the exception of agents and host, which have already been reviewed.

Epidemiology is a science of rates. The expected frequency of any infectious disease must be calculated so that

EPIDEMIOLOGY OF INFECTIOUS DISEASES

- ➤ Epidemiology is the study of factors, events, and circumstances that influence the transmission of infectious diseases in human populations.
- ➤ Epidemiology focuses on the incidence (number of new cases) and prevalence (number of active cases at any given time) of an infectious disease; the source of infection, its portal of entry, site of infection, and virulence factors of the infecting organism; and the signs and symptoms of the infection and its course.
- ➤ The ultimate goals of epidemiologic studies are the interruption of the spread of infectious diseases and their eradication.

gradual or abrupt changes in frequency can be observed. The term *incidence* is used to describe the number of new cases of an infectious disease that occur within a defined population (*e.g.*, per 100,000 persons) over an established period of time (*e.g.*, monthly, quarterly, yearly). Disease *prevalence* indicates the number of active cases at any given time. A disease is considered *endemic* in a particular geographic region if the incidence and prevalence are expected and relatively stable. An *epidemic* describes an abrupt and unexpected increase in the incidence of disease over endemic rates. A *pandemic* refers to the spread of disease beyond continental boundaries. The advent of rapid worldwide travel increased the likelihood of pandemic transmission of pathogenic microorganisms.

As an illustration of these principles, an outbreak of a suspected arboviral (virus transmitted by an insect) encephalitis (inflammation of the brain) was recognized in the New York City metropolitan area in the fall of 1999. Beginning in August, local health officials noted an increased incidence of encephalitis; by the end of September, 17 confirmed and 20 probable cases with four deaths were reported in the area. Studies of antibodies produced by the infected individuals suggested that the illnesses were caused by St. Louis encephalitis virus, which is classified as a flavivirus, is endemic in the United States, and is transmitted from infected birds and rodents to humans by mosquitoes. During the same time period, public health workers also noted increased deaths among several New York City bird populations, particularly crows. The birds also developed meningoencephalitis and myocarditis (inflammation of the heart). Tissue samples from the birds were sent to the National Veterinary Services Laboratory in Ames, Iowa, and to the Centers for Disease Control and Prevention (CDC) in Atlanta. Much to the researchers' surprise, the virus isolated from the patients and birds in New York City appeared to be West Nile virus (WNV), a virus endemic to Europe, Africa, and the Middle East that had never been isolated in the United States before. Therefore, the outbreak of WNV encephalitis was not only an epidemic but also a pandemic because the disease crossed continental borders for the first time.

PORTAL OF ENTRY

The portal of entry refers to the process by which a pathogen enters the body, gains access to susceptible tissues, and causes disease. Among the potential modes of transmission are penetration, direct contact, ingestion, and inhalation.

Penetration

Any disruption in the integrity of the body's surface barrier such as skin or mucous membranes is a potential site for invasion of microorganisms. The break may be the result of an accidental injury resulting in abrasions, burns, or penetrating wounds; medical procedures such as surgery or catheterization; a primary infectious process that produces surface lesions such as chickenpox or impetigo; or direct inoculation from intravenous drug use or from animal or arthropod bites. The latter mode of transmission can be extremely dangerous because large numbers of organisms can gain access directly into vital sites, thus bypassing the host's primary immune defense systems.

Direct Contact

Some pathogens are transmitted directly from infected tissue or secretions to exposed, intact mucous membranes without a prerequisite for damaged mucosal barriers. This is especially true of certain sexually transmitted diseases (STDs) such as gonorrhea, syphilis, chlamydia, and herpes, for which exposure of uninfected membranes to pathogens occurs during intimate contact.

The transmission of STDs is not limited to sexual contact. *Vertical transmission* of these agents, from mother to child, can occur across the placenta or during birth when the mucous membranes of the child come in contact with infected vaginal secretions of the mother. When an infectious disease is transmitted from mother to child during gestation or birth, it is classified as a *congenital infection.* The most frequently observed congenital infections include the parasite *Toxoplasma gondii,* other infections (most commonly syphilis), rubella, cytomegalovirus, and herpes simplex viruses (the so-called *TORCH* infections), varicella-zoster (chickenpox), parvovirus B19, group B streptococci (*Streptococcus agalactiae*), and HIV. Of these, cytomegalovirus is by far the most common cause of congenital infection in the United States, affecting nearly 1% of all newborns. However, more than 6000 HIV-infected women give birth each year in the United States, and the numbers are likely far greater in developing nations. With a 13% to 30% chance of vertical transmission, HIV is rapidly gaining in stature as a congenitally transmitted infection.

The severity of congenital defects associated with these infections depends greatly on the gestational age of the fetus when transmission occurs, but most of these agents can cause profound mental retardation and neurosensory deficits, including blindness and hearing loss. HIV rarely produces overt signs and symptoms in the infected newborn, and it sometimes takes years for the effects of the illness to manifest.

Ingestion

The entry of pathogenic microorganisms or their toxic products through the oral cavity and gastrointestinal tract represents one of the more efficient means of disease transmission in humans. Many bacterial, viral, and parasitic infections, including cholera, typhoid fever, dysentery (amebic and bacillary), food poisoning, traveler's diarrhea, cryptosporidiosis, and hepatitis A, are initiated through the ingestion of contaminated food and water. This mechanism of transmission necessitates that an infectious agent survives the low pH and enzyme activity of gastric secretions and the peristaltic action of the intestines in numbers sufficient to establish infection to be deemed an *infectious dose.* Ingested pathogens also must compete successfully with the normal bacterial flora of the bowel for nutritional needs. Persons with reduced gastric acidity (called *achlorhydria*) due to disease or medication are more susceptible to infection by this route because the number of ingested microorganisms surviving the gastric environment is greater. Ingestion has also been postulated as a means of transmission of HIV infection from mother to child through breast-feeding.

Inhalation

The respiratory tract of healthy persons is equipped with a multitiered defense system to prevent potential pathogens from entering the lungs. The surface of the respiratory tree is lined with a layer of mucus that is continuously swept up and away from the lungs and toward the mouth by the beating motion of ciliated epithelial cells. Humidification of inspired air increases the size of aerosolized particles, which are effectively filtered by the mucous membranes of the upper respiratory tract. Coughing also aids in the removal of particulate matter from the lower respiratory tract. Respiratory secretions contain antibodies and enzymes capable of inactivating infectious agents. Particulate matter and microorganisms that ultimately reach the lung are cleared by phagocytic cells.

Despite this impressive array of protective mechanisms, a number of pathogens can invade the human body through the respiratory tract, including agents of bacterial pneumonia (*Streptococcus pneumoniae, Legionella pneumophila*), meningitis and sepsis (*N. meningitidis* and *Haemophilus influenzae*), tuberculosis, and the viruses responsible for measles, mumps, chickenpox, influenza, and the common cold. Defective pulmonary function or mucociliary clearance caused by noninfectious processes such as cystic fibrosis, emphysema, or smoking can increase the risk for inhalation-acquired diseases.

The portal of entry does not dictate the site of infection. Ingested pathogens may penetrate the intestinal mucosa, disseminate through the circulatory system, and cause diseases in other organs such as the lung or liver. Whatever the mechanisms of entry, the transmission of infectious agents is directly related to the number of infectious agents absorbed by the host.

SOURCE

The source of an infectious disease refers to the location, host, object, or substance from which the infectious agent was acquired: essentially the who, what, where, and when of disease transmission. The source may be endogenous (acquired from the host's own microbial flora, as would be the case in an opportunistic infection) or exogenous (acquired from sources in the external environment such as the water, food, soil, or air). The infectious agent can originate from another human being, as from mother to child during gestation (congenital infections) or birth (perinatal infections). Zoonoses are a category of infectious diseases passed from other animal species to humans. Examples of zoonoses include cat-scratch disease, rabies, and visceral or cutaneous larval migrans. The spread of infectious diseases, including Lyme disease, malaria, trypanosomiasis, and arboviral encephalitis viruses such as West Nile and St. Louis encephalitis viruses, through biting arthropod vectors has already been mentioned.

Source can denote a place. For instance, infections that develop in patients while they are hospitalized are called *nosocomial,* and those that are acquired outside of health care facilities are called *community acquired.* The source may also pertain to the body substance that is the most likely vehicle for transmission, such as feces, blood, body fluids, respiratory secretions, and urine. Infections can be transmitted from person to person through shared inanimate objects (fomites) contaminated with infected body fluids. An example of this mechanism of transmission would include the spread of HIV and hepatitis B virus through the use of shared syringes by intravenous drug users. Infection can also be spread through a complex combination of source, portal of entry, and vector. The well-publicized 1993 outbreak of hantavirus pulmonary syndrome in the southwestern United States is a prime example. This viral illness was transmitted to humans by inhalation of dust contaminated with saliva, feces, and urine of infected rodents.

SYMPTOMATOLOGY

The term *symptomatology* refers to the collection of signs and symptoms expressed by the host during the disease course. This is also known as the *clinical picture* or *disease presentation* and can be characteristic of any given infectious agent. In terms of pathophysiology, symptoms are the outward expression of the struggle between invading organisms and the retaliatory inflammatory and immune responses of the host. The symptoms of an infectious disease may be specific and reflect the site of infection (*e.g.,* diarrhea, rash, convulsions, hemorrhage, pneumonia). Conversely, symptoms such as fever, myalgia, headache, and lethargy are relatively nonspecific and can be shared by a number of diverse infectious diseases. The symptoms of a diseased host can be obvious, as in the cases of chickenpox or measles. Other covert symptoms, such as hepatitis or an increased white blood cell count, may require laboratory testing to detect. Accurate recognition and documentation of symptomatology can aid in the diagnosis of an infectious disease.

DISEASE COURSE

The course of any infectious disease can be divided into several distinguishable stages after the point of time in which the potential pathogen enters the host. These stages are the incubation period, the prodromal stage, the acute stage, the convalescent stage, and the resolution stage (Fig. 18-6). The stages are based on the progression and intensity of the host's symptoms over time. The duration of each phase and the pattern of the overall illness can be specific for different pathogens, thereby aiding in the diagnosis of an infectious disease.

The incubation period is the phase during which the pathogen begins active replication without producing recognizable symptoms in the host. The incubation period may be short, as in the case of salmonellosis (6 to 24 hours), or prolonged, such as that of hepatitis B (50 to 180 days) or HIV (months to years). The duration of the incubation period can be influenced by additional factors, including the general health of the host, the portal of entry, and the infectious dose of the pathogen.

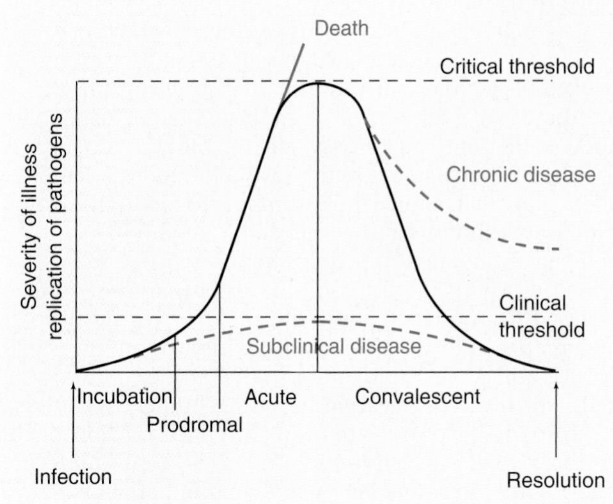

FIGURE 18-6 The stages of a primary infectious disease as they appear in relation to the severity of symptoms and the numbers of infectious agents. The clinical threshold corresponds with the initial expression of recognizable symptoms whereas the critical threshold represents the peak of disease intensity.

The hallmark of the *prodromal stage* is the initial appearance of symptoms in the host, although the clinical presentation during this time may be only a vague sense of malaise. The host may experience mild fever, myalgia, headache, and fatigue. These are constitutional changes shared by a great number of disease processes. The duration of the prodromal stage can vary considerably from host to host.

The *acute stage* is the period during which the host experiences the maximum impact of the infectious process corresponding to rapid proliferation and dissemination of the pathogen. During this phase, toxic byproducts of microbial metabolism, cell lysis, and the immune response mounted by the host combine to produce tissue damage and inflammation. The symptoms of the host are pronounced and more specific than in the prodromal stage, usually typifying the pathogen and sites of involvement.

The *convalescent period* is characterized by the containment of infection, progressive elimination of the pathogen, repair of damaged tissue, and resolution of associated symptoms. Similar to the incubation period, the time required for complete convalescence may be days, weeks, or months, depending on the type of pathogen and the voracity of the host's immune response. The *resolution* is the total elimination of a pathogen from the body without residual signs or symptoms of disease.

Several notable exceptions of the classic presentations of an infectious process have been recognized. Chronic infectious diseases have a markedly protracted and sometimes irregular course. The host may experience symptoms of the infectious process continuously or sporadically for months or years without a convalescent phase. In contrast, *subclinical* or *subacute illness* progresses from infection to resolution without clinically apparent symptoms. A disease is called *insidious* if the prodromal phase is protracted; a fulminant illness is characterized by abrupt onset of symptoms with little or no prodrome. Fatal infections are variants of the typical disease course.

SITE OF INFECTION

Inflammation of an anatomic location is usually designated by adding the suffix *-itis* to the name of the involved tissue (*e.g.,* bronchitis, infection of the bronchi and bronchioles; encephalitis, brain infection; carditis, infection of the heart). These are general terms, however, and they apply equally to inflammation from infectious and noninfectious causes. The suffix *-emia* is used to designate the presence of a substance in the blood; for example, *bacteremia, viremia,* and *fungemia* describe the presence of these infectious agents in the bloodstream. The term *sepsis,* or *septicemia,* refers to the presence of microbial toxins in the blood.

The site of an infectious disease is determined ultimately by the type of pathogen, the portal of entry, and the competence of the host's immunologic defense system. Many pathogenic microorganisms are restricted in their capacity to invade the human body. *Mycoplasma pneumoniae,* influenza viruses, and *Legionella pneumophila* rarely cause disease outside the respiratory tract; infections caused by *Neisseria gonorrhoeae* are generally confined to the genitourinary tract; and shigellosis and giardiasis seldom extend beyond the gastrointestinal tract. These are considered localized infectious diseases. The bacterium *Helicobacter pylori* is an extreme example of a site-specific pathogen. *H. pylori* is a significant cause of gastric ulcers and has not been implicated in disease processes elsewhere in the human body. Bacteria such as *Neisseria meningitidis*—a prominent pathogen of children and young adults; *Salmonella typhi*—the cause of typhoid fever; and *Borrelia burgdorferi*—the agent of Lyme disease, tend to disseminate from the primary site of infection to involve other locations and organ systems. These are examples of systemic pathogens. Most systemic infections disseminate throughout the body by way of the circulatory system.

An *abscess* is a localized pocket of infection composed of devitalized tissue, microorganisms, and the host's phagocytic white blood cells—in essence, a stalemate in the infectious process. In this case, the dissemination of the pathogen has been contained by the host, but white cell function within the toxic environment of the abscess is hampered, and the elimination of microorganisms is retarded. Abscesses usually must be surgically drained to effect a complete cure. Similarly, infections of biomedical implants such as catheters, artificial heart valves, and prosthetic bone implants are seldom cured by the host's immune response and antimicrobial therapy. The infecting organism colonizes the surface of the implant producing a dense matrix of cells, host proteins, and capsular material, called a *biofilm,* necessitating the removal of the device.

VIRULENCE FACTORS

Virulence factors are substances or products generated by infectious agents that enhance their ability to cause disease. Although the number and type of microbial products that fit this description are numerous, they can generally be grouped into four categories: toxins, adhesion factors, evasive factors, and invasive factors (Table 18-3).

Toxins

Toxins are substances that alter or destroy the normal function of the host or host's cells. Toxin production is a trait chiefly monopolized by bacterial pathogens, although certain fungal and protozoan pathogens also elaborate substances toxic to humans. Bacterial toxins have a diverse spectrum of activity and exert their effects on a wide variety of host target cells. For classification purposes, however, the bacterial toxins can be divided into two main types: *exotoxins* and *endotoxins.*

Exotoxins are proteins released from the bacterial cell during growth. Bacterial exotoxins enzymatically inactivate or modify key cellular constituents, leading to cell death or dysfunction. Diphtheria toxin, for example, inhibits cellular protein synthesis; botulism toxin decreases the release of neurotransmitter from cholinergic neurons, causing flaccid paralysis; tetanus toxin decreases the release of neurotransmitter from inhibitory neurons, producing spastic paralysis; and cholera toxin induces fluid secretion into the lumen of the intestine, causing diarrhea. Other examples of exotoxin-induced diseases include pertussis (whooping cough), anthrax, traveler's diarrhea, toxic shock syndrome, and a host of food-borne illnesses (*i.e.,* food poisoning).

Bacterial exotoxins that produce vomiting and diarrhea are sometimes referred to as *enterotoxins.* There has been a resurgent interest in streptococcal pyrogenic exotoxin A (SPEA), an exotoxin produced by certain strains of group A, beta-hemolytic streptococci (*Streptococcus pyogenes*) that causes a life-threatening toxic shock–like syndrome similar to the disease associated with tampon use produced by *Staphylococcus aureus.* The streptococcal form of intoxication is sometimes called Henson's disease because it was this infection that caused the death of the famous puppeteer Jim Henson. Other exotoxins that have gained notoriety include the Shiga toxins produced by *Escherichia coli* O157:H7 and other select strains. The ingestion of undercooked hamburger meat or unpasteurized fruit juices contaminated with this organism produces hemorrhagic colitis and a sometimes fatal illness called hemolytic-uremic syndrome (HUS), characterized by vascular endothelial damage, acute renal failure, and thrombocytopenia. HUS occurs primarily in infants and young children who have not developed antibodies to the Shiga toxins.

Endotoxins do not contain protein, are not actively released from the bacterium during growth, and have no enzymatic activity. Rather, endotoxins are complex molecules composed of lipid and polysaccharides found in the cell wall of gram-negative bacteria. Studies of different endotoxins have indicated that the lipid portion of the endotoxin confers the toxic properties to the molecule. Endotoxins are potent activators of a number of regulatory systems in humans. A small amount of endotoxin in the circulatory system (endotoxemia) can induce clotting, bleeding, inflammation, hypotension, and fever. The sum of the physiologic reactions to endotoxins is sometimes called *endotoxic shock.*

Adhesion Factors

No interaction between microorganisms and humans can progress to infection or disease if the pathogen is unable to attach to and colonize the host. The process of microbial attachment may be site specific (*e.g.,* mucous membranes, skin surfaces), cell specific (*e.g.,* T lymphocytes, respiratory epithelium), or nonspecific (*e.g.,* moist areas, charged surfaces). In any of these cases, adhesion requires a positive interaction between the surfaces of host cells and the infectious agent.

The site to which microorganisms adhere is called a *receptor,* and the reciprocal molecule or substance that binds to the receptor is called a *ligand* or *adhesin.* Receptors may

TABLE 18-3 Examples of Virulence Factors Produced by Pathogenic Microorganisms

Factor	Category	Organism	Effect on Host
Cholera toxin	Exotoxin	*Vibrio-cholerae* (bacterium)	Secretory diarrhea
Diphtheria toxin	Exotoxin	*Corynebacterium diphtheriae* (bacterium)	Inhibits protein synthesis
Lipopolysaccharide	Endotoxin	Many gram-negative bacteria	Fever, hypotension, shock
Toxic shock toxin	Enterotoxin	*Staphylococcus aureus* (bacterium)	Rash, diarrhea, vomiting, hepatitis
Hemagglutinin	Adherence	Influenza virus	Establishment of infection
Pili	Adherence	*Neisseria gonorrhoeae* (bacterium)	Establishment of infection
Leukocidin	Evasive	*S. aureus*	Kills phagocytes
IgA protease	Evasive	*Haemophilus influenzae* (bacterium)	Inactivates antibody
Capsule	Evasive	*Cryptococcus neoformans* (yeast)	Prevents phagocytosis
Collagenase	Invasive	*Pseudomonas aeruginosa* (bacterium)	Penetration of tissue
Protease	Invasive	*Aspergillus* (mold)	Penetration of tissue
Phospholipase	Invasive	*Clostridium perfringens* (bacterium)	Penetration of tissue
Botulinum toxin	Exotoxin	*Clostridium botulinum* (bacterium)	Neuroparalysis, inhibits acetylcholine release
Pneumolysin	Exotoxin	*Streptococcus pneumoniae*	Inhibition of respiratory ciliated and phagocytic cell function

be proteins, carbohydrates, lipids, or complex molecules composed of all three. Similarly, ligands may be simple or complex molecules and, in some cases, highly specific structures. Ligands that bind to specific carbohydrates are called *lectins*. Certain bacteria produce hairlike structures protruding from the cell surface called *pili* or *fimbriae,* which anchor the organism to receptors on host cell membranes to establish an infection. Many viral agents, including influenza, mumps, measles, and adenovirus, produce filamentous appendages or spikes called *hemagglutinins,* which recognize carbohydrate receptors on the surfaces of specific cells in the upper respiratory tract of the host.

After initial attachment, a number of bacterial agents become embedded in a gelatinous matrix of polysaccharides called a slime or mucous layer. The slime layer serves two purposes: it anchors the agent firmly to host tissue surfaces, and it protects the agent from the immunologic defenses of the host.

Evasive Factors

A number of factors produced by microorganisms enhance virulence by evading various components of the host's immune system. Extracellular polysaccharides, including capsules, slime, and mucous layers, discourage engulfment and killing of pathogens by the phagocytic white blood cells (*i.e.,* neutrophils and macrophages) of the host. Encapsulated organisms such as *Streptococcus agalactiae, Streptococcus pneumoniae, N. meningitidis,* and (before the vaccine) *H. influenza* type b are a cause of significant morbidity and mortality in neonates and children who lack protective anticapsular antibodies. Certain bacterial, fungal, and parasitic pathogens avoid phagocytosis by excreting leukocidin C toxins that deplete the host of neutrophils and macrophages by causing specific and lethal damage to the cytoplasmic membrane of white blood cells. Other pathogens, such as the bacterial agents of listeriosis and Legionnaires' disease, are adapted to survive and reproduce within phagocytic white blood cells after ingestion, avoiding or neutralizing the usually lethal products contained within the lysosomes of the cell.

Other unique strategies employed by pathogenic microbes to evade immunologic surveillance have evolved solely to avoid recognition by host antibodies. Strains of *S. aureus* produce a surface protein (protein A) that immobilizes immunoglobulin G (IgG), holding the antigen-binding region harmlessly away from the organisms. This pathogen also secretes a unique enzyme called coagulase. Coagulase converts soluble human coagulation factors into a solid clot, which envelops and protects the organism from phagocytic host cells and antibodies. *H. influenzae* and *N. gonorrhoeae* secrete enzymes that cleave and inactivate secretory immunoglobulin A, neutralizing the primary defense of the respiratory and genital tracts at the site of infection. *Helicobacter pylori,* the infectious cause of gastritis and gastric ulcers, produces a urease enzyme on its outer cell wall. The urease converts gastric urea into ammonia, thus neutralizing the acidic environment of the stomach and allowing the organism to survive in this hostile environment.

Borrelia species, including the agents of Lyme disease and relapsing fever, alter surface antigens during the disease course to avoid immunologic detection. It appears that the ingenuity to devise strategic defense systems and stealth technologies is not limited to humans. Viruses such as HIV impair the function of immunoregulatory cells. Although this property increases the virulence of these agents, it is not considered a virulence factor in the true sense of the definition.

Invasive Factors

Invasive factors are products produced by infectious agents that facilitate the penetration of anatomic barriers and host tissue. Most invasive factors are enzymes capable of destroying cellular membranes (*e.g.,* phospholipases), connective tissue (*e.g.,* elastases, collagenases), intercellular matrices (*e.g.,* hyaluronidase), and structural protein complexes (*e.g.,* proteases). It is the combined effects of invasive factors, toxins, and antimicrobial and inflammatory substances released by host cells to counter infection that mediate the tissue damage and pathophysiology of infectious diseases.

In summary, epidemiology is the study of factors, events, and circumstances that influence the transmission of disease. *Incidence* refers to the number of new cases of an infectious disease that occurs in a defined population, and *prevalence* to the number of active cases that are present at any given time. Infectious diseases are considered endemic in a geographic area if the incidence and prevalence are expected and relatively stable. An epidemic refers to an abrupt and unexpected increase in the incidence of a disease over endemic rates, and a pandemic to the spread of disease beyond continental boundaries.

The ultimate goal of epidemiology and epidemiologic studies is to devise strategies to interrupt or eliminate the spread of infectious disease. To accomplish this, infectious diseases are classified according to incidence, portal of entry, source, symptoms, disease course, site of infection, and virulence factors.

Diagnosis and Treatment of Infectious Diseases

After completing this section of the chapter, you should be able to meet the following objectives:

- State the two criteria used in the diagnosis of an infectious disease
- Explain the differences in culture, serology, and antigen, metabolite, or molecular detection methods for diagnosis of infectious disease
- Cite three general intervention methods that can be used in treatment of infectious illnesses
- State four basic mechanisms by which antibiotics exert their action
- Differentiate bactericidal from bacteriostatic

DIAGNOSIS

The diagnosis of an infectious disease requires two criteria: the recovery of a probable pathogen or evidence of its presence from the infected sites of a diseased host, and accurate documentation of clinical signs and symptoms (symptomatology) compatible with an infectious process. In the laboratory, the diagnosis of an infectious agent is accomplished using three basic techniques: culture, serology, or the detection of characteristic antigens, genomic sequences, or metabolites produced by the pathogen.

Culture refers to the propagation of a microorganism outside of the body, usually on or in artificial growth media such as agar plates or broth (Fig. 18-7). The specimen from the diseased host is inoculated into broth or onto the surface of an agar plate, and the culture is placed in a controlled environment such as an incubator until the growth of microorganisms becomes detectable. In the case of a bacterial pathogen, identification is based on microscopic appearance and Gram's stain reaction, shape, texture, and color (*i.e.*, morphology) of the colonies and by a panel of reactions that fingerprint salient biochemical characteristics of the organism. Certain bacteria, such as *Mycobacterium leprae,* the agent of leprosy, and *T. pallidum,* the syphilis spirochete, do not grow on artificial media and require additional methods of identification. Fungi and mycoplasmas are cultured in much the same way as bacteria but with more reliance on microscopic and colonial morphology for identification.

Chlamydiae, rickettsiae, and all human viruses are obligate intracellular pathogens. As a result, the propagation of these agents in the laboratory requires the inoculation of eukaryotic cells grown in culture (cell cultures). A cell culture consists of a flask containing a single layer, or monolayer, of eukaryotic cells covering the bottom and overlaid with broth containing essential nutrients and growth factors. When a virus infects and replicates within cultured eukaryotic cells, it produces pathologic changes in the appearance of the cell called *cytopathic effect* (CPE) (Fig. 18-8). The CPE can be detected microscopically, and the pattern and extent of cellular destruction are often characteristic of a particular virus.

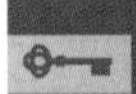

DIAGNOSIS AND TREATMENT OF INFECTIOUS DISEASES

- The definitive diagnosis of an infectious disease requires recovery and identification of the infecting organism by microscopic identification of the agent in stains of specimens or sections of tissue, culture isolation and identification of the agents, demonstration of antibody- or cell-mediated immune responses to an infectious agent, or DNA or RNA identification of infectious agents.
- Treatment of infectious disease is aimed at eliminating the infectious organism and promoting recovery of the infected person. Treatment is provided through the use of antimicrobial agents, immunotherapy, and, when necessary, surgical interventions.
- Prevention of infectious disease is accomplished through the use of immunization methods.

Although culture media have been developed for the growth of certain human protozoa and helminths in the

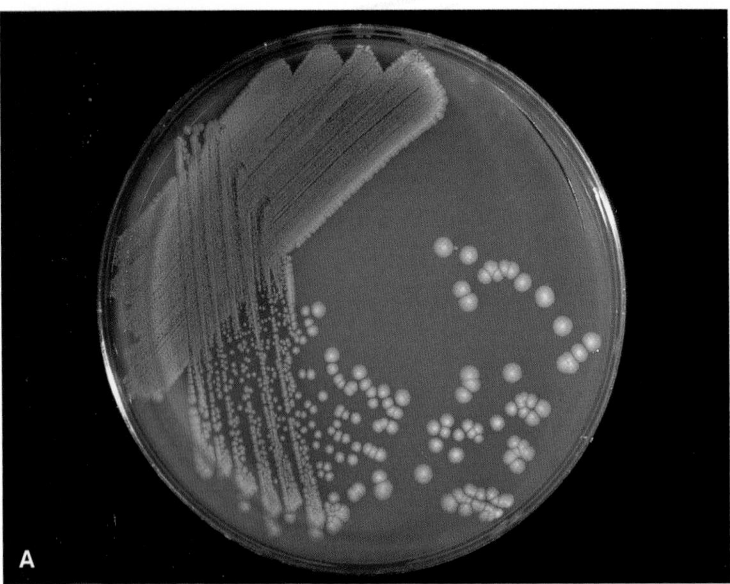

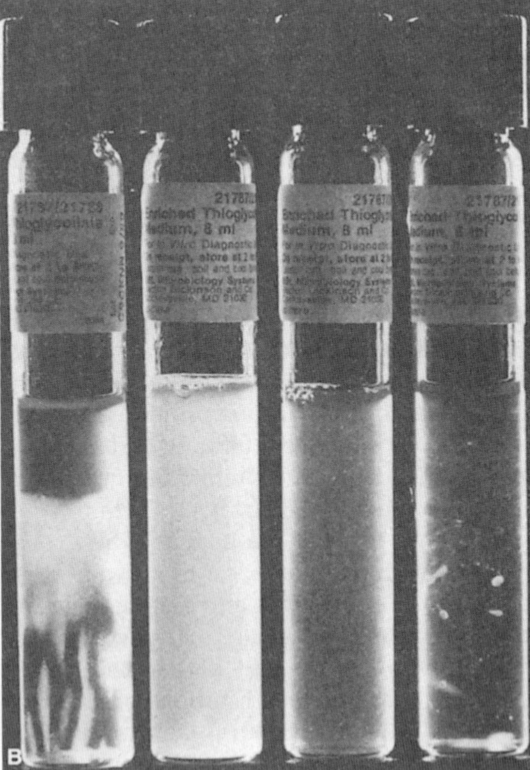

FIGURE 18-7 Variability of the macroscopic appearance of bacterial cultured on solid, agar-containing medium (**A**) and liquid broth medium (**B**). On solid surfaces, bacteria form distinct colonies as demonstrated by the β-hemolytic streptococcus (*Streptococcus pyogenes*) on sheep blood agar (**A**). Bacteria cultured in broth form a variety of growth patterns, ranging from particulate to homogenous, turbid suspensions. Anaerobic bacteria cultured in liquid medium tend to grow best at the bottom of the tube, where the concentration of molecular oxygen is lowest. (**A,** © Science Source/Photo Researchers)

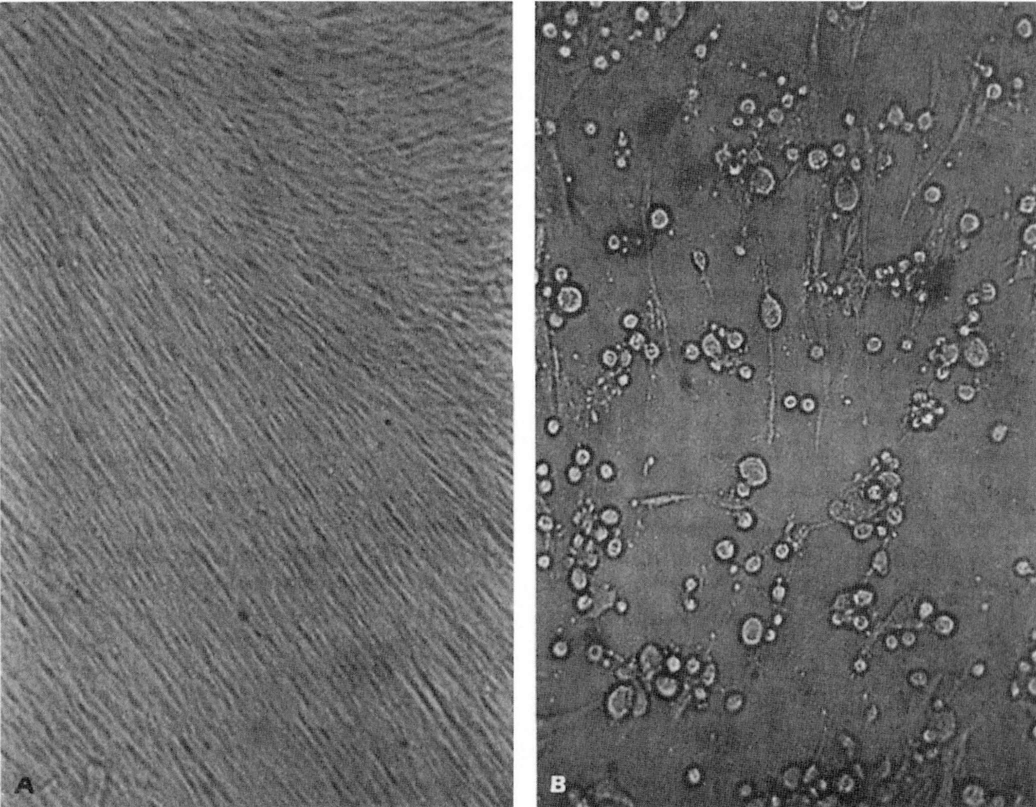

FIGURE 18-8 The microscopic appearance of a monolayer of uninfected human fibroblasts grown in cell culture (**A**) and the same cells after infection with herpes simplex virus (**B**), demonstrating the cytopathic effect caused by viral replication and concomitant cell lysis.

laboratory, the diagnosis of parasitic infectious diseases has traditionally relied on microscopic, or in the case of worms, visible identification of organisms, cysts, or ova directly from infected patient specimens.

Serology, literally the study of serum, is an indirect means of identifying infectious agents by measuring serum antibodies in the diseased host. A tentative diagnosis can be made if the antibody level, also called *antibody titer,* against a specific pathogen rises during the acute phase of the disease and falls during convalescence. Serologic identification of an infectious agent is not as accurate as culture, but it may be a useful adjunct, especially for the diagnosis of diseases caused by pathogens such as the hepatitis B virus that cannot be cultured. The measurement of antibody titers has another advantage in that specific antibody types, such as IgM and IgG, are produced by the host during different phases of an infectious process. IgM-specific antibodies generally rise and fall during the acute phase of the disease, whereas the synthesis of the IgG class of antibodies increases during the acute phase and remains elevated until or beyond resolution. Measurements of class-specific antibodies are also useful in the diagnosis of congenital infections. IgM antibodies do not cross the placenta, but certain IgG antibodies are transferred passively from mother to child during the final trimester of gestation. Consequently, an elevation of pathogen-specific IgM antibodies found in the serum of a neonate must have originated from the child and therefore indicates congenital infection. A similarly increased IgG titer in the neonate does not differentiate congenital from maternal infection.

The technology of *direct antigen detection* has evolved rapidly over the past decade and in the process has revolutionized the diagnosis of certain infectious diseases. Antigen detection incorporates features of culture and serology but reduces by a fraction the time required for diagnosis. In principle, this method relies on purified antibodies to detect antigens of infectious agents in specimens obtained from the diseased host. The source of antibodies used for antigen detection can be animals immunized against a particular pathogen or *hybridomas.* Hybridomas are created by fusing normal antibody-producing spleen cells from an immunized animal with malignant myeloma cells, which synthesize large quantities of antibody. The result is a cell that produces an antibody called a *monoclonal antibody,* which is highly specific for a single antigen and a single pathogen. Regardless of the source, the antibodies are labeled with a substance that allows microscopic or overt detection when bound to the pathogen or its products. Generally, the three types of labels used for this purpose are fluorescent dyes, enzymes, and particles such as latex beads. Fluorescent antibodies allow visualization of an infectious agent with the aid of a fluorescent microscope. Depending on the type of fluorescent dye used, the organism may appear a bright green or orange color against a black background, making detection extremely easy. Enzyme-labeled antibodies function in a similar manner. The enzyme is capable of converting a colorless compound into a colored substance, thereby permitting detection of antibody bound to an infectious agent without the use of a fluorescent microscope. Particles coated with antibodies clump together, or agglutinate, when the appropriate antigen is present in a specimen. Particle agglutination is especially useful when examining infected body fluids such as urine, serum, or spinal fluid.

The identification of infectious agents through the detection of DNA or RNA sequences unique to a single agent has undergone rapid development and use during the past few years. Several techniques have been devised to accomplish this goal, each having different degrees of sensitivity regarding the number of organisms that need to be present in a specimen for detection. The first of these methods is called *DNA probe hybridization*. Small fragments of DNA are cut from the genome of a specific pathogen and labeled with compounds (photo-emitting chemicals or antigens) that allow detection. The labeled DNA probes are added to specimens from an infected host. If the pathogen is present, the probe attaches to the complementary strand of DNA on the genome of the infectious agent, permitting rapid diagnosis. The use of labeled probes has allowed visualization of particular agents within and around individual cells in histologic sections of tissue.

A second and more sensitive method of DNA detection to be developed is called the *polymerase chain reaction* (PCR) (Fig. 18-9). This method incorporates two unique reagents: a specific pair of oligonucleotides (usually more than 25 nucleotides long) called *primers* and a heat-stable DNA polymerase. To perform the assay, the primers are added to the specimen containing the suspect pathogen, and the sample is heated to melt the DNA in the specimen and then allowed to cool. The primers locate and bind only to the complementary target DNA of the pathogen in question. The heat-stable polymerase begins to replicate the DNA from the point at which the primers attached, similar to two trains approaching one another on separate but converging tracks. After the initial cycle, DNA polymerization ceases at the point where the primers were located, producing a strand of DNA with a distinct size, depending on the distance separating the two primers. The specimen is heated again, and the process starts anew. After many cycles of heating, cooling, and polymerization, a large number of uniformly sized DNA fragments are produced only if the specific pathogen (or its DNA) is present in the specimen. The polymerized DNA fragments are separated by electrophoresis and visualized with a dye or identification by hybridization by a specific probe.

PCR is an extremely useful and powerful tool. In some circumstances, this method can detect as little as one virus or bacterium in a single specimen. This method also allows for the diagnosis of infections caused by microorganisms that are impossible or difficult to grow in culture.

Several variations of molecular gene detection techniques in addition to PCR have been developed and incorporated into diagnostic kits for use in the clinical laboratory, including ligase chain reaction (LCR), transcription-mediated amplification (TMA), strand displacement amplification, branched chain DNA signal amplification (bDNA), and hybrid capture assays. Many of the newer gene detection technologies have been adapted for quantitation of the target DNA or RNA in patient specimens, such as HIV and hepatitis C virus in serum or plasma of the infected patient. If the therapy is effective, viral replication is suppressed, and the viral load (level of viral genome) in the peripheral blood is low. Conversely, if mutations in the viral genome lead to resistant strains or if the antiviral therapy is ineffective, viral replication and the patient's viral load rise, indicating a need to change the therapeutic approach.

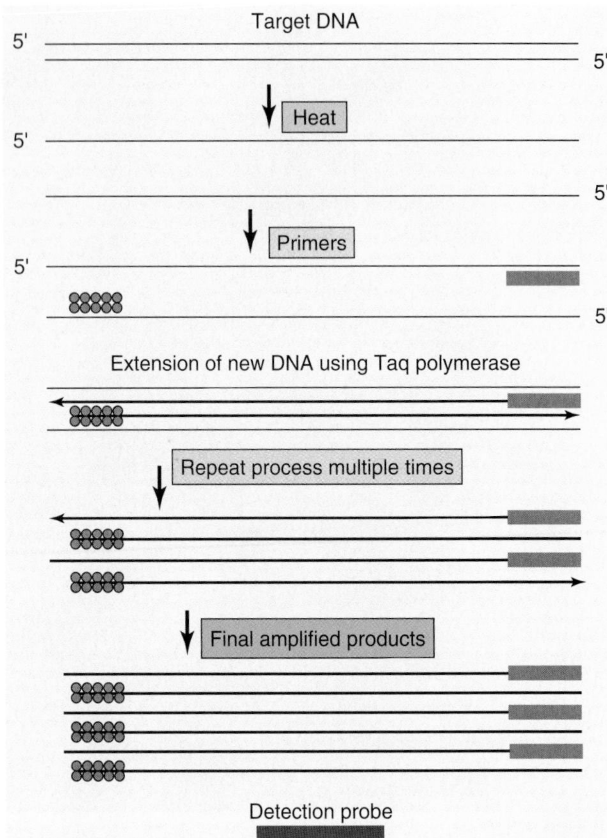

FIGURE 18-9 The polymerase chain reaction is depicted. The target DNA is first melted using heat (generally around 94°C) to separate the strands of DNA. Primers that recognize specific sequences within the target DNA are allowed to bind as the reaction cools. Using a unique, thermostable DNA polymerase called Taq and an abundance of deoxynucleoside triphosphates, new DNA strands are amplified from the point of the primer attachment. The process is repeated many times (called cycles) until millions of copies of DNA are produced, all of which have the same length defined by the distance (in base pairs) between the primer binding sites. These copies are then detected by electrophoresis and staining or through the use of labeled DNA probes that, similar to the primers, recognize a specific sequence located within the amplified section of DNA.

TREATMENT

The goal of treatment for an infectious disease is complete removal of the pathogen from the host and the restoration of normal physiologic function to damaged tissues. Most infectious diseases of humans are self-limiting in that they require little or no medical therapy for a complete cure. When an infectious process gains the upper hand and therapeutic intervention is essential, the choice of treatment may be medicinal through the use of antimicrobial agents; immunologic with antibody preparations, vaccines, or substances that stimulate and improve the host's immune function; or surgical by removing infected tissues. The decision of which therapeutic modality or combination of therapies to use is based on the extent, urgency, and location of the disease process, the pathogen, and the availability of effective antimicrobial agents.

Antimicrobial Agents

The use of chemicals, potions, and elixirs in the treatment of infectious diseases dates back to the earliest records of human medicine. More than 2000 years ago, Greek and Chinese physicians recognized that certain substances were useful for preventing or curing wound infections. Although the biologic activity of these compounds was not understood, some may have inadvertently contained byproducts of molds that resemble modern antibiotics. From that time until the late 1800s, when the relation between infection and microorganisms was finally accepted, the evolution of antiinfective therapy was less than explosive. It was not until the advent of World War II, after the introduction of sulfonamides and penicillin, that the development of antimicrobial compounds matured into a science of great consequence. Today, the comprehensive list of effective antiinfective agents is burgeoning. Most antimicrobial compounds can be categorized roughly according to mechanism of antiinfective activity, chemical structure, and target pathogen (*e.g.*, antibacterial, antiviral, antifungal, or antiparasitic agents).

Antibacterial Agents. Antibacterial agents are generally called antibiotics. Most antibiotics are actually produced by other microorganisms, primarily bacteria and fungi, as byproducts of metabolism and usually are only effective against other prokaryotic organisms. An antibiotic is considered *bactericidal* if it causes irreversible and lethal damage to the bacterial pathogen and *bacteriostatic* if its inhibitory effects on bacterial growth are reversed when the agent is eliminated. Antibiotics can be classified into families of compounds with related chemical structure and activity (Table 18-4).

Not all antibiotics are effective against all pathogenic bacteria. Some agents are only effective against gram-negative bacteria, and others are specific for gram-positive organisms. The so-called broad-spectrum antibiotics, such as the newest class of cephalosporin, are active against a wide variety of gram-positive and gram-negative bacteria. Members of the *Mycobacterium* genus, including *Mycobacterium tuberculosis,* are extremely resistant to the effects of the major classes of antibiotics and require an entirely different spectrum of agents for therapy. The four basic mechanisms of the antibiotic action are interference with a

TABLE 18-4 Classification and Activity of Antibacterial Agents (Antibiotics)

Family	Example	Target Site	Side Effects
Penicillins	Ampicillin	Cell wall	Allergic reactions
Cephalosporins	Cephalexin	Cell wall	Allergic reactions
Monobactams	Aztreonam	Cell wall	Rash
Aminoglycosides	Tobramycin	Ribosomes (protein synthesis)	Hearing loss Nephrotoxicity
Tetracyclines	Doxycycline	Ribosomes (protein synthesis)	Gastrointestinal irritation Allergic reactions Teeth and bone dysplasia
Macrolides	Clindamycin	Ribosomes (protein synthesis)	Colitis Allergic reactions
Sulfonamides	Sulfadiazine	Folic acid synthesis	Allergic reactions Anemia Gastrointestinal irritation
Glycopeptides	Vancomycin	Ribosomes (protein synthesis)	Allergic reactions Hearing loss Nephrotoxicity
Quinolones	Ciprofloxacin	DNA synthesis	Gastrointestinal irritation
Miscellaneous	Chloramphenicol Rifampin Trimethoprim	Ribosomes (protein synthesis) Ribosomes (protein synthesis) Folic acid synthesis	Anemia Hepatotoxicity Allergic reactions Same as sulfonamides
Oxazolidinone	Linezolid	Ribosomes (protein synthesis)	Diarrhea, thrombocytopenia
Carbapenem	Imipenem	Cell wall	Nausea, diarrhea
Streptogramin	Quinupristin/dalfopristin	Ribosomes (protein synthesis)	Muscle and joint aches

specific step in bacterial cell wall synthesis (*e.g.*, penicillins, cephalosporins, glycopeptides, monobactams, carbapenems); inhibition of bacterial protein synthesis (*e.g.*, aminoglycosides, macrolides, ketolides, tetracyclines, chloramphenicol, oxazolidinones, streptogramins, and rifampin); interruption of nucleic acid synthesis (*e.g.*, fluoroquinolones, nalidixic acid); and interference with normal metabolism (*e.g.*, sulfonamides, trimethoprim).

Despite lack of antibiotic activity against eukaryotic cells, many agents can cause unwanted or toxic side effects in humans, including allergic responses (penicillins, cephalosporins, sulfonamides, glycopeptides), hearing and kidney impairment (aminoglycosides), and liver or bone marrow toxicity (chloramphenicol, fluoroquinolones). Of greater concern is the increasing prevalence of bacteria resistant to the effects of antibiotics. The ways in which bacteria acquire resistance to antibiotics are becoming as numerous as the number of antibiotics. Bacterial resistance mechanisms include the production of enzymes that inactivate antibiotics such as β-lactamases, genetic mutations that alter antibiotic binding sites, alternative metabolic pathways that bypass antibiotic activity, and changes in the filtration qualities of the bacterial cell wall that prevent access of antibiotics to the target site within the organism. It is the continuous search for a better mousetrap that makes antiinfective therapy such a fascinating aspect of infectious diseases.

Antiviral Agents. Until recently, few effective antiviral agents were available for treating human infections. The reason for this is host toxicity; viral replication requires the use of eukaryotic host cell enzymes, and the drugs that effectively interrupt viral replication are likely to interfere with host cell reproduction as well. However, in response to the AIDS epidemic, there has been massive, albeit delayed, development of antiretroviral agents. Almost all antiviral compounds are synthetic, and with few exceptions, the primary target of antiviral compounds is viral RNA or DNA synthesis. Agents such as acyclovir, ganciclovir, vidarabine, and ribavirin mimic the nucleoside building blocks of RNA and DNA. During active viral replication, the nucleoside analogs inhibit the viral DNA polymerase, preventing duplication of the viral genome and spread of infectious viral progeny to other susceptible host cells. Similar to the specificity of antibiotics, antiviral agents may be active against RNA viruses only, DNA viruses only, or occasionally both. Other nucleoside analogs such as zidovudine, lamivudine, didanosine, stavudine, and zalcitabine and nonnucleoside inhibitors including nevirapine, efavirenz, and delavirdine were developed specifically for the treatment of AIDS by targeting the HIV-specific enzyme, reverse transcriptase, for inhibition. This key enzyme is essential for viral replication and has no counterpart in the infected eukaryotic host cells.

Another class of antiviral agents, developed solely for the treatment of HIV infections, is called *protease inhibitors* (*e.g.*, indinavir, ritonavir, and saquinavir). These drugs inhibit an HIV-specific enzyme that is necessary for late maturation events in the virus life cycle.

Experimental approaches to antiviral therapy include compounds that inhibit viral attachment to susceptible host cells, drugs that prevent uncoating of the viral genome once inside the host cell, and agents that directly inhibit viral DNA polymerase like foscarnet. An example of drugs that prevent attachment is enfuvirtide—a peptide that binds to the docking glycopeptide (gp41) of HIV-1 and prevents its binding and fusion to the target CD4 lymphocytes (see Chapter 22). Recently, a new class of antiviral agents has been developed and released that specifically inhibits influenza virus neuraminidase B, which is an essential enzyme for viral replication. Two agents within this class, zanamivir and oseltamivir, have been approved for treatment of both influenza A and B.

Although the treatment of viral infections with antimicrobial agents is a relatively recent endeavor, reports of viral mutations resulting in resistant strains have become increasingly more common. This is especially troubling in the case of HIV, in which resistance to relatively new antiviral agents, including nucleoside analogs and protease inhibitors, has already been described, prompting the need for combination or alternating therapy with multiple antiretroviral agents.

Antifungal Agents. The target site of the two most important families of antifungal agents is the cytoplasmic membrane of yeasts or molds. Fungal membranes differ from human cell membranes in that they contain the sterol ergosterol instead of cholesterol. The polyene family of antifungal compounds (*e.g.*, amphotericin B, nystatin) preferentially bind to ergosterol and form holes in the cytoplasmic membrane, causing leakage of the fungal cell contents and, eventually, lysis of the cell. The imidazole class of drugs (*e.g.*, fluconazole, itraconazole, voriconazole) inhibits the synthesis of ergosterol, thereby damaging the integrity of the fungal cytoplasmic membrane. Both types of drugs bind to a certain extent to the cholesterol component of host cell membranes and elicit a variety of toxic side effects in treated patients. The nucleoside analog 5-fluorocytosine (5-FC) disrupts fungal RNA and DNA synthesis but without the toxicity associated with the polyene and imidazole drugs. Unfortunately, 5-FC demonstrates little or no antifungal activity against molds or dimorphic fungi and is primarily reserved for infections caused by yeasts.

A novel class of antifungal compounds called *echinocandins* has received considerable attention because these drugs inhibit the synthesis of β-1,3-glucan, a major cell wall polysaccharide that is found in fungi, including *Candida albicans*, *Aspergillus* species, and *Pneumocystis carinii*. *Caspofungin* is the first of these inhibitors to be available for treatment of patients with candidiasis or invasive aspergillosis that is refractory to treatment with other antifungal agents.

Antiparasitic Agents. Because of the extreme diversity of human parasites and their growth cycles, a review of antiparasitic therapies and agents would be highly impractical and lengthy. Similar to other infectious diseases caused by eukaryotic microorganisms, treatment of parasitic illnesses is based on exploiting essential components of the parasite's metabolism or cellular anatomy that are not shared by the host. Any relatedness between the target site of the parasite and the cells of the host increases the likelihood of toxic reactions in the host.

Continued development of improved antiparasitic agents suffers greatly from economic considerations. Parasitic diseases of humans are primarily the scourge of poor, developing nations of the world. As a result, financial incentives to produce more effective therapies are nonexistent. Resistance among human parasites to standard, effective therapy is also a major concern. In Africa, Asia, and South America, the incidence of chloroquine-resistant malaria (*Plasmodium falciparum*) is on the rise. Resistant strains require more complicated, expensive, and potentially toxic therapy with a combination of agents.

Immunotherapy

An exciting approach to the treatment of infectious diseases is immunotherapy. This strategy involves supplementing or stimulating the host's immune response so that the spread of a pathogen is limited or reversed. Several products are available for this purpose, including intravenous immune globulin (IVIG) and cytokines. IVIG is a pooled preparation of antibodies obtained from normal, healthy immune human donors that is infused as an intravenous solution. In theory, pathogen-specific antibodies present in the infusion facilitate neutralization, phagocytosis, and clearance of infectious agents above and beyond the capabilities of the diseased host. Hyperimmune immunoglobulin preparations, which are also commercially available, contain high titers of antibodies against specific pathogens, including hepatitis B virus, cytomegalovirus, rabies, and varicella-zoster virus.

Cytokines are substances produced by human white blood cells that, in small quantities, stimulate white cell replication, phagocytosis, antibody production, and the induction of fever, inflammation, and tissue repair—all of which counteract infectious agents and hasten recovery. With the advent of genetic engineering and cloning, many cytokines, including interferons and interleukins, have been produced in the laboratory and are being evaluated experimentally as antiinfective agents. As we learn more about the action of cytokines, we are beginning to appreciate that some of the adverse reactions associated with infectious processes result from our own inflammatory response. Interventional therapies designed to inactivate certain cytokines, such as tumor necrosis factor, have proved to be helpful in animal models of infection. It is not unlikely that therapies based on the regulation of the inflammatory response will become widely used in human medicine over the next few years.

One of the most efficient but often overlooked means of preventing infectious diseases is immunization. Proper and timely adherence to recommended vaccination schedules in children and boosters in adults effectively reduces the senseless spread of vaccine-preventable illnesses such as measles, mumps, pertussis, and rubella, which still occur in the United States with alarming frequency. New strategies for the development of vaccines carried by harmless viral vectors are currently being developed that, someday, might lead to inexpensive and effective oral immunization against HIV, hepatitis C, malaria, and other potentially lethal infectious diseases.

Surgical Intervention

Before the discovery of antimicrobial agents, surgical removal of infected tissues, organs, or limbs was occasionally the only option available to prevent the demise of the infected host. Today, medicinal therapy with antibiotics and other antiinfective agents is an effective solution for most infectious diseases. However, surgical intervention is still an important option for cases in which the pathogen is resistant to available treatments. Surgical interventions may be used to hasten the recovery process by providing access to an infected site by antimicrobial agents (drainage of an abscess), cleaning of the site (débridement), or removing infected organs or tissue (*e.g.*, appendectomy). In some situations, surgery may be the only means of effecting a complete cure, as in the case of endocarditis most commonly affecting infected heart valves, in which the diseased valve must be replaced with a mechanical or biologic valve to restore normal function. In other situations, surgical containment of a rapidly progressing infectious process such as gas gangrene may be the only means of saving a person's life.

In summary, the ultimate outcome of any interaction between microorganisms and the human host is decided by a complex and ever-changing set of variables that take into account the overall health and physiologic function of the host and the virulence and infectious dose of the microbe. In many instances, disease is an inevitable consequence, but with continued advancement of science and technology, the vast number of cases can be eliminated or rapidly cured with appropriate therapy. It is the intent of those who study infectious diseases to understand thoroughly the pathogen, the disease course, the mechanisms of transmission, and the host response to infection. This knowledge will lead to development of improved diagnostic techniques, revolutionary approaches to antiinfective therapy, and eradication or control of microscopic agents that cause frightening devastation and loss of life throughout the world.

Bioterrorism and Emerging Global Infectious Diseases

After completing this section of the chapter, you should be able to meet the following objectives:

- List the infectious agents considered to be in the highest level of bioterrorism threat
- Describe the effect of international travel on the spread of infection
- State an important concept in containment of infections due to bioterrorism and global travel

BIOTERRORISM

In October of 2001, less than 1 month after the tragedy of September 11, the world became instantly acquainted with the term *bioterrorism*. By the end of November of that year,

22 cases of human anthrax (11 cutaneous and 11 inhalation) had been identified, resulting in five deaths, and all cases were associated with exposure to four intentionally contaminated envelopes delivered through the U.S. Postal Service. Although the possibility of such an attack had been discussed in a workshop hosted by the Centers for Disease Control and Prevention (CDC) 3 years earlier, the reality of the 2001 outbreak brought a new sense of awareness concerning the use of microorganisms as weapons.

Anthrax is an ancient disease caused by the cutaneous inoculation, inhalation, or ingestion of the spores of *Bacillus anthracis*—gram-positive bacilli. Anthrax is more commonly known as a disease of herbivores that can be transmitted to humans through contact with infected secretions, soil, or animal products. It is a rare disease in the United States; thus, the sudden increase in cases over a short period of time was a chilling indication that the spread of the organism had been intentional. Fortunately, the number of deaths was limited thanks to prompt recognition of cases by private physicians and public health personnel and rapid institution of antimicrobial prophylaxis to exposed individuals.

To prepare for the possibility of secondary bioterrorist attacks, the CDC along with other federal, state, and local agencies, has created the laboratory response network (LRN). The LRN is a four-tiered structure (A through D) consisting of laboratories with ever-increasing expertise, responsibility, and biocontainment facilities allowing for the rapid and coordinated detection and identification of bioterrorism events under safe working conditions. Further, potential agents of bioterrorism have been categorized into three levels (A, B, C) based on risk of use, transmissibility, invasiveness, and rate of mortality. The agents considered to be in the highest biothreat level include *B. anthracis, Yersinia pestis* (the cause of plague), *Francisella tularensis* (the cause of tularemia), smallpox (variola major virus), and several hemorrhagic fever viruses (Ebola, Marburg, Lassa, and Junin). The toxin of the anaerobic gram-positive organism *Clostridium botulinum* that causes neuromuscular paralysis termed *botulism* is also listed as a category A agent. Interestingly, purified *C. botulinum* toxins A and B are finding increasing use under the trade names of Botox, Myobloc, and Neurobloc for various medicinal and cosmetic purposes. The category B agents include agents of food-borne and water-borne disease (*Salmonella and Shigella* species, *Vibrio cholera, Escherichia coli* O157:H7), agents of zoonotic infections (*Brucella* species, *Coxiella burnetii, Burkholderia mallei*), viral encephalitides (Venezuelan, Western, and Eastern equine encephalitis viruses), as well as toxins from *Staphylococcus aureus, Clostridium perfringens,* and *Ricinus communis* (the castor bean). Category C agents are defined as emerging pathogens and potential risks for the future even though many of these organisms are causes of ancient diseases. Category C agents include *Mycobacterium tuberculosis,* Nipah virus, Hantavirus, tick-borne and yellow fever viruses, and the only protozoan of the group, *Cryptosporidium parvum.* An excellent website is available through the CDC entitled the "CDC Public Health Emergency Preparedness & Response Site" that provides detailed information on agents of bioterrorism, emergency contacts, and contingency plans in the event of an outbreak (www.bt.cdc.gov).

The potential for bioterrorism using smallpox virus pilfered from frozen stocks maintained in unsecured laboratory facilities has reinvigorated a national vaccination program in the United States that ended with the last reported human case of smallpox in 1978. Because the availability of smallpox vaccine is limited, a tiered approach to vaccination has been undertaken to protect individuals most likely to encounter sentinel cases of the disease should an outbreak occur (*e.g.,* emergency room personnel, infectious disease physicians, laboratory personnel, and public health workers). Efforts are also underway to engineer and rapidly manufacture a safer form of the vaccine so as to avoid the side effects associated with the older vaccinia virus vaccine.

EMERGING GLOBAL INFECTIOUS DISEASES

Aided by a global market and the ease of international travel, the past 5 years has witnessed the importation and emergence of a host of novel infectious diseases. During the late summer and early fall of 1999, West Nile virus (WNV, an arthropod-borne *Flavivirus*) was identified as the cause of an epidemic involving 56 patients in the New York City area. This outbreak, which led to seven deaths (primarily in elderly people), marked the first time that WNV had been recognized in the Western Hemisphere since its discovery in Uganda nearly 60 years earlier. Because WNV is a mosquito-borne disease and is transmitted to a number of susceptible avian (*e.g.,* blue jays, crows, and hawks) and equine hosts, the potential for rapid and sustained spread of the disease across the United States was appreciated early on. By the fall of 2002, a national surveillance network had detected WNV activity in 2289 counties from 44 states including Los Angeles County, California and had identified more than 3000 human cases. The disease ranges in intensity from nonspecific febrile illness to fulminate meningoencephalitis. In 2002 alone, 3389 cases of WNV-associated illness were identified in the United States with 201 deaths, making this the largest arboviral meningoencephalitis outbreak ever described in the Western Hemisphere. Efforts to prevent further spread of the disease are currently centered on surveillance of WNV-associated illness in birds, humans, and other mammals as well as mosquito control.

In the winter of 2003, the Ministry of Health of China reported 305 cases of a mysterious and virulent respiratory tract illness that had recently appeared in Guangdong province in Southern China over the previous 4 months. The illness was highly transmissible as evidenced by the spread of the disease to household contacts of sick individuals and medical personnel caring for patients with the disease. In a very short period of time, patients with compatible symptoms were recognized in Hong Kong and Vietnam. The illness was called *severe acute respiratory syndrome* (SARS), and the World Health Organization (WHO) promptly issued a global alert and started international surveillance for patients with typical symptomatology with a history of travel to the endemic region. As of June 2003, more than 8000 cases of SARS from 29 countries and 809 deaths were reported to WHO. In a remarkable feat of molecular technology, the etiology of SARS was quickly determined to be a novel coronavirus possibly of mammal or avian origin, and its entire genome was sequenced by the end of May 2003. Because of the intense effort by WHO in conjunction with international health agencies, the SARS epidemic was held in check (temporary or permanent) through the use of intense infection control strategies, and by the summer of 2003, most travel restrictions to countries with high levels of endemic disease were lifted.

In May 2003, a child was seen in central Wisconsin for fever, lymphadenopathy, and a papular rash. Electron microscopic examination of tissue from one of the patient's skin lesions revealed a virus that morphologically resembled poxvirus, obviously generating some concern because of the awareness of the potential for bioterrorism using smallpox virus. However, the same virus was identified from a lymph node biopsy of the patient's ill pet prairie dog. Additional testing of the patient and the prairie dog specimens indicated that the virus was a monkeypox virus, one of the orthopoxvirus family of viruses. By the beginning of June, 53 possible cases of monkeypox infection were being followed in Wisconsin, Illinois, and Indiana. Epidemiologic investigations conducted by state and federal health care agencies identified the potential source of the virus as nine different species of small mammals, including Gambian giant rats that had been imported from Ghana in April and were housed in common facilities with prairie dogs. A number of these animals were then shipped to a pet distributor in Illinois and subsequently sold to the public.

These three scenarios highlight the rapidity with which novel or exotic diseases can be introduced into nonindigenous regions of the world and to a susceptible population. Although great strides in molecular microbiology have allowed for the rapid identification of new or rare microorganisms, the potential devastation in terms of human life and economic loss is great, underscoring the need to maintain resources for public health surveillance and intervention. To gain more detail in these intriguing cases of infectious detective work, please refer to these excellent websites: www.who.int/en/, www.cdc.gov/mmwr/week/cvol.html, www.cdc.gov/eid.

In summary, the ultimate outcome of any interaction between microorganisms and the human host is decided by a complex and ever-changing set of variables that take into account the overall health and physiologic function of the host and the virulence and infectious dose of the microbe. In many instances, disease is an inevitable consequence, but with continued advancement of science and technology, the vast number of cases can be eliminated or rapidly cured with appropriate therapy. It is the intent of those who study infectious diseases to understand thoroughly the pathogen, the disease course, the mechanisms of transmission, and the host response to infection. This knowledge will lead to development of improved diagnostic techniques, revolutionary approaches to antiinfective therapy, and eradication or control of microscopic agents that cause frightening devastation and loss of life throughout the world.

REVIEW EXERCISES

Newborn infants who have not yet developed an intestinal flora are routinely given an intramuscular injection of vitamin K to prevent bleeding due to a deficiency in vitamin K–dependent coagulation factors.

A. Use the concept of mutalism to explain why.

Microorganisms are only capable of causing infection if they can grow at the temperature of the infected body site.

A. Using this concept, explain the different sites of fungal infections due to the dermatophyte fungal species that causes tinea pedis (athlete's foot) and *Candida albicans,* which causes infections of the mouth (thrush) and female genitalia (vulvovaginitis).

Given the ever-growing threat of global infectious diseases, such as severe acute respiratory syndrome (SARS):

A. What is one of the most important functions of health care professionals in terms of controlling the spread of such infections?

Bibliography

Bush K., Jacoby G.A., Medeiros A.A. (1995). A functional classification scheme for β-lactamases and its correlation with molecular structure. *Antimicrobial Agents and Chemotherapy 39,* 1211–1233.

Butler J.C., Peters C.J. (1994). Hantaviruses and hantavirus pulmonary syndrome. *Clinical Infectious Diseases 19,* 387–395.

Carpenter C.C.J., Fischl M.A., Hammer S.M., et al. (1996). Antiviral therapy for HIV infection in 1996. *Journal of the American Medical Association 276,* 146–154.

Centers for Disease Control and Prevention. (1999). Outbreak of West Nile-like viral encephalitis. *Morbidity and Mortality Weekly Report 48,* 845–849.

CDC. (1999). Outbreak of West Nile-like viral encephalitis—New York, 1999. *Morbidity and Mortality Weekly Report 48,* 845–849.

CDC. (2002). Provisional surveillance summary of the West Nile Virus epidemic—United States, January–November 2002. *Morbidity and Mortality Weekly Report 51,* 1129–1133.

CDC. (2003). Update: Severe acute respiratory syndrome—worldwide and United States, 2003. *Morbidity and Mortality Weekly Report 52,* 664–665.

CDC. (2003). Multistate outbreak of monkeypox—Illinois, Indiana, and Wisconsin, 2003. *Morbidity and Mortality Weekly Report 52,* 537–540.

Dumler J.S., Bakken J.S. (1995). Ehrlichial diseases in humans: Emerging tick-borne infections. *Clinical Infectious Diseases 20,* 1102–1110.

Dunne W.M., Jr. (2002). "Bacterial adhesion: Seen any good biofilms lately?" *Clinical Microbiology Review 15,* 155–166.

Gold H.S., Moellering R.C., Jr. (1996). Drug resistance: Antimicrobial-drug resistance. *New England Journal of Medicine 335,* 1445–1453.

Jacobsen H., Hanggi M., Ott M., et al. (1996). In vivo resistance to a human immunodeficiency virus type 1 proteinase inhibitor: Mutations, kinetics, and frequencies. *Journal of Infectious Diseases 173,* 1379–1387.

Jernigan D.M., Raghunathan P.L., Bell B.P., et al. (2001). Investigation of bioterrorism-related anthrax, United States, 2001: Epidemiologic findings. *Emerg Infect Dis 8,* 1019–1028.

Krogfelt K.A. (1991). Bacterial adhesion: Genetics, biogenetics, and role in pathogenesis of fimbrial adhesions of *Escherichia coli*. *Review of Infectious Disease 13,* 721–735.

Livermore D.M. (1995). β-Lactamases in laboratory and clinical resistance. *Clinical Microbiology Review 8,* 557–584.

Moore S.S. (1996). Pattern and predictability of emerging infections. *Hospital Practice 31,* 85–108.

O'Brien K.K., Higdon M.L., Halverson J.J. (2003). Recognition and management of bioterrorism infections. *American Family Physician 67*(9), 1927–1934.

Peiris J.S.M., Lai S.T., Poon L.L.M., et al. (2003). Coronavirus as a possible cause of severe acute respiratory syndrome. *Lancet 361,* 1319–1325.

Rosenthal N. (1994). Tools of the trade—recombinant DNA. *New England Journal of Medicine 331,* 315–317.

Ruan Y.J., Wei C.L., Ling A.E., et al. (2003). Comparative full-length genome sequence analysis of 14 SARS coronavirus isolates and common mutations associated with putative origins of infection. *Lancet 361,* 1779–1785.

Ryan E.T., Wilson M.E., Kain K.C. (2002). Illness after international travel. *New England Journal of Medicine 347*(7), 505–516.

Tang Y.W., Persing D.H. (1999). Molecular detection and identification of microorganisms. In Murray P.R., Baron E.J., Pfaller M.A., et al. (Eds.), *Manual of clinical microbiology* (7th ed., pp. 215–244). Washington, DC: American Society for Microbiology.

Tyler K.L. (2000). Prions and prion diseases of the central nervous system (neurodegenerative diseases). In Mandell G.L., Bennett J.E., Dolin R. (Eds.), *Mandell, Douglas, and Bennett's principles and practice of infectious diseases* (5th ed., pp. 1971–1985). Philadelphia: Churchill Livingstone.

White N.J. (1996). Current concepts: The treatment of malaria. *New England Journal of Medicine* 335, 800–806.

CHAPTER

19

The Immune Response

Cynthia Sommer

The immune system is clearly essential for survival. It constantly defends the body against bacteria, viruses, and other foreign substances it encounters. It also defends against abnormal cells and molecules that periodically develop in the body, such as cancer cells. An essential aspect of the immune response is the ability to recognize almost limitless numbers of foreign invaders and nonself substances, distinguishing them from self molecules that are native to the body. Although the immune response normally is protective, it also can produce undesirable effects such as when the response is excessive, as in allergies, or when it recognizes self tissue as foreign, as in autoimmune disease.

The major focus of this chapter is to present an overview of the immune cells, molecules, and tissues of the adaptive immune system and to describe the normal mechanisms used to protect the body against foreign invaders.

Immune System

After completing this section of the chapter, you should be able to meet the following objectives:

- ✦ State the properties associated with adaptive or specific immunity
- ✦ Define and describe the characteristics of an antigen or immunogen
- ✦ Characterize the significance and function of major histocompatibility complex molecules
- ✦ Describe the antigen-presenting functions of monocytes-macrophages and dendritic cells
- ✦ Contrast and compare the development of the T and B lymphocytes
- ✦ Describe the activation and function of T and B lymphocytes
- ✦ Describe the function and characteristics of natural killer cells
- ✦ State the function of the five classes of immunoglobulins
- ✦ Differentiate between the central and peripheral lymphoid structures
- ✦ Describe the properties of cytokines and their impact on an immune response
- ✦ Compare passive and active immunity
- ✦ Characterize the role of the complement system in the immune response

The term *immunity* has come to mean the protection from disease and, more specifically, infectious disease. The collective, coordinated response of the cells and molecules of the immune system is called the *immune response.* Although the relationship between microbes and infectious diseases dates far back in history, it has only been within the past 50 to 60 years that an understanding of the cellular and biochemical mechanisms involved in the immune response have begun to emerge. Advances in cell culture techniques, immunochemistry, recombinant DNA technology, and creation of genetically altered animals such as "transgenic" and "knockout" mice have transformed immunology from a largely descriptive science to one of immune phenomena that can be explained in structural and biochemical terms.

INNATE AND ADAPTIVE IMMUNE DEFENSES

There are two types of immune defenses: the early reactions of innate immunity and the later responses of adaptive immunity (Table 19-1). *Innate,* or *nonspecific, immunity* is the natural resistance with which a person is born. It provides resistance through several physical, chemical, and cellular approaches. Microbes first encounter the epithelial layers, physical barriers that line our skin and mucous membranes. Subsequent general defenses include secreted chemical signals (cytokines), antimicrobial substances, fever, and phagocytic activity associated with the inflammatory response. The phagocytes express cell surface receptors that can bind and respond to common molecular patterns expressed on the surface of invading microbes. Through these approaches, innate immunity can prevent the colonization, entry, and spread of microbes.

Adaptive, or *specific, immunity* is the second line of defense, responding less rapidly than innate immunity but more effectively. Adaptive immunity responds through a focused recognition and amplified response to each unique type of foreign invader or molecule. The components of the adaptive immune system are white blood cells called *lymphocytes* and their products. Foreign substances that elicit specific responses are called *antigens.* There are two types of adaptive immune responses: humoral and cell-mediated immunity. *Humoral immunity* is mediated by molecules in the blood and is the principal defense against extracellular microbes and toxins. *Cell-mediated immunity,* or *cellular immunity,* is mediated by specific T lymphocytes and defends against intracellular microbes such as viruses. In contrast to innate immunity, adaptive immunity exhibits exact or specific recognition of the microbe, can amplify and sustain its responses, and has the unique ability to "remember" the pathogen and quickly produce a heightened immune response on subsequent encounters with the same agent. By convention, the terms immune responses and immune system usually refer to adaptive immunity.

Innate and adaptive immune responses form a dynamic network in which numerous cells and molecules function cooperatively. Innate immunity provides a rapid response and serves to control or contain an infection while the adaptive or specific immune responses are being produced. Innate immunity does not, however, eliminate all infections and threats. It has limitations in that the same level of response is produced on each encounter with a pathogen, and some microbes have evolved resistance to the cells and molecules. However, the innate immune response to microbes stimulates the adaptive immune response and influences the nature of the response. Also, adaptive immune responses use many of the effector mechanisms of innate immunity to eliminate microbes, and they often function by enhancing the antimicrobial effects of the innate immunity.

ANTIGENS

Before discussing the cells and responses inherent to immunity, it is important to understand the substances that elicit a response from the host. *Antigens,* or *immunogens,* are substances foreign to the host that can stimulate an immune response. These foreign molecules are recognized by receptors on immune cells and by proteins, called *antibodies* or *immunoglobulins,* that are secreted in response to the antigen. Antigens include bacteria, fungi, viruses, protozoa, and parasites. Nonmicrobial agents such as plant pollens, poison ivy resin, insect venom, and transplanted organs can also act as antigens. Most antigens are macromolecules, such as proteins and polysaccharides, although lipids and nucleic acids occasionally can serve as antigens.

Antigens, which in general are large and chemically complex, are biologically degraded into smaller chemical units or peptides. These discrete, immunologically active sites on antigens are called *antigenic determinants,* or *epitopes*

TABLE 19-1 Comparison of Innate and Adaptive Immune Responses

	Innate	Adaptive
Time of response	Rapid (minutes to hours)	Slower (days to weeks)
Diversity	Limited to groups of microbes	Very large; cell for each unique antigen
Microbe recognition	General patterns on microbes; nonspecific	Specific to microbe and antigen
Nonself-recognition	Yes	Yes
Response to repeated infections	Similar each exposure	Immunologic memory; more rapid and efficient with subsequent exposure
Defenses	Barriers (skin, mucous membranes), phagocytes, antimicrobial molecules; inflammation, fever	Cell killing; tagging of antigen by antibody for removal
Cells and molecules	Phagocytes (macrophages, neutrophils), natural killer cells, dendritic cells	T and B lymphocytes

COMPONENTS OF THE IMMUNE SYSTEM

- The immune system consists of immune cells; the central immune structures (the bone marrow and thymus), where immune cells are produced and mature; and the peripheral immune structures (lymph nodes, spleen, and other accessory structures), where the immune cells interact with antigen.
- The immune cells consist of the lymphocytes (T and B lymphocytes), which are the primary cells of the immune system, and the accessory cells such as the macrophages, which aid in processing and presentation of antigens to the lymphocytes.
- Cytokines are molecules that form a communication link between immune cells and other tissues and organs of the body.
- Recognition of self from nonself by the immune cells depends on a system of MHC membrane molecules that differentiate viral-infected and abnormal cells from normal cells (MHC I) and allow appropriate interactions among immune cells (MHC II).

(Fig. 19-1). It is the unique molecular shape of an epitope that is recognized by a specific immunoglobulin receptor found on the surface of the lymphocyte or by an antigen-binding site of a secreted antibody. A single antigen may contain multiple antigenic determinants, each stimulating a distinct clone of lymphocytes to produce a unique type of antibody. For example, different proteins that comprise a virus may function as unique antigens, each of which contains several antigenic determinants. Hundreds of antigenic determinants are found on structures such as the bacterial cell wall.

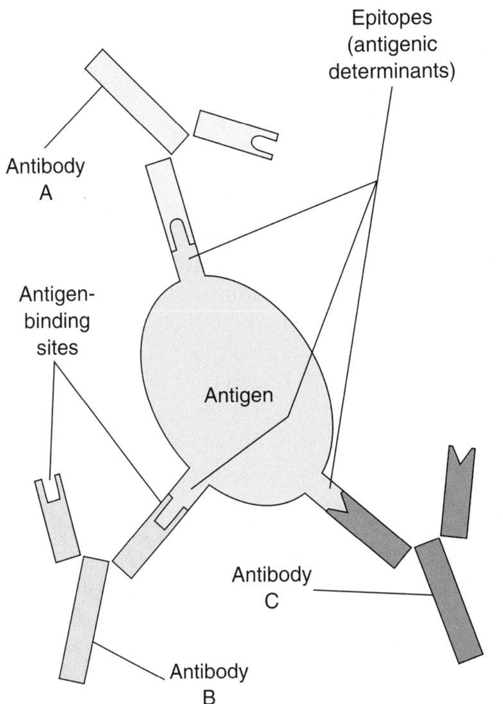

FIGURE 19-1 Multiple epitopes on a complex antigen being recognized by their respective (**A, B, C**) antibodies.

Smaller substances (molecular masses <10,000 daltons) usually are unable to stimulate an adequate immune response by themselves. When these low-molecular-weight compounds, known as *haptens,* combine with larger protein molecules, they function as antigens. The proteins act as carrier molecules for the haptens to form antigenic hapten–carrier complexes. An allergic response to the antibiotic penicillin is an example of a medically important reaction due to hapten–carrier complexes. Penicillin (molecular mass of approximately 350 daltons) is normally a nonantigenic molecule. However, in some individuals, it can chemically combine with body proteins to form larger complexes that can then generate a potentially harmful immune allergic response.

IMMUNE CELLS

The principal cells of the immune system are the lymphocytes, antigen-presenting cells, and effector cells. Lymphocytes are the cells that specifically recognize and respond to foreign antigens. Accessory cells, such as macrophages and dendritic cells, function as antigen-presenting cells by the processing of a complex antigen into epitopes required for the activation of lymphocytes. Functionally, there are two types of immune cells: regulatory cells and effector cells. The *regulatory cells* assist in orchestrating and controlling the immune response. For example, helper T lymphocytes activate other lymphocytes and phagocytes. The final stages of the immune response are accomplished with the elimination of the antigen by *effector cells*. Activated T lymphocytes, mononuclear phagocytes, and other leukocytes function as effector cells in different immune responses.

Lymphocytes represent 25% to 35% of blood leukocytes, and 99% of the lymphocytes reside in the lymph. Like other blood cells, lymphocytes are generated from stem cells in the bone marrow (Fig. 19-2). Undifferentiated immature lymphocytes congregate in the central lymphoid tissues, where they develop into distinct types of mature lymphocytes. One class of lymphocyte, the *B lymphocytes* (B cells), matures in the bone marrow and is essential for *humoral, or antibody-mediated, immunity*. The other class of lymphocyte, the *T lymphocytes* (T cells), completes its maturation in the thymus and functions in the peripheral tissues to produce *cell-mediated immunity*, as well as aiding in antibody production. Approximately 60% to 70% of blood lymphocytes are T cells, and 10% to 20% are B cells. The various types of lymphocytes are distinguished by their function and response to antigen, their cell membrane molecules and receptors, their types of secreted proteins, and their tissue location. High concentrations of mature T and B lymphocytes are found in the lymph nodes, spleen, skin, and mucosal tissues, where they can respond to antigen.

The key trigger for the activation of B and T cells is the recognition of the antigen by unique surface receptors. The

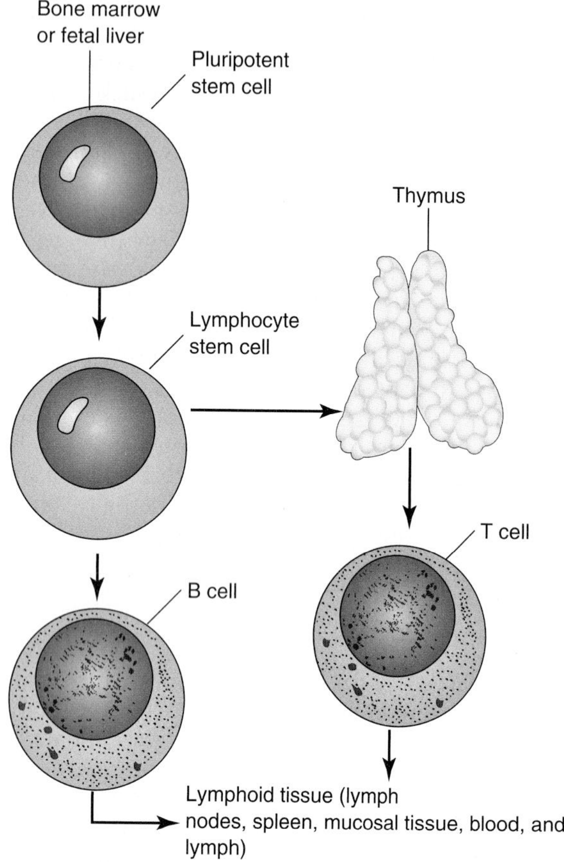

FIGURE 19-2 Pathway for T- and B-cell differentiation.

B-cell antigen receptor consists of membrane-bound immunoglobulin molecules that can bind a specific epitope. The T-cell receptor recognizes a processed antigen peptide in association with a self-recognition protein, called a *major histocompatibility complex* (MHC) molecule (to be discussed). The appropriate recognition of MHC and self peptides or MHC associated with foreign peptides is essential for lymphocytes to differentiate "self" from "foreign."

The immune system enlists specialized *antigen-presenting cells* (APCs), such as macrophages and dendritic cells, to ensure the appropriate processing and presentation of antigen. On recognition of antigen and after additional stimulation by various secreted signaling molecules called *cytokines,* the B and T lymphocytes divide several times to form populations or clones of cells that continue to differentiate into several types of effector and memory cells. These effector cells and molecules defend the body in an immune response (Fig. 19-3). In humoral or antibody-mediated immunity, activated B cells produce effector cells called *plasma cells,* which secrete protein molecules called *antibodies,* or *immunoglobulins.* The binding of antibodies can neutralize the biologic impact of the microbes and cause subsequent aggregation to ensure their removal. Phagocytic cells can more efficiently bind, engulf, and digest antigen–antibody aggregates or immune complexes than they can antigen alone.

T and B cells display additional membrane molecules called *clusters of differentiation* (CD) molecules. These molecules aid the function of immune cells and also serve to define functionally distinct subsets of cells, such as $CD4^+$ helper T cells and $CD8^+$ cytotoxic T cells. The many cell surface CD molecules detected on immune cells have allowed scientists to identify distinct subsets of lymphocytes and study both the normal and abnormal developmental processes displayed by these cells. In cell-mediated immunity, regulatory $CD4^+$ helper T cells enhance the response of other T cells, and effector cytotoxic T lymphocytes ($CD8^+$) destroy cellular antigens such as tumor cells and virus-infected cells (see Fig. 19-3).

T and B lymphocytes possess all of the key properties associated with the adaptive immune response—specificity, diversity, memory, and self- and nonself-recognition. These cells can exactly recognize a particular microorganism or foreign molecule. Each lymphocyte targets a specific antigen and differentiates that invader from other substances that may be similar. The approximately 10^{12} lymphocytes in the body have tremendous diversity. They can respond to the millions of different kinds of antigens encountered daily. This diversity occurs because an enormous variety of lymphocyte populations have been programmed during development, each to respond to a different antigen. After lymphocytes have been stimulated by their antigen, they can acquire a memory response. The memory T and B lymphocytes that are generated remain in the body for a long time and can respond more rapidly on repeat exposure than naïve cells (see Fig. 19-3). Because of this heightened state of immune reactivity, the immune system usually can respond to commonly encountered microorganisms so efficiently that we are unaware of the response.

Major Histocompatibility Complex Molecules

An essential feature of adaptive or specific immunity is the ability to discriminate between the body's own molecules and foreign antigens. Key recognition molecules essential for distinguishing self from nonself are the cell surface MHC molecules. These proteins, which in humans are coded by closely linked genes on chromosome 6, were first identified because of their role in organ and tissue transplantation. When cells are transplanted between individuals who are not identical for their MHC molecules, the immune system produces a vigorous immune response leading to rejection of the transferred cells or organs. MHC molecules did not evolve to reject transplanted tissues, a situation not encountered in nature. Rather, these molecules are essential for correct cell-to-cell interactions among immune and body cells.

The MHC molecules involved in self-recognition and cell-to-cell communication fall into two classes, class I and class II (Fig. 19-4). *Class I MHC* (MHC-1) molecules are cell surface glycoproteins that interact with the antigen receptor and the CD8 molecule on cytotoxic T lymphocytes. Class I MHC molecules are found on nearly all nucleated cells in the body and are capable of alerting the immune system of any cell changes due to viruses, intracellular bacteria, or cancer.

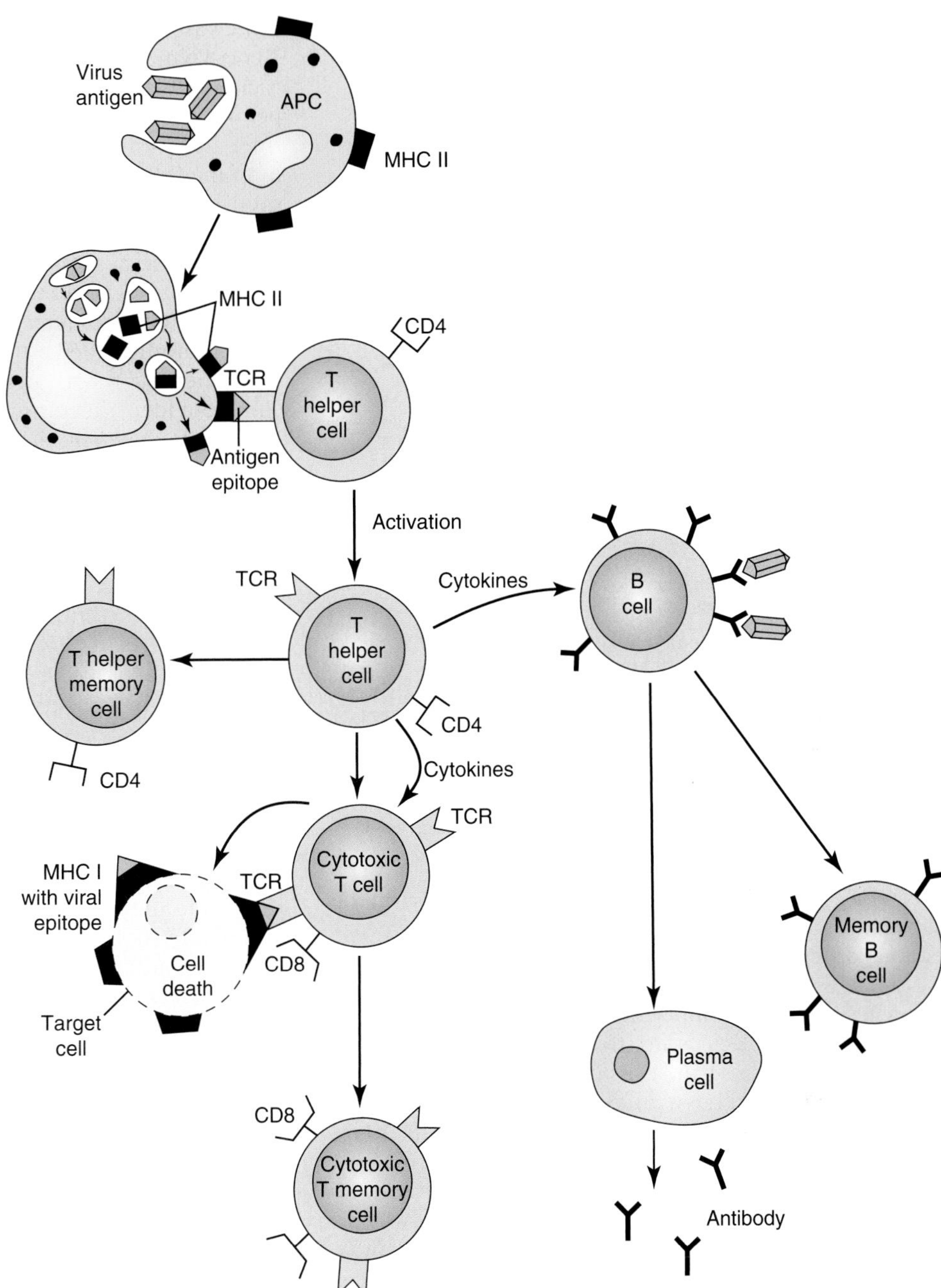

FIGURE 19-3 Pathway for immune cell participation in an immune response.

The class I MHC molecule contains a groove that accommodates a peptide fragment of antigen. Cytotoxic T cells can become activated only when they are presented with the foreign antigen peptide associated with the class I MHC molecule. Antigen peptides associate with class I molecules in cells that are infected by intracellular pathogens such as a virus. As the virus multiplies, small peptides from degraded virus proteins associate with class I MHC molecules and are then transported to the infected cell membrane. This complex communicates to the cytotoxic T cell that the cell must be destroyed for the overall survival of the host. *Class II MHC* molecules, which are found primarily on APCs such as macrophages, dendritic cells, and B lymphocytes, communicate with the antigen receptor and CD4 molecule on helper T lymphocytes.

Class II MHC molecules also have a groove or cleft that binds a fragment of antigen from pathogens that have been engulfed and digested during the process of phagocytosis. The engulfed pathogen is degraded into peptides in cytoplasmic vesicles and then complexed with class II MHC molecules. Helper T cells recognize these complexes on the surface of APCs and then become activated. These triggered helper T cells multiply quickly and direct other immune cells to respond to the invading pathogen through the

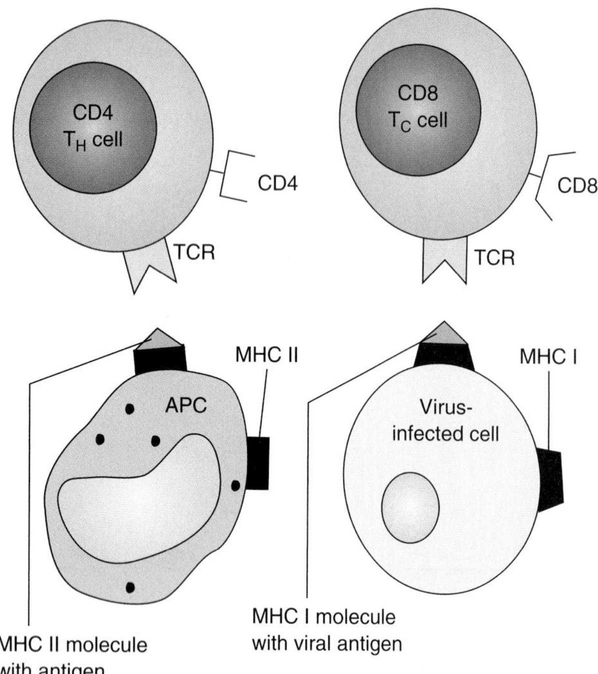

FIGURE 19-4 Recognition by a T-cell receptor (TCR) on a CD4 helper T (T_H) cell of an epitope associated with class II MHC molecule on an antigen-presenting (APC) cell, and CD8 cytotoxic (T_C) T cell with class I MHC molecule on a virus-infected cell.

secretion of cytokines. A third group of genes located on the same chromosome near the class I and class II MHC genes encode other proteins involved in the immune response. Complement and cytokines important for signaling an immune response are examples of the third class of molecules. These secreted molecules are structurally and functionally unrelated to the class I and class II MHC molecules.

Each individual has a unique collection of MHC proteins, and a variety of MHC molecules can exist in a population. Thus, MHC molecules are both polygenic and polymorphic. The MHC genes are the most polymorphic genes known. Because of the number of MHC genes and the possibility of several alleles for each gene, it is almost impossible for any two individuals to be identical, except if they are identical twins. In contrast to the receptors on T and B lymphocytes that bind a unique antigen molecule, each MHC protein can bind a broad spectrum of antigen peptides. The antigen fragments bound to MHC molecules then allow for proper recognition of self and nonself by immune cells, and a subsequent appropriate immune response results.

Human MHC proteins are called *human leukocyte antigens* (HLA) because they were first detected on white blood cells. Because these molecules play a role in transplant rejection and are detected by immunologic tests, they are commonly called antigens. More recently, analysis of the genes for the HLA molecules has ensured a more complete identification of the potential antigens present in an individual. The classic human class I MHC molecules are divided into types called HLA-A, HLA-B, and HLA-C, and the class II MHC molecules are identified as HLA-DR, HLA-DP, and HLA-DQ (Table 19-2). Additional, less well-studied, nonclassic MHC genes have been described and shown to influence other immune interactions. Each of the gene loci that describe HLA molecules can be occupied by multiple alleles or alternate genes. For example, there are more than 120 possible genes for the A locus and 250 genes for the B locus. The genes and their expressed molecule are designated by a letter and numbers (*i.e.*, HLA-B27).

Because the class I and II MHC genes are closely linked on one chromosome, the combination of HLA genes usually is inherited as a unit, called a *haplotype*. Each person inherits a chromosome from each parent and therefore has two HLA haplotypes. The identification or typing of HLA molecules is important in tissue or organ transplantation, forensics, and paternity evaluations. In organ or tissue transplantation, the closer the matching of HLA types, the greater is the probability of identical antigens and the lower the chance of rejection.

Monocytes, Macrophages, and Dendritic Cells

Monocytes, tissue macrophages, and most dendritic cells arise from a common precursor in the bone marrow. Monocytes and macrophages are key members of the mononuclear phagocytic system. The monocytes migrate from the blood to various tissues where they mature into the major tissue phagocyte, the macrophages. Macrophages are char-

TABLE 19-2 Properties of Class I and II MHC Molecules

Properties	HLA Antigens	Distribution	Functions
Class I MHC	HLA-A, HLA-B, HLA-C	Virtually all nucleated cells	Present processed antigen to cytotoxic $CD8^+$ T cells; restrict cytolysis to virus-infected cells, tumor cells, and transplanted cells
Class II MHC	HLA-DR, HLA-DP, HLA-DQ	Immune cells, antigen-presenting cells, B cells, and macrophages	Present processed antigenic fragments to $CD4^+$ T cells; necessary for effective interaction among immune cells

HLA, human leukocyte antigen; MHC, major histocompatibility complex.

acterized as large cells with extensive cytoplasm and numerous vacuoles. As the general scavenger cells of the body, macrophages can be fixed in a tissue or can be free to migrate from an organ to lymphoid tissues. The tissue macrophages are scattered in connective tissue or clustered in organs such as the lung (*i.e.,* alveolar macrophages), liver (*i.e.,* Kupffer's cells), spleen, lymph nodes, peritoneum, central nervous system (*i.e.,* microglial cells), and other areas.

Macrophages are activated to engulf and digest antigens that associate with their cell membrane. The initial attachment of the microbe to the phagocyte can be aided by antibody or complement-coated microbes or by pathogen-associated molecular pattern receptors (*i.e.,* Toll-like receptors) that are integral to innate immune recognition. On phagocyte membranes, the family of Toll-like receptors (so-called because they correspond in structure to a *Drosophila* protein called Toll) recognizes general chemical patterns common to groups of microbes such as the lipopolysaccharides of gram-negative bacteria or the lipoteichoic acids found in gram-positive bacteria. Once the microbe is ingested, the cell generates digestive enzymes and toxic oxygen and nitrogen products (*i.e.,* hydrogen peroxide or nitric oxide) through metabolic pathways. The phagocytic killing of microorganisms helps to contain infectious agents until adaptive immunity can be marshaled. In addition to phagocytosis, macrophages function early in the immune response to amplify the inflammatory response and initiate adaptive immunity. Macrophages direct these processes through the secretion of cytokines (*e.g.,* tumor necrosis factor [TNF], interleukin-1) that signal inflammation and activation of lymphocytes.

Activated macrophages also influence adaptive immunity as APCs that break down complex antigens into peptide fragments for association with class II MHC molecules (Fig. 19-5). Macrophages can then present these complexes to the helper T cell so that self- and nonself-recognition and activation of the immune response can occur. Macrophages also function at the end of an immune response as effector cells in both humoral and cell-mediated immune responses. Macrophages can remove antigen–antibody aggregates or, under the influence of T-cell cytokines, can destroy virus-infected cells or tumor cells.

Dendritic cells share with the macrophage the important task of presenting processed antigen to T lymphocytes. These distinctive, star-shaped cells with long extensions of their cytoplasmic membrane provide an extensive surface rich in class II MHC molecules and other membrane molecules important for initiation of adaptive immunity. Dendritic cells are found in most tissues where antigen enters the body and in the peripheral lymphoid tissues where they function as potent APCs. In these different environments, dendritic cells can acquire specialized functions and appearances, as do macrophages. Langerhans' cells are specialized dendritic cells in the skin, whereas follicular dendritic cells are found in the lymph nodes. Langerhans' cells are constantly surveying the skin for antigen and can transport foreign material to a nearby lymph node. Skin dendritic cells and macrophages also are involved in cell-mediated immune reactions of the skin such as delayed allergic contact hypersensitivity.

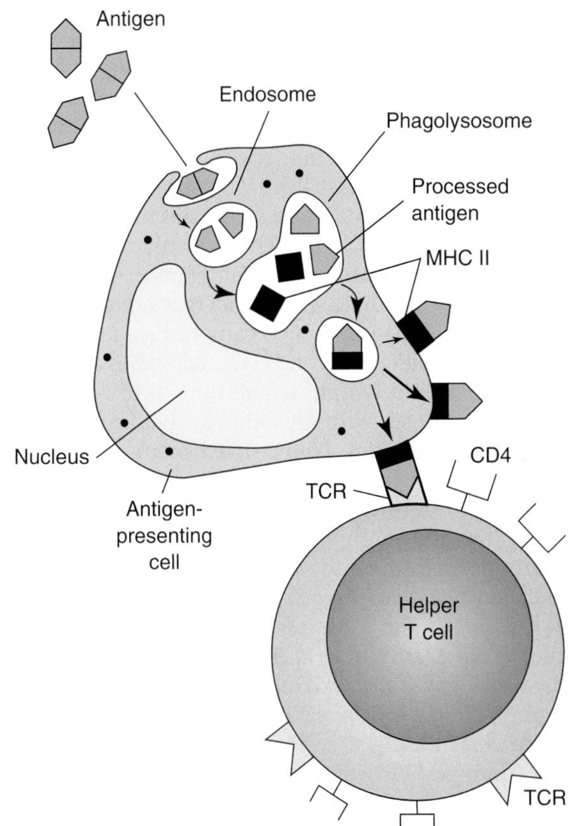

FIGURE 19-5 Processing and presentation of antigen to helper T cell by an antigen-presenting cell (APC).

B Lymphocytes

The B lymphocytes are responsible for humoral immunity. Humoral immunity provides for elimination of bacterial invaders, neutralization of bacterial toxins, prevention of viral infection, and immediate allergic responses (see Chapter 21).

B lymphocytes can be identified by the presence of membrane immunoglobulin that functions as the antigen receptor, class II MHC proteins, complement receptors, and specific CD molecules. During the maturation of B cells in the bone marrow, stem cells change into immature precursor (pre-B) cells. A rearrangement of immunoglobulin genes produces in each cell a unique membrane receptor and secreted effector antibody (*e.g.,* immunoglobulin M [IgM] or IgD). This stage of maturation is programmed into the B cells and does not require antigen; it is an antigen-independent process. The various stages of maturation can be defined by the presence of a partial or complete immunoglobulin receptor and the type of CD molecules. The mature B cell leaves the bone marrow, enters the circulation, and migrates to the various peripheral lymphoid tissues, where it is stimulated to respond to a specific antigen.

The commitment of a B-cell line to a specific antigen is evident by the expression of the membrane immunoglobulin antigen receptor molecule. B cells that encounter antigen complementary to their surface immunoglobulin receptor and receive T-cell help undergo a series of changes that transform the B cells into antibody-secreting plasma cells or into memory B cells (Fig. 19-6). B lymphocytes also can function as APCs by ingesting the surface immunoglobulin–antigen complex, processing the antigen into small peptides, and presenting the peptide, now complexed to the class II MHC molecules, at its cell membrane. The antigen peptide–class II MHC complex is recognized through cell-to-cell contact and stimulates the helper T cells to secrete various cytokines. These cytokines trigger the multiplication and maturation of antigen-activated B cells. The activated B cell divides and undergoes terminal maturation into a plasma cell, which can produce thousands of antibody molecules per second. The antibodies are released into the blood and lymph, where they bind and remove their unique antigen with the help of other immune effector cells and molecules. Longer-lived memory B cells are generated and distributed into the peripheral tissues in preparation for subsequent antigen exposure.

Immunoglobulins. Antibodies comprise a class of proteins called *immunoglobulins*. The immunoglobulins have been divided into five classes: IgG, IgA, IgM, IgD, and IgE (Table 19-3), each with a different role in the immune defense strategy. Immunoglobulins have a characteristic four-polypeptide structure consisting of at least two identical antigen-binding sites (Fig. 19-7). Each immunoglobulin is composed of two identical light (L) chains and two identical heavy (H) chains to form a Y-shaped molecule. The two forked ends of the immunoglobulin molecule bind antigen and are called *Fab* (*i.e.,* antigen-binding) fragments, and the tail of the molecule, which is called the *Fc* fragment, determines the biologic properties that are characteristic of a particular class of immunoglobulins. The amino acid sequence of the heavy and light chains shows constant (C) regions and variable (V) regions. The *constant regions* have sequences of amino acids that vary little among the antibodies of a particular class of immunoglobulin. The constant regions allow separation of immunoglobulins into classes (*e.g.,* IgM, IgG) and allow each class of antibody to interact with certain effector cells and molecules. For example, IgG can tag an antigen for recognition and destruction by phagocytes. The *variable regions* contain the antigen-binding sites of the molecule. The wide variation in the amino acid sequence of the variable regions seen from antibody to antibody allows this region to recognize its complementary epitope. A unique amino acid sequence in this region determines a distinctive three-dimensional pocket that is complementary to the antigen, allowing recognition and binding. Each B-cell clone produces antibody with one specific antigen-binding variable region or domain. During the course of the immune response, class switching (*e.g.,* from IgM to IgG) can occur, causing the B-cell clone to produce one of the following antibody types.

IgG (gamma globulin) is the most abundant of the circulating immunoglobulins. It is present in body fluids and readily enters the tissues. IgG is the only immunoglobulin that crosses the placenta and can transfer immunity from the mother to the fetus. This class of immunoglobulin protects against bacteria, toxins, and viruses in body fluids and activates the complement system. There are four subclasses of IgG (*i.e.,* IgG1, IgG2, IgG3, and IgG4) that have some restrictions in their response to certain types of antigens. For example, IgG2 appears to be responsive to bacteria that are encapsulated with a polysaccharide layer, such as *Streptococcus pneumoniae, Haemophilus influenzae,* and *Neisseria meningitidis.*

IgA, a secretory immunoglobulin, is found in saliva, tears, colostrum (*i.e.,* first milk of a nursing mother), and bronchial, gastrointestinal, prostatic, and vaginal secretions. This dimeric secretory immunoglobulin is considered a primary defense against local infections in mucosal tissues. IgA prevents the attachment of viruses and bacteria to epithelial cells.

IgM is a macromolecule that forms a polymer of five basic immunoglobulin units. It cannot cross the placenta and does not transfer maternal immunity. It is the first circulating immunoglobulin to appear in response to an antigen and is the first antibody type made by a newborn. This is diagnostically useful because the presence of IgM suggests

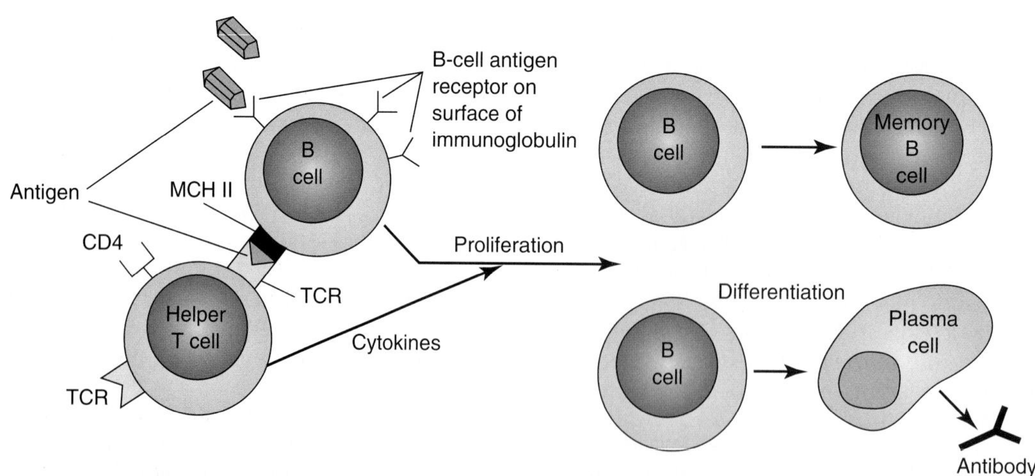

FIGURE 19-6 Pathway for B-cell differentiation.

TABLE 19-3 Classes and Characteristics of Immunoglobulins

Figure	Class	Percentage of Total	Characteristics
	IgG	75.0	Displays antiviral, antitoxin, and antibacterial properties; only Ig that crosses the placenta; responsible for protection of newborn; activates complement and binds to macrophages
J	IgA	15.0	Predominant Ig in body secretions, such as saliva, nasal and respiratory secretions, and breast milk; protects mucous membranes
	IgM	10.0	Forms the natural antibodies such as those for ABO blood antigens; prominent in early immune responses; activates complement
	IgD	0.2	Found on B lymphocytes; needed for maturation of B cells
	IgE	0.004	Binds to mast cells and basophils; involved in parasitic infections, allergic and hypersensitivity reactions

a current infection in the infant by a specific pathogen. The identification of newborn IgM rather than maternally transferred IgG to the specific pathogen is indicative of an in utero or newborn infection.

IgD is found primarily on the cell membranes of B lymphocytes. It serves as an antigen receptor for initiating the differentiation of B cells.

IgE is involved in inflammation, allergic responses, and combating parasitic infections. It binds to mast cells and basophils. The binding of antigen to mast cell– or basophil-bound IgE triggers these cells to release histamine and other mediators important in inflammation and allergies.

T Lymphocytes

T lymphocytes function in the activation of other T cells and B cells, in the control of intracellular viral infections, in the rejection of foreign tissue grafts, and in delayed hypersensitivity reactions (see Chapter 21). Collectively, these immune responses are called *cell-mediated,* or *cellular, immunity*. Besides the ability to respond to cell-associated antigens, the T cell is integral to immunity because it regulates self-recognition and amplifies the response of B and T lymphocytes.

T lymphocytes arise from bone marrow stem cells, but unlike B cells, pre-T cells migrate to the thymus for their maturation. There, the immature T lymphocytes undergo rearrangement of the genes needed for expression of a unique T-cell antigen receptor similar to but distinct from the B-cell receptor. The T-cell receptor (TCR) is composed of two polypeptides that fold to form a groove that recognizes processed antigen peptide–MHC complexes (Fig. 19-8). The TCR–antigen–MHC complex is further stabilized by the $CD4^+$ molecule on the helper T cell or by the $CD8^+$ molecules on the cytotoxic T cells. The TCR is associated

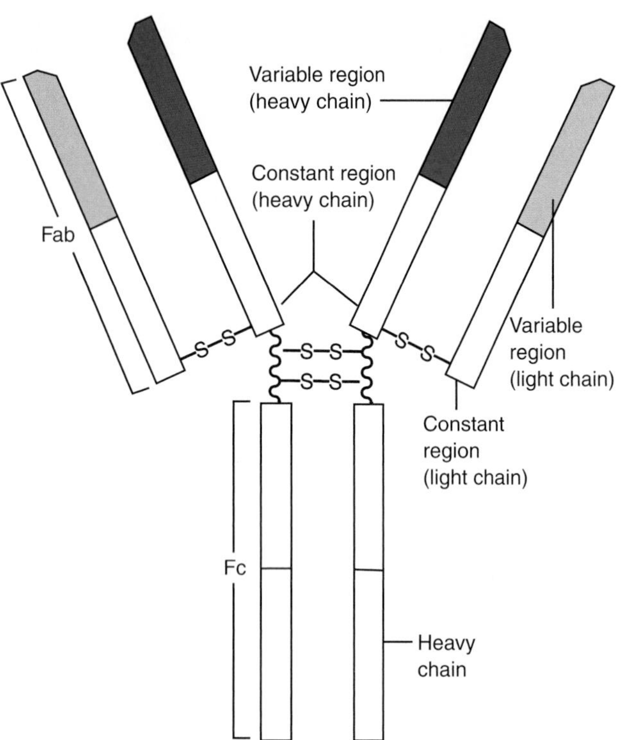

FIGURE 19-7 Schematic model of an IgG molecule showing the constant and variable regions of the light and dark chains.

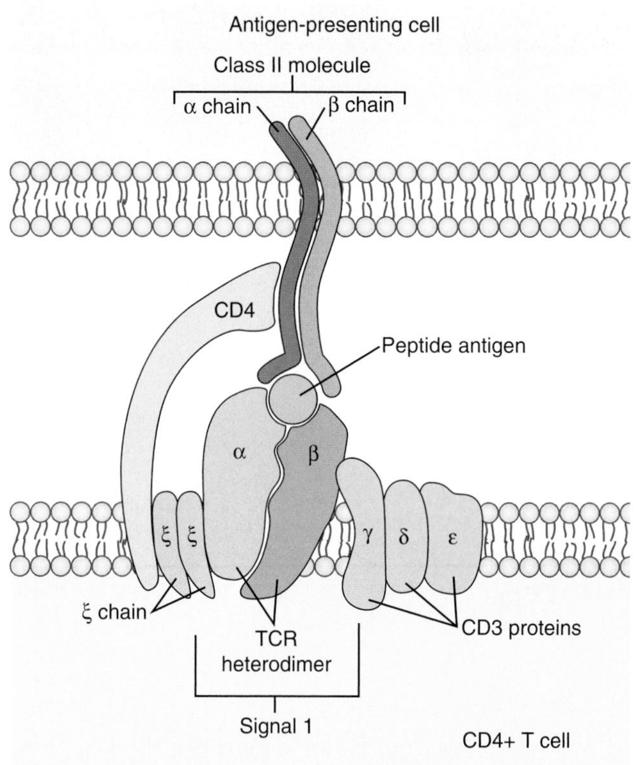

FIGURE 19-8 The T-cell receptor (TCR) on a CD4+ T cell and its interaction with the class II major histocompatibility complex (MHC) molecule on the antigen-presenting cell. Notice that the αβ-TCR heterodimer recognizes a peptide fragment of antigen bound to the MHC class II molecule. The CD4 molecule binds to nonpolymorphic portion of the class II molecule stabilizing the interaction. The CD3 proteins associated with the TCR aid in cell signaling. (Adapted from Kumar V., Cotran R.S., Robbins S.L. (2003). *Robbins basic pathology* (p. 106). Philadelphia: W.B. Saunders)

with other surface molecules known as the *CD3 complex* that aid cell signaling. Maturation of subpopulations of T cells (*i.e.,* $CD4^+$ and $CD8^+$) also occurs in the thymus. Mature T cells migrate to the peripheral lymphoid tissues and, on encountering antigen, multiply and differentiate into memory T cells and various effector T cells.

Helper T Cells. The $CD4^+$ helper T cell (T_H) serves as a master regulator for the immune system. Activation of helper T cells depends on the recognition of antigen in association with class II MHC molecules. Once activated, the cytokines they secrete will influence the function of nearly all other cells of the immune system. These cytokines activate and regulate B cells, cytotoxic T lymphocytes, natural killer (NK) cells, macrophages, and other immune cells. The activated helper T cell can differentiate into distinct subpopulations of helper T cells (*i.e.,* T_H1 or T_H2) based on the cytokines secreted by the APC at the site of activation (Table 19-4). The cytokine interleukin-12 (IL-12) produced by macrophages and dendritic cells directs the maturation of helper T cells toward T_H1 cells, whereas IL-4 produced by mast cells and T cells induce differentiation toward T_H2 cells. The distinct pattern of cytokine secreted by mature T_H1 and T_H2 cells determines whether a humoral or cell-mediated response will occur. Activated T_H1 cells characteristically produce the cytokines IL-2 and interferon-γ (IFN-γ), whereas T_H2 cells produce IL-4 and IL-5. In most immune responses, a balanced response of T_H1 and T_H2 cells occurs; however, extensive immunization can skew the response to one or the other subset. For example, the extensive exposure to an allergen in atopic individuals has been shown to shift the naïve helper T cell toward a T_H2 response with the production of the cytokines that influence IgE production and mast cell priming. An appreciation of these processes has led to clinical research suggesting that redirection of an allergic T_H2 response to a nonallergic T_H1 response can occur in atopic individuals through modified immunization protocols.

T Cytotoxic Cells. Activated $CD8^+$ cytotoxic T (Tc) cells become cytotoxic T lymphocytes (CTLs) after recognition of class I MHC–antigen complexes on target cell surfaces, such as body cells infected by viruses or transformed by cancer (Fig. 19-9). The recognition of class I MHC–antigen complexes on infected target cells ensures that neighboring uninfected host cells, which express class I MHC molecules alone or with self peptide, are not indiscriminately destroyed. The $CD8^+$ cytotoxic T lymphocytes destroy target cells by releasing cytolytic enzymes, toxic cytokines, and pore-forming molecules (*i.e.,* perforins) or through programmed cell death of the target cell through triggering membrane molecules and intracellular apoptosis. Apopto-

TABLE 19-4 Comparison of Properties of Helper T Cell Subtypes 1 (T_H1) and 2 (T_H2)

	T_H1	T_H2
Stimulus for differentiation to T_H subtype	Microbes	Allergens and parasitic worms
Cells and cytokines influencing T_H subtype maturation	Macrophages, NK cells, IL-12	Mast cells, IL-4
Cytokines secreted by T_H subtype	IFN-γ	IL-4, IL-5
Function of T_H subtype	Enhances inflammation and cell-mediated immunity; activates macrophages	Enhances B cells and antibody response; promotes secretion of IgE

NK, natural killer; IL, interleukin; IFN, interferon; IgE, immunoglobulin E.

sis is a conserved cell process for the controlled elimination of excessive, dangerous, or damaged cells (see Chapter 5). In addition, the perforin proteins can produce pores in the target cell membrane, allowing entry of toxic molecules and loss of cell constituents. The $CD8^+$ T cells are especially important in controlling replicating viruses and intracellular bacteria because antibody cannot readily penetrate the membrane of living cells.

Cell-mediated immunity involves both $CD4^+$ and $CD8^+$ T lymphocytes. Activated $CD4^+$ helper T cells release various cytokines (*i.e.*, IFN-γ) that recruit and activate other lymphocytes, macrophages, and inflammatory cells.

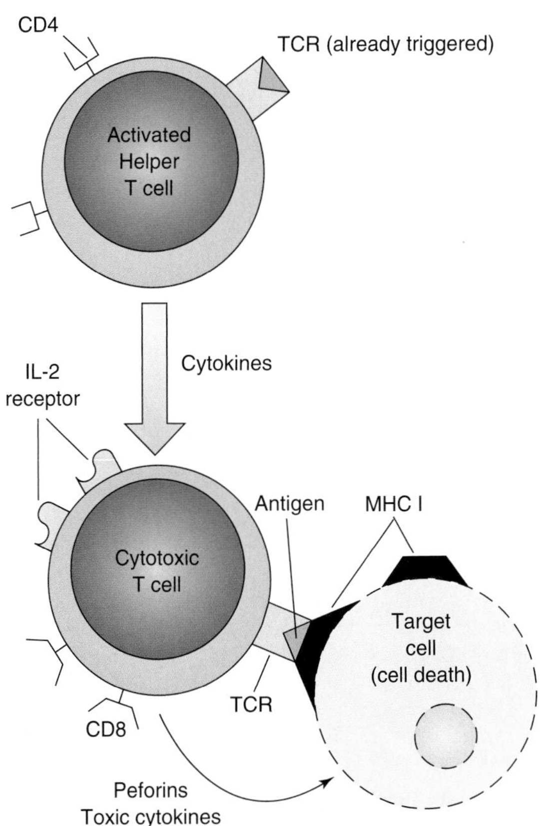

FIGURE 19-9 Destruction of target cell by cytotoxic T cell. Cytokines released from the activated helper T cell enhance the potential of the cytotoxic T cell in destruction of the target cell.

Cytokines (*e.g.*, IL-8) can induce positive migration or chemotaxis of several types of inflammatory cells, including macrophages, neutrophils, and basophils. Activation of macrophages ensures enhanced phagocytic, metabolic, and enzymatic potential, resulting in more efficient destruction of infected cells. This type of defense is important against intracellular pathogens such as *Mycobacterium* species and *Listeria monocytogenes.*

A similar sequence of T-cell and macrophage activation, but with sustained inflammation, is elicited in delayed hypersensitivity reactions. Contact dermatitis due to a poison ivy reaction or dye sensitivity is an example of delayed or cell-mediated hypersensitivity caused by hapten–carrier complexes.

Natural Killer Cells

Natural killer cells are lymphocytes that are functionally and phenotypically distinct from T cells, B cells, and monocyte-macrophages. The NK cell is an effector cell important in innate immunity that can kill tumor cells, virus-infected cells, or intracellular microbes. These cells are called *natural killer cells* because, unlike cytotoxic T cells, they do not need to recognize a specific antigen before being activated. Both NK cells and cytotoxic T cells kill after contact with a target cell. The NK cell is programmed to kill foreign cells automatically, in contrast to the $CD8^+$ T cell, which needs to be activated to become cytotoxic. However, programmed killing is inhibited in the NK cell if its cell membrane receptors contact MHC self molecules on normal host cells.

NK cells appear as large, granular lymphocytes with an indented nucleus and abundant, pale cytoplasm containing red granules. These cells characteristically express CD16 and CD94 cell surface molecules but lack the typical T-cell markers (*i.e.*, TCR, CD4). The mechanism of NK cytotoxicity is similar to T-cell cytotoxicity in that it depends on production of pore-forming proteins (*i.e.*, NK perforins), enzymes, and toxic cytokines. NK cell activity can be enhanced in vitro on exposure to IL-2, a phenomenon called *lymphokine-activated killer* activity. NK cells also participate in *antibody-dependent cellular cytotoxicity,* a mechanism by which a cytotoxic effector cell can kill an antibody-coated target cell. The role of NK cells is believed to be one of immune surveillance for cancerous or virus-infected cells.

LYMPHOID ORGANS

The cells of the immune system are present in large numbers in the central and peripheral lymphoid organs. These organs and tissues are widely distributed in the body and provide different, but often overlapping, functions (Fig. 19-10). The central lymphoid organs, the bone marrow and the thymus, provide the environment for immune cell production and maturation. The peripheral lymphoid organs function to trap and process antigen and promote its interaction with mature immune cells. Lymph nodes, spleen, tonsils, appendix, Peyer's patches in the intestine, and mucosa-associated lymphoid tissues in the respiratory, gastrointestinal, and reproductive systems compose the peripheral lymphoid organs. The lymphoid organs are connected by networks of lymph channels, blood vessels, and capillaries. The immune cells continuously circulate through the various tissues and organs to seek out and destroy foreign material. The structure and organization of the cellular components of the peripheral lymphoid tissues ensures that the rare antigen-specific B and T cells will see each other and the antigen peptide– and MHC-coated APCs (*e.g.*, dendritic cells).

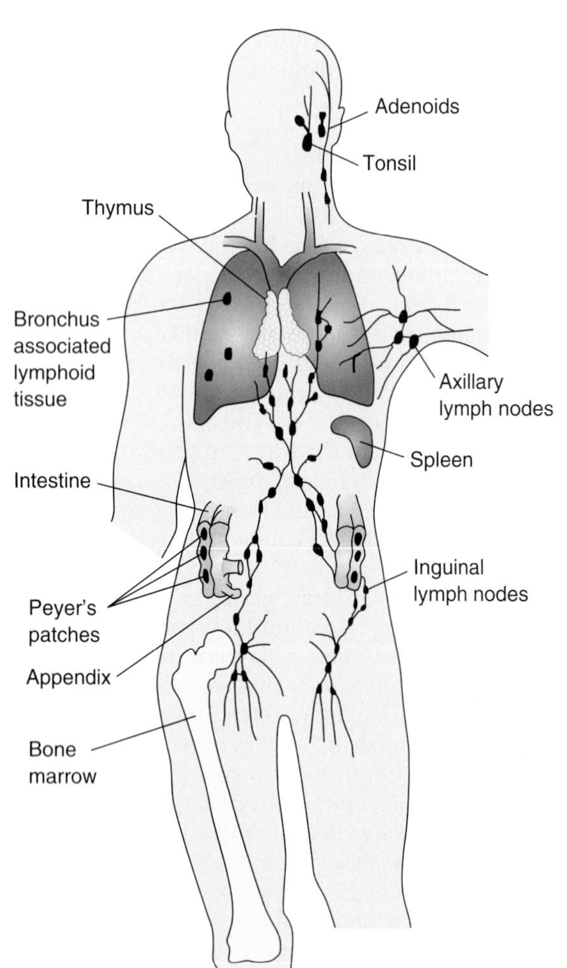

FIGURE 19-10 Central and peripheral lymphoid organs and tissues.

Thymus

The thymus is an elongated, bilobed structure that is located in the neck region above the heart. Each lobe is surrounded by a connective tissue capsule layer and is divided into lobules. Each lobule is composed of two compartments: an outer area or cortex, which is densely packed with thymocytes or immature T lymphocytes, and an inner, less dense area or medulla that contains fewer but more mature lymphocytes. The medulla also contains dendritic cells, macrophages, and the distinctive morphologic structure of the thymus, Hassall's corpuscles (Fig. 19-11).

The function of the thymus is central to the development of the immune system because it generates mature immunocompetent T lymphocytes. The thymus is a fully developed organ at birth, weighing approximately 15 to 20 g. At puberty, when the immune cells are well established in peripheral lymphoid tissues, the thymus begins slowly regressing and is replaced by adipose tissue. Nevertheless, some thymus tissue persists into old age. Precursor T (pre-T) cells enter the thymus as functionally and phenotypically immature T cells. They progressively develop into mature T cells as they transverse the organ from the cortical to medullary areas. Rapid cell multiplication, maturation, and selection occur in the cortex under the influence of the microenvironment, thymic hormones, and cytokines. Cortical thymocytes undergo TCR gene rearrangement and

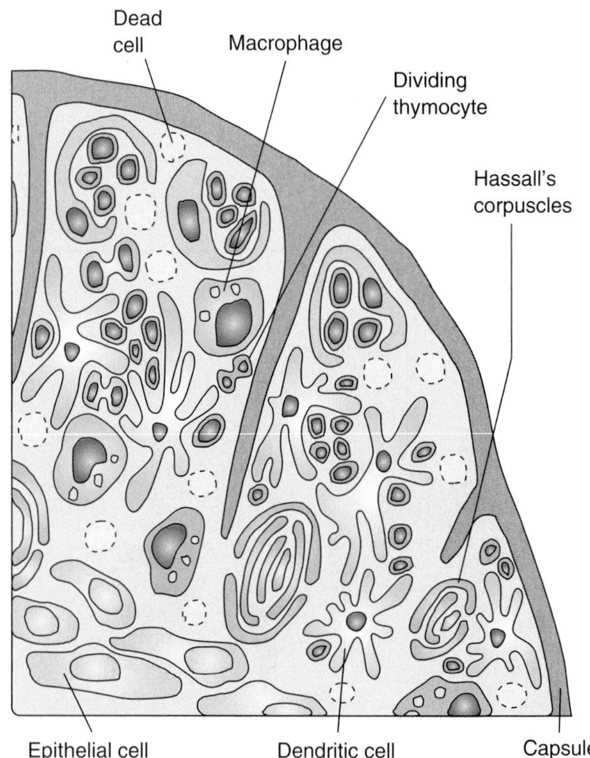

FIGURE 19-11 Structural features of the thymus gland. The thymus gland is divided into lobules containing an outer cortex densely packed with dividing thymocytes or premature T cells and an inner medulla that contains mature T lymphocytes, macrophages, dendritic cells, and Hassall's corpuscles.

TCR and $CD4^+/CD8^+$ surface expression. More than 95% of the thymocytes die in the cortex and never leave the thymus because in the random rearrangement of genes, cells are produced with inappropriate receptors. Only those T cells able to recognize foreign antigen and not react to self (*i.e.*, MHC or self antigens) are allowed to mature. This process is called *thymic selection*. The thymus must be extremely thorough in eliminating self-reactive cells to ensure that autoimmune reactivity and disease do not result. Mature immunocompetent helper T and cytotoxic T cells leave the thymus in 2 to 3 days and enter the peripheral lymphoid tissues through the bloodstream.

Impairment of thymic function can occur in immunologic deficiency disorders. If the thymus is removed from certain animals at birth or is congenitally absent, as is seen in certain human conditions, the result is a decrease in the number of lymphocytes in the blood and a marked depletion or absence of T lymphocytes in the circulation and peripheral lymphoid tissues.

Lymph Nodes

Lymph nodes are small aggregates of lymphoid tissue located along lymphatic vessels throughout the body. Each lymph node processes lymph from a discrete, adjacent anatomic site. Many lymph nodes are in the axillae and groin and along the great vessels of the neck, thorax, and abdomen. These lymph nodes are located along the lymph ducts, which lead from the tissues to the thoracic duct. Lymph nodes have two functions: removal of foreign material from lymph before it enters the bloodstream and serving as centers for proliferation and response of immune cells.

A lymph node is a bean-shaped tissue surrounded by a connective tissue capsule. Lymph enters the node through afferent lymph channels that penetrate the capsule, and the lymph leaves through the efferent lymph vessels located in the deep indentation of the hilus. Lymphocytes and macrophages flow slowly through the node, which allows trapping and interaction of antigen and immune cells. The reticular meshwork serves as a surface on which macrophages and dendritic cells can more easily present antigens.

A lymph node is divided into several specialized areas: an outer cortex, a paracortex, and inner medulla (Fig. 19-12). The T lymphocytes are more abundant in the paracortex of the node, and the B lymphocytes are more abundant in the follicles and germinal centers located in the outer cortex. The T lymphocytes proliferate on antigenic stimulation and migrate to the follicles, where they interact with B lymphocytes. These activated follicles become germinal centers, containing macrophages, follicular dendritic cells, and maturing T and B cells. Activated B cells then migrate to the medulla, where they complete their

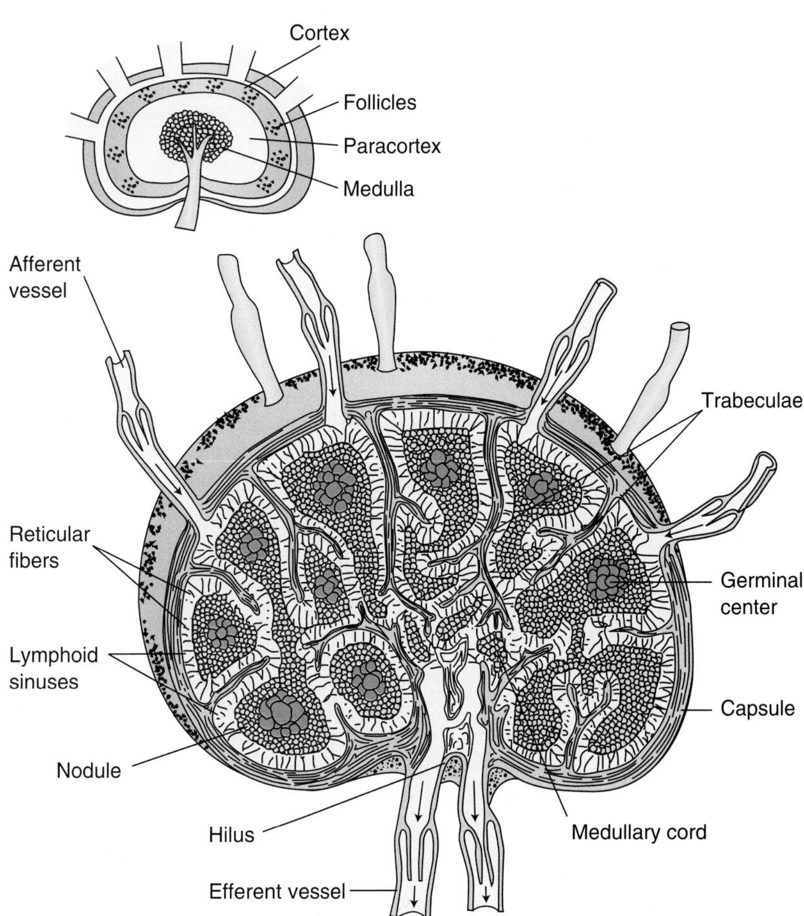

FIGURE 19-12 Structural features of a lymph node.

maturation into plasma cells. These cells stay localized in the lymph node but release large quantities of antibodies into the circulation.

Spleen

The spleen is a large, ovoid secondary lymphoid organ located high in the left abdominal cavity. The spleen filters antigens from the blood and is important in response to systemic infections. The spleen is composed of red and white pulp. The red pulp is well supplied with arteries and is the area where senescent and injured red blood cells are removed. The white pulp contains concentrated areas of B and T lymphocytes permeated by macrophages and dendritic cells. The lymphocytes (primarily T cells) that surround the central arterioles form the area called the *periarterial lymphoid sheath.* The diffuse marginal zone contains follicles and germinal centers rich in B cells and separates the white pulp from the red pulp. A sequence of activation events similar to that seen in the lymph nodes occurs in the spleen.

Other Secondary Lymphoid Tissues

Other secondary lymphoid tissues include the *mucosa-associated lymphoid tissues.* These nonencapsulated clusters of lymphoid tissues are located around mucosal membranes lining the respiratory, digestive, and urogenital tract. These gateways into the body must contain the immune cells needed to respond to a large and diverse population of microorganisms. In some tissues, the lymphocytes are organized in loose clusters, but in other tissues such as the tonsils, Peyer's patches in the intestine, and the appendix, organized structures are evident (see Fig. 19-10). These tissues contain all the necessary cell components (*i.e.,* T cells, B cells, macrophages, and dendritic cells) for an immune response. Because of the continuous stimulation of the lymphocytes in these tissues by microorganisms constantly entering the body, large numbers of plasma cells are evident. Immunity at the mucosal layers helps to exclude many pathogens and thus protects the vulnerable internal organs.

CYTOKINES AND THE IMMUNE RESPONSE

Cytokines are low-molecular-weight regulatory proteins that are produced during all phases of an immune response. These molecules can be named for the general cell type that produces them (*e.g.,* lymphokines, monokines). More specifically, they are named by an international nomenclature (*i.e.,* IL-1 to IL-30) or for the biologic property that was first ascribed to them. For example, *interferons* (IFNs) were named because they interfered with virus multiplication.

Cytokines are made primarily by and act predominantly on immune cells. These intercellular signaling molecules are very potent, act at very low concentrations, and usually regulate neighboring cells. Cytokines modulate reactions of the host to foreign antigens or injurious agents by regulating the movement, proliferation, and differentiation of leukocytes and other cells (Table 19-5). Cytokines are synthesized by many cell types but are made primarily by activated T_H lymphocytes and macrophages. Cytokines

TABLE 19-5 Characteristic Biologic Properties of Human Cytokines

Cytokines	Biologic Activity
Interleukin-1 (alpha and beta)	Wide variety of biologic effects; activates endothelium and lymphocytes; induces fever and acute phase response; stimulates neutrophil production
Interleukin-2	Growth factor for activated T cells; induces synthesis of other cytokines, activates cytotoxic T lymphocytes and NK cells
Interleukin-3	Growth factor for progenitor hematopoietic cells
Interleukin-4	Promotes growth and survival of T, B, and mast cell; causes T_H2 cell differentiation; activates B cells and eosinophils and induces IgE-type responses
Interleukin-5	Induces eosinophil growth and differentiation; induces IgA production in B cells
Interleukin-6	Stimulates the liver to produce acute-phase response; induces proliferation of antibody-producing cells
Interleukin-7	Stimulates pre-B cells and thymocyte development and proliferation
Interleukin-8	Chemoattracts neutrophils and T lymphocytes; regulates lymphocyte homing and neutrophil infiltration
Interleukin-10	Decreases inflammation by inhibiting T_H1 cells and release of IL-12 from macrophages
Interleukin-12	Induces T_H1 cell differentiation and IFN-γ synthesis by T and NK cells. Enhances NK cytotoxicity.
Interferon-γ	Activates macrophages; increases expression of class I and II and MHC antigen processing and presentation.
Interferon (type I α and β)	Exerts antiviral activity in body cells; induces class I antigen expression; activates NK cells
Tumor necrosis factor (α)	Induces inflammation, fever, and acute-phase response; activates neutrophils and endothelial cells; kills cells through apoptosis.
Colony-stimulating factors (CSFs)	Promotes neutrophil, eosinophil, and macrophage maturation and growth; activates mature granulocytes; promotes growth and maturation of monocytes
Granulocyte-macrophage CSF	Promotes growth and maturation of neutrophils
Macrophage CSF	Promotes growth and maturation of monocytes

Ig, immunoglobulin; IL, interleukin; IFN, interferon; NK, natural killer; MHC, major histocompatibility complex.

commonly affect more than one cell type and have more than one biologic effect. For example, IFN-γ inhibits virus replication and is a potent activator of macrophages and NK cells. Specific cytokines can have biologic activities that overlap. Maximization of the immune response and protection against detrimental mutations in a single cytokine are possible benefits of this redundancy.

The production of cytokines often occurs in a cascade in which one cytokine affects the production of subsequent cytokines or cytokine receptors. Some cytokines function as antagonists to inhibit the biologic effects of earlier cytokines. This pattern of expression and feedback ensures appropriate control of cytokine synthesis and subsequently of the immune response. Excessive cytokine production can have serious adverse effects, including those associated with septic shock, food poisoning, and types of cancer.

Cytokines generate their responses by binding to specific receptors on their target cells. Many cytokine receptors share a common structural shape and a cytoplasmic tail that interacts with a family of signaling proteins (Janus kinases [JAKs]). These signaling molecules then interact with cytoplasmic intermediary molecules (signal transducers and activators of transcription [STATs]) that are responsible for the induction of the genes for cell responses. Most cytokines are released at cell-to-cell interfaces, where they bind to receptors on nearby cells. The biologic responses associated with cytokines are also regulated by the time of expression of the cytokine receptor. The short half-life of cytokines ensures that excessive immune responses and systemic activation do not occur.

The biologic properties of cytokines fall into several major functional groups. One group of cytokines (*e.g.*, IL-1, IL-6, TNF) mediates inflammation by producing fever and the acute-phase response and by attracting and activating phagocytes (*e.g.*, IL-8, IFN-γ). Other cytokines are maturation factors for the hematopoiesis of white or red blood cells (*e.g.*, IL-3, granulocyte-macrophage colony-stimulating factor [GM-CSF]) (see Chapter 14). Recombinant CSF molecules are being used to increase the success rates of bone marrow transplantations. Most of the IL cytokines and IFN-γ function in adaptive immunity as cell communication molecules among T cells, B cells, macrophages, and other immune cells. The availability of recombinant cytokines offers the possibility of several clinical therapies whereby stimulation or inhibition of the immune response or cell production is desirable. IL-2 therapy for several malignancies has led to some clinical success.

Cytokines in Innate Immunity and Inflammation

Interleukin-1, IL-6, and TNF are the major mediators of the early inflammatory response. In concert, they can stimulate the production of acute-phase proteins by the liver, mobilize neutrophils to the site of insult, direct the hypothalamus for a fever response, and increase the adhesion molecules on the vascular epithelium. Depending on the concentration of these cytokines, the biologic changes can be seen as local inflammation (low concentration), systemic inflammation (moderate concentration), or even septic shock (high concentration). The major source of IL-1, IL-6, and TNF includes macrophages and dendritic and endothelial cells. TNF is a potent cytokine with multiple immunologic and inflammatory effects. It was first identified (and so named) as a substance in the serum of animals treated with bacterial endotoxin that caused hemorrhagic necrosis in certain tumors and later as a circulating mediator of the wasting syndrome seen in chronic inflammation. New inhibitors of TNF or its receptors have been used to control the chronic inflammation associated with rheumatoid arthritis and inflammatory bowel disease.

Other mediators in innate immunity include IFNs and IL-12. Type I IFNs (alpha and beta) also play a role in innate immunity by controlling virus infection. Type I IFNs interact with receptors on neighboring cells to stimulate the translation of an antiviral protein that affects viral synthesis and its spread to uninfected cells. The actions of type I IFNs are not pathogen specific; they are effective against different types of viruses and intracellular parasites. IL-12 is a key inducer of adaptive cell-mediated immunity and indirectly of inflammation and can influence the cytolytic potential of cytotoxic T and NK cells.

Cytokines in Adaptive Immunity

Cytokines activate the immune cells in adaptive immune responses to undergo proliferation and differentiation and to ensure their appropriate development into effector and memory cells. The cytokines secreted by T_H1 and T_H2 cells are essential for these processes. Key cytokines in adaptive immunity are IL-2, IL-4, IL-5, and IFN-γ.

IL-2 is necessary for the proliferation and function of helper T, cytotoxic T, B, and NK cells. IL-2 interacts with T lymphocytes by binding to specific membrane receptors that are present on activated T cells but not on resting T cells. The expression of high-affinity IL-2 receptors can be triggered by specific antigen peptide–class II MHC interactions and other stimulatory signals. Sustained T-cell amplification relies on the presence of both IL-2 and IL-2 receptors; if either is missing, cell proliferation ceases. Severe combined immunodeficiency diseases have been associated with mutations in IL-2 and the IL-2 receptor, thereby documenting the importance of these molecules. Cyclosporine and tacrolimus are drugs used to prevent rejection of heart, kidney, and liver transplants, and function primarily by inhibiting the synthesis of IL-2.

IL-4 is the major regulatory molecule for the development of T_H2 cells, which direct B cells in the class switching needed to produce IgE antibodies. IL-4 can further expand T_H2 cell populations in an autocrine manner and at the same time inhibits T_H1-directed cell-mediated immunity. The detrimental impact of increased IL-4 on excessive IgE production is evident in allergic individuals. IL-5 is an activator of eosinophils, which work with IgE antibodies in their protective role of controlling parasitic helminth infections.

IFN-γ is the key macrophage-activating cytokine and aids both adaptive cell-mediated immunity and innate immune responses. Macrophages and NK cells are activated by IFN-γ to kill microbes more efficiently. The adaptive immune response is regulated by IFN-γ through maturation of T_H2 cells and inhibition of the proliferation of T_H2 cells.

Cytokines in Hematopoiesis

Colony-stimulating factors are cytokines that stimulate bone marrow pluripotent stem cells and progenitor or precursor cells to produce large numbers of platelets, erythrocytes, lymphocytes, neutrophils, monocytes, eosinophils, basophils, and dendritic cells. The colony-stimulating factors were named according to the type of target cell on which they act (see Table 19-5). GM-CSF acts on the granulocyte-monocyte progenitor cells to produce monocytes, neutrophils, and dendritic cells; G-CSF more specifically induces neutrophil proliferation; and M-CSF specifically directs the mononuclear phagocyte progenitor. Other cytokines, including IL-3, IL-7, and IL-11, also influence hematopoiesis.

IMMUNITY AND THE IMMUNE RESPONSE

Adaptive, or specific, immune responses are designed to protect the body against potentially harmful foreign substances, infections, and other sources of nonself antigens. It is the specific protection that is induced following exposure to antigens (active immunity) or through transfer of protective antibodies against an antigen (passive immunity).

Active immunity is acquired through immunization or actually having a disease. It is called *active immunity* because it depends on a response to the antigen by the person's immune system. Active immunity, although long lasting once established, requires a few days to weeks after a first exposure before the immune response is sufficiently developed to contribute to the destruction of the pathogen. However, the immune system usually is able to react within hours to subsequent exposure to the same agent because of the presence of memory B and T lymphocytes and circulating antibodies. The process of acquiring the ability to respond to an antigen after administration by vaccines is known as *immunization.* An acquired immune response can improve on repeated exposures to an injected antigen or a natural infection. The immune response describes the interaction between an antigen (*i.e.,* immunogen) and an antibody (*i.e.,* immunoglobulin) or reactive T lymphocyte.

Passive immunity is immunity transferred from another source. An infant receives passive immunity naturally from the transfer of antibodies from its mother in utero and through the mother's breast milk. Maternal IgG crosses the placenta and protects the newborn during the first few months of life. Normally, an infant has few infectious diseases during the first 3 to 6 months owing to the protection provided by the mother's antibodies. Passive immunity also can be artificially provided by the transfer of antibodies produced by other people or animals. Some protection against infectious disease can be provided by the injection of hyperimmune serum, which contains high concentrations of antibodies for a specific disease, or immune serum or gamma globulin, which contains a pool of antibodies from many individuals providing protection against many infectious agents. Passive immunity produces only short-term protection that lasts weeks to months.

THE IMMUNE RESPONSE

- The immune response involves a complex series of interactions between components of the immune system and the antigens of a foreign pathogen.
- Passive immunity represents a temporary type of immunity that is transferred from another source (in utero transfer of antibodies from mother to infant).
- Active immunity depends on a response by the person's immune system and is acquired through immunization or actually having a disease.
- Humoral immunity consists of protection provided by the B lymphocyte-derived plasma cells, which produce antibodies that travel in the blood and interact with circulating and cell surface antigens.
- Cell-mediated immunity consists of protection provided by cytotoxic T lymphocytes, which protect against virus-infected or cancer cells.

Humoral Immunity

Humoral immunity depends on maturation of B lymphocytes into plasma cells, which produce and secrete antibodies. The combination of antigen with antibody can result in several effector responses, such as precipitation of antigen–antibody complexes, agglutination or clumping of cells, neutralization of bacterial toxins and viruses, lysis and destruction of pathogens or cells, adherence of antigen to immune cells, facilitation of phagocytosis, and complement activation. For example, antibodies can neutralize a virus by blocking the sites on the virus that it uses to bind to the host cell, thereby negating its ability to infect the cell.

Two types of responses occur in the development of humoral immunity: a primary and a secondary response (Fig. 19-13). A *primary immune response* occurs when the

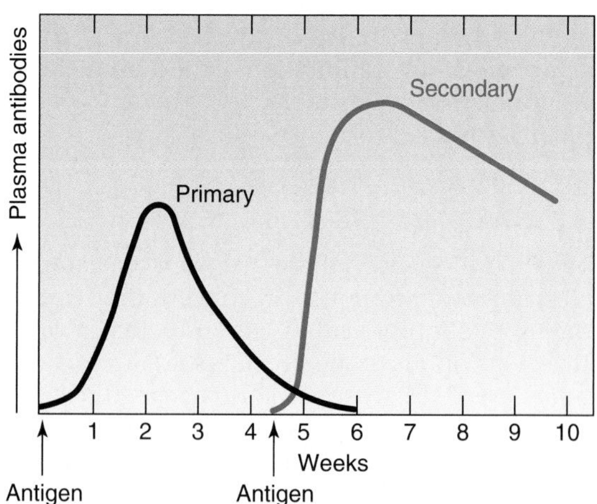

FIGURE 19-13 Primary and secondary or memory phases of the humoral immune response to the same antigen.

antigen is first introduced into the body. During this primary response, there is a latent period or lag before the antibody can be detected in the serum. This latent period involves the processing of antigen by the APCs and recognition by helper T cells. The antigen receptors on helper T cells recognize the antigenic peptide–class II MHC complex, become activated, and produce cytokines to further stimulate and direct the immune system. In humoral immunity, activated helper T cells trigger B cells to proliferate and differentiate into a clone of plasma cells that produce antibody. This activation process takes 1 to 2 weeks, but once generated, detectable antibody continues to rise for a few weeks. Recovery from many infectious diseases occurs at the time during the primary response when the antibody concentration is reaching its peak. The *secondary* or *memory response* occurs on second or subsequent exposures to the antigen. During the secondary response, the rise in antibody occurs sooner and reaches a higher level because of available memory cells.

During the primary response, B cells are activated to proliferate and differentiate into antibody-secreting plasma cells. A fraction of activated B cells does not differentiate into plasma cells but forms a pool of memory B cells. During the secondary response, the memory cells recognize the antigen and respond more efficiently to produce the specific antibody. The booster immunization given for some diseases, such as tetanus, makes use of the memory response. For a person who has been previously immunized, administration of a booster shot causes an almost immediate rise in antibody to a level sufficient to prevent development of the disease. Activated T cells can also generate primary and secondary cell-mediated immune response and the concurrent development of T memory cells.

Cell-Mediated Immunity

Cell-mediated immunity provides protection against viruses, intracellular bacteria, and cancer cells. In cell-mediated immunity, the actions of T lymphocytes and effector macrophages predominate. The most aggressive phagocyte, the macrophage, becomes activated after exposure to T-cell cytokines, especially IFN-γ. As in humoral immunity, the initial stages of cell-mediated immunity are directed by an APC displaying the antigen peptide–class II MHC complex to the helper T cell. Helper T cells become activated after antigen recognition and by induction with IL-12. The activated helper T cell then synthesizes IL-2 and IL-4. These molecules drive the multiplication of clones of helper T cells, which amplify the response. Further differentiation of the helper T cells leads to production of additional cytokines (*e.g.*, IFN-γ), which enhance the activity of cytotoxic T cells and effector macrophages. A cell-mediated immune response usually occurs through the cytotoxic activity of cytotoxic T cells and the enhanced engulfment and killing by macrophages.

Complement System

The complement system is a primary effector system for both innate and adaptive humoral immune responses. The activation of this system results in enhanced inflammatory responses, lysis of foreign cells, and increased phagocytosis. The complement system, like the blood coagulation system, consists of a group of proteins that are present in the circulation as functionally inactive precursors (Fig. 19-14). These proteins, mainly proteolytic enzymes, make up 10% to 15% of the plasma protein fraction. For a complement reaction to occur, the complement components must be activated in the proper sequence. Uncontrolled activation of

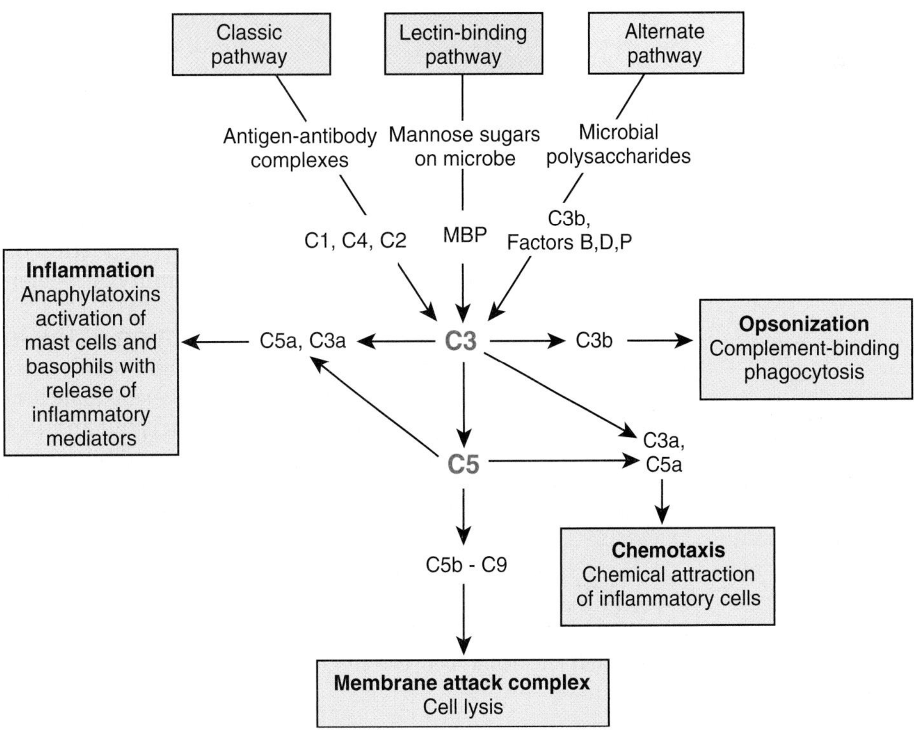

FIGURE 19-14 Classic, lectin, and alternative complement pathways.

the complement system is prevented by inhibitor proteins and the instability of the activated complement proteins at each step of the process.

There are three parallel but independent mechanisms for recognizing microorganisms that result in the activation of the complement system: the classic, the alternate, and the lectin-mediated pathways. All three pathways of activation generate a series of enzymatic reactions that proteolytically cleave successive complement proteins in the pathway. The consequence is the deposition of some complement protein fragments on the pathogen surface, thereby producing tags for better recognition by the receptors on phagocytic cells. Other complement fragments are released into the tissue fluids to stimulate further the inflammatory response.

The *classic pathway* of complement activation is initiated by antibody bound to epitopes on the surface of microbes or through soluble immune complexes (Fig. 19-15). The alternate and the lectin pathways do not use antibodies and are part of the innate immune defenses. The alternate pathway of complement activation is initiated by the interaction of complement proteins (*i.e.,* C3b) with certain polysaccharide molecules characteristic of bacterial surfaces. The lectin-mediated pathway is initiated following the binding of a mannose-binding protein to mannose-containing molecules commonly present on the surface of bacteria and yeast.

The activation of the three pathways produces similar effects on C3 and subsequent complement proteins.

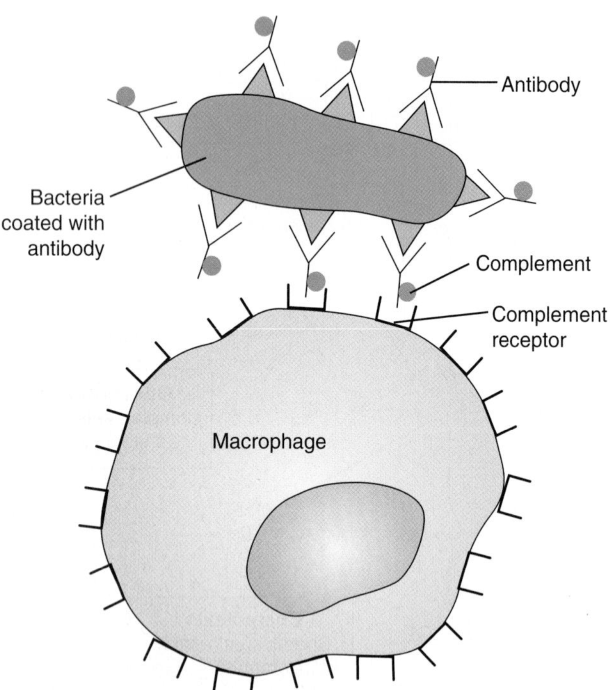

FIGURE 19-15 Complement-mediated interaction between macrophage and bacterium.

The classic pathway of complement activation was the first discovered and is the best studied. The major proteins of the classic system are designated by a numbering system from C1 to C9. The classic pathway is triggered when complement-fixing antibodies, such as IgG or IgM, bind to antigens. The immune complexes with complement trigger a series of enzyme reactions that act in a cascade fashion to generate modified or split complement proteins (*e.g.,* C3b, C3a, and C5a). C3 has a central role in the complement pathways because it is integral to all three pathways. The triggering of C3 initiates several mechanisms for microbial destruction. One result of activation of C3 is the formation of the membrane attack complex formed by C5 to C9. Several structurally modulated complement proteins bind to form pores in the membrane of foreign cells that lead to eventual cell lysis.

The alternate and lectin pathways are activated by microbial surface molecules and substitute other molecules for the proteins in the first two steps of the classic complement pathway. The alternate pathway uses proteins B, D, and P for activation, whereas the lectin pathway uses mannose-binding protein and accessory proteins. Both pathways require the presence of C3b and subsequent complement proteins to generate biologic effects similar to those of the classic complement pathway.

Whatever the mechanism of activation of the complement system, the effects of complement fixation and activation range from cell lysis to direct mediation of the inflammatory process (Table 19-6). First, complement has been shown to mediate the lytic destruction of many kinds of cells, including red blood cells, platelets, and bacteria. All complement pathways may induce cytolysis. Second, a major biologic function of complement activation is opsonization—the coating of antigen–antibody complexes with complement proteins such that antigens are engulfed and cleared more efficiently by macrophages. Third, chemotactic complement products (C3a and C5a) can trigger an influx of leukocytes. These white blood cells remain fixed in the area of complement activation through cell receptor attachment to specific sites on C3b and C4b molecules. Fourth, production of anaphylatoxin (C3a and C5a) can activate mast cells and basophils to release biologically active mediators (*e.g.,* histamine) that produce contraction of smooth muscle, increased vascular permeability, and edema.

Regulation of the Immune Response

Self-regulation is an essential property of the immune system. An inadequate immune response may lead to immunodeficiency, but an inappropriate or excessive response may lead to conditions varying from allergic reactions to autoimmune diseases. This regulation is not well understood and involves all aspects of the immune response, including antigen, antibody, cytokines, regulatory T cells, and the neuroendocrine system.

With each exposure to antigen, the immune system must determine the branch of the immune system to be activated and the extent and duration of the immune response. After exposure to an antigen, the immune response

TABLE 19-6 Complement-Mediated Immune Responses

Response	Complement Products	Effects
Cytolysis	C5b–C9	Lysis and destruction of cell membranes of body cells or pathogens
Opsonization	C3b, C5b	Targeting of the antigen so that it can be easily engulfed and digested by the macrophages and other phagocytic cells
Chemotaxis	C3a, C5a	Chemical attraction of neutrophils and phagocytic cells to the antigen
Anaphylaxis	C3a, C5a	Activation of mast cells and basophils with release of inflammatory mediators that produce smooth muscle contraction and increased vascular permeability

to that antigen develops after a brief lag, reaches a peak, and then recedes. Normal immune responses are self-limited because the response eliminates the antigen, and the products of the response, such as cytokines and antibodies, have a short or limited life span and are secreted only for brief periods after antigen recognition. Evidence suggests that cytokine feedback from the helper T or regulatory cells controls several aspects of the immune response.

Another facet of immune self-regulation is inhibition of immune responses by tolerance. The term *tolerance* is used to define the ability of the immune system to be nonreactive to self antigens while producing immunity to foreign agents. Tolerance to self antigens protects an individual from harmful autoimmune reactions. Exposure of an individual to foreign antigens may lead to tolerance and the inability to respond to potential pathogens that cause infection. Tolerance exists not only to self tissues but also to maternal-fetal tissues. Special regulation of the immune system is evident in defined privileged sites such as the brain, testes, ovaries, and eyes. Immune damage in these areas could result in serious consequences to the individual and the species.

In summary, immunity is the resistance to a disease that is provided by the immune system. Immune mechanisms can be divided into two types: adaptive, or specific, and innate, or nonspecific, immunity. Innate immunity is the first line of defense against microbial agents. It can distinguish between self and nonself through recognition of conserved patterns on microbes but cannot differentiate among unique antigens. Adaptive, or specific, immunity involves humoral and cellular mechanisms that respond to a unique antigen, can amplify and sustain its responses, distinguish self from nonself, and remember the antigen to produce a heightened response quickly on subsequent encounters with the same agent.

Antigens are substances foreign to the host that can stimulate an immune response. They have antigenic determinant sites or epitopes, which the immune system recognizes with specific receptors that distinguish the antigens as nonself and as unique foreign molecules.

The principal cells of the immune system are the lymphocytes, antigen-presenting cells, and effector cells that eliminate the antigen. There are two classes of lymphocytes: T lymphocytes and B lymphocytes. B lymphocytes differentiate into plasma cells that produce antibodies and provide for the elimination of microbes in the extracellular fluids (humoral immunity). T lymphocytes differentiate into regulatory (helper T cells) and effector (cytotoxic T cells) cells. Natural killer cells are lymphocytes that are functionally and phenotypically distinct from T cell, B cells, and monocyte-macrophages. They are nonspecific in their action and their recognition of antigen without being activated. Antigen-presenting cells consist of monocytes, tissue macrophages, and dendritic cells. They engulf and process antigens and present them to helper T cells.

Central to the identity of the immune cells are the CD molecules that distinguish between the different immune cells and their level of differentiation. The regulatory $CD4^+$ helper cells serve as a trigger for the immune response and are essential to the differentiation of B cells into antibody-producing plasma cells and into the differentiation of T lymphocytes into effector $CD8^+$ cytotoxic T cells that eliminate intracellular microbes such as viruses. The cell surface MHC molecules are key recognition molecules that the immune system uses in distinguishing self from nonself. Class I MHC molecules, which are present on almost all cells, interact with cytotoxic $CD8^+$ T cells in the destruction of cells that have been affected by intracellular pathogens or cancer. Class II MHC molecules, which are found on immune cells, aid in receptor communication between different members of the immune system.

Immunity can be acquired actively through immunization or by having a disease (active immunity) or by receiving antibodies or immune cells from another source (passive immunity). The humoral immune response involves secreted antibodies produced by activated B lymphocytes. Cell-mediated immunity depends on T-cell responses to cellular antigens.

The immune cells and their effector responses rely upon chemical messengers and signal systems. Cytokines are low-molecular-weight proteins that are produced during all phases of the immune response and serve as a communication system for coordinating the functions of the various members of the immune system. The complement system, which is a primary effector system for both the innate and adaptive immune system, consists of a group of proteins that present in the circulation as functionally inactive precursors. The effector functions of activated members of the complement system include (1) cell lysis, (2) chemotaxis with recruitment of inflammatory cells, (3) opsonization or coating of antigen–antibody complexes so that they can be more efficiently cleared by phagocytes, and (4) anaphylaxis or activation of mast cells and basophils to produce contraction of smooth muscle, increased vascular permeability, and edema.

Developmental Aspects of the Immune System

After completing this section of the chapter, you should be able to meet the following objectives:

- ✦ Explain the transfer of passive immunity from mother to fetus and from mother to infant during breast-feeding
- ✦ Characterize the development of active immunity in the infant and small child
- ✦ Describe changes in the immune response that occur with aging

Embryologically, the immune system develops in several stages, beginning at 5 to 6 weeks as the fetal liver becomes active in hematopoiesis. Development of the primary lymphoid organs (*i.e.*, thymus and bone marrow) begins during the middle of the first trimester and proceeds rapidly. Secondary lymphoid organs (*i.e.*, spleen, lymph nodes, and mucosa-associated lymphoid tissues) develop soon after. These secondary lymphoid organs are rather small but well developed at birth and mature rapidly following exposure to microbes during the postnatal period. The thymus at birth is the largest lymphoid tissue relative to body size and normally is approximately two thirds its mature weight, which it achieves during the first year of life.

TRANSFER OF IMMUNITY FROM MOTHER TO INFANT

Protection of a newborn against antigens occurs through transfer of maternal antibodies. Maternal IgG antibodies cross the placenta during fetal development and remain functional in the newborn for the first months of life (Fig. 19-16). IgG is the only class of immunoglobulins to cross the placenta. Levels of maternal IgG decrease significantly during the first 3 to 6 months of life, while infant synthesis of immunoglobulins increases. Maternally transmitted IgG is effective against most microorganisms and viruses. The largest amount of IgG crosses the placenta during the last weeks of pregnancy and is stored in fetal tissues, and infants born prematurely may be deficient. Because of transfer of IgG antibodies to the fetus, an infant born to a mother infected with HIV has a positive HIV antibody test result, although the child may not be infected with the virus.

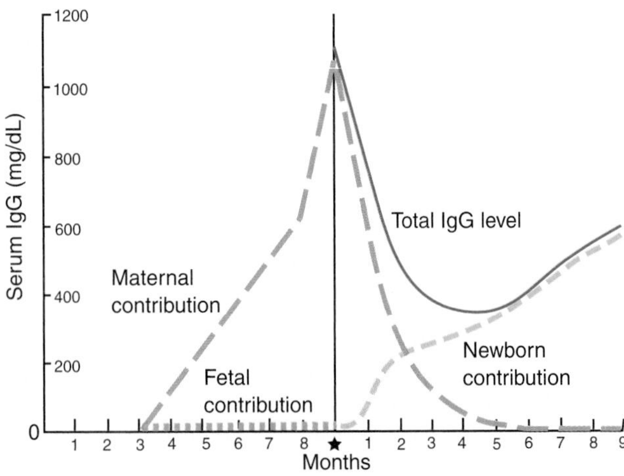

FIGURE 19-16 Maternal/neonatal serum immunoglobulin levels. (From Allansmith M., McClellan B.H., Butterworth M., Maloney, J.R. [1968]. *Journal of Pediatrics 72*, 289)

Cord blood does not normally contain IgM or IgA. If present, these antibodies are of fetal origin and represent exposure to intrauterine infection. The infant begins producing IgM antibodies shortly after birth, in response to the immense antigenic stimulation of his or her new environment. Premature infants appear to be able to produce IgM as well as term infants. At approximately 6 days of age, the IgM rises sharply, and this rise continues until approximately 1 year of age, when the adult level is achieved.

Serum IgA normally is first detected at approximately 13 days after birth. The level increases during early childhood until adult levels are reached between the sixth and seventh year. Maternal IgA also is transferred to the infant in colostrum, or milk, by breast-feeding. These antibodies provide local immunity for the intestinal system and have been shown to decrease diarrheal infections in underdeveloped countries. These evolutionary adaptations of the immune system have increased the survival of our species and optimized the development of other important organs in the early months of life.

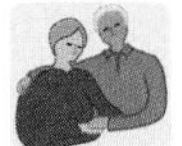

IMMUNE RESPONSE IN ELDERLY PERSONS

Aging is characterized by a declining ability to adapt to environmental stresses. One of the factors thought to contribute to this problem is a decline in immune responsiveness. This includes changes in cell-mediated and humoral immune responses. Elderly persons tend to be more susceptible to infections than younger persons, have more evidence of autoimmune and immune complex disorders, and have a higher incidence of cancer. Experimental evidence suggests that vaccination is less successful in inducing immunization in older persons than younger adults. However, the effect of altered immune function on the health of elderly persons is clouded by the fact that age-related changes or disease may affect the immune response.

The alterations in immune function that occur with advanced age are not fully understood. There is a decrease in the size of the thymus gland, which is thought to affect T-cell function. The size of the gland begins to decline shortly after sexual maturity, and by 50 years of age, it usually has diminished to 15% or less of its maximum size. There are conflicting reports regarding age-related changes in the peripheral lymphocytes. The suggestion of a biologic clock in T cells that determines the number of times it divides may regulate cell number with age. Some researchers have reported a decrease in the absolute number of lymphocytes, and others have found little change, if any. The most common finding is a slight decrease in the proportion of T cells to other lymphocytes and a decrease in $CD4^+$ and $CD8^+$ cells.

More evident are altered responses of the immune cells to antigen stimulation; increasing proportions of lymphocytes become unresponsive, whereas the remainder continue to function relatively normally. T and B cells show deficiencies in activation. In the T-cell types, the $CD4^+$ subset is most severely affected. Evidence indicates that aged T cells have a decreased rate of synthesis of the cytokines that drive the proliferation of lymphocytes and a diminished expression of the receptors that interact with those cytokines. For example, it has been shown that IL-2, IL-4, and IL-12 levels decrease with aging. Although B-cell function is compromised with age, the range of antigens that can be recognized is not diminished. If anything, the repertoire, including outgrowths of autoreactive B-cell clones, is increased to the extent that B cells begin to recognize some self antigens as foreign antigens. This may be the basis for the increased incidence of autoimmune disease in elderly persons.

In summary, a newborn is protected against antigens in early life by passive transfer of maternal antibodies through the placenta (IgG) and in colostrum (IgA) through breast-feeding. Some changes are seen with aging, including an increase in autoimmune diseases. The impact of alterations in immune function that occur with aging is not fully understood.

REVIEW EXERCISES

A nursing student is working in a community clinic as a volunteer. Each time she enters the clinic she suffers bouts of sneezing and runny eyes. She has a history of mold allergy, and her younger brother has asthma. Analysis at the allergy clinic indicates a strong reaction to latex. She is recommended to avoid exposure to all forms of latex.

A. What class of immunoglobulin and what type of mediator cells are responsible for the symptoms expressed in this individual?

B. What types of helper T cell and cytokines direct the expression of this humoral immune response?

C. Is this an example of active or passive immunity? Is this likely to be a primary or secondary immune response?

A young child, 5 months of age, presents with thrush, a yeast infection of the mouth. He has also had recurrent bouts of otitis media during the past 2 months. His tonsils are very small. Laboratory analysis indicates a low lymphocyte count and no T lymphocytes. Further analysis indicates a genetic mutation in the T cell receptor molecule complex (TCR–CD3) that affected maturation of all T cells. The final diagnosis is severe combined immunodeficiency disease. Bone marrow transplantation is being pursued with cells from his HLA-matched sibling.

A. Why were infections not present in the first few month of life in this child?

B. What would be the impact of an absence of T cells on both humoral and cell-mediated immunity?

C. Why would it not be advisable to administer a live virus vaccine to this child?

Bibliography

Abbas A.K., Litchman A.H. (2003). *Cellular and molecular immunology* (5th ed.). Philadelphia: W.B. Saunders.

Ahmed R., Gray D. (1996). Immunological memory and protective immunity: Understanding their relation. *Science 272,* 54–60.

Benjamini E., Cioco R., Sunshine G. (2003). *Immunology: A short course* (5th ed.). New York: John Wiley & Sons.

Chaplin D.D. (2003). Overview of the Immune Response. *Journal of Allergy and Clinical Immunology 111,* S442–S459.

Fearon D., Locksley R.M. (1996). The instructive role of innate immunity in the acquired immune response. *Science 272,* 50–54.

Goldsby R.A., Kindt T.J., Osborne B.A., Kuby J. (2003). *Immunology* (5th ed.). San Francisco: W.H. Freeman.

Janeway C.A. Jr., Travers P., Walport M., Shlomchik M. (2001). *Immunobiology: The immune system in health and disease* (5th ed.). New York: Garland Publishing.

Klein J., Sato A. (2000). The HLA system. *New England Journal of Medicine 343,* 702–709 and 782–786.

Levinson W., Jawetz E. (2002). *Medical microbiology and immunology* (7th ed.) East Norwalk, CT: McGraw-Hill/Appleton and Lange.

Lui Y.J. (2001). Dendritic cell subsets and lineages and their functions in innate and adaptive immunity. *Cell 106,* 259–262.

Nairn R., Helbert M. (2002). *Immunology for medical students.* New York: Mosby/Elsevier.

Natarajan K., Dimasi N., Wang J., et al. (2002). Structure and function of natural killer cell receptors: Multiple molecular solutions to self, nonself discrimination. *Annual Review of Immunology 20,* 853–885.

Parham P. (2000). *The immune system.* New York: Garland Publishing.

Roitt I., Rabson A. (2002). *Really essential immunology.* London: Blackwell Science.

Russell J.H., Ley T.J. (2002). Lymphocyte mediated cytotoxicity. *Annual Review of Immunology 20,* 323–370.

Sunyer J.O., Boshra H., Lorenzo G., et al. (2003). Evolution of complement as an effector system in innate and adaptive immunity. *Immunologic Research 27,* 549–564.

Szabo S.J., Sullivan B.M., Peng S.L., Glimcher L.H. (2003). Molecular mechanisms regulating T_H1 immune responses. *Annual Review of Immunology 21,* 713–758.

Takeda K., Kaisho T., Akira S. (2003). Toll-like receptors. *Annual Review of Immunology, 21,* 335–376.

Underhill D.M., Ozinski A. (2002). Phagocytosis of microbes: Complexity in action. *Annual Review of Immunology 20,* 825–852.

Walport M.J. (2001). Complement. *New England Journal of Medicine 344,* 1058–1066, 1141–1144.

CHAPTER 20

Inflammation and Healing

The ability of the body to sustain injury, resist attack by microbial agents, and repair damaged tissue is dependent on the inflammatory reaction, the immune response, and tissue repair and wound healing. Inflammation is a protective response intended to eliminate the initial cause of cell injury as well as the necrotic cells and tissues resulting from that injury. It accomplishes this by diluting, destroying, or otherwise neutralizing the harmful agents. It then sets the stage for the events that will eventually heal and reconstitute the sites of injury. Thus, inflammation is intimately interwoven with the repair processes in which damaged tissue is replaced by regeneration of parenchymal cells or by filling in the residual defects with fibrous scar tissue.

This chapter focuses on the manifestations of acute and chronic inflammation, tissue repair, and wound healing. The immune response is discussed in Chapter 19.

The Inflammatory Response

After completing this section of the chapter, you should be able to meet the following objectives:

- State the purpose of inflammation
- State the five cardinal signs of acute inflammation and describe the physiologic mechanisms involved in production of these signs
- Compare the hemodynamic and cellular phases of the inflammatory response
- Contrast acute and chronic inflammation
- List four types of inflammatory mediators and state their function
- Name and describe the five types of inflammatory exudates
- Define the characteristics of an acute-phase response

Inflammation is the reaction of vascularized tissue to local injury. The causes of inflammation are many and varied. It commonly results from an immune response to infectious microorganisms. Other causes of inflammation are trauma, surgery, caustic chemicals, extremes of heat and cold, and ischemic damage to body tissues.

The inflammatory response, first described more than 2000 years ago, has evoked renewed interest during the past several decades. As a result, a number of diseases are now known to have a basis in the inflammatory response. For example, the role of the inflammatory response in producing the incapacitating effects of bronchial asthma and the crippling effects of rheumatoid arthritis has been well established. There is also emerging evidence that the inflammatory response may play a role in the pathogenesis of a number of other diseases, such as atherosclerosis and Alzheimer's disease. Thus, what was once narrowly viewed as a local response to injury is today becoming an engaging problem in inflammatory mediators as well as a multibillion dollar market for the antiinflammatory drugs produced by the pharmaceutical industry.

Inflammatory conditions are named by adding the suffix *-itis* to the affected organ or system. For example, *appendicitis* refers to inflammation of the appendix, *pericarditis* to inflammation of the pericardium, and *neuritis* to inflammation of a nerve. More descriptive expressions of the inflammatory process might indicate whether the process was acute or chronic and what type of exudate was formed (*e.g.*, acute fibrinous pericarditis).

Inflammation is commonly divided into two basic patterns: acute and chronic. Acute inflammation is of relatively short duration, lasting from a few minutes to several days. Chronic inflammation is of a longer duration, lasting for days to years. These basic forms of inflammation often overlap, however, and many factors may influence their course.

THE INFLAMMATORY RESPONSE

- Inflammation represents the response of body tissue to immune reactions, injury, or ischemic damage.
- The classic response to inflammation includes redness, swelling, heat, pain or discomfort, and loss of function.
- The manifestations of an acute inflammatory response can be attributed to the immediate vascular changes that occur (vasodilation and increased capillary permeability), the influx of inflammatory cells such as neutrophils, and, in some cases, the widespread effects of inflammatory mediators, which produce fever and other systemic signs and symptoms.
- The manifestations of chronic inflammation are due to infiltration with macrophages, lymphocytes, and fibroblasts, leading to persistent inflammation, fibroblast proliferation, and scar formation.

ACUTE INFLAMMATION

Acute inflammation is the early (almost immediate) response to injury. It is nonspecific and may be evoked by any injury short of one that is immediately fatal. It is usually of short duration, typically occurs before the immune response becomes established, and is aimed primarily at removing the injurious agent and limiting the extent of tissue damage.

Cardinal Signs

The classic description of acute inflammation has been handed down through the ages. In the first century AD, the Roman physician Celsus described the local reaction of injury in terms now known as the *cardinal signs* of inflammation.[1] These signs are *rubor* (redness), *tumor* (swelling), *calor* (heat), and *dolor* (pain). In the second century AD, the Greek physician Galen added a fifth cardinal sign, *functio laesa* (loss of function). These signs and symptoms, which are apparent when inflammation occurs on the surface of the body, may not be present when internal organs are involved. Inflammation of the lung, for example, usually does not cause pain unless the pleura, where pain receptors are located, is affected. Also, an increase in heat is uncommon in inflammation involving internal organs where tissues are normally maintained at core temperature.

In addition to the cardinal signs that appear at the site of injury, systemic manifestations (*e.g.*, fever) may occur as chemical mediators produced at the site of inflammation gain entrance to the circulatory system. The constellation of systemic manifestations that may occur during an acute inflammation is known as the *acute-phase response* (to be discussed). At times, acute local inflammation may lead to a body-wide response (the systemic inflammatory response), which can spiral out of control, leading to deadly sepsis (see Chapter 28).

Acute inflammation involves two major components: the vascular and cellular stages.[1-3] At the biochemical level, the inflammatory mediators, acting together or in sequence, amplify the initial response and influence its evolution by regulating the subsequent vascular and cellular responses.

Vascular Stage

The vascular, or hemodynamic, changes that occur with inflammation begin almost immediately after injury and are initiated by a momentary constriction of small blood vessels in the area. This vasoconstriction is followed rapidly by vasodilation of the arterioles and venules that supply the area (Fig. 20-1). As a result, the area becomes congested, causing the redness (erythema) and warmth associated with acute inflammation. Accompanying this hyperemic response is an increase in capillary permeability, which causes fluid to move into the tissues and cause swelling (*i.e.*, edema), pain, and impaired function. The exudation or movement of fluid out of the capillaries and into the tissue spaces dilutes the offending agent. As fluid moves out of the capillaries, stagnation of flow and clotting of blood in the small capillaries occurs at the site of injury. This aids in localizing the spread of infectious microorganisms.

Depending on the severity of injury, the vascular changes that occur with inflammation follow one of three patterns of responses.[3] The first is an immediate transient response, which occurs with minor injury. The second is an immediate sustained response, which occurs with more serious injury and continues for several days and damages the vessels in the area. The third is a delayed hemodynamic response, which involves an increase in capillary permeability that occurs 4 to 24 hours after injury. A delayed response often accompanies radiation types of injuries, such as sunburn.

Cellular Stage

The cellular stage of acute inflammation is marked by movement of phagocytic white blood cells (leukocytes) into the area of injury. Two types of leukocytes participate in the acute inflammatory response: granulocytes and monocytes. Although attention has focused on the recruitment of leukocytes from the blood, a rapid response also

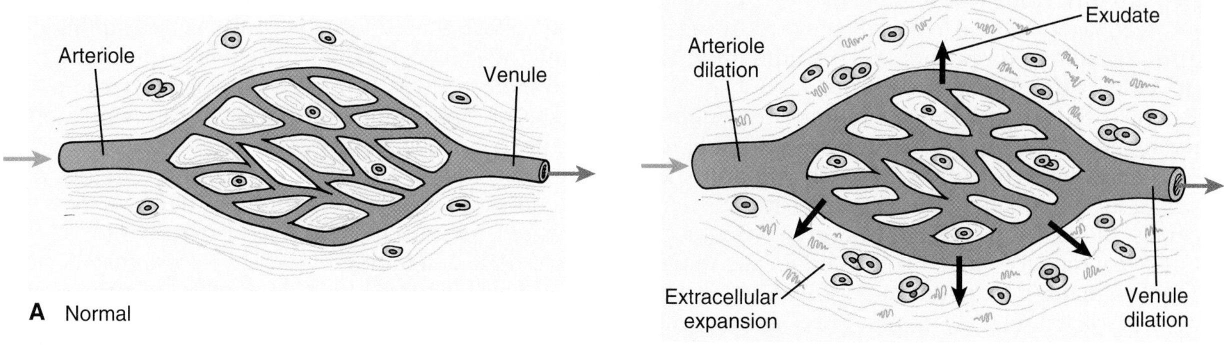

FIGURE 20-1 Vascular phase of acute inflammation. (**A**) Normal capillary bed. (**B**) Acute inflammation with vascular dilation causing increased redness (erythema) and heat (calor), movement of fluid into the interstitial spaces (swelling), and extravasation of plasma proteins into the extracellular spaces (exudate).

requires the release of chemical mediators from sentinel cells (mast cells and macrophages) that are pre-positioned in the tissues.[4]

Granulocytes. Granulocytes are identifiable because of their characteristic cytoplasmic granules. These white blood cells have distinctive multilobed nuclei. The granulocytes are divided into three types (*i.e.*, neutrophils, eosinophils, and basophils) according to the staining properties of the granules when treated with a Wright or Giemsa polychrome stain (Fig. 20-2).

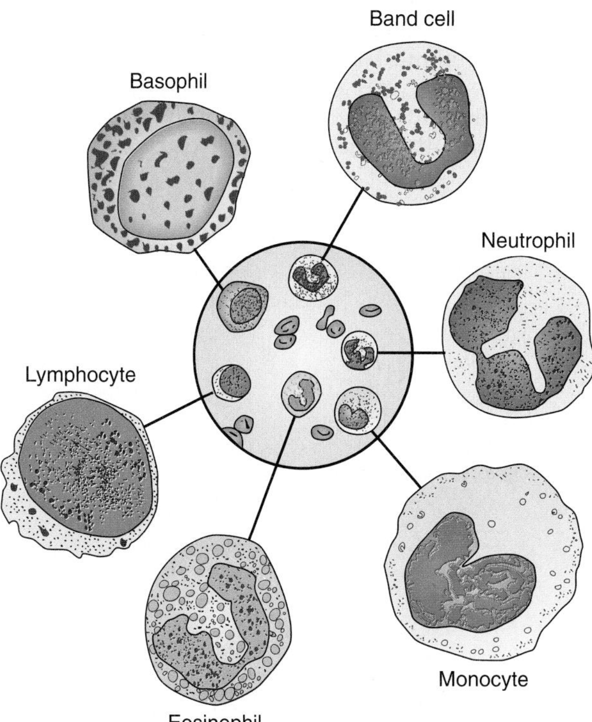

FIGURE 20-2 White blood cells.

The *neutrophil* is the primary phagocyte that arrives early at the site of inflammation, usually within 90 minutes of injury. Its cytoplasmic granules, which resist staining and remain a neutral color, contain enzymes and other antibacterial substances that are used in destroying and degrading the engulfed particles. Neutrophils also have oxygen-dependent metabolic pathways that generate toxic oxygen (*e.g.*, hydrogen peroxide) and nitrogen (*e.g.*, nitric oxide) products. Because these white blood cells have nuclei that are divided into three to five lobes, they often are called *polymorphonuclear neutrophils* (PMNs) or *segmented neutrophils* (segs). The neutrophil count in the blood often increases greatly during the inflammatory process, especially with bacterial infections. After being released from the bone marrow, circulating neutrophils have a life span of only approximately 10 hours and therefore must be constantly replaced if their numbers are to remain adequate. This requires an increase in circulating white blood cells, a condition called *leukocytosis.* With excessive demand for phagocytes, immature forms of neutrophils are released from the bone marrow. These immature cells often are called *bands* because of the horseshoe shape of their nuclei.

The cytoplasmic granules of the *eosinophils* stain red with the acid dye eosin. These granulocytes increase in the blood during allergic reactions and parasitic infections. The granules of eosinophils contain a protein that is highly toxic to large parasitic worms that cannot be phagocytized. They also regulate inflammation and allergic reactions by controlling the release of specific chemical mediators during these processes.

The granules of the *basophils,* which stain blue with a basic dye, contain histamine and other bioactive mediators of inflammation. The basophils are involved in producing the symptoms associated with inflammation and allergic reactions.

Mononuclear Phagocytes. The monocytes are the largest of the white blood cells and constitute 3% to 8% of the total blood leukocytes. The circulating life span of the monocyte is three to four times longer than that of the granulocytes, and they also survive for a longer time in the tissues. These longer-lived phagocytes help to destroy the causative agent, aid in the signaling processes of specific immunity, and serve to resolve the inflammatory process.

The monocytes, which migrate in increased numbers into the tissues in response to inflammatory stimuli, mature into macrophages. Within 24 hours, mononuclear cells arrive at the inflammatory site, and by 48 hours, monocytes and macrophages are the predominant cell types. The macrophages engulf larger and greater quantities of foreign material than the neutrophils. They also migrate to the local lymph nodes to prime specific immunity. These leukocytes play an important role in chronic inflammation, where they can surround and wall off foreign material that cannot be digested.

Mast Cells. The mast cell, which is widely distributed in connective tissues throughout the body, is very similar in many of its properties to the basophil. Mast cells are particularly prevalent along mucosal surfaces of the lung and gastrointestinal tract and the dermis of the skin. This distribution places the mast cell in a sentinel position between environmental antigens and the host for a variety of acute and chronic inflammatory conditions.[2] Sensitized mast cells, which are "armed" with immunoglobulin E (IgE), play a central role in allergic and hypersensitivity responses (see Chapter 21).

Leukocyte Response. The sequence of events in the cellular response to inflammation includes leukocyte: (1) margination, (2) emigration, (4) chemotaxis, and (3) phagocytosis (Fig. 20-3). During the early stages of the inflammatory response, fluid leaves the capillaries, causing blood viscosity to increase. The release of chemical mediators and cytokines affect the endothelial cells of the capillaries and cause the leukocytes to increase their expression of adhesion molecules. As this occurs, the leukocytes slow their migration and begin pavementing or moving along the periphery of the blood vessels.

Emigration is a mechanism by which the leukocytes extend pseudopodia, pass through the capillary walls by ameboid movement, and then migrate into the tissue spaces. The emigration of leukocytes also may be accompanied by an escape of red blood cells. Once they have exited the capillary, the leukocytes wander through the tissue guided by secreted cytokines, bacterial and cellular debris, and complement fragments (*e.g.*, C3a, C5a). The process by which leukocytes migrate in response to a chemical signal is called *chemotaxis*.

During the next and final stage of the cellular response, the neutrophils and macrophages engulf and degrade the bacteria and cellular debris in a process called *phagocytosis*. Phagocytosis involves three distinct steps: (1) opsonization plus attachment, (2) engulfment, and (3) intracellular killing (Fig. 20-4). Contact of the bacteria or antigen with the phagocyte cell membrane is essential for trapping the agent and triggering the final steps of phagocytosis. If the antigen is coated with antibody or complement, its adherence is increased because of binding to complement. The enhanced binding of an antigen due to antibody or complement is called *opsonization* (see Chapter 19). Engulfment follows the recognition of the agent as foreign. Cytoplasmic extensions (pseudopods) surround and enclose the particle in a membrane-bounded phagocytic vesicle or phagosome. In the cell cytoplasm, the phagosome merges with a lysosome containing antibacterial molecules and enzymes that can digest the microbe.

Intracellular killing of pathogens is accomplished through several mechanisms, including enzymes, defensins, and toxic oxygen and nitrogen products produced by oxygen-dependent metabolic pathways. The metabolic burst pathways that generate toxic oxygen and nitrogen products (*i.e.*, nitric oxide, peroxyonitrites, hydrogen per-

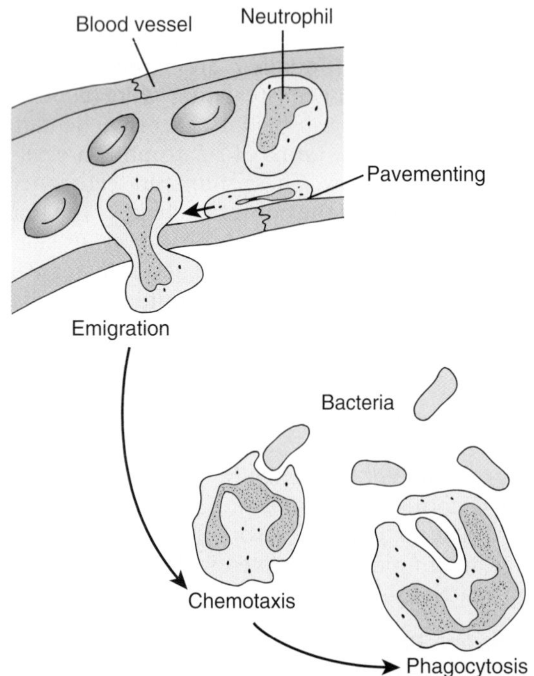

FIGURE 20-3 Cellular phase of acute inflammation. Neutrophil margination, emigration, chemotaxis, and phagocytosis.

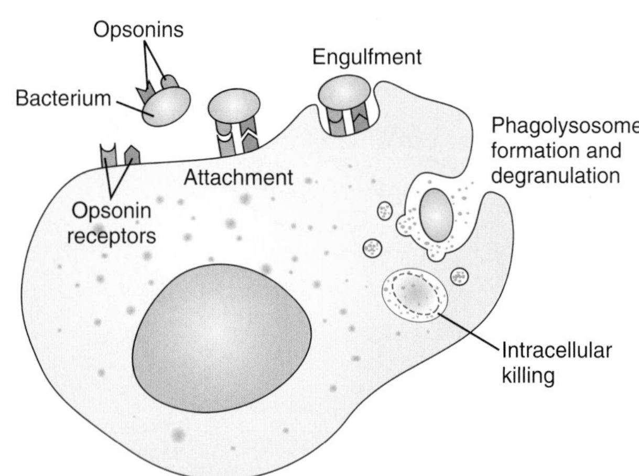

FIGURE 20-4 Phagocytosis of a particle (*e.g.*, bacterium): opsonization, attachment, engulfment, and intracellular killing.

oxide, and hypochlorous acid) require oxygen and metabolic enzymes such as myeloperoxidase, NADPH oxidase, and nitric oxide synthetase. Individuals born with genetic defects in some of these enzymes have immunodeficiency conditions that make them susceptible to repeated bacterial infection.

Inflammatory Mediators

Although inflammation is precipitated by injury, its signs and symptoms are produced by chemical mediators. Mediators can be classified by function: (1) those with vasoactive and smooth muscle–constricting properties such as histamine, prostaglandins, leukotrienes, and platelet-activating factor (PAF); (2) chemotactic factors such as complement fragments and cytokines; (3) plasma proteases that can activate complement and components of the clotting system; and (4) reactive molecules and cytokines liberated from leukocytes, which when released into the extracellular environment can damage the surrounding tissue (Table 20-1). Nitric oxide, which is produced by a variety of cells, plays multiple roles in inflammation, including smooth muscle relaxation, antagonism of platelet functions (adhesion, aggregation, and degranulation), reduction of leukocyte recruitment, and the killing of microbial agents by phagocytic cells.

Histamine. Histamine is widely distributed throughout the body. It is found in high concentration in circulating platelets and basophils. Preformed histamine is found in high concentrations in mast cells and is released in response to a variety of stimuli, including trauma and immune reactions involving binding of IgE antibodies. It is one of the first mediators of an inflammatory response. Histamine causes dilation and increased permeability of capillaries. Antihistamine drugs inhibit this immediate, transient response.

Plasma Proteases. The plasma proteases consist of the kinins, activated complement proteins, and clotting factors. One kinin, bradykinin, causes increased capillary permeability and pain. The clotting system (see Chapter 15) contributes to the vascular phase of inflammation, mainly through fibrinopeptides that are formed during the final steps of the clotting process. The complement system consists of a cascade of plasma proteins that plays an important role in both immunity and inflammation. Complement fragments contribute to the inflammatory response by (1) causing vasodilation and increasing vascular permeability; (2) promoting leukocyte activation, adhesion, and chemotaxis; and (3) augmenting phagocytosis (see Chapter 19).

Arachidonic Acid Metabolites. Arachidonic acid is a 20-carbon unsaturated fatty acid found in phospholipids of cell membranes. Release of arachidonic acid by phospholipases initiates a series of complex reactions that lead to the production of prostaglandins, leukotrienes, and other mediators of inflammation. The synthesis of inflammatory mediators follows one of two pathways: the cyclooxygenase pathway, which culminates in the synthesis of the prostaglandins, and the lipoxygenase pathway, which culminates in the synthesis of the leukotrienes (Fig. 20-5).

Several prostaglandins are synthesized from arachidonic acid through the cyclooxygenase metabolic pathway. The stable prostaglandins (PGE_1 and PGE_2) induce inflammation and potentiate the effects of histamine and other inflammatory mediators. The prostaglandin thromboxane A_2 promotes platelet aggregation and vasoconstriction. Aspirin and the nonsteroidal antiinflammatory drugs (NSAIDs) reduce inflammation by inactivating the first enzyme in the cyclooxygenase pathway for prostaglandin synthesis.

Like the prostaglandins, the leukotrienes are formed from arachidonic acid, but through the lipoxygenase pathway. Histamine and leukotrienes are complementary in action in that they have similar functions. Histamine is produced rapidly and transiently while the more potent leukotrienes are being synthesized. The leukotrienes also have been reported to affect the permeability of the postcapillary venules, the adhesion properties of endothelial cells, and the chemotaxis and extravasation of neutrophils, eosinophils, and monocytes. Leukotrienes C_4, D_4, and E_4, collectively known as the *slow-reacting substance of anaphylaxis* (SRS-A), cause slow and sustained constriction of the bronchioles and are important inflammatory mediators in bronchial asthma and anaphylaxis.

Platelet-activating Factor. Platelet-activating factor (PAF), which is generated from a complex lipid stored in cell membranes, affects a variety of cell types and induces platelet

TABLE 20-1 Signs of Inflammation and Corresponding Chemical Mediator

Inflammatory Response	Chemical Mediator
Swelling, redness, and tissue warmth (vasodilation and increased capillary permeability)	Histamine, prostaglandins, leukotrienes, bradykinin, platelet-activating factor
Tissue damage	Lysosomal enzymes and products released from neutrophils, macrophages, and other inflammatory cells
Chemotaxis	Complement fragments
Pain	Prostaglandins Bradykinin
Fever	Interleukin-1, interleukin-6 tumor necrosis factor
Leukocytosis	Interleukin-1, other cytokines

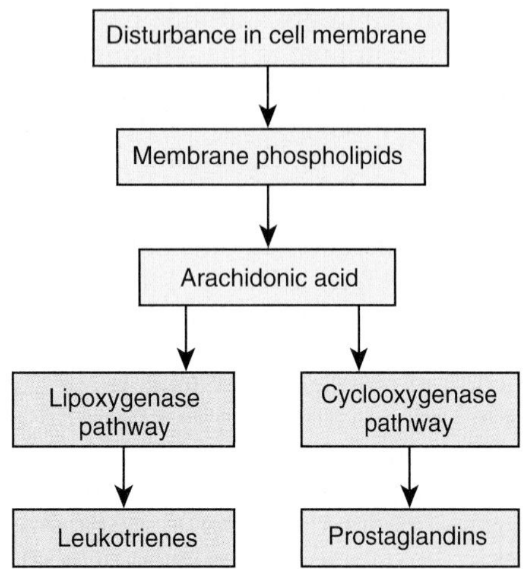

FIGURE 20-5 The cyclooxygenase and lipoxygenase pathways.

aggregation. It activates neutrophils and is a potent eosinophil chemoattractant. When injected into the skin, PAF causes a wheal-and-flare reaction and the leukocyte infiltrate characteristic of immediate hypersensitivity reactions. When inhaled, PAF causes bronchospasm, eosinophil infiltration, and nonspecific bronchial hyperreactivity.

Cytokines. Cytokines are polypeptide products of many cell types (but primarily lymphocytes and macrophages) that modulate the function of other cell types. They include the colony-stimulating factors that direct the growth of immature marrow precursor cells and the interleukins (ILs), interferons (IFNs), and tumor necrosis factor (TNF) that are important in the inflammatory response. The actions of the various cytokines are summarized in Chapter 19, Table 19-5.

CHRONIC INFLAMMATION

In contrast to acute inflammation, which is usually self-limited and of short duration, chronic inflammation is self-perpetuating and may last for weeks, months, or even years. It may develop as the result of a recurrent or progressive acute inflammatory process or from low-grade, smoldering responses that fail to evoke an acute response.

Characteristic of chronic inflammation is an infiltration by mononuclear cells (macrophages) and lymphocytes instead of the influx of neutrophils commonly seen in acute inflammation. Chronic inflammation also involves the proliferation of fibroblasts instead of exudates. As a result, the risk for scarring and deformity usually is considered greater than in acute inflammation. Agents that evoke chronic inflammation typically are low-grade, persistent irritants that are unable to penetrate deeply or spread rapidly. Among the causes of chronic inflammation are foreign bodies such as talc, silica, asbestos, and surgical suture materials. Many viruses provoke chronic inflammatory responses, as do certain bacteria, fungi, and larger parasites of moderate to low virulence. Examples are the tubercle bacillus, the treponema of syphilis, and the actinomyces. The presence of injured tissue such as that surrounding a healing fracture also may incite chronic inflammation. Immunologic mechanisms are thought to play an important role in chronic inflammation. The two patterns of chronic inflammation are a nonspecific chronic inflammation and granulomatous inflammation.

Nonspecific Chronic Inflammation

Nonspecific chronic inflammation involves a diffuse accumulation of macrophages and lymphocytes at the site of injury. Ongoing chemotaxis causes macrophages to infiltrate the inflamed site, where they accumulate owing to prolonged survival and immobilization. These mechanisms lead to fibroblast proliferation, with subsequent scar formation that in many cases replaces the normal connective tissue or the functional parenchymal tissues of the involved structures. For example, scar tissue resulting from chronic inflammation of the bowel causes narrowing of the bowel lumen.

Granulomatous Inflammation

A granulomatous lesion is a distinctive form of chronic inflammation. A *granuloma* typically is a small, 1- to 2-mm lesion in which there is a massing of macrophages surrounded by lymphocytes. These modified macrophages resemble epithelial cells and sometimes are called *epithelioid cells*. Like other macrophages, these epithelioid cells are derived originally from blood monocytes. Granulomatous inflammation is associated with foreign bodies such as splinters, sutures, silica, and asbestos and with microorganisms that cause tuberculosis, syphilis, sarcoidosis, deep fungal infections, and brucellosis. These types of agents have one thing in common: they are poorly digested and usually are not easily controlled by other inflammatory mechanisms. The epithelioid cells in granulomatous inflammation may clump in a mass or coalesce, forming a multinucleated giant cell that attempts to surround the foreign agent (Fig. 20-6). A dense membrane of connective tissue eventually encapsulates the lesion and isolates it. These cells are often referred to as foreign-body giant cells.

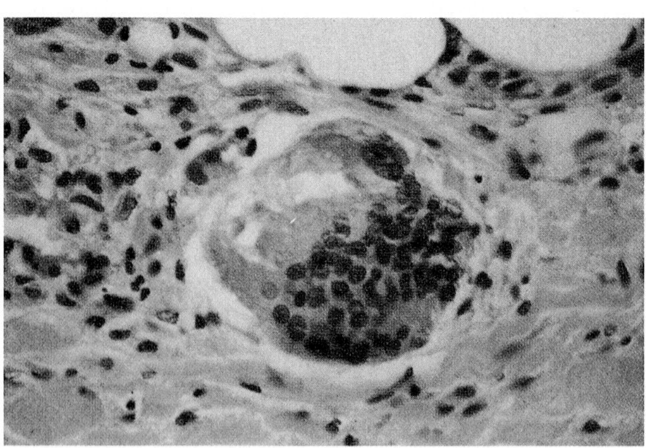

FIGURE 20-6 Foreign-body giant cell. The numerous nuclei are randomly arranged in the cytoplasm. (Rubin E., Farber J. L. [1999]. *Pathology* [3rd ed., p. 40]. Philadelphia: Lippincott-Raven)

A *tubercle* is a granulomatous inflammatory response to *Mycobacterium tuberculosis* infection. Peculiar to the tuberculosis granuloma is the presence of a caseous (cheesy) necrotic center.

LOCAL MANIFESTATIONS OF INFLAMMATION

The local manifestations of acute and chronic inflammation are dependent on its cause and the particular tissue involved. These manifestations can range from swelling and the formation of exudates to abscess formation or ulceration.

Characteristically, the acute inflammatory response involves production of exudates. These exudates vary in terms of fluid, plasma proteins, and cell count. Acute inflammation can produce serous, hemorrhagic, fibrinous, membranous, or purulent exudates. Inflammatory exudates often are composed of a combination of these types. *Serous exudates* are watery fluids low in protein content that result from plasma entering the inflammatory site. *Hemorrhagic exudates* occur when there is severe tissue injury that causes damage to blood vessels or when there is significant leakage of red cells from the capillaries. *Fibrinous exudates* contain large amounts of fibrinogen and form a thick and sticky meshwork, much like the fibers of a blood clot. *Membranous* or *pseudomembranous exudates* develop on mucous membrane surfaces and are composed of necrotic cells enmeshed in a fibropurulent exudate.

A *purulent* or *suppurative exudate* contains pus, which is composed of degraded white blood cells, proteins, and tissue debris. Certain microorganisms, such as staphylococci, are more likely to induce localized suppurative inflammation than others. An abscess is a localized area of inflammation containing a purulent exudate (Fig. 20-7). Abscesses typically have a central necrotic core containing purulent exudates surrounded by a layer of neutrophils.[2] Fibroblasts may eventually enter the area and wall off the abscess. Because antimicrobial agents cannot penetrate the abscess wall, surgical incision and drainage may be required to effect a cure.

An *ulceration* refers to a site of inflammation where an epithelial surface (*e.g.*, skin or gastrointestinal epithelium) has become necrotic and eroded, often with associated subepithelial inflammation. Ulceration may occur as the result of traumatic injury to the epithelial surface (*e.g.*, peptic ulcer) or because of vascular compromise (*e.g.*, foot ulcers associated with diabetes). In chronic lesions where there is repeated insult, the area surrounding the ulcer develops fibroblastic proliferation, scarring, and accumulation of chronic inflammatory cells.[2]

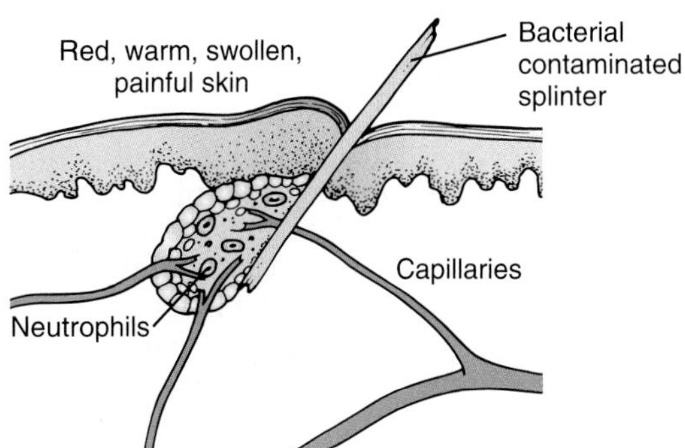

A Inflammation
Capillary dilation, fluid exudation, neutrophil migration

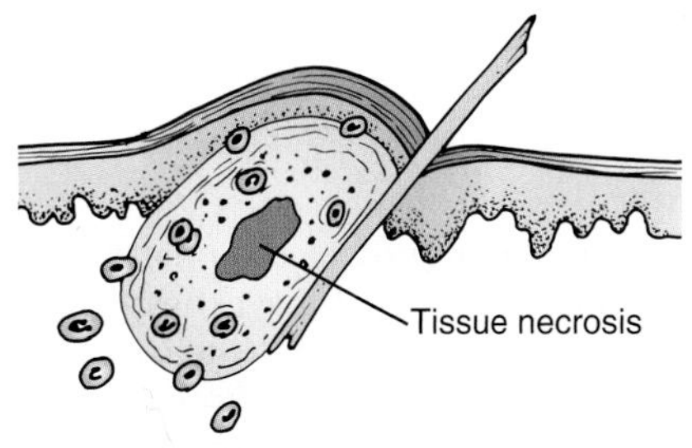

B Suppuration
Development of suppurative or purulent exudate containing degraded neutrophils and tissue debris

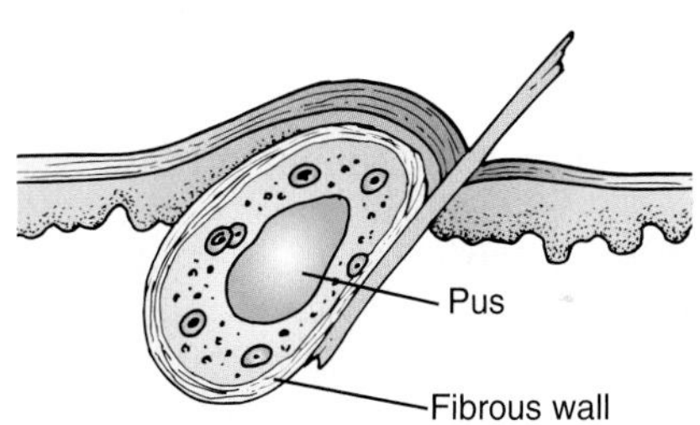

C Abscess formation
Walling off of the area of purulent (pus) exudate to form an abscess

FIGURE 20-7 Abscess formation. (**A**) Bacterial invasion and development of inflammation. (**B**) Continued bacterial growth, neutrophil migration, liquefaction tissue necrosis, and development of a purulent exudate. (**C**) Walling off of the inflamed area with its purulent exudate to form an abscess.

SYSTEMIC MANIFESTATIONS OF INFLAMMATION

Under optimal conditions, the inflammatory response remains confined to a localized area. In some cases, however, local injury can result in prominent systemic manifestations as inflammatory mediators are released into the circulation. The most prominent systemic manifestations of inflammation are the acute-phase response, alterations in white blood cell count (leukocytosis or leukopenia), and fever. Sepsis and septic shock, also called the *systemic inflammatory response,* represent the severe systemic manifestations of inflammation (see Chapter 28).

Acute-Phase Response

Along with the cellular responses that occur during the inflammatory response, a constellation of systemic effects called the *acute-phase response* occurs. The acute-phase response, which usually begins within hours or days of the onset of inflammation or infection, includes changes in the concentrations of plasma proteins, increased erythrocyte sedimentation rate, fever, increased numbers of leukocytes, skeletal muscle catabolism, and negative nitrogen balance. These responses are generated by the release of cytokines, particularly IL-1, IL-6, and TNF-α. These cytokines affect the thermoregulatory center in the hypothalamus to produce fever, the most obvious sign of the acute-phase response. IL-1 and other cytokines induce an increase in the number and immaturity of circulating neutrophils by stimulating their production in the bone marrow. Lethargy, a common feature of the acute-phase response, results from the effects of IL-1 and TNF-α on the central nervous system. The metabolic changes, including skeletal muscle catabolism, provide amino acids that can be used in the immune response and for tissue repair. In general, the acute-phase response serves to coordinate the various changes in body activity to enable an optimal host response.

Acute-Phase Proteins. During the acute-phase response, the liver dramatically increases the synthesis of acute-phase proteins, such as fibrinogen and C-reactive protein (CRP), that serve several different nonspecific defense functions. Increased plasma levels of some acute-phase proteins are reflected in an accelerated erythrocyte sedimentation rate (ESR).

CRP, first described in 1930, is the classic acute-phase reactant. It was originally named *C precipitant* or *C-reactive substance* because it precipitated with the C fraction (C-polypeptide) of pneumococci. Ultimately, it was determined to be a protein; hence, its permanent designation became *C-reactive protein.*[5] The complete amino acid sequence of CRP has been described, and it can be accurately measured in the laboratory. Everyone maintains a low level of CRP; this level rises when there is an acute inflammatory response, sometimes to a factor of 500 or more. The function of CRP is thought to be protective, in that it binds to the surface of invading microorganisms and targets them for destruction by complement and phagocytosis. It is also thought to have an antiinflammatory function, neutralizing antiinflammatory cytokines, proteases, and oxidants released into the blood from inflamed tissues. Recent interest has focused on the use of CRP as a predictor of risk in cardiovascular events in persons with coronary heart disease.[6,7]

The ESR, which measures the rate at which erythrocytes settle out of anticoagulated blood, is used as a qualitative index to monitor the activity of many inflammatory diseases. The presence of increased levels of acute-phase proteins is associated with an increase in the ESR. The increased levels of acute-phase proteins are thought to dampen the repulsive effects of like charges on red blood cells, causing them to clump or aggregate, forming stacks (rouleau formation).

White Blood Cell Response (Leukocytosis and Leukopenia)

Leukocytosis, or the increase in white blood cells, is a common feature of the inflammatory response, especially that caused by bacterial infection. The white blood cell count commonly increases to 15,000 to 20,000 cells/μL (normal, 4000 to 10,000 cells/μL) in acute inflammatory conditions. After being released from the bone marrow, circulating neutrophils have a life span of only about 10 hours and therefore must be constantly replaced if their numbers are to be adequate. With excessive demand for phagocytes, immature forms of neutrophils (bands) are released from the bone marrow. The phase, which is referred to as a *shift to the left* in a white blood cell differential count, refers to the increase in immature neutrophils seen in severe infections.

Bacterial infections produce a relatively selective increase in neutrophils (neutrophilia), whereas parasitic and allergic responses induce eosinophilia. Viral infections tend to produce a decrease in neutrophils (neutropenia) and an increase in lymphocytes (lymphocytosis).[3] Leukopenia is also encountered in infections that overwhelm persons with other debilitating diseases, such as cancer.

Lymphadenitis

Localized acute and chronic inflammation may lead to a reaction in the lymph nodes that drain the affected area. This response represents a nonspecific response to mediators released from the injured tissue or an immunologic response to a specific antigen. Painful palpable nodes are more commonly associated with inflammatory processes, whereas nonpainful lymph nodes are more characteristic of neoplasms.[1]

In summary, inflammation describes a local response to tissue injury and can present as an acute or chronic condition. The classic signs of inflammation are redness, swelling, local heat, pain, and loss of function. It involves a hemodynamic phase during which blood flow and capillary permeability are increased, and a cellular phase during which phagocytic white blood cells move into the area to engulf and degrade the inciting agent. The inflammatory response is orchestrated by chemical mediators such as histamine, prostaglandins, PAF, complement fragments, and reactive molecules that are liberated by leukocytes.

In contrast to acute inflammation, which is self-limiting, chronic inflammation is prolonged and usually is caused by persistent irritants, most of which are insoluble and resistant to phagocytosis and other inflammatory mechanisms. Chronic inflammation involves the presence of mononuclear cells (lymphocytes and macrophages) rather than granulocytes.

The local manifestations of acute and chronic inflammation depend on the agent and extent of injury. Acute inflammation may involve the production of exudates containing serous fluid (serous exudate), red blood cells (hemorrhagic exudate), fibrinogen (fibrinous exudate), or tissue debris and white blood cell breakdown products (purulent exudate). *Ulceration* occurs at the site of inflammation where an epithelial surface (skin or mucous membranes) has become necrotic and eroded. In chronic lesions where there is repeated insult, the area surrounding the ulcer develops fibroblastic proliferation, scarring, and accumulation of chronic inflammatory cells.

The systemic manifestations of inflammation include the systemic effects of the acute-phase response, such as an increased ESR, fever, and lethargy; increased levels of CRP and other acute-phase proteins; and leukocytosis or, in some cases, leukopenia. These responses are mediated by release of cytokines such as IL-1, TNF-α, and IL-6. Localized acute and chronic inflammation may lead to a reaction in the lymph nodes and enlargement of the lymph nodes that drain the affected area.

Tissue Repair and Wound Healing

After completing this section of the chapter, you should be able to meet the following objectives:

- Define the terms *parenchymal* and *stromal* as they relate to the tissues of an organ
- Compare labile, stable, and permanent cell types in terms of their capacity for regeneration
- Describe healing by primary and secondary intention
- Explain the effects of soluble mediators and the extracellular matrix on tissue repair and wound healing
- Trace the wound-healing process through the inflammatory, proliferative, and remodeling phases
- Explain the effect of malnutrition; ischemia and oxygen deprivation; impaired immune and inflammatory responses; and infection, wound separation, and foreign bodies on wound healing
- Discuss the effect of age on wound healing

TISSUE REPAIR

Tissue repair, which overlaps the inflammatory process, is a response to tissue injury and represents an attempt to maintain normal body structure and function. It can take the form of regeneration in which the injured cells are replaced with cells of the same type, sometimes leaving no residual trace of previous injury, or it can take the form of replacement by connective tissue, which leaves a permanent scar. Both regeneration and repair by connective tissue replacement are determined by similar mechanisms involving cell migration, proliferation, and differentiation as well as interaction with the extracellular matrix.

Tissue Regeneration

Body organs and tissues are composed of two types of structures: parenchymal and stromal. The parenchymal (*i.e.*, from the Greek for "anything poured in") tissues contain the functioning cells of an organ or body part (*e.g.*, hepatocytes, renal tubular cells). The stromal tissues (*i.e.*, from the Greek for "something laid out to lie on") consist of the supporting connective tissues, blood vessels, extracellular matrix, and nerve fibers.

Tissue regeneration involves repair of the injured tissue with cells of the same parenchymal type, leaving little or no evidence of the previous injury. It is dependent on cell proliferation and the ability of the cells to enter and move through the cell cycle (see Chapter 8).

Cell proliferation and the ability to regenerate vary with the tissue and cell type. Body cells are divided into three types according to their ability to undergo regeneration: labile, stable, or permanent cells.[8,9]

Labile cells are those that continue to divide and replicate throughout life, replacing cells that are continually being destroyed. Labile cells can be found in tissues that have a daily turnover of cells. They include the surface epithelial cells of the skin, oral cavity, vagina, and cervix; the columnar epithelium of the gastrointestinal tract, uterus, and fallopian tubes; the transitional epithelium of the urinary tract; and bone marrow cells.

Stable cells are those that normally stop dividing when growth ceases. These cells are capable, however, of undergoing regeneration when confronted with an appropriate stimulus. For stable cells to regenerate and restore tissues to their original state, the supporting stromal framework must be present. When this framework has been destroyed, the replacement of tissues is haphazard. The hepatocytes of the liver are one form of stable cell, and the importance of the supporting framework to regeneration is evidenced by two forms of liver disease. In some types of viral hepatitis, there is selective destruction of the parenchymal liver cells, whereas the cells of the supporting tissue remain unharmed. After the disease has subsided, the injured cells regenerate, and liver function returns to normal. In cirrhosis of the liver, disorganized bands of fibrous tissue form and replace the normal supporting architecture of the liver, causing disordered replacement of liver cells and disturbance of hepatic blood flow and liver function.

Permanent or *fixed cells* cannot undergo mitotic division. The fixed cells include nerve cells, skeletal cells, and cardiac muscle cells. These cells cannot regenerate; once destroyed, they are replaced with fibrous scar tissue that lacks the functional characteristics of the destroyed parenchymal cells. For example, the scar tissue that develops in the heart (Fig. 20-8) after a heart attack cannot conduct impulses or contract to pump blood.

TISSUE REPAIR AND WOUND HEALING

- Injured tissues can be repaired by regeneration of the injured tissue cells with cells of the same tissue or parenchymal type, or by connective repair processes in which scar tissue is used to effect healing.
- Regeneration is limited to tissues with cells that are able to undergo mitosis.
- Connective tissue repair occurs by primary or secondary intention and involves the inflammatory phase, the proliferative phase, and remodeling phases of the wound healing process.
- Wound healing is impaired by conditions that diminish blood flow and oxygen delivery, restrict nutrients and other materials needed for healing, and depress the inflammatory and immune responses; and by infection, wound separation, and the presence of foreign bodies.

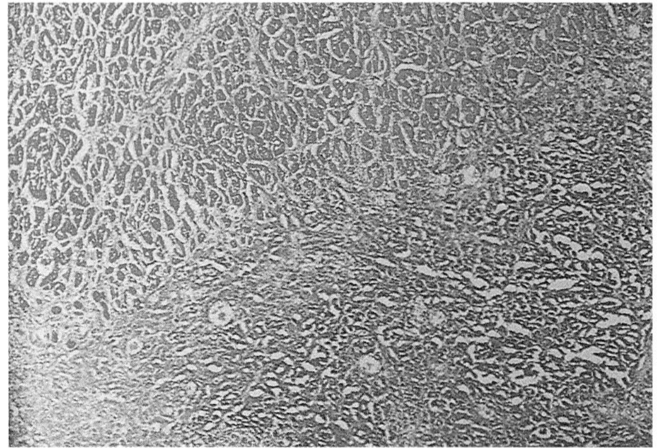

FIGURE 20-8 Healed myocardial infarct. Tissues with permanent cells are replaced with scar tissue only. (Rubin E., Farber J. L. [1999]. *Pathology* [3rd ed., p. 102]. Philadelphia: Lippincott-Raven)

Extracellular Matrix

The *extracellular matrix* (ECM), which is secreted locally, assembles into a network of spaces surrounding tissue cells (see Chapter 4). There are three basic components of the ECM: fibrous structural proteins (*e.g.,* collagen and elastin fibers), water-hydrated gels (*e.g.,* proteoglycans and hyaluronan) that permit resilience and lubrication, and adhesive glycoproteins (*e.g.,* fibronectin and laminin) that connect the matrix elements one to another and to cells.[8,9] The ECM occurs in two basic forms: (1) the *basement membrane* that surrounds epithelial, endothelial, and smooth muscle cells; and (2) the *interstitial matrix* that is present in the spaces between cells in connective tissue and between the epithelium and supporting cells of blood vessels.

The ECM provides turgor to soft tissue and rigidity to bone; it supplies the substratum for cell adhesion; it is involved in the regulation of growth, movement, and differentiation of the cells surrounding it; and it provides for the storage and presentation of regulatory molecules. For example, fibroblast growth factor (FGF) is excreted and stored in the basement membrane of normal tissues. The ECM also provides the scaffolding for tissue renewal. Although the cells in many tissues are capable of regeneration, injury does not always result in restitution of normal structure unless the ECM is intact. The integrity of the underlying basement membrane, in particular, is critical to the regeneration of tissue. When the basement membrane is disrupted, cells proliferate in a haphazard way, resulting in disorganized and nonfunctional tissues.

Fibrous Tissue Repair

Severe or persistent injury with damage to both the parenchymal cells and ECM leads to a situation in which the repair cannot be accomplished with regeneration alone. Under these conditions, repair occurs by replacement with connective tissue, a process that involves formation of granulation tissue and development of scar tissue.

Granulation Tissue. Granulation tissue is a highly vascular connective tissue that contains newly formed capillaries, proliferating fibroblasts, and residual inflammatory cells. The development of granulation tissue involves the growth of new capillaries (angiogenesis), fibrogenesis, and involution to the formation of scar tissue.

Angiogenesis involves the generation and sprouting of new blood vessels from preexisting vessels. These sprouting capillaries tend to protrude from the surface of the wound as minute red granules, imparting the name *granulation tissue.* Eventually, portions of the new capillary bed differentiate into arterioles and venules. There are four steps in development of a new capillary vessel: (1) proteolytic degradation of the parent vessel basement membrane, allowing for formation of a capillary sprout; (2) migration of endothelial cells from the original capillary toward an angiogenic stimuli; (3) proliferation of the endothelial cells behind the leading edge of the migrating cells; and (4) maturation of the endothelial cells and proliferation of pericytes (for capillaries) and smooth muscle cells (for larger vessels).

Fibrogenesis involves the influx of activated fibroblasts. Activated fibroblasts secrete ECM components, including fibronectin, hyaluronic acid, proteoglycans, and collagen. Fibronectin and hyaluronic acid are the first to be deposited in the healing wound, and proteoglycans appear later. Because the proteoglycans are hydrophilic, their accumulation contributes to the edematous appearance of the wound. The initiation of collagen synthesis contributes to subsequent formation of scar tissue.

Development of Scar Tissue. Scar formation builds on the granulation tissue framework of new vessels and loose ECM. The process occurs in two phases: (1) emigration and proliferation of fibroblasts into the site of injury, and (2) deposition of ECM by these cells. As healing progresses, the number of proliferating fibroblasts and new vessels decreases, and there is increased synthesis and deposition of collagen. Collagen synthesis is important to the development of strength in the healing wound site. Ultimately, the granulation tissue scaffolding evolves into a scar composed of largely inactive spindle-shaped fibroblasts, dense collagen fibers, fragments of elastic tissue, and other ECM components. As the scar matures, vascular regeneration eventually transforms the highly vascular granulation tissue into a pale, largely avascular scar.

Regulation of the Healing Process

Regulation of the healing process is determined by the action of chemical mediators and growth factors that mediate the healing process as well as interactions between the extracellular and cell matrix.

Chemical Mediators and Growth Factors. Considerable research has contributed to the understanding of chemical mediators and growth factors that orchestrate the healing process. These chemical mediators and growth factors are released in an orderly manner from many of the cells that participate in tissue regeneration and the healing process. Growth factors act as chemoattractants, enhancing the migration of white blood cells and fibroblasts to the wound site, and others act as mitogens, causing increased proliferation of cells that participate in the healing process.[10,11]

The chemical mediators include the interleukins, interferons, tumor necrosis factor, and arachidonic acid derivatives (prostaglandins and leukotrienes) that participate in the inflammatory response. The growth factors are hormone-like molecules that interact with specific cell surface receptors to control processes involved in tissue repair and wound healing. They may act on adjacent cells or on the cell producing the growth factor. Some growth factors are transported through plasma to more distant sites and thus act as endocrine factors.

The growth factors are named for their tissue of origin (*e.g.,* platelet-derived growth factor [PDGF], fibroblast growth factor [FGF]), their biological activity (*e.g.,* transforming growth factor [TGF]), or the cells on which they act (*e.g.,* epithelial growth factor [EGF]). The growth factors control the proliferation, differentiation, and metabolism of cells during each of the three phases of wound healing. They assist in regulating the inflammatory process, serve as chemoattractants for neutrophils, monocytes (macrophages), fibroblasts, and epithelial cells; stimulate angiogenesis; and contribute to the generation of the ECM.

Extracellular Matrix and Cell Matrix Interactions. The transition from granulation tissue to scar tissue involves shifts in the composition of the ECM with continued ECM synthesis and degradation. In the transitional process, the matrix components are degraded by ECM enzymes (proteases) that are secreted locally by a variety of cells (fibroblasts, macrophages, neutrophils, synovial cells, and epithelial cells). Many of these proteases are matrix metalloproteases (MMPs), so named because they depend on zinc for their activity.[12] Some of the metalloproteases, such as the collagenases, are highly specific, cleaving particular proteins at a small number of sites. This allows for the structural integrity of the ECM to be retained, whereas cell migration can be greatly facilitated by a small amount of proteolysis. It is particularly important in débridement of injured tissue and in remodeling of the ECM necessary for wound repair.[8,9]

Because of their potential to produce havoc in tissues, the actions of the MMPs are tightly controlled. They are typically elaborated in an inactive form that must be first activated by certain chemicals or proteases that are likely to be present at the site of injury, and they are rapidly inactivated by tissue inhibitors. Recent research has focused on the unregulated action of the metalloproteases in disorders such as cartilage matrix breakdown in arthritis and neuroinflammation in multiple sclerosis.[12]

WOUND HEALING

Injured tissues are repaired by regeneration of parenchymal cells or by connective tissue repair in which scar tissue is substituted for the parenchymal cells of the injured tissue. The primary objective of the healing process is to fill the gap created by tissue destruction and to restore the structural continuity of the injured part. When regeneration cannot occur, healing by replacement with a connective scar tissue provides the means for maintaining this continuity. Although scar tissue fills the gap created by tissue death, it does not repair the structure with functioning parenchymal cells. Because the regenerative capabilities of most tissues are limited, wound healing usually involves some connective tissue repair. The following discussion particularly addresses skin wounds.

Healing by Primary and Secondary Intention

Depending on the extent of tissue loss, wound closure and healing occur by *primary* or *secondary* intention (Fig. 20-9). A sutured surgical incision is an example of healing by primary intention. Larger wounds (*e.g.,* burns and large surface wounds) that have a greater loss of tissue and contamination, heal by secondary intention. Healing by secondary intention is slower than healing by primary intention and results in the formation of larger amounts of scar tissue. A wound that might otherwise have healed by primary intention may become infected and heal by secondary intention.

Phases of Wound Healing

Wound healing is commonly divided into three phases: (1) the inflammatory phase, (2) the proliferative phase, and (3) the maturational or remodeling phase.[8,9,13–16] The duration of the phases is fairly predictable in wounds healing by primary intention. In wounds healing by secondary intention, the process depends on the extent of injury and the healing environment.

Inflammatory Phase. The inflammatory phase of wound healing begins at the time of injury and is a critical period because it prepares the wound environment for healing (Fig. 20-10). It includes hemostasis (see Chapter 15) and the vascular and cellular phases of inflammation. Hemostatic processes are activated immediately at the time of injury. There is constriction of injured blood vessels and initiation of blood clotting by way of platelet activation and aggregation. After a brief period of constriction, these

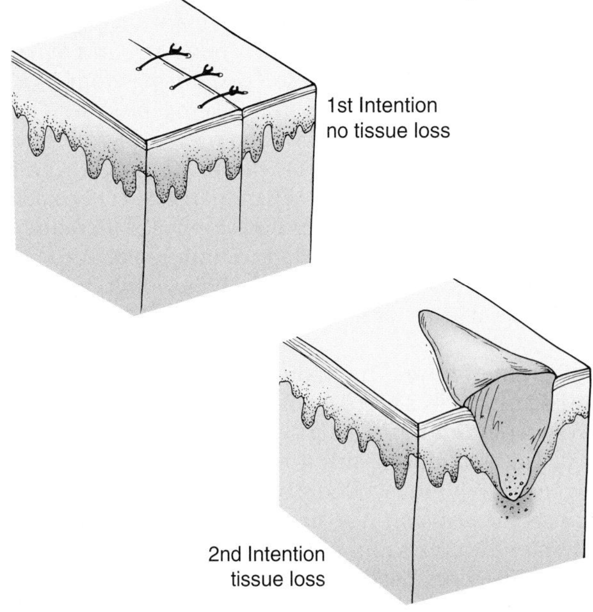

FIGURE 20-9 Healing of a skin wound by first and second intention.

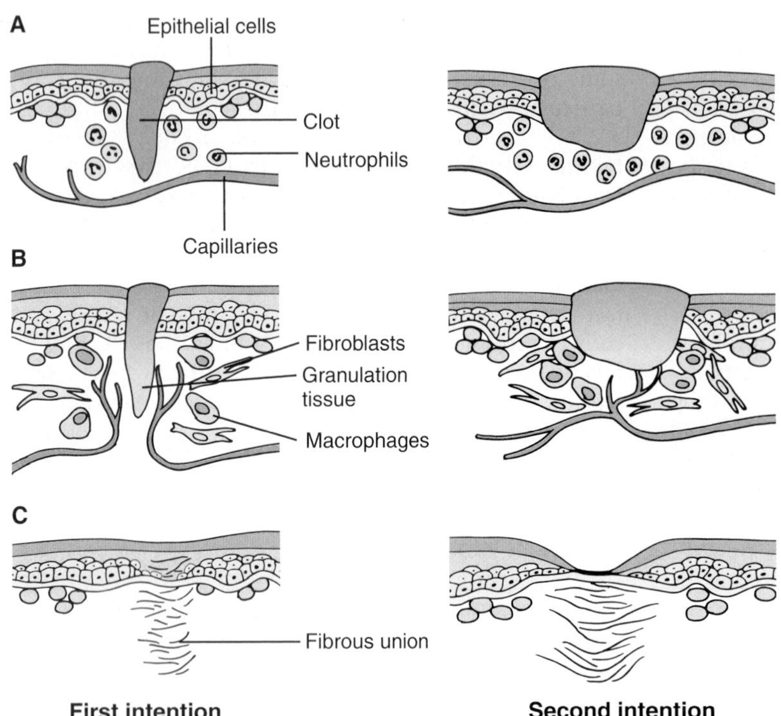

FIGURE 20-10 The phases in healing of a skin wound by primary and secondary intention. (**A**) The inflammatory phase with formation of a blood clot and migration of neutrophils. (**B**) The proliferative phase with migration of macrophages and fibroblasts, proliferation of vascular endothelial cells, and development of granulation tissue. (**C**) Remodeling stage with development of the fibrous scar, disappearance of increased vascularity, and exit of inflammatory cells.

same vessels dilate, and capillaries increase their permeability, allowing plasma and blood components to leak into the injured area. In small surface wounds, the clot loses fluid and becomes a hard, desiccated scab that protects the area.

The cellular phase of inflammation follows and is evidenced by the migration of phagocytic white blood cells that digest and remove invading organisms, fibrin, extracellular debris, and other foreign matter. The neutrophils are the first cells to arrive and are usually gone by day 3 or 4. They ingest bacteria and cellular debris. After approximately 24 hours, macrophages, which are larger and less specific phagocytic cells, enter the wound area and remain for an extended period. These cells, arising from blood monocytes, are essential to the healing process. Their functions include phagocytosis and release of growth factors that stimulate epithelial cell growth, angiogenesis, and attraction of fibroblasts. When a large defect occurs in deeper tissues, neutrophils and macrophages are required to remove the debris and facilitate wound closure. Although a wound may heal in the absence of neutrophils, it cannot heal in the absence of macrophages.

Proliferative Phase. The proliferative phase of healing usually begins within 2 to 3 days of injury and may last as long as 3 weeks in wounds healing by primary intention. The primary processes during this time focus on the building of new tissue to fill the wound space. The key cell during this phase is the *fibroblast.* The fibroblast is a connective tissue cell that synthesizes and secretes collagen and other intercellular elements needed for wound healing. Fibroblasts also produce a family of growth factors that induce angiogenesis and endothelial cell proliferation and migration.

As early as 24 to 48 hours after injury, fibroblasts and vascular endothelial cells begin proliferating to form the granulation tissue that serves as the foundation for scar tissue development. This tissue is fragile and bleeds easily because of the numerous, newly developed capillary buds. Wounds that heal by secondary intention have more necrotic debris and exudate that must be removed, and they involve larger amounts of granulation tissue. The newly formed blood vessels are leaky and allow plasma proteins and white blood cells to leak into the tissues.

The final component of the proliferative phase is epithelialization, which is the migration, proliferation, and differentiation of the epithelial cells at the wound edges to form a new surface layer that is similar to that destroyed by the injury. In wounds that heal by primary intention, these epidermal cells proliferate and seal the wound within 24 to 48 hours.[9] Because epithelial cell migration requires a moist vascular wound surface and is impeded by a dry or necrotic wound surface, epithelialization is delayed in open wounds until a bed of granulation tissue has formed. When a scab has formed on the wound, the epithelial cells migrate between it and the underlying viable tissue; when a significant portion of the wound has been covered with epithelial tissue, the scab lifts off.

At times, excessive granulation tissue, sometimes referred to as *proud flesh,* may form and extend above the edges of the wound, preventing reepithelialization from taking place. Surgical removal or chemical cauterization of the defect allows healing to proceed.

As the proliferative phase progresses, there is continued accumulation of collagen and proliferation of fibroblasts. Collagen synthesis reaches a peak within 5 to 7 days and continues for several weeks, depending on wound size. By the second week, the white blood cells have largely left the area, the edema has diminished, and the wound begins to blanch as the small blood vessels become thrombosed and degenerate.

Remodeling Phase. The third phase of wound healing, the remodeling process, begins approximately 3 weeks after injury and can continue for 6 months or longer, depending on the extent of the wound. As the term implies, there is continued remodeling of scar tissue by simultaneous synthesis of collagen by fibroblasts and lysis by collagenase enzymes. As a result of these two processes, the architecture of the scar becomes reoriented to increase the tensile strength of the wound.

Most wounds do not regain the full tensile strength of unwounded skin after healing is completed. Carefully sutured wounds immediately after surgery have approximately 70% of the strength of unwounded skin, largely because of the placement of the sutures. This allows persons to move about freely after surgery without fear of wound separation. When the sutures are removed, usually at the end of the first week, wound strength is approximately 10%. It increases rapidly over the next 4 weeks and then slows, reaching a plateau of approximately 70% to 80% of the tensile strength of unwounded skin at the end of 3 months.[9] An injury that heals by secondary intention undergoes wound contraction during the proliferative and remodeling phases. As a result, the scar that forms is considerably smaller than the original wound. Cosmetically, this may be desirable because it reduces the size of the visible defect. However, contraction of scar tissue over joints and other body structures tends to limit movement and cause deformities. As a result of loss of elasticity, scar tissue that is stretched fails to return to its original length.

An abnormality in healing by scar tissue repair is *keloid* formation. Keloids are tumor-like masses caused by excess production of scar tissue (Fig. 20-11). The tendency toward development of keloids is more common in African Americans and seems to have a genetic basis.

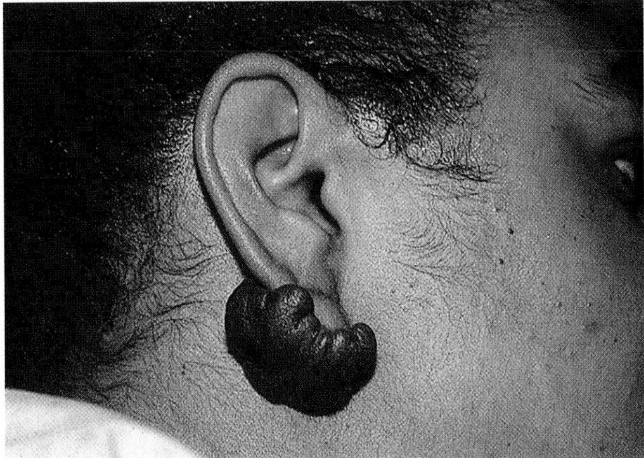

FIGURE 20-11 Keloid. A light-skinned black woman with keloid that developed following ear piercing. (Rubin E., Farber J. L. [1999]. *Pathology* [3rd ed., p. 99]. Philadelphia: Lippincott-Raven)

Factors That Affect Wound Healing

Many local and systemic factors influence wound healing. Although there are many factors that impair healing, science has found a few ways to hasten the normal process of wound repair. Among the causes of impaired wound healing are malnutrition; impaired blood flow and oxygen delivery; impaired inflammatory and immune responses; infection, wound separation, and foreign bodies; and age effects.

Malnutrition. Successful wound healing depends in part on adequate stores of proteins, carbohydrates, fats, vitamins, and minerals. It is well recognized that malnutrition slows the healing process, causing wounds to heal inadequately or incompletely.[17–19] Protein deficiencies prolong the inflammatory phase of healing and impair fibroblast proliferation, collagen and protein matrix synthesis, angiogenesis, and wound remodeling. Carbohydrates are needed as an energy source for white blood cells. Carbohydrates also have a protein-sparing effect and help to prevent the use of amino acids for fuel when they are needed for the healing process. Fats are essential constituents of cell membranes and are needed for the synthesis of new cells.

Although most vitamins are essential cofactors for the daily functions of the body, vitamins A and C play an essential role in the healing process. Vitamin C is needed for collagen synthesis. In vitamin C deficiency, improper sequencing of amino acids occurs, proper linking of amino acids does not take place, the byproducts of collagen synthesis are not removed from the cell, new wounds do not heal properly, and old wounds may fall apart. Administration of vitamin C rapidly restores the healing process to normal. Vitamin A functions in stimulating and supporting epithelialization, capillary formation, and collagen synthesis. Vitamin A also has been shown to counteract the anti-inflammatory effects of corticosteroid drugs and can be used to reverse these effects in persons who are on chronic steroid therapy. The B vitamins are important cofactors in enzymatic reactions that contribute to the wound-healing process. All are water soluble, and with the exception of vitamin B_{12}, which is stored in the liver, almost all must be replaced daily. Vitamin K plays an indirect role in wound healing by preventing bleeding disorders that contribute to hematoma formation and subsequent infection.

The role of minerals in wound healing is less clearly defined. The macrominerals, including sodium, potassium, calcium, and phosphorus, as well as the microminerals, such as copper and zinc, must be present for normal cell function. Zinc is a cofactor in a variety of enzyme systems responsible for cell proliferation. In animal studies, zinc has been found to aid in reepithelialization.

Blood Flow and Oxygen Delivery. For healing to occur, wounds must have adequate blood flow to supply the necessary nutrients and to remove the resulting waste, local toxins, bacteria, and other debris. Impaired wound healing due to poor blood flow may occur as a result of wound conditions (*e.g.*, swelling) or preexisting health problems. Arterial disease and venous pathology are well-documented causes of impaired wound healing. In situations of trauma, a decrease in blood volume may cause a reduction in blood flow to injured tissues.

Molecular oxygen is required for collagen synthesis. It has been shown that even a temporary lack of oxygen can result in the formation of less stable collagen.[20,21] Wounds in ischemic tissue become infected more frequently than wounds in well vascularized tissue. PMNs and macrophages require oxygen for destruction of microorganisms that have invaded the area. Although these cells can accomplish phagocytosis in a relatively anoxic environment, they cannot digest bacteria.

Hyperbaric oxygen is a treatment in which 100% oxygen is delivered at greater than two times the normal atmospheric pressure at sea level.[22] The goal is to increase oxygen delivery to tissues by increasing the partial pressure of oxygen dissolved in the plasma. An increase in tissue oxygen tension by hyperbaric oxygen enhances wound healing by a number of mechanisms, including the increased killing of bacteria by neutrophils, impaired growth of anaerobic bacteria, and promotion of angiogenesis and fibroblast activity. Hyperbaric oxygen is currently reserved for the treatment of problem wounds in which hypoxia and infection interfere with healing.

Impaired Inflammatory and Immune Responses. Inflammatory and immune mechanisms function in wound healing. Inflammation is essential to the first phase of wound healing, and immune mechanisms prevent infections that impair wound healing. Among the conditions that impair inflammation and immune function are disorders of phagocytic function, diabetes mellitus, and therapeutic administration of corticosteroid drugs.

Phagocytic disorders can be divided into extrinsic and intrinsic defects. Extrinsic disorders are those that impair attraction of phagocytic cells to the wound site, prevent engulfment of bacteria and foreign agents by the phagocytic cells (*i.e.*, opsonization), or cause suppression of the total number of phagocytic cells (*e.g.*, immunosuppressive agents). Intrinsic phagocytic disorders are the result of enzymatic deficiencies in the metabolic pathway for destroying the ingested bacteria by the phagocytic cell. The intrinsic phagocytic disorders include chronic granulomatous disease (see Chapter 21), an X-linked inherited disease in which there is a deficiency of myeloperoxidase and nicotinamide adenine dinucleotide phosphate (NADPH)-dependent oxidase enzymes. Deficiencies of these compounds prevent generation of hydrogen superoxide and hydrogen peroxide needed for killing bacteria.

Wound healing is a problem in persons with diabetes mellitus, particularly those who have poorly controlled blood glucose levels.[23,24] Studies have shown delayed wound healing, poor collagen formation, and poor tensile strength in diabetic animals. Of particular importance is the effect of hyperglycemia on phagocytic function. Neutrophils, for example, have diminished chemotactic and phagocytic function, including engulfment and intracellular killing of bacteria, when exposed to altered glucose levels. Small blood vessel disease is also common among persons with diabetes, impairing the delivery of inflammatory cells, oxygen, and nutrients to the wound site.

The therapeutic administration of corticosteroid drugs decreases the inflammatory process and may delay the healing process. These hormones decrease capillary permeability during the early stages of inflammation, impair the phagocytic property of the leukocytes, and inhibit fibroblast proliferation and function.

Infection, Wound Separation, and Foreign Bodies. Wound contamination, wound separation, and foreign bodies delay wound healing. Infection impairs all dimensions of wound healing.[25] It prolongs the inflammatory phase, impairs the formation of granulation tissue, and inhibits proliferation of fibroblasts and deposition of collagen fibers. All wounds are contaminated at the time of injury. Although body defenses can handle the invasion of microorganisms at the time of wounding, badly contaminated wounds can overwhelm host defenses. Trauma and existing impairment of host defenses also can contribute to the development of wound infections.

Approximation of the wound edges (*i.e.*, suturing of an incision type of wound) greatly enhances healing and prevents infection. Epithelialization of a wound with closely approximated edges occurs within 1 to 2 days. Large, gaping wounds tend to heal more slowly because it is often impossible to effect wound closure with this type of wound. Mechanical factors such as increased local pressure or torsion can cause wounds to pull apart, or *dehisce.* Foreign bodies tend to invite bacterial contamination and delay healing. Fragments of wood, steel, glass, and other compounds may have entered the wound at the site of injury and can be difficult to locate when the wound is treated. Sutures are also foreign bodies, and although needed for the closure of surgical wounds, they are an impediment to healing. This is why sutures are removed as soon as possible after surgery. Wound infections are of special concern in persons with implantation of foreign bodies such as orthopedic devices (*e.g.*, pins, stabilization devices), cardiac pacemakers, and shunt catheters. These infections are difficult to treat and may require removal of the device.

Bite Wounds. Animal and human bites are particularly troublesome in terms of infection.[26,27] The animal inflicting the bite, the location of the bite, and the type of injury are all important determinants of whether the wound becomes infected. Approximately 28% to 80% of all cat bites become infected. Dog bites, for unclear reasons, become infected only approximately 3% to 18% of the time. Bites inflicted by children are usually superficial and seldom become infected, whereas bites inflicted by adults have a much higher rate of infection. Puncture wounds are more likely to become infected than lacerations, probably because lacerations are easier to irrigate and débride.

Treatment of bite wounds involves vigorous irrigation and cleansing as well as débridement or removal of necrotic tissue. Whether bite wounds are closed with sutures to promote healing by primary intention depends on the location of the bite and whether the wound is already infected. Wounds that are not infected and require closure for mechanical or cosmetic reasons may be sutured. Wounds of the hand are not usually sutured because closed-space infection of the hand can produce loss of function. Antibiotics are usually administered prophylactically to persons with high-risk bites (*e.g.*, cat bites in any location and human or animal bites to the hand). All persons with bites should be evaluated to determine whether tetanus or rabies prophylaxis is needed.

Effect of Age. Wound healing in the pediatric population follows a course similar to that in the adult population.[28] The child has a greater capacity for repair than the adult but may lack the reserves needed to ensure proper healing. Such lack is evidenced by an easily upset electrolyte balance, sudden elevation or lowering of temperature, and rapid spread of infection. The neonate and small child may have an immature immune system with no antigenic experience with organisms that contaminate wounds. The younger the child, the more likely is the development of immune depression.

Successful wound healing also depends on adequate nutrition. Children need sufficient calories to maintain growth and promote wound healing. The premature infant is often born with immature organ systems and minimal energy stores but high metabolic requirements—a condition that predisposes to impaired wound healing.

A number of structural and functional changes have been reported to occur in aging skin, including a decrease in dermal thickness, a decline in collagen content, and a loss of elasticity.[29] The observed changes in skin that occur with aging are complicated by the effects of sun exposure. Because the effects of sun exposure are cumulative, older persons show more changes in skin structure.

Wound healing is thought to be progressively impaired with aging. The elderly have reduced collagen and fibroblast synthesis, impaired wound contraction, and slower reepithelialization of open wounds.[30] Although wound healing may be delayed, most wounds heal, even in debilitated elderly persons undergoing major surgical procedures.

Elderly people are more vulnerable to chronic wounds, chiefly pressure, diabetic, and ischemic ulcers, than are younger persons, and these wounds heal more slowly. However, these wounds are more likely to be caused by other disorders, such as immobility, diabetes mellitus, or vascular disease, rather than by aging.

In summary, the ability of tissues to repair damage due to injury depends on the body's ability to replace the parenchymal cells and to organize them as they were originally. Regeneration describes the process by which tissue is replaced with cells of a similar type and function. Healing by regeneration is limited to tissue with cells that are able to divide and replace the injured cells. Body cells are divided into types according to their ability to regenerate: labile cells, such as the epithelial cells of the skin and gastrointestinal tract, which continue to regenerate throughout life; stable cells, such as those in the liver, which normally do not divide but are capable of regeneration when confronted with an appropriate stimulus; and permanent or fixed cells, such as nerve cells, which are unable to regenerate. Scar tissue repair involves the substitution of fibrous connective tissue for injured tissue that cannot be repaired by regeneration.

Wound healing occurs by primary and secondary intention and is commonly divided into three phases: the inflammatory phase, the proliferative phase, and the maturational or remodeling phase. In wounds healing by primary intention, the duration of the phases is fairly predictable. In wounds healing by secondary intention, the process depends on the extent of injury and the healing environment. Wound healing can be impaired or complicated by factors such as malnutrition; restricted blood flow and oxygen delivery; diminished inflammatory and immune responses; and infection, wound separation, and the presence of foreign bodies.

REVIEW EXERCISES

A 15-year-old boy presents with a temperature of 38°C (100.5°F) and an elevated white blood cell count of 13,000/μL with an increase in neutrophils. A tentative diagnosis of appendicitis is made.

A. Explain the significance of pain as it relates to the inflammatory response.

B. What is the cause of the fever and elevated white blood cell count?

C. What would be the preferred treatment for this boy?

Aspirin and other NSAIDs are used to control the manifestations of chronic inflammatory disorders such as arthritis.

A. Explain their mechanism of action in controlling the inflammatory response.

Following a heart attack, the area of heart muscle that has become necrotic because of lack of blood flow undergoes healing by replacement with scar tissue.

A. Compare the function of the healed area of the heart with that of the normal surrounding heart muscle.

A 35-year-old man comes in with a large abscess on his leg. He tells you he injured his leg while doing repair work on his house and he thinks there might be a wood sliver in the infected area.

A. Explain the events that participate in formation of an abscess.

B. He is told that incision and drainage of the lesion will be needed if healing is to take place. Explain.

C. He is reluctant to have the procedure done and asks whether an antibiotic would work as well. Explain why antibiotics alone are usually not effective in eliminating the microorganisms contained in an abscess.

References

1. Fantone J. C., Ward P. A. (1999). Inflammation. In Rubin E., Farber J. L. *Pathology* (3rd ed., pp. 37–75). Philadelphia: Lippincott-Raven.

2. Mitchell R. N., Cotran R. V. (2003). Acute and chronic inflammation. In Kumar V., Cotran R. S., Robbins S. *Basic pathology* (7th ed., pp. 61–59). Philadelphia: W. B. Saunders.
3. Chandrasoma P., Taylor C. R. (1998). Concise pathology (3rd ed., pp. 31–92). Stamford T: Appleton & Lange.
4. Nathan C. (2002). Points of control in inflammation. *Nature 420,* 848–852.
5. Gewurz H. (1982). Biology of C-reactive protein and the acute phase response. *Hospital Practice 17*(6), 67–81.
6. Haverkate F., Thompson S. G., Pyke S. D., et al. (1997). Production of C-reactive protein and risk of coronary events in stable and unstable angina. *Lancet 349,* 462–466.
7. Ridker P. M., Hennekens C. H., Buring J. E., et al. (2000). C-reactive protein and other markers of inflammation in prediction of cardiovascular disease in women. *New England Journal of Medicine 342,* 836–843.
8. Martinez-Hernandez A. (1999). Repair, regeneration, and fibrosis. In Rubin E., Farber J. L. *Pathology* (3rd ed., pp. 77–103). Philadelphia: Lippincott-Raven.
9. Mitchell R. N., Cotran R. S. (2003). Tissue repair: Cell regeneration and fibrosis. In Kumar V., Cotran R., Robbins S. *Basic pathology* (7th ed., pp. 61–78). Philadelphia: W. B. Saunders.
10. Steed D. L. (1997). The role of growth factors in wound healing. *Surgical Clinics of North America 77*(3), 575–585.
11. Robson M. C. (2003). Cytokine manipulation of the wound. *Clinical Plastic Surgery 30,* 57–65.
12. Parks W. C. (1999). Metric metalloproteinases in repair. *Wound Repair and Regeneration 7,* 423–432.
13. Singer A. J., Clark R. A. F. (1999). Cutaneous wound healing. *New England Journal of Medicine 341*(10), 738–746.
14. Monaco J. L., Lawrence W. T. (2003). Acute wound healing: An overview. *Clinical Plastic Surgery 30,* 1–12.
15. Waldrop J., Doughty D. (2000). Wound-healing physiology. In Bryant R. A. *Acute and chronic wounds* (2nd ed., pp. 17–35). St. Louis: Mosby.
16. Waldorf H., Fewkes J. (1995). Wound healing. *Advances in Dermatology 10,* 77–95.
17. Harding K. G., Morris H. L., Patel K. G. (2002). Healing chronic wounds. *British Medical Journal 324,* 160–163.
18. Burns J. L. Mancoll J. S., Phillips L. G. (2003). Impairments of wound healing. *Clinical Plastic Surgery 30,* 47–56.
19. Albina J. E. (1995). Nutrition and wound healing. *Journal of Parenteral and Enteral Nutrition 18,* 367–376.
20. Whitney J. D. (1990). The influence of tissue oxygenation and perfusion on wound healing. *Clinical Issues in Critical Care Nursing 1,* 578–584.
21. Whitney J. D. (1989). Physiologic effects of tissue oxygenation on wound healing. *Heart and Lung 18,* 466–474.
22. Zamboni W. A., Browder L. K., Martinez J. (2003). Hyperbaric oxygen and wound healing. *Clinics in Plastic Surgery 30,* 67–75.
23. King L. (2000). Impaired wound healing in patients with diabetes. *Nursing Standards 15*(38), 39–45.
24. Greenhalgh D. G. (2003). Wound healing and diabetes mellitus. *Clinics in Plastic Surgery 30,* 37–45.
25. Hunt T. K., Hopf H. W. (1977). Wound healing and wound infection. *Surgical Clinics of North America 77,* 587–605.
26. Fleisher G. R. (1999). The management of bite wounds. *New England Journal of Medicine 340,* 138–140.
27. Talan D. A., Citron D. M., Abrahamian F. M., et al. (1999). Bacteriologic analysis of infected dog and cat bites. *New England Journal of Medicine 340,* 85–92.
28. Garvin G. (1990). Wound healing in pediatrics. *Nursing Clinics of North America 25,* 181–191.
29. Boynton P. R., Jaworski D., Paustian C. (1999). Meeting the challenges of healing chronic wounds in older adults. *Nursing Clinics of North America 34*(4), 921–932.
30. Thomas D. R. (2001). Age-related changes in wound healing. *Drugs & Aging 18*(8), 607–620.

CHAPTER 21

Alterations in the Immune Response

The immune system is a multifaceted defense network that has evolved to protect against invading microorganisms, prevent the proliferation of cancer cells, and mediate the healing of damaged tissue. Under normal conditions, the immune response deters or prevents disease. Occasionally, however, the inadequate, inappropriate, or misdirected activation of the immune system can lead to debilitating or life-threatening illnesses, typified by immunodeficiency states, allergic or hypersensitivity reactions, transplantation rejection, and autoimmune disorders.

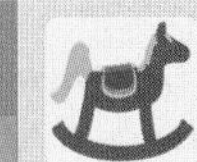

Immunodeficiency Disease

After completing this section of the chapter, you should be able to meet the following objectives:

- State the difference between primary and secondary immunodeficiency states
- Compare and contrast immunodeficiency disorders caused by B-cell and T-cell disorders
- State the function of the complement system and relate to the manifestations of hereditary angioneurotic edema
- State the proposed mechanisms of dysfunction and manifestations in primary disorders of phagocytosis

Immunodeficiency can be defined as an abnormality in one or more branches of the immune system that renders a person susceptible to diseases normally prevented by an intact immune system. Four major categories of immune mechanisms defend the body against infectious or neoplastic disease: humoral or antibody-mediated immunity (*i.e.,* B lymphocytes), cell-mediated immunity (*i.e.,* T lymphocytes), the complement system, and phagocytosis (*i.e.,* neutrophils and macrophages). Humoral and cell-mediated immunodeficiencies represent disorders of adaptive or specific immunity; and complement and phagocytic immunodeficiencies, disorders of innate or nonspecific immunity (see Chapter 19).

Immunodeficiency states can be classified as primary (*i.e.,* congenital or inherited) or secondary (acquired later in life). Secondary immunodeficiency can be the result of malnutrition, infection (*e.g.,* acquired immunodeficiency syndrome [AIDS]), neoplastic disease (*e.g.*, lymphoma), or immunosuppressive therapy (*e.g.*, corticosteroids or transplant rejection medications). Regardless of the cause, primary and secondary deficiencies can produce the same spectrum of disease. The severity and symptomatology of the various immunodeficiencies depend on the disorder and extent of immune system involvement. The various categories of immunodeficiency are summarized in Chart 21-1. AIDS is discussed in Chapter 22.

Until recently, little was known about the causes of primary immunodeficiency diseases. However, this has changed with recent advances in genetic technology.[1–3] To date, more than 100 primary immunodeficiency syndromes have been identified, and specific molecular defects have been identified in more than one third of these diseases.[4] Most are recessive traits, several of which are caused by mutations in genes on the X chromosome and others by mutations on autosomal chromosomes. Many of these disorders have been traced to mutations affecting signaling pathways (*e.g.*, cytokines and cytokine signaling, receptor subunits, and metabolic pathways) that dictate immune cell development and their function.[5]

CHART 21-1

Immunodeficiency States

Humoral (B-Cell) Immunodeficiency

Primary
- Transient hypogammaglobulinemia of infancy
- X-linked hypogammaglobulinemia
- Common variable immunodeficiency
- Selective deficiency of IgG, IgA, IgM

Secondary
- Increased loss of immunoglobulins (nephrotic syndrome)*

Cellular (T-Cell) Immunodeficiency

Primary
- Congenital thymic aplasia (DiGeorge syndrome)
- Abnormal T-cell production (Nezelof syndrome)

Secondary
- Malignant disease (Hodgkin's disease and others)
- Transient suppression of T-cell production and function due to an acute viral infection such as measles
- AIDS
- Purine nucleoside phosphorylase or adenosine deaminase deficiency

Combined B-Cell and T-Cell Immunodeficiency

Primary
- Severe combined immunodeficiency (autosomal or sex-linked recessive)
- Wiskott-Aldrich syndrome (immunodeficiency, thrombocytopenia, and eczema)
- Ataxia-telangiectasia

Secondary
- Irradiation
- Immune suppressant and cytotoxic drugs
- Aging

Complement Disorders

Primary
- Angioneurotic edema (complement 1 inactivator deficiency)
- Selective deficiency in a complement component

Secondary
- Acquired disorders that involve complement utilization

Phagocytic Dysfunction

Primary
- Chronic granulomatous disease
- Glucose-6-phosphate dehydrogenase deficiency
- Job syndrome
- Chédiak-Higashi syndrome
- CD11/CD18 deficiency

Secondary
- Drug induced (corticosteroid and immunosuppressive therapy)
- Diabetes mellitus

*Examples are not inclusive.

HUMORAL (B-CELL) IMMUNODEFICIENCIES

Humoral immunodeficiencies involve B-cell function and immunoglobulin or antibody production. Defects in humoral immunity increase the risk for recurrent pyogenic infections, including those caused by *Streptococcus pneumoniae, Haemophilus influenzae, Staphylococcus aureus,* and gram-negative organisms such as *Pseudomonas* species. Humoral immunity usually is not as important in defending against intracellular bacteria (mycobacteria), fungi, and protozoa. Viral infections, with the exception of the enteroviruses that cause gastrointestinal infections, rely on cell-mediated immunity and usually are handled normally.

Transient Hypogammaglobulinemia of Infancy

During the first few months of life, infants are protected from infection by immunoglobulin G (IgG) class antibodies that have been transferred from the maternal circulation during fetal life. IgA, IgM, IgD, and IgE do not normally cross the placenta. The presence of elevated levels of IgA or IgM in the infant cord blood suggests premature antibody production in response to an intrauterine infection. An infant's level of maternal IgG gradually declines over a period of approximately 6 months (see Fig. 19-16 in Chapter 19). Concomitant with the loss of maternal antibody, the infant's immature humoral immune system begins to function, and between the ages of 1 and 2 years, the child's antibody production reaches adult levels.

Any abnormality that blocks or prevents the maturation of B lymphocyte stem cells can produce a state of immunodeficiency. For example, certain infants may experience a delay in the maturation process of B cells that leads to a prolonged deficiency in IgG levels (IgM and IgA levels are normal) beyond 6 months of age. The total number and antigenic response of circulating B cells is normal,

PRIMARY IMMUNODEFICIENCY DISORDERS

- Primary immunodeficiency disorders are congenital or inherited abnormalities of immune function that render a person susceptible to diseases normally prevented by an intact immune system.
- Disorders of B-cell function impair the ability to produce antibodies and defend against microorganisms and toxins that circulate in body fluids (IgM and IgG) or enter the body through the mucosal surface of the respiratory or gastrointestinal tract (IgA). Persons with primary B-cell immunodeficiency are particularly prone to pyogenic infections due to encapsulated organisms.
- Disorders of T-cell function impair the ability to orchestrate the immune response ($CD4^+$ helper T cells) and to protect against fungal, protozoan, viral, and intracellular bacterial infections ($CD8^+$ cytotoxic T cells). T cells also play an important role in surveillance against oncogenic viruses and tumor; hence, persons with impaired T-cell function are at increased risk for certain types of cancers.
- Combined T-cell and B-cell immunodeficiency states affect all aspects of immune function. Severe combined immunodeficiency represents a life-threatening absence of immune function that requires bone marrow or stem cell transplantation for survival.

but the chemical communication between B and T cells that leads to clonal proliferation of antibody-producing plasma cells seems to be reduced.[6] This condition is referred to as *transient hypogammaglobulinemia of infancy*. The result of this condition usually is limited to repeated bouts of upper respiratory and middle ear infections. This condition usually resolves by the time the child is 2 to 4 years of age.

Primary Humoral Immunodeficiency Disorders

Primary humoral immunodeficiency disorders are genetic disorders of the B lymphocytes. They are the most frequent type of primary immunodeficiencies, accounting for 70% of all primary immunodeficiency disorders.[7] Immunoglobulin production depends on the differentiation of stem cells to mature B lymphocytes and the generation of immunoglobulin-producing plasma cells (Fig. 21-1). This maturation cycle initially involves the production of surface IgM, migration from the marrow to the peripheral lymphoid tissue, and switching to the specialized production of IgG, IgA, IgD, IgE, or IgM antibodies after antigenic stimulation. Primary humoral immunodeficiency disorders can interrupt the production of one or all of the immunoglobulins.

X-Linked Agammaglobulinemia. X-linked or Bruton's agammaglobulinemia is a recessive trait that affects only males.[3,4,6] As the name implies, persons with this disorder have essentially undetectable levels of all serum immunoglobulins. Therefore, they are susceptible to meningitis and recurrent otitis media and to sinus and pulmonary

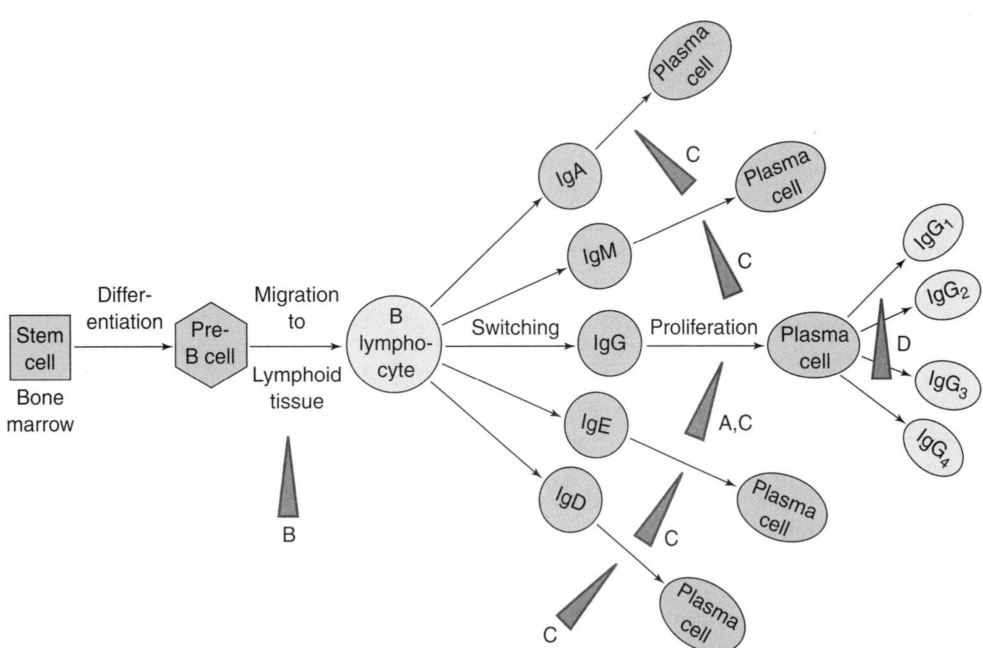

FIGURE 21-1 Stem cells to mature immunoglobulin-secreting plasma cells. *Arrows* indicate the stage of the maturation process that is interrupted in (**A**) transient hypoglobulinemia, (**B**) X-linked hypogammaglobulinemia, (**C**) common variable immunodeficiency, and (**D**) IgG subclass deficiency.

infections with encapsulated organisms such as *S. pneumoniae, H. influenzae* type b, *S. aureus,* and *Neisseria meningitidis.*[3] Many boys with this disorder have severe tooth decay.

The central defect in this syndrome is a genetic mutation that blocks the differentiation of pre-B cells, creating an absence of mature circulating B cells and plasma cells. T lymphocytes, however, are normal in number and function. Symptoms of the disorder usually coincide with the loss of maternal antibodies. A clue to the presence of the disorder is the failure of an infection to respond completely and promptly to antibiotic therapy.

Diagnosis is based on demonstration of low or absent serum immunoglobulins. Therapy consists of prophylaxis with intravenous immunoglobulin and prompt antimicrobial therapy for suspected infections. The prognosis of this condition depends on the prompt recognition and treatment of infections. Chronic pulmonary disease is an ever-present danger.

Common Variable Immunodeficiency. Another disorder of B-cell maturation, which is similar to X-linked agammaglobulinemia, is a condition called *common variable immunodeficiency.* In this syndrome, the terminal differentiation of mature B cells to plasma cells is blocked. The result is markedly reduced serum immunoglobulin levels, normal numbers of circulating B lymphocytes, and a complete absence of germinal centers and plasma cells in lymph nodes and the spleen.

The symptomatology of common variable immunodeficiency is similar to that of X-linked agammaglobulinemia (*i.e.,* recurrent otitis media and sinus and pulmonary infections with encapsulated organisms), but the onset of symptoms occurs much later, usually between the ages of 15 and 35 years, and distribution of disease between the sexes is equal. Persons with late-onset hypogammaglobulinemia also have an increased tendency toward development of chronic lung disease, autoimmune disorders, hepatitis, gastric carcinoma, and chronic diarrhea with associated intestinal malabsorption. Approximately one half of persons with the disorder have evidence of abnormal T-cell immunity, suggesting that this syndrome is a complex immunodeficiency. Treatment methods for late-onset hypogammaglobulinemia are similar to those used for X-linked hypogammaglobulinemia.

Selective IgA Deficiency. Selective IgA deficiency is the most common type of immunoglobulin deficiency, affecting 1 in 400 to 1 in 1000 persons.[3] The syndrome is characterized by moderate to marked reduction in levels of serum and secretory IgA. It's likely caused by a block in the pathway that promotes terminal differentiation of mature B cells to IgA-secreting plasma cells. The occurrence of IgA deficiency in both males and females and in members of successive generations within families suggests autosomal inheritance with variable expressivity. The disorder has also been noted in persons treated with certain drugs (*e.g.,* phenytoin, sulfasalazine), suggesting that environmental factors may trigger the disorder.[4]

Approximately two thirds of persons with selective IgA deficiency have no overt symptoms, presumably because IgG and IgM levels are normal and compensate for the defect. At least 50% of affected children overcome the deficiency by the age of 14 years. Persons with markedly reduced levels of IgA often experience repeated upper respiratory and gastrointestinal infections and have increased incidence of allergic manifestations, such as asthma, and autoimmune disorders. Persons with IgA deficiency also can develop antibodies against IgA, which can lead to severe anaphylactic reactions when blood components containing IgA are given.[4] Therefore, only specially washed erythrocytes from normal donors or erythrocytes from IgA-deficient donors should be used.

There is no treatment available for selective IgA deficiency unless there is a concomitant reduction in IgG levels. Administration of IgA immunoglobulin is of little benefit because it has a short half-life and is not secreted across the mucosa. There also is the risk for anaphylactic reactions associated with IgA antibodies in the immunoglobulin.

Immunoglobulin G Subclass Deficiency. An IgG subclass deficiency can affect one or more of IgG subtypes, despite normal levels or elevated serum concentrations of IgG. As discussed in Chapter 19, IgG immunoglobulins can be divided into four subclasses (IgG1 through IgG4) based on structure and function. Most circulating IgG belongs to the IgG1 (70%) and IgG2 (20%) subclasses. In general, antibodies directed against protein antigens belong to the IgG1 and IgG3 subclasses, and antibodies directed against carbohydrate and polysaccharide antigens are primarily IgG2 subclass. As a result, persons who are deficient in IgG2 subclass antibodies can be at greater risk for development of sinusitis, otitis media, and pneumonia caused by polysaccharide-encapsulated microorganisms such as *S. pneumoniae, H. influenzae* type b, and *N. meningitidis.*

Children with mild forms of the deficiency can be treated with prophylactic antibiotics to prevent repeated infections. Intravenous immune globulin can be given to children with severe manifestations of this deficiency. The use of polysaccharide vaccines conjugated to protein carriers rather than the protein conjugated to protein carriers that would stimulate an IgG1 response can provide protection against some of these infections.

Secondary Humoral Immunodeficiency Disorders

Secondary deficiencies in humoral immunity can develop as a consequence of selective loss of immunoglobulins through the gastrointestinal or genitourinary tracts. Such is the case in persons with nephrotic syndrome who, because of abnormal glomerular filtration, lose serum IgA and IgG in their urine. Because of its larger molecular size, IgM is not filtered into the urine, and serum levels remain normal.

CELL-MEDIATED (T-CELL) IMMUNODEFICIENCIES

Unlike the B-cell lineage or immunodeficiency, in which a well-defined series of differentiation steps ultimately leads to the production of immunoglobulins, mature T lymphocytes are composed of distinct subpopulations whose immunologic assignments are diverse. T cells can be functionally divided into two subtypes ($CD4^+$ helper and $CD8^+$ cytotoxic T cells). Collectively, T lymphocytes protect against fungal, protozoan, viral, and intracellular bacterial infections; control malignant cell proliferation; and are responsible for coordinating the overall immune response.

Primary Cell-Mediated Immunodeficiency Disorders

In general, persons with cell-mediated immunodeficiency disorders have infections or other clinical problems that are more severe than antibody disorders. Children with defects in this branch of the immune response rarely survive beyond infancy or childhood. However, exceptions are being recognized as newer T-cell defects, such as the X-linked hyper-IgM syndrome, are identified. Other more recently identified primary T-cell immunodeficiency disorders result from defective expression of the T-cell receptor (TCR) complex, defective cytokine production, and defects in T-cell activation.

For children with fatal forms of T-cell defects, transplantation of thymic tissue or major histocompatibility complex (MHC)–compatible bone marrow is currently the treatment of choice.[4] Stem cell transplantation (to be discussed), an alternative to bone marrow transplantation, has also proved useful in treating some disorders. The major risk to recipients of bone marrow transplantation is that of graft-versus-host disease. Gene replacement therapy remains a distant goal for most immunodeficiencies at present. The main obstacles to this type of therapy are purifying self-renewing stem cells, which are the ideal target for introduction of the replacement gene, and lack of methods for introducing the genes into the stem cell.

DiGeorge Syndrome. DiGeorge syndrome stems from an embryonic developmental defect. The defect is thought to occur before the 12th week of gestation, when the thymus, parathyroid gland, and parts of the head, neck, and heart are developing. The disorder affects both sexes. Because familial occurrence is rare, it seems unlikely that the disorder is inherited. Formerly thought to be caused by a variety of factors, including extrinsic teratogens, this defect has been traced to microdeletion of a gene on chromosome 22 (22q11).[2,6–9]

Infants born with this defect have partial or complete failure of development of the thymus and parathyroid glands and have congenital defects of the head, neck, and heart. The extent of immune and parathyroid abnormalities is highly variable, as are the other defects. Occasionally, a child has no heart defect. In some children, the thymus is not absent but is in an abnormal location and is extremely small. These infants can have partial DiGeorge syndrome, in which hypertrophy of the thymus occurs with development of normal immune function. The facial disorders can include hypertelorism (*i.e.,* increased distance between the eyes); micrognathia (*i.e.,* fish mouth); low-set, posteriorly angulated ears; split uvula; and high-arched palate (Fig. 21-2). Urinary tract abnormalities also are common. The most frequent presenting sign is hypocalcemia and tetany that develops in the first 24 hours of

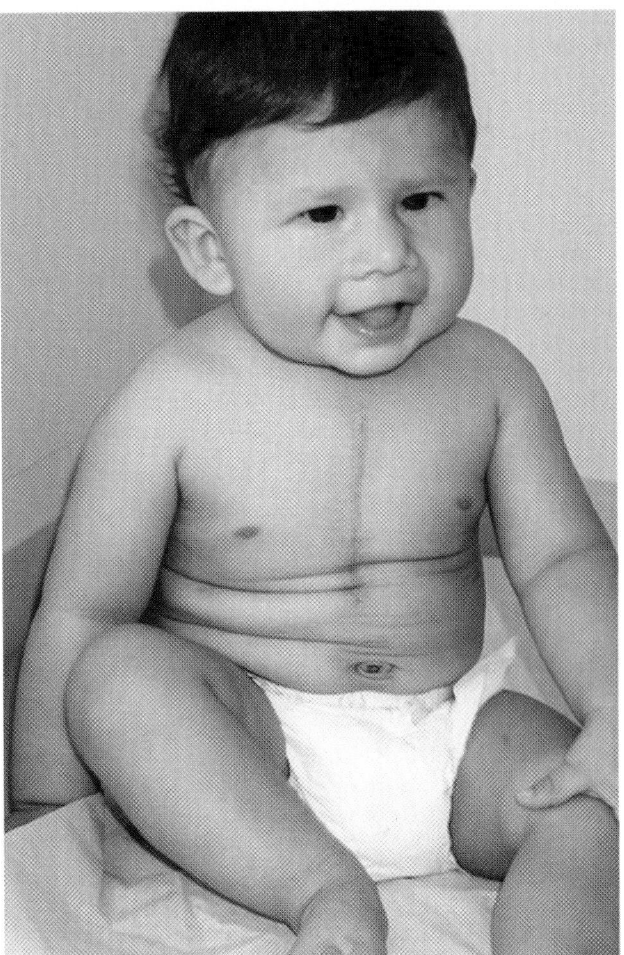

FIGURE 21-2 An infant with DiGeorge syndrome. The surgical scar on the chest indicates repair of heart disease caused by truncus arteriosus or interrupted aortic arch, which is common in this syndrome. The infant also has the facial features of a child with DiGeorge syndrome, as illustrated by hypertelorism, low-set ears, hypoplastic mandible, and bowing upward of the upper lip. (From Roberts R. *Atlas of Infectious Diseases.* Edited by Gerald Mandell (series editor), Catherine M. Wilfert. © 1998 Current Medicine, Inc.)

life. It is caused by the absence of the parathyroid gland and is resistant to standard therapy.

Children who survive the immediate neonatal period may have recurrent or chronic infections because of impaired T-cell immunity. Children also may have an absence of immunoglobulin production, caused by a lack of helper T-cell function. For children who do require treatment, thymus transplantation can be performed to reconstitute T-cell immunity. Bone marrow transplantation also has been successfully used to restore normal T-cell populations. If blood transfusions are needed, as during corrective heart surgery, special processing is required to prevent graft-versus-host disease.

X-Linked Immunodeficiency With Hyper-IgM. The X-linked immunodeficiency of hyper-IgM, also known as the *hyper-IgM syndrome,* is characterized by low IgG and IgA levels with normal or, more frequently, high IgM concentrations. Being X-linked, the disorder is confined to males. Formerly classified as a B-cell defect, it now has been traced to a T-cell defect. The disorder results from the inability of T cells to signal B cells to undergo isotype switching to IgG and IgA; thus, they produce only IgM.[8]

Like boys with X-linked agammaglobulinemia, affected boys become symptomatic during the first and second years of life. They have recurrent pyogenic infections, including otitis media, sinusitis, tonsillitis, and pneumonia. They are also more susceptible to *Pneumocystis carinii* infection. Thymic-dependent lymphoid tissues and T-cell function usually are normal, as are B-cell counts. Hemolytic anemia and thrombocytopenia may occur, and transient, persistent, or cyclic neutropenia is a common feature.[8] The frequency of autoimmune disorders is higher than with other immunoglobulin deficiency disorders.[8]

Secondary Cell-Mediated Immunodeficiency Disorders

Secondary deficiencies of T-cell function are more common than primary deficiencies and have been described in conjunction with acute viral infections (*e.g.*, measles virus, cytomegalovirus) and with certain malignancies such as Hodgkin's disease and other lymphomas. In the case of viruses, direct infection of specific T-lymphocyte subpopulations (*e.g.*, helper cells) by lymphotropic viruses such as the human immunodeficiency virus (HIV) and human herpesvirus type 6 can lead to loss of cellular function and selective subtype depletion with a concomitant loss of immunologic function associated with that subtype. Persons with neoplastic disorders can have impaired T-cell function based on unregulated multiplication or dysfunction of one particular subclone of T cells. The outward expression of this may be an increased susceptibility to infections caused by normally harmless pathogens (*i.e.*, opportunistic infections) or failure to generate delayed-type hypersensitivity reactions (*i.e.*, anergy). Persons with anergy have a diminished or absent reaction to a battery of skin test antigens, including *Candida* and the tuberculin test, even when infected with *Mycobacterium tuberculosis*. In persons with anergy, a negative skin test result for tuberculosis can mean a true lack of exposure to tuberculosis or indicate the person's inability to mount an appropriate T-cell response (see Chapter 30).

COMBINED T-CELL AND B-CELL IMMUNODEFICIENCIES

Disorders that affect both B and T lymphocytes, with resultant defects in both humoral and cell-mediated immunity, fall under the broad classification of combined immunodeficiency syndrome (CIDS). A single mutation in any one of the many genes that influence lymphocyte development or response, including lymphocyte receptors, cytokines, or major histocompatibility antigens, can lead to combined immunodeficiency. Regardless of the affected gene, the net result is a disruption in the normal communication system of B and T lymphocytes and deregulation of the immune response. The spectrum of disease resulting from combined immunodeficiency disorders ranges from mild to severe to ultimately fatal forms.

Severe Combined Immunodeficiency

The most pronounced form of the combined immunodeficiencies often is referred to as *severe combined immunodeficiency syndrome* (SCIDS). SCIDS is caused by diverse genetic mutations that lead to absence of all immune function and, in some cases, a lack of natural killer (NK) cells.[4,8] Affected infants have a disease course that resembles AIDS, with failure to thrive, chronic diarrhea, and opportunistic infections that usually lead to death by the age of 2 years. If recognized at birth or within the first 3 months of life, 95% of infants can be successfully treated with bone marrow or stem cell transplantation.[4] A family history of similarly affected relatives occurs in approximately 50% of cases.[8] Both X-linked and autosomal recessive inheritance are involved.

X-linked SCIDS. Approximately 50% of SCIDS are X linked and due to mutations in the gene encoding the common gamma chain (γ_c) shared by receptors for many of the cytokines that direct the differentiation and maturation of both T and B lymphocytes.[1] These mutations are recessive, so that heterozygous females are usually normal carriers of the gene, whereas males who inherit the abnormal chromosome manifest the disease.

Children with this disorder appear similar to those with other forms of SCIDS except for having uniformly low percentages of T and NK cells and an elevated percentage of B cells. However, the B cells do not produce immunoglobulin in a normal manner because of a lack of T-cell help.

The recent successful correction of T and NK cell defects using gene transfer therapy (insertion of exogenous genetic material into the infant's bone marrow cells) offers hope that this method will eventually become the treatment of choice for this form of SCIDS.[9]

Autosomal Recessive SCIDS. About 50% of persons with SCIDS show an autosomal recessive pattern of inheritance, and about half of these are due to a deficiency in adenosine deaminase (ADA) deficiency.[1] Absence of this enzyme leads to accumulation of toxic metabolites that kill dividing and resting T cells.

Infants with ADA-deficiency SCIDS usually have a much more profound lymphopenia than do infants with other forms of SCIDS. The absolute numbers of both T and B cells are very low (usually <500/mm³). Although the number of NK cells is low, their function is normal. Other distinguishing features of the ADA deficiency include the presence of rib cage deformity and numerous skeletal deformities.

Bone marrow transplantation has been successful in treating children with ADA-negative SCIDS.[4,8,9] Enzyme replacement therapy also may be used in the management of persons with this form of SCIDS.[4,9] However, it should not be used if bone marrow transplantation is anticipated because it can predispose to graft rejection.[4,9]

Combined Immunodeficiency

Combined immunodeficiency syndrome (CIDS) is distinguished from SCIDS by the presence of low, but not absent, T-cell function. Although antibody-forming capacity is impaired in most cases, it is not absent. Like SCIDS, however, CIDS is a syndrome of diverse genetic causes and is often associated with other disorders such as ataxia-telangiectasis and Wiskott-Aldrich syndrome (eczema and thrombocytopenia). An autosomal pattern of inheritance is common.

Children with CIDS are prone to develop recurrent pulmonary infections, failure to thrive, oral and cutaneous candidiasis, chronic diarrhea, recurrent skin infections, gram-negative sepsis, and urinary tract infections. Although they usually survive longer than children with SCIDS, they fail to thrive and often die early in life.

Ataxia-Telangiectasia

Ataxia-telangiectasia is a complex syndrome of neurologic, immunologic, endocrinologic, hepatic, and cutaneous abnormalities. It is an autosomal recessive disorder that is thought to result from the mutation of a single gene located on the long arm of chromosome 11 (11q22–23).[8,9] As the name implies, this syndrome is heralded by worsening cerebellar ataxia (*i.e.,* poor muscle coordination) and the appearance of telangiectases (*i.e.,* lesions consisting of dilated capillaries and arterioles) on skin and conjunctival surfaces (Fig. 21-3). The ataxia usually goes unnoticed until the toddler begins to walk; the telangiectases develop thereafter, especially on skin surfaces exposed to the sun. The ataxia progresses slowly and relentlessly to severe disability. Intellectual development is normal at first but seems to stop at the 10-year level in many of these children.

Children with ataxia-telangiectasia have deficiencies in both cellular and humoral immunity, including reduced levels of IgA, IgE, and IgG2, absolute lymphopenia, and a decrease in the ratio of $CD4^+$ helper T cells to $CD8^+$ suppressor T cells. Approximately 70% have an IgA deficiency, and approximately half also have an IgG subclass deficiency. There is increased susceptibility to recurrent upper and lower respiratory tract infections (particularly those caused by encapsulated bacteria) and an increased risk for the development of malignancies. Death from malignant lymphoma is common.

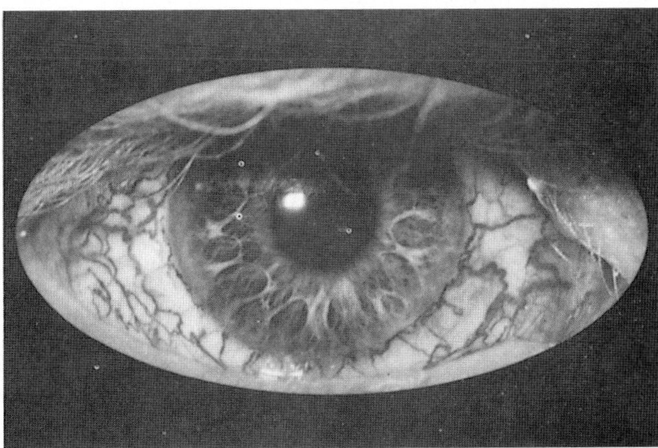

FIGURE 21-3 Striking telangiectasis on the bulbar conjunctiva of a 22-year-old patient with ataxia-telangiectasia. These dilated vessels typically appear between the ages of 2 and 5 years. (From Oski F.A. [Ed.]. [1990]. *Principles and practice of pediatrics.* Philadelphia: J.B. Lippincott)

Wiskott-Aldrich Syndrome

Wiskott-Aldrich syndrome is an X-linked recessive disorder that becomes symptomatic during the first year of life.[8,9] Infants with this syndrome are plagued by eczema, low platelet counts, and susceptibility to bacterial infections. Bleeding episodes or symptoms due to infection usually begin within the first 6 months of life. Abnormalities of humoral immunity include decreased serum levels of IgM and markedly elevated serum IgA and IgE concentrations. T-cell dysfunction initially is mild but progressively deteriorates, and patients become increasingly susceptible to the development of malignancies of the mononuclear phagocytic system, including Hodgkin's lymphoma and leukemia. Children with Wiskott-Aldrich syndrome typically are unable to produce antibody to polysaccharide antigens and therefore are susceptible to infections caused by encapsulated microorganisms. They also are prone to septicemia and meningitis with these organisms. Varicella infection can be lethal to children with this condition.

Bone marrow transplantation has been successful in children with Wiskott-Aldrich syndrome. Splenectomy may be used to control the thrombocytopenia in situations in which bone marrow transplantation cannot be done.

DISORDERS OF THE COMPLEMENT SYSTEM

The complement system is an integral part of the innate or nonspecific immune response (see Chapter 19). The activation of the complement network through the classic, lectin-mediated, or alternative pathways promotes chemotaxis, opsonization, and phagocytosis of invasive pathogens, bacteriolysis, and anaphylactic reactions. Thus, alterations in normal levels of complement or the absence of a particular complement component can lead to enhanced susceptibility to infectious diseases and immune-mediated disorders such as hemolytic anemia and collagen vascular disorders. As with B- and T-cell deficiencies, complement disorders can be classified as primary if the deficiency is inherited or secondary if the condition develops because of another disease process.

Primary Disorders of the Complement System

Most primary disorders of the complement system are transmitted as autosomal recessive traits and can involve one or more complement components (the complement components are designated by "C" and enzyme subcomponents by "q," "r," and "s"). Deficiencies of C1r, C1rs, C4, C2, C3, C5, C6, C7, C8, and C9 are transmitted as autosomal codominant traits, in which each parent transmits a gene that codes for half the serum level of the component.[10,11] Because 50% activity is sufficient to prevent disease, persons who are heterozygous and have one normally functioning gene seldom have problems.

In general, persons with deficiencies in factors C1 (C1q, r, and s) and C4 are not necessarily at increased risk for recurrent infections because the lectin-mediated and alternative pathways can be activated normally through C3. However, many of them acquire autoimmune diseases, particularly lupus-like syndromes. Persons with primary deficiency of C1q have a high incidence of systemic lupus erythematosus (SLE), an SLE-like syndrome without typical SLE serology, a chronic rash with underlying vasculitis on biopsy, or membranoproliferative glomerulonephritis.[10,11] Like persons with C1q deficiency, persons with C1r, C1r/C1s, C4, C2, and C3 deficiencies have a high incidence of vasculitis syndromes, especially SLE or SLE-like syndrome.

A C2 deficiency causes a susceptibility to multiple and potentially life-threatening infections caused by encapsulated bacteria, especially *S. pneumoniae*. Similarly, persons with C3 deficiency are predisposed to infections that trigger the lectin-mediated or alternate pathway (*e.g.*, those caused by encapsulated bacteria and *S. aureus*) because of their inability to opsonize and lyse bacteria. Although persons with deficiencies in the terminal components of complement (C5 through C9) are susceptible to repeated episodes of meningitis and sepsis caused by *N. meningitidis* or systemic gonococcal disease, they are less likely to have autoimmune disorders than persons with other complement deficiencies.[11]

Only supportive measures are available for treatment of primary disorders of the complement system. Measures to prevent bacterial infections are important. The affected person and close contacts should be immunized with vaccines for *S. pneumoniae, H. influenzae,* and *N. meningitidis.*

Hereditary Angioneurotic Edema. Hereditary angioneurotic edema is a particularly interesting form of complement deficiency.[12,13] Persons with this disorder do not produce a functional C1 inhibitor. Activation of the classic complement pathway is uncontrolled, leading to increased breakdown of C4 and C2 with concomitant release of C-kinin, a vasodilator. This causes episodic attacks of localized edema involving the face, neck, joints, abdomen, and sites of trauma. Swelling of the subcutaneous tissues, especially of the face, can be disfiguring, and swelling of the gastric mucosa causes nausea, vomiting, and diarrhea. If the trachea or larynx is involved, the episode can prove fatal. The attacks associated with this inherited disease usually begin before the age of 2 years and become progressively worse with age. Symptoms can last from 1 to 4 days, and most persons with the disorder have more than one attack a month. Adults with hereditary angioneurotic edema can be treated with danazol, a synthetic androgen with weak virilizing and mild anabolic potential. The drug, given orally, increases C1 inhibitor levels and prevents attacks.[10] A vapor-heated C1 inhibitor concentrate has been developed. This concentrate can be used to prevent and treat an acute attack of hereditary angioneurotic edema.[13,14]

Secondary Disorders of the Complement System

Secondary complement deficiencies also can occur in persons with functionally normal complement systems because of rapid activation and turnover of complement components (as is seen in immune complex disease) or reduced synthesis of components, as would be the case in chronic cirrhosis of the liver or malnutrition.

DISORDERS OF PHAGOCYTOSIS

The phagocytic system is composed primarily of polymorphonuclear leukocytes (*i.e.,* neutrophils and eosinophils) and mononuclear phagocytes (*i.e.,* circulating monocytes and tissue and fixed [spleen] macrophages). The primary purpose of phagocytic cells is to migrate to the site of infection (*i.e.,* chemotaxis), aggregate around the affected tissue (*i.e.,* adherence), envelope invading microorganisms or foreign substances (*i.e.,* phagocytosis), and generate microbicidal substances (*e.g.,* enzymes or byproducts of metabolism) to kill the ingested pathogens. A defect in any of these functions or a reduction in the absolute number of available cells can disrupt the phagocytic system. Persons with phagocytic disorders are particularly prone to infections by bacteria and often by *Candida* species and filamentous fungi, although the types of pathogens vary with different disorders.[15] As with other alterations in immune function, defects in phagocytosis can be primary or secondary disorders.

Primary Disorders of Phagocytosis

The best known of the primary disorders of phagocytosis is chronic granulomatous disease (CGD). CGD represents a group of inherited disorders that greatly reduce or inactivate the ability of phagocytic cells to produce the so-called *respiratory burst* that results in the generation of toxic derivatives of oxygen (superoxide anion and hydrogen peroxide).[16,17] These oxygen species participate in creating an intracellular environment that kills ingested microorganisms. Recurrent infections, along with granulomatous lesions, in persons with CGD are thought to be due to persistence of viable microorganisms in impaired phagocytic cells. Other aspects of phagocyte function, such as engulfment of microorganisms, are normal. About two thirds of persons with CGD are males who inherit their disorder as a result of mutations in the X-chromosome; about one third inherit CGD as a result of mutations on chromosome 7; and a small number (about 5%) result from mutations on chromosome 1.

Children with CGD are subject to chronic and acute infections of the skin, liver, lung, and other soft tissues despite aggressive antibiotic therapy. Severe facial acne and painful inflammation of the nares are common. Organisms responsible for the infections include *S. aureus, Serratia marcescens, Pseudomonas cepacia, Escherichia coli, Candida albicans,* and *Aspergillus* species.[16,17] These infections usually begin during the first 2 years of life. The disorder is diagnosed by examining the ability of a person's phagocytes to reduce a yellow dye (*i.e.,* nitroblue tetrazolium) to a blue compound during active respiration. Bone marrow transplantation is the only known cure for CGD. Supportive care includes the use of recombinant interferon-γ and prophylactic antibiotic therapy.

Secondary Disorders of Phagocytosis

Secondary deficiencies of the phagocytic system can be caused by a number of circumstances, such as deficiencies of opsonins, which coat the surface of a foreign substance and enhance phagocytosis, and deficiencies of chemotactic factors (*e.g.*, antibody and complement), which coat the surface of microorganisms and promote increased migration of phagocytes to the site of infection and stimulate phagocytosis. Deficiencies of either of these factors reduce the overall effectiveness of phagocytes. Drugs that impair or prevent inflammation and T-cell function, such as corticosteroids or cyclosporine, also alter phagocytic response through modulation of cytokines.

Persons with diabetes mellitus also demonstrate poor phagocytic function, primarily because of altered chemotaxis. The reason for this dysfunction is not understood, but it is unrelated to the person's age or the severity of the metabolic disorder. Apparently, this is a separate genetic disorder that is coinherited at a higher frequency among persons with diabetes and among family members.

HIV infection and AIDS represent another form of acquired or secondary deficiency of phagocytic function. However, in this case, the deficiency is due to direct infection and destruction of helper T cells and monocytes–macrophages by the virus (see Chapter 22).

STEM CELL TRANSPLANTATION

Many of the primary immunodeficiency disorders in which the defect has been traced to the stem cell can be cured with allogeneic stem cell transplantation from an unaffected donor.[18] These include disorders such as SCIDS, Wiskott-Aldrich syndrome, and chronic granulomatous disease.

It has been shown that stem cells can repopulate the bone marrow and reestablish hematopoiesis. For the procedure to be effective, the bone marrow cells of the host are destroyed by myeloablative doses of chemotherapy. The exception is children with SCIDS. Because of the profound cellular immune defect that is present in children with SCIDS, pretransplantation myeloablation may not be necessary.[18] After transplantation, a lineage-specific chimeric state usually develops in these children, in which the T-cell component is of donor origin and the B-cell component, although variable, remains largely of host origin.[18] Chronic immunoglobulin therapy may be necessary for transplant recipients who primarily retain B cells of host origin.

Stem cells can be collected from the bone marrow or peripheral blood. Donors with identical HLA types (*i.e.*, matched for at least three of the six HLA loci) are associated with the least risk for graft-versus-host disease or graft rejection. HLA-matched siblings usually produce the best results. Stem cell aspiration from the bone marrow is the most common form of allograft collection. Only a few (<1 in 100,000) nucleated bone marrow cells are true hematopoietic stem cells. These stem cells are separated from other bone marrow cells before transplantation. Peripheral blood offers a less invasive method for obtaining stem cells. Hematopoietic growth factors, such as granulocyte colony-stimulating factor, often are used to induce stem cells to move out of the bone marrow into the blood. Many of these stem cells can be collected from the blood using leukapheresis, a process that separates the stem cells from other blood cells. A third potential source of stem cells is umbilical cord blood. Umbilical cord blood is a rich source of primitive hematopoietic blood. Up to 250 mL of umbilical cord blood can be collected at the time of delivery without producing detrimental effects to the mother and newborn. Although reliable engraftment of bone marrow can be achieved in children, it is uncertain whether cord blood contains enough stem cells to engraft adult recipients.[18]

In summary, immunodeficiency is defined as an absolute or partial loss of the normal immune response, which places a person in a state of compromise and increases the risk for development of infections or malignant complications. Immunodeficiency states can affect one or more of the four main components of the immune response: antibody or humoral (B-cell) immunity, cellular or T-cell immunity, the complement system, and the phagocytic system. The variety of defects known to involve the immune response can be classified as primary (*i.e.*, endogenous or inherited) or secondary (*i.e.*, caused by exogenous factors, such as drugs or infection). The extent to which any or all of these components are compromised dictates the severity of the immunodeficiency.

Hypersensitivity Disorders

After completing this section of the chapter, you should be able to meet the following objectives:

- Differentiate between adaptive immune responses that protect against microbial agents and hypersensitivity responses
- Describe the immune mechanisms involved in a type I, type II, type III, and type IV hypersensitivity reaction
- Describe the pathogenesis of allergic rhinitis, food allergy, serum sickness, Arthus reaction, contact dermatitis, and hypersensitivity pneumonitis
- Characterize the differences in latex allergy caused by a type I, IgE-mediated hypersensitivity response and that caused by a type IV, cell-mediated response

Hypersensitivity disorders refer to excessive or inappropriate activation of the immune system. Although activation of the immune system normally leads to production of antibodies and T-cell responses that protect the body against attack by microorganisms, it is also capable of causing tissue injury and disease. Disorders caused by immune responses are collectively referred to as *hypersensitivity reactions*. The term hypersensitivity arose from the observation that a person who has been exposed to an antigen is exquisitely "sensitive" to subsequent encounters with the antigen.[19]

Historically, hypersensitivity disorders have been subdivided into four types: type I, immediate hypersensitivity disorders; type II, antibody-mediated disorders; type III, immune complex-mediated immune disorders; and type IV, T-cell–mediated disorders[1,19] (Table 21-1). These categories

TABLE 21-1 Classification of Hypersensitivity Responses

Type of Hypersensitivity	Immune Mechanism	Mechanism of Injury
Type I, immediate hypersensitivity	IgE antibody	Release of mast cell mediators
Type II, antibody mediated	IgM, IgG antibodies against cell surface or extracellular matrix	Complement-mediated opsonization and phagocytosis of cells
Type III, immune complex mediated	Formation of immune complexes involving circulating antigens and IgM or IgG antibodies	Complement-mediated recruitment and activation of inflammatory cells
Type IV, T-cell mediated	$CD4^+$ T cells (delayed-type hypersensitivity, or $CD8^+$ cytotoxic T-cell–mediated cytolysis)	Macrophage activation of cytokine-mediated inflammation; direct target cell killing, cytokine-mediated inflammation

differ in terms of the type of immune response causing the injury and the nature and location of the antigen that is the target of the response. Latex allergy is a disorder that can result from an IgE-mediated or T-cell–mediated hypersensitivity response. It is discussed separately at the end of this section. Transplant rejections and autoimmune disorders (discussed separately) may also be regarded as hypersensitivity responses.

TYPE I, IMMEDIATE HYPERSENSITIVITY DISORDERS

Type I reactions are IgE-mediated hypersensitivity reactions that begin rapidly, often within minutes of antigen challenge. These types of reactions to antigens are often referred to as *allergic reactions*. In the context of an allergic response, the antigens usually are referred to as *allergens*.

ALLERGIC AND HYPERSENSITIVITY DISORDERS

- Hypersensitivity disorders result from immune responses to exogenous and endogenous antigens that produce inflammation and cause tissue damage.
- Type I hypersensitivity is an IgE-mediated immune response that leads to the release of inflammatory mediators for sensitized mast cells.
- Type II disorders involve humoral antibodies that participate directly in injuring cells by predisposing them to phagocytosis or lysis.
- Type III disorders result in generation of immune complexes in which humoral antibodies bind antigen and activate complement. The fractions of complement attract inflammatory cells that release tissue-damaging products.
- Type IV disorders involve tissue damage in which cell-mediated immune responses with sensitized T lymphocytes cause cell and tissue injury.

Typical allergens include the protein in pollen, house dust mites, animal dander, foods, and chemicals like the antibiotic penicillin. Exposure to the allergen can be through inhalation, ingestion, injection, or skin contact. Depending on the portal of entry, type I reactions may occur as a local or atopic reaction that is merely annoying (*e.g.,* seasonal rhinitis) or severely debilitating (asthma), or as a systemic and potentially life-threatening reaction (anaphylaxis).

Two types of cells are central to a type I hypersensitivity reaction: helper T subtype 2 (T_H2) cells and mast cells or basophils.[1,19,20] There are two subsets of helper T cells (T_H1 and T_H2) that develop from the same precursor $CD4^+$ T lymphocyte (see Chapter 19). T_H1 cells differentiate in response to microbes and stimulate the differentiation of B cells into IgM- and IgG-producing plasma cells. T_H2 differentiation occurs in response to allergens and hellminths (intestinal parasites).[1] Cytokines (*i.e.,* interleukin-4 [IL-4], IL-5, IL-13) secreted by T_H2 cells stimulate differentiation of B cells into IgE-producing plasma cells, act as growth factors for mast cells, and recruit and activate eosinophils.

Mast cells, which are tissue cells, and basophils, which are blood cells, are derived from hematopoietic (blood) precursor cells. Mast cells normally are distributed throughout connective tissue, especially in areas beneath the skin and mucous membranes of the respiratory, gastrointestinal, and genitourinary tracts, and adjacent to blood and lymph vessels.[21,22] This location places mast cells near surfaces that are exposed to environmental antigens and parasites. Microscopically, mast cells vary in shape, have round nuclei, and have membrane-bound mediator-containing granules and lipid bodies. Mast cells in different parts of the body and even in a single site can have significant differences in mediator content and sensitivity to agents that produce mast cell degranulation. For example, skin mast cells differ from lung mast cells in being more sensitive to morphine, substance P, and other neuropeptides and in the ideal temperature at which degranulation occurs (30°C in skin versus 37°C in the lungs).[23]

Type I hypersensitivity reactions begin with mast cell or basophil sensitization. During the sensitization or priming stage, allergen-specific IgE antibodies attach to receptors on the surface of mast cells and basophils. With subsequent exposure, the sensitizing allergen binds to the cell-associated

IgE and triggers a series of events that ultimately lead to degranulation of the sensitized mast cells or basophils, causing release of their preformed mediators (Fig. 21-4). Mast cells are also the source of lipid-derived membrane products (*e.g.*, prostaglandins and leukotrienes) and cytokines that participate in the continued response to the allergen.

Many type I hypersensitivity reactions such as bronchial asthma have two well-defined phases: (1) a primary or initial-phase response characterized by vasodilation, vascular leakage, and smooth muscle contraction; and (2) a secondary or late-phase response characterized by more intense infiltration of tissues with eosinophils and other acute and chronic inflammatory cells as well as tissue destruction in the form of epithelial cell damage.

The primary or initial-phase response usually occurs within 5 to 30 minutes of exposure to antigen and subsides within 60 minutes. It is mediated by mast cell degranulation and the release of preformed mediators. These mediators include histamine, acetylcholine, adenosine, chemotactic mediators, and enzymes such as chymase and trypsin that lead to generation of kinins. Histamine is a potent vasodilator that increases the permeability of capillaries and venules and causes smooth muscle contraction and bronchial constriction. Acetylcholine produces bronchial smooth muscle contraction and dilation of small blood vessels. The kinins,

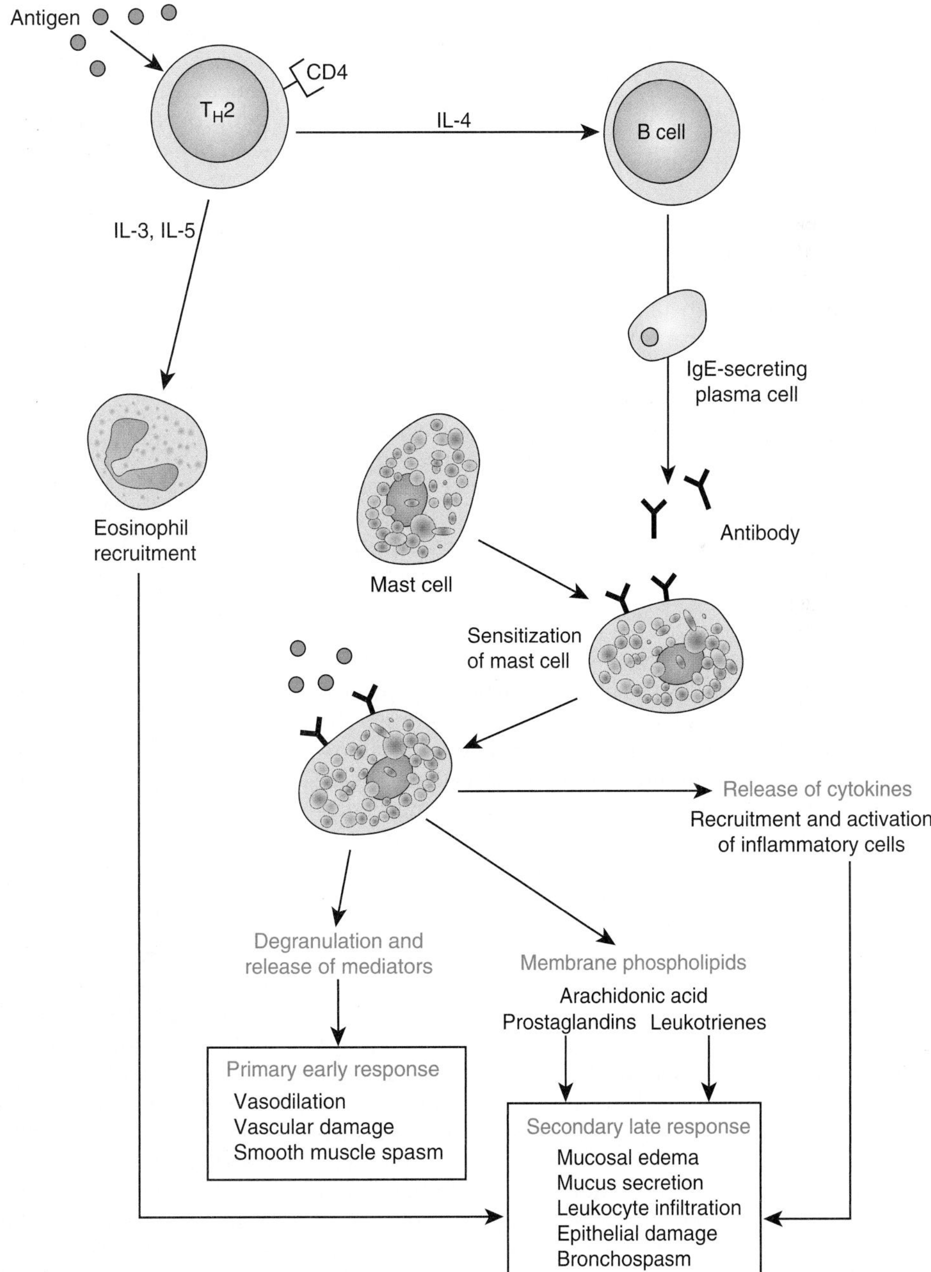

FIGURE 21-4 Type I, IgE-mediated hypersensitivity reaction. The stimulation of B cell differentiation by an antigen-stimulated T_H2 cell leads to plasma cell production of IGE and mast cell sensitization. Subsequent binding of the antigen produces degranulation of the sensitized mast cell with release of preformed mediators that leads to a primary early response. T_H2 cell recruitment of eosinophils along with the release of cytokines and membrane phospholipids from the mast cell leads to a secondary late response.

which are a group of potent inflammatory peptides, require activation through enzymatic modification. Once activated, these peptide mediators produce vasodilation and smooth muscle contraction.

The secondary or late-phase response sets in about 2 to 8 hours later and lasts for several days. It results from the action of lipid mediators and cytokines involved in the inflammatory response. The lipid mediators are derived from mast cell membrane phospholipids, which are broken down to form arachidonic acid. Arachidonic acid, in turn, is the parent compound from which the leukotrienes and prostaglandins are synthesized (see Chapter 20). The leukotrienes and prostaglandins produce responses similar to histamine and acetylcholine, although their effects are delayed and prolonged by comparison. Mast cells also produce cytokines and chemotactic factors that prompt the influx of eosinophils and leukocytes to the site of allergen contact, contributing to the inflammatory response.

At this point, it is important to note that not all IgE-mediated responses produce discomfort and disease. Type I hypersensitivity, particularly the late-phase response, plays a protective role in control of parasitic infections. IgE antibodies serve to damage directly the larvae of these parasites by recruiting inflammatory cells and causing antibody-dependent cell-mediated cytotoxicity. This type of type I hypersensitivity reaction is particularly important in developing countries, where much of the population is infected with intestinal parasites.

Anaphylactic (Systemic) Reactions

Anaphylaxis is a systemic life-threatening hypersensitivity reaction characterized by edema in many tissues and a fall in blood pressure secondary to vasodilation (see the section on Anaphylactic Shock in Chapter 28). It results from the intravascular presence of antigen introduced by injection, insect sting, or absorption across the epithelial surface of the skin or gastrointestinal mucosa.

Atopic (Local) Reactions

Local or atopic reactions usually occur when the antigen is confined to a particular site by virtue of exposure. The term *atopic* refers to a genetically determined hypersensitivity to common environmental allergens mediated by an IgE–mast cell reaction. Persons with atopic disorders commonly are allergic to more than one, and often many, environmental allergens. The most common atopic disorders are urticaria (hives), allergic rhinitis (hay fever), atopic dermatitis, food allergies, and some forms of asthma. The discussion in this section focuses on allergic rhinitis and food allergy. Allergic asthma is discussed in Chapter 31 and atopic dermatitis in Chapter 61.

Atopic disorders tend to run in families and affect approximately 1 in 10 persons in the United States.[19] The genetic basis of atopy is unclear; however, linkage studies suggest an association with cytokine genes on chromosome 5q that regulate the expression of circulating IgE.[19] Persons with atopic allergic conditions tend to have high serum levels of IgE and increased numbers of basophils and mast cells. Although the IgE-triggered response is likely a key factor in the pathophysiology of atopic allergic disorders, it is not the only factor and may not be responsible for conditions such as atopic dermatitis and certain forms of asthma.

Allergic Rhinitis. Allergic rhinitis (*i.e.,* allergic rhinoconjunctivitis) is characterized by symptoms of sneezing, itching, and watery discharge from the eyes and nose. Allergic rhinitis not only produces nasal symptoms but also frequently is associated with other chronic airway disorders, such as sinusitis and bronchial asthma.[24,25] Severe attacks may be accompanied by systemic malaise, fatigue, and muscle soreness from sneezing. Fever is absent. Sinus obstruction may cause headache. Typical allergens include pollens from ragweed, grasses, trees, and weeds; fungal spores; house dust mites; animal dander; and feathers. Allergic rhinitis can be divided into perennial and seasonal types depending on the chronology of symptoms. Persons with the perennial type of allergic rhinitis experience symptoms throughout the year, while those with seasonal allergic rhinitis (*i.e.,* hay fever) are plagued with intense symptoms in conjunction with periods of high allergen (*e.g.,* pollens, fungal spores) exposure. Symptoms that become worse at night suggest a household allergen, and symptoms that disappear on weekends suggest occupational exposure.

Diagnosis depends on a careful history and physical examination, microscopic identification of an increased number of eosinophils on a nasal smear, and skin testing to identify the offending allergens. Treatment is symptomatic in most cases and includes the use of oral antihistamines and decongestants.[25] Intranasal corticosteroids often are effective when used appropriately. Intranasal cromolyn, a drug that stabilizes mast cells and prevents their degranulation, may be useful, especially when administered before expected contact with an offending allergen. The anticholinergic agent ipratropium, which is available as a nasal spray, also may be used. When possible, avoidance of the offending allergen is recommended. A program of specific immunotherapy (allergy shots) may be used when symptoms are particularly bothersome. Desensitization involves frequent (usually weekly) injections of the offending antigens.[24–26] The antigens, which are given in increasing doses, stimulate production of high levels of IgG, which acts as a blocking antibody by combining with the antigen before it can combine with the cell-bound IgE antibodies. Recent studies suggest a possible role for sublingual-swallow immunotherapy or local nasal immunotherapy.[26]

Food Allergies. Virtually any food can produce atopic or nonatopic allergies. The primary target of food allergy may be the skin, the gastrointestinal tract, or the respiratory system. The foods most commonly causing these reactions in children are milk, eggs, peanuts, soy, tree nuts, fish, and shellfish foods (*i.e.,* crustaceans and mollusks).[27] In adults, they are peanuts,[28] shellfish, and fish.[27] The allergenicity of a food may be changed by heating or cooking. A person may be allergic to drinking milk but may not have symptoms when milk is included in cooked foods. Both acute reactions (hives and anaphylaxis) and chronic reactions (asthma, atopic dermatitis, and gastrointestinal disorders) can occur. Anaphylaxis occurs as a multiorgan response associated with IgE-mediated hypersensitivity. The foods most responsible for anaphylaxis are peanuts, tree nuts (*e.g.*, walnuts, almonds, pecans, cashews, hazelnuts), and shellfish. One form of food-associated anaphylaxis occurs with exercise.[27,29] Food-associated, exercise-induced anaphylaxis may occur when exercise follows ingestion of a particular food to which IgE sensitivity has been demonstrated, or it may occur after ingestion of any food. Exercise without ingestion of the incriminated food does not produce symptoms.

Food allergies can occur at any age but, similar to atopic dermatitis and rhinitis, they tend to manifest during childhood. The allergic response is thought to occur after contact between specific food allergens and sensitized mast cells found in the intestinal mucosa causes local and systemic release of histamine and other mediators of the allergic response. In this disorder, allergens usually are food proteins and partially digested food products. Carbohydrates, lipids, or food additives, such as preservatives, colorings, or flavorings, also are potential allergens. Closely related food groups can contain common cross-reacting allergens. For example, some persons are allergic to all legumes (*i.e.*, beans, peas, and peanuts).

Diagnosis of food allergies usually is based on careful food history and provocative diet testing. Provocative testing involves careful elimination of a suspected allergen from the diet for a period of time to see if the symptoms disappear and reintroducing the food to see if the symptoms reappear. Only one food should be tested at a time. Treatment focuses on avoidance of the food or foods responsible for the allergy. However, avoidance may be difficult for persons who are exquisitely sensitive to a particular food protein because foods may be contaminated with the protein during processing or handling of the food. For example, contamination may occur when chocolate candies without peanuts are processed with the same equipment used for making candies with peanuts. Even using the same spatula to serve cookies with and without peanuts can cause enough contamination to produce a severe reaction.

TYPE II, ANTIBODY-MEDIATED DISORDERS

Type II hypersensitivity reactions are mediated by IgG or IgM antibodies directed against target antigens on the surface of cells or other tissue components (Fig. 21-5). The antigens may be endogenous antigens that are present on the membranes of body cells or exogenous antigens that are adsorbed on the membrane surface. Examples of type II reactions include mismatched blood transfusion reactions, hemolytic disease of the newborn due to ABO or Rh incompatibility (see Chapter 16), and certain drug reactions. In the latter, the binding of certain drugs or drug metabolites to the surface of red or white blood cells elicits an antibody response that lyses the drug-coated cell. Lytic drug reactions can produce transient anemia, leukopenia, or thrombocytopenia, which are corrected by the removal of the offending drug.

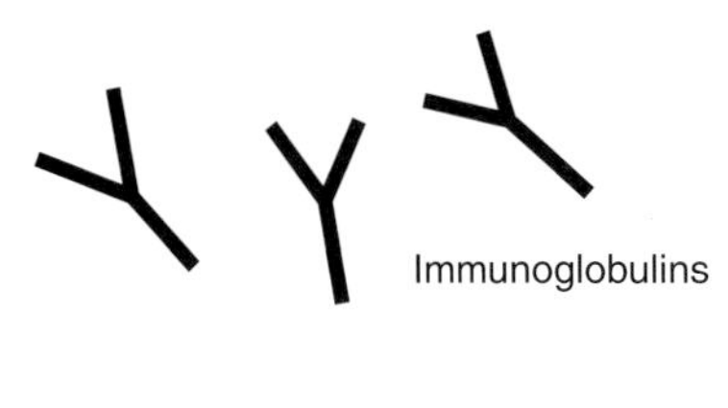

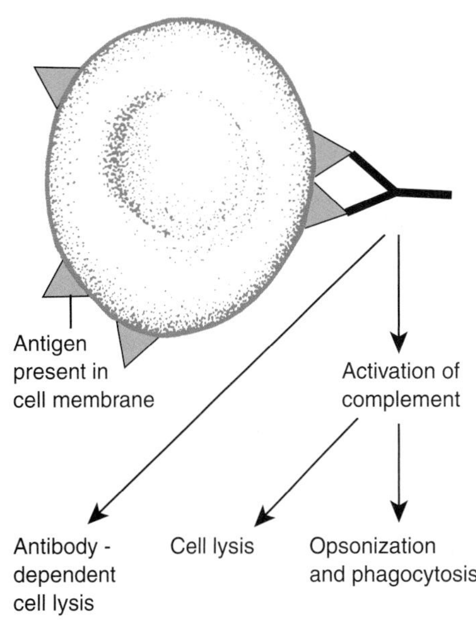

FIGURE 21-5 Type II, antibody-mediated reactions involve formation of immunoglobins (IgG and IgM) against cell surface antigens. The antigen-antibody response leads to (1) complement-mediated mechanisms of cell injury or to (2) antibody cytotoxicity that does not require the complement system.

TYPE III, IMMUNE COMPLEX-MEDIATED DISORDERS

Type III hypersensitivity disorders are mediated by the formation of insoluble antigen–antibody complexes that activate complement (Fig. 21-6). Activation of complement by the immune complex generates chemotactic and vasoactive mediators that cause tissue damage by a variety of mechanisms, including alterations in blood flow, increased vascular permeability, and the destructive action of inflammatory cells. Immune complexes formed in the circulation produce damage when they come in contact with the vessel lining or are deposited in tissues, including the glomeruli in the kidney, skin venules, lung, and joint synovium. Once deposited, the immune complexes elicit an inflammatory response by activating complement, thereby leading to chemotactic recruitment of neutrophils and other inflammatory cells.

Type III reactions are responsible for the vasculitis seen in certain autoimmune diseases such as SLE or the kidney damage seen with acute glomerulonephritis. Unlike type II reactions, in which the damage is caused by direct and specific binding of antibody to tissue, the harmful effects of type III reactions are indirect (*i.e.*, secondary to the inflammatory response induced by activated complement).

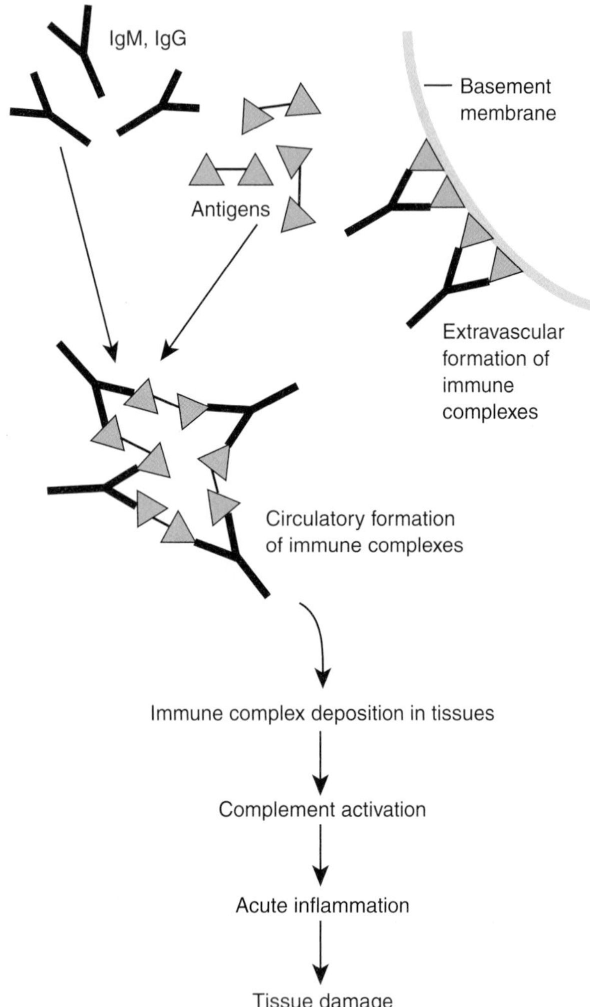

FIGURE 21-6 Type III, immune complex-mediated reactions involve complement-activating IgG and IgM immunoglobulins with formation of blood-borne immune complexes that are eventually deposited in tissues. Complement activation at the site of immune complex deposition leads to recruitment of leukocytes, which are eventually responsible for tissue injury.

Immune complex disorders can present with systemic manifestations, as in serum sickness, or as a local reaction, as in the Arthus reaction.

Systemic Immune Complex Disorders

Serum sickness has become the prototype for systemic immune complex disorders. The term *serum sickness* was originally coined to describe a syndrome consisting of rash, lymphadenopathy, arthralgias, and occasionally neurologic disorders that appeared 7 or more days after injections of horse antisera (tetanus). Although this therapy is not used today, the name remains. The most common contemporary causes of this allergic disorder include antibiotics (especially penicillin), various foods, drugs, and insect venoms. Serum sickness is triggered by the deposition of insoluble antigen–antibody (IgM and IgG) complexes in blood vessels, joints, heart, and kidney tissue. The deposited complexes activate complement, increase vascular permeability, and recruit phagocytic cells, all of which can promote focal tissue damage and edema. The signs and symptoms include urticaria, patchy or generalized rash, extensive edema (usually of the face, neck, and joints), and fever. In most cases, the damage is temporary, and symptoms resolve within a few days. However, a prolonged and continuous exposure to the sensitizing antigen can lead to irreversible damage. In previously sensitized persons, severe and even fatal forms of serum sickness may occur immediately or within several days after the sensitizing drug or serum is administered.

Treatment of serum sickness usually is directed toward removal of the sensitizing antigen and providing symptom relief. This may include aspirin for joint pain and antihistamines for pruritus. Systemic corticosteroids may be used for severe reactions.

Localized Immune Complex Reactions

The *Arthus reaction* is a term used by pathologists and immunologists to describe localized tissue necrosis (usually in the skin) caused by immune complexes. In the laboratory, an Arthus reaction can be produced by injecting an antigen preparation into the skin of an immune animal with high levels of circulating antibody. Within 4 to 10 hours, a red, raised lesion appears on the skin at the site of the injection.[19] An ulcer often forms in the center of the lesion. It is thought that the injected antigen diffuses into local blood vessels, where it comes in contact with specific antibody (IgG) to incite a localized vasculitis (*i.e.,* inflammation of a blood vessel). Tissue sections of Arthus lesions show deposited immunoglobulin, complement, and fibrinolytic products in blood vessels. If the blood vessel bursts, hemorrhage into surrounding tissue occurs. Should fibrinolytic products occlude the vessel, the oxygen supply to the surrounding tissue is interrupted, causing cell death and tissue necrosis.

TYPE IV, T-CELL–MEDIATED HYPERSENSITIVITY DISORDERS

Type IV hypersensitivity reactions involve T-cell–mediated rather than antibody-mediated immune responses.[19] Cell-mediated immunity is the principal mechanism of response to a variety of microorganisms, including intracellular pathogens such as *Mycobacterium tuberculosis* and viruses, as well as extracellular agents such as fungi, protozoa, and parasites. It can also lead to cell death and tissue injury in response to chemical antigens (contact dermatitis), organic substances (hypersensitivity pneumonia), or self antigens (autoimmunity).

Type IV hypersensitivity reactions, which are mediated by specifically sensitized T lymphocytes, can be divided into two basic types: direct cell-mediated cytotoxicity and delayed-type hypersensitivity (Fig. 21-7).

Direct Cell-Mediated Cytotoxicity

In direct cell-mediated cytotoxicity, $CD8^+$ cytolytic T lymphocytes (CTLs) directly kill the antigen-presenting target cells. CTLs responses in viral infection can lead to tissue in-

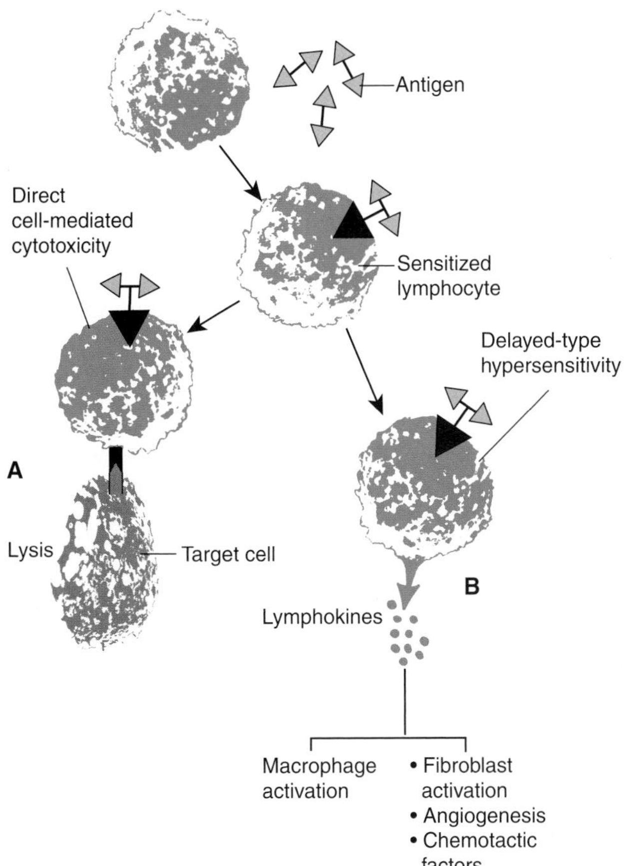

FIGURE 21-7 Type IV, direct cell-mediated cytotoxicity (**A**) or delayed-type hypersensitivity (**B**) reactions involve sensitization of T lymphocytes with the subsequent formation of cytotoxic T cells that lyse target cells or T cells that release cell-damaging lymphokines.

jury by killing infected target cells even if the virus itself has no cytotoxic effects.[19] Some viruses directly injure infected cells and are said to be cytopathic, whereas other noncytopathic viruses do not. Because CTLs cannot distinguish between cytopathic and noncytopathic viruses, they kill virtually all infected cells regardless of whether the infection is harmful or not. In certain forms of hepatitis, for example, the destruction of liver cells is due to the host CTL response and not the virus.

Delayed-Type Hypersensitivity Disorders

In delayed-type hypersensitivity (DTH), T_H1 cells secrete immunoregulatory and proinflammatory cytokines.[19] Some of the cytokines promote differentiation and activation of macrophages that function as phagocytic and antigen-presenting cells (APCs). Chronic DTH reactions often lead to fibrosis as a result of the secretion of cytokines and growth factors by the macrophages.

The best-known type of DTH hypersensitivity response is the reaction to the tuberculin test, in which inactivated tuberculin or purified protein derivative is injected under the skin. In a person who has been sensitized by previous infection, a local area of redness and induration develops within 8 to 12 hours, reaching a peak in 24 to 72 hours. The tuberculin reaction is characterized by perivascular accumulation of $CD4^+$ T_H1 cells and, to a lesser extent, macrophages. Local secretion of cytokines by these mononuclear inflammatory cells leads to increased microvascular permeability, giving rise to swelling and fibrosis. A positive tuberculin test indicates that a person has had sufficient exposure to the *M. tuberculosis* organism to incite a hypersensitivity reaction; it does not mean that the person has tuberculosis.

The sequence of events in DTH, as demonstrated by the tuberculin reaction, begins with the first exposure to the tuberculin bacilli. $CD4^+$ lymphocytes recognize the peptide antigens of the tuberculin bacilli in association with class II MHC antigens on the surface of monocytes and antigen-presenting cells that have processed the mycobacterial antigens. This process leads to sensitized $CD4^+$ cells of the T_H1 type that remain in the circulation for years. Subsequent injection of tuberculin into such an individual results in the secretion of T_H1 cytokines that are ultimately responsible for the DTH response.

Allergic Contact Dermatitis. Allergic contact dermatitis is a DTH hypersensitivity response confined to the skin that is initiated by reexposure to an allergen to which a person had previously become sensitized (*e.g.*, cosmetics, hair dyes, metals, topical drugs). Contact dermatitis usually consists of erythematous macules, papules, and vesicles (*i.e.*, blisters). The affected area often becomes swollen and warm, with exudation, crusting, and development of a secondary infection. The location of the lesions often provides a clue about the nature of the antigen causing the disorder. The most common form of this condition is the dermatitis that follows an intimate encounter with poison ivy or poison oak antigens, although many other substances can trigger a reaction.

The mechanism of events leading to prior sensitization to an antigen is not completely understood. It is likely that sensitization follows transdermal transport of an antigen, with subsequent presentation to T lymphocytes. Subpopulations of sensitized lymphocytes are distributed throughout the body so that subsequent cutaneous exposure to the offending antigen promotes a localized reaction regardless of the initial site of contact. The severity of the reaction associated with contact dermatitis ranges from mild to intense, depending on the person and the allergen. Because this condition follows the pathway of a DTH response, the reaction does not become apparent for at least 12 hours and usually more than 24 hours after exposure. Depending on the antigen and the duration of exposure, the reaction may last from days to weeks and is typified by erythematous, vesicular, or papular lesions associated with intense pruritus and weeping.

Diagnosis of contact dermatitis is made by observing the distribution of lesions on the skin surface and associating a particular pattern with exposure to possible allergens. If a particular allergen is suspected, a patch test can be used to confirm the suspicion. For this, the suspected allergen is applied to a gauze or patch that is taped to a hair-free surface for 48 hours. The patch is removed, and the surface is inspected daily for a response. Treatment usually is limited to removal of the irritant and application of topical preparations (*e.g.*, ointments, corticosteroid creams) to relieve symptomatic skin lesions and prevent secondary bacterial infections. Severe reactions may require systemic corticosteroid therapy.

Hypersensitivity Pneumonitis. Hypersensitivity pneumonitis, which is associated with exposure to inhaled organic dusts or related occupational antigens, is another example of a DTH reaction. The disorder is thought to involve a susceptible host and activation of pulmonary T cells, followed by the release of cytokine mediators of inflammation.[30] The inflammatory response that ensues (usually several hours after exposure) produces labored breathing, dry cough, chills and fever, headache, and malaise. The symptoms usually subside within hours after the sensitizing antigens are removed. A primary example of hypersensitivity pneumonitis is "farmer's lung," a condition resulting from exposure to moldy hay. Other sensitizing antigens include tree bark, sawdust, animal danders, and *Actinomycetes* bacteria that are occasionally found in humidifiers, hot tubs, and swimming pools. Exposure to small amounts of antigen for a long period may lead to chronic lung disease with minimal reversibility. This can happen to persons exposed to avian or animal antigens or a contaminated home air humidifier.[30]

The most important element in the diagnosis of hypersensitivity pneumonitis is to obtain a good history (occupational and otherwise) of exposure to possible antigens. Skin tests, when available, and serum tests for precipitating antibody can be done. Occasionally, direct observation of the person's work and other environments may help to establish a diagnosis. Treatment consists of identifying and avoiding the offending antigens. Severe forms of the disorder may be treated with systemic corticosteroid therapy.

LATEX ALLERGY

With the advent of HIV and other blood-borne diseases, the use of natural latex gloves has spiraled. Between 1988 and 1992, an estimated 11.8 billion examining gloves and 1.8 billion surgical gloves were used in the United States.[31] Along with the expanded use of latex gloves have come increased reports of latex allergy among health care workers. It has been estimated that 10% to 17% of health care workers have already been sensitized, and more than 2% have occupational asthma as a result of exposure.[31] Other persons at high risk for sensitization are those with prolonged exposure to latex, including persons who have undergone repeated surgeries.

Exposure to latex may occur by cutaneous, mucous membrane, inhalation, internal tissue, or intravascular routes. Most severe reactions have resulted from latex proteins coming in contact with the mucous membranes of the mouth, vagina, urethra, or rectum. Although their allergen content is not very high, condoms can cause severe reactions because they come in contact with the mucous membranes.[32] Children with meningomyelocele (spina bifida) who undergo frequent examinations and treatments involving the mucosal surface of the bladder or rectum are at particular risk for development of latex allergy.[31,33,34] A large number of latex products are used in dentistry, and oral mucosal contact is common during dental procedures. Anaphylactic reactions have been caused by exposure of the internal organs to the surgeon's gloves during surgery.

Natural rubber latex is derived from the milky sap of the *Heva brasiliensis* plant or rubber tree.[32] Various accelerants, curing agents, antioxidants, and stabilizers are added to the liquid latex during the manufacturing process. Cornstarch powder is applied to the gloves during the manufacturing process to prevent stickiness and give the gloves a smooth feel. Allergic reactions to latex products can be triggered by the latex proteins or by the additives used in the manufacturing process. The cornstarch glove powder has an important role in the allergic response. Latex proteins are readily absorbed by glove powder and become airborne during removal of the gloves. High-exposure areas such as operating rooms where powdered gloves are used contain sufficiently high levels of aerosolized latex to produce symptoms in sensitized persons.

The allergy to latex products can involve a type I, IgE-mediated hypersensitivity reaction or a type IV, T cell-mediated response. Irritant dermatitis, which can result from glove use, is an entirely nonimmunologic response and should not be regarded as an allergy.[32] The distinction between the type I and type IV reactions to latex products is not always clear. Affected individuals may experience both types of reactions. The most common type of reaction to latex gloves is contact dermatitis caused by a type IV, DTH response to the chemical additives used to process most gloves. It usually develops 48 to 96 hours after direct contact with latex additives. It often affects the dorsum of the hands and is characterized by a vesicular rash. When glove contact is continued, the area becomes crusted and thickened.

The type 1, IgE-mediated hypersensitivity reactions occur in response to the latex proteins. They may manifest as urticaria, rhinoconjunctivitis, asthma, or anaphylaxis. They are less common but far more serious than type IV responses. Persons with latex allergy commonly show cross-sensitivity to bananas, avocado, kiwi, tomatoes, and chestnuts, probably because latex proteins are similar to proteins in these products.[31,33] These foods have been responsible for anaphylactic reactions in latex-sensitive persons.

Diagnosis of latex allergy often is based on careful history and evidence of skin reactions due to latex exposure. Symptoms after use of a rubber condom or diaphragm should raise suspicion of latex allergy. Because many of the reported reactions to latex gloves have been the result of a nonimmunologic dermatitis, it is important to differentiate between nonallergic and allergic types of dermatitis. Latex skin-prick testing can be done, but it should be done in an allergy center familiar with the test and with equipment available to treat possible anaphylactic reactions. Serum tests for latex-specific IgE antibodies also can be done. However, these tests may give false-positive or false-negative results. Thus, at this time, diagnosis usually is based on latex-specific symptoms of IgE-mediated reactions to latex exposure.[33]

Treatment of latex allergy consists of avoiding latex exposure. Use of powder-free gloves can reduce the amount of airborne latex particles. Health care workers with severe and life-threatening allergy may be forced to change employment. Patients at high risk for latex allergy (*e.g.*, children with spina bifida, health care workers with atopy) should be offered clinical testing for latex allergy before undergoing procedures that expose them to natural rubber latex. All surgical or other procedures on persons with latex allergy should be done in a latex-free environment.

In summary, hypersensitivity disorders are responses to environmental, food, or drug antigens that would not affect most of the population. There are four basic categories of hypersensitivity responses: (1) type I responses, which are mediated by the IgE class immunoglobulins and include anaphylactic shock, hay fever, and bronchial asthma; (2) type II antibody-mediated reactions, which are mediated by IgG antibodies directed against antigens on the surface of cells such as those on the red cells of donor blood, which cause hemolytic transfusion reactions; (3) type III reactions, which involve IgG and IgM antibodies and result from the formation of insoluble antigen–antibody complexes that become deposited in blood vessels or in the kidney and cause localized tissue injury; and (4) type IV, T-cell–mediated responses in which sensitized T lymphocytes promote an inflammatory response when presented with the sensitizing antigen.

T_H2 cells and mast cells play a pivotal role in the pathogenesis of type I reactions. Exposure to antigen stimulates the production of T_H2 cells, which secrete cytokines that cause B cells to produce IgE. The antigen-specific IgE binds to mast cells and basophils, sensitizing them to the antigen. Once mast cells and basophils have become sensitized, the individual is primed to develop a type I hypersensitivity response. Type II and type III hypersensitivity responses involve T_H1 cells and IgG and IgM antibodies.

Latex allergy can involve a type I, IgE-mediated reaction or a type IV, cell-mediated response. The most common type of allergic reaction to latex gloves is a contact dermatitis caused by a type IV, delayed-type hypersensitivity reaction to rubber additives. The type I, IgE-mediated response to the latex protein is less common but can cause far more serious anaphylactic reactions.

Transplantation Immunopathology

After completing this section of the chapter, you should be able to meet the following objectives:

- Discuss the rationale for matching of human leukocyte antigen in organ transplantation
- Compare the immune mechanisms involved in host-versus-graft and graft-versus-host transplant rejection

Not too many years ago, transplantation of solid organs (*e.g.*, liver, kidney, heart) and bone marrow was considered experimental and reserved for persons for whom alternative methods of therapy were exhausted and survival was unlikely. However, with a greater understanding of humoral and cellular immune regulation, the development of immunosuppressive drugs such as cyclosporine, and an appreciation of the role of the major histocompatibility complex (MHC) antigens, transplantation has become nearly routine, and the subsequent success rate has been greatly enhanced.

The cell surface antigens that determine whether transplanted tissue is recognized as foreign are the MHC or *human leukocyte antigens* (HLA) (see Chapter 19). Transplanted tissue can be categorized as *allogeneic* if the donor and recipient are related or unrelated but share similar HLA types, *syngeneic* if the donor and recipient are identical twins, and *autologous* if donor and recipient are the same person. Donors of solid organ transplants can be living or dead (cadaver) and related or unrelated (heterologous). When cells bearing foreign MHC antigens are transplanted, the recipient's immune system can attempt to eliminate the donor cells, a process referred to as *host-versus-graft disease* (HVGD). Conversely, the cellular immune system of the transplanted tissue can attack unrelated recipient tissue, causing *graft-versus-host disease* (GVHD) (Fig. 21-8). The likelihood of rejection varies indirectly with the degree of MHC or HLA relatedness between donor and recipient.

HOST-VERSUS-GRAFT DISEASE

In HVGD, the immune cells of the transplant recipient attack the donor cells of the transplanted organ. HVGD usually is limited to allogeneic organ transplants, although even HLA-identical siblings may differ in some minor HLA loci, which can evoke slow rejection. Rejection due to HVGD is a complex process that involves a cell-mediated immune response and circulating antibodies. Although many cells may participate in the process of acute transplant rejection, only the T lymphocytes seem to be absolutely required.[35] The activation of $CD4^+$ helper T cells and $CD8^+$ cytotoxic T cells is triggered in response to the donor's HLA antigens. Activation of $CD4^+$ helper T cells leads to proliferation of B-cell–mediated antibody production and T-cell–mediated DTH or CTL hypersensitivity reactions. There are three basic patterns of transplant rejection: hyperacute, acute, and chronic.[1,19]

A *hyperacute reaction* occurs almost immediately after transplantation. In kidney transplants, it can often be seen at the time of surgery. As soon as blood flow from the recipient to the donor kidney begins, it takes on a cyanotic, mottled appearance. At other times, the reaction may take hours or days to develop. The hyperacute response is produced by existing recipient antibodies to graft antigens that initiate a type III, Arthus-type hypersensitivity reaction in the blood vessels of the graft. These antibodies usually have developed in response to previous blood transfusions, pregnancies in which the mother makes antibodies to fetal antigens, or infections with bacteria or viruses possessing antigens that mimic MHC antigens of the donor.

Acute rejection usually occurs within the first few months after transplantation and is evidenced by signs of organ failure. It also may occur suddenly months or even

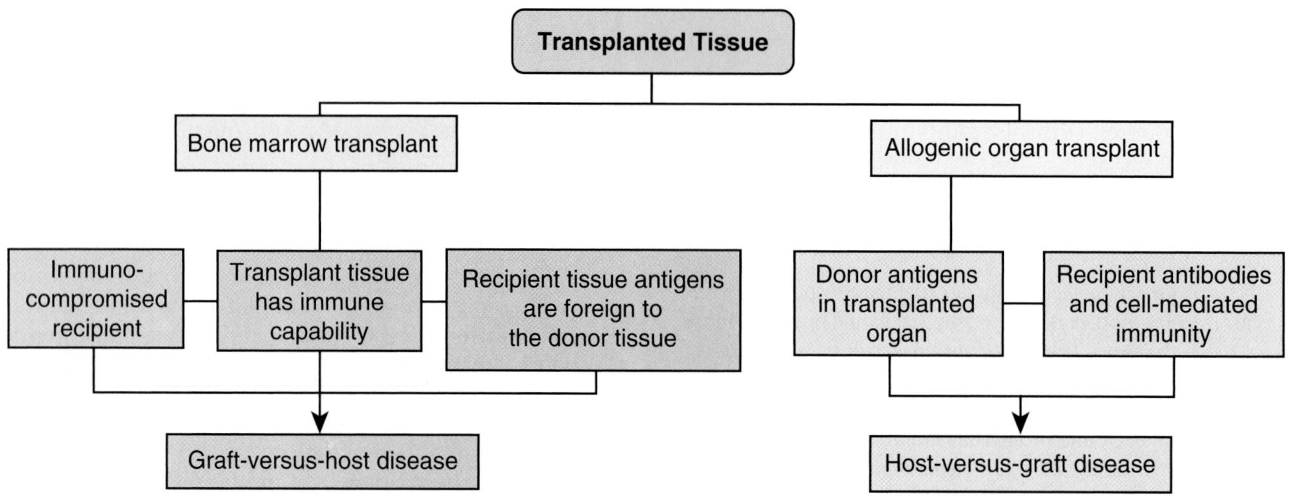

FIGURE 21-8 Mechanism of graft-versus-host disease in bone marrow transplantation and host-versus-graft disease in allogenic organ transplantation.

years later, after immunosuppression has been used and terminated. T lymphocytes play a central role in acute rejection, responding to antigens in the graft tissue. The activated T cells cause direct lysis of graft cells and recruit and activate inflammatory cells that injure the graft. In vascularized grafts such as kidney grafts, the endothelial cells of blood vessels are the earliest targets of acute rejection.

Chronic host-versus-graft rejection occurs over a prolonged period. It manifests with dense intimal fibrosis of blood vessels of the transplanted organ. In renal transplantation, it is characterized by a gradual rise in serum creatinine over a period of 4 to 6 months. The actual mechanism of this type of response is unclear but may include release of cytokines that stimulate fibrosis.

GRAFT-VERSUS-HOST DISEASE

Graft-versus-host disease occurs when immunologically competent cells or precursors are transplanted into recipients who are immunologically compromised. Although GVHD occurs most often in persons who have undergone allogenic bone marrow transplantation, it may also follow transplantation of organs rich in lymphoid tissue (*e.g.,* the liver) or follow transfusions with nonirradiated blood.[19,36,37]

Three basic requirements are necessary for GVHD to develop: the transplant must have a functional cellular immune component; the recipient tissue must bear antigens foreign to the donor tissue; and the recipient immunity must be compromised to the point that it cannot destroy the transplanted cells.[1,19,36] The primary agents of GVHD are the donor immunocompetent T cells derived from the donor marrow and the recipient tissue that they recognize as foreign and react against.[19] GVHD results in activation of both $CD4^+$ and $CD8^+$ T cells with ultimate generation of type IV, cell-mediated DTH and CTL hypersensitivity reactions. The greater the difference in tissue antigens between the donor and recipient, the greater is the likelihood of GVHD.

GVHD can occur as an acute or chronic reaction. Acute GVHD, which develops within days to weeks after transplantation, affects the epithelial cells of the skin, liver, and gastrointestinal tract.[19,36] The organ most commonly affected in acute GVHD is the skin. There is development of a pruritic, maculopapular rash, which begins on the palms and soles and frequently extends over the entire body, with subsequent desquamation. Involvement of the gastrointestinal tract usually parallels the development of skin and liver involvement. Gastrointestinal symptoms include nausea, bloody diarrhea, and abdominal pain. GVHD of the liver is heralded by painless jaundice, hyperbilirubinemia, and abnormal liver function tests. Liver involvement can progress to development of venoocclusive disease with extrahepatic biliary obstruction, sepsis, and coma. Venoocclusive disease is characterized by obliteration of the small hepatic veins and venules. In acute venoocclusive disease, there is striking centrilobular congestion and hepatocellular necrosis. As the disease progresses, connective tissue is deposited in the lumen of venules, and the centrilobular congestion becomes less evident. The incidence of venoocclusive disease approaches 25% of recipients of allogenic marrow transplants, with mortality rates higher than 30%.[38]

GVHD is considered chronic if symptoms persist or begin 100 days or more after transplantation. Chronic GVHD may follow acute GVHD, or it may develop insidiously. Although persons who develop chronic GVHD are profoundly immunocompromised, they may develop skin lesions resembling systemic sclerosis (discussed in Chapter 59) and manifestations mimicking other autoimmune diseases.

A second type of GVHD can follow the transplantation of genetically identical tissue (*i.e.,* syngeneic or autologous). This type of GVHD stems from the use of pretreatment conditioning regimens (*e.g.*, total-body irradiation or treatment with cytotoxic drugs). The conditioning therapy disrupts the normal immune surveillance system and allows "rogue" autoreactive T cells to proliferate and attack native tissue. This type of GVHD usually is self-limited and not severe.

GVHD can be prevented by blocking any of the steps of pathogenesis. For example, donor T cells can be selectively removed from the transplanted tissue or destroyed using various treatments such as monoclonal antibodies with attached toxins, equivalent to heat-seeking missiles. Alternatively, immunosuppressive or anti-inflammatory drugs such as cyclosporine and tacrolimus or glucocorticoids can be used to block T-cell activation and the action of cytokines.

In summary, organ and bone marrow transplantation has been enhanced by a greater understanding of humoral and cellular immune regulation, the development of immunosuppressive drugs (*e.g.*, cyclosporine or tacrolimus), and an appreciation of the role of the MHC antigens. The likelihood of rejection varies with the degree of HLA (or MHC) relatedness between donor and recipient. A rejection can involve an attempt by the recipient's immune system to eliminate the donor cells, as in HVGD, or an attack by the cellular immunity of the transplanted tissue on the unrelated recipient tissue, as in GVHD.

Autoimmune Disease

After completing this section of the chapter, you should be able to meet the following objectives:

- Relate the mechanisms of self-tolerance to the possible explanations for development of autoimmune disease
- Name four or more diseases attributed to autoimmunity
- Describe three or more postulated mechanisms underlying autoimmune disease
- State the criteria for establishing an autoimmune basis for a disease

Autoimmune diseases represent a group of disorders that are caused by a breakdown in the ability of the immune system to differentiate between self and nonself antigens. Autoimmune diseases can affect almost any cell or tissue in the body. Some autoimmune disorders, such as Hashimoto's thyroiditis, are tissue specific; others, such as SLE, affect multiple organs and systems. Chart 21-2 lists some of the probable autoimmune diseases. Many of these disorders are discussed elsewhere in this book.

CHART 21-2

*Probable Autoimmune Disease**

Systemic

Mixed connective tissue disease
Polymyositis-dermatomyositis
Rheumatoid arthritis
Scleroderma
Sjögren's syndrome
Systemic lupus erythematosus

Blood

Autoimmune hemolytic anemia
Autoimmune neutropenia and lymphopenia
Idiopathic thrombocytopenic purpura

Other Organs

Acute idiopathic polyneuritis
Atrophic gastritis and pernicious anemia
Autoimmune adrenalitis
Goodpasture's syndrome
Hashimoto's thyroiditis
Type 1 diabetes mellitus
Myasthenia gravis
Premature gonadal (ovarian) failure
Primary biliary cirrhosis
Sympathetic ophthalmia
Temporal arteritis
Thyrotoxicosis (Graves' disease)
Crohn disease, ulcerative colitis

*Examples are not inclusive.

IMMUNOLOGIC TOLERANCE

To function properly, the immune system must be able to differentiate foreign antigens from self antigens. The ability of the immune system to differentiate self from nonself is called *self-tolerance*. It is the HLA antigens encoded by MHC genes that serve as recognition markers of self and nonself for the immune system (see Chapter 19). To elicit an immune response, an antigen must first be processed by an antigen-presenting cell (APC), such as a macrophage, which then presents the antigenic determinants along with an MHC II molecule to a $CD4^+$ helper T cell. The dual recognition of the MHC–antigen complex by the T-cell receptor (TCR) of the $CD4^+$ helper cell acts like a security check. Similar recognition checks occur between $CD8^+$ cytotoxic T cells and the class I MHC–antigen complex of tissue cells that have been targeted for elimination. A number of chemical messengers (*e.g.*, interleukins) and costimulatory signals are essential to the activation of immune responses and the preservation of self-tolerance.

The mechanisms postulated to explain the tolerant state include central tolerance and peripheral tolerance.[19] *Central tolerance* refers to the elimination of self-reactive T cells and B cells in the central lymphoid organs (*i.e.*, the thymus for T cells and the bone marrow for B cells). *Peripheral tolerance* derives from the deletion or inactivation of autoreactive T cells or B cells that escaped elimination in the central lymphoid organs. *Anergy* represents the state of immunologic tolerance to specific antigens. It may take the form of diminished immediate hypersensitivity, delayed-type hypersensitivity, or both.

IMMUNOLOGIC TOLERANCE

- Immunologic tolerance is the ability of the immune system to differentiate self from nonself. It results from central and peripheral mechanisms that delete self-reactive immune cells that cause autoimmunity or render their response ineffective in destroying self-cells and self-tissue.
- Central tolerance involves the elimination of self-reactive T and B cells in the central lymphoid organs. Self-reactive T cells are deleted in the thymus and self-reactive B cells in the bone marrow.
- Peripheral tolerance derives from the deletion or inactivation of self-reactive T and B cells that escaped deletion in the central lymphoid organs. It involves mechanisms such as receptor editing, absence of necessary costimulatory signals, production of immunologic ignorance by separating self-reactive immune cells from target tissues, and the presence of suppressor immune cells.

B-Cell Tolerance

Loss of self-tolerance with development of autoantibodies is characteristic of a number of autoimmune disorders. For example, hyperthyroidism in Graves' disease is due to autoantibodies to the thyroid-stimulating hormone receptor (see Chapter 42). Several mechanisms are available to filter autoreactive B cells out of the B-cell population: clonal deletion of immature B cells in the bone marrow; deletion of autoreactive B cells in the spleen or lymph nodes; functional inactivation or anergy; and receptor editing, a process that changes the specificity of a B-cell receptor when autoantigen is encountered.[39] There is increasing evidence that B-cell tolerance is predominantly due to help from T cells.[39]

T-Cell Tolerance

The central mechanisms of T-cell tolerance involve the deletion of self-reactive T cells in the thymus (Fig. 21-9). T cells develop from bone marrow–derived progenitor cells that migrate to the thymus, where they encounter self-peptides bound to MHC molecules. T cells that display the host's MHC antigens and TCRs for a nonself antigen are allowed to mature in the thymus (*i.e.*, positive selection). T cells that have a high affinity for host cells are sorted out and undergo apoptosis and die in the process (*i.e.*, negative selection). The deletion of self-reactive T cells in the thymus requires the presence of autoantigens. Because many autoantigens are not present in the thymus, self-reactive T cells may escape the thymus, requiring the need for peripheral mechanisms that participate in T-cell tolerance.

Several peripheral mechanisms are available to control the responsiveness of the self-reactive T cells in the periphery. Sometimes, the host antigens are not available in the appropriate immunologic form or are separated from the T cells (*e.g.*, by the blood–brain barrier) so that corresponding T cells remain *immunologically ignorant* of their presence.[39] In other cases, the autoreactive T cell encounters its corresponding antigen in the absence of the costimulatory signals that are necessary for its activation. The peripheral activation of T cells requires two signals: recognition of the peptide antigen in association with the MHC molecules on the APCs and a set of secondary costimulatory signals. Because costimulatory signals are not strongly expressed on most normal tissues, the encounter of the autoreactive T cells and their specific target antigens frequently results in anergy.[19]

Another mechanism involves the apoptotic death of autoreactive T cells.[39,40] This type of apoptosis is mediated by an apoptotic cell surface receptor (called Fas) that is present on the T cell and a soluble membrane messenger molecule (Fas ligand) that binds to the apoptotic receptor and activates the death program. The expression of the apoptotic Fas receptor is markedly increased in activated T cells; thus, coexpression of the Fas messenger molecule by the same cohort of activated autoreactive T cells may serve to induce their death.

Suppressor T cells with the ability to down-regulate the function of autoreactive T cells are also thought to play an essential role in peripheral T-cell tolerance. These cells are believed to be a distinct subset of CD4+ T cells.[41] The mechanism by which these T cells exert their suppressor function is unclear. They may secrete cytokines that suppress the activity of self-reactive immune cells.

MECHANISMS OF AUTOIMMUNE DISEASE

There are multiple explanations for the loss of self-tolerance and formation of autoantibodies or failure to recognize host antigens as self. Among the possible mechanisms responsible for development of autoimmune disease are aberrations in immune cell function or antigen structure. Heredity and gender may play a role in the development of autoimmunity. Because of the complexity of the immune system, it seems unlikely that autoimmune disorders arise from a single defect.

Failure of Self-Tolerance

Autoimmune disorders can result from one or more mechanisms producing loss of self-tolerance. Immunologic cells are undoubtedly involved in the tissue injury that results, but the precise mechanisms involved in initiating the response is largely unknown. More than one defect might be present in each disease, and each mechanism may be involved in more than one disease. Among the proposed mechanisms involved in loss of self-tolerance are failure of T-cell–mediated suppression, breakdown of T-cell anergy, disorders of MHC–antigen receptor/complex interactions, release of sequestered antigens, molecular mimicry, and superantigens.

Failure of T-Cell–Mediated Suppression. Disorders of immune regulatory or surveillance function can result from failure to delete autoreactive immune cells or suppress the immune response.[19,39] Because T cells regulate the immune response, an increasing ratio of CD4+ helper T cells to CD8+ suppressor T cells may lead to the development of autoimmune disorders.

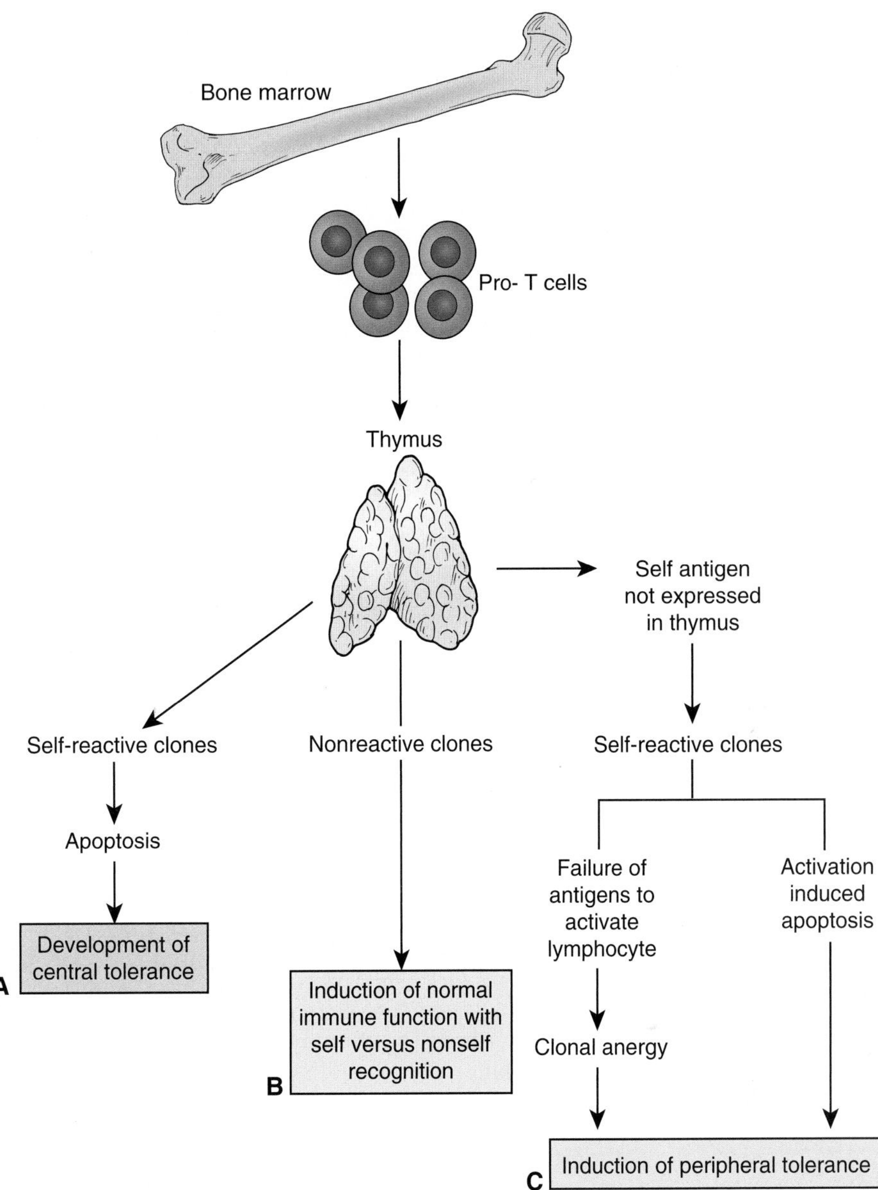

FIGURE 21-9 Development of immunologic tolerance. (**A**) Development of central tolerance with deletion of self-reactive T lymphocytes in the thymus. (**B**) Nonreactive lymphocytes with development of normal immune function. (**C**) Induction of peripheral tolerance in self-reactive cells that are not eliminated in the thymus.

Breakdown in T-Cell Anergy. T-cell anergy involves the prolonged or irreversible inactivation of T cells under certain conditions. Activation of antigen-specific CD4+ helper T cells requires two signals: recognition of the antigen in association with class II MHC molecules on the surface of the APCs and a set of costimulatory signals provided by the APCs. If the second costimulatory signal is not delivered, the T cell becomes anergic. Most normal tissues do not express the costimulatory molecules and thus are protected from autoreactive T cells. This protection can be broken if the normal cells that do not express the costimulatory molecules are induced to do so. Some inductions can occur after an infection, or in situations in which there is tissue necrosis and local inflammation. For example, up-regulation of the costimulator molecule B7-1 has been observed in the central nervous system of persons with multiple sclerosis, in the synovium of persons with rheumatoid arthritis, and in the skin of persons with psoriasis.[1]

Disorders in MHC–Antigen Complex/Receptor Interactions. The immune system normally recognizes antigen in the context of MHC–antigen complex and TCR interactions. Aberrations in any of these three components of the immune response—antigen structure, TCR recognition of antigen, or MHC antigen presentation—have the potential for initiating an autoimmune response.

There are many ways in which chemical or microbial antigens can be modified to evoke an altered immune response, leading to an autoimmune disorder. Autoantigenic drugs and viruses can be complexed to a carrier that is recognized by nontolerant CD4+ helper T cells as foreign. Virus-encoded antigens expressed on the cell surface can serve as carriers for self antigens. In this case, the self antigen would appear as a hapten for which an immune response could be induced.

Partial degradation of self antigens also may occur. For example, partially degraded collagen or enzymatically altered thyroglobulin or gamma globulin may be sufficiently foreign to promote an autoimmune response.

Release of Sequestered Antigens. Normally, the body does not produce antibodies against self antigens. Thus, any self antigen that was completely sequestered during development and then reintroduced to the immune system is likely to be regarded as foreign. Among the sequestered tissues that could be regarded as foreign are spermatozoa and ocular antigens such as those found in uveal tissue. Posttraumatic uveitis and orchiditis after vasectomy may fall into this category.

Molecular Mimicry. It is possible that certain autoimmune disorders are caused by molecular mimicry, in which a foreign antigen so closely resembles a self antigen that antibodies produced against the former react with the latter.[42,43] A humoral or cellular response can be mounted against antigenically altered or injured tissue, creating an immune process. In rheumatic fever and acute glomerulonephritis, for example, a protein in the cell wall of group A β-hemolytic streptococci has considerable similarity with antigens in heart and kidney tissue, respectively. After infection, antibodies directed against the microorganism cause a classic case of mistaken identity, which leads to inflammation of the heart or kidney. Certain drugs, when bound to host proteins or glycoproteins, form a complex to which a humoral response is directed with substantial cross-reactivity to the original self protein. The antihypertensive agent methyldopa can bind to surface antigens on red cells to induce an antibody-mediated hemolytic anemia.

Not everyone exposed to group A β-hemolytic streptococci has an autoimmune reaction. The reason that only certain persons are targeted for autoimmune reactions to a particular self-mimicry molecule may be determined by differences in HLA types. The HLA type determines exactly which fragments of a pathogen are displayed on the cell surface for presentation to T cells. One individual's HLA may bind self-mimicry molecules for presentation to T cells, and another's HLA type may not. In the spondyloarthropathies, particularly Reiter's syndrome and reactive arthritis, there is a clear relationship between arthritis and a prior bacterial infection, combined with the inherited HLA-B27 antigens.[43]

Superantigens. Superantigens are a family of related substances, including staphylococcal and streptococcal exotoxins, which can short-circuit the normal sequence of events in an immune response, leading to inappropriate activation of $CD4^+$ helper T cells. Superantigens do not require processing and presentation of antigen by APCs to induce a T-cell response.[44,45] Instead, they are able to interact with a TCR outside the normal antigen-binding site. Normally, only a small percentage of the T-cell population (0.01%) is stimulated by the presence of processed antigens on the surface of macrophages; however, superantigens can interact with 5% to 30% of T cells.[44] Superantigens directly link the class II MHC complex molecules of APCs such as macrophages to TCRs, causing a massive release of T-cell inflammatory cytokines, primarily IL-2 and tumor necrosis factor-α (TNF-α), and an uncontrolled proliferation of T cells. At least one disease in adults, toxic shock syndrome, is mediated by superantigens. Kawasaki disease in children (see Chapter 26) probably has a similar cause.

Heredity and Gender

Genetic factors can increase the incidence and severity of autoimmune diseases,[46] as shown by the familial clustering of several autoimmune diseases and the observation that certain inherited HLA types occur more frequently in persons with a variety of immunologic and lymphoproliferative disorders. For example, 90% of persons with ankylosing spondylitis carry the HLA-B27 antigen, as compared with 7% of persons without the disease.[19] Other HLA-associated diseases are Reiter's syndrome and HLA-B27, rheumatoid arthritis and HLA-DR4, and systemic lupus erythematosus (SLE) and HLA-DR3 (see Chapter 59). The molecular basis for these associations is unknown. Because autoimmunity does not develop in all persons with genetic predisposition, it appears that other factors, such as a "trigger event," interact to precipitate the altered immune state. The event or events that trigger the development of an autoimmune response are unknown. It has been suggested that the trigger may be a virus or other microorganism, a chemical substance, or a self antigen from a body tissue that has been hidden from the immune system during development.

A number of autoimmune disorders, such as SLE, occur more commonly in women than men, suggesting that estrogens may play a role in the development of autoimmune disease. Evidence suggests that estrogens stimulate and androgens suppress the immune response.[47] For example, estrogen stimulates a DNA sequence that promotes the production of interferon-γ, which is thought to assist in the induction of an autoimmune response.

DIAGNOSIS AND TREATMENT OF AUTOIMMUNE DISEASE

Suggested criteria for determining that a disorder is an autoimmune disorder include evidence of an autoimmune reaction, determination that the immunologic findings are not secondary to another condition, and the lack of other identified causes for the disorder. Currently, the diagnosis of autoimmune disease is based primarily on clinical findings and serologic testing. In the future, it is likely that autoimmune disorders will be diagnosed by directly identifying the genes responsible for the condition.

The basis for most serologic assays is the demonstration of antibodies directed against tissue antigens or cellular components. For example, a child with chronic or acute history of fever, arthritis, and a macular rash along with high levels of antinuclear antibody has a probable diagnosis of SLE. The detection of autoantibodies in the laboratory usually is accomplished by one of three methods: indirect fluorescent antibody assays (IFA), enzyme-linked immunosorbent assay (ELISA), or particle agglutination of some kind. The rationale behind each of these methods is similar: the patient's serum is diluted and allowed to react with an antigen-coated surface (*i.e.*, whole, fixed cells for the detection of antinuclear antibodies). In the cases of IFA and ELISA, a second "labeled" antibody is added, which binds to the patient's antibody and forms a visible reaction. Particle agglutination assays are much simpler. The binding of the patient's antibody to antigen-coated particles causes a visible agglutination reaction. For most serologic assays, the patient's serum is serially diluted until it no longer produces a visible reaction (*e.g.,* 1:100 dilution). This is called a *positive titer.* Healthy persons sometimes have low titers of antibody against cellular and tissue antigens, but the titers usually are far lower than in patients with autoimmune disease.

Treatment of autoimmune disease is based on the tissue or organ that is involved, the effector mechanism involved, and the magnitude and chronicity of the effector processes. Ideally, treatment should focus on the mechanism underlying the autoimmune disorder. Corticosteroids and immunosuppressive drugs may be used to arrest or reverse the downhill course of some autoimmune disorders. Purging autoreactive cells from the immune repertoire, through the use of plasmapheresis, is also an option in some severe cases of autoimmunity.[40]

Recent research has focused on the cytokines involved in the inflammatory response that accompanies many of the autoimmune disorders. Notably, interferon-β for multiple sclerosis and TNF-α antibodies (*e.g.,* infliximab) for rheumatoid arthritis and Crohn disease are the first new treatments for autoimmunity approved by the Food and Drug Administration in the past 20 years.[40] Finally, research into the development of vaccines to target critical pathways in the emergence of autoimmune responses is ongoing.

In summary, autoimmune diseases represent a disruption in self-tolerance that results in damage to body tissues by the immune system. Autoimmune diseases can affect almost any cell or tissue of the body. The ability of the immune system to differentiate self from nonself is called *self-tolerance.* Normally, self-tolerance is maintained through central and peripheral mechanisms that delete autoreactive B or T cells or otherwise suppress or inactivate immune responses that would be destructive to host tissues. Defects in any of these mechanisms could impair self-tolerance and predispose to development of autoimmune disease.

The ability of the immune system to differentiate foreign from self antigens is the responsibility of HLA encoded by MHC genes. Antigen is presented to receptors of T cells in combination with MHC molecules. Among the possible mechanisms responsible for development of autoimmune disease are failure of T-cell–mediated immune suppression, aberrations in MHC–antigen–TCR interactions, molecular mimicry, and superantigens.

Suggested criteria for determining that a disorder results from an autoimmune disorder are evidence of an autoimmune reaction, determination that the immunologic findings are not secondary to another condition, and the lack of other identifiable causes for the disorder.

REVIEW EXERCISES

A 20-year-old woman has been diagnosed with IgA deficiency. She has been plagued with frequent bouts of bronchitis and sinus infections.

A. Why are these types of infections particularly prominent in persons with an IgA deficiency?

B. The patient has been told that she needs to be aware that she could have a severe reaction if given unwashed blood transfusions. Explain.

Persons with impaired cellular immunity may not respond to the tuberculin test, even when infected with *Mycobacterium tuberculosis.*

A. Explain.

A 32-year-old man presents in the allergy clinic with complaints of allergic rhinitis or hay fever. His major complaints are those of nasal pruritus (itching), nasal congestion with profuse watery drainage, sneezing, and eye irritation. The physical examination reveals edematous and inflamed nasal mucosa and redness of the ocular conjunctiva. He relates that this happens every fall during "ragweed season."

A. Explain the immunologic mechanisms that are responsible for this man's symptoms.

B. What type of diagnostic tests might be used?

C. What type of treatments might be used to relieve his symptoms?

Persons with intestinal parasites and those with allergies may both have elevated levels of eosinophils in their blood.

A. Explain.

References

1. Abbas A.K., Lichtman A.H. (2003). Cellular and molecular immunology (5th ed., pp. 453–464) Philadelphia: W.B. Saunders.
2. Shyur S., Hill H.R. (1996). Recent advances in the genetics of primary immunodeficiency syndromes. *Journal of Pediatrics 129,* 8–24.
3. Buckley R.H. (2000). Primary immunodeficiency diseases due to defects in lymphocytes. *New England Journal of Medicine 343,* 1313–1324.
4. Buckley R. (2004). T-, B-, and NK-cell systems. In Behrman R.E., Kliegman R.M., Jenson H.B. (Eds.), *Nelson textbook of pediatrics* (17th ed., pp. 683–700). Philadelphia: W.B. Saunders.
5. Candotti, F., Notarangelo L., Visconti R., O'Shea J. (2001). Molecular aspects of primary immunodeficiencies: Lessons from cytokine and other signaling pathways. *Journal of Clinical Investigation 109,* 1261–1269.
6. Sorensen R.U., Moore C. (2000). Antibody deficiency syndromes. *Pediatric Clinics of North America 47,* 1225–1252.
7. Ten R.M. (1998). Primary immunodeficiencies. *Mayo Clinic Proceedings 73,* 865–872.
8. Elder M.E. (2000). T-cell immunodeficiencies. *Pediatric Clinics of North America 47,* 1253–1274.
9. Buckley R.H. (2002). Primary cellular immunodeficiency. *Journal of Allergy and Clinical Immunology 109,* 747–757.

10. Johnston R.B. Jr. (2004). The complement system. In Behrman R.E., Kliegman R.M., Jensen H.B. (Eds.), *Nelson textbook of pediatrics* (17th ed., pp. 725–731). Philadelphia: W.B Saunders.
11. Frank M.M. (2000). Complement deficiencies. *Pediatric Clinics of North America 47,* 1339–1353.
12. Cotten H.R. (1987). Hereditary angioneurotic edema, 1887–1987. *New England Journal of Medicine 317,* 43–45.
13. Cicardi M., Agostoni A. (1996). Hereditary angioedema. *New England Journal of Medicine 334,* 1666–1667.
14. Waytes A.T., Rosen F.S., Frank M.M. (1996). Treatment of hereditary angioedema with a vapor-heated C1 inhibitor concentrate. *New England Journal of Medicine 334,* 1630–1634.
15. Segal B.H., Holland S.M. (2000). Primary phagocytic disorders of childhood. *Pediatric Clinics of North America 47,* 1311–1333.
16. Boxer L.A. (2004). Disorders of phagocyte function. In Behrman R.E., Kliegman R.M., Jensen H.B. (Eds.), *Nelson textbook of pediatrics* (17th ed., pp. 701–717). Philadelphia: W.B. Saunders.
17. Lekstrom-Himes J.A., Gallin J.I. (2000). Immunodeficiency diseases caused by defects in phagocytes. *New England Journal of Medicine 343,* 1703–1714.
18. Horwitz M.E. (2000). Stem-cell transplantation for inherited immunodeficiency disorders. *Pediatric Clinics of North America 47,* 1371–1384.
19. Mitchell R.N., Kumar V. (2003). Diseases of immunity. In Kumar V., Cotran R.S., Robbins S.L. *Robbins basic pathology* (7th ed., pp. 103–164). Philadelphia: W.B. Saunders.
20. Kay A.B. (2001). Allergy and allergic disease (first of two parts). *New England Journal of Medicine 344,* 30–37.
21. Galli S.J. (1993). New concepts about the mast cell. *New England Journal of Medicine 328,* 257–265.
22. Benoist C., Mathias D. (2003). Mast cells in autoimmune disease. *Nature 420*(6917), 875–878.
23. Johnson K.J., Chensue S.W., Ward P.A. (1999). In Rubin E., Farber J.L. (Eds.), *Pathology* (3rd ed., pp. 114–127). Philadelphia: Lippincott-Raven.
24. Kay A.B. (2001). Allergy and allergic disease (second of two parts). *New England Journal of Medicine 344,* 109–113.
25. Jackler R.K., Kaplan M.J. (2003). Ear, nose, and throat. In Tierney L.M., McPhee S.J., Papadakis M.A. (Eds.), *Current medical diagnosis and treatment* (40th ed., pp. 195–196). New York: Lange Medical Books/McGraw-Hill.
26. Rachelefsky G.S. (1999). National guidelines need to manage rhinitis and prevent complications. *Annals of Allergy, Asthma, and Immunology 82,* 296–305.
27. Sicherer S.H. (1999). Manifestations of food allergy: Evaluation and management. *American Family Physician 57,* 93–102.
28. Sampson H.A. (2002). Peanut allergy. *New England Journal of Medicine 346,* 1294–1299.
29. Sampson H.A. (1998). Fatal food-induced anaphylaxis. *Allergy 53*(Suppl. 46), 125–130.
30. Salvaggio J.E. (1995). The identification of hypersensitivity pneumonitis. *Hospital Practice 30*(5), 57–66.
31. Sussman G.L. (1995). Allergy to latex rubber. *Annals of Internal Medicine 122,* 43–46.
32. Zucker-Pinchoff B., Stadtmauer G.J. (2002). Latex allergy. *Mount Sinai Journal of Medicine 69,* 88–95.
33. Reddy S. (1998). Latex allergy. *American Family Physician 57,* 93–102.
34. Poley G.E., Slater J.E. (2000). Latex allergy. *Journal of Allergy and Clinical Immunology 105,* 1054–1062.
35. Lin H., Kauffman M., McBride M.A., et al. (1998). Center-specific graft and patient survival rate. *Journal of the American Medical Association 280,* 1153–1160.
36. Saveigh M.H., Turka L.A. (1998). The role of T-cell costimulatory activation pathways in transplant rejection. *New England Journal of Medicine 338,* 1813–1821.
37. Vogelsang G.B., Lee L., Bensen-Kennedy D.M. (2003). Pathogenesis and treatment of graft-versus-host disease after bone marrow transplant. *Annual Review of Medicine 54,* 29–52.
38. Crawford J.M. (2003). The liver and biliary tract. In Kumar V., Cotran R.S., Robbins S.L. *Robbins basic pathology* (7th ed., p. 625). Philadelphia: W.B. Saunders.
39. Kamradt T., Mitchison N.A. (2001). Advances in immunology: Tolerance and autoimmunity. *New England Journal of Medicine 344,* 655–664.
40. Davidson A., Diamond B. (2001). Autoimmune disease. *New England Journal of Medicine 345,* 340–350.
41. Chatenoud L., Salomon B., Bluestone J.A. (2001). Suppressor T cells—they're back and critical to the regulation of autoimmunity. *Immunological Reviews 182,* 149–163.
42. Rose N.R. (1997). Autoimmune disease: Tracing the shared threads. *Hospital Practice 32*(4), 147–154.
43. Albert L.J., Inman R.D. (1999). Molecular mimicry and autoimmunity. *New England Journal of Medicine 341,* 2068–2074.
44. Kotzin B.L. (1994). Superantigens and their role in disease. *Hospital Practice 29*(11), 59–70.
45. Llewelyn M., Cohen J. (2001). Superantigens antagonist peptides. *Critical Care 5,* 53–55.
46. Theofilopoulos A.N. (1995). The basis of autoimmunity. Part II: Genetic predisposition. *Immunology Today 16,* 150–158.
47. Cutolo M., Sulli A., Seriolo S., et al. (1995). Estrogens, the immune response and autoimmunity. *Clinical and Experimental Rheumatology 13,* 217–226.

CHAPTER 22

Acquired Immunodeficiency Syndrome

Kathleen A. Sweeney

The acquired immunodeficiency syndrome (AIDS) is a disease caused by infection with the human immunodeficiency virus (HIV) and is characterized by profound immunosuppression with associated opportunistic infections, malignancies, wasting, and central nervous system degeneration. Because the disease affects an exceptionally high proportion of the population throughout the world, it is often referred to as a *pandemic*.[1]

The AIDS Epidemic and Transmission of HIV Infection

After completing this section of the chapter, you should be able to meet the following objectives:

- Briefly trace the history of the AIDS epidemic
- State the virus responsible for AIDS and explain how it differs from most other viruses
- Describe the mechanisms of HIV transmission and relate them to the need for public awareness and concern regarding the spread of AIDS

As a national and global epidemic, the degree of morbidity and mortality caused by HIV, as well as its impact on health care resources and the economy, is tremendous—and unrelenting. At the end of 2002, it was estimated that there were 42 million people worldwide living with HIV/AIDS and that more than 25 million had died of the infection[2] (Table 22-1). During the same year, 5 million people were newly infected with the virus, and for the first time, women and young people 15 to 24 years of age accounted for 50% of HIV infections. Because the reporting of cases is not uniform throughout the world, many countries may not be accurately represented in this number. Projections for the next 10 years suggest that there will be 100 million people infected with HIV.

Most of the new infections worldwide are in people younger than 25 years of age who live in developing countries. Sub-Saharan Africa has been hardest hit by HIV. There are 29.4 million people living with HIV in Africa, with a reported 3.5 million new infections in 2002. There are countries in Africa where more than 30% of the adults are infected with HIV. Because of the large number of infected people in Africa, the life expectancy is expected to drop from 59 years to 45 years by 2005.[3] Eastern Europe and central Asia have the world's fastest growing HIV population.[2] In the United States, there had been more than 816,000 cases and more than 467,000 deaths from HIV at the end of 2000, with racial and ethnic minorities being disproportionately affected.[3] Although blacks and Hispanics

TABLE 22-1 Estimated Number of Adults and Children Living With HIV/AIDS, New Infections, and Deaths at the End of 2002

	Living With	Newly Infected	Deaths
North America	980,000	45,000	15,000
Sub-Saharan Africa	29,400,000	3,500,000	2,400,000
Eastern Europe and Central Asia	1,200,000	250,000	25,000
East Asia and Pacific	1,200,000	270,000	45,000
South and South East Asia	6,000,000	700,000	440,000
Western Europe	570,000	30,000	8,000
Caribbean	440,000	60,000	42,000
Latin America	1,500,000	150,000	60,000
Australia and New Zealand	15,000	500	<100
Total	42 million	5 million	3.1 million

(Data from UNAIDS: AIDS epidemic update—December 2002.) Available online at www.unaids.org/worldaidsday/2002/press/epiupdate.html.

represent a minority of the population in the United States, they account for 55% of HIV infections.[4]

EMERGENCE OF THE AIDS EPIDEMIC

Compared with other human pathogens, HIV evolved very recently. In 1981, clinicians in New York, San Francisco, and Los Angeles recognized a new immunodeficiency syndrome in homosexual men. Initially, the syndrome was called GRIDS, for "gay-related immunodeficiency syndrome." By the end of 1981, there had been several hundred cases reported, and the name was changed to acquired immunodeficiency syndrome, or AIDS.[5] It soon became apparent that this disease was not confined to one segment of the population, but was also occurring in intravenous drug users, hemophiliacs, blood transfusion recipients, infants born to infected mothers, and high-risk heterosexuals. Studies of these diverse groups led to the conclusion that AIDS was an infectious disease spread by blood, sexual contact, and perinatally from mother to child.

An understanding of the virology of AIDS progressed with amazing efficiency; within 3 years of the first cases being recognized, the virus that causes AIDS had been identified. The virus was initially known by various names, including human T-cell lymphotropic virus type 3 (HTLV-III), lymphadenopathy-associated virus (LAV), and AIDS-associated retrovirus (ARV).[6] In 1986, the name *human immunodeficiency virus* became internationally accepted.[7,8]

TRANSMISSION OF HIV INFECTION

HIV is a retrovirus that selectively attacks the $CD4^+$ T lymphocytes, the immune cells responsible for orchestrating and coordinating the immune response to infection. As a consequence, persons with HIV infection have a deteriorating immune system, and thus are more susceptible to severe infections with ordinarily harmless organisms.

HIV is transmitted from one person to another through sexual contact, blood-to-blood contact, or perinatally. It is not transmitted through casual contact. Several studies involving more than 1000 uninfected, nonsexual household contacts with persons with HIV infection (including siblings, parents, and children) have shown no evidence of casual transmission.[9] HIV is not spread by mosquitoes or other insect vectors.[7] Transmission can occur when infected blood, semen, or vaginal secretions from one person are deposited onto a mucous membrane or into the bloodstream of another person.

Sexual contact is the most frequent way that HIV is transmitted. Worldwide, 75% to 85% of HIV infections are transmitted through unprotected sex.[10] HIV is present in semen and vaginal fluids. There is risk for transmitting HIV when these fluids come in contact with a part of the body that lets them enter the bloodstream. This can include the vaginal mucosa, anal mucosa, and wounds or sores on the skin.[10] Contact with semen occurs during vaginal and anal sexual intercourse, oral sex (*i.e.,* fellatio), and donor insemination. Exposure to vaginal or cervical secretions occurs during vaginal intercourse and oral sex (*i.e.,* cunnilingus). Condoms are highly effective in preventing the transmission of HIV. In most cities in the United States, sexual transmission of HIV is primarily related to vaginal or anal intercourse. In the United States, about 45% of HIV infections are among men who have sex with men, and 11% are from heterosexual contact.[3] In the developing world, heterosexual transmission is the major route of HIV infection.[6]

THE AIDS EPIDEMIC AND TRANSMISSION OF HIV

- Acquired immunodeficiency disease (AIDS) is caused by the human immunodeficiency virus (HIV).
- HIV is transmitted through blood, semen, vaginal fluids, and breast milk.
- Persons with HIV are infectious even when asymptomatic.

Because HIV is found in blood, the use of needles, syringes, and other drug injection paraphernalia is a direct route for transmission. Of the reported cases of AIDS in the United States, almost 25% occurred among persons who injected drugs.[3] HIV-infected injecting drug users can pass the virus to their needle-sharing and sex partners and, in the case of pregnant women, to their offspring.[7] Although alcohol, cocaine, and other noninjected drugs do not directly transmit infection, their use alters perception of risk and reduces inhibitions about engaging in behaviors that pose a high risk for transmitting HIV infection.

Transfusions of whole blood, plasma, platelets, or blood cells before 1985 resulted in the transmission of HIV. Since 1985, all blood donations in the United States have been screened for HIV, and this is no longer a transmission risk. The clotting factor used by persons with hemophilia is derived from the pooled plasma of hundreds of donors. Before HIV testing of plasma donors was implemented in 1985, the virus was transmitted to persons with hemophilia through infusions of these clotting factors.[7] Seventy percent to 80% of hemophiliacs who were treated with factor before 1985 became infected. Other blood products, such as gamma globulin and hepatitis B immune globulin, have not been implicated in the transmission of HIV.

Transmission from mother to infant is the most common way that children become infected with HIV. HIV may be transmitted from infected women to their offspring in utero, during labor and delivery, or through breastfeeding.[11] Ninety percent of infected children acquired the virus from their mother. The risk for transmission of HIV from mother to infant is approximately 25%, with estimates ranging from 15% to 45% depending on what country they live in.[12]

Occupational HIV infection among health care workers is uncommon. Through June 2000, the Centers for Disease Control and Prevention (CDC) had received only 56 documented occupational HIV infections in the United States.[13] Fewer than 20 additional cases of occupational infections have been reported from outside the United States through the 1990s.[14] Universal Blood and Body Fluid Precautions should be used in encounters with all patients in the health care setting because HIV status is not always known. Occupational risk for infection of health care workers most often is associated with percutaneous inoculation (*i.e.*, needle stick) of blood from a patient with HIV. Transmission is associated with the size of the needle, amount of blood present, depth of the injury, type of fluid contamination, stage of illness of the patient, and viral load of the patient. The average risk for HIV infection from percutaneous exposure to HIV-infected blood is about 0.3%, and about 0.9% after a mucous membrane exposure.[13]

People with other sexually transmitted diseases (STDs) are at increased risk for HIV infection. The risk for HIV transmission is increased in the presence of genital ulcerative STDs (*i.e.*, syphilis, herpes simplex virus infection, and chancroid) and nonulcerative STDs (*i.e.*, gonorrhea, chlamydial infection, and trichomoniasis). HIV increases the duration and recurrence of STD lesions, treatment failures, and atypical presentation of genital ulcerative diseases as a result of suppression of the immune system.

The HIV-infected person is infectious even when no symptoms are present. The point at which an infected person converts from being negative for the presence of HIV antibodies in the blood to being positive is called *seroconversion*. Seroconversion typically occurs within 1 to 3 months after exposure to HIV but can take up to 6 months.[15] An HIV-infected person can occasionally transmit the virus to others even before seroconversion. The time after infection and before seroconversion is known as the *window period*. During the window period, a person's HIV antibody test will be negative. Rarely, infection can occur from transfused blood that was screened for HIV antibody and found negative because the donor was recently infected and still in the window period. Consequently, the U.S. Food and Drug Administration (FDA) requires blood collection centers to screen potential donors through interviews designed to identify behaviors known to present risk for HIV infection.

In summary, AIDS is an infectious disease of the immune system caused by the HIV retrovirus that causes profound immunosuppression. First described in June 1981, the disease is one of the leading causes of morbidity and mortality worldwide. The severity of the clinical disease and the absence of a cure or preventive vaccine have increased public awareness and concern. In the most recent years, the greatest increase in incidence of the disease has been in women and young people 15 to 24 years of age.

HIV is transmitted from one person to another through sexual contact, through blood-to-blood contact, or perinatally. Transmission occurs when the infected blood, semen, or vaginal secretions from one person are deposited onto a mucous membrane or into the bloodstream of another person. The primary routes of transmission are through sexual intercourse, through intravenous drug use, and from mother to infant. Blood transfusions and other blood products continue to be routes of transmission in some underdeveloped countries. Occupational exposure in health care settings accounts for only a tiny percentage of HIV transmission. HIV infection is not transmitted through casual contact or by insect vectors. There is growing evidence of an association between HIV infection and other STDs. Infected individuals can transmit the virus to others before their own infections can be detected by antibody tests.

Pathophysiology and Clinical Course

After completing this section of the chapter, you should be able to meet the following objectives:

- Describe the structure of HIV and trace its entry and steps in replication within the CD4+ T lymphocyte
- Describe the alterations in immune function that occur in persons with AIDS
- Describe the CDC HIV/AIDS classification system

- ✦ Relate the altered immune function in persons with HIV infection and AIDS to the development of opportunistic infections, malignant tumors, nervous system manifestations, the wasting syndrome, and metabolic disorders

MOLECULAR AND BIOLOGIC FEATURES OF HIV

HIV is a member of the lentivirus family of animal retroviruses.[16,17] Lentiviruses, including feline immunodeficiency virus, simian immunodeficiency virus, and the visna virus of sheep, are capable of long-term latency and short-term cytopathic effects. They can all produce slowly progressive fatal diseases that include wasting syndromes and central nervous system (CNS) degeneration. Two genetically different but antigenically related forms of HIV, HIV-1 and HIV-2, have been isolated in people with AIDS. HIV-1 is the type most associated with AIDS in the United States, Europe, and Central Africa, whereas HIV-2 causes a similar disease principally in West Africa. HIV-2 appears to be transmitted in the same manner as HIV-1; it can also cause immunodeficiency as evidenced by a reduction in the number of CD4+ T cells and the development of AIDS. Although the spectrum of disease for HIV-2 is similar to that of HIV-1, it spreads more slowly and causes disease more slowly than HIV-1. Specific tests are now available for HIV-2, and blood collected for transfusion is routinely screened for HIV-2. The ensuing discussion focuses on HIV-1.

The human immunodeficiency virus infects a limited number of cell types in the body, including a subset of lymphocytes called CD4+ T lymphocytes (also known as *helper T cells* or *CD4+ T cells*), macrophages, and dendritic cells[7] (see Chapter 19). The CD4+ T cells are necessary for normal immune function. Among other functions, the CD4+ T cell recognizes foreign antigens and helps activate antibody-producing B lymphocytes.[7] The CD4+ T cells also orchestrate cell-mediated immunity, in which cytotoxic CD8+ T cells and natural killer (NK) cells directly destroy virus-infected cells, tubercular bacillus, and foreign antigens. The phagocytic function of monocytes and macrophages is also influenced by CD4+ T cells.

Like other retroviruses, HIV carries its genetic information in ribonucleic acid (RNA) rather than deoxyribonucleic acid (DNA). The HIV virion is spherical in shape and contains an electron-dense core surrounded by a lipid membrane or envelope (Fig. 22-1). The virus core contains the

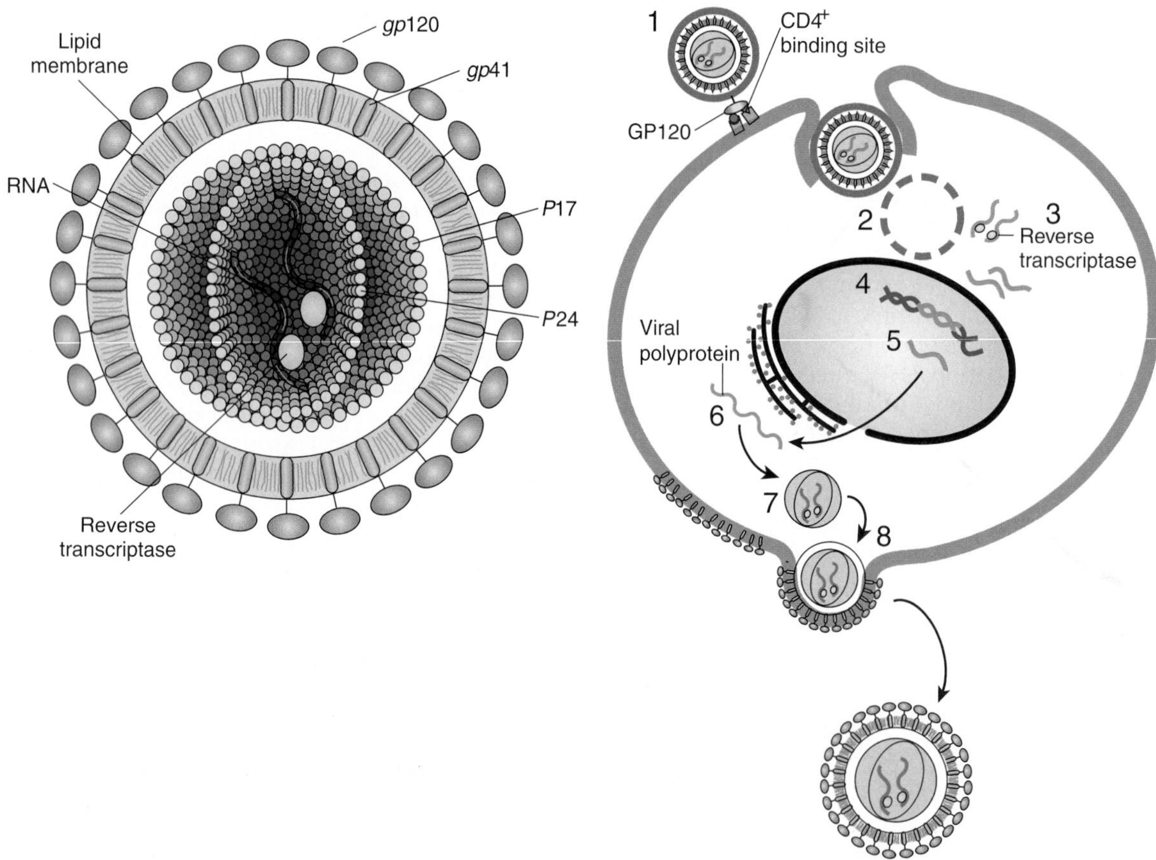

FIGURE 22-1 Life cycle of the HIV-1: (**1**) Attachment of the HIV virus to CD4+ receptor; (**2**) internalization and uncoating of the virus with viral RNA and reverse transcriptase; (**3**) reverse transcription, which produces a mirror image of the viral RNA and double-stranded DNA molecule; (**4**) integration of viral DNA into host DNA using the integrase enzyme; (**5**) transcription of the inserted viral DNA to produce viral messenger RNA; (**6**) translation of viral messenger RNA to create viral polyprotein; (**7**) cleavage of viral polyprotein into individual viral proteins that make up the new virus; and (**8**) assembly and release of the new virus from the host cell.

major capsid protein p24, two copies of the genomic RNA, and three viral enzymes (protease, reverse transcriptase, and integrase). Because p24 is the most readily detected antigen, it is the target for the antibodies used in screening for HIV infection. The viral core is surrounded by a matrix protein called p17, which lies beneath the viral envelope. The viral envelope is studded with two viral glycoproteins, gp120 and gp41, which are critical for the infection of cells.

Replication of HIV occurs in eight steps[16,17] (see Fig. 22-1). Each of these steps provides insights into the development of methods used for preventing or treating the infection. The *first step* involves the binding of the virus to the CD4+ T cell. Once HIV has entered the bloodstream, it attaches to the surface of a CD4+ T cell by binding to a CD4 receptor that has a high affinity for HIV. However, binding to the CD4 receptor is not sufficient for infection; the virus must also bind with other surface molecules (chemokine coreceptors) that bind the gp120 and gp41 envelope glycoproteins. This process is known as *attachment.* The *second step* allows for the internalization of the virus. After attachment, the viral envelope peptides fuse to the CD4+ T cell membrane. Fusion results in an *uncoating* of the virus, allowing the contents of the viral core (the two single strands of viral RNA and the reverse transcriptase, integrase, and protease enzymes) to enter the host cell. The chemokine coreceptors are critical components of the HIV infection process. It has recently been found that people with defective coreceptors are more resistant to developing HIV, despite repeated exposure.[17]

The *third step* consists of DNA synthesis. In order for the HIV to reproduce, it must change its RNA into DNA. It does this by using the *reverse transcriptase* enzyme. Reverse transcriptase makes a copy of the viral RNA, and then in reverse makes another mirror-image copy. The result is double-stranded DNA that carries instructions for viral replication. The *fourth step* is called *integration.* During integration, the new DNA enters the nucleus of the CD4+ T cell and, with the help of the enzyme integrase, is inserted into the cell's original DNA. The *fifth step* involves *transcription* of the double-stranded viral DNA to form a single-stranded messenger RNA (mRNA) with the instructions for building new viruses. Transcription involves activation of the T cell and induction of host cell transcription factors. The *sixth step* includes translation of mRNA. During *translation,* ribosomal RNA (rRNA) uses the instructions in the mRNA to create a chain of proteins and enzymes called a *polyprotein.* These polyproteins contain the components needed for the next stages in the construction of new viruses. The *seventh step* is called *cleavage.* During cleavage, the protease enzyme cuts the polyprotein chain into the individual proteins that will make up the new viruses. Finally, during the *eighth step,* the proteins and viral RNA are assembled into new HIV viruses and released from the CD4+ T cell.

HIV replication involves the killing of the CD4+ T cell and the release of copies of the HIV into the bloodstream. These viral particles, or *virions,* invade other CD4+ T cells, allowing the infection to progress. Every day, millions of infected CD4+ T cells are destroyed, releasing billions of viral particles into the bloodstream; but each day, nearly all the CD4+ T cells are replaced, and nearly all the viral particles are destroyed. The problem is that over years, the CD4+ cell count gradually decreases through this process, and the number of viruses detected in the blood of persons infected with HIV increases.[18]

Until the CD4+ cell count falls to a very low level, a person infected with HIV can remain asymptomatic, although active viral replication is still taking place and serologic tests can identify antibodies to HIV.[19] These antibodies, unfortunately, do not convey protection against the virus. Although symptoms are not evident, the infection proceeds on a microbiologic level, including the invasion and selective destruction of CD4+ T cells. The continual decline of CD4+ T cells, which are pivotal cells in the immune response, strips the person with HIV of protection against common organisms and cancerous cells.[18]

PATHOPHYSIOLOGY OF AIDS

- The HIV is a retrovirus that destroys the body's immune system by taking over and destroying CD4+ T cells.
- In the process of taking over the CD4+ T cell, the virus attaches to receptors on the CD4+ cell, fuses to and enters the cell, incorporates its RNA into the cell's DNA, and then uses the CD4+ cell's DNA to reproduce large amounts of HIV, which are released into the blood.
- The three phases of HIV are primary HIV acute infection; latency, during which there are no signs or symptoms of disease; and overt AIDS, during which the CD4+ cell count falls to low levels and signs of opportunistic infections and other disease manifestations develop.
- As the CD4+ T-cell count decreases, the body becomes susceptible to opportunistic infections.

CLASSIFICATION AND PHASES OF HIV INFECTION

HIV Infection and AIDS Case Definition Classification

Effective January 1, 1993, the CDC implemented a new classification system for HIV infection and a new AIDS case definition for adolescents and adults that emphasizes the clinical importance of the CD4+ cell count in the categorization of HIV-related clinical conditions.[20] The new classification system defines three categories that correspond to CD4+ cell counts per microliter (µL) of blood: *category 1:* >500 cells/µL, *category 2:* 200 to 400 cells/µL, and *category 3:* <200 cells/µL (Fig. 22-2).

There also are three clinical categories. *Clinical category A* includes persons who are asymptomatic or have persistent generalized lymphadenopathy or symptoms of primary HIV infection (*i.e.,* acute seroconversion illness). *Clinical category B* includes persons with symptoms of immune deficiency not serious enough to be AIDS defining. *Clinical category C* includes AIDS-defining illnesses that are listed in the AIDS surveillance case definition shown in Chart 22-1. Each HIV-infected person has a CD4+ cell count category and a clinical category. The combination of these two categorizations, CD4+ cell count categories 1,

CD4+ cell count (u/L)

AIDS defining clinical category	Category 1 >500 cells	Category 2 200–400	Category 3 <200 cells
Category A No defining criteria			
Category B Symptoms not severe enough to be AIDS defining			
Category C AIDS illness or illnesses present			

Equals AIDS defined

FIGURE 22-2 HIV classification for adolescents and adults.

2, and 3 and clinical categories A, B, and C, can guide clinical and therapeutic decisions in the management of HIV infection (see Fig. 22-2). According to the 1993 case definition, persons in category 3 or category C are considered to have AIDS.

Phases of HIV Infection

The typical course of HIV is defined by three phases, which usually occur over a period of 8 to 12 years. The three phases are the primary infection phase, chronic asymptomatic or latency phase, and overt AIDS phase[21] (Fig. 22-3).

Many persons, when they are initially infected with HIV, have an acute mononucleosis-like syndrome known as primary infection. This acute phase may include fever, fatigue, myalgias, sore throat, night sweats, gastrointestinal problems, lymphadenopathy, maculopapular rash, and headache (Chart 22-2). Fever and rash are the symptoms most commonly associated with primary infection.[22] During primary infection, there is an increase in viral replication, which leads to very high viral loads, sometimes greater than 1,000,000 copies/mL, and a decrease in the $CD4^+$ cell count. The signs and symptoms of primary HIV infection usually appear 2 to 4 weeks after exposure to HIV and last a few days to 2 weeks.[21] After several weeks, the immune system acts to control viral replication and reduces the viral load to a lower level, where it often remains for several years.

People who are diagnosed with HIV while they are in the primary infection phase appear to have a unique opportunity for treatment. It seems possible that if started early, treatment may reduce the number of long-living HIV-infected cells (*e.g.,* $CD4^+$ memory cells).[23] Early therapy may also protect the functioning of HIV-infected $CD4^+$ T cells and cytotoxic T cells. Finally, early treatment can help maintain a homogeneous viral population that will be better controlled by antiretroviral therapy and the immune system.

CHART 22-1

Conditions Included in the 1993 AIDS Surveillance Case Definition

Candidiasis of bronchi, trachea, or lungs
Candidiasis, esophageal
Cervical cancer, invasive*
Coccidioidomycosis, disseminated or extrapulmonary
Cryptococcosis, extrapulmonary
Cryptosporidiosis, chronic intestinal (>1 month's duration)
Cytomegalovirus disease (other than liver, spleen, or nodes)
Cytomegalovirus retinitis (with loss of vision)
Encephalopathy, HIV-related
Herpes simplex: chronic ulcer(s) (>1 month's duration) or bronchitis, pneumonitis, or esophagitis
Histoplasmosis, disseminated or extrapulmonary
Isosporiasis, chronic intestinal (>1 month's duration)
Kaposi's sarcoma
Lymphoma, Burkitt's (or equivalent term)
Lymphoma, immunoblastic (or equivalent term)
Lymphoma, primary, of brain
Mycobacterium avium-intracellulare complex or *M. kansasii,* disseminated or extrapulmonary
Mycobacterium tuberculosis, any site (pulmonary* or extrapulmonary)
Mycobacterium, other species or unidentified species, disseminated or extrapulmonary
Pneumocystis carinii pneumonia
Pneumonia, recurrent*
Progressive multifocal leukoencephalopathy
Salmonella septicemia, recurrent
Toxoplasmosis of brain
Wasting syndrome due to HIV

*Added to the 1993 expansion of the AIDS surveillance case definition.
(Centers for Disease Control and Prevention. [1992]. 1993 Revised classification system for HIV infection and expanded surveillance case definition for AIDS among adolescents and adults. *Morbidity and Mortality Weekly Report* 41 [RR-17], 19)

The primary phase is followed by a latent period during which the person has no signs or symptoms of illness. The median time of the latent period is about 10 years. During this time, the $CD4^+$ cell count falls gradually from the normal range of 800 to 1000 cells/µL to 200 cells/µL or lower.[24] Lymphadenopathy develops in some persons with HIV infection during this phase.[24] Persistent generalized lymphadenopathy usually is defined as lymph nodes that are chronically swollen for more than 3 months in at least two locations, not including the groin. The lymph nodes may be sore or visible externally.

The third phase, overt AIDS, occurs when a person has a $CD4^+$ cell count of less than 200 cells/µL or an AIDS-defining illness.[21] Without antiretroviral therapy, this phase can lead to death within 2 to 3 years. The risk for death and opportunistic infection increases significantly when the $CD4^+$ cell count reaches this level.

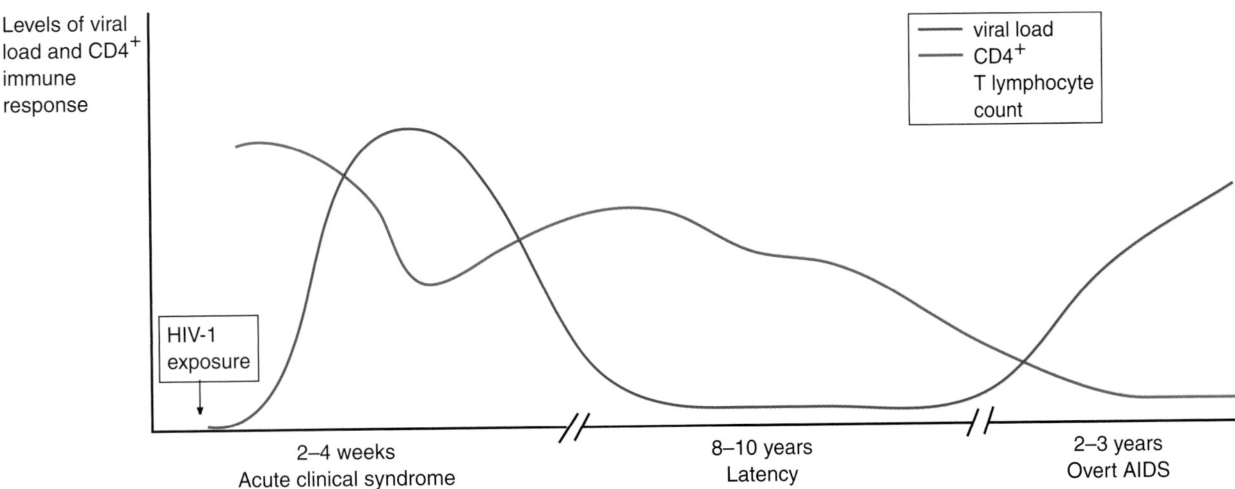

FIGURE 22-3 Viral load and $CD4^+$ cell count during the phases of HIV.

CLINICAL COURSE

The clinical course of HIV varies from person to person. Most—60% to 70%—of those infected with HIV acquire AIDS 10 to 11 years after infection. These people are the *typical progressors.*[21] Another 10% to 20% of those infected progress rapidly. They acquire AIDS in less than 5 years and are called *rapid progressors.* The final 5% to 15% are *slow progressors,* who do not progress to AIDS for more than 15 years. There is a subset of slow progressors, called *long-term nonprogressors,* who account for 1% of all HIV infections. These people have been infected for at least 8 years, are antiretroviral naïve, have high $CD4^+$ cell counts, and usually have very low viral loads (Fig. 22-4).

Opportunistic Infections

Opportunistic infections begin to occur as the immune system becomes severely compromised. The number of $CD4^+$ T cells directly correlates with the risk for developing opportunistic infections. Once the $CD4^+$ cell count drops below 200 cells/μL, the risk for developing an opportunistic infection is 33% after 1 year and 58% after 2 years.[25]

CHART 22-2

Signs and Symptoms of Acute HIV Infection

- Fever
- Fatigue
- Rash
- Headache
- Lymphadenopathy
- Pharyngitis
- Arthralgia
- Myalgia
- Night sweats
- Gastrointestinal problems
- Aseptic meningitis
- Oral or genital ulcers

Opportunistic infections involve common organisms that normally do not produce infection unless there is impaired immune function. Although a person with AIDS may live for many years after the first serious illness, as the immune system fails, these opportunistic illnesses become progressively more severe and difficult to treat.

Most opportunistic infections can be categorized as bacterial, fungal, protozoal, or viral. Bacterial opportunistic infections include bacterial pneumonia, tuberculosis, salmonellosis, and *Mycobacterium avium–intracellulare* complex (MAC) infection. Fungal opportunistic infections include candidiasis, coccidioidomycosis, cryptococcosis, and histoplasmosis. Protozoal opportunistic infections include cryptosporidiosis, isosporiasis, pneumocystiasis, and toxoplasmosis. Viral infections include cytomegalovirus (CMV), herpes, and progressive multifocal leukoencephalopathy (PML).

In the United States, the most common opportunistic infections are *Pneumocystis carinii* pneumonia (PCP), oropharyngeal or esophageal candidiasis (thrush), CMV, and infections caused by MAC.[25]

Respiratory Manifestations

The most common causes of respiratory disease in persons with HIV infection are PCP and pulmonary tuberculosis (TB).[26] Other organisms that cause opportunistic pulmonary infections in persons with AIDS include CMV, MAC, *Toxoplasma gondii,* and *Cryptococcus neoformans.* Pneumonia also may occur because of more common bacterial pulmonary pathogens, including *Streptococcus pneumoniae, Haemophilus influenzae,* and *Legionella pneumophila.* Some persons may become infected with multiple organisms. Kaposi's sarcoma (to be discussed) also can occur in the lungs.

Pneumocystis carinii *Pneumonia.* *P. carinii* pneumonia was the most common presenting manifestation of AIDS during the first decade of the epidemic. Since highly active antiretroviral therapy (HAART) and prophylaxis for PCP were instituted, the incidence has decreased.[27] PCP still is common in people who do not know their HIV status, in those who choose not to treat their HIV, and in those with

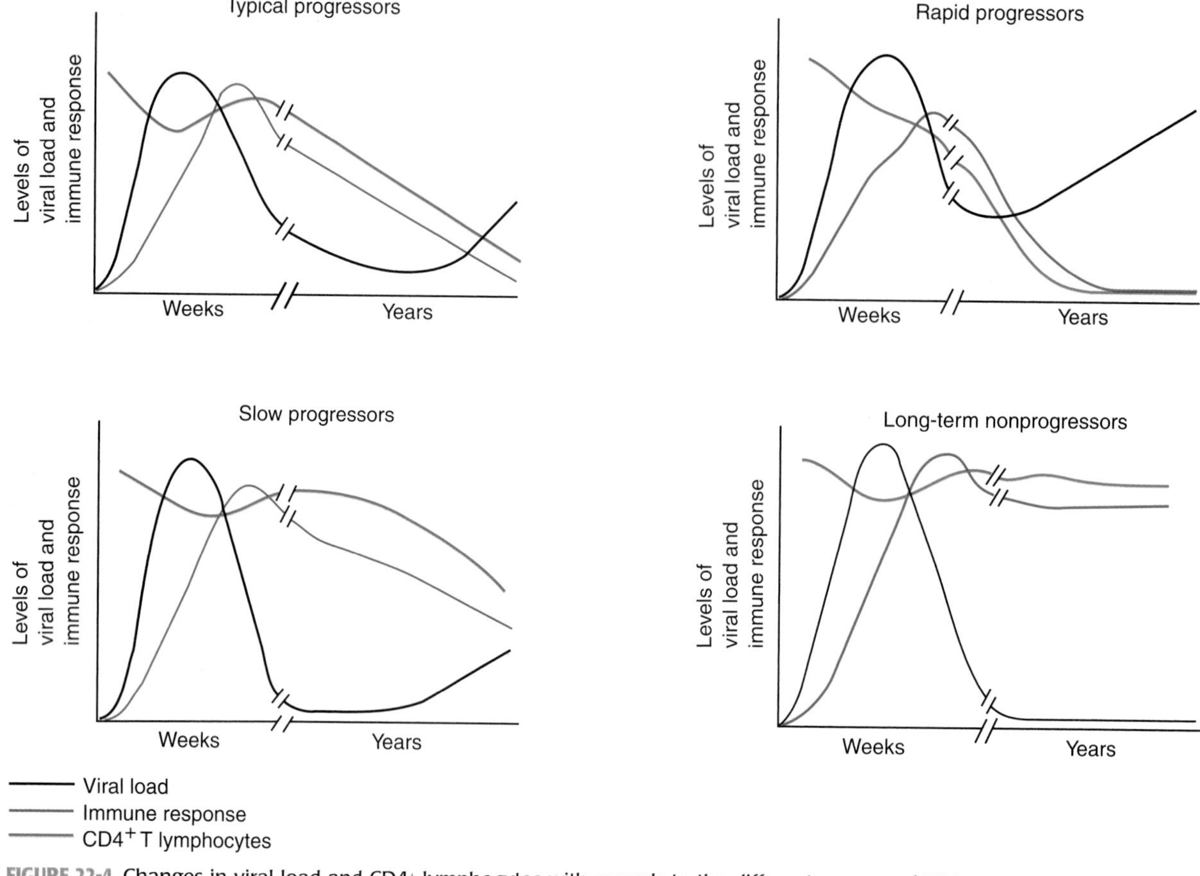

FIGURE 22-4 Changes in viral load and CD4+ lymphocytes with regards to the different courses of HIV. (Adapted from Rizzardi G.P., Pantaleo G. [1999]. *The immunopathogenesis of HIV-1 infection.* In Armstrong D., Cohen J. [Eds.], *Infectious diseases.* London: Harcourt)

poor access to health care. The best predictor of PCP is a CD4+ cell count below 200 cell/μL,[28] and it is at this point that prophylaxis with trimethoprim-sulfamethoxazole is started.[27] PCP is caused by *P. carinii,* an organism that is common in soil, houses, and many other places in the environment. In persons with healthy immune systems, *P. carinii* does not cause infection or disease. In persons with HIV, *P. carinii* can multiply quickly in the lungs and cause pneumonia. As the disease progresses, the alveoli become filled with foamy protein-rich fluid causing impairment of gas exchange (Fig. 22-5).

The symptoms of PCP may be acute or gradually progressive. Patients may present with complaints of a mild cough, fever, shortness of breath, and weight loss. Physical examination may demonstrate only fever and tachypnea, and breath sounds may be normal. The chest x-ray film may show interstitial infiltrates, but in 5% of cases, the x-ray may be negative.[28] Diagnosis of PCP is made on recognition of the organism in pulmonary secretions. This can be done through examination of induced sputum, bronchoalveolar lavage, occasionally bronchoscopy, and rarely, lung biopsy.[27]

Mycobacterium tuberculosis. Tuberculosis is the leading cause of death in people with HIV worldwide. More than 80,000 people are coinfected with HIV and TB in North America and another 5 million in the rest of the world.[29] TB cases in the United States decreased from the 1950s until 1985; then, in 1986, the number of TB cases began to increase (see Chapter 30). A number of factors contributed to this increase, including changes in immigration patterns and increased numbers of people living in group settings like prisons, shelters, and nursing homes, but the most profound factor is HIV infection. TB is often the first manifestation of HIV infection.

The lungs are the most common site of *M. tuberculosis* infection, but extrapulmonary infection of the kidney, bone marrow, and other organs also occurs in people with HIV. Whether a person has pulmonary or extrapulmonary TB, most patients present with fever, night sweats, cough, and weight loss. Persons infected with *M. tuberculosis* (*i.e.,* those with positive tuberculin skin tests) are more likely to develop reactivated TB if they become infected with HIV. Coinfected individuals are also more likely to have a rapidly progressive form of TB. Equally important, HIV-infected persons with TB coinfection usually have an increase in viral load, which decreases the success of TB therapy. They also have an increased number of other opportunistic infections and an increased mortality rate.

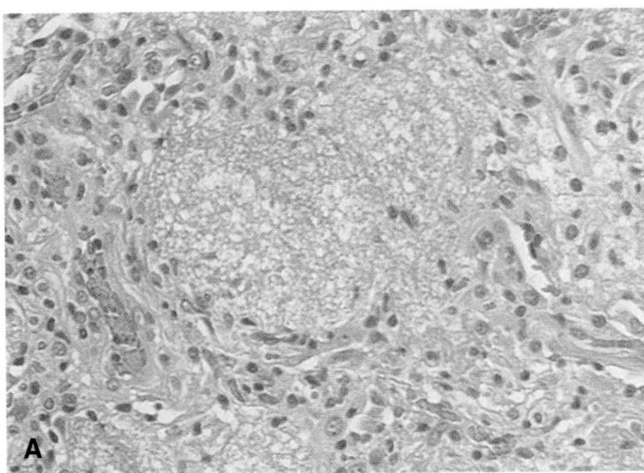

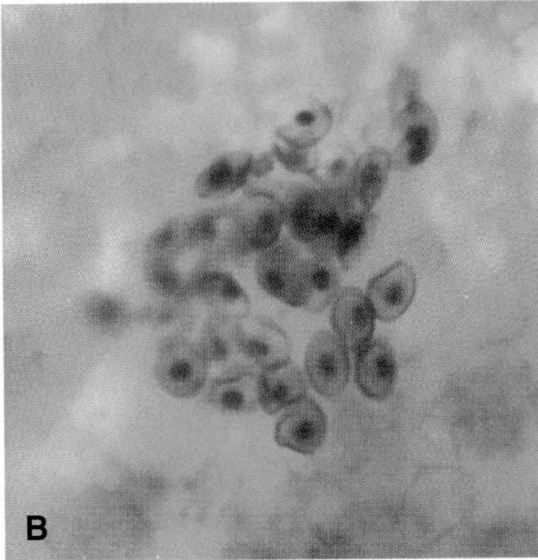

FIGURE 22-5 *Pneumocystis carinii* pneumonia. (**A**) The alveoli are filled with a foamy exudate, and the interstitium is thickened and contains a chronic inflammatory infiltrate. (**B**) A centrifuged bronchoalveolar lavage specimen impregnated with silver shows a cluster of *Pneumocystis carinii* cysts. (From Rubin E., Farber J.L. [1994]. *Pathology* [2nd ed.]. Philadelphia: J.B. Lippincott)

Since the late 1960s, most persons with TB have responded well to therapy. However, in 1991, there were outbreaks of multidrug-resistant (MDR) TB.[29] Many cases of drug-resistant TB occur in HIV-infected persons. A survey of MDR TB in eight metropolitan areas in the United States found that 38% of HIV-infected people with TB in New York had MDR TB, as compared with 18% of HIV-uninfected individuals with TB. Originally, mortality rates from MDR TB among HIV-infected persons were high, and the survival time was only approximately 2 months. Now, because of earlier recognition and therapy, the survival time is approximately 7 months.

Gastrointestinal Manifestations

Diseases of the gastrointestinal tract are some of the most frequent complications of HIV and AIDS. Esophageal candidiasis (thrush), CMV infection, and herpes simplex virus infection are common opportunistic infections that cause esophagitis in people with HIV.[30] Persons experiencing these infections usually complain of painful swallowing or retrosternal pain. The clinical presentation can range from asymptomatic to a complete inability to swallow and dehydration. Endoscopy or barium esophagography is required for definitive diagnosis.

Diarrhea or gastroenteritis is a common complaint in persons with HIV. The most common protozoal infection that causes diarrhea is *Cryptosporidium parvum*. The clinical features of cryptosporidiosis can range from mild diarrhea to severe, watery diarrhea with a loss of up to several liters of water per day. The most severe form usually occurs in persons with a $CD4^+$ cell count of less than 50 cells/µL, and also can include malabsorption, electrolyte disturbances, dehydration, and weight loss.[21] Other organisms that cause gastroenteritis and diarrhea are *Salmonella, Shigella, and Giardia* species, CMV, *Clostridium difficile, Escherichia coli,* and microsporida.[30] These organisms are identified by examination of stool cultures or endoscopy.

Nervous System Manifestations

Human immunodeficiency virus infection, particularly in its late stages of severe immunocompromise, leaves the nervous system vulnerable to an array of neurologic disorders, including AIDS dementia complex (ADC), toxoplasmosis, and PML. These disorders can affect the peripheral or central nervous system (CNS) and contribute to the morbidity and mortality of persons with HIV.

AIDS Dementia Complex. AIDS dementia complex, or HIV-associated dementia, is a syndrome of cognitive and motor dysfunction.[31] ADC is caused by HIV itself, rather than an opportunistic infection, and usually is a late complication of HIV. The clinical features of ADC are impairment of attention and concentration, slowing of mental speed and agility, slowing of motor speed, and apathetic behavior. The diagnosis of ADC can be based on these clinical findings. Treatment of ADC consists of HAART therapy to decrease symptoms, but there is no cure.

Toxoplasmosis. Toxoplasmosis is a common opportunistic infection in persons with AIDS. The organism responsible, *T. gondii,* is a parasite that most often affects the CNS.[32] Toxoplasmosis usually is a reactivation of a latent *T. gondii* infection that has been dormant in the CNS. The typical presentation includes fever, headaches, and neurologic dysfunction, including confusion and lethargy, visual disturbances, and seizures. Computed tomography scans or magnetic resonance imaging (MRI) should be performed immediately to detect the presence of neurologic lesions. Prophylactic treatment with trimethoprim-sulfamethoxazole is effective against *T. gondii* when the $CD4^+$ cell count falls below 200 cells/µL. Since the use of trimethoprim-sulfamethoxazole and HAART was put into practice, the incidence of toxoplasmosis has decreased.[31]

Progressive Multifocal Leukoencephalopathy. *Progressive multifocal leukoencephalopathy* is a demyelinating disease of the white matter of the brain caused by the JC virus, a DNA papovavirus that attacks the oligodendrocytes.[31] PML advances slowly, and it can be weeks to months before the patient seeks medical care. PML is characterized by progressive limb weakness, sensory loss, difficulty controlling the digits, visual disturbances, subtle alterations in mental status,[33] hemiparesis, ataxia, diplopia, and seizures.[34] The mortality rate is high, and the average survival time is 2 to 4 months. Diagnosis is based on clinical findings and an MRI, and confirmed by the presence of the JC virus.[33] There is no proven cure for PML, but improvement can occur after starting HAART.[34]

Cancers and Malignancies

Persons with AIDS have a high incidence of certain malignancies, especially Kaposi's sarcoma (KS), non-Hodgkin's lymphoma, and noninvasive cervical carcinoma. It has been reported that KS or lymphoma is likely to develop in as many as 30% to 40% of people with HIV.[35] The increased incidence of malignancies probably is a function of impaired cell-mediated immunity.

Kaposi's Sarcoma. Kaposi's sarcoma is a malignancy of the endothelial cells that line small blood vessels.[36] An opportunistic cancer, KS occurs in immunosuppressed persons (*e.g.*, transplant recipients or persons with AIDS). KS was one of the first opportunistic cancers associated with AIDS and remains the most frequent malignancy related to HIV. It is 2000 times more common in people infected with HIV than in the rest of the population.[35] Before 1981, most cases of KS were found in North America among elderly men of Mediterranean or Eastern European Jewish descent and in Africa among young black adults and children.[37]

There is evidence linking KS to a herpesvirus (herpesvirus-8, also called KS-associated herpes virus [KSHV]).[37] More than 95% of KS lesions, regardless of the source or clinical subtype, have reportedly been found to be infected with KSHV. The virus is readily transmitted through homosexual and heterosexual activities. Maternal–infant transmission also occurs. The virus has been detected in saliva from infected persons, and other modes of transmission are suspected.

The lesions of KS can be found on the skin and in the oral cavity, gastrointestinal tract, and lungs. More than 50% of people with skin lesions also have gastrointestinal lesions. The disease usually begins as one or more macules, papules, or violet skin lesions that enlarge and become darker (Fig. 22-6). They may enlarge to form raised plaques or tumors. These irregularly shaped tumors can be from one eighth of an inch to silver dollar size. Tumor nodules frequently are located on the trunk, neck, and head, especially the tip of the nose. They usually are painless in the early stages, but discomfort may develop as the tumor develops. Invasion of internal organs, including the lungs, gastrointestinal tract, and lymphatic system, commonly occurs. Gastrointestinal tract KS is often asymptomatic but can cause pain, bleeding, or obstruction.[35] Pulmonary KS usually is a late development of the disease and causes dyspnea, cough, and hemoptysis.[36] The tumors may obstruct organ function or rupture and cause internal bleeding. The progression of KS may be slow or rapid.

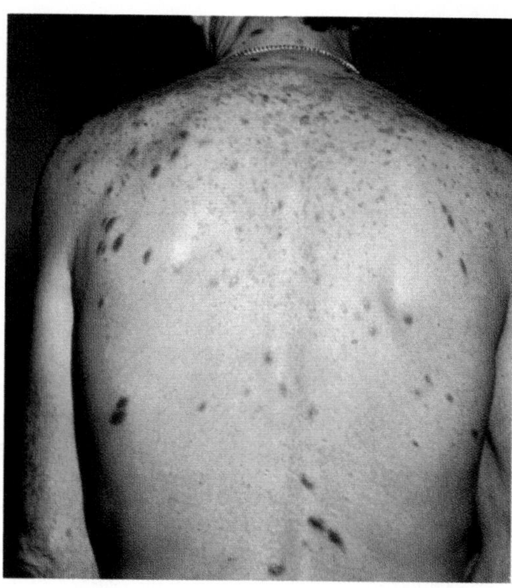

FIGURE 22-6 Disseminated Kaposi's sarcoma. Multiple red to brown papules distributed along the skin lines in a man with AIDS. (Hall J.C. [2000]. *Sauer's manual of skin* [8th ed., p. 197]. Philadelphia: Lippincott Williams & Wilkins)

A presumptive diagnosis of KS usually is made based on visual identification of red or violet skin or oral lesions.[35] Biopsy of at least one lesion must be done to establish the diagnosis and to distinguish the KS from other skin lesions that may resemble it. Diagnosis of gastrointestinal or pulmonary KS is more difficult because endoscopy and bronchoscopy are needed for diagnosis. Effective HAART, local therapy with liquid nitrogen or vinblastine, chemotherapy, radiation, and interferon injections are the most common therapies.[36] These therapies are only palliative and are not a cure. However, with evidence that links KS to a herpesvirus, there is hope that effective therapies will be developed for preventing KS in persons at risk.[37]

Non-Hodgkin's Lymphoma. Non-Hodgkin's lymphoma (see Chapter 17) develops in 3% to 4% of people with HIV infection.[35] The clinical features are fever, night sweats, and weight loss. Because the manifestations of non-Hodgkin's lymphoma are similar to those of other opportunistic infections, diagnosis often is difficult. Diagnosis can be made by biopsy of the affected tissue. Treatment includes aggressive combination chemotherapy that includes intrathecal chemotherapy. The prognosis for those with non-Hodgkin's lymphoma is poor, with survival ranging from 4 to 20 months.

Noninvasive Cervical Carcinoma. Women with HIV infection experience a higher incidence of cervical dysplasia than non–HIV-infected women.[38,39] These lesions are usually a slowly developing precursor to cervical carcinoma and progress rapidly in women with HIV infection. Cervical carcinoma results from infection with human papillomavirus.[39] In addition to the rapid progression from mild dysplasia to carcinoma in situ, women with HIV infection may be less responsive to standard treatments and have a poorer prognosis than uninfected women.[38] Occurrence of cervical dysplasia is detected by Papanicolaou smear and cervical colposcopy.

Wasting Syndrome

In 1997, wasting became an AIDS-defining illness. The syndrome is common in persons with HIV infection or AIDS. Wasting is characterized by involuntary weight loss of at least 10% of baseline body weight in the presence of diarrhea, more than two stools per day, or chronic weakness and a fever.[40] This diagnosis is made when no other opportunistic infections or neoplasms can be identified as causing these symptoms. Factors that contribute to wasting are anorexia, metabolic abnormalities, endocrine dysfunction, malabsorption, and cytokine dysregulation. Treatment for wasting includes nutritional interventions such as oral supplements or parenteral nutrition. There also are numerous pharmacologic agents used to treat appetite suppression including appetite stimulants (*e.g.,* cannabinoids and megestrol acetate).

Metabolic and Morphologic Disorders

A wide range of metabolic and morphologic disorders is associated with HIV infection, including lipodystrophy and mitochondrial disorders, hypercholesterolemia, hypertriglyceridemia, insulin resistance, and impaired glucose tolerance. Metabolic complications among people with HIV on HAART have been increasing during the past five years.[41] Diabetes is now seen in 0.5% to 4.4% of people on HAART. Insulin resistance is seen in as many as 55% of patients receiving protease inhibitors (PIs). It is still not known why insulin resistance occurs in people with HIV. Treatment of insulin resistance is the same as for people without HIV: a healthy balanced diet, exercise, and weight loss if needed (see Chapter 43).

Lipid abnormalities such as increases in triglycerides and cholesterol are also becoming more common in persons with HIV. Most protease inhibitors (PIs) have been shown to increase LDL and triglycerides.[41] Before beginning antiretroviral therapy, a fasting lipid panel should be drawn, then repeated in 3 to 6 months, and then repeated yearly. Currently, treatment of these lipid abnormalities includes use of the dietary guidelines recommended by the National Cholesterol Education Program (NCEP).[42] There is evidence to indicate that switching from a PI-containing to a non–PI-containing regimen is beneficial. The statins (*e.g.,* atorvastatin, fluvastatin, pravastatin, simvastatin, discussed in Chapter 24) are the recommended medication to manage hypercholesterolemia, although caution must be used because there can be drug-metabolizing interactions between the PIs, nonnucleoside reverse transcriptase inhibitors (NNRTIs), and statins. Because increased triglycerides can lead to pancreatitis, the fibric acid derivatives (*e.g.,* gemfibrozil and fenofibrate) may be prescribed as a means of decreasing triglyceride levels.

Lipodystrophy. A metabolic disorder called *lipodystrophy* is one of the newest group of problems for those infected with HIV. Lipodystrophy related to HIV includes symptoms that fall into two categories: changes in body appearance and metabolic changes.[43] The alterations in body appearance are an increase in abdominal girth, buffalo hump development (abnormal distribution of fat in the supraclavicular area), wasting of fat from the face and extremities, and breast enlargement in men and women. The metabolic changes include elevated serum cholesterol and triglyceride levels and insulin resistance. Originally attributed to the use of protease inhibitors, the pathogenesis of lipodystrophy is still not understood. It may be due to protease inhibitor therapy or nucleoside reverse transcriptase inhibitor therapy, or may arise simply because people are living longer with HIV.

There is no case definition for lipodystrophy; thus, diagnosis is based on patient complaints, clinical monitoring of triglycerides and cholesterol, and body shape.[43] Recently, the European Evaluation Agency, which is the European equivalent of the FDA, began a study to come up with a case definition of lipodystrophy.[41] They isolated 10 factors that define lipodystrophy: being female, being older than age 40, having HIV for more than 4 years, reaching CDC stage C AIDS classification, and having a wide anion gap, low HDL levels, increased waist-to-hip ratio, high visceral adipose tissue (VAT)–to–subcutaneous adipose tissue (SAT) ratio, increased trunk-to-limb fat ratio, and decreased percentage of leg fat.

There is no consensus on the best treatment for lipodystrophy. Preliminary studies suggest that recombinant human growth hormone (RHGH) decreases VAT and SAT, although its use has been associated with a high frequency of adverse affects.[41] Metformin, an oral antidiabetic drug, has also been used, and patients have experienced increased glucose tolerance, a decrease in weight, and a decrease in waist circumference. Some authorities recommend switching to a non–protease inhibitor–based HAART regimen. The problem with this is that although triglycerides and cholesterol decrease,[43] and there is some resolution to the fat redistribution, viral load can increase and become detectable.[44] Liposuction has been used with some success for patients with breast enlargement.[43] Many clinicians initiate lipid-lowering therapy.[45] The long-term consequences of these metabolic changes need to be carefully evaluated, and management guidelines need to be developed.

Mitochondrial Disorders. The mitochondria control many of the oxidative chemical reactions that release energy from glucose and other organic molecules.[43] The mitochondria transform this newly released energy into adenosine triphosphate (ATP), which cells use as an energy source. In the absence of normal mitochondrial function, cells revert to anaerobic metabolism with generation of lactic acid. The mitochondrial disorders seen in persons with HIV are caused by antiretroviral therapy, in particular, nucleoside reverse transcriptase inhibitors (NRTIs). Patients often present with nonspecific gastrointestinal symptoms, including nausea, vomiting, and abdominal pain. On examination, they can have hepatomegaly with normal liver function test results. The only laboratory abnormality may be lactic acidosis. Mitochondrial dysfunction is the most feared complication of antiretroviral therapy. This fear is due to the condition's unpredictability, its fatality in half of presenting patients, the nonspecific presenting symptoms, and the prevalence of elevated lactate levels in 8% to 22% of patients who are asymptomatic.[46]

In summary, HIV is a retrovirus that infects the body's CD4+ T cells and macrophages. The integration of viral RNA into the DNA of infected cells allows the virus to replicate, thereby infecting and eventually producing a profound loss of CD4+ cells from the peripheral blood.

The course of infection occurs in three phases: an acute mononucleosis-like infection that occurs shortly after infection, a latent phase that may last years, and an overt AIDS phase that occurs when the CD4+ cell count falls to 200 cells/µL or less. The AIDS phase is marked by the onset of opportunistic infections and cancers. These opportunistic pathologies can affect the respiratory, gastrointestinal, nervous, and other body systems causing conditions such as pneumonia, esophagitis, diarrhea, gastroenteritis, tumors, wasting syndrome, dementia, seizures, motor deficits, and metabolic disorders.

Prevention, Diagnosis, and Treatment

After completing this section of the chapter, you should be able to meet the following objectives:

- Discuss the transmission of HIV
- Describe preventive strategies to decrease the transmission of HIV
- Explain the possible significance of a positive antibody test for HIV infection
- Differentiate between the enzyme immunoassay (enzyme-linked immunosorbent assay) and Western blot antibody detection tests for HIV infection
- Describe the methods used in the early management of HIV infection
- Compare the actions of the reverse transcriptase inhibitors (*e.g.,* nucleoside reverse transcriptase inhibitors, nucleotide analog reverse transcriptase inhibitors), nonnucleoside reverse transcriptase inhibitors, protease inhibitors, and fusion inhibitors in terms of controlling HIV replication
- Enumerate some of the psychosocial issues associated with HIV/AIDS

Since the first description of AIDS, considerable strides have been made in understanding the pathophysiology of the disease. The virus and its mechanism of action, HIV antibody screening tests, and some treatment methods were discovered within a few years after the recognition of the first cases. Further progress in understanding the pathophysiology of AIDS and the development of more powerful treatments continues to be made.

PREVENTION

Because there is no cure for HIV or AIDS, adopting risk-free or low-risk behavior is the best protection against the disease. Abstinence or long-term, mutually monogamous sexual relationships between two uninfected partners are the best ways to avoid HIV infection and other STDs. Correct and consistent use of latex condoms can provide protection from HIV by not allowing contact with semen or vaginal secretions during intercourse.[10] Natural or lambskin condoms do not provide the same protection from HIV as latex because of the larger pores in the material. Only water-based lubricants should be used with condoms; petroleum (oil-based) products weaken the structure of the latex.

Injection of drugs provides another opportunity for HIV transmission. Avoiding recreational drug use and particularly avoiding the practice of using syringes that may have been used by another person are important to HIV prevention. Medical and public health authorities recommend that persons who inject drugs use a new sterile syringe for each injection or, if this is not possible, clean their syringes thoroughly with a household bleach mixture. Other substances that alter inhibitions can lead to risky sexual behavior and increase the risk for exposure to HIV. For example, smoking cocaine (*i.e.,* "crack") heightens the perception of sexual arousal, and this can influence the user to practice unsafe sexual behavior.[47] The addictive nature of many recreational drugs can lead to an increase in the frequency of unsafe sexual behavior and the number of partners as the user engages in sex exchanged for money or drugs. Persons concerned about their risk should be encouraged to get information and counseling and to be tested to find out their infection status.

Public health programs in the United States have been profoundly affected by the HIV epidemic. Although standard methods for disease intervention and statistical analysis are applied to HIV, public health programs have become more responsive to community concerns, confidentiality, and long-term follow-up of clients as a direct result of the HIV epidemic. Testing for HIV antibodies and counseling have become widely available in the United States. Whenever HIV testing is performed, pretest and posttest counseling should be offered. HIV prevention counseling should be culturally competent, sensitive to issues of sexual identity, developmentally appropriate, and linguistically relevant.[12]

The essential elements of any HIV prevention or counseling interaction include a personalized risk assessment and prevention plan.[48] Education and behavioral intervention continue to be the mainstays of HIV prevention programs. Individual risk assessment and education regarding HIV transmission and possible prevention techniques or skills are delivered to persons in clinical settings and to those at high risk for infection in community settings. Community-wide education is provided in schools, in the workplace, and in the media. Training for professionals can have an impact on the spread of HIV and is an important element of prevention. The constant addition of new information on HIV makes prevention an ever-changing and challenging endeavor.

DIAGNOSTIC METHODS

The diagnostic methods used for HIV infection include laboratory methods to determine infection and clinical methods to evaluate the progression of the disease. The most accurate and inexpensive method for identifying HIV is the HIV antibody test. The first commercial assays for HIV were introduced in 1985 to screen donated blood.

Since then, use of antibody detection tests has been expanded to include evaluating persons at increased risk for HIV infection. The HIV antibody test procedure consists of screening with an *enzyme immunoassay* (EIA), also known as *enzyme-linked immunosorbent assay* (ELISA), followed by a confirmatory test, the *Western blot* assay, which is performed if the EIA is positive.[49] EIA tests are used first because they are less expensive and are quicker to perform. In light of the psychosocial issues related to HIV and AIDS, sensitivity and confidentiality must be maintained whenever testing is implemented. Counseling before and after testing to allay fears, provide accurate information, ensure appropriate follow-up testing, and provide referral to needed medical and psychosocial services is essential.

The EIA detects antibodies produced in response to HIV infection.[19] In an EIA test, when blood is added, antibodies to HIV bind to HIV antigens. The antigen–antibody complex is then detected using an antihuman immunoglobulin G (IgG) antibody conjugated to an enzyme like alkaline phosphatase. A substrate is then added from which the enzyme produces a color reaction. Color development, indicating the amount of HIV antibodies found, is measured. The test is considered reactive, or positive, if color is produced, and negative, or nonreactive, if there is no color. EIA tests have high false-positive rates; thus, samples that are repeatedly reactive are tested by a confirmatory test such as the Western blot.

The Western blot test is more specific than the EIA, and in the case of a false-positive EIA test result, the Western blot test can identify the person as uninfected. The Western blot is a more sensitive assay that looks for the presence of antibodies to specific viral antigens.[19] For the test, HIV antigens are separated by electrophoresis based on their weight, and then transferred to nitrocellulose paper and arranged in strips, with larger proteins at the top and smaller proteins at the bottom. The serum sample is then added. If HIV antibodies are present, they bind with the specific viral antigen on the paper. An enzyme and substrate then are added to produce a color reaction as in the EIA test. If there are no colored bands present, the test is negative. A test is positive when certain combinations of bands are present. A test can be indeterminate if there are bands present but they do not meet the criteria for a positive test result. An indeterminate or false-positive test result can occur during the window period before seroconversion. When a serum antibody test result is reactive or borderline by EIA and positive by Western blot, the person is considered to be infected with HIV. When an EIA is reactive, and the Western blot is negative, the person in not infected with HIV. Both tests are important because, in some situations, misinformation can be generated by EIA testing alone because there are many situations that can produce a false-positive (Chart 22-3) or a false-negative ELISA result. The Western blot test therefore is essential to determine which persons with positive EIA tests are truly infected.

Millions of HIV antibody tests are performed in the United States each year. New technology has led to new forms of testing, like the oral test, home testing kits, and the new rapid blood test. Oral fluids contain antibodies to HIV. In the late 1990s, the FDA approved the OraSure test.[19] The OraSure uses a cotton swab, which is inserted into the mouth for 2 minutes, placed in a transport container with preservative, and then sent to a laboratory for EIA and Western blot testing. Home HIV testing kits can be bought over the counter. The kits, approved by the FDA, allow persons to collect their own blood sample through a finger-stick process, mail the specimen to a laboratory for EIA and confirmatory Western Blot tests, and receive results by telephone in 3 to 7 days. In November 2002, the FDA approved the Ora Quick Rapid HIV-1 Antibody Test.[50] The Ora Quick uses a whole blood specimen from a finger stick and can provide results in about 20 minutes. Reactive, or positive, test results require confirmation using Western blot testing. A person with a reactive result needs to be told that the preliminary test was positive, but they need a confirmatory test. The use of a rapid test should facilitate people receiving the results of their HIV test more regularly because they do not need to return for their test results 2 weeks later.

CHART 22-3

Causes of False-Positive or False-Negative HIV ELISA Test Results

False-Positive Results

- Hematologic malignant disorders (*e.g.*, malignant melanoma)
- DNA viral infections (*e.g.*, infectious mononucleosis [Epstein-Barr virus])
- Autoimmune disorders
- Primary biliary cirrhosis
- Immunizations (influenza, hepatitis)
- Passive transfer of HIV antibodies (mother to infant)
- Antibodies to class II leukocytes
- Chronic renal failure/renal transplant
- Stevens-Johnson syndrome
- Positive rapid plasma reagin test

False-Negative Results

- "Window" period after infection
- Immunosuppression therapy
- Replacement transfusion
- B-cell dysfunction
- Bone marrow transplant
- Contamination of specimen with starch powder from gloves
- Use of kits that detect primary antibody to the p24 viral core protein

Polymerase chain reaction (PCR) is a technique for detecting HIV DNA (see Chapter 18). PCR detects the presence of the virus rather than the antibody to the virus, which the EIA and Western blot tests detect.[51] PCR is useful in diagnosing HIV infection in infants born to infected mothers because these infants have their mothers' HIV antibody regardless of whether or not the infants are infected. Because the amount of viral DNA in the HIV-infected cell is small compared with the amount of human DNA, direct detection of viral genetic material is difficult.

PCR is a method for amplifying the viral DNA up to 1 million times or more to increase the probability of detection.

EARLY MANAGEMENT

The management of HIV infection has changed dramatically since the mid-1990s. This change is due to a better understanding of the pathogenesis of HIV, the emergence of viral load testing, and the increased number of medications available to fight the virus. After HIV infection is confirmed, a baseline evaluation should be done.[52] This evaluation should include a complete history and physical examination and baseline laboratory tests. Routine follow-up care of a stable, asymptomatic HIV-infected patient should include a history and physical examination along with CD4+ cell count and viral load testing every 3 to 4 months. Persons who are symptomatic may need to be seen more frequently.

Therapeutic interventions are determined by the level of disease activity based on the viral load, the degree of immunodeficiency based on the CD4+ cell count, and the appearance of specific opportunistic infections. The current guidelines released July 14, 2003 recommend that antiretroviral therapy be initiated when a person's CD4+ cell count is less than 350 cells/μl or the viral load is greater than 55,000 copies/mL.[53] As HIV progresses, prophylaxis and treatment of opportunistic infections becomes very important.[52] Prophylaxis is different for every opportunistic infection and depends on the person's CD4+ cell count. Early recognition of HIV is becoming more common, and medical intervention in the early stages may delay life-threatening symptoms and slow the spread of disease.

Because of frequent advances in the management of HIV infection, primary care providers must be prepared to update their knowledge of diagnosis, testing, evaluation, and medical intervention. The CDC, the Department of Health and Human Services, and the U.S. Public Health Service regularly issue guidelines to assist clinicians in caring for persons with HIV disease.

TREATMENT

There is no cure for HIV. The medications that are currently available to treat HIV decrease the amount of HIV in the body, but they do not get rid of the HIV virus. The treatment of HIV is one of the most rapidly evolving fields in medicine. Because different drugs act on different stages of the replication cycle, optimal treatment includes a combination of at least three drugs, often referred to as HAART.[54] The goal of HAART is a sustained suppression of HIV replication, resulting in an undetectable viral load and an increasing CD4+ cell count. In general, antiviral therapies are prescribed to slow the progression to AIDS and improve the overall survival time of persons with HIV infection.

The first drug that was approved by the FDA for the treatment of HIV was zidovudine, which came out in 1987.[54] Since then, an increasing number of therapeutics have been approved by the FDA for treatment of HIV infection. There currently are five different types of HIV antiretroviral medications: nucleoside reverse transcriptase inhibitors; nucleotide analog reverse transcriptase inhibitors; nonnucleoside reverse transcriptase inhibitors; protease inhibitors; and the newest class, fusion inhibitors (Table 22-2). Each type of agent attempts to interrupt viral replication at a different point.

Reverse transcriptase inhibitors inhibit HIV replication by acting on the enzyme reverse transcriptase.[55] Three types of HIV medications work on this enzyme: nucleoside reverse transcriptase inhibitors, nucleotide analog reverse transcriptase inhibitors, and nonnucleoside reverse transcriptase inhibitors. *Nucleoside reverse transcriptase inhibitors* and *nucleotide analog reverse transcriptase inhibitors* act by blocking the elongation of the DNA chain by stopping more nucleosides from being added. *Nonnucleoside reverse transcriptase inhibitors* work by binding to the reverse transcriptase enzyme so that it cannot copy the virus's RNA into DNA (see Fig. 22-1).

Protease inhibitors bind to the protease enzyme and inhibit its action.[52] This inhibition prevents the cleavage of the polyprotein chain into individual proteins, which would be used to construct the new virus. Because the information inside the nucleus is not put together properly, the new viruses that are released into the body are immature and noninfectious (see Fig. 22-1).

The newest class of antiretroviral therapy consists of the *fusion inhibitors*. These prevent HIV from fusing with the CD4+ cell, thus blocking the HIV from inserting its genetic information into the CD4+ T cell[56] (see Fig. 22-1). The FDA approved the first of this class in March 2003. It is a subcutaneous injection given twice daily.

Many other HIV medications are currently under investigation, including two new classes of drugs—entry inhibitors and integrase inhibitors. Entry inhibitors, which include fusion inhibitors as well as receptor blockers, block the receptors on the CD4+ T cells so that the HIV cannot attach to the CD4+ T cell.[57] Integrase inhibitors prevent the HIV DNA from being integrated into the host genome.

Finding a vaccine for HIV is also being investigated. There are currently two types of vaccines being examined.[58] First, there is a vaccine that would prevent infection. This vaccine would be given to someone who is HIV negative, with the goal of preventing infection if exposed to HIV. These vaccines have focused on stimulating the development of neutralizing antibodies to prevent HIV infection. The second type of vaccine would be used in people who are already infected with HIV. The goal of these vaccines would be to better control the HIV viremia by lowering the viral load set point, changing the viral load trajectories, or preserving immune function for longer periods of time. These vaccines have focused on boosting the body's cellular immune responses and preparing the cytotoxic T cells for lysis of HIV-infected cells.

Opportunistic infections occur as a consequence of immunodeficiency, which is caused by the progressive loss of CD4+ T cells. Drugs and vaccines commonly are used for the prevention and treatment of opportunistic infections and conditions, including PCP, toxoplasma, MAC,[59] candidal, CMV, influenza, hepatitis B, and *S. pneu-*

TABLE 22-2 Antiviral Medications Used in the Treatment of HIV Infection

Medication (Generic Name and Initials) by Classification	Medication (Trade Name)	Dosing Schedule
Nucleoside Reverse Inhibitors		
Zidovudine (AZT)	Retrovir	Twice daily
Didanosine (ddl)	Videx	Twice daily
Didanosine (ddl) enteric coated	Videx EC	Once daily
Lamivudine (3TC)	Epivir	Twice daily
Stavudine (d4T)	Zerit	Twice daily
Abacavir	Ziagen	Twice daily
Zalcitabine (ddC)	Hivid	Every 8 hours
AZT and 3TC	Combivir	Twice daily
AZT, 3TC, and abacavir	Trizir	Twice daily
Emtricitabine (FTC)	Emtiriva	Once daily
Nucleoside Analog Reverse Transcriptase Inhibitors		
Tenofovir (TNV)	Viread	Once daily
Nonnucleoside Reverse Transcriptase Inhibitors		
Nevirapine (NVP)	Viramune	Twice daily
Efavirenz (EFV)	Sustiva	Once daily
Delavirdine (DLV)	Rescriptor	Three times daily
Protease Inhibitors		
Saquinavir (SAQ)	Invirase, Fortovase	Every 8 hours
Ritonavir (RTV)	Novir	Every 12 hours
Indinavir (IDV)	Crixivan	Every 8 hours
Nelfinavir (NLF)	Viracept	Every 12 hours
Amprenavir (APV)	Agenerase	Every 12 hours
Lopinavir/ritonavir	Kaletra	Every 12 hours
Atazanavir	Reyataz	Once a day
Fusion Inhibitors		
Enfuvirtide (T-20)	Fuzeon	Every 12 hours

moniae infections.[60,61] Prophylactic medications are used once an individual's CD4+ cell count has dropped below a certain level that indicates his or her immune system is no longer able to fight off opportunistic infections.

Persons with HIV should be advised to avoid infections as much as possible and seek evaluation promptly when they occur. Immunization is important because persons infected with HIV are at risk for contracting other infectious diseases. Some of these diseases can be avoided by vaccination while the immune system's responsiveness is relatively intact.[62] Persons with asymptomatic HIV infection should be vaccinated against measles, mumps, and rubella. Pneumococcal vaccine should be given once, as soon as possible after HIV infection is diagnosed and then a booster should be given at 5 years, and influenza vaccine should be given yearly. Live-virus vaccines should not be given to persons with HIV infection.

PSYCHOSOCIAL ISSUES

HIV and AIDS affect all spheres of life.[63] The psychological effects of HIV infection or AIDS may be just as significant as the physical effects. The dramatic impact of this illness is compounded by complex reactions on the part of the person with HIV or AIDS; his or her partner, friends, and family; members of the health care team; and the community. These reactions may be influenced by inadequate information, fear of contagion, shame, prejudices, and condemnation of risk behaviors.[64] Acknowledging a diagnosis of AIDS may be the first indication to family and colleagues of an otherwise hidden lifestyle (*i.e.,* homosexuality or drug use). This increases the strain on relationships with important support persons. Shock is a common reaction people have when they are diagnosed with HIV, often followed by anger at themselves or others and denial or guilt. In addition to the fear and grief associated with death, the person with HIV or AIDS also may experience uncertainty and may feel helpless, hopeless, stigmatized, and out of control.[63]

Many people with HIV have preexisting mental health conditions like depression or anxiety disorders as well as alcohol and other drug problems (AODA). Appropriate diagnosis and treatment should be made available when mental health or AODA problems are evident. Diagnosis and treatment of cognitive and affective disorders are essential parts of ongoing care for the HIV-infected person.[63] The emotional stress, feelings of isolation, and sadness experienced by the person with HIV or AIDS can be overwhelming. Most persons, however, manage to learn to cope and live with their HIV infection. Persons with the disease must have as much information and control as possible. They should be encouraged to direct their energies in a positive manner and continue with their social and group activities as long as such activities are helpful. Appropriate social support systems (*e.g.*, AIDS service organizations, community groups, religious organizations) should be called on to assist whenever possible. When they learn they can live with HIV infection, many persons acquire a positive outlook based on living their lives to the fullest.

In summary, because there is no cure for HIV, risk-free or low-risk behavior is the best protection against HIV infection. Abstinence or long-term, mutually monogamous sexual relationships between two uninfected partners, use of condoms, avoiding drug use, and the use of sterile syringes are essential to stopping the spread of HIV.

HIV is diagnosed using the EIA together with the Western blot assay antibody detection tests. The emotional stress, feelings of isolation, and sadness experienced by the person with HIV or AIDS can be overwhelming, but most persons adjust to living with HIV infection. Diagnosis and treatment of cognitive and affective disorders are an essential part of ongoing care for the HIV-infected person. Appropriate treatment should be made available when alcohol or other drug dependence is noted.

The management of HIV/AIDS incorporates the use of HAART therapy, early recognition and treatment of opportunistic infections and other clinical disorders, as well as acknowledgment and support of the psychosocial issues that are an ongoing concern for those who are infected with the virus.

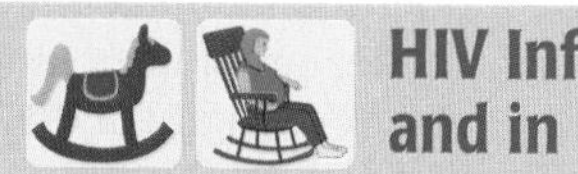

HIV Infection in Pregnancy and in Infants and Children

After completing this section of the chapter, you should be able to meet the following objectives:

- Discuss the vertical transmission of HIV from mother to child and recommended prevention measures
- Cite problems with the diagnosis of HIV infection in the infant
- Compare the progress of HIV infection in infants and children with HIV infection in adults

Early in the AIDS epidemic, children who contracted HIV could have become infected through blood products or perinatally. Now, almost all of the children who become infected with HIV at a young age in the United States get HIV perinatally. Infected women may transmit the virus to their offspring in utero, during labor and delivery, or through breast milk.[65] The risk for transmission is increased if the mother has advanced HIV disease as evidenced by low $CD4^+$ cell counts, high levels of HIV in her blood (high viral load), or prolonged time from rupture of membranes to delivery; if the mother breast-feeds the child[12]; or if there is increased exposure of the fetus to maternal blood.[66]

Diagnosis of HIV infection in children born to HIV-infected mothers is complicated by the presence of maternal HIV IgG antibody, which crosses the placenta to the fetus.[12] Consequently, infants born to HIV-infected women can be HIV antibody positive by ELISA for up to 18 months of age even though they are not HIV infected. PCR testing for HIV DNA is used most often to diagnose HIV in infants younger than 18 months of age. Two positive PCR tests for HIV DNA are needed to diagnose a child with HIV. Children born to mothers with HIV infection are considered uninfected if they become HIV antibody negative after 6 months of age, have no other laboratory evidence of HIV infection, and have not met the surveillance case definition criteria for AIDS in children.

The landmark PACTG 076 trial of 1994 found that perinatal transmission could be lowered by two thirds, from 26% to 8%, by administering zidovudine to the mother during pregnancy, labor, and delivery and to the infant when it is born.[11] The U.S. Public Health Service therefore recommends that HIV counseling and testing should be offered to all pregnant women.[67] The recommendations also stress that women who test positive for HIV antibodies should be informed of the perinatal prevention benefits of zidovudine therapy and offered HAART therapy, which often includes zidovudine. This is done because it has now been found that women receiving antiretroviral therapy who also have a viral load of less than 1000 copies/mL have very low rates of perinatal transmission. Benefits of voluntary testing for mothers and newborns include reduced morbidity because of intensive treatment and supportive health care, the opportunity for early antiviral therapy for mother and child, and information regarding the risk for transmission from breast milk.[65]

Because pregnant women in less developed countries do not always have access to zidovudine, studies are being conducted in Africa to determine whether any other simple and less expensive antiretroviral regimen can be used to decrease transmission from mother to infant. One such study, HIVNET 012, looked at single-dose nevirapine com-

HIV INFECTION IN PREGNANCY AND IN INFANTS AND CHILDREN

- HIV can be passed from mother to infant during labor and delivery or through breast-feeding.
- The course of HIV infection is different for children than adults.

pared with zidovudine. It found that nevirapine lowered the risk for HIV transmission by almost 50%.[68]

Children have a very different pattern of HIV infection than adults. Failure to thrive, CNS abnormalities, and developmental delays are the most prominent primary manifestations of HIV infection in children.[12] Children born infected with HIV usually weigh less and are shorter than noninfected infants. A major cause of early mortality for HIV-infected children is PCP. As opposed to adults, in whom PCP occurs in the late stages, PCP occurs early in children, with the peak age of onset at 3 to 6 months. For this reason, prophylaxis with trimethoprim-sulfamethoxazole is started by 4 to 6 weeks for all infants born to HIV-infected mothers, regardless of their CD4+ cell count or infection status.

In summary, infected women may transmit the virus to their offspring in utero, during labor and delivery, or through breast milk. It is recommended that all pregnant women get tested for HIV. Diagnosis of HIV infection in children born to HIV-infected mothers is complicated by the presence of maternal HIV antibody, which crosses the placenta to the fetus. This antibody usually disappears within 18 months in uninfected children. Administration of zidovudine to the mother during pregnancy, labor, and delivery and to the infant when it is born can decrease perinatal transmission.

REVIEW EXERCISES

A 29-year-old woman presents to the clinic for her initial obstetric visit, about 10 weeks into her pregnancy.

A. This woman is in a monogamous relationship. Should an HIV test be a part of her initial blood work? Why?

B. The woman's HIV test comes back positive. What should be done to decrease the risk for her passing on HIV to her baby?

C. The baby is born, and its initial antibody test is positive. Does this mean the baby is infected? How is the diagnosis of HIV in a baby younger than 18 months made, and why is this different than the diagnosis for adults?

A 40-year-old man presents to the clinic very short of breath, and on x-ray and examination, he is diagnosed with *Pneumocystis carinii* pneumonia (PCP). His provider performs an HIV test, and the results are positive. Upon further testing, the man's CD4+ count is found to be 100 cells/μL, and his viral load is 250,000 copies/mL.

A. Why did the provider perform an HIV test after the man was diagnosed with PCP?

B. Is there a way to prevent PCP?

C. What classification does this man fall into based on his CD4+ count and symptomatology, and why?

References

1. Quinn, T.C. (2003). World AIDS day: Reflections on the pandemic. *The Hopkins HIV Report 15*(1), 12–14.
2. UNAIDS (2002). AIDS epidemic update, December 2002. [On-line.] Available: www.unaids.org/worldaidsday/2002/press/Epiupdate.html.
3. Electronic reference from the Centers for Disease Control and Prevention. (2002). [On-line.] Available: www.CDC.gov/stats. Retrieved June 23, 2003.
4. Wisconsin Department of Health and Family Services. (2000). *Wisconsin AIDS/HIV update*. Madison, WI: Author.
5. Quinn T.C. (2001). The global HIV pandemic: Lessons from the past and glimpses into the future. *The Hopkins HIV Report 13*(1), 4–5, 16.
6. Montagnier L., Alizon M. (1986). The human immune deficiency virus (HIV): An update. In Gluckman J.C., Vilmer E. (Eds.), *Proceedings of the Second International Conference on AIDS* (p. 13). Paris: Elsevier.
7. Friedland G.H., Klein R.S. (1987). Transmission of the human immunodeficiency virus. *New England Journal of Medicine 317,* 1125–1135.
8. Sepkowitz K.A. (2001). AIDS—The first 20 years. *New England Journal of Medicine 344*(23), 1764–1772.
9. Gershon R.R.M., Vlahov D., Nelson K.E. (1990). The risk of transmission of HIV-1 through non-percutaneous, non-sexual modes: A review. *AIDS 4,* 645–650.
10. Colpin H. (1999). Prevention of HIV transmission through behavioral changes and sexual means. In Armstrong D., Cohen J. (Eds.), *Infectious diseases* (Section 5, Chapter 2, pp. 1–4). London: Harcourt.
11. Connor E.M., Sperling R.S., Gelber R., et al. (1994). Reduction of maternal-infant transmission of human immunodeficiency virus type 1 with zidovudine treatment. *New England Journal of Medicine 331,* 1173–1180.
12. Havens P.L. (1999). Pediatric AIDS. In Armstrong D., Cohen J. (Eds.), *Infectious diseases* (Section 5, Chapter 20). London: Harcourt.
13. Center for Disease Control and Prevention. (2001). Update U.S. Public Health Service guidelines for the management of occupational exposures to HBV, HCV, and HIV and recommendations for post exposure prophylaxis. *Morbidity and Mortality Weekly Report 50* (RR-11), 1–43.
14. Henderson D.K. (1999). Preventing occupational infections with HIV in health care settings. In Armstrong D., Cohen J. (Eds.), *Infectious diseases* (Section 5, Chapter 3, pp. 1–10). London: Harcourt.
15. Hirschel B. (1999). Primary HIV infection. In Armstrong D., Cohen J. (Eds.), *Infectious diseases* (Section 5, Chapter 8, pp. 1–4). London: Harcourt.
16. Abbas A.K., Lichtman A.H. (2003). *Cellular and molecular immunology* (5th ed., pp. 464–476). Philadelphia: W.B. Saunders.
17. Mitchell R.N., Kumar V. (2003). Diseases of immunity. In Kumar V., Cotran R.S., Robbins S.L. (Eds.), *Robbins basic pathology* (7th ed., pp. 147–158). Philadelphia: W.B. Saunders.
18. Fauci A.S. (1988). The human immunodeficiency virus: Infectivity and mechanisms of pathogenesis. *Science 239,* 617–622.
19. Holodniy M. (1999). Establishing the diagnosis of HIV infection. In Dolin R., Masur H., Saag M.S. (Eds.), *AIDS therapy* (pp. 3–14). Philadelphia: Churchill Livingstone.
20. Centers for Disease Control and Prevention. (1992). 1993 Revised classification system for HIV infection and expanded surveillance case definition for AIDS among adolescents

and adults. *Morbidity and Mortality Weekly Report 41*(RR-17), 1–23.

21. Rizzardi G.P., Pantaleo G. (1999). The immunopathogenesis of HIV-sa1 infection. In Armstrong D., Cohen J. (Eds.), *Infectious diseases* (Section 5, Chapter 6, pp. 1–12). London: Harcourt.
22. Braun, J. (2002). Antibody-negative but HIV-RNA positive. Is PHI your differential? *The PRN Notebook*. Special Edition, 3–7.
23. Markowitz, M. (2002). The treatment of PHI (part I): The hope of eradication. *The PRN Notebook*. Special Edition, 16–19.
24. Pantaleo G., Graziosi C., Fauci A.S. (1993). The immunopathogenesis of human immunodeficiency virus infection. *New England Journal of Medicine 328,* 327–335.
25. Clumeck N., Dewit S. (1999). Prevention of opportunistic infections in the presence of HIV infection. In Armstrong D., Cohen J. (Eds.), *Infectious diseases* (Section 5, Chapter 9). London: Harcourt.
26. Dolin R., Masur H., Saag M.S. (Eds.). (1999). *AIDS therapy*. Philadelphia: Churchill Livingstone.
27. Masur H. (1999). *Pneumocystis*. In Dolin R., Masur H., Saag M.S. (Eds.), *AIDS therapy* (pp. 291–306). Philadelphia: Churchill Livingstone.
28. Girard P.M. (1999). *Pneumocystis carinii* pneumonia. In Armstrong D., Cohen J. (Eds.), *Infectious diseases* (Section 5, Chapter 10, pp. 1–4). London: Harcourt.
29. Gordin F. (1999). *Mycobacterium tuberculosis*. In Dolin R., Masur H., Saag M.S. (Eds.), *AIDS therapy* (pp. 359–374). Philadelphia: Churchill Livingstone.
30. Wilcox C.M., Monkemuller K.E. (1999). Gastrointestinal disease. In Dolin R., Masur H., Saag M.S. (Eds.), *AIDS therapy* (pp. 752–765). Philadelphia: Churchill Livingstone.
31. Price R.W. (1999). Neurologic disease. In Dolin R., Masur H., Saag M.S. (Eds.), *AIDS therapy* (pp. 620–638). Philadelphia: Churchill Livingstone.
32. Katlama C. (1999). Parasitic infections. In Armstrong D., Cohen J. (Eds.), *Infectious diseases* (Section 5, Chapter 13, pp. 1–4). London: Harcourt.
33. Hall C.D. (1999). JC virus neurologic infection. In Dolin R., Masur H., Saag M.S. (Eds.), *AIDS therapy* (pp. 565–572). Philadelphia: Churchill Livingstone.
34. Murphy M.E., Polisky B. (1999). Viral infection. In Armstrong D., Cohen J. (Eds.), *Infectious diseases* (Section 5, Chapter 11). London: Harcourt.
35. Tirelli U., Vaccher E. (1999). Neoplastic disease. In Armstrong D., Cohen J. (Eds.), *Infectious diseases* (Section 5, Chapter 15, pp. 1–4). London: Harcourt.
36. Krown S.E. (1999). Kaposi sarcoma. In Dolin R., Masur H., Saag M.S. (Eds.), *AIDS therapy* (pp. 580–591). Philadelphia: Churchill Livingstone.
37. Anteman K., Chang Y. (2000). Kaposi's sarcoma. *New England Journal of Medicine 342,* 1027–1038.
38. Centers for Disease Control. (1990). Risk of cervical disease in HIV infected women. *Morbidity and Mortality Weekly Report 39,* 846–849.
39. Bonnez W. (1999). Sexually transmitted human papillomavirus infection. In Dolin R., Masur H., Saag M.S. (Eds.), *AIDS therapy* (pp. 530–564). Philadelphia: Churchill Livingstone.
40. Von Ruenn J.H., Mulligan K. (1999). Wasting syndrome. In Dolin R., Masur H., Saag M.S. (Eds.), *AIDS therapy* (pp. 607–619). Philadelphia: Churchill Livingstone.
41. Mulligan K., Kotler D.P. (2003). Metabolic and morphologic complications in HIV disease: What's new? *The PRN Notebook* 8(1), 11–20.
42. National Institute of Health Expert Panel (2001). *Third Report of the National Cholesterol Education Program (NCEP) Expert Panel on Detection, Evaluation, and Treatment of High Blood Cholesterol in Adults (Adult Treatment Panel III).* (NIH Publication No. 01–3670). Bethesda, MD: Author.
43. Chaisson R.E., Triesman G.J. (2000). *Antiretroviral therapy in perspective: Managing drug side effects to improve patient outcomes* (Vol. I). Connecticut: Scientific Exchange.
44. Lyon D., Truban E. (2000). HIV-related lipodystrophy: A clinical syndrome with implications for nursing practice. *Journal of the Association of Nurses in AIDS Care 11*(2), 36–42.
45. Lo J.C., Schambelan M. (1999). Endocrine disease. In Dolin R., Masur H., Saag M.S. (Eds.), *AIDS therapy* (pp. 740–751). Philadelphia: Churchill Livingstone.
46. Lucas, G.M. (2000). Report from the 38th IDSA: Preserving the immune response to HIV, HAART, and long-term toxicities. *The Hopkins HIV Report 12*(5), 1, 6, 12.
47. Edlin B.R., Irwin K.L., Faruque S., et al., and the Multicenter Crack Cocaine and HIV Infection Study Team. (1994). Intersecting epidemics: Crack cocaine use and HIV infection among inner-city young adults. *New England Journal of Medicine 331,* 1422–1427.
48. Centers for Disease Control and Prevention. (1998). Public health service task force recommendations for the use of antiretroviral drugs in pregnant women infected with HIV-1 for maternal health and for reducing perinatal HIV-1 transmission in the United States. *Morbidity and Mortality Weekly Report 47*(RR-2), 1–30.
49. Brun-Vezinet F., Simon F. (1999). Diagnostic tests for HIV infection. In Armstrong D., Cohen J. (Eds.), *Infectious diseases* (Section 5, Chapter 23, pp. 1–10). London: Harcourt.
50. Centers for Disease Control and Prevention. (2002). Notice to readers: Approval of a new rapid test for HIV antibody. *Morbidity and Mortality Weekly Report 51*(46), 1051–1052.
51. Rogers M.F., Ou C.Y., Kilbourne B., Schochetman G. (1991). Advances and problems in the diagnosis of human immunodeficiency virus infection in infants. *Pediatric Infectious Disease Journal 10,* 523–531.
52. Montaner J.S.G., Montesorri V. (1999). Principles of management. In Armstrong D., Cohen J. (Eds.), *Infectious diseases* (Section 5, Chapter 25, pp. 1–2). London: Harcourt.
53. Panel on Clinical Practices for Treatment of HIV infection convened by the Department of Health and Human Services. (2003). Guidelines for the use of antiretroviral agents in HIV-1 infected adults and adolescents. [On-line.] Available: www.aidsinfo.nih.gov/guidelines.
54. Vella S., Floridia M. (1999). Antiretroviral therapy. In Armstrong D., Cohen J. (Eds.), *Infectious diseases* (Section 5, Chapter 26, pp. 1–10). London: Harcourt.
55. Merck & Co., Inc. (1999). *The HIV life cycle* (brochure). West Point, PA: Author.
56. Hammer, S.M. (2003). The view from the pipeline: The 2003 review of experimental antiretrovirals. *PRN Notebook 8*(1), 3–10.
57. Project Inform. (2003). New hope from new classes of therapy. *PI Perspective 35,* 8–10.
58. Beyer C. (2003). The HIV/AIDS vaccine research effort: An update. *The Hopkins HIV Report 15*(1), 6–7.
59. Powderly W.G. (1999). Opportunistic infection prophylaxis in the era of highly active antiretroviral therapy. In Armstrong D., Cohen J. (Eds.), *Infectious diseases* (Section 5, Chapter 19, pp. 1–2). London: Harcourt.
60. Sande M.A., Gilbert D.N., Moellering, R.C. (Eds.). (2000). *The Sanford guide to HIV/AIDS therapy* (9th ed.). Hyde Park, VT: Antiretroviral Therapy.

61. Bartlett J.G., Gallant J.E. (2000). *2000–2001 Medical management of HIV infection.* Baltimore, MD: Johns Hopkins University Press.
62. Maenza J.R., Chaisson R.E. (1999). Bacterial infections in HIV disease. In Armstrong D., Cohen J. (Eds.), *Infectious diseases* (Section 5, Chapter 14, pp. 1–6). London: Harcourt.
63. O'Brien A.M., Oerlemans-Bunn M., Blachfield J.C. (1987). Nursing the AIDS patient at home. *AIDS Patient Care 1,* 21.
64. Lippman S.W., James W.A., Frierson R.L. (1993). AIDS and the family: Implications for counseling. *AIDS Care 5,* 71–78.
65. U.S. Public Health Service. (2000). *Revised public health service recommendations for human immunodeficiency virus screening of pregnant women.* Washington, DC: Author.
66. Boyer P., Dillon M., Navaie M., et al. (1994). Factors predictive of maternal-fetal transmission of HIV-1. *Journal of the American Medical Association 271,* 1925–1930.
67. U.S. Public Health Service. (2002). U.S. Public Health Service task force recommendations for the use of antiretroviral drugs in pregnant HIV-1 infected women for maternal health and interventions to reduce perinatal transmission in the United States. *Morbidity and Mortality Weekly Report 51*(RR-18), 1–40.
68. Guay L., Muskoe P., Fleming T., et al. (1999). Intrapartum and neonatal single-dose nevirapine compared with zidovudine for prevention of mother-to-child transmission of HIV-1 in Kampala, Uganda: HIVNET 012 randomised trial. *Lancet 354,* 795–802.

UNIT

VI

Cardiovascular Function

Of all body systems, the heart and circulation presented the most difficult puzzle to solve. From the fifth century BC, theories about blood and its movement were linked to the concept of the four elements (fire, earth, air, and water) and the *pneuma*, or life force. According to the Greek physician Galen (AD 130–200), the starting point of the circulatory system was the gut, where food was made into "chyle" and then carried to the liver where it was converted into blood. From the liver, which was believed to be the center of the circulation, a small amount of blood was sent to the heart and lungs where heat from the heart and pneuma from the air were added, producing an ultimate concoction of "vital spirits" that was carried in the arteries to all parts of the body.

It was not until the work of the English physician William Harvey (1578–1657) that answers to the mysteries of the circulation began to emerge. It was he who first proposed that blood traveled in a circuitous route through the body, being pumped by the active phase of the heart's contraction, not relaxation as had previously been believed. In his studies, Harvey showed that a cut artery in an animal spurts during the heart's contraction. He also demonstrated that the atria of the heart had the same relationship to the ventricles as the ventricles do to the arteries and that blood from the heart was circulated through the lungs, where it was oxygenated. As strange as it may seem today, these concepts were so revolutionary to Harvey's contemporaries that the world's basic understanding of how the body functions was thrown into turmoil.

CHAPTER

23

Control of Cardiovascular Function

The main function of the *circulatory system,* which consists of the heart and blood vessels, is transport. The circulatory system delivers oxygen and nutrients needed for metabolic processes to the tissues, carries waste products from cellular metabolism to the kidneys and other excretory organs for elimination, and circulates electrolytes and hormones needed to regulate body function. This process of nutrient delivery is carried out with exquisite precision so that the blood flow to each tissue of the body is exactly matched to tissue need. The circulatory system also plays an important role in body temperature regulation, which relies on the circulatory system for transport of core heat to the periphery, where it can be dissipated into the external environment. Transport of various immune substances that contribute to the body's defense mechanisms is also an important circulatory function. The purpose of this chapter is to discuss the organization of the circulatory system, the function of the heart as a pump, the anatomy and circulatory function of the blood vessels, neural control of circulatory function, and the microcirculation and lymphatic system.

Organization of the Circulatory System

After you have completed this section of the chapter, you should be able to meet the following objectives:

- Compare the functions and distribution of blood flow and blood pressure in the systemic and pulmonary circulations
- State the relation between blood volume and blood pressure in the circulatory system

PULMONARY AND SYSTEMIC CIRCULATIONS

The circulatory system can be divided into two parts: the *pulmonary circulation,* which moves blood through the lungs and creates a link with the gas exchange function of the respiratory system, and the *systemic circulation,* which supplies all the other tissues of the body (Fig. 23-1). The blood that is in the heart and pulmonary circulation is sometimes referred to as the *central circulation,* and that outside the central circulation as the *peripheral circulation.*

Both the pulmonary and systemic circulations have a pump, an arterial system, capillaries, and a venous system. Arteries and arterioles function as a distribution system to move blood to the tissues. Capillaries serve as an exchange system where transfer of gases, nutrients, and wastes takes place. Venules and veins serve as collection and storage vessels that return blood to the heart. The pulmonary circulation consists of the right heart, the pulmonary artery, the pulmonary capillaries, and the pulmonary veins. The large pulmonary vessels are unique in that the pulmonary artery is the only artery that carries venous blood, and the pulmonary veins are the only veins that carry arterial blood. The systemic circulation consists of the left heart, the aorta and its branches, the capillaries that supply the brain and peripheral tissues, and the systemic venous system and the vena cava. The veins from the lower portion of the body converge into the inferior vena cava, and those from the head and upper extremities converge into the superior vena cava. The inferior vena cava and superior vena cava empty into the right heart.

FUNCTIONAL ORGANIZATION OF THE CIRCULATORY SYSTEM

- The circulatory system consists of the heart, which pumps blood; the arterial system, which distributes oxygenated blood to the tissues; the venous system, which collects deoxygenated blood from the tissues and returns it to the heart; and the capillaries, where exchange of gases, nutrients, and wastes takes place.
- The circulatory system is divided into two parts: the low-pressure pulmonary circulation, linking circulation and gas exchange in the lungs, and the high-pressure systemic circulation, providing oxygen and nutrients to the tissues.
- Blood flows down a pressure gradient from the high-pressure arterial circulation to the low-pressure venous circulation.
- The circulation is a closed system, so the output of the right and left heart must be equal over time for effective functioning of the circulation.

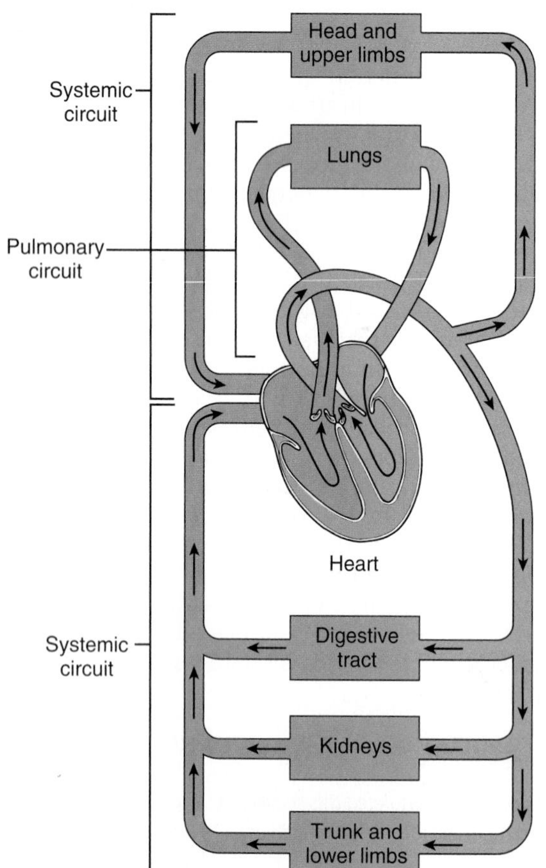

FIGURE 23-1 Systemic and pulmonary circulations. The right side of the heart pumps blood to the lungs, and the left side of the heart pumps blood to the systemic circulation.

Although the pulmonary and systemic systems function similarly, they have some important differences. The pulmonary circulation is the smaller of the two and functions with a much lower pressure. Because the pulmonary circulation is located in the chest near the heart, it functions as a low-pressure system with a mean arterial pressure of approximately 12 mm Hg. The low pressure of the pulmonary circulation allows blood to move through the lungs more slowly, which is important for gas exchange. Because the systemic circulation must transport blood to distant parts of the body, often against the effects of gravity, it functions as a high-pressure system, with a mean arterial pressure of 90 to 100 mm Hg.

The circulatory system is a closed system in which the heart consists of two pumps in series: one to propel blood through the lungs (*i.e.,* pulmonary circulation) and the other to propel blood to all other tissues of the body (*i.e.,* systemic circulation). Unidirectional flow through the heart is ensured by the heart valves. Both sides of the heart are further divided into two chambers, an *atrium* and a *ventricle.* The atria function as collection chambers for blood returning to the heart and as auxiliary pumps that assist in filling the ventricles. The ventricles are the main pumping chambers of the heart. The right ventricle pumps blood through the pulmonary artery to the lungs, and the left ventricle pumps blood through the aorta into the systemic circulation. The ventricular chambers of the right and left heart have inlet and outlet valves that act reciprocally (*i.e.,* one set of valves is open while the other is closed) to control the direction of blood flow through the cardiac chambers.

The effective function of the circulatory system requires that the outputs of both sides of the heart pump the same amount of blood over time. If the output of the left heart were to fall below that of the right heart, blood would accumulate in the pulmonary circulation. Likewise, if the right heart were to pump less effectively than the left heart, blood would accumulate in the systemic circulation. However, the left and right heart seldom ejects exactly the same amount of blood with each beat. This is because blood return to the heart is affected by activities of daily living such as taking a deep breath or moving from the seated to standing position. These beat-by-beat variations in cardiac output are accommodated by the storage capabilities of the venous system that allow for temporary changes in volume. Fluid accumulation occurs only when the storage capacity of the venous system has been exceeded.

VOLUME AND PRESSURE DISTRIBUTION

Blood flow in the circulatory system depends on a blood volume that is sufficient to fill the blood vessels and a pressure difference across the system that provides the force to move blood forward. The total blood volume is a function of age and body weight, ranging from 85 to 90 mL/kg in the neonate and from 70 to 75 mL/kg in the adult. As shown in Figure 23-2, approximately 4% of the blood at any given time is in the left heart, 16% is in the arteries and arterioles, 4% is in the capillaries, 64% is in the venules and veins, and 4% is in the right heart. The arteries and arterioles, which have thick, elastic walls and function as a distribution system, have the highest pressure. The capillaries are small, thin-walled vessels that link the arterial and venous sides of the circulation. Because of their small size and large surface area, the capillaries contain the smallest amount of blood. The venules and veins, which contain the largest amount of blood, are thin-walled, distensible vessels that function as a reservoir to collect blood from the capillaries and return it to the right heart.

Blood moves from the arterial to the venous side of the circulation along a pressure difference, moving from an area of higher pressure to one of lower pressure. The pressure distribution in the different parts of the circulation is almost an inverse of the volume distribution (see Fig. 23-2). The pressure in the arterial side of the circulation, which contains only approximately one sixth of the blood volume, is much greater than the pressure on the venous side of the circulation, which contains approximately two thirds of the blood. This pressure and volume distribution is due in large part to the structure and relative elasticity of the arteries and veins. It is the pressure difference between the arterial and venous sides of the circulation (approximately 84 mm Hg) that provides the driving force for flow of blood in the systemic circulation. The pulmonary circulation has a similar arterial-venous pressure difference, albeit of a lesser magnitude, that facilitates blood flow.

Because the pulmonary and systemic circulations are connected and function as a closed system, blood can be shifted from one circulation to the other. In the pulmonary circulation, the blood volume (approximately 450 mL in the adult) can vary from as low as 50% of normal to as high as 200% of normal. An increase in intrathoracic pressure, which impedes venous return to the right heart, can produce a transient shift from the central to the systemic circulation of as much as 250 mL of blood. Body position also affects the distribution of blood volume. In the recumbent position, approximately 25% to 30% of the total blood volume is in the central circulation. On standing,

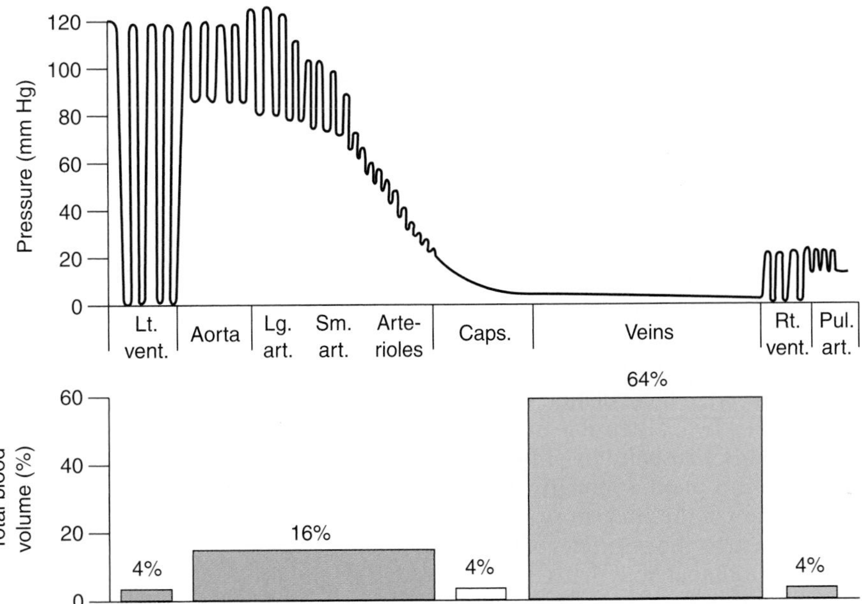

FIGURE 23-2 Pressure and volume distribution in the systemic circulation. The graphs show the inverse relation between internal pressure and volume in different portions of the circulatory system. (Smith J. J., Kampine J. P. [1990]. *Circulatory physiology: The essentials* [3rd ed.]. Baltimore: Williams & Wilkins)

this blood is rapidly displaced to the lower part of the body because of the force of gravity. Because the volume of the systemic circulation is approximately seven times that of the pulmonary circulation, a shift of blood from one system to the other has a much greater effect in the pulmonary than in the systemic circulation.

In summary, the circulatory system functions as a transport system that circulates nutrients and other materials to the tissues and removes waste products. The circulatory system can be divided into two parts: the systemic and the pulmonary circulation. The heart pumps blood throughout the system, and the blood vessels serve as tubes through which blood flows. The arterial system carries fluids from the heart to the tissues, and the veins carry them back to the heart. The cardiovascular system is a closed system with a right and left heart connected in series. The systemic circulation, which is served by the left heart, supplies all the tissues except the lungs, which are served by the right heart and the pulmonary circulation. Blood moves throughout the circulation along a pressure gradient, moving from the high-pressure arterial system to the low-pressure venous system. In the circulatory system, pressure is inversely related to volume. The pressure on the arterial side of the circulation, which contains only approximately one sixth of the blood volume, is much greater than the pressure on the venous side of the circulation, which contains approximately two thirds of the blood.

Principles of Blood Flow

After you have completed this section of the chapter, you should be able to meet the following objectives:

- Define the term *hemodynamics* and describe the effects of blood pressure; vessel radius, length, and cross-sectional area; and blood viscosity on the characteristics of blood flow
- Use Laplace's law to explain the effect of radius size on the pressure and wall tension in a vessel
- Use the term *compliance* to describe the characteristics of arterial and venous blood vessels

The term *hemodynamics* (*hemo* means "blood," and *dynamic* refers to the relation between motion and forces) describes the physical principles governing pressure, flow, and resistance as they relate to the cardiovascular system. The hemodynamics of the circulatory system is complex. The heart is an intermittent pump, and as a result, blood flow in the arterial circulation is pulsatile. The blood vessels are branched, distensible tubes of various dimensions. The blood is a suspension of blood cells, platelets, lipid globules, and plasma proteins. Despite this complexity, the function of the circulatory system can, at least in part, be explained by the principles of basic fluid mechanics that apply to nonbiologic systems, such as household plumbing systems.

HEMODYNAMICS

- Blood flow is directly related to the difference in pressure between the inlet and outlet of a vessel and is inversely related to the resistance to flow through that vessel. Resistance to flow through a vessel is inversely related to the fourth power of the vessel radius (r^4). Small decreases in vessel radius cause large increases in resistance to flow.
- At any given intraluminal pressure, the tension in a vessel wall (the force that opposes the intraluminal pressure) is greater in the vessel with the greater radius.
- Compliance (C) is defined by the equation C = V/P. A given change in volume (V) causes less of an increase in transmural pressure (P) in a more compliant vessel. A vein is 24 times more compliant than its corresponding artery.

PRESSURE, FLOW, AND RESISTANCE

The most important factors governing the function of the circulatory system are *volume, pressure, resistance,* and *flow.* Optimal function requires a volume that is sufficient to fill the vascular compartment and a pressure that is sufficient to ensure blood flow to all body tissues.

Blood flow is determined by two factors: a pressure difference between the two ends of a vessel or group of vessels and the resistance that blood must overcome as it moves through the vessel or vessels (Fig. 23-3). The relation between pressure, resistance, and flow is expressed by the equation F = P/R, in which F is the blood flow, P is the difference in pressure between the two ends of the system, and R is the resistance to flow through the system.

The total resistance that the blood encounters as it flows through the systemic circulation is referred to as the *peripheral vascular resistance* (PVR) or, sometimes, as the *systemic vascular resistance.* In the systemic circulation, blood flow is determined by the cardiac output (CO) and PVR. The PVR cannot be measured directly. Instead, it is estimated by rearranging the variables in the previous equation (PVR = P/CO),

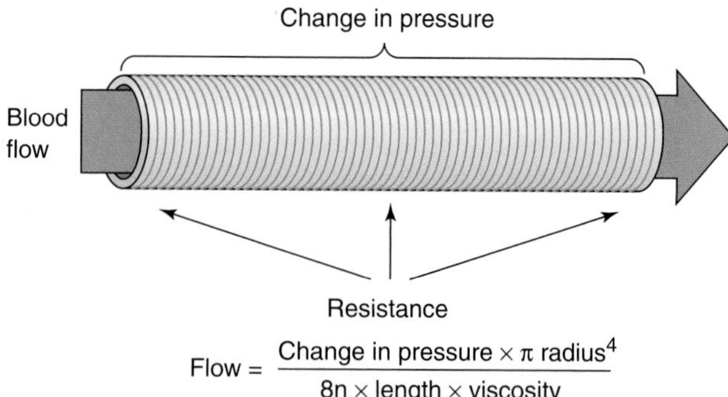

$$\text{Flow} = \frac{\text{Change in pressure} \times \pi \text{ radius}^4}{8n \times \text{length} \times \text{viscosity}}$$

FIGURE 23-3 Factors that affect blood flow (Poiseuille's law). Increasing the pressure difference between the two ends of the vessel increases flow. Flow diminishes as resistance increases. Resistance is directly proportional to blood viscosity and the length of the vessel and inversely proportional to the fourth power of the radius.

in which P represents the pressure difference between the aortic or mean arterial pressure (approximately 100 mm Hg) and right atrial pressure (approximately 0 mm Hg). The flow (F) or cardiac output is approximately 100 mL/second at rest. The PVR is therefore 100/100 or 1 peripheral resistance unit (PRU). The total resistance in the pulmonary circulation is only approximately 0.12 PRU. In this case, the blood flow is the same as in the systemic circulation, but the pressure difference between the pulmonary artery and left atrium (16 mm Hg versus 4 mm Hg) is much less.

A helpful equation ($F = \Delta P \times \pi \times r^4/8n \times L \times \text{viscosity}$) for understanding factors that affect blood flow was derived by the French physician Poiseuille more than a century ago (see Fig. 23-3). According to this equation, the two most important determinants of flow in the circulatory system are a difference in pressure (ΔP) and the vessel radius to the fourth power (r^4). The length (L) of vessels does not usually change, and 8n is a constant that does not change. Because flow is directly related to the fourth power of the radius, small changes in vessel radius can produce large changes in flow to an organ or tissue. For example, if the pressure difference remains constant, the rate of flow is 16 times greater in a vessel with a radius of 2 mm than in a vessel with a radius of 1 mm.

According to Poiseuille's equation, blood flow is also affected by the viscosity of blood. Viscosity is the resistance to flow caused by the friction of molecules in a fluid. The viscosity of a fluid is largely related to its thickness. The more particles that are present in a solution, the greater the frictional forces that develop between the molecules. Unlike water that flows through plumbing pipes, blood is a nonhomogeneous liquid. It contains blood cells, platelets, fat globules, and plasma proteins that increase its viscosity. The red blood cells, which constitute 40% to 45% of the formed elements of the blood, largely determine the viscosity of the blood. When measured in relation to water, the relative viscosity of plasma is 1.5, and at a normal hematocrit of 42% to 45%, that of whole blood is 3.0. Under special conditions, temperature may affect viscosity. There is a 2% rise in viscosity for each 1°C decrease in body temperature, a fact that helps explain the sluggish blood flow seen in persons with hypothermia.

CROSS-SECTIONAL AREA AND VELOCITY OF FLOW

Velocity is a distance measurement; it refers to the speed or linear movement with time (centimeters per second) with which blood flows through a vessel. *Flow* is a volume measurement (milliliters per second); it is determined by the cross-sectional area of a vessel and the velocity of flow (Fig. 23-4). When the flow through a given segment of the circulatory system is constant—as it must be for continuous flow—the velocity is inversely proportional to the cross-sectional area of the vessel (*i.e.,* the smaller the cross-sectional area, the greater the velocity of flow). This phenomenon can be compared with cars moving from a two-lane to a single-lane section of a highway. To keep traffic moving at its original pace, cars would have to double their speed in the single-lane section of the highway. So it is with flow in the circulatory system.

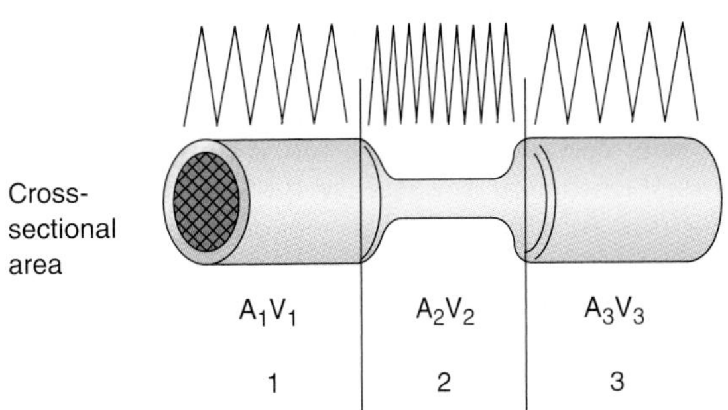

FIGURE 23-4 Effect of cross-sectional area (A) on velocity (V) of flow. In section 1, velocity is low because of an increase in cross-sectional area. In section 2, velocity is increased because of a decrease in cross-sectional area. In section 3, velocity is again reduced because of an increase in cross-sectional area. Flow is assumed to be constant.

The linear velocity of blood flow in the circulatory system varies widely from 30 to 35 cm/second in the aorta to 0.2 to 0.3 mm/second in the capillaries. This is because even though each individual capillary is very small, the total cross-sectional area of all the systemic capillaries greatly exceeds the cross-sectional area of other parts of the circulation. As a result of this large surface area, the slower movement of blood allows ample time for exchange of nutrients, gases, and metabolites between the tissues and the blood.

LAMINAR AND TURBULENT FLOW

Blood flow normally is *laminar,* with the blood components arranged in layers so that the plasma is adjacent to the smooth, slippery endothelial surface of the blood vessel, and the blood cells, including the platelets, are in the center or *axis* of the bloodstream (Fig. 23-5, vessel A). This

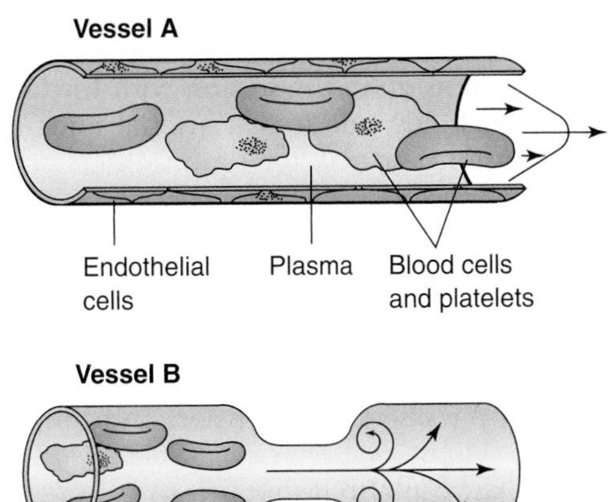

FIGURE 23-5 Laminar and turbulent flow in blood vessels. Vessel A shows streamlined or laminar flow in which the plasma layer is adjacent to the vessel endothelial layer and blood cells are in the center of the bloodstream. Vessel B shows turbulent flow in which the axial location of the platelets and other blood cells is disturbed.

arrangement reduces friction by allowing the blood layers to slide smoothly over one another, with the axial layer having the most rapid rate of flow.

Under certain conditions, blood flow switches from laminar to turbulent flow (see Fig. 23-5, vessel B). *Turbulent* flow is flow in which blood moves crosswise and lengthwise along a vessel in a manner similar to the eddy currents seen in a rapidly flowing river at a point of obstruction. Turbulent flow is influenced by a number of conditions, including high velocity of flow, change in vessel diameter, and low blood viscosity. The tendency for turbulence to occur increases in direct proportion to the velocity of flow. Imagine the chaos as cars from a two- or three-lane highway converge on a single-lane section of the highway. The same type of thing happens in blood vessels that have been narrowed by disease processes, such as atherosclerosis. Low blood viscosity allows the blood to move faster and accounts for the transient occurrence of heart murmurs in some persons who are severely anemic. Turbulent flow predisposes to clot formation as platelets and other coagulation factors come in contact with the endothelial lining of the vessel. Turbulent flow often can be heard through a stethoscope. An audible murmur in a blood vessel experiencing turbulent flow is referred to as a *bruit.*

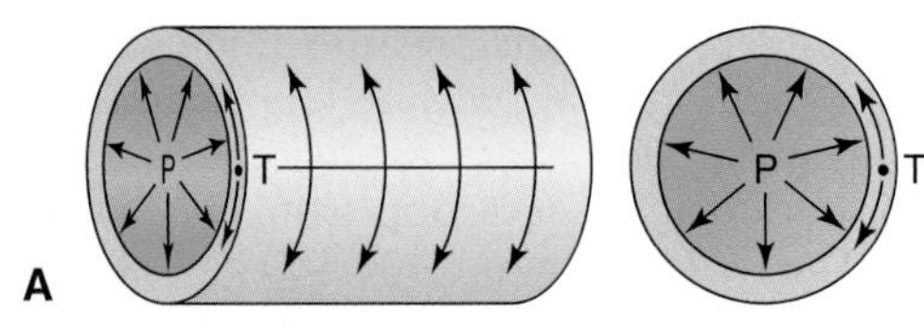

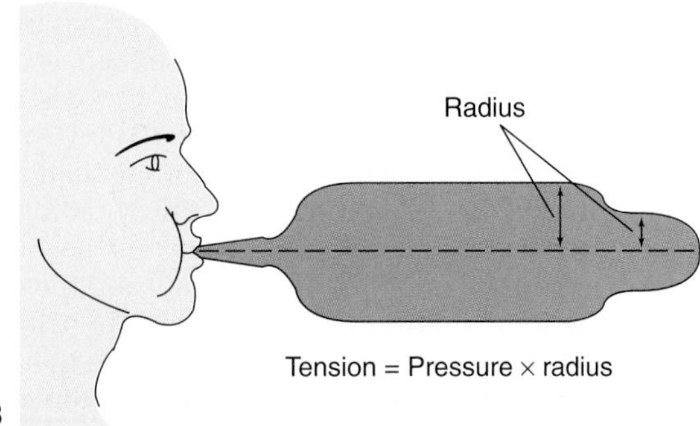

FIGURE 23-6 Laplace's law relates pressure (P), tension (T), and radius in a cylindrical blood vessel. **(A)** The pressure expanding the vessel is equal to the wall tension multiplied by the vessel radius. **(B)** Effect of the radius of a cylinder on tension. In a balloon, the tension in the wall is proportional to the radius because the pressure is the same everywhere inside the balloon. The tension is lower in the portion of the balloon with the smaller radius. (Rhoades R. A., Tanner G. A. [1996]. *Medical physiology* [p. 627]. Boston: Little, Brown)

WALL TENSION, RADIUS, AND PRESSURE

In a blood vessel, *wall tension* is the force in the vessel wall that opposes the distending pressure inside the vessel. The French astronomer and mathematician Pierre de Laplace described the relationship among wall tension, pressure, and the radius of a vessel or sphere more than 200 years ago. This relationship, which has come to be known as *Laplace's law,* can be expressed by the equation, $T = P \times r$, in which T represents wall tension, P the intraluminal pressure, and r the vessel radius (Fig. 23-6A). Accordingly, the internal pressure expands the vessel until it is exactly balanced by the tension in the vessel wall. This correlation can be compared with a partially inflated long balloon (see Fig. 23-6B). Because the pressure is equal throughout, the tension in the part of the balloon with the smaller radius is less than the tension in the section with the larger radius. The same holds true for an arterial aneurysm in which the tension and risk for rupture increase as the aneurysm grows in size (see Chapter 24).

Laplace's law was later expanded to include wall thickness, with wall tension being inversely related to wall thickness ($T = P \times r/\text{wall thickness}$). Thus, the thicker the vessel wall, the lower the tension, and vice versa. In hypertension, arterial vessel walls hypertrophy and become thicker, thereby reducing the tension and minimizing wall stress.

Laplace's law can also be applied to the pressure required to maintain the patency of small blood vessels. Provided that the thickness of a vessel wall remains constant, it takes more pressure to overcome wall tension and to keep a vessel open as its radius decreases in size ($P = T/r$). The critical closing pressure refers to the point at which vessels collapse so that blood can no longer flow through them. In circulatory shock, for example, there is a decrease in blood volume and vessel radii, along with a drop in blood pressure. As a result, many of the small vessels collapse as blood pressure drops to the point at which it can no longer overcome the wall tension. The collapse of peripheral veins often makes it difficult to insert venous lines that are needed for fluid and blood replacement.

DISTENTION AND COMPLIANCE

Compliance refers to the total quantity of blood that can be stored in a given portion of the circulation for each millimeter rise in pressure. Compliance (C) is defined by the equation, $C = V/P$, in which V is the change in volume and P is the change in distending pressure. The distending pressure is the difference between the pressure inside the vessel and the pressure outside the vessel. This is called the *transmural pressure.* As compliance increases, there is less change in transmural pressure with any given change in volume.

Compliance reflects the *distensibility* of the blood vessel (*i.e.,* increase in volume/increase in pressure × original volume). The distensibility of the arteries allows them to accommodate the pulsatile output of the heart. The most distensible of all vessels are the veins, which can increase their volume with only slight changes in pressure, allowing them to function as a reservoir for storing large quantities of blood that can be returned to the circulation when it is needed.

In summary, blood flow is controlled by many of the same mechanisms that control fluid flow in nonbiologic systems. It is influenced by vessel length, pressure differences, vessel radius, blood viscosity, cross-sectional area, and wall tension. The rate of flow is directly related to the pressure difference between the two ends of the vessel and the vessel radius and inversely related to vessel length and blood viscosity. The cross-sectional area of a vessel influences the velocity of flow; as the cross-sectional area decreases, the velocity is increased, and vice versa. Laminar blood flow is flow in which there is layering of blood components in the center of the bloodstream. This reduces frictional forces and prevents clotting factors from coming in contact with the vessel wall. In contrast to laminar flow, turbulent flow is disordered flow, in which the blood moves crosswise and lengthwise in blood vessels. The relation between wall tension, transmural pressure, and radius is described by Laplace's law, which states that wall tension becomes greater as the radius increases. Wall tension is also affected by wall thickness; it increases as the wall becomes thinner and decreases as the wall becomes thicker.

The Heart as a Pump

After you have completed this section of the chapter, you should be able to meet the following objectives:

- Describe the structural components and function of the pericardium, myocardium, endocardium, and the heart valves and fibrous skeleton
- Draw a figure of the cardiac cycle, incorporating volume, pressure, phonocardiographic, and electrocardiographic changes that occur during atrial and ventricular systole and diastole
- Define the terms *preload* and *afterload*
- State the formula for calculating the cardiac output and explain the effects that venous return, cardiac contractility, and heart rate have on cardiac output
- Describe the cardiac reserve and relate it to the Frank-Starling mechanism

The heart is a four-chambered muscular pump approximately the size of a man's fist that beats an average of 70 times each minute, 24 hours each day, 365 days each year for a lifetime. In 1 day, this pump moves more than 1800 gallons of blood throughout the body, and the work performed by the heart over a lifetime would lift 30 tons to a height of 30,000 ft.

FUNCTIONAL ANATOMY OF THE HEART

The heart is located between the lungs in the mediastinal space of the intrathoracic cavity in a loose-fitting sac called the *pericardium*. It is suspended by the great vessels, with its broader side (*i.e.*, base) facing upward and its tip (*i.e.*, apex) pointing downward, forward, and to the left. The heart is positioned obliquely, so that the right side of the heart is almost fully in front of the left side of the heart, with only a small portion of the lateral left ventricle on the frontal plane of the heart (Fig. 23-7). When the hand is placed on the thorax, the main impact of the heart's contraction is felt against the chest wall at a point between the fifth and sixth ribs, a little below the nipple and approximately 3 inches to the left of the midline. This is called the *point of maximum impulse*.

The wall of the heart is composed of an outer epicardium, which lines the pericardial cavity; the myocardium or muscle layer; and the smooth endocardium, which lines the chambers of the heart. A fibrous skeleton supports the valvular structures of the heart. The interatrial and interventricular septa divide the heart into a right and a left pump, each composed of two muscular chambers: a thin-walled atrium, which serves as a reservoir for blood coming into the heart, and a thick-walled ventricle, which pumps blood out of the heart. The increased thickness of the left ventricular wall results from the additional work this ventricle is required to perform.

THE HEART

- The heart is a four-chambered pump consisting of two atria (the right atrium, which receives blood returning to the heart from the systemic circulation, and the left atrium, which receives oxygenated blood from the lungs) and two ventricles (a right ventricle, which pumps blood to the lungs, and a left ventricle, which pumps blood into the systemic circulation).
- Heart valves control the direction of blood flow from the atria to the ventricles (the atrioventricular valves), from the right side of the heart to the lungs (pulmonic valve), and from the left side of the heart to the systemic circulation (aortic valve).
- The myocardium, or muscle layer of the atria and ventricles, produces the pumping action of the heart. Intercalated disks between cardiac muscle cells contain gap junctions that allow for immediate communication of electrical signals from one cell to another so the cardiac muscle acts as a single unit, or syncytium.
- The cardiac cycle is divided into two major periods: systole, when the ventricles are contracting, and diastole, when the ventricles are relaxed and filling.
- The cardiac output or amount of blood that the heart pumps each minute is determined by the amount of blood pumped with each beat (stroke volume) and the number of times the heart beats each minute (heart rate). Cardiac reserve refers to the maximum percentage of increase in cardiac output that can be achieved above the normal resting level.
- The work of the heart is determined by the volume of blood it pumps out (preload) and the pressure that it must generate to pump the blood out of the heart (afterload).

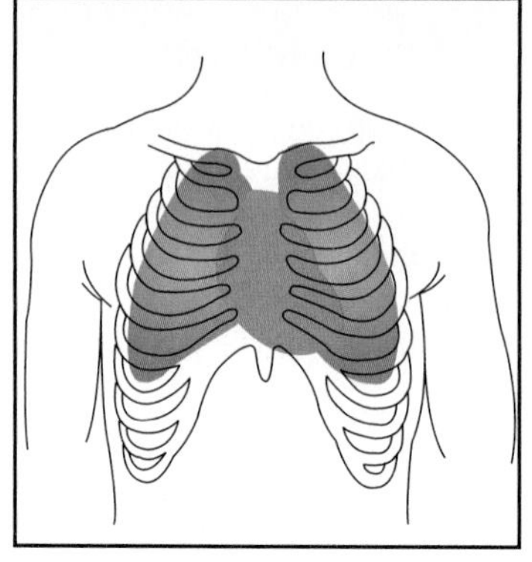

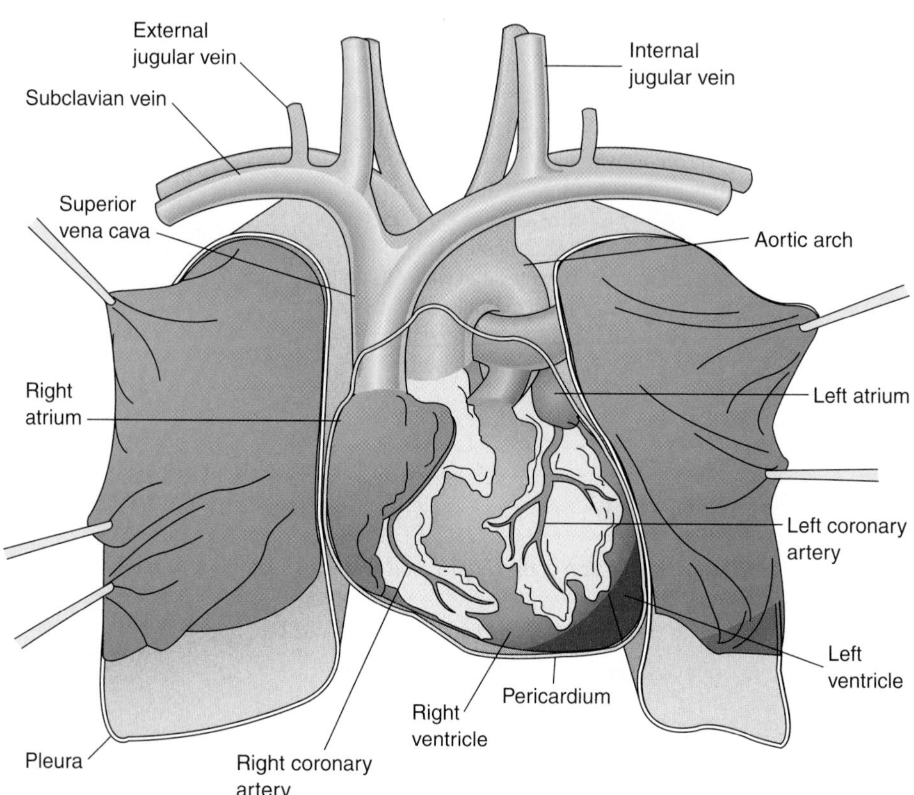

FIGURE 23-7 Anterior view of the heart and great vessels and their relationship to lungs and skeletal structures of the chest cage (*upper left box*).

Pericardium

The pericardium forms a fibrous covering around the heart, holding it in a fixed position in the thorax and providing physical protection and a barrier to infection. The pericardium consists of a tough outer fibrous layer and a thin inner serous layer. The outer fibrous layer is attached to the great vessels that enter and leave the heart, the sternum, and the diaphragm. The fibrous pericardium is highly resistant to distention; it prevents acute dilation of the heart chambers and exerts a restraining effect on the left ventricle. The inner serous layer consists of a visceral layer and a parietal layer. The visceral layer, also known as the *epicardium,* covers the entire heart and great vessels and then folds over to form the parietal layer that lines the fibrous pericardium (Fig. 23-8). Between the visceral and parietal layers is the *pericardial cavity,* a potential space that contains 30 to 50 mL of serous fluid. This fluid acts as a lubricant to minimize friction as the heart contracts and relaxes.

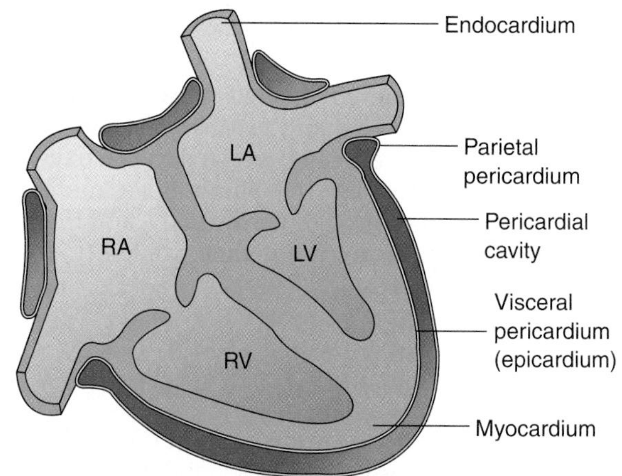

FIGURE 23-8 Layers of the heart, showing the visceral pericardium, the pericardial cavity, and the parietal pericardium. RA, right atrium; LA, left atrium; RV, right ventricle; LV, left ventricle.

Myocardium

The myocardium, or muscular portion of the heart, forms the wall of the atria and ventricles. Cardiac muscle cells, like skeletal muscle, are striated and composed of *sarcomeres* that contain actin and myosin filaments (see Chapter 4, Fig. 4-24). They are smaller and more compact than skeletal muscle cells and contain many large mitochondria, reflecting their continuous energy needs. The extracellular matrix of cardiac muscle is filled with a loose connective tissue, called the *endomysium,* containing numerous capillaries that support the function of the contracting muscle cells.

Cardiac muscle contracts much like skeletal muscle, except the contractions are involuntary, and the duration of contraction is much longer (see Chapter 4). Unlike the orderly longitudinal arrangement of skeletal muscle fibers, cardiac muscle cells are arranged as an interconnecting latticework, with their fibers dividing, recombining, and then dividing again (Fig. 23-9A). The fibers are separated from neighboring cardiac muscle cells by dense structures called *intercalated disks.* The intercalated disks, which are unique to cardiac muscle, contain gap junctions consisting of intramembrane proteins surrounding a core channel that serves as a low-resistance pathway for the passage of ions and electrical impulses from one cardiac cell to another (see Fig. 23-9B). The myocardium therefore behaves as a single unit, or *syncytium,* rather than as a group of isolated units, as does skeletal muscle. When one myocardial cell becomes excited, the impulse travels rapidly so that the heart can beat as a unit.

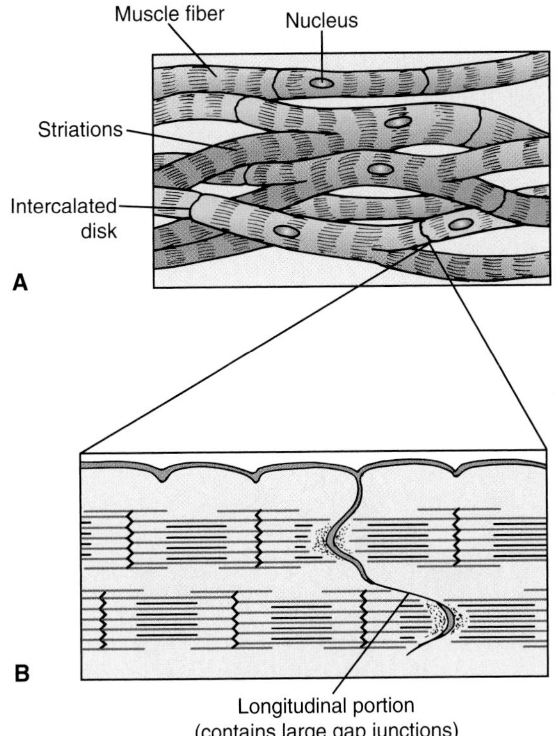

FIGURE 23-9 **(A)** Cardiac muscle fibers showing the branching structure. **(B)** Area indicated where cell junctions lie in the intercalated disks.

As in skeletal muscle, cardiac muscle contraction involves actin and myosin filaments, which interact and slide along one another during muscle contraction. However, compared with skeletal muscle cells, cardiac muscle cells have less well-defined sarcoplasmic reticulum for storing calcium, and the distance from the cell membrane to the myofibrils is shorter. Because less calcium can be stored in the muscle cells, cardiac muscle relies more heavily than skeletal muscle on an influx of extracellular calcium ions for contraction. Extracellular calcium, which enters through channels in the cell membrane and T tubules of the muscle cell, triggers the release of intracellular calcium from the sarcoplasmic reticulum, and it participates in muscle contraction. Muscle relaxation results from cessation of calcium release, its removal from the actin-myosin sites, and its energy-dependent reuptake from the cytoplasm into the sarcoplasmic reticulum and other storage sites. The cardiac drug, digoxin, increases cardiac contractility through an increase in intracellular calcium concentration.

Endocardium

The endocardium is a thin, three-layered membrane that lines the heart. The innermost layer consists of smooth endothelial cells supported by a thin layer of connective tissue. The endothelial lining of the endocardium is continuous with the lining of the blood vessels that enter and leave the heart. The middle layer consists of dense connective tissue with elastic fibers. The outer layer, composed of irregularly arranged connective tissue cells, contains blood vessels and branches of the conduction system and is continuous with the myocardium.

Heart Valves and Fibrous Skeleton

An important structural feature of the heart is its fibrous skeleton, which consists of four interconnecting valve rings and surrounding connective tissue. It separates the atria and ventricles and forms a rigid support for attachment of the valves and insertion of the cardiac muscle (Fig. 23-10). The tops of the valve rings are attached to the muscle tissue of the atria, pulmonary trunks, aorta, and valve rings. The bottoms are attached to the ventricular walls.

There are four heart valves: two atrioventricular (*i.e.,* tricuspid and mitral) valves and two semilunar (*i.e.,* pulmonic and aortic) valves (Fig. 23-11). For the heart to function effectively, blood must move through the valves that separate its chambers in a *orthograde,* or forward, direction (Fig. 23-12).

The atrioventricular (AV) valves control the flow of blood between the atria and the ventricles. The thin edges of the AV valves form cusps, two on the left side of the heart (*i.e., bicuspid valve*) and three on the right side (*i.e., tricuspid valve*). The bicuspid valve is also known as the *mitral* valve. The AV valves are supported by the papillary muscles, which project from the wall of the ventricles, and the *chordae tendineae,* which attach to the valve (Fig 23-13). Contraction of the papillary muscles at the onset of systole

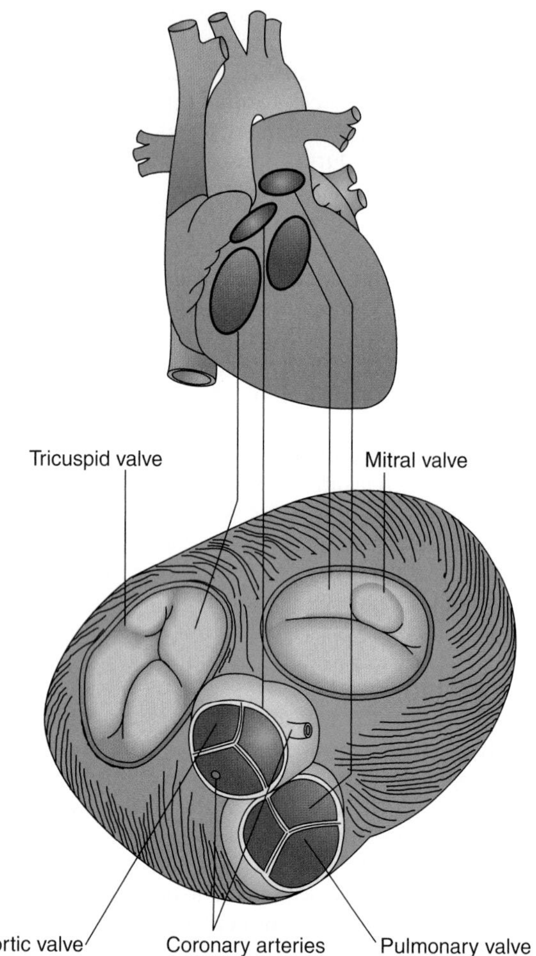

FIGURE 23-10 Fibrous skeleton of the heart, which forms the four interconnecting valve rings and support for attachment of the valves and insertion of cardiac muscle.

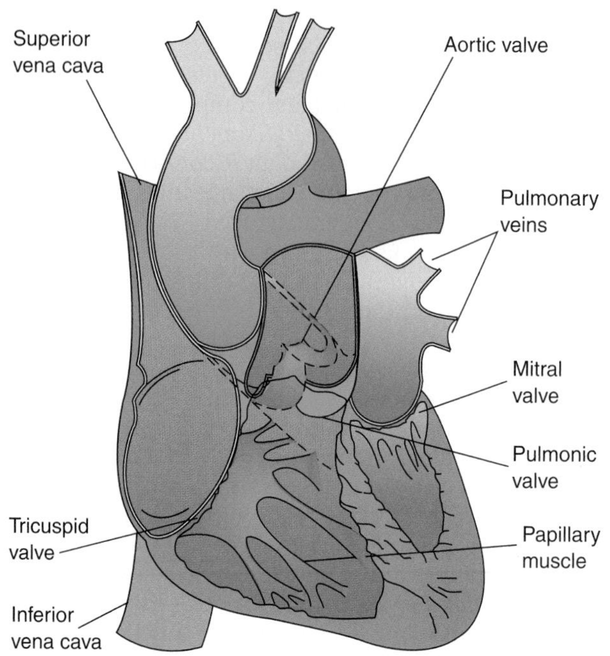

FIGURE 23-11 Valvular structures of the heart. The atrioventricular valves are in an open position, and the semilunar valves are closed. There are no valves to control the flow of blood at the inflow channels (*i.e.,* vena cava and pulmonary veins) to the heart.

ensures closure by producing tension on the leaflets of the AV valves before the full force of ventricular contraction pushes against them. The chordae tendineae are cordlike structures that support the AV valves and prevent them from everting into the atria during systole.

The *semilunar* valves control the movement of blood out of the ventricles. The *aortic* valve controls the flow of blood into the aorta; the *pulmonic* valve controls blood flow into the pulmonary artery. The aortic and pulmonic valves often are referred to as the semilunar valves because their flaps are shaped like half-moons. The pulmonic and the aortic valve have three small, teacup-shaped leaflets (Fig. 23-14B). These cuplike structures collect the *retrograde,* or backward, flow of blood that occurs toward the end of systole, enhancing closure. For the development of a perfect seal along the free edges of the semilunar valves, each valve cusp must have a triangular shape, which is facilitated by a nodular thickening at the apex of each leaflet (see Fig. 23-14A). The openings for the coronary arteries are located in the aorta just above the aortic valve.

There are no valves at the atrial sites (*i.e.,* venae cavae and pulmonary veins) where blood enters the heart. This means that excess blood is pushed back into the veins when the atria become distended. For example, the jugular veins typically become prominent in severe right-sided heart failure when they normally should be flat or collapsed. Likewise, the pulmonary venous system becomes congested when outflow from the left atrium is impeded.

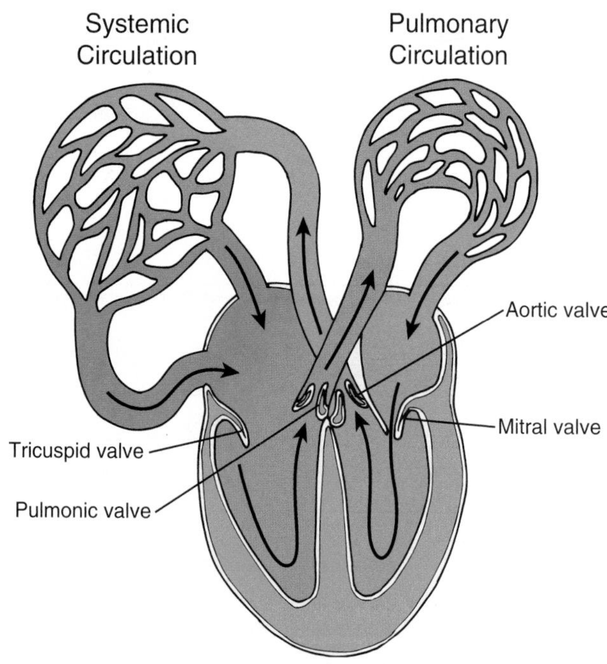

FIGURE 23-12 Unidirectional flow of blood through the heart valves.

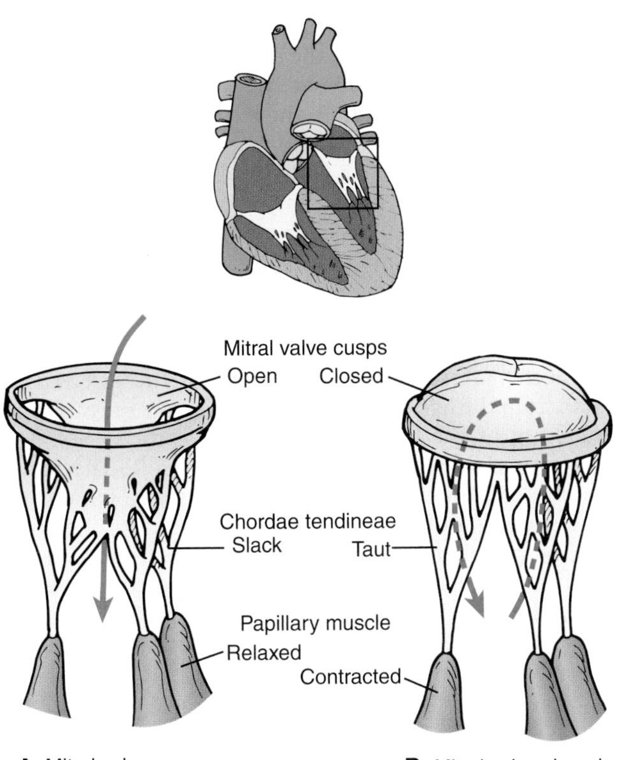

FIGURE 23-13 The mitral AV valve showing the papillary muscles and chordae tendineae. (**A**) The open mitral valve with relaxed papillary muscles and slack chordae tendineae. (**B**) The closed mitral valve with contracted papillary muscles and taut chordae tendineae that prevent the valve cusps from everting into the atria.

CARDIAC CYCLE

The term *cardiac cycle* is used to describe the rhythmic pumping action of the heart. The cardiac cycle is divided into two parts: *systole,* the period during which the ventricles are contracting, and *diastole,* the period during which the ventricles are relaxed and filling with blood. Simultaneous changes occur in left atrial pressure, left ventricular pressure, aortic pressure, ventricular volume, the electrocardiogram (ECG), and heart sounds during the cardiac cycle (Fig. 23-15).

The electrical activity, recorded on the ECG, precedes the mechanical events of the cardiac cycle. The small, rounded P wave of the ECG represents depolarization of the sinoatrial node (*i.e.,* pacemaker of the heart), the atrial conduction tissue, and the atrial muscle mass. The QRS complex registers the depolarization of the ventricular conduction system and the ventricular muscle mass. The T wave on the ECG occurs during the last half of systole and represents repolarization of the ventricles. The cardiac conduction system and the ECG are discussed in detail in Chapter 27.

Ventricular Systole and Diastole

Ventricular systole is divided into two periods: the isovolumetric contraction period and the ejection period. The *isovolumetric contraction period,* which begins with the closure of the AV valves and occurrence of the first heart sound, heralds the onset of systole. Immediately after closure of the AV valves, there is an additional 0.02 to 0.03 second during which the semilunar outlet (pulmonic and aortic) valves remain closed. During this period (see Fig. 23-15), the ventricular pressures rise abruptly because all of the valves are closed and no blood is leaving the heart. The ventricles continue to contract until left ventricular pressure is slightly higher than aortic pressure, and right ventricular pressure is higher than pulmonary artery pressure. At this point, the semilunar valves open, signaling the onset of the *ejection period.* Approximately 60% of the stroke volume is ejected during the first quarter of systole, and the remaining 40% is ejected during the next two quarters of systole. Little blood is ejected from the heart during the last quarter of systole, although the ventricle remains contracted.

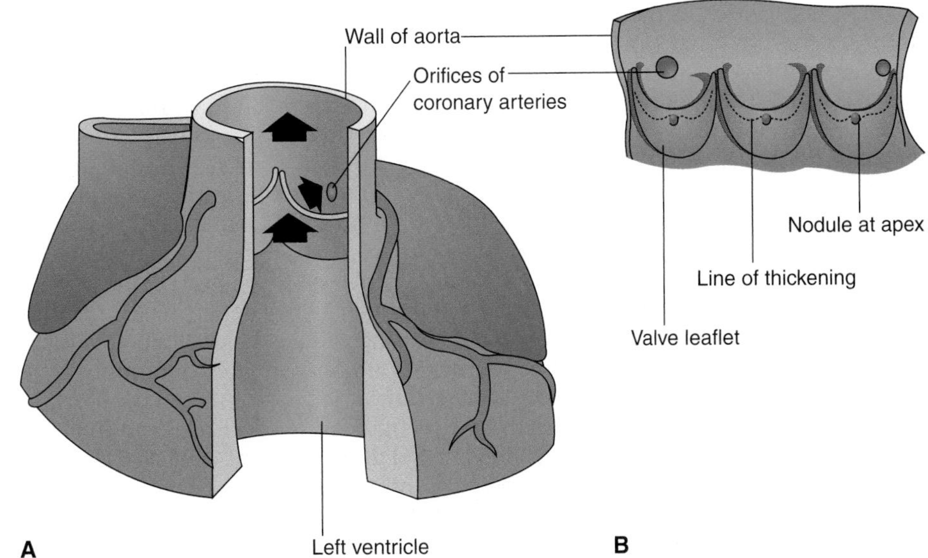

FIGURE 23-14 Diagram of the aortic valve. (**A**) The position of the aorta at the base of the ascending aorta is indicated. (**B**) The appearance of the three leaflets of the aortic valve when the aorta is cut open and spread out, flat. (Cormack D. H. [1987]. *Ham's histology* [9th ed.]. Philadelphia: J. B. Lippincott)

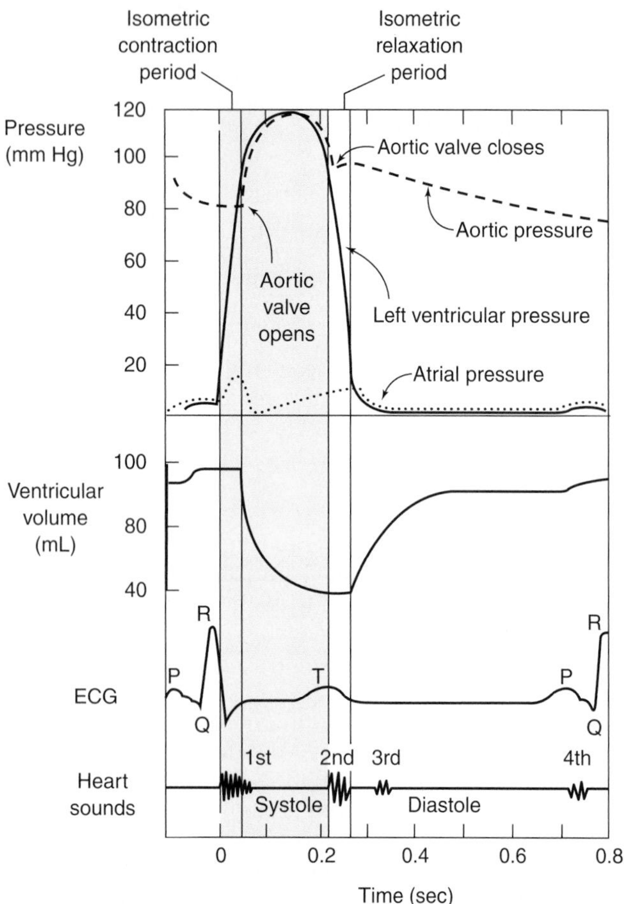

FIGURE 23-15 The cardiac cycle. Changes in aortic pressure, left ventricular pressure, left atrial pressure, left ventricular volume, the electrocardiogram (ECG), and heart sounds.

At the end of systole, the ventricles relax, causing a precipitous fall in intraventricular pressures. As this occurs, blood from the large arteries flows back toward the ventricles, causing the aortic and pulmonic valves to snap shut—an event that is marked by the second heart sound. After closure of the semilunar valves, the ventricles continue to relax for another 0.03 to 0.06 second (the *isovolumetric relaxation period*). During this time, both the semilunar and AV valves are closed, and the ventricular volume remains the same, as the ventricular pressure drops (see Fig 23-15).

Ventricular diastole is marked by ventricular filling. When ventricular pressure becomes less than atrial pressure, the AV valves open, and blood that has been accumulating in the atria during systole flows into the ventricles. Most of ventricular filling occurs during the first third of diastole, which is called the *rapid filling period.* During the middle third of diastole, inflow into the ventricles is almost at a standstill. The last third of diastole is marked by atrial contraction, which gives an additional thrust to ventricular filling. When audible, the third heart sound is heard during the rapid filling period of diastole as blood flows into a distended or noncompliant ventricle. A fourth heart sound occurs during the last third of diastole as the atria contract.

During diastole, the ventricles increase their volume to approximately 120 mL (*i.e.,* the *end-diastolic volume*), and at the end of systole, approximately 50 mL of blood (*i.e.,* the *end-systolic volume*) remains in the ventricles (see Fig. 23-15). The difference between the end-diastolic and end-systolic volumes (approximately 70 mL) is called the *stroke volume.* The *ejection fraction,* which is the stroke volume divided by the end-diastolic volume, represents the fraction or percentage of the diastolic volume that is ejected from the heart during systole.

Aortic Pressure

The aortic pressure reflects changes in the ejection of blood from the left ventricle. There is a rise in pressure and stretching of the elastic fibers in the aorta as blood is ejected into the aorta at the onset of systole. The aortic pressure continues to rise and then begins to fall during the last quarter of systole as blood flows out of the aorta into the peripheral vessels. The *incisura,* or notch, in the aortic pressure tracing represents closure of the aortic valve. The aorta is highly elastic and as such stretches during systole to accommodate the blood that is being ejected from the left heart during systole. During diastole, the recoil of the elastic fibers in the aorta serves to maintain the aortic pressure.

Atrial Filling and Contraction

Atrial contraction occurs during the last third of diastole. There are three main atrial pressure waves that occur during the cardiac cycle. The *a* wave is caused by atrial contraction. The *c* wave occurs as the ventricles begin to contract, and their increased pressure causes the AV valves to bulge into the atria. The *v* wave results from a slow buildup of blood in the atria toward the end of systole when the AV valves are still closed. The right atrial pressure waves are transmitted to the internal jugular veins as pulsations. These pulsations can be observed visually and may be used to assess cardiac function. For example, exaggerated *a* waves occur when the volume of the right atrium is increased because of impaired emptying into the right ventricle.

Because there are no valves between the junctions of the central veins (*i.e.,* venae cavae and pulmonary veins) and the atria, atrial filling occurs during both systole and diastole. During normal quiet breathing, right atrial pressure usually varies between −2 and +2 mm Hg. It is this low atrial pressure that maintains the movement of blood from the systemic circulation into the right atrium and from the pulmonary veins into the left atrium. Right atrial pressure is regulated by a balance between the ability of the heart to move blood out of the right heart and through the left heart into the systemic circulation and the tendency of blood to flow from the peripheral circulation into the right atrium.

When the heart pumps strongly, right atrial pressure is decreased and atrial filling is enhanced. Right atrial pressure is also affected by changes in intrathoracic pressure. It is decreased during inspiration when intrathoracic pressure becomes more negative, and it is increased during coughing or forced expiration when intrathoracic pressure becomes more positive. Venous return is a reflection of the amount of blood in the systemic circulation that is available for return to the right heart and the force that moves blood back to the right side of the heart. Venous return is increased when the blood volume is expanded or when right atrial pressure falls, and it is decreased in hypovolemic shock or when right atrial pressure rises.

Although the main function of the atria is to store blood as it enters the heart, these chambers also act as pumps that aid in ventricular filling. This function becomes more important during periods of increased activity when the diastolic filling time is decreased because of an increase in heart rate or when heart disease impairs ventricular filling. In these two situations, the cardiac output would fall drastically were it not for the action of the atria. It has been estimated that atrial contraction can contribute as much as 30% to cardiac reserve during periods of increased need, while having little or no effect on cardiac output during rest.

REGULATION OF CARDIAC PERFORMANCE

The efficiency of the heart as a pump often is measured in terms of *cardiac output* or the amount of blood the heart pumps each minute. The cardiac output (CO) is the product of the *stroke volume* (SV) and the *heart rate* (HR) and can be expressed by the equation: CO = SV × HR. The cardiac output varies with body size and the metabolic needs of the tissues. It increases with physical activity and decreases during rest and sleep. The average cardiac output in normal adults ranges from 3.5 to 8.0 L/min. In the highly trained athlete, this value can increase to levels as high as 32 L/min during maximum exercise.

The *cardiac reserve* refers to the maximum percentage of increase in cardiac output that can be achieved above the normal resting level. The normal young adult has a cardiac reserve of approximately 300% to 400%. The heart's ability to increase its output according to body needs mainly depends on four factors: the *preload,* or ventricular filling; the *afterload,* or resistance to ejection of blood from the heart; *cardiac contractility;* and the *heart rate.* Cardiac performance is influenced by the work demands of the heart and the ability of the coronary circulation to meet its metabolic needs.

Preload

The preload represents the volume work of the heart. It is called the *preload* because it is the work imposed on the heart before the contraction begins. Preload represents the amount of blood that the heart must pump with each beat and is largely determined by the venous return to the heart and the accompanying stretch of the muscle fibers.

The anatomic arrangement of the actin and myosin filaments in the myocardial muscle fibers is such that the tension or force of contraction is greatest when the muscle fibers are stretched just before the heart begins to contract. The maximum force of contraction and cardiac output is achieved when venous return produces an increase in left ventricular end-diastolic filling (*i.e.,* preload) such that the muscle fibers are stretched approximately two and one-half times their normal resting length (Fig. 23-16). When the muscle fibers are stretched to this degree, there is optimal overlap of the actin and myosin filaments and number of *cross-bridge attachments* needed for maximal contraction.

The increased force of contraction that accompanies an increase in ventricular end-diastolic volume is referred to as the *Frank-Starling mechanism* or Starling's law of the heart. The Frank-Starling mechanism allows the heart to adjust its pumping ability to accommodate various levels of venous return. Cardiac output is less when decreased filling causes excessive overlap of the actin and myosin filaments or when the filaments are pulled too far apart because of excessive filling (see Fig. 25-16).

Afterload

The afterload is the pressure or tension work of the heart. It is the pressure that the heart must generate to move blood into the aorta. It is called the *afterload* because it is the work presented to the heart after the contraction has commenced. The systemic arterial blood pressure is the main source of afterload work for the left heart, and the pulmonary arterial pressure is the main source of afterload

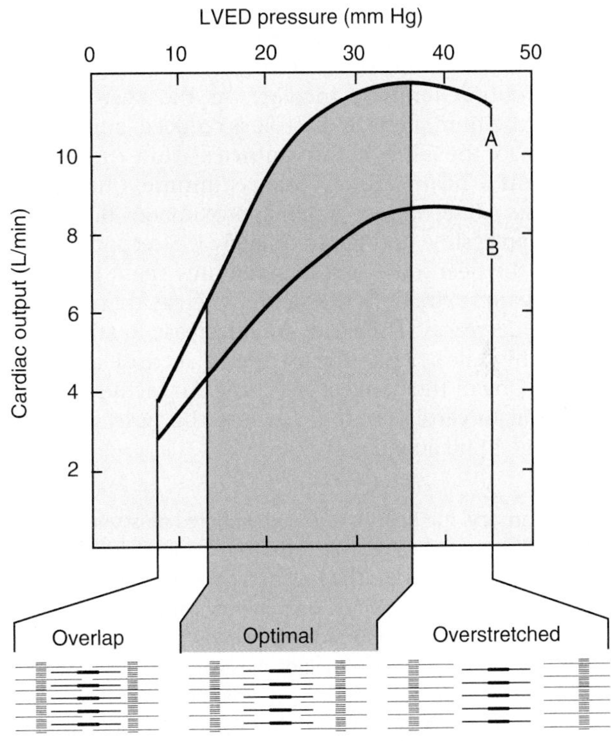

FIGURE 23-16 **(Top)** Starling ventricular function curve in normal heart. An increase in left ventricular end-diastolic (LVED) pressure produces an increase in cardiac output (*curve B*) by means of the Frank-Starling mechanism. The maximum force of contraction and increased stroke volume are achieved when diastolic filling causes the muscle fibers to be stretched about two and one half times their resting length. In *curve A,* an increase in cardiac contractility produces an increase in cardiac output without a change in LVED volume and pressure. **(Bottom)** Stretching of the actin and myosin filaments at the different LVED filling pressures.

work for the right heart. The afterload work of the left ventricle is increased with narrowing (*i.e.,* stenosis) of the aortic valve. For example, in the late stages of aortic stenosis, the left ventricle may need to generate systolic pressures up to 300 mm Hg to move blood through the diseased valve.

Cardiac Contractility

Cardiac contractility refers to the ability of the heart to change its force of contraction without changing its resting (*i.e.,* diastolic) length. The contractile state of the myocardial muscle is determined by biochemical and biophysical properties that govern the actin and myosin interactions in the myocardial cells. It is strongly influenced by the number of calcium ions that are available to participate in the contractile process.

An *inotropic* influence is one that modifies the contractile state of the myocardium independent of the Frank-Starling mechanism (see Fig. 23-16, top curve). For instance, sympathetic stimulation produces a positive inotropic effect by increasing the calcium that is available for interaction between the actin and myosin filaments. Hypoxia exerts a negative inotropic effect by interfering with the generation of adenosine triphosphate (ATP), which is needed for muscle contraction.

Heart Rate

The heart rate determines the frequency with which blood is ejected from the heart. Therefore, as heart rate increases, cardiac output tends to increase. As the heart rate increases, the time spent in diastole is reduced, and there is less time for the filling of the ventricles before the onset of systole. At a heart rate of 75 beats/minute, one cardiac cycle lasts 0.8 second, of which approximately 0.3 second is spent in systole and approximately 0.5 second in diastole. As the heart rate increases, the time spent in systole remains approximately the same, whereas that spent in diastole decreases. This leads to a decrease in stroke volume; at high heart rates, it may cause a decrease in cardiac output. One of the dangers of ventricular tachycardia is a reduction in cardiac output because the heart does not have time to fill adequately.

In summary, the heart is a four-chambered muscular pump that lies in the pericardial sac within the mediastinal space of the intrathoracic cavity. The wall of the heart is composed of an outer epicardium, which lines the pericardial cavity; a fibrous skeleton; the myocardium, or muscle layer; and the smooth endocardium, which lines the chambers of the heart. The four heart valves control the direction of blood flow.

The cardiac cycle describes the pumping action of the heart. It is divided into two parts: systole, during which the ventricles contract and blood is ejected from the heart, and diastole, during which the ventricles are relaxed and blood is filling the heart. The stroke volume (approximately 70 mL) represents the difference between the end-diastolic volume (approximately 120 mL) and the end-systolic volume (approximately 50 mL). The electrical activity of the heart, as represented on the ECG, precedes the mechanical events of the cardiac cycle. The heart sounds signal the closing of the heart valves during the cardiac cycle. Atrial contraction occurs during the last third of diastole. Although the main function of the atria is to store blood as it enters the heart, atrial contraction acts to increase cardiac output during periods of increased activity when the filling time is reduced or in disease conditions in which ventricular filling is impaired.

The heart's ability to increase its output according to body needs depends on the preload, or filling of the ventricles (*i.e.,* end-diastolic volume); the afterload, or resistance to ejection of blood from the heart; cardiac contractility, which is determined by the interaction of the actin and myosin filaments of cardiac muscle fibers; and the heart rate, which determines the frequency with which blood is ejected from the heart. The maximum force of cardiac contraction occurs when an increase in preload stretches muscle fibers of the heart to approximately two and one-half times their resting length (*i.e.,* Frank-Starling mechanism).

Blood Vessels and the Systemic Circulation

After you have completed this section of the chapter, you should be able to meet the following objectives:

- ✦ Compare the structure and function of arteries, arterioles, veins, and capillaries
- ✦ Describe the structure and function of vascular smooth muscle
- ✦ Use the equation, blood pressure = cardiac output × peripheral vascular resistance, to explain the regulation of arterial blood pressure
- ✦ Describe mechanisms involved in short-term and long-term regulation of blood pressure
- ✦ Define autoregulation and characterize mechanisms responsible for short-term and long-term regulation of blood flow

The vascular system functions in the delivery of oxygen and nutrients and removal of wastes from the tissues. It consists of arteries and arterioles, the capillaries, and the venules and veins. Although blood vessels are often compared with a system of plumbing pipes, this analogy serves as only a starting point. Blood vessels are dynamic structures that constrict and relax to adjust blood pressure and flow to meet the varying needs of the many different tissue types and organ systems. Structures such as the heart, brain, liver, and kidneys require a large and continuous flow to carry out their vital functions. In other tissues such as the skin and skeletal muscle, the need for blood flow varies with the level of function. For example, there is a need for increased blood flow to the skin during fever and for increased skeletal muscle blood flow during exercise.

BLOOD VESSELS

All blood vessels, except the capillaries, have walls composed of three layers, or coats, called *tunicae* (Fig. 23-17). The *tunica externa,* or *tunica adventitia,* is the outermost cov-

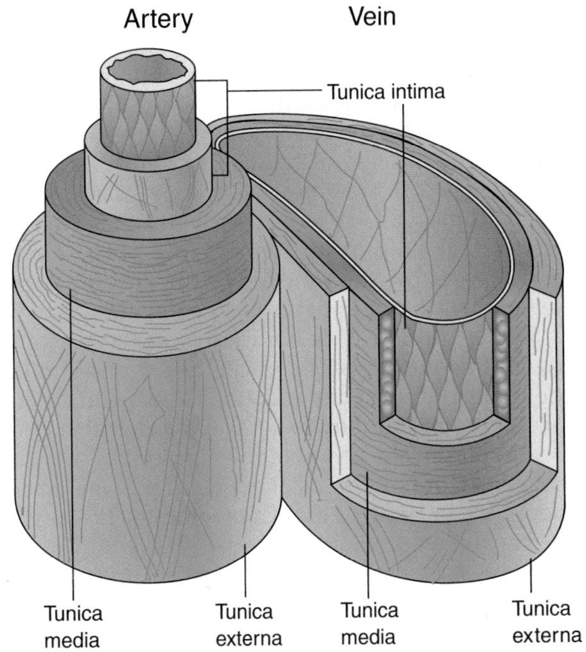

FIGURE 23-17 Medium-sized artery and vein, showing the relative thickness of the three layers.

ering of the vessel. This layer is composed of fibrous and connective tissues that support the vessel. The *tunica media,* or middle layer, is largely a smooth muscle layer that constricts to regulate and control the diameter of the vessel. The *tunica intima,* or inner layer, has an elastic layer that joins the media and a thin layer of endothelial cells that lie adjacent to the blood. The endothelial layer provides a smooth and slippery inner surface for the vessel. This smooth inner lining, as long as it remains intact, prevents platelet adherence and blood clotting. The layers of the different types of blood vessels vary with vessel function. The walls of the arterioles, which control blood pressure, have large amounts of smooth muscle. Veins are thin-walled, distensible, and collapsible vessels. Capillaries are single-cell–thick vessels designed for the exchange of gases, nutrients, and waste materials.

Vascular Smooth Muscle

Smooth muscle contracts slowly and generates high forces for long periods with low energy requirements; it uses only 1/10 to 1/300 the energy of skeletal muscle. These characteristics are important in structures, such as blood vessels, that must maintain their tone day in and day out.

Compared with skeletal and cardiac muscle, smooth muscle has less well-developed sarcoplasmic reticulum for storing intracellular calcium, and it has very few fast sodium channels. Depolarization of smooth muscle instead relies largely on extracellular calcium, which enters through calcium channels in the muscle membrane. Sympathetic nervous system control of vascular smooth muscle tone occurs by way of receptor-activated opening and closing of the calcium channels. In general, α-adrenergic receptors are excitatory in that they cause the channels to open and produce vasoconstriction; and β-adrenergic receptors are inhibitory in that they cause the channels to close and produce vasodilation. Calcium channel blocking drugs cause vasodilation by blocking calcium entry through the calcium channels.

Smooth muscle contraction and relaxation also occur in response to local tissue factors such as lack of oxygen, increased hydrogen ion concentrations, and excess carbon dioxide. Nitric oxide, formerly known as the *endothelial relaxing factor,* acts locally to produce smooth muscle relaxation and regulate blood flow. These factors are discussed more fully in the section on local control of blood flow.

ARTERIAL SYSTEM

The arterial system consists of the large and medium-sized arteries and the arterioles. Arteries are thick-walled vessels with large amounts of elastic fibers. The elasticity of these vessels allows them to stretch during cardiac systole, when the heart contracts and blood enters the circulation, and to recoil during diastole, when the heart relaxes. The arterioles, which are predominantly smooth muscle, serve as resistance vessels for the circulatory system. They act as

THE VASCULAR SYSTEM AND CONTROL OF BLOOD FLOW

- The vascular system, which consists of the arterial system, the venous system, and the capillaries, functions in the delivery of oxygen and nutrients and in the removal of wastes from the tissues.
- The arterial system is a high-pressure system that delivers blood to the tissues. It relies on the intermittent ejection of blood from the left ventricle and the generation of arterial pressure pulsations or waves that move blood toward the capillaries where the exchange of gases, nutrients, and wastes occur.
- The venous system is a low-pressure system that collects blood from the capillaries. It relies on the presence of valves in the veins of the extremities to prevent retrograde flow and on the milking action of the skeletal muscles that surround the veins to return blood to the right heart.
- Local control of blood flow is regulated by local mechanisms that match blood flow to the metabolic needs of the tissue. Over the short term, the tissues autoregulate flow through the synthesis of vasodilators and vasoconstrictors derived from the tissue, smooth muscle, or endothelial cells; over the long term, blood flow is regulated by creation of a collateral circulation.
- Neural control of circulatory function occurs through the sympathetic and parasympathetic divisions of the autonomic nervous system. Sympathetic stimulation increases heart rate, cardiac contractility, and vessel tone (vascular resistance), whereas parasympathetic stimulation decreases heart rate.

control valves through which blood is released as it moves into the capillaries. Changes in the activity of sympathetic fibers that innervate these vessels cause them to constrict or to relax as needed to maintain blood pressure.

Arterial Pressure Pulse

The arterial blood pressure, often referred to simply as the *blood pressure,* results from the intermittent ejection of blood from the left ventricle into the aorta at the onset of systole. It rises during systole as the left ventricle contracts and falls as the heart relaxes during diastole. This creates an *impulse* or *pressure wave* that is transmitted from molecule to molecule along the length of the vessel (Fig. 23-18). In the aorta, this pressure wave is transmitted at a velocity of 4 to 6 m/second, which is approximately 20 times faster than the flow of blood. These pressure waves are similar to those created by splashing water in a basin or tub. When taking a pulse, it is the pressure pulses that are felt, and it is the pressure pulses that produce the Korotkoff sounds heard during blood pressure measurement. The tip or maximum deflection of the pressure pulse coincides with the systolic blood pressure, and the minimum point of deflection coincides with the diastolic pressure.

As the pressure wave moves out through the aorta into the arteries, it changes as it collides with reflected waves from the periphery. Just as the waves created by splashing water in a tub increase in amplitude as they hit the edge of the tub and reverse their direction of movement, the pressure pulse increases as it moves to the peripheral arteries. This is why the systolic pressure is higher in the medium-sized arteries than in the aorta even though the diastolic pressure is lower. With peripheral arterial disease, there is a delay in the transmission of the reflected wave so that the pulse decreases rather than increases in amplitude.

After its initial amplification, the pressure pulse becomes smaller and smaller as it moves through the smaller arteries and arterioles, until it disappears almost entirely in the capillaries. This damping of the pressure pulse is caused by the resistance and distensibility characteristics of these vessels. The increased resistance of these small vessels impedes the transmission of the pressure waves; however, their distensibility is great enough so that any small change in flow does not cause a pressure change. Although the pressure pulses usually are not transmitted to the capillaries, there are situations in which this does occur. For example, injury to a finger or other area of the body often results in a throbbing sensation. In this case, extreme dilatation of the small vessels in the injured area produces a reduction in the dampening of the pressure pulse. Capillary pulsations also occur in conditions that cause exaggeration of aortic pressure pulses, such as aortic regurgitation or patent ductus arteriosus (see Chapter 26).

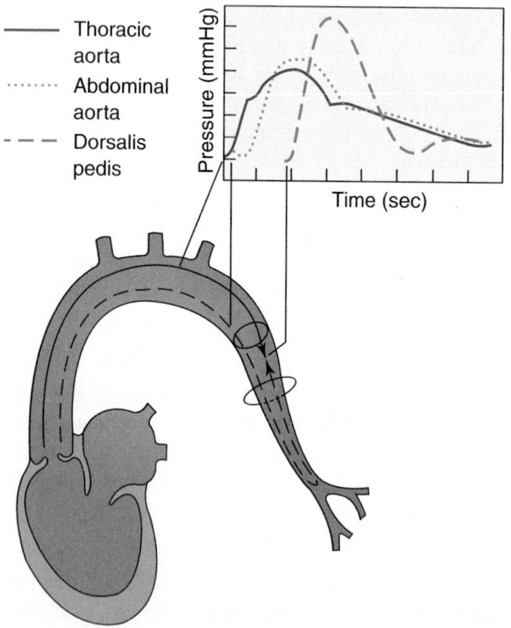

FIGURE 23-18 Amplification of the arterial pressure wave as it moves forward in the peripheral arteries. This amplification occurs as a forward-moving pressure wave merges with a backward-moving reflected pressure wave. **(Inset)** The amplitude of the pressure pulse increases in the thoracic aorta, abdominal aorta, and dorsalis pedis.

VENOUS SYSTEM

The veins and venules are thin-walled, distensible, and collapsible vessels. The venules collect blood from the capillaries, and the veins transport blood back to the heart. The veins are capable of enlarging and storing large quantities of blood, which can be made available to the circulation as needed. Even though the veins are thin walled, they are muscular. This allows them to contract or expand to accommodate varying amounts of blood. Veins are innervated by the sympathetic nervous system. When blood is lost from the circulation, the veins constrict as a means of maintaining intravascular volume.

The venous system is a low-pressure system, and when a person is in the upright position, blood flow in the venous system must oppose the effects of gravity. Valves in the veins of extremities prevent retrograde flow (Fig. 23-19),

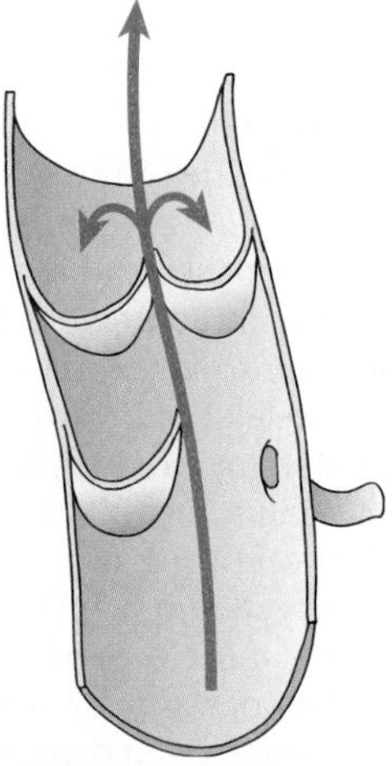

FIGURE 23-19 Portion of a femoral vein opened, to show the valves. The direction of flow is upward.

and with the help of skeletal muscles that surround and intermittently compress the veins in a milking manner, blood is moved forward to the heart. Their pressure ranges from approximately 10 mm Hg at the end of the venules to approximately 0 mm Hg at the entrance of the vena cava into the heart. There are no valves in the abdominal or thoracic veins, and blood flow in these veins is heavily influenced by the pressure in the abdominal and thoracic cavities, respectively.

CAPILLARIES

Capillaries are microscopic, single-cell–thick vessels that connect the arterial and venous segments of the circulation. In each person, there are approximately 10 billion capillaries, with a total surface area of 500 to 700 m^2. The capillary wall is composed of a single layer of endothelial cells surrounded by a basement membrane (Fig. 23-20).

Intracellular junctions join the capillary endothelial cells; these are called the *capillary pores*. Lipid-soluble materials diffuse directly through the capillary cell membrane. Water and water-soluble materials leave and enter the capillary through the capillary pores. The size of the capillary pores varies with capillary function. In the brain, the endothelial cells are joined by tight junctions that form the blood–brain barrier. This prevents substances that would alter neural excitability from leaving the capillary. In organs that process blood contents, such as the liver, capillaries have large pores so that substances can pass easily through the capillary wall. In the kidneys, the glomerular capillaries have small openings called *fenestrations* that pass directly through the middle of the endothelial cells.

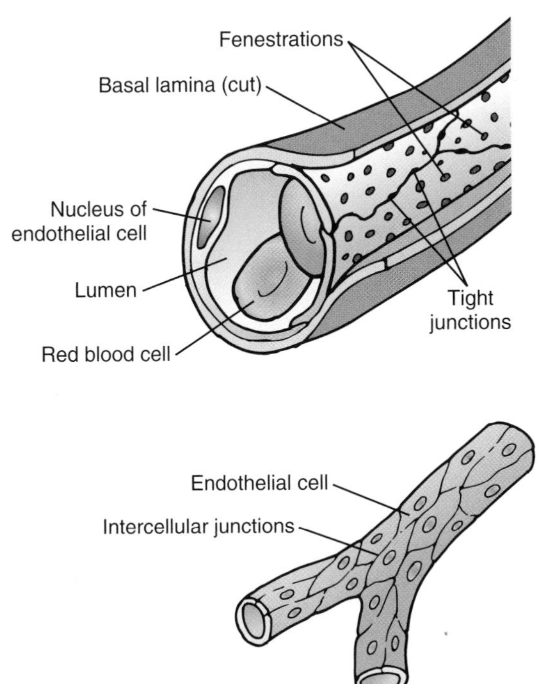

FIGURE 23-20 Endothelial cells and intercellular cement in a section of capillary.

Fenestrated capillary walls are consistent with the filtration function of the glomerulus.

LOCAL CONTROL OF BLOOD FLOW

Tissue blood flow is regulated on a minute-to-minute basis in relation to tissue needs and on a longer-term basis through the development of collateral circulation. Neural mechanisms regulate the cardiac output and blood pressure needed to support these local mechanisms.

Short-Term Autoregulation

Local control of blood flow is governed largely by the nutritional needs of the tissue. For example, blood flow to organs such as the heart, brain, and kidneys remains relatively constant, although blood pressure may vary over a range of 60 to 180 mm Hg (Fig. 23-21). The ability of the tissues to regulate their own blood flow over a wide range of pressures is called *autoregulation*. Autoregulation of blood flow is mediated by changes in blood vessel tone due to changes in flow through the vessel or by local tissue factors, such as lack of oxygen or accumulation of tissue metabolites (*i.e.*, potassium, lactic acid, or adenosine, which is a breakdown product of ATP). Local control is particularly important in tissues such as skeletal muscle, which has blood flow requirements that vary according to the level of activity.

An increase in local blood flow is called *hyperemia*. The ability of tissues to increase blood flow in situations of increased activity, such as exercise, is called *functional hyperemia*. When the blood supply to an area has been occluded and then restored, local blood flow through the tissues increases within seconds to restore the metabolic equilibrium of the tissues. This increased flow is called *reactive hyperemia*. The transient redness seen on an arm after leaning on a hard surface is an example of reactive hyperemia. Local control mechanisms rely on a continuous flow from the

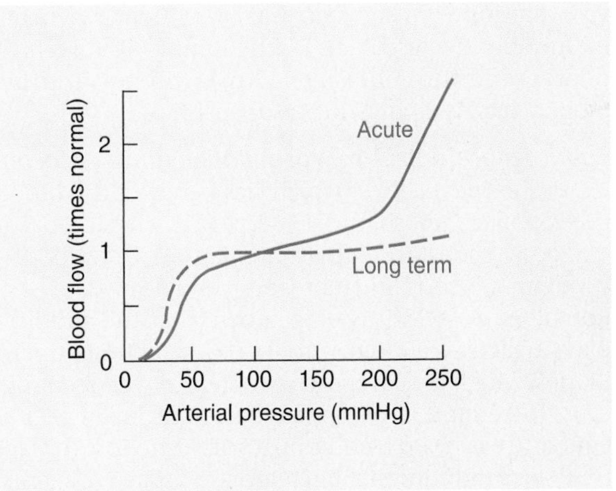

FIGURE 23-21 Effect of increasing arterial pressure on blood flow through a muscle. The *solid curve* shows the effect if pressure is raised over a few minutes. The *dashed curve* shows the effect if the arterial pressure is raised slowly over many weeks. (Guyton A. C., Hall J. E. [1996]. *Textbook of medical physiology* [9th ed., p. 203]. Philadelphia: W. B. Saunders)

main arteries; therefore, hyperemia cannot occur when the arteries that supply the capillary beds are narrowed. For example, if a major coronary artery becomes occluded, the opening of channels supplied by that vessel cannot restore blood flow.

Tissue Factors Contributing to Local Control of Blood Flow. Vasodilator substances, formed in tissues in response to a need for increased blood flow, also aid in the local control of blood flow. The most important of these are histamine, serotonin (*i.e.,* 5-hydroxytryptamine), kinins, and prostaglandins.

Histamine increases blood flow. Most blood vessels contain histamine in mast cells and non–mast cell stores; when these tissues are injured, histamine is released. In certain tissues, such as skeletal muscle, the activity of the mast cells is mediated by the sympathetic nervous system; when sympathetic control is withdrawn, the mast cells release histamine. Vasodilation then results from increased histamine and the withdrawal of vasoconstrictor activity.

Serotonin is liberated from aggregating platelets during the clotting process; it causes vasoconstriction and plays a major role in control of bleeding. Serotonin is found in brain and lung tissues, and there is some speculation that it may be involved in the vascular spasm associated with some allergic pulmonary reactions and migraine headaches.

The *kinins* (*i.e.,* kallidins and bradykinin) are liberated from the globulin kininogen, which is present in body fluids. The kinins cause relaxation of arteriolar smooth muscle, increase capillary permeability, and constrict the venules. In exocrine glands, the formation of kinins contributes to the vasodilation needed for glandular secretion.

Prostaglandins are synthesized from constituents of the cell membrane (*i.e.,* the long-chain fatty acid *arachidonic acid*). Tissue injury incites the release of arachidonic acid from the cell membrane, which initiates prostaglandin synthesis. There are several prostaglandins (*e.g.,* E_2, F_2, I_2), which are subgrouped according to their chemical characteristics; some produce vasoconstriction, and some produce vasodilation. Prostacyclin (PGI_2), which is synthesized mainly by the vascular endothelium, is a powerful vasodilator, and thromboxane (TXA_2), which is synthesized by platelets, is a powerful vasoconstrictor.

Endothelial Control of Vasodilation and Vasoconstriction. The *endothelium,* which lies between the blood and the vascular smooth muscle, serves as a physical barrier for vasoactive substances that circulate in the blood. Once thought to be nothing more than a single layer of cells that line blood vessels, it is now known that the endothelium plays an active role in controlling vascular function. In capillaries, which are composed of a single layer of endothelial cells, the endothelium is active in transporting cell nutrients and wastes. In addition to its function in capillary transport, the endothelium removes vasoactive agents such as norepinephrine from the blood, and it produces enzymes that convert precursor molecules to active products (*e.g.,* angiotensin I to angiotensin II in lung vessels).

One of the important functions of the normal endothelium is to synthesize and release factors that control vessel dilation. Of particular importance was the discovery, first reported in the early 1980s, that the intact endothelium was able to produce a factor that caused relaxation of vascular smooth muscle. This factor was originally named *endothelium-derived relaxing factor* and is now known to be *nitric oxide.* Many other cell types produce nitric oxide. In these tissues, nitric oxide has other functions, including modulation of nerve activity in the nervous system.

The normal endothelium maintains a continuous release of nitric oxide, which is formed from L-arginine through the action of an enzyme called *nitric oxide synthase* (Fig. 23-22). The production of nitric oxide can be stimulated by a variety of endothelial *agonists,* including acetylcholine, bradykinin, histamine, and thrombin. *Shear stress* on the endothelium resulting from an increase in blood flow or blood pressure also stimulates nitric oxide production and vessel relaxation. Nitric oxide also inhibits platelet aggregation and secretion of platelet contents, many of which cause vasoconstriction. The fact that nitric oxide is released into the vessel lumen (to inactivate platelets) and away from the lumen (to relax smooth muscle) suggests that it protects against both thrombosis and vasoconstriction. It has been suggested that the tendency toward vasoconstriction that characterizes atherosclerotic vessels may be related to impaired vasodilator function due to disruption of the vessel endothelial layer.

In addition to nitric oxide, the endothelium also produces other vasodilating substances such as the prostaglandin *prostacyclin,* which produces vasodilation and inhibits platelet aggregation. The endothelium also produces a number of vasoconstrictor substances, including *angiotensin II,* vasoconstrictor prostaglandins, and a family of peptides called *endothelins.* There are at least three endothelins. Endothelin-1, made by human endothelial cells, is the most potent endogenous vasoconstrictor known. Receptors for endothelins also have been identified.

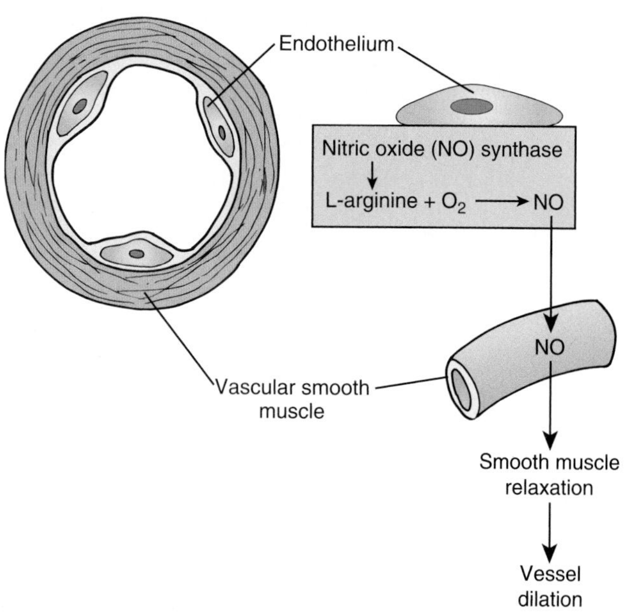

FIGURE 23-22 Function of nitric oxide in smooth muscle relaxation.

Long-Term Regulation

Collateral circulation is a mechanism for the long-term regulation of local blood flow. In the heart and other vital structures, anastomotic channels exist between some of the smaller arteries. These channels permit perfusion of an area by more than one artery. When one artery becomes occluded, these anastomotic channels increase in size, allowing blood from a patent artery to perfuse the area supplied by the occluded vessel. For example, persons with extensive obstruction of a coronary blood vessel may rely on collateral circulation to meet the oxygen needs of the myocardial tissue normally supplied by that vessel. As with other long-term compensatory mechanisms, the recruitment of collateral circulation is most efficient when obstruction to flow is gradual rather than sudden.

In summary, the walls of all blood vessels, except the capillaries, are composed of three layers: the tunica externa, tunica media, and tunica intima. The layers of the vessel vary with its function. Arteries are thick-walled vessels with large amounts of elastic fibers. The walls of the arterioles, which control blood pressure, have large amounts of smooth muscle. Veins are thin-walled, distensible, and collapsible vessels. Venous flow is designed to return blood to the heart. It is a low-pressure system and relies on venous valves and the action of muscle pumps to offset the effects of gravity. Capillaries are single-cell–thick vessels designed for the exchange of gases, nutrients, and waste materials.

The delivery of blood to the tissues of the body is dependent on pressure pulses that are generated by the intermittent ejection of blood from the left ventricle into the distensible aorta and large arteries of the arterial system. The combination of distensibility of the arteries and their resistance to flow reduces the pressure pulsations so that there are almost no pulsations and blood flow is almost constant by the time blood reaches the capillaries.

The mechanisms that control blood flow are designed to ensure adequate delivery of blood to the capillaries in the microcirculation, where the exchange of cellular nutrients and wastes occurs. Local control is governed largely by the needs of the tissues and is regulated by local tissue factors such as lack of oxygen and the accumulation of metabolites. Hyperemia is a local increase in blood flow that occurs after a temporary occlusion of blood flow. It is a compensatory mechanism that decreases the oxygen debt of the deprived tissues. Collateral circulation is a mechanism for long-term regulation of local blood flow that involves the development of collateral vessels.

Neural Control of Circulatory Function

After you have completed this section of the chapter, you should be able to meet the following objectives:

- Describe the roles of the medullary vasomotor and cardioinhibitory centers in controlling the function of the heart and blood vessels
- Describe the autonomic nervous system innervation of the circulatory system and the effect of the sympathetic and parasympathetic nervous system on cardiovascular function.
- Describe the distribution of sympathetic and parasympathetic nervous system in the innervation of the circulatory system and their effects on heart rate and cardiac contractility
- Relate the role of the central nervous system in terms of regulating circulatory function

The neural control centers for the integration and modulation of cardiac function and blood pressure are located bilaterally in the medulla oblongata. The medullary cardiovascular neurons are grouped into three distinct pools that lead to sympathetic innervation of the heart and blood vessels and parasympathetic innervation of the heart. The first two, which control sympathetic-mediated acceleration of heart rate and blood vessel tone, are called the *vasomotor center.* The third, which controls parasympathetic-mediated slowing of heart rate, is called the *cardioinhibitory center.* These brain stem centers receive information from many areas of the nervous system, including the hypothalamus. The arterial baroreceptors and chemoreceptors provide the medullary cardiovascular center with continuous information regarding changes in blood pressure (see Chapter 25).

AUTONOMIC NERVOUS SYSTEM REGULATION

The neural control of the circulatory system occurs primarily through the *sympathetic* and *parasympathetic* divisions of the autonomic nervous system (ANS). The ANS contributes to the control of cardiovascular function through modulation of cardiac (*i.e.,* heart rate and cardiac contractility) and vascular (*i.e.,* peripheral vascular resistance) function.

Autonomic Regulation of Cardiac Function

The heart is innervated by the parasympathetic and sympathetic nervous systems. Parasympathetic innervation of the heart is achieved by means of the *vagus nerve.* The parasympathetic outflow to the heart originates from the vagal nucleus in the medulla. The axons of these neurons pass to the heart in the cardiac branches of the vagus nerve. The effect of vagal stimulation on heart function is largely limited to heart rate, with increased vagal activity producing a slowing of the pulse. Sympathetic outflow to the heart and blood vessels arises from neurons located in the reticular formation of the brain stem. The axons of these neurons exit the thoracic segments of the spinal cord to synapse with the postganglionic neurons that innervate the heart. Cardiac sympathetic fibers are widely distributed to the sinoatrial and AV nodes and the myocardium. Increased sympathetic activity produces an increase in the heart rate and the velocity and force of cardiac contraction.

Autonomic Regulation of Vascular Function

The sympathetic nervous system serves as the final common pathway for controlling the smooth muscle tone of the blood vessels. Most of the sympathetic preganglionic fibers that control vessel function originate in the vasomotor center of the brain stem, travel down the spinal cord, and exit in the thoracic and lumbar (T1 to L2) segments. The sympathetic neurons that supply the blood vessels maintain them in a state of tonic activity, so that even under resting conditions, the blood vessels are partially constricted. Vessel constriction and relaxation are accomplished by altering this basal input. Increasing sympathetic activity causes constriction of some vessels, such as those of the skin, the gastrointestinal tract, and the kidneys. Blood vessels in skeletal muscle are supplied by both vasoconstrictor and vasodilator fibers. Activation of sympathetic vasodilator fibers causes vessel relaxation and provides the muscles with increased blood flow during exercise. Although the parasympathetic nervous system contributes to the regulation of heart function, it has little or no control over blood vessels.

Autonomic Neurotransmitters

The actions of the ANS are mediated by chemical neurotransmitters. *Acetylcholine* is the postganglionic neurotransmitter for parasympathetic neurons, and *norepinephrine* is the main neurotransmitter for postganglionic sympathetic neurons. Sympathetic neurons also respond to epinephrine, which is released into the bloodstream by the adrenal medulla. The neurotransmitter *dopamine* can also act as a neurotransmitter for some sympathetic neurons. The synthesis, release, and inactivation of the autonomic neurotransmitters are discussed in Chapter 49.

CENTRAL NERVOUS SYSTEM RESPONSES

It is not surprising that the central nervous system (CNS), which plays an essential role in regulating vasomotor tone and blood pressure, would have a mechanism for controlling the blood flow to the cardiovascular centers that control circulatory function. When the blood flow to the brain has been sufficiently interrupted to cause ischemia of the vasomotor center, these vasomotor neurons become strongly excited, causing massive vasoconstriction as a means of raising the blood pressure to levels as high as the heart can pump against. This response is called the *CNS ischemic response,* and it can raise the blood pressure to levels as high as 270 mm Hg for as long as 10 minutes. The CNS ischemic response is a last-ditch stand to preserve the blood flow to vital brain centers; it does not become activated until blood pressure has fallen to at least 60 mm Hg, and it is most effective in the range of 15 to 20 mm Hg. If the cerebral circulation is not reestablished within 3 to 10 minutes, the neurons of the vasomotor center cease to function, so that the tonic impulses to the blood vessels stop, and the blood pressure falls precipitously.

The *Cushing reflex* is a special type of CNS reflex resulting from an increase in intracranial pressure. When the intracranial pressure rises to levels that equal intra-arterial pressure, blood vessels to the vasomotor center become compressed, initiating the CNS ischemic response. The purpose of this reflex is to produce a rise in arterial pressure to levels above intracranial pressure so that the blood flow to the vasomotor center can be reestablished. Should the intracranial pressure rise to the point that the blood supply to the vasomotor center becomes inadequate, vasoconstrictor tone is lost, and the blood pressure begins to fall. The elevation in blood pressure associated with the Cushing reflex is usually of short duration and should be considered a protective homeostatic mechanism. The brain and other cerebral structures are located within the rigid confines of the skull, with no room for expansion, and any increase in intracranial pressure tends to compress the blood vessels that supply the brain.

In summary, the neural control centers for the regulation of cardiac function and blood pressure are located in the reticular formation of the lower pons and medulla of the brain stem, where the integration and modulation of ANS responses occur. These brain stem centers receive information from many areas of the nervous system, including the hypothalamus. Both the parasympathetic and sympathetic nervous systems innervate the heart. The parasympathetic nervous system functions in regulating heart rate through the vagus nerve, with increased vagal activity producing a slowing of heart rate. The sympathetic nervous system has an excitatory influence on heart rate and contractility, and it serves as the final common pathway for controlling the smooth muscle tone of the blood vessels.

The Microcirculation and Lymphatic System

After you have completed this section of the chapter, you should be able to meet the following objectives:

- Describe the structure and function of the microcirculation
- Relate the effects of the capillary pressure, interstitial fluid pressure, capillary colloidal osmotic pressure, and interstitial colloidal osmotic pressure to the exchange of fluids at the capillary level
- Describe the structures of the lymphatic system and relate them to the role of the lymphatics in controlling interstitial fluid volume
- Define the term *edema*

The capillaries, venules, and arterioles of the circulatory system are collectively referred to as the *microcirculation.* It is here that exchange of gases, nutrients, and metabolites takes place between the tissues and the circulating blood.

THE MICROCIRCULATION

Blood enters the microcirculation through an arteriole, passes through the capillaries, and leaves by way of a small venule. The metarterioles serve as thoroughfare channels that link arterioles and capillaries (Fig. 23-23). Small cuffs of smooth muscle, the precapillary sphincters, are positioned

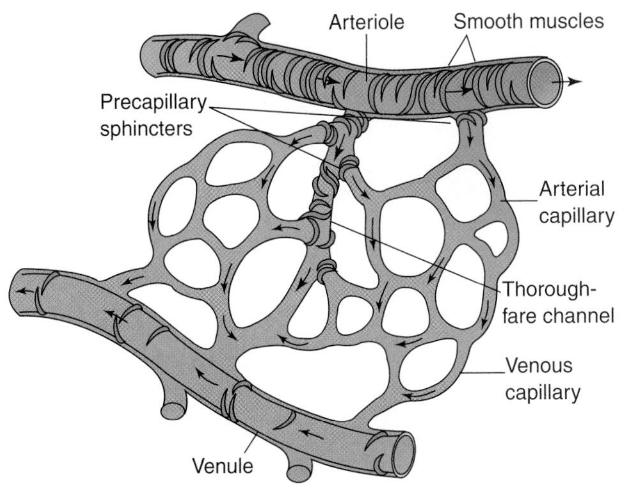

FIGURE 23-23 Capillary bed. Precapillary sphincters control the flow of blood through the capillary network. Thoroughfare channels (*i.e.*, arteriovenous shunts) allow blood to move directly from the arteriole into the venule without moving through nutrient channels of the capillary.

at the arterial end of the capillary. The smooth muscle tone of the arterioles, venules, and precapillary sphincters serves to control blood flow through the capillary bed. Depending on venous pressure, blood flows through the capillary channels when the precapillary sphincters are open.

Blood flow through capillary channels, designed for exchange of nutrients and metabolites, is called *nutrient flow*. In some parts of the microcirculation, blood flow bypasses the nutrient capillary bed, moving through a connection called an *arteriovenous shunt,* which directly connects an arteriole and a venule. This type of blood flow is called *nonnutrient flow* because it does not allow for nutrient exchange. Nonnutrient channels are common in the skin and are important in terms of heat exchange and temperature regulation.

The lymphatic system represents an accessory system that removes excess fluid, including osmotically active proteins, and large particles from the interstitial spaces and returns them to the circulation. Because of their size, these proteins and large particles cannot be reabsorbed into the venous capillaries. The removal of proteins from the interstitial spaces is an essential function, without which death would occur in approximately 24 hours.

CAPILLARY–INTERSTITIAL FLUID EXCHANGE

Approximately one sixth of the body consists of spaces between body cells called the *interstitium*. The interstitium is supported by *collagen* and *elastin* fibers and filled with *proteoglycan* (sugar-protein) molecules that combine with water to form a tissue gel. The tissue gel acts like a sponge to entrap the interstitial fluid and provide for even distribution of the fluid to all the cells, even those that are most distant from the capillary. Although most of the fluid is entrapped in the tissue gel, small "trickles" of free fluid develop between the proteoglycan molecules. Normally, only a small amount of free fluid is present. In a condition called *edema,* in which excess fluid is present in the interstitial spaces, the amount of free fluid can expand tremendously.

Four forces determine the movement of fluid between capillaries and the interstitial spaces: (1) the *intracapillary fluid pressure,* (2) the *interstitial fluid pressure,* (3) the *plasma colloidal osmotic pressure,* and (4) the *interstitial colloidal osmotic pressure*. Water moves between the capillary and the tissue by the processes of filtration and osmosis. *Filtration* is the movement of water across the capillary wall due to differences in fluid pressures between the capillary and the tissue. *Osmosis* is the movement of water across the capillary wall due to differences in osmotic pressure between the capillary and the tissue.

The intracapillary and tissue pressures can be viewed as pushing pressures that force fluid out of the capillary or interstitial space and the osmotic pressures as pulling pressures that draw fluid into the capillary or interstitium. The intracapillary pressure causes fluids to move through the capillary pores into the interstitial spaces, and the capillary colloidal osmotic pressure pulls the fluids back into the capillary. Also important to this exchange mechanism is the lymphatic system, which returns osmotically active proteins and excess interstitial fluids to the circulatory system.

Normally, the movement of fluid between the capillary bed and the interstitial spaces is continuous. As E. H. Starling pointed out more than a century ago, a state of equilibrium exists as long as equal amounts of fluid enter and leave the interstitial spaces (Fig. 23-24). The forces that contribute to the Starling equilibrium are illustrated in Figure 23-25. In the diagram, the capillary fluid pressure is 28 mm Hg. The capillary pressure, along with a negative interstitial pressure (3 mm Hg) and an interstitial colloidal osmotic pressure (8 mm Hg), contributes to the outward movement of fluid. Plasma proteins and other nondiffusible particles that remain in the capillary exert an osmotic pressure (28 mm Hg) that pulls fluids back into the venous end of the capillary. This yields a total outward pushing pressure of approximately 39 mm Hg and an inward pulling pressure of 28 mm Hg at the arterial end of the capillary. On the venous end, the outward pushing pressures drop to 21 mm Hg, and the inward pulling forces remain at 28 mm Hg. A slight imbalance in forces (*i.e.*, 11 mm Hg outward forces and 7 mm Hg inward forces) causes slightly more filtration of fluid into interstitial spaces than is pulled back into the capillary; it is this fluid that is returned to the circulation by the lymphatic system.

Capillary Filtration Pressure

The intracapillary fluid pressure, also called the *capillary filtration pressure,* is the force that pushes water through the capillary pores into the interstitial spaces. Capillary filtration pressure reflects the arterial pressure, the venous pressure, and the hydrostatic effects of gravity. The pressure at the arterial end of the capillary is normally higher than the pressure at its venous end because arterial pressure decreases as blood moves away from the heart. If arterial

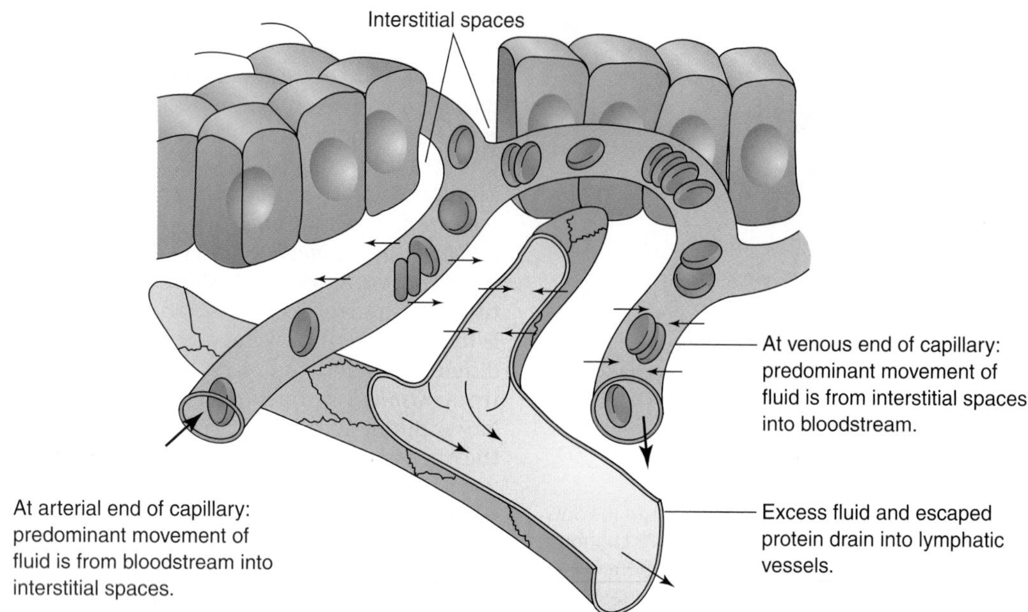
Interstitial spaces
At venous end of capillary: predominant movement of fluid is from interstitial spaces into bloodstream.
Excess fluid and escaped protein drain into lymphatic vessels.
At arterial end of capillary: predominant movement of fluid is from bloodstream into interstitial spaces.

FIGURE 23-24 Exchanges through capillary membranes in the formation and removal of interstitial fluid.

pressure changes, capillary pressure changes, which in turn affects the movement of water across the membrane. For example, if arterial pressure falls owing to hemorrhage, the movement of water out of the capillaries into the tissues decreases, helping to maintain vascular volume. Capillary pressure also reflects changes in capillary volume. For example, intracapillary fluid pressure can be expected to increase when the tone of the precapillary sphincters and the arterioles that supply the capillary bed is decreased. The swelling that occurs with inflammation develops because of a histamine-induced dilatation of the precapillary sphincters and arterioles that supply the affected area. Venous pressure can be transmitted back to the capillary, thereby increasing intracapillary fluid pressure and the outward movement of fluid. For example, venous thrombosis can obstruct venous flow, producing an increase in venous and capillary pressures.

The pressure due to gravity is called the *hydrostatic pressure*. In a person in the standing position, the weight of the blood in the vascular column causes an increase of

Outward Forces	
Capillary pressure	28 mm Hg
Negative interstitial pressure	3 mm Hg
Interstitial colloidal osmotic pressure	8 mm Hg
Total forces	39 mm Hg
Inward Forces	
Plasma colloidal osmotic pressure	28 mm Hg
Total forces	28 mm Hg
Summation of Forces	
Outward	39 mm Hg
Inward	28 mm Hg
Net outward force	11 mm Hg

Inward Forces	
Plasma colloidal osmotic pressure	28 mm Hg
Total forces	28 mm Hg
Outward Forces	
Capillary pressure	10 mm Hg
Negative interstitial pressure	3 mm Hg
Interstitial colloidal osmotic pressure	8 mm Hg
Total forces	21 mm Hg
Summation of Forces	
Inward	28 mm Hg
Outward	21 mm Hg
Net inward force	7 mm Hg

FIGURE 23-25 Inward and outward forces in the capillary.

1 mm Hg in pressure for every 13.6 mm of distance below the level of the heart. The hydrostatic pressure in the veins of an adult man can reach a level of 90 mm Hg. This pressure is then transmitted to the capillary bed. Gravity has no effect on blood pressure in a person in the recumbent position because the blood vessels are then at the level of the heart. Because of the passive nature of pressure in the capillary bed, the terms *capillary fluid pressure* and *hydrostatic pressure* are often used interchangeably.

Interstitial Fluid Pressure

The interstitial fluid pressure reflects the pressure exerted on the interstitial fluids. It can be positive or negative. In some organs, such as the kidneys, which are encased in a tough fibrous capsule, the interstitial fluid pressure is positive, thereby opposing filtration of fluid out of the capillaries. Atmospheric pressure is usually negative in relation to capillary pressure. In the skin exposed to atmospheric pressure, the interstitial pressure is usually several millimeters of mercury less than capillary pressures. A negative interstitial fluid pressure increases the outward forces that influence the movement of fluid out of the capillary into the interstitium.

Capillary Colloidal Osmotic Pressure

The capillary colloidal osmotic pressure reflects the osmotic effect of the plasma proteins in drawing fluid into the capillary. Osmosis is the movement of water across a semipermeable membrane along its concentration gradient, moving from the side of the membrane that has the greatest number of particles to the one that has the least number. A colloid solution is one in which there are evenly dispersed particles, much as cream particles become dispersed when milk is homogenized. The term *colloidal osmotic pressure* is used to differentiate the osmotic effects of the particles in a colloidal solution from those of the dissolved crystalloids such as sodium. The pressure units (millimeters of mercury) used for measuring osmotic pressure represent the mechanical pressure or force that would be needed to oppose the osmotic movement of water.

The plasma proteins are large molecules that disperse in the blood and occasionally escape into the tissue spaces. Because the capillary membrane is almost impermeable to the plasma proteins, these particles exert a force that draws fluid into the capillary and offsets the pushing force of the capillary filtration pressure. The plasma contains a mixture of plasma proteins, including albumin, the globulins, and fibrinogen. Albumin, which is the smallest and most abundant of the plasma proteins, accounts for approximately 70% of the total osmotic pressure. It is the number, not the size, of the particles in solution that controls the osmotic pressure. One gram of albumin (molecular weight of 69,000) contains almost six times as many molecules as 1 g of fibrinogen (molecular weight of 400,000). (Normal values for the plasma proteins are albumin, 4.5 g/dL; globulins, 2.5 g/dL; and fibrinogen, 0.3 g/dL.)

Tissue Colloidal Osmotic Pressure

Although the size of the capillary pores prevents most plasma proteins from leaving the capillary, small amounts do leak into the interstitial spaces to exert an osmotic force that favors movement of capillary fluid into the interstitium. This amount is often increased in conditions such as inflammation that increase capillary permeability. The lymphatic system is responsible for removing proteins from the interstitium. In the absence of a functioning lymphatic system, tissue colloidal osmotic pressure increases, causing fluid to accumulate. Normally, a few white blood cells, plasma proteins, and other large molecules enter the interstitial spaces; these cells and molecules, which are too large to reenter the capillary, rely on the loosely structured wall of the lymphatic vessels for return to the vascular compartment.

THE LYMPHATIC SYSTEM

The lymphatic system, commonly called the *lymphatics,* serves almost all body tissues, except cartilage, bone, epithelial tissue, and tissues of the CNS. Most of these tissues, however, have prelymphatic channels that eventually flow into areas supplied by the lymphatics. Lymph is derived from interstitial fluids that flow through the lymph channels. It contains plasma proteins and other osmotically active particles that rely on the lymphatics for movement back into the circulatory system. When lymph flow is obstructed, a condition called *lymphedema* occurs. Involvement of lymph structures by malignant tumors and removal of lymph nodes at the time of cancer surgery are common causes of lymphedema. The lymphatic system is also the main route for absorption of nutrients, particularly fats, from the gastrointestinal tract. The lymph system also filters the fluid at the lymph nodes and removes foreign particles such as bacteria.

The lymphatic system is made up of vessels similar to those of the circulatory system. These vessels commonly travel with an arteriole or venule or with its companion artery and vein. The terminal lymphatic vessels are made up of a single layer of connective tissue with an endothelial lining and resemble blood capillaries. The lymphatic vessels lack tight junctions and are loosely anchored to the surrounding tissues by fine filaments (Fig. 23-26). The loose junctions permit the entry of large particles, and the filaments hold the vessels open under conditions of edema, when the pressure of the surrounding tissues would otherwise cause them to collapse. The lymph capillaries drain into larger lymph vessels that ultimately empty into the right and left thoracic ducts (Fig. 23-27). The thoracic ducts empty into the circulation at the junctions of the subclavian and internal jugular veins.

Although the divisions are not as distinct as in the circulatory system, the larger lymph vessels show evidence of having intimal, medial, and adventitial layers similar to blood vessels. The intima of these channels contain elastic tissue and an endothelial layer, and the larger collecting lymph channels contain smooth muscle in their medial layer. Contraction of this smooth muscle assists in propelling lymph fluid toward the thorax. External compression of the lymph channels by pulsating blood vessels in the vicinity and active and passive movements of body

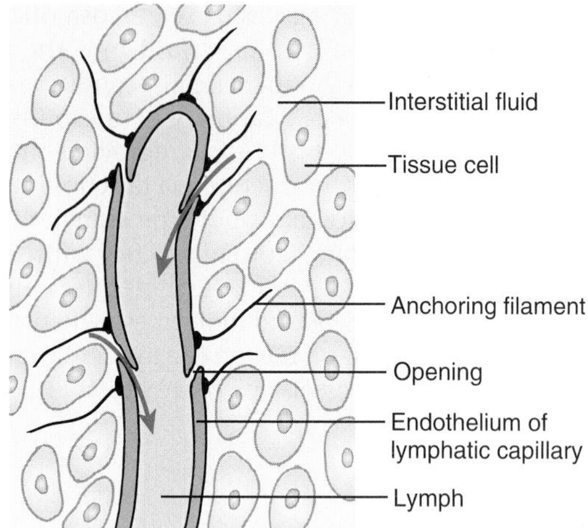

FIGURE 23-26 Special structure of the lymphatic capillaries that permits passage of substances of high molecular weight back into the lymph.

parts also aid in forward propulsion of lymph fluid. The rate of flow through the lymphatic system by way of all of the various lymph channels, approximately 120 mL/hour, is determined by the interstitial fluid pressure and the activity of lymph pumps.

EDEMA

Edema refers to excess interstitial fluid in the tissues (see Chapter 33). Edema can result from an imbalance of any of the factors that control movement of water between the vascular compartment and the tissue spaces. It can occur because of a disproportionate increase in capillary fluid pressure or permeability, decreased capillary colloidal osmotic pressure, or impaired lymph flow. Edema is not a disease but rather the manifestation of altered physiologic function, and it can occur in healthy and sick individuals. In hot weather, the superficial blood vessels dilate, and sodium and water retention increases, which causes swelling of the hands and feet. Edema of the ankles and feet becomes more pronounced during prolonged periods of standing, when the forces of gravity are superimposed on the heat-induced vasodilation and increased extracellular fluid volume. Pulmonary edema, which develops with severe impairment of left ventricular function, is a severe, life-threatening event.

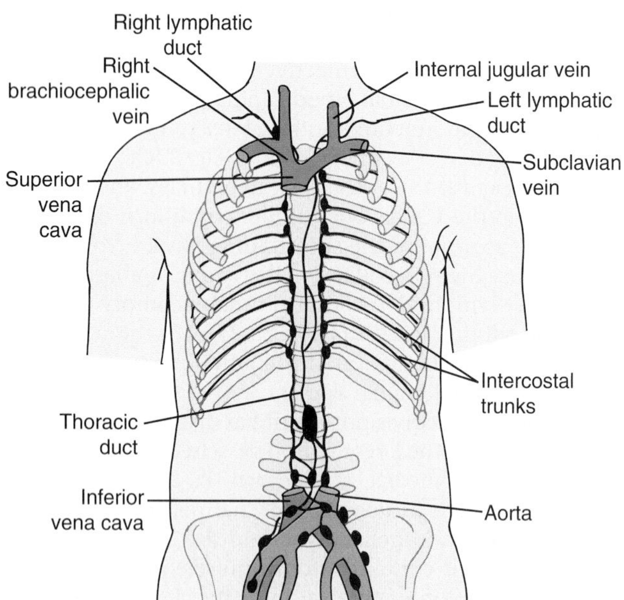

FIGURE 23-27 This diagram shows the course of the thoracic duct and right and left lymphatic ducts. Deep lymphatic vessels and nodes are also shown.

In summary, exchange of fluids between the vascular compartment and the interstitial spaces occurs at the capillary level. The capillary filtration pressure pushes fluids out of the capillaries, and the colloidal osmotic pressure exerted by the plasma proteins pulls fluids back into the capillaries. Albumin, which is the smallest and most abundant of the plasma proteins, provides the major osmotic force for return of fluid to the vascular compartment. Normally, slightly more fluid leaves the capillary bed than can be reabsorbed. This excess fluid is returned to the circulation by way of the lymphatic channels.

REVIEW EXERCISES

In persons with atherosclerosis of the coronary arteries, symptoms of ischemia do not usually occur until the vessel has been 75% occluded.

A. Use Poiseuille's law to explain.

Once an arterial aneurysm has begun to form, it continues to enlarge as the result of the increased tension in its wall.

A. Explain the continued increase in size using Laplace's law.

B. Using information related to cross-sectional area and velocity of flow, explain why there is stasis of blood flow with the tendency to form clots in aneurysms with a large cross-sectional area.

Use events in the cardiac cycle depicted in Figure 23-15 to explain:

A. The effect of hypertension on the isovolumetric contraction period.

B. The effect of an increase in heart rate on the time spent in diastole.

C. The effect of an increase in the isovolumetric relaxation period on the diastolic filling of the ventricle.

Use the Frank-Starling ventricular function curve depicted in Figure 23-16 to explain the changes in cardiac output that occur as a result of changes in respiratory effort.

A. What happens to cardiac output during increased inspiratory effort in which a marked decrease in intrathoracic pressure produces an increase in venous return to the right heart?

B. What happens to cardiac output during increased expiratory effort in which a marked increase in intrathoracic pressure produces a decrease in venous return to the right heart?

C. Given these changes in cardiac output that occur during increased respiratory effort, what would you propose as one of the functions of the Frank-Starling curve?

Bibliography

Berne R. M., Levy M. N. (2001). *Cardiovascular physiology* (8th ed). St. Louis: C. V. Mosby.

Feletou M., Vanhoutte P. M. (1999). The alternative: EDHF. *Journal of Molecular and Cellular Cardiology 31,* 15–22.

Guyton A. C., Hall J. E. (2000). *Medical physiology* (10th ed., pp. 144–222). Philadelphia: W. B. Saunders.

Johansen K. (1982). Aneurysms. *Scientific American 247*(1), 110–118.

McCormack D. H. (1987). *Ham's histology* (9th ed., p. 448). Philadelphia: J. B. Lippincott.

Rhoades R. S., Tanner G. A. (2003). *Medical physiology* (2nd ed. pp. 191–308). Boston: Little, Brown.

Smith J. J., Kampine J. P. (1989). *Circulatory physiology* (3rd ed.). Baltimore: Williams & Wilkins.

Vanhoutte P. M. (1999). How to assess endothelial function in human blood vessels. *Journal of Hypertension 17,* 1047–1058.

CHAPTER

24

Disorders of Blood Flow in the Systemic Circulation

Glenn Matfin and Carol M. Porth

Blood flow in the arterial and venous systems depends on a system of patent blood vessels and adequate perfusion pressure. Unlike disorders of the respiratory system or central circulation that cause hypoxia and impair oxygenation of tissues throughout the body, the effects of blood vessel disease usually are limited to local tissues supplied by a particular vessel or group of vessels. With arterial disorders, there is decreased blood flow to the tissues along with impaired delivery of oxygen and nutrients. Venous disorders interfere with the outflow of blood from the capillaries, removal of tissue wastes, and return of blood to the heart.

Disturbances in blood flow can result from pathologic changes in the vessel wall (*i.e.*, atherosclerosis and vasculitis), acute vessel obstruction due to thrombus or embolus, vasospasm (*i.e.*, Raynaud's phenomenon), abnormal vessel dilation (*i.e.*, arterial aneurysms or varicose veins), or compression of blood vessels by extravascular forces (*i.e.*, tumors, edema, or firm surfaces such as those associated with pressure ulcers).

This chapter is organized into three sections: disorders of the arterial circulation, disorders of the venous circulation, and disorders of blood vessel compression.

Disorders of the Arterial Circulation

After you have completed this section of the chapter, you should be able to meet the following objectives:

- List the five types of lipoproteins and state their function in terms of lipid transport and development of atherosclerosis
- Describe the role of low-density lipoprotein receptors in removal of cholesterol from the blood
- Cite the criteria for diagnosis of hypercholesterolemia
- List the vessels most commonly affected by atherosclerosis and describe the vessel changes that occur
- Describe possible mechanisms involved in the development of atherosclerosis
- List risk factors in atherosclerosis
- Describe the role of inflammation in the development of atherosclerosis and how it can be assessed clinically
- State the signs and symptoms of acute arterial occlusion
- Describe the pathology associated with the vasculitides and relate it to four disease conditions associated with vasculitis
- Compare the mechanisms and manifestations of ischemia associated with atherosclerotic peripheral

vascular disease, Raynaud's phenomenon, and thromboangiitis obliterans (*i.e.*, Buerger's disease)

✦ Distinguish between the pathology and manifestations of aortic aneurysms and dissection of the aorta

The arterial system distributes blood to all the tissues in the body. There are three types of arteries: large elastic arteries, including the aorta and its distal branches; medium-sized arteries, such as the coronary and renal arteries; and small arteries and arterioles that pass through the tissues. The large arteries function mainly in transport of blood. The medium-sized arteries are composed predominantly of circular and spirally arranged smooth muscle cells. Distribution of blood flow to the various organs and tissues of the body is controlled by contraction and relaxation of the smooth muscle of these vessels. The small arteries and arterioles regulate capillary blood flow. Each of these different types of arteries tends to be affected by different disease processes.

Pathology of the arterial system affects body function by impairing blood flow. The effect of impaired blood flow on the body depends on the structures involved and the extent of altered flow. The term *ischemia* (*i.e.*, holding back of blood) denotes a reduction in arterial flow to a level that is insufficient to meet the oxygen demands of the tissues. *Infarction* refers to an area of ischemic necrosis in an organ produced by occlusion of its arterial blood supply or its venous drainage. The discussion in this section focuses on blood lipids and hypercholesterolemia, atherosclerosis, vasculitis, arterial disease of the extremities, and arterial aneurysms.

DISORDERS OF THE ARTERIAL CIRCULATION

- The arterial system delivers oxygen and nutrients to the tissues.
- Disorders of the arterial circulation produce ischemia owing to narrowing of blood vessels, thrombus formation associated with platelet adhesion, and weakening of the vessel wall.
- Atherosclerosis is a progressive disease characterized by the formation of fibrofatty plaques in the intima of large and medium-sized vessels, including the aorta, coronary arteries, and cerebral vessels. The major risk factors for atherosclerosis are hypercholesterolemia and inflammation.
- Vasculitis is an inflammation of the blood vessel wall resulting in vascular tissue injury and necrosis. Arteries, capillaries, and veins may be affected. The inflammatory process may be initiated by direct injury, infectious agents, or immune processes.
- Aneurysms represent an abnormal localized dilatation of an artery due to a weakness in the vessel wall. As the aneurysm increases in size, the tension in the wall of the vessel increases and it may rupture. The increased size of the vessel also may exert pressure on adjacent structures.

HYPERLIPIDEMIA

Triglycerides, phospholipids, and cholesterol, which are classified as lipids, are chemical substances composed of long-chain hydrocarbon fatty acids. Triglycerides, which are used in energy metabolism, are combinations of three fatty acids condensed with a single glycerol molecule. Phospholipids, which contain a phosphate group, are important structural constituents of lipoproteins, blood clotting components, the myelin sheath, and cell membranes. Although cholesterol is not composed of fatty acids, its steroid nucleus is synthesized from fatty acids; thus, its chemical activity is similar to that of other lipid substances.[1]

Elevated levels of blood cholesterol (*hypercholesterolemia*) are implicated in the development of atherosclerosis with its attendant risk for heart attack and stroke. This is a major public health issue that is underscored by striking statistics released by the American Heart Association. An estimated 41.3 million Americans have high serum cholesterol levels that could contribute to a heart attack, stroke, or other cardiovascular event associated with atherosclerosis,[2] and more than 100 million Americans have cholesterol levels that are considered borderline high.

Lipoproteins

Because cholesterol and triglyceride are insoluble in plasma, they are encapsulated by special fat-carrying proteins called *lipoproteins* for transport in the blood. There are five types of lipoproteins, classified by their densities as measured by ultracentrifugation: chylomicrons, very–low-density lipoprotein (VLDL), intermediate-density lipoprotein (IDL), low-density lipoprotein (LDL), and high-density lipoprotein (HDL). VLDL carries large amounts of triglycerides that have a lower density than cholesterol. LDL is the main carrier of cholesterol, whereas HDL actually is 50% protein (Fig. 24-1).

Each type of lipoprotein consists of a large molecular complex of lipids combined with proteins called *apoproteins*.[3,4] The major lipid constituents are cholesterol esters, triglycerides, nonesterified cholesterol, and phospholipids. The insoluble cholesterol esters and triglycerides are located in the hydrophobic core of the lipoprotein macromolecule, surrounded by the soluble phospholipids, nonesterified cholesterol, and apoproteins (Fig. 24-2). Nonesterified cholesterol and phospholipids provide a negative charge that allows the lipoprotein to be soluble in plasma.

There are four major classes of apoproteins: A (*i.e.*, A-I, A-II, and A-IV), B (*e.g.*, B-48, B-100), C (*i.e.*, C-I, C-II, and C-III), and E.[3,4] The apoproteins control the interactions and ultimate metabolic fate of the lipoproteins. Some of the apoproteins activate the lipolytic enzymes that facilitate the removal of lipids from the lipoproteins; others serve as a reactive site that cellular receptors can recognize and use in the endocytosis and metabolism of the lipoproteins. The major apoprotein in LDL is B-100. HDL is associated with A-I and A-II. Research findings suggest that genetic defects in apoproteins may be involved in hyperlipidemia and accelerated atherosclerosis.[3–6]

There are two sites of lipoprotein synthesis: the small intestine and the liver. The chylomicrons, which are the largest of the lipoprotein molecules, are synthesized in the

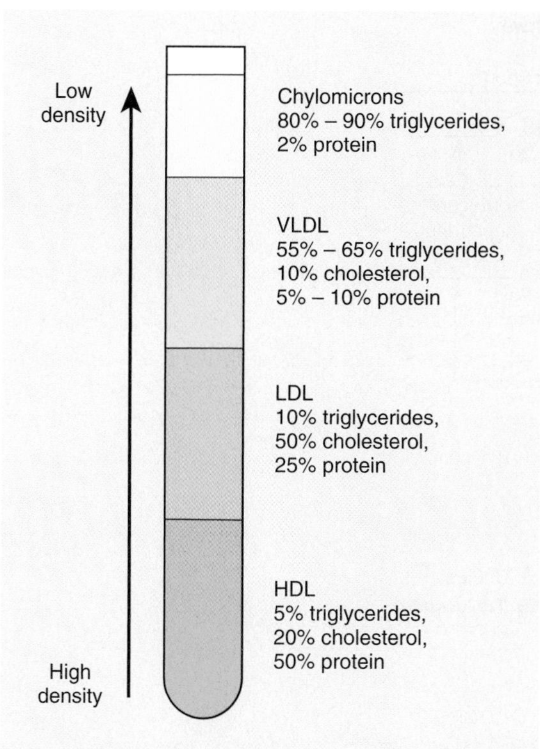

FIGURE 24-1 Lipoproteins are named based on their protein content, which is measured in density. Because fats are less dense than proteins, as the proportion of triglycerides decreases, the density increases.

wall of the small intestine. They are involved in the transport of dietary (exogenous pathway) triglycerides and cholesterol that have been absorbed from the gastrointestinal tract (Fig. 24-3). Chylomicrons transfer their triglycerides to the cells of adipose and skeletal muscle tissue. The remnant chylomicron particles, which contain cholesterol, are then taken up by the liver, and the cholesterol is used in the synthesis of VLDL or is excreted in the bile.

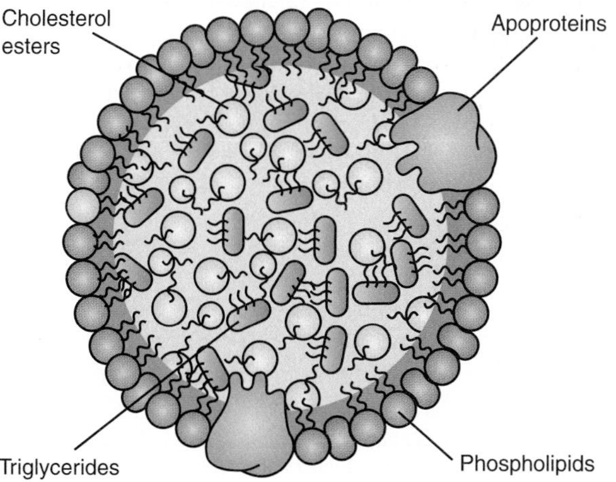

FIGURE 24-2 General structure of a lipoprotein. The cholesterol esters and triglycerides are located in the hydrophobic core of the macromolecule, surrounded by phospholipids and apoproteins.

The liver synthesizes and releases VLDL and HDL. The VLDLs contain large amounts of triglycerides and lesser amounts of cholesterol esters.[7] They provide the primary pathway for transport of the endogenous triglycerides produced in the liver, as opposed to those obtained from the diet (see Fig. 24-3). Like chylomicrons, VLDLs carry their triglycerides to fat and muscle cells, where the triglycerides are removed. The resulting IDL fragments are reduced in triglyceride content and enriched in cholesterol. They are taken to the liver and recycled to form VLDL, or converted to LDL in the vascular compartment. IDLs are the main source of LDL.

LDL, sometimes called the *bad cholesterol,* is the main carrier of cholesterol. The LDL is removed from the circulation by either LDL receptors or by nonreceptor mechanisms involving scavenger cells such as monocytes or macrophages. Approximately 70% of LDL is removed by way of the LDL receptor-dependent pathway.[7] Approximately 75% are located on hepatocytes; thus, the liver plays an extremely important role in LDL metabolism. Receptor-mediated removal involves binding of LDL to cell surface receptors, followed by *endocytosis,* a phagocytic process in which LDL is engulfed and moved into the cell in the form of a membrane-covered endocytic vesicle. Within the cell, the endocytic vesicles fuse with lysosomes, and the LDL molecule is enzymatically degraded, causing free cholesterol to be released into the cytoplasm.

Other, nonhepatic tissues (*i.e.,* adrenal glands, smooth muscle cells, endothelial cells, and lymphoid cells) also use the receptor-dependent pathway to obtain cholesterol needed for membrane and hormone synthesis. These tissues can control their cholesterol intake by adding or removing LDL receptors. The remaining LDL is removed by non–receptor-dependent mechanisms, including ingestion by phagocytic monocytes and macrophages. These scavenger cells have receptors that bind LDL that has been oxidized or chemically modified. The amount of LDL that is removed by the scavenger pathway is directly related to the plasma cholesterol level. When there is a decrease in LDL receptors or when LDL levels exceed receptor availability, the amount of LDL that is removed by scavenger cells is greatly increased. The uptake of LDL by macrophages in the arterial wall can result in the accumulation of insoluble cholesterol esters, the formation of foam cells, and the development of atherosclerosis.

HDL is synthesized in the liver and often is referred to as the *good cholesterol.* HDL participates in the reverse transport of cholesterol, that is, carrying cholesterol from the peripheral tissues back to the liver. Epidemiologic studies show an inverse relation between HDL levels and the development of atherosclerosis.[8,9] It is thought that HDL, which is low in cholesterol and rich in surface phospholipids, facilitates the clearance of cholesterol from atheromatous plaques and transports it to the liver, where it may be excreted rather than reused in the formation of VLDL. The mechanism whereby HDL takes up cholesterol from peripheral cells has recently been elucidated. A lipid transporter (adenosine triphosphate [ATP]-binding cassette transporter A class 1, or ABCA1) promotes the movement of cholesterol from peripheral cells to lipid-poor

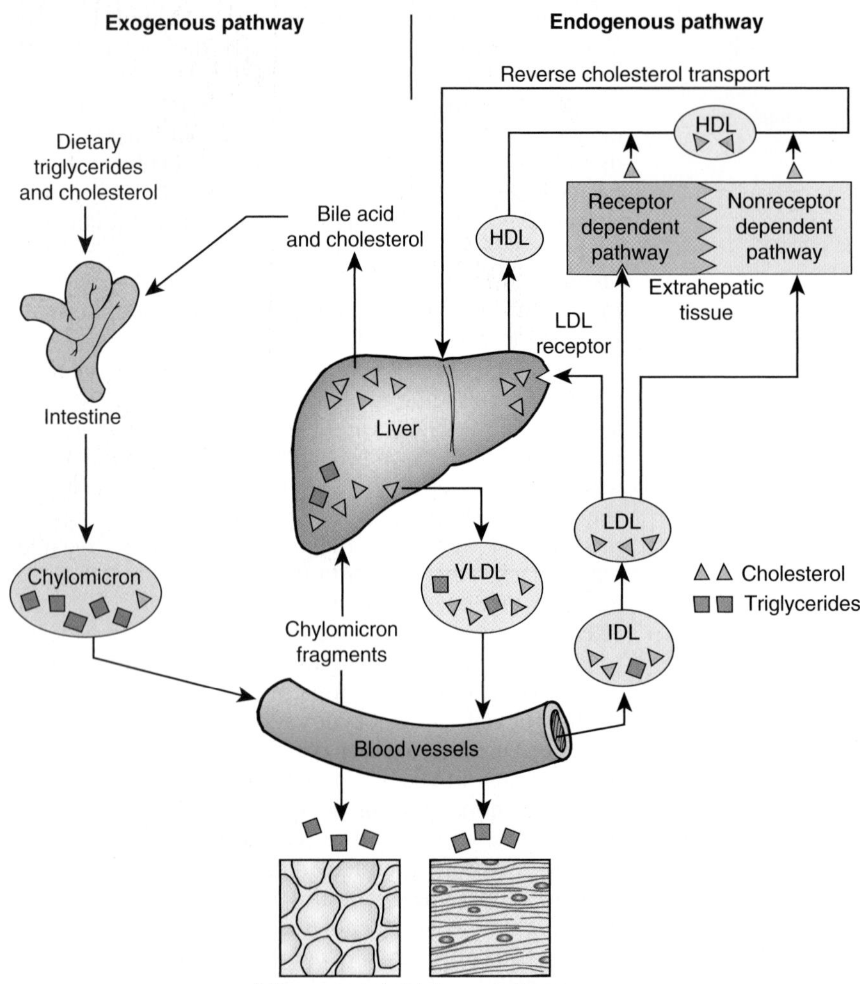

FIGURE 24-3 Schematic representation of the exogenous and endogenous pathways for triglyceride and cholesterol transport.

HDL.[10] Defects in this system (resulting from mutations in the ABCA1 transporter) are responsible for Tangier disease, which is characterized by accelerated atherosclerosis and little or no HDL. HDL also is believed to inhibit cellular uptake of LDL. It has been observed that regular exercise and moderate alcohol consumption increase HDL levels. Smoking and the metabolic syndrome (see Chapter 43), which are in themselves risk factors for atherosclerosis, are associated with decreased levels of HDL.[7,9]

Hypercholesterolemia

The *Third Report of the National Cholesterol Education Program (NCEP) Expert Panel on Detection, Evaluation, and Treatment of High Blood Cholesterol in Adults* includes a classification system for hyperlipidemia that describes optimal to very high levels of LDL cholesterol, desirable to high levels of total cholesterol, and low and high levels of HDL cholesterol[11] (Table 24-1). The NCEP recommends that all adults 20 years of age and older should have a fasting lipoprotein profile (total cholesterol, LDL cholesterol, HDL cholesterol, and triglycerides) measured once every 5 years. If testing is done in the nonfasting state, only the total cho-

TABLE 24-1	NCEP Adult Treatment Panel III Classification of LDL, Total, and HDL Cholesterol (mg/dL)
LDL Cholesterol	
<100	Optimal
100–129	Near optimal/above optimal
130–159	Borderline high
160–189	High
≥190	Very high
Total Cholesterol	
<200	Desirable
200–239	Borderline high
≥240	High
HDL Cholesterol	
<40	Low
≥60	High

(National Institutes of Health Expert Panel [2001]. *Third report of the National Cholesterol Education Program [NCEP] Expert Panel on Detection, Evaluation, and Treatment of High Blood Cholesterol in Adults [Adult Treatment Panel III].* [NIH Publication No. 01–3670]. Bethesda, MD: National Institutes of Health) lesterol and HDL are considered useful. A follow-up lipoprotein profile should be done on persons with nonfasting total cholesterol levels of 200 mg/dL or greater, or HDL levels of less than 40 mg/dL. Lipoprotein measurements are particularly important in persons at high risk for development of coronary heart disease (CHD).

Serum cholesterol levels may be elevated as a result of an increase in any of the lipoproteins—the chylomicrons, VLDL, IDL, LDL, or HDL. The commonly used classification system for hyperlipidemia is based on the type of lipoprotein involved (Table 24-2). Three factors—nutrition, genetics, and metabolic diseases—can raise blood lipid levels. Most cases of elevated levels of cholesterol are probably multifactorial. Some persons may have increased sensitivity to dietary cholesterol, others have a lack of LDL receptors, and still others have an altered synthesis of the apoproteins, including oversynthesis of apoprotein B-100, the major apoprotein in LDL.

Hypercholesterolemia can be classified as primary or secondary hypercholesterolemia. *Primary hypercholesterolemia* describes elevated cholesterol levels that develop independent of other health problems or lifestyle behaviors. *Secondary hypercholesterolemia* is associated with other health problems and behaviors.

Many types of primary hypercholesterolemia have a genetic basis. There may be a defective synthesis of the apoproteins, a lack of receptors, defective receptors, or defects in the handling of cholesterol in the cell that are genetically determined.[3,5] For example, the LDL receptor is deficient or defective in the genetic disorder known as *familial hypercholesterolemia (type 2A)*. This autosomal dominant type of hyperlipoproteinemia results from a mutation in the gene specifying the receptor for LDL. More than 600 different mutations in the LDL receptor have been described.[5] Because most of the circulating cholesterol is removed by receptor-dependent mechanisms, blood cholesterol levels are markedly elevated in persons with this disorder. The disorder is probably one of the most common of all mendelian disorders; the frequency of heterozygotes is 1 in 500 persons in the general population.[5] Plasma LDL levels in heterozygotes range between 250 and 500 mg/dL, whereas in homozygotes, LDL cholesterol levels may rise to 1000 mg/dL. Although heterozygotes commonly have an elevated cholesterol level from birth, they do not develop symptoms until adult life, when they develop *xanthomas* (*i.e.*, cholesterol deposits) along the tendons, and atherosclerosis appears (Fig. 24-4). Myocardial infarction before 40 years of age is common. Homozygotes are much more severely affected; they have cutaneous xanthomas in childhood and may experience myocardial infarction by as early as 1 to 2 years of age.

Causes of secondary hyperlipoproteinemia include obesity with high-calorie intake and diabetes mellitus. High-calorie diets increase the production of VLDL, with triglyceride elevation and high conversion of VLDL to LDL. Excess ingestion of cholesterol may reduce the formation of LDL receptors and thereby decrease LDL removal. Diets that are high in triglycerides and saturated fats increase cholesterol synthesis and suppress LDL receptor activity. In diabetes mellitus and the metabolic syndrome, typical dyslipidemia is seen with elevation of triglycerides, low HDL, and minimal or modest elevation of LDL.[9,11]

Management of Hyperlipidemia. The NCEP continues to identify reduction in LDL cholesterol as the primary target for cholesterol-lowering therapy, particularly in people at risk for CHD. The major risk factors for CHD, exclusive of LDL cholesterol levels, that modify LDL cholesterol goals include cigarette smoking, hypertension, family history of premature CHD in a first-degree relative, age (men, 45 years and older; women, 55 years and older), and HDL cholesterol levels of less than 40 mg/dL (Chart 24-1). Accordingly, the NCEP recommends that persons with CHD or

TABLE 24-2 Classification of Hyperlipoproteinemias and Their Genetic Basis

Type	Familiar Name	Lipoprotein Abnormality	Known Underlying Genetic Defects
1	Exogenous dietary hypertriglyceridemia	Elevated chylomicrons and triglycerides	Mutation in lipoprotein lipase gene
2a	Familial hypercholesterolemia	Elevated LDL cholesterol	Mutation in LDL receptor gene or in apoprotein B gene
2b	Combined hyperlipidemia	Elevated LDL, VLDL, and triglycerides	Mutation in LDL receptor gene or apoprotein B gene
3	Remnant hyperlipidemia	Increased remnants (chylomicrons), IDL triglycerides, and cholesterol	Mutation in apolipoprotein E gene
4	Endogenous hypertriglyceridemia	Elevated VLDL and triglycerides	Unknown
5	Mixed hypertriglyceridemia	Elevated VLDL, chylomicrons, and cholesterol; triglycerides greatly elevated	Mutation in apolipoprotein C-II gene

IDL, intermediate-density lipoprotein; LDL, low-density lipoprotein; VLDL, very–low-density lipoprotein.
(Data developed from Cotran R.S., Kumar V., Robbins S.L. [1994]. *Robbins pathologic basis of disease* [5th ed., pp. 481–482]. Philadelphia: W.B. Saunders; and Gotto A.M. [1988]. Lipoprotein metabolism and etiology of hyperlipidemia. *Hospital Practice*, 23[Suppl. 1], 4)

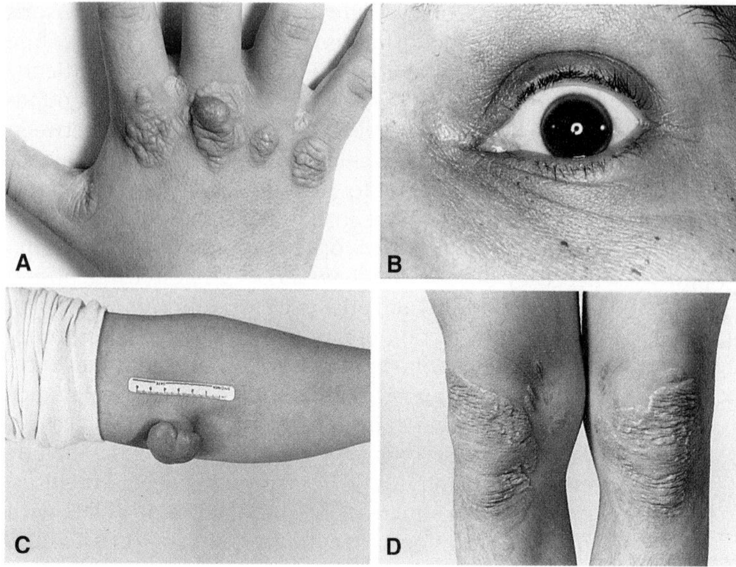

FIGURE 24-4 Xanthomas in the skin and tendons (**A, C, D**). Arcus lipoides represents the deposition of lipids in the peripheral cornea (**B**). (Rubin E., Farber J. L. [1999]. *Pathology* [3rd ed., p. 506]. Philadelphia: Lippincott-Raven)

CHD equivalents (other forms of atherosclerotic disease or diabetes) should have an LDL cholesterol goal of less than 100 mg/dL; those with two or more of the major risk factors should have an LDL cholesterol goal of 130 mg/dL; and those with zero or no major risk factors should have an LDL cholesterol goal of 160 mg/dL or lower.[11] The management of hypercholesterolemia focuses on dietary and therapeutic lifestyle changes; when these are unsuccessful, pharmacologic treatment may be necessary. Therapeutic lifestyle changes include an increased emphasis on physical activity, dietary measures to reduce LDL cholesterol levels, smoking cessation, and weight reduction for people who are overweight.

Three dietary elements affect cholesterol and its lipoprotein fractions: (1) excess calorie intake, (2) saturated fats, and (3) cholesterol. Excess calories consistently lower HDL and less consistently elevate LDL. Saturated fats in the diet can strongly influence cholesterol levels. Each 1% of saturated fat relative to caloric intake increases the cholesterol level an average of 2.8 mg/dL.[12] Depending on individual differences, it raises the VLDL and the LDL. Dietary cholesterol tends to increase LDL cholesterol. On average, each 100 mg/dL of ingested cholesterol raises the serum cholesterol 8 to 10 mg/dL.[12]

The aims of dietary therapy are to reduce total and LDL cholesterol levels, to increase HDL cholesterol by reduction in total calories, and to reduce the percentage of total calories from saturated fat and cholesterol. The American Heart Association (AHA) has issued new dietary guidelines that focus on an overall plan of healthy food choices and increased physical activity to decrease the risk for development of cardiovascular disease.[13] The specific guidelines are intended to assist the general public in the maintenance of a body mass index lower than 25 (weight in kilograms divided by body surface area in square meters), to achieve and maintain a low total cholesterol and LDL and a high HDL, and to maintain a blood pressure within normal limits. In general, the dietary guidelines emphasize an increased intake of fruits, vegetables, and fish, and decreased intake of fat, cholesterol, and salt. For persons who already have an elevated LDL, the AHA recommends that the upper limit of saturated fat intake be less than 7% of the total daily intake. However, even with strict adherence to the diet, drug therapy is usually necessary. Clinical data suggest

CHART 24-1

Risk Factors in Coronary Heart Disease Other Than Low-Density Lipoproteins

Positive Risk Factors

Age
- Men: ≥45 years
- Women: ≥55 years or premature menopause without estrogen replacement therapy

Family history of premature coronary heart disease (definite myocardial infarction or sudden death before 55 years of age in father or other male first-degree relative, or before 65 years of age in mother or other female first-degree relative)

Current cigarette smoking

Hypertension (≥140/90 mm Hg* or on antihypertensive medication)

Low HDL cholesterol (<40 mg/dL*)

Diabetes mellitus

C-reactive protein (CRP)

Negative Risk Factor

High HDL cholesterol (≥60 mg/dL)

HDL, high-density lipoprotein.
*Confirmed by measurements on several occasions.
(Modified from National Institutes of Health Expert Panel [2001]. *Third Report of the National Cholesterol Program [NCEP] Expert Panel on Detection, Evaluation, and Treatment of High Blood Cholesterol in Adults* [Adult Treatment Panel III]. [NIH Publication No. 01-3670]. Bethesda, MD: National Institutes of Health.)

that drug therapy may be efficacious even for those with normal LDL cholesterol.[14] The Heart Protection Study recently showed cardiovascular benefit from statin therapy (to be discussed) in patients who had a baseline LDL level of less than 100 mg/dL.[14] This also suggests that some of the cardioprotective effects of the statin drugs (to be discussed) are related not just to LDL lowering but also to their antiinflammatory effects.[15,16]

Lipid-lowering drugs ultimately work by affecting cholesterol production, decreasing cholesterol absorption from the intestine, increasing intravascular breakdown, or removing cholesterol from the bloodstream. Drugs that act directly to decrease cholesterol levels also have the beneficial effect of further lowering cholesterol levels by stimulating the production of additional LDL receptors. Unless lipid levels are severely elevated, it is recommended that a minimum of 3 months of intensive diet therapy be undertaken before drug therapy is considered.[11]

Five types of medications are available for treating hypercholesterolemia: 3-hydroxy-3-methylglutaryl coenzyme A (HMG CoA) reductase inhibitors (statins), bile acid–binding resins, cholesterol absorption inhibitor agents, niacin and its congeners, and the fibrates.[9] Inhibitors of HMG CoA reductase (*e.g.,* atorvastatin, rosuvastatin, fluvastatin, lovastatin, pravastatin, simvastatin), a key enzyme in the cholesterol biosynthetic pathway, can reduce or block the hepatic synthesis of cholesterol and are the cornerstone of LDL-reducing therapy. Statins also reduce triglyceride levels.

The bile acid–binding resins (cholestyramine, colestipol, and colesevelam) bind and sequester cholesterol-containing bile acids in the intestine and result in a decrease in serum cholesterol levels, due to increased uptake of cholesterol by the liver to synthesize more bile acids. These agents are typically used as adjuncts to statin therapy for patients requiring further reduction in LDL. The cholesterol absorption inhibitor (ezetimibe) was recently approved by the U.S. Food and Drug Administration (FDA). It interferes with the absorption of cholesterol, and when used as monotherapy, it reduces LDL by 15% to 20%.[9]

Nicotinic acid, a niacin congener, blocks the synthesis and release of VLDL by the liver, thereby lowering not only VLDL levels but also IDL and LDL levels. Nicotinic acid also increases HDL concentrations up to 30%. The fibrates (fenofibrate and gemfibrozil) decrease the synthesis of VLDL from chylomicron fragments and enhance the intravascular lipolysis of VLDL and IDL. The resulting decrease in triglycerides and increase in HDL with these agents are especially important in the treatment of the metabolic syndrome.[9]

ATHEROSCLEROSIS

Atherosclerosis is a type of arteriosclerosis or hardening of the arteries. The term *atherosclerosis,* which comes from the Greek words *atheros* (meaning "gruel" or "paste") and *sclerosis* (meaning "hardness"), denotes the formation of fibrofatty lesions in the intimal lining of the large and medium-sized arteries, such as the aorta and its branches, the coronary arteries, and the large vessels that supply the brain (Fig. 24-5).

Although there has been a gradual decline in deaths from atherosclerosis over the past several decades, CHD remains the leading cause of death among men and women in the United States.[2] The reported decline in death rate probably reflects new and improved methods of medical treatment and improved health care practices resulting from an increased public awareness of the factors that predispose to the development of this disorder. The major complications of atherosclerosis, including ischemic heart disease, stroke, and peripheral vascular disease, account for more than 40% of the deaths in the United States.[17]

Atherosclerosis begins as an insidious process, and clinical manifestations of the disease typically do not become

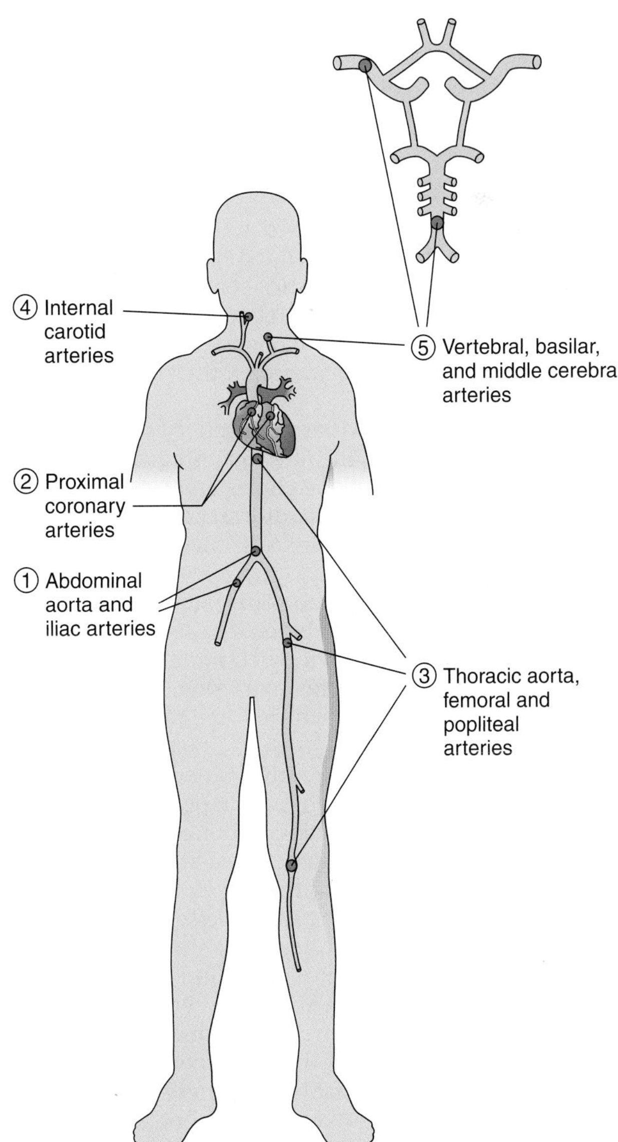

FIGURE 24-5 Sites of severe atherosclerosis in order of frequency. (Rubin E., Farber J. L. [1999]. *Pathology* [3rd ed., p. 508]. Philadelphia: Lippincott-Raven)

evident for 20 to 40 years or longer. Fibrous plaques commonly begin to appear in the arteries of Americans in their 20s. Necropsy findings from 300 American soldiers (average age of 22 years) killed during the Korean War indicated that 77% had gross evidence of atherosclerosis.[18]

Risk Factors

The cause or causes of atherosclerosis have not been determined with certainty. Epidemiologic studies have, however, identified predisposing risk factors, which are listed in Chart 24-1.[3,9,11,15,16,19,20] In terms of health care behaviors, some of these risk factors can be affected by a change in behavior, and others cannot.

The major risk factor for atherosclerosis is hypercholesterolemia. Nonlipid risk factors, such as increasing age, family history of premature CHD, and male sex, cannot be changed. The tendency to the development of atherosclerosis appears to run in families. Persons who come from families with a strong history of heart disease or stroke due to atherosclerosis are at greater risk for developing atherosclerosis than those with a negative family history. Several genetically determined alterations in lipoprotein and cholesterol metabolism have been identified, and it seems likely that others will be identified in the future.[5] The incidence of atherosclerosis increases with age. Other factors being equal, men are at greater risk for developing CHD than are premenopausal women, probably because of the protective effects of natural estrogens. After menopause, the incidence of atherosclerotic-related diseases in women increases, and by the seventh to eighth decade of life, the frequency of myocardial infarction in the two sexes tends to equalize.[7]

The major risk factors that can be affected by a change in health care behaviors include cigarette smoking, obesity, hypertension, high blood cholesterol levels, and diabetes mellitus (traditional cardiovascular risk factors). Cigarette smoking is closely linked with CHD and sudden death. One hypothesis is that components of cigarette smoke may be toxic, causing oxidative insult and damage to the endothelial lining of blood vessels.[21] Endothelial dysfunction may be worsened by cigarette smoke, which is why cessation of smoking by high-risk individuals often is followed within a few years by reduced risk for ischemic heart disease.

Obesity, type 2 diabetes, high blood pressure, and high blood cholesterol levels often can be controlled with a change in health care behaviors and medications. There is evidence that elevated serum cholesterol not only contributes to development of atherosclerotic lesions that block arteries but also interferes with vessel relaxation.[21,22] Observational research indicates that a linear relation exists between serum cholesterol levels and coronary heart disease; a 10% decrease in serum cholesterol is associated with a 20% decrease in coronary heart disease.[23]

However, not all atherothrombotic vascular disease can be explained by the established genetic and environmental risk factors. Other, so-called nontraditional, cardiovascular risk factors can be associated with an increased risk for developing atherosclerosis, including C-reactive protein (CRP), serum homocysteine, serum lipoprotein (a), infectious agents, and endothelial dysfunction.

Considerable interest in the role of inflammation in the etiology of atherosclerosis has emerged during the past few years.[9,15,16,19,20] In particular, CRP is now considered a major risk factor marker.[24,25] CRP is a serum marker for systemic inflammation (see Chapter 20). Several prospective studies have indicated that elevated CRP levels are associated with vascular disease. The pathophysiologic role of CRP in atherosclerosis has not yet been defined. Measurement of high-sensitivity CRP (hs-CRP) may be a better predictor of cardiovascular risk than lipid measurement alone.[25] Indeed, approximately 50% of myocardial infarction patients have a normal LDL.[15] In the Heart Protection study, statin therapy decreased cardiovascular complications even in patients with normal LDL. This was thought to be due to the antiinflammatory effects of these agents. Inflammation (as assessed by a decrease in hs-CRP) can be reduced by using certain lifestyle changes and by drugs (including statins, fibrates, and thiazolidinediones [glitazones]). Because CRP is an acute-phase reactant, major infections, trauma, or acute hospitalization can elevate CRP levels (usually 100-fold or more). CRP levels to determine cardiovascular risk should be performed when the patient is clinically stable. If the level remains markedly elevated, an alternative source of systemic inflammation should be considered.[25]

Homocysteine is derived from the metabolism of dietary methionine, an amino acid that is abundant in animal protein. The normal metabolism of homocysteine requires adequate levels of folate, vitamin B_6, vitamin B_{12}, and riboflavin. Evidence is growing that an increased plasma level of homocysteine (>15 μmol/L) is an independent and dose-related risk factor for development of atherosclerosis. Homocysteine inhibits elements of the anticoagulant cascade and is associated with endothelial damage, which is thought to be an important first step in the development of atherosclerosis.[3,20,26] Factors tending to increase plasma levels of homocysteine include lower serum levels of folate and vitamins B_6 and B_{12}, genetic defects in homocysteine metabolism, renal impairment, malignancies, increasing age, male sex, and menopause.[13,26] Supplementation with folic acid, vitamin B_6, and vitamin B_{12} to decrease plasma homocysteine levels can be used, especially in persons with premature cardiovascular disease.[26]

Lipoprotein (a) is similar to LDL in composition and is an independent risk factor for the development of premature CHD in men. Lipoprotein (a) can cause atherosclerosis by binding to macrophages through a high-affinity receptor that promotes foam cell formation and the deposition of cholesterol in atherosclerotic plaques. Lipoprotein (a) levels should be determined in persons who have premature coronary artery disease or a positive family history.[20] There also has been increased interest in the possible connection between infectious agents (*Chlamydia pneumoniae,* herpesvirus hominis, cytomegalovirus) and the development of vascular disease. The presence of these organisms in atheromatous lesions has been demonstrated by immunocytochemistry, but no cause-and-effect relationship has been established. The organisms may play a role in atherosclerotic development by initiating and enhancing the inflammatory response.[27]

Of recent interest is the role of endothelial dysfunction as a key variable in the pathogenesis of atherosclerosis and its complications. Endothelial function reflects a balance between factors such as nitric oxide (NO), which promotes vasodilatation and inhibits inflammation and vascular smooth muscle proliferation, and endothelial-derived contracting factors, which increase shear stress and promote the development of atherosclerosis.[21] Current evidence suggests that endothelial status is not determined solely by individual risk factor such as lipids, hypertension, and smoking, but by an integrated index of all the atherogenic and atheroprotective factors present in an individual, including known and as yet unknown variables and genetic predisposition.

Mechanisms of Development

The lesions associated with atherosclerosis are of three types: the fatty streak, the fibrous atheromatous plaque, and the complicated lesion. The latter two are responsible for the clinically significant manifestations of the disease.

Fatty streaks are thin, flat, yellow intimal discolorations that progressively enlarge by becoming thicker and slightly elevated as they grow in length (Fig. 24-6). Histologically, they consist of macrophages and smooth muscle cells that have become distended with lipid to form foam cells. Fatty streaks are present in children, often in the first year of life.[3,7] This occurs regardless of geographic setting, sex, or race. They increase in number until about 20 years of age and then remain static or regress. There is controversy about whether fatty streaks, in and of themselves, are precursors of atherosclerotic lesions.

The *fibrous atheromatous plaque* is the basic lesion of clinical atherosclerosis. It is characterized by the accumulation of intracellular and extracellular lipids, proliferation of vascular smooth muscle cells, and formation of scar tissue. The lesions begin as a gray to pearly white elevated thickening of the vessel intima with a core of extracellular lipid (mainly cholesterol, which usually is complexed to proteins) covered by a fibrous cap of connective tissue and smooth muscle (Fig. 24-7). As the lesions increase in size, they encroach on the lumen of the artery and eventually may occlude the vessel or predispose to thrombus formation, causing a reduction of blood flow.

The more advanced and complicated lesions contain hemorrhage, ulceration, and scar tissue deposits. Thrombosis is the most important complication of atherosclerosis. It is caused by slowing and turbulence of blood flow in the region of the plaque and ulceration of the plaque. The thrombus may cause occlusion of small vessels in the heart and brain. Aneurysms may develop in arteries weakened by extensive plaque formation.

Although the risk factors associated with atherosclerosis have been identified through epidemiologic studies, many unanswered questions remain regarding the mechanisms by which these risk factors contribute to the development of atherosclerosis. The vascular endothelial layer, which consists of a single layer of cells with cell-to-cell attachments, normally serves as a selective barrier that protects the subendothelial layers by interacting with blood cells and other blood components. One hypothesis of plaque formation suggests that injury to the endothelial vessel layer is the initiating factor in the development of atherosclerosis[3,7] (Fig. 24-8). A number of factors are regarded as possible injurious agents, including products associated with smoking, immune mechanisms, and mechanical stress such as that associated with hypertension. The fact that atherosclerotic lesions tend to form where vessels branch or where there is turbulent flow suggests that hemodynamic factors also play a role.

Hyperlipidemia, particularly LDL with its high cholesterol content, is also believed to play an active role in the pathogenesis of the atherosclerotic lesion. Interactions between the endothelial layer of the vessel wall and white blood cells, particularly the monocytes (blood macrophages), normally occur throughout life; these interactions increase when blood cholesterol levels are elevated. One

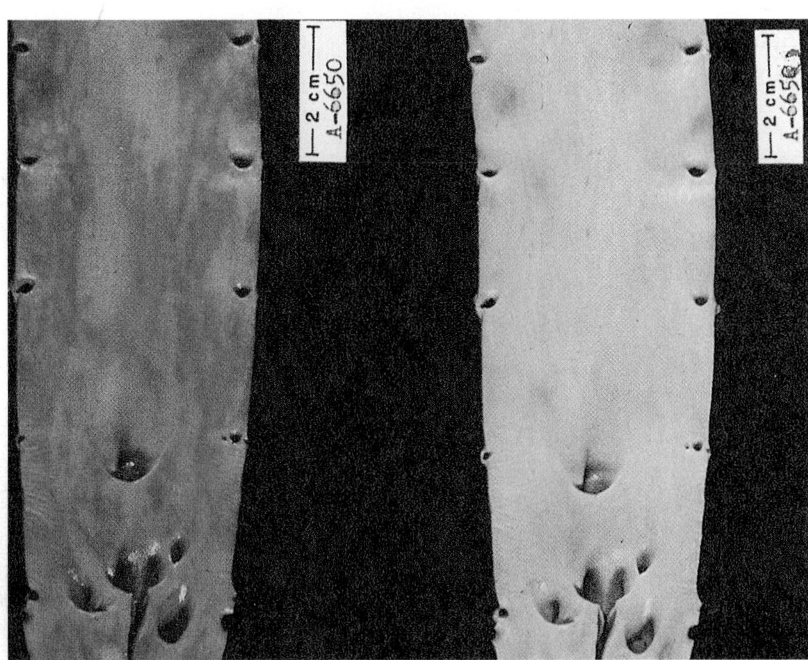

FIGURE 24-6 Fatty streaks of atherosclerosis. The aorta of a young man shows numerous fatty streaks on the luminal surface when stained with Sudan red. (Rubin E., Farber J. L. [1999]. *Pathology* [3rd ed., p. 496]. Philadelphia: Lippincott-Raven)

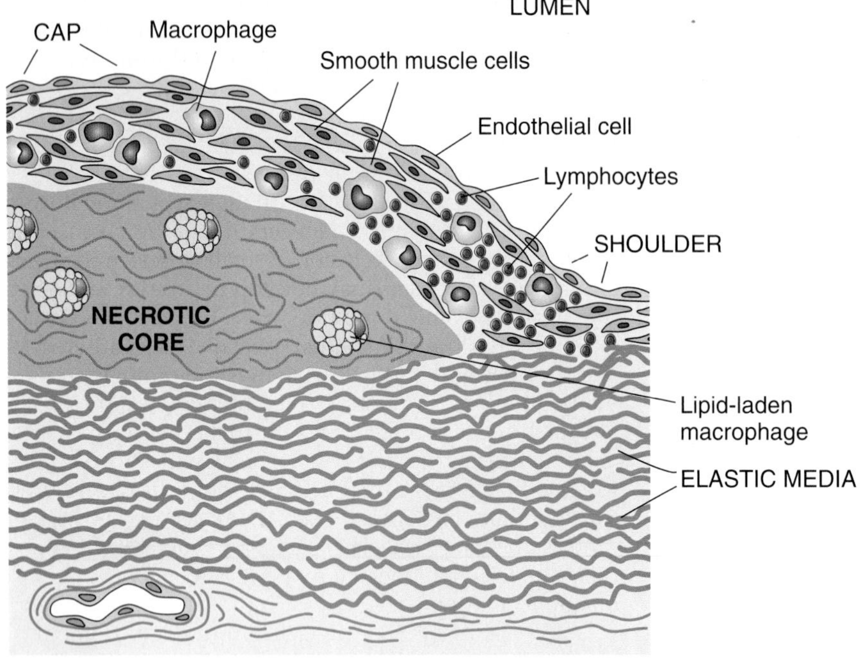

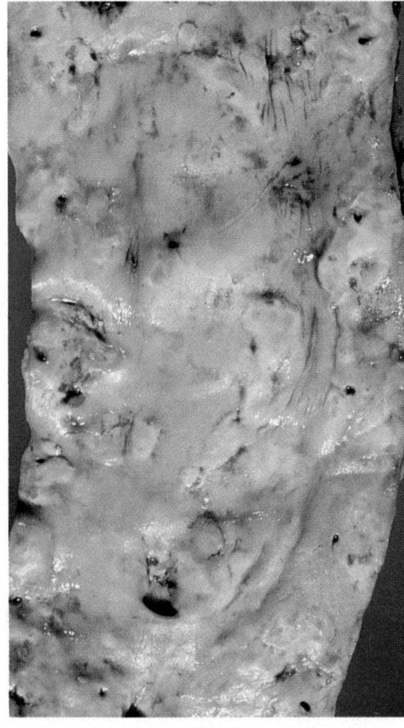

FIGURE 24-7 Fibrofatty plaque of atherosclerosis. (**A**) In this fully developed fibrous plaque, the core contains lipid-filled macrophages and necrotic smooth muscle cell debris. The "fibrous" cap is composed largely of smooth muscle cells, which produce collagen, small amounts of elastin, and glycosaminoglycans. Also shown are infiltrating macrophages and lymphocytes. Note that the endothelium over the surface of the fibrous cap frequently appears intact. (**B**) The aorta shows discrete raised, tan plaques. Focal plaque ulcerations are also evident. (Rubin E., Farber J. L. [1999]. *Pathology* [3rd ed., p. 497]. Philadelphia: Lippincott-Raven)

of the earliest responses to elevated cholesterol levels is the attachment of monocytes to the endothelium[24] (see Fig. 24-8). The monocytes have been observed to emigrate through the cell-to-cell attachments of the endothelial layer into the subendothelial spaces, where they are transformed into macrophages.

Activated macrophages release free radicals that oxidize LDL. Oxidized LDL is toxic to the endothelium, causing endothelial loss and exposure of the subendothelial tissue to blood components. This leads to platelet adhesion and aggregation and fibrin deposition. Platelets and activated macrophages release various factors that are thought to promote growth factors that modulate the proliferation of smooth muscle cells and deposition of extracellular matrix in the lesions[3,7] (see Fig. 24-8). Activated macrophages also ingest oxidized LDL to become foam cells, which are

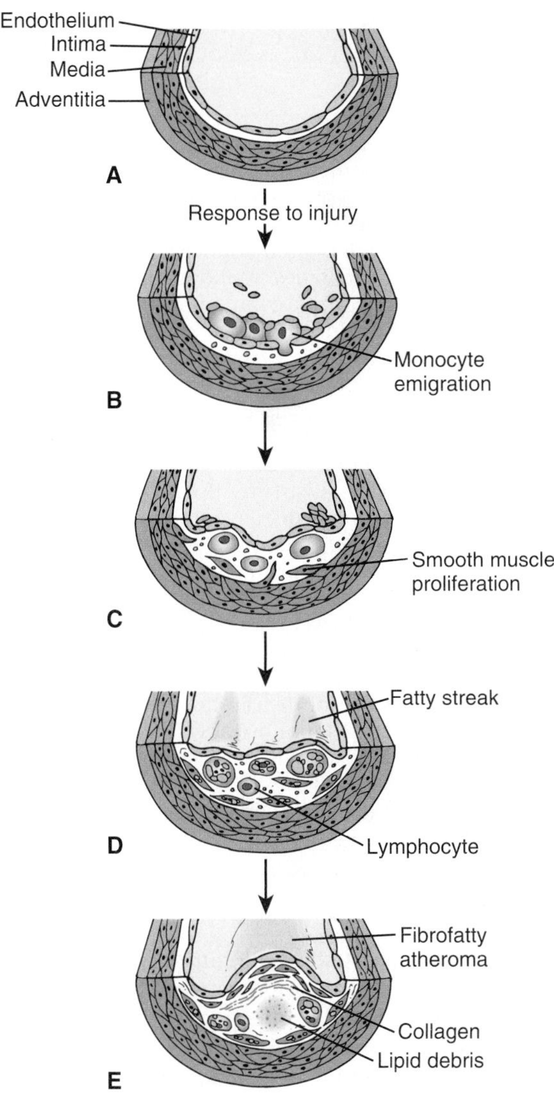

FIGURE 24-8 Response to injury hypothesis: (**A**) normal, (**B**) endothelial dysfunction (*e.g.,* increased permeability and leukocyte adhesion) with monocyte emigration and platelet adhesion, (**C**) smooth muscle cell emigration from the media into the intima, (**D**) macrophage engulfment of lipid and accumulation of lipids in the intima, (**E**) smooth muscle proliferation, collagen and other extracellular matrix deposition, and development of atheromatous plaque with a lipid core. (Modified from Kumar V., Cotran R. S., Robbins S. L. [2003]. *Robbins basic pathology* [7th ed., p. 335]. Philadelphia: W. B. Saunders, with permission from Elsevier Science)

present in all stages of atherosclerotic plaque formation. Lipids released from necrotic foam cells accumulate to form the lipid core of unstable plaques. Unstable plaques typically have features of endothelial erosion (plaque erosion) or fissuring (plaque fissuring), or the presence of fresh thrombosis. They are characterized histologically by a large central lipid core, inflammatory infiltrate, and a thin fibrous cap.[28] These "vulnerable plaques" are at risk for rupture (plaque rupture), often at the shoulder of the plaque (see Fig. 24-7A) where the fibrous cap is thinnest (due to the presence of local inflammatory cells and mediators that degrade the cap) and the mechanical stresses highest.[24] Thus, "active" atherosclerosis is associated with evidence of inflammation both systemically (which can be assessed using hs-CRP) and at the level of the arterial wall.

Clinical Manifestations

The clinical manifestations of atherosclerosis depend on the vessels involved and the extent of vessel obstruction. Atherosclerotic lesions produce their effects through narrowing of the vessel and production of ischemia; sudden vessel obstruction due to plaque hemorrhage or rupture; thrombosis and formation of emboli resulting from damage to the vessel endothelium; and aneurysm formation due to weakening of the vessel wall.[7] In larger vessels, such as the aorta, the important complications are those of thrombus formation and weakening of the vessel wall. In medium-sized arteries, such as the coronary and cerebral arteries, ischemia and infarction due to vessel occlusion are more common. Although atherosclerosis can affect any organ or tissue, the arteries supplying the heart, brain, kidneys, lower extremities, and small intestine are most frequently involved.

VASCULITIS

The vasculitides are a group of vascular disorders that cause inflammatory injury and necrosis of the blood vessel wall (*i.e.,* vasculitis). The vasculitides, which are a common pathway for tissue and organ involvement in many different disease conditions, involve the endothelial cells and smooth muscle cells of the arterial wall.[29,30] Vessels of any type (arteries, veins, and capillaries) in virtually any organ can be affected. Because they may affect veins and capillaries, the terms *vasculitis, angiitis,* and *arteritis* often are used interchangeably. Clinical manifestations often include fever, myalgia, arthralgia, and malaise. Vasculitis may result from direct injury to the vessel, infectious agents, or immune processes, or may be secondary to other disease states such as systemic lupus erythematosus. Physical agents such as cold (*i.e.,* frostbite), irradiation (*i.e.,* sunburn), mechanical injury, and toxins may secondarily cause vessel damage, often leading to necrosis of the vessels. Small vessel vasculitides are sometimes associated with *antineutrophil cytoplasmic antibodies* (ANCAs). ANCAs are antibodies directed against certain proteins in the cytoplasm of neutrophils. These autoantibodies may cause endothelial damage.[3] Serum ANCA titers, which can correlate with disease activity, may serve as a useful quantitative diagnostic marker for these disorders.

The vasculitides are commonly classified based on etiology, pathologic findings, and prognosis. One classification system divides the conditions into three groups: (1) small vessel, (2) medium-sized vessel, and (3) large vessel vasculitides[3,7] (Table 24-3). Small vessel refers to small arteries (ANCA-associated disease only), arterioles, venules, and capillaries; medium vessels refer to medium-sized and small arteries and arterioles; and large vessel refers to the aorta and its major tributaries. The small vessel vasculitides are involved in a number of different diseases, most of which are mediated by type III immune complex hypersensitivity reaction (see Chapter 21). They

TABLE 24-3 Classification of the Vasculitides

Group	Examples	Characteristics
Small vessel vasculitis	Microscopic polyangiitis	Necrotizing vasculitis with few or no immune deposits affecting medium and small blood vessels, including capillaries, venules, arterioles; necrotizing glomerulonephritis and involvement of the pulmonary capillaries is common.
	Wegener granulomatosis	Granulomatous inflammation involving the respiratory tract and necrotizing vasculitis affecting capillaries, venules, arterioles, and arteries; necrotizing glomerulonephritis common.
	Churg-Strauss syndrome	Eosinophil-rich and granulomatous inflammation involving the respiratory tract and necrotizing vasculitis affecting small to medium-sized vessels associated with asthma and blood eosinophilia.
Medium-sized vessel vasculitis	Polyarteritis nodosa	Necrotizing inflammation of medium-sized or small arteries without vasculitis in arteries, capillaries, or venules; usually associated with underlying disease or environmental agents.
	Kawasaki disease	Involves large, medium-sized, and small arteries (frequently the coronaries) and is associated with mucocutaneous lymph node syndrome. Usually occurs in small children.
	Thromboangiitis obliterans	Segmental, thrombosing, acute and chronic inflammation of the medium-sized and small arteries, principally the tibial and radial arteries, sometimes extending to the veins and nerves of the extremities; occurs almost exclusively in men who are heavy smokers.
Large vessel vasculitis	Giant cell (temporal) arteritis	Granulomatous inflammation of aorta and its major branches with predilection for extracranial vessels of the carotid artery; infiltration of vessel wall with giant cells and mononuclear cells; usually occurs in people older than 50 years and is often associated with polymyalgia rheumatica.
	Takayasu arteritis	Granulomatous inflammation of the aorta and its branches; usually occurs in people younger than 50 years.

commonly involve the skin and are often a complication of an underlying disease (*i.e.,* vasculitis associated with neoplasms or connective tissue disease) and exposure to environmental agents (*i.e.,* serum sickness and urticarial vasculitis). ANCA-positive small vessel vasculitides include microscopic polyangiitis, Wegener's granulomatosis, and Churg-Strauss syndrome. These ANCA-positive vasculitides are treated by similar regimens.[31]

Medium-sized vessel vasculitides produce necrotizing damage to medium-sized muscular arteries of major organ systems. This group includes polyarteritis nodosa, Kawasaki disease (discussed in Chapter 26), and thromboangiitis obliterans (discussed in the section on arterial diseases of the extremities). Large vessel vasculitides involve large elastic arteries. They include giant cell (temporal) arteritis, polymyalgia rheumatica (discussed in Chapter 59), and Takayasu arteritis. The following discussion focuses on two of the vasculitides: polyarteritis nodosa and giant cell (temporal) arteritis.

Polyarteritis Nodosa

Polyarteritis nodosa, so named because of the numerous nodules found along the course of muscular arteries, is a primary multisystem inflammatory disease of smaller and medium-sized blood vessels, especially those of the kidney, liver, intestine, peripheral nerve, skin, and muscle. The disease is seen more commonly in men than women.

The cause of polyarteritis nodosa remains unknown. It can occur in drug abusers and may be associated with use of certain drugs such as allopurinol and the sulfonamides. There is an association between polyarteritis nodosa and hepatitis B and C infection, with 10% to 30% of persons with the disease having antibodies to hepatitis B or C in their serum. Other associations include serous otitis media, hairy cell leukemia, and hyposensitization therapy for allergies. Persons with connective tissue diseases such as systemic lupus erythematosus, rheumatoid arthritis, and primary Sjögren's syndrome may have manifestations similar to those of primary polyarteritis nodosa.

The onset of polyarteritis nodosa usually is abrupt, with complaints of anorexia, weight loss, fever, and fatigue often accompanied by signs of organ involvement. The kidney is the most frequently affected organ, and hypertension is a common manifestation of the disorder. Gastrointestinal involvement may manifest as abdominal pain, nausea, vomiting, or diarrhea. Myalgia, arthralgia, and arthritis are common, as are peripheral neuropathies such as paresthesias, pain, and weakness. Central nervous system complications include thrombotic and hemorrhagic stroke. Cardiac manifestations result from involvement of the coronary arteries. Skin lesions also may occur and are highly variable. They include reddish blue, mottled areas of discoloration of the skin of the extremities called *livedo reticularis,* purpura (*i.e.,* black and blue discoloration from bleeding into the skin), urticaria (*i.e.,* hives), and ulcers.

Laboratory findings, although variable, include an elevated erythrocyte sedimentation rate, leukocytosis, anemia, and signs of organ involvement such as hematuria and abnormal liver function tests. The diagnosis is confirmed through biopsy specimens demonstrating necrotizing vasculitis of the small and large arteries. Treatment involves use of high-dose corticosteroid therapy and often cytotoxic immunosuppressant agents (*e.g.*, azathioprine, cyclophosphamide). Before the availability of corticosteroids and immunosuppressive agents, the disease commonly was fatal. With the use of these agents, the 5-year survival rate is greater than 50%.[32] After the disease is under control, treatment usually is continued for 18 to 24 months and then gradually tapered.[29]

Giant Cell Temporal Arteritis

Temporal arteritis (*i.e.*, giant cell arteritis), the most common of the vasculitides, is a focal inflammatory condition of medium-sized and large arteries. It predominantly affects branches of arteries originating from the aortic arch, including the superficial temporal, vertebral, ophthalmic, and posterior ciliary arteries. The disorder progresses to involve the entire artery wall with focal necrosis and granulomatous inflammation involving multinucleated giant cells. It is more common in elderly persons, with a 2:1 female-to-male ratio. The cause is unknown, although an autoimmune origin has been suggested.[33]

The disorder often is insidious in onset and may be heralded by the sudden onset of headache, tenderness over the artery, swelling and redness of the overlying skin, blurred vision or diplopia, and facial pain. Almost one half of affected persons have systemic involvement in the form of polymyalgia rheumatica. Up to 10% of patients with giant cell arteritis go on to develop aortic aneurysm (especially thoracic).

Diagnosis is based on the clinical manifestations, a characteristically elevated erythrocyte sedimentation rate and CRP, and temporal artery biopsy. Treatment includes use of high-dose corticosteroids. Before persons with the disorder were treated with corticosteroids, blindness developed in almost 80% of cases due to involvement of the posterior ciliary artery.

ARTERIAL DISEASE OF THE EXTREMITIES

Disorders of the circulation in the extremities often are referred to as *peripheral vascular disorders*. In many respects, the disorders that affect arteries in the extremities are the same as those affecting the coronary and cerebral arteries in that they produce ischemia, pain, impaired function, and in some cases infarction and tissue necrosis. Not only are the effects similar, but also the pathologic conditions that impair circulation in the extremities are identical. This section focuses on acute arterial occlusion of the extremities, atherosclerotic occlusive disease, thromboangiitis obliterans, and Raynaud's disease and Raynaud's phenomenon.

Acute Arterial Occlusion

Acute arterial occlusion is a sudden event that interrupts arterial flow to the affected tissues or organ. Most acute arterial occlusions are the result of an embolus or a thrombus. Rarely, the tips of catheters that have been inserted into a vessel can break off and become emboli. Although much less common than emboli and thrombus, trauma or arterial spasm caused by arterial cannulation can be another cause of acute arterial occlusion.

An embolus is a freely moving particle such as a blood clot that breaks loose and travels in the larger vessels of the circulation until lodging in a smaller vessel and occluding blood flow. Most emboli arise in the heart and are caused by conditions that cause blood clots to develop on the wall of a heart chamber or valve surface. Emboli usually are a complication of heart disease: ischemic heart disease with or without infarction, atrial fibrillation, or rheumatic heart disease. Prosthetic heart valves can be another source of emboli. Other types of emboli are fat emboli that originate from bone marrow of fractured bones, air emboli from the lung, and amniotic fluid emboli that develop during childbirth. Acute arterial embolism is associated with a 5% to 25% risk for affected limb loss and a 25% to 30% increase in hospital mortality. Heart disease is responsible for more than half of these deaths.

A thrombus is a blood clot that forms on the wall of a vessel and continues to grow until reaching a size that obstructs blood flow. These thrombi often arise as the result of erosion or rupture of the fibrous cap of an arteriosclerotic plaque.

Manifestations. The signs and symptoms of acute arterial occlusion depend on the artery involved and the adequacy of the collateral circulation. Emboli tend to lodge in bifurcations of the major arteries, including the aorta and iliac, femoral, and popliteal arteries. The presentation of acute arterial embolism is often described as that of the seven Ps: (1) pistol shot (acute onset); (2) pallor; (3) polar (cold); (4) pulselessness; (5) pain; (6) paresthesia; and (7) paralysis. Occlusion in an extremity causes sudden onset of acute pain with numbness, tingling, weakness, pallor, and coldness. There often is a sharp line of demarcation between the oxygenated tissue above the line of obstruction and that below the line of obstruction. Pulses are absent below the level of the occlusion. These changes are followed rapidly by cyanosis, mottling, and loss of sensory, reflex, and motor function. Tissue death occurs unless blood flow is restored.

Diagnosis and Treatment. Diagnosis of acute arterial occlusion is based on signs of impaired blood flow. It uses visual assessment, palpation of pulses, and methods to assess blood flow. Treatment of acute arterial occlusion is aimed at restoring blood flow. An embolectomy—surgical removal of the embolus—is the optimal therapy when a large artery is occluded.

Thrombolytic therapy (*i.e.*, streptokinase or tissue plasminogen activator) may be used in an attempt to dissolve the clot. Anticoagulant therapy (*i.e.*, heparin) usually is given to prevent extension of the embolus and to prevent progression of the original thrombus. Application of cold should be avoided, and the extremity should be protected from injury resulting from hard surfaces and overlying bedclothes.

Atherosclerotic Occlusive Disease

Atherosclerosis is an important cause of peripheral vascular disease (PVD) and is seen most commonly in the vessels of the lower extremities. The condition is sometimes referred

CLINICAL APPLICATION

Assessment of Arterial Flow in the Extremities

The methods for assessing arterial blood flow and detecting arterial disease include monitoring of capillary refill time and peripheral pulses. Angiography, Doppler ultrasound flow studies, and magnetic resonance imaging (MRI) may be used for a more definitive diagnosis.

Capillary refill time is an indicator of the efficiency of the microcirculation. It is measured by depressing the nail bed of a finger or toe until the underlying skin blanches. The refill time is normal if the capillary vessels refill within 3 seconds after pressure is released. The volume of the peripheral pulses and capillary refill time are useful indirect methods for assessing peripheral perfusion. Peripheral pulses can be palpated over vessels in the head, neck (*i.e.*, carotid), and extremities. In situations associated with potential vessel spasm or thrombosis, it may be necessary to check only for the presence of pulses. In many situations, however, the pulse volume (weak and thready to strong and bounding) provides useful information about vascular volume and the condition of the arterial circulation. Arterial auscultation is used to listen to the flow of blood with a stethoscope. The term *bruit* is used to describe an audible murmur heard over a peripheral artery. It is caused by turbulent blood flow and is suggestive of obstructive arterial disease.

Doppler ultrasound flow studies use reflected ultrasound waves, which are transmitted back to the skin surface from a blood vessel, to determine the direction and velocity of blood flow. Doppler studies can be used to assess the patency of a given blood vessel. They are useful in studying blood flow in the carotid arteries, abdominal vessels, fetal blood vessels, and peripheral blood vessels.

MRI is a noninvasive technique that can be used to study blood flow. The method uses a magnetic field to align the charges on blood components as they move through blood vessels. The aligned charges emit measurable radiofrequency signals, which can be detected electronically and recorded.

to as *arteriosclerosis obliterans.* The superficial femoral and popliteal arteries are the most commonly affected vessels. When lesions develop in the lower leg and foot, the tibial, common peroneal, or pedal vessels are the arteries most commonly affected. The disease is seen most commonly in men in their 60s and 70s.[34–36] At least one in five of the population older than 65 years of age has PVD.[36] The risk factors for this disorder are similar to those for atherosclerosis. Cigarette smoking contributes to the progress of the atherosclerosis of the lower extremities and to the development of symptoms of ischemia. Persons with diabetes mellitus develop more extensive and rapidly progressive vascular disease than do nondiabetic individuals.

Manifestations. As with atherosclerosis in other locations, the signs and symptoms of vessel occlusion are gradual. Usually, there is at least a 50% narrowing of the vessel before symptoms of ischemia arise. The primary symptom of chronic obstructive arterial disease is *intermittent claudication* or pain with walking.[34,36] Typically, persons with the disorder complain of calf pain because the gastrocnemius muscle has the highest oxygen consumption of any muscle group in the leg during walking. Some persons may complain of a vague aching feeling or numbness, rather than pain. Other activities, such as swimming, bicycling, and climbing stairs, use other muscle groups and may not incite the same degree of discomfort as walking. Intermittent claudication affects at least 1 in 20 people older than 65 years of age.[36] Other signs of ischemia include atrophic changes and thinning of the skin and subcutaneous tissues of the lower leg and diminution in the size of the leg muscles. The foot often is cool, and the popliteal and pedal pulses are weak or absent. Limb color blanches with elevation of the leg because of the effects of gravity on perfusion pressure and becomes deep red when the leg is in the dependent position because of an autoregulatory increase in blood flow and a gravitational increase in perfusion pressure.

When blood flow is reduced to the extent that it no longer meets the minimal needs of resting muscle and nerves, ischemic pain at rest, ulceration, and gangrene develop. As tissue necrosis develops, there typically is severe pain in the region of skin breakdown, which is worse at night with limb elevation and is improved with standing.[34]

Diagnosis and Treatment. Diagnostic methods include inspection of the limbs for signs of chronic low-grade ischemia such as subcutaneous atrophy, brittle toenails, hair loss, pallor, coolness, or dependent rubor. Palpation of the femoral, popliteal, posterior tibial, and dorsalis pedis pulses allows for an estimation of the level and degree of obstruction. The ratio of ankle-to-arm (*i.e.*, tibial and brachial arteries) systolic blood pressure is used to detect significant obstruction, with a ratio of less than 0.9 indicating occlusion. Normally, systolic pressure in the ankle exceeds that in the brachial artery because systolic pressure and pulse pressure tend to increase as the pressure wave moves away from the heart (see Chapter 31). Blood pressures may be taken at various levels on the leg to determine the level of obstruction. A Doppler ultrasound stethoscope may be used for detecting pulses and measuring blood pressure. Ultrasound imaging, magnetic resonance imaging (MRI) arteriography, spiral computed tomography (CT) arteriography, and invasive contrast angiography may also be used as diagnostic methods.[34–36]

The two goals of treatment in persons with PVD are (1) to decrease their considerable cardiovascular risk and (2) to reduce symptoms. Patients should be evaluated for coexisting coronary and cerebrovascular atherosclerosis. The risk for death, mainly from coronary and cerebrovascular events, is high (5% to 10% per year).[36] The other cardiovascular risk factors that should be addressed include smoking cessation, hypertension, lipid lowering, and diabetes. Antiplatelet agents (aspirin, clopidogrel, or both) reduce vascular death in patients with PVD by about 25%.[36] Other medications that are useful include angiotensin-converting enzyme (ACE) inhibitors (even in normotensive patients), cilostazol (a phosphodiesterase inhibitor), and pentoxifylline (an adenosine diphosphate [ADP] receptor antagonist). The tissues of extremities affected by atherosclerosis are easily injured and slow to heal. Treatment includes measures directed at protection of the affected tissues and preservation of functional capacity. Walking (slowly) to the point of claudication usually is encouraged because it increases collateral circulation.

Percutaneous or surgical intervention is typically reserved for the patient with disabling claudication or limb-threatening ischemia. Surgery (*i.e.,* femoropopliteal bypass grafting using a section of saphenous vein) may be indicated in severe cases. In persons with diabetes, the peroneal arteries between the knees and ankles commonly are involved, making revascularization difficult. Thromboendarterectomy with removal of the occluding core of atherosclerotic tissue may be done if the section of diseased vessel is short. Percutaneous transluminal angioplasty and stent placement, in which a balloon catheter is inserted into the area of stenosis and the balloon inflated to increase vessel diameter, is another form of treatment.[34–36]

Thromboangiitis Obliterans

Thromboangiitis obliterans, or Buerger's disease, is an inflammatory (*i.e.,* vasculitis) arterial disorder that causes thrombus formation. The disorder affects the medium-sized arteries, usually the plantar and digital vessels in the foot and lower leg. Arteries in the arm and hand also may be affected. Although primarily an arterial disorder, the inflammatory process often extends to involve adjacent veins and nerves. Usually it is a disease of men between the ages of 25 and 40 years who are heavy cigarette smokers, but it is now also being reported with increasing frequency in young female smokers. The pathogenesis of Buerger's disease remains speculative, although cigarette smoking and in some instances tobacco chewing seem to be involved. It has been suggested that the tobacco may trigger an immune response in susceptible persons or may unmask a clotting defect, either of which could incite an inflammatory reaction of the vessel wall.[37]

Manifestations. Pain is the predominant symptom of the disorder. It usually is related to distal arterial ischemia. During the early stages of the disease, there is intermittent claudication in the arch of the foot and the digits. In severe cases, pain is present even when the person is at rest. The impaired circulation increases sensitivity to cold. The peripheral pulses are diminished or absent, and there are changes in the color of the extremity. In moderately advanced cases, the extremity becomes cyanotic when the person assumes a dependent position, and the digits may turn reddish blue even when in a nondependent position. With lack of blood flow, the skin assumes a thin, shiny look, and hair growth and skin nutrition suffer. Chronic ischemia causes thick, malformed nails. If the disease continues to progress, tissues eventually ulcerate, and gangrenous changes arise that may necessitate amputation.

Diagnosis and Treatment. Diagnostic methods are similar to those for atherosclerotic disease of the lower extremities. As part of the treatment program for thromboangiitis obliterans, it is mandatory that the person stop smoking cigarettes or using tobacco. Even passive smoking and nicotine replacement therapy should be eliminated. Other treatment measures are of secondary importance and focus on methods for producing vasodilation and preventing tissue injury. Sympathectomy may be done to alleviate the vasospastic manifestations of the disease.

Raynaud's Disease and Phenomenon

Raynaud's disease or phenomenon is a functional disorder caused by intense vasospasm of the arteries and arterioles in the fingers and, less often, the toes. This is a common disorder affecting 10% of the population. The disorder is divided into two types: the primary type, called *Raynaud's disease,* occurs without demonstrable cause, and the secondary type, called *Raynaud's phenomenon,* is associated with other disease states or known causes of vasospasm.[38–40]

Vasospasm implies an excessive vasoconstrictor response to stimuli that normally produce only moderate vasoconstriction. In contrast to other regional circulations that are supplied by vasodilator and vasoconstrictor fibers, the cutaneous vessels of the fingers and toes are innervated only by sympathetic vasoconstrictor fibers. In these vessels, vasodilation occurs by withdrawal of sympathetic stimulation. Cooling of specific body parts such as the head, neck, and trunk produces a sympathetic-mediated reduction in digital blood flow, as does emotional stress.

Raynaud's disease is seen in otherwise healthy young women, and it often is precipitated by exposure to cold or by strong emotions and usually is limited to the fingers. It also follows a more benign course than Raynaud's phenomenon, seldom causing tissue necrosis. The cause of vasospasm in primary Raynaud's disease is unknown. Hyperreactivity of the sympathetic nervous system has been suggested as a contributing cause.[38] Raynaud's phenomenon is associated with previous vessel injury such as frostbite, occupational trauma associated with the use of heavy vibrating tools, collagen diseases, neurologic disorders, and chronic arterial occlusive disorders. Another occupation-related cause is the exposure to alternating hot and cold temperatures such as that experienced by butchers and food preparers.[38] Raynaud's phenomenon often is the first symptom of collagen diseases. It occurs in almost 100% of scleroderma cases and can precede the diagnosis of scleroderma by many years.[40]

Manifestations. In Raynaud's disease and Raynaud's phenomenon, ischemia due to vasospasm causes changes in skin color that progress from pallor to cyanosis, a sensation of cold, and changes in sensory perception, such as numbness and tingling. The color changes usually are first noticed in the tips of the fingers, later moving into one or more of the distal phalanges (Fig. 24-9). After the ischemic episode, there is a period of hyperemia with intense redness, throbbing, and paresthesias. The period of hyperemia is followed by a return to normal color. Although all of the fingers usually are affected symmetrically, the involvement may affect only one or two digits. In some cases, only a portion of the digit is affected.

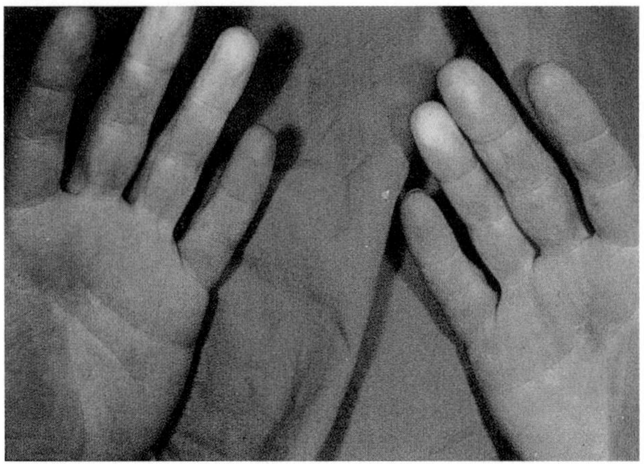

FIGURE 24-9 Raynaud's phenomenon. The tips of the fingers show marked pallor. (Rubin E., Farber J. L. [1999]. *Pathology* [3rd ed., p. 514]. Philadelphia: Lippincott-Raven)

In severe, progressive cases usually associated with Raynaud's phenomenon, trophic changes may develop. The nails may become brittle, and the skin over the tips of the affected fingers may thicken. Nutritional impairment of these structures may give rise to arthritis. Ulceration and superficial gangrene of the fingers, although infrequent, may occur.

Diagnosis and Treatment. The initial diagnosis is based on history of vasospastic attacks supported by other evidence of the disorder. Immersion of the hand in cold water may be used to initiate an attack as an aid to diagnosis. Laser Doppler flow velocimetry may be used to quantify digital blood flow during changes in temperature. Raynaud's disease is differentiated from Raynaud's phenomenon by excluding secondary disorders known to cause vasospasm.[40]

Treatment measures are directed toward eliminating factors that cause vasospasm and protecting the digits from trauma during an ischemic episode. Abstinence from smoking and protection from cold are priorities. The entire body must be protected from cold, not just the extremities. Avoidance of emotional stress is another important factor in controlling the disorder because anxiety and stress may precipitate a vascular spasm in predisposed persons. Biofeedback training may be helpful in persons with Raynaud's disease but does not seem to be as effective for those with Raynaud's phenomenon. Vasoconstrictor medications, such as the decongestants contained in allergy and cold preparations, should be avoided. Treatment with vasodilator drugs may be indicated, particularly if episodes are frequent because frequency encourages the potential for development of thrombosis and gangrene. The calcium channel-blocking drugs (*e.g.*, diltiazem, nifedipine, and nicardipine) decrease the severity and frequency of attacks. Prazosin, an α-adrenergic receptor-blocking drug, also may be used. The selective serotonin reuptake inhibitor (SSRI) fluoxetine may be useful in about 20% of patients. Analogs of prostacyclin (prostaglandin vasodilator) are being investigated as well. Surgical interruption of sympathetic nerve pathways (sympathectomy) may be used for persons with severe symptoms.[40]

ANEURYSMS AND DISSECTION

An *aneurysm* is an abnormal localized dilatation of a blood vessel. Aneurysms can occur in arteries and veins, but they are most common in the aorta. There are two types of aneurysms: true aneurysms and false aneurysms. A *true aneurysm* is one in which the aneurysm is bounded by a complete vessel wall and an increase in diameter of 50%.[41] The blood in a true aneurysm remains within the vascular compartment. A *false aneurysm* or *pseudoaneurysm* represents a localized dissection or tear in the inner wall of the artery with formation of an extravascular hematoma that causes vessel enlargement. Unlike true aneurysms, false aneurysms are bounded only by the outer layers of the vessel wall or supporting tissues.

Aneurysms can assume several forms and may be classified according to their cause, location, and anatomic features (Fig. 24-10). A *berry aneurysm* consists of a small, spherical dilatation of the vessel at a bifurcation.[3] This type of aneurysm usually is found in the circle of Willis in the cerebral circulation. A *fusiform aneurysm* involves the entire circumference of the vessel and is characterized by a gradual and progressive dilatation of the vessel. These aneurysms, which vary in diameter (up to 20 cm) and length, may involve the entire ascending and transverse portions of the thoracic aorta or may extend over large segments of the abdominal aorta. A *saccular aneurysm* extends over part of the circumference of the vessel and appears saclike. A *dissecting aneurysm* is a false aneurysm resulting from a tear in the intimal layer of the vessel that allows blood to enter the vessel wall, dissecting its layers to create a blood-filled cavity.

The weakness that leads to aneurysm formation may be caused by several factors, including congenital defects, trauma, infections, and atherosclerosis. Once initiated, the aneurysm grows larger as the tension in the vessel increases. This is because the tension in the wall of a vessel is equal to the pressure multiplied by the radius (*i.e.*, tension = pressure × radius; see Chapter 23). In this case, the pressure in the segment of the vessel affected by the aneurysm does not change but remains the same as that of adjacent portions of the vessel. As an aneurysm increases in diameter, the tension in the wall of the vessel increases in direct proportion to its increased size. If untreated, the aneurysm may rupture because of the increased tension. Even an unruptured aneurysm can cause damage by exerting pressure on adjacent structures and interrupting blood flow.

Aortic Aneurysms

Aortic aneurysms may involve any part of the aorta: the ascending aorta, aortic arch, descending aorta, thoracoabdominal aorta, or abdominal aorta. Multiple aneurysms may be present. The two most common causes of aortic aneurysms are atherosclerosis and degeneration of the vessel media. Half of the people with aortic aneurysms have hypertension.[3] Population-based studies suggest that up to 9% of persons older than 65 years of age have unsuspected and asymptomatic abdominal aortic aneurysms and that ruptured abdominal aortic aneurysms cause at least 15,000 deaths each year in the United States.[42]

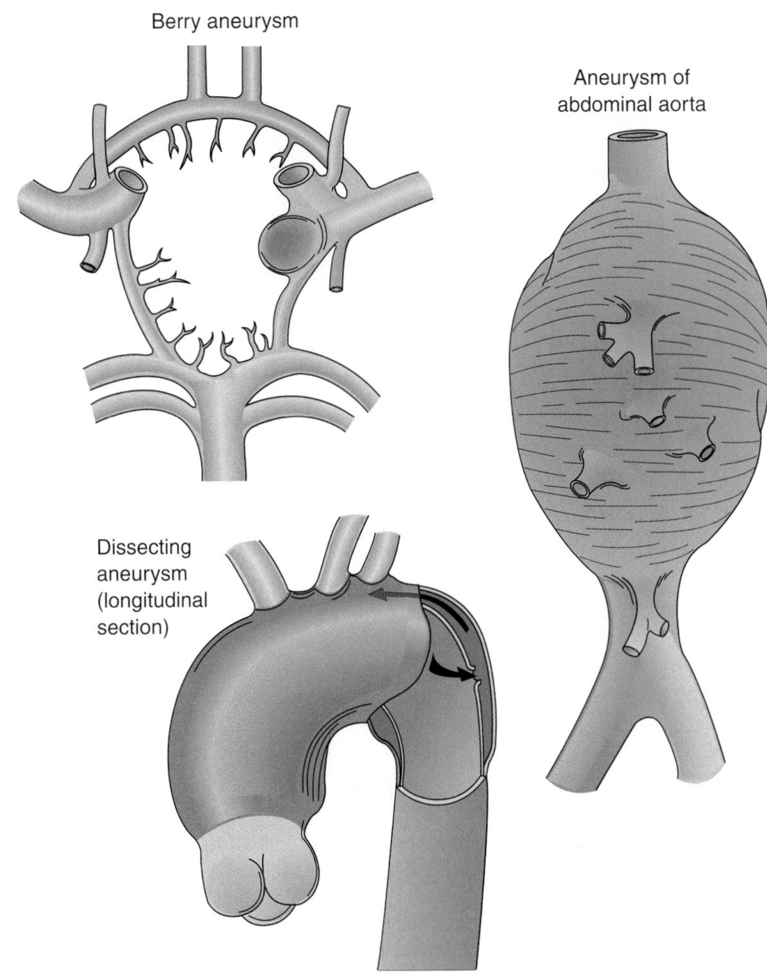

FIGURE 24-10 Three forms of aneurysms—berry aneurysm in the circle of Willis, fusiform-type aneurysm of the abdominal aorta, and a dissecting aortic aneurysm.

Manifestations. The signs and symptoms of aortic aneurysms depend on the size and location. An aneurysm also may be asymptomatic, with the first evidence of its presence being associated with vessel rupture. Aneurysms of the thoracic aorta are less common than abdominal aortic aneurysms. They account for less than 10% of aortic aneurysms and may present with substernal, back, and neck pain. There also may be dyspnea, stridor, or a brassy cough caused by pressure on the trachea. Hoarseness may result from pressure on the recurrent laryngeal nerve, and there may be difficulty swallowing because of pressure on the esophagus.[43] The aneurysm also may compress the superior vena cava, causing distention of neck veins and edema of the face and neck.

Abdominal aortic aneurysms are located most commonly below the level of the renal artery (>90%) and involve the bifurcation of the aorta and proximal end of the common iliac arteries.[3,7] The infrarenal aorta is normally 2 cm in diameter; an aneurysm is defined as an aortic diameter of more than 3 cm. They can involve any part of the vessel circumference (saccular) or extend to involve the entire circumference (fusiform). Most abdominal aneurysms are asymptomatic. Because an aneurysm is of arterial origin, a pulsating mass may provide the first evidence of the disorder. Typically, aneurysms larger than 4 cm are palpable. The mass may be discovered during a routine physical examination, or the affected person may complain of its presence. Calcification, which frequently exists on the wall of the aneurysm, may be detected during abdominal radiologic examination. Pain may be present and varies from mild midabdominal or lumbar discomfort to severe abdominal and back pain. As the aneurysm expands, it may compress the lumbar nerve roots, causing lower back pain that radiates to the posterior aspects of the legs. The aneurysm may extend to and impinge on the renal, iliac, mesenteric, or vertebral arteries that supply the spinal cord. An abdominal aneurysm also may cause erosion of vertebrae. Stasis of blood favors thrombus formation along the wall of the vessel (Fig. 24-11), and peripheral emboli may develop, causing symptomatic arterial insufficiency.

With thoracic and abdominal aneurysms, the most dreaded complication is rupture. The likelihood of rupture correlates with increasing aneurysm size. The risk for rupture rises from less than 2% for small abdominal aneurysms (those less than 4 cm in diameter) to 5% to 10% per year for aneurysms larger than 5 cm in diameter.[7]

Diagnosis and Treatment. Diagnostic methods include use of ultrasound imaging, echocardiography, CT scans, and

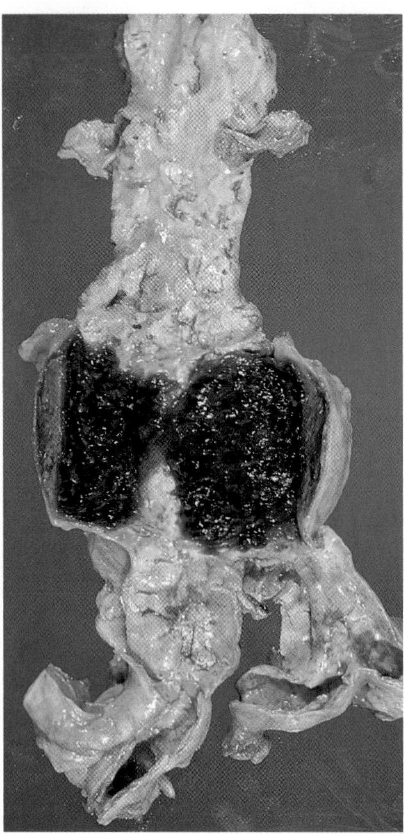

FIGURE 24-11 Atherosclerotic aneurysm of the abdominal aorta. The aneurysm has been opened longitudinally to reveal a large thrombus in the lumen. The aorta and common iliac arteries display complicated lesions of atherosclerosis. (Rubin E., Farber J. L. [1999]. *Pathology* [3rd ed., p. 521]. Philadelphia: Lippincott-Raven)

MRI. Surgical repair, in which the involved section of the aorta is replaced with a synthetic graft of woven Dacron, frequently is the treatment of choice.[41,43]

Aortic Dissection

Aortic dissection (dissecting aneurysm) is an acute, life-threatening condition. It involves hemorrhage into the vessel wall with longitudinal tearing of the vessel wall to form a blood-filled channel. Unlike atherosclerotic aneurysms, aortic dissection often occurs without evidence of previous vessel dilation. The dissection can originate anywhere along the length of the aorta. Two thirds of dissections involve the ascending aorta.[44] The second most common site is the thoracic aorta just distal to the origin of the subclavian artery.

Aortic dissection is caused by conditions that weaken or cause degenerative changes in the elastic and smooth muscle of the layers of the aorta. It is most common in the 40- to 60-year-old age group and more prevalent in men than in women.[7] There are two risk factors that predispose to dissection: hypertension and degeneration of the medial layer of the vessel wall. There is a history of hypertension in most cases.[7] Aortic dissection also is associated with connective tissue diseases, such as Marfan's syndrome. It also may occur during pregnancy because of changes in the aorta that occur during this time. Other factors that predispose to dissection are congenital defects of the aortic valve (*i.e.*, bicuspid or unicuspid valve structures) and aortic coarctation. Aortic dissection is a potential complication of cardiac surgery or catheterization. Surgically related dissection may occur at the points where the aorta has been incised or cross-clamped; it also has been reported at the site where the saphenous vein was sutured to the aorta during coronary artery bypass surgery.

There are several systems for classifying dissecting aortic aneurysms. The Stanford system uses two classifications, type A and type B. Those in the ascending aorta, regardless of the site of the primary tear, are designated type A; and those not involving the ascending aorta are designated type B. Approximately 60% of thoracic aortic dissections are of the type A variety, and 40% are type B. Dissections usually extend distally from the intimal tear. When the ascending aorta is involved, expansion of the wall of the aorta may impair closure of the aortic valve. There also is the risk for aortic rupture with blood moving into the pericardium and compressing the heart. Although the length of dissection varies, it is possible for the abdominal aorta to be involved with progression into the renal, iliac, or femoral arteries. Partial or complete occlusion of the arteries that arise from the aortic arch or the intercostal or lumbar arteries may lead to stroke, ischemic peripheral neuropathy, or impaired blood flow to the spinal cord.

Manifestations. A major symptom of a dissecting aneurysm is the abrupt presence of excruciating pain, described as tearing or ripping. The location of the pain may point to the site of dissection.[7] Pain associated with dissection of the ascending aorta frequently is located in the anterior chest, and pain associated with dissection of the descending aorta often is located in the back. In the early stages, blood pressure typically is moderately or markedly elevated. Later, the blood pressure and the pulse rate become unobtainable in one or both arms as the dissection disrupts arterial flow to the arms. Syncope, hemiplegia, or paralysis of the lower extremities may occur because of occlusion of blood vessels that supply the brain or spinal cord. Heart failure may develop when the aortic valve is involved.

Diagnosis and Treatment. Diagnosis of aortic dissection is based on history and physical examination. Aortic angiography, transesophageal echocardiography, CT scans, and MRI studies aid in the diagnosis.

The treatment of dissecting aortic aneurysm may be medical or surgical. Aortic dissection is a life-threatening emergency situation; persons with a probable diagnosis are stabilized medically even before the diagnosis is confirmed. Two important factors that participate in propagating the dissection are high blood pressure and the steepness of the pulse wave. Without intervention, these forces continue to cause extension of the dissection. Medical treatment therefore focuses on control of hypertension and the use of drugs that lessen the force of systolic blood ejection from the heart. Two commonly used drugs, given in combination, are intravenous sodium nitroprusside and a β-adrenergic receptor blockers. Surgical treatment consists of resection of the involved segment of the aorta and replacement with a prosthetic graft. The mortality rate due to untreated dissecting aneurysm is high, exceeding 50% within the first 48 hours and 80% within 6 weeks.[45]

In summary, the arterial system distributes blood to all the tissues of the body, and lesions of the arterial system exert their effects through ischemia or impaired blood flow. There are two types of arterial disorders: diseases such as atherosclerosis, vasculitis, and peripheral arterial diseases that obstruct blood flow, and disorders such as aneurysms that weaken the vessel wall.

Cholesterol relies on lipoproteins (LDLs and HDLs) for transport in the blood. The LDLs, which are atherogenic, carry cholesterol to the peripheral tissues. The HDLs, which are protective, remove cholesterol from the tissues and carry it back to the liver for disposal (reverse cholesterol transport). LDL receptors play a major role in removing cholesterol from the blood; persons with reduced numbers of receptors are at particularly high risk for development of atherosclerosis.

Atherosclerosis, a leading cause of death in the United States, affects large and medium-sized arteries, such as the coronary and cerebral arteries. It has an insidious onset, and its lesions usually are far advanced before symptoms appear. Although the mechanisms of atherosclerosis are uncertain, risk factors associated with its development have been identified. These include factors such as heredity, sex, and age, which cannot be controlled; factors such as smoking, high blood pressure, high serum cholesterol levels, diabetes, obesity, and inflammation, which can be controlled or modified; and other contributing factors such as lack of exercise and stress.

The vasculitides are a group of vascular disorders characterized by vasculitis or inflammation and necrosis of the blood vessels in various tissues and organs of the body. They can be caused by injury to the vessel, infectious agents, or immune processes, or they can occur secondary to other disease states such as systemic lupus erythematosus.

Occlusive disorders interrupt arterial flow of blood and interfere with the delivery of oxygen and nutrients to the tissues. Occlusion of flow can result from a thrombus, emboli, vessel compression, vasospasm, or structural changes in the vessel. Peripheral arterial diseases affect blood vessels outside the heart and thorax. They include Raynaud's disease or phenomenon, caused by vessel spasm, and thromboangiitis obliterans (Buerger's disease), characterized by an inflammatory process that involves medium-sized arteries.

Aneurysms are localized areas of vessel dilation caused by weakness of the arterial wall. A berry aneurysm, most often found in the circle of Willis in the brain circulation, consists of a small, spherical vessel dilation. Fusiform and saccular aneurysms, most often found in the thoracic and abdominal aorta, are characterized by gradual and progressive enlargement of the aorta. They can involve part of the vessel circumference (saccular) or extend to involve the entire circumference of the vessel (fusiform). Aortic dissection is an acute, life-threatening condition. It involves hemorrhage into the vessel wall with longitudinal tearing (dissection) of the vessel wall to form a blood-filled channel. The most serious consequence of aneurysms is rupture.

Disorders of the Venous Circulation

After you have completed this section of the chapter, you should be able to meet the following objectives:

- Describe venous return of blood from the lower extremities, including the function of the muscle pumps and the effects of gravity, and relate to the development of varicose veins
- Differentiate primary from secondary varicose veins
- Characterize the pathology of venous insufficiency and relate to the development of stasis dermatitis and venous ulcers
- List the four most common causes of lower leg ulcer
- Cite risk factors associated with venous thrombosis and describe the manifestation of the disorder and its treatment

Veins are low-pressure, thin-walled vessels that rely on the ancillary action of skeletal muscle pumps and changes in abdominal and intrathoracic pressure to return blood to the heart. Unlike the arterial system, the venous system is equipped with valves that prevent retrograde flow of blood. Although its structure enables the venous system to serve as a storage area for blood, it also renders the system susceptible to problems related to stasis and venous insufficiency. This section focuses on three common problems of the venous system: varicose veins, venous insufficiency, and venous thrombosis.

VENOUS CIRCULATION OF THE LOWER EXTREMITIES

The venous system in the legs consists of two components: the superficial veins (*i.e.,* saphenous vein and its tributaries) and the deep venous channels (Fig. 24-12). Perforating or communicating veins connect these two systems. Blood from the skin and subcutaneous tissues in the leg collects in the superficial veins and is then transported across the communicating veins into the deeper venous channels for return to the heart. Venous valves prevent the retrograde flow of blood and play an important role in the function of the venous system. Although these valves are irregularly located along the length of the veins, they almost always are found at junctions where the communicating veins merge with the larger deep veins and where two veins meet. The number of venous valves differs somewhat from one person to another, as does the structural competence, factors that may help to explain the familial predisposition to development of varicose veins.

The action of the leg muscles assists in moving venous blood from the lower extremities back to the heart. When a person walks, the action of the leg muscles serves to increase flow in the deep venous channels and return venous blood to the heart (Fig. 24-13). The function of the so-called *muscle pump,* located in the gastrocnemius and soleus muscles of the lower extremities, can be compared with pumping action of the heart.[46] During muscle contraction, which is similar to systole, valves in the communicating channels

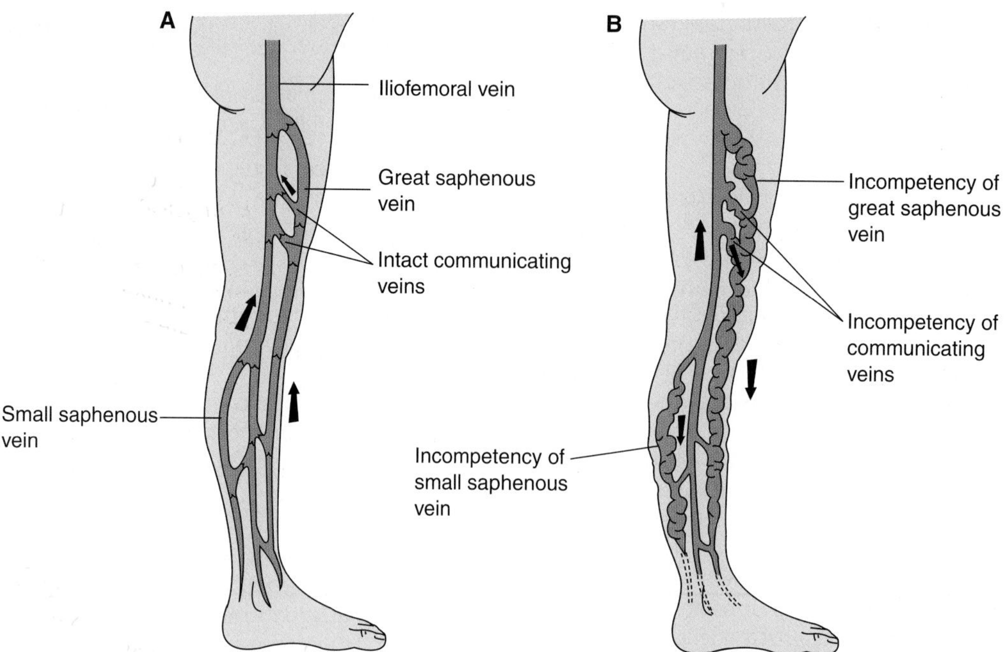

FIGURE 24-12 Superficial and deep venous channels of the leg. (**A**) Normal venous structures and flow patterns. (**B**) Varicosities in the superficial venous system are the result of incompetent valves in the communicating veins. The arrows in both views indicate the direction of blood flow. (Modified from Abramson D. I. [1974]. *Vascular disorders of the extremities* [2nd ed.]. New York: Harper & Row)

close to prevent backward flow of blood into the superficial system, as blood in the deep veins is moved forward by the action of the contracting muscles. During relaxation, which is similar to diastole, the communicating valves open, allowing blood from the superficial veins to move into the deep veins.

DISORDERS OF THE VENOUS CIRCULATION

- Veins are thin-walled, distensible vessels that collect blood from the tissues and return it to the heart. The venous system is a low-pressure system that relies on the pumping action of the skeletal muscles to move blood forward and the presence of venous valves to prevent retrograde flow.
- Disorders of the venous system produce congestion of the affected tissues and predispose to clot formation because of stagnation of flow and activation of the clotting system.
- Varicose veins are dilated and tortuous veins that result from a sustained increase in pressure that causes the venous valves to become incompetent, allowing for reflux of blood and vein engorgement.
- Thrombophlebitis refers to thrombus formation in a vein and the accompanying inflammatory response in the vessel wall as a result of conditions that obstruct or slow blood flow, increase the activity of the coagulation system, or cause vessel injury. Deep vein thrombosis may be a precursor to pulmonary embolism.

DISORDERS OF THE VENOUS CIRCULATION

Varicose Veins

Varicose, or dilated, tortuous veins of the lower extremities are common and often lead to secondary problems of venous insufficiency (see Fig. 24-12). Varicose veins are described as being primary or secondary. Primary varicose veins originate in the superficial saphenous veins, and sec-

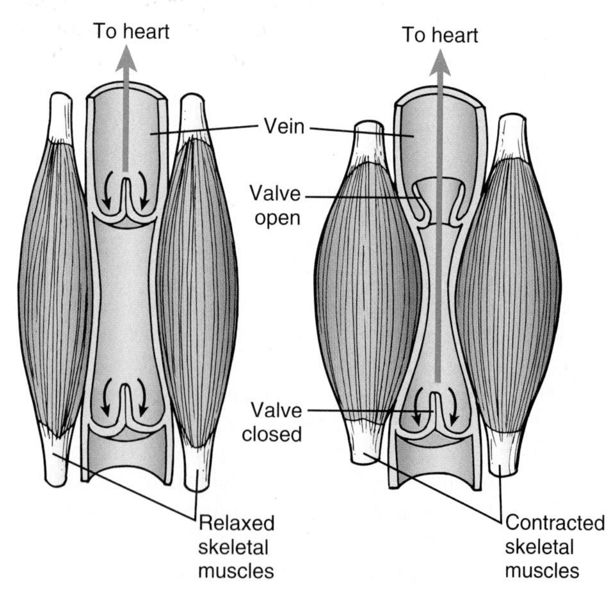

FIGURE 24-13 The skeletal muscle pumps and their function in promoting blood flow in the deep and superficial calf vessels of the leg.

ondary varicose veins result from impaired flow in the deep venous channels. Approximately 80% to 90% of venous blood from the lower extremities is transported through the deep channels. The development of secondary varicose veins becomes inevitable when flow in these deep channels is impaired or blocked. The most common cause of secondary varicose veins is deep vein thrombosis. Other causes include congenital or acquired arteriovenous fistulas, congenital venous malformations, and pressure on the abdominal veins caused by pregnancy or a tumor.

The prevalence of varicose veins in Western populations is about 25% to 30% in women and 10% to 20% in men. The condition is more common after 50 years of age and in obese persons, and it occurs more often in women, probably because of venous stasis caused by pregnancy.[3] More than 50% of persons with primary varicose veins have a family history of the disorder, suggesting that heredity may play a role.

Mechanisms of Development. Prolonged standing and increased intraabdominal pressure are important contributing factors in the development of primary varicose veins. Prolonged standing increases venous pressure and causes dilatation and stretching of the vessel wall. One of the most important factors in the elevation of venous pressure is the hydrostatic effect associated with the standing position. When a person is in the erect position, the full weight of the venous columns of blood is transmitted to the leg veins. The effects of gravity are compounded in persons who stand for long periods without using their leg muscles to assist in pumping blood back to the heart.

Because there are no valves in the inferior vena cava or common iliac veins, blood in the abdominal veins must be supported by the valves located in the external iliac or femoral veins. When intraabdominal pressure increases, as it does during pregnancy, or when the valves in these two veins are absent or defective, the stress on the saphenofemoral junction is increased. The high incidence of varicose veins in women who have been pregnant also suggests a hormonal effect on venous smooth muscle contributing to venous dilatation and valvular incompetence. Lifting also increases intraabdominal pressure and decreases flow of blood through the abdominal veins. Occupations that require repeated heavy lifting also predispose to development of varicose veins.

Prolonged exposure to increased pressure causes the venous valves to become incompetent so that they no longer close properly. When this happens, the reflux of blood causes further venous enlargement, pulling the valve leaflet apart and causing more valvular incompetence in sections of adjacent distal veins. Another consideration in the development of varicose veins is the fact that the superficial veins have only subcutaneous fat and superficial fascia for support, but the deep venous channels are supported by muscle, bone, and connective tissue. Obesity reduces the support provided by the superficial fascia and tissues, increasing the risk for development of varicose veins.

Manifestations. The signs and symptoms associated with primary varicose veins vary. Most women with superficial varicose veins complain of their unsightly appearance. In many cases, aching in the lower extremities and edema, especially after long periods of standing, may occur. The edema usually subsides at night when the legs are elevated. When the communicating veins are incompetent, symptoms are more common.

Diagnosis and Treatment. The diagnosis of varicose veins often can be made after physical inspection. Several procedures are used to assess the extent of venous involvement associated with varicose veins. In one of these, Trendelenburg's test, a tourniquet is applied to the affected leg while it is elevated and the veins are empty. The person then assumes the standing position, and the tourniquet is removed. If the superficial veins are involved, the veins distend quickly. To assess the deep channels, the tourniquet is applied while the person is standing and the veins are filled. The person then lies down, and the affected leg is elevated. Emptying of the superficial veins indicates that the deep channels are patent. The Doppler ultrasonic flow probe also may be used to assess the flow in the large vessels. Angiographic studies using a radiopaque contrast medium also are used to assess venous function.

After the venous channels have been repeatedly stretched and the valves rendered incompetent, little can be done to restore normal venous tone and function. Ideally, measures should be taken to prevent the development and progression of varicose veins. These measures center on avoiding activities such as continued standing that produce prolonged elevation of venous pressure. Treatment measures for varicose veins focus on improving venous flow and preventing tissue injury. When correctly fitted, elastic support stockings or leggings compress the superficial veins and prevent distention. The most precise control is afforded by prescription stockings, measured to fit properly. These stockings should be applied before the standing position is assumed, when the leg veins are empty.

Sclerotherapy, which often is used in the treatment of small residual varicosities, involves the injection of a sclerosing agent into the collapsed superficial veins to produce fibrosis of the vessel lumen. Surgical treatment consists of removing the varicosities and the incompetent perforating veins, but it is limited to persons with patent deep venous channels.

Chronic Venous Insufficiency

The term *venous insufficiency* refers to the physiologic consequences of deep vein thrombosis (DVT), valvular incompetence, or a combination of both conditions. The most common cause is DVT, which causes deformity of the valve leaflets, rendering them incapable of closure. In the presence of valvular incompetence, effective unidirectional flow of blood and emptying of the deep veins cannot occur. The muscle pumps also are ineffective, often driving blood in retrograde directions. Secondary failure of the communicating and superficial veins subjects the subcutaneous tissues to high pressures.

With venous insufficiency, there are signs and symptoms associated with impaired blood flow. In contrast to the ischemia caused by arterial insufficiency, venous insufficiency leads to tissue congestion, edema, and eventual impairment of tissue nutrition.[46] The edema is exacerbated by long periods of standing. Necrosis of subcutaneous fat deposits occurs, followed by skin atrophy. Brown pigmentation of the skin caused by hemosiderin deposits resulting from the breakdown of red blood cells is common. Secondary lymphatic insufficiency occurs, with progressive sclerosis of the lymph channels in the face of increased demand for clearance of interstitial fluid.

In advanced venous insufficiency, impaired tissue nutrition causes stasis dermatitis and the development of stasis or venous ulcers (Fig. 24-14). Stasis dermatitis is characterized by the presence of thin, shiny, bluish brown, irregularly pigmented desquamative skin that lacks the support of the underlying subcutaneous tissues. Minor injury leads to relatively painless ulcerations that are difficult to heal. The lower part of the leg is particularly prone to development of stasis dermatitis and venous ulcers. Most lesions are located medially over the ankle and lower leg, with the highest frequency just above the medial malleolus. Venous insufficiency is the most common cause of lower leg ulcers, accounting for nearly 80% of all cases.[47] The other common causes of lower extremity ulcers are arterial insufficiency, neuropathy (often due to diabetes), and pressure ulcers. Of the approximately 7 million people in the United States with venous insufficiency, about 1 million will develop leg ulcers. Treatment of venous ulcers includes compression therapy with dressings and inelastic or elastic bandages. Medications that help include aspirin and pentoxifylline. Occasionally, skin grafting is required for large or slow-healing venous ulcers. Growth factors (which are administered topically or by perilesional injection) may also be warranted.[47] Persons with long-standing venous insufficiency may also experience stiffening of the ankle joint and loss of muscle mass and strength.

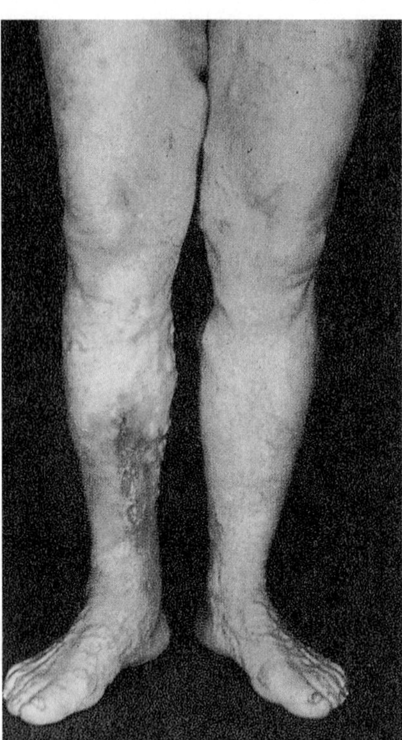

FIGURE 24-14 Varicose veins of the legs. Severe varicosities of the superficial leg veins have led to stasis dermatitis and secondary ulcerations. (Rubin E., Farber J. L. [1999]. *Pathology* [3rd ed., p. 525]. Philadelphia: Lippincott-Raven)

Venous Thrombosis

The term *venous thrombosis,* or *thrombophlebitis,* describes the presence of thrombus in a vein and the accompanying inflammatory response in the vessel wall. Thrombi can develop in the superficial or the deep veins. DVT most commonly occurs in the lower extremities. DVT of the lower extremity is a serious disorder, complicated by pulmonary embolism (see Chapter 31), recurrent episodes of DVT, and development of chronic venous insufficiency. Most postoperative thrombi arise in the soleal sinuses or the large veins draining the gastrocnemius muscles.[48] Isolated calf thrombi often are asymptomatic. If left untreated, they may extend to the larger, more proximal veins, with an increased risk for pulmonary emboli.

In 1846, Virchow described the triad that has come to be associated with venous thrombosis: stasis of blood, increased blood coagulability, and vessel wall injury.[49] Risk factors for venous thrombosis are summarized in Chart 24-2. Stasis of blood occurs with immobility of an extremity or the entire body. Bed rest and immobilization are associated with decreased blood flow, venous pooling in the lower extremities, and increased risk for DVT. Persons who are immobilized by a hip fracture, joint replacement, or

CHART 24-2

*Risk Factors Associated With Venous Thrombosis**

Venous Stasis

Bed rest
Immobility
Spinal cord injury
Acute myocardial infarction
Congestive heart failure
Shock
Venous obstruction

Hyperreactivity of Blood Coagulation

Genetic factors
Stress and trauma
Pregnancy
Childbirth
Oral contraceptive and hormone replacement use
Dehydration
Cancer
Antiphospholipid syndrome
Hyperhomocysteinemia

Vascular Trauma

Indwelling venous catheters
Surgery
Massive trauma or infection
Fractured hip
Orthopedic surgery

*Many of these disorders involve more than one mechanism.

spinal cord injury are particularly vulnerable to DVT. The risk for DVT is increased in situations of impaired cardiac function. This may account for the relatively high incidence in persons with acute myocardial infarction and congestive heart failure. Elderly persons are more susceptible than younger persons, probably because disorders that produce venous stasis occur more frequently in older persons. Long airplane travel poses a particular threat in persons predisposed to DVT because of prolonged sitting and increased blood viscosity due to dehydration.[50]

Hypercoagulability is a homeostatic mechanism designed to increase clot formation, and conditions that increase the concentration or activation of clotting factors predispose to DVT. Thrombosis also can be caused by inherited or acquired deficiencies in certain plasma proteins that normally inhibit thrombus formation, such as antithrombin III, protein C, and protein S.[51] However, the most common inherited risk factors are the factor V Leiden and the prothrombin gene mutations.[5] The postpartum state is associated with increased levels of fibrinogen, prothrombin, and other coagulation factors. The use of oral contraceptives and hormone replacement therapy appears to increase coagulability and predispose to venous thrombosis, a risk that is further increased in women who smoke. Certain cancers are associated with increased clotting tendencies, and although the reason for this is largely unknown, substances that promote blood coagulation may be in the tumor cells or be released from the tissues because of the cancerous growth. Immune interactions with cancer cells can result in the release of cytokines, which can cause endothelial damage and predispose to thrombosis.[52] Aggressive antitumor therapy can also cause vascular damage. When body fluid is lost because of injury or disease, the resulting hemoconcentration causes clotting factors to become more concentrated. Other important risk factors include the antiphospholipid syndrome and hyperhomocysteinemia.[53]

Vessel injury can result from a trauma situation or from surgical intervention. It also may occur secondary to infection or inflammation of the vessel wall. Persons undergoing hip surgery and total hip replacement are at particular risk because of trauma to the femoral and iliac veins and, in the case of hip replacement, thermal damage from heat generated by the polymerization of the acrylic cement that is used in the procedure.[48] Venous catheters are another source of vascular injury.

Manifestations. Many persons with venous thrombosis are asymptomatic, probably because the vein is not totally occluded or because of collateral circulation.[54] When present, the most common signs and symptoms of venous thrombosis are those related to the inflammatory process: pain, swelling, and deep muscle tenderness. Fever, general malaise, and an elevated white blood cell count and sedimentation rate are accompanying indications of inflammation. There may be tenderness and pain along the vein. Swelling may vary from minimal to maximal. As many as 50% of DVT cases are asymptomatic.

The site of thrombus formation determines the location of the physical findings. The most common site is in the venous sinuses in the soleus muscle and posterior tibial and peroneal veins (Fig. 24-15). Swelling in these cases

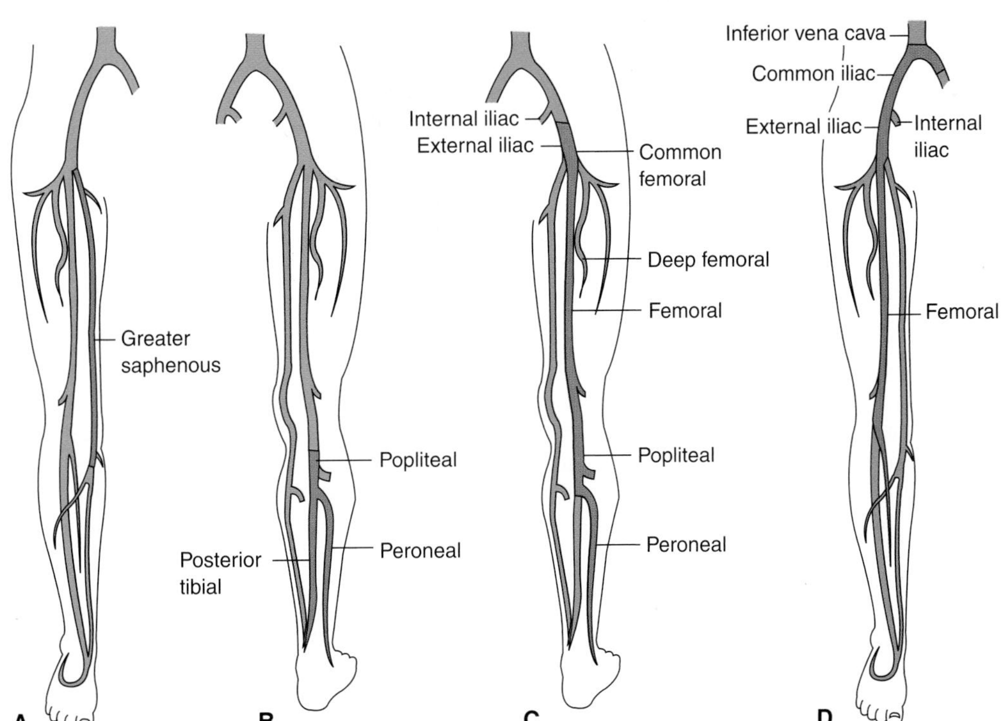

FIGURE 24-15 Common sites of venous thrombosis. (**A**) Superficial thrombophlebitis. (**B**) Most common form of deep thrombophlebitis. (**C** and **D**) Deep thrombophlebitis from the calf to iliac veins. (Haller J. A. Jr. [1967]. *Deep thrombophlebitis: Pathophysiology and treatment.* Philadelphia: W. B. Saunders)

involves the foot and ankle, although it may be slight or absent. Calf pain and tenderness are common. Femoral vein thrombosis with calf thrombosis produces pain and tenderness in the distal thigh and popliteal area. Thrombi in ileofemoral veins produce the most profound manifestations, with swelling, pain, and tenderness of the entire extremity. With DVT in the calf veins, active dorsiflexion produces calf pain (*i.e.,* Homans sign).

Diagnosis and Treatment. The risk for pulmonary embolism emphasizes the need for early detection and treatment of DVT. Several tests are useful for this purpose: ascending venography, ultrasonography (*e.g.,* real-time, B-mode, duplex), and plasma D-dimer assessment.[55]

Whenever possible, venous thrombosis should be prevented in preference to being treated. Early ambulation after childbirth and surgery is one measure that decreases the risk for thrombus formation. Exercising the legs and wearing support stockings improve venous flow. A further precautionary measure is to avoid assuming body positions that favor venous pooling. Antiembolism stockings of the proper fit and length should be used routinely in persons at risk for DVT. Another strategy used for immobile persons at risk for developing DVT is a sequential pneumatic compression device. This consists of a plastic sleeve that encircles the legs and provides alternating periods of compression on the lower extremity. When properly used, these devices enhance venous emptying to augment flow and reduce stasis. Prophylactic anticoagulation often is used in persons who are at high risk for development of venous thrombi.

The objectives of treatment of venous thrombosis are to prevent the formation of additional thrombi, prevent extension and embolization of existing thrombi, and minimize venous valve damage. A 15- to 20-degree elevation of the legs prevents stasis. It is important that the entire lower extremity or extremities be carefully extended to avoid acute flexion of the knee or hip. Heat often is applied to the leg to relieve venospasm and to aid in the resolution of the inflammatory process. Bed rest usually is maintained until local tenderness and swelling have subsided. Gradual ambulation with elastic support is then permitted. Standing and sitting increase venous pressure and are to be avoided. Elastic support is needed for 3 to 6 months to permit recanalization and collateralization and to prevent venous insufficiency.

Anticoagulation therapy (*i.e.,* heparin and warfarin) is used to treat and prevent venous thrombosis. Treatment typically is initiated with continuous infusion or subcutaneous injections of heparin. Subcutaneous injections of low-molecular-weight heparin may be given on an outpatient basis. This usually is followed by prophylactic therapy with oral anticoagulants to prevent further thrombus formation.[56] The mechanisms of action of the anticoagulant drugs are discussed in Chapter 15. Thrombolytic therapy (*i.e.,* streptokinase, urokinase, or tissue plasminogen activator) may be used in an attempt to dissolve the clot.

Surgical removal of the thrombus may be undertaken in selected cases. Percutaneous (through the skin) insertion of intracaval filters may be done in persons at high risk for developing pulmonary emboli. This procedure prevents large clots from moving through the vessel. However, although filters prevent pulmonary embolus developing, an increase in thrombosis occurs at the site of the filter in the absence of anticoagulation.

In summary, the storage function of the venous system renders it susceptible to venous insufficiency, stasis, and thrombus formation. Varicose veins occur with prolonged distention and stretching of the superficial veins owing to venous insufficiency. Varicosities can arise because of defects in the superficial veins (*i.e.,* primary varicose veins) or because of impaired blood flow in the deep venous channels (*i.e.,* secondary varicose veins). Venous insufficiency reflects chronic venous stasis resulting from valvular incompetence. It is associated with stasis dermatitis and stasis or venous ulcers. Venous thrombosis describes the presence of thrombus in a vein and the accompanying inflammatory response in the vessel wall. It is associated with vessel injury, stasis of venous flow, and hypercoagulability states. Thrombi can develop in the superficial or the deep veins (*i.e.,* DVT). Thrombus formation in deep veins is a precursor to venous insufficiency and embolus formation.

Disorders of Blood Flow Due to Extravascular Forces

After you have completed this section of the chapter, you should be able to meet the following objectives:

- Describe the principles of tissue blood flow
- State five possible causes of compartment syndrome
- Explain why pulses and capillary refill time are not good assessment measures for compartment syndrome
- Cite two causes of pressure ulcers
- Explain how shearing forces contribute to ischemic skin damage
- List four measures that contribute to the prevention of pressure ulcers

PRINCIPLES OF BLOOD FLOW

The previous sections of this chapter have focused on disruption in blood flow resulting from disorders affecting blood vessels of the arterial and venous circulations. Disruption of blood flow can also occur when external forces compress blood flow in otherwise healthy vessels.

Blood flow to the tissues occurs along a pressure gradient, moving from the arterial to capillaries and then to the venous side of the circulation. For blood to move through the vessels of the systemic circulation, arterial pressure must be greater than venous pressure, and the arterial and venous pressures must be greater than the external pressure of the surrounding tissues. Injury or infections that cause swelling can compromise tissue blood flow, particularly in parts of the body where the skin or other supporting tissues cannot expand to accommodate the increased volume. In other situations, external pressure may compress the tissues

DISORDERS OF BLOOD FLOW DUE TO EXTRAVASCULAR FORCES

- Blood flow requires that arterial pressure is greater than venous pressure, and that arterial, venous, and capillary pressures are greater than the pressure surrounding the vessels.
- Compartment syndrome describes a condition of increased pressure in an anatomic space that cannot expand. The increased pressure may compromise blood flow to the tissue, resulting in ischemic damage. Causes include decreases in compartment size (*i.e.*, cast) or increases in compartment volume (*i.e.*, internal bleeding or edema).
- Pressure ulcers are ischemic lesions of the skin and underlying tissues caused by compression of blood vessels due to external pressure, such as that exerted by the weight of the body on the bed or chair surface. Prevention of pressure ulcers is preferable to treatment. Frequent position changes and meticulous skin care are essential components of prevention.

and the blood vessels. Two conditions in which external pressure compromises tissue blood flow are compartment syndrome and pressure ulcers.

Compartment Syndrome

The muscles and nerves of an extremity are enclosed in a tough, inelastic fascial envelope called a *muscle compartment* (Fig. 24-16). *Compartment syndrome* describes a condition of increased pressure in a limited anatomic space, usually a muscle compartment, that impairs circulation and produces ischemic tissue injury.[57] If the pressure in the compartment is sufficiently high, tissue circulation is compromised, causing the death of nerve and muscle cells. Permanent loss of function and limb contracture may occur. The amount of pressure required to produce a compartment syndrome depends on many factors, including the duration of the pressure elevation, the metabolic rate of the tissues, vascular tone, and local blood pressure. Less tissue pressure is required to stop circulation when hypotension or vasoconstriction is present.

Intracompartmental pressures of 30 to 40 mm Hg (normal is approximately 6 mm Hg) are considered sufficient to impair capillary blood flow.[58] Nerve dysfunction (*i.e.*, paresthesia and hypoesthesia) develops within 30 minutes of ischemia, and muscle dysfunction within 2 to 4 hours; irreversible loss of function (*e.g.*, contractures, sensory aberrations, muscle weakness) begins after 12 to 24 hours of total ischemia.[59] Prompt diagnosis and decompression are essential to reinstate capillary pressure and prevent permanent disability.

Causes. Compartment syndrome can result from: (1) a decrease in compartment size or (2) an increase in the volume of its contents (Chart 24-3). The most common causes are crushing injuries, fractures, contusions, snake bites, postischemic swelling after arterial injury or thrombosis, severe exercise, limb compression due to drug or alcohol overdose, and venous occlusion.

Among the causes of decreased compartment size are constrictive dressings and casts, closure of fascial defects, and thermal injuries or frostbite. Splitting a cast or releasing the dressing usually is sufficient to relieve most of the pressure. The appearance of a muscle hernia or fascial defect may be the result of increased compartmental pressure. This commonly is seen in persons with chronic exercise-related compartment syndrome. Surgical closure of the hernia decreases compartmental size and may result in an acute compartment syndrome. In persons with circumferential third-degree burns, the inelastic and constricting eschar decreases the size of the underlying compartments. Burns also are associated with the formation of massive edema and an increase in compartment volume. The combination of the two problems may lead to necrosis of the underlying

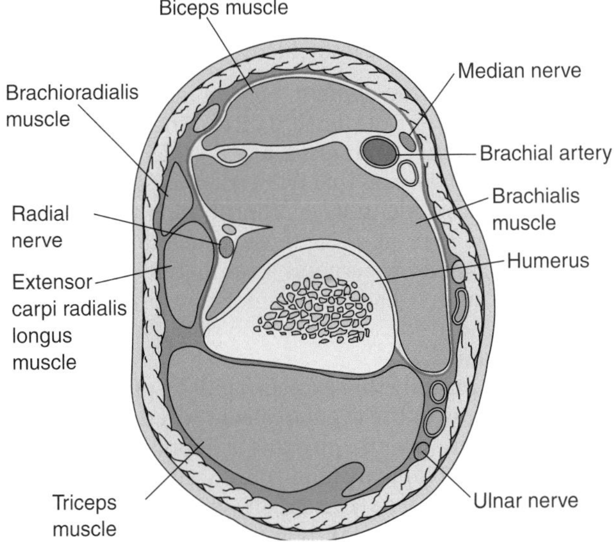

FIGURE 24-16 Distal anterior arm muscle compartment, showing the location of fascia, muscles, nerves, and blood vessels.

CHART 24-3

Causes of Compartment Syndrome

Decreased Compartment Size

Constrictive dressings and casts
Infiltration of intravenous fluids
Thermal injury and frostbite
Surgical closure of fascial defects

Increased Compartment Volume

Fractures and orthopedic surgery
Trauma and bleeding
Postischemic injury
Severe exercise
Prolonged immobilization with limb compression (*e.g.*, drug overdose)
Thermal injury and frostbite
Intravenous infiltration

neuromuscular tissues. Frostbite produces neuromuscular injury for similar reasons.

Increased compartment volume can be caused by postischemic swelling, trauma, vascular injury and bleeding, infiltration of intravenous infusions, and venous obstruction. One of the most important causes of compartment syndrome is bleeding and edema caused by fractures and osteotomies (see Chapter 57). Contusions and soft tissue injury also are common causes of compartment syndrome. Bleeding can occur as a complication of arterial punctures, particularly in persons with bleeding disorders and in those who are receiving anticoagulant drugs. Infiltration of intravenous fluids also can restrict compartment size and cause compartment ischemia and postischemic swelling. Increased compartment volume may follow ischemic events, such as arterial occlusion, that are of sufficient duration to produce capillary damage, causing increased capillary permeability and edema. During unattended coma caused by drug overdose or carbon monoxide poisoning, high compartment pressures are produced when an extremity is compressed by the weight of the overlying head or torso. Exercise may produce acute or chronic elevations in compartment pressure.

Diagnosis and Treatment. It is important that a person at risk for development of compartment syndrome be identified and that proper assessment methods be instituted. Assessment should include pain assessment, examination of sensory (*i.e.,* light touch and two-point discrimination) and motor function (*i.e.,* movement and muscle strength), test of passive stretch, and palpation of the muscle compartments.

The most important symptom of compartment syndrome is unrelenting pain, usually described as a deep, throbbing sensation, that is greater than that expected for the primary problem, such as fracture or contusion. Pain with passive stretch is a common finding. Tenseness and tenderness of the involved compartment are specific symptoms of compartment syndrome. The skin over the compartment may become taut, shiny, warm, and red. Paresthesias progressing to anesthesia occur secondary to nerve involvement. Muscle weakness results from muscle ischemia. Although peripheral pulses and capillary refill time are parts of a complete assessment, they frequently are normal in the presence of compartment syndrome because the major arteries are located outside the muscle compartments. Although edema may make it difficult to palpate the pulse, the increased compartment pressure seldom is sufficient to occlude flow in a major artery. Doppler methods usually confirm the existence of a pulse. Direct measurements of tissue pressure can be obtained using a needle or wick catheter inserted into the muscle compartment. This method is particularly useful in persons who are unresponsive and in those with nerve deficits.

Compartment decompression is recommended when pressures rise to 30 mm Hg.

Treatment consists of reducing compartmental pressures. This entails cast splitting or removal of restrictive dressings. These procedures often are sufficient to relieve most of the underlying pressure and symptoms. Limb elevation is not recommended when compartment syndrome is suspected. Although elevation is widely used to promote venous drainage of an injured extremity, it may be detrimental in compartment syndrome. Because venous pressure must exceed tissue pressure, elevation of an extremity cannot augment venous drainage after intracompartmental pressures are elevated. When an extremity is elevated, its arterial pressure falls because of the effects of gravity. Blood flow to an extremity can be arrested because of diminution of arterial pressure in the elevated extremity.

When compartment syndrome cannot be relieved by the measures described, a fasciotomy may become necessary. During this procedure, the fascia is incised longitudinally and separated so that the compartment volume can expand and blood flow can be reestablished. Because of potential problems with wound infection and closure, this procedure is performed as a last resort.

Pressure Ulcers

Pressure ulcers are ischemic lesions of the skin and underlying structures caused by external pressure that impairs the flow of blood and lymph. Pressure ulcers often are referred to as *decubitus ulcers* or *bedsores*. The word *decubitus* comes from the Latin term meaning "lying down." However, a pressure ulcer may result from pressure exerted in the seated or the lying position. Pressure ulcers are most likely to develop over a bony prominence, but they may occur on any part of the body that is subjected to external pressure, friction, or shearing forces.

The reported prevalence of pressure ulcers in hospital settings in the United States is approximately 8%,[60] and in skilled care and nursing home settings, it ranges from 2.4% to 23%.[61,62] Several subpopulations are at particular risk, including persons with quadriplegia, those with impaired nutrition, elderly persons with restricted activity and hip fractures, and persons in the critical care setting. About 95% of pressure ulcers occur in the lower part of the body.[63] The sacrum is the most frequent site, followed by the heel. The prevention and treatment of pressure ulcers is a public health issue and is addressed in *Healthy People 2010,* a national public health policy statement, which has set a target of a 50% decrease in prevalence of pressure ulcers in nursing home residents.[64]

Mechanisms of Development. Several factors contribute to the development of pressure ulcers, including (1) external pressure that compresses blood vessels and (2) friction and shearing forces that tear and injure blood vessels. Other risk factors identified as contributing to the development of pressure ulcers are those related to sensory perception (*i.e.,* ability to respond meaningfully to pressure-related discomfort), level of skin moisture, urine and fecal continence, nutrition and hydration status, mobility, and circulatory status.

External pressure that exceeds capillary pressure interrupts blood flow in the capillary beds. When the pressure between a bony prominence and a support surface exceeds the normal capillary filling pressure of approximately 32 mm Hg, capillary flow essentially is obstructed.[65] If this pressure is applied constantly for 2 hours, oxygen deprivation coupled with an accumulation of metabolic end products leads to irreversible tissue damage. Dependent on host factors, such as tissue metabolism, tissue damage may occur in a lesser amount of time. The same amount of pressure causes more damage when it is distributed over a small area than when it is distributed over a larger area. Approximately 7 lb of pressure per square inch of tissue surface is sufficient to obstruct blood flow. If a person weighing 70 kg with a total surface area of 1.8 m^2 were in the supine position, with pressure evenly distributed, the pressure at any given point would be 5.7 mm Hg.[66]

Whether a person is sitting or lying down, the weight of the body is borne by tissues covering the bony prominences. Ninety-six percent of pressure ulcers are located on the lower part of the body, most often over the sacrum, the coccygeal areas, the ischial tuberosities, and the greater trochanter.[67] Pressure over a bony area is transmitted from the surface to the underlying dense bone, compressing all of the intervening tissue. As a result, the greatest pressure occurs at the surface of the bone and dissipates outward in a conelike manner toward the surface of the skin (Fig. 24-17). Thus, extensive underlying tissue damage can be present when a small superficial skin lesion is first noticed.

Altering the distribution of pressure from one skin area to another prevents tissue injury. Pressure ulcers most commonly occur in persons with conditions in which normal sensation and movement to effect redistribution of body weight are impaired, such as spinal cord injury. Normally, persons unconsciously shift their weight to redistribute pressure on the skin and underlying tissues. During the night, for example, they turn in their sleep, preventing ischemic injury of tissues that overlie the bony prominences that support the weight of the body; the same is true for sitting for any length of time. The movements needed to shift the body weight are made unconsciously, and only when movement is restricted do they become aware of discomfort.

Shearing forces are caused by the sliding of one tissue layer over another with stretching and angulation of blood vessels, causing injury and thrombosis. Injury caused by shearing forces commonly occurs when the head of the bed is elevated, causing the torso to slide down toward the foot of the bed. When this happens, friction and perspiration cause the skin and superficial fascia to remain fixed against the bed linens while the deep fascia and skeleton slide downward. The same thing can happen when a person sitting up in a chair slides downward. Another source of shearing forces is pulling rather than lifting a person up in bed. In this case, the skin remains fixed to the sheet while the fascia and muscles are pulled upward.

Prevention. The prevention of pressure ulcers is preferable to treatment. In 1992, a special panel of the Agency for Health Care Policy and Research (AHCPR; now the Agency for Healthcare Research and Quality), the Panel for the Prediction and Prevention of Pressure Ulcers in Adults, released the *Clinical Practice Guidelines for Pressure Ulcers in Adults*.[68] The panel recommended four overall goals: (1) identifying at-risk persons who need preventative measures and the specific factors placing them at risk; (2) maintaining and improving tissue tolerance to pressure in order to prevent injury; (3) protecting against the adverse effects of external mechanical forces (*i.e.*, pressure, friction, and shear); and (4) reducing the incidence of pressure ulcers through educational programs.[68] A 1994 publication of the AHCPR made specific recommendations for assessment of the person with pressure ulcers, management of tissue load, ulcer care, managing bacterial colonization and infection, operative repair, and education and quality control.[69]

Methods for preventing pressure ulcers include frequent position change, meticulous skin care, and frequent and careful observation to detect early signs of skin breakdown. All persons at risk for pressure ulcers should have systematic skin inspection done at least once each day, with particular attention to bony prominences.[68] Bed linens should be kept clean, dry, and wrinkle free. The skin should be cleaned at the time of urine and fecal soiling with a mild cleaning agent that minimizes irritation and skin dryness. When soiling of the skin cannot be controlled, it is recommended that absorbent underpads or briefs be used to present a quick-drying surface for the skin.

Frequent change of position prevents tissue injury due to pressure. Persons who are in bed and at risk for development of pressure ulcers should be repositioned at least every 2 hours if this is consistent with the overall treatment goals. It is recommended that persons who are in a chair or wheelchair be repositioned every hour or put back to bed. Persons who are able to shift their weight should be advised to do so every 15 minutes.

Special pads and mattresses that distribute weight more evenly may be used. Silicone-filled pads, egg-crate cushions, turning frames, flotation pads, air-fluidized beds, and

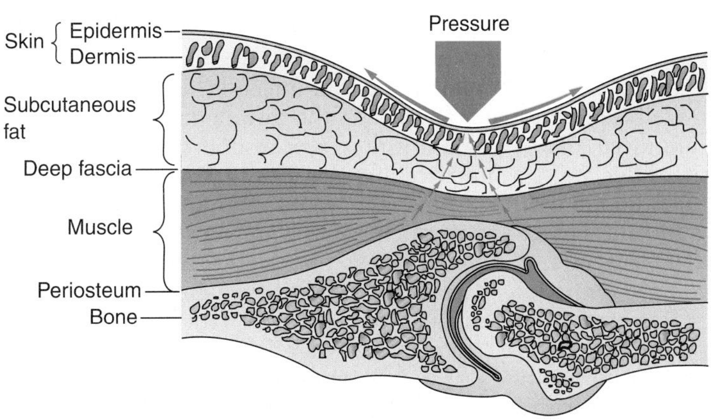

FIGURE 24-17 Pressure over a bony prominence compresses all intervening soft tissue, with a resulting wide, three-dimensional pressure gradient that causes various degrees of ischemia and damage. (Shea J. D. [1975]. Pressure sores: Classification and management. *Clinical Orthopaedics and Related Research* 112, 90)

other devices minimize contact pressure. Adequate exposure of the skin to air is necessary to avoid the buildup of heat and perspiration. Care should be taken to maintain the person at a position of 30 to 40 degrees to minimize slipping and shearing forces from sliding against the sheets. It also is important that the person be lifted and not dragged across the sheet. A lifting sheet works well for this purpose. Elevation of the ankles and heels off the sheets with foam pads can reduce skin breakdown in these areas of the body. The use of air cushions (*i.e.,* donuts) is not recommended. Casts, braces, and splints can exert extreme pressure on underlying tissues, and persons with these devices require special attention to avoid skin breakdown.

Adequate hydration and nutrition are important. Adequate hydration of the stratum corneum appears to protect the skin against mechanical insult.[68] The skin should be kept clean and protected from environmental factors that cause drying. The level of skin hydration decreases with decreasing ambient air temperature, particularly when the relative humidity of the ambient air is low.[68] Dry skin should be treated with moisturizers. The prevention of dehydration also improves the circulation. It also decreases the concentration of urine, thereby minimizing skin irritation in persons who are incontinent, and it reduces urinary problems that contribute to incontinence.

Staging and Treatment. Pressure ulcers can be staged according to four categories.[68,70–72] *Stage I* ulcers represent an intact skin with areas of persistent redness in lightly pigmented skin or persistent red, blue, or purple hues in darker pigmented skin.[73] *Stage II* ulcers represent a partial-thickness loss of skin involving the epidermis or dermis, or both. The ulcer is superficial and presents clinically as an abrasion, a blister, or a shallow crater. *Stage III* ulcers represent a full-thickness skin loss with damage and necrosis of the underlying subcutaneous tissue that may extend down to but not through underlying fascia. The ulcer manifests as a deep crater with or without undermining of adjacent tissue. *Stage IV* ulcers represent full-thickness skin loss with extensive damage and necrosis of the underlying subcutaneous tissues that may extend to involve muscle, bone, or other supporting structures (*e.g.,* tendon or joint capsule).

These staging criteria have limitations. Identification of stage I pressure ulcers may be difficult in persons with darkly pigmented skin, and when eschar is present. Accurate staging of the pressure ulcer may be difficult until the eschar has sloughed or the wound has been débrided.

After skin breakdown has occurred, special treatment measures are needed to prevent further ischemic damage, reduce bacterial contamination and infection, and promote healing. A major advance in the treatment of pressure ulcers has occurred in the area of wound dressings that offer moist wound healing. Dry dressings favor the formation of a dry crust over the wound, through which granulation tissue and advancing epithelium must burrow as it heals the area. Moist dressings, on the other hand, encourage formation of granulation and epithelialization.[74]

Treatment methods are selected based on the stage of the ulcer.[65,69] Stage I ulcers usually are treated with frequent turning and measures to remove pressure. Stage II or III ulcers with little exudate are treated with petroleum gauze, semipermeable, or occlusive dressings to maintain a moist healing environment. Transparent semipermeable dressings (*e.g.,* Op-Site, Tegaderm) allow wound visibility and seal in the body's own defenses against invasion—leukocytes, plasma, fibrin, and growth factors. Stage III ulcers usually require débridement (*i.e.,* removal of necrotic tissue and eschar). This can be done surgically, with wet-to-dry dressings, through the use of proteolytic enzymes (*e.g.,* fibrinolysin-desoxyribonuclease [Elase], streptokinase-streptodornase [Varidase]), or autolytic débridement, which involves the use of synthetic dressings to cover the wound and allow devitalized tissues to self-digest from enzymes normally present in wound fluids.[65] Stage IV wounds often require packing to obliterate dead space and are covered with nonadherent dressings. Care is taken to avoid overpacking the wound because it may produce pressure and cause additional tissue damage. Dressings usually are changed every 8 to 12 hours, depending on severity, degree of infection, and amount of exudate. Stage IV ulcers may require surgical interventions, such as skin grafts or myocutaneous flaps.

There has been recent interest in the use of growth factors in the healing of pressure ulcers.[75] Growth factors provide a means by which cells communicate with each other and can have profound effects on cell proliferation, migration, and extracellular matrix synthesis.[75] Becaplermin, a topical preparation of recombinant human platelet-derived growth factor, is used in the treatment of neuropathic lower extremity ulcers. Granulocyte-macrophage colony-stimulating factor (GM-CSF) promotes healing of venous leg ulcers and is safe.[75] There is hope that growth factors may prove beneficial in the treatment of pressure ulcers.

In summary, blood flow in the circulatory system is brought about by pressure differences between the arterial and venous systems and a transmural pressure (*i.e.,* internal minus external) that holds the vessel open. Under certain conditions, such as compartment syndrome and pressure ulcers, increases in external pressures can exceed intravascular pressure and interrupt blood flow. Compartment syndrome is a condition of increased pressure in a muscle compartment that compromises blood flow and potentially leads to death of nerve and muscle tissues. It can result from a decrease in compartment size (*e.g.,* constrictive dressings, closure of fascial defects, thermal injury, frostbite) or an increase in compartment volume (*e.g.,* postischemic swelling, fractures, contusion and soft tissue trauma, bleeding caused by vascular injury, venous congestion).

Pressure ulcers are caused by ischemia of the skin and underlying tissues. They result from external pressure, which disrupts blood flow, or shearing forces, which cause stretching and injury to blood vessels. Pressure ulcers are divided into four stages, according to the depth of tissue involvement. The prevention of pressure ulcers is preferable to treatment. The goals of prevention should include identifying at-risk persons who need prevention and the specific factors placing them at risk; maintaining and improving tissue tolerance to pressure to prevent injury; protecting against the adverse effects of external mechanical forces (*i.e.,* pressure, friction, and shear), and reducing the incidence of pressure ulcers through educational programs.

REVIEW EXERCISES

The *Third Report of the National Cholesterol Education Program (NCEP) Expert Panel on Detection, Evaluation, and Treatment of High Blood Cholesterol in Adults* recommends that a person's HDL should be above 40 mg/dL.

A. Explain the protective role of HDL in prevention of atherosclerosis.

A 55-year-old male executive has a history of ischemic heart disease. His cholesterol level is normal. He is otherwise well. He has recently read in the media about "inflammation" and the heart. He requests further evaluation.

A. Which test might be done?

B. Define low-, medium-, and high-risk in terms of the test performed.

C. Are there other factors that might influence the test results?

A 72-year-old woman complains of a 3-week history of severe right-sided headache accompanied by tenderness to the touch over the right temporal area. She denies any visual disturbance. Investigations reveal a markedly elevated erythrocyte sedimentation rate.

A. What is the likely diagnosis?

B. What is the pathology underlying the diagnosis?

C. What is best way of confirming the diagnosis?

D. What are the outcomes of the disorder if left untreated?

E. Which medication should be started immediately?

A 34-year-old otherwise healthy woman complains of episodes lasting several hours in which her fingers become pale and numb. This is followed by a period of time during which the fingers become red, throbbing, and painful.

A. What do you think is causing this woman's symptoms?

B. The patient relates that the episodes often occur when her fingers become cold or when she becomes upset. Explain the possible underlying mechanisms.

C. What types of measures could be used to treat this woman?

References

1. Guyton A., Hall J. E. (2000). *Textbook of medical physiology* (10th ed., pp. 781–790). Philadelphia: W. B. Saunders.
2. American Heart Association. (2002). Cholesterol statistics for professionals. [On-line]. Available: www.americanheart.org/cholesterol.
3. Rubin E., Farber J. L. (Eds.) (1999). *Pathology* (3rd ed., pp. 491–509, 520–522). Philadelphia: Lippincott-Raven.
4. Beisiegel U. (1998). Lipoprotein metabolism. *European Heart Journal 19*(Suppl. A), A20–A23.
5. Nabel E. G. (2003). Genomic medicine: Cardiovascular disease. *New England Journal of Medicine 349,* 60–72.
6. Lusis A. J. (2000). Atherosclerosis. *Nature 407,* 233–241.
7. Schoen F. J., Cotran R. S. (2003). Blood vessels. In Cotran R. S., Kumar V., Collins T. (Eds.), *Pathologic basis of disease* (7th ed., pp. 325–360). Philadelphia: W. B. Saunders.
8. Harper C. R., Jacobson T. A. (1999). New perspectives on the management of low levels of high-density lipoprotein cholesterol. *Archives of Internal Medicine 159,* 1049–1057.
9. Kreisberg R. A., Oberman A. (2003). Medical management of hyperlipidemia/dyslipidemia. *Journal of Clinical Endocrinology and Metabolism 88,* 2445–2461.
10. Oram J. F. (2002). ATP-binding cassette transporter A1 and cholesterol trafficking. *Current Opinions in Lipidology 13,* 373–381.
11. National Institute of Health Expert Panel (2001). *Third report of the National Cholesterol Education Program (NCEP) Expert Panel on Detection, Evaluation, and Treatment of High Blood Cholesterol in Adults (Adult Treatment Panel III).* (NIH Publication No. 01–3670). Bethesda, MD: National Institutes of Health.
12. Goldberg R. B. (1988). Dietary modification of cholesterol levels. *Consultant 28*(Suppl. 6), 35–41.
13. AHA Dietary Guidelines. (2000). Revision 2000: A statement for healthcare professionals from the Nutrition Committee of the American Heart Association. *Circulation 102,* 2284–2299.
14. MRC/BHF. (2002). Heart protection study of cholesterol lowering with simvastatin in 20,536 high risk individuals. *Lancet 360,* 7–22.
15. Sinatra S. T. (2003). Is cholesterol lowering with statins the gold standard for treating patients with cardiovascular risk and disease? *Southern Medical Journal 96,* 220–223.
16. Steinberg D. (2002). Atherogenesis in perspective: hypercholesterolemia and inflammation as partners in Crime. *Nature Medicine 8,* 1211–1217.
17. American Heart Association. (2002). Heart Facts 2002: All Americans. [On-line]. Available: www.americanheart.org.
18. Enos W. F., Beyer J. C., Holmes R. F. (1955). Pathogenesis of coronary artery disease in American soldiers killed in Korea. *JAMA 158,* 912.
19. Ross R. (1999). Mechanisms of disease: Atherosclerosis—an inflammatory disease. *New England Journal of Medicine 340,* 115–126.
20. Kullo I. J., Gau G. T., Tajik A. J. (2000). Novel risk factors for atherosclerosis. *Mayo Clinic Proceedings 75,* 369–380.
21. Glasser S. P., Selwyn A. P., Ganz P. (1996). Atherosclerosis: Risk factors and the vascular endothelium. *American Heart Journal 31,* 379–384.
22. Levine G. N., Keaney J. F., Vita J. A. (1995). Cholesterol reduction in cardiovascular disease. *New England Journal of Medicine 332,* 512–521.
23. Gaziano J. M., Hebert P. R., Hennekens C. H. (1996). Cholesterol reduction: Weighing the benefits and risks. *Annals of Internal Medicine 124,* 914–918.
24. Libby P., Ridker P. M., Maseri A. (2003). Inflammation and atherosclerosis. *Circulation 105,* 1135–1143.
25. Ridker P. M. (2003). Clinical application of C-reactive protein for cardiovascular disease detection and prevention. *Circulation 107,* 363–369.
26. Hankey G. J., Eikelboom J. W. (1999). Homocysteine and vascular disease. *Lancet 354,* 407–413.
27. Fong I. W. (2000). Emerging relations between infectious diseases and coronary artery disease and atherosclerosis. *Canadian Medical Association Journal 163,* 49–56.
28. Maseri A., Fuster V. (2003). Is there a vulnerable plaque? *Circulation 107,* 2068–2071.

29. Savage C. O. S., Harper L., Cockwell P., et al. (2000). Vasculitis. Clinical review: ABC of arterial and vascular disease. *British Medical Journal 320,* 1325–1328.
30. Gross W. L., Trabandt A., Reinhold-Keller E. (2000). Diagnosis and evaluation of vasculitis. *Rheumatology 39,* 245–252.
31. Longford C. A. (2003). Treatment of ANCA-associated vasculitis. *New England Journal of Medicine 349,* 3–5.
32. Jayne D. (2000). Evidence-based treatment of systemic vasculitis. *Rheumatology 39,* 585–595.
33. Weyand C. M., Goronzy J. J. (2003). Medium- and large-vessel vasculitis. *New England Journal of Medicine 349,* 160–169.
34. Bartholomew J. R., Gray B. H. (1999). Large artery occlusive disease. *Rheumatic Disease Clinics of North America 25,* 669–686.
35. Carter S. A. (1999). Peripheral arterial disease. *Canadian Journal of Cardiology 15*(Suppl. G), 106G–109G.
36. Burns P., Gough S., Bradbury A. W. (2003). The management of peripheral artery disease in primary care. *British Medical Journal 326,* 584–588.
37. Olin J. W. (2000). Thromboangiitis obliterans (Buerger's disease). *New England Journal of Medicine 343,* 864–869.
38. Belch, J. (1997). Raynaud's phenomenon. *Cardiovascular Research 33,* 25–30.
39. Pope J. (2003). Raynaud's phenomenon. *Clinical Evidence Concise 9,* 254–255.
40. Ho M., Belch J. (1998). Raynaud's phenomenon: State of the art. *Scandinavian Journal of Rheumatology 27,* 319–322.
41. Thompson M. M., Bell P. R. F. (2000). Arterial aneurysms. Clinical review: ABC of arterial and venous disease. *British Medical Journal 320,* 1193–1196.
42. Thompson R. W. (2002). Detection and management of small aortic aneurysms. *New England Journal of Medicine 346*(19), 1484–1486.
43. Creager M. A., Halperin J. L., Whittemore A. D. (1992). Aneurysm disease of the aorta and its branches. In Loscalzo J., Creager M. A., Dzau V. J. (Eds.), *Vascular medicine: A textbook of vascular biology and diseases* (pp. 903–923). Boston: Little, Brown.
44. Coady M. A., Rizzo J. A., Goldstein L. J., Elefteriades J. A. (1999). Natural history, pathogenesis, and etiology of thoracic aortic aneurysms and dissections. *Cardiology Clinics of North America 17,* 615–635.
45. House-Fancher M. A. (1996). Aortic dissection. Pathophysiology, diagnosis, and acute care management. *AACN Clinical Issues 6*(3), 602–614.
46. Alguire P. C., Mathes B. M. (1997). Chronic venous insufficiency and venous ulceration. *Journal of General Internal Medicine 12,* 374–383.
47. de Araujo T., Valencia I., Federman D. G., et al. (2003). Managing the patient with venous ulcers. *Annals of Internal Medicine 138,* 326–334.
48. Weinmann E. E., Salzman E. W. (1994). Deep-vein thrombosis. *New England Journal of Medicine 331,* 1630–1641.
49. Virchow R. (1846). Weinere untersuchungen uber die verstropfung der lungenrarterie und ihre folgen. *Beitrage zur Experimentelle Pathologie und Physiologie 2,* 21.
50. Schurr J. H., Machin S. J., Bailey-King S., et al. (2001). Frequency and prevention of symptomless deep-vein thrombosis in long-haul flights. *Lancet 357,* 1485–1489.
51. Sheppard D. R. (2000). Activated protein C resistance: The most common risk factor for venous thromboembolism. *Journal of the American Board of Family Practice 13,* 111–115.
52. Bick R. L. (2003). Cancer-associated thrombosis. *New England Journal of Medicine 349,* 109–111.
53. Levine J. S., Branch D. W., Rauch J. (2002). The antiphospholipid syndrome. *New England Journal of Medicine 346,* 752–763.
54. Gorman W. P., Davis K. R., Donnelly R. (2000). Swollen lower limb—1: General assessment and deep vein thrombosis: Clinical review: ABC of arterial and venous disease. *British Medical Journal 320,* 1453–1456.
55. Kelly J., Hunt B. J. (2002). Role of D-dimers in diagnosis of venous thromboembolism. *Lancet 359,* 456–458.
56. Schafer A. I. (2003). Warfarin for venous thromboembolism—walking the dosing tightrope. *New England Journal of Medicine 348,* 1478–1480.
57. Kalb R. L. (1999). Preventing the sequelae of compartment syndrome. *Hospital Practice 34*(1), 105–107.
58. Matsen F. (1975). Compartment syndrome: A unified concept. *Clinical Orthopaedics and Related Research 113,* 8–13.
59. Ashton H. (1962). Critical closing pressure in human peripheral vascular beds. *Clinical Science 22, 79.*
60. Cullum N., Nelson E. A., Nixon J. (2003). Pressure sores. *Clinical Evidence Concise 9,* 408–409.
61. Langema D. K., Olson B., Hunter S., et al. (1989). Incidence and prediction of pressure ulcers in five patient care settings, extended care, home health, and hospice in one locale. *Decubitus 2*(2), 42.
62. Young L. (1989). Pressure ulcer prevalence and associated patient characteristics in one long-term facility. *Decubitus 2*(2), 52.
63. Thomas D. R. (2001). Prevention and treatment of pressure ulcers: What works? What doesn't. *Cleveland Clinic Journal of Medicine 68,* 704–707, 710–714, 717–722.
64. National Institutes of Health. *Healthy people 2010.* [On-line]. Available: www.health.gov/healthypeople.
65. Patterson J. A., Bennett R. G. (1995). Prevention and treatment of pressure sores. *Journal of the American Geriatric Society 43,* 919–927.
66. Beland I., Passos J. Y. (1981). *Clinical nursing* (4th ed., p. 1112). New York: Macmillan.
67. Reuler J. B., Cooney T. G. (1981). The pressure sore: Pathophysiology and principles of management. *Annals of Internal Medicine 94,* 661–666.
68. Panel for the Prediction and Prevention of Pressure Ulcers in Adults. (1992). *Pressure ulcers in adults: Prediction and prevention.* Clinical practice guideline. No. 3. AHCPR publication no. 92-0047. Rockville, MD: Agency for Health Care Policy and Research, Public Health Service, U.S. Department of Health and Human Services.
69. Bergstrom N., Bennett M. A., Carlson C. E., et al. (1994). *Treatment of pressure ulcers.* Clinical practice guideline. No. 15. AHCPR Publication No. 95-0652. Rockville, MD: U.S. Department of Health and Human Services. Public Health Service, Agency for Health Care Policy and Research.
70. Norton D. (1989). Calculating the risk: Reflections on the Norton Scale. *Decubitus 2*(3), 24–31.
71. Braden B. J. (1989). Clinical utility of the Braden scale for predicting pressure ulcer risk. *Decubitus 2*(3), 44–46, 50–51.
72. National Pressure Ulcer Advisory Panel. (1989). Pressure ulcers, incidence, economics, and risk assessment: Consensus Development Conference Statement. *Decubitus 2*(2), 24–28.
73. Henderson C. T., Ayello E. A., Sussman C., et al. (1997). Draft Definition of stage I pressure ulcers: Inclusion of persons with darkly pigmented skin. National Pressure Ulcer Advisory Panel. *Advances in Wound Care 10,* 16–19.
74. Findlay D. (1996). Practical management of pressure ulcers. *American Family Physician 54,* 1519–1528.
75. Bernabei R., Landi F., Bonini S., et al. (1999). Effect of topical application of nerve-growth factor on pressure ulcers. *Lancet 354,* 307.

CHAPTER 25

Disorders of Blood Pressure Regulation

Blood pressure is probably one of the most variable but best regulated functions of the body. The purpose of the control of blood pressure is to keep blood flow constant to vital organs such as the heart, brain, and kidneys. Without constant flow to these organs, death ensues in seconds, minutes, or days. Although a decrease in flow produces an immediate threat to life, the continuous elevation of blood pressure that occurs with hypertension is a contributor to premature death and disability due to its effects on the heart, blood vessels, and kidneys.

The discussion in this chapter focuses on determinants of blood pressure and conditions of altered arterial pressure—hypertension and orthostatic hypotension.

The Arterial Blood Pressure

After you have completed this section of the chapter, you should be able to meet the following objectives:

- ✦ Define the terms *arterial blood pressure, systolic blood pressure, diastolic blood pressure, pulse pressure,* and *mean arterial blood pressure*
- ✦ Explain how cardiac output and peripheral vascular resistance interact in determining systolic and diastolic blood pressure
- ✦ Describe the neural, humoral, and renal mechanisms for short-term and long-term regulation of blood pressure
- ✦ Describe the requirements for accurate and reliable blood pressure measurement in terms of cuff size, method for determining cuff inflation pressure, deflation rate, and need for observer preparation in measurement method
- ✦ State the rationale for use of self-measurement and ambulatory measurement of blood pressure

The arterial blood pressure reflects the rhythmic ejection of blood from the left ventricle into the aorta. It rises during systole as the left ventricle contracts and falls as the heart relaxes during diastole, giving rise to a pressure pulse (see Chapter 23). The contour of the arterial pressure tracing shown in Figure 25-1 is typical of the pressure changes that occur in the large arteries of the systemic circulation. There is a rapid rise in the pulse contour during left ventricular

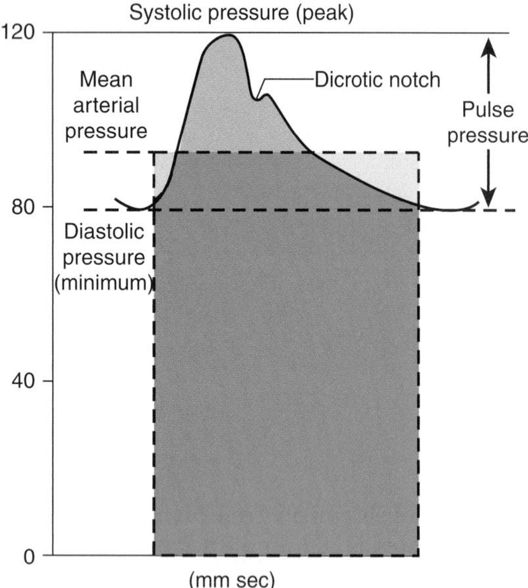

FIGURE 25-1 Intraarterial pressure tracing made from the brachial artery. Pulse pressure is the difference between systolic and diastolic pressures. The darker area represents the mean arterial pressure, which can be calculated by using the formula of mean arterial pressure = diastolic pressure + pulse pressure/3.

contraction, followed by a slower rise to peak pressure. Approximately 70% of the blood that leaves the left ventricle is ejected during the first one third of systole; this accounts for the rapid rise in the pressure contour. The end of systole is marked by a brief downward deflection and formation of the dicrotic notch, which occurs when ventricular pressure falls below that in the aorta. The sudden closure of the aortic valve is associated with a small rise in pressure caused by continued contraction of the aorta and other large vessels against the closed valve. As the ventricles relax and blood flows into the peripheral vessels during diastole, the arterial pressure falls rapidly at first and then declines slowly as the driving force decreases.

In healthy adults, the pressure at the height of the pressure pulse, called the *systolic pressure,* ideally is less than 120 mm Hg, and the lowest pressure, called the *diastolic pressure,* is less than 80 mm Hg. The difference between the systolic and diastolic pressure (approximately 40 mm Hg) is called the *pulse pressure.* It reflects the magnitude or height of the pressure pulse. The *mean arterial pressure* (approximately 90 to 100 mm Hg), depicted by the darker area under the pressure tracing in Figure 25-1, represents the average pressure in the arterial system during ventricular contraction and relaxation.

DETERMINANTS OF BLOOD PRESSURE

The systolic and diastolic components of blood pressure are determined by the cardiac output and the peripheral vascular resistance and can be expressed as the product of the two (blood pressure = cardiac output × peripheral vascular resistance). The cardiac output is the product of the stroke volume (amount of blood that the heart ejects with each beat) and the heart rate or number of times the heart beats each minute. The peripheral vascular resistance reflects changes in the radius of the arterioles as well as the viscosity or thickness of the blood. The arterioles often are referred to as the resistance vessels because they can selectively constrict or relax to control the resistance to outflow of blood into the capillaries. The body maintains its blood pressure by adjusting the cardiac output to compensate for changes in peripheral vascular resistance and changes the peripheral vascular resistance to compensate for changes in cardiac output.

In hypertension and disease conditions that affect blood pressure, changes in blood pressure usually are described in terms of systolic, diastolic, pulse pressure, and mean arterial pressure. These pressures are influenced by the stroke volume, the rapidity with which blood is ejected from the heart, the elastic properties of the aorta and large arteries and their ability to accept the various amounts of blood as it is ejected from the heart, and the properties of the resistance vessels that control the runoff of blood into the smaller vessels and capillaries that connect the arterial and venous circulation.[1]

Systolic Blood Pressure

The *systolic blood pressure* reflects the rhythmic ejection of blood into the aorta (Fig. 25-2). As blood is ejected from the left ventricle into the aorta, it stretches the vessel wall and produces a rise in aortic pressure. The extent to which the systolic pressure rises or falls with each cardiac cycle is determined by the amount of blood ejected into the aorta with each heart beat (*i.e., stroke volume*), the velocity of ejection, and the elastic properties of the aorta. Systolic pressure increases when there is a rapid ejection of a large stroke volume or when the stroke volume is ejected into a

DETERMINANTS OF BLOOD PRESSURE

- The arterial blood pressure represents the pressure of the blood as it moves through the arterial system. It reaches its peak (systolic pressure) as blood is ejected from the heart during systole and its lowest level (diastolic pressure) as the heart relaxes during diastole.
- Blood pressure is determined by the cardiac output (stroke volume × heart rate) and the resistance that the blood encounters as it moves through the peripheral vessels (peripheral vascular resistance).
- The systolic blood pressure is largely determined by the characteristics of the stroke volume being ejected from the heart and the ability of the aorta to stretch and accommodate the stroke volume.
- The diastolic pressure is largely determined by the energy that is stored in the aorta as its elastic fibers are stretched during systole and by the resistance to the runoff of blood from the peripheral blood vessels.

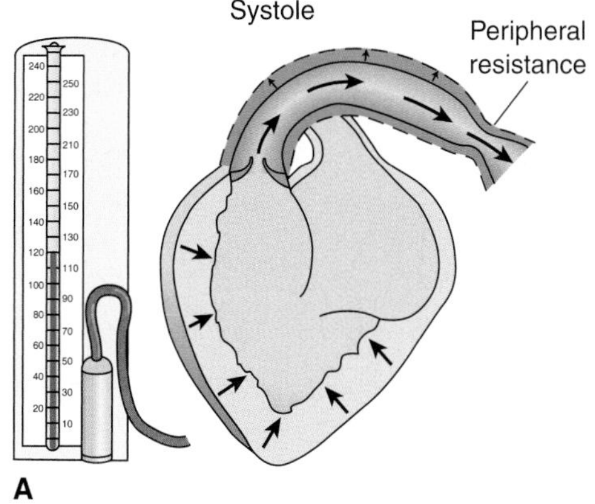

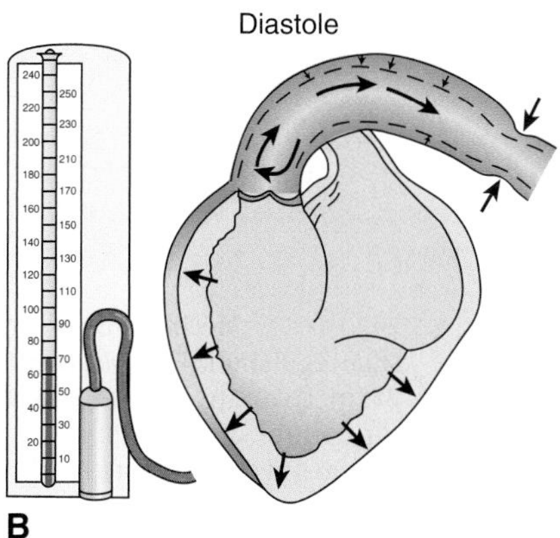

FIGURE 25-2 Diagram of the left side of the heart and aorta. (**A**) Systolic blood pressure represents the ejection of blood into the aorta during ventricular systole; it reflects the stroke volume, the distensibility of the aorta, and the velocity with which blood is ejected from the heart. (**B**) Diastolic blood pressure represents the pressure in the arterial system during diastole; it is largely determined by the peripheral vascular resistance.

rigid aorta. Only approximately one third of the ejected blood leaves the aorta during ventricular systole. The elastic walls of the aorta normally stretch to accommodate the varying amounts of blood that are ejected into the aorta; this prevents the pressure from rising excessively during systole and serves to maintain the pressure during diastole. In some elderly persons, the elastic fibers of the aorta lose some of their resiliency, and the aorta becomes more rigid. When this occurs, the aorta is less able to stretch and buffer the pressure that is generated as blood is ejected into the aorta, resulting in an elevated systolic pressure.

Diastolic Blood Pressure

The *diastolic blood pressure* is maintained by the energy that has been stored in the elastic walls of the aorta during systole (see Fig. 25-2). The level at which the diastolic pressure is maintained depends on the condition of the aorta and large arteries and their ability to stretch and store energy, the competency of the aortic valve, and the resistance of the arterioles that control the outflow of blood into the capillaries of the microcirculation. The larger arteries are located between the outlet of the aorta and the arterioles, which control the runoff of blood from the arterial circulation. When there is an increase in peripheral vascular resistance, as with sympathetic stimulation, diastolic blood pressure rises. With arteriosclerosis, the smaller arteries may become rigid and unable to accept the runoff of blood from the aorta without producing an increase in diastolic pressure. Closure of the aortic valve at the onset of diastole is essential to the maintenance of the diastolic pressure. When there is incomplete closure of the aortic valve, as in aortic regurgitation (see Chapter 26), the diastolic pressure drops as blood flows backward into the left ventricle rather than moving forward into the arterial system.

Pulse Pressure

The *pulse pressure* is the difference between the systolic and diastolic pressures. It reflects the pulsatile nature of arterial blood flow and is an important component of blood pressure. During the rapid ejection period of ventricular systole, the volume of blood that is ejected into the aorta exceeds the amount that is already in the arterial system. The pulse pressure reflects this difference. The pulse pressure rises when additional amounts of blood are ejected into the arterial circulation, and it falls when the resistance to outflow is decreased. In hypovolemic shock, the pulse pressure declines because of a decrease in stroke volume and systolic pressure. This occurs despite an increase in peripheral vascular resistance, which maintains the diastolic pressure.

Mean Arterial Pressure

The *mean arterial blood pressure* represents the average blood pressure in the systemic circulation. Mean arterial pressure can be estimated by adding one third of the pulse pressure to the diastolic pressure (*i.e.,* diastolic blood pressure + pulse pressure/3). Hemodynamic monitoring equipment in intensive and coronary care units measures or computes mean arterial pressure automatically. Because it is a good indicator of tissue perfusion, the mean arterial pressure often is monitored, along with systolic and diastolic blood pressures, in critically ill patients.

MECHANISMS OF BLOOD PRESSURE REGULATION

Although different tissues in the body are able to regulate their own blood flow, it is necessary for the arterial pressure to remain relatively constant as blood shifts from one area of the body to another. The mechanisms used to regulate the arterial pressure depend on whether short-term or long-term adaptation is needed. The mechanisms of blood pressure regulation are illustrated in Figure 25-3.

Short-Term Regulation

The mechanisms for short-term regulation of blood pressure, those occurring over minutes or hours, are intended

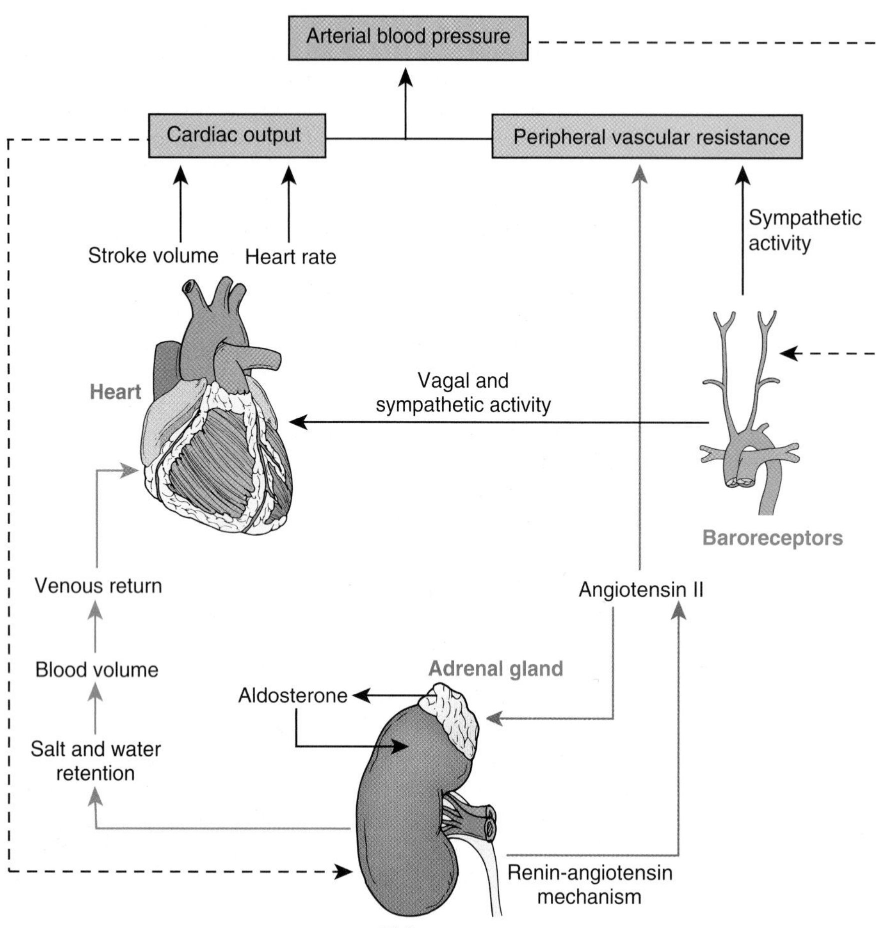

FIGURE 25-3 Mechanisms of blood pressure regulation. The *solid lines* represent the mechanisms for renal and baroreceptor control of blood pressure through changes in cardiac output and peripheral vascular resistance. The *dashed lines* represent the stimulus for regulation of blood pressure by the baroreceptors and the kidneys.

to correct temporary imbalances in blood pressure, such as occur during physical exercise and changes in body position. These mechanisms also are responsible for maintenance of blood pressure at survival levels during life-threatening situations. The short-term regulation of blood pressure relies mainly on neural and hormonal mechanisms, the most rapid of which are the neural mechanisms.

Neural Mechanisms. The neural control centers for the regulation of blood pressure is located in the reticular formation of the lower pons and medulla of the brain where integration and modulation of autonomic nervous system (ANS) responses occur.[2] This area of the brain contains the vasomotor and cardiac control centers and is often collectively referred to as the *cardiovascular center.* The cardiovascular center transmits parasympathetic impulses to the heart through the vagus nerve and transmits sympathetic impulses to the heart and blood vessels through the spinal cord and peripheral sympathetic nerves. Vagal stimulation of the heart produces a slowing of heart rate, while sympathetic stimulation produces an increase in heart rate and cardiac contractility. Blood vessels are selectively innervated by the sympathetic nervous system. Increased sympathetic activity produces constriction of the small arteries and arterioles with a resultant increase in peripheral vascular resistance.

The ANS control of blood pressure is mediated through intrinsic circulatory reflexes, extrinsic reflexes, and higher neural control centers. The *intrinsic reflexes,* including the *baroreflex* and *chemoreceptor-mediated reflex,* are located in the circulatory system and are essential for rapid and short-term regulation of blood pressure. The sensors for *extrinsic reflexes* are found outside the circulation. They include blood pressure responses associated with factors such as pain and cold. The neural pathways for these reactions are more diffuse, and their responses are less consistent than those of the intrinsic reflexes. Many of these responses are channeled through the hypothalamus, which plays an essential role in the control of sympathetic nervous system responses. Among higher-center responses are those caused by changes in mood and emotion.

The *baroreceptors* are pressure-sensitive receptors located in the walls of blood vessels and the heart. The carotid and aortic baroreceptors are located in strategic positions between the heart and the brain (Fig. 25-4). They respond to changes in the stretch of the vessel wall by sending impulses to cardiovascular centers in the brain stem to effect appropriate changes in heart rate and vascular smooth muscle tone. For example, the fall in blood pressure that

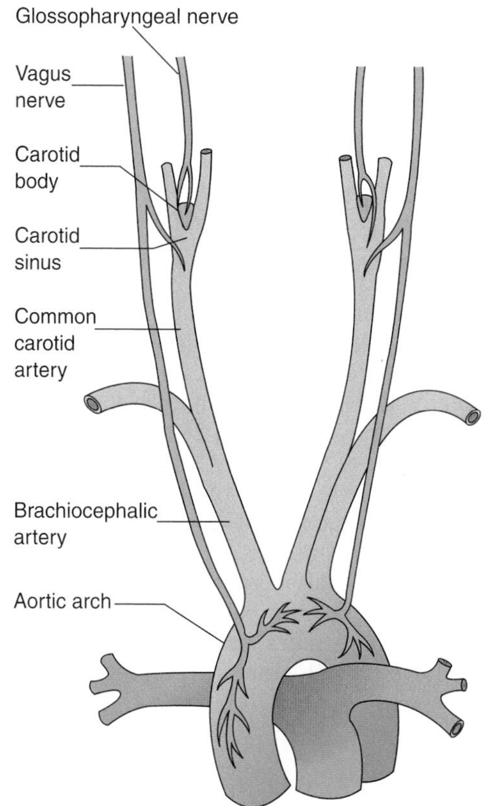

FIGURE 25-4 Location and innervation of the aortic arch and carotid sinus baroreceptors and the carotid body chemoreceptors.

occurs on moving from the lying to the standing position produces a decrease in the stretch of the baroreceptors with a resultant increase in heart rate and sympathetically induced vasoconstriction that causes an increase in peripheral vascular resistance.

The *arterial chemoreceptors* are sensitive to changes in the oxygen, carbon dioxide, and hydrogen ion content of the blood. They are located in the carotid bodies, which lie in the bifurcation of the two common carotids, and in the aortic bodies of the aorta (see Fig. 25-4). Because of their location, these chemoreceptors are always in close contact with the arterial blood. Although the main function of the chemoreceptors is to regulate ventilation, they also communicate with cardiovascular centers in the brain stem and can induce widespread vasoconstriction. Whenever the arterial pressure drops below a critical level, the chemoreceptors are stimulated because of diminished oxygen supply and a buildup of carbon dioxide and hydrogen ions. In persons with chronic lung disease, systemic and pulmonary hypertension may develop because of hypoxemia (see Chapter 31).

Humoral Mechanisms. A number of hormones and humoral mechanisms contribute to blood pressure regulation, including the *renin-angiotensin-aldosterone mechanism* and *vasopressin*. Other humoral substances, such as epinephrine, a sympathetic neurotransmitter released from the adrenal gland, have the effect of directly stimulating an increase in heart rate, cardiac contractility, and vascular tone.

The *renin-angiotensin-aldosterone mechanism* plays a central role in blood pressure regulation. Renin is an enzyme that is synthesized, stored, and released by the kidneys in response to an increase in sympathetic nervous system activity or a decrease in blood pressure, extracellular fluid volume, or extracellular sodium concentration. Most of the renin that is released leaves the kidney and enters the bloodstream, where it acts enzymatically to convert an inactive circulating plasma protein called *angiotensinogen* to angiotensin I (Fig. 25-5). Angiotensin I travels to the small blood vessels of the lung, where it is converted to angiotensin II by the angiotensin-converting enzyme that is present in the endothelium of the lung vessels. Although angiotensin II has a half-life of several minutes, renin persists in the circulation for 30 minutes to 1 hour and continues to cause production of angiotensin II during this time.

Angiotensin II functions in both the short-term and long-term regulation of blood pressure. It is a strong vasoconstrictor, particularly of arterioles and to a lesser extent of veins. The vasoconstrictor response produces an increase in peripheral vascular resistance (and blood pressure) and functions in the short-term regulation of blood pressure. A second major function of angiotensin II, stimulation of aldosterone secretion from the adrenal gland, contributes to the long-term regulation of blood pressure by increasing salt and water retention by the kidney. It also acts directly on the kidney to decrease the elimination of salt and water.

Vasopressin, also known as antidiuretic hormone (ADH), is released from the posterior pituitary gland in response to decreases in blood volume and blood pressure, an increase in the osmolality of body fluids, and other stimuli. The antidiuretic actions of vasopressin are discussed in Chapter 33. Vasopressin has a direct vasoconstrictor effect on blood vessels, particularly those of the splanchnic circulation that supplies the abdominal viscera. However, long-term increases in vasopressin cannot maintain volume expansion or hypertension, and vasopressin does not enhance hypertension produced by sodium-retaining hormones or other vasoconstricting substances. It has been suggested that vasopressin plays a permissive role in hypertension through its fluid-retaining properties or as a neurotransmitter that serves to modify ANS function.

Long-Term Regulation

Long-term mechanisms control the daily, weekly, and monthly regulation of blood pressure. Although the neural and hormonal mechanisms involved in the short-term regulation of blood pressure act rapidly, they are unable to maintain their effectiveness over time. Instead, the long-term regulation of blood pressure is largely vested in the kidneys and their role in the regulation of extracellular fluid volume.[2]

Renal Mechanism. The role that the kidneys play in blood pressure regulation is emphasized by the fact that many

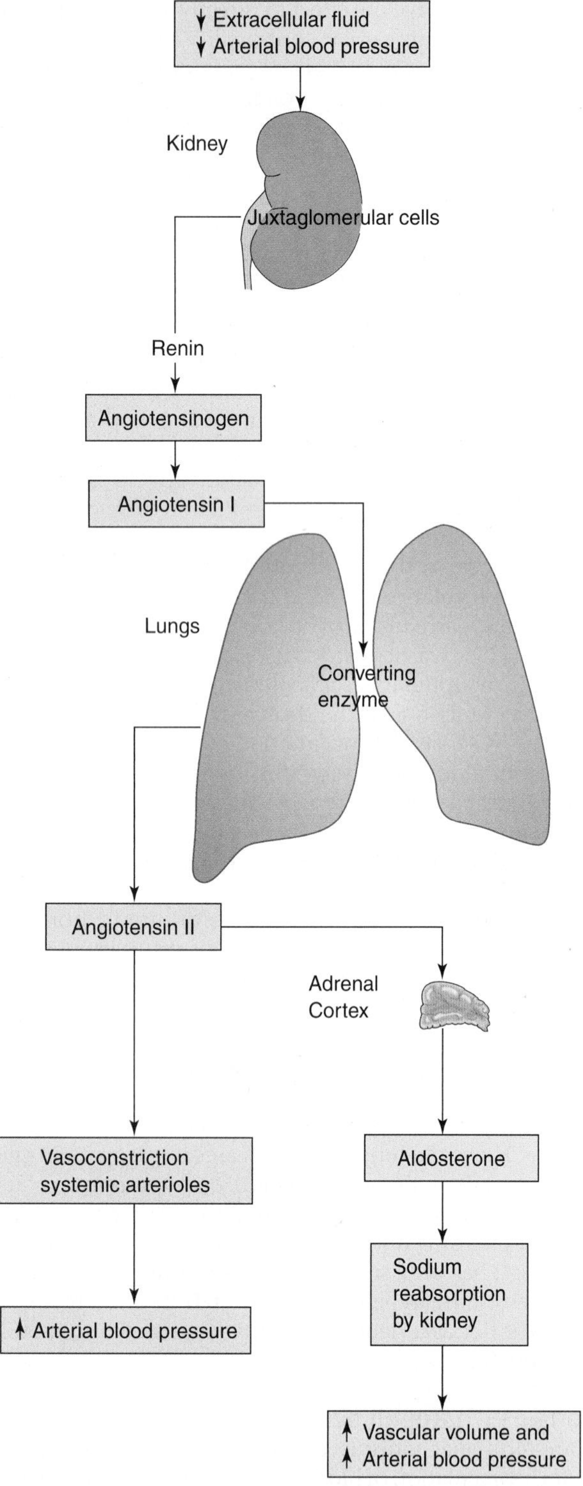

FIGURE 25-5 Control of blood pressure by the renin-angiotensin-aldosterone system. Renin enzymatically converts the plasma protein angiotensinogen to angiotensin I; angiotensin-converting enzyme in the lung converts angiotensin I to angiotensin II; and angiotensin II produces vasoconstriction and increases salt and water retention through direct action on the kidney and through increased aldosterone secretion by the adrenal cortex.

hypertension medications produce their blood pressure–lowering effects by increasing salt and water elimination.

According to the late Arthur Guyton, a noted physiologist, the extracellular fluid volume and the arterial blood pressure are regulated around an equilibrium point, which represents the normal pressure for a given individual (Fig. 25-6). When the body contains an excess of extracellular fluid, the arterial pressure rises, and the rate at which water (*i.e., pressure diuresis*) and salt (*i.e., pressure natriuresis*) are excreted by the kidney is increased.[2] Accordingly, there are two ways that arterial pressure can be increased using this model: one is by shifting the elimination of salt and water to a higher pressure level (see Fig. 25-6A), and the second is by changing the extracellular fluid level at which diuresis and natriuresis occur (see Fig. 25-6B).

The function of the kidney in the long-term regulation of blood pressure can be influenced by a number of factors. For example, excess sympathetic nerve activity or the release of vasoconstrictor substances can alter the transmission of arterial pressure to the kidney. Similarly, changes in neural and humoral control of kidney function can shift the diuresis-natriuresis process to a higher fluid or pressure level, thereby initiating an increase in arterial pressure.

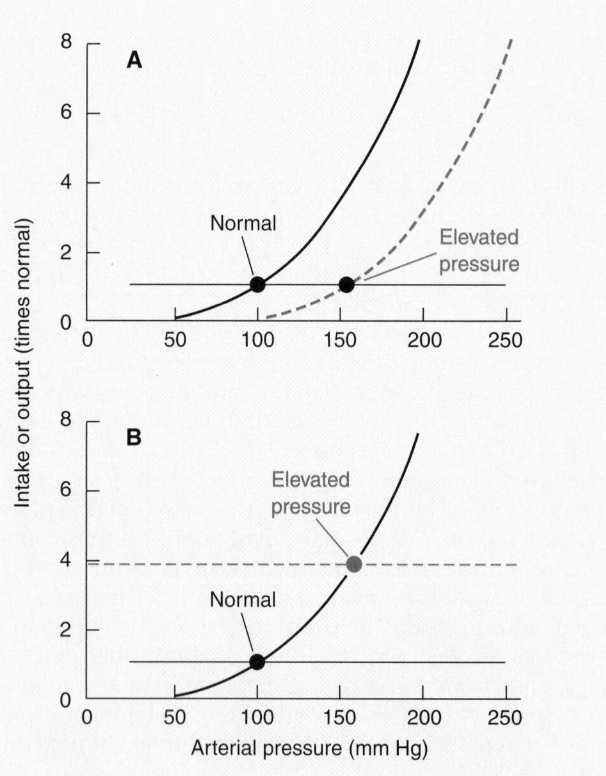

FIGURE 25-6 Two ways in which the arterial pressure can be increased: (**A**) by shifting the renal output curve in the right-hand direction toward a higher pressure level and (**B**) by increasing the intake level of salt and water. (Guyton A. C., Hall J. E. [1996]. *Textbook of medical physiology* [9th ed., p. 223]. Philadelphia: W. B. Saunders)

Extracellular Fluid Volume. There are several ways that extracellular fluid volume regulates blood pressure. One is through a direct effect on cardiac output, and another is indirect, resulting from autoregulation of blood flow and its effect on peripheral vascular resistance (Fig. 25-7). Autoregulatory mechanisms function in distributing blood flow to the various tissues of the body according to their metabolic needs (see Chapter 23). When the blood flow to a specific tissue bed is excessive, local blood vessels constrict, and when the flow is deficient, the local vessels dilate. In situations of increased blood volume and cardiac output, all of the tissues of the body are exposed to the same increase in flow. This results in a generalized constriction of arterioles and an increase in the peripheral vascular resistance (and blood pressure).

CIRCADIAN RHYTHMS IN BLOOD PRESSURE

Normal changes in blood pressure follow a characteristic circadian pattern. Blood pressure tends to be highest in the early morning, shortly after arising from sleep, and then decreases gradually throughout the day, reaching its lowest point at approximately 2:00 to 5:00 AM. In healthy normotensive people, mean intraarterial pressure falls by approximately 20% from waking to sleeping hours.[3]

BLOOD PRESSURE MEASUREMENT

Arterial blood pressure measurements usually are obtained by the *indirect auscultatory method,* which uses a sphygmomanometer and a stethoscope. In the measurement of blood pressure, a cuff that contains an inflatable rubber bladder is placed around the upper arm. It is important that the bladder of the cuff be appropriate for the arm size. The width of the bladder should be at least 40% of arm circumference and the length at least 80% of arm circumference.[4,5] Undercuffing (using a cuff with a bladder that is small) can cause an overestimation of blood pressure.[6] This is because a cuff that is too small results in an uneven distribution of pressure across the arm, such that a greater cuff pressure is needed to occlude blood flow. Likewise, overcuffing (using a cuff with a bladder that is too large) can cause an underestimation of blood pressure.

The bladder of the cuff is inflated to a point at which its pressure exceeds that of the artery, occluding the blood flow. This should be done by palpation before the actual pressure is measured to get the palpated systolic pressure. By inflating the pressure in the cuff to a level of 30 mm Hg above the palpated pressure, the observer can be certain that the cuff pressure is high enough to avoid missing the auscultatory gap. This pressure (palpated pressure + 30 mm Hg) is called the *maximum inflation level.*[4] The

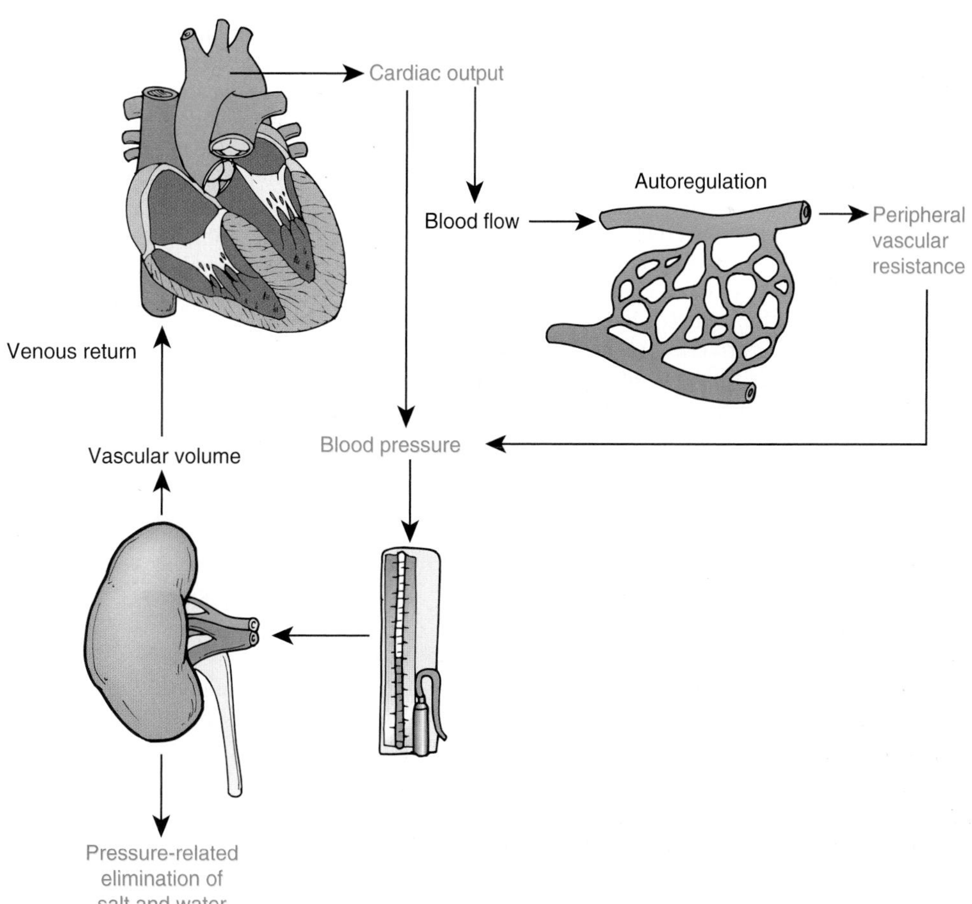

FIGURE 25-7 Effect of extracellular fluid volume on cardiac output, peripheral vascular resistance, blood pressure, and elimination of salt and water by the kidney.

cuff is then slowly deflated at 2 mm/s. The accuracy of the reading can be no greater than the rate of deflation. At the point where the pressure in the vessel again exceeds the pressure in the cuff, a small amount of blood squirts through the partially obstructed artery. The sounds generated by the turbulent flow are called the *Korotkoff (K) sounds* (Chart 25-1). These low-pitched sounds are best heard with the bell of the stethoscope. Blood pressure is recorded in terms of systolic and diastolic pressures (*e.g.*, 120/70 mm Hg) unless sounds are heard to zero, then three readings are required (122/64/0 or K1/K4/K5). Systolic pressure is defined as the first of at least two regular Korotkoff sounds. Diastolic pressure is recorded as the last sound heard (K5) unless sounds are heard to zero, in which case, the muffling sound of K4 is used.

Automated or *semiautomated methods* of blood pressure measurement use a microphone, arterial pressure pulse sensor (oscillometric method), or Doppler equipment for detecting the equivalent of the Korotkoff sounds. Oscillometric measurement depends on the detection of pulsatile oscillations of the brachial artery in the blood pressure cuff.[7] In contrast to the auscultatory method, this method determines the mean arterial pressure based on the amplitude of the arterial pulsations and then uses an algorithm to calculate the systolic and diastolic pressures.

Blood pressures obtained by automated devices are usually less accurate than those obtained by trained observers using the auscultatory method, and it is recommended that their use be limited to situations in which frequent and less accurate measures of blood pressure trends are needed. They should not be used for the diagnosis and management of hypertension.[4] Automated devices are useful for the self-monitoring of blood pressure and for 24-hour ambulatory monitoring of blood pressure.[8]

Intraarterial methods provide for direct measurement of blood pressure. Intraarterial measurement requires the insertion of a catheter into a peripheral artery, or it may be obtained at the time of cardiac catheterization in the aortic root. The arterial catheter is connected to a pressure transducer, which converts pressure into a digital signal that can be measured, displayed, and recorded. This type of blood pressure monitoring usually is restricted to intensive care units.

CHART 25-1

Korotkoff Sounds

Phase I	Period marked by the first tapping sounds, which gradually increase in intensity
Phase II	Period during which a murmur or swishing sound is heard
Phase III	Period during which sounds are crisper and greater in intensity
Phase IV	Period marked by distinct, abrupt muffling or by a soft blowing sound
Phase V	Point at which sounds disappear

CLINICAL APPLICATION

Ambulatory and Home Blood Pressure Monitoring

The use of ambulatory and home (self) blood pressure monitoring equipment has grown dramatically. Ambulatory and self blood pressure monitoring equipment should meet the testing standards of the Association for Advancement of Medical Instrumentation or the British Hypertension Society.[8] Ambulatory blood pressure units are fully automatic, small, and easy to use. Typically, they take a blood pressure reading every 15 to 30 minutes throughout the day and night while the person goes about her or his normal activities. The readings are stored and then downloaded onto a personal computer for analysis. Many of the ambulatory blood pressure measuring devices are equipped with "event buttons" that allow persons to obtain a blood pressure reading when they feel dizzy or have other symptoms associated with blood pressure changes.

Home monitoring equipment is sold in pharmacies and medical supply stores throughout the country and is available in many styles and prices. It is important that automated devices have been certified as accurate and reliable because not all devices on the market are considered acceptable.[4] The equipment should be a validated electronic device or an aneroid monitor, should use an appropriate-sized inflatable cuff, and should be checked once each year for accuracy. *Self-measurement of blood pressure* may provide valuable information outside the clinician's office regarding a person's blood pressure and response to treatment. It can help distinguish white-coat hypertension, a condition in which the blood pressure is consistently elevated in the health care provider's office but normal at other times, and it can be used to assess the response to treatment methods for hypertension.[7]

In summary, the alternating contraction and relaxation of the heart produce a pressure pulse that moves the blood through the circulatory system. The elastic walls of the aorta stretch during systole and relax during diastole to maintain the diastolic pressure. The pressure pulse is responsible for the Korotkoff sounds heard when blood pressure is measured using a blood pressure cuff, and it is this impulse that is felt when the pulse is taken. Systolic pressure denotes the highest point of the pulse pressure, and diastolic denotes the lowest point. The pulse pressure is the difference between these two pressures. The mean arterial pressure reflects the average pressure throughout the cardiac cycle. It can be estimated by adding one third of the pulse pressure to the diastolic pressure.

Physical (*i.e.*, blood volume and the elastic properties of the blood vessels) and physiologic (*i.e.*, cardiac output and peripheral vascular resistance) factors influence mean arterial blood pressure. Systolic pressure is determined primarily by the characteristics of the stroke volume, whereas diastolic pressure is determined largely by the conditions of the arteries and arterioles and their abilities to accept the runoff of blood from the aorta. The pulse pressure reflects the pulsatile nature of the arterial blood flow and is an important component of blood pressure. The mean arterial blood pressure represents the average blood pressure in the systemic circulation. It can be estimated by adding one third of the pulse pressure to the diastolic blood pressure.

The regulation of blood pressure involves both short-term and long-term mechanisms. The short-term mechanisms are responsible for regulating blood pressure on a minute-by-minute or hour-by-hour basis during activities such as physical exercise and changes in body position. These mechanisms also are responsible for the maintenance of blood pressure at survival levels during life-threatening situations. The short-term regulation of blood pressure relies mainly on neural and hormonal mechanisms, the most rapid of which are the neural mechanisms. The long-term mechanisms, those maintaining blood pressure over days, weeks, and even years, are largely vested in the kidney and the regulation of extracellular fluid volume. When the body contains excess extracellular fluid, the blood pressure rises, and the rate at which water (pressure diuresis) and salt (pressure natriuresis) are excreted by the kidney is increased.

Normal changes in blood pressure follow a characteristic circadian pattern, being highest in the early morning, decreasing gradually throughout the day, and reaching its lowest point at approximately 2:00 to 5:00 AM.

Arterial blood pressure measurements usually are obtained by the indirect auscultatory method, which uses a sphygmomanometer and a stethoscope. Automated or semiautomated methods of blood pressure measurement use a microphone, arterial pressure pulse sensor (oscillometric method), or Doppler equipment for detecting the equivalent of the Korotkoff sounds. Self-measurement of blood pressure may provide valuable information outside the clinician's office regarding a person's blood pressure and response to treatment. Accurate blood pressure measurement, whether by auscultatory or automated methods, requires the use of accurately calibrated equipment, a properly fitted cuff, and proper level of cuff inflation and timing for deflation of the blood pressure cuff.

Hypertension

After you have completed this section of the chapter, you should be able to meet the following objectives:

- Cite the definition of hypertension put forth by the seventh report of the Joint National Committee on Detection, Evaluation, and Treatment of Hypertension
- Differentiate essential, systolic, secondary, and malignant forms of hypertension
- Describe the possible influence of genetics, age, race, obesity, diet and sodium intake, and alcohol consumption on the development of essential hypertension
- Cite the risks of hypertension in terms of target organ damage
- Describe behavior modification strategies used in the prevention and treatment of hypertension
- List the different categories of drugs used to treat hypertension and state their mechanisms of action in the treatment of high blood pressure
- Explain the changes in blood pressure that accompany normal pregnancy and describe the four types of hypertension that can occur during pregnancy
- Cite the criteria for the diagnosis of high blood pressure in children
- Define systolic hypertension and relate the circulatory changes that occur with aging that predispose to the development of systolic hypertension

Hypertension, or high blood pressure, is probably the most common of all health problems in adults and is the leading risk factor for cardiovascular disorders. It affects approximately 50 million individuals in the United States and approximately 1 billion worldwide.[9] Hypertension is more common in younger men compared with younger women, in blacks compared with whites, in persons from lower socioeconomic groups, and in older persons. Men have higher blood pressures than women up until the time of menopause, at which point women quickly lose their protection. The prevalence of hypertension increases with age. Recent data from the Framingham study suggest that persons who are normotensive at age 55 have a 90% lifetime risk for developing hypertension.[10] Thus, the problem of hypertension can be expected to become even greater with the aging of the "baby-boomer" population. Hypertension commonly is divided into the categories of primary and secondary hypertension. In primary hypertension, often called *essential hypertension,* the chronic elevation in blood pressure occurs without evidence of other disease. In secondary hypertension, the elevation of blood pressure results from some other disorder, such as kidney disease. Malignant hypertension, as the name implies, is an accelerated form of hypertension.

ESSENTIAL HYPERTENSION

The seventh report of the Joint National Committee on Detection, Evaluation, and Treatment of High Blood Pressure (JNC-7) of the National Institutes of Health was published in 2003.[9] According to the JNC-7 recommendations, a systolic pressure of less than 120 mm Hg and a diastolic pressure of less than 80 mm Hg are normal, and systolic pressures between 120 and 139 mm Hg and diastolic pressures between 80 and 89 mm Hg are considered prehypertensive (Table 25-1). A diagnosis of hypertension is made if the systolic blood pressure is 140 mm Hg or higher and the diastolic blood pressure is 90 mm Hg or higher. For adults with diabetes mellitus, the blood pressure goal has been lowered to less than 130/80 mm Hg.[11] Hypertension is further divided into stages 1 and 2 based on systolic and

HYPERTENSION

- Hypertension represents an elevation in systolic and/or diastolic blood pressure.
- Essential hypertension is characterized by a chronic elevation in blood pressure that occurs without evidence of other disease, and secondary hypertension by an elevation of blood pressure that results from some other disorder, such as kidney disease.
- The pathogenesis of essential hypertension is thought to reside with the kidney and its role regulating vascular volume through salt and water elimination; the renin-angiotensin-aldosterone system through its effects on blood vessel tone, regulation of renal blood flow, and salt metabolism; and the sympathetic nervous system, which regulates the tone of the resistance vessels. The medications that are used in the treatment of hypertension exert their effects through one or more of these regulatory mechanisms.
- Uncontrolled hypertension produces increased demands on the heart, resulting in left ventricular hypertrophy and heart failure, and on the vessels of the arterial system, leading to atherosclerosis, kidney disease, and stroke.

diastolic blood pressure measurements (see Table 25-1). Systolic hypertension (to be discussed) is defined as a systolic pressure of 140 mm Hg or greater and a diastolic pressure less than 90 mm Hg.

Risk Factors

Although the cause or causes of essential hypertension are largely unknown, several risk factors have been implicated as contributing to its development. These risk factors include family history of hypertension, race, and age-related increases in blood pressure.[12] Another factor that is thought to contribute to hypertension is the insulin resistance and resultant hyperinsulinemia that occurs in persons with metabolic abnormalities such as those that occur with obesity and type 2 diabetes.

Family History. The inclusion of heredity as a contributing factor in the development of hypertension is supported by the fact that hypertension is seen most frequently among persons with a family history of hypertension. The strength of the prediction depends on the definition of positive family history and the age of the person at risk.[13] Persons with two or more first-degree relatives with hypertension before age 55 years have a 3.8 times greater risk for development of hypertension before age 50 years than persons without a family history.[14] At the same time, older persons in families with a strong family history of developing hypertension at a later age have a risk similar to that of the general population, suggesting they do not share the genetic predisposition associated with early-onset hypertension. The inherited predisposition does not seem to rely on other risk factors, but when they are present, the risk apparently is additive.

The pattern of heredity is unclear; it is unknown whether a single gene or multiple genes are involved. Whatever the explanation, the higher incidence of hypertension among close family members seems significant enough to be presented as a case for recommending that persons from these high-risk families be encouraged to participate in hypertensive screening programs on a regular basis.

Age-Related Changes in Blood Pressure. Maturation and growth are known to cause predictable increases in blood pressure. For example, in the newborn, arterial blood pressure normally is only approximately 50 mm Hg systolic and 40 mm Hg diastolic. Sequentially, blood pressure increases with physical growth from a value of 78 mm Hg systolic at 10 days of age to 120 mm Hg at the end of adolescence. Systolic blood pressure continues to undergo a slow rate of increase throughout adult life, whereas diastolic pressure increases until 50 years of age and then declines from the sixth decade onward.[15,16]

Race. Hypertension not only is more prevalent in African Americans than whites, it is more severe. The Third National Health and Nutrition Survey (NHANES) III, 1988 to 1991, reported that diastolic blood pressures were significantly greater for African Americans than for white men and women 35 years of age and older, and that systolic pressures of African-American women at every age were greater than those of white women.[17,18] Hypertension tends to occur earlier in African Americans than in whites, and it often is not treated early enough or aggressively enough. Blacks also tend to experience greater cardiovascular and renal damage at any level of pressure.[18] Unfor-

TABLE 25-1 Classification of Blood Pressure for Adults

Blood Pressure Classification	Systolic Blood Pressure (mm Hg)	Diastolic Blood Pressure (mm Hg)
Normal	<120	and <80
Prehypertensive	120–139	or 80–89
Stage 1 hypertension	140–159	or 90–99
Stage 2 hypertension	≥160	Or ≥100

(Modified from National Heart, Lung, and Blood Institute. [2003]. *The seventh report of the National Committee on Detection, Evaluation, and Treatment of High Blood Pressure.* Publication No. 03–5233. Bethesda, MD: NIH) tunately, there is less information regarding hypertension in other racial groups, including Native Americans, Asians and Pacific Islanders, and Hispanics.

The reasons for the increased incidence of hypertension among African Americans are unknown. Studies have shown that many African-American persons with hypertension have lower renin levels than white persons with hypertension.[19] They also do not respond to increased salt intake by increasing their renal excretion of sodium at normal levels of arterial blood pressure. Instead, sodium elimination requires a higher level of blood pressure. These changes in sodium excretion have been linked to what has been called a *salt-thrifty gene*. It has been suggested that the genetic trait may have developed as an evolutionary adaptation to the severe demands for sodium conservation in the western African environment and the slavery environment of the Western Hemisphere. In both environments, survival under conditions of heavy exertion in a warm climate along with salt and water deprivation depended on the body's ability to conserve sodium.[20]

Evidence suggests that blacks, when provided equal access to diagnosis and treatment, can achieve overall reductions in blood pressure and experience fewer cardiovascular complications similar to whites. Barriers that limit access to the health care system include inadequate financial support, inconveniently located health care facilities, long waiting times, and inaccessibility to culturally relevant health education about hypertension. With the high prevalence of salt sensitivity, obesity, and smoking among blacks, health education and lifestyle modifications are particularly important.

Insulin Resistance and Metabolic Abnormalities. Insulin resistance and an accompanying compensatory hyperinsulinemia have been suggested as possible etiologic links to the development of hypertension and associated metabolic disturbances such as impaired glucose tolerance, type 2 diabetes, hyperlipidemias, and obesity.[21] This clustering of cardiovascular risk factors has been named the *insulin resistance syndrome, cardiovascular dysmetabolic syndrome,* or *metabolic syndrome X* (see Chapter 43).[22]

In persons with obesity and type 2 diabetes, the defect appears to be in the ability of insulin to stimulate the uptake and disposal of glucose by skeletal muscle.[23] It has been suggested that the insulin-mediated increase in sympathetic activity is directed at increasing the metabolic rate as a means of burning the calories that cannot be stored because of insulin resistance. Unfortunately, the increase in sympathetic activity also contributes to the development of hypertension by stimulating the heart, blood vessels, and kidney.

Insulin resistance may be a genetic or acquired trait. For example, it has been shown that insulin-mediated glucose disposal declines by 30% to 40% in persons who are 40% over ideal weight. Nonpharmacologic interventions, such as caloric restriction, weight loss, and exercise, tend to decrease insulin resistance, sympathetic nervous system activity, and blood pressure.[23]

Circadian Variations (Dippers Versus Nondippers). The term *dippers* is used to refer to persons with a normal circadian blood pressure profile in which blood pressure falls during the night, and *nondippers* for persons whose 24-hour blood pressure profile is flattened. Ambulatory blood pressure monitoring can be used to determine alterations in a person's circadian blood pressure profile. Changes in the normal circadian blood pressure profile may occur in a number of conditions, including malignant hypertension, Cushing syndrome, preeclampsia, orthostatic hypotension, congestive heart failure, and sleep apnea.[3] There is increasing evidence that alterations in the normal nocturnal decline in blood pressure may contribute to the development of target-organ damage in persons with hypertension.

Lifestyle Factors

Lifestyle factors can contribute to the development of hypertension by interacting with the risk factors. These lifestyle factors include high sodium intake, excessive calorie intake and obesity, physical inactivity, excessive alcohol consumption, and low intake of potassium. Oral contraceptive drugs also may increase blood pressure in predisposed women. Although stress can raise blood pressure acutely, there is less evidence linking it to chronic elevations in blood pressure. Smoking and a diet high in saturated fats and cholesterol, although not identified as primary risk factors for hypertension, are independent risk factors for coronary heart disease and should be avoided.

High Salt Intake. Increased salt intake has long been suspected as an etiologic factor in the development of hypertension.[24] Just how increased salt intake contributes to the development of hypertension is still unclear. It may be that salt causes an elevation in blood volume, increases the sensitivity of cardiovascular or renal mechanisms to adrenergic influences, or exerts its effects through some other mechanism such as the renin-angiotensin-aldosterone mechanism. Regardless of the mechanism, numerous studies have shown that a reduction in salt intake can lower blood pressure.[25] The strongest data come from the INTERSALT study, which measured 24-hour urine sodium excretion (an indirect measure of salt intake) in 10,079 men and women 20 to 59 years of age in 52 locations around the world. In all 52 sites, there was a positive correlation between sodium excretion and both systolic and diastolic blood pressure. Furthermore, the association of sodium and blood pressure was greatest for older (40 to 59 years) subjects when compared with younger (20 to 39 years) subjects in the study.[26]

At present, salt intake among adults in the United States and United Kingdom averages at least 9 g/day, with large numbers of people consuming 12 g/day or more.[26] This is far in excess of the maximal intake of 6 g/day for adults recommended by the American Heart Association.[27] Approximately 75% of salt intake comes from salt added in the processing and manufacturing of food; 15% from the discretionary addition in cooking and at the table; and 10% from the natural sodium content of food.[24–26]

The Dietary Approaches to Stop Hypertension (DASH) diet is a nutritional plan that emphasizes fruits, vegetables, low-fat dairy products, whole grains, poultry, fish, and nuts, and is reduced in fat, red meat, sweets, and sugar-containing beverages. Results from studies using the low-sodium

DASH diet have shown significant reductions in systolic and diastolic blood pressures.[28,29]

Obesity. Excessive weight commonly is associated with hypertension. Weight reduction of as little as 4.5 kg (10 lb) can produce a decrease in blood pressure in a large proportion of overweight people with hypertension.[9] It has been suggested that fat distribution might be a more critical indicator of hypertension risk than actual overweight. The waist-to-hip ratio commonly is used to differentiate central or upper body obesity (*i.e.*, fat cell deposits in the abdomen) from peripheral or lower body obesity with fat cell deposits in the buttocks and legs (see Chapter 11). Studies have found an association between hypertension and increased waist-to-hip ratio (*i.e.*, central obesity), even when body mass index and skinfold thickness are taken into account.[30,31] Abdominal or visceral fat seems to be more insulin resistant than fat deposited over the buttocks and legs.

Excess Alcohol Consumption. Regular alcohol drinking plays a role in the development of hypertension. The effect is seen with different types of alcoholic drinks, in men and women, and in a variety of ethnic groups.[32,33] One of the first reports of a link between alcohol consumption and hypertension came from the Oakland–San Francisco Kaiser Permanente Medical Care Program study that correlated known drinking patterns and blood pressure levels of 84,000 persons.[34] This study revealed that the regular consumption of three or more drinks per day increases the risk for hypertension. Systolic pressures were more markedly affected than diastolic pressures. Blood pressure may improve or return to normal when alcohol consumption is decreased or eliminated. The mechanism whereby alcohol exerts its effect on blood pressure is unclear. It has been suggested that lifestyle factors such as obesity and lack of exercise may be accompanying factors.

Dietary Intake of Potassium, Calcium, and Magnesium. Low levels of dietary potassium have also been linked to increased blood pressure.[35,36] The strongest evidence comes from the previously described INTERSALT study. In this study, a 60 mmol/day or greater urinary excretion of potassium (an indirect measure of potassium intake) was associated with a reduction in systolic pressure of 3.4 mm Hg or more and a decrease in diastolic pressure of 1.9 mm Hg or more.[36] Various mechanisms have been proposed to explain the influence of potassium on blood pressure. These include a purported change in the ratio of sodium to potassium in the diet, a direct natriuretic effect, and suppression of the renin-angiotensin system. In terms of food intake, a diet high in potassium usually is low in sodium. One of the major benefits of increased potassium intake is increased elimination of sodium (natriuretic effect) through the renin-angiotensin-aldosterone mechanism.

The associations between high blood pressure and calcium and magnesium levels also have been investigated. Although there have been reports of high blood pressure in persons with low calcium intake or lowering of blood pressure with increased calcium intake, the link between low calcium and magnesium intake and hypertension is inconclusive.[37]

Oral Contraceptive Drugs. Oral contraceptives cause a mild increase in blood pressure in many women and overt hypertension in approximately 5%.[38] Why this occurs is largely unknown, although it has been suggested that estrogen and progesterone are responsible for the effect. Various contraceptive drugs contain different amounts and combinations of estrogen and progestational agents, and these differences may contribute to the occurrence of hypertension in some women but not others. Fortunately, the hypertension associated with oral contraceptives usually disappears after the drug has been discontinued, although it may take as long as 6 months for this to happen. However, in some women, the blood pressure may not return to normal; they may be at risk for developing hypertension. The risk for hypertension-associated cardiovascular complications is found primarily in women older than 35 years of age and in those who smoke.

Stress. Physical and emotional stresses undoubtedly contribute to transient alterations in blood pressure. Studies in which arterial blood pressure was continually monitored on a 24-hour basis as persons performed their normal activities showed marked fluctuations in pressure associated with normal life stresses—increasing during periods of physical discomfort and family crisis and declining during rest and sleep.[39] However, the role of transient stress-related episodes of hypertension in the production of chronically elevated pressures seen in essential hypertension remains speculative. It may be that vascular smooth muscle hypertrophies with increased activity in a manner similar to that of skeletal muscle, or that the central integrative pathways in the brain become adapted to the frequent stress-related input.

Psychological techniques involving biofeedback, relaxation, and transcendental meditation have emerged as possible methods for controlling blood pressure. However, there is a lack of well-designed research studies validating the efficacy of these techniques as a primary treatment for hypertension.

Systolic Hypertension

Essential hypertension may be classified as systolic/diastolic hypertension in which both the systolic and diastolic pressures are elevated; as diastolic hypertension in which the diastolic pressure is selectively elevated; or as systolic hypertension in which the systolic pressure is selectively elevated. The JNC-7 report defined systolic hypertension as a systolic pressure of 140 mm Hg or greater and a diastolic pressure of less than 90 mm Hg, indicating a need for increased recognition and control of isolated systolic hypertension.[9] Historically, diastolic hypertension was thought to confer a greater risk for cardiovascular events than systolic hypertension.[9] However, there is mounting evidence that elevated systolic blood pressure is at least as important, if not more so, than diastolic hypertension.[40–42] In a recent study that used data from the Framingham Offspring cohort to arrive at a hypertension classification based on the JNC-6 stages, it was found that systolic pressure alone correctly classified 95% of persons 60 years of age or younger and 99% of those older than 60 years of age.[43]

There are two aspects of systolic hypertension that confer increased risk for cardiovascular events—one is the actual elevation in systolic pressure and the other is the disproportionate rise in pulse pressure. Elevated pressures during systole favor the development of left ventricular hypertrophy, increased myocardial oxygen demands, and eventual left heart failure. At the same time, the absolute or relative lowering of diastolic pressure is a limiting factor in coronary perfusion because coronary perfusion is greatest during diastole. Elevated levels of pulse pressure produce greater stretch of arteries, causing damage to the elastic elements of the vessel and thus predisposing to aneurysms and development of the intimal damage that leads to atherosclerosis and thrombosis.[44]

Manifestations

Essential hypertension is typically an asymptomatic disorder. When symptoms do occur, they are usually related to the long-term effects of hypertension on other organ systems such as the kidneys, heart, eyes, and blood vessels.

The 2003 JNC-7 report used the term *target-organ damage* to describe the heart, brain, peripheral vascular, kidney, and retinal complications associated with hypertension (Chart 25-2).[9] The excess morbidity and mortality related to hypertension is progressive over the whole range of systolic and diastolic pressures. Target-organ damage varies markedly among persons with similar levels of hypertension.

Hypertension is a major risk factor for atherosclerosis; it predisposes to all major atherosclerotic cardiovascular disorders, including heart failure, stroke, coronary artery disease, and peripheral artery disease. The risk for coronary artery disease and stroke depends to a great extent on other risk factors, such as obesity, smoking, and elevated cholesterol levels. The risk for stroke occurring in persons with hypertension occurs over an eightfold range, depending on the number of associated risk factors. Cerebrovascular complications are more closely related to systolic than diastolic hypertension. The incidence of these complications is greatly reduced by antihypertensive therapy.

CHART 25-2

Target Organ Damage

Heart
- Left ventricular hypertrophy
- Angina or prior myocardial infarction
- Prior coronary revascularization
- Heart failure

Brain
- Stroke or transient ischemic attack

Chronic kidney disease
Peripheral vascular disease
Retinopathy

(National Heart, Lung, and Blood Institute. [2003]. *The seventh report of the National Committee on Detection, Evaluation, and Treatment of High Blood Pressure.* Publication No. 03-5233. Bethesda, MD: NIH)

Hypertension increases the workload of the left ventricle by increasing the pressure against which the heart must pump as it ejects blood into the systemic circulation. As the workload of the heart increases, the left ventricular wall hypertrophies to compensate for the increased pressure work. The prevalence of left ventricular hypertrophy increases with age and is highest in persons with blood pressures over 160/95 mm Hg. It was observed in 12% to 20% of persons with mild hypertension and in 50% of asymptomatic persons with mild to moderate hypertension.[40] Despite its adaptive advantage, left ventricular hypertrophy is a major risk factor for ischemic heart disease, cardiac dysrhythmias, sudden death, and congestive heart failure. Hypertensive left ventricular hypertrophy regresses with therapy. Regression is most closely related to systolic pressure reduction and does not appear to reflect the particular type of medication used.

Hypertension also can lead to nephrosclerosis, a common cause of renal insufficiency (see Chapter 35). Hypertensive kidney disease is more common in blacks than whites. Hypertension also plays an important role in accelerating the course of other types of kidney disease, particularly diabetic nephropathy. Because of the risk for diabetic nephropathy, the American Diabetes Association recommends that persons with diabetes maintain their blood pressure at levels less than 130/80 mm Hg (see Chapter 43).

Diagnosis

Unlike disorders of other body systems that are diagnosed by methods such as x-rays and tissue examination, hypertension and other blood pressure disorders are determined by repeated blood pressure measurement. Accurate and reliable blood pressure measurements require that the blood pressure equipment be properly maintained and calibrated and that the persons taking the blood pressures are adequately prepared in blood pressure measurement. The increased availability of hypertensive screening clinics provides one of the best means for early detection. Laboratory tests, x-ray films, and other diagnostic tests usually are done to exclude secondary hypertension and determine the presence or extent of target-organ disease.

The JNC-6 report emphasized that obtaining one elevated blood pressure reading should not constitute the diagnosis of hypertension. The diagnosis of hypertension in a person who is not taking antihypertensive medications should be based on the average of at least two or more blood pressure readings taken at each of two or more visits after an initial screening visit.[9] Blood pressure measurements should be taken when the person is relaxed and has rested for at least 5 minutes and has not smoked or ingested caffeine within 30 minutes. At least two measurements should be made at each visit in the same arm while the person is seated in a chair (rather than on the exam table) with the feet on the floor and arm supported at heart level. If the first two readings differ by more than 5 mm Hg, additional readings should be taken. Both the systolic and diastolic pressures should be recorded. The appearance of the first K sound (phase 1) is used to define systolic pressure, and the disappearance of the K sounds (phase 5) is used to define the diastolic pressure.[3] Because blood pressure in many individuals is highly variable, blood pressure should be measured on different occasions over a period of several months before a diagnosis of hypertension is made unless the pressure is extremely elevated or associated with symptoms.

Treatment

The main objective for treatment of essential hypertension is to achieve and maintain arterial blood pressure below 140/90 mm Hg, with the goal of preventing morbidity and mortality. In persons with hypertension and diabetes or renal disease, the goal is below 130/80 mg Hg. The JNC-7 report contains a treatment algorithm for hypertension that includes lifestyle modification and, when necessary, guidelines for the use of pharmacologic agents to achieve and maintain blood pressure within an optimal range (Fig. 25-8).[9]

For persons with secondary hypertension, efforts are made to correct or control the disease condition causing the hypertension. Antihypertensive medications and other measures supplement the treatment of the underlying disease.

Lifestyle Modification. Lifestyle modification has been shown to reduce blood pressure, enhance antihypertensive drug therapy, and prevent cardiovascular risk. Major lifestyle modifications shown to lower blood pressure include weight reduction in persons who are overweight or obese, regular physical activity, adoption of the DASH eating plan, reduction of dietary sodium intake, and moderation in alcohol intake.[9] Although nicotine has not been associated with long-term elevations in blood pressure as in essential hypertension, it has been shown to increase the risk for heart disease. The fact that smoking and hypertension are major cardiovascular risk factors should be reason enough to encourage the hypertensive smoker to quit.

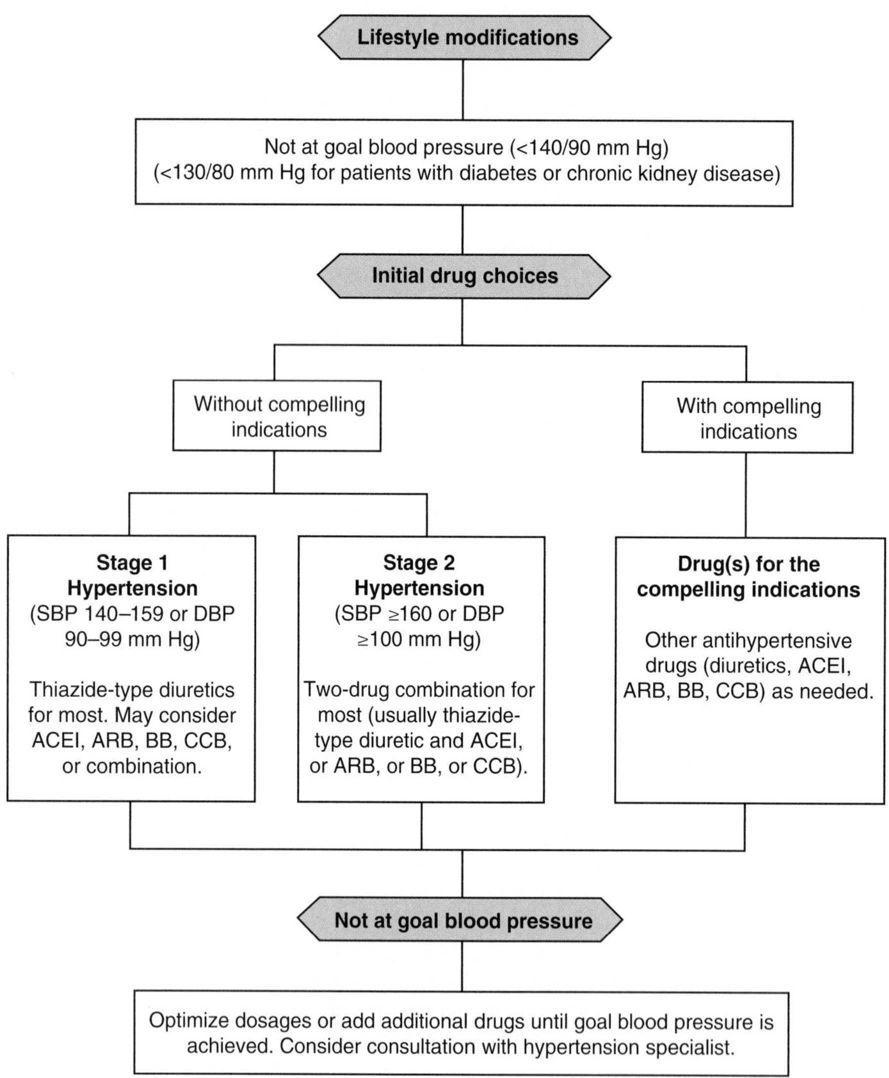

FIGURE 25-8 Algorithm for treatment of hypertension. (National Heart, Lung, and Blood Institute. [2003]. *The seventh report of the National Committee on Detection, Evaluation, and Treatment of High Blood Pressure.* Publication No. 03-5233. Bethesda, MD: NIH)

Table 25-2 summarizes the recommended lifestyle modifications and their effects in terms of reducing systolic blood pressure.

There is conflicting evidence about the direct effects of dietary fats on blood pressure. As with smoking, the interactive effects of saturated fats and high blood pressure as cardiovascular risk factors would seem to warrant dietary modification to reduce the intake of foods high in cholesterol and saturated fats.

Pharmacologic Treatment. The decision to initiate pharmacologic treatment is based on the severity of the hypertension, the presence of target-organ disease, and the existence of other conditions and risk factors. Drug selection is based on the stage of hypertension. Among the drugs used in the treatment of hypertension are diuretics, β-adrenergic blockers, angiotensin-converting enzyme (ACE) inhibitors or angiotensin II receptor blockers, the calcium channel blockers, central α_2-adrenergic agonists, α_1-adrenergic receptor blockers, and vasodilators. The JNC-7 treatment algorithm recommends that thiazide-type diuretics should be used as initial treatment for most persons with hypertension, either alone or in combination with one of the other classes of drugs (β-adrenergic blockers, ACE inhibitors, angiotensin II receptor blockers, calcium channel blockers) shown to be beneficial in randomized controlled outcome trials (see Fig. 25-8).[9] If the drug is not tolerated or is contraindicated, JNC-7 recommends that one of the other classes proven to reduce cardiovascular events should be used instead. JNC-7 suggests that most persons with hypertension will require two or more antihypertensive drugs to achieve their blood pressure goals.[9]

Diuretics, such as the thiazides, loop diuretics, and the aldosterone antagonist (potassium-sparing) diuretics, lower blood pressure initially by decreasing vascular volume (by suppressing renal reabsorption of sodium and increasing salt and water excretion) and cardiac output (see Fig. 25-3). With continued therapy, a reduction in peripheral vascular resistance becomes a major mechanism of blood pressure reduction.

The *β-adrenergic blockers* are effective in hypertension because they decrease heart rate and cardiac output. These agents also decrease renin release, thereby decreasing the effect of the renin-angiotensin-aldosterone mechanism on blood pressure. There are two types of β-adrenergic receptors: β_1 and β_2. The β_1-blocking drugs are cardioselective, exerting their effects on the heart, whereas the β_2-adrenergic receptor blockers affect bronchodilation, relaxation of skeletal blood vessels, and other β-mediated functions. Both cardioselective (β_1) and nonselective (β_1 and β_2) β-adrenergic blockers are used in the treatment of hypertension.

The *ACE inhibitors* act by inhibiting the conversion of angiotensin I to angiotensin II, thus decreasing angiotensin II levels and reducing its effect on vasoconstriction, aldosterone levels, intrarenal blood flow, and the glomerular filtration rate. They also inhibit the degradation of bradykinin. The ACE inhibitors are increasingly used as the initial medication in mild to moderate hypertension. Because of their effect on the renin-angiotensin system, these drugs are contraindicated in persons with renal artery stenosis, in which the renin-angiotensin mechanism functions as a compensatory mechanism to maintain adequate renal perfusion. Because they inhibit aldosterone secretion, these agents also can increase serum potassium levels and cause hyperkalemia. A relative newcomer to the field of antihypertensive medications is the angiotensin II receptor–blocking drug class. Because they do not inhibit bradykinin degradation in the lungs, they are less likely to produce a cough, which is a frequent side effect of ACE inhibitors.

TABLE 25-2 Lifestyle Modifications to Manage Hypertension*†

Modification	Recommendation	Approximate Systolic Blood Pressure Reduction (mm Hg)
Weight reduction	Maintain normal body weight (BMI, 18.5–24.9 kg/m^2)	5–20 mm Hg/10 kg weight loss
Adopt DASH eating plan	Consume a diet rich in fruits, vegetables, and low-fat diary products with a reduced content of saturated and total fat	8–14 mm Hg
Dietary sodium reduction	Reduce dietary sodium intake to no more than 100 mmol per day (2.4 g sodium or 6 g sodium chloride)	2–8 mm Hg
Physical activity	Engage in regular aerobic physical activity such as brisk walking (at least 30 minutes per day, most days of the week)	4–9 mm Hg
Moderation of alcohol consumption	Limit consumption to no more than 2 drinks (1 oz or 30 mL ethanol; *e.g.,* 24 oz beer, 10 oz wine, or 3 oz 80-proof whiskey) per day in most men and 1 drink per day in women and lighter-weight persons	2–4 mm Hg

DASH, Dietary Approaches to Stop Hypertension; BMI, body mass index.
*For overall cardiovascular reduction, stop smoking.
†The effects of implementing these modifications is dose and time dependent, and could be greater for some individuals.
(National Heart, Lung, and Blood Institute. [2003]. *The seventh report of the National Committee on Detection, Evaluation, and Treatment of High Blood Pressure.* Publication No. 03–5233. Bethesda, MD: NIH)

The *calcium channel receptor-blocking drugs* inhibit the movement of calcium into cardiac and vascular smooth muscle. They probably reduce blood pressure by several mechanisms, including a reduction of smooth muscle tone in the venous and arterial systems. Each of the different agents in this group acts in a slightly different way. Some calcium blockers have a direct myocardial effect that reduces the cardiac output through a decrease in cardiac contractility and heart rate. Other calcium channel blockers influence venous tone and reduce the cardiac output through a decrease in venous return. Still others influence arterial vascular smooth muscle by inhibiting calcium transport across the cell membrane channels or inhibiting the vascular response to norepinephrine or angiotensin.

The *centrally acting adrenergic agonists* block sympathetic outflow from the central nervous system. These agents are α_2-adrenergic agonists that act in a negative-feedback manner to decrease sympathetic outflow from presynaptic sympathetic neurons in the central nervous system. The α_2-adrenergic agonists are effective as a single therapy for some persons, but they often are used as second- or third-line agents because of the high incidence of side effects. One of the agents, clonidine, is available as a transdermal patch that is replaced weekly.

The *α_1-adrenergic receptor antagonists* block postsynaptic α_1 receptors and reduce the effect of the sympathetic nervous system on the vascular smooth muscle tone of the blood vessels that regulate the peripheral vascular resistance. These drugs produce a pronounced decrease in blood pressure after the first dose; therefore, treatment is initiated with a smaller dose given at bedtime. Postdosing palpitations, headache, and nervousness may continue with chronic treatment. These agents usually are more effective when used in combination with other agents.

The *direct-acting smooth muscle vasodilators* promote a decrease in peripheral vascular resistance by producing relaxation of vascular smooth muscle, particularly of the arterioles. These drugs often produce initial stimulation of the sympathetic nervous system and tachycardia and salt and water retention as a result of the decreased filling of the vascular compartment. Vasodilators work best in combination with other antihypertensive drugs that oppose the compensatory cardiovascular responses.

Treatment Strategies. Factors considered when hypertensive drugs are prescribed are the person's lifestyle (*i.e.*, someone with a busy schedule may have problems with medications that must be taken two or three times each day); demographics (*e.g.*, some drugs are more effective in elderly or African-American persons); motivation for adhering to the drug regimen (*e.g.*, some drugs can produce undesirable and even life-threatening consequences if discontinued abruptly); other disease conditions and therapies; and potential for side effects (*e.g.*, some drugs may impair sexual functioning or mental acuity; others have not been proved safe for women of childbearing age). Particular caution should be used in persons who are at risk for orthostatic hypotension (*e.g.*, those with diabetes, ANS dysfunction, and some older individuals). Another factor to be considered is the cost of the drug in relation to financial resources. There is wide variation in the prices of antihypertensive medications that should be considered when medications are prescribed. This is particularly important for low-income persons with moderate to severe hypertension because keeping costs at an affordable level may be the key to compliance.

SECONDARY HYPERTENSION

Only 5% to 10% of hypertensive cases are classified as secondary hypertension (*i.e.*, hypertension due to another disease condition).[45,46] Unlike essential hypertension, many of the conditions causing secondary hypertension can be corrected or cured by surgery or specific medical treatment. Secondary hypertension tends to be seen in persons younger than 30 and older than 50 years of age.[46] Renal artery stenosis and coarctation of the aorta are more common in younger persons. Cocaine, amphetamines, and other illicit drugs can cause significant hypertension, as can sympathomimetic agents (decongestants, anorectics), erythropoietin, and licorice (including some chewing tobacco). Obstructive sleep apnea (see Chapter 13) is an independent risk factor for hypertension. At least one half of persons with obstructive sleep apnea have hypertension.[45]

Among the most common causes of secondary hypertension are kidney disease (*i.e.*, renovascular hypertension), adrenal cortical disorders, pheochromocytoma, coarctation of the aorta, and sleep apnea. To avoid duplication in descriptions, the mechanisms associated with elevations of blood pressure in these disorders are discussed briefly, and a more detailed discussion of specific disease disorders is reserved for other sections of this book.

Renal Hypertension

With the dominant role that the kidney assumes in blood pressure regulation, it is not surprising that the largest single cause of secondary hypertension is renal disease. Most acute kidney disorders result in decreased urine formation, retention of salt and water, and hypertension. This includes acute glomerulonephritis, acute renal failure, and acute urinary tract obstruction. Hypertension also is common among persons with chronic pyelonephritis, polycystic kidney disease, diabetic nephropathy, and end-stage renal disease, regardless of cause. In older persons, the sudden onset of secondary hypertension often is associated with atherosclerotic disease of the renal blood vessels.

Renovascular hypertension refers to hypertension caused by reduced renal blood flow and activation of the renin-angiotensin-aldosterone mechanism. It is the most common cause of secondary hypertension, accounting for 1% to 2% of all cases of hypertension. The reduced renal blood flow that occurs with renovascular disease causes the affected kidney to release excessive amounts of renin, increasing circulating levels of angiotensin II. Angiotensin II, in turn, acts as a vasoconstrictor to increase peripheral vascular resistance and as a stimulus for increasing aldosterone levels and sodium retention by the kidney. One or both of the kidneys may be affected. When the renal artery of only one kidney is involved, the unaffected kidney is subjected to the detrimental effects of the elevated blood pressure so that the affected kidney can maintain its function.

There are two major types of renovascular disease: atherosclerotic artery stenosis and fibromuscular dysplasia.[47,48] Atherosclerotic artery stenosis accounts for 70% to 90% of cases and is seen most often in older persons, particularly those with diabetes, aortoiliac occlusive disease, coronary artery disease, or hypertension. Fibromuscular dysplasia is more common in women and tends to occur in younger age groups, often persons in their third decade. Genetic factors may be involved, and the incidence tends to increase with risk factors such as smoking and hyperlipidemia.

Renal artery stenosis should be suspected when hypertension develops in a previously normotensive person older than 50 (*i.e.,* atherosclerotic form) or younger than 30 (*i.e.,* fibromuscular hyperplasia) years of age, or when accelerated hypertension occurs in a person with previously controlled hypertension. Hypokalemia (due to increased aldosterone levels), the presence of an abdominal bruit, the absence of a family history of hypertension, and a duration of hypertension of less than 1 year help to distinguish renovascular hypertension from essential hypertension. Because renal blood flow depends on the increased blood pressure generated by the renin-angiotensin system, administration of ACE inhibitors can cause a rapid decline in renal function.

Diagnostic tests may include studies to assess overall renal function, physiologic studies to assess the renin-angiotensin system, perfusion studies to assess renal blood flow, and imaging studies to identify renal artery stenosis.[48] Methods to assess the renin-angiotensin response include the measurement of renin and sodium levels before and after oral administration of captopril, an ACE inhibitor. The captopril renal scintigram (scan) also can be used to assess renal blood flow. This test is based on the assumption that captopril can decrease renal blood flow, thereby decreasing the uptake of the radionuclide by the affected kidney. Renal arteriography remains the definitive test for identifying renal artery disease. Renal artery duplex ultrasonography or contrast-enhanced magnetic resonance imaging (MRI) also may be used.

The goal of treatment is to control the blood pressure and stabilize renal function. Angioplasty or revascularization has been shown to be an effective long-term treatment for the disorder. ACE inhibitors may be used in medical management of renal stenosis. However, these agents must be used with caution because of their ability to produce marked hypotension and renal dysfunction.

Disorders of Adrenocorticosteroid Hormones

Increased levels of adrenocorticosteroid hormones also can give rise to hypertension. Primary hyperaldosteronism (excess production of aldosterone due to adrenocortical hyperplasia or adenoma) and excess levels of glucocorticoid (Cushing's disease or syndrome) tend to raise the blood pressure (see Chapter 42). These hormones facilitate salt and water retention by the kidney; the hypertension that accompanies excessive levels of either hormone probably is related to this factor. For patients with primary hyperaldosteronism, a salt-restricted diet often produces a reduction in blood pressure. Because aldosterone acts on the distal renal tubule to increase sodium absorption in exchange for potassium elimination in the urine, persons with hyperaldosteronism usually have decreased potassium levels. Potassium-sparing diuretics, such as spironolactone, which is an aldosterone antagonist, often are used in the medical management of persons with the disorder.[48]

Licorice is an extract from the roots of the *Glycyrrhiza glabra* plant that has been used in medicine since ancient times. European licorice (not licorice flavoring) is associated with sodium retention, edema, hypertension, and hypokalemia. Licorice is an effective analog of the steroid 11 β-dehydrogenase enzyme that modulates access to the aldosterone receptor in the kidney.[30] It produces a syndrome similar to primary hyperaldosteronism.

Pheochromocytoma

A pheochromocytoma is a tumor of chromaffin tissue, which contains sympathetic nerve cells that stain with chromium salts. The tumor is most commonly located in the adrenal medulla but can arise in other sites, such as sympathetic ganglia, where there is chromaffin tissue.[48,49] Although only 0.1% to 0.5% of persons with hypertension have an underlying pheochromocytoma, the disorder can cause serious hypertensive crises. The tumors are malignant 8% to 10% of the time.

Like adrenal medullary cells, the tumor cells of a pheochromocytoma produce and secrete the catecholamines epinephrine and norepinephrine. The hypertension that develops is a result of the massive release of these catecholamines. Their release may be paroxysmal rather than continuous, causing periodic episodes of headache, excessive sweating, and palpitations. Headache is the most common symptom and can be quite severe. Nervousness, tremor, facial pallor, weakness, fatigue, and weight loss occur less frequently. Marked variability in blood pressure between episodes is typical. Approximately 50% of persons with pheochromocytoma have paroxysmal episodes of hypertension, sometimes to dangerously high levels. The other 50% have sustained hypertension, and some even may be normotensive.[50]

Several tests are available to differentiate hypertension due to pheochromocytoma from other forms of hypertension. The most commonly used diagnostic measure is the determination of urinary catecholamines and their metabolites. Although measurement of plasma catecholamines also may be used, other conditions can cause catecholamines to be elevated. After the presence of a pheochromocytoma has been established, the tumor needs to be located. Computed tomographic (CT) scans or MRI may be used for this purpose. Surgical removal of operable tumors is usually curative.[50]

Coarctation of the Aorta

Coarctation represents a narrowing of the aorta. In the adult form of coarctation, the narrowing most commonly occurs just distal to the origin of the subclavian arteries[51] (see Chapter 26). Because of the narrowing, blood flow to the lower parts of the body and kidneys is reduced. In the infantile form of coarctation, the narrowing occurs proximal to the ductus arteriosus, in which case heart failure and other problems may occur. Many affected children die within their first year of life.

In the adult form of coarctation, an increase in cardiac output may result from renal compensatory mechanisms. The ejection of a large stroke volume into a narrowed aorta with limited ability to accept the runoff results in an increase in systolic blood pressure and blood flow to the upper part of the body. Blood pressure in the lower extremities may be normal, although it frequently is low. It has been suggested that the increase in cardiac output and maintenance of the pressure to the lower part of the body is achieved through the renin-angiotensin-aldosterone mechanism in response to a decrease in renal blood flow. Pulse pressure in the legs almost always is narrowed, and the femoral pulses are weak. Because the aortic capacity is diminished, there usually is a marked increase in pressure (measured in the arms) during exercise, when the stroke volume and heart rate are exaggerated. For this reason, blood pressures in both arms and one leg should be determined; a pressure that is 20 mm Hg more in the arms than in the legs suggests coarctation of the aorta. Involvement of the left subclavian artery or an anomalous origin of the right subclavian may produce decreased or absent left or right brachial pulses, respectively. Palpation of both brachial pulses and measurement of blood pressure in both arms are important.

Treatment consists of surgical repair or balloon angioplasty. Although balloon angioplasty is a relatively recent form of treatment, it has been used in children and adults with good results. However, there are few data on long-term follow-up.

MALIGNANT HYPERTENSION

A small number of persons with secondary hypertension develop an accelerated and potentially fatal form of the disease: malignant hypertension. This usually is a disease of younger persons, particularly young African-American men, women with toxemia of pregnancy, and persons with renal and collagen diseases.

Malignant hypertension is characterized by sudden marked elevations in blood pressure, with diastolic values above 120 mm Hg complicated by evidence of acute or rapidly progressive life-threatening organ dysfunction.[52] There may be intense arterial spasm of the cerebral arteries with hypertensive encephalopathy. Cerebral vasoconstriction probably is an exaggerated homeostatic response designed to protect the brain from excesses of blood pressure and flow. The regulatory mechanisms often are insufficient to protect the capillaries, and cerebral edema frequently develops. As it advances, papilledema (*i.e.,* swelling of the optic nerve at its point of entrance into the eye) ensues, giving evidence of the effects of pressure on the optic nerve and retinal vessels. The patient may have headache, restlessness, confusion, stupor, motor and sensory deficits, and visual disturbances. In severe cases, convulsions and coma follow.

Prolonged and severe exposure to exaggerated levels of blood pressure in malignant hypertension injures the walls of the arterioles, and intravascular coagulation and fragmentation of red blood cells may occur. The renal blood vessels are particularly vulnerable to hypertensive damage. Renal damage due to vascular changes probably is the most important prognostic determinant in malignant hypertension. Elevated levels of blood urea nitrogen and serum creatinine, metabolic acidosis, hypocalcemia, and proteinuria provide evidence of renal impairment.

The complications associated with a hypertensive crisis demand immediate and rigorous medical treatment in an intensive care unit with continuous monitoring of arterial blood pressure. With proper therapy, the death rate from this cause can be markedly reduced, as can additional episodes. Because chronic hypertension is associated with autoregulatory changes in coronary artery, cerebral artery, and kidney blood flow, care should be taken to avoid excessively rapid decreases in blood pressure, which can lead to hypoperfusion and ischemic injury. Therefore, the goal of initial treatment measures should be to obtain a partial reduction in blood pressure to a safer, noncritical level, rather than to normotensive levels.[52]

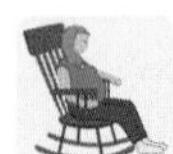

HIGH BLOOD PRESSURE IN PREGNANCY

Hypertensive disorders complicate 6% to 8% of pregnancies. They are the second leading cause, after embolism, of maternal mortality in the United States, accounting for almost 15% of such deaths.[37] Hypertensive disorders also contribute to stillbirths and neonatal morbidity and mortality. Premature separation of the placenta (abruptio placentae) is reported to complicate up to 10% of hypertensive pregnancies.[53] The incidence of hypertensive disorders of pregnancy increases with maternal age and is more common in African-American women.[53]

Classification

In 2000, the National Institutes of Health Working Group on High Blood Pressure in Pregnancy published a revised classification system for high blood pressure in pregnancy that included chronic hypertension, preeclampsia-eclampsia, preeclampsia superimposed on chronic hypertension, and gestational hypertension[54] (Table 25-3).

Chronic Hypertension. Chronic hypertension is considered as hypertension that is unrelated to the pregnancy. It is defined as a history of high blood pressure before pregnancy, identification of hypertension before 20 weeks of pregnancy, and hypertension that persists after pregnancy. Hypertension is defined as a systolic pressure of 140 mm Hg or higher or a diastolic pressure of 90 mm Hg or higher. Hypertension that is diagnosed for the first time during pregnancy and does not resolve after pregnancy also is classified as chronic hypertension.

In women with chronic hypertension, blood pressure often decreases in early pregnancy and increases during the last trimester (3 months) of pregnancy, resembling preeclampsia. Consequently, women with undiagnosed chronic hypertension who do not present for medical care until the later months of pregnancy may be incorrectly

TABLE 25-3 Classification of High Blood Pressure in Pregnancy

Classification	Description
Gestational hypertension	Blood pressure elevation, without proteinuria, that is detected for the first time during midpregnancy and returns to normal by 12 weeks postpartum.
Chronic hypertension	Blood pressure ≥140 mm Hg systolic or ≥90 mm Hg diastolic that is present and observable before the 20th week of pregnancy. Hypertension that is diagnosed for the first time during pregnancy and does not resolve after pregnancy also is classified as chronic hypertension.
Preeclampsia-eclampsia	Pregnancy-specific syndrome of blood pressure elevation (blood pressure >140 mm Hg systolic or >90 mm Hg diastolic) that occurs after the first 20 weeks of pregnancy and is accompanied by proteinuria (urinary excretion of 0.3 g protein in a 24-hour specimen).
Preeclampsia superimposed on chronic hypertension	Chronic hypertension (blood pressure ≥140 mm Hg systolic or ≥90 mm Hg diastolic prior to 20th week of pregnancy) with superimposed proteinuria and with or without signs of the preeclampsia syndrome

(Developed using information from National Institutes of Health. [2000]. *Working group report on high blood pressure in pregnancy*. NIH publication no. 00-3029. Bethesda, MD: Author. Available: http://www.nhlbi.gov/health/prof/heart/hbp/hbp_preg.htm)

diagnosed as having preeclampsia. Women with chronic hypertension are at increased risk for the development of preeclampsia.

Preeclampsia-Eclampsia. Preeclampsia-eclampsia is a pregnancy-specific syndrome that usually occurs after 20 weeks of gestation. It is defined as an elevation in blood pressure (systolic blood pressure >140 mm Hg or diastolic pressure >90 mm Hg) and proteinuria (≥300 g in 24 hours) developing after 20 weeks of gestation. The Working Group recommends that K5 be used for determining diastolic pressure. Edema, which previously was included in definitions of preeclampsia, was excluded from this most recent definition. The presence of a systolic blood pressure of 160 mm Hg or higher or a diastolic pressure of 110 mm Hg or higher; hyperproteinuria greater than 2 g in 24 hours; serum creatinine greater than 1.2 mg/dL; platelet counts less than 100,000 cells/mm^3; elevated liver enzymes (alanine aminotransferase [ALT] or aspartate aminotransferase [AST]); persistent headache or cerebral or visual disturbances; and persistent epigastric pain serve to reinforce the diagnosis.[54] Eclampsia is the occurrence, in a woman with preeclampsia, of seizures that cannot be attributed to other causes.[54]

Preeclampsia occurs primarily during first pregnancies and during subsequent pregnancies in women with multiple fetuses, diabetes mellitus, or coexisting renal disease. It is associated with a condition called a *hydatidiform mole* (*i.e.*, abnormal pregnancy caused by a pathologic ovum, resulting in a mass of cysts). Women with chronic hypertension who become pregnant have an increased risk for preeclampsia and adverse neonatal outcomes, particularly when associated with proteinuria early in pregnancy.[55] Of interest is the reversal of the diurnal pattern of blood pressure in preeclamptic hypertension; it often is highest during the night.[56]

Pregnancy-induced hypertension is thought to involve a decrease in placental blood flow leading to the release of toxic mediators that alter the function of endothelial cells in blood vessels throughout the body, including those of the kidney, brain, liver, and heart.[55,57] The endothelial changes result in signs and symptoms of preeclampsia and, in more severe cases, of intravascular clotting and hypoperfusion of vital organs. There is risk for development of disseminated intravascular coagulation, cerebral hemorrhage, hepatic failure, and acute renal failure. Thrombocytopenia is the most common hematologic complication of preeclampsia. Platelet counts of less than 100,000/mm^3 signal serious disease. The cause of thrombocytopenia has been ascribed to platelet deposition at the site of endothelial injury. The renal changes that occur with preeclampsia include a decrease in glomerular filtration rate and renal blood flow. Sodium excretion may be impaired, although this is variable. Edema may or may not be present. Some of the severest forms of preeclampsia occur in the absence of edema. Even when there is extensive edema, the plasma volume usually is lower than that of normal pregnancy. Liver damage, when it occurs, may range from mild hepatocellular necrosis with elevation of liver enzymes to the more ominous hemolysis, elevated liver function tests, and low platelet count (HELLP) syndrome that is associated with significant maternal mortality. Eclampsia, the convulsive stage of preeclampsia, is a significant cause of maternal mortality. The pathogenesis of eclampsia remains unclear and has been attributed to both increased coagulability and fibrin deposition in the cerebral vessels.

Defining the causes of pregnancy-induced hypertension is difficult because of the normal circulatory changes that occur during pregnancy. Blood pressure normally decreases during the first trimester, reaches its lowest point during the second trimester, and gradually rises during the third trimester. The fact that there is a 40% to 60% increase in cardiac output during early pregnancy suggests the decrease in blood pressure that occurs during the first part of pregnancy results from a decrease in peripheral vascular resistance. Because the cardiac output remains high throughout pregnancy, the gradual rise in blood pressure that begins during the second trimester probably represents a return of the peripheral vascular resistance to normal. Pregnancy normally is accompanied by increased levels of renin, angiotensin I and II, estrogen, progesterone, prolactin, and aldosterone, all of which may alter vascular reactivity. Women who develop preeclampsia are thought to be particularly sensitive to the vasoconstrictor responses of the renin-angiotensin-aldosterone system. They also are particularly responsive to other vasoconstrictors, including the catecholamines and vasopressin. It has been proposed that some of the sensitivity may be caused by a prostacyclin-thromboxane imbalance. Thromboxane is a prostaglandin with vasoconstrictor properties, and prostacyclin is a prostaglandin with vasodilator properties. Emerging evidence suggests that insulin resistance, including gestational diabetes, polycystic ovary syndrome, and obesity, may predispose to hypertensive disorders in pregnancy.[57]

Preeclampsia Superimposed on Chronic Hypertension. Preeclampsia may occur in women who already are hypertensive, in which case the prognosis for the mother and fetus tends to be worse than for either condition alone. Superimposed preeclampsia should be considered in women with hypertension before 20 weeks of gestation who develop new-onset proteinuria; women with hypertension and proteinuria before 20 weeks of gestation; women with previously well-controlled hypertension who develop a sudden increase in blood pressure; and women with chronic hypertension who develop thrombocytopenia or an increase in serum ALT or AST to abnormal levels.

Gestational Hypertension. Gestational hypertension represents a blood pressure elevation without proteinuria that is detected for the first time after midpregnancy. It includes women with preeclampsia syndrome who have not yet manifested proteinuria as well as women who do not have the syndrome. The hypertension may be accompanied by other signs of the syndrome. The final determination that a woman does not have the preeclampsia syndrome is made only postpartum. If preeclampsia has not developed and blood pressure has returned to normal by 12 weeks postpartum, the condition is considered to be gestational hypertension. If blood pressure elevation persists, a diagnosis of chronic hypertension is made.

Diagnosis and Treatment

Early prenatal care is important in the detection of high blood pressure during pregnancy. It is recommended that all pregnant women, including those with hypertension, refrain from alcohol and tobacco use. Salt restriction usually is not recommended during pregnancy because pregnant women with hypertension tend to have lower plasma volumes than normotensive pregnant women and because the severity of hypertension may reflect the degree of volume contraction. The exception is women with preexisting hypertension who have been following a salt-restricted diet.

In women with preeclampsia, delivery of the fetus is curative. The timing of delivery becomes a difficult decision in preterm pregnancies because the welfare of both the mother and the infant must be taken into account. Bed rest is a traditional therapy. Antihypertensive medications, when required, must be carefully chosen because of their potential effects on uteroplacental blood flow and on the fetus. For example, the ACE inhibitors can cause injury and even death of the fetus when given during the second and third trimesters of pregnancy.

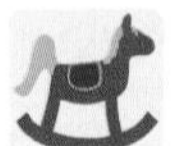

HIGH BLOOD PRESSURE IN CHILDREN

Blood pressure is known to rise from infancy to late adolescence. The average systolic blood pressure at 1 day of age is approximately 70 mm Hg and increases to approximately 85 mm Hg at 1 month of age.[58,59] In premature infants, during the first 3 to 6 hours of life, the limits of systolic and diastolic blood pressure are shown to be independent of birth weight and gestational age, but tend to correlate with low Apgar scores and maternal hypertension.[58,59] During the preschool years, blood pressure begins to follow a pattern that tends to be maintained as the child grows older. This pattern continues into adolescence and adulthood, suggesting that the roots of essential hypertension are established early in life. A familial influence on blood pressure often can be identified early in life. Children of parents with high blood pressure tend to have higher blood pressures than children with normotensive parents.

Blood pressure norms for children and adolescents are based on age, height, and gender-specific percentiles. In 1977, the Task Force on Hypertension in Children published its first recommendations on blood pressure measurement and control in children. Several updates have followed, and in 1996, the Task Force included height as a variable in the determination of blood pressure[60] (Table 25-4). The Task Force also recommended the continued classification of blood pressure into three ranges: normal (*i.e.,* systolic and diastolic pressures below the 90th percentile for age, height, and sex); high normal (*i.e.,* systolic or diastolic blood pressures between the 90th and 95th percentiles for age, height, and sex); and high blood pressures or hypertension (*i.e.,* average systolic and diastolic blood pressures equal to or greater than the 95th percentile for age, height, and sex on at least three occasions).[60] High blood pressure in children and adolescents has been further defined as significant hypertension (*i.e.,* blood pressure between the 95th and 99th percentiles for age and sex) and severe hypertension (*i.e.,* blood pressure above the 99th percentile for age and sex).

Secondary hypertension is the most common form of high blood pressure in infants and children. In later childhood and adolescence, essential hypertension is more common. Approximately 75% to 80% of secondary hypertension in children is caused by kidney abnormalities.[61] Coarctation of the aorta is another cause of hypertension in children and adolescents. Endocrine causes of hypertension, such as pheochromocytoma and adrenal cortical disorders, are rare. Hypertension in infants is associated most commonly with high umbilical catheterization and renal artery obstruction due to thrombosis.[62] Most cases of

TABLE 25-4 The 90th and 95th Percentiles of Systolic and Diastolic Blood Pressure for Boys and Girls 1 to 16 Years of Age by Percentiles for Height*

Blood Pressure Percentiles	Age (yr)	Height Percentile for Boys				Height Percentile for Girls			
		5th	25th	75th	95th	5th	25th	75th	95th
Systolic Pressure									
90th	1	94	97	100	102	97	99	102	104
95th		98	101	104	106	101	103	105	107
90th	3	100	103	107	109	100	102	104	106
95th		104	107	111	113	104	105	108	110
90th	6	105	108	111	114	104	106	109	111
95th		109	112	115	117	108	110	112	114
90th	10	110	113	117	119	112	114	116	118
95th		114	117	121	123	116	117	120	122
90th	13	117	120	124	126	118	119	122	124
95th		121	124	128	130	121	123	126	128
90th	16	125	128	132	134	122	123	126	128
95th		129	132	136	138	125	127	130	132
Diastolic Pressure									
90th	1	50	52	54	55	53	53	55	56
95th		55	56	58	59	57	57	59	60
90th	3	59	60	62	63	61	61	63	64
95th		63	64	66	67	65	65	67	68
90th	6	67	69	70	72	67	68	69	71
95th		72	73	75	76	71	72	73	75
90th	10	73	74	76	78	73	73	75	76
95th		77	79	80	82	77	77	79	80
90th	13	75	76	78	80	76	77	78	80
95th		79	81	83	84	80	81	82	84
90th	16	79	80	82	83	79	79	81	82
95th		83	84	86	87	83	83	85	86

*The height percentiles were determined with standard growth curves. (Data adapted from National Heart, Lung, and Blood Institute. [1996]. Update of the 1987 Task Force Report of the Second Task Force on High Blood Pressure in Children and Adolescents. A working group report from the National High Blood Pressure Education Program. *Pediatrics* 98, 653-654. Available: http://www.nhibi.nih.gov/health/prof/heart/hbp/hbp_ped.htm)

essential hypertension are associated with obesity or a family history of hypertension.

A number of drugs of abuse, therapeutic agents, and toxins also may increase blood pressure. Alcohol should be considered as a risk factor in adolescents. Oral contraceptives may be a cause of hypertension in adolescent females. The nephrotoxicity of the drug cyclosporine, an immunosuppressant used in transplant therapy, may cause hypertension in children after bone marrow, heart, kidney, or liver transplantation. The coadministration of glucocorticosteroid drugs appears to increase the incidence of hypertension.

Diagnosis and Treatment

The Task Force recommended that children 3 years of age through adolescence should have their blood pressure taken once each year and that phase V Korotkoff sounds be used for determining diastolic pressure for children of all ages. Systolic pressure is determined by the onset of the "tapping" Korotkoff sounds.[61] As with adults, blood pressure should be obtained using the proper-sized cuff and a well-functioning manometer. Repeated measurements over time, rather than a single, isolated determination, are required to establish consistent and significant observations.

Accurate blood pressure measurements often are difficult to obtain in infants and children who are restless; errors are easily generated in Korotkoff sounds if heavy pressure is exerted on the stethoscope. The Task Force recommended the use of auscultatory methods of blood pressure measurement in children, rather than automated methods. Automated methods are acceptable in infants, in the intensive care unit, and in children in whom auscultation is difficult. Ambulatory blood pressure monitoring may be indicated in some children, particularly those suspected of having abnormalities in the circadian blood pressure pattern.

Children with high blood pressure, significant high blood pressure, or severe high blood pressure should be referred for medical evaluation and treatment as indicated. Treatment includes nonpharmacologic methods and, if necessary, pharmacologic therapy. The Task Force suggested use of the stepped-care approach for drug treatment of children who require antihypertensive medications.[60]

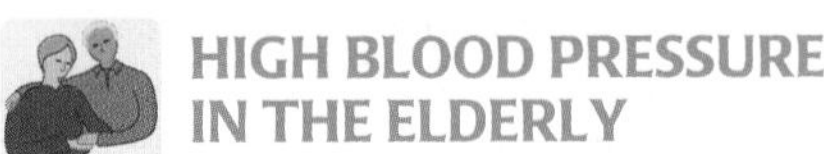

HIGH BLOOD PRESSURE IN THE ELDERLY

The prevalence of hypertension in the elderly population (65 to 74 years of age) of the United States ranges from 60% for whites to 71% for African Americans.[63] The most common type of hypertension in elderly persons is isolated systolic hypertension, in which systolic pressure is elevated while diastolic pressure remains within normal range. The *Clinical Advisory Statement* intended to advance and clarify the JNC-6 guidelines on the importance of systolic pressure in older Americans, issued by the Coordinating Committee of the National High Blood Pressure Education Program in 2000, reaffirmed the importance of lifelong maintenance of a blood pressure of 140/90 mm Hg or less.[64] The Committee further emphasized that the use of age-adjusted blood pressure targets is inappropriate, including the unsubstantiated but persistent clinical folklore that it is acceptable for the systolic blood pressure to be 100 plus the person's age.

Systolic blood pressure rises almost linearly between 30 and 84 years of age, whereas diastolic pressure rises until 50 years of age and then levels off or decreases.[9] Among the aging processes that contribute to an increase in blood pressure are a stiffening of the large arteries, particularly the aorta; decreased baroreceptor sensitivity; increased peripheral vascular resistance; and decreased renal blood flow. With aging, the elastin fibers in the walls of the arteries are gradually replaced by collagen fibers that render the vessels stiffer and less compliant.[65] Differences in the central and peripheral arteries relate to the fact that the larger vessels contain more elastin, whereas the peripheral resistance vessels have more smooth muscle and less elastin. Because of increased wall stiffness, the aorta and large arteries are less able to buffer the rise in systolic pressure that occurs as blood is ejected from the left heart, and they are less able to store the energy needed to maintain the diastolic pressure. As a result, the systolic pressure increases, the diastolic pressure remains unchanged or actually decreases, and the pulse pressure or difference between the systolic pressure and diastolic pressure widens.

Isolated systolic hypertension is recognized as an important risk factor for cardiovascular morbidity and mortality in older persons.[65,66] Stroke is two to three times more common in elderly hypertensive people than in age-matched normotensive subjects. Treatment of hypertension in the elderly has beneficial effects in terms of reducing the incidence of cardiovascular events such as stroke. The Systolic Hypertension in the Elderly Program (SHEP) showed reductions of 36% in stroke and 27% in myocardial infarction in persons who were treated for hypertension compared with those who were not.[67]

Diagnosis and Treatment

The recommendations for measurement of blood pressure in elderly persons are similar to those for the rest of the population. Blood pressure variability is particularly prevalent among older persons, and it therefore is especially important to obtain six to nine measurements (*i.e.,* two or three readings on two or three occasions) to establish a diagnosis of hypertension. The effects of food, position, and other environmental factors also are exaggerated in older persons. Special care also is warranted when the blood pressure is being taken because blood pressure measurement methods can produce pressures that are too low (*i.e.,* auscultatory gap) or falsely elevated (*i.e.,* pseudohypertension). In some elderly persons with hypertension, a silent interval, called the *auscultatory gap,* may occur between the end of the first and beginning of the third phases of the Korotkoff sounds, providing the potential for underestimating the systolic pressure, sometimes by as much as 50 mm Hg. Because the gap occurs only with auscultation, it is recommended that a preliminary determination of systolic blood pressure be made by palpation and the cuff inflated 30 mm Hg above this value for auscultatory measurement of blood pressure. It also is recommended that the cuff be deflated slowly to avoid missing the first Korotkoff sounds. In some older persons, the indirect measurement using a blood pressure cuff and the Korotkoff sounds has been shown to give falsely elevated readings compared with the direct intraarterial method. This is because excessive cuff pressure is needed to compress the rigid vessels of older persons. Pseudohypertension should be suspected in older persons with hypertension in whom the radial or brachial artery remains palpable but pulseless at higher cuff pressures.

Although sitting has become the standard position for blood pressure measurement, it is recommended that blood pressure also be taken in the supine and standing positions in the elderly. There often is a transient decrease in blood pressure on standing, after which baroreflex-mediated increases in heart rate and peripheral vascular resistance (*i.e.,* vascular constriction) usually return blood pressure to normal values. Because these reflexes often are less responsive in elderly persons and may be impaired by hypertensive medications, it has been recommended that blood pressure be measured in the supine position and 2 to 5 minutes after assumption of the standing position. This should be done during pretreatment examinations and during follow-up examinations after treatment has been instituted. This approach can detect the complication of postural hypotension, which can occur with some medications.

Despite the proven benefits of reducing elevated systolic blood pressure levels, many older persons remain untreated or are inadequately treated. The treatment of hypertension in the elderly is similar to that for younger age groups. However, blood pressure should be reduced slowly and cautiously. When possible, appropriate lifestyle modification measures should be tried first. Antihypertensive medications should be prescribed carefully because the older person may have impaired baroreflex sensitivity and renal function. Usually, medications are initiated at smaller doses, and doses are increased more gradually. Health care providers must be alert to the hazards of adverse drug interactions in older persons, who may be taking multiple medications, including over-the-counter drugs.

In summary, hypertension probably is one of the most common cardiovascular disorders. It may occur as a primary disorder (*i.e.,* essential hypertension) or as a symptom of some other disease (*i.e.,* secondary hypertension). Causes of secondary hypertension include renal disorders and adrenal cortical disorders such as hyperaldosteronism and Cushing's disease, which increase salt and water retention; pheochromocytomas, which increase catecholamine levels; and coarctation of the aorta, which produces a compensatory increase in blood pressure.

The incidence of essential hypertension increases with age. The condition is seen more frequently among African Americans, and it is linked to a family history of high blood pressure, obesity, and increased salt intake. Uncontrolled hypertension increases the risk for heart disease, renal complications, retinopathy, and stroke. Because hypertension occurs as a silent disorder, screening programs provide an effective means of early detection. The importance of screening lies in the fact that hypertension usually can be controlled and its complications prevented or minimized with appropriate treatment measures. Treatment of essential hypertension focuses on nonpharmacologic methods such as weight reduction, reduction of sodium intake, regular physical activity, modification of alcohol intake, and smoking cessation. The decision to initiate pharmacologic treatment is based on the severity of the hypertension, the presence of target-organ disease, and the existence of other conditions and risk factors. Among the drugs used in the treatment of hypertension are diuretics, adrenergic inhibitors, vasodilators, ACE inhibitors, and calcium channel blockers.

Hypertension that occurs during pregnancy can be divided into four categories: chronic hypertension, preeclampsia-eclampsia, chronic hypertension with superimposed preeclampsia-eclampsia, and gestational hypertension. Preeclampsia-eclampsia is hypertension that develops after 20 weeks' gestation and is accompanied by proteinuria. This form of hypertension, which is thought to result from impaired placental perfusion along with the release of toxic vasoactive substances that alter blood vessel tone and blood clotting mechanisms, poses a particular threat to the mother and the fetus.

Blood pressure is known to rise from infancy to late adolescence. During childhood, blood pressure is influenced by growth and maturation; therefore, blood pressure norms have been established using percentiles specific to age and height, race, and sex to identify children for further follow-up and treatment. Although hypertension occurs infrequently in children, it is recommended that children 3 years of age through adolescence should have their blood pressure taken once each year.

The most common type of hypertension in elderly persons is isolated systolic hypertension (systolic pressure ≥140 mm Hg and diastolic pressure <90 mm Hg). Its pathogenesis is related to the loss of elastin fibers in the aorta and the inability of the aorta to stretch during systole. Untreated systolic hypertension is recognized as an important risk factor for stroke and other cardiovascular morbidity and mortality in older persons. Indirect blood pressure measurements can be falsely elevated because of sclerotic blood vessels that require excessive cuff pressures, or blood pressure may be underestimated because of an auscultatory gap.

ORTHOSTATIC HYPOTENSION

- Orthostatic hypotension represents an abnormal decrease in blood pressure on assumption of the upright position that results from a decrease in venous return to the heart, due to pooling of blood in the lower part of the body, or from an inadequate circulatory response to decreased cardiac output and a decrease in blood pressure.
- Orthostatic hypotension is accompanied by a decrease in cerebral perfusion that causes a feeling of light-headedness, dizziness, and, in some cases, fainting. It poses a particular threat for falls in the elderly.
- It can be caused by conditions that decrease vascular volume (dehydration), impair muscle pump function (bed rest and spinal cord injury), or interfere with the cardiovascular reflexes (medications that decrease heart rate or cause vasodilation, disorders of the autonomic nervous system, effects of aging on baroreflex function).

Orthostatic Hypotension

After you have completed this section of the chapter, you should be able to meet the following objectives:

- Define the term *orthostatic hypotension*
- Explain how fluid deficit, medications, aging, disorders of the ANS, and bed rest contribute to the development of orthostatic hypotension

Orthostatic or postural hypotension is an abnormal drop in blood pressure on assumption of the standing position. In the absence of normal circulatory reflexes or blood volume, blood pools in the lower part of the body when the standing position is assumed, cardiac output and blood pressure fall, and blood flow to the brain is inadequate. Dizziness, syncope (*i.e.,* fainting), or both may occur. Some authorities differentiate between *orthostatic hypotension,* which is characterized by a rapid decrease in blood pressure and the inability to stand for more than 1 to 2 minutes, and *orthostatic intolerance,* which generally occurs in younger persons and is characterized by a delayed decrease in blood pressure.[68] Rather than inability to stand, persons with orthostatic intolerance complain of dizziness, visual changes, head and neck discomfort, poor concentration while standing, palpitations, tremor, anxiety, presyncope, and in some cases syncope. This text uses orthostatic hypotension to indicate both types of postural hypotension.

After the assumption of the upright posture from the supine position, approximately 500 to 700 mL of blood is momentarily shifted to the lower part of the body, with an accompanying decrease in central blood volume and arterial pressure.[69,70] Normally, this decrease in blood pressure is transient, lasting through several cardiac cycles, because the baroreceptors located in the thorax and carotid sinus area sense the decreased pressure and initiate reflex constriction of the veins and arterioles and an increase in heart rate, which brings blood pressure back to normal (Fig. 25-9). The initial adjustment to orthostatic stress is mediated exclusively by the ANS.[68] Within a few minutes of standing, blood levels of antidiuretic hormone and sympathetic neuromediators increase as a secondary means of ensuring maintenance of normal blood pressure in the standing position. Under normal conditions, the renin-angiotensin-aldosterone system is also activated when the standing position is assumed, and even more so in situations of hypotensive orthostatic stress. Muscle movement in the lower extremities also aids venous return to the heart by pumping blood out of the legs. The unconscious slight body and leg movement during standing (postural sway) is recognized as an important factor in moving venous blood back

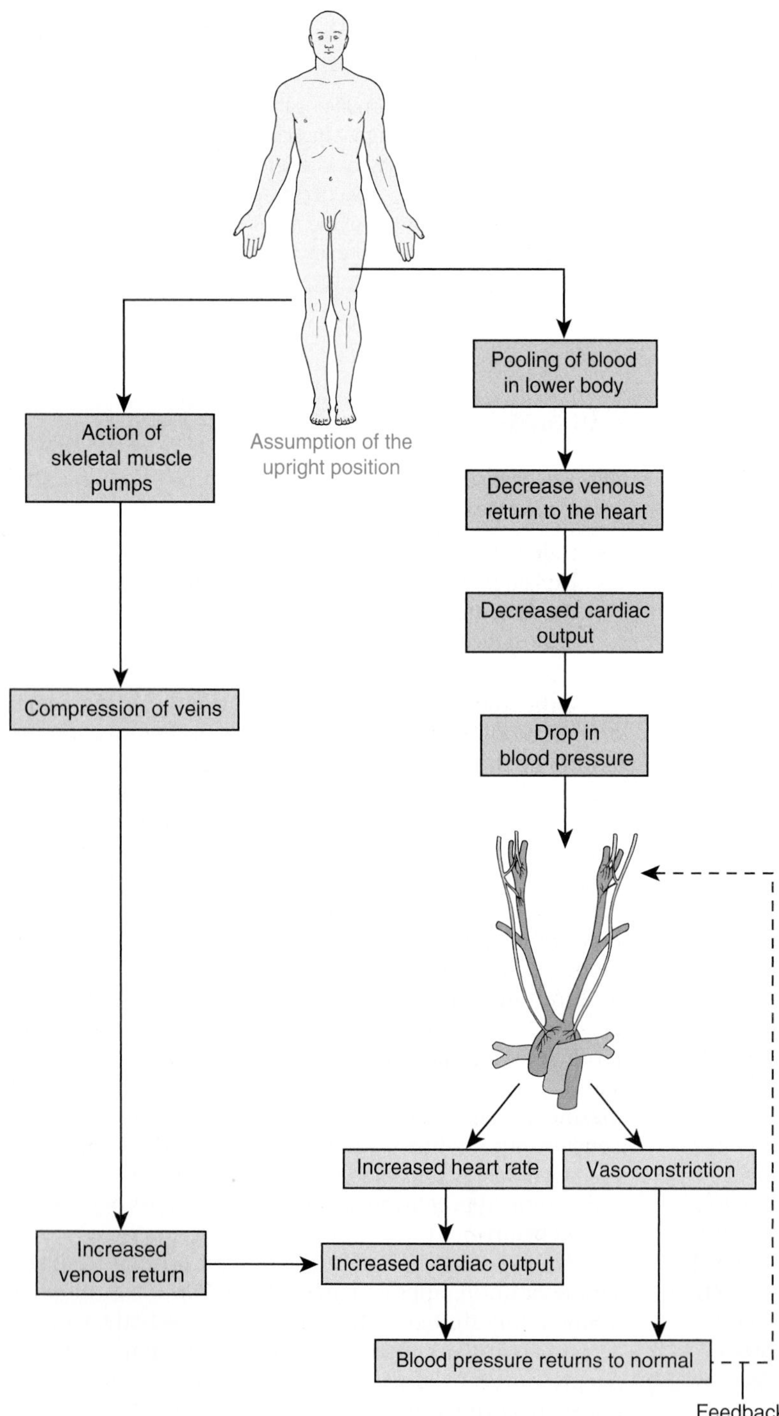

FIGURE 25-9 Mechanisms of blood control upon immediate assumption of the upright position.

to the heart.[71] Crossing the legs, which involves contraction of the agonist and antagonist muscles, has been shown to be a simple and effective way of increasing cardiac output and, therefore, blood pressure. When leg crossing is practiced routinely by persons with autonomic failure, standing systolic and diastolic pressures can be increased by approximately 20/10 mm Hg.[71]

In persons with healthy blood vessels and normal ANS function, cerebral blood flow usually is not reduced on assumption of the upright position unless arterial pressure falls below 70 mm Hg. The strategic location of the arterial baroreceptors between the heart and brain is designed to ensure that the arterial pressure is maintained within a range sufficient to prevent a reduction in cerebral blood flow.

CLASSIFICATION

Although there is no firm agreement on the definition of orthostatic hypotension, many authorities consider a fall in blood pressure equal to or greater than 20 mm Hg systolic or 10 mm Hg diastolic as indicative of orthostatic hypotension.[72] The presence of orthostatic symptoms (*e.g.,* dizziness, syncope) may be more relevant to the diagnosis of orthostatic hypotension than the numeric decrease in blood pressure.[73] A diagnosis of chronic orthostatic hypotension is characterized by signs of sympathetic activation, a heart rate increase of equal to or greater than 30 beats/minute, and plasma norepinephrine equal to or greater than 600 pg/mL.[74]

CAUSES

A wide variety of conditions, acute and chronic, are associated with orthostatic hypotension. These include reduced blood volume, drug-induced hypotension, altered vascular responses associated with aging, bed rest, and ANS dysfunction.

Reduced Blood Volume

Orthostatic hypotension often is an early sign of reduced blood volume or fluid deficit. When blood volume is decreased, the vascular compartment is only partially filled; although cardiac output may be adequate when a person is in the recumbent position, it often decreases to the point of causing weakness and fainting when the person assumes the standing position. Common causes of orthostatic hypotension related to hypovolemia are excessive use of diuretics, excessive diaphoresis, loss of gastrointestinal fluids through vomiting and diarrhea, and loss of fluid volume associated with prolonged bed rest.

Drug-Induced Hypotension

Antihypertensive drugs and psychotropic drugs are the most common cause of chronic orthostatic hypotension. In most cases, the orthostatic hypotension is well tolerated. However, if the hypotension causes lightheadedness or syncope, the dosage of the drug is usually reduced or a different drug substituted.[73]

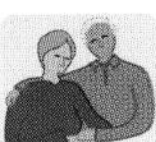

Aging

Weakness and dizziness on standing are common complaints of elderly persons. The Cardiovascular Health Study reports a 16.2% prevalence of asymptomatic orthostatic hypotension among persons 65 years of age and older.[75] Orthostatic hypotension was associated with systolic hypertension, major electrocardiographic abnormalities, and carotid artery stenosis. Because cerebral blood flow primarily depends on systolic pressure, patients with impaired cerebral circulation may experience symptoms of weakness, ataxia, dizziness, and syncope when their arterial pressure falls even slightly. This may happen in older persons who are immobilized for brief periods or whose blood volume is decreased owing to inadequate fluid intake or overzealous use of diuretics.

Postprandial blood pressure often decreases in elderly persons.[76] The greatest postprandial changes occur after a high-carbohydrate meal.[77] Although the mechanism responsible for these changes is not fully understood, it is thought to result from glucose-mediated impairment of baroreflex sensitivity and increased splanchnic blood flow mediated by insulin and vasoactive gastrointestinal hormones.

Bed Rest

Prolonged bed rest promotes a reduction in plasma volume, a decrease in venous tone, failure of peripheral vasoconstriction, and weakness of the skeletal muscles that support the veins and assist in returning blood to the heart (see Chapter 12). Physical deconditioning follows even short periods of bed rest. After 3 to 4 days, the blood volume is decreased.[78] Loss of vascular and skeletal muscle tone is less predictable but probably becomes maximal after approximately 2 weeks of bed rest. Orthostatic intolerance is a recognized problem of space flight—a potential risk after reentry into the earth's gravitational field.

Disorders of Autonomic Nervous System Function

The sympathetic nervous system plays an essential role in adjustment to the upright position. Sympathetic stimulation increases heart rate and cardiac contractility and causes constriction of peripheral veins and arterioles. Orthostatic hypotension caused by altered autonomic function is common in peripheral neuropathies associated with diabetes mellitus, after injury or disease of the spinal cord, or as the result of a cerebral vascular accident in which sympathetic outflow from the brain stem is disrupted. The American Autonomic Society and the American Academy of Neurology have distinguished three forms of primary ANS dysfunction: (1) pure autonomic failure, which is defined as a sporadic, idiopathic cause of persistent orthostatic hypotension and other manifestations of autonomic failure such as urinary retention, impotence, or decreased sweating; (2) Parkinson disease with autonomic failure; and (3) multiple-system atrophy (Shy-Drager syndrome).[79,80] Shy-Drager syndrome usually develops in middle to late life as orthostatic hypotension associated with uncoordinated movements, urinary incontinence, constipation, and other signs of neurologic deficits referable to the corticospinal, extrapyramidal, corticobulbar, and cerebellar systems.

DIAGNOSIS AND TREATMENT

Orthostatic hypotension can be assessed with the blood pressure cuff. A reading should be made when the patient is supine, immediately after assumption of the seated or upright position, and at 2- to 3-minute intervals for 5 minutes. Because it takes approximately 5 to 10 minutes for the blood pressure to stabilize after lying down, it is recommended that the patient be supine for this period before standing. It is strongly recommended that a second person be available when blood pressure is measured in the standing position to prevent injury should the patient become faint. A tilt table also can be used for this purpose. With a tilt table, the recumbent patient can be moved to a head-up position without voluntary movement when the table is tilted. The tilt table also has the advantage of rapidly and safely returning persons with a profound postural drop in blood pressure to the horizontal position.

Persons with a drop in blood pressure to orthostatic levels should be evaluated to determine the cause and seriousness of the condition. A history should be taken to elicit information about symptoms, particularly dizziness and history of syncope and falls; medical conditions, particularly those such as diabetes mellitus that predispose to orthostatic hypotension; use of prescription and over-the-counter drugs; and symptoms of ANS dysfunction, such as impotence or bladder dysfunction. A physical examination should document blood pressure in both arms and the heart rate while in the supine, sitting, and standing positions and should note the occurrence of symptoms. Noninvasive, 24-hour ambulatory blood pressure monitoring may be used to determine blood pressure responses to other stimuli of daily life, such as food ingestion and exertion.

Treatment of orthostatic hypotension usually is directed toward alleviating the cause or, if this is not possible, toward helping people learn ways to cope with the disorder and prevent falls and injuries. Medications that predispose to postural hypotension should be avoided. Correcting the fluid deficit and trying a different antihypertensive medication are examples of measures designed to correct the cause. Measures designed to help persons prevent symptomatic orthostatic drops in blood pressure include gradual ambulation to allow the circulatory system to adjust (*i.e.*, sitting on the edge of the bed for several minutes and moving the legs to initiate skeletal muscle pump function before standing); avoidance of situations that encourage excessive vasodilation (*e.g.*, drinking alcohol, exercising vigorously in a warm environment); and avoidance of excess diuresis (*e.g.*, use of diuretics), diaphoresis, or loss of body fluids. Tight-fitting elastic support hose or an abdominal support garment may help prevent pooling of blood in the lower extremities and abdomen.

Pharmacologic treatment may be used when nonpharmacologic methods are unsuccessful. A number of types of drugs can be used for this purpose.[72] Mineralocorticoids (*e.g.*, fludrocortisone) can be used to reduce salt and water loss and probably increase α-adrenergic sensitivity. Vasopressin-2 receptor agonists (desmopressin as a nasal spray) may be used to reduce nocturnal polyuria. Sympathomimetic drugs that act directly on the resistance vessels (phenylephrine, noradrenaline, clonidine) or on the capacitance vessels (*e.g.*, dihydroergotamine) may be used. Many of these agents have undesirable side effects. Octreotide, a somatostatin analog that inhibits the release of vasodilatory gastrointestinal peptides, may prove useful in persons with postprandial hypotension.

In summary, orthostatic hypotension refers to an abnormal decrease in systolic and diastolic blood pressures that occurs on assumption of the upright position. An important consideration in orthostatic hypotension is the occurrence of dizziness and syncope. Among the factors that contribute to its occurrence are decreased fluid volume, medications, aging, defective function of the ANS, and the effects of immobility. Diagnosis of orthostatic hypotension includes blood pressure measurement in the supine and upright positions, a history of symptomatology, medication use, and disease conditions that contribute to a postural drop in blood pressure. Treatment includes correcting the reversible causes and assisting the person to compensate for the disorder and prevent falls and injuries.

REVIEW EXERCISES

A 47-year-old African-American man, who is an executive in a law firm, had his blood pressure taken at a screening program and had been told that his pressure was 142/90 mm Hg. His father and older brother have hypertension, and his paternal grandparents had a history of stroke and myocardial infarction. The patient enjoys salty foods and routinely uses a salt shaker to add salt to meals his wife prepares, drinks about 4 beers while watching television in the evening, and gained 15 pounds in the past year. Although his family has encouraged him to engage in physical activities with them, he states he is too either too busy or too tired.

A. According to JNC-7 guidelines, into what category does the patient's blood pressure fall?

B. What are his risk factors for hypertension?

C. Explain how an increased salt intake might contribute to an increase in blood pressure.

D. What lifestyle changes would you suggest to the patient? Explain the rationale for your suggestions.

A 36-year-old woman enters the clinic complaining of headache and not feeling well. Her blood pressure is 175/90 mm Hg. Her renal tests are abnormal, and follow-up tests confirm that she has a stricture of the left renal artery.

A. Would this woman's hypertension be classified as primary or secondary?

B. Explain the physiologic mechanisms underlying her blood pressure elevation.

A 75-year-old woman, who resides in an extended care facility, has multiple health problems, including diabetes, hypertension, and heart failure. Lately, she has been feeling dizzy when she stands up, and she has almost fallen on several occasions. Her family is concerned and wants to know why this is happening and what they can do to prevent her from falling and breaking her hip.

A. How would you go about assessing this woman for orthostatic hypotension?

B. What are the causes of orthostatic hypotension in elderly persons?

C. How might this woman's medical conditions and their treatment contribute to her orthostatic hypotension?

D. The woman tells you that she feels particularly dizzy after she has eaten, yet the staff insists that she sit up and socialize with the other residents even though she would rather lie down and rest until the dizziness goes away. Explain the possible reason for her dizziness and what measures might be used to counteract the dizziness.

E. The woman recently had an episode of vomiting and diarrhea on an extremely hot day. She told her family that she was so dizzy that she was sure she would fall. Explain why her dizziness was more severe under these conditions and what might be done to alleviate the situation.

References

1. Smith J. J., Kampine J. P. (1990). Circulatory physiology (3rd ed., pp. 89–109). Baltimore: Williams & Wilkins.
2. Guyton A. C., Hall J. E. (2000). *Textbook of medical physiology* (10th ed., pp. 195–209). Philadelphia: W. B. Saunders.
3. Verdecchia P., Schillaci G., Porcella C. (1991). Dippers versus non-dippers. *Hypertension 9*(Suppl. 8), S42–S44.
4. Grim C. E., Grim C. M. (2001). Accurate and reliable blood pressure measurement in the clinic and home: The key to hypertension control. In Hollenberg N. (Ed.), *Hypertension: Mechanisms and management* (3rd ed., pp. 315–324). Philadelphia: Current Medicine.
5. Grim C. M., Grim C. E. (2000). Manual blood pressure measurement: Still the gold standard. In Weber M. A. (Ed.), *Hypertension medicine* (pp. 131–145). Totowa, NJ: Humana Press.
6. O'Brien E. (1996). Review: A century of confusion; which bladder for accurate blood pressure measurement? *Journal of Human Hypertension 10,* 565–572.
7. White W. B. (2003). Ambulatory and home blood pressure monitoring. In Izzo J. L., Black H. R. (Eds.), *Hypertension primer* (3rd ed. pp. 330–334). Dallas: American Heart Association.
8. Pickering T. (1995). American Society for Blood Pressure Ad Hoc Panel: Recommendations for use of home (self) and ambulatory blood pressure monitoring. *Journal of Hypertension 9,* 1–11.
9. National Heart, Lung, and Blood Institute. (2003). The seventh report of the Joint National Committee on Detection, Evaluation, and Treatment of High Blood Pressure. U.S. Department of Health and Human Services (NIH Publication 03-5233).
10. Vassan R. S., Larson M. G., Leip E. P., et al. (2001). Assessment of frequency of progression to hypertension in nonhypertensive participants in the Framingham Heart Study: a cohort study. *Lancet 358,* 1682–1686.
11. American Diabetes Association. (2001). Summary of revisions for the 2001 clinical practice recommendations. *Diabetes Care 24*(Suppl. 1), 1.
12. Staesen J. A., Wang J., Blanchi G., Birkenhäger W. H. (2003). Essential hypertension. *Lancet 361,* 1629–1641.
13. Hunt S. C. (2003). Genetics and family history of hypertension. In Izzo J. L., Black H. R. (Eds.). *Hypertension primer* (pp. 218–221). Dallas: American Heart Association.
14. Williams R. R., Hunt S. C., Hasstedt S. J., et al. (1991). Are there interactions and relations between genetic and environmental factors predisposing to high blood pressure? *Hypertension 18*(Suppl. I), S29–S37.
15. Franklin S. S., Milagros J. J., Wong N. D., et al. (2001). Predominance of isolated systolic hypertension among middle-aged and elderly US hypertensives. *Hypertension 37,* 869–874.
16. Burt V. L., Whelton P., Rocella E. J., et al. (1995). Prevalence of hypertension in the US population: Results from the Third National Health and Nutrition Examination Survey, 1988–91. *Hypertension 25,* 305–313.
17. Gillum R. F. (1996). Epidemiology of hypertension in African American women. *American Heart Journal 131,* 385–395.
18. Grim C. E., Henry J. P., Myers H. (1995). High blood pressure in blacks: Salt, slavery, survival, stress, and racism. In Laragh J. H., Brenner B. M. (Eds.), *Hypertension: Pathophysiology, diagnosis, and management* (pp. 171–207). New York: Raven Press.
19. Blaustein M. P., Grim C. E. (1991). The pathogenesis of hypertension: Black-white differences. *Cardiovascular Clinics 21*(3), 97–114.
20. Wilson T. W., Grim C. E. (1991). Biohistory of slavery and blood pressure differences in blacks today: A hypothesis. *Hypertension 17*(Suppl. I), I122–I128.
21. Ward K. D., Sparrow D., Landsberg L. (1996). Influence of insulin, sympathetic nervous system activity, and obesity on blood pressure: The Normative Aging Study. *Journal of Hypertension 14,* 301–306.
22. Steinberg H. O. (2003). Insulin resistance and hypertension. In Izzo J. L., Black H. R. (Ed). *Hypertension Primer* (3rd ed., pp. 131–132). Dallas: American Heart Association.
23. Reaven G. M., Lithell H., Landsberg L. (1996). Hypertension and associated metabolic abnormalities: The role of insulin resistance and the sympathoadrenal system. *New England Journal of Medicine 334,* 374–381.
24. Wilson T. W., Grim C. E. (2000). Sodium and hypertension. In Kiple K (Ed.), *The Cambridge world history of food and nutrition* (pp. 848–856). Cambridge: Cambridge University Press.
25. Kaplan N. M. (2000). Evidence in favor of moderate dietary sodium reduction. *American Journal of Hypertension 13*(9), 8–13.
26. Elliott P., Stamler S., Nichols R., Dyer A. R., et al. (1996). Intersalt revisited: Further analyses of 24 hour sodium excretion and blood pressure within and across populations. *British Medical Journal 312,* 1249–1253.
27. Kotchen T. A., McCarron D. A. (1998). Dietary electrolytes and blood pressure: A statement for healthcare professionals

from the American Heart Association Nutrition Committee. *Circulation 98,* 613–617.
28. Conlin P. R., Chow D., Miller E. R. III, et al. (2000). The effect of dietary pattern on blood pressure control in hypertensive patients: Results from the Dietary Approaches to Stop Hypertension (DASH) trial. *Journal of Hypertension 13,* 949–953.
29. Sacks F. M., Svetkey L. P., Vollmer W. M., et al. (2001). Effects on blood pressure of reduced sodium and the Dietary Approaches to Stop Hypertension (DASH) diet. *New England Journal of Medicine 344,* 3–10.
30. Cassano P. A., Segal M. R., Vokonas P. S., Weiss S. T. (1990). Body fat distribution, blood pressure, and hypertension: A prospective study of men in the normative aging study. *Annals of Epidemiology 1,* 33–48.
31. Peiris A. N., Sothmann M. S., Hoffmann R. G., et al. (1989). Obesity, fat distribution, and cardiovascular risk. *Annals of Internal Medicine 110,* 867–872.
32. Fuchs F. D., Chambless L. E., Whelton P. K., et al. (2001). Alcohol consumption and the incidence of hypertension. *Hypertension 37,* 1242–1250.
33. Marmot M. G., Elliott P., Shipley M. J., et al. (1994). Alcohol and blood pressure: The INTERSALT study. *British Medical Journal 308,* 1263–1267.
34. Klatsky A. L., Freidman G. D., Siegelaub A. B. (1977). Alcohol consumption and blood pressure. *New England Journal of Medicine 296,* 1194–1200.
35. Whelton P. K. (2003). Potassium and blood pressure. In Izzo J. L., Black H. R. (Eds.), *Hypertension primer* (3rd ed., pp. 280–283). Dallas: American Heart Association.
36. Intersalt Cooperative Research Group. (1988). Intersalt: An international study of electrolyte excretion and blood pressure. Results of 24 hour urinary sodium and potassium excretion. *British Medical Journal 297,* 319–328.
37. Sacks F. M., Willett W. C., Smith A., et al. (1998). Effect on blood pressure of potassium, calcium, and magnesium in women with low habitual intake. *Hypertension 31,* 131–138.
38. Kaplan N. M. (1995). The treatment of hypertension in women. *Archives of Internal Medicine 155,* 563–567.
39. Pickering T., Harshfield G. A., Kleinert H. D., et al. (1982). Blood pressure during normal daily activities, sleep, and exercise. *Journal of the American Medical Association 247,* 992–996.
40. Frohlich E. D., Chobanian A. B., Devereux R. G., et al. (1992). The heart in hypertension. *New England Journal of Medicine 327,* 998–1008.
41. Black H. R., Kuller L. H., O'Rourke M. F., et al. (1999). The first report of the Systolic and Pulse Pressure (SYPP) working group. *Journal of Hypertension 17*(Suppl. 5), S3–S14.
42. Alderman M. H. (1999). A new model of risk implications of increasing pulse pressure and systolic blood pressure in cardiovascular disease. *Journal of Hypertension 17*(Suppl. 5), S23–S28.
43. Lloyd-Jones D. M., Evans J. C., Larson M. G., et al. (1999). Differential impact of systolic and diastolic blood pressure level on JNC-VI staging. *Hypertension 34,* 381–385.
44. Benetos A. (1999). Pulse pressure and cardiovascular risk. *Journal of Hypertension 17*(Suppl. 5), S21–S24.
45. Ram C. V. (1994). Secondary hypertension: Workup and correction. *Hospital Practice 4,* 137–155.
46. Onusko E. (2003). Diagnosing secondary hypertension. *American Family Physician 67,* 67–74.
47. Safian R. D., Textor S. C. (2001). Renal-artery stenosis. *New England Journal of Medicine 344,* 431–442.
48. Kaplan N. N. (2001). Hypertension and atherosclerotic cardiovascular disease. Hypertension: Mechanisms and diagnosis. In Braunwald E., Zipes D. P., Libby P. (Ed.), *Heart disease: A textbook of cardiovascular disease* (6th ed., pp. 958–968). Philadelphia: W. B. Saunders.
49. Gomez-Sanchez C. E., Gomez-Sanchez E. P., Yamakita N. (1995). Endocrine causes of hypertension. *Seminars in Nephrology 15,* 106–115.
50. Venkata C., Ram S., Fierro-Carrion G. A. (1995). Pheochromocytoma. *Seminars in Nephrology 15,* 126–137.
51. Roa P. S. (1995). Coarctation of the aorta. *Seminars in Nephrology 15,* 87–105.
52. Vidt D. G. (2003). Treatment of hypertensive emergencies and urgencies. In Izzo J. L., Black H. R. (Eds.), *Hypertension primer* (3rd ed., pp. 462–455). Dallas: American Heart Association.
53. Chames M. C., Sibal B. M. (2001). When chronic hypertension complicates pregnancy. *Contemporary OB/GYN Archive* April 2 [On-line.] Available: http://ahgyn.pdf.net/public.htm. Accessed 5/14/01/.
54. Gifford R. W. Jr. (Chair) (2000). *National High Blood Pressure Working Group report on high blood pressure in pregnancy.* NIH publication no. 00-3029. Bethesda, MD: National Institutes of Health.
55. Sibai B. M., Lindheimer M., Hauth J., et al. (1998). Risk factors for preeclampsia, abruptio placentae, and adverse neonatal outcomes among women with chronic hypertension. *New England Journal of Medicine 339,* 667–671.
56. Olofsson P. (1995). Characteristics of a reversed circadian blood pressure rhythm in pregnant women with hypertension. *Journal of Human Hypertension 9,* 565–570.
57. Solomon C. G. (2001). Hypertension in pregnancy: A manifestation of insulin resistance syndrome. *Hypertension 37,* 232–239.
58. Sinaiko A. R. (1996). Hypertension in children (Review). *New England Journal of Medicine 335,* 1968–1973.
59. Bartosh S. M., Aronson A. J. (1999). Childhood hypertension. *Pediatric Clinics of North America 46,* 235–251.
60. National Heart, Lung and Blood Institute. (1996). Update of the 1987 Task Force Report of the Second Task Force on High Blood Pressure in Children and Adolescents: A working group report from the National High Blood Pressure Education Program. *Pediatrics 88,* 649–658.
61. Sorof J. M., Portman R. J. (2000). Ambulatory blood pressure monitoring in the pediatric patient. *Journal of Pediatrics 136,* 578–586.
62. Behrman R. E., Kliegman R. M., Arvin A. M. (2004). Systemic hypertension. In Behrman R. E., Kliegman R. M., Jenson H. B. (Eds.), *Nelson textbook of pediatrics* (17th ed., pp. 1592–1598). Philadelphia: W. B. Saunders.
63. National High Blood Pressure Education Program Working Group. (1994). National High Blood Pressure Education Working Group report on hypertension in the elderly. *Hypertension 23,* 275–285.
64. Izzo J. L., Levy D., Black H. R. (2000). Clinical advisory statement: Importance of systolic blood pressure in older Americans. *Hypertension 35,* 1021–1024.
65. Franklin S. S., Larson M. G., Khan S. A., et al. (2001). Does the relation of blood pressure to coronary heart disease risk change with aging? *Circulation 103,* 1245–1250.
66. Black H. R. (1999). Isolated hypertension in the elderly: Lessons from clinical trials and future directions. *Journal of Hypertension 17*(Suppl. 5), S49–S54.
67. SHEP Cooperative Research Group. (1991). Prevention of stroke by antihypertensive drug treatment in older persons with isolated systolic hypertension. *Journal of the American Medical Association 265,* 3255–3264.
68. Goldstein D. S. (Moderator), Robertson D., Murray E., Straus S. E., Eisenhofer G. (Discussants). (2002). NIH Conference. Disautonomias: Clinical disorders of the autonomic nervous system. *Annals of Internal Medicine 137,* 753–763.
69. Smith J. J., Porth C. J. M. (1990). Age and the response to orthostatic stress. In Smith J. J. (Ed.), *Circulatory response to the upright posture* (pp. 121–138). Boca Raton, FL: CRC Press.

70. Smit A. A. J., Halliwatt J. R., Low P. A., Wieling W. (1999). Pathophysiological basis of orthostatic hypotension in autonomic failure. *Journal of Physiology 591*(1), 1–10.
71. Van Lieshout J. J., Ten Harkel A. D. J., Weiling W. (1992). Physical maneuvers for combating orthostatic dizziness in autonomic failure. *Lancet 339,* 897–898.
72. Mathias C. J., Kimber J. R. (1999). Postural hypotension: Causes, clinical features, investigation, and management. *Annual Review of Medicine 50,* 317–336.
73. Robertson D. (2003). Treatment of orthostatic disorders and baroreflex failure. In Izzo J. L., Black H. R. (Eds.), *Hypertension primer* (3rd ed., pp. 479–482). Dallas: American Heart Association.
74. Kochar M. S. (1990). Orthostatic hypotension. In Smith J. J. (Ed.), *Circulatory response to the upright posture* (pp. 170–179). Boca Raton, FL: CRC Press.
75. Rutan G. H., Hermanson B., Bild D. E., et al. (1992). Orthostatic hypotension in older adults: The Cardiovascular Study. *Hypertension 19,* 508–519.
76. Jansen R. W. M. M., Lipsitz L. A. (1995). Postprandial hypotension: Epidemiology, pathophysiology, and clinical management. *Annals of Internal Medicine 122,* 286–295.
77. Potter J. F., Heseltine D., Matthews J., et al. (1989). Effects of meal composition on the postprandial blood pressure, catecholamine and insulin changes in elderly subjects. *Clinical Science 77,* 265–272.
78. Taylor H. L., Henschel A., Broek J., et al. (1949). Effects of bed rest on cardiovascular function and work performance. *Journal of Applied Physiology 11,* 223–239.
79. American Autonomic Society and American Academy of Neurologists. (1996). Consensus statement of the definition of orthostatic hypotension, pure autonomic failure, and multiple system atrophy. *Neurology 46,* 1470.
80. Goldstein D. S., Holmes C., Cannon R. O. III, et al. (1997). Sympathetic cardioneuropathy in dysautonomias. *New England Journal of Medicine 336,* 696–702.

CHAPTER

26

Disorders of Cardiac Function

Cardiovascular disease is the number one cause of death in the United States. Coronary heart disease caused more than one out of every five deaths in the United States in 2000.[1] Of the 681,000 deaths that occurred that year, 50.6% of deaths were in males and 49.4% were in females. The American Heart Association (AHA) has stated that if cardiovascular disease were eliminated, life expectancy would increase by almost 7 years.[1] It is projected that by 2020, cardiovascular disease will, for the first time in human history, be the most common cause of death worldwide.[2]

In an attempt to focus on common heart problems that affect persons in all age groups, this chapter is organized into six sections: disorders of the pericardium, coronary heart disease, disorders of the myocardium, infectious and immunologic disorders, valvular heart disease, and heart disease in infants and children.

Disorders of the Pericardium

After completing this section of the chapter, you should be able to meet the following objectives:

- Describe the function of the pericardium
- Describe the physiology of pericardial effusion
- Relate the cardiac compression that occurs with cardiac tamponade to the clinical manifestations of the disorder, including pulsus paradoxus
- Compare the manifestations of acute pericarditis with those of chronic pericarditis with effusion and constrictive pericarditis

The pericardium is a double-layered serous membrane that isolates the heart from other thoracic structures, maintains its position in the thorax, and prevents it from overfilling. The pericardium also contributes to coupling the distensibility between the two ventricles during diastole so that they both fill equally.[3] The two layers of the pericardium are separated by a thin layer of serous fluid, which prevents frictional forces from developing as the inner visceral layer, or epicardium, comes in contact with the outer parietal layer of the fibrous pericardium. The mechanisms that control the movement of fluid between the capillaries and the pericardial space are the same as those that control fluid movement between the capillaries and the interstitial spaces of other body tissues (see Chapter 23).

TYPES OF PERICARDIAL DISORDERS

The pericardium is subject to many of the same pathologic processes (*e.g.*, congenital disorders, infections, trauma, immune mechanisms, and neoplastic disease) that affect other structures of the body. Pericardial disorders frequently are associated with or result from another disease in the heart or the surrounding structures (Chart 26-1).

DISORDERS OF THE PERICARDIUM

- The pericardium isolates the heart from other thoracic structures, maintains its position in the thorax, and prevents it from overfilling.
- The two layers of the pericardium are separated by a thin layer of serous fluid, which prevents frictional forces from developing between the visceral and parietal layers of the pericardium.
- Disorders that produce inflammation of the pericardium interfere with the friction-reducing properties of the pericardial fluid and produce pain.
- Disorders that increase the fluid volume of the pericardial sac interfere with cardiac filling and produce a subsequent reduction in cardiac output.

CHART 26-1

Classification of Disorders of the Pericardium

Inflammation

Acute inflammatory pericarditis

1. Infectious
   Viral (echovirus, coxsackievirus, and others)
   Bacterial (*e.g.*, tuberculosis, *Staphylococcus*, *Streptococcus*)
   Fungal
2. Immune and collagen disorders
   Rheumatic fever
   Rheumatoid arthritis
   Systemic lupus erythematosus
3. Metabolic disorders
   Uremia and dialysis
   Myxedema
4. Ischemia and tissue injury
   Myocardial infarction
   Cardiac surgery
   Chest trauma
5. Physical and chemical agents
   Radiation therapy
   Untoward reactions to drugs, such as hydralazine, procainamide, and anticoagulants

Chronic inflammatory pericarditis
   Can be associated with most of the agents causing an acute inflammatory response

Neoplastic Disease

1. Primary
2. Secondary (*e.g.*, carcinoma of the lung or breast, lymphoma)

Congenital Disorders

1. Complete or partial absence of the pericardium
2. Congenital pericardial cysts

Pericardial Effusion

Pericardial effusion refers to the accumulation of fluid in the pericardial cavity. It may develop as the result of injury, inflammation, or altered capillary filtration pressures. Its major threat is compression of the heart chambers. The amount of fluid, the rapidity with which it accumulates, and the elasticity of the pericardium determine the effect the effusion has on cardiac function. Small pericardial effusions may produce no symptoms or abnormal clinical findings. Even a large effusion that develops slowly may cause few or no symptoms, provided the pericardium is able to stretch and avoid compressing the heart. However, a sudden accumulation of even 200 mL may raise intracardiac pressure to levels that seriously limit the venous return to the heart. Symptoms of cardiac compression also may occur with relatively small accumulations of fluid when the pericardium has become thickened by scar tissue or neoplastic infiltrations.

Cardiac Tamponade. Cardiac tamponade is a life-threatening, slow or rapid compression of the heart due to the accumulation of fluid, pus, or blood in the pericardial sac.[3,4] It can occur as the result of conditions such as trauma, cardiac surgery, cancer, uremia, or cardiac rupture due to myocardial infarction. The seriousness of cardiac tamponade results from increased intracardiac pressure, progressive limitation of ventricular diastolic filling, and reduction in stroke volume and cardiac output. The severity of the condition depends on the amount of fluid that is present and the rate at which it accumulated. A rapid accumulation of fluid results in an elevation of central venous pressure, jugular venous distention, a decline in venous return to the heart, a decrease in cardiac output despite an increase in heart rate, a fall in systolic blood pressure, and signs of circulatory shock. The heart sounds may become difficult to hear owing to the insulating effects of the pericardial fluid and reduced cardiac function. Persons in whom cardiac tamponade develops slowly usually appear acutely ill, but not to the extreme seen in those with rapidly developing tamponade, and the major complaint usually is dyspnea.

A key diagnostic finding is *pulsus paradoxus,* conventionally defined as a 10 mm Hg or more fall in arterial blood pressure during normal breathing.[3,4] Normally, the decrease in intrathoracic pressure that occurs during inspiration accelerates venous flow, increasing right atrial and right ventricular filling. This causes the interventricular septum to bulge to the left, producing a slight decrease in left ventricular filling, stroke volume output, and systolic blood pressure. In cardiac tamponade, the left ventricle is compressed from within by movement of the interventricular septum and from without by fluid in the pericardium (Fig. 26-1). This produces a marked decrease in left ventricular filling and left ventricular stroke volume output, often within a beat of the beginning of inspiration. Pulsus paradoxus is determined by palpation or cuff sphygmomanometry. When present, the arterial pulse, as palpated at the carotid or femoral artery, is reduced or absent during inspiration. Palpation provides only a gross estimate of the degree of pulsus paradoxus. It is more sensitively estimated when the blood pressure cuff is used to compare the Korotkoff sounds during inspiration and expiration.

The echocardiogram is a rapid, accurate, and widely used method of evaluating pericardial effusion. Aspiration and laboratory evaluation of the pericardial fluid may be used to identify the causative agent. Cardiac catheterization may be used to determine the hemodynamic effects of pericardial effusion and cardiac tamponade. Pericardiocentesis or removal of fluid from the pericardial sac, often with a needle inserted through the chest wall, may be an emergency lifesaving measure in severe cardiac tamponade. Surgical treatment may be required for traumatic lesions of the heart.

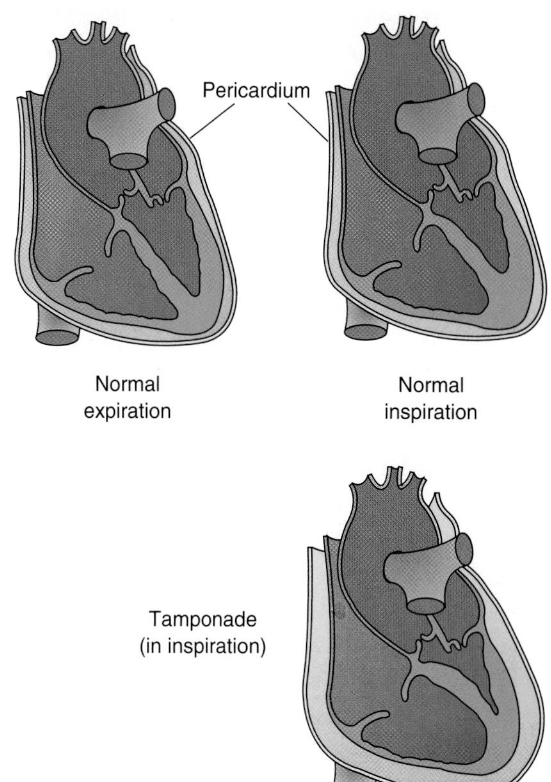

FIGURE 26-1 Effects of respiration and cardiac tamponade on ventricular filling and cardiac output. During inspiration venous flow into the right heart increases, causing the interventricular septum to bulge into the left ventricle. This produces a decrease in left ventricular volume, with a subsequent decrease in stroke volume output. In cardiac tamponade, the fluid in the pericardial sac produces further compression of the left ventricle, causing an exaggeration of the normal inspiratory decrease in stroke volume and systolic blood pressure.

Pericarditis

Pericarditis represents an acute inflammatory process of the pericardium.[3,5] It can result from a number of diverse causes. Most forms of pericarditis occur secondary to other systemic or cardiac diseases. Primary pericarditis is unusual and is usually of viral origin. Most cases of pericarditis evoke an acute inflammatory process. Exceptions are tuberculosis and fungal infections, which often produce a chronic pericarditis.

Acute Pericarditis. Acute pericarditis can be classified according to cause (*e.g.,* infections, trauma, rheumatic fever) or the nature of the exudate (*e.g.,* serous, fibrinous, purulent, hemorrhagic). Like other inflammatory conditions, acute pericarditis often is associated with increased capillary permeability. The capillaries that supply the serous pericardium become permeable, allowing plasma proteins, including fibrinogen, to leave the capillaries and enter the pericardial space. This results in an exudate that varies in type and amount according to the causative agent. Acute pericarditis frequently is associated with a fibrinous (fibrin-containing) exudate (Fig. 26-2), which heals by resolution or progresses to deposition of scar tissue and formation of adhesions between the layers of the serous pericardium. Inflammation also may involve the superficial myocardium and the adjacent pleura.

Viral infection (especially infections with the coxsackieviruses and echoviruses, but also influenza, Epstein-Barr, varicella, hepatitis, mumps, and human immunodeficiency virus [HIV]) is the most common cause of acute pericarditis. Acute viral pericarditis is seen more frequently in men than in women and often is preceded by a prodromal phase

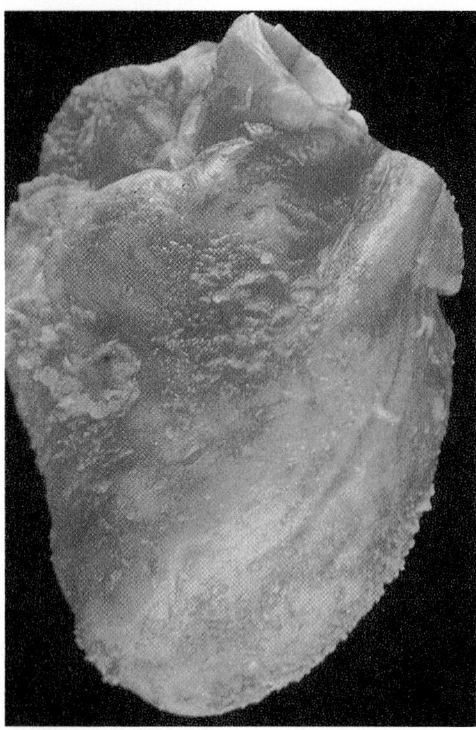

FIGURE 26-2 Fibrinous pericarditis. The heart of a patient who died in uremia displays a shaggy, fibrinous exudate covering the visceral pericardium. (Rubin E., Farber J.L. [1999]. *Pathology* [3rd ed., p. 585]. Philadelphia: Lippincott-Raven).

during which fever, malaise, and other flulike symptoms are present. In some cases, a well-defined infection elsewhere in the body, such as an upper respiratory tract infection, precedes the onset of pericarditis and is the primary site of infection. Although the acute symptoms usually subside in several weeks, easy fatigability often continues for several months. In many cases, the condition is self-limited, resolving in 2 to 6 weeks; but in other cases, pericarditis from the same cause may persist and produce recurrent subacute or chronic disease.

Other causes of pericarditis are rheumatic fever, postpericardiotomy syndrome, post-traumatic pericarditis, metabolic disorders (*e.g.*, uremia, myxedema), and pericarditis associated with connective tissue diseases (*e.g.*, systemic lupus erythematosus, rheumatoid arthritis). With the increased use of open-heart surgery in the treatment of various heart disorders, the postpericardiotomy syndrome has become a commonly recognized form of pericarditis. Pericarditis with effusion is a common complication in persons with renal failure, in those with untreated uremia, and in those being treated with hemodialysis. Irradiation may initiate a subacute pericarditis, with an onset usually within the first year of therapy. It is most commonly associated with high doses of radiation delivered to areas near the heart.

The manifestations of acute pericarditis include a triad of chest pain, pericardial friction rub, and electrocardiographic (ECG) changes. The clinical findings may vary according to the causative agent. Nearly all persons with acute pericarditis have chest pain. The pain usually is abrupt in onset, occurs in the precordial area, and is described as sharp. It may radiate to the neck, back, abdomen, or side. It typically is worse with deep breathing, coughing, swallowing, and positional changes because of changes in venous return and cardiac filling. Many persons seek relief by sitting up and leaning forward. Only a small portion of the pericardium, the outer layer of the lower parietal pericardium below the fifth and sixth intercostal spaces, is sensitive to pain. This means that pericardial pain probably results from inflammation of the surrounding structures, particularly the pleura.

Diagnosis of acute pericarditis is based on clinical manifestations, ECG, chest radiography, and echocardiography. A pericardial friction rub, which is often described as leathery or close to the ear, results from the rubbing and friction between the inflamed pericardial surfaces. Because it results from the rubbing together of the inflamed pericardial surfaces, large effusions are unlikely to produce a friction rub. The ECG changes in pericarditis typically show ST-segment elevations and PR-segment depression, but unlike myocardial infarction, the T waves are not inverted.[5]

Treatment depends on the cause. When infection is present, antibiotics specific for the causative agent usually are prescribed. Antiinflammatory drugs such as aspirin and nonsteroidal antiinflammatory agents (NSAIDs) may be given to minimize the inflammatory response and the accompanying undesirable effects.

Chronic Pericarditis With Effusion. Chronic pericarditis with effusion is characterized by an increase in inflammatory exudate that continues beyond the acute period. In some cases, the exudate persists for several years. In most cases of chronic pericarditis, no specific pathogen can be identified. The process commonly is associated with other forms of heart disease, such as rheumatic fever, congenital heart lesions, or hypertensive heart disease. Systemic diseases, such as lupus erythematosus, rheumatoid arthritis, scleroderma, and myxedema, also are causes of chronic pericarditis, as are metabolic disturbances associated with acute and chronic renal failure. Unlike acute pericarditis, the signs and symptoms of chronic pericarditis often are minimal; often, the disease is detected for the first time on routine chest x-ray films. As the condition progresses, the fluid may accumulate and compress the adjacent cardiac structures and impair cardiac filling.

Constrictive Pericarditis. In constrictive pericarditis, fibrous scar tissue develops between the visceral and parietal layers of the serous pericardium. In time, the scar tissue contracts and interferes with diastolic filling of the heart, at which point cardiac output and cardiac reserve become fixed. Ascites is a prominent early finding and may be accompanied by pedal edema, dyspnea on exertion, and fatigue. The jugular veins also are distended. Kussmaul's sign is an inspiratory distention of the jugular veins caused by the inability of the right atrium, encased in its rigid pericardium, to accommodate the increase in venous return that occurs with inspiration. In chronic constrictive pericarditis, surgical removal or resection of the pericardium (*i.e.*, pericardiectomy) is often the treatment of choice.

In summary, the pericardium is a two-layered membranous sac that isolates the heart from other thoracic structures, maintains its position in the thorax, and prevents it from overfilling. The mechanisms that control the movement of fluid between the capillaries and the space that separates the two layers of the pericardium are the same as those that control fluid movement between the capillaries and the interstitial spaces of other body tissues.

Disorders of the pericardium include pericardial effusion, cardiac tamponade, acute and chronic pericarditis, and constrictive pericarditis. The major threat of pericardial disease is compression of the heart chambers. Pericardial effusion refers to the presence of an exudate in the pericardial cavity. It can increase intracardiac pressure, compress the heart, and interfere with venous return to the heart. The amount of exudate, the rapidity with which it accumulates, and the elasticity of the pericardium determine the effect the effusion has on cardiac function. Cardiac tamponade is a life-threatening cardiac compression resulting from excess fluid in the pericardial sac. Acute pericarditis is characterized by chest pain, ECG changes, and a friction rub. Among its causes are infections, uremia, rheumatic fever, connective tissue diseases, and myocardial infarction. Chronic pericarditis with effusion is characterized by an increase in inflammatory exudate that continues beyond the acute period. In constrictive pericarditis, scar tissue develops between the visceral and parietal layers of the serous pericardium. In time, the scar tissue contracts and interferes with cardiac filling.

Coronary Heart Disease

After completing this section of the chapter, you should be able to meet the following objectives:

- Describe blood flow in the coronary circulation and relate it to the metabolic needs of the heart
- Characterize the pathogenesis of atherosclerosis in terms of fixed atherosclerotic lesions, unstable plaque, and thrombosis with obstruction
- Define the term *acute coronary syndromes* and distinguish among chronic stable angina, unstable angina, non–ST-segment elevation myocardial infarction, and ST-segment elevation myocardial infarction in terms of pathology, symptomatology, ECG changes, and serum cardiac markers
- Compare the diagnostic measures and treatment goals for stable angina and the acute coronary syndromes

The term *coronary heart disease* (CHD) describes heart disease caused by impaired coronary blood flow. In most cases, CHD is caused by atherosclerosis. Diseases of the coronary arteries can cause angina, myocardial infarction or heart attack, cardiac arrhythmias, conduction defects, heart failure, and sudden death. Heart attack is the largest killer of American men and women, claiming more than 218,000 lives annually.[1] Each year, 1.5 million Americans have new or recurrent heart attacks, and one third of those die within the first hour, usually as the result of cardiac arrest resulting from ventricular fibrillation.

Over the past 50 years, there have been phenomenal advances in understanding the pathogenesis of CHD and in the development of diagnostic techniques and treatment methods for the disease. However, declines in morbidity and mortality have failed to keep pace with these scientific advances, probably because many of the outcomes are more dependent on lifestyle factors and age than on scientific advances.

CORONARY CIRCULATION

Coronary Arteries and Control of Coronary Blood Flow

There are two main coronary arteries, the left and the right, which arise from the coronary sinus just above the aortic valve (Fig. 26-3). The left coronary artery extends for approximately 3.5 cm as the *left main coronary artery* and then divides into the left anterior descending and circumflex branches. The *left anterior descending artery* passes down through the groove between the two ventricles, giving off diagonal branches, which supply the left ventricle, and perforating branches, which supply the anterior portion of the interventricular septum and the anterior papillary muscle of the left ventricle. The *circumflex branch* of the left coronary artery passes to the left and moves posteriorly in the groove that separates the left atrium and ventricle, giving off branches that supply the left lateral wall of the left ventricle. The *right coronary artery* lies in the right atrioventricular (AV) groove, and its branches supply the right ventricle. The right coronary artery usually moves to the back of the heart, where it forms the *posterior descending artery,* which supplies the posterior portion of the heart (the interventricular septum, AV node, and posterior papillary muscle). The sinoatrial node usually is supplied by the right coronary artery. In 10% to 20% of persons, the left circumflex rather than the right coronary artery moves posteriorly to form the posterior descending artery.

Although there are no connections between the large coronary arteries, there are anastomotic channels that join the small arteries (Fig. 26-4). With gradual occlusion of the larger vessels, the smaller collateral vessels increase in size and provide alternative channels for blood flow. One of the reasons CHD does not produce symptoms until it is far advanced is that the collateral channels develop at the same time the atherosclerotic changes are occurring.

The openings for the coronary arteries originate in the root of the aorta just outside the aortic valve; thus, the primary factor responsible for perfusion of the coronary arteries is the aortic blood pressure. Changes in aortic pressure produce parallel changes in coronary blood flow.

In addition to generating the aortic pressure that moves blood through the coronary vessels, the contracting heart muscle influences its own blood supply by compressing the intramyocardial and subendocardial blood vessels.[6] The large epicardial coronary arteries lie on the surface of the heart, with the smaller intramyocardial coronary arteries branching off and penetrating the myocardium before merging with a network or plexus of subendocardial vessels.

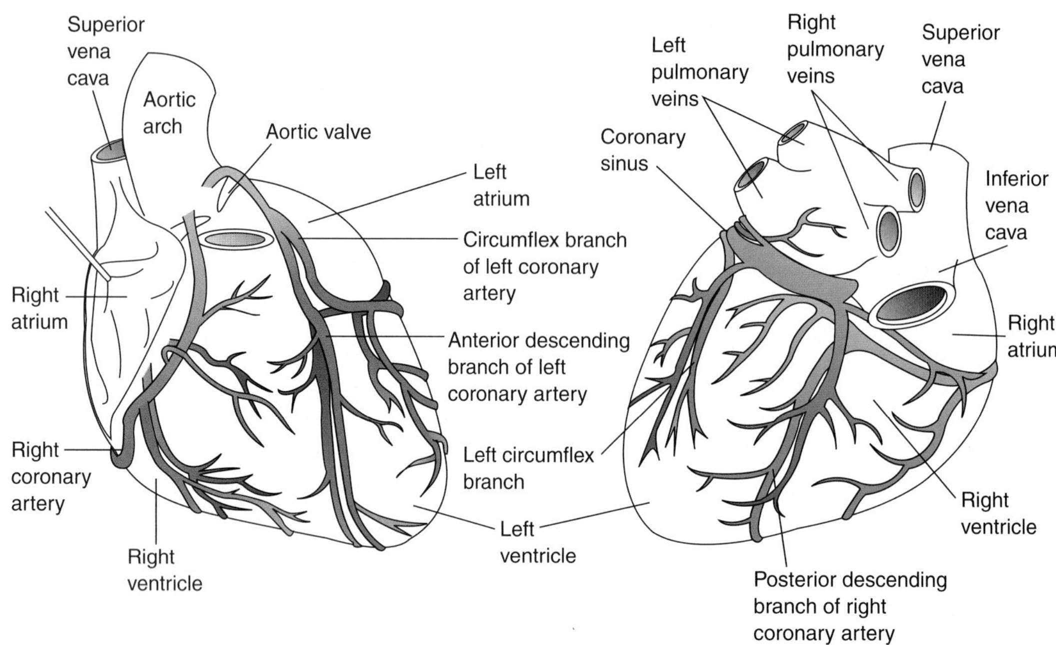

FIGURE 26-3 Coronary arteries and some of the coronary sinus veins.

During systole, contraction of the cardiac muscle compresses the intramyocardial vessels that supply the vessels of the subendocardial plexus, and the increased pressure in the ventricle causes further compression of these vessels (Fig. 26-5). As a result, blood flow through the subendocardial vessels is less during systole than in the outer coronary vessels. To compensate, the subendocardial vessels are far more extensive than the outermost arteries, allowing a disproportionate increase in subendocardial flow during diastole. Because blood flow mainly occurs during diastole, there is a risk for subendocardial ischemia and infarction when diastolic pressure is low and when there is an elevation in diastolic intraventricular pressure sufficient to compress the vessels in the subendocardial plexus.[6,7] Intramyocardial blood flow also is affected by heart rate because at rapid heart rates, the time spent in diastole is greatly reduced.

Heart muscle relies primarily on fatty acids and aerobic metabolism to meet its energy needs. Although the heart can engage in anaerobic metabolism, this process relies on the continuous delivery of glucose and results in the formation of large amounts of lactic acid. Blood flow usually is regulated by the need of the cardiac muscle for oxygen. Even under normal resting conditions, the heart extracts

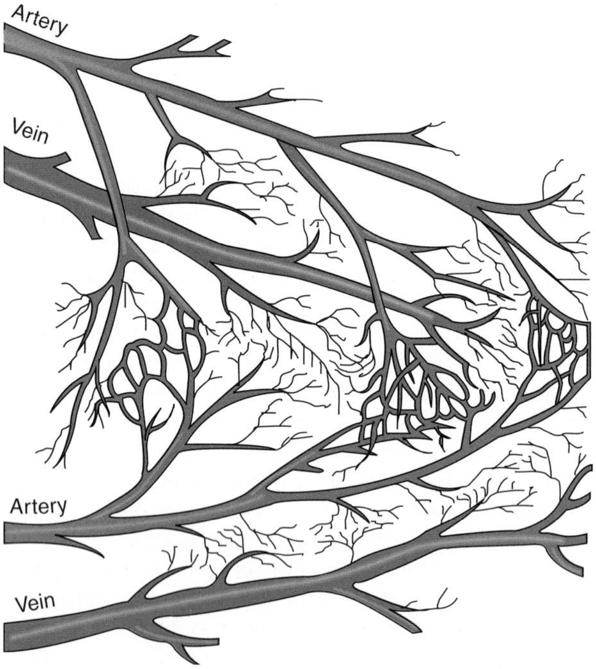

FIGURE 26-4 Anastomoses of the smaller coronary arterial vessels. (Guyton A.C., Hall J.E. [1996]. *Textbook of medical physiology* [9th ed., p. 260]. Philadelphia: W.B. Saunders).

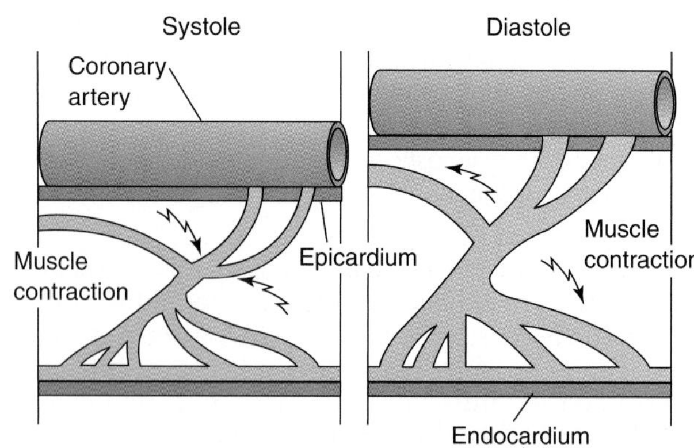

FIGURE 26-5 The compressing effect of the contracting myocardium on intramyocardial blood vessels and subendocardial blood flow during systole and diastole.

and uses 60% to 80% of oxygen in blood flowing through the coronary arteries, compared with the 25% to 30% extracted by skeletal muscle. Because there is little oxygen reserve in the blood, the coronary arteries must increase their flow to meet the metabolic needs of the myocardium during periods of increased activity. The normal resting blood flow through the coronary arteries averages approximately 225 mL/minute.[6] During strenuous exercise, coronary flow may increase fourfold to fivefold to meet the energy requirements of the heart.

One of the major determinants of coronary blood flow is the metabolic activity of the heart. Although the link between cardiac metabolic rate and coronary blood flow remains unsettled, it appears to result from the release of metabolic mediators that are generated as a result of a decrease in the ratio of oxygen supply to oxygen demand. Numerous agents, referred to as *metabolites,* are thought to act as mediators for the vasodilation that accompanies increased cardiac work. These substances, which include potassium ions, lactic acid, carbon dioxide, and adenosine, are released from working myocardial cells. Of these substances, adenosine has the greatest vasodilator action and is perhaps the critical mediator of local metabolic regulation.[6,7]

The endothelial cells that line blood vessels, including the coronaries, normally form a barrier between the blood and the arterial wall, and they have antithrombogenic properties that inhibit platelet aggregation and clot formation. They also synthesize several substances that, when released, can affect relaxation or constriction of the smooth muscle in the vessel wall. The most important of these is *nitric oxide* (see Chapter 23). Most vasodilators and vasodilating stimuli exert their effects through nitric oxide. The synthesis and release of nitric oxide is stimulated by products from aggregating platelets, thrombin, products of mast cells, and increased shear force, which is responsible for the so-called flow-mediated vasodilation.[7] Only a few vasodilators act independently of the endothelium to produce vasodilation. These include the nitrate vasodilator drugs (*e.g.,* nitroglycerin).

The endothelium also is the source of vasoconstricting factors, the best known of which are the endothelins. Although there are several endothelins, endothelin-1 (ET-1) seems to be important in producing vasoconstriction. The formation of ET-1 is stimulated by thrombin, epinephrine, and vasopressin. Plasma levels of ET-1 are reportedly elevated in atherosclerosis, acute myocardial infarction, congestive heart failure, and hypertension. ET-1 also is reportedly produced by activated macrophages in atherosclerotic lesions of persons with acute ischemic coronary disease and plaque rupture.[7] Unlike nitric oxide, which is released rapidly in response to vasodilator stimuli and is then inactivated within seconds, ET-1–mediated vasoconstriction is slow in onset and lasts for minutes or hours.[7]

Assessment of Coronary Blood Flow and Myocardial Perfusion

Among the methods used in the evaluation of coronary blood flow and myocardial perfusion are ECG, echocardiogram, exercise stress testing, and nuclear cardiovascular imaging methods.

Electrocardiography. The ECG is the most frequently used method for detecting myocardial ischemia, injury, or infarction due to CHD. During the period of impaired blood flow, injured and ischemic cells revert to anaerobic metabolism, with a resultant increase in lactic acid production, much of which is released into the local extracellular fluid. With myocardial infarction, the necrotic cells become electrically inactive, and their membranes become disrupted, such that their intracellular contents, including potassium, are released into the surrounding extracellular fluid. This causes local areas of hyperkalemia, which can affect the resting membrane potentials of functioning myocardial cells. As a result of membrane injury and local changes in extracellular potassium and pH levels, some parts of the infarcted myocardium are unable to conduct or generate impulses, other areas are more difficult to excite, and still others are overly excitable. These different levels of membrane excitability set the stage for development of arrhythmias and conduction defects after myocardial infarction. Each of these zones in the infarcted area conducts impulses differently. These changes in impulse conduction can be detected on the ECG and are the basis for detecting myocardial ischemia and infarction.

The ECG pattern also is used to detect arrhythmias that manifest as a result of myocardial ischemia due to CHD, and it can provide evidence of old myocardial infarction. Continuous ambulatory ECG monitoring can be done using a Holter monitor (see Chapter 27).

Ambulatory ECG monitoring often is done to detect transient ST-segment and T-wave changes that occur and are not accompanied by symptoms (*i.e.,* silent ischemia). Another method, called *signal-averaged* or *high-resolution ECG,* accentuates the QRS complex so that low-amplitude afterpotentials that correlate with high risk for ventricular dysrhythmias and sudden death can be detected.

Echocardiography. The term *echocardiography* refers to a group of tests that use ultrasound to examine the heart and record information in the form of echoes. An ultrasound signal has a frequency greater than 20,000 Hz (cycles per second) and is inaudible to the human ear. Echocardiography uses ultrasound signals in the range of 2 to 5 million Hz.[8] The ultrasound signal is reflected (*i.e.,* echoes) whenever there is a change in the resistance to transmission of the sound beam. Thus, it is possible to create a moving image of the internal structures of the heart because the chest wall, blood, and different heart structures all reflect ultrasound differently. The echocardiogram is useful for determining ventricular dimensions and valve movements, obtaining data on the movement of the left ventricular wall and septum, estimating diastolic and systolic volumes, and viewing the motion of individual segments of the left ventricular wall during systole and diastole. It also can be used for studying valvular disease and detecting pericardial effusion.

There are several types of echocardiography tests: M-mode, two-dimensional, Doppler, and esophageal echocardiography.[8] *M-mode echocardiography,* which was the earliest form of cardiac ultrasonography, uses a stationary ultrasonic beam to produce a one-dimensional or "ice-pick" view of the heart. *Two-dimensional echocardiography* uses a moving ultrasonic beam to produce an integrated view of the heart comprising multiple pie-shaped images. *Doppler echocardiography* uses ultrasound to record blood flow within the heart. *Transesophageal echocardiography* uses a two-dimensional echocardiography transducer placed at the end of a flexible endoscope to obtain echocardiographic images from the esophagus. Placement of the transducer into the esophagus allows echocardiographic images of cardiac structures to be obtained from different viewpoints, rather than only from the surface of the chest. Transesophageal echocardiography is particularly useful in assessing valve function.

Stress Testing. Exercise stress testing is a means of observing cardiac function under stress. Two types of tests commonly are used: the motorized treadmill and the bicycle ergometer. Pharmacologic stress testing may be used to simulate the stress of exercise in persons who cannot participate in active forms of exercise.

Treadmill exercise, which is the most commonly used method of cardiovascular stress testing, requires higher levels of myocardial performance than other forms of exercise. Bicycle exercise does not require as high a level of myocardial oxygen demand as treadmill walking, and the person can become fatigued before myocardial ischemia is reached. Blood pressure is monitored during both types of exercise testing and the ECG pattern recorded for the purpose of determining heart rate and detecting myocardial ischemic changes. Chest pain, severe shortness of breath, arrhythmias, ST-segment changes on the ECG, or a decrease in blood pressure suggests CHD, and if one or more of these signs or symptoms is present, the test usually is terminated.

Some persons are unable to undergo exercise stress testing owing to orthopedic, neurologic, peripheral vascular, or other conditions that preclude use of the treadmill or exercise bicycle. These persons can be evaluated for the presence of significant CHD by use of pharmacologic vasodilation in combination with nuclear myocardial imaging techniques. The intravenous infusion of either dipyridamole or adenosine can be used. Dipyridamole blocks the uptake of adenosine, an endogenous vasodilator, and increases coronary blood flow three to five times above baseline levels. In persons with significant CHD, the resistance vessels distal to the stenosis already are maximally dilated to maintain normal resting flow. In these persons, further vasodilation does not produce an increase in blood flow. Intravenous injection of adenosine has comparable effects.

Nuclear Cardiology Imaging. Nuclear cardiology imaging techniques involve the use of radionuclides (*i.e.,* radioactive substances) and essentially are noninvasive. Four types of nuclear cardiology tests commonly are used: myocardial perfusion imaging, infarct imaging, radionuclide angiocardiography, and positron-emission tomography. With all four tests, a scintillation (gamma) camera is used to record radiation emitted from the radionuclide. Single-photon emission computed tomography (SPECT), which uses a multiple head camera to obtain a series of planar images over a 180- to 360-degree arc around the thorax, is the most widely used imaging technique at present.[9]

Myocardial perfusion imaging is used to visualize the regional distribution of blood flow. *Myocardial perfusion scintigraphy* uses thallium-201 or one of the newer technetium-based agents that are extracted from the blood and taken up by functioning myocardial cells. Thallium-201, an analog of potassium, is distributed to the myocardium in proportion to the magnitude of blood flow. After injection, an external detection device describes the distribution of the radioactive material. An ischemic area appears as a "cold spot" that lacks radioactive uptake. The most important application of this technique has been its use during stress testing for evaluation of ischemic heart disease.

Radionuclide angiocardiography provides actual visualization of the ventricular structures during systole and diastole and provides a means for evaluating ventricular function during rest and exercise stress testing. A radioisotope such as technetium-labeled albumin, which does not leave the capillaries but remains in the blood and is not bound to the myocardium, is used for this type of imaging. This type of nuclear imaging can be used to determine right and left ventricular volumes, ejection fractions, regional wall motion, and cardiac contractility. This method also is useful in the diagnosis of intracardiac shunts.

Acute infarct imaging uses a radionuclide that is taken up by the cells in the infarcted zone. With this method, the damaged myocardium is visualized as a "hot spot," or positive area, of increased uptake of the radionuclide. Its usefulness usually is limited by an 18- to 26-hour lag after acute infarction before the test becomes positive, and it has limited sensitivity for small, nontransmural infarcts.

Positron-emission tomography (PET) uses positron-emitting agents to demonstrate either perfusion or metabolism of the myocardium. The radioisotopes used as positron emitters are naturally occurring low-atomic-weight atoms (*e.g.,* carbon [C], nitrogen [N], oxygen [O]) that are the predominant constituents of organic compounds such as glucose.[9] During ischemia, cardiac muscle shifts from fatty acid to glucose metabolism. Thus, a radioactive tracer such as fluorodeoxyglucose (FDG) can be used to distinguish transiently dysfunctional ("stunned") myocardium from scar tissue by showing persistent glucose metabolism in areas of reduced blood flow.

Cardiac Catheterization. Cardiac catheterization involves the passage of flexible catheters into the great vessels and chambers of the heart. In right heart catheterization, the catheters are inserted into a peripheral vein (usually the basilic or femoral) and then advanced into the right heart. The left heart catheter is inserted retrograde through a peripheral artery (usually the brachial or femoral) into the aorta and left heart. The cardiac catheterization laboratory, where the procedure is done, is equipped for viewing and recording fluoroscopic images of the heart and vessels in the chest and for measuring pressures in the heart and great vessels. It also has equipment for cardiac output studies and for obtaining samples of blood for blood gas analysis. Angiographic studies are done by injecting a radiographic contrast medium into the heart so that an outline of the moving structures can be visualized and filmed. Coronary arteriography involves the injection of a radiographic contrast medium into the coronary arteries; this permits visualization of lesions in these vessels.

Coronary Atherosclerosis and the Pathogenesis of Coronary Artery Disease

Atherosclerosis (discussed in Chapter 24) is by far the most common cause of CHD, and atherosclerotic plaque disruption is the most frequent cause of myocardial infarction and sudden death. More than 90% of persons with CHD have coronary atherosclerosis.[10] Most, if not all, have one or more lesions causing at least 75% reduction in cross-sectional area, the point at which augmented blood flow provided by compensatory vasodilation no longer is able to keep pace with even moderate increases in the metabolic demands of the myocardium.[10]

Atherosclerosis can affect one or all three of the major epicardial coronary arteries and their branches. Clinically significant lesions may be located anywhere in these vessels but tend to predominate in the first several centimeters of the left anterior descending and left circumflex or the entire length of the right coronary artery.[10] Sometimes, the major secondary branches also are involved.

Stable Versus Unstable Plaque. There are two types of atherosclerotic lesions: the fixed or stable plaque, which obstructs blood flow, and the unstable or vulnerable plaque, which can rupture and cause platelet adhesion and thrombus formation. The fixed or stable plaque is commonly implicated in stable angina and the unstable plaque in unstable angina and myocardial infarction. There are three major determinants of plaque vulnerability to rupture: (1) the size of the lipid-rich core and the stability and thickness of its fibrous cap, (2) the presence of inflammation with plaque degradation, and (3) the lack of smooth muscle cells with impaired healing and plaque stabilization[11–13] (Fig. 26-6). Plaques with a thin fibrous cap overlaying a large lipid core are at high risk for rupture.

Although plaque rupture may occur spontaneously, it is often triggered by hemodynamic factors such as blood flow characteristics and vessel tension. For example, a sudden surge of sympathetic activity with an increase in blood pressure, heart rate, force of cardiac contraction, and coronary blood flow is thought to increase the risk for plaque disruption.[11] Indeed, many people with myocardial infarction report a trigger event, most often emotional stress or physical activity.[11,13] Plaque rupture also has a diurnal variation, occurring most frequently during the first hour of arising, suggesting that physiologic factors such as surges in coronary artery tone and blood pressure may promote atherosclerotic plaque disruption and subsequent platelet deposition.[13] It has been suggested that the sympathetic nervous system is activated on arising, resulting in changes in platelet aggregation and fibrinolytic activity that tend to favor thrombosis. This diurnal variation in plaque rupture can be minimized by β-adrenergic blockers and aspirin.[13]

Thrombosis and Vessel Occlusion. Local thrombosis occurring after plaque disruption results from complex interactions among its lipid core, smooth muscle cells, macrophages, and collagen. The lipid core provides a stimulus for platelet aggregation and thrombus formation.[14] Both smooth muscle and foam cells in the lipid core contribute

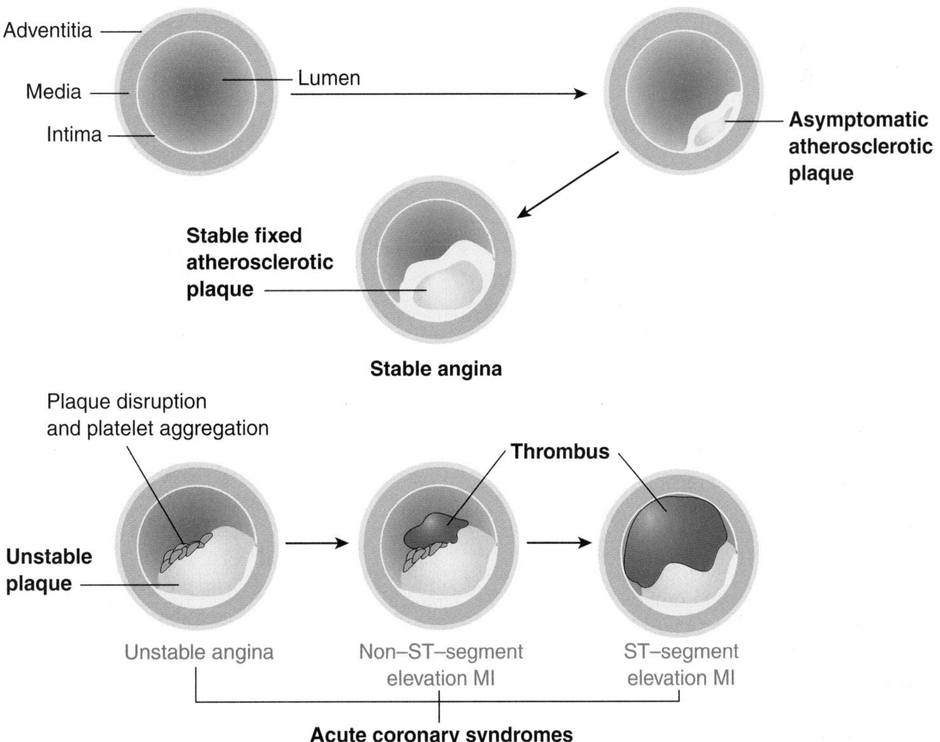

FIGURE 26-6 Atherosclerotic plaque. Stable fixed atherosclerotic plaque in stable angina and the unstable plaque with plaque disruption and platelet aggregation in the acute coronary syndromes.

to the expression of tissue factor in unstable plaques. Once exposed to blood, tissue factor initiates the extrinsic coagulation pathway, resulting in the local generation of thrombin and deposition of fibrin (see Chapter 15).

Platelets play an important role in linking plaque disruption to acute CHD. As a part of the response to plaque disruption, platelets adhere to the endothelium and release substances (adenosine diphosphate [ADP], thromboxane A_2, and thrombin) that promote further aggregation of platelets and thrombus formation. The platelet membrane, which contains glycoprotein receptors that bind fibrinogen and link platelets together, contributes to thrombus formation. Platelet adhesion and aggregation occur in several steps (Fig. 26-7). First, release of ADP, thromboxane A_2, and thrombin initiates the aggregation process. Second, glycoprotein IIb/IIIa receptors on the platelet surface are activated. Third, fibrinogen binds to the activated glycoprotein receptors, forming bridges between adjacent platelets.

There are two types of thrombi formed as a result of plaque disruption—white platelet-containing thrombi and red fibrin-containing thrombi. The thrombi in unstable angina have been characterized as grayish white and presumably platelet rich.[15] Red thrombi, which develop with vessel occlusion in myocardial infarction, are rich in fibrin and red blood cells superimposed on the platelet component and extended by the stasis of blood flow.

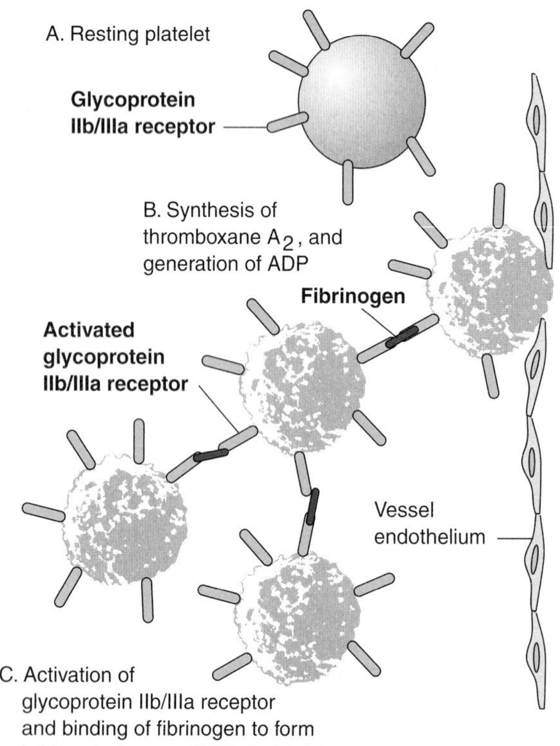

FIGURE 26-7 Steps in development of the platelet clot: (**A**) Resting platelet; (**B**) synthesis of thromboxane A_2 (inhibited by aspirin) and generation of adenosine diphosphate (ADP) (inhibited by ticlopidine and clopidogrel) that leads to platelet adhesion and aggregation; and (**C**) activation of glycoprotein IIb/IIIa receptors, which bind fibrinogen, form bridges between adjacent platelet (blocked by glycoprotein receptor IIb/IIIa antagonists).

Antiplatelet and Anticoagulant Therapy. Studies relating plaque disruption, platelet aggregation, and thrombus formation to CHD have led to the use of antiplatelet drugs for preventing platelet aggregation at the site of plaque disruption. The site of action of antiplatelet drugs is described in Figure 26-7. Anticoagulation therapy, which targets the coagulation pathway and formation of the fibrin clot, involves the use of unfractionated and low-molecular-weight heparin (see Chapter 15).

Aspirin is the preferred antiplatelet agent for preventing platelet aggregation in persons with CHD. Aspirin acts by inhibiting synthesis of the prostaglandin, thromboxane A_2. The actions of aspirin (*i.e.,* acetylsalicylic acid) are related to the presence of the acetyl group, which irreversibly acetylates the critical platelet enzyme, cyclooxygenase, which is required for thromboxane A_2 synthesis. Because the action is irreversible, the effect of aspirin on platelet function lasts for the lifetime of the platelet—approximately 8 to 10 days. *Ticlopidine* and *clopidogrel* are other antiplatelet agents that may be used when aspirin is contraindicated.[16] Ticlopidine and clopidogrel achieve their antiplatelet effects by irreversibly inhibiting the binding of ADP to its receptor on the platelets. Unlike aspirin, these drugs have no effect on prostaglandin synthesis.

Another class of antiplatelet agents is the platelet receptor antagonists. In contrast to aspirin and ticlopidine or clopidogrel, which target a single step in the aggregation process, the platelet glycoprotein IIb/IIIa receptor inhibitors (*e.g.,* tirofiban, eptifibatide, abciximab) block the receptor involved in the final common pathway for platelet adhesion, activation, and aggregation. These agents are usually used for the treatment of persons with acute coronary syndrome, including those who are undergoing percutaneous coronary intervention.

CHRONIC ISCHEMIC HEART DISEASE

Coronary heart disease is commonly divided into two types of disorders: chronic ischemic heart disease and the acute coronary syndromes (Fig. 26-8). There are three types of chronic ischemic heart disease: chronic stable angina, silent myocardial ischemia, and variant or vasospastic angina. The acute coronary syndromes represent the spectrum of ischemic coronary disease ranging from unstable angina through myocardial infarction.

The term *ischemia* means "to suppress or withhold blood flow." Myocardial ischemia occurs when the ability of the coronary arteries to supply blood is inadequate to meet the metabolic demands of the heart. Limitations in coronary blood flow most commonly are the result of atherosclerosis, with vasospasm and thrombosis as contributing factors. The metabolic demands of the heart are increased with everyday activities such as mental stress, exercise, and exposure to cold. In certain disease states such as thyrotoxicosis, the metabolic demands may be so excessive that the blood flow may be inadequate despite normal coronary arteries. In other situations, such as aor-

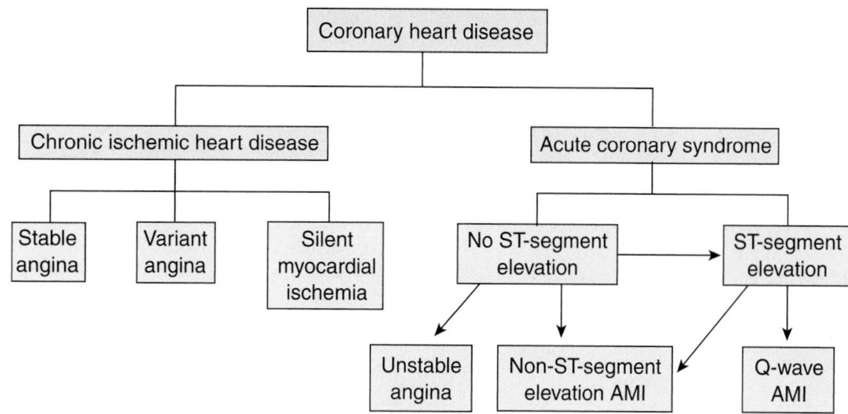

FIGURE 26-8 Types of coronary heart disease. AMI, acute myocardial infarction.

tic stenosis, the coronary arteries may not be diseased, but the perfusion pressure may be insufficient to provide adequate blood flow.

Stable Angina

The term *angina* is derived from a Latin word meaning "to choke." Angina pectoris is a symptomatic paroxysmal chest pain or pressure sensation associated with transient myocardial ischemia. Chronic stable angina is associated with a fixed coronary obstruction that produces a disparity between coronary blood flow and metabolic demands of the myocardium. Stable angina is the initial manifestation of ischemic heart disease in approximately half of persons with CHD.[16] Although most persons with stable angina have atherosclerotic heart disease, angina does not develop in a considerable number of persons with advanced coronary atherosclerosis. This probably is because of their sedentary lifestyle, the development of adequate collateral circulation, or the inability of these persons to perceive pain. In many instances, myocardial infarction occurs without a history of angina.

Angina pectoris usually is precipitated by situations that increase the work demands of the heart, such as physical exertion, exposure to cold, and emotional stress. The pain typically is described as a constricting, squeezing, or suffocating sensation. It usually is steady, increasing in intensity only at the onset and end of the attack. The pain of angina commonly is located in the precordial or substernal area of the chest; it is similar to myocardial infarction in that it may radiate to the left shoulder, jaw, arm, or other areas of the chest (Fig. 26-9). In some persons, the arm or shoulder pain may be confused with arthritis; in others, epigastric pain is confused with indigestion. Angina commonly is categorized according to whether it occurs with exercise or during rest and is of new onset or of increasing severity. The Canadian Cardiovascular Society Classification (CCSC) system can be used to grade the severity of anginal pain and discomfort[17] (Table 26-1).

Typically, chronic stable angina is provoked by exertion or emotional stress and relieved within minutes by rest or the use of nitroglycerin. A delay of more than 5 to 10 minutes before relief is obtained suggests that the

ISCHEMIC HEART DISEASE

- The term *ischemic heart disease* refers to disorders of myocardial blood flow due to stable or unstable coronary atherosclerotic plaques.
- Stable atherosclerotic plaques produce fixed obstruction of coronary blood flow with myocardial ischemia occurring during periods of increased metabolic need, such as in stable angina.
- Unstable atherosclerotic plaques tend to fissure or rupture, causing platelet aggregation and potential for thrombus formation with production of a spectrum of acute coronary syndromes of increasing severity, ranging from unstable angina, to non–ST-segment elevation myocardial infarction, to ST-segment elevation myocardial infarction.

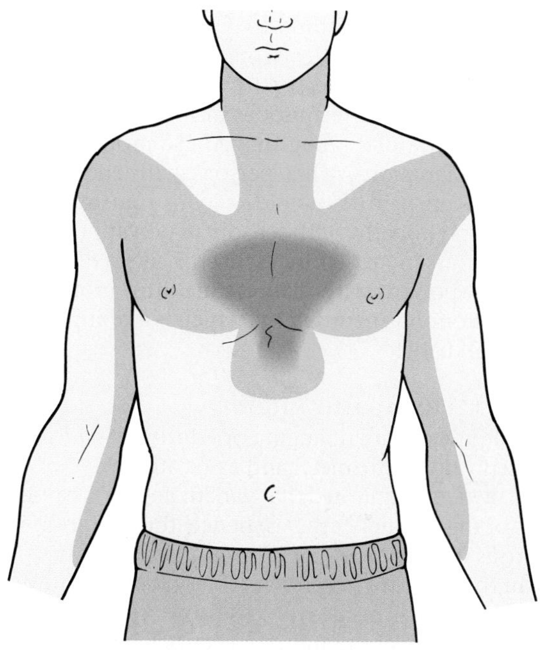

FIGURE 26-9 Areas of pain due to angina.

TABLE 26-1 Canadian Cardiovascular Society Classification for Angina

Class	Description of Stage
Class I	Ordinary physical activity, such as walking or climbing stairs, does not cause angina. Angina occurs with strenuous, rapid, or prolonged exertion at work or recreation.
Class II	Slight limitation of ordinary activity. Angina occurs on walking or climbing stairs rapidly, walking uphill, walking or stair climbing after meals, or in cold, in wind, under emotional stress, or only during the few hours after awakening. Walking more than two blocks on the level and climbing more than one flight of ordinary stairs at a normal pace and in normal conditions can elicit angina.
Class III	Marked limitations of ordinary physical activity. Angina occurs on walking one to two blocks on the level and climbing one flight of stairs in normal conditions and at a normal pace.
Class IV	Inability to carry on any physical activity without discomfort—anginal symptoms may be present at rest.

(From Campeau L. [1976]. Grading of angina pectoris [letter]. *Circulation* 54, 522–523. Copyright 1976, American Heart Association, Inc. Used with permission.)

symptoms are not due to ischemia or that they are due to severe ischemia.[18] Angina that occurs at rest, is of new onset, or is increasing in intensity or duration denotes an increased risk for myocardial infarction and should be evaluated using the criteria for acute coronary syndromes (discussed later).

Silent Myocardial Ischemia

Silent myocardial ischemia occurs in the absence of anginal pain. The factors that cause silent myocardial ischemia appear to be the same as those responsible for angina: impaired blood flow from the effects of coronary atherosclerosis or vasospasm. Silent myocardial ischemia affects three populations—persons who are asymptomatic without other evidence of CHD, persons who have had a myocardial infarct and continue to have episodes of silent ischemia, and persons with angina who also have episodes of silent ischemia.[19] The reason for the painless episodes of ischemia is unclear. The episodes may be shorter and involve less myocardial tissue than those producing pain. Another explanation is that persons with silent angina have defects in pain threshold or pain transmission, or autonomic neuropathy with sensory denervation. There is evidence of an increased incidence of silent myocardial ischemia in persons with diabetes mellitus, probably the result of autonomic neuropathy, which is a common complication of diabetes.[20]

Variant or Vasospastic Angina

The syndrome of variant angina or *Prinzmetal's angina* was first described by Prinzmetal and associates in 1959.[21] Subsequent evidence indicated that variant angina is caused by spasms of the coronary arteries; hence, the condition is referred to as *vasospastic angina*. In most instances, the spasms occur in the presence of coronary artery stenosis; however, variant angina has occurred in the absence of visible disease. Unlike stable angina that occurs with exertion or stress, variant angina usually occurs during rest or with minimal exercise and frequently occurs nocturnally (between midnight and 8:00 AM).[18] The mechanism of coronary vasospasm is uncertain. It has been suggested that it may result from hyperactive sympathetic nervous system responses, from a defect in the handling of calcium in vascular smooth muscle, from an alteration in nitric oxide production, or from an imbalance between endothelium-derived relaxing and contracting factors.

Arrhythmias often occur when the pain is severe, and most persons are aware of their presence during an attack. ECG changes are significant if recorded during an attack. These abnormalities include ST-segment elevation or depression, T-wave peaking, inversion of U waves, and rhythm disturbances. Persons with variant angina who have serious arrhythmias during spontaneous episodes of pain are at a higher risk for sudden death.

Diagnosis and Treatment

Diagnosis. The diagnosis of angina is based on a detailed pain history and the presence of risk factors. Noncoronary causes of chest pain, such as that due to esophageal reflux or musculoskeletal disorders, should be ruled out. ECG, echocardiography, exercise stress testing or pharmacologic imaging studies, and coronary angiography may be used to confirm the diagnosis. Because the resting ECG is often normal, exercise testing is often used in evaluating persons with angina. Ischemia that is not present at rest is detected by precipitation of typical chest pain or ST-segment changes on the ECG. Continuous ECG monitoring or ambulatory Holter monitoring may be used in diagnosis of variant angina. Ergonovine, a nonspecific vasoconstrictor, may be administered during cardiac catheterization to evoke an attack of variant angina and demonstrate the presence and location of coronary vasospasm.

Treatment. The treatment goals for stable angina are directed toward prevention of myocardial infarction and symptom reduction.[16] Both nonpharmacologic and pharmacologic treatment methods are used. Coronary artery bypass surgery or percutaneous transluminal coronary angioplasty (PTCA) may be indicated in persons with significant coronary artery occlusion.

Nonpharmacologic methods are aimed at symptom control and lifestyle modifications to lower risk factors for coronary disease. They include smoking cessation in persons who smoke, stress reduction, a regular exercise program, limiting dietary intake of cholesterol and saturated fats, weight reduction if obesity is present, and avoidance of cold or other stresses that produce vasoconstriction. Immediate cessation of activity often is sufficient to abort an anginal attack. Sitting down or standing quietly may be preferable to lying down because these positions decrease preload by producing pooling of blood in the lower extremities.

The pharmacologic treatment of angina includes the use of antiplatelet drugs, β-adrenergic–blocking drugs in the absence of contraindications, calcium antagonists or long-acting nitrates when β-adrenergic blockers are contraindicated, sublingual nitroglycerin or nitroglycerin spray for immediate relief of anginal pain, and lipid-lowering therapy in persons with elevated low-density lipoprotein (LDL) cholesterol levels.[16]

The *β-adrenergic–blocking drugs* act as antagonists that block β-receptor–mediated functions of the sympathetic nervous system. There are two types of β receptors, β_1 and β_2. The β_1 receptors are found primarily in the heart, and β_2 receptors are found in smooth muscle in other parts of the body (*e.g.,* bronchial smooth muscle and skeletal muscle blood vessels). In angina, the primary benefits of β-adrenergic–blocking drugs are derived from their effects on β_1 receptors in the heart that decrease cardiac work and myocardial oxygen consumption.

The *calcium channel–blocking drugs* sometimes are called *calcium antagonists.* Free intracellular calcium serves to link many membrane-initiated events with cellular responses, such as action potential generation and muscle contraction. Vascular smooth muscle lacks the sarcoplasmic reticulum and other structures necessary for adequate intracellular storage of calcium; instead, it relies on the influx of calcium from the extracellular fluid into the cell to initiate and sustain contraction. In cardiac muscle, the slow inward calcium current contributes to the plateau of the action potential and to cardiac contractility. The slow calcium current is particularly important in the pacemaker activity of the sinoatrial node and the conduction properties of the AV node. The therapeutic effect of the calcium antagonists results from coronary and peripheral artery dilatation and decreased myocardial metabolism associated with the decrease in myocardial contractility.

Nitroglycerin (glycerol trinitrate) and *long-acting nitrates* (*e.g.,* isosorbide dinitrate and isosorbide mononitrate) are used to relieve anginal pain and silent myocardial ischemia. They are vasodilating drugs that relax venous and arterial vessels. Venous dilation decreases venous return to the heart (*i.e.,* preload), thereby reducing ventricular volume and compression of the subendocardial vessels. These drugs also decrease the tension in the wall of the left ventricle so that less pressure is needed to pump blood. Relaxation of the arteries reduces the pressure against which the heart must pump (*i.e.,* afterload). In addition to their vasodilator effects, the nitrates are thought to have an inhibitory effect on platelet activation and aggregation that may contribute to their beneficial effects in persons with CHD. Nitroglycerin is absorbed into the portal circulation and destroyed by the liver when it is taken orally; therefore, it is administered by methods such as sublingual pills or sprays or with topical ointments or patches that bypass the portal circulation.

Persons with variant angina usually respond to treatment with calcium antagonists. These agents, along with short- and long-term nitrates, are the mainstay of treatment of variant angina. Because the two drugs act through different mechanisms, their beneficial effects may be additive.

ACUTE CORONARY SYNDROMES

The term *acute coronary syndrome* (ACS) has recently been accepted to describe the spectrum of acute ischemic heart diseases that include unstable angina, non–ST-segment elevation (non–Q-wave), myocardial infarction, and ST-segment elevation (Q-wave) myocardial infarction.[22–25] Persons with ST-segment elevation on ECG are usually found to have complete coronary occlusion on angiography, and many ultimately have Q-wave myocardial infarction. Persons without ST-segment elevation are those in which thrombotic coronary occlusion is subtotal or intermittent.

Determinants of ACS Status

Persons with an ACS are routinely classified as low risk or high risk for infarction based on presenting characteristics, ECG variables, serum cardiac markers, and the timing of presentation.

ECG Changes. The classic ECG changes that occur with ACS involve T-wave inversion, ST-segment elevation, and development of an abnormal Q wave[26] (Fig. 26-10). These changes vary considerably depending on the duration of the ischemic event (acute versus evolving), its extent (subendocardial versus transmural), and its location (anterior versus inferior posterior). Because these changes usually occur over time and are seen on the ECG leads that view the involved area of the myocardium, provision for continuous 12-lead ECG monitoring is usually indicated.

The repolarization phase of the action potential (T wave and ST segment on the ECG) is usually the first to be involved during myocardial ischemia and injury. As the involved area becomes ischemic, myocardial repolarization is altered, causing changes in the T wave. This is usually represented by T-wave inversion, although a hyperacute T-wave elevation may occur as the earliest sign of infarction. ST-segment changes occur with ischemia that produces myocardial injury. Normally, the ST segment of the ECG is nearly isoelectric (*e.g.,* flat along the baseline) because healthy myocardial cells attain the same potential during early repolarization. Acute severe ischemia reduces the resting membrane potential and shortens the duration of the action potential in the ischemic area. These changes create a voltage difference between the normal and ischemic areas of the myocardium that leads to a current of

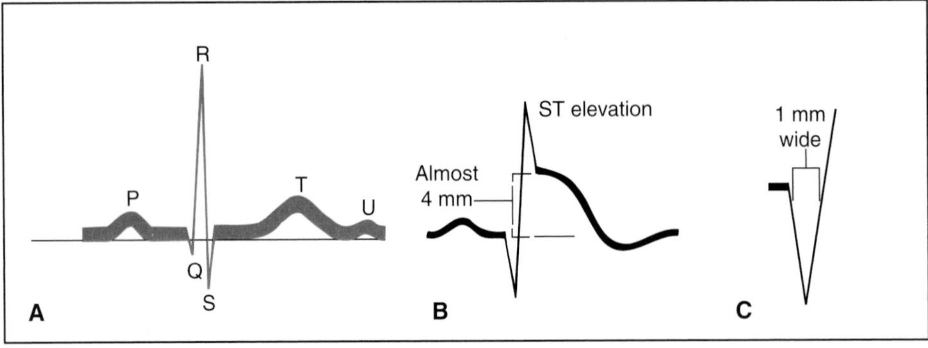

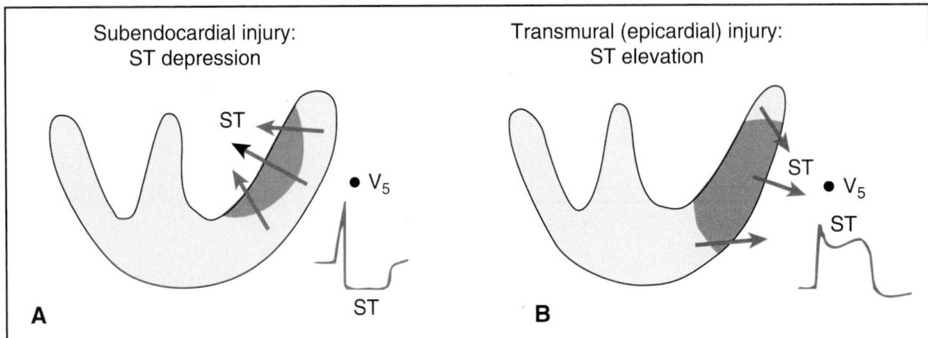

FIGURE 26-10 **(Top)** (**A**) ECG tracing showing normal P, Q,R,S, and T waves. (**B**) ST elevation with acute ischemia. (**C**) Q wave with acute myocardial infarction. **(Bottom)** Current-of-injury patterns with acute ischemia. With predominant subendocardial ischemia (**A**), the resultant ST segment is directed toward the inner layer of the affected ventricle and the ventricular cavity. Overlying leads therefore record ST-segment depression. With ischemia involving the outer ventricular layer (**B**) (transmural or epicardial injury), the ST vector is directed outward. Overlying leads record ST-segment elevation. (*Bottom* adapted from Braunwald E., Zipes D.P., Libby P. [2002]. *Heart disease: A textbook of cardiovascular medicine* [6th ed., p. 108]. Philadelphia: W.B. Saunders.)

injury between these regions. It is these currents of injury that are represented on the surface ECG as a deviation of the ST segment. When the acute injury is transmural, the overall ST vector is shifted in the direction of the outer epicardium, resulting in ST-segment elevation[26] (see Fig. 26-10). When the injury is confined primarily to the subendocardium, the overall ST segment shifts toward the inner ventricular layer, resulting in an overall depression of the ST segment.

With actual infarction, depolarization (QRS) changes often follow the T-wave and ST-segment abnormalities. With Q-wave infarction, abnormal Q waves develop because there is no depolarizing current conduction from the necrotic tissue.

Serum Markers. The serum markers for acute myocardial infarction (AMI) include myoglobin, creatine kinase MB (CK-MB), and troponin I (TnI) and troponin T (TnT).[27] As the myocardial cells become necrotic, their intracellular enzymes begin to diffuse into the surrounding interstitium and then into the blood. The rate at which the enzymes appear in the blood depends on their intracellular location, their molecular weight, and local blood flow. For example, they may appear at an earlier than predicted time in patients who have undergone successful reperfusion therapy.

Creatine kinase (CK) is an intracellular enzyme found in muscle cells. CK exceeds normal range within 4 to 8 hours of myocardial injury and declines to normal within 2 to 3 days.[27] There are three isoenzymes of CK, with the MB isoenzyme being highly specific for injury to myocardial tissue.

Myoglobin is an oxygen-carrying protein, similar to hemoglobin, which is normally present in cardiac and skeletal muscle. It is a small molecule that is released quickly from infarcted myocardial tissue and becomes elevated within 1 hour after myocardial cell death, with peak levels reached within 4 to 8 hours.[27] Because myoglobin is present in both cardiac and skeletal muscle, it is not cardiac specific.

The *troponin* complex, which is part of the actin filament, consists of three subunits (*i.e.*, TnC, TnT, and TnI) that regulate the calcium-mediated actin–myosin contractile process in striated muscle. TnI and TnT, which are present in cardiac muscle, begin to rise within 3 hours after the onset of myocardial infarction and may remain elevated for 3 to 4 days after the event.[27] It is thought that cardiac troponin assays are more capable of detecting episodes of myocardial infarction in which cell damage is below that detected by CK-MB level.

There has been recent interest in early markers that become elevated before other markers of myocardial injury or in their absence. One such marker is C-reactive protein (CRP), a widely studied inflammatory marker that has been associated with increased risk for recurrent events across the spectrum of acute coronary syndromes, independent of myocardial cell necrosis.[28] B-type natriuretic peptide (BNP), another marker, is currently used for diagnosis, assessment of severity, and prognosis of congestive heart failure. BNP is a natriuretic and vasodilative peptide that is synthesized in the ventricular myocardium and released into circulation in response to ventricular dilation and pressure overload. In one study, a single measurement of BNP, obtained

40 hours after onset of ischemic symptoms, predicted the risk for death in patients who had AMI with ST-segment elevation, AMI without ST-segment elevation, or unstable angina, as well as the risk for new or progressive congestive heart failure and new or recurrent AMI.[29]

Unstable Angina/Non–ST-Segment Elevation Myocardial Infarction

Unstable angina is considered to be a clinical syndrome of myocardial ischemia ranging between stable angina and myocardial infarction. It most frequently results from atherosclerotic plaque disruption, platelet aggregation, and secondary hemostasis. Coronary vasoconstriction may also play a role. Unstable angina may occur as a primary disorder (*i.e.*, progression of variant or stable angina); as a secondary disorder due to a noncoronary condition (*e.g.*, anemia, infection, cocaine use); or as a postinfarction angina that develops within 2 weeks of an AMI.[30] Cocaine can induce myocardial ischemia through increased myocardial oxygen demand or decreased oxygen supply from coronary artery spasm or thrombosis and can cause unstable angina and myocardial infarction.[31]

In contrast to stable angina, the pain associated with unstable angina has a more persistent and severe course and is characterized by at least one of three features: (1) it occurs at rest (or with minimal exertion) usually lasting more than 20 minutes (if not interrupted by nitroglycerin); (2) it is severe and described as frank pain and of new onset (*i.e.*, within 1 month); and (3) it occurs with a pattern that is more severe, prolonged, or frequent than previously experienced.[30]

The diagnosis of unstable angina/non–ST-segment elevation myocardial infarction is based on pain severity and presenting symptoms, hemodynamic stability, ECG findings, and serum cardiac markers. Guidelines developed by the American College of Cardiology and AHA (ACC/AHA) Task Force on Practice Guidelines for Management of Patients with Unstable Angina and Non–ST-Segment Elevation Myocardial Infarction indicate that the two conditions are similar but of different severity.[32] They differ primarily in whether the ischemia is severe enough to cause sufficient myocardial damage to release detectable quantities of serum cardiac markers. Persons who have no evidence of serum markers for myocardial damage are considered to have unstable angina, whereas a diagnosis of non–ST-segment elevation myocardial infarction is indicated if a serum marker of myocardial injury is present.

ST-Segment Elevation Myocardial Infarction

Acute myocardial infarction or ST-segment elevation myocardial infarction, also known as a *heart attack,* is characterized by the ischemic death of myocardial tissue associated with atherosclerotic disease of the coronary arteries. The area of infarction is determined by the coronary artery that is affected and by its distribution of blood flow. Approximately 30% to 40% of infarcts affect the right coronary artery, 40% to 50% affect the left anterior descending artery, and the remaining 15% to 20% affect the left circumflex artery.[10]

Manifestations. ST-segment elevation AMI may occur as an abrupt-onset event or as a progression from unstable angina/non–ST-segment elevation myocardial infarction.

The onset of AMI usually is abrupt, with pain as the significant symptom. The pain typically is severe and crushing, often described as being constricting, suffocating, or like "someone sitting on my chest." The pain usually is substernal, radiating to the left arm, neck, or jaw, although it may be experienced in other areas of the chest. Unlike that of angina, the pain associated with AMI is more prolonged and not relieved by rest or nitroglycerin, and narcotics frequently are required. Women often experience atypical ischemic-type chest discomfort, whereas elderly persons may complain of shortness of breath more frequently than chest pain.[32]

Gastrointestinal complaints are common. There may be a sensation of epigastric distress; nausea and vomiting may occur. These symptoms are thought to be related to the severity of the pain and vagal stimulation. The epigastric distress may be mistaken for indigestion, and the patient may seek relief with antacids or other home remedies, which only delays getting medical attention. Complaints of fatigue and weakness, especially of the arms and legs, are common. Pain and sympathetic stimulation combine to give rise to tachycardia, anxiety, restlessness, and feelings of impending doom. The skin often is pale, cool, and moist. Impairment of myocardial function may lead to hypotension and shock.

Sudden death from AMI is death that occurs within 1 hour of symptom onset. It usually is attributed to fatal arrhythmias, which may occur without evidence of infarction. Approximately 30% to 50% of persons with AMI die of ventricular fibrillation within the first few hours after symptoms begin. Early hospitalization after onset of symptoms greatly improves chances of averting sudden death because appropriate resuscitation facilities are immediately available when the ventricular arrhythmia occurs.

Pathologic Changes. The extent of the infarct depends on the location and extent of occlusion, amount of heart tissue supplied by the vessel, duration of the occlusion, metabolic needs of the affected tissue, extent of collateral circulation, and other factors such as heart rate, blood pressure, and cardiac rhythm. An infarct may involve the endocardium, myocardium, epicardium, or a combination of these. *Transmural infarcts* involve the full thickness of the ventricular wall and most commonly occur when there is obstruction of a single artery. *Subendocardial infarcts* involve the inner one third to one half of the ventricular wall and occur more frequently in the presence of severely narrowed but still patent arteries. Most infarcts are transmural, involving the free wall of the left ventricle and the interventricular septum (Fig. 26-11).

The principal biochemical consequence of AMI is the conversion from aerobic to anaerobic metabolism with inadequate production of energy to sustain normal myocardial function. As a result, a striking loss of contractile function occurs within 60 seconds of AMI onset. Changes in cell structure (*i.e.*, glycogen depletion and mitochondrial

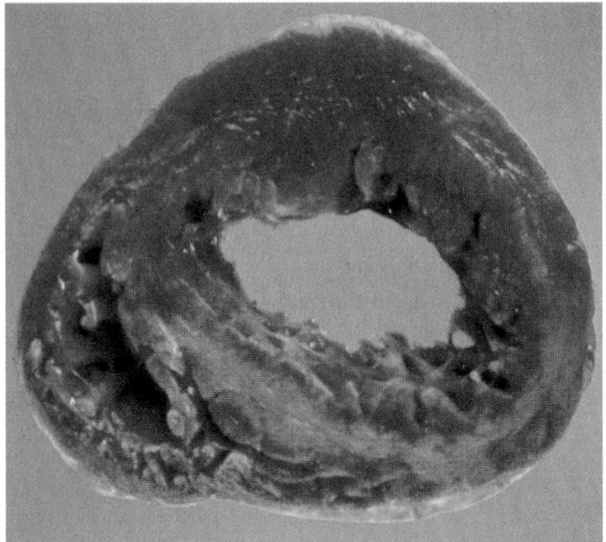

FIGURE 26-11 Acute myocardial infarct. A cross section of the ventricles of a man who died a few days after the onset of severe chest pain shows a transmural infarct in the posterior and septal regions of the left ventricle. The necrotic myocardium is soft, yellowish, and sharply demarcated. (Rubin E., Farber J.L. [1999]. *Pathology* [3rd ed., p. 558]. Philadelphia: Lippincott-Raven)

swelling) develop within several minutes. These early changes are reversible if blood flow is restored.

Although gross tissue changes are not apparent for hours after onset of an AMI, the ischemic area ceases to function within a matter of minutes, and irreversible damage to cells occurs in approximately 40 minutes. Irreversible myocardial cell death (necrosis) occurs after 20 to 40 minutes of severe ischemia.[10] Microvascular injury occurs in approximately 1 hour and follows irreversible cell injury. The term *reperfusion* refers to reestablishment of blood flow through use of thrombolytic therapy. Early reperfusion (within 15 to 20 minutes) after onset of ischemia can prevent necrosis. Reperfusion after a longer interval can salvage some of the myocardial cells that would have died owing to longer periods of ischemia. It also may prevent microvascular injury that occurs over a longer period. Even though much of the viable myocardium existing at the time of reflow ultimately recovers, critical abnormalities in biochemical function may persist, causing impaired ventricular function. The recovering area of the heart is often referred to as a *stunned myocardium*. Because myocardial function is lost before cell death occurs, a stunned myocardium may not be capable of sustaining life, and persons with large areas of dysfunctional myocardium may require life support until the stunned regions regain their function.[10]

Medical Management of ACS

The medical management of ACS depends on the extent of ischemia or infarction. Because the specific diagnosis of AMI often is difficult to make at the time of entry into the health care system, the immediate management of all cases of ACS in general is the same. Commonly indicated treatment regimens include administration of oxygen by nasal prongs, analgesic agents, aspirin, β-adrenergic blockers, and nitrates.[32] Persons with ECG evidence of infarction should receive immediate reperfusion therapy with thrombolytic agents or PTCA.[32]

ECG monitoring should be instituted, and a 12-lead ECG should be performed. The typical ECG changes may not be present immediately after the onset of symptoms, except as arrhythmias. Diagnostic ECG tracings (*i.e.,* ST-segment elevation, prolongation of the Q wave, and inversion of the T wave) are absent in about half of patients with AMI who present with chest pain.[32] Premature ventricular contractions are common arrhythmias after myocardial infarction. The occurrence of other arrhythmias and conduction defects depends on the areas of the heart and conduction pathways that are included in the infarct.

The administration of oxygen augments the oxygen content of inspired air and increases the oxygen saturation of hemoglobin. Arterial oxygen levels may fall precipitously after AMI, and oxygen administration helps to maintain the oxygen content of the blood perfusing the coronary circulation.

The severe pain of myocardial infarction gives rise to anxiety and recruitment of autonomic nervous system responses, both of which increase the work demands of the heart. Although a number of analgesic agents have been used to treat the pain of AMI, morphine is usually the drug of choice.[32] The reduction in anxiety that accompanies the administration of morphine contributes to a decrease in restlessness and autonomic nervous system activity, with a subsequent decrease in the metabolic demands of the heart. It is commonly given intravenously because of the rapid onset of action and because the intravenous route does not elevate enzyme levels. The intravenous route also bypasses the variable rate of absorption of subcutaneous or intramuscular sites, which often are underperfused because of the decrease in cardiac output that occurs after infarction. Sublingual nitroglycerin is given because of its vasodilating effect and ability to relieve coronary pain. The vasodilating effects of the drug decrease venous return (*i.e.,* reduce preload) and arterial blood pressure (*i.e.,* reduce afterload), thereby reducing oxygen consumption. Intravenous nitroglycerin may be given to limit infarction size and is most effective if given within 4 hours of symptom onset.

Because sympathetic nervous system activity increases the metabolic demands of the myocardium, β-adrenergic–blocking drugs may be used to reduce sympathetic stimulation of the heart after myocardial infarction. These drugs decrease myocardial contractility and cardiac workload, alter resting myocardial membrane potentials and decrease arrhythmia frequency, and may aid in redistributing coronary artery blood flow and improving myocardial blood flow.

Platelets play a major role in the thrombotic response to rupture of a coronary plaque; therefore, inhibition of platelet aggregation is an important aspect in the early treatment of AMI. Although several antiplatelet regimens have been evaluated, the agent most tested has been aspirin, and this is the drug for which the most compelling evidence of benefit exists.[33] Aspirin inhibits platelet aggregation and is thought to promote reperfusion and reduce the likelihood of rethrombosis. The glycoprotein IIb/IIIa receptor inhibitors may be used in persons who have non–ST-segment elevation AMI provided they do not have a major contraindication due to bleeding risk. Low-molecular-weight heparin may be used to prevent thrombin generation.

Thrombolytic Therapy. Thrombolytic drugs dissolve blood and platelet clots and are used to reduce mortality and limit infarct size. These agents interact with plasminogen to generate plasmin, which lyses fibrin clots and digests clotting factors V and VIII, prothrombin, and fibrinogen (see Chapter 15). The best results occur if treatment is initiated within 60 to 90 minutes of symptom onset.[32] The magnitude of benefit declines after this period, but it is possible that some benefit can be achieved for up to 12 hours after the onset of pain. The person must be a low-risk candidate for complications caused by bleeding.

Revascularization Interventions. Revascularization interventions include percutaneous coronary intervention and coronary artery bypass surgery. These interventions are increasingly being used on an emergency basis as a primary intervention to relieve coronary artery obstruction caused by atherosclerotic lesions.

Percutaneous coronary intervention (PCI) includes PTCA, stent implantation, atherectomy, and thrombectomy.[34] Balloon PTCA involves dilatation of a stenotic atherosclerotic plaque with an inflatable balloon (Fig. 26-12). The procedure is done under local anesthesia in the cardiac catheterization laboratory and is similar to cardiac catheterization for coronary angiography. During the procedure, a double-lumen balloon dilatation catheter is introduced percutaneously into the femoral or brachial artery and advanced under fluoroscopic view into the stenotic area of the affected coronary vessel. There, it is used to expand the coronary lumen by stretching and tearing the atherosclerotic plaque and to a lesser extent by distributing the plaque along its longitudinal axis.[34] Acute complications of PTCA include thrombosis and vessel dissection; longer-term complications involve restenosis of the dilated vessel. Refinements in the balloon catheters have resulted in decreased risk for vessel perforation and ischemic complications. Measures to reduce thrombosis during angioplasty also decrease the risk for death and myocardial infarction.

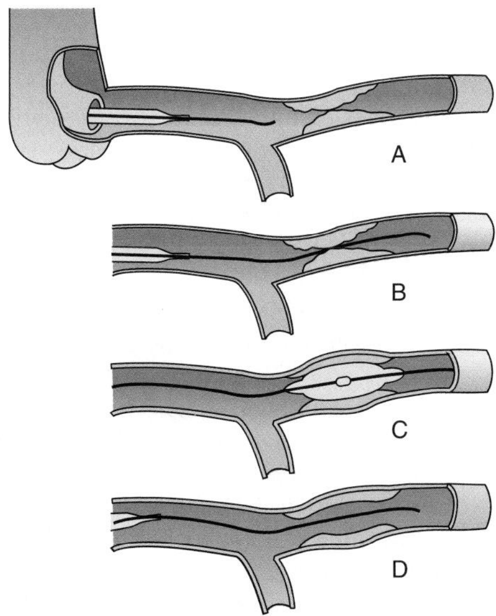

FIGURE 26-12 (**A**) PTCA dilation catheter and guidewire exiting the guiding catheter. (**B**) Guidewire advanced across the stenosis. (**C**) Dilation catheter advanced across the stenosis and inflated. (**D**) Dilation catheter pulled back to assess luminal diameter. (Reprinted with permission of Advanced Cardiovascular Systems [ACS], Inc., Santa Clara, CA)

Because of the risk for restenosis, a stent may be inserted into the dilated vessel at the time of PTCA. *Coronary stents* are fenestrated, stainless steel tubes that can be inserted into a coronary artery and then expanded to prevent vessel restenosis.[34] Stents also are used to prevent abrupt vessel closure caused by vessel dissection that can occur as a complication of PTCA. Stenting is used in high-risk situations that are not likely to be managed successfully by PTCA alone. Persons undergoing stent procedures are treated with antiplatelet and anticoagulant drugs to prevent thrombosis, which is a major risk after the procedure. Adjunctive blockade of the platelet glycoprotein IIb/IIIa receptor may be used to prevent thrombosis and complications associated with PTCA.

A relatively new approach to the prevention of coronary restenosis after balloon angioplasty and stent placement is the use of localized intracoronary radiation. Two approaches to intracoronary radiation—endoluminal beta irradiation and localized intracoronary gamma radiation—were approved by the U.S. Food and Drug Administration (FDA) in November 2000.[35,36] The procedure, also known as *brachytherapy,* is credited with inhibiting cell proliferation and vascular lesion formation and preventing constrictive arterial remodeling. The radiation source can be impregnated into stents, or the radiation can be delivered by a radiation catheter containing a sealed source of radiation (radioactive seeds, wire, or ribbon) that is inserted into the treatment site and then removed.[35]

Atherectomy (*i.e.,* cutting of the atherosclerotic plaque with a high-speed circular blade from within the vessel) is being tested as a mechanical technique to remove atherosclerotic tissue during angioplasty. Laser angioplasty devices also are being tested.[34] Thrombectomy (removal of the thrombus) involves the use of a special catheter device to fracture the thrombus into small pieces and then pull the fracture fragments into the catheter tip so they can be propelled proximally and removed.

Coronary artery bypass grafting (CABG) may be the treatment of choice for people with significant CHD who do not respond to medical treatment and who are not suitable candidates for PCI. It may also be indicated as a treatment for AMI, in which case the surgery should be done within 4 to 6 hours of symptom onset if possible.

CABG involves revascularization of the affected myocardium by placing a saphenous vein graft between the aorta and the affected coronary artery distal to the site of occlusion, or by using the internal mammary artery as a means of revascularizing the left anterior descending artery or its branches. Figure 26-13 shows the placement of a saphenous vein graft and a mammary artery graft. One to

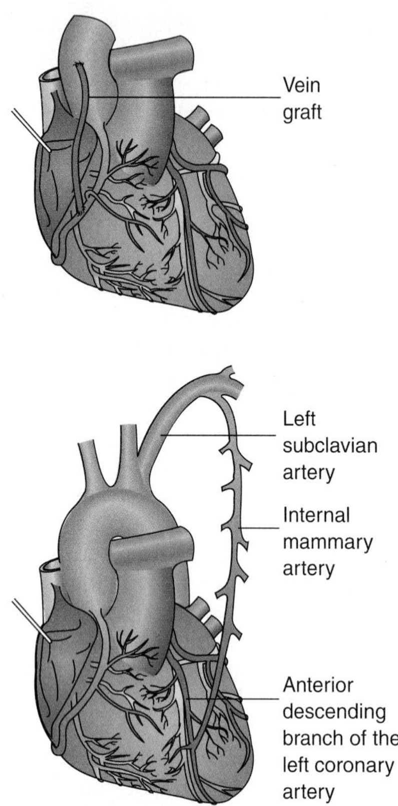

FIGURE 26-13 Coronary artery revascularization. (**Top**) Saphenous vein bypass graft. The vein segment is sutured to the ascending aorta and the right coronary artery at a point distal to the occluding lesion. (**Bottom**) Mammary artery bypass. The mammary artery is anastomosed to the anterior descending left coronary artery, bypassing the obstructing lesion.

five distal anastomoses commonly are done. Although it cannot be documented that this surgery significantly alters the progress of the disease, it does relieve pain, and patients may have more productive lives.[27]

Myocardial Postinfarction Recovery Period

After a myocardial infarction, there usually are three zones of tissue damage: a zone of myocardial tissue that becomes necrotic because of an absolute lack of blood flow; a surrounding zone of injured cells, some of which will recover; and an outer zone in which cells are ischemic and can be salvaged if blood flow can be reestablished (Fig. 26-14). The boundaries of these zones may change with time after the infarction and with the success of treatment measures to reestablish blood flow. If blood flow can be restored within the 20- to 40-minute time frame, loss of cell viability does not occur or is minimal. The progression of ischemic necrosis usually begins in the subendocardial area of the heart and extends through the myocardium to involve progressively more of the transmural thickness of the ischemic zone.

Myocardial cells that undergo necrosis are gradually replaced with scar tissue (Table 26-2). An acute inflammatory response develops in the area of necrosis approximately 2 to 3 days after infarction. Thereafter, macrophages begin removing the necrotic tissue; the damaged area is gradually replaced with an ingrowth of highly vascularized granulation tissue, which gradually becomes less vascular and more fibrous.[10] At approximately 4 to 7 days, the center of the infarcted area is soft and yellow; if rupture of the ventricle, interventricular septum, or valve structures occurs, it usually happens at this time. Replacement of the necrotic myocardial tissue usually is complete by the seventh week. Areas of the myocardium that have been replaced with scar tissue lack the ability to contract and initiate or conduct action potentials.

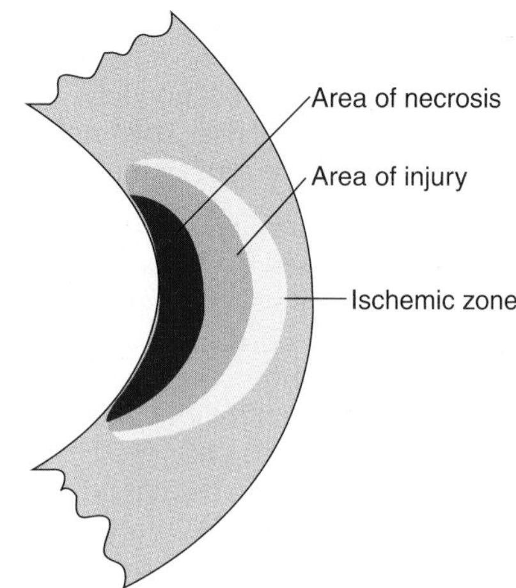

FIGURE 26-14 Areas of tissue damage after myocardial infarction.

Complications. The stages of recovery from AMI are closely related to the size of the infarct and the changes that have taken place in the infarcted area. Fibrous scar tissue lacks the contractile, elastic, and conductive properties of normal myocardial cells; the residual effects and the complications are determined essentially by the extent and location of the injury. Among the complications of AMI are sudden death, heart failure and cardiogenic shock, pericarditis and Dressler's syndrome, thromboemboli, rupture of the heart, and ventricular aneurysms. Depending on its severity, myocardial infarction has the potential for compromising the pumping action of the heart. Heart failure and cardiogenic shock (see Chapter 28) are dreaded complications of AMI.

Pericarditis may complicate the course of AMI. It usually appears on the second or third day after infarction. The person experiences a new type of pain that is sharp and stabbing and is aggravated with deep inspiration and positional changes. A pericardial friction rub may or may not be heard in all persons who have postinfarction pericarditis, and it often is transitory, usually resolving uneventfully. *Dressler's syndrome* describes the signs and symptoms associated with pericarditis, pleurisy, and pneumonitis: fever, chest pain, dyspnea, and abnormal laboratory test results (*i.e.,* elevated white blood cell count and sedimentation rate) and ECG findings. The symptoms may arise between 1 day and several weeks after infarction and are thought to represent a hypersensitivity response to tissue necrosis. Antiinflammatory agents or corticosteroid drugs may be used to reduce the inflammatory response.

TABLE 26-2 Tissues Changes After Myocardial Infarction

Time After Onset	Type of Injury and Gross Tissue Changes
0–0.5 hours	Reversible injury
1–2 hours	Onset of irreversible injury
4–12 hours	Beginning of coagulation necrosis
18–24 hours	Continued coagulation necrosis; gross pallor of infarcted tissue
1–3 days	Total coagulation necrosis; continued gross pallor of infarcted area and sometimes hyperemia due to onset of acute inflammatory process
3–7 days	Infarcted area becomes soft with a yellow-brown center and hyperemic edges
7–10 days	Maximally soft and yellow with vascularized edges; fibroblastic activity at edges denotes beginning of scar tissue generation
8th week	Scar tissue replacement complete

(Developed from information in Cotran R.S., Kumar V., Collins T. [1999]. *Robbins pathologic basis of disease* [6th ed., pp. 555–560]. Philadelphia: W.B. Saunders.)

Thromboemboli are a potential complication of AMI, arising as venous thrombi or occasionally as clots from the wall of the ventricle. Immobility and impaired cardiac function contribute to stasis of blood in the venous system. Elastic stockings, along with active and passive leg exercises, usually are included in the postinfarction treatment plan as a means of preventing thrombus formation. If a clot is detected on the wall of the ventricle (usually by echocardiography), treatment with anticoagulants is indicated.

Dreaded complications of AMI are rupture of the myocardium, the interventricular septum, or a papillary muscle. Myocardial rupture, occurring on the fourth to seventh day after AMI when the injured ventricular tissue is soft and weak, often is fatal. Necrosis of the septal wall or papillary muscle may lead to the rupture of either of these structures, with worsening of ventricular performance. Surgical repair usually is indicated, but whenever possible, it is delayed until the heart has had time to recover from the initial infarction. Vasodilator therapy and the aortic balloon counterpulsation pump may provide supportive assistance during this period.

An aneurysm is an outpouching of the ventricular wall. Scar tissue does not have the characteristics of normal myocardial tissue; when a large section of ventricular muscle is replaced by scar tissue, an aneurysm may develop (Fig. 26-15). This section of the myocardium does not contract with the rest of the ventricle during systole. Instead, it diminishes the pumping efficiency of the heart and increases the work of the left ventricle, predisposing the patient to heart failure. Ischemia in the surrounding area predisposes the patient to development of arrhythmias, and stasis of blood in the aneurysm can lead to thrombus formation. Surgical resection often is corrective.

Cardiac Rehabilitation Programs

Rehabilitation programs for persons with ACS incorporate rest, exercise, and risk factor modification. Modifying the diet to include foods that are low in salt and cholesterol and easy to digest is another treatment measure used to decrease cardiac work. Stool softeners may be prescribed to prevent constipation and avoid straining with defecation.

An exercise program is an integral part of a cardiac rehabilitation program. It includes activities such as walking, swimming, and bicycling. These exercises involve changes in muscle length and rhythmic contractions of muscle groups. Most exercise programs are individually designed to meet each person's physical and psychological needs. The goal of the exercise program is to increase the maximal oxygen consumption by the muscle tissues, so that these persons are able to perform more work at a lower heart rate and blood pressure. In addition to exercise, cardiac risk factor modification incorporates strategies for smoking cessation, weight loss, stress reduction, and control of hypertension and diabetes.

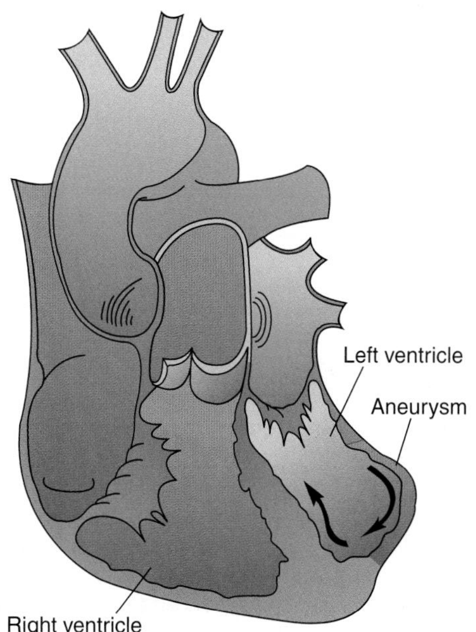

FIGURE 26-15 Paradoxical movement of a ventricular aneurysm during systole.

In summary, CHD is a disorder of impaired coronary blood flow, usually caused by atherosclerosis. Myocardial ischemia occurs when there is a disparity between coronary blood flow and the metabolic needs of the heart. Ischemia can be present as a chronic ischemic heart disease and as an ACS. Diagnostic methods for CHD include ECG methods, exercise testing, nuclear imaging studies, and angiographic studies in the cardiac catheterization laboratory.

The chronic ischemic heart diseases include chronic stable angina, silent myocardial ischemia, and variant angina. Chronic stable angina is associated with a fixed atherosclerotic obstruction and pain that is precipitated by increased work demands on the heart and relieved by rest. Silent myocardial ischemia occurs without symptoms. Variant angina results from spasms of the coronary arteries. Treatment includes nonpharmacologic methods, such as pacing of activities and avoidance of activities that cause angina, and the use of pharmacologic agents, including aspirin, β-adrenergic blockers, calcium channel blockers, and nitrates. Revascularization procedures include PCI along with the use of coronary artery stents and CABG.

ACS results from unstable atherosclerotic plaques, platelet aggregation, and thrombus formation. These syndromes include unstable angina, non–ST-segment elevation AMI, and ST-segment elevation AMI. Unstable angina is an accelerated form of angina in which the pain occurs more frequently, is more severe, and lasts longer than in chronic stable angina. AMI refers to the ischemic death of myocardial tissue associated with obstructed blood flow in the coronary arteries due to plaque disruption and occlusion of blood flow. Non–ST-segment and ST-segment elevation AMI differ in terms of extent of myocardial damage. The complications of AMI include potentially fatal arrhythmias, heart failure and cardiogenic shock, pericarditis, thromboemboli, rupture of cardiac structures, and ventricular aneurysms. Diagnostic methods include the use of ECG monitoring and serum cardiac markers. Treatment goals focus on reestablishment of myocardial blood flow through rapid recanalization of the occluded coronary artery, prevention of clot extension through use of aspirin and other antiplatelet and antithrombotic agents, alleviation of pain, measures such as administration of oxygen to increase the oxygen saturation of hemoglobin, and the use of vasodilators to reduce the work demands of the heart.

Myocardial Disease

After completing this section of the chapter, you should be able to meet the following objectives:

- ✦ Define and cite selected causes of myocarditis
- ✦ Characterize the pathogenesis and possible outcomes of viral myocarditis
- ✦ Define the term *cardiomyopathy* and compare the heart changes that occur with dilated, hypertrophic, and constrictive cardiomyopathies, and arrhythmogenic right ventricular cardiomyopathy

Myocardial diseases, including myocarditis and the primary cardiomyopathies, are disorders originating in the myocardium, but not from cardiovascular disease. Both myocarditis and the cardiomyopathies are causes of sudden death and heart failure. Of the more than 3 million persons in the United States who have heart failure, approximately 25% of cases result from idiopathic dilated cardiomyopathy.[35]

MYOCARDITIS

The term *myocarditis* is used to describe an inflammation of the heart muscle and conduction system without evidence of myocardial infarction.[36–38] Viruses are the most important cause of myocarditis in North America and Europe.[37] *Coxsackieviruses A* and *B* and other enteroviruses probably account for most of the cases. Myocarditis is a frequent pathologic cardiac finding in persons with acquired immunodeficiency syndrome (AIDS), although it is unclear whether it is due to the human immunodeficiency virus (HIV) itself or to a secondary infection. Other causes of myocarditis are radiation therapy, hypersensitivity reactions, or exposure to chemical or physical agents that induce acute myocardial necrosis and secondary inflammatory changes. A drug that is increasingly associated with myocarditis is cocaine, probably owing to its vasoconstrictive properties.[37]

Myocardial injury due to infectious agents is thought to result from necrosis caused by direct invasion of the offending organism, toxic effects of exogenous toxins or endotoxins produced by a systemic pathogen, or destruction of cardiac tissue by immunologic mechanisms initiated by the infectious agent. The immunologic response may be directed at foreign antigens of the infectious agent that share molecular characteristics with those of the host cardiac myocytes (*i.e.,* molecular mimicry; see Chapter 21), providing a continuous stimulus for the immune response even after the infectious agent has been cleared from the body.

The *manifestations of myocarditis* vary from an absence of symptoms to profound heart failure or sudden death. When viral myocarditis occurs in children or young adults, it often is asymptomatic. Acute symptomatic myocarditis typically manifests as a flulike syndrome with malaise, low-grade fever, and tachycardia that is more pronounced than would be expected for the level of fever present. There commonly is a history of an upper respiratory tract or gastrointestinal tract infection, followed by a latent period of several days. Cardiac auscultation may reveal an S_3 ventricular gallop rhythm and a transient pericardial or pleurocardial rub. In approximately one half of the cases, myocarditis is transient, and symptoms subside within 1 to 2 months. In other cases, fulminant heart failure and life-threatening arrhythmias develop, causing sudden death. Still others progress to subacute and chronic disease.

The *diagnosis* of myocarditis can be suggested by clinical manifestations. The ECG changes of acute myocarditis include conduction disturbances such as ventricular arrhythmias, AV junctional block, ST-segment elevation, T-wave inversion, and transient Q waves. Serum creatinine kinase often is elevated. Troponin T or troponin I, or both, may be elevated, providing evidence of myocardial cell damage.[37] Confirmation of active myocarditis requires endomyocardial biopsy.

Treatment measures focus on symptom management and prevention of myocardial damage. Bed rest is necessary, and activity restriction must be maintained until fever and cardiac symptoms subside to decrease the myocardial workload. Activity is gradually increased but kept at a sedentary level for 6 months to 1 year. The restriction includes the avoidance of swimming, jogging, weight lifting, and carrying heavy objects. The use of corticosteroids and immunosuppressant drugs such as azathioprine and cyclosporine remains controversial. There is some evidence that people with acute fulminant myocarditis may benefit from short-term circulatory support with left ventricular assist devices.[37] The use of the antiviral agent, interferon-alfa, for treatment of enterovirus-positive forms of myocarditis is under study.[37] Although treatment of myocarditis is successful in many persons, some progress to congestive heart failure and can expect only a limited life span. For these persons, heart transplantation becomes an alternative.

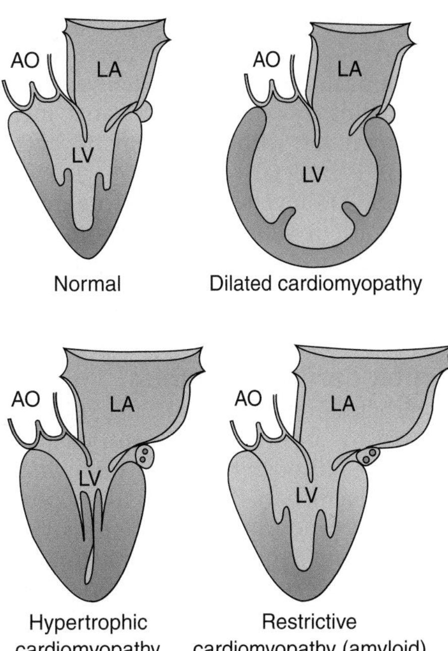

FIGURE 26-16 The various types of cardiomyopathies compared with the normal heart. (Roberts W.C., Ferrans V.J. [1975]. Pathologic anatomy of the cardiomyopathies. *Human Pathology 6,* 289)

CARDIOMYOPATHIES

The cardiomyopathies are a group of disorders that affect the heart muscle. They can develop as primary or secondary disorders.[39] The primary cardiomyopathies, which are discussed in this chapter, are heart muscle diseases of unknown origin. Secondary cardiomyopathies are conditions in which the cardiac abnormality results from another cardiovascular disease, such as myocardial infarction. The onset of the primary cardiomyopathies often is silent, and symptoms do not occur until the disease is well advanced. The diagnosis is suspected when a young, previously healthy, normotensive person experiences cardiomegaly and heart failure.

In 1989, the International Society and Federation of Cardiology and the World Health Organization categorized the primary cardiomyopathies into three groups: dilated, hypertrophic, and restrictive[40] (Fig. 26-16). This classification was enlarged in 1996 to include arrhythmogenic right ventricular cardiomyopathy.[41] Peripartum cardiomyopathy is a disorder of pregnancy.

Dilated Cardiomyopathies

Dilated cardiomyopathies are characterized by progressive cardiac hypertrophy and dilation and impaired pumping ability of one or both ventricles. Although all four chambers of the heart are affected, the ventricles are more dilated than the atria. Because of the wall thinning that accompanies dilation, the thickness of the ventricular wall often is less than would be expected for the amount of hypertrophy present.[42] Mural thrombi are common and may be a source of thromboemboli. The cardiac valves are intrinsically normal. Microscopically, there is evidence of scarring and atrophy of myocardial cells.

Dilated cardiomyopathy may result from a number of different myocardial insults, including infectious myocarditis, alcohol and other toxic agents, metabolic influences, neuromuscular diseases, and immunologic disorders. Genetic influences have been documented in some cases. One study found that 20% of affected persons have first-degree relatives with myocardial dysfunction.[43] These disorders can be inherited in an autosomal dominant, autosomal recessive, or X-linked inheritance pattern. High alcohol consumption is another cause of cardiomyopathy. It accounts for 3.8% of all cardiomyopathy cases and is reported to be the second-leading cause of a dilated cardiomyopathy.[44] Often, the cause is unknown; these cases are appropriately designated *idiopathic dilated cardiomyopathy*.

The most common initial manifestations of dilated cardiomyopathy are those related to heart failure. There is a profound reduction in the left ventricular ejection fraction (*i.e.*, ratio of stroke volume to end-diastolic volume) to 40% or less, compared with a normal value of approximately 67%. After symptoms have developed, the course of the disorder is distinguished by worsening of heart failure, development of mural thrombi, and ventricular arrhythmias.[45] The most striking symptoms of dilated cardiomyopathy are dyspnea on exertion, paroxysmal nocturnal dyspnea, orthopnea, weakness, fatigue, ascites, and peripheral edema. On physical examination, an enlarged apical beat with the presence of a third and fourth heart sound and a murmur associated with regurgitation of one or both AV valves frequently are found. The systolic blood pressure is normal or low, and the peripheral pulses often are of low amplitude. Pulsus alternans, in which the pulse regularly alternates between weaker and stronger volume, may be present. Basilar rales frequently are detected. Sinus tachycardia, atrial fibrillation, and complex ventricular arrhythmias leading to sudden cardiac death are common.

The treatment of dilated cardiomyopathy is directed toward relieving the symptoms of heart failure and reducing the workload of the heart (see Chapter 28). Digoxin, diuretics, and afterload-reducing drugs are used to improve myocardial contractility and decrease left ventricular filling pressures. Avoiding myocardial depressants, including alcohol, and pacing rest with asymptomatic levels of exercise or activity is imperative. Proper electrolyte balance and implantable cardioverter-defibrillators are effective in controlling recurrent ventricular arrhythmias associated with dilated cardiomyopathy. In persons with severe heart failure that is refractory to treatment, cardiac transplantation may be considered.

Hypertrophic Cardiomyopathies

Hypertrophic cardiomyopathy is characterized by an abnormality that involves excessive ventricular growth or hypertrophy.[46–48] Although the hypertrophy may be symmetric, the involvement of the ventricular septum often is disproportionate, producing intermittent left ventricular outflow obstruction. Synonyms for this disorder include *idiopathic hypertrophic subaortic stenosis* and *asymmetric septal hypertrophy*.

Symptomatic hypertrophic cardiomyopathy commonly is a disease of young adulthood and is the most common cause of sudden cardiac death in the young.[46] The cause of the disorder is unknown, although it often is of familial origin, with the disorder being inherited as an autosomal dominant trait. Molecular studies of the genetic alterations responsible for hypertrophic cardiomyopathy suggest that the disease is caused by mutation in one of 10 genes encoding the proteins of the cardiac sarcomeres (*i.e.*, muscle fibers).[47] Three of the mutant genes predominate: the β-myosin heavy chain, cardiac troponin T, and myosin-binding protein C. The other genes account for a minority of cases. The prognosis of persons with different myosin mutations varies greatly; some mutations are relatively benign, whereas others are associated with premature death.

A distinctive microscopic finding in hypertrophic cardiomyopathy is myofibril disarray (Fig. 26-17). Instead of the normal parallel arrangement of myofibrils, the myofibrils branch off at random angles, sometimes at right angles to an adjacent fiber with which they connect. Small bundles of fibers may course haphazardly through normally arranged muscle fibers.[10,48] These disordered fibers may produce abnormal movements of the ventricles, with uncoordinated contraction and impaired relaxation. Arrhythmias and premature sudden death are common with this disorder.

The manifestations of hypertrophic cardiomyopathy are variable; for reasons that are unclear, some persons with the disorder remain stable for many years and gradually acquire more symptoms as the disease progresses, but others experience sudden cardiac death as first evidence of the disease.[46,47] Atrial fibrillation is a common precursor to sudden death in those who die of arrhythmias. Dyspnea is the most common symptom associated with a gradual elevation in left ventricular diastolic pressure resulting from impaired ventricular filling and increased wall stiffness due to ventricular hypertrophy. Because of the obstruction to outflow from the left ventricle, increasingly greater levels of ventricular pressure are needed to eject blood into the aorta, limiting cardiac output. Chest pain, fatigue, and syncope are common and worsen during exertion.

Diagnosis of hypertrophic cardiomyopathy is usually based on history and physical examination. It may be first suspected because of a heart murmur (occasionally discovered during sports preparation examination), positive family history, or ECG findings.[47] Clinical diagnosis is usually

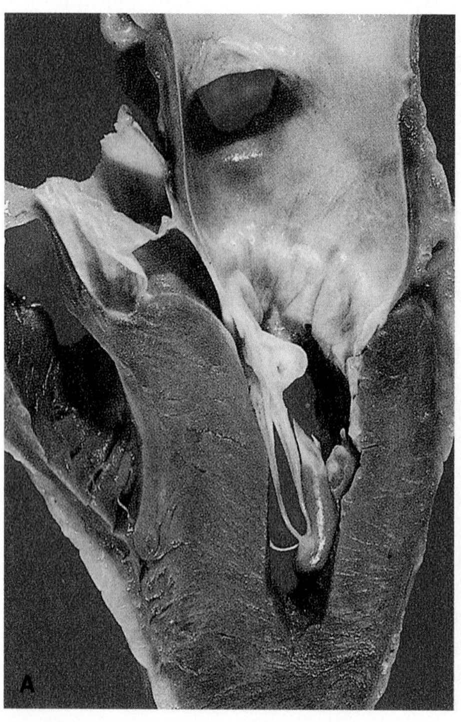

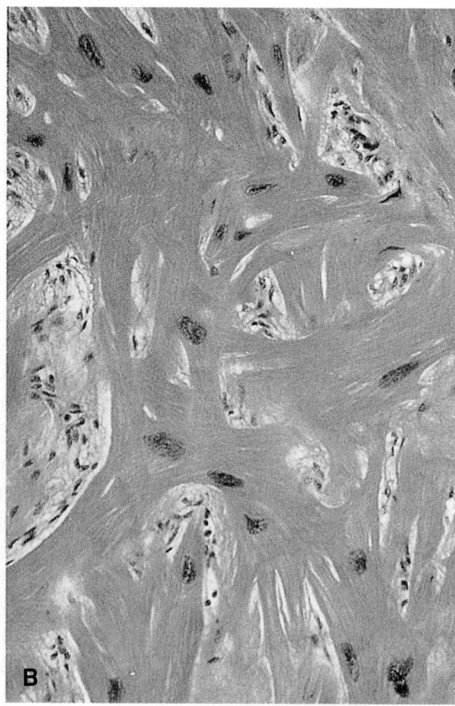

FIGURE 26-17 Hypertrophic cardiomyopathy. (**A**) The heart has been opened to show striking asymmetric left ventricular hypertrophy. The interventricular septum is thicker than the free wall of the ventricle and impinges on the outflow tract. (**B**) A section of the myocardium shows myocardial fiber disarray characterized by oblique and often perpendicular orientation of adjacent hypertrophic myocytes. (Rubin E., Farber J.L. [1999]. *Pathology* [3rd ed., p. 580]. Philadelphia: Lippincott-Raven)

established through echocardiography. Screening of first-degree relatives should be encouraged once a diagnosis is made. However, not all people harboring the gene express the clinical features of the gene mutation, such as echocardiographic evidence of left ventricular hypertrophy. For example, it is not unusual for children younger than 13 years to carry the gene without evidence of left ventricular hypertrophy. This is because substantial left ventricular remodeling with spontaneous appearance of hypertrophic cardiomyopathy occurs with accelerated rate of growth during adolescence, and morphologic expression of the gene is usually completed by about 17 to 18 years of age.[47]

The treatment of hypertrophic cardiomyopathy includes medical and surgical management. The goal of medical management is to decrease the risk for sudden death and relieve the symptoms associated with the disorder. Drugs that block the β-adrenergic receptors may be used in persons with chest pain, arrhythmias, or dyspnea.[47,49,50] These drugs reduce the heart rate and improve myocardial function by allowing more time for ventricular filling and reducing ventricular stiffness. The calcium channel–blocking drug verapamil may be used as an alternative to the β-adrenergic blockers. Increased calcium uptake and increased intracellular calcium content are associated with an increased contractile state, a characteristic finding in patients with hypertrophic cardiomyopathy. Most persons with hypertrophic cardiomyopathy should undergo a risk stratification assessment using echocardiography, 24- to 48-hour Holter ECGs, and exercise testing.[47] An implantable cardioverter-defibrillator may be used in persons at high risk for developing lethal arrhythmias.[47,49]

Surgical treatment may be used if severe symptoms persist despite medical treatment. It involves incision of the septum (*i.e.*, myotomy) with or without the removal of part of the tissue (*i.e.*, myectomy). It is accompanied by all the risks of open-heart surgery.

Restrictive Cardiomyopathies

Of the three categories of cardiomyopathies, the restrictive type is the least common in Western countries. With this form of cardiomyopathy, ventricular filling is restricted because of excessive rigidity of the ventricular walls, although the contractile properties of the heart remain relatively normal. The condition is endemic in parts of Africa, India, South and Central America, and Asia.[51] Outside the tropics, the most common causes of restrictive cardiomyopathy are endocardial infiltrations such as amyloidosis. Amyloid infiltrations of the heart are common in the elderly. The idiopathic form of the disorder may have a familial origin.

Symptoms of restrictive cardiomyopathy include dyspnea, paroxysmal nocturnal dyspnea, orthopnea, peripheral edema, ascites, fatigue, and weakness. The manifestations of restrictive cardiomyopathy resemble those of constrictive pericarditis. In the advanced form of the disease, all the signs of heart failure are present except cardiomegaly.

Arrhythmogenic Right Ventricular Cardiomyopathy

In arrhythmogenic right ventricular cardiomyopathy, right ventricular myocardium is replaced with a fibrofatty deposit. This condition frequently has a familial predisposition, with an autosomal dominant inheritance pattern. Sudden death due to arrhythmias is common, particularly in the young.[41]

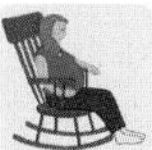

Peripartum Cardiomyopathy

Peripartum cardiomyopathy refers to left ventricular dysfunction developing in the last month before delivery to 5 months postpartum. The condition is relatively rare, with an estimated incidence of 1 per 3000 to 4000 live births.[52] Risk factors for peripartum cardiomyopathy include advanced maternal age, African-American race, multifetal pregnancies, preeclampsia, and gestational hypertension.[52] The reported mortality rate ranges from 18% to 56%. Survivors may not recover completely and may require heart transplantation.

The cause of peripartum cardiomyopathy is uncertain. A number of causes have been proposed, including myocarditis, an abnormal immune response to pregnancy, maladaptive response to the hemodynamic stresses of pregnancy, or prolonged inhibition of contractions in premature labor. There is more evidence for myocarditis as a cause than for other purported etiologies.[53]

The signs and symptoms resemble those of dilated cardiomyopathy. Because many women experience dyspnea, fatigue, and pedal edema during the last month of normal pregnancy, the symptoms may be ignored and the diagnosis delayed. The diagnosis is based on echocardiography studies, ECG, and other tests of cardiac function. Treatment methods are similar to those used in dilated cardiomyopathy.

There are two possible outcomes of peripartum cardiomyopathy. In approximately one half of cases, the heart returns to normal within 6 months, and the chances for long-term survival are good. In these women, heart failure returns only during subsequent pregnancies. In the other one half of cases, cardiomegaly persists, the prognosis is poor, and death is probable if another pregnancy occurs. In women with cardiomyopathy from documented viral myocarditis, the likelihood of recurrence is low.

In summary, myocardial disorders represent a diverse group of disorders of myocardial muscle cells, not related to coronary artery disease. Myocarditis is an acute inflammation of cardiac muscle cells, most often of viral origin. Myocardial injury from myocarditis is thought to result from necrosis due to direct invasion of the offending organism, toxic effects of exogenous toxins or endotoxins produced by a systemic pathogen, and destruction of cardiac tissue by immunologic mechanisms initiated by the infectious agent. Although the disease usually is benign and self-limited, it can result in sudden death or chronic heart failure, for which heart transplantation may be considered.

The cardiomyopathies represent disorders of the heart muscle. Cardiomyopathies may manifest as primary or secondary disorders. There are four main types of primary cardiomyopathies: dilated cardiomyopathy, in which fibrosis and atrophy of myocardial cells produces progressive dilation and impaired pumping ability of the heart; hypertrophic cardiomyopathy, characterized by myocardial hypertrophy, abnormal diastolic filling, and in many cases intermittent left ventricular outflow obstruction; restrictive cardiomyopathy, in which there is excessive rigidity of the ventricular wall; and arrhythmogenic right ventricular cardiomyopathy. Peripartum cardiomyopathy occurs during pregnancy. The cause of many of the primary cardiomyopathies is unknown. The disease is suspected when cardiomegaly and heart failure develop in a young, previously healthy person.

Infectious and Immunologic Disorders

After completing this section of the chapter, you should be able to meet the following objectives:

- Distinguish between the role of infectious organisms and the immune system in rheumatic fever and infective endocarditis
- Compare the effects of rheumatic fever and bacterial endocarditis on cardiac structures and their function
- Describe the relation between the infective vegetations associated with infective endocarditis and the extracardiac manifestations of the disease
- Explain measures that can be used to prevent infective endocarditis

INFECTIVE ENDOCARDITIS

Infective endocarditis is a relatively uncommon, life-threatening infection of the endocardial surface of the heart, including the heart valves. It is characterized by colonization or invasion of the heart valves and the mural endocardium by a microbial agent, leading to the formation of bulky, friable vegetations and destruction of underlying cardiac tissues.[10] Because bacteria are the most frequent infecting organisms, the condition may be referred to as *bacterial endocarditis*. Despite important advances in antimicrobial therapy and improved ability to diagnose and treat complications, infective endocarditis continues to produce substantial morbidity and mortality.

Although anyone can contract infective endocarditis, the infection usually develops in people with preexisting heart defects. Heart valves are involved most commonly, but the lesions may affect a septal defect or the endocardial surface of the heart wall. Factors that determine the clinical presentation and outcome of infective endocarditis are the nature of the infecting organism and the presence of preexisting heart defects. Because endocarditis in intravenous drug users and infections acquired during heart surgery have special features, the source of the infection also is important.

Predisposing Factors

For infective endocarditis to develop, two independent factors normally are required: a damaged endocardial surface and a portal of entry by which the organism gains access to the circulatory system. The presence of valvular disease, prosthetic heart valves, or congenital heart defects provides an environment conducive to bacterial growth.[10,54,55] In persons with preexisting valvular or endocardial defects, simple gum massage or an innocuous oral lesion may afford the pathogenic bacteria access to the bloodstream. Transient bacteremia may emerge in the course of seemingly minor health problems, such as an upper respiratory tract infection, a skin lesion, or a dental procedure.

Although infective endocarditis usually occurs in persons with preexisting heart lesions, it also can develop in normal hearts of intravenous drug abusers. The risk for infective endocarditis is increased among intravenous drug users to an incidence of 2% to 5% per patient year, which is several times greater than that for persons with rheumatic heart disease and prosthetic heart valves.[54] The mode of infection is a contaminated drug solution or a needle contaminated with skin flora. Intravenous drug abuse is the most common source of right-sided (tricuspid) lesions. Although staphylococcal infections are common, intravenous drug users may be infected with unusual organisms, such as gram-negative bacilli, yeasts, and fungi.

In hospitalized patients, infective endocarditis may arise as a complication of infected intravascular or urinary tract catheters. Infective endocarditis also may complicate prosthetic heart valve replacement. It can develop as an early infection that follows surgery or as a later infection that results from the long-term presence of the prosthesis. Infections of prosthetic valves account for 10% to 30% of cases of infectious endocarditis.[54]

Depending on the duration of the disease, presenting manifestations, and complications, cases of infective endocarditis can be classified as acute, subacute, or chronic. Acute infective endocarditis is usually caused by *Staphylococcus aureus*.[54] *S. aureus* in particular produces a rapidly progressive and destructive form of the disease. Subacute endocarditis is usually caused by less virulent organisms such as *Streptococcus viridans*, coagulase-negative staphylococci, enterococci, and other gram-negative bacilli.[54] Certain low-virulence organisms such as *Legionella* and *Brucella* may produce a chronic form of the disease.

The pathophysiology of infective endocarditis involves the formation of intracardiac vegetative lesions that have local and distant systemic effects. The vegetative lesion that is characteristic of infective endocarditis consists of a collection of infectious organisms and cellular debris enmeshed in the fibrin strands of clotted blood. The infectious loci continuously release bacteria into the bloodstream and are a source of persistent bacteremia. These lesions may be singular or multiple, may grow to be as large as several centimeters, and usually are found loosely attached to the free edges of the valve surface[48] (Fig. 26-18). As the lesions grow, they cause valve destruction, leading to valvular regurgitation, ring abscesses with heart block, and valve perforation. The loose organization of these lesions permits the organisms and fragments of the lesions to form emboli and travel in the bloodstream. The fragments may lodge in small blood vessels, causing small hemorrhages, abscesses, and infarction of tissue. The bacteremia also can initiate immune responses thought to be

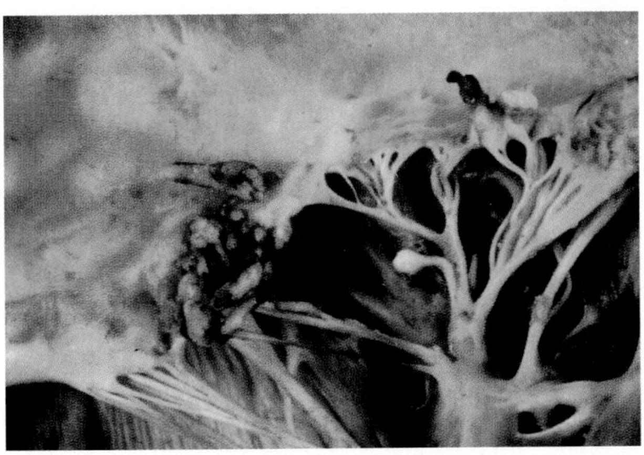

FIGURE 26-18 Bacterial endocarditis. The mitral valve shows destructive vegetations, which have eroded through the free margin of the valve leaflet. (Rubin E., Farber J.L. [1999]. *Pathology* [3rd ed., p. 572]. Philadelphia: Lippincott-Raven)

responsible for the skin manifestations, arthritis, glomerulonephritis, and other immune disorders associated with the condition.

Manifestations

The signs and symptoms of infective endocarditis include fever and signs of systemic infection, change in the character of an existing heart murmur, and evidence of embolic distribution of the vegetative lesions. In the acute form, the fever usually is spiking and accompanied by chills. In the subacute form, the fever usually is of low grade and gradual onset, and frequently is accompanied by other systemic signs of inflammation, such as anorexia, malaise, and lethargy. Small petechial hemorrhages frequently result when emboli lodge in the small vessels of the skin, nail beds, and mucous membranes. Splinter hemorrhages (*i.e.,* dark-red lines) under the nails of the fingers and toes are common. Cough, dyspnea, arthralgia or arthritis, diarrhea, and abdominal or flank pain may occur as the result of systemic emboli.

The clinical course of infective endocarditis is determined by the extent of heart damage, the type of organism involved, the site of infection (*i.e.,* right or left side of the heart), and whether embolization from the site of infection occurs. Destruction of infected heart valves is common with certain forms of organisms, such as *S. aureus.* Peripheral embolization can lead to metastatic infections and abscess formation; these are particularly serious when they affect organs such as the brain and kidneys. In right-sided endocarditis, which usually involves the tricuspid valve, septic emboli travel to the lung, causing infarction and lung abscesses.

Diagnosis and Treatment

The blood culture is the most definitive diagnostic procedure and is essential to guide treatment. At least six cultures should be obtained to increase the probability of obtaining a positive culture. The optimal time to obtain cultures is during a chill, just before a temperature rise. Positive cultures usually are obtainable for infections caused by gram-positive cocci, but cultures may fail to grow gram-negative organisms or fungi. The echocardiogram is useful in detecting underlying valvular disease. Transesophageal echocardiography is rapid and noninvasive and has proved useful for detecting vegetations.

The Duke University criteria can be used in making a definitive diagnosis of infective endocarditis. A diagnosis of infective endocarditis using the Duke criteria requires the presence of two major criteria, one major and three minor criteria, or five minor criteria.[56] The two major criteria are persistently positive blood cultures (at least two positive cultures separated by 12 hours, or all of three or the majority of four or more separate cultures, with the first and last drawn at least 1 hour apart) and evidence of endocardial involvement as demonstrated by a positive echocardiogram or new valvular regurgitation. The six minor criteria are a predisposing heart condition; fever; vascular phenomena such as emboli, mycotic aneurysm, or intracranial hemorrhage; immunologic phenomena such as glomerulonephritis or rheumatoid factor; positive blood cultures not meeting the major criteria; and a positive echocardiogram not meeting the major criteria.

Treatment of infective endocarditis focuses on identifying and eliminating the causative microorganism, minimizing the residual cardiac effects, and treating the pathologic effects of the emboli. Antibiotic therapy is used to eradicate the pathogen. Blood cultures are used to identify the causative organism and determine the most appropriate antibiotic regimen.

Of great importance is the prevention of infective endocarditis in persons with prosthetic heart valves, previous bacterial endocarditis, certain congenital heart defects, and other known risk factors.[57] Prevention can be accomplished largely through prophylactic administration of an antibiotic before dental and other procedures that may cause bacteremia.[57]

RHEUMATIC HEART DISEASE

Rheumatic fever is an acute, immune-mediated, multisystem inflammatory disease that follows a group A (β-hemolytic) streptococcal (GAS) throat infection. The most serious aspect of rheumatic fever is the development of chronic valvular disorders that produce permanent cardiac dysfunction and sometimes cause fatal heart failure years later. In the United States and other industrialized countries, the incidence of rheumatic fever and prevalence of rheumatic heart disease have markedly declined in the past 40 to 50 years.[58] This decline has been attributed to the introduction of antimicrobial agents for improved treatment of GAS pharyngitis, increased access to medical care, and improved economic standards, along with better and less crowded housing. Unfortunately, rheumatic fever and rheumatic heart disease continue to be major health problems in many underdeveloped countries, where inadequate health care, poor nutrition, and crowded living conditions still prevail.

Rheumatic fever is primarily a disease of school-aged children. The incidence of acute rheumatic fever peaks between 5 and 15 years of age.[10] The disease usually follows an inciting GAS throat infection by 1 to 4 weeks. Rheumatic fever and its cardiac complications can be prevented by antibiotic treatment of the initial GAS throat infection.

The pathogenesis of rheumatic fever is unclear. The time frame for development of symptoms in relation to the sore throat and the presence of antibodies to the GAS organism strongly suggests an immunologic origin. Like other immunologic phenomena, rheumatic fever requires an initial sensitizing exposure to the offending streptococcal agent, and the risk for recurrence is high after each subsequent exposure. Although only a small percentage (*e.g.*, 3%) of persons with untreated GAS pharyngitis develop rheumatic fever, the incidence of recurrence with a subsequent untreated infection is substantially greater (about 50%).[58] These observations and more recent studies suggest a familial predisposition to development of the disease.[58]

Manifestations

Rheumatic fever can manifest as an acute, recurrent, or chronic disorder. The *acute stage* of rheumatic fever includes a history of an initiating streptococcal infection and subsequent involvement of the mesenchymal connective tissue of the heart, blood vessels, joints, and subcutaneous tissues. Common to all is a lesion called the *Aschoff body*,[10] which is a localized area of tissue necrosis surrounded by immune cells. The *recurrent phase* usually involves extension of the cardiac effects of the disease. The *chronic phase* of rheumatic fever is characterized by permanent deformity of the heart valves and is a common cause of mitral valve stenosis. Chronic rheumatic heart disease usually does not appear until at least 10 years after the initial attack, sometimes decades later.

Clinical Course

Most children with rheumatic fever have a history of sore throat, headache, fever, abdominal pain, nausea, vomiting, swollen glands (usually at the angle of the jaw), and other signs and symptoms of streptococcal infection. Other clinical features associated with an acute episode of rheumatic fever are related to the acute inflammatory process and the structures involved in the disease process. The course of the disease is characterized by a constellation of findings that includes carditis, migratory polyarthritis of the large joints, erythema marginatum, subcutaneous nodules, and Sydenham's chorea.[58]

Carditis. Acute rheumatic carditis, which complicates the acute phase of rheumatic fever, may progress to chronic valvular disorders. The carditis can affect the pericardium, myocardium, or endocardium, and all of these layers of the heart usually are involved. Both the pericarditis and myocarditis usually are self-limited manifestations of the acute stage of rheumatic fever. The involvement of the endocardium and valvular structures produces the permanent and disabling effects of rheumatic fever. Although any of the four valves can be involved, the mitral and aortic valves are affected most often. During the acute inflammatory stage of the disease, the valvular structures become red and swollen; small vegetative lesions develop on the valve leaflets. The acute inflammatory changes gradually proceed to development of fibrous scar tissue, which tends to contract and cause deformity of the valve leaflets and shortening of the chordae tendineae. In some cases, the edges or commissures of the valve leaflets fuse together as healing occurs.

The manifestations of acute rheumatic carditis include a heart murmur in a child without a previous history of rheumatic fever, change in the character of a murmur in a person with a previous history of the disease, cardiomegaly or enlargement of the heart, friction rub or other signs of pericarditis, and congestive heart failure in a child without discernible cause.

Arthritis, Erythema Marginatum, Subacute Nodes, and Chorea. Although not a cause of permanent disability, polyarthritis is the most common finding in rheumatic fever. The arthritis involves the larger joints, particularly the knees, ankles, elbows, and wrists, and almost always is migratory, affecting one joint and then moving to another. In untreated cases, the arthritis lasts approximately 4 weeks. A striking feature of rheumatic arthritis is the dramatic response (usually within 48 hours) to salicylates.

Erythema marginatum lesions are maplike, macular areas most commonly seen on the trunk or inner aspects of the upper arm and thigh. Skin lesions are present only in approximately 10% of patients who have rheumatic fever; they are transitory and disappear during the course of the disease.

The subcutaneous nodules are 1 to 4 cm in diameter. They are hard, painless, and freely movable and usually overlie the extensor muscles of the wrist, elbow, ankle, and knee joints. Subcutaneous nodules are rare, but when present, they occur most often in persons with carditis.

Chorea (*i.e.*, Sydenham's chorea), sometimes called *St. Vitus' dance,* is the major central nervous system manifestation. It is seen most frequently in girls. There typically is an insidious onset of irritability and other behavior problems. The child often is fidgety, cries easily, begins to walk clumsily, and drops things. The choreic movements are spontaneous, rapid, purposeless, jerking movements that interfere with voluntary activities. Facial grimaces are common, and even speech may be affected. The chorea is self-limited, usually running its course within a matter of weeks or months.

Diagnosis and Treatment

The diagnosis of rheumatic fever is based on the Jones criteria, which were initially proposed in 1955 and revised in 1984 and 1992 by a committee of the AHA.[59] The criteria group the signs and symptoms into major and minor categories. The presence of two major signs (*i.e.*, carditis, polyarthritis, chorea, erythema marginatum, and subcutaneous nodules) or one major and two minor signs (*i.e.*, arthralgia, fever, elevated levels of acute-phase reactants, and prolonged PR interval) accompanied by evidence of a preceding GAS infection indicates a high probability of rheumatic fever.

Elevated levels of acute-phase reactants are not specific for rheumatic fever but provide evidence of an acute inflammatory response. The erythrocyte sedimentation rate, C-reactive protein, and white blood cell count commonly are used; unless corticosteroids or salicylates have been used, the results of these tests almost always are elevated in persons who present with polyarthritis, carditis, or chorea. These tests also are used to determine when the acute phase of the illness has subsided. A prolonged PR interval on the ECG is a nonspecific finding. It does not correlate with the ultimate development of chronic rheumatic heart disease.

Echocardiography and Doppler ultrasound (echo-Doppler) may be used to identify cardiac lesions in persons who do not show typical signs of cardiac involvement during an attack of rheumatic fever.

Prevention. Prevention of initial episodes of acute rheumatic fever requires accurate recognition and proper antibiotic treatment of GAS pharyngitis. Evidence of a streptococcal infection is established through the use of throat cultures, antigen tests, and antibodies to products liberated by the streptococci.[60,61] It takes several days to obtain the results of a throat culture. The development of rapid tests for direct detection of GAS antigens has provided at least a partial solution for this problem. Both the throat culture and the rapid antigen tests are highly specific for GAS infection but are limited in terms of their sensitivity (*e.g.*, the person may have a negative test result but have a streptococcal infection), and a negative antigen test result should be confirmed with a throat culture when a streptococcal infection is suspected.[60] GAS elaborates a large number of extracellular products, including streptolysin O and deoxyribonuclease B. The antibodies to these products are measured for retrospective confirmation of recent streptococcal infections in persons thought to have acute rheumatic fever. Penicillin (or another antibiotic in penicillin-sensitive patients) is the treatment of choice for GAS infection.[60]

Treatment. Treatment of acute rheumatic fever is designed to control the acute inflammatory process and prevent cardiac complications and recurrence of the disease. During the acute phase, prevention of residual cardiac effects is of primary concern; antibiotics, antiinflammatory drugs, and selective restriction of physical activities are prescribed. Penicillin also is the antibiotic of choice for treating the acute illness. Salicylates and corticosteroids also are widely used.[58]

The person who has had an attack of rheumatic fever is at high risk for recurrence after subsequent GAS throat infections. Penicillin is the treatment of choice for secondary prophylaxis, but sulfadiazine or erythromycin may be used in penicillin-allergic individuals.[58] The duration of prophylaxis depends on whether residual valvular disease is present or absent. It is recommended that persons with persistent valvular disease receive prophylaxis for at least 10 years after the last episode of acute rheumatic fever.[58]

Secondary prevention and compliance with a plan for prophylactic administration of penicillin require that the patient and family understand the rationale for such measures and the measures themselves. Patients also need to be instructed to report possible streptococcal infections to their physicians. They should be instructed to inform their dentists about the disease so that they can be adequately protected during dental procedures that may traumatize the oral mucosa.

In summary, infective endocarditis involves the invasion of the endocardium by pathogens that produce vegetative lesions on the endocardial surface. The loose organization of these lesions permits the organisms and fragments of the lesions to be disseminated throughout the systemic circulation. The condition can be caused by several organisms. Two predisposing factors contribute to the development of infective endocarditis: a damaged endocardium and a portal of entry through which the organisms gain access to the bloodstream.

Rheumatic fever, which is associated with an antecedent GAS throat infection, is an important cause of heart disease. Its most serious and disabling effects result from involvement of the heart valves. Because there is no single laboratory test, sign, or symptom that is pathognomonic of acute rheumatic fever, the Jones criteria are used to establish the diagnosis during the acute stage of the disease.

Valvular Heart Disease

After completing this section of the chapter, you should be able to meet the following objectives:

- State the function of the heart valves and relate alterations in hemodynamic function of the heart that occur with valvular disease
- Compare the effects of stenotic and regurgitant mitral and aortic valvular heart disease on cardiovascular function
- Compare the methods of and diagnostic information obtained from cardiac auscultation, phonocardiography, and echocardiography as they relate to valvular heart disease

The past three decades have brought remarkable advances in the treatment and outlook for people with valvular heart disease. This is undoubtedly due to improved methods for noninvasive monitoring of ventricular function, improvement in prosthetic valves, advances in valve reconstruction procedures, and the development of useful guidelines to improve the timing of surgical interventions.[62–64] Nonetheless, valvular heart disease continues to produce considerable mortality and morbidity. In 2003, valvular heart disease contributed to 42,300 deaths in the United States and accounted for 93,000 hospitalizations.[1]

HEMODYNAMIC DERANGEMENTS

The function of the heart valves is to promote directional flow of blood through the chambers of the heart. Dysfunction of the heart valves can result from a number of disorders, including congenital defects, trauma, ischemic damage, degenerative changes, and inflammation.

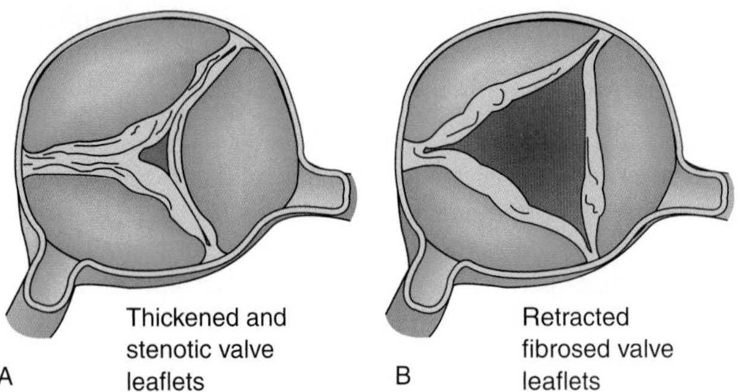

FIGURE 26-19 Disease of the aortic valve as viewed from the aorta. (**A**) Stenosis of the valve opening. (**B**) An incompetent or regurgitant valve that is unable to close completely.

Although any of the four heart valves can become diseased, the most commonly affected are the mitral and aortic valves. Disorders of the pulmonary and tricuspid valves are uncommon, probably because of the low pressure in the right side of the heart.

The heart valves consist of thin leaflets of tough, flexible, endothelium-covered fibrous tissue firmly attached at the base to the fibrous valve rings (see Chapter 23). Capillaries and smooth muscle are present at the base of the leaflet but do not extend up into the valve. The leaflets of the heart valves may be injured or become the site of an inflammatory process that can deform their line of closure. Healing of the valve leaflets often is associated with increased collagen content and scarring, causing the leaflets to shorten and become stiffer. The edges of the valve leaflets can heal together so that the valve does not open or close properly.

Two types of mechanical disruptions occur with valvular heart disease: narrowing of the valve opening so that it does not open properly and distortion of the valve so that it does not close properly (Fig. 26-19). *Stenosis* refers to a narrowing of the valve orifice and failure of the valve leaflets to open normally. Blood flow through a normal valve can increase by five to seven times the resting volume; consequently, valvular stenosis must be severe before it causes problems. Significant narrowing of the valve orifice increases the resistance to blood flow through the valve, converting the normally smooth laminar flow to a less efficient turbulent flow. This increases the volume and work of the chamber emptying through the narrowed valve—the left atrium in the case of mitral stenosis and the left ventricle in aortic stenosis. Symptoms usually are noticed first during situations of increased flow, such as exercise. An *incompetent* or *regurgitant valve* permits backward flow to occur when the valve should be closed—flowing back into the left ventricle during diastole when the aortic valve is affected and back into the left atrium during systole when the mitral valve is diseased.

The effect that valvular heart disease has on cardiac function is related to alterations in blood flow across the valve and to the resultant increase in work demands on the heart that the disorder generates. Many valvular heart defects are characterized by heart murmurs resulting from turbulent blood flow through a diseased valve. Disorders in valve flow and heart chamber size for mitral and aortic valve disorders are illustrated in Figure 26-20.

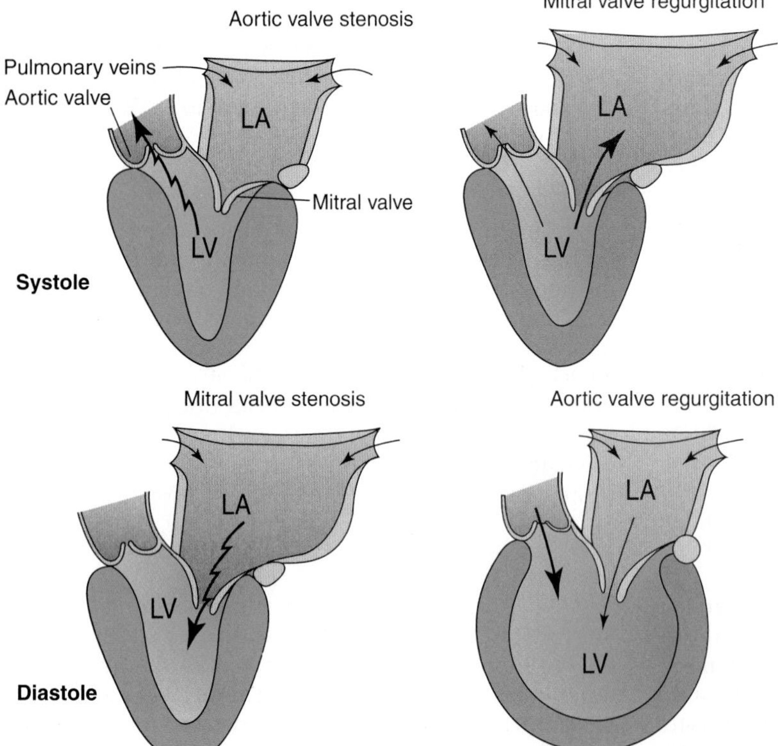

FIGURE 26-20 Alterations in hemodynamic function that accompany aortic valve stenosis, mitral valve regurgitation, mitral valve stenosis, and aortic valve regurgitation. *Thin arrows* indicate direction of normal flow, and *thick arrows* the direction of abnormal flow.

VALVULAR HEART DISEASE

- The heart valves determine the direction of blood flow through the heart chambers.
- Valvular heart defects exert their effects by obstructing flow of blood (stenotic valve disorder) or allowing backward flow of blood (regurgitant valve disorders).
- Stenotic valvular defects produce distention of the heart chamber that empties blood through the diseased valve and impaired filling of the chamber that receives blood that moves through the valve.
- Regurgitant valves allow blood to move back through the valve when it should be closed. This produces distention and places increased work demands on the chamber ejecting blood through the diseased valve.

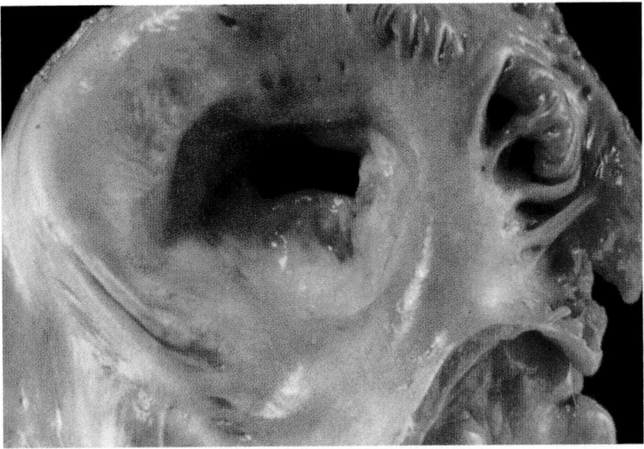

FIGURE 26-21 Chronic rheumatic valvulitis. A view of the mitral valve from the left atrium shows rigid, thickened, and fused leaflets with a narrow orifice, creating the characteristic "fish mouth" appearance of the rheumatic mitral stenosis. (Rubin E., Farber J.L. [1999]. *Pathology* [3rd ed., p. 570]. Philadelphia: Lippincott-Raven)

MITRAL VALVE DISORDERS

The mitral valve controls the directional flow of blood between the left atrium and the left ventricle. The edges or cusps of the AV valves are thinner than those of the semilunar valves; they are anchored to the papillary muscles by the chordae tendineae. During much of systole, the mitral valve is subjected to the high pressure generated by the left ventricle as it pumps blood into the systemic circulation. During this period of increased pressure, the chordae tendineae prevent the eversion of the valve leaflets into the left atrium (see Chapter 23, Fig. 23-13).

Mitral Valve Stenosis

Mitral valve stenosis represents the incomplete opening of the mitral valve during diastole with left atrial distention and impaired filling of the left ventricle. Mitral valve stenosis most commonly is the result of rheumatic fever.[65] Less frequently, the defect is congenital and manifests during infancy or early childhood. Mitral valve stenosis is a continuous, progressive, lifelong disorder, consisting of a slow, stable course in the early years and progressive acceleration in later years.

Mitral valve stenosis is characterized by fibrous replacement of valvular tissue, along with stiffness and fusion of the valve apparatus (Fig. 26-21). Typically, the mitral cusps fuse at the edges, and involvement of the chordae tendineae causes shortening, which pulls the valvular structures more deeply into the ventricles. As the resistance to flow through the valve increases, the left atrium becomes dilated and left atrial pressure rises. The increased left atrial pressure eventually is transmitted to the pulmonary venous system, causing pulmonary congestion.

The rate of flow across the valve depends on the size of the valve orifice, the driving pressure (*i.e.*, atrial minus ventricular pressure), and the time available for flow during diastole. The normal mitral valve area is 4 to 5 cm^2. Narrowing of the valve area to less than 2 cm^2 must occur before mild symptoms begin to develop.[65] As the condition progresses, symptoms of decreased cardiac output occur during extreme exertion or other situations that cause tachycardia and thereby reduce diastolic filling time. In the late stages of the disease, pulmonary vascular resistance increases with the development of pulmonary hypertension; this increases the pressure against which the right heart must pump and eventually leads to right-sided heart failure.

The signs and symptoms of mitral valve stenosis depend on the severity of the obstruction and are related to the elevation in left atrial pressure and pulmonary congestion, decreased cardiac output owing to impaired left ventricular filling, and left atrial enlargement with development of atrial arrhythmias and mural thrombi. The symptoms are those of pulmonary congestion, including nocturnal paroxysmal dyspnea and orthopnea. Palpitations, chest pain, weakness, and fatigue are common complaints. Premature atrial beats, paroxysmal atrial tachycardia, and atrial fibrillation may occur as a result of distention of the left atrium. Atrial fibrillation develops in 30% to 40% of persons with symptomatic mitral stenosis.[65] Together, the fibrillation and distention predispose to mural thrombus formation. The risk for arterial embolization, particularly stroke, is significantly increased in persons with atrial fibrillation.

The murmur of mitral valve stenosis is heard during diastole when blood is flowing through the constricted valve orifice; it is characteristically a low-pitched, rumbling murmur, best heard at the apex of the heart. The first heart sound often is accentuated and somewhat delayed because of the increased left atrial pressure; an opening snap may precede the diastolic murmur as a result of the elevation in left atrial pressure.

Medical treatment of mitral valve stenosis is aimed at relieving signs of decreased cardiac output and pulmonary congestion. Anticoagulation therapy is used to prevent systemic embolization in persons with atrial fibrillation. Three different procedures can be used to correct valve function: percutaneous mitral balloon valvuloplasty, mitral valve repair, and mitral valve replacement. Percutaneous balloon valvuloplasty, which emerged in the 1980s, has become an accepted alternative to surgical treatments in selected people.

Mitral Valve Regurgitation

Mitral valve regurgitation is characterized by incomplete closure of the mitral valve, with the left ventricular stroke volume being divided between the forward stroke volume that moves into the aorta and the regurgitant stroke volume that moves back into the left atrium during systole (see Fig. 26-20). Mitral valve regurgitation can result from many processes. Rheumatic heart disease is associated with a rigid and thickened valve that does not open or close completely. In addition to rheumatic disease, mitral regurgitation can result from rupture of the chordae tendineae or papillary muscles, papillary muscle dysfunction, or stretching of the valve structures due to dilatation of the left ventricle or valve orifice. Mitral valve prolapse is a common cause of mitral valve regurgitation.

Acute mitral valve regurgitation may occur abruptly, such as with papillary muscle dysfunction after myocardial infarction, valve perforation in infective endocarditis, or ruptured chordae tendineae in mitral valve prolapse. In acute severe mitral regurgitation, acute volume overload increases left ventricular preload, allowing a modest increase in left ventricular stroke volume. However, the forward stroke volume (that moving through the aorta into the systemic circulation) is reduced, and the regurgitant stroke volume leads to a rapid rise in left atrial pressure and pulmonary edema. Acute mitral valve prolapse almost always is symptomatic; if severe, mitral valve replacement often is indicated.

The hemodynamic changes that occur with chronic mitral valve regurgitation occur more slowly, allowing for recruitment of compensatory mechanisms. An increase in left ventricular end-diastolic volume permits an increase in total stroke volume, with restoration of forward flow into the aorta. Augmented preload and reduced or normal afterload (provided by unloading the left ventricle into the left atrium) facilitates left ventricular ejection. At the same time, a gradual increase in left atrial size allows for accommodation of the regurgitant volume at a lower filling pressure.

The increased volume of work associated with mitral regurgitation is relatively well tolerated, and many persons with the disorder remain asymptomatic for many years, with the average interval of 16 years from diagnosis to onset of symptoms.[66] The degree of left ventricular enlargement reflects the severity of regurgitation. As the disorder progresses, left ventricular function becomes impaired, the forward (aortic) stroke volume decreases, and the left atrial pressure increases, with the subsequent development of pulmonary congestion. Mitral regurgitation, like mitral stenosis, predisposes to atrial fibrillation.

A characteristic feature of mitral valve regurgitation is an enlarged left ventricle, a hyperdynamic left ventricular impulse, and a pansystolic (throughout systole) murmur. Valvular surgery may be indicated for persons with severe regurgitant disease.

Mitral Valve Prolapse

Sometimes referred to as the *floppy mitral valve syndrome,* mitral valve prolapse occurs in 2.4% to 7% of the general population.[67] The disorder is seen more frequently in women than in men and may have a familial basis. Although the cause of the disorder usually is unknown, it has been associated with Marfan's syndrome, osteogenesis imperfecta, and other connective tissue disorders and with cardiac, hematologic, neuroendocrine, metabolic, and psychological disorders.

Pathologic findings in persons with mitral valve prolapse include a myxedematous (mucinous) degeneration of mitral valve leaflets that causes them to become enlarged and floppy so that they prolapse or balloon back into the left atrium during systole[48] (Fig. 26-22). Secondary fibrotic changes reflect the stresses and injury that the ballooning movements impose on the valve. Certain forms of mitral valve prolapse may arise from disorders of the myocardium that result in abnormal movement of the ventricular wall or papillary muscle; this places undue stress on the mitral valve.

Most persons with mitral valve prolapse are asymptomatic, and the disorder is discovered during a routine physical examination. A minority of persons have chest pain mimicking angina, dyspnea, fatigue, anxiety, palpitations, and light-headedness. Unlike angina, the chest pain often is prolonged, ill defined, and not associated with exercise or exertion. The pain has been attributed to ischemia resulting from traction of the prolapsing valve leaflets. The anxiety, palpitations, and arrhythmias may result from abnormal autonomic nervous system function that commonly accompanies the disorder. Rare cases of sudden death have been reported in persons with mitral valve prolapse, mainly those with a family history of similar occurrences.

The disorder is characterized by a spectrum of auscultatory findings, ranging from a silent form to one or more midsystolic clicks followed by a late systolic murmur. Various abnormal ECG changes can occur. Arrhythmias may be brought out by exercise stress testing or detected on

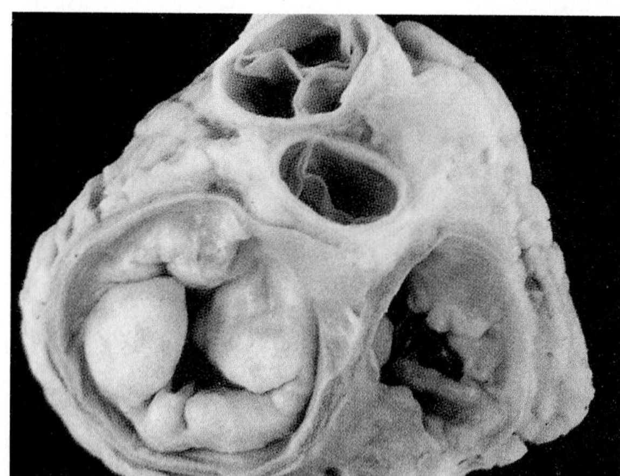

FIGURE 26-22 Mitral valve prolapse. A view of the mitral valve from the left atrium shows redundant and deformed leaflets that billow into the left atrial cavity. (Rubin E., Farber J.L. [1999]. *Pathology* [3rd ed., p. 574]. Philadelphia: Lippincott-Raven)

24-hour ECG monitoring. Echocardiographic studies have become a method for the diagnosis of mitral valve prolapse, and the availability of this technique undoubtedly has contributed to increased recognition of the problem, particularly in its asymptomatic form.

The treatment of mitral valve prolapse focuses on the relief of symptoms and the prevention of complications.[63,64] Persons with palpitations and mild tachyarrhythmias or increased adrenergic symptoms and those with chest discomfort, anxiety, and fatigue often respond to therapy with the β-adrenergic–blocking drugs. In many cases, the cessation of stimulants such as caffeine, alcohol, and cigarettes may be sufficient to control symptoms. Infective endocarditis is an uncommon complication in persons with a murmur; antibiotic prophylaxis usually is recommended before dental or surgical procedures associated with bacteremia. Persons with severe valve dysfunction may require valve surgery.

AORTIC VALVE DISORDERS

The aortic valve is located between the aorta and left ventricle. The aortic valve has three cusps and sometimes is referred to as the *aortic semilunar valve* because its leaflets are crescent or moon shaped (see Chapter 23, Fig. 23-10). The aortic valve has no chordae tendineae. Although their structures are similar, the cusps of the aortic valve are thicker than those of the mitral valve. The middle layer of the aortic valve is thickened near the middle, where the three leaflets meet, ensuring a tight seal. Between the thickened tissue and their free margins, the leaflets are more thin and flimsy.

An important aspect of the aortic valve is the location of the orifices for the two main coronary arteries, which are located behind the valve and at right angles to the direction of blood flow. It is the lateral pressure in the aorta that propels blood into the coronary arteries (Fig. 26-23). During the ejection phase of the cardiac cycle, the lateral pressure is diminished by conversion of potential energy to kinetic energy as blood moves forward into the aorta. This process is grossly exaggerated in aortic stenosis because of the high flow velocities.

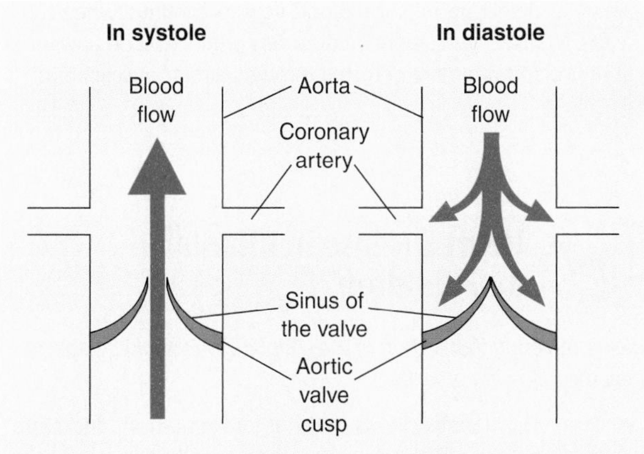

FIGURE 26-23 Location of the orifices for the coronary arteries in relation to the aortic valve and the direction of blood flow during systole and diastole.

Aortic Valve Stenosis

Aortic valve stenosis is characterized by increased resistance to ejection of blood from the left ventricle into the aorta (see Fig. 26-20). Because of the increased resistance, the work demands on the left ventricle are increased, and the volume of blood ejected into the systemic circulation is decreased. The most common causes of aortic stenosis are rheumatic fever and congenital valve malformations. Congenital malformations may result in unicuspid, bicuspid, or misshaped valve leaflets. In elderly persons, stenosis may be related to degenerative atherosclerotic changes of the valve leaflets. Approximately 25% of persons older than 65 years of age and 35% of those older than 70 years of age have echocardiographic evidence of sclerosis, with 2% to 3% having evidence of aortic stenosis.[68]

The progression of aortic stenosis varies widely among individuals. The progression may be more rapid in persons with degenerative calcific disease than in those with congenital or rheumatic disease. The aortic valve must be reduced to approximately one fourth its normal size before critical changes in cardiac function occur.[69] Significant obstruction to aortic outflow causes a decrease in stroke volume, along with a reduction in systolic blood pressure and pulse pressure. Because of the narrowed valve opening, it takes longer for the heart to eject blood; the heart rate often is slow, and the pulse is of low amplitude. There is a soft, absent, or paradoxically split S_2 sound and a harsh systolic ejection murmur that is heard best along the left sternal border.

Persons with aortic stenosis tend to be asymptomatic for many years despite severe obstruction. Eventually, symptoms of angina, syncope, and heart failure develop. Angina occurs in approximately two thirds of persons with advanced aortic stenosis and is similar to that observed in CHD. Syncope (fainting) is most commonly due to the reduced cerebral circulation that occurs during exertion when the arterial pressure declines consequent to vasodilation in the presence of a fixed cardiac output. Exertional hypotension may cause "graying out" spells or dizziness on exercise.[65] Dyspnea, marked fatigability, peripheral cyanosis, and other signs of low-output heart failure usually are not prominent until late in the course of the disease.

Both percutaneous balloon valvuloplasty and aortic valve replacement are used in the treatment of aortic stenosis. Percutaneous balloon valvuloplasty may be used to treat aortic stenosis in adolescents and young adults. In most adults with aortic valve stenosis, aortic valve replacement is the most effective treatment.

Aortic Valve Regurgitation

Aortic regurgitation is the result of an incompetent aortic valve that allows blood to flow back to the left ventricle during diastole (see Fig. 26-20). As a result, the left ventricle must increase its stroke volume to include blood entering from the lungs as well as that leaking back through the regurgitant valve. This defect may result from conditions that cause scarring of the valve leaflets or from enlargement of the valve orifice to the extent that the valve leaflets no longer meet. Rheumatic fever ranks first on the list of causes of aortic regurgitation; failure of a prosthetic valve is another cause.

Acute aortic regurgitation is characterized by the presentation of a sudden, large regurgitant volume to a left ventricle of normal size that has not had time to adapt to the volume overload. It is caused most commonly by disorders such as infective endocarditis, trauma, or aortic dissection. Although the heart responds with use of the Frank-Starling mechanisms and an increase in heart rate, these compensatory mechanisms fail to maintain the cardiac output. As a result, there is severe elevation in left ventricular end-diastolic pressure, which is transmitted to the left atrium and pulmonary veins, culminating in pulmonary edema. A decrease in cardiac output leads to sympathetic stimulation and a resultant increase in heart rate and peripheral vascular resistance that cause the regurgitation to worsen. Death from pulmonary edema, ventricular arrhythmias, or circulatory collapse is common in severe acute aortic regurgitation.

Chronic aortic regurgitation, which usually has a gradual onset, represents a condition of combined left ventricular volume and pressure overload. As the valve deformity increases, regurgitant flow into the left ventricle increases, diastolic blood pressure falls, and the left ventricle progressively enlarges. Hemodynamically, the increase in left ventricular volume results in the ejection of a large stroke volume that usually is adequate to maintain the forward cardiac output until late in the course of the disease. Most persons remain asymptomatic during this compensated phase, which may last decades. The only sign for many years may be soft systolic aortic murmur.

As the disease progresses, signs and symptoms of left ventricular failure begin to appear. These include exertional dyspnea, orthopnea, and paroxysmal nocturnal dyspnea. In aortic regurgitation, failure of aortic valve closure during diastole causes an abnormal drop in diastolic pressure. Because coronary blood flow is greatest during diastole, the drop in diastolic pressure produces a decrease in coronary perfusion. Although angina is rare, it may occur when the heart rate and diastolic pressure fall to low levels. Persons with severe aortic regurgitation often complain of an uncomfortable awareness of heartbeat, particularly when lying down, and chest discomfort due to pounding of the heart against the chest wall. Tachycardia, occurring with emotional stress or exertion, may produce palpitations, head pounding, and premature ventricular contractions.

The major physical findings relate to the widening of the arterial pulse pressure. The pulse has a rapid rise and fall (Corrigan's pulse), with an elevated systolic pressure and low diastolic pressure owing to the large stroke volume and rapid diastolic runoff of blood back into the left ventricle. Korotkoff sounds may persist to zero, even though intraarterial pressure rarely falls below 30 mm Hg.[65] The large stroke volume and wide pulse pressure may result in prominent carotid pulsations in the neck, throbbing peripheral pulses, and a left ventricular impulse that causes the chest to move with each beat. The hyperkinetic pulse of more severe aortic regurgitation, called a *water-hammer pulse,* is characterized by distention and quick collapse of the artery. In persons with severe aortic stenosis, the head may bob with each heartbeat (*i.e.,* de Musset's sign). The turbulence of flow across the aortic valve during diastole produces a high-pitched or blowing sound.

Treatment includes medical management of heart failure and associated problems. Surgery (valve replacement or repair) usually is indicated once aortic regurgitation causes symptoms.

DIAGNOSIS AND TREATMENT

Valvular defects usually are detected through cardiac auscultation (*i.e.,* heart sounds). Diagnosis is aided by phonocardiography, echocardiography, and cardiac catheterization. A phonocardiogram (a permanent recording of the heart sounds) is obtained by placing a high-fidelity microphone on the chest wall over the heart while a recording is made. An ECG tracing usually is made simultaneously for timing purposes.

The treatment of valvular defects consists of medical management of heart failure and associated problems and surgical intervention to repair or replace the defective valve. Surgical valve repair or replacement depends on the valve that is involved and the extent of deformity. Valvular replacement with a prosthetic device or a homograft usually is reserved for severe disease because the ideal substitute valve has not yet been invented. Percutaneous balloon valvuloplasty involves the opening of a stenotic valve by guiding an inflated balloon through the valve orifice. The procedure is done in the cardiac catheterization laboratory and involves the insertion of a balloon catheter into the heart by way of a peripheral blood vessel.

In summary, dysfunction of the heart valves can result from a number of disorders, including congenital defects, trauma, ischemic heart disease, degenerative changes, and inflammation. Rheumatic endocarditis is a common cause. Valvular heart disease produces its effects through disturbances of blood flow. A stenotic valvular defect is one that causes a decrease in blood flow through a valve, resulting in impaired emptying and increased work demands on the heart chamber that empties blood across the diseased valve. A regurgitant valvular defect permits the blood flow to continue when the valve is closed. Valvular heart disorders produce blood flow turbulence and often are detected through cardiac auscultation.

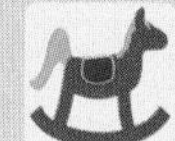

Heart Disease in Infants and Children

After completing this section of the chapter, you should be able to meet the following objectives:

- Trace the flow of blood in the fetal circulation, and state the function of the foramen ovale and ductus arteriosus
- State the changes in circulatory function that occur at birth
- Compare the effects of left-to-right and right-to-left shunts on the pulmonary circulation and production of cyanosis

- Describe the anatomic defects and altered patterns of blood flow in children with atrial septal defects, ventricular septal defects, endocardial cushion defects, pulmonary stenosis, tetralogy of Fallot, patent ductus arteriosus, transposition of the great vessels, and coarctation of the aorta
- Compare the role of infectious organisms in Kawasaki disease to that of the immune system
- Describe the manifestations related to each phase—acute, subacute, and convalescent phase—of Kawasaki disease

Approximately 40,000 infants are born each year with a congenital heart defect.[1] Kawasaki disease is another disorder of children. Along with end-stage renal disease, it ranks as the second cause of death (behind accidents) in children younger than 15 years.[1]

Advances in diagnostic methods and surgical treatment have greatly increased the long-term survival and outcomes for children born with congenital heart defects. The diagnosis is now established within the first week of life in 40% to 50% of infants and in the first month in 50% to 60% of infants.[70] Surgical correction of many of these defects is now possible, often within the first weeks of life.

EMBRYONIC DEVELOPMENT OF THE HEART

The heart is the first functioning organ in the embryo; its first pulsatile movements begin during the third week after conception. This early development of the heart is essential to the rapidly growing embryo as a means of circulating nutrients and removing waste products. Most of the development of the heart and blood vessels occurs between the third and eighth weeks of embryonic life.

The developing heart begins as two endothelial tubes that fuse into a single tubular structure.[70,71] The early heart structures develop as the tubular heart elongates and forms alternate dilations and constrictions. A single atrium and ventricle along with the bulbus cordis develop first. This is followed by formation of the truncus arteriosus and the sinus venosus, a large venous sinus that receives blood from the embryo and developing placenta (Fig. 26-24). The early pulsatile movements of the heart begin in the sinus venosus and move blood out of the heart by way of the bulbus cordis, truncus arteriosus, and aortic arches.

A differential growth rate in the early cardiac structures, along with fixation of the heart at the venous and arterial ends, causes the tubular heart to bend over on itself. As the heart bends, the atrium and the sinus venosus come to lie behind the bulbus cordis, truncus arteriosus, and ventricle. This looping of the primitive heart results in the heart's alignment in the left side of the chest with the atrium located behind the ventricle. Malrotation during formation of the ventricular loop can cause various malpositions, such as dextroposition of the heart.

The embryonic heart undergoes further development as partitioning of the chambers occurs. Partitioning of the AV canal, atrium, and ventricle begins in the fourth week and essentially is complete by the fifth week. The separation of the heart begins as tissue bundles, called the *endocardial cushions,* form in the midportion of the dorsal and ventral walls of the heart in the region of the AV canal and begin to grow inward. Until the separation begins, a single AV canal exists between the atria and the ventricles. As the endocardial cushions enlarge, they meet and fuse to form separate right and left AV canals (Fig. 26-25). The mitral and tricuspid valves develop in these canals. The endocardial cushions also contribute to formation of parts of the atrial and ventricular septum. Defects in endocardial cushion formation can result in atrial and ventricular septal defects, complete AV canal defects, and anomalies of the mitral and tricuspid valves.

Compartmentalization of the ventricles begins with the growth of the interventricular septum from the floor of the ventricle moving upward toward the endocardial cushions. Fusion of the endocardial cushions with the interventricular septum usually is completed by the end of the seventh week.

Partitioning of the atrial septum is more complex and occurs in two stages, beginning with the formation of a thin, crescent-shaped membrane called the *septum primum* that emerges from the anterosuperior portion of the heart and grows toward the endocardial cushions, leaving an

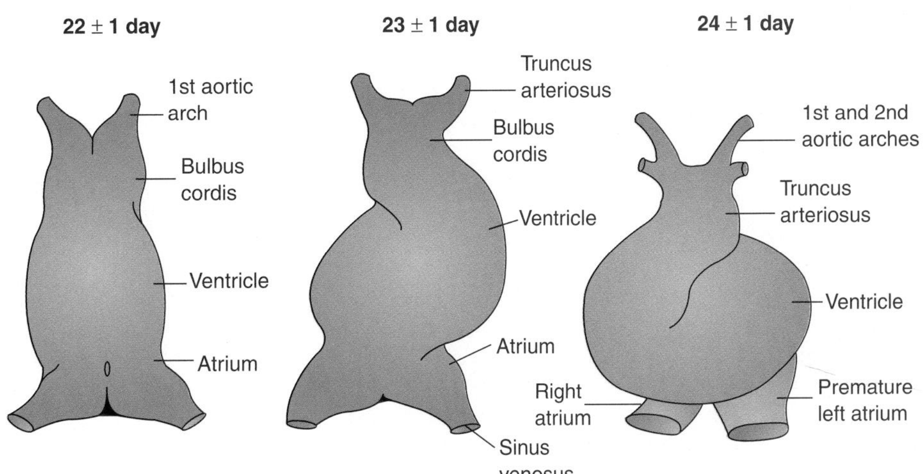

FIGURE 26-24 Ventral view of the developing heart (20–25 days). (Adapted from Moore K.L. [1977]. *The developing human* [2nd ed.]. Philadelphia: W.B. Saunders)

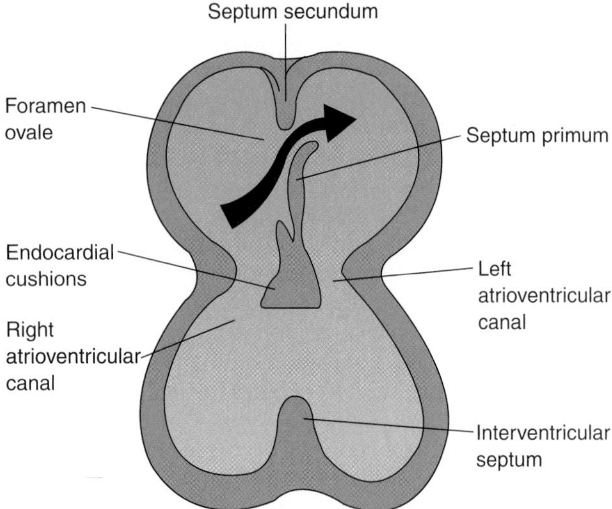

FIGURE 26-25 Development of the endocardial cushions, right and left atrioventricular canals, interventricular septum, and septum primum and septum secundum of the foramen ovale. Note that blood from the right atrium flows through the foramen ovale to the left atrium.

opening called the *foramen primum* between its lower edge and the endocardial cushions. A second membrane, called the *septum secundum,* also begins to grow from the upper wall of the atrium on the right side of the septum primum. As this membrane grows toward the endocardial cushions, it gradually overlaps an opening in the upper part of the septum primum, forming an oval opening with a flap-type valve called the *foramen ovale* (see Fig. 26-25). The upper part of the septum primum gradually disappears; the remaining part becomes the valve of the foramen ovale. The foramen ovale forms a communicating channel between the two upper chambers of the heart. This opening, which closes shortly after birth, allows blood from the umbilical vein to pass directly into the left heart, bypassing the lungs. An *ostium secundum defect,* which is one type of atrial septal defect, is thought to result from excessive absorption of the septum primum.

To complete the transformation into a four-chambered heart, provision must be made for separating the blood pumped from the right side of the heart, which is to be diverted into the pulmonary circulation, from the blood pumped from the left side of the heart, which is to be pumped to the systemic circulation. This separation of blood flow is accomplished by developmental changes in the outflow channels of the tubular heart, the *bulbus cordis* and the *truncus arteriosus,* which undergo spiral twisting and vertical partitioning (Fig. 26-26). As these vessels spiral and divide, the location of the aorta becomes posterior and to the right of the pulmonary artery. Impaired spiraling during this stage of development can lead to defects such as *transposition of the great vessels.*

In the process of forming a separate pulmonary trunk and aorta, a vessel called the *ductus arteriosus* develops. This vessel, which connects the pulmonary artery and the aorta, allows blood entering the pulmonary trunk to be shunted into the aorta as a means of bypassing the lungs. Like the foramen ovale, the ductus arteriosus usually closes shortly after birth.

FETAL AND PERINATAL CIRCULATION

The fetal circulation is different anatomically and physiologically than the postnatal circulation. Before birth, oxygenation of blood occurs by way of the placenta, and after birth, it occurs by way of the lungs. The fetus is maintained in a low-oxygen state (PO_2, 30 to 35 mm Hg; 60% to 70% saturation).[70–72] To compensate, fetal cardiac output is higher than at any other time in life (400 to 500 mL/kg/minute). Also, the pulmonary vessels in the fetus are markedly constricted owing to the fluid-filled lungs and the heightened hypoxic stimulus for vasoconstriction that is present in the fetus. As a result, blood flow through the lungs is less than at any other time in life.

In the fetus, blood enters the circulation through the umbilical vein and returns to the placenta by way of the two umbilical arteries (Fig. 26-27). A vessel called the *ductus venosum* allows blood from the umbilical vein to bypass the hepatic circulation and pass directly into the inferior vena cava. From the inferior vena cava, blood flows into

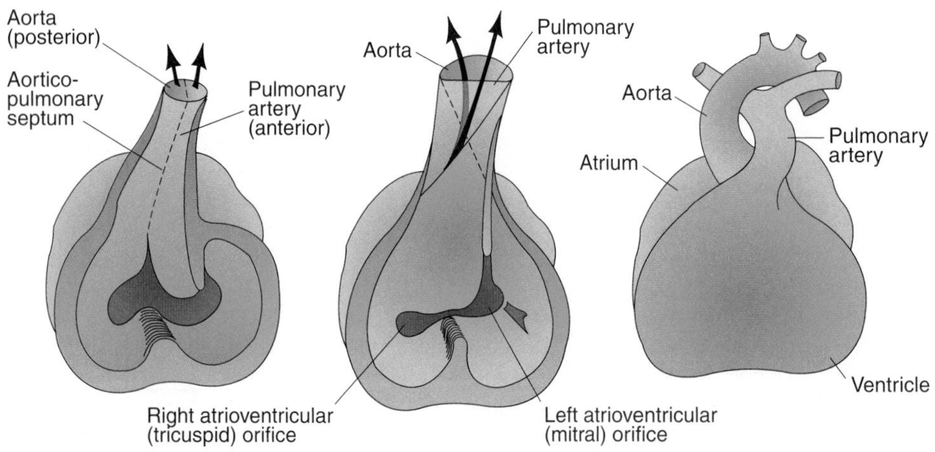

FIGURE 26-26 Separation and twisting of the truncus arteriosus to form the pulmonary artery and aorta.

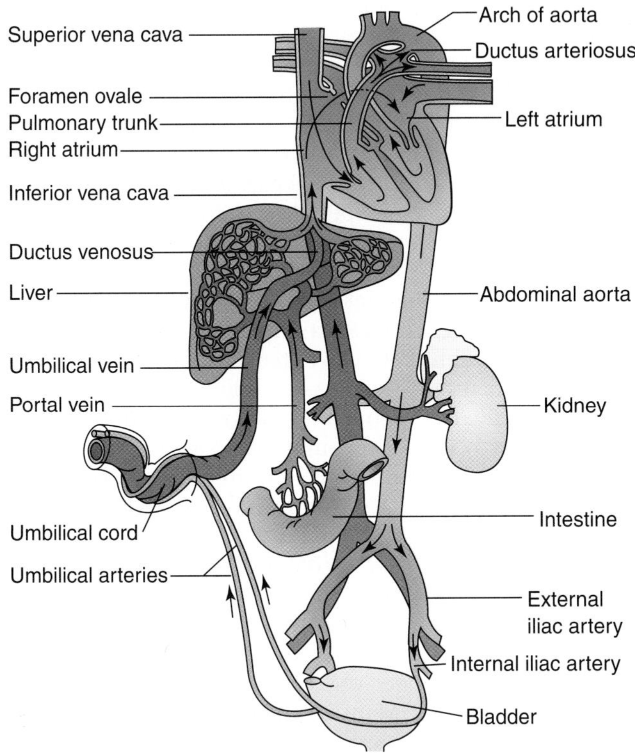

FIGURE 26-27 Fetal circulation.

the right atrium and then moves through the foramen ovale into the left atrium. It then passes into the left ventricle and is ejected into the ascending aorta to perfuse the head and upper extremities. In this way, the best-oxygenated blood from the placenta is used to perfuse the brain. At the same time, venous blood from the head and upper extremities returns to the right side of the heart by way of the superior vena cava, moves into the right ventricle, and is ejected into the pulmonary artery. Because of the very high pulmonary vascular resistance that is present, blood ejected into the pulmonary artery gets diverted through the ductus arteriosus into the descending aorta. This blood perfuses the lower extremities and is returned to the placenta by way of the umbilical arteries.

At birth, the infant takes its first breath and switches from placental to pulmonary oxygenation of the blood. The most dramatic alterations in the circulation after birth are the elimination of the low-resistance placental vascular bed and the marked pulmonary vasodilation that is produced by initiation of ventilation. The pressure in the pulmonary circulation and the right side of the heart falls as fetal lung fluid is replaced by air and as lung expansion decreases the pressure transmitted to the pulmonary blood vessels. With lung inflation, the alveolar oxygen tension increases, causing reversal of the hypoxemia-induced pulmonary vasoconstriction of the fetal circulation. Cord clamping and removal of the low-resistance placental circulation produce an increase in systemic vascular resistance and a resultant increase in left ventricular pressure. The resultant decrease in right atrial pressure and increase in left atrial pressure produce closure of the foramen ovale. Reversal of the fetal hypoxemic state also produces constriction of ductal smooth muscle, contributing to closure of the ductus arteriosus. The foramen ovale and the ductus arteriosus normally close within the first day of life, effectively separating the pulmonary and systemic circulations.

After the initial precipitous fall in pulmonary vascular resistance, a more gradual decrease in pulmonary vascular resistance is related to regression of the medial smooth muscle layer in the pulmonary arteries. During the first 2 to 9 weeks of life, gradual thinning of the smooth muscle layer results in further decreases in pulmonary vascular resistance. By the time a healthy, term infant is several weeks old, the pulmonary vascular resistance has fallen to adult levels.

Several factors, including prematurity, alveolar hypoxia, lung disease, and congenital heart defects, may affect postnatal pulmonary vascular development.[72] If an infant is born prematurely, the smooth muscle layers of the pulmonary vasculature may develop incompletely or regress in a shorter period. Much of the development of the smooth muscle layer in the pulmonary arterioles occurs during the latter part of gestation; as a result, infants who are born prematurely have less medial smooth muscle. These infants follow the same pattern of smooth muscle regression, but because less muscle exists, the muscle layer may regress in a shorter period. The pulmonary vascular smooth muscle in premature infants also may be less responsive to hypoxia. For these reasons, a premature infant may demonstrate a larger decrease in pulmonary vascular resistance and a resultant shunting of blood from the aorta through the ductus arteriosus to the pulmonary artery within hours of birth.

Hypoxia during the first days of life may also delay or prevent the normal decrease in pulmonary vascular resistance. During this period, the pulmonary arteries remain highly reactive and can constrict in response to hypoxia, acidosis, hyperinflation of the alveoli, and hypothermia. Alveolar hypoxia is one of the most potent stimuli of pulmonary vasoconstriction and pulmonary hypertension in the neonate.

CONGENITAL HEART DEFECTS

The major development of the fetal heart occurs between the fourth and seventh weeks of gestation, and most congenital heart defects arise during this time. The development of the heart may be altered by environmental, genetic, and chromosomal influences.

Most congenital heart defects are thought to be multifactorial in origin, resulting from an interaction between a genetic predisposition toward development of a heart defect and environmental influences. Infants born to parents with congenital heart defects or with siblings who have congenital heart defects are at higher risk. Some heart defects, such as coarctation of the aorta, atrial septal defect of the secundum type, pulmonary valve stenosis, and certain ventricular septal defects, have a stronger familial predisposition than others.

Approximately 13% of children with congenital heart disease have an associated chromosomal abnormality. Heart disease is found in 90% of children with trisomy 18, 50% of those with trisomy 21, and 40% of those with Turner's syndrome.[70] Another 2% to 4% of cases result from adverse maternal conditions and teratogenic influences, including maternal diabetes, congenital rubella, maternal alcohol ingestion, and treatment with anticonvulsant drugs.

Ultrasound technology now allows examination of fetal development and function in utero.[70,73] Diagnostic images of the fetal heart can be obtained as early as 16 weeks of gestation. Echocardiography of the fetus allows for differentiation among heart defects in the fetus. Among the disorders that can be diagnosed with certainty by fetal echocardiography are hypoplastic left heart syndrome, aortic valve stenosis, hypertrophic cardiomyopathy, pulmonic valve stenosis, AV septal defect, transposition of the great arteries, and patent ductus arteriosus.[73]

Depending on the type of defect, children with congenital heart disease experience various signs and symptoms associated with altered heart action, heart failure, pulmonary vascular disorders, and difficulty in supplying the peripheral tissues with oxygen and other nutrients.

Acyanotic and Cyanotic Disorders

Congenital heart defects produce their effects through abnormal shunting of blood and alterations in pulmonary blood flow. They commonly are classified as congenital heart disease with cyanosis or congenital heart disease with little or no cyanosis.[70,73,74] Left-to-right shunts commonly are categorized as acyanotic disorders and right-to-left shunts with obstruction as cyanotic disorders. Of the congenital defects discussed in this chapter, patent ductus arteriosus, atrial and ventricular septal defects, endocardial cushion defects, pulmonary valve stenosis, and coarctation of the aorta are considered defects with little or no cyanosis; tetralogy of Fallot and transposition of the great vessels are considered defects with cyanosis.

Shunting of blood refers to the diverting of blood flow from one system to the other—from the arterial to the venous system (*i.e.,* left-to-right shunt) or from the venous to the arterial system (*i.e.,* right-to-left shunt). The shunting of blood in congenital heart defects is determined by the presence of an abnormal opening between the right and left circulations and the degree of resistance to flow through the opening.

A right-to-left shunt results in unoxygenated blood moving from the right side of the heart into the left side of the heart and then being ejected into the systemic circulation. Cyanosis develops when sufficient unoxygenated blood mixes with oxygenated blood in the left side of the heart. In left-to-right shunt, blood intended for ejection into the systemic circulation is recirculated through the right side of the heart and back through the lungs; this increased volume distends the right side of the heart and pulmonary circulation and increases the workload placed on the right ventricle. A child with a septal defect that causes left-to-right shunting usually has an enlarged right side of the heart and pulmonary blood vessels.

The vascular resistance of the systemic and pulmonary circulations may influence the direction of shunting. Because of the high pulmonary vascular resistance in the neonate, atrial and septal defects usually do not produce significant shunt or symptoms during the first weeks of life. As the pulmonary vascular smooth muscle regresses in the neonate, the resistance in the pulmonary circulation normally falls below that of the systemic circulation; in uncomplicated atrial or ventricular septal defects, blood shunts from the left side of the heart to the right. In more complicated ventricular septal defects, increased resistance to outflow may affect the pattern of shunting. For example, defects that increase resistance to aortic outflow (*e.g.,* aortic valve stenosis, coarctation of the aorta) increase left-to-right shunting, and defects that obstruct pulmonary outflow (*e.g.,* pulmonary valve stenosis, increased pulmonary vascular resistance) increase right-to-left shunting. Crying may increase right-to-left shunting in infants with septal defects by increasing pulmonary vascular resistance. This may be one of the reasons some infants with congenital heart defects become cyanotic during crying.

Changes in Pulmonary Vascular Resistance and Blood Flow

In contrast to the arterioles in the systemic circulation, the mature pulmonary arterioles are thin-walled vessels, and they can accommodate various levels of stroke volume from the right heart. Many of the complications of congenital heart disorders result from their effect on the pulmonary circulation, which may be exposed to an increase or a decrease in blood flow.

In a term infant who has a congenital heart defect that produces markedly increased pulmonary blood flow (*e.g.,* ventricular septal defect), the increased flow stimulates pulmonary vasoconstriction and prevents normal thinning of pulmonary vascular smooth muscle. These conditions delay or reduce the normal decrease in pulmonary vascular resistance. As a result, symptoms related to increased pulmonary blood flow often are not apparent until the infant is 4 to 12 weeks of age.

Congenital heart defects that persistently increase pulmonary blood flow or pulmonary vascular resistance have the potential of causing pulmonary hypertension and producing pathologic changes in the pulmonary vasculature. When shunting of systemic blood flow into the pulmonary circulation threatens permanent injury to the pulmonary vessels, a surgical procedure may be done in an attempt to reduce the flow by increasing resistance to outflow from the right ventricle. This procedure, called *pulmonary banding,* consists of placing a constrictive band around the main pulmonary artery.[70] The banding technique is used as a temporary measure to alleviate the symptoms and protect the pulmonary vessels in anticipation of later surgical repair of the defect.

Some congenital heart defects, such as pulmonary valve stenosis, decrease pulmonary blood flow, producing inadequate oxygenation of blood. The affected child may experience fatigue, exertional dyspnea, impaired growth, and even syncope.

Manifestations and Treatment

Congenital heart defects manifest with numerous signs and symptoms. Some defects, such as patent ductus arteriosus and small ventricular septal defects, close spontaneously, and in other, less severe defects, there are no signs and symptoms. The disorder typically is discovered during a routine health examination. Pulmonary congestion, cardiac failure, and decreased peripheral perfusion are the chief concerns in children with more severe defects. Such defects often cause problems shortly after birth or early in infancy. The child may exhibit cyanosis, respiratory difficulty, and fatigability and is likely to have difficulty with feeding and failure to thrive. A generalized cyanosis that persists longer than 3 hours after birth suggests congenital heart disease.

One technique for evaluating the infant consists of administering 100% oxygen for 10 minutes. If the infant "pinks up," the cyanosis probably was caused by respiratory problems. Because infant cyanosis may appear as duskiness, it is important to assess the color of the mucous membranes, fingernails, toenails, tongue, and lips. Pulmonary congestion in the infant causes an increase in respiratory rate, orthopnea, grunting, wheezing, coughing, and crackles. The infant whose peripheral perfusion is markedly decreased may appear to be in a shocklike state.

The manifestations and treatment of heart failure in the infant and young child are similar to those in the adult, but the infant's small size and limited physical reserve make the manifestations more serious and treatment more difficult. The treatment plan usually includes supportive therapy designed to help the infant compensate for the limitations in cardiac reserve and to prevent complications. Surgical intervention often is required for severe defects; it may be done in the early weeks of life or, conditions permitting, delayed until the child is older. A discussion of congestive heart failure in children is presented in Chapter 28.

Most children with structural congenital heart disease and those who have had corrective surgery are at risk for development of infectious endocarditis. These children should receive prophylactic antibiotic therapy during periods of increased risk for bacteremia.

Types of Defects

Congenital heart defects can affect almost any of the cardiac structures or central blood vessels. Defects include communication defects between heart chambers, interrupted development of the heart chambers or valve structures, malposition of heart chambers and great vessels, and altered closure of fetal communication channels. The particular defect reflects the embryo's stage of development at the time it occurred. Some congenital heart disorders, such as tetralogy of Fallot, involve several defects. The development of the heart is simultaneous and sequential; a heart defect may reflect the multiple developmental events that were occurring simultaneously or sequentially. At least 35 types of defects have been identified, the most common being patent ductus arteriosus (6% to 8%), atrial septal defects (6% to 8%), and ventricular septal defects (25% to 30%).[70]

Patent Ductus Arteriosus. Patent ductus arteriosus results from persistence of the fetal ductus beyond the prenatal period. In fetal life, the ductus arteriosus is the vital link by which blood from the right side of the heart bypasses the lungs and enters the systemic circulation (Fig. 26-28G). After birth, this passage no longer is needed, and it usually closes during the first 24 to 72 hours. The physiologic stimulus and mechanisms associated with permanent closure of the ductus are not entirely known, but the fact that infant hypoxia predisposes to a delayed closure suggests that the increase in arterial oxygen levels that occurs immediately after birth plays a role. Additional factors that contribute to closure are a fall in endogenous levels of prostaglandins and adenosine and the release of vasoactive substances. After constriction, the lumen of the ductus becomes permanently sealed with fibrous tissue within 2 to 3 weeks. Ductal closure may be delayed or prevented in very premature infants, probably as a result of a combination of factors, including decreased medial smooth muscle in the ductus wall, decreased constrictive response to oxygen, and increased circulating levels of prostaglandins, which have a vasodilating effect. Hemodynamically significant patent ductus arteriosus is observed in approximately one third of infants with birth weights less than 1500 g.[73] Ductal closure also may be delayed in infants with congenital heart defects that produce a decrease in oxygen tension.

As is true of other heart and circulatory defects, patency of the ductus arteriosus may vary; the size of the opening may be small, medium, or large. After the infant's pulmonary vascular resistance falls, the patent ductus arteriosus provides for a continuous runoff of aortic blood into the pulmonary artery, causing a decrease in aortic diastolic and mean arterial pressure and a widening of the pulse pressure. With a large patent ductus, the runoff is continuous, resulting in increased pulmonary blood flow, pulmonary congestion, and increased resistance against which the right side of the heart must pump. Increased pulmonary venous return and increased work demands may lead to left ventricular failure.

Patent ductus arteriosus can be treated either pharmacologically or surgically. Indomethacin, an inhibitor of prostaglandin synthesis, can be used to induce closure of a patent ductus arteriosus. Indomethacin has been associated with several adverse effects in newborns, including alterations in renal function and gastrointestinal complications. Recent studies suggest that ibuprofen, another prostaglandin inhibitor, may be equally effective in promoting closure and may produce fewer side effects.[75] Surgical closure can be accomplished using a transcatheter or a thoracoscopic approach. Transcatheter closure, using a Teflon plug, occlusive umbrella, or intravascular coil, is done in the cardiac catheterization laboratory.[70,73] The thoracoscopic surgical technique, which is used to ligate the ductus, allows closure to be accomplished without thoracotomy.

The function of the ductus arteriosus in providing a right-to-left shunt in prenatal life has prompted the surgical creation of an aortic-pulmonary shunt as a means of improving pulmonary blood flow in children with severe pulmonary outflow disorders. Research has focused on the role of type E prostaglandins in maintaining the patency of the ductus. By injecting prostaglandin E into the umbilical vein of infants who require a ductal shunt, closure has been delayed or prevented.

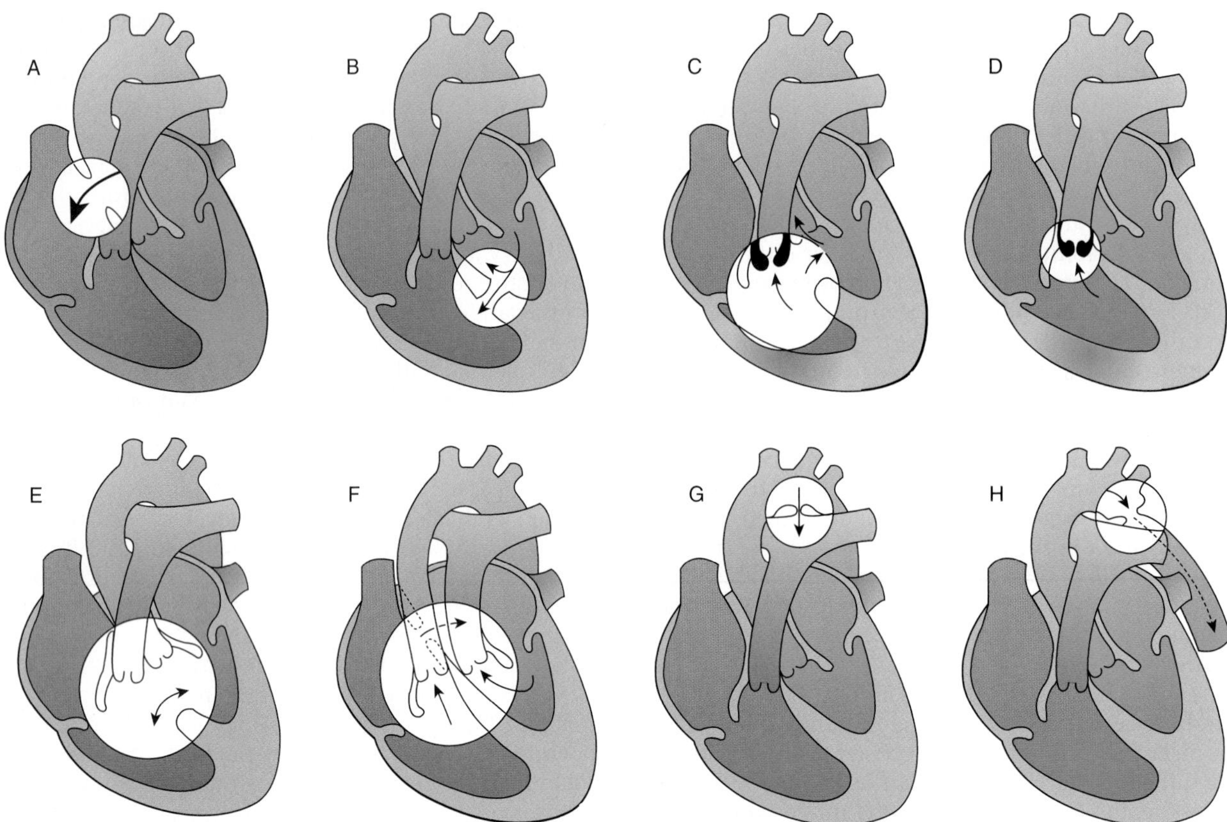

FIGURE 26-28 Congenital heart defects. (**A**) Atrial septal defect. Blood is shunted from left to right. (**B**) Ventricular septal defect. Blood is usually shunted from left to right. (**C**) Tetralogy of Fallot. This involves a ventricular septal defect, dextroposition of the aorta, right ventricular outflow obstruction, and right ventricular hypertrophy. Blood is shunted from right to left. (**D**) Pulmonary stenosis, with decreased pulmonary blood flow and right ventricular hypertrophy. (**E**) Endocardial cushion defects. Blood flows between the chambers of the heart. (**F**) Transposition of the great vessels. The pulmonary artery is attached to the left side of the heart and the aorta to the right side. (**G**) Patent ductus arteriosus. The high-pressure blood of the aorta is shunted back to the pulmonary artery. (**H**) Postductal coarctation of the aorta.

Atrial Septal Defects. In atrial septal defects, a hole in the atrial septum persists as a result of improper septal formation (see Fig. 26-28A). Two common types of atrial septal defects are those that involve the ostium secundum (most common) and those that involve the ostium primum (with endocardial cushion defects). The defect occurs more frequently in females than males. It may be single or multiple and varies from a small, asymptomatic opening to a large, symptomatic opening.

Most atrial septal defects are small and discovered inadvertently during a routine physical examination.[76] In the case of an isolated septal defect that is large enough to allow shunting, the flow of blood usually is from the left side to the right side of the heart because of the more compliant right ventricle and because the pulmonary vascular resistance is lower than the systemic vascular resistance. This produces right ventricular volume overload and increased pulmonary blood flow. The increased volume of blood that must be ejected from the right heart also prolongs closure of the pulmonary valve and produces a separation (*i.e.,* fixed splitting) of the aortic and pulmonary components of the second heart sound. Most children with atrial septal defects are asymptomatic. Adolescents and young adults may experience atrial fibrillation or atrial flutter and palpations because of atrial dilation.

Because spontaneous closure occurs in some children, surgical treatment usually is delayed until the child is of school age. Transcatheter closure in the cardiac catheterization laboratory has proved effective. This procedure uses a double-umbrella catheter, with an umbrella placed on each side of the defect.[73] It often is used in children who have complex congenital heart defects that require multistage surgical procedures. This approach can eliminate one surgical procedure. Surgical closure may be necessary when the defect does not close spontaneously or transcatheter closure is not deemed appropriate.

Ventricular Septal Defects. A ventricular septal defect is an opening in the ventricular septum that results from an imperfect separation of the ventricles during early fetal development (see Fig. 26-28B). Ventricular septal defects are the most common form of congenital heart defect, accounting for 20% to 30% of congenital heart disorders.[70] Ventricular septal defect may be the only cardiac defect, or it may be one of multiple cardiac anomalies.

The ventricular septum originates from two sources: the interventricular groove of the folded tubular heart that gives rise to the muscular part of the septum, and the endocardial cushions that extend to form the membranous portion of the septum. The upper membranous portion of the septum is the last area to close, and it is here that most defects occur.

Depending on the size of the opening, the signs and symptoms of a ventricular septal defect may range from an asymptomatic murmur to congestive heart failure. If the defect is small, it allows a small shunt and small increases in pulmonary blood flow. These defects produce few symptoms, and approximately one third close spontaneously.[70,73] With medium-sized defects, a larger shunt occurs, producing a larger increase in pulmonary blood flow (*i.e.,* twice as much blood may pass through the pulmonary circulation as through the systemic circulation). The increased pulmonary flow most often occurs under relatively low pressure. Most of the children with such defects are asymptomatic and have a low risk for development of pulmonary vascular disease.

Children with large defects have a large amount of pulmonary blood flow. Because the defect is nonrestrictive, the pressure in the left and right sides of the heart is equalized, and blood is shunted from the left side of the heart into the pulmonary artery under high pressures that are sufficient to produce pulmonary hypertension. In these children, left-to-right shunting through the ventricular defect is lessened when pulmonary and systemic circulations offer equal resistance to flow. The child's symptoms improve during this time. As the child's pulmonary vascular resistance increases further, a right-to-left shunt develops, and the child demonstrates cyanosis. This reversal of the direction of shunt flow is called *Eisenmenger's syndrome.*

Most infants with a ventricular septal defect are asymptomatic during early infancy because the higher pulmonary vascular resistance prevents shunting from occurring. After an infant's pulmonary vascular resistance falls and a shunt develops, a characteristic systolic murmur develops. The infant with a large, uncomplicated ventricular septal defect usually is asymptomatic until pulmonary vascular resistance begins to fall at approximately 4 to 25 weeks of age. After a large shunt develops, the mother reports that the infant breathes rapidly, feeds poorly, and is diaphoretic (*i.e.,* signs of congestive heart failure). Right-to-left shunting produces cyanosis.

The treatment of a ventricular septal defect depends on the size of the defect and accompanying hemodynamic derangements. Children with small or medium-sized defects are followed closely in the hope that the defect will close spontaneously. Prophylactic antibiotic therapy is given during periods of increased risk for bacteremia. Cardiac catheterization may be performed in children with medium-sized or large defects who become symptomatic to document the location of the lesion, identify any associated heart defects, and determine the pulmonary vascular resistance. Congestive heart failure is treated medically. Surgical intervention is required for infants who do not respond to medical management. When possible, surgical closure of the defect is performed. Pulmonary artery banding may be done in cases of complex congenital defects with the risk for pulmonary vascular involvement, in children with defects that are not amenable to medical or surgical treatment, or when the ventricular defect is only one of several defects present. The pulmonary band is removed when the ventricular defect is closed during open-heart surgery at a later time.

Endocardial Cushion Defects. The endocardial cushions form the AV canals, the upper part of the ventricular septum, and the lower part of the atrial septum. Endocardial cushion defects are responsible for approximately 5% of all congenital heart defects. As many as 50% of children with Down syndrome have endocardial cushion defects.[70]

Because endocardial cushions contribute to multiple aspects of heart development, several variations with this type of defect are possible. The terms most commonly used to categorize endocardial cushion defects are *partial* and *complete AV canal defects.* In partial AV canal defects, the two AV valve rings are complete and separate. The most common type of partial AV canal defect is an ostium primum defect, with a cleft in the mitral valve. In complete canal defect, there is a common AV valve orifice along with defects in both the atrial and ventricular septal tissue. Many variations of these two forms of endocardial cushion defect are possible (see Fig. 26-28E). Ebstein's anomaly is a defect in endocardial cushion development characterized by displacement of tricuspid valvular tissue into the ventricle. The displaced tricuspid leaflets are attached directly to the right ventricular endocardial surface or to shortened or malformed chordae tendineae.

The direction and magnitude of a shunt in a child with endocardial cushion defects are determined by the combination of defects and the child's pulmonary and systemic vascular resistance. The hemodynamic effects of an isolated ostium primum defect are those of the previously described atrial septal defect. These children are largely asymptomatic during childhood. If a ventricular septal defect is present, pulmonary blood flow is increased after pulmonary vascular resistance falls. Many children with ventricular septal defects have effort intolerance, easy fatigability, and recurrent infections, particularly when the shunt is large. The larger the defect, the greater is the shunt and the higher is the pressure in the pulmonary vascular system.

With complete AV canal defects, congestive heart failure and intercurrent pulmonary infections appear early in infancy. There is left-to-right shunting and transatrial and transventricular mixing of blood. Pulmonary hypertension and increased pulmonary vascular resistance are common. Cyanosis develops with progressive shunting.

The treatment for endocardial cushion defects is determined by the severity of the defect. With an ostium primum defect, surgical repair usually is planned on an elective basis before the child enters school. Palliative or corrective surgery is required in infants with complete AV canal defects who have congestive heart failure and do not respond to medical treatment. Total surgical repair of complete AV canal defects can be accomplished with low operative risk.

Pulmonary Stenosis. Pulmonary stenosis may occur as an isolated valvular lesion or in conjunction with more complex defects, such as tetralogy of Fallot. In isolated valvular defects, the pulmonary cusps may be absent or malformed, or they may remain fused at their commissural edges; often, there are coexisting abnormalities.

Pulmonary valvular defects usually cause some impairment of pulmonary blood flow and increase the workload imposed on the right side of the heart (see Fig. 26-28D). Most children with pulmonic valve stenosis have mild to moderate stenosis that does not increase in severity. These children are largely asymptomatic. Severe defects are manifested by marked impairment of pulmonary blood flow that begins during infancy and is likely to become more severe as the child grows. Cyanosis develops in approximately one third of children younger than 2 years of age.[72] The ductus arteriosus may provide the vital accessory route for perfusing the lungs in infants with severe stenosis. When pulmonary stenosis is extreme, increased pressures in the right side of the heart may delay closure of the foramen ovale.

Treatment measures designed to maintain the patency of the ductus arteriosus may be used as a palliative measure to maintain or increase pulmonary blood flow in infants with severe pulmonary stenosis. Pulmonary valvotomy often is the treatment of choice. Transcatheter balloon valvuloplasty may be used in some infants with moderate degrees of obstruction. Introduction of an expandable intravascular stent may be used to prevent restenosis.[70]

Tetralogy of Fallot. As the name implies, tetralogy of Fallot consists of four associated congenital heart defects: (1) a ventricular septal defect involving the membranous septum and the anterior portion of the muscular septum; (2) dextroposition or shifting to the right of the aorta, so that it overrides the right ventricle and is in communication with the septal defect; (3) obstruction or narrowing of the pulmonary outflow channel, including pulmonic valve stenosis, a decrease in the size of the pulmonary trunk, or both; and (4) hypertrophy of the right ventricle because of the increased work required to pump blood through the obstructed pulmonary channels[70,73,77] (see Fig. 26-28C).

Most children with tetralogy of Fallot display some degree of cyanosis—hence the term *blue babies*. The cyanosis develops as the result of decreased pulmonary blood flow and because the right-to-left shunt causes mixing of unoxygenated blood with the oxygenated blood, which is ejected into the systemic circulation. Hypercyanotic attacks ("tet spells") may occur during the first months of life. These spells typically occur in the morning during crying, feeding, or defecating. These activities increase the infant's oxygen requirements. Crying and defecating may further increase pulmonary vascular resistance, thereby increasing right-to-left shunting and decreasing pulmonary blood flow. With the hypercyanotic spell, the infant becomes acutely cyanotic, hyperpneic, irritable, and diaphoretic. Later in the spell, the infant becomes limp and may lose consciousness. Placing the infant in the knee-chest position increases systemic vascular resistance, which increases pulmonary blood flow and decreases right-to-left shunting. During a hypercyanotic spell, toddlers and older children may spontaneously assume the squatting position, which functions like the knee-chest position to relieve the spell.[72]

Total surgical correction is ultimately advised for all children with tetralogy of Fallot. Early definitive repair, even in infancy, is currently advocated in most centers that are experienced in intracardiac surgery in infants.[73] Obstruction of right ventricular outflow through the pulmonic valve and into the pulmonary arteries is an important determinant in assessing whether primary correction is undertaken during infancy. Marked hypoplasia of the pulmonary arteries is a relative contraindication for early corrective surgery, in which case palliative surgery designed to increase pulmonary blood flow is usually recommended. The most popular procedures use the subclavian artery or prosthetic material to create a shunt between the aorta and pulmonary artery. Balloon dilation of the pulmonary valve may also afford palliation in some infants. Total correction is then carried out later in childhood.

Transposition of the Great Vessels. In complete transposition of the great vessels, the aorta originates in the right ventricle, and the pulmonary artery originates in the left ventricle (see Fig. 26-28F). The defect is more common in infants whose mothers have diabetes and in boys. In infants born with this defect, survival depends on communication between the right and left sides of the heart in the form of a patent ductus arteriosus or septal defect. Prostaglandin E_1 may be administered in an effort to maintain the patency of the ductus arteriosus. Balloon atrial septostomy may be done to increase the blood flow between the two sides of the heart. In this procedure, a balloon-tipped catheter is inserted into the heart through the vena cava and then passed through the foramen ovale into the left atrium. The balloon is then inflated and brought back through the foramen ovale, enlarging the opening as it goes.

Corrective surgery is essential for long-term survival.[70] An arterial switch procedure (*i.e.*, Jatene operation) may be done. This procedure, which corrects the relation of the systemic and pulmonary blood flows, is preferably performed in the first 2 to 3 weeks of life, before postnatal reduction in pulmonary vascular resistance. An atrial (venous) switch procedure (*i.e.*, Mustard or Senning operation) is performed on older children. Both of these procedures reverse the blood flow at the atrial level by the surgical formation of intraatrial baffles. The atrial switch procedures have a much higher long-term morbidity and are done when conditions prevent performance of the arterial switch procedure.

Coarctation of the Aorta. Coarctation of the aorta is a localized narrowing of the aorta, proximal (preductal or coarctation of infancy) or distal (postductal) to the ductus (see Fig. 26-28H). Approximately 98% of coarctations are postductal. The anomaly occurs twice as often in males as in females. Coarctation of the aorta may be a feature of Turner's syndrome (see Chapter 7).

The classic sign of coarctation of the aorta is a disparity in pulsations and blood pressures in the arms and legs. The femoral, popliteal, and dorsalis pedis pulsations are weak or delayed compared with the bounding pulses of the arms and carotid vessels. The systolic blood pressure in the legs obtained by the cuff method normally is 10 to 20 mm Hg higher than in the arms.[70] In coarctation, the pressure is lower and may be difficult to obtain. The differential in blood pressure is common in children older than 1 year of age, approximately 90% of whom have hypertension in the upper extremities greater than the 95th percentile for age (see Chapter 25).

Children with significant coarctation should be treated surgically; the optimal age for surgery is 2 to 4 years. If untreated, most persons with coarctation of the aorta die between 20 and 40 years of age. The common serious complications are related to the hypertensive state. In some centers, balloon valvoplasty has been used for treatment of unoperated coarctation. This method is still being developed, and ongoing clinical trials are needed to determine its long-term effectiveness and possible complications.[70]

In preductal or infantile coarctation, the ductus remains open and shunts blood from the pulmonary artery through the ductus arteriosus into the aorta. It frequently is seen with other cardiac anomalies and carries a high mortality rate. Because of the position of the defect, blood flow throughout the systemic circulation is reduced, and heart failure develops in the affected infant at an early age because of the increased workload imposed on the left ventricle. Medical and surgical methods are used to treat these infants.

KAWASAKI DISEASE

Kawasaki disease, also known as *mucocutaneous lymph node syndrome,* is an acute febrile disease of young children. First described in Japan in 1967 by Dr. Tomisaku Kawasaki, the disease affects the skin, brain, eyes, joints, liver, lymph nodes, and heart.[78–80] The disease can produce aneurysmal disease of the coronary arteries and is the most common cause of acquired heart disease in young children. More than 3500 children with Kawasaki disease are hospitalized annually in the United States.[79] Although first reported in Japanese children, the disease affects children of many races, occurs worldwide, and is increasing in frequency.

The disease is characterized by a vasculitis (*i.e.,* inflammation of the blood vessels) that begins in the small vessels (*i.e.,* arterioles, venules, and capillaries) and progresses to involve some of the larger arteries, such as the coronaries. The cause of Kawasaki disease is unknown, but it is thought to be of immunologic origin. Immunologic abnormalities that include increased activation of helper T cells and increased levels of immune mediators and antibodies that destroy endothelial cells have been detected during the acute phase of the disease. It has been hypothesized that some unknown antigen, possibly a common infectious agent, triggers the immune response in a genetically predisposed child.

Manifestations and Clinical Course

The course of the disease is triphasic and includes an acute febrile phase that lasts approximately 7 to 14 days; a subacute phase that follows the acute phase and lasts from days 10 through 24; and a convalescent phase that follows the subacute stage and continues until the signs of the acute-phase inflammatory response have subsided and the signs of the illness have disappeared.

The *acute phase* begins with an abrupt onset of fever, followed by conjunctivitis, rash, involvement of the oral mucosa, redness and swelling of the hands and feet, and enlarged cervical lymph nodes. The fever typically is high, reaching 40°C (104°F) or more, has an erratic spiking pattern, is unresponsive to antibiotics, and persists for 5 or more days. The conjunctivitis, which is bilateral, begins shortly after the onset of fever, persists throughout the febrile course of the disease, and may last as long as 3 to 5 weeks. There is no exudate, discharge, or conjunctival ulceration, differentiating it from many other types of conjunctivitis. The rash usually is deeply erythematous and may take several forms, the most common of which is a nonpruritic urticarial rash with large erythematous plaques, or a measles-type rash. Although the rash usually is generalized, it may be accentuated centrally or peripherally. Some children have a perianal rash with a diaper-like distribution (see Fig. 26-29). Oropharyngeal manifestations include fissuring of the lips, diffuse erythema of the oropharynx, and hypertrophic papillae of the tongue, creating a "strawberry" appearance. The hands and feet become swollen and painful, and have reddened palms and soles. The rash, oropharyngeal manifestations, and changes in hands and feet appear within 1 to 3 days of fever onset and usually disappear as the fever subsides. Lymph node involvement is the least constant feature of the disease. It is cervical and unilateral, with a single, firm, enlarged lymph node mass that usually is larger than 1.5 cm in diameter.

The *subacute phase* begins with defervescence and lasts until all signs of the disease have disappeared. During the subacute phase, desquamation (*i.e.,* peeling) of the skin of the fingers and toe tips begins and progresses to involve the entire surface of the palms and soles. Patchy peeling of skin areas other than the hands and feet may occur in some children. The *convalescent stage* persists from the complete resolution of symptoms until all signs of inflammation have disappeared. This usually takes approximately 8 weeks.

In addition to the major manifestations that occur during the acute stage of the illness, there are several associated, less specific characteristics of the disease, including arthritis, urethritis and pyuria, gastrointestinal manifestations (*e.g.,* diarrhea, abdominal pain), hepatitis, and hydrops of the gallbladder. Arthritis or arthralgia occurs in approximately 30% of children with the disease, characterized by symmetric joint swelling that involves large and small joints. Central nervous system involvement occurs in almost all children and is characterized by pronounced irritability and lability of mood.

Cardiac involvement is the most important manifestation of Kawasaki disease. Coronary vasculitis develops in between 10% and 40% of children within the first 2 weeks of the illness, manifested by dilatation and aneurysm formation in the coronary arteries, as seen on two-dimensional echocardiography. The manifestations of coronary artery involvement include signs and symptoms of myocardial ischemia or, rarely, overt myocardial infarction or rupture of the aneurysm. Pericarditis, myocarditis, endocarditis, heart failure, and arrhythmias also may develop.

Diagnosis and Treatment

As with rheumatic fever, the diagnosis of Kawasaki disease is based on clinical findings because no specific laboratory test for the disease exists. The AHA Council on Cardiovascular Disease in the Young, Committee on Rheumatic Fever, Endocarditis, and Kawasaki Disease has established guidelines for diagnosis of the disease.[81] According to these guidelines, a diagnosis of Kawasaki disease is confirmed by the presence of a fever that lasts 5 or more days without another more reasonable explanation and by at least four of the following five acute-stage manifestations of the disease (Fig. 26-29): changes in the extremities (an acute erythema and edema of the hands, followed by membranous desquamation of fingertips during the convalescent period); polymorphous exanthema (skin eruption involving the trunk and extremities); bilateral, painless bulbar conjunctival infection without exudate; changes in the lips and oral cavity (*e.g.*, erythema and cracking of the lips, strawberry tongue, diffuse infection of the oral and pharyngeal mucosae); and cervical lymphadenopathy (≥1.5 cm in diameter). Chest radiographs, ECG tests, and two-dimensional echocardiography are used to detect coronary artery involvement and follow its progress. Coronary angiography may be used to determine the extent of coronary artery involvement.

Intravenous gamma globulin and aspirin are considered the best therapy for prevention of coronary artery abnormalities in children with Kawasaki disease.[79,80] During the acute phase of the illness, aspirin usually is given in larger doses and for its antiinflammatory and antipyretic effects. After the fever is controlled, the aspirin dose is lowered, and the drug is given for its anti–platelet-aggregating effects.

Recommendations for cardiac follow-up evaluation (*i.e.*, stress testing and sometimes coronary angiography) are based on the level of coronary artery changes. Anticoagulant therapy may be recommended for children with multiple or large coronary aneurysms. Some restrictions in

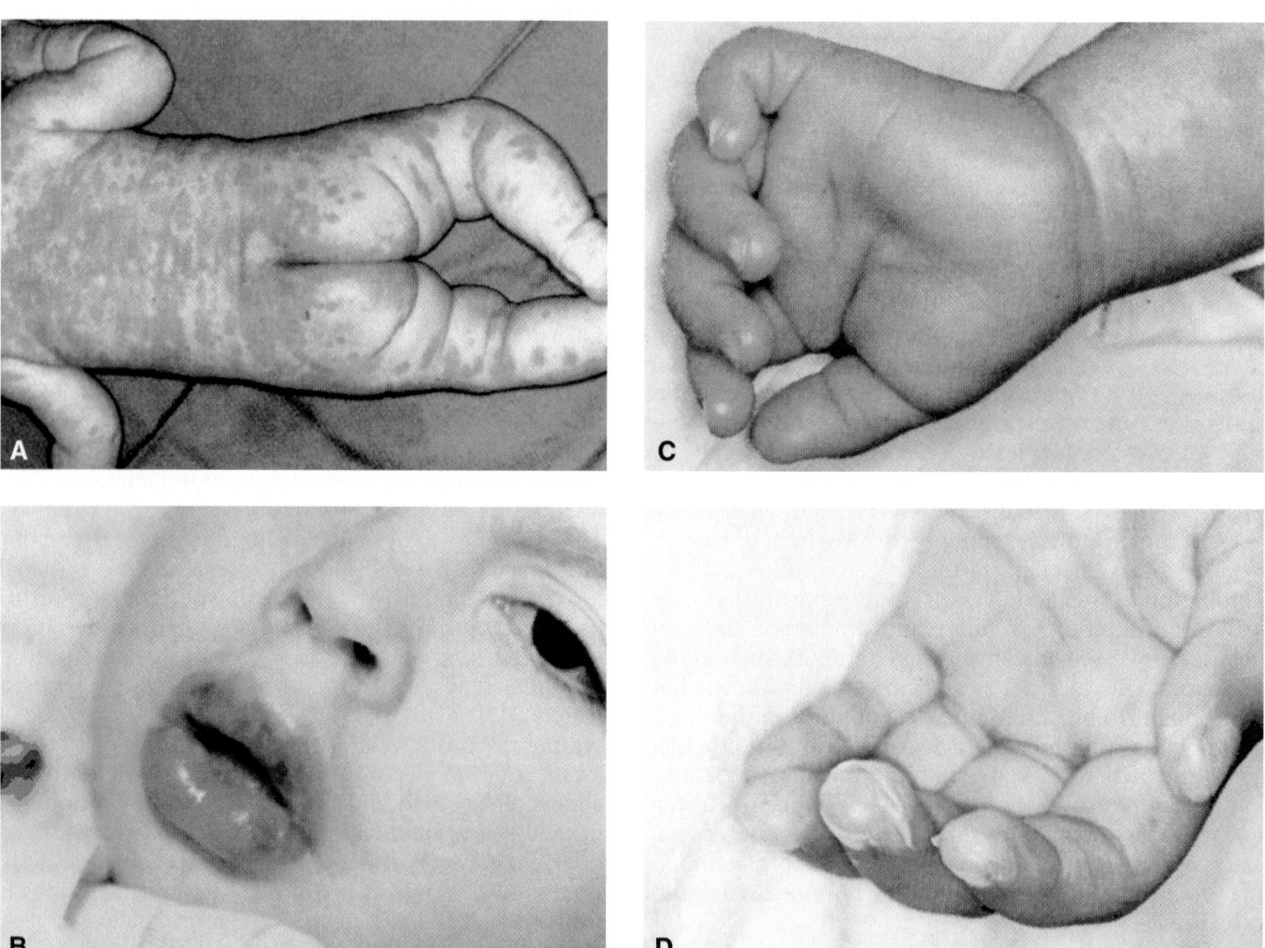

FIGURE 26-29 Kawasaki disease. (**A**) Rash of Kawasaki disease in a 7-month-old child on the 4th day of illness; (**B**) conjunctival injection, lip edema in a 2-year-old boy on the 6th day of illness; (**C**) erythema and edematous hand of a 1½-year-old girl on the 6th day of illness; and (**D**) periungual desquamation in a 3-year-old child on the 12th day of illness. (From The Council on Cardiovascular Disease in Young, Committee on Rheumatic Fever, Endocarditis, and Kawasaki Disease. (2001). Diagnostic guidelines for Kawasaki disease. *Circulation 103,* 335–336)

activities such as competitive sports may be advised for children with significant coronary artery abnormalities.

In summary, congenital heart defects arise during fetal heart development, which occurs during week 3 through 8 following conception, and reflect the stage of development at the time the causative event occurred. Several factors contribute to the development of congenital heart defects, including genetic and chromosomal influences, viruses, and environmental agents such as drugs and radiation. The cause of the defect often is unknown.

Congenital heart defects may produce no effects, or they may markedly affect cardiac function. The defects may produce shunting of blood from the right to the left side of the heart or from the left to the right side of the heart. Left-to-right shunts typically increase the volume of the right side of the heart and pulmonary circulation, and right-to-left shunts transfer unoxygenated blood from the right side of the heart to the left side, diluting the oxygen content of blood that is being ejected into the systemic circulation and causing cyanosis. The direction and degree of shunt depend on the size of the defect that connects the two sides of the heart and the difference in resistance between the two sides of the circulation. Congenital heart defects often are classified as defects that produce cyanosis and those that produce little or no cyanosis. Depending on the severity of the defect, congenital heart defects may be treated medically or surgically. Medical and surgical treatment often is indicated in children with severe defects.

Kawasaki disease is an acute febrile disease of young children that affects the skin, brain, eyes, joints, liver, lymph nodes, and heart. The disease can produce aneurysmal disease of the coronary arteries and is the most common cause of acquired heart disease in young children.

REVIEW EXERCISES

A 40-year-old man presents in the emergency department complaining of substernal chest pain that is also felt in his left shoulder. He is short of breath and nauseated. His blood pressure is 148/90 mm Hg and his heart rate is 110 mm Hg. His ECG shows an ST-elevation with T-wave inversion. He is given aspirin, morphine, and oxygen. Blood tests reveal elevated CK-MB and troponin I.

A. What is the probable cause of the man's symptoms?

B. Explain the origin of the left arm pain, nausea, and increased heart rate.

C. What is the significance of the ST-segment changes and elevation in CK-MB and troponin I?

D. Relate the actions of aspirin, morphine, and oxygen to the treatment of this man's condition.

A 50-year-old woman presents with complaints of nocturnal paroxysmal dyspnea and orthopnea, palpitations, and fatigue. An echocardiogram demonstrates a thickened, immobile mitral valve with anterior and posterior leaflets moving together; slow early diastolic filling of the ventricle, and left atrial enlargement.

A. What is the probable cause of this woman's symptoms?

B. Explain the pathologic significance of the slow early diastolic filling, distended left atrium, and palpitations.

C. Given the echocardiogram data, what type of cardiac murmur would you expect to find in this woman?

D. Which circulation (systemic or pulmonary) would you expect to be affected as this woman's mitral valve disorder progresses?

A 4-month-old male infant is brought into the pediatric clinic by his mother. She reports that over the past several weeks the baby's lips and mouth and his fingernails and toenails have turned a bluish gray color. She also states that he seems to tire easily and that even nursing seems to wear him out. Lately, he has had several spells during which he has suddenly turned blue, has had difficulty breathing, and has been very irritable. During one of these spells, he turned limp and seemed to have passed out for a short time. An echocardiogram reveals a thickening of the right ventricular wall with overriding of the aorta, a large subaortic ventricular septal defect, and a narrowing of the pulmonary outflow with stenosis of the pulmonary valve.

A. What is this infant's probable diagnosis?

B. Describe the shunting of blood that occurs with this disorder and its relationship to the development of cyanosis.

C. The mother is instructed regarding the placement of the infant in the knee-chest position when he has one of the spells during which he becomes blue and irritable. How does this position help to relieve the cyanosis and impaired oxygenation of tissues?

D. The surgical creation of a shunt between the aorta and pulmonary artery may be performed as a palliative procedure for infants with marked hypoplasia of the pulmonary artery, with corrective surgery performed later in childhood. Explain how this procedure increases blood flow to the lungs.

References

1. American Heart Association. (2003). *Heart diseases and stroke statistics—2003 Update.* Dallas, TX: Author.
2. Hoyert D.L., Kochanek K.D., Murphy S.L. (1999). Deaths: Final data for 1997. *National Vital Statistics Report 47*(19), 1–104.
3. Spodick D.H. (2001). Pericardial diseases. In Braunwald E., Zipes D.P., Libby D. (Eds.), *Heart disease: A textbook of cardiovascular medicine* (6th ed., vol. 2, pp. 1823–1855). Philadelphia: W.B. Saunders.
4. Spodick. D.H. (2003). Acute cardiac tamponade. *New England Journal of Medicine 349,* 684–690.
5. Krishan K.G., Walling A.D. (2002). Diagnosing pericarditis. *American Family Physician 66,* 1695–1702.

6. Guyton A., Hall J.E. (2000). *Textbook of medical physiology* (10th ed., pp. 226–229). Philadelphia: W.B. Saunders.
7. Ganz P., Ganz W. (2001). Coronary blood flow and myocardial ischemia. In Braunwald E., Zipes D.D., Libbey D. (Ed.), *Heart disease: A textbook of cardiovascular medicine* (6th ed., pp. 1087–1108). Philadelphia: W.B. Saunders.
8. Armstrong W.F., Flagenbaum H. (2001). Echocardiography. In Braunwald E., Zipes D.D., Libbey D. (Eds.), *Heart disease: A textbook of cardiovascular medicine* (6th ed., pp. 160–161). Philadelphia: W.B. Saunders.
9. Wachers F.H. Th., Soufer R., Zaret B.L. (2001). Nuclear cardiology. In Braunwald E., Zipes D.D., Libbey D. (Eds.), *Heart disease: A textbook of cardiovascular medicine* (6th ed., pp. 273–314). Philadelphia: W.B. Saunders.
10. Cotran R.S., Kumar V., Collins T. (1999). *Robbins pathologic basis of disease* (6th ed., pp. 528, 566–656, 570–576). Philadelphia: W.B. Saunders.
11. Kullo I.J., Edwards W.D., Schwartz R.S. (1998). Vulnerable plaque: Pathophysiology and clinical implications. *Annals of Internal Medicine 129,* 1050–1060.
12. Falk E. (1999). Stable versus unstable atherosclerosis: Clinical aspects. *American Heart Journal 138,* S421–S425.
13. Forrester J.S. (2000). Role of plaque rupture in acute coronary syndromes. *American Journal of Cardiology 86*(Suppl.) 15J–23J.
14. Yeghiazarians Y., Braunstein J.B., Askari A., Stone P.H. (2000). Unstable angina pectoris. *New England Journal of Medicine 342,* 101–114.
15. Ambrose J.A., Dangas G. (2000). Unstable angina: Current concepts of pathogenesis and treatment. *Archives of Internal Medicine 160,* 25–35.
16. Gibbons R.J., Abrams J., Chatterjee K., et al. Members of the Committee to Update the 1999 Guidelines. (2002). ACC/AHA 2002 guideline update for the management of patients with chronic stable angina: A report of the American College of Cardiology/American Heart Association Task Force on Practice Guidelines. [On-line.] Available: www.acc.org/clinical/guidelines/stable/stable.pdf.
17. Champeau L. (1976). Grading of angina pectoris [Letter]. *Circulation 54,* 522–523.
18. Gersh B.J., Braunwald E., Bonow R.O. (2001). Chronic coronary artery disease. In Braunwald E., Zipes D.D., Libbey D. (Eds.), *Heart disease: A textbook of cardiovascular medicine* (6th ed., pp. 1272–1352). Philadelphia: W.B. Saunders.
19. Cohn P.F. (1994). Silent myocardial ischemia: To treat or not to treat. *Hospital Practice 29*(6), 107–116.
20. Chiariello M., Indolfi C. (1996). Silent myocardial ischemia in patients with diabetes mellitus. *Circulation 93,* 2089–2091.
21. Prinzmetal M., Kennamer, R., Merliss R., et al. (1959). A variant form of angina pectoris. *American Journal of Medicine 27,* 375–388.
22. Braunwald E., Antman E.M., Beasley J.W., et al., and Committee members. (2002). ACC/AHA guideline update for the management of patients with unstable angina and non-ST-segment elevation myocardial infarction—2002: Executive summary and recommendations. *Circulation 106,* 1893–1900.
23. Cannon C.C., Braunwald E. (2001). Unstable angina. In Braunwald E., Zipes D.D., Libbey D. (Eds.), *Heart disease: A textbook of cardiovascular medicine* (6th ed., pp. 1232–1255). Philadelphia: W.B. Saunders.
24. Fullwood J., Butler G., Smith T., et al. (2000). New strategies in management of acute coronary syndromes. *Nursing Clinics of North America 35,* 877–896.
25. Lincoff A.M. (2000). Gusto IV: Expanding therapeutic options in acute coronary syndromes. *American Heart Journal 140,* S104–S114.
26. Mirvis D.M., Goldberger A.L. (2001). Electrocardiography. In Braunwald E., Zipes D.D., Libbey D. (Eds.), *Heart disease: A textbook of cardiovascular medicine* (6th ed., pp. 106–118). Philadelphia: W.B. Saunders.
27. Antman E.M., Braunwald E. (2001). Acute myocardial infarction. In Braunwald E., Zipes D.D., Libbey D. (Eds.), *Heart disease: A textbook of cardiovascular medicine* (6th ed., pp. 1114–1207). Philadelphia: W.B. Saunders.
28. DeLemos J.A., Morrow D.A., Bentley J.H., et al. (2001). The prognostic value of B-type natriuretic peptide in patients with acute coronary syndrome. *New England Journal of Medicine 345,* 1014–1021.
29. Rabbini L.R. (2001). Acute coronary syndromes—beyond myocyte necrosis. *New England Journal of Medicine 345,* 1057–1058.
30. Cannon C.P., Braunwald E. (2001). Unstable angina. In Braunwald E., Zipes D.D., Libbey D. (Eds.), *Heart disease: A textbook of cardiovascular medicine* (6th ed., pp. 1232–1271). Philadelphia: W.B. Saunders.
31. Kloner R.A., Rezkalla S.H. (2003). Cocaine and the heart. *New England Journal of Medicine 348,* 487–488.
32. Ryan T.J., Antman E.M., Brooks N.H., et al., and Committee members. (1999). 1999 Update: ACC/AHA guidelines for the management of acute myocardial infarction: Executive summary and recommendation. A report of the American College of Cardiology/American Heart Association Task Force on Practice Guidelines (Committee on Management of Acute Myocardial Infarction). *Journal of the American College of Cardiology 28,* 1328–1428.
33. Collins R., Petro R., Baigent C., Sleight P. (1997). Aspirin, heparin, and fibrinolytic therapy in suspected acute myocardial infarction. *New England Journal of Medicine 336,* 847–860.
34. Popma J.J., Kuntz R.E. (2001). Percutaneous coronary and valvular intervention. In Braunwald E., Zipes D.D., Libbey D. (Eds.), *Heart disease: A textbook of cardiovascular medicine* (6th ed., pp. 1364–1365). Philadelphia: W.B. Saunders.
35. Shepard R., Eisenberg M.J. (2001). Intracoronary radiotherapy for restenosis. *New England Journal of Medicine 344,* 295–296.
36. Sapirstein W., Zuckerman B., Dillard J. (2001). FDA approval of coronary-artery brachytherapy. *New England Journal of Medicine 344,* 297–298.
37. Brown C.A., O'Connell J.B. (1995). Myocarditis and idiopathic dilated cardiomyopathy. *American Journal of Medicine 99,* 309–314.
38. Feldman A.M., McNamara D. (2000). Myocarditis. *New England Journal of Medicine 343,* 1388–1398.
39. Wyne J., Braunwald E. (2001). The cardiomyopathies and myocarditides. In Braunwald E., Zipes D.D., Libbey D. (Eds.), *Heart disease: A textbook of cardiovascular medicine* (6th ed., pp. 1751–1806). Philadelphia: W.B. Saunders.
40. Bradenburg R.O., Chazo J.E., Cherian G., et al., Committee members. (1982). Report of WHO/ISF Task Force on the Definition and Classification of Cardiomyopathies. *British Heart Journal 44,* 672–673.
41. Richardson P., Rapporteur W., McKenna W., et al. (1996). Report of the 1995 World Health Organization/International Society and Federation of Cardiology Task Force on Definition and Classification of Cardiomyopathies. *Circulation 93,* 841–842.
42. Dec G.W., Fuster V. (1994). Idiopathic dilated cardiomyopathy. *New England Journal of Medicine 331,* 1564–1575.
43. Mohan S., Parker M., Wehbi M., Douglass P. (2002). Idiopathic dilated cardiomyopathy: A common but mystifying cause of heart failure. *Cleveland Clinic Journal of Medicine 69*(6), 481–487.
44. Manolio T.A., Baughman K.I., Rodeheffer R., et al. (1992). Prevalence and etiology of idiopathic dilated cardiomy-

opathy (Summary of the National Heart, Lung, and Blood Institute Workshop). *American Journal of Cardiology 69,* 1458.
45. Piano M.R. (2002). Alcoholic cardiomyopathy. *Chest 121,* 1638–1650.
46. Roberts R., Sigwart U. (2001). New Concepts in hypertrophic cardiomyopathies, Part I and Part II. *Circulation 104,* 2113–2116, 2249–2252.
47. Maron B.J. (2002). Hypertrophic cardiomyopathy. *JAMA 287,* 1308–1320.
48. Jennings R.B., Steinburger C. Jr. (2001). The heart. In Rubin E. (Ed.), *Essential pathology* (3rd ed., pp 303–304, 299–300). Philadelphia: Lippincott Williams & Wilkins.
49. Spirito P., Seidman C.E., McKenna W.J., Maron B.J. (1997). The management of hypertrophic cardiomyopathy. *New England Journal of Medicine 336,* 775–783.
50. Golledge P., Knight C.J. (2001). Current management of hypertrophic cardiomyopathy. *Hospital Medicine 62*(2), 79–82.
51. Kushwaha S.S., Fallon J.T., Fuster V. (1997). Restrictive cardiomyopathy. *New England Journal of Medicine 336,* 267–274.
52. Pearson G.D., Veille J., Rahimtoola S., et al. (2000). Peripartum cardiomyopathy: National Heart, Lung, and Blood Institute and Office of Rare Diseases (National Institutes of Health) Workshop Recommendations and Review. *Journal of the American Medical Association 283,* 83–88.
53. Felker G.M., Jaeger C.J., Kodas E., et al. (2000). Myocarditis and long-term survival in peripartum cardiomyopathy. *American Heart Journal 140,* 785–791.
54. Karchmer A.W. (2001). Infective endocarditis. In Braunwald E., Zipes D.D., Libbey D. (Eds.), *Heart disease: A textbook of cardiovascular medicine* (6th ed., pp. 1723–1750). Philadelphia: W.B. Saunders.
55. Mylonakis E., Calderwood S.B. (2001). Infective endocarditis in adults. *New England Journal of Medicine 345,* 1318–1330.
56. Durack D.T., Lukes A.S., Bright D.K. (1994). New criteria for diagnosis of infective endocarditis. *American Journal of Medicine 96,* 200–209.
57. American Heart Association Advisory and Coordinating Committee. (1998). Diagnosis and management of infective endocarditis and its complications. *Circulation 98,* 2936–2948.
58. Ad Hoc Committee to Revise Jones Criteria (Modified) of the Council on Rheumatic Fever and Congenital Heart Disease of the American Heart Association. (1984). Jones criteria (revised) for guidance in the diagnosis of rheumatic fever. *Circulation 69,* 203A–208A.
59. Dajani A. (2001). Rheumatic fever. In Braunwald E., Zipes D.D., Libbey D. (Eds.), *Heart disease: A textbook of cardiovascular medicine* (6th ed., pp. 2192–2198). Philadelphia: W.B. Saunders.
60. Dajani A., Taubert K., Ferrieri P., et al., and other Committee members. (1995). Treatment of acute streptococcal pharyngitis and prevention of rheumatic fever: A statement for health professionals. [On-line.] Available: www.americanheart.org/Scientific/statements.
61. Narula J., Chandrasekhar Y., Rahimtoola S. (1999). Diagnosis of active rheumatic carditis. *Circulation 100,* 1576–1581.
62. Bonow R.O., Carabello B., deLeon A.D. Jr., et. al., for the Committee on Management of Patients with Valvular Heart Disease. (1998). Guideline for the management of patients with valvular heart disease: Executive summary. A report of the American College of Cardiology/American Heart Association Task Force on Guidelines. *Circulation 98,* 1949–1984.
63. Carabello B.A., Crawford F.A. (1997). Valvular heart disease. *New England Journal of Medicine 337,* 32–41.
64. Shipton B., Wahba H. (2001). Valvular heart disease: Review and update. *American Family Physician 63,* 2201–2208.
65. Braunwald E. (2001). Valvular heart disease. In Braunwald E., Zipes D.D., Libbey D. (Eds.), *Heart disease: A textbook of cardiovascular medicine* (6th ed., pp. 1643–1722). Philadelphia: W.B. Saunders.
66. Otto C.M. (2001). Evaluation and management of chronic mitral regurgitation. *New England Journal of Medicine 345,* 740–746.
67. Playford D., Weyman A.E. (2001). Mitral valve prolapse: Time for a fresh look. *Reviews in Cardiovascular Medicine 2,* 73–76.
68. Massie B.M., Amidon T.M. (2003). Heart. In Tierney L.M., McPhee S.J., Papadakis M.A. (Eds.), *Current medical diagnosis and treatment* (42nd ed., pp. 322–332). New York: Lange Medical Books/McGraw-Hill.
69. Carbello B.A. (2002). Aortic stenosis. *New England Journal of Medicine 346,* 677–682.
70. Bernstein D. (2004). The cardiovascular system. In Behrman R.E., Kliegman R.M., Jenson H.B. (Eds.), *Nelson textbook of pediatrics* (17th ed., pp. 1475–1555). Philadelphia: Saunders.
71. Moore K.L. (2001). *The developing human* (7th ed., pp. 329–379). Philadelphia: W.B. Saunders.
72. Hazinski M.F. (1992). *Nursing care of the critically ill child* (2nd ed., pp. 112–131, 271–361). St. Louis: Mosby-Year Book.
73. Friedman W.F., Silverman N. (2001). Congenital heart disease in infancy and childhood. In Braunwald E., Zipes D.D., Libbey D. (Eds.), *Heart disease: A textbook of cardiovascular medicine* (6th ed., pp. 1505–1591). Philadelphia: Saunders.
74. Nouri S. (1997). Congenital heart defects: Cyanotic and acyanotic. *Pediatric Annals 26,* 92–98.
75. Van Overmeire B., Smets K., Lecoutere D., et al. (2000). A comparison of ibuprofen and indomethacin for closure of patent ductus arteriosus. *New England Journal of Medicine 343,* 674–681.
76. Driscoll D.J. (1999). Left-to-right shunt lesions. *Pediatric Clinics of North America 46,* 355–368.
77. Waldman J.D., Wernly J.A. (1999). Cyanotic congenital heart disease with decreased pulmonary blood flow in children. *Pediatric Clinics of North America 46,* 385–404.
78. Shulman S.T., DeInocencio J., Hirsch R. (1995). Kawasaki disease. *Pediatric Clinics of North America 42,* 1205–1222.
79. Taubert K.A., Stanford S.T. (1999). Kawasaki disease. *American Family Physician 59,* 3093–3108.
80. Lueng D.Y.M., Meissner H.C. (2001). The many faces of Kawasaki syndrome. *Hospital Practice 35*(1), 77–94.
81. Council on Cardiovascular Disease in the Young, Committee on Rheumatic Fever, Endocarditis, and Kawasaki Disease. American Heart Association. *Circulation 103,* 335–336.

CHAPTER

27

Cardiac Conduction and Rhythm Disorders

Jill M. White Winters

Heart muscle is unique among other muscles in that it is capable of generating and rapidly conducting its own electrical impulses or action potentials. These action potentials result in excitation of muscle fibers throughout the myocardium. Impulse formation and conduction result in weak electrical currents that spread through the entire body. These impulses are recorded on an electrocardiogram. Disorders of cardiac impulse generation and conduction range from benign arrhythmias that are merely annoying to those causing serious disruption of heart function and sudden cardiac death.

Cardiac Conduction System

After completing this section of the chapter, you should be able to meet the following objectives:

- Describe the cardiac conduction system and relate it to the mechanical functioning of the heart
- Characterize the four phases of a cardiac action potential and differentiate between the fast and slow responses
- Draw an ECG tracing and state the origin of the component parts of the tracing
- Provide rationale for the importance of careful lead placement and monitoring of ischemic events

In certain areas of the heart, the myocardial cells have been modified to form the specialized cells of the conduction system. Although most myocardial cells are capable of initiating and conducting impulses, it is the conduction system that maintains the pumping efficiency of the heart. Specialized pacemaker cells generate impulses at a faster rate than other types of heart tissue, and the conduction tissue transmits these impulses at a more rapid rate than other cardiac cell types. Because of these properties, the conduction system usually controls the rhythm of the heart. Blood reaches the conduction tissues by way of the coronary blood vessels. Coronary heart disease that interrupts blood flow through the vessels supplying tissues of the conduction system can induce serious and sometimes fatal disturbances in cardiac rhythm.

The specialized excitatory and conduction system of the heart consists of the sinoatrial (SA) node, in which the normal rhythmic impulse is generated; the internodal pathways between the atria and the ventricles; the atrioventricular (AV) node and bundle of His, which conduct the impulse from the atria to the ventricles; and the Purkinje fibers, which conduct the impulses to all parts of the ventricle (Fig. 27-1).

The SA node, which has the fastest intrinsic rate of firing (60 to 100 beats per minute), normally serves as the pacemaker of the heart. It is a spindle-shaped strip of specialized muscle tissue, about 10 to 20 mm in length and 2 to 3 mm wide, located in the posterior wall of the right

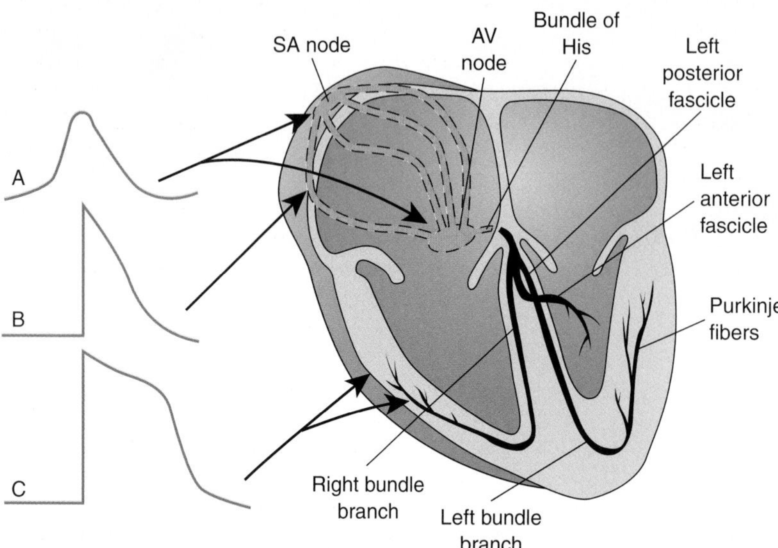

FIGURE 27-1 Conduction system of the heart and action potentials. (**A**) Action potential of sinoatrial (SA) and atrioventricular (AV) nodes; (**B**) atrial muscle action potential; (**C**) action potential of ventricular muscle and Purkinje fibers.

atrium just below of the opening of the superior vena cava and less than 1 mm from the epicardial surface.[1] Blood supply to the SA node is provided by means of the circumflex artery. It has been suggested that no single cell in the SA node serves as the pacemaker, but rather that sinus nodal cells discharge synchronously because of mutual entrainment.[2] As a result, the firing of faster-discharging cells is slowed down by slower-discharging cells, and the firing rate of slower-discharging cells is sped up by faster-discharging cells, resulting in a synchronization of their firing rate.

Impulses originating in the SA node travel through the atria to the AV node. Because of the anatomic location of the SA node, the progression of atrial depolarization occurs in an inferior, leftward, and somewhat posterior direction, and the right atrium is depolarized slightly before the left atrium.[3] There are three internodal pathways between the SA node and the AV node, including the anterior (Bachmann's), middle (Wenckebach's), and posterior (Thorel's) internodal tracts. These three tracts anastomose proximal to the AV node. Interatrial conduction appears to be accomplished through Bachmann's bundle. This large muscle bundle originates along the anterior border of the SA node and travels posteriorly around the aorta to the left atrium.[4]

The heart essentially has two conduction systems: one that controls atrial activity and one that controls ventricular activity. The AV node connects the two conduction systems and provides one-way conduction between the atria and ventricles. The AV node is a compact ovoid structure measuring approximately $1 \times 3 \times 5$ mm, which is located slightly beneath the right atrial endocardium, anterior to the opening of the coronary sinus, and immediately above the insertion of the septal leaflet of the tricuspid valve.[1,4] In 85% to 90% of people, blood supply to the AV node is provided by the right coronary artery.[1] The AV node is divided into three functional regions: the AN, or transitional, zone between the atria and the rest of the node; the middle N, or nodal, zone; and the NH, or upper, zone of the ventricular conduction system.[5] Within the AN portion of the node, atrial fibers connect with very small junctional fibers of the node itself. The velocity of conduction through the AN and N fibers is very slow (approximately one half that of normal cardiac muscle), which greatly delays transmission of the impulse.[5,6] A further delay occurs as the impulse travels through the nodal region into the NH region, which connects with the *bundle of His* (also called the *AV bundle*). This delay provides a mechanical advantage whereby the atria complete their ejection of blood before ventricular contraction begins. Under normal circumstances, the AV node provides the only connection between the atrial and

CARDIAC CONDUCTION SYSTEM

- The cardiac conduction system controls the rate and direction of electrical impulse conduction in the heart.
- Normally, impulses are generated in the SA node, which has the fastest rate of firing, and travel via the AV node to the Purkinje system in the ventricles.
- Cardiac action potentials are divided into five phases: phase 0, or the rapid upstroke of the action potential; phase 1, or early repolarization; phase 2, or the plateau; phase 3, or final repolarization period; and phase 4, or diastolic repolarization period.
- Cardiac muscle has two types of ion channels that function in producing the voltage changes that occur during the depolarization phase of the action potential: the fast sodium channels and the slow calcium channels.
- There are two types of cardiac action potentials: the fast response, which occurs in atrial and ventricular muscle cells and the Purkinje conduction system and uses the fast sodium channels; and the slow response of the SA and AV nodes, which uses the slow calcium channels.

ventricular conduction systems. The atria and ventricles would beat independently of each other if the transmission of impulses through the AV node were blocked.

The *Purkinje system,* which supplies the ventricles, has large fibers that allow for rapid conduction and almost simultaneous excitation of the entire right and left ventricles (0.06 second).[6] This rapid rate of conduction throughout the Purkinje system is necessary for the swift and efficient ejection of blood from the heart. The fibers of the Purkinje system originate in the AV node and proceed to form the bundle of His, which extends through the fibrous tissue between the valves of the heart and into the ventricular system. Because of its proximity to the aortic valve and the mitral valve ring, the bundle of His is predisposed to inflammation and deposits of calcified debris that can interfere with impulse conduction.[6] The bundle of His penetrates into the ventricles and almost immediately divides into *right* and *left bundle branches* that straddle the interventricular septum. Branches from the anterior and posterior descending coronary arteries provide blood supply for the His bundle, making this conduction site less susceptible to ischemic damage, unless the damage is extensive.[1] The bundle branches move through the subendocardial tissues toward the papillary muscles and then subdivide into the Purkinje fibers, which branch out and supply the outer walls of the ventricles. The main trunk of the left bundle branch extends for approximately 1 to 2 cm before fanning out as it enters the septal area and divides further into two segments: the *left posterior* and *anterior fascicles.* The left bundle branch is supplied with blood from both the left anterior descending artery and the posterior descending artery (formed from the right coronary artery), whereas the right bundle branch receives its blood from both the right and left anterior descending coronary arterial systems.[1]

The AV nodal fibers, when not stimulated, discharge at an intrinsic discharge rate of 40 to 60 times a minute, and the Purkinje fibers discharge at 15 to 40 times per minute. Although the AV node and Purkinje system have the ability to control the rhythm of the heart, they do not normally do so because the discharge rate of the SA node is considerably faster. Each time the SA node discharges, its impulses are conducted into the AV node and Purkinje fibers, causing them to fire. The AV node can assume the pacemaker function of the heart should the SA node fail to discharge, and the Purkinje system can assume the pacemaker function of the ventricles should the AV node fail to conduct impulses from the atria to the ventricles. Should this occur, the heart rate will reflect the intrinsic firing rate of these structures.

ACTION POTENTIALS

A stimulus delivered to excitable tissues (*i.e.,* muscles, nerves) evokes an electrical event called an *action potential* (see Chapter 4). The electrical events that normally take place in the heart are responsible for initiating each cardiac contraction. An action potential can be divided into three phases: the resting or unexcited state, depolarization, and repolarization.

The inside of a cardiac cell, like all living cells, contains a negative electrical charge compared with the outside of the cell. During the *resting state,* the membrane is relatively permeable to potassium but much less so to sodium and calcium.[6] Charges of opposite polarity become aligned along the membrane (positive on the outside and negative on the inside; Fig. 27-2).

Depolarization occurs when the cell membrane suddenly becomes selectively permeable to current-carrying ions such as sodium. Sodium ions enter the cell and result in a sharp rise of the intracellular potential to positivity.

Repolarization involves reestablishment of the resting membrane potential. It is a complex and somewhat slower process, involving the outward flow of electrical charges and the return of membrane potential to its resting state.[7] During repolarization, the membrane conductance or permeability for potassium greatly increases, allowing the positively charged potassium ions to move outward across the membrane. This outward movement of potassium removes positive charges from inside the cell; thus, the membrane again becomes negative on the inside and positive on the outside. The sodium-potassium membrane pump also assists in repolarization by pumping positively charged sodium ions out across the cell membrane.[8]

Cardiac Action Potential

The action potential in cardiac muscle is typically divided into five phases: *phase 0*—upstroke or rapid depolarization, *phase 1*—early repolarization period, *phase 2*—plateau, *phase 3*—final rapid repolarization period, and *phase 4*—diastolic depolarization (Fig. 27-3). Cardiac muscle has three types of membrane ion channels that contribute to the voltage changes that occur during the phases of the cardiac action potential. They are the *fast sodium channels,* the *slow calcium channels,* and the *potassium channels.*

During *phase 0,* in atrial and ventricular muscle and in the Purkinje system, the fast sodium channels in the cell membrane are stimulated to open, resulting in the rapid influx of sodium. The action potentials in the normal SA and AV nodes have a much slower upstroke and are mediated predominantly by the slow calcium currents. The point at which the sodium gates open is called the *depolarization*

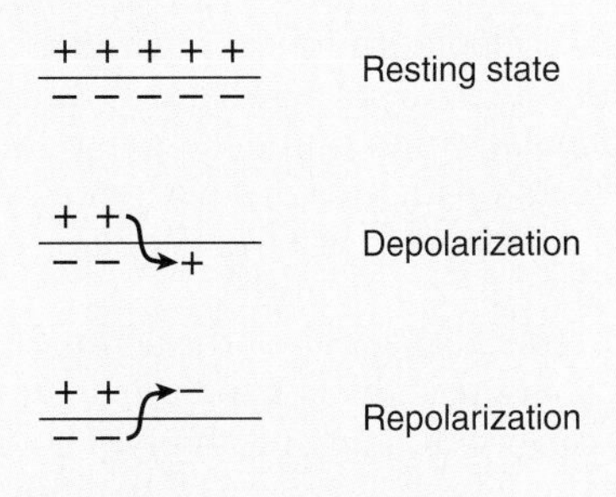

FIGURE 27-2 The flow of charge during impulse generation in excitable tissue. During the resting state, opposite charges are separated by the cell membrane. Depolarization represents the flow of charge across the membrane, and repolarization denotes the return of the membrane potential to its resting state.

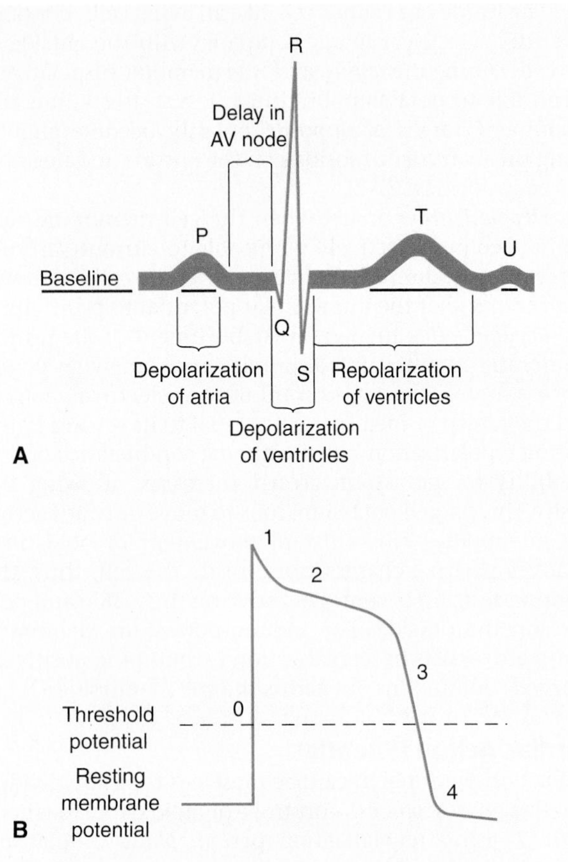

FIGURE 27-3 Relation between (**A**) the electrocardiogram and (**B**) phases of the ventricular action potential.

threshold. When the cell has reached this threshold, a rapid influx of sodium occurs. The exterior of the cell now is negatively charged in relation to the highly positive interior of the cell. This rapid influx of sodium produces a rapid, positively directed change in the transmembrane potential, resulting in the electrical spike and overshoot during phase 0 of the action potential.[7] The membrane potential shifts from a resting membrane potential of approximately −90 millivolts (mV) to +20 mV (Fig. 27-4). The rapid depolarization that constitutes phase 0 is responsible for the QRS complex on the electrocardiogram (ECG) (see Fig. 27-3). Depolarization of a cardiac cell tends to cause adjacent cells to depolarize because the voltage spike of the cell's depolarization stimulates the sodium channels in nearby cells to open. Therefore, when a cardiac cell is stimulated to depolarize, a wave of depolarization is propagated across the heart, cell by cell.

Phase 1 occurs at the peak of the action potential and signifies inactivation of the fast sodium channels with an abrupt decrease in sodium permeability. The slight downward slope is thought to be caused by the influx of a small amount of negatively charged chloride ions and efflux of potassium.[1] The decrease in intracellular positivity reduces the membrane potential to a level near 0 mV, from which the plateau, or phase 2, arises.

Phase 2 represents the plateau of the action potential. If potassium permeability increased to its resting level at this time, as it does in nerve fibers or skeletal muscle, the cell would repolarize rapidly. Instead, potassium permeability is low, allowing the membrane to remain depolarized throughout the phase 2 plateau. A concomitant influx of calcium into the cell through slow channels contributes to the phase 2 plateau.[7] Calcium ions entering the muscle during this phase also play a key role in the contractile process.[1] These unique features of the phase 2 plateau in these cells cause the action potential of cardiac muscle (several hundred milliseconds) to last 3 to 15 times longer than that of skeletal muscle and cause a corresponding increased period of contraction.[6] The phase 2 plateau coincides with the ST segment of the ECG.

Phase 3 reflects final rapid repolarization and begins with the downslope of the action potential. During the phase 3 repolarization period, the slow channels close, and the influx of calcium and sodium ceases. There is a sharp rise in potassium permeability, contributing to the rapid outward movement of potassium and reestablishment of the resting membrane potential (−90 mV). At the conclusion of phase 3, the distribution of potassium and sodium returns membrane to the normal resting state. The T wave on the ECG corresponds with phase 3 of the action potential.

Phase 4 represents the resting membrane potential. During phase 4, the activity of the sodium-potassium pump contributes to maintenance of the resting membrane potential by transporting sodium out of the cell and moving potassium back in. Phase 4 corresponds to diastole.

The Fast and Slow Response. There are two main types of action potentials in the heart—the fast response and the slow response (see Fig. 27-4). The *fast response* occurs in the normal myocardial cells of the atria, the ventricles, and the Purkinje fibers. It is characterized by the opening of voltage-dependent sodium channels called the *fast sodium channels.* The fast-response cardiac cells do not normally initiate cardiac action potentials. Instead, impulses originating in the specialized cells of the SA node are conducted to the fast-response myocardial cells, where they effect a change in membrane potential to the threshold level. On reaching threshold, the voltage-dependent *sodium* channels open to initiate the rapid upstroke of the phase 1 action potential. The amplitude and the rate of rise of phase 1 are important to the conduction velocity of the fast response. Myocardial fibers with a fast response are capable of conducting electrical activity at relatively rapid rates (0.5 to 5.0 m/second), thereby providing a high safety factor for conduction.[9]

The *slow response* occurs in the SA node, which is the natural pacemaker of the heart, and in the conduction fibers of the AV node (see Fig. 27-4). The hallmark of these pacemaker cells is a spontaneous phase 4 depolarization. The membrane permeability of these cells allows a slow inward leak of current to occur through the slow channels during phase 4. This leak continues until the threshold for firing is reached, at which point the cell spontaneously depolarizes. Under normal conditions, the slow response,

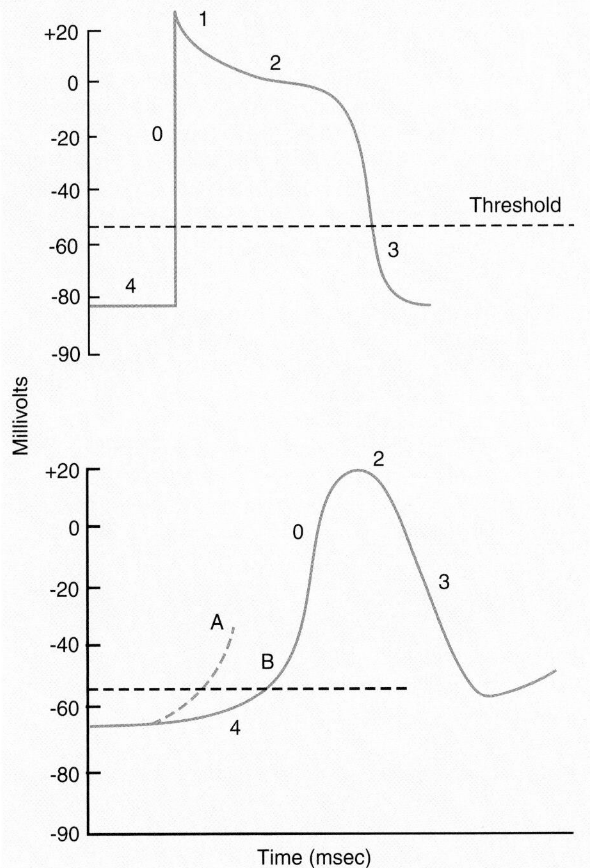

FIGURE 27-4 Changes in action potential recorded from a fast response in cardiac muscle cell (**top**) and from a slow response recorded in the sinoatrial and atrioventricular nodes (**bottom**). The phases of the action potential are identified by numbers: phase 4, resting membrane potential; phase 0, depolarization; phase 1, brief period of repolarization; phase 2, plateau; phase 3, repolarization. The slow response is characterized by a slow, spontaneous rise in the phase 4 membrane potential to threshold levels; it has a lesser amplitude and shorter duration than the fast response. Increased automaticity *(A)* occurs when the rate of phase 4 depolarization is increased.

sometimes referred to as the *calcium current,* does not contribute significantly to myocardial depolarization in the atria and ventricles. Its primary role in normal atrial and ventricular cells is to provide for the entrance of calcium for the excitation-contraction mechanism that couples the electrical activity with muscle contraction.

The rate of pacemaker cell discharge varies with the resting membrane potential and the slope of phase 4 depolarization (see Fig. 27-4). Catecholamines (*i.e.,* epinephrine and norepinephrine) increase the heart rate by increasing the slope or rate of phase 4 depolarization. Acetylcholine, which is released during vagal stimulation of the heart, slows the heart rate by decreasing the slope of phase 4.

The fast response of atrial and ventricular muscle can be converted to a slow pacemaker response under certain conditions. For example, such conversions may occur spontaneously in individuals with severe coronary artery disease, in areas of the heart where blood supply has been markedly compromised or curtailed. Impulses generated by these cells can lead to ectopic beats and serious arrhythmias.

Absolute and Relative Refractory Periods

The pumping action of the heart requires alternating contraction and relaxation. There is a period in the action potential curve during which no stimuli can generate another action potential (Fig. 27-5). This period, which is known as the *absolute refractory period,* includes phases 0, 1, 2, and part of phase 3. During this time, the cell cannot depolarize again under any circumstances. When repolarization has returned the membrane potential to below threshold, although not to the resting membrane potential (–90 mV), the cell is capable of responding to a greater-than-normal stimulus. This condition is referred to as the *relative refractory period.* The relative refractory period begins when the transmembrane potential in phase 3 reaches the threshold potential level and ends just before the terminal portion of phase 3. After the relative refractory period is a short period, called the *supernormal excitatory period,* during which a weak stimulus can evoke a response. The supernormal excitatory period extends from the terminal portion of phase 3 until the beginning of phase 4. It is during this period that cardiac arrhythmias develop.

In skeletal muscle, the refractory period is very short compared with the duration of contraction, such that a second contraction can be initiated before the first is over, resulting in a summated tetanized contraction. In cardiac muscle, the absolute refractory period is almost as long as the contraction, and a second contraction cannot be stimulated until the first is over. The longer length of the

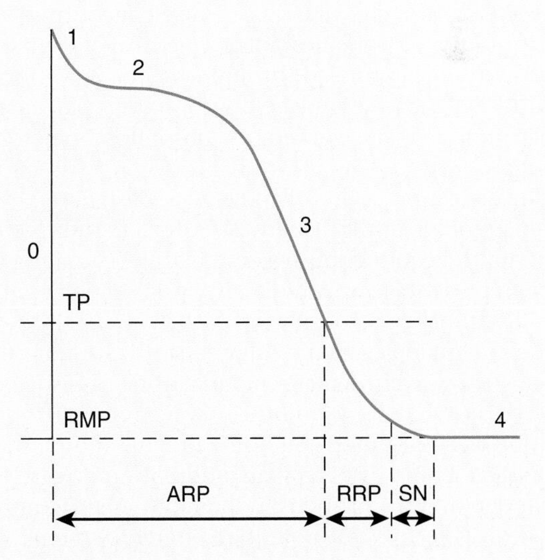

FIGURE 27-5 Diagram of an action potential of a ventricular muscle cell, showing the threshold potential (TP), resting membrane potential (RMP), absolute refractory period (ARP), relative refractory period (RRP), and supernormal (SN) period.

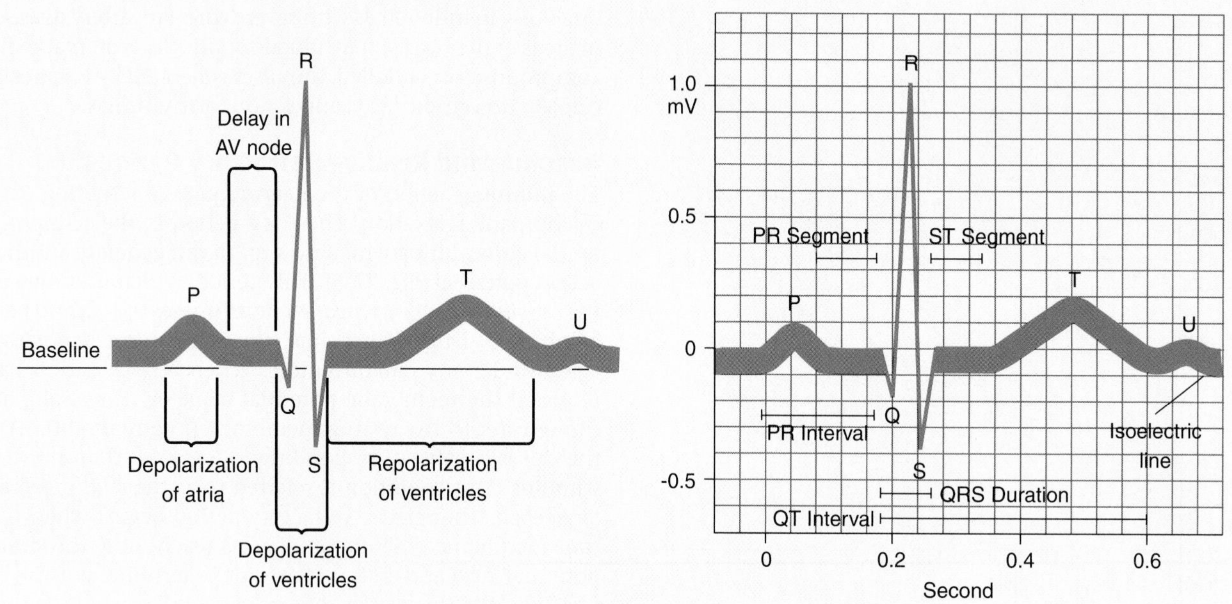

FIGURE 27-6 Diagram of the electrocardiogram (lead II) and representative depolarization and repolarization of the atria and ventricle. The P wave represents atrial depolarization, the QRS complex ventricular depolarization, and the T wave ventricular repolarization. Atrial repolarization occurs during ventricular depolarization and is hidden under the QRS complex.

absolute refractory period of cardiac muscle is important in maintaining the alternating contraction and relaxation that is essential to the pumping action of the heart and for the prevention of fatal arrhythmias.

ELECTROCARDIOGRAPHY

The electrocardiogram (ECG) is a graphic recording of the electrical activity of the heart. The electrical currents generated by the heart spread through the body to the skin, where they can be sensed by appropriately placed electrodes, amplified, and viewed on an oscilloscope or chart recorder.

The deflection points of an ECG are designated by the letters P, Q, R, S, and T. Figure 27-6 depicts the electrical activity of the conduction system on an ECG tracing. The P wave represents the SA node and atrial depolarization; the QRS complex (*i.e.*, beginning of the Q wave to the end of the S wave) depicts ventricular depolarization; and the T wave portrays ventricular repolarization. The isoelectric line between the P wave and the Q wave represents depolarization of the AV node, bundle branches, and Purkinje system (Fig. 27-7). Atrial repolarization occurs during ventricular depolarization and is hidden in the QRS complex.

The ECG records the potential difference in charge (in millivolts) between two electrodes as depolarization and repolarization waves move through the heart and are conducted to the skin surface. The shape of the recorder tracing is determined by the direction in which the impulse spreads through the heart muscle in relation to electrode placement. A depolarization wave that moves toward the recording electrode registers as a positive, or upward, deflection. Conversely, if the impulse moves away from the recording electrode, the deflection is downward, or negative. When there is no flow of charge between electrodes, the potential is zero, and a straight line is recorded at the baseline of the chart.

The ECG recorder is much like a camera in that it can record different views of the electrical activity of the heart,

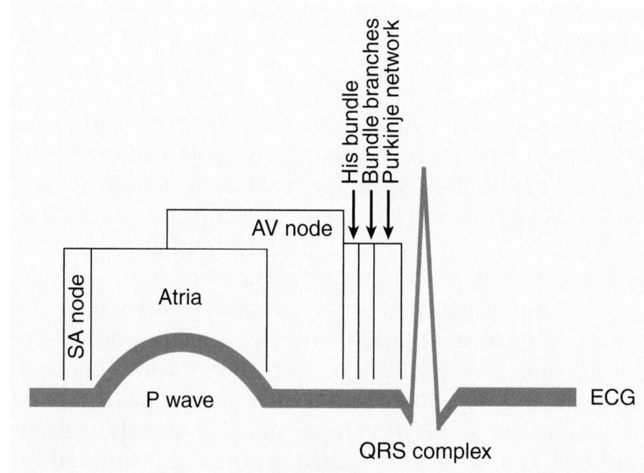

FIGURE 27-7 Tissues depolarized by a wave of activation commencing in the sinoatrial (SA) node are shown in a series of blocks superimposed on the deflections of the electrocardiogram (ECG). (Katz A.M. [1992]. *Physiology of the heart* [p. 483]. New York: Raven Press)

depending on where the recording electrode is placed. The horizontal axis of the ECG measures time (seconds), and the vertical axis measures the amplitude of the impulse (millivolts). Each heavy vertical line represents 0.2 second, and each thin line represents 0.04 second (see Fig. 27-6). The widths of ECG complexes are commonly referred to in terms of duration of time. On the vertical axis, each heavy horizontal line represents 0.5 mV. The connections of the ECG are arranged such that an upright deflection indicates a positive potential and a downward deflection indicates a negative potential. Although the vertical axis determines amplitude in terms of voltage, these values frequently are communicated as millimeters of positive or negative deflection rather than in millivolts.

Conventionally, 12 leads (6 limb leads and 6 chest leads) are recorded for a diagnostic ECG, each providing a unique view of the electrical forces of the heart from a different position on the body's surface. The six limb leads view the electrical forces as they pass through the heart on the frontal or vertical plane. The electrodes are attached to the four extremities or representative areas on the body near the shoulders and lower chest or abdomen. The electrical potential recorded from any one extremity should be the same no matter where the electrode is placed on the extremity. The six chest leads provide a view of the electrical forces as they pass through the heart on the horizontal plane. They are moved to different positions on the chest, including the right and left sternal borders and the left anterior surface. The right lower extremity lead is used as a ground electrode. When indicated, additional electrodes may be applied to other areas of the body, such as the back or right anterior chest.

The goals of continuous bedside cardiac monitoring have shifted from simple heart rate and arrhythmia monitoring to identification of ST-segment changes, advanced arrhythmia identification, diagnosis, and treatment. Many diagnostic criteria are lead specific. The monitoring leads selected must maximize the potential for accurately identifying anticipated arrhythmias and ischemic events on the basis of the patient's underlying clinical situation.

When monitoring patients with wide QRS-complex tachycardia (discussed later), the use of 12-lead ECG monitoring systems is considered optimal. For example, Drew and Scheinman[10] found that the use of 12-lead ECG monitoring systems resulted in more than 90% accuracy when diagnosing wide QRS arrhythmias; whereas the use of lead II, a limb lead commonly used for continuous monitoring, resulted in only 34% being correctly identified.

Although accurate ECG placement and lead selection are an important aspect of ECG monitoring, two national surveys conducted in 1991 and 1995, respectively,[11,12] identified two common errors: inaccurate electrode placement and inappropriate lead selection for individual clinical situations. Improper lead placement can significantly change QRS morphology, resulting in misdiagnosis of cardiac arrhythmias.[13] Inappropriate lead selection can also result in conduction defects being missed.

In persons with acute coronary syndrome (ACS), including unstable angina and ST-segment elevation and non–ST-segment elevation myocardial infarction, careful cardiac ECG monitoring is imperative[14] (see Chapter 26). Persons with ACS are at risk for developing extension of an infarcted area, ongoing myocardial ischemia, and life-threatening arrhythmias. Research has revealed that 80% to 90% of ECG-detected ischemic events are clinically silent.[15,16] Thus, ECG monitoring is more sensitive than a patient's report of symptoms for identifying transient ongoing myocardial ischemia. ECG monitoring also provides for more accurate and timely detection of ischemic events, essential for treatment options such as reperfusion strategies.[17] It is recommended that all 12 ECG leads be used for monitoring patients with ACS because ischemic changes that occur may be evident in different leads at different times.

In summary, the rhythmic contraction and relaxation of the heart rely on the specialized cells of the heart's conduction system. Specialized cells in the SA node have the fastest inherent rate of impulse generation and act as the pacemaker of the heart. Impulses from the SA node travel through the atria to the AV node and then to the AV bundle and the ventricular Purkinje system. The AV node provides the only connection between the atrial and ventricular conduction systems. The atria and the ventricles function independently of each other when AV node conduction is blocked.

The action potential of cardiac muscle is divided into five phases: phase 0 represents depolarization and is characterized by the rapid upstroke of the action potential; phase 1 is characterized by a brief period of repolarization; phase 2 consists of a plateau, which prolongs the duration of the action potential; phase 3 represents repolarization; and phase 4 is the resting membrane potential. After an action potential, there is a refractory period during which the membrane is resistant to a second stimulus. During the absolute refractory period, the membrane is insensitive to stimulation. This period is followed by the relative refractory period, during which a more intense stimulus is needed to initiate an action potential. The relative refractory period is followed by a supernormal excitatory period, during which a weak stimulus can evoke a response.

The ECG provides a means for monitoring the electrical activity of the heart. Conventionally, 12 leads (6 limb leads and 6 chest leads) are recorded for a diagnostic ECG, each providing a unique view of the electrical forces of the heart from a different position on the body's surface. This allows for advanced arrhythmia interpretation, detection of wide QRS-complex tachycardia, and early identification of ischemic and infarction changes in persons with ACS.

Disorders of Cardiac Rhythm and Conduction

After completing this section of the chapter, you should be able to meet the following objectives:

- Describe the possible mechanisms for arrhythmia generation
- Compare sinus arrhythmias with atrial arrhythmias

- Characterize the effects of atrial flutter and atrial fibrillation on heart rhythm
- Describe the significance of long QT syndrome
- Describe the characteristics of first-, second-, and third-degree heart block
- Compare the effects of premature ventricular contractions, ventricular tachycardia, and ventricular fibrillation on cardiac function
- Cite the types of cardiac conditions that can be diagnosed using the ECG
- Describe the methods used in diagnosis of cardiac arrhythmias
- Explain the mechanisms, criteria for use, and benefits of antiarrhythmic drugs, internal cardioverter-defibrillator therapy, ablation therapy, and surgical procedures in the treatment of persons with recurrent, symptomatic arrhythmias

There are two types of disorders of the cardiac conduction system: disorders of rhythm and disorders of impulse conduction. The terms *dysrhythmia* and *arrhythmia* have sometimes been used interchangeably to describe disorders of cardiac rhythm. Marriott[18] has pointed out that the term *arrhythmia* was originally based on the usage of the alpha privative (the prefix *a-*) to imply "imperfection in" as opposed to "absence of" cardiac rhythms. However, Marriott further pointed out that the term dysrhythmia has not been generally accepted, and conventional use of the term *arrhythmia* continues. Therefore, the term *arrhythmia* will be used throughout this chapter.

There are many causes of cardiac arrhythmias and conductions disorders, including congenital defects or degenerative changes in the conduction system, myocardial ischemia and infarction, fluid and electrolyte imbalances, and the effects of drug ingestion. Arrhythmias are not necessarily pathologic; they can occur in both healthy and diseased hearts. Disturbances in cardiac rhythms exert their harmful effects by interfering with the heart's pumping ability. Excessively rapid heart rates (tachyarrhythmias) reduce the diastolic filling time, causing a subsequent decrease in the stroke volume output and in coronary perfusion while increasing the myocardial oxygen needs. Abnormally slow heart rates (bradyarrhythmias) may impair the blood flow to vital organs such as the brain.

MECHANISMS OF ARRHYTHMIAS AND CONDUCTION DISORDERS

The specialized cells in the conduction system manifest four inherent properties that contribute to the genesis of all cardiac rhythms, both normal and abnormal. They are automaticity, excitability, conductivity, and refractoriness. An alteration in any of these four properties may produce arrhythmias or conduction defects.

The ability of certain cells in the conduction system to initiate an impulse or action potential spontaneously is referred to as *automaticity*. The SA node has an inherent discharge rate of 60 to 100 times per minute. It normally acts as the pacemaker of the heart because it reaches the threshold for excitation before other parts of the conduction system have recovered sufficiently to be depolarized. If the SA node fires more slowly or SA node conduction is blocked, another site that is capable of automaticity takes over as pacemaker. Other regions that are capable of automaticity include the atrial fibers that have plateau-type action potentials, the AV node, the bundle of His, and the bundle branch Purkinje fibers. These pacemakers have a slower rate of discharge than the SA node. The AV node has an inherent firing rate of 40 to 60 times per minute, and the Purkinje system fires at a rate of 20 to 40 times per minute. The SA node may be functioning properly, but because of additional precipitating factors, other cardiac cells can assume accelerated properties of automaticity and begin to initiate impulses. These additional factors might include injury, hypoxia, electrolyte disturbances, enlargement or hypertrophy of the atria or ventricles, and exposure to certain chemicals or drugs.

An *ectopic pacemaker* is an excitable focus outside the normally functioning SA node. These pacemakers can reside in other parts of the conduction system or in muscle cells of the atria or ventricles. A premature contraction occurs when an ectopic pacemaker initiates a beat. Premature contractions do not follow the normal conduction pathways, they are not coupled with normal mechanical events, and they often render the heart refractory or incapable of responding to the next normal impulse arising in the SA node. They occur without incident in persons with healthy hearts in response to sympathetic nervous system stimulation or other stimulants such as caffeine. In the diseased heart, premature contractions may lead to more serious arrhythmias.

Excitability describes the ability of a cell to respond to an impulse and generate an action potential. Myocardial cells that have been injured or replaced by scar tissue do

PHYSIOLOGIC BASIS OF ARRHYTHMIA GENERATION

- Cardiac arrhythmias represent disorders of cardiac rhythm related to alterations in automaticity, excitability, conductivity, or refractoriness of specialized cells in the conduction system of the heart.
- Automaticity refers to the ability of pacemaker cells in the heart to spontaneously generate an action potential. Normally, the SA node is the pacemaker of the heart because of its intrinsic automaticity.
- Excitability is the ability of cardiac tissue to respond to an impulse and generate an action potential.
- Conductivity and refractoriness represent the ability of cardiac tissue to conduct action potentials.
- Whereas conductivity relates to the ability of cardiac tissue to conduct impulses, refractoriness represents temporary interruptions in conductivity related to the repolarization phase of the action potential.

not possess normal excitability. For example, during the acute phase of an ischemic event, involved cells become depolarized. These ischemic cells remain electrically coupled to the adjacent nonischemic area; current from the ischemic zone can induce reexcitation of cells in the nonischemic zone.

Conductivity is the ability to conduct impulses, and *refractoriness* refers to the extent to which the cell is able to respond to an incoming stimulus. The refractory period of cardiac muscle is the interval in the repolarization period during which an excitable cell has not recovered sufficiently to be reexcited. Disturbances in conductivity or refractoriness predispose to arrhythmias.

Almost all tachyarrhythmias are the result of a phenomenon known as *reentry*.[5,19–21] Under normal conditions, an electrical impulse is conducted through the heart in an orderly, sequential manner. The electrical impulse then dies out and does not reenter adjacent tissue because that tissue has already been depolarized and is refractory to immediate stimulation. However, fibers that were not activated during the initial wave of depolarization can recover excitability before the initial impulse dies out, and they may serve as a link to reexcite areas of the heart that were just discharged and have recovered from the initial depolarization.[1,19] This activity disrupts the normal conduction sequence. For reentry to occur, there must be areas of slow conduction and unidirectional conduction block (Fig. 27-8). For previously depolarized areas to repolarize adequately to conduct an impulse again, slow conduction is necessary. Unidirectional block is necessary to provide a one-way route for the original impulse to reenter, thereby blocking other impulses entering from the opposite direction from extinguishing the reentrant circuit. Reentry requires a triggering stimulus such as an extrasystole. If sufficient time has elapsed for the refractory period in the reentered area to end, a self-perpetuating, circuitous movement can be initiated.[1]

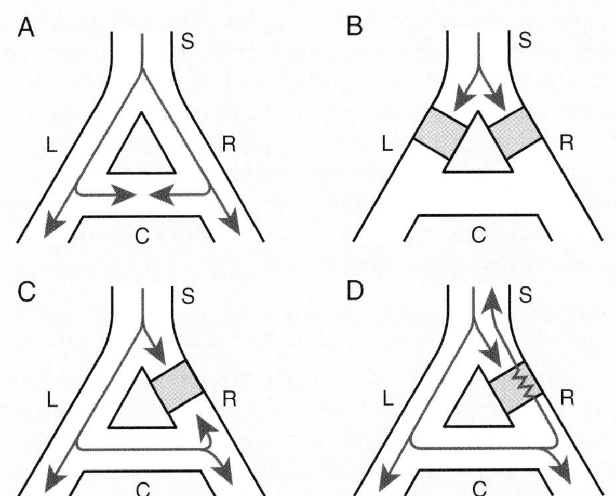

FIGURE 27-8 The role of unidirectional block in reentry. (**A**) An excitation wave traveling down a single bundle (S) of fibers continues down the left (L) and right (R) branches. The depolarization wave enters the connecting branch (C) from both ends and is extinguished at the zone of collision. (**B**) The wave is blocked in the L and R branches. (**C**) Bidirectional block exists in branch R. (**D**) The antegrade impulse is blocked, but the retrograde impulse is conducted through and reenters bundle S. (Berne R.M., Levy M.N. [1988]. *Physiology* [2nd ed., p. 417]. St. Louis: C.V. Mosby)

Reentry may occur anywhere in the conduction system. The functional components of a reentry circuit can be large and include an entire specialized conduction system, or the circuit can be microscopic. It can include myocardial tissue, AV nodal cells, junctional tissue, or the ventricles. Factors contributing to the development of a reentrant circuit include ischemia, infarction, and elevated serum potassium levels.[22] Scar tissue interrupts the normally low-resistance paths between viable myocardial cells, slowing conduction, promoting asynchronous myocardial activation, and predisposing to unidirectional conduction block. Specially filtered signal-averaged electrocardiography can be used to detect the resultant late potentials. Effects of drugs such as epinephrine can produce a shortened refractory period, thereby increasing the likelihood of reentrant arrhythmias.

There are several forms of reentry. The first is anatomic reentry. It consists of an excitation wave that travels in a set pathway.[1,23] Arrhythmias that arise as a result of anatomic reentry are paroxysmal supraventricular tachycardias, as seen in Wolff-Parkinson-White syndrome, atrial fibrillation, atrial flutter, AV nodal reentry, and some ventricular tachycardias. Functional reentry does not rely on an anatomic structure to circle; rather, it depends on the local differences in conduction velocity.[1,23] Spiral reentry is the most common form of this type of reentry.[24] It is initiated by a wave of electrical current that does not propagate naturally in its normal plane after meeting refractory tissue. The broken end of the wave curls, forms a vortex, and permanently rotates. This phenomenon suppresses normal pacemaker activity and can result in atrial fibrillation.[23] Arrhythmias observed with functional reentry are likely to be polymorphic because of charging circuits.[1] Reflection is sometimes considered another form of reentry that can occur in parallel pathways of myocardial tissue or the Purkinje network. With reflection, the cardiac impulse reaches the depressed segment, triggers the surrounding tissue, and then returns in a retrograde direction through the severely depressed region. Reflection differs from true reentry in that the impulse travels along the same pathway in both directions and does not require a circuit.[1]

TYPES OF ARRHYTHMIAS

Sinus Node Arrhythmias

In a healthy heart driven by sinus node discharge, the heart rate ranges between 60 and 100 beats per minute. On the ECG, a P wave may be observed to precede every QRS complex. Historically, normal sinus rhythm has been considered the "normal" rhythm of a healthy heart. In normal sinus rhythm, a P wave precedes each QRS complex, and the RR intervals, which are used to measure heart rate, remain relatively constant over time (Fig. 27-9). Alterations in the function of the SA node lead to changes in rate or rhythm of the heartbeat.

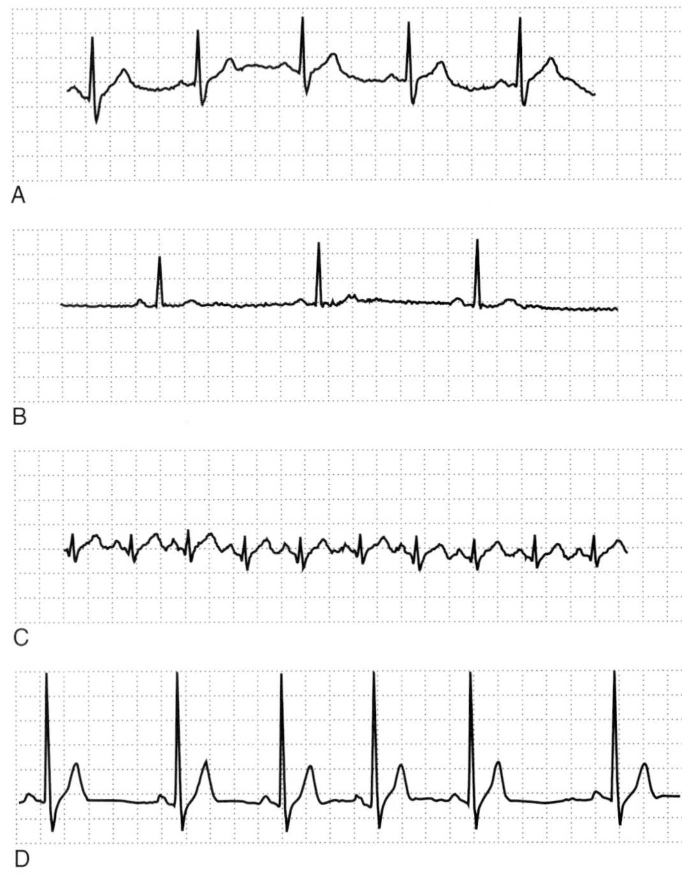

FIGURE 27-9 Electrocardiographic (ECG) tracings of rhythms originating in the sinus node. (**A**) Normal sinus rhythm (60 to 100 beats per minute). (**B**) Sinus bradycardia (<60 beats per minute). (**C**) Sinus tachycardia (>100 beats per minute). (**D**) Respiratory sinus arrhythmia, characterized by gradually lengthening and shortening of RR intervals.

Years ago, it was believed that sinus rhythm should be regular; that is, all RR intervals should be equal. Today, it is accepted that a more optimal rhythm is respiratory sinus arrhythmia. Respiratory sinus arrhythmia is a cardiac rhythm characterized by gradual lengthening and shortening of RR intervals (see Fig. 27-9). This variation in cardiac cycles is related to intrathoracic pressure changes that occur with respiration and resultant alterations in autonomic control of the SA node. Inspiration causes acceleration of the heart rate, and expiration causes slowing. Respiratory sinus arrhythmia accounts for most heart rate variability in healthy individuals. Decreased heart rate variability has been associated with altered health states, including myocardial infarction, congestive heart failure, hypertension, diabetes mellitus, and prematurity in infants.

Sinus Bradycardia. Sinus bradycardia describes a slow (<60 beats per minute) heart rate (see Fig. 27-9). In sinus bradycardia, a P wave precedes each QRS. A normal P wave and PR interval (0.12 to 0.20 second) indicate that the impulse originated in the SA node rather than in another area of the conduction system that has a slower inherent rate. Vagal stimulation decreases the firing rate of the SA node and conduction through the AV node to cause a decrease in heart rate. This rhythm may be normal in trained athletes, who maintain a large stroke volume, and during sleep. Sinus bradycardia may be an indicator of poor prognosis when it occurs in conjunction with acute myocardial infarction, particularly if associated with hypotension.

Sinus Tachycardia. Sinus tachycardia refers to a rapid heart rate (>100 beats per minute) that has its origin in the SA node (see Fig. 27-9). A normal P wave and PR interval should precede each QRS complex. The mechanism of sinus tachycardia is enhanced automaticity related to sympathetic stimulation or withdrawal of vagal tone. Sinus tachycardia is a normal response during fever and exercise and in situations that incite sympathetic stimulation. It may be associated with congestive heart failure, myocardial infarction, and hyperthyroidism. Pharmacologic agents such as atropine, isoproterenol, epinephrine, and quinidine also can cause sinus tachycardia.

Sinus Arrest. Sinus arrest refers to failure of the SA node to discharge and results in an irregular pulse. An escape rhythm develops as another pacemaker takes over. Sinus arrest may result in prolonged periods of asystole and often predisposes to other arrhythmias. Causes of sinus arrest include disease of the SA node, digitalis toxicity, myocardial infarction, acute myocarditis, excessive vagal tone, quinidine, acetylcholine, and hyperkalemia or hypokalemia.[25]

Sick Sinus Syndrome. Sick sinus syndrome is a term that describes a number of forms of cardiac impulse formation and intra-atrial and AV conduction abnormalities.[26–28] The syndrome most frequently is the result of total or subtotal destruction of the SA node, areas of nodal–atrial discontinuity, inflammatory or degenerative changes of the nerves and ganglia surrounding the node, or pathologic changes in the atrial wall.[28] In addition, occlusion of the sinus node artery may be a significant contributing factor. Approximately 40% of adults with sick sinus syndrome also have coronary heart disease.[29] In children, the syndrome is most commonly associated with congenital heart defects, particularly following corrective cardiac surgery.[28]

The arrhythmias associated with sick sinus syndrome include spontaneous persistent sinus bradycardia that is not drug induced or appropriate for the physiologic circumstances, prolonged sinus pauses, combinations of SA and AV node conduction disturbances, or alternating paroxysms of rapid regular or irregular atrial tachyarrhythmias and periods of slow atrial and ventricular rates (bradycardia-tachycardia syndrome).[30] Most commonly, the term *sick sinus syndrome* is used to refer to the bradycardia-tachycardia syndrome. The bradycardia is caused by disease of the sinus node (or other intraatrial conduction pathways), and the tachycardia is caused by paroxysmal atrial or junctional arrhythmias. Individuals with this syndrome often are asymptomatic. Ironically, the development of atrial fibrillation may alleviate symptoms in persons who are symptomatic because heart rate can be controlled more consistently under these circumstances.[27]

The most common manifestations of sick sinus syndrome are lightheadedness, dizziness, and syncope, symptoms related to the bradyarrhythmias.[29,31] When patients with sick sinus syndrome experience palpitations, they are generally the result of tachyarrhythmias and are suggestive of the presence of bradycardia-tachycardia syndrome.[29]

Treatment depends on the rhythm problem and frequently involves the implantation of a permanent pacemaker. Pacing for the bradycardia, combined with drug therapy to treat the tachycardia, is often required in bradycardia-tachycardia syndrome.[28] Medications that affect SA node discharge must be cautiously used.

Arrhythmias of Atrial Origin

Impulses from the SA node pass through the conductive pathways in the atria to the AV node. Arrhythmias of atrial origin include premature atrial contractions, paroxysmal supraventricular tachycardia, atrial flutter, and atrial fibrillation (Fig. 27-10).

Premature Atrial Contractions. Premature atrial contractions (PACs) are contractions that originate in the atrial conduction pathways or atrial muscle cells and occur before the next expected SA node impulse. This impulse to contract usually is transmitted to the ventricle and back to the SA node. The location of the ectopic focus determines the configuration of the P wave. In general, the closer the ectopic focus is to the SA node, the more the ectopic complex resembles a normal sinus complex. The retrograde transmission to the SA node often interrupts the timing of the next sinus beat, such that a pause occurs between the two normally conducted beats. In healthy individuals, PACs may be the result of stress, tobacco, or caffeine. They also have been associated with myocardial infarction, digitalis toxicity, low serum potassium or magnesium levels, and hypoxia.

Paroxysmal Supraventricular Tachycardia. Paroxysmal supraventricular tachycardia is sometimes referred to as *paroxysmal atrial tachycardia.* This term includes all

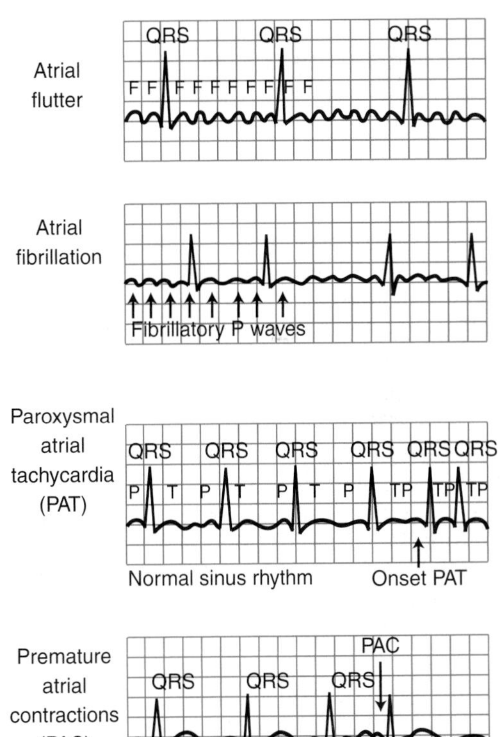

FIGURE 27-10 Electrocardiographic tracings of atrial arrhythmias. Atrial flutter *(first tracing)* is characterized by the atrial flutter (F) waves occurring at a rate of 240 to 450 beats per minute. The ventricular rate remains regular because of the conduction of every sixth atrial contraction. Atrial fibrillation *(second tracing)* has grossly disorganized atrial electrical activity that is irregular with respect to rate and rhythm. The ventricular response is irregular, and no distinct P waves are visible. The *third tracing* illustrates paroxysmal atrial tachycardia (PAT), preceded by a normal sinus rhythm. The *fourth tracing* illustrates premature atrial complexes (PAC).

SUPRAVENTRICULAR AND VENTRICULAR ARRHYTHMIAS

- Supraventricular arrhythmias represent disorders of atrial rhythm or conduction.
- Atrioventricular nodal and junctional arrhythmias result from disruption in conduction of impulses from the atria to the ventricles.
- Ventricular arrhythmias represent disorders of ventricular rhythm or conduction.
- Because the ventricles are pumping chambers of the heart, arrhythmias that produce an abnormally slow (*e.g.*, heart block) or rapid ventricular rate (*e.g.*, ventricular tachycardia or fibrillation) are potentially life threatening.

tachyarrhythmias that originate above the bifurcation of the bundle of His and have a sudden onset and termination. They may be the result of AV nodal reentry, Wolff-Parkinson-White syndrome (caused by an accessory conduction pathway between the atria and ventricles), or intraatrial or sinus node reentry. Paroxysmal supraventricular tachycardias tend to be recurrent and of short duration.

Atrial Flutter. Atrial flutter is a rapid atrial ectopic tachycardia, with an atrial rate that ranges from 240 to 450 beats per minute. There are two types of atrial flutter.[27] Type I flutter (classic) is the result of a reentry mechanism in the right atrium and can be entrained and interrupted with atrial pacing techniques. The atrial rate in typical type I flutter usually is in the vicinity of 300 beats per minute, but it can range from 240 to 340 beats per minute. The mechanism of type II flutter is unknown. With type II flutter, the atrial rate ranges from 350 to 450 beats per minute. On the ECG, atrial flutter generates a defined sawtooth pattern in leads II, III, aVF, and V_1.[32] The ventricular response rate and regularity are variable and depend on the AV conduction sequence. When regular, the ventricular response rate usually is a defined fraction of the atrial rate (*i.e.*, when conduction from the atria to the ventricles is 2:1, an atrial flutter rate of 300 would result in a ventricular response rate of 150 beats per minute). The QRS complex may be normal or abnormal, depending on the presence or absence of preexisting intraventricular conduction defects or aberrant ventricular conduction.

Atrial flutter rarely is seen in normal, healthy individuals. It may be seen in persons of any age in the presence of underlying atrial abnormalities. Subgroups that are at particularly high risk for development of atrial flutter include children, adolescents, and young adults who have undergone corrective surgery for complex congenital heart diseases.[27]

Atrial Fibrillation. Atrial fibrillation is characterized by chaotic impulses propagating in different directions and causing disorganized atrial depolarizations without effective atrial contraction.[33] In most cases, multiple, small reentrant circuits are constantly arising in the atria, colliding, being extinguished, and arising again. Fibrillation occurs when the atrial cells cannot repolarize in time for the next incoming stimulus. Atrial fibrillation is characterized on the ECG by a grossly disorganized pattern of atrial electrical activity that is irregular with respect to rate and rhythm and the absence of discernible P waves. Atrial activity is depicted by fibrillatory (f) waves of varying amplitude, duration, and morphology. These f waves appear as random oscillation of the baseline. Because of the random conduction through the AV node, QRS complexes appear in an irregular pattern.

Atrial fibrillation is the only common arrhythmia in which the ventricular rate is rapid and the rhythm irregular.[34] The atrial rate typically ranges from 400 to 600 beats per minute, with many impulses blocked at the AV node. The ventricular response is completely irregular, ranging from 80 to 180 beats per minute in the untreated state. Because of changes in stroke volumes resulting from varying periods of diastolic filling, not all ventricular beats produce a palpable pulse. The difference between the apical rate and the palpable peripheral pulses is called the *pulse deficit.* The pulse deficit may increase when the ventricular rate is high.

Atrial fibrillation may appear paroxysmally or as a chronic phenomenon.[31] It can be seen in persons without any apparent disease, or it may occur in individuals with coronary artery disease, mitral valve disease, ischemic heart disease, hypertension, myocardial infarction, pericarditis, congestive heart failure, digitalis toxicity, and hyperthyroidism. Spontaneous conversion to sinus rhythm within 24 hours of atrial fibrillation is common, occurring in up to two thirds of persons with the disorder.[33] Once the duration exceeds 24 hours, the likelihood of conversion decreases, and after 1 week of persistent arrhythmia, spontaneous conversion is rare.[33]

Atrial fibrillation is the most common chronic arrhythmia with an incidence and prevalence that increases with age. The incidence of chronic atrial fibrillation doubles with each decade of life and ranges from 2 or 3 new cases per 1000 population per year between the ages of 55 and 64 years, to 35 new cases per 1000 per year between the ages of 85 and 95 years.[33]

The symptoms of chronic atrial fibrillation vary. Some people have minimal symptoms, and others have severe symptoms, particularly at the onset of the arrhythmia. The symptoms may range from palpitations to acute pulmonary edema. Fatigue and other nonspecific symptoms are common in the elderly. The condition predisposes individuals to thrombus formation in the atria, with subsequent risk for embolic stroke.

The treatment of atrial fibrillation is dependent on its cause, recency of onset, and persistence of the arrhythmia. Anticoagulant medications may be used to prevent embolic stroke, and medications (*e.g.*, digitalis, beta blockers) may be used to control the ventricular rate in persons with persistent atrial fibrillation.[33,34] Cardioversion may be considered in some persons, particularly those with pulmonary edema or unstable cardiac status. Because conversion to sinus rhythm is associated with increased risk for thromboembolism, anticoagulation therapy is usually administered for at least 3 weeks before cardioversion is attempted in persons in whom the duration of atrial fibrillation is unknown or exceeds 2 to 3 days.[33] Transesophageal echocardiography can be used to detect atrial thrombus, and transesophageal echo-guided cardioversion provides a means of ensuring that atrial thrombus is not present when cardioversion is attempted. Anticoagulant medication is usually continued after cardioversion.

Junctional Arrhythmias

The AV node can act as a pacemaker in the event the SA node fails to initiate an impulse. Junctional rhythms can be transient or permanent, and they usually have a rate of 40 to 60 beats per minute. Junctional fibers in the AV node or bundle of His also can serve as ectopic pacemakers, producing premature junctional complexes. Another rhythm originating in the junctional tissues is nonparoxysmal junctional tachycardia. This rhythm usually is of gradual onset and termination. However, it may occur abruptly if the dominant pacemaker slows sufficiently. The rate associated with junctional tachycardia ranges from 70 to 130 beats per minute, but it may be faster.[1] The P waves may precede, be buried in, or follow the QRS complexes, depending on the site of the originating impulses. The clinical significance of nonparoxysmal junctional tachycardia is the same as for atrial tachycardias. Catheter ablation therapy has been used successfully to treat some individuals with recurrent or intractable junctional tachycardia. Nonparoxysmal junctional tachycardia is observed most frequently in individuals with underlying heart disease, such as inferior wall myocardial infarction or myocarditis, or after open-heart surgery. It also may be present in persons with digitalis toxicity.

Disorders of Ventricular Conduction and Rhythm

The junctional fibers in the AV node join with the bundle of His, which divides to form the right and left bundle branches. The bundle branches continue to divide and form the Purkinje fibers, which supply the walls of the ventricles (see Fig. 27-1). As the cardiac impulse leaves the junctional fibers, it travels through the AV bundle. Next, the impulse moves down the right and left bundle branches that lie beneath the endocardium on either side of the septum. It then spreads out through the walls of the ventricles. Interruption of impulse conduction through the bundle branches is called *bundle branch block*. These blocks usually do not cause alterations in the rhythm of the heartbeat. Instead, a bundle branch block interrupts the normal progression of depolarization, causing the ventricles to depolarize one after the other because the impulses must travel through muscle tissue rather than through the specialized conduction tissue.[35] This prolonged conduction causes the QRS complex to be wider than the normal 0.04 to 0.10 second. The left bundle branch bifurcates into the left anterior and posterior fascicles. An interruption of one of these fascicles is referred to as a *hemiblock*.

Long QT Syndrome and Torsades de Pointes

The *long QT syndrome* (LQTS) is characterized by prolongation of the QT interval that may result in a characteristic type of polymorphic ventricular tachycardia called *torsades de pointes* and sudden cardiac death.[36–38] Torsades de pointes (twisting or rotating around a point) is a specific type of ventricular tachycardia (Fig. 27-11). The term refers to the polarity of the QRS complex, which swings from positive to negative and vice versa. The QRS abnormality is characterized by large, bizarre, polymorphic, multiformed QRS complexes that vary, often from beat to beat, in amplitude and direction, at, as well as in, rotation of the complexes around the isoelectric line. The rate of tachycardia is 100 to 180 beats per minute but can be as fast as 200 to 300 beats per minute. The rhythm is highly unstable and may terminate in ventricular fibrillation or revert to sinus rhythm.

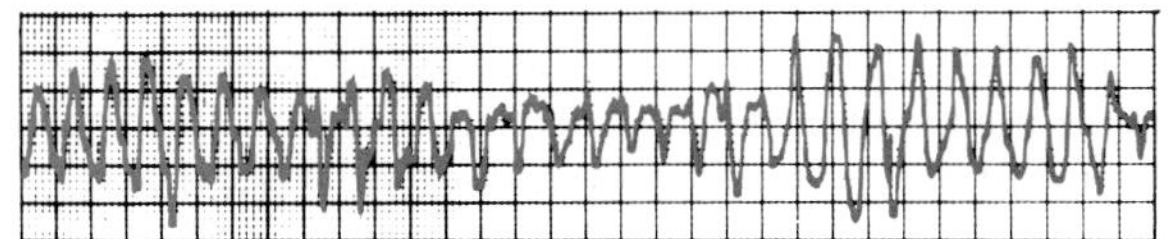

FIGURE 27-11 Torsades de pointes. (From Hudak C.M., Gallo B.M., Morton P.G. (1998). Critical care nursing: A holistic approach [7th ed., p. 216]. Philadelphia: Lippincott-Raven)

LQTS is caused by various agents and conditions that reduce the magnitude of outward repolarizing potassium currents, enhance the magnitude of the inward depolarizing sodium and calcium currents, or both. Thus, there is delayed repolarization of the ventricles with development of early depolarizing afterpotentials that initiate the arrhythmia. Typically, the QT interval is measured in a lead in which the T wave is prominent and its end is easily distinguished, such as V_2 or V_3. Because the QT interval shortens with tachycardia and lengthens with bradycardia, it is typically corrected for heart rate and is noted as QT_c.[39–42] Nonetheless, a QT_c greater than 440 msec in men and greater than 460 msec in women has been linked with episodes of sudden arrhythmia death syndrome. In addition, T-wave morphology frequently is abnormal in patients with LQTS.[1,43]

LQTS has been classified into hereditary and acquired forms, both of which are associated with the development of torsades de pointes and sudden cardiac death. The hereditary forms of LQTS are caused by disorders of membrane ion-channel proteins, with either potassium channel defects or sodium channel defects.[1] In some cases, the disorder may result from a gene defect that alters the function of a single ion channel. The gene mutations that result in congenital LQTS have been identified on chromosomes 3, 4, 7, 11, and 21.[44] The hereditary forms of LQTS are typically considered adrenergic dependent because they are generally triggered by increased activity of the sympathetic nervous system.[36]

Acquired LQTS has been linked to a variety of conditions, including cocaine use, exposure to organophosphorous compounds, electrolyte imbalances, marked bradycardia, myocardial infarction, subarachnoid hemorrhage, autonomic neuropathy, human immunodeficiency virus (HIV) infection, and protein-sparing fasting.[36,37,38,45] Medications linked to LQTS include digitalis, antiarrhythmic agents (*e.g.,* amiodarone, procainamide, and quinidine), verapamil (calcium channel blocker), haloperidol (antipsychotic agent), and erythromycin (antibiotic).[37] The acquired forms of LQTS are often classified as pause dependent because the torsades associated with them generally occurs at slow heart rates or in response to short-long-short RR-interval sequences. Treatment of acquired forms of LQTS is primarily directed at identifying and withdrawing the offending agent, although emergency-type measures that modulate the function of transmembrane ion currents can be lifesaving.

Ventricular Arrhythmias

Arrhythmias that arise in the ventricles commonly are considered more serious than those that arise in the atria because they afford the potential for interfering with the pumping action of the heart.

Premature Ventricular Contractions. A premature ventricular contraction (PVC) is caused by a ventricular ectopic pacemaker. After a PVC, the ventricle usually is unable to repolarize sufficiently to respond to the next impulse that arises in the SA node. This delay is commonly referred to as a *compensatory pause,* which occurs while the ventricle waits to reestablish its previous rhythm (Fig. 27-12). When a PVC occurs, the diastolic volume usually is insufficient for ejection of blood into the arterial system. As a result, PVCs usually do not produce a palpable pulse, or the pulse amplitude is significantly diminished. In the absence of heart disease, PVCs typically are not clinically significant. The incidence of PVCs is greatest with ischemia, acute myocardial infarction, history of myocardial infarction, ventricular hypertrophy, infection, increased sympathetic nervous system activity, or increased heart rate.[46] PVCs also can be the result of electrolyte disturbances or medications.

A special pattern of PVC called *ventricular bigeminy* is a condition in which each normal beat is followed by or paired with a PVC. This pattern often is an indication of digitalis toxicity or heart disease. The occurrence of frequent PVCs in the diseased heart predisposes the patient to the development of other, more serious arrhythmias, including ventricular tachycardia and ventricular fibrillation.

Ventricular Tachycardia. Ventricular tachycardia describes a cardiac rhythm originating distal to the bifurcation of the bundle of His, in the specialized conduction system in ventricular muscle, or both.[1] It is characterized by a ventricular rate of 70 to 250 beats per minute, and the onset can be sudden or insidious. Usually, ventricular tachycardia is exhibited electrocardiographically by wide, tall, bizarre-looking QRS complexes that persist longer than 0.10 second (see Fig. 27-12). QRS complexes can be uniform in appearance, or they can vary randomly, in a repetitive manner (*e.g.,* torsades de pointes), in an alternating pattern (*e.g.,* bidirectional), or in a stable but changing fashion. Ventricular tachycardia can be sustained, lasting more than 30 seconds and requiring intervention, or it can be nonsustained and stop spontaneously. This rhythm is dangerous because it eliminates atrial kick and can cause a reduction in diastolic filling time to the point at which cardiac output is severely diminished or nonexistent.

Ventricular Flutter and Fibrillation. These arrhythmias represent severe derangements of cardiac rhythm that terminate fatally within minutes unless corrective measures are taken promptly. The ECG pattern in ventricular flutter has a sine wave appearance with large oscillations occurring at a rate of 150 to 300 per minute.[38] In ventricular fibrillation, the ventricle quivers but does not contract. The classic ECG pattern of ventricular fibrillation is that of gross disorganization without identifiable waveforms or intervals (see Fig. 27-12). When the ventricles do not contract, there is no cardiac output, and there are no palpable or audible pulses. The immediate defibrillation using a nonsynchronized DC electrical shock is mandatory for ventricular fibrillation and for ventricular flutter that has caused loss of consciousness.[28]

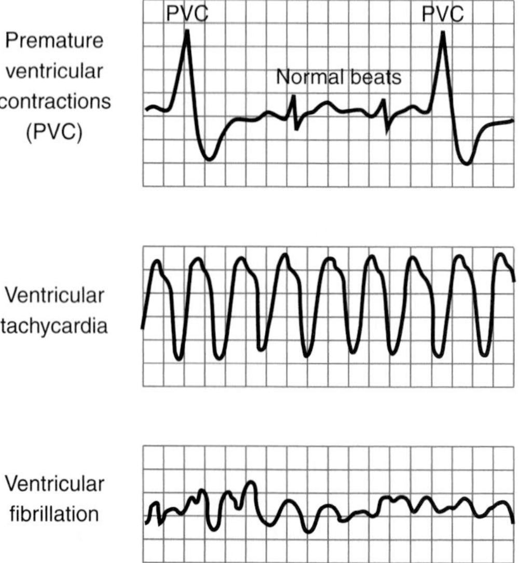

FIGURE 27-12 Electrocardiographic (ECG) tracings of ventricular arrhythmias. Premature ventricular contractions (PVCs) (*top tracing*) originate from an ectopic focus in the ventricles, causing a distortion of the QRS complex. Because the ventricle usually cannot repolarize sufficiently to respond to the next impulse that arises in the sinoatrial node, a PVC frequently is followed by a compensatory pause. Ventricular tachycardia (*middle tracing*) is characterized by a rapid ventricular rate of 70 to 250 beats per minute and the absence of P waves. In ventricular fibrillation (*bottom tracing*), there are no regular or effective ventricular contractions, and the ECG tracing is totally disorganized.

Disorders of Atrioventricular Conduction

Under normal conditions, the AV junction, which consists of the AV node with its connections to the entering atrial internodal pathways, the AV bundle, and the nonbranching portion of the bundle of His, provides the only connection for transmission of impulses between the atrial and ventricular conduction systems. Junctional fibers in the AV node have high-resistance characteristics that cause a delay in the transmission of impulses from the atria to the ventricles. This delay provides optimal timing for atrial contribution to ventricular filling and protects the ventricles from abnormally rapid rates that arise in the atria. Conduction defects of the AV node are most commonly associated with fibrosis or scar tissue in fibers of the conduction system. Conduction defects also may result from medications, including digoxin, β-adrenergic–blocking agents, calcium channel–blocking agents, and class 1A antiarrhythmic agents.[47] Additional contributing factors include electrolyte imbalances, inflammatory disease, or cardiac surgery.

Heart block refers to abnormalities of impulse conduction. It may be normal, physiologic (*e.g.,* vagal tone), or pathologic. It may occur in the AV nodal fibers or in the AV bundle (*i.e.,* bundle of His), which is continuous with the Purkinje conduction system that supplies the ventricles. The PR interval on the ECG corresponds with the time it takes for the cardiac impulse to travel from the SA node to the ventricular pathways. Normally, the PR interval ranges from 0.12 to 0.20 second.

First-Degree AV Block. First-degree AV block is characterized by a prolonged PR interval (exceeds 0.20 second) (Fig. 27-13). The prolonged PR interval indicates delayed AV conduction, but all atrial impulses are conducted to the ventricles. This condition usually produces a regular atrial and ventricular rhythm. Clinically significant PR interval prolongation can result from conduction delays in the AV node itself, the His-Purkinje system, or both.[1] When the QRS complex is normal in contour and duration, the AV delay almost always occurs in the AV node and rarely in the bundle of His. In contrast, when the QRS complex is prolonged, showing a bundle branch block pattern, conduction delays may be in the AV node or the His-Purkinje system. First-degree block may be the result of disease in the AV node such as ischemia or infarction, or of infections such as rheumatic fever or myocarditis.[48–50] Isolated first-degree heart block usually is not symptomatic, and temporary or permanent cardiac pacing is not indicated.

Second-Degree AV Block. Second-degree AV block is characterized by intermittent failure of conduction of one or more impulses from the atria to the ventricles. The nonconducted P wave can appear intermittently or frequently. A distinguishing feature of second-degree AV block is that conducted P waves relate to QRS complexes with recurring PR intervals; that is, the association of P waves with QRS complexes is not random.[1] Second-degree AV block has been divided into two types: type I (*i.e.,* Mobitz type I or Wenckebach's phenomenon) and type II (*i.e.,* Mobitz type II). A *Mobitz type I* AV block is characterized by progressive lengthening of the PR interval until an impulse is blocked and the sequence begins again. It frequently occurs in persons with inferior wall myocardial infarction, particularly with concomitant right ventricular infarction.[1] The condition usually is associated with an adequate ventricular rate and rarely is symptomatic. It usually is transient and does not require temporary pacing. [27] In the *Mobitz type II* AV block, an intermittent block of atrial impulses occurs, with a constant PR interval (see Fig. 27-13). It frequently accompanies anterior wall myocardial infarction and can require temporary or permanent pacing. This condition is associated with a high mortality rate. In addition, Mobitz type II AV block is associated with other types of organic heart disease and often progresses to complete heart block.

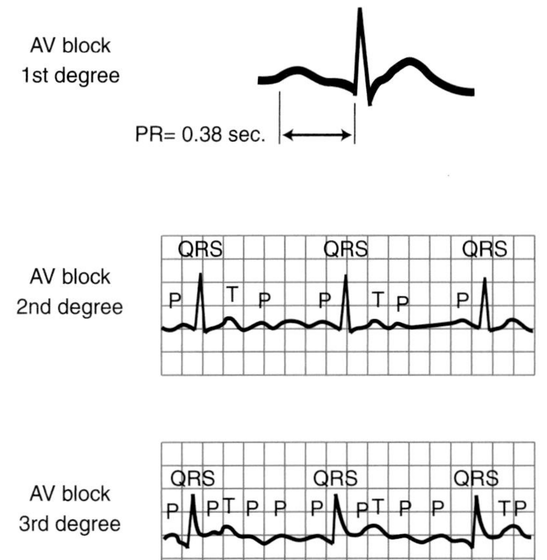

FIGURE 27-13 Electrocardiographic changes that occur with alterations in atrioventricular (AV) node conduction. The *top tracing* shows the prolongation of the PR interval, which is characteristic of first-degree AV block. The *middle tracing* illustrates Mobitz type II second-degree AV block, in which the conduction of one or more P waves is blocked. In third-degree AV block (*bottom tracing*), complete block in conduction of impulses through the AV node occurs, and the atria and ventricles develop their own rates of impulse generation.

Third-Degree AV Block. Third-degree, or complete, AV block occurs when the conduction link for all impulses from the SA node and atria through the AV node is blocked, resulting in depolarization of the atria and ventricles being controlled by separate pacemakers (see Fig. 27-13). The atrial pacemaker can be sinus or ectopic in origin. The ventricular pacemaker usually is located just below the region of the block. The atria usually continue to beat at a normal rate, and the ventricles develop their own rate, which normally is slow (30 to 40 beats per minute). The atrial and ventricular rates are regular but dissociated. Third-degree AV block can result from an interruption at the level of the AV node, in the bundle of His, or in the Purkinje system. Third-degree blocks at the level of the AV node usually are congenital, whereas blocks in the Purkinje system usually are acquired. Normal QRS complexes, with rates ranging from 40 to 60 complexes per minute, usually are displayed on the ECG when the block occurs proximal to the bundle of His.

Complete heart block causes a decrease in cardiac output with possible periods of syncope (fainting), known as a *Stokes-Adams attack.*[1] Other symptoms include dizziness, fatigue, exercise intolerance, or episodes of acute heart failure. Most persons with complete heart block require a permanent cardiac pacemaker.

DIAGNOSTIC METHODS

The diagnosis of disorders of cardiac rhythm and conduction usually is made on the basis of the surface ECG. Further clarification of conduction defects and cardiac arrhythmias can be obtained using electrophysiologic studies.

A resting surface ECG records the impulses originating in the heart as they are recorded at the body surface. These impulses are recorded for a limited time and during periods of inactivity. Although there are no complications related to the procedure, errors related to misdiagnosis may result in iatrogenic heart disease.[3] The resting ECG is the first approach to the clinical diagnosis of disorders of cardiac rhythm and conduction but it is limited to events that occur during the period the ECG is being monitored.

Signal-Averaged Electrocardiogram

Signal-averaged ECG is a special type of ECG that is used to detect ventricular late action potentials that are thought to originate from slow-conducting areas of the myocardium. Ventricular late action potentials are low-amplitude, high-frequency waveforms in the terminal QRS complex, and they persist for tens of milliseconds into the ST segment.[51] The presence of late potentials indicates high risk for development of ventricular tachycardia and sudden cardiac death. These late potentials are detectable from leads of the surface ECG when signal averaging is performed.

The intent of signal averaging is reduction of noise that makes surface ECG analysis more difficult to interpret. This technique averages together multiple samples of QRS waveforms and creates a tracing that is an average of all the repetitive signals. Signal averaging can be carried out by using either temporal or spatial averaging. Both approaches are based on the assumption that the noise is random and that the signal of interest is coherent and repetitive. [52] As a result, when several inputs that represent the same event are combined, the coherent signal will be reinforced, and the noise will cancel itself.

Temporal averaging is frequently referred to as signal averaging. Most studies use temporal averaging as opposed to spatial averaging because it affords greater noise reduction. Six standard bipolar orthogonal leads and one ground are typically used over a large number of beats (generally 100 or more). Theoretically, this method allows for noise reduction by a factor of 10 or more.[52] The implicit assumption underlying signal averaging is that the waveform is repetitive and can be captured without loss of beat-to-beat synchronization.

Spatial averaging uses from 4 to 16 electrodes,[53] and the inputs are averaged to provide noise reduction. The degree of noise reduction is limited by the number of electrodes that can be placed, the potential that closely spaced electrodes will respond to a common noise source and not cancel effectively, and the theoretical limit of a two-fold to four-fold reduction in noise.[52] The advantage of using spatial averaging is that it enhances one's ability to provide a signal-averaged ECG from a single beat, thereby permitting beat-to-beat analysis of transient events and complex arrhythmias.

Signal averaging is a computer-based process. Each electrode input is amplified, its voltage is sampled or measured at intervals of 1 msec or less, and each sample is converted into a digital number with at least 12-bit precision.[54] The ECG waveform is converted from an analog waveform to digital numbers that become a computer-readable ECG.

Holter Monitoring

Holter monitoring is one form of long-term monitoring during which a person wears a device that digitally records two or three ECG leads for up to 48 hours. During this time, the person keeps a diary of his or her activities or symptoms, which later are correlated with the ECG recording. Most recording devices also have an event marker button that can be pressed when the individual experiences symptoms, which assists the technician or physician in correlating the diary, symptoms, and ECG changes during analysis. Holter monitoring is useful for documenting arrhythmias, conduction abnormalities, and ST-segment changes. The interpretative accuracy of long-term Holter recordings varies with the system used and clinician expertise. Most computer software packages used to scan Holter recordings are sufficiently accurate to meet clinical demand. The majority of patients who have ischemic heart disease exhibit premature ventricular complexes, particularly those who have recently experienced myocardial infarction.[55] The frequency of premature ventricular complexes increases progressively over the first several weeks, and it decreases approximately 6 months after infarction. Holter recordings also are used to determine antiarrhythmic drug efficacy, episodes of myocardial ischemia, and heart rate variability.

Intermittent ECG recorders also are used in the diagnosis of arrhythmias and conduction defects. There are two basic types of recorders that perform this type of monitoring.[56] The first continuously monitors rhythm and is programmed to recognize abnormalities. In the second variety, the unit does not continuously monitor the ECG and therefore cannot automatically recognize abnormalities. This latter form relies on the person to activate the unit when he or she is symptomatic. The data are stored in memory or transmitted telephonically to an electrocardiographic receiver, where they are recorded. These types of ECG recordings are useful in persons who have transient symptoms.

Exercise Stress Testing

The exercise stress test elicits the body's response to measured increases in acute exercise (see Chapter 26). This technique provides information about changes in heart rate, blood pressure, respiration, and perceived level of exercise. It is useful in determining exercise-induced alterations in hemodynamic response and ischemic-type ECG ST-segment changes, and it can detect and classify disturbances in cardiac rhythm and conduction associated with exercise. These changes are indicative of a poorer prognosis in persons with known coronary disease and recent myocardial infarction.

Electrophysiologic Studies

An electrophysiologic study involves the passage of two or more electrode catheters into the right side of the heart. These catheters are inserted into the femoral, subclavian, internal jugular, or antecubital veins and positioned with fluoroscopy into the high right atrium near the sinus node, the area of the His bundle, the coronary sinus that lies in the posterior AV groove, and into the right ventricle.[7] The electrode catheters are used to stimulate the heart and record intracardiac ECGs. During the study, overdrive pacing, cardioversion, or defibrillation may be necessary to terminate tachycardia induced during the stimulation procedures.

Electrophysiologic studies are performed for diagnostic or therapeutic purposes. A diagnostic study is performed to determine a person's potential for arrhythmia formation. Electrophysiologic testing also defines reproducible arrhythmia induction characteristics and, as a result, can be used to evaluate the therapeutic efficacy of a particular treatment modality. Diagnostic studies can locate arrhythmia foci for therapeutic intervention as well.

Therapeutic electrophysiologic studies are used as interventions. These interventions may include pacing a person out of tachycardia or ablation therapy. Both types of electrophysiologic testing may be done repeatedly to test patient responses to drugs, devices such as implantable defibrillators, and surgical interventions used in the treatment of arrhythmias.

Risks associated with electrophysiologic studies are small.[57] Most electrophysiologic studies do not involve left-sided heart access, and therefore the risk for myocardial infarction, stroke, or systemic embolism is less than observed with coronary arteriography. The addition of therapeutic maneuvers, such as ablation therapy, to the procedure increases the risk for complications.[58] Predictors of major complications include an ejection fraction of less than 35% and multiple ablation targets.[59]

QT Dispersion

A hallmark of reentrant arrhythmias is heterogeneity in refractoriness and conduction velocity. An index of the heterogeneity of ventricular refractoriness is found by examining the differences in the length of QT intervals using the surface ECG. The most common index used to examine QT dispersion is the difference between the longest and shortest QT_c interval on the 12-lead ECG. Unusually high QT dispersion has been associated with the risk for life-threatening arrhythmias in a variety of disorders,[60] but these results have been inconsistent.[61,62] Many different techniques exist for determining QT dispersion, often making it difficult to compare results of various studies. The utility of QT dispersion is not established as yet.[28]

TREATMENT

The treatment of cardiac rhythm or conduction disorders is directed toward controlling the arrhythmia, correcting the cause, and preventing more serious or fatal arrhythmias. Correction may involve simply adjusting an electrolyte disturbance or withholding a medication such as digitalis. Preventing more serious arrhythmias often involves drug therapy, electrical stimulation, or surgical intervention.

Pharmacologic Treatment

Antiarrhythmic drugs act by modifying disordered formation and conduction of impulses that induce cardiac muscle contraction. These drugs are classified into four major groups according to the drug's effect on the action potential of the cardiac cells. Although drugs in one category have similar effects on conduction, they may vary significantly in their hemodynamic effects.

Class I drugs act by blocking the fast sodium channels. The drugs affect impulse conduction, excitability, and automaticity to various degrees and therefore have been divided further into three groups: IA, IB, and IC. Class IA drugs (*e.g.,* quinidine, procainamide, disopyramide) decrease automaticity by depressing phase 4 of the action potential, decrease conductivity by moderately prolonging phase 0, and prolong repolarization by extending phase 3 of the action potential. Because these drugs are effective in suppressing ectopic foci and in treating reentrant arrhythmias, they are used for supraventricular and ventricular arrhythmias. Class IB drugs (*e.g.,* lidocaine, phenytoin, mexiletine) decrease automaticity by depressing phase 4 of the action potential, have little effect on conductivity, decrease refractoriness by decreasing phase 2, and shorten repolarization by decreasing phase 3. Drugs in this group are used for treating ventricular arrhythmias only and have little or no effect on myocardial contractility. Class IC drugs (*e.g.,* flecainide, propafenone, moricizine) decrease conductivity by markedly depressing phase 0 of the action potential but have little effect on refractoriness or repolarization. Drugs in this class are used for life-threatening ventricular arrhythmias and supraventricular tachycardias.

Class II agents (*e.g.,* propranolol, nadolol, atenolol, timolol, acebutolol, metoprolol, pindolol, esmolol) are β-adrenergic–blocking drugs that act by blunting the effect of sympathetic nervous system stimulation on the heart. These drugs decrease automaticity by depressing phase 4 of the action potential; they also decrease heart rate and cardiac contractility. These medications are effective for treatment of supraventricular arrhythmias and tachyarrhythmias secondary to excessive sympathetic activity, but they are not very effective in treating severe arrhythmias such as recurrent ventricular tachycardia.[63]

Class III drugs (*e.g.,* amiodarone, bretylium, sotalol) act by extending the action potential and refractoriness. These agents are used in the treatment of serious ventricular arrhythmias.[28]

Class IV drugs (*e.g.,* verapamil, diltiazem, nifedipine, bepridil, nitrendipine, felodipine, isradipine, nicardipine) act by blocking the slow calcium channels, thereby depressing phase 4 and lengthening phases 1 and 2. By blocking the release of intracellular calcium ions, these agents reduce the force of myocardial contractility, thereby decreasing myocardial oxygen demand. These drugs are used to slow the ventricular response in atrial tachycardias and to terminate reentrant paroxysmal supraventricular tachycardias when the AV node functions as a reentrant pathway.[28]

Two other types of antiarrhythmic drugs, the cardiac glycosides and adenosine, are not included in this classification schema. The cardiac glycosides (*i.e.,* digitalis drugs) slow the heart rate and are used in the management of arrhythmias such as atrial tachycardia, atrial flutter, and atrial fibrillation. Adenosine, an endogenous nucleoside that is present in every cell, is used for emergency intravenous treatment of paroxysmal supraventricular tachycardia involving the AV node. It interrupts AV node conduction and slows SA node firing.

Electrical Interventions

The correction of conduction defects, bradycardias, and tachycardias can involve the use of an electronic pacemaker, cardioversion, or defibrillation. Electrical interventions can be used in emergency and elective situations.

Efforts directed at cardiac electrostimulation date back more than a century. During this time, tremendous strides have been made in the effectiveness of cardiac pacing. A cardiac pacemaker is an electronic device that delivers an electrical stimulus to the heart. It is used to initiate heartbeats in situations in which the normal pacemaker of the heart is defective, with certain types of AV heart block, symptomatic bradycardia in which the rate of cardiac contraction and consequent cardiac output is inadequate to perfuse vital tissues, as well as other cardiac arrhythmias. A pacemaker may be used as a temporary or a permanent measure. Pacemakers can pace the atria, the ventricles, or the atria and ventricles sequentially, or overdrive pacing can be used. Overdrive pacing is used to treat recurrent ventricular tachycardia and reentrant atrial or ventricular tachyarrhythmias, and to terminate atrial flutter.

Temporary pacemakers are useful for treatment of symptomatic bradycardias and to perform overdrive pacing. They can be placed transcutaneously, transvenously, or epicardially. External temporary pacing, also known as *transcutaneous pacing,* involves the placement of large patch electrodes on the anterior and posterior chest wall, which then are connected by a cable to an external pulse generator. Many defibrillators today have transcutaneous pacing capabilities as well. Internal temporary pacing, also known as *transvenous pacing,* involves the passage of a venous catheter with electrodes on its tip into the right atrium or ventricle, where it is wedged against the endocardium. The electrode then is attached to an external pulse generator. This procedure is performed under fluoroscopic or electrocardiographic direction. During open thoracotomy procedures, epicardial pacing wires sometimes are placed. These wires are brought out directly through the chest wall and also can be attached to an external pulse generator, if necessary.

Permanent cardiac pacemakers may become necessary for a variety of reasons. Permanent pacemakers require implantation of pacing wires into the epicardium and a pulse generator. The pulse generator typically weighs approximately 25 to 40 g.[64] Ongoing evaluation of the pacemaker's sensing and firing capabilities is necessary.

Synchronized cardioversion is used to terminate tachycardias due to reentry, such as atrial fibrillation and most forms of ventricular tachycardia, and defibrillation is used as a life-saving intervention in ventricular fibrillation. The discharge of electrical energy that is synchronized with the R wave of the ECG is referred to as *synchronized cardioversion,* and unsynchronized discharge is known as *defibrillation.* The goal of both of these techniques is to provide an electrical pulse to the heart in such a way as to depolarize the heart completely during passage of the current. This electrical current interrupts the disorganized impulses, allowing the SA node to regain control of the heart. Defibrillation and synchronized cardioversion can be delivered externally through large patch electrodes on the chest or internally through small paddle electrodes placed directly on the myocardium, patch electrodes sewn into the epicardium, or transvenous wires placed in the right ventricle. Electrical devices that combine antitachycardial pacing, cardioversion, defibrillation, and bradycardial pacing are under investigation.

Automatic implantable cardioverter-defibrillators (AICDs) are being used successfully to treat individuals with life-threatening ventricular tachyarrhythmias by the use of intrathoracic electrical countershock.[65] Reliable sensing and detection of ventricular tachyarrhythmias is essential for proper functioning of the AICD. Sensing and detection are accomplished by means of endocardial leads. The AICD responds to ventricular tachyarrhythmias by delivering an electrical shock between intrathoracic electrodes within 10 to 20 seconds of its onset. This time frame provides nearly a 100% likelihood of reversal of the arrhythmia, supporting the utility of this device as a reliable and effective means of preventing sudden cardiac death in survivors of out-of-hospital cardiac arrest.

Ablation and Surgical Interventions

Ablation therapy is used for treating recurrent, life-threatening supraventricular and ventricular tachyarrhythmias. It involves localized destruction, isolation, or excision of cardiac tissue that is considered to be arrhythmogenic.[7,28] Ablative therapy may be performed by catheter or surgical techniques. Radiofrequency ablation uses radiofrequency energy waves to destroy defective or aberrant electrical conduction pathways. Cryoablation is the direct application of an extremely cold probe to arrhythmogenic cardiac tissue that causes freezing and necrosis of defective or aberrant electrical conduction pathways. The major complication with surgical ablation techniques is the perioperative mortality rate of 5% to 15%.[7] There also has been a high morbidity rate reported.

Additional surgical interventions such as coronary artery bypass surgery, ventriculotomy, and endocardial resection may be used to improve myocardial oxygenation, remove arrhythmogenic foci, or alter electrical conduction pathways. Coronary artery bypass surgery improves myocardial oxygenation by increasing blood supply to the myocardium. Ventriculotomy involves the removal of aneurysm tissue and the resuturing of the myocardial walls to eliminate the paradoxical ventricular movement and the foci of arrhythmias. In endocardial resection, endocardial tissue that has been identified as arrhythmogenic through the use of electrophysiologic testing or intraoperative mapping is surgically removed. Ventriculotomy and endocardial resection have been performed with cryoablation or laser ablation as an adjunctive therapy.[28] Other surgical techniques, including transvenous electrocoagulation[66] and laser ablation,[67] are under investigation as potential treatment modalities for recurrent tachycardias.

In summary, disorders of cardiac rhythm arise as the result of disturbances in impulse generation or conduction in the heart. Normal sinus rhythm and respiratory sinus arrhythmia (*i.e.,* heart rate speeds up and slows down in concert with respiratory cycle) are considered normal cardiac rhythms. Cardiac arrhythmias are not necessarily pathologic; they occur in healthy and diseased hearts. Sinus arrhythmias originate in the SA node. They include sinus bradycardia (heart rate <60 beats per minute); sinus tachycardia (heart rate >100 beats per minute); sinus arrest, in which there are prolonged periods of asystole; and sick sinus syndrome, a condition characterized by periods of bradycardia alternating with tachycardia.

Atrial arrhythmias arise from alterations in impulse generation that occur in the conduction pathways or muscle of the atria. They include atrial premature contractions, atrial flutter (*i.e.,* atrial depolarization rate of 240 to 450 beats per minute), and atrial fibrillation (*i.e.*, grossly disorganized atrial depolarization that is irregular with regard to rate and rhythm). Atrial arrhythmias often go unnoticed unless they are transmitted to the ventricles.

Arrhythmias that arise in the ventricles commonly are considered more serious than those that arise in the atria because they afford the potential for interfering with the pumping action of the heart. The long QT syndrome represents a prolongation of the QT interval that may result in torsades de pointes and sudden cardiac death. PVCs are caused by a ventricular ectopic pacemaker. Ventricular tachycardia is characterized by a ventricular rate of 70 to 250 beats per minute. Ventricular fibrillation (*e.g.*, ventricular rate >350 beats per minute) is a fatal arrhythmia unless it is successfully treated with defibrillation.

Alterations in the conduction of impulses through the AV node lead to disturbances in the transmission of impulses from the atria to the ventricles. There can be a delay in transmission (*i.e.*, first-degree heart block), failure to conduct one or more impulses (*i.e.*, second-degree heart block), or complete failure to conduct impulses between the atria and the ventricles (*i.e.*, third-degree heart block). Conduction disorders of the bundle of His and Purkinje system, called *bundle branch blocks*, cause a widening of and changes in the configuration of the QRS complex of the ECG.

The diagnosis of disorders of cardiac rhythm and conduction typically is accomplished using surface ECG recordings or electrophysiologic studies. Surface electrodes can be used to obtain a 12-lead ECG; signal-averaged electrocardiographic studies in which multiple samples of QRS waves are averaged to detect ventricular late action potentials; and Holter monitoring, which provides continuous ECG recordings for up to 48 hours. Electrophysiologic studies use electrode catheters inserted into the right heart by way of a peripheral vein as a means of directly stimulating the heart while obtaining an intracardiac ECG recording.

Both electrical devices and medications are used in the treatment of arrhythmias and conduction disorders. Temporary and permanent cardiac pacemakers are used to treat symptomatic bradycardias or to provide overdrive pacing procedures. Defibrillation is used to treat ventricular fibrillation. Synchronized cardioversion procedures are carried out to treat atrial fibrillation and ventricular tachycardia. These can be external or internally implanted devices. They deliver an electrical charge to the myocardium in order to depolarize the heart completely, supplying the SA node with an opportunity to take over as the primary pacemaker of the heart. Radiofrequency ablation and cryoablation therapy are used to destroy specific irritable foci in the heart. Surgical procedures can be performed to excise irritable or dysfunctional tissue, replace cardiac valves, or provide better blood supply to the myocardial muscle wall.

REVIEW EXERCISES

A 63-year-old woman with a history of congestive heart failure comes to the clinic complaining of feeling tired. Her heart rate is 97 beats per minute, and the rhythm is irregularly irregular.

A. What type of arrhythmia do you think she might be having? What would it look like if you were to obtain an ECG?

B. What causes this irregularity?

C. Why do you think she is feeling tired?

D. What are some of the concerns with this type of arrhythmia?

A 42-year-old man appears at the urgent care center with complaints of chest discomfort, shortness of breath, and generally not feeling well. You assess vital signs and find that he has a temperature of 99.2°F, blood pressure of 166/90 mm HG, pulse of 87 beats per minute and slightly irregular, and respiratory rate of 26 breaths per minute. You perform an ECG and find that he is experiencing an ischemic episode in his anterior leads.

A. You attach him to a cardiac monitor and see that his underlying rhythm is normal sinus rhythm, but he is having frequent premature contractions that are more than 0.10 sec in duration. You suspect that these are what type of premature contractions?

B. What would you expect his pulse to feel like?

C. What type of ECG monitoring is indicated for this man?

D. What do you think the etiology of this arrhythmia might be? How might it be treated?

References

1. Rubart M., Zipes D.P. (2001). Genesis of cardiac arrhythmias: Electrophysiological considerations. In Braunwald E. (Ed.), *Heart disease: A textbook of cardiovascular medicine* (6th ed., pp. 659–699). Philadelphia: W.B. Saunders.
2. Anumonwo J.M.B., Jalife J. (1994). Cellular and subcellular mechanisms of pacemaker activity initiation and synchronization in the heart. In Zipes D.P., Jalife J. (Eds.), *Cardiac electrophysiology: From cell to bedside* (2nd ed., p. 151). Philadelphia: W.B. Saunders.
3. Castellanos A., Iterian A., Myerburg R.J. (2001). The resting electrocardiogram. In Fuster V., Alexander R.W., et al. (Eds.), *Hurst's the heart* (10th ed., pp. 281–314). New York: McGraw-Hill.
4. Malouf J.F., Edwards W.D., Tajik A.J. (2001). Functional anatomy of the heart. In Fuster V., Alexander R.W., King S.B., et al. (Eds.), *Hurst's the heart* (10 ed., pp. 19–62). New York: McGraw-Hill.
5. Berne R.M., Levy M.N. (2001). *Cardiovascular physiology* (8th ed., pp. 1–51). St. Louis: Mosby.
6. Guyton A.C., Hall J.E. (2001). *Textbook of medical physiology* (10th ed., pp. 107–113). Philadelphia: W.B. Saunders.
7. Fogoros R.N. (1999). *Electrophysiologic testing* (3rd ed.). Malden, MA: Blackwell Science.
8. Katz A.M. (2001). *Physiology of the heart* (3rd ed.). Philadelphia: Lippincott Williams & Wilkins.
9. Wit A.L., Friedman P.L. (1975). Basis for ventricular arrhythmias accompanying myocardial infarction. *Archives of Internal Medicine 135*, 459–472.
10. Drew B.J., Scheinman M.M. (1995). ECG criteria to distinguish between aberrantly conducted supraventricular tachycardia and ventricular tachycardia: Practical aspects for the

immediate care setting. *Pacing and Clinical Electrophysiology 18*(12 Pt 1), 2194–2208.
11. Drew B.J., Ide B., Sparacino P.S. (1991). Accuracy of bedside electrocardiographic monitoring: a report on current practices of critical care nurses. *Heart and Lung 20,* 597–607.
12. Thomason T.R., Riegel B., Carlson B., Gocka I. (1995). Monitoring electrocardiographic changes: results of a national survey. *Journal of Cardiovascular Nursing 9,* 1–9.
13. Drew B.J. (2002). Celebrating the 100th birthday of the electrocardiogram: Lessons learned from research in cardiac monitoring. *American Journal of Critical Care 11,* 378–388.
14. Mirvis D.M., Goldberger A.L. (2001). Electrocardiography. In Braunwald E., Zipes D.P., Libby P (Eds.), *Heart disease: A textbook of cardiovascular medicine* (6th ed., pp. 106–110). Philadelphia: W.B. Saunders.
15. Adams M.G., Pelter M.M., Wung S., et al. (1999). Frequency of silent myocardial ischemia with 12-lead ST segment monitoring in the coronary care unit: Are there sex differences? *Heart & Lung 28,* 81–86.
16. Drew B.J., Pelter M.M., Adams M.G., et al. (1998). 12-Lead ST-segment monitoring vs single-lead maximum ST-segment monitoring for detecting ongoing ischemia in patients with unstable coronary syndromes. *American Journal of Critical Care 7,* 355–363.
17. Drew B.J., Krucoff M.W. (1999). Multilead ST-segment monitoring in patients with acute coronary syndromes: a consensus statement for healthcare professionals. ST-Segment Monitoring Practice Guideline International Working Group. *American Journal of Critical Care 8,* 372–386.
18. Marriott H.J.L. (1984). Arrhythmia versus dysrhythmia. *American Journal of Cardiology 53,* 628.
19. Haines D.E., DiMarco J.P. (1990). Sustained intraatrial reentrant tachycardia: clinical, electrocardiographic and electrophysiologic characteristics and long-term follow-up. *Journal of the American College of Cardiology 15,* 1345–1354.
20. El-Sherif N. (2000). Reentrant mechanisms in ventricular arrhythmias. In Zipes D.P., Jalife J. (Eds.), *Cardiac electrophysiology: From cell to bedside* (2nd ed., p. 567). Philadelphia: W.B. Saunders.
21. Waldo A.L., Wit A.L. (2001). Mechanisms of cardiac arrhythmias and conduction disturbances. In Fuster V., Alexander R.W., King S.B., et al. (Eds.), *Hurst's the heart* (10th ed., pp. 751–796). New York: McGraw-Hill.
22. Kay G.N., Bubien R.S. (1992). *Clinical management of cardiac arrhythmias.* Gaithersburg, MD: Aspen.
23. Conover M. (2003). Mechanisms of arrhythmias. In Conover M. (Ed.), *Understanding electrocardiography* (8th ed., pp. 25–31). St. Louis: Mosby.
24. Beaumont J., Jalife, J. (2000). Rotors and spiral waves in two dimension. In Zipes, D.P., Jalife J. (Eds.), *Cardiac electrophysiology: From cell to bedside* (2nd ed., pp. 327–335). Philadelphia: W.B. Saunders.
25. Kyriakidis M., Barbetseas J., Antonopoulos A., et al. (1992). Early atrial arrhythmias in acute myocardial infarction. Role of the sinus node artery. *Chest 101,* 944–947.
26. Kastor J.A. (2000). Sick sinus syndrome. In Kastor J.A. (Ed.), *Arrhythmias* (2nd ed., pp. 566–591). Philadelphia: W.B. Saunders.
27. Myerburg R.J., Kloosterman, E.M., Castellanos A. (2001). Recognition, clinical assessment, and management of arrhythmias and conduction disturbances. In Fuster V., Alexander R.W., King S.B., et al. (Eds.), *Hurst's the heart* (10th ed., pp. 797–874). New York: McGraw-Hill.
28. Miller J.M., Zipes D.P. (2001). Management of the patient with cardiac arrhythmias. In Braunwald E. (Ed.), *Heart disease: A textbook of cardiovascular medicine* (6th ed., pp. 700–767). Philadelphia: W.B. Saunders.
29. Rubenstein J.J., Schulman C.L., Yurchak P.M., DeSanctis R.W. (1972). Clinical spectrum of the sick sinus syndrome. *Circulation 46,* 5–13.
30. Marriott H.J.L., Conover, M.B. (1998). *Advanced concepts in arrhythmias* (3rd ed.). St. Louis: Mosby.
31. Brignole M., Menozzi C., Bottoni N., et al. (1995). Mechanisms of syncope caused by transient bradycardia and the diagnostic value of electrophysiologic testing and cardiovascular reflexivity maneuvers. *American Journal of Cardiology 76,* 273–278.
32. Surawicz B., Knilans T.K. (2001). *Chou's electrocardiography in clinical practice* (5th ed.). Philadelphia: W.B. Saunders.
33. Falk R.H. (2001). Atrial fibrillation. *New England Journal of Medicine 344,* 1067–1078.
34. Massie B.M., Amidon T.M. (2003). The heart. In Tierney L.M., McPhee S.J., Papadakis M.A. (Eds.), *Current medical diagnosis and treatment* (42nd ed., pp. 369–372). New York, McGraw-Hill.
35. Menzel L.K., White J.M. (1996). Electrocardiogram interpretation. In Clochesy J.M., Breu C., Cardin S., et al. (Eds.), *Critical care nursing* (2nd ed., pp. 127–166). Philadelphia: W.B. Saunders.
36. Khan I.A. (2002). Long QT syndrome: Diagnosis and management. *American Heart Journal 143,* 7–14.
37. Tan H.L., Hou C.J.Y, Lauer M.R., Sung R.J. (1995). Electrophysiologic mechanisms of the long QT interval syndromes and torsade de pointes: Review. *Annals of Internal Medicine 122,* 701–714.
38. Olgin J.E., Zipes D.P. (2001). Specific arrhythmias: Diagnosis and treatment. In Braunwald E. (Ed.), *Heart disease: A textbook of cardiovascular medicine* (6th ed., pp. 867–871). Philadelphia: W.B. Saunders.
39. Bazett J.C. (1920). An analysis of time relations of electrocardiograms. *Heart 7,* 353–367.
40. Sagie A., Larson M.G., Goldberg R.J., et al. (1992). An improved method for adjusting the QT interval for heart rate (the Framingham Heart Study). *American Journal of Cardiology 70,* 797–801.
41. Hodges M. (1997). Rate correction of the QT interval. *Cardiac Electrophysiology Review 1,* 360–363.
42. Smetana P, Batchvarov V, Hnatkova K, et al. (2003). Circadian rhythm of the corrected QT interval: Impact of different heart rate correction models. *Pacing and Clinical Electrophysiology 26*(1 Pt 2), 383–386.
43. Schwartz P.J., Priori, S.G., Napolitano, C. (2000). The long QT syndrome. In Zipes, D.P. Jalife, J. (Eds.), *Cardiac electrophysiology: From cell to bedside* (2nd ed., pp. 597–615). Philadelphia: W.B. Saunders.
44. Vincent G.M. (2000). Long QT syndrome. *Cardiology Clinics 18,* 309–325.
45. Kocheril A.G., Bokhari S.A., Batsford W.P., Sinusas A.J. (1997). Long QTc and torsades de pointes in human immunodeficiency virus disease. *Pacing and Clinical Electrophysiology 20,* 2810–2816.
46. Bigger J.T., Jr. (2000). Ventricular premature complexes. In Kastor J.A. (Ed.), *Arrhythmias* (2nd ed., pp. 310–325). Philadelphia: W.B. Saunders.
47. Moungey S.J. (1994). Patients with sinus node dysfunction or atrioventricular blocks. *Critical Care Nursing Clinics of North America 6,* 55–68.
48. Phillips R.E., Feeney M.A. (1990). *The cardiac rhythms: A systematic approach to interpretation* (3rd ed.). Philadelphia: W.B. Saunders.
49. Rosenfeld L.E. (1988). Bradyarrhythmias, abnormalities of conduction, and indications for pacing in acute myocardial infarction. *Cardiology Clinics 6,* 49–61.
50. Wellens H.J.J. (1993). Right ventricular infarction. *New England Journal of Medicine 8,* 1036–1038.

51. Walter P.F. (1994). Technique of signal-averaged electrocardiography. In Schlant R.C., Alexander R.W., O'Rourke R.A., et al. (Eds.), *Hurst's the heart* (8th ed., pp. 893–904). New York: McGraw-Hill.
52. Conover E.L. (2003). Signal-averaged ECG and fast Fourier transform analysis. In Conover M. (2003). *Understanding electrocardiography* (8th ed., pp. 447–454). St. Louis: Mosby.
53. Flowers N.C., Shvartsman V., Kennelly B.M., et al. (1981). Surface recording of His-Purkinje activity on an every-beat basis without digital averaging. *Circulation 63,* 948–952.
54. Gomes J.A., Cain M.E., Buxton A.E., et al. (2001). Prediction of long-term outcomes by signal-averaged electrocardiography in patients with unsustained ventricular tachycardia, coronary artery disease, and left ventricular dysfunction. *Circulation 104,* 436–441.
55. Manolio T.A., Furberg C.D., Rautaharju P.M., et al. (1994). Cardiac arrhythmias on 24-h ambulatory electrocardiography in older women and men: The Cardiovascular Health Study. *Journal of the American College of Cardiology 23,* 916–925.
56. Noble R.J., Prystowsky, E.N. (2001). Long-term continuous electrocardiographic recording. In Fuster V., Alexander R.W., King S.B., et al. (Eds.), *Hurst's the heart* (10th ed., pp. 875–884). New York: McGraw-Hill.
57. Horowitz L.N., Kay H.R., Kutalek S.P., et al. (1987). Risks and complications of clinical cardiac electrophysiologic studies: A prospective analysis of 1,000 consecutive patients. *Journal of the American College of Cardiology 9,* 1261–1268.
58. Zhou L., Keane D., Reed G., Ruskin J. (1999). Thromboembolic complications of cardiac radiofrequency catheter ablation: A review of the reported incidence, pathogenesis and current research directions. *Journal of Cardiovascular Electrophysiology 10,* 611–620.
59. Calkins H., Wharton J.M., Epstein A.E., et al. (1998). Safety and efficacy of catheter ablation of ventricular tachycardia using the cooled ablation system: Final report. *Pacing and Clinical Electrophysiology 21,* 843.
60. Spargias K.S., Lindsay S.J., Kawar G.I., et al. (1999). QT dispersion as a predictor of long-term mortality in patients with acute myocardial infarction and clinical evidence of heart failure. *European Heart Journal 20,* 1158–1165.
61. Gang Y., Ono T., Hnatkova K., et al. (2003). QT dispersion has no prognostic value in patients with symptomatic heart failure: an ELITE II substudy. *Pacing and Clinical Electrophysiology 26*(1 Pt 2), 394–400.
62. Zabel M., Klingenheben T., Franz M.R., Hohnloser S.H. (1998). Assessment of QT dispersion for prediction of mortality or arrhythmic events after myocardial infarction: Results of a prospective, long-term follow-up study. *Circulation 97,* 2543–2550.
63. Woosley R.L. (2001). Antiarrhythmic drugs. In Fuster V., Alexander R.W., King S.B., et al. (Eds.), *Hurst's the heart* (10th ed., pp. 899–924). New York: McGraw-Hill.
64. Mitrani R.D., Myerburg R.J., Castellanos A. (2001). Cardiac pacemakers. In Fuster V., Alexander R.W., King S.B., et al. (Eds.), *Hurst's the heart* (10th ed., pp. 963–994). New York: McGraw-Hill.
65. O'Callaghan P.A., Ruskin J.N. (2001). The implantable cardioverter defibrillator. In Fuster V., Alexander R.W., King S.B., et al. (Eds.), *Hurst's the heart* (10th ed., pp. 945–962). New York: McGraw-Hill.
66. Lanzotti ME, De Ponti R, Tritto M, et al. (2002). Successful treatment of anteroseptal accessory pathways by transvenous cryomapping and cryoablation. *Italian Heart Journal 3,* 128–132.
67. d'Avila A., Splinter R., Svenson R.H., et al. (2002). New perspectives on catheter-based ablation of ventricular tachycardia complicating Chagas' disease: Experimental evidence of the efficacy of near infrared lasers for catheter ablation of Chagas' VT. *Journal of Interventional Cardiac Electrophysiology 7,* 23–38.

CHAPTER

28

Heart Failure and Circulatory Shock

Adequate perfusion of body tissues depends on the pumping ability of the heart, a vascular system that transports blood to the cells and back to the heart, sufficient blood to fill the circulatory system, and tissues that are able to extract and use oxygen and nutrients from the blood. Impaired pumping ability of the heart and circulatory shock are separate conditions that reflect failure of the circulatory system. Both conditions exhibit common compensatory mechanisms even though they differ in terms of pathogenesis and causes.

Heart Failure

After completing this section of the chapter, you should be able to meet the following objectives:

- ✦ Explain the effect of the cardiac reserve on symptom development in heart failure
- ✦ Define the terms *preload, afterload,* and *cardiac contractility*
- ✦ Explain how increased Frank-Starling mechanism, sympathetic activity, the renin-angiotensin-aldosterone mechanism, the natriuretic peptides, the endothelins, and myocardial hypertrophy and remodeling contribute to the initial adaptation to heart failure and then to its progression
- ✦ Differentiate high-output versus low-output heart failure, systolic versus diastolic heart failure, and right-sided versus left-sided heart failure
- ✦ Describe the physiologic mechanisms underlying the manifestations of congestive heart failure
- ✦ Describe the methods used in diagnosis and assessment of cardiac function in persons with heart failure
- ✦ Relate the actions of diuretics, digoxin, angiotensin-converting enzyme inhibitors, and β-adrenergic–blocking drugs to the treatment of heart failure
- ✦ Relate the effect of left ventricular failure to the development of and manifestations of pulmonary edema
- ✦ Describe the pathophysiology of cardiogenic shock
- ✦ Compare the indications for use of ventricular support devices, heart transplantation, and cardiomyoplasty in treatment of heart failure

Heart failure affects an estimated 5 million Americans, with approximately 550,000 new cases diagnosed each year.[1] Although morbidity and mortality rates from other cardiovascular diseases have decreased over the past several decades, the incidence of heart failure is increasing at an alarming rate. This change undoubtedly reflects improved treatment methods and increased survival from other forms of heart disease. Despite advances in treatment, 80% of men and 79% of women younger than age 65 who have heart failure will die within 8 years.[1]

This section of the chapter is divided into four parts: pathophysiology of heart failure, congestive heart failure, acute pulmonary edema, and cardiogenic shock.

PHYSIOLOGY OF HEART FAILURE

The heart has the amazing capacity to adjust its pumping ability to meet the varying needs of the body. During sleep, its output declines, and during exercise, it increases markedly. The ability to increase cardiac output during increased activity is called the *cardiac reserve*. For example, competitive swimmers and long-distance runners have large cardiac reserves. During exercise, the cardiac output of these athletes rapidly increases to as much as five to six times their resting level. In sharp contrast with healthy athletes, persons with heart failure often use their cardiac reserve at rest. For them, just climbing a flight of stairs may cause shortness of breath because they have exceeded their cardiac reserve.

The pathophysiology of heart failure involves an interaction between two factors: a decrease in pumping ability of the heart with a consequent decrease in the cardiac reserve and the adaptive mechanisms that serve to maintain the cardiac output while also contributing to the progression of heart failure.

Cardiac Output

The cardiac output is the amount of blood that the heart pumps each minute. It reflects how often the heart beats each minute (heart rate) and how much blood the heart pumps with each beat (stroke volume) and can be expressed as the product of the heart rate and stroke volume: cardiac output = heart rate × stroke volume. The heart rate is regulated by a balance between the activity of the sympathetic nervous system, which produces an increase in heart rate, and the parasympathetic nervous system, which slows it down, whereas the stroke volume is a function of preload, afterload, and cardiac contractility.

Preload and Afterload. The work that the heart performs consists mainly of ejecting blood that has returned to the ventricles during diastole into the pulmonary or systemic circulations. As with skeletal muscle, the work of cardiac muscle is determined by what is called *loading conditions*—the stretch imposed by the load (*i.e.,* blood volume) and the force that the muscle must generate to move the load. The terms *preload* and *afterload* often are used to describe the workload of the heart.

Preload reflects the loading condition of the heart at the end of diastole just before the onset of systole. It is the volume of blood stretching the resting heart muscle and is determined mainly by the venous return to the heart. For any given cardiac cycle, the maximum volume of blood filling the ventricle is present at the end of diastole. Known as the *end-diastolic volume,* this volume causes the tension in the wall of the ventricles and the pressure in the ventricles to rise. End-diastolic pressure can be measured clinically, providing an estimate of preload status. Within limits, as end-diastolic volume or preload increases, the stroke volume increases in accord with the Frank-Starling mechanism (see Chapter 23, Fig. 23-16). In heart failure, the ventricles may become overstretched because of excessive filling. When this happens, intraventricular pressure rises, and stroke volume may decrease. Preload may be excessively elevated in conditions such as myocardial infarction, in which the ventricles become distended because of impaired pumping ability; in valvular heart disease, such as aortic regurgitation, in which a portion of the ejected systolic volume moves back into the ventricle and is added to the diastolic volume; and in renal failure, in which an increase in blood volume produces an increase in venous return.

Afterload represents the force that the contracting heart must generate to eject blood from the filled heart. The main components of afterload are the systemic (peripheral) vascular resistance and ventricular wall tension. When the systemic vascular resistance is elevated, as with arterial hypertension or aortic stenosis, an increased intraventricular pressure must be generated first to open the aortic valve and then, during the ejection period, to move blood out of the heart and into the systemic circulation. This equates to an increase in ventricular wall stress or tension. As a result, excessive afterload may impair ventricular ejection and increase wall tension if the ventricles cannot generate sufficient pressure.

Cardiac Contractility. Cardiac contractility refers to the mechanical performance of the heart—the ability of the contractile elements (actin and myosin filaments) of the heart muscle to interact with and shorten against a load. The ejec-

HEART FAILURE

- The function of the heart is to move deoxygenated blood from the venous system through the right heart into the pulmonary circulation, and to move the oxygenated blood from the pulmonary circulation through the left heart into the arterial system.
- To function effectively, the right and left hearts must maintain an equal output.
- Right heart failure represents failure of the right heart to pump blood forward into the pulmonary circulation; blood backs up in the systemic circulation, causing peripheral edema and congestion of the abdominal organs.
- Left heart failure represents failure of the left heart to move blood from the pulmonary circulation into the system circulation; blood backs up in the pulmonary circulation.

tion of blood from the heart during systole depends on cardiac contractility. Contractility increases cardiac output independent of preload filling and muscle stretch.

An *inotropic influence* is one that increases cardiac contractility. Sympathetic stimulation increases the strength of cardiac contraction (*i.e.,* positive inotropic action), and hypoxia and ischemia decrease contractility (*i.e.,* negative inotropic effect). The drug digitalis, which is classified as an inotropic agent, increases cardiac contractility such that the heart is able to eject more blood at any level of preload filling. A decrease in cardiac contractility can result from loss of functional muscle tissue due to myocardial infarction or from conditions such as cardiomyopathy that diffusely affect the myocardium.

Adaptive Mechanisms

In heart failure, the cardiac reserve is largely maintained through compensatory or adaptive mechanisms such as the Frank-Starling mechanism; activation of neurohumoral influences such as the sympathetic nervous system, the renin-angiotensin-aldosterone mechanism, natriuretic peptides, and locally produced vasoactive substances; and myocardial hypertrophy and remodeling (Fig. 28-1). The first two of these adaptations occur rapidly over minutes to hours of myocardial dysfunction and may be adequate to maintain the overall pumping performance of the heart at relatively normal levels. Myocardial hypertrophy and remodeling occur slowly over weeks to months and play an important role in the long-term adaptation to hemodynamic overload. These adaptive mechanisms contribute not only to the adaptation of the failing heart but also to the pathophysiology of heart failure.

Frank-Starling Mechanism. The Frank-Starling mechanism increases stroke volume by means of an increase in ventricular end-diastolic volume (Fig. 28-2). With increased diastolic filling, there is increased stretching of the myocardial fibers, more optimal approximation of the actin and myosin filaments, and a resultant increase in the force of the next contraction. In the normally functioning heart, the Frank-Starling mechanism serves to match the outputs of the two ventricles.

In heart failure, the Frank-Starling mechanism helps to support the cardiac output. Cardiac output may be normal at rest in persons with heart failure because of increased ventricular end-diastolic volume and the Frank-Starling mechanism. However, this mechanism becomes ineffective when the heart becomes overfilled and the muscle fibers are overstretched. With deterioration of myocardial function, the ventricular function curve depicted in Figure 28-2 flattens, and when an increase in cardiac output is needed, as occurs with increased physical activity, there is a lesser increase in cardiac output at any given increase in left ventricular end-diastolic volume or pressure. In this situation, the maximal increase in cardiac output that can be achieved may severely limit activity, while at the same time producing an elevation in left ventricular and pulmonary capillary pressure and development of dyspnea and pulmonary congestion. At the point at which the heart becomes overfilled to the extent that actin and myosin filaments cannot produce an effective contraction,

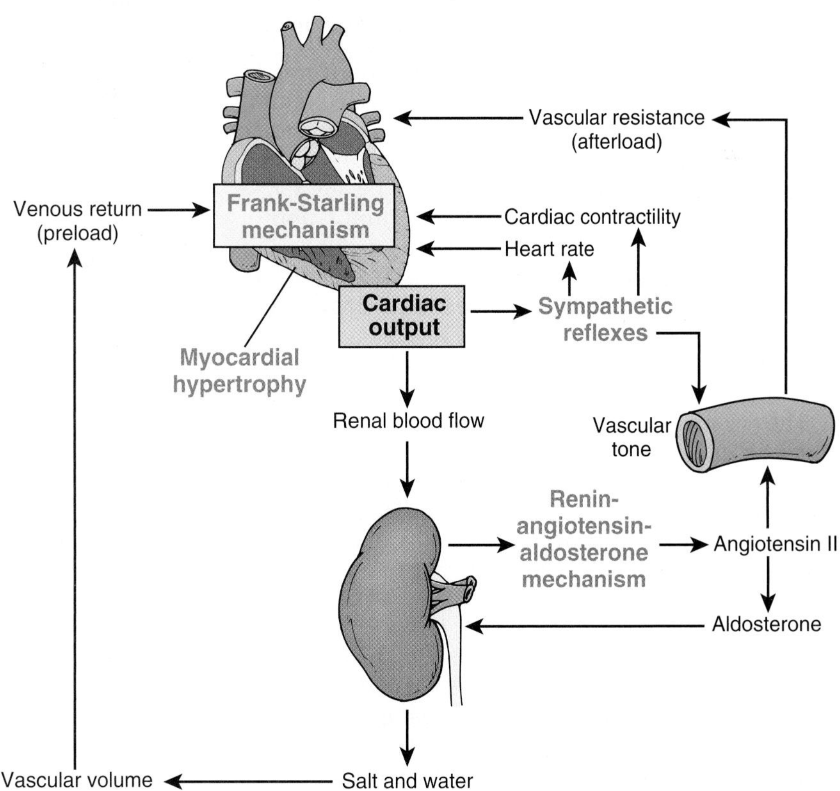

FIGURE 28-1 Compensatory mechanisms in heart failure. The Frank-Starling mechanism, sympathetic reflexes, renin-angiotensin-aldosterone mechanism, and myocardial hypertrophy function in maintaining the cardiac output for the failing heart.

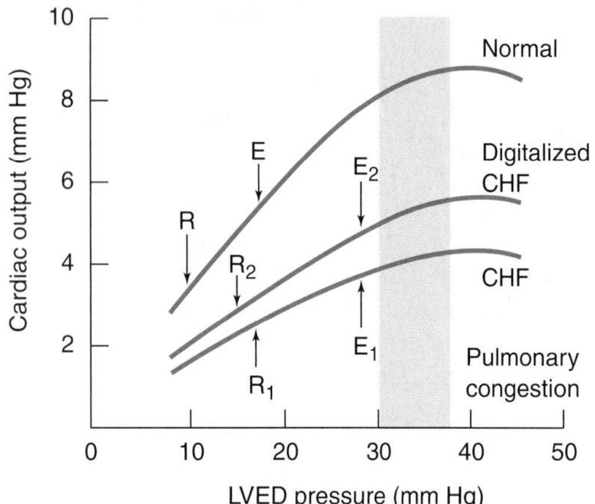

FIGURE 28-2 Frank-Starling curves. R, resting; E, exercise; LVED, left ventricular end-diastolic; CHF, congestive heart failure. (Iseri L.T., Benvenuti D.J. [1983]. Pathogenesis and management of congestive heart failure—revisited. *American Heart Journal 105* [2], 346)

further increases in ventricular filling may produce a decrease in cardiac output.

An important determinant of myocardial energy consumption is ventricular wall tension. Overfilling of the ventricle produces a decrease in wall thickness and an increase in wall tension. Because increased wall tension increases myocardial oxygen requirements, it can produce ischemia and further impairment of cardiac function. The use of diuretics in persons with heart failure helps to reduce vascular volume and ventricular filling, thereby unloading the heart and reducing ventricular wall tension.

Sympathetic Nervous System Activity. Stimulation of the sympathetic nervous system plays an important role in the compensatory response to decreased cardiac output and to the pathogenesis of heart failure.[2–5] Both cardiac sympathetic tone and catecholamine (epinephrine and norepinephrine) levels are elevated during the late stages of most forms of heart failure. By direct stimulation of heart rate and cardiac contractility and by regulation of vascular tone, the sympathetic nervous system helps to maintain perfusion of the various organs, particularly the heart and brain. In persons with more severe heart failure, blood is diverted to the more critical cerebral and coronary circulations.

The negative aspects of increased sympathetic activity include an increase in systemic vascular resistance and the afterload against which the heart must pump. Excessive sympathetic stimulation also may result in decreased blood flow to skin, skeletal muscle, kidneys, and abdominal organs. This not only decreases tissue perfusion but also contributes to an increase in systemic vascular resistance and afterload stress of the heart.

There also is evidence that prolonged sympathetic stimulation may exhaust myocardial stores of norepinephrine and may lead to down-regulation and a reduction in β-adrenergic receptors.[2] Moreover, these effects adversely affect the balance between oxygen supply and demand in persons in whom this ratio is precariously balanced. The catecholamines also may contribute to the high rate of sudden death by promoting arrhythmias.[6]

Renin-Angiotensin-Aldosterone Mechanism. One of the most important effects of a lowered cardiac output in heart failure is a reduction in renal blood flow and glomerular filtration rate, which leads to salt and water retention. Normally, the kidneys receive approximately 25% of the cardiac output, but this may be decreased to as low as 8% to 10% in persons with heart failure. With decreased renal blood flow, there is a progressive increase in renin secretion by the kidneys along with parallel increases in circulating levels of angiotensin II. The increased concentration of angiotensin II contributes to a generalized and excessive vasoconstriction and provides a powerful stimulus for aldosterone production by the adrenal cortex (see Chapter 25). Aldosterone increases tubular reabsorption of sodium, with an accompanying increase in water retention. Because aldosterone is metabolized in the liver, its levels are further increased when heart failure causes liver congestion. Angiotensin II also increases the level of antidiuretic hormone (ADH), which serves as a vasoconstrictor and inhibitor of water excretion[7] (see Chapter 33). In addition to their individual effects on salt and water balance, angiotensin II and aldosterone are also involved in regulating the inflammatory and reparative processes that follow tissue injury.[8] In this capacity, they stimulate cytokine production, inflammatory cell (*e.g.*, neutrophils and macrophages) adhesion, and chemotaxis; activate macrophages at sites of injury and repair; and stimulate the growth of fibroblasts and the synthesis of collagen fibers.

Aldosterone-synthesizing enzymes have recently been demonstrated in endothelial and vascular smooth muscle cells as well as in the adrenal gland, suggesting that these cells are capable of both producing aldosterone and responding to it.[8,9] Thus, the progression of heart failure may be augmented by aldosterone-mediated vascular remodeling in the heart and other organs. In the recent international (Randomized Aldactone Evaluation Study [RALES]) trial involving more than 1600 patients with moderately severe to severe heart failure, there was a 30% decrease in mortality from any cause among patients treated with standard therapy plus spironolactone (an aldosterone antagonist) as compared with those who received a placebo plus standard therapy.[10]

Natriuretic Peptides. The natriuretic peptide family consists of three peptides: atrial natriuretic peptide, brain natriuretic peptide, and C-type natriuretic peptide.[11,12] Atrial natriuretic peptide (ANP), which is released from atrial cells in response to increased atrial stretch and pressure, produces rapid and transient natriuresis, diuresis, and moderate loss of potassium in the urine. It also inhibits aldosterone and renin secretion, acts as an antagonist to angiotensin II, and inhibits the release of norepinephrine from presynaptic nerve terminals. Brain natriuretic peptide (BNP), so named because it was originally found in extracts of porcine brain, is stored mainly in the ventricular cells and is responsive to increased ventricular filling pressures. BNP has cardiovascular effects similar to ANP. The role of C-type natriuretic peptide (CNP), which is found primarily in vascular tissue, has not as yet been clarified.

Circulating levels of both ANP and BNP are reportedly elevated in persons with congestive heart failure. The concentrations are correlated with the extent of ventricular dysfunction, increasing up to 30-fold in persons with advanced heart disease.[11] Reliable assays of BNP are now available and are used clinically in the diagnosis of heart failure. Human BNP, synthesized by recombinant DNA technology, is now available for treatment of persons with acutely decompensated heart failure (discussed later).

Endothelin. The endothelins, released from the endothelial cells throughout the circulation, are potent vasoconstrictors. Other actions of the endothelins include induction of vascular smooth muscle cell proliferation and myocyte hypertrophy. Thus far, four endothelin peptides (endothelin-1 [ET-1], ET-2, ET-3, and ET-4) have been identified.[13] There are at least two types of endothelin receptors—type A and type B.[2,13,14] Plasma ET-1 levels correlate directly with pulmonary vascular resistance, and it is thought that the peptide may play a role in mediating pulmonary hypertension in persons with heart failure.[2] An endothelin receptor antagonist is now available for use in the treatment of persons with pulmonary arterial hypertension due to severe heart failure.

Myocardial Hypertrophy and Remodeling. The development of myocardial hypertrophy constitutes one of the principle mechanisms by which the heart compensates for an increase in workload.[2–4] Although ventricular hypertrophy improves the work performance of the heart, it also is an important risk factor for subsequent cardiac morbidity and mortality. Inappropriate hypertrophy and remodeling can result in changes in structure (muscle mass, chamber dilation) and function (impaired systolic or diastolic function) that often lead to further pump dysfunction and hemodynamic overload.

It is now recognized that myocardial hypertrophy and remodeling involve a series of complex events at both the molecular and cellular levels.[15] The myocardium is composed of myocytes, or muscle cells, and nonmyocytes. The myocytes are the functional units of cardiac muscle. Their growth is limited by an increment in cell size, as opposed to an increase in cell number. The nonmyocytes include cardiac macrophages, fibroblasts, vascular smooth muscle cells, and endothelial cells. These cells, which are present in the interstitial space and remain capable of an increase in cell number, provide support for the myocytes. They also determine many of the inappropriate changes that occur during myocardial hypertrophy. For example, uncontrolled cardiac fibroblast growth is associated with increased synthesis of collagen fibers, myocardial fibrosis, and ventricular wall stiffness.

Recent interest has focused on the type of hypertrophy that develops in persons with heart failure. At the cellular level, cardiac muscle cells respond to stimuli from stress placed on the ventricular wall by pressure and volume overload by initiating several different processes that lead to hypertrophy.[15] These include stimuli that produce *symmetric hypertrophy* with a proportionate increase in muscle length and width, as occurs in athletes; *concentric hypertrophy* with an increase in wall thickness, as occurs in hypertension; and *eccentric hypertrophy* with a disproportionate increase in muscle length, as occurs in dilated cardiomyopathy[2] (Fig. 28-3). When the primary stimulus for hypertrophy is *pressure overload,* the increase in wall stress leads to parallel replication of myofibrils, thickening of the individual myocytes, and concentric hypertrophy. Concentric hypertrophy may preserve systolic function for a period of time, but eventually the work performed by the ventricle exceeds the vascular reserve, predisposing to ischemia. When the primary stimulus is *ventricular volume overload,* increased diastolic wall stress leads to replication of myofibrils in series, elongation of the cardiac muscle cells, and eccentric hypertrophy. Eccentric hypertrophy leads to a decrease in ventricular wall thickness with an increase in diastolic volume and wall tension.

The stimuli for hypertrophy and remodeling are thought to reflect not only the mechanical stress placed on the myocytes but also growth signals provided by the release of substances such as angiotensin II, ANP, and ET-1. Further research into the signals that cause specific

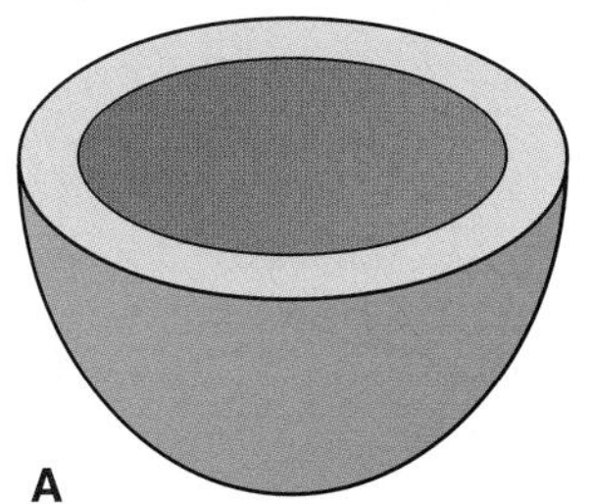

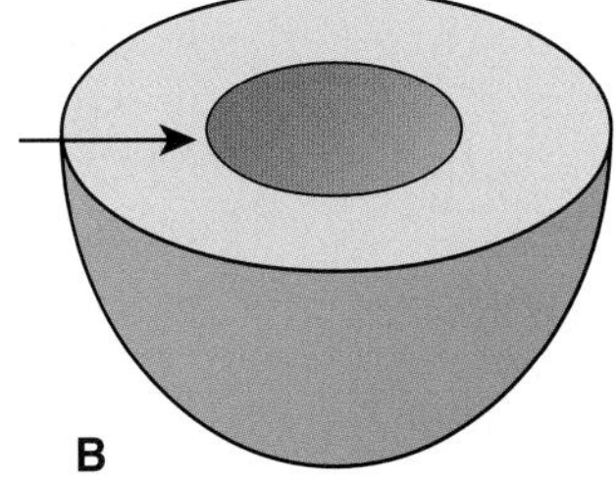

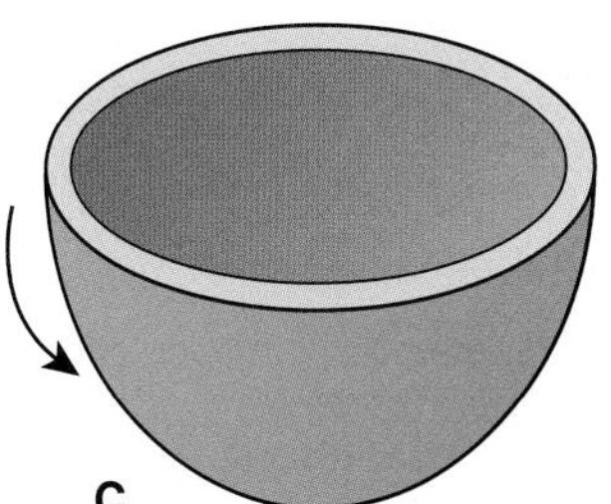

FIGURE 28-3 Different types of myocardial hypertrophy: **(A)** Normal symmetric hypertrophy with proportionate increases in myocardial wall thickness and length; **(B)** concentric hypertrophy with a disproportionate increase in wall thickness; and **(C)** eccentric hypertrophy with a disproportionate decrease in wall thickness and ventricular dilatation.

features of inappropriate myocardial hypertrophy and remodeling will hopefully lead to the identification of targets whose actions can be interrupted or modified.

CONGESTIVE HEART FAILURE

Heart failure occurs when the pumping ability of the heart becomes impaired. Congestive heart failure (CHF) is heart failure that is accompanied by congestion of body tissues. After an initial compensatory period, the clinical manifestations of heart failure become complicated by pulmonary or systemic venous congestion.

Heart failure may be caused by a variety of conditions, including acute myocardial infarction, hypertension, or degenerative conditions of the heart muscle known collectively as *cardiomyopathies*. Heart failure also may occur because of excessive work demands, such as occurs with hypermetabolic states, or with volume overload, such as occurs with renal failure. Either of these states may exceed the work capacity of even a healthy heart. In persons with asymptomatic heart disease, heart failure may be precipitated by an unrelated illness or stress. Table 28-1 lists major causes of heart failure. Heart failure may be described as high-output or low-output failure, systolic or diastolic failure, and right-sided or left-sided failure.

High-Output Versus Low-Output Failure

High- and low-output heart failure are described in terms of cardiac output. *High-output failure* is an uncommon type of heart failure that is caused by an excessive need for cardiac output. With high-output failure, the function of the heart may be supranormal but inadequate owing to excessive metabolic needs. Causes of high-output failure include severe anemia, thyrotoxicosis, conditions that cause arteriovenous shunting, and Paget's disease. High-output failure tends to be specifically treatable.

Low-output failure is caused by disorders that impair the pumping ability of the heart, such as ischemic heart disease and cardiomyopathy. As a result, treatment options tend to be more limited and focus primarily on symptom management, with attempts to slow the natural progress of the etiologic disease state.

TABLE 28-1 Causes of Heart Failure

Impaired Cardiac Function	Excess Work Demands
Myocardial Disease	**Increased Pressure Work**
Cardiomyopathies	Systemic hypertension
Myocarditis	Pulmonary hypertension
Coronary insufficiency	Coarctation of the aorta
Myocardial infarction	
Valvular Heart Disease	**Increased Volume Work**
Stenotic valvular disease	Arteriovenous shunt
Regurgitant valvular disease	Excessive administration of intravenous fluids
Congenital Heart Defects	**Increased Perfusion Work**
	Thyrotoxicosis
	Anemia
Constrictive Pericarditis	

Systolic Versus Diastolic Failure

Until recently, CHF was viewed mainly in terms of backward and forward failure. *Backward failure* represented failure of one of the ventricles to empty the heart effectively, such that blood backs up in the venous system, causing congestion. *Forward failure* was characterized by impaired forward movement of blood into the arterial system emerging from the heart.

A more recent classification separates the pathophysiology of congestive failure into two categories—systolic dysfunction and diastolic dysfunction. With systolic dysfunction, there is impaired ejection of blood from the heart during systole; with diastolic dysfunction, there is impaired filling of the ventricles during diastole (Fig. 28-4). Many persons with heart failure fall into an intermediate category, with combined elements of both systolic and diastolic failure.[16]

Systolic Dysfunction. Systolic dysfunction involves a decrease in cardiac contractility and ejection fraction. It commonly results from conditions that impair the contractile performance of the heart (*e.g.,* ischemic heart disease and cardiomyopathy), produce a volume overload (*e.g.,* valvular insufficiency and anemia), or generate a pressure overload (*e.g.,* hypertension and valvular stenosis) on the heart.

A normal heart ejects approximately 65% of the blood that is present in the ventricle at the end of diastole when it contracts. This is called the *ejection fraction.* In systolic heart failure, the ejection fraction declines progressively with increasing degrees of myocardial dysfunction. In very severe forms of heart failure, the ejection fraction may drop

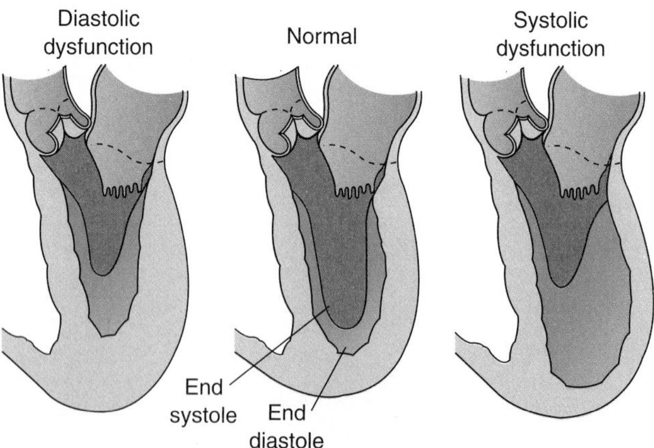

FIGURE 28-4 Congestive heart failure due to systolic and diastolic dysfunction. The ejection fraction represents the difference between the end-diastolic and end-systolic volumes. Normal systolic and diastolic function with normal ejection fraction (**middle**); diastolic dysfunction with decreased ejection fraction due to decreased diastolic filling (**left**); systolic dysfunction with decreased ejection fraction due to impaired systolic function (**right**).

to a single-digit percentage. With a decrease in ejection fraction, there is a resultant increase in diastolic volume, ventricular dilation, and ventricular wall tension and a rise in ventricular end-diastolic pressure. The symptoms of persons with systolic dysfunction result mainly from reductions in ejection fraction and cardiac output.

Diastolic Dysfunction. Diastolic dysfunction, which reportedly accounts for approximately 40% of all cases of CHF, is characterized by a smaller ventricular chamber size, ventricular hypertrophy, and poor ventricular compliance (*i.e.,* ability to stretch during filling).[17,18] Because of impaired filling, congestive symptoms tend to predominate in diastolic dysfunction. Among the conditions that cause diastolic dysfunction are those that restrict diastolic filling (*e.g.,* mitral stenosis), those that increase ventricular wall thickness and reduce chamber size (*e.g.,* myocardial hypertrophy due to lung disease and hypertrophic cardiomyopathy), and those that delay diastolic relaxation (*e.g.,* aging, ischemic heart disease). Aging often is accompanied by a delay in relaxation of the heart during diastole; diastolic filling begins while the ventricle is still stiff and resistant to stretching to accept an increase in volume.[19] A similar delay occurs with myocardial ischemia, resulting from a lack of energy to break the rigor bonds that form between the actin and myosin filaments of the contracting cardiac muscle. Because tachycardia produces a decrease in diastolic filling time, persons with diastolic dysfunction often become symptomatic during activities and situations that increase heart rate.

Right-Sided Versus Left-Sided Heart Failure

Heart failure also can be classified according to the side of the heart (right or left) that is affected. An important feature of the circulatory system is that the right and left ventricles act as two pumps that are connected in series. To function effectively, the right and left ventricles must maintain an equal output. Although the initial event that leads to heart failure may be primarily right sided or left sided in origin, long-term heart failure usually involves both sides. To understand the physiologic mechanisms associated with heart failure, right- and left-sided failure are considered separately (Fig. 28-5).

Right-Sided Heart Failure. The right heart pumps deoxygenated blood from the systemic circulation into the pulmonary circulation. Consequently, when the right heart fails, there is accumulation or damming back of blood in the systemic venous system. This causes an increase in right atrial, right ventricular end-diastolic, and systemic venous pressures.

A major effect of right-sided heart failure is the development of peripheral edema (see Fig. 28-5). Because of the effects of gravity, the edema is most pronounced in the dependent parts of the body—in the lower extremities when the person is in the upright position and in the area over the sacrum when the person is supine. The accumulation of edema fluid is evidenced by a gain in weight (*i.e.,* 1 pint of accumulated fluid results in a 1-lb weight gain). Daily measurement of weight can be used as a means of assessing fluid accumulation in a patient with chronic CHF. As

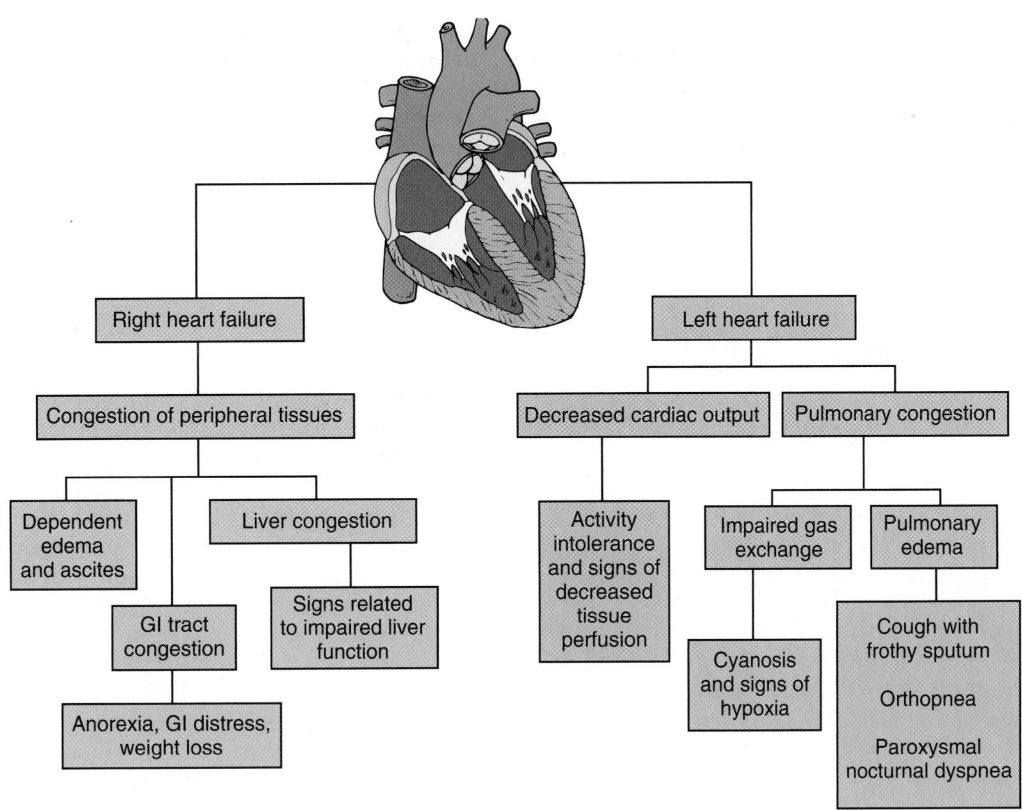

FIGURE 28-5 Manifestations of left- and right-sided heart failure.

a rule, a weight gain of more than 2 lb in 24 hours or 5 lb in 1 week is considered a sign of worsening failure.

Right-sided heart failure also produces congestion of the viscera. As venous distention progresses, blood backs up in the hepatic veins that drain into the inferior vena cava, and the liver becomes engorged. This may cause hepatomegaly and right upper quadrant pain. In severe and prolonged right-sided failure, liver function is impaired, and hepatic cells may die. Congestion of the portal circulation also may lead to engorgement of the spleen and the development of ascites. Congestion of the gastrointestinal tract may interfere with digestion and absorption of nutrients, causing anorexia and abdominal discomfort. The jugular veins, which are above the level of the heart, are normally collapsed in the standing position or when sitting with the head at higher than a 30-degree angle. In severe right-sided failure, the external jugular veins become distended and can be visualized when the person is sitting up or standing.

The causes of right-sided heart failure include conditions that restrict blood flow into the lungs. Stenosis or regurgitation of the tricuspid or pulmonic valves, right ventricular infarction, cardiomyopathy, and persistent left-sided failure are common causes. Acute or chronic pulmonary disease, such as severe pneumonia, pulmonary embolus, or pulmonary hypertension, can cause right heart failure, referred to as *cor pulmonale*.

Left-Sided Heart Failure. The left side of the heart moves blood from the low-pressure pulmonary circulation into the high-pressure arterial side of the systemic circulation. With impairment of left heart function, there is a decrease in cardiac output, an increase in left atrial and left ventricular end-diastolic pressures, and congestion in the pulmonary circulation (see Fig. 28-5). When the pulmonary capillary filtration pressure (normally approximately 10 mm Hg) exceeds the capillary osmotic pressure (normally approximately 25 mm Hg), there is a shift of intravascular fluid into the interstitium of the lung and development of pulmonary edema (Fig. 28-6). An episode of pulmonary edema often occurs at night, after the person has been reclining for some time and the gravitational forces have been removed from the circulatory system. It is then that the edema fluid that had been sequestered in the lower extremities during the day is returned to the vascular compartment and redistributed to the pulmonary circulation.

The most common causes of left-sided heart failure are acute myocardial infarction and cardiomyopathy. Left-sided heart failure and pulmonary congestion can develop very rapidly in persons with acute myocardial infarction. Even when the infarcted area is small, there may be a surrounding area of ischemic tissue. This may result in a large area of nonpumping ventricle and rapid onset of pulmonary edema. Stenosis or regurgitation of the aortic or mitral valves also creates the level of left-sided backflow that results in pulmonary congestion. Pulmonary edema also may develop during rapid infusion of intravenous fluids or blood transfusions in an elderly person or in a person with limited cardiac reserve.

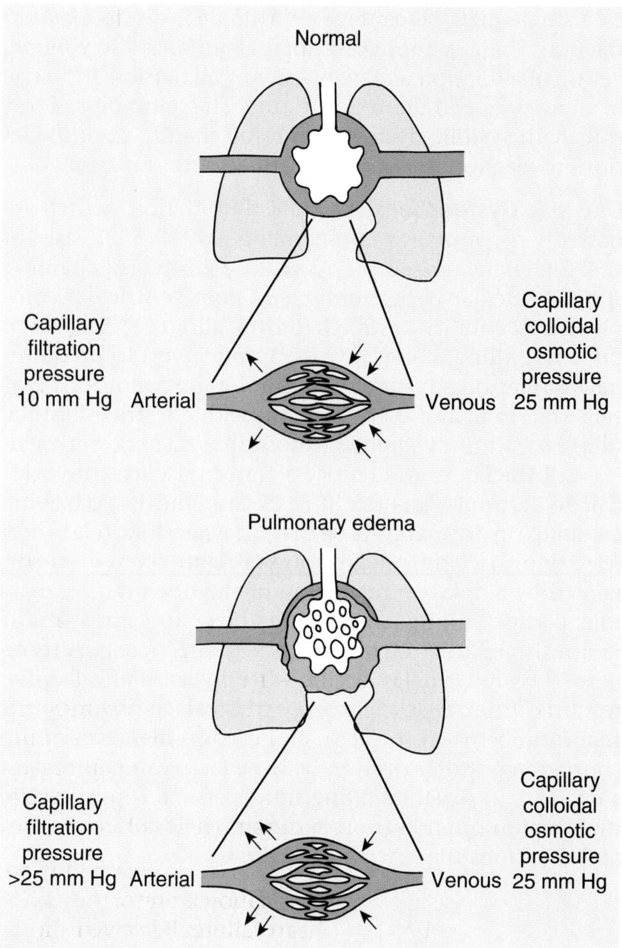

FIGURE 28-6 Mechanism of respiratory symptoms in left-sided heart failure. Normal exchange of fluid in the pulmonary capillaries (**top**). The capillary filtration pressure that moves fluid out of the capillary into the lung is less than the capillary colloidal osmotic pressure that pulls fluid back into the capillary. Development of pulmonary edema (**bottom**) occurs when the capillary filtration pressure exceeds the capillary colloidal osmotic pressure that pulls fluid back into the capillary.

Manifestations of Congestive Heart Failure

The manifestations of heart failure depend on the extent and type of cardiac dysfunction that is present and the rapidity with which it develops. A person with previously stable compensated heart failure may develop signs of heart failure for the first time when the condition has advanced to a critical point, such as with a progressive increase in pulmonary hypertension in a person with mitral valve regurgitation. Overt heart failure also may be precipitated by conditions such as infection, emotional stress, uncontrolled hypertension, administration of fluid overload, or inappropriate reduction in therapy.[16] Many persons with serious underlying heart disease, regardless of whether they have previously experienced heart failure, may be relatively asymptomatic as long as they carefully adhere to their treatment regimen. A dietary excess of sodium is a frequent cause of sudden cardiac decompensation.

The manifestations of heart failure reflect the physiologic effects of the impaired pumping ability of the heart, decreased renal blood flow, and activation of the sympathetic compensatory mechanisms. The severity and progression of symptoms depend on the extent and type of dysfunction that is present (systolic vs. diastolic failure). The signs and symptoms include fluid retention and edema, shortness of breath and other respiratory manifestations, fatigue and limited exercise tolerance, cachexia and malnutrition, and cyanosis. Distention of the jugular veins may be present in right-sided failure. Persons with severe heart failure may exhibit diaphoresis and tachycardia.

Fluid Retention and Edema. Many of the manifestations of CHF result from the increased capillary pressures that develop in the peripheral circulation in right-sided heart failure and in the pulmonary circulation in left-sided heart failure. The increased capillary pressure reflects an overfilling of the vascular system because of increased salt and water retention and venous congestion resulting from the impaired pumping ability of the heart.

Nocturia is a nightly increase in urine output that occurs relatively early in the course of CHF. It results from the return to the circulation of edema fluids from the dependent parts of the body when the person assumes the supine position for the night. As a result, the cardiac output, renal blood flow, glomerular filtration, and urine output increase. Oliguria is a late sign related to a severely reduced cardiac output and resultant renal failure.

Respiratory Manifestations. Shortness of breath due to congestion of the pulmonary circulation is one of the major manifestations of left-sided heart failure. Perceived shortness of breath (*i.e.*, breathlessness) is called *dyspnea*. Dyspnea related to an increase in activity is called *exertional dyspnea*. *Orthopnea* is shortness of breath that occurs when a person is supine. The gravitational forces that cause fluid to become sequestered in the lower legs and feet when the person is standing or sitting are removed when a person with CHF assumes the supine position; fluid from the legs and dependent parts of the body is mobilized and redistributed to an already distended pulmonary circulation. *Paroxysmal nocturnal dyspnea* is a sudden attack of dyspnea that occurs during sleep. It disrupts sleep, and the person awakens with a feeling of extreme suffocation that resolves when he or she sits up. Initially, the experience may be interpreted as awakening from a bad dream.

A subtle and often overlooked symptom of heart failure is a chronic dry, nonproductive cough, which becomes worse when the person is lying down. Bronchospasm due to congestion of the bronchial mucosa may cause wheezing and difficulty in breathing. This condition is sometimes referred to as *cardiac asthma*.

Cheyne-Stokes respiration, also known as *periodic breathing*, is characterized by a slow waxing and waning of respiration. The person breathes deeply for a period when the arterial carbon dioxide pressure (PCO_2) is high and then slightly or not at all when the PCO_2 falls. In persons with left-sided heart failure, the condition is thought to be caused by a prolongation of the heart-to-brain circulation, particularly in persons with hypertension and associated cerebral vascular disease. Cheyne-Stokes breathing may contribute to daytime sleepiness, and occasionally the person awakens at night with dyspnea precipitated by Cheyne-Stokes breathing.[16]

Fatigue and Limited Exercise Tolerance. Fatigue and limb weakness often accompany diminished output from the left ventricle. Cardiac fatigue is different from general fatigue in that it usually is not present in the morning but appears and progresses as activity increases during the day. In acute or severe left-sided failure, cardiac output may fall to levels that are insufficient for providing the brain with adequate oxygen, and there are indications of mental confusion and disturbed behavior. Confusion, impairment of memory, anxiety, restlessness, and insomnia are common in elderly persons with advanced heart failure, particularly in those with cerebral atherosclerosis. These very symptoms may confuse the diagnosis of heart failure in the elderly because of the myriad other causes associated with aging.

Cachexia and Malnutrition. Cardiac cachexia is a condition of malnutrition and tissue wasting that occurs in persons with end-stage heart failure. A number of factors probably contribute to its development, including the fatigue and depression that interfere with food intake, the congestion of the liver and gastrointestinal structures that impairs digestion and absorption and produces feelings of fullness, and the circulating toxins and mediators released from poorly perfused tissues that impair appetite and contribute to tissue wasting.

Cyanosis. Cyanosis is the bluish discoloration of the skin and mucous membranes caused by excess desaturated hemoglobin in the blood; it often is a late sign of heart failure. Cyanosis may be central, caused by arterial desaturation resulting from impaired pulmonary gas exchange, or peripheral, caused by venous desaturation resulting from extensive extraction of oxygen at the capillary level. Central cyanosis is caused by conditions that impair oxygenation of the arterial blood, such as pulmonary edema, left heart failure, or right-to-left shunting. Peripheral cyanosis is caused by conditions such as low-output failure that cause delivery of poorly oxygenated blood to the peripheral tissues, or by conditions such as peripheral vasoconstriction that cause excessive removal of oxygen from the blood. Central cyanosis is best monitored in the lips and mucous membranes because these areas are not subject to conditions such as cold that cause peripheral cyanosis. Persons with right-sided or left-sided heart failure may develop cyanosis especially around the lips and in the peripheral parts of the extremities.

Diagnostic Methods

Diagnostic methods in heart failure are directed toward establishing the cause of the disorder and determining the extent of the dysfunction.[20] Because heart failure represents the failure of the heart as a pump and can occur in the course of a number of heart diseases or other systemic disorders, the diagnosis of heart failure often is based on signs and symptoms related to the failing heart itself, such as shortness of breath and fatigue. The functional classification of the New York Heart Association (NYHA) is one guide to classifying the extent of dysfunction (Table 28-2).

The diagnostic methods include history and physical examination, laboratory studies, electrocardiography, chest radiography, and echocardiography. The history should include information related to dyspnea, cough, nocturia, generalized fatigue, and other signs and symptoms of heart failure. A complete physical examination includes assessment of heart rate, heart sounds, blood pressure, jugular veins for venous congestion, lungs for signs of pulmonary congestion, and lower extremities for edema. Laboratory tests are used in the diagnosis of anemia and electrolyte imbalances and to detect signs of chronic liver congestion. Measurements of BNP are increasingly being used to confirm the diagnosis of heart failure; to evaluate the severity of left ventricular compromise and estimate the prognosis and predict future cardiac events, such as sudden death; and to evaluate the effectiveness of treatment.[21,22]

Echocardiography plays a key role in assessing the anatomic and functional abnormalities in CHF, which include the size and function of cardiac valves, the motion of both ventricles, and the ventricular ejection fraction.[22,23] Electrocardiographic findings may indicate atrial or ventricular hypertrophy, underlying disorders of cardiac rhythm, or conduction abnormalities such as right or left bundle branch block. Radionuclide angiography and cardiac catheterization are other diagnostic tests used to detect the underlying causes of heart failure, such as heart defects and cardiomyopathy. Chest radiographs provide information about the size and shape of the heart and pulmonary vasculature. The cardiac silhouette can be used to detect cardiac hypertrophy and dilatation. X-ray films can indicate the relative severity of the failure by revealing whether pulmonary edema is predominantly vascular, interstitial, or advanced to the alveolar and bronchial stages.

TABLE 28-2 New York Heart Association Functional Classification of Patients With Heart Disease

Classification	Characteristics
Class I	Patients with cardiac disease but without the resulting limitations in physical activity. Ordinary activity does not cause undue fatigue, palpitation, dyspnea, or anginal pain.
Class II	Patients with heart disease resulting in slight limitations of physical activity. They are comfortable at rest. Ordinary physical activity results in fatigue, palpitation, dyspnea, or anginal pain.
Class III	Patients with cardiac disease resulting in marked limitation of physical activity. They are comfortable at rest. Less than ordinary physical activity causes fatigue, palpitation, dyspnea, or anginal pain.
Class IV	Patients with cardiac disease resulting in inability to carry on any physical activity without discomfort. The symptoms of cardiac insufficiency or of the anginal syndrome may be present even at rest. If any physical activity is undertaken, discomfort increases.

(From Criteria Committee of the New York Heart Association. [1964]. *Diseases of the heart and blood vessels: Nomenclature and criteria for diagnosis* [6th ed., pp. 112–113]. Boston: Little, Brown)

Invasive hemodynamic monitoring often is used in the management of acute, life-threatening episodes of heart failure. These monitoring methods include central venous pressure (CVP), pulmonary capillary wedge pressure (PCWP), thermodilution cardiac output measurements, and intra-arterial measurements of blood pressure.

CVP reflects the amount of blood returning to the heart. Measurements of CVP are best obtained by means of a catheter inserted into the right atrium through a peripheral vein, or by means of the right atrial port (opening) in a pulmonary artery catheter. This pressure is decreased in hypovolemia and increased in right heart failure. The changes that occur in CVP over time usually are more significant than the absolute numeric values obtained during a single reading.

PCWP is obtained by means of a flow-directed, balloon-tipped pulmonary artery (Swan-Ganz) catheter. This catheter is introduced through a peripheral or central vein and then advanced into the right atrium. The balloon is then inflated with air, enabling the catheter to float through the right ventricle into the pulmonary artery until it becomes wedged in a small pulmonary vessel (Fig. 28-7). After the catheter is in place, the balloon is deflated and then inflated only when the PCWP is being measured. Continuous inflation of the balloon with its accompanying occlusion of a small pulmonary artery would cause necrosis of pulmonary tissue. With the balloon inflated,

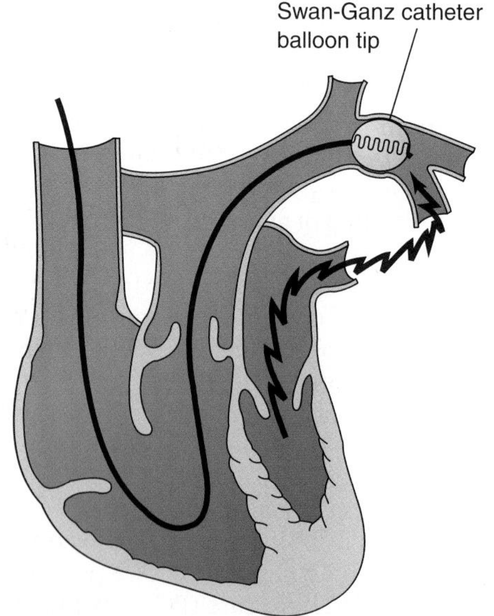

FIGURE 28-7 Swan-Ganz balloon-tipped catheter positioned in a pulmonary capillary. The pulmonary capillary wedge pressure, which reflects the left ventricular diastolic pressure, is measured with the balloon inflated.

the catheter monitors pulmonary capillary pressures in direct communication with pressures from the left heart, thus providing a means of assessing the pumping ability of the left heart.

One type of pulmonary artery catheter is equipped with a thermistor probe to obtain *thermodilution measurements* of cardiac output. A known amount of solution of a known temperature (iced or room temperature) is injected into the right atrium through an opening in the catheter, and the temperature of the blood is measured downstream in the pulmonary artery by means of a thermistor probe located at the end of that catheter. A microcomputer calculates the cardiac output from the time-temperature curve resulting from the rate of change of the temperature of the blood that flows past the thermistor. Catheters with oximeters built into their tips that permit continuous monitoring of oxygen saturation (SvO_2) also are available, as are catheters that provide continuous output data.

Intra-arterial blood pressure monitoring provides a means for continuous monitoring of blood pressure. It is used in persons with acute heart failure when aggressive intravenous drug therapy or a mechanical assist device is required. Measurements are obtained through the use of a small catheter inserted into a peripheral artery, usually the radial artery. The catheter is connected to a pressure transducer, and beat-by-beat measurements of blood pressure are recorded. The monitoring system displays the contour of the pressure waveform and a digital reading of the systolic, diastolic, and mean arterial pressures along with heart rate and rhythm. Continuous digital display of respiratory rate and core temperature from the thermistor located at the end of the pulmonary artery catheter also may be warranted.

Treatment Methods

The goals of treatment for chronic heart failure are directed toward relieving the symptoms and improving the quality of life, with a long-term goal of slowing, halting, or reversing the cardiac dysfunction.[3,22,24,25] Treatment measures include correction of reversible causes such as anemia or thyrotoxicosis, surgical repair of a ventricular defect or an improperly functioning valve, pharmacologic and nonpharmacologic control of afterload stresses such as hypertension, modification of activities and lifestyle to a level consistent with the functional limitations of a reduced cardiac reserve, and the use of medications to improve cardiac function and limit excessive compensatory mechanisms. Restriction of salt intake and diuretic therapy facilitate the excretion of edema fluid. Counseling, health teaching, and ongoing evaluation programs help persons with heart failure to manage and cope with their treatment regimen.

In severe heart failure, restriction of activity, including bed rest if necessary, often facilitates temporary recompensation of cardiac function. However, there is no convincing evidence that continued bed rest is of benefit. Carefully designed and managed exercise programs for patients with CHF are well tolerated and beneficial to patients with stable NYHA class I to III heart failure.[26,27]

Pharmacologic Treatment. Once heart failure is moderate to severe, polypharmacy becomes a management standard and often includes diuretics, digoxin, angiotensin-converting enzyme (ACE) inhibitors, and β-adrenergic–blocking agents.[28–30] The choice of pharmacologic agents is determined by problems caused by the disorder (*i.e.,* systolic or diastolic dysfunction) and those brought about by activation of compensatory mechanisms (*e.g.,* excess fluid retention, inappropriate activation of sympathetic mechanisms).

Diuretics are among the most frequently prescribed medications for heart failure. They promote the excretion of edema fluid and help to sustain cardiac output and tissue perfusion by reducing preload and allowing the heart to operate at a more optimal part of the Frank-Starling curve. Thiazide and loop diuretics are used. In emergencies, such as acute pulmonary edema, loop diuretics such as furosemide can be administered intravenously. When given intravenously, these drugs act quickly to reduce venous return through vasodilatation so that right ventricular output and pulmonary vascular pressures are decreased. This response to intravenous drug administration is extrarenal and precedes the onset of diuresis.

Digitalis has been a recognized treatment for CHF for more than 200 years. The various forms of digitalis are called *cardiac glycosides.* They improve cardiac function by increasing the force and strength of ventricular contraction. By decreasing sinoatrial node activity and decreasing conduction through the atrioventricular node, they also slow the heart rate and increase diastolic filling time. Although not a diuretic, digitalis promotes urine output by improving cardiac output and renal blood flow. The digitalis drugs act by binding to sodium-potassium adenosine triphosphatase (ATPase) on the cell membrane and inhibiting the sodium-potassium pump. When intracellular sodium is increased because of inhibition of the sodium-potassium pump by digitalis, the exchange of intracellular calcium for extracellular sodium is inhibited; as a result, more calcium is available to activate the myocardial actin–myosin contractile apparatus. The role of digitalis in the treatment of heart failure is controversial and has been studied in clinical trials over the past several decades. Although the results of these studies remain controversial, there seems to be a growing consensus that although it does not necessarily reduce mortality rates, digitalis prevents clinical deterioration and hospitalization and improves exercise tolerance.[31,32]

The *ACE inhibitors,* which prevent the conversion of angiotensin I to angiotensin II, have been effectively used in the treatment of heart failure. In heart failure, renin activity frequently is elevated because of decreased renal blood flow. The net result is an increase in angiotensin II, which causes vasoconstriction and increased aldosterone production with a subsequent increase in salt and water retention by the kidney. Both mechanisms increase the workload of the heart. The newer angiotensin II receptor blockers have the advantage of not causing a cough, which is a troublesome side effect of the ACE inhibitors for many persons. The results of the previously mentioned RALES trial suggest that the aldosterone antagonist, spironolactone, may be beneficial for persons with moderately severe to severe heart failure.[10]

Large clinical trials have shown that long-term therapy with β-adrenergic–blocking agents reduces morbidity and mortality in persons with CHF.[24,29,33] Left ventricular dysfunction is associated with activation of the renin-angiotensin-aldosterone and sympathetic nervous systems. Chronic elevation of norepinephrine levels has been shown to cause cardiac muscle cell death and progressive left ventricular dysfunction and is associated with poor prognosis in heart failure. Until recently, β-blockers were thought to be contraindicated in left ventricular systolic dysfunction because of their negative inotropic effects. Large clinical trials involving more than 10,000 patients, most of whom had stable NYHA class II and III heart failure, have demonstrated significant reductions in the overall mortality rate with treatment with various β blockers. Several β-blockers (*i.e.*, carvedilol, metoprolol, and bisoprolol) are used in the treatment of heart failure. The ongoing Carvedilol and Metoprolol European Trial (COMET) is designed to evaluate the relative benefits of these agents.[29]

The new agent, nesiritide, a recombinant form of human B-type natriuretic peptide, has recently been approved for treatment of acute and decompensated heart failure.[34,35] The drug, which has the same structure as the endogenous natriuretic peptide, is a potent vasodilator that reduces ventricular filling pressures and improves cardiac output. Because it must be given intravenously in a closely supervised clinical setting, it is usually reserved for patients with severe heart failure who do not respond to other forms of therapy.

Cardiac Resynchronization. Some patients with heart failure due to systolic dysfunction have abnormal intraventricular conduction that results in dyssynchronous and ineffective contractions.[36] Cardiac resynchronization therapy involves the placement of pacing leads into the right and left ventricles as a means of resynchronizing the contraction of the two ventricles. Results of studies with up to 6 months of follow-up data have reported an increase in ejection fraction and improvement in symptoms and exercise tolerance. Definitive data on more long-term morbidity and mortality are not yet available.

ACUTE PULMONARY EDEMA

Acute pulmonary edema is the most dramatic symptom of left heart failure. It is a life-threatening condition in which capillary fluid moves into the alveoli. The accumulated fluid in the alveoli and respiratory airways causes lung stiffness, makes lung expansion more difficult, and impairs the gas exchange function of the lung. With the decreased ability of the lungs to oxygenate the blood, the hemoglobin leaves the pulmonary circulation without being fully oxygenated, resulting in shortness of breath and cyanosis.

Manifestations

Acute pulmonary edema usually is a terrifying experience. The person usually is seen sitting and gasping for air, in obvious apprehension. The pulse is rapid, the skin is moist and cool, and the lips and nail beds are cyanotic. As the lung edema worsens and oxygen supply to the brain drops, confusion and stupor appear. Dyspnea and air hunger are accompanied by a cough productive of frothy (resembling beaten egg whites) and often blood-tinged sputum—the effect of air mixing with serum albumin and red blood cells that have moved into the alveoli. The movement of air through the alveolar fluid produces fine crepitant sounds called *crackles,* which can be heard through a stethoscope placed on the chest. As fluid moves into the larger airways, the breathing becomes louder. The crackles heard earlier become louder and coarser. In the terminal stage, the breathing pattern is called the *death rattle.* Persons with severe pulmonary edema literally drown in their own secretions.

Treatment

Treatment of acute pulmonary edema is directed toward reducing the fluid volume in the pulmonary circulation. This can be accomplished by reducing the amount of blood that the right heart delivers to the lungs or by improving the work performance of the left heart. Several measures can decrease the blood volume in the pulmonary circulation; the seriousness of the pulmonary edema determines which are used. One of the simplest measures to relieve orthopnea is assumption of the seated position. For many persons, sitting up or standing is almost instinctive and may be sufficient to relieve the symptoms associated with mild accumulation of fluid.

Measures to improve left heart performance focus on decreasing the preload by reducing the filling pressure of the left ventricle and on reducing the afterload against which the left heart must pump. This can be accomplished through the use of diuretics, vasodilator drugs, treatment of arrhythmias that impair cardiac function, and improvement of the contractile properties of the left ventricle with digitalis. Rapid digitalization can be accomplished with intravenous administration of the drug. Although its mechanisms of action are unclear, morphine sulfate usually is the drug of choice in acute pulmonary edema. Morphine relieves anxiety and depresses the pulmonary reflexes that cause spasm of the pulmonary vessels. It also increases venous pooling by vasodilatation.

Oxygen therapy increases the oxygen content of the blood and helps relieve anxiety. Positive-pressure breathing increases the intra-alveolar pressure, opposes the capillary filtration pressure in the pulmonary capillaries, and sometimes is used as a temporary measure to decrease the amount of fluid moving into the alveoli. Positive-pressure breathing can be administered through a specially designed, continuous positive airway pressure mask. In the most severe cases, however, endotracheal intubation and mechanical ventilation may be necessary.

CARDIOGENIC SHOCK

Cardiogenic shock implies failure of the heart to pump blood adequately. Cardiogenic shock can occur relatively quickly because of the damage to the heart that occurs during myocardial infarction; ineffective pumping caused by cardiac arrhythmias; mechanical defects that may occur as a complication of myocardial infarction, such as ventricular septal defect; ventricular aneurysm; acute disruption of valvular function; or problems associated with open-heart surgery. Cardiogenic shock also may ensue as an end-stage condition of coronary artery disease or cardiomyopathy.

The most common cause of cardiogenic shock is myocardial infarction. Most patients who die of cardiogenic shock have lost at least 40% of the contracting muscle of the left ventricle because of a recent infarct or a combination of recent and old infarcts.[37,38] Cardiogenic shock can follow other types of shock associated with inadequate coronary blood flow, or it can develop because substances released from ischemic tissues impair cardiac function. One such substance, myocardial depressant factor, is thought to be released into the circulation during severe shock. Myocardial depressant factor produces reversible (although often severe) myocardial depression, ventricular dilation, and decreased left ventricular ejection fraction and diastolic pressure.[39]

In all cases of cardiogenic shock, there is failure to eject blood from the heart, hypotension, and inadequate cardiac output. Increased systemic vascular resistance often contributes to the deterioration of cardiac function by increasing afterload or the resistance to ventricular systole. The filling pressure, or preload of the heart, also is increased as blood returning to the heart is added to blood that previously returned but was not pumped forward, resulting in an increase in end-systolic ventricular volume. Increased resistance to ventricular systole (*i.e.,* afterload), combined with decreased myocardial contractility, causes the increased end-systolic ventricular volume and increased preload, which further complicate cardiac status.

Manifestations

The signs and symptoms of cardiogenic shock are consistent with those of extreme heart failure. The lips, nail beds, and skin are cyanotic because of stagnation of blood flow and increased extraction of oxygen from the hemoglobin as it passes through the capillary bed. The CVP and PCWP rise as a result of volume overload caused by the pumping failure of the heart.

Treatment

Treatment of cardiogenic shock requires a precarious balance between improving cardiac output, reducing the workload and oxygen needs of the myocardium, and preserving coronary perfusion. Fluid volume must be regulated within a level that maintains the filling pressure (*i.e.,* venous return) of the heart and maximum use of the Frank-Starling mechanism without causing pulmonary congestion.

Pharmacologic treatment includes the use of vasodilators such as nitroprusside and nitroglycerin. Nitroprusside causes arterial and venous dilatation, producing a decrease in venous return to the heart, with a reduction in arterial resistance against which the left heart must pump. Nitroglycerin focuses its effects on the venous vascular beds until, at high doses, it begins to dilate the arterial beds as well. The arterial pressure is maintained by an increased ventricular stroke volume ejected against a lowered systemic vascular resistance; this allows blood to be redistributed from the pulmonary vascular bed to the systemic circulation. Catecholamines increase cardiac contractility but must be used with caution because they also produce vasoconstriction and increased work of the heart by increasing afterload.

The *intra-aortic balloon pump* provides a means of increasing aortic diastolic pressure and enhances coronary and peripheral blood flow without increasing systolic pressure and the afterload, against which the left ventricle must pump.[40] The device, which pumps in synchrony with the heart, consists of a 10-inch long balloon that is inserted through a catheter into the descending aorta (Fig. 28-8). The balloon is positioned so that the distal tip lies approximately 1 inch from the aortic arch. The balloon is filled with helium and is timed to inflate during ventricular diastole and deflate just before ventricular systole. Diastolic inflation creates a pressure wave in the ascending aorta that increases coronary artery flow and a less intense wave in the lower aorta that enhances organ perfusion. The sudden balloon deflation at the onset of systole lowers the resistance to ejection of blood from the left ventricle, thereby increasing the heart's pumping efficiency and decreasing myocardial oxygen consumption.

When cardiogenic shock is caused by myocardial infarction, several aggressive interventions can be used successfully. The rapid and aggressive administration of a thrombolytic agent to dissolve intracoronary thrombi has been shown to improve aortic pressure and survival significantly.[41] Another alternative includes emergent direct percutaneous transluminal angioplasty (see Chapter 26).

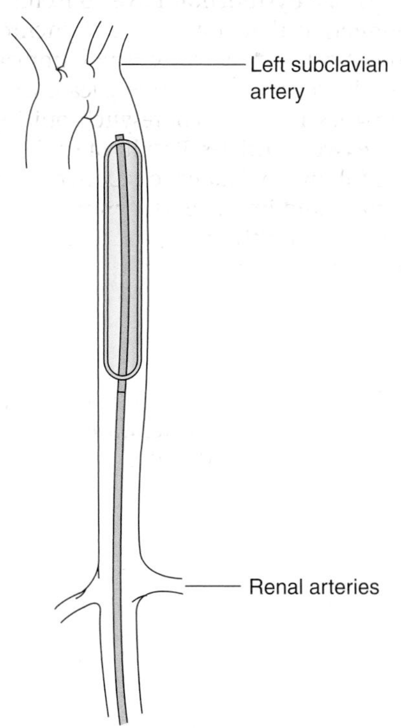

FIGURE 28-8 Aortic balloon pump. (Hudak C.M., Gallo B.M. [1994]. *Critical care nursing* [6th ed.]. Philadelphia: J.B. Lippincott)

MECHANICAL SUPPORT AND HEART TRANSPLANTATION

Refractory heart failure reflects deterioration in cardiac function that is unresponsive to medical or surgical interventions. With improved methods of treatment, more people are reaching a point at which a cure is unachievable and death is imminent without mechanical support or heart transplantation.

Since the early 1960s, significant progress has been made in improving the efficacy of *ventricular assist devices* (VADs), which are mechanical pumps used to support ventricular function. VADs are used to decrease the workload of the myocardium while maintaining cardiac output and systemic arterial pressure. This decreases the workload on the ventricle and allows it to rest and recover. Most VADs require an invasive open chest procedure for implantation. They may be used in patients who fail or have difficulty being weaned from cardiopulmonary bypass after cardiac surgery; those who develop cardiogenic shock after myocardial infarction; those with end-stage cardiomyopathy; and those who are awaiting cardiac transplantation. Earlier and more aggressive use of VADs as a bridge to transplantation has been shown to increase survival.[40,42] VADs that allow the patient to be mobile and managed at home are beginning to be considered as long-term or permanent support for treatment of end-stage heart failure, rather than simply as a bridge to transplantation. VADs can be used to support the function of the left ventricle, right ventricle, or both.

Heart transplantation remains the treatment of choice for end-stage cardiac failure. The number of successful heart transplantations has been steadily climbing, with more than 2800 procedures performed per year. Patients with heart transplants who are treated with triple-immunosuppressant therapy have 5-year survival rates of 75% in men and 62% in women.[43] Despite the overall success of heart transplantation, donor availability and complications from infection, rejection, and immunosuppression drug therapy remain problems.

The current technique for orthotopic heart transplantation (the most common) was described in 1960 by Lower and Shumway.[43] The procedure is performed by placing the recipient on cardiopulmonary bypass and excising the diseased heart. The method involves retaining a large portion of the posterior wall of the right and left atrium in the recipient and attaching the donor heart with relatively long sutures (Fig. 28-9). Pacing wires are loosely attached to the right ventricle to assist with temporary pacing of the heartbeat in the event of bradycardia in the immediate postoperative phase.

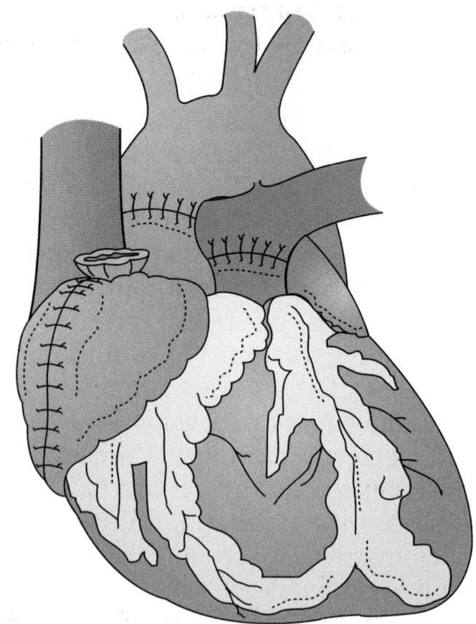

FIGURE 28-9 Orthotopic heart transplantation and sites of donor heart attachment.

An alternative to heart transplantation is a procedure called *cardiomyoplasty*.[44] This procedure involves fashioning one of the patient's latissimus dorsi back muscles into a wrap that embraces the heart. The muscle is native tissue; thus, rejection is not a problem. Because the proximal end of the muscle remains intact, perfusion is optimal with enhanced potential for healing and performance. A pacemaker, which is placed between the heart and the back muscle, stimulates the muscle to contract. After several weeks of rest and healing, the skeletal muscle is gradually stimulated by the pacemaker to condition it in a necessary transformation into a more fatigue-resistant type of muscle tissue. Although more work is needed to identify the optimal way to wrap the muscle and condition it for maximum ventricular assist, cardiomyoplasty provides an alternative to transplantation for some persons, particularly when a donor heart is not available.

In summary, heart failure occurs when the heart fails to pump sufficient blood to meet the metabolic needs of body tissues. The physiology of heart failure reflects an interplay between a decrease in cardiac output that accompanies impaired function of the failing heart and the compensatory mechanisms designed to preserve the cardiac reserve. Adaptive mechanisms include the Frank-Starling mechanism, sympathetic nervous system activation, the renin-angiotensin-aldosterone mechanism, natriuretic peptides, the endothelins, and myocardial hypertrophy, and remodeling. In the failing heart, early decreases in cardiac function may go unnoticed because these compensatory mechanisms maintain the cardiac output. This is called *compensated heart failure.* Unfortunately, the mechanisms were not intended for long-term use, and in severe and prolonged decompensated heart failure, the compensatory mechanisms no longer are effective, and instead contribute to the progression of cardiac heart failure.

Heart failure may be described as high-output or low-output failure, systolic or diastolic failure, and right-sided or left-sided failure. With high-output failure, the function of the heart may be supranormal but inadequate because of excessive metabolic needs, and low-output failure is caused by disorders that impair the pumping ability of the heart. With systolic dysfunction, there is impaired ejection of blood from the heart during systole; with diastolic dysfunction, there is impaired filling of the heart during diastole. Right-sided failure is characterized by congestion in the peripheral circulation, and left-sided failure by congestion in the pulmonary circulation.

The manifestations of heart failure include edema, nocturia, fatigue and impaired exercise tolerance, cyanosis, signs of increased sympathetic nervous system activity, and impaired gastrointestinal function and malnutrition. In right-sided failure, there is dependent edema of the lower parts of the body, engorgement of the liver, and ascites. In left-sided failure, shortness of breath and chronic, nonproductive cough are common.

The diagnostic methods in heart failure are directed toward establishing the cause and extent of the disorder. Treatment is directed toward correcting the cause whenever possible, improving cardiac function, maintaining the fluid volume within a compensatory level, and developing an activity pattern consistent with individual limitations in cardiac reserve. Among the medications used in the treatment of heart failure are diuretics, digoxin, ACE inhibitors, and β-blockers.

Acute pulmonary edema is a life-threatening condition in which the accumulation of fluid in the interstitium of the lung and alveoli interferes with lung expansion and gas exchange. It is characterized by extreme breathlessness, crackles, frothy sputum, cyanosis, and signs of hypoxemia. In cardiogenic shock, there is failure to eject blood from the heart, hypotension, inadequate cardiac output, and impaired perfusion of peripheral tissues. Mechanical support devices, including the intra-aortic balloon pump (for acute failure) and the VAD, sustain life in persons with severe heart failure. Heart transplantation remains the treatment of choice for many persons with end-stage heart failure.

Circulatory Failure (Shock)

After completing this section of the chapter, you should be able to meet the following objectives:

- State a clinical definition of shock
- Compare the chief characteristics of hypovolemic shock, obstructive shock, and distributive shock
- Describe the compensatory mechanisms that occur and relate them to the stages and manifestations of hypovolemic shock
- State the causes of obstructive shock
- Compare the pathophysiology of neurogenic shock, anaphylactic shock, and septic shock as they relate to the pathophysiology of distributive shock
- Describe the complications of shock as they relate to the lung, kidney, gastrointestinal tract, and blood clotting
- State the rationale for treatment measures to correct and reverse shock
- Define multiple organ dysfunction syndrome and cite its significance in shock

The functions of the circulatory system are to perfuse body tissues and supply them with oxygen. Adequate perfusion of body tissues depends on the pumping ability of the heart, a vascular system that transports blood to the cells and back to the heart, sufficient blood to fill the vascular system, and tissues that are able to use and extract oxygen and nutrients from the blood.

Circulatory shock can be described as a failure of the vascular system to supply the peripheral tissues and organs of the body with an adequate blood supply. It is not a specific disease but a syndrome that can occur in the course of many life-threatening traumatic conditions or disease states. It can be caused by a decrease in blood volume (hypovolemic shock), obstruction of blood flow through the circulatory system (obstructive shock), or vasodilation with redistribution of blood flow (distributive shock). These three main types of shock are summarized in Chart 28-1 and depicted in Figure 28-10. Cardiogenic shock, which results from failure of the heart as a pump, was discussed earlier in the chapter. As with heart failure, circulatory shock produces compensatory physiologic responses that eventually decompensate into various shock states if the condition is not properly treated in a timely manner.

HYPOVOLEMIC SHOCK

Hypovolemic shock is characterized by diminished blood volume such that there is inadequate filling of the vascular compartment (see Fig. 28-10). It occurs when there is an acute loss of 15% to 20% of the circulating blood volume. The decrease may be caused by an external loss of whole blood (*e.g.*, hemorrhage), plasma (*e.g.*, severe burns), or extracellular fluid (*e.g.*, gastrointestinal fluids lost in vomiting or diarrhea). Hypovolemic shock also can result from an internal hemorrhage or from third-space losses, when extracellular fluid is shifted from the vascular compartment to the interstitial space or compartment.

Physiology of Hypovolemic Shock

Hypovolemic shock has been the most widely studied type of shock and usually serves as a prototype in discussions of the manifestations of shock. Figure 28-11 shows the effect of removing blood from the circulatory system during approximately 30 minutes.[45] Approximately 10% can be removed without changing the cardiac output or

CHART 28-1

Classification of Circulatory Shock

Hypovolemic

Loss of whole blood
Loss of plasma
Loss of extracellular fluid

Obstructive

Inability of the heart to fill properly (cardiac tamponade)
Obstruction to outflow from the heart (pulmonary embolus, cardiac myxoma, pneumothorax, or dissecting aneurysm)

Distributive

Loss of sympathetic vasomotor tone
Presence of vasodilating substances in the blood (anaphylactic shock)
Presence of inflammatory mediators (septic shock)

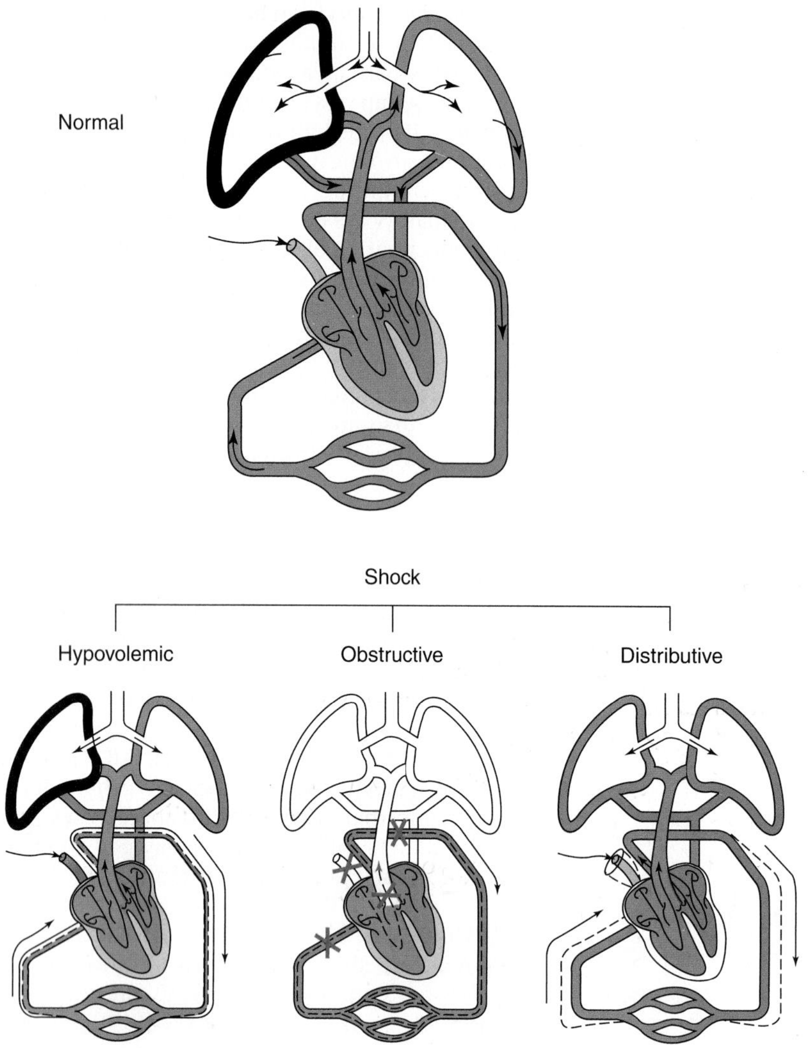

Normal

Shock

Hypovolemic

Obstructive

Distributive

FIGURE 28-10 Types of shock.

CIRCULATORY SHOCK

- Circulatory shock represents the inability of the circulation to adequately perfuse the tissues of the body.
- It can result from a loss of fluid from the vascular compartment (hypovolemic shock), obstruction of flow through the vascular compartment (obstructive shock), or an increase in the size of the vascular compartment that interferes with the distribution of blood (distributive shock).
- The manifestations of shock reflect both the impaired perfusion of body tissues and the body's attempt to maintain tissue perfusion through conservation of water by the kidney, translocation of fluid from extracellular to the intravascular compartment, and activation of sympathetic nervous system mechanisms that increase heart rate and divert blood from less to more essential body tissues.

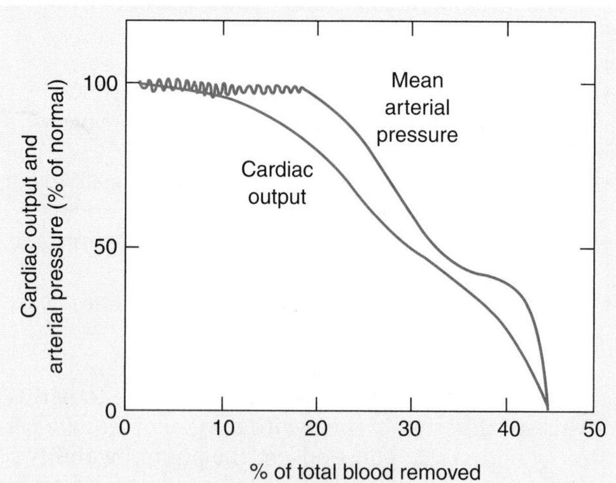

FIGURE 28-11 Effect of hemorrhage on cardiac output and arterial pressure. (Guyton A.C. [1986]. *Textbook of medical physiology* [7th ed.]. Philadelphia: W.B. Saunders)

arterial pressure. The average blood donor loses a pint of blood without experiencing adverse effects. As increasing amounts of blood (10% to 25%) are removed, the cardiac output falls, but the arterial pressure is maintained because of sympathetic-mediated increases in heart rate and vasoconstriction. Blood pressure is the product of cardiac output and systemic vascular resistance (also known as the peripheral vascular resistance); thus, an increase in systemic vascular resistance can maintain the blood pressure in the presence of decreased cardiac output for a short period of time. Cardiac output and tissue perfusion decrease before signs of hypotension occur. Cardiac output and arterial pressure fall to zero when approximately 35% to 45% of the total blood volume has been removed.[45]

Compensatory Mechanisms. Without compensatory mechanisms to maintain cardiac output and blood pressure, the loss of vascular volume would result in a rapid progression from the initial to the progressive and irreversible stages of shock. The most immediate of the compensatory mechanisms are the sympathetic-mediated responses designed to maintain cardiac output and blood pressure. Within seconds after the onset of hemorrhage or the loss of blood volume, tachycardia, increased cardiac contractility, vasoconstriction, and other signs of sympathetic and adrenal medullary activity appear. The sympathetic vasoconstrictor response affects the arterioles and the veins. Arteriolar constriction helps to maintain blood pressure by increasing the systemic vascular resistance, and venous constriction mobilizes blood that has been stored in the capacitance side of the circulation as a means of increasing venous return to the heart. There is considerable capacity for blood storage in the large veins of the abdomen and liver. Approximately 350 mL of blood that can be mobilized in shock is stored in the liver. Sympathetic stimulation does not cause constriction of the cerebral and coronary vessels, and blood flow through the heart and brain is maintained at essentially normal levels as long as the mean arterial pressure remains above 70 mm Hg.[45]

During the early stages of hypovolemic shock, vasoconstriction causes a reduction in the size of the vascular compartment and an increase in systemic vascular resistance. This response usually is all that is needed when the injury is slight, and blood loss is arrested at this point. As hypovolemic shock progresses, there are further increases in heart rate and cardiac contractility, and vasoconstriction becomes more intense. There is vasoconstriction of the blood vessels that supply the skin, skeletal muscles, kidneys, and abdominal organs, with a resultant decrease in blood flow and conversion to anaerobic metabolism with lactic acid formation.

Compensatory mechanisms designed to restore blood volume include absorption of fluid from the interstitial spaces, conservation of salt and water by the kidneys, and thirst. Extracellular fluid is distributed between the interstitial spaces and the vascular compartment. When there is a loss of vascular volume, capillary pressures decrease, and water is drawn into the vascular compartment from the interstitial spaces. The maintenance of vascular volume is further enhanced by renal mechanisms that conserve fluid. A decrease in renal blood flow and glomerular filtration rate results in activation of the renin-angiotensin-aldosterone mechanism, which produces an increase in sodium reabsorption by the kidney. The decrease in blood volume also stimulates centers in the hypothalamus that regulate ADH release and thirst. A decrease in blood volume of 5% to 10% is sufficient to stimulate ADH release and thirst.[46] ADH, also known as *vasopressin,* constricts the peripheral arteries and veins and greatly increases water retention by the kidneys. While more sensitive to changes in serum osmolality, a decrease of 10% to 15% in blood volume serves as a strong stimulus for thirst.[46]

The compensatory mechanisms that the body recruits in hypovolemic and other forms of circulatory shock were not intended for long-term use. When injury is severe or its effects prolonged, the compensatory mechanisms begin to exert their own detrimental effects. The intense vasoconstriction causes a decrease in tissue perfusion, impaired cellular metabolism, release of vasoactive inflammatory mediators such as histamine, liberation of lactic acid, and cell death. After circulatory function has been reestablished, whether the shock will be irreversible or the patient will survive is determined largely at the cellular level.

Cellular Function. Shock ultimately exerts its effect at the cellular level with failure of the circulation to supply the cell with the oxygen and nutrients needed for production of adenosine triphosphate (ATP). The cell uses ATP for a number of purposes, including operation of the sodium-potassium membrane pump that moves sodium out of the cell and potassium back into the cell. The cell uses two pathways to convert nutrients to energy (see Chapter 4). The first is the anaerobic (nonoxygen) glycolytic pathway, which is located in the cytoplasm. Glycolysis converts glucose to ATP and pyruvate. The second pathway is the aerobic (oxygen-dependent) pathway, called the *citric acid cycle,* which is located in the mitochondria. When oxygen is available, pyruvate from the glycolytic pathway moves into the mitochondria and enters the citric acid cycle, where it is transformed into ATP and the metabolic byproducts carbon dioxide and water. Fatty acids and proteins also can be metabolized in the mitochondrial pathway. When oxygen is lacking, pyruvate does not enter the citric acid cycle; instead, it is converted to lactic acid.

In severe shock, cellular metabolic processes are essentially anaerobic, which means that excess amounts of lactic acid accumulate in the cellular and the extracellular compartment. The anaerobic pathway, although allowing energy production to continue in the absence of oxygen, is relatively inefficient and produces significantly less ATP than does the aerobic pathway. Without sufficient energy production, normal cell function cannot be maintained, and the activity of the sodium-potassium membrane pump is impaired. As a result, sodium chloride accumulates in cells, and potassium is lost from cells. The cells then swell, and their membranes become more permeable. Mitochondrial activity becomes severely depressed, and lysosomal membranes rupture, resulting in the release of enzymes that cause further intracellular destruction. This is followed by cell death and the release of intracellular contents into the extracellular spaces. The resultant changes in the microcirculation reduce the chance of recovery.

Clinical Course

Stages. The progression of hypovolemic shock can be divided into four stages. During the *initial stage,* the circulatory blood volume is decreased, but not enough to cause serious effects. The *second stage* is the compensatory stage; although the circulating blood volume is reduced, compensatory mechanisms are able to maintain blood pressure and tissue perfusion at a level sufficient to prevent cell damage. The *third stage* is the progressive stage or stage of decompensated shock. At this point, unfavorable signs begin to appear: the blood pressure begins to fall, blood flow to the heart and brain is impaired, capillary permeability is increased, fluid begins to leave the capillaries, blood flow becomes sluggish, and the cells and their enzyme systems are damaged. The *fourth stage* is the final, irreversible stage. In irreversible shock, even though the blood volume may be restored and vital signs stabilized, death ensues eventually. Although the factors that determine recovery from severe shock have not been clearly identified, it appears that they are related to blood flow at the level of the microcirculation. The severity of and clinical findings associated with hypovolemic shock are summarized in Table 28-3.

Manifestations. The signs and symptoms of hypovolemic shock depend on shock stage and are closely related to low peripheral blood flow and excessive sympathetic stimulation. They include thirst, an increase in heart rate, cool and clammy skin, a decrease in arterial blood pressure, a decrease in urine output, and changes in mentation. Laboratory tests of hemoglobin and hematocrit provide information regarding the severity of blood loss or hemoconcentration due to dehydration. Serum lactate and arterial pH provide information about the severity of acidosis.

Thirst is an early symptom in hypovolemic shock. Although the underlying cause is not fully understood, it probably is related to decreased blood volume and increased serum osmolality (see Chapter 33). An increase in heart rate often is another early sign of shock. As shock progresses, the pulse becomes weak and thready, indicating vasoconstriction and a reduction in filling of the vascular compartment.

Arterial blood pressure is decreased in moderate to severe shock (see Fig. 28-11). However, blood pressure measurements may not prove useful in the early diagnosis of shock. This is because compensatory mechanisms tend to preserve blood pressure until shock is relatively far advanced. Furthermore, an adequate arterial pressure does not ensure adequate perfusion and oxygenation of vital organs at the cellular level. This does not imply that blood pressure should not be closely monitored in patients at risk for development of shock, but it does indicate the need for other assessment measures. Blood pressure often is measured intraarterially in persons with severe shock because auscultatory (cuff and stethoscope) or oscillometric

TABLE 28-3 Correlation of Clinical Findings and the Magnitude of Volume Deficit in Hemorrhagic Shock

Severity of Shock	Clinical Findings	Percentage of Reduction in Blood Volume (mL)
None	None; normal blood donation	≤10 (500)*
Mild	Minimal tachycardia Slight decrease in blood pressure Mild evidence of peripheral vasoconstriction with cool hands and feet	15–25 (750–1250)
Moderate	Tachycardia, 100–120 beats per minute Decrease in pulse pressure Systolic pressure, 90–100 mm Hg Restlessness Increased sweating Pallor Oliguria	25–35 (1250–1750)
Severe	Tachycardia over 120 beats per minute Blood pressure below 60 mm Hg systolic and frequently unobtainable by cuff Mental stupor Extreme pallor, cold extremities Anuria	Up to 50 (2500)

*Based on blood volume of 7% in a 70-kg male of medium build.
(Adapted from Weil M., Shubin H. [1967]. *Diagnosis and treatment of shock* [p. 118]. Baltimore: Williams & Wilkins)

(automatic blood pressure machines) methods may not always provide an accurate measurement. The Doppler method, in which blood pressure is measured noninvasively by ultrasound, may provide a more accurate estimate of Korotkoff sounds when they are no longer audible through the stethoscope. In some instances, this method may be used as an alternative to continuous intraarterial monitoring.

As shock progresses, the respirations become rapid and deep. Decreased intravascular volume results in decreased venous return to the heart and a decrease in CVP. When shock becomes severe, the peripheral veins collapse, making it difficult to insert peripheral venous lines. Sympathetic stimulation also leads to intense vasoconstriction of the skin vessels and activation of the sweat glands. As a result, the skin is cool and moist. When shock is caused by hemorrhage, the loss of red blood cells leaves the skin and mucous membranes looking pale.

Urine output decreases very quickly in hypovolemic and other forms of shock. Compensatory mechanisms decrease renal blood flow as a means of diverting blood flow to the heart and brain. Oliguria of 20 mL/hour or less indicates severe shock and inadequate renal perfusion. Continuous measurement of urine output is essential for assessing the circulatory status of the person in shock.

Restlessness and apprehension are common behaviors in early shock. As the shock progresses and blood flow to the brain decreases, restlessness is replaced by apathy and stupor. If shock is unchecked, the apathy progresses to coma. Coma caused by blood loss alone and not related to head injury or other factors is an unfavorable sign.

Treatment. The treatment of hypovolemic shock is directed toward correcting or controlling the underlying cause and improving tissue perfusion. Persons who have sustained blood loss are commonly placed in supine position with the legs elevated to maximize cerebral blood flow. Oxygen is administered to persons with signs of hypoxemia. Because subcutaneous administration is unpredictable, pain medications usually are administered intravenously. Frequent measurements of heart rate and cardiac rhythm, blood pressure, and urine flow are used to assess the severity of circulatory compromise and to monitor treatment.

In hypovolemic shock, the goal of treatment is to restore vascular volume. This can be accomplished through intravenous administration of fluids and blood. The crystalloids (*e.g.,* isotonic saline) are readily available for emergencies and mass casualties. They often are effective, at least temporarily, when given in adequate doses. Plasma expanders, including dextrans and colloidal albumin solutions, have a high molecular weight, do not necessitate blood typing, and remain in the circulation for longer periods than the crystalloids, such as glucose and saline. The dextrans must be used with caution because they may induce serious or fatal reactions, including anaphylaxis. Blood or blood products (packed or frozen red cells) are administered based on hematocrit and hemodynamic findings. Fluids and blood are best administered based on volume indicators such as CVP and PCWP. This is particularly important in pediatric patients, whose fluid balance allows less variation from normal before compromise to tissue perfusion results, and who may respond better to hypertonic saline than to other crystalloid or colloid solutions.[47]

Vasoactive drugs (*e.g.,* adrenergic agents) are agents capable of constricting or dilating blood vessels. Considerable controversy exists about the advantages or disadvantages related to the use of these drugs. There are two types of adrenergic receptors for the sympathetic nervous system: α and β. The β receptors are further subdivided into β_1 and β_2 receptors. In the cardiorespiratory system, stimulation of the α receptors causes vasoconstriction; stimulation of β_1 receptors causes an increase in heart rate and the force of myocardial contraction; and stimulation of β_2 receptors produces vasodilatation of the skeletal muscle beds and relaxation of the bronchioles.

As a general rule, the adrenergic drugs are not used as a primary form of therapy in shock. An increase in blood pressure produced by vasopressor drugs usually has little effect on the underlying cause of shock and in many cases may be detrimental. These agents are given only when hypotension persists after volume deficits have been corrected. Dopamine, which induces a more favorable array of α- and β-receptor actions than many of the other adrenergic drugs, may be used in the treatment of severe and prolonged shock. Dopamine is thought to increase blood flow to the kidneys, liver, and other abdominal organs while maintaining vasoconstriction of less vital structures, such as the skin and skeletal muscles, when given in low doses. In severe shock, higher doses may be needed to maintain blood pressure. After dopamine administration exceeds this low-dose range, it has vasoconstrictive effects on blood flow to the kidneys and abdominal organs that are similar to those of epinephrine.

OBSTRUCTIVE SHOCK

The term *obstructive shock* is used to describe circulatory shock that results from mechanical obstruction of the flow of blood through the central circulation (great veins, heart, or lungs; see Fig. 28-10). Obstructive shock may be caused by a number of conditions, including dissecting aortic aneurysm, cardiac tamponade, pneumothorax, atrial myxoma, or evisceration of abdominal contents into the thoracic cavity because of a ruptured hemidiaphragm. The most frequent cause of obstructive shock is pulmonary embolism.

The primary physiologic results of obstructive shock are elevated right heart pressure and impaired venous return to the heart. The signs of right heart failure are seen, including elevation of CVP and jugular venous distention. Treatment modalities focus on correcting the cause of the disorder, frequently with surgical interventions such as pulmonary embolectomy, pericardiocentesis (*i.e.,* removal of fluid from the pericardial sac) for cardiac tamponade, or the insertion of a chest tube for correction of a tension pneumothorax or hemothorax. In select cases of pulmonary embolus, thrombolytic drugs may be used to dissolve the clots causing the obstruction.

DISTRIBUTIVE SHOCK

Distributive or vasodilatory shock is characterized by loss of blood vessel tone, enlargement of the vascular compartment, and displacement of the vascular volume away from the heart and central circulation.[48] With distributive shock, the capacity of the vascular compartment expands to the extent that a normal volume of blood does not fill the circulatory system (see Fig. 28-10). Venous return is decreased in distributive shock, which leads to a diminished cardiac output but not a decrease in total blood volume; this type of shock is also referred to as *normovolemic shock.* Loss of vessel tone has two main causes: a decrease in the sympathetic control of vasomotor tone and the presence of vasodilator substances in the blood. It can also occur as a complication of vessel damage resulting from prolonged and severe hypotension due to hemorrhage, known as irreversible or late-phase hemorrhagic shock.[48] Three shock states share the basic circulatory pattern of distributive shock: neurogenic shock, anaphylactic shock, and septic shock.

Neurogenic Shock

Neurogenic shock describes shock caused by decreased sympathetic control of blood vessel tone due to a defect in the vasomotor center in the brain stem or the sympathetic outflow to the blood vessels. Output from the vasomotor center can be interrupted by brain injury, the depressant action of drugs, general anesthesia, hypoxia, or lack of glucose (*e.g.,* insulin reaction). Fainting due to emotional causes is a transient form of neurogenic shock. Spinal anesthesia or spinal cord injury above the midthoracic region can interrupt the transmission of outflow from the vasomotor center. The term *spinal shock* is used to describe the neurogenic shock that occurs in persons with spinal cord injury. Many general anesthetic agents can cause a neurogenic shock-like reaction, especially during induction, because of interference with sympathetic nervous system function. In contrast to hypovolemic shock, the heart rate in neurogenic shock often is slower than normal, and the skin is dry and warm. This type of distributive shock is rare and usually transitory.

Anaphylactic Shock

Anaphylaxis is a clinical syndrome that represents the most severe systemic allergic reaction.[49,50] It results from an immunologically mediated reaction in which vasodilator substances such as histamine are released into the blood (see Chapter 21). These substances cause vasodilatation of arterioles and venules along with a marked increase in capillary permeability. The vascular response in anaphylaxis is often accompanied by life-threatening laryngeal edema and bronchospasm, circulatory collapse, contraction of gastrointestinal and uterine smooth muscle, and urticaria or angioedema.

Among the most frequent causes of anaphylactic shock are reactions to drugs, such as penicillin; foods, such as nuts and shellfish; and insect venoms. The most common cause is stings from insects of the order Hymenoptera (*i.e.,* bees, wasps, and fire ants). Latex allergy has also caused life-threatening anaphylaxis in a growing segment of the population. Health care workers and others who are exposed to latex are developing latex sensitivities that range from mild urticaria, contact dermatitis, and mild respiratory distress to anaphylactic shock.[51] Children with spina bifida are at extreme risk for this increasingly serious allergy (see Chapter 21).

The onset of anaphylaxis depends on the sensitivity of the person and the rate and quantity of antigen exposure. Anaphylactic shock often develops suddenly; death can occur within a matter of minutes unless appropriate medical intervention is promptly instituted. Signs and symptoms associated with impending anaphylactic shock include abdominal cramps; apprehension; burning and warm sensation of the skin, itching, and urticaria (*i.e.,* hives); and coughing, choking, wheezing, chest tightness, and difficulty in breathing. After blood begins to pool peripherally, there is a precipitous drop in blood pressure, and the pulse becomes so weak that it is difficult to detect. Life-threatening airway obstruction may ensue as a result of laryngeal edema or bronchial spasm.

Treatment includes immediate discontinuance of the inciting agent or institution of measures to decrease its absorption (*e.g.,* application of ice to a beesting); close monitoring of cardiovascular and respiratory function; and maintenance of adequate respiratory gas exchange, cardiac output, and tissue perfusion. Epinephrine constricts the blood vessels and relaxes the smooth muscle in the bronchioles; it usually is the first drug to be given to a patient believed to be experiencing an anaphylactic reaction. Other treatment measures include the administration of oxygen, antihistaminic drugs, and corticosteroids. Resuscitation measures may be required.

The prevention of anaphylactic shock is preferable to treatment. Once a person has been sensitized to an antigen, the risk for repeated anaphylactic reactions with subsequent exposure is high. All health care providers should question patients regarding previous drug reactions and inform patients as to the name of the medication they are to receive before it is administered or prescribed. Persons with known hypersensitivities should carry some form of medical identification to alert medical personnel if they become unconscious or unable to relate this information. Persons who are at risk for anaphylaxis should be provided with emergency medications (*e.g.,* epinephrine autoinjector) and instructed in procedures to follow in case they are inadvertently exposed to the offending antigen. In some situations, it may be medically necessary to administer agents known to cause anaphylaxis. Protocols that have been developed to prevent or decrease the severity of the reaction involve pharmacologic pretreatment to block or blunt the reaction.

Sepsis and Septic Shock

Septic shock, which is the most common type of vasodilatory shock, is associated with severe infection and the systemic response to infection.[48] It is associated most frequently with gram-negative bacteremia, although it can be caused by gram-positive bacilli and other microorganisms such as fungi, which carry an even greater risk for mortality.[52] Unlike other types of shock, septic shock commonly is associated with pathologic complications, such as pulmonary insufficiency, disseminated intravascular coagulation, and multiple organ dysfunction syndrome.

Severe sepsis accompanied by acute organ dysfunction is a frequently occurring condition in critically ill patients, affecting approximately 750,000 Americans annually and causing more than 200,000 deaths.[53,54] The growing incidence has been attributed to an increased awareness of the diagnosis, increased numbers of immunocompromised patients, increased use of invasive procedures, increased number of resistant organisms, and an increased number of elderly patients.[55] Despite advances in treatment methods, the mortality rate remains approximately 40%.[56]

Septic shock has been described in the context of what has been termed the *systemic inflammatory response syndrome.* Although usually associated with infection, the systemic inflammatory response syndrome can be initiated by noninfectious disorders such as acute trauma and pancreatitis.[52] To enable recognition, description, and classification of persons with sepsis, the American College of Chest Physicians and the Society of Critical Care Medicine published consensus terminology to describe and define the clinical manifestations and progression of sepsis[57] (Chart 28-2).

CHART 28-2

Definitions of Sepsis and Septic Shock

Infection: Microbial phenomenon characterized by an inflammatory response to the presence of microorganisms and the invasion of normally sterile host tissue by these organisms.

Bacteremia: The presence of viable bacteria in the blood.

Systemic inflammatory response syndrome: The systemic inflammatory response to a variety of severe clinical insults. The response is manifested by two or more of the following conditions:

Temperature >38°C or <36°C

Heart rate >90 beats per minute

Respiratory rate >20 breaths per minute or $PaCO_2$ <32 mm Hg (pH <4.3)

WBC >12,000 cells/mm^3, <4000 cells/mm^3, or 10% immature (band) forms

Sepsis: The systemic response to infection. This systemic response is manifested by two or more of the above conditions (temperature, heart rate, respiratory rate, and WBC) as a result of infection.

Severe sepsis: Sepsis associated with organ dysfunction, hypoperfusion, or hypotension. Hypoperfusion and perfusion abnormalities may include, but are not limited to, lactic acidosis, oliguria, or an acute alteration in mental status.

Septic shock: Sepsis with hypotension, despite adequate fluid resuscitation, along with the presence of perfusion abnormalities that may include, but are not limited to, lactic acidosis, oliguria, or an acute alteration in mental status. Patients who are on inotropic or vasopressor agents may not be hypotensive at the time that perfusion abnormalities are measured.

Hypotension: A systolic blood pressure of <90 mm Hg or a reduction of >40 mm Hg from baseline in the absence of other causes of hypotension.

Multiple organ dysfunction syndrome: Presence of altered organ function in an acutely ill patient such that homeostasis cannot be maintained without intervention.

(From American College of Chest Physicians/Society of Critical Care Medicine Consensus Conference. [1992]. Definitions for sepsis and organ failure and guidelines for use of innovative therapies in sepsis. *Critical Care Medicine* 20 [6], 866)

Mechanisms. The mechanisms of sepsis and septic shock are thought to be related to mediators of the inflammatory response.[52–56,58] Although the immune system and the inflammatory response are designed to overcome infection and eliminate bacterial breakdown products, the unregulated release of inflammatory mediators or cytokines (see Chapter 20) may elicit toxic reactions, resulting in the potentially fatal sepsis syndrome. The most widely investigated cytokines have been tumor necrosis factor-α (TNF-α), interleukin-1, and interleukin-8, which usually are proinflammatory, and interleukin-6 and interleukin-10, which tend to be anti-inflammatory. A trigger such as a microbial toxin stimulates the release of TNF-α and interleukin-1, which in turn promotes endothelial cell–leukocyte adhesion, release of cell-damaging proteases and prostaglandins, and activation of the clotting cascade. The prostaglandins, thromboxane A_2 (a vasoconstrictor), prostacyclin (a vasodilator), and prostaglandin E_2, participate in the generation of fever, tachycardia, ventilation-perfusion abnormalities, and lactic acidosis. Interleukin-8, a neutrophil chemotaxin, may have a particularly important role in perpetuating tissue inflammation. Interleukin-6 and interleukin-10, which have anti-inflammatory actions and perhaps are counter-regulatory, augment the acute-phase response and consequent generation of additional proinflammatory mediators.[59]

In addition to inducing the release of inflammatory mediators, the sepsis-producing endotoxins may induce tissue damage by directly activating pathways such as the coagulation cascade, the complement cascade, vessel injury, or release of vasodilating prostaglandins.[59] Thus, the processes that result in the sepsis syndrome are complex consequences of microbial products that profoundly dysregulate the release of inflammatory mediators and the regulation of several important inflammatory and coagulation pathways.

Manifestations. Septic shock typically manifests with fever, vasodilatation, and warm, flushed skin. Mild hyperventilation, respiratory alkalosis, and abrupt changes in personality and behavior due to reduction in cerebral blood flow may be the earliest signs and symptoms of septic shock. These manifestations, which are thought to be a primary response to the bacteremia, commonly precede the usual signs and symptoms of sepsis by several hours or days. Unlike other forms of shock (*i.e.,* cardiogenic, hypovolemic, and obstructive) that are characterized by a compensatory increase in systemic vascular resistance, septic shock often presents with hypovolemia because of arterial and venous dilatation and leakage of plasma into the interstitial spaces.

Aggressive treatment of the hypovolemia in septic shock usually leads to a decrease in systemic vascular resistance and an increase in cardiac output. In the past, this hyperdynamic pattern of response was thought to be present early in shock and was called *warm shock*. A second pattern of *cold shock* accompanied by a low cardiac output and cold extremities was thought to indicate the late stages of septic shock and a poor prognosis. With the development of refined resuscitation methods and better hemodynamic monitoring systems, approximately 90% of patients in septic shock demonstrate a hyperdynamic response with high cardiac output and low systemic vascular resistance.[59] Despite the fact that the cardiac output is normal or increased, cardiac function is depressed, the heart becomes dilated, and the ejection fraction decreases.

Treatment. The treatment of sepsis and septic shock focuses on the control of the causative agent and support of the circulation. Although control of the source of infection is important and the use of antibiotics specific to the infectious agent essential, antibiotics do not treat the inflammatory response to the infection.[60] The cardiovascular status of the patient must be supported to maintain oxygen delivery to the cells. Swift and aggressive fluid administration is needed to compensate for third spacing, and equally aggressive use of vasopressor agents is needed to counteract the vasodilation caused by endotoxins. Monitoring of central venous pressure, mean arterial pressure, urine output, and laboratory measurements of serum lactate, base deficit, and pH is used to evaluate for the progression of sepsis and adequacy of treatment.[54,60]

Among the more recent advances in the treatment of sepsis are the use of intensive insulin therapy for hyperglycemia[54] and the administration of recombinant human activated protein C.[54,60] It has been demonstrated that intensive insulin therapy that maintained blood glucose levels at 80 to 110 mg/dL resulted in lower mortality and morbidity than did conventional therapy that maintained blood glucose levels at 180 to 200 mg/dL.[61] The protective mechanism of insulin in sepsis is unknown. The phagocytic function of neutrophils is impaired in hyperglycemia, suggesting that this may be one of the reasons. Insulin also prevents apoptotic cell death by numerous stimuli, suggesting a second reason. Recombinant human activated protein C, a naturally occurring anticoagulant that acts by inactivating coagulation factors Va and VIII (see Chapter 15), is the first anti-inflammatory agent that has proved effective in the treatment of sepsis.[62,63] In addition to its anticoagulant actions, activated protein C has direct anti-inflammatory properties, including blocking the production of cytokines by monocytes and blocking cell adhesion. Activated protein C also has antiapoptotic actions that may contribute to its effectiveness. The use of corticosteroids, once considered a mainstay in the treatment of sepsis, remains controversial. The use of high doses of corticosteroids, in particular, has not been shown to improve survival and may worsen outcomes by increasing the risk for secondary infections.

COMPLICATIONS OF SHOCK

Wiggers, a noted circulatory physiologist, stated, "Shock not only stops the machine, but it wrecks the machinery."[64] Many body systems are wrecked by severe shock. Five major complications of severe shock are shock lung, acute renal failure, gastrointestinal ulceration, disseminated intravascular coagulation, and multiple organ dysfunction syndrome. The complications of shock are serious and often fatal.

Acute Respiratory Distress Syndrome

Acute respiratory distress syndrome (ARDS) is a potentially lethal form of respiratory failure that can follow severe shock (see Chapter 31). The mortality rate remains at greater than 50% despite advances in mechanical ventilation.[65]

The symptoms of ARDS usually do not develop until 24 to 48 hours after the initial trauma; in some instances, they occur later. The respiratory rate and effort of breathing increase. Arterial blood gas analysis establishes the presence of profound hypoxemia with hypercapnia, resulting from impaired matching of ventilation and perfusion and from the greatly reduced diffusion of blood gases across the thickened alveolar membranes.

The exact cause of ARDS is unknown. Neutrophils are thought to play a key role in the pathogenesis of ARDS. A cytokine-mediated activation and accumulation of neutrophils in the pulmonary vasculature and subsequent endothelial injury is thought to cause leaking of fluid and plasma proteins into the interstitium and alveolar spaces.[65,66] The fluid leakage impairs gas exchange and makes the lung stiffer and more difficult to inflate. Abnormalities in the production, composition, and function of surfactant may contribute to alveolar collapse and gas exchange abnormalities.[66]

Interventions for ARDS focus on increasing the oxygen concentration in the inspired air and supporting ventilation mechanically to optimize gas exchange while avoiding oxygen toxicity and preventing further lung injury.[65–67] Despite the delivery of high levels of oxygen using high-pressure mechanical ventilatory support and positive end-expiratory pressure, many persons with ARDS remain hypoxic, often with a fatal outcome.

Inhaled nitrous oxide is under investigation in the treatment of ARDS. Nitrous oxide appears to improve gas exchange but has not been demonstrated to significantly decrease mortality.[65,66] New interventions have focused on more aggressive treatment of the underlying cause, with the first line of treatment remaining supportive care.

Acute Renal Failure

The renal tubules are particularly vulnerable to ischemia, and acute renal failure is one important late cause of death in severe shock. Sepsis and trauma account for most cases of acute renal failure. The endotoxins implicated in septic shock are powerful vasoconstrictors that are capable of activating the sympathetic nervous system and causing intravascular clotting. They have been shown to trigger all the separate physiologic mechanisms that contribute to the onset of acute renal failure. The degree of renal damage is related to the severity and duration of shock. The normal kidney is able to tolerate severe ischemia for 15 to 20 minutes. The renal lesion most frequently seen after severe shock is acute tubular necrosis. Acute tubular necrosis usually is reversible, although return to normal renal function may require weeks or months (see Chapter 36). Continuous monitoring of urine output during shock provides a means of assessing renal blood flow. Frequent monitoring of serum creatinine and blood urea nitrogen levels also provides valuable information regarding renal status.

Gastrointestinal Complications

The gastrointestinal tract is particularly vulnerable to ischemia because of the changes in distribution of blood flow to its mucosal surface. In shock, there is widespread constriction of blood vessels that supply the gastrointestinal tract, causing a redistribution of blood flow that severely diminishes mucosal perfusion. Superficial mucosal lesions of the stomach and duodenum can develop within hours of severe trauma, sepsis, or burn.

Bleeding is a common symptom of gastrointestinal ulceration caused by shock. Hemorrhage has its onset usually within 2 to 10 days after the original insult and often begins without warning. Poor perfusion in the gastrointestinal tract has been credited with allowing intestinal bacteria to enter the bloodstream, thereby contributing to the development of sepsis and shock.[68]

Histamine type 2 receptor antagonists, proton-pump inhibitors, or sucralfate may be given prophylactically to prevent gastrointestinal ulcerations caused by shock.[68] Nasogastric tubes, when attached to intermittent suction, also help to diminish the accumulation of hydrogen ions in the stomach.

Disseminated Intravascular Coagulation

Disseminated intravascular coagulation (DIC) is characterized by widespread activation of the coagulation system with resultant formation of fibrin clots and thrombotic occlusion of small and mid-sized vessels (see Chapter 15). The systemic formation of fibrin results from increased generation of thrombin, the simultaneous suppression of physiologic anticoagulation mechanisms, and the delayed removal of fibrin as a consequence of impaired fibrinolysis. Clinically overt DIC is reported to occur in as many as 30% to 50% of persons with sepsis and septic shock.[69] As with other systemic inflammatory responses, the derangement of coagulation and fibrinolysis is thought to be mediated by inflammatory mediators.

The contribution of DIC to morbidity and mortality in sepsis depends on the underlying clinical condition and the intensity of the coagulation disorder. Depletion of the platelets and coagulation factors increases the risk for bleeding. Deposition of fibrin in the vasculature of organs contributes to ischemic damage and organ failure. In a large number of clinical trials, the occurrence of DIC appeared to be associated with an unfavorable outcome and was an independent predictor of mortality.[69] However, it remains uncertain whether DIC was a predictor of unfavorable outcome or merely a marker of the seriousness of the underlying condition causing the DIC.

The management of sepsis-induced DIC focuses on treatment of the underlying disorder and measures to interrupt the coagulation process. Anticoagulation therapy and administration of platelets and plasma may be used. The use of antithrombin III, a coagulation inhibitor, is under investigation. Clinical trails have shown modest to marked reductions in mortality based on the dose of antithrombin III that was used.[69] Other therapeutic options, aimed at interrupting the intrinsic coagulation pathway at the point at which tissue factor complexes with factor VIIa, also are being investigated.[69]

Multiple Organ Dysfunction Syndrome

Multiple organ dysfunction syndrome (MODS) represents the presence of altered organ function in an acutely ill patient such that homeostasis cannot be maintained without intervention. As the name implies, MODS commonly affects multiple organ systems, including the kidneys, lungs, liver, brain, and heart. MODS is a particularly life-threatening complication of shock, especially septic shock. It has been reported as the most frequent cause of death in the noncoronary intensive care unit. Mortality rates vary from 30% to 100%, depending on the number of organs involved.[70] Mortality rates increase with an increased number of organs failing. A high mortality rate is associated with failure of the brain, liver, kidney, and lung. The pathogenesis of MODS is not clearly understood, and current management therefore is primarily supportive. Major risk factors for the development of MODS are sepsis, shock, prolonged periods of hypotension, hepatic dysfunction, trauma, infarcted bowel, advanced age, and alcohol abuse.[70] Interventions for multiple organ failure are focused on support of the affected organs.

In summary, circulatory shock is an acute emergency in which body tissues are deprived of oxygen and cellular nutrients or are unable to use these materials in their metabolic processes. Circulatory shock may develop because there is not enough blood in the circulatory system (*i.e.*, hypovolemic shock), blood flow or venous return is obstructed (*i.e.*, obstructive shock), or the tissues are unable to use oxygen and nutrients (*i.e.*, distributive shock). Three types of shock share the basic circulatory pattern of distributive shock: neurogenic shock, anaphylactic shock, and septic shock. Septic shock, which is the most common of these three types, is associated with a severe, overwhelming infection and has a mortality rate of approximately 40%.

The manifestations of hypovolemic shock, which serves as a prototype for circulatory shock, are related to low peripheral blood flow and excessive sympathetic stimulation. The low peripheral blood flow produces thirst, changes in skin temperature, a decrease in blood pressure, an increase in heart rate, decreased venous pressure, decreased urine output, and changes in the sensorium. The intense vasoconstriction that serves to maintain blood flow to the heart and brain causes a decrease in tissue perfusion, impaired cellular metabolism, liberation of lactic acid, and, eventually, cell death. Whether the shock will be irreversible or the patient will survive is determined largely by changes that occur at the cellular level.

The complications of shock result from the deprivation of blood flow to vital organs or systems, such as the lungs, kidneys, gastrointestinal tract, and blood coagulation system. ARDS produces lung changes that occur with shock. It is characterized by changes in the permeability of the alveolar-capillary membrane with the development of interstitial edema and severe hypoxia that does not respond to oxygen therapy. The renal tubules are particularly vulnerable to ischemia, and acute renal failure is an important complication of shock. Gastrointestinal ischemia may lead to gastrointestinal bleeding and increased permeability to the intestinal bacteria, which cause further sepsis and shock. DIC is characterized by formation of small clots in the circulation. It is thought to be caused by inappropriate activation of the coagulation cascade because of toxins or other products released as a result of the shock state. Multiple organ failure, perhaps the most ominous complication of shock, rapidly depletes the body's ability to compensate and recover from a shock state.

Circulatory Failure in Children and the Elderly

After completing this section of the chapter, you should be able to meet the following objectives:

- Describe the manifestations of heart failure in infants and children
- Cite how the aging process affects heart failure in the elderly
- State how the signs and symptoms of heart failure may differ between younger and older adults

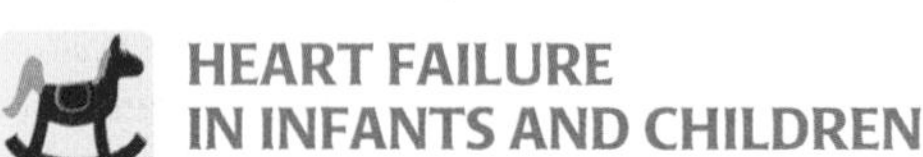

HEART FAILURE IN INFANTS AND CHILDREN

As in adults, heart failure in infants and children results from the inability of the heart to maintain the cardiac output required to sustain metabolic demands.[71–73] Congenital heart defects are the most common cause of CHF during childhood. Surgical correction of congenital heart defects may cause CHF as a result of intraoperative manipulation of the heart and resection of heart tissue, with subsequent alterations in pressure, flow, and vascular resistance .[57] Usually, the heart failure that results is acute and resolves after the effects of the surgical procedure have subsided. Chronic congestive failure occasionally is observed in children with severe chronic anemia, inflammatory heart disease, end-stage congenital heart disease, or cardiomyopathy. Chart 28-3 lists some of the more common causes of heart failure in children. Inflammatory heart disorders (*e.g.*, myocarditis, rheumatic fever, bacterial endocarditis, Kawasaki's disease), cardiomyopathy, and congenital heart disorders are discussed in Chapter 26.

CHART 28-3

Causes of Heart Failure in Children

Newborn Period

- Congenital heart defects
  - Severe left ventricular outflow disorders
    - Hypoplastic left heart
    - Critical aortic stenosis or coarctation of the aorta
  - Large arteriovenous shunts
    - Ventricular septal defects
    - Patent ductus arteriosus
  - Transposition of the great vessels
- Heart muscle dysfunction (secondary)
  - Asphyxia
  - Sepsis
  - Hypoglycemia
- Hematologic disorders (*e.g.*, anemia)

Infants 1 to 6 Months

- Congenital heart disease
  - Large arteriovenous shunts (ventricular septal defect)
- Heart muscle dysfunction
  - Myocarditis
  - Cardiomyopathy
- Pulmonary abnormalities
  - Bronchopulmonary dysplasia
  - Persistent pulmonary hypertension

Toddlers, Children, and Adolescents

- Acquired heart disease
  - Cardiomyopathy
  - Viral myocarditis
  - Rheumatic fever
  - Endocarditis
  - Systemic disease
    - Sepsis
    - Kawasaki's disease
    - Renal disease
    - Sickle cell disease
- Congenital heart defects
  - Nonsurgically treated disorders
  - Surgically treated disorders

Manifestations

Many of the signs and symptoms of heart failure in infants and children are similar to those in adults. They include fatigue, effort intolerance, cough, anorexia, and abdominal pain. A subtle sign of cardiorespiratory distress in infants and children is a change in disposition or responsiveness, including irritability or lethargy. Sympathetic stimulation produces peripheral vasoconstriction and diaphoresis. Decreased renal blood flow often results in a urine output of less than 0.5 to 1.0 mL/kg/hour, despite adequate fluid intake.[74] When right ventricular function is impaired, systemic venous congestion develops. Hepatomegaly due to liver congestion often is one of the first signs of systemic venous congestion in infants and children. However, dependent edema or ascites rarely is seen unless the CVP is extremely high. Because of their short, fat necks, jugular venous distention is difficult to detect in infants; it is not a reliable sign until the child is of school age or older.

A third heart sound, or gallop rhythm, is a common finding in infants and children with heart failure. It results from rapid filling of a noncompliant ventricle. However, it is difficult to distinguish at high heart rates.

Most commonly, children develop interstitial rather than alveolar pulmonary edema. This reduces lung compliance and increases the work of breathing, causing tachypnea and increased respiratory effort. Older children display use of accessory muscles (*i.e.,* scapular and sternocleidomastoid). Head bobbing and nasal flaring may be observed in infants. Signs of respiratory distress often are the first and most noticeable indication of CHF in infants and young children. Pulmonary congestion may be mistaken for bronchiolitis or lower respiratory tract infection. The infant or young child with respiratory distress often grunts with expiration. This grunting effort (essentially, exhaling against a closed glottis) is an instinctive effort to increase end-expiratory pressures and prevent collapse of small airways and the development of atelectasis. Respiratory crackles (*i.e.,* rales) are uncommon in infants and usually suggest development of a respiratory tract infection. Wheezes may be heard, particularly if there is a large left-to-right shunt.

Infants with heart failure often have increased respiratory problems during feeding.[70,74] The history is one of prolonged feeding with excessive respiratory effort and fatigue. Weight gain is slow owing to high energy requirements and low calorie intake. Other frequent manifestations of heart failure in infants are excessive sweating (due to increased sympathetic tone), particularly over the head and neck, and repeated lower respiratory tract infections. Peripheral perfusion usually is poor, with cool extremities; tachycardia is common (resting heart rate >150 beats per minute); and respiratory rate is increased (resting rate >50 breaths per minute).[74]

Diagnosis and Treatment

Diagnosis of congestive failure in infants and children is based on symptomatology, chest radiographic films, electrocardiographic findings, echocardiographic techniques to assess cardiac structures and ventricular function (*i.e.,* end-systolic and end-diastolic diameters), arterial blood gases to determine intracardiac shunting and ventilation-perfusion inequalities, and other laboratory studies to determine anemia and electrolyte imbalances.

Treatment of congestive failure in infants and children includes measures aimed at improving cardiac function and eliminating excess intravascular fluid. Oxygen delivery must be supported and oxygen demands controlled or minimized. Whenever possible, the cause of the disorder is corrected (*e.g.,* medical treatment of sepsis and anemia, surgical correction of congenital heart defects). With congenital anomalies that are amenable to surgery, medical treatment often is needed for a time before surgery and usually is continued in the immediate postoperative period. For many children, only medical management can be provided.

Medical management of heart failure in infants and children is similar to that in adults, although it is tailored to the special developmental needs of the child. Inotropic agents such as digitalis often are used to increase cardiac contractility. Diuretics may be given to reduce preload, and vasodilating drugs may be used to manipulate the afterload. Drug doses must be carefully tailored to control for the child's weight and conditions such as reduced renal function. Daily weighing and accurate measurement of intake and output are imperative during acute episodes of failure.

Most children feel better in the semiupright position. An infant seat is useful for infants with chronic CHF. Activity restrictions usually are designed to allow children to be as active as possible within the limitations of their heart disease. Infants with congestive failure often have problems feeding. Small, frequent feedings usually are more successful than larger, less frequent feedings. Severely ill infants may lack sufficient strength to suck and may need to be tube fed.

The treatment of heart failure in children should be designed to allow optimal physical and psychosocial development. It requires the full involvement of the parents, who often are the primary care providers; therefore, parent education and support is essential.

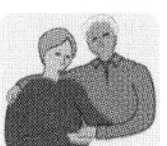

HEART FAILURE IN THE ELDERLY

Congestive heart failure is one of the most common causes of disability in the elderly and is the most frequent hospital discharge diagnosis for the elderly. More than 75% of patients with CHF are older than 65 years of age. CHF also is a major cause of chronic disability, and annual expenditures exceed $10 billion.[75] Among the factors that have contributed to the increased numbers of older people with CHF are the improved therapies for ischemic and hypertensive heart disease.[75] Thus, persons who would have died from acute myocardial disease 20 years ago are now surviving, but with residual left ventricular dysfunction. Similarly, improved blood pressure control has led to a 60% decline in stroke mortality rates, yet these same people remain at risk for CHF as a complication of hypertension. Also, advances in treatment of other diseases have contributed indirectly to the rising prevalence of CHF in the older population.

Coronary heart disease, hypertension, and valvular heart disease (particularly aortic stenosis and mitral regurgitation) are common causes of CHF in older adults.[75,76] Although the pathophysiology of CHF is similar in younger and older persons, elderly persons tend to develop cardiac failure when confronted with stresses that would not produce failure in younger persons. There are four principal changes associated with cardiovascular aging that impair the ability to respond to stress.[75] First, reduced responsiveness to β-adrenergic stimulation limits the heart's capacity maximally to increase heart rate and contractility. A second major effect of aging is increased vascular stiffness, which results in an increased resistance to left ventricular ejection (afterload) and contributes to the development of systolic hypertension in the elderly. Third, in addition to increased vascular stiffness, the heart itself becomes stiffer and less compliant with age. The changes in diastolic stiffness result in important alterations in diastolic filling and atrial function. A reduction in ventricular filling not only affects cardiac output but also produces an elevation in diastolic pressure that is transmitted back to the left atrium, where it stretches the muscle wall and predisposes to atrial ectopic beats and atrial fibrillation. The fourth major effect of cardiovascular aging is altered myocardial metabolism at the level of the mitochondria. Although older mitochondria may be able to generate sufficient ATP to meet the normal energy needs of the heart, they may not be able to respond under stress.

Manifestations

The manifestations of CHF in elderly persons often are masked by other disease conditions.[77] Nocturia is an early symptom but may be caused by other conditions such as prostatic hypertrophy. Dyspnea on exertion may result from lung disease, lack of exercise, and deconditioning. Lower extremity edema commonly is caused by venous insufficiency.

Among the acute manifestations of CHF in the elderly are increasing lethargy and confusion, probably the result of impaired cerebral perfusion. Activity intolerance is common. Instead of dyspnea, the prominent sign may be restlessness. Impaired perfusion of the gastrointestinal tract is a common cause of anorexia and profound loss of lean body mass. Loss of lean body mass may be masked by edema.

The elderly also maintain a precarious balance between the managed symptom state and acute symptom exacerbation. During the managed symptom state, they are relatively symptom free while adhering to their treatment regimen. Acute symptom exacerbation, often requiring emergency medical treatment, can be precipitated by seemingly minor conditions such as poor compliance with sodium restriction, infection, or stress. Failure to seek medical care promptly is a common cause of progressive acceleration of symptoms.

Diagnosis and Treatment

The diagnosis of heart failure in the elderly is based on the history, physical examination, chest radiograph, and electrocardiographic findings.[77] However, the presenting symptoms of CHF often are difficult to evaluate. Symptoms of dyspnea on exertion are often attributed to a sign of "getting older" or deconditioning from other diseases. Ankle edema is not unusual in the elderly because the skin turgor decreases and the elderly tend to be more sedentary with the legs in a dependent position.

Treatment of CHF in the elderly involves many of the same methods as in younger persons. Activities are restricted to a level that is commensurate with the cardiac reserve. Seldom is bed rest recommended or advised. Bed rest causes rapid deconditioning of skeletal muscles and increases the risk for complications such as orthostatic hypotension and thromboemboli. Instead, carefully prescribed exercise programs can help to maintain activity tolerance. Even walking around a room usually is preferable to continuous bed rest. Sodium restriction usually is indicated.

Age- and disease-related changes increase the likelihood of adverse drug reactions and drug–drug interactions. Drug dosages and the number of drugs prescribed should be kept to a minimum. Compliance with drug regimens often is difficult; the simpler the regimen, the more likely it is that the older person will comply. In general, the treatment plan for the elderly person with CHF must be put in the context of his or her overall needs. An improvement in the quality of life may take precedence over increasing the length of survival.

In summary, the mechanisms of heart failure in children and the elderly are similar to those in adults. However, the causes and manifestations may differ because of age. In children, CHF is seen most commonly during infancy and immediately after heart surgery. It can be caused by congenital and acquired heart defects and is characterized by fatigue, effort intolerance, cough, anorexia, abdominal pain, and impaired growth. Treatment of CHF in children includes correction of the underlying cause whenever possible. For congenital anomalies that are amenable to surgery, medical treatment often is needed for a time before surgery and usually is continued in the immediate postoperative period. For many children, only medical management can be provided.

In elderly people, age-related changes in cardiovascular functioning contribute to CHF but are not in themselves sufficient to cause heart failure. The manifestations of congestive failure often are different and superimposed on other disease conditions; therefore, CHF often is more difficult to diagnose in the elderly than in younger persons. Because the elderly are more susceptible to adverse drug reactions and have more problems with compliance, the number of drugs prescribed is kept to a minimum, and the drug regimen is kept as simple as possible.

REVIEW EXERCISES

A 75-year-old woman with long-standing hypertension and angina due to coronary heart disease presents with ankle edema, nocturia, increased shortness of breath with activity, and a chronic nonproductive cough. Her blood pressure is 170/80 mm Hg, and her heart rate is 92 beats per minute. Electrocardiograph and chest x-ray reports indicate the presence of left ventricular hypertrophy.

A. Relate the presence of uncontrolled hypertension and coronary artery disease to the development of heart failure in this woman.

B. Explain the significance of left ventricular hypertrophy in terms of both a compensatory mechanism and a pathologic mechanism in the progression of heart failure.

C. Use Figure 28-2 to explain this woman's symptoms, including shortness of breath and nonproductive cough.

A 26-year-old man is admitted to the emergency room with excessive blood loss following an automobile injury. He is alert and anxious, his skin is cool and moist, his heart rate is 135 beats per minute, and his blood pressure 100/85 mm Hg. He is receiving intravenous fluids, which were started at the scene of the accident by an emergency medical technician. He has been typed and cross-matched for blood transfusions, and a urinary catheter has been inserted to monitor his urine output. His urine output has been less than 10 mL since admission, and his blood pressure has dropped to 85/70 mm Hg. Efforts to control his bleeding have been unsuccessful, and he is being prepared for emergency surgery.

A. Use information regarding the compensatory mechanisms in circulatory shock to explain this man's presenting symptoms, including urine output.

B. Use Figure 26-12 to hypothesize on this man's blood loss and maintenance of blood pressure.

C. The treatment of hypovolemic shock is usually directed at maintaining the circulatory volume through fluid resuscitation rather than maintaining the blood pressure through the use of vasoactive medications. Explain.

References

1. American Heart Association. (2003). *Heart disease and stroke statistics—2003 update.* Dallas: American Heart Association.
2. Colucci W.C., Braunwald E. (2001). Pathophysiology of heart failure. In Braunwald E., Zipes D.P., Libbey P. (Eds.), *Heart disease: A textbook of cardiovascular medicine* (6th ed., pp. 503–553). Philadelphia: W.B. Saunders.
3. Jessup M., Brozena S. (2003). Heart failure. *New England Journal of Medicine 348,* 2007–2018.
4. Francis G.S., Tang W.H.W. (2003). Pathophysiology of congestive heart failure. *Reviews in Cardiovascular Medicine 4*(Suppl 2), S14–S20.
5. Braunwald E., Bristow M.R. (2000). Congestive heart failure: Fifty years of progress. *Circulation 102,* IV-14–V-23.
6. Mark A.L. (1995). Sympathetic dysregulation in heart failure: Mechanisms and therapy. *Clinical Cardiology 18*(3 Suppl. I), I3–I8.
7. Schrier R.W., Abraham W.T. (1999). Hormones and hemodynamics in heart failure. *New England Journal of Medicine 341,* 577–584.
8. Weber K.T. (2001). Aldosterone in congestive heart failure. *New England Journal of Medicine 345,* 1689–1697.
9. Rajagopalan S., Pitt B. (2003). Aldosterone as a target in congestive heart failure. *Medical Clinics of North America 87,* 441–457.
10. Pitt B., Zannad F., Remme W.J., et al. (1999). The effect of spironolactone on morbidity and mortality in patients with severe heart failure. *New England Journal of Medicine 341,* 709–717.
11. Levin E.R., Gardner D.G., Samson W.K. (1998). Natriuretic peptides. *New England Journal of Medicine 339,* 321–328.
12. Baughman K.L. (2002). B-type natriuretic peptide–A window to the heart. *New England Journal of Medicine 347,* 158–159.
13. Spieker L.E., Lüscher T.F. (2003). Will endothelin receptor antagonists have a role in heart failure? *Medical Clinics of North America 87,* 259–474.
14. Piano M.R., Bondmass M., Schwertz D.W. (1998). The molecular and cellular pathophysiology of heart failure. *Heart and Lung 27,* 3–19.
15. Hunter J.J., Chien K.R. (1999). Signaling pathways for cardiac hypertrophy and failure. *New England Journal of Medicine 341,* 1276–1284.
16. Braunwald E., Colucci W.S., Grossman W. (2001). Clinical aspects of high output heart failure: High output heart failure; pulmonary edema. In Braunwald E., Zipes D.P., Libbey P. (Eds.), *Heart disease: A textbook of cardiovascular medicine* (6th ed., pp. 503–553). Philadelphia: W.B. Saunders.
17. Weinberger H.D. (1999). Diagnosis and treatment of diastolic heart failure. *Hospital Practice 34*(3), 115–126.
18. Angeja B.G., Grossman W. (2003). Evaluation and management of diastolic heart failure. *Circulation 107,* 659–663.
19. Tresch D.D., McGough M.F. (1995). Heart failure with normal systolic function: A common disorder in older people. *Journal of the American Geriatric Society 49*(9), 1035–1042.
20. Shamsham F., Mitchell J. (2000). Essentials of the diagnosis of heart failure. *American Family Physician 61,* 1319–1328.
21. Maisel A.S., Krishnaswamy P., Nowak R.M., et al. (2002). Rapid measurement of B-type natriuretic peptide in the emergency diagnosis of heart failure. *New England Journal of Medicine 347,* 161–167.
22. Hunt S.A. (Chair). (2001) ACC/AHA Guidelines for the evaluation and management of chronic heart failure in the adult: Executive summary. *Circulation 104,* 2996–3007.
23. Vitarelli A., Gheorghiade M. (2000). Transthoracic and transesophageal echocardiogram in the hemodynamic assessment of patients with CHF. *American Journal of Cardiology 86,* 366–406.
24. Parker W.R., Anderson A.S. (2001). Slowing the progression of CHF. *Postgraduate Medicine 109*(3), 36–45.
25. Hoyt R.E., Bowling L.S. (2001). Reducing readmission for congestive heart failure. *American Family Physician 63,* 1593–1600.
26. Wielenga R.P., Huisveld A., Bol E., et al. (1999). Safety and effects of physical training in chronic heart failure: Results of the chronic heart failure and graded exercise study. *European Heart Journal 20*(12), 872–879.
27. Piña H.L. (Chair Writing Group). (2003). Exercise and heart failure: A statement from the American Heart Association Committee on exercise, rehabilitation, and prevention. *Circulation 107,* 1210–1225.
28. Stanek B. (2000). Optimizing management of patients with advanced heart failure: The importance of preventing progression. *Drugs and Aging 16,* 87–106.
29. Fruedenberger R.S., Gottlieb S.S., Robinson S.W., Fisher M.L. (1999). A four-part regimen for clinical heart failure. *Hospital Practice 34*(9), 51–64.
30. Katz A.M., Silverman D.I. (2000). Treatment of heart failure. *Hospital Practice 35*(12B), 19–26.
31. Haji S.A., Movahed A. (2000). Update on digoxin therapy in congestive heart failure. *American Family Physician 62,* 409–416.
32. Dee W.J. (2003). Digoxin remains useful in the management of chronic heart failure. *Medical Clinics of North America 87,* 317–337.
33. Ramahi T.M. (2000). Beta blocker therapy for chronic heart failure. *American Family Physician 62,* 2267–2274.
34. Young J.B. (2001). New therapeutic choices in management of acute heart failure. *Reviews in Cardiovascular Medicine 2*(Suppl 2), S19–24.
35. Hachey D.M., Smith T. (2003). Use of nesiritide to treat acute decompensated heart failure. *Critical Care Nurse 23,* 53–55.
36. Albert N.M. (2003). Cardiac resynchronization therapy through biventricular pacing in patients with heart failure and ventricular dyssynchrony. *Critical Care Nurse 23* (June Suppl), 2–13.
37. Antman E.M., Braunwald E. (2001). Myocardial infarction. In Braunwald E., Zipes D.P., Libbey P. (Eds.), *Heart disease: A text-*

book of cardiovascular medicine (6th ed., pp. 1178–1182). Philadelphia: W.B. Saunders.

38. Califf R.M., Bengton J.R. (1994). Cardiogenic shock. *New England Journal of Medicine 330,* 1724–1730.
39. Hollenberg S.M., Kavinsky C.J., Parrillo J.E. (1999). Cardiogenic shock. *Annals of Internal Medicine 131,* 47–59.
40. Richenbacher W.E., Pierce W.S. (2001). Treatment of heart failure: Assisted circulation. In Braunwald E., Zipes D.P., Libbey P. (Eds.), *Heart disease: A textbook of cardiovascular medicine* (6th ed., pp. 600–614). Philadelphia: W.B. Saunders.
41. Garber P.J., Mathieson A.L., Ducas J., et al. (1995). Thrombolytic therapy for cardiogenic shock: Effect of increased intrathoracic pressure and rapid tPA administration. *Canadian Journal of Cardiology 11*(1), 30–36.
42. Mussivand T. (1999). Mechanical circulatory devices for the treatment of heart failure. *Journal of Cardiac Surgery 14,* 218–228.
43. Miniati D.N. Robbins R.C., Reitz B.A. (2001). Heart and heart-lung transplantation. In Braunwald E., Zipes D.P., Libbey P. (Eds.), *Heart disease: A textbook of cardiovascular medicine* (6th ed., pp. 615–634). Philadelphia: W.B. Saunders.
44. Futterman L.G., Lemberg L. (1996). Cardiomyoplasty: A potential alternative to cardiac transplantation. *American Journal of Critical Care 5*(1), 80–86.
45. Guyton A.C., Hall J.E. (2000). *Textbook of medical physiology* (10th ed., pp. 253–262). Philadelphia: W.B. Saunders.
46. Berne R.M., Levy M.N. (2000). *Principles of physiology* (3rd ed., p. 437). St. Louis: Mosby.
47. Taylor G., Myers S, Kurth C.D., et al. (1996). Hypertonic saline improves brain resuscitation in pediatric model of head injury and hemorrhagic shock. *Journal of Pediatric Surgery 31*(1), 65–70.
48. Landry D.W., Oliver J.A. (2001). The pathogenesis of vasodilatory shock. *New England Journal of Medicine 345,* 588–595.
49. Bochner B.S., Lichtenstein L.M. (1991). Anaphylaxis. *New England Journal of Medicine 324,* 1785–1790.
50. Ellis A.K., Day J.H. (2003). Diagnosis and management of anaphylaxis. *Canadian Medical Association Journal 169,* 307–312.
51. Stankiewicz J., Ruta W., Gorski P. (1995). Latex allergy. *International Journal of Occupational Medicine and Environmental Health 8,* 139–148.
52. Parrillo J.E. (1995). Pathogenetic mechanisms of septic shock. *New England Journal of Medicine 328,* 1471–1477.
53. Sommers M.S. (2003). The cellular basis of septic shock. *Critical Care Nursing Clinics of North America 15,* 13–25.
54. Hotchkiss R.S., Karl I.E. (2003). The pathogenesis and treatment of sepsis. *New England Journal of Medicine 348,* 138–150.
55. Balk R.A. (2000). Severe sepsis and septic shock. *Critical Care Clinics 16,* 179–191.
56. Carcillo J.A., Cunnin R.E. (1997). Septic shock. *Critical Care Clinics 13,* 553–574.
57. Members of the American College of Chest Physicians/Society of Critical Care Medicine Consensus Conference Committee. (1992). American College of Chest Physicians/Society of Critical Care Medicine consensus conference: Definitions of sepsis and organ failure and guidelines for the use of innovative therapies in sepsis. *Critical Care Medicine 20,* 864–874.
58. Glauser M.P. (2000). Pathologic basis of sepsis: Considerations for future strategies of intervention. *Critical Care Medicine 28*(9 Suppl.), S4–S8.
59. Wheeler A.P., Bernard G.R. (1999). Treating patients with severe sepsis. *New England Journal of Medicine 340,* 207–214.
60. Ahrens T. (2003). Severe sepsis management: Are we doing enough. *Critical Care Nurse* (Suppl #5), 2–15.
61. VanDenBerghe G., Wouters P., Weekers F., et al. (2001). Intensive insulin therapy in critically ill patients. *New England Journal of Medicine 345,* 1359–1367.
62. Bernard G.R., Vincent J., Laterre P., et al. (2001). Efficacy and safety of recombinant human activated protein C for severe sepsis. *New England Journal of Medicine 344,* 699–709.
63. Matthay M.A. (2001). Severe sepsis—A new treatment with both anticoagulant and antiinflammatory properties. *New England Journal of Medicine 344,* 759–762.
64. Smith J.J., Kampine J.P. (1980). *Circulatory physiology* (p. 298). Baltimore: Williams & Wilkins.
65. Fein A.M., Calalang-Colucci M.G. (2000). Acute lung injury and acute respiratory distress syndrome in sepsis and septic shock. *Critical Care Clinics 4,* 289–317.
66. Ware L.B., Mattay M.A. (2000). The acute respiratory distress syndrome. *New England Journal of Medicine 342,* 1334–1349.
67. Sessler C.N. (1998). Mechanical ventilation of patients with acute lung injury. *Critical Care Clinics of North America 14,* 707–729.
68. Fink M. (1991). Gastrointestinal mucosal injury in experimental models of shock, trauma and sepsis. *Critical Care Medicine 19,* 627–641.
69. Levi M., Ten Cate H.T. (1999). Disseminated intravascular coagulation. *New England Journal of Medicine 341,* 586–592.
70. Balk R.A. (2000), Pathogenesis and management of multiple organ dysfunction or failure in acute sepsis and septic shock. *Critical Care Clinics 16,* 337–352.
71. Bernstein D. (2004). Heart failure. In Behrman R.E., Kliegman R.M., Nelson W., Jenson H.B. (Eds.), *Nelson textbook of pediatrics* (17th ed., pp. 1582–1587). Philadelphia: W.B. Saunders.
72. Kay J.D., Colan S.D., Graham T.P. (2001). Congestive heart failure in pediatric patients. *American Heart Journal 142,* 923–928.
73. O'Laughlin M.P. (1999). Congestive heart failure in children. *Pediatric Clinics of North America 46,* 263–273.
74. Hazinski F.H. (1992). *Nursing care of the critically ill child* (2nd ed., pp. 156–170). St. Louis: C.V. Mosby.
75. Rich M.W. (1997). Epidemiology, pathophysiology, and etiology of congestive heart failure in older adults. *Journal of the American Geriatrics Society 45,* 968–974.
76. Cheitlin M.D., Zipes D.P. (2001). Cardiovascular disease in the elderly. In Braunwald E., Zipes D.P., Libbey P. (Eds.), *Heart disease: A textbook of cardiovascular medicine.* (6th ed., pp. 2019–2037). Philadelphia: W.B. Saunders.
77. Abdelhafiz A.H. (2002). Heart failure in older people: Causes, diagnosis, and treatment. *Age and Aging 31,* 29–36.

UNIT
VII

Respiratory Function

In the early studies of the body, there is almost no mention of the lungs or respiratory passages. Although the pneuma, or "vital spirits," of the body were closely related to the air and vapors of the universe, the lungs and air passages were almost disregarded. It was not until the circulation of blood had been charted that real progress in understanding the respiratory system took place.

A major step in the understanding of respiration began with the work of Robert Boyle (1627–1691), an Irish scholar. Using an air pump, Boyle proved that a candle would not burn and a small bird or mouse could not live inside a jar from which the air had been removed. Scientists at this time believed that when something burned, air lost a mysterious substance called *phlogiston*. It was the British clergyman Joseph Priestley (1733–1804) who discovered that a gas made by heating oxide of mercury supported combustion. He called this gas, which later became known as oxygen, *dephlogisticated* air. Priestley showed that a mouse lived longer in a given volume of dephlogisticated air than it did in ordinary air. Antoine Lavoisier (1743–1794), a French chemist, confirmed that oxygen was present in inspired air and carbon dioxide in expired air and gave oxygen its name. In 1791, just 16 years after Priestley's discovery of oxygen, it was shown that blood contained both oxygen and carbon dioxide. From this point on, a detailed understanding of the respiratory system and its function proceeded rapidly.

CHAPTER

29

Control of Respiratory Function

Respiration provides the body with a means of gas exchange. It is the process whereby oxygen from the air is transferred to the blood and carbon dioxide is eliminated from the body. Respiration can be divided into three parts: ventilation, or the movement of air between the atmosphere and the respiratory portion of the lungs; perfusion, or the flow of blood through the lungs; and diffusion, or the transfer of gases between the air-filled spaces in the lungs and the blood. The nervous system controls the movement of the respiratory muscles and adjusts the rate of breathing so that it matches the needs of the body during various levels of activity.

The content in this chapter focuses on the structure and function of the respiratory system as it relates to these aspects of respiration. The function of the red blood cell in the transport of oxygen is discussed in Chapter 16.

Structural Organization of the Respiratory System

After completing this section of the chapter, you should be able to meet the following objectives:

- State the difference between the conducting and the respiratory airways
- Trace the movement of air through the airways, beginning in the nose and oropharynx and moving into the respiratory tissues of the lung
- Describe the function of the mucociliary blanket
- Define the term *water vapor pressure* and cite the source of water for humidification of air as it moves through the airways
- Compare the supporting structures of the large and small airways in terms of cartilaginous and smooth muscle support
- Differentiate the function of the bronchial and pulmonary circulations that supply the lungs
- State the function of the two types of alveolar cells

The respiratory system consists of the air passages and the lungs. Functionally, the respiratory system can be divided into two parts: the *conducting airways,* through which

CONDUCTING AND RESPIRATORY AIRWAYS

- Respiration requires ventilation, or movement of gases into and out of the lungs; perfusion, or movement of blood through the lungs; and diffusion of gases between the lungs and the blood.
- Ventilation depends on conducting airways, including the nasopharynx and oropharynx, larynx, and tracheobronchial tree, which move air into and out of the lungs but do not participate in gas exchange.
- Gas exchange takes place in the respiratory airways of the lungs, where gases diffuse across the alveolar-capillary membrane as they are exchanged between the lungs and the blood that flows through the pulmonary capillaries.

air moves as it passes between the atmosphere and the lungs, and the *respiratory tissues* of the lungs, where gas exchange takes place.

THE CONDUCTING AIRWAYS

The conducting airways consist of the nasal passages, mouth and pharynx, larynx, trachea, bronchi, and bronchioles (Fig. 29-1). The air we breathe is warmed, filtered, and moistened as it moves through these structures. Heat is transferred to the air from the blood flowing through the walls of the respiratory passages; the mucociliary blanket removes foreign materials; and water from the mucous membranes is used to moisten the air. The conducting airways are lined with a pseudostratified columnar epithelium that contains a mosaic of mucus-secreting goblet cells and cells that contain hairlike projections called *cilia* (Fig. 29-2). The epithelial layer gradually becomes thinner as it moves from the pseudostratified epithelium of the bronchi to the cuboidal epithelium of the bronchioles and then to the squamous epithelium of the alveoli. The mucus produced by the goblet cells in the conducting airways forms a layer, called the *mucociliary blanket,* that protects the respiratory system by entrapping dust and other foreign particles that enter the airways. The cilia, which constantly are in motion, move the mucociliary blanket with its entrapped particles toward the oropharynx, from which it is expectorated or swallowed. The function of the mucociliary blanket in clearing the lower airways and alveoli is optimal at normal oxygen levels and is impaired in situations of low and high oxygen levels. Clearance is facilitated by coughing. It is impaired by drying, such as breathing heated but unhumidified indoor air during winter. Cigarette smoking slows down or paralyzes the motility of the cilia. This slowing allows the residue from tobacco smoke, dust, and other particles to accumulate in the lungs, decreasing the efficiency of this pulmonary defense system. There also is evidence that smoking causes hyperplasia of the goblet cells, with a resultant increase in respiratory tract secretions and increased susceptibility to respiratory tract infections. As discussed in Chapter 31, these changes are thought to contribute to the development of chronic bronchitis and emphysema.

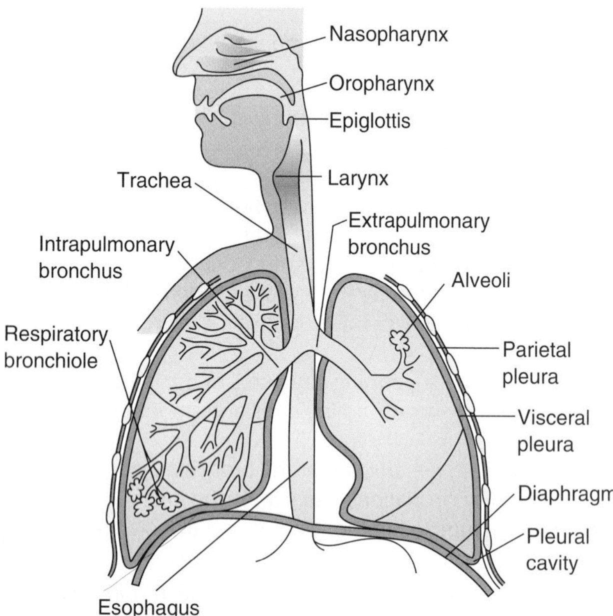

FIGURE 29-1 Structures of the respiratory system.

The airways are kept moist by water contained in the mucous layer. Moisture is added to the air as it moves through the conducting airways. The capacity of the air to contain moisture or water vapor without condensation increases as the temperature rises. Thus, the air in the alveoli, which is maintained at body temperature, usually contains considerably more water vapor than the atmospheric-temperature air that we breathe. The difference between the water vapor contained in the air we breathe and that found in the alveoli is drawn from the moist surface of the mucous membranes that line the conducting airways and is a source of insensible water loss. Under normal conditions, approximately 1 pint of water per day is lost in humidifying the air breathed. During fever, the water vapor in the lungs increases, causing more water to be lost from the respiratory mucosa. Also, fever usually is accompanied by an increase in respiratory rate so that more air passes through the airways, withdrawing moisture from its mucosal surface. As a result, respiratory secretions thicken, preventing free movement of the cilia and impairing the protective function of the mucociliary defense system. This is particularly true in persons whose water intake is inadequate.

Nasopharyngeal Airways

The nose is the preferred route for the entrance of air into the respiratory tract during normal breathing. As air passes through the nasal passages, it is filtered, warmed, and humidified. The outer nasal passages are lined with coarse hairs, which filter and trap dust and other large particles from the air. The upper portion of the nasal cavity is lined with mucous membrane that contains a rich network

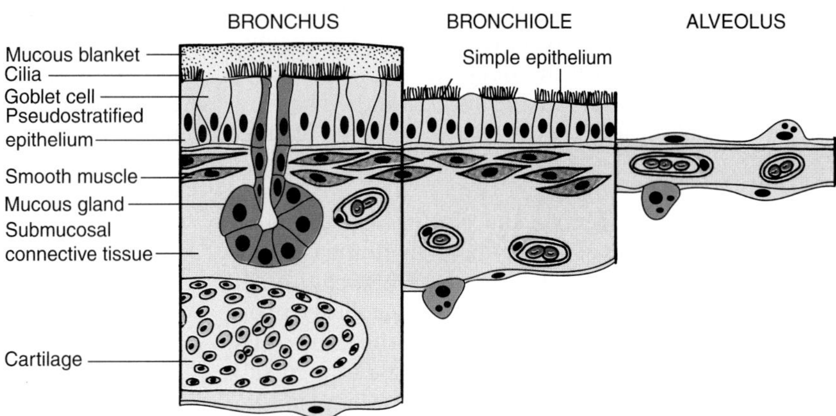

FIGURE 29-2 Airway wall structure: bronchus, bronchiole, and alveolus. The bronchial wall contains pseudostratified epithelium, smooth muscle cells, mucous glands, connective tissue, and cartilage. In smaller bronchioles, a simple epithelium is found, cartilage is absent, and the wall is thinner. The alveolar wall is designed for gas exchange, rather than structural support. (From Weibel E. R., Taylor R. C. [1988]. Design and structure of the human lung. In Fishman A. P. [Ed.]. *Pulmonary diseases and disorders*, Vol. 1. [p. 14] New York: McGraw-Hill)

of small blood vessels; this portion of the nasal cavity supplies warmth and moisture to the air we breathe.

The mouth serves as an alternative airway when the nasal passages are plugged or when there is a need for the exchange of large amounts of air, as occurs during exercise. The oropharynx extends posteriorly from the soft palate to the epiglottis. The oropharynx is the only opening between the nose and mouth and the lungs. Both swallowed food on its way to the esophagus and air on its way to the larynx pass through it. Obstruction of the oropharynx leads to immediate cessation of ventilation. Neural control of the tongue and pharyngeal muscles may be impaired in coma and certain types of neurologic disease. In these conditions, the tongue falls back into the pharynx and obstructs the airway, particularly if the person is lying on his or her back. Swelling of the pharyngeal structures caused by injury, infection, or severe allergic reaction also predisposes a person to airway obstruction, as does the presence of a foreign body.

Laryngotracheal Airways

The larynx connects the oropharynx with the trachea. The walls of the larynx are supported by firm cartilaginous structures that prevent collapse during inspiration. The functions of the larynx can be divided into two categories: those associated with speech and those associated with protecting the lungs from substances other than air. The larynx is located in a strategic position between the upper airways and the lungs and sometimes is referred to as the "watchdog of the lungs."

The epiglottis, which is located above the larynx, is a large, leaf-shaped piece of cartilage that is covered with epithelium. During swallowing, the free edges of the epiglottis move downward to cover the larynx, thus routing liquids and foods into the esophagus.

The cavity of the larynx is divided into two pairs of two-by-two folds of mucous membrane stretching from front to back with an opening in the midline (Fig. 29-3).

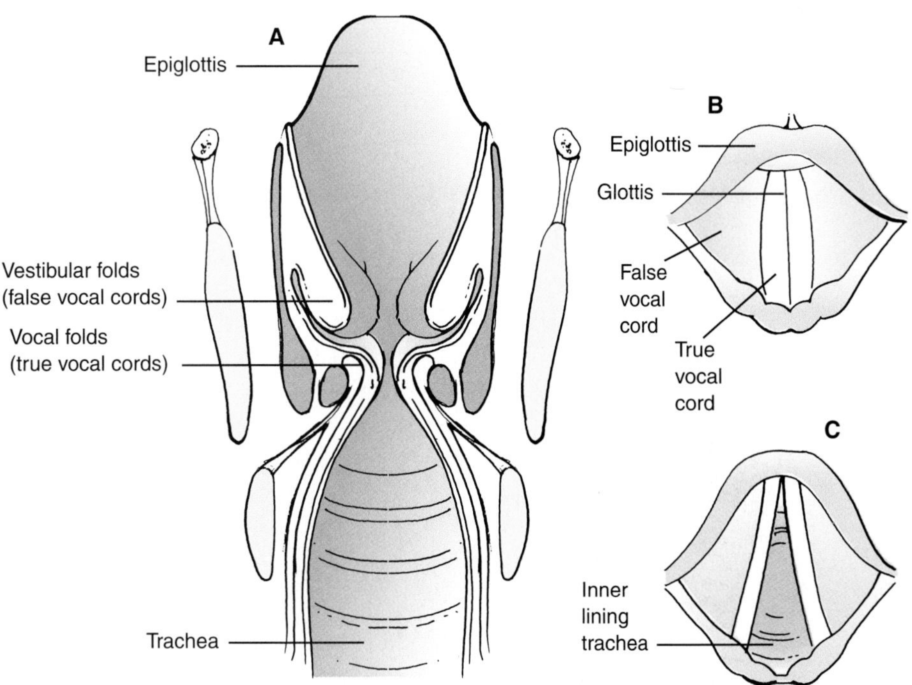

FIGURE 29-3 (**A**) Coronal section showing the position of the epiglottis, the vestibular folds (false vocal cords), the vocal folds (true vocal cords), and glottis. (**B**) Vocal cords viewed from above with the glottis closed and (**C**) with the glottis open.

The upper pair of folds, called the *vestibular folds,* has a protective function. The lower pair of folds has cordlike margins; they are termed the *vocal folds* because their vibrations are required for making vocal sounds. The vocal folds and the elongated opening between them are called the *glottis.* A complex set of muscles controls the opening and closing of the glottis.

In addition to opening and closing the glottis for speech, the vocal folds of the larynx can perform a sphincter function in closing off the airways. When confronted with substances other than air, the laryngeal muscles contract and close off the airway. At the same time, the cough reflex is initiated as a means of removing a foreign substance from the airway. This protective mechanism prevents food and fluids from being pulled into the lungs where they can cause serious problems.

During defecation and urination, inhaled air is temporarily held in the lungs by closing the glottis. The intraabdominal muscles then contract, causing both intraabdominal and intrathoracic pressures to rise. These collective actions are called the *Valsalva maneuver.* By producing an increase in intrathoracic pressure, the Valsalva maneuver decreases the return of blood to the heart, thereby inciting a series of circulatory reflexes. A tachycardia, or increase in heart rate, develops during the maneuver as the circulatory system compensates for the decrease in blood return to the heart. On termination of the maneuver, a short period of bradycardia, or decreased heart rate, occurs as blood that has been dammed back in the venous circulation returns to the heart.

Tracheobronchial Tree

The tracheobronchial tree, which consists of the trachea, bronchi, and bronchioles, can be viewed as a system of branching tubes (Fig. 29-4). The trachea, or windpipe, is a continuous tube that connects the larynx and the major bronchi of the lungs. The walls of the trachea are supported by horseshoe-shaped cartilages, which prevent it from collapsing when the pressure in the thorax becomes negative.

The trachea is located anterior to the esophagus and extends to superior border of the fifth thoracic vertebra where it divides to form the right and the left primary bronchi. Each bronchus enters the lung through a slit called the *hilus.* The point at which the trachea divides is called the *carina.* The carina is heavily innervated with sensory neurons, and coughing and bronchospasm result when this area is stimulated, as during tracheal suctioning. The right primary bronchus is shorter and wider and continues at a more vertical angle with the trachea than the left primary bronchus, which is longer and narrower and forms a more acute angle with the trachea. The anatomic differences between the two bronchi also make it easier for foreign bodies to enter the right main bronchus than the left.

On entering the lungs, the primary bronchi divide into secondary, or lobular, bronchi, which supply each of the lobes of the lungs (the right lung has three lobes; the left has two). The secondary bronchi continue to branch, forming the still smaller tertiary bronchi, which divide into the bronchioles. Bronchioles, in turn, branch repeatedly until they become the terminal bronchioles, the smallest of the conducting airways. This extensive branching is similar to a tree whose branches become smaller and more numerous as they divide. In all, there are approximately 23 levels of branching, beginning with the conducting airways and ending with the respiratory airways, where gas exchange takes place (Fig. 29-5).

The right middle lobe bronchus is of relatively small diameter and length and sometimes bends sharply near its bifurcation. It is surrounded by a collar of lymph nodes that

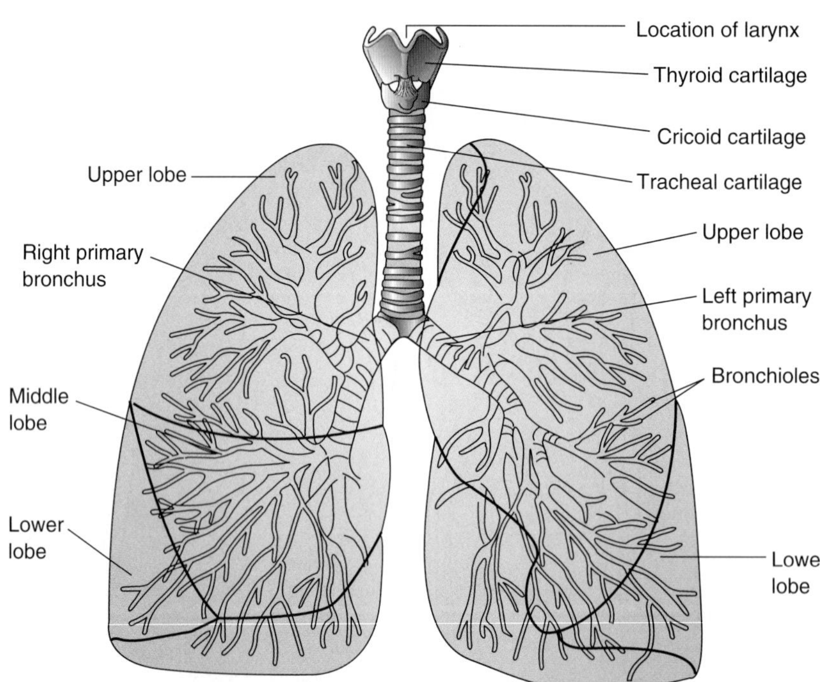

FIGURE 29-4 Larynx, trachea, and bronchial tree (anterior view).

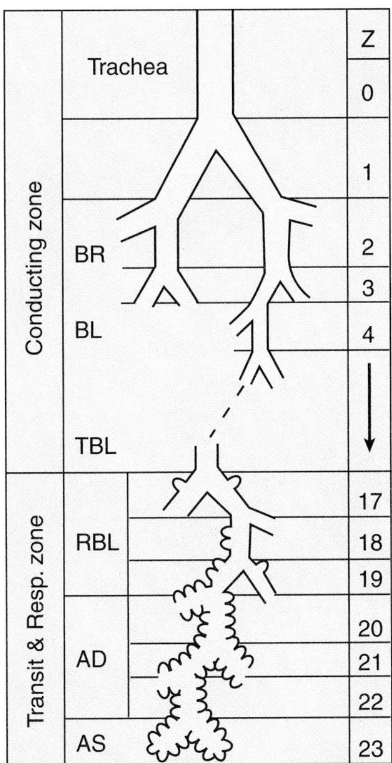

FIGURE 29-5 Idealization of the human airways. The first 16 generations of branching (Z) make up the conducting airways, and the last seven constitute the respiratory zone (or transitional and respiratory zone). BR, bronchus; BL, bronchiole; TBL, terminal bronchiole; RBL, respiratory bronchiole; AD, alveolar ducts; AS, alveolar sacs. (Weibel E. R. [1962]. *Morphometry of the human lung* [p. 111]. Berlin: Springer-Verlag)

drain the middle and the lower lobe and is particularly subject to obstruction. The secondary bronchi divide to form the tertiary segmental bronchi, which supply the bronchopulmonary segments of the lung. There are 10 segments in the right lung and 9 segments in the left lung (Fig. 29-6). These segments are identified according to their location in the lung (*e.g.,* the apical segment of the right upper lobe) and are the smallest named units in the lung. Lung lesions such as atelectasis and pneumonia often are localized to a particular bronchopulmonary segment.

The structure of the primary bronchi is similar to that of the trachea, in that these airways are supported by cartilaginous rings. As the bronchi move into the lungs, irregular plates of cartilage replace the horseshoe-shaped cartilage rings. These cartilaginous plates gradually become thinner and then disappear at the level of the respiratory bronchioles. Between the cartilaginous support and the mucosal surface are two crisscrossing layers of smooth muscle that wind in opposite directions (Fig. 29-7). Bronchospasm, or contraction of these muscles, causes narrowing of the bronchioles and impairs air flow.

THE LUNGS AND RESPIRATORY AIRWAYS

The lungs are soft, spongy, cone-shaped organs located side by side in the chest cavity (see Fig. 29-1). They are separated from each other by the *mediastinum* (*i.e.,* the space between the lungs) and its contents—the heart, blood vessels, lymph nodes, nerve fibers, thymus gland, and esophagus. The upper part of the lung, which lies against the top of the thoracic cavity, is called the *apex,* and the lower part, which lies against the diaphragm, is called the *base.* The lungs are divided into lobes: three in the right lung and two in the left (see Fig. 29-4).

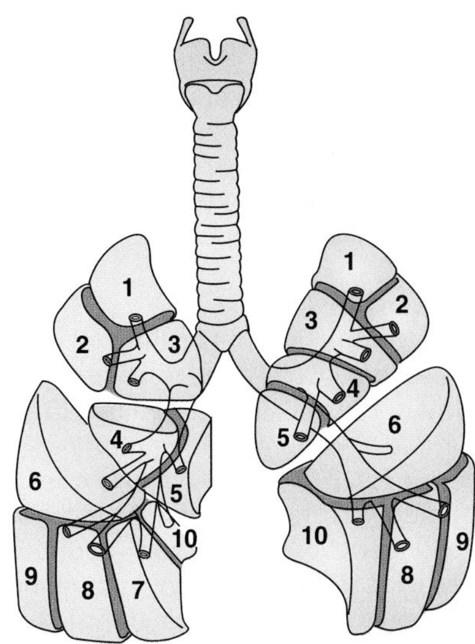

FIGURE 29-6 Bronchopulmonary segments of the human lung. Left and right upper lobes: (*1*) apical, (*2*) posterior, (*3*) anterior, (*4*) superior lingular, and (*5*) inferior lingular segments. Right middle lobe: (*4*) lateral and (*5*) medial segments. Lower lobes: (*6*) superior (apical), (*7*) medial-basal, (*8*) anterior-basal, (*9*) lateral-basal, and (*10*) posterior-basal segments. The medial-basal segment (*7*) is absent in the left lung. (Fishman A. P. [1980]. *Assessment of pulmonary function* [p. 19]. New York: McGraw-Hill)

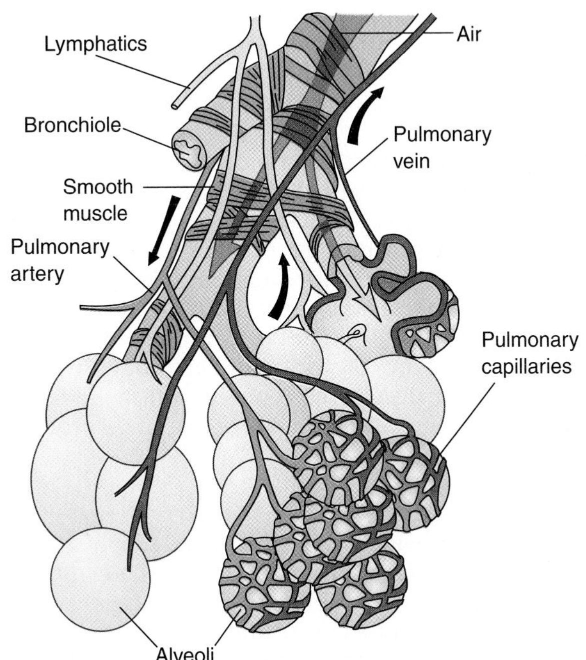

FIGURE 29-7 Lobule of the lung, showing the bronchial smooth muscle fibers, pulmonary blood vessels, and lymphatics.

The lungs are the functional structures of the respiratory system. In addition to their gas exchange function, they inactivate vasoactive substances such as bradykinin; they convert angiotensin I to angiotensin II; and they serve as a reservoir for blood storage. Heparin-producing cells are particularly abundant in the capillaries of the lung, where small clots may be trapped.

Respiratory Lobules

The gas exchange function of the lung takes place in the lobules of the lungs. Each lobule, which is the smallest functional unit of the lung, is supplied by a branch of a terminal bronchiole, an arteriole, the pulmonary capillaries, and a venule (see Fig. 29-7). Gas exchange takes place in the terminal respiratory bronchioles and the alveolar ducts and sacs. Blood enters the lobules through a pulmonary artery and exits through a pulmonary vein. Lymphatic structures surround the lobule and aid in the removal of plasma proteins and other particles from the interstitial spaces.

Unlike the larger bronchi, the respiratory bronchioles are lined with simple epithelium rather than ciliated pseudostratified epithelium (see Fig. 29-2). The respiratory bronchioles also lack the cartilaginous support of the larger airways. Instead, they are attached to the elastic spongework of tissue that contains the alveolar air spaces. When the air spaces become stretched during inspiration, the bronchioles are pulled open by expansion of the surrounding tissue.

The alveolar sacs are cup-shaped, thin-walled structures that are separated from each other by thin alveolar septa. A single network of capillaries occupies most of the septa, so that blood is exposed to air on both sides. There are approximately 300 million alveoli in the adult lung, with a total surface area of approximately 50 to 100 m^2. Unlike the bronchioles, which are tubes with their own separate walls, the alveoli are interconnecting spaces that have no separate walls (Fig. 29-8). As a result of this arrangement, there is a continual mixing of air in the alveolar structures. Small holes in the alveolar walls, the pores of Kohn, probably contribute to the mixing of air under certain conditions.

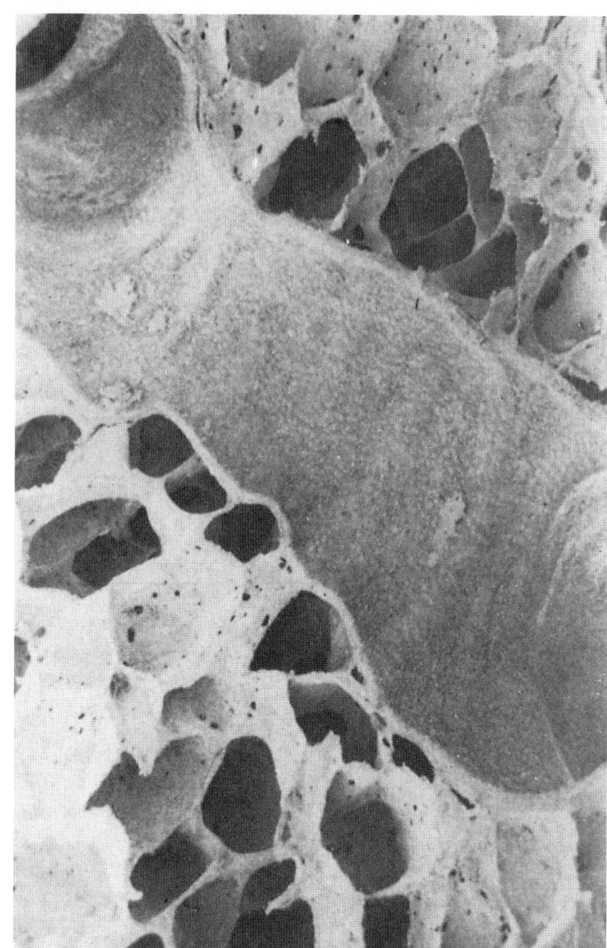

FIGURE 29-8 Close-up of a cross section of a small bronchus and surrounding alveoli. (Courtesy of Janice A. Nowell, University of California, Santa Cruz)

The alveolar structures are composed of two types of cells: type I alveolar cells and type II alveolar cells (Fig. 29-9). The type I alveolar cells are flat squamous epithelial cells across which gas exchange takes place. The type II alveolar cells produce surfactant, a lipoprotein substance that decreases the surface tension in the alveoli. This action allows for greater ease of lung inflation and helps to prevent the collapse of smaller airways. The alveoli also contain alveolar macrophages, which are responsible for the removal of offending substances from the alveolar epithelium.

Lung Circulation

The lungs are provided with a dual blood supply, the pulmonary and bronchial circulations. The pulmonary circulation arises from the pulmonary artery and provides for the gas exchange function of the lungs. Deoxygenated blood leaves the right heart through the pulmonary artery, which divides into a left pulmonary artery that enters the left lung and a right pulmonary artery that enters the right lung. Return of oxygenated blood to the heart occurs by way of the pulmonary veins, which empty into the left atrium.

The bronchial circulation distributes blood to the conducting airways and supporting structures of the lung. The bronchial circulation has a secondary function of warming and humidifying incoming air as it moves through the conducting airways. The bronchial arteries arise from the thoracic aorta and enter the lungs with the major bronchi, dividing and subdividing along with the bronchi as they move out into the lung, supplying them and other lung structures with oxygen. The capillaries of the bronchial circulation drain into the bronchial veins, the larger of which empties into the vena cava. The smaller of the bronchial veins empties into the pulmonary veins. This blood is unoxygenated because the bronchial circulation does not participate in gas exchange. As a result, this blood dilutes the oxygenated blood returning to the left side of the heart.

The bronchial blood vessels are the only ones that undergo angiogenesis (formation of new vessels) and

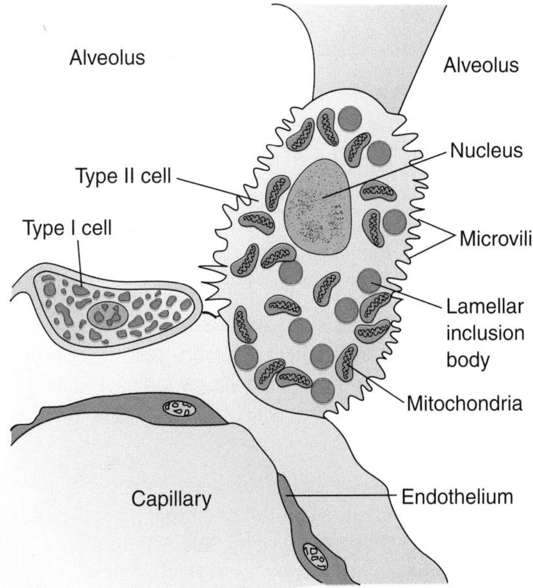

FIGURE 29-9 Schematic drawing of the two types of alveolar cells and their relation to alveoli and capillaries. Alveolar type I cells comprise most of the alveolar surface. Alveolar type II cells are located in the corner between two adjacent alveoli. Also shown are endothelial cells that line the pulmonary capillaries. (Rhoades R. A., Tanner G. A. [1996]. *Medical physiology* [p. 362]. Boston: Little, Brown)

develop collateral circulation when vessels in the pulmonary circulation are obstructed, as in pulmonary embolism. The development of new blood vessels helps to keep lung tissue alive until the pulmonary circulation can be restored.

PLEURA

A thin, transparent, double-layered serous membrane, called the *pleura,* lines the thoracic cavity and encases the lungs. The outer parietal layer lies adjacent to the chest wall, and the inner visceral layer adheres to the outer surface of the lung (see Fig. 29-1). The parietal pleura forms part of the mediastinum and lines the inner wall of the thoracic or chest cavity. A thin film of serous fluid separates the two pleural layers, and this allows the two layers to glide over each other and yet hold together, so that there is no separation between the lungs and the chest wall. The pleural cavity is a potential space in which serous fluid or inflammatory exudate can accumulate. The term *pleural effusion* is used to describe an abnormal collection of fluid or exudate in the pleural cavity.

In summary, the respiratory system consists of the air passages and the lungs, where gas exchange takes place. Functionally, the air passages of the respiratory system can be structurally divided into two parts: the conducting airways, through which air moves as it passes into and out of the lungs, and the respiratory tissues, where gas exchange actually takes place. The conducting airways include the nasal passages, mouth and nasopharynx, larynx, and tracheobronchial tree. Air is warmed, filtered, and humidified as it passes through these structures.

The lungs are the functional structures of the respiratory system. In addition to their gas exchange function, they inactivate vasoactive substances such as bradykinin; they convert angiotensin I to angiotensin II; and they serve as a reservoir for blood. The lobules, which are the functional units of the lung, consist of the respiratory bronchioles, alveoli, and pulmonary capillaries. It is here that gas exchange takes place. Oxygen from the alveoli diffuses across the alveolar capillary membrane into the blood, and carbon dioxide from the blood diffuses into the alveoli.

The lungs are provided with a dual blood supply: the pulmonary circulation provides for the gas exchange function of the lungs and the bronchial circulation distributes blood to the conducting airways and supporting structures of the lung. The lungs are encased in a thin, transparent, double-layered serous membrane called the *pleura.*

Exchange of Gases Between the Atmosphere and the Lungs

After completing this section of the chapter, you should be able to meet the following objectives:

- Describe the basic properties of gases in relation to their partial pressures and their pressures in relation to volume and temperature
- State the definitions of intrathoracic, intrapleural, and intra-alveolar pressures, and state how each of these pressures changes in relation to atmospheric pressure during inspiration and expiration
- State a definition of lung compliance
- Use Laplace's law to explain the need for surfactant in maintaining the inflation of small alveoli
- State the major determinant of airway resistance
- Explain why increasing lung volume (*e.g.,* taking deep breaths) reduces airway resistance
- Define inspiratory reserve, expiratory reserve, vital capacity, and residual volume
- Describe the method for measuring $FEV_{1.0}$

BASIC PROPERTIES OF GASES

The air we breathe is made up of a mixture of gases, mainly nitrogen and oxygen. These gases exert a combined pressure called the *atmospheric pressure.* The pressure at sea level, which is defined as one atmosphere, is 760 millimeters of mercury (mm Hg), or 14.7 pounds per square inch (PSI). When measuring respiratory pressures, atmospheric pressure is assigned a value of 0. A respiratory pressure of +15 mm Hg means that the pressure is 15 mm Hg above atmospheric pressure, and a respiratory pressure of −15 mm Hg is 15 mm Hg less than atmospheric pressure. Respiratory pressures often are expressed in centimeters of water (cm H_2O) because of the small pressures involved (1 mm Hg = 1.35 cm H_2O pressure).

The pressure exerted by a single gas in a mixture is called the *partial pressure*. The capital letter "P" followed by the chemical symbol of the gas (PO_2) is used to denote its partial pressure. The law of partial pressures states that the total pressure of a mixture of gases, as in the atmosphere, is equal to the sum of the partial pressures of the different gases in the mixture. If the concentration of oxygen at 760 mm Hg (1 atmosphere) is 20%, its partial pressure is 152 mm Hg (760×0.20).

Water vapor is different from other types of gases; its partial pressure is affected by temperature but not atmospheric pressure. The relative humidity refers to the percentage of moisture in the air compared with the amount that the air can hold without causing condensation (100% saturation). Warm air holds more moisture than cold air. This is the reason that precipitation in the form of rain or snow commonly occurs when the relative humidity is high and there is a sudden drop in atmospheric temperature. The air in the alveoli, which is 100% saturated at normal body temperature, has a water vapor pressure of 47 mm Hg. The water vapor pressure must be included in the sum of the total pressure of the gases in the alveoli (*i.e.*, the total pressure of the other gases in the alveoli is 760 – 47 = 713 mm Hg).

Air moves between the atmosphere and the lungs because of a pressure difference. According to the laws of physics, the pressure of a gas varies inversely with the volume of its container, provided the temperature remains constant. If equal amounts of a gas are placed in two different-sized containers, the pressure of the gas in the smaller container is greater than the pressure in the larger container. The movement of gases is always from the container with the greater pressure to the one with the lesser pressure. The chest cavity can be viewed as a volume container. During inspiration, the size of the chest cavity increases, and air moves into the lungs; during expiration, air moves out as the size of the chest cavity decreases.

VENTILATION AND THE MECHANICS OF BREATHING

Ventilation is concerned with the movement of gases into and out of the lungs. There is nothing mystical about ventilation. It is purely a mechanical event that obeys the laws of physics as they relate to the behavior of gases. It relies on a system of open airways and the respiratory pressures created as the movements of the respiratory muscles change the size of the chest cage. The degree to which the lungs inflate and deflate depends on the respiratory pressures inflating the lung, compliance of the lungs, and airway resistance.

Respiratory Pressures

The pressure inside the airways and alveoli of the lungs is called the *intrapulmonary pressure* or *alveolar pressure*. The gases in this area of the lungs are in communication with atmospheric pressure (Fig. 29-10). When the glottis is open and air is not moving into or out of the lungs, as occurs just before inspiration or expiration, the intrapulmonary pressure is zero or equal to atmospheric pressure.

The pressure in the pleural cavity is called the *intrapleural pressure*. The intrapleural pressure is always negative in relation to alveolar pressure, approximately –4 mm Hg between breaths when the glottis is open and the alveolar spaces are open to the atmosphere. The lungs and the chest wall have elastic properties, each pulling in the opposite direction. If removed from the chest, the lungs would contract to a smaller size, and the chest wall, if freed from the lungs, would expand. The opposing forces of the chest wall

VENTILATION AND GAS EXCHANGE

- Ventilation refers to the movement of gases into and out of the lungs through a system of open airways and along a pressure gradient resulting from a change in chest volume.
- During inspiration, air is drawn into the lungs as the respiratory muscles expand the chest cavity; during expiration, air moves out of the lungs as the chest muscles recoil and the chest cavity becomes smaller.
- The ease with which air is moved into and out of the lung depends on the resistance of the airways, which is inversely related to the fourth power of the airway radius, and lung compliance, or the ease with which the lungs can be inflated.
- The minute volume, which is determined by the metabolic needs of the body, is the amount of air that is exchanged each minute. It is the product of the tidal volume or amount of air exchanged with each breath multiplied by the respiratory rate.

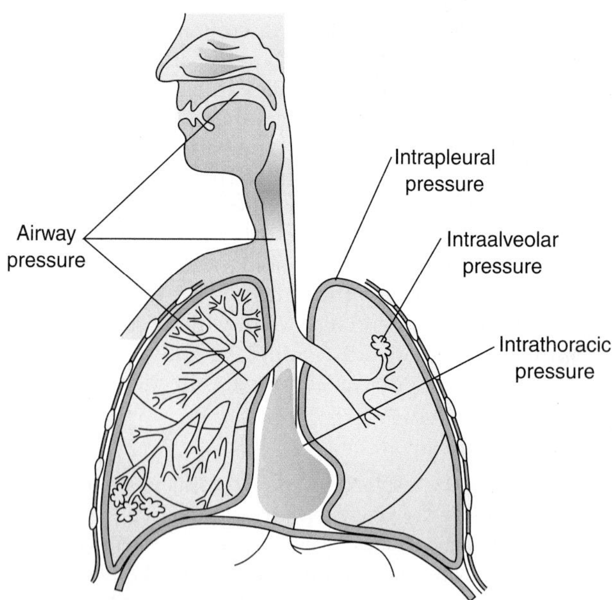

FIGURE 29-10 Partitioning of respiratory pressures.

and lungs create a pull against the visceral and parietal layers of the pleura, causing the pressure in the pleural cavity to become negative. During inspiration, the elastic recoil of the lungs increases, causing intrapleural pressure to become more negative than during expiration. Without the negative intrapleural pressure holding the lungs against the chest wall, their elastic recoil properties would cause them to collapse. Although intrapleural pressure is negative in relation to alveolar pressure, it may become positive in relation to atmospheric pressure (*e.g.*, during forced expiration and coughing).

The *intrathoracic pressure* is the pressure in the thoracic cavity. It is essentially equal to intrapleural pressure and is the pressure to which the lungs, heart, and great vessels are exposed. Forced expiration against a closed glottis compresses the air in the thoracic cavity and produces marked increases in intrathoracic pressure and intrapleural pressure.

The Chest Cage and Respiratory Muscles

The lungs and major airways share the chest cavity with the heart, great vessels, and esophagus. The chest cavity is a closed compartment bounded on the top by the neck muscles and at the bottom by the diaphragm. The outer walls of the chest cavity are formed by 12 pairs of ribs, the sternum, the thoracic vertebrae, and the intercostal muscles that lie between the ribs. Mechanically, the act of breathing depends on the fact that the chest cavity is a closed compartment whose only opening to the external atmosphere is through the trachea.

Ventilation consists of inspiration and expiration. During *inspiration,* the size of the chest cavity increases, the intrathoracic pressure becomes more negative, and air is drawn into the lungs. *Expiration* occurs as the elastic components of the chest wall and lung structures that were stretched during inspiration recoil, causing the size of the chest cavity to decrease and the pressure in the chest cavity to increase. The diaphragm is the principal muscle of inspiration. When the diaphragm contracts, the abdominal contents are forced downward, and the chest expands from top to bottom (Fig. 29-11). During normal levels of inspiration, the diaphragm moves approximately 1 cm, but this can be increased to 10 cm on forced inspiration. The diaphragm is innervated by the phrenic nerve roots, which arise from the cervical level of the spinal cord, mainly from C4 but also from C3 and C5. Paralysis of one side of the diaphragm causes the chest to move up on that side rather than down during inspiration because of the negative pressure in the chest. This is called *paradoxical movement.*

The external intercostal muscles, which also aid in inspiration, connect to the adjacent ribs and slope downward and forward (Fig. 29-12). When they contract, they raise the ribs and rotate them slightly so that the sternum is pushed forward; this enlarges the chest from side to side and from front to back. The intercostal muscles receive their innervation from nerves that exit the central nervous system at the thoracic level of the spinal cord. Paralysis of these muscles usually does not have a serious effect on respiration because of the effectiveness of the diaphragm.

The accessory muscles of inspiration include the scalene muscles and the sternocleidomastoid muscles. The scalene muscles elevate the first two ribs, and the sternocleidomastoid muscles raise the sternum to increase the size of the chest cavity. These muscles contribute little to

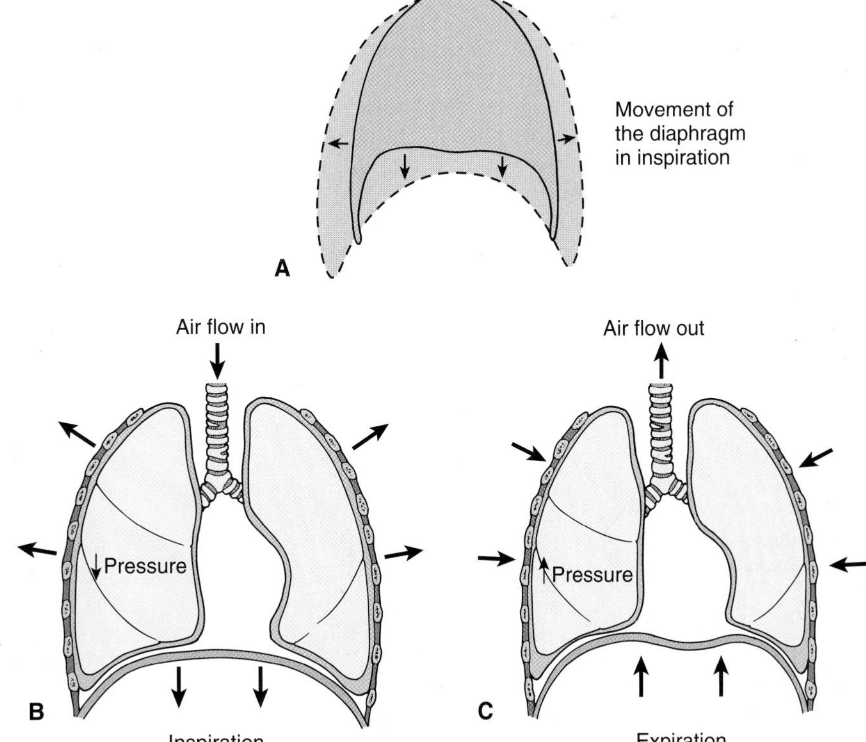

FIGURE 29-11 Movement of the diaphragm and changes in chest volume and pressure during inspiration and expiration. (**A**) Movement of diaphragm and expansion of the chest cavity during inspiration. (**B**) During inspiration, contraction of the diaphragm and expansion of the chest cavity produce a decrease in intrathoracic pressure, causing air to move into the lungs. (**C**) During expiration, relaxation of the diaphragm and chest cavity produce an increase in intrathoracic pressure, causing air to move out of the lungs.

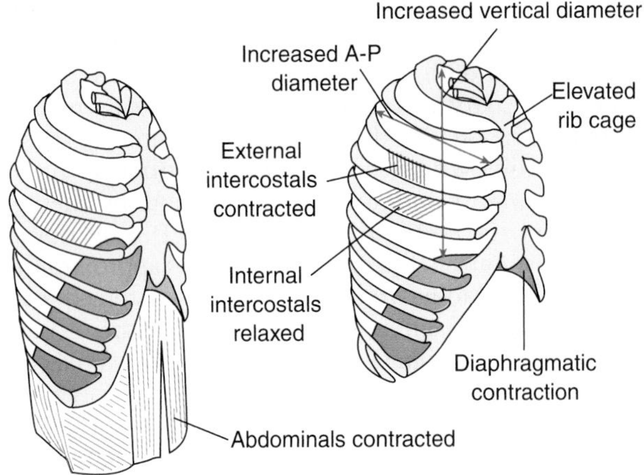

FIGURE 29-12 Expansion and contraction of the thoracic cage during expiration and inspiration, demonstrating especially diaphragmatic contraction, elevation of the rib cage, and function of the intercostals. (Guyton A. C., Hall J. E. [2000]. *Textbook of medical physiology* [10th ed., p. 433]. Philadelphia: W. B. Saunders)

quiet breathing but contract vigorously during exercise. For the accessory muscles to assist in ventilation, they must be stabilized in some way. For example, persons with bronchial asthma often brace their arms against a firm object during an attack as a means of stabilizing their shoulders so that the attached accessory muscles can exert their full effect on ventilation. The head commonly is bent backward so that the scalene and sternocleidomastoid muscles can elevate the ribs more effectively. Other muscles that play a minor role in inspiration are the alae nasi, which produce flaring of the nostrils during obstructed breathing.

Expiration is largely passive. It occurs as the elastic components of the chest wall and lung structures that were stretched during inspiration recoil, causing air to leave the lungs as the intrathoracic pressure increases. When needed, the abdominal and the internal intercostal muscles can be used to increase expiratory effort (see Fig. 29-12). The increase in intra-abdominal pressure that accompanies the forceful contraction of the abdominal muscles pushes the diaphragm upward and results in an increase in intrathoracic pressure. The internal intercostal muscles move inward, which pulls the chest downward, increasing expiratory effort.

Lung Compliance

Lung compliance refers to the ease with which the lungs can be inflated. It is determined by the elastin and collagen fibers of the lung, its water content, and surface tension. Compliance can be appreciated by comparing the ease of blowing up a noncompliant new balloon that is stiff and resistant with a compliant one that has been previously blown up and stretched. Specifically, lung compliance (C) describes the change in lung volume (ΔV) that can be accomplished with a given change in respiratory pressure (ΔP).

$$C = \Delta V/\Delta P$$

The normal compliance of both lungs in the average adult is approximately 200 mL/cm H_2O. This means that every time the transpulmonary pressure increases by 1 cm/H_2O, the lung volume expands by 200 mL. It would take more pressure to move the same amount of air into a noncompliant lung.

Changes in Elastin and Collagen Composition of Lung Tissue. Lung tissue is made up of elastin and collagen fibers. The elastin fibers are easily stretched and increase the ease of lung inflation, whereas the collagen fibers resist stretching and make lung inflation more difficult. In lung diseases such as interstitial lung disease and pulmonary fibrosis, the lungs become stiff and noncompliant as the elastin fibers are replaced with scar tissue. Pulmonary congestion and edema produce a reversible decrease in pulmonary compliance.

Elastic recoil describes the ability of the elastic components of the lung to recoil to their original position after having been stretched. Overstretching the airways, as occurs with emphysema, causes the elastic components of the lung to lose their recoil, making the lung easier to inflate but more difficult to deflate because of its inability to recoil.

Surface Tension. An important factor in lung compliance is the *surface tension* in the alveoli. The alveoli are lined with a thin film of liquid, and it is at the interface between this liquid film and the alveolar air that surface tension develops. This is because the forces that hold the liquid film molecules together are stronger than those that hold the air molecules in the alveoli together. As an example, it is surface tension that holds the water molecules in a raindrop together. In the alveoli, excess surface tension causes the liquid film to contract, making lung inflation more difficult.

The pressure in the alveoli (which are modeled as spheres with open airways projecting from them) can be predicted using Laplace's law (pressure = 2 × surface tension/radius). If the surface tension were equal throughout the lungs, the alveoli with the smallest radii would have the greatest pressure, and this would cause them to empty into the larger alveoli (Fig. 29-13). The reason this does not occur

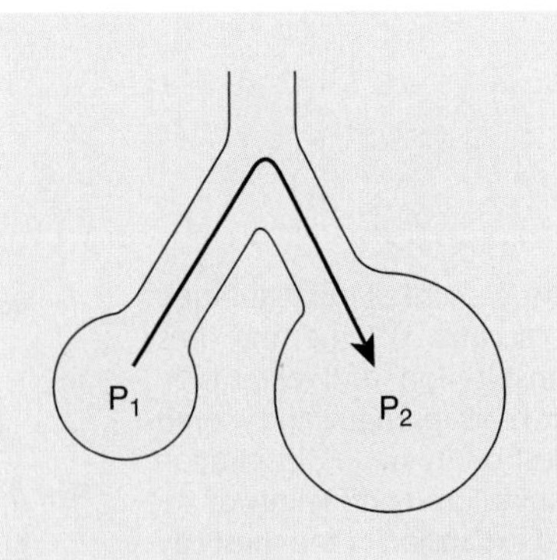

FIGURE 29-13 Law of Laplace (P = 2 T/r, P = pressure, T = tension, r = radius). The effect of the radius on the pressure and movement of gases in the alveolar structures is depicted. Air moves from P_1 with a small radius and higher pressure to P_2 with its larger radius and lower pressure.

is because of special surface tension–lowering molecules, called *surfactant,* that line the inner surface of the alveoli.

Surfactant is a complex mixture of lipoproteins (largely phospholipids) and small amounts of carbohydrates that is synthesized in the type II alveolar cells. The surfactant molecule has two ends: a hydrophobic (water-insoluble) tail and a hydrophilic (water-soluble) head (Fig. 29-14). The hydrophilic head of the surfactant molecule attaches to the liquid molecules and the hydrophobic tail to the gas molecules, interrupting the intermolecular forces that are responsible for creating the surface tension.

Surfactant exerts four important effects on lung inflation: it lowers the surface tension; it increases lung compliance and ease of inflation; it provides for stability and more even inflation of the alveoli; and it assists in preventing pulmonary edema by keeping the alveoli dry. Without surfactant, lung inflation would be extremely difficult, requiring intrapleural pressures of –20 to –30 mm Hg, compared with the pressures of –3 to –5 mm Hg that normally are needed. The surfactant molecules are more densely packed in the small alveoli than in larger alveoli, where the density of the molecules is less. Therefore, surfactant reduces the surface tension more effectively in the small alveoli, which have the greatest tendency to collapse, providing for stability and more even distribution of ventilation. Surfactant also helps to keep the alveoli dry and prevent pulmonary edema. This is because water is pulled out of the pulmonary capillaries into the alveoli when increased surface tension causes the alveoli to contract.

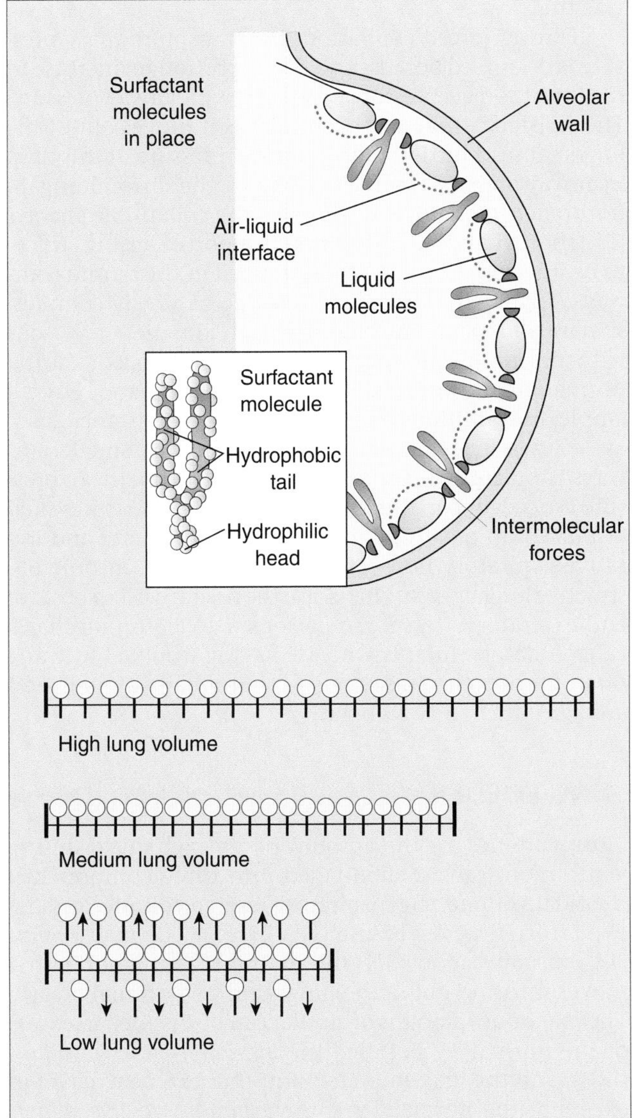

FIGURE 29-14 (Top) Alveolar wall depicting surface tension resulting from the intramolecular forces in the air–liquid film interface; the surfactant molecule with its hydrophobic tail and hydrophilic head; and its function in reducing surface tension by disrupting the intermolecular forces. **(Bottom)** The surface concentration of surfactant molecules at high, medium, and low lung volumes.

The type II alveolar cells that produce surfactant do not begin to mature until the 26th to 28th week of gestation; consequently, many premature infants have difficulty producing sufficient amounts of surfactant. This can lead to alveolar collapse and severe respiratory distress. This condition, called *infant respiratory distress syndrome,* is the single most common cause of respiratory disease in premature infants. Surfactant dysfunction also is possible in the adult. This usually occurs as the result of severe injury or infection and can contribute to the development of a condition called *adult respiratory distress syndrome* (see Chapter 31).

Airway Resistance

The volume of air that moves into and out of the air exchange portion of the lungs is directly related to the pressure difference between the lungs and the atmosphere and inversely related to the resistance that the air encounters as it moves through the airways.

Airway resistance is the ratio of the pressure driving inspiration or expiration to airflow. The French physician Jean Léonard Marie Poiseuille first described the pressure-flow characteristics of laminar flow in a straight circular tube, a correlation that has become known as *Poiseuille's law.* According to Poiseuille's law, the resistance to flow is inversely related to the fourth power of the radius ($R = 1/r^4$). If the radius is reduced by one half, the resistance increases 16-fold ($2 \times 2 \times 2 \times 2 = 16$).

Airway resistance normally is so small that only small changes in pressure are needed to move large volumes of air into the lungs. For example, the average pressure change that is needed to move a normal breath of 500 mL of air into the lungs is approximately 1 to 2 cm H_2O. Because the resistance of the airways is inversely proportional to the fourth power of the radius, small changes in airway caliber, such as those caused by pulmonary secretions or bronchospasm, can produce a marked increase in airway resistance. For persons with these conditions to maintain the same rate of airflow as before the onset of increased airway resistance, an increase in driving pressure (*i.e.,* respiratory effort) is needed.

Airway resistance is greatly affected by lung volumes, being less during inspiration than during expiration. This is because elastic-type fibers connect the outside of the airways to the surrounding lung tissues. As a result, these airways are pulled open as the lungs expand during inspiration, and they become narrower as the lungs deflate during expiration (Fig. 29-15). This is one of the reasons that persons with conditions that increase airway resistance, such as bronchial asthma, usually have less difficulty during inspiration than during expiration.

Laminar Versus Turbulent Flow. Airflow can be laminar or turbulent, depending on the velocity and pattern of flow. Laminar, or streamlined, airflow occurs at low flow rates in which the airstream is parallel to the sides of the airway. With laminar flow, the air at the periphery must overcome the resistance to flow, and as a result, the air in the center of the airway moves faster.

Turbulent flow is disorganized flow in which the molecules of the gas move laterally, collide with one another, and change their velocities. Whether turbulence develops depends on the radius of the airways, the interaction of the gas molecules, and the velocity of airflow. It is most likely to occur when the radius of the airways is large and the velocity of flow is high. Turbulent flow occurs regularly in the trachea. Turbulence of airflow accounts for the respiratory sounds that are heard during chest auscultation (*i.e.*, listening to chest sounds using a stethoscope).

In the bronchial tree with its many branches, laminar airflow probably occurs only in the very small airways, where the velocity of flow is low. Because the small airways contribute little resistance to airflow, they constitute a silent zone. In small airway disease (*e.g.*, chronic obstructive pulmonary disease), it is probable that considerable abnormalities are present before the usual measurements of airway resistance can detect them.

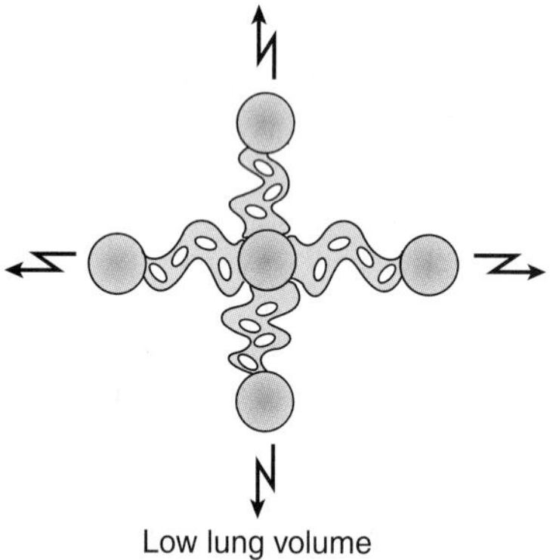

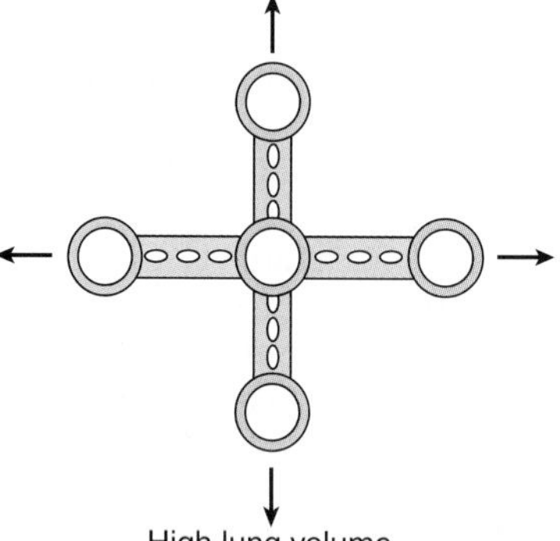

FIGURE 29-15 Interaction of tissue forces on airways during low and high lung volumes. At low lung volumes, the tissue forces tend to fold and place less tension on the airways and they become smaller; during high lung volumes, the tissue forces are stretched and pull the airways open.

Airway Compression. Airflow through the collapsible airways in the lungs depends on the distending airway (intrapulmonary) pressures that hold the airways open and the external (intrapleural or intrathoracic) pressures that surround and compress the airways. The difference between these two pressures (intrathoracic pressure minus airway pressure) is called the *transpulmonary pressure*. For airflow to occur, the distending pressure inside the airways must be greater than the compressing pressure outside the airways.

During forced expiration, the transpulmonary pressure is decreased because of a disproportionate increase in the intrathoracic pressure compared with airway pressure. The resistance that air encounters as it moves out of the lungs causes a further drop in airway pressure. If this drop in airway pressure is sufficiently great, the surrounding intrathoracic pressure will compress the collapsible airways (*i.e.*, those that lack cartilaginous support), causing airflow to be interrupted and air to be trapped in the terminal airways (Fig. 29-16). Although this type of airway compression usually is seen only during forced expiration in persons with normal respiratory function, it may occur during normal breathing in persons with lung diseases. For example, in conditions that increase airway resistance, such as emphysema, the pressure drop along the smaller airways is magnified, and an increase in intra-airway pressure is needed to maintain airway patency. Measures such as pursed-lip breathing increase airway pressure and improve expiratory flow rates in persons with chronic obstructive lung disease. This is also the basis for using positive end-expiratory pressure in persons who are on mechanical ventilators. Infants who are having trouble breathing often grunt to increase their expiratory airway pressures and keep their airways open.

LUNG VOLUMES

Lung volumes, or the amount of air exchanged during ventilation, can be subdivided into three components: the tidal volume, the inspiratory reserve volume, and the expiratory reserve volume (Fig. 29-17). The *tidal volume* (TV), usually about 500 mL, is the amount of air that moves into and out of the lungs during a normal breath. The maximum amount of air that can be inspired in excess of the normal TV is called the *inspiratory reserve volume* (IRV), and the maximum amount that can be exhaled in excess of the normal TV is the *expiratory reserve volume* (ERV). Approximately 1200 mL of air always remains in the lungs after forced expiration; this air is the *residual volume* (RV). The RV increases with age because there is more trapping of air in the lungs at the end of expiration. These volumes can be measured using an instrument called a *spirometer*.

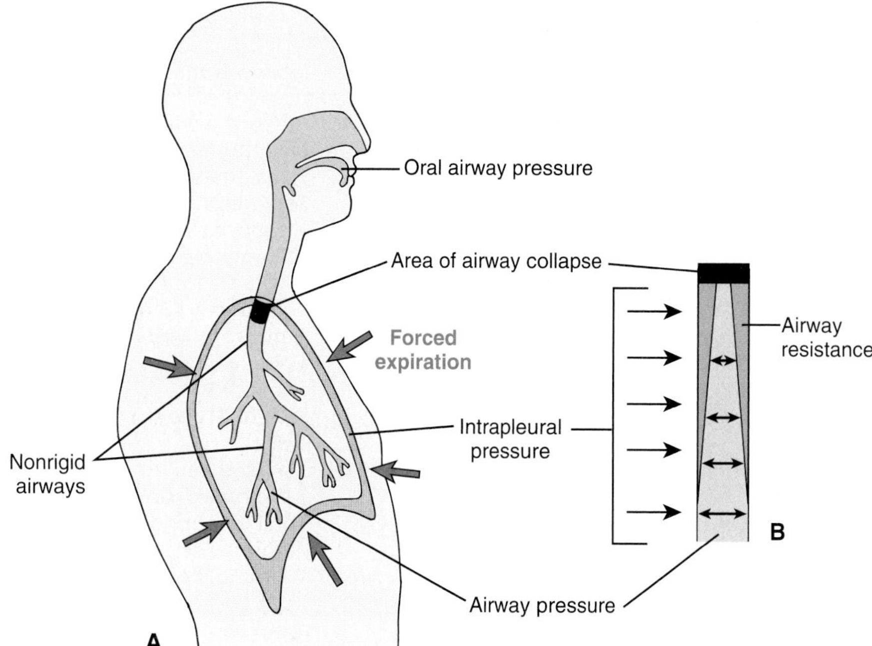

FIGURE 29-16 Mechanism that limits maximal expiratory flow rate. (**A**) Airway patency and airflow in the nonrigid airways of the lungs rely on a transpulmonary pressure gradient in which airway pressure is greater than intrapleural pressure. (**B**) Airway resistance normally produces a drop in airway pressure as air moves out of the lungs. The increased airway pressure that occurs with forced expiration produces airway collapse in the nonrigid airways at the point where intrapleural pressure exceeds airway pressure.

Lung capacities include two or more lung volumes. The *vital capacity* equals the IRV plus the TV plus the ERV and is the amount of air that can be exhaled from the point of maximal inspiration. The *inspiratory capacity* equals the TV plus the IRV. It is the amount of air a person can breathe in beginning at the normal expiratory level and distending the lungs to the maximal amount. The *functional residual capacity* is the sum of the RV and ERV; it is the volume of air that remains in the lungs at the end of normal expiration. The *total lung capacity* is the sum of all the volumes in the lungs. The RV cannot be measured with the spirometer because this air cannot be expressed from the lungs. It is measured by indirect methods, such as the helium dilution method, the nitrogen washout techniques, or body plethysmography. Lung volumes and capacities are summarized in Table 29-1.

Pulmonary Function Studies

The previously described lung volumes and capacities are anatomic or static measures, determined by lung volumes and measured without relation to time. The spirometer also is used to measure dynamic lung function (*i.e.*, ventilation with respect to time); these tests often are used in assessing pulmonary function. Pulmonary function measures include maximum voluntary ventilation, forced vital capacity, forced expiratory volumes and flow rates, and forced inspiratory flow rates (Table 29-2). Pulmonary function is measured for various clinical purposes, including diagnosis of respiratory disease, preoperative surgical and anesthetic risk evaluation, and symptom and disability evaluation for legal or insurance purposes. The tests also are used for evaluating dyspnea, cough, wheezing, and abnormal radiologic or laboratory findings.

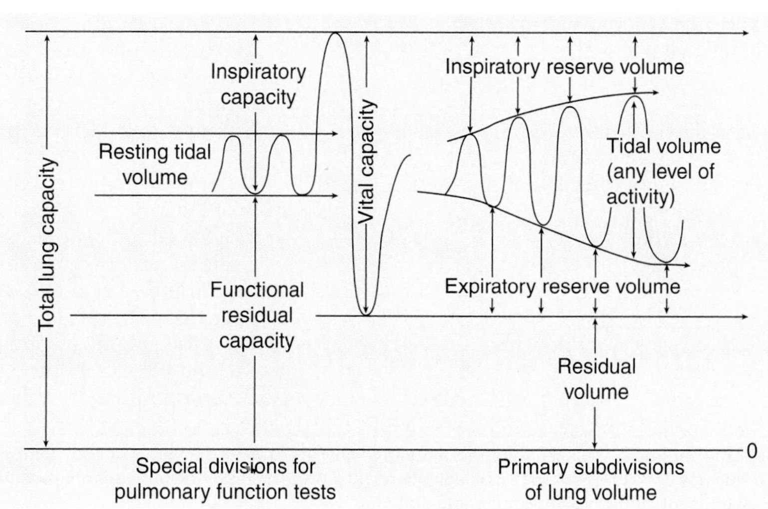

FIGURE 29-17 A tracing of respiratory volumes and capacities made with the use of a spirometer.

TABLE 29-1 Lung Volumes and Capacities

Volume	Symbol	Measurement
Tidal volume (about 500 mL at rest)	TV	Amount of air that moves into and out of the lungs with each breath
Inspiratory reserve volume (about 3000 mL)	IRV	Maximum amount of air that can be inhaled from the point of maximal expiration
Expiratory reserve volume (about 1100 mL)	ERV	Maximum volume of air that can be exhaled from the resting end-expiratory level
Residual volume (about 1200 mL)	RV	Volume of air remaining in the lungs after maximal expiration. This volume cannot be measured with the spirometer; it is measured indirectly using methods such as the helium dilution method, the nitrogen washout technique, or body plethysmography.
Functional residual capacity (about 2300 mL)	FRC	Volume of air remaining in the lungs at end-expiration (sum of RV and ERV)
Inspiratory capacity (about 3500 mL)	IC	Sum of IRV and TV
Vital capacity (about 4600 mL)	VC	Maximal amount of air that can be exhaled from the point of maximal inspiration
Total lung capacity (about 5800 mL)	TLC	Total amount of air that the lungs can hold; it is the sum of all the volume components after maximal inspiration. This value is about 20% to 25% less in females than in males.

The *maximum voluntary ventilation* measures the volume of air that a person can move into and out of the lungs during maximum effort lasting for 12 to 15 seconds. This measurement usually is converted to liters per minute. The *forced expiratory vital capacity* (FVC) involves full inspiration to total lung capacity followed by forceful maximal expiration. Obstruction of airways produces an FVC that is lower than that observed with more slowly performed vital capacity measurements. The *forced expiratory volume* (FEV) is the expiratory volume achieved in a given time period. The $FEV_{1.0}$ is the forced expiratory volume that can be exhaled in 1 second. The $FEV_{1.0}$ frequently is expressed as a percentage of the FVC. The $FEV_{1.0}$ and FVC are used in the diagnosis of obstructive lung disorders.

The *forced inspiratory vital flow* (FIF) measures the respiratory response during rapid maximal inspiration. Calculation of airflow during the middle half of inspiration ($FIF_{25\%-75\%}$) relative to the forced midexpiratory flow rate ($FEF_{25\%-75\%}$) is used as a measure of respiratory muscle dysfunction because inspiratory flow depends more on effort than does expiration.

TABLE 29-2 Pulmonary Function Tests

Test	Symbol	Measurement*
Maximal voluntary ventilation	MVV	Maximum amount of air that can be breathed in a given time
Forced vital capacity	FVC	Maximum amount of air that can be rapidly and forcefully exhaled from the lungs after full inspiration. The expired volume is plotted against time.
Forced expiratory volume achieved in 1 second	$FEV_{1.0}$	Volume of air expired in the first second of FVC
Percentage of forced vital capacity	$FEV_{1.0}/FVC\%$	Volume of air expired in the first second, expressed as a percentage of FVC
Forced midexpiratory flow rate	$FEF_{25\%-75\%}$	The forced midexpiratory flow rate determined by locating the points on the volume-time curve recording obtained during FVC corresponding to 25% and 75% of FVC and drawing a straight line through these points. The slope of this line represents the average midexpiratory flow rate.
Forced inspiratory flow rate	$FIF_{25\%-75\%}$	FIF is the volume inspired from RV at the point of measurement. $FIF_{25\%-75\%}$ is the slope of a line between the points on the volume pressure tracing corresponding to 25% and 75% of the inspired volume.

*By convention, all the lung volumes and rates of flow are expressed in terms of body temperature and pressure and saturated with water vapor (BTPS), which allows for a comparison of the pulmonary function data from laboratories with different ambient temperatures and altitudes.

EFFICIENCY AND THE WORK OF BREATHING

The *minute volume,* or total ventilation, is the amount of air that is exchanged in 1 minute. It is determined by the metabolic needs of the body. The minute volume is equal to the TV multiplied by the respiratory rate, which is normally about 6000 mL (500 mL TV × respiratory rate of 12 breaths/minute) during normal activity. The efficiency of breathing is determined by matching the TV and respiratory rate in a manner that provides an optimal minute volume while minimizing the work of breathing.

The work of breathing is determined by the amount of effort required to move air through the conducting airways and by the ease of lung expansion, or compliance. Expansion of the lungs is difficult for persons with stiff and noncompliant lungs; they usually find it easier to breathe if they keep their TV low and breathe at a more rapid rate (*e.g.,* 300 × 20 = 6000 mL) to achieve their minute volume and meet their oxygen needs. In contrast, persons with obstructive airway disease usually find it less difficult to inflate their lungs but expend more energy in moving air through the airways. As a result, these persons take deeper breaths and breathe at a slower rate (*e.g.,* 600 × 10 = 6000 mL) to achieve their oxygen needs.

In summary, the movement of air between the atmosphere and the lungs follows the laws of physics as they relate to gases. The air in the alveoli contains a mixture of gases, including nitrogen, oxygen, carbon dioxide, and water vapor. With the exception of water vapor, each gas exerts a pressure that is determined by the atmospheric pressure and the concentration of the gas in the mixture. Water vapor pressure is affected by temperature but not atmospheric pressure. Air moves into the lungs along a pressure gradient. The pressure inside the airways and alveoli of the lungs is called *intrapulmonary* (or *alveolar*) *pressure;* the pressure in the pleural cavity is called *pleural pressure;* and the pressure in the thoracic cavity is called *intrathoracic pressure.*

Breathing is the movement of gases between the atmosphere and the lungs. It requires a system of open airways and pressure changes resulting from the action of the respiratory muscles in changing the volume of the chest cage. The diaphragm is the principal muscle of inspiration, assisted by the external intercostal muscles. The scalene and sternocleidomastoid muscles elevate the ribs and act as accessory muscles for inspiration. Expiration is largely passive, aided by the elastic recoil of the respiratory muscles that were stretched during inspiration. When needed, the abdominal and internal intercostal muscles can be used to increase expiratory effort.

Lung compliance describes the ease with which the lungs can be inflated. It reflects the elasticity of the lung tissue and the surface tension in the alveoli. Surfactant molecules, produced by type II alveolar cells, reduce the surface tension in the lungs and thereby increase lung compliance. Airway resistance refers to the impediment to flow that the air encounters as it moves through the airways.

Lung volumes and lung capacities reflect the amount of air that is exchanged during normal and forced breathing. The tidal volume (TV) is the amount of air that moves into and out of the lungs during normal breathing; the inspiratory reserve volume (IRV) is maximum amount of air that can be inspired in excess of the normal TV; and the expiratory reserve volume (ERV) is the maximum amount that can be exhaled in excess of the normal TV. The residual volume is the amount of air that remains in the lungs after forced expiration. Lung capacities include two or more lung volumes. The vital capacity equals the IRV plus the TV plus the ERV and is the amount of air that can be exhaled from the point of maximal inspiration. The minute volume, which is determined by the metabolic needs of the body, is the amount of air that is exchanged in 1 minute (*i.e.,* respiratory rate and TV).

Exchange and Transport of Gases

After completing this section of the chapter, you should be able to meet the following objectives:

- Trace the exchange of gases between the air in the alveoli and the blood in the pulmonary capillaries
- Differentiate between pulmonary and alveolar ventilation
- Explain why ventilation and perfusion must be matched
- Cite the difference between dead air space and shunt
- List four factors that affect the diffusion of gases in the alveoli
- Explain the difference between PO_2 and hemoglobin-bound oxygen and O_2 saturation and content
- Explain the significance of a shift to the right and a shift to the left in the oxygen–hemoglobin dissociation curve

The primary functions of the lungs are oxygenation of the blood and removal of carbon dioxide. Pulmonary gas exchange is conventionally divided into three processes: ventilation, or the flow of gases into and out of the alveoli of the lungs; perfusion, or flow of blood in the adjacent pulmonary capillaries; and diffusion, or transfer of gases between the alveoli and the pulmonary capillaries. The efficiency of gas exchange requires that alveolar ventilation occur adjacent to perfused pulmonary capillaries.

VENTILATION

Ventilation refers to the exchange of gases in the respiratory system. There are two types of ventilation: pulmonary and alveolar. *Pulmonary ventilation* refers to the total exchange of gases between the atmosphere and the lungs. *Alveolar ventilation* is the exchange of gases within the gas exchange portion of the lungs. Ventilation requires a system of open airways and a pressure difference that moves air into and out of the lungs. It is affected by body position and lung volume as well as by disease conditions that affect the heart and respiratory systems.

Distribution of Ventilation

The distribution of ventilation between the apex and base of the lung varies with body position and the weight of the lung and the effects of gravity on intrapleural pressure. Compliance reflects the change in volume that occurs with a change in pressure. It is less in fully expanded alveoli, which have difficulty accommodating more air, and greater in alveoli that are less inflated. In the seated or standing position, gravity exerts a downward pull on the lung, causing intrapleural pressure at the apex of the lung to become more negative than that at the base of the lung (Fig. 29-18). As a result, the alveoli at the apex of the lung are more fully expanded and less compliant than those at the base of the lung. The same holds true for lung compliance in the dependent portions of the lung in the supine or lateral position. In the supine position, ventilation in the lowermost (posterior) parts of the lung exceeds that in the uppermost (anterior) parts. In the lateral position (*i.e.,* lying on the side), the dependent lung is better ventilated.

The distribution of ventilation also is affected by lung volumes. During full inspiration in the seated or standing position, the airways are pulled open, and air moves into the more compliant portions of the lower lung. At low lung volumes, the opposite occurs. At functional residual capacity, the pleural pressure at the base of the lung exceeds airway pressure compressing the airways, so that ventilation is greatly reduced. In contrast, the airways in the apex of the lung remain open, and this area of the lung is well ventilated.

Even at low lung volumes, some air remains in the alveoli of the lower portion of the lungs, preventing their collapse. According to Laplace's law (discussed previously), the pressure needed to overcome the tension in the wall of a sphere or an elastic tube is inversely related to its radius; therefore, the small airways close first, trapping some gas in the alveoli. There may be increased trapping of air in the alveoli of the lower part of the lungs in older persons and in those with lung disease (*e.g.,* emphysema). This condition is thought to result from a loss in the elastic recoil properties of the lungs, so that the intrapleural pressure, created by the elastic recoil of the lung and chest wall, becomes less negative. In these persons, airway closure occurs at the end of normal instead of low lung volumes, trapping larger amounts of air.

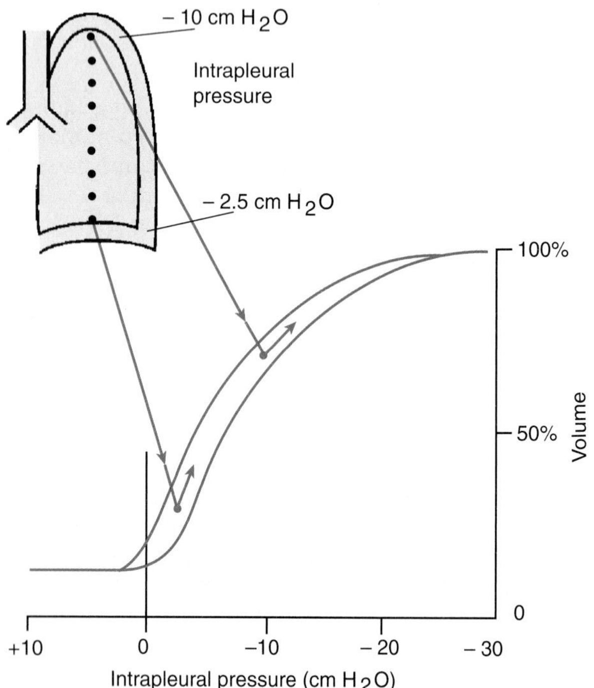

FIGURE 29-18 Explanation of the regional differences in ventilation down the lung; the intrapleural pressure is less negative at the base than at the apex. As a consequence, the basal lung is relatively compressed in its resting state but expands more on inspiration than the apex. (West J. B. [2001]. *Pulmonary physiology and pathophysiology* [p. 43]. Lippincott Williams & Wilkins)

PERFUSION

The primary functions of the pulmonary circulation are to perfuse or provide blood flow to the gas exchange portion of the lung and to facilitate gas exchange. The pulmonary circulation serves several important functions in addition to gas exchange. It filters all the blood that moves from the right to the left side of the circulation; it removes most of the thromboemboli that might form; and it serves as a reservoir of blood for the left side of the heart.

The gas exchange function of the lungs requires a continuous flow of blood through the respiratory portion of the lungs. Deoxygenated blood enters the lung through the pulmonary artery, which has its origin in the right side of the heart and enters the lung at the hilus, along with the primary bronchus. The pulmonary arteries branch in a manner similar to that of the airways. The small pulmonary arteries accompany the bronchi as they move down the lobules and branch to supply the capillary network that surrounds the alveoli (see Fig. 29-7). The meshwork of capillaries in the respiratory portion of the lungs is so dense that the flow in these vessels often is described as being similar to a sheet of blood. The oxygenated capillary blood is collected in the small pulmonary veins of the lobules; it then moves to the larger veins to be collected in the four large pulmonary veins that empty into the left atrium.

The pulmonary blood vessels are thinner, more compliant, and offer less resistance to flow than those in the systemic circulation, and the pressures in the pulmonary system are much lower (*e.g.,* 22/8 mm Hg versus 120/70 mm Hg). The low pressure and low resistance of the pulmonary circulation accommodate the delivery of varying amounts of blood from the systemic circulation without producing signs and symptoms of congestion. The volume in the pulmonary circulation is approximately 500 mL, with approximately 100 mL of this volume located in the pulmonary capillary bed. When the output of the right ventricle and input of the left ventricle are equal, pulmonary blood flow remains constant. Small differences between input and output can result in large changes in pulmonary volume if the differences continue for many heartbeats. The movement of blood through the pulmonary capillary bed requires that the mean pulmonary arterial pressure be greater than the mean pulmonary venous pressure. Pulmonary venous pressure increases in left-sided heart failure, allowing blood to accumulate in the pulmonary capillary bed and to cause pulmonary edema (see Chapter 28).

Distribution of Blood Flow and Body Position

As with ventilation, the distribution of pulmonary blood flow is affected by body position and gravity. In the upright position, the distance of the upper apices of the lung above the level of the heart may exceed the perfusion capabilities of the mean pulmonary arterial pressure (approximately 12 mm Hg); therefore, blood flow in the upper part of the lungs is less than that in the base or bottom part of the lungs (Fig. 29-19). In the supine position, the lungs and the heart are at the same level, and blood flow to the apices and base of the lungs becomes more uniform. In this position, blood flow to the posterior or dependent portions (*e.g.*, bottom of the lung when lying on the side) exceeds flow in the anterior or nondependent portions of the lungs.

Hypoxia-induced Vasoconstriction

The blood vessels in the pulmonary circulation undergo marked vasoconstriction when they are exposed to hypoxia. The precise mechanism for this response is unclear. When alveolar oxygen levels drop below 60 mm Hg, marked vasoconstriction may occur, and at very low oxygen levels, the local flow may be almost abolished. In regional hypoxia, as occurs with atelectasis, vasoconstriction is localized to a specific region of the lung. Vasoconstriction has the effect of directing blood flow away from the hypoxic regions of the lungs. When alveolar hypoxia no longer exists, blood flow is restored.

Generalized hypoxia causes vasoconstriction throughout the lung. Generalized vasoconstriction occurs when the partial pressure of oxygen is decreased at high altitudes, or it can occur in persons with chronic hypoxia due to lung disease. Prolonged hypoxia can lead to pulmonary hypertension and increased workload on the right heart. A low blood pH also produces vasoconstriction, especially when alveolar hypoxia is present (*e.g.*, during circulatory shock).

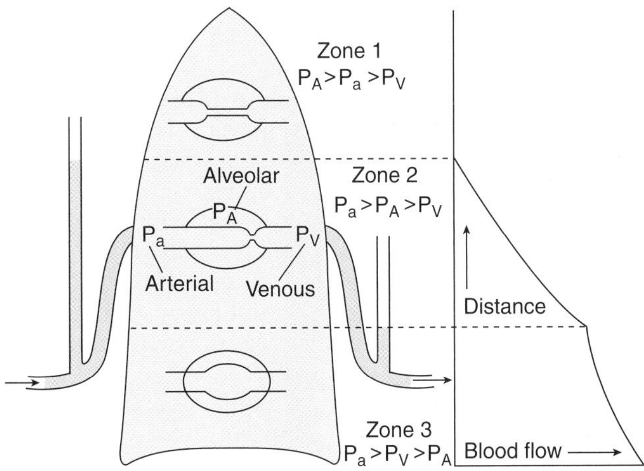

FIGURE 29-19 The uneven distribution of blood flow in the lung results from different pressures affecting the capillaries, which are affected by body position and gravity. (West J. B. [2000]. *Respiratory physiology: The essentials* [p. 29]. Philadelphia: Lippincott Williams & Wilkins)

DIFFUSION

There are two types of air movement in the lung: bulk flow and diffusion. Bulk flow occurs in the conducting airways and is controlled by pressure differences between the mouth and the airways in the lung. Diffusion refers to the movement of gases in the alveoli and across the alveolar capillary membrane. Gas diffusion in the lung can be described by *Fick's law*. Fick's law states that the volume of a gas ($\dot{V}$gas) diffusing across the membrane per unit time is directly proportional to the partial pressure difference of the gas ($P_1 - P_2$), the surface area (SA) of the membrane, and the diffusion coefficient (D) and is inversely proportional to the thickness (T) of the membrane:

$$\dot{V}\text{gas} = \frac{(P_1 - P_2) \times SA \times D}{T}$$

Several factors influence diffusion of gases in the lung. The administration of high concentrations of oxygen increases the difference in partial pressure between the two sides of the membrane and increases the diffusion of the gas. Diseases that destroy lung tissue (*i.e.*, surface area for diffusion) or increase the thickness of the alveolar-capillary membrane adversely influence the diffusing capacity of the lungs. The removal of one lung, for example, reduces the diffusing capacity by one half. The thickness of the alveolar-capillary membrane and the distance for diffusion are increased in persons with pulmonary edema or pneumonia. The characteristics of the gas and its molecular weight and solubility constitute the diffusion coefficient and determine how rapidly the gas diffuses through the respiratory membranes. For example, carbon dioxide diffuses 20 times more rapidly than oxygen because of its greater solubility in the respiratory membranes. The factors that affect alveolar-capillary gas exchange are summarized in Table 29-3.

MATCHING OF VENTILATION AND PERFUSION

The gas exchange properties of the lung depend on matching ventilation and perfusion, ensuring that equal amounts of air and blood are entering the respiratory portion of the lungs. Two factors may interfere with the matching of ventilation and perfusion: dead air space and shunt.

Dead Air Space

Dead space refers to the volume of air that must be moved with each breath but does not participate in gas exchange. The movement of air through dead space contributes to the work of breathing but not to gas exchange.

There are two types of dead air space: that contained in the conducting airways, called the *anatomic dead space,*

TABLE 29-3 Factors Affecting Alveolar-Capillary Gas Exchange

Factors Affecting Gas Exchange	Examples
Surface area available for diffusion	Removal of a lung or diseases such as emphysema and chronic bronchitis, which destroy lung tissue or cause mismatching of ventilation and perfusion
Thickness of the alveolar-capillary membrane	Conditions such as pneumonia, interstitial lung disease, and pulmonary edema, which increase membrane thickness
Partial pressure of alveolar gases	Ascent to high altitudes where the partial pressure of oxygen is reduced. In the opposite direction, increasing the partial pressure of a gas in the inspired air (*e.g.*, oxygen therapy) increases the gradient for diffusion
Solubility and molecular weight of the gas	Carbon dioxide, which is more soluble in the cell membranes, diffuses across the alveolar-capillary membrane more rapidly than oxygen.

and that contained in the respiratory portion of the lung, called the *alveolar dead space*. The volume of anatomic airway dead space is fixed at approximately 150 to 200 mL, depending on body size. It constitutes air contained in the nose, pharynx, trachea, and bronchi. The creation of a tracheostomy decreases anatomic dead space ventilation because air does not have to move through the nasal and oral airways. Alveolar dead space, normally about 5 to 10 mL, constitutes alveolar air that does not participate in gas exchange. When alveoli are ventilated but deprived of blood flow, they do not contribute to gas exchange and thereby constitute alveolar dead space.

The *physiologic dead space* includes the anatomic dead space plus alveolar dead space. In persons with normal respiratory function, physiologic dead space is about the same as anatomic dead space. Only in lung disease does physiologic dead space increase. Alveolar ventilation is equal to the minute ventilation minus the physiologic dead space ventilation.

MATCHING OF VENTILATION AND PERFUSION

- Exchange of gases between the air in the alveoli and the blood in pulmonary capillaries requires a matching of ventilation and perfusion.
- Two factors interfere with matching of ventilation and perfusion: dead air space and shunt.
- Dead air space refers to the volume of air that is moved with each breath but does not participate in gas exchange. Anatomic dead space is that contained in the conducting airways that normally do not participate in gas exchange. Alveolar dead space results from alveoli that are ventilated but not perfused.
- Shunt refers to blood that moves from the right to the left side of the circulation without being oxygenated. With an anatomic shunt, blood moves from the venous to the arterial side of the circulation without going through the lungs. Physiologic shunting results from blood moving through unventilated parts of the lung.
- The blood oxygen level reflects the mixing of blood from alveolar dead space and physiologic shunting areas as it moves into the pulmonary veins.

Shunt

Shunt refers to blood that moves from the right to the left side of the circulation without being oxygenated. As with dead air space, there are two types of shunts: physiologic and anatomic. In an *anatomic shunt,* blood moves from the venous to the arterial side of the circulation without moving through the lungs. Anatomic intracardiac shunting of blood due to congenital heart defects is discussed in Chapter 26. In a *physiologic shunt,* there is mismatching of ventilation and perfusion with the lung, resulting in insufficient ventilation to provide the oxygen needed to oxygenate the blood flowing through the alveolar capillaries. Physiologic shunting of blood usually results from destructive lung disease that impairs ventilation or from heart failure that interferes with movement of blood through sections of the lungs.

Mismatching of Ventilation and Perfusion

Both dead air space and shunt produce a mismatching of ventilation and perfusion as depicted in Figure 29-20. With shunt (depicted on the left), there is perfusion without ventilation, resulting in a low ventilation–perfusion ratio. It occurs in conditions such as atelectasis in which there is airway obstruction (see Chapter 31). With dead air space (depicted on the right), there is ventilation without perfusion, resulting in a high ventilation–perfusion ratio. It occurs with conditions such as pulmonary embolism, which impairs blood flow to a part of the lung. The arterial blood leaving the pulmonary circulation reflects mixing of blood from normally ventilated and perfused areas of the lung as well as areas that are not ventilated (dead air space) or perfused (shunt). Many of the conditions that cause mismatching of ventilation and perfusion involve both dead air space and shunt. In chronic obstructive lung disease, for example, there may be impaired ventilation in one area of the lung and impaired perfusion in another area.

GAS TRANSPORT

Although the lungs are responsible for the exchange of gases, it is the blood that transports these gases between the lungs and body tissues. The blood carries oxygen and

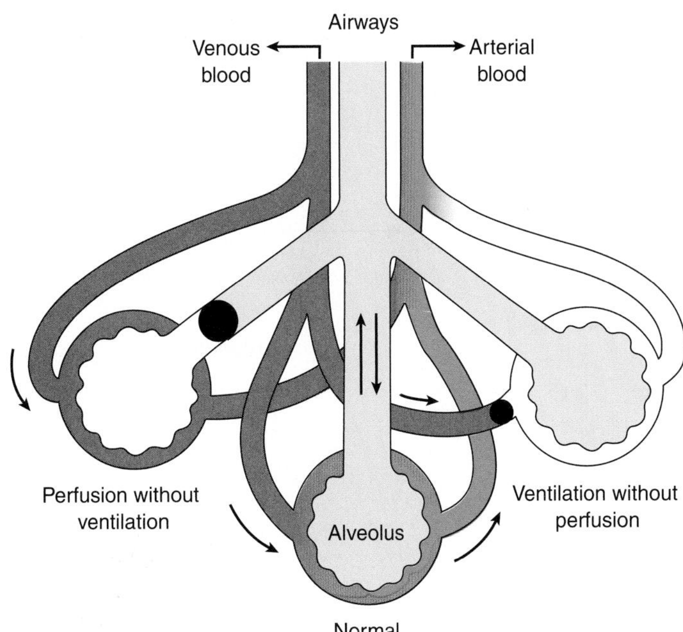

FIGURE 29-20 Matching of ventilation and perfusion. **(Center)** Normal matching of ventilation and perfusion; **(left)** perfusion without ventilation (*i.e.*, shunt); **(right)** ventilation without perfusion (*i.e.*, dead air space).

carbon dioxide in the dissolved state and in combination with hemoglobin. Carbon dioxide also is converted to bicarbonate and transported in that form.

The amount of a gas that can dissolve in plasma is determined by two factors: the solubility of the gas in the plasma and the partial pressure of the gas in the alveoli. In the clinical setting, blood gas measurements are used to determine the level of the partial pressure of oxygen (PO_2) and carbon dioxide (PCO_2) in the blood. Arterial blood commonly is used for measuring blood gases. Venous blood is not used because venous levels of oxygen and carbon dioxide reflect the metabolic demands of the tissues rather than the gas exchange function of the lungs. The PO_2 of arterial blood normally is above 80 mm Hg, and the PCO_2 is in the range of 35 to 45 mm Hg. Normally, the arterial blood gases are the same or nearly the same as the partial pressure of the gases in the alveoli. The arterial PO_2 often is written PaO_2, and the alveolar PO_2 as PAO_2, with the same types of designations being used for PCO_2. This text uses PO_2 and PCO_2 to designate both arterial and alveolar levels of the gases.

OXYGEN TRANSPORT

- Oxygen is transported in chemical combination with hemoglobin and as a gas dissolved in the plasma.
- Hemoglobin, which is the main transporter for oxygen, binds oxygen as it passes through the lungs and releases it as it moves through the tissues.
- The amount of oxygen that is carried as a dissolved gas is determined by the partial pressure of the gas in the lungs.
- The oxygen content of the blood, or the amount of oxygen that is available to the tissues, represents the total amount of oxygen carried by the hemoglobin (hemoglobin concentration [g/dL] multiplied by its saturation) plus the amount of oxygen that is carried in the dissolved state.

Oxygen Transport

Oxygen is transported in two forms: in chemical combination with hemoglobin and in the dissolved state. The hemoglobin in red blood cells serves as a transport vehicle for oxygen. It binds oxygen in the pulmonary capillaries and releases it in the tissue capillaries. As oxygen moves into or out of the red blood cells, it dissolves in the plasma (Fig. 29-21). It is the dissolved form of oxygen that leaves the capillary, crosses cell membranes, and participates in cell metabolism.

Dissolved Oxygen. The partial pressure of oxygen (PO_2) represents the level of dissolved oxygen in plasma. The amount of gas that can be dissolved in a liquid depends on the solubility of the gas and its pressure. The solubility of oxygen in plasma is fixed and very small. For every 1 mm Hg of PO_2 present in the alveoli, 0.003 mL of oxygen becomes dissolved in 100 mL of plasma. This means that at a normal alveolar PO_2 of 100 mm Hg, the blood carries only 0.3 mL of dissolved oxygen in each 100 mL of plasma. This amount (approximately 1%) is very small compared with the amount that can be carried in an equal amount of blood when oxygen is attached to hemoglobin.

Although the amount of oxygen carried in plasma under normal conditions is small, it can become a lifesaving mode of transport in carbon monoxide poisoning, when most of the hemoglobin sites are occupied by carbon monoxide and are unavailable for transport of oxygen. The use of a hyperbaric chamber, in which 100% oxygen can be administered at high atmospheric pressures, increases the amount of oxygen that can be carried in the dissolved state.

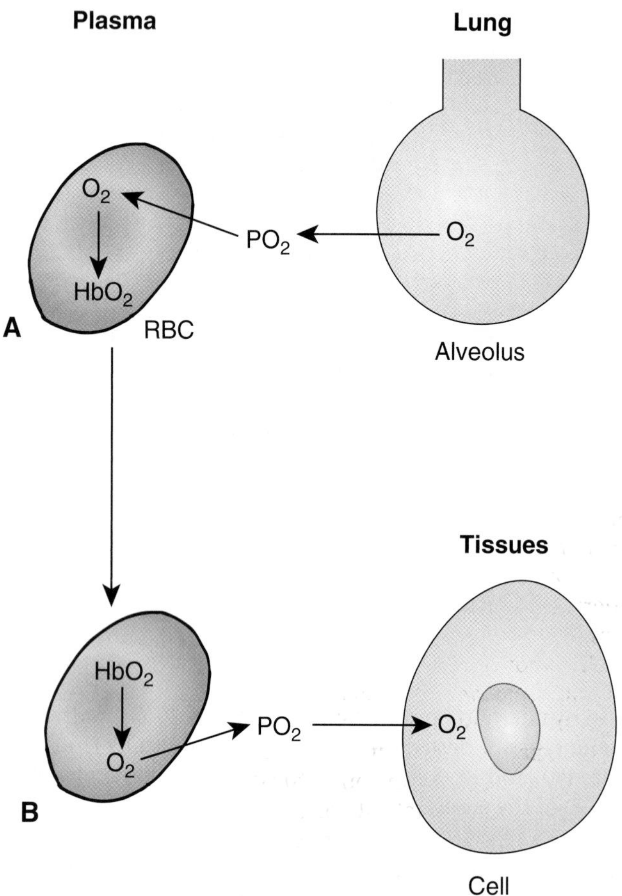

FIGURE 29-21 Transport of oxygen. (**A**) In the lung, oxygen (O_2) moves across the alveolar membrane, becomes dissolved in the plasma (PO_2), and then moves into the red blood cell (RBC) where it attaches to the hemoglobin molecule (HbO_2) for transport to the tissues. (**B**) In the tissues, O_2 dissociates from hemoglobin and leaves the RBC, becomes dissolved in the plasma (PO_2), and then moves into tissue cells where it is used in the production of energy substrates.

Hemoglobin Transport. Hemoglobin is a highly efficient carrier of oxygen, and approximately 98% to 99% of the oxygen used by body tissues is carried in this manner. Hemoglobin with bound oxygen is called *oxyhemoglobin,* and when oxygen is removed, it is called *deoxygenated* or *reduced hemoglobin.* Each gram of hemoglobin carries approximately 1.34 mL of oxygen when it is fully saturated. This means that a person with a hemoglobin of 14 g/100 mL carries 18.8 mL of oxygen per 100 mL of blood. In the lungs, oxygen moves across the alveolar-capillary membrane, through the plasma, and into the red blood cell, where it forms a loose and reversible bond with the hemoglobin molecule. In normal lungs, this process is rapid, so that even with a fast heart rate, the hemoglobin is almost completely saturated with oxygen during the short time it spends in the pulmonary capillaries.

The oxygenated hemoglobin is transported in the arterial blood to the peripheral capillaries, where the oxygen is released and made available to the tissues for use in cell metabolism. As the oxygen moves out of the capillaries in response to the needs of the tissues, the hemoglobin saturation, which usually is approximately 95% to 97% as the blood leaves the left side of the heart, drops to approximately 75% as the mixed venous blood returns to the right side of the heart.

Binding Affinity of Hemoglobin for Oxygen. Oxygen that remains bound to hemoglobin cannot participate in tissue metabolism. The efficiency of the hemoglobin transport system depends on the ability of the hemoglobin molecule to bind oxygen in the lungs and release it as it is needed in the tissues. The affinity of hemoglobin refers to its capacity to bind oxygen. Hemoglobin binds oxygen more readily when its affinity is increased and releases it more readily when its affinity is decreased.

As described in Chapter 16, the hemoglobin molecule is composed of four polypeptide chains with an iron-containing heme group. Because oxygen binds to the iron atom, each hemoglobin molecule can bind four molecules of oxygen when it is fully saturated. Oxygen binds cooperatively with the heme groups on the hemoglobin molecule. After the first molecule of oxygen binds to hemoglobin, the molecule undergoes a change in shape. As a result, the second and third molecules bind more readily, and binding of the fourth molecule is even easier. In a like manner, the unloading of the first oxygen molecule enhances the unloading of the next molecule, and so on. Thus, the affinity of hemoglobin for oxygen changes with oxygen saturation.

Hemoglobin's affinity for oxygen is also influenced by pH, carbon dioxide concentration, and temperature. Hemoglobin binds oxygen more strongly under conditions of increased pH (alkalosis), decreased carbon dioxide concentration, and decreased body temperature and releases it more readily under conditions of decreased pH (acidosis), increased carbon dioxide concentration, and fever. Conditions that decrease affinity and favor unloading of oxygen reflect the level of tissue metabolism and need for oxygen. For example, increased tissue metabolism generates carbon dioxide and metabolic acids and thereby decreases the affinity of hemoglobin for oxygen. Heat also is a byproduct of tissue metabolism, explaining the effect of fever on oxygen binding.

Red blood cells contain a metabolic intermediate called *2,3-diphosphoglycerate* (2,3-DPG) that also affects the affinity of hemoglobin for oxygen. An increase in 2,3-DPG enhances unloading of oxygen from hemoglobin at the tissue level. An increase in 2,3-DPG occurs with exercise and the hypoxia that occurs with high altitude and chronic lung disease.

Oxygen–Hemoglobin Dissociation Curve. The relation between the oxygen carried in combination with hemoglobin and the PO_2 of the blood is described by the *oxygen–hemoglobin dissociation curve,* which is shown in Figure 29-22. The *x* axis of the graph depicts the PO_2 or dissolved oxygen; the left *y* axis, hemoglobin saturation; and the right y axis, the oxygen content. The PO_2 reflects the partial pressure of the gas in the lung (*i.e.,* the PO_2 is approximately 100 mm Hg when room air is being breathed, but can rise to 200 mm Hg or higher when oxygen enriched

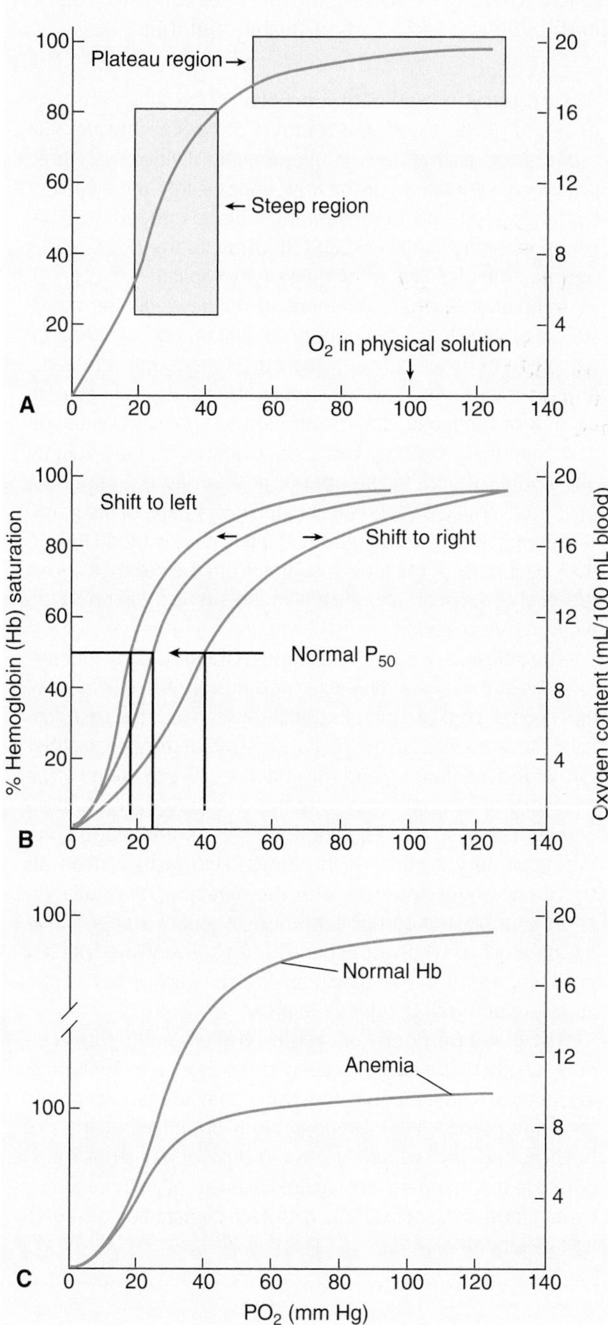

FIGURE 29-22 Oxygen–hemoglobin dissociation curve. (**A**) Left boxed area represents the steep portion of the curve where oxygen is released from hemoglobin (Hb) to the tissues, and the top boxed area the plateau of the curve where oxygen is loaded onto hemoglobin in the lung. (**B**) The effect of body temperature, arterial PCO_2, and pH on hemoglobin affinity for oxygen as indicated by a shift in the curve and position of the P_{50}. A shift of the curve to the right due to an increase in temperature, PCO_2, or decreased pH favors release of oxygen to the tissues. A decrease in temperature, PCO_2, or increase in pH shifts the curve to the left and has the opposite effect. The P_{50} is the partial pressure of oxygen required to saturate 50% of hemoglobin with oxygen. (**C**) Effect of anemia on the oxygen-carrying capacity of blood. The hemoglobin can be completely saturated, but the oxygen content of the blood is reduced.

air is breathed). The hemoglobin saturation reflects the amount of oxygen that is carried by the hemoglobin.

The S-shaped oxygen dissociation curve has a flat top portion representing binding of oxygen by the hemoglobin in the lungs and a steep portion representing its release into the tissue capillaries (see Fig. 29-22A). The S shape of the curve reflects the effect that oxygen saturation has on the conformation of the hemoglobin molecule and its affinity for oxygen. At approximately 100 mm Hg PO_2, a plateau occurs, at which point the hemoglobin is approximately 98% saturated. Increasing the alveolar PO_2 above this level does not increase the hemoglobin saturation. Even at high altitudes, when the partial pressure of oxygen is considerably decreased, the hemoglobin remains relatively well saturated. At 60 mm Hg PO_2, for example, the hemoglobin is still approximately 89% saturated.

The steep portion of the dissociation curve—between 60 and 40 mm Hg—represents the removal of oxygen from the hemoglobin as it moves through the tissue capillaries. This portion of the curve reflects the fact that there is considerable transfer of oxygen from hemoglobin to the tissues with only a small drop in PO_2, thereby ensuring a gradient for oxygen to move into body cells. The tissues normally remove approximately 5 mL of oxygen per 100 mL of blood, and the hemoglobin of mixed venous blood is approximately 75% saturated as it returns to the right side of the heart. In this portion of the dissociation curve (saturation <75%), the rate at which oxygen is released from hemoglobin is determined largely by tissue uptake. During strenuous exercise, for example, the muscle cells may remove as much as 15 mL of oxygen per 100 mL of blood from hemoglobin.

Hemoglobin can be regarded as a buffer system that regulates the delivery of oxygen to the tissues. In order to function as a buffer system, the affinity of hemoglobin for oxygen must change with the metabolic needs of the tissues. This change is represented by a shift to the right or left in the dissociation curve (see Fig. 29-22B). A shift to the right indicates that the tissue PO_2 is greater for any given level of hemoglobin saturation and represents reduced affinity of the hemoglobin for oxygen at any given PO_2. It usually is caused by conditions such as fever or acidosis or by an increase in PCO_2, which reflects increased tissue metabolism. High altitude and conditions such as pulmonary insufficiency, heart failure, and severe anemia also cause the oxygen dissociation curve to shift to the right. A shift to the left in the oxygen dissociation curve represents an increased affinity of hemoglobin for oxygen and occurs in situations associated with a decrease in tissue metabolism, such as alkalosis, decreased body temperature, and decreased PCO_2 levels. The degree of shift can be determined by the P_{50}, or the partial pressure of oxygen that is needed to achieve a 50% saturation of hemoglobin. Returning to Figure 29-22B, the dissociation curve on the left has a P_{50} of approximately 20 mm Hg; the normal curve, a P_{50} of 26; and the curve on the right, a P_{50} of 39 mm Hg.

The oxygen content of the blood (measured in milliliters per 100 milliliters of blood) represents the total amount of oxygen carried in the blood, including the dissolved oxygen and that carried by the hemoglobin (see

Fig. 29-22C). It is the oxygen content of the blood rather than the PO_2 or hemoglobin saturation that determines the amount of oxygen that is carried in the blood and delivered to the tissues. An anemic person may have a normal PO_2 and hemoglobin saturation level but decreased oxygen content because of the lower amount of hemoglobin for binding oxygen.

Carbon Dioxide Transport

Carbon dioxide is transported in the blood in three forms (see Chapter 34, Fig. 34-2): as dissolved carbon dioxide (10%), attached to hemoglobin (30%), and as bicarbonate (60%). Acid-base balance is influenced by the amount of dissolved carbon dioxide and the bicarbonate level in the blood.

As carbon dioxide is formed during the metabolic process, it diffuses out of cells into the tissue spaces and then into the capillaries. The amount of dissolved carbon dioxide that can be carried in plasma is determined by the partial pressure of the gas and its solubility coefficient (0.03 mL/100 mL/1 mm Hg PCO_2). Carbon dioxide is 20 times more soluble in plasma than oxygen. Thus, the dissolved state plays a greater role in transport of carbon dioxide compared with oxygen.

Most of the carbon dioxide diffuses into the red blood cells, where it either forms carbonic acid or combines with hemoglobin. *Carbonic acid* (H_2CO_3) is formed when carbon dioxide combines with water ($CO_2 + H_2O = H^+ + HCO_3^-$). The process is catalyzed by an enzyme called *carbonic anhydrase,* which is present in large quantities in red blood cells. Carbonic anhydrase increases the rate of the reaction between carbon dioxide and water approximately 5000-fold. Carbonic acid readily ionizes to form bicarbonate (HCO_3^-) and hydrogen (H^+) ions. The hydrogen ions combine with the hemoglobin, which is a powerful acid-base buffer, and the bicarbonate ion diffuses into plasma in exchange for a chloride ion. This exchange is made possible by a special bicarbonate-chloride carrier protein in the red blood cell membrane. As a result of the bicarbonate-chloride shift, the chloride and water content of the red blood cell is greater in venous blood than in arterial blood.

In addition to the carbonic anhydrase–mediated reaction with water, carbon dioxide reacts directly with hemoglobin to form *carbaminohemoglobin.* The combination of carbon dioxide and hemoglobin is a reversible reaction that involves a loose bond, which allows transport of carbon dioxide from tissues to the lungs, where it is released into the alveoli for exchange with the external environment. The release of oxygen from hemoglobin in the tissues enhances the binding of carbon dioxide to hemoglobin; in the lungs, the combining of oxygen with hemoglobin displaces carbon dioxide. The binding of carbon dioxide to hemoglobin is determined by the acidic nature of hemoglobin. Binding with carbon dioxide causes the hemoglobin to become a stronger acid. In the lungs, the highly acidic hemoglobin has a lesser tendency to form carbaminohemoglobin, and carbon dioxide is released from hemoglobin into the alveoli. In the tissues, the release of oxygen from hemoglobin causes hemoglobin to become less acid, thereby increasing its ability to combine with carbon dioxide and form carbaminohemoglobin.

In summary, the primary functions of the lungs are oxygenation of the blood and removal of carbon dioxide. Pulmonary gas exchange is conventionally divided into three processes: ventilation, or the flow of gases into the alveoli of the lungs; perfusion, or movement of blood through the adjacent pulmonary capillaries; and diffusion, or transfer of gases between the alveoli and the pulmonary capillaries.

Ventilation is the movement of air between the atmosphere and the lungs. Pulmonary ventilation refers to the total exchange of gases between the atmosphere and the lungs, and alveolar ventilation to ventilation in the gas exchange portion of the lungs. The distribution of alveolar ventilation and pulmonary capillary blood flow varies with lung volume and body position. In the upright position and at high lung volumes, ventilation is greatest in the lower parts of the lungs. The upright position also produces a decrease in blood flow to the upper parts of the lung, resulting from the distance above the level of the heart and the low mean arterial pressure in the pulmonary circulation.

The diffusion of gases in the lungs is influenced by four factors: the surface area available for diffusion; the thickness of the alveolar-capillary membrane, through which the gases diffuse; the differences in the partial pressure of the gas on either side of the membrane; and the characteristics of the gas. The efficiency of gas exchange requires matching of ventilation and perfusion, so that equal amounts of air and blood enter the respiratory portion of the lungs. Two factors—dead air space and shunt—interfere with the matching of ventilation and perfusion and do not contribute to gas exchange. Dead air space occurs when areas of the lungs are ventilated but not perfused. Shunt is the condition under which areas of the lungs are perfused but not ventilated.

The blood transports oxygen to the cells and returns carbon dioxide to the lungs. Oxygen is transported in two forms: in chemical combination with hemoglobin and physically dissolved in plasma (PO_2). Hemoglobin is an efficient carrier of oxygen, and approximately 98% to 99% of oxygen is transported in this manner. Carbon dioxide is carried in three forms: carbaminohemoglobin (30%), dissolved carbon dioxide (10%), and bicarbonate (60%).

Control of Breathing

After completing this section of the chapter, you should be able to meet the following objectives:

- Compare the neural control of the respiratory muscles, which control breathing, with that of cardiac muscle, which controls the pumping action of the heart
- Describe the function of the chemoreceptors and lung receptors in the regulation of ventilation
- Trace the integration of the cough reflex from stimulus to explosive expulsion of air that constitutes the cough

- Describe the type of periodic breathing known as Cheyne-Stokes breathing
- Define dyspnea and list three types of conditions in which dyspnea occurs

Unlike the heart, which has inherent rhythmic properties and can beat independently of the nervous system, the muscles that control respiration require continuous input from the nervous system. Movement of the diaphragm, intercostal muscles, sternocleidomastoid, and other accessory muscles that control ventilation is integrated by neurons located in the pons and medulla. These neurons are collectively referred to as the *respiratory center* (Fig. 29-23).

RESPIRATORY CENTER

The respiratory center consists of two dense, bilateral aggregates of respiratory neurons involved in initiating inspiration and expiration and incorporating afferent impulses into motor responses of the respiratory muscles. The first, or dorsal, group of neurons in the respiratory center is concerned primarily with inspiration. These neurons control the activity of the phrenic nerves that innervate the diaphragm and drive the second, or ventral, group of respiratory neurons. They are thought to integrate sensory input from the lungs and airways into the ventilatory response. The second group of neurons, which contains inspiratory and expiratory neurons, controls the spinal motor neurons of the intercostal and abdominal muscles.

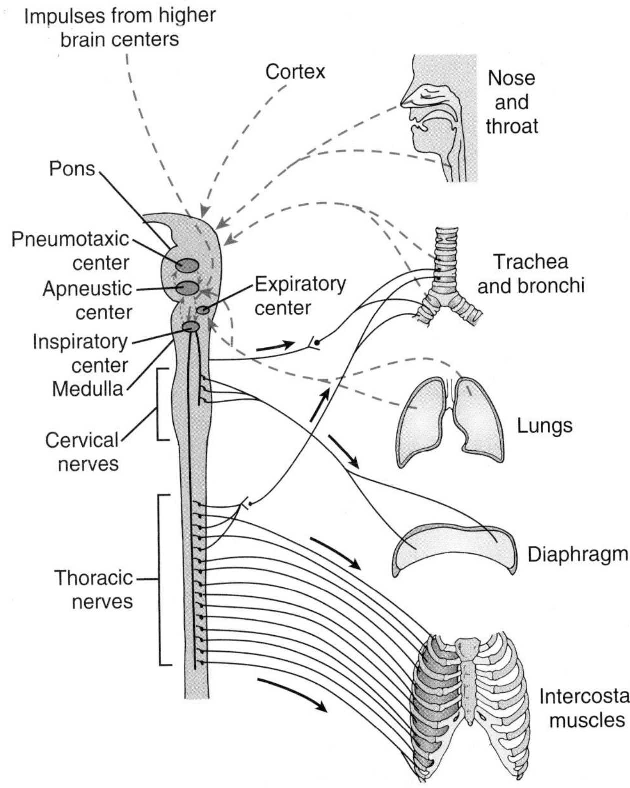

FIGURE 29-23 Schematic representation of activity in the respiratory center. Impulses traveling over afferent neurons activate central neurons, which activate efferent neurons that supply the muscles of respiration. Respiratory movements can be altered by a variety of stimuli.

The pacemaker properties of the respiratory center result from the cycling of the two groups of respiratory neurons: the *pneumotaxic center* in the upper pons and the *apneustic center* in the lower pons. These two groups of neurons contribute to the function of the respiratory center in the medulla. The apneustic center has an excitatory effect on inspiration, tending to prolong inspiration. The pneumotaxic center switches inspiration off, assisting in the control of respiratory rate and inspiratory volume. Brain injury that damages the connection between the pneumotaxic and apneustic centers results in an irregular breathing pattern that consists of prolonged inspiratory gasps interrupted by expiratory efforts.

Axons from the neurons in the respiratory center cross in the midline and descend in the ventrolateral columns of the spinal cord. The tracts that control expiration and inspiration are spatially separated in the cord, as are the tracts that transmit specialized reflexes (*i.e.*, coughing and hiccupping) and voluntary control of ventilation. Only at the level of the spinal cord are the respiratory impulses integrated to produce a reflex response. The neural control of ventilation is illustrated in Figure 29-23.

The control of breathing has automatic and voluntary components. The automatic regulation of ventilation is controlled by input from two types of sensors or receptors: chemoreceptors and lung receptors. Chemoreceptors monitor blood levels of oxygen, carbon dioxide, and pH and adjust ventilation to meet the changing metabolic needs of the body. Lung receptors monitor breathing patterns and lung function. Voluntary regulation of ventilation integrates breathing with voluntary acts such as speaking, blowing, and singing. These acts, which are initiated by the motor and premotor cortex, cause a temporary suspension of automatic breathing. The automatic and voluntary components of respiration are regulated by afferent impulses that come to the respiratory center from a number of sources. Afferent input from higher brain centers is evidenced by the fact that a person can consciously alter the depth and rate of respiration. Fever, pain, and emotion exert their influence through lower brain centers. Vagal afferents from sensory receptors in the lungs and airways are integrated in the dorsal area of the respiratory center. It has been suggested that alterations in the control of automatic and voluntary regulation of breathing may contribute to various forms of sleep apnea (see Chapter 13).

CHEMORECEPTORS

Tissue needs for oxygen and the removal of carbon dioxide are regulated by chemoreceptors that monitor blood levels of these gases. Input from these sensors is transmitted to the respiratory center, and ventilation is adjusted to maintain the arterial blood gases within a normal range.

There are two types of chemoreceptors: central and peripheral. The most important chemoreceptors for sensing changes in blood carbon dioxide content are the *central chemoreceptors*. These receptors are located in chemosensitive regions near the respiratory center in the medulla and are bathed in cerebrospinal fluid. Although the central chemoreceptors monitor carbon dioxide levels, the actual stimulus for these receptors is provided by hydrogen ions in the cerebrospinal fluid. This fluid is separated from the blood by the blood–brain barrier, which permits free diffusion of carbon dioxide but not bicarbonate or hydrogen ions. The carbon dioxide combines rapidly with water to form carbonic acid, which dissociates into hydrogen and bicarbonate ions. The carbon dioxide content in the blood regulates ventilation through its effect on the pH of the extracellular fluid of the brain. The central chemoreceptors are extremely sensitive to short-term changes in carbon dioxide. The effect of an increase in plasma carbon dioxide levels on ventilation reaches its peak within a minute or so and then declines if the carbon dioxide level remains elevated. Long-term elevation of the carbon dioxide level prompts a compensatory increase in bicarbonate secretion into the cerebrospinal fluid, which acts as a buffer for the hydrogen ions. Thus, persons with chronically elevated levels of carbon dioxide no longer respond to this stimulus for increased ventilation but rely on the stimulus provided by a decrease in blood oxygen levels.

The *peripheral chemoreceptors* are located in the carotid and aortic bodies, which are found at the bifurcation of the common carotid arteries and in the arch of the aorta, respectively. These chemoreceptors monitor arterial blood oxygen levels. Although the peripheral chemoreceptors also monitor carbon dioxide, they play a much more important role in monitoring oxygen levels. These receptors exert little control over ventilation until the PO_2 has dropped below 60 mm Hg. Hypoxia is the main stimulus for ventilation in persons with chronic hypercapnia. If these patients are given oxygen therapy at a level sufficient to increase the PO_2 above that needed to stimulate the peripheral chemoreceptors, their ventilation may be seriously depressed.

LUNG RECEPTORS

Lung and chest wall receptors provide information on the status of breathing in terms of airway resistance and lung expansion. There are three types of lung receptors: stretch, irritant, and juxtacapillary receptors.

Stretch receptors are located in the smooth muscle layers of the conducting airways. They respond to changes in pressure in the walls of the airways. When the lungs are inflated, these receptors inhibit inspiration and promote expiration (*i.e., Hering-Breuer reflex*). They are important in establishing breathing patterns and minimizing the work of breathing by adjusting respiratory rate and TV to accommodate changes in lung compliance and airway resistance.

The *irritant receptors* are located between the airway epithelial cells. They are stimulated by noxious gases, cigarette smoke, inhaled dust, and cold air. Stimulation of the irritant receptors leads to airway constriction and a pattern of rapid, shallow breathing. This pattern of breathing probably protects respiratory tissues from the damaging effects of toxic inhalants. It also is thought that the mechanical stimulation of these receptors may ensure more uniform lung expansion by initiating periodic sighing and yawning. It is possible that these receptors are involved in the bronchoconstriction response that occurs in some persons with bronchial asthma.

The *juxtacapillary* or *J receptors* are located in the alveolar wall, close to the pulmonary capillaries. It is thought that these receptors sense lung congestion. These receptors may be responsible for the rapid, shallow breathing that occurs with pulmonary edema, pulmonary embolism, and pneumonia.

COUGH REFLEX

Coughing is a neurally mediated reflex that protects the lungs from accumulation of secretions and from entry of irritating and destructive substances. It is one of the primary defense mechanisms of the respiratory tract. The cough reflex is initiated by receptors located in the tracheobronchial wall; these receptors are extremely sensitive to irritating substances and to the presence of excess secretions. Afferent impulses from these receptors are transmitted through the vagus to the medullary center, which integrates the cough response.

Coughing itself requires the rapid inspiration of a large volume of air (usually about 2.5 L), followed by rapid closure of the glottis and forceful contraction of the abdominal and expiratory muscles. As these muscles contract, intrathoracic pressures are elevated to levels of 100 mm Hg or more. The rapid opening of the glottis at this point leads to an explosive expulsion of air.

Many conditions can interfere with the cough reflex and its protective function. The reflex is impaired in persons whose abdominal or respiratory muscles are weak. This problem can be caused by disease conditions that lead to muscle weakness or paralysis, by prolonged inactivity, or as an outcome of surgery involving these muscles. Bed rest interferes with expansion of the chest and limits the amount of air that can be taken into the lungs in preparation for coughing, making the cough weak and ineffective. Disease conditions that prevent effective closure of the glottis and laryngeal muscles interfere with production of the marked increase in intrathoracic pressure that is needed for effective coughing. The presence of a nasogastric tube, for example, may prevent closure of the upper airway structures and may fatigue the receptors for the cough reflex that are located in the area. The cough reflex also is impaired when there is depressed function of the medullary centers in the brain that integrate the cough reflex. Interruption of the central integration aspect of the cough reflex can arise as the result of disease of this part of the brain or the action of drugs that depress the cough center.

Although the cough reflex is a protective mechanism, frequent and prolonged coughing can be exhausting and painful and can exert undesirable effects on the cardiovascular and respiratory systems and on the elastic tissues of the lungs. This is particularly true in young children and elderly persons.

DYSPNEA

Dyspnea is a subjective sensation or a person's perception of difficulty in breathing that includes the perception of labored breathing and the reaction to that sensation. The terms *dyspnea, breathlessness,* and *shortness of breath* often are used interchangeably. Dyspnea is observed in at least three major cardiopulmonary disease states: primary lung diseases such as pneumonia, asthma, and emphysema; heart disease that is characterized by pulmonary congestion; and neuromuscular disorders such as myasthenia gravis and muscular dystrophy that affect the respiratory muscles. Although dyspnea commonly is associated with respiratory disease, it also occurs during exercise, particularly in untrained persons.

The cause of dyspnea is unknown. Four types of mechanisms have been proposed to explain the sensation: stimulation of lung receptors; increased sensitivity to changes in ventilation perceived through central nervous system mechanisms; reduced ventilatory capacity or breathing reserve; and stimulation of neural receptors in the muscle fibers of the intercostals and diaphragm. The first of the suggested mechanisms is stimulation of lung receptors. These receptors are stimulated by the contraction of bronchial smooth muscle, the stretch of the bronchial wall, pulmonary congestion, and conditions that decrease lung compliance. The second category of proposed mechanisms focuses on central nervous system mechanisms that transmit information to the cortex regarding respiratory muscle weakness or a discrepancy between the increased effort of breathing and inadequate respiratory muscle contraction. The third type of mechanism focuses on a reduction in ventilatory capacity or breathing reserve. A reduction in breathing reserve (*i.e.,* maximum voluntary ventilation) to less than 65% to 75% usually correlates well with dyspnea. The fourth possible mechanism is stimulation of muscle and joint receptors in the chest wall because of a discrepancy in the tension generated by these muscles and the tidal volume that results. These receptors, once stimulated, transmit signals that bring about an awareness of the breathing discrepancy. Like other subjective symptoms, such as fatigue and pain, dyspnea is difficult to quantify because it relies on a person's perception of the problem.

The most common method for measuring dyspnea is a retrospective determination of the level of daily activity at which a person experiences dyspnea. Several scales are available for this use. One of these uses four grades of dyspnea to evaluate disability. The visual analog scale may be used to assess breathing difficulty that occurs with a given activity, such as walking a certain distance. The visual analog scale consists of a line (often 10 cm in length) with descriptors such as "easy to breathe" on one end and "very difficult to breathe" on the other. The person being assessed selects a point on the scale that describes his or her perceived dyspnea. It also can be used to assess dyspnea over time.

The treatment of dyspnea depends on the cause. For example, persons with impaired respiratory function may require oxygen therapy, and those with pulmonary edema may require measures to improve heart function. Methods to decrease anxiety, breathing retraining, and energy conservation measures may be used to decrease the subjective sensation of dyspnea.

In summary, the respiratory system requires continuous input from the nervous system. Movement of the diaphragm, intercostal muscles, and other respiratory muscles is controlled by neurons of the respiratory center located in the pons and medulla. The control of breathing has automatic and voluntary components. The automatic regulation of ventilation is controlled by two types of receptors: lung receptors, which protect respiratory structures, and chemoreceptors, which monitor the gas exchange function of the lungs by sensing changes in blood levels of carbon dioxide, oxygen, and pH. There are three types of lung receptors: stretch receptors, which monitor lung inflation; irritant receptors, which protect against the damaging effects of toxic inhalants; and J receptors, which are thought to sense lung congestion. There are two groups of chemoreceptors: central and peripheral. The central chemoreceptors are the most important in sensing changes in carbon dioxide levels, and the peripheral chemoreceptors function in sensing arterial blood oxygen levels.

Voluntary respiratory control is needed for integrating breathing and actions such as speaking, blowing, and singing. These acts, which are initiated by the motor and premotor cortex, cause temporary suspension of automatic breathing. The cough reflex protects the lungs from the accumulation of secretions and from the entry of irritating and destructive substances; it is one of the primary defense mechanisms of the respiratory tract. Dyspnea is a subjective sensation of difficulty in breathing.

REVIEW EXERCISES

Use the solubility coefficient for oxygen and the oxygen dissociation curve depicted in Figure 29-22 to answer the following questions:

A. What is the hemoglobin saturation at a high altitude in which the barometric pressure is 500 mm Hg (consider oxygen to represent 21% of the total gases)?

B. It is usually recommended that the hemoglobin saturation of persons with chronic lung disease be maintained at about 89% when they are receiving supplemental low-flow oxygen. What would their PO_2 be at this level of hemoglobin saturation, and what is the rationale for keeping the PO_2 at this level?

C. What is the oxygen content of a person with a hemoglobin of 6 g/dL who is breathing room air?

D. What is the oxygen content of a person with carbon monoxide poisoning who is receiving 100% oxygen at 3 atmospheres pressure in a hyperbaric chamber? Consider that most of the person's hemoglobin is saturated with carbon monoxide.

Bibliography

Berne R. M., Levy M. N. (2000). *Principles of physiology* (3rd ed., pp. 302–352). St. Louis: C. V. Mosby.

Caminiti S. P., Young S. (1991). The pulmonary surfactant system. *Hospital Practice 26*(1), 87–100.

Carrieri-Kohlman V., Stulbarg (2003). Dyspnea. In Carreri-Kohlman V., Lindsey A. M., West C. M. (Eds.), *Pathophysiological phenomena in nursing* (3rd ed., pp. 179–207). Philadelphia: W. B. Saunders.

Crapo R. O. (1994). Pulmonary function testing. *New England Journal of Medicine 331*, 25–30.

Fishman A. P. (1980). *Assessment of pulmonary function*. New York: McGraw-Hill.

Gartner L. P., Hiatt J. L. (2001). *Color textbook of histology* (2nd ed., pp. 343–364). Philadelphia: W. B. Saunders.

Guyton A., Hall J. E. (2000). *Textbook of medical physiology* (10th ed., pp. 432–482). Philadelphia: W. B. Saunders.

Moore K. L., Dalley A. F. (1999). *Clinically oriented anatomy* (4th ed., pp. 79–115). Philadelphia: Lippincott Williams & Wilkins.

Rhoades R. A., Tanner G. A. (2003). *Medical physiology* (2nd ed., pp. 309–375). Philadelphia: Lippincott Williams & Wilkins.

West J. B. (2000). *Respiratory physiology: The essentials*. Philadelphia: Lippincott Williams & Wilkins.

CHAPTER 30

Respiratory Tract Infections, Neoplasms, and Childhood Disorders

Respiratory illnesses represent one of the more common reasons for visits to the physician, admission to the hospital, and forced inactivity among all age groups. The common cold, although not usually serious, results in missed work and school days. Pneumonia is the sixth leading cause of death in the United States, particularly among the elderly and those with compromised immune function. Tuberculosis remains one of the deadliest diseases in the world. It has been estimated that between 19% and 43% of the world's population is infected with tuberculosis. Although the rate of tuberculosis infection in the United States has declined slightly since its resurgence in the early 1990s, there remain a large number of people who are infected; without effective treatment for latent infection, new cases can be expected to emerge from within this group. Lung cancer remains the leading cause of cancer death in the United States.

Respiratory Tract Infections

After completing this section of the chapter, you should be able to meet the following objectives:

- Describe the transmission of the common cold from one person to another
- Relate the characteristics of the influenza virus to its contagious properties and the need for a yearly "flu shot."
- Describe the causes, manifestations, and treatment of acute and chronic sinusitis
- Differentiate among community-acquired pneumonia, hospital-acquired pneumonia, and pneumonia in immunocompromised persons in terms of pathogens, manifestations, and prognosis

- Differentiate between primary tuberculosis and reactivated tuberculosis on the basis of their pathophysiology
- State the mechanism for the transmission of fungal infections of the lung

Respiratory tract infections can involve the upper respiratory tract (*i.e.*, nose, oropharynx, and larynx), the lower respiratory tract (*i.e.*, lower airways and lungs), or the upper and lower airways. The discussion in this section of the chapter focuses on the common cold, influenza, pneumonia, tuberculosis, and fungal infections of the lung. Acute respiratory infections in children are discussed in the last section of the chapter.

The respiratory tract is susceptible to infectious processes caused by many different types of microorganisms. For the most part, the signs and symptoms of respiratory tract infections depend on the function of the structure involved, the severity of the infectious process, and the person's age and general health status.

Viruses are the most frequent cause of respiratory tract infections. They can cause infections ranging from a self-limited cold to life-threatening pneumonia. Moreover, viral infections can damage bronchial epithelium, obstruct airways, and lead to secondary bacterial infections. Each viral species has its own pattern of respiratory tract involvement. The rhinoviruses grow best at 33°C to 35°C and remain strictly confined to the upper respiratory tract.[1] The influenza viruses can infect the upper and lower respiratory tracts. Measles and chickenpox viruses "pass through" the respiratory tract and do not cause respiratory symptoms until secondary viremic spread has occurred. Other microorganisms, such as bacteria (*e.g.*, pneumococci, staphylococci), mycobacteria (*e.g.*, *Mycobacterium tuberculosis*), fungi (*e.g.*, histoplasmosis, coccidioidomycosis, blastomycosis), and opportunistic organisms (*e.g.*, *Pneumocystis carinii*), also produce infections of the lung, many of which produce significant morbidity and mortality.

THE COMMON COLD

The common cold is a viral infection of the upper respiratory tract. It occurs more frequently than any other respiratory tract infection. Most adults have two to four colds per year; the average school child may have up to 10 per year.[2] The condition usually begins with a feeling of dryness and stuffiness affecting mainly the nasopharynx; it is accompanied by excessive production of nasal secretions and lacrimation, or tearing of the eyes. Usually, the secretions remain clear and watery. The mucous membranes of the upper respiratory tract become reddened, swollen, and bathed in secretions. Involvement of the pharynx and larynx causes sore throat and hoarseness. The affected person may experience headache and generalized malaise. In severe cases, there may be chills, fever, and exhaustion. The disease process is usually self-limited, lasting approximately 7 days.

Initially thought to be caused by either a single "cold virus" or a group of them, the common cold is now recognized to be associated with a number of viruses.[3,4] The most common of these are the rhinoviruses, parainfluenza viruses, respiratory syncytial virus, coronaviruses, and adenoviruses. The season of the year, age, and prior exposure are important factors in the type of virus causing the infection and the type of symptoms that occur. For example, outbreaks of colds due to rhinoviruses are most common in early fall and late spring; those due to respiratory syncytial virus peak in the winter and spring months; and infections due to the adenoviruses and coronaviruses are more frequent during the winter and spring months. Infections resulting from respiratory syncytial virus and parainfluenza viruses are most common and severe in children younger than 3 years of age. Infections occur less frequently and with milder symptoms with increasing age. Parainfluenza viruses often produce lower respiratory symptoms with first infections, but less severe upper respiratory symptoms with reinfections. The rhinoviruses are the most common cause of colds in persons between 5 and 40 years of age. There are more than 100 serotypes of rhinovirus.[4,5] Although people acquire lifetime immunity to an individual serotype, it would take a long time to become immune to all serotypes.

The cold viruses are rapidly spread from person to person. Children are the major reservoir of cold viruses, often acquiring a new virus from another child in school or day care.[3] The first step in the spreading of the common cold is the shedding of viruses, the area of greatest potential being the nasal mucosa. The fingers are the greatest source of spread, and the nasal mucosa and conjunctival surface of the eyes are the most common portals of entry of the virus. The most highly contagious period is during the first 3 days after the onset of symptoms, and the incubation period is approximately 5 days. Cold viruses have been found to survive for more than 5 hours on the skin and hard surfaces, such as plastic countertops.[4,5] Aerosol spread of colds through coughing and sneezing is much less important than the spread by fingers picking up the virus from contaminated surfaces and carrying it to the nasal membranes and eyes.[6] This suggests that careful attention to hand washing is one of the most important preventive measures for avoiding the common cold. Host defenses also influence the development of the common cold. Psychological stress, which is thought to influence immune function, is reported to increase the risk for development of a cold.[7]

Many over-the-counter (OTC) remedies are available for treating the common cold. Because the common cold is an acute and self-limited illness in persons who are otherwise healthy, symptomatic treatment with rest and antipyretic drugs is usually all that is needed. Antibiotics are ineffective against viral infections and are not recommended. There is some controversy about the use of vitamin C to reduce the incidence and severity of colds and influenza. Some studies have found vitamin C intake to be beneficial, and others have found it to be of questionable value.[8] Zinc lozenges are also marketed as an OTC remedy for colds. As with vitamin C, some studies have shown the lozenges to be beneficial, and others have not.[8,9]

Antihistamines are popular OTC drugs because of their action in drying nasal secretions. However, they may dry up bronchial secretions and worsen the cough, and they may cause dizziness, drowsiness, and impaired judgment.

As with vitamin C, there is no evidence that they shorten the duration of the cold. Decongestant drugs (*i.e.,* sympathomimetic agents) are available in OTC nasal sprays, drops, and oral cold medications. These drugs constrict the blood vessels in the swollen nasal mucosa and reduce nasal swelling. Rebound nasal swelling can occur with indiscriminate use of nasal drops and sprays. Oral preparations containing decongestants may cause systemic vasoconstriction and elevation of blood pressure when given in doses large enough to relieve nasal congestion, and they should be avoided by persons with hypertension, heart disease, hyperthyroidism, diabetes mellitus, or other health problems.

Efforts to develop vaccines against the cold viruses have been largely unsuccessful, mainly because of the number of viruses involved and their large array of serotypes. Recently, investigators have isolated a receptor (intracellular adhesion molecule-1) on the respiratory epithelial cells that is the site of attachment for most of the rhinovirus serotypes. Identification of this receptor molecule provides a target for development of pharmacologic interventions. A recombinant, soluble form of a glycoprotein, known as *tremacamra,* has been developed to inhibit adhesion of the rhinovirus to the receptor and thus reduce the severity of infection in exposed persons.[10]

RHINOSINUSITIS

Rhinitis refers to inflammation of the nasal mucosa and sinusitis to inflammation of the paranasal sinuses. The paranasal sinuses are air cells that are connected by narrow openings or *ostia* with the superior, middle, and inferior nasal turbinates of the nasal cavity (Fig. 30-1). Each sinus is named for the bone in which it occurs—frontal, ethmoid, sphenoid, and maxillary. The *maxillary sinus* is inferior to the bony orbit and superior to the hard palate, and its opening is located superiorly and medially in the sinus, a location that impedes drainage. The *frontal sinuses* open into the middle meatus of the nasal cavity. The *sphenoid sinus* is just anterior to the pituitary fossa behind the posterior ethmoid sinuses, and its paired openings drain into the sphenoethmoidal recess at the top of the nasal cavity. The *ethmoid sinuses* comprise 3 to 15 air cells on each side, with each maintaining a separate path to the nasal chamber.

The sinus mucosa is similar to that of the respiratory tract and nasal passages. Ciliated mucous membranes help move fluid and microorganisms out of the sinuses and into the nasal cavity. Nasal swelling that obstructs the sinus openings and impairs mucociliary function is thought to be a major cause of sinus infections. The lower oxygen content in the sinuses facilitates the growth of organisms, impairs local defenses, and alters the function of immune cells.

The most common causes of rhinosinusitis are conditions that obstruct the narrow ostia that drain the sinuses. Most commonly, rhinosinusitis develops when upper respiratory tract infection or allergic rhinitis narrows the ostia and obstructs flow of mucus. Nasal polyps also can obstruct the sinus opening and facilitate sinus infection. Infections associated with nasal polyps can be self-perpetuating because constant irritation from infection can facilitate growth of the polyps. Barotrauma caused

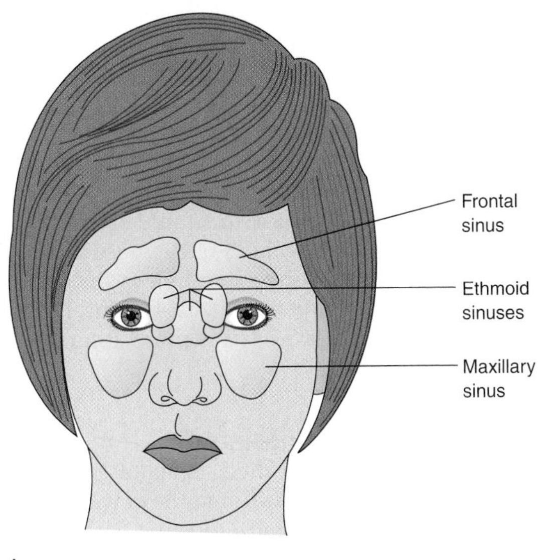

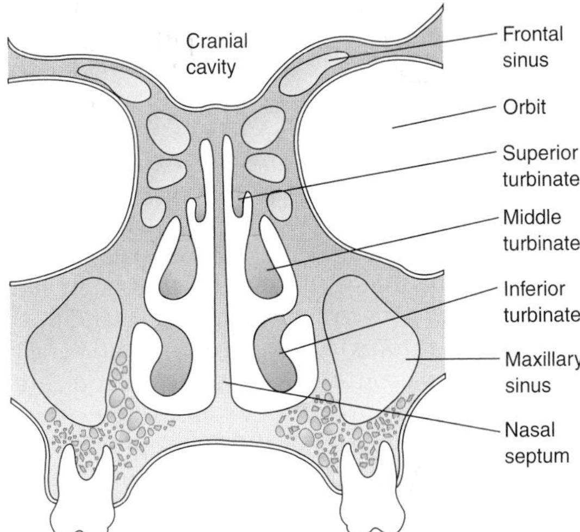

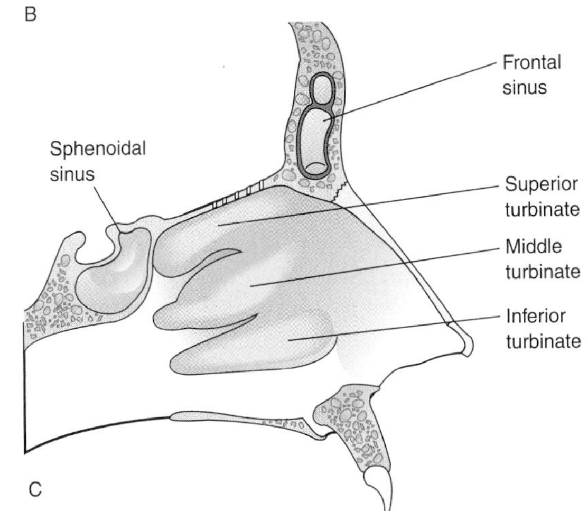

FIGURE 30-1 Paranasal sinuses. **(A)** Frontal view; **(B)** cross-section of nasal cavity, anterior view; **(C)** lateral wall, left nasal cavity. (Courtesy of Carole Russell Hilmer, C.M.I.)

by changes in barometric pressure, as occurs in airline pilots and flight attendants, may lead to impaired sinus ventilation and clearance of secretions. Swimming, diving, and abuse of nasal decongestants are other causes of sinus irritation and impaired drainage.

Historically, acute sinusitis was considered a bacterial infection that most commonly developed as a complication of a viral upper respiratory tract infection or rhinitis. Because the mucous membranes of the nose and sinuses are contiguous, current understanding is that sinus involvement occurs regularly with a viral rhinitis, indicating that the term *acute rhinosinusitis* is more accurate in describing the infection.[11,12]

Acute and Chronic Rhinosinusitis

Rhinosinusitis can be classified as acute, subacute, or chronic.[11–13] Acute rhinosinusitis may be of viral, bacterial, or mixed viral-bacterial origin and may last from 5 to 7 days, as in the case of acute viral rhinosinusitis, or up to 4 weeks, as in the case of acute bacterial rhinosinusitis. Subacute rhinosinusitis lasts from 4 weeks to less than 12 weeks, whereas chronic rhinosinusitis lasts beyond 12 weeks.

The symptoms of acute viral rhinosinusitis usually resolve within 5 to 7 days without medical treatment. Acute bacterial rhinosinusitis is suggested by symptoms that worsen after 5 days or persist beyond 10 days or symptoms that are out of proportion to those usually associated with a viral upper respiratory tract infection. Symptoms often are difficult to differentiate from those of the common cold and allergic rhinitis. They include facial pain, headache, purulent nasal discharge, decreased sense of smell, and fever. A history of a preceding common cold and the presence of purulent rhinitis, pain on bending, unilateral maxillary pain, and pain in the teeth are common findings with involvement of the maxillary sinuses. Recurrent acute rhinosinusitis is defined as four or more episodes of acute disease within a 12-month period.

In persons with chronic rhinosinusitis, the only symptoms may be those such as nasal obstruction, a sense of fullness in the ears, postnasal drip, hoarseness, chronic cough, loss of taste and smell, or unpleasant breath.[14] Sinus pain often is absent; instead, the person may complain of a headache that is dull and constant. Persons who are immunocompromised, such as those with leukemia, aplastic anemia, a bone marrow transplant, primary immunodeficiency disease, or human immunodeficiency virus (HIV) infection, often present with fever of unknown origin, rhinorrhea, or facial edema. Often, other signs of inflammation such as purulent drainage are absent.

Persons with chronic rhinosinusitis may have superimposed bouts of acute rhinosinusitis. The epithelial changes that occur during acute and subacute forms of rhinosinusitis usually are reversible, but the mucosal changes that occur with chronic rhinosinusitis often are irreversible.

Etiology. In adults, acute bacterial rhinosinusitis most commonly results from infection with *Haemophilus influenzae* or *Streptococcus pneumoniae*.[11–13] In chronic rhinosinusitis, anaerobic organisms, including species of *Peptostreptococcus*, *Fusobacterium*, and *Prevotella*, tend to predominate, alone or in combination with aerobes such as the *Streptococcus* species or *Staphylococcus aureus*. In immunocompromised persons, such as those with HIV infection, the sinuses may become infected with gram-negative species and opportunistic fungi. In this group, particularly those with leukopenia, the disease may have a fulminant and even fatal course.

Hospital-acquired rhinosinusitis is more often caused by different microbial agents than community-acquired rhinosinusitis. In the hospital, *S. aureus*, *Pseudomonas* species, *Klebsiella* species, and other gram-negative organisms predominate. Hospital-acquired infections are commonly polymicrobial. Predisposing factors include irritation from endotracheal tubes, nasogastric tubes, and nasal packing and the use of corticosteroids and other immunosuppressant drugs.

Diagnosis and Treatment. The diagnosis of rhinosinusitis usually is based on symptom history and a physical examination that includes inspection of the nose and throat. Headache due to sinusitis needs to be differentiated from other types of headache. Sinusitis headache usually is exaggerated by bending forward, coughing, or sneezing. Diagnostic nasal endoscopy, which is done in the office of an otolaryngologist, provides a clear view of the anterior nasal cavity and sinus openings.[11] It is usually indicated in persons with rhinosinusitis who do not respond to therapy as expected. Sinus radiographs and computed tomography (CT) scans may be used. CT scans usually are reserved for diagnosis of chronic rhinosinusitis or to exclude complications. Magnetic resonance imagining (MRI) is expensive and reserved for cases of suspected neoplasms or intracranial lesions.[14]

Treatment of rhinosinusitis includes appropriate antibiotic therapy, depending on whether the infection is community acquired or hospital acquired, or occurs in an immunocompromised person. The duration of antibiotic therapy is longer for chronic rhinosinusitis than for acute rhinosinusitis. In addition to antibiotic therapy, the treatment of acute rhinosinusitis includes measures to promote adequate drainage by reducing nasal congestion. Oral and topical decongestants and antihistamines may be used for this purpose. Oral decongestants constrict nasal blood vessels, decrease tissue congestion, and facilitate drainage. The use of intranasal decongestants should be limited to 3 to 5 days to prevent rebound vasodilatation.[13] The use of antihistamines is controversial, particularly for acute rhinosinusitis, because they can dry up secretions and thereby decrease drainage. Mucolytic agents such as guaifenesin may be used to thin secretions. Topical corticosteroids may be used to decrease inflammation in persons with allergic rhinitis or rhinosinusitis. Nonpharmacologic measures include saline nasal sprays and steam inhalations.

Surgical intervention directed at correcting obstruction of the ostiomeatal openings may be indicated in persons with chronic rhinosinusitis that is resistant to other forms of therapy. Indications for surgical intervention include obstructive nasal polyps and obstructive nasal deformities.

Complications. Because of the sinuses' proximity to the brain and orbital wall, sinusitis can lead to intracranial and orbital wall complications. Intracranial complications are seen most commonly with infection of the frontal and ethmoid sinuses because of their proximity to the dura and drainage of the veins from the frontal sinus into the dural sinus. Orbital complications can range from edema of the eyelids to orbital cellulitis and subperiosteal abscess formation. Orbital involvement can result in exophthalmos, edema of the ocular conjunctiva, and visual impairment. Involvement of nerves supplying the extraocular muscles can lead to ophthalmoplegia. In persons with ethmoid sinusitis, infection can extend to the nasolacrimal gland, causing obstruction and tearing.

Allergic Rhinoconjunctivitis

Allergic rhinosinusitis occurs in conjunction with allergic rhinitis. The mucosal changes are the same as those seen in allergic rhinitis. Symptoms usually consist of nasal stuffiness, itching and burning of the nose, frequent bouts of sneezing, recurrent frontal headache, and a watery nasal discharge. Headache located in the frontal area between the eyes is a common symptom. Treatment includes oral antihistamines, nasal decongestants, and intranasal cromolyn. Persistent symptoms may be treated with nasal corticosteroids and severe symptoms with oral corticosteroids.[15]

Hypersensitivity to aspirin is present in 5% to 10% of persons with bronchial asthma and is associated with chronic rhinosinusitis and nasal polyps; the constellation of aspirin hypersensitivity, nasal polyps, and asthma is often referred to as the *aspirin triad*.[16] A positive history of aspirin hypersensitivity, which is the hallmark for the syndrome, is a significant and reliable indicator of chronic rhinosinusitis, nasal polyps, and persistent asthma requiring higher than normal medication requirements. The mechanism of the hypersensitivity reaction is not immunologic, but is related to the inhibition of cyclooxygenase, an enzyme necessary for prostaglandin synthesis. Avoidance of aspirin and all nonsteroidal anti-inflammatory drugs (NSAIDs) is a necessary part of the treatment program. Careful management of the rhinosinusitis is a prerequisite for improvement of bronchial symptoms. Topical corticosteroids are highly effective in relieving the symptoms. Dependent upon the stage of the disease, surgery may be used to remove the polyps. However, surgery does not affect the underlying inflammatory process; topical steroid therapy is also necessary following surgery.

INFLUENZA

Influenza is a viral infection that is arguably the most important cause of acute upper respiratory tract infection in humans. Until the advent of acquired immunodeficiency syndrome (AIDS), it was the last uncontrolled pandemic killer of humans. In the United States, approximately 36,000 persons die each year of influenza-related illness during nonpandemic years.[17] Rates of infection are highest among children, but rates of serious illness and death are highest among persons who are 65 years of age or older.

The viruses that cause influenza belong to the *orthomyxoviridae* family, which consists of a segmented, single-stranded ribonucleic acid (RNA) genome.[18] There are two types of influenza viruses that cause epidemics in humans: types A and B. Type A, which is most common and causes the most severe disease, is further divided into subtypes based on two surface antigens: hemagglutinin (H) and neuraminidase (N). Influenza B has not been categorized into subtypes.[17,18] Influenza A differs in its ability to infect multiple species, including avian and mammalian species. Although avian strains occasionally cause outbreaks of disease in humans, a reassortment of human and avian influenza usually occurs in an intermediate host such as pigs. In this setting, a virus is produced that contains determinants of human infection as well as avian characteristics to which humans may not be immune. It is noteworthy that many of the pandemics of the past were thought to arise in Asia, where large human populations live in close proximity to ducks, chickens, and pigs, thus facilitating the phenomenon of viral reassortment.[19] The current nomenclature for influenza A provides the host of origin, the geographic location of the first isolation, the year of isolation, the surface antigen, and the strain number (*e.g.*, equine/Miami/1/63/H3N8).[18]

As with many viral respiratory tract infections, influenza is more contagious than bacterial respiratory tract infections. Transmission is by aerosol or direct contact. Inhalation of as few as three infective particles can transmit the infection.[20] Most infected people develop symptoms of the disease, increasing the likelihood of contagion. Young children are most likely to become infected and also to spread the infection. Contagion of influenza results from the ability of the virus to develop new subtypes that the population is not protected against. New variants result from frequent mutations or antigenic changes in the H and N surface antigens. An *antigenic shift,* which involves a major change in either antigen, may lead to epidemic or pandemic infection. Lesser changes, called *antigenic drift,* find the population partially protected by cross-reacting antibodies. Influenza B undergoes less frequent shifts than influenza A.

The incubation period for influenza is 1 to 4 days, with 2 days being the average. Persons become infectious starting 1 day before their symptoms begin and remain infectious through approximately 5 days after illness onset.[17] Children can be infectious for greater than 10 days, and young children can shed virus for up to 6 days before their illness onset. Severely immunocompromised persons can shed virus for weeks or months.

The influenza viruses can cause three types of infections: an uncomplicated rhinotracheitis, viral pneumonia, and a respiratory viral infection followed by a bacterial infection. In the early stages, the symptoms of influenza often are indistinguishable from other viral infections. There is an abrupt onset of fever and chills, malaise, muscle aching, headache, profuse watery nasal discharge, nonproductive cough, and sore throat.[17,21,22] One distinguishing feature of an influenza viral infection is the rapid onset, sometimes in as little as 1 to 2 minutes, of profound malaise. The symptoms of uncomplicated rhinotracheitis usually peak by days 3 to 5 and disappear by days 7 to 10. The infection causes necrosis and shedding of the serous and ciliated cells that line the respiratory tract, leaving gaping holes between the underlying basal cells and allowing extracellular fluid to escape. This is the reason for the "runny nose" that is characteristic of this phase of the infection. During recovery, the serous cells are replaced more rapidly than the ciliated cells. Mucus is produced, but the ciliated cells are unable to move it adequately; people recovering from influenza must continue to blow their nose and cough to clear the airways.

Primary viral pneumonia occurs as a complication of influenza, most frequently in the elderly or in persons with cardiopulmonary disease, but has been reported in pregnant women and in healthy immunocompetent people. It typically develops within 1 day after onset of influenza and is characterized by rapid progression of fever, tachypnea, tachycardia, cyanosis, and hypotension.[22,23] The clinical course of influenza pneumonia progresses rapidly. It can cause hypoxemia and death within a few days of onset. Survivors often develop diffuse pulmonary fibrosis.[23]

Secondary complications typically include sinusitis, otitis media, bronchitis, and bacterial pneumonia. Reye's syndrome (fatty liver with encephalitis) is a rare complication of influenza, particularly in young children.[23] It is most commonly associated with aspirin use during a viral infection such as influenza. Persons who develop secondary bacterial pneumonia usually report that they were beginning to feel better when they experienced a return of fever, shaking chills, pleuritic chest pain, and productive cough. The most common causes of secondary bacterial pneumonia are *Streptococcus pneumoniae, Staphylococcus aureus, Haemophilus influenzae,* and *Moraxella catarrhalis*. This form of pneumonia commonly produces less cyanosis and tachypnea and is usually milder than primary influenza pneumonia. Influenza-related deaths can result from pneumonia as well as exacerbations of cardiopulmonary conditions and other disease. Older adults account for 90% or more of deaths attributed to pneumonia.[17]

Diagnosis and Treatment

The appropriate treatment of people with influenza depends on accurate and timely diagnosis. The early diagnosis can reduce the inappropriate use of antibiotics and provide the opportunity for use of an antiviral drug. Rapid diagnostic tests, which are available for use in outpatient settings, allow health care providers to diagnose influenza more accurately, consider treatment options more carefully, and monitor influenza type and its prevalence in their community.[24]

The goals of treatment for influenza are designed to limit the infection to the upper respiratory tract. The symptomatic approach for treatment of uncomplicated influenza rhinotracheitis focuses on rest, keeping warm, and drinking large amounts of liquids. Analgesics and cough medications can also be used. Rest decreases the oxygen requirements of the body and reduces the respiratory rate and the chance of spreading the virus from the upper to lower respiratory tract. Keeping warm helps maintain the respiratory epithelium at a core body temperature of 37°C (or higher if fever is present), thereby inhibiting viral replication, which is optimal at 35°C. Drinking large amounts of liquids ensures that the function of the epithelial lining of the respiratory tract is not further compromised by dehydration. Antiviral medications may be indicated in some persons. Antibacterial antibiotics should be reserved for bacterial complications. The use of aspirin to treat fever should be avoided in children.

Antiviral Drugs. Four antiviral drugs are available for treatment of influenza: amantadine, rimantadine, zanamivir, and oseltamivir.[25,26] The first-generation antiviral drugs amantadine and rimantadine are similarly effective against influenza A but not influenza B. These agents inhibit the uncoating of viral RNA in the host cells and prevent its replication. Both drugs are effective in prevention of influenza A in high-risk groups and in treatment of persons who acquire the disease. Unfortunately, resistance to the drugs develops rapidly and strains that are resistant to amantadine also are resistant to rimantadine. Amantadine stimulates release of catecholamines, which can produce central nervous system side effects such as anxiety, depression, and insomnia.

The second-generation antiviral drugs zanamivir and oseltamivir are inhibitors of neuraminidase, a viral glycoprotein that is necessary for viral replication and release. These drugs, which have been approved for treatment of acute uncomplicated influenza infection, are effective against both influenza A and B viruses. Zanamivir and oseltamivir result in less resistance than amantadine and rimantadine. Zanamivir is administered intranasally and oseltamivir is administered orally. Zanamivir can cause bronchospasm and is not recommended for persons with asthma or chronic obstructive lung disease. To be effective, the antiviral drugs should be initiated within 30 hours after onset of symptoms.

Influenza Immunization. Because influenza is so highly contagious, prevention relies primarily on vaccination.[27,28] Currently, there are two types of influenza vaccines available: the trivalent inactivated influenza vaccine (TIIV), which was developed in the 1940s, and the live, attenuated influenza vaccine (LAIV), which was approved for use in 2003.[29] The formulation of the vaccines must be changed yearly in response to antigenic changes in the influenza virus. The Centers for Disease Control and Prevention (CDC) Advisory Committee on Immunization Practices (ACIP) annually updates its recommendations for the composition of the vaccine.

The TIIV, which is administered by injection, has become the mainstay for prevention of influenza. It has proved to be inexpensive and effective in reducing illness caused by influenza.

Immunization is recommended for high-risk groups who, because of their age or underlying health problems, are unable to cope well with the infection and often require medical attention, including hospitalization. The effectiveness of the influenza vaccine in preventing and lessening the effects of influenza infection depend primarily on the age and immunocompetence of the recipient and the match between the virus strains included in the vaccine and those that circulate during the influenza season.[17] When there is a good match, the vaccine is effective in preventing the illness in approximately 70% to 90% of healthy persons younger than 65 years of age.[17]

The ACIP recommends annual immunization using inactivated influenza vaccine to prevent or minimize the effect of influenza infections in any person 6 months of age or older who is at high risk for complications of influenza.[17] Groups at highest risk for complications include persons 50 years of age or older; residents of nursing homes or other chronic care facilities housing persons of any age with chronic medical conditions; adults or children with chronic disorders of the pulmonary or cardiovascular systems, including children with asthma; adults and children who have required regular medical follow-up or hospitalization during the preceding year because of chronic metabolic diseases (*e.g.*, diabetes mellitus), renal dysfunction, hemoglobinopathies (*e.g.*, sickle cell anemia), or immunosuppression (including immunosuppression caused by medications or by HIV infection); children or teenagers (6 months to 18 years) who are receiving long-term aspirin therapy (because of the risk for development of Reye's syndrome); and women who will be in the second or third trimester of pregnancy during the influenza season. Because the influenza vaccine is an inactivated vaccine, it is thought to be safe during pregnancy.[17] Immunization also is recommended for groups (*e.g.*, household members, health care workers) who live with or care for persons who are at high risk for development of influenza complications. It is believed that the protection of persons in the high-risk groups can be improved by reducing the chances of exposure to influenza from household contacts and health care providers. Vaccination is contraindicated for persons who have a history of anaphylactic hypersensitivity to egg or other components of the vaccine.

The LAIV, which is administered intranasally, has been approved for use in healthy persons aged 5 to 49 years.[29] The LAIVs are in use in Russia and have been in development in the United States since the 1960s. The LAIVs are cold-adapted viruses that replicate efficiently in the 25°C temperatures of the nasopharynx, inducing protective immunity against viruses included in the vaccine, but replicate inefficiently at 38°C to 39°C of the lower airways.

PNEUMONIAS

The term *pneumonia* describes inflammation of parenchymal structures of the lung, such as the alveoli and the bronchioles. An estimated 2 to 3 million cases occur annually in the United States each year.[30,31] Pneumonia is the sixth leading cause of death in the United States and the most common cause of death from infectious disease.[32,33] Etiologic agents include infectious and noninfectious agents. Although much less common than infectious pneumonia, inhalation of irritating fumes or aspiration of gastric contents can result in severe pneumonia.

Although antibiotics have significantly reduced the mortality rate from pneumonias, these diseases remain an important immediate cause of death of the elderly and persons with debilitating diseases. There have been subtle changes in the spectrum of microorganisms that cause infectious pneumonias, including a decrease in pneumonias caused by *S. pneumoniae* and an increase in pneumonias caused by other microorganisms such as *Pseudomonas*, *Candida* and other fungi, and nonspecific viruses. Many of these pneumonias occur in persons with impaired immune defenses, including persons who are on immunosuppressant drugs to prevent rejection of a bone marrow or organ transplant. *P. carinii* pneumonia, a virulent type of infection, is associated with AIDS (see Chapter 22).

Pathogenesis

Bacteria commonly enter the lower airways but do not normally cause pneumonia because of extensive defense mechanisms. When pneumonia does occur, it usually is because of an exceedingly virulent organism, large inoculum, or impaired host defenses. In nonhospitalized persons, bacteria reach the lung by one of four routes: inhalation from the ambient air, aspiration from the previously colonized upper airway, direct spread from contiguous infected sites, or hematogenous spread. Critically ill patients may acquire organisms from colonized nasogastric tubes or from an endotracheal tube.

Most of the agents that cause pneumonia and lower respiratory tract infections are aspirated from the tracheobronchial tree or inhaled into the lung along with the air breathed. Most persons unknowingly aspirate small amounts of organisms that have colonized their upper airways, particularly during sleep. Normally, these organisms do not cause infection because of the small numbers that are aspirated and because of the respiratory tract's defense mechanisms (Table 30-1). After bacteria reach the lower airways, they encounter a number of host defenses that prevent them from entering the lung and causing pneumonia. Loss of the cough reflex, damage to the ciliated endothelium that lines the respiratory tract, or impaired immune defenses predispose to colonization and infection of the lower respiratory system. Immune defenses include the bronchial-associated lymphoid tissue, phagocytic cells (*i.e.*, polymorphonuclear cells and macrophages), immunoglobulins (*i.e.*, IgA and IgG), and T-cell–mediated cellular

PNEUMONIAS

- Pneumonias are respiratory disorders involving inflammation of the lung structures, such as the alveoli and bronchioles.
- Pneumonia can be caused by infectious agents such as bacteria and viruses and noninfectious agents such as gastric secretions that are aspirated into the lungs.
- The development of pneumonia is facilitated by an exceedingly virulent organism, large inoculum, and impaired host defenses.
- Pneumonias due to infectious agents commonly are classified according to the source of infection (community- vs. hospital-acquired) and according to the immune status of the host (pneumonia in the immunocompromised person).

TABLE 30-1 Respiratory Defense Mechanisms and Conditions That Impair Their Effectiveness

Defense Mechanism	Function	Factors That Impair Effectiveness
Nasopharyngeal defenses	Remove particles from the air; contact with surface lysosomes and immunoglobulins (IgA) protects against infection	IgA deficiency state, hay fever, common cold, trauma to the nose
Glottic and cough reflexes	Protect against aspiration into tracheobronchial tree	Loss of cough reflex due to stroke or neural lesion, neuromuscular disease, abdominal or chest surgery, depression of the cough reflex due to sedation or anesthesia, presence of a nasogastric tube (tends to cause adaptation of afferent receptors)
Mucociliary blanket	Removes secretions, microorganisms, and particles from the respiratory tract	Smoking, viral diseases, chilling, inhalation of irritating gases
Pulmonary macrophages	Remove microorganisms and foreign particles from the lung	Chilling, alcohol intoxication, smoking, hypoxia

immunity (see Chapter 19). Bacterial adherence also plays a role in colonization of the lower airways. The epithelial cells of critically and chronically ill persons are more receptive to binding microorganisms that cause pneumonia. Other clinical risk factors favoring colonization of the tracheobronchial tree include antibiotic therapy that alters the normal bacterial flora, diabetes, smoking, chronic bronchitis, and viral infection.

Until recently, pneumonias have been classified as typical (*i.e.,* bacterial) or atypical (*i.e.,* viral or mycoplasmal) pneumonias. Bacterial pneumonia results from infection by bacteria that multiply extracellularly in the alveoli and cause inflammation and exudation of fluid into the air-filled spaces of the alveoli (Fig. 30-2A). It is characterized by chills and fever, severe malaise, purulent sputum, elevated white blood cell counts, and patchy or lobar infiltrates seen on the chest radiograph. Atypical pneumonias produce patchy inflammatory changes that are confined to the alveolar septum and the interstitium of the lung (see Fig. 30-2B). They produce less striking symptoms and physical findings than bacterial pneumonia; there is a lack of alveolar infiltration and purulent sputum, leukocytosis, and lobar consolidation on the radiograph.

Because of the overlap in symptomatology and changing spectrum of infectious organisms involved, pneumonias are increasingly being classified as community-acquired and hospital-acquired pneumonias. Persons with compromised immune function constitute a special concern in both categories.

Community-Acquired Pneumonia

The term *community-acquired pneumonia* is used to describe infections from organisms found in the community rather than in the hospital or nursing home. It is defined as an infection that begins outside the hospital or is diagnosed within 48 hours after admission to the hospital in a person who has not resided in a long-term care facility for 14 days or more before admission.[30]

The most common cause of infection in all categories is *S. pneumoniae*.[34] Other common pathogens include *Haemophilus influenzae, S. aureus,* and gram-negative bacilli. Less common agents are *Moraxella catarrhalis, Klebsiella pneumoniae,* and *Neisseria meningitidis. Legionella* species, *Mycoplasma pneumoniae,* and *Chlamydia pneumoniae* (strain TWAR), sometimes called *atypical agents,* account for 20% to 40% of all cases.[32] Common viral causes of community-acquired pneumonia include the influenza virus, respiratory syncytial virus, adenovirus, and parainfluenza virus.

There are several different systems for classifying community-acquired pneumonia based on factors such as age, preexisting health care status, and severity of illness. Guidelines developed by the American Thoracic Society divide persons with community-acquired pneumonia into four categories based on severity of illness, presence of coexisting disease, age, and need for hospitalization.[35] The categories are (1) persons without cardiopulmonary disease or other modifying factors that can be treated on an outpatient basis; (2) persons with cardiopulmonary disease (congestive heart failure or chronic obstructive pulmonary disease) or other modifying factors (risk factors for drug-resistant *S. pneumoniae* or gram-negative bacteria) who can be treated on an outpatient basis; (3) persons who require hospitalization but not admission to the intensive care unit (ICU), including those with cardiopulmonary disease, those with other modifying factors such as coming from a nursing home, or those requiring special therapy because of the type of infectious organism causing the infection; and (4) persons who require admission to the ICU either because of cardiopulmonary disease or type of infectious organism causing the infection. The infecting organisms can remain confined to the lungs, as in persons in the first category, or they can cause bacteremia and sepsis. The mortality rate for persons in the first category is low (1% to 2%) compared with the fourth category, which requires admission to the intensive care unit and for which the mortality rate can be as high as 25%.[35]

The signs and symptoms of pneumonia vary from fever, general malaise, chest discomfort, and a cough to those of respiratory compromise with a respiratory rate above 30 breaths per minute, signs of hemoglobin desaturation

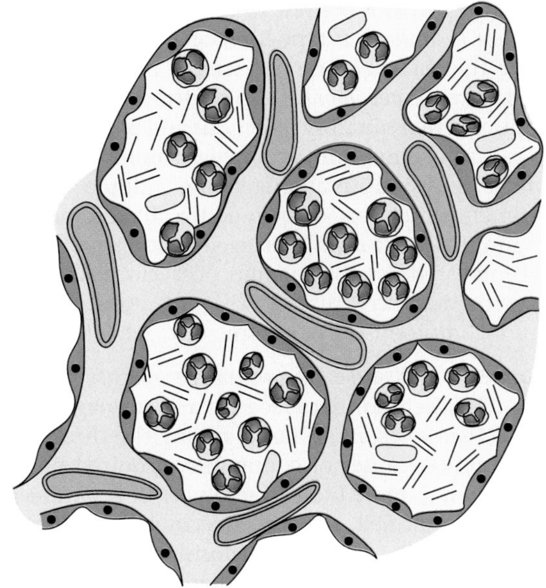

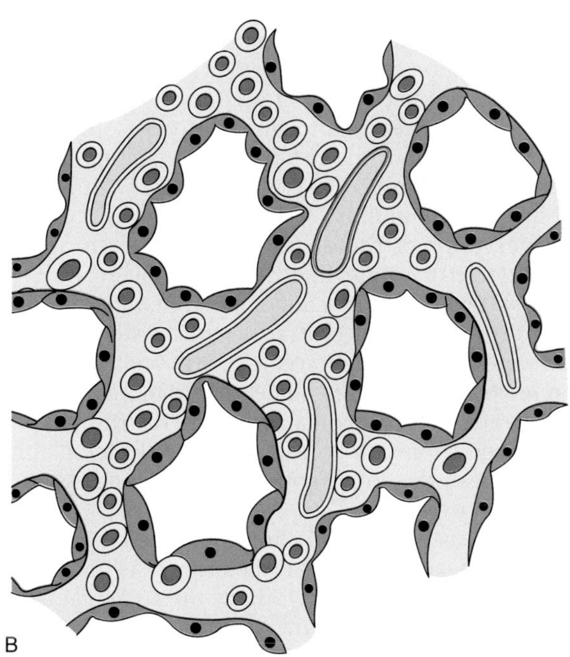

FIGURE 30-2 Location of inflammatory processes in (**A**) typical and (**B**) atypical forms of pneumonia.

and respiratory failure, and evidence of sepsis or shock (see Chapter 28).

The type and extent of tests used in diagnosis depend on the severity of illness. In persons younger than 65 years of age and without coexisting disease, the diagnosis usually is based on history and physical examination, chest radiographs, and knowledge of the microorganisms currently causing infections in the community. Sputum specimens may be obtained for staining procedures and culture. Blood cultures may be done for persons requiring hospitalization. Diagnostic measures may include procedures such as fiberoptic bronchoscopy, which is done to obtain samples of lower respiratory tract secretions for identifying the pathogen, particularly in severely ill persons and those who are unresponsive to antimicrobial therapy. Thoracentesis may be used to obtain specimens of pleural fluid when the infection extends into the pleural cavity.

Treatment involves the use of appropriate antibiotic therapy. Empiric therapy, based on knowledge regarding an antibiotic's spectrum of action and ability to penetrate bronchopulmonary secretions, often is used for persons with community-acquired pneumonia who do not require hospitalization. Hospitalization and more intensive care may be required depending on the person's age, preexisting health status, and severity of the infection.

Pneumococcal Pneumonia. *S. pneumoniae* (pneumococcus) remains the most common cause of bacterial pneumonia. *S. pneumoniae* colonizes the upper respiratory system and, in addition to pneumonia and lower respiratory tract infections, the organism is an important cause of upper respiratory infections, including sinusitis and otitis media, and of disseminated invasive infections such as bacteremia and meningitis.[36] Worldwide it is among the leading causes of illness and death of young children, persons with other health problems, and the elderly worldwide.

S. pneumoniae is a gram-positive diplococcus, possessing a capsule of polysaccharide. There are 90 serologically distinct types of *S. pneumoniae* based on the antigenic properties of their capsular polysaccharides. The virulence of the pneumococcus is a function of its capsule, which prevents or delays digestion by phagocytes. The polysaccharide is an antigen that primarily elicits a B-cell response with antibody production. In the absence of antibody, clearance of the pneumococci from the body relies on the reticuloendothelial system, with the macrophages in the spleen playing a major role in elimination of the organism.[37] This, along with the spleen's role in antibody production, increases the risk for pneumococcal bacteremia in persons who are anatomically or functionally asplenic, such as children with sickle cell disease. The initial step in the pathogenesis of pneumococcal infection is the attachment and colonization of the organism to the mucus and cells of the nasopharynx. Colonization does not equate with signs of infection. Perfectly healthy people can be colonized and carry the organism without evidence of infection. The spread of particular strains of pneumococci, particularly antibiotic-resistant strains, is largely by healthy colonized individuals. The factors that permit the pneumococci to spread beyond the nasopharynx vary depending on the virulence of the organism, impaired host defense mechanisms, and the existence of preceding viral infection. Viral and other infections damage the surface cells or increase mucus production, protecting pneumococci from phagocytosis. In the alveoli, the pneumococci initially adhere to the alveolar wall, causing an outpouring of red cells and leukocytes, which results in consolidation of the lung. They reach the bloodstream through lymphatic drainage.

The signs and symptoms of pneumococcal pneumonia vary widely, depending on the age and health status of the infected person. In previously healthy persons, the onset usually is sudden and is characterized by malaise, severe shaking chill, and fever. The temperature may go as high as 106°F. During the initial or congestive stage, coughing brings up watery sputum, and breath sounds are limited, with fine crackles. As the disease progresses, the character of the sputum changes; it may be blood tinged or rust colored to purulent. Pleuritic pain, a sharp pain that is more severe with respiratory movements, is common. With antibiotic therapy, fever usually subsides in approximately 48 to 72 hours, and recovery is uneventful. Elderly persons are less likely to experience marked elevations in temperature; in these persons, the only sign of pneumonia may be a loss of appetite and deterioration in mental status.

Treatment includes the use of antibiotics that are effective against *S. pneumoniae.* In the past, *S. pneumoniae* was uniformly susceptible to penicillin. However, penicillin-resistant and multidrug-resistant strains have been emerging in the United States and other countries.[37]

Pneumococcal pneumonia can be prevented through immunization. A 23-valent pneumococcal vaccine, composed of antigens from 23 types of *S. pneumoniae* capsular polysaccharides, is used. The capsular polysaccharides induce antibodies primarily by T-cell–independent mechanisms. Because the immune system of children younger than 2 years of age is immature, the antibody response to most pneumococcal capsular polysaccharides usually is poor or inconsistent.[38] The vaccine is recommended for persons 65 years of age or older and persons aged 2 to 65 years with chronic illnesses, particularly cardiovascular and pulmonary diseases, diabetes mellitus, and alcoholism, who sustain increased morbidity with respiratory infections. Immunization also is recommended for immunocompromised persons 2 years of age or older, including those with sickle cell disease, splenectomy, Hodgkin's disease, multiple myeloma, renal failure, nephrotic syndrome, organ transplantation, and HIV infection.[38] Immunization is recommended for residents in special environments or social settings in which the risk for invasive pneumococcal disease is increased (*e.g.,* Alaskan Natives, certain Native American populations) and for residents of nursing homes and long-term care facilities.

A single dose of pneumococcal vaccine usually confers some lifetime immunity. Serotype antibody levels decline after 5 to 10 years and decrease more rapidly in some groups than others.[38] Although not currently recommended for immunocompetent people who received the 23-valent vaccine, a second dose of vaccine is recommended for persons older than 65 years of age if 5 years or more have elapsed since the previous vaccine was given and if the person was younger than 65 years at the time of vaccination.[38] Revaccination also is recommended for immunocompromised persons 10 to 64 years of age and those with anatomic or functional asplenia (*i.e.,* splenectomy or sickle cell disease) if more than 5 years have elapsed since the previous dose and after 3 years if the person is younger than 10 years of age.[38]

In 2000, a 7-valent pneumococcal polysaccharide–protein conjugate vaccine (Prevnar) was licensed for use among infants and children.[39] Although the 23-valent vaccines are effective in older children, they do not prevent infection in children 2 years of age or younger, the age group with the highest rate of infection. With the success of *H. influenzae* type B vaccine, *S. pneumoniae* has become the leading cause of bacterial meningitis in the United States. *S. pneumoniae* also contributes substantially to noninvasive respiratory infections and is the most common cause of community-acquired pneumonia, acute otitis media, and sinusitis among young children. The ACIP recommends that vaccine be used for all children aged 2 to 23 months and for children aged 24 to 49 months who are at increased risk for pneumococcal disease (*e.g.,* children with sickle cell disease, HIV infection, and other immunocompromising or chronic medical conditions).[39]

Legionnaire's Disease. Legionnaire's disease is a form of bronchopneumonia caused by a gram-negative rod, *Legionella pneumophila.* It ranks among the three or four most common causes of community-acquired pneumonia.[30] Although more than 14 serotypes of *L. pneumophila* have been identified, serotype 1 accounts for more than 80% of reported cases of legionellosis.[40] The organism frequently is found in water, particularly in warm, standing water. The disease was first recognized and received its name after an epidemic of severe and, for some, fatal pneumonia that developed among delegates to the 1976 American Legion convention held in a Philadelphia hotel. The spread of infection was traced to a water-cooled air-conditioning system. Although healthy persons can contract the infection, the risk is greatest among smokers, persons with chronic diseases, and those with impaired cell-mediated immunity.[30,40,41]

Symptoms of the disease typically begin approximately 2 to 10 days after infection, with malaise, weakness, lethargy, fever, and dry cough. Other manifestations include disturbances of central nervous system function, gastrointestinal tract involvement, arthralgias, and elevation in body temperature, sometimes to more than 104°F. The presence of pneumonia along with diarrhea, hyponatremia, and confusion is characteristic of *Legionella* pneumonia. The disease causes consolidation of lung tissues and impairs gas exchange.

Diagnosis is based on clinical manifestations, radiologic studies, and specialized laboratory tests to detect the presence of the organism. Of these, the *Legionella* urinary antigen test is a relatively inexpensive, rapid test that detects antigens of *L. pneumophila* in the urine.[41] The urine test usually is easier to obtain because people with legionellosis often have a nonproductive cough and the test results remain positive for weeks despite antibiotic therapy. The test is available as both a radioimmunoassay and an enzyme immunoassay. The possible disadvantage of the urine test is that it detects only *L. pneumophila* serogroup 1. Culture methods permit identification of other serotypes.[40]

Treatment consists of administration of antibiotics that are known to be effective against *L. pneumophila.* Delay in instituting antibiotic therapy significantly increases mortality rates; therefore, antibiotics known to be effective against *L. pneumophila* should be included in the treatment regimen for severe community-acquired pneumonia.[40]

Mycoplasma and Viral Pneumonias. Mycoplasmas and viruses tend to cause atypical or interstitial pneumonias.[1] The mycoplasmas are the smallest free-living agents of disease, having characteristics of viruses and bacteria. The influenza virus is the most common cause of viral pneumonia. Less common offenders are parainfluenza and respiratory syncytial viruses. Other viruses sometimes are implicated, including the measles and chickenpox viruses.

The clinical course among persons with mycoplasmal and viral pneumonias varies widely from a mild infection (*e.g.*, influenza types A and B, adenovirus) that masquerades as a chest cold to a more serious and even fatal outcome (*e.g.*, chickenpox pneumonia). The symptoms may remain confined to fever, headache, and muscle aches and pains. Cough, when present, is characteristically dry, hacking, and nonproductive. Viruses impair the respiratory tract defenses and predispose to secondary bacterial infections with the development of lobar or bronchopneumonia. Some viruses such as herpes simplex, varicella, and adenovirus may be associated with necrosis of the alveolar epithelium and acute inflammation.

Hospital-Acquired Pneumonia

Hospital-acquired, or nosocomial, pneumonia is defined as a lower respiratory tract infection that was not present or incubating on admission to the hospital. Usually, infections occurring 48 hours or more after admission are considered hospital acquired.[30,42] Hospital-acquired pneumonia is the second most common cause of hospital-acquired infection and has a mortality rate of 20% to 50%.[30] Persons requiring mechanical ventilation are particularly at risk, as are those with compromised immune function, chronic lung disease, and airway instrumentation, such as endotracheal intubation or tracheotomy.

Ninety percent of infections are bacterial. The organisms are those present in the hospital environment and include *Pseudomonas aeruginosa, S. aureus, Enterobacter* species, *Klebsiella* species, *Escherichia coli,* and *Serratia.* The organisms that are responsible for hospital-acquired pneumonias are different from those responsible for community-acquired pneumonias, and many of them have acquired antibiotic resistance and are more difficult to treat.

Pneumonia in Immunocompromised Persons

Pneumonia in immunocompromised persons remains a major source of morbidity and mortality. The term *immunocompromised host* usually is applied to persons with a variety of underlying defects in host defenses. It includes persons with primary and acquired immunodeficiency states, those who have undergone bone marrow or organ transplantation, persons with solid organ or hematologic cancers, and those on corticosteroid and other immunosuppressant drugs.[43] Although almost all types of microorganisms can cause pulmonary infection in immunocompromised persons, certain types of immunologic defects tend to favor certain types of infections. Defects in humoral immunity predispose to bacterial infections against which antibodies play an important role; whereas defects in cellular immunity predispose to infections caused by viruses, fungi, mycobacteria, and protozoa. Neutropenia and impaired granulocyte function, as occurs in persons with leukemia, chemotherapy, and bone marrow metaplasia, predispose to infections caused by *S. aureus, Aspergillus,* gram-negative bacilli, and *Candida.* The time course of infection often provides a hint to the type of agent involved. A fulminant pneumonia usually is caused by bacterial infection, while an insidious onset usually is indicative of a viral, fungal, protozoal, or mycobacterial infection.

TUBERCULOSIS

Tuberculosis is the world's foremost cause of death from a single infectious agent, causing 26% of avoidable deaths in developing countries.[44–47] It is estimated that each year more than 8 million new cases of tuberculosis occur worldwide and approximately 3 million persons die of the disease.[47] In the United States, there were approximately 15,000 new cases and 750 deaths attributed to tuberculosis in 2001.[44] With the introduction of antibiotics in the 1950s, the United States and other Western countries enjoyed a long decline in the number of infections until the mid-1980s. Since that time, the rate of infection has increased, particularly among HIV-infected people. In the United States, the biggest increase in new cases was from 1985 to 1993, after which the rate of cases reported yearly has again declined. In part, this decline reflects the impact of resources to assist state and local control efforts, wider screening and prevention programs, and increased support for prevention programs among HIV-infected persons.[44] Tuberculosis is more common among foreign-born persons from countries with a high incidence of tuberculosis and among residents of high-risk congregate settings such as correctional facilities, drug treatment facilities, and homeless shelters. Outbreaks of a drug-resistant form of tuberculosis have emerged, complicating the selection of drugs and affecting the duration of treatment.

TUBERCULOSIS

- Tuberculosis is an infectious disease caused by *Mycobacterium tuberculosis,* a rod-shaped, aerobic bacteria that is resistant to destruction and can persist in necrotic and calcified lesions for prolonged periods and remain capable of reinstating growth.
- The organism is spread by inhaling the mycobacterium-containing droplet nuclei that circulate in the air. Overcrowded living conditions increase the risk of tuberculosis spread.
- The tubercle bacillus has no known antigens to stimulate an early immunoglobulin response; instead, the host mounts a delayed-type cell-mediated immune response.
- The cell-mediated response plays a dominant role in walling off the tubercle bacilli and preventing the development of active tuberculosis. People with impaired cell-mediated immunity are more likely to develop active tuberculosis when infected.
- A positive tuberculin skin test results from a cell-mediated immune response and implies that a person has been infected with *M. tuberculosis* and has mounted a cell-mediated immune response. It does not mean that the person has active tuberculosis.

Etiology

Tuberculosis is an infectious disease caused by the mycobacterium, *M. tuberculosis*. The mycobacteria are slender, rod-shaped, aerobic bacteria that do not form spores. They are similar to other bacterial organisms except for an outer waxy capsule that makes them more resistant to destruction; the organism can persist in old necrotic and calcified lesions and remain capable of reinitiating growth. The waxy coat also causes the organism to retain red dye when treated with acid in acid-fast staining.[34,44] Thus, the mycobacteria are often referred to as *acid-fast bacilli*. Although *M. tuberculosis* can infect practically any organ of the body, the lungs are most frequently involved. The tubercle bacilli are strict aerobes that thrive in an oxygen-rich environment. This explains their tendency to cause disease in the upper lobe or upper parts of the lower lobe of the lung, where the ventilation and oxygen content are greatest.

Two forms of tuberculosis pose a particular threat to humans: *M. tuberculosis hominis* (human tuberculosis) and *M. tuberculosis bovis* (bovine tuberculosis). Human tuberculosis is an airborne infection spread by minute, invisible particles, called *droplet nuclei,* that are harbored in the respiratory secretions of persons with active tuberculosis. Coughing, sneezing, and talking all create respiratory droplets; these droplets evaporate, leaving the organisms (droplet nuclei), which remain suspended in the air and are circulated by air currents. Living under crowded and confined conditions increases the risk for spread of the disease. Bovine tuberculosis is acquired by drinking milk from infected cows, and it initially affects the gastrointestinal tract. This form of tuberculosis has been virtually eradicated in North America and other developed countries as a result of rigorous controls on dairy herds and the pasteurization of milk. Other mycobacterium, including *M. avium–intracellulare* complex, are much less virulent than *M. hominis* and *M. bovis* and rarely cause disease except in severely immunosuppressed persons, such as those with HIV infection.[34]

The pathogenesis of tuberculosis in a previously unexposed immunocompetent person is centered on the development of a cell-mediated immune response that confers resistance to the organism and development of tissue hypersensitivity to the tubercular antigens.[34] The destructive nature of the disease, such as caseating necrosis and cavitation, result from the hypersensitivity immune response rather than the destructive capabilities of the tubercle bacillus. Tuberculosis can manifest as a primary or reactivated infection.

Primary Tuberculosis

Primary tuberculosis occurs in a person lacking previous contact with the tubercle bacillus. It typically is initiated as a result of inhaling droplet nuclei that contain the tubercle bacillus[34,44] (Fig. 30-3). Inhaled droplet nuclei pass down the bronchial tree without settling on the epithelium and implant in a respiratory bronchiole or alveolus beyond the mucociliary system. Soon after entering the lung, the bacilli are surrounded and engulfed by macrophages. *M. tuberculosis* has no known endotoxins or exotoxins; therefore, there is no early immunoglobulin response to infection.

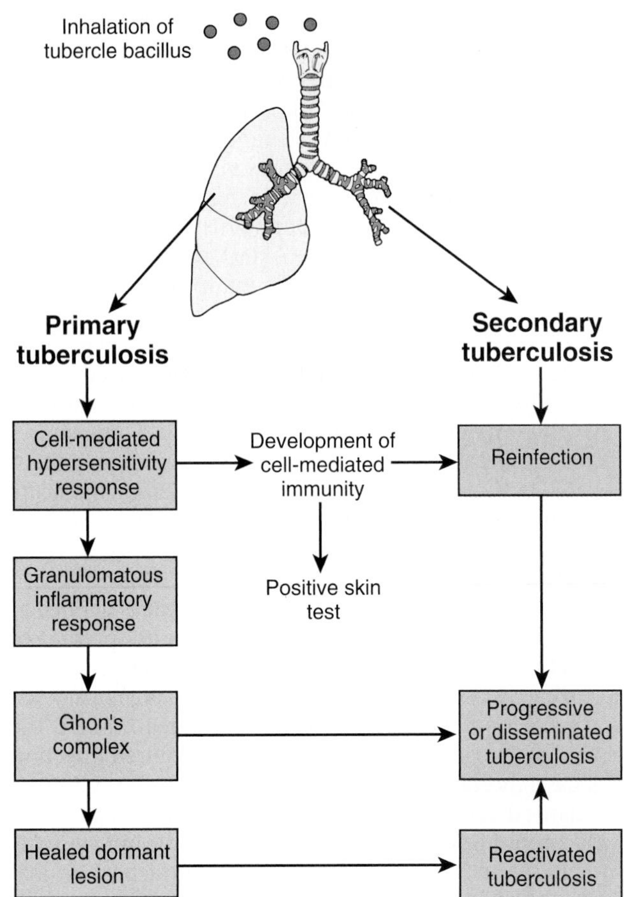

FIGURE 30-3 Pathogenesis of TB Infection.

The tubercle bacillus grows slowly, dividing every 25 to 32 hours in the macrophage. As the bacilli multiply, the macrophages degrade some mycobacteria and present antigen to the T lymphocytes for development of a cell-mediated immune response. The organisms grow for 2 to 12 weeks until they reach sufficient numbers to elicit a cellular immune response. In persons with intact cell-mediated immunity, this action is followed by the development of a single, gray-white, circumscribed granulomatous lesion, called a *Ghon's focus,* that contains the tubercle bacilli, modified macrophages, and other immune cells.[45] Within 2 to 3 weeks, the central portion of the Ghon's focus undergoes soft, caseous (cheeselike) necrosis. This occurs at approximately the time that the tuberculin test result becomes positive, suggesting that the necrosis is caused by the cell-mediated hypersensitivity immune response (see Chapter 21). During this same period, tubercle bacilli, free or inside macrophages, drain along the lymph channels to the tracheobronchial lymph nodes of the affected lung and there evoke the formation of caseous granulomas. The combination of the primary lung lesion and lymph node granulomas is called *Ghon's complex* (Fig. 30-4).

In most people, infection with *M. tuberculosis* is initially contained by the cell-mediated immune response of the host, and the infection remains latent.[46] However,

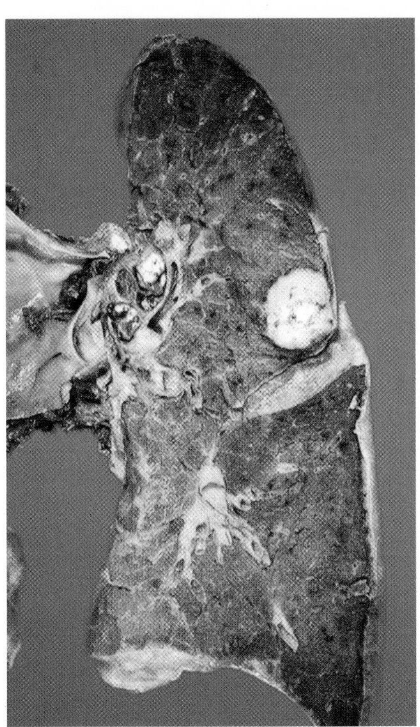

FIGURE 30-4 Primary tuberculosis. A healed Ghon's complex is represented by a subpleural nodule and involved hilar lymph nodes. (From Rubin E., Farber J.L. [1994]. *Pathology* [2nd ed.]. Philadelphia: J.B. Lippincott)

latent tuberculosis infection has the potential to develop into active tuberculosis at any time, and persons with active tuberculosis become sources of infection. Treatment of latent tuberculosis greatly reduces the likelihood that active tuberculosis will develop.

Primary tuberculosis usually is asymptomatic, with the only evidence of the disease being a positive tuberculin skin test result and calcified lesions seen on the chest radiograph. Occasionally, primary tuberculosis may progress, causing more extensive destruction of lung tissue and spreading through the airways and lymphatics to multiple sites within the lung. As the disease spreads, the organism gains access to the sputum, allowing the person to infect others. People with HIV infection and others with disorders of cell-mediated immunity are more likely to acquire active tuberculosis if they become infected.

In rare instances, tuberculosis may erode into a blood vessel, giving rise to hematogenic dissemination. *Miliary tuberculosis* describes minute lesions, resembling millet seeds, resulting from this type of dissemination that can involve almost any organ, particularly the brain, meninges, liver, kidney, and bone marrow.

Secondary Tuberculosis

Secondary tuberculosis represents either reinfection from inhaled droplet nuclei or reactivation of a previously healed primary lesion (see Fig. 30-3). It often occurs in situations of impaired body defense mechanisms. The partial immunity that follows primary tuberculosis affords protection against reinfection and to some extent aids in localizing the disease should reactivation occur. In secondary tuberculosis, the cell-mediated hypersensitivity reaction can be an aggravating factor, as evidenced by the frequency of cavitation and bronchial dissemination. The cavities may coalesce to a size of up to 10 to 15 cm in diameter[44] (Fig. 30-5). Pleural effusion and tuberculous empyema are common as the disease progresses.

Persons with secondary tuberculosis commonly present with low-grade fevers, night sweats, easy fatigability, anorexia, and weight loss. A cough initially is dry but later becomes productive with purulent and sometimes blood-tinged sputum. Dyspnea and orthopnea develop as the disease advances.

Diagnosis

The most frequently used screening methods for pulmonary tuberculosis are the tuberculin skin tests and chest radiographic studies. The tuberculin skin test measures delayed hypersensitivity (*i.e.*, cell-mediated, type IV) that follows exposure to the tubercle bacillus. Persons who become tuberculin positive usually remain so for the remainder of their lives. A positive reaction to the skin test does not mean that a person has active tuberculosis, only that there has been exposure to the bacillus and that cell-mediated immunity to the organism has developed. False-positive and false-negative skin test reactions can occur. False-positive reactions often result from cross-reactions with nontuberculosis mycobacteria, such as *M. avium–intracellulare* complex.[47] Because the hypersensitivity response to the tuberculin test depends on cell-mediated immunity, a false-negative test result can occur because of immunodeficiency states that result from HIV infection, immunosuppressive therapy, lymphoreticular malignancies, or aging. This is called *anergy*. In the immunocompromised person, a negative tuberculin test result can mean that the person has a true lack of exposure to tuberculosis or is unable to mount an immune response to the test. Because of the problem with anergy in persons with HIV infection and other immunocompromised states, the use of control tests is recommended. Three antigens that can be

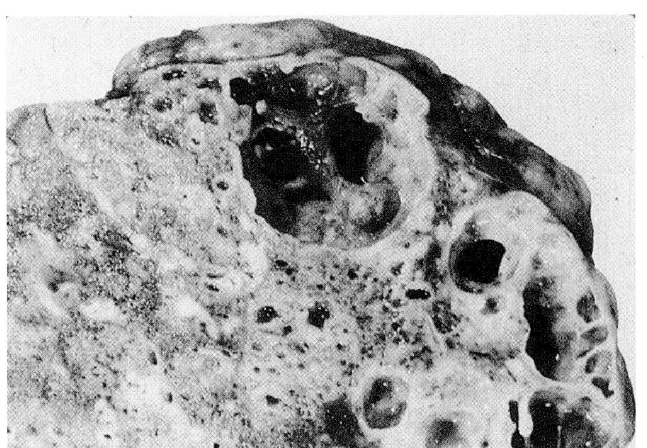

FIGURE 30-5 Cavitary tuberculosis in the apex of the left upper lobe of the lung. (Rubin E., Farber J.L. [1999]. *Pathology* [3rd ed., p. 607]. Philadelphia: Lippincott-Raven)

used for control testing are *Candida,* mumps virus, and tetanus toxoid. Most healthy persons in the population have been exposed to these antigens and will display a positive response to these control tests.[47]

A two-step testing procedure, which uses a "boosting" phenomenon, may be used to increase the reaction to a subsequent tuberculin test in persons who have been infected with tuberculosis.[47] If the first test result of the two-step procedure is negative, a second test is administered 1 week later. If the second test result is negative, the person is considered to be uninfected or anergic. If the second test result is positive, it is assumed to have occurred because of a boosted response. The boosted effect can last for 1 year or longer. Use of the two-step test procedure for employee health or institutional screening can reduce the likelihood that a boosted response in a subsequent test will not be interpreted as a recent infection.

Diagnosis of active pulmonary tuberculosis requires identification of the organism in respiratory tract secretions. Bacteriologic studies (*i.e.,* acid-fast stain and cultures) of early-sputum specimens, gastric aspirations, or bronchial washings obtained during fiberoptic bronchoscopy may be used. The polymerase chain reaction allows rapid detection of *M. tuberculosis* and differentiation from other mycobacteria (see Chapter 18). Genotyping can be done to identify different strains of *M. tuberculosis.* It can be used to evaluate second episodes of tuberculosis to determine whether the second episode was due to relapse or reinfection. Genotyping also permits the evaluation of isolates with different patterns of drug susceptibility.[48] In addition, genotyping is useful in investigating outbreaks of infection and determining sites and patterns of *M. tuberculosis* transmission in communities.

Treatment

Two groups meet the criteria established for the use of antimycobacterial therapy for tuberculosis: persons with active tuberculosis and those who have had contact with cases of active tuberculosis and who are at risk for development of an active form of the disease.

The primary drugs used in the treatment of tuberculosis are isoniazid (INH), rifampin, pyrazinamide (PZA), ethambutol, and streptomycin.[49] INH is remarkably potent against the tubercle bacillus and probably is the most widely used drug for tuberculosis. Although its exact mechanism of action is unknown, it apparently combines with an enzyme that is needed by the INH-susceptible strains of the tubercle bacillus. Resistance to the drug develops rapidly, and combination with other effective drugs delays the development of resistance. Rifampin inhibits RNA synthesis in the bacillus. Although ethambutol and PZA are known to inhibit the growth of the tubercle bacillus, their mechanisms of action are largely unknown. Streptomycin, the first drug found to be effective against tuberculosis, must be given by injection, which limits its usefulness, particularly in long-term therapy. However, it remains an important drug in tuberculosis therapy and is used primarily in persons with severe, possibly life-threatening forms of tuberculosis.

Treatment of active tuberculosis requires the use of multiple drugs. Tuberculosis is an unusual disease in that chemotherapy is required for a relatively long period of time. The tubercle bacillus is an aerobic organism that multiplies slowly and remains relatively dormant in oxygen-poor caseous material. It undergoes a high rate of mutation and tends to acquire resistance to any one drug. For this reason, multidrug regimens are used for treating persons with active tuberculosis. Drug susceptibility tests are used to guide treatment in drug-resistant forms of the disease.

Prophylactic treatment is used for persons who are infected with *M. tuberculosis* but do not have active disease.[49] This group includes persons with a positive skin test who have had close contact with active cases of tuberculosis; have converted from a negative to positive skin test result within 2 years; have a history of untreated or inadequately treated tuberculosis; have chest radiographs with evidence of tuberculosis but no bacteriologic evidence of the active disease; have special risk factors such as silicosis, diabetes mellitus, prolonged corticosteroid therapy, immunosuppression therapy, end-stage renal disease, chronic malnutrition from any cause, or hematologic or reticuloendothelial cancers; have a positive HIV test result or have AIDS; or are 35 years of age or younger with a positive reaction of unknown duration. These persons are considered to harbor a small number of microorganisms and usually are treated with INH.

Outbreaks of multidrug-resistant tuberculosis have posed a problem for the prophylactic treatment of exposed persons, including health care workers.[50] Most exposed persons who have contracted active multidrug-resistant tuberculosis were infected with the HIV virus; the fatality rate among these persons is high, at 80%.[51] Various treatment protocols are recommended, depending on the type of resistant strain that is identified.

Success of chemotherapy for prophylaxis and treatment of tuberculosis depends on strict adherence to a lengthy drug regimen. This often is a problem, particularly for asymptomatic persons with tuberculosis infections and for poorly motivated groups such as intravenous drug users. Directly observed therapy, which requires that a health care worker observe while the person takes the antituberculosis drug, is recommended for some persons and for some types of treatment protocols.[49]

First administered to humans in 1921, the bacillus Calmette-Guérin (BCG) vaccine is used to prevent the development of tuberculosis in persons who are at high risk for infection. BCG is an attenuated strain of *M. tuberculosis bovis.* It is administered only to persons who have a negative tuberculin skin test result. The vaccine, which is given intradermally, produces a local reaction that can last as long as 3 months and may result in scarring at the injection site. Persons who have been vaccinated with BCG usually have a positive tuberculin skin test result that wanes with time and is unlikely to persist beyond 10 years. The CDC recommends that use of the BCG vaccine in the United States be reserved for high-risk groups, such as infants and children, who reside in settings in which the likelihood of *M. tuberculosis* transmission and infection is high and for health care workers in whom the risk for transmission of multidrug-resistant strains of the bacterium are high. The vaccine is not recommended for children and adults infected with HIV.[52]

Today, more than 70 years after its development, BCG remains the only tuberculosis vaccine available. Worldwide, the vaccine is used as a major method of prevention for tuberculosis. Although it is currently delivered to approximately 90% of all neonates in developing countries through the Expanded Programme on Immunization, the disease continues to cause more than 2 to 3 million deaths annually, suggesting the need for more effective vaccines.[53] Currently, several candidate vaccines are being prepared or are already in the early stages of human testing.

FUNGAL INFECTIONS

Fungi are classified as yeasts and molds. Yeasts are round and grow by budding. Molds form tubular structures called hyphae and grow by branching and forming spores (see Chapter 18). Some fungi are *dimorphic,* meaning that they grow as yeasts at body temperatures and as molds at room temperatures. A simple classification of mycoses that cause human disease divides them into superficial, cutaneous, subcutaneous, or deep (systemic) mycoses. The superficial, cutaneous, or subcutaneous mycoses cause disease of the skin, hair, and nails. Deep fungal infections may produce pulmonary and systemic infections and are sometimes fatal. They are caused by virulent fungi that live free in nature or soil or in decaying organic matter and are frequently limited to certain geographic regions. The most common of these are the dimorphic fungi, which include *Histoplasma capsulatum* (histoplasmosis), *Coccidioides immitis* (coccidioidomycosis), and *Blastomyces dermatitidis* (blastomycosis). These fungi form infectious spores, which enter the body by way of the respiratory system. Most people who become infected with these fungi develop only minor symptoms, or none at all; only a small minority develops serious disease.

The host's cell-mediated immune response is paramount in controlling such infections. Pathologic fungi generally produce no toxins. In the host, they induce a delayed cell-mediated hypersensitivity response to their chemical constituents (see Chapter 21). Cellular immunity is mediated by antigen-specific T lymphocytes and cytokine-activated macrophages that assume fungicidal properties. The primary pulmonary lesions consist of aggregates of macrophages stuffed with organisms, with similar lesions developing in the lymph nodes that drain the area. These lesions develop into granulomas complete with giant cells and may develop central necrosis and calcification resembling that of primary tuberculosis.

Although most fungal infections are asymptomatic, they can be severe or even fatal in persons who have experienced a heavy exposure, have underlying immune deficiencies, or develop progressive disease that is not recognized or treated. Immunocompromised persons, particularly those with HIV, are particularly prone to developing disseminated infection.

Histoplasmosis

Histoplasmosis is caused by the dimorphic fungus *H. capsulatum* and is one of the most common fungal infections in the United States. Most cases occur along the major river valleys of the Midwest—the Ohio, the Mississippi, and the Missouri.[54,55] The organism grows in soil and other areas that have been enriched with bird excreta: old chicken houses, pigeon lofts, barns, and trees where birds roost. The infection is acquired by inhaling the fungal spores that are released when the dirt or dust from the infected areas is disturbed. The spores convert to the parasitic yeast phase when exposed to body temperature in the alveoli. They are then carried to the regional lymphatics and from there are disseminated throughout the body in the bloodstream. Dissemination occurs during the first several weeks of infection before specific immunity has developed. After 2 to 3 weeks, cellular immunity develops, establishing the body's ability to control the infection.

The manifestations of histoplasmosis are strikingly similar to those of tuberculosis. Depending on the host's resistance and immunocompetence, the disease usually takes one of four forms: latent asymptomatic disease, self-limited primary disease, chronic pulmonary disease, or disseminated infection. The average incubation period for the infection is approximately 14 days.

Latent asymptomatic histoplasmosis is characterized by evidence of healed lesions in the lungs or hilar lymph nodes. Primary pulmonary histoplasmosis occurs in otherwise healthy persons as a mild, self-limited, febrile respiratory infection. Its symptoms include muscle and joint pains and a nonproductive cough. Erythema nodosum (*i.e.,* subcutaneous nodules) or erythema multiforme (*i.e.,* hivelike lesions) sometimes appears. During this stage of the disease, chest radiographs usually show single or multiple infiltrates.

Chronic histoplasmosis resembles reactivation tuberculosis. Infiltration of the upper lobes of one or both lungs occurs with cavitation. This form of the disease is more common in middle-aged men who smoke and in persons with chronic lung disease. The most common manifestations are a productive cough, fever, night sweats, and weight loss. In many persons, the disease is self-limited. In others, there is progressive destruction of lung tissue and dissemination of the disease.

Disseminated histoplasmosis can follow primary or chronic histoplasmosis but most often develops as an acute and fulminating infection in the very old or the very young or in persons with compromised immune function. Although the macrophages of the reticuloendothelial system can remove the fungi from the bloodstream, they are unable to destroy them. Characteristically, this form of the disease produces a high fever, generalized lymph node enlargement, hepatosplenomegaly, muscle wasting, anemia, leukopenia, and thrombocytopenia. There may be hoarseness, ulcerations of the mouth and tongue, nausea, vomiting, diarrhea, and abdominal pain. Often, meningitis becomes a dominant feature of the disease.

A number of laboratory tests, including cultures, fungal stain, antigen detection, and serologic tests for antibodies, are used in the diagnosis of histoplasmosis. The type of test that is used depends on the type of involvement that is present. In pulmonary disease, sputum culture is rarely positive; whereas blood or bone marrow cultures from immunocompromised people with acute disseminated disease are positive in 80% to 90% of cases.

Antigen tests can be performed on blood, urine, cerebral spinal fluid, or bronchoalveolar lavage fluid. A urine antigen assay is particularly useful in detecting disseminated histoplasmosis.

The antifungal drug, itraconazole, usually is the drug of choice for treatment of persons with disease severe enough to require treatment or those with compromised immune function who are at risk for the development of disseminated disease.[54,55] Amphotericin B, which is administered intravenously, usually is the drug of choice in severe disease. Persons with HIV-related histoplasmosis usually require lifelong suppression therapy with itraconazole.

Coccidioidomycosis

Coccidioidomycosis is a common fungal infection caused by inhaling the spores of *C. immitis*.[55–58] The disease resembles tuberculosis, and its mechanisms of infection are similar to those of histoplasmosis. It is most prevalent in the southwestern United States, principally in parts of California, Arizona, Nevada, New Mexico, and Texas. Because of its prevalence in the San Joaquin Valley, the disease is sometimes referred to as *San Joaquin fever* or *valley fever*. The *C. immitis* organism lives in soil and can establish new sites in the soil. Events such as dust storms and digging for construction have been associated with increased incidence of the disease.

The disease most commonly occurs as an acute, primary, self-limited pulmonary infection with or without systemic involvement, but in some cases, it progresses to a disseminated disease. The incubation period is 10 to 30 days. About 40% of infected persons develop symptoms of primary coccidioidomycosis.[55] The symptoms are usually those of a respiratory tract infection with fever, cough, and pleuritic pain. Erythema nodosum may occur 2 to 20 days after onset of symptoms. The skin lesions usually are accompanied by arthralgias or arthritis without effusion, particularly of the ankles and knees. The terms *desert bumps* and *desert arthritis* are used to describe these manifestations. The presence of skin and joint manifestations indicates strong host defenses because persons who have had such manifestations seldom acquire disseminated disease.

Disseminated disease occurs in approximately 0.5% to 1% of infected persons. Commonly affected structures in disseminated disease are the lymph nodes, meninges, spleen, liver, kidney, skin, and adrenal glands. Meningitis is the most common cause of death. Persons with diabetes or compromised immune function, infants, and members of dark-skinned races tend to localize the disease poorly and are at higher risk for disseminated disease. In HIV-infected persons in endemic areas, coccidioidomycosis is now a common opportunistic infection.

Radiologic studies, including chest radiographic studies and bone scans, are useful in determining disease but cannot distinguish coccidioidomycosis from other pulmonary diseases. A definitive diagnosis requires microscopic or serologic evidence that *C. immitis* is present in body tissues or fluids. *C. immitis* spherules can be visualized in specially stained biopsy specimens. Serologic tests can be done for immunoglobulin M (IgM) and IgG antibody detection.

Treatment depends on the severity of infection. Persons without associated risk factors such as HIV infection or without specific evidence of progressive disease usually can be managed without antifungal therapy. The oral antifungal drugs itraconazole and fluconazole are used for treatment of less severe forms of infection. Intravenous amphotericin B is used in the treatment of persons with progressive disease. Long-term treatment is often required.

Blastomycosis

Blastomycosis is a fungal infection caused by inhaling the spores of *B. dermatitidis*. The disease is most commonly found in the southern and north central United States, especially in areas bordering the Mississippi and Ohio River basins and the Great Lakes.[55,59] *B. dermatitidis* is most commonly found in soil containing decayed vegetation or decomposed wood. The disease occurs most often in men infected during occupational or recreational outdoor activities.

The infection is characterized by local suppurative and granulomatous lesions of the lungs and skin. The symptoms of acute infection, which are similar to those of acute histoplasmosis, include fever, cough, aching joints and muscles, and, uncommonly, pleuritic pain. In contrast to histoplasmosis, the cough in blastomycosis often is productive, and the sputum is purulent. Acute pulmonary infections may be self-limited or progressive. In persons with overwhelming pulmonary disease, diffuse interalveolar infiltrates and evidence of acute respiratory distress syndrome may develop (see Chapter 31). Extrapulmonary spread most commonly involves the skin, bones, or prostate. These lesions may provide the first evidence of the disease.

The diagnosis of blastomycosis is more difficult than that of histoplasmosis. Visualization of the yeast in the sputum after application of 10% potassium hydroxide provides a presumptive diagnosis. When this fails, cultural isolation of the fungus often is attempted.

Treatment of the progressive or disseminated form of the disease includes the use of itraconazole or amphotericin B.[55] Most persons with blastomycosis are identified and treated before the development of overwhelming or fatal disease.

In summary, respiratory infections are the most common cause of respiratory illness. They include the common cold, influenza, pneumonias, tuberculosis, and fungal infections. The common cold occurs more frequently than any other respiratory infection. The fingers are the usual source of transmission, and the most common portals of entry are the nasal mucosa and the conjunctiva of the eye. The influenza virus causes three syndromes: an uncomplicated rhinotracheitis, a respiratory viral infection followed by a bacterial infection, and viral pneumonia. The contagiousness of influenza results from the ability of the virus to mutate and form subtypes that the population is not protected against.

Pneumonia describes an infection of the parenchymal tissues of the lung. Loss of the cough reflex, damage to the ciliated endothelium that lines the respiratory tract, or impaired immune defenses predispose to pneumonia. Pneumonia is being increasingly classified as community acquired or hospital acquired. Persons with compromised immune function constitute a special concern in both categories. Community-acquired pneumonia involves infections from organisms that are present more often in the community than in the hospital or nursing home. The most common cause of community-acquired pneumonia is *S. pneumoniae.* Hospital-acquired (nosocomial) pneumonia is defined as a lower respiratory tract infection occurring 48 hours or more after admission. Hospital-acquired pneumonia is the second most common cause of hospital-acquired infection. Legionnaire's disease is a form of bronchopneumonia caused by the gram-negative bacillus *L. pneumophila.* Viral or atypical pneumonia can occur as a primary infection, such as that caused by influenza virus, or as a complication of other viral infections, such as measles or chickenpox. Viral and atypical pneumonias involve the interstitium of the lung and often masquerade as chest colds.

Tuberculosis is a chronic respiratory infection caused by *M. tuberculosis,* which is spread by minute, invisible particles called *droplet nuclei.* Tuberculosis is a particular threat among HIV-infected persons, foreign-born persons from countries with a high incidence of tuberculosis, and residents of high-risk congregate settings such as correctional facilities, drug treatment facilities, and homeless shelters. The tubercle bacillus incites a distinctive chronic inflammatory response referred to as *granulomatous inflammation.* The destructiveness of the disease results from the cell-mediated hypersensitivity response that the bacillus evokes rather than its inherent destructive capabilities. Cell-mediated immunity and hypersensitivity reactions contribute to the evolution of the disease. The treatment of tuberculosis has been complicated by outbreaks of drug-resistant forms of the disease.

Infections caused by the fungi *H. capsulatum* (histoplasmosis), *C. immitis* (coccidioidomycosis), and *B. dermatitidis* (blastomycosis) produce pulmonary manifestations that resemble tuberculosis. These infections are common but seldom serious unless they produce progressive destruction of lung tissue or the infection disseminates to organs and tissues outside the lungs.

Cancer of the Lung

After completing this section of the chapter, you should be able to meet the following objectives:

- Cite risk factors associated with lung cancer
- Differentiate between small cell lung cancer and non–small cell lung cancer in terms of histopathology, prognosis, and treatment methods
- Describe the manifestations of lung cancer and list two symptoms of lung cancer that are related to the invasion of the mediastinum
- Define the term *paraneoplastic* and cite three paraneoplastic manifestations of lung cancer
- Characterize the effect of age on treatment of lung cancer

Lung cancer is the leading cause of cancer deaths among men and women in the United States. In 2004, it was responsible for the deaths of approximately 93,000 men and 80,500 women.[60] The increases in lung cancer incidence and deaths over the past 50 years have coincided closely with the increase in cigarette smoking over the same period. Between 1980 and 1998, lung cancer mortality rates decreased for persons younger than 55 years and increased for those older than 65 years, reflecting generational patterns in smoking prevalence.[61,62] Because lung cancer usually is far advanced before it is discovered, the prognosis in general is poor. The overall 5-year survival rate is 13% to 15%, a dismal statistic that has not changed since the late 1960s.

Most (about 95%) primary lung tumors arise from the bronchial epithelium (bronchogenic carcinoma). The remaining 5% are a miscellaneous group that includes bronchial carcinoid tumors (neuroendocrine tumors), bronchial gland tumors, fibrosarcomas, and lymphomas. The lung is also a frequent site of metastasis from cancers in other parts of the body.

BRONCHOGENIC CARCINOMA

Bronchogenic carcinomas are aggressive, locally invasive, and widely metastatic tumors that arise from the epithelial lining of the major bronchi. These tumors begin as small mucosal lesions that may follow one of several patterns of growth. They may form intraluminal masses that invade the bronchial mucosa and infiltrate the peribronchial connective tissue, or they may form large, bulky masses that extend into the adjacent lung tissue. Some large tumors undergo central necrosis and acquire local areas of hemorrhage, and some invade the pleural cavity and chest wall and spread to adjacent intrathoracic structures.[34] All varieties of bronchogenic carcinomas, especially small cell lung carcinoma, have the capacity to synthesize bioactive products and produce paraneoplastic syndromes (see Chapter 8).

Bronchogenic carcinomas can be subdivided into four major categories: squamous cell lung carcinoma (25% to 40%), adenocarcinoma (20% to 40%), small cell carcinoma (20% to 25%), and large cell carcinoma (10% to 15%).[34] For purposes of staging and treatment, bronchogenic cancers are commonly identified as small cell lung cancer (SCLC) or non–small cell lung cancer (NSCLC). The key reason for this classification is that all SCLCs have metastasized by the time of diagnosis and hence are not amenable to cancer surgery. They are usually best treated with chemotherapy, with or without radiation.

Small Cell Lung Cancers

The SCLCs are characterized by a distinctive cell type—small round to oval cells that are approximately the size of a lymphocyte.[34] The cells grow in clusters that exhibit neither glandular nor squamous organization. Electron microscopic studies demonstrate the presence of neurosecretory granules in some of the tumor cells similar to those found in the bronchial epithelium of the fetus or neonate. The presence of these granules, the ability of some of these tumors to secrete polypeptide hormones, and the presence of neuroendocrine markers such as neuron-specific enolase and parathormone-like and other hormonally active products suggest that these tumors may arise from the neuroendocrine cells of the bronchial epithelium. This cell type has the strongest association with cigarette smoking and is rarely observed in someone who has not smoked.[63]

The SCLCs are highly malignant, tend to infiltrate widely, disseminate early in their course, and rarely are resectable. About 70% have detectable metastasis at the time of diagnosis.[64] Brain metastases are particularly common with SCLC and may provide the first evidence of the tumor. Without treatment, one half of persons with SCLC die within 12 to 15 weeks.

This type of lung cancer is associated with several types of paraneoplastic syndrome, including the syndrome of inappropriate antidiuretic hormone (SIADH; see Chapter 33), Cushing's syndrome associated with ectopic production of adrenocorticotropic hormone (ACTH), and the Eaton-Lambert syndrome of neuromuscular disorder (see Chapter 8).[61]

Non–Small Cell Lung Cancers

The NSCLCs include squamous cell carcinomas, adenocarcinomas, and large cell carcinomas. As with the SCLCs, these cancers have the capacity to synthesize bioactive products and produce paraneoplastic syndromes.

Squamous Cell Carcinoma. Squamous cell carcinoma is found most commonly in men and is closely correlated with a smoking history. Squamous cell carcinoma tends to originate in the central bronchi as an intraluminal growth and is thus more amenable to early detection through cytologic examination of the sputum than other forms of lung cancer (Fig. 30-6). It tends to spread centrally into major bronchi and hilar lymph nodes and disseminates outside the thorax later than other types of bronchogenic cancers. Squamous cell carcinoma is associated with the paraneoplastic syndromes that produce hypercalcemia.

Adenocarcinoma. Currently, adenocarcinoma is the most common type of lung cancer found in North America. Its association with cigarette smoking is weaker than for squamous cell carcinoma. It is the most common type of lung cancer in women and nonsmokers.

Adenocarcinomas can have their origin in either the bronchiolar or alveolar tissues of the lung. These tumors tend to be located more peripherally than squamous cell sarcomas and sometimes are associated with areas of scarring (Fig. 30-7). The scars may be due to old infarcts, metallic foreign bodies, wounds, and granulomatous infections such as tuberculosis. In general, adenocarcinomas have a poorer stage-for-stage prognosis than squamous cell carcinomas.

Large Cell Cancer. Large cell carcinomas have large polygonal cells. They constitute a group of neoplasms that are highly anaplastic and difficult to categorize as squamous cell or adenocarcinoma. They tend to occur in the periphery of the lung, invading subsegmental bronchi and larger airways. They have a poor prognosis because of their tendency to spread to distant sites early in their course.

ETIOLOGY AND PATHOGENESIS

As with other cancers, bronchogenic carcinoma arises by stepwise accumulation of abnormalities that result in transformation of benign bronchial epithelium into neoplastic tissue (see Chapter 8). A common genetic abnormality is a loss of genetic material from chromosome 3. Several of the regions on this chromosome are altered to varying degrees in precancerous lung lesions. The SCLCs are also characterized by high frequency of *TP53* and *RB* tumor suppressor gene mutations. With respect to prognosis, over-expression of *HER-2/neu* (see Chapter 8) predicts a worse outcome with respect to adenocarcinomas. Alterations in the expression

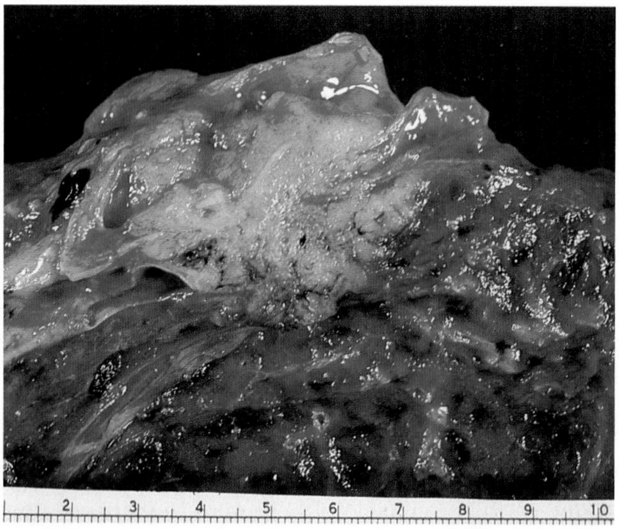

FIGURE 30-6 Squamous cell carcinoma of the lung. Tumor mass arising from a proximal branch of the left main-stem bronchus (*arrow*) has occluded the bronchial lumen and metastasized to the regional lymph nodes. (Rubin E., Farber J.L. [1999]. *Pathology* [3rd ed., p. 656]. Philadelphia: Lippincott-Raven)

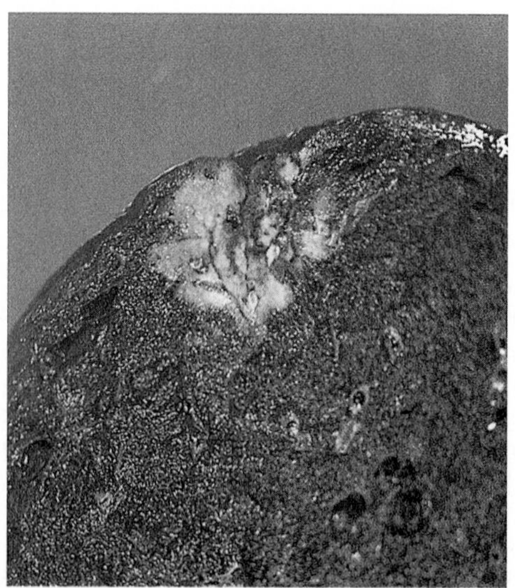

FIGURE 30-7 Adenocarcinoma of the lung. A peripheral tumor in the upper right lobe of the lung. (Rubin E., Farber J.L. [1999]. *Pathology* [3rd ed., p. 657]. Philadelphia: Lippincott-Raven)

of retinoic acid receptors may also contribute to the carcinogenesis of lung cancer. It is anticipated that some of these molecular defects may serve as targets for the design of novel cancer treatments.

At the end of the 20th century, lung cancer had emerged as one of the leading causes of preventable death.[65] It was a rare disease at the beginning of the century, but exposure to new etiologic agents such as cigarette smoke and increased life span have combined to make it one of the leading causes of death. Although tobacco has been widely used throughout the world for centuries, the present pandemic of lung cancer followed the introduction of manufactured cigarettes with addictive properties that resulted in a new pattern of sustained exposure of the lung to inhaled carcinogens.[65] The risk for lung cancer among cigarette smokers increases with duration of smoking and the number of cigarettes smoked per day. Cigarette smokers can benefit at any age from smoking cessation. However, even for periods of abstinence greater than 40 years, the risk for lung cancer among former smokers remains elevated compared with that of nonsmokers.[65]

Industrial hazards also contribute to the incidence of lung cancer. A commonly recognized hazard is exposure to asbestos, with the mean risk for lung cancer being significantly greater in asbestos workers than in the general population. Tobacco smoke contributes heavily to the development of lung cancer in persons exposed to asbestos; the risk in this population group is estimated to be 60 to 90 times greater than that for nonsmokers.[65]

There is also evidence to suggest that lung cancer may aggregate in some families. This occurrence may be due to a genetic predispostion, with the trait being expressed only in the presence of its major predisposing factor: cigarette smoking.[61]

Epidemiologic studies demonstrate a reduction in lung cancer in persons who consume large amounts of fruits and vegetables, a benefit theoretically related to high levels of beta-carotene, vitamin A, and other antioxidants. Newer ongoing chemopreventive efforts are using agents selectively directed at some of these molecular targets.

MANIFESTATIONS

The manifestations of lung cancer are extremely variable, depending on the location of the tumor, the presence of distant metastasis, and the occurrence of paraneoplastic syndromes. Often, the malignancy develops insidiously, giving little or no warning of its presence. Because its symptoms are similar to those associated with smoking and chronic bronchitis, they often are disregarded.

The manifestations of lung cancer can be divided into three categories: those due to involvement of the lung and adjacent structures, the effects of local spread and metastasis, and the nonmetastatic paraneoplastic manifestations involving endocrine, neurologic, and connective tissue function. As with other cancers, lung cancer also causes nonspecific symptoms such as anorexia and weight loss.

Many of the manifestations of lung cancers result from local irritation and obstruction of the airways and from invasion of the mediastinum and pleural space. The earliest symptoms usually are chronic cough, shortness of breath, and wheezing because of airway irritation and obstruction. Hemoptysis (*i.e.,* blood in the sputum) occurs when the lesion erodes blood vessels. Pain receptors in the chest are limited to the parietal pleura, mediastinum, larger blood vessels, and peribronchial afferent vagal fibers. Dull, intermittent, poorly localized retrosternal pain is common in tumors that involve the mediastinum. Pain becomes persistent, localized, and more severe when the disease invades the pleura.

Tumors that invade the mediastinum may cause hoarseness because of the involvement of the recurrent laryngeal nerve and cause difficulty in swallowing because of compression of the esophagus. An uncommon complication called the *superior vena cava syndrome* can occur in some persons with mediastinal involvement. Interruption of blood flow in this vessel usually results from compression by the tumor or involved lymph nodes. The disorder can interfere with venous drainage from the head, neck, and chest wall. The outcome is determined by the speed with which the disorder develops and the adequacy of the collateral circulation.

Tumors adjacent to the visceral pleura often insidiously produce pleural effusion. This effusion can compress the lung and cause atelectasis and dyspnea. It is less likely to cause fever, pleural friction rub, or pain than pleural effusion resulting from other causes.

Metastatic spread occurs by way of lymph channels and the vascular system. Metastases already exist in 50% of patients presenting with evidence of lung cancer and develop eventually in about 90% of patients. The most common sites of these metastases are the brain, bone, and liver.

Paraneoplastic disorders are those that are unrelated to metastasis. These include hypercalcemia from secretion of parathyroid-like peptide, Cushing's syndrome from ACTH secretion, SIADH, neuromuscular syndromes (*e.g.,* Eaton-Lambert syndrome), and hematologic disorders (*e.g.,* migratory thrombophlebitis, nonbacterial endocarditis, disseminated intravascular coagulation). Neurologic or muscular symptoms can develop 6 months to 4 years before the lung tumor is detected. One of the more common of these problems is weakness and wasting of the proximal muscles of the pelvic and shoulder girdles, with decreased deep tendon reflexes but without sensory changes. Hypercalcemia is seen most often in persons with squamous cell carcinoma, hematologic syndromes in persons with adenocarcinomas, and the remaining syndromes in persons with small cell neoplasms. Manifestations of the paraneoplastic syndrome may precede the onset of other signs of lung cancer and may lead to discovery of an occult tumor.

DIAGNOSIS AND TREATMENT

The diagnosis of lung cancer is based on a careful history and physical examination and on other tests such as chest radiography, bronchoscopy, cytologic studies (Papanicolaou's [Pap] test) of the sputum or bronchial washings, percutaneous needle biopsy of lung tissue, and scalene lymph node biopsy.[61] CT scans, MRI studies, and ultrasonography are used to locate lesions and evaluate the extent of the disease. Positron-emission tomography (PET) is a noninvasive alternative for identifying metastatic lesions in the mediastinum or distant sites. Persons with SCLC should also have a CT scan or MRI of the brain for detection of metastasis.

Like other types of cancer, lung cancers also are classified according to cell type (*i.e.*, squamous cell carcinoma, adenocarcinoma, and large cell carcinoma) and staged according to the TNM system (see Chapter 8).

Treatment methods for NSCLC include surgery, radiation therapy, and chemotherapy.[61] These treatments may be used singly or in combination. Surgery is used for the removal of small, localized NSCLC tumors. It can involve a lobectomy, pneumonectomy, or segmental resection of the lung. Radiation therapy can be used as a definitive or main treatment modality, as part of a combined treatment plan, or for palliation of symptoms. Because of the frequency of metastases, chemotherapy often is used in treating lung cancer. Combination chemotherapy, which uses a regimen of several drugs, usually is used. New targeted treatments are under development with the goal of increasing survival and ultimately providing a cure for this type of cancer.

Therapy for SCLC is based on chemotherapy and radiotherapy.[61,63,64] Advances in the use of combination chemotherapy, along with thoracic irradiation, have improved the outlook for persons with SCLC. Because SCLC may metastasize to the brain, prophylactic cranial irradiation is often indicated. In most persons who achieve a complete remission from SCLC, the brain is the most frequent site of relapse. About half of such persons develop clinical metastasis within 3 years. Newer combination chemotherapy regimens and targeted therapies are being developed in hopes of providing treatment alternatives that increase survival and produce fewer treatment liabilities.

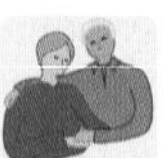

Management of Lung Cancer in Older Adults

At the time of diagnosis, most people with lung cancer are older than 65 years and have stage III or IV disease.[61,62] Knowledge about the optimal treatment for older persons is limited because of underrepresentation in clinical trials and failure to evaluate younger versus older persons in randomized clinical trials. At present, it is recommended that the elderly should be treated based on their general physiologic rather than chronologic age. This includes an evaluation of functional status (ability to be independent in daily tasks at home and in the community), coexisting medical conditions, nutritional status, cognition, psychological functioning, social support, and medication review. Those with good performance status and normal renal and hematologic parameters may be treated surgically or receive standard chemoradiation for limited-stage disease and combination chemotherapy for extensive-stage disease.

Surgery remains the mainstay for older persons with stages I to III NSCLC. Curative resection is feasible in older persons. The challenge for surgical treatment for older persons is age-related physiologic changes in cardiovascular and respiratory systems that may affect tolerance to surgery.

Radiation can be given with curative intent for older persons who are not surgical candidates. It may also be used for palliation of cancer-related symptoms. Evidence suggests that treatment tolerance and efficacy of thoracic radiation is similar in younger and older patients. Age is reported to have no effect on acute or late radiation toxicity, including nausea, dyspnea, esophagitis, or weakness. Older patients are more likely, however, to experience weight loss as compared with younger patients.[61]

Chemotherapy is the mainstay of treatment of SCLC. Older persons with good performance status may receive standard chemotherapy for limited disease and combination chemotherapy for extensive-stage disease. Some older persons may require dose reductions or be unable to complete the full chemotherapy course.[61]

In summary, cancer of the lung is a leading cause of death among men and women in the United States. Recently, there has been a greater increase in incidence and mortality of lung cancer in persons older than 65 years of age. Because lung cancer develops insidiously, it often is far advanced before it is diagnosed; a fact that is used to explain the poor 5-year survival rate. The increased death rate from lung cancer has coincided with an increase in cigarette smoking. Industrial hazards, such as exposure to asbestos, increase the risk for development of lung cancer. Bronchogenic carcinoma, which accounts for 95% of all primary lung cancers, can be subdivided into four major categories: squamous cell carcinoma, adenocarcinoma, large cell carcinoma, and small cell carcinoma. For purposes of staging and treatment, bronchogenic carcinoma is divided into small cell lung cancer and non–small cell lung cancer. The main reason for this is that almost all small cell lung cancers have metastasized at the time of diagnosis and are not amenable to surgical resection.

The manifestations of lung cancer can be attributed to the involvement of the lung and adjacent structures, the effects of local spread and metastasis, and paraneoplastic syndromes involving endocrine, neurologic, and hematologic dysfunction. As with other cancers, lung cancer causes nonspecific symptoms such as anorexia and weight loss. Treatment methods for lung cancer include surgery, irradiation, and chemotherapy. The current increase in lung cancer among the elderly has required a rethinking of the treatment strategies for this age group, with the trend being to base treatment on physiologic rather than chronologic age.

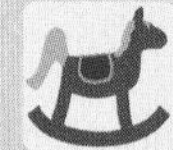

Respiratory Disorders in Children

After completing this section of the chapter, you should be able to meet the following objectives:

- Trace the development of the respiratory tract through the five stages of embryonic and fetal development
- Cite the function of surfactant in lung function in the neonate
- Cite the possible cause and manifestations of respiratory distress syndrome and bronchopulmonary dysplasia

- ✦ Describe the physiologic basis for sternal and chest wall retractions and grunting, stridor, and wheezing as signs of respiratory distress in infants and small children
- ✦ Compare croup, epiglottitis, and bronchiolitis in terms of incidence by age, site of infection, and signs and symptoms
- ✦ List the signs of impending respiratory failure in small children

Acute respiratory disease is the most common cause of illness in infancy and childhood, accounting for 50% of illness in children younger than 5 years of age and 30% of illness in children between 5 and 12 years of age.[66] This section focuses on (1) lung development, with an emphasis on the developmental basis for lung disorders in children; (2) respiratory disorders in the neonate; and (3) respiratory infections in children. A discussion of bronchial asthma in children and cystic fibrosis is included in Chapter 31.

LUNG DEVELOPMENT

Although other body systems are physiologically ready for extrauterine life as early as 25 weeks of gestation, the lungs require much longer. Immaturity of the respiratory system is a major cause of morbidity and mortality in infants born prematurely. Even at birth, the lungs are not fully mature, and additional growth and maturation continue well into childhood.

Lung development may be divided into five stages: embryonic period, pseudoglandular period, canicular period, saccular period, and alveolar period.[67,68] The development of the respiratory system begins with the embryonic period (weeks 4 to 6 of gestation), during which a rudimentary lung bud branches from the esophagus to begin formation of the airways and alveolar spaces (Fig. 30-8). The lung bud divides into two lung buds that grow laterally; the right bud gives rise to two secondary buds and the

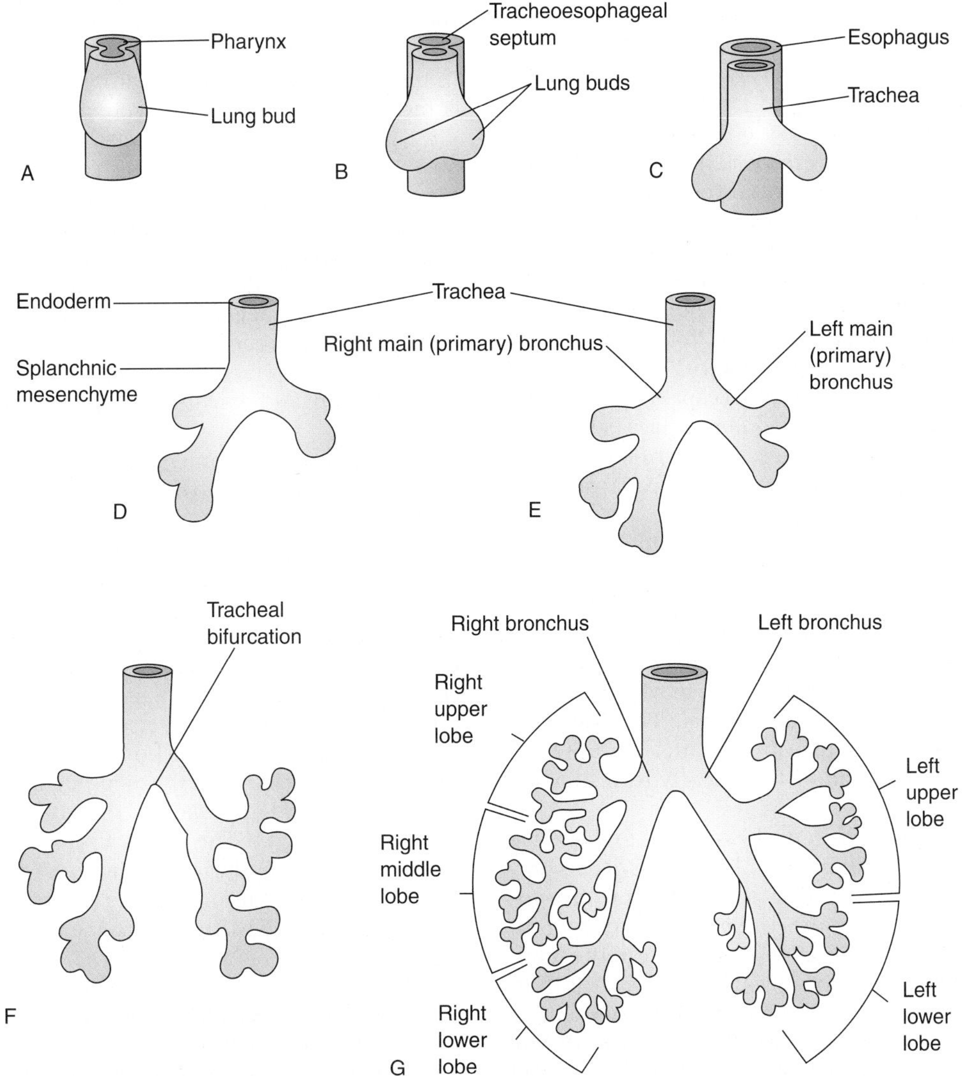

FIGURE 30-8 Drawings of ventral views illustrating successive stages in the development of the bronchi and lungs. **(A–C)** 4 weeks, **(D, E)** 5 weeks, **(F)** 6 weeks, **(G)** 8 weeks. (Moore K. [1993]. *The developing human* [5th ed.]. Philadelphia: W.B. Saunders)

left bud to one secondary bud. Consequently, at maturity, there are three main (primary) bronchi and three lung lobes on the right and only two main bronchi and two lung lobes on the left. Each secondary lung bud subsequently undergoes continuous branching. The tertiary (segmental) bronchi (10 in the right lung and 8 or 9 in the left lung) begin to form during the seventh week.

During the pseudo-glandular period (weeks 5 to 16), the lungs resemble a gland. During this period, the conducting airways are formed. At 17 weeks, all of the major elements of the lung have formed except the gas exchange structures. Respiration is not possible because the airways end in blind tubes.

The canicular period (weeks 17 to 27) marks the formation of the primitive alveoli. The lumina of the bronchi and bronchioles become much larger, and the lung tissue becomes more highly vascularized. By the 24th week, each bronchiole has given rise to two or more respiratory bronchioles. Respiration is possible at this time because some primitive alveoli have developed at the ends of the bronchioles.[67]

The saccular period (weeks 27 to 35) is devoted to the development of the terminal alveolar sacs, which facilitate gas exchange. During this period, the terminal sacs thin out, and capillaries begin to bulge into the terminal sacs. These thin cells are known as type I alveolar cells. By the 25th to 28th week, sufficient terminal sacs are present to permit survival. Before this time, the premature lungs are incapable of adequate gas exchange. It is not so much the presence of the thin alveolar epithelium as it is the adequate matching of pulmonary vasculature to it that is critical to survival.[67] Type II alveolar cells begin to develop at approximately 24 weeks. These cells produce surfactant, a substance capable of lowering the surface tension of the air–alveoli interface (see Chapter 29). By the 28th to 30th week, sufficient amounts of surfactant are available to prevent alveolar collapse when breathing begins.

The alveolar period (late fetal to early childhood) marks the maturation and expansion of the alveoli. Starting as early as 30 weeks and usually by 36 weeks, the saccular structures become alveoli. Alveolar development is characterized by thinning of the pulmonary interstitium and the appearance of a single-capillary network, in which one capillary bulges into each terminal alveolar sac. By the late fetal period, the lungs are capable of respiration because the alveolar-capillary membrane is sufficiently thin to allow for gas exchange.

Although transformation of the lungs from glandlike structures to highly vascular, alveoli-like organs occurs during the late fetal period, mature alveoli do not form for some time after birth. The growth of the lung during infancy and early childhood involves an increase in the number rather than the size of the alveoli. Only one eighth to one sixth of the adult number of alveoli are present at birth. There is a relative slowing of alveolar growth during the first 3 months after birth, and this is followed by a rapid increase in alveolar number during the rest of the first year of life, reaching approximately the adult number of 300 million alveoli by 8 years of age.[67]

Development of Breathing in the Fetus and Neonate

The fetal lung is a secretory organ, and fluids and electrolytes are secreted into the potential air spaces. This fluid appears to be important in stimulating alveolar development. For the fetus to complete the transition from intrauterine to extrauterine life, this fluid must be cleared from the lung soon after birth. Presumably with the onset of labor, the secretion of fluid ceases. During the birth process, pressure on the fetal thorax causes the fluid to be expelled from the mouth and nose. When the lungs expand after birth, the fluid moves into the tissues surrounding the alveoli and is then absorbed into the pulmonary capillaries or removed by the lymphatic system.

Fetal breathing movements occur in utero. These movements are irregular in rate and amplitude, ranging from 30 to 70 breaths per minute, and become more rapid as gestation advances. Because they are rapid and shallow, these movements do not result in movement of fluid into or out of the fetal lung. Instead, they are thought to condition the respiratory muscles and stimulate lung development. The breathing movements in the fetus become more rapid in response to an increase in carbon dioxide levels and become slower in response to hypoxia.

The major difference between respiration in the fetus and the neonate is that there is complete separation between gas exchange and breathing movements in the fetus. The gas supply and exchange depend entirely on maternal mechanisms controlling placental circulation. At birth, dependence on the placental circulation is terminated, and the infant must integrate the two previously separate functions of gas exchange and respiratory movements. Within seconds of clamping the umbilical cord, the infant takes its first breath, and rhythmic breathing begins and persists for life.

Effective ventilation requires coordinated interaction between the muscles of the upper airways, including those of the pharynx and larynx, the diaphragm, and the intercostal muscles of the chest wall. In infants, a specific sequence of upper airway nerve and muscle activity occurs before and early in inspiration: the tongue moves forward to prevent airway obstruction, and the vocal cord abducts, reducing laryngeal resistance. By moving downward, the action of the diaphragm increases chest volume in both the longitudinal and transverse directions. In the infant, the diaphragm inserts more horizontally than in the adult. As a result, contraction of the diaphragm tends to draw the lower ribs inward, especially if the infant is placed in the horizontal position. The function of the intercostal muscles is to lift the ribs during inspiration. In the infant, however, the intercostal muscles are not fully developed, so they function largely to stabilize the chest rather than lift the chest wall.

The chest wall of the neonate is highly compliant; although this is advantageous during the birth process in that it allows for marked distortion to occur without damaging chest structures, it has implications for ventilation during the postnatal period. A striking characteristic of neonatal breathing is the paradoxical inward movement of the upper chest during inspiration, especially during active sleep. This occurs because of decreased activity of the intercostal muscles during active sleep, which allows the contracting diaphragm to pull the highly compliant chest wall inward. Under circumstances such as crying, the intercostal muscles of the neonate function together with the diaphragm to splint the chest wall and prevent its collapse.

Normally, the infant's lungs also are compliant; this is advantageous to the infant with its compliant chest cage because it takes only small changes in inspiratory pressure to inflate a compliant lung. When respiratory disease develops, lung compliance is reduced, and it takes more effort to inflate the lungs. The diaphragm must generate more negative pressure; as a result, the compliant chest wall structures are sucked inward. *Retractions* are abnormal inward movements of the chest wall during inspiration; they may occur intercostally (between the ribs), in the substernal or epigastric area, and in the supraclavicular spaces. Because the chest wall of the infant is compliant, substernal retractions become more obvious with small changes in lung function. Retractions can indicate airway obstruction or atelectasis.

Also influencing the effectiveness of ventilation in the neonate are the intrinsic mechanical properties of the diaphragm. Although much uncertainty remains regarding the functioning of the respiratory muscles in the neonate, it seems that these muscles, particularly in the preterm infant, are undeveloped and poorly adapted for high workloads. The underdeveloped sarcoplasmic reticulum of the premature infant results in an increased contraction and relaxation time. This increased relaxation time may be an important factor in impeding blood flow and limiting oxidative metabolism during increased muscle function.[68]

Airway Resistance

Normal lung inflation requires uninterrupted movement of air through the extrathoracic airways (*i.e.*, nose, pharynx, larynx, and upper trachea) and intrathoracic airways (*i.e.*, bronchi and bronchioles). The neonate (0 to 4 weeks of age) breathes predominantly through the nose and does not adapt well to mouth breathing. Any obstruction of the nose or nasopharynx may increase upper airway resistance and increase the work of breathing.

The airways of the infant and small child are much smaller than those of the adult. Because the resistance to airflow is directly related to the fourth power of the radius (resistance = $1/r^4$), relatively small amounts of mucus secretion, edema, or airway constriction can produce marked changes in airway resistance and airflow. Nasal flaring is a method that infants use to take in more air. This method of breathing increases the size of the nares and decreases the resistance of the small airways.

Normally, the extrathoracic airways in the infant narrow during inspiration and widen during expiration, and the intrathoracic airways widen during inspiration and narrow during expiration.[69] This occurs because the pressure inside the extrathoracic airways reflects the intrapleural pressures that are generated during breathing, whereas the pressure outside the airways is similar to atmospheric pressure. Thus, during inspiration, the pressure inside becomes more negative, causing the airways to narrow, and during expiration it becomes more positive, causing them to widen. In contrast to the extrathoracic airways, the pressure outside the intrathoracic airways is equal to the intrapleural pressure. These airways widen during inspiration as the surrounding intrapleural pressure becomes more negative and pulls them open, and they narrow during expiration as the surrounding pressure becomes more positive.

Lung Volumes and Gas Exchange

The functional residual capacity, which is the air left in the lungs at the end of normal expiration, plays an important role in the gas exchange of the infant. In the infant, the functional residual capacity occurs at a higher lung volume than in the older child or adult.[70] This higher end-expiratory volume results from a more rapid respiratory rate, which leaves less time for expiration. However, the increased residual volume is important to the neonate because it holds the airways open throughout all phases of respiration; it favors the reabsorption of intrapulmonary fluids; and it maintains more uniform lung expansion and enhances gas exchange. During sleep, the tone of the upper airway muscles is reduced, so that the time spent in expiration is shorter and the intercostal activity that stabilizes the chest wall is less; this produces a lower end-expiratory volume and less optimal gas exchange during active sleep.[70]

Control of Ventilation

Fetal blood oxygen (PO_2) levels normally range from 25 to 30 mm Hg, and carbon dioxide (PCO_2) levels range from 45 to 50 mm Hg, independent of any respiratory movements. Any decrease in oxygen levels induces quiet sleep in the fetus with subsequent cessation of breathing movements, both of which lead to a decrease in oxygen consumption. Switching to oxygen derived from the aerated lung at birth causes an immediate increase in PO_2 to approximately 50 mm Hg; within a few hours, it increases to approximately 70 mm Hg.[69] These levels, which greatly exceed fetal levels, cause the chemoreceptors (see Chapter 29) to become silent for several days. Although the infant's PO_2 may fluctuate during this critical time, the chemoreceptors do not respond appropriately. It is not until several days after birth that the chemoreceptors "reset" their PO_2 threshold; only then do they become the major controller of breathing. However, the response seems to be biphasic, with an initial hyperventilation followed by a decreased respiratory rate and even apnea. In normal neonates, particularly in preterm infants, breathing patterns and respiratory reflexes depend on the arousal state.[70] Periodic breathing and apnea are characteristic of premature infants and reflect patterns of fetal breathing. The fact that they occur with sleep and disappear during wakefulness underscores the importance of arousal.

ALTERATIONS IN BREATHING

Most lung diseases in children produce decreased lung compliance and manifestations of restrictive lung disease, or they increase airway resistance. Children with restrictive lung disease breathe at faster rates, and their respiratory excursions are shallow. Grunting is an audible noise emitted during expiration. An expiratory grunt is common as the child tries to raise the functional residual capacity by closing the glottis at the end of expiration. Grunting is a sign of labored breathing that usually is caused by decreased lung compliance or lung volume; it may serve as a compensatory mechanism for lung dysfunction by increasing lung volume and improving arterial oxygenation.

The pressure needed to overcome airway resistance depends on the rate of airflow as it moves into and out of the lungs; the need is greatest during periods of high flow. Because airway resistance increases the work of breathing, children with obstructive disease take slower, deeper breaths. When the obstruction is in the extrathoracic airways, inspiration is more prolonged than expiration, and an audible "crowing sound" called an *inspiratory stridor* commonly is produced. When the obstruction is in the intrathoracic airways, expiration is prolonged, and the child makes use of the accessory expiratory muscles.

When obstruction of the extrathoracic airways occurs, as in croup, the pressures distal to the point of obstruction must become more negative to overcome the resistance; this causes collapse of the distal airways, and the increased turbulence of air moving through the obstructed airways produces an audible crowing sound called *stridor.* With intrathoracic airway obstruction, as occurs with bronchiolitis and bronchial asthma, the intrapleural pressure becomes more positive during expiration because of air trapping; this causes collapse of intrathoracic airways and produces an audible wheezing or whistling sound during expiration.

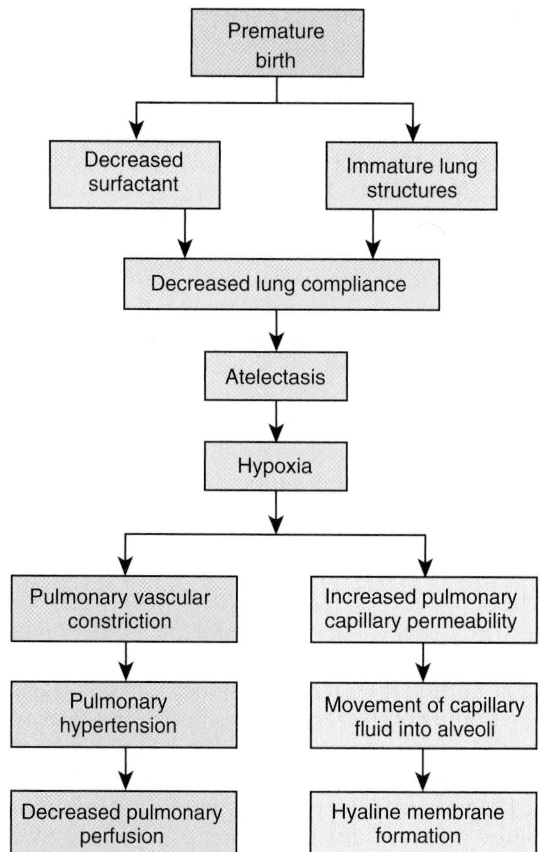

FIGURE 30-9 Pathogenesis of respiratory distress syndrome (RDS) in the infant.

RESPIRATORY DISORDERS IN THE NEONATE

The neonatal period is one of transition from placental dependency to air breathing. This transition requires functioning of the surfactant system, conditioning of the respiratory muscles, and establishment of parallel pulmonary and systemic circulations. Respiratory disorders develop in infants who are born prematurely or who have other problems that impair this transition. Among the respiratory disorders of the neonate are the respiratory distress syndrome, bronchopulmonary dysplasia, and persistent fetal circulation (*i.e.,* delayed closure of the ductus arteriosus and foramen ovale).

Respiratory Distress Syndrome

Respiratory distress syndrome (RDS), also known as *hyaline membrane disease,* is one of the most common causes of respiratory disease in premature infants. In these infants, pulmonary immaturity, together with surfactant deficiency, leads to alveolar collapse (Fig. 30-9). The type II alveolar cells that produce surfactant do not begin to mature until approximately the 25th to 28th weeks of gestation, and consequently, many premature infants are born with poorly functioning type II alveolar cells and have difficulty producing sufficient amounts of surfactant. The incidence of RDS is higher among preterm male infants, white infants, infants of diabetic mothers, and those subjected to asphyxia, cold stress, precipitous deliveries, and delivery by cesarean section (when performed before the 38th week of gestation).

Surfactant synthesis is influenced by several hormones, including insulin and cortisol. Insulin tends to inhibit surfactant production; this explains why infants of insulin-dependent diabetic mothers are at increased risk for development of RDS. Cortisol can accelerate maturation of type II cells and formation of surfactant. The reason that premature infants born by cesarean section presumably are at greater risk for development of RDS is because they are not subjected to the stress of vaginal delivery, which is thought to increase the infants' cortisol levels. These observations have led to administration of corticosteroid drugs before delivery to mothers with infants at high risk for development of RDS.[71]

Surfactant reduces the surface tension in the alveoli, thereby equalizing the retractive forces in the large and small alveoli and reducing the amount of pressure needed to inflate and hold the alveoli open. Without surfactant, the large alveoli remain inflated, whereas the small alveoli become difficult to inflate. At birth, the first breath requires high inspiratory pressures to expand the lungs. With normal levels of surfactant, the lungs retain up to 40% of the residual volume after the first breath, and subsequent breaths require far lower inspiratory pressures.[1] With a surfactant deficiency, the lungs collapse between breaths, making the infant work as hard with each successive breath as with the first breath. The airless portions of the lungs become stiff and noncompliant. A hyaline membrane forms inside the alveoli as protein- and fibrin-rich fluids are pulled into the alveolar spaces. The fibrin-hyaline membrane constitutes a barrier to gas exchange, leading to hypoxemia and carbon dioxide retention, a condition that further impairs surfactant production.

Infants with RDS present with multiple signs of respiratory distress, usually within the first 24 hours of birth. Central cyanosis is a prominent sign. Breathing becomes more difficult, and retractions occur as the infant's soft chest wall is pulled in as the diaphragm descends. Grunting sounds occur during expiration. As the tidal volume drops because of atelectasis, the respiration rate increases (usually to 60 to 120 breaths/min) in an effort to maintain normal minute ventilation. Fatigue may develop rapidly because of the increased work of breathing. The stiff lung of infants with RDS also increases resistance to blood flow in the pulmonary circulation. As a result, a hemodynamically significant patent ductus arteriosus may develop in infants with RDS (see Chapter 26).

The basic principles of treatment for infants with suspected RDS focus on the provision of supportive care, including gentle handling and minimal disturbance.[71] An isolette or radiant warmer is used to prevent hypothermia and increased oxygen consumption. Continuous cardiorespiratory monitoring is needed. Monitoring of blood glucose and prevention of hypoglycemia are also recommended. Oxygen levels can be assessed through an arterial line (umbilical) or by a transcutaneous oxygen sensor. Treatment includes administration of supplemental oxygen, continuous positive airway pressure through nasal prongs, and often assisted mechanical ventilation.

Exogenous surfactant therapy is used to prevent and treat RDS.[71] There are two types of surfactants available in the United States: natural surfactants prepared from animal sources and synthetic surfactants. The surfactants are suspended in saline and administered into the airways, usually through an endotracheal tube. The treatment often is initiated soon after birth in infants who are at high risk for RDS.

Bronchopulmonary Dysplasia

Bronchopulmonary dysplasia (BPD) is a chronic lung disease that develops in premature infants who were treated with mechanical ventilation, mainly for RDS. The condition is considered to be present if the neonate is oxygen dependent at 36 weeks after gestation. The disorder is thought to be a response of the premature lung to early injury. High inspired oxygen concentration and injury from positive-pressure ventilation (*i.e.*, barotrauma) have been implicated. Newer therapies such as administration of surfactants, high-frequency ventilation, and prenatal or postnatal administration of corticosteroids may have altered the severity of BPD, but the condition remains a major health problem.[72–74]

BPD is characterized by chronic respiratory distress, persistent hypoxemia when breathing room air, reduced lung compliance, increased airway resistance, and severe expiratory flow limitation. There is a mismatching of ventilation and perfusion with development of hypoxemia and hypercapnia. Pulmonary vascular resistance may be increased and pulmonary hypertension and cor pulmonale (*i.e.*, right heart failure associated with lung disease) may develop. The infant with BPD may have tachycardia, shallow breathing, chest retractions, cough, barrel chest, and poor weight gain. Clubbing of the fingers occurs in children with severe disease. In infants with right heart failure, tachycardia, tachypnea, hepatomegaly, and periorbital edema develop.

The treatment of BPD includes mechanical ventilation and administration of adequate oxygenation. Weaning from ventilation is accomplished gradually, and some infants may require ventilation at home. Rapid lung growth occurs during the first year of life, and lung function usually improves.

Adequate nutrition is essential for recovery of infants with BPD. There has been an interest in the protective effect of polyunsaturated fatty acids, vitamin A, and other nutrients such as inositol (a sulfur-containing amino acid), and selenium in preventing lung injury in high-risk premature infants.[74] Research into the effects of some of these dietary substances is ongoing. Other areas of investigation include developmental influences such as glucocorticoid hormones, which accelerate the maturation of lung tissue, increase surfactant production and lung compliance, reduce vascular permeability, and increase lung water clearance.

Most adolescents and young adults who had severe BPD during infancy have some degree of pulmonary dysfunction, consisting of airway obstruction, airway hyperreactivity, or hyperinflation.

RESPIRATORY INFECTIONS IN CHILDREN

In children, respiratory tract infections are common, and although they are troublesome, they usually are not serious. Frequent infections occur because the immune system of infants and small children has not been exposed to many common pathogens; consequently, they tend to contract infections with each new exposure. Although most of these infections are not serious, the small size of an infant or child's airways tends to foster impaired airflow and obstruction. For example, an infection that causes only sore throat and hoarseness in an adult may result in serious airway obstruction in a small child.

Upper Airway Infections

Two serious upper respiratory tract infections are relatively common during early childhood—croup and epiglottitis. Croup is the more common one, and it usually is benign and self-limited. Epiglottitis is a rapidly progressive and life-threatening condition. The site of involvement is illustrated in Figure 30-10, and the characteristics of both infections are described in Table 30-2.

Obstruction of the upper airways because of infection tends to exert its greatest effect during the inspiratory phase of respiration. Movement of air through an obstructed

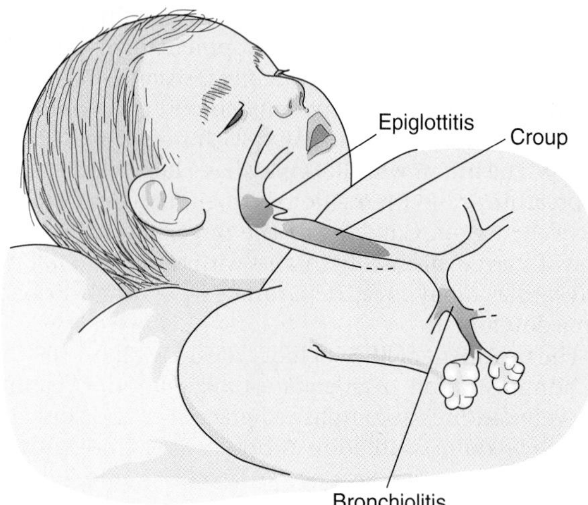

FIGURE 30-10 Location of airway obstruction in epiglottitis, acute laryngotracheobronchitis (croup), and bronchiolitis. (Courtesy of Carole Russell Hilmer, C.M.I.)

upper airway, particularly the vocal cords in the larynx, causes stridor.[75] Impairment of the expiratory phase of respiration also can occur, causing wheezing. With mild to moderate obstruction, inspiratory stridor is more prominent than expiratory wheezing because the airways tend to dilate with expiration. When the swelling and obstruction become severe, the airways no longer can dilate during expiration, and both stridor and wheezing occur.

Cartilaginous support of the trachea and the larynx is poorly developed in infants and small children. These structures are soft and tend to collapse when the airway is obstructed and the child cries, causing the inspiratory pressures to become more negative. When this happens, the stridor and inspiratory effort are increased. The phenomenon of airway collapse in the small child is analogous to what happens when a thick beverage, such as a milkshake, is drunk through a soft paper or plastic straw. The straw collapses when the negative pressure produced by the sucking effort exceeds the flow of liquid through the straw.

Viral Croup. Croup is characterized by inspiratory stridor, hoarseness, and a barking cough. The British use the term *croup* to describe the cry of the crow or raven, and this is undoubtedly how the term originated.

Viral croup, more appropriately called *acute laryngotracheobronchitis,* is a viral infection that affects the larynx, trachea, and bronchi. The parainfluenza viruses account for approximately 75% all cases; the remaining 25% are caused by adenoviruses, respiratory syncytial virus, influenza A and B viruses, and measles virus.[75–78] Viral croup usually is seen in children 3 months to 5 years of age. The condition may affect the entire laryngotracheal tree, but because the subglottic area is the narrowest part of the respiratory tree in this age group, the obstruction usually is greatest in this area. For example, the subglottic airway in the 1- to 2-year-old child is approximately 6.5 mm in diameter, and 1 mm of edema can reduce the cross-sectional area by 50%.[75]

Although the respiratory manifestations of croup often appear suddenly, they usually are preceded by upper respiratory infections that cause rhinorrhea (*i.e.,* runny nose), coryza (*i.e.,* common cold), hoarseness, and a low-grade fever. In most children, the manifestation of croup advances only to stridor and slight dyspnea before they begin to recover. The symptoms usually subside when the child is exposed to moist air. For example, letting the bathroom shower run and then taking the child into the bathroom often brings prompt and dramatic relief of symptoms. Exposure to cold air also seems to relieve the airway spasm;

TABLE 30-2 Characteristics of Epiglottitis, Croup, and Bronchiolitis in Small Children

Characteristics	Epiglottitis	Croup	Bronchiolitis
Common causative agent	*Haemophilus influenzae* type B bacterium	Mainly parainfluenza virus	Respiratory syncytial virus
Most commonly affected age group	2–7 years (peak 3–5 years)	3 months to 5 years	Less than 2 years (most severe in infants younger than 6 months)
Onset and preceding history	Sudden onset	Usually follows symptoms of a cold	Preceded by stuffy nose and other signs
Prominent features	Child appears very sick and toxic Sits with mouth open and chin thrust forward Low-pitched stridor, difficulty swallowing, fever, drooling, anxiety *Danger of airway obstruction and asphyxia*	Stridor and a wet, barking cough Usually occurs at night Relieved by exposure to cold or moist air	Breathlessness, rapid, shallow breathing, wheezing, cough, and retractions of lower ribs and sternum during inspiration
Usual treatment	Hospitalization Intubation or tracheotomy Treatment with appropriate antibiotic	Mist tent or vaporizer Administration of oxygen	Supportive treatment, administration of oxygen and hydration

often, the severe symptoms are relieved simply because the child is exposed to cold air on the way to the hospital emergency room. Viral croup does not respond to antibiotics; expectorants, bronchodilating agents, and antihistamines are not helpful. The child should be disturbed as little as possible and carefully monitored for signs of respiratory distress.

Airway obstruction may progress in some children. As obstruction increases, the stridor becomes continuous and is associated with nasal flaring with substernal and intercostal retractions. Agitation and crying aggravate the signs and symptoms, and the child prefers to sit up or be held upright. In the cyanotic, pale, or obstructed child, any manipulation of the pharynx, including use of a tongue depressor, can cause cardiorespiratory arrest and should be done only in a medical setting that has the facilities for emergency airway management. Other treatments may be required when a humidifier or mist tent is ineffective. One method is to administer a racemic mixture of epinephrine (L-epinephrine and D-epinephrine) by positive-pressure breathing through a face mask.[75] Establishment of an artificial airway may become necessary in severe airway obstruction.

Spasmodic Croup. Spasmodic croup manifests with symptoms similar to those of acute viral croup. Because the child is afebrile and lacks other manifestations of the viral prodrome, it is thought that it may have an allergic origin. Spasmodic croup characteristically occurs at night and tends to recur with respiratory tract infections. The episode usually lasts several hours and may recur several nights in a row.

Most children with spasmodic croup can be effectively managed at home. An environment of high humidification (*i.e.*, cold-water room humidifier or taking the child into a bathroom with a warm, running shower) lessens irritation and prevents drying of secretions.

Epiglottitis. Acute epiglottitis is a dramatic, potentially fatal condition most often caused by the *H. influenzae* type B bacterium. It is seen less commonly since the widespread use of immunization against *H. influenzae* type B. The condition usually occurs in children 2 to 7 years of age, with a peak incidence at approximately 3.5 years.[75] It is characterized by inflammatory edema of the supraglottic area, including the epiglottis and pharyngeal structures, that comes on suddenly, bringing danger of airway obstruction and asphyxia.[75,76] Within a matter of hours, epiglottitis may progress to complete obstruction of the airway and death unless adequate treatment is instituted.

The child appears pale, toxic, and lethargic and assumes a distinctive position—sitting up with the mouth open and the chin thrust forward. The child has difficulty in swallowing, a muffled voice, drooling, fever, and extreme anxiety. Moderate to severe respiratory distress is evident. There is inspiratory and sometimes expiratory stridor, flaring of the nares, and inspiratory retractions of the suprasternal notch and supraclavicular and intercostal spaces. Usually, no other family members are ill with acute respiratory disease.

The child with epiglottitis requires immediate hospitalization. Immediate establishment of an airway by endotracheal tube or tracheotomy usually is needed. If epiglottitis is suspected, the child should never be forced to lie down because this causes the epiglottis to fall backward and may lead to complete airway obstruction. Examination of the throat with a tongue blade or other instrument may cause cardiopulmonary arrest and should be done only by medical personnel experienced in intubation of small children. It also is unwise to attempt any procedure, such as drawing blood, that would heighten the child's anxiety, because this also could precipitate airway spasm and cause death. Recovery from epiglottitis usually is rapid and uneventful after an adequate airway has been established and appropriate antibiotic therapy has been initiated.

Epiglottitis can occur in adults as well as children. The incidence is low (an estimated 9.7 cases per 1 million persons) but appears to be increasing. In adults, epiglottitis may present with acute respiratory compromise or as a milder form of disease. Although the causative agent or agents have not been identified, *H. influenzae* does not appear to be a primary causative agent in adults. Airway closure is less of a threat in adults; it does occur, however, and provision for emergency tracheotomy should be available.[79]

Lower Airway Infections

Lower airway infections produce air trapping with prolonged expiration. Wheezing results from bronchospasm, mucosal inflammation, and edema. The child presents with increased expiratory effort, increased respiratory rate, and wheezing. If the infection is severe, there also are marked intercostal retractions and signs of impending respiratory failure.

Acute bronchiolitis is a viral infection of the lower airways, most commonly caused by the respiratory syncytial virus.[76,78,80] Other viruses, such as parainfluenza-3 virus and some adenoviruses, as well as mycoplasma, also are causative. The infection produces inflammatory obstruction of the small airways and necrosis of the cells lining the lower airways. It occurs during the first 2 years of life, with a peak incidence between 3 to 6 months of age. The source of infection usually is a family member with a minor respiratory illness. Older children and adults tolerate bronchiolar edema much better than infants and do not manifest the clinical picture of bronchiolitis. Because the resistance to airflow in a tube is related to the fourth power of the radius, even minor swelling of bronchioles in an infant can produce profound changes in airflow.

Most affected infants in whom bronchiolitis develops have a history of a mild upper respiratory tract infection. These symptoms usually last several days and may be accompanied by fever and diminished appetite. There is then a gradual development of respiratory distress, characterized by a wheezy cough, dyspnea, and irritability. The infant usually is able to take in sufficient air but has trouble exhaling it. Air becomes trapped in the lung distal to the site of obstruction and interferes with gas exchange. Hypoxemia and, in severe cases, hypercapnia may develop. Airway obstruction may produce air trapping and hyperinflation of the lungs or collapse of the alveoli. Infants with acute bronchiolitis have a typical appearance, marked by breathlessness with rapid respirations, a distressing cough, and retractions of the lower ribs and sternum. Crying and feeding exaggerate these signs. Wheezing and crackles may or may not be present, depending on the degree of airway obstruction. In infants with severe airway obstruction, wheezing decreases as the airflow diminishes. Usually, the most critical phase of the disease is the first 48 to 72 hours. Cyanosis, pallor, listlessness, and sudden diminution or absence of breath sounds indicate impending respiratory failure. The characteristics of bronchiolitis are described in Table 30-2.

Infants with respiratory distress usually are hospitalized. Treatment is supportive and includes administration of humidified oxygen to relieve hypoxia. Elevation of the head facilitates respiratory movements and avoids airway compression. Handling is kept at a minimum to avoid tiring. Because the infection is viral, antibiotics are not effective and are given only for a secondary bacterial infection. Dehydration may occur as the result of increased insensible water losses because of the rapid respiratory rate and feeding difficulties, and measures to ensure adequate hydration are needed. Recovery usually begins after the first 48 to 72 hours and usually is rapid and complete.

Signs of Impending Respiratory Failure

Respiratory problems of infants and small children often are of sudden origin, and recovery usually is rapid and complete. Children are at risk for the development of airway obstruction and respiratory failure resulting from obstructive disorders or lung infection. The child with epiglottitis is at risk for airway obstruction. The child with bronchiolitis is at risk for respiratory failure resulting from impaired gas exchange. Children with impending respiratory failure due to airway or lung disease have rapid breathing; exaggerated use of the accessory muscles; retractions, which are more pronounced in the child than in the adult because of more compliant chest; nasal flaring; and grunting during expiration.[81] The signs and symptoms of impending respiratory failure are listed in Chart 30-1.

CHART 30-1

Signs of Respiratory Distress and Impending Respiratory Failure in the Infant and Small Child

Severe increase in respiratory effort, including severe retractions or grunting, decreased chest movement
Cyanosis that is not relieved by administration of oxygen (40%)
Heart rate of 150 beats per minute or greater or bradycardia
Very rapid breathing (rate 60 per minute in the newborn to 6 months or above 30 per minute in children 6 months to 2 years)
Very depressed breathing (rate 20 per minute or below)
Retractions of the supraclavicular area, sternum, epigastrium, and intercostal spaces
Extreme anxiety and agitation
Fatigue
Decreased level of consciousness

Respiratory failure due to central nervous system conditions such as narcotic overdose or brain tumor usually cause a decreased ventilatory drive and hypoventilation.

In summary, acute respiratory disease is the most common cause of illness in infancy and childhood, accounting for 50% of illnesses in children younger than 5 years of age and 30% of illnesses in children between 5 and 12 years of age. Although other body systems are physiologically ready for extrauterine life as early as 25 weeks of gestation, the lungs take longer. Immaturity of the respiratory system is a major cause of morbidity and mortality in premature infants.

Lung development may be divided into five stages: embryonic period, pseudoglandular period, canicular period, saccular period, and alveolar period. The first three phases are devoted to development of the conducting airways, and the last two phases are devoted to development of the gas exchange portion of the lung. By the 25th to 28th weeks of gestation, sufficient terminal air sacs are present to permit survival. It is also during this period that type II alveolar cells, which produce surfactant, begin to function. Lung development is incomplete at birth; an infant is born with only one eighth to one sixth the adult number of alveoli. Alveoli continue to be formed during early childhood, reaching the adult number of 300 million alveoli by 8 years of age.

Children with restrictive lung disease breathe at faster rates, and their respiratory excursions are shallow. An expiratory grunt is common as the child tries to raise the functional residual capacity by closing the glottis at the end of expiration. Obstruction of the extrathoracic airways often produces turbulence of airflow and an audible inspiratory crowing sound called *stridor,* and obstruction of the intrathoracic airways produces an audible expiratory wheezing or whistling sound. RDS is one of the most common causes of respiratory disease in premature infants. In these infants, pulmonary immaturity, together with surfactant deficiency, leads to alveolar collapse. BPD is a chronic pulmonary disease that develops in premature infants who were treated with mechanical ventilation.

Because of the small size of the airway of infants and children, respiratory tract infections in these groups often are more serious. Infections that may cause only a sore throat and hoarseness in the adult may produce serious obstruction in the child. Among the respiratory tract infections that affect small children are croup, epiglottitis, and bronchiolitis. Epiglottitis is a life-threatening supraglottic infection that may cause airway obstruction and asphyxia.

REVIEW EXERCISES

It is flu season, and although you had a flu shot last year, you have not had one this year. Imagine yourself having an abrupt onset of fever, chills, malaise, muscle aching, and nasal stuffiness.

A. Which of these symptoms would lead you to believe you are coming down with the flu?

B. Because you hate to miss classes, you decide to go to the student health center to get an antibiotic. After being seen by a health professional, you are told that antibiotics are ineffective against the flu virus, and you are instructed not to attend classes but instead to go home, take acetaminophen for your fever, go to bed and stay warm, and drink a lot of fluids. Explain the rationale for each of these recommendations.

C. Explain why last year's flu shot did not protect you during this year's flu season. There is current concern about the possibility of an influenza pandemic such as that occurring during the 1917–1918 season. What is the rationale for this concern?

Bacterial (*e.g., Streptococcus pneumoniae*) pneumonia is commonly manifested by a cough productive of sputum, whereas with atypical (*e.g, Mycoplasma pneumoniae*) pneumonia, the cough is usually nonproductive or absent.

A. Explain.

A 4-month-old infant is admitted to the pediatric intensive care unit with a diagnosis of bronchiolitis. The infant is tachypneic, with wheezing, nasal flaring, and retractions of the lower sternum and intercostal spaces during inspiration.

A. What is the usual pathogen in bronchiolitis? Would this infection be treated with an antibiotic?

B. Explain the physiologic mechanism involved in the retraction of the lower sternum and intercostal spaces during inspiration.

C. What would be the signs of impending respiratory failure in this infant?

References

1. Cotran R.S., Kumar V., Collins T. (Eds.). (1999). *Robbins' pathologic basis of disease* (6th ed., pp. 347–348, 471–473, 741–753). Philadelphia: W.B. Saunders.
2. Kirkpatrick G.L. (1996). The common cold. *Primary Care 23,* 657–673.
3. Turner R.B., Hayden G.F., Szilagy P.G. (2004). In Behrman R.E., Kliegman R.M., Jenson H.B. (Eds.), *Nelson textbook of pediatrics* (17th ed., pp. 1389–1391). Philadelphia: W.B. Saunders.
4. Heikkinen T., Järvinsen A. (2003). The common cold. *Lancet 361,* 51–59.
5. Greenberg S.B. (2003). Respiratory consequences of rhinovirus infection. *Archives of Internal Medicine 163,* 278–284.
6. Goldman D.A. (2000). Transmission of viral respiratory tract infections in the home. *Pediatric Infectious Disease Journal 19,* S97–S107.
7. Cohen S., Tyrerell D.A.J., Smith A.P. (1991). Psychological stress and susceptibility to the common cold. *New England Journal of Medicine 325,* 606–612.
8. Mossad S.B. (1998). Treatment of the common cold. *British Medical Journal 317,* 33–36.
9. Mossad S.B., Maknin M.L., Medendorp S.V., Mason P. (1996). Zinc gluconate lozenges for treating the common cold. *Annals of Internal Medicine 125,* 81–88.
10. Turner R.B., Wecker M.T., Pohl G., et al. (1999). Efficacy of tremacamra, a soluble intercellular adhesion molecule 1, for experimental rhinovirus infection. *Journal of the American Medical Association 281,* 1797–1804.
11. Osguthorpe J.D. (2001). Adult rhinosinusitis: Diagnosis and management. *American Family Physician 63*(1), 69–76.
12. Dykewicz M.S. (2003). Rhinitis and sinusitis. *Journal Allergy and Clinical Immunology 111,* S520–S539.
13. Winstead W. (2003). Rhinosinusitis. *Primary Care in Clinical Office Practice 30,* 137–154.
14. Lockey R.F. (1996). Management of chronic sinusitis. *Hospital Practice 31*(3), 141–151.
15. Hollingsworth H.M. (1996). Allergic rhinoconjunctivitis: Current therapy. *Hospital Practice 31*(6), 61–73.
16. Dykewicz M.S. (2003). Rhinitis and sinusitis. *Journal of Allergy and Clinical Immunology 111,* S520–529.
17. Advisory Committee on Immunization Practices. (2003). Prevention and control of influenza: Recommendations of the Advisory Committee on Immunization Practices (ACIP). *Morbidity and Mortality Weekly Report 52*(RR-8), 1–20.
18. Moorman J.P. (2003). Viral characteristics of influenza. *Southern Medical Journal 98*(8), 758–761.
19. Webby R.J., Webster R.G. (2003) Are we ready for pandemic influenza? *Science 302,* 1519–1522.
20. Musher D.M. (2003). How contagious are common respiratory infections? *New England Journal of Medicine 348,* 1256–1266.
21. Shorman M., Moorman J.P. (2003). Clinical manifestations and diagnosis of influenza. *Southern Medical Journal 96*(8), 737–739.
22. Olshaker J.S. (2003). Influenza. *Emergency Clinics of North America 21,* 353–361.
23. Khater F., Moorman J.P. (2003). Complications of influenza. *Southern Medical Journal 96*(8), 740–743.
24. Montal N.J. (2003). An office-based approach to influenza: Clinical diagnosis and laboratory testing. *American Family Physician 67,* 111–118.
25. Stiver G. (2003). The treatment of influenza with antiviral drugs. *Canadian Medical Association Journal 168*(1), 49–57.
26. Myers J.W. (2003). Influenza therapy. *Southern Medical Journal 96*(8), 744–749.
27. Palese P., Garcia-Sastre A. (2002). Influenza vaccines: Present and future. *Journal Clinical Investigation 110,* 9–13.
28. Lee P.P. (2003). Prevention and control of influenza. *Southern Medical Journal 96*(8), 751–757.
29. Advisory Committee on Immunization Practices. (2003). Using live attenuated influenza vaccine for prevention and control of influenza. *Morbidity and Mortality Weekly Report 52*(RR-13), 1–8.
30. Chestnutt M.S., Prendergast T.J. (2003). Lung. In Tierney L.M., McPhee S.J., Papadakis M.A. (Eds.), *Current medical diagnosis and treatment* (42nd ed., pp. 246–256). New York: Lange Medical Books/McGraw-Hill.
31. Marrie T.J. (1998). Community-acquired pneumonia: Etiology, treatment. *Infectious Disease Clinics of North America 12,* 723–739.
32. Halm E.A., Teirstein A.S. (2002). Management of community-acquired pneumonia. *New England Journal of Medicine 347*(25), 2039–2045.
33. Ramirez J.A. (2003). Community-acquired pneumonia in adults. *Primary Care Clinics and Office Practice 30,* 155–171.
34. Maitra A., Kumar V. (2003). The lung and upper respiratory tract. In Kumar V., Cotran R.S., Robbins S.L. *Robbins basic pathology* (7th ed., 478–495). Philadelphia: W.B. Saunders.
35. Neiderman M.S., Mandell L.A. Co-chair. (2001). American Thoracic Society guidelines for the initial management of adults with community-acquired pneumonia. *American Journal Respiratory Critical Care Medicine 163,* 1730–1754.
36. Centers for Disease Control and Prevention. (1996). Prevention of pneumococcal disease: Recommendations of the Advisory Committee on Immunization Practices (ACIP). *Morbidity and Mortality Weekly Report 46*(RR-8), 1–24.

37. Catterall J.R. (1999). *Streptococcus pneumoniae. Thorax 54,* 929–937.
38. Centers for Disease Control and Prevention. (1996). Defining the public health impact of drug-resistant *Streptococcus pneumoniae. Morbidity and Mortality Weekly Report 45*(RR-1), 1–20.
39. Centers for Disease Control and Prevention. (2000). Preventing pneumococcal disease among infants and small children: Recommendations of the Advisory Committee on Immunization Practices (ACIP). *Morbidity and Mortality Weekly Report 46*(RR-9), 1–38.
40. Chambers H.F. (2003). Infectious diseases: Bacterial and chlamydial. In Tierney L.M., McPhee S.J., Papadakis M.A. (Eds.), *Current medical diagnosis and treatment* (42nd ed., pp. 1369–1370). New York: Lange Medical Books/McGraw-Hill.
41. Stout J.E., Yu V.C. (1997). Legionellosis. *New England Journal of Medicine 337,* 682–688.
42. McEachen R., Campbell G.D. (1998). Hospital-acquired pneumonia: Epidemiology, etiology, and treatment. *Infectious Disease Clinics of North America 12*(3), 761–779.
43. Collin B.A., Ramphal R. (1998). Pneumonia in the compromised host including cancer patients and transplant patients. *Infectious Disease Clinics of North America 12*(3), 781–801.
44. American Lung Association Research and Scientific Affairs Epidemiology and Statistics Unit. (2003). Trends in tuberculosis morbidity and mortality. [On-line]. Available: http://www.lungusa.org.
45. Travis W.D., Farber J.L., Rubin E. (1999). The respiratory system. In Rubin E., Farber J.E. (Eds.), *Pathology* (3rd ed., pp. 606–608). Philadelphia: Lippincott-Raven.
46. Jasmer R.M., Nahid P., Hopewell P.C. (2002). Latent tuberculosis infection. *New England Journal of Medicine 347*(23), 1860–1866.
47. American Thoracic Society and Centers for Disease Control and Prevention. (2000). Diagnostic standards and classification of tuberculosis in adults and children. *American Review of Respiratory Disease 161,* 1376–1395.
48. Barnes P.F., Cave M.D. (2003). Molecular epidemiology of tuberculosis. *New England Journal of Medicine 349,* 1149–1156.
49. American Thoracic Society, Centers for Disease Control and Prevention, and Infectious Diseases Society of America. (2003). Treatment of tuberculosis. *Morbidity and Mortality Weekly Report 52*(RR-11), 1–14.
50. Spiegler P., Ilowitz J. (1999). Multiple-drug-resistant tuberculosis: Parts 1 and 2. *Emergency Medicine 31*(6, 7), 10–23.
51. Havlir D.V., Barnes P.F. (1999). Tuberculosis in patients with human immunodeficiency virus infection. *New England Journal of Medicine 380,* 367–372.
52. Centers for Disease Control and Prevention. (1996). The role of BCG vaccine in the prevention and control of tuberculosis in the United States. *Morbidity and Mortality Weekly Report 45*(RR-4), 1–19.
53. Ginsberg A.M. (2002). What's new in tuberculosis vaccines? *Bulletin of the World Health Organization 80,* 483–488.
54. Wheat L.J., Kauffman C.A. (2003). Histoplasmosis. *Infectious Disease Clinics of North America 17,* 1–19.
55. Hamill R.J. (2003). Infectious disease: Mycotic. In Tierney L.M., McPhee S.J., Papadakis M.A. (Eds.), *Current medical diagnosis and treatment* (42nd ed., pp. 1482–1494). New York: Lange Medical Books/McGraw-Hill.
56. Galgiani J.N. (1999). Coccidioidomycosis: A regional disease of national importance. *Annals of Internal Medicine 130,* 293–300.
57. Vaz A., Pineda-Roman M., Thomas A.R., Carlson R.W. (1998). Coccidioidomycosis: An update. *Hospital Practice 33*(9), 105–120.
58. Chiller T.M., Galgianna J.N., Stevens D.A. (2003). Coccidioidomycosis. *Infectious Disease Clinics of North America 17,* 41–57.
59. Bradsher R.W., Chapman S.W., Pappas P.G. (2003). Blastocytosis. *Infectious Disease Clinics of North America 17,* 21–40.
60. American Cancer Society. (2004). Lung cancer: Overview. [On-line]. Available: http://www.cancer.org.
61. Thomas C.R., Williams T.E., Cobos E., Turris A.T. III (2001). Lung cancer. In Lenhard R.E., Osteen R.T., Gansler T. *The American Cancer Society's clinical oncology* (pp. 269–295). Atlanta: American Cancer Society.
62. Hurria A. (2003). Management of lung cancer in older adults. *CA: A Cancer Journal for Clinicians 53,* 325–341.
63. Oklund S.H., Jett J.R. (2002). Small cell lung cancer: Current therapy and promising new regimens. *Oncologist 7,* 234–238.
64. Walker S. (2003). Updates in small cell lung cancer treatment. *Clinical Journal of Oncology Nursing 7*(5), 563–568.
65. Alberg A.J., Samet J.M. (2003). Epidemiology of lung cancer. *Chest 123*(Suppl. 1), 21S–44S.
66. Zander J., Hazinski M.F. (1992). Pulmonary disorders. In Hazinski M.F. (Ed.), *Nursing care of the critically ill child* (2nd ed., pp. 395–407). Philadelphia: W.B. Saunders.
67. Moore K., Persaud T.V.N. (2003). *The developing human* (6th ed., pp. 242–253). Philadelphia: W.B. Saunders.
68. Haddad G.G., Fontán J.J.P. (2004). Development of the respiratory system. In Behrman R.E., Kliegman R.M., Jensen H.L. (Eds.), *Nelson textbook of pediatrics* (17th ed., pp. 1362–1370). Philadelphia: W.B. Saunders.
69. Fontán J.J.P., Haddad G.G. (2000). Respiratory pathophysiology. In Behrman R.E., Kliegman R.M., Jensen H.L. (Eds.), *Nelson textbook of pediatrics* (16th ed., pp. 1237–1240). Philadelphia: W.B. Saunders.
70. Oski F.A. (Ed.). (1994). *Principles and practices of pediatrics* (2nd ed., pp. 336–339, 365–370). Philadelphia: J.B. Lippincott.
71. Stoll B.J., Kliegman R.M. (2000). The fetus and neonatal infant. In Behrman R.E., Kliegman R.M., Jensen H.L. (Eds.), *Nelson textbook of pediatrics* (16th ed., pp. 498–505). Philadelphia: W.B. Saunders.
72. McColley S.A. (1998). Bronchopulmonary dysplasia. *Pediatric Clinics of North America 45,* 573–585.
73. Alexander K.C., Leung M.B.B.C., Cho H. (1999). Diagnosis of stridor in children. *American Family Physician 60,* 2289–2296.
74. Jobe A.H., Bancalari E. (2001). Bronchopulmonary dysplasia. *American Journal of Respiratory Critical Care 163,* 1723–1729.
75. Roosevelt G.E. (2004). Acute inflammatory upper airway obstruction. In Behrman R.E., Kiegman R.M., Jensen H.L. (Eds.), *Nelson textbook of pediatrics* (17th ed., pp. 1405–1409). Philadelphia: W.B. Saunders.
76. Rotta A.T., Wiryawan B. (2003). Respiratory emergencies in children. *Respiratory Care 48*(3), 248–258.
77. Klassen T.P. (1999). Croup: A current perspective. *Pediatric Clinics of North American 46*(6), 1167–1177.
78. Wright R.B., Pomerantz W.J., Luria J.W. (2002). New approaches to respiratory infections in children. *Emergency Medical Clinics of North America 20*(1), 93–111.
79. Baker A.S., Eavey R.D. (1986). Adult supraglottitis (epiglottitis). *New England Journal of Medicine 314,* 1185–1186.
80. Goodman D. (2004). Bronchitis. In Behrman R.E., Kliegman R.M., Jensen H.L. (Eds.), *Nelson textbook of pediatrics* (17th ed., pp. 1414–1417). Philadelphia: W.B. Saunders.
81. Frankel L.R. (2004). Respiratory distress and failure. In Behrman R.E., Kliegman R.M., Jensen H.L. (Eds.), *Nelson textbook of pediatrics* (17th ed., pp. 301–306). Philadelphia: W.B. Saunders.

CHAPTER 31

Disorders of Ventilation and Gas Exchange

The major function of the lungs is to oxygenate and remove carbon dioxide from the blood as a means of supporting the metabolic functions of body cells. The gas exchange function of the lungs depends on a system of open airways, expansion of the lungs, an adequate area for gas diffusion, and blood flow that carries the gases to the rest of the body. This chapter focuses on diseases that disrupt ventilation and pulmonary gas exchange.

Disorders of Lung Inflation

After completing this section of the chapter, you should be able to meet the following objectives:

- ✦ State the characteristics of pleural pain and differentiate it from other types of chest pain
- ✦ Differentiate among the causes and manifestations of spontaneous pneumothorax, secondary pneumothorax, and tension pneumothorax
- ✦ Characterize the pathogenesis and manifestations of pleural effusion
- ✦ Describe the causes and manifestations of atelectasis

Air entering through the airways inflates the lung, and the negative pressure in the pleural cavity keeps the lung from collapsing. Disorders of lung inflation are caused by conditions that produce lung compression or lung collapse. There can be compression of the lung by an accumulation of fluid in the intrapleural space, complete collapse of an entire lung as in pneumothorax, or collapse of a segment of the lung as in atelectasis.

DISORDERS OF THE PLEURA

The pleura is a thin, double-layered membrane that encases the lungs. The inner visceral layer lies adjacent to the lung; the outer parietal layer lines the inner aspect of the chest wall, the superior aspect of the diaphragm, and the mediastinum. The visceral and parietal pleurae are separated by a thin layer of serous fluid, and the potential space between these two layers is called the *pleural* or *thoracic cavity* (Fig. 31-1). The right and left pleural cavities are separated by the mediastinum, which contains the heart and other thoracic structures.

Both the chest wall and the lungs have elastic properties. Because of these elastic properties, there is a tendency for the chest wall to expand and move outward and for the lungs to recoil or move inward and collapse (see Chapter 29). As a result of these two opposing forces, the pressure in the pleural cavity becomes negative in relation to alveolar pressure. It is the negative pressure in the pleural cavity that holds the lungs against the chest wall and keeps them from collapsing. Disorders of the pleura include pain, pleural effusion, and pneumothorax.

Pleural Pain

Pain is a frequent symptom of *pleuritis* (also called *pleurisy*) or inflammation of the pleura. Pleuritis is common in infectious processes such as viral respiratory infections or pneumonia that extend to involve the pleura. Most commonly, the pain is abrupt in onset, such that the person experiencing it can cite almost to the minute when the pain started. It usually is unilateral and tends to be localized to the lower and lateral part of the chest. When the central part of the diaphragm is irritated, the pain may be referred to the shoulder. The pain is usually made worse by chest movements, such as deep breathing and coughing, that exaggerate pressure changes in the pleural cavity and increase movement of the inflamed or injured pleural surfaces. Because deep breathing is painful, tidal volumes usually are kept small, and breathing becomes more rapid. Reflex splinting of the chest muscles may occur, causing a lesser respiratory excursion on the affected side.

It is important to differentiate pleural pain from pain produced by other conditions, such as musculoskeletal strain of chest muscles, bronchial irritation, and myocardial disease. Musculoskeletal pain may occur as the result of frequent, forceful coughing. This type of pain usually is bilateral and located in the inferior portions of the rib cage, where the abdominal muscles insert into the anterior rib cage. It is made worse by movements associated with contraction of the abdominal muscles. The pain associated with irritation of the bronchi usually is substernal and dull in character rather than sharp. It is made worse with coughing but is not affected by deep breathing. Myocardial pain, which is discussed in Chapter 26, usually is located in the substernal area and is not affected by respiratory movements.

Analgesics and nonsteroidal anti-inflammatory drugs (*e.g.*, indomethacin) may be used for pleural pain. Although these agents reduce awareness of pleural pain, they do not entirely relieve the discomfort associated with deep breathing and coughing.

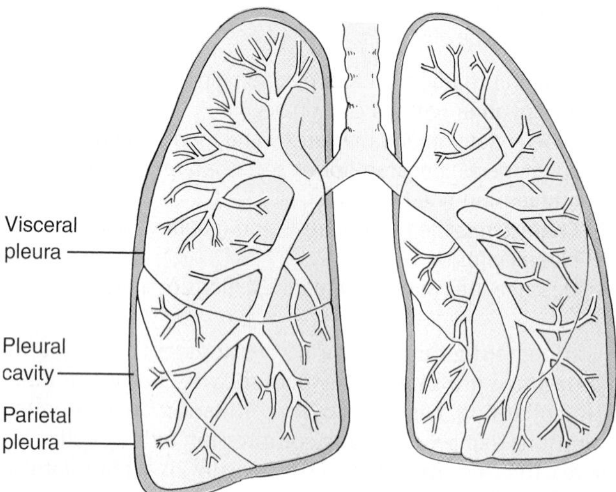

FIGURE 31-1 The parietal and visceral pleura and pleural cavity, which is the site of fluid accumulation in pleural effusions.

Pleural Effusion

Pleural effusion refers to an abnormal collection of fluid in the pleural cavity (see Fig. 31-1). The fluid may be a transudate, exudate, purulent drainage (empyema), chyle, or blood. Normally, only a thin layer (<10 to 20 mL) of serous fluid separates the visceral and parietal layers of the pleural cavity. Like fluid developing in other transcellular spaces in the body, pleural effusion occurs when the rate of fluid formation exceeds the rate of its removal (see Chapter 33). Five mechanisms have been linked to the abnormal collection of fluid in the pleural cavity: (1) increased capillary pressure, as in congestive heart failure; (2) increased capillary permeability, which occurs with inflammatory conditions; (3) decreased colloidal osmotic pressure, such as the hypoalbuminemia occurring with liver disease and nephrosis; (4) increased negative intrapleural pressure, which develops with atelectasis; and (5) impaired lymphatic drainage of the pleural space, which results from obstructive processes such as mediastinal carcinoma.

A transudate consists of serous fluid. The accumulation of a serous transudate in the pleural cavity often is referred to as *hydrothorax*. The condition may be unilateral or bilateral. The most common cause of hydrothorax is congestive heart failure. Other causes are renal failure, nephrosis, liver failure, and malignancy.

An exudate is a pleural fluid having one or more of the following characteristics: a pleural fluid protein to serum protein ratio greater than 0.5; a pleural fluid lactate dehydrogenase (LDH) to serum LDH ratio greater than 0.6; and pleural fluid LDH greater than two thirds the upper limit of normal serum LDH.[1] LDH is an enzyme that is released from inflamed and injured pleural tissue. Because measurements of LDH are easily obtained from a sample of pleural fluid, it is a useful marker for diagnosis of exudative pleural disorders. Conditions that produce exudative pleural effusions are infections, pulmonary infarction, malignancies, rheumatoid arthritis, and lupus erythematosus.

Empyema refers to pus in the pleural cavity. It is caused by direct infection of the pleural space from an adjacent bacterial pneumonia, rupture of a lung abscess into the pleural space, invasion from a subdiaphragmatic infection, or infection associated with trauma.

Chylothorax is the effusion of lymph in the thoracic cavity.[2] Chyle, a milky fluid containing chylomicrons, is found in the lymph fluid originating in the gastrointestinal tract. The thoracic duct transports chyle to the central circulation. Chylothorax also results from trauma, inflammation, or malignant infiltration obstructing chyle transport from the thoracic duct into the central circulation. It is the most common cause of pleural effusion in the fetus and neonate, resulting from congenital malformation of the thoracic duct or lymph channels.[2] Chylothorax also can occur as a complication of intrathoracic surgical procedures and use of the great veins for total parenteral nutrition and hemodynamic monitoring.

Hemothorax is the presence of blood in the thoracic cavity. Bleeding may arise from chest injury, a complication of chest surgery, malignancies, or rupture of a great vessel such as an aortic aneurysm. Hemothorax may be classified as minimal, moderate, or large.[3] A minimal hemothorax involves the presence of 300 to 500 mL of blood in the pleural space. Small amounts of blood usually are absorbed from the pleural space, and a minimal hemothorax usually clears in 10 to 14 days without complication. A moderate hemothorax (500 to 1000 mL of blood) fills approximately one third of the pleural space and may produce signs of lung compression and loss of intravascular volume. It requires immediate drainage and replacement of intravascular fluids. A large hemothorax fills one half or more of one side of the chest; it indicates the presence of 1000 mL or more of blood in the thorax and usually is caused by bleeding from a high-pressure vessel such as an intercostal or mammary artery. It requires immediate drainage and, if the bleeding continues, surgery to control the bleeding. One of the complications of untreated moderate or large hemothorax is fibrothorax—the fusion of the pleural surfaces by fibrin, hyalin, and connective tissue—and in some cases, calcification of the fibrous tissue, which restricts lung expansion.

Manifestations. The manifestations of pleural effusion vary with the cause. Hemothorax may be accompanied by signs of blood loss, and empyema by fever and other signs of inflammation. Fluid in the pleural cavity acts as a space-occupying mass; it causes a decrease in lung expansion on the affected side that is proportional to the amount of fluid collected. The effusion may cause a mediastinal shift toward the contralateral side of the chest with a decrease in lung volume on that side as well as the side with the pneumothorax. Characteristic signs of pleural effusion are dullness or flatness to percussion and diminished breath sounds. Dyspnea, the most common symptom, occurs when fluid compresses the lung, resulting in decreased ventilation. Pleuritic pain usually occurs only when inflammation is present, although constant discomfort may be felt with large effusions. Mild hypoxemia may occur and usually is corrected with supplemental oxygen.

Diagnosis and Treatment. Diagnosis of pleural effusion is based on chest radiographs, chest ultrasound, and computed tomography (CT). Thoracentesis is the aspiration of fluid from the pleural space. It can be used to obtain a sample of pleural fluid for diagnosis, or it can be used for therapeutic purposes. The treatment of pleural effusion is directed at the cause of the disorder. With large effusions, thoracentesis may be used to remove fluid from the intrapleural space and allow for reexpansion of the lung. A palliative method used for treatment of pleural effusions caused by a malignancy is the injection of a sclerosing agent into the pleural cavity. This method of treatment causes obliteration of the pleural space and prevents the reaccumulation of fluid. Open surgical drainage may be necessary in cases of continued effusion.

Pneumothorax

Normally, the pleural cavity is free of air and contains only a thin layer of fluid. When air enters the pleural cavity, it is called *pneumothorax*. Pneumothorax causes partial or complete collapse of the affected lung. Pneumothorax can occur without an obvious cause or injury (*i.e.*, spontaneous pneumothorax) or as a result of direct injury to the chest or major airways (*i.e.*, traumatic pneumothorax). Tension pneumothorax describes a life-threatening condition of excessive pressure in the pleural cavity.

Spontaneous Pneumothorax. Spontaneous pneumothorax occurs when an air-filled bleb, or blister, on the lung surface ruptures. Rupture of these blebs allows atmospheric air from the airways to enter the pleural cavity (Fig. 31-2). Because alveolar pressure normally is greater than pleural pressure, air flows from the alveoli into the pleural space, causing the involved portion of the lung to collapse as a

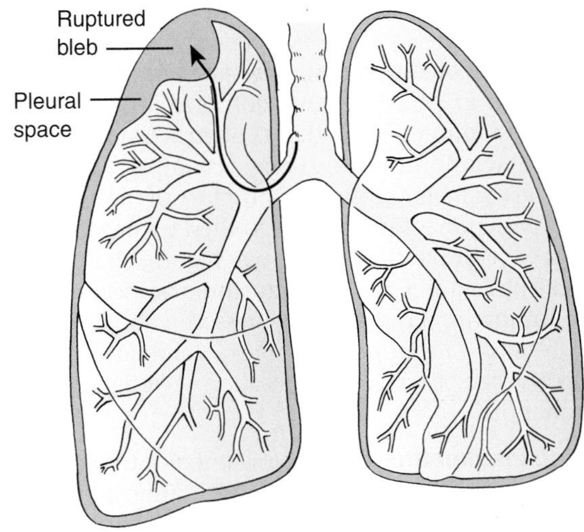

FIGURE 31-2 Mechanisms for development of spontaneous pneumothorax.

result of its own recoil. Air continues to flow into the pleural space until a pressure gradient no longer exists or until the decline in lung size causes the leak to seal. Spontaneous pneumothoraces can be divided into primary and secondary pneumothoraces.[4] Primary spontaneous pneumothorax occurs in otherwise healthy persons. Secondary spontaneous pneumothorax occurs in persons with underlying lung disease.

What causes the air-filled blebs responsible for primary spontaneous pneumothorax and the reasons why they rupture are largely unknown. In primary spontaneous pneumothorax, these blebs usually are located at the top of the lungs. The condition is seen most often in tall boys and young men between 10 and 30 years of age.[4] It has been suggested that the difference in pleural pressure from the top to the bottom of the lung is greater in tall persons and that this difference in pressure may contribute to the development of blebs. Another factor that has been associated with primary spontaneous pneumothorax is smoking. Disease of the small airways related to smoking probably contributes to the condition.

Secondary spontaneous pneumothoraces usually are more serious because they occur in persons with lung disease. They are associated with many different types of lung conditions that cause trapping of gases and destruction of lung tissue, including asthma, tuberculosis, cystic fibrosis, sarcoidosis, bronchogenic carcinoma, and metastatic pleural diseases. The most common cause of secondary spontaneous pneumothorax is emphysema.

Catamenial pneumothorax occurs in relation to the menstrual cycle and usually is recurrent.[4] It typically occurs in women who are 30 to 40 years of age and have a history of endometriosis. It usually affects the right lung and develops within 72 hours of onset of menses. Although the cause of catamenial pneumothorax is unknown, it has been suggested that air may gain access to the peritoneal cavity during menstruation and then enter the pleural cavity through a diaphragmatic defect. Pleural and diaphragmatic endometriosis also have been implicated as causes of the condition.

Traumatic Pneumothorax. Traumatic pneumothorax may be caused by penetrating or nonpenetrating injuries. Fractured or dislocated ribs that penetrate the pleura are the most common cause of pneumothorax from nonpenetrating chest injuries. Hemothorax often accompanies these injuries. Pneumothorax also may accompany fracture of the trachea or major bronchus or rupture of the esophagus. Persons with pneumothorax due to chest trauma frequently have other complications and may require chest surgery. Medical procedures such as transthoracic needle aspirations, intubation, and positive-pressure ventilation occasionally may cause pneumothorax. Traumatic pneumothorax also can occur as a complication of cardiopulmonary resuscitation.

Tension Pneumothorax. Tension pneumothorax occurs when the intrapleural pressure exceeds atmospheric pressure. It is a life-threatening condition and occurs when injury to the chest or respiratory structures permits air to enter but not leave the pleural space (Fig. 31-3). This results in a rapid increase in pressure in the chest with compression atelectasis of the unaffected lung, a shift in the mediastinum to the opposite side of the chest, and compression of the vena cava with impairment of venous return to the heart.[5] Although tension pneumothorax can develop in persons with spontaneous pneumothoraces, it is seen most often in persons with traumatic pneumothoraces. It also may result from mechanical ventilation.

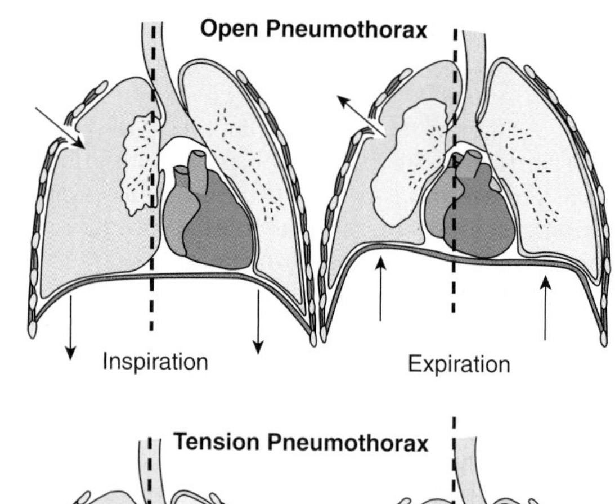

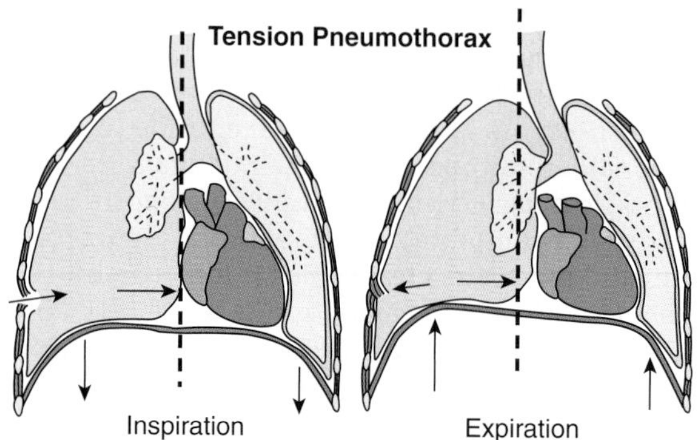

FIGURE 31-3 Open or communicating pneumothorax (**top**) and tension pneumothorax (**bottom**). In an open pneumothorax, air enters the chest during inspiration and exits during expiration. There may be slight inflation of the affected lung due to a decrease in pressure as air moves out of the chest. In tension pneumothorax, air can enter but not leave the chest. As the pressure in the chest increases, the heart and great vessels are compressed and the mediastinal structures are shifted toward the opposite side of the chest. The trachea is pushed from its normal midline position toward the opposite side of the chest, and the unaffected lung is compressed.

Manifestations. The manifestations of pneumothorax depend on its size and the integrity of the underlying lung. In spontaneous pneumothorax, manifestations of the disorder include development of ipsilateral chest pain in an otherwise healthy person. There is an almost immediate increase in respiratory rate, often accompanied by dyspnea that occurs as a result of the activation of receptors that monitor lung volume. Heart rate is increased. Asymmetry of the chest may occur because of the air trapped in the pleural cavity on the affected side. This asymmetry may be evidenced during inspiration as a lag in the movement of the affected side, with inspiration being delayed until the unaffected lung reaches the same level of pressure as the lung with the air trapped in the pleural space. Percussion of the chest produces a more hyperresonant sound, and breath sounds are decreased or absent over the area of the pneumothorax. With tension pneumothorax, the structures in the mediastinal space shift toward the opposite side of the chest (see Fig. 31-3). When this occurs, the position of the trachea, normally located in the midline of the neck, deviates with the mediastinum. The position of the trachea can be used as a means of assessing for a mediastinal shift. There may be distention of the neck veins and subcutaneous emphysema (*i.e.,* air bubbles in the subcutaneous tissues of the chest and neck) and clinical signs of shock.

Hypoxemia usually develops immediately after a large pneumothorax, followed by vasoconstriction of the blood vessels in the affected lung, causing the blood flow to shift to the unaffected lung. In persons with primary spontaneous pneumothorax, this mechanism usually returns oxygen saturation to normal within 24 hours. Hypoxemia usually is more serious in persons with underlying lung disease in whom secondary spontaneous pneumothorax develops. In these persons, the hypoxemia caused by the partial or total loss of lung function can be life threatening.

Diagnosis and Treatment. Diagnosis of pneumothorax can be confirmed by chest radiograph or CT scan. Blood gas analysis may be done to determine the effect of the condition on blood oxygen levels.

Treatment of pneumothorax varies with the cause and extent of the disorder. Even without treatment, air in the pleural space usually reabsorbs after the pleural leak seals. In small spontaneous pneumothoraces, the air usually reabsorbs spontaneously, and only observation and follow-up chest radiographs are required. Supplemental oxygen may be used to increase the rate at which the air is reabsorbed. In larger pneumothoraces, the air is removed by needle aspiration or a closed drainage system used with or without an aspiration pump. This type of drainage system uses a one-way valve or a tube submerged in water to allow air to exit the pleural space and prevent it from reentering the chest. In secondary pneumothorax, surgical closure of the chest wall defect, ruptured airway, or perforated esophagus may be required.

Emergency treatment of tension pneumothorax involves the prompt insertion of a large-bore needle or chest tube into the affected side of the chest along with one-way valve drainage or continuous chest suction to aid in lung reexpansion. Sucking chest wounds, which allow air to pass in and out of the chest cavity, should be treated by promptly covering the area with an airtight covering (*e.g.,* Vaseline gauze, firm piece of plastic). Chest tubes are inserted as soon as possible.

Because of the risk for recurrence, persons with primary spontaneous pneumothorax should be advised against cigarette smoking, exposure to high altitudes, flying in nonpressurized aircraft, and scuba diving.

ATELECTASIS

Atelectasis means "imperfect expansion"; it refers to the incomplete expansion of a lung or portion of a lung. It can be caused by airway obstruction, lung compression such as occurs in pneumothorax or pleural effusion, or the increased recoil of the lung due to loss of pulmonary surfactant (see Chapter 29). The disorder may be present at birth (*i.e.,* primary atelectasis), or it may develop in the neonatal period or later in life (*i.e.,* acquired or secondary atelectasis).

Primary Atelectasis

Primary atelectasis of the newborn implies that the lung has never been inflated. It is seen most frequently in premature and high-risk infants (Fig. 31-4).

Secondary Atelectasis

A secondary form of atelectasis can occur in infants who established respiration and subsequently experienced impairment of lung expansion. Among the causes of secondary atelectasis in the newborn is the respiratory distress syndrome associated with lack of surfactant and airway obstruction due to aspiration of amniotic fluid or blood.

Acquired atelectasis occurs mainly in adults. It is caused most commonly by airway obstruction and lung compression (Fig. 31-5). Obstruction can be caused by a mucus plug in the airway or by external compression by fluid, tumor mass, exudate, or other matter in the area surrounding the airway. A small segment of lung or an entire lung lobe may be involved in obstructive atelectasis. Complete obstruction of an airway is followed by the absorption of air from the dependent alveoli and collapse of that portion of the lung. Breathing high concentrations of oxygen, such as while on a ventilator, increases the rate at

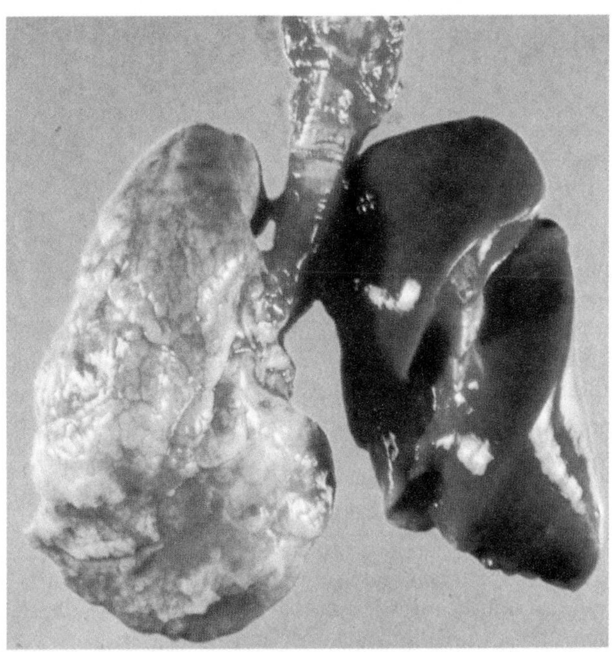

FIGURE 31-4 Atelectasis. The right lung of an infant (left side of photo) is pale and expanded by air, whereas the left lung is collapsed. (Rubin E., Farber J.L. [1994]. *Pathology* [2nd ed.]. Philadelphia: J.B. Lippincott)

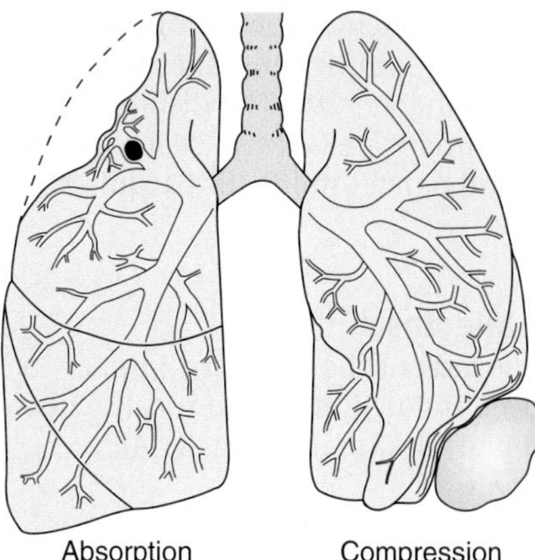

FIGURE 31-5 Atelectasis caused by airway obstruction and absorption of air from the involved lung area on the *left* and by compression of lung tissue on the *right*.

which gases are absorbed from the alveoli and predisposes to atelectasis.

The danger of obstructive atelectasis increases after surgery. Anesthesia, pain, administration of narcotics, and immobility tend to promote retention of viscid bronchial secretions and hence airway obstruction. Encouraging a patient to take deep breaths and cough, frequent changes of position, adequate hydration, and early ambulation decrease the likelihood of atelectasis developing.

Another cause of atelectasis is compression of lung tissue. It occurs when the pleural cavity is partially or completely filled with fluid, exudate, blood, a tumor mass, or air. It is observed most commonly in persons with pleural effusion from congestive heart failure or cancer.

Manifestations. The clinical manifestations of atelectasis include tachypnea, tachycardia, dyspnea, cyanosis, signs of hypoxemia, diminished chest expansion, absence of breath sounds, and intercostal retractions. Fever and other signs of infection may develop. Both chest expansion and breath sounds are decreased on the affected side. There may be intercostal retraction (pulling in of the intercostal spaces) over the involved area during inspiration. If the collapsed area is large, the mediastinum and trachea shift to the affected side. Signs of respiratory distress are proportional to the extent of lung collapse. In compression atelectasis, the mediastinum shifts away from the affected lung.

Diagnosis and Treatment. The diagnosis of atelectasis is based on signs and symptoms. Chest radiographs are used to confirm the diagnosis. CT scans may be used to show the exact location of the obstruction.

Treatment depends on the cause and extent of lung involvement. It is directed at reducing the airway obstruction or lung compression and at reinflating the collapsed area of the lung. Ambulation and body positions that favor increased lung expansion are used when appropriate. Administration of oxygen may be needed to treat the hypoxemia. Bronchoscopy may be used as a diagnostic and treatment method.

In summary, disorders of the pleura include pleuritis and pain, pleural effusion, and pneumothorax. Pain is commonly associated with conditions that produce inflammation of the pleura. Characteristically, it is unilateral, abrupt in onset, and exaggerated by respiratory movements. Pleural effusion refers to the abnormal accumulation of fluid in the pleural cavity. The fluid may be a transudate (*i.e.,* hydrothorax), exudate (*i.e.,* empyema), blood (*i.e.,* hemothorax), or chyle (*i.e.,* chylothorax). Pneumothorax refers to an accumulation of air in the pleural cavity with the partial or complete collapse of the lung. It can result from rupture of an air-filled bleb on the lung surface or from penetrating or nonpenetrating injuries. A tension pneumothorax is a life-threatening event in which air progressively accumulates in the thorax, collapsing the lung on the injured side and progressively shifting the mediastinum to the opposite side of the thorax, producing severe cardiorespiratory impairment.

Atelectasis refers to an incomplete expansion of the lung. The disorder may be present at birth (*i.e.,* primary atelectasis), or it may develop in the neonatal period or later in life (*i.e.,* acquired or secondary atelectasis). Primary atelectasis occurs most often in premature and high-risk infants. Acquired atelectasis occurs mainly in adults and is caused most commonly by a mucus plug in the airway or by external compression by fluid, tumor mass, exudate, or other matter in the area surrounding the airway.

Obstructive Airway Disorders

After completing this section of the chapter, you should be able to meet the following objectives:

- Describe the physiology of bronchial smooth muscle as it relates to airway disease
- Describe the interaction between heredity, alterations in the immune response, and environmental agents in the pathogenesis of bronchial asthma
- Characterize the acute- or early-phase and late-phase responses in the pathogenesis of bronchial asthma and relate them to current methods for treatment of the disorder
- Explain the changes in pulmonary function studies that occur with airway disease
- Explain the distinction between chronic bronchitis and emphysema in terms of pathology and clinical manifestations
- State the chief manifestations of bronchiectasis
- Describe the genetic abnormality responsible for cystic fibrosis and state the disorder's effect on lung function

Obstructive airway disorders are caused by disorders that limit expiratory airflow. Bronchial asthma represents a reversible form of airway disease caused by narrowing of airways due to bronchospasm, inflammation, and increased airway secretions. Chronic obstructive airway disease can be caused by a variety of airway disorders, including chronic bronchitis, emphysema, bronchiectasis, and cystic fibrosis.

PHYSIOLOGY OF AIRWAY DISEASE

Air moves through the upper airways (*i.e.*, trachea and major bronchi) into the lower or pulmonary airways (*i.e.*, bronchi and alveoli), which are located in the lung. In the pulmonary airways, the cartilaginous layer that provides support for the trachea and major bronchi gradually disappears and is replaced with crisscrossing strips of smooth muscle (see Chapter 29). The contraction and relaxation of the smooth muscle layer, which is innervated by the autonomic nervous system, controls the diameter of the airways and consequent resistance to airflow. Parasympathetic stimulation, through the vagus nerve and cholinergic receptors, produces bronchial constriction; and sympathetic stimulation, through β_2-adrenergic receptors, increases bronchodilation. Normally, a slight vagally mediated bronchoconstrictor tone predominates. When there is need for increased airflow, as during exercise, the bronchoconstrictor effects of the parasympathetic nervous system are inhibited, and the bronchodilator effects of the sympathetic nervous system are stimulated.

Bronchial smooth muscle also responds to inflammatory mediators, such as histamine, that act directly on bronchial smooth muscle cells to produce constriction. During an antigen–antibody response, inflammatory mediators are released by a special type of cell, called the *mast cell,* which is present in the airways. The binding of immunoglobulin E (IgE) to specific receptors on sensitized mast cells prepares them for release of the inflammatory mediators during an allergic reaction (see Chapter 21).

BRONCHIAL ASTHMA

Bronchial asthma is a chronic disorder of the airways that causes episodes of airway obstruction, bronchial hyperresponsiveness, and airway inflammation that usually are reversible.[6,7] According to 2001 data, an estimated 20.3 million Americans (6.3 million children) have been diagnosed with asthma.[8] Although the prevalence rates for asthma have increased over the past several decades, the mortality rate and hospitalizations due to asthma have plateaued during the past few years, indicating a higher level of disease management.[8]

AIRWAY DISORDERS

- Airway disorders involve the movement of gases into and out of the lung. They involve bronchial smooth muscle tone, mucosal injury, and obstruction due to secretions.
- The tone of the bronchial smooth muscles surrounding the airways determines airway radius, and the presence or absence of airway secretions influences airway patency.
- Bronchial smooth muscle is innervated by the autonomic nervous system–the parasympathetic nervous system produces bronchoconstriction and the sympathetic nervous system produces bronchodilation.
- Inflammatory mediators that are released in response to environmental irritants, immune responses, and infectious agents increase airway responsiveness by producing bronchospasm, increasing mucus secretion, and producing injury to the mucosal lining of the airways.

Definition and Pathogenesis

The National Heart, Lung, and Blood Institute's Second Expert Panel on the Management of Asthma defined bronchial asthma as "a chronic inflammatory disorder of the airways in which many cells and cellular elements play a role, in particular, mast cells, eosinophils, T lymphocytes, and epithelial cells."[6] This inflammatory process produces recurrent episodes of airway obstruction, characterized by wheezing, breathlessness, chest tightness, and a cough that often is worse at night and in the early morning. These episodes, which usually are reversible either spontaneously or with treatment, also cause an associated increase in bronchial responsiveness to a variety of stimuli.[6]

The pathophysiology of asthma involves a genetic (atopy) predisposition coupled with environmental factors (viruses, allergens, and occupational exposure). In susceptible persons, an asthma attack can be triggered by a variety of stimuli that do not normally cause symptoms. Based on their mechanism of response, these triggers can be divided into two categories—bronchospastic or inflammatory. Bronchospastic triggers depend on the existing level of airway responsiveness. They do not normally increase airway responsiveness but produce symptoms in persons who already are predisposed to bronchospasm. Bronchospastic triggers include cold air, exercise, emotional upset, and exposure to bronchial irritants such as cigarette smoke. Inflammatory triggers exert their effects through the inflammatory response. They cause inflammation and prime the airways so they are hyperresponsive to allergic and nonallergic stimuli.

The mechanisms whereby the bronchospastic and inflammatory triggers produce their effects can be further divided into the early- or acute-phase response and the late-phase response.[9,10] The *early-* or *acute-phase response* results in immediate bronchoconstriction on exposure to an inhaled antigen or irritant (Fig. 31-6). The symptoms of the acute response, which usually develop within 10 to 20 minutes, are caused by the release of chemical mediators from IgE-coated mast cells. In the case of airborne antigens, the reaction occurs when antigen binds to sensitized mast cells on the mucosal surface of the airways. Mediator release results in opening of the mucosal intercellular junctions and enhancement of antigen movement to the more prevalent submucosal mast cells (Fig. 31-7). In addition, there is bronchoconstriction due to direct stimulation of parasympathetic receptors, mucosal edema due to increased vascular permeability, and increased mucus secretions. The acute response usually can be inhibited or reversed by bronchodilators, such as β_2-adrenergic agonists, but not by the anti-inflammatory actions of the corticosteroids.

The *late-phase response* develops 4 to 8 hours after exposure to an asthmatic trigger.[9] The late-phase response

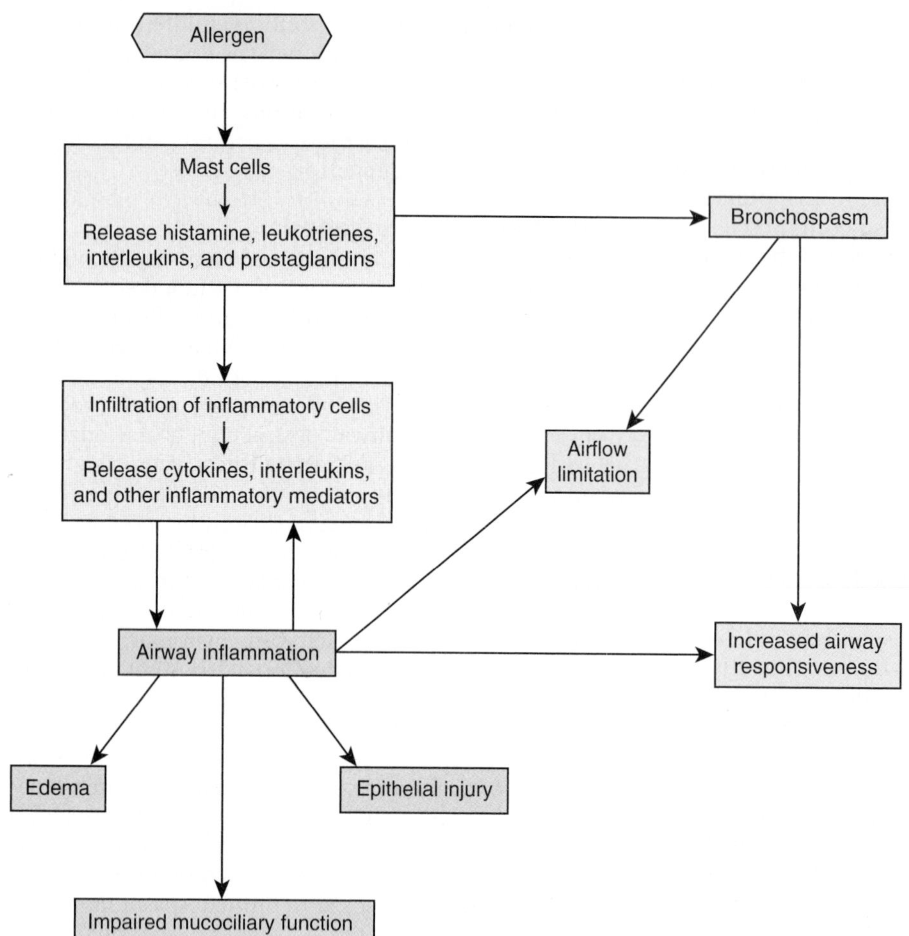

FIGURE 31-6 Mechanisms of early- and late-phase Ig-E mediated bronchospasm.

involves inflammation and increased airway responsiveness that prolong the asthma attack and set into motion a vicious cycle of exacerbations. Typically, the response reaches a maximum within a few hours and may last for days or even weeks. An initial trigger in the late-phase response causes the release of inflammatory mediators from mast cells, macrophages, and epithelial cells. These substances induce the migration and activation of other inflammatory cells (*e.g.*, basophils, eosinophils, neutrophils), which then produce epithelial injury and edema, changes in mucociliary function and reduced clearance of respiratory tract secretions, and increased airway responsiveness (see Fig. 31-7). Responsiveness to cholinergic mediators often is heightened, suggesting changes in parasympathetic control of airway function. Chronic inflammation can lead to airway remodeling, in which case airflow limitations may be only partially reversible.[7]

Recent interest has focused on the role of the T lymphocytes in the pathogenesis of bronchial asthma. It is now known that there are two subsets of T helper cells (T_H1 and T_H2) that develop from the same precursor $CD4^+$ T lymphocyte.[7,11–13] T_H1 cells differentiate in response to microbes and stimulate the differentiation of B cells into IgM- and IgG-producing plasma cells. T_H2 cells, on the other hand, respond to allergens and helminths (intestinal parasites) and stimulate the differentiation of B cells into IgE-producing plasma cells. Cytokines (*i.e.*, interleukin-4 [IL-4], IL-5, IL-6, IL-9, and IL-13) secreted by T_H2 cells stimulate differentiation of B cells into IgE-producing plasma cells, act as growth factors for mast cells, and recruit and activate eosinophils[7,11] (see Chapter 21, Fig. 21-4).

The current "hygiene hypothesis" may explain some of the dramatic increase in asthma prevalence in the westernized world. This hypothesis is based on the assumption that the immune system in newborn infants is skewed toward T_H2 responses; following birth, environmental stimuli such as infections stimulate T_H1 responses and bring the T_H1 and T_H2 responses into proper balance.[7,11] There is evidence that the incidence of asthma is reduced in situations that favor the development of T_H1 cell responses—infection with certain organisms (*e.g.*, *Mycobacterium tuberculosis*, measles, or hepatitis A); exposure to other children (*e.g.*, having older siblings and being enrolled in day care); and less frequent use of antibiotics.[7,11] The absence of these lifestyle events in genetically predisposed persons is thought to favor the persistence of T_H2 cell responses and set the stage for production of IgE antibodies in response to environmental allergens such as house dust mite and animal dander.

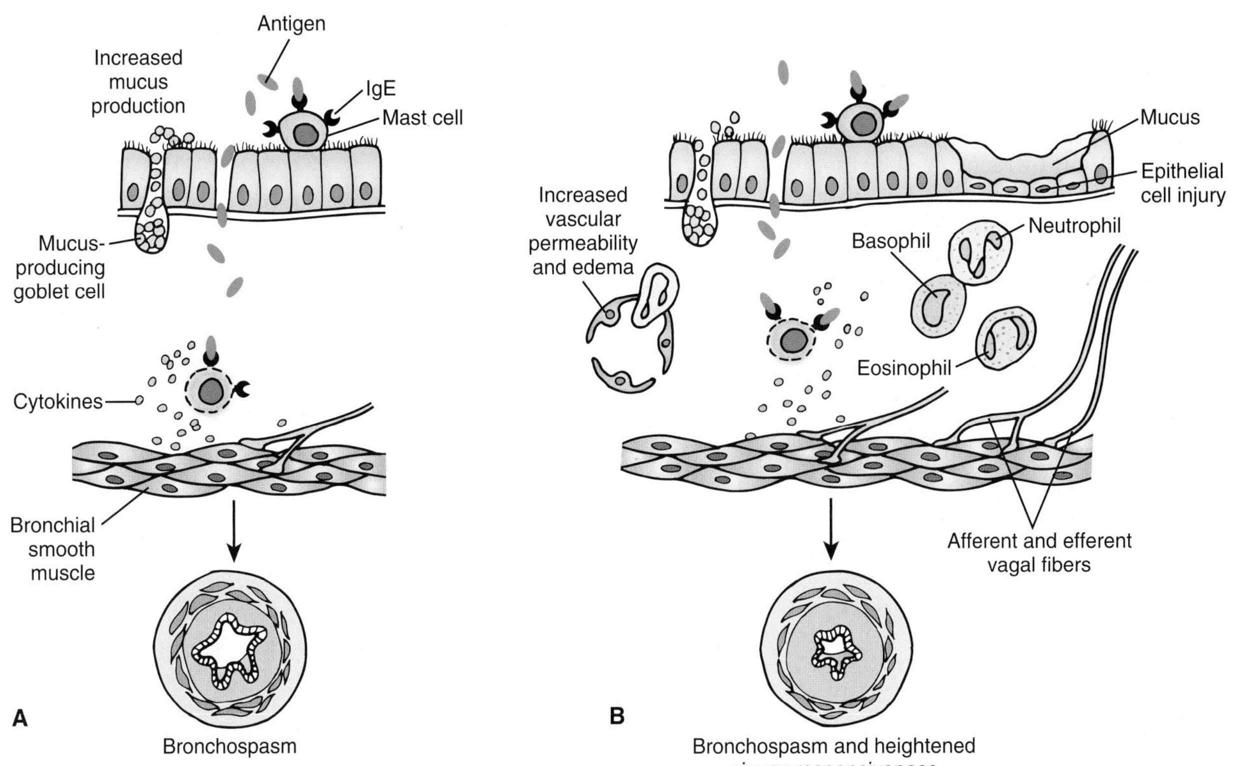

FIGURE 31-7 The pathogenesis of bronchial asthma. (**A**) The acute or early-phase response. On exposure to an antigen, the immediate reaction is triggered by an IgE-mediated release of chemical mediators from sensitized mast cells. The release of chemical mediators results in increased mucus secretion, opening of mucosal intercellular junctions with increased antigen exposure of submucosal mast cells, and bronchoconstriction. (**B**) The late-phase response involves release of inflammatory mediators from mast cells, macrophages, basophils, neutrophils, and eosinophils; epithelial cell injury and edema, decreased mucociliary function, and accumulation of mucus; and increased airway responsiveness.

Causes of Asthma

The causes of asthma involve a complex interaction between genetic (atopy) and environmental factors. Factors that can contribute to the development of an asthmatic attack include allergens, respiratory tract infections, exercise, drugs and chemicals, hormonal changes and emotional upsets, airborne pollutants, and gastroesophageal reflux.

Bronchial asthma with an atopic component usually has its onset in childhood or adolescence and is seen in persons with a family history of allergies. Among the airborne allergens implicated in asthma are house dust mite allergens, cockroach allergens, animal dander, pollens, and molds. Persons with atopic asthma often have other allergic disorders, such as hay fever, hives, and eczema.

Respiratory tract infections, especially those caused by viruses, may produce their effects by causing epithelial damage and stimulating the production of IgE antibodies directed toward the viral antigens. In addition to precipitating an asthmatic attack, viral respiratory infections increase airway responsiveness to other asthma triggers that may persist for weeks beyond the original infection.

Exercise-induced asthma occurs in 40% to 90% of persons with bronchial asthma.[14] The cause of exercise-induced asthma is unclear. One possible cause is the loss of heat and water from the tracheobronchial tree because of the need for warming and humidifying of large volumes of air.[15] The response is commonly exaggerated when the person exercises in a cold environment. Wearing a mask over the nose and mouth often minimizes the attack or prevents it. A proper warm-up period also is important.

Inhaled irritants, such as tobacco smoke and strong odors, are thought to induce bronchospasm by way of irritant receptors and a vagal reflex. Exposure to parental smoking has been reported to increase asthma severity in children.[16] High doses of irritant gases such as sulfur dioxide, nitrogen dioxide, and ozone may induce inflammatory exacerbations of airway responsiveness (*e.g.*, smog-related asthma). Occupational asthma is stimulated by fumes and gases (*e.g.*, epoxy resins, plastics, toluene), organic and chemical dusts (*i.e.*, wood, cotton, platinum), and other chemicals (*e.g.*, formaldehyde) in the workplace.[17]

There is a small group of asthmatic patients in whom aspirin and nonsteroidal anti-inflammatory drugs (NSAIDs) are associated with asthmatic attacks, nasal polyps, and recurrent episodes of rhinitis.[18,19] An addition to the list of chemicals that can provoke an asthmatic attack are the sulfites used in food processing and as a preservative added to beer, wine, and fresh vegetables. Nonselective β-blocking drugs (*e.g.*, propranolol), including those used in ophthalmic preparations (*e.g.*, timolol, betaxolol), also can produce asthma symptoms by blocking the vasodilating effects of sympathetic neurotransmitters.

Both emotional factors and changes in hormone levels are thought to contribute to an increase in asthma symptoms. Emotional factors produce bronchospasm by way of vagal pathways. They can act as a bronchospastic trigger, or they can increase airway responsiveness to other triggers through noninflammatory mechanisms. The role of sex hormones in asthma is unclear, although there is much circumstantial evidence to suggest that they may be important. Up to 40% of women with asthma report a premenstrual increase in asthma symptoms.[20] Female sex hormones have a regulatory role on β_2-adrenergic function, and it has been suggested that abnormal regulation may be a possible mechanism for premenstrual asthma.[20]

Symptoms of gastroesophageal reflux are common in both adults and children with asthma, suggesting that reflux of gastric secretions may act as a bronchospastic trigger. Reflux during sleep can contribute to nocturnal asthma.[6]

Manifestations

Persons with asthma exhibit a wide range of signs and symptoms, from episodic wheezing and feelings of chest tightness to an acute, immobilizing attack. The attacks differ from person to person, and between attacks, many persons are symptom free. Attacks may occur spontaneously or in response to various triggers, respiratory infections, emotional stress, or weather changes. Asthma is often worse at night. Nocturnal asthma attacks usually occur at approximately 4:00 AM because of the occurrence of the late response to allergens inhaled during the evening and because of circadian variations in bronchial reactivity.[21]

During an asthmatic attack, the airways narrow because of bronchospasm, edema of the bronchial mucosa, and mucus plugging. Expiration becomes prolonged because of progressive airway obstruction. The amount of air that can be forcibly expired in 1 second (forced expiratory volume in 1 second [$FEV_{1.0}$]) and the peak expiratory flow rate (PEF), measured in liters per second, are decreased. A fall in the PEF to levels below 50% of the predicted value during an acute asthmatic attack indicates a severe exacerbation and the need for emergency room treatment.[6]

During a prolonged attack, air becomes trapped behind the occluded and narrowed airways causing hyperinflation of the lungs. This produces an increase in the residual volume (RV) along with a decrease in the inspiratory reserve capacity (tidal volume + inspiratory reserve volume [IRC]) and forced vital capacity (FVC), such that the person breathes close to his or her functional residual capacity (residual volume + expiratory reserve volume) (Fig. 31-8). As a result, more energy is needed to overcome the tension already present in the lungs, and the accessory muscles (*i.e.*, sternocleidomastoid muscles) are used to maintain ventilation and gas exchange. This causes dyspnea and fatigue. Because air is trapped in the alveoli and inspiration is occurring at higher residual lung volumes, the cough becomes less effective. As the condition progresses, the effectiveness of alveolar ventilation declines, and mismatching of ventilation and perfusion occurs, causing hypoxemia and hypercapnia. Pulmonary vascular resistance may increase as a result of the hypoxemia and hyperinflation, leading to a rise in pulmonary artery pressure and increased work demands on the right heart.

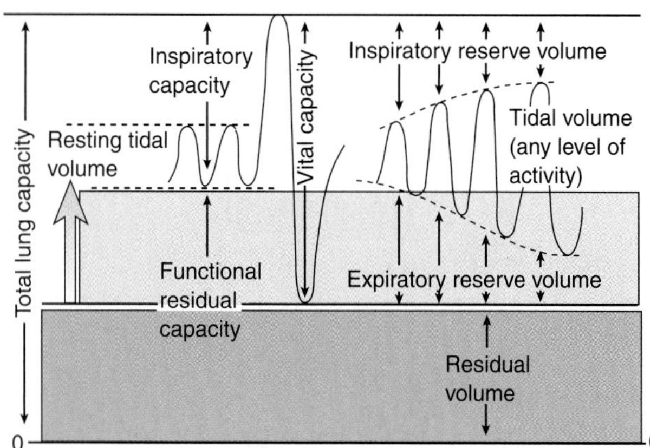

FIGURE 31-8 A spirometry tracing. Residual volume during normal respiratory function (*dark blue*) and the effect of air trapping during an asthmatic attack on residual lung volume and inspiratory and expiratory reserve volumes (*light blue*).

The physical signs of bronchial asthma vary with the severity of the attack. A mild attack may produce a feeling of chest tightness, a slight increase in respiratory rate with prolonged expiration, and mild wheezing. A cough may accompany the wheezing. More severe attacks are accompanied by use of the accessory muscles, distant breath sounds due to air trapping, and loud wheezing. As the condition progresses, fatigue develops, the skin becomes moist, and anxiety and apprehension are obvious. Dyspnea may be severe, and often the person is able to speak only one or two words before taking a breath. At the point at which airflow is markedly decreased, breath sounds become inaudible with diminished wheezing, and the cough becomes ineffective despite being repetitive and hacking. This point often marks the onset of respiratory failure.

Diagnosis and Treatment

Diagnosis. The diagnosis of asthma is based on a careful history and physical examination, laboratory findings, and pulmonary function studies (see Chapter 29). Spirometry provides a means for measuring FVC, $FEV_{1.0}$, PEF, tidal volume, expiratory reserve, and IRC. The level of airway responsiveness can be measured by inhalation challenge tests using methacholine (a cholinergic agonist), histamine, or exposure to a nonpharmacologic agent such as cold air.

Small, inexpensive, portable meters that measure PEF are available. Although not intended for use in diagnosis of asthma, they can be used in clinics and physicians' offices and in the home to provide frequent measures of flow rates. Day–night (circadian) variations in asthma symptoms and PEF variability can be used to indicate the severity of bronchial hyperresponsiveness. The person's best performance is established from readings taken over several weeks. This often is referred to as the individual's *personal best* and is used as a reference to indicate changes in respiratory function.[6]

Treatment. The Expert Panel of the National Asthma Education and Prevention Program (NAEPP) has developed classification systems intended for use in directing asthma treatment and identifying persons at high risk for development of life-threatening asthma attacks[6,7] (Table 31-1). Based on these classifications systems, the panel recommends two categories for management and treatment of asthma: control of factors contributing to asthma severity and pharmacologic treatment.[6,7]

Measures to control factors contributing to asthma severity are aimed at prevention of exposure to irritants and factors that increase asthma symptoms and precipitate asthma exacerbations. They include education of the patient and family regarding measures used in avoiding exposure to irritants and allergens that are known to induce or trigger an attack. A careful history often is needed to identify all the contributory factors. Factors such as nasal polyps, a history of aspirin sensitivity, and gastroesophageal reflux should be considered. Annual influenza vaccination is recommended for persons with persistent asthma.

Relaxation techniques and controlled breathing often help to allay the panic and anxiety that aggravate breathing difficulties. The hyperventilation that often accompanies anxiety and panic is known to act as an asthmatic trigger. In a child, measures to encourage independence as it relates to symptom control, along with those directed at helping to develop a positive self-concept, are essential.

A program of desensitization may be undertaken in persons with persistent asthma who react to allergens, such as house dust mites, that cannot be avoided. This involves the injection of selected antigens (based on skin tests) to stimulate the production of IgG antibodies that block the IgE response. A course of allergen immunotherapy is typically of 3 to 5 years' duration.[6]

Pharmacologic treatment is used to prevent or treat reversible airway obstruction and airway hyperresponsiveness caused by the inflammatory process. The Expert Panel recommends a stepwise approach to pharmacologic therapy based on frequency and severity of disease symptoms.[7] The medications used in the treatment of asthma include those with bronchodilator and anti-inflammatory actions. They are categorized into two general categories: quick-relief medications and long-term control medications.

The *quick-relief medications* include the short-acting β_2-adrenergic agonists, anticholinergic agents, and systemic corticosteroids. The short-acting β_2-adrenergic agonists (*e.g.*, albuterol, bitolterol, pirbuterol, terbutaline) relax bronchial smooth muscle and provide prompt relief of symptoms, usually within 30 minutes. They are administered by inhalation (*i.e.*, metered-dose inhaler [MDI] or nebulizer). The short-acting β_2-agonists are used for treating acute attacks of asthma but are not recommended for daily use because of concern over safety.[6] The increasing use of

TABLE 31-1 Classification of Asthma Severity

	Symptoms	Nighttime Symptoms	Lung Function
Mild intermittent	Symptoms ≤2 times a week Asymptomatic and normal PEF between exacerbations Exacerbations brief (from a few hours to a few days); intensity may vary	≤2 times a month	$FEV_{1.0}$ or PEF ≥80% predicted PEF variability <20%
Mild persistent	Symptoms >2 times a week but <1 time a day Exacerbations may affect activity	>2 times a month	$FEV_{1.0}$ or PEF ≥80% predicted PEF variability 20%–30%
Moderate persistent	Daily symptoms Daily use of inhaled short-acting β_2-agonist Exacerbations affect activity Exacerbations ≥2 times a week; may last days	>1 time a week	$FEV_{1.0}$ or PEF >60%–<80% predicted PEF variability >30%
Severe persistent	Continual symptoms Limited physical activity Frequent exacerbations	Frequent	$FEV_{1.0}$ or PEF ≤60% predicted PEF variability >30%

$FEV_{1.0}$, forced expiratory volume in 1 second; PEF, peak expiratory flow rate.
(Adapted from National Asthma Education and Prevention Program. [2003]. *Expert Panel report 2: Guidelines for the diagnosis and management of asthma: Update of selected topics—2002.* National Institutes of Health publication no. 02-5074. Bethesda, MD: National Institutes of Health.)

short-acting β_2-agonists or use of more than one canister in a month indicates inadequate control of asthma. The anticholinergic drugs (*e.g.*, ipratropium) block the postganglionic efferent vagal pathways that cause bronchoconstriction. These drugs, which are administered by inhalation, produce bronchodilation by direct action on the large airways and do not change the composition or viscosity of the bronchial mucus. It is thought that they may provide some additive benefit for treatment of asthma exacerbations when administered with inhaled β_2-agonists.[6] A short course of systemic corticosteroids, administered orally or parenterally, may be used for treating the inflammatory reaction associated with the late-phase response. Although their onset of action is slow (>4 hours), systemic corticosteroids often are used in the treatment of moderate to severe exacerbations because of their action in preventing the progression of the exacerbation, speeding recovery, and preventing early relapses.[6]

The *long-term medications* are taken on a daily basis to achieve and maintain control of persistent asthma symptoms. They include anti-inflammatory agents, long-acting bronchodilators, and leukotriene modifiers. The Expert Panel defines anti-inflammatory medications as "those that cause a reduction in markers of airway inflammation in airway tissues and airway secretions (*e.g.*, eosinophils, mast cells, activated lymphocytes, macrophages, cytokines or inflammatory mediators) and thus decrease the intensity of airway hyperresponsiveness."[7] The corticosteroids are considered the most effective anti-inflammatory agents for use in long-term treatment of asthma. Inhaled corticosteroids that are administered by MDI usually are preferred because of minimal systemic absorption and degree of disruption in hypothalamic-pituitary-adrenal function. In severe cases, oral or parenterally administered corticosteroids may be necessary.

The anti-inflammatory agents sodium cromolyn and nedocromil are also used to prevent an asthmatic attack. These agents act by stabilizing mast cells, thereby preventing release of the inflammatory mediators that cause an asthmatic attack. They are used prophylactically to prevent early and late responses. They are of no benefit when taken during an attack.

The long-acting β_2-agonists, which are available in inhalation (*e.g.*, salmeterol, formoterol) or oral (*e.g.*, albuterol sustained release) forms, act by relaxing bronchial smooth muscle. They are used as an adjunct to anti-inflammatory medications for providing long-term control of symptoms, especially nocturnal symptoms, and for preventing exercise-induced bronchospasm. The long-acting β_2-agonists have a duration of action of at least 12 hours and should not be used to treat acute symptoms or exacerbations.[7]

Theophylline, a methylxanthine, is a bronchodilator that acts by relaxing bronchial smooth muscle. The sustained-release form of the drug is used as an adjuvant therapy and is particularly useful in relieving nighttime symptoms. It may be used as an alternative, but not preferred, medication in long-term preventative therapy when there are issues concerning adherence with regimens using inhaled medications or when cost is a factor. Because elimination of the drug varies widely among persons, blood levels are required to ensure that the therapeutic, but not toxic dose, is achieved.[7]

A newer group of drugs called the *leukotriene modifiers* have become available for use in the treatment of asthma.[22] The leukotrienes are potent biochemical mediators released from mast cells that cause bronchoconstriction, increased mucus secretion, and attraction and activation of inflammatory cells in the airways of people with asthma. There are two types of leukotriene modifiers: (1) those that act by inhibiting 5-lipoxygenase (*e.g.*, zileuton), an enzyme required for leukotriene synthesis; and (2) those that act as receptor antagonists (*e.g.*, zafirlukast and montelukast) by inhibiting the binding of leukotrienes to their receptor in the target tissues. A particular advantage of the leukotriene modifiers is that they are taken orally.

Severe Asthma

Severe or refractory asthma represents a subgroup (probably less than 5%) of persons with asthma who have more troublesome disease as evidenced by high medication requirements to maintain good disease control or continue to have persistent symptoms despite high medication use.[23,24] These persons are at increased risk for fatal or near fatal asthma.

Severe or refractory asthma has been defined as persistent asthma that requires continuous high-dose inhaled or oral corticosteroids for more than 50% of the previous year, obstructive lung function and evidence of disease exacerbations or instability, and need for additional medications.[23,24] In the population of persons with refractory asthma, approximately 10% have been hospitalized, 20% have been seen in the emergency room, and 40% have required an increase in corticosteroid dose.[24]

Little is known about the causes of severe asthma. Among the proposed risk factors are genetic predisposition, continued allergen or tobacco exposure, infection, intercurrent sinusitis or gastroesophageal reflux disease, and lack of compliance or adherence with treatment measures.[24] It has been proposed that because asthma is a disease involving multiple genes, certain factors such as mutations in genes regulating cytokines (*e.g.*, IL-4), growth factors, or mutations in receptors for primary treatments of asthma (β_2 or glucocorticoid) could be involved. Environmental factors include both allergen and tobacco exposure, with the strongest response occurring in response to house dust, cockroach, and *Alternaria* (a mold) exposure. Infections may also play a role. Respiratory syncytial virus infections are implicated in children, and pathogens such as *Mycoplasma* and *Chlamydia* may play a role in adults. Gastroesophageal reflux and chronic sinusitis may also play a role.

Fatal and near-fatal asthma attacks, although uncommon, have increased during the past several decades.[25] Most asthma deaths have occurred outside the hospital. Persons at highest risk are those with previous exacerbations resulting in respiratory failure, respiratory acidosis, and the need for intubation.[26] Although the cause of death during an acute asthmatic attack is largely unknown, both cardiac dysrhythmias and asphyxia due to severe airway obstruction have been implicated. It has been suggested that an underestimation of the severity of the attack may be a contributing factor. Deterioration often occurs rapidly during an acute attack, and underestimation of its severity may lead to a life-threatening delay in seeking medical attention. Frequent and repetitive use of β_2-agonist inhalers (more than twice in a month) far in excess of the recommended doses may temporarily blunt symptoms and mask the severity of the condition. It has been suggested that persons who have fatal or near-fatal asthmatic attacks may have impaired perception of dyspnea and its severity.[27,28] Thus, they may not realize the severity of their condition and may not take the appropriate measures in terms of securing appropriate emergency treatment.

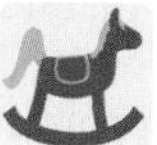

Bronchial Asthma in Children

Asthma is a leading cause of chronic illness in children and is responsible for a significant number of lost school days. It is the most frequent admitting diagnosis in children's hospitals. In 1998, as many as 8.65 children (12.1%) were reported to have physician or health care professional diagnosis of asthma at some time during childhood.[29] Asthma may have its onset at any age; 80% of children are symptomatic by 6 years of age.[29,30] Asthma is more prevalent in black than white children and results in more frequent disability and more frequent hospitalizations in black children.[30]

As with adults, asthma in children commonly is associated with an IgE-related reaction. It has been suggested that IgE directed against respiratory viruses in particular may be important in the pathogenesis of wheezing illnesses in infants (*i.e.*, bronchiolitis), which often precedes the onset of asthma. The RSV and parainfluenza viruses are the most commonly involved.[29,31] Other contributing factors include exposure to environmental allergens such as pet dander, dust mite antigens, and cockroach allergens. Exposure to environmental tobacco smoke also may contribute to asthma in children. Of particular concern is the effect of in utero exposure to maternal smoking on lung function in infants and children.[32,33]

The signs and symptoms of asthma in infants and small children vary with the stage and severity of an attack. Because airway patency decreases at night, many children have acute signs of asthma at this time. Often, previously well infants and children develop what may seem to be a cold with rhinorrhea, rapidly followed by irritability, a tight and nonproductive cough, wheezing, tachypnea, dyspnea with prolonged expiration, and use of accessory muscles of respiration. Cyanosis, hyperinflation of the chest, and tachycardia indicate increasing severity of the attack. Wheezing may be absent in children with extreme respiratory distress. The symptoms may progress rapidly and require a trip to the emergency room or hospitalization.

The Expert Panel of the National Asthma Education and Prevention Program has developed guidelines for management of asthma in infants and children younger than 5 years of age and for adults and children older than 5 years of age.[7,34] As with adults and older children, the Expert Panel recommends a stepwise approach to diagnosing and managing asthma in infants and children younger than 5 years of age. The anti-inflammatory agents cromolyn and nedocromil are recommended as an initial therapy for mild to moderate persistent asthma in infants and children. Inhaled short-acting β_2-agonists may be used for mild intermittent symptoms or exacerbations. More severe symptoms may require the use of inhaled corticosteroids. Systemic corticosteroids may be required during an episode of severe disease. Growth velocity should be monitored in children and adolescents receiving long-term corticosteroid therapy by any route because these drugs may suppress growth.[7]

Special delivery systems for administration of inhalation medications are available for infants and small children, including nebulizers with face masks and spacers and holding chambers for use with an MDI. For children younger than 2 years of age, nebulizer therapy usually is preferred. Children between 3 and 5 years of age may begin using an MDI with a spacer and holding chamber. The child's caregiver should be carefully instructed in the appropriate use of these devices.

The Expert Panel recommends that adolescents (and younger children when appropriate) be directly involved in developing their asthma management plans. Active participation in physical activities, exercise, and sports should be encouraged.

CHRONIC OBSTRUCTIVE PULMONARY DISEASE

Chronic obstructive pulmonary disease (COPD) denotes a group of respiratory disorders characterized by chronic and recurrent obstruction of airflow in the pulmonary airways.[35] Airflow obstruction usually is progressive and is accompanied by inflammatory responses to noxious particles or gases.[35–37] COPD is a leading cause of morbidity and mortality worldwide. It has been estimated that approximately 14 million Americans have COPD. The prevalence, morbidity, and mortality vary among different groups within countries but in general are related to cigarette smoking. In the United States, COPD now represents the fourth leading cause of death in the United States, with more than 117,000 deaths reported in 2000.[38] The death rate from COPD is low among people younger than 35 years, but then increases with age, reflecting the cumulative effects of smoking.[37]

Etiology and Pathogenesis

The risk factors for COPD include both host and environmental factors. The most common cause of COPD is smoking.[35–37] Thus, the disease is largely preventable. Unfortunately, clinical findings are almost always absent during the early stages of COPD, and by the time symptoms appear, the disease usually is far advanced. For smokers with early signs of airway disease, there is hope that early recognition, combined with appropriate treatment and smoking cessation, may prevent or delay the usually relentless progression of the disease. A second, less common host factor is a hereditary deficiency in α_1-antitrypsin. Other predisposing factors are asthma and airway hyperresponsiveness and conditions occurring during infancy or early childhood that impair lung growth.

The mechanisms involved in the pathogenesis of COPD usually are multiple and include inflammation and fibrosis of the bronchial wall, hypertrophy of the submucosal glands and hypersecretion of mucus, and loss of elastic lung fibers and alveolar tissue[39] (Fig. 31-9). Inflammation and fibrosis of the bronchial wall, along with excess mucus secretion, obstruct airflow and cause mismatching of ventilation and perfusion. Destruction of alveolar tissue decreases the surface area for gas exchange, and loss of elastic fibers leads to airway collapse. Normally, recoil of the elastic fibers that were stretched during inspiration provides the force needed to move air out of the lung during expiration. Because the elastic fibers are attached to the airways, they also provide radial traction to hold the airways open during expiration. In persons with COPD, the loss of elastic fibers impairs the expiratory flow rate, increases air trapping, and predisposes to airway collapse.

The term *chronic obstructive pulmonary disease* encompasses two types of obstructive airway disease: *emphysema,* with enlargement of air spaces and destruction of lung tissue, and *chronic obstructive bronchitis,* with obstruction of small airways.

Emphysema. Emphysema is characterized by a loss of lung elasticity and abnormal enlargement of the air spaces distal to the terminal bronchioles, with destruction of the alveolar walls and capillary beds (see Fig. 31-9). Enlargement of the air spaces leads to hyperinflation of the lungs and produces an increase in total lung capacity (TLC). Two of the recognized causes of emphysema are smoking, which incites lung injury, and an inherited deficiency of *α_1-antitrypsin,* an antiprotease enzyme that protects the lung from injury. Genetic factors, other than an inherited α_1-antitrypsin deficiency, also may play a role in smokers who develop COPD at an early age.[39]

Emphysema is thought to result from the breakdown of elastin and other alveolar wall components by enzymes, called *proteases,* that digest proteins. These proteases, particularly elastase, which is an enzyme that digests elastin, are released from polymorphonuclear leukocytes (*i.e.,* neutrophils), alveolar macrophages, and other inflammatory cells.[35] Normally, the lung is protected by antiprotease enzymes including α_1-antitrypsin. Cigarette smoke and other irritants stimulate the movement of inflammatory cells into the lungs, resulting in increased release of elastase and other proteases. In smokers in whom COPD develops, antiprotease production and release may be inadequate to neutralize the excess protease production such that the process of elastic tissue destruction goes unchecked (Fig. 31-10).

A hereditary deficiency in α_1-antitrypsin accounts for approximately 1% of all cases of COPD and is more common in young persons with emphysema.[35] The type and amount of α_1-antitrypsin that a person has is determined by a pair of codominant genes referred to as *PI* (protein inhibitor) genes. An α_1-antitrypsin deficiency is inherited as an autosomal recessive disorder. There are more than 75 mutations of the gene. One of these, the *PIZ* variant, which occurs in 5% of the population, causes the most serious deficiency in α_1-antitrypsin. It is most common in persons of Scandinavian descent and is rare in Jews, blacks, and Japanese.[39] Homozygotes who carry two defective *PIZ* genes have only about 15% to 20% of the normal plasma concentration of α_1-antitrypsin. Almost all persons who have emphysema before the age of 40 years have an α_1-antitrypsin deficiency. Smoking and repeated respiratory tract infections, which also decrease α_1-antitrypsin levels, contribute to the risk for emphysema in persons with an α_1-antitrypsin deficiency. Laboratory methods

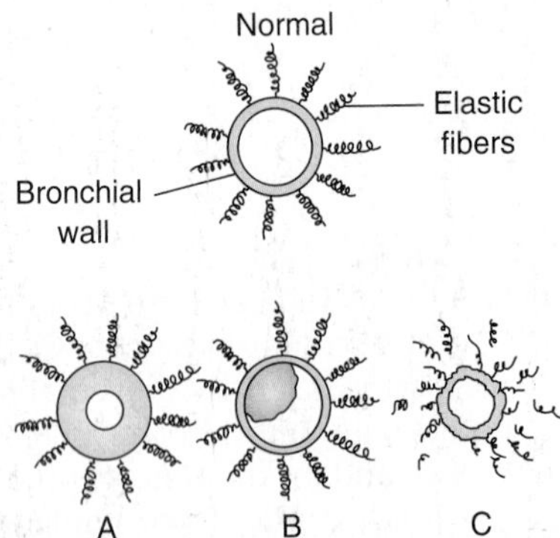

FIGURE 31-9 Mechanisms of airflow obstruction in chronic obstructive lung disease. (**Top**) The normal bronchial airway with elastic fibers that provide traction and hold the airway open. (**Bottom**) Obstruction of the airway caused by (**A**) hypertrophy of the bronchial wall, (**B**) inflammation and hypersecretion of mucus, and (**C**) loss of elastic fibers that hold the airway open.

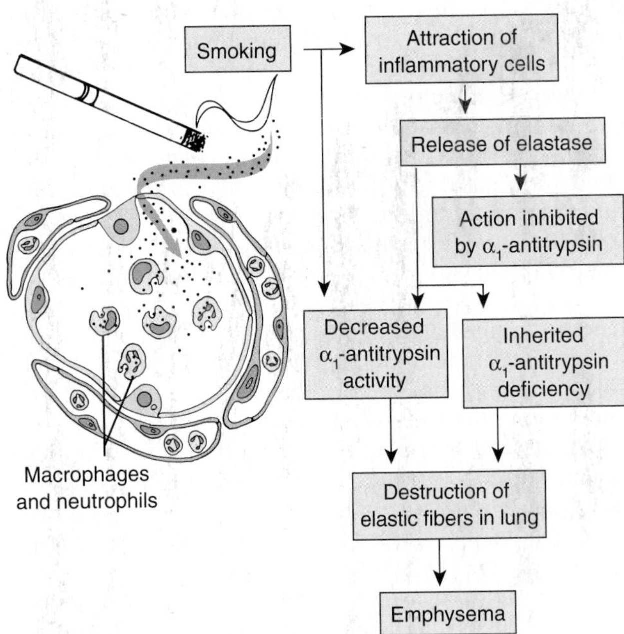

FIGURE 31-10 Smoking and protease–antiprotease mechanisms of emphysema. Smoking inhibits α_1-antitrypsin and favors the recruitment of macrophages and neutrophils and release of elastase, with elastic tissue destruction in the lung and development of emphysema.

are available for measuring α_1-antitrypsin levels. Human α_1-antitrypsin is available for replacement therapy in persons with a hereditary deficiency of the enzyme. The preparation is administered once weekly by intravenous infusion.[1]

There are two commonly recognized types of emphysema: centriacinar and panacinar (Fig. 31-11). The centriacinar type affects the bronchioles in the central part of the respiratory lobule, with initial preservation of the alveolar ducts and sacs[39] (Fig. 31-12). It is the most common type of emphysema and is seen predominantly in male smokers. The panacinar type produces initial involvement of the peripheral alveoli and later extends to involve the more central bronchioles. This type of emphysema is more common in persons with α_1-antitrypsin deficiency. It also is found in smokers in association with centrilobular emphysema. In such cases, panacinar changes are seen in the lower parts of the lung and the centriacinar changes in the upper parts of the lung.

Chronic Bronchitis. In chronic bronchitis, airway obstruction is caused by inflammation of the major and small airways. There is edema and hyperplasia of submucosal glands and excess mucus excretion into the bronchial tree.[39] A history of a chronic productive cough of more than 3 months' duration for more than 2 consecutive years is necessary for diagnosis of chronic bronchitis.[37] Typically, the cough has been present for many years, with a gradual increase in acute exacerbations that produce frankly purulent sputum. Chronic bronchitis without airflow obstruction often is referred to as *simple bronchitis* and chronic bronchitis with airflow obstruction as *chronic obstructive bronchitis*. The outlook for persons with simple bronchitis is good, compared with the premature morbidity and mortality associated with chronic obstructive bronchitis.

Chronic bronchitis is seen most commonly in middle-aged men and is associated with chronic irritation from smoking and recurrent infections. In the United States, smoking is the most important cause of chronic bronchitis. Viral and bacterial infections are common in persons with chronic bronchitis and are thought to be a result rather than a cause of the problem.

Clinical Manifestations

The clinical manifestations of COPD represent a progressive change in respiratory function, ranging from cough and sputum production to severe respiratory impairment. The mnemonics "pink puffer" and "blue bloater" have been used to differentiate the clinical manifestations of emphysema and chronic obstructive bronchitis.[1] In practice, differentiation between the two types is often difficult. This is because persons with COPD often have some degree of both emphysema and chronic bronchitis. A major difference between the pink puffers and the blue bloaters is the respiratory responsiveness to the hypoxic stimuli. With pulmonary emphysema, there is a proportionate loss of ventilation and perfusion area in the lung. These persons are pink puffers, or fighters able to overventilate and thus maintain relatively normal blood gas levels until late in the disease. Chronic obstructive bronchitis is characterized by excessive bronchial secretions and airway obstruction that causes mismatching of ventilation and perfusion. Thus, persons with chronic bronchitis are unable to compensate by increasing their ventilation; instead, hypoxemia and cyanosis develop. These are the blue bloaters, or nonfighters.

Persons with emphysema have marked dyspnea and struggle to maintain normal blood gas levels with increased ventilatory effort, including prominent use of the accessory muscles. The seated position, which stabilizes chest structures and allows for maximum chest expansion and use of accessory muscles, is preferred. With loss

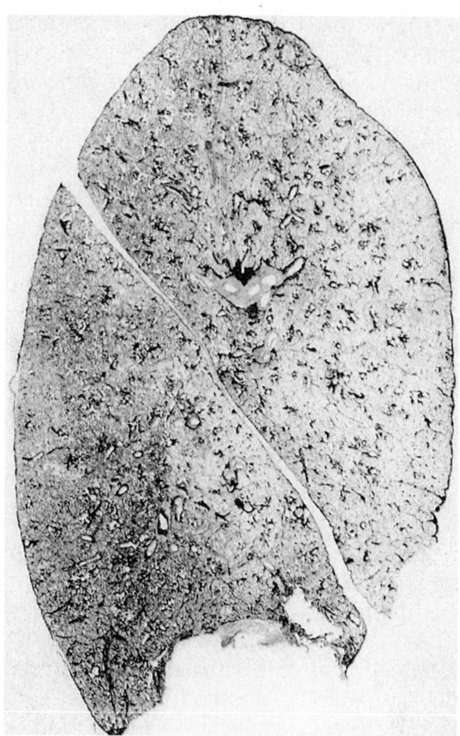

FIGURE 31-12 Centrilobular emphysema. A whole mount of the left lung of a smoker with mild emphysema shows enlarged air spaces scattered throughout both lobes, which represent destruction of terminal bronchioles in the central part of the pulmonary lobule. These abnormal spaces are surrounded by intact pulmonary parenchyma. (Rubin E., Farber J.L. [1999]. *Pathology* [3rd ed., p. 628]. Philadelphia: Lippincott-Raven)

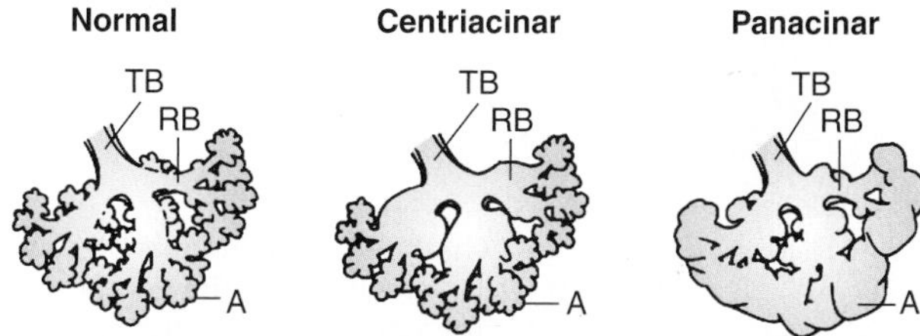

FIGURE 31-11 Centriacinar and panacinar emphysema. In centriacinar emphysema, the destruction is confined to the terminal (TB) and respiratory bronchioles (RB). In panacinar emphysema, the peripheral alveoli (A) are also involved. (West J.B. [1997]. *Pulmonary pathophysiology* [5th ed., p. 53]. Philadelphia: Lippincott-Raven)

of lung elasticity and hyperinflation of the lungs, the airways often collapse during expiration because pressure in surrounding lung tissues exceeds airway pressure. Air becomes trapped in lungs, producing an increase in the anteroposterior dimensions of the chest, the so-called *barrel chest* that is typical of persons with emphysema (Fig. 31-13). Expiration often is accomplished through pursed lips. Pursed-lip breathing, which increases the resistance to the outflow of air, helps to prevent airway collapse by increasing airway pressure. The work of breathing is greatly increased in persons with emphysema, and eating often is difficult. As a result, there often is considerable weight loss.

Chronic bronchitis is characterized by shortness of breath with a progressive decrease in exercise tolerance. As the disease progresses, breathing becomes increasingly more labored, even at rest. The expiratory phase of respiration is prolonged, and expiratory wheezes and crackles can be heard on auscultation. In contrast to persons with emphysema, those with chronic obstructive bronchitis are unable to maintain normal blood gases by increasing their breathing effort. Hypoxemia, hypercapnia, and cyanosis develop, reflecting an imbalance between ventilation and perfusion. Hypoxemia, in which arterial PO_2 levels fall below 55 mm Hg, causes reflex vasoconstriction of the pulmonary vessels and further impairment of gas exchange in the lung. Hypoxemia also stimulates red blood cell production, causing polycythemia. As a result, persons with chronic obstructive bronchitis develop pulmonary hypertension and, eventually, right-sided heart failure with peripheral edema (*i.e.,* cor pulmonale).

Persons with combined forms of COPD characteristically seek medical attention in the fifth or sixth decade of life, complaining of cough, sputum production, and shortness of breath. The symptoms typically have existed to some extent for 10 years or longer. The productive cough usually occurs in the morning. Dyspnea becomes more severe as the disease progresses. Frequent exacerbations of infection and respiratory insufficiency are common, causing absence from work and eventual disability. The late stages of COPD are characterized by pulmonary hypertension, cor pulmonale, recurrent respiratory infections, and chronic respiratory failure. Death usually occurs during an exacerbation of illness associated with infection and respiratory failure.

Diagnosis and Treatment

Diagnosis. The diagnosis of COPD is based on a careful history and physical examination, pulmonary function studies, chest radiographs, and laboratory tests. Airway obstruction prolongs the expiratory phase of respiration and affords the potential for impaired gas exchange because of mismatching of ventilation and perfusion. The FVC is the amount of air that can be forcibly exhaled after maximal inspiration. In an adult with normal respiratory function, this should be achieved in 4 to 6 seconds. In patients with chronic lung disease, the time required for FVC is in-

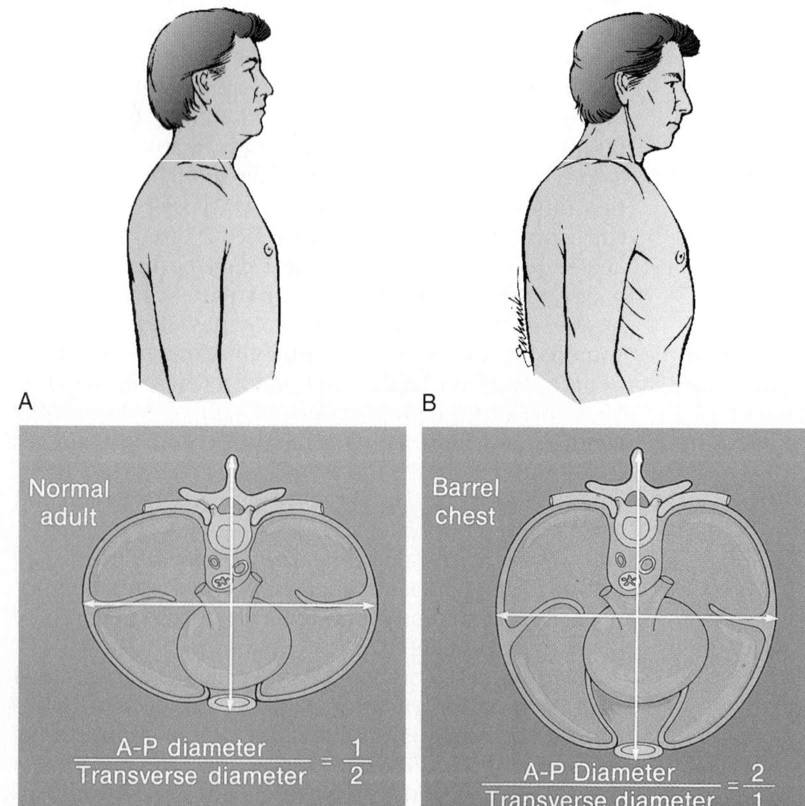

FIGURE 31-13 Characteristics of normal chest wall and chest wall in emphysema. The normal chest wall and its cross-section are illustrated on the left (**A**). The barrel-shaped chest of emphysema and its cross-section are illustrated on the right (**B**). (Smeltzer S.C., Bare B.G. [2000]. *Medical-surgical nursing.* [9th ed., p. 454]. Philadelphia: Lippincott Williams & Wilkins)

creased, the $FEV_{1.0}$ is decreased, and the ratio of $FEV_{1.0}$ to FVC is decreased. In severe disease, the FVC is markedly reduced. Lung volume measurements reveal a marked increase in RV, an increase in TLC, and elevation of the RV to TLC ratio. These and other measurements of expiratory flow are determined by spirometry and are used in the diagnosis of COPD (see Chapter 29, Fig. 29-17). Spirometry measurements can be used in staging disease severity. For example, an $FEV_{1.0}$-to-FVC ratio of less than 70% with an $FEV_{1.0}$ of 80% or more, with or without symptoms, indicates mild disease; and a $FEV_{1.0}$-to-FVC ratio of less than 70% with an $FEV_{1.0}$ of less than 50%, with or without symptoms, indicates severe disease.[36]

Other diagnostic measures become important as the disease advances. Measures of exercise tolerance, nutritional status, hemoglobin saturation, and arterial blood gases can be used to assess the overall impact of COPD on health status and to direct treatment.

Treatment. The treatment of COPD depends on the stage of the disease and often requires an interdisciplinary approach. Education of persons with COPD and their families is a key to successful management of the disease. Psychosocial rehabilitation must be individualized to meet the specific needs of persons with COPD and their families. These needs vary with age, occupation, financial resources, social and recreational interests, and interpersonal and family relationships.

Smoking cessation is the only measure that slows the progression of the disease. Nicotine replacement therapy (gum, transdermal patches, or inhaler) or the noradrenergic antidepressant drug bupropion may be used to reduce withdrawal symptoms. Persons in more advanced stages of the disease often require measures to maintain and improve physical and psychosocial functioning, pharmacologic interventions, and oxygen therapy. Avoidance of cigarette smoke and other environmental airway irritants is a must. Wearing a cold-weather mask often prevents dyspnea and bronchospasm due to cold air and wind exposure.

Respiratory tract infections can prove life threatening to persons with severe COPD. A person with COPD should avoid exposure to others with known respiratory tract infections and should avoid attending large gatherings during periods of the year when influenza or respiratory tract infections are prevalent. Immunization for influenza and pneumococcal infections decreases the likelihood of their occurrence. Although antibiotics are used to treat acute exacerbations of COPD due to bacterial infection, there is no evidence that the prophylactic use of antibiotics prevents acute exacerbations.[35]

Because persons with COPD expend so much effort on breathing, many find it difficult to chew their food and manage the effort of a large meal. This situation, combined with impaired diaphragm descent, air swallowing, and medications that cause anorexia and nausea, impairs nutrition and promotes weight loss. Undernutrition (body weight <90% of ideal weight) affects approximately 25% of persons with COPD.[40] Specifically, nutrition depletion is associated with decreased exercise capacity, dyspnea, fatigue, and increased susceptibility to respiratory infections. Small, frequent, nutritious, and easily swallowed feedings aid in maintaining good nutrition and preventing weight loss. Excess carbohydrates in the diet can increase carbon dioxide production and arterial carbon dioxide levels. However, it usually is not a problem unless a high-carbohydrate diet is followed.

Maintaining and improving physical and psychosocial functioning is an important part of the treatment program for persons with COPD. A long-term pulmonary rehabilitation program can significantly reduce episodes of hospitalization and add measurably to a person's ability to manage and cope with his or her impairment in a positive way. This program includes breathing exercises that focus on restoring the function of the diaphragm, reducing the work of breathing, and improving gas exchange. Physical conditioning with appropriate exercise training increases maximal oxygen consumption and reduces ventilatory effort and heart rate for a given workload. Work simplification and energy conservation strategies may be needed when impairment is severe.

The pharmacologic treatment of COPD includes the use of bronchodilators, including inhaled adrenergic and anticholinergic agents.[35–37] Inhaled β_2-adrenergic agonists have been the mainstay of treatment of COPD for many years. It has been suggested that long-acting inhaled β_2-adrenergic agonists may be even more effective than the short-acting forms of the drug. In addition to their action as bronchodilators, the long-acting β_2-adrenergic agonists are thought to reduce the adherence of bacteria such as *Haemophilus influenzae* to airway epithelial cells, thereby reducing the risk for infective exacerbations.[35] The anticholinergic drugs (*e.g.*, ipratropium), which are administered by inhalation, produce bronchodilation by blocking parasympathetic cholinergic receptors that produce contraction of bronchial smooth muscle. They also reduce the volume of sputum without altering its viscosity. Because the drugs have a slower onset and longer duration of action, they usually are used on a regular basis rather than on an as-needed basis. Inhalers that combine an anticholinergic drug with a β_2-adrenergic agonist are available.

Oral theophylline may be used in treatment of persons who fail to respond to inhaled bronchodilators. The long-acting theophylline preparations may be used to reduce overnight declines in respiratory function. There also is evidence that theophylline may improve respiratory muscle function, increase mucociliary clearance, and improve central respiratory drive.[31] When theophylline is prescribed, blood levels are used as a guide in arriving at an effective dose schedule.

Although inhaled corticosteroids often are used in treatment of COPD, there is controversy regarding their usefulness. There is evidence that inflammation in COPD is not suppressed by inhaled or oral corticosteroids.[35] An explanation for this lack of effect may be related to the fact that corticosteroids prolong the action of neutrophils and hence do not suppress the neutrophilic inflammation seen in COPD. Because corticosteroids are useful in relieving asthma symptoms, they may benefit persons with asthma concomitant with COPD. Inhaled corticosteroids also may be beneficial in treating acute exacerbations of COPD, minimizing the undesirable effects that often accompany systemic use.

Oxygen therapy is prescribed for selected persons with significant hypoxemia (arterial PO_2 <55 mm Hg). Administration of continuous low-flow (1 to 2 L/minute) oxygen to maintain arterial PO_2 levels between 55 and 65 mm Hg decreases dyspnea and pulmonary hypertension and improves neuropsychological function and activity tolerance. The overall goal of oxygen therapy is to maintain a hemoglobin oxygen saturation of at least 90%.[36] Oxygen usually is administered using a nasal cannula. Portable oxygen administration units, which allow mobility and the performance of activities of daily living, usually are used. Transtracheal oxygen, delivered by a small-diameter percutaneous catheter placed in the trachea, can be used to increase oxygen delivery and decrease ventilatory effort. It is particularly useful in persons with high oxygen requirements.[35] It also can be used to increase ambulation by eliminating the need to wear a nasal cannula. Oxygen administration in persons with severe COPD must be undertaken with a certain amount of caution. The flow rate (in liters per minute) usually is titrated to provide an arterial PO_2 of 55 to 65 mm Hg. Because the ventilatory drive associated with hypoxic stimulation of the peripheral chemoreceptors does not occur until the arterial PO_2 has been reduced to about 60 mm Hg or less, increasing the arterial PO_2 above 60 mm Hg tends to depress the hypoxic stimulus for ventilation and often leads to hypoventilation and carbon dioxide retention.

Lung reduction surgery or bullectomy may prove useful in a limited number of cases. Lung volume reduction surgery involves the resection of the most distended areas of the lung as a means of improving respiratory function. The procedure is designed to reduce the overall volume of the lung, reshape the configuration of the lung, and improve elastic recoil and its effects on the airways and the diaphragm. Although the procedure still is experimental, early results have demonstrated improvement in the 6-minute walk, dyspnea index, and quality-of-life assessment.[41] Bullectomy is a surgical procedure that involves the removal of large emphysematous bullae that compress adjacent lung tissue and cause dyspnea.

Lung transplantation is becoming an alternative treatment for persons with severe lung disease, limited life expectancy without transplantation, adequate functioning of other organ systems, and a good social support system.

BRONCHIECTASIS

Bronchiectasis is an uncommon type of COPD characterized by a permanent dilation of the bronchi and bronchioles caused by destruction of the muscle and elastic supporting tissue resulting from a vicious cycle of infection and inflammation[39,42,43] (Fig. 31-14). It is not a primary disease but is secondary to persisting infection or obstruction.[10] In the past, bronchiectasis often followed a necrotizing bacterial pneumonia that frequently complicated measles, pertussis, or influenza. Tuberculosis was also

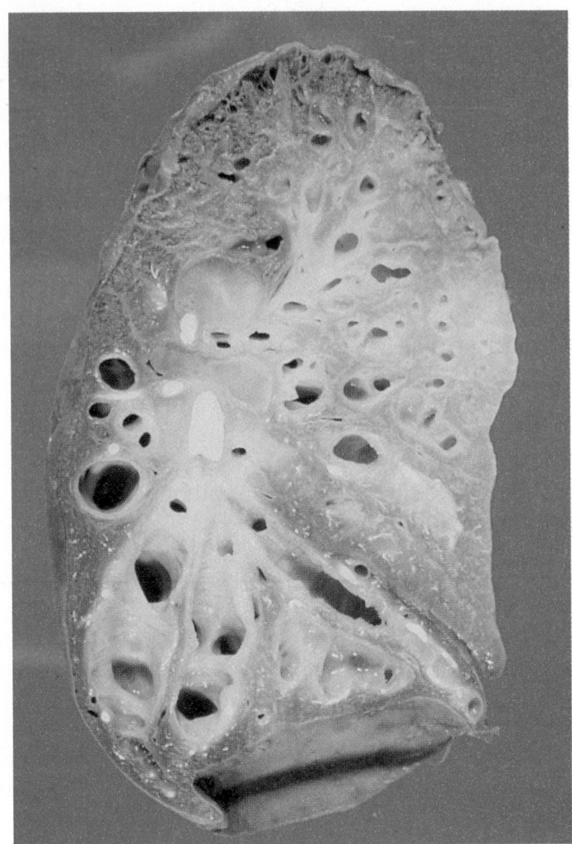

FIGURE 31-14 Bronchiectasis. The resected upper lobe shows widely dilated bronchi, with thickening of the bronchial walls and collapse and fibrosis of the pulmonary parenchyma. (Rubin E., Farber J.L. [1999]. *Pathology* [3rd ed., p. 601]. Philadelphia: Lippincott-Raven)

commonly associated with bronchiectasis. Thus, with the advent of antibiotics that more effectively treat respiratory infections such as tuberculosis and immunizations against pertussis and measles, there has been a marked decrease in the prevalence of bronchiectasis.

Bronchiectasis can present in either of two forms: a local obstructive process involving a lobe or segment of a lung or a diffuse process involving much of both lungs.[43] Two processes are critical to the pathogenesis of both types of bronchiectasis: obstruction and chronic persistent infection.[10] Regardless of which may come first, both cause damage to the bronchial walls, leading to weakening and dilation. Normal clearance mechanisms are hampered by obstruction, allowing infection to develop, and persistent necrotizing infection in the bronchi or bronchioles may cause obstructive secretions.

Localized bronchiectasis can affect any area of the lung, the area being determined by the site of obstruction or infection. Obstructive bronchiectasis is confined to a segment of the lung distal to a mechanical obstruction. It is most commonly caused by conditions such as tumors, foreign bodies, and mucus plugs that produce atelectasis and infection due to obstructed drainage of bronchial secretions. Generalized bronchiectasis is due largely to inherited impairments of host mechanisms or acquired disorders that permit introduction of infectious organisms into the airways. They include inherited conditions such as cystic fibrosis, in which airway obstruction is caused by impairment of normal mucociliary function; congenital and acquired immunodeficiency states, which predispose to respiratory tract infections; lung infection (*e.g.,* tuberculosis, fungal infections, lung abscess); and exposure to toxic gases that cause airway obstruction. Generalized bronchiectasis usually is bilateral and most commonly affects the lower lobes.

Bronchiectasis is associated with an assortment of abnormalities that profoundly affect respiratory function, including atelectasis, obstruction of the smaller airways, and diffuse bronchitis. Affected persons have recurrent bronchopulmonary infection; coughing; production of copious amounts of foul-smelling, purulent sputum; and hemoptysis. Weight loss and anemia are common. The physiologic abnormalities that occur in bronchiectasis are similar to those seen in chronic bronchitis and emphysema. As in the latter two conditions, chronic bronchial obstruction leads to marked dyspnea and cyanosis. Clubbing of the fingers, which is not seen in other types of obstructive lung diseases, is common in moderate to advanced bronchiectasis.

Diagnosis is based on history and imaging studies. The condition often is evident on chest radiographs. High-resolution CT scanning of the chest allows for definitive diagnosis. Accuracy of diagnosis is important because interventional bronchoscopy or surgery may be palliative or curative in some obstructive forms of the disease.

Treatment consists of early recognition and treatment of infection along with regular postural drainage and chest physical therapy. Persons with this disorder benefit from many of the rehabilitation and treatment measures used for chronic bronchitis and emphysema.

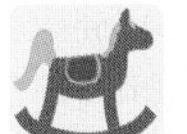

CYSTIC FIBROSIS

Cystic fibrosis (CF), which is the major cause of severe chronic respiratory disease in children, is an autosomal recessive disorder involving fluid secretion in the exocrine glands in the epithelial lining of the respiratory, gastrointestinal, and reproductive tracts.[44–46] In addition to chronic respiratory disease, CF is manifested by pancreatic exocrine deficiency and elevation of sodium chloride in the sweat. Nasal polyps, sinus infections, pancreatitis, and cholelithiasis also are common. Excessive loss of sodium in the sweat predisposes young children to salt depletion episodes. Most males with cystic fibrosis have congenital bilateral absence of the vas deferens with azoospermia.

Cystic fibrosis is caused by mutations in a single gene on the long arm of chromosome 7 that encodes for the cystic fibrosis transmembrane regulator (CFTR), which functions as a chloride (Cl^-) channel in epithelial cell membranes. The disease affects approximately 30,000 children and adults in the United States, and more than 10 million persons are asymptomatic carriers of the defective gene.[47] The gene is rare in African blacks and Asians. Homozygotes (*i.e.,* persons with two defective genes) have all or substantially all of the clinical symptoms of the disease, compared with heterozygotes, who are carriers of the disease but have no recognizable symptoms.

Although a large number of mutations in the CFTR gene have been identified, only 22 have been identified with any degree of frequency. The most common and first identified mutation, which involves a three base pair deletion that codes for phenylalanine, accounts for 70% of CF cases in whites. Mutations in the CFTR gene render the epithelial membrane relatively impermeable to the chloride ion. The impact on transport function is relatively tissue specific. In the sweat glands, the concentration of sodium (Na^+) and Cl^- secreted into the lumen of the gland remains unaffected, whereas the reabsorption of Cl^- through the CFTR and accompanying reabsorption of Na^+ in the ducts of the gland fail to occur. This accounts for the high concentration of NaCl in the sweat of persons with CF.[48] In the normal airway epithelium, Cl^- is secreted into airway lumen through the CFTR. The impaired transport of Cl^- ultimately leads to a series of secondary events, including increased absorption of Na^+ and water from the airways into the blood. This lowers the water content of the mucociliary blanket coating the respiratory epithelium, causing it to become more viscid. The resulting dehydration of the mucous layer leads to defective mucociliary function and accumulation of viscid secretions that obstruct the airways and predispose to recurrent pulmonary infections. Similar transport abnormalities and pathophysiologic events take place in the pancreatic and biliary ducts and in the vas deferens in males.

Respiratory manifestations of CF are caused by an accumulation of viscid mucus in the bronchi, impaired mucociliary clearance, and lung infections. Chronic bronchiolitis and bronchitis are the initial lung manifestations, but after months and years, structural changes in the bronchial wall lead to bronchiectasis. In addition to airway obstruction, the basic genetic defect that occurs with CF predisposes to chronic infection with a surprising small number of organisms, the most common being *Pseudomonas aeruginosa,* followed by *Staphylococcus aureus, Haemophilus influenza,* and *Stenotrophomonas maltophilia.*[46] Soon after birth, initial infection with bacterial pathogens occurs and is associated with an excessive neutrophilic inflammatory response that seems to occur independent of infection. Recent studies suggest that because of the Cl^- channel defect, the epithelium consumes more oxygen than normal; thus, creating an anaerobic environment.[48] The normally aerobic *P. aeruginosa* responds to the change by assuming a mucoid phenotype that is resistant to phagocytosis by neutrophils. Even with intensive antibiotic regimens, the mucoid *P. aeruginosa* cannot be eradicated, probably because of poor penetration of antibiotics into anaerobic sputum plugs and development of antibiotic-resistant strains of the organism.

Pancreatic function is abnormal in approximately 80% to 90% of affected persons.[49] Steatorrhea, diarrhea, and abdominal pain and discomfort are common. In the newborn, meconium ileus may cause intestinal obstruction. The degree of pancreatic involvement is highly variable.

In some children, the defect is relatively mild, and in others, the involvement is severe and impairs intestinal absorption. In addition to exocrine pancreatic insufficiency, hyperglycemia may occur, especially after 10 years of age, when approximately 8% of persons with cystic fibrosis develop diabetes mellitus.[48]

Early diagnosis and treatment are important in delaying the onset and severity of chronic illness in children with CF. Diagnosis is based on the presence of respiratory and gastrointestinal manifestations typical of cystic fibrosis, a history of cystic fibrosis in a sibling, or a positive newborn screening test. Confirmatory laboratory tests include the sweat test, assessment of bioelectrical properties of respiratory epithelia by measurement of transepithelial potential differences in the nasal membrane, and genetic tests for CFTR gene mutations.[49] The *sweat test,* using pilocarpine iontophoresis to collect the sweat followed by chemical analysis of its chloride content, remains the standard approach to diagnosis. Newborns with cystic fibrosis have elevated blood levels of immunoreactive trypsinogen, presumably because of secretory obstruction in the pancreas. *Newborn screening* consists of a test for determination of immunoreactive trypsinogen. The test can be done on blood spots collected for routine newborn screening tests.

At present, there are no approved treatments for correcting the genetic defects in CF or to reverse the ion transport abnormalities associated with the dysfunctional CFTR. Thus, treatment measures are directed toward slowing the progression of secondary organ dysfunction and sequelae such as chronic lung infection and pancreatic insufficiency. They include the use of antibiotics to prevent and manage infections; the use of chest physical therapy (chest percussion and postural drainage) and mucolytic agents to prevent airway obstruction; and pancreatic enzyme replacement and nutritional therapy. Routine laboratory evaluations are key to assessing pulmonary function and response to therapeutic interventions. These studies include radiologic examinations, pulmonary function testing, and microbiologic cultures of respiratory secretions.

Appropriate antibiotic therapy directed against bacterial pathogens isolated from the respiratory tract is an essential component in the management of CF lung disease. Antibiotics are initially used to prevent colonization with *P. aeruginosa;* they are used as maintenance therapy once the airways are colonized with *P. aeruginosa* and other organisms such as *S. aureus;* and they are administered as aggressive treatment during acute exacerbations of pulmonary symptoms caused by infections.[45] To avoid adverse effects and to obtain high airway concentrations, the inhalation route is often used. Indications for oral antibiotics include the presence of respiratory tract symptoms and identification of pathogenic organisms in respiratory tract cultures. Intravenous antibiotics are used for progressive and unrelenting symptoms.

The abnormal viscosity of airway secretions is attributed largely to the presence of polymorphonuclear white blood cells and their degradation products. A purified recombinant human deoxyribonuclease (rhDNase), an enzyme that breaks down these products, has been developed.[44,45,49] Clinical trials have shown that the drug, which is administered by inhalation, can improve pulmonary symptoms and reduce the frequency of respiratory exacerbations. Although many persons benefit from the therapy, the drug is costly, and recommendations for its use are evolving.

Up to 90% of patients with CF have complete loss of exocrine pancreas function and inadequate digestion of fats and proteins. They require diet adjustment, pancreatic enzyme replacement, and supplemental vitamins and minerals. Many individuals with CF have higher than normal caloric need because of the increased work of breathing and perhaps because of the increased metabolic activity related to the basic defect. Pancreatic enzyme dosage and product type are individualized for each patient. Enteric-coated, pH-sensitive enzyme microspheres are available. A low-fat, high-protein, high-calorie diet was generally recommended in the past. With the advent of improved pancreatic enzyme products, however, normal amounts of fat in the diet are usually tolerated and preferred.[48]

Progress of the disease is variable. Improved medical management has led to longer survival. Today, nearly 40% of people with CF are 18 years of age or older.[46] Lung transplantation is being used as a treatment for persons with end-stage lung disease. Current hopes reside in research that would make gene therapy a feasible alternative for persons with the disease.

In summary, obstructive ventilatory disorders are characterized by airway obstruction and limitation in expiratory airflow. Bronchial asthma is a chronic inflammatory disorder of the airways, characterized by airway hyperreactivity and episodic attacks of airway narrowing. An asthmatic attack can be triggered by a variety of stimuli including allergens, respiratory tract infections, exercise, drugs and chemicals, airborne pollutants, and gastroesophageal reflux. Based on their mechanism of response, these triggers can be divided into two types: bronchospastic and inflammatory. Bronchospastic triggers depend on the level of airway responsiveness. There are two types of responses in persons with asthma: the acute- or early-phase response and the late-phase response. The acute-phase response results in immediate bronchoconstriction on exposure to an inhaled antigen and usually subsides within 90 minutes. The late-phase response usually develops 3 to 5 hours after exposure to an asthmatic trigger; it involves inflammation and increased airway responsiveness that prolong the attack and cause a vicious cycle of exacerbations.

COPD describes a group of conditions characterized by obstruction to airflow in the lungs. Among the conditions associated with COPD are emphysema, chronic bronchitis, and bronchiectasis. Emphysema is characterized by a loss of lung elasticity, abnormal, permanent enlargement of the air spaces distal to the terminal bronchioles, and hyperinflation of the lungs. Chronic bronchitis is caused by inflammation of major and small airways and is characterized by edema and hyperplasia of submucosal glands and excess mucus secretion into the bronchial tree. A history of a chronic productive cough that has persisted for at least 3 months and for at least 2 consecutive years in the absence of other disease is necessary for the diagnosis of chronic bronchitis. Emphysema and chronic bronchitis are manifested by eventual mismatching of ventilation and perfusion. As the condition advances, signs of respiratory distress and impaired gas exchange become evident, with development of hypercapnia and hypoxemia. Bronchiectasis is a less common form of COPD that is characterized by an abnormal dilatation of the large bronchi associated with infection and destruction of the bronchial walls.

Cystic fibrosis is an autosomal recessive genetic disorder manifested by chronic lung disease, pancreatic exocrine deficiency, and elevation of sodium chloride in the sweat. The disorder is caused by a mutation of a single gene on the long arm of chromosome 7 that codes for the cystic fibrosis transmembrane regulator (CFTR), which functions in the transepithelial transport of the chloride ion. The defect causes exocrine gland secretions to become exceedingly viscid, and it promotes colonization of the respiratory tract with *P. aeruginosa* and other organisms such as *S. aureus.* Accumulation of viscid mucus in the bronchi, impaired mucociliary function, and infection contribute to the development of chronic lung disease and a decrease in life expectancy.

Interstitial Lung Diseases

After completing this section of the chapter, you should be able to meet the following objectives:

- State the difference between chronic obstructive pulmonary diseases and interstitial lung diseases
- Cite the characteristics of occupational dusts that determine their pathogenicity in terms of the production of pneumoconiosis
- Characterize the organ involvement in sarcoidosis

The diffuse interstitial lung diseases are a diverse group of lung disorders that produce similar inflammatory and fibrotic changes in the interstitium or interalveolar septa of the lung. They include sarcoidosis, occupational lung diseases, hypersensitivity pneumonitis, and lung diseases caused by exposure to toxic drugs (*e.g.,* amiodarone) and radiation.[10,50] The disorders may be acute or insidious in onset; they may be rapidly progressive, slowly progressive, or static in their course. Because they result in a stiff and noncompliant lung, they are commonly classified as fibrotic or restrictive lung disorders.

The most common of the interstitial lung diseases are those caused by exposure to occupational and environmental inhalants, and sarcoidosis, the cause of which is unknown. Idiopathic pulmonary fibrosis refers to a lung disease of unknown origin characterized by diffuse interstitial fibrosis, which in advanced cases results in severe hypoxemia and cyanosis.[51] Examples of interstitial lung diseases and their causes are listed in Chart 31-1.

In contrast to the obstructive lung diseases, which primarily involve the airways of the lung, the interstitial lung disorders exert their effects on the collagen and elastic connective tissue found between the airways and the blood vessels of the lung. Many of these diseases also involve the airways, arteries, and veins. In general, these lung diseases share a pattern of lung dysfunction that includes diminished lung volumes, reduced diffusing capacity of the lung, and varying degrees of hypoxemia.

Current theory suggests that most interstitial lung diseases, regardless of the causes, have a common pathogenesis. It is thought that these disorders are initiated by some type of injury to the alveolar epithelium, followed by an

INTERSTITIAL OR RESTRICTIVE LUNG DISEASES

- Interstitial lung diseases result from inflammatory conditions that affect the interalveolar structures of the lung and produce lung fibrosis and a stiff lung.
- A stiff and noncompliant lung is difficult to inflate, increasing the work of breathing and causing decreased exercise tolerance due to hypoxemia.
- Because of the increased effort needed for lung expansion, persons with interstitial lung disease tend to take small but more frequent breaths.

CHART 31-1

*Causes of Interstitial Lung Diseases**

Occupational and Environmental Inhalants

Inorganic dusts
- Asbestosis
- Silicosis
- Coal miner's pneumoconiosis

Organic dusts
- Hypersensitivity pneumonitis

Gases and fumes
- Ammonia, phosgene, sulfur dioxide

Drugs and Therapeutic Agents

Cancer chemotherapeutic agents
- Busulfan
- Bleomycin
- Methotrexate

Ionizing radiation

Immunologic Lung Disease

Sarcoidosis

Collagen vascular diseases
- Systemic lupus erythematosus
- Rheumatoid arthritis
- Scleroderma
- Dermatomyositis-polymyositis

Miscellaneous

Postacute respiratory distress syndrome

Idiopathic pulmonary fibrosis

*This list is not intended to be inclusive.

inflammatory process that involves the alveoli and interstitium of the lung. An accumulation of inflammatory and immune cells causes continued damage to lung tissue and replacement of normal functioning lung tissue with fibrous scar tissue.

In general, the interstitial lung diseases are characterized by clinical changes consistent with restrictive rather than obstructive changes in the lung. Persons with interstitial lung diseases have dyspnea, tachypnea, and eventual cyanosis, without evidence of wheezing or signs of airway obstruction. Usually, there is an insidious onset of breathlessness that initially occurs during exercise and may progress to the point at which the person is totally incapacitated. Typically, a person with a restrictive lung disease breathes with a pattern of rapid, shallow respirations. This tachypneic pattern of breathing, in which the respiratory rate is increased and the tidal volume is decreased, reduces the work of breathing because it takes less work to move air through the airways at an increased rate than it does to stretch a stiff lung to accommodate a larger tidal volume. A nonproductive cough may develop, particularly with continued exposure to the inhaled irritant. Clubbing of the fingers and toes may develop.

Lung volumes, including vital capacity and TLC, are reduced in interstitial lung disease. In contrast to COPD, in which expiratory flow rates are reduced, the $FEV_{1.0}$ usually is preserved, even though the ratio between the $FEV_{1.0}$ and FVC may increase. Although resting arterial blood gases usually are normal early in the course of the disease, arterial oxygen levels may fall during exercise, and in cases of advanced disease, hypoxemia often is present, even at rest. In the late stages of the disease, hypercapnia and respiratory acidosis develop. The impaired diffusion of gases that occurs in persons with interstitial lung disease is thought to be caused by an increase in physiologic dead space resulting from unventilated regions of the lung.

The diagnosis of interstitial lung disease requires a careful personal and family history, with particular emphasis on exposure to environmental, occupational, and other injurious agents. Chest radiographs may be used as an initial diagnostic method, and serial chest films often are used to follow the progress of the disease. A biopsy specimen for histologic study and culture may be obtained by surgical incision or bronchoscopy using a fiberoptic bronchoscope. In bronchoalveolar lavage, fluid is instilled into the alveoli through a bronchoscope and then removed by suction to obtain inflammatory and immune cells for laboratory study. Gallium lung scans often are used to detect and quantify the chronic alveolitis that occurs in interstitial lung disease. Gallium does not localize in normal lung tissue, but uptake of the radionuclide is increased in interstitial lung disease and other diffuse lung diseases.

The treatment goals for persons with interstitial lung disease focus on identifying and removing the injurious agent, suppressing the inflammatory response, preventing progression of the disease, and providing supportive therapy for persons with advanced disease. In general, the treatment measures vary with the type of lung disease. Corticosteroid drugs frequently are used to suppress the inflammatory response. Many of the supportive treatment measures used in the late stages of the disease, such as oxygen therapy and measures to prevent infection, are similar to those discussed for persons with COPD.

OCCUPATIONAL LUNG DISEASE

The occupational lung diseases can be divided into two major groups: the pneumoconioses and the hypersensitivity diseases.[52] The *pneumoconioses* are caused by the inhalation of inorganic dusts and particulate matter. The *hypersensitivity diseases* result from the inhalation of organic dusts and related occupational antigens. A third type of occupational lung disease, byssinosis, a disease that affects cotton workers, has characteristics of the pneumoconioses and hypersensitivity lung disease.

Among the pneumoconioses are silicosis, found in hard-rock miners, foundry workers, sandblasters, pottery makers, and workers in the slate industry; coal miner's pneumoconiosis; asbestosis, found in asbestos miners, manufacturers of asbestos products, and installers and removers of asbestos insulation; talcosis, found in talc miners or millers and infants and small children who accidentally inhale powder containing talc; and berylliosis, found in ore extraction workers and alloy production workers. The danger of exposure to asbestos dust is not confined to the workplace. The dust pervades the general environment because it was used in the construction of buildings and in other applications before its health hazards were realized. It has been mixed into paints and plaster, wrapped around water and heating pipes, used to insulate hair dryers, and woven into theater curtains, hot pads, and ironing board covers.

Important etiologic determinants in the development of the pneumoconioses are the size of the dust particle, its chemical nature and ability to incite lung destruction, and the concentration of dust and the length of exposure to it. The most dangerous particles are those in the range of 1 to 5 μm.[53] These small particles are carried through the inspired air into the alveolar structures, whereas larger particles are trapped in the nose or mucous linings of the airways and removed by the mucociliary blanket. Exceptions are asbestos and talc particles, which range in size from 30 to 60 μm but find their way into the alveoli because of their density.

All particles in the alveoli must be cleared by the lung macrophages. Macrophages are thought to transport engulfed particles from the small bronchioles and the alveoli, which have neither cilia nor mucus-secreting cells, to the mucociliary escalator or to the lymphatic channels for removal from the lung. This clearing function is hampered when the function of the macrophage is impaired by factors such as cigarette smoking, consumption of alcohol, and hypersensitivity reactions. This helps to explain the increased incidence of lung disease among smokers exposed to asbestos. In silicosis, the ingestion of silica particles leads to the destruction of the lung macrophages and the release of substances resulting in inflammation and fibrosis.[43] Tuberculosis and other diseases caused by mycobacteria are common in persons with silicosis. Because the macrophages are responsible for protecting the lungs from tuberculosis, the destruction of macrophages accounts for an increased susceptibility to tuberculosis in persons with silicosis.

The concentration of some dusts in the environment strongly influences their effects on the lung. For example, acute silicosis is seen only in persons whose occupations entail intense exposure to silica dust over a short period. It is seen in sandblasters, who use a high-speed jet of sand to clean and polish bricks and the insides of corroded tanks; in tunnelers; and in rock drillers, particularly if they drill through sandstone. Acute silicosis is a rapidly progressive disease, usually leading to severe disability and death within 5 years of diagnosis. In contrast to acute silicosis, which is caused by exposure to extremely high concentrations of silica dust, the symptoms related to chronic, low-level exposure to silica dust often do not begin to develop until after many years of exposure, and then the symptoms often are insidious in onset and slow to progress.

The hypersensitivity occupational lung disorders (*e.g.*, hypersensitivity pneumonitis) are caused by intense and often prolonged exposure to inhaled organic dusts and related occupational antigens. Affected persons have a heightened sensitivity to the antigen. The most common forms of hypersensitivity pneumonitis are farmer's lung, which results from exposure to moldy hay; pigeon breeder's lung, provoked by exposure to the serum, excreta, or feathers of birds; bagassosis, from contaminated sugar cane; and humidifier or air conditioner lung, caused by mold in the water reservoirs of these appliances. Unlike bronchial asthma, this type of hypersensitivity reaction involves primarily the alveoli. These disorders cause progressive fibrotic lung disease, which can be prevented by the removal of the environmental agent.

SARCOIDOSIS

Sarcoidosis is a multisystem granulomatous disorder that primarily affects the lungs and lymphatic systems of the body.[54–58] The disease predominantly affects adults younger than 40 years of age, although it can occur in older persons. The incidence of sarcoidosis in the United States is approximately 5.9 of 100,000 persons per year for men and 6.3 of 100,000 persons per year for women.[54] It is more common among African Americans and whites living in the southeastern part of the country.

The cause of sarcoidosis remains obscure. It is thought that the disorder may result from exposure of genetically predisposed persons to specific environmental agents.[56,57] Support for a genetic influence comes from epidemiologic studies that have demonstrated the higher incidence in American blacks and Scandinavian populations. Additional evidence comes from familial clustering of the disease. Analysis of HLA genes located within the major histocompatibility complex also suggests that unique HLA genes can be linked to disease susceptibility and prognosis. Despite advances, including the identification of sarcoidosis genetic factors, a specific etiologic agent has yet to be identified. Multiple lines of evidence suggest that the inciting agent triggers an immune response that is dependent on host susceptibility and characterized by chronic inflammation, monocyte recruitment, and granuloma formation.

Sarcoidosis has variable manifestations and an unpredictable course of progression in which any organ system can be affected. The three systems that most commonly manifest symptoms are the lungs, the skin, and the eyes. More than 40% of persons with sarcoidosis report nonspecific symptoms such as fever, sweating, anorexia, weight loss, fatigue, and myalgia. Although only approximately 60% of persons with sarcoidosis have respiratory symptoms, almost all have abnormalities on chest radiography. In approximately 25% of cases, the disease is detected first on a routine chest radiogram. Overall, approximately 50% have permanent pulmonary abnormalities, and 5% to 15% have progressive pulmonary fibrosis.[55] Pulmonary involvement in sarcoidosis is primarily an interstitial lung disease. Approximately one third to one half of persons with chronic sarcoidosis have skin lesions, most of which are granulomatous. Ocular disease, usually in the form of chorioretinitis, affects approximately 20% of persons with the disease. Hepatic involvement, due to the presence of granulomas, is present in approximately 20% of persons at some time during the course of the disease. Cardiac sarcoidosis occurs in approximately 3% to 5% of persons. It often manifests as bundle branch block, tachyarrhythmias, or bradyarrhythmias.[58] Bone sarcoidosis affects approximately 3% to 4% of persons and is associated with soft tissue swelling and joint stiffness and pain.[55] Kidney and liver involvement also are infrequent accompaniments of the disorder.

The diagnosis of sarcoidosis is based on history and physical examination, tests to exclude other diseases, chest radiography, and biopsy to obtain confirmation of noncaseating granuloma.[54–58]

The treatment of sarcoidosis is directed at interrupting the granulomatous inflammatory process that is characteristic of the disease and managing the associated complications. When treatment is indicated, corticosteroid drugs are used. These agents produce clearing of the lung, as seen on the chest radiograph, and improve pulmonary function, but it is not known whether they affect the long-term outcome of the disease.

In summary, the interstitial lung diseases are characterized by fibrosis and decreased compliance of the lung. They include the occupational lung diseases, lung diseases caused by toxic drugs and radiation, and lung diseases of unknown origin, such as idiopathic pulmonary fibrosis and sarcoidosis. These disorders are thought to result from an inflammatory process that begins in the alveoli and extends to involve the interstitial tissues of the lung. Unlike COPD, which affects the airways, interstitial lung diseases affect the supporting collagen and elastic tissues that lie between the airways and blood vessels. These lung diseases decrease lung volumes, reduce the diffusing capacity of the lung, and cause various degrees of hypoxia. Because lung compliance is reduced, persons with this form of lung disease have a rapid, shallow breathing pattern.

Pulmonary Vascular Disorders

After completing this section of the chapter, you should be able to meet the following objectives:

- ✦ State the most common cause of pulmonary embolism and the clinical manifestations of the disorder
- ✦ Describe the physiology of pulmonary arterial hypertension and state three causes of secondary pulmonary hypertension
- ✦ Describe the alterations in cardiovascular function that are characteristic of cor pulmonale
- ✦ Describe the pathologic lung changes that occur in acute respiratory distress syndrome and relate them to the clinical manifestations of the disorder

As blood moves through the lung, blood oxygen levels are raised, and carbon dioxide is removed. These processes depend on the matching of ventilation (*i.e.,* gas exchange) and perfusion (*i.e.,* blood flow). This section discusses three major problems of the pulmonary circulation: pulmonary embolism, pulmonary hypertension, and acute respiratory distress syndrome. Pulmonary edema, another major problem of the pulmonary circulation, is discussed in Chapter 28.

PULMONARY EMBOLISM

Pulmonary embolism develops when a blood-borne substance lodges in a branch of the pulmonary artery and obstructs the flow. The embolism may consist of a thrombus (Fig. 31-15), air that has accidentally been injected during intravenous infusion, fat that has been mobilized from the bone marrow after a fracture or from a traumatized fat depot (see Chapter 58), or amniotic fluid that has entered the maternal circulation after rupture of the membranes at the time of delivery. In the United States, 50,000 to 100,000 deaths occur each year as the result of pulmonary emboli.[59,60] The overall mortality rate for pulmonary embolism continues to be high—15% to 17.5%.

DISORDERS OF THE PULMONARY VASCULAR SYSTEM

- ➤ The pulmonary circulation, which links the peripheral venous system with the peripheral arterial system, functions as a conduit for gas exchange. Pulmonary emboli are blood clots that originate in the peripheral venous system and become lodged in the pulmonary vessels as they move through the lungs.
- ➤ The pulmonary circulation is a low-pressure system located between the right and left heart. Pulmonary hypertension can be caused by an elevation in left atrial pressure, increased pulmonary blood flow, or increased pulmonary vascular resistance resulting from stimuli such as hypoxia.

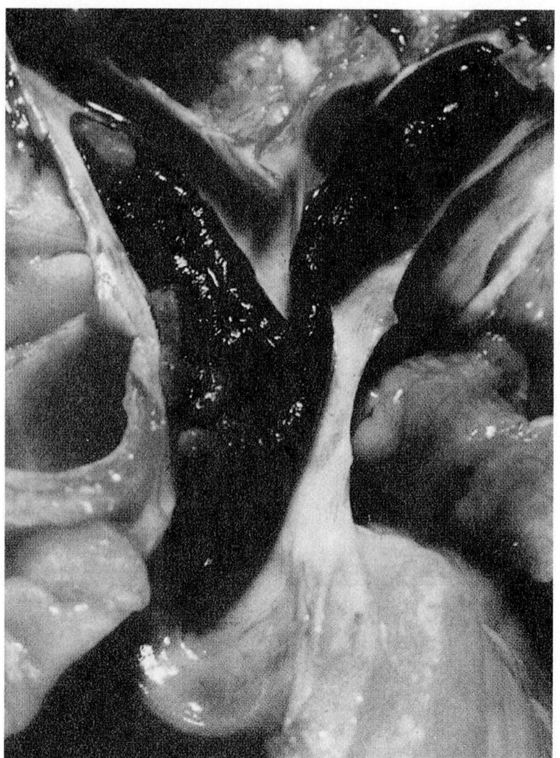

FIGURE 31-15 Pulmonary embolism. The main pulmonary and its bifurcation have opened to reveal a large saddle embolus. (Rubin E., Farber J.L. [1999]. *Pathology* [3rd ed., p. 289]. Philadelphia: Lippincott-Raven)

Almost all pulmonary emboli arise from deep vein thrombosis (DVT) in the lower extremities (see Chapter 24). The presence of thrombosis in the deep veins of the legs or pelvis often is unsuspected until embolism occurs. The effects of emboli on the pulmonary circulation are related to mechanical obstruction of the pulmonary circulation and neurohumoral reflexes causing vasoconstriction. Obstruction of pulmonary blood flow causes reflex bronchoconstriction in the affected area of the lung, wasted ventilation and impaired gas exchange, and loss of alveolar surfactant. Pulmonary hypertension and right heart failure may develop when there is massive vasoconstriction because of a large embolus. Although small areas of infarction may occur, frank pulmonary infarction is uncommon.

Persons at risk for developing DVT also are at risk for developing thromboemboli. Among the physiologic factors that contribute to venous thrombosis are venous stasis, venous endothelial injury, and hypercoagulability states.[59,60] Venous stasis and venous endothelial injury can result from prolonged bed rest, trauma, surgery, childbirth, fractures of the hip and femur, myocardial infarction and congestive heart failure, and spinal cord injury. Persons undergoing orthopedic surgery and gynecologic cancer surgery are at particular risk, as are bedridden patients in an intensive care unit. Cancer cells can produce thrombin and synthesize procoagulation factors, increasing the risk for thromboembolism. Use of oral contraceptives, pregnancy, and hormone replacement therapy are thought to increase the resistance to endogenous anticoagulants. The risk for pulmonary embolism among users of oral contraceptives is approximately three times the risk in nonusers.[59] Women who smoke are at particular risk.

Manifestations

The manifestations of pulmonary embolism depend on the size and location of the obstruction. Chest pain, dyspnea, and increased respiratory rate are the most frequent signs and symptoms of pulmonary embolism. Pulmonary infarction often causes pleuritic pain that changes with respiration; it is more severe on inspiration and less severe on expiration. Moderate hypoxemia without carbon dioxide retention occurs as a result of impaired gas exchange. Small emboli that become lodged in the peripheral branches of the pulmonary artery may exert little effect and go unrecognized. However, repeated small emboli gradually reduce the size of the pulmonary capillary bed, resulting in pulmonary hypertension. Moderate-sized emboli often present with breathlessness accompanied by pleuritic pain, apprehension, slight fever, and cough productive of blood-streaked sputum. Tachycardia often is detected, and the breathing pattern is rapid and shallow. Patients with massive emboli usually present with sudden collapse, crushing substernal chest pain, shock, and sometimes loss of consciousness. The pulse is rapid and weak, the blood pressure is low, the neck veins are distended, and the skin is cyanotic and diaphoretic. Massive pulmonary emboli often are fatal.

Diagnosis and Treatment

The diagnosis of pulmonary embolism is based on clinical signs and symptoms, blood gas determinations, venous thrombosis studies, D-dimer testing, lung scans, helical CT scans of the chest, and, in selected cases, pulmonary angiography.[61,62] Laboratory studies and radiologic films are useful in ruling out other conditions that might give rise to similar symptoms. Because emboli can cause an increase in pulmonary vascular resistance, the electrocardiogram (ECG) may be used to detect signs of right heart strain. There has been recent interest in combining several noninvasive methods (lower limb compression ultrasonography, D-dimer measurements, and clinical assessment measures) as a means of establishing a diagnosis of pulmonary embolism.

Because almost all pulmonary emboli originate from DVT, venous studies such as *lower limb compression ultrasonography, impedance plethysmography,* and *contrast venography* often are used as initial diagnostic procedures. Of these, lower limb compression ultrasonography has become an important noninvasive means for detecting DVT.

D-dimer testing involves the measurement of plasma D-dimer, a degradation product of coagulation factors that have been activated as the result of a thromboembolic event. The *ventilation-perfusion scan* uses radiolabeled albumin, which is injected intravenously, and a radiolabeled gas, which is inhaled. A scintillation (gamma) camera is used to scan the various lung segments for blood flow and distribution of the radiolabeled gas. Ventilation-perfusion scans are useful only when their results are either normal or indicate a high probability of pulmonary embolism. *Helical (spiral) CT angiography* requires administration of an intravenous radiocontrast media. It is sensitive for the detection of emboli in the proximal pulmonary arteries and provides another method of diagnosis. *Pulmonary angiography* involves the passage of a venous catheter through the right heart and into the pulmonary artery under fluoroscopy. Although it remains the most accurate method of diagnosis, it is an invasive procedure; therefore, its use is reserved for selected cases. An embolectomy sometimes is performed during this procedure.

The treatment goals for pulmonary emboli focus on preventing DVT and the development of thromboemboli, protecting the lungs from exposure to thromboemboli when they occur, and in the case of large and life-threatening pulmonary emboli, sustaining life and restoring pulmonary blood flow. Prevention focuses on identification of persons at risk, avoidance of venous stasis and hypercoagulability states, and early detection of venous thrombosis.

For patients at risk, graded compression elastic stockings and intermittent pneumatic compression (IPC) boots can be used to prevent venous stasis. Both of these devices are safe and practical ways to prevent venous thrombosis. IPC boots provide intermittent inflation of air-filled sleeves that prevent venous stasis. Some devices produce sequential gradient compression that moves blood upward in the leg.

Pharmacologic prophylaxis involves the use of anticoagulant drugs. Anticoagulant therapy may be used to decrease the likelihood of deep vein thrombosis, thromboembolism, and fatal pulmonary embolism after major surgical procedures. Low-molecular-weight heparin, which can be administered subcutaneously on an outpatient basis, often is used. Warfarin, an oral anticoagulation drug, may be used for persons with long-term risk for developing thromboemboli.

Surgical interruption of the vena cava often is indicated when pulmonary embolism poses a life-threatening risk. There are two surgical procedures for protecting the lung from thromboemboli: venous ligation to prevent the embolus from traveling to the lung, and vena caval plication. The plication, done with a suture or by insertion of a clip, filter, or sieve, permits blood to flow while trapping the embolus. Percutaneous transjugular placement of a filter has become the preferred mode of inferior vena caval interruption.

Thrombolytic therapy using streptokinase, urokinase, or recombinant tissue plasminogen activator may be indicated in persons with multiple or large emboli. Thrombolytic therapy is followed by administration of heparin and then warfarin. Restoration of blood flow in persons with life-threatening pulmonary emboli can be accomplished through the surgical removal of the embolus or emboli.

PULMONARY HYPERTENSION

The pulmonary circulation is a low-pressure system designed to accommodate varying amounts of blood delivered from the right heart and to facilitate gas exchange.

The main pulmonary artery and major branches are relatively thin-walled, compliant vessels. The distal pulmonary arterioles also are thin walled and have the capacity to dilate, collapse, or constrict depending on the presence of vasoactive substances released from the endothelial cells of the vessel, neurohumoral influences, flow velocity, oxygen tension, and alveolar ventilation.

The term *pulmonary hypertension* describes the elevation of pressure in the pulmonary arterial system. The normal mean pulmonary artery pressure is approximately 15 mm Hg (*e.g.,* 28 mm Hg systolic/8 mm Hg diastolic). Pulmonary artery hypertension can be caused by an elevation in left atrial pressure, increased pulmonary blood flow, or increased pulmonary vascular resistance. Because of the increased pressure in the pulmonary circulation, pulmonary hypertension increases the workload of the right heart. Although pulmonary hypertension can develop as a primary disorder, most cases develop secondary to some other condition.

Secondary Pulmonary Hypertension

Secondary pulmonary hypertension refers to an increase in pulmonary pressures associated with other disease conditions, usually cardiac or pulmonary. Secondary causes, or mechanisms, of pulmonary hypertension can be divided into three major categories: pulmonary venous pressure elevation, increased pulmonary blood flow and pulmonary vascular obstruction, and hypoxemia.[63] Often more than one factor, such as COPD, heart failure, and sleep apnea, contributes to the elevation in pulmonary pressures.

Elevation of pulmonary venous pressure is common in conditions such as mitral valve stenosis and left ventricular heart failure, in which an elevated left atrial pressure is transmitted to the pulmonary circulation. Continued increases in left atrial pressure can lead to medial hypertrophy and intimal thickening of the small pulmonary arteries, causing sustained hypertension.

Increased pulmonary blood flow results from increased flow through left-to-right shunts in congenital heart diseases such as atrial or ventricular septal defects and patent ductus arteriosus. If the high-flow state is allowed to continue, morphologic changes occur in the pulmonary vessels, leading to sustained pulmonary hypertension. The pulmonary vascular changes that occur with congenital heart disorders are discussed in Chapter 26. Pulmonary emboli are common causes of obstructed flow in the pulmonary circulation.[64] Once initiated, the pulmonary hypertension is self-perpetuating because of hypertrophy and proliferation of vascular smooth muscle.

Hypoxemia is also a common cause of pulmonary hypertension. Unlike the vessels in the systemic circulation, most of which dilate in response to hypoxemia and hypercapnia, the pulmonary vessels constrict. The stimulus for constriction seems to originate in the air spaces near the smaller branches of the pulmonary arteries. In situations in which certain regions of the lung are hypoventilated, the response is adaptive in that it diverts blood flow away from the poorly ventilated areas to more adequately ventilated portions of the lung. This effect, however, becomes less beneficial as more and more areas of the lung become poorly ventilated. Pulmonary hypertension is a common problem in persons with advanced chronic bronchitis and emphysema. It also may develop at high altitudes in persons with normal lungs. Persons who experience marked hypoxemia during sleep (*i.e.,* those with sleep apnea) often experience marked elevations in pulmonary arterial pressure.

The signs and symptoms of secondary pulmonary hypertension reflect not only the underlying cause but also the effect that the elevated pressures have on right heart function and oxygen transport. Dyspnea and fatigue are common. Peripheral edema, ascites, and signs of right heart failure (cor pulmonale, discussed later) develop as the condition progresses.

Diagnosis is based on radiographic findings, echocardiography, and Doppler ultrasonography. Precise measurement of pulmonary pressures can be obtained only through right heart cardiac catheterization. Treatment measures are directed toward the underlying disorder. Vasodilator therapy may be indicated for some persons.

Primary Pulmonary Hypertension

Primary pulmonary hypertension is a relatively rare and rapidly progressive form of pulmonary hypertension that often leads to right ventricular failure and death within a few years. Estimates of incidence range from 1 to 2 cases per million people in the general population.[65,66] The disease can occur at any age, and familial occurrences have been reported. Persons with the disorder usually have a steadily progressive downhill course, with death occurring in 3 to 4 years. Overall, the 5-year survival rate of untreated primary pulmonary hypertension is approximately 20%.[66]

Primary pulmonary hypertension is thought to be associated with a number of factors, including an autosomal dominant genetic predisposition along with an exogenous trigger. Triggers include low oxygen levels that occur at high altitudes, exposure to certain drugs, human immunodeficiency virus (HIV) infection, and autoimmune disorders. Studies of a rare familial form of the disease point to a mutation in the transforming growth factor-β (TGF-β) superfamily of receptors as being responsible for the thickening of the vessel wall.[67,68] Mutations in these receptors are thought to prevent TGF-β and related molecules from exerting an inhibitory effect on smooth muscle and endothelial cell proliferation. Studies also suggest that acquired defects in TGF-β receptor signaling may be important in nonfamilial forms of the disease.[67] Studies of TGF-β receptor abnormalities are under way, and insights into relevant mechanisms of function are likely to emerge during the next several years. A potent endogenous peptide, endothelin-1, is also thought to have a role in pulmonary hypertension.[67] Endothelin-1 acts on two receptors—endothelin-A and endothelin-B receptors. Activation of endothelin-B receptors causes vasodilation, and activation of endothelin-A receptors results in vasoconstriction and smooth muscle growth. Although plasma endothelin levels are increased in patients with primary pulmonary hypertension, it is not clear whether the peptide has a primary role in development of the disease or whether it is a secondary mediator that perpetuates the condition.

Primary pulmonary hypertension is characterized by endothelial damage, coagulation abnormalities, and marked intimal fibrosis leading to obliteration or obstruction of the pulmonary arteries and arterioles. Most of the manifestations of the disorder are attributable to increased work demands on the right heart and a decrease in cardiac output. Symptoms are the same as those for secondary hypertension. The most obvious are dyspnea and fatigue that is out of proportion to other signs of a person's well-being.

The diagnosis of primary pulmonary hypertension is based on an absence of disorders that cause secondary hypertension and mean pulmonary artery pressures greater than 25 mm Hg at rest or 30 mm Hg with exercise.

Treatment consists of measures to improve right heart function to reduce fatigue and peripheral edema. Supplemental oxygen may be used to increase exercise tolerance. The calcium channel blockers (nifedipine and diltiazem) may be effective early in the course of the disease but offer little in advanced stages. More advanced disease has been managed with epoprostenol, a prostacyclin that has potent pulmonary vasodilator effects.[65,66] Because of its short half-life (3 to 5 minutes), the drug must be administered by continuous infusion through an indwelling catheter with an automatic ambulatory pump. Properties of the drug other than its vasodilating effects include inhibition of platelet aggregation and beneficial vascular remodeling effects. This agent often improves symptoms, sometimes dramatically, in persons who have not responded to other vasodilators. Bosentan, an oral endothelin antagonist, has proved to be effective in treating moderate to severe primary pulmonary hypertension and may become the treatment of choice for all stages of the disease.[67] Lung transplantation may be an alternative for persons who do not respond to other forms of treatment.

Cor Pulmonale

The term *cor pulmonale* refers to right heart failure resulting from primary lung disease and long-standing primary or secondary pulmonary hypertension. It involves hypertrophy and the eventual failure of the right ventricle. The manifestations of cor pulmonale include the signs and symptoms of the primary lung disease and the signs of right-sided heart failure (see Chapter 28). Signs of right-sided heart failure include venous congestion, peripheral edema, shortness of breath, and a productive cough, which becomes worse during periods of heart failure. Plethora (*i.e.*, redness), cyanosis, and warm, moist skin may result from the compensatory polycythemia and desaturation of arterial blood that accompany chronic lung disease. Drowsiness and altered consciousness may occur as the result of carbon dioxide retention. Management of cor pulmonale focuses on the treatment of the lung disease and heart failure. Low-flow oxygen therapy may be used to reduce the pulmonary hypertension and polycythemia associated with severe hypoxemia caused by chronic lung disease.

ACUTE RESPIRATORY DISTRESS SYNDROME

Acute respiratory distress syndrome (ARDS), first described in 1967, is a devastating syndrome of acute lung injury. Initially called the *adult respiratory distress syndrome,* it is now called the *acute respiratory distress syndrome* because it also affects children. ARDS affects approximately 150,000 to 200,000 persons each year; at least 50% to 60% of these persons die, despite the most sophisticated intensive care.[69–73] The disorder is the final common pathway through which many serious localized and systemic disorders produce diffuse injury to the alveolar-capillary membrane.

ARDS may result from a number of conditions, including aspiration of gastric contents, major trauma (with or without fat emboli), sepsis secondary to pulmonary or nonpulmonary infections, acute pancreatitis, hematologic disorders, metabolic events, and reactions to drugs and toxins[69–73] (Chart 31-2).

Although a number of conditions may lead to ARDS, they all produce similar pathologic lung changes that include diffuse epithelial cell injury with increased permeability of the alveolar-capillary membrane (Fig. 31-16). The increased permeability permits fluid, plasma proteins, and blood cells to move out of the vascular compartment into the interstitium and alveoli of the lung. Alveolar cell damage leads to accumulation of edema fluid, surfactant inactivation, and formation of a hyaline membrane that is impervious to gas exchange. As the disease progresses, the work of breathing becomes greatly increased as the lung stiffens and becomes more difficult to inflate. There is increased intrapulmonary shunting of blood, impaired gas exchange, and profound hypoxia. Gas exchange is further compromised by alveolar collapse resulting from abnormalities in surfactant production. When injury to the

CHART 31-2

*Conditions in Which ARDS Can Develop**

Aspiration

Near drowning
Aspiration gastric contents

Drugs, Toxins, Therapeutic Agents

Heroin
Inhaled gases (*e.g.*, smoke, ammonia)
Breathing high concentrations of oxygen
Radiation

Infections

Gram-negative septicemia
Other bacterial infections
Viral infections

Trauma and Shock

Burns
Fat embolism
Chest trauma

*This list is not intended to be inclusive.

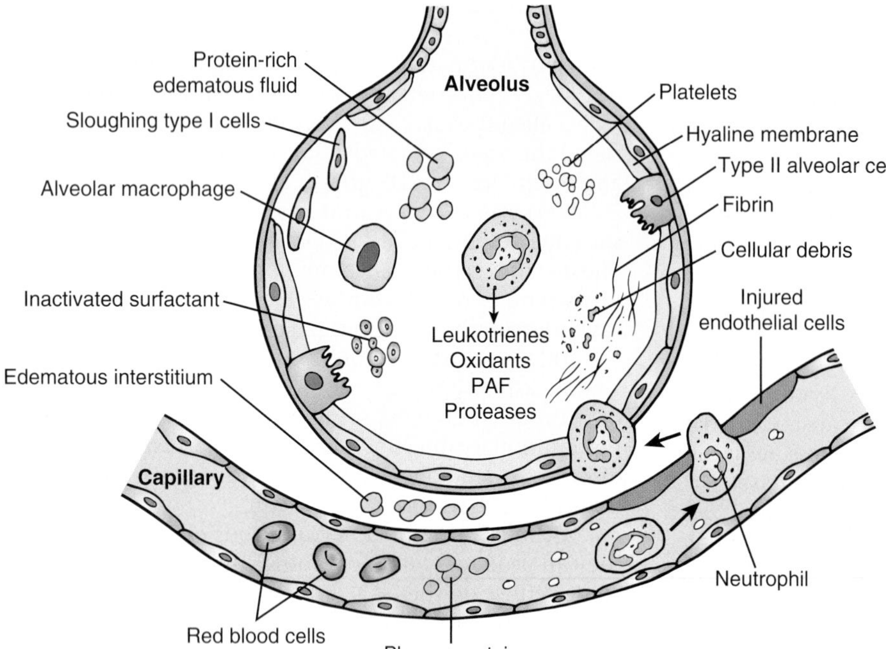

FIGURE 31-16 The mechanism of lung changes in ARDS. Injury and increased permeability of the alveolar capillary membrane allow fluid, protein, cellular debris, platelets, and blood cells to move out of the vascular compartment and enter the interstitium and alveoli. Activated neutrophils release a variety of products that damage the alveolar cells and lead to edema, surfactant inactivation, and formation of a hyaline membrane.

alveolar epithelium is severe, disorganized epithelial repair may lead to fibrosis.

The pathogenesis of ARDS is unclear. Neutrophils accumulate early in the course of the disorder and are thought to play a role in the pathogenesis of ARDS. Activated neutrophils synthesize and release a variety of products, including proteolytic enzymes, toxic oxygen species, and phospholipid products that increase the inflammatory response and cause injury to the capillary endothelium and alveolar epithelium.

Clinically, ARDS is marked by a rapid onset, usually within 12 to 18 hours of the initiating event, of respiratory distress, an increase in respiratory rate, and signs of respiratory failure. Chest radiography shows diffuse bilateral consolidation of the lung tissue. Marked hypoxemia occurs that is refractory to treatment with supplemental oxygen therapy. Many persons with ARDS demonstrate multiple organ failure, particularly involving the kidneys, gastrointestinal system, central nervous system, and cardiovascular system.

The treatment goals in ARDS are to supply oxygen to vital organs and provide supportive care until the condition causing the pathologic process has been reversed and the lungs have had a chance to heal. Assisted ventilation using high concentrations of oxygen may be required to overcome the hypoxia. Positive end-expiratory pressure breathing, which increases the pressure in the airways during expiration, may be used to assist in reinflating the collapsed areas of the lung and to improve the matching of ventilation and perfusion.

Most survivors of ARDS are left with some pulmonary symptoms (cough, dyspnea, sputum production) that may improve over time. Mild abnormalities of oxygenation, diffusing capacity, and lung mechanics persist in some individuals.

In summary, pulmonary vascular disorders include pulmonary embolism and pulmonary hypertension. Pulmonary embolism develops when a blood-borne substance lodges in a branch of the pulmonary artery and obstructs blood flow. The embolus can consist of a thrombus, air, fat, or amniotic fluid. The most common form is a thromboembolus arising from the deep venous channels of the lower extremities. Pulmonary hypertension is the elevation of pulmonary arterial pressure. It can be caused by an elevated left atrial pressure, increased pulmonary blood flow, or increased pulmonary vascular resistance secondary to lung disease. The term *cor pulmonale* describes right heart failure caused by primary pulmonary disease and long-standing pulmonary hypertension.

ARDS is a devastating syndrome of acute lung injury resulting from a number of serious localized and systemic disorders that damage the alveolar-capillary membrane of the lung. It results in interstitial edema of lung tissue, an increase in surface tension caused by inactivation of surfactant, collapse of the alveolar structures, a stiff and noncompliant lung that is difficult to inflate, and impaired diffusion of the respiratory gases with severe hypoxia that is resistant to oxygen therapy.

Respiratory Failure

After completing this section of the chapter, you should be able to meet the following objectives:

- Define the terms *hypoxia, hypoxemia,* and *hypercapnia*
- State a general definition for respiratory failure
- Characterize the mechanisms whereby respiratory disorders cause hypoxemia and hypercapnia

- ✦ Compare the manifestations of hypoxia and hypercapnia
- ✦ Describe the treatment of respiratory failure

The function of the respiratory system is to add oxygen to the blood and remove carbon dioxide. To accomplish this task, the respiratory system moves air into and out of the lung, provides for the transfer of the gases from the air to the blood, and moves blood through the lung so that gas exchange can take place. When respiratory function is impaired, the blood is not completely oxygenated, and carbon dioxide is not fully removed.

CAUSES

Respiratory failure is a condition in which the lungs fail to oxygenate the blood adequately and prevent carbon dioxide retention. It is not a specific disease, but rather is the result of a number of conditions that impair ventilation, compromise the matching of ventilation and perfusion, or disrupt blood flow in the lung. These conditions include impaired ventilation caused by impaired function of the respiratory center, airway obstruction, weakness and paralysis of the respiratory muscles, chest wall deformities, and disease of the airways and lungs. It may occur in previously healthy persons as the result of acute disease or trauma involving the respiratory system, or it may develop in the course of a chronic neuromuscular or respiratory disease. The causes of respiratory failure are summarized in Chart 31-3.

The common result of respiratory failure is hypoxemia and hypercapnia. The term *hypoxia* refers to a reduction in oxygen supply to the tissues; *hypoxemia,* to a low level of oxygen in the blood; and *hypercapnia* (sometimes referred to as *hypercarbia*), to excess carbon dioxide in the blood. Hypoxia and hypercapnia can manifest as acute and chronic conditions, and hypoxia may exist without hypercapnia, or the two conditions may coexist. The abbreviation PO_2 often is used to indicate the partial pressure of oxygen in arterial blood, and the abbreviation PCO_2, the partial pressure of carbon dioxide.

CHART 31-3

*Causes of Respiratory Failure**

Impaired Ventilation

Upper airway obstruction
- Infection (*e.g.,* epiglottitis)
- Foreign body
- Laryngospasm
- Tumors

Weakness or paralysis of respiratory muscles
- Brain injury
- Drug overdose
- Guillain-Barré syndrome
- Muscular dystrophy
- Spinal cord injury

Chest wall injury

Impaired Matching of Ventilation and Perfusion

Chronic obstructive pulmonary disease
Restrictive lung disease
Severe pneumonia
Atelectasis

Impaired Diffusion

Pulmonary edema
Acute respiratory distress syndrome

*This list is not intended to be inclusive.

DISORDERS OF BLOOD GASES IN RESPIRATORY FAILURE

- ➤ Respiratory failure represents failure of the lungs to adequately oxygenate the blood and prevent carbon dioxide retention.
- ➤ Hypoxemia results from decreased concentration of oxygen in the inspired air, airway diseases that impair ventilation, respiratory disorders that impair ventilation and/or perfusion, and cardiovascular disorders that impair movement of blood through the respiratory portions of the lung.
- ➤ Carbon dioxide retention is characteristic of conditions that produce hypoventilation. Conditions such as acute respiratory distress syndrome that impede the diffusion of gases in the lung impair the oxygenation of blood but do not interfere with the elimination of carbon dioxide.

Various types of respiratory failure are associated with different degrees of hypoxemia or hypercapnia. For example, pure hypoventilation, as occurs in conditions such as drug overdose, favors retention of CO_2. Severe ventilation-perfusion mismatching with alveolar ventilation that is inadequate to maintain arterial PO_2 levels results in hypoxemia that is more severe in relation to the hypercapnia than occurs with pure hypoventilation. This pattern of respiratory failure is seen most commonly in persons with advanced COPD. In this situation, the breathing of high concentrations of oxygen increases both the PO_2 and the PCO_2. Persons with interstitial lung disease may develop severe hypoxemia but not hypercapnia because of increased ventilation. In persons with ARDS, the degree of hypoxemia is usually severe, whereas the arterial PCO_2 is low because of the greater diffusing capacity of carbon dioxide. In this case, administration of oxygen can produce an increase in PO_2 without producing an increase in PCO_2.

Hypoventilation

Hypoventilation occurs when the volume of "fresh" air moving into and out of the lung is significantly reduced. Hypoventilation is commonly caused by conditions outside the lung such as depression of the respiratory center (*e.g.,* drug overdose), diseases of the nerves supplying the respiratory muscles (*e.g.,* Guillain-Barré syndrome), disorders of the respiratory muscles (*e.g.,* muscular dystrophy), or thoracic cage disorders (*e.g.,* severe scoliosis or crushed chest).

Hypoventilation has two important effects on arterial blood gases. First, it almost always causes an increase in PCO_2. The rise in PCO_2 is directly related to the level of ventilation. Reducing the ventilation by one half causes a doubling of the PCO_2. Thus, the PCO_2 level is a good diagnostic measure for hypoventilation.[74] Second, hypoxemia that is caused by hypoventilation can be readily abolished by increasing the oxygen content of the inspired air. In fact, pure hypoventilation does not cause large decreases in PO_2. The PO_2 falls by approximately 1 mm Hg for every 1 mm Hg rise in PCO_2. Hypoventilation sufficient to double the PCO_2 from 40 to 80 mm Hg decreases the PO_2 from 100 to 60 mm Hg.[74]

Ventilation-Perfusion Mismatching

The mismatching of ventilation and perfusion occurs when areas of the lung are ventilated but not perfused or when areas are perfused but not ventilated. Usually, the hypoxemia seen in situations of ventilation-perfusion mismatching is more severe in relation to hypercapnia than that seen in hypoventilation. Severe mismatching of ventilation and perfusion often is seen in persons with advanced COPD. These disorders contribute to the retention of carbon dioxide by reducing the effective alveolar ventilation, even when total ventilation is maintained. This occurs because a region of the lung is not perfused and gas exchange cannot take place or because an area of the lung is not being ventilated. Maintaining a high ventilation rate effectively prevents hypercapnia but also increases the work of breathing.

The hypoxemia associated with ventilation-perfusion disorders often is exaggerated by conditions such as hypoventilation and decreased cardiac output. For example, sedation can cause hypoventilation in persons with severe COPD, resulting in further impairment of ventilation. Likewise, a decrease in cardiac output because of myocardial infarction can exaggerate the ventilation-perfusion impairment in a person with mild pulmonary edema.

The beneficial effect of oxygen administration on PO_2 levels in ventilation-perfusion disorders depends on the degree of mismatching that is present. Because oxygen administration increases the diffusion gradient in ventilated portions of the lung, it usually is effective in raising arterial PO_2 levels. However, it may also decrease the respiratory drive and produce an increase in PCO_2.

Impaired Diffusion

Diffusion impairment describes a condition in which gas exchange between the alveoli and the red blood cells is impeded because of an increase in the distance for diffusion or a decrease in the permeability of the alveolar capillary membrane to movement of gases. It most commonly occurs in conditions such as interstitial lung disease, ARDS, pulmonary edema, and pneumonia.

Hypoxemia resulting from impaired diffusion can be partially or completely corrected by the administration of high concentrations of oxygen. In this case, the high concentration of oxygen serves to overcome the resistance to diffusion by establishing a large alveolar-to-capillary diffusion gradient. The elimination of carbon dioxide, which has a diffusion capacity about 20 times that of oxygen, is generally unaffected by diffusion abnormalities.

MANIFESTATIONS

Respiratory failure is manifested by varying degrees of hypoxemia and hypercapnia. There is no absolute definition of the levels of PO_2 and PCO_2 that indicate respiratory failure. As a general rule, *respiratory failure* refers to a PO_2 level of 50 mm Hg or less and a PCO_2 level greater than 50 mm Hg.[74] These values are not reliable when dealing with persons who have chronic lung disease because many of these persons are alert and functioning with blood gas levels outside this range.

Hypoxemia

Hypoxemia refers to a reduction in blood oxygen levels. Hypoxemia can result from an inadequate amount of oxygen in the air, disease of the respiratory system, or alterations in circulatory function. The mechanisms whereby respiratory disorders lead to a significant reduction in PO_2 are hypoventilation, impaired diffusion of gases, shunt, and mismatching of ventilation and perfusion[74] (see Chapter 29). Another cause of hypoxemia, reduction of the partial pressure of oxygen in the inspired air, occurs only under special circumstances, such as at high altitudes. Often, more than one mechanism contributes to hypoxemia in a person with respiratory or cardiac disease.

Manifestations. Hypoxemia produces its effects through tissue hypoxia and the compensatory mechanisms that the body uses to adapt to the lowered oxygen level. Body tissues vary considerably in their vulnerability to hypoxia; those with the greatest need are the nervous system and heart. Cessation of blood flow to the cerebral cortex results in loss of consciousness within 10 to 20 seconds. If the PO_2 of the tissues falls below a critical level, aerobic metabolism ceases, and anaerobic metabolism takes over, with formation and release of lactic acid.

The signs and symptoms of hypoxia can be grouped into two categories: those resulting from impaired function of vital centers and those resulting from activation of compensatory mechanisms. Mild hypoxemia produces few manifestations. There may be slight impairment of mental performance and visual acuity and sometimes hyperventilation. This is because hemoglobin saturation still is approximately 90% when the PO_2 is only 60 mm Hg (see Chapter 29, Fig. 29-22). More pronounced hypoxemia may produce personality changes, restlessness, agitated or combative behavior, uncoordinated muscle movements, euphoria, impaired judgment, delirium, and eventually, stupor and coma. Recruitment of sympathetic nervous system compensatory mechanisms produces an increase in heart rate, peripheral vasoconstriction, diaphoresis, and a mild increase in blood pressure. Profound acute hypoxemia can cause convulsions, retinal hemorrhages, and permanent brain damage. Hypotension and bradycardia often are preterminal events in persons with hypoxemia, indicating the failure of compensatory mechanisms.

The body compensates for hypoxemia by increased ventilation, pulmonary vasoconstriction, and increased production of red blood cells. Hyperventilation results from the hypoxic stimulation of the chemoreceptors. Increased production of red blood cells results from the release of erythropoietin from the kidneys in response to hypoxia (see Chapter 16). Polycythemia increases the red blood cell concentration and the oxygen-carrying capacity of the blood. Pulmonary vasoconstriction occurs as a local response to alveolar hypoxia; it increases pulmonary arterial pressure and improves the matching of ventilation and blood flow. Other adaptive mechanisms include a shift to the right in the oxygen dissociation curve as a means of increasing oxygen release to the tissues (see Chapter 29).

In conditions of chronic hypoxemia, the manifestations may be insidious in onset and attributed to other causes, particularly in chronic lung disease. Decreased sensory function, such as impaired vision or fewer complaints of pain, may be an early sign of worsening hypoxemia. This is probably because the involved sensory neurons have the same need for high levels of oxygen, as do other parts of the nervous system. Pulmonary hypertension is common because of associated alveolar hypoxia.

Cyanosis refers to the bluish discoloration of the skin and mucous membranes that results from an excessive concentration of reduced or deoxygenated hemoglobin in the small blood vessels. It usually is most marked in the lips, nail beds, ears, and cheeks. The degree of cyanosis is modified by the amount of cutaneous pigment, skin thickness, and the state of the cutaneous capillaries. Cyanosis is more difficult to distinguish in persons with dark skin and in areas of the body with increased skin thickness.

Although cyanosis may be evident in persons with respiratory failure, it often is a late sign. A concentration of approximately 5 g/dL of deoxygenated hemoglobin is required in the circulating blood for cyanosis.[75] The absolute quantity of reduced hemoglobin, rather than the relative quantity, is important in producing cyanosis. Persons with anemia and low hemoglobin levels are less likely to exhibit cyanosis (because they have less hemoglobin to deoxygenate), even though they may be relatively hypoxic because of their decreased ability to transport oxygen, than persons who have high hemoglobin concentrations. Someone with a high hemoglobin level because of polycythemia may be cyanotic without being hypoxic.

Cyanosis can be divided into two types: central or peripheral. *Central cyanosis* is evident in the tongue and lips. It is caused by an increased amount of deoxygenated hemoglobin or an abnormal hemoglobin derivative in the arterial blood. Abnormal hemoglobin derivatives include *methemoglobin,* in which the nitrite ion reacts with hemoglobin. Because methemoglobin has a low affinity for oxygen, large doses of nitrites can result in cyanosis and tissue hypoxia. Although nitrites are used in treating angina, the therapeutic dose is too small to cause cyanosis. Sodium nitrite is used as a curing agent for meat. In nursing infants, the intestinal flora is capable of converting significant amounts of inorganic nitrate (*e.g.,* from well water) into nitrite ion.[76]

Peripheral cyanosis occurs in the extremities and on the tip of the nose or ears. It is caused by slowing of blood flow to an area of the body, with increased extraction of oxygen from the blood. It results from vasoconstriction and diminished peripheral blood flow, as occurs with cold exposure, shock, congestive heart failure, and peripheral vascular disease. Acute arterial obstruction in an extremity, such as occurs with an embolus or arterial spasm (*i.e.,* Raynaud's phenomenon, discussed in Chapter 24), usually presents with pallor and coldness, although there may be cyanosis.

Diagnosis. Diagnosis of hypoxemia is based on clinical observation and diagnostic measures of oxygen levels. The analysis of arterial blood gases provides a direct measure of the oxygen content of the blood and is a good indicator of the lungs' ability to oxygenate the blood. Continuous mixed venous oxygen saturation ($S\bar{V}O_2$) can be monitored using a special type of pulmonary artery catheter.[77] This method, which measures the mixed venous blood that is being returned to the lungs, reflects the use of oxygen by the peripheral tissues. Arterial blood gases and $S\bar{V}O_2$ often are monitored in critically ill patients. Both measurements are invasive and require direct sampling of the patient's blood through a peripheral arterial catheter (for blood gases) or a pulmonary artery catheter (for $S\bar{V}O_2$).

Noninvasive measurements of arterial oxygen saturation of hemoglobin can be obtained using an instrument called the *pulse oximeter.* The pulse oximeter uses light-emitting diodes and combines plethysmography (*i.e.,* changes in light absorbance and vasodilatation) with spectrophotometry.[78,79] Spectrophotometry uses a red-wavelength light that passes through oxygenated hemoglobin and is absorbed by deoxygenated hemoglobin and an infrared-wavelength light that is absorbed by oxygenated hemoglobin and passes through deoxygenated hemoglobin. Sensors that can be placed on the ear, finger, toe, or forehead are available. These methods, although not as accurate as the invasive methods, provide a means for continuous monitoring of oxygen levels and are useful indicators of respiratory and circulatory status. The pulse oximeters cannot distinguish between oxygen-carrying hemoglobin and carbon monoxide–carrying hemoglobin. In addition, the pulse oximeter cannot detect elevated levels of methemoglobin.

Hypercapnia

Hypercapnia refers to an increase in the carbon dioxide content of the arterial blood.[80] The diagnosis of hypercapnia is based on physiologic manifestations, arterial pH, and arterial blood gas levels. The carbon dioxide level in the arterial blood, or PCO_2, is proportional to carbon dioxide production and inversely related to alveolar ventilation. The diffusing capacity of carbon dioxide is

20 times that of oxygen; therefore, hypercapnia is observed only in situations of hypoventilation sufficient to cause hypoxia.[75]

Hypercapnia can occur in a number of disorders that cause hypoventilation or mismatching of ventilation and perfusion. Hypoventilation is a cause of hypercapnia in respiratory failure due to depression of the respiratory center in drug overdose, neuromuscular diseases such as Guillain-Barré syndrome, or chest wall deformities such as seen with severe scoliosis. Hypercapnia due to ventilation-perfusion inequalities is seen most commonly in persons with COPD. Conditions that increase carbon dioxide production, such as an increase in metabolic rate or a high-carbohydrate diet, can contribute to the degree of hypercapnia that occurs in persons with impaired respiratory function.

Impaired Neural Control. The function of the respiratory center, which controls the activity of the muscles of respiration, is a crucial determinant of ventilation and elimination of carbon dioxide. It is composed of widely dispersed groups of neurons located in the medulla oblongata and pons (see Chapter 29). The activity of the respiratory center is regulated by chemoreceptors that monitor changes in the chemical composition of the blood. The most important chemoreceptors in terms of the minute-by-minute control of ventilation are the central chemoreceptors that respond to changes in the hydrogen ion (H^+) concentration of the cerebrospinal fluid. Although the blood–brain barrier is impermeable to H^+ ions, CO_2 crosses it with ease. The CO_2, in turn, reacts with water to form carbonic acid, which dissociates to form H^+ and bicarbonate (HCO_3^-) ions. When the CO_2 content of the blood rises, CO_2 crosses the blood–brain barrier, liberating H^+ ions that stimulate the central chemoreceptors. The excitation of the respiratory center due to CO_2 is greatest during the first 1 to 2 days that blood levels are elevated, but it gradually declines over the next 1 to 2 days.[80] Part of this decline results from renal compensatory mechanisms that readjust the blood pH by increasing blood bicarbonate levels.

In persons with respiratory problems that cause chronic hypoxia and hypercapnia, the peripheral chemoreceptors become the driving force for ventilation. These chemoreceptors, which are located in the bifurcation of the common carotid arteries and in the aortic arch, respond to changes in PO_2. Administration of high-flow oxygen to these persons can abolish the input from these peripheral receptors, causing a decrease in alveolar ventilation and a further rise in PCO_2 levels.

Respiratory Muscle Fatigue. Respiratory muscle fatigue can contribute to carbon dioxide retention in persons with various primary respiratory diseases and in those with neuromuscular disorders. In these persons, respiratory muscle fatigue develops when energy requirements exceed the energy supply. A number of factors increase energy requirements or decrease the energy supply. The energy demands of the respiratory muscles are increased by high levels of ventilation or by factors that increase the work of breathing, such as high levels of airway resistance. The energy supply depends on blood flow and the oxygen content of the blood. Low cardiac output, anemia, and decreased oxygen saturation contribute to a decreased energy supply and increase the likelihood of respiratory muscle fatigue. With malnutrition, the energy stores of the muscles are diminished, and there may be structural changes in the muscle as well. Electrolyte imbalances, especially hypokalemia and hypophosphatemia, contribute to respiratory muscle weakness.

Increased Carbon Dioxide Production. Disorders of carbon dioxide retention may be exaggerated by changes in metabolic rate or intake of carbon dioxide–generating foods. Changes in the metabolic rate resulting from an increase in activity level, fever, or disease can have profound effects on carbon dioxide production. Alveolar ventilation usually rises proportionally with these changes, and hypercapnia occurs only when this increase is inappropriate. Carbon dioxide production also increases with carbohydrate metabolism.

The respiratory quotient (RQ), which is the ratio of carbon dioxide production to oxygen consumption ($RQ = CO_2$ production/O_2 consumption), varies with the type of food metabolized. A characteristic of carbohydrate metabolism is an RQ of 1.0, with equal amounts of carbon dioxide being produced and oxygen being consumed. Because fats contain less oxygen than carbohydrates, their oxidation produces less carbon dioxide ($RQ = 0.7$). The metabolism of pure proteins ($RQ = 0.81$) results in the production of more carbon dioxide than the metabolism of fat but less than the metabolism of carbohydrates. The type of food that is eaten or the types of nutrients that are delivered through enteral feedings (*i.e.*, through a tube placed in the small intestine) or parenteral nutrition (*i.e.*, through a venous catheter placed in the central vena cava) may influence PCO_2 levels. Portable devices and metabolic carts that use indirect calorimetry to determine the RQ and energy requirements are available for use in the clinical setting.[75]

In persons who receive a high glucose load in association with total parenteral nutrition, the RQ can rise to a level of 1.0 or more.[81] Persons with adequate respiratory function can increase their alveolar ventilation proportional to the increase in carbon dioxide production. Hypercapnic respiratory failure can occur in persons who cannot adequately increase their ventilation. It has been suggested that such persons receive a larger proportion of nonprotein calories in the form of fat emulsions because these emulsions are associated with a lower rate of carbon dioxide production.[81]

Manifestations. Hypercapnia affects a number of body functions, including renal function, neural function, cardiovascular function, and acid-base balance. Elevated levels of PCO_2 produce a decrease in pH and respiratory acidosis (see Chapter 34). The body normally compensates for an increase in PCO_2 by increasing renal bicarbonate retention. As long as the pH is in an acceptable range, the main complications of hypercapnia are those resulting from the accompanying hypoxia. Because the body adapts to chronic increases in blood levels of carbon dioxide, persons with chronic hypercapnia may not have symptoms until the PCO_2 becomes markedly elevated.

Carbon dioxide has a direct vasodilating effect on many blood vessels and a sedative effect on the nervous system. Raised levels of PCO_2 greatly increase cerebral blood flow, causing headache, increased cerebral spinal fluid pressure, and sometimes papilledema. There is headache due to dilation of the cerebral vessels; the conjunctivae are hyperemic; and the skin is warm and flushed. Hypercapnia has nervous system effects similar to those of an anesthetic—hence the term *carbon dioxide narcosis*. There is progressive somnolence, disorientation, and, if the condition is untreated, coma. Mild to moderate increases in blood pressure are common. Air hunger and rapid breathing occur when alveolar PCO_2 levels rise to approximately 60 to 75 mm Hg; as PCO_2 levels reach 80 to 100 mm Hg, the person becomes lethargic and sometimes semicomatose. Anesthesia and death can result when PCO_2 levels reach 100 to 150 mm Hg.[75]

TREATMENT

The treatment of respiratory failure focuses on correcting the problem causing impaired gas exchange when possible and on relieving the hypoxemia and hypercapnia. A number of treatment modalities are available, including the establishment of an airway, use of bronchodilating drugs, and antibiotics for respiratory infections. Controlled oxygen therapy and mechanical ventilation are used in treating blood gas abnormalities associated with respiratory failure.

Decreasing the Work of Breathing and Improving Respiratory Muscle Function

Therapy for hypercapnia is directed at decreasing the work of breathing and improving the ventilation-perfusion balance. Intermittent rest therapy, such as nocturnal negative-pressure ventilation, applied to hypercapnic patients with chronic obstructive disease or chest wall disease may be effective in increasing the strength and endurance of the respiratory muscles and improving the PCO_2. Respiratory muscle retraining aimed at improving the respiratory muscles, their endurance, or both has been used to improve exercise tolerance and diminish the likelihood of respiratory fatigue.

Oxygen Therapy

Oxygen may be delivered by nasal cannula or mask. It also may be administered directly into an endotracheal or tracheostomy tube in persons who are being ventilated. A high-flow administration system is one in which the flow rate and reserve capacity are sufficient to provide all the inspired air.[77] A low-flow oxygen system delivers less than the total inspired air.[77] The oxygen must be humidified as it is being administered. The concentration of oxygen that is being administered (usually determined by the flow rate) is based on the PO_2. The rate must be carefully monitored in persons with chronic lung disease because increases in PO_2 above 60 mm Hg are likely to depress the ventilatory drive. There also is the danger of oxygen toxicity with high concentrations of oxygen. Continuous breathing of oxygen at high concentrations can lead to diffuse parenchymal lung injury. Persons with healthy lungs begin to experience respiratory symptoms such as cough, sore throat, substernal distress, nasal congestion, and painful inspiration after breathing pure oxygen for 24 hours.[74]

Mechanical Ventilation

When alveolar ventilation is inadequate to maintain PO_2 or PCO_2 levels because of respiratory or neurologic failure, mechanical ventilation may be lifesaving. Usually a nasotracheal, orotracheal, or tracheotomy tube is inserted into the trachea to provide the patient with the airway needed for mechanical ventilation. There has been recent interest in noninvasive forms of mechanical ventilation that use a face mask to deliver positive-pressure ventilation.[82,83]

There are two basic types of positive-pressure mechanical ventilators: pressure-cycled units and volume-cycled units.[84] The pressure-cycled unit delivers a tidal volume determined by the airway pressure while the flow rate is being controlled. The volume-cycled ventilator delivers a preselected tidal volume while the pressure is monitored. The tidal volume and respiratory rate are adjusted to maintain ventilation at a given minute volume. Ventilators are capable of functioning in assist-control mode, in which the ventilator delivers a breath triggered by the patient or independently if such an effort does not occur; an intermittent mandatory ventilation, in which the patient receives periodic positive-pressure ventilation from the ventilator at a preset volume and rate; and pressure-support ventilation, in which the ventilator delivers a set pressure rather than volume to augment each spontaneous respiratory effort. Ventilators also can be programmed to supply positive end-expiratory pressure or continuous positive airway pressure in spontaneously breathing patients.

A third type of ventilator uses negative pressure to expand the chest. These ventilators do not require an artificial airway. The early negative-pressure ventilator, known as the *iron lung*, consisted of a large tank that enclosed all of the body except the head.[75] It was used extensively to ventilate patients with bulbar poliomyelitis. A modification of the iron lung is the cuirass ventilator that fits over the thorax. Negative-pressure ventilators no longer are used in treatment of acute respiratory failure, but occasionally are used for persons with chronic neuromuscular disorders who need to be ventilated for months or years.

In summary, the lungs enable inhaled air to come in proximity to the blood flowing through the pulmonary capillaries, so that the exchange of gases between the internal environment of the body and the external environment can take place. Respiratory failure is a condition in which the lungs fail to oxygenate the blood adequately or prevent undue retention of carbon dioxide. The causes of respiratory failure are many. It may arise acutely in persons with previously healthy lungs, or it may be superimposed on chronic lung disease. Respiratory failure is defined as a PO_2 of 50 mm Hg or less and a PCO_2 of 50 mm Hg or more.

Hypoxia refers to an acute or chronic reduction in tissue oxygenation. It can occur as the result of hypoventilation, diffusion impairment, shunt, and ventilation-perfusion impairment. Acute hypoxia incites sympathetic nervous system responses such as tachycardia and produces symptoms that are similar to those of alcohol intoxication. In conditions of chronic hypoxia, the manifestations may be insidious in onset and attributed to other causes, particularly in chronic lung disease. The development of cyanosis requires a concentration of 5 g/dL of deoxygenated hemoglobin.

Hypercapnia refers to an increase in carbon dioxide levels. In the clinical setting, four factors contribute to hypercapnia: alterations in carbon dioxide production, disturbance in the gas exchange function of the lungs, abnormalities in respiratory function of the chest wall and respiratory muscles, and changes in neural control of respiration. The manifestations of hypercapnia consist of those associated with the vasodilation of blood vessels, including those in the brain, and depression of the central nervous system (*e.g.*, carbon dioxide narcosis).

REVIEW EXERCISES

A 30-year-old man is brought into the emergency room with a knife wound to the chest. On visual inspection, asymmetry of chest movement during inspiration, displacement of the trachea, and absence of breath sounds on the side of the wound are noted. His neck veins are distended, and his pulse is rapid and thready. A rapid diagnosis of tension pneumothorax is made.

A. Explain the observed respiratory and cardiovascular function in terms of the impaired lung expansion and air that has entered the chest as a result of the injury.

B. What type of emergent treatment is necessary to save this man's life?

A 10-year-old boy, who is having an acute asthmatic attack, is brought into the emergency room by his parents. The boy is observed to be sitting up and struggling to breathe. His breathing is accompanied by use of the accessory muscles, a weak cough, and audible wheezing sounds. His pulse is rapid and weak and both heart and breath sounds are distant on auscultation. His parents relate that his asthma began to worsen after he developed a "cold" and now he doesn't even get relief from his "albuterol" inhaler.

A. Explain the changes in physiologic function underlying this boy's signs and symptoms.

B. What is the most probable reason for the progression of this boy's asthma in terms of the early and late phase response?

C. The boy is treated with a systemic corticosteroid and inhaled anticholinergic and β_2-adrenergic agonist and then transferred to the intensive care unit. Explain the action of each of these medications in terms of relieving this boy's symptoms.

References

1. Chestnut M.S., Prendergast T.J. (2003). Lung. In Tierney L.M., McPhee S.J., Papadakis M.A. (Eds.), *Current medical diagnosis and treatment* (42nd ed., pp. 299–302, 339–344, COPD). New York: Lange Medical Books/McGraw-Hill.
2. Romero S. (2000). Nontraumatic chylothorax. *Current Opinion in Pulmonary Medicine 6,* 287–291.
3. Guenther C.A., Welch M.H. (1982). *Pulmonary medicine* (2nd ed., 524–526). Philadelphia: J.B. Lippincott.
4. Sahn S.A., Heffner J.E. (2000). Spontaneous pneumothorax. *New England Journal of Medicine 342,* 868–874.
5. Light R.W. (2001). Disorders of the pleura, mediastinum, and diaphragm. In Braunwald E., Fauci A.S., Kasper D., et al. (Eds.), *Harrison's principles of internal medicine* (15th ed., pp. 1513–1515). New York: McGraw-Hill.
6. National Asthma Education and Prevention Program. (1997). *Expert Panel report 2: Guidelines for the diagnosis and management of asthma.* Bethesda, MD: National Institutes of Health, National Heart, Lung, and Blood Institute. NIH Publication 98-4051.
7. National Asthma Education and Prevention Program. (2003). *Expert Panel report: Guidelines for the diagnosis and management of asthma: Update of selected topics—2002.* Bethesda, MD: National Institutes of Health, National Heart, Lung, and Blood Institute. NIH Publication 02-5074.
8. American Lung Association. (2003). *Trends in asthma morbidity and mortality.* [On-line]. Available: http://lungusa.org/data.
9. Elias J.A., Lee C.G., Zheng T., et al. (2003). New insights into the pathogenesis of asthma. *Journal of Clinical Investigation 111,* 291–297.
10. Maitra A., Kumar V. (2003). The lung and upper respiratory tract. In Kumar R.S., Cotran R.S., Robbins S.L. *Robbins basic pathology* (7th ed., pp. 453–478). Philadelphia: W.B. Saunders.
11. Fireman P. (2003). Understanding asthma pathophysiology. *Allergy and Asthma Proceedings 24*(2), 79–83.
12. Busse W.W., Lemanske R.F. (2001). Asthma. *New England Journal of Medicine 344*(5), 350–362.
13. Jarjour N.N., Kelly E.A.B. (2002). Pathogenesis of asthma. *Medical Clinics of North America 86,* 925–936.
14. McFadden E.R., Gilbert I.A. (1994). Exercise-induced asthma. *New England Journal of Medicine 330,* 1362–1366.
15. Roberts J.A. (1988). Exercise-induced asthma in athletes. *Sports Medicine 6,* 193–195.
16. Young S., LeSouef P.N., Geelhoed G.C., et al. (1991). The influence of a family history of asthma and parental smoking on airway responsiveness in early infancy. *New England Journal of Medicine 324,* 1168–1173.
17. Chan-Yeung M., Malo J. (1995). Occupational asthma. *New England Journal of Medicine 333,* 107–112.
18. Babu K.S., Salvi S.S. (2000). Aspirin and asthma. *Chest 118,* 1470–1476.

19. Szczeklik A., Nizankowska E. (2000). Clinical features and diagnosis of aspirin induced asthma. *Thorax 55*(Suppl. 2), S42–S44.
20. Tan K.S., McFarlane L.C., Lipworth B.J. (1997). Loss of normal cyclical B_2 adrenoreceptor regulation and increased premenstrual responsiveness to adenosine monophosphate in stable female asthmatic patients. *Thorax 52,* 608–611.
21. Dubuske D.M. (1994). Asthma: Diagnosis and management of nocturnal symptoms. *Comprehensive Therapy 20,* 628–639.
22. Drazen J.M., Israel E., O'Bryne P.M. (1999). Treatment of asthma with drugs modifying the leukotriene pathway. *New England Journal of Medicine 340,* 197–204.
23. Wenzel S. (Chair). (2000). Proceedings of the ATS workshop on refractory asthma. *American Journal of Respiratory Critical Care Medicine 162,* 2341–2351.
24. Wenzel S. (2003). Severe asthma. *Mount Sinai Journal of Medicine 70*(3), 185–190.
25. Papiris S., Kotanidou A., Malagari K., Roussos C. (2002). Clinical review: Severe asthma. *Critical Care 6,* 30–44.
26. Macklem P. (1996). Fatal asthma. *Annual Review of Medicine 47,* 161–168.
27. Barnes P.J. (1994). Blunted perception and death from asthma. *New England Journal of Medicine 330,* 1383–1384.
28. Magadle R., Berar-Yanay N., Weiner P. (2002). The risk of hospitalization and near-fatal and fatal asthma in relation to the perception of dyspnea. *Chest 121,* 329–333.
29. Lui A.H., Spahn J.D., Leung D.Y.M. (2004). Childhood asthma. In Behrman R.E., Kliegman R.M., Jenson H.B. *Nelson textbook of pediatrics* (16th ed., pp. 760–774). Philadelphia: W.B. Saunders.
30. Kemp J.P., Kemp J.A. (2001). Management of asthma in children. *American Family Physician 63*(7), 1341–1348.
31. Gern J.E., Lemanske R.F. (2003). Infectious triggers of pediatric asthma. *Pediatric Clinics of North America 50,* 555–575.
32. Gilliland F.D., Berhane K., McConnell R., et al. (2000). Maternal smoking during pregnancy, environmental tobacco smoke exposure and childhood lung function. *Thorax 55,* 271–276.
33. Stein R.T., Holberg C.J., Sherrill D., et al. (1999). Influence of parental smoking on respiratory symptoms during the first decade of life: The Tucson Children's Respiratory Study. *American Journal of Epidemiology 149,* 1030–1037.
34. Szefler S.J. (2003). Identifying the child in need of asthma therapy. *Pediatric Clinics of North American 50,* 577–591.
35. Barnes P.J. (2000). Chronic obstructive pulmonary disease. *New England Journal of Medicine 343,* 269–280.
36. Pawels R.A., Buist A.S., Calverley P.M.A., et al. (2003). Global strategy for the diagnosis, management, and prevention of chronic obstructive pulmonary disease: NHLBI/WHO Global initiative for chronic obstructive lung disease (GOLD) Workshop Update. [On-line]. Available: http://www.goldcopd.com.
37. Calverley P.M.A., Walker P. (2003). Chronic obstructive pulmonary disease. *Lancet 362,* 1053–1061.
38. American Lung Association. (2003). *Trends in chronic bronchitis and emphysema: Morbidity and mortality.* [On-line]. Available: http://lungusa.org/data.
39. Travis W.D., Farber J.L., Rubin E. (1999). The respiratory system. In Rubin E., Farber J.L. (Eds.), *Pathology* (3rd ed., pp. 600–601, 623–630). Philadelphia: Lippincott-Raven.
40. Berry J.K., Baum C.L. (2001). Malnutrition in chronic obstructive pulmonary disease. *AACN Clinical Issues 18*(2), 210–219.
41. Rogers R.M., Sciurba F.C., Keenan R.J. (1996). Lung reduction surgery in chronic obstructive lung disease. *Medical Clinics of North America 80,* 623–643.
42. Barker A.F. (2002). Bronchiectasis. *New England Journal of Medicine 346*(18), 1383–1393.
43. Mysliwiec V., Pina J.S. (1999). Bronchiectasis: The "other" obstructive lung disease. *Postgraduate Medicine 106,* 123–131.
44. Ratjen F. (2003). Cystic fibrosis. *Lancet 361,* 681–689.
45. Gibsen R.L., Burns J.L., Ramsey B.W. (2003). Pathophysiology and management of pulmonary infections in cystic fibrosis. *American Journal Respiratory Critical Care Medicine 168,* 918–951.
46. Cystic Fibrosis Foundation. (2003). *Facts about cystic fibrosis.* [On-line]. Available: http://www.cff.org/facts.htm.
47. Maitra A., Kumar V. (2003). Genetic and pediatric diseases. In Kumar V., Cotran R., Robbins S.L. (Eds.), *Robbins basic pathology* (7th ed., pp. 248–251). Philadelphia: W.B. Saunders.
48. Stern R.C. (1997). The diagnosis of cystic fibrosis. *New England Journal of Medicine 336,* 487–491.
49. Boat T.F. (2004). Cystic fibrosis. In Behrman R.E., Kliegman R.M., Jensen H.B. (Eds.), *Nelson textbook of pediatrics* (17th ed., pp. 1437–1450). Philadelphia: W.B. Saunders.
50. Gross F.H.Y. (2002). Overview of pulmonary fibrosis. *Chest 122*(6 Suppl), 334S–335S.
51. Gross T.J., Hunninghake G.W. (2001). Idiopathic pulmonary fibrosis. *New England Journal of Medicine 345*(7), 517–525.
52. Kushner W.G., Stark P. (2003). Occupational lung disease. *Postgraduate Medicine 113*(4), 81–88.
53. Kumar V., Cotran R.S., Robbins S.L. (2003). *Robbins basic pathology* (7th ed., pp. 268–274). Philadelphia: W.B. Saunders.
54. American Thoracic Society. (1999). Statement on sarcoidosis. *American Journal of Respiratory and Critical Care Medicine 160,* 736–755.
55. Newman L.S., Rose C.S., Maier L.A. (1997). Sarcoidosis. *New England Journal of Medicine 336,* 1224–1233.
56. Thomas K.W., Hunninghake G.W. (2003). Sarcoidosis. *JAMA 289*(24), 3300–3303.
57. Baughman R.P. (2003). Sarcoidosis. *Lancet 361,* 111–118.
58. Belfer M.H., Stevens R.W. (1998). Sarcoidosis: A primary care review. *American Family Physician 58*(9), 2041–2050.
59. Goldhaber S.Z. (1998). Pulmonary embolism. *New England Journal of Medicine 339,* 93–104.
60. Sadosty A.T., Boie E.T., Stead L.G. (2003). Pulmonary embolism. *Emergency Clinics of North America 21,* 363–384.
61. Kearon C. (2003). Diagnosis of pulmonary embolism. *Canadian Medical Association Journal 168*(2), 183–194.
62. Olin J.W. (2002). Pulmonary embolism. *Reviews in Cardiovascular Medicine 3*(Suppl 2), S68–S75.
63. Richardi M.J., Rubenfire M. (1999). How to manage secondary pulmonary hypertension. *Postgraduate Medicine 105*(2), 183–190.
64. Fedullo P.F., Auger W.R., Kerr K.M., Rubin L. (2001). Chronic thromboembolic pulmonary hypertension. *New England Journal of Medicine 345*(20), 1465–1472.
65. Rubin L.J. (1997). Primary pulmonary hypertension. *New England Journal of Medicine 336,* 111–117.
66. Newman J.H., Wheeler I., Barst R.J., et al. (2001). Mutations in the gene for bone morphogenic protein receptor II as a cause of primary pulmonary hypertension in large kindred. *New England Journal of Medicine 345,* 319–324.
67. Richardi M.J., Rubenfire M. (1999). How to manage primary pulmonary hypertension. *Postgraduate Medicine 105*(2), 45–56.
68. Newman J.H. (2002). Treatment of pulmonary hypertension: The next generation. *New England Journal of Medicine 346*(12), 933–935.
69. Kollef M.H., Schuster D.P. (1995). The acute respiratory distress syndrome. *New England Journal of Medicine 332,* 27–36.
70. Ware L.B., Matthay M.A. (2000). The acute respiratory distress syndrome. *New England Journal of Medicine 342,* 1334–1348.
71. Mortellitti M.P., Manning H.L. (2002). Acute respiratory distress syndrome. *American Family Physician 65*(9), 1823–1830.
72. Udobi K., Childs E., Touther K. (2003). Acute respiratory distress syndrome. *American Family Physician 67*(2), 315–322.

73. Fulkerson W.J., MacIntyre N., Stamler J., Crapo J.D. (1996). Pathogenesis and treatment of adult respiratory distress syndrome. *Archives of Internal Medicine 156,* 29–38.
74. West J.B. (1998). *Pulmonary pathophysiology: The essentials* (5th ed., pp. 18–40, 132–142, 151). Philadelphia: Lippincott-Raven.
75. Guyton A.C., Hall J.E. (2000). *Textbook of medical physiology* (10th ed., pp. 477–478, 491–492, 804). Philadelphia: W.B. Saunders.
76. Katzung B.G. (2001). *Basic and clinical pharmacology* (8th ed., p. 186). New York: Lange Medical Books/McGraw-Hill.
77. Hudak C.M., Gallo B.M., Morton P.G. (1998). *Critical care nursing* (7th ed., pp. 449–455, 476–489). Philadelphia: Lippincott Williams & Wilkins.
78. St. John R.E., Thomson P.D. (1999). Noninvasive respiratory monitoring. *Critical Care Nursing Clinics of North America 11,* 423–434.
79. Grap M.J. (2002). Pulse oximetry. *Critical Care Nurse 22*(3), 69–74.
80. Weinberger S.E., Schwartzstein R.M., Weiss J.W. (1989). Hypercapnia. *New England Journal of Medicine 321,* 1223–1230.
81. St. John R.E., Eisenberg P. (1991). Nutrition and use of metabolic assessment in the ventilator-dependent patient. *AACN Clinical Issues in Critical Care Nursing 2,* 453–462.
82. Hillberg R.E., Johnson D.C. (1997). Current concepts: Noninvasive ventilation. *New England Journal of Medicine 337,* 1746–1752.
83. American Thoracic Society. (2001). International consensus conference in intensive care medicine: Noninvasive positive pressure ventilation in acute respiratory failure. *American Journal of Respiratory and Critical Care Medicine 163,* 283–291.
84. Tobin M.J. (2001). Advances in mechanical ventilation. *New England Journal of Medicine 344*(26), 1986–1996..

UNIT VIII

Renal Function and Fluids and Electrolytes

Throughout the earlier part of the Middle Ages, one of the major concerns of the physician was examination of the urine. Many physicians of this time thought that most diseases could be diagnosed by careful examination of the urine. Numerous illustrations taken from this period show early physicians holding up flasks of urine to study its color, cloudiness, and other properties. It was thought that if the cloudiness was at the top of the urine, the problem was in the head, and if it was at the bottom, the problem was in the legs.

From the 16th century on, anatomists began to acquire a fairly good understanding of the gross structure of the kidney, ureters, and bladder. The first great discovery of the minute structures of the kidney was made by Marcello Malphigi (1628–1694), one of the earliest microscopists, who described the ball-shaped structure of the glomerulus. The work of Malphigi was followed by that of Sir William Bowman (1816–1892), who described the urine collecting capsule of the nephron, Bowman's capsule. Bowman also described the relationship between the glomerulus and the tubules. German pathologist Friedrich Henle (1809–1885) described the long U-shaped loop, called the loop of Henle, that contributes to the concentrating abilities of the kidney. Once this structure of the kidney was established, other scientists began to focus on the chemical composition of urine and on the function of the kidney in the regulation of blood pressure.

CHAPTER

32

Control of Renal Function

It is no exaggeration to say that the composition of the blood is determined not so much by what the mouth takes in as by what the kidneys keep.

—Homer Smith, *From Fish to Philosopher*

The kidneys are remarkable organs. Each is smaller than a person's fist, but in a single day, the two organs process approximately 1700 L of blood and combine its waste products into approximately 1.5 L of urine. As part of their function, the kidneys filter physiologically essential substances, such as sodium and potassium ions, from the blood and selectively reabsorb those substances that are needed to maintain the normal composition of internal body fluids. Substances that are not needed for this purpose or are in excess pass into the urine. In regulating the volume and composition of body fluids, the kidneys perform excretory and endocrine functions. The renin-angiotensin mechanism participates in the regulation of blood pressure and the maintenance of circulating blood volume, and erythropoietin stimulates red blood cell production. The discussion in this chapter focuses on the structure and function of the kidneys, tests of renal function, and the physiologic action of diuretics.

Kidney Structure and Function

After you have completed this section of the chapter, you should be able to meet the following objectives:

- Describe the location and gross structure of the kidney
- Explain why the kidney receives such a large percentage of the cardiac output and describe the mechanisms for regulating renal blood flow
- Explain the structure and function of the glomerulus and tubular components of the nephron
- Explain the function of sodium in terms of tubular transport mechanisms
- Describe how the kidney produces a concentrated or dilute urine
- Describe the elimination functions of the kidney
- Characterize the function of the juxtaglomerular complex
- Explain the endocrine functions of the kidney

GROSS STRUCTURE AND LOCATION

The kidneys are paired, bean-shaped organs that lie outside the peritoneal cavity in the back of the upper abdomen, one on each side of the vertebral column at the level of the

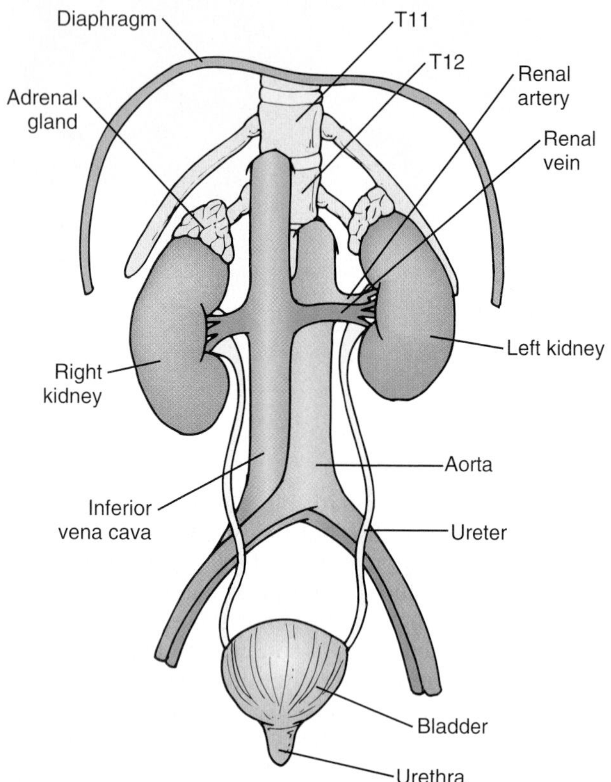

FIGURE 32-1 Kidneys, ureters, and bladder. (The right kidney is usually lower than the left.)

12th thoracic to 3rd lumbar vertebrae (Fig. 32-1). The right kidney normally is situated lower than the left, presumably because of the position of the liver. In the adult, each kidney is approximately 10 to 12 cm long, 5 to 6 cm wide, and 2.5 cm deep and weighs approximately 113 to 170 g. The medial border of the kidney is indented by a deep fissure called the *hilus*. It is here that blood vessels and nerves enter and leave the kidney. The ureters, which connect the kidneys to the bladder, also enter the kidney at the hilus.

The kidney is a multilobular structure, composed of up to 18 lobes. Each lobule is composed of nephrons, which are the functional units of the kidney. Each nephron has a glomerulus that filters the blood and a system of tubular structures that selectively reabsorb material from the filtrate back into the blood and secrete materials from the blood into the filtrate as urine is being formed.

On longitudinal section, a kidney can be divided into an outer cortex and an inner medulla (Fig. 32-2). The cortex, which is reddish brown, contains the glomeruli and convoluted tubules of the nephron and blood vessels. The medulla consists of light-colored, cone-shaped masses—the renal pyramids—that are divided by the columns of the cortex (*i.e.*, columns of Bertin) that extend into the medulla. Each pyramid, topped by a region of cortex, forms a lobe of the kidney. The apices of the pyramids form the papillae (*i.e.*, 8 to 18 per kidney, corresponding to the number of lobes), which are perforated by the openings of the collecting ducts. The renal pelvis is a wide, funnel-shaped structure at the upper end of the ureter. It is made up of the calyces or cuplike structures that drain the upper and lower halves of the kidney.

The kidney is ensheathed in a fibrous external capsule and surrounded by a mass of fatty connective tissue, especially at its ends and borders. The adipose tissue protects the kidney from mechanical blows, and it assists, together with the attached blood vessels and fascia, in holding the kidney in place. Although the kidneys are relatively well protected, they may be bruised by blows to the loin or by compression between the lower ribs and the ilium. Because the kidneys are outside the peritoneal cavity, injury and rupture do not produce the same threat of peritoneal involvement as the rupture of organs such as the liver or spleen.

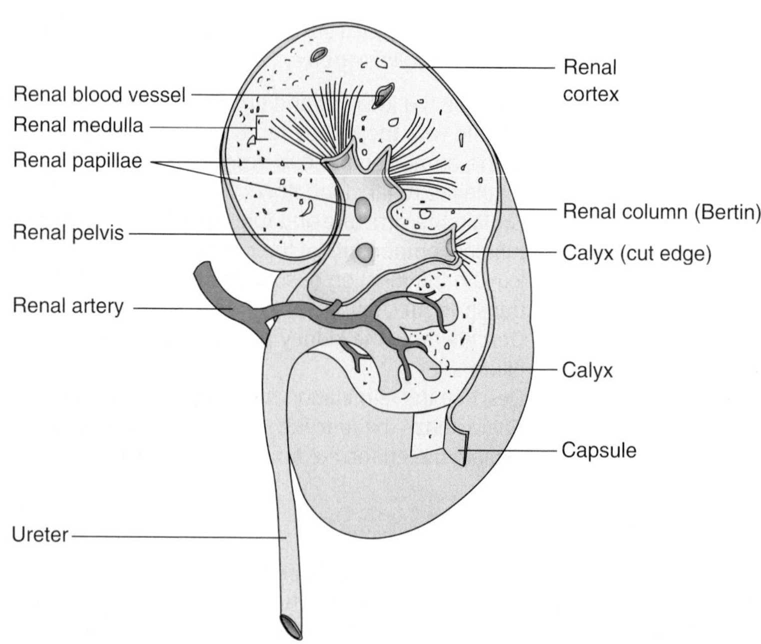

FIGURE 32-2 Internal structure of the kidney.

RENAL BLOOD SUPPLY

Each kidney is supplied by a single renal artery that arises on either side of the aorta. As the renal artery approaches the kidney, it divides into five segmental arteries that enter the hilus of the kidney. In the kidney, each segmental artery branches into several lobular arteries that supply the upper, middle, and lower parts of the kidney. The lobar arteries further subdivide to form the interlobular arteries at the level of the cortical medullary junction (Fig. 32-3). These arteries give off branches, called the arcuate arteries, that arch across the top of the pyramids. Small intralobular arteries radiate from the arcuate arteries to supply the cortex of the kidney. The afferent arterioles that supply the glomeruli arise from the intralobular arteries.

The nephron is supplied by two capillary systems: the glomerulus and the peritubular capillary network (Fig. 32-4). The glomerulus is a unique, high-pressure capillary filtration system located between two arterioles—the afferent and the efferent arterioles—that selectively dilate or constrict to regulate glomerular capillary pressure. The peritubular capillary network is a low-pressure reabsorptive system that originates from the efferent arteriole. These capillaries surround all portions of the tubules, an arrangement that permits rapid movement of solutes and water between the fluid in the tubular lumen and the blood in the capillaries. The medullary nephrons are supplied with two types of capillaries: the peritubular capillaries, which are similar to those in the cortex, and the vasa recta, which are long, straight capillaries. The vasa recta accompany the long loops of Henle in the medullary portion of the kidney to assist in exchange of substances flowing in and out of that portion of the kidney. The peritubular capillaries rejoin to form the venous channels by which blood leaves the kidneys and empties into the inferior vena cava.

Although nearly all the blood flow to the kidneys passes through the cortex, less than 10% is directed to the medulla, and only approximately 1% goes to the papillae.

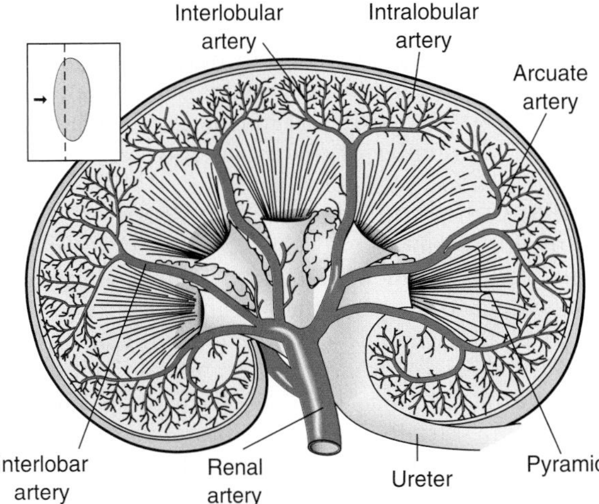

FIGURE 32-3 Simplified illustration of the arterial supply of the kidney. (Cormack D. H. [1987]. *Ham's histology* [9th ed.]. Philadelphia: J. B. Lippincott)

Under conditions of decreased perfusion or increased sympathetic nervous system stimulation, blood flow is redistributed away from the cortex toward the medulla. This redistribution of blood flow decreases glomerular filtration while maintaining the urine concentrating ability of the kidneys, a factor that is important during conditions such as shock.

THE NEPHRON

Each kidney is composed of more than 1 million tiny, closely packed functional units called *nephrons*. Each nephron consists of a glomerulus, where blood is filtered, and a tubular component. Here, water, electrolytes, and other substances needed to maintain the constancy of the internal environment are reabsorbed into the bloodstream while other unneeded materials are secreted into the tubular filtrate for elimination (see Fig. 32-4).

The Glomerulus

The glomerulus consists of a compact tuft of capillaries encased in a thin, double-walled capsule, called *Bowman's capsule*. Blood flows into the glomerular capillaries from the afferent arteriole and flows out of the glomerular capillaries into the efferent arteriole, which leads into the peritubular capillaries. Fluid and particles from the blood are filtered through the capillary membrane into a fluid-filled space in Bowman's capsule, called *Bowman's space*. The portion of the blood that is filtered into the capsule space is called the *filtrate*. The mass of capillaries and its surrounding epithelial capsule are collectively referred to as the *renal corpuscle* (Fig. 32-5A).

The glomerular capillary membrane is composed of three layers: the capillary endothelial layer, the basement membrane, and the single-celled capsular epithelial layer (see Fig. 32-5B). The endothelial layer lines the glomerulus and interfaces with blood as it moves through the capillary. This layer contains many small perforations, called *fenestrations*.

The epithelial layer that covers the glomerulus is continuous with the epithelium that lines Bowman's capsule. The cells of the epithelial layer have unusual octopus-like structures that possess a large number of extensions, or *foot processes* (*i.e., podocytes*), which are embedded in the basement membrane (see Fig. 32-5B). These foot processes form *slit pores* through which the glomerular filtrate passes. The basement membrane consists of a homogeneous acellular meshwork of collagen fibers, glycoproteins, and mucopolysaccharides (see Fig. 32-5C). Because the endothelial and epithelial layers of the glomerular capillary have porous structures, the basement membrane determines the permeability of the glomerular capillary membrane. The spaces between the fibers that make up the basement membrane represent the pores of a filter and determine the size-dependent permeability barrier of the glomerulus. The size of the pores in the basement membrane normally prevents red blood cells and plasma proteins from passing through the glomerular membrane into the filtrate. There is evidence that the epithelium plays a major role in producing the basement membrane components, and it is

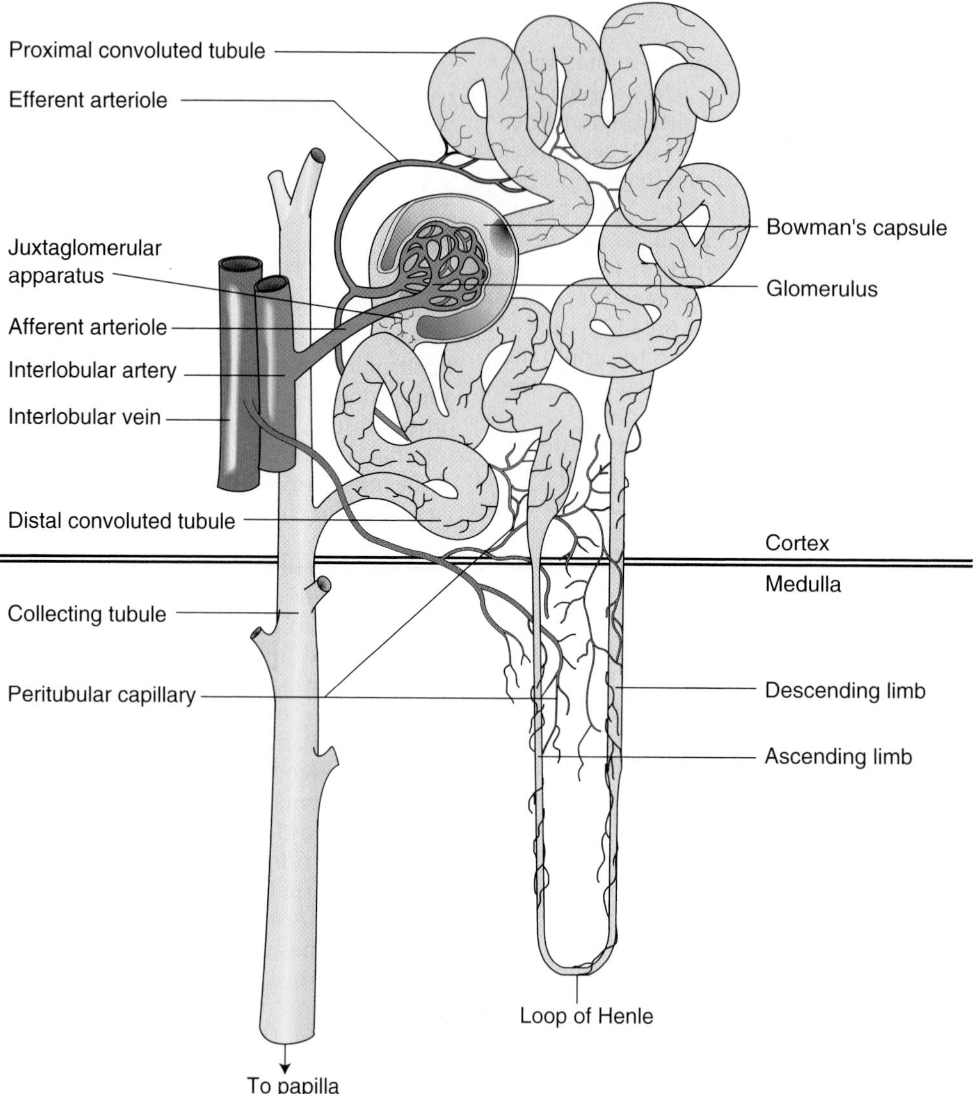

FIGURE 32-4 Nephron, showing the glomerular and tubular structures along with the blood supply.

probable that the epithelial cells are active in forming new basement membrane material throughout life. Alterations in the structure and function of the glomerular basement membrane are responsible for the leakage of proteins and blood cells into the filtrate that occurs in many forms of glomerular disease.

Another important component of the glomerulus is the *mesangium.* In some areas, the capillary endothelium and the basement membrane do not completely surround each capillary. Instead, the mesangial cells, which lie between the capillary tufts, provide support for the glomerulus in these areas (see Fig. 32-5B). The mesangial cells produce an intercellular substance similar to that of the basement membrane. This substance covers the endothelial cells where they are not covered by basement membrane. The mesangial cells possess (or can develop) phagocytic properties and remove macromolecular materials that enter the intercapillary spaces. Mesangial cells also exhibit contractile properties in response to neurohumoral substances and are thought to contribute to the regulation of blood flow through the glomerulus. In normal glomeruli, the mesangial area is narrow and contains only a small number of cells. Mesangial hyperplasia and increased mesangial matrix occur in a number of glomerular diseases.

Tubular Components of the Nephron

The nephron tubule is divided into four segments: a highly coiled segment called the *proximal convoluted tubule,* which drains Bowman's capsule; a thin, looped structure called the *loop of Henle;* a distal coiled portion called the *distal convoluted tubule;* and the final segment called the *collecting tubule,* which joins with several tubules to collect the filtrate. The filtrate passes through each of these segments before reaching the pelvis of the kidney.

Nephrons can be roughly grouped into two categories. Approximately 85% of the nephrons originate in the superficial part of the cortex and are called *cortical nephrons.* They have short, thick loops of Henle that penetrate only a short

THE NEPHRON

- The nephron, which is the functional unit of the kidney, is composed of a vascular component, which connects to the circulatory system, and a tubular component, which has connections to both the circulatory system and the elimination functions of the kidney.
- The vascular component of the nephron consists of two arterioles closely associated with two capillary beds: the glomerulus (where water-soluble nutrients, wastes, and other small particles are filtered into the blood) and the peritubular capillaries (which surround the tubular structures).
- The tubular portion of the nephron processes the glomerular filtrate (urine), facilitating the reabsorption of substances from the tubular fluid into the peritubular capillaries and the secretion of substances from the peritubular capillaries into the urine filtrate.

distance into the medulla. The remaining 15% are called *juxtamedullary nephrons*. They originate deeper in the cortex and have longer and thinner loops of Henle that penetrate the entire length of the medulla. The juxtamedullary nephrons are largely concerned with urine concentration.

The proximal tubule is a highly coiled structure that dips toward the renal pelvis to become the descending limb of the loop of Henle. The ascending loop of Henle returns to the region of the renal corpuscle, where it becomes the distal tubule. The distal convoluted tubule, which begins at the juxtaglomerular complex, is divided into two segments: the *diluting segment* and the *late distal tubule*. The late distal tubule fuses with the collecting tubule. Like the distal tubule, the collecting duct is divided into two segments: the *cortical collecting tubule* and the *inner medullary collecting tubule*.

Throughout its course, the tubule is composed of a single layer of epithelial cells resting on a basement membrane. The structure of the epithelial cells varies with tubular function. The cells of the proximal tubule have a fine villous structure that increases the surface area for reabsorption; they also are rich in mitochondria, which support active transport processes. The epithelial layer of the thin segment of the loop of Henle has few mitochondria, indicating minimal metabolic activity and passive reabsorptive function.

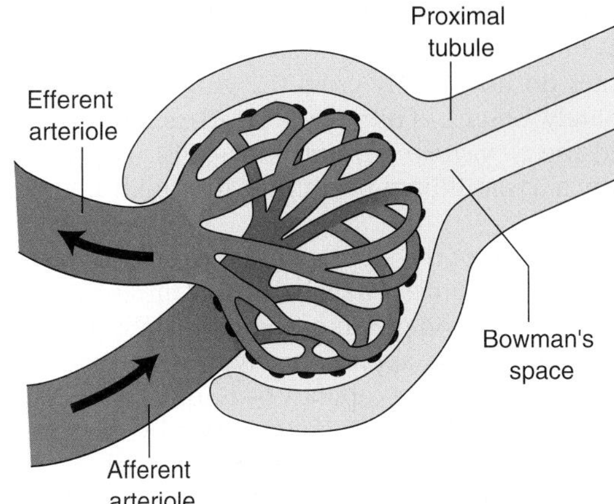

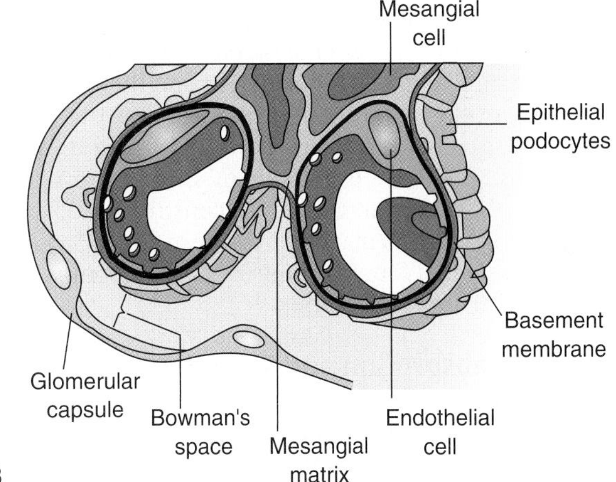

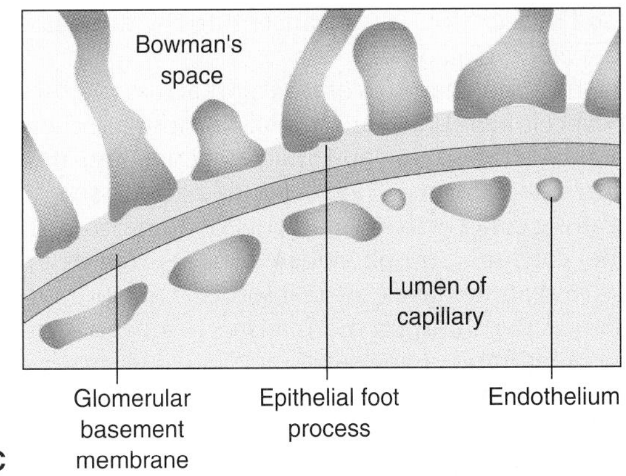

FIGURE 32-5 Renal corpuscle. (**A**) Structures of the glomerulus. (**B**) Position of the mesangial cells in relation to the capillary loops and Bowman's capsule. (**C**) Cross-section of the glomerular membrane, showing the position of the endothelium, basement membrane, and epithelial foot processes.

URINE FORMATION

Urine formation involves the filtration of blood by the glomerulus to form an *ultrafiltrate of urine* and the tubular reabsorption of electrolytes and nutrients needed to maintain the constancy of the internal environment while eliminating waste materials.

Glomerular Filtration

Urine formation begins with the filtration of essentially protein-free plasma through the glomerular capillaries into Bowman's space. The movement of fluid through the glomerular capillaries is determined by the same factors (*i.e.*, capillary filtration pressure, colloidal osmotic pressure, and capillary permeability) that affect fluid movement through other capillaries in the body (see Chapter 33). The glomerular filtrate has a chemical composition similar to plasma, but it contains almost no proteins because large molecules do not readily cross the glomerular wall. Approximately 125 mL of filtrate is formed each minute. This is called the *glomerular filtration rate* (GFR). This rate can vary from a few milliliters per minute to as high as 200 mL/minute.

The location of the glomerulus between two arterioles allows for maintenance of a high-pressure filtration system. The capillary filtration pressure (approximately 60 mm Hg) in the glomerulus is approximately two to three times higher than that of other capillary beds in the body. The filtration pressure and the GFR are regulated by the constriction and relaxation of the afferent and efferent arterioles. Constriction of the efferent arteriole increases resistance to outflow from the glomeruli and increases the glomerular pressure and the GFR. Constriction of the afferent arteriole causes a reduction in the renal blood flow, glomerular filtration pressure, and GFR. The afferent and the efferent arterioles are innervated by the sympathetic nervous system and are sensitive to vasoactive hormones, such as angiotensin II, as well. During periods of strong sympathetic stimulation, as occurs during shock, constriction of the afferent arteriole causes a marked decrease in renal blood flow and thus glomerular filtration pressure. Consequently, urine output can fall almost to zero.

Tubular Reabsorption and Secretion

From Bowman's capsule, the glomerular filtrate moves into the tubular segments of the nephron. In its movement through the lumen of the tubular segments, the glomerular filtrate is changed considerably by the tubular transport of water and solutes. Tubular transport can result in reabsorption of substances from the tubular fluid into the blood or secretion of substances into the tubular fluid from the blood (Fig. 32-6).

The basic mechanisms of transport across the tubular epithelial cell membrane are similar to those of other cell membranes in the body and include active and passive transport mechanisms. Water and urea are passively absorbed along concentration gradients. Sodium, potassium, chloride, calcium, and phosphate ions, as well as urate, glucose, and amino acids, are reabsorbed using primary or secondary active transport mechanisms to move across the tubular membrane. Some substances, such as hydrogen, potassium, and urate ions, are secreted into the tubular fluids. Under normal conditions, only approximately 1 mL of the 125 mL of glomerular filtrate that is formed each minute is excreted in the urine. The other 124 mL is reabsorbed in the tubules. This means that the average output of urine is approximately 60 mL/hour.

Renal tubular cells have two membrane surfaces through which substances must pass as they are reabsorbed from the tubular fluid. The side of the cell that is in contact with the tubular lumen and tubular filtrate is called the *luminal membrane*. The outside membrane that lies adjacent to the interstitial fluid is called the *basolateral membrane*. In most cases, substances move from the tubular filtrate into the tubular cell along a concentration gradient, but they require facilitated transport or carrier systems to move

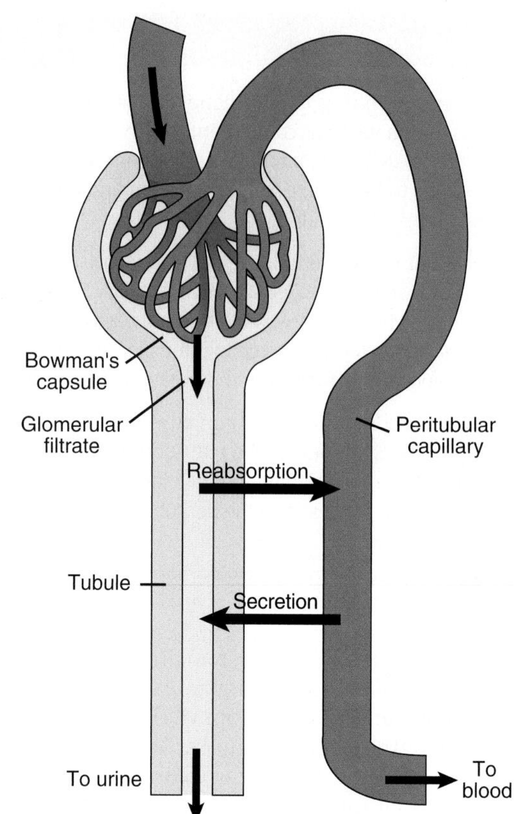

FIGURE 32-6 Reabsorption and secretion of substances between the renal tubules and peritubular capillaries.

across the basolateral membrane into the interstitial fluid, where they are absorbed into the peritubular capillaries.

The bulk of energy used by the kidney is for active sodium transport mechanisms that facilitate sodium reabsorption and cotransport of other electrolytes and substances such as glucose and amino acids. This is called *secondary active transport* or *cotransport* (Fig. 32-7). Secondary active transport depends on the energy-dependent sodium–potassium adenosine triphosphatase (ATPase) pump on the basolateral side of renal tubular cells. The pump maintains a low intracellular sodium concentration that facilitates the downhill (*i.e.,* from a higher to lower concentration) movement of sodium from the filtrate across the luminal membrane. Cotransport uses a carrier system in which the downhill movement of one substance such as sodium is coupled to the uphill movement (*i.e.,* from a lower to higher concentration) of another substance such as glucose or an amino acid. A few substances, such as hydrogen, are secreted into the tubule using countertransport, in which the movement of one substance, such as sodium, enables the movement of a second substance in the opposite direction.

Proximal Tubule. Approximately 65% of all reabsorptive and secretory processes that occur in the tubular system take place in the proximal tubule. There is almost complete reabsorption of nutritionally important substances, such as glucose, amino acids, lactate, and water-soluble vitamins. Electrolytes, such as sodium, potassium, chloride,

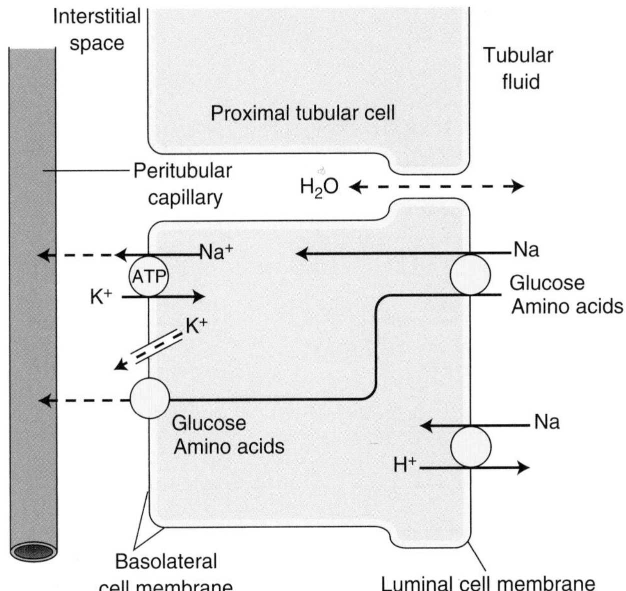

FIGURE 32-7 Mechanism for secondary active transport or cotransport of glucose and amino acids in the proximal tubule. The energy-dependent sodium-potassium pump on the basal lateral surface of the cell maintains a low intracellular gradient that facilitates the downhill movement of sodium and glucose or amino acids (cotransport) from the tubular lumen into the tubular cell and then into the peritubular capillary.

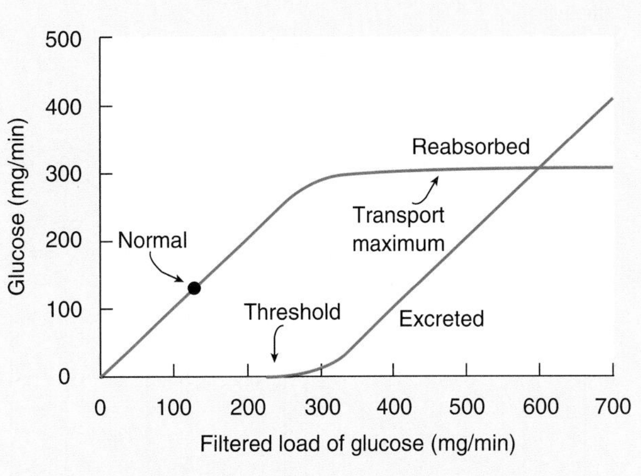

FIGURE 32-8 Relations among the filtered load (plasma concentration of glucose × GFR) of glucose, the rate of glucose reabsorption by the renal tubules, and the rate of glucose excretion in the urine. The *transport maximum* is the maximum rate at which glucose can be reabsorbed from the tubules. The *threshold* for glucose refers to the filtered load of glucose at which glucose first begins to appear in the urine. (Guyton A., Hall J. E. [1996]. *Textbook of medical physiology* [9th ed., p. 335]. Philadelphia: W. B. Saunders)

and bicarbonate, are 65% to 80% reabsorbed. As these solutes move into the tubular cells, their concentration in the tubular lumen decreases, providing a concentration gradient for the osmotic reabsorption of water and urea. The proximal tubule is highly permeable to water, and the osmotic movement of water occurs so rapidly that the concentration difference of solutes on either side of the membrane seldom is more than a few milliosmoles.

Many substances, such as glucose, are freely filtered in the glomerulus and reabsorbed by energy-dependent cotransport carrier mechanisms. The maximum amount of substance that these transport systems can reabsorb per unit of time is called the *transport maximum.* The transport maximum is related to the number of carrier proteins that are available for transport and usually is sufficient to ensure that all of a filtered substance such as glucose can be reabsorbed rather than being eliminated in the urine. The plasma level at which the substance appears in the urine is called the *renal threshold* (Fig. 32-8). Under some circumstances, the amount of substance filtered in the glomerulus exceeds the transport maximum. For example, when the blood glucose level is elevated in uncontrolled diabetes mellitus, the amount that is filtered in the glomerulus often exceeds the transport maximum (approximately 320 mg/minute), and glucose spills into the urine.

The Loop of Henle. The loop of Henle is divided into three segments: the thin descending segment, the thin ascending segment, and the thick ascending segment. Each of these segments has special structural and functional properties.

Fluid that enters the loop of Henle is iso-osmotic to plasma, but it becomes hypo-osmotic as it moves through the loop. The thin descending limb is highly permeable to water and moderately permeable to urea, sodium, and other ions. The ascending limb, in contrast to the descending limb, is impermeable to water. As fluid moves down the descending limb, water is reabsorbed until the osmolality of the tubular fluid reaches an equilibrium with the interstitial fluid, which is more hypertonic. In the ascending limb, which is impermeable to water, solutes are reabsorbed, but water cannot follow; as a result, the tubular fluid becomes more and more dilute, often reaching an osmolality of 100 mOsm/kg of H_2O as it enters the distal convoluted tubule, compared with the 285 mOsm/kg of H_2O in plasma (Fig. 32-9).

The thick segment of the loop of Henle begins in the ascending limb where the epithelial cells become thickened. As with the thin ascending limb, this segment is impermeable to water. The thick segment contains a $Na^+/K^+–2Cl^-$ cotransport system. This system involves the cotransport of a positively charged sodium and a positively charged potassium ion accompanied by two negatively charged chloride ions (Fig. 32-10). The gradient for the operation of this cotransport system is provided by the basolateral sodium–potassium pump, which maintains a low intracellular sodium concentration. The repetitive reabsorption of sodium chloride from the thick ascending limb of Henle and the continued inflow of new sodium chloride from the proximal tubule into the loop of Henle serve to trap solutes in the medullary interstitium, contributing to the high osmolality in this part of the nephron. Approximately 20% to 25% of the filtered load of sodium, potassium, and chloride is reabsorbed in the thick loop of Henle.

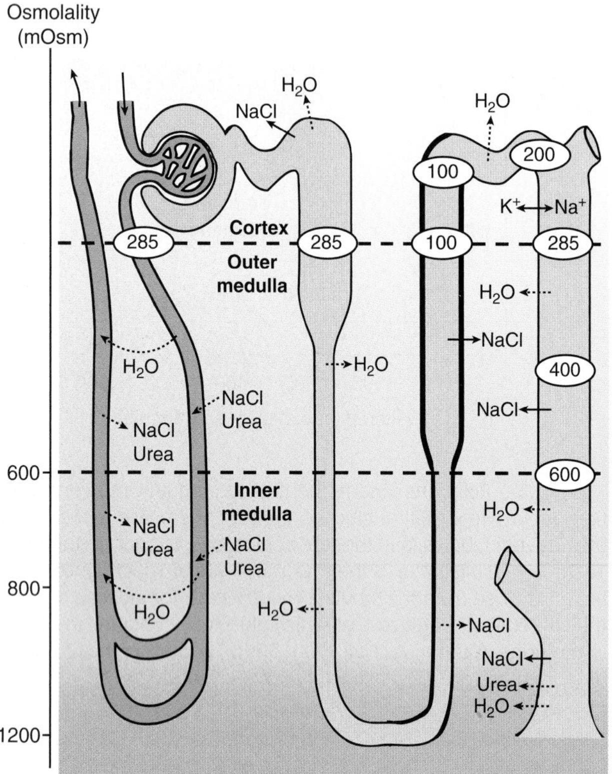

FIGURE 32-9 Summary of movements of ions, urea, and water in the kidney during production of a maximally concentrated urine (1200 mOsm/kg H_2O). *Numbers in ovals* give osmolality of the urine filtrate and medullary interstitium in mOsm/kg H_2O. *Solid arrows* indicate active transport; *dashed arrows* indicate passive transport. The heavy outlining along the ascending limb of Henle's loop indicates a decreased water permeability in that tubule segment. Note the osmotic gradient in the medulla from the outer to the inner medulla. (Adapted from Rhoades R. A., Tanner G. A. [1996]. *Medical physiology* [p. 441]. Boston: Little, Brown)

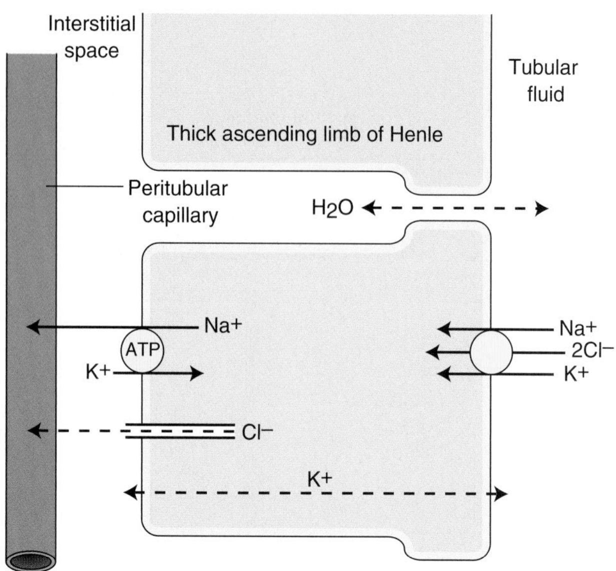

FIGURE 32-10 Sodium, chloride, and potassium reabsorption in the thick segment of the loop of Henle.

Movement of these ions out of the tubule leads to the development of a transmembrane potential that favors the passive reabsorption of small divalent cations such as calcium and magnesium.

Sodium reabsorption occurs in the proximal tubule, the thick ascending loop of Henle, and the distal tubule, where aldosterone regulates sodium and potassium exchange.

In approximately one fifth of the juxtamedullary nephrons, the loops of Henle and special hairpin-shaped capillaries called the *vasa recta* descend into the medullary portion of the kidney. A countercurrent mechanism controls water and solute movement so that water is kept out of the peritubular area and sodium and urea are retained (see Fig. 32-9). The term *countercurrent* refers to a flow of fluids in opposite directions in adjacent structures. There is an exchange of solutes between the adjacent descending and ascending loops of Henle and between the ascending and descending sections of the vasa recta. Because of these exchange processes, a high concentration of osmotically active particles (approximately 1200 mOsm/kg of H_2O) collects in the interstitium of the kidney medulla. The presence of these osmotically active particles in the interstitium surrounding the medullary collecting tubules facilitates the antidiuretic hormone (ADH)–mediated reabsorption of water (see following discussion).

Distal Convoluted Tubule. Like the thick ascending loop of Henle, the distal convoluted tubule is relatively impermeable to water, and reabsorption of sodium chloride from this segment further dilutes the tubular fluid (see Fig. 32-9). Sodium reabsorption occurs through a sodium and chloride cotransport mechanism. Approximately 10% of filtered sodium chloride is reabsorbed in this section of the tubule. Unlike the thick ascending loop of Henle, neither calcium nor magnesium is passively absorbed in this segment of the tubule. Instead, calcium ions are actively reabsorbed in a process that is largely regulated by parathyroid hormone and possibly by vitamin D.

The thick ascending loop of Henle, the distal tubule, and the cortical collecting tubule are often referred to as the *diluting segment* of the tubule. As solutes are reabsorbed from these segments, the urine becomes more and more dilute, often reaching an osmolar concentration that is equal to or less than that of plasma. This allows excretion of free water from the body.

Late Distal Tubule and Cortical Collecting Tubule. The late distal tubule and the cortical collecting tubule constitute the site where aldosterone exerts its action on sodium and potassium reabsorption. Although responsible for only 2% to 5% of sodium chloride reabsorption, this site is largely responsible for determining the final sodium concentration of the urine. The late distal tubule with the cortical collecting tubule also is the major site for regulation of potassium excretion by the kidney. When the body is confronted with a potassium excess, as occurs with a diet high in potassium content, the amount of potassium secreted at this site may exceed the amount filtered in the glomerulus.

The mechanism for sodium reabsorption and potassium secretion by this section of the kidney is distinct from other tubular segments. This tubular segment is composed of two types of cells: the *principal cells* and the *intercalated cells*. The principal cells reabsorb sodium and water from the tubular filtrate and secrete potassium into the tubular filtrate. The intercalated cells reabsorb potassium and secrete hydrogen ions into the tubular filtrate. The principal cells use separate channels for transport of sodium and potassium rather than cotransport mechanisms (Fig. 32-11). Aldosterone is thought to exert its effect on sodium and potassium excretion by increasing the number of ion channels and the function of the basolateral sodium–potassium pump.

Medullary Collecting Duct. The epithelium of the inner medullary collecting duct is well designed to resist extreme changes in the osmotic or pH characteristics of tubular fluid, and it is here that the urine becomes highly concentrated, highly diluted, highly alkaline, or highly acidic. During periods of water excess or dehydration, the kidneys play a major role in maintaining water balance.

ADH exerts its effect in the medullary collecting duct. ADH maintains extracellular volume by returning water to the vascular compartment and leads to the production of a concentrated urine by removing water from the tubular filtrate. Osmoreceptors in the hypothalamus sense the increase in osmolality of extracellular fluids and stimulate the release of ADH from the posterior pituitary gland (see Chapter 33). The permeability of the collecting ducts to water is determined mainly by the concentration of ADH. In exerting its effect, ADH, also known as *vasopressin,* binds to vasopressin receptors on the basolateral side of the tubular cells (Fig. 32-12). Binding of ADH to the vasopressin receptors causes water channels, known as *aquaporin-2*

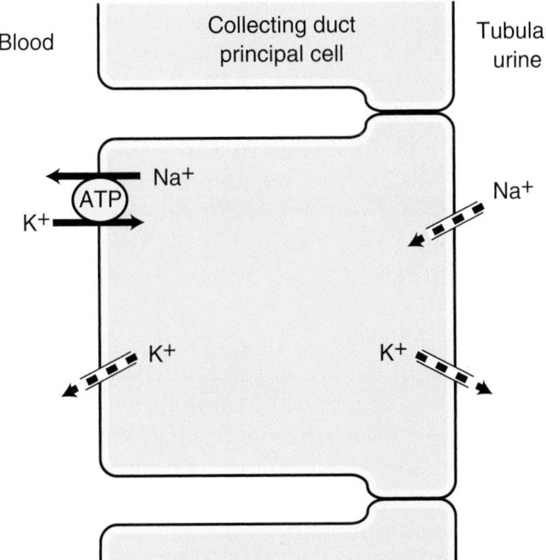

FIGURE 32-11 Model for ion transport of sodium and potassium by collecting duct principal cells. (Rhoades R. A., Tanner G. A. [1996]. *Medical physiology* [p. 438]. Boston: Little, Brown)

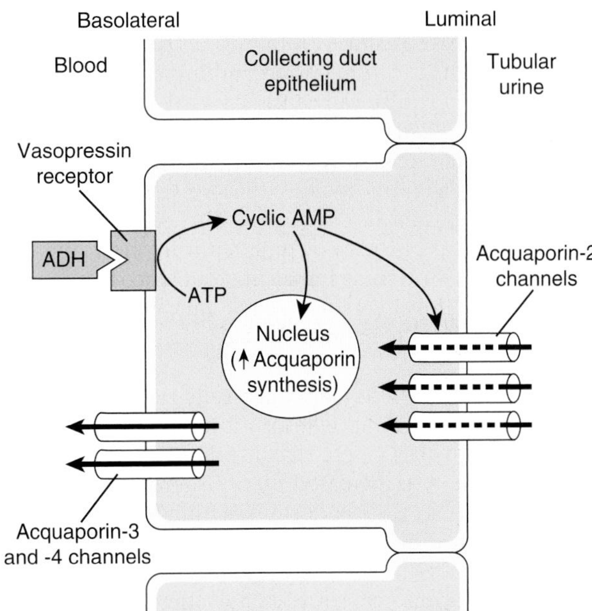

FIGURE 32-12 Model for the action of antidiuretic hormone (ADH) on the epithelium of the collecting duct. The ADH receptor is on the basolateral side, but the water permeability increase occurs on the luminal side. (Adapted from Rhoades R. A., Tanner G. A. [1996]. *Medical physiology* [p. 439]. Boston: Little, Brown)

channels, to move into the luminal side of the tubular cell membrane, producing a marked increase in water permeability. At the basolateral side of the membrane, water exits the tubular cell through aquaporin-3 and aquaporin-4 cells into the hyperosmotic interstitium of the medullary area, where it enters the peritubular capillaries for return to the vascular system. In the absence of ADH, the inserted aquaporin channels are removed, the tubular cells lose their water permeability, and dilute urine is formed.

Action of Diuretics

Diuretics are drugs that increase urine production. Most diuretics (loop, thiazide, and potassium sparing) act by decreasing the reabsorption of sodium (and water) by the kidney. Approximately 25% to 30% of sodium is reabsorbed in the thick ascending loop of Henle, approximately 10% in the distal convoluted tubule, and 2% to 5% in the late distal and cortical collecting tubule. The effectiveness of a diuretic is determined by its site of action.

Loop diuretics exert their effect in the thick ascending loop of Henle. Because of their site of action, these drugs are the most effective diuretic agents available. These drugs inhibit the coupled $Na^+/K^+–2Cl^-$ transport system on the luminal side of the ascending limb of Henle. By inhibiting this transport system, they reduce the reabsorption of NaCl, decrease potassium reabsorption, and increase calcium and magnesium elimination. Prolonged use can cause significant loss of magnesium in some persons. Because calcium is actively reabsorbed in the distal convoluted tubule, loop diuretics usually do not cause hypocalcemia. Impairment of sodium reabsorption in the loop of Henle causes a decrease in the osmolarity of the interstitial fluid surrounding the collecting ducts and further impedes the kidneys' ability to concentrate urine. The loop diuretics may increase uric acid retention and impair glucose tolerance. These drugs also can cause hypovolemia.

The *thiazide diuretics* act by preventing the reabsorption of NaCl in the distal convoluted tubule. Because of their site of action, the thiazide diuretics are less effective than loop diuretics in terms of effecting diuresis. The thiazides produce increased losses of potassium in the urine, uric acid retention, and some impairment in glucose tolerance. Thiazide diuretics also reduce peripheral vascular resistance and therefore often are prescribed as a first-line antihypertensive treatment.

The *aldosterone antagonists,* also called *potassium-sparing diuretics,* reduce sodium reabsorption and increase potassium secretion in the late distal tubule and cortical collecting tubule site regulated by aldosterone. Because of their site of action, the aldosterone antagonists have the least effect on diuresis compared with the loop diuretics and the thiazide diuretics. They have the advantage of increasing potassium reabsorption and thereby eliminating the risk for hypokalemia. These agents also tend to interfere with secretion of hydrogen ions in the collecting duct, explaining in part the metabolic acidosis sometimes seen with the use of these agents.

There are two types of potassium-sparing diuretics: those that act as direct aldosterone antagonists and those that act independently of aldosterone. The first type (*e.g.,* spironolactone) binds to the mineralocorticoid receptor on the basolateral side of the tubular cell, preventing aldosterone from binding and exerting its effects. The second type (*e.g.,* triamterene, amiloride) does not bind to the receptor, but instead directly interferes with sodium entry through the sodium-selective ion channels on the luminal side of the tubular cell.

REGULATION OF RENAL BLOOD FLOW

In the adult, the kidneys are perfused with 1000 to 1300 mL of blood per minute, or 20% to 25% of the cardiac output. This large blood flow is mainly needed to ensure a sufficient GFR for the removal of waste products from the blood, rather than for the metabolic needs of the kidney. Feedback mechanisms, both intrinsic (*e.g.,* autoregulation, local hormones) and extrinsic (*e.g.,* sympathetic nervous system, blood-borne hormones), normally keep blood flow and GFR constant despite changes in arterial blood pressure.

Neural and Humoral Control Mechanisms

The kidney is richly innervated by the sympathetic nervous system. Increased sympathetic activity causes constriction of the afferent and efferent arterioles and thus a decrease in renal blood flow. Intense sympathetic stimulation such as occurs in shock and trauma can produce marked decreases in renal blood flow and GFR, even to the extent of causing blood flow to cease altogether.

Several humoral substances, including angiotensin II, ADH, and endothelins, cause vasoconstriction of renal vessels. The endothelins are a group of peptides released from damaged endothelial cells in the kidney and other tissues. Although not thought to be important regulators of renal blood flow during everyday activities, endothelin I, which is released by renal endothelial cells, may play a role in reduction of blood flow in conditions such as postischemic acute renal failure (see Chapter 36).

Other substances such as dopamine, nitric oxide, and prostaglandins (*i.e.,* E_2 and I_2) produce vasodilation. Nitric oxide, a vasodilator produced by the vascular endothelium, appears to be important in preventing excessive vasoconstriction of renal blood vessels and allowing normal excretion of sodium and water. Prostaglandins are a group of mediators of cell function that are produced locally and exert their effects locally. Although prostaglandins do not appear to be of major importance in regulating renal blood flow and GFR under normal conditions, they may protect the kidneys against the vasoconstricting effects of sympathetic stimulation and angiotensin II. Aspirin and nonsteroidal antiinflammatory drugs that inhibit prostaglandin synthesis may cause reduction in renal blood flow and GFR under certain conditions.

Autoregulation

The constancy of renal blood flow is maintained by a process called *autoregulation* (see Chapter 23). Normally, autoregulation of blood flow is designed to maintain blood flow at a level consistent with the metabolic needs of the tissues. In the kidney, autoregulation of blood flow also must allow for precise regulation of renal excretion of water and solutes. For autoregulation to occur, the resistance to blood flow through the kidneys must be varied in direct proportion to the arterial pressure. The exact mechanisms responsible for the intrarenal regulation of blood flow are unclear. One of the proposed mechanisms is a direct effect on vascular smooth muscle that causes the blood vessels to relax when there is an increase in blood pressure and to constrict when there is a decrease in pressure. A second proposed mechanism is the juxtaglomerular complex.

The Juxtaglomerular Complex. The juxtaglomerular complex is thought to represent a feedback control system that links changes in the GFR with renal blood flow. The juxtaglomerular complex is located at the site where the distal tubule extends back to the glomerulus and then passes between the afferent and efferent arteriole (Fig. 32-13). The distal tubular site that is nearest the glomerulus is characterized by densely nucleated cells called the *macula densa.* In the adjacent afferent arteriole, the smooth muscle cells of the media are modified as special secretory cells called *juxtaglomerular cells.* These cells contain granules of inactive renin, an enzyme that functions in the conversion of angiotensinogen to angiotensin. Renin functions by means of angiotensin II to produce vasoconstriction of the efferent arteriole as a means of preventing serious decreases in GFR. Angiotensin II also increases sodium reabsorption indirectly by stimulating aldosterone secretion from the adrenal gland and directly by increasing sodium reabsorption by the proximal tubule cells.

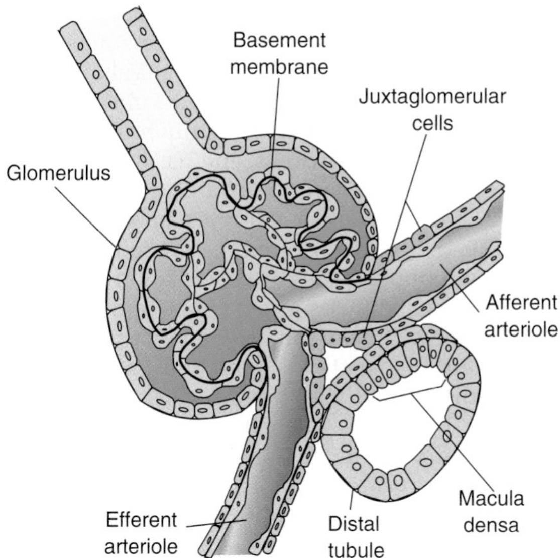

FIGURE 32-13 Juxtaglomerular apparatus, showing the close contact of the distal tubule with the afferent arteriole, the macula densa, and the juxtaglomerular cells.

Because of its location between the afferent and efferent arteriole, the juxtaglomerular complex is thought to play an essential feedback role in linking the level of arterial blood pressure and renal blood flow to the GFR and the composition of the distal tubular fluid. The juxtaglomerular complex monitors the systemic blood pressure by sensing the stretch of the afferent arteriole, and it monitors the concentration of sodium chloride in the tubular filtrate as it passes through the macula densa. This information is then used in determining how much renin should be released to keep the arterial blood pressure within its normal range and maintain a relatively constant GFR.

Effect of Increased Protein and Glucose Load. Although renal blood flow and glomerular filtration are relatively stable under most conditions, two conditions can increase renal blood flow and glomerular filtration. These are an increased amount of protein in the diet and an increase in blood glucose. With ingestion of a high-protein diet, renal blood flow increases 20% to 30% within 1 to 2 hours. Although the exact mechanism for this increase is uncertain, it is thought to be related to the fact that amino acids and sodium are absorbed together in the proximal tubule (secondary active transport). As a result, delivery of sodium to the macula densa is decreased, which elicits an increase in renal blood flow through the juxtaglomerular complex feedback mechanism. The resultant increase in blood flow and GFR allows sodium excretion to be maintained at a near-normal level while increasing the excretion of the waste products of protein metabolism, such as urea. The same mechanism is thought to explain the large increases in renal blood flow and GFR that occur with high blood glucose levels in persons with uncontrolled diabetes mellitus.

ELIMINATION FUNCTIONS OF THE KIDNEY

Renal Clearance

Renal clearance is the volume of plasma that is completely cleared each minute of any substance that finds its way into the urine. It is determined by the ability of the substance to be filtered in the glomeruli and the capacity of the renal tubules to reabsorb or secrete the substance. Every substance has its own clearance rate, the units of which are always in volume of plasma cleared per unit of time. It can be determined by measuring the amount of a substance that is excreted in the urine (*i.e.*, urine concentration × urine flow rate in milliliters per minute) and dividing by its plasma concentration. Inulin, a large polysaccharide, is freely filtered in the glomeruli and neither reabsorbed nor secreted by the tubular cells. After intravenous injection, the amount that appears in the urine is equal to the amount that is filtered in the glomeruli (*i.e.*, the clearance rate is equal to the GFR). Because of these properties, inulin can be used as a laboratory measure of the GFR. Some substances, such as urea, are freely filtered in the glomeruli, but the volume that is cleared from the plasma is less than the GFR, indicating that at least some of the substance is being reabsorbed. At normal plasma levels, glucose has a clearance of zero because it is reabsorbed in the tubules and none appears in the urine.

Regulation of Sodium and Potassium Elimination

Elimination of sodium and potassium is regulated by the GFR and by humoral agents that control their reabsorption. Aldosterone functions in the regulation of sodium and potassium elimination. Atrial natriuretic peptide (ANP) contributes to the regulation of sodium elimination.

Aldosterone. Sodium reabsorption in the distal tubule and collecting duct is highly variable and depends on the presence of aldosterone, a hormone secreted by the adrenal gland. In the presence of aldosterone, almost all the sodium in the distal tubular fluid is reabsorbed, and the urine essentially becomes sodium free. In the absence of aldosterone, virtually no sodium is reabsorbed from the distal tubule. The remarkable ability of the distal tubular and collecting duct cells to alter sodium reabsorption in relation to changes in aldosterone allows the kidneys to excrete urine with sodium levels that range from a few tenths of a gram to 40 g/day.

Like sodium, potassium is freely filtered in the glomerulus, but unlike sodium, potassium is reabsorbed from and secreted into the tubular fluid. The secretion of potassium into the tubular fluid occurs in the distal tubule and, like that of sodium, is regulated by aldosterone. Only approximately 70 mEq of potassium is delivered to the distal tubule each day, but the average person consumes this much or more potassium in the diet. Excess potassium that is not filtered in the glomerulus and delivered to the collecting tubule therefore must be secreted (*i.e.*, transported from the blood) into the tubular fluid for elimination from the body.

In the absence of aldosterone (as in Addison disease; see Chapter 42), potassium secretion becomes minimal. In these circumstances, potassium reabsorption exceeds secretion, and blood levels of potassium increase.

Atrial Natriuretic Peptide. Atrial natriuretic peptide, discovered in 1981, is a hormone believed to have an important role in salt and water excretion by the kidney. It is synthesized in muscle cells of the atria of the heart and released when the atria are stretched. The actions of ANP include vasodilation of the afferent and efferent arterioles, which results in an increase in renal blood flow and GFR. ANP inhibits aldosterone secretion by the adrenal gland and sodium reabsorption from the collecting tubules through its action on aldosterone and through direct action on the tubular cells. It also inhibits ADH release from the posterior pituitary gland, thereby increasing excretion of water by the kidneys. ANP also has vasodilator properties. Whether these effects are sufficient to produce long-term changes in blood pressure is uncertain.

Regulation of pH

The kidneys regulate body pH by conserving base bicarbonate and eliminating hydrogen ions (H^+). Neither the blood buffer systems nor the respiratory control mechanisms for carbon dioxide elimination can eliminate hydrogen ions from the body. This is accomplished by the kidneys. The average North American diet results in the liberation of 40 to 80 mmol of hydrogen ions each day. Virtually all the hydrogen ions excreted in the urine are secreted into the tubular fluid by means of tubular secretory mechanisms. The lowest tubular fluid pH that can be achieved is 4.4 to 4.5. The ability of the kidneys to excrete hydrogen ions depends on buffers in the urine that combine with the hydrogen ion. The three major urine buffers are bicarbonate (HCO_3^-), phosphate (HPO_4^-), and ammonia (NH_3). Bicarbonate ions, which are present in the urine filtrate, combine with hydrogen ions that have been secreted into the tubular fluid; this results in the formation of carbon dioxide and water. The carbon dioxide is then absorbed into the tubular cells, and bicarbonate is regenerated. The phosphate ion is a metabolic end product that is filtered into the tubular fluid; it combines with a secreted hydrogen ion and is not reabsorbed. Ammonia is synthesized in tubular cells by deamination of the amino acid glutamine; it diffuses into the tubular fluid and combines with the hydrogen ion. An important aspect of this buffer system is that the deamination process increases whenever the body's hydrogen ion concentration remains elevated for 1 to 2 days. These mechanisms for pH regulation are described more fully in Chapter 34.

THE FUNCTIONS OF THE KIDNEY

- The kidney regulates the composition and pH of body fluids through the reabsorption and elimination or conservation of sodium, potassium, hydrogen, chloride, and bicarbonate ions.
- It functions in the elimination of metabolic wastes (urea, uric acid, creatinine) and drugs and their metabolites.
- It serves to regulate the osmolality of the extracellular fluid through the action of antidiuretic hormone (ADH).
- It plays a central role in blood pressure regulation through the renin-angiotensin-aldosterone mechanism and the regulation of salt and water elimination.
- It contributes to the metabolic functions of the skeletal system through activation of vitamin D and regulation of calcium and phosphate conservation and elimination.
- It controls the production of red blood cells in the bone marrow through the production of erythropoietin.

pH-Dependent Elimination of Organic Ions

The proximal tubule actively secretes large amounts of different organic anions. Foreign anions (*e.g.*, salicylates, penicillin) and endogenously produced anions (*e.g.*, bile acids, uric acid) are actively secreted into the tubular fluid. Most of the anions that are secreted use the same transport system, allowing the kidneys to rid the body of many different drugs and environmental agents. Because the same transport system is shared by different anions, there is competition for transport such that elevated levels of one substance tend to inhibit the secretion of other anions. The proximal tubules also possess an active transport system for organic cations that is analogous to that for organic anions.

Uric Acid Elimination

Uric acid is a product of purine metabolism (see Chapter 59). Excessively high blood levels (*i.e.*, hyperuricemia) can cause gout, and excessive levels in the urine can cause kidney stones. Uric acid is freely filtered in the glomerulus and is reabsorbed and then secreted back into the proximal tubules. Uric acid is one of the anions that use the previously described anion transport system in the proximal tubule. Tubular reabsorption normally exceeds secretion, and the net effect is removal of uric acid from the filtrate. Although the rate of reabsorption exceeds secretion, the secretory process is homeostatically controlled to maintain a constant plasma level. Many persons with elevated uric acid levels secrete less uric acid than do persons with normal uric acid levels.

Uric acid uses the same transport systems as other anions, such as aspirin, sulfinpyrazone, and probenecid. Small doses of aspirin compete with uric acid for secretion into the tubular fluid and reduce uric acid secretion, and large doses compete with uric acid for reabsorption and increase uric acid excretion in the urine. Because of its effect on uric acid secretion, aspirin is not recommended for treatment of gouty arthritis. Thiazide and loop diuretics (*i.e.*, furosemide and ethacrynic acid) also can cause hyperuricemia and gouty arthritis, presumably through a decrease in extracellular fluid volume and enhanced uric acid reabsorption.

Urea Elimination

Urea is an end product of protein metabolism. The normal adult produces 25 to 30 g/day; the quantity rises when a high-protein diet is consumed, when there is excessive tissue breakdown, or in the presence of gastrointestinal bleeding. With gastrointestinal bleeding, the blood proteins are broken down to form ammonia in the intestine; the ammonia is then absorbed into the portal circulation and converted to urea by the liver before being released into the bloodstream. The kidneys, in their role as regulators of blood urea nitrogen (BUN) levels, filter urea in the glomeruli and then reabsorb it in the tubules. This enables maintenance of a normal BUN, which is in the range of 8 to 25 mg/dL (2.9 to 8.9 mmol/L). During periods of dehydration, the blood volume and GFR drop, and BUN levels increase. The renal tubules are permeable to urea, which means that the longer the tubular fluid remains in the kidneys, the greater is the reabsorption of urea into the blood. Only small amounts of urea are reabsorbed into the blood when the GFR is high, but relatively large amounts of urea are returned to the blood when the GFR is reduced.

Drug Elimination

Many drugs are eliminated in the urine. These drugs are selectively filtered in the glomerulus and reabsorbed or secreted into the tubular fluid. Only drugs that are not bound to plasma proteins are filtered in the glomerulus and therefore able to be eliminated by the kidneys.

Many drugs are weak acids or weak bases and are present in the renal tubular fluid partly as water-soluble ions and partly as nonionized lipid-soluble molecules. The nonionized lipid-soluble form of a drug diffuses more readily through the lipid membrane of the tubule and then back into the bloodstream, whereas the water-soluble ionized form remains in the urine filtrate. The ratio of ionized to nonionized drug depends on the pH of the urine. For example, aspirin is highly ionized in alkaline urine and in this form is rapidly excreted in the urine. Aspirin is largely nonionized in acid urine and is reabsorbed rather than excreted. Alkaline or acid diuresis may be used to increase elimination of drugs in the urine, particularly in situations of drug overdose.

ENDOCRINE FUNCTIONS OF THE KIDNEY

In addition to their function in regulating body fluids and electrolytes, the kidneys function as an endocrine organ in that they produce chemical mediators that travel through the blood to distant sites where they exert their actions. The kidneys participate in control of blood pressure by way of the renin-angiotensin mechanism, in calcium metabolism by activating vitamin D, and in regulating red blood cell production through the synthesis of erythropoietin.

The Renin-Angiotensin-Aldosterone Mechanism

The renin-angiotensin-aldosterone mechanism plays an important part in short-term and long-term regulation of blood pressure (see Chapter 25). Renin is an enzyme that is synthesized and stored in the juxtaglomerular cells of the kidney. This enzyme is thought to be released in response to a decrease in renal blood flow or a change in the composition of the distal tubular fluid, or as the result of sympathetic nervous system stimulation. Renin itself has no direct effect on blood pressure. Rather, it acts enzymatically to convert a circulating plasma protein called *angiotensinogen* to angiotensin I (see Chapter 25, Fig. 25-5). Angiotensin I, which has few vasoconstrictor properties, leaves the kidneys and enters the circulation; as it is circulated through the lungs, *angiotensin-converting enzyme* catalyzes the conversion of angiotensin I to angiotensin II. Angiotensin II is a potent vasoconstrictor, and it acts directly on the kidneys to decrease salt and water excretion. Both mechanisms have relatively short periods of action. Angiotensin II also stimulates aldosterone secretion by the adrenal gland. Aldosterone acts on the distal tubule to increase sodium reabsorption and exerts a longer-term effect on the maintenance of blood pressure. Renin also functions by means of angiotensin II to produce constriction of the efferent arteriole as a means of preventing a serious decrease in glomerular filtration pressure.

Erythropoietin

Erythropoietin is a polypeptide hormone that regulates the differentiation of red blood cells in the bone marrow (see Chapter 16). Between 89% and 95% of erythropoietin is formed in the kidneys. The synthesis of erythropoietin is stimulated by tissue hypoxia, which may be brought about by anemia, residence at high altitudes, or impaired oxygenation of tissues due to cardiac or pulmonary disease. Persons with end-stage kidney disease often are anemic because of an inability of the kidneys to produce erythropoietin. This anemia usually is managed by the administration of epoetin-alfa, a synthetic form of erythropoietin produced through DNA technology, to stimulate erythropoiesis.

Vitamin D

Activation of vitamin D occurs in the kidneys. Vitamin D increases calcium absorption from the gastrointestinal tract and helps to regulate calcium deposition in bone. It also has a weak stimulatory effect on renal calcium absorption. Although vitamin D is not synthesized and released from an endocrine gland, it often is considered as a hormone because of its pathway of molecular activation and mechanism of action.

Vitamin D exists in several forms: natural vitamin D (cholecalciferol), which results from ultraviolet irradiation of the skin, and synthetic vitamin D (ergocalciferol), which is derived from irradiation of ergosterol. The active form of vitamin D is 1,25-dihydroxycholecalciferol. Cholecalciferol and ergocalciferol must undergo chemical transformation to become active: first to 25-hydroxycholecalciferol in the liver and then to 1,25-dihydroxycholecalciferol in the kidneys. Persons with end-stage renal disease are unable to transform vitamin D to its active form and must rely on pharmacologic preparations of the active vitamin (calcitriol) for maintaining mineralization of their bones.

In summary, the kidneys perform excretory and endocrine functions. In the process of excreting wastes, the kidneys filter the blood and then selectively reabsorb those materials that are needed to maintain a stable internal environment. The kidneys rid the body of metabolic wastes, regulate fluid volume and the concentration of electrolytes, assist in maintaining acid-base balance, aid in regulation of blood pressure through the renin-angiotensin-aldosterone mechanism and control of extracellular fluid volume, regulate red blood cell production through erythropoietin, and aid in calcium metabolism by activating vitamin D.

The nephron is the functional unit of the kidney. It is composed of a glomerulus, which filters the blood, and a tubular component, where electrolytes and other substances needed to maintain the constancy of the internal environment are reabsorbed into the bloodstream while unneeded materials are secreted into the tubular filtrate for elimination. Urine concentration occurs in the collecting tubules under the influence of ADH. ADH maintains extracellular volume by returning water to the vascular compartment, producing a concentrated urine by removing water from the tubular filtrate.

The GFR is the amount of filtrate that is formed each minute as blood moves through the glomeruli. It is regulated by the arterial blood pressure and renal blood flow in the normally functioning kidney. The juxtaglomerular complex is thought to represent a feedback control system that links changes in the GFR with renal blood flow. Renal clearance is the volume of plasma that is completely cleared each minute of any substance that finds its way into the urine. It is determined by the ability of the substance to be filtered in the glomeruli and the capacity of the renal tubules to reabsorb or secrete the substance.

Tests of Renal Function

After you have completed this section of the chapter, you should be able to meet the following objectives:

- ✦ Describe the characteristics of normal urine
- ✦ Explain the significance of casts in the urine
- ✦ Explain the value of urine specific gravity in evaluating renal function
- ✦ Explain the concept of the GFR
- ✦ Explain the value of serum creatinine levels in evaluating renal function
- ✦ Describe the methods used in cystoscopic examination of the urinary tract, ultrasound studies of the urinary tract, computed tomographic scans, magnetic resonance imaging studies, excretory urography, and renal angiography

The function of the kidneys is to filter the blood, selectively reabsorb those substances that are needed to maintain the constancy of body fluid, and excrete metabolic wastes. The composition of urine and blood provides valuable information about the adequacy of renal function. Radiologic tests, endoscopy, and renal biopsy afford means for viewing the gross and microscopic structures of the kidneys and urinary system.

URINALYSIS

Urine is a clear, amber-colored fluid that is approximately 95% water and 5% dissolved solids. The kidneys normally produce approximately 1.5 L of urine each day. Normal urine contains metabolic wastes and few or no plasma proteins, blood cells, or glucose molecules.

Urine tests can be performed on a single urine specimen or on a 24-hour urine specimen. First-voided morning specimens are useful for qualitative protein and specific gravity testing. A freshly voided specimen is most reliable. Urine specimens that have been left standing may contain lysed red blood cells, disintegrating *casts,* and rapidly multiplying bacteria. Table 32-1 describes urinalysis values for normal urine.

Casts are molds of the distal nephron lumen. A gel-like substance called *Tamm-Horsfall mucoprotein,* which is formed in the tubular epithelium, is the major protein constituent of urinary casts. Casts composed of this gel but devoid of cells are called *hyaline casts*. These casts develop when the protein concentration of the urine is high (as in nephrotic syndrome), urine osmolality is high, and urine pH is low. The inclusion of granules or cells in the matrix of the protein gel leads to the formation of various other types of casts.

Because of the glomerular capillary filtration barrier, less than 150 mg of protein is excreted in the urine over

TABLE 32-1 Normal Values for Routine Urinalysis

General Characteristics and Measurements	Chemical Determinations	Microscopic Examination of Sediment
Color: yellow-amber—indicates a high specific gravity and small output of urine Turbidity: clear to slightly hazy Specific gravity: 1.010–1.025 with a normal fluid intake pH: 4.6–4.8—average person has a pH of about 6 (acid)	Glucose: negative Ketones: negative Blood: negative Protein: negative Bilirubin: negative Urobilinogen: 0.1–1 Nitrate for bacteria: negative Leukocyte esterase: negative	Casts negative: occasional hyaline casts Red blood cells: negative or rare Crystals: negative White blood cells; negative or rare Epithelial cells: few

(From Fischbach F. [1992]. *A manual of laboratory diagnostic tests* [p. 148]. Philadelphia: J.B. Lippincott)

24 hours in a healthy person. Qualitative and quantitative tests to determine urinary protein content are important tools to assess the extent of glomerular disease. pH-sensitive reagent strips are used to test for the presence of proteins, whereas immunoassay methods are used to test for microalbuminuria.

The *specific gravity* (or osmolality) of urine varies with its concentration of solutes. Urine specific gravity provides a valuable index of the hydration status and functional ability of the kidneys. Although there are more sophisticated methods for measuring specific gravity, it can be measured easily using an inexpensive piece of equipment called a *urinometer*. Healthy kidneys can produce a concentrated urine with a specific gravity of 1.030 to 1.040. During periods of marked hydration, the specific gravity can approach 1.000. With diminished renal function, there is a loss of renal concentrating ability, and the urine specific gravity may fall to levels of 1.006 to 1.010 (usual range is 1.010 to 1.025 with normal fluid intake). These low levels are particularly significant if they occur during periods that follow a decrease in water intake (*e.g.*, during the first urine specimen on arising in the morning).

GLOMERULAR FILTRATION RATE

The GFR provides a gauge of renal function. It can be measured clinically by collecting timed samples of blood and urine. *Creatinine*, a byproduct of creatine metabolism by the muscle, is filtered by the kidneys but not reabsorbed in the renal tubule. Creatinine levels in the blood and urine can be used to measure GFR. The clearance rate for creatinine is the amount that is completely cleared by the kidneys in 1 minute. The formula is expressed as $C = UV/P$, in which C is the clearance rate (mL/minute), U is the urine concentration (mg/dL), V is the urine volume excreted (mL/minute or 24 hours), and P is plasma concentration (mg/dL).

Normal creatinine clearance is 115 to 125 mL/minute. This value is corrected for body surface area, which reflects the muscle mass where creatinine metabolism takes place. The test may be done on a 24-hour basis, with blood being drawn when the urine collection is completed. In another method, two 1-hour urine specimens are collected, and a blood sample is drawn in between.

BLOOD TESTS

Blood tests can provide valuable information about the kidneys' ability to remove metabolic wastes from the blood and maintain normal electrolyte and pH composition of the blood. Normal blood values are listed in Table 32-2. Serum levels of potassium, phosphate, BUN, and creatinine increase in renal failure. Serum pH, calcium, and bicarbonate levels decrease in renal failure. The effect of renal failure on the concentration of serum electrolytes and metabolic end products is discussed in Chapter 36.

Serum Creatinine

Serum creatinine levels reflect the glomerular filtration rate. Because these measurements are easily obtained and relatively inexpensive, they often are used as a screening measure of renal function. Creatinine is a product of creatine metabolism in muscles; its formation and release are relatively constant and proportional to the amount of muscle mass present. Creatinine is freely filtered in the glomeruli, is not reabsorbed from the tubules into the blood, and is only minimally secreted into the tubules from the blood; therefore, its blood values depend closely on the GFR.

The normal creatinine value is approximately 0.6 mg/dL of blood for a woman with a small frame, approximately 1.0 mg/dL of blood for a normal adult man, and approximately 1.2 mg/dL of blood (50 to 100 mmol/L) for a muscular man. Because both muscle mass and GFR decline with age, serum creatinine values should be adjusted in the elderly to account for the changes (see Chapter 36). A normal serum creatinine level usually indicates normal renal function. In addition to its use in calculating the GFR, the serum creatinine level is used in estimating the functional capacity of the kidneys (Fig. 32-14). If the value doubles, the GFR—and renal function—probably has fallen to one half of its normal state. A rise in the serum creatinine level to three times its normal value suggests that there is a 75% loss of renal function, and with creatinine values of 10 mg/dL

TABLE 32-2 Normal Blood Chemistry Levels

Substance	Normal Value*
Blood urea nitrogen	8.0–20.0 mg/dL (2.9–7.1 mmol/L)
Creatinine	0.6–1.2 mg/dL (50–100 mmol/L)
Sodium	135–145 mEq/L (135–148 mmol/L)
Chloride	98–106 mEq/L (98–106 mmol/L)
Potassium	3.5–5 mEq/L (3.5–5 mmol/L)
Carbon dioxide (CO_2 content)	24–29 mEq/L (24–29 mmol/L)
Calcium	8.5–10.5 mg/dL (2.1–2.6 mmol/L)
Phosphate	2.5–4.5 mg/dL (0.77–1.45 mmol/L)
Uric acid	1.4–7.4 mg/dL (0.154–0.42 mmol/L)
pH	7.35–7.45

*Values may vary among laboratories, depending on the method of analysis used.

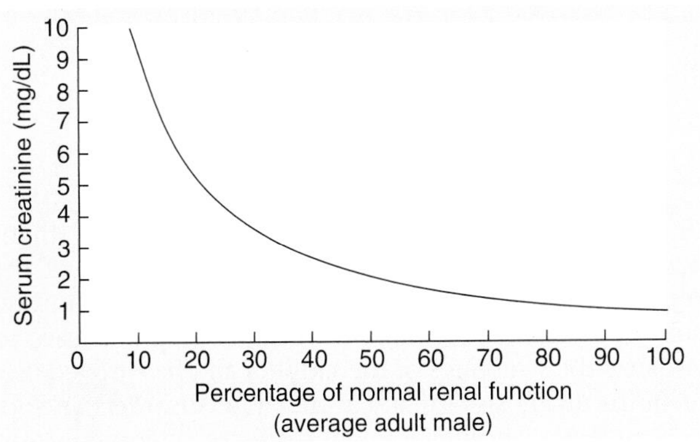

FIGURE 32-14 Relation between the percentage of renal function and serum creatinine levels.

or more, it can be assumed that approximately 90% of renal function has been lost.

Recently, it has been proposed that another serum protein, *cystatin-C* (a cysteine protease inhibitor), could be useful as a marker of GFR because it has a stable production rate, is freely filtered at the glomerulus, and in several studies to date has shown a greater sensitivity in detecting a decreased GFR. Further clinical studies are needed to determine the clinical efficacy of cystatin-C as a marker and to determine whether there is an advantage in its use compared with creatinine.

Blood Urea Nitrogen

Urea is formed in the liver as a byproduct of protein metabolism and is eliminated entirely by the kidneys. BUN therefore is related to the GFR but, unlike creatinine, also is influenced by protein intake, gastrointestinal bleeding, and hydration status. Increased protein intake and gastrointestinal bleeding increase urea by means of protein metabolism. In gastrointestinal bleeding, the blood is broken down by the intestinal flora, and the nitrogenous waste is absorbed into the portal vein and transported to the liver, where it is converted to urea. During dehydration, elevated BUN levels result from increased concentration. Approximately two thirds of renal function must be lost before a significant rise in the BUN level occurs.

The BUN is less specific for renal insufficiency than creatinine, but the *BUN–creatinine ratio* may provide useful diagnostic information. The ratio normally is approximately 10:1. Ratios greater than 15:1 represent prerenal conditions, such as congestive heart failure and upper gastrointestinal tract bleeding, that produce an increase in BUN but not in creatinine. A ratio of less than 10:1 occurs in persons with liver disease and in those who receive a low-protein diet or chronic dialysis because BUN is more readily dialyzable than creatinine.

CYSTOSCOPY

Cystoscopy provides a means for direct visualization of the urethra, bladder, and ureteral orifices. It relies on the use of a cystoscope, an instrument with a lighted lens. The cystoscope is inserted through the urethra into the bladder. Biopsy specimens, lesions, small stones, and foreign bodies can be removed from the bladder. Urethroscopy may be used to remove stones from the ureter and aid in the treatment of ureteral disorders such as ureteral strictures.

ULTRASONOGRAPHY

Ultrasound studies use the reflection of ultrasonic (high-frequency) waves to visualize the deep structures of the body. The procedure is painless and noninvasive and requires no patient preparation. Ultrasonography is used to visualize the structures of the kidneys and has proved useful in the diagnosis of many urinary tract disorders, including congenital anomalies, renal abscesses, hydronephrosis, and kidney stones. It can differentiate a renal cyst from a renal tumor. The use of ultrasonography also enables accurate placement of needles for renal biopsy and catheters for percutaneous nephrostomy.

RADIOLOGIC AND OTHER IMAGING STUDIES

Radiologic studies include a simple flat plate (radiograph) of the kidneys, ureters, and bladder that can be used to determine the size, shape, and position of the kidneys and observe any radiopaque stones that may be in the kidney pelvis or ureters. In excretory urography, or *intravenous pyelography,* a radiopaque dye is injected into a peripheral vein; the dye is then filtered by the glomerulus and excreted into the urine, and x-ray films are taken as it moves through the kidneys and ureters.

Urography is used to detect space-occupying lesions of the kidneys, pyelonephritis, hydronephrosis, vesicoureteral reflux, and kidney stones. Some persons are allergic to the dye used for urography and may have an anaphylactic reaction after its administration. Every person undergoing urography studies should be questioned about previous reactions to the dye or to similar dyes. If the test is considered essential in such persons, premedication with antihistamines and corticosteroids may be used. The dye also reduces renal blood flow; acute renal failure can occur, particularly in persons with vascular disease or preexisting renal insufficiency.

Other diagnostic tests include computed tomographic (CT) scans, magnetic resonance imaging (MRI), radionuclide imaging, and renal angiography. CT scans may be used to outline the kidneys and detect renal masses and tumors. MRI is becoming readily available and is used in imaging the kidneys, retroperitoneum, and urinary bladder. It is particularly useful in evaluating vascular abnormalities in and around the kidneys. Radionuclide imaging involves the injection of a radioactive material that subsequently is detected externally by a scintillation camera, which detects the radioactive emissions. Radionuclide imaging is used to evaluate renal function and structures as well as the ureters and bladder. It is particularly useful in evaluating the function of kidney transplants. Renal angiography provides x-ray pictures of the blood vessels that supply the kidneys. It involves the injection of a radiopaque dye directly into the renal artery. A catheter usually is introduced through the femoral artery and advanced under fluoroscopic view into the abdominal aorta. The catheter tip then is maneuvered into the renal artery, and the dye is injected. This test is used to evaluate persons suspected of having renal artery stenosis, abnormalities of renal blood vessels, or vascular damage to the renal arteries after trauma.

In summary, urinalysis and blood tests that measure levels of byproducts of metabolism and electrolytes provide information about renal function. Cystoscopic examinations can be used for direct visualization of the urethra, bladder, and ureters. Ultrasonography can be used to determine kidney size, and renal radionuclide imaging can be used to evaluate the kidney structures. Radiologic methods such as excretory urography provide a means by which kidney structures such as the renal calyces, pelvis, ureters, and bladder can be outlined.

REVIEW EXERCISES

A 60-year-old woman with a diagnosis of hypertension is being treated with a thiazide diuretic.

A. What diuretic effect would you expect the woman to have based on the percentage of sodium reaching the site where the diuretic exerted its action?

B. What type of effects might be expected in terms of renal losses of potassium and calcium?

A 54-year-old man, seen by his physician for elevated blood pressure, was found to have a serum creatinine of 2.5. He complains that he has been urinating more frequently than usual, and his first-morning urine specimen reveals a dilute urine with a specific gravity of 1.010.

A. Explain the elevation of serum creatinine in terms of renal function.

B. Explain the inability of persons with early renal failure to produce a concentrated urine as evidenced by the frequency of urination and the low specific gravity of the patient's first-morning urine specimen.

A 10-year-old boy with bed-wetting was placed on an ADH nasal spray at bedtime as a means of treating the disorder.

A. Explain the rationale for the use of this treatment of ADH on urine output.

Bibliography

Cormack D. H. (1993). *Essential histology* (pp. 322–333). Philadelphia: J. B. Lippincott.

Guyton A. C., Hall J. E. (2000). *Textbook of medical physiology* (10th ed., pp. 279–311). Philadelphia: W. B. Saunders.

Koeppen B. M., Stanton B. A. (2001). *Renal physiology* (3rd ed.). St. Louis: Mosby.

Price C. P., Finney H. (2000). Developments in the assessment of glomerular filtration rate. *Clinica Chimica Acta 297,* 55–66.

Rahn K. H., Heidenreich S., Bruckner D. (1999). How to assess glomerular function and damage in humans. *Journal of Hypertension 17,* 309–317.

Rhoades R. A., Tanner G. A. (2003). *Medical physiology* (pp. 377–402). Philadelphia: Lippincott Williams & Wilkins.

Smith H. (1953). *From fish to philosopher* (p. 4). Boston: Little, Brown.

Vander A. J. (1995). *Renal physiology* (5th ed.). New York: McGraw-Hill.

CHAPTER 33

Disorders of Fluid and Electrolyte Balance

Glenn Matfin and Carol M. Porth

Fluids and electrolytes are present in body cells, in the tissue spaces between the cells, and in the blood that fills the vascular compartment. Body fluids transport gases, nutrients, and wastes, help generate the electrical activity needed to power body functions, take part in the transforming of food into energy, and otherwise maintain the overall function of the body. Although fluid volume and composition remain relatively constant in the presence of a wide range of changes in intake and output, conditions such as environmental stresses and disease can increase fluid loss, impair its intake, and otherwise interfere with mechanisms that regulate fluid volume, composition, and distribution.

This chapter is divided into four sections: (1) the composition and compartmental distribution of body fluids, (2) sodium and water balance, (3) potassium balance, and (4) calcium, phosphate, and magnesium balance. The mechanisms of edema formation are discussed in the section on composition and compartmentalization of body fluids.

Composition and Compartmental Distribution of Body Fluids

After you have completed this section of the chapter, you should be able to meet the following objectives:

- Define the terms *electrolyte, ion,* and *nonelectrolyte*
- Differentiate intracellular from extracellular compartments in terms of distribution and composition of water, electrolytes, and other osmotically active solutes

- Cite the rationale for the use of concentration rather than absolute values in describing electrolyte content of body fluids
- Relate the concept of a concentration gradient to the processes of diffusion and osmosis
- Differentiate between effective and ineffective osmoles in determining the tonicity of a solution
- Describe the control of cell volume and the effect of isotonic, hypotonic, and hypertonic solutions on cell size
- Describe factors that control fluid exchange between the vascular and interstitial fluid compartments and relate them to the development of edema and third spacing of extracellular fluids
- Describe the manifestations and treatment of edema

Body fluids are distributed between the intracellular fluid (ICF) and extracellular fluid (ECF) compartments. The *ICF compartment* consists of fluid contained within all of the billions of cells in the body. It is the larger of the two compartments, with approximately two thirds of the body water in healthy adults. The remaining one third of body water is in the *ECF compartment,* which contains all the fluids outside the cells, including those in the interstitial or tissue spaces and blood vessels (Fig. 33-1). The ECF, including the plasma and interstitial fluids, contains large amounts of sodium and chloride, moderate amounts of bicarbonate, but only small quantities of potassium, magnesium, calcium, and phosphate. In contrast to the ECF, the ICF contains almost no calcium; small amounts of sodium, chloride, bicarbonate, and phosphate; moderate amounts of magnesium; and large amounts of potassium (Table 33-1). It is the ECF levels of electrolytes in the blood or blood plasma that are measured clinically. Although blood levels usually are representative of the total body levels of an electrolyte, this is not always the case, particularly with potassium, which is approximately 28 times more concentrated inside the cell than outside.

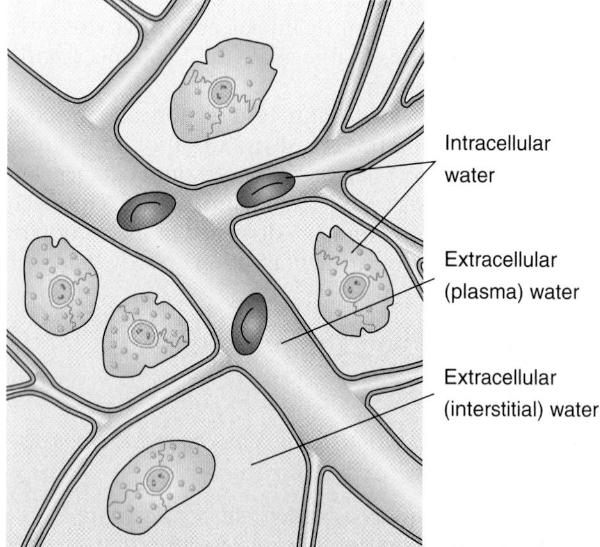

FIGURE 33-1 Distribution of body water. The extracellular space includes the vascular compartment and the interstitial spaces.

TABLE 33-1 Concentrations of Extracellular and Intracellular Electrolytes in Adults

Electrolyte	Extracellular Concentration*	Intracellular Concentration*
Sodium	135–145 mEq/L	10–14 mEq/L
Potassium	3.5–5.0 mEq/L	140–150 mEq/L
Chloride	98–106 mEq/L	3–4 mEq/L
Bicarbonate	24–31 mEq/L	7–10 mEq/L
Calcium	8.5–10.5 mg/dL	<1 mEq/L
Phosphate/ phosphorus	2.5–4.5 mg/dL	4 mEq/kg†
Magnesium	1.8–3.0 mg/dL	40 mEq/kg†

*Values may vary among laboratories, depending on the method of analysis used.
†Values vary among various tissues and with nutritional status.

The cell membrane serves as the primary barrier to the movement of substances between the ECF and ICF compartments. Lipid-soluble substances such as gases (*i.e.,* oxygen and carbon dioxide), which dissolve in the lipid bilayer of the cell membrane, pass directly through the membrane. Many ions, such as sodium (Na^+) and potassium (K^+) rely on transport mechanisms such as the Na^+/K^+ pump that is located in the cell membrane for movement across the membrane (see Chapter 4). Because the Na^+/K^+ pump relies on adenosine triphosphate (ATP) and the enzyme ATPase for energy, it is often referred to as the Na^+/K^+-ATPase membrane pump. Water crosses the cell membrane by osmosis using special protein channels called *aquaporins.*

INTRODUCTORY CONCEPTS

Dissociation of Electrolytes

Body fluids contain water and electrolytes. Electrolytes are substances that dissociate in solution to form charged particles, or *ions.* For example, a sodium chloride (NaCl) molecule dissociates to form a positively charged Na^+ and a negatively charged Cl^- ion. Particles that do not dissociate into ions such as glucose and urea are called *nonelectrolytes.* Positively charged ions are called *cations* because they are attracted to the cathode of a wet electric cell, and negatively charged ions are called *anions* because they are attracted to the anode. The ions found in body fluids carry one charge (*i.e.,* monovalent ion) or two charges (*i.e.,* divalent ion). Because of their attraction forces, positively charged cations are always accompanied by negatively charged anions. The distribution of electrolytes between body compartments is influenced by their electrical charge. However, one cation may be exchanged for another, provided it carries the same charge. For example, a positively charged H^+ ion may be exchanged for a positively charged K^+ ion, and a negatively charged bicarbonate (HCO_3^-) ion may be exchanged for another negatively charged Cl^- anion.

Diffusion and Osmosis

Diffusion. *Diffusion* is the movement of charged or uncharged particles along a concentration gradient. All molecules and ions, including water and dissolved molecules, are in constant random motion. It is the motion of these particles, each colliding with one another, that supplies the energy for diffusion. Because there are more molecules in constant motion in a concentrated solution, particles move from an area of higher concentration to one of lower concentration.

Osmosis. *Osmosis* is the movement of water across a semipermeable membrane (*i.e.,* one that is permeable to water but impermeable to most solutes). As with particles, water diffuses down its concentration gradient, moving from the side of the membrane with the lesser number of particles and greater concentration of water to the side with the greater number of particles and lesser concentration of water (Fig. 33-2). As water moves across the semipermeable membrane, it generates a pressure called the *osmotic pressure.* The osmotic pressure represents the pressure (measured in millimeters of mercury [mm Hg]) needed to oppose the movement of water across the membrane.

The osmotic activity that nondiffusible particles exert in pulling water from one side of the semipermeable membrane to the other is measured by a unit called an *osmole.* The osmole is derived from the gram molecular weight of a substance (*i.e.,* 1 gram molecular weight of a nondiffusible and nonionizable substance is equal to 1 osmole). In the clinical setting, osmotic activity usually is expressed in milliosmoles (one thousandth of an osmole) per liter. Each nondiffusible particle, large or small, is equally effective in its ability to pull water through a semipermeable membrane. Thus, it is the number, rather than the size, of the nondiffusible particles that determines the osmotic activity of a solution.

The osmotic activity of a solution may be expressed in terms of either its osmolarity or osmolality. *Osmolarity* refers to the osmolar concentration in 1 L of solution (mOsm/L) and *osmolality* to the osmolar concentration in 1 kg of water (mOsm/kg of H_2O). Osmolarity is usually used when referring to fluids outside the body and osmolality for describing fluids inside the body. Because 1 L of

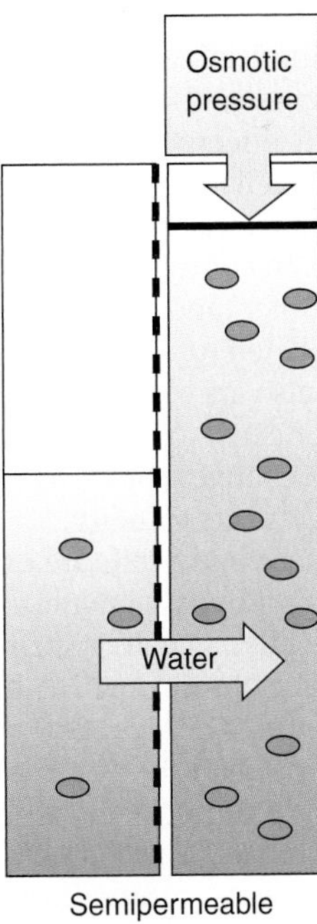

FIGURE 33-2 Movement of water across a semipermeable membrane. Water moves from the side that has fewer nondiffusible particles to the side that has more. The osmotic pressure is equal to the hydrostatic pressure needed to oppose water movement across the membrane.

CLINICAL APPLICATION

Measurement Units

The amount of electrolytes and solutes in body fluids is expressed as a concentration or amount of solute in a given volume of fluid, such as milligrams per deciliter (mg/dL), milliequivalents per liter (mEq/L), or millimoles per liter (mmol/L). The *milligrams per deciliter* measurement unit expresses the weight of the solute in one tenth of a liter (dL) or 100 mL of solution. The concentration of electrolytes, such as calcium, phosphate, and magnesium, is often expressed in mg/dL.

The *milliequivalent* is used to express the charge equivalency for a given weight of an electrolyte. Electroneutrality requires that the total number of cations in the body equals the total number of anions. When cations and anions combine, they do so according to their ionic charge, not according to their atomic weight. Thus, 1 mEq of sodium has the same number of charges as 1 mEq of chloride, regardless of molecular weight (although sodium is positive and chloride is negative). The number of milliequivalents of an electrolyte in a liter of solution can be derived from the following equation:

$$\text{mEq} = \frac{\text{mg/100 mL} \times 10 \times \text{valence}}{\text{atomic weight}}$$

The Système Internationale (SI) units express electrolyte content of body fluids in *millimoles per liter* (mmol/L). A millimole is one thousandth of a mole, or the molecular weight of a substance expressed in milligrams. The number of millimoles of an electrolyte in a liter of solution can be calculated using the following equation:

$$\text{mmol/L} = \frac{\text{mEq/L}}{\text{valence}}$$

For monovalent electrolytes such as sodium and potassium, the mmol and mEq values are identical. For example 140 mEq is equal to 140 mmol of sodium.

water weighs 1 kg, the terms *osmolarity* and *osmolality* are often used interchangeably.

The predominant osmotically active particles in the ECF are Na^+ and its attendant anions (Cl^- and HCO_3^-), which together account for 90% to 95% of the osmotic pressure. Blood urea nitrogen (BUN) and glucose, which also are osmotically active, account for less than 5% of the total osmotic pressure in the extracellular compartment. This can change, however, as when blood glucose levels are elevated in persons with diabetes mellitus or when BUN levels change rapidly in persons with renal failure. Serum osmolality, which normally ranges between 275 and 295 mOsm/kg, can be calculated using the following equation:

$$\text{Osmolality (mOsm/kg)} = 2[\text{Na}^+(\text{mmol/L})] + \frac{\text{glucose (mg/dl)*}}{18} + \frac{\text{BUN (mg/dl)*}}{2.8}$$

**1 mOsm of glucose equal 180 mg / L,*

and 1 mOsm of urea equals 28 mg / L

Ordinarily, the calculated and measured osmolality are within 10 mOsm of one another. The difference between the calculated and measured osmolality is called the *osmolar gap*. An osmolar gap larger than 10 mOsm suggests the presence of an unmeasured, osmotically active substance such as alcohol, acetone, or mannitol.

Tonicity. A change in water content causes cells to swell or shrink. The term *tonicity* refers to the tension or effect that the effective osmotic pressure of a solution with impermeable solutes exerts on cell size because of water movement across the cell membrane. An effective osmole is one that exerts an osmotic force and cannot permeate the cell membrane, whereas an ineffective osmole is one that exerts an osmotic force but crosses the cell membrane. Tonicity is determined solely by effective solutes such as glucose that cannot penetrate the cell membrane, thereby producing an osmotic force that pulls water into or out of the cell, causing it to change size. In contrast, urea, which is osmotically active but lipid soluble, tends to distribute equally across the cell membrane. Therefore, when ECF levels of urea are elevated, ICF levels also are elevated. Urea is therefore considered to be an ineffective osmole. It is only when extracellular levels of urea change rapidly, as during hemodialysis treatment, that urea affects tonicity.

Solutions to which body cells are exposed can be classified as isotonic, hypotonic, or hypertonic depending on whether they cause cells to swell or shrink (Fig. 33-3). Cells placed in an isotonic solution, which has the same effective osmolality as the ICF (*i.e.*, 280 mOsm/L), neither shrink nor swell. An example of an isotonic solution is 0.9% sodium chloride. When cells are placed in a hypotonic solution, which has a lower effective osmolality than the ICF, they swell as water moves into the cell, and when they are placed in a hypertonic solution, which has a greater effective osmolality than the ICF, they shrink as water is pulled out of the cell. However, an iso-osmotic solution is not necessarily isotonic. For example, the intravenous administration of a solution of 5% dextrose in water, which is iso-osmotic, is equivalent to the infusion of a hypotonic solution of distilled water because the glucose is rapidly metabolized to carbon dioxide and water.

CLINICAL APPLICATION

Urine Osmolality

Urine osmolality reflects the kidneys' ability to produce a concentrated or diluted urine based on serum osmolality and the need for water conservation or excretion. The ratio of urine osmolality to serum osmolality in a 24-hour urine sample normally exceeds 1:1, and after a period of overnight water deprivation, it should be greater than 3:1. A dehydrated person (one who has a loss of water) may have a urine–serum ratio that approaches 4:1. In these persons, urine osmolality may exceed 1000 mOsm/kg H_2O. In those who have difficulty concentrating their urine (*e.g.*, those with diabetes insipidus or chronic renal failure), the urine–serum ratio often is less than or equal to 1:1.

Urine specific gravity compares the weight of urine with that of water, providing an index for solute concentration. Water is considered to be 1.000. A change in specific gravity of 1.010 to 1.020 is an increase of 400 mOsm/kg H_2O. In the sodium-depleted state, the kidneys usually try to conserve sodium, urine specific gravity is normal, and urine sodium and chloride concentrations are low.

COMPARTMENTAL DISTRIBUTION OF BODY FLUIDS

Body water is distributed between the ICF and ECF compartments. In the adult, the fluid in the ICF compartment constitutes approximately 40% of body weight.[1] The fluid

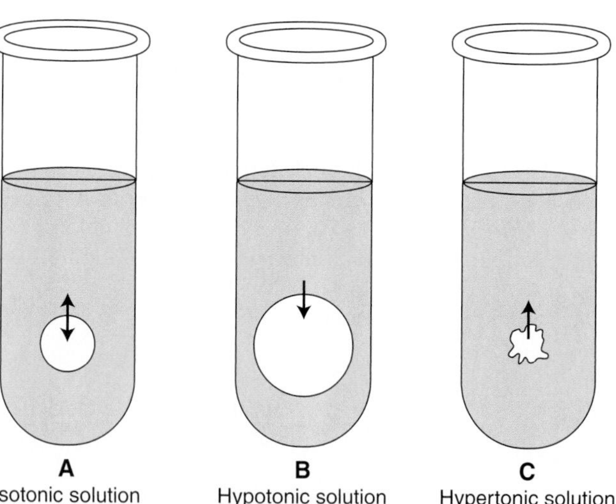

FIGURE 33-3 Osmosis. Red cells undergo no change in size in isotonic solutions (**A**). They increase in size in hypotonic solutions (**B**) and decrease in size in hypertonic solutions (**C**).

in the ECF compartment is further divided into two major subdivisions: the plasma compartment, which constitutes approximately 4% of body weight, and the interstitial fluid compartment, which constitutes approximately 15% of body weight (Fig. 33-4).

A third, usually minor, subdivision of the ECF compartment is the transcellular compartment, which is defined as being separated by a layer of epithelium. It includes the cerebrospinal fluid and fluid contained in the various body spaces, such as the peritoneal, pleural, and pericardial cavities; the joint spaces; and the gastrointestinal tract. Normally, only approximately 1% of ECF is in the transcellular space. This amount can increase considerably in conditions such as ascites, in which large amounts of fluid are sequestered in the peritoneal cavity. When the transcellular fluid compartment becomes considerably enlarged, it is referred to as a *third space* because this fluid is not readily available for exchange with the rest of the ECF.

Intracellular Fluid Volume

The ICF volume is regulated by proteins and organic compounds in the ICF and by solutes that move between the ECF and ICF. The membrane in most cells is freely permeable to water; therefore, water moves between the ECF and ICF fluid as a result of osmosis. In contrast, osmotically active proteins and other organic compounds cannot pass through the membrane. Water entry into the cell is regulated by these osmotically active substances as well as by solutes such as sodium and potassium that pass through the cell membrane. Many of the intracellular proteins are negatively charged and attract positively charged ions such as the K^+ ion, accounting for its higher concentration in the ICF. The Na^+ ion, which has a greater concentration in the ECF, tends to enter the cell by diffusion. The Na^+ ion is osmotically active, and its entry would, if left unchecked, pull water into the cell until it ruptured. The reason this does not occur is because the Na^+/K^+-ATPase membrane pump continuously removes three Na^+ ions from the cell for every two K^+ ions that are moved back into the cell. Situations that impair the function of the Na^+/K^+-ATPase pump, such as hypoxia, cause cells to swell because of an accumulation of Na^+ ions. Other ions, such as Ca^{2+} and H^+, are exchanged by similar transport systems.

Intracellular volume is also affected by the concentration of osmotically active substances in the ECF that cannot cross the cell membrane. In diabetes mellitus, for example, glucose cannot enter the cell, and its increased concentration in the ECF pulls water out of the cell.

Extracellular Fluid Volume

The ECF volume is divided between the vascular and interstitial fluid compartments. The vascular compartment contains blood, which is essential to the transport of substances such as electrolytes, gases, nutrients, and waste products throughout the body. Interstitial fluid acts as a transport vehicle for gases, nutrients, wastes, and other materials that move between the vascular compartment and body cells. Interstitial fluid also provides a reservoir from which vascular volume can be maintained during periods of hemorrhage or loss of vascular volume. A tissue gel, which is a spongelike material composed of large quantities of mucopolysaccharides, fills the tissue spaces and aids in even distribution of interstitial fluid. Normally, most of the fluid in the interstitium is in gel form. The tissue gel is supported by collagen fibers that hold the gel in place. The tissue gel, which has a firmer consistency than water, opposes the outflow of water from the capillaries and prevents the accumulation of free water in the interstitial spaces.

CAPILLARY–INTERSTITIAL FLUID EXCHANGE

The transfer of water between the vascular and interstitial compartments occurs at the capillary level and is governed by the Starling forces described in Chapter 23. Four forces control the movement of water between the capillary and interstitial spaces (Fig. 33-5): (1) the capillary filtration pressure, which pushes water out of the capillary into the

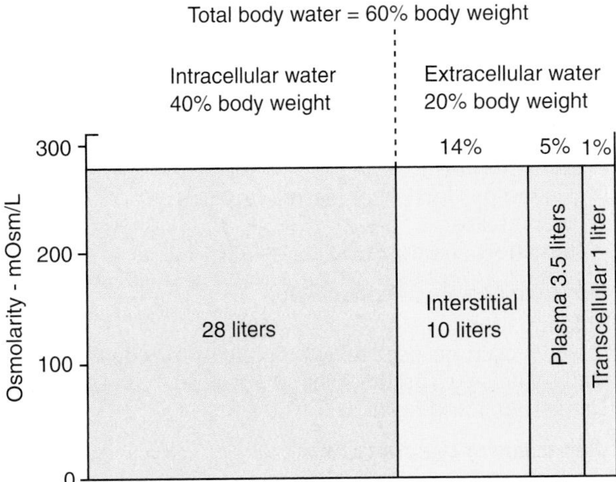

FIGURE 33-4 Approximate size of body compartments in a 70-kg adult.

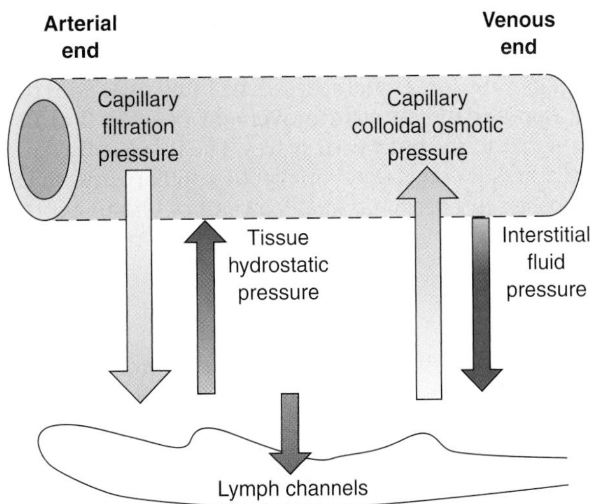

FIGURE 33-5 Exchange of fluid at the capillary level.

interstitial spaces; (2) the capillary colloidal osmotic pressure, which pulls water back into the capillary; (3) the interstitial fluid pressure, which opposes the movement of water out of the capillary; and (4) the tissue colloidal osmotic pressure, which pulls water out of the capillary into the interstitial spaces. Normally, the combination of these four forces is such that only a small excess of fluid remains in the interstitial compartment. This excess fluid is removed from the interstitium by the lymphatic system and returned to the systemic circulation.

Capillary filtration refers to the movement of water through capillary pores because of a mechanical rather than an osmotic force. The capillary filtration pressure, sometimes called the *capillary hydrostatic pressure,* is the pressure pushing water out of the capillary into the interstitial spaces. It reflects the arterial and venous pressures, the precapillary (arterioles) and postcapillary (venules) resistances, and the force of gravity.[2] A rise in arterial or venous pressure increases capillary pressure. A decrease in arterial resistance or increase in venous resistance increases capillary pressure, and an increase in arterial resistance or decrease in venous resistance decreases capillary pressure. The force of gravity increases capillary pressure in the dependent parts of the body. In a person who is standing absolutely still, the weight of blood in the vascular column causes an increase of 1 mm Hg in pressure for every 13.6 mm of distance from the heart.[2] This pressure results from the weight of water and is therefore called *hydrostatic pressure.* For example, the hydrostatic pressure in the veins of an adult man can reach 90 mm Hg. This pressure is then transmitted to the capillaries.

The capillary colloidal osmotic pressure is the osmotic pressure generated by the plasma proteins that are too large to pass through the pores of the capillary wall. The term *colloidal osmotic pressure* differentiates this type of osmotic pressure from the osmotic pressure that develops at the cell membrane from the presence of electrolytes and nonelectrolytes. Because plasma proteins do not normally penetrate the capillary pores and because their concentration is greater in the plasma than in the interstitial fluids, it is capillary colloidal osmotic pressure that pulls fluids back into the capillary.

The interstitial fluid pressure and the tissue colloidal osmotic pressure contribute to movement of water into and out of the interstitial spaces. The interstitial fluid pressure opposes the outward movement of water from the capillary into the interstitial spaces. The tissue colloidal osmotic pressure pulls water out of the capillary into the tissue spaces. It reflects the small amount of plasma proteins that normally escape from the capillary to enter the interstitial spaces.

Edema

Edema can be defined as palpable swelling produced by expansion of the interstitial fluid volume. Edema does not become evident until the interstitial volume has been increased by 2.5 to 3 L.[3]

Causes. The physiologic mechanisms that contribute to edema formation include factors that (1) increase the capillary filtration pressure, (2) decrease the capillary colloidal osmotic pressure, (3) increase capillary permeability, or (4) produce obstruction to lymph flow. The causes of edema are summarized in Chart 33-1.

Increased Capillary Filtration Pressure. As the capillary filtration pressure rises, the movement of vascular fluid into the interstitial spaces increases. Among the factors that increase capillary pressure are (1) increased arterial pressure or decreased resistance to flow through the precapillary sphincters, (2) an increase in venous pressure or increased resistance to outflow at the postcapillary sphincter, and (3) capillary distention due to increased vascular volume.

Edema can be either localized or generalized. The localized edema that occurs with urticaria (*i.e.,* hives) or other allergic or inflammatory conditions results from the release of histamine and other inflammatory mediators that cause dilation of the precapillary sphincters and arterioles that supply the swollen lesions. Thrombophlebitis obstructs venous flow, producing an elevation of venous pressure and edema of the affected part, usually one of the lower extremities.

Generalized edema is common in conditions such as congestive heart failure that produce fluid retention and

CHART 33-1

Causes of Edema

Increased Capillary Pressure

Increased vascular volume
- Heart failure
- Kidney disease
- Premenstrual sodium retention
- Pregnancy
- Environmental heat stress
- Thiazolidinedione (Glitazone) therapy

Venous obstruction
- Liver disease with portal vein obstruction
- Acute pulmonary edema
- Venous thrombosis (thrombophlebitis)

Decreased arteriolar resistance
- Calcium channel–blocking drug responses

Decreased Colloidal Osmotic Pressure

Increased loss of plasma proteins
- Protein-losing kidney diseases
- Extensive burns

Decreased production of plasma proteins
- Liver disease
- Starvation, malnutrition

Increased Capillary Permeability

Inflammation
Allergic reactions (*e.g.,* hives, angioneurotic edema)
Malignancy (*e.g.,* ascites, pleural effusion)
Tissue injury and burns

Obstruction of Lymphatic Flow

Malignant obstruction of lymphatic structures
Surgical removal of lymph nodes

venous congestion. In right-sided heart failure, blood dams up throughout the entire venous system, causing organ congestion and edema of the dependent extremities. Decreased sodium and water excretion by the kidneys leads to an increase in extracellular volume, with an increase in capillary volume and pressure and subsequent movement of fluid into the tissue spaces. The swelling of hands and feet that occurs in healthy persons during hot weather results from vasodilation of superficial blood vessels along with sodium and water retention.

Because of the effects of gravity, edema resulting from increased capillary pressure commonly causes fluid to accumulate in the dependent parts of the body, a condition referred to as *dependent edema*. For example, edema of the ankles and feet becomes more pronounced during prolonged periods of standing.

Decreased Capillary Colloidal Osmotic Pressure. Plasma proteins exert the osmotic force needed to pull fluid back into the capillary from the tissue spaces. The plasma proteins constitute a mixture of proteins, including albumin, globulins, and fibrinogen. Albumin, the smallest of the plasma proteins, has a molecular weight of 69,000; globulins have molecular weights of approximately 140,000; and fibrinogen has a molecular weight of 400,000.[2] Because of its lower molecular weight, 1 g of albumin has approximately twice as many osmotically active molecules as 1 g of globulin and almost six times as many osmotically active molecules as 1 g of fibrinogen. Also, the concentration of albumin (approximately 4.5 g/dL) is greater than that of the globulins (2.5 g/dL) and fibrinogen (0.3 mg/dL).

Edema due to decreased capillary colloidal osmotic pressure usually is the result of inadequate production or abnormal loss of plasma proteins, mainly albumin. The plasma proteins are synthesized in the liver. In persons with severe liver failure, impaired synthesis of albumin results in a decrease in colloidal osmotic pressure. In starvation and malnutrition, edema develops because there is a lack of amino acids needed in plasma protein synthesis.

The most common site of plasma protein loss is the kidney. In kidney diseases such as nephrosis, the glomerular capillaries become permeable to the plasma proteins, particularly albumin, which is the smallest of the proteins. When this happens, large amounts of albumin are filtered out of the blood and lost in the urine. An excessive loss of plasma proteins also occurs when large areas of skin are injured or destroyed. Edema is a common problem during the early stages of a burn, resulting from capillary injury and loss of plasma proteins.

Because the plasma proteins are evenly distributed throughout the body and are not affected by the force of gravity, edema due to a decrease in capillary colloidal osmotic pressure tends to affect tissues in nondependent as well as dependent parts of the body. There is swelling of the face as well as the legs and feet.

Increased Capillary Permeability. When the capillary pores become enlarged or the integrity of the capillary wall is damaged, capillary permeability is increased. When this happens, plasma proteins and other osmotically active particles leak into the interstitial spaces, increasing the tissue colloidal osmotic pressure and thereby contributing to the accumulation of interstitial fluid. Among the conditions that increase capillary permeability are burn injury, capillary congestion, inflammation, and immune responses.

Obstruction of Lymph Flow. Osmotically active plasma proteins and other large particles that cannot be reabsorbed through the pores in the capillary membrane rely on the lymphatic system for movement back into the circulatory system. Edema due to impaired lymph flow is commonly referred to as *lymphedema*. Malignant involvement of lymph structures and removal of lymph nodes at the time of cancer surgery are common causes of lymphedema. Another cause of lymphedema is infection involving the lymphatic channels and lymph nodes.

Manifestations. The effects of edema are determined largely by its location. Edema of the brain, larynx, or lungs is an acute, life-threatening condition. Although not life threatening, edema may interfere with movement, limiting joint motion. Swelling of the ankles and feet often is insidious in onset and may or may not be associated with disease. At the tissue level, edema increases the distance for diffusion of oxygen, nutrients, and wastes. Edematous tissues usually are more susceptible to injury and development of ischemic tissue damage, including pressure ulcers. Edema can also compress blood vessels. The skin of a severely swollen finger can act as a tourniquet, shutting off the blood flow to the finger. Edema can also be disfiguring, causing psychological effects and disturbances in self-concept. Edema often causes a distortion of body features and creates problems in obtaining proper-fitting clothing and shoes.

Pitting edema occurs when the accumulation of interstitial fluid exceeds the absorptive capacity of the tissue gel. In this form of edema, the tissue water becomes mobile and can be translocated with pressure exerted by a finger. Nonpitting edema usually reflects a condition in which plasma proteins have accumulated in the tissue spaces and coagulated. The area often is firm and discolored. Brawny edema is a type of nonpitting edema in which the skin thickens and hardens. Nonpitting edema most frequently is seen after local infection or trauma.

Assessment and Treatment. Methods for assessing edema include daily weight, visual assessment, measurement of the affected part, and application of finger pressure to assess for pitting edema. Daily weight performed at the same time each day with the same amount of clothing provides a useful index of water gain (1 L of water weighs 2.2 pounds) due to edema. Visual inspection and measurement of the circumference of an extremity can also be used to assess the degree of swelling. This is particularly useful when swelling is due to thrombophlebitis. Finger pressure can be used to assess the degree of pitting edema. If an indentation remains after the finger has been removed, pitting edema is identified. It is evaluated on a scale of +1 (minimal) to +4 (severe) (Fig. 33-6).

Treatment of edema usually is directed toward maintaining life when the swelling involves vital structures, correcting or controlling the cause, and preventing tissue

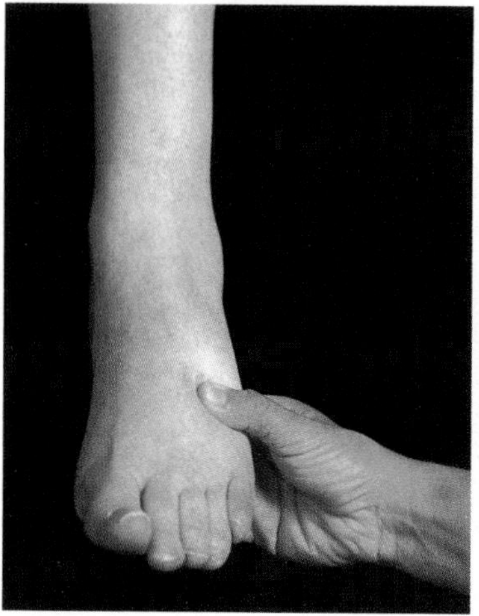
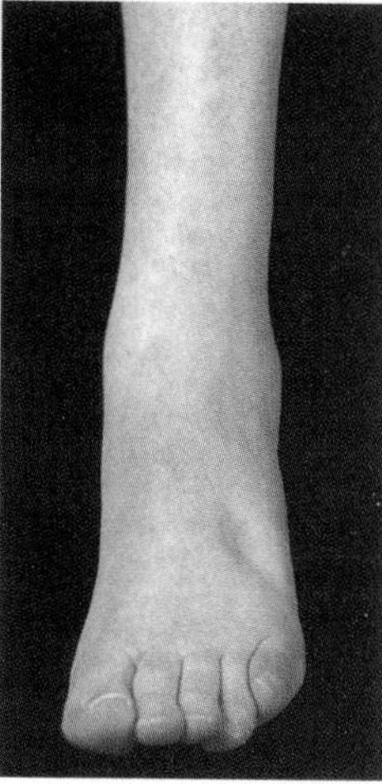

FIGURE 33-6 3 + pitting edema of the left foot. (Used with permission from Bates B. [1995]. *Bates' guide to physical examination and history taking* [6th ed., p. 438]. Philadelphia: Lippincott Williams & Wilkins)

injury. Diuretic therapy commonly is used to treat edema. Edema of the lower extremities may respond to simple measures such as elevating the feet.

Elastic support stockings and sleeves increase interstitial fluid pressure and resistance to outward movement of fluid from the capillary into the tissue spaces. These support devices typically are prescribed for patients with conditions such as lymphatic or venous obstruction and are most efficient if applied before the tissue spaces have filled with fluid—in the morning, for example, before the effects of gravity have caused fluid to move into the ankles.

Serum albumin levels can be measured, as can the colloidal osmotic pressure of the plasma (normally approximately 25.4 mm Hg). Albumin can be administered intravenously to raise the plasma colloidal osmotic pressure when edema is caused by hypoalbuminemia.

Third-Space Accumulation

Third spacing represents the loss or trapping of ECF into the transcellular space. The serous cavities are part of the transcellular compartment (*i.e.*, third-space) located in strategic body areas where there is continual movement of body structures—the pericardial sac, the peritoneal cavity, and the pleural cavity. The exchange of ECF between the capillaries, the interstitial spaces, and the transcellular space of the serous cavity uses the same mechanisms as capillaries elsewhere in the body. The serous cavities are closely linked with lymphatic drainage systems. The milking action of the moving structures, such as the lungs, continually forces fluid and plasma proteins back into the circulation, keeping these cavities empty. Any obstruction to lymph flow causes fluid accumulation in the serous cavities. As with edema fluid, third-space fluids represent an accumulation or trapping of body fluids that contribute to body weight but not to fluid reserve or function.

The prefix *hydro-* may be used to indicate the presence of excessive fluid, as in *hydrothorax,* which means excessive fluid in the pleural cavity. The accumulation of fluid in the peritoneal cavity is called *ascites*. The transudation of fluid into the serous cavities is also referred to as *effusion.* Effusion can contain blood, plasma proteins, inflammatory cells (*i.e.,* pus), and ECF.

In summary, body fluids are distributed between the ICF and ECF compartments of the body. Two thirds of body fluids are contained in the body cells of the ICF compartment, and one third is contained in the vascular compartment, interstitial spaces, and third-space areas of the ECF compartment. Body fluids contain water, charged particles called *electrolytes,* and noncharged particles called *nonelectrolytes.* ICF has high concentrations of potassium, calcium, phosphates, and magnesium, and ECF has high concentrations of sodium, chloride, and bicarbonate. Electrolytes and nonelectrolytes move by diffusion across cell membranes that separate the ICF and ECF compartments. Water moves by osmosis across semipermeable membranes, moving from the side of the membrane that has the lesser number of particles and greater concentration of water to the side that has the greater number of particles and lesser concentration of water. The osmotic tension or effect that a solution exerts on cell volume in terms of causing the cell to swell or shrink is called *tonicity.*

ICF volume is regulated by the large numbers of proteins and other inorganic solutes that cannot cross the cell's membrane and solutes such as sodium, potassium, and glucose that selectively move between the ICF and ECF dependent on concentration gradients and transport mechanisms. ECF volume, which is distributed between the vascular and interstitial compartments, is regulated by the elimination of sodium and water by the kidney.

Edema represents an increase in interstitial fluid volume. The physiologic mechanisms that predispose to edema formation are increased capillary filtration pressure, decreased capillary colloidal osmotic pressure, increased capillary permeability, and obstruction of lymphatic flow. The effect that edema exerts on body function is determined by its location; cerebral edema can be a life-threatening situation, but swollen feet can be a normal discomfort that accompanies hot weather. Fluid can also accumulate in the transcellular compartment—the joint spaces, pericardial sac, peritoneal cavity, and pleural cavity. Because this fluid is not easily exchanged with the rest of the ECF, it is often referred to as third-space fluid.

Sodium and Water Balance

After you have completed this section of the chapter, you should be able to meet the following objectives:

- State the functions and physiologic mechanisms controlling body water levels and sodium concentration
- Describe the relationship between body water and the extracellular sodium concentration
- Describe measures that can be used in assessing sodium concentration and body fluid levels
- Compare and contrast the causes, manifestations, and treatment of isotonic fluid volume deficit, isotonic fluid

volume excess, hyponatremia with water excess, and hypernatremia with water deficit
- Describe the causes, manifestations, and treatment of psychogenic polydipsia
- Describe the relationship between antidiuretic hormone and aquaporin-2 in water reabsorption in the kidney
- Compare the pathology, manifestations, and treatment of diabetes insipidus and the syndrome of inappropriate antidiuretic hormone

The movement of body fluids between the ICF and ECF compartments occurs at the cell membrane and depends on regulation of ECF water and sodium. Water provides approximately 90% to 93% of the volume of body fluids and sodium salts approximately 90% to 95% of extracellular solutes. Normally, equivalent changes in sodium and water are such that the volume and osmolality of ECF are maintained within a normal range. Because it is the concentration of sodium (in milligrams per liter) that controls ECF osmolality, changes in sodium are usually accompanied by proportionate changes in water volume.

Protection of the circulatory volume can be viewed as the single most important characteristic of body fluid homeostasis. In situations in which multiple physiologic variables are threatened simultaneously, the homeostatic response protects the vascular volume even at the expense of aggravating another electrolyte disorder.[4] For example, a volume-depleted person who is given water but no sodium retains water and becomes hyponatremic as a means of avoiding circulatory collapse. Two mechanisms protect the ECF (and vascular fluid) volume: (1) alterations in hemodynamic variables such as vasoconstriction and an increase in heart rate, and (2) alterations in sodium and water balance. Both mechanisms serve to maintain filling of the vascular compartment. Tachycardia, peripheral arterial vasoconstriction, and venoconstriction occur within minutes of external fluid losses, whereas salt and water retention take hours to become effective.

WATER BALANCE

- Protection of blood volume and filling of the vascular compartment can be viewed as the single most important characteristic of body fluid homeostasis.
- Two homeostatic mechanisms protect the vascular volume component of the extracellular fluid compartment: (1) the immediate recruitment of hemodynamic responses such as increased heart rate and vasoconstriction that function to maintain blood flow to vital organs, and (2) more long-term alterations in sodium and water balance that function to restore extracellular fluid volume.
- In situations where multiple physiologic functions are threatened simultaneously, homeostatic mechanisms strive to protect the volume of the vascular compartment at the expense of aggravating other electrolyte disorders.

Alterations of sodium and water balance can be divided into two main categories: (1) isotonic contraction or expansion of ECF volume, and (2) hypotonic dilution (dilutional hyponatremia) or hypertonic concentration (hypernatremia) of extracellular sodium brought about by changes in extracellular water (Fig. 33-7). Isotonic disorders usually are confined to the ECF compartment producing a contraction (fluid volume deficit) or expansion (fluid volume excess) of the interstitial and vascular fluids. Disorders of sodium concentration produce a change in the osmolality of the ECF with movement of water from the ECF compartment into the ICF compartment (hyponatremia) or from the ICF compartment into the ECF fluid compartment (hypernatremia) (Fig. 33-8).

REGULATION OF SODIUM BALANCE

Sodium is the most abundant cation in the body, averaging approximately 60 mEq/kg of body weight.[5] Most of the body's sodium is in the ECF compartment (135 to 145 mEq/L), with only a small amount (10 to 14 mEq/L) located in the ICF compartment. The resting cell membrane is relatively impermeable to sodium. Sodium that enters the cell is transported out of the cell against an electrochemical gradient by the energy-dependent Na^+/K^+-ATPase membrane pump.

Sodium functions mainly in regulating extracellular and vascular volume. As the major cation in the ECF compartment, Na^+ and its attendant anions (Cl^- and HCO_3^-) account for approximately 90% to 95% of the osmotic activity in the ECF. Because sodium is part of the sodium bicarbonate molecule, it is important in regulating acid-base balance. As a current-carrying ion, Na^+ contributes to the function of the nervous system and other excitable tissue.

Gains and Losses

Sodium normally enters the body through the gastrointestinal tract and is eliminated by the kidneys or lost from the gastrointestinal tract or skin. Sodium intake normally is derived from dietary sources. Body needs for sodium usually can be met by as little as 500 mg/day. In the United States, the average salt intake is approximately 6 to 15 g/day, or 12 to 30 times the daily requirement. Dietary intake, which frequently exceeds the amount needed by the body, is often influenced by culture and food preferences rather than need. As package labels indicate, many commercially prepared foods and soft drinks contain considerable amounts of sodium. Other sources of sodium are intravenous saline infusions and medications that contain sodium. An often-forgotten source of sodium is the sodium bicarbonate or other sodium-containing home remedies or over-the-counter medications used to treat upset stomach or other ailments.

Most sodium losses occur through the kidney. The kidneys are extremely efficient in regulating sodium output, and when sodium intake is limited or conservation of sodium is needed, the kidneys are able to reabsorb almost all the sodium that has been filtered by the glomerulus. This results in an essentially sodium-free urine. Conversely, urinary losses of sodium increase as intake increases.

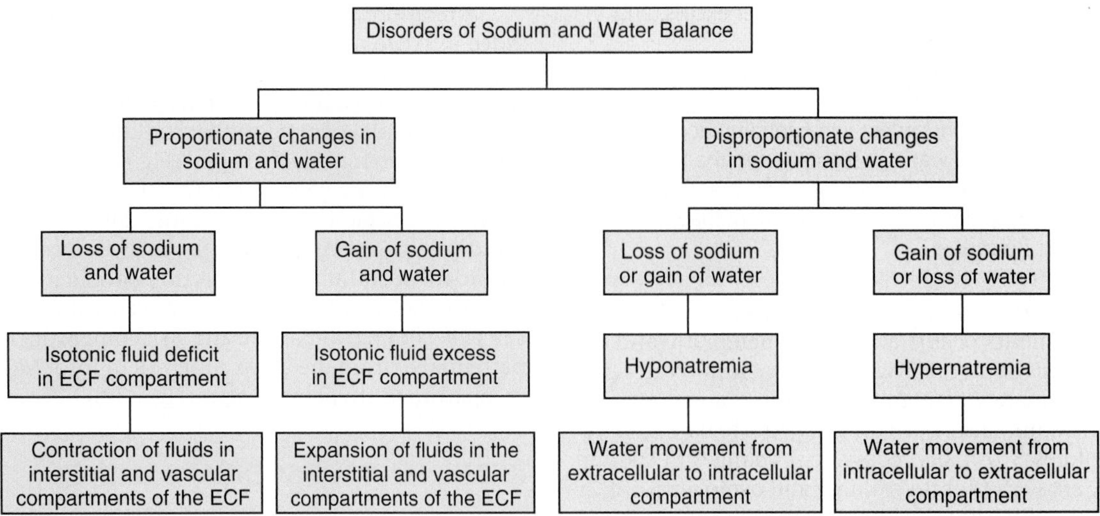

FIGURE 33-7 The effect of proportionate and disproportionate changes in sodium and water balance on extracellular sodium concentration.

Usually, less than 10% of sodium intake is lost through the gastrointestinal tract and skin. Although the sodium concentration of fluids in the upper part of the gastrointestinal tract approaches that of the ECF, sodium is reabsorbed as the fluids move through the lower part of the bowel, so that the concentration of sodium in the stool is only approximately 40 mEq/L. Sodium losses increase with conditions such as vomiting, diarrhea, fistula drainage, and gastrointestinal suction that remove sodium from the upper gastrointestinal tract. Irrigation of gastrointestinal tubes with distilled water removes sodium from the gastrointestinal tract, as do repeated tap-water enemas.

Excessive amounts of sodium can also be lost through the skin. Sweat losses, which usually are negligible, can in-

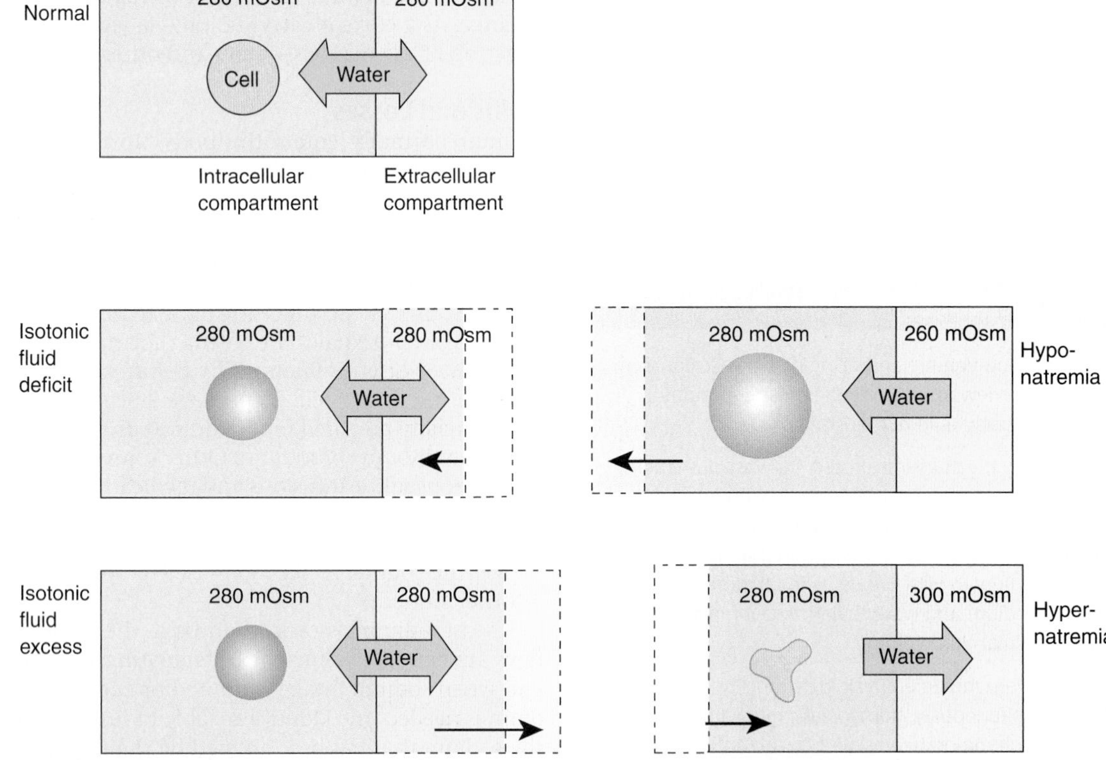

FIGURE 33-8 The effect of isotonic fluid volume excess and deficit and of hyponatremia and hypernatremia on movement of water between the extracellular and intracellular fluid compartment.

SODIUM BALANCE

- Water provides about 90% to 93% of the volume of body fluids and sodium salts approximately 90% to 95% of the solutes in the extracellular compartment. Together they serve to regulate the distribution of fluid between the intracellular and extracellular compartments.
- All gains or losses of sodium and water occur through the extracellular fluid compartment.
- Isotonic changes in body fluids that result from proportionate gains or losses of sodium and water are largely confined to the extracellular compartment.
- In contrast, changes in the tonicity of extracellular fluid brought about by disproportionate losses or gains of sodium or water are transmitted to the intracellular compartment, causing water to move into or out of body cells.

crease greatly during exercise and periods of exposure to a hot environment. A person who sweats profusely can lose as much as 15 to 30 g of sodium per day. Fortunately, this amount decreases to as little as 3 to 5 g/day with acclimatization to the heat.[2] Loss of skin integrity, such as occurs in extensive burns, also leads to excessive skin losses of sodium.

Mechanisms of Regulation

The kidney is the main regulator of sodium. The kidney monitors arterial pressure and retains sodium when arterial pressure is decreased and eliminates it when arterial pressure is increased. The rate at which the kidney excretes or conserves sodium is coordinated by the sympathetic nervous system and the renin-angiotensin-aldosterone system (RAAS). Another possible regulator of sodium excretion by the kidney is atrial natriuretic peptide (ANP), which is released from cells in the atria of the heart. ANP, which is released in response to atrial stretch and overfilling, increases sodium excretion by the kidney (see Chapter 32). Although ANP acts at several sites in the kidney to increase sodium excretion, its role in regulating sodium balance remains uncertain.[3]

The Sympathetic Nervous System. The sympathetic nervous system responds to changes in arterial pressure and blood volume by adjusting the glomerular filtration rate and thus the rate at which sodium is filtered from the blood. Sympathetic activity also regulates tubular reabsorption of sodium and renin release.

The Renin-Angiotensin-Aldosterone System. The RAAS exerts its action through angiotensin II and aldosterone. Renin is a small protein enzyme that is released by the kidney in response to changes in arterial pressure, the glomerular filtration rate, and the amount of sodium in the tubular fluid. Most of the renin that is released leaves the kidney and enters the bloodstream, where it interacts enzymatically to convert a circulating plasma protein called *angiotensinogen* to angiotensin I (see Chapter 25, Fig. 25-5). Angiotensin I is rapidly converted to angiotensin II by the angiotensin-converting enzyme in the small blood vessels of the lung. Angiotensin II acts directly on the renal tubules to increase sodium reabsorption. It also acts to constrict renal blood vessels, thereby decreasing the glomerular filtration rate and slowing renal blood flow so that less sodium is filtered and more is reabsorbed. Angiotensin II is also a powerful regulator of aldosterone, a hormone secreted by the adrenal cortex. Aldosterone acts at the level of the cortical collecting tubules of the kidneys to increase sodium reabsorption while increasing potassium elimination.

The sodium-retaining action of aldosterone can be inhibited by blocking the actions of aldosterone with potassium-sparing diuretics (*e.g.*, spironolactone, amiloride, triamterene, and eplerenone), by suppressing renin release (*e.g.*, β-adrenergic blockers), by inhibiting the conversion of angiotensin I to angiotensin II (*e.g.*, angiotensin-converting enzyme inhibitors), or by blocking the action of angiotensin II on the angiotensin receptor (angiotensin II receptor blockers [ARBs], *e.g.*, losartan, valsartan, irbesartan, and candesartan).[6]

REGULATION OF WATER BALANCE

Total body water (TBW) varies with gender and weight. These differences can be explained by differences in body fat, which is essentially water free. In men, body water approximates 60% of body weight during young adulthood and decreases to approximately 50% in old age; in young women, it is approximately 50%, and in elderly women, approximately 40%.[7] Obesity produces further decreases in body water, sometimes reducing these levels to values as low as 30% to 40% of body weight in adults (Fig. 33-9).

Infants and young children have a greater water content than adults. TBW constitutes approximately 75% to

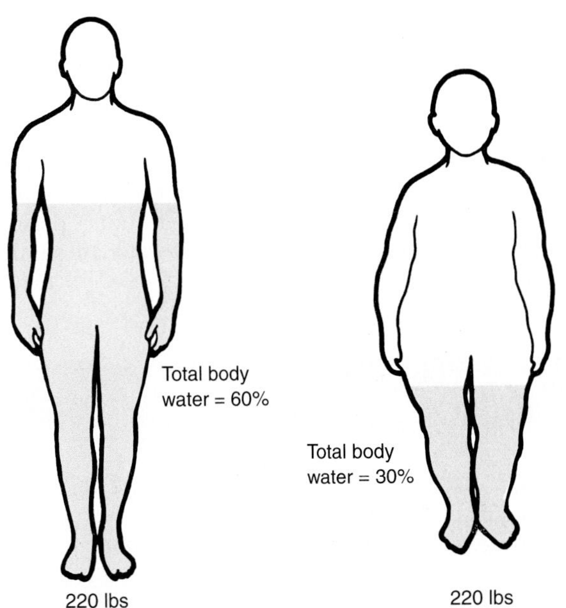

FIGURE 33-9 Body composition of a lean and an obese individual. (Adapted with permission from Statland H. [1963]. *Fluids and electrolytes in practice* [3rd ed.]. Philadelphia: J. B. Lippincott)

80% of body weight in full-term infants and is even greater in premature infants. In addition to having proportionately more body water than adults have, infants have relatively more water in their ECF compartment and a greater water turnover. Infants have more than half of their TBW in the ECF compartment, whereas adults have only approximately one third.[8] The greater ECF water content and water turnover of an infant can be explained in terms of its higher metabolic rate, larger surface area in relation to body mass, and its inability to concentrate its urine because of immature kidney structures. Because ECF is more readily lost from the body, infants are more vulnerable to fluid deficit than are older children and adults. As an infant grows older, TBW decreases, and by the second year of life, the percentages and distribution of body water approach those of an adult.[8]

Gains and Losses

Regardless of age, all healthy persons require approximately 100 mL of water per 100 calories metabolized for dissolving and eliminating metabolic wastes. This means that a person who expends 1800 calories for energy requires approximately 1800 mL of water for metabolic purposes. The metabolic rate increases with fever; it rises approximately 12% for every 1°C (7% for every 1°F) increase in body temperature.[2] Fever also increases the respiratory rate, resulting in additional loss of water vapor through the lungs.

The main source of water gain is through oral intake and metabolism of nutrients. Water, including that obtained from liquids and solid foods, is absorbed from the gastrointestinal tract. Tube feedings and parenterally administered fluids are also a source of water gain. Metabolic processes also generate a small amount of water. The amount of water gained from these processes varies from 150 to 300 mL/day, depending on metabolic rate.

Normally, the largest loss of water occurs through the kidneys, with lesser amounts being lost through the skin, lungs, and gastrointestinal tract. Even when oral or parenteral fluids are withheld, the kidneys continue to produce urine as a means of ridding the body of metabolic wastes. The urine output that is required to eliminate these wastes is called the *obligatory urine output.* The obligatory urine loss is approximately 300 to 500 mL/day. Water losses that occur through the skin and lungs are referred to as *insensible water losses* because they occur without a person's awareness. The gains and losses of body water are summarized in Table 33-2.

TABLE 33-2 Sources of Body Water Gains and Losses in the Adult

Gains		Losses	
Oral intake		Urine	1500 mL
As water	1000 mL	Insensible losses	
In food	1300 mL	Lungs	300 mL
Water of oxidation	200 mL	Skin	500 mL
		Feces	200 mL
Total	2500 mL	Total	2500 mL

Mechanisms of Regulation

There are two main physiologic mechanisms that assist in regulating body water: thirst and antidiuretic hormone (ADH). Thirst is primarily a regulator of water intake and ADH a regulator of water output. Both mechanisms respond to changes in extracellular osmolality and volume (Fig. 33-10).

Thirst. Like appetite and eating, thirst and drinking behavior are two separate entities.[9] Thirst is a conscious sensation of the need to obtain and drink fluids high in water content. Drinking of water or other fluids often occurs as the result of habit or for reasons other than those related to thirst. Most people drink without being thirsty, and water is consumed before it is needed. As a result, thirst is basically an emergency response. It usu-

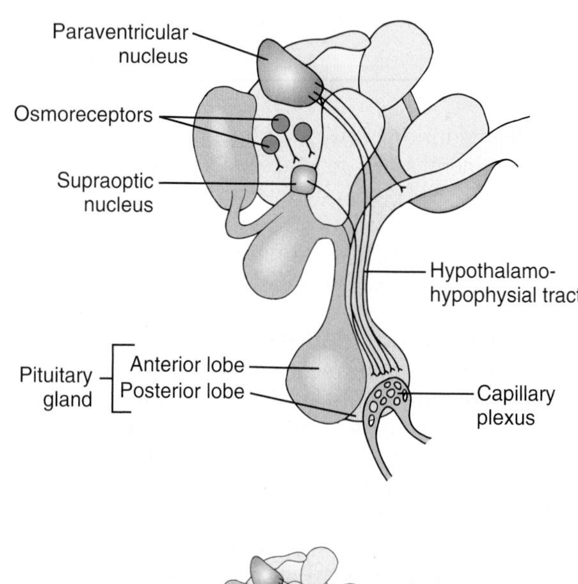

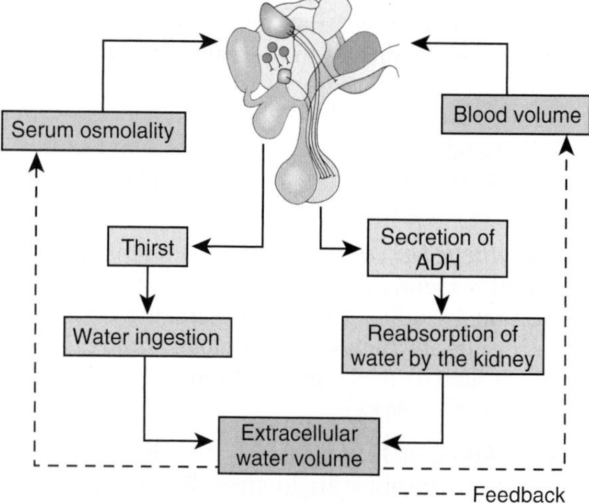

FIGURE 33-10 (Top) Sagittal section through the pituitary and anterior hypothalamus. Antidiuretic hormone (ADH) is formed primarily in the supraoptic nucleus and to a lesser extent in the paraventricular nucleus of the hypothalamus. It is then transported down the hypothalamohypophysial tract and stored in secretory granules in the posterior pituitary, where it can be released into the blood. **(Bottom)** Pathways for regulation of extracellular water volume by thirst and antidiuretic hormone.

ally occurs only when the need for water has not been anticipated.

Thirst is controlled by the thirst center in the hypothalamus. There are two stimuli for true thirst based on water need: (1) cellular dehydration caused by an increase in extracellular osmolality, and (2) a decrease in blood volume, which may or may not be associated with a decrease in serum osmolality. Sensory neurons, called *osmoreceptors,* which are located in or near the thirst center in the hypothalamus, respond to changes in extracellular osmolality by swelling or shrinking (see Fig. 33-10). Thirst normally develops when there is as little as a 1% to 2% change in serum osmolality.[10] Stretch receptors in the vascular system that are sensitive to changes in arterial blood pressure (high-pressure baroreceptors located in the carotid sinus and aorta) and central blood volume (low-pressure baroreceptors located in the left atrium and major thoracic veins) also aid in the regulation of thirst. Thirst is one of the earliest symptoms of hemorrhage and is often present before other signs of blood loss appear.

Dryness of the mouth, such as the thirst a lecturer experiences during speaking, produces a sensation of thirst that is not necessarily associated with the body's hydration status. Thirst sensation also occurs in those who breathe through their mouths, such as smokers and persons with chronic respiratory disease or hyperventilation syndrome.

A third important stimulus for thirst is angiotensin II, which becomes increased in response to low blood volume and low blood pressure. The renin-angiotensin mechanism contributes to nonosmotic thirst. This system is considered a backup system for thirst should other systems fail. Because it is a backup system, it probably does not contribute to the regulation of normal thirst. However, elevated levels of angiotensin II may lead to thirst in conditions, such as chronic renal failure and congestive heart failure, in which renin levels may be elevated. Thirst and elevated renin levels are also found in persons with primary hyperaldosteronism and in those with secondary hyperaldosteronism accompanying anorexia nervosa, hemorrhage, and sodium depletion.

Adipsia and Hypodipsia. Adipsia represents an absence, and hypodipsia a decrease, in the ability to sense thirst. There is evidence that thirst is decreased and water intake reduced in elderly persons, despite higher plasma sodium and osmolality levels.[11–12] The inability to perceive and respond to thirst is compounded in elderly persons who have had a stroke and may be further influenced by confusion and sensory disturbances.

Polydipsia. Polydipsia, or excessive thirst, is normal when it accompanies conditions of water deficit. Increased thirst and drinking behavior can be classified into three categories: symptomatic or true thirst, inappropriate or false thirst that occurs despite normal levels of body water and serum osmolality, and compulsive water drinking. Symptomatic thirst develops when there is a loss of body water and resolves after the loss has been replaced. Among the most common causes of symptomatic thirst are water losses associated with diarrhea, vomiting, diabetes mellitus, and diabetes insipidus. Inappropriate or excessive thirst may persist despite adequate hydration. It is a common complaint in persons with renal failure and congestive heart failure. Although the cause of thirst in these persons is unclear, it may result from increased angiotensin levels. Thirst is also a common complaint in persons with dry mouth caused by decreased salivary function or treatment with drugs with an anticholinergic action (*e.g.,* antihistamines, atropine) that lead to decreased salivary flow.

Psychogenic polydipsia involves compulsive water drinking and is usually seen in persons with psychiatric disorders, most commonly schizophrenia. Persons with the disorder drink large amounts of water and excrete large amounts of urine. The cause of excessive water drinking in these persons is uncertain. It has been suggested that the compulsive water drinking may share the same pathology as the psychosis because persons with the disorder often increase their water drinking during periods of exacerbation of their psychotic symptoms.[13] The condition may be compounded by antipsychotic medications that increase ADH levels and interfere with water excretion by the kidneys. Cigarette smoking, which is common among persons with psychiatric disorders, also stimulates ADH secretion.

Excessive water ingestion coupled with impaired water excretion (or rapid ingestion at a rate that exceeds renal excretion) in persons with psychogenic polydipsia can lead to water intoxication (see Hyponatremia).

Treatment usually consists of water restriction and behavioral measures aimed at decreasing water consumption. Measurements of body weight can be used to provide an estimate of water consumption.[14]

Antidiuretic Hormone. The reabsorption of water by the kidneys is regulated by ADH, also known as *vasopressin.* ADH is synthesized by cells in the supraoptic and paraventricular nuclei of the hypothalamus[15] (see Fig. 33-10). ADH from neurons in the supraoptic and paraventricular nuclei is transported along a neural pathway (*i.e.,* hypothalamo-hypophysial tract) to the neurohypophysis (*i.e.,* posterior pituitary) and then stored for future release.

ADH exerts its effects through two types of vasopressin (V) receptors—V_1 and V_2 receptors. V_1 receptors, which are located in vascular smooth muscle, cause vasoconstriction—hence the name *vasopressin.* Although ADH can increase blood pressure through V_1 receptors, this response occurs only when ADH levels are very high. The V_2 receptors, which are located on the tubular cells of the cortical collecting duct, control water reabsorption by the kidney. Binding of ADH to the V_2 receptors increases water reabsorption by increasing the permeability of the collecting duct to water (*i.e.,* the antidiuretic effect). In the absence of ADH, the permeability of the collecting duct to water is very low, and reabsorption of water decreases, leading to polyuria.

The mechanism whereby ADH causes water reabsorption has recently been elucidated. ADH stimulates V_2 receptors (and through cyclic AMP) results in the movement of water channels known as aquaporins.[16] Aquaporin-2 water channels move from the cytoplasm of cells in the collecting duct to the luminal surface of these cells (see Chapter 32, Fig. 32-12). The aquaporin-2 channels then allow free movement of water from the tubular lumen into the cell along a concentration gradient. At the basolateral membrane, water exits the cell through aquaporin-3 and -4 water channels. The basolateral water channels are continually being synthesized and always present. However, in the absence of ADH, the aquaporin-2 channels readily move out of the apical membrane so that water is no longer transferred out of the collecting duct. The synthesis of aquaporin-2, as well as the movement in and out of the collecting duct membrane, is regulated by ADH stimulation.

As with thirst, ADH levels are controlled by extracellular volume and osmolality. Osmoreceptors in the hypothalamus sense changes in extracellular osmolality and stimulate the production and release of ADH. A small increase in serum osmolality of 1% is sufficient to cause ADH release.[17] Likewise, stretch receptors that are sensitive to changes in blood pressure and central blood volume aid in the regulation of ADH release. A blood volume decrease of 5% to 10% produces a maximal increase in ADH levels.[17] As with many other homeostatic mechanisms, acute conditions produce greater changes in ADH levels than do chronic conditions; long-term changes in blood volume or blood pressure may exist without affecting ADH levels.

The effect of changes in glucose concentration on ADH secretion depends on the presence or absence of insulin. In nondiabetic persons, insulin facilitates glucose entry into the osmoreceptors, rendering it an ineffective osmole. In contrast, glucose stimulates ADH secretion in persons with diabetes, presumably because insulin is required for glucose uptake by the osmoreceptors.[5]

Responsiveness to osmolality changes with age, with older persons being more responsive to changes in serum osmolality.[7] Osmoregulation is also altered in normal pregnancy and the menstrual cycle. Plasma sodium concentration normally falls by an average of 5 mEq/L and serum osmolality by 10 mOsm/kg within 5 to 8 weeks of conception, and then remains stable for the duration of pregnancy.[5] This change represents a resetting of the osmotic threshold for ADH and an increase in the ECF volume that accompanies pregnancy. Rapid catabolism of ADH (vasopressin) can also occur during pregnancy due to the production of a vasopressinase.[15] A decrease in plasma osmolality of 2 to 3 mOsm/kg occurs during the ovulatory luteal phase of the menstrual cycle in healthy young women.[5]

The abnormal synthesis and release of ADH occurs in a number of stress situations. Severe pain, nausea, trauma, surgery, certain anesthetic agents, and some analgesic drugs increase ADH levels. Nausea is a potent stimulus of ADH secretion; it can increase ADH levels 10 to 1000 times those required for maximal diuresis.[15] The stimulus is mediated by the chemoreceptor trigger zone in the medulla oblongata, which then relays the impulse to the supraoptic and paraventricular nuclei in the hypothalamus. Afferent input from the gastrointestinal tract also may be important in some circumstances. Among the drugs that affect ADH are nicotine, which stimulates its release, and alcohol, which inhibits it (Table 33-3). Two important conditions alter ADH levels: diabetes insipidus and inappropriate secretion of ADH.

TABLE 33-3 Drugs That Affect Antidiuretic Hormone Levels*

Drugs That Decrease ADH Levels/Action	Drugs That Increase ADH Levels/Action
Amphotericin B	Anticancer drugs (vincristine and cyclophosphamide)
Demeclocycline	Carbamazepine
Ethanol	Chlorpropamide
Foscarnet	Clofibrate
Lithium	General anesthetics (most)
Morphine antagonists	Narcotics (morphine and meperidine)
	Nicotine
	Nonsteroidal anti-inflammatory drugs
	Phenothiazine antipsychotic drugs
	Selective serotonin reuptake inhibitors
	Thiazide diuretics (chlorothiazide)
	Thiothixene (antipsychotic drug)
	Tricyclic antidepressants

ADH, antidiuretic hormone
*List not inclusive.

Diabetes Insipidus. Diabetes insipidus, which means "tasteless diabetes," as opposed to diabetes mellitus, or "sweet diabetes," is caused by a deficiency of or a decreased response to ADH. Diabetes insipidus is characterized by excessive urination of a dilute urine (polyuria, usually greater than 2 L/day) and polydipsia.

There are two types of diabetes insipidus: central or neurogenic diabetes insipidus, which occurs because of a defect in the synthesis or release of ADH, and nephrogenic diabetes insipidus, which occurs because the kidneys do not respond to ADH.[15,18] In neurogenic diabetes insipidus, loss of 75% to 80% of ADH-secretory neurons is necessary before polyuria becomes evident. Most persons with neurogenic diabetes insipidus have an incomplete form of the disorder and retain some ability to concentrate their urine. Temporary neurogenic diabetes insipidus may follow head injury or surgery near the hypothalamohypophysial tract. Nephrogenic diabetes insipidus is characterized by impairment of urine-concentrating ability and free-water conservation. It may occur as a genetic trait that affects the V_2 receptor that binds ADH or in the aquaporin-2 protein that forms the water channels in the collecting tubules. Other acquired causes of nephrogenic diabetes insipidus are drugs such as lithium[19] and electrolyte disorders such as potassium depletion or chronic hypercalcemia. Lithium and the electrolyte disorders are thought to interfere with the postreceptor actions of ADH on the permeability of the collecting ducts.

Persons with diabetes insipidus are unable to concentrate their urine during periods of water restriction; they excrete large volumes of urine, usually 3 to 20 L/day, depending on the degree of ADH deficiency or renal insensitivity to ADH. This large urine output is accompanied by excessive thirst. As long as the thirst mechanism is normal and fluid is readily available, there is little or no alteration in the fluid levels in persons with diabetes insipidus. The danger arises when the condition develops in someone who is unable to communicate the need for water or is unable to secure the needed water. In such cases, inadequate fluid intake rapidly leads to hypertonic dehydration and increased serum osmolality.

Diagnosis of diabetes insipidus usually starts by attempting to document the total 24-hour urine output. Also, it must be documented that an osmotic diuresis is not caused by glucose or such disorders as renal disease. Further evaluation is based on measurement of ADH levels along with plasma and urine osmolality before and after a period of fluid deprivation or hypertonic saline infusion. Persons with neurogenic diabetes insipidus do not increase their ADH levels in response to increased plasma osmolality. Another diagnostic approach is to conduct a carefully monitored trial of a pharmacologic form of ADH. Persons with nephrogenic diabetes insipidus do not respond to pharmacologic preparations of the hormone. When central diabetes insipidus is suspected, diagnostic methods such as skull x-ray studies and magnetic resonance imaging (MRI) of the pituitary-hypothalamic area are used to determine the cause of the disorder. MRI studies localize the normal posterior pituitary as a high-intensity signal on T_1-weighted images. Research reports indicate that the "bright spot" is related to the content of stored ADH. This high-intensity signal is present in most (but not all) normal subjects and is absent in most (but not all) patients with diabetes insipidus.[15]

The management of central diabetes insipidus depends on the cause and severity of the disorder. Many persons with incomplete neurogenic diabetes insipidus maintain near-normal water balance when permitted to ingest water in response to thirst. Pharmacologic preparations of ADH are available for persons who cannot be managed by conservative measures. The preferred drug for treating chronic diabetes insipidus is desmopressin acetate (DDAVP). It usually is given orally but is also available in parenteral and nasal forms. The oral antidiabetic agent chlorpropamide may be used to stimulate ADH release in partial neurogenic diabetes insipidus. It usually is reserved for special cases because of its ability to cause hypoglycemia. Both neurogenic and nephrogenic forms of the disorder respond partially to the thiazide diuretics (*e.g.,* hydrochlorothiazide). These diuretics are thought to act by increasing sodium excretion by the kidneys, which lowers the glomerular filtration rate and increases reabsorption of water in the proximal tubule.

Syndrome of Inappropriate Antidiuretic Hormone. The syndrome of inappropriate antidiuretic hormone (SIADH) results from a failure of the negative feedback system that regulates the release and inhibition of ADH.[20] In persons with this syndrome, ADH secretion continues even when serum osmolality is decreased; this causes marked retention of water in excess of sodium and dilutional hyponatremia (see Hyponatremia). An increase in the glomerular filtration rate resulting from an increased plasma volume causes further increases in sodium loss by suppressing the renin-angiotensin mechanism. Urine osmolality is high, and serum osmolality is low. Urine output decreases despite adequate or increased fluid intake. Hematocrit and the plasma sodium and BUN levels are all decreased because of the expansion of the ECF volume. The diagnosis of SIADH should only be considered if the five cardinal features are fulfilled: (1) hypotonic hyponatremia, (2) natriuresis, (3) urine osmolality in excess of plasma osmolality, (4) absence of edema and volume depletion, and (5) normal renal and adrenal function.[20]

SIADH can be caused by a number of conditions; however, the major causes are neoplasia, neurologic diseases, lung diseases, and a variety of pharmacologic agents. Tumors, particularly bronchogenic carcinomas and cancers of the lymphoid tissue, prostate, and pancreas, are known to produce and release ADH independent of normal hypothalamic control mechanisms. Other intrathoracic conditions, such as advanced tuberculosis, severe pneumonia, and positive-pressure breathing, also cause SIADH. The suggested mechanism for SIADH in positive-pressure ventilation is activation of baroreceptors (*e.g.,* aortic baroreceptors, cardiopulmonary receptors) that respond to marked changes in intrathoracic pressure. Disease and injury to the central nervous system (CNS) can cause direct pressure on or direct involvement of the hypothalamic–posterior pituitary structures. Examples include brain tumors, hydrocephalus, head injury, meningitis, and encephalitis. Other stimuli, such as surgery, pain, stress, and temperature changes, are capable of stimulating ADH release through the limbic system. Human immunodeficiency virus infection is frequently associated with SIADH. It has been reported that up to 35% of persons with acquired immunodeficiency syndrome who are admitted to the acute care setting have SIADH related to *Pneumocystis carinii* pneumonia, CNS infections, or malignancies.[21]

Drugs induce SIADH in different ways; some drugs are thought to increase hypothalamic production and release, and others are believed to act directly on the renal tubules to enhance the action of ADH.

SIADH may occur as a transient condition, as in a stress situation, or as a chronic condition, resulting from disorders such as lung tumors. The manifestations of SIADH are those of dilutional hyponatremia. The severity of symptoms usually is proportional to the extent of sodium depletion and water intoxication.

The treatment of SIADH depends on its severity. In mild cases, treatment consists of fluid restriction. If fluid restriction is not sufficient, diuretics such as mannitol and furosemide (Lasix) may be given to promote diuresis and free-water clearance. Lithium and the antibiotic demeclocycline inhibit the action of ADH on the renal collecting ducts and sometimes are used in treating the disorder. In cases of severe water intoxication, a hypertonic (*e.g.,* 3%) sodium chloride solution may be administered intravenously. New antagonists to the antidiuretic action of ADH (aquaretics) offer a new therapeutic approach.[20]

ALTERATIONS IN ISOTONIC FLUID VOLUME

Isotonic fluid volume disorders represent an expansion or contraction of the ECF brought about by proportionate changes in both sodium and water.

Isotonic Fluid Volume Deficit

Fluid volume deficit is characterized by a decrease in the ECF, including the circulating blood volume. The term *isotonic fluid volume deficit* is used to differentiate the type of fluid deficit in which there are proportionate losses in sodium and water from water deficit and the hyperosmolar state associated with hypernatremia. Unless other fluid and electrolyte imbalances are present, the concentration of plasma electrolytes remains essentially unchanged. When the effective circulating blood volume is compromised, the condition is often referred to as *hypovolemia.*

Causes. Isotonic fluid volume deficit results when water and electrolytes are lost in isotonic proportions (Table 33-4). It is almost always caused by a loss of body fluids and is often accompanied by a decrease in fluid intake. It can occur because of a loss of gastrointestinal fluids, polyuria, or sweating due to fever and exercise. Fluid intake may be reduced because of a lack of access to fluids, impaired thirst, unconsciousness, oral trauma, impaired swallowing, or neuromuscular problems that prevent fluid access.

In a single day, 8 to 10 L of ECF is secreted into the gastrointestinal tract. Most of it is reabsorbed in the ileum and proximal colon, and only approximately 150 to 200 mL/day is eliminated in the feces. Vomiting and diarrhea interrupt the reabsorption process and, in some situations, lead to increased secretion of fluid into the intestinal tract. In Asiatic cholera, death can occur within a matter of hours as the cholera organism causes excessive amounts of fluid to be secreted into the bowel. These fluids are then lost as vomitus or excreted as diarrheal fluid. Gastrointestinal suction, fistulas, and drainage tubes can remove large amounts of fluid from the gastrointestinal tract.

Excess sodium and water losses also can occur through the kidney. Certain forms of kidney disease are characterized by salt wasting due to impaired sodium reabsorption. Fluid volume deficit also can result from osmotic diuresis or injudicious use of diuretic therapy. Glucose in the urine filtrate prevents reabsorption of water by the renal tubules, causing a loss of sodium and water. In Addison disease, a condition of chronic adrenocortical insufficiency, there is unregulated loss of sodium in the urine with a resultant loss of ECF (see Chapter 42). This is accompanied by increased potassium retention.

The skin acts as an exchange surface for heat and as a vapor barrier to prevent water from leaving the body. Body surface losses of sodium and water increase when there is excessive sweating or when large areas of skin have been damaged. Hot weather and fever increase sweating. In hot weather, water losses through sweating may be increased by as much as 1 to 3 L/hour, depending on acclimatization.[2] The respiratory rate and sweating usually are in-

TABLE 33-4 Causes and Manifestations of Isotonic Fluid Volume Deficit

Causes	Manifestations
Inadequate Fluid Intake	**Acute Weight Loss (% body weight)**
Oral trauma or inability to swallow	Mild fluid volume deficit: 2%
Inability to obtain fluids (*e.g.*, impaired mobility)	Moderate fluid volume deficit: 2%–5%
Impaired thirst sensation	Severe fluid deficit: 8% or greater
Therapeutic withholding of fluids	**Compensatory Increase in Antidiuretic Hormone**
Unconsciousness or inability to express thirst	Decreased urine output
	Increased osmolality and specific gravity
Excessive Gastrointestinal Fluid Losses	**Increased Serum Osmolality**
Vomiting	Thirst
Diarrhea	Increased hematocrit and blood urea nitrogen
Gastrointestinal suction	
Draining gastrointestinal fistula	**Decreased Vascular Volume**
Excessive Renal Losses	Postural hypotension
Diuretic therapy	Tachycardia, weak and thready pulse
Osmotic diuresis (hyperglycemia)	Decreased vein filling and increased vein refill time
Adrenal insufficiency (Addison's disease)	Hypotension and shock
Salt-wasting kidney disease	
Excessive Skin Losses	**Decreased Extracellular Fluid Volume**
Fever	Depressed fontanel in an infant
Exposure to hot environment	Sunken eyes and soft eyeballs
Burns and wounds that remove skin	**Impaired Temperature Regulation**
Third-Space Losses	Elevated body temperature
Intestinal obstruction	
Edema	
Ascites	
Burns (first several days)	

creased as body temperature rises. As much as 3 L of water may be lost in a single day as a result of fever. Burns are another cause of excess fluid loss. Evaporative losses can increase 10-fold with severe burns, to 3 to 5 L/day.[2]

Third-space losses cause sequestering of ECF in the serous cavities, extracellular spaces in injured tissues, or lumen of the gut. Because the fluid remains in the body, fluid volume deficit caused by third spacing does not usually cause weight loss.

Manifestations. The manifestations of fluid volume deficit reflect a decrease in ECF volume. They include thirst, loss of body weight, signs of water conservation by the kidney, impaired temperature regulation, and signs of reduced interstitial and vascular volume (see Table 33-4).

A loss in fluid volume is accompanied by a decrease in body weight. One liter of water weighs 1 kg (2.2 lb). A mild ECF deficit exists when weight loss equals 2% of body weight. In a person who weighs 68 kg (150 lb), this percentage of weight loss equals 1.4 L of water. A moderate deficit equates to a 5% loss in weight and a severe deficit to an 8% or greater loss in weight.[8] To be accurate, weight must be measured at the same time each day with the person wearing the same amount of clothing. Because ECF is trapped in the body in persons with third-space losses, their body weight may not decrease.

Thirst is a common symptom of fluid deficit, although it is not always present in early stages of isotonic fluid deficit. It develops as the effective circulating volume decreases to a point sufficient to stimulate the thirst mechanism. Urine output decreases and urine osmolality and specific gravity increase as ADH levels rise because of a decrease in vascular volume. Although there is an isotonic loss of fluid from the vascular compartment, blood components such as red blood cells and BUN become more concentrated.

The fluid content of body tissues decreases as fluid is removed from the interstitial spaces. The eyes assume a sunken appearance and feel softer than normal as the fluid content in the anterior chamber of the eye is decreased. Fluids add resiliency to the skin and underlying tissues that is referred to as *skin* or *tissue turgor.* Tissue turgor is assessed by pinching a fold of skin between the thumb and forefinger. The skin should immediately return to its original configuration when the fingers are released. A loss of 3% to 5% of body water in children causes the resiliency of the skin to be lost, and the tissue remains raised for several seconds. Decreased tissue turgor is less predictive of fluid deficit in older persons (>65 years of age) because of the loss of tissue elasticity. In infants, fluid deficit may be evidenced by depression of the anterior fontanel due to a decrease in cerebrospinal fluid. There may be a rise in body temperature that accompanies fluid volume deficit. Interstitial fluids insulate the body against changes in the external temperature, and vascular fluids transport heat from the inner core of the body to the periphery, where it can be released into the external environment.

Arterial and venous volumes decline during periods of fluid deficit, as does filling of the capillary circulation. As the volume in the arterial system declines, the blood pressure decreases, heart rate increases, and the pulse becomes weak and thready. Postural hypotension is an early sign of fluid deficit, characterized by a blood pressure that is at least 10 mm Hg lower when the patient is sitting or standing than when the patient is lying down. When volume depletion becomes severe, signs of hypovolemic shock and vascular collapse appear (see Chapter 28). On the venous side of the circulation, the veins become less prominent, and venous refill time increases.

Diagnosis and Treatment. Diagnosis of fluid volume deficit is based on a history of conditions that predispose to sodium and water losses, weight loss, and observations of altered physiologic function indicative of decreased fluid volume. Intake and output measurements afford a means for assessing fluid balance. Although these measurements provide insight into the causes of fluid imbalance, they often are inadequate in measuring actual losses and gains because accurate measurements of intake and output often are difficult to obtain, and insensible losses are difficult to estimate.

Measurement of heart rate and blood pressure provides useful information about vascular volume. A simple test to determine venous refill time consists of compressing the distal end of a vein on the dorsal aspect of the hand when it is not in the dependent position. The vein is then emptied by "milking" the blood toward the heart. The vein should refill almost immediately when the occluding finger is removed. When venous volume is decreased, as occurs in fluid deficit, venous refill time increases. Capillary refill time is also increased. Capillary refill can be assessed by applying pressure to a fingernail for 5 seconds and then releasing the pressure and observing the time (normally 1 to 2 seconds) that it takes for the color to return to normal.[8]

Treatment of fluid volume deficit consists of fluid replacement and measures to correct the underlying cause. Usually, isotonic electrolyte solutions are used for fluid replacement. Acute hypovolemia and hypovolemic shock can cause renal damage; therefore, prompt assessment of the degree of fluid deficit and adequate measures to resolve the deficit and treat the underlying cause are essential (see Chapter 28).

Isotonic Fluid Volume Excess

Fluid volume excess represents an isotonic expansion of the ECF compartment. It occurs secondary to an increase in total body sodium, which in turn leads to an increase in body water. Fluid volume excess involves an increase in interstitial and vascular volumes. Although increased fluid volume is usually the result of a disease condition, this is not always true. For example, a compensatory isotonic expansion of body fluids can occur in healthy persons during hot weather as a mechanism for increasing body heat loss.

Causes. Isotonic fluid volume excess almost always results from an increase in total body sodium that is accompanied by a proportionate increase in body water. Although it can occur as the result of excessive sodium intake, it is most commonly caused by a decrease in sodium and water elimination by the kidney. Among the causes of decreased sodium and water elimination are disorders of renal function, heart failure, liver failure, and corticosteroid excess (Table 33-5).

Heart failure produces a decrease in renal blood flow and a compensatory increase in sodium and water retention (see Chapter 28). Persons with severe congestive heart failure maintain a precarious balance between sodium and water intake and output. Even small increases in sodium intake can precipitate a state of fluid volume excess and a worsening of heart failure. A condition called *circulatory overload* results from an increase in intravascular blood volume; it can occur during infusion of intravenous fluids or transfusion of blood if the amount or rate of administration is excessive. Elderly persons and those with heart disease require careful observation because even small amounts of intravenous fluid or blood may overload the circulatory system. Liver failure (*e.g.*, cirrhosis of the liver) impairs aldosterone metabolism and alters renal perfusion, leading to increased salt and water retention.

Cushing's syndrome is a condition of glucocorticoid excess (see Chapter 42). Because cortisol, the most active of the glucocorticoids, has weak mineralocorticoid activity, Cushing's syndrome predisposes to increased sodium retention. The fact that cortisol increases salt and water retention also helps to explain why edema and hypertension may develop in persons who are being treated with corticosteroid drugs.

Manifestations. Isotonic fluid volume excess is manifested by an increase in interstitial and vascular fluids. It is characterized by weight gain over a short period of time. Mild fluid volume excess represents a 2% gain in weight; moderate fluid volume excess, a 5% gain in weight; and severe fluid volume excess, a gain of 8% or more in weight[8] (see Table 33-5). Edema is characteristic of isotonic fluid excess. When the fluid excess accumulates gradually, as often happens in debilitating diseases and starvation, edema fluid may mask the loss of tissue mass. The edema associated with ECF excess may be generalized, or it may be confined to dependent areas of the body, such as the legs and feet. The eyelids often are puffy when the person awakens. There may be a decrease in BUN and hematocrit as a result of dilution due to expansion of the plasma volume. An increase in vascular volume may be evidenced by distended neck veins, slow-emptying peripheral veins, a full and bounding pulse, and an increase in central venous pressure. When excess fluid accumulates in the lungs (*i.e.*, pulmonary edema), there are complaints of shortness of breath and difficult breathing, respiratory crackles, and a productive cough (see Chapter 28). Ascites and pleural effusion may occur with severe fluid volume excess.

Diagnosis and Treatment. Diagnosis of fluid volume excess is usually based on a history of factors that predispose to sodium and water retention, weight gain, and manifestations such as edema and cardiovascular symptoms indicative of an expanded ECF volume.

The treatment of fluid volume excess focuses on providing a more favorable balance between sodium and water intake and output. A sodium-restricted diet is often prescribed as a means of decreasing extracellular sodium and water levels. Diuretic therapy is commonly used to increase sodium elimination. When there is a need for intravenous fluid administration or transfusion of blood components, the procedure requires careful monitoring to prevent fluid overload.

ALTERATIONS IN SODIUM CONCENTRATION

The normal plasma concentration of sodium ranges from 135 to 145 mEq/L (135 to 145 mmol/L). Plasma sodium values reflect the sodium concentration (or dilution of sodium by extracellular water) expressed in milliequivalents or millimoles per liter, rather than an absolute amount. Because sodium and its attendant anions account for 90% to 95% of the osmolality of ECF, serum osmolality (normal

TABLE 33-5 Causes and Manifestations of Isotonic Fluid Volume Excess

Causes	Manifestations
Inadequate Sodium and Water Elimination	**Acute Weight Gain (% body weight)**
Congestive heart failure	Mild fluid volume excess: 2%
Renal failure	Moderate fluid volume excess: 5%
Increased corticosteroid levels	Severe fluid volume excess: 8% or greater
Hyperaldosteronism	**Increased Interstitial Fluid Volume**
Cushing's disease	Dependent and generalized edema
Liver failure (*e.g.*, cirrhosis)	**Increased Vascular Volume**
Excessive Sodium Intake in Relation to Output	Full and bounding pulse
Excessive dietary intake	Venous distention
Excessive ingestion of sodium-containing medications or home remedies	Pulmonary edema
Excessive administration of sodium-containing parenteral fluids	Shortness of breath
Excessive Fluid Intake in Relation to Output	Crackles
Ingestion of fluid in excess of elimination	Dyspnea
Administration of parenteral fluids or blood at an excessive rate	Cough

range, 275 to 295 mOsm/kg) usually changes with changes in plasma sodium concentration.

Hyponatremia

Hyponatremia represents a decrease in plasma sodium concentration below 135 mEq/L (135 mmol/L). Unlike hypernatremia, which is always associated with hypertonicity, hyponatremia may be associated with high, normal, or low tonicity because of the effects of other osmotically active particles in the ECF such as glucose.[20–23]

Hypertonic (translocational) hyponatremia results from an osmotic shift of water from ICF to the ECF as occurs with hyperglycemia. In this case, the sodium in the ECF becomes diluted as water moves out of cells in response to the osmotic effects of the elevated blood glucose level. There is approximately a 1.7mEq/L decrease in plasma sodium for every 100 mg/dL rise in plasma glucose above the normal level (100 mg/dL).[22] A normotonic hyponatremia, termed *pseudohyponatremia,* can be detected in plasma samples from persons with hyperlipidemia and hyperproteinemia because of laboratory methods. This disturbance is caused by laboratory methods that include excess lipids or proteins in the water volume of the sample, causing an artifactual dilution of sodium. The increased availability of direct measurement of plasma sodium by ion-specific electrodes has helped to eliminate this laboratory artifact.

Hypotonic (dilutional) is by far the most common form of hyponatremia. It is caused by water retention and characterized by a decrease in serum osmolality. Dilutional hyponatremia can present as a hypervolemic, euvolemic, or hypovolemic condition. Hypervolemic hyponatremia involves an increase in ECF volume and is seen when hyponatremic conditions are accompanied by edema-forming disorders such as congestive heart failure, cirrhosis, and advanced kidney disease.

Euvolemic hyponatremia represents a retention of water with dilution of sodium while maintaining the ECF volume within a normal range. It is usually the result of inappropriate thirst or SIADH. Hypovolemic hyponatremia occurs when water is lost along with sodium, but to a lesser extent. It occurs with diuretic use, excessive sweating in hot weather, and vomiting and diarrhea.

Causes. Hypotonic, or dilutional, hyponatremia represents a decreased sodium concentration and tonicity of the ECF (Table 33-6). The most common causes of acute dilutional hyponatremia in adults are drug therapy (diuretics and drugs that increase ADH levels), inappropriate fluid replacement during heat exposure or following heavy exercise, SIADH, and polydipsia in persons with psychotic disorder.

Among the causes of hypovolemic hyponatremia is the loss of salt and water from excessive sweating in hot weather, particularly during heavy exercise; hyponatremia develops when water rather than electrolyte-containing liquids is used to replace the fluids lost in sweating. Another potential cause of hypovolemic hyponatremia is the loss

TABLE 33-6 Causes and Manifestations of Hyponatremia

Causes	Manifestations
Excessive Sodium Losses and Replacement with Tap Water or Sodium-Free Losses	**Laboratory Values**
Exercise- or heat-induced sweating and replacement with sodium-free fluids	Serum sodium level below 135 mEq/L (135 mmol/L)
Gastrointestinal losses	Decreased serum osmolality
Vomiting, diarrhea	Dilution of blood components, including hematocrit, blood urea nitrogen
Renal losses	**Signs Related to Hypo-osmolality of Extracellular Fluids and Movement of Water Into Brain Cells and Neuromuscular Tissue**
Diuresis	Muscle cramps
Excessive Water Intake in Relation to Output	Weakness
Excessively diluted infant formula	Headache
Excessive administration of sodium-free parenteral solutions	Depression
Repeated irrigation of body cavities with sodium-free solutions	Apprehension, feeling of impending doom
Irrigation of gastrointestinal tube with distilled water	Personality changes
Tap water enemas	Lethargy
Use of nonelectrolyte irrigating solutions during prostate surgery	Stupor, coma
Kidney disorders that impair water elimination	**Gastrointestinal Manifestations**
Increased ADH levels	Anorexia, nausea, vomiting
Trauma, stress, pain	Abdominal cramps, diarrhea
Syndrome of inappropriate ADH	**Increased Intracellular Fluid**
Use of medications that increase ADH	Fingerprint edema
Psychogenic polydipsia	

ADH, antidiuretic hormone

of sodium from the gastrointestinal tract due to repeated tap-water enemas or frequent gastrointestinal irrigations with distilled water. Iso-osmotic fluid loss, as in vomiting or diarrhea, does not usually lower plasma sodium levels unless these losses are replaced with disproportionate amounts of orally ingested or parenterally administered water. Gastrointestinal fluid loss and ingestion of excessively diluted formula are common causes of acute hyponatremia in infants and children.

Hypovolemic hyponatremia is a common complication of adrenal insufficiency and is due to the effects of aldosterone and cortisol deficiency (see Chapter 42). A lack of aldosterone increases renal losses of sodium, and a cortisol deficiency leads to increased release of ADH with water retention.

The risk for euvolemic hyponatremia is increased during the postoperative period. During this time, ADH levels are often high, producing an increase in water reabsorption by the kidney (see SIADH). Although these elevated levels usually resolve in about 72 hours, they can persist for up to 5 days. The hyponatremia becomes exaggerated when electrolyte-free fluids (*e.g.*, 5% glucose in water) are used for fluid replacement. Excessive water drinking during this period can also increase the risk for hyponatremia.

Manifestations. The manifestations of hypotonic hyponatremia are largely related to sodium dilution (see Table 33-6). Serum osmolality is decreased, and cellular swelling occurs owing to the movement of water from the ECF to the ICF compartment. The manifestations of hyponatremia depend on the rapidity of onset and the severity of the sodium dilution. The signs and symptoms may be acute, as in severe water intoxication, or more insidious in onset and less severe, as in chronic hyponatremia. Because of water movement, hyponatremia causes ICF hypo-osmolality, which is responsible for many of the clinical manifestations of the disorder.[23]

Fingerprint edema is a sign of excess intracellular water. This phenomenon is demonstrated by pressing the finger firmly over the bony surface of the sternum for 15 to 30 seconds. When excess intracellular water is present, a fingerprint similar to that observed when pressing on a piece of modeling clay is seen.

Muscle cramps, weakness, and fatigue reflect the hypo-osmolality of skeletal muscle cells and are often early signs of hyponatremia. These effects commonly are observed in persons with hyponatremia that occurs during heavy exercise in hot weather. Gastrointestinal manifestations such as nausea and vomiting, abdominal cramps, and diarrhea may develop. The brain and nervous system are the most seriously affected by increases in intracellular water. Symptoms include apathy, lethargy, and headache, which can progress to disorientation, confusion, gross motor weakness, and depression of deep tendon reflexes. Seizures and coma occur when plasma sodium levels reach extremely low levels. These severe effects, which are caused by brain swelling, may be irreversible.[23] If the condition develops slowly, signs and symptoms do not develop until plasma sodium levels approach 125 mEq/L. Progressive neurologic symptoms occur when the plasma sodium falls below this level. The term *water intoxication* is often used to describe the neurologic effects of acute hypotonic hyponatremia.

Diagnosis and Treatment. Diagnosis of hyponatremia is based on laboratory reports of decreased sodium concentration, the presence of conditions that predispose to sodium loss or water retention, and signs and symptoms indicative of the disorder.

The treatment of hyponatremia with water excess focuses on the underlying cause. When hyponatremia is caused by water intoxication, limiting water intake or discontinuing medications that contribute to SIADH may be sufficient. The administration of a saline solution orally or intravenously may be needed when hyponatremia is caused by sodium deficiency. Symptomatic hyponatremia (*i.e.*, neurologic manifestations) is often treated with hypertonic saline solution and a loop diuretic, such as furosemide, to increase water elimination. This combination allows for correction of plasma sodium levels while ridding the body of excess water.

There is concern about the rapidity with which plasma sodium levels are corrected, particularly in persons with chronic symptomatic hyponatremia. Cells, particularly those in the brain, tend to defend against changes in cell volume caused by increased ECF osmolality by synthesizing amino acids and other osmotically active organic solutes.[24] Because these solutes cannot cross the cell membrane, they confine their osmotic activity to the ICF compartment. In contrast to electrolytes and other solutes that disturb cell function and harm cells by altering the resting membrane potential or disrupting metabolic processes when they are present in large amounts, these organic osmoles have unique biochemical properties that allow them to accumulate in high concentrations without disrupting cell structure or function. In the case of prolonged water intoxication, brain cells reduce their concentration of organic osmoles as a means of preventing an increase in cell volume. It takes several days for brain cells to restore the organic osmoles lost during hyponatremia.[15] Rapid changes in serum osmolality when brain cells have already undergone volume regulation may cause a dramatic change in brain cell volume. One of the reported effects of rapid treatment of hyponatremia is an osmotic demyelinating condition called *central pontine myelosis,* which produces serious neurologic sequelae and sometimes causes death.[15,20]

Hypernatremia

Hypernatremia implies a plasma sodium level above 145 mEq/L and a serum osmolality greater than 295 mOsm/kg. Because sodium is functionally an impermeable solute, it contributes to tonicity and induces movement of water across cell membranes. Hypernatremia is characterized by hypertonicity of ECF and almost always causes cellular dehydration.[25]

Causes. Hypernatremia represents a deficit of water in relation to the body's sodium stores. It can be caused by net loss of water or sodium gain. Net water loss can occur through the urine, gastrointestinal tract, lungs, or skin. A defect in thirst or inability to obtain or drink water can interfere with water replacement. Rapid ingestion or infusion of sodium with insufficient time or opportunity for water ingestion can produce a disproportionate gain in sodium (Table 33-7).

Hypernatremia almost always follows a loss of body fluids that have a lower than normal concentration of sodium, so that water is lost in excess of sodium. This can result from increased losses from the respiratory tract during fever or strenuous exercise, from watery diarrhea, or when osmotically active tube feedings are given with inadequate amounts of water. With pure water loss, each body fluid compartment loses an equal percentage of its volume. Because approximately one third of the water is in the extracellular compartment, compared with the two thirds in the intracellular compartment, more actual water volume is lost from the ICF than the ECF compartment.[7]

Normally, water deficit stimulates thirst and increases water intake. Therefore, hypernatremia is more likely to occur in infants and in persons who cannot express their thirst or obtain water to drink. With hypodipsia, or impaired thirst, the need for fluid intake does not activate the thirst response. Hypodipsia is particularly prevalent among the elderly population. In persons with diabetes insipidus, hypernatremia can develop when thirst is impaired or access to water is impeded. The therapeutic administration of sodium-containing solutions may also cause hypernatremia. For example, the administration of sodium bicarbonate during cardiopulmonary resuscitation increases body sodium levels because the sodium concentration of each 50-mL ampule of 7.5% sodium bicarbonate contains 892 mEq of sodium.[5] Hypertonic saline solution intended for intraamniotic instillation for therapeutic abortion may inadvertently be injected intravenously, causing hypernatremia. Rarely, salt intake occurs rapidly, as in taking excess salt tablets or during near-drowning in salt water.

Manifestations. The clinical manifestations of hypernatremia caused by water loss are largely those of ECF loss and cellular dehydration (see Table 33-7). The severity of signs and symptoms is greatest when the increase in plasma sodium is large and occurs rapidly. Body weight is decreased in proportion to the amount of water that has been lost. Because blood plasma is roughly 90% to 93% water, the concentrations of blood cells and other blood components increase as ECF water decreases.

Thirst is an early symptom of water deficit, occurring when water losses are equal to 0.5% of body water. Urine output is decreased and urine osmolality increased because of renal water-conserving mechanisms. Body temperature frequently is elevated, and the skin becomes warm and flushed. The vascular volume decreases, the pulse becomes rapid and thready, and the blood pressure drops. Hypernatremia produces an increase in serum osmolality

TABLE 33-7 Causes and Manifestations of Hypernatremia

Causes	Manifestations
Excessive Water Losses	**Laboratory Values**
Watery diarrhea	Serum sodium level above 145 mEq/L (145 mmol/L)
Excessive sweating	Increased serum osmolality
Increased respirations due to conditions such as tracheobronchitis	Increased hematocrit and blood urea nitrogen
Hypertonic tube feedings	**Thirst and Signs of Increased ADH Levels**
Diabetes insipidus	Polydipsia
Decreased Water Intake	Oliguria or anuria
Unavailability of water	High urine specific gravity
Oral trauma or inability to swallow	**Intracellular Dehydration**
Impaired thirst sensation	Dry skin and mucous membranes
Withholding water for therapeutic reasons	Decreased tissue turgor
Unconsciousness or inability to express thirst	Tongue rough and fissured
Excessive Sodium Intake	Decreased salivation and lacrimation
Rapid or excessive administration of sodium-containing parenteral solutions	**Signs Related to Hyperosmolality of Extracellular Fluids and Movement of Water Out of Brain Cells**
Near-drowning in salt water	Headache
	Agitation and restlessness
	Decreased reflexes
	Seizures and coma
	Extracellular Dehydration and Decreased Vascular Volume
	Tachycardia
	Weak and thready pulse
	Decreased blood pressure
	Vascular collapse

and results in water being pulled out of body cells. As a result, the skin and mucous membranes become dry, and salivation and lacrimation are decreased. The mouth becomes dry and sticky, and the tongue becomes rough and fissured. Swallowing is difficult. The subcutaneous tissues assume a firm, rubbery texture. Most significantly, water is pulled out of the cells in the CNS, causing decreased reflexes, agitation, headache, and restlessness. Coma and seizures may develop as hypernatremia progresses.

Diagnosis and Treatment. The diagnosis of hypernatremia is based on history, physical examination findings indicative of dehydration, and results of laboratory tests. The treatment of hypernatremia includes measures to treat the underlying cause of the disorder and fluid replacement therapy to treat the accompanying dehydration. Replacement fluids can be given orally or intravenously. The oral route is preferable. Oral glucose–electrolyte replacement solutions are available for the treatment of infants with diarrhea.[26–28] Until recently, these solutions were used only early in diarrheal illness or as a first step in reestablishing oral intake after parenteral replacement therapy. These solutions are now widely available in grocery stores and pharmacies for use in the treatment of diarrhea and other dehydrating disorders in infants and young children. They are particularly important in developing countries, where the availability of intravenous fluids is limited, and diarrhea is a leading cause of death among children.

The composition of the oral rehydration solution recommended by the Diarrheal Disease Control Center of the World Health Organization (WHO) contains glucose (2.0 g/L), sodium (90 mEq/L), potassium (20 mEq/L), chloride (80 mEq/L), and bicarbonate (30 mEq/L).[27] It is recommended that ingredients be supplied in preweighed packets. Using teaspoons or other household items for measuring the ingredients often is inaccurate and is not recommended. Glucose is preferred to sucrose (*i.e.,* table sugar), which is a disaccharide and must be broken down before it can be absorbed. Commercially available preparations usually contain less sodium and chloride (*e.g.,* 45 to 50 mEq/L of sodium, 35 to 45 mEq/L of chloride) than the WHO formulation, with citrate being substituted for bicarbonate. Although cola drinks commonly are recommended as a remedy for dehydration caused by acute diarrhea, their electrolyte content often is inadequate for replacement purposes, and their high sugar content may complicate the situation by inducing an osmotic diarrhea.[27,29] Sport drinks usually contain more sodium and sugar than the oral rehydration solutions. Intravenous replacement solutions continue to be the treatment of choice for severe fluid deficit.

One of the serious aspects of fluid volume deficit is dehydration of brain and nerve cells. Serum osmolality should be corrected slowly in cases of chronic hypernatremia. This is because brain cells synthesize osmotically active organic solutes to protect against volume changes. These organic solutes serve to produce a gradual increase in intracellular osmolality, allowing osmotic flow of water back into the cell and restoring cell volume. This response begins within 4 to 6 hours of increased serum osmolality and takes several days to become fully effective.[5] Changes in brain water content are greatest during acute hypernatremia but only slightly reduced in chronic hypernatremia. If hypernatremia is corrected too rapidly before the organic osmoles have had a chance to dissipate, the plasma may become relatively hypotonic in relation to brain cell osmolality. When this occurs, water moves into the brain cells, causing cerebral edema and potentially severe neurologic impairment.

In summary, body fluids are distributed between the ICF and ECF compartments. Regulation of fluid volume, solute concentration, and distribution between the two compartments depends on water and sodium balance. Water provides approximately 90% to 93% of fluid volume, and sodium salts approximately 90% to 95% of ECF solutes. Body water is regulated by thirst, which controls water intake, and by ADH, which controls urine concentration and renal output. Sodium is largely regulated by the kidney under the influence of the sympathetic nervous system and the RAAS.

Alterations of salt and water balance can be divided into two main categories: (1) isotonic contraction or expansion of ECF volume brought about by proportionate losses of sodium and water, and (2) hypotonic dilution (dilutional hyponatremia) or hypertonic concentration (hypernatremia) of extracellular sodium brought about by disproportionate increases or decreases in extracellular water.

Isotonic fluid volume deficit is characterized by a reduction in ECF volume. It causes thirst, decreased vascular volume and circulatory function, decreased urine output, and increased urine specific gravity. Isotonic fluid volume excess is characterized by an increase in ECF volume. It is manifested by signs of increased vascular volume and edema.

Alterations in ECF sodium concentration are brought about by a disproportionate gain (hyponatremia) or loss (hypernatremia) of water. As the major cation in the ECF compartment, sodium controls the ECF osmolality and its effect on cell volume. Hypotonic hyponatremia is characterized by water being pulled into the cell from the ECF compartment, causing cells to swell. It is manifested by muscle cramps and weakness; nausea, vomiting, abdominal cramps, and diarrhea; and CNS signs such as lethargy, headache, depression of deep tendon reflexes, and in severe cases, seizure and coma. Hypernatremia is characterized by ICF water being pulled into the ECF compartment, causing cells to shrink. It is manifested by thirst and decreased urine output; dry mouth and decreased tissue turgor; signs of decreased vascular volume (tachycardia, weak and thready pulse); and CNS signs such as decreased reflexes, agitation, headache, and in severe cases, seizures and coma.

Potassium Balance

After you have completed this section of the chapter, you should be able to meet the following objectives:

- Characterize the distribution of potassium in the body and explain how extracellular potassium levels are regulated in relation to body gains and losses

- State the causes of hypokalemia and hyperkalemia in terms of altered intake, output, and transcellular shifts
- Relate the functions of potassium to the manifestations of hypokalemia and hyperkalemia
- Describe methods of diagnosis and treatment of hypokalemia and hyperkalemia

REGULATION OF POTASSIUM BALANCE

Potassium is the second most abundant cation in the body and the major cation in the ICF compartment. Approximately 98% of body potassium is contained within body cells, with an intracellular concentration of 140 to 150 mEq/L.[30] The potassium content of the ECF (3.5 to 5.0 mEq/L) is considerably less. Because potassium is an intracellular ion, total body stores of potassium are related to body size and muscle mass. In adults, total body potassium ranges from 50 to 55 mmol/kg of body weight.[31] Approximately 65% to 75% of potassium is in muscle.[32] Thus, potassium content declines with age, mainly as a result of a decrease in muscle mass.

Gains and Losses

Potassium intake is normally derived from dietary sources. In healthy persons, potassium balance usually can be maintained by a daily dietary intake of 50 to 100 mEq. Additional amounts of potassium are needed during periods of trauma and stress. The kidneys are the main source of potassium loss. Approximately 80% to 90% of potassium losses occur in the urine, with the remainder being lost in stools or sweat.

Mechanisms of Regulation

Normally, the ECF concentration of potassium is precisely regulated at about 4.2 mEq/mL. The precise control is necessary because many cell functions are sensitive to even small changes in ECF potassium levels. An increase in potassium of only 0.3 to 0.4 mEq/L can cause serious cardiac dysrhythmias and even death.

Plasma potassium is largely regulated through two mechanisms: (1) renal mechanisms that conserve or eliminate potassium, and (2) a transcellular shift between the intracellular and extracellular compartments. Normally, it takes 6 to 8 hours to eliminate 50% of potassium intake.[5] To avoid an increase in ECF potassium during this time, excess potassium is temporarily shifted in cells such as those of muscle, liver, red blood cells, and bone.

Renal Regulation. The major route for potassium elimination is the kidney. Unlike other electrolytes, the regulation of potassium elimination is controlled by secretion from the blood into the tubular filtrate rather than through reabsorption from the tubular filtrate into the blood. Potassium is filtered in the glomerulus, reabsorbed along with sodium and water in the proximal tubule and with sodium and chloride in the thick ascending loop of Henle, and then secreted into the late distal and cortical collecting tubules for elimination in the urine. The latter mechanism serves to "fine-tune" the concentration of potassium in the ECF.

> **POTASSIUM BALANCE**
>
> - Potassium is mainly an intracellular ion with only a small, but vital, amount being present in the extracellular fluids.
> - The distribution of potassium between the intracellular and extracellular compartments regulates electrical membrane potentials controlling the excitability of nerve and muscle cells as well as contractility of skeletal, cardiac, and smooth muscle tissue.
> - Because of its vital role in regulating neuromuscular excitability, potassium regulation must be extremely efficient. Even a 1% to 2% addition of potassium to the extracellular fluid compartment can elevate serum levels to dangerously high levels.
> - Two major mechanisms function in the control of serum potassium: (1) renal mechanisms that conserve or eliminate potassium, and (2) transcellular buffer systems that remove potassium from and release it into the serum as needed. Conditions that disrupt the function of either mechanism can result in serious alteration in serum potassium levels.

Aldosterone plays an essential role in regulating potassium elimination by the kidney. The effects of aldosterone on potassium elimination are mediated through a sodium–potassium exchange system located in the late distal and cortical collecting tubules of the kidney. In the presence of aldosterone, sodium is transported back into the blood, and potassium is secreted in the tubular filtrate for elimination in the urine. The rate of aldosterone secretion by the adrenal gland is strongly controlled by plasma potassium levels. For example, an increase of less than 1 mEq/L of potassium causes aldosterone levels to triple.[2] The effect of plasma potassium on aldosterone secretion is an example of the powerful feedback regulation of potassium elimination. In the absence of aldosterone, as occurs in persons with Addison disease, renal elimination of potassium is impaired, causing plasma potassium levels to rise to dangerously high levels. Aldosterone is often referred to as a *mineralocorticoid hormone* because of its effect on sodium and potassium. The term *mineralocorticoid activity* also is used to describe the aldosterone-like actions of other adrenocortical hormones, such as cortisol.

There is also a potassium–hydrogen ion exchange mechanism in the cortical collecting tubules of the kidney (see Chapter 32). When plasma potassium levels are increased, potassium ions (K^+) are secreted into the urine, and hydrogen ions (H^+) are reabsorbed into the blood, producing a decrease in pH and metabolic acidosis. Conversely, when potassium levels are low, K^+ ions are reabsorbed, and H^+ ions are secreted in the urine, leading to metabolic alkalosis.

Extracellular–Intracellular Shifts. The transcellular shift of potassium between the ECF and ICF compartments allows potassium to move into body cells when plasma levels are high and move out when the plasma levels are low. This movement is controlled by the function of the Na^+/K^+-ATPase membrane pump and the permeability of ion channels in the cell membrane.

Both insulin and β-adrenergic catecholamines (*e.g.,* epinephrine) increase cellular uptake of potassium by increasing the activity of the Na^+/K^+-ATPase membrane pump (Fig. 33-11). Studies indicate that insulin deficiency impedes cellular uptake of potassium and that insulin excess increases uptake. The plasma potassium concentration directly affects insulin release from beta cells in the pancreas. An increase in potassium levels stimulates insulin release, and a decrease inhibits its release, suggesting a potassium–insulin regulatory feedback mechanism.[32,33] The catecholamines, particularly epinephrine, facilitate the movement of potassium into muscle tissue. The action of epinephrine on potassium transport is additive to that of insulin.

The osmolality of the ECF also influences transcellular shifts in potassium. Acute increases in serum osmolality cause potassium to move out of cells. When serum osmolality increases because of the presence of impermeable extracellular solutes such as mannitol or glucose (without insulin), water leaves the cell. The loss of cell water produces an increase in ICF potassium concentration, causing potassium to diffuse out of the cell. There is usually a 1.0- to 1.5-mEq/L rise in plasma potassium that occurs in response to an acute 10% increase in serum osmolality.[5] A hyperosmolality-induced increase in plasma potassium is usually counteracted by the opposing actions of insulin and epinephrine. The reverse condition, hypo-osmolality, usually occurs more slowly and does not affect plasma potassium levels.

The exchange of K^+ and H^+ ions between the ICF and ECF plays a significant role in regulating the ECF concentration of both ions. In acidosis, H^+ ions move into the cell as a means of preventing large changes in ECF pH. As H^+ ions move into the cell, other positively charged ions, such as K^+, must move out as a means of maintaining electrical neutrality. The plasma potassium concentration rises 0.7 mEq/L for each 0.1-unit fall in plasma pH.[5] The pH-related shifts in ICF to ECF potassium are more pronounced when changes in pH are caused by nonorganic acids (*i.e.,* hyperchloremic acidosis associated with diarrhea and renal failure), in which the companion anion, chloride, cannot permeate the cell membrane and remains outside the cell as a companion for the K^+ ion. In contrast, acidosis due to accumulation of organic acids (*i.e.,* lactic acidosis and ketoacidosis) has little effect on potassium because the companion anion is able to enter the cell. Although there is increased movement of potassium out of the cell in diabetic ketoacidosis, it is more likely related to the effects of insulin deficiency and the hyperosmolality of the ECF. Respiratory acidosis and alkalosis cause little change in plasma potassium concentration. Metabolic alkalosis tends to have a smaller opposite effect: H^+ ions move out of the cell as K^+ ions move in. Plasma potassium concentrations fall by approximately 0.3 mEq/L for each 0.1-unit increase in plasma pH.[5]

Exercise also produces compartmental shifts in potassium. Repeated muscle contraction releases potassium into the ECF. Although the increase usually is small with modest exercise, it can be considerable during exhaustive exercise. Even the repeated clenching and unclenching of the fist during a blood draw can cause potassium to move out of cells and artificially elevate plasma potassium levels.

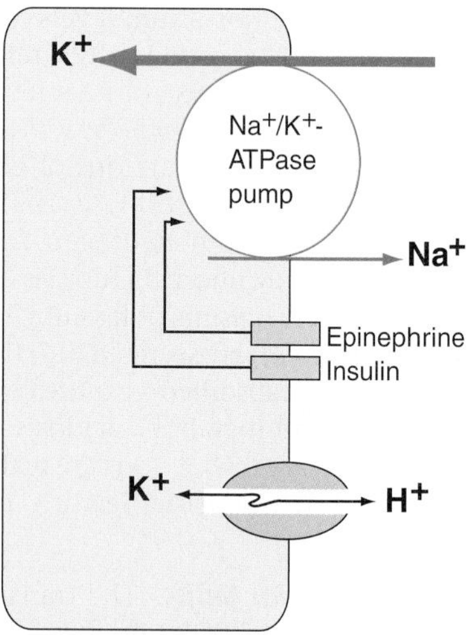

FIGURE 33-11 Mechanisms regulating transcellular shifts in potassium.

ALTERATIONS IN POTASSIUM BALANCE

As the major intracellular cation, potassium is critical to many body functions. It is involved in a wide range of body functions, including the maintenance of the osmotic integrity of cells, acid-base balance, and the kidney's ability to concentrate urine. Potassium is necessary for growth, and it contributes to the intricate chemical reactions that transform carbohydrates into energy, change glucose into glycogen, and convert amino acids to proteins. Potassium also plays a critical role in conducting nerve impulses and the excitability of skeletal, cardiac, and smooth muscle. It does this by regulating the resting membrane potential (see Chapter 4), the opening of the sodium channels that control the flow of current during the action potential, and the rate of membrane repolarization. Changes in nerve and muscle excitability are particularly important in the heart, where alterations in serum potassium can produce serious dysrhythmias and conduction defects. Changes in plasma potassium also affect skeletal muscles and the smooth muscle in blood vessels and the gastrointestinal tract.

The *resting membrane potential* is determined by the ratio of intracellular to extracellular potassium (Fig. 33-12). A decrease in serum potassium causes the resting membrane potential to become more negative (hyperpolarization), moving further from the threshold for excitation. Thus, it takes a greater stimulus to reach threshold and open the sodium channels that are responsible for the action potential. An increase in serum potassium has the opposite effect; it causes the resting membrane potential to become more positive (hypopolarized), moving closer

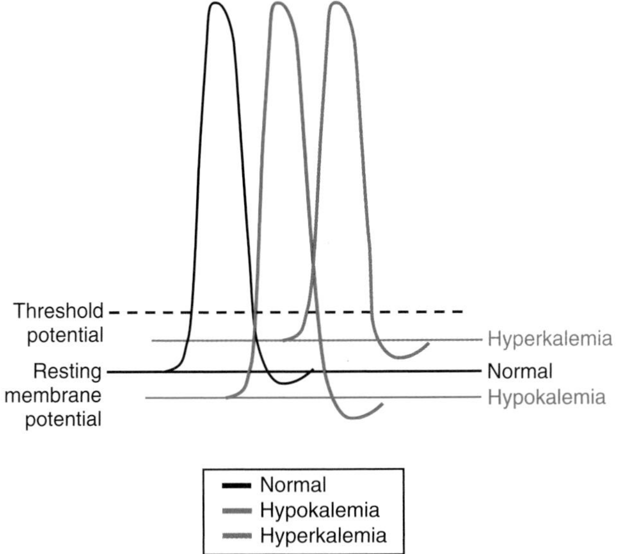

FIGURE 33-12 Effect of changes in serum hypokalemia (*red*) and hyperkalemia (*blue*) on the resting membrane potential, activation and opening of the sodium channels at threshold potential, and the rate of repolarization during a nerve action potential.

to threshold. The activation and opening of the sodium channels, which control the flow of current during an action potential, are also affected by potassium levels. With severe hyperkalemia, the resting membrane approaches the threshold potential, causing sustained subthreshold depolarization. This inactivates the sodium channels and produces a net decrease in excitability. The *rate of repolarization* also varies with plasma potassium levels. It is more rapid in hyperkalemia and delayed in hypokalemia. Both the inactivation of the sodium channels and the rate of membrane repolarization are important clinically because they predispose to conduction defects or dysrhythmias in the heart (see Chapter 27).

Hypokalemia

Hypokalemia refers to a decrease in plasma potassium levels below 3.5 mEq/L (3.5 mmol/L). Because of transcellular shifts, temporary changes in plasma potassium may occur as the result of movement between the ICF and ECF compartments.

Causes. The causes of potassium deficit can be grouped into three categories: (1) inadequate intake; (2) excessive gastrointestinal, renal, and skin losses; and (3) redistribution between the ICF and ECF compartments (Table 33-8).

TABLE 33-8 Causes and Manifestations of Hypokalemia

Causes	Manifestations
Inadequate Intake Diet deficient in potassium Inability to eat Administration of potassium-free parenteral solutions **Excessive Renal Losses** Diuretic therapy (except potassium-sparing diuretics) Diuretic phase of renal failure Increased mineralocorticoid levels Primary hyperaldosteronism Treatment with corticosteroid drugs **Excessive Gastrointestinal Losses** Vomiting Diarrhea Gastrointestinal suction Draining gastrointestinal fistula **Transcompartmental Shift** Administration of β-adrenergic agonist (*e.g.*, albuterol) Administration of insulin for treatment of diabetic ketoacidosis Alkalosis, metabolic or respiratory	**Laboratory Values** Serum potassium less than 3.5 mEq/L (3.5 mmol/L) **Impaired Ability to Concentrate Urine** Polyuria Urine with low osmolality and specific gravity Polydipsia **Gastrointestinal Manifestations** Anorexia, nausea, vomiting Abdominal distention Paralytic ileus **Neuromuscular Manifestations** Muscle flabbiness, weakness, and fatigue Muscle cramps and tenderness Paresthesias Paralysis **Cardiovascular Manifestations** Postural hypotension Increased sensitivity to digitalis toxicity Changes in electrocardiogram Cardiac dysrhythmias **Central Nervous System Manifestations** Confusion Depression **Acid-Base Disorders** Metabolic alkalosis

Inadequate Intake. *Inadequate intake* is a frequent cause of hypokalemia. A potassium intake of at least 10 to 30 mEq/day is needed to compensate for obligatory urine losses.[5,32] A person on a potassium-free diet continues to lose approximately 5 to 15 mEq of potassium daily. Insufficient dietary intake may result from the inability to obtain or ingest food or from a diet that is low in potassium-containing foods. Potassium intake is often inadequate in persons on fad diets and those who have eating disorders. Elderly persons are particularly likely to have potassium deficits. Many have poor eating habits as a consequence of living alone; they may have limited income, which makes buying foods high in potassium difficult; they may have difficulty chewing many foods that have a high potassium content because of poorly fitting dentures; or they may have problems with swallowing. Also, many medical problems in elderly persons require treatment with drugs, such as diuretics, that increase potassium losses.

Excessive Losses. The kidneys are the main source of potassium loss. Approximately 80% to 90% of potassium losses occur in the urine, with the remaining losses occurring in the stool and sweat. The kidneys do not have the homeostatic mechanisms needed to conserve potassium during periods of insufficient intake. After trauma and in stress situations, urinary losses of potassium are greatly increased, sometimes approaching levels of 150 to 200 mEq/L.[33] This means that a potassium deficit can develop rather quickly if intake is inadequate. Renal losses also can be increased by medications, metabolic alkalosis, magnesium depletion, and increased levels of aldosterone. Some antibiotics, particularly amphotericin B and gentamicin, are impermeable anions that require the presence of positively charged cations for elimination in the urine; this causes potassium wasting.

Diuretic therapy, with the exception of potassium-sparing diuretics, is the most common cause of hypokalemia. Both thiazide and loop diuretics increase the loss of potassium in the urine. The degree of hypokalemia is directly related to diuretic dose and is greater when sodium intake is higher.[32] Magnesium depletion causes renal potassium wasting. Magnesium deficiency often coexists with potassium depletion due to diuretic therapy or disease processes such as diarrhea. Importantly, the ability to correct potassium deficiency is impaired when magnesium deficiency is present.

Renal losses of potassium are accentuated by aldosterone and cortisol. Increased potassium losses occur in situations such as trauma and surgery that produce a stress-related increase in these hormones. Primary aldosteronism is caused by a tumor in the cells of the adrenal cortex (in the zona glomerulosa) that secrete aldosterone. Excess secretion of aldosterone by the tumor cells causes severe potassium losses and a decrease in plasma potassium levels. Licorice-induced hypokalemia results from inhibition of the enzyme that inactivates cortisol. Cortisol binds to aldosterone receptors and exerts aldosterone-like effects on potassium elimination.

Although potassium losses from the skin and the gastrointestinal tract usually are minimal, these losses can become excessive under certain conditions. For example, burns increase surface losses of potassium. Losses due to sweating increase in persons who are acclimated to a hot climate, partly because increased secretion of aldosterone during heat acclimatization increases the loss of potassium in urine and sweat. Gastrointestinal losses also can become excessive; this occurs with vomiting and diarrhea and when gastrointestinal suction is being used. The potassium content of liquid stools, for example, is approximately 40 to 60 mEq/L.

Transcellular Shifts. Because of the high ratio of intracellular to extracellular potassium, a redistribution of potassium from the ECF to the ICF compartment can produce a marked decrease in the plasma concentration (see Fig. 33-11). One cause of potassium redistribution is insulin. After insulin administration, there is increased movement of glucose and potassium into cells. This is one of the reasons that potassium deficit often develops during treatment of diabetic ketoacidosis. β-Adrenergic agonists, such as pseudoephedrine and albuterol, have a similar effect on potassium distribution. For example, a standard dose of nebulized albuterol (a bronchodilator) reduces plasma potassium by 0.2 to 0.4 mEq/L, and a second dose taken within 1 hour reduces it by almost 1 mEq/L.[32] Ingestion of excess doses of pseudoephedrine, an over-the-counter decongestant, can cause severe hypokalemia. Theophylline and caffeine, although not catecholamines, may increase Na^+/K^+-ATPase membrane pump activity by inhibiting phosphodiesterase. Severe hypokalemia is a common manifestation of theophylline toxicity.[32]

Manifestations. The manifestations of hypokalemia include alterations in renal, gastrointestinal, cardiovascular, and skeletal muscle function (see Table 33-8). These manifestations reflect both the intracellular functions of potassium as well as the body's attempt to regulate ECF potassium levels within the very narrow range needed to maintain the normal electrical activity of excitable tissues such as nerve and muscle cells. The signs and symptoms of potassium deficit seldom develop until the plasma potassium level has fallen below 3.0 mEq/L. They are typically gradual in onset; therefore, the disorder may go undetected for some time.

The renal processes that conserve potassium during hypokalemia interfere with the kidney's ability to concentrate urine. Urine output and plasma osmolality are increased, urine specific gravity is decreased, and complaints of polyuria, nocturia, and thirst are common. Metabolic alkalosis and renal chloride wasting are signs of severe hypokalemia.

There are numerous signs and symptoms associated with gastrointestinal function, including anorexia, nausea, and vomiting. Atony of the gastrointestinal smooth muscle can cause constipation, abdominal distention, and, in severe hypokalemia, paralytic ileus. When gastrointestinal symptoms occur gradually and are not severe, they often impair potassium intake and exaggerate the condition.

The most serious effects of hypokalemia are those affecting cardiovascular function. Postural hypotension is common. Digitalis toxicity can be provoked in persons treated with this drug, and there is an increased risk for ventricular dysrhythmias, particularly in persons with underlying heart disease. Potassium and digitalis compounds compete for binding to sites on the Na^+/K^+-ATPase membrane pump. In hypokalemia, more sites are available for digitalis to bind to and exert its action. The dangers associated with digitalis toxicity are compounded in persons who are receiving diuretics that increase urinary losses of potassium.

Most persons with plasma potassium levels below 3.0 mEq/L demonstrate electrocardiographic (ECG) changes typical of hypokalemia. These changes include prolongation of the PR interval, depression of the ST segment, flattening of the T wave, and appearance of a prominent U wave (Fig. 33-13). Normally, potassium leaves the cell during the repolarization phase of the action potential, returning the membrane potential to its normal resting value. Hypokalemia produces a decrease in potassium efflux that prolongs the rate of repolarization and lengthens the relative refractory period. The U wave normally may be present on the ECG but should be of lower amplitude than the T wave. With hypokalemia, the amplitude of the T wave decreases as the U-wave amplitude increases. Although these ECG changes usually are not serious, they may predispose to sinus bradycardia and ectopic ventricular dysrhythmias. The reader is referred to Chapter 27 for additional information on the ECG and cardiac dysrhythmias.

Complaints of weakness, fatigue, and muscle cramps, particularly during exercise, are common in moderate hypokalemia (plasma potassium, 3.0 to 2.5 mEq/L). Muscle paralysis with life-threatening respiratory insufficiency can occur with severe hypokalemia (plasma potassium <2.5 mEq/L). Leg muscles, particularly the quadriceps, are most prominently affected. Some persons complain of muscle tenderness and paresthesias rather than weakness. In chronic potassium deficiency, muscle atrophy may contribute to muscle weakness. At least three defects in skeletal muscle function occur with potassium deficiency: alterations in the resting membrane potential, alterations in glycogen synthesis and storage, and impaired ability to increase blood flow during strenuous exercise.[34] In hypokalemia, the resting membrane potential becomes more negative, resulting in a decrease in neuromuscular excitability (see Chapter 4). Normal concentrations of intracellular potassium are necessary for glycogen synthesis in muscle cells. Therefore, hypokalemia can interfere with muscle metabolism, especially under exercise conditions that rely heavily on anaerobic pathways that use glycogen as fuel. Potassium released from muscle normally contributes to the autoregulation of blood flow during exercise. Thus, potassium deficiency is thought to lead to impaired blood flow with increased risk for ischemic injury to muscle cells during intense physical exercise.[34]

In a rare condition called *hypokalemic familial periodic paralysis,* episodes of hypokalemia cause attacks of flaccid paralysis that last 6 to 48 hours if untreated.[3] The paralysis may be precipitated by situations that cause severe hypokalemia by producing an intracellular shift in potassium, such as ingestion of a high-carbohydrate meal or administration of insulin, epinephrine, or glucocorticoid drugs. The paralysis often can be reversed by potassium replacement therapy. A similar condition can occur with poorly controlled hyperthyroidism (thyrotoxic hypokalemic periodic paralysis), especially in Asian patients. Treatment is with potassium replacement and appropriate therapy for the underlying thyroid disorder.[35]

Treatment. When possible, hypokalemia caused by potassium deficit is treated by increasing the intake of foods high in potassium content—meats, dried fruits, fruit juices (particularly orange juice), and bananas. Oral potassium supplements are prescribed for persons whose intake of potassium is insufficient in relation to losses. This is particularly true of persons who are receiving diuretic therapy and those who are taking digitalis.

Potassium may be given intravenously when the oral route is not tolerated or when rapid replacement is needed. Magnesium deficiency may impair potassium correction; in such cases, magnesium replacement is indicated.[36] The rapid infusion of a concentrated potassium solution can cause death from cardiac arrest. Health personnel who assume responsibility for administering intravenous solutions that contain potassium should be fully aware of all the precautions pertaining to their dilution and flow rate.

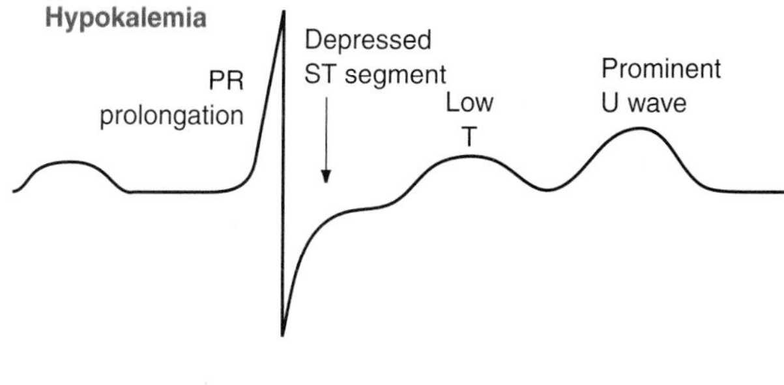

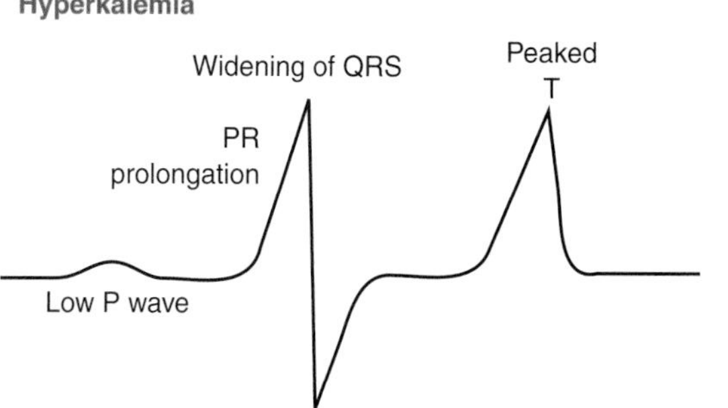

FIGURE 33-13 Electrocardiographic changes with hyperkalemia and hypokalemia.

Hyperkalemia

Hyperkalemia refers to an increase in plasma levels of potassium in excess of 5.0 mEq/L (5.0 mmol/L). It seldom occurs in healthy persons because the body is extremely effective in preventing excess potassium accumulation in the ECF.

Causes. The three major causes of potassium excess are decreased renal elimination, excessively rapid administration, and movement of potassium from the intracellular to extracellular compartment (Table 33-9). A pseudohyperkalemia can occur secondary to release of potassium from intracellular stores after a blood sample has been collected, hemolysis of red blood cells from excessive agitation of a blood sample, traumatic venipuncture, or prolonged application of a tourniquet during venipuncture.[37]

The most common cause of hyperkalemia is decreased renal function. Chronic hyperkalemia is almost always associated with renal failure. Usually, the glomerular filtration rate must decline to less than 10 mL/minute before hyperkalemia develops. Some renal disorders, such as sickle cell nephropathy, lead nephropathy, and systemic lupus nephritis, can selectively impair tubular secretion of potassium without causing renal failure. As discussed previously, acidosis diminishes potassium elimination by the kidney. Persons with acute renal failure accompanied by lactic acidosis or ketoacidosis are at increased risk for development of hyperkalemia. Correcting the acidosis usually helps to correct the hyperkalemia.[37]

Aldosterone acts at the level of the distal tubular sodium–potassium exchange system to increase potassium excretion while facilitating sodium reabsorption. A decrease in aldosterone-mediated potassium elimination can result from adrenal insufficiency (*i.e.*, Addison's disease), depression of aldosterone release due to a decrease in renin or angiotensin II, or impaired ability of the kidneys to respond to aldosterone. Potassium-sparing diuretics (*e.g.*, spironolactone, amiloride, triamterene, eplerenone) can produce hyperkalemia by means of the latter mechanism. Because of their ability to decrease aldosterone levels, angiotensin-converting enzyme inhibitors and angiotensin II receptor blockers can also produce an increase in plasma potassium levels.

Potassium excess can result from excessive oral ingestion or intravenous administration of potassium. It is difficult to increase potassium intake to the point of causing hyperkalemia when renal function is adequate and the aldosterone sodium–potassium exchange system is functioning. An exception to this rule is the intravenous route of administration. In some cases, severe and fatal incidents of hyperkalemia have occurred when intravenous potassium solutions were infused too rapidly. Because the kidneys control potassium elimination, intravenous solutions that contain potassium should never be started until urine output has been assessed and renal function has been deemed to be adequate.

The movement of potassium out of body cells into the ECF also can lead to elevated plasma potassium levels. Tissue injury causes release of intracellular potassium into the ECF compartment. For example, burns and crushing injuries cause cell death and release of potassium into the ECF. The same injuries often diminish renal function, which contributes to the development of hyperkalemia. Transient hyperkalemia may be induced during extreme exercise or seizures, when muscle cells are permeable to potassium. In a rare autosomal dominant disorder called *hyperkalemic periodic paralysis,* hyperkalemia may cause transient periods of muscle weakness and paralysis after exercise, cold exposure, or other situations that cause potassium to move out of the cells. In contrast to hypokalemic periodic paralysis, the episodes are mild, lasting less than 2 hours.[3]

Manifestations. The signs and symptoms of potassium excess are closely related to the alterations in neuromuscular excitability (see Table 33-9). The effect that potassium has on membrane excitability is determined by the ratio of K^+ ions inside the cell membrane to those outside the cell membrane. As the ECF potassium concentration rises, there is a decrease in the potassium ratio. This change produces an initial increase in membrane excitability because it brings the resting membrane potential closer to the threshold potential, such that a lesser stimulus is needed for depolarization. However, with persistent depolarization, as occurs with severe hyperkalemia, the Na^+ ion channels

TABLE 33-9 Causes and Manifestations of Hyperkalemia

Causes	Manifestations
Excessive Intake	**Laboratory Values**
Excessive oral intake	Serum potassium above 5.0 mEq/L (5.0 mmol/L)
Treatment with oral potassium supplements	**Gastrointestinal Manifestations**
Excessive or rapid infusion of potassium-containing parenteral fluids	Nausea and vomiting
Release From Intracellular Compartment	Intestinal cramps
Tissue trauma	Diarrhea
Burns	**Neuromuscular Manifestations**
Crushing injuries	Paresthesias
Extreme exercise or seizures	Weakness, dizziness
Inadequate Elimination by Kidneys	Muscle cramps
Renal failure	**Cardiovascular Manifestations**
Adrenal insufficiency (Addison's disease)	Changes in electrocardiogram
Treatment with potassium-sparing diuretics	Risk of cardiac arrest with severe excess
Treatment with angiotensin-converting enzyme inhibitors	

become inactivated, producing a net decrease in excitability.[38] The neuromuscular manifestations of potassium excess usually are absent until the plasma concentration exceeds 6 mEq/L. The first symptom associated with hyperkalemia typically is paresthesia. There may be complaints of generalized muscle weakness or dyspnea secondary to respiratory muscle weakness.

The most serious effect of hyperkalemia is on the heart. As potassium levels increase, disturbances in cardiac conduction occur. The earliest changes are peaked, narrow T waves and widening of the QRS complex. If plasma levels continue to rise, the PR interval becomes prolonged and is followed by disappearance of P waves (see Fig. 33-13). The heart rate may be slow. Ventricular fibrillation and cardiac arrest are terminal events. Detrimental effects of hyperkalemia on the heart are most pronounced when the plasma potassium level rises rapidly.

Diagnosis and Treatment. Diagnosis of hyperkalemia is based on complete history, physical examination to detect muscle weakness and signs of volume depletion, plasma potassium levels, and ECG findings. The history should include questions about dietary intake, use of potassium-sparing diuretics, history of kidney disease, and recurrent episodes of muscle weakness.

The treatment of potassium excess varies with the degree of increase in plasma potassium and whether there are ECG and neuromuscular manifestations. Calcium antagonizes the potassium-induced decrease in membrane excitability, restoring excitability toward normal. Plasma potassium levels affect the resting membrane potential, whereas plasma calcium levels affect the threshold potential. In persons with severe hyperkalemia, calcium gluconate (10 mL of a 10% solution) is given intravenously over a period of 2 to 3 minutes.[38] The protective effect of calcium administration is usually rather rapid and should be used only in persons in whom the P wave is absent or the QRS is widened. Insulin lowers plasma potassium concentration by driving potassium into cells. Intravenous infusions of insulin and glucose are used for this purpose.

Less emergent measures focus on decreasing or curtailing intake or absorption, increasing renal excretion, and increasing cellular uptake. Decreased intake can be achieved by restricting dietary sources of potassium. The major ingredient in most salt substitutes is potassium chloride, and such substitutes should not be given to patients with renal problems. Increasing potassium output often is more difficult. Patients with renal failure may require hemodialysis or peritoneal dialysis to reduce plasma potassium levels. Sodium polystyrene sulfonate, a cation exchange resin, also may be used to remove K^+ ions from the colon. The sodium ions in the resin are exchanged for K^+ ions, and then the potassium-containing resin is eliminated in the stool.

In summary, potassium is the major ICF cation. It contributes to the maintenance of intracellular osmolality, is necessary for normal neuromuscular function, and influences acid-base balance. Potassium is ingested in the diet and eliminated through the kidney. Because potassium is poorly conserved by the kidney, an adequate daily intake is needed. A transcellular shift can produce a redistribution of potassium between the extracellular and intracellular compartments, causing blood levels to increase or decrease.

Hypokalemia represents a decrease in plasma potassium levels below 3.5 mEq/L. It can result from inadequate intake, excessive losses, or redistribution between the ICF and ECF compartments. The manifestations of potassium deficit include alterations in renal, skeletal muscle, gastrointestinal, and cardiovascular function, reflecting the crucial role of potassium in cell metabolism and neuromuscular function.

Hyperkalemia represents an increase in plasma potassium greater than 5.0 mEq/L. It seldom occurs in healthy persons because the body is extremely effective in preventing excess potassium accumulation in the ECF. The major causes of potassium excess are decreased renal elimination of potassium, excessively rapid intravenous administration of potassium, and a transcellular shift of potassium out of the cell to the ECF compartment. The most serious effect of hyperkalemia is cardiac arrest.

Calcium, Phosphate, and Magnesium Balance

After you have completed this section of the chapter, you should be able to meet the following objectives:

- Describe the associations among intestinal absorption, renal elimination, bone stores, and the functions of vitamin D and parathyroid hormone in regulating calcium, phosphate, and magnesium levels
- State the difference between ionized and bound or chelated forms of calcium in terms of physiologic function
- Describe the mechanisms of calcium gain and loss and relate them to the causes of hypocalcemia and hypercalcemia
- Relate the functions of calcium to the manifestations of hypocalcemia and hypercalcemia
- Describe the mechanisms of phosphate gain and loss and relate them to causes of hypophosphatemia and hyperphosphatemia
- Relate the functions of phosphate to the manifestations of hypophosphatemia and hyperphosphatemia
- Describe the mechanisms of magnesium gain and loss and relate them to the causes of hypomagnesemia and hypermagnesemia
- Relate the functions of magnesium to the manifestations of hypomagnesemia and hypermagnesemia

MECHANISMS REGULATING CALCIUM, PHOSPHATE, AND MAGNESIUM BALANCE

Calcium, phosphate, and magnesium are the major divalent cations in the body. They are ingested in the diet, absorbed from the intestine, filtered in the glomerulus of the kidney, reabsorbed in the renal tubules, and eliminated in the urine. Approximately 99% of calcium, 85% of phosphate, and 50% to 60% of magnesium is found in bone. Most of the remaining calcium (approximately 1%), phosphate (approximately 14%), and magnesium (approximately 40% to 50%) is located inside cells. Only a small amount of these three ions is present in ECF. This small, but vital, amount of ECF calcium, phosphate, and magnesium is directly or indirectly regulated by vitamin D and parathyroid hormone (PTH). Calcitonin, a hormone produced by C cells in the thyroid, is thought to act on the kidney and bone to remove calcium from the extracellular circulation. The role of vitamin D, PTH, and calcitonin on skeletal function is discussed further in Chapters 56 and 58.

Vitamin D

Although classified as a vitamin, vitamin D functions as a hormone. It acts to sustain normal plasma levels of calcium and phosphate by increasing their absorption from the intestine, and it also is necessary for normal bone formation. Vitamin D is synthesized by ultraviolet irradiation of 7-dehydrocholesterol, which is present in the skin or obtained from foods in the diet, many of which are fortified with vitamin D. The synthesized or ingested forms of vitamin D are essentially prohormones that lack biologic activity and must undergo metabolic transformation to achieve potency. Once vitamin D enters the circulation from the skin or intestine, it is concentrated in the liver. There, it is hydroxylated to form 25-hydroxyvitamin D [25-$(OH)D_3$]. It is then transported to the kidney, where it is transformed into active 1,25-$(OH)_2D_3$. The major action of the activated form of vitamin D, also called *calcitriol,* is to increase the absorption of calcium from the intestine. Calcitriol also sensitizes bone to the resorptive actions of PTH. There is also recent evidence that vitamin D controls parathyroid gland growth and suppresses the synthesis and secretion of PTH.[39] The formation of 1,25-$(OH)_2D_3$ in the kidneys is regulated in feedback fashion by plasma calcium and phosphate levels. Low calcium levels lead to an increase in PTH, which then increases vitamin D activation. A lowering of plasma phosphate levels also augment vitamin D activation. Additional control of renal activation of vitamin D is exerted by a negative feedback loop that monitors 1,25-$(OH)_2D_3$ levels.

Parathyroid Hormone

Parathyroid hormone (PTH), a major regulator of plasma calcium and phosphate, is secreted by the parathyroid glands. There are four parathyroid glands located on the dorsal surface of the thyroid gland. The dominant regulator of PTH is the plasma calcium concentration. A unique calcium receptor on the parathyroid cell membrane (extracellular calcium-sensing receptor) responds rapidly to changes in plasma calcium levels.[40] When the plasma calcium level is high, PTH is inhibited, and the calcium is deposited in the bones. When the level is low, PTH secretion is increased, and calcium is mobilized from the bones. The response to a decrease in plasma calcium is prompt, occurring within seconds. Phosphate does not exert a direct effect on PTH secretion. Instead, it acts indirectly by complexing with calcium and decreasing plasma calcium concentration.

The secretion, synthesis, and action of PTH are also influenced by magnesium. Magnesium serves as a cofactor in the generation of cellular energy and is important in the function of second messenger systems. Magnesium's effects on the synthesis and release of PTH are thought to be mediated through these mechanisms.[41] Because of its function in regulating PTH release, severe and prolonged hypomagnesemia can markedly inhibit PTH levels.

The main function of PTH is to maintain the calcium concentration of the ECF. It performs this function by promoting the release of calcium from bone, increasing the activation of vitamin D as a means of enhancing intestinal absorption of calcium, and stimulating calcium conservation by the kidney while increasing phosphate excretion (Fig. 33-14).

PTH acts on bone to accelerate the mobilization and transfer of calcium to the ECF. The skeletal response to PTH is a two-step process. There is an immediate response in which calcium that is present in bone fluid is released into the ECF, and there is a second, more slowly developing response in which completely mineralized bone is resorbed,

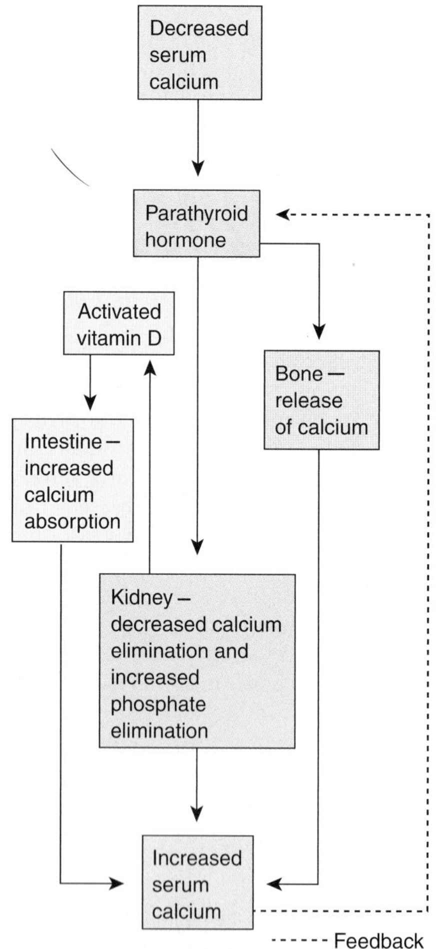

FIGURE 33-14 Regulation of serum calcium concentration by parathyroid hormone.

resulting in the release of both calcium and phosphate. The actions of PTH in terms of bone resorption require normal levels of both vitamin D and magnesium. The activation of vitamin D by the kidney is enhanced by the presence of PTH; it is through the activation of vitamin D that PTH increases intestinal absorption of calcium and phosphate. PTH also acts directly on the kidney to increase tubular reabsorption of calcium and magnesium while increasing phosphate elimination. The accompanying increase in phosphate elimination ensures that calcium released from bone does not produce hyperphosphatemia and increase the risk for soft tissue deposition of calcium-phosphate crystals.

Hypoparathyroidism. Hypoparathyroidism reflects deficient PTH secretion, resulting in hypocalcemia. PTH deficiency may be caused by a congenital absence of all of the parathyroid glands, as in DiGeorge syndrome. An acquired deficiency of PTH may occur after neck surgery, particularly if the surgery involves removal of a parathyroid adenoma, thyroidectomy, or bilateral neck resection for cancer. A transient form of PTH deficiency, occurring within 1 to 2 days and lasting up to 5 days, may occur after thyroid surgery owing to parathyroid gland suppression.[8] Hypoparathyroidism also may have an autoimmune origin. Antiparathyroid antibodies have been detected in some persons with hypoparathyroidism, particularly those with multiple endocrine disorders. Other causes of hypoparathyroidism include heavy metal damage such as occurs with Wilson disease, metastatic tumors, and infection. Functional impairment of parathyroid function occurs with magnesium deficiency. Correction of the hypomagnesemia results in rapid disappearance of the condition.

Manifestations of acute hypoparathyroidism, which result from a decrease in plasma calcium, include tetany with muscle cramps, carpopedal spasm, and convulsions (see Hypocalcemia). Paresthesias, such as tingling of the circumoral area and in the hands and feet, are almost always present. Low calcium levels may cause prolongation of the QT interval, resistance to digitalis, hypotension, and refractory heart failure. Symptoms of chronic PTH deficiency include lethargy, anxiety state, and personality changes. There may be blurring of vision because of cataracts, which develop over a number of years. Extrapyramidal signs, such as those seen with Parkinson disease, may occur because of calcification of the basal ganglia. Successful treatment of the hypocalcemia may improve the disorder and is sometimes associated with decreases in basal ganglia calcification on x-ray. Teeth may be defective if the disorder occurs during childhood.

Diagnosis of hypoparathyroidism is based on low plasma calcium levels, high plasma phosphate levels, and low plasma PTH levels. Plasma magnesium levels usually are measured to rule out hypomagnesemia as a cause of the disorder.

Acute hypoparathyroid tetany is treated with intravenous calcium gluconate followed by oral administration of calcium salts and vitamin D. Magnesium supplementation is used when the disorder is caused by magnesium deficiency. Persons with chronic hypoparathyroidism are treated with oral calcium and vitamin D. Plasma calcium levels are monitored at regular intervals (at least every 3 months) as a means of maintaining plasma calcium within a slightly low but asymptomatic range. Maintaining plasma calcium within this range helps to prevent hypercalciuria and kidney damage.

Pseudohypoparathyroidism is a rare familial disorder characterized by target tissue resistance to PTH. It is characterized by hypocalcemia, increased parathyroid function, and a variety of congenital defects in the growth and development of the skeleton, including short stature and short metacarpal and metatarsal bones. There are variants in the disorder, with some persons having the pseudohypoparathyroidism with the congenital defects and others having the congenital defects with normal calcium and phosphate levels. The manifestations of the disorder are due primarily to chronic hypocalcemia. Treatment is similar to that for hypoparathyroidism.

Hyperparathyroidism. Hyperparathyroidism is caused by hypersecretion of PTH. Hyperparathyroidism can manifest as a primary disorder caused by hyperplasia (15%), an adenoma (85%), and rarely carcinoma of the parathyroid glands or as a secondary disorder seen in persons with renal failure or chronic malabsorption of calcium. Parathyroid adenomas and hyperplasia can occur in several distinct familial diseases (including multiple endocrine neoplasia [MEN], type 1 and 2a).

Primary hyperparathyroidism is seen more commonly after 50 years of age and is more common in women than men (3:1). This disorder is relatively common with an incidence of 1 in 500 to 1000. Primary hyperparathyroidism causes hypercalcemia and an increase in calcium in the urine filtrate, resulting in hypercalciuria and the potential for development of kidney stones. Chronic bone resorption may produce diffuse demineralization, pathologic fractures, and cystic bone lesions. A dual-energy x-ray absorptiometry [DEXA] bone scan should be performed to assess bone mineral density. Signs and symptoms of the disorder are related to skeletal abnormalities, exposure of the kidney to high calcium levels, and elevated plasma calcium levels (see Hypercalcemia). At the present time, most patients with primary hyperparathyroidism manifest an asymptomatic disorder that is discovered in the course of routine biochemical testing.

Diagnostic procedures, which include plasma calcium and intact PTH levels, are used to differentiate between the two most common causes of hypercalcemia: primary hyperparathyroidism and hypercalcemia of malignancy. Assays of intact PTH employ two antibodies that bind to different sites on the PTH and are designed to measure the intact, biologically active hormone, specifically. In primary hyperparathyroidism, the intact PTH levels will be elevated in 75% to 90% of affected persons or will be inappropriately "normal" in the face of hypercalcemia when they should be suppressed. In hypercalcemia of malignancy, the intact PTH levels are suppressed. Imaging studies of the parathyroid area may be used to identify a parathyroid adenoma. The radioisotopic imaging technetium-sestamibi scan is preferred. However, the role of imaging studies before and during surgery is the topic of much debate.[42] Parathyroid surgery is usually the treatment of choice.

Secondary hyperparathyroidism involves hyperplasia of the parathyroid glands and occurs primarily in persons with renal failure (see Chapter 36). In early renal failure, an increase in PTH results from decreased plasma calcium and activated vitamin D levels. As the disease progresses, there is a decrease in vitamin D and calcium receptors, making the parathyroid glands more resistant to vitamin D and calcium.[43,44] At this point, elevated phosphate levels induce hyperplasia of the parathyroid glands independent of calcium and activated vitamin D.

The bone disease seen in persons with secondary hyperparathyroidism due to renal failure is known as *renal osteodystrophy* (see Chapter 36). Treatment includes resolving the hypercalcemia with large fluid intake. Persons with mild disease are advised to keep active and drink adequate fluids. They also are advised to avoid calcium-containing antacids, vitamin D, and thiazide diuretics, which increase reabsorption of calcium by the kidney. Parathyroidectomy may be indicated in persons with symptomatic hyperparathyroidism, kidney stones, or bone disease. Avoiding hyperphosphatemia may prevent renal osteodystrophies caused by secondary hyperparathyroidism in renal failure. Calcium acetate or a newer calcium-free agent (sevelamer HCl [Renagel]) can be given with meals to bind phosphate.[45] Calcitriol, the activated form of vitamin D, may be used to control parathyroid growth and suppress the synthesis and secretion of PTH. However, because of its potent effect on intestinal absorption and bone mobilization, calcitriol can cause hypercalcemia. Newer analogs of activated vitamin D are being developed that retain the ability to suppress parathyroid function while having minimal effects on calcium or phosphate reabsorption.[39] Calcimimetics, which increase the sensitivity of the parathyroid calcium-sensing receptor to extracellular calcium, are being developed to control primary and secondary hyperparathyroidism.[40]

ALTERATIONS IN CALCIUM BALANCE

Calcium enters the body through the gastrointestinal tract, is absorbed from the intestine under the influence of vitamin D, is stored in bone, and is excreted by the kidney. Approximately 99% of body calcium is found in bone, where it provides the strength and stability for the skeletal system and serves as an exchangeable source to maintain extracellular calcium levels. Most of the remaining calcium (approximately 1%) is located inside cells, and only approximately 0.1% to 0.2% (approximately 8.5 to 10.5 mg/dL) of the remaining calcium is present in the ECF. The extracellular concentrations of calcium and phosphate are reciprocally regulated such that calcium levels fall when phosphate levels are high, and vice versa. Normal plasma levels of calcium (8.5 to 10.5 mg/dL in adults) and phosphate (2.5 to 4.5 mg/dL in adults) are regulated so that the product of the two concentrations ($[Ca^{2+}] \times [PO_4^{2-}]$) is normally maintained below 70.[43] Maintenance of the calcium × phosphate product within this range is important in preventing the deposition of $CaPO_4$ salts in soft tissue, damaging the kidneys, blood vessels, heart, and lungs.

The ECF calcium exists in three forms: protein bound, complexed, and ionized. Approximately 40% of ECF calcium is bound to plasma proteins, mostly albumin, and cannot diffuse or pass through the capillary wall to leave the vascular compartment (Fig. 33-15). Another 10% is complexed (*i.e.,* chelated) with substances such as citrate, phosphate, and sulfate. This form is not ionized. The remaining 50% of ECF calcium is present in the ionized form. It is the ionized form of calcium that is free to leave the vascular compartment and participate in cellular functions. The total plasma calcium level fluctuates with changes in plasma albumin and pH. As a rule, the total plasma calcium level is decreased 0.75 to 1.0 mg/dL for every 1g/dL decrease from normal in the plasma albumin level, and by 0.16 mg/dL for each 0.1-unit rise in pH.[5]

Ionized calcium serves a number of functions. It participates in many enzyme reactions; exerts an important effect on membrane potentials and neuronal excitability; is necessary for contraction in skeletal, cardiac, and smooth muscle; participates in the release of hormones, neurotransmitters, and other chemical messengers; influences cardiac contractility and automaticity by way of slow calcium channels; and is essential for blood clotting. The use of calcium channel blockers in circulatory disorders demonstrates the importance of the Ca^{2+} ions in the normal function of the heart and blood vessels. Calcium is required for all but the first two steps of the intrinsic pathway for blood coagulation. Because of its ability to bind calcium, citrate often is used to prevent clotting in blood that is to be used for transfusions.

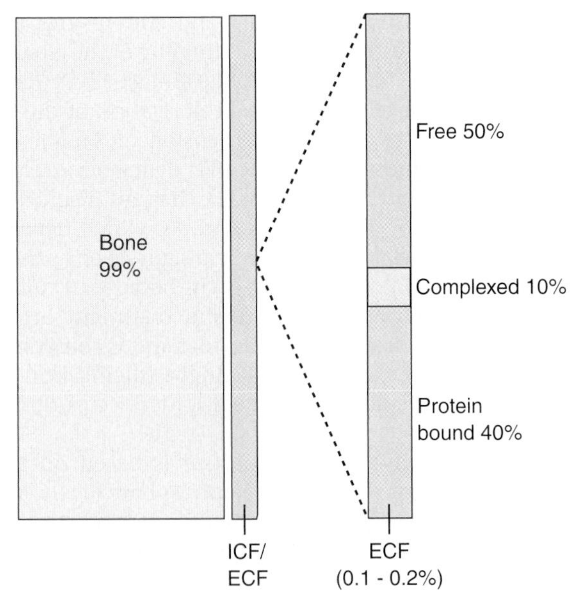

FIGURE 33-15 Distribution of body calcium between the bone and the intracellular and extracellular fluids. The percentages of free, complexed, and protein-bound calcium in extracellular fluids are indicated.

CALCIUM BALANCE

- About 99% of body calcium is stored in bone; 1% is located inside cells; and 0.1% is found in the extracellular fluid.
- Extracellular fluid calcium levels are made up of free (ionized), complexed, and protein-bound fractions. Only the ionized Ca^{2+} plays an essential role in neuromuscular and cardiac excitability.
- Serum calcium levels are regulated by parathyroid hormone and by renal mechanisms in which serum levels of calcium and phosphate are reciprocally regulated to prevent the damaging deposition of calcium phosphate crystals in the soft tissues of the body.

Gains and Losses

The major sources of calcium are milk and milk products. Only 30% to 50% of dietary calcium is absorbed from the duodenum and upper jejunum; the remainder is eliminated in the stool. There is a calcium influx of approximately 150 mg/day into the intestine from the blood. Net absorption of calcium is equal to the amount that is absorbed from the intestine less the amount that moves into the intestine. Calcium balance can become negative when dietary intake (and calcium absorption) is less than intestinal secretion. A dietary intake of less than 400 mg/day can be associated with negative calcium balance.[5]

Calcium is stored in bone and excreted by the kidney. Approximately 60% to 65% of filtered calcium is passively reabsorbed in the proximal tubule, driven by the reabsorption of sodium chloride; 15% to 20% is reabsorbed in the thick ascending loop of Henle, driven by the Na^+/K^+-$2Cl^-$ cotransport system; and 5% to 10% is reabsorbed in the distal convoluted tubule (see Chapter 32). The distal convoluted tubule is an important regulatory site for controlling the amount of calcium that enters the urine. PTH and possibly vitamin D stimulate calcium reabsorption in this segment of the nephron. Other factors that may influence calcium reabsorption in the distal convoluted tubule are phosphate levels and glucose and insulin levels. Thiazide diuretics, which exert their effects in the distal convoluted tubule, enhance calcium reabsorption.

Hypocalcemia

Hypocalcemia represents a plasma calcium level of less than 8.5 mg/dL. Hypocalcemia occurs in many forms of critical illness and has affected as many as 70% to 90% of patients in intensive care units.[46]

Causes. The causes of hypocalcemia can be divided into four categories: (1) impaired ability to mobilize calcium bone stores, (2) abnormal losses of calcium from the kidney, (3) increased protein binding or chelation such that greater proportions of calcium are in the nonionized form, and (4) soft tissue sequestration (Table 33-10). Pseudohypocalcemia is caused by hypoalbuminemia. It results in

TABLE 33-10 Causes and Manifestations of Hypocalcemia

Causes	Manifestations
Impaired Ability to Mobilize Calcium From Bone	**Laboratory Values**
Hypoparathyroidism	Serum calcium level below 8.5 mg/dL
Resistance to the actions of parathyroid hormone	**Neuromuscular Manifestations (Increased Neuromuscular Excitability)**
Hypomagnesemia	Paresthesias, especially numbness and tingling
Decreased Intake or Absorption	Skeletal muscle cramps
Malabsorption	Abdominal spasms and cramps
Vitamin D deficiency	Hyperactive reflexes
Failure to activate	Carpopedal spasm
Liver disease	Tetany
Kidney disease	Laryngeal spasm
Medications that impair activation of vitamin D (*e.g.*, phenytoin)	Positive Chvostek's and Trousseau's signs
Abnormal Renal Losses	**Cardiovascular Manifestations**
Renal failure and hyperphosphatemia	Hypotension
Increased Protein Binding or Chelation	Signs of cardiac insufficiency
Increased pH	Failure to respond to drugs that act by calcium-mediated mechanisms
Increased fatty acids	Prolongation of QT interval predisposes to ventricular dysrhythmias
Rapid transfusion of citrated blood	**Skeletal Manifestations (Chronic Deficiency)**
Increased Sequestration	Osteomalacia
Acute pancreatitis	Bone pain, deformities, fracture

a decrease in protein-bound, rather than ionized, calcium and usually is asymptomatic.[47,48]

Plasma calcium exists in a dynamic equilibrium with calcium in bone. The ability to mobilize calcium from bone depends on adequate levels of PTH. Decreased levels of PTH may result from primary or secondary forms of hypoparathyroidism. Suppression of PTH release may also occur when vitamin D levels are elevated. The activated form of vitamin D (calcitriol) can be used to suppress the secondary hyperparathyroidism that occurs in persons with kidney failure. Magnesium deficiency inhibits PTH release and impairs the action of PTH on bone resorption. This form of hypocalcemia is difficult to treat with calcium supplementation alone and requires correction of the magnesium deficiency.

There is an inverse relation between calcium and phosphate excretion by the kidneys. Phosphate elimination is impaired in renal failure, causing plasma calcium levels to decrease. Hypocalcemia and hyperphosphatemia occur when the glomerular filtration rate falls below 25 to 30 mL/minute (normal is 100 to 120 mL/minute).

Only the ionized form of calcium is able to leave the capillary and participate in body functions. A change in pH alters the proportion of calcium that is in the bound and ionized forms. An acid pH decreases binding of calcium to protein, causing a proportionate increase in ionized calcium, whereas total plasma calcium remains unchanged. An alkaline pH has the opposite effect. As an example, hyperventilation sufficient to cause respiratory alkalosis can produce tetany because of increased protein binding of calcium. Free fatty acids increase binding of calcium to albumin, causing a reduction in ionized calcium. Elevations in free fatty acids sufficient to alter calcium binding may occur during stressful situations that cause elevations of epinephrine, glucagon, growth hormone, and adrenocorticotropic hormone levels. Heparin, β-adrenergic drugs (*i.e.*, epinephrine, isoproterenol, and norepinephrine), and alcohol can also produce elevations in free fatty acid levels sufficient to increase calcium binding.

Citrate, which is often used as an anticoagulant in blood transfusions, complexes with calcium. Theoretically, excess citrate in donor blood could combine with the calcium in a recipient's blood, producing a sharp drop in ionized calcium. This normally does not occur because the liver removes the citrate within a matter of minutes. When blood transfusions are administered at a slow rate, there is little danger of hypocalcemia caused by citrate binding.[2]

Hypocalcemia is a common finding in a patient with acute pancreatitis. Inflammation of the pancreas causes release of proteolytic and lipolytic enzymes. It is thought that the Ca^{2+} combines with free fatty acids released by lipolysis in the pancreas, forming soaps and removing calcium from the circulation.

Calcium deficit due to dietary deficiency exerts its effects on bone stores rather than extracellular calcium levels. A dietary deficiency of vitamin D is seldom seen today because many foods are fortified with vitamin D. Vitamin D deficiency is more likely to occur in malabsorption states, such as biliary obstruction, pancreatic insufficiency, and celiac disease, in which the ability to absorb fat and fat-soluble vitamins is impaired. Failure to activate vitamin D is another cause of hypocalcemia. Anticonvulsant medications, particularly phenytoin, can impair initial activation of vitamin D in the liver. The final step in activation of vitamin D is impaired in persons with renal failure (see Chapter 36). Fortunately, the activated form of vitamin D, calcitriol, has been synthesized and is available for use in the treatment of calcium deficiency in persons with renal failure.

Manifestations. Hypocalcemia can manifest as an acute or chronic condition. The manifestations of acute hypocalcemia reflect the increased neuromuscular excitability and cardiovascular effects of a decrease in ionized calcium (see Table 33-10). Ionized calcium stabilizes neuromuscular excitability, thereby making nerve cells less sensitive to stimuli. Nerves exposed to low ionized calcium levels show decreased thresholds for excitation, repetitive responses to a single stimulus, and, in extreme cases, continuous activity. The severity of the manifestations depends on the underlying cause, rapidity of onset, accompanying electrolyte disorders, and extracellular pH. Increased neuromuscular excitability can manifest as paresthesias (*i.e.*, tingling around the mouth and in the hands and feet) and tetany (*i.e.*, muscle spasms of the muscles of the face, hands, and feet). Severe hypocalcemia can lead to laryngeal spasm, seizures, and even death.

Cardiovascular effects of acute hypocalcemia include hypotension, cardiac insufficiency, cardiac dysrhythmias (particularly heart block and ventricular fibrillation), and failure to respond to drugs such as digitalis, norepinephrine, and dopamine that act through calcium-mediated mechanisms.

Chronic hypocalcemia is often accompanied by skeletal manifestations and skin changes. There may be bone pain, fragility, deformities, and fractures. The skin may be dry and scaling, the nails brittle, and the hair dry. Development of cataracts is common. A person with chronic hypocalcemia may also present with mild diffuse brain disease mimicking depression, dementia, or psychoses.

Chvostek's and Trousseau's tests can be used to assess for an increase in neuromuscular excitability and tetany.[8] Chvostek's sign is elicited by tapping the face just below the temple at the point where the facial nerve emerges. Tapping the face over the facial nerve causes spasm of the lip, nose, or face when the test result is positive. An inflated blood pressure cuff is used to test for Trousseau's sign. The cuff is inflated above systolic blood pressure for 3 minutes. Contraction of the fingers and hands (*i.e.*, carpopedal spasm) indicates the presence of tetany (Fig. 33-16).

Treatment. Acute hypocalcemia is an emergency situation, requiring prompt treatment. An intravenous infusion containing calcium (*e.g.*, calcium gluconate, calcium gluceptate, calcium chloride) is used when tetany or acute symptoms are present or anticipated because of a decrease in the plasma calcium level.

Chronic hypocalcemia is treated with oral intake of calcium. One glass of milk contains approximately 300 mg of calcium. Oral calcium supplements of carbonate, gluconate, or lactate salts may be used. In some cases, long-term treatment may require the use of vitamin D preparations. The active form of vitamin D is administered when the liver or

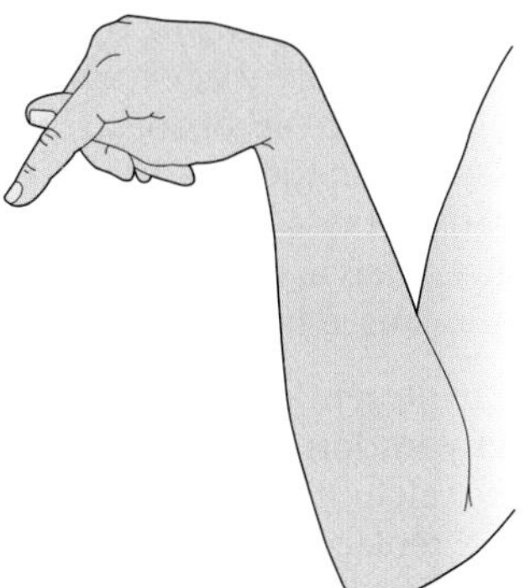

FIGURE 33-16 Trousseau's sign. Ischemia-induced carpal spasm can occur with hypocalcemia or hypomagnesemia. (Smeltzer S. C., Bare B. G. [2003]. *Medical-surgical nursing* (10th ed., p. 271). Philadelphia: Lippincott Williams & Wilkins)

kidney mechanisms needed for hormone activation are impaired.

Hypercalcemia

Hypercalcemia represents a total plasma calcium concentration of greater than 10.5 mg/dL. Falsely elevated levels of calcium can result from prolonged drawing of blood with an excessively tight tourniquet. Increased plasma proteins (*e.g.*, hyperalbuminemia, hyperglobulinemia) may elevate the total plasma calcium but not affect the ionized calcium concentration.

Causes. A plasma calcium excess (*i.e.*, hypercalcemia) results when calcium movement into the circulation overwhelms the calcium regulatory hormones or the ability of the kidney to remove excess calcium ions (Table 33-11). The two most common causes of hypercalcemia are increased bone resorption due to neoplasms and hyperparathyroidism.[49] These two etiologies account for more than 90% of all patients with hypercalcemia. Hypercalcemia is a common complication of malignancy, occurring in approximately 10% to 20% of persons with advanced disease.[50] A number of malignant tumors, including carcinoma of the lungs, have been associated with hypercalcemia. Some tumors destroy the bone, but others produce humoral agents that stimulate osteoclastic activity, increase bone resorption, or inhibit bone formation. Approximately 80% of patients with hypercalcemia of malignancy produce PTH-related protein (PTH-rP).[50] PTH-rP is an important factor in skeletal development in utero. PTH and PTH-rP have marked homology, or structural similarity, at

TABLE 33-11 Causes and Manifestations of Hypercalcemia

Causes	Manifestations
Increased Intestinal Absorption Excessive vitamin D Excessive calcium in the diet Milk-alkali syndrome **Increased Bone Resorption** Increased levels of parathyroid hormone Malignant neoplasms Prolonged immobilization **Decreased Elimination** Thiazide diuretics Lithium therapy	**Laboratory Values** Serum calcium level above 10.5 mg/dL **Impaired Ability to Concentrate Urine and Exposure of Kidney to Increased Concentration of Calcium** Polyuria Polydipsia Flank pain Signs of acute and chronic renal insufficiency Signs of kidney stones **Gastrointestinal Manifestations** Anorexia Nausea, vomiting Constipation **Neuromuscular Manifestations (Decreased Neuromuscular Excitability)** Muscle weakness and atrophy Ataxia, loss of muscle tone **Skeletal Manifestations** Osteopenia Osteoporosis **Central Nervous System Manifestations** Lethargy Personality and behavioral changes Stupor and coma **Cardiovascular Manifestations** Hypertension Shortening of the QT interval Atrioventricular block on electrocardiogram

their amino terminal ends, with 8 of the first 13 amino acids in the same positions. This homology results in both PTH and PTH-rP binding to the same receptor (PTH/PTH-rP receptor). PTH-rP is produced by several tumors, including cancers of the lung, breast, kidney, head and neck, and ovary.[50]

Less frequent causes of hypercalcemia are prolonged immobilization, increased intestinal absorption of calcium, excessive doses of vitamin D, and the effects of drugs such as lithium and thiazide diuretics. Prolonged immobilization and lack of weight bearing cause demineralization of bone and release of calcium into the bloodstream. Intestinal absorption of calcium can be increased by excessive doses of vitamin D or as a result of a condition called the *milk-alkali syndrome.* The milk-alkali syndrome is caused by excessive ingestion of calcium (often in the form of milk) and absorbable antacids. Because of the advent of nonabsorbable antacids, the condition is seen less frequently than in the past, but it may occur in women who are overzealous in taking calcium preparations for osteoporosis prevention. The condition is thought to be initiated by mild hypercalcemia leading to increased sodium excretion along with a decrease in ECF volume and glomerular filtration rate. The decreased glomerular filtration rate leads to alkalosis and increased calcium reabsorption by the kidney. Discontinuance of the antacid repairs the alkalosis and increases calcium elimination.

A variety of drugs elevate calcium levels. The use of lithium to treat bipolar disorders has caused hypercalcemia and hyperparathyroidism. The thiazide diuretics increase calcium reabsorption in the distal convoluted tubule of the kidney. Although the thiazide diuretics seldom cause hypercalcemia, they can unmask hypercalcemia from other causes such as underlying bone disorders and conditions that increase bone resorption.

Manifestations. The signs and symptoms associated with calcium excess originate from three sources: changes in neural excitability, alterations in smooth and cardiac muscle function, and exposure of the kidneys to high concentrations of calcium (see Table 33-11).

Neural excitability is decreased in patients with hypercalcemia. There may be a dulling of consciousness, stupor, weakness, and muscle flaccidity. Behavioral changes may range from subtle alterations in personality to acute psychoses.

The heart responds to elevated levels of calcium with increased contractility and ventricular dysrhythmias. Digitalis accentuates these responses. Gastrointestinal symptoms reflect a decrease in smooth muscle activity and include constipation, anorexia, nausea, and vomiting. Pancreatitis is another potential complication of hypercalcemia and is probably related to stones in the pancreatic ducts.

High calcium concentrations in the urine impair the ability of the kidneys to concentrate urine by interfering with the action of ADH (an example of nephrogenic diabetes insipidus). This causes salt and water diuresis and an increased sensation of thirst. Hypercalciuria also predisposes to the development of renal calculi.

Hypercalcemic crisis describes an acute increase in the plasma calcium level.[49] Malignant disease and hyperparathyroidism are the major causes of hypercalcemic crisis. In hypercalcemic crisis, polyuria, excessive thirst, volume depletion, fever, altered levels of consciousness, azotemia (*i.e.,* nitrogenous wastes in the blood), and a disturbed mental state accompany other signs of calcium excess. Symptomatic hypercalcemia is associated with a high mortality rate; death often is caused by cardiac arrest.

Treatment. The treatment of calcium excess usually is directed toward rehydration and measures to increase urinary excretion of calcium and inhibit release of calcium from bone.[49] Fluid replacement is needed in situations of volume depletion. The excretion of sodium is accompanied by calcium excretion. Diuretics and sodium chloride can be administered to increase urinary elimination of calcium after the ECF volume has been restored. Loop diuretics commonly are used rather than thiazide diuretics, which increase calcium reabsorption. Initial lowering of calcium levels is followed by measures to inhibit bone reabsorption. Drugs that are used to inhibit calcium mobilization include bisphosphonates, calcitonin, mithramycin, glucocorticosteroids, and gallium nitrate. The bisphosphonates (*e.g.,* etidronate, pamidronate, zoledronate, alendronate, risedronate) act mainly by inhibiting osteoclastic activity. These agents provide a significant reduction in calcium levels with relatively few side effects. Calcitonin inhibits osteoclastic activity, thereby decreasing resorption. The corticosteroids and mithramycin inhibit bone resorption and are used to treat hypercalcemia associated with cancer. The long-term use of mithramycin, an antineoplastic drug, is limited because of its potential for nephrotoxicity and hepatotoxicity. Gallium nitrate is highly effective in the treatment of severe hypercalcemia associated with malignancy. It is a chemical compound that inhibits bone resorption, although the precise mechanism of action is unclear. Dialysis can be used in hypercalcemic patients with renal failure and in heart failure patients in whom fluid overload is a concern.

ALTERATIONS IN PHOSPHATE BALANCE

Phosphorus is mainly an intracellular anion. It is the fourth most abundant element in the body after carbon, nitrogen, and calcium. Phosphate is essential to many bodily functions. It plays a major role in bone formation; is essential to certain metabolic processes, including the formation of ATP and the enzymes needed for metabolism of glucose, fat, and protein; is a necessary component of several vital parts of the cell, being incorporated into the nucleic acids of DNA and RNA and the phospholipids of the cell membrane; and serves as an acid-base buffer in the ECF and in the renal excretion of hydrogen ions. Delivery of oxygen by the red blood cell depends on organic phosphates in ATP and 2,3-diphosphoglycerate. Phosphate is also needed for normal function of other blood cells, including the white blood cells and platelets.

Approximately 85% of phosphate is contained in bone, and most of the remainder (14%) is located in cells. Only approximately 1% is in the ECF compartment, and of that, only a minute proportion is in the plasma. ECF phosphorus exists mainly as phosphate, although laboratory measurements are often reported as elemental phosphorus.[51] Most of the intracellular phosphorus (approximately 90%) is in the organic form (*e.g.,* nucleic acids, phosphoproteins, ATP). Entry of phosphate into cells is enhanced after glucose uptake because phosphorus is incorporated into the phosphorylated intermediates of glucose metabolism. Cell injury or atrophy leads to a loss of cell components that contain organic phosphate; regeneration of these cellular components results in withdrawal of inorganic phosphate from the extracellular compartment.

In the adult, the normal plasma phosphate level ranges from 2.5 to 4.5 mg/dL. These values are slightly higher in infants (3.7 to 8.5 mg/dL) and children (4.0 to 5.4 mg/dL), probably because of increased growth hormone and decreased gonadal hormones. Changing the plasma phosphate levels to as high as three to four times the normal value does not seem to have an immediate effect on body function.

PHOSPHATE BALANCE

- Approximately 85% of the phosphorus is contained in bone. Most of the remaining phosphorus is incorporated into organic compounds such as nucleic acids, high-energy compounds (*e.g.,* ATP), and coenzymes that are critically important for cell function.
- Many of the manifestations of hypophosphatemia are related to a decrease in cell energy due to ATP depletion.
- Serum phosphate levels are regulated by the kidneys, which eliminate or conserve phosphate as serum levels change. Serum levels of calcium and phosphate are reciprocally regulated to prevent the damaging deposition of calcium phosphate crystals in the soft tissues of the body. Many of the manifestations of hyperphosphatemia reflect a decrease in serum calcium levels.

Gains and Losses

Phosphate is ingested in the diet and eliminated in the urine. Phosphate is derived from many dietary sources, including milk and meats. Approximately 80% of ingested phosphate is absorbed in the intestine, primarily in the jejunum. Absorption is diminished by concurrent ingestion of substances that bind phosphate, including calcium, magnesium, and aluminum.

The overall elimination of phosphate by the kidney involves glomerular filtration and tubular reabsorption. Essentially all of the phosphate that is present in the plasma is filtered in the glomerulus. Renal elimination of phosphate is then regulated by an overflow mechanism in which the amount of phosphate lost in the urine is directly related to phosphate concentrations in the blood. Essentially all the filtered phosphate is reabsorbed when phosphate levels are low. When plasma phosphate levels rise above a critical level, the rate of phosphate loss in the urine reflects the excess plasma phosphate levels. Phosphate is reabsorbed from the filtrate into the proximal tubular epithelial cells through the action of a sodium-phosphate cotransporter, NPT2a. PTH also plays a significant role in regulating phosphate concentration. It does this by promoting bone resorption, which dumps large amounts of phosphate into the ECF, and it increases the renal threshold for phosphate reabsorption. Thus, whenever PTH is increased, tubular phosphate reabsorption is decreased, and more phosphate is lost in the urine (because PTH decreases the synthesis and expression of the NPT2a transporter on the luminal surface of the proximal tubular cell).

Hypophosphatemia

Hypophosphatemia is commonly defined by a plasma phosphorus level of less than 2.5 mg/dL in adults; it is considered severe at concentration of less than 1.0 mEq/L.[51] Hypophosphatemia may occur despite normal body phosphate stores as a result of movement from the ECF into the ICF compartment. Serious depletion of phosphate may exist with low, normal, or high plasma concentrations.

Causes. The most common causes of hypophosphatemia are depletion of phosphate because of insufficient intestinal absorption, transcompartmental shifts, and increased renal losses (Table 33-12). Often, more than one of these mechanisms is active. Unless food intake is severely restricted, dietary intake and intestinal absorption of phosphorus are usually adequate. Intestinal absorption may be inhibited by administration of glucocorticoids, high dietary levels of magnesium, and hypothyroidism. Prolonged ingestion of antacids may also interfere with intestinal absorption. Antacids that contain aluminum hydroxide, aluminum carbonate, and calcium carbonate bind with phosphate, causing increased phosphate losses in the stool. Because of their ability to bind phosphate, calcium-based antacids are sometimes used therapeutically to decrease phosphate levels in persons with chronic renal failure.

Alcoholism is a common cause of hypophosphatemia. The mechanisms underlying hypophosphatemia in the person addicted to alcohol may be related to malnutrition, increased renal excretion rates, or hypomagnesemia. Malnutrition and diabetic ketoacidosis increase phosphate excretion and phosphate loss from the body. Refeeding of malnourished patients increases the incorporation of phosphate into nucleic acids and phosphorylated compounds in the cell. The same thing happens when diabetic ketoacidosis is reversed with insulin therapy. Urinary losses of phosphate may be caused by drugs, such as theophylline, corticosteroids, and loop diuretics, that increase renal excretion.

Hypophosphatemia can occur during prolonged courses of glucose administration or hyperalimentation. Glucose administration causes insulin release, with transport of glucose and phosphorus into the cell. The catabolic events that occur with diabetic ketoacidosis also deplete phosphate stores. However, hypophosphatemia does not become apparent until insulin and fluid replacement have reversed dehydration and glucose has started to move back into the cell. Administration of hyperalimentation solutions without adequate phosphorus can cause a rapid influx

TABLE 33-12 Causes and Manifestations of Hypophosphatemia

Causes	Manifestations
Decreased Intestinal Absorption	**Laboratory Values**
Antacids (aluminum and calcium)	Serum levels below 2.5 mg/dL in adults and 4.0 mg/dL in children
Severe diarrhea	
Lack of vitamin D	**Neural Manifestations**
Increased Renal Elimination	Intention tremor
Alkalosis	Ataxia
Hyperparathyroidism	Paresthesias
Diabetic ketoacidosis	Confusion, stupor, coma
Renal tubular absorption defects	Seizures
Malnutrition and Intracellular Shifts	**Musculoskeletal Manifestations**
Alcoholism	Muscle weakness
Total parenteral hyperalimentation	Joint stiffness
Recovery from malnutrition	Bone pain
Administration of insulin during recovery from diabetic ketoacidosis	Osteomalacia
	Blood Disorders
	Hemolytic anemia
	Platelet dysfunction with bleeding disorders
	Impaired white blood cell function

of phosphorus into the body's muscle mass, particularly if treatment is initiated after a period of tissue catabolism. Because only a small amount of total body phosphorus is in the extracellular compartment, even a small redistribution between the extracellular and intracellular compartments can cause hypophosphatemia, even though total phosphate levels have not changed.

Respiratory alkalosis due to prolonged hyperventilation can produce hypophosphatemia through decreased levels of ionized calcium from increased protein binding, increased PTH release, and increased phosphate excretion. Clinical conditions associated with hyperventilation include gram-negative septicemia, alcohol withdrawal, heat stroke, and primary hyperventilation.[51,52]

Manifestations. Many of the manifestations of phosphorus deficiency result from a decrease in cellular energy stores due to deficiency in ATP and impaired oxygen transport due to a decrease in red blood cell 2,3-diphosphoglycerate (see Chapter 16). Hypophosphatemia results in altered neural function, disturbed musculoskeletal function, and hematologic disorders (see Table 33-12).

Red blood cell metabolism is impaired by phosphate deficiency; the cells become rigid, undergo increased hemolysis, and have diminished ATP and 2,3-diphosphoglycerate levels. Chemotaxis and phagocytosis by white blood cells are impaired. Platelet function also is disturbed. Respiratory insufficiency resulting from impaired function of the respiratory muscles can develop in patients with severe hypophosphatemia.

Neural manifestations include intention tremors, paresthesia, hyporeflexia, stupor, coma, and seizures. Anorexia and dysphagia can occur. Muscle weakness, which is common in hypophosphatemia, is related to a reduction in 2,3-diphosphoglycerate. Chronic phosphate depletion interferes with mineralization of newly formed bone matrix. In growing children, this process causes abnormal endochondral growth and clinical manifestations of rickets. In adults, the condition leads to joint stiffness, bone pain, and skeletal deformities consistent with osteomalacia (see Chapter 58).

Treatment. The treatment of hypophosphatemia is replacement therapy. This may be accomplished with dietary sources high in phosphate (one glassful of milk contains approximately 250 mg of phosphate) or with oral or intravenous replacement solutions. Phosphate supplements usually are contraindicated in hypercalcemia and renal failure because of the increased risk for extracellular calcifications that occur when the calcium × phosphate product exceeds that needed for precipitation of calcium phosphate.

Hyperphosphatemia

Hyperphosphatemia represents a plasma phosphorus concentration in excess of 4.5 mg/dL in adults. Growing children normally have plasma phosphate levels higher than those of adults.

Causes. Hyperphosphatemia results from failure of the kidneys to excrete excess phosphate, rapid redistribution of intracellular phosphate to the extracellular compartment, and excessive intake of phosphate.[52] The most common cause of hyperphosphatemia is impaired renal function (Table 33-13).

Hyperphosphatemia is a common electrolyte disorder in persons with chronic renal failure. A reduction in glomerular filtration rate to less than 30 to 50 mL/minute results in a reduction of phosphate elimination. The increase in phosphate levels in persons with end-stage renal disease occurs despite compensatory increases in PTH. Recent studies have shown an increase in soft tissue calcification (vascular and cardiac calcification especially) and mortality

TABLE 33-13 Causes and Manifestations of Hyperphosphatemia

Causes	Manifestations
Acute Phosphate Overload	**Laboratory Values**
Laxatives and enemas containing phosphate	Serum levels above 4.5 mg/dL in adults and 5.4 mg/dL in children
Intravenous phosphate supplementation	(ectopic calcification when Ca × PO_4 > 60)
Intracellular-to-Extracellular Shift	**Neuromuscular Manifestations (Reciprocal Decrease in Serum Calcium)**
Massive trauma	Paresthesias
Heat stroke	Tetany
Seizures	**Cardiovascular Manifestations**
Rhabdomyolysis	Hypotension
Tumor lysis syndrome	Cardiac dysrhythmias
Potassium deficiency	
Impaired Elimination	
Kidney failure	
Hypoparathyroidism	

among patients with end-stage renal disease with hyperphosphatemia.[44,45] Release of intracellular phosphate can result from conditions such as massive tissue injury, rhabdomyolysis, heat stroke, potassium deficiency, and seizures. Chemotherapy can raise plasma phosphate levels because of the rapid destruction of tumor cells (tumor lysis syndrome).

The administration of excess phosphate-containing antacids, laxatives, or enemas can be another cause of hyperphosphatemia, especially when there is a decrease in vascular volume and a reduced glomerular filtration rate. Phosphate-containing laxatives and enemas predispose to hypovolemia and a decreased glomerular filtration rate by inducing diarrhea, thereby increasing the risk for hypophosphatemia. Serious and even fatal hyperphosphatemia has resulted from administration of Fleet Phospho-Soda enterally[53] or as an enema.

Manifestations. Hyperphosphatemia is accompanied by a decrease in plasma calcium. Many of the signs and symptoms of phosphate excess are related to a calcium deficit (see Table 33-13). Ectopic calcifications may develop when the calcium × phosphate concentration product exceeds 60.

Treatment. The treatment of hyperphosphatemia is directed at the cause of the disorder. Dietary restriction of foods that are high in phosphate may be used. Calcium-based phosphate binders are useful in chronic hyperphosphatemia. However, sevelamer, a recently approved calcium- and aluminium-free phosphate binder, is as effective as a calcium-based binder but without its adverse manifestations, such as elevation of the calcium × phosphate product, hypercalcemia, and vascular and cardiac calcifications.[45] Hemodialysis is used to reduce phosphate levels in persons with end-stage renal disease.

ALTERATIONS IN MAGNESIUM BALANCE

Magnesium is the second most abundant intracellular cation. The average adult has approximately 24 g of magnesium distributed throughout the body.[53] Of the total magnesium content, approximately 50% to 60% is stored in bone, 39% to 49% is contained in the body cells, and the remaining 1% is dispersed in the ECF.[54–57] Approximately 20% to 30% of ECF magnesium is protein bound, and only a small fraction of ICF magnesium (15% to 30%) is exchangeable with the ECF. The normal plasma concentration of magnesium is 1.8 to 2.7 mg/dL.

Only recently has the importance of magnesium to the overall function of the body been recognized. Magnesium acts as a cofactor in many intracellular enzyme reactions, including those related to transfer of phosphate groups. It is essential to all reactions that require ATP, for every step related to replication and transcription of DNA, and for the translation of messenger RNA. It is required for cellular energy metabolism, functioning of the sodium–potassium membrane pump, membrane stabilization, nerve conduction, ion transport, and calcium channel activity. Magnesium binds to calcium receptors, and it has been suggested that alterations in magnesium levels may exert their effects through calcium-mediated mechanisms. Magnesium may bind competitively to calcium-binding sites, producing the appropriate response; it may compete with calcium for a binding site but not exert an effect; or it may alter the distribution of calcium by interfering with its movement across the cell membrane.

Gains and Losses

Magnesium is ingested in the diet, absorbed from the intestine, and excreted by the kidneys. Intestinal absorption is not closely regulated, and approximately 25% to 65% of dietary magnesium is absorbed. Magnesium is contained in all green vegetables, grains, nuts, meats, and seafood. Magnesium is also present in much of the groundwater in North America.

The kidney is the principal organ of magnesium regulation. Magnesium is a unique electrolyte in that only approximately 30% to 40% of the filtered amount is reabsorbed in the proximal tubule. The greatest quantity, approximately 50% to 70%, is reabsorbed in the thick ascending loop of Henle. The distal tubule, which reabsorbs

MAGNESIUM BALANCE

- Most of the body's magnesium is located within cells, where it functions in regulation of enzyme activity, generation of ATP, and calcium transport. Magnesium is necessary for parathyroid hormone function and hypomagnesemia is a common cause of hypocalcemia.
- Elimination of magnesium occurs mainly through the kidney, which adjusts urinary excretion as a means of maintaining serum magnesium levels. Diuretics tend to disrupt renal regulatory mechanisms and increase urinary losses of magnesium.
- There is an interdependency between intracellular concentrations of magnesium and potassium such that a decrease in one is accompanied by a decrease in the other. Magnesium deficiency contributes to cardiac dysrhythmias that occur with hypokalemia.

a small amount of magnesium, is the major site of magnesium regulation. Magnesium reabsorption is decreased in the presence of increased plasma levels, stimulated by PTH, and inhibited by increased calcium levels. The major driving force for magnesium absorption in the thick ascending loop of Henle is the $Na^+/K^+\text{-}2Cl^-$ cotransport system (see Chapter 32). Inhibition of this transport system by loop diuretics lowers magnesium reabsorption.

Hypomagnesemia

Hypomagnesemia represents a plasma magnesium concentration of less than 1.8 mg/dL.[58] It is seen in conditions that limit intake or increase intestinal or renal losses, and it is a common finding in emergency departments and critical care patients.

Causes. Magnesium deficiency can result from insufficient intake, excessive losses, or movement between the ECF and ICF compartments (Table 33-14). It can result from conditions that directly limit intake, such as malnutrition, starvation, or prolonged maintenance of magnesium-free parenteral nutrition. Other conditions, such as diarrhea, malabsorption syndromes, prolonged nasogastric suction, and laxative abuse, decrease intestinal absorption. Excessive calcium intake impairs intestinal absorption of magnesium by competing for the same transport site. Another common cause of magnesium deficiency is chronic alcoholism. Many factors contribute to hypomagnesemia in alcoholism, including low intake and gastrointestinal losses from diarrhea. The effects of hypomagnesemia are exaggerated by other electrolyte disorders, such as hypokalemia, hypocalcemia, and metabolic acidosis. There also is evidence that alcohol inhibits reabsorption of magnesium by the kidney.[54]

Although the kidneys are able to defend against hypermagnesemia, they are less able to conserve magnesium and prevent hypomagnesemia. Urine losses are increased in diabetic ketoacidosis, hyperparathyroidism, and hyperaldosteronism. Some drugs increase renal losses of magnesium, including diuretics (particularly loop diuretics) and nephrotoxic drugs such as aminoglycoside antibiotics, cyclosporine, cisplatin, and amphotericin B.

Relative hypomagnesemia may also develop in conditions that promote movement of magnesium between the extracellular and intracellular compartments, including rapid administration of glucose, insulin-containing parenteral solutions, and alkalosis. Although transient, these conditions can cause serious alterations in body function.

Manifestations. Magnesium deficiency usually occurs in conjunction with hypocalcemia and hypokalemia, producing a number of related neurologic and cardiovascular manifestations (see Table 33-14). Hypocalcemia is typical of severe hypomagnesemia. Most persons with

TABLE 33-14 Causes and Manifestations of Hypomagnesemia

Causes	Manifestations
Impaired Intake or Absorption	**Laboratory Values**
Alcoholism	Serum magnesium level less than 1.8 mg/dL
Malnutrition or starvation	**Neuromuscular Manifestations**
Malabsorption	Personality change
Small bowel bypass surgery	Athetoid or choreiform movements
Parenteral hyperalimentation with inadequate amounts of magnesium	Nystagmus
High dietary intake of calcium without concomitant amounts of magnesium	Tetany
Increased Losses	Positive Babinski's, Chvostek's, Trousseau's signs
Diuretic therapy	**Cardiovascular Manifestations**
Hyperparathyroidism	Tachycardia
Hyperaldosteronism	Hypertension
Diabetic ketoacidosis	Cardiac dysrhythmias
Magnesium-wasting kidney disease	

hypomagnesemia-related hypocalcemia have decreased PTH levels, probably as a result of impaired magnesium-dependent mechanisms that control PTH release and synthesis. There is also evidence that hypomagnesemia decreases both the PTH-dependent and PTH-independent release of calcium from bone. In hypomagnesemia, magnesium ions (Mg^{2+}) are released from bone in exchange for increased uptake of calcium from the ECF.

Hypokalemia also is a typical feature of hypomagnesemia. It leads to a reduction in intracellular potassium and impairs the ability of the kidney to conserve potassium. When hypomagnesemia is present, hypokalemia is unresponsive to potassium replacement therapy.

Magnesium is vital to carbohydrate metabolism and the generation of both aerobic and anaerobic metabolisms. Many of the manifestations of magnesium deficit are due to related electrolyte disorders such as hypokalemia and hypocalcemia. Hypocalcemia may be evidenced by personality changes and neuromuscular irritability along with tremors, athetoid or choreiform movements, and positive Chvostek's or Trousseau's signs (see Fig. 33-16). Cardiovascular manifestations include tachycardia, hypertension, and ventricular dysrhythmias. There may be ECG changes such as widening of the QRS complex, appearance of peak T waves, prolongation of PR interval, T-wave inversion, and appearance of U waves. Ventricular dysrhythmias, particularly in the presence of digitalis, may be difficult to treat unless magnesium levels are normalized.

Persistent magnesium deficiency has been implicated as a risk factor for osteoporosis and osteomalacia, particularly in persons with chronic alcoholism, diabetes mellitus, and malabsorption syndrome.

Treatment. Hypomagnesemia is treated with magnesium replacement. The route of administration depends on the severity of the condition. Symptomatic, moderate to severe magnesium deficiency is treated by parenteral administration. Treatment must be continued for several days to replace stored and plasma levels. In conditions of chronic intestinal or renal loss, maintenance support with oral magnesium may be required. Patients with any degree of renal failure must be carefully monitored to prevent magnesium excess. Magnesium often is used therapeutically to treat cardiac dysrhythmia, myocardial infarct, angina, and pregnancy complicated by preeclampsia or eclampsia. Caution to prevent hypermagnesemia is essential.

Hypermagnesemia

Hypermagnesemia represents a plasma magnesium concentration in excess of 2.7 mg/dL. Because of the ability of the normal kidney to excrete magnesium, hypermagnesemia is rare.

Causes. When hypermagnesemia does occur, it usually is related to renal insufficiency and the injudicious use of magnesium-containing medications such as antacids, mineral supplements, and laxatives (Table 33-15). Elderly persons are particularly at risk because they have age-related reductions in renal function and tend to consume more magnesium-containing medications. Magnesium sulfate is used to treat toxemia of pregnancy and premature labor; in these cases, careful monitoring for signs of hypermagnesemia is essential.

Manifestations. Hypermagnesemia affects neuromuscular and cardiovascular function (see Table 33-15). Because magnesium tends to suppress PTH secretion, hypocalcemia may accompany hypermagnesemia. The signs and symptoms occur only when plasma magnesium levels exceed 4.9 mg/dL (2 mmol/L). Deep tendon reflexes begin to decrease as magnesium plasma levels exceed 4 mEq/L.[58]

Hypermagnesemia diminishes neuromuscular function, causing hyporeflexia, muscle weakness, and confusion. Magnesium decreases acetylcholine release at the myoneural junction and may cause neuromuscular blockade and respiratory paralysis. Cardiovascular effects are related to the calcium channel–blocking effects of magnesium. Blood pressure is decreased, and the ECG shows an increase in the PR interval, a shortening of the QT interval, T-wave abnormalities, and prolongation of the QRS and PR intervals. Hypotension due to vasodilation and cardiac dysrhythmias can occur with moderate hypermagnesemia (<10 mg/dL), and confusion and coma can occur with severe

TABLE 33-15 Causes and Manifestations of Hypermagnesemia

Causes	Manifestations
Excessive Intake	**Laboratory Values**
Intravenous administration of magnesium for treatment of preeclampsia	Serum values in excess of 2.7 mg/dL
Excessive use of oral magnesium-containing medications	**Neuromuscular Manifestations**
Decreased Excretion	Lethargy
Kidney disease	Hyporeflexia
Glomerulonephritis	Confusion
Tubulointerstitial kidney disease	Coma
Acute renal failure	**Cardiovascular Manifestations**
	Hypotension
	Cardiac dysrhythmias
	Cardiac arrest

hypermagnesemia (≥10 mg/dL). Very severe hypermagnesemia (>15 mg/dL) may cause cardiac arrest.

Treatment. The treatment of hypermagnesemia includes cessation of magnesium administration. Calcium is a direct antagonist of magnesium, and intravenous administration of calcium may be used. Peritoneal dialysis or hemodialysis may be required.

In summary, calcium, phosphate, and magnesium are major divalent ions in the body. Calcium is a major divalent cation. Approximately 99% of body calcium is found in bone; less than 1% is found in the ECF compartment. The calcium in bone is in dynamic equilibrium with ECF calcium. Of the three forms of ECF calcium (*i.e.*, protein bound, complexed, and ionized), only the ionized form can cross the cell membrane and contribute to cellular function. Ionized calcium has a number of functions. It contributes to neuromuscular function, plays a vital role in the blood-clotting process, and participates in a number of enzyme reactions. Alterations in ionized calcium levels produce neural effects; neural excitability is increased in hypocalcemia and decreased in hypercalcemia.

Phosphate is largely an ICF anion. It is incorporated into the nucleic acids and ATP. The most common causes of altered levels of ECF phosphate are alterations in intestinal absorption, transcompartmental shifts, and disorders of renal elimination. Phosphate deficit causes signs and symptoms of neural dysfunction, disturbed musculoskeletal function, and hematologic disorders. Most of these manifestations result from a decrease in cellular energy stores from a deficiency in ATP and oxygen transport by 2,3-diphosphoglycerate in the red blood cell. Phosphate excess occurs with renal failure and PTH deficit; it is associated with decreased serum calcium levels.

Magnesium is the second most abundant ICF cation. It acts as a cofactor in many enzyme reactions and affects neuromuscular function in the same manner as the Ca^{2+}. Magnesium deficiency can result from insufficient intake, excessive losses, or movement between the ECF and ICF compartments. Hypomagnesemia impairs PTH release and the actions of PTH; it leads to a reduction in ICF potassium and impairs the ability of the kidney to conserve potassium. The signs and symptoms of hypomagnesemia are therefore similar to those of hypocalcemia. Hypermagnesemia usually is related to renal insufficiency and the injudicious use of magnesium-containing medications such as antacids, mineral supplements, or laxatives. It can cause neuromuscular dysfunction with hyporeflexia, muscle weakness, and confusion. Magnesium decreases acetylcholine release at the myoneural junction and may cause neuromuscular blockade and respiratory paralysis.

REVIEW EXERCISES

A 40-year-old man with advanced acquired immunodeficiency syndrome (AIDS) presents with an acute chest infection. Investigations confirm a diagnosis of *P. carinii* pneumonia. Although he is being treated appropriately, his serum sodium level is 118 mEq/L. Tests of adrenal function are normal.

A. What is the likely cause of his electrolyte disturbance?

B. What are the five cardinal features of this condition?

A 70-year-old woman who is taking furosemide (a loop diuretic) for congestive heart failure complains of weakness, fatigue, and cramping of the muscles in her legs. Her serum potassium is 2.0 mEq, and her serum sodium is 140 mEq/L. She also complains that she notices a "strange heartbeat" at times.

A. What is the likely cause of this woman's symptoms?

B. An ECG shows depressed ST segment and low T-wave changes. Explain the physiologic mechanism underlying these changes.

C. What would be the treatment for this woman?

A 50-year-old woman presents with symptomatic hypercalcemia. She has a recent history of breast cancer treatment.

A. How do you evaluate this person with increased serum calcium levels?

B. What is the significance of the recent history of malignancy?

C. What further tests may be indicated?

References

1. Krieger J.N., Sherrad D.J. (1991). *Practical fluid and electrolytes* (pp. 104–105). Norwalk, CT: Appleton & Lange.
2. Guyton A., Hall J.E. (2000). *Textbook of medical physiology* (10th ed., pp. 158–171, 264–278, 322–345, 820–826). Philadelphia: W.B. Saunders.
3. Rose B.D., Post T.W. (2001). *Clinical physiology of acid-base and electrolyte disorders* (5th ed., pp. 187–190, 478–479, 547, 841–842, 896–897). New York: McGraw-Hill.
4. Kokko J.P. (1996). Disorders of fluid volume, electrolyte, and acid-base balance. In Bennett J.C., Plum F. (Eds.), *Cecil textbook of medicine* (20th ed., p. 525–543). Philadelphia: W.B. Saunders.
5. Cogan M.G. (1991). *Fluid and electrolytes* (pp. 43, 112–123, 80–84, 1, 100–111, 125–130, 242–245). Norwalk, CT: Appleton & Lange.
6. Brewster U.C., Selaro J.F., Perazella M.A. (2003). The renin-angiotensin-aldosterone system: cardiorenal effects and implications for renal and cardiovascular disease states. *American Journal of Medical Sciences 326*, 15–24.
7. Stearns R.H., Spital A., Clark E.C. (1996). Disorders of water balance. In Kokko J., Tannen R.L. (Eds.), *Fluids and electrolytes* (3rd ed., pp. 65, 69, 95). Philadelphia: W.B. Saunders.
8. Metheney N.M. (2000). *Fluid and electrolyte balance* (4th ed., pp. 3, 18, 47, 56, 256). Philadelphia: Lippincott Williams & Wilkins.
9. Porth C.J.M., Erickson M. (1992). Physiology of thirst and drinking: Implications for nursing practice. *Heart and Lung 21*, 273–284.
10. Ayus J.C., Arieff A.I. (1996). Abnormalities of water metabolism in the elderly. *Seminars in Nephrology 16*(4), 277–288.
11. Rolls B., Phillips P.A. (1990). Aging and disturbances of thirst and fluid balance. *Nutrition Reviews 48*(3), 137–143.

12. Kugler J.P., Hustead T. (2000). Hyponatremia and hypernatremia in the elderly. *American Family Physician 61,* 3623–3630.
13. Illowsky B.P., Kirch D.G. (1988). Polydipsia and hyponatremia in psychiatric patients. *American Journal of Psychiatry 145,* 675–683.
14. Vieweg W.V.R. (1994). Treatment strategies for polydipsia-hyponatremia syndrome. *Journal of Clinical Psychiatry 55*(4), 154–159.
15. Robertson A.G., Verbalis J.G. (2003). The posterior pituitary gland. *Williams textbook of Endocrinology* (10th ed., pp. 281–329). Philadelphia: W.B. Saunders.
16. Ishikara S., Schrier R.W. (2003). Pathophysiological roles of arginine vasopressin and aquaporin-2 in impaired water excretion. *Clinical Endocrinology 58,* 1–17.
17. Berne R.M., Levy M. (2000). *Principles of physiology* (3rd ed., p. 438). St. Louis: Mosby.
18. Holzman E.J., Ausiello D.A. (1994). Nephrogenic diabetes insipidus: Causes revealed. *Hospital Practice 29*(3), 89–104.
19. Bendz H., Aurell M. (1999). Drug-induced diabetes insipidus. *Drug Safety 21,* 449–456.
20. Baylis P. (2003). The syndrome of inappropriate antidiuretic hormone secretion. *International Journal of Biochemistry and Cellular Biology 35,* 1495–1499.
21. Kumar S., Beri T. (1998). Sodium. *Lancet 352,* 220–228.
22. Adrogue H.J., Madias N.E. (2000). Hyponatremia. *New England Journal of Medicine 343,* 1581–1589.
23. Oh M.S., Carroll H.J. (1992). Disorders of sodium metabolism: Hypernatremia and hyponatremia. *Critical Care Medicine 20,* 94–103.
24. McManus M.L., Churchwell K.B., Strange K. (1995). Regulation of cell volume in health and disease. *New England Journal of Medicine 333,* 1260–1266.
25. Adrogue H.J., Madias N.E. (2000). Hypernatremia. *New England Journal of Medicine 342,* 1493–1499.
26. Casteel H.B., Fiedorek S.C. (1990). Oral rehydration therapy. *Pediatric Clinics of North America 37,* 295–311.
27. Behrman R.E., Kliegman R.M., Jenson H.B. (2000). *Nelson textbook of pediatrics* (16th ed., pp. 215–218). Philadelphia: W.B. Saunders.
28. Meyers A. (1995). Modern management of acute diarrhea and dehydration in children. *American Family Physician 51*(5), 1103–1118.
29. Weisman Z. (1986). Cola drinks and rehydration in acute diarrhea [Letter]. *New England Journal of Medicine 315,* 768.
30. Gennari F.J. (2002). Disorders of potassium homeostasis—hypokalemia and hyperkalemia. *Critical Care Clinics of North America 18,* 273–288.
31. Mandel A.K. (1997). Hypokalemia and hyperkalemia. *Medical Clinics of North America 81,* 611–639.
32. Gennari F.J. (1998). Hypokalemia. *New England Journal of Medicine 339,* 451–458.
33. Tannen R.L. (1996). Potassium disorders. In Kokko J., Tannen R.L. (Eds.). *Fluids and electrolytes* (3rd ed., pp. 116–118). Philadelphia: W.B. Saunders.
34. Knochel J.P. (1982). Neuromuscular manifestations of electrolyte disorders. *American Journal of Medicine 72*(3), 521–535.
35. Matfin G., Durand D., D'Agostino A., Adelman H. (1998). Thyrotoxic hypokalemic periodic paralysis. *Hospital Practice 1,* 23–26.
36. Whang G., Whang G.G., Ryan M.P. (1992). Refractory potassium repletion: A consequence of magnesium deficiency. *Archives of Internal Medicine 152*(1), 40–45.
37. Clark B.A., Brown R.S. (1995). Potassium homeostasis and hyperkalemic syndromes. *Endocrinology and Metabolic Clinics of North America 24,* 573–590.
38. Peterson L.N., Levi M. (2003). Disorders of potassium metabolism. In Schrier R.W. *Renal and Electrolyte Disorders* (6th ed., pp. 171–212). Philadelphia: Lippincott Williams & Wilkins.
39. Slatopolsky E., Finch J., Brown A. (2003). New vitamin D analogs. *Kidney International 85,* 83–87.
40. Quarles L.D. (2003). Extracellular calcium-sensing receptors in the parathyroid gland, kidney, and other tissues. *Current Opinions in Nephrology and Hypertension 12,* 349–355.
41. Korbin S.M., Goldfarb S. (1990). Magnesium deficiency. *Seminars in Nephrology 10,* 525–535.
42. Clark O.H. (2003). How should patients with primary hyperparathyroidism be treated? *Journal of Clinical Endocrinology and Metabolism 88,* 3011–3014.
43. Llach F. (1999). Hyperphosphemia in end-stage renal disease patients: Pathological consequences. *Kidney International 56*(Suppl. 73), S31–S37.
44. Goodman W.G. (2003). Medical management of secondary hyperparathyroidism in chronic renal failure. *Nephrology, Dialysis and Transplantation 18*(Suppl 3), S2–S8.
45. Hervas J.G., Prados D., Cerezo S. (2003). Treatment of hyperphosphatemia with sevelamer hydrochloride in hemodialysis patients. *Kidney International 85,* 69–72.
46. Zaloga G.F. (1992). Hypocalcemia in critically ill patients. *Critical Care Medicine 20,* 251–262.
47. Yucha C.B., Toto K.H. (1994). Calcium and phosphorous derangements. *Critical Care Clinics of North America 6,* 747–765.
48. Reber R.M., Heath H. (1995). Hypocalcemic emergencies. *Medical Clinics of North America 79,* 93–165.
49. Carroll M.F., Schade D.S. (2003). A practical approach to hypercalcemia. *American Family Physician 67,* 1959–1966.
50. Strewler G.J. (2000). The physiology of parathyroid hormone-related protein. *New England Journal of Medicine 342,* 177–185.
51. Dennis V.W. (1996). Phosphate disorders. In Kokko J., Tannen R.L. (Eds.), *Fluids and electrolytes* (3rd ed., pp. 359–382). Philadelphia: W.B. Saunders.
52. Weisinger J., Bellorin-Font E. (1998). Magnesium and phosphate. *Lancet 352,* 391–396.
53. Fass R., Do S., Hixson L.J. (1993). Fatal hyperphosphatemia following Fleet Phospho-Soda in patient with colonic ileus. *American Journal of Gastroenterology 88*(6), 929–932.
54. Workman L. (1992). Magnesium and phosphorus: The neglected electrolytes. *ACCN Clinical Issues 3,* 655–663.
55. Swain R., Kaplan-Machlis B. (1999). Magnesium for the next millennium. *Southern Medical Journal 92,* 1040–1046.
56. Nadler J.L., Rude R.K. (1995). Disorders of magnesium metabolism. *Endocrinology and Metabolism Clinics of North America 24,* 623–639.
57. Rude R.K. (1998). Magnesium deficiency: A cause for heterogeneous disease in humans. *Journal of Bone and Mineral Metabolism 13,* 749–755.
58. Topf J.M., Murray P.T. (2003). Hypomagnesemia and hypermagnesemia. *Reviews in Endocrine and Metabolic Disorders 4,* 195–206.

CHAPTER

34

Disorders of Acid-Base Balance

Metabolic activities of the body require the precise regulation of acid-base balance, which is reflected in the pH of extracellular fluids. Membrane excitability, enzyme systems, and chemical reactions depend on acid-base balance being regulated within a narrow physiologic range to function in an optimal way. Many conditions, pathologic or otherwise, can alter body pH. This chapter has been organized into two sections: mechanisms of acid-base balance and disorders of acid-base balance.

Mechanisms of Acid-Base Balance

After you have completed this section of the chapter, you should be able to meet the following objectives:

- Characterize an acid and a base
- Cite the source of metabolic acids
- Describe the three forms of carbon dioxide transport and their contribution to acid-base balance
- Define pH and use the Henderson-Hasselbalch equation to calculate the pH and to compare compensatory mechanisms for regulating pH
- Describe the intracellular and extracellular mechanisms for buffering changes in body pH
- Compare the role of the kidneys and respiratory system in regulation of acid-base balance
- Explain how potassium and hydrogen ions and how bicarbonate and chloride ions interact in pH regulation

Normally, the concentration of body acids and bases is regulated so that the pH of extracellular body fluids is maintained within a very narrow range of 7.35 to 7.45. This balance is maintained through mechanisms that generate, buffer, and eliminate acids and bases. This section of the chapter focuses on acid-base chemistry, the production and regulation of metabolic acids and bicarbonate, calculation of pH, and laboratory tests of acid-base balance.

ACID-BASE CHEMISTRY

An *acid* is a molecule that can release a hydrogen ion (H^+), and a *base* is a molecule that can accept or combine with an hydrogen ion.[1,2] When an acid (HA) is added to water, it dissociates reversibly to form H^+ and anions (A^-); for example, $HA \rightleftharpoons H^+ + A^-$. The degree to which an acid dissociates and acts as a H^+ ion donor determines whether it is a strong or weak acid. *Strong acids,* such as sulfuric acid, dissociate completely; *weak acids,* such as acetic acid, dissociate only to a limited extent. The same is true of a base and its ability to dissociate and accept an H^+ ion. Most

MECHANISMS OF ACID-BASE BALANCE

- The pH is determined by the ratio of the bicarbonate (HCO_3^-) base to the volatile carbonic acid ($H_2CO_3 \rightleftharpoons H^+ + HCO_3^-$). At a normal pH of 7.4, the ratio is 20:1.
- The pH is regulated by extracellular (carbonic acid [H_2CO_3]/bicarbonate [HCO_3^-]) and intracellular (proteins) systems that buffer changes in pH that would otherwise occur because of the metabolic production of volatile (CO_2) and nonvolatile (*i.e.*, sulfuric and phosphoric) acids.
- The respiratory system regulates the concentration of the volatile carbonic acid ($CO_2 + H_2O \rightleftharpoons H_2CO_3 \rightleftharpoons H^+ + HCO_3^-$) by changing the rate and depth of respiration.
- The kidneys regulate the plasma concentration of HCO_3^- by two processes: reabsorption of the filtered HCO_3^- and generation of new HCO_3^- or the elimination of H^+ ions that have been buffered by tubular systems (phosphate and ammonia) to maintain a luminal pH of at least 4.5.

of the body's acids and bases are weak acids and bases; the most important are *carbonic acid* (H_2CO_3), which is a weak acid derived from carbon dioxide (CO_2), and *bicarbonate* (HCO_3^-), which is a weak base.

The concentration of the H^+ ion in body fluids is low compared with other ions. For example, the sodium ion (Na^+) is present at a concentration approximately 1 million times that of the H^+ ion. Because of its low concentration in body fluids, the H^+ ion is commonly expressed in terms of pH. Specifically, *pH* represents the negative logarithm (p) of the H^+ ion concentration in milliequivalents per liter; a pH value of 7.0 implies an H^+ ion concentration of 10^{-7} (0.0000001) equivalents per liter (mEq/L). The pH is inversely related to the H^+ ion concentration; a low pH indicates a high concentration of H^+ ions, and a high pH indicates a low concentration of H^+ ions.

The *dissociation constant* (K) is used to describe the degree to which an acid or base dissociates. The symbol pK_a refers to the negative logarithm of the dissociation constant for an acid and represents the pH at which the acid is 50% dissociated.[1] Use of a negative logarithm for the dissociation constant allows pH to be expressed as a positive value. Each acid in an aqueous solution has a characteristic pK_a that varies slightly with temperature and pH. At normal body temperature, the pK_a for the HCO_3^- buffer system of the extracellular fluid compartment is 6.1.

METABOLIC ACID AND BICARBONATE PRODUCTION

Acids are continuously generated as byproducts of metabolic processes. Physiologically, these acids fall into two groups: the *volatile acid* H_2CO_3 and all other *nonvolatile* or *fixed acids*.

The difference between the two types of acids arises because H_2CO_3 is in equilibrium with the volatile gas CO_2, which leaves the body by way of the lungs (Fig. 34-1). The concentration of H_2CO_3 is therefore determined by the lungs and their respiratory capacity. The *fixed acids* (*e.g.*, sulfuric, hydrochloric, phosphoric) are *nonvolatile* and are not eliminated by the lungs. Instead, they are buffered by body proteins or extracellular buffers, such as HCO_3^-, and then excreted by the kidney.

Carbon Dioxide and Bicarbonate Production

Body metabolism results in the production of approximately 15,000 mmol of CO_2 each day.[1] Carbon dioxide is transported in the circulation in three forms: attached to hemoglobin, as dissolved CO_2 in the plasma, and as HCO_3^- (Fig. 34-2). Collectively, dissolved CO_2 and HCO_3^- constitute approximately 77% of the CO_2 that is transported in the extracellular fluid; the remaining CO_2 travels attached to hemoglobin.[2] Although CO_2 is not an acid, a small percentage of the gas combines with water in the bloodstream to form H_2CO_3.

The reaction that generates H_2CO_3 from CO_2 and water is catalyzed by an enzyme called *carbonic anhydrase,* which is present in large quantities in red blood cells, renal tubular cells, and other tissues in the body. The rate of the reaction between CO_2 and water is increased approximately 5000 times by the presence of carbonic anhydrase. Were it not for this enzyme, the reaction would occur too slowly to be of any significance.

Because it is almost impossible to measure H_2CO_3, dissolved CO_2 measurements are commonly substituted when calculating pH. The H_2CO_3 content of the blood can be calculated by multiplying the partial pressure of CO_2 (PCO_2) by its solubility coefficient, which is 0.03. This means that the concentration of H_2CO_3 in arterial blood, which normally has a PCO_2 of approximately 40 mm Hg, is 1.2 mEq/L ($40 \times 0.03 = 1.2$).

Production of Noncarbonic Acids and Bases

The metabolism of dietary proteins and other substances results in the generation of noncarbonic acids and bases.[1] Oxidation of the sulfur-containing amino acids (*e.g.*, methionine, cysteine, cystine) results in the production of sulfuric acid. Oxidation of arginine and lysine produces hydrochloric acid, and oxidation of phosphorus-containing nucleic acids yields phosphoric acid. Incomplete oxidation of glucose results in the formation of lactic acid, and incomplete oxidation of fats results in the production of ketoacids. The major source of base is the metabolism of amino acids such as aspartate and glutamate and the metabolism of certain organic anions (*e.g.*, citrate, lactate, acetate). Acid production normally exceeds base production, with the net effect being the addition of approximately 1 mmol/kg body weight of nonvolatile or fixed acid to the body each day.[1] A vegetarian diet, which contains large amounts of organic anions, results in the net production of base.

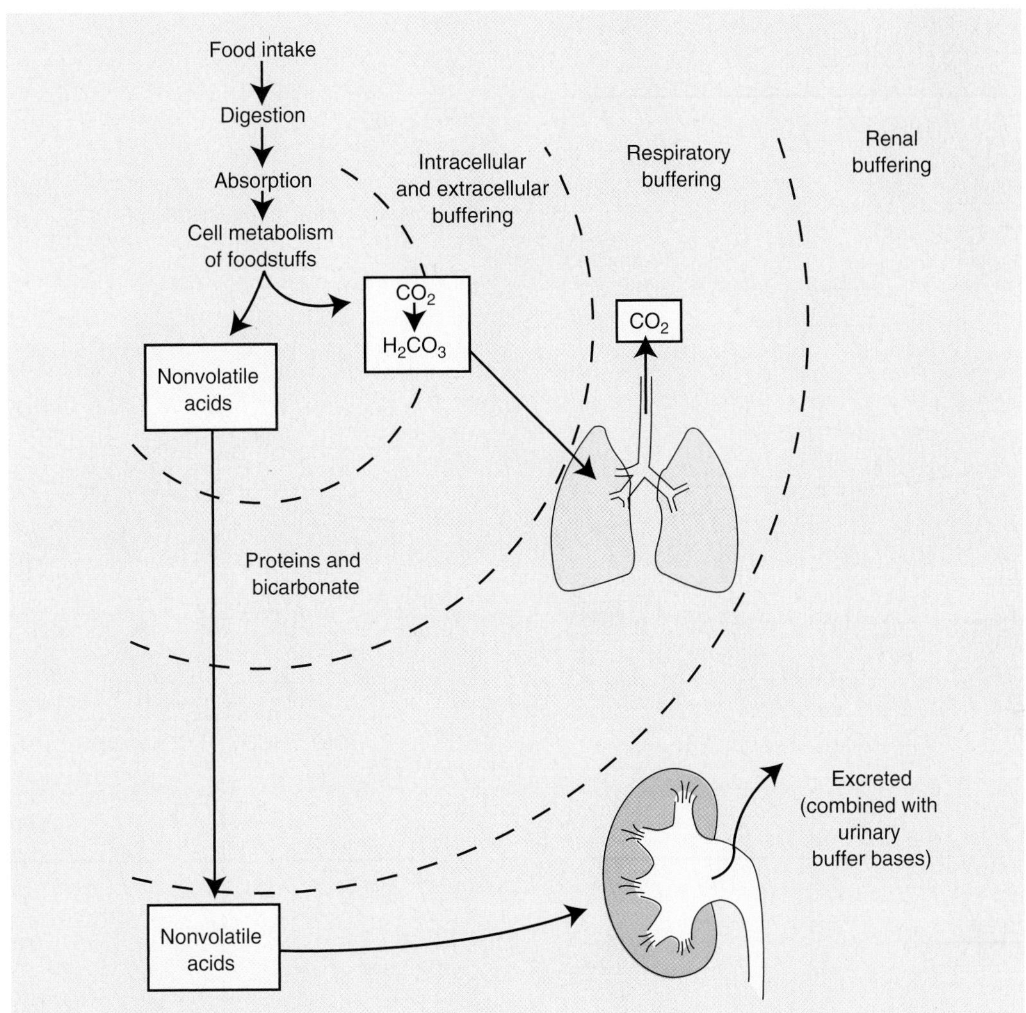

FIGURE 34-1 The role of intracellular and extracellular buffer, respiratory, and renal mechanisms in maintaining normal blood pH. (Rhoades R. A., Tanner G. A. [1996]. *Medical physiology* [p. 468]. Boston: Little, Brown)

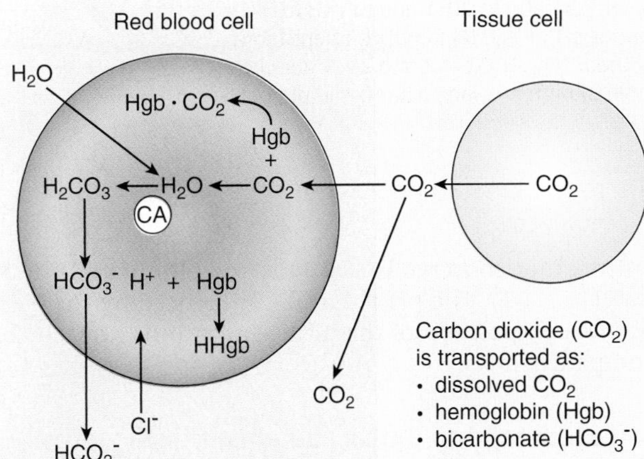

FIGURE 34-2 Mechanisms of carbon dioxide transport. CA, carbonic anhydrase.

CALCULATION OF pH

The plasma pH can be calculated using an equation called the *Henderson-Hasselbalch equation.* This equation uses the negative logarithm of the dissociation constant and the logarithm of the HCO_3^- to CO_2 (HCO_3^-/CO_2) ratio to calculate pH: pH = pK_a (6.1) + $\log_{10}$ $HCO_3^-/(0.03 \times CO_2)$. It should be noted that it is the ratio rather than the absolute values for bicarbonate and dissolved CO_2 that determines pH (*e.g.,* when the ratio is 20:1, pH = 7.4). Plasma pH decreases when the ratio is less than 20:1, and it increases when the ratio is greater than 20:1 (Fig. 34-3).

Because it is the ratio rather than the absolute values of HCO_3^- or CO_2 that determines pH, the pH can remain within relatively normal values as long as changes in HCO_3^- are accompanied by similar changes in CO_2, or vice versa. For example, the pH will remain at 7.4 when plasma HCO_3^- has increased from 24 to 48 mEq/L as long as CO_2

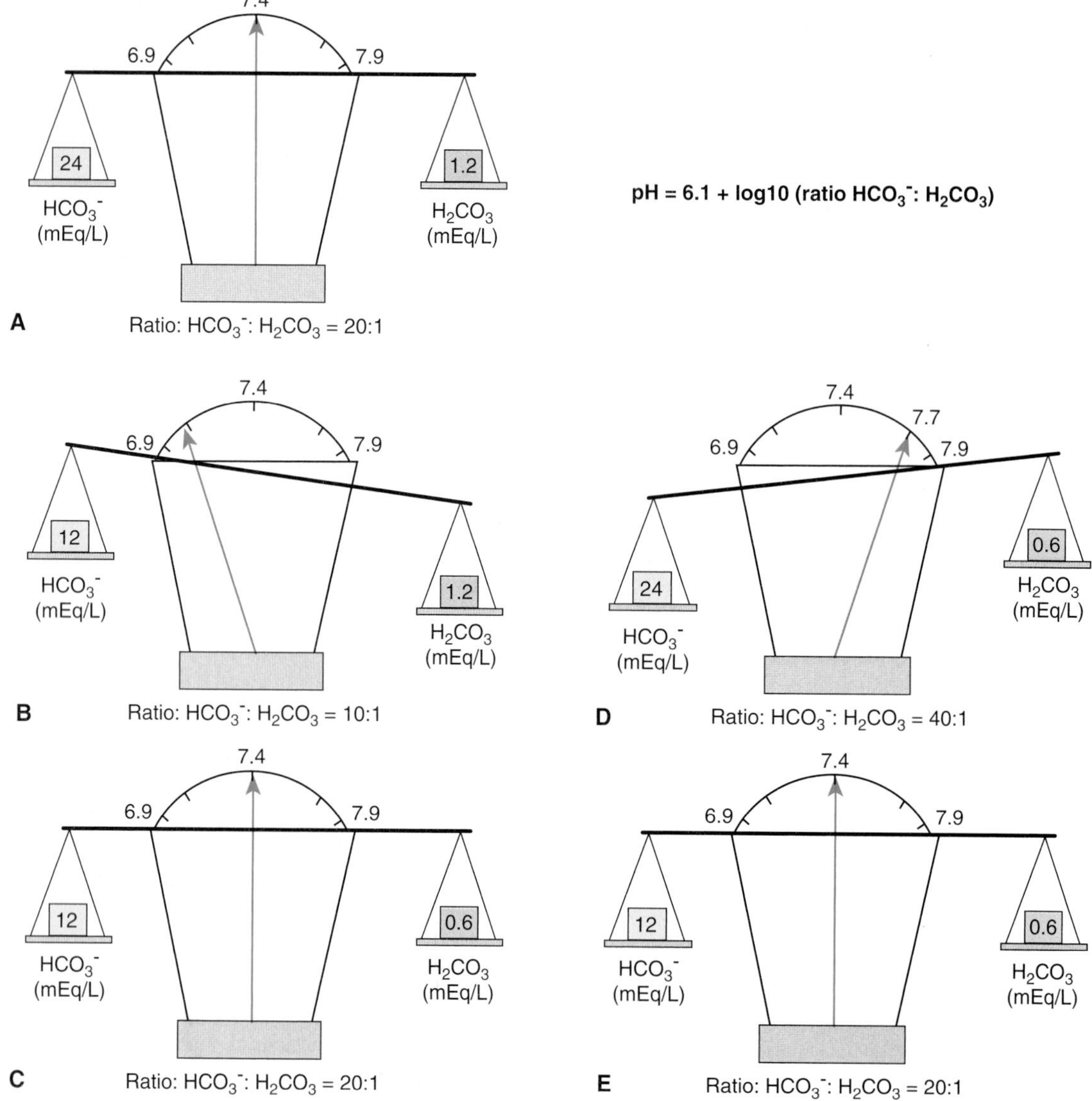

FIGURE 34-3 Normal and compensated states of pH and acid-base balance represented as a balance scale. (**A**) When the ratio of bicarbonate (HCO_3^-) to carbonic acid (H_2CO_3, arterial $CO_2 \times .03$) = 20:1, the pH = 7.4. (**B**) Metabolic acidosis with an HCO_3^-:H_3CO_3 ratio of 10:1 and a pH of 7.1. (**C**) Respiratory compensation lowers the H_3CO_3 to 0.6 mEq/L and returns the HCO_3^-:H_3CO_3 ratio to 20:1 and the pH to 7.4. (**D**) Respiratory alkalosis with an HCO_3^-:H_3CO_3 ratio of 40:1 and a pH of 7.7. (**E**) Renal compensation eliminates HCO_3^-, reducing serum levels to 12 mEq/L, returning the HCO_3^-:H_3CO_3 ratio to 20:1 and the pH to 7.4. Normally, these compensatory mechanisms are capable of buffering large changes in pH, but do not return the pH completely to normal, as illustrated here.

levels are also doubled (see Fig. 34-3). Likewise, the pH will remain at 7.4 when plasma HCO_3^- has decreased from 24 to 12 mEq/L as long as CO_2 levels are reduced by one half.

REGULATION OF pH

The pH of body fluids is regulated by intracellular and extracellular buffering systems that prevent large changes in the extracellular pH from occurring through respiratory mechanisms that eliminate CO_2 and by renal mechanisms that conserve HCO_3^- ions and eliminate H^+ ions (see Fig. 34-1). The pH is further influenced by the electrolyte composition of the intracellular and extracellular compartments.

Intracellular and Extracellular Buffer Systems

The moment-by-moment regulation of pH depends on intracellular and extracellular buffer systems. A *buffer system* consists of a weak acid and the base salt of that acid or of a weak base and its acid salt. In the process of preventing large changes in pH, the system trades a strong acid for a weak acid or a strong base for a weak base.

The two major buffer systems that protect the pH of body fluids are proteins and the bicarbonate buffer system.[3,4] These buffer systems are immediately available to combine with excess acids or bases and prevent large changes in pH from occurring during the time it takes for respiratory and renal mechanisms to become effective. Bone also represents an important site for buffering of acids and bases.[3] Although it is difficult to measure, it has been estimated that 40% of acute acid-base buffering occurs in bone.[1] The role of bone buffers is even higher in chronic acid-base disorders. One consequence of bone buffering is the release of calcium from bone and increased renal excretion of calcium. In addition to causing demineralization of bone, it also predisposes to kidney stones.

Protein Buffer Systems. Proteins are the largest buffer system in the body. Proteins are amphoteric, meaning that they can function as acids or bases. They contain many ionizable groups that can release or bind H^+. The protein buffers are largely located in cells, and H^+ ions and CO_2 diffuse across cell membranes for buffering by intracellular proteins. Albumin and plasma globulins are the major protein buffers in the vascular compartment.

Bicarbonate Buffer System. The bicarbonate buffer system uses H_2CO_3 as its weak acid and a bicarbonate salt such as sodium bicarbonate ($NaHCO_3$) as its weak base. It substitutes the weak H_2CO_3 for a strong acid such as hydrochloric acid ($HCl + NaHCO_3 \rightleftharpoons H_2CO_3 + NaCl$) or the weak bicarbonate base for a strong base such as sodium hydroxide ($NaOH + H_2CO_3 \rightleftharpoons NaHCO_3 + H_2O$). The HCO_3^-/CO_2 buffer system is a particularly efficient system because the buffer components can be readily added or removed from the body.[2,5] Metabolism provides an ample supply of CO_2, which can replace any H_2CO_3 that is lost when excess base is added, and CO_2 can be readily eliminated when excess acid is added. Likewise, the kidney can conserve or form new HCO_3^- when excess acid is added, and it can excrete HCO_3^- when excess base is added.

Plasma Potassium–Hydrogen Exchange. Potassium ions (K^+) and H^+ ions interact in important ways in the regulation of acid-base balance. Both ions are positively charged, and both ions move freely between the intracellular and extracellular compartments. In situations of acidosis, excess H^+ ions move into the intracellular compartment for buffering. When this happens, another cation, in this case the K^+ ion, must leave the cell and move into the extracellular fluid. When extracellular potassium levels fall, K^+ ions move out of the cell and are replaced by H^+ ions. Thus, alterations in extracellular potassium levels can affect acid-base balance, and changes in acid-base balance can influence extracellular potassium levels. Potassium shifts tend to be more pronounced in metabolic acidosis than respiratory acidosis.[5,6] Also, metabolic acidosis caused by an accumulation of nonorganic acids (*e.g.,* HCl that occurs in diarrhea, phosphoric acid that occurs in renal failure) produces a greater increase in extracellular potassium than does acidosis caused by an accumulation of organic acids (*e.g.,* lactic acid, ketoacids).

Respiratory Control Mechanisms

The second line of defense against acid-base disturbances is the control of CO_2 by the respiratory system. Excess CO_2 or excess H^+ ions in the blood mainly act directly on the respiratory center in the brain to control ventilation. Although H^+ ions do not easily cross the blood–brain barrier, CO_2 crosses with ease and in the process reacts with water to form carbonic acid, which dissociates into H^+ and HCO_3^- ions. It is the H^+ ion that stimulates the respiratory center, causing an increase or decrease in ventilation.

The respiratory control of pH is rapid, occurring within minutes, and is maximal within 12 to 24 hours.[1] Although the respiratory response is rapid, it does not completely return the pH to normal. It is only about 50% to 75% effective as a buffer system. This means that if the pH falls from 7.4 to 7.0, the respiratory system can return the pH to a value of about 7.2 to 7.3.[2] In acting rapidly, however, it prevents large changes in pH from occurring while waiting for the much more slowly reacting kidneys to respond.

Although CO_2 readily crosses the blood–brain barrier, there is a lag for entry of the HCO_3^- ion. Thus, blood pH and HCO_3^- levels drop more rapidly than cerebrospinal fluid (CSF) levels. In metabolic acidosis, for example, in which there is a primary decrease in HCO_3^- ions, there is often a 12- to 24-hour delay in maximal respiratory response.[1] Likewise, when metabolic acid-base disorders are corrected rapidly, the respiratory response may persist because of a delay in CSF adjustments.

Renal Control Mechanisms

The kidneys regulate acid-base balance by excreting either an acidic or an alkaline urine. Excreting an acidic urine reduces the amount of acid in the extracellular fluid, and excreting an alkaline urine removes base from the extracellular fluid. The renal mechanisms for regulating acid-base balance cannot adjust the pH within minutes, as respiratory mechanisms can, but they continue to function for days until the pH has returned to normal or near-normal range.

Hydrogen Ion Elimination and Bicarbonate Conservation. The kidney regulates pH by excreting excess H^+ ions and reabsorbing or regenerating HCO_3^- ions. Bicarbonate is freely filtered in the glomerulus (approximately 4500 mEq/day) and reabsorbed in the tubules.[5] Loss of even small amounts of HCO_3^- impairs the body's ability to buffer its daily load of metabolic acids. Because H^+ ions are not filtered in adequate amounts to maintain acid-base balance, they are secreted from blood in the peritubular capillaries into the urine filtrate in the renal tubules.

Most of the H^+ ion secretion and reabsorption of HCO_3^- ions takes place in the proximal tubule. The process begins with a coupled Na^+/H^+ transport system in which a H^+ ion is secreted into the tubular fluid and a Na^+ ion is reabsorbed into the tubular cell (Fig. 34-4). The secreted H^+ ion combines with a filtered HCO_3^- ion to yield CO_2 and H_2O. The water is eliminated in the urine, and the CO_2 diffuses into the tubular cell, where it combines with water, in a carbonic anhydrase–mediated reaction to form a HCO_3^- ion and a H^+ ion. The HCO_3^- ion is then reabsorbed into the blood along with the Na^+ ion, and the newly generated H^+

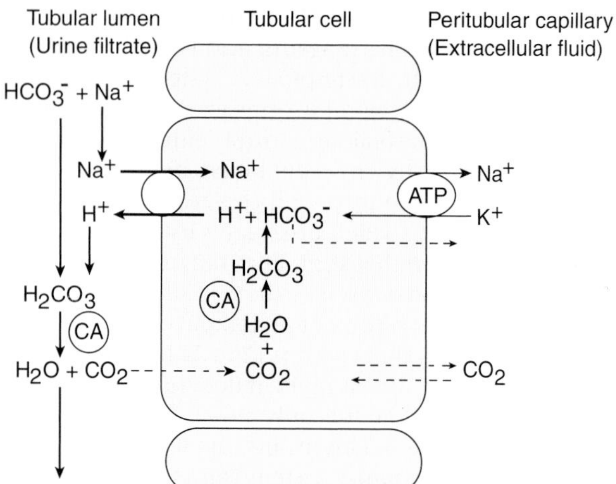

FIGURE 34-4 Hydrogen ion (H^+) secretion and bicarbonate ion (HCO_3^-) reabsorption in a renal tubular cell. Carbon dioxide (CO_2) diffuses from the blood or urine filtrate into the tubular cell, where it combines with water in a carbonic anhydrase-catalyzed reaction that yields carbonic acid (H_2CO_3). The H_2CO_3 dissociates to form H^+ and HCO_3^-. The H^+ is secreted into the tubular fluid in exchange for Na^+. The Na^+ and HCO_3^- enter the extracellular fluid.

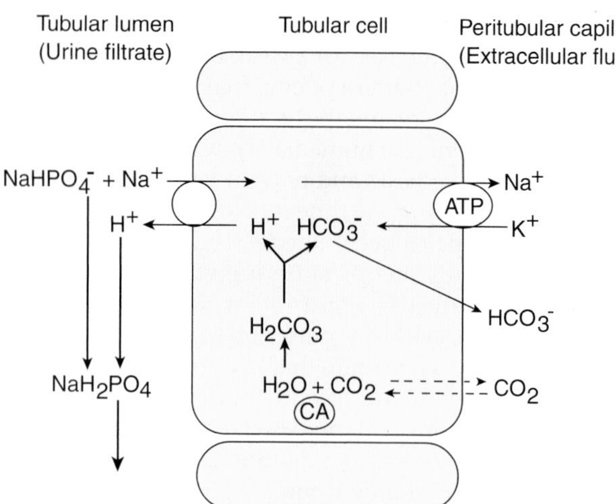

FIGURE 34-5 The renal phosphate buffer system. The monohydrogen phosphate ion (HPO_4^{2-}) enters the renal tubular fluid in the glomerulus. A H^+ combines with the HPO_4^{2-} to form $H_2PO_4^-$ and is then excreted into the urine in combination with Na^+. The HCO_3^- moves into the extracellular fluid along with the Na^+ that was exchanged during secretion of the H^+.

ion is secreted into the tubular fluid to begin another cycle. Normally, only a few of the secreted H^+ ions remain in the tubular fluid because the secretion of H^+ ions is roughly equivalent to the number of HCO_3^- ions that are filtered in the glomerulus.

Tubular Buffer Systems. Because an extremely acidic urine would be damaging to structures in the urinary tract, the pH of the urine is maintained within a range from 4.5 to 8.0. This limits the number of unbuffered H^+ ions that can be excreted by the kidney. When the number of free H^+ ions secreted into the tubular fluid threatens to cause the pH of the urine to become too acidic, they must be carried in some other form. This is accomplished by combining H^+ ions with intratubular buffers before they are excreted in the urine. There are two important intratubular buffer systems: the phosphate buffer system and the ammonia buffer system.

The *phosphate buffer system* uses HPO_4^{2-} and $H_2PO_4^-$ that are present in the tubular filtrate. Both become concentrated in the tubular fluid because of their relatively poor absorption and because of reabsorption of water from the tubular fluid. The combination of H^+ with HPO_4^{2-} to form $H_2PO_4^-$ allows the kidneys to increase their secretion of H^+ ions (Fig. 34-5).

Another important but more complex buffer system is the *ammonia buffer system*. The excretion of H^+ and generation of HCO_3^- by the ammonia buffer system occurs in three major steps: (1) the synthesis of ammonium (NH_4^+) from the amino acid glutamine in the proximal tubule, thick ascending loop of Henle, and distal tubules; (2) the reabsorption and recycling of NH_3 within the medullary portion of the kidney; and (3) the buffering of H^+ ions by NH_3 in the collecting tubules.[1,2] The metabolism of glutamate in the proximal tubule results in the formation of two NH_4^+ and two HCO_3^- ions (Fig. 34-6A). The two NH_4^+ ions are secreted into the tubular fluid by a countertransport mechanism in exchange for a Na^+ ion. The two HCO_3^- ions move out of the tubular cell along with the reabsorbed Na^+ ion to enter the peritubular capillaries system. Thus, for each molecule of glutamine metabolized in the proximal tubule, two NH_4^+ ions are secreted into the tubular filtrate, and two HCO_3^- ions are reabsorbed into the blood. The HCO_3^- generated by this process constitutes new HCO_3^-. A second buffering mechanism involves the recycling of NH_4^+ by tubular cells in the medullary portion of the kidney. Here, NH_4^+ is converted to NH_3 and secreted into the tubular lumen. In the collecting tubules, H^+ ions that are secreted into the tubular lumen combine with NH_3 to form NH_4^+ ions (see Fig. 34-6B). However, this part of the tubule is relatively impermeable to NH_4^+; therefore, once the H^+ has reacted with NH_3 to NH_4^+, it becomes trapped in the tubular lumen and is eliminated in the urine. In the process of being converted to NH_3, the H^+ from the recycled NH_4^+ promotes the reabsorption of HCO_3^- by combining with HCO_3^- delivered from the proximal tubule. Thus, an additional new HCO_3^- is generated and added to the blood for each NH_4^+ that is recycled.

One of the most important features of the ammonia buffer system is that it is subject to physiologic control. Under normal conditions, the amount of H^+ ion eliminated by the ammonia buffer system is about 50% of the acid excreted and new HCO_3^- regenerated. However, with chronic acidosis, it can become the dominant mechanism for H^+ excretion and new HCO_3^- generation.

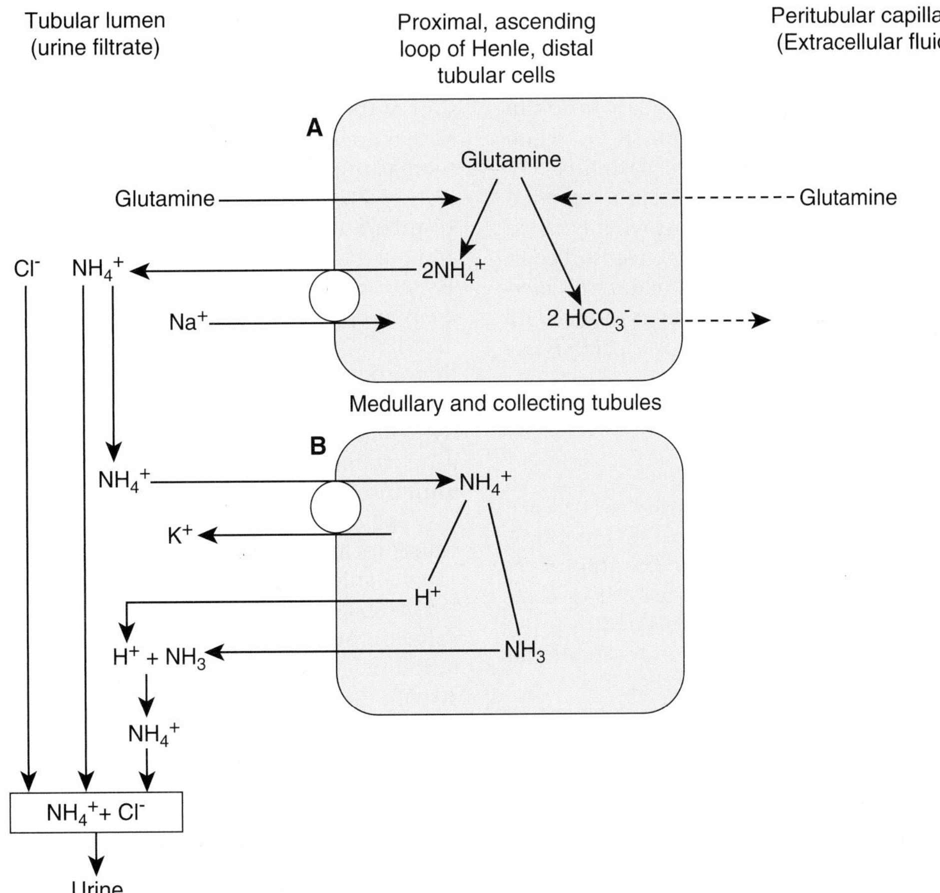

FIGURE 34-6 The ammonia buffer systems. (**A**) In the proximal, ascending loop of Henle, and distal tubule, two ammonium (NH_4^+) ions and two bicarbonate (HCO_3^-) ions are synthesized from the amino acid glutamine. The two NH_4^+ are secreted into the tubular fluid in exchange for a two sodium (Na^+) ions and are either eliminated in the urine as ammonium chloride (NH_4Cl) or recycled in the medullary nephrons. The two HCO_3^- ions, which represent new HCO_3^- are returned to the circulation. (**B**) A second NH_4^+ exchange system occurs in the collecting tubules where secreted hydrogen (H^+) ions combine with ammonia (NH_3) from recycled NH_4^+ and are then eliminated in the urine as NH_4Cl.

Hydrogen and Potassium Ions Compete for Elimination in the Urine. Plasma K^+ levels influence renal elimination of H^+ ions, and vice versa. When plasma K^+ levels fall, there is movement of K^+ ions from body cells into the extracellular fluid and a reciprocal movement of H^+ ions from the extracellular fluid into body cells. In the kidney, these movements lower the intracellular pH of tubular cells, causing an increase in H^+ ion secretion. Potassium depletion also stimulates ammonia synthesis by the kidney as a means of buffering the excess H^+ ions. The net result is an increased reabsorption of the filtered HCO_3^- ions and the development of metabolic alkalosis. An elevation in plasma K^+ levels has the opposite effect. Plasma K^+ levels are similarly altered by acid-base balance. Acidosis tends to increase H^+ ion elimination and decrease K^+ ion elimination, with a resultant increase in plasma potassium levels. Alkalosis has the opposite effect.

Aldosterone also influences H^+ ion elimination by the kidney. It acts in the collecting duct to stimulate H^+ ion secretion indirectly, while increasing Na^+ ion reabsorption and K^+ ion secretion (see Chapter 32). Hyperaldosteronism tends to lead to a decrease in plasma K^+ levels and increased pH and alkalosis because of increased H^+ ion secretion. Hypoaldosteronism has the opposite effect. It leads to increased K^+ levels, decreased H^+ ion secretion, and acidosis.

Influence of Sodium Chloride–Bicarbonate Exchange on pH. Body sodium levels can indirectly influence acid-base balance by way of the Cl^-/HCO_3^- exchange system. Sodium reabsorption in the kidneys requires the reabsorption of an accompanying anion. The two major anions in the extracellular fluid are Cl^- and HCO_3^-.

One of the mechanisms that the kidneys use in regulating the pH of the extracellular fluids is to conserve or eliminate HCO_3^- ions; in the process, it often is necessary to shuffle anions. Chloride is the most abundant anion in the extracellular fluid and can substitute for HCO_3^- when an anion shift is needed. As an example, plasma HCO_3^- levels normally increase as hydrochloric acid is secreted into the stomach after a heavy meal, causing what is called the *postprandial alkaline tide.* Later, as the Cl^- is reabsorbed in the small intestine, the pH returns to normal. *Hypochloremic alkalosis* refers to an increase in pH that is induced by a decrease in plasma Cl^- levels. *Hyperchloremic acidosis* occurs when excess levels of Cl^- are present.

LABORATORY TESTS

Laboratory tests that are used in assessing acid-base balance include those for arterial blood gases and pH, CO_2 content and HCO_3^- levels, base excess or deficit, and the anion gap. Although useful in determining whether acidosis or alkalosis is present, the pH of the blood as measured by a pH meter or electrode provides little information about the cause of an acid-base disorder.

Carbon Dioxide and Bicarbonate Levels

The PCO_2 of the arterial blood gases provides a means of assessing the respiratory component of acid-base balance. Arterial blood gases are used because venous blood gases are highly variable, depending on metabolic demands of the various tissues that empty into the vein from where the sample is being drawn. The dissolved CO_2 levels can be determined from arterial blood gas measurements using the PCO_2 and the solubility coefficient for CO_2 (normal arterial PCO_2 is 38 to 42 mm Hg). Arterial blood gases also provide a measure of blood oxygen (PO_2) levels. This can be important in assessing respiratory function.

Laboratory tests include measurements of the CO_2 content and HCO_3^- in the blood. The CO_2 content that is included in these measurements is different from the PCO_2 that is measured in blood gases. Instead, it refers to the total CO_2 content of blood, including that contained in HCO_3^-. More than 70% of the CO_2 in the blood is in the form of bicarbonate. The CO_2 content is determined by adding a strong acid to a plasma sample and measuring the amount of CO_2 generated. The plasma HCO_3^- concentration is then determined from the total CO_2 content of the blood. The normal range of values for venous HCO_3^- concentration is 24 to 29 mEq/L (24 to 29 mmol/L).

Base Excess or Deficit

Base excess or deficit measures the level of all the buffer systems of the blood—hemoglobin, protein, phosphate, and HCO_3^-. The base excess or deficit describes the amount of a fixed acid or base that must be added to a blood sample to achieve a pH of 7.4 (normal ± 3.0 mEq/L).[1] For practical purposes, base excess or deficit is a measurement of bicarbonate excess or deficit. Base excess indicates metabolic alkalosis, and base deficit indicates metabolic acidosis.

Anion Gap

The anion gap describes the difference between the plasma concentration of the major measured cation (Na^+) and the sum of the measured anions (Cl^- and HCO_3^-). This difference represents the concentration of unmeasured anions, such as phosphates, sulfates, organic acids, and proteins (Fig. 34-7). Normally, the anion gap ranges between 8 and 12 mEq/L (a value of 16 mEq/L is normal if both sodium and potassium concentrations are used in the calculation). The anion gap is increased in conditions such as lactic acidosis and ketoacidosis that result from elevated levels of metabolic acids. A low anion gap is found in conditions that produce a fall in unmeasured anions (primarily albumin) or rise in unmeasured cations. The latter can occur in hyperkalemia, hypercalcemia, hypermagnesemia, lithium intoxication, or multiple myeloma, in which an abnormal immunoglobulin is produced.[1]

The anion gap of urine can also be measured. It uses values for the measurable cations (Na^+ and K^+) and measurable anion (Cl^-) to provide an estimate of ammonium (NH_4^+) excretion. Because ammonium is a cation, the value of the anion gap becomes more negative as the ammonium level increases. In normal persons secreting 20 to 40 mmol of ammonium per liter, the urine anion gap is close to zero. In metabolic acidosis, the amount of unmeasurable NH_4^+ should increase if renal excretion of H^+ is intact; as a result, the urine anion gap should become more negative.

In summary, normal body function depends on the precise regulation of acid-base balance. The pH of the extracellular fluid is normally maintained within the narrow physiologic range of 7.35 to 7.45. Metabolic processes produce volatile and fixed or nonvolatile metabolic acids that must be buffered and eliminated from the body. The volatile acid, H_2CO_3, is in equilibrium with dissolved CO_2, which is eliminated through

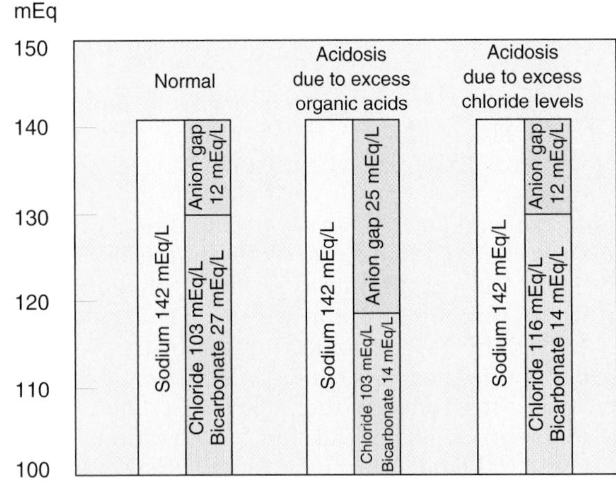

FIGURE 34-7 The anion gap in acidosis due to excess metabolic acids and excess plasma chloride levels. Unmeasured anions such as phosphates, sulfates, and organic acids increase the anion gap because they replace bicarbonate. This assumes there is no change in sodium content.

the lungs. The nonvolatile metabolic acids, most of which are excreted by the kidneys, are derived mainly from protein metabolism and incomplete carbohydrate and fat metabolism. It is the ratio of the HCO_3^- ion concentration to dissolved CO_2 (H_2CO_3 concentration) that determines body pH. When this ratio is 20:1, the pH is 7.4.

The ability of the body to maintain pH within the normal physiologic range depends on intracellular and extracellular mechanisms for buffering excess H^+ and HCO_3^- ions and on the respiratory and renal mechanisms for eliminating or conserving excess acids and bases. Proteins are the most important intracellular buffers, and the HCO_3^- buffer system includes the most important extracellular buffers. The respiratory system contributes to the regulation of pH by controlling the elimination of CO_2. The kidney aids in regulation of pH by eliminating H^+ ions or conserving HCO_3^- ions. In the process of eliminating H^+ ions, it uses the phosphate and ammonia buffer systems. Body pH is also affected by the distribution of exchangeable cations (K^+ and H^+) and anions (Cl^- and HCO_3^-).

Laboratory tests that are used in assessing acid-base balance include arterial blood gas measurements, CO_2 content and HCO_3^- levels, base excess or deficit, and the anion gap. The base excess or deficit describes the amount of a fixed acid or base that must be added to a blood sample to achieve a pH of 7.4. The anion gap describes the difference between the plasma concentration of the major measured cation (Na^+) and the sum of the measured anions (Cl^- and HCO_3^-). This difference represents the concentration of unmeasured anions, such as phosphates, sulfates, organic acids, and proteins, that are present.

Disorders of Acid-Base Balance

After you have completed this section of the chapter, you should be able to meet the following objectives:

- Differentiate the terms *acidemia, alkalemia, acidosis,* and *alkalosis*
- Describe a clinical situation involving an acid-base disorder in which primary and compensatory mechanisms might be active
- Define metabolic acidosis, metabolic alkalosis, respiratory acidosis, and respiratory alkalosis
- Explain the use of the plasma anion gap in differentiating types of metabolic acidosis
- List common causes of metabolic and respiratory acidosis and metabolic and respiratory alkalosis
- Contrast and compare the clinical manifestations and treatment of metabolic and respiratory acidosis and of metabolic and respiratory alkalosis

The terms *acidosis* and *alkalosis* describe the clinical conditions that arise as a result of changes in dissolved CO_2 and HCO_3^- concentrations. An alkali represents a combination of one or more alkali metals such as sodium or potassium with a highly basic ion such as a hydroxyl ion (OH^-). Sodium bicarbonate is the main alkali in the extracellular fluid. Although the definitions differ somewhat, the terms *alkali* and *base* are often used interchangeably. Hence, the term *alkalosis* has come to mean the opposite of *acidosis*.

METABOLIC VERSUS RESPIRATORY ACID-BASE DISORDERS

There are two types of acid-base disorders: metabolic and respiratory (Table 34-1). *Metabolic disorders* produce an alteration in bicarbonate concentration and result from the addition or loss of nonvolatile acid or alkali to or from the extracellular fluid. A reduction in pH due to a decrease in HCO_3^- is called *metabolic acidosis,* and an elevated pH due to increased HCO_3^- levels is called *metabolic alkalosis. Respiratory disorders* involve an alteration in the PCO_2, reflecting an increase or decrease in alveolar ventilation. *Respiratory acidosis* is characterized by a decrease in pH, reflecting a decrease in ventilation and an increase in PCO_2. *Respiratory alkalosis* involves an increase in pH, resulting from an increase in alveolar ventilation and a decrease in PCO_2.

PRIMARY VERSUS COMPENSATORY MECHANISMS

Acidosis and alkalosis typically involve a *primary* or *initiating event* and a *compensatory* or *adaptive state* that results from homeostatic mechanisms that attempt to correct or prevent large changes in pH. For example, a person may have a primary metabolic acidosis as a result of overproduction of

TABLE 34-1 Summary of Acid-Base Imbalances

Acid-Base Imbalance	Primary Disturbance	Respiratory Compensation	Renal Compensation
Metabolic acidosis	Decrease in bicarbonate	Hyperventilation to decrease PCO_2	If no renal disease, increased H^+ excretion and increased HCO_3^- reabsorption
Metabolic alkalosis	Increase in bicarbonate	Hypoventilation to increase PCO_2	If no renal disease, decreased H^+ excretion and decreased HCO_3^- reabsorption
Respiratory acidosis	Increase in PCO_2	None	Increased H^+ excretion and increased HCO_3^- reabsorption
Respiratory alkalosis	Decrease in PCO_2	None	Decreased H^+ excretion and decreased HCO_3^- reabsorption

ketoacids and respiratory alkalosis because of a compensatory increase in ventilation (see Table 34-1). *Compensatory mechanisms* adjust the pH toward a more normal level without correcting the underlying cause of the disorder (see Fig. 34-3). A mixed acid-base disorder is one in which there is both a primary and a compensatory change in acid-base balance. The respiratory mechanisms, which compensate by increasing or decreasing ventilation, are rapid but seldom able to return the pH to normal because as the pH returns toward normal, the respiratory stimulus is lost. The kidneys compensate by conserving HCO_3^- or H^+ ions. It normally takes longer to recruit renal compensatory mechanisms than it does respiratory compensatory mechanisms. Renal mechanisms are more efficient, however, because they continue to operate until the pH has returned to a normal or near-normal value.

Compensatory mechanisms provide a means to control pH when correction is impossible or cannot be immediately achieved. Often, compensatory mechanisms are interim measures that permit survival while the body attempts to correct the primary disorder. Compensation requires the use of mechanisms that are different from those that caused the primary disorder. In other words, the lungs cannot compensate for respiratory acidosis that is caused by lung disease, nor can the kidneys compensate for metabolic acidosis that occurs because of renal failure. The body can, however, use renal mechanisms to compensate for respiratory-induced changes in pH, and it can use respiratory mechanisms to compensate for metabolically induced changes in acid-base balance. Because compensatory mechanisms become more effective with time, there are often differences between the level of pH change that is present in acute and chronic acid-base disorders.

METABOLIC ACIDOSIS

Metabolic acidosis involves a primary deficit in base HCO_3^- along with a decrease in plasma pH. In metabolic acidosis, the body compensates for the decrease in pH by increasing the respiratory rate in an effort to decrease CO_2 and H_2CO_3 levels. The PCO_2 can be expected to fall by 1 to 1.5 mm Hg for each 1 mEq/L fall in HCO_3^-.[3,4]

Causes

Metabolic acidosis can be caused by one of four mechanisms: increased production of nonvolatile metabolic acids, decreased acid secretion by the kidney, excessive loss of bicarbonate, or an increase in Cl^-.[7–9] The anion gap is often useful in determining the cause of the metabolic acidosis (Chart 34-1). The presence of excess metabolic acids produces an increase in the anion gap as sodium bicarbonate is replaced by the sodium salt of the offending acid (*e.g.*, sodium lactate). When acidosis results from increased chloride levels (*e.g.*, hyperchloremic acidosis), the anion gap remains within normal levels. The causes of metabolic acidosis are summarized in Table 34-2.

Increased Production of Metabolic Acids. Metabolic acids increase when there is an accumulation of lactic acid, overproduction of ketoacids, or drug or chemical anion ingestion.

METABOLIC ACID-BASE IMBALANCE

- Metabolic acid-base disorders represent a primary change in the plasma HCO_3^- ion concentration.
- Metabolic acidosis can be defined as a decrease in plasma HCO_3^- and a pH that is caused by an excess of production or accumulation of fixed acids or loss of HCO_3^- ion. Compensatory responses include an increase in ventilation and elimination of CO_2 and the reabsorption and generation of bicarbonate by the kidney.
- Metabolic alkalosis can be defined as an increase in plasma HCO_3^- and pH that is initiated by excess H^+ ion loss or HCO_3^- ion gain and maintained by conditions that impair the ability of the kidney to excrete the excess HCO_3^- ion. Compensatory responses include a decreased respiratory rate with retention of PCO_2 and increased elimination of HCO_3^- by the kidney.

Lactic Acidosis. Acute lactic acidosis is one of the most common types of metabolic acidosis.8 Lactic acidosis develops when there is excess production of lactic acid or diminished lactic acid removal from the blood. Lactic acid is produced by the anaerobic metabolism of glucose. Virtually all tissues can produce lactic acid under appropriate cir-

CHART 34-1

The Anion Gap in Differential Diagnosis of Metabolic Acidosis

Decreased Anion Gap (<8 mEq/L)

Hypoalbuminemia (decrease in unmeasured anions)
Multiple myeloma (increase in unmeasured cationic IgG paraproteins)
Increased unmeasured cations (hyperkalemia, hypercalcemia, hypermagnesemia, lithium intoxication)

Increased Anion Gap (>12 mEq/L)

Presence of unmeasured metabolic anion
- Diabetic ketoacidosis
- Alcoholic ketoacidosis
- Lactic acidosis
- Starvation
- Renal insufficiency

Presence of drug or chemical anion
- Salicylate poisoning
- Methanol poisoning
- Ethylene glycol poisoning

Normal Anion Gap (8–12 mEq/L)

Loss of bicarbonate
- Diarrhea
- Pancreatic fluid loss
- Ileostomy (unadapted)

Chloride retention
- Renal tubular acidosis
- Ileal loop bladder
- Parenteral nutrition (arginine and lysine)

TABLE 34-2 Metabolic Acidosis

Causes	Manifestations
Excess Metabolic Acids (Increased Anion Gap)	**Blood pH, HCO_3^-, CO_2**
Excessive production of metabolic acids	pH decreased
Lactic acidosis	HCO_3^- (primary) decreased
Diabetic ketoacidosis	PCO_2 (compensatory) decreased
Alcoholic ketoacidosis	**Gastrointestinal Function**
Fasting and starvation	Anorexia
Poisoning (*e.g.*, salicylate, methanol, ethylene glycol)	Nausea and vomiting
Impaired elimination of metabolic acids	Abdominal pain
Kidney failure or dysfunction	**Neural Function**
Excessive Bicarbonate Loss (Normal Anion Gap)	Weakness
Loss of intestinal secretions	Lethargy
Diarrhea	General malaise
Intestinal suction	Confusion
Intestinal or biliary fistula	Stupor
Increased renal losses	Coma
Renal tubular acidosis	Depression of vital functions
Treatment with carbonic anhydrase inhibitors	**Cardiovascular Function**
Hypoaldosteronism	Peripheral vasodilation
Increased Chloride Levels (Normal Anion Gap)	Decreased heart rate
Excessive reabsorption of chloride by the kidney	Cardiac dysrhythmias
Sodium chloride infusions	**Skin**
Treatment with ammonium chloride	Warm and flushed
Parenteral hyperalimentation	**Skeletal System**
	Bone disease (*e.g.*, chronic acidosis)
	Signs of Compensation
	Increased rate and depth of respiration (*i.e.*, Kussmaul breathing)
	Hyperkalemia
	Acid urine
	Increased ammonia in urine

cumstances. Tissues such as red blood cells, intestine, and skeletal muscle do so under normal conditions. Excess lactate is produced with vigorous exercise, during which there is a local disproportion between oxygen supply and demand in the contracting muscles. The liver and, to a lesser extent, the kidney normally remove lactic acid from the blood and use it for energy or convert it back to glucose.

Most cases of lactic acidosis are caused by inadequate oxygen delivery, as in shock or cardiac arrest.[8] Such conditions increase lactic acid production, and they impair lactic acid clearance because of poor liver perfusion. Mortality rates are high for persons with lactic acidosis because of shock and tissue hypoxia.[8]

Lactic acidosis is also associated with disorders in which tissue hypoxia does not appear to be present. It has been reported in patients with leukemia, lymphomas, and other cancers; those with poorly controlled diabetes; and patients with severe liver failure. Mechanisms causing lactic acidosis in these conditions are poorly understood. Some conditions, such as neoplasms, may produce local increases in tissue metabolism and lactate production or interfere with blood flow to noncancerous cells. Ethanol produces a slight elevation in lactic acid, but clinically significant lactic acidosis does not occur in alcohol intoxication unless other problems, such as liver failure, are present.

Lactic acidosis may also occur in mitochondrial disorders that impair oxidative metabolism. Lactic acidosis occurs in genetic mitochondrial disorders that impair lactate metabolism.[10,11] One of these disorders, referred to by the acronym MELAS, involves mitochondrial encephalopathy (ME), lactic acidosis (LA), and strokelike episodes (S). Children with the disorder function normally for the first few years of their lives and then begin to display impaired motor and cognitive development. The mitochondrial defect also leads to short stature, seizure disorders, and multiple strokes. Lowering the plasma lactate level of children with severe lactic acidosis may result in marked clinical improvement. A variety of drugs can also produce life-threatening lactic acidosis by inhibiting mitochondrial function. These drugs include the biguanide antidiabetic drugs and the antiretroviral nucleoside analogs that are used to treat acquired immunodeficiency syndrome (AIDS).[8]

A unique form of lactic acidosis, called D-lactic acidosis, can occur in persons with intestinal disorders that involve the generation and absorption of D-lactic acid (L-lactic acid is the usual cause of lactic acidosis). D-Lactic acidosis can occur in persons with jejunoileal bypass, small bowel resection, or short bowel syndrome, in which there is impaired reabsorption of carbohydrate in the small intestine.[8,12] In these cases, the unabsorbed carbohydrate is delivered to the colon, where it is converted to D-lactic acid by an overgrowth of gram-positive anaerobes. Persons with D-lactic acidosis experience episodic periods of metabolic acidosis often brought on by eating a meal high in carbohydrates. Manifestations include confusion, cerebellar ataxia, slurred speech, and loss of memory. They may complain of feeling (or may appear) intoxicated. Treatment includes use of antimicrobial agents to decrease the number of D-lactic acid–producing microorganisms in the bowel along with a low-carbohydrate diet.

Ketoacidosis. Ketoacids (*i.e.,* acetoacetic and β-hydroxybutyric acid), produced in the liver from fatty acids, are the source of fuel for many body tissues. An overproduction of ketoacids occurs when carbohydrate stores are inadequate or when the body cannot use available carbohydrates as a fuel. Under these conditions, fatty acids are mobilized from adipose tissue and delivered to the liver, where they are converted to ketones. Ketoacidosis develops when ketone production exceeds tissue use.

The most common cause of ketoacidosis is uncontrolled diabetes mellitus, in which an insulin deficiency leads to the release of fatty acids from adipose cells with subsequent production of excess ketoacids (see Chapter 43). Ketoacidosis may also develop as the result of fasting or food deprivation, during which the lack of carbohydrates produces a self-limited state of ketoacidosis. The self-limited nature of ketoacidosis results from a decrease in insulin, which further suppresses the release of fatty acids from fat cells.

Ketones are also formed during the oxidation of alcohol, a process that occurs in the liver. A condition called *alcoholic ketoacidosis* can develop in persons who engage in excess alcohol consumption.[13] It usually follows prolonged alcohol ingestion, particularly if accompanied by decreased food intake and vomiting—conditions that result in using fatty acids as an energy source. The ketoacids responsible for alcoholic ketoacidosis are formed in part as a result of alcohol metabolism. Ketone formation may be further enhanced by the hypoglycemia that results from alcohol-induced inhibition of glucose synthesis (*i.e.,* gluconeogenesis) by the liver and impaired ketone elimination by the kidneys because of dehydration. An extracellular fluid volume deficit caused by vomiting and decreased fluid intake often contributes to the acidosis. Numerous other factors, such as elevations in cortisol, growth hormone, glucagon, and catecholamines, mediate free fatty acid release and thereby contribute to the development of alcoholic ketoacidosis.

Salicylate Toxicity. Salicylates are another potential source of metabolic acids. Aspirin (acetylsalicylic acid) is rapidly converted to salicylic acid in the body. Although aspirin is the most common cause of salicylate toxicity, other salicylate preparations such as methyl salicylate, sodium salicylate, and salicylic acid may be involved. Salicylate overdose produces serious toxic effects, including death. A fatal overdose can occur with as little as 10 to 30 g in adults and 3 g in children.[1]

A variety of acid-base disturbances occur with salicylate toxicity. The salicylates cross the blood–brain barrier and directly stimulate the respiratory center, causing hyperventilation and respiratory alkalosis. The kidneys compensate by secreting increased amounts of HCO_3^-, K^+, and Na^+, thereby contributing to the development of metabolic acidosis. Salicylates also interfere with carbohydrate metabolism, which results in increased production of metabolic acids.

One of the treatments for salicylate toxicity is *alkalinization* of the plasma. Salicylic acid, which is a weak acid, exists in equilibrium with the alkaline salicylate anion. It is the salicylic acid that is toxic because of its ability to cross cell membranes and enter brain cells. The salicylate anion crosses membranes poorly and is less toxic. With alkalinization of the extracellular fluids, the ratio of salicylic acid to salicylate is greatly reduced. This allows salicylic acid to move out of cells into the extracellular fluid along a concentration gradient. The renal elimination of salicylates follows a similar pattern when the urine is alkalinized.

Methanol and Ethylene Glycol Toxicity. Ingestion of methanol and ethylene glycol results in the production of metabolic acids and causes metabolic acidosis. Both produce an osmolar gap because of their small size and osmotic properties. Methanol (wood alcohol) is a component of shellac, varnish, deicing solutions, sterno, and other commercial products. Methanol can be absorbed through the skin or gastrointestinal tract or inhaled through the lungs. A dose as small as 30 mL can be fatal.14 In addition to metabolic acidosis, methanol produces severe optic nerve and central nervous system toxicity. Organ system damage occurs after a 24-hour period in which methanol is converted to formaldehyde and formic acid.

Ethylene glycol is a solvent found in products ranging from antifreeze and deicing solutions to carpet and fabric cleaners. It tastes sweet and is intoxicating, factors that contribute to its abuse potential. A lethal dose is approximately 100 mL.[15,16] It is rapidly absorbed from the intestine, making treatment with gastric lavage and syrup of ipecac ineffective. Acidosis occurs as ethylene glycol is converted to oxalic and lactic acid. Manifestations of ethylene glycol toxicity occur in three stages: neurologic symptoms ranging from drunkenness to coma, which appear during the first 12 hours; cardiorespiratory disorders such as tachycardia and pulmonary edema; and flank pain and renal failure caused by plugging of the tubules with oxalate crystals (from excess oxalic acid production).[16]

The enzyme *alcohol dehydrogenase* metabolizes methanol and ethylene glycol into toxic metabolites. This is the same enzyme that is used in the metabolism of ethanol. Because alcohol dehydrogenase has an affinity for ethanol 10 times its affinity for methanol or ethylene glycol, intravenous or oral ethanol is used as an antidote for methanol and ethylene glycol poisoning.[1] Extracellular volume expansion and hemodialysis are also used. Fomepizole, with specific indications for ethylene glycol poisoning, was recently approved by the U.S. Food and Drug Administration.[15,17] In a manner similar to ethanol, it is thought to act as an inhibitor of alcohol dehydrogenase, thereby preventing the formation of the toxic ethylene glycol metabolites.

Decreased Renal Function. Kidney disease is the most common cause of chronic metabolic acidosis. The kidneys normally conserve HCO_3^- and secrete H^+ ions into the urine as a means of regulating acid-base balance. In renal failure, there is loss of glomerular and tubular function, with retention of nitrogenous wastes and metabolic acids. In a condition called *renal tubular acidosis,* glomerular function is normal, but the tubular secretion of H^+ or reabsorption of HCO_3^- is abnormal (see Chapter 35).

Increased Bicarbonate Losses. Increased HCO_3^- losses occur with the loss of bicarbonate-rich body fluids or with impaired conservation of HCO_3^- by the kidney. Intestinal secretions have a high HCO_3^- concentration. Consequently, excessive loss of HCO_3^- ions occur with severe diarrhea; small bowel, pancreatic, or biliary fistula drainage; ileostomy drainage; and intestinal suction. In diarrhea of microbial origin, HCO_3^- is also secreted into the bowel as a means of neutralizing the metabolic acids produced by the microorganisms causing the diarrhea. Creation of an ileal bladder, which is done for conditions such as neurogenic bladder or surgical removal of the bladder because of cancer, involves the implantation of the ureters into a short, isolated loop of ileum that serves as a conduit for urine collection. With this procedure, contact time between the urine and ileal bladder is normally too short for significant anion exchange, and HCO_3^- is lost in the urine.[1]

Hyperchloremic Acidosis. Hyperchloremic acidosis occurs when Cl^- ion levels are increased. Because Cl^- and HCO_3^- are anions, the HCO_3^- ion concentration decreases when there is an increase in Cl^- ions. Hyperchloremic acidosis can occur as the result of abnormal absorption of chloride by the kidneys or as a result of treatment with chloride-containing medications (*i.e.,* sodium chloride, amino acid–chloride hyperalimentation solutions, and ammonium chloride). Ammonium chloride is broken down into NH_4^+ and Cl^-. The ammonium ion is converted to urea in the liver, leaving the Cl^- ion free to react with H^+ to form HCl. The administration of intravenous sodium chloride or parenteral hyperalimentation solutions that contain an amino acid–chloride combination can cause acidosis in a similar manner.[18] With hyperchloremic acidosis, the anion gap is within the normal range, whereas the chloride levels are increased, and bicarbonate levels are decreased.

Manifestations

Metabolic acidosis is characterized by an increased extracellular H^+ ion concentration with a decrease in pH (<7.35) and a decrease in HCO_3^- levels (<24 mEq/L). Acidosis typically produces a compensatory increase in respiratory rate with a decrease in PCO_2.

The manifestations of metabolic acidosis fall into three categories: signs and symptoms of the disorder causing the acidosis, changes in body function related to recruitment of compensatory mechanisms, and alterations in cardiovascular, neurologic, and musculoskeletal function resulting from the decreased pH (see Table 34-2). The signs and symptoms of metabolic acidosis usually begin to appear when the plasma HCO_3^- concentration falls to 20 mEq/L or less. A fall in pH to less than 7.0 to 7.10 can reduce cardiac contractility and predispose to potentially fatal cardiac dysrhythmias.[1]

Metabolic acidosis is seldom a primary disorder; it usually develops during the course of another disease. The manifestations of metabolic acidosis frequently are superimposed on the symptoms of the contributing health problem. With diabetic ketoacidosis, which is a common cause of metabolic acidosis, there is an increase in blood and urine glucose and a characteristic smell of ketones to the breath. In metabolic acidosis that accompanies renal failure, blood urea nitrogen levels are elevated, and other tests of renal function yield abnormal results.

Manifestations related to respiratory and renal compensatory mechanisms usually occur early in the course of metabolic acidosis. In situations of acute metabolic acidosis, the respiratory system compensates for a decrease in pH by increasing ventilation to reduce PCO_2; this is accomplished through deep and rapid respirations. In diabetic ketoacidosis, this breathing pattern is referred to as *Kussmaul breathing.* For descriptive purposes, it can be said that Kussmaul breathing resembles the hyperpnea of exercise—the person breathes as though he or she had been running. There may be complaints of difficult breathing or dyspnea with exertion; with severe acidosis, dyspnea may be present even at rest. Respiratory compensation for acute acidosis tends to be somewhat greater than for chronic acidosis. When kidney function is normal, H^+ ion excretion increases promptly in response to acidosis, and the urine becomes more acid.

Changes in pH have a direct effect on body function that can produce signs and symptoms common to most types of metabolic acidosis, regardless of cause. A person with metabolic acidosis often complains of weakness, fatigue, general malaise, and a dull headache. The person also may have anorexia, nausea, vomiting, and abdominal pain. Tissue turgor is impaired, and the skin is dry when fluid deficit accompanies acidosis. In persons with undiagnosed diabetes mellitus, the nausea, vomiting, and abdominal symptoms may be misinterpreted as being caused by gastrointestinal flu or other abdominal disease, such as appendicitis. Acidosis depresses neuronal excitability and decreases binding of calcium to plasma proteins so that more free calcium is available to decrease neural activity. As acidosis progresses, the level of consciousness declines, and stupor and coma develop. The skin is often warm and flushed because skin vessels become less responsive to sympathetic stimulation and lose tone.

When the pH falls to 7.0 to 7.1, cardiac contractility and cardiac output decrease, the heart becomes less responsive to catecholamines (*i.e.,* epinephrine and norepinephrine), and dysrhythmias, including fatal ventricular dysrhythmias, can develop. A decrease in ventricular function may be particularly important in perpetuating shock-induced lactic acidosis, and partial correction of the acidemia may be necessary before tissue perfusion can be restored.[1]

Chronic acidemia, as in renal failure, can lead to a variety of musculoskeletal problems, some of which result from the release of calcium and phosphate during bone buffering of excess H^+ ions.[19] Of particular importance is impaired growth in children. In infants and children, acidemia may be associated with a variety of nonspecific symptoms such as anorexia, weight loss, muscle weakness, and listlessness.[1,14] Muscle weakness and listlessness may result from alterations in muscle metabolism.

Treatment

The treatment of metabolic acidosis focuses on correcting the condition that caused the disorder and restoring the fluids and electrolytes that have been lost from the body. The treatment of diabetic ketoacidosis is discussed in Chapter 43.

The use of supplemental sodium bicarbonate ($NaHCO_3$) may be indicated in the treatment of some forms of normal anion gap acidosis. However, its use in treatment of metabolic acidosis with an increased anion gap is controversial, particularly in cases of impaired tissue perfusion.[4,20] In most patients with cardiac arrest, shock, or sepsis, impaired oxygen delivery is the primary cause of lactic acidosis. In these situations, the administration of large amounts of $NaHCO_3$ does not improve oxygen delivery and may produce hypernatremia, hyperosmolality, and decreased oxygen release by hemoglobin because of a shift in the oxygen dissociation curve.[20]

METABOLIC ALKALOSIS

Metabolic alkalosis is a systemic disorder caused by an increase in pH due to a primary excess of plasma HCO_3^- ions.[21,22] It can be caused by a loss of H^+ ions, net gain in HCO_3^- ions, or loss of Cl^- ions in excess of HCO_3^- ions. Metabolic alkalosis is reported to be the second most common acid-base disorder in hospitalized adults, accounting for about 32% of all acid-base disorders.[22]

Causes

Most of the body's plasma HCO_3^- is obtained from three sources: from CO_2 that is produced during metabolic processes, from reabsorption of filtered HCO_3^-, or from generation of new HCO_3^- by the kidney. Usually, HCO_3^- production and renal reabsorption are balanced in a manner that prevents alkalosis from occurring. The proximal tubule reabsorbs 99.9% of the filtered HCO_3^-. When the plasma levels of HCO_3^- rise above the threshold for tubular reabsorption, the excess is excreted in the urine. Many of the conditions that increase plasma HCO_3^- also raise the level for HCO_3^- reabsorption; thus, an increase in HCO_3^- contributes not only to the generation of metabolic alkalosis but also to its maintenance.

Metabolic alkalosis involves both the factors that generate the loss of H^+ or gain of HCO_3^- ions and those that maintain it by interfering with excretion of the excess HCO_3^- (Table 34-3). Factors that serve to maintain metabolic alkalosis include extracellular fluid volume contraction accompanied by hypokalemia and hypochloremia and mineralocorticoid (aldosterone) excess.

TABLE 34-3 Metabolic Alkalosis

Causes	Manifestations
Excessive Gain of Bicarbonate or Alkali	**Blood pH, HCO_3^-, CO_2**
Ingestion or administration of sodium bicarbonate	pH increased
Administration of hyperalimentation solutions containing acetate	HCO_3^- (primary) increased
Administration of parenteral solutions containing lactate	PCO_2 (compensatory) increased
Administration of citrate-containing blood transfusions	**Neural Function**
Excessive Loss of Hydrogen Ions	Confusion
Vomiting	Hyperactive reflexes
Gastric suction	Tetany
Binge-purge syndrome	Convulsions
Potassium deficit	**Cardiovascular Function**
Diuretic therapy	Hypotension
Hyperaldosteronism	Dysrhythmias
Milk-alkali syndrome	**Respiratory Function**
Increased Bicarbonate Retention	Respiratory acidosis due to decreased respiratory rate
Loss of chloride with bicarbonate retention	**Signs of Compensation**
Volume Contraction	Decreased rate and depth of respiration
Loss of body fluids	Increased urine pH
Diuretic therapy	

Excess Alkali Intake. Excessive alkali ingestion, as in the use of bicarbonate-containing antacids (*e.g.,* Alka-Seltzer) or $NaHCO_3$ administration during cardiopulmonary resuscitation, can cause metabolic alkalosis. Other sources of alkali intake are acetate in hyperalimentation solutions, lactate in parenteral solutions such as Ringer's lactate, and citrate used in blood transfusions. A condition called the *milk-alkali syndrome* may develop in persons who consume excessive amounts of milk along with an antacid such as calcium carbonate. In this case, the carbonate raises the plasma HCO_3^- while the hypercalcemia prevents the excretion of excess HCO_3^-. The most common cause at present is the use of calcium carbonate as a phosphate buffer in persons with renal failure.

Hydrogen, Chloride, and Potassium Ion Loss Associated With Bicarbonate Ion Retention. Vomiting, removal of gastric secretions through use of nasogastric suction, and low potassium levels resulting from diuretic therapy are the most common causes of metabolic alkalosis in hospitalized patients. The binge and purge syndrome, or self-induced vomiting, also is associated with metabolic alkalosis.[22] Gastric secretions contain high concentrations of HCl and lesser concentrations of potassium chloride (KCL). As Cl^- is taken from the blood and secreted into the stomach with the H^+ ion, it is replaced by HCO_3^-. Under normal conditions, each 1 mEq of H^+ ion that is secreted into the stomach generates 1 mEq of plasma HCO_3^-.[22] Because the entry of acid into the duodenum stimulates an equal amount of pancreatic HCO_3^- secretion, the increase in plasma HCO_3^- concentration is usually transient, and pH returns to normal within a matter of hours. However, loss of H^+ and Cl^- ions from the stomach due to vomiting or gastric suction stimulates continued production of gastric acid and thus the addition of more bicarbonate into the blood.

Maintenance of Metabolic Alkalosis by Volume Contraction, Hypokalemia, and Hypochloremia. Vomiting also results in the loss of water, sodium, and potassium (Fig. 34-8). The resultant volume depletion and hypokalemia maintain the generated metabolic alkalosis by increasing the renal reabsorption of HCO_3^- ion. Administration of diuretics (e.g., loop and thiazide diuretics) is often associated with metabolic alkalosis. Loop diuretics decrease Na^+, K^+, and Cl^- reabsorption, leading to volume contraction and hypokalemia. The thiazide diuretics increase renal K^+ loss, leading to increased HCO_3^- reabsorption.

Extracellular volume depletion is one of the most important factors affecting HCO_3^- reabsorption in the proximal tubule. A decrease in extracellular fluid volume activates the renin-angiotensin-aldosterone system, which increases Na^+ reabsorption as a means of maintaining extracellular fluid volume. The reabsorption of Na^+ requires concomitant anion reabsorption; because there is a Cl^- deficit, HCO_3^- is reabsorbed along with Na^+.

Hypokalemia is a potent stimulus for H^+ secretion and HCO_3^- reabsorption. The mechanisms by which hypokalemia increases HCO_3^- reabsorption are likely the effects of tubular K^+/H^+ ion exchange. In hypokalemia, K^+ moves out of the tubular cell into the blood and is replaced by the H^+ ion. This results in intracellular acidosis and increased HCO_3^- reabsorption. For some unknown reason, severe hypokalemia may cause a reduction in Cl^- reabsorption by the distal tubule.[1] As a result, Na^+ reabsorption at this site is associated with greater tubular electronegativity and greater tendency to H^+ secretion.

It has been proposed recently that hypochloremia and the reduced delivery of Cl^- to the distal tubule of the kidney are responsible for maintaining metabolic alkalosis, rather than volume depletion per se. A low intraluminal concentration of Cl^- ion is interpreted by the kidney as a sign of low extracellular fluid volume, thereby serving as a stimulus for activation of the renin-angiotensin-aldosterone system. Low intraluminal concentrations of Cl^- ion also reduce the driving force for bicarbonate reabsorption.[22]

Metabolic alkalosis can also result from excessive adrenocorticosteroid hormones (*e.g.,* hyperaldosteronism, Cushing's syndrome). The hormone aldosterone increases H^+ ion secretion as it increases Na^+ and HCO_3^- ion reabsorption. In hyperaldosteronism, the concurrent loss of K^+ in the urine serves to perpetuate the alkalosis.

Chronic respiratory acidosis produces a compensatory loss of H^+ and Cl^- ions in the urine along with HCO_3^- retention. When respiratory acidosis is corrected abruptly, as with mechanical ventilation, a "posthypercapneic" metabolic alkalosis may develop because of a rapid drop in PCO_2; however, the concentration of HCO_3^- ions, which are eliminated renally, remains elevated.

Manifestations

Metabolic alkalosis is characterized by a plasma pH above 7.45, plasma HCO_3^- level above 29 mEq/L (29 mmol/L), and base excess above 3.0 mEq/L (3 mmol/L) (see Table 34-3). Persons with metabolic alkalosis often are asymptomatic or have signs related to volume depletion or hypokalemia. Neurologic signs and symptoms (*e.g.,* hyperexcitability) occur less frequently with metabolic alkalosis than with other acid-base disorders because the HCO_3^- ion enters the CSF more slowly than CO_2. When neurologic manifestations do occur, as in acute and severe metabolic alkalosis, they include mental confusion, hyperactive reflexes, tetany, and carpopedal spasm. Metabolic alkalosis also leads to a compensatory hypoventilation with development of various degrees of hypoxemia and respiratory acidosis. Significant morbidity occurs with severe metabolic alkalosis (pH >7.55), including respiratory failure, dysrhythmias, seizures, and coma.

Treatment

The treatment of metabolic alkalosis usually is directed toward correcting the cause of the condition. A chloride deficit requires correction. Potassium chloride usually is the treatment of choice for metabolic alkalosis when there is an accompanying K^+ deficit. When KCl is used as a therapy, the Cl^- anion replaces the HCO_3^- anion, and correcting the potassium deficit allows the kidney to conserve the

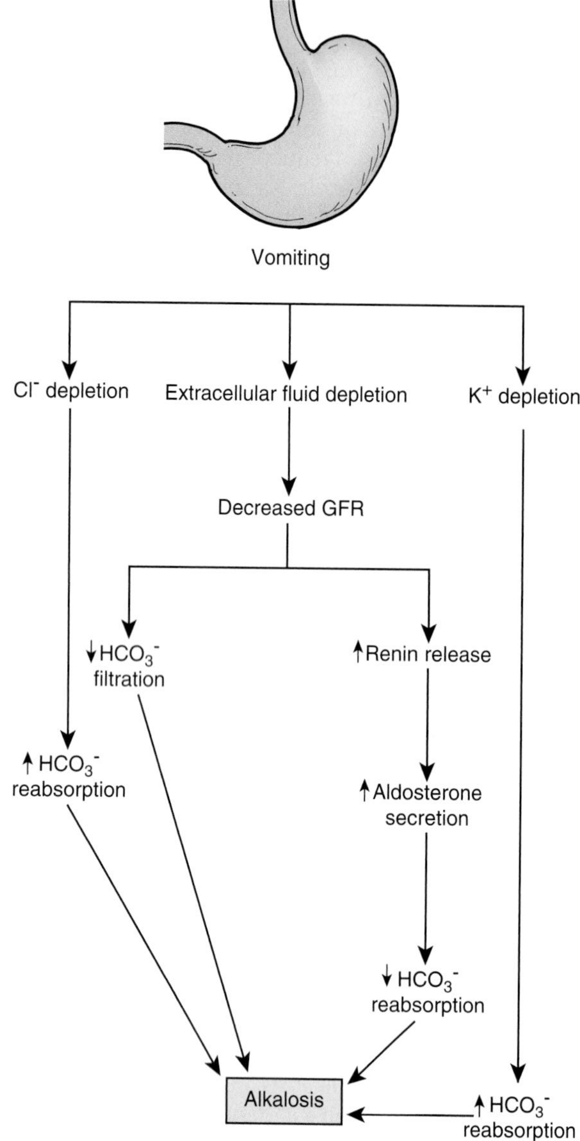

FIGURE 34-8 Renal mechanisms for generating and maintaining metabolic alkalosis following depletion of extracellular fluid volume, chloride (Cl^-), and potassium (K^+) due to vomiting. HCO_3^-, bicarbonate; GFR, glomerular filtration rate.

H^+ ion while eliminating the K^+ ion. Fluid replacement with normal saline or one half normal saline often is used in the treatment of patients with volume contraction alkalosis.

RESPIRATORY ACIDOSIS

Respiratory acidosis occurs in conditions that impair alveolar ventilation and cause an increase in plasma PCO_2, also known as *hypercapnia,* along with a decrease in pH. Respiratory acidosis can occur as an acute or chronic disorder. Acute respiratory failure is associated with a rapid rise in arterial PCO_2 with a minimal increase in plasma HCO_3^- and large decrease in pH. Chronic respiratory acidosis is characterized by a sustained increase in arterial PCO_2, resulting in renal adaptation and a more marked increase in plasma HCO_3^-.[23–26]

Causes

Respiratory acidosis occurs in acute or chronic conditions that impair effective alveolar ventilation and cause an accumulation of PCO_2 (Table 34-4). Impaired ventilation can occur as the result of decreased respiratory drive, lung disease, or disorders of chest wall and respiratory muscle. Less commonly, it results from excess CO_2 production.

Acute Disorders of Ventilation. Acute respiratory acidosis can be caused by impaired function of the respiratory center in the medulla (as in narcotic overdose), lung disease, chest injury, weakness of the respiratory muscles, or airway obstruction. Almost all persons with acute respiratory acidosis are hypoxemic if they are breathing room air. In many cases, signs of hypoxemia develop before those of respiratory acidosis because CO_2 diffuses across the alveolar capillary membrane 20 times more rapidly than oxygen.[1,2]

Chronic Disorders of Ventilation. Chronic respiratory acidosis is a relatively common disturbance in patients with chronic obstructive lung disease (see Chapter 31). In these persons, the persistent elevation of PCO_2 stimulates renal H^+ ion secretion and HCO_3^- reabsorption. The effectiveness of these compensatory mechanisms can often return the pH to near-normal values as long as oxygen levels are maintained within a range that does not unduly suppress chemoreceptor control of respirations.

An acute episode of respiratory acidosis can develop in patients with chronic lung disease who have chronically elevated PCO_2 levels. This is sometimes called *carbon dioxide narcosis.* In these persons, the medullary respiratory center has become adapted to the elevated levels of CO_2 and no longer responds to increases in PCO_2. Instead, the oxygen content of their blood becomes the major stimulus for respiration. When oxygen is administered at a flow rate that suppresses this stimulus, the rate and depth of respiration decrease, and the CO_2 content of the blood increases.

Increased Carbon Dioxide Production. Carbon dioxide is a product of the body's metabolic processes, generating a substantial amount of acid that must be excreted by the lungs or kidney to prevent acidosis. An increase in CO_2 production can result from numerous processes, including exercise, fever, sepsis, and burns. For example, CO_2 production increases by approximately 13% for each 1°C rise in temperature above normal.[27] Nutrition also affects the production of carbon dioxide. A carbohydrate-rich diet produces larger amounts of CO_2 than one containing reasonable amounts of protein and fat. Although excess carbon dioxide production can lead to an increase in PCO_2, it seldom does. In cases of healthy persons, an increase in CO_2 is usually matched by an increase in CO_2 elimination by the lungs. In contrast, persons with respiratory diseases may be unable to eliminate the excess CO_2.

RESPIRATORY ACID-BASE IMBALANCE

- Respiratory acid-base imbalances are due to a primary disturbance in PCO_2, reflecting an increase or decrease in alveolar ventilation.
- Respiratory acidosis, or hypercapnia, represents an increase in PCO_2 and a decrease in plasma pH, resulting from a decrease in effective alveolar ventilation. Compensatory mechanisms include increased conservation and generation of HCO_3^- and elimination of H^+ by the kidney.
- Respiratory alkalosis, or hypocapnia, represents a decrease in PCO_2 and an increase in plasma pH, resulting from increased alveolar ventilation. Compensatory mechanisms include increased elimination of HCO_3^- and conservation of H^+ by the kidney.

Manifestations

Respiratory acidosis is associated with a plasma pH below 7.35 and an arterial PCO_2 above 50 mm Hg (see Table 34-4). The signs and symptoms of respiratory acidosis depend on the rapidity of onset and whether the condition is acute or chronic. Because respiratory acidosis often is accompanied by hypoxemia, the manifestations of respiratory acidosis often are intermixed with those of oxygen deficit. Carbon dioxide readily crosses the blood–brain barrier, exerting its effects by changing the pH of brain fluids. Elevated levels of CO_2 produce vasodilation of cerebral blood vessels. Headache, blurred vision, irritability, muscle twitching, and psychological disturbances can occur with acute respiratory acidosis. If the condition is severe and prolonged, it can cause an increase in CSF pressure and papilledema. Impaired consciousness, ranging from lethargy to coma, develops as the PCO_2 rises. Paralysis of extremities may occur, and there may be respiratory depression. Less severe forms of acidosis often are accompanied by warm and flushed skin, weakness, and tachycardia.

Treatment

The treatment of acute and chronic respiratory acidosis is directed toward improving ventilation. In severe cases, mechanical ventilation may be necessary. The treatment of respiratory acidosis due to respiratory failure is discussed in Chapter 31.

RESPIRATORY ALKALOSIS

Respiratory alkalosis is a systemic acid-base disorder characterized by a primary decrease in plasma PCO_2, also referred to as *hypocapnia*, which produces an elevation in pH and a subsequent decrease in HCO_3^-.[25,27,28] Because respiratory alkalosis can occur suddenly, a compensatory decrease in bicarbonate level may not occur before respiratory correction has taken place.

Causes

Respiratory alkalosis is caused by hyperventilation or a respiratory rate in excess of that needed to maintain normal

TABLE 34-4 Causes and Manifestations of Respiratory Acidosis

Causes	Manifestations
Depression of Respiratory Center	**Blood pH, CO_2, HCO_3^-**
Drug overdose	pH decreased
Head injury	PCO_2 (primary) increased
	HCO_3^- (compensatory) increased
Lung Disease	
Bronchial asthma	**Neural Function**
Emphysema	Dilation of cerebral vessels and depression of neural function
Chronic bronchitis	Headache
Pneumonia	Weakness
Pulmonary edema	Behavior changes
Respiratory distress syndrome	Confusion
	Depression
Airway Obstruction, Disorders of Chest Wall and Respiratory Muscles	Paranoia
Paralysis of respiratory muscles	Hallucinations
Chest injuries	Tremors
Kyphoscoliosis	Paralysis
Extreme obesity	Stupor and coma
Treatment with paralytic drugs	
	Skin
Breathing Air With High CO_2 Content	Skin warm and flushed
	Signs of Compensation
	Acid urine

plasma PCO_2 levels (Table 34-5). It may occur as the result of central stimulation of the medullary respiratory center or stimulation of peripheral (*e.g.*, carotid chemoreceptor) pathways to the medullary respiratory center.[25]

Mechanical ventilation may produce respiratory alkalosis if the rate and tidal volume are set so that CO_2 elimination exceeds CO_2 production. Carbon dioxide crosses the alveolar capillary membrane 20 times more rapidly than oxygen. Therefore, the increased minute ventilation may be necessary to maintain adequate oxygen levels while producing a concomitant decrease in CO_2 levels. In some cases, respiratory alkalosis may be induced medically as a means of controlling disorders such as severe intracranial hypertension.[27]

Central stimulation of the medullary respiratory center occurs with anxiety, pain, pregnancy, febrile states, sepsis, encephalitis, and salicylate toxicity. Respiratory alkalosis has long been recognized as a common acid-base disorder in critically ill patients and is a consistent finding in both septic shock and the systemic inflammatory response syndrome[27] (see Chapter 28). Progesterone increases ventilation in women; during the progesterone phase of the menstrual cycle, normal women increase their PCO_2 values by 2 to 4 mm Hg and their pH by 0.01 to .02.[3] Women also develop substantial hypocapnia during pregnancy, most notably during the last trimester, with PCO_2 values of 29 to 32 mm Hg.[3,27]

One of the most common causes of respiratory alkalosis is the hyperventilation syndrome, which is characterized by recurring episodes of overbreathing often associated with anxiety. Persons experiencing panic attacks frequently present in the emergency room with manifestations of acute respiratory alkalosis.

Hypoxemia exerts its effect on pH through the peripheral chemoreceptors in the carotid bodies. Stimulation of peripheral chemoreceptors occurs in conditions that cause hypoxemia with relatively unimpaired CO_2 transport such as exposure to high altitudes, asthma, and respiratory disorders that decrease lung compliance.

Manifestations

Respiratory alkalosis manifests with a decrease in PCO_2 and a deficit in H_2CO_3 (see Table 34-5). In respiratory alkalosis, the pH is above 7.45, arterial PCO_2 is below 35 mm Hg, and plasma HCO_3^- levels usually are below 24 mEq/L (24 mmol/L).

The signs and symptoms of respiratory alkalosis are associated with hyperexcitability of the nervous system and a decrease in cerebral blood flow. Alkalosis increases protein binding of extracellular calcium. This reduces ionized calcium levels, causing an increase in neuromuscular excitability. A decrease in the CO_2 content of the blood causes constriction of cerebral blood vessels. Because CO_2 crosses the blood–brain barrier rather quickly, the manifestations of acute respiratory alkalosis are usually of sudden onset. The person often experiences light-headedness, dizziness, tingling, and numbness of the fingers and toes. These manifestations may be accompanied by sweating, palpitations, panic, air hunger, and dyspnea. Chvostek's and Trousseau's signs may be positive (see Chapter 33), and tetany and convulsions may occur. Because CO_2 provides the stimulus for short-term regulation of respiration, short periods of apnea may occur in persons with acute episodes of hyperventilation.

Treatment

The treatment of respiratory alkalosis focuses on measures to correct the underlying cause. Hypoxia may be corrected by administration of supplemental oxygen. Changing ventilator settings may be used to prevent or treat respiratory alkalosis in persons who are being mechanically ventilated. Persons with hyperventilation syndrome may benefit from reassurance, rebreathing from a paper bag during symptomatic attacks, and attention to the psychological stress.

TABLE 34-5 Causes and Manifestations of Respiratory Alkalosis

Causes	Manifestations
Excessive Ventilation	**Blood pH, CO_2, HCO_3^-**
Anxiety and psychogenic hyperventilation	pH increased
Hypoxia and reflex stimulation of ventilation	PCO_2 (primary) decreased
Lung disease that reflexly stimulates ventilation	HCO_3^- (compensatory) decreased
Stimulation of respiratory center	**Neural Function**
Elevated blood ammonia level	Constriction of cerebral vessels and increased neuronal excitability
Salicylate toxicity	Dizziness, panic, light-headedness
Encephalitis	Tetany
Fever	Numbness and tingling of fingers and toes
Mechanical ventilation	Positive Chvostek's and Trousseau's signs
	Seizures
	Cardiovascular Function
	Cardiac dysrhythmias

In summary, acidosis describes a decrease in pH, and alkalosis describes an increase in pH. Acid-base disorders may be caused by alterations in the body's volatile acids (*i.e.,* respiratory acidosis or respiratory alkalosis) or nonvolatile or fixed acids (*i.e.,* metabolic acidosis or metabolic alkalosis). Acidosis and alkalosis typically involve a primary or initiating event and a compensatory or adaptive state that results from homeostatic mechanisms that attempt to prevent or correct large changes in pH. A mixed acid-base disorder is one in which there is both a primary and a compensatory change in acid-base balance.

Metabolic acidosis is defined as a decrease in pH due to a decrease in the HCO_3^- ion, and metabolic alkalosis as an increase in pH due to an increase in the HCO_3^- ion. It is caused by an increased production of nonvolatile metabolic acids such as lactic acids or ketoacids, decreased acid excretion by the kidney, excessive loss of HCO_3^- as in diarrhea, or an increase in Cl^- ion. Metabolic acidosis may present with an increase in anion gap in which sodium bicarbonate is replaced by the sodium salt of the defending anion or with a normal anion gap as when HCO_3^- is replaced by Cl^-. Metabolic alkalosis involves factors related to the generation of a loss of H^+ ion or gain of HCO_3^- ion and those that serve to maintain it by interfering with the excretion of excess HCO_3^-. Factors that serve to maintain the alkalosis include decreased glomerular filtration rate, extracellular volume contraction, hypokalemia, hypochloremia, and aldosterone excess.

Respiratory acidosis reflects an increase in PCO_2 levels and is caused by conditions that impair alveolar ventilation. It can occur as an acute disorder in which there is a rapid rise in PCO_2, a minimal increase in plasma HCO_3^-, and a large decrease in pH. Respiratory alkalosis is caused by conditions that cause hyperventilation and a reduction in PCO_2 levels. Because respiratory alkalosis often occurs suddenly, a compensatory decrease in HCO_3^- levels may not occur before correction has been accomplished.

The signs and symptoms of acidosis and alkalosis reflect alterations in body function associated with the disorder causing the acid-base disturbance, the effect of the change of pH on body function, and the body's attempt to correct and maintain the pH within a normal physiologic range. In general, neuromuscular excitability is decreased in acidosis and increased in alkalosis.

REVIEW EXERCISES

A 34-year-old woman with diabetes is admitted to the emergency in a stuporous state. Her skin is flushed and warm, her breath has a sweet odor, her pulse is rapid and weak, and her respirations are rapid and deep. Her initial laboratory tests indicate a blood sugar of 320 mg/dL, serum bicarbonate of 12 mEq/L (normal, 24 to 27 mEq/L), and a pH of 7.1.

A. What is the most likely cause of her lowered pH and bicarbonate levels?

B. How would you account for her rapid and deep respirations?

C. Using the Henderson-Hasselbalch equation and the solubility coefficient for carbon dioxide that is given in this chapter, what would you expect her PCO_2 to be?

D. How would you explain her warm, flushed skin and stuporous mental state?

A 65-year-old man with chronic obstructive lung disease has been using low-flow oxygen therapy because of difficulty in maintaining adequate oxygenation of his blood. He has recently had a severe respiratory tract infection and has had increasing difficulty breathing. He is admitted to the emergency room because he has become increasingly lethargic and his wife has had trouble arousing him. She relates that he had "turned his oxygen way up" because of difficulty breathing.

A. What is the most likely cause of this man's problem?

B. How would you explain the lethargy and difficulty in arousal?

C. Blood gases, drawn on admission to the emergency room, indicated a PO_2 of 85 mm Hg and a PCO_2 of 90 mm Hg. His serum bicarbonate levels were 34 mEq/L. What is his pH?

D. What would be the main goal of his treatment in terms of acid-base balance?

References

1. Rose B. D. (2001). *Clinical physiology of acid-base and electrolyte disorders* (5th ed., pp. 302, 325–364, 578–647, 669). New York: McGraw-Hill.
2. Guyton A., Hall J. E. (2000). *Textbook of medical physiology* (10th ed., pp. 346–363). Philadelphia: W. B. Saunders.
3. Adrogu'e H. E., Adrogu'e H. J. (2001). Acid-base physiology. *Respiratory Care 46,* 328–341.
4. Shapiro J. I., Kaehny W. D. (2003). Pathogenesis and management of metabolic acidosis and alkalosis. In Schrier R. W. (ed). *Renal and electrolyte disorders* (pp.115–153). Philadelphia: Lippincott Williams & Wilkins.
5. Rhoades R. A., Tanner G. A. (1996). *Medical physiology* (pp. 465–483). Boston: Little, Brown.
6. Metheny N. M. (2000). *Fluid and electrolyte balance* (4th ed., p. 162). Philadelphia: J. B. Lippincott.
7. Kraut J. A., Madias N. E. (2001). Approach to patients with acid-base disorders. *Respiratory Care 46,* 392–402.
8. Adrogue H. J., Madias N. E. (1998). Management of life-threatening acid-base disorders: First of two parts. *New England Journal of Medicine 338,* 26–34.
9. Gauthier P. M., Szerlip H. M. (2002). Metabolic acidosis in the intensive care unit. *Critical Care Medicine 18,* 289–308.
10. Swenson E. R. (2001). Metabolic acidosis. *Respiratory Care 46,* 342–353.
11. Rothman S. M. (1999). Mutations of the mitochondrial genome: Clinical overview and possible pathophysiology of cell damage. *Biochemical Society Symposia 66,* 111–122.
12. Howell N. (1999). Human mitochondrial diseases: Answering questions and questioning answers. *International Review of Cytology 186,* 49–116.
13. Uribarri J., Oh M. S., Carroll H. J. (1998). D-Lactic acidosis: A review of clinical presentation, biochemical features and pathophysiological mechanisms. *Medicine (Baltimore) 77*(2), 73–82.

14. Umpierrez G. E., DiGirolamo M., Tuvlin J. A., et al. (2000). Differences in metabolic and hormonal milieu in diabetic and alcohol-induced ketoacidosis. *Journal of Critical Care 15*(2), 52–59.
15. Meyer R. J., Beard M. E., Ardagh M. W., Henderson S. (2000). Methanol poisoning. *New Zealand Medical Journal 113*(1102), 3–11.
16. Scalley RD., Smart M. L., Archie T. E. (2002). Treatment of ethylene glycol poisoning. *American Family Physician 66,* 807–812.
17. Egbert P. A., Abraham K. (1999). Ethylene glycol intoxication: Pathophysiology, diagnosis, and emergency management. *ANNA Journal 26,* 295–300.
18. Brent J., McMartin K., Phillips S. (2001). Fomepizole for treatment of methanol poisoning. *New England Journal of Medicine 344,* 424–429.
19. Powers F. (1999). The role of chloride in acid-base balance. *Journal of Intravenous Nursing 22,* 286–291.
20. Alpern R. J., Sakhaee K. (1997). The clinical spectrum of chronic metabolic acidosis: Homeostatic mechanisms produce significant morbidity. *American Journal of Kidney Diseases 29,* 291–302.
21. Forsythe S. M., Schmidt G. A. (2000). Sodium bicarbonate for the treatment of lactic acidosis. *Chest 117,* 260–267.
22. Khanna A., Kurtzman N. A. (2001). Metabolic alkalosis. *Respiratory Care 46,* 354–365.
23. Galla J. H. (2000). Metabolic alkalosis. *Journal of the American Society of Nephrology 11,* 369–375.
24. Adrogue H. J., Madias N. E. (1998). Management of life-threatening acid-base disorders. *New England Journal of Medicine 338,* 107–111.
25. Kaehny W. D. (2003). Pathogenesis and management of respiratory and mixed acid-base disorders. In Schrier R. W. (ed). *Renal and electrolyte disorders* (pp. 154–170). Philadelphia: Lippincott Williams & Wilkins.
26. Epstein S. K., Singh N. (2001). Respiratory acidosis. *Respiratory Care 46,* 366–383.
27. Laffey J. H., Kavenaugh B. P. (2002). Hypocapnia. *New England Journal of Medicine 347,* 43–53.
28. Foste G. T., Vaziri N. D., Sassoon C. S. H. (2001). Respiratory alkalosis. *Respiratory Care 46,* 384–391.

CHAPTER

35

Disorders of Renal Function

More than 20 million North Americans, or one in nine adults, have chronic kidney disease.[1] Kidney and urologic disease continue to be major causes of work loss, physician visits, and hospitalizations among men and women. Each year, kidney stones result in 1 million physician office visits and 300,000 hospitalizations, and urinary tract infections (UTIs) result in 8.3 million office visits and 1.6 million hospitalizations.[1]

The kidneys are subject to many of the same types of disorders that affect other body structures, including developmental defects, infections, altered immune responses, and neoplasms. The kidneys filter blood from all parts of the body, and although many forms of kidney disease originate in the kidneys, others develop secondary to disorders such as hypertension, diabetes mellitus, and systemic lupus erythematosus (SLE). The content in this chapter focuses on congenital disorders of the kidneys, obstructive disorders, UTIs, disorders of glomerular function, tubulointerstitial disorders, and neoplasms of the kidneys. Acute and chronic renal failure is discussed in Chapter 36.

Congenital Disorders of the Kidneys

After completing this section of the chapter, you should be able to meet the following objectives:

- Define the terms *agenesis, dysgenesis,* and *hypoplasia* as they refer to the development of the kidney
- Cite the effect of urinary obstruction in the fetus
- Describe the genetic basis for renal cystic disease, the pathology of the disorder, and its signs and symptoms

Some abnormality of the kidneys and ureters occurs in approximately 3% to 4% of newborn infants.[2] Anomalies in shape and position are the most common. Less common are disorders involving a decrease in renal mass (*e.g.*, agenesis, hypogenesis) or a change in renal structure (*e.g.*, renal cysts). Many fetal anomalies can be detected before birth by ultrasonography. In the normal fetus, the kidneys can be visualized as early as 12 weeks.

AGENESIS AND HYPOPLASIA

The kidneys begin to develop early in the fifth week of gestation and start to function approximately 3 weeks later. Formation of urine is thought to begin in the 9th to 12th weeks of gestation; by the 32nd week, fetal production of urine reaches approximately 28 mL/hour.[3] Urine is the main constituent of amniotic fluid. The relative amount of amniotic fluid can provide information about the status of fetal renal function. In pregnancies that involve infants with nonfunctional kidneys or outflow obstruction of urine from the kidneys, the amount of amniotic fluid is small—a condition called *oligohydramnios*. The condition causes compression of the developing fetus and is often associated with impaired development of fetal structures.[2]

The term *dysgenesis* refers to a failure of an organ to develop normally. *Agenesis* is the complete failure of an organ to develop. Total agenesis of both kidneys is incompatible with extrauterine life. Infants are stillborn or die shortly after birth of pulmonary hypoplasia. Newborns with renal agenesis often have characteristic facial features, termed *Potter's syndrome*.[4] The eyes are widely separated and have epicanthic folds, the ears are low set, the nose is broad and flat, the chin is receding, and limb defects often are present.[4,5] Other causes of neonatal renal failure with the Potter phenotype include cystic renal dysplasia, obstructive uropathy, and autosomal recessive polycystic disease. Unilateral agenesis is an uncommon anomaly that is compatible with life if no other abnormality is present. The opposite kidney usually is enlarged as a result of compensatory hypertrophy.

In *renal hypoplasia,* the kidneys do not develop to normal size. Like agenesis, hypoplasia more commonly affects only one kidney. When both kidneys are affected, there is progressive development of renal failure. It has been suggested that true hypoplasia is extremely rare; most cases probably represent acquired scarring due to vascular, infectious, or other kidney diseases rather than an underlying developmental failure.[5,6]

ALTERATIONS IN KIDNEY POSITION AND FORM

The development of the kidneys during embryonic life can result in kidneys that lie outside their normal position, usually just above the pelvic brim or within the pelvis. Because of the abnormal position, kinking of the ureters and obstruction of urine flow may occur.

One of the most common alterations in kidney form is an abnormality called a *horseshoe kidney*. This abnormality occurs in approximately 1 of every 500 to 1000 persons.[4,5] In this disorder, the upper or lower poles of the two kidneys are fused, producing a horseshoe-shaped structure that is continuous along the midline of the body anterior to the great vessels. Most horseshoe kidneys are fused at the lower pole[6] (Fig. 35-1). The condition usually does not cause problems unless there is an associated defect in the renal pelvis or other urinary structures that obstructs urine flow.

CYSTIC DISEASE OF THE KIDNEY

Renal cysts are fluid-filled sacs or segments of a dilated nephron. The cysts may be single or multiple and can vary in size from microscopic to several centimeters in diameter. There are four basic types of renal cystic disease: polycystic kidney disease, medullary sponge kidney, acquired cystic disease, and simple kidney cysts. Although some types of cysts are not congenital, they are included in this section.

Renal cystic disease is thought to result from tubular obstructions that increase intratubular pressure or from changes in the basement membrane of the renal tubules that predispose to cystic dilatation. After a cyst begins to form, continued fluid accumulation contributes to its persistent growth. Renal cystic diseases probably exert their effects by compressing renal blood vessels, producing degeneration of functional renal tissue and obstructing tubular flow.

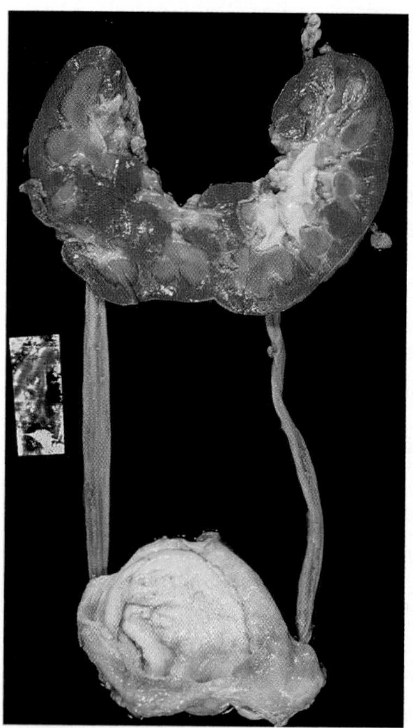

FIGURE 35-1 Horseshoe kidney. The kidneys are fused at the lower poles. (Rubin E., Farber J.L. [1999]. *Pathology* [3rd ed., p. 865]. Philadelphia: Lippincott-Raven)

Simple and Acquired Renal Cysts

Simple cysts are a common disorder of the kidney. The cysts may be single or multiple, unilateral or bilateral, and they usually are less than 1 cm in diameter, although they may grow larger. Most simple cysts do not produce signs or symptoms or compromise renal function. When symptomatic, they may cause flank pain, hematuria, infection, and hypertension related to ischemia-produced stimulation of the renin-angiotensin system. They are most common in older persons. Although the cysts are benign, they may be confused clinically with renal cell carcinoma.

An acquired form of renal cystic disease occurs in persons with end-stage renal failure who have undergone prolonged dialysis treatment. The cysts, which measure 0.2 to 2 cm in diameter, probably develop as a result of tubular obstruction.[5] Although the condition is largely asymptomatic, the cysts may bleed, causing hematuria. Tumors, usually adenomas but occasionally adenosarcomas, may develop in the walls of these cysts.

Medullary Cystic Disease

Two major types of cystic disease involve the medullary portion of the kidney: medullary sponge kidney and nephronophthisis–medullary cystic disease complex.[5,6] *Medullary sponge kidney* is characterized by small (<5 mm in diameter), multiple cystic dilations of the collecting ducts of the medulla. The disorder does not cause progressive renal failure; it does, however, produce urinary stasis and predisposes to kidney infections and kidney stones. The disease usually is asymptomatic in young adults. Symptomatic disease usually develops between the ages of 30 and 60 years, when affected persons begin to have flank pain, dysuria, hematuria, and "gravel" in the urine as a result of stone formation in the cysts.[6]

Nephronophthisis–medullary cystic disease complex is a group of related diseases characterized by renal medullary cysts, sclerotic kidneys, and renal failure. Approximately 85% of cases have a hereditary basis. Symptoms usually develop during childhood, and the disorder accounts for 10% to 20% of renal failure in children. Polyuria, polydipsia, and enuresis (bed-wetting), which are early manifestations of the disorder, reflect impaired ability of the kidneys to concentrate urine.[5,6]

Polycystic Kidney Disease

The most common form of renal cystic disease is polycystic kidney disease, which is the result of a hereditary trait. It is one of the most common hereditary diseases in the United States, affecting more than 600,000 Americans.[1] There are two types of inherited polycystic disease: autosomal recessive and autosomal dominant.

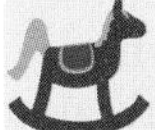

Autosomal Recessive Polycystic Kidney Disease. Autosomal recessive polycystic kidney disease, which is present at birth, is rare compared with the adult variety.[5,6] The disorder is inherited as a recessive trait, meaning that both parents are carriers of the gene and that there is a one in four chance of the parents having another child with the disorder. Because the condition is present at birth, it formerly was called *infantile* or *childhood polycystic disease.* The condition is bilateral, and significant renal dysfunction usually is present, accompanied by variable degrees of liver fibrosis and portal hypertension. The disorder can be diagnosed by ultrasonography.

There is no known treatment for the disease. Approximately 75% of infants die in the perinatal period, often because the large kidneys compromise expansion of the lungs.[6] Some children may present with less severe kidney problems and more severe liver disease.

Autosomal Dominant Polycystic Kidney Disease. Autosomal dominant polycystic kidney disease (ADPKD), also called *adult polycystic kidney disease,* is a systemic disorder that primarily affects the kidneys. The disease, which is inherited as an autosomal trait, results in the formation of fluid-filled cysts in both kidneys with the threat of progression to chronic renal failure. Other manifestations of the disease include hypertension, cardiovascular abnormalities, cerebral aneurysms, and cyst formation in other organs such as the liver and pancreas.

Two mutant genes have been implicated in most cases of the disorder.[5–8] A polycystic kidney disease gene called *PKD1,* located on chromosome 16, is responsible for approximately 85% of cases. It encodes a large membrane protein called *polycystin 1* that has domains similar to proteins involved in cell-to-cell and cell-to–extracellular matrix interactions. A second gene, called *PKD2,* is located on chromosome 4. It encodes for a product called *polycystin 2,* which is an integral membrane protein that is similar to certain calcium and sodium channel proteins as well as a portion of polycystin 1. Although the two mutations produce almost identical disease phenotypes, disease progression is typically more rapid in people with ADPKD type 1 disease than those with ADPKD type 2 disease.[7,8]

The link between the genetic defect in the polycystin proteins and the formation of the fluid-filled cysts in the kidney has not been fully established. It is thought that the membrane proteins may play a role in cell-to-cell matrix interactions that are important in tubular epithelial cell growth and differentiation.[5] Accordingly, it is hypothesized that cysts develop as a result of an abnormality in cell differentiation, increased transepithelial fluid secretion, and formation of an abnormal extracellular matrix that allows the cyst to grow and separate from adjacent tubules. In addition, cyst fluids have been shown to harbor mediators that enhance fluid secretion and induce inflammation, resulting in further enlargement of the cysts and the interstitial fibrosis that is characteristic of progressive polycystic kidney disease.

It is interesting to note that although the mutant ADPKD gene is present in all tubular cells of affected persons, cysts develop in only some tubules. Progression of the disease is characterized by tubular dilatation with cyst formation interspersed among normally functioning nephrons. Fluid collects in the cyst while it is still part of the tubular lumen, or it is secreted into the cyst after it has separated from the tubule. As the fluid accumulates, the cysts gradually increase in size, with some becoming as large as 5 cm in diameter.[5,6] The kidneys of persons with polycystic kidney disease eventually become enlarged because of the presence of multiple cysts (Fig. 35-2). Cysts also may be found in the liver and, less commonly, the pancreas and spleen. Mitral valve prolapse and other valvular heart diseases occur in 20% to 25% of persons, but are largely asymptomatic. Most persons with polycystic disease also have colonic diverticula. One of the most devastating extrarenal manifestations is a weakness in the walls of the cerebral arteries that can lead to aneurysm formation. Approximately 20% of persons with polycystic kidney disease have an associated aneurysm, and subarachnoid hemorrhage is a frequent cause of death.[6]

The manifestations of ADPKD include pain from the enlarging cysts that may reach debilitating levels, episodes of gross hematuria from bleeding into a cyst, infected cysts from ascending UTI, and hypertension resulting from compression of intrarenal blood vessels with activation of the renin-angiotensin mechanism.[9,10] Renal colic caused by kidney stones occurs in about 20% of persons with ADPKD.[10] The progress of the disease is slow, and end-stage renal disease is uncommon before 40 years of age.

Ultrasound usually is the preferred technique for diagnosis of symptomatic patients and for screening of asymptomatic family members.[9] The ability to detect cysts increases with age; 80% to 90% of affected persons older than age 20 have detectable cysts. Computed tomography (CT) may be used for detection of small cysts. Genetic linkage studies are now available for diagnosis of ADPKD, but are usually reserved for cases in which radiographic imaging is negative and the need for a definitive diagnosis is essential, such as when screening family members for potential kidney donation.[9]

The treatment of ADPKD is largely supportive and aimed at delaying the progression of the disease. Control of hypertension and prevention of ascending urinary tract infections are important. Pain is a common complaint of persons with ADPKD, and a systematic approach is needed to differentiate the etiology of the pain and define an approach for management.[10] Dialysis and kidney transplantation are reserved for those who progress to end-stage renal disease.

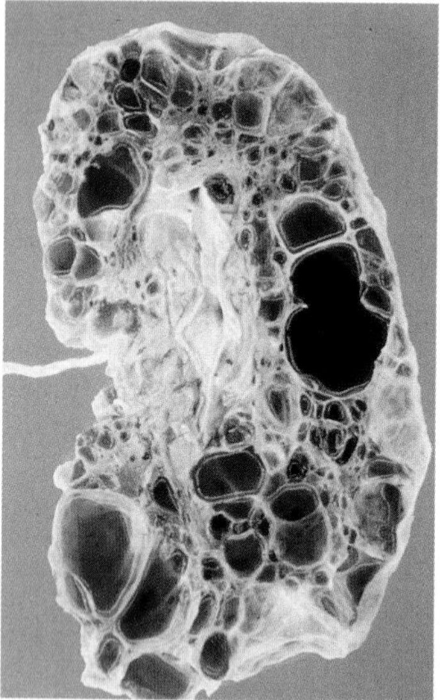

FIGURE 35-2 Adult polycystic disease. The kidney is enlarged, and the parenchyma is almost entirely replaced by cysts of varying size. (Rubin E., Farber J.L. [1999]. *Pathology* [3rd ed., p. 867]. Philadelphia: Lippincott-Raven)

In summary, approximately 10% of infants are born with potentially significant malformations of the urinary system. These abnormalities can range from bilateral renal agenesis, which is incompatible with life, to hypogenesis of one kidney, which usually causes no problems unless the function of the remaining kidney is impaired. The developmental process can result in kidneys that lie outside their normal position. Because of the abnormal position, kinking of the ureters and obstruction of urine flow can occur.

Renal cystic disease is a condition in which there is dilatation of tubular structures with cyst formation. Cysts may be single or multiple. Polycystic kidney disease is an inherited form of renal cystic disease; it can be inherited as an autosomal recessive or an autosomal dominant trait. Autosomal recessive polycystic kidney disease is rare and usually presents as severe renal dysfunction during infancy. Autosomal dominant polycystic disease usually does not become symptomatic until later in life, often after 40 years of age. The disease, which involves mutations in a polycystin gene, results in the formation of fluid-filled cysts in both kidneys with the threat of progression to chronic renal failure. Other manifestations of the disease include hypertension, cardiovascular abnormalities, cerebral aneurysms, and cysts in other organs such as the liver and pancreas.

Obstructive Disorders

After completing this section of the chapter, you should be able to meet the following objectives:

- List common causes of urinary tract obstruction
- Describe the effects of urinary tract obstruction on renal structure and function
- Cite three theories that are used to explain the formation of kidney stones
- Explain the mechanisms of pain and infection that occur with kidney stones
- Describe methods used in the diagnosis and treatment of kidney stones

Urinary obstruction can occur in persons of any age and can involve any level of the urinary tract from the urethra to the renal pelvis (Fig. 35-3). The conditions that cause urinary tract obstruction include developmental defects, calculi (*i.e.,* stones), pregnancy, benign prostatic hyperplasia, scar tissue resulting from infection and inflammation, tumors, and neurologic disorders such as spinal cord injury. The causes of urinary tract obstructions are summarized in Table 35-1.

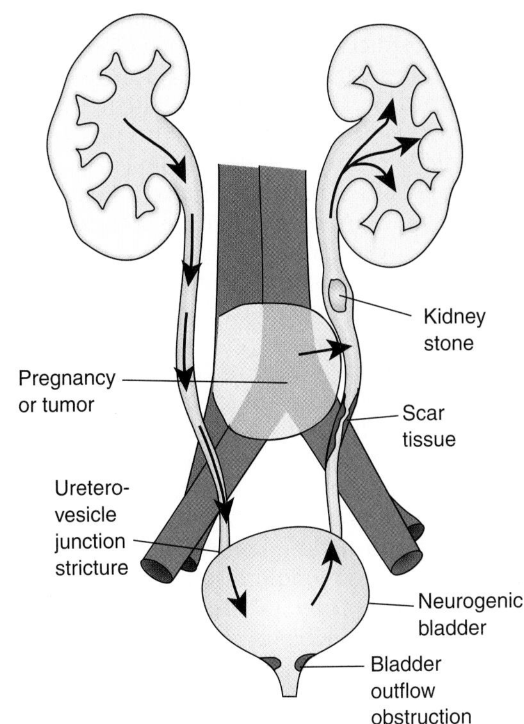

FIGURE 35-3 Locations and causes of urinary tract obstruction.

MECHANISMS OF RENAL DAMAGE

The destructive effects of urinary obstruction on kidney structures are determined by the degree (*i.e.,* partial vs. complete, unilateral vs. bilateral) and the duration of the obstruction. The two most damaging effects of urinary obstruction are stasis of urine, which predisposes to infection and stone formation, and development of backpressure, which interferes with renal blood flow and destroys kidney tissue.

TABLE 35-1 Causes of Urinary Tract Obstruction

Level of Obstruction	Cause
Renal pelvis	Renal calculi Papillary necrosis
Ureter	Renal calculi Pregnancy Tumors that compress the ureter Ureteral stricture Congenital disorders of the ureterovesical junction and ureteropelvic junction strictures
Bladder and urethra	Bladder cancer Neurogenic bladder Bladder stones Prostatic hyperplasia or cancer Urethral strictures Congenital urethral defects

A common complication of urinary tract obstruction is infection. Stagnation of urine predisposes to infection, which may spread throughout the urinary tract. When present, urinary calculi serve as foreign bodies and contribute to the infection. Once established, the infection is difficult to treat. It often is caused by urea-splitting organisms (*e.g., Proteus,* staphylococci) that increase ammonia production and cause the urine to become alkaline.[11] Calcium salts precipitate more readily in stagnant alkaline urine; thus, urinary tract obstructions also predispose to stone formation.

In situations of marked or complete obstruction, backpressure develops because of a combination of continued glomerular filtration and impedance to urinary flow. Prolonged or severe partial obstruction causes irreversible kidney damage. Depending on the degree of obstruction, pressure builds up, beginning at the site of obstruction and moving backward from the ureter or renal pelvis into the calices and collecting tubules. Typically, the most severe effects occur at the level of the papillae because these structures are subjected to the greatest pressure. Damage to the nephrons and other functional components of the kidney is caused by compression from increased intrapelvic pressure and ischemia from disturbances in blood flow. Experiments have shown recovery of renal function after release of complete obstruction of up to 4 weeks' duration. Irreversible damage, however, can begin as early as 7 days.[11]

Dilatation of the ureters and renal pelves occurs with prolonged urinary tract obstruction. When the obstruction is in the distal ureter, the increased pressure dilates the proximal ureter, a condition called *hydroureter* (Fig. 35-4). Hydroureter also is a complication of bladder outflow obstruction due to prostatic hyperplasia (see Chapter 45). With increasing pressure, the ureteral wall becomes severely stretched and loses its ability to undergo peristaltic contractions. In extreme cases, the ureter may become so dilated that it resembles a loop of bowel. *Hydronephrosis* refers to urine-filled dilatation of the renal pelvis and calices. The degree of hydronephrosis depends on the duration, degree, and site of obstruction. Bilateral hydronephrosis occurs only when the obstruction is below the level of the ureters. If the obstruction occurs at the level of the ureters or above, hydronephrosis is unilateral. The kidney eventually is destroyed and appears as a thin-walled shell that is filled with fluid (Fig. 35-5).

Manifestations

The manifestations of urinary obstruction depend on the site of obstruction, the cause, and the rapidity with which the condition developed. Most commonly, the person has pain, signs and symptoms of UTI, and manifestations of renal dysfunction, such as an impaired ability to concentrate urine. Changes in urine output may be misleading because output may be normal or even high in cases of partial obstruction.

Pain, which often is the factor that causes a person to seek medical attention, is the result of distention of the bladder, collecting system, or renal capsule. Its severity is related most closely to the rate rather than the degree of distention. Pain most often occurs with acute obstruction,

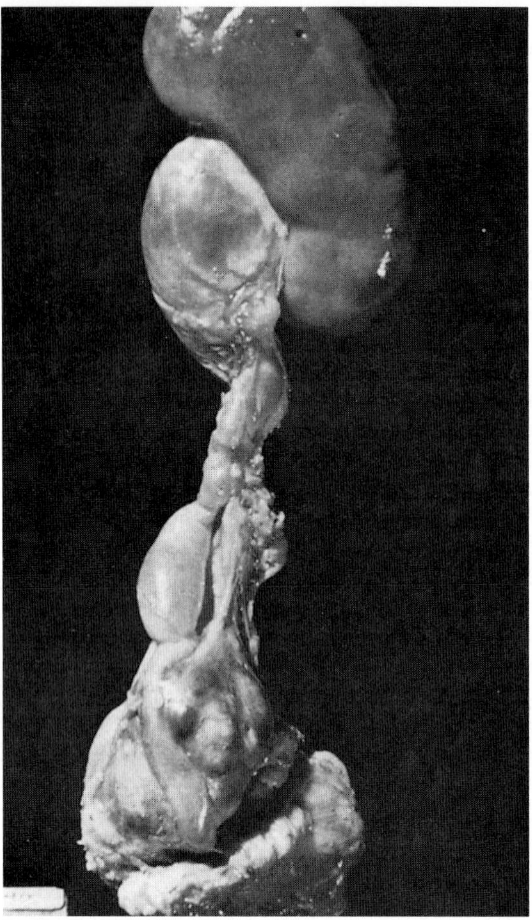

FIGURE 35-4 Hydroureter caused by ureteral obstruction in a woman with cancer of the uterus.

in which the distention of urinary structures is rapid. This is in contrast to chronic obstruction, in which distention is gradual and may not cause pain. Instead, gradual obstruction may produce only vague abdominal or back discomfort. When pain occurs, it is related to the site of obstruction. Obstruction of the renal pelvis or upper ureter causes pain and tenderness over the flank area. With lower levels of obstruction, the pain may radiate to the testes in the male or the labia in the female. With partial obstruction, particularly of the ureteropelvic junction, pain may occur during periods of high fluid intake, when a high rate of urine flow causes an acute distention of the renal pelvis. Because of its visceral innervation, ureteral obstruction may produce reflex impairment of gastrointestinal tract peristalsis and motility with abdominal distention and, in severe cases, paralytic ileus.

Hypertension is an occasional complication of urinary tract obstruction. It is more common in cases of unilateral obstruction in which renin secretion is enhanced, probably secondary to impaired renal blood flow. In these circumstances, removal of the obstruction often leads to a reduction in blood pressure. When hypertension accompanies bilateral obstruction, renin levels usually are normal, and the elevated blood pressure probably is volume related. The relief of bilateral obstruction leads to a loss of volume and a decrease in blood pressure. In some cases, relieving the obstruction does not correct the hypertension.

Diagnosis and Treatment

Early diagnosis of urinary tract obstruction is important because the condition usually is treatable and a delay in therapy may result in permanent damage to the kidneys. Diagnostic methods vary with the symptoms. Ultrasonography has proved to be the single most useful noninvasive diagnostic modality for urinary obstruction. Radiologic methods, CT scans, and intravenous urography may also be used. Other diagnostic methods, such as urinalysis, are used to determine the extent of renal involvement and the presence of infection.

Treatment of urinary obstruction depends on the cause. Urinary stone removal may be necessary, or surgical treatment of structural defects may be indicated.

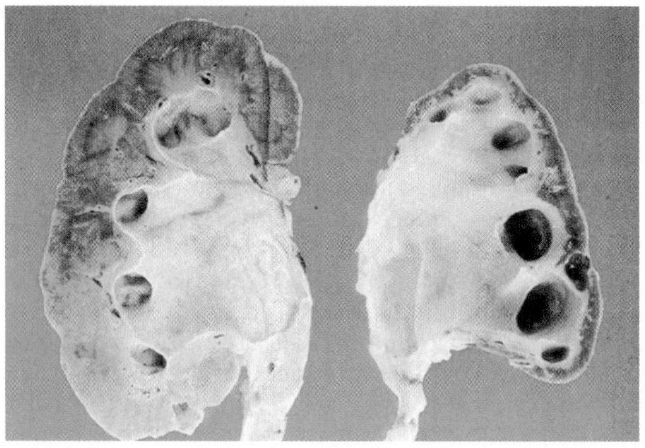

FIGURE 35-5 Hydronephrosis. Bilateral urinary tract obstruction has led to conspicuous dilatation of the ureters, pelves, and calices. The kidney on the right shows severe cortical atrophy. (Rubin E., Farber J.L. [1999]. *Pathology* [3rd ed., p. 910]. Philadelphia: Lippincott-Raven)

RENAL CALCULI

The term *nephrolithiasis* refers to kidney stones. The most common cause of upper urinary tract obstruction is urinary calculi. Although stones can form in any part of the urinary tract, most develop in the kidneys. Urinary stones are the third most common disorder of the urinary tract, exceeded only by UTIs and prostate disorders.[12] Men are two to three times more likely to develop stones than women.[13]

Kidney stones are crystalline structures made up of materials that the kidneys normally excrete in the urine. The etiology of urinary stone formation is complex, and not all aspects are well understood. It is thought to encompass a number of factors, including increases in blood and urinary levels of stone components and interactions among the components; anatomic changes in urinary tract structures; metabolic and endocrine influences; dietary and intestinal absorption factors; and UTI. To add to the mystery of stone formation is the fact that although both kidneys are exposed to the same urinary constituents, kid-

KIDNEY STONES

- Kidney stones are crystalline structures that form from components of the urine.
- Stones require a nidus to form and a urinary environment that supports continued crystallization of stone components.
- The development of kidney stones is influenced by the concentration of stone components in the urine, the ability of the stone components to complex and form stones, and the presence of substances that inhibit stone formation.

ney stones tend to form in only one kidney. Three major theories are used to explain stone formation: the saturation theory, the matrix theory, and the inhibitor deficiency theory.[14–17] One or more of these theories may apply to stone formation in the same person.

Kidney stones require a nidus, or nucleus, to form and a urinary environment that supports continued precipitation of stone components to grow. The *saturation theory* states that the risk for stone formation is increased when the urine is supersaturated with stone components (*e.g.,* calcium salts, uric acid, magnesium ammonium phosphate, cystine). Supersaturation depends on urinary pH, solute concentration, ionic strength, and complexation. The greater the concentration of two ions, the more likely they are to precipitate. Complexation influences the availability of specific ions. For example, sodium complexes with oxalate and decreases its free ionic form.

The *matrix theory* proposes that organic materials, such as mucopolysaccharides derived from the epithelial cells that line the tubules, act as a nidus for stone formation. This theory is based on the observation that organic matrix materials can be found in all layers of kidney stones. It is not known whether the matrix material contributes to the initiation of stone formation or the material is merely entrapped as the stone forms.

Proteins produced by the kidney inhibit all phases of crystallization. The *inhibitor theory* suggests that persons who have a deficiency of proteins that inhibit stone formation in their urine are at increased risk for stone formation. Kidney cells produce at least three proteins that are thought to slow the rate of calcium oxalate crystallization: nephrocalcin, Tamm-Horsfall mucoprotein, and uropontin.[14,15,18] Nephrocalcin inhibits nucleation, aggregation, and growth of calcium oxalate stones. *Tamm-Horsfall mucoprotein* is thought to exert a minor effect on crystal aggregation. Uropontin inhibits the growth of calcium oxalate crystals. Much of the information about the function of organic inhibitors in terms of stone formation is still experimental. Nonorganic substances also can act as inhibitors of stone formation. For example, citrate is a key factor affecting development of calcium stones. It complexes with calcium, thereby decreasing the concentration of ionic calcium. Citrate is a normal byproduct of the citric acid cycle in renal cells; metabolic stimuli that consume this product (as with metabolic acidosis due to fasting or hypokalemia) reduce the urinary concentration of citrate. Citrate supplementation (potassium citrate) may be used in the treatment of some forms of hypocitraturic kidney stones.[12]

Types of Stones

There are four basic types of kidney stones: calcium stones (*i.e.,* oxalate or phosphate), magnesium ammonium phosphate stones, uric acid stones, and cystine stones. The causes and treatment measures for each of these types of renal stones are described in Table 35-2.

TABLE 35-2 Composition, Contributing Factors, and Treatment of Kidney Stones

Type of Stone	Contributing Factors	Treatment
Calcium (oxalate and phosphate)	Hypercalcemia and hypercalciuria Immobilization Hyperparathyroidism Vitamin D intoxication Diffuse bone disease Milk-alkali syndrome Renal tubular acidosis Hyperoxaluria	Treatment of underlying conditions Increased fluid intake Thiazide diuretics Dietary restriction of foods high in oxalate
Magnesium ammonium phosphate (struvite)	Urinary tract infections	Treatment of urinary tract infection Acidification of the urine Increased fluid intake
Uric acid (urate)	Formed in acid urine with pH of approximately 5.5 Gout High-purine diet	Increased fluid intake Allopurinol for hyperuricuria Alkalinization of urine
Cystine	Cystinuria (inherited disorder of amino acid metabolism)	Increased fluid intake Alkalinization of urine

Most kidney stones (70% to 80%) are calcium stones—calcium oxalate, calcium phosphate, or a combination of the two materials. Calcium stones usually are associated with increased concentrations of calcium in the blood and urine. Excessive bone resorption caused by immobility, bone disease, hyperparathyroidism, and renal tubular acidosis all are contributing conditions. High oxalate concentrations in the blood and urine predispose to formation of calcium oxalate stones.

Magnesium ammonium phosphate stones, also called *struvite stones,* form only in alkaline urine and in the presence of bacteria that possess an enzyme called *urease,* which splits the urea in the urine into ammonia and carbon dioxide. The ammonia that is formed takes up a hydrogen ion to become an ammonium ion, increasing the pH of the urine so that it becomes more alkaline. Because phosphate levels are increased in alkaline urine and because magnesium always is present in the urine, struvite stones form. These stones enlarge as the bacterial count grows, and they can increase in size until they fill an entire renal pelvis (Fig. 35-6). Because of their shape, they often are called *staghorn stones.* Staghorn stones almost always are associated with UTIs and persistently alkaline urine. Because these stones act as a foreign body, treatment of the infection often is difficult. Struvite stones usually are too large to be passed and require lithotripsy or surgical removal.

Uric acid stones develop in conditions of gout and high concentrations of uric acid in the urine. Hyperuricosuria also may contribute to calcium stone formation by acting as a nucleus for calcium oxalate stone formation. Unlike radiopaque calcium stones, uric acid stones are not visible on x-ray films. Uric acid stones form most readily in urine with a pH of 5.1 to 5.9.[14] Thus, these stones can be treated by raising the urinary pH to 6 to 6.5 with potassium alkali salts.

Cystine stones are rare. They are seen in cystinuria, which results from a genetic defect in renal transport of cystine. These stones resemble struvite stones except that infection is unlikely to be present.

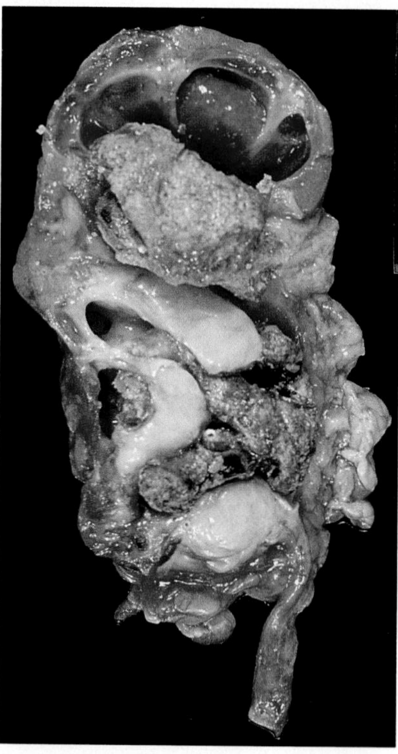

FIGURE 35-6 Staghorn calculi. The kidney shows hydronephrosis and stones that are casts of the dilated calices. (Rubin E., Farber J.L. [1999]. *Pathology* [3rd ed., p. 909]. Philadelphia: Lippincott-Raven)

Manifestations

One of the major manifestations of kidney stones is pain. Depending on location, there are two types of pain associated with kidney stones: renal colic and noncolicky renal pain.[12,13] *Renal colic* is the term used to describe the colicky pain that accompanies stretching of the collecting system or ureter. The symptoms of renal colic are caused by stones 1 to 5 mm in diameter that can move into the ureter and obstruct flow. Classic ureteral colic is manifested by acute, intermittent, and excruciating pain in the flank and upper outer quadrant of the abdomen on the affected side. The pain may radiate to the lower abdominal quadrant, bladder area, perineum, or scrotum in the male. The skin may be cool and clammy, and nausea and vomiting are common. Noncolicky pain is caused by stones that produce distention of the renal calices or renal pelvis. The pain usually is a dull, deep ache in flank or back that can vary in intensity from mild to severe. The pain is often exaggerated by drinking large amounts of fluid.

Diagnosis and Treatment

Patients with kidney stones often present with acute renal colic, and the diagnosis is based on symptomatology and diagnostic tests, which include urinalysis, plain film radiography, intravenous pyelography, and abdominal ultrasonography.[13] Urinalysis provides information related to hematuria, infection, the presence of stone-forming crystals, and urine pH. At least 90% of stones are radiopaque and readily visible on a plain radiograph of the abdomen. Intravenous pyelography uses an intravenously injected contrast medium that is filtered in the glomeruli to visualize the collecting system and the ureters of the kidneys. Abdominal ultrasound is highly sensitive to hydronephrosis, which may be a manifestation of ureteral obstruction. Retrograde urography and CT scanning also may be used. A new imaging technique called *nuclear scintigraphy* uses bisphosphonate markers as a means of imaging stones.[12] The method has been credited with identifying stones that are too small to be detected by other methods.

Treatment of acute renal colic usually is supportive. Pain relief may be needed during acute phases of obstruction, and antibiotic therapy may be necessary to treat urinary infections. Most stones that are less than 5 mm in diameter pass spontaneously. All urine should be strained during an attack in the hope of retrieving the stone for chemical analysis and determination of type. This information, along with a careful history and laboratory tests, provides the basis for long-term preventive measures.

A major goal of treatment in persons who have passed kidney stones or have had them removed is to prevent their recurrence. Prevention requires investigation into the cause of stone formation using urine tests, blood chemistries, and stone analysis. Underlying disease conditions, such as hyperparathyroidism, are treated. Adequate fluid intake reduces the concentration of stone-forming crystals in the urine and needs to be encouraged. Depending on the type of stone that is formed, dietary changes, medications, or both may be used to alter the concentration of stone-forming elements in the urine. For example, persons who form calcium oxalate stones may need to decrease their intake of foods that are high in oxalate (*e.g.,* spinach, Swiss chard, cocoa, chocolate, pecans, peanuts). Calcium supplementation with calcium salts such as calcium carbonate and calcium phosphate also may be used to bind oxalate in the intestine and decrease its absorption. Thiazide diuretics lower urinary calcium by increasing tubular reabsorption so that less remains in the urine. Drugs that bind calcium in the gut (*e.g.,* cellulose phosphate) may be used to inhibit calcium absorption and urinary excretion.

Measures to change the pH of the urine also can influence kidney stone formation. In persons who lose the ability to lower the pH of (or acidify) their urine, there is an increase in the divalent and trivalent forms of urine phosphate that combine with calcium to form calcium phosphate stones. The formation of uric acid stones is increased in acid urine; stone formation can be reduced by raising the pH of urine to 6.0 to 6.5 with potassium alkali (*e.g.,* potassium citrate) salts. Table 35-2 summarizes measures for preventing the recurrence of different types of kidney stones.

In some cases, stone removal may be necessary. Several methods are available for removing kidney stones: ureteroscopic removal, percutaneous removal, and extracorporeal lithotripsy. All these procedures eliminate the need for an open surgical procedure, which is another form of treatment. Open stone surgery may be required to remove large calculi or those that are resistant to other forms of removal.

Ureteroscopic removal involves the passage of an instrument through the urethra into the bladder and then into the ureter. The development of high-quality optics has improved the ease with which this procedure is performed and its outcome. The procedure, which is performed under fluoroscopic guidance, involves the use of various instruments for dilating the ureter and for grasping, fragmenting, and removing the stone. Preprocedure radiologic studies using a contrast medium (*i.e.,* excretory urography) are done to determine the position of the stone and direct the placement of the ureteroscope.

Percutaneous nephrolithotomy is the treatment of choice for removal of renal or proximal ureteral calculi. It involves the insertion through the flank of a small-gauge needle into the collecting system of the kidney; the needle tract is then dilated, and an instrument called a *nephroscope* is inserted into the renal pelvis. The procedure is performed under fluoroscopic guidance. Preprocedure radiologic and ultrasonographic examinations of the kidney and ureter are used in determining the placement of the nephroscope. Stones up to 1 cm in diameter can be removed through this method. Larger stones must be broken up with an electrohydraulic or ultrasonic lithotriptor (*i.e.,* stone breaker).

A nonsurgical treatment called *extracorporeal shock-wave lithotripsy,* introduced in Germany in 1980, received U.S. Food and Drug Administration approval in 1984 for treatment of stones primarily in the renal calyx and pelvis and the upper third of the ureter. The procedure uses acoustic shock waves to fragment calculi into sandlike particles that are passed in the urine over the next few days. Because of the large amount of stone particles that are generated during the procedure, a ureteral stent (*i.e.,* tubelike device used to hold the ureter open) may be inserted to ensure adequate urine drainage.

In summary, obstruction of urine flow can occur at any level of the urinary tract. Among the causes of urinary tract obstruction are developmental defects, pregnancy, infection and inflammation, kidney stones, neurologic defects, and prostatic hypertrophy. Obstructive disorders produce stasis of urine, increasing the risk for infection and calculi formation and resulting in backpressure that is damaging to kidney structures.

Kidney stones are a major cause of upper urinary tract obstruction. There are four types of kidney stones: calcium (*i.e.,* oxalate and phosphate) stones, which are associated with increased serum calcium levels; magnesium ammonium phosphate (*i.e.,* struvite) stones, which are associated with UTIs; uric acid stones, which are related to elevated uric acid levels; and cystine stones, which are seen in cystinuria. A major goal of treatment for persons who have passed kidney stones or have had them removed is to identify stone composition and prevent their recurrence. Treatment measures depend on stone type and include adequate fluid intake to prevent urine saturation, dietary modification to decrease intake of stone-forming constituents, treatment of UTI, measures to change urine pH, and the use of diuretics that decrease the calcium concentration of urine.

Urinary Tract Infections

After completing this section of the chapter, you should be able to meet the following objectives:

- Cite the organisms most responsible for UTIs and state why urinary catheters, obstruction, and reflux predispose to infections
- List three physiologic mechanisms that protect against UTIs
- Compare the signs and symptoms of upper and lower UTIs
- Describe factors that predispose to UTIs in children, sexually active women, pregnant women, and older adults
- Compare the manifestations of UTIs in different age groups, including infants, toddlers, adolescents, adults, and older adults
- Cite measures used in the diagnosis and treatment of UTIs

Urinary tract infections are the second most common type of bacterial infections seen by health care providers, respiratory tract infections being the first. Each year, more than 8 million people are diagnosed with UTIs. According to the 1997 National Ambulatory Medical Care Survey, UTI accounted for nearly 7 million office visits and 1 million emergency room visits, resulting in 100,000 hospitalizations.[19]

ETIOLOGIC FACTORS

UTIs can include several distinct entities, including asymptomatic bacteriuria, symptomatic infections, lower UTIs such as cystitis, and upper UTIs such as pyelonephritis. Because of their ability to cause renal damage, upper UTIs are considered more serious than lower UTIs.

Most uncomplicated UTIs are caused by *Escherichia coli.* Other uropathic pathogens include *Staphylococcus saprophyticus* in uncomplicated UTIs, and both non–*E. coli* gram-negative rods (*Proteus mirabilis, Klebsiella pneumoniae,* and *Enterobacter, Pseudomonas,* and *Serratia* species) and gram-positive cocci (*Staphylococcus aureus,* group B streptococci) in complicated UTIs.[20–22] Most UTIs are caused by bacteria that enter through the urethra. Bacteria can also enter through the bloodstream, usually in immunocompromised persons and neonates. Although the distal portion of the urethra often contains pathogens, the urine formed in the kidneys and found in the bladder normally is sterile or free of bacteria. This is because of the *washout phenomenon,* in which urine from the bladder normally washes bacteria out of the urethra. When a UTI occurs, it is usually from bacteria that have colonized the urethra, vagina, or perianal area.

There is an increased risk for UTI in persons with urinary obstruction and reflux; in people with neurogenic disorders that impair bladder emptying; in women who are sexually active, especially if they use a diaphragm or spermicide for contraception; in postmenopausal women; in men with diseases of the prostate; and in elderly persons. Instrumentation and urinary catheterization are the most common predisposing factors for nosocomial UTIs. UTIs occur more commonly in women with diabetes than in women without the disease. People with diabetes are also at increased risk for complications associated with UTIs, including pyelonephritis, and they are more susceptible to fungal infections (particularly, *Candida* species) and infections with gram-negative pathogens other than *E. coli,* both of which are accompanied by increased severity and unusual manifestations.[23]

URINARY TRACT INFECTIONS

- Urinary tract infections involve both the lower and upper urinary tract structures.
- In lower urinary tract infections, the infecting pathogens tend to propagate in the urine and cause irritative voiding symptoms, often with minimal systemic signs of infection.
- Upper urinary tract infections tend to invade the tissues of the kidney pelvis, inciting an acute inflammatory response with marked systemic manifestations of infection.

Host–Agent Interactions

Because certain people tend to be predisposed to development of UTIs, considerable interest has been focused on host–pathogen interactions and factors that increase the risk for UTI.

Host Defenses. In the development of a UTI, host defenses are matched against the virulence of the pathogen. The host defenses of the bladder have several components, including the washout phenomenon, in which bacteria are removed from the bladder and urethra during voiding; the protective mucin layer that lines the bladder and protects against bacterial invasion; and local immune responses. In the ureters, peristaltic movements facilitate the movement of urine from the renal pelvis through the ureters and into the bladder. Immune mechanisms, particularly secretory immunoglobulin A (IgA), appear to provide an important antibacterial defense. Phagocytic blood cells further assist in the removal of bacteria from the urinary tract.

There has been a growing appreciation of the protective function of the bladder's mucin layer.[22] It is thought that the epithelial cells that line the bladder synthesize protective substances that subsequently become incorporated into the mucin layer that adheres to the bladder wall. One theory proposes that the mucin layer acts by binding water, which then constitutes a protective barrier between the bacteria and the bladder epithelium. Elderly and postmenopausal women produce less mucin than younger women, suggesting that estrogen may play a role in mucin production in women.

Other important host factors include the normal flora of the periurethral area in women and prostate secretions in men. In women, the normal flora of the periurethral area, which consists of organisms such as lactobacillus, provides defense against the colonization of uropathic bacteria. Alterations in the periurethral environment, such as occurs with a decrease in estrogen levels during menopause or the use of antibiotics, can alter the protective periurethral flora, allowing uropathogens to colonize and enter the urinary tract. In men, the prostatic fluid has antimicrobial properties that protect the urethra from colonization.

Pathogen Virulence. Not all bacteria are capable of infecting the urinary tract. Of the many strains of *E. coli* and other uropathogens, only those with adherence properties are able to infect the urinary tract. These bacteria have fine protein filaments that help them adhere to receptors on the lining of urinary tract structures.[22] These filaments are called *pili* or *fimbriae.* Among the factors that contribute to bacterial virulence, the type of *pili* that the bacteria possess may be the most important. Bacteria with certain types of *pili* are associated primarily with cystitis, and those with other types are associated with a high incidence of pyelonephritis. The bacteria associated with pyelonephritis are thought to have *pili* that bind to carbohydrates that are specific to the surfaces of epithelial cells in this part of the urinary tract.

Obstruction and Reflux

Obstruction and reflux are important contributing factors in the development of UTIs. Any microorganisms that enter the bladder normally are washed out during voiding. When outflow is obstructed, urine remains in the bladder and acts as a medium for microbial growth; the microorganisms in the contaminated urine can then ascend along the ureters to infect the kidneys. The presence of residual urine correlates closely with bacteriuria and with its recurrence after treatment. Another aspect of bladder outflow obstruction and bladder distention is increased intravesicular pressure, which compresses blood vessels in the bladder wall, leading to a decrease in the mucosal defenses of the bladder.

In UTIs associated with stasis of urine flow, the obstruction may be anatomic or functional. Anatomic obstructions include urinary tract stones, prostatic hyperplasia, pregnancy, and malformations of the ureterovesical junction. Functional obstructions include neurogenic bladder, infrequent voiding, detrusor (bladder) muscle instability, and constipation.

Reflux occurs when urine from the urethra moves into the bladder (*i.e.*, urethrovesical reflux) or from the bladder into the ureters (*i.e.*, vesicoureteral reflux). In women, *urethrovesical reflux* can occur during activities such as coughing or squatting, in which an increase in intra-abdominal pressure causes the urine to be squeezed into the urethra and then to flow back into the bladder as the pressure decreases. This also can happen when voiding is abruptly interrupted. Because the urethral orifice frequently is contaminated with bacteria, the reflux mechanism may cause bacteria to be drawn back into the bladder.

A second type of reflux mechanism, *vesicoureteral reflux*, occurs at the level of the bladder and ureter. Normally, the distal portion of the ureter courses between the muscle layer and the mucosal surface of the bladder wall, forming a flap. The flap is compressed against the bladder wall during micturition, preventing urine from being forced into the ureter (Fig. 35-7). In persons with vesicoureteral reflux, the ureter enters the bladder at an approximate right angle such that urine is forced into the ureter during micturition. It is seen most commonly in children with UTIs and is believed to result from congenital defects in length, diameter, muscle structure, or innervation of the submucosal segment of the ureter. Vesicoureteral reflux also is seen in adults with obstruction to bladder outflow, primarily due to increased bladder volume and pressure.

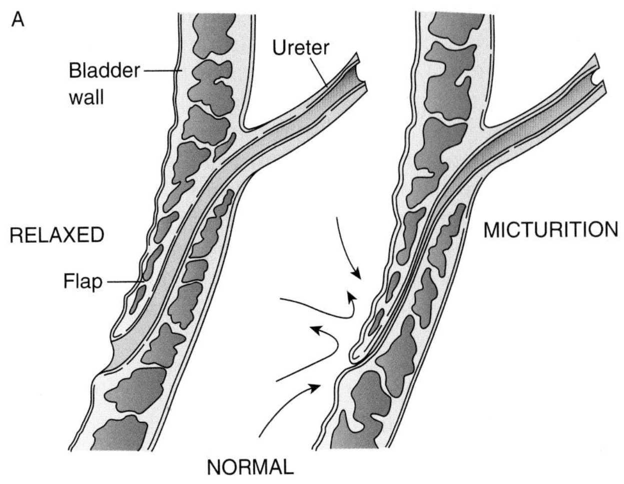

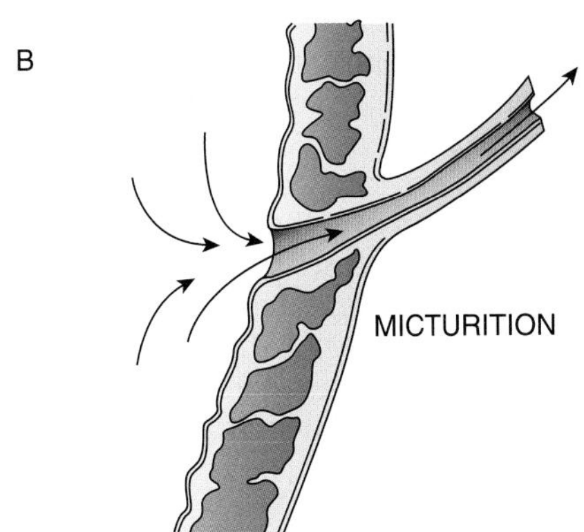

FIGURE 35-7 Anatomic features of the bladder and kidney in pyelonephritis caused by vesicoureteral reflux. Bladder. (**A**) In the normal bladder, the distal portion of the intravesical ureter courses between the mucosa and the muscularis of the bladder. A mucosal flap is thus formed. On micturition, the elevated intravesicular pressure compresses the flap against the bladder wall, thereby occluding the lumen. (**B**) Persons with a congenitally short intravesical ureter have no mucosal flap, because the entry of the ureter into the bladder approaches a right angle. Thus, micturition forces urine into the ureter. (Rubin E., Farber J.L. [1999]. *Pathology* [3rd ed., p. 903]. Philadelphia: Lippincott-Raven) (Courtesy of Dmitri Karetnikov, artist)

Catheter-Induced Infection

Urinary catheters are tubes made of latex or plastic. They are inserted through the urethra into the bladder for the purpose of draining urine. They are a source of urethral irritation and provide a means for entry of microorganisms into the urinary tract.

Catheter-associated bacteriuria remains the most frequent cause of gram-negative septicemia in hospitalized patients. Studies have shown that bacteria adhere to the surface of the catheter and initiate the growth of a biofilm that then covers the surface of the catheter.[24] The biofilm tends to protect the bacteria from the action of antibiotics and makes treatment difficult. A closed drainage system (*i.e.*, closed to air and other sources of contamination) and careful attention to perineal hygiene (*i.e.*, cleaning the area around the urethral meatus) help to prevent infections in persons who require an indwelling catheter. Careful hand washing and early detection and treatment of UTIs also are essential.

MANIFESTATIONS

The manifestations of UTI depend on whether the infection involves the lower (bladder) or upper (kidney) urinary tract and whether the infection is acute or chronic. Most UTIs are acute uncomplicated bladder infections that occur in women. Upper UTIs are less common and occur more frequently in children and adults with urinary tract obstructions or other predisposing conditions such as diabetes.

An acute episode of cystitis (bladder infection) is characterized by frequency of urination (sometimes as often as every 20 minutes), lower abdominal or back discomfort, and burning and pain on urination (*i.e.,* dysuria). Occasionally, the urine is cloudy and foul smelling. In adults, fever and other signs of infection usually are absent. If there are no complications, the symptoms disappear within 48 hours of treatment. The symptoms of cystitis also may represent urethritis caused by *Chlamydia trachomatis, Neisseria gonorrhoeae,* or herpes simplex virus, or vaginitis attributable to *Trichomonas vaginalis* or *Candida* species (see Chapter 48).

Upper UTIs affect the parenchyma and pelvis of the kidney (pyelonephritis). They tend to produce more systemic signs of infection than lower UTIs because of closer proximity to the vascular compartment and blood cells (*e.g.,* neutrophils) that incite the inflammatory response. Acute pyelonephritis tends to present with an abrupt onset of shaking chills, moderate to high fever, and constant ache in the loin area of the back that is unilateral or bilateral.[22] Lower urinary tract symptoms, including dysuria, frequency, and urgency, also are common. There may be significant malaise, and the person usually looks and feels ill. Nausea and vomiting may occur along with abdominal pain. Palpation or percussion over the costovertebral angle on the affected side usually causes pain. Chronic pyelonephritis, which results from repeated kidney infections that cause scarring and atrophy of the kidney, often is asymptomatic, and the condition is detected during evaluation for complications associated with renal insufficiency, such as hypertension.

DIAGNOSIS AND TREATMENT

Diagnosis

The diagnosis of UTI usually is based on symptoms and on examination of the urine for the presence of microorganisms. When necessary, x-ray films, ultrasonography, and CT and renal scans are used to identify contributing factors, such as obstruction.

Microscopic urine tests are used to establish the presence of bacteria and blood cells in the urine.[22] A commonly accepted criterion for diagnosis of a UTI is the presence of 10^5 or more bacteria per milliliter of urine.[22] Colonization usually is defined as the multiplication of microorganisms in or on a host without apparent evidence of invasiveness or tissue injury. Pyuria (the presence of less than five to eight leukocytes per high-power field) indicates a host response to infection rather than asymptomatic bacterial colonization. A Gram stain may be done to determine the type of organism that is present (gram positive or gram negative).

Chemical screening (urine dipstick) for markers of infection may provide useful information but is less sensitive than microscopic analysis. Bacteria reduce nitrates in the urine to nitrites, providing a means for chemical analysis. Similarly, activated leukocytes secrete leukocyte esterase, which can be detected chemically. These two chemical tests have sensitivities ranging from 80% and rarely are positive in the absence of infection.[11] Therefore, they are commonly used as a screening tool in persons with symptoms of UTI. The tests are relatively inexpensive, easy to perform, and can be done in the clinic setting or even in the home. A urine culture confirms the presence of pathogenic bacteria in urine specimens, allows for their identification, and permits the determination of their sensitivity to specific antibiotics.

Treatment

The treatment of UTI is based on the type of infection that is present (lower or upper UTI), the pathogen causing the infection, and the presence of contributing host–agent factors. Other considerations include whether the infection is acute, recurrent, or chronic.

Acute Urinary Tract Infections. Most acute lower UTIs, which occur mainly in women and are generally caused by *E. coli,* are treated successfully with a short course of antimicrobial therapy. Forcing fluids may relieve signs and symptoms, and this approach is used as an adjunct to antimicrobial treatment. For several decades, first-line therapy for acute uncomplicated UTI has been a 3-day regimen of trimethoprim-sulfamethoxazole (TMP-SMX).[25] However, there is increasing resistance among commonly acquired *E. coli* infections to TMP-SMX in many parts of the United States, varying from 22% to 39% depending on geographic location.[26] The resistance of *E. coli* to TMP-SMX is often accompanied by resistance to other antimicrobial drugs, including ampicillin, cephalothin, and tetracycline. Thus, selection of a therapeutic agent must now take into account the geographic location and susceptibility of the bacteria to the different antimicrobial agents.

Because there is risk for permanent kidney damage with pyelonephritis, these infections are treated more aggressively. Treatment with an appropriate antimicrobial agent usually is continued for 10 to 14 days. Hospitalization may be recommended during the early stages of infection until a response to treatment is observed.[27]

Recurrent Urinary Tract Infections. Recurrent lower UTIs are those that recur after treatment. They are due either to bacterial persistence or reinfection. Bacterial persistence usually is curable by removal of the infectious source (*e.g.,* urinary catheter or infected bladder stones). Reinfection is managed principally through education regarding pathogen transmission and prevention measures. Cranberry juice or blueberry juice has been suggested as a preventive measure for persons with frequent UTIs. Studies suggest that these juices reduce bacterial adherence to the epithelial lining of the urinary tract.[28,29] Because of their mechanism of action, these juices are used more appropriately in prevention rather than treatment of an established UTI.

Chronic Urinary Tract Infections. Chronic UTIs are more difficult to treat. Because they often are associated with obstructive uropathy or reflux flow of urine, diagnostic tests usually are performed to detect such abnormalities. When possible, the condition causing the reflux flow or obstruction is corrected. Most persons with recurrent UTIs are treated with antimicrobial agents for 10 to 14 days in doses sufficient to maintain high urine levels of the drug, and they are examined for obstruction or other causes of infection. Men in particular should be investigated for obstructive disorders or a prostatic focus of infection.

INFECTIONS IN SPECIAL POPULATIONS

Urinary tract infections affect persons of all ages. In infants, they occur more often in boys than in girls. After the first year of life, however, UTIs are more frequent in females because of the shorter length of the urethra and because the vaginal vestibule can be easily contaminated with fecal flora. Approximately half of all adult women have at least one UTI during their lifetime.[30] In men, the longer length of the urethra and the antibacterial properties of the prostatic fluid provide some protection from ascending UTIs until approximately 50 years of age. After this age, prostatic hypertrophy becomes more common, and with it may come obstruction and increased risk for UTI (see Chapter 45).

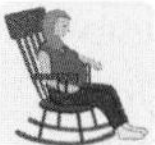

Urinary Tract Infections in Women

In women, the urethra is short and close to the vagina and rectum, offering little protection against entry of microorganisms into the bladder. There is a peak incidence of these infections in the 15- to 24-year-old age group, suggesting that hormonal and anatomic changes associated with puberty and sexual activity contribute to UTIs.

The role of sexual activity in the development of urethritis and cystitis is controversial. The well-documented "honeymoon cystitis" suggests that sexual activity may contribute to such infections in susceptible women. The anterior urethra usually is colonized with bacteria; urethral massage or sexual intercourse can force these bacteria back into the bladder. Using a diaphragm and spermicide enhances the susceptibility to infection.[30,31] A nonpharmacologic approach to the treatment of frequent UTIs associated with sexual intercourse is to increase fluid intake before intercourse and to void soon after intercourse. This procedure uses the washout phenomenon to remove bacteria from the bladder.

Pregnant women are at increased risk for UTIs. Normal changes in the functioning of the urinary tract that occur during pregnancy predispose to UTIs.[32] These changes involve the collecting system of the kidneys and include dilatation of the renal calices, pelves, and ureters that begins during the first trimester and becomes most pronounced during the third trimester. This dilatation of the upper urinary system is accompanied by a reduction in the peristaltic activity of the ureters that is thought to result from the muscle-relaxing effects of progesterone-like hormones and mechanical obstruction from the enlarging uterus. In addition to the changes in the kidneys and ureters, the bladder becomes displaced from its pelvic position to a more abdominal position, producing further changes in ureteral position.

Asymptomatic UTIs are common, with a prevalence rate of 10% in pregnant women. The complications of asymptomatic UTIs during pregnancy include persistent bacteriuria, acute and chronic pyelonephritis, toxemia of pregnancy, and premature delivery. Evidence suggests that few women become bacteriuric during pregnancy. Rather, it appears that symptomatic UTIs during pregnancy reflect preexisting asymptomatic bacteriuria and that changes occurring during pregnancy simply permit the prior urinary colonization to lead to symptomatic infection and invasion of the kidneys.[33] Untreated asymptomatic bacteriuria leads to symptomatic cystitis in approximately 30% of pregnant women.[33] Because bacteriuria may occur as an asymptomatic condition in pregnant women, the American College of Obstetrics and Gynecology recommends that a urine culture be obtained at the first prenatal visit.[34] A repeat culture should be obtained during the third trimester. Women with bacteriuria should be followed closely, and infections should be properly treated to prevent complications. The choice of antimicrobial agent should address the common infecting organisms and should be safe for the mother and fetus.

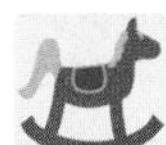

Urinary Tract Infections in Children

Urinary tract infections occur in as many as 3% to 5% of female and 1% of male children.[4,35] In girls, the average age at first diagnosis is 5 years or younger, with peaks during infancy and toilet training. In boys, most UTIs occur during the first year of life; they are more common in uncircumcised than in circumcised boys. Children who are at increased risk for bacteriuria or symptomatic UTIs are premature infants discharged from neonatal intensive care units; children with systemic or immunologic disease or urinary tract abnormalities such as neurogenic bladder or vesicoureteral reflux; those with a family history of UTI or urinary tract anomalies with reflux; and girls younger than 5 years of age with a history of UTI.[4,35]

UTIs in children frequently involve the upper urinary tract (pyelonephritis). In children in whom renal development is not complete, pyelonephritis can lead to renal scarring and permanent kidney damage. It has been reported that more than 75% of children younger than 5 years of age with febrile UTIs have pyelonephritis, and that renal scarring occurs in 27% to 64% of children with pyelonephritis.[36] Most UTIs that lead to scarring and diminished kidney growth occur in children younger than 4 years, especially infants younger than 1 year of age. The incidence of scarring is greatest in children with gross vesicoureteral reflux or obstruction, in children with recurrent UTIs, and in those with a delay in treatment.

Unlike adults, children frequently do not present with the typical signs of a UTI.[36,37] Many neonates with UTIs have bacteremia and may show signs and symptoms of septicemia, including fever, hypothermia, apneic spells, poor skin perfusion, abdominal distention, diarrhea, vomiting, lethargy, and irritability. Older infants may present with feeding problems, failure to thrive, diarrhea, vomiting, fever, and foul-smelling urine. Toddlers often present with abdominal pain, vomiting, diarrhea, abnormal voiding patterns, foul-smelling urine, fever, and poor growth. In older children with lower UTIs, the classic features—enuresis, frequency, dysuria, and suprapubic discomfort—are more common. Fever is a common sign of UTI in children, and the possibility of UTI should be considered in children with unexplained fever.

Diagnosis is based on a careful history of voiding patterns and symptomatology; physical examination to determine fever, hypertension, abdominal or suprapubic tenderness, and other manifestations of UTI; and urinalysis to determine bacteriuria, pyuria, proteinuria, and hematuria. A positive urine culture that is obtained correctly is essential for the diagnosis. Additional diagnostic methods may be needed to determine the cause of the disorder. Vesicoureteral reflux is the most commonly associated abnormality in UTIs, and reflux nephropathy is an important cause of end-stage renal disease in children and adolescents. Children with a relatively uncomplicated first UTI may turn out to have significant reflux. Therefore, even a single documented UTI in a child requires careful diagnosis. Urinary symptoms in the absence of bacteriuria suggest vaginitis, urethritis, sexual molestation, the use of irritating bubble baths, pinworms, or viral cystitis. In adolescent girls, a history of dysuria and vaginal discharge makes vaginitis or vulvitis a consideration.

The approach to treatment is based on the clinical severity of the infection, the site of infection (*i.e.*, lower versus upper urinary tract), the risk for sepsis, and the presence of structural abnormalities. The immediate treatment of infants and young children is essential. Most infants with symptomatic UTIs and many children with clinical evidence of acute upper UTIs require hospitalization and intravenous antibiotic therapy. Follow-up is essential for children with febrile UTIs to ensure resolution of the infection. Follow-up urine cultures often are done at the end of treatment. Imaging studies often are recommended for all children after first UTIs to detect renal scarring, vesicoureteral reflux, or other abnormalities.[36,38]

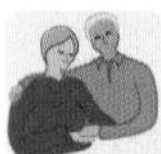

Urinary Tract Infections in the Elderly

Urinary tract infections are relatively common in elderly persons.[35] They are the second most common form of infection, after respiratory tract infections, among otherwise healthy community-dwelling elderly. It is particularly prevalent in elderly living in nursing homes or extended-care facilities.

Most of these infections follow invasion of the urinary tract by the ascending route. Several factors predispose elderly persons to UTIs: immobility resulting in poor bladder emptying, bladder outflow obstruction caused by prostatic hyperplasia or kidney stones, bladder ischemia caused by urine retention, senile vaginitis, constipation, and diminished bactericidal activity of urine and prostatic secretions. Added to these risks are other health problems that necessitate instrumentation of the urinary tract. UTIs develop in 1% of ambulatory patients after a single catheterization and within 3 to 4 days in essentially all patients with indwelling catheters.[39]

Elderly persons with bacteriuria have varying symptoms, ranging from the absence of symptoms to the presence of typical UTI symptoms. Even when symptoms of lower UTIs are present, they may be difficult to interpret because elderly persons without UTIs commonly experience urgency, frequency, and incontinence. Alternatively, elderly persons may have vague symptoms such as anorexia, fatigue, weakness, or change in mental status. Even with more serious upper UTIs (*e.g.*, pyelonephritis), the classic signs of infection such as fever, chills, flank pain, and tenderness may be altered or absent in elderly persons.[35] Sometimes, no symptoms occur until the infection is far advanced.

In summary, UTI is the second most common type of bacterial infection seen by health care professionals. Infections can range from simple bacteriuria to severe kidney infections that cause irreversible kidney damage. Predisposition to infection is determined by host defenses and pathogen virulence. Host defenses include the washout phenomenon associated with voiding, the protective mucin lining of the bladder, and the local immune defenses. Pathogen virulence is enhanced by the presence of pili that facilitate adherence to structures in the urinary tract.

Most UTIs ascend from the urethra and bladder. A number of factors interact in determining the predisposition to development of UTIs, including urinary tract obstruction, urine stasis and reflux, pregnancy-induced changes in urinary tract function, age-related changes in the urinary tract, changes in the protective mechanisms of the bladder and ureters, impaired immune function, and virulence of the pathogen. Urinary tract catheters and urinary instrumentation contribute to the incidence of UTIs. Early diagnosis and treatment of UTI are essential to preventing permanent kidney damage.

Disorders of Glomerular Function

After completing this section of the chapter, you should be able to meet the following objectives:

- ✦ Describe the two types of immune mechanisms involved in glomerular disorders
- ✦ Use the terms *proliferation, sclerosis, membranous, diffuse, focal, segmental,* and *mesangial* to explain changes in glomerular structure that occur with glomerulonephritis
- ✦ Relate the proteinuria, hematuria, pyuria, oliguria, edema, hypertension, and azotemia that occur with glomerulonephritis to changes in glomerular structure
- ✦ Differentiate the pathology and manifestations of the nephrotic syndrome from those of the nephritic syndrome

The glomeruli are tufts of capillaries that lie between the afferent and efferent arterioles. The capillaries of the glomeruli are arranged in lobules and supported by a stalk consisting of mesangial cells and a basement membrane–like extracellular matrix (Fig. 35-8). The glomerular capillary membrane is composed of three structural layers that constitute its permeability characteristics: an endothelial cell layer lining the capillary, a basement membrane made up of a network of matrix proteins, and a layer of epithelial cells forming the outer surface of the capillary and lining

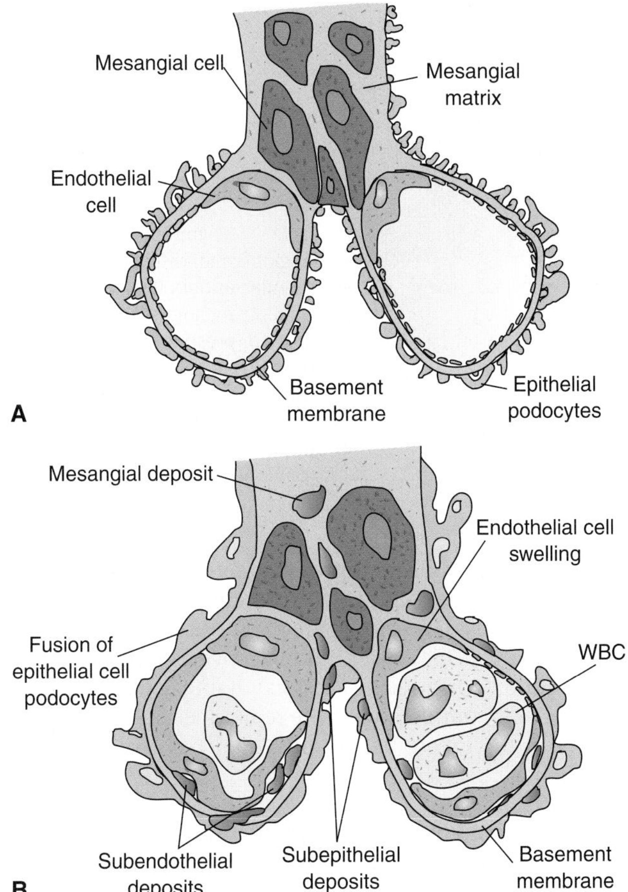

FIGURE 35-8 Schematic representation of glomerulus. (**A**) Normal; (**B**) localization of immune deposits (mesangial, subendothelial, subepithelial) and changes in glomerular architecture associated with injury. (Whitley K., Keane W.F., & Vernier R.L. [1984]. Acute glomerulonephritis: A clinical overview. *Medical Clinics of North America 68* [2], 263)

Bowman's capsule (see Chapter 32, Fig. 32-5). The epithelial cells are attached to the basement membrane by discrete cytoplasmic extensions, the foot processes (*i.e.*, podocytes). In the glomeruli, blood is filtered, and the urine filtrate formed. The capillary membrane is selectively permeable: it allows water, electrolytes, and dissolved particles, such as glucose and amino acids, to leave the capillary and enter Bowman's space and prevents larger particles, such as plasma proteins and blood cells, from leaving the blood.

MECHANISMS OF GLOMERULAR INJURY

Glomerulonephritis, an inflammatory process that involves glomerular structures, is the leading cause of chronic renal failure in the United States, accounting for one half of persons with end-stage renal disease.[40] There are many causes of glomerular disease. The disease may occur as a primary condition in which the glomerular abnormality is the only disease present, or it may occur as a secondary condition in which the glomerular abnormality results from another disease, such as diabetes mellitus or SLE. An understanding of the various forms of glomerular disease has emerged only recently. Much of this knowledge can be attributed to advances in immunobiology and electron microscopy, development of animal models, and increased use of renal biopsy during the early stages of glomerular disease.

Glomerulonephritis is characterized by hematuria with red cell casts, a diminished glomerular filtration rate (GFR), azotemia (presence of nitrogenous wastes in the blood), oliguria, and hypertension. It is caused by diseases that provoke a proliferative inflammatory response of the endothelial, mesangial, or epithelial cells of the glomeruli. The inflammatory process damages the capillary wall, permitting red blood cells to escape into the urine and producing hemodynamic changes that decrease the GFR.

Although little is known about the causative agents or triggering events that produce glomerular disease, most cases of primary and many cases of secondary glomerular disease probably have an immune origin.[5,6,40–42] Two types of immune mechanisms have been implicated in the development of glomerular disease: injury resulting from antibodies reacting with fixed glomerular antigens, and injury resulting from circulating antigen–antibody complexes that become trapped in the glomerular membrane (Fig. 35-9). Antigens responsible for development of the immune response may be of endogenous origin, such as auto-antibodies to DNA in SLE, or they may be of exogenous origin, such as streptococcal membrane antigens in poststreptococcal glomerulonephritis. Frequently, the source of the antigen is unknown.

SPECIFIC TYPES OF GLOMERULAR DISEASE

The cellular changes that occur with glomerular disease include proliferative, sclerotic, and membranous changes. The term *proliferative* refers to an increase in the cellular components of the glomerulus, regardless of origin; *sclerotic* to an increase in the noncellular components of the glomerulus, primarily collagen; and *membranous* to an increase in the thickness of the glomerular capillary wall, often caused by immune complex deposition. Glomerular changes can be *diffuse,* involving all glomeruli and all parts of the glomeruli; *focal,* in which only some glomeruli are affected and others are essentially normal; *segmental,* involving only a certain segment of each glomeruli; or *mesangial,* affecting only the mesangial cell. Figure 35-8 shows changes associated with various types of glomerular disease.

Among the different types of glomerular diseases are acute proliferative glomerulonephritis, rapidly progressive glomerulonephritis, nephrotic syndrome, membranous glomerulonephritis, minimal change disease (lipoid nephrosis), focal segmental glomerulosclerosis, IgA nephropathy, and chronic glomerulonephritis.

Acute Proliferative Glomerulonephritis

The most commonly recognized form of acute glomerulonephritis is diffuse proliferative glomerulonephritis, which follows infections caused by strains of group A β-hemolytic streptococci. Diffuse proliferative glomerulonephritis also may occur after infections by other organisms, including

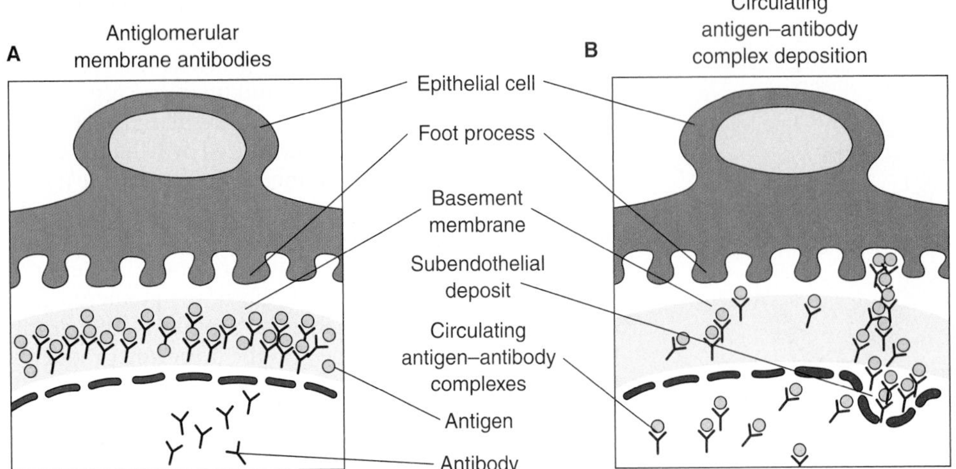

FIGURE 35-9 Immune mechanisms of glomerular disease. (**A**) Antiglomerular antibodies leave the circulation and interact with antigens that are present in the basement membrane of the glomerulus. (**B**) Antigen–antibody complexes circulating in the blood become trapped as they are filtered in the glomerulus.

staphylococci and a number of viral agents, such as those responsible for mumps, measles, and chickenpox. With this type of glomerulonephritis, the inflammatory response is caused by an immune reaction that occurs when circulating immune complexes become entrapped in the glomerular capillary membrane. Proliferation of the endothelial cells lining the glomerular capillary (*i.e.*, endocapillary form of the disease) and the mesangial cells lying between the endothelium and the epithelium follows (see Fig. 35-8). The capillary membrane swells and becomes permeable to plasma proteins and blood cells. Although the disease is seen primarily in children, adults of any age can be affected.

The classic case of poststreptococcal glomerulonephritis follows a streptococcal infection by approximately 7 to 12 days—the time needed for the development of antibodies.[40] Oliguria, which develops as the GFR decreases, is one of the first symptoms. Proteinuria and hematuria follow because of increased glomerular capillary wall permeability. The red blood cells are degraded by materials in the urine, and cola-colored urine may be the first sign of the disorder. Sodium and water retention gives rise to edema, particularly of the face and hands, and hypertension. Important laboratory findings include an elevated streptococcal exoenzyme (antistreptolysin O) titer, a decline in C3 complement (see Chapter 19), and cryoglobulins (*i.e.*, large immune complexes) in the serum.

Treatment of acute poststreptococcal glomerulonephritis is largely symptomatic. The acute symptoms usually begin to subside in approximately 10 days to 2 weeks, although in some children, the proteinuria may persist for several months. The immediate prognosis is favorable, and approximately 95% of children recover spontaneously.[5] The outlook for adults is less favorable; approximately 60% recover completely. In the remainder of cases, the lesions eventually resolve, but there may be permanent kidney damage.

GLOMERULAR DISORDERS

- Glomerular disorders affect the glomerular capillary structures that filter material from the blood.
- Nephritic syndromes are caused by diseases that produce proliferative inflammatory responses that decrease the permeability of the glomerular capillary membrane.
- The nephrotic syndrome is caused by disorders that increase the permeability of the glomerular capillary membrane, causing massive loss of protein in the urine.

Rapidly Progressive Glomerulonephritis

Rapidly progressive glomerulonephritis is a clinical syndrome characterized by signs of severe glomerular injury that does not have a specific cause. As its name indicates, this type of glomerulonephritis is rapidly progressive, often within a matter of months. The disorder involves focal and segmental proliferation of glomerular cells and recruitment of monocytes (macrophages) with formation of crescent-shaped structures that obliterate Bowman's space.[5] Rapidly proliferative glomerulonephritis may be caused by a number of immunologic disorders, some systemic and others restricted to the kidney. Among the diseases associated with this form of glomerulonephritis are immune complex disorders such as SLE, the small vessel vasculitides (*e.g.*, microscopic polyangiitis), and an immune disorder condition called *Goodpasture's syndrome.*

Goodpasture's syndrome, which is caused by antibodies to the glomerular basement membrane (GBM), accounts for approximately 5% of cases of rapidly progressive glomerulonephritis. It is a rare disease and is associated with a triad of pulmonary hemorrhage, iron-deficiency anemia, and glomerulonephritis. All of these manifestations result from anti-GBM antibody deposition in the lungs and glomeruli. The cause of the disorder is unknown, although influenza infection and exposure to hydrocarbon solvent (found in paints and dyes) have been implicated in some persons, as have various drugs and cancers. There is a high prevalence of certain human leukocyte antigen subtypes (*e.g.*, HLA-DRB1), suggesting a genetic predisposition.[5] Treatment includes plasmapheresis to remove circulating anti-GBM antibodies and immunosuppressive therapy (*i.e.*, corticosteroids and cyclophosphamide) to inhibit antibody production.

Nephrotic Syndrome

Nephrotic syndrome is not a specific glomerular disease but a constellation of clinical findings that result from increased glomerular permeability to the plasma proteins (Fig. 35-10). The glomerular derangements that occur with nephrosis can develop as a primary disorder or secondary to changes caused by systemic diseases such as diabetes mellitus, amyloidosis, and SLE. Among the primary glomerular lesions leading to nephrotic syndrome are minimal change disease (lipoid nephrosis), focal segmental glomerulosclerosis, and membranous glomerulonephritis. The relative frequency of these causes varies with age. In children younger than 15 years of age, nephrotic syndrome almost always is caused by primary idiopathic glomerular disease, whereas in adults, it often is a secondary disorder.[5,43]

The nephrotic syndrome is characterized by massive proteinuria (>3.5 g/day) and lipiduria (*e.g.,* free fat, oval bodies, fatty casts), along with an associated hypoalbuminemia (<3 g/dL), generalized edema, and hyperlipidemia (cholesterol >300 mg/dL).[6,44–47] The initiating event in the development of nephrosis is a derangement in the glomerular membrane that causes increased permeability to plasma proteins. The glomerular membrane acts as a size and charge barrier through which the glomerular filtrate must pass. Any increased permeability allows protein to escape from the plasma into the glomerular filtrate.

Generalized edema, which is a hallmark of nephrosis, results from salt and water retention and a loss of serum albumin below that needed to maintain the colloid osmotic pressure of the vascular compartment.[5] The sodium and water retention appears to be due to several factors, including a compensatory increase in aldosterone, stimulation of the sympathetic nervous system, and a reduction in secretion of natriuretic factors. Initially, the edema presents in dependent parts of the body such as the lower extremities, but becomes more generalized as the disease progresses. Dyspnea due to pulmonary edema, pleural effusions, and diaphragmatic compromise due to ascites can develop in persons with nephrotic syndrome.

Although the largest proportion of plasma protein loss is in albumin, globulins also are lost. As a result, persons with nephrosis are particularly vulnerable to infections, particularly those caused by staphylococci and pneumococci.[5] This decreased resistance to infection probably is related to loss of both immunoglobulins and low-molecular-weight complement components in the urine. Many binding proteins also are lost in the urine. Consequently, the plasma levels of many ions (iron, copper, zinc), hormones (thyroid and sex hormones), and drugs may be low because of decreased binding proteins. Many drugs require protein binding for transport. Hypoalbuminemia reduces the number of available protein-binding sites, thereby producing a potential increase in the amount of free (active) drug that is available.[44]

Thrombotic complications also have evolved as a risk in persons with nephrotic syndrome.[43] These disorders reflect a disruption in the function of the coagulation system brought about by a loss of coagulation and anticoagulation factors. Renal vein thrombosis, once thought to be a cause of the disorder, is more likely a consequence of the hypercoagulable state.[5] Other thrombotic complications include deep vein thrombosis and pulmonary emboli.

The hyperlipidemia that occurs in persons with nephrosis is characterized by elevated levels of triglycerides and low-density lipoproteins (LDLs). Levels of high-density lipoproteins (HDLs) usually are normal. It is thought that these abnormalities are related, at least in part, to increased synthesis of lipoproteins in the liver secondary to a compensatory increase in albumin production.[43] Because of the elevated LDL levels, persons with nephrotic syndrome are at increased risk for development of atherosclerosis.

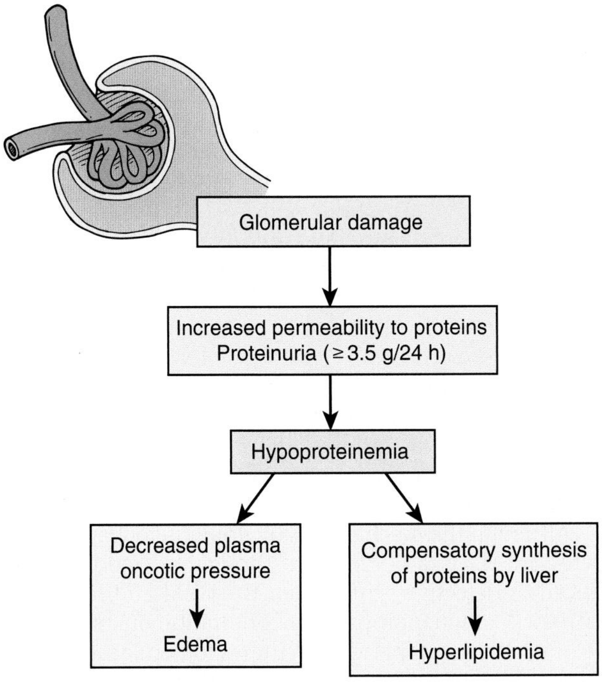

FIGURE 35-10 Pathophysiology of the nephrotic syndrome.

Membranous Glomerulonephritis. Membranous glomerulonephritis is the most common cause of primary nephrosis in adults, most commonly in their sixth or seventh decade. The disorder is caused by diffuse thickening of the GBM due to deposition of immune complexes. The disorder may be idiopathic or associated with a number of disorders, including autoimmune diseases such as SLE, infections such as chronic hepatitis B, metabolic disorders such as diabetes mellitus and thyroiditis, and use of certain drugs such as gold compounds, penicillamine, and captopril.[5] Because of the presence of immunoglobulins and complement in the subendothelial deposits, it is thought that the disease represents a chronic antigen–antibody complex–mediated disorder.

The disorder is treated with corticosteroids. Cytotoxic drugs may be added to the treatment regimen. The progress of the disease is variable; approximately one half of persons sustain a slow but progressive loss of renal function.

Minimal Change Disease (Lipoid Nephrosis). Minimal change disease is characterized by diffuse loss (through fusion) of the foot processes from the epithelial layer of the glomerular membrane. The peak incidence is between 2 and 6 years of age. The cause of minimal change nephrosis is unknown; however, children in whom the disease develops often have a history of recent upper respiratory infections or of receiving routine immunizations.[5] Although minimal change disease does not progress to renal failure, it can cause significant complications, including predisposition to infection with gram-positive organisms, a tendency toward thromboembolic events, hyperlipidemia, and protein malnutrition. There usually is a dramatic response to corticosteroid therapy.[5,43]

Focal Segmental Glomerulosclerosis. Focal segmental glomerulosclerosis is characterized by sclerosis (*i.e.*, increased collagen deposition) of some but not all glomeruli, and in the affected glomeruli, only a portion of the glomerular tuft is involved.[48] Although focal segmental sclerosis often is an idiopathic syndrome, it may be associated with reduced oxygen in the blood (*e.g.*, sickle cell disease and cyanotic congenital heart disease), human immunodeficiency virus (HIV) infection, or intravenous drug abuse, or it may be a secondary event reflecting glomerular scarring due to other forms of glomerulonephritis or reflux nephropathy.[5,6] The presence of hypertension and decreased renal function distinguishes focal sclerosis from minimal change disease. The disorder usually is treated with corticosteroids. Most persons with the disorder progress to end-stage renal disease within 5 to 10 years.

Immunoglobulin A Nephropathy

Immunoglobulin A nephropathy (*i.e.*, Buerger's disease) is a primary glomerulonephritis characterized by the presence of glomerular IgA immune complex deposits. It can occur at any age, but most commonly occurs with clinical onset in the second and third decades of life.[49] The disease occurs more commonly in males than females and is the most common cause of glomerular nephritis in Asians.

The disorder is characterized by the deposition of IgA-containing immune complexes in the mesangium of the glomerulus. Once deposited in the kidney, the immune complexes are associated with glomerular inflammation. The cause of the disorder is unknown. Some persons with the disorder have elevated serum IgA levels. Recent studies have focused on potential abnormalities of the IgA molecule as a factor in the pathogenesis of the disorder.[49]

Early in the disease, many persons with the disorder have no obvious symptoms and are unaware of the problem. In these persons, IgA nephropathy is suspected during routine screening or examination for another condition. In other persons, the disorder presents with gross hematuria that is preceded by upper respiratory tract infection, gastrointestinal tract symptoms, or a flulike illness. The hematuria usually lasts 2 to 6 days. Approximately one half of the persons with gross hematuria have a single episode; the remainder have gradual progression of glomerular disease with recurrent episodes of hematuria and mild proteinuria. Progression usually is slow, extending over several decades.

There is no satisfactory treatment for IgA nephropathy. The role of immunosuppressive drugs such as steroids and cytotoxic drugs is not clear. There has been recent interest in the use of omega-3 fatty acids (fish oil) in delaying the progression of the disease. Evidence suggests that the daily use of fish oil in the diet may retard the progress of the disease, particularly in persons with mildly impaired renal function.[49]

CHRONIC GLOMERULONEPHRITIS

Chronic glomerulonephritis represents the chronic phase of a number of specific types of glomerulonephritis.[5] Some forms of glomerulonephritis (*e.g.*, poststreptococcal glomerulonephritis) undergo complete resolution, whereas others progress at variable rates to chronic glomerulonephritis. Some persons who present with chronic glomerulonephritis have no history of glomerular disease. These cases may represent the end result of relatively asymptomatic forms of glomerulonephritis. Histologically, the condition is characterized by small kidneys with sclerosed glomeruli. In most cases, chronic glomerulonephritis develops insidiously and slowly progresses to end-stage renal disease over a period of years (see Chapter 36).

GLOMERULAR LESIONS ASSOCIATED WITH SYSTEMIC DISEASE

Many immunologic, metabolic, or hereditary systemic diseases are associated with glomerular injury. In some diseases, such as SLE and diabetes mellitus, the glomerular involvement may be a major clinical manifestation. The glomerular lesions associated with diabetes mellitus and hypertension are discussed in this chapter.

Diabetic Glomerulosclerosis

Diabetic nephropathy, or kidney disease, is a major complication of diabetes mellitus. It affects approximately 30% of persons with type 1 diabetes and accounts for 20% of deaths in diabetic patients younger than 40 years of age.[5]

The glomerulus is the most commonly affected structure in diabetic nephropathy, evidenced by three glomerular syndromes: nonnephrotic proteinuria, nephrotic syndrome, and renal failure. Widespread thickening of the glomerular capillary basement membrane occurs in almost all persons with diabetes and can occur without evidence of proteinuria.[5] This is followed by a diffuse increase in mesangial matrix, with mild proliferation of mesangial cells. As the disease progresses, the mesangial cells impinge on the capillary lumen, drastically reducing the surface area for glomerular filtration. In nodular glomerulosclerosis, also known as *Kimmelstiel-Wilson syndrome,* there is nodular deposition of hyaline in the mesangial portion of the glomerulus. As the sclerotic process progresses in the diffuse and nodular forms of glomerulosclerosis, there is complete obliteration of the glomerulus, with impairment of renal function.

Although the mechanisms of glomerular change in diabetes are uncertain, they are thought to represent enhanced or defective synthesis of the GBM and mesangial matrix with an inappropriate incorporation of glucose into the noncellular components of these glomerular structures. Alternatively, hemodynamic changes that occur secondary to elevated blood glucose levels may contribute to the initiation and progression of diabetic glomerulosclerosis. It has been hypothesized that elevations in blood glucose produce an increase in GFR and glomerular intracapillary pressure that leads to an enlargement of glomerular capillary pores by a mechanism that is at least partly mediated by angiotensin II. This enlargement impairs the size-selective function of the membrane so that the protein content of the glomerular filtrate increases, which in turn requires increased endocytosis of protein by the tubular endothelial cells, a process that ultimately leads to nephron destruction and progressive deterioration of renal function.[50,51]

The clinical manifestations of diabetic glomerulosclerosis are closely linked to those of diabetes. The increased GFR that occurs in persons with early alterations in renal function is associated with *microalbuminuria,* defined as urinary albumin excretion greater than 30 mg/24 hours and no more than 300 mg/24 hours.[51,52] Microalbuminuria is an important predictor of future diabetic nephropathies.[5,51] In many cases, these early changes in glomerular function can be reversed by careful control of blood glucose levels[50,51] (see Chapter 43). Inhibition of angiotensin by angiotensin-converting enzyme inhibitors (*e.g.,* captopril) has been shown to have a beneficial effect, possibly by reversing increased glomerular pressure.[6,51] Hypertension and cigarette smoking have been implicated in the progression of diabetic nephropathy. Thus, control of high blood pressure and smoking cessation are recommended as primary and secondary prevention strategies in persons with diabetes.

Hypertensive Glomerular Disease

Hypertension can be viewed as both a cause and an effect of kidney disease. Most persons with advanced kidney disease have hypertension, and many persons with long-standing hypertension eventually sustain changes in kidney function. Renal failure and azotemia occur in 1% to 5% of persons with long-standing hypertension (see Chapter 25). Hypertension is associated with a number of changes in glomerular structures, including sclerotic changes. As the glomerular vascular structures thicken and perfusion diminishes, the blood supply to the nephron decreases, causing the kidneys to lose some of their ability to concentrate the urine. This may be evidenced by nocturia. Blood urea nitrogen levels also may become elevated, particularly during periods of water deprivation. Proteinuria may occur as a result of changes in glomerular structure.

In summary, diseases of the glomerulus disrupt glomerular filtration and alter the permeability of glomerular capillary membrane to plasma proteins and blood cells. *Glomerulonephritis* is a term used to describe a group of diseases that result in inflammation and injury of the glomerulus. These diseases disrupt the capillary membrane and cause proteinuria, hematuria, pyuria, oliguria, edema, hypertension, and azotemia. Almost all types of glomerulonephritis are caused by immune mechanisms.

Glomerular diseases have been grouped into two categories: the nephritic and the nephrotic syndromes. The nephritic syndrome evokes an inflammatory response in the glomeruli and is characterized by hematuria with red cell casts in the urine, a diminished GFR, azotemia, oliguria, and hypertension. The nephrotic syndrome affects the integrity of the glomerular capillary membrane and is characterized by massive proteinuria, hypoalbuminemia, generalized edema, lipiduria, and hyperlipidemia. Both conditions can lead to progressive loss of glomerular function and eventual development of end-stage renal disease. Among the secondary causes of glomerular kidney disease are diabetes and hypertension. Kidney disease is a major complication of diabetes mellitus and is thought to be related to hemodynamic changes associated with defective synthesis of glomerular structures that occurs secondary to increased blood glucose levels. Hypertension is closely linked with kidney disease, and kidney disease can be a cause or effect of elevated blood pressure.

Tubulointerstitial Disorders

After completing this section of the chapter, you should be able to meet the following objectives:

- Cite a definition of tubulointerstitial kidney disease
- Differentiate between the defects in tubular function that occur in proximal and distal tubular acidosis
- Explain the pathogenesis of kidney damage in pyelonephritis
- Explain the vulnerability of the kidneys to injury caused by drugs and toxins

Several disorders affect renal tubular structures, including the proximal and distal tubules. Most of these disorders also affect the interstitial tissue that surrounds the tubules. These disorders, which sometimes are referred to as *tubulointerstitial disorders,* include acute tubular necrosis (see Chapter 36), renal tubular acidosis, pyelonephritis, and the effects of drugs and toxins.

Tubulointerstitial renal diseases may be divided into acute and chronic disorders. The acute disorders are characterized by their sudden onset and by signs and symptoms of interstitial edema; they include acute pyelonephritis and acute hypersensitivity reaction to drugs. The chronic disorders produce interstitial fibrosis, atrophy, and mononuclear infiltrates; most persons are asymptomatic until late in the course of the disease. In the early stages, tubulointerstitial diseases commonly are manifested by fluid and electrolyte imbalances that reflect subtle changes in tubular function. These manifestations can include inability to concentrate urine, as evidenced by polyuria and nocturia; interference with acidification of urine, resulting in metabolic acidosis; and diminished tubular reabsorption of sodium and other substances.[5]

RENAL TUBULAR ACIDOSIS

Renal tubular acidosis (RTA) refers to a group of tubular defects in reabsorption of bicarbonate ions (HCO_3^-) or excretion of hydrogen ions (H^+) that result in acidosis and its subsequent complications, including metabolic bone disease, kidney stones, and growth failure in children. There are two main types of RTA: proximal tubular disorders that affect bicarbonate reabsorption, and distal tubular defects that affect the secretion of fixed metabolic acids.[53,54] A third type of RTA results from aldosterone deficiency or resistance to its action that leads to impaired reabsorption of sodium ions (Na^+) with decreased elimination of H^+ and potassium ions (K^+) (see Chapter 34). Renal acidosis also occurs in renal failure (see Chapter 36).

Proximal Renal Tubular Acidosis. Proximal RTA involves a defect in proximal tubular reabsorption of HCO_3^-, the nephron site where 85% of filtered HCO_3^- is reabsorbed (see Chapter 32). With the onset of impaired tubular HCO_3^- absorption, there is a loss of HCO_3^- in the urine that reduces plasma HCO_3^- levels. The concomitant loss of Na^+ in the urine leads to contraction of the extracellular fluid volume with increased aldosterone secretion and a resultant decrease in serum K^+ levels (see Chapter 33). With proximal tubular defects in acid-base regulation, the distal tubular sites for secretion of the fixed acids into the urine continue to function, and the reabsorption of HCO_3^- eventually resumes, albeit at a lower level of serum HCO_3^-. Whenever serum levels rise above this decreased level, HCO_3^- is lost in the urine. Persons with proximal RTA generally have plasma HCO_3^- levels greater than 15 mEq/L and seldom develop severe acidosis.

Proximal RTA may occur as a hereditary or acquired disorder and may involve an isolated defect in HCO_3^- reabsorption or accompany other defects in proximal tubular function (Fanconi's syndrome). Isolated defects in HCO_3^- reabsorption are relatively rare. The term *Fanconi's syndrome* is used to describe a generalized proximal tubular dysfunction in which the RTA is accompanied by impaired reabsorption of glucose, amino acids, phosphate, and uric acid. Children with Fanconi's syndrome are likely to have growth retardation, rickets, osteomalacia, and abnormal vitamin D metabolism in addition to mild acidosis associated with proximal RTA.

Children and infants with proximal RTA require alkali therapy because of the high incidence of growth retardation due to acidemia. Potassium supplements are also needed because of increased loss of potassium that occurs with alkali therapy. Adults may also require alkali therapy. Vitamin D and phosphate are appropriate treatments for rickets and hypophosphatemia.

Distal Renal Tubular Acidosis. Distal RTA has its origin in the distal convoluted tubule and the collecting duct where about 15% of the filtered bicarbonate is reabsorbed. The clinical syndrome of distal RTA includes hypokalemia, hyperchloremic metabolic acidosis, inability to acidify the urine, nephrocalcinosis, and nephrolithiasis. Additional features include osteomalacia or rickets.

Distal tubular RTA results from distal tubular defect in H^+ secretion with failure to acidify the urine. Because the secretion of H^+ in the distal tubules is linked to sodium reabsorption, failure to secrete H^+ results in a net loss of sodium bicarbonate in the urine. This results in contraction of fluids in the extracellular fluid compartment, a compensatory increase in aldosterone levels, and development of hypokalemia. The persistent acidosis, which requires buffering by the skeletal system, causes calcium to be released from bone. Increased losses of calcium in the urine lead to increased levels of parathyroid hormone, osteomalacia, bone pain, impaired growth in children, and development of kidney stones and nephrocalcinosis.

Long-term treatment of distal RTA requires alkali supplementation. Greater amounts are needed for children because of the need for base deposition in growing bone and because bicarbonate wastage is greater in children than in adults. Alkali therapy will generally allow for correction of potassium wasting and hypokalemia. It also decreases the calcium concentration in the urine and increases citrate excretion, both of which serve to decrease the incidence of nephrocalcinosis and nephrolithiasis.[54]

PYELONEPHRITIS

Pyelonephritis refers to an inflammation of the kidney parenchyma and renal pelvis. There are two forms of pyelonephritis: acute and chronic.

Acute Pyelonephritis

Acute pyelonephritis represents a patchy interstitial infectious inflammatory process, with abscess formation and tubular necrosis. Gram-negative bacteria, including *E. coli* and *Proteus, Klebsiella, Enterobacter,* and *Pseudomonas* species, are the most common causative agents. Gram-positive bacteria are less commonly seen but include *Enterococcus faecalis* and *S. aureus.* The infection usually ascends from the lower urinary tract, with the exception of *S. aureus,* which is usually spread through the bloodstream. Factors that contribute to the development of acute pyelonephritis are catheterization and urinary instrumentation, vesicoureteral reflux, pregnancy, and neurogenic bladder. A second less frequent and more serious type of acute pyelonephritis, called *necrotizing pyelonephritis,* is characterized by necrosis of the renal papillae. It is particularly common in persons with diabetes and may also be a complication of acute pyelonephritis when there is significant urinary tract obstruction.

The onset of acute pyelonephritis typically is abrupt, with chills, fever, headache, back pain, tenderness over the costovertebral angle, and general malaise. It usually is accompanied by symptoms of bladder irritation, such as dysuria, frequency, and urgency. Pyuria occurs but is not diagnostic because it also occurs in lower UTIs. The development of necrotizing papillitis is associated with a much poorer prognosis. These persons have evidence of overwhelming sepsis with frequent development of renal failure.

Acute pyelonephritis is treated with appropriate antimicrobial drugs. Unless obstruction or other complications occur, the symptoms usually disappear within several days. Hospitalization during initial treatment may be necessary. Depending on the cause, recurrent infections are possible.

Chronic Pyelonephritis

Chronic pyelonephritis represents a progressive process. There is scarring and deformation of the renal calices and pelvis[5] (Fig. 35-11). The disorder appears to involve a bacterial infection superimposed on obstructive abnormalities or vesicoureteral reflux. Chronic obstructive pyelonephritis is associated with recurrent bouts of inflammation and scarring, which eventually lead to chronic pyelonephritis. Reflux, which is the most common cause of chronic pyelonephritis, results from superimposition of infection on congenital vesicoureteral reflux or intrarenal reflux. Reflux may be unilateral with involvement of a single kidney or bilateral leading to scarring and atrophy of both kidneys with the eventual development of chronic renal insufficiency.

Chronic pyelonephritis may cause many of the same symptoms as acute pyelonephritis, or its onset may be insidious. Loss of tubular function and of the ability to concentrate urine give rise to polyuria and nocturia, and mild proteinuria is common. Severe hypertension often is a contributing factor in the progress of the disease. Chronic pyelonephritis is a significant cause of renal failure. It is thought to be responsible for 11% to 20% of all cases of end-stage renal disease.[5]

DRUG-RELATED NEPHROPATHIES

Drug-related nephropathies involve functional or structural changes in the kidneys that occur after exposure to a drug. The kidneys are exposed to a high rate of delivery of any substance in the blood because of their large blood flow and high filtration pressure. The kidneys also are active in the metabolic transformation of drugs and therefore are exposed to a number of toxic metabolites. The tolerance to drugs varies with age and depends on renal function, state of hydration, blood pressure, and the pH of the urine. Because of a decrease in physiologic function, elderly persons are particularly susceptible to kidney damage caused by drugs and toxins. The dangers of nephrotoxicity are increased when two or more drugs capable of producing kidney damage are given at the same time.

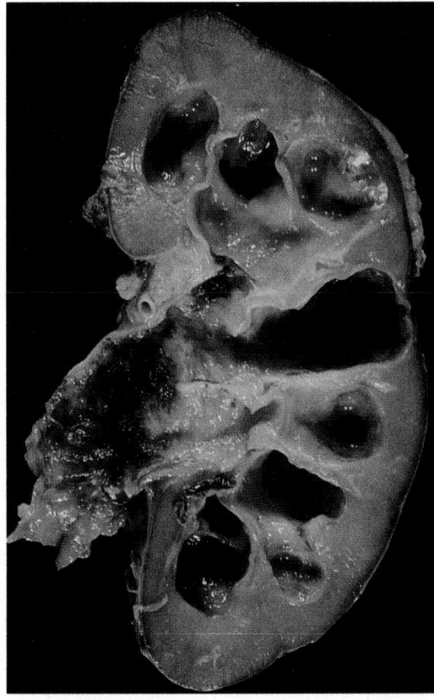

FIGURE 35-11 Chronic pyelonephritis. Marked dilatation of calices caused by inflammatory destruction of papillae, with atrophy and scarring of the overlying cortex. (Rubin E., Farber J.L. [1999]. *Pathology* [3rd ed., p. 905] Philadelphia: Lippincott-Raven)

Drugs and toxic substances can damage the kidneys by causing a decrease in renal blood flow; obstructing urine flow; directly damaging tubulointerstitial structures; or producing hypersensitivity reactions.[55]

Some drugs such as diuretics, high-molecular-weight radiocontrast media, the immunosuppressive drugs cyclosporine and tacrolimus, and the nonsteroidal antiinflammatory drugs can cause acute prerenal failure by decreasing renal blood flow (see Chapter 36). Persons at risk are those who already have compromised renal blood flow. Other drugs such as sulfonamides and vitamin C (due to oxalate crystals) can form crystals that cause kidney damage by obstructing urine flow within the tubules.

Acute drug-related hypersensitivity reactions produce tubulointerstitial nephritis, with damage to the tubules and interstitium. This condition was observed initially in persons who were sensitive to the sulfonamide drugs; currently, it is observed most often with the use of methicillin and other synthetic antibiotics, and with the use of furosemide and the thiazide diuretics in persons sensitive to these drugs. The condition begins approximately 15 days (range, 2 to 40 days) after exposure to the drug.[56] At the onset, there is fever, eosinophilia, hematuria, mild proteinuria, and in approximately one fourth of cases, a rash. In approximately 50% of cases, signs and symptoms of acute renal failure develop. Withdrawal of the drug commonly is followed by complete recovery, but there may be permanent damage in some persons, usually in older persons. Drug nephritis may not be recognized in its early stage because it is uncommon.

Chronic analgesic nephritis, which is associated with analgesic abuse, causes interstitial nephritis with renal papillary necrosis. When first observed, it was attributed to phenacetin, a then-common ingredient of over-the-counter medications containing aspirin, phenacetin, and caffeine. Although phenacetin is no longer contained in these preparations, it has been suggested that other ingredients, such as aspirin and acetaminophen, also may contribute to the disorder. How much analgesic it takes to produce papillary necrosis is unknown.

Nonsteroidal anti-inflammatory drugs (NSAIDs) also have the potential for damaging renal structures, including medullary interstitial cells. Prostaglandins (particularly PGI_2 and PGE_2) contribute to regulation of tubular blood flow.[56] The deleterious effects of NSAIDs on the kidney are thought to result from their ability to inhibit prostaglandin synthesis. Persons who are particularly at risk are the elderly because of age-related changes in renal function, persons who are dehydrated or have a decrease in blood volume, and persons with preexisting kidney disease or renal insufficiency.

In summary, tubulointerstitial diseases affect the tubules and the surrounding interstitium of the kidneys. These disorders include renal tubular acidosis, chronic pyelonephritis, and the effects of drugs and toxins. Renal tubular acidosis describes a form of systemic acidosis that results from tubular defects in bicarbonate reabsorption or hydrogen ion secretion. Pyelonephritis, or infection of the kidney and kidney pelvis, can occur as an acute or a chronic condition. Acute pyelonephritis typically is caused by ascending bladder infections or infections that come from the bloodstream; it usually is successfully treated with appropriate antimicrobial drugs. Chronic pyelonephritis is a progressive disease that produces scarring and deformation of the renal calices and pelvis. Drug-induced impairment of tubulointerstitial structure and function usually is the result of direct toxic injury, decreased blood flow, or hypersensitivity reactions.

Neoplasms

After completing this section of the chapter, you should be able to meet the following objectives:

- Characterize Wilms' tumor in terms of age of onset, possible oncogenic origin, manifestations, and treatment
- Cite the risk factors for renal cell carcinoma, describe the manifestations, and explain why the 5-year survival rate has been so low

There are two major groups of renal neoplasms: embryonic kidney tumors (*i.e.*, Wilms' tumor), which occur during childhood, and adult kidney cancers.

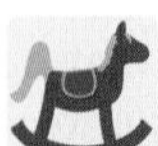

WILMS' TUMOR

Wilms' tumor (*i.e.*, nephroblastoma) is one of the most common primary neoplasms of young children. The median age at time of diagnosis of unilateral Wilms' tumor is approximately 3 to 5 years.[57,58] Classically, the tumor is composed of all three embryonic cell types: blastemic, stromal, and epithelial. An important feature of Wilms' tumor is its association with other congenital anomalies, the most frequent being those affecting genitourinary structures. Several chromosomal abnormalities have been associated with Wilms' tumor. Deletions involving at least two loci on chromosome 11 have been found in approximately 20% of children with Wilms' tumor.[57]

Wilms' tumor usually is a solitary mass that occurs in any part of the kidney. It usually is sharply demarcated and variably encapsulated. The tumors grow to a large size, distorting kidney structure. The tumors usually are staged using the Wilms' Tumor Study Group classification.[57] Stage I tumors are limited to the kidney and can be excised with the capsular surface intact. Stage II tumors extend into the kidney but can be excised. In stage III, extension of the tumor is confined to the abdomen, and in stage IV, hematogenous metastasis most commonly involves the lung. Bilateral kidney involvement occurs in 5% to 10% of cases.

The common presenting signs are a large asymptomatic abdominal mass and hypertension. The tumor is often discovered inadvertently, and it is not uncommon for the mother to discover it while bathing the child. Some children may present with abdominal pain, vomiting, or both. Microscopic and gross hematuria is present in 10% to 25% of children. CT scans are used to confirm the diagnosis.

Treatment involves surgery, chemotherapy, and sometimes radiation therapy. Long-term survival rates have increased to greater than 80% with an aggressive treatment plan.[57,58]

ADULT KIDNEY CANCER

Adult kidney cancer accounts for 2% to 3% of all new cancers. Men are affected about twice as often as women, and the mean age at time of diagnosis is about 60 years.[59] The increased use of imaging procedures such as ultrasonography, CT scanning, and magnetic resonance imaging (MRI) has contributed significantly to earlier diagnosis and more accurate staging of kidney cancers.[60]

Renal cell carcinoma originates in the renal cortex and accounts for approximately 80% to 85% of kidney tumors, with transitional or squamous cell cancers of the renal pelvis accounting for most of the remaining cancers.[61] The cause of renal cell carcinoma remains unclear. Some of these tumors may occur as a result of chronic irritation associated with kidney stones. Epidemiologic evidence suggests a correlation between smoking and kidney cancer. Obesity also is a risk factor, particularly in women.[61] Additional risk factors include occupational exposure to petroleum products, heavy metals, and asbestos. The risk for renal cell carcinoma also is increased in persons with acquired cystic kidney disease associated with chronic renal insufficiency.[60,61] Most cases of renal cell carcinoma occur without a recognizable hereditary pattern. However, there are several rare forms of renal cell cancer that are characterized by an autosomal dominant pattern of inheritance, young age at onset (third and fourth decade), and bilateral or multifocal tumors.[60,61]

Kidney cancer is largely a silent disorder during its early stages, and symptoms usually denote advanced disease. Presenting features include hematuria, costovertebral pain, presence of a palpable flank mass, polycythemia, and fever. Hematuria, which occurs in 70% to 90% of cases, is the most reliable sign. It is, however, intermittent and may be microscopic; as a result, the tumor may reach considerable size before it is detected. In approximately one third of cases, metastases are present at the time of diagnosis.

Kidney cancer is suspected when there are findings of hematuria and a renal mass. Ultrasonography, CT scanning, excretory urography, and renal angiography are used to confirm the diagnosis. MRI with intravenous gadolinium may be used when involvement of the inferior vena cava is suspected.

Surgery (radical nephrectomy with lymph node dissection) is the treatment of choice for all resectable tumors. Nephron-sparing surgery may be done when both kidneys are involved or when the contralateral kidney is threatened by an associated disease such as hypertension or diabetes mellitus. Single-agent and combination chemotherapy have been used with limited success. Immunotherapy involving interferon-alfa and interleukin-2 has been used with some success.[61] The 5-year survival rate for stage I disease ranges from 65% to 85%; 45% to 80% for stage II disease; 15% to 35% for stage III disease; and 0% to 10% for stage IV disease.[60]

In summary, there are two major groups of renal neoplasms: embryonic kidney tumors (*i.e.,* Wilms' tumor) that occur during childhood and adult renal cell carcinomas. Wilms' tumor is the most common malignant tumor of children. The most common presenting signs are a large abdominal mass and hypertension. Treatment is surgery, chemotherapy, and sometimes radiation therapy. The long-term survival rate for children with Wilms' tumor is approximately 90% with an aggressive plan of treatment.

Adult kidney cancers account for 2% of all cancers. Renal cell carcinoma is the most frequent type of kidney cancer. These tumors are characterized by a lack of early warning signs, diverse clinical manifestations, and resistance to chemotherapy and radiation therapy. Because of the lack of early warning signs, the tumors often are far advanced at the time of diagnosis. Diagnostic methods include ultrasonography and CT scans. The treatment of choice is surgical resection. Prognosis depends on the stage of the cancer; the 5-year survival rate for stage I tumors is 65% to 85%, and for stage IV tumors, it is 0% to 10%.

REVIEW EXERCISES

A 6-year-old boy is diagnosed with glomerulonephritis secondary to a streptococcal throat infection. He had been diagnosed with nephrotic syndrome several months ago. At this time, the following manifestations are noted: a decrease in urine output, increasing lethargy, hyperventilation, and generalized edema. Trace amounts of protein are detected in his urine. Blood analysis reveals the following: pH = 7.35, HCO_3 = 18 mEq/L, hematocrit = 29%, Na = 132 mEq/L, K = 5.6 mEq/L, BUN = 62 mg/dL, creatinine = 4.1 mg/dL, albumin = 2 g/dL.

A. What is the probable cause of this boy's glomerular disease?

B. Use the lab values in the appendix to interpret his lab values. Which values are significant and why?

C. Is he progressing to uremia? How can you tell?

A 26-year-old woman makes an appointment with her health care provider complaining of urinary frequency, urgency, and burning. She reports that her urine is cloudy and smells abnormal. Her urine is cultured, and she is given a prescription for antibiotics.

A. What is the most likely cause of the woman's symptoms?

B. What microorganism is most likely responsible for the infection?

C. What factors may have predisposed to this disorder?

D. What could this woman do to prevent future infection?

References

1. National Kidney Foundation. (2003). *Fact Sheets: The problem of kidney and urologic diseases.* [On-line]. Available: http://www.kidney.org.
2. Moore K.L., Persaud T.V.N. (2003). *The developing human: Clinically oriented embryology* (7th ed., pp. 288–296). Philadelphia: W.B. Saunders.
3. Stewart C.L., Jose P.A. (1991). Transitional nephrology. *Urologic Clinics of North America 18,* 143–149.
4. Elder J.S. (2004). Urologic disorders in infants and children. In Behrman R.E., Kliegman R.M., Jenson H.B. (Eds.), *Nelson textbook of pediatrics* (17th ed., pp. 1783–1785, 1785–1789). Philadelphia: W.B. Saunders.
5. Cotran R.S., Kumar V., Collins T. (1999). *Robbins pathologic basis of disease* (6th ed., pp. 936–965, 971–979). Philadelphia: W.B. Saunders.
6. Jennette J.C., Spargo B.H. (1999). The kidney. In Rubin E., Farber J.L. (Eds.), *Pathology* (3rd ed., pp. 865–893, 902–907, 913–917). Philadelphia: Lippincott-Raven.
7. Sutters M., Germino G.G. (2003). Autosomal dominant polycystic kidney disease: Molecular genetics and pathophysiology. *Journal of Laboratory and Clinical Medicine 141,* 91–110.
8. Peters D.J.M., Breuning M.H. (2001). Autosomal dominant polycystic kidney disease: Modification of disease progression. *Lancet 358,* 1439–1444.
9. Martinez J.R., Grantham J.J. (1995). Polycystic kidney disease: Etiology, pathogenesis, and treatment. *Disease-a-Month 41*(11), 696–765.
10. Bajwa Z.H., Gupta S., Warfield C.A., Steinman T.I. (2001). Pain management in polycystic kidney disease. *Kidney International 60,* 1631–1644.
11. Tanagho E.A. (2004). Urinary obstruction and stasis. In Tanagho E.A., McAninch J.W. (Eds.), *Smith's general urology* (16th ed., p. 175). New York: Lange Medical Books/McGraw-Hill.
12. Stoller M.L. (2004). Urinary stone disease. In Tanagho E.A., McAninch J.W. (Eds.), *Smith's general urology* (16th ed., pp. 256–290). New York: Lange Medical Books/McGraw-Hill.
13. Portis A.J., Sundram C.P. (2002). Diagnosis and initial management of kidney stones. *American Family Physician 63*(7), 1329–1338.
14. Coe F.L., Parks J.H., Asplin J.R. (1992). The pathogenesis and treatment of kidney stones. *New England Journal of Medicine 327,* 1141–1152.
15. Ross A.R., Iliescu E.A., Wilson J.W.L (2002). Nephrology. I. Investigation and treatment of recurrent kidney stones. *Canadian Medical Association Journal 166*(2), 213–218.
16. Mandel N. (1996). Mechanisms of stone formation. *Seminars in Nephrology 16,* 364–374.
17. Scheinman S.J. (2000). New insights into causes and treatments of kidney stones. *Hospital Practice 35*(3), 49–56, 67–68.
18. Worchester E.M. (1996). Inhibitors of stone formation. *Seminars in Nephrology 16,* 474–486.

19. Schappert S.M. (1999). Ambulatory care visits to physician offices, hospital outpatient departments, and emergency departments, United States, 1997. *Vital Health Statistics 13,* i–iv, 1–39.
20. Stamm W.E. (2002). Scientific and clinical challenges in the management of urinary tract infections. *American Journal of Medicine 113*(1A), 1S–4S.
21. Ronald A. (2002). The etiology of urinary tract infections: Traditional and emerging pathogens. *American Journal of Medicine 113*(1A), 14S–19S.
22. Nguyen H.T. (2004). Bacterial infections of the genitourinary tract. In Tanagho E.A., McAninch J.W. (Eds.), *Smith's general urology* (16th ed., pp. 203–227). New York: Lange Medical Books/McGraw-Hill.
23. Stapleton A. (2002). Urinary tract infections in patients with diabetes. *American Journal of Medicine 113*(1A), 80S–84S.
24. Stamm W.E., Hooton T.M. (1993). Management of urinary tract infections in adults. *New England Journal of Medicine 328,* 1328–1334.
25. Nicolle L.E. (2002). Urinary tract infections: Traditional pharmacologic therapies. *American Journal of Medicine 113*(1A), 35S–44S.
26. Manges A.R., Johnson J.R., Foxman B., et al. (2001). Widespread distribution of urinary tract infections caused by multidrug resistant *Escherichia coli* colonal group. *New England Journal of Medicine 345,* 1007–1013.
27. Roberts J.A. (1999). Management of pyelonephritis and upper urinary tract infections. *Urologic Clinics of North America 26,* 753–763.
28. Ofek I., Goldhar J., Zafriri D., Lis H., et al. (1991). Anti-*Escherichia coli* adhesin activity of cranberry and blueberry juices. *New England Journal of Medicine 324,* 1599.
29. Lowe F.C., Fagelman E. (2001). Cranberry juice and urinary tract infections: What is the evidence? *Urology 57,* 407–413.
30. Fihn S.D. (2003). Acute uncomplicated urinary tract infections in women. *New England Journal of Medicine 349*(3), 259–266.
31. Hooton T.M., Scholes D., Hughes J.P., et al. (1996). A prospective study of risk factors for symptomatic urinary tract infections in young women. *New England Journal of Medicine 335,* 468–474.
32. Fihn S.D. (2003). Acute uncomplicated urinary tract infections in women. *New England Journal of Medicine 349*(3), 259–266.
33. Delzell J.E., Lefevre M.L. (2000). Urinary tract infections during pregnancy. *American Family Physician 61,* 713–721.
34. American College of Obstetricians and Gynecologists. (1998). *Antimicrobial therapy for obstetric patients* (pp. 8–10). ACOG Educational Bulletin no. 245. Washington, DC: Author.
35. Shortliffe L.M., McCue J.D. (2002). Urinary tract infections at the age extremes: Pediatrics and geriatrics. *American Journal of Medicine 113*(1A), 55S–66S.
36. Shaw K.N., Gorelick M.H. (1999). Urinary tract infections in children. *Pediatric Clinics of North America 46,* 1111–1122.
37. Bartkowski D.P. (2001). Recognizing UTIs in infants and children. *Postgraduate Medicine 109,* 171–181.
38. Johnson C.E. (1999). New advances in childhood urinary tract infections. *Pediatrics in Review 20,* 335–342.
39. Mouton C.P., Pierce B., Espino D.V. (2001). Common infections in older adults. *American Family Physician 63,* 257–268.
40. Hricik D.E., Chung-Park M., Sedor J.R. (1998). Glomerulonephritis. *New England Journal of Medicine 339,* 888–899.
41. Couser W.O. (1999). Glomerulonephritis. *Lancet 35,* 1509–1515.
42. Glassock R.J. (2003). The glomerulopathies. In Shrier R.W. *Renal and electrolyte disorders* (6th ed., pp. 633–670). Philadelphia: Lippincott Williams & Wilkins.
43. Eddy A.A., Symons J.M. (2003). Nephrotic syndrome in childhood. *Lancet 362,* 629–639.
44. Vincenti F.G., Amend W.J.C. (2004). Diagnosis of medical renal diseases. In Tanagho E.A., McAninch J.W. (Eds.), *Smith's general urology* (16th ed., pp. 527–537). New York: Lange Medical Books/McGraw-Hill.
45. Orth S.R., Ritz E. (1998). The nephrotic syndrome. *New England Journal of Medicine 339,* 1202–1211.
46. Kaysen G.A. (2003). Proteinuria and the nephrotic syndrome. In Shrier R.W. *Renal and electrolyte disorders* (6th ed., pp. 580–622). Philadelphia: Lippincott Williams & Wilkins.
47. Jennette J.C., Falk R.J. (1997). Diagnosis and management of glomerular disease. *Medical Clinics of North America 81*(3), 653–675.
48. Devarajan P., Spitzer A. (2002). Toward a biological characterization of focal segmental glomerulonephritis. *American Journal of Kidney Diseases 39*(3), 625–636.
49. Donadio J.V., Grande J.P. (2002). IgA nephropathy. *New England Journal of Medicine 347*(1), 738–748.
50. Dunfee T.P. (1995). The changing management of diabetic nephropathy. *Hospital Practice 30*(5), 45–55.
51. Remuzzi G., Bertani T. (1998). Pathophysiology of progressive nephropathies. *New England Journal of Medicine 339,* 1448–1455.
52. Parving H.-H., Østerby R., Ritz E. (2000). Diabetic nephropathy. In Brenner B.M. (Ed.), *Brenner and Rector's the kidney* (6th ed., pp. 1731–1753). Philadelphia: W.B. Saunders.
53. Soriano J.R. (2002). Renal tubular acidosis. *Journal of the American Society Nephrology 13,* 2160–2170.
54. Kurtzman N.A. (2000). Renal tubular acidosis syndromes. *Southern Medical Journal 93*(11), 1042–1052.
55. Guo S., Nzerue C. (2002). How to prevent, recognize, and treat drug-induced nephrotoxicity. *Cleveland Clinic Journal of Medicine 69*(4), 289–297.
56. Palmer B., Hendrich W.L. (1995). Clinical acute renal failure with nonsteroidal anti-inflammatory drugs. *Seminars in Nephrology 15,* 214–227.
57. Jaffe N., Huff V. (2004). Neoplasms of the kidney. In Behrman R.E., Kiegman R.M., Jenson H.B. (Eds.), *Nelson textbook of pediatrics* (17th ed., pp. 1711–1714). Philadelphia: W.B. Saunders.
58. Marcus K.C. (2001). Pediatric solid tumors. In Lenhard R.E., Osteen R.T., Gansler T. (Eds.), *The American Cancer Society's clinical oncology* (pp. 588–590). Atlanta: American Cancer Society.
59. Bostwick, D.G. (2001). Renal cell carcinoma. In Lenhard R.E., Osteen R.T., Gansler T. (Eds.), *The American Cancer Society's clinical oncology* (pp. 415–419). Atlanta: American Cancer Society.
60. Chow W.H., Devesa S.S., Warren J.L., Fraumeni J.F. (1999). Rising incidence of renal cell cancer in the United States. *Journal of the American Medical Association 281,* 1628–1631.
61. Motzer R.J., Bander N.H., Nanus D.M. (1997). Medical progress: Renal-cell carcinoma. *New England Journal of Medicine 335,* 865–875.

CHAPTER

36

Renal Failure

Renal failure is a condition in which the kidneys fail to remove metabolic end products from the blood and regulate the fluid, electrolyte, and pH balance of the extracellular fluids. The underlying cause may be renal disease, systemic disease, or urologic defects of nonrenal origin. Renal failure can occur as an acute or a chronic disorder. Acute renal failure is abrupt in onset and often is reversible if recognized early and treated appropriately. In contrast, chronic renal failure is the end result of irreparable damage to the kidneys. It develops slowly, usually over the course of a number of years.

Acute Renal Failure

After completing this section of the chapter, you should be able to meet the following objectives:

- Distinguish between acute and chronic renal failure in terms of causes, treatment, and outcome
- Differentiate the prerenal, intrinsic, and postrenal forms of acute renal failure in terms of the mechanisms of development and manifestations
- Cite the two most common causes of acute tubular necrosis and describe the course of the disease in terms of the initiation, maintenance, and recovery phases

Acute renal failure represents a rapid decline in renal function sufficient to increase blood levels of nitrogenous wastes and impair fluid and electrolyte balance. Unlike chronic renal failure, acute renal failure is potentially reversible if the precipitating factors can be corrected or removed before permanent kidney damage has occurred.

Acute renal failure is a common threat to seriously ill persons in intensive care units, with a mortality rate ranging from 40% to 75%.[1,2] Although treatment methods such as dialysis and renal replacement methods are effective in correcting life-threatening fluid and electrolyte disorders, the mortality rate from acute renal failure has not changed substantially since the 1960s. This probably is because acute renal failure is seen more often in older persons than before, and because it frequently is superimposed on other life-threatening conditions, such as trauma, shock, and sepsis.

The most common indicator of acute renal failure is *azotemia,* an accumulation of nitrogenous wastes (urea nitrogen, uric acid, and creatinine) in the blood. In acute renal failure, the glomerular filtration rate (GFR) is decreased. As a result, excretion of nitrogenous wastes is reduced, and fluid and electrolyte balance cannot be maintained.

ACUTE RENAL FAILURE

- Acute renal failure is caused by conditions that produce an acute shutdown in renal function.
- It can result from decreased blood flow to the kidney (prerenal failure), disorders that disrupt the structures in the kidney (intrinsic or intrarenal failure), or disorders that interfere with the elimination of urine from the kidney (postrenal failure).
- Acute renal failure, although it causes an accumulation of products normally cleared by the kidney, is a reversible process if the factors causing the condition can be corrected.

CHART 36-1

Causes of Acute Renal Failure

Prerenal

Hypovolemia
  Hemorrhage
  Dehydration
  Excessive loss of gastrointestinal tract fluids
  Excessive loss of fluid due to burn injury
Decreased vascular filling
  Anaphylactic shock
  Septic shock
Heart failure and cardiogenic shock
Decreased renal perfusion due to vasoactive mediators, drugs, diagnostic agents

Intrinsic or intrarenal

Acute tubular necrosis
  Prolonged renal ischemia
  Exposure to nephrotoxic drugs, heavy metals, and organic solvents
  Intratubular obstruction resulting from hemoglobinuria, myoglobinuria, myeloma light chains, or uric acid casts
  Acute renal disease (acute glomerulonephritis, pyelonephritis)

Postrenal

Bilateral ureteral obstruction
Bladder outlet obstruction

TYPES OF ACUTE RENAL FAILURE

Acute renal failure can be caused by several types of conditions, including a decrease in blood flow without ischemic injury; ischemic, toxic, or obstructive tubular injury; and obstruction of urinary tract outflow. The causes of acute renal failure commonly are categorized as prerenal, intrinsic, and postrenal[1–6] (Fig. 36-1). Collectively, prerenal and intrinsic causes account for 80% to 90% of cases of acute renal failure.[3] Causes of renal failure within these categories are summarized in Chart 36-1.

Prerenal Failure

Prerenal failure, the most common form of acute renal failure, is characterized by a marked decrease in renal blood flow. It is reversible if the cause of the decreased renal blood flow can be identified and corrected before kidney damage occurs. Causes of prerenal failure include profound depletion of vascular volume (*e.g.,* hemorrhage, loss of extracellular fluid volume), impaired perfusion due to heart failure and cardiogenic shock, and decreased vascular filling because of increased vascular capacity (*e.g.,* anaphylaxis or sepsis). Elderly persons are particularly at risk because of their predisposition to hypovolemia and their high prevalence of renal vascular disorders.

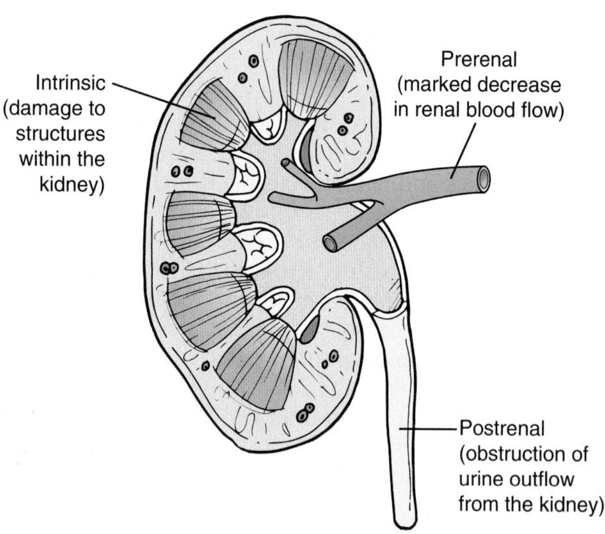

FIGURE 36-1 Types of acute renal failure.

Some vasoactive mediators, drugs, and diagnostic agents stimulate intense intrarenal vasoconstriction and induce glomerular hypoperfusion and prerenal failure.[3–5] Examples include hypercalcemia, endotoxins, radiocontrast agents such as those used for cardiac catheterization, cyclosporine (an immunosuppressant drug that is used to prevent transplant rejection), amphotericin B (an antifungal agent), epinephrine, and high doses of dopamine.[3] Many of these drugs also cause acute tubular necrosis (discussed later). In addition, several commonly used classes of drugs impair renal adaptive mechanisms and can convert compensated renal hypoperfusion into prerenal failure. Angiotensin-converting enzyme (ACE) inhibitors reduce the effects of renin on renal blood flow; when combined with diuretics, they may cause prerenal failure in persons with decreased blood flow due to large or small vessel renal vascular disease. Prostaglandins have a vasodilatory effect on renal blood vessels. Nonsteroidal anti-inflammatory drugs (NSAIDs) reduce renal blood flow through inhibition of prostaglandin synthesis. In some persons with diminished renal perfusion, NSAIDs can precipitate prerenal failure. A new class of NSAIDs that selectively inhibit the cyclooxygenase type 2 (COX-2) isoform of the enzyme have become widely available for clinical use. Although the NSAIDS that selectively inhibit COX-2 are less toxic to the gastrointestinal tract, they appear to exert the same effect on the kidney as the conventional nonselective NSAIDS.[6]

Normally, the kidneys receive 20% to 25% of the cardiac output.[7] This large blood supply is required to remove metabolic wastes and regulate body fluids and electrolytes. Fortunately, the normal kidney can tolerate relatively large reductions in blood flow before renal damage occurs. As renal blood flow is reduced, the GFR decreases, the amount of sodium and other substances that is filtered by the glomeruli is reduced, and the need for energy-dependent mechanisms to reabsorb these substance is reduced (see Chapter 32). As the GFR and urine output approach zero, oxygen consumption by the kidney approximates that required to keep renal tubular cells alive.[7] When blood flow falls below this level, which is about 20% of normal, ischemic changes occur. Because of their high metabolic rate, the tubular epithelial cells are most vulnerable to ischemic injury. Improperly treated, prolonged renal hypoperfusion can lead to ischemic tubular necrosis with significant morbidity and mortality.

Acute renal failure is manifested by a sharp decrease in urine output and a disproportionate elevation of blood urea nitrogen (BUN) in relation to serum creatinine levels. The kidney normally responds to a decrease in the GFR with a decrease in urine output. Thus, an early sign of prerenal failure is a sharp decrease in urine output. A low fractional excretion of sodium (<1%) suggests that oliguria is due to decreased renal perfusion and that the nephrons are responding appropriately by decreasing the excretion of filtered sodium in an attempt to preserve vascular volume. BUN levels also depend on the GFR. A low GFR allows more time for small particles such as urea to be reabsorbed into the blood. Creatinine, which is larger and nondiffusible, remains in the tubular fluid, and the total amount of creatinine that is filtered, although small, is excreted in the urine. Thus, there also is a disproportionate elevation in the ratio of BUN to serum creatinine to greater than 15:1 to 20:1 (normal, approximately 10:1).[1]

Postrenal Failure

Postrenal failure results from obstruction of urine outflow from the kidneys. The obstruction can occur in the ureter (*i.e.*, calculi and strictures), bladder (*i.e.*, tumors or neurogenic bladder), or urethra (*i.e.*, prostatic hypertrophy). Prostatic hyperplasia is the most common underlying problem. Because both ureters must be occluded to produce renal failure, obstruction of the bladder rarely causes acute renal failure unless one of the kidneys already is damaged or a person has only one kidney. The treatment of acute postrenal failure consists of treating the underlying cause of obstruction so that urine flow can be reestablished before permanent nephron damage occurs.

Intrinsic Renal Failure

Intrinsic or intrarenal renal failure results from conditions that cause damage to structures within the kidney—glomerular, tubular, or interstitial. The major causes of intrarenal failure are ischemia associated with prerenal failure, toxic insult to the tubular structures of the nephron, and intratubular obstruction. Acute glomerulonephritis and acute pyelonephritis also are intrarenal causes of acute renal failure. Injury to the tubules (acute tubular necrosis) is most common and often is ischemic or toxic in origin.

Acute Tubular Necrosis. Acute tubular necrosis (ATN) is characterized by destruction of tubular epithelial cells with acute suppression of renal function (Fig. 36-2). ATN can be caused by a variety of conditions, including acute tubular damage due to ischemia, the nephrotoxic effects of drugs, tubular obstruction, and toxins from a massive infection.[3,6,8] Tubular epithelial cells are particularly sensitive to ischemia and also are vulnerable to toxins. The tubular injury that occurs in ATN frequently is reversible. The process depends on the recovery of the injured cells, removal of the necrotic cells and intratubular casts, and regeneration of renal cells to restore the normal continuity of the tubular epithelium. If, however, the ischemia is severe enough to cause cortical necrosis, irreversible renal failure occurs.

Ischemic ATN occurs most frequently in persons who have major surgery, severe hypovolemia, overwhelming sepsis, trauma, and burns.[3] Sepsis produces ischemia by provoking a combination of systemic vasodilation and intrarenal hypoperfusion. In addition, sepsis results in the generation of toxins that sensitize renal tubular cells to the damaging effects of ischemia.[6,8] ATN complicating trauma and burns frequently is multifactorial in origin and due to

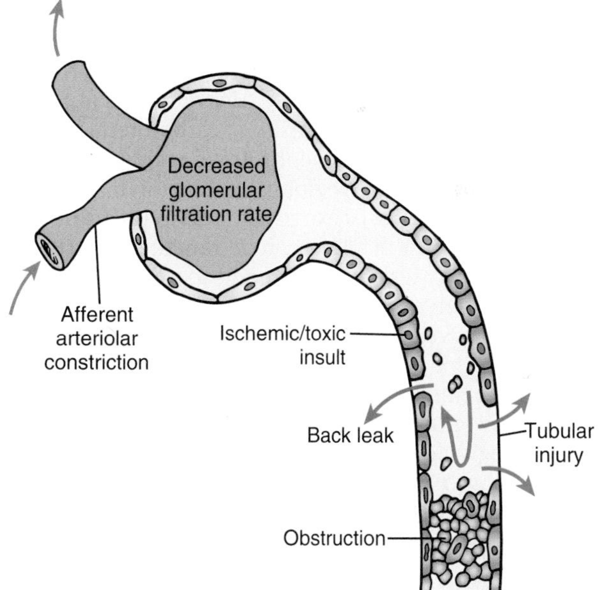

FIGURE 36-2 Pathogenesis of acute tubular necrosis. Sloughing and necrosis of tubular epithelial cells lead to obstruction and increased intraluminal pressure, which reduce glomerular filtration. Afferent arteriolar vasconstriction, caused in part by tubuloglomerular feedback, results in decreased glomerular capillary filtration pressure. Tubular injury and increased intraluminal pressure cause fluid to move from the tubular lumen into the interstitium (backleak). (Modified from: Rubin E., Farber J.L. [1999]. *Pathology* [3rd ed., p. 901]. Philadelphia: Lippincott-Raven)

the combined effects of hypovolemia and myoglobinuria or other toxins released from damaged tissue. In contrast to prerenal failure, the GFR does not improve with the restoration of renal blood flow in acute renal failure caused by ischemic ATN.

Nephrotoxic ATN complicates the administration of or exposure to many structurally diverse drugs and other toxic agents. Nephrotoxic agents cause renal injury by inducing varying combinations of renal vasoconstriction, direct tubular damage, or intratubular obstruction. The kidney is particularly vulnerable to nephrotic injury because of its rich blood supply and ability to concentrate toxins to high levels in the medullary portion of the kidney. In addition, the kidney is an important site for metabolic processes that transform relatively harmless agents into toxic metabolites. Pharmacologic agents that are directly toxic to the renal tubule include antimicrobials such as the aminoglycosides, chemotherapeutic agents such as cisplatin and ifosfamide, and the radiocontrast agents.[5,6,8] Several factors contribute to aminoglycoside nephrotoxicity, including a decrease in the GFR, preexisting renal disease, hypovolemia, and concurrent administration of other drugs that have a nephrotoxic effect. Nonoliguric ATN occurs in 10% to 30% of courses of aminoglycoside therapy, even when the blood levels of the drug are within therapeutic range.[3] Cisplatin accumulates in proximal tubule cells, inducing mitochondrial injury and inhibition of adenosine triphosphatase (ATP) activity and solute transport. ATN complicates up to 70% of courses of cisplatin therapy. Radiocontrast media–induced nephrotoxicity is thought to result from direct tubular toxicity and renal ischemia.[9,10] The risk for renal damage caused by radiocontrast media is greatest in elderly persons, in persons with diabetes mellitus, and in persons who, for various reasons, are susceptible to kidney disease. Heavy metals (*e.g.*, lead, mercury) and organic solvents (*e.g.*, carbon tetrachloride, ethylene glycol) are other nephrotoxic agents.

The presence of myoglobin, hemoglobin, uric acid, myeloma light chains, or excess uric acid in the urine is the most frequent cause of ATN due to intratubular obstruction. Both myeloma cast nephropathy and acute urate nephropathy usually are seen in the setting of widespread malignancy or massive tumor destruction by therapeutic agents.[3] Hemoglobinuria results from blood transfusion reactions and other hemolytic crises. Skeletal and cardiac muscles contain myoglobin, which accounts for their rubiginous color. Myoglobin corresponds to hemoglobin in function, serving as an oxygen reservoir in the muscle fibers. Myoglobin normally is not found in the serum or urine. It has a low molecular weight of 17,000 daltons; if it escapes into the circulation, it is rapidly filtered in the glomerulus. Myoglobinuria most commonly results from muscle trauma but may result from extreme exertion, hyperthermia, sepsis, prolonged seizures, potassium or phosphate depletion, and alcoholism or drug abuse. Both myoglobin and hemoglobin discolor the urine, which may range from the color of tea to red, brown, or black.

The course of ATN can be divided into three phases: the onset or initiating phase, the maintenance phase, and the recovery or convalescent phase.[3] The *onset* or *initiating phase,* which lasts hours or days, is the time from the onset of the precipitating event (*e.g.,* ischemic phase of prerenal failure or toxin exposure) until tubular injury occurs.

The *maintenance phase* of ATN is characterized by a marked decrease in the GFR, causing sudden retention of endogenous metabolites such as urea, potassium, sulfate, and creatinine that normally are cleared by the kidneys. The urine output usually is lowest at this point. Fluid retention gives rise to edema, water intoxication, and pulmonary congestion. If the period of oliguria is prolonged, hypertension frequently develops and with it signs of uremia. When untreated, the neurologic manifestations of uremia progress from neuromuscular irritability to seizures, somnolence, coma, and death. Hyperkalemia usually is asymptomatic until serum levels of potassium rise above 6.0 to 6.5 mEq/L, at which point characteristic electrocardiographic changes and symptoms of muscle weakness are seen.

Formerly, most patients with ATN were oliguric. During the past several decades, a nonoliguric form of ATN has become increasingly prevalent. Persons with nonoliguric failure have higher levels of glomerular filtration and excrete more nitrogenous waste, water, and electrolytes in their urine than persons with acute oliguric renal failure. Abnormalities in blood chemistry levels usually are milder and cause fewer complications. The decrease in oliguric ATN probably reflects new approaches to the treatment of poor cardiac performance and circulatory failure that focus on vigorous plasma volume expansion and the selective use of dopamine and other drugs to improve renal blood flow. Dopamine has renal vasodilator properties and inhibits sodium reabsorption in the proximal tubule, thereby decreasing the work demands of the nephron.

The *recovery phase* is the period during which repair of renal tissue takes place. Its onset usually is heralded by a gradual increase in urine output and a fall in serum creatinine, indicating that the nephrons have recovered to the point at which urine excretion is possible. Diuresis often occurs before renal function has fully returned to normal. Consequently, BUN and serum creatinine, potassium, and phosphate levels may remain elevated or continue to rise even though urine output is increased. In some cases, the diuresis may result from impaired nephron function and may cause excessive loss of water and electrolytes. Eventually, renal tubular function is restored with improvement in concentrating ability. At about the same time, the BUN and creatinine begin to return to normal. In some cases, mild to moderate kidney damage persists.

DIAGNOSIS AND TREATMENT

Given the high morbidity and mortality rates associated with acute renal failure, attention should be focused on prevention and early diagnosis. This includes assessment measures to identify persons at risk for development of acute renal failure, including those with preexisting renal insufficiency and diabetes. These persons are particularly at risk for development of acute renal failure due to nephrotoxic drugs such as aminoglycosides and contrast agents, or to drugs such as the NSAIDs that alter intrarenal hemodynamics. Elderly persons are susceptible to all forms of acute renal failure because of the effects of aging on renal reserve.

Careful observation of urine output is essential for persons at risk for development of acute renal failure. Urine tests that measure urine osmolality, urinary sodium concentration, and fractional excretion of sodium help differentiate prerenal azotemia, in which the reabsorptive capacity of the tubular cells is maintained, from tubular necrosis, in which these functions are lost. One of the earliest manifestations of tubular damage is the inability to concentrate the urine.

Further diagnostic information that can be obtained from the urinalysis includes evidence of proteinuria, hemoglobinuria, and casts or crystals in the urine. Blood tests for BUN and creatinine provide information regarding the ability to remove nitrogenous wastes from the blood. It also is important to exclude urinary obstruction.

A major concern in the treatment of acute renal failure is identifying and correcting the cause (*e.g.*, improving renal perfusion, discontinuing nephrotoxic drugs). Fluids are carefully regulated in an effort to maintain normal fluid volume and electrolyte concentrations. Adequate caloric intake is needed to prevent the breakdown of body proteins, which increases nitrogenous wastes. Parenteral hyperalimentation may be used for this purpose. Because secondary infections are a major cause of death in persons with acute renal failure, constant effort is needed to prevent and treat such infections.

Dialysis or continuous renal replacement therapy (CRRT) may be indicated when nitrogenous wastes and the water and electrolyte balance cannot be kept under control by other means. Venovenous or arteriovenous CRRT has emerged as a method for treating acute renal failure in patients too hemodynamically unstable to tolerate hemodialysis.[11] An associated advantage of the continuous renal replacement therapies is the ability to administer nutritional support. The disadvantages are the need for prolonged anticoagulation and continuous sophisticated monitoring.

In summary, acute renal failure is an acute, reversible suppression of kidney function. It is a common threat to seriously ill persons in intensive care units, with a mortality rate of 40% to 75%. Acute renal failure is characterized by an accumulation of nitrogenous wastes in the blood (*i.e.*, azotemia) and alterations in body fluids and electrolytes. Acute renal failure is classified as prerenal, intrinsic or intrarenal, or postrenal in origin. Prerenal failure is caused by decreased blood flow to the kidneys; postrenal failure by obstruction to urine output; and intrinsic renal failure by disorders in the kidney itself. ATN, due to ischemia or nephrotoxic agents, is a common cause of acute intrinsic renal failure. ATN typically progresses through three phases: the initiation phase, during which tubular injury is induced; the maintenance phase, during which the GFR falls, nitrogenous wastes accumulate, and urine output decreases; and the recovery or reparative phase, during which the GFR, urine output, and blood levels of nitrogenous wastes return to normal.

Because of the high morbidity and mortality rates associated with acute renal failure, identification of persons at risk is important to clinical decision making. Acute renal failure often is reversible, making early identification and correction of the underlying cause (*e.g.*, improving renal perfusion, discontinuing nephrotoxic drugs) important. Treatment includes the judicious administration of fluids and dialysis or CRRT.

Chronic Renal Failure

After completing this section of the chapter, you should be able to meet the following objectives:

- State the definitions of renal impairment, renal insufficiency, renal failure, and end-stage renal disease
- List the common problems associated with end-stage renal disease, including alterations in fluid and electrolyte balance and disorders of skeletal, hematologic, cardiovascular, immune, neurologic, skin, and sexual function, and explain their physiologic significance
- State the basis for adverse drug reactions in patients with end-stage renal disease
- Describe the scientific principles underlying dialysis treatment, and compare hemodialysis with peritoneal dialysis
- Cite the complications of kidney transplantation
- State the goals for dietary management of persons with end-stage renal disease

Unlike acute renal failure, chronic renal failure represents progressive and irreversible destruction of kidney structures. As recently as 1965, many patients with chronic renal failure progressed to the final stages of the disease and then died. The high mortality rate was associated with limitations in the treatment of renal disease and with the tremendous cost of ongoing treatment. In 1972, federal support began for dialysis and transplantation through a Medicare entitlement program.[12] Technologic advances in renal replacement therapy (*i.e.*, dialysis therapy and transplantation) have improved the outcomes for persons with renal failure. The number of persons with kidney failure who are treated with dialysis and transplantation is projected to increase from 340,000 in 1999 to 651,000 in 2010.[13]

Chronic renal failure can result from a number of conditions that cause permanent loss of nephrons, including diabetes, hypertension, glomerulonephritis, and polycystic kidney disease.[13–15] Diabetic kidney disease is the largest single cause of kidney failure in the United States.[13]

STAGES OF PROGRESSION

Regardless of cause, chronic renal failure results in loss of renal cells with progressive deterioration of glomerular filtration, tubular reabsorptive capacity, and endocrine functions of the kidneys.[14] All forms of renal failure are characterized by a reduction in the GFR, reflecting a corresponding reduction in the number of functional nephrons. The rate of nephron destruction differs from case to case, ranging from several months to many years.

CHRONIC RENAL FAILURE

- Chronic renal failure represents the end result of conditions that greatly reduce renal function by destroying renal nephrons and producing a marked decrease in the glomerular filtration rate (GFR).
- Because of the remarkable ability of the kidneys to adapt, signs of renal failure do not appear until 50% or more of the renal functional tissue has been destroyed. After this, signs of renal failure begin to appear as renal function moves from renal insufficiency (GFR 5% to 20% normal), to renal failure with a GFR of less than 5% of normal or a need for renal replacement therapy (dialysis or kidney transplantation).
- The manifestations of chronic renal failure represent the inability of the kidney to perform its normal functions in terms of regulating fluid and electrolyte balance, controlling blood pressure through fluid volume and the renin-angiotensin system, eliminating nitrogenous and other waste products, governing the red blood cell count through erythropoietin synthesis, and directing parathyroid and skeletal function through phosphate elimination and activation of vitamin D.

The progression of chronic renal failure usually occurs in four stages: diminished renal reserve, renal insufficiency, renal failure, and end-stage renal disease.[8] Typically, the signs and symptoms of chronic renal failure occur gradually and do not become evident until the disease is far advanced. This is because of the amazing compensatory ability of the kidneys. As kidney structures are destroyed, the remaining nephrons undergo structural and functional hypertrophy, each increasing its function as a means of compensating for those that have been lost (Fig. 36-3). It is only when the few remaining nephrons are destroyed that the manifestations of renal failure become evident.

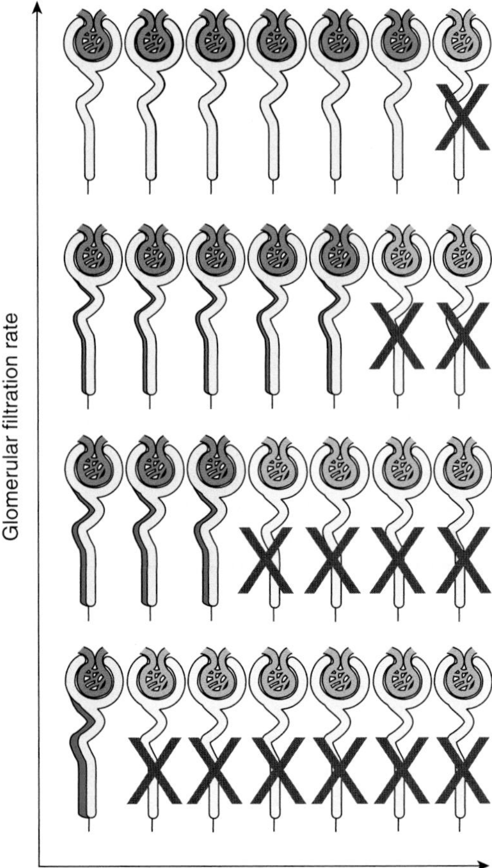

FIGURE 36-3 Relation of renal function and nephron mass. Each kidney contains 1 million tiny nephrons. A proportional relation exists between the number of nephrons affected by disease and the resulting glomerular filtration rate.

Diminished Renal Reserve

The GFR is considered the best measure of overall function of the kidney. The normal level of GFR varies with age, sex, and body size. The normal GFR for young healthy adults is approximately 120 to 130 mL/minute (1.73 mL/minute per mm^2).[13] Diminished renal reserve occurs when the GFR drops to approximately 50% of normal. At this point, the serum BUN and creatinine levels still are normal, and no symptoms of impaired renal function are evident. This is supported by the fact that many persons survive an entire lifetime with only one kidney. Because of the diminished reserve, the risk for development of azotemia increases with an additional renal insult, such as that due to nephrotoxic drugs.

Renal Insufficiency

Renal insufficiency represents a reduction in the GFR to 20% to 50% of normal. The kidneys initially have tremendous adaptive capabilities. As nephrons are destroyed, the remaining nephrons undergo changes to compensate for those that are lost. In the process, each of the remaining nephrons must filter more solute particles from the blood. Because the solute particles are osmotically active, they cause additional water to be lost in the urine. One of the earliest symptoms of renal insufficiency is *isosthenuria,* or polyuria with urine that is almost isotonic with plasma.[8] It is during this stage that azotemia, anemia, and hypertension also begin to appear.

Conservative treatment during this stage includes measures to retard deterioration of renal function and assist the body in managing the effects of impaired function. Urinary tract infections should be treated promptly, and medication with renal damaging potential should be avoided. Blood pressure control is important, as is control of blood sugar in persons with diabetes. Smoking cessation is recommended, particularly in persons with diabetic nephropathy.[14,15] Because the kidneys have difficulty eliminating the waste products of protein metabolism, a restricted-protein diet usually produces fewer uremic symptoms and slows progression of renal failure. The few remaining nephrons that constitute the functional reserve of the kidneys can be easily disrupted, after which renal failure progresses rapidly.

Renal Failure and End-Stage Renal Disease

Renal failure develops when the GFR is less than 20% of normal. At this point, the kidneys cannot regulate volume and solute composition, and edema, metabolic acidosis, and hyperkalemia develop. Overt uremia may ensue with neurologic, gastrointestinal, and cardiovascular manifestations.

End-stage renal disease (ESRD) occurs when the GFR is less than 5% of normal. Histologic findings of an end-stage kidney include a reduction in renal capillaries and scarring in the glomeruli. Atrophy and fibrosis are evident in the tubules. The mass of the kidneys usually is reduced. At this final phase of renal failure, treatment with dialysis or transplantation is necessary for survival.

The National Kidney Foundation Practice Guidelines, published in 2003, define renal failure "as either (1) a GFR of less than 15 mL/min per 1.73 m^2, which is accompanied by most signs and symptoms of uremia, or (2) a need to start renal replacement therapy (dialysis or transplantation)."[13] These guidelines point out that ESRD is an administrative term in the United States that indicates a person is treated with dialysis and transplantation, which is a condition for payment of health care by the Medicare ESRD program.[13]

CLINICAL MANIFESTATIONS

The manifestations of chronic renal failure include an accumulation of nitrogenous wastes; alterations in water, electrolyte, and acid-base balance; mineral and skeletal disorders; anemia and coagulation disorders; hypertension and alterations in cardiovascular function; gastrointestinal disorders; neurologic complications; disorders of skin integrity; and immunologic disorders[16] (Fig. 36-4). There currently are four target populations that comprise the entire population of persons with chronic renal failure: persons with chronic renal insufficiency, those with renal failure being treated with hemodialysis, those being treated with peritoneal dialysis, and renal transplant recipients. The manifestations of renal failure are determined largely by the extent of renal function that is present, coexisting disease conditions, and the type of renal replacement therapy that the person is receiving.

Accumulation of Nitrogenous Wastes

The accumulation of nitrogenous wastes is an early sign of renal failure, usually occurring before other symptoms become evident. Urea is one of the first nitrogenous wastes

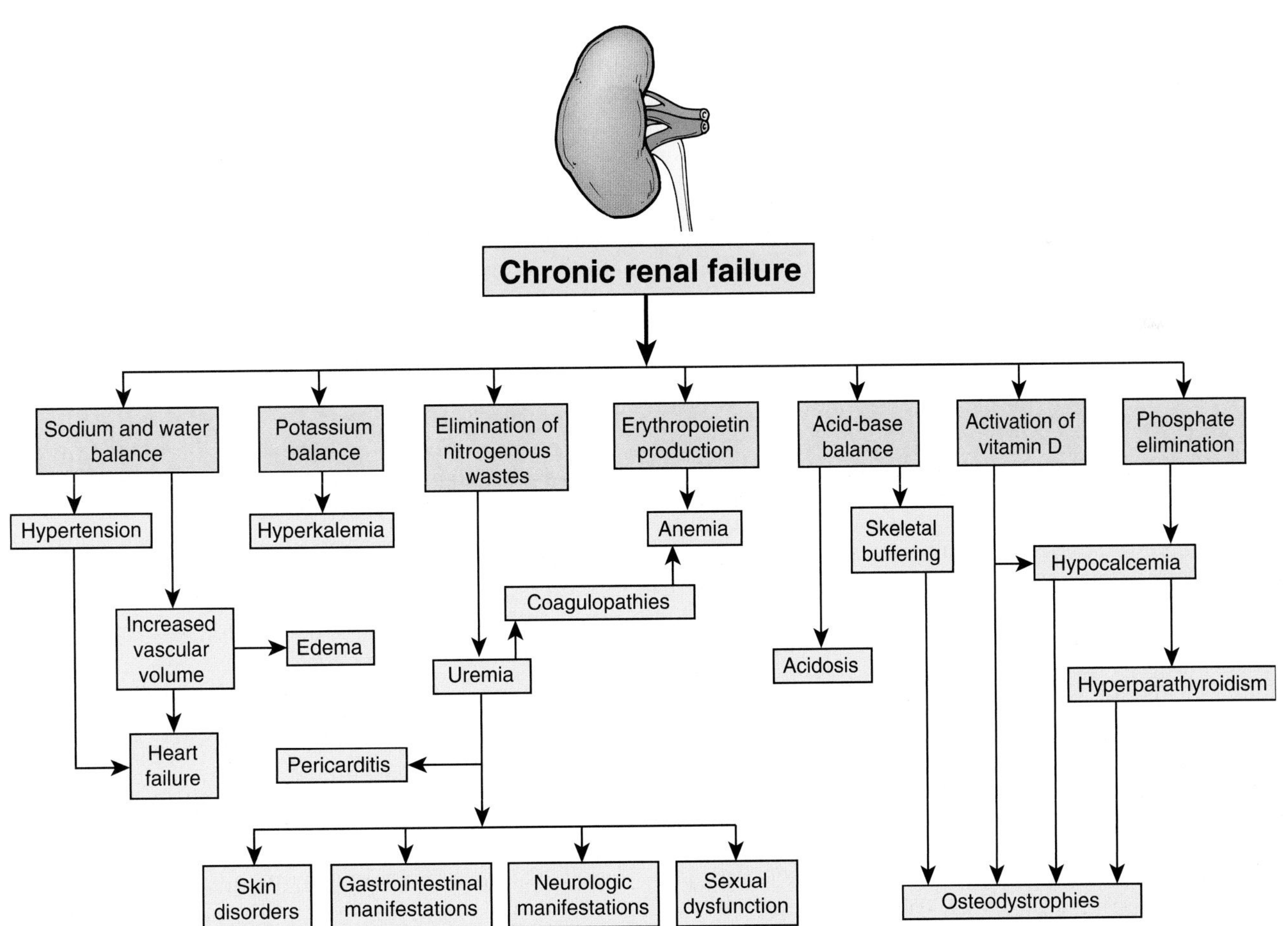

FIGURE 36-4 Manifestations of chronic renal failure.

to accumulate in the blood, and the BUN level becomes increasingly elevated as renal failure progresses. The normal concentration of urea in the plasma is approximately 20 mg/dL. In renal failure, this level may rise to as high as 800 mg/dL. Creatinine, a by-product of muscle metabolism, is freely filtered in the glomerulus and is not reabsorbed in the renal tubules. Creatinine is produced at a relatively constant rate, and any creatinine that is filtered in the glomerulus is lost in the urine rather than being reabsorbed into the blood. Thus, serum creatinine can be used as an indirect method for assessing the GFR and the extent of renal damage that has occurred in renal failure (see Chapter 32).

Uremia, which literally means "urine in the blood," is the term used to describe the clinical manifestations of renal failure. Few symptoms of uremia appear until at least two thirds of the nephrons have been destroyed. Uremia differs from azotemia, which merely indicates the accumulation of nitrogenous wastes in the blood and can occur without symptoms. The uremic state includes signs and symptoms of altered fluid, electrolyte, and acid-base balance; alterations in regulatory functions (*e.g.,* hypertension, anemia, osteodystrophy); and the effects of uremia on body function (*e.g.,* uremic encephalopathy, peripheral neuropathy, pruritus). At this stage, virtually every organ and structure in the body is affected. The symptoms at the onset of uremia (*e.g.,* weakness, fatigue, nausea, apathy) often are subtle. More severe symptoms include extreme weakness, frequent vomiting, lethargy, and confusion. Without treatment, coma and death follow.

Disorders of Water, Electrolyte, and Acid-Base Balance

Sodium and Water Balance. The kidneys function in the regulation of extracellular fluid volume. They do this by either eliminating or conserving sodium and water. Chronic renal failure can produce dehydration or fluid overload, depending on the pathology of the renal disease. In addition to volume regulation, the ability of the kidneys to concentrate the urine is diminished. In renal failure, the specific gravity of the urine becomes fixed (1.008 to 1.012) and varies little from voiding to voiding. Polyuria and nocturia are common.

As renal function declines further, the ability to regulate sodium excretion is reduced. The kidneys normally tolerate large variations in sodium intake while maintaining normal serum sodium levels. In chronic renal failure, they lose the ability to regulate sodium excretion. There is impaired ability to adjust to a sudden reduction in sodium intake and poor tolerance of an acute sodium overload. Volume depletion with an accompanying decrease in the GFR can occur with a restricted sodium intake or excess sodium loss caused by diarrhea or vomiting. Salt wasting is a common problem in advanced renal failure because of impaired tubular reabsorption of sodium. Increasing sodium intake in persons with chronic renal failure often improves the GFR and whatever renal function remains. In patients with associated hypertension, the possibility of increasing blood pressure or production of congestive heart failure often excludes supplemental sodium intake.

Potassium Balance. Approximately 90% of potassium excretion is through the kidneys. In renal failure, potassium excretion by each nephron increases as the kidneys adapt to a decrease in the GFR. As a result, hyperkalemia usually does not develop until renal function is severely compromised. Because of this adaptive mechanism, it usually is not necessary to restrict potassium intake in patients with chronic renal failure until the GFR has dropped below 10 mL/minute.[16] In patients with chronic renal failure, hyperkalemia often results from failure to follow dietary potassium restrictions and ingestion of medications that contain potassium, or from an endogenous release of potassium, as in trauma or infection.

Acid-Base Balance. The kidneys normally regulate blood pH by eliminating hydrogen ions produced in metabolic processes and regenerating bicarbonate. This is achieved through hydrogen ion secretion, sodium and bicarbonate reabsorption, and the production of ammonia, which acts as a buffer for titratable acids (see Chapter 34). With a decline in renal function, these mechanisms become impaired, and metabolic acidosis results. In chronic renal failure, acidosis seems to stabilize as the disease progresses, probably as a result of the tremendous buffering capacity of bone. However, this buffering action is thought to increase bone resorption and contribute to the skeletal disorders that occur in persons with chronic renal failure.

Mineral and Bone Disorders

Abnormalities of calcium, phosphate, and vitamin D metabolism occur early in the course of chronic renal failure.[17] The regulation of serum phosphate levels requires a daily urinary excretion of an amount equal to that ingested in the diet. With deteriorating renal function, phosphate excretion is impaired, and as a result, serum phosphate levels rise. At the same time, serum calcium levels, which are inversely regulated in relation to serum phosphate levels, fall (see Chapter 33). In turn, the drop in serum calcium stimulates parathyroid hormone (PTH) release, with a resultant increase in calcium resorption from bone. Most persons with ESRD develop a secondary hyperparathyroidism, the result of chronic stimulation of the parathyroid glands. Although serum calcium levels are maintained through increased PTH function, this adjustment is accomplished at the expense of the skeletal system and other body organs.

Vitamin D synthesis also is impaired in renal failure. The kidneys regulate vitamin D activity by converting the inactive form of vitamin D [25(OH) vitamin D_3] to its active form (1,25-OH_2 vitamin D_3). Decreased levels of active vitamin D lead to a decrease in intestinal absorption of calcium with a resultant increase in PTH levels. Vitamin D also regulates osteoblast differentiation, thereby affecting bone matrix formation and mineralization.

Skeletal Disorders. The term *renal osteodystrophy* is used to describe the skeletal complications of ESRD.[17,18] Several factors are thought to contribute to the development of renal osteodystrophy, including elevated serum phosphate levels, decreased serum calcium levels, impaired renal activation of vitamin D, and hyperparathyroidism. The skeletal changes that occur with renal failure have been divided into two major types of disorders: high-turnover and low-turnover osteodystrophy.[8] Inherent to both of these conditions is abnormal reabsorption and defective remodeling of bone (see Chapter 58).

High–bone-turnover osteodystrophy, sometimes referred to as *osteitis fibrosa*,[18] is characterized by increased bone resorption and formation, with bone resorption predominating. The disorder is associated with secondary hyperparathyroidism; altered vitamin D metabolism, along with resistance to the action of vitamin D; and impaired regulation of locally produced growth factors and inhibitors. There is an increase in both osteoblast and osteoclast numbers and activity. Although the osteoblasts produce excessive amounts of bone matrix, mineralization fails to keep pace, and there is a decrease in bone density and formation of porous and coarse-fibered bone. Cortical bone is affected more severely than cancellous bone. Marrow fibrosis is another component of osteitis fibrosa; it occurs in areas of increased bone cell activity. In advanced stages of the disorder, cysts may develop in the bone, a condition called *osteitis fibrosa cystica*.[18]

Low–bone-turnover osteodystrophy is characterized by decreased numbers of osteoblasts and low or reduced numbers of osteoclasts, a low rate of bone turnover, and an accumulation of unmineralized bone matrix.[19] There are two forms of low-turnover osteodystrophy: osteomalacia and adynamic osteodystrophy. *Osteomalacia* is characterized by a slow rate of bone formation and defects in bone mineralization. Several factors are thought to contribute to the development of osteomalacia in renal failure, including decreased levels of 25(OH) vitamin D_3, the precursor of activated 1,25-OH_2 vitamin D_3, and metabolic acidosis. It is thought that 25(OH) vitamin D_3 deficiency is a major risk factor for defective bone mineralization, completely independent of 1,25-OH_2 vitamin D_3 levels.[16] Metabolic acidosis is thought to have a direct effect on both osteoblastic and osteoclastic activity, as well as on the mineralization process, by decreasing the availability of trivalent phosphate.[16] Until the 1980s, osteomalacia in renal failure resulted mainly from aluminum intoxication. Aluminum intoxication causes decreased and defective mineralization of bone by existing osteoblasts and more long-term inhibition of osteoblast differentiation. During the 1970s and 1980s, it was discovered that accumulation of aluminum from water used in dialysis and aluminum salts used as phosphate binders caused osteomalacia and adynamic bone disease.[19] This discovery led to a change in the composition of dialysis solutions and substitution of calcium carbonate for aluminum salts as phosphate binders. As a result, the prevalence of osteomalacia in persons with ESRD is declining.

The second type of low-turnover osteodystrophy, *adynamic osteodystrophy*, is characterized by a low number of osteoblasts, the osteoclast number being normal or reduced.[19] In persons with adynamic bone disease, bone remodeling is greatly reduced, and the bone surfaces become hypocellular. Adynamic bone disease is associated with an increased fracture rate. The disease is associated with a "relative hyperparathyroidism." It has been suggested that hypersecretion of PTH may be necessary to maintain normal rates of bone formation in persons with ESRD. Thus, this form of renal osteodystrophy is seen more commonly in persons with ESRD who do not have secondary hyperparathyroidism (*i.e.*, those who have been treated with parathyroidectomy) or have been overtreated with calcium and vitamin D.

The symptoms of renal osteodystrophy, which occur late in the disease, include bone tenderness and muscle weakness. Proximal muscle weakness in the lower extremities is common, making it difficult to get out of a chair or climb stairs.[17] Fractures are more common with low-turnover osteomalacia and adynamic renal bone disease.

Early treatment of hyperphosphatemia and hypocalcemia is important to prevent or slow long-term skeletal complications.[20,21] Milk products and other foods high in phosphorus content are restricted in the diet. Phosphate-binding antacids (aluminum salts, calcium carbonate, or calcium acetate) may be prescribed to decrease absorption of phosphate from the gastrointestinal tract. Calcium-containing phosphate binders can lead to hypercalcemia, thus worsening soft tissue calcification, especially in persons receiving vitamin D therapy. Aluminum-containing antacids can contribute to the development of osteodystrophy. To avoid these side effects, a new, well-tolerated aluminum- and calcium-free binder (sevelamer) has been developed. Sevelamer is a hydrogel that is resistant to digestive degradation and not absorbed.

Activated forms of vitamin D (*e.g.*, calcitriol) and calcium supplements often are used to facilitate intestinal absorption of calcium, increase serum calcium levels, and prevent parathyroid gland overactivity. Although calcitriol is effective in controlling PTH overproduction and improving bone structure, its stimulatory effects on intestinal absorption of both calcium and phosphorus, combined with its suppressive effects on bone turnover, predispose to hypercalcemia and hyperphosphatemia and an increase in the calcium-phosphate ($Ca \times P$) product (see Chapter 33). Hypercalcemia and an elevated $Ca \times P$ product increase the risk for metastatic calcification, a complication associated with cardiac dysfunction and death; the risk is greater in patients who are also taking calcium-based phosphate binders.[21,22] Several vitamin D analogs (paricalcitol, doxercalciferol) that prevent hyperactivity of the parathyroid gland without induction of hypercalcemia and hyperphosphatemia have recently become available.[21]

Hematologic Disorders

Anemia. Chronic anemia is the most profound hematologic alteration that accompanies renal failure. Anemia first appears when the GFR falls below 40 mL/minute, and is present in most persons with ESRD.[23] Nephrologists have defined clinically significant anemia as a hemoglobin level of less than 10 g/dL and a hematocrit of less than 30%, in the absence of erythropoietin therapy.[24] An analysis of patients beginning dialysis in the United States found that 67% had a hematocrit of less than 30%, and 51% had a hematocrit of less than 28%.[25]

The kidneys are the primary site for the production of the hormone *erythropoietin,* which controls red blood cell production. In renal failure, erythropoietin production usually is insufficient to stimulate adequate red blood cell production by the bone marrow. The accumulation of uremic toxins further suppresses red cell production in the bone marrow, and the cells that are produced have a shortened life span. Iron is essential for erythropoiesis. Many persons on maintenance hemodialysis also are iron deficient because of blood sampling and accidental loss of blood during dialysis. Other causes of iron deficiency include factors such as anorexia and dietary restrictions that limit intake.

When untreated, anemia causes or contributes to weakness, fatigue, depression, insomnia, and decreased cognitive function. There also is an increasing concern regarding the physiologic effects of anemia on cardiovascular function. The anemia of renal failure produces a decrease in blood viscosity and a compensatory increase in heart rate. The decreased blood viscosity also exacerbates peripheral vasodilatation and contributes to decreased vascular resistance. Cardiac output increases in a compensatory fashion to maintain tissue perfusion. Echocardiographic studies after initiation of chronic dialysis have shown ventricular dilatation with compensatory left ventricular hypertrophy.[23] Anemia also limits myocardial oxygen supply, particularly in persons with coronary heart disease, leading to angina pectoris and other ischemic events.[24] Thus, anemia, when coupled with hypertension, may be a major contributing factor to the development of left ventricular dysfunction and congestive heart failure in persons with ESRD.

A remarkable advance in medical management of ESRD occurred with the availability of recombinant human erythropoietin (rhEPO). Since its approval by the U.S. Food and Drug Administration in June 1989, rhEPO therapy has been used to maintain hematocrit levels in the range of 28% to 33%, with an upper limit of 36%. It currently is recommended that the hematocrit be maintained at the higher target range of 33% to 36% (hemoglobin, 11 to 12 g/dL).[26,27] Secondary benefits of treating anemia with rhEPO, previously attributed to the correction of uremia, include improvement in appetite, energy level, sexual function, skin color, and hair and nail growth, and reduced cold intolerance. Because worsening of hypertension and seizures have occurred when the hematocrit was raised too suddenly, frequent measurements of hematocrit are necessary.

Because iron deficiency is common among persons with chronic renal failure, iron supplementation often is needed. Iron can be given orally or intravenously. Intravenous iron (iron dextran and ferric sodium gluconate) is used for treatment of persons who are not able to maintain adequate iron status with oral iron. Because intravenously administered iron may cause serious immediate and delayed hypersensitivity reactions, including life-threatening anaphylactic reactions, care is required when prescribing and administering these drugs.[26,27]

Coagulopathies. Bleeding disorders are manifested by epistaxis, menorrhagia, gastrointestinal bleeding, and bruising of the skin and subcutaneous tissues. Although platelet production often is normal in ESRD, platelet function is impaired. Coagulative function improves with dialysis but does not completely normalize, suggesting that uremia contributes to the problem. Anemia may accentuate the problem by changing the position of the platelets with respect to the vessel wall. Normally, the red cells occupy the center of the bloodstream, and the platelets are in the skimming layer along the endothelial surface. In anemia, the platelets become dispersed, impairing the platelet–endothelial cell adherence needed to initiate hemostasis.[28]

Cardiovascular Disorders

Cardiovascular disease is the major cause of death in patients with ESRD. The overall mortality rate from cardiovascular disease in people with renal failure is 30 times that of the general population. Even after stratification for age, the incidence of cardiovascular disease remains 10 to 20 times higher in persons with ESRD than in the general population.[29]

Hypertension. Hypertension commonly is an early manifestation of chronic renal failure. The mechanisms that produce hypertension in ESRD are multifactorial; they include an increased vascular volume, elevation of peripheral vascular resistance, decreased levels of renal vasodilator prostaglandins, and increased activity of the renin-angiotensin system.[30]

Early identification and aggressive treatment of hypertension has been shown to slow the rate of renal impairment in many types of renal disease. Treatment involves salt and water restriction and the use of antihypertensive medications to control blood pressure. Many persons with renal insufficiency need to take several antihypertensive medications to control blood pressure (see Chapter 25).

Heart Disease. The spectrum of cardiovascular disease includes left ventricular hypertrophy and ischemic heart disease. Congestive heart failure and pulmonary edema tend to occur in the late stages of renal failure. Coexisting conditions that have been identified as contributing to the burden of cardiovascular disease include hypertension, anemia, diabetes mellitus, dyslipidemia, and coagulopathies. Anemia, in particular, has been correlated with the presence of left ventricular hypertrophy. PTH also may play a role in the pathogenesis of cardiomyopathy in renal failure.

People with renal failure tend to have an increased prevalence of left ventricular dysfunction, with both depressed left ventricular ejection fraction, as in systolic dysfunction, and impaired ventricular filling, as in diastolic failure[31,32] (see Chapter 28). Multiple factors lead to development of left ventricular dysfunction, including extracellular fluid overload, shunting of blood through an arteriovenous fistula for dialysis, and anemia. These abnormalities, coupled with the hypertension that often is present, cause increased myocardial work and oxygen demand, with eventual development of heart failure.

Pericarditis. Pericarditis occurs in approximately 20% of persons receiving chronic dialysis.[33] It can result from metabolic toxins associated with the uremic state or from dialysis. The manifestations of uremic pericarditis resemble those of viral pericarditis, with all its potential complications, including cardiac tamponade (see Chapter 26).

The presenting signs include mild to severe chest pain with respiratory accentuation and a pericardial friction rub. Fever is variable in the absence of infection and is more common in dialysis than uremic pericarditis.

Gastrointestinal Disorders

Anorexia, nausea, and vomiting are common in patients with uremia, along with a metallic taste in the mouth that further depresses the appetite. Early-morning nausea is common. Ulceration and bleeding of the gastrointestinal mucosa may develop, and hiccups are common. A possible cause of nausea and vomiting is the decomposition of urea by intestinal flora, resulting in a high concentration of ammonia. PTH increases gastric acid secretion and contributes to gastrointestinal problems. Nausea and vomiting often improve with restriction of dietary protein and after initiation of dialysis, and disappear after kidney transplantation.

Disorders of Neural Function

Many persons with chronic renal failure have alterations in peripheral and central nervous system function. Peripheral neuropathy, or involvement of the peripheral nerves, affects the lower limbs more frequently than the upper limbs. It is symmetric and affects both sensory and motor function. Neuropathy is caused by atrophy and demyelination of nerve fibers, possibly caused by uremic toxins. Restless legs syndrome is a manifestation of peripheral nerve involvement and can be seen in as many as two thirds of patients on dialysis. This syndrome is characterized by creeping, prickling, and itching sensations that typically are more intense at rest. Temporary relief is obtained by moving the legs. A burning sensation of the feet, which may be followed by muscle weakness and atrophy, is a manifestation of uremia.

The central nervous system disturbances in uremia are similar to those caused by other metabolic and toxic disorders. Sometimes referred to as *uremic encephalopathy,* the condition is poorly understood and may result, at least in part, from an excess of toxic organic acids that alter neural function. Electrolyte abnormalities, such as sodium shifts, also may contribute. The manifestations are more closely related to the progress of the uremic disorder than to the level of the metabolic end products. Reductions in alertness and awareness are the earliest and most significant indications of uremic encephalopathy. These often are followed by an inability to fix attention, loss of recent memory, and perceptual errors in identifying persons and objects. Delirium and coma occur late in the course; seizures are the preterminal event.

Disorders of motor function commonly accompany the neurologic manifestations of uremic encephalopathy. During the early stages, there often is difficulty in performing fine movements of the extremities; the gait becomes unsteady and clumsy with tremulousness of movement. Asterixis (dorsiflexion movements of the hands and feet) typically occurs as the disease progresses. It can be elicited by having the person hyperextend his or her arms at the elbow and wrist with the fingers spread apart. If asterixis is present, this position causes side-to-side flapping movements of the fingers.

Altered Immune Function

Infection is a common complication and cause of hospitalization and death of patients with chronic renal failure. Immunologic abnormalities decrease the efficiency of the immune response to infection. All aspects of inflammation and immune function may be affected adversely by the high levels of urea and metabolic wastes, including a decrease in granulocyte count, impaired humoral and cell-mediated immunity, and defective phagocyte function. The acute inflammatory response and delayed-type hypersensitivity response are impaired. Although persons with ESRD have normal humoral responses to vaccines, a more aggressive immunization program may be needed. Skin and mucosal barriers to infection also may be defective. In persons who are maintained on dialysis, vascular access devices are common portals of entry for pathogens. Many persons with ESRD fail to mount a fever with infection, making the diagnosis more difficult.

Disorders of Skin Integrity

Skin manifestations are common in persons with renal failure. The skin often is pale owing to anemia and may have a sallow, yellow-brown hue. The skin and mucous membranes often are dry, and subcutaneous bruising is common. Skin dryness is caused by a reduction in perspiration owing to the decreased size of sweat glands and the diminished activity of oil glands. Pruritus is common; it results from the high serum phosphate levels and the development of phosphate crystals that occur with hyperparathyroidism. Severe scratching and repeated needlesticks, especially with hemodialysis, break the skin integrity and increase the risk for infection. In the advanced stages of untreated renal failure, urea crystals may precipitate on the skin as a result of the high urea concentration in body fluids. The fingernails may become thin and brittle, with a dark band just behind the leading edge of the nail, followed by a white band. This appearance is known as *Terry's nails.*

Sexual Dysfunction

The cause of sexual dysfunction in men and women with chronic renal failure is unclear. The cause probably is multifactorial and may result from high levels of uremic toxins, neuropathy, altered endocrine function, psychological factors, and medications (*e.g.,* antihypertensive drugs). Alterations in physiologic sexual responses, reproductive ability, and libido are common.

Impotence occurs in as many as 56% of male patients on dialysis.[34] Derangements of the pituitary and gonadal hormones, such as decreases in testosterone levels and increases in prolactin and luteinizing hormone levels, are common and cause erectile difficulties and decreased spermatocyte counts. Loss of libido may result from chronic anemia and decreased testosterone levels. Several drugs, such as exogenous testosterone and bromocriptine, have been used in an attempt to return hormone levels to normal.

Impaired sexual function in women is manifested by abnormal levels of progesterone, luteinizing hormone, and prolactin. Hypofertility, menstrual abnormalities, decreased vaginal lubrication, and various orgasmic problems have been described.[35] Amenorrhea is common among women who are on dialysis therapy.

Elimination of Drugs

The kidneys are responsible for the elimination of many drugs and their metabolites.[9] Renal failure and its treatment can interfere with the absorption, distribution, and elimination of drugs. The administration of large quantities of phosphate-binding antacids to control hyperphosphatemia and hypocalcemia in patients with advanced renal failure interferes with the absorption of some drugs. Many drugs are bound to plasma proteins, such as albumin, for transport in the body; the unbound portion of the drug is available to act at the various receptor sites and is free to be metabolized. A decrease in plasma proteins, particularly albumin, that occurs in many persons with renal failure results in less protein-bound drug and greater amounts of free drug.

In the process of metabolism, some drugs form intermediate metabolites that are toxic if not eliminated. Some pathways of drug metabolism, such as hydrolysis, are slowed with uremia. In persons with diabetes, for example, insulin requirements may be reduced as renal function deteriorates. Decreased elimination by the kidneys allows drugs or their metabolites to accumulate in the body and requires that drug dosages be adjusted accordingly. Some drugs contain unwanted nitrogen, sodium, potassium, and magnesium and must be avoided in patients with renal failure. Penicillin, for example, contains potassium. Nitrofurantoin and ammonium chloride add to the body's nitrogen pool. Many antacids contain magnesium. Because of problems with drug dosing and elimination, persons with renal failure should be cautioned against the use of over-the-counter remedies.

TREATMENT

During the past several decades, an increasing number of persons have required renal replacement therapy with dialysis or transplantation. The growing volume is largely attributable to the improvement in treatment and more liberal policies regarding who is treated. Between 1980 and 1992, there was a twofold reported increase in treatment for renal failure.[36] In 2000, almost 275,053 persons were maintained by dialysis therapy in the United States, and another 14,311 underwent kidney transplantation.[37]

Medical Management

Chronic renal failure can be treated by conservative management of renal insufficiency and by renal replacement therapy with dialysis or transplantation. Conservative treatment consists of measures to prevent or retard deterioration in remaining renal function and to assist the body in compensating for the existing impairment. Interventions that have been shown to significantly retard the progression of chronic renal insufficiency include dietary protein restriction and blood pressure normalization. Various interventions are used to compensate for reduced renal function and correct the resulting anemia, hypocalcemia, and acidosis. These interventions often are used in conjunction with dialysis therapy for patients with ESRD.

Dialysis and Transplantation

Dialysis or renal replacement therapy is indicated when advanced uremia or serious electrolyte imbalances are present. The choice between dialysis and transplantation is dictated by age, related health problems, donor availability, and personal preference. Although transplantation often is the treatment preference, dialysis plays a critical role as a treatment method for ESRD. It is life sustaining for persons who are not candidates for transplantation or who are awaiting transplantation. There are two broad categories of dialysis: hemodialysis and peritoneal dialysis.

Hemodialysis. The basic principles of hemodialysis have remained unchanged over the years, although new technology has improved the efficiency and speed of dialysis.[38,39] A hemodialysis system, or artificial kidney, consists of three parts: a blood compartment, a dialysis fluid compartment, and a cellophane membrane that separates the two compartments. There are several types of dialyzers; all incorporate these parts, and all function in a similar manner.

The cellophane membrane is semipermeable, permitting all molecules except blood cells and plasma proteins to move freely in both directions—from the blood into the dialyzing solution and from the dialyzing solution into the blood. The direction of flow is determined by the concentration of the substances contained in the two solutions. The waste products and excess electrolytes in the blood normally diffuse into the dialyzing solution. If there is a need to replace or add substances, such as bicarbonate, to the blood, these can be added to the dialyzing solution (Fig. 36-5).

During dialysis, blood moves from an artery through the tubing and blood chamber in the dialysis machine and then back into the body through a vein. Access to the vascular system is accomplished through an external arteriovenous shunt (*i.e.*, tubing implanted into an artery and a vein) or, more commonly, through an internal arteriovenous fistula (*i.e.*, anastomosis of a vein to an artery, usually in the forearm). Heparin is used to prevent clotting during the dialysis treatment; it can be administered continuously or intermittently. Problems that may occur during dialysis, depending on the rates of blood flow and solute removal, include hypotension, nausea, vomiting, muscle cramps, headache, chest pain, and disequilibrium syndrome.

Most persons are dialyzed three times each week for 3 to 4 hours; treatment is determined by kinetic profiles, referred to as Kt/V values, which consider dialyzer size, dialysate, flow rate, time of dialysis, and body size.[40] Many dialysis centers provide the option for patients to learn how to perform hemodialysis at home.

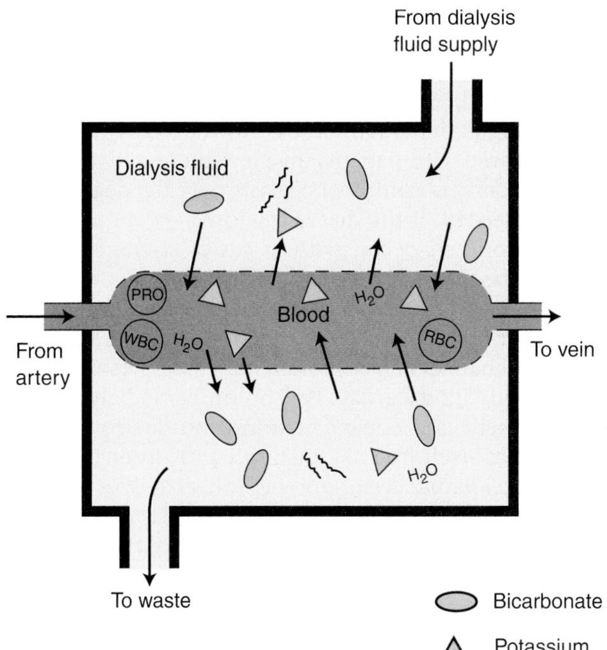

FIGURE 36-5 Schematic diagram of a hemodialysis system. The blood compartment and dialysis solution compartment are separated by a cellophane membrane. This membrane is porous enough to allow all the constituents, except the plasma proteins and blood cells, to diffuse between the two compartments.

Peritoneal Dialysis. Peritoneal dialysis was introduced in the mid-1970s. Improvements in technology and the ability to deliver adequate dialysis resulted in improved outcomes and the acceptance of peritoneal dialysis as a renal replacement therapy.

The same principles of diffusion, osmosis, and ultrafiltration that apply to hemodialysis apply to peritoneal dialysis. The thin serous membrane of the peritoneal cavity serves as the dialyzing membrane. A Silastic catheter is surgically implanted in the peritoneal cavity below the umbilicus to provide access. The catheter is tunneled through subcutaneous tissue and exits on the side of the abdomen (Fig. 36-6). The dialysis process involves instilling a sterile dialyzing solution (usually 2 L) through the catheter over a period of approximately 10 minutes. The solution then is allowed to remain, or dwell, in the peritoneal cavity for a prescribed amount of time, during which the metabolic end products and extracellular fluid diffuse into the dialysis solution. At the end of the dwell time, the dialysis fluid is drained out of the peritoneal cavity by gravity into a sterile bag. Glucose in the dialysis solution accounts for water removal. Commercial dialysis solution is available in 1.5%, 2.5%, and 4.25% dextrose concentrations. Solutions with higher dextrose levels increase osmosis, causing more fluid to be removed. As with hemodialysis, Kt/V values are used to evaluate adequacy of peritoneal dialysis.

Peritoneal dialysis can be performed at home or in a center, by an automated or manual system, and on an intermittent or continuous basis—all with variations in the number of exchanges and in dwell time. Individual preference, manual ability, lifestyle, knowledge of the procedure, and physiologic response to treatment are used to determine the dialysis schedule. The most common method is continuous ambulatory peritoneal dialysis (CAPD), a self-care procedure in which the person manages the dialysis procedure and the type of solution (*i.e.,* dextrose concentration) used at home. CAPD involves instilling dialysate into the peritoneal cavity and rolling up the bag and tubing and securing them under clothing during the dwell. After the dwell time is completed (4 to 6 hours during the day), the bag is unrolled and lowered, allowing the waste-containing dialysis solution to drain from the peritoneal cavity into the bag. Each exchange, which involves draining the solution and infusing a new solution, requires approximately 30 to 45 minutes. Four exchanges usually are performed each day. The continuous rather than intermittent nature of CAPD ensures that the rapid fluctuations in extracellular fluid volume associated with hemodialysis are avoided, and dietary restrictions can be liberalized somewhat.

Potential problems with peritoneal dialysis include infection, catheter malfunction, dehydration caused by excessive fluid removal, hyperglycemia, and hernia. The most serious complication is infection, which can occur at the catheter exit site, in the subcutaneous tunnel, or in the peritoneal cavity (*i.e.,* peritonitis).

Transplantation. Greatly improved success rates have made kidney transplantation the treatment of choice for many patients with chronic renal failure. The availability of donor organs continues to limit the number of transplantations performed each year. Donor organs are obtained from cadavers and living related donors (*e.g.,* parent, sibling). Transplants from living nonrelated donors (*e.g.,* spouse) have

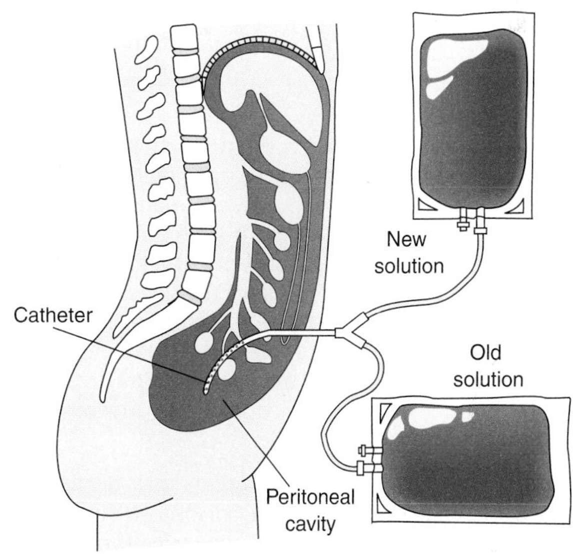

FIGURE 36-6 Peritoneal dialysis. A semipermeable membrane, richly supplied with small blood vessels, lines the peritoneal cavity. With dialysate dwelling in the peritoneal cavity, waste products diffuse from the network of blood cells into the dialysate.

been used in cases of suitable ABO and tissue compatibility. Of the transplantations performed in 2000, 8884 were from cadaver donors, 4052 were from living related donors, and 1375 were from living unrelated donors.[37] The 1-year graft survival rates for cadaver transplants were 95.0%, and for living related donors, 98.1%.[37]

The success of transplantation depends primarily on the degree of histocompatibility, adequate organ preservation, and immunologic management.[41] Maintenance immunosuppressive therapy typically consists of corticosteroids, azathioprine, and cyclosporine (or tacrolimus [FK506] or sirolimus). Interleukin-2, a cytokine, plays an essential role in T- and B-cell activation (see Chapter 19). Cyclosporine and tacrolimus inhibit interleukin-2 synthesis, and sirolimus inhibits the T-cell response to interleukin. Genetically engineered antibodies that selectively target interleukin receptors also are available. Monoclonal antibodies such as OKT-3 (directed against the CD3 T-cell receptor) and antilymphocyte antibodies may be used as induction therapy. Because of the increased number of effective immunosuppressive agents that have become available, lower corticosteroid doses are used, resulting in reduced cushingoid effects after transplantation.

Rejection, which is categorized as acute and chronic, can occur at any time (see Chapter 21). Acute rejection most commonly occurs during the first several months after transplantation and involves a cellular response with the proliferation of T lymphocytes. Chronic rejection can occur months to years after transplantation. Because chronic rejection is caused by both cellular and humoral immunity, it does not respond to increased immunosuppressive therapy.

Maintenance immunosuppressive therapy and increased use of immunosuppression to treat rejection predispose the person to a spectrum of infectious complications. Prophylactic antimicrobials may be prescribed to decrease the incidence of common infections, such as candidiasis, herpesvirus infections, and *Pneumocystis carinii* pneumonia. Other infections, such as cytomegalovirus infection and aspergillosis, are seen with chronic immunosuppression.

Dietary Management

A major component in the treatment of chronic renal failure is dietary management. The goal of dietary treatment is to provide optimum nutrition while maintaining tolerable levels of metabolic wastes. The specific diet prescription depends on the type and severity of renal disease and on the dialysis modality. Because of the severe restrictions placed on food and fluid intake, these diets may be complicated and unappetizing. After kidney transplantation, some dietary restrictions still may be necessary, even when renal function is normal, to control the adverse effects from immunosuppressive medication.

Protein. Restriction of dietary proteins may decrease the progress of renal impairment in persons with advanced renal disease. Proteins are broken down to form nitrogenous wastes, and reducing the amount of protein in the diet lowers the BUN and reduces symptoms. Moreover, a high-protein diet is high in phosphates and inorganic acids. The Modification of Diet in Renal Disease (MDRD) Study, which was conducted in 15 university hospital outpatient nephrology clinics and included 255 patients between the ages of 18 and 70 years, demonstrated a slower decline in GFR among patients randomized to the very-low-protein diet compared with patients on a low-protein diet.[42]

Considerable controversy exists over the degree of restriction needed. If the diet is too low in protein, protein malnutrition can occur, with a loss of strength, muscle mass, and body weight. Results of the MDRD Study indicate that protein requirements can be met by providing 0.6 g of protein per kilogram of body weight per day (g/kg/day).[43] The maintenance dietary protein intake for persons on hemodialysis is 1.2 g/kg/day. Persons on hemodialysis experience protein and energy malnutrition due to anorexia from uremia itself, the dialysis procedure, intercurrent illness, and acidemia. Persons on peritoneal dialysis have significant protein losses, ranging from 5 to 15 g/day, through dialysis and require a dietary protein intake of 1.2 to 1.3 g/kg/day.[44] At least 50% of the protein intake should consist of proteins of high biologic value, such as those in eggs, lean meat, and milk, which are rich in essential amino acids. Proteins with a high biologic value are believed to promote the reuse of endogenous nitrogen, decreasing the amount of nitrogenous wastes that are produced and ameliorating the symptoms of uremia. In reusing nitrogen, the proteins ingested in the diet are broken down into their constituent amino acids and recycled in the synthesis of protein required by the body. In contrast to proteins with a high biologic value, fewer than half of the amino acids in cereal proteins are reused. Amino acids that are not reused to build body proteins are broken down and form the end products of protein metabolism, such as urea.

Carbohydrates, Fat, and Calories. With renal failure, adequate calories in the form of carbohydrates and fat are required to meet energy needs. This is particularly important when the protein content of the diet is severely restricted. If sufficient calories are not available, the limited protein in the diet goes into energy production, or body tissue itself is used for energy purposes. Caloric intake for persons on CAPD includes food intake and calories absorbed from the dialysis solution. A 2-L bag of 1.5% dialysate solution equals 105 calories, and a 4.25% solution delivers 289 calories.

Potassium. When the GFR falls to extremely low levels in ESRD or when undergoing hemodialysis therapy, dietary restriction of potassium becomes mandatory. Using salt substitutes that contain potassium, or ingesting fruits, fruit juice, chocolate, potatoes, or other high-potassium foods can cause hyperkalemia. Most persons on CAPD do not need to limit potassium intake and often may even need to increase intake.

Sodium and Fluid Intake. The sodium and fluid restrictions depend on the kidneys' ability to excrete sodium and water and must be individually determined. Renal disease of glomerular origin is more likely to contribute to sodium retention, whereas tubular dysfunction causes salt wasting. Fluid intake in excess of what the kidneys can excrete causes circulatory overload, edema, and water intoxication. Thirst is a common problem among patients on hemodialysis, often resulting in large weight gains between treatments. Inadequate intake, on the other hand, causes volume depletion and hypotension and can cause further decreases in the already compromised GFR. It is common practice to allow a daily fluid intake of 500 to 800 mL, which is equal to insensible water loss plus a quantity equal to the 24-hour urine output.

In summary, chronic renal failure results from the destructive effects of many forms of renal disease. Regardless of the cause, the consequences of nephron destruction in ESRD are alterations in the filtration, reabsorption, and endocrine functions of the kidneys. The progression of chronic renal failure usually occurs in four stages: diminished renal reserve, renal insufficiency, renal failure, and ESRD. Renal insufficiency represents a reduction in the GFR to approximately 20% to 50% of normal; renal failure, a reduction to less than 20% to 25% of normal; and ESRD, a decrease in GFR to less than 5% of normal.

End-stage renal disease affects almost every body system. It causes an accumulation of nitrogenous wastes (*i.e.*, azotemia), alters sodium and water excretion, and alters regulation of body levels of potassium, phosphate, calcium, and magnesium. It also causes skeletal disorders, anemia, alterations in cardiovascular function, neurologic disturbances, gastrointestinal dysfunction, and discomforting skin changes.

The treatment of ESRD can be divided into two types: conservative management of renal insufficiency and renal replacement therapy with dialysis or transplantation. Conservative treatment consists of measures to prevent or retard deterioration in remaining renal function and to assist the body in compensating for the existing impairment. Interventions that have been shown to retard significantly the progression of chronic renal insufficiency include dietary protein restriction and blood pressure normalization. Activated vitamin D can be used to increase calcium absorption and control secondary hyperparathyroidism. Recombinant human erythropoietin is used to treat the profound anemia that occurs in persons with ESRD.

Renal Failure in Children and Elderly Persons

After completing this section of the chapter, you should be able to meet the following objectives:

- List the causes of renal failure in children and describe the special problems of children with ESRD
- State why renal failure is so common in the elderly and describe measures to prevent or delay the onset of ESRD in this population
- Describe the treatment of ESRD in children and the elderly

Although the spectrum of renal disease among children and elderly persons is similar to that of adults, several unique issues affecting these groups warrant further discussion.

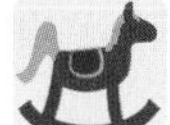

CHRONIC RENAL FAILURE IN CHILDREN

The true incidence of chronic renal failure in infants and children is unknown. Available data suggest that 1% to 2% of patients with chronic renal failure are in the pediatric age range.[44] The causes of chronic renal failure in children include congenital malformations, inherited disorders, acquired diseases, and metabolic syndromes. The underlying cause correlates closely with the age of the child. In children younger than 5 years of age, chronic renal failure is commonly the result of congenital malformations such renal dysplasia or obstructive uropathy.[45] After 5 years of age, acquired diseases (*e.g.*, glomerulonephritis) and inherited disorders (*e.g.*, familial juvenile nephronophthisis) predominate.[45] Chronic renal failure related to metabolic disorders such as hyperoxaluria and inherited disorders such as polycystic kidney disease may present throughout childhood.[45]

The stages of progression of chronic renal failure in children is similar to that for adults: mild reduction of GFR to 60 to 89 mL/minute per 1.73 m^2; moderate reduction of GFR to 30 to 59 mL/minute per 1.73 m^2; severe reduction in GFR to 15 to 29 mL/minute per 1.73 m^2; and kidney failure with a GFR of less than 15 mL/minute per 1.73 m^2, with a need for renal replacement therapy. Because the GFR is much lower in infancy and undergoes gradual changes in relation to body size during the first 2 years of age, these values apply only to children older than 2 years of age.[46]

The manifestations of chronic renal failure in children are quite varied and dependent on the underlying disease condition. Features of renal disease that are marked during childhood include severe growth impairment, developmental delay, delay in sexual maturation, bone abnormalities, and development of psychosocial problems. Critical growth periods occur during the first 2 years of life and during adolescence. Physical growth and cognitive development occur at a slower rate as consequences of renal disease, especially among children with congenital renal disease.[47] Puberty usually occurs at a later age in children with renal failure, partly because of endocrine abnormalities. Renal osteodystrophy is more common and extensive in children than in adults because of the presence of open epiphyses. As a result, metaphyseal fractures, bone pain, impaired bone growth, short stature, and osteitis fibrosa cystica occur with greater frequency. Some hereditary renal diseases, such as medullary cystic disease, have patterns of skeletal involvement that further complicate the problems of renal osteodystrophy. Factors related to impaired growth include deficient nutrition, anemia, renal osteodystrophy, chronic acidosis, and cases of nephrotic syndrome that require high-dose corticosteroid therapy.

Success of treatment depends on the level of bone maturation at the initiation of therapy. Nutrition is believed to be the most important determinant during infancy.[48] During childhood, growth hormone is important, and gonadotropic hormones become important during puberty.[48] Parental heights provide a means of assessing growth potential (see Chapter 42). For many children, catch-up growth is important because a growth deficit frequently is established during the first months of life. Recombinant human growth hormone therapy has been used to improve growth in children with ESRD.[48,49] Success of treatment depends on the level of bone maturation at the initiation of therapy.

All forms of renal replacement therapy can be safely and reliably used for children. Children typically are treated with CAPD or transplantation to optimize growth and development.[45] An alternative to CAPD is continuous cyclic peritoneal dialysis. The procedure reverses the schedule of CAPD by providing the exchanges at night rather than during the day. The exchanges are performed automatically during sleep by a simple cycler machine. Renal transplantation is considered the best alternative for children.[44,45] Early transplantation in young children is regarded as the best way to promote physical growth, improve cognitive function, and foster psychosocial development.[50–51] Immunosuppressive therapy in children is similar to that used in adults. All of these immunosuppressive agents have side effects, including increased risk for infection. Corticosteroids, which have been the mainstay of chronic immunosuppressive therapy for decades, carry the risk for hypertension, orthopedic complications (especially aseptic necrosis), cataracts, and growth retardation.

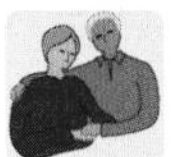

CHRONIC RENAL FAILURE IN ELDERLY PERSONS

Since the mid-1980s, there have been increasing numbers of elderly persons accepted to ESRD programs. In 1998, 20.6% of persons being treated for ESRD were 65 to 74 years of age, and 12.9% were older than 75 years of age.[52] Among elderly persons, the presentation and course of renal failure may be altered because of age-related changes in the kidneys and concurrent medical conditions.

Normal aging is associated with a decline in the GFR and subsequently with reduced homeostatic regulation under stressful conditions.[53] This reduction in GFR makes elderly persons more susceptible to the detrimental effects of nephrotoxic drugs, such as radiographic contrast compounds. The reduction in GFR related to aging is not accompanied by a parallel rise in the serum creatinine level because the serum creatinine level, which results from muscle metabolism, is significantly reduced in elderly persons because of diminished muscle mass and other age-related changes. Evaluation of renal function in elderly persons should include a measurement of creatinine clearance along with the serum creatinine level. The Cockroft and Gault equation can be used to provide an estimate of GFR and of renal function with allowance for age (see the accompanying box).

The prevalence of chronic disease affecting the cerebrovascular, cardiovascular, and skeletal systems is higher in this age group. Because of concurrent disease, the presenting symptoms of renal disease in elderly persons may be less typical than those observed in younger adults. For example, congestive heart failure and hypertension may be the dominant clinical features with the onset of acute glomerulonephritis, whereas oliguria and discolored urine more often are the first signs in younger adults. The course of renal failure may be more complicated in older patients with numerous chronic diseases.

Treatment options for chronic renal failure in elderly patients include hemodialysis, peritoneal dialysis, transplantation, and acceptance of death from uremia. Neither hemodialysis nor peritoneal dialysis has proved to be superior in the elderly. The mode of renal replacement therapy should be individualized, taking into account underlying medical and psychosocial factors. Age alone should not preclude renal transplantation.[54] With increasing experience, many transplantation centers have increased the age for acceptance on transplant waiting lists. Reluctance to provide transplantation as an alternative may have been due, at least in part, to the scarcity of available organs and the view that younger persons are more likely to benefit for a longer time.[51] The general reduction in T-cell function that occurs with aging has been suggested as a beneficial effect that increases transplant graft survival.

Prediction of Creatinine Clearance Using Serum Clearance*

$$\text{Creatine clearance (ml/minute)} = \frac{(140 - \text{age}) \times (\text{body weight in kg})}{72 \times \text{serum creatine in mg/dl}}$$

*The equation result should be multiplied by a factor of 0.85 for women.

(From Cockroft D.W., Gault M.H. [1976]. Prediction of creatinine clearance from serum creatinine. *Nephron* 16, 31.)

In summary, available data suggest that 1% to 2% of patients with chronic renal failure are in the pediatric age range. The causes of renal failure include congenital malformations (*e.g.,* renal dysplasia and obstructive uropathy), inherited disorders (*e.g.,* polycystic kidney disease), acquired diseases (*e.g.,* glomerulonephritis), and metabolic syndromes (*e.g.,* hyperoxaluria). Problems associated with renal failure in children include growth impairment, delay in sexual maturation, and more extensive bone abnormalities than in adults. Although all forms of renal replacement therapy can be safely and reliably used for children, CAPD or transplantation optimize growth and development.

Adults 65 years of age and older account for close to one half of the new cases of ESRD each year. Normal aging is associated with a decline in the GFR, which makes elderly persons more susceptible to the detrimental effects of nephrotoxic drugs and other conditions that compromise renal function. Treatment options for chronic renal failure in elderly patients are similar to those for younger persons.

REVIEW EXERCISES

A 55-year-old man with diabetes and coronary heart disease, who had undergone cardiac catheterization with use of radiocontrast agent 2 days ago, is admitted to the emergency department with a flulike syndrome including chills, nausea, vomiting, abdominal pain, fatigue, and pulmonary congestion. His serum creatinine is elevated, and he has protein in his urine. He is admitted to the intensive care unit with a tentative diagnosis of acute renal failure due to radiocontrast nephropathy.

A. Radiocontrast agents are thought to exert their effects through decreased renal perfusion and through direct toxic effects on renal tubular structures. Explain how each of these phenomena contributes to the development of acute renal failure.

B. Explain the elevated serum creatinine, proteinuria, and presence of pulmonary congestion.

Chronic renal failure is accompanied by hyperphosphatemia, hypocalcemia, impaired activation of vitamin D, hyperparathyroidism, and skeletal complications.

A. Explain the impaired activation of vitamin D and its consequences on calcium and phosphate homeostasis, parathyroid function, and mineralization of bone in persons with renal failure.

B. Explain the possible complications of the administration of activated forms of vitamin D on parathyroid function and the calcium and phosphate homeostasis (*e.g.,* calcium × phosphate product).

References

1. Singri N., Ahya S.N., Levin M.L. (2003). Acute renal failure. *Journal of the American Medical Association 289*(6), 747–751.
2. Albright R.C. Jr. (2001). Acute renal failure: A practical update. *Mayo Clinic Proceedings 76,* 67–74.
3. Brady H.R., Brenner B.M., Clarkson M.R., Liebman W. (2000). Acute renal failure. In Brenner B.M. (Eds.), *Brenner and Rector's the kidney* (6th ed., pp. 1201–1247). Philadelphia: W.B. Saunders.
4. Thadhani R., Pascual M., Bonventre J.V. (1996). Acute renal failure. *New England Journal of Medicine 334,* 1448–1460.
5. Nally J.V. (2002). Acute renal failure in hospitalized patients. *Cleveland Clinic Journal of Medicine 69*(7), 569–574.
6. Abernethy V.E., Lieberthal W. (2002). Acute renal failure in the critically ill patient. *Critical Care Clinics 18,* 203–222.
7. Guyton A., Hall J.E. (2000). *Textbook of medical physiology* (10th ed., pp. 369–371, 373–378). Philadelphia: W.B. Saunders.
8. Cotran R.S., Kumar V., Collins T. (1999). *Robbins pathologic basis of disease* (6th ed., pp. 932–933, 969–971, 1229). Philadelphia: W.B. Saunders.
9. Gerlach A.T., Pickworth K.K. (2000). Contrast medium-induced nephrotoxicity: Pathophysiology and prevention. *Pharmacotherapy 20,* 540–548.
10. Maddox T.G. (2002). Adverse reactions to contrast material: Recognition, prevention, and treatment. *American Family Physician 66*(7), 1229–1234.
11. Forni L.G., Hilton P.J. (1997). Continuous hemofiltration in the treatment of acute renal failure. *New England Journal of Medicine 336,* 1303–1309.
12. Rettig R.A. (1996). The social contract and the treatment of permanent renal failure. *Journal of the American Medical Association 274,* 1123–1126.
13. Levey A.S., Coresh J., Balk E., et al. (2003). National Kidney Foundation practice guidelines for chronic kidney disease: Evaluation, classification, and stratification. *Annals of Internal Medicine 139,* 137–147.
14. Yu H.T. (2003). Progression of chronic renal failure. *Archives of Internal Medicine 163,* 1417–1429.
15. Parmar M.S. (2002). Chronic renal disease. *British Medical Journal 325,* 85–90.
16. Skorecki K., Green J., Brenner B.M. (2001). Chronic renal failure. In Braunwald E., Fauci A.S., Kasper D.L., et al. (Eds.), *Harrison's principles of internal medicine* (17th ed., pp. 1551–1572). New York: McGraw-Hill.
17. Llach F., Bover J. (2000). Renal osteodystrophies. In Brenner B.M. (Ed.), *Brenner and Rector's the kidney* (6th ed., pp. 2103–2135). Philadelphia: W.B. Saunders.
18. Hrusks K.A., Teitelbaum S.L. (1995). Renal osteodystrophy. *New England Journal of Medicine 333,* 166–174.
19. Couttenye M.M., D'Haese P.C., Verschoren W.J., et al. (1999). Low bone turnover in patients with renal failure. *Kidney International 56*(7 Suppl. 73), S70–S76.
20. Slatopolsky E., Brown A., Dusso A. (2000). Role of phosphorous in pathogenesis of secondary hyperthyroidism. *American Journal of Kidney Diseases 37*(1 Suppl 2), S54–S57.
21. Albaaj F., Hutchison A.J. (2003). Hyperphosphatemia in renal failure. *Drugs 63*(6), 577–596.
22. Drüeke T.B. (2001). Control of secondary hyperthyroidism by vitamin D derivatives. *American Journal of Kidney Diseases 37* (1 Suppl. 2), S58–S61.
23. Tong E.M., Nissenson A.R. (2001). Erythropoietin and anemia. *Seminars in Nephrology 21,* 190–203.
24. Besarab A., Levin A. (2000). Defining a renal anemia management period. *American Journal of Kidney Diseases 36*(6 Suppl. 3), S13–S23.
25. Obrador G.T., Ruthazer R., Aora P., et al. (1999). Prevalence of and factors associated with suboptimal care before initiation of dialysis in the United States. *Journal of the American Society of Nephrologists 10,* 1793–1800.
26. Kautz A.T., Obrader G.T., Pereira B.J.G. (2000). Anemia management in patients with chronic renal failure. *American Journal of Kidney Diseases 36*(6 Suppl. 3), S39–S49.
27. National Kidney Foundation. (2001). NKF-KDOQ Clinical practice guidelines for anemia in chronic renal failure. Target hemoglobin/hematocrit. *American Journal of Kidney Diseases 37*(1 Suppl. 1), S182–238.
28. Eberst M.E., Berkowitz L.R. (1993). Hemostasis in renal disease: Pathophysiology and management. *American Journal of Medicine 96,* 168–179.
29. National Kidney Foundation Task Force on Cardiovascular Disease. (1998). Controlling the epidemic of cardiovascular disease in chronic renal disease. *American Journal of Kidney Diseases 32,* 853–906.
30. Preston R.A., Singer I., Epstein M. (1996). Renal parenchymal hypertension. *Archives of Internal Medicine 156,* 602–611.
31. Levin A., Foley R.N. (2000). Cardiovascular disease in chronic renal failure. *American Journal of Kidney Diseases 36*(6 Suppl. 3), S24–S30.
32. Al-Ahmad A., Sarnak M.J., Salem D.N., Konstam M.A. (2001). Cause and management of heart failure in patients with chronic renal disease. *Seminars in Nephrology 21,* 3–12.

33. Gunukula S., Spodick D.H. (2001). Pericardial disease in renal failure. *Seminars in Nephrology 21,* 52–56.
34. Rickus M.A. (1987). Sexual dysfunction in the female ESRD patient. *American Nephrology Nurses' Association Journal 14,* 185–186.
35. Foulks C.J., Cushner H.M. (1986). Sexual dysfunction in the male dialysis patient: Pathogenesis, evaluation, and therapy. *American Journal of Kidney Diseases 8,* 211–212.
36. Agodaoa L.Y., Eggers P.W. (1995). Renal replacement therapy in the United States: Data from the United States Renal Data System. *American Journal of Kidney Diseases 25,* 119–133.
37. National Kidney and Urologic Diseases Information Clearinghouse. (2003). *Kidney and urologic diseases statistics in the United States.* [On-line]. Available: http://www.niddk.gov/health/kidney/pubs/kustats/kustats.htm
38. Ifudu O. (1998). Care of patients undergoing hemodialysis. *New England Journal of Medicine 339,* 1054–1062.
39. Daelemans R.A., D'Haese P.C., BeBroe M.E. (2001). Dialysis. *Seminars in Nephrology 21,* 204–212.
40. Renal Physicians' Association, Working Committee on Clinical Practice Guidelines. (1993). *Clinical practice guidelines on adequacy of hemodialysis.* Washington, DC: Author.
41. Ramanathan V., Goral S., Helderman J.H. (2001). Renal transplantation. *Seminars in Nephrology 21,* 213–219.
42. Levey A.S., Adler S., Caggiula A.W., et al. (1996). Effects of dietary protein restriction on the progression of advanced renal disease in the modification of diet in renal disease study. *American Journal of Kidney Diseases 27,* 652–663.
43. National Kidney Foundation. (2000). *Clinical practice guidelines for nutrition in chronic renal failure.* [On-line]. Available: http://www.kidney.org/professionals/kdoqi/guidelines_updates/doqi_nut.html.
44. Chan J.C.M., Williams D.M., Roth K.S. (2002). Kidney failure in infants and children. *Pediatrics in Review 23*(2), 47–60.
45. Vogt B.A., Avner E.D. (2004). Renal failure. In Behrman R.E., Kliegman R.M., Jensen H.B. (Eds.), *Nelson textbook of pediatrics* (17th ed., pp. 1767–1775). Philadelphia: Saunders.
46. Hogg R.J., Furth S., Lemley K.V., et al. (2003). National Kidney Foundation's kidney disease outcomes quality initiative clinical practice guidelines for chronic kidney disease in children and adolescents: Evaluation, classification, and stratification. *Pediatrics 111*(6), 1416–1423.
47. Hanna J.D., Krieg R.J., Scheinman J.I., Chan J.C.M. (1996). Effects of uremia on growth in children. *Seminars in Nephrology 16,* 230–241.
48. Abitbol C., Chan J.C.M., Trachtman H., et al. (1996). Growth in children with moderate renal insufficiency: Measurement, evaluation, and treatment. *Journal of Pediatrics 129,* S3–S7.
49. Haffner D., Schaffer F., Nissel R., et al. (Study Group for Growth Hormone Treatment in Chronic Renal Failure). (2000). Effect of growth hormone treatment on the adult height of children with chronic renal failure. *New England Journal of Medicine 343,* 923–930.
50. Bereket G., Fine R.N. (1995). Pediatric renal transplantation. *Pediatric Clinics of North America 42,* 1603–1627.
51. Urizar R.E. (2004). Renal transplantation. In Behrman R.E., Kliegman R.M., Jensen H.B. (Eds.), *Nelson textbook of pediatrics* (17th ed., pp. 1775–1782). Philadelphia: W.B. Saunders.
52. National Kidney Foundation. (2000). *End stage renal disease.* [On-line]. Available: http://www.kidney.org/general/news/esrd/cfm.
53. Choudhury D., Raj D.S.D., Palmer B., Levi M. (2000). Effect of aging on renal function and disease. In Brenner B.M. (Ed.), *Brenner and Rector's the kidney* (6th ed., pp. 2187–2210). Philadelphia: W.B. Saunders.
54. Davison A.M. (1998). Renal disease in the elderly. *Nephron 80,* 6–16.

CHAPTER

37

Disorders of Urine Elimination

Although the kidneys control the formation of urine and regulate the composition of body fluids, it is the bladder that stores urine and controls its elimination from the body. Alterations in the storage and expulsion functions of the bladder can result in incontinence, with its accompanying social and hygienic problems, or obstruction of urinary flow, which has deleterious effects on ureteral and, ultimately, renal function. The discussion in this chapter focuses on normal control of urine elimination, urinary obstruction and stasis, neurogenic bladder, incontinence, and bladder cancer. Urinary tract infections are discussed in Chapter 35.

Control of Urine Elimination

After completing this section of the chapter, you should be able to meet the following objectives:

- ✦ Trace the innervation of the bladder and control of micturition from the detrusor muscle and external sphincter, the micturition centers in the sacral and thoracolumbar cord, the pontine micturition center, and the cerebral cortex
- ✦ Explain the mechanism of low-pressure urine storage in the bladder
- ✦ List at least three classes of autonomic drugs and explain their potential effect on bladder function
- ✦ Describe at least three urodynamic studies that can be used to assess bladder function

The bladder, also known as the *urinary vesicle,* is a freely movable organ located behind the pelvic bone in the male and in front of the vagina in the female. It consists of two parts: the fundus, or body, and the neck, or posterior urethra. In the man, the urethra continues anteriorly through the penis. Urine passes from the kidneys to the bladder through the ureters, which are 4 to 5 mm in diameter and approximately 30 cm long. The ureters enter the bladder bilaterally at a location toward its base and close to the urethra (Fig. 37-1). The triangular area that is bounded by the ureters and the urethra is called the *trigone.* There are no valves at the ureteral openings, but as the pressure of the urine in the bladder rises, the ends of the ureters are compressed against the bladder wall to prevent the backflow of urine.

BLADDER STRUCTURE

The bladder is composed of four layers. The first is an outer serosal layer, which covers the upper surface and is contin-

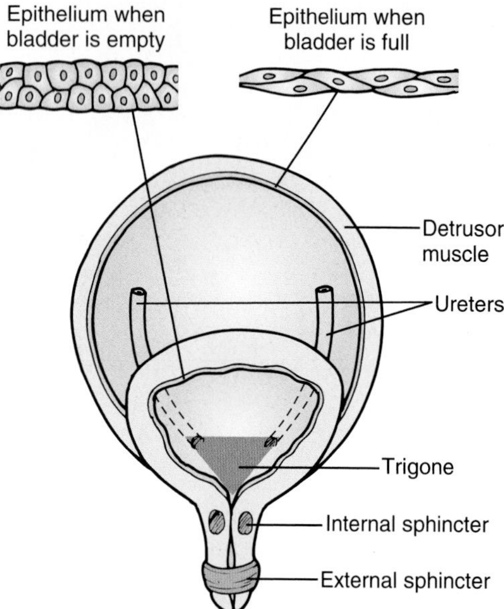

FIGURE 37-1 Diagram of the bladder, showing the detrusor muscle, ureters, trigone area, and urethral orifice. Note the flattening of epithelial cells when the bladder is full and the wall is stretched.

uous with the peritoneum. The second is a network of smooth muscle fibers called the *detrusor muscle.* The third is a submucosal layer of loose connective tissue, and the fourth is an inner mucosal lining of transitional epithelium.

The tonicity of the urine often is quite different from that of the blood, and the transitional epithelial lining of the bladder acts as an effective barrier to prevent the passage of water between the bladder contents and the blood. The inner layers of the bladder form smooth folds, or rugae. As the bladder expands during filling, these rugae spread out to form a single layer without disrupting the integrity of the epithelial lining.

BLADDER FUNCTION

- The functions of the bladder are storage and emptying of urine.
- The control of the storage and emptying functions of the bladder involves both involuntary (autonomic nervous system) and voluntary (somatic nervous system) control.
- The parasympathetic nervous system promotes bladder emptying. It produces contraction of the smooth muscle of the bladder wall and relaxation of the internal sphincter.
- The sympathetic nervous system promotes bladder filling. It produces relaxation of the smooth muscle of the bladder wall and contraction of the internal sphincter.
- The striated muscles in the external sphincter and pelvic floor, which are innervated by the somatic nervous system, provide for the voluntary control of urination and maintenance of continence.

The detrusor muscle is the muscle of micturition (passage of urine). When it contracts, urine is expelled from the bladder. The abdominal muscles play a secondary role in micturition. Their contraction increases intra-abdominal pressure, which further increases intravesicular pressure.

Muscles in the bladder neck, sometimes referred to as the *internal sphincter,* are a continuation of the detrusor muscle. They run down obliquely behind the proximal urethra, forming the posterior urethra in males and the entire urethra in females. When the bladder is relaxed, these circular muscle fibers are closed and act as a sphincter. When the detrusor muscle contracts, the sphincter is pulled open by the changes that occur in bladder shape. In the female, the urethra (2.5 to 3.5 cm) is shorter than in the male (16.5 to 18.5 cm), and usually affords less resistance to urine outflow.

Another muscle important to bladder function is the *external sphincter,* a circular muscle composed of striated muscle fibers that surrounds the urethra distal to the base of the bladder. The external sphincter operates as a reserve mechanism to stop micturition when it is occurring and to maintain continence in the face of unusually high bladder pressure. The skeletal muscle of the pelvic floor also contributes to the support of the bladder and the maintenance of continence.

NEURAL CONTROL OF BLADDER FUNCTION

The control of bladder emptying is unique in that it involves both involuntary autonomic nervous system (ANS) reflexes and some voluntary control. The excitatory input to the bladder that causes bladder emptying is controlled by the parasympathetic nervous system. The sympathetic nervous system relaxes the bladder smooth muscle. There are three main levels of neurologic control for bladder function: the spinal cord reflex centers, the micturition center in the pons, and the cortical and subcortical centers.

Spinal Cord Centers

The centers for reflex control of micturition are located in the sacral (S1 through S4) and thoracolumbar (T11 through L2) segments of the spinal cord[1–3] (Fig. 37-2). The parasympathetic lower motor neurons (LMNs) for the detrusor muscle of the bladder are located in the sacral segments of the spinal cord; their axons travel to the bladder by way of the *pelvic nerve.* LMNs for the external sphincter also are located in the sacral segments of the spinal cord. These LMNs receive their control from the motor cortex by way of the corticospinal tract and send impulses to the external sphincter through the *pudendal nerve.* The bladder neck and trigone area of the bladder, because of their different embryonic origin, receive sympathetic outflow from the thoracolumbar (T11 to L2) segments of the spinal cord. The seminal vesicles, ampulla of the vas, and vas deferens also receive sympathetic innervation from the thoracolumbar segments of the cord.

The afferent input from the bladder and urethra is carried to the central nervous system (CNS) by means of fibers that travel with the parasympathetic (pelvic), so-

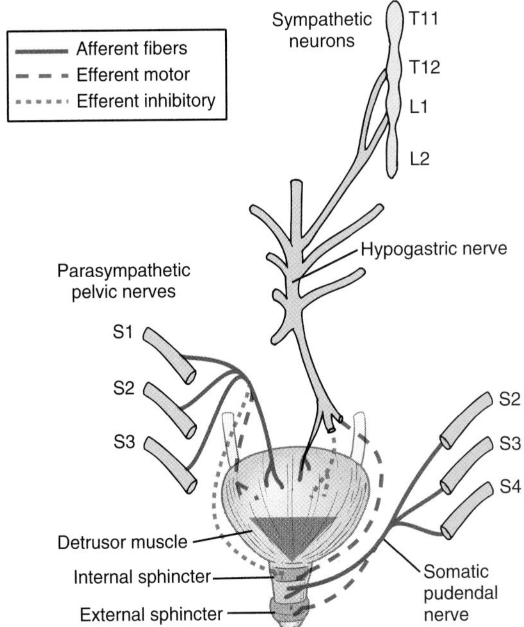

FIGURE 37-2 Nerve supply to the bladder and the urethra.

matic (pudendal), and sympathetic (hypogastric) nerves. The pelvic nerve carries sensory fibers from the stretch receptors in the bladder wall; the pudendal nerve carries sensory fibers from the external sphincter and pelvic muscles; and the hypogastric nerve carries sensory fibers from the trigone area.[3]

Pontine Micturition Center

The immediate coordination of the normal micturition reflex occurs in the micturition center in the pons, facilitated by descending input from the forebrain and ascending input from the reflex centers in the spinal cord[1,2] (Fig. 37-3). This center is thought to coordinate the activity of the detrusor muscle and the external sphincter. As bladder filling occurs, ascending spinal afferents relay this information to the micturition center, which also receives important descending information from the forebrain concerning behavioral cues for bladder emptying. Descending pathways from the pontine micturition center produce coordinated inhibition or relaxation of the external sphincter. Disruption of pontine control of micturition, as in spinal cord injury, results in uninhibited spinal reflex-controlled contraction of the bladder without relaxation of the external sphincter, a condition known as *detrusor-sphincter dyssynergia.*

Cortical and Subcortical Centers

Cortical brain centers enable inhibition of the micturition center in the pons and conscious control of urination. Neural influences from the subcortical centers in the basal ganglia, which are conveyed by extrapyramidal pathways, modulate the contractile response. They modify and delay the detrusor contractile response during filling and then modulate the expulsive activity of the bladder to facilitate complete emptying.

Micturition and Maintenance of Continence

To maintain continence, or retention of urine, the bladder must function as a low-pressure storage system; the pressure in the bladder must remain lower than urethral pressure. To ensure that this condition is met, the increase in intravesicular pressure that accompanies bladder filling is almost imperceptible. An increase in bladder volume from 10 to 400 mL may be accompanied by only a 5 cm H_2O increase in pressure.[1] Sustained elevations in intravesicular pressures (>40 to 50 cm H_2O) often are associated with vesicoureteral reflux (*i.e.,* backflow of urine from the bladder into the ureter) and the development of ureteral dilatation (see Chapter 35). Although the pressure in the bladder is maintained at low levels, sphincter pressure remains high (45 to 65 cm H_2O) as a means of preventing loss of urine as the bladder fills.

Micturition, or the act of bladder emptying, involves both sensory and motor functions associated with bladder emptying. When the bladder is distended to 150 to 250 mL in the adult, the sensation of fullness is transmitted to the spinal cord and then to the cerebral cortex, allowing for conscious inhibition of the micturition reflex.[4] During the act of micturition, the detrusor muscle of the bladder fundus and bladder neck contract down on the urine; the ureteral orifices are forced shut; the bladder neck is widened and shortened as it is pulled up by the globular muscles in the bladder fundus; the resistance of the internal sphincter in the bladder neck is decreased; and the external sphincter relaxes as urine moves out of the bladder.

Pharmacology of Micturition

The ANS and its neuromediators play a central role in micturition. Parasympathetic innervation of the bladder is mediated by the neurotransmitter acetylcholine. Two types of cholinergic receptors affect various aspects of micturition: nicotinic and muscarinic. *Nicotinic* (N) receptors are found in the synapses between the preganglionic and postganglionic neurons of the sympathetic and the parasympathetic system, as well as in the neuromuscular end plates of the striated muscle fibers of the external sphincter and pelvic muscles. *Muscarinic* (M) receptors are found in the postganglionic parasympathetic endings of the detrusor muscle. Several subtypes of M receptors have been identified. The M_2 and M_3 receptors appear predominantly to mediate detrusor contraction and internal sphincter contraction. The M_3 receptor also mediates salivary secretion and bowel activity.[5] The identification of receptor subtypes has facilitated the development of medications that selectively target bladder structures while minimizing other, undesired effects.

Although sympathetic innervation is not essential to the act of micturition, it allows the bladder to store a large volume without the involuntary escape of urine—a mechanism that is consistent with the fight-or-flight function subserved by the sympathetic nervous system. The bladder is supplied with α_1- and β_2-adrenergic receptors. The β_2-adrenergic receptors are found in the detrusor muscle; they produce relaxation of the detrusor muscle, increasing the bladder volume at which the micturition reflex is triggered.

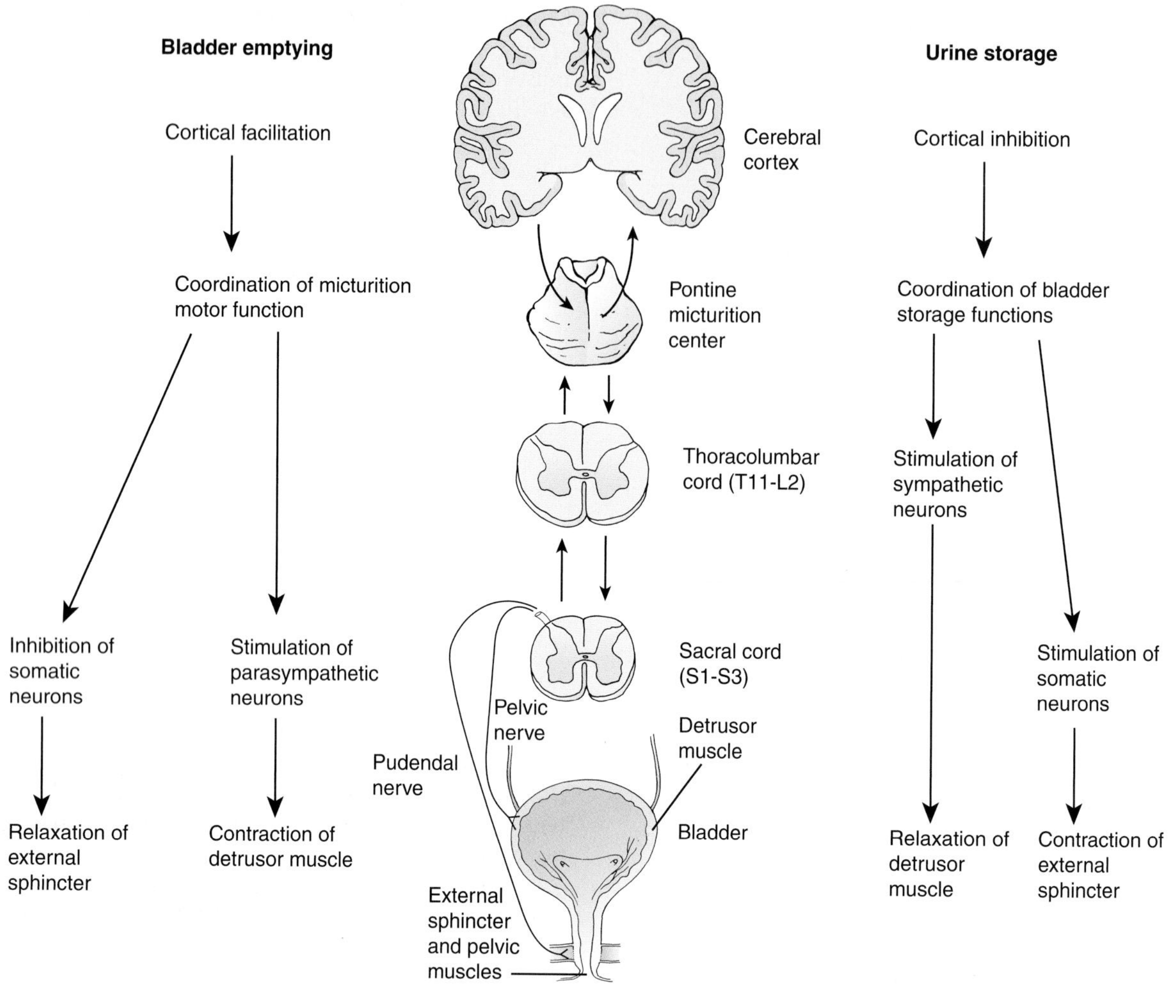

FIGURE 37-3 Pathways and central nervous system centers involved in the control of bladder (**left**) emptying and (**right**) storage functions. Efferent pathways for micturition (**left**) and urine storage (**right**).

The α_1-adrenergic receptors are found in the trigone area, including the intramural ureteral musculature, bladder neck, and internal sphincter. The activation of α_1 receptors produces contraction of these muscles. Sympathetic activity ceases when the micturition reflex is activated. During male ejaculation, which is mediated by the sympathetic nervous system, the musculature of the trigone area and that of the bladder neck and prostatic urethra contract and prevent the backflow of seminal fluid into the bladder.

Because of their effects on bladder function, drugs that selectively activate or block ANS outflow or receptor activity can alter urine elimination. Table 37-1 describes the action of drug groups that can impair bladder function or can be used in the treatment of micturition disorders. Many of the nonprescription cold preparations contain α-adrenergic agonists and antihistamine agents that have anticholinergic properties. These drugs can cause urinary retention. Many of the antidepressant and antipsychotic drugs also have anticholinergic actions that influence urination.

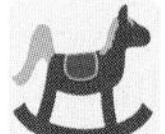

Continence in Children

In infants and young children, micturition is an involuntary act that is triggered by a spinal cord reflex; when the bladder fills to a given capacity, the detrusor muscle contracts, and the external sphincter relaxes. As the child grows, the bladder gradually enlarges, with an increase in capacity, in ounces, that approximates the age of the child plus 2.[6] This formula applies up to ages 12 to 14 years. As the bladder grows and increases in capacity, the tone of the external sphincter muscle increases. Toilet training begins at about 2 to 3 years of age when the child becomes conscious of the need to urinate. Conscious control of bladder function depends on (1) normal bladder growth, (2) myelination of the ascending afferents that signal awareness of bladder filling, (3) development of cortical control and descending communication with the sacral micturition center, (4) ability to consciously tighten the external sphincter to prevent incontinence, (5) and motivation of the child to stay dry. Girls typically achieve continence before boys,

TABLE 37-1 Action of Drug Groups on Bladder Function

Function	Drug Groups	Mechanism of Action
Detrusor Muscle		
Increased tone and contraction	Cholinergic drugs	Stimulate parasympathetic receptors that cause detrusor contraction
Inhibition of detrusor muscle relaxation during filling	β_2-Adrenergic–blocking drugs	Block β_2 receptors that produce detrusor muscle relaxation
Decreased tone	Anticholinergic drugs and drugs with an anticholinergic action	Block the muscarinic receptors that cause detrusor muscle contraction
	Calcium channel–blocking drugs	May interfere with influx of calcium to support contraction of detrusor smooth muscle
Internal Bladder Sphincter		
Increased tone	α_1-Adrenergic agonists	Activate α_1 receptors that produce contraction of the smooth muscle of the internal sphincter
Decreased tone	α_1-Adrenergic–blocking drugs	Block contraction of the smooth muscle of the internal sphincter
External Sphincter		
Decreased tone	Skeletal muscle relaxants	Decrease the tone of the external sphincter by acting at the level of the spinal cord or by interfering with release of calcium in muscle fiber

and bowel control is typically achieved before bladder control. By 5 years of age, 90% to 95% of children are continent during the day and 80% to 85% are continent at night.[6]

DIAGNOSTIC METHODS OF EVALUATING BLADDER FUNCTION

Bladder structure and function can be assessed by a number of methods.[7] Reports or observations of frequency, hesitancy, straining to urinate or void, and a weak or interrupted stream are suggestive of outflow obstruction. Palpation and percussion provide information about bladder distention.

Physical Examination

Postvoid residual (PVR) urine volume provides information about bladder emptying. It can be estimated by abdominal palpation and percussion. Catheterization and ultrasonography can be used to obtain specific measurements of PVR. A PVR value of less than 50 mL is considered adequate bladder emptying, and more than 200 mL indicates inadequate bladder emptying.[8]

Pelvic examination is used in women to assess perineal skin condition, perivaginal muscle tone, genital atrophy, pelvic prolapse (*e.g.*, cystocele, rectocele, uterine prolapse), pelvic mass, or other conditions that may impair bladder function. Bimanual examination (*i.e.*, pelvic and abdominal palpation) can be used to assess PVR volume. Rectal examination is used to test for perineal sensation, sphincter tone, fecal impaction, and rectal mass. It is used to assess the contour of the prostate in men.

Laboratory and Radiologic Studies

Urine tests provide information about kidney function and urinary tract infections. The presence of bacteriuria or pyuria suggests urinary tract infection and the possibility of urinary tract obstruction. Blood tests (*i.e.*, blood urea nitrogen and creatinine) provide information about renal function.

Bladder structures can be visualized indirectly by taking x-ray films of the abdomen and by using excretory urography (which involves the use of a radiopaque dye, computed tomographic (CT) scanning, magnetic resonance imaging (MRI), or ultrasonography. Cystoscopy enables direct visualization of the urethra, bladder, and ureteral orifices.

Ultrasound Bladder Scan

The ultrasound bladder scan provides a noninvasive method for estimating bladder volume.[9] The device measures ultrasonic reflections to differentiate the urinary bladder from the surrounding tissue. A computer system calculates and displays bladder volume. The device can be used to determine the need for catheterization, for evaluation and diagnosis of urinary retention, to measure PVR volumes, and for facilitating volume-dependent or time-dependent catheterization or toileting programs.

Urodynamic Studies

Urodynamic studies are used to study bladder function and voiding problems. Three aspects of bladder function can be assessed by urodynamic studies: bladder, urethral, and intra-abdominal pressure changes; characteristics of urine flow; and the activity of the striated muscles of the external sphincter and pelvic floor. Specific urodynamic tests include uroflowmetry, cystometry, urethral pressure profile, and sphincter electromyography (EMG). It often is advantageous to evaluate several components of bladder function simultaneously.

Uroflowmetry. Uroflowmetry measures the flow rate (milliliters per minute) during urination.[7] It commonly is done using a weight-recording device located at the bottom of a commode receptacle unit. As the person being tested voids, the weight of the commode receptacle unit increases. This weight change is electronically recorded and then analyzed using weight (converted to milliliters) and time.

Cystometry. Cystometry is used to measure bladder pressure during filling and voiding. It provides valuable information about total bladder capacity, intravesicular pressures during bladder filling, the ability to perceive bladder fullness and the desire to urinate, the ability of the bladder to contract and sustain a contraction, uninhibited bladder contractions, and the ability to inhibit urination. The test can be done by allowing physiologic filling of the bladder with urine and recording intravesicular pressure throughout a voiding cycle, or by filling the bladder with water and measuring intravesicular pressure against the volume of water instilled into the bladder.[7]

In a normally functioning bladder, the sensation of bladder fullness is first perceived when the bladder contains 100 to 200 mL of urine while bladder pressure remains constant at approximately 8 to 15 cm H_2O. The desire to void occurs when the bladder is full (normal capacity is approximately 400 to 500 mL). At this point, a definite sensation of fullness occurs, the pressure rises sharply to 40 to 100 cm H_2O, and voiding occurs around the catheter.[7] Urinary continence requires that urethral pressure exceed bladder pressure. Bladder pressure usually rises 30 to 40 cm H_2O during voiding. If the urethral resistance is high because of obstruction, greater pressure is required, a condition that can be detected by cystometry.

Urethral Pressure Profile. The urethral pressure profile is used to evaluate the intraluminal pressure changes along the length of the urethra with the bladder at rest.[7] It provides information about smooth muscle activity along the length of the urethra. This test can be done using the infusion method (most commonly used), the membrane catheter method, or the microtip transducer. The infusion method involves the insertion of a small double-lumen urethral catheter, followed by the infusion of water into the bladder and measurement of the changes in urethral pressure as the catheter is slowly withdrawn.

Sphincter Electromyography. Sphincter EMG allows the activity of the striated (voluntary) muscles of the perineal area to be studied. Activity is recorded using an anal plug electrode, a catheter electrode, adhesive skin electrodes, or needle electrodes.[7] Electrode placement is based on the muscle groups that need to be tested. The test usually is done along with urodynamic tests such as the cystometrogram and uroflow studies.

In summary, although the kidneys function in the formation of urine and the regulation of body fluids, it is the bladder that stores and controls the elimination of urine. Micturition is a function of the peripheral ANS, subject to facilitation or inhibition from higher neurologic centers. The parasympathetic nervous system controls the motor function of the bladder detrusor muscle and the tone of the internal sphincter; its cell bodies are located in the sacral spinal cord and communicate with the bladder through the pelvic nerve. Efferent sympathetic control originates at the level of segments T11 through L2 of the spinal cord and produces relaxation of the detrusor muscle and contraction of the internal sphincter. Skeletal muscle found in the external sphincter and the pelvic muscles that support the bladder are supplied by the pudendal nerve, which exits the spinal cord at the level of segments S2 through S4. The micturition center in the brain stem coordinates the action of the detrusor muscle and the external sphincter, whereas cortical centers permit conscious control of micturition.

Bladder function can be evaluated using urodynamic studies that measure bladder, urethral, and abdominal pressures; urine flow characteristics; and skeletal muscle activity of the external sphincter.

Alterations in Bladder Function

After completing this section of the chapter, you should be able to meet the following objectives:

- ✦ Describe the causes of and compensatory changes that occur with urinary tract obstruction
- ✦ Differentiate lesions that produce storage dysfunction associated with spastic bladder from those that produce emptying dysfunction associated with flaccid bladder in terms of the level of the lesions and their effects on bladder function
- ✦ Cite the pathology and causes of nonrelaxing external sphincter
- ✦ Describe methods used in treatment of neurogenic bladder
- ✦ Define *incontinence* and list the categories of this condition
- ✦ List the treatable causes of incontinence in the elderly
- ✦ Describe behavioral, pharmacologic, and surgical methods used in treatment of incontinence

Alterations in bladder function include urinary obstruction with retention or stasis of urine and urinary incontinence with involuntary loss of urine. Although the two conditions have almost opposite effects on urination, they can have similar causes. Both can result from structural changes in the bladder, urethra, or surrounding organs or from impairment of neurologic control of bladder function.

URINARY OBSTRUCTION AND STASIS

In lower urinary tract obstruction and stasis, urine is produced normally by the kidneys but is retained in the bladder. Obstructions are classified according to cause (congenital or acquired), degree (partial or complete), duration (acute or chronic), and level (upper or lower urinary tract).[10] Because it has the potential to produce vesicoureteral reflux and cause kidney damage, urinary obstruction and stasis is a serious disorder.

Congenital narrowing of the external meatus (*i.e.*, meatal stenosis) is more common in boys, and obstructive disorders of the posterior urethra are more common in girls. Another common cause of congenital obstruction is the damage to sacral nerves that occurs in spina bifida and meningomyelocele.

The acquired causes of lower urinary tract obstruction and stasis are numerous. In males, the most important cause of urinary obstruction is external compression of the urethra caused by the enlargement of the prostate gland. Gonorrhea and other sexually transmitted diseases contribute to the incidence of infection-produced urethral strictures. Bladder tumors and secondary invasion of the bladder by tumors arising in structures that surround the bladder and urethra can compress the bladder neck or urethra and cause obstruction. Constipation and fecal impaction can compress the urethra and produce urethral obstruction. This can be a particular problem in elderly persons.

Compensatory and Decompensatory Changes

The body compensates for the obstruction of urine outflow with mechanisms designed to prevent urine retention. These mechanisms can be divided into two stages: a compensatory stage and a decompensatory stage.[10] The degree to which these changes occur and their effect on bladder structure and urinary function depend on the extent of the obstruction, the rapidity with which it occurs, and the presence of other contributing factors, such as neurologic impairment and infection.

During the early stage of obstruction, the bladder begins to hypertrophy and becomes hypersensitive to afferent stimuli arising from bladder filling. The ability to suppress urination is diminished, and bladder contraction can become so strong that it virtually produces bladder spasm. There is urgency, sometimes to the point of incontinence, and frequency during the day and at night.

With continuation and progression of the obstruction, compensatory changes begin to occur. There is further hypertrophy of the bladder muscle, the thickness of the bladder wall may double, and the pressure generated by detrusor contraction can increase from a normal 20 to 40 cm H_2O to 50 to 100 cm H_2O to overcome the resistance from the obstruction. As the force needed to expel urine from the bladder increases, compensatory mechanisms may become ineffective, causing muscle fatigue before complete emptying can be accomplished. After a few minutes, voiding can again be initiated and completed, accounting for the frequency of urination.

The inner bladder surface forms smooth folds. With continued outflow obstruction, this smooth surface is replaced with coarsely woven structures (*i.e.*, hypertrophied smooth muscle fibers) called *trabeculae*. Small pockets of mucosal tissue, called *cellules*, commonly develop between the trabecular ridges. These pockets form diverticula when they extend between the actual fibers of the bladder muscle (Fig. 37-4). Because the diverticula have no muscle, they are unable to contract and expel their urine into the bladder, and secondary infections caused by stasis are common.

Along with hypertrophy of the bladder wall, there is hypertrophy of the trigone area and the interureteric ridge, which is located between the two ureters. This causes backpressure on the ureters, the development of hydroureters (*i.e.*, dilated, urine-filled ureters), and eventually, kidney damage. Stasis of urine predisposes to urinary tract infections.

When compensatory mechanisms no longer are effective, signs of decompensation begin to occur. The period of detrusor muscle contraction becomes too short to completely expel the urine, and residual urine remains in the bladder. At this point, the symptoms of obstruction—frequency of urination, hesitancy, need to strain to initiate

NEUROGENIC BLADDER DISORDERS

- Neurogenic disorders of the bladder commonly are manifested by a spastic bladder dysfunction, in which there is failure to store urine, or as flaccid bladder dysfunction, in which bladder emptying is impaired.
- Spastic bladder dysfunction results from neurologic lesions above the level of the sacral cord that allow neurons in the micturition center to function reflexively without control from higher central nervous system centers.
- Flaccid bladder dysfunction results from neurologic disorders affecting the motor neurons in the sacral cord or peripheral nerves that control detrusor muscle contraction and bladder emptying.

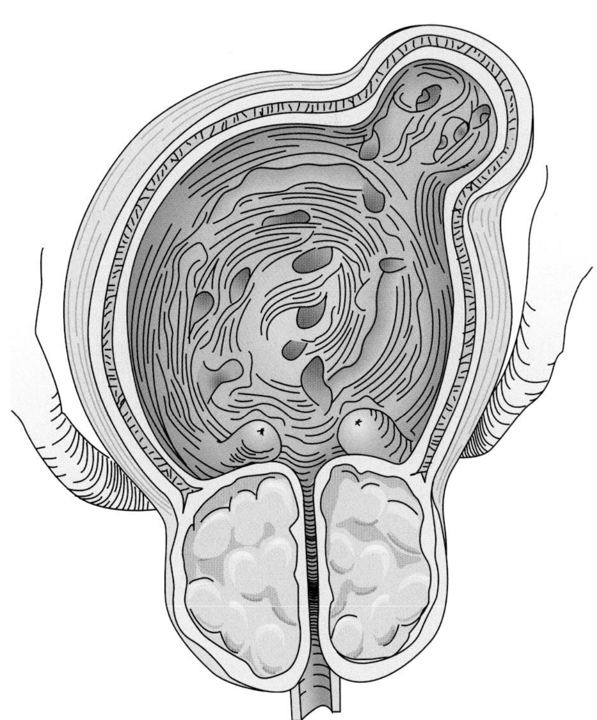

FIGURE 37-4 Destructive changes of the bladder wall with development of diverticula caused by benign prostatic hypertrophy.

CHART 37-1

Signs of Outflow Obstruction and Urine Retention

Bladder distention
Hesitancy
Straining when initiating urination
Small and weak stream
Frequency
Feeling of incomplete bladder emptying
Overflow incontinence

urination, a weak and small stream, and termination of the stream before the bladder is completely emptied—become pronounced. With progressive decompensation, the bladder may become severely overstretched with residual urine volume of 1000 to 3000 ml.[10] At this point, it loses its power of contraction and overflow incontinence occurs. The signs of urine retention are summarized in Chart 37-1.

Treatment

The immediate treatment of lower urinary obstruction and stasis is directed toward relief of bladder distention. This usually is accomplished through urinary catheterization (discussed later in this chapter). Constipation or fecal impaction should be corrected. Long-term treatment is directed toward correcting the problem causing the obstruction.

NEUROGENIC BLADDER DISORDERS

The urinary bladder is unique in that it is probably the only autonomically innervated visceral organ that is under CNS control. The neural control of bladder function can be interrupted at any level. It can be interrupted at the level of the peripheral nerves that connect the bladder to the reflex micturition center in the sacral cord, the ascending and descending tracts in the spinal cord, the pontine micturition center, or the cortical centers that are involved in voluntary control of micturition.[11,12] Neurogenic disorders of bladder function commonly are manifested in one of two ways: failure to store urine (spastic bladder dysfunction) or failure to empty (flaccid bladder dysfunction).[11] Spastic bladder dysfunction usually results from neurologic lesions located above the level of the sacral micturition reflexes, whereas flaccid bladder dysfunction results from lesions at the level of sacral reflexes or the peripheral nerves that innervate the bladder. In addition to disorders of detrusor muscle function, disruption of micturition occurs when the neurologic control of external sphincter function is disrupted. Some disorders, such as stroke and Parkinson's disease, may affect both the storage and emptying functions of the bladder. Table 37-2 describes the characteristics of neurogenic bladder according to the level of the lesion.

Spastic Bladder: Failure to Store Urine

Failure to store urine results from conditions that cause reflex bladder spasm and a decrease in bladder volume. It commonly is caused by conditions that produce partial or extensive neural damage above the micturition reflex center in the sacral cord (see Fig. 37-3). As a result, bladder function is regulated by segmental reflexes, without control from higher brain centers. The degree of bladder spasticity and dysfunction depends on the level and extent of neurologic dysfunction. Usually, both the ANS neurons controlling bladder function and the somatic neurons controlling the function of the striated muscles in the external sphincter are affected. In some cases, there is a detrusor-

TABLE 37-2 Types and Characteristics of Neurogenic Bladder

Level of Lesion	Change in Bladder Function	Common Causes
Sensory cortex, motor cortex, or corticospinal tract	Loss of ability to perceive bladder filling; low-volume, physiologically normal micturition that occurs suddenly and is difficult to inhibit	Stroke and advanced age
Basal ganglia or extrapyramidal tract	Detrusor contractions are elicited suddenly without warning and are difficult to control; bladder contraction is shorter than normal and does not produce full bladder emptying	Parkinson's disease
Pontine micturition center or communicating tracts in the spinal cord	Storage reflexes are provoked during filling, and external sphincter responses are heightened; uninhibited bladder contractions occur at a lower volume than normal and do not continue until the bladder is emptied; antagonistic activity occurs between the detrusor muscle and the external sphincter	Spinal cord injury
Sacral cord or nerve roots	Areflexic bladder fills but does not contract; loss of external sphincter tone occurs when the lesion affects the α-adrenergic motor neurons or pudendal nerve	Injury to sacral cord or spinal roots
Pelvic nerve	Increased filling and impaired sphincter control cause increased intravesicular pressure	Radical pelvic surgery
Autonomic peripheral sensory pathways	Bladder overfilling occurs owing to a loss of ability to perceive bladder filling	Diabetic neuropathies, multiple sclerosis

sphincter dyssynergia with uncoordinated contraction and relaxation of the detrusor and external sphincter muscles. The most common causes of spastic bladder dysfunction are spinal cord lesions such as spinal cord injury, herniated intervertebral disk, vascular lesions, tumors, and myelitis. Other neurologic conditions that affect voiding are stroke, multiple sclerosis, and brain tumors.

Bladder Dysfunction Caused by Spinal Cord Injury. One of the most common types of spinal cord lesions is spinal cord injury (see Chapter 51). The immediate and early effects of spinal cord injury on bladder function are quite different from those that follow recovery from the initial injury. During the period immediately after spinal cord injury, a state of spinal shock develops, during which all the reflexes, including the micturition reflex, are depressed. During this stage, the bladder becomes atonic and cannot contract. Catheterization is necessary to prevent injury to urinary structures associated with overdistention of the bladder. Aseptic intermittent catheterization is the preferred method of catheterization. Depression of reflexes lasts from a few weeks to 6 months (usually 2 to 3 months), after which the spinal reflexes return and become hyperactive.

After the acute stage of spinal cord injury, the micturition response changes from a long-tract reflex to a segmental reflex. Because the sacral reflex arc remains intact, stimuli generated by bladder stretch receptors during filling produce frequent spontaneous contractions of the detrusor muscle. This creates a small, hyperactive bladder subject to high-pressure and short-duration uninhibited bladder contractions. Voiding is interrupted, involuntary, or incomplete. Dilation of the internal sphincter and spasticity of the external sphincter and perineal muscles innervated by upper motoneurons occur, producing resistance to bladder emptying. Hypertrophy of the trigone develops, often leading to vesicoureteral reflux and risk for renal damage.

Spastic bladder due to spinal cord injuries at the cervical level is often accompanied by a condition known as autonomic hyperreflexia (see Chapter 51). Because the injury occurs above the CNS control of sympathetic reflexes in the spinal cord, severe hypertension, bradycardia, and sweating can be triggered by insertion of a catheter or mild overdistention of the bladder.

Uninhibited Neurogenic Bladder. A mild form of reflex neurogenic bladder, sometimes called *uninhibited bladder,* can develop after a stroke, during the early stages of multiple sclerosis, or as a result of lesions located in the inhibitory centers of the cortex or the pyramidal tract. With this type of disorder, the sacral reflex arc and sensation are retained, the urine stream is normal, and there is no residual urine. Bladder capacity is diminished, however, because of increased detrusor muscle tone and spasticity.

Detrusor-Sphincter Dyssynergia. Depending on the level of the lesion, the coordinated activity of the detrusor muscle and the external sphincter may be affected. Lesions that affect the micturition center in the pons or impair communication between this center and spinal cord centers interrupt the coordinated activity of the detrusor muscle and the external sphincter. This is called *detrusor-sphincter dyssynergia.* Instead of relaxing during micturition, the external sphincter becomes more constricted. This condition can lead to elevated intravesicular pressures, vesicoureteral reflux, and kidney damage.

Treatment. Among the methods used to treat spastic bladder and detrusor-sphincter dyssynergia are the use of anticholinergic medications to decrease bladder hyperactivity and urinary catheterization to produce bladder emptying (discussed later). A sphincterotomy (surgical resection of the external sphincter) or implantable urethral stent may be used to decrease outflow resistance in a person who cannot be managed with medications and catheterization procedures. An alternative to surgical resection of the external sphincter is the injection of botulinum-A toxin to produce paralysis of the striated muscles in the external sphincter. The effects of the injection last from 3 to 9 months, after which the injection must be repeated.[11]

Flaccid Bladder: Failure to Empty Urine

Failure to empty the bladder can be due to flaccid bladder dysfunction, peripheral neuropathies that interrupt afferent or efferent communication between the bladder and the spinal cord, or conditions that prevent relaxation of the external sphincter (see Fig. 37-3).

Flaccid Bladder Dysfunction. Detrusor muscle areflexia, or flaccid neurogenic bladder, occurs when there is injury to the micturition center of the sacral cord, the cauda equina, or the sacral roots that supply the bladder.[12] Atony of the detrusor muscle and loss of the perception of bladder fullness permit the overstretching of the detrusor muscle that contributes to weak and ineffective bladder contractions. External sphincter tone and perineal muscle tone are diminished. Voluntary urination does not occur, but fairly efficient emptying usually can be achieved by increased intra-abdominal pressure or manual suprapubic pressure. Among the causes of flaccid neurogenic bladder are trauma, tumors, and congenital anomalies (*e.g.,* spina bifida, meningomyelocele).

Bladder Dysfunction Caused by Peripheral Neuropathies. In addition to CNS lesions and conditions that disrupt bladder function, disorders of the peripheral (pelvic, pudendal, and hypogastric) neurons that supply the bladder can occur. These neuropathies can selectively interrupt sensory or motor pathways for the bladder or involve both pathways.

Bladder atony with dysfunction is a frequent complication of diabetes mellitus.[13,14] The disorder initially affects the sensory axons of the urinary bladder without involvement of the pudendal nerve. This leads to large residual volumes after micturition, sometimes complicated by infection. There frequently is a need for straining, accompanied by hesitation, weakness of the stream, dribbling, and a sensation of incomplete bladder emptying.[14] The chief complications are vesicoureteral reflux and ascending urinary tract infection. Because persons with diabetes are already at risk for development of glomerular disease (see Chapter 35), reflux can have serious effects on kidney function. Treatment consists of client education, including the need for frequent voiding (*e.g.,* every 3 to 4 hours while awake), use of abdominal compression to effect more complete bladder emptying, and intermittent catheterization when necessary.[12]

Nonrelaxing External Sphincter

Another condition that affects micturition and bladder function is the nonrelaxing external sphincter. This condition usually is related to a delay in maturation, developmental regression, psychomotor disorders, or locally irritative lesions. Inadequate relaxation of the external sphincter can be the result of anxiety or depression. Any local irritation can produce spasms of the sphincter by means of afferent sensory input from the pudendal nerve; included are vaginitis, perineal inflammation, and inflammation or irritation of the urethra. In men, chronic prostatitis contributes to the impaired relaxation of the external sphincter.

Treatment

The goals of treatment for neurogenic bladder disorders focus on preventing bladder overdistention, urinary tract infections, and potentially life-threatening renal damage and reducing the undesirable social and psychological effects of the disorder. The methods used in treatment of neurogenic bladder disorders are individualized based on the type of neurologic lesion that is involved; information obtained through the health history, including fluid intake; report or observation of voiding patterns; presence of other health problems; urodynamic studies when indicated; and the ability of the person to participate in the treatment. Treatment methods include catheterization, bladder training, pharmacologic manipulation of bladder function, and surgery.

Catheterization. Catheterization involves the insertion of a small-diameter latex or silicone tube into the bladder through the urethra.[15] The catheter may be inserted on a one-time basis to relieve temporary bladder distention, left indwelling (*i.e.*, retention catheter), or inserted intermittently. With acute overdistention of the bladder, usually no more than 1000 mL of urine is removed from the bladder at one time. The theory behind this limitation is that removing more than this amount at one time releases pressure on the pelvic blood vessels and predisposes to alterations in circulatory function.

Permanent indwelling catheters sometimes are used when there is urine retention or incontinence in persons who are ill or debilitated or when conservative or surgical methods for the correction of incontinence are not feasible. The use of permanent indwelling bladder catheters in patients with spinal cord injury has been shown to produce a number of complications, including urinary tract infections, urethral irritation and injury, pyelonephritis, and kidney stones.

Intermittent catheterization is used to treat urine retention or incomplete emptying secondary to various neurologic or obstructive disorders.[15] Properly used, it prevents bladder overdistention and urethral irritation, allows more freedom of activity, and provides periodic distention of the bladder to prevent muscle atony. It often is used with pharmacologic manipulation to achieve continence; when possible, it is learned and managed as a self-care procedure (*i.e.*, intermittent self-catheterization).[16] It may be carried out as an aseptic (sterile) or a clean procedure. Aseptic intermittent catheterization is used in persons with spinal shock and in those who need short-term catheterization.

The clean procedure typically is used for self-catheterization. It is performed at 3- to 4-hour intervals to prevent overdistention of the bladder. The best results are obtained if only 300 to 400 mL is allowed to collect in the bladder between catheterizations. The use of the clean instead of the sterile procedure has been defended on the basis that most urinary tract infections are caused by some underlying abnormality of the urinary tract that leads to impaired mucosal resistance to bacterial infection, the most common cause of which is decreased blood flow because of bladder overdistention.[15]

Bladder Retraining. Bladder retraining differs with the type of disorder.[17] Methods used to supplement bladder retraining include monitoring fluid intake to prevent urinary tract infections and control urine volume and osmolality, developing scheduled times for urination, and using body positions that facilitate micturition.

Among the considerations when monitoring fluid intake is the need to ensure adequate fluid intake to prevent unduly concentrated urine, which may serve to stimulate afferent neurons of the micturition reflex. In hyperreflexive bladder or detrusor-sphincter dyssynergia, the stimulation of afferent nerve endings by irritating urinary constituents results in increased vesicular pressures, vesicoureteral reflux, and overflow incontinence. Fluid intake must be balanced to prevent bladder overdistention from occurring during the night. Adequate fluid intake also is needed to prevent urinary tract infections, the irritating effects of which increase bladder irritability and the risk for urinary incontinence and renal damage. Developing scheduled times for urinating prevents overdistention of the bladder.

The methods used for bladder retraining depend on the type of lesion causing the disorder. In spastic neurogenic bladder, methods designed to trigger the sacral micturition reflex are used; in flaccid neurogenic bladder, manual methods that increase intravesicular pressure are used. Trigger voiding methods include manual stimulation of the afferent loop of the micturition reflex through such maneuvers as tapping the suprapubic area, pulling on the pubic hairs, stroking the glans penis, or rubbing the thighs. Credé's method, which is done with the person in a sitting position, consists of applying pressure with four fingers of one hand or both hands to the suprapubic area as a means of increasing intravesicular pressure. The use of Valsalva's maneuver (*i.e.*, bearing down by exhaling against a closed glottis) increases intra-abdominal pressure and aids in bladder emptying. This maneuver is repeated until the bladder is empty. For the best results, the patient must cooperate fully with the procedures and, if possible, learn to perform them independently.

Biofeedback methods have been useful for teaching some aspects of bladder control. They involve the use of EMG or cystometry as a feedback signal for training a person to control the function of the external sphincter or raise intravesicular pressure enough to overcome outflow resistance.

Pharmacologic Manipulation. Pharmacologic manipulation includes the use of drugs to alter the contractile properties of the bladder, decrease the outflow resistance of the internal sphincter, and relax the external sphincter. The usefulness of drug therapy often is evaluated during cystometric studies. Anticholinergic drugs, such as tolterodine (Detrol), oxybutynin (Ditropan), and propantheline (generic; Pro-Banthine), decrease detrusor muscle tone and increase bladder capacity in persons with spastic bladder dysfunction.[12,18] Cholinergic drugs that stimulate parasympathetic receptors, such as bethanechol chloride (generic; Urecholine), provide increased bladder tonus and may prove helpful in the symptomatic treatment of milder forms of flaccid neurogenic bladder. Muscle relaxants, such as diazepam (Valium) and baclofen (Lioresal), may be used to decrease the tone of the external sphincter. A nasal spray preparation of desmopressin (DDAVP), a synthetic antidiuretic hormone, can be used to treat persons with nighttime frequency due to spastic bladder symptoms.

Surgical Procedures. Among the surgical procedures used in the management of neurogenic bladder are sphincterectomy, reconstruction of the sphincter, nerve resection of the sacral reflex nerves that cause spasticity or the pudendal nerve that controls the external sphincter, and urinary diversion. Urinary diversion can be done by creating an ileal or a colon loop into which the ureters are anastomosed; the distal end of the loop is brought out and attached to the abdominal wall. Other procedures include the attachment of the ureters to the skin of the abdominal wall or the attachment of the ureters to the sigmoid colon, with the rectum serving as a receptacle for the urine.

Extensive research is being conducted on methods of restoring voluntary control of the storage and evacuation functions of the bladder through the use of implanted electrodes. Single and multiple electrodes can be placed on selected nerves and then coupled to a subcutaneous receiver.[12]

URINARY INCONTINENCE

The Urinary Incontinence Guideline Panel defines urinary incontinence as an involuntary loss of urine that is sufficient to be a problem.[19] This panel was convened by the Agency for Health Care Policy and Research in 1992 and again in 1996 for the purpose of developing specific guidelines to improve the care of persons with urinary incontinence.[19]

Urinary incontinence affects approximately 13 million Americans. Many body functions decline with age, and incontinence, although not a normal accompaniment of the aging process, is seen with increased frequency in elderly persons.[19] For elderly persons living in the community, the prevalence of incontinence ranges from 15% to 35%,[20,21] with women being affected twice as often as men.[20] The increase in health problems often seen in elderly persons probably contributes to the greater frequency of incontinence. Despite the prevalence of incontinence, most affected persons do not seek help for it, primarily because of embarrassment or because they are not aware that help is available.

Incontinence can be caused by a number of conditions. It can occur without the person's knowledge; at other times, the person may be aware of the condition but be unable to prevent it. The Urinary Incontinence Guideline Panel has identified four main types of incontinence: stress incontinence, urge incontinence, overflow incontinence, and mixed incontinence, which is a combination of stress and urge incontinence.[19] Recently, the term *overactive bladder* has been designated as a term to replace *urge incontinence*.[20] Table 37-3 summarizes the characteristics of stress incontinence, urge incontinence/overactive bladder, and overflow incontinence.

Incontinence may occur as a transient and correctable phenomenon, or it may not be totally correctable and

INCONTINENCE

- Incontinence represents the involuntary loss of urine due to increased bladder pressures (overactive bladder with urge incontinence or overflow incontinence) or decreased ability of the vesicourethral sphincter to prevent the escape of urine (stress incontinence).
- Stress incontinence is caused by the decreased ability of the vesicourethral sphincter to prevent the escape of urine during activities, such as lifting and coughing, that raise bladder pressure above the sphincter closing pressure.
- Overactive bladder/urge incontinence is caused by neurogenic or myogenic disorders that result in hyperactive bladder contractions.
- Overflow incontinence results from overfilling of the bladder with escape of urine.

TABLE 37-3 Types and Characteristics of Urinary Incontinence

Type	Characteristics
Stress	Involuntary loss of urine associated with activities, such as coughing, that increase intra-abdominal pressure
Overactive bladder/ urge incontinence	Urgency and frequency associated with hyperactivity of the detrusor muscle; may or may not involve involuntary loss of urine
Overflow	Involuntary loss of urine when intravesicular pressure exceeds maximal urethral pressure in the absence of detrusor activity

occur with various degrees of frequency. Among the transient causes of urinary incontinence are confusional states; medications that alter bladder function or perception of bladder filling and the need to urinate; diuretics and conditions that increase bladder filling; restricted mobility; and stool impaction.[22]

Stress Incontinence

Stress incontinence is the involuntary loss of urine during coughing, laughing, sneezing, or lifting that increases intra-abdominal pressure. With severe urinary stress incontinence, any strain or increase in bladder pressure leads to urinary leakage.

In women, the angle between the bladder and the posterior proximal urethra (*i.e.*, urethrovesical junction) is important to continence.[23] This angle normally is 90 to 100 degrees, with at least one third of the bladder base contributing to the angle when not voiding[24] (Fig. 37-5). During the first stage of voiding, this angle is lost as the bladder descends. In women, diminution of muscle tone associated with normal aging, childbirth, or surgical procedures can cause weakness of the pelvic floor muscles and result in stress incontinence by obliterating the critical posterior urethrovesical angle. In these women, loss of the posterior urethrovesical angle, descent and funneling of the bladder neck, and backward and downward rotation of the bladder occur, so that the bladder and urethra are already in an anatomic position for the first stage of voiding. Any activity that causes downward pressure on the bladder is sufficient to allow the urine to escape involuntarily.

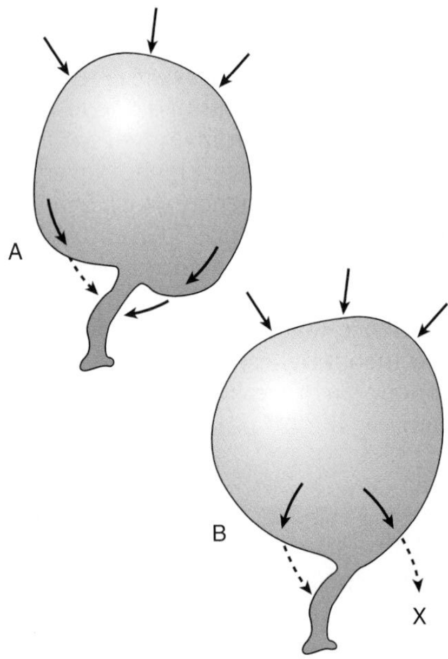

FIGURE 37-5 Importance of the posterior urethrovesical (PU-V) angle to the continence mechanism. **(A)** In the presence of the normal PU-V angle, sudden changes in intra-abdominal pressure are transmitted optimally (indicated by the *arrows with dotted lines*) to all sides of the proximal urethra. In this way, intraurethral pressure is maintained higher than the simultaneously elevated intravesicular pressure. This prevents loss of urine with sudden stress. **(B)** Loss of the PU-V angle results in displacement of the vesicle neck to the most dependent portion of the bladder, preventing the equal transmission of sudden increases in intra-abdominal pressure to the lumen of the proximal urethra. Thus, the pressure in the region of the vesicle neck rises considerably more than the intraurethral pressure just beyond it, and stress incontinence occurs. (Green J.T., Jr. [1968]. *Obstetrical and Gynecological Survey* 23, 603. Reprinted with permission)

Another cause of stress incontinence is intrinsic urethral deficiency, which may result from congenital sphincter weakness, as occurs with meningomyelocele. It also may be acquired as a result of trauma, irradiation, or sacral cord lesion. Stress incontinence in men may result from a congenital defect or from trauma or surgery to the bladder outlet, as occurs with prostatectomy. Neurologic dysfunction, as occurs with impaired sympathetic innervation of the bladder neck, impaired pelvic nerve innervation to the intrinsic sphincter, or impaired pudendal nerve innervation to the external sphincter, may also be a contributing factor.

Overactive Bladder/Urge Incontinence

The Urinary Incontinence Guideline Panel has defined urge incontinence as the involuntary loss of urine associated with a strong desire to void (urgency).[19] To expand the number and types of patients eligible for clinical trials, the U.S. Food and Drug Administration adopted the term *overactive bladder* to describe the clinical syndrome that describes not only urge incontinence but also urgency, frequency, dysuria, and nocturia.[20] Although overactive bladder often is associated with urge incontinence, it can occur without incontinence.[18]

Although some cases of overactive bladder result from specific conditions such as acute or chronic urinary tract infections, in many cases, the cause is unknown. Regardless of the primary cause of overactive bladder, two types of mechanisms are thought to contribute to its symptomatology: those involving CNS control of bladder sensation and emptying (neurogenic), and those involving the smooth muscle of the bladder itself (myogenic).[18]

The CNS functions as an on-off switching circuit for voluntary control of bladder function. Therefore, neurologic damage to central inhibitory pathways or sensitization of peripheral afferent terminals in the bladder may trigger bladder overactivity owing to uncontrolled voiding reflexes. Neurogenic causes of overactive bladder include stroke, Parkinson's disease, and multiple sclerosis. Other neurogenic causes of overactive bladder include increased peripheral afferent activity or increased peripheral sensitivity to efferent impulses.

Myogenic causes of overactive bladder are thought to result from spontaneous elevations in bladder pressure arising from changes in the properties of the smooth muscle of the bladder itself. One example is overactive bladder associated with bladder outlet obstruction. It is hypothesized that the sustained increase in intravesicular pressure that occurs with the outlet obstruction causes a partial destruction of the efferent nerve endings that control bladder excitability.[18] The result is urgency and frequency of urination due to spontaneous bladder contractions resulting from detrusor muscle hyperexcitability. Disorders of detrusor muscle structure and excitability also can occur as the result of the aging process or disease conditions such as diabetes mellitus. Overactive bladder symptoms usually are exaggerated by incomplete bladder emptying.

In persons with overactive bladder, urge incontinence may occur because the interval between knowing the bladder needs to be emptied and being able to stop it from emptying may be less than the time needed to reach the lavatory. Musculoskeletal disorders, such as arthritis and joint instability, also may prevent an otherwise continent person from reaching the toilet in time. Drugs such as hypnotics, tranquilizers, and sedatives can interfere with the conscious inhibition of voiding, leading to urge incontinence. Diuretics, particularly in elderly persons, increase the flow of urine and may contribute to incontinence, particularly in persons with diminished bladder capacity and in those who have difficulty reaching the toilet.

Treatment methods for overactive bladder include the use of behavioral methods and pharmacologic agents. Behavioral methods include fluid management, modification of voiding frequency, and bladder retraining.[25] Bladder retraining and biofeedback techniques seek to reestablish cortical control over bladder function by having the person ignore urgency and respond only to cortical signals during waking hours. Two newer anticholinergic medications, tolterodine (Detrol) and extended-release oxybutynin (Ditropan XL), may be used to inhibit detrusor muscle hyperactivity and thereby increase overall bladder capacity.[18,25,26]

Overflow Incontinence

Overflow incontinence is an involuntary loss of urine that occurs when intravesicular pressure exceeds the maximal urethral pressure because of bladder distention in the absence of detrusor activity. It can occur with retention of urine owing to nervous system lesions or obstruction of the bladder neck. With this type of incontinence, the bladder is distended, and small amounts of urine are passed, particularly at night. In males, one of the most common causes of obstructive incontinence is enlargement of the prostate gland. Another cause that commonly is overlooked is fecal impaction (*i.e.,* dry, hard feces in the rectum). When a large bolus of stool forms in the rectum, it can push against the urethra and block the flow of urine.

The Standardization Sub-Committee of the International Continence Committee recommends that the term *overflow incontinence* should no longer be used, indicating that the term is confusing and lacking definition.[27] Instead, it suggests that more specific terms such as *reduced urethral function* or *overactivity/low bladder compliance* be used.

Other Causes of Incontinence

Another cause of incontinence is decreased bladder compliance or distensibility. This abnormal bladder condition may result from radiation therapy, radical pelvic surgery, or interstitial cystitis. Many persons with this disorder have severe urgency related to bladder hypersensitivity that results in loss of bladder elasticity, such that any small increase in bladder volume or detrusor function causes a sharp rise in bladder pressure and severe urgency.

Incontinence also may be caused by factors outside the lower urinary tract, such as the inability to locate, reach, or receive assistance in reaching an appropriate place to void.[14] This may be a particular problem for elderly persons, who may have problems with mobility and manual dexterity or find themselves in unfamiliar surroundings. It occurs when a person cannot find or reach the bathroom or manipulate clothing quickly enough. Failing vision may contribute to the problem. Embarrassment in front of other persons at having to use the bathroom, particularly if the timing seems inappropriate, may cause a person to delay emptying the bladder and may lead to incontinence.

Treatment with drugs such as diuretics may cause the bladder to fill more rapidly than usual, making it difficult to reach the bathroom in time if there are problems with mobility or if a bathroom is not readily available. Night sedation may cause a person to sleep through the signal that normally would waken a person so that he or she could get up and empty the bladder and avoid wetting the bed.

Diagnosis and Treatment

Urinary incontinence is a frequent and major health problem. It increases social isolation, frequently leads to institutionalization of elderly persons, and predisposes to infections and skin breakdown.

Urinary incontinence is not a single disease but a symptom with many possible causes. As a symptom, it requires full investigation to establish its cause. This usually is accomplished through a careful history, physical examination, blood tests, and urinalysis.[20,22] A voiding record (*i.e.,* diary) may be used to determine the frequency, timing, amount of voiding, and other factors associated with the incontinence.[20] Because many drugs affect bladder function, a full drug history is essential. Estimation of PVR volume is recommended for all persons with incontinence. Provocative stress testing is done when stress incontinence is suspected. This test is done by having the person relax and then cough vigorously while the examiner observes for urine loss. The test usually is done in the lithotomy position; if no leakage is observed, it is repeated in the standing position.[20] Urodynamic studies may be needed to provide information about urinary pressures and urine flow rates.

Treatment or management depends on the type of incontinence, accompanying health problems, and the person's age. Exercises to strengthen the pelvic muscles and surgical correction of pelvic relaxation disorders often are used for women with stress incontinence. Noncatheter devices to obstruct urine flow or collect urine as it is passed may be used when urine flow cannot be controlled. Indwelling catheters (discussed earlier), although a solution to the problem of urinary incontinence, usually are considered only after all other treatment methods have failed. In some types of incontinence, such as that associated with spinal cord injury or meningomyelocele, self-catheterization provides the means for controlling urine elimination.

Treatment of Stress Incontinence. Stress incontinence can be treated by physiotherapeutic measures, surgery, or a combination of the two. Surgical correction of cystocele and pelvic relaxation disorders may be needed for women.

Active muscle-tensing exercises of the pelvic muscles may prove effective.[20,28,29] These exercises were first advocated by Kegel, and they commonly are called *Kegel's exercises.*[30] Two groups of muscles are strengthened: those of the back part of the pelvic floor (*i.e.,* muscles used to contract the anus and control the passing of stool) and the front muscles of the pelvic floor (*i.e.,* muscles used to stop the flow of urine during voiding). In learning the exercises, a woman concentrates on identifying the muscle groups and learning how to control contraction. After this has been accomplished, she can start an exercise program that consists of slowly contracting the muscles, beginning at the front and working to the back while counting to four and then releasing. The exercises can be done while sitting or standing and usually are performed in repetitions of 10, three times each day. A vaginal cone, a tampon-like device, may be used to enhance the benefits of the exercise. The cone is placed in the vagina, and the woman instructed to hold it in place by contracting the proper inner muscles.[31]

The α-adrenergic agonist drugs, such as pseudoephedrine, increase sympathetic relaxation of the detrusor muscle and internal sphincter tone and may be used in treating stress incontinence.[20] Imipramine, a tricyclic antidepressant agent that has α-adrenergic and anticholinergic properties, has proved useful in some women. Surgical intervention may be considered when other treatment methods have proved ineffective. Three types of surgical procedures are used: procedures that increase outlet resistance, surgeries that decrease detrusor muscle instability, and operations that remove outflow obstruction to reduce overflow incontinence and detrusor muscle instability. A new development for the treatment of stress incontinence is the tension-free vaginal tape procedure.[32] The procedure, which is minimally invasive and performed under local anesthesia, involves recreating suburethral support with a polypropylene mesh, without repositioning the bladder or urethra. Initial results from the procedure appear to be promising, with one study reporting a 90% cure rate.[32]

Another minimally invasive procedure for the treatment of stress incontinence is periurethral injection of a bulking agent (glutaraldehyde cross-linked bovine collagen or carbon-coated beads). Both of these agents typically require multiple treatment sessions to achieve cure.[20,23]

Noncatheter Devices. Two types of noncatheter devices commonly are used in the management of urinary incontinence: one obstructs flow, and the other collects urine as it is passed. Obstruction of urine flow is achieved by compressing the urethra or stimulating contraction of the pelvic floor muscles. Penile clamps are available that occlude the urethra without obstructing blood circulation to the penis. Clamps must be removed at 3-hour intervals to empty the bladder. Complications such as penile and urethral erosion can occur if clamps are used incorrectly. In females, compression of the urethra usually is accomplished by intravaginal devices.

Surgically implanted artificial sphincters are available for use in males and females. These devices consist of an inflatable cuff that surrounds the proximal urethra. The cuff is connected by tubing to an implanted fluid reservoir and an inflation bulb. Pressing the bulb, which is placed in the scrotum in males, inflates the cuff. It is emptied in a similar manner.

When urinary incontinence cannot be prevented, various types of urine collection devices or protective pads are used. Men can be fitted with collection devices (*i.e.,* condom or sheath urinals) that are worn over the penis and attached to a container at the bedside or fastened to the body. There are no effective external collection devices for women. Pants and pads usually are used. Dribbling bags (males) and pads (females) in which the urine changes to a nonpourable gel are available for occasional dribbling but are unsuitable for considerable wetting.

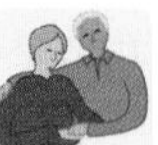

Special Needs of Elderly Persons

Urinary incontinence is a common problem in elderly persons. An estimated 15% to 30% of community-dwelling elders and 50% of institutionalized elders have severe urinary incontinence.[21,33] The economic and social costs of incontinence are staggering. Annually, more than $3 billion is spent managing incontinence in nursing homes alone.[34]

Many factors contribute to incontinence in elderly persons, a number of which can be altered. More than half of normal elderly persons experience nocturia. The overall capacity of the bladder is reduced, as is the urethral closing pressure.[21] Detrusor muscle function also tends to decline with aging; thus, there is a trend toward a reduction in the strength of bladder contraction and impairment in emptying that leads to larger PVR volumes.[2,21,35] It has been proposed that many of these changes are due to degenerative detrusor muscle changes rather than neurologic changes, as was once thought. The combination of involuntary detrusor contraction (detrusor hyperactivity) leading to urge incontinence, along with impaired contractile function, leads to incomplete bladder emptying. Pelvic relaxation disorders are also more frequent in older than in younger women, and prostatic hypertrophy is more common in older than in younger men.

Furthermore, advancing age often results in restricted mobility, an increasing number of medications being taken, comorbid illness, infection, and stool impaction, all of which can precipitate urinary incontinence.[21,35] Many elderly persons have difficulty getting to the toilet in time. This can be caused by arthritis that makes walking or removing clothing difficult or by failing vision that makes trips to the bathroom precarious, especially in new and unfamiliar surroundings.

Medication prescribed for other health problems may prevent a healthy bladder from functioning normally.[21,23,35] Potent, fast-acting diuretics are known for their ability to cause urge incontinence. Psychoactive drugs, such as tranquilizers and sedatives, may diminish normal attention to bladder clues. Impaired thirst or limited access to fluids predisposes to constipation with urethral obstruction and overflow incontinence and to concentrated and infected urine, which increases bladder excitability.

Diagnosis and Treatment. According to Stanton, "there are two guiding principles in management of incontinence in the elderly. First, growing old does not imply becoming incontinent, and second, incontinence should not be left untreated just because the patient is old."[36]

The treatment of urinary incontinence in elderly persons requires a thorough history and physical examination to determine the cause of the problem. A voiding history is important. A voiding diary provides a means for the person to provide objective information about the number of bathroom visits, the number of protective pads used, and even the volume of urine voided. A medication history is also important because medications can affect bladder function.[21]

There are many nonurologic conditions that predispose to urinary incontinence. The transient and often treatable causes of urinary incontinence in elderly persons may best be remembered with the acronym DIAPPERS, in which the D stands for dementia/dementias, I for infection (urinary or vaginal), A for atrophic vaginitis, P for pharmaceutical agents, P for psychological causes, E for endocrine conditions (diabetes), R for restricted mobility, and S for stool impaction.[37] These eight transient causes of incontinence should be identified and treated before other treatment options are considered.

Treatment may involve changes in the physical environment so that the older person can reach the bathroom more easily or remove clothing more quickly. Habit training with regularly scheduled toileting—usually every 2 to 4 hours—often is effective. Many elderly persons who void on a regular schedule can gradually increase the interval between toileting while improving their ability to suppress bladder instability. The treatment plan may require dietary changes to prevent constipation or a plan to promote adequate fluid intake to ensure adequate bladder filling and prevent urinary stasis and symptomatic urinary tract infections.

In summary, alterations in bladder function include urinary obstruction with retention of urine, neurogenic bladder, and urinary incontinence with involuntary loss of urine. Urine retention occurs when the outflow of urine from the bladder is obstructed because of urethral obstruction or impaired bladder innervation. Urethral obstruction causes bladder irritability, detrusor muscle hypertrophy, trabeculation and the formation of diverticula, development of hydroureters, and eventually, renal failure.

Neurogenic bladder is caused by interruption in the innervation of the bladder. It can result in spastic bladder dysfunction caused by failure of the bladder to fill or flaccid bladder dysfunction caused by failure of the bladder to empty. Spastic bladder dysfunction usually results from neurologic lesions that are above the level of the sacral micturition reflex center; flaccid bladder dysfunction results from lesions at the level of the sacral micturition reflexes or peripheral innervation of the bladder. A third type of neurogenic disorder involves a nonrelaxing external sphincter.

Urinary incontinence is the involuntary loss of urine in amounts sufficient to be a problem. It may manifest as stress incontinence, in which the loss of urine occurs as a result of coughing, sneezing, laughing, or lifting; overactive bladder, characterized by frequency and urgency associated with hyperactive bladder contractions; or overflow incontinence, which results when intravesicular pressure exceeds the maximal urethral pressure because of bladder distention. Other causes of incontinence include a small, contracted bladder or external environmental conditions that make it difficult to access proper toileting facilities. The acronym DIAPPERS—D (dementia) I (infection) A (atrophic vaginitis) P (pharmaceutical) P (psychological) E (endocrine) R (restricted mobility) S (stool impaction) emphasizes the transient and often treatable causes of incontinence in the elderly.

The treatment of urinary obstruction, neurogenic bladder, and incontinence requires careful diagnosis to determine the cause and contributing factors. Treatment methods include correction of the underlying cause, such as obstruction due to prostatic hyperplasia; pharmacologic methods to improve bladder and external sphincter tone; behavior methods that focus on bladder and habit training; exercises to improve pelvic floor function; and the use of catheters and urine collection devices.

Cancer of the Bladder

After completing this section of the chapter, you should be able to meet the following objectives:

- Discuss the difference between superficial and invasive bladder cancer in terms of bladder involvement, extension of the disease, and prognosis
- State the most common sign of bladder cancer

Bladder cancer is the most frequent form of urinary tract cancer in the United States, accounting for more than 57,700 new cases and 12,500 deaths each year.[38] It is three times more common in men than women and has an average age of onset of 65 years. Its incidence is higher in whites than African Americans.[39]

Approximately 90% of bladder cancers are derived from the transitional (urothelial) cells that line the bladder.[40–42] These tumors can range from low-grade noninvasive tumors to high-grade tumors that invade the bladder wall and metastasize frequently. The low-grade tumors, which may recur after resection, have an excellent prognosis, with only a small number (2% to 10%) progressing to higher-grade tumors.[41,42] The high-grade tumors tend to have greater invasive and metastatic potential and are potentially fatal in approximately 60% of cases within 10 years of diagnosis.[40]

ETIOLOGY AND PATHOPHYSIOLOGY

Although the cause of bladder cancer is unknown, evidence suggests that its origin is related to local influences, such as carcinogens that are excreted in the urine and stored in the bladder. These include the breakdown products of aromatic amines used in the dye industry, products used in the manufacture of rubber, textiles, paint, chemicals, and petroleum.[42] Smoking also deserves attention.[41,42] Fifty percent to 80% of bladder cancers in men are associated with cigarette smoking.[40] Chronic bladder infections and bladder stones also increase the risk for bladder cancer. Bladder cancer is more frequent among persons harboring the parasite *Schistosoma haematobium* in their bladder.[40]

The parasite is endemic in Egypt and Sudan. It is not known whether the parasite excretes a carcinogen or produces its effects through irritation of the bladder.

MANIFESTATIONS

The most common sign of bladder cancer is painless hematuria.[38,39,42] Gross hematuria is a presenting sign in 75% of persons with the disease, and microscopic hematuria is present in most others. Frequency, urgency, and dysuria occasionally accompany the hematuria. Because hematuria often is intermittent, the diagnosis may be delayed. Periodic urine cytology is recommended for all persons who are at high risk for the development of bladder cancer because of exposure to urinary tract carcinogens. Ureteral invasion leading to bacterial and obstructive renal disease and dissemination of the cancer are potential complications and ultimate causes of death. The prognosis depends on the histologic grade of the cancer and the stage of the disease at the time of diagnosis.

DIAGNOSIS AND TREATMENT

Diagnostic methods include cytologic studies, excretory urography, cystoscopy, and biopsy. Ultrasonography, CT scans, and MRI are used as aids for staging the tumor. Cytologic studies performed on biopsy tissues or cells obtained from bladder washings may be used to detect the presence of malignant cells.[39,42] A technique called *flow cytometry* is helpful in screening persons at high risk for the disease and for monitoring the results of therapy. In flow cytometry, the interaction between fluorochromes or dyes with DNA causes the emission of high-intensity light similar to that produced by a laser.[39] Flow cytometry can be carried out on biopsy specimens, bladder washings, or cytologic preparations.

The treatment of bladder cancer depends on the extent of the lesion and the health of the patient. Endoscopic resection usually is done for diagnostic purposes and may be used as a treatment for superficial lesions. Diathermy (*i.e.*, electrocautery) may be used to remove the tumors. Segmental surgical resection may be used for removing a large single lesion. When the tumor is invasive, cystectomy with resection of the pelvic lymph nodes frequently is the treatment of choice. In males, the prostate and seminal vesicles often are removed as well. Until the 1980s, most men who underwent radical cystectomy became impotent. Newer surgical approaches designed to preserve erectile function now are being used. Cystectomy requires urinary diversion, an alternative reservoir, usually created from the ileum (*e.g.*, an ileal loop), that is designed to collect the urine. Traditionally, the ileostomy reservoir drains urine continuously into an external collecting device. External beam radiation therapy is an alternative to radical cystectomy in some patients with deeply infiltrating bladder cancer.[39]

Although a number of chemotherapeutic drugs have been used in the treatment of bladder cancer, no chemotherapeutic regimens for the disease have been established. Perhaps of more importance is the increasing use of intravesicular chemotherapy, in which the cytotoxic drug is instilled directly into the bladder, thereby avoiding the side effects of systemic therapy. These drugs can be instilled prophylactically after surgical resection of all demonstrable tumor or therapeutically in the presence of residual disease. Among the chemotherapeutic drugs that have been used for this purpose are thiotepa, mitomycin C, and doxorubicin (Adriamycin).[39] The intervesicular administration of bacillus Calmette-Guérin (BCG) vaccine, made from a strain of *Mycobacterium bovis* that formerly was used to protect against tuberculosis, causes a significant reduction in the rate of relapse and prolongs relapse-free interval in persons with cancer in situ. The vaccine is thought to act as a nonspecific stimulator of cell-mediated immunity. It is not known whether the effects of BCG are immunologic or include a component of direct toxicity. Several strains of this agent exist, and it is not known which is the most active and least toxic.

In summary, cancer of the bladder is the most common cause of urinary tract cancer in the United States. Bladder cancers fall into two major groups: low-grade noninvasive tumors, and high-grade invasive tumors that are associated with metastasis and a worse prognosis. Although the cause of cancer of the bladder is unknown, evidence suggests that carcinogens excreted in the urine may play a role. Microscopic and gross, painless hematuria are the most frequent presenting signs of bladder cancer. The methods used in treatment of bladder cancer depend on the cytologic grade of the tumor and the lesion's degree of invasiveness. The methods include surgical removal of the tumor, radiation therapy, and chemotherapy. In many cases, chemotherapeutic or immunotherapeutic agents can be instilled directly into the bladder, thereby avoiding the side effects of systemic therapy.

REVIEW EXERCISES

A 23-year-old man is recovering after the acute phase of a cervical (C6) spinal cord injury with complete loss of motor and sensory function below the level of injury. He is now experiencing spastic bladder contractions with involuntary and incomplete urination. Urodynamic studies reveal spastic contraction of the external sphincter with urine retention and high bladder pressures.

A. Explain the reason for the involuntary urination and incomplete emptying of the bladder despite high bladder pressures.

B. What are possible complications associated with overdistention and high pressure within the bladder?

A 66-year-old woman complains of leakage of urine during coughing, sneezing, laughing, or squatting down.

A. Explain the source of this woman's problem.

B. One of the recommended treatments for stress incontinence is use of Kegel's exercises, which focus on strengthening the muscles of the pelvic floor. Explain how these exercises contribute to the control of urine leakage in women with stress incontinence.

References

1. Kandel E.R., Schwartz J.H., Jessel T.M. (2000). *Principles of neural science* (4th ed.). New York: McGraw-Hill.
2. Fowler C.J. (1999). Neurological disorders of micturition and their treatment. *Brain 122,* 1213–1231.
3. Guyton A.C., Hall J.E. (2000). *Textbook of medical physiology* (10th ed., pp. 364–367). Philadelphia: W.B. Saunders.
4. Rhoades R.A., Tanner G.A. (2003). *Medical physiology* (2nd ed., pp. 423–424). Philadelphia: Lippincott Williams & Wilkins.
5. Dmochowski R.R., Appell R.A. (2000). Advances in pharmacologic management of overactive bladder. *Urology 56*(Suppl. 6A), 41–49.
6. Elder J.S. (2004). Voiding dysfunction. In Behrman R.E., Kliegman R.M., Jenson H.B. (Eds.), *Nelson textbook of pediatrics* (17th ed., pp. 1808–1809). Philadelphia: W.B. Saunders.
7. Tanagho E.A. (2004). Urodynamic studies. In Tanagho E.A., McAninch J.W. (Eds.), *Smith's general urology* (16th ed., pp. 453–472). New York: Lange Medical Books/McGraw-Hill.
8. Fantl J.A., Newman D.K., Colling J., et al., for the Public Health Service, Agency for Health Care Policy and Research. (1996). *Urinary incontinence in adults: Acute and chronic management.* Clinical Practice Guideline no. 2, 1996 update. AHCPR publication no. 96-0682. Rockville, MD: U.S. Department of Health and Human Services.
9. Schott-Baer F.D., Reaume L. (2001). Accuracy of ultrasound estimates of urine volume. *Urological Nursing 21*(3), 193–195.
10. Tanagho E.A. (2004). Urinary obstruction and stasis. In Tanagho E.A., McAninch J.W. (Eds.), *Smith's general urology* (16th ed., pp. 175–187). New York: Lange Medical Books/McGraw-Hill.
11. Elliott D.S., Boone T.B. (2000). Recent advances in management of neurogenic bladder. *Urology 56*(Suppl. 6A), 76–81.
12. Tanagho E.A., Lue T.F. (2000). Neuropathic bladder disorders. In Tanagho E.A., McAninch J.W. (Eds.), *Smith's general urology* (16th ed., pp. 435–452). New York: Lange Medical Books/McGraw-Hill.
13. Sasaki K., Yoshimura N., Chancellor M.B. (2003). Implication of diabetes mellitus in urology. *Urological Clinics of North America 30*(1), 1–12.
14. Vinik A.I., Maser R.E., Mitchell B.D., Freeman R. (2003). Diabetic autonomic neuropathy. *Diabetes Care 26*(5), 1553–1579.
15. Cravens D.D., Zwieg S. (2000). Urinary catheter management. *American Family Physician 61,* 369–376.
16. Barton R. (2000). Intermittent self-catheterization. *Nursing Standard 15*(9), 47–52.
17. Addison R., Lopez J. (2001). Bladder retraining. *Nursing Times 97*(5), 45–46.
18. Dmochowski R.R., Appell R.A. (2000). Advancements in pharmacologic management of overactive bladder. *Urology 56*(Suppl. 6A), 41–49.
19. Agency for Health Care Policy and Research (AHCPR). Public Health Service, U.S. Department of Heath and Human Services. (1996). *Urinary incontinence in adults: Acute and chronic management.* Clinical Practice Guideline (AHCPR Pub. No 96-0682). Washington D.C.: U.S. Government Printing Office.
20. Culligan P.J., Heit M. (2000). Urinary incontinence in women: Evaluation and management. *American Family Physician 62,* 2433–2452.
21. Klausner A.P., Vapnek J.M. (2003). Urinary incontinence in the geriatric population. *Mount Sinai Journal of Medicine 70*(1), 54–61.
22. Gray M., Burns S.M. (1996). Continence management. *Critical Care Clinics of North America 8,* 29–38.
23. Tanagho E.A. (2004). Urinary incontinence. In Tanagho E.A., McAninch J.W. (Eds.), *Smith's general urology* (17th ed., pp. 473–491). New York: Lange Medical Books/McGraw-Hill.
24. Green T.H. (1975). Urinary stress incontinence: Differential diagnosis, pathophysiology, and management. *American Journal of Obstetrics and Gynecology 122,* 368–382.
25. Wein A.J. (2001). Putting overactive bladder into clinical perspective. *Patient Care for the Nurse Practitioner* (Spring Suppl.), 1–5.
26. Roberts R.R. (2001). Current management strategies for overactive bladder. *Patient Care for the Nurse Practitioner* (Spring Suppl.), 22–30.
27. Abrams P., Cardozo L., Fall M., et al. (2003). The standardization of terminology in lower urinary tract function: Report of the standardization sub-committee of the International Continence Society. *Urology 61,* 37–49.
28. Wells T.J., Brink C.A., Kiokno A.C., et al. (1991). Pelvic muscle exercise for stress urinary incontinence in elderly women. *Journal of the American Geriatrics Society 39,* 785–791.
29. Thakar R., Stanton S. (2000). Management of urinary incontinence in women. *British Medical Journal 321,* 1326–1330.
30. Kegel A.H. (1948). Progressive resistance exercises in the functional restoration of the perineal muscles. *American Journal of Obstetrics and Gynecology 56,* 238–248.
31. Boourcier A.P., Jurat J.C. (1995). Nonsurgical therapy for stress incontinence. *Urologic Clinics of North America 22,* 613–627.
32. Carlin B.I., Klutke J.J., Klutke C.G. (2000). The tension-free vaginal tape procedure for treatment of stress incontinence in the female patient. *Urology 56*(Suppl. 6A), 28–31.
33. Lee S.Y., Phanumus D., Fields S.D. (2000). Urinary incontinence: A primary guide to managing acute and chronic symptoms in older adults. *Geriatrics 55*(11), 65–71.
34. Weiss B.D. (1998). Diagnostic evaluation of urinary incontinence in geriatric patients. *American Family Physician 57,* 2675–2684, 2688–2690.
35. Dubeau C.E. (2002). The continuum of urinary incontinence in an aging population. *Geriatrics 57*(Suppl 1), 12–17.
36. Stanton S.L. (1984). Surgical management of female incontinence. In Brocklehurst J.C. (Ed.), *Urology in the elderly* (p. 93). New York: Churchill Livingstone.
37. Resnick N.M., Yalla S.V. (1998). Geriatric incontinence and voiding dysfunction. In Walsh P.C., Retik A.B., Vaughan E.D., Wein A.J. (Eds.), *Campbell's urology* (7th ed., p. 1045). Philadelphia: W.B. Saunders.
38. American Cancer Society (2003). Bladder cancer: Overview. [On-line]. Available: http://www.cancer.org/cancerinfo.
39. Grossfeld G.D., Carroll P. (2004). Urothelial carcinoma: Cancers of the bladder, ureter, and renal pelvis. In Tanagho E.A., McAninch J.W. (Eds.), *Smith's general urology* (16th ed., pp. 324–345). New York: Lange Medical Books/McGraw-Hill.
40. Cotran R.S., Kumar V., Collins T. (1999). *Robbins pathologic basis of disease* (6th ed., pp. 1003–1008). Philadelphia: W.B. Saunders.
41. Lee R., Droller M.J. (2000). The natural history of bladder cancer. *Urologic Clinics of North America 27*(1), 1–13.
42. Murphy G.P. (2001). Urologic and male genital cancer. In Lenhard R.E., Osteen R.T., Gansler T. (Eds.), *Clinical oncology* (pp. 408–415). Atlanta: American Cancer Society.

UNIT

IX

Gastrointestinal Function

The study of the gastrointestinal system aroused none of the philosophical interest that surrounded the elements, humors, and pneuma of Galen's time. During ancient times, the gut was thought merely to provide the chyle that was turned into blood by the liver. Although the structures of the gut had been fairly well described, perhaps owing to observations made during the slaughtering of animals, it was not until the 18th and 19th centuries that the function of the gastrointestinal tract began to unfold.

One of the breakthroughs in gastrointestinal physiology came as the result of an accident. In 1822, William Beaumont (1785–1853), a self-trained surgeon in the United States Army, was called upon to render aid to Alexis St. Martin, a Canadian traveler who had suffered a large gunshot wound to the chest and abdomen. Although not expected to live, young St. Martin rallied and his wounds healed; however, he was left with a permanent fistula that opened to his stomach. Beaumont became intrigued with this patient's unique defect, using this living laboratory to study the process of digestion. He would have St. Martin swallow different types of food and then collect the stomach contents by means of a tube passed into the fistula. Beaumont described the movement of the stomach, and he confirmed the presence of hydrochloric acid and a ferment, later shown to be the result of the protein-breaking enzyme pepsin. Because of an unfortunate accident, both Beaumont and St. Martin gained a place in the history of gastrointestinal physiology.

CHAPTER 38

Control of Gastrointestinal Function

The digestive system is an amazing structure. In this system, enzymes and hormones are produced, vitamins are synthesized and stored, and food is dismantled and then reassembled. Nutrients, vitamins, minerals, electrolytes, and water enter the body through the gastrointestinal tract. Wastes are collected and eliminated efficiently.

Structurally, the gastrointestinal tract is a long, hollow tube with its lumen inside the body and its wall acting as an interface between the internal and external environments. The wall does not normally allow harmful agents to enter the body, nor does it permit body fluids and other materials to escape. The process of digestion and absorption of nutrients requires an intact and healthy gastrointestinal tract epithelial lining that can resist the effects of its own digestive secretions. The process also involves movement of materials through the gastrointestinal tract at a rate that facilitates absorption, and it requires the presence of enzymes for the digestion and absorption of nutrients.

As a matter of semantics, the gastrointestinal tract also is referred to as the *digestive tract*, the *alimentary canal*, and, at times, the *gut*. The intestinal portion also may be called the *bowel*. For the purposes of this text, the liver and the pancreas (discussed in Chapter 40), which produce secretions that aid in digestion, are considered *accessory organs*.

Structure and Organization of the Gastrointestinal Tract

After completing this section of the chapter, you should be able to meet the following objectives:

- Describe the physiologic function of the four parts of the digestive system
- List the five layers of the digestive tract and describe their function
- Characterize the function of the intramural neural plexuses in control of gastrointestinal function

In the digestive tract, food and other materials move slowly along its length as they are systematically broken down into ions and molecules that can be absorbed into the body. In the large intestine, unabsorbed nutrients and wastes are collected for later elimination. Although the gastrointestinal tract is located inside the body, it is a long, hollow tube, the lumen (*i.e.*, hollow center) of which is an extension of the external environment. Nutrients do not become part of the internal environment until they have passed through the intestinal wall and have entered the blood or lymph channels.

For simplicity and understanding, the digestive system can be divided into four parts (Fig. 38-1). The upper part—the mouth, esophagus, and stomach—acts as an intake source and receptacle through which food passes and in which initial digestive processes take place. The middle portion consists of the small intestine—the duodenum, jejunum, and ileum. Most digestive and absorptive processes occur in the small intestine. The lower segment—the

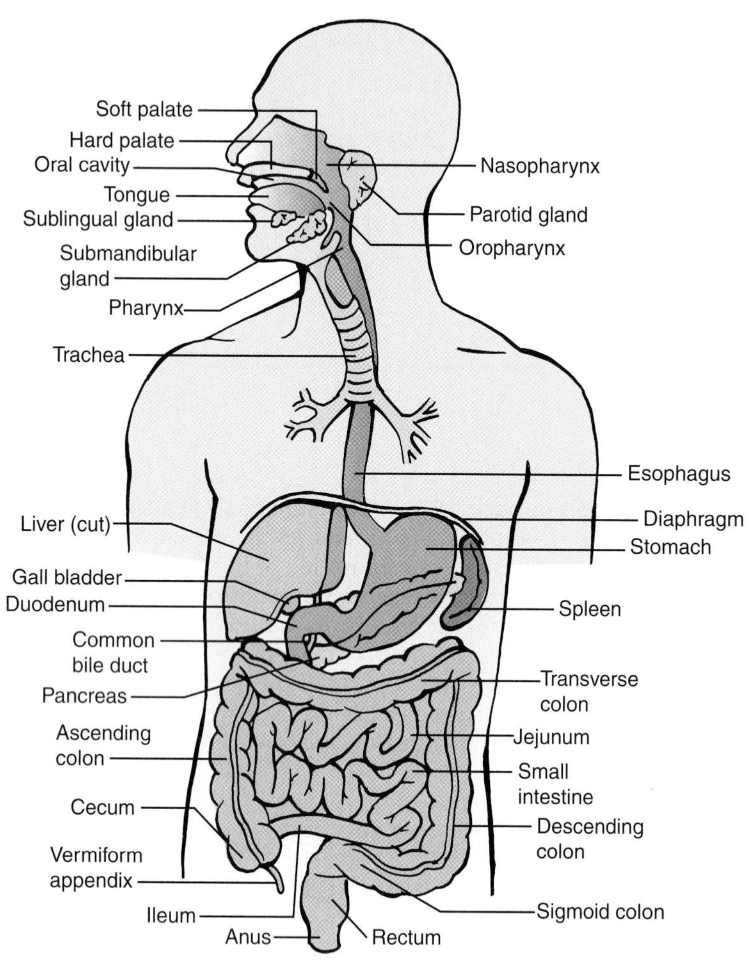

FIGURE 38-1 The digestive system.

cecum, colon, and rectum—serves as a storage channel for the efficient elimination of waste. The fourth part consists of the accessory organs—the salivary glands, liver, and pancreas. These structures produce digestive secretions that help dismantle foods and regulate the use and storage of nutrients. The discussion in this chapter focuses on the first three parts of the gastrointestinal tract. The liver and pancreas are discussed in Chapter 40.

UPPER GASTROINTESTINAL TRACT

The mouth forms the entryway into the gastrointestinal tract for food; it contains the teeth, used in the mastication of food, and the tongue and other structures needed to direct food toward the pharyngeal structures and the esophagus.

The esophagus begins at the lower end of the pharynx. It receives food from the pharynx, and in the process of swallowing, a series of peristaltic contractions moves the food into the stomach. The esophagus is a muscular, collapsible tube, approximately 25 cm (10 in) long, that lies behind the trachea. The muscular walls of the upper third of the esophagus are skeletal-type striated muscle; these muscle fibers are gradually replaced by smooth muscle fibers until, at the lower third of the esophagus, the muscle layer is entirely smooth muscle.

STRUCTURE AND FUNCTION OF THE GASTROINTESTINAL TRACT

- The gastrointestinal tract is a long, hollow tube that extends from the mouth to the anus; food and fluids that enter the gastrointestinal tract do not become part of the internal environment until they have been broken down and absorbed into the blood or lymph channels.
- The wall of the gastrointestinal tract is essentially a five-layered tube: an inner mucosal layer; a supporting submucosal layer of connective tissue; a fourth and fifth layer of circular and longitudinal smooth muscle that functions to propel its contents in a proximal-to-distal direction; and an outer, two-layered peritoneum that encloses and prevents friction between the continuously moving segments of the intestine.
- The nutrients contained in ingested foods and fluids must be broken down into molecules that can be absorbed across the wall of the intestine. Gastric acids and pepsin from the stomach begin the digestive process: bile from the liver, digestive enzymes from the pancreas, and brush border enzymes break carbohydrates, fats, and proteins into molecules that can be absorbed from the intestine.

The upper and lower ends of the esophagus function as sphincters. The upper sphincter is formed by a thickening of the striated muscle; it prevents air from entering the esophagus during respiration. The lower sphincter, which is not identifiable anatomically, occurs at a point 1 to 2 cm (0.4 to 0.8 in) from where the esophagus joins the stomach. The lower sphincter prevents gastric reflux into the esophagus.

The stomach is a pouchlike structure that lies in the upper part of the abdomen and serves as a food storage reservoir during the early stages of digestion. Although the residual volume of the stomach is only approximately 50 mL, it can increase to almost 1000 mL before the intraluminal pressure begins to rise. The esophagus opens into the stomach through an opening called the *cardiac orifice,* so named because of its proximity to the heart. The part of the stomach that lies above and to the left of the cardiac orifice is called the *fundus,* the central portion is called the *body,* the orifice encircled by a ringlike muscle that opens into the small intestine is called the *pylorus,* and the portion between the body and pylorus is called the *antrum* (Fig. 38-2). The presence of a true pyloric sphincter is controversial. Regardless of whether an actual sphincter exists, contractions of the smooth muscle in the pyloric area control the rate of gastric emptying.

MIDDLE GASTROINTESTINAL TRACT

The small intestine, which forms the middle portion of the digestive tract, consists of three subdivisions: the duodenum, the jejunum, and the ileum. The duodenum, which is approximately 22 cm (10 in) long, connects the stomach to the jejunum and contains the opening for the common bile duct and the main pancreatic duct. Bile and pancreatic juices enter the intestine through these ducts. It is in the jejunum and ileum, which together are approximately 7 m (23 ft) long and must be folded onto themselves to fit into the abdominal cavity, that food is digested and absorbed.

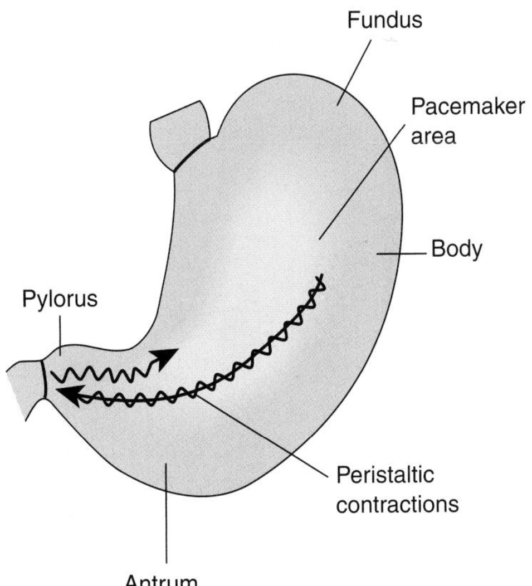

FIGURE 38-2 Structures of the stomach, showing the pacemaker area and the direction of chyme movement resulting from peristaltic contractions.

LOWER GASTROINTESTINAL TRACT

The large intestine, which forms the lower gastrointestinal tract, is approximately 1.5 m (4.5 to 5 ft) long and 6 to 7 cm (2.4 to 2.7 in) in diameter. It is divided into the cecum, colon, rectum, and anal canal. The cecum is a blind pouch that projects down at the junction of the ileum and the colon. The ileocecal valve lies at the upper border of the cecum and prevents the return of feces from the cecum into the small intestine. The appendix arises from the cecum approximately 2.5 cm (1 in) from the ileocecal valve. The colon is further divided into ascending, transverse, descending, and sigmoid portions. The ascending colon extends from the cecum to the undersurface of the liver, where it turns abruptly to form the right colic (hepatic) flexure. The transverse colon crosses the upper half of the abdominal cavity from right to left and then curves sharply downward beneath the lower end of the spleen, forming the left colic (splenic) flexure. The descending colon extends from the colic flexure to the rectum. The rectum extends from the sigmoid colon to the anus. The anal canal passes between the two medial borders of the levator ani muscles. Powerful sphincter muscles guard against fecal incontinence.

GASTROINTESTINAL WALL STRUCTURE

The digestive tract, below the upper third of the esophagus, is essentially a five-layered tube (Fig. 38-3). The inner luminal layer, or *mucosal layer,* is so named because its cells produce mucus that lubricates and protects the inner surface of the alimentary canal. The epithelial cells in this layer have a rapid turnover rate and are replaced every 4 to 5 days. Approximately 250 g of these cells are shed each day in the stool. Because of the regenerative capabilities of the mucosal layer, injury to this layer of tissue heals rapidly without leaving scar tissue. The *submucosal layer* consists of connective tissue. This layer contains blood vessels, nerves, and structures responsible for secreting digestive enzymes.

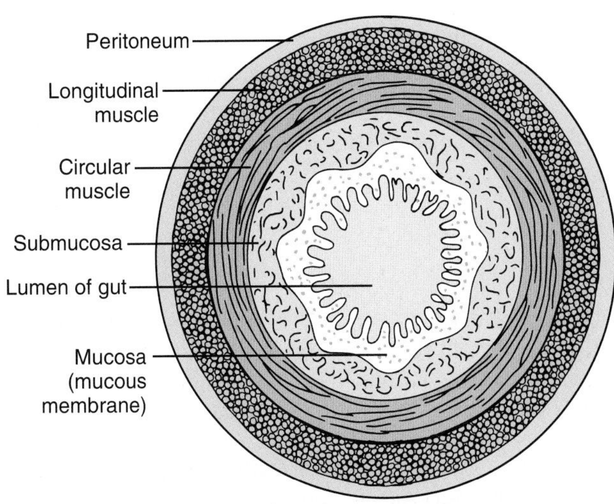

FIGURE 38-3 Transverse section of the digestive system. (Thomson J.S. [1977]. *Core textbook of anatomy.* Philadelphia: J.B. Lippincott)

The third and fourth layers, the *circular* and *longitudinal muscle layers,* facilitate movement of the contents of the gastrointestinal tract. The outer muscularis is enveloped by a thin connective tissue layer that may or may not be surrounded by the simple squamous epithelium of the visceral peritoneum. If the region of the digestive tract is intraperitoneal, it is invested in the peritoneum.

The peritoneum is the largest serous membrane in the body, having a surface area approximately equal to that of the skin. The peritoneal membrane is composed of two layers, a thin layer of simple squamous epithelial cells resting on a layer of connective tissue. If the epithelial layer is injured because of surgery or inflammation, there is danger that adhesions (*i.e.,* fibrous scar tissue bands) may form, causing sections of the viscera to heal together. Adhesions can alter the position and movement of the abdominal viscera.

The peritoneal cavity is a potential space formed between what is called the *parietal peritoneum* and the *visceral peritoneum.* The parietal peritoneum comes in contact with and is loosely attached to the abdominal wall, whereas the abdominal organs are in contact with the visceral peritoneum. The connective tissue layer of the peritoneum forms the parietal and the visceral peritoneum, and the smooth, epithelial cell layer of the membrane lines the cavity. The adjacent membrane layers in the peritoneal cavity are separated by a thin layer of serous fluid. This fluid forms a moist and slippery surface that prevents friction between the continuously moving abdominal structures. In certain pathologic states, the amount of fluid in the potential space of the peritoneal cavity is increased, causing a condition called *ascites.*

The jejunum and ileum are suspended by a double-layered fold of peritoneum called the *mesentery* (Fig. 38-4). The mesentery contains the blood vessels, nerves, and lymphatic vessels that supply the intestinal wall. The mesentery is gathered in folds that attach to the dorsal abdominal wall along a short line of insertion, giving a fan-shaped appearance, with the intestines at the edge. A filmy, double fold of peritoneal membrane called the *greater omentum* extends from the stomach to cover the transverse colon and folds of the intestine (Fig. 38-5). The greater omentum protects the intestines from cold. It always contains some fat, which in obese persons can be a considerable amount. The omentum also controls the spread of infection from gastrointestinal contents. In the case of infection, the omentum adheres to the inflamed area so that the infection is less likely to enter the peritoneal cavity. The lesser omentum extends between the transverse fissure of the liver and the lesser curvature of the stomach.

In summary, the gastrointestinal tract is a long, hollow tube, the lumen of which is an extension of the external environment. The digestive tract can be divided into four parts: an upper part, consisting of the mouth, esophagus, and stomach; a middle part, consisting of the small intestine; a lower part, consisting of the cecum, colon, and rectum; and the accessory organs, consisting of the salivary glands, the liver, and the pancreas. Throughout its length, except for the mouth, throat, and upper esophagus, the gastrointestinal tract is composed of five layers: an inner mucosal layer, a submucosal layer, a layer of circular smooth muscle fibers, a layer of longitudinal smooth muscle fibers, and an outer serosal layer that forms the peritoneum and is continuous with the mesentery.

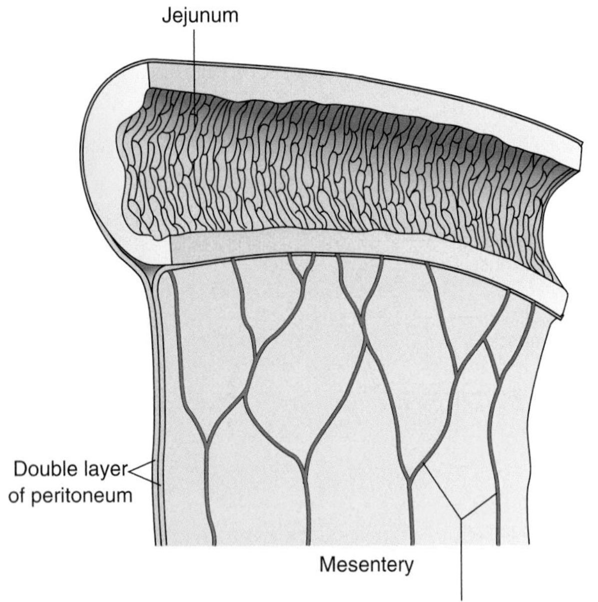

FIGURE 38-4 The attachment of the mesentery to the small bowel. (Thomson J.S. [1977]. *Core textbook of anatomy.* Philadelphia: J.B. Lippincott)

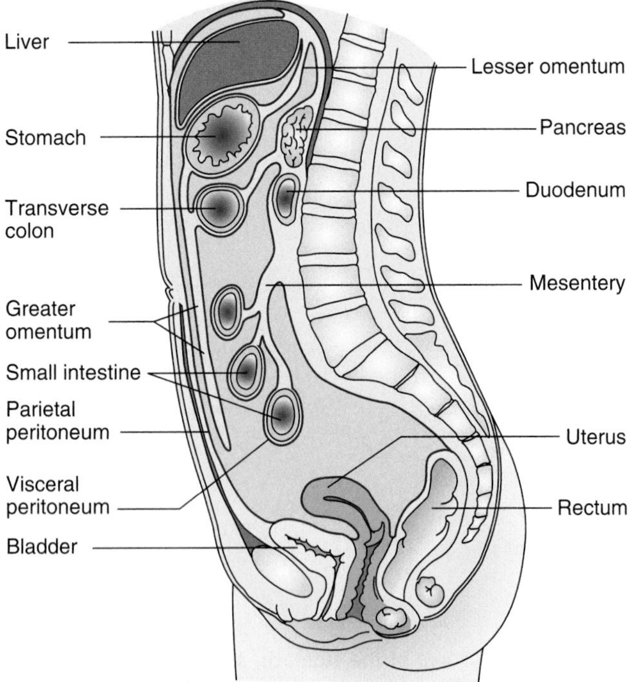

FIGURE 38-5 Reflections of the peritoneum as seen in sagittal section.

Motility

After completing this section of the chapter, you should be able to meet the following objectives:

- ✦ Compare the effects of parasympathetic and sympathetic activity on the motility and secretory function of the gastrointestinal tract
- ✦ Differentiate tonic and peristaltic movements in the gastrointestinal tract
- ✦ Trace a bolus of food through the stages of swallowing
- ✦ Describe the action of the internal and external sphincters in the control of defecation

The motility of the gastrointestinal tract propels food products and fluids along its length, from mouth to anus, in a manner that facilitates digestion and absorption. Except in the pharynx and upper third of the esophagus, smooth muscle provides the contractile force for gastrointestinal motility (the actions of smooth muscle are discussed in Chapter 4). The rhythmic movements of the digestive tract are self-perpetuating, much like the activity of the heart, and are influenced by local, humoral (*i.e.*, bloodborne), and neural influences. The ability to initiate impulses is a property of the smooth muscle itself. Impulses are conducted from one muscle fiber to another.

The movements of the gastrointestinal tract are tonic and rhythmic. The tonic movements are continuous movements that last for minutes or even hours. Tonic contractions occur at sphincters. The rhythmic movements consist of intermittent contractions that are responsible for mixing and moving food along the digestive tract. Peristaltic movements are rhythmic propulsive movements that occur when the smooth muscle layer constricts, forming a contractile band that forces the intraluminal contents forward. During peristalsis, the segment that lies distal to, or ahead of, the contracted portion relaxes, and the contents move forward with ease. Normal peristalsis always moves in the direction from the mouth toward the anus.

NEURAL CONTROL MECHANISMS

Gastrointestinal function is controlled by the *enteric nervous system,* which lies entirely within the wall of the gastrointestinal tract, and by the parasympathetic and sympathetic divisions of the autonomic nervous system (ANS). The intramural neurons (*i.e.*, those contained within the wall of the gastrointestinal tract) consist of two networks, the myenteric and submucosal plexuses. Both plexuses are aggregates of ganglionic cells that extend along the length of the gastrointestinal wall. The myenteric (Auerbach's) plexus is located between the circular muscle and longitudinal muscle layers, and the submucosal (Meissner's) plexus is between the mucosal layer and the circular muscle layers (Fig. 38-6). The activity of the neurons in the myenteric and submucosal plexuses is regulated by local influences, by input from the ANS, and by interconnecting fibers that transmit information between the two plexuses. The myenteric plexus consists mainly of a linear chain of interconnecting neurons that extends the full length of the

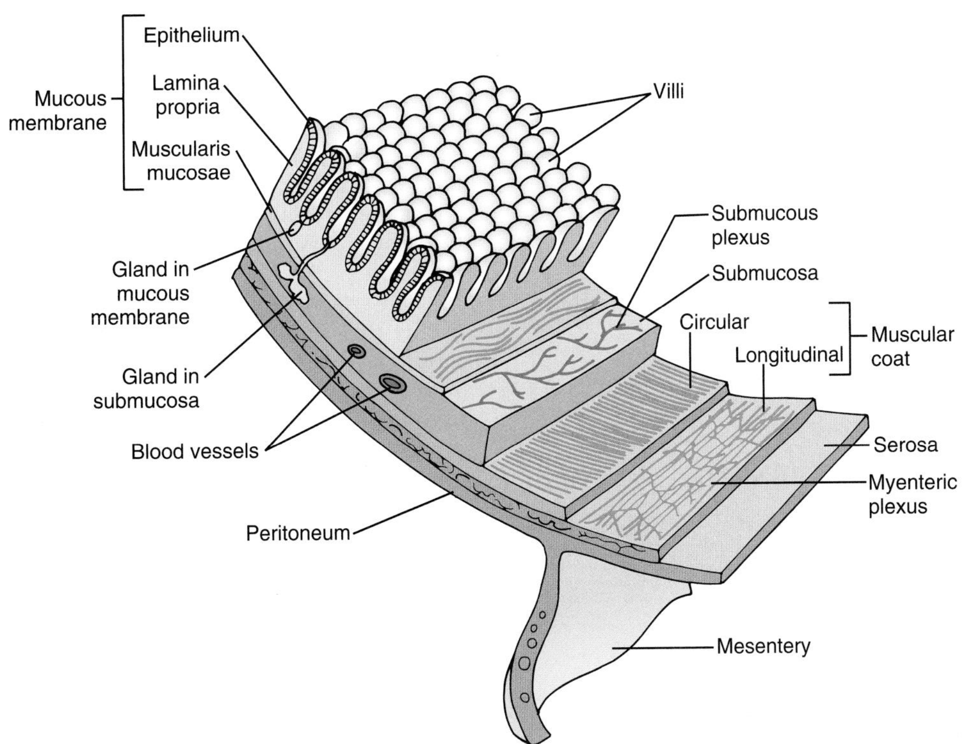

FIGURE 38-6 Diagram of the four main layers of the wall of the digestive tube: mucosa, submucosa, muscular, and serosa (below the diaphragm).

gastrointestinal tract. Because it extends all the way down the intestinal wall and because it lies between the two muscle layers, it is concerned mainly with motility along the length of the gut. The submucosal plexus, which lies between the mucosal and muscle layers of the intestinal wall, is mainly concerned with controlling the function of each segment of the intestinal tract. It integrates signals received from the mucosal layer into local control of motility, intestinal secretions, and absorption of nutrients.

The digestive tract contains two types of afferent fibers: those with cell bodies located in the nervous system and those with cell bodies located in the intramural plexuses. The first group has receptors in the mucosal epithelium and in the muscle layers; their fibers pass centrally in vagal and sympathetic fibers. The second group is located in the intramural plexus and exerts local control over motility.

Efferent parasympathetic innervation to the stomach, small intestine, cecum, ascending colon, and transverse colon occurs by way of the vagus nerve (Fig. 38-7). The remainder of the colon is innervated by parasympathetic fibers that exit the sacral segments of the spinal cord by way of the pelvic nerve. Preganglionic parasympathetic fibers can synapse with intramural plexus neurons, or they can act directly on intestinal smooth muscle. Most parasympathetic fibers are excitatory. Numerous vagovagal reflexes influence motility and secretions of the digestive tract.

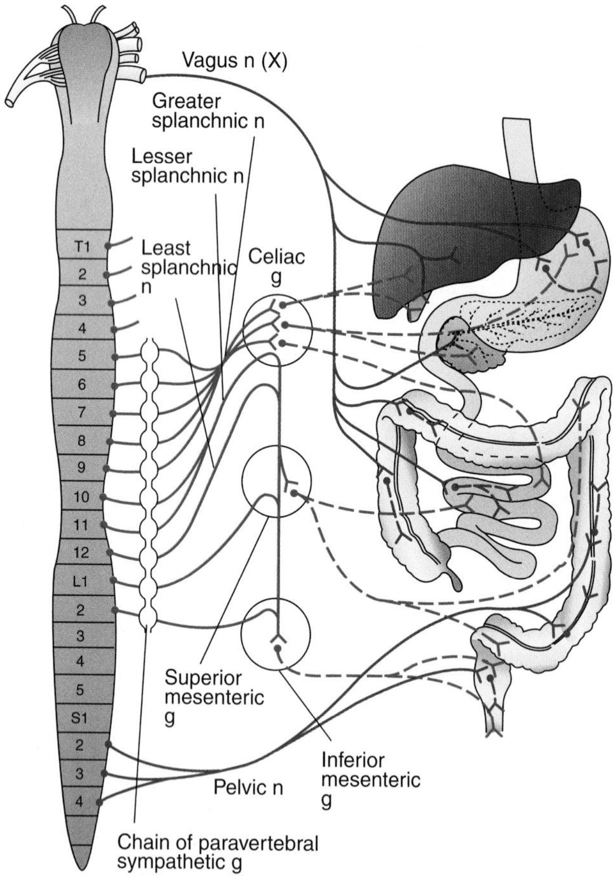

FIGURE 38-7 The autonomic innervation of the gastrointestinal tract (g, ganglion; n, nerve).

Efferent sympathetic innervation of the gastrointestinal tract occurs through the thoracic chain of sympathetic ganglia and the celiac, superior mesenteric, and inferior mesenteric ganglia. The sympathetic nervous system exerts several effects on gastrointestinal function. It controls the extent of mucus secretion by the mucosal glands, reduces motility by inhibiting the activity of intramural plexus neurons, enhances sphincter function, and increases the vascular smooth muscle tone of the blood vessels that supply the gastrointestinal tract. The effect of the sympathetic stimulation is to block the release of the excitatory neuromediators in the intramural plexuses, inhibiting gastrointestinal motility. Sympathetic control of gastrointestinal function is largely mediated by activity in the intramural plexuses. For example, when gastric motility is enhanced because of increased vagal activity, stimulation of sympathetic centers in the hypothalamus promptly and often completely inhibits motility. The sympathetic fibers that supply the lower esophageal, pyloric, and internal and external anal sphincters are largely excitatory, but their role in controlling these sphincters is poorly understood.

Intramural plexus neurons also communicate with receptors in the mucosal and muscle layers. Mechanoreceptors monitor the stretch and distention of the gastrointestinal tract wall, and chemoreceptors monitor the chemical composition (*i.e.,* osmolality, pH, and digestive products of protein and fat metabolism) of its contents. These receptors can communicate directly with ganglionic cells in the intramural plexuses or with visceral afferent fibers that influence ANS control of gastrointestinal function.

CHEWING AND SWALLOWING

Chewing begins the digestive process; it breaks the food into particles of a size that can be swallowed, lubricates it by mixing it with saliva, and mixes starch-containing food with salivary amylase. Although chewing usually is considered a voluntary act, it can be carried out involuntarily by a person who has lost the function of the cerebral cortex.

The swallowing reflex is a rigidly ordered sequence of events that results in the propulsion of food from the mouth to the stomach through the esophagus. Although swallowing is initiated as a voluntary activity, it becomes involuntary as food or fluid reaches the pharynx. Sensory impulses for the reflex begin at tactile receptors in the pharynx and esophagus and are integrated with the motor components of the response in an area of the reticular formation of the medulla and lower pons called the *swallowing center.* The motor impulses for the oral and pharyngeal phases of swallowing are carried in the trigeminal (V), glossopharyngeal (IX), vagus (X), and hypoglossal (XII) cranial nerves, and impulses for the esophageal phase are carried by the vagus nerve. Diseases that disrupt these brain centers or their cranial nerves disrupt the coordination of swallowing and predispose an individual to food and fluid lodging in the trachea and bronchi, leading to risk for asphyxiation or aspiration pneumonia.

Swallowing consists of three phases: an oral, or voluntary phase; a pharyngeal phase; and an esophageal phase. During the *oral phase,* the bolus is collected at the back of the mouth so the tongue can lift the food upward until it touches the posterior wall of the pharynx. At this point, the *pharyngeal phase* of swallowing is initiated. The soft palate is pulled upward, the palatopharyngeal folds are pulled together so that food does not enter the nasopharynx, the vocal cords are pulled together, and the epiglottis is moved so that it covers the larynx. Respiration is inhibited, and the bolus is moved backward into the esophagus by constrictive movements of the pharynx. Although the striated muscles of the pharynx are involved in the second stage of swallowing, it is an involuntary stage.

The third phase of swallowing is the *esophageal stage.* As food enters the esophagus and stretches its walls, local and central nervous system reflexes that initiate peristalsis are triggered. There are two types of peristalsis—primary and secondary. Primary peristalsis is controlled by the swallowing center in the brain stem and begins when food enters the esophagus. Secondary peristalsis is partially mediated by smooth muscle fibers in the esophagus and occurs when primary peristalsis is inadequate to move food through the esophagus. Peristalsis begins at the site of distention and moves downward. Before the peristaltic wave reaches the stomach, the lower esophageal sphincter relaxes to allow the bolus of food to enter the stomach. The pressure in the lower esophageal sphincter normally is greater than that in the stomach, an important factor in preventing the reflux of gastric contents. The lower esophageal sphincter is innervated by the vagus nerve. Increased levels of parasympathetic stimulation increase the constriction of the sphincter. The hormone gastrin also increases constriction of the sphincter. Gastrin provides the major stimulus for gastric acid production, and its action on the lower esophageal sphincter protects the esophageal mucosa when gastric acid levels are elevated.

GASTRIC MOTILITY

The stomach serves as a reservoir for ingested solids and liquids. Motility of the stomach results in the churning and grinding of solid foods and regulates the emptying of the gastric contents, or chyme, into the duodenum. Peristaltic mixing and churning contractions begin in a pacemaker area in the middle of the stomach and move toward the antrum (see Fig. 38-2). They occur at a frequency of three to five contractions per minute, each with a duration of 2 to 20 seconds. As the peristaltic wave approaches the antrum, it speeds up, and the entire terminal 5 to 10 cm of the antrum contracts, occluding the pyloric opening. Contraction of the antrum reverses the movement of the chyme, returning the larger particles to the body of the stomach for further churning and kneading. Because the pylorus is contracted during antral contraction, the gastric contents are emptied into the duodenum between contractions.

Although the pylorus does not contain a true anatomic sphincter, it does function as a physiologic sphincter to prevent the backflow of gastric contents and allow them to flow into the duodenum at a rate commensurate with the ability of the duodenum to accept them. This is important because the regurgitation of bile salts and duodenal contents can damage the mucosal surface of the antrum and lead to gastric ulcers. Likewise, the duodenal mucosa can be damaged by the rapid influx of highly acid gastric contents.

Like other parts of the gastrointestinal tract, the stomach is richly innervated by the enteric nervous system and its connections with the sympathetic and parasympathetic nervous systems. Axons from the intramural plexuses innervate the smooth muscles and glands of the stomach. Parasympathetic innervation is provided by the vagus nerve and sympathetic innervation by the celiac ganglia. The emptying of the stomach is regulated by hormonal and neural mechanisms. The hormones cholecystokinin and gastric inhibitory peptide, which are thought to control gastric emptying, are released in response to the pH and the osmolar and fatty acid composition of the chyme. Local and central circuitry are involved in the neural control of gastric emptying. Afferent receptor fibers synapse with the neurons in the intramural plexus or trigger intrinsic reflexes by means of vagal or sympathetic pathways that participate in extrinsic reflexes.

Disorders of gastric motility can occur when the rate is too slow or too fast. A rate that is too slow leads to gastric retention. It can be caused by obstruction or gastric atony. Obstruction can result from the formation of scar tissue in the pyloric area after a peptic ulcer. Another example of obstruction is hypertrophic pyloric stenosis, which can occur in infants with an abnormally thick muscularis layer in the terminal pylorus. Myotomy, or surgical incision of the muscular ring, may be done to relieve the obstruction. Gastric atony can occur as a complication of visceral neuropathies in diabetes mellitus. Surgical procedures that disrupt vagal activity also can result in gastric atony. Abnormally fast emptying occurs in the dumping syndrome, which is a consequence of certain types of gastric operations. This condition is characterized by the rapid dumping of highly acidic and hyperosmotic gastric secretions into the duodenum and jejunum.

SMALL INTESTINE MOTILITY

The small intestine is the major site for the digestion and absorption of food; its movements are mixing and propulsive. Regular peristaltic movements begin in the duodenum near the entry sites of the common duct and the main hepatic duct. A series of local pacemakers maintains the frequency of intestinal contraction. The peristaltic movements (approximately 12 per minute in the jejunum) become less frequent as they move further from the pylorus, becoming approximately 9 per minute in the ileum.

The peristaltic contractions produce segmentation waves and propulsive movements through the muscles of the small intestine. With segmentation waves, slow contractions of circular muscle occlude the lumen and drive the contents forward and backward. Most of the contractions that produce segmentation waves are local events involving only 1 to 4 cm at a time. They function mainly to mix the chyme with the digestive enzymes from the pancreas and to ensure adequate exposure of all parts of the chyme to the mucosal surface of the intestine, where absorption takes place. The frequency of segmenting activity increases after a meal. Presumably, it is stimulated by receptors in the stomach and intestine.

Propulsive movements occur with synchronized activity in a section 10 to 20 cm long. They are accomplished by contraction of the proximal, or orad, portion of the intestine with the sequential relaxation of its distal, or anal, portion. After material has been propelled to the ileocecal junction by peristaltic movement, stretching of the distal ileum produces a local reflex that relaxes the sphincter and allows fluid to squirt into the cecum.

Motility disturbances of the small bowel are common, and auscultation of the abdomen can be used to assess bowel activity. Inflammatory changes increase motility. In many instances, it is not certain whether changes in motility occur because of inflammation or secondary to toxins and unabsorbed materials. Delayed passage of materials in the small intestine also can be a problem. Transient interruption of intestinal motility often occurs after gastrointestinal surgery. Intubation with suction often is required to remove the accumulating intestinal contents and gases until activity is resumed.

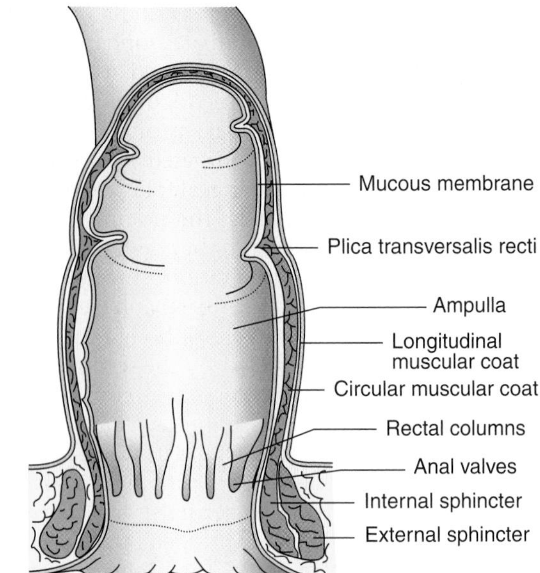

FIGURE 38-8 Interior of the rectum and anal canal.

COLONIC MOTILITY

The storage function of the colon dictates that movements in this section of the gut are different from those in the small intestine. Movements in the colon are of two types. First are the segmental mixing movements, called *haustrations,* so named because they occur within sacculations called *haustra.* These movements produce a local digging-type action, which ensures that all portions of the fecal mass are exposed to the intestinal surface. Second are the propulsive mass movements, in which a large segment of the colon (≥20 cm) contracts as a unit, moving the fecal contents forward as a unit. Mass movements last approximately 30 seconds, followed by a 2- to 3-minute period of relaxation, after which another contraction occurs. A series of mass movements lasts only for 10 to 30 minutes and may occur only several times a day. Defecation normally is initiated by the mass movements.

DEFECATION

Defecation is controlled by the action of two sphincters, the internal and external anal sphincters (Fig. 38-8). The internal sphincter is a circular thickening of smooth muscle, several centimeters long, that lies inside the anus. The external sphincter, which is composed of striated voluntary muscle, surrounds the internal sphincter. The external sphincter is controlled by nerve fibers in the pudendal nerve, which is part of the somatic nervous system and therefore under voluntary control. Defecation is controlled by defecation reflexes. One of these reflexes is the intrinsic myenteric reflex mediated by the local enteric nervous system. It is initiated by distention of the rectal wall, with initiation of reflex peristaltic waves that spread through the descending colon, sigmoid colon, and rectum. A second defecation reflex, the parasympathetic reflex, is integrated at the level of the sacral cord. When the nerve endings in the rectum are stimulated, signals are transmitted first to the sacral cord and then reflexly back to the descending colon, sigmoid colon, rectum, and anus by way of the pelvic nerves (see Fig. 38-7). These impulses greatly increase peristaltic movements as well as relax the internal sphincter.

To prevent involuntary defecation from occurring, the external anal sphincter is under the conscious control of the cortex. As afferent impulses arrive at the sacral cord, signaling the presence of a distended rectum, messages are transmitted to the cortex. If defecation is inappropriate, the cortex initiates impulses that constrict the external sphincter and inhibit efferent parasympathetic activity. Normally, the afferent impulses in this reflex loop fatigue easily, and the urge to defecate soon ceases. At a more convenient time, contraction of the abdominal muscles compresses the contents in the large bowel, reinitiating afferent impulses to the cord.

In summary, motility of the gastrointestinal tract propels food products and fluids along its length from mouth to anus. Although the activity of gastrointestinal smooth muscle is self-propagating and can continue without input from the nervous system, its rate and strength of contractions are regulated by a network of intramural neurons that receive input from the ANS and local receptors that monitor wall stretch and the chemical composition of luminal contents. Parasympathetic innervation occurs by means of the vagus nerve and nerve fibers from sacral segments of the spinal cord; it increases gastrointestinal motility. Sympathetic activity occurs by way of thoracolumbar output from the spinal cord, its paravertebral ganglia, and celiac, superior mesenteric, and inferior mesenteric ganglia. Sympathetic stimulation enhances sphincter function and reduces motility by inhibiting the activity of intramural plexus neurons.

Secretory and Digestive Functions

After completing this section of the chapter, you should be able to meet the following objectives:

- State the source and function of water and electrolytes that are secreted in digestive secretions
- Explain the protective function of saliva
- Describe the function of the gastric secretions in the process of digestion
- List three major gastrointestinal hormones and cite their function
- Describe the site of gastric acid and pepsin production and secretion in the stomach
- Describe the function of the gastric mucosal barrier
- Describe the functions of the secretions of the small and the large intestine

Each day, approximately 7000 mL of fluid is secreted into the gastrointestinal tract (Table 38-1). Approximately 50 to 200 mL of this fluid leaves the body in the stool; the remainder is reabsorbed in the small and large intestines. These secretions are mainly water and have sodium and potassium concentrations similar to those of extracellular fluid. Because water and electrolytes for digestive tract secretions are derived from the extracellular fluid compartment, excessive secretion or impaired absorption can lead to extracellular fluid deficit.

CONTROL OF SECRETORY FUNCTIONS

The secretory and digestive functions of the gut are influenced by local, humoral, and neural influences. Neural control of gastrointestinal secretory activity is mediated through the ANS. Secretory activity, like motility, is increased with parasympathetic stimulation and inhibited with sympathetic activity. Many of the local influences, including pH, osmolality, and chyme, consistently act as stimuli for neural and humoral mechanisms.

GASTROINTESTINAL HORMONES

The gastrointestinal tract is the largest endocrine organ in the body. It produces hormones that pass from the portal circulation into the general circulation and then back to the digestive tract, where they exert their actions. Among the hormones produced by the gastrointestinal tract are gastrin, secretin, and cholecystokinin (CCK). These hormones influence motility and the secretion of electrolytes, enzymes, and other hormones. The gastrointestinal tract hormones and their functions are summarized in Table 38-2.

The primary function of *gastrin* is the stimulation of gastric acid secretion. Gastrin also has trophic, or growth-producing, effect on the mucosa of the small intestine, colon, and oxyntic (acid-secreting) gland area of the stomach. Removal of the tissue that produces gastrin results in atrophy of these structures. This atrophy can be reversed by the administration of exogenous gastrin. *Secretin* is secreted by S cells in the mucosa of the duodenum and jejunum in an inactive form called prosecretin. When an acid chyme with a pH of less than 4.5 to 5.0 enters the intestine, secretin is activated and absorbed into the blood. Secretin causes the pancreas to secrete large quantities of fluid with a high bicarbonate concentration and low chloride concentration.

The primary function of *cholecystokinin* is stimulation of pancreatic enzyme secretion. CCK also regulates gallbladder contraction and gastric emptying. CCK potentiates the action of secretin, increasing the pancreatic bicarbonate response to low circulating levels of secretin. In addition to its effects on the pancreas, CCK secretion stimulates biliary secretion of fluid and bicarbonate.

Two other hormones that contribute to gastrointestinal function are gastric inhibitory peptide and motilin. *Gastric inhibitory peptide,* which is released from the intestinal mucosa in response to increased concentration of glucose and fats, inhibits gastric acid secretion, gastric motility, and gastric emptying. *Motilin,* which stimulates intestinal motility and contributes to the control of the interdigestive actions of the intestinal neurons, is released from the upper small intestine.

Other neural peptides are found in the neurons of the gut. These include *vasoactive intestinal peptide* (VIP), *gastrin-releasing peptide* (GRP), and the *enkephalins*. Gastrointestinal muscle is innervated by VIP-containing neurons. VIP mediates relaxation of gastrointestinal smooth muscle and is thought also to cause relaxation of vascular smooth muscle. GRP-containing neurons are located in the gastric mucosa and function in the release of gastrin. The action of the enkephalins, which exert their function through opioid receptors (see Chapter 50), is to slow the transit of material through the gut and inhibit intestinal secretions. The combination of these actions probably accounts for the effectiveness of selected opioid drugs in treating diarrhea.

Histamine and somatostatin are paracrine agents that act at receptors close to the site of release. *Somatostatin* inhibits gastrin release and gastric acid secretion. *Histamine,* which is released in response to gastrin, stimulates gastric acid secretion by the parietal cells. Histamine also potentiates the action of gastrin and acetylcholine on gastric acid secretion. Histamine type 2 (H_2) antagonists reduce gastric acid secretion by blocking H_2 receptors.

TABLE 38-1 Secretions of the Gastrointestinal Tract

Secretions	Amount Daily (mL)
Salivary	1200
Gastric	2000
Pancreatic	1200
Biliary	700
Intestinal	2000
Total	7100

TABLE 38-2 Major Gastrointestinal Hormones and Their Actions

Hormone	Site of Secretion	Stimulus for Secretion	Action
Cholecystokinin	Duodenum, jejunum	Amino acids	Stimulates contraction of the gallbladder; stimulates secretion of pancreatic enzymes; slows gastric emptying
Gastrin	Antrum of the stomach, duodenum	Vagal stimulation; epinephrine; neutral amino acids; calcium-containing fluids such as milk; and alcohol. Secretion is inhibited by acid contents in the antrum of the stomach (below pH 2.5)	Stimulates secretion of gastric acid and pepsinogen; increases gastric blood flow; stimulates gastric smooth muscle contraction; stimulates growth of gastric, small intestine, and colon mucosa
Secretin	Duodenum	Acid pH or chyme entering duodenum (below pH 3.0)	Stimulates secretion of bicarbonate-containing solution by pancreas and liver

SALIVARY SECRETIONS

Saliva is secreted by the salivary glands. The salivary glands consist of the parotid, submaxillary, sublingual, and buccal glands. Saliva has three functions. The first is protection and lubrication. Saliva is rich in mucus, which protects the oral mucosa and coats the food as it passes through the mouth, pharynx, and esophagus. The sublingual and buccal glands produce only mucus-type secretions. The second function of saliva is its protective antimicrobial action. The saliva cleans the mouth and contains the enzyme lysozyme, which has an antibacterial action. Third, saliva contains ptyalin and amylase, which initiate the digestion of dietary starches. Secretions from the salivary glands are primarily regulated by the ANS. Parasympathetic stimulation increases flow, and sympathetic stimulation decreases flow. The dry mouth that accompanies anxiety attests to the effects of sympathetic activity on salivary secretions.

Mumps, or parotitis, is an infection of the parotid glands. Although most of us associate mumps with the contagious viral form of the disease, inflammation of the parotid glands can occur in the seriously ill person who does not receive adequate oral hygiene and who is unable to take fluids orally. Potassium iodide increases the secretory activity of the salivary glands, including the parotid glands. In a small percentage of persons, parotid swelling may occur in the course of treatment with this drug.

GASTRIC SECRETIONS

In addition to mucus-secreting cells that line the entire surface of the stomach, the stomach mucosa has two types of glands: oxyntic (or gastric) glands and pyloric glands. The *oxyntic glands* are located in the proximal 80% (body and fundus) of the stomach. They secrete hydrochloric acid (HCl), pepsinogen, intrinsic factor, and mucus. The *pyloric glands* are located in the distal 20%, or antrum, of the stomach. The pyloric glands secret mainly mucus, some pepsinogen, and the hormone gastrin.

The oxyntic gland area of the stomach is composed of glands and pits (Fig. 38-9). The surface area and gastric pits are lined with mucus-producing epithelial cells. The bases of the gastric pits contain the parietal cells, which secrete hydrochloric acid and intrinsic factor, and the chief cells, which secrete large quantities of pepsinogen. There are approximately 1 billion parietal cells in the stomach; together, they produce and secrete approximately 20 mEq of hydrochloric acid in several hundred milliliters of gastric juice each hour. The pepsinogen that is secreted by the chief cells is rapidly converted to pepsin when exposed to the low pH of the gastric juices. Gastric intrinsic factor, which is produced by the parietal cells, is necessary for the absorption of vitamin B_{12}.

One of the important characteristics of the gastric mucosa is resistance to the highly acidic secretions that it produces. When the gastric mucosa is damaged by aspirin, nonsteroidal antiinflammatory drugs (NSAIDs), ethyl alcohol, or bile salts, this impermeability is disrupted, and hydrogen ions move into the tissue. This is called *breaking the mucosal barrier,* and substances that alter gastric mucosal permeability are called *barrier breakers*. As the hydrogen ions accumulate in the mucosal cells, intracellular pH decreases, enzymatic reactions become impaired, and cellular structures are disrupted. The result is local ischemia, vascular stasis, hypoxia, and tissue necrosis. The mucosal surface is further protected by prostaglandins. Aspirin and NSAIDs inhibit prostaglandin synthesis, which also impairs the integrity of the mucosal surface.

Parasympathetic stimulation (through the vagus nerve) and gastrin increase gastric secretions. Histamine increases gastric acid secretions. Research and clinical use of the H_2 receptor antagonists suggest that histamine may be the final common pathway for gastric acid production. Gastric acid secretion and its relation to peptic ulcer are discussed in Chapter 39.

Cells in the fundus of the stomach also secrete gastric lipase, an enzyme that breaks dietary fats into fatty acids and diglycerides. Because pancreatic lipase is produced in great excess, the absence of gastric lipase would not normally alter fat digestion. However, the contribution of gastric lipase may be significant in newborns and persons with pancreatic lipase deficiency or inactivation.

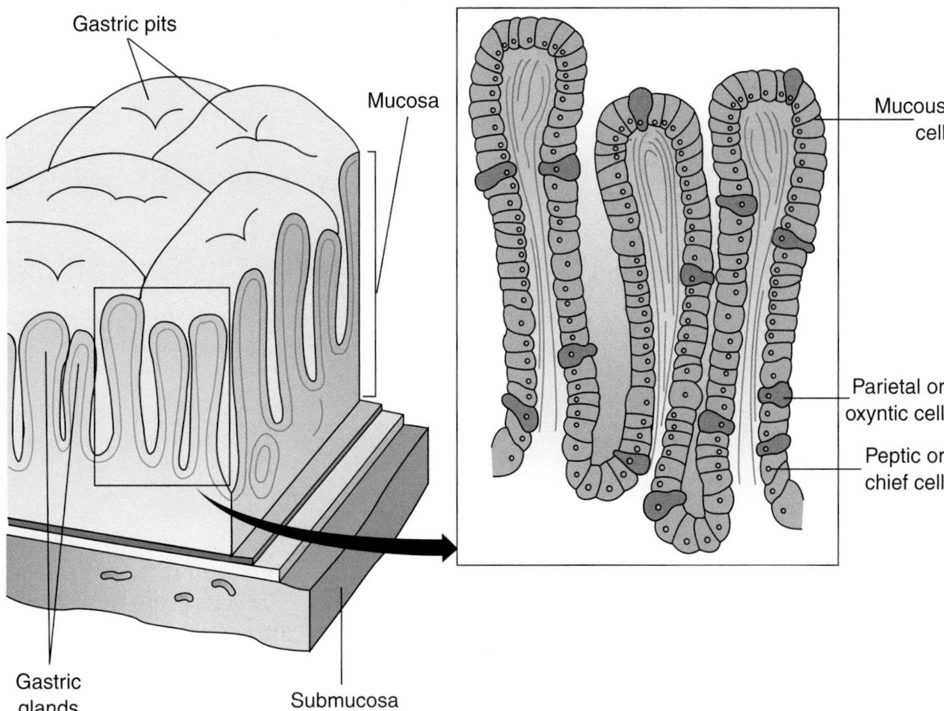

FIGURE 38-9 Gastric pit from body of the stomach.

INTESTINAL SECRETIONS

The small intestine secretes digestive juices and receives secretions from the liver and pancreas (see Chapter 40). Digestive enzymes from the pancreas (*e.g.*, amylase, lipases, proteases) contribute to carbohydrate, fat, and protein digestion. Bile salts from the liver perform an important function in the actual absorption of lipolytic products (*e.g.*, fatty acids, lysophospholipids, cholesterol, fat-soluble vitamins) from the intestine. An extensive array of mucus-producing glands, called *Brunner's glands,* are concentrated at the site where the contents from the stomach and secretions from the liver and pancreas enter the duodenum. These glands secrete large amounts of alkaline mucus, which protects the duodenum from the acid content in the gastric chyme and from the action of the digestive enzymes. The activity of Brunner's glands is strongly influenced by ANS activity. For example, sympathetic stimulation causes a marked decrease in mucus production, leaving this area more susceptible to irritation. Between 75% and 80% of peptic ulcers occur at this site.

In addition to mucus, the intestinal mucosa produces two other types of secretions. The first is a serous fluid (pH 6.5 to 7.5) secreted by specialized cells (*i.e.*, crypts of Lieberkühn) in the intestinal mucosal layer. This fluid, which is produced at the rate of 2000 mL/day, acts as a vehicle for absorption. The second type of secretion consists of surface enzymes that aid absorption. These enzymes are the peptidases, or enzymes that separate amino acids, and the disaccharidases, or enzymes that split sugars.

The large intestine usually secretes only mucus. ANS activity strongly influences mucus production in the bowel, as in other parts of the digestive tract. During intense parasympathetic stimulation, mucus secretion may increase to the point that the stool contains large amounts of obvious mucus. Although the bowel normally does not secrete water or electrolytes, these substances are lost in large quantities when the bowel becomes irritated or inflamed.

In summary, the secretions of the gastrointestinal tract include saliva, gastric juices, bile, and pancreatic and intestinal secretions. Each day, more than 7000 mL of fluid is secreted into the digestive tract; all but 50 to 200 mL of this fluid is reabsorbed. Water, derived from the extracellular fluid compartment, is the major component of gastrointestinal tract secretions. Neural, humoral, and local mechanisms contribute to the control of these secretions. The parasympathetic nervous system increases secretion, and sympathetic activity exerts an inhibitory effect. In addition to secreting fluids containing digestive enzymes, the gastrointestinal tract produces and secretes hormones, such as gastrin, secretin, and CCK, that contribute to the control of gastrointestinal function.

Digestion and Absorption

After completing this section of the chapter, you should be able to meet the following objectives:

- Differentiate digestion from absorption
- Relate the characteristics of the small intestine to its absorptive function
- Explain the function of intestinal brush border enzymes
- Compare the digestion and absorption of carbohydrates, fats, and proteins

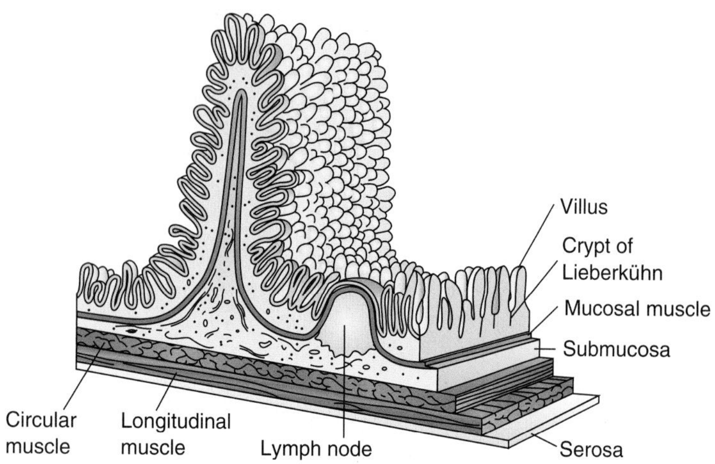

FIGURE 38-10 The mucous membrane of the small intestine. Note the numerous villi on a circular fold.

The digestion, or breakdown of foods, begins in the mouth with the action of salivary α-amylase, continues in the stomach, and is finalized in the small intestine. The absorption of nutrients takes place mainly in the small intestine. Only a relatively few substances, including alcohol, are absorbed from the stomach.

Digestion is the process of dismantling foods into their constituent parts. Digestion requires hydrolysis, enzyme cleavage, and fat emulsification. Hydrolysis is breakdown of a compound that involves a chemical reaction with water. The importance of hydrolysis to digestion is evidenced by the amount of water (7 to 8 L) that is secreted into the gastrointestinal tract daily. The intestinal mucosa is impermeable to most large molecules. Most proteins, fats, and carbohydrates must be broken down into smaller particles before they can be absorbed. Although some digestion of carbohydrates, proteins, and fats takes place in the stomach, the final breakdown of these substances occurs in the small intestine. The breakdown of fats to free fatty acids and monoglycerides takes place entirely in the small intestine. The liver, with its production of bile, and the pancreas, which supplies a number of digestive enzymes, play important roles in digestion.

Absorption is the process of moving nutrients and other materials from the external environment of the gastrointestinal tract into the internal environment. Absorption is accomplished by active transport and diffusion. The absorptive function of the large intestine focuses mainly on water reabsorption. A number of substances require a specific carrier or transport system. For example, vitamin B_{12} is not absorbed in the absence of intrinsic factor, which is secreted by the parietal cells of the stomach. Transport of amino acids and glucose occurs mainly in the presence of sodium. Water is absorbed passively along an osmotic gradient.

The distinguishing characteristic of the small intestine is its large surface area, which in the adult is estimated to be approximately 250 m^2. Anatomic features that contribute to this enlarged surface area are the circular folds that extend into the lumen of the intestine and the villi, which are finger-like projections of mucous membrane, numbering as many as 25,000, that line the entire small intestine (Fig. 38-10). Each villus is equipped with an artery, vein, and lymph vessel (*i.e.,* lacteal), which bring blood to the surface of the intestine and transport the nutrients and other materials that have passed into the blood from the lumen of the intestine (Fig. 38-11). Fats rely largely on the lymphatics for absorption.

Each villus is covered with cells called *enterocytes* that contribute to the absorptive and digestive functions of the small bowel, and goblet cells that provide mucus. The crypts of Lieberkühn are glandular structures that open into the spaces between the villi. The enterocytes have a life span of approximately 4 to 5 days, and it is believed that replacement cells differentiate from progenitor cells located in the area of the crypts. The maturing enterocytes migrate up the villus and eventually are extruded from the tip.

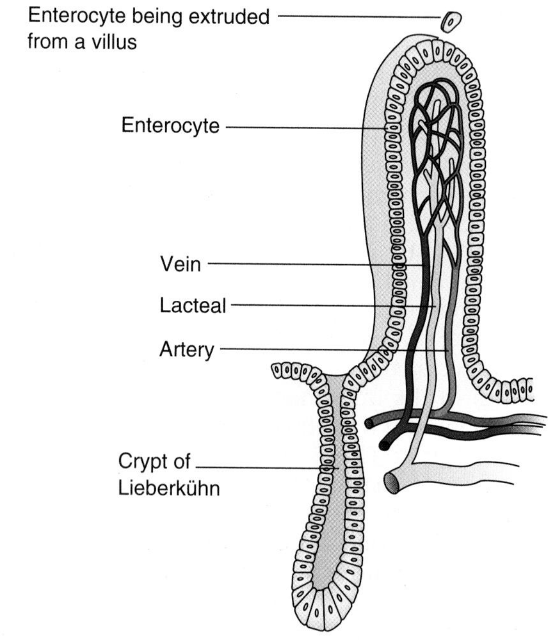

FIGURE 38-11 A single villus from the small intestine.

TABLE 38-3 Enzymes Used in Digestion of Carbohydrates

Dietary Carbohydrates	Enzyme	Monosaccharides Produced
Lactose	Lactase	Glucose and galactose
Sucrose	Sucrase	Fructose and glucose
Starch	Amylase	Maltose, maltotriase, and α-dextrins
Maltose and maltotriose	Maltase	Glucose and glucose
α-Dextrins	α-Dextrimase	Glucose and glucose

The enterocytes secrete enzymes that aid in the digestion of carbohydrates and proteins. These enzymes are called *brush border enzymes* because they adhere to the border of the villus structures. In this way, they have access to the carbohydrates and protein molecules as they come in contact with the absorptive surface of the intestine. This mechanism of secretion places the enzymes where they are needed and eliminates the need to produce enough enzymes to mix with the entire contents that fill the lumen of the small bowel. The digested molecules diffuse through the membrane or are actively transported across the mucosal surface to enter the blood or, in the case of fatty acids, the lacteal. These molecules are then transported through the portal vein or lymphatics into the systemic circulation.

CARBOHYDRATE ABSORPTION

Carbohydrates must be broken down into monosaccharides, or single sugars, before they can be absorbed from the small intestine. The average daily intake of carbohydrate in the American diet is approximately 350 to 400 g. Starch makes up approximately 50% of this total, sucrose (*i.e.,* table sugar) approximately 30%, lactose (*i.e.,* milk sugar) approximately 6%, and maltose approximately 1.5%.

Digestion of starch begins in the mouth with the action of amylase. Pancreatic secretions also contain an amylase. Amylase breaks down starch into several disaccharides, including maltose, isomaltose, and α-dextrins. The brush border enzymes convert the disaccharides into monosaccharides that can be absorbed (Table 38-3). Sucrose yields glucose and fructose, lactose is converted to glucose and galactose, and maltose is converted to two glucose molecules. When the disaccharides are not broken down to monosaccharides, they cannot be absorbed but remain as osmotically active particles in the contents of the digestive system, causing diarrhea. Persons who are deficient in lactase, the enzyme that breaks down lactose, experience diarrhea when they drink milk or eat dairy products.

Fructose is transported across the intestinal mucosa by facilitated diffusion, which does not require energy expenditure. In this case, fructose moves along a concentration gradient. Glucose and galactose are transported by way of a sodium-dependent carrier system that uses adenosine triphosphate (ATP) as an energy source (Fig. 38-12). Water absorption from the intestine is linked to absorption of osmotically active particles, such as glucose and sodium. It follows that an important consideration in facilitating the transport of water across the intestine (and decreasing diarrhea) after temporary disruption in bowel function is to include sodium and glucose in the fluids that are taken.

FAT ABSORPTION

The average adult eats approximately 60 to 100 g of fat daily, principally as triglycerides containing long-chain fatty acids. These triglycerides are broken down by gastric and pancreatic lipase. Bile salts act as a carrier system for the fatty acids and fat-soluble vitamins A, D, E, and K by forming micelles, which transport these substances to the surface of intestinal villi, where they are absorbed. The major site of fat absorption is the upper jejunum. Medium-chain triglycerides, with 6 to 10 carbon atoms in their structures, are absorbed better than longer-chain fatty acids because they are more completely broken down by pancreatic lipase and they form micelles more easily. Because they are easily absorbed, medium-chain triglycerides often are used in the treatment of persons with malabsorption syndrome. The absorption of vitamins A, D, E, and K, which are fat-soluble vitamins, requires bile salts.

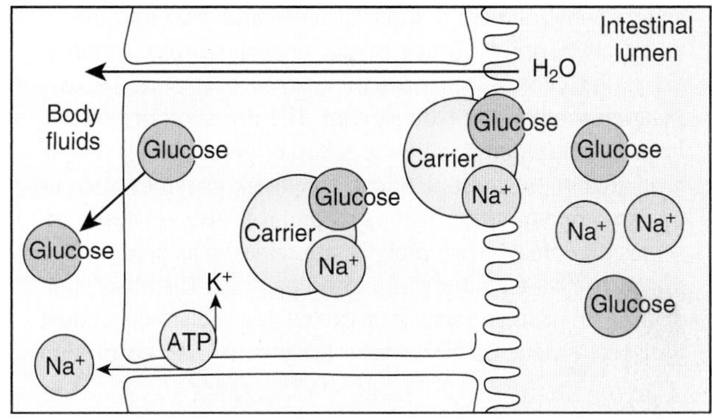

FIGURE 38-12 The hypothetical sodium-dependent transport system for glucose. Both sodium and glucose must attach to the transport carrier before either can be transported into the cell. The concentration of glucose builds up in the intestinal cell until a diffusion gradient develops, causing glucose to move into the body fluids. Sodium is transported out of the cell by the energy-dependent (ATP) sodium pump. This creates the gradient needed to operate the transport system.

Fat that is not absorbed in the intestine is excreted in the stool. *Steatorrhea* is the term used to describe fatty stools. It usually indicates that there is 20 g or more of fat in a 24-hour stool sample. Normally, a chemical test is done on a 72-hour stool collection, during which time the diet is restricted to 80 to 100 g of fat per day.

PROTEIN ABSORPTION

Protein digestion begins in the stomach with the action of pepsin. Pepsinogen, the enzyme precursor of pepsin, is secreted by the chief cells in response to a meal and acid pH. Acid in the stomach is required for the conversion of pepsinogen to pepsin. Pepsin is inactivated when it enters the intestine by the alkaline pH.

Proteins are broken down further by pancreatic enzymes, such as trypsin, chymotrypsin, carboxypeptidase, and elastase. As with pepsin, the pancreatic enzymes are secreted as precursor molecules. Trypsinogen, which lacks enzymatic activity, is activated by an enzyme located on the brush border cells of the duodenal enterocytes. Activated trypsin activates additional trypsinogen molecules and other pancreatic precursor proteolytic enzymes. The amino acids are liberated intramurally or on the surface of the villi by brush border enzymes that degrade proteins into peptides that are one, two, or three amino acids long. Similar to glucose, many amino acids are transported across the mucosal membrane in a sodium-linked process that uses ATP as an energy source. Some amino acids are absorbed by facilitated diffusion processes that do not require sodium.

In summary, the digestion and absorption of foodstuffs take place mainly in the small intestine. Digestion is the process of dismantling foods into their constituent parts. Digestion requires hydrolysis, enzyme cleavage, and fat emulsification. Proteins, fats, carbohydrates, and other components of the diet are broken down into molecules that can be transported from the intestinal lumen into the body fluids. Absorption is the process of moving nutrients and other materials from the external environment of the gastrointestinal tract into the internal environment. Brush border enzymes break carbohydrates into monosaccharides that can be transported across the intestine into the bloodstream. The digestion of proteins begins in the stomach with the action of pepsin and is further facilitated in the intestine by the pancreatic enzymes, such as trypsin, chymotrypsin, carboxypeptidase, and elastase. Enzymes that break down proteins are released as proenzymes that are activated in the gastrointestinal tract. The absorption of glucose and amino acids is facilitated by a sodium-dependent transport system. Fat in the diet is broken down by gastric and pancreatic lipase into triglycerides containing medium- and long-chain fatty acids. Bile salts form micelles that transport these substances to the surface of intestinal villi, where they are absorbed.

REVIEW EXERCISES

Persons receiving chemotherapeutic agents, which interfere with mitosis of cancer cells as well as the cells of other rapidly proliferating tissues in the body, often experience disorders such as ulcerations in the mucosal tissues of the mouth and other parts of the gastrointestinal tract. These disorders are resolved once the chemotherapy treatment has been completed.

A. Explain.

People with gastroesophageal reflux (movement of gastric contents into the esophagus) often complain of heartburn that becomes worse as the pressure in the stomach increases.

A. Use information on hormonal control of gastric emptying to explain why eating a meal high in fat content would increase gastric reflux.

Infections of the gastrointestinal tract, such as the "GI flu," often cause profound diarrhea.

A. Describe the neural mechanisms involved in the increase in gastrointestinal motility that produces the diarrhea.

People with lactase deficiency often experience bloating and diarrhea.

A. Explain.

Bibliography

Berne R.M., Levy M.N. (2000). *Principles of physiology* (3rd ed., pp. 354–405). St. Louis: C.V. Mosby.

Gershon M.D. (1999). The enteric nervous system: A second brain. *Hospital Practice 34*(7), 31–52.

Guyton A.C., Hall J.E. (2000). *Textbook of medical physiology* (10th ed., pp. 718–770). Philadelphia: W.B. Saunders.

Johnson L.R. (2001). *Gastrointestinal physiology* (6th ed.). St. Louis: C.V. Mosby.

Moore K.L., Dalley A.F. (1999). *Clinically oriented anatomy* (4th ed., pp. 209–271). Philadelphia: Lippincott Williams & Wilkins.

Rhoades R.A., Tanner G.A. (2004). *Medical physiology* (2nd ed., pp. 449–511). Boston: Little, Brown.

CHAPTER

39

Disorders of Gastrointestinal Function

Gastrointestinal disorders are not cited as the leading cause of death in the United States, nor do they receive the same publicity as heart disease and cancer. However, according to government reports, digestive diseases rank third in the total economic burden of illness, resulting in considerable human suffering, personal expenditures for treatment, lost working hours, and a drain on the nation's economy. It has been estimated that 60 to 70 million people in the United States have a digestive disease, and more than 10 million (13%) of all hospitalizations are for digestive disorders.[1] Even more important is the fact that proper nutrition or a change in health practices could prevent or minimize many of these disorders.

Manifestations of Gastrointestinal Disorders

After completing this section of the chapter, you should be able to meet the following objectives:

- Describe the physiologic mechanisms involved in anorexia, nausea, and vomiting
- Characterize the appearance of blood in vomitus and stool according to the site and extent of bleeding

Several signs and symptoms are common to many types of gastrointestinal disorders. These include anorexia, nausea, vomiting, and gastrointestinal bleeding. Because they occur with so many gastrointestinal disorders, they are discussed separately as an introduction to the content that follows.

ANOREXIA, NAUSEA, AND VOMITING

Anorexia, nausea, and vomiting are physiologic responses that are common to many gastrointestinal disorders. These responses are protective to the extent that they signal the presence of disease and, in the case of vomiting, remove noxious agents from the gastrointestinal tract. They also can contribute to impaired intake or loss of fluids and nutrients.

Anorexia represents a loss of appetite. Several factors influence appetite. One is hunger, which is stimulated by contractions of the empty stomach. Appetite or the desire for food intake is regulated by the hypothalamus and other associated centers in the brain. Smell plays an important role, as evidenced by the fact that appetite can be stimulated or suppressed by the smell of food. Loss of appetite is associated with emotional factors, such as fear, depression, frustration, and anxiety. Many drugs and disease states cause anorexia. In uremia, for example, the accumulation of nitrogenous wastes in the blood contributes to the development of anorexia. Anorexia often is a forerunner of nausea, and most conditions that cause nausea and vomiting also produce anorexia.

Nausea is an ill-defined and unpleasant subjective sensation. It is the conscious sensation resulting from stimulation of the medullary vomiting center that often precedes or accompanies vomiting. Nausea usually is preceded by anorexia, and stimuli such as foods and drugs that cause anorexia in small doses usually produce nausea when given in larger doses. A common cause of nausea is distention of the duodenum, or upper small intestinal tract. Nausea frequently is accompanied by autonomic nervous system manifestations such as watery salivation and vasoconstriction with pallor, sweating, and tachycardia. Nausea may function as an early warning signal of disease.

Vomiting, or emesis, is the sudden and forceful oral expulsion of the contents of the stomach. It usually is preceded by nausea. The contents that are vomited are called *vomitus*. Vomiting, as a basic physiologic protective mechanism, limits the possibility of damage from ingested noxious agents by emptying the contents of the stomach and portions of the small intestine. Nausea and vomiting may represent a total-body response to drug therapy, including overdosage, toxicity, and side effects.

Vomiting appears to involve two functionally distinct medullary centers: the vomiting center and the chemoreceptor trigger zone. The act of vomiting is integrated by the vomiting center, which is located in the dorsal portion of the reticular formation of the medulla near the sensory nuclei of the vagus. The chemoreceptor trigger zone is located in a small area on the floor of the fourth ventricle, where it is exposed to both blood and cerebrospinal fluid. It is thought to mediate the emetic effects of blood-borne drugs and toxins.

The act of vomiting consists of taking a deep breath, closing the airways, and producing a strong, forceful contraction of the diaphragm and abdominal muscles along with relaxation of the gastroesophageal sphincter. Respiration ceases during the act of vomiting. Vomiting may be accompanied by dizziness, light-headedness, decrease in blood pressure, and bradycardia.

The vomiting center receives input from the gastrointestinal tract and other organs; from the cerebral cortex; from the vestibular apparatus, which is responsible for motion sickness; and from the chemoreceptor trigger zone, which is activated by many drugs and endogenous and exogenous toxins. Hypoxia exerts a direct effect on the vomiting center, producing nausea and vomiting. This direct effect probably accounts for the vomiting that occurs during periods of decreased cardiac output, shock, environmental hypoxia, and brain ischemia caused by increased intracranial pressure. Inflammation of any of the intra-abdominal organs, including the liver, gallbladder, or urinary tract, can cause vomiting because of the stimulation of the visceral afferent pathways that communicate with the vomiting center. Distention or irritation of the gastrointestinal tract also causes vomiting through the stimulation of visceral afferent neurons.

Several neurotransmitters and receptor subtypes are implicated as neuromediators in nausea and vomiting. Dopamine, serotonin (*i.e.*, 5-HT_3), and opioid receptors are found in the gastrointestinal tract and in the vomiting and chemoreceptor trigger zone. Dopamine antagonists such as prochlorperazine depress vomiting caused by stimulation of the chemoreceptor trigger zone. Serotonin is believed to be involved in the nausea and emesis associated with cancer chemotherapy and radiation therapy.[2,3] Serotonin antagonists (*e.g.*, dolasetron, granisetron, ondansetron) are effective in treating the nausea and vomiting associated with these stimuli. Motion sickness appears to be a central nervous system (CNS) response to vestibular stimuli. Norepinephrine and acetylcholine receptors are located in the vestibular center. The acetylcholine receptors are thought to mediate the impulses responsible for exciting the vomiting center; norepinephrine receptors may have a stabilizing influence that resists motion sickness. Many of the motion sickness drugs (*e.g.*, dimenhydrinate and meclizine) have a strong CNS anticholinergic effect and act on the receptors in the vomiting center and areas related to the vestibular system.

GASTROINTESTINAL TRACT BLEEDING

Bleeding from the gastrointestinal tract can be evidenced by blood that appears in the vomitus or the feces. It can result from disease or trauma to the gastrointestinal structures (*e.g.*, peptic ulcers), blood vessel abnormalities (*e.g.*, esophageal varices, hemorrhoids), or disorders in blood clotting.

Blood in the stomach usually is irritating and causes vomiting. Hematemesis refers to blood in the vomitus. It may be bright red or have a "coffee-ground" appearance because of the action of the digestive enzymes.

Blood that appears in the stool may range in color from bright red to tarry black. Bright red blood usually indicates that the bleeding is from the lower bowel. When it coats the stool, it often is the result of bleeding hemorrhoids.

The word *melena* comes from the Greek word for "black" and refers to the passage of black and tarry stools. These stools have a characteristic odor that is not easily forgotten. Tarry stools usually indicate that the source of the bleeding is above the level of the ileocecal valve, although this is not always the case. Approximately 150 to 200 mL of blood must be present in the stomach to produce a single tarry stool; acute blood loss may produce melena for up to 3 days.[4] With hypermotility of the gastrointestinal tract, bright red blood may be present in the stools even though the bleeding is from the upper gastrointestinal tract.

Occult, or hidden, blood can only be detected by chemical means. It can be caused by gastritis, peptic ulcer, or lesions of the intestine. Occult bleeding can be detected by guaiac-based stool tests that make use of the pseudoperoxidase activity of hemoglobin. Guaiac turns blue after oxidation by oxidants or peroxidases in the presence of an oxygen donor such as hydrogen peroxide. The likelihood that a guaiac-based test result will be positive is directly proportional to the quantity of fecal heme, which in turn is related to the size and location of the bleeding lesion. Many factors influence guaiac-based tests, including ingestion of vitamin C and dietary factors such as nonhuman heme derived from eating meat or peroxidases from dietary sources.

The blood urea nitrogen (BUN) level frequently is elevated after hematemesis or melena. This results from the breakdown of the blood by the digestive enzymes and the absorption of the nitrogenous end products into the blood. The BUN level usually reaches a peak within 24 hours after the gastrointestinal hemorrhage. It is not elevated when the bleeding is in the colon because digestion does not take place at this level of the digestive system.

In summary, the signs and symptoms of many gastrointestinal tract disorders are manifested by anorexia, nausea, and vomiting. Anorexia, or loss of appetite, may occur alone or may accompany nausea and vomiting. Nausea, which is an ill-defined, unpleasant sensation, signals the stimulation of the medullary vomiting center. It often precedes vomiting and frequently is accompanied by autonomic responses such as salivation and vasoconstriction with pallor, sweating, and tachycardia. The act of vomiting, which is integrated by the vomiting center, involves the forceful oral expulsion of the gastric contents. It is a basic physiologic mechanism that rids the gastrointestinal tract of noxious agents. Disorders that disrupt the integrity of the gastrointestinal tract often cause bleeding, which can be manifested as blood in the vomitus (*i.e.,* hematemesis) or as blood in the stool (*i.e.,* melena).

Disorders of the Esophagus

After completing this section of the chapter, you should be able to meet the following objectives:

- ✦ Define dysphagia, odynophagia, and achalasia
- ✦ Relate the pathophysiology of gastroesophageal reflux to measures used in diagnosis and treatment of the disorder in adults and children
- ✦ State the reason for the poor prognosis associated with esophageal cancer

The esophagus is a tube that connects the oropharynx with the stomach. It lies posterior to the trachea and larynx and extends through the mediastinum, intersecting the diaphragm at the level of the 11th thoracic vertebra.

The esophagus functions primarily as a conduit for passage of food from the pharynx to the stomach, and the structures of its walls are designed for this purpose: the smooth muscle layers provide the peristaltic movements needed to move food along its length, and the epithelial layer secretes mucus, which protects its surface and aids in lubricating food. There are sphincters at either end of the esophagus: an upper esophageal sphincter and a lower esophageal sphincter. The upper esophageal, or pharyngoesophageal, sphincter consists of a circular layer of striated muscle, the cricopharyngeal muscle. The lower esophageal, or gastroesophageal, sphincter is an area approximately 3 cm above the junction with the stomach. The circular muscle in this area normally remains tonically constricted, creating a zone of high pressure that serves to prevent reflux of gastric contents into the esophagus.[5] During swallowing, there is "receptive relaxation" of the lower esophageal sphincter, which allows easy propulsion of the esophageal contents into the stomach. The lower esophageal sphincter passes through an opening, or hiatus, in the diaphragm as it joins with the stomach, which is located in the abdomen. The portion of the diaphragm that surrounds the lower esophageal sphincter helps to maintain the zone of high pressure needed to prevent reflux of stomach contents.[6]

DYSPHAGIA

The act of swallowing depends on the coordinated action of the tongue and pharynx. These structures are innervated by cranial nerves V, IX, X, and XII. *Dysphagia* refers to difficulty in swallowing. If swallowing is painful, it is referred to as *odynophagia.* Dysphagia can result from altered nerve function or from disorders that produce narrowing of the esophagus. Lesions of the CNS, such as a stroke, often involve the cranial nerves that control swallowing. Strictures and cancer of the esophagus and strictures resulting from scarring can reduce the size of the esophageal lumen and make swallowing difficult. Scleroderma, an autoimmune disease that causes fibrous replacement of tissues in the muscularis layer of the gastrointestinal tract, is another important cause of dysphagia.[7] Persons with dysphagia usually complain of choking, coughing, or an abnormal sensation of food sticking in the back of the throat or upper chest when they swallow.

In a condition called *achalasia,* the lower esophageal sphincter fails to relax; food that has been swallowed has difficulty passing into the stomach, and the esophagus above the lower esophageal sphincter becomes enlarged. One or several meals may lodge in the esophagus and pass slowly into the stomach over time. There is danger of aspiration of esophageal contents into the lungs when the person lies down.

Endoscopy, barium esophagoscopy, and videoradiography may be used to determine the site and extent of the swallowing disorder. Esophageal manometry, a procedure in which a small pressure-sensing catheter is inserted into the esophagus, may be done to measure pressures in different parts of the esophagus. Treatment of swallowing disorders depends on the cause and type of altered function that is present. Treatment of dysphagia often involves a multidisciplinary team of health professionals, including a speech therapist. Mechanical dilatation or surgical procedures may be done to enlarge the lower esophageal sphincter in persons with esophageal strictures.

ESOPHAGEAL DIVERTICULUM

A diverticulum of the esophagus is an outpouching of the esophageal wall caused by a weakness of the muscularis layer. An esophageal diverticulum tends to retain food. Complaints that the food stops before it reaches the stomach are common, as are reports of gurgling, belching, coughing, and foul-smelling breath. The trapped food may cause esophagitis and ulceration. Because the condition usually is progressive, correction of the defect requires surgical intervention.

TEARS (MALLORY-WEISS SYNDROME)

Longitudinal tears in the esophagus at the esophagogastric junction are termed *Mallory-Weiss tears*.[8] They are most often encountered in chronic alcoholics after a bout of severe retching or vomiting, but may also occur during acute illness with severe vomiting. The presumed pathogenesis is inadequate relaxation of the esophageal sphincter during vomiting, with stretching and tearing of the esophageal junction at the moment of propulsive expulsion of gastric contents. Tears may involve only the mucosa or may penetrate the wall of the esophagus. Infection may lead to inflammatory ulcer or mediastinitis.

Esophageal lacerations account for 5% to 10% of all upper gastrointestinal bleeding episodes.[8] Most often, bleeding is not severe and does not require surgical intervention. Severe bleeding usually responds to vasoconstrictive medications, transfusions, and balloon compression. Healing is usually prompt, with minimal or no residual effects.

GASTROESOPHAGEAL REFLUX

The term *reflux* refers to backward or return movement. In the context of gastroesophageal reflux, it refers to the backward movement of gastric contents into the esophagus, a condition that causes heartburn. It probably is the most common disorder originating in the gastrointestinal tract. Most persons experience heartburn occasionally as a result of reflux. Such symptoms usually occur soon after eating, are short lived, and seldom cause more serious problems. However, for some persons, persistent heartburn can represent reflux disease with esophagitis.

The lower esophageal sphincter regulates the flow of food from the esophagus into the stomach. Both internal and external mechanisms function in maintaining the antireflux function of the lower esophageal sphincter.[6,9,10] The circular muscles of the distal esophagus constitute the internal mechanisms, and the portion of the diaphragm that surrounds the esophagus constitutes the external mechanism. The oblique muscles of the stomach, located below the lower esophageal sphincter, form a flap that contributes to the antireflux function of the internal sphincter. Relaxation of the lower esophageal sphincter is a brain stem reflex that is mediated by the vagus nerve in response to a number of afferent stimuli. Transient relaxation with reflux is common after meals. Gastric distention and meals high in fat increase the frequency of relaxation. Normally, refluxed material is returned to the stomach by secondary peristaltic waves in the esophagus and swallowed saliva neutralizes and washes away the refluxed acid.

Gastroesophageal reflux is thought to be associated with a weak or incompetent lower esophageal sphincter that allows reflux to occur, the irritant effects of the refluxate, and the decreased clearance of the refluxed acid from the esophagus after it has occurred.[11] In most cases, reflux occurs during transient relaxation of the esophagus. Delayed gastric emptying also may contribute to reflux by increasing gastric volume and pressure with greater chance for reflux. Esophageal mucosal injury is related to the destructive nature of the refluxate and the amount of time it is in contact with mucosa. Acidic gastric fluids (pH <4.0) are particularly damaging. The gastroesophageal reflux normally is cleared and neutralized by esophageal peristalsis and salivary bicarbonate. Decreased salivation and salivary buffering capacity may contribute to impaired clearing of acid reflux from the esophagus. There is controversy regarding the importance of hiatal hernia (*i.e.,* herniation of the stomach through an enlarged hiatus in the diaphragm) in the pathogenesis of reflux disease. Small hiatal hernias are common and considered to be of no significance in asymptomatic people. However, in cases of severe erosive esophagitis in which gastroesophageal reflux and large hiatal hernia coexist, the hernia may retard esophageal acid clearance and contribute to the disorder.[6,11,12]

Reflux esophagitis involves mucosal injury to the esophagus, hyperemia, and inflammation. The most frequent symptom of gastroesophageal reflux is heartburn. It frequently is severe, occurring 30 to 60 minutes after eating. It often is made worse by bending at the waist and recumbency and usually is relieved by sitting upright. The severity of heartburn is not indicative of the extent of mucosal injury; only a small percentage of people who complain of heartburn have mucosal injury. Often, the heartburn occurs during the night. Antacids give prompt, although transient, relief. Other symptoms include belching and chest pain. The pain usually is located in the epigastric or retrosternal area and often radiates to the throat, shoulder, or back. Because of its location, the pain may be confused with angina. The reflux of gastric contents also may produce respiratory symptoms such as wheezing, chronic cough, and hoarseness. There is considerable evidence linking gastroesophageal reflux with bronchial asthma.[13,14] The proposed mechanisms of reflux-associated asthma and chronic cough include microaspiration and macroaspiration, laryngeal injury, and vagal-mediated bronchospasm.

Complications can result from persistent reflux, which produces a cycle of mucosal damage that causes hyperemia, edema, and erosion of the luminal surface. These complications include strictures and a condition called

Barrett's esophagus.[11,15] Strictures are caused by a combination of scar tissue, spasm, and edema. They produce narrowing of the esophagus and cause dysphagia when the lumen becomes sufficiently constricted. Barrett's esophagus is characterized by a reparative process in which the squamous mucosa that normally lines the esophagus gradually is replaced by columnar epithelium resembling that in the stomach or intestines.[11,15] It is associated with increased risk for development of esophageal cancer.

Diagnosis of gastroesophageal reflux depends on a history of reflux symptomatology and selective use of diagnostic methods, including radiographic studies using a contrast medium such as barium, esophagoscopy, and ambulatory esophageal pH monitoring.[12,16] Esophagoscopy involves the passage of a flexible fiberoptic endoscope into the esophagus for the purpose of visualizing the lumen of the upper gastrointestinal tract. It also permits performance of a biopsy, if indicated. For 24-hour pH monitoring, a small tube with a pH electrode is passed through the nose and down into the esophagus. Data from the electrode are recorded in a small, lightweight box worn on a belt around the waist and later are analyzed by computer. The box has a button that the person can press to indicate episodes of heartburn or pain; these can be correlated with episodes of acid reflux.

The treatment of gastroesophageal reflux usually focuses on conservative measures. These measures include avoidance of positions and conditions that increase gastric reflux.[16] Avoidance of large meals and foods that reduce lower esophageal sphincter tone (*e.g.*, caffeine, fats, chocolate), alcohol, and smoking is recommended. It is recommended that meals be eaten sitting up and that the recumbent position be avoided for several hours after a meal. Bending for long periods should be avoided because it tends to increase intra-abdominal pressure and cause gastric reflux. Sleeping with the head elevated helps to prevent reflux during the night. This is best accomplished by placing blocks under the head of the bed or by using a wedge-shaped bolster to elevate the head and shoulders by at least 6 inches. Weight loss usually is recommended in overweight people.

Antacids or a combination of antacids and alginic acid also are recommended for mild disease. Alginic acid produces a foam when it comes in contact with gastric acid; if reflux occurs, the foam rather than the acid rises into the esophagus. Histamine-2 receptor (H_2)–blocking antagonists (*i.e.*, cimetidine, ranitidine, nizatidine, famotidine), which inhibit gastric acid production, often are recommended when additional treatment is needed.[12] The proton-pump inhibitors (*e.g.*, omeprazole, lansoprazole, rabeprazole, pantoprazole, esomeprazole) act by inhibiting the gastric proton pump, which regulates the final pathway for acid secretion. These agents may be used for persons who continue to have daytime symptoms, recurrent strictures, or large esophageal ulcerations. Promotility agents (*e.g.*, metoclopramide) may be used to increase lower esophageal pressure and enhance esophageal clearance.[12] Metoclopramide is a dopamine antagonist that may cause neuropsychiatric side effects, limiting its use. Surgical treatment may be indicated in some people.

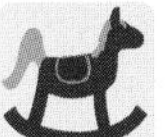

Gastroesophageal Reflux in Children

Gastroesophageal reflux is a common problem in infants and children. The small reservoir capacity of an infant's esophagus, coupled with frequent spontaneous reductions in sphincter pressure, contributes to reflux. Regurgitation of at least one episode a day occurs in as many as half of infants aged 0 to 3 months. By 6 months of age, it becomes less frequent, and it abates by 2 years of age as the child assumes a more upright posture and eats solid foods.[17,18] Although many infants have minor degrees of reflux, complications occur in 1 of every 300 to 500 children.[17] The condition occurs more frequently in children with cerebral palsy, Down syndrome, and other neurologic disorders.

In most cases, infants with simple reflux are thriving and healthy, and symptoms resolve between 9 and 24 months of age. Pathologic reflux is classified into three categories: (1) regurgitation and malnutrition, (2) esophagitis, and (3) respiratory problems. Symptoms of esophagitis include evidence of pain when swallowing, hematemesis, anemia due to esophageal bleeding, heartburn, irritability, and sudden or inconsolable crying. Parents often report feeding problems in their infants.[17] These infants often are irritable and demonstrate early satiety. Sometimes the problems progress to actual resistance to feeding. Tilting of the head to one side and arching of the back may be noted in children with severe reflux. The head positioning is thought to represent an attempt to protect the airway or reduce the pain-associated reflux. Sometimes regurgitation is associated with dental caries and recurrent otalgia. The ear pain is thought to occur through referral from the vagus nerve in the esophagus to the ear. A variety of respiratory symptoms are caused by damage to the respiratory mucosa when gastric reflux enters the esophagus. Reflux may cause coughing, hoarseness, bronchospasm and wheezing, apnea, and bradycardia.[17,18]

Diagnosis of gastroesophageal reflux in infants and children often is based on parental and clinical observations. The diagnosis may be confirmed by esophageal pH probe studies or barium fluoroscopic esophagography. In severe cases, esophagoscopy may be used to demonstrate reflux and obtain a biopsy.

Various treatment methods are available for infants and children with gastroesophageal reflux. Small, frequent feedings are recommended because of the association between gastric volume and transient relaxation of the esophagus. Thickening an infant's feedings with cereal tends to decrease the volume of reflux, decrease crying and energy expenditure, and increase the calorie density of the formula.[17,18] In infants, positioning on the left side seems to decrease reflux. In older infants and children, raising the head of the bed and keeping the child upright may help. Medications usually are not added to the treatment regimen until pathologic reflux has been documented by diagnostic testing. Antacids are the most commonly used antireflux therapy and are readily available over the counter. H_2-receptor antagonists and proton-pump inhibitors may be used in children with persistent reflux. Promotility agents may be used in selected cases.

CANCER OF THE ESOPHAGUS

Carcinoma of the esophagus accounts for approximately 6% of all gastrointestinal cancers. This disease is more common in older persons, with a mean age at diagnosis of 67 years. It is more frequent in men than women and is the seventh leading cause of cancer death among men, particularly black men.[19]

There are two types of esophageal cancers: squamous cell carcinoma and adenocarcinoma. Most squamous cell esophageal carcinomas are attributable to alcohol and tobacco use. Worldwide squamous cell carcinomas constitute 90% of esophageal cancers, but in the United States, there has been an exponential increase in adenocarcinomas associated with Barrett's esophagus. These tumors usually arise from dysplastic changes that occur in the histologic environment of Barrett's esophagus. Endoscopic surveillance in people with Barrett's esophagus provides the means for detecting adenocarcinoma at an earlier stage when it is most amenable to curative surgical resection.[19] Whereas adenocarcinomas are usually found in the distal esophagus and may invade the adjacent upper part of the stomach, squamous cell carcinomas usually occur in the middle and lower third of the esophagus.[19]

Dysphagia is by far the most frequent complaint of persons with esophageal cancer. It is apparent first with ingestion of bulky food, later with soft food, and finally with liquids. Unfortunately, it is a late manifestation of the disease. Weight loss, anorexia, fatigue, and pain on swallowing also may occur.

Treatment of esophageal cancer depends on tumor stage. Surgical resection provides a means of cure when done in early disease and palliation when done in late disease. Radiation may be used as an alternative to surgery. Chemotherapy may be used preoperatively to decrease the size of the tumor, or it may be used along with irradiation and surgery in an effort to increase survival.[19]

The prognosis for persons with cancer of the esophagus, although poor, has improved. Even with modern forms of therapy, however, the long-term survival is limited because, in many cases, the disease has already metastasized by the time the diagnosis is made.

In summary, the esophagus is a tube that connects the oropharynx with the stomach; it functions primarily as a conduit for passage of food from the pharynx to the stomach. Dysphagia refers to difficulty in swallowing; it can result from altered nerve function or from disorders that produce narrowing of the esophagus. A diverticulum of the esophagus is an outpouching of the esophageal wall caused by a weakness of the muscularis layer. Longitudinal tears (Mallory-Weiss tears) at the esophagogastric junction can occur with severe bouts of retching or vomiting. They are most often encountered in chronic alcoholics, but may also occur during acute illness with severe vomiting.

Gastrointestinal reflux refers to the backward movement of gastric contents into the esophagus, a condition that causes heartburn. Although most persons experience occasional esophageal reflux and heartburn, persistent reflux can cause esophagitis. Complications can result from persistent reflux, which produces a cycle of mucosal damage that causes hyperemia, edema, and erosion of the luminal surface. Persistent reflux can result in Barrett's esophagus, a condition associated with increased risk for development of esophageal cancer. Gastroesophageal reflux is a common problem in infants and children. Reflux commonly corrects itself with age, and symptoms abate in most children by 2 years of age. Although many infants have minor degrees of reflux, some infants and small children have significant reflux that interferes with feeding, causes esophagitis, and results in respiratory symptoms and other complications.

Carcinoma of the esophagus, which accounts for 6% of all cancers, is more common in older persons (mean age, 67 years) and is more frequent in men than women. There are two types of esophageal cancer: squamous cell carcinomas and adenocarcinomas. Most squamous cell carcinomas are attributable to alcohol and tobacco use, whereas adenocarcinomas are more closely linked to esophageal reflux and Barrett's esophagus.

Disorders of the Stomach

After completing this section of the chapter, you should be able to meet the following objectives:

- Describe the factors that contribute to the gastric mucosal barrier
- Characterize the proposed role of *Helicobacter pylori* in the development of chronic gastritis and peptic ulcer and cite methods for diagnosing the infection
- Differentiate between the causes and manifestations of acute and chronic gastritis
- Describe the predisposing factors in development of peptic ulcer and cite the three complications of peptic ulcer
- Describe the goals for pharmacologic treatment of peptic ulcer disease
- Cite the etiologic factors in ulcer formation related to Zollinger-Ellison syndrome and stress ulcer
- List risk factors associated with gastric cancer

The stomach is a reservoir for contents entering the digestive tract. It lies in the upper abdomen, anterior to the pancreas, splenic vessels, and left kidney. Anteriorly, the stomach is bounded by the anterior abdominal wall and the left inferior lobe of the liver. While in the stomach, food is churned and mixed with hydrochloric acid and pepsin before being released into the small intestine. Normally, the mucosal surface of the stomach provides a barrier that protects it from the hydrochloric acid and pepsin contained in gastric secretions. Disorders of the stomach include gastritis, peptic ulcer, and gastric carcinoma.

GASTRIC MUCOSAL BARRIER

The stomach lining usually is impermeable to the acid it secretes, a property that allows the stomach to contain acid and pepsin without having its wall digested. Several factors contribute to the protection of the gastric mucosa, including an impermeable epithelial cell surface covering, mechanisms for the selective transport of hydrogen and bicarbonate ions, and the characteristics of gastric mucus.[20] These mechanisms are collectively referred to as the *gastric mucosal barrier*.

The gastric epithelial cells are connected by tight junctions that prevent acid penetration, and they are covered with an impermeable hydrophobic lipid layer that prevents diffusion of ionized water-soluble molecules. Aspirin, which is nonionized and lipid soluble in acid solutions, rapidly diffuses across this lipid layer, increasing mucosal permeability and damaging epithelial cells.[21] Gastric irritation and occult bleeding due to gastric irritation occur in a significant number of persons who take aspirin on a regular basis (Fig. 39-1). Alcohol, which also is lipid soluble, disrupts the mucosal barrier; when aspirin and alcohol are taken in combination, as they often are, there is increased risk for gastric irritation. Bile acids also attack the lipid components of the mucosal barrier and afford the potential for gastric irritation when there is reflux of duodenal contents into the stomach.

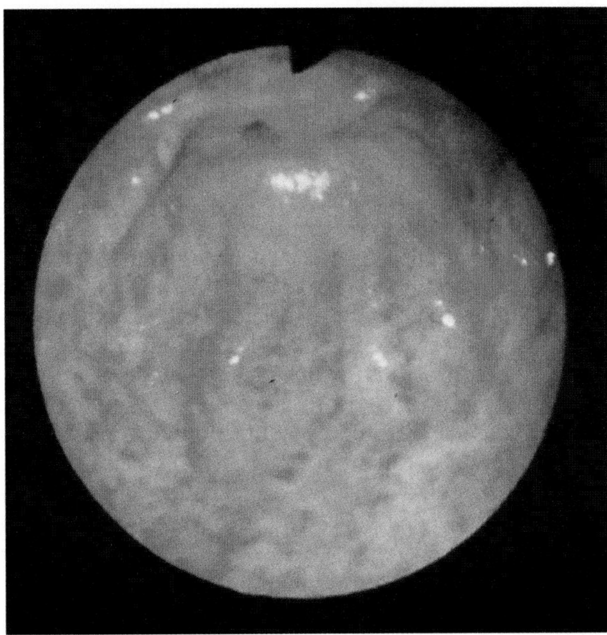

FIGURE 39-1 Erosive gastritis. This endoscopic view of the stomach in a patient who was ingesting aspirin reveals acute hemorrhagic lesions. (From Rubin E., Farber J.L. [1999]. *Pathology* [3rd ed., p. 683]. Philadelphia: Lippincott-Raven)

Normally, the secretion of hydrochloric acid by the parietal cells of the stomach is accompanied by secretion of bicarbonate ions (HCO_3^-). For every hydrogen ion (H^+) that is secreted, an HCO_3^- ion is produced, and as long as HCO_3^- production is equal to H^+ secretion, mucosal injury does not occur. Changes in gastric blood flow, as in shock, tend to decrease HCO_3^- production. This is particularly true in situations in which decreased blood flow is accompanied by acidosis. Aspirin and the nonsteroidal anti-inflammatory drugs (NSAIDs), such as indomethacin and ibuprofen, also impair HCO_3^- secretion.

The mucus that protects the gastric mucosa is of two types: water insoluble and water soluble.[20] Water-insoluble mucus forms a thin, stable gel that adheres to the gastric mucosal surface and provides protection from the proteolytic (protein-digesting) actions of pepsin. It also forms an unstirred layer that traps bicarbonate, forming an alkaline interface between the luminal contents of the stomach and its mucosal surface. The water-soluble mucus is washed from the mucosal surface and mixes with the luminal contents; its viscid nature makes it a lubricant that prevents mechanical damage to the mucosal surface. In addition to their effects on mucosal permeability and bicarbonate production, damaging agents such as aspirin and the NSAIDs inhibit and modify the characteristics of gastric mucus.

Prostaglandins, chemical messengers derived from cell membrane lipids, play an important role in protecting the gastrointestinal mucosa from injury. The prostaglandins probably exert their effect through improved blood flow, increased bicarbonate ion secretion, and enhanced mucus production. The fact that drugs such as aspirin and the NSAIDs inhibit prostaglandin synthesis may contribute to their ability to produce gastric irritation.[21]

DISRUPTION OF THE GASTRIC MUCOSA AND ULCER DEVELOPMENT

- The stomach is protected by a mucosal barrier that prevents gastric secretions and other destructive agents from injuring the epithelial and deeper layers of the stomach wall.
- The integrity of the mucosal layer is maintained by tight cellular junctions and the presence of a protective mucus layer.
- Prostaglandins serve as chemical messengers that protect the stomach lining by improving blood flow, increasing bicarbonate secretion, and enhancing mucus production.
- Two of the major causes of gastric irritation and ulcer formation are aspirin or nonsteroidal anti-inflammatory drugs (NSAIDs) and infection with *H. pylori.*
- Aspirin and NSAIDs exert their destructive effects by irritating the stomach and inhibiting prostaglandin synthesis.
- *H. pylori* is an infectious agent that thrives in the acid environment of the stomach and disrupts the mucosal barrier that protects the stomach from the harmful effects of its digestive enzymes.

GASTRITIS

Gastritis refers to inflammation of the gastric mucosa. There are many causes of gastritis, most of which can be grouped under the headings of acute or chronic gastritis.

Acute Gastritis

Acute gastritis refers to a transient inflammation of the gastric mucosa. It is most commonly associated with local irritants such as bacterial endotoxins, alcohol, and aspirin. Depending on the severity of the disorder, the mucosal response may vary from moderate edema and hyperemia to hemorrhagic erosion of the gastric mucosa.

The complaints of persons with acute gastritis vary. Persons with aspirin-related gastritis can be totally unaware of the condition or may complain only of heartburn or sour stomach. Gastritis associated with excessive alcohol consumption is a different situation; it often causes transient gastric distress, which may lead to vomiting and, in more severe situations, to bleeding and hematemesis. Gastritis caused by the toxins of infectious organisms, such as the staphylococcal enterotoxins, usually has an abrupt and violent onset, with gastric distress and vomiting ensuing approximately 5 hours after the ingestion of a contaminated food source. Acute gastritis usually is a self-limiting disorder, with complete regeneration and healing occurring within several days.

Chronic Gastritis

Chronic gastritis is a separate entity from acute gastritis. It is characterized by the absence of grossly visible erosions and the presence of chronic inflammatory changes leading eventually to atrophy of the glandular epithelium of the stomach. There are three major types of chronic gastritis: *Helicobacter pylori* gastritis, autoimmune gastritis and multifocal atrophic gastritis, and chemical gastropathy.[22]

***Helicobacter pylori* Gastritis.** *H. pylori* infection is the most common cause of chronic gastritis in the United States. Infection occurs worldwide, but the prevalence varies greatly among countries and population groups within countries. The prevalence among middle-aged adults is more than 80% in many developing countries, as compared with 20% to 50% in industrialized countries.[23] It has been suggested that transmission in industrialized countries is largely person to person by contaminated vomitus, saliva, or feces, whereas additional transmission routes such as water may be important in developing countries. In industrialized countries, the rate of infection with *H. pylori* has decreased substantially over the past several decades owing to improved sanitation. Thus, the reported increase in prevalence that occurs with age (*e.g.*, >50% in American adults older than 50 years) has been credited to a cohort effect reflecting intense transmission when members of earlier birth cohorts were children.[23]

H. pylori gastritis is a chronic inflammatory disease of the antrum and body of the stomach. It is the most common type of chronic nonerosive gastritis in the United States. Chronic infection with *H. pylori* can lead to gastric atrophy, peptic ulcer, and is associated with increased risk for gastric adenocarcinoma and low-grade B-cell gastric lymphoma.[8,23,24]

H. pylori are small, curved, gram-negative rods (protobacteria) that can colonize the mucus-secreting epithelial cells of the stomach[23,24] (Fig. 39-2). *H. pylori* have multiple flagella, which allow them to move through the mucous layer of the stomach, and they secrete urease, which enables them to produce sufficient ammonia to buffer the acidity of their immediate environment. These properties help to explain why the organism is able to survive in the acidic environment of the stomach. *H. pylori* produce enzymes and toxins that have the capacity to interfere with the local protection of the gastric mucosa against acid, produce intense inflammation, and elicit an immune response. There is increased production of proinflammatory cytokines that serve to recruit and activate neutrophils. Several *H. pylori* proteins are immunogenic, and they evoke an intense immune response in the mucosa. Both T and B cells can be seen in the chronic gastritis caused by *H. pylori*. Although the role of T and B cells in causing epithelial injury has not been established, T-cell–driven activation of B cells may be involved in the pathogenesis of gastric lymphomas.[8]

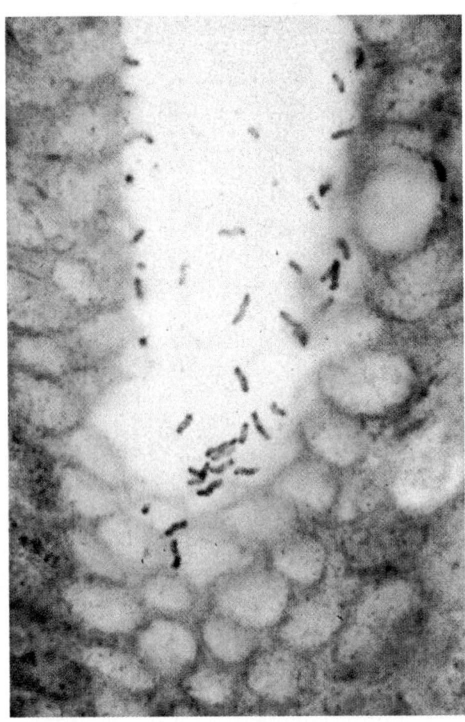

FIGURE 39-2 Infective gastritis. *H. pylori* appears on silver staining as small, curved rods on the surface of the gastric mucosa. (From Rubin E., Farber J.L. [1999]. *Pathology* [3rd ed., p. 687]. Philadelphia: Lippincott-Raven)

Why some people with *H. pylori* infection develop clinical disease and others do not is unclear. Scientists are studying the different strains of the bacteria in an attempt to establish whether certain strains are more virulent than others and whether host and environmental factors contribute to the development of clinical disease.[8]

Methods for establishing the presence of *H. pylori* infection include the C urea breath test using a radioactive carbon isotope (^{13}C or ^{14}C), the stool antigen test, and an endoscopic biopsy for urease testing.[23,24] Blood tests to obtain serologic titers of *H. pylori* antibodies also can be done. The serologic test can establish that a person has been infected with *H. pylori*, but it cannot distinguish how recently the infection occurred.

The goal for *H. pylori* treatment is the complete elimination of the organism. Treatment requires combination therapy that includes two antibiotics and bismuth or a proton-pump inhibitor.[23,24] *H. pylori* mutates rapidly to develop antibiotic resistant strains. The combination of two or more antimicrobial agents increases the rates of cure and reduces the risk for developing resistant strains. The antibiotics that have shown the greatest efficacy against *H. pylori* are clarithromycin, metronidazole, amoxicillin, and tetracycline. The proton pump inhibitors have direct antimicrobial properties against *H. pylori,* and by raising the intragastric pH, they suppress bacterial growth and optimize antibiotic efficacy. Bismuth has a direct antibacterial effect against *H. pylori.*

Autoimmune Gastritis and Multifocal Atrophic Gastritis. Autoimmune gastritis is the least common form of chronic gastritis. It typically involves the fundus and the body of the stomach and is associated with pernicious anemia. Most persons with the disorder have circulating antibodies to parietal cells and intrinsic factor, and hence this form of chronic gastritis is considered to be of autoimmune origin. Autoimmune destruction of the parietal cells leads to hypochlorhydria or achlorhydria, a high intragastric pH, and hypergastrinemia. Pernicious anemia is a megaloblastic anemia that is caused by malabsorption of vitamin B_{12} resulting from a deficiency of intrinsic factor (see Chapter 16). This type of chronic gastritis frequently is associated with other autoimmune disorders such as Hashimoto's thyroiditis and Addison's disease.

Multifocal atrophic gastritis is a disorder of unknown etiology. It is more common than autoimmune gastritis and is seen more frequently in whites than in other races. It is particularly common in Asia, Scandinavia, and parts of Europe and Latin America. Multifocal atrophic gastritis typically affects the antrum and adjacent areas of the stomach. As with autoimmune gastritis, it is associated with reduced gastric acid secretion, but achlorhydria and pernicious anemia are less common.

Chronic autoimmune gastritis and multifocal atrophic gastritis cause few symptoms related directly to gastric function. Persons with autoimmune chronic gastritis may develop signs of pernicious anemia. More important is the development of peptic ulcer and increased risk for peptic ulcer and gastric carcinoma. Approximately 2% to 4% of persons with atrophic gastritis eventually develop gastric carcinoma.[8]

Chemical Gastropathy. Chemical gastropathy is a chronic gastric injury resulting from reflux of alkaline duodenal contents, pancreatic secretions, and bile into the stomach. It is most commonly seen in persons who have had gastroduodenostomy or gastrojejunostomy surgery. A milder form may occur in persons with gastric ulcer, gallbladder disease, or various motility disorders of the distal stomach.

ULCER DISEASE

Peptic Ulcer Disease

Peptic ulcer is a term used to describe a group of ulcerative disorders that occur in areas of the upper gastrointestinal tract that are exposed to acid-pepsin secretions. The most common forms of peptic ulcer are duodenal and gastric ulcers. Peptic ulcer disease, with its remissions and exacerbations, represents a chronic health problem. Approximately 10% of the population have or will develop peptic ulcer.[8] Duodenal ulcers occur five times more commonly than gastric ulcers. Ulcers in the duodenum occur at any age and frequently are seen in early adulthood. Gastric ulcers tend to affect the older age group, with a peak incidence between 55 and 70 years of age.[12] Both types of ulcer affect men three to four times more frequently than women.

A peptic ulcer can affect one or all layers of the stomach or duodenum (Fig. 39-3). The ulcer may penetrate only the mucosal surface, or it may extend into the smooth muscle layers. Occasionally, an ulcer penetrates the outer wall of the stomach or duodenum. Spontaneous remissions and exacerbations are common. Healing of the muscularis layer involves replacement with scar tissue; although the mucosal layers that cover the scarred muscle layer regenerate, the regeneration often is less than perfect, which contributes to repeated episodes of ulceration.

Since the early 1980s, there has been a radical shift in thinking regarding the cause of peptic ulcer. No longer is peptic ulcer thought to result from a genetic predisposition, stress, or dietary indiscretions. Most cases of peptic ulcer are caused by *H. pylori* infection.[23,24] The second most common cause of peptic ulcer is NSAID and aspirin use.

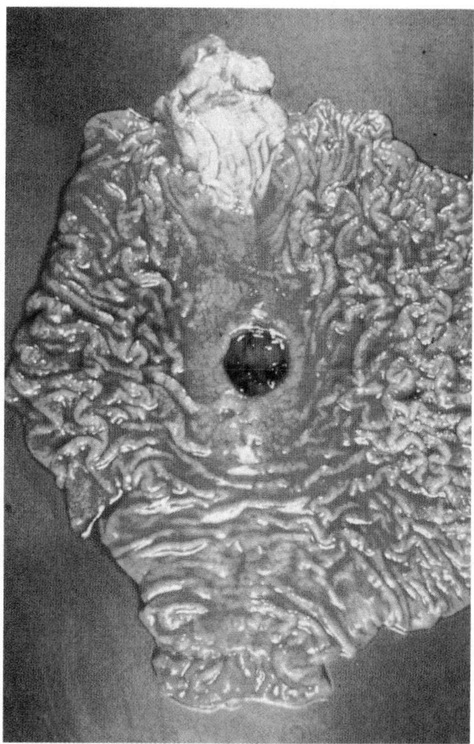

FIGURE 39-3 Gastric ulcer. The stomach has been opened to reveal a sharply demarcated, deep peptic ulcer on the lesser curvature. (From Rubin E., Farber J.L. [1999]. *Pathology* [3rd ed., p. 693]. Philadelphia: Lippincott-Raven)

Much of the familial aggregation of peptic ulcer that formerly was credited to genetic factors in the development of peptic ulcer probably is due to intrafamilial infection with *H. pylori* rather than genetic susceptibility.

There is a 10% to 20% prevalence of gastric ulcers and a 2% to 5% prevalence of duodenal ulcers among chronic NSAID users.[12] Aspirin appears to be the most ulcerogenic of the NSAIDs. Ulcer development in NSAID users is dose dependent, but some risk occurs even with aspirin doses of 81 mg/day.[12] The pathogenesis of NSAID-induced ulcers is thought to involve mucosal injury and inhibition of prostaglandin synthesis. In contrast to peptic ulcer from other causes, NSAID-induced gastric injury often is without symptoms, and life-threatening complications can occur without warning. There is reportedly less gastric irritation with the newer class of NSAIDs that selectively inhibit cyclooxygenase 2 (COX-2 selective NSAIDs), the principal enzyme involved in prostaglandin synthesis at the site of inflammation, than with the nonselective NSAIDs that also inhibit COX-1, the enzyme involved in prostaglandin production in the gastric mucosa.

Manifestations. The clinical manifestations of uncomplicated peptic ulcer focus on discomfort and pain. The pain, which is described as burning, gnawing, or cramplike, usually is rhythmic and frequently occurs when the stomach is empty—between meals and at 1 or 2 o'clock in the morning. The pain usually is located over a small area near the midline in the epigastrium near the xiphoid and may radiate below the costal margins, into the back, or rarely, to the right shoulder. Superficial and deep epigastric tenderness and voluntary muscle guarding may occur with more extensive lesions. An additional characteristic of ulcer pain is periodicity. The pain tends to recur at intervals of weeks or months. During an exacerbation, it occurs daily for a period of several weeks and then remits until the next recurrence. Characteristically, the pain is relieved by food or antacids.

Complications. The complications of peptic ulcer include hemorrhage, obstruction, and perforation. Hemorrhage is caused by bleeding from granulation tissue or from erosion of an ulcer into an artery or vein. It occurs in up to 10% to 20% of persons with peptic ulcer.[12] Evidence of bleeding may consist of hematemesis or melena. Bleeding may be sudden, severe, and without warning, or it may be insidious, producing only occult blood in the stool. Up to 20% of persons with bleeding ulcers have no antecedent symptoms of pain; this is particularly true in persons receiving NSAIDs. Acute hemorrhage is evidenced by the sudden onset of weakness, dizziness, thirst, cold and moist skin, the desire to defecate, and the passage of loose, tarry, or even red stools and coffee-ground emesis. Signs of circulatory shock develop depending on the amount of blood lost.

Obstruction is caused by edema, spasm, or contraction of scar tissue and interference with the free passage of gastric contents through the pylorus or adjacent areas. There is a feeling of epigastric fullness and heaviness after meals. With severe obstruction, there is vomiting of undigested food.

Perforation occurs when an ulcer erodes through all the layers of the stomach or duodenum wall. Perforation develops in approximately 5% of persons with peptic ulcers, usually from ulcers on the anterior wall of the stomach or duodenum.[12] With perforation, gastrointestinal contents enter the peritoneum and cause peritonitis, or penetrate adjacent structures such as the pancreas. Radiation of the pain into the back, severe night distress, and inadequate pain relief from eating foods or taking antacids in persons with a long history of peptic ulcer may signify perforation. Peritonitis is discussed as a separate topic near the end of this chapter.

Diagnosis. Diagnostic procedures for peptic ulcer include history taking, laboratory tests, radiologic imaging, and endoscopic examination. The history should include careful attention to aspirin and NSAID use. Peptic ulcer should be differentiated from other causes of epigastric pain. Laboratory findings of hypochromic anemia and occult blood in the stools indicate bleeding.

Endoscopy (*i.e.,* gastroscopy and duodenoscopy) can be used to visualize the ulcer area and obtain biopsy specimens to test for *H. pylori* and exclude malignant disease. X-ray studies with a contrast medium such as barium are used to detect the presence of an ulcer crater and to exclude gastric carcinoma.

Treatment. The treatment of peptic ulcer has changed dramatically over the past several years and now aims to eradicate the cause and effect a permanent cure for the disease. Pharmacologic treatment focuses on eradicating *H. pylori,* relieving ulcer symptoms, and healing the ulcer crater. Acid-neutralizing, acid-inhibiting drugs and mucosal protective agents are used to relieve symptoms and promote healing of the ulcer crater. There is no evidence that special diets are beneficial in treating peptic ulcer. Aspirin and NSAID use should be avoided when possible.

There are two pharmacologic methods for reducing gastric acid content. The first involves the neutralization of gastric acid through the use of antacids, and the second a decrease in gastric acid production through the use of H_2-receptor antagonists or proton-pump inhibitors. Essentially three types of antacids are used to reduce gastric acidity: calcium carbonate, aluminum hydroxide, and magnesium hydroxide. Many antacids contain a combination of ingredients, such as magnesium aluminum hydroxide. *Calcium preparations* are constipating and may cause hypercalcemia and the milk-alkali syndrome. There also is evidence that oral calcium preparations increase gastric acid secretion after their buffering effect has been depleted. *Magnesium hydroxide* is a potent antacid that also has laxative effects. Approximately 5% to 10% of the magnesium in this preparation is absorbed from the intestine; because magnesium is excreted through the kidneys, this formulation should not be used in persons with renal failure. *Aluminum hydroxide* reacts with hydrochloric acid to form aluminum chloride. It combines with phosphate in the intestine, and prolonged use may lead to phosphate depletion and osteoporosis. Because antacids can decrease the absorption, bioavailability, and renal elimination of a number of drugs, this should be considered when antacids are administered with other medications.

Histamine is the major physiologic mediator for hydrochloric acid secretion. The H_2-receptor antagonists block gastric acid secretion stimulated by histamine, gastrin, and acetylcholine. The volume of gastric secretion and the concentration of pepsin also are reduced. The proton-pump inhibitors block the final stage of hydrogen ion secretion by blocking the action of the gastric parietal cell proton pump (H^+-K^+-ATPase).

Among the agents that enhance mucosal defenses are sucralfate and prostaglandin analogs. The drug sucralfate, which is a complex salt of sucrose-containing aluminum and sulfate, selectively binds to necrotic ulcer tissue and serves as a barrier to acid, pepsin, and bile. Sucralfate also can directly absorb bile salts. The drug is not absorbed systemically. The drug requires an acid pH for activation and should not be administered with antacids or an H_2 antagonist. Misoprostol, a prostaglandin analog, promotes ulcer healing by stimulating mucus and bicarbonate secretion and by modestly inhibiting acid secretion. It is used as a prophylactic agent to prevent NSAID-induced peptic ulcers. The drug causes dose-dependent diarrhea, and because of its stimulant effect on the uterus, it is contraindicated in women of childbearing age.

The current surgical management of peptic ulcer disease is largely limited to treatment of complications. When surgery is needed, it usually is performed using minimally invasive methods. With bleeding ulcers, hemostasis often can be achieved by endoscopic methods, and endoscopic balloon dilation often is effective in relieving outflow obstruction.

Zollinger-Ellison Syndrome

The Zollinger-Ellison syndrome is a rare condition caused by a gastrin-secreting tumor (gastrinoma). In persons with this disorder, gastric acid secretion reaches such levels that ulceration becomes inevitable.[25] The tumors may be single or multiple; although most tumors are located in the pancreas, a few develop in the submucosa of the stomach or duodenum. More than two thirds of gastrinomas are malignant.[26] The increased gastric secretions cause symptoms related to peptic ulcer. Diarrhea may result from hypersecretion or from the inactivation of intestinal lipase and impaired fat digestion that occurs with a decrease in intestinal pH.

Hypergastrinemia may also occur in an autosomal dominant disorder called the *multiple endocrine neoplasia type 1* (MEN 1) syndrome. The syndrome is characterized by hyperparathyroidism and multiple endocrine tumors, including gastrinomas. Approximately 20% of gastrinomas are due to MEN 1.

The diagnosis of the Zollinger-Ellison syndrome is based on elevated serum gastrin and basal gastric acid levels and elimination of the MEN 1 syndrome as a cause of the disorder. Proton-pump inhibitors are used to control gastric acid secretion. Computed tomography (CT), abdominal ultrasonography, and selective angiography are used to localize the tumor and determine whether metastatic disease is present. Surgical removal is indicated when the tumor is malignant and has not metastasized.

Stress Ulcers

A stress ulcer, sometimes called *Curling's ulcer,* refers to gastrointestinal ulcerations that develop in relation to major physiologic stress.[8] Persons at high risk for development of stress ulcers include those with large-surface-area burns, trauma, sepsis, acute respiratory distress syndrome, severe liver failure, and major surgical procedures. These lesions occur most often in the fundus of the stomach and proximal duodenum and are thought to result from ischemia, tissue acidosis, and bile salts entering the stomach in critically ill persons with decreased gastrointestinal tract motility.[8,27,28] Another form of stress ulcer, called *Cushing ulcer,* consists of gastric, duodenal, and esophageal ulcers arising in persons with intracranial injury, operations, or tumors. They are thought to be caused by hypersecretion of gastric acid resulting from stimulation of vagal nuclei by increased intracranial pressure. These ulcers are associated with a high incidence of perforation.[27]

Persons admitted to hospital intensive care units are at particular risk for the development of stress ulcers.[11] They usually are manifested by painless upper gastrointestinal tract bleeding. Monitoring and maintaining the gastric pH at 3.5 or higher helps to prevent the development of stress ulcers. H_2-receptor antagonists, proton-pump inhibitors, and sucralfate are used in the prevention and treatment of stress ulcers.

CANCER OF THE STOMACH

Although its incidence has decreased during the past 50 years, stomach cancer is the seventh most frequent cause of cancer mortality in the United States. In 2004, approximately 22,710 Americans were diagnosed with stomach cancer, and 11,780 died of the disease.[28] The disease is much more common in other countries and regions, principally Japan, Central Europe, the Scandinavian countries, South and Central America, the Soviet Union, China, and Korea. It is the major cause of cancer death worldwide.

Among the factors that increase the risk for gastric cancer are a genetic predisposition, carcinogenic factors in the diet (*e.g., N*-nitroso compounds and benzopyrene found in smoked and preserved foods), autoimmune gastritis, and gastric adenomas or polyps. The incidence of stomach cancer in the United States has decreased fourfold since 1930, presumably because of improved storage of food with decreased consumption of salted, smoked, and preserved foods.[12] Infection with *H. pylori* appears to serve as a cofactor in some types of gastric carcinomas.[12]

Between 50% and 60% of gastric cancers occur in the pyloric region or adjacent to the antrum. Compared with a benign ulcer, which has smooth margins and is concentrically shaped, gastric cancers tend to be larger, are irregularly shaped, and have irregular margins.

Unfortunately, stomach cancers often are asymptomatic until late in their course. Symptoms, when they do occur, usually are vague and include indigestion, anorexia, weight loss, vague epigastric pain, vomiting, and an abdominal mass.

Diagnosis of gastric cancer is accomplished by means of a variety of techniques, including barium x-ray studies, endoscopic studies with biopsy, and cytologic studies (*e.g.*, Papanicolaou smear) of gastric secretions. Cytologic studies can prove particularly useful as routine screening tests for persons with atrophic gastritis or gastric polyps. CT and endoscopic ultrasonography often are used to delineate the spread of a diagnosed stomach cancer.

Surgery in the form of radical subtotal gastrectomy usually is the treatment of choice.[29] Irradiation and chemotherapy have not proved particularly useful as primary treatment modalities in stomach cancer. These methods usually are used for palliative purposes or to control metastatic spread of the disease.

In summary, disorders of the stomach include gastritis, peptic ulcer, and cancer of the stomach. Gastritis refers to inflammation of the gastric mucosa. Acute gastritis refers to a transient inflammation of the gastric mucosa; it is associated most commonly with local irritants such as bacterial endotoxins, caffeine, alcohol, and aspirin. Chronic gastritis is characterized by the absence of grossly visible erosions and the presence of chronic inflammatory changes leading eventually to atrophy of the glandular epithelium of the stomach. There are three main types of chronic gastritis: *H. pylori* gastritis, autoimmune gastritis and multifocal atrophic gastritis, and chemical gastropathy. *H. pylori* is an "S"-shaped bacterium that colonizes the mucus-secreting epithelial cells of the stomach. Infection increases the risk for chronic gastritis, peptic ulcer, gastric carcinoma, and low-grade B-cell gastric lymphoma. Treatment of the *H. pylori* involves the use of multidrug therapy aimed at increasing the pH of gastric secretions and antimicrobial agents designed to eradicate the organism.

Peptic ulcer is a term used to describe a group of ulcerative disorders that occur in areas of the upper gastrointestinal tract that are exposed to acid-pepsin secretions, most commonly the duodenum and stomach. There are two main causes of peptic ulcer: *H. pylori* infection and aspirin or NSAID use. The treatment of peptic ulcer focuses on eradication of *H. pylori*, avoidance of gastric irritation from NSAIDs, and conventional pharmacologic treatment directed at symptom relief and ulcer healing.

The Zollinger-Ellison syndrome is a rare condition caused by a gastrin-secreting tumor, in which gastric acid secretion reaches such levels that ulceration becomes inevitable. Stress ulcers, also called *Curling's ulcers,* occur in relation to major physiologic stresses such as burns and trauma and are thought to result from ischemia, tissue acidosis, and bile salts entering the stomach in critically ill persons with decreased gastrointestinal tract motility. Another form of stress ulcer, Cushing ulcer, occurs in persons with intracranial trauma or surgery and is thought to be caused by hypersecretion of gastric acid resulting from stimulation of vagal nuclei by increased intracranial pressure.

Although the incidence of cancer of the stomach has declined during the past 50 years, it remains the seventh leading cause of death in the United States. Because there are few early symptoms with this form of cancer, the disease often is far advanced at the time of diagnosis.

Disorders of the Small and Large Intestines

After completing this section of the chapter, you should be able to meet the following objectives:

- ✦ State the diagnostic criteria for irritable bowel syndrome
- ✦ Compare the characteristics of Crohn disease and ulcerative colitis
- ✦ Relate the use of a high-fiber diet in the treatment of diverticular disease to the etiologic factors for the condition
- ✦ Describe the common causes of infectious enterocolitis
- ✦ Describe the rationale for the symptoms associated with appendicitis
- ✦ Compare the causes and manifestations of small-volume diarrhea and large-volume diarrhea
- ✦ Explain why a failure to respond to the defecation urge may result in constipation
- ✦ Differentiate between mechanical and paralytic intestinal obstruction in terms of cause and manifestations
- ✦ Describe the characteristics of the peritoneum that increase its vulnerability to and protect it against the effects of peritonitis
- ✦ List conditions that cause malabsorption by impaired intraluminal malabsorption, mucosal malabsorption, and lymphatic obstruction
- ✦ List the risk factors associated with colorectal cancer and cite the screening methods for detection

There are many similarities in conditions that disrupt the integrity and function of the small and large intestine. The walls of the small and large intestines consist of five layers (see Chapter 38, Fig. 38-3): an outer serosal layer; a muscularis layer, which is divided into a layer of circular and a layer of longitudinal muscle fibers; a submucosal layer; and an inner mucosal layer, which lines the lumen of the intestine. Among the conditions that cause altered intestinal function are irritable bowel disease, inflammatory bowel disease, diverticulitis, appendicitis, alterations in bowel motility (*i.e.*, diarrhea, constipation, and bowel obstruction), malabsorption syndrome, and cancer of the colon and rectum.

IRRITABLE BOWEL SYNDROME

The term *irritable bowel syndrome* is used to describe a functional gastrointestinal disorder characterized by a variable combination of chronic and recurrent intestinal symptoms not explained by structural or biochemical abnormalities. There is evidence to suggest that 10% to 20% of people in Western countries have the disorder, although most do not seek medical attention.[30]

Irritable bowel disease is characterized by persistent or recurrent symptoms of abdominal pain, altered bowel function, and varying complaints of flatulence, bloatedness, nausea and anorexia, constipation or diarrhea, and anxiety or depression. A hallmark of irritable bowel syndrome is abdominal pain that is relieved by defecation and associated with a change in consistency or frequency of stools. Abdominal pain usually is intermittent, cramping, and in the lower abdomen. It does not usually occur at night or interfere with sleep. The condition is believed to result from dysregulation of intestinal motor and sensory functions modulated by the CNS.[30–32] Persons with irritable bowel syndrome tend to experience increased motility and abnormal intestinal contractions in response to psychological and physiologic stress. The role that psychological factors play in the disease is uncertain. Although changes in intestinal activity are normal responses to stress, these responses appear to be exaggerated in persons with irritable bowel syndrome. Women tend to be affected more often than men. Menarche often is associated with onset of the disorder. Women frequently notice an exacerbation of symptoms during the premenstrual period, suggesting a hormonal component.

Because irritable bowel syndrome lacks anatomic or physiologic markers, diagnosis is usually based on signs and symptoms of abdominal pain or discomfort, bloating, constipation, diarrhea, or an alteration between both. A commonly used set of diagnostic criteria require continuous or recurrent symptoms of at least 12 weeks' duration (which may be nonconsecutive) of abdominal discomfort or pain in the preceding 12 months with two of three accompanying features: relief with defecation, onset associated with a change in bowel frequency, and onset associated with a change in form (appearance) of stool.[33] Other symptoms that support the diagnosis of irritable bowel syndrome include abnormal stool frequency (>3 times per day or <3 times per week), abnormal stool form (lumpy and hard or loose and watery), abnormal stool passage (straining, urgency, or feeling of incomplete evacuation), passage of mucus, bloating, or feeling of abdominal distention.[33] A history of lactose intolerance should be considered because intolerance to lactose and other sugars may be a precipitating factor in some persons. The acute onset of symptoms raises the likelihood of organic disease, as does weight loss, anemia, fever, occult blood in the stool, nighttime symptoms, or signs and symptoms of malabsorption. These signs and symptoms require additional investigation.[30–32]

The treatment of irritable bowel syndrome focuses on methods of stress management, particularly those related to symptom production. Reassurance is important. Usually, no special diet is indicated, although adequate fiber intake usually is recommended. Avoidance of offending dietary substances such as fatty and gas-producing foods, alcohol, and caffeine-containing beverages may be beneficial. Various pharmacologic agents, including antispasmodic and anticholinergic drugs, have been used with varying success in treatment of the disorder. Alosetron, a 5-HT_3 antagonist, was the first specific drug to be approved by the U.S. Food and Drug Administration (FDA) for the treatment of irritable bowel disease. It acts by reducing intestinal secretion, decreasing visceral afferent nerve activity (thereby reducing abdominal pain), and reducing intestinal motility. The drug, which was indicated for treatment of women with the severe diarrhea form of the disease, was removed from the market in late 2000 because of serious side effects and then reintroduced in 2002 under a restricted prescribing program.[30–32]

INFLAMMATORY BOWEL DISEASE

The term *inflammatory bowel disease* is used to designate two related inflammatory intestinal disorders: Crohn disease and ulcerative colitis. The prevalence of these diseases ranges from 300,000 to 500,000.[34] Although the two diseases differ sufficiently to be distinguishable, they have many features in common. Both diseases produce inflammation of the bowel, both lack confirming evidence of a proven causative agent, both have a pattern of familial occurrence, and both can be accompanied by systemic manifestations.[35] The distinguishing characteristics of Crohn disease and ulcerative colitis are summarized in Table 39-1.

The clinical manifestations of both Crohn disease and ulcerative colitis are ultimately the result of activation of inflammatory cells with elaboration of inflammatory mediators that cause nonspecific tissue damage. Both diseases are characterized by remissions and exacerbations of diarrhea, fecal urgency, and weight loss. Acute complications such as

TABLE 39-1 Differentiating Characteristics of Crohn Disease and Ulcerative Colitis

Characteristic	Crohn Disease	Ulcerative Colitis
Types of inflammation	Granulomatous	Ulcerative and exudative
Level of involvement	Primarily submucosal	Primarily mucosal
Extent of involvement	Skip lesions	Continuous
Areas of involvement	Primarily ileum, secondarily colon	Primarily rectum and left colon
Diarrhea	Common	Common
Rectal bleeding	Rare	Common
Fistulas	Common	Rare
Strictures	Common	Rare
Perianal abscesses	Common	Rare
Development of cancer	Uncommon	Relatively common

intestinal obstruction may develop during periods of fulminant disease.

A number of systemic manifestations have been identified in persons with Crohn disease and ulcerative colitis. These include axial arthritis affecting the spine and sacroiliac joints and oligoarticular arthritis affecting the large joints of the arms and legs; inflammatory conditions of the eye, usually uveitis; skin lesions, especially erythema nodosum; stomatitis; and autoimmune anemia, hypercoagulability of blood, and sclerosing cholangitis. Occasionally, these systemic manifestations may herald the recurrence of intestinal disease. In children, growth retardation may occur, particularly if the symptoms are prolonged and nutrient intake has been poor.

The causes of Crohn disease and ulcerative colitis are largely unknown. One of the common beliefs is that genetic factors predispose to some form of autoimmune reaction, possibly triggered by a relatively innocuous environmental agent such as a dietary antigen or microbial agent. The sites affected by inflammatory bowel disease, the distal ileum and the colon, are awash with bacteria. Although it is unlikely that inflammatory bowel disease is caused by microbes, it seems likely that microbes may provide the antigen trigger for an unregulated immune response. Interestingly, smoking tobacco has the opposite effect on the two forms of inflammatory bowel disease. It predisposes to development of Crohn disease, yet is associated with a reduced incidence of ulcerative colitis. Smoking also increases the likelihood of disease exaggeration and need for surgery in people with Crohn disease.[35]

The genetic basis of inflammatory bowel disease has long been suspected. Approximately 15% of persons with inflammatory bowel disease have affected first-degree relatives.[36] Genetic factors seem to be more important in Crohn disease than ulcerative colitis. A genetic susceptibility locus for Crohn disease has been mapped to the *IBD1* locus on chromosome 16.[8,37,38] The product of the implicated gene, *NOD2,* activates a nuclear factor in macrophages in response to bacterial lipopolysaccharides exposure. Activated macrophages produce a potent mixture of inflammatory mediators, including interleukin-1 (IL-1), IL-6, and tumor necrosis factor (TNF) that are thought to be key to the inflammatory response that occurs in Crohn disease. Although the *IBD1* gene may account for only a limited number of cases of Crohn disease, the discovery of the gene provides the first molecular evidence to support a genetic basis for the disease, and the functional properties of the gene provide the first evidence for a linkage between enteric bacteria and the inflammatory basis of the disease.[8]

Accumulating evidence also suggests that both Crohn disease and ulcerative colitis are associated with profound disorders of mucosal immunity. A large number of immunologic abnormalities have been noted in persons with Crohn disease and ulcerative colitis. In keeping with an underlying immunologic dysfunction, both Crohn disease and ulcerative colitis have been linked to specific major histocompatibility (HLA) class II alleles. Ulcerative colitis has been associated with HLA-D2 and Crohn disease with HLA-DR1 and –DQw5 alleles, suggesting that the two diseases are genetically distinct.[8]

Crohn Disease

Crohn disease is a recurrent, granulomatous type of inflammatory response that can affect any area of the gastrointestinal tract from the mouth to the anus. In nearly 30% of persons with disease, the lesions are restricted to the small intestine; in 30%, only the large bowel is affected; and in the remaining 40%, the large bowel and small bowel are affected.[8] It is a slowly progressive, relentless, and often disabling disease. The prevalence of Crohn disease is greatest in the United States, Great Britain, and the Scandinavian countries. The disease usually strikes people in their 20s or 30s, with women being affected slightly more often than men.

A characteristic feature of Crohn disease is the sharply demarcated, granulomatous lesions that are surrounded by normal-appearing mucosal tissue. When the lesions are multiple, they often are referred to as *skip lesions* because they are interspersed between what appear to be normal segments of the bowel. All the layers of the bowel are involved, with the submucosal layer affected to the greatest extent. The surface of the inflamed bowel usually has a characteristic "cobblestone" appearance resulting from the fissures and crevices that develop and that are surrounded by areas of submucosal edema[8] (Fig. 39-4). There usually is a relative sparing of the smooth muscle layers of the bowel, with marked inflammatory and fibrotic changes of the submucosal layer. The bowel wall, after a time, often becomes thickened and inflexible; its appearance has been likened to a lead pipe or rubber hose. The adjacent mesentery may become inflamed, and the regional lymph nodes and channels may become enlarged.

The clinical course of Crohn disease is variable; often, there are periods of exacerbations and remissions, with symptoms being related to the location of the lesions. The principal symptoms include intermittent diarrhea, colicky pain (usually in the lower right quadrant), weight loss, fluid and electrolyte disorders, malaise, and low-grade fever.[38,39] Because Crohn disease affects the submucosal layer to a greater extent than the mucosal layer, there is less bloody diarrhea than with ulcerative colitis. Ulcera-

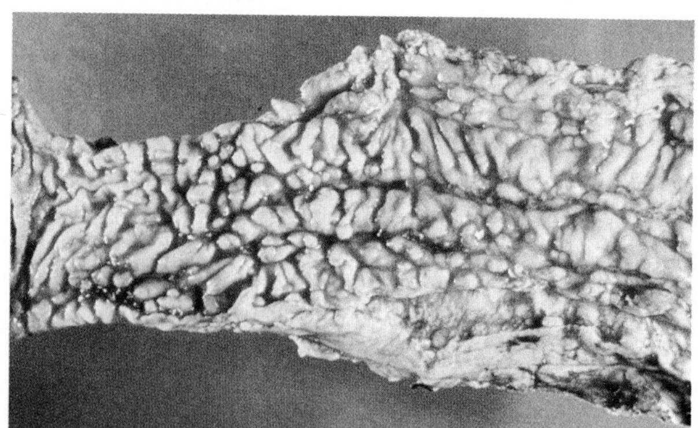

FIGURE 39-4 Crohn disease. The mucosal surface of the colon displays a "cobblestone" appearance owing to the presence of linear ulcerations and edema and inflammation of the intervening tissue. (From Rubin E., Farber J.L. [1999]. *Pathology* [3rd ed., p. 728]. Philadelphia: Lippincott-Raven)

tion of the perianal skin is common, largely because of the severity of the diarrhea. The absorptive surface of the intestine may be disrupted; nutritional deficiencies may occur, related to the specific segment of the intestine that is involved. When Crohn disease occurs in childhood, one of its major manifestations may be retardation of growth and physical development.[22]

Complications of Crohn disease include fistula formation, abdominal abscess formation, and intestinal obstruction. Fistulas are tubelike passages that form connections between different sites in the gastrointestinal tract. They also may develop between other sites, including the bladder, vagina, urethra, and skin. Perineal fistulas that originate in the ileum are relatively common. Fistulas between segments of the gastrointestinal tract may lead to malabsorption, syndromes of bacterial overgrowth, and diarrhea. They also can become infected and cause abscess formation.

Diagnosis and Treatment. The diagnosis of Crohn disease requires a thorough history and physical examination. Sigmoidoscopy is used for direct visualization of the affected areas and to obtain biopsies. Measures are taken to exclude infectious agents as the cause of the disorder. This usually is accomplished by the use of stool cultures and examination of fresh stool specimens for ova and parasites. In persons suspected of having Crohn disease, radiocontrast studies provide a means for determining the extent of involvement of the small bowel and establishing the presence and nature of fistulas. CT scans may be used to detect an inflammatory mass or abscess.

Treatment methods focus on terminating the inflammatory response and promoting healing, maintaining adequate nutrition, and preventing and treating complications. Several medications have been successful in suppressing the inflammatory reaction, including the corticosteroids, sulfasalazine, metronidazole, 6-mercaptopurine, and cyclosporine. Surgical resection of damaged bowel, drainage of abscesses, or repair of fistula tracts may be necessary.

Sulfasalazine is a topically active agent that has a variety of anti-inflammatory effects. The beneficial effects of the sulfasalazine are attributable to one component of the drug, 5-aminosalicylic acid (5-ASA). Agents containing 5-ASA affect multiple sites in the arachidonic acid pathway critical to the pathogenesis of inflammation. Sulfasalazine contains 5-ASA with sulfapyridine linked to an azo bond. The drug is poorly absorbed from the intestine, and the azo linkage is broken down by the bacterial flora in the ileum and colon to release 5-ASA. Metronidazole is an antibiotic used to treat bacterial overgrowth in the small intestine. Immunosuppressive drugs such as cyclosporine and azathioprine or its active derivative, 6-mercaptopurine, also may be used.

In 1999, the FDA approved the drug infliximab for treatment of moderate to severe Crohn disease that does not respond to standard therapies or for the treatment of open draining fistulas.[40] Infliximab is the first treatment approved specifically for Crohn disease. It is a monoclonal antibody that targets the destruction of TNF, a mediator of the inflammatory response that is known to be important in granulomatous inflammatory processes such as Crohn disease.

Nutritional deficiencies are common in Crohn disease because of diarrhea, steatorrhea, and other malabsorption problems. A nutritious diet that is high in calories, vitamins, and proteins is recommended. Because fats often aggravate the diarrhea, it is recommended that they be avoided. Elemental diets, which are nutritionally balanced but residue free and bulk free, may be given during the acute phase of the illness. These diets are largely absorbed in the jejunum and allow the inflamed bowel to rest. Total parenteral nutrition (*i.e.*, parenteral hyperalimentation) consists of intravenous administration of hypertonic glucose solutions to which amino acids and fats may be added. This form of nutritional therapy may be needed when food cannot be absorbed from the intestine. Because of the hypertonicity of these solutions, they must be administered through a large-diameter central vein.

Ulcerative Colitis

Ulcerative colitis is a nonspecific inflammatory condition of the colon. The disease is more common in the United States and Western countries. The disease may arise at any age, with a peak incidence between ages 20 and 25 years.[8] Unlike Crohn disease, which can affect various sites in the gastrointestinal tract, ulcerative colitis is confined to the rectum and colon. The disease usually begins in the rectum and spreads proximally, affecting primarily the mucosal layer, although it can extend into the submucosal layer. The length of proximal extension varies. It may involve the rectum alone (ulcerative proctitis), the rectum and sigmoid colon (proctosigmoiditis), or the entire colon (pancolitis). The inflammatory process tends to be confluent and continuous instead of skipping areas, as it does in Crohn disease.

Characteristic of the disease are the lesions that form in the crypts of Lieberkühn in the base of the mucosal layer (see Chapter 38, Fig. 38-11). The inflammatory process leads to the formation of pinpoint mucosal hemorrhages, which in time suppurate and develop into *crypt abscesses.* These inflammatory lesions may become necrotic and ulcerate. Although the ulcerations usually are superficial, they often extend, causing large denuded areas (Fig. 39-5). As a result of the inflammatory process, the mucosal layer often develops tonguelike projections that resemble polyps and therefore are called *pseudopolyps.* The bowel wall thickens in response to repeated episodes of colitis.

Diarrhea, which is the characteristic manifestation of ulcerative colitis, varies according to the severity of the disease. There may be up to 30 to 40 bowel movements a day. Because ulcerative colitis affects the mucosal layer of the bowel, the stools typically contain blood and mucus. Nocturnal diarrhea usually occurs when daytime symptoms are severe. There may be mild abdominal cramping and fecal incontinence. Anorexia, weakness, and fatigability are common.

Ulcerative colitis usually follows a course of remissions and exacerbations. The severity of the disease varies from mild to fulminating. Accordingly, the disease has been divided into three types: mild chronic, chronic intermittent,

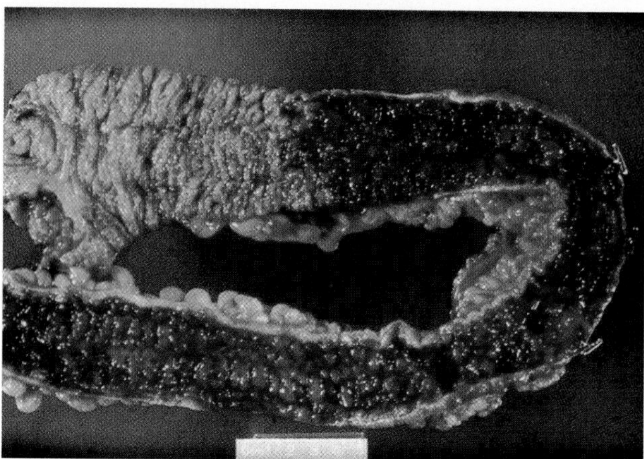

FIGURE 39-5 Ulcerative colitis. Prominent erythema and ulceration of the colon begin in the ascending colon and are most severe in the rectosigmoid area. (From Rubin E., Farber J.L. [1999]. *Pathology* [3rd ed., p. 731]. Philadelphia: Lippincott-Raven)

and acute fulminating. The most common form of the disease is the mild chronic from, in which bleeding and diarrhea are mild and systemic signs are minimal or absent. This form of the disease usually can be managed conservatively. The chronic intermittent form continues after the initial attack. Compared with the milder form, more of the colon surface usually is involved with the chronic intermittent form, and there are more systemic signs and complications. In approximately 15% of affected persons, the disease assumes a more fulminant course, involves the entire colon, and manifests with severe, bloody diarrhea, fever, and acute abdominal pain. These persons are at risk for development of toxic megacolon, which is characterized by dilatation of the colon and signs of systemic toxicity. It results from extension of the inflammatory response, with involvement of neural and vascular components of the bowel. Contributing factors include use of laxatives, narcotics, and anticholinergic drugs and the presence of hypokalemia.

Cancer of the colon is one of the feared complications of ulcerative colitis. The risk for development of cancer among persons who have had pancolitis for 10 years or more is 20 to 30 times that of the general population.[8]

Diagnosis and Treatment. Diagnosis of ulcerative colitis is based on history and physical examination. The diagnosis usually is confirmed by proctosigmoidoscopy.

Treatment depends on the extent of the disease and severity of symptoms. It includes measures to control the acute manifestations of the disease and prevent recurrence. Some people with mild to moderate symptoms are able to control their symptoms simply by avoiding caffeine, lactose (milk), highly spiced foods, and gas-forming foods. Fiber supplements may be used to decrease diarrhea and rectal symptoms.

The medications used in the treatment of ulcerative colitis are similar to those used in the treatment of Crohn disease. They include the use of nonabsorbable 5-ASA compounds (*e.g.,* mesalamine, olsalazine).[38] The corticosteroids are used selectively to lessen the acute inflammatory response. Many of these medications can be administered rectally by suppository or enema. Immunosuppressant drugs, such as cyclosporine, may be used to treat persons with severe colitis.

Surgical treatment (*i.e.,* removal of the rectum and entire colon) with the creation of an ileostomy or ilioanal anastomosis may be required for those persons with ulcerative colitis who do not respond to conservative methods of treatment.

INFECTIOUS ENTEROCOLITIS

A number of microbial agents can infect the intestine, including viruses, bacteria, and protozoa. Most infections are spread by oral–fecal route, often through contaminated water or food.

Viral Infection

Most viral infections affect the superficial epithelium of the small intestine, destroying these cells and disrupting their absorptive function. Repopulation of the small intestine villi with immature enterocytes and preservation of crypt secretory cells leads to net secretion of water and electrolytes compounded by incomplete absorption of nutrients and osmotic diarrhea. Symptomatic disease is caused by several distinct viruses, including the rotavirus, which most commonly affects children ages 6 to 24 months; caliciviruses, previously referred to as the Norwalk family of viruses, which are responsible for most cases of nonbacterial gastroenteritis in older children and adults; and adenoviruses, which are another common cause of diarrhea in children.[8]

Rotavirus. Worldwide, rotavirus is estimated to cause more than 125 million cases of diarrhea in children younger than 5 years of age. In the United States, the disease causes 3 million cases of diarrhea, 50,000 hospitalizations, and 20 to 40 deaths.[41] The disease tends to be most severe in children ages 3 to 24 months of age. Infants younger than 3 months of age are relatively protected by transplacental antibodies and possibly by breast-feeding. The virus is spread through a fecal–oral route, and outbreaks are common in children in day care centers. The virus is shed before and for days after clinical illness. Very few infectious virions are needed to cause disease in a susceptible host.

Rotavirus infection typically begins after an incubation period of less than 24 hours, with mild to moderate fever, and vomiting, followed by onset of frequent, watery stools. The fever and vomiting usually disappear on about the second day, but the diarrhea continues for 5 to 7 days. Dehydration may develop rapidly, particularly in infants.

Treatment is largely supportive. Avoiding and treating dehydration are the main goals. An oral vaccine for rotavirus was licensed in 1998 but was withdrawn from the market within less than a year when several infants developed intussusception after receiving the vaccine. Several new rotavirus vaccines are under development.[41]

Bacterial Infection

Bacterial infections exert their effects through the ingestion of organisms that proliferate within the gut lumen and elaborate an enterotoxin or that invade and destroy the epithelial cells of the intestine. Some forms of food poisoning result from the ingestion of preformed bacterial toxins, one of the major offenders being the toxins of *Staphylococcus aureus*.

In general, bacterial infections produce more severe effects than viral infections. The complications of bacterial enterocolitis result from massive fluid loss or destruction of intestinal mucosa and include dehydration, sepsis, and perforation. Two particularly serious forms of bacterial enterocolitis are *Clostridium difficile* and *Escherichia coli* O157:H7.

Clostridium difficile Colitis. *C. difficile* colitis is associated with antibiotic therapy.[42,43] *C. difficile* is a gram-positive, spore-forming bacillus that is part of normal flora in 1% to 3% of humans.[43] The spores are resistant to the acid environment of the stomach and convert to vegetative forms in the colon. Treatment with broad-spectrum antibiotics predisposes to disruption of the normal protective bacterial flora of the colon, leading to colonization by *C. difficile* along with the release of toxins that cause mucosal damage and inflammation. Almost any antibiotic may cause *C. difficile* colitis, but broad-spectrum antibiotics with activity against gram-negative enteric bacteria are the most frequent agents. After antibiotic therapy has made the bowel susceptible to infection, colonization by *C. difficile* occurs by the oral–fecal route. *C. difficile* infection usually is acquired in the hospital, where the organism is commonly encountered.

In general, *C. difficile* is noninvasive. Development of *C. difficile* colitis and diarrhea requires an alteration in the normal gut flora, acquisition and germination of the spores, overgrowth of *C. difficile,* and toxin production. The toxins bind to mucosa and damage the intestinal mucosa, causing hemorrhage, inflammation, and necrosis. The toxins also interfere with protein synthesis, attract inflammatory cells, increase capillary permeability, and stimulate intestinal peristalsis. The infection commonly manifests with diarrhea that is mild to moderate and sometimes is accompanied by lower abdominal cramping. Typically, symptoms begin within 1 to 2 weeks (range, 1 day to 6 weeks),[43] although they can be delayed for weeks. In most cases, systemic manifestations are absent, and the symptoms subside after the antibiotic has been discontinued.

A more severe form of colitis, *pseudomembranous colitis,* is characterized by an adherent inflammatory membrane overlying the areas of mucosal injury. It is a life-threatening form of the disease. Persons with the disease are acutely ill, with lethargy, fever, tachycardia, abdominal pain and distention, and dehydration. The smooth muscle tone of the colon may be lost, resulting in toxic dilatation of the colon. Prompt therapy is needed to prevent perforation of the bowel.

Diagnostic findings include a history of antibiotic use and laboratory tests that confirm the presence of *C. difficile* toxins in the stool. Treatment includes the immediate discontinuation of antibiotic therapy. Specific treatment aimed at eradicating *C. difficile* is used when symptoms are severe or persistent. Metronidazole is the drug of first choice, with vancomycin being reserved for persons who cannot tolerate metronidazole or do not respond to the drug. Both drugs are given orally.[42,43] Metronidazole is absorbed from the upper gastrointestinal tract and may cause side effects. Vancomycin is poorly absorbed, and its actions are limited to the gastrointestinal tract.

Escherichia coli O157:H7 Infection. *E. coli* O157:H7 has become recognized as an important cause of epidemic and sporadic colitis.[44] *E. coli* O157:H7 is a strain of *E. coli* found in feces and contaminated milk of healthy dairy and beef cattle, but it also has been found in contaminated pork, poultry, and lamb. Infection usually is by food-borne transmission, often by ingesting undercooked hamburger. The organism also can be transferred to nonmeat products such as fruits and vegetables. Person-to-person transmission may occur, particularly in nursing homes, day care settings, and hospitals. The very young and the very old are particularly at risk for the infection and its complications.

The infection may cause no symptoms or cause a variety of manifestations, including acute, nonbloody diarrhea, hemorrhagic colitis, hemolytic-uremic syndrome, and thrombotic thrombocytopenic purpura. The infection often presents with abdominal cramping and watery diarrhea and subsequently may progress to bloody diarrhea. The diarrhea commonly lasts 3 to 7 days or longer, with 10 to 12 diarrheal episodes per day. Fever occurs in up to one third of the cases.

An important aspect of the disease is the production of toxins and the ability to produce toxemia. The two complications of the infection, hemolytic-uremic syndrome and thrombotic thrombocytopenic purpura, reflect the effects of toxins. Hemolytic-uremic syndrome is characterized by hemolytic anemia, thrombocytopenia, and renal failure. It occurs predominantly in infants and young children and is the most common cause of acute renal failure in children.[44] It has a mortality rate of 5% to 10%, and one third of the survivors are left with permanent disability. Thrombotic thrombocytopenic purpura is manifested by thrombocytopenia, renal failure, fever, and neurologic manifestations. It often is regarded as the severe end of the disease that leads to hemolytic-uremic syndrome plus neurologic problems.

No specific therapy is available for *E. coli* O157:H7 infection. Treatment is largely symptomatic and directed toward treating the effects of complications. Antibiotics have not proved useful and may even be harmful, extending the duration of bloody diarrhea.

Because of the seriousness of the infection and its complications, education of the public about techniques for decreasing primary transmission of the infection from animal sources is important. Undercooked meats and unpasteurized milk are sources of transmission. The FDA recommends a minimal internal temperature of 155°F for cooked hamburger. Food handlers and consumers should be aware of the proper methods for handling uncooked meat to prevent cross-contamination of other foods. Particular attention should be paid to hygiene in day care centers and nursing homes, where the spread of infection to the very young and very old may result in severe complications.[44]

Protozoal Infection

Amebiasis refers to an infection by *Entamoeba histolytica* that involves the colon and occasionally the liver.[45,46] Humans are the only known reservoir for *E. histolytica,* which reproduce in the colon and pass in the feces. Although *E. histolytica* infection occurs worldwide, it is more common and more severe in tropical and subtropical areas, where crowding and poor sanitation prevail. Intestinal amebiasis ranges from completely asymptomatic infection to serious dysenteric disease.

E. histolytica has three distinct stages: the trophozoites (ameboid form), the precyst, and the cyst.[45] The trophozoites thrive in the colon and feed on bacteria and human cells. They may colonize any portion of the large bowel, but the area of maximum disease is usually the cecum. Persons with symptomatic disease pass both cysts and trophozoites in their feces, but the latter survive only briefly outside the body. Only the cysts are infectious because they survive gastric acidity, which destroys the trophozoites. Once established, the trophozoites invade the crypts of colonic glands and burrow down into the submucosa; the organism then fans out to create a flask-shaped ulcer with a narrow neck and broad base. In about 40% of cases, parasites penetrate the portal vein and embolize the liver to produce solitary and less often multiple discrete hepatic abscesses that may range in size from a few millimeters to 15 cm or more.[46]

The incubation period is 8 to 10 days.[45] Manifestations include abdominal discomfort, tenderness, cramps, and fever, often accompanied by nausea, vomiting, and passage of malodorous flatus. There may be frequent passage of liquid stools containing bloody mucus, but the duration of diarrhea is not usually so prolonged as to cause dehydration. The infection often persists for months or years, causing emaciation and anemia. In severe cases, massive destruction of the colonic mucosa may lead to hemorrhage, perforation, or peritonitis. Treatment includes use of the antimicrobial agent metronidazole, which acts against the trophozoites, and diloxanide furoate, which is effective against the cysts.[45]

DIVERTICULAR DISEASE

Diverticulosis is a condition in which the mucosal layer of the colon herniates through the muscularis layer.[47,48] There are often multiple diverticula, most of which occur in the sigmoid colon (Fig. 39-6). Diverticular disease is common in Western society, affecting approximately 5% to 10% of the population older than 45 years of age and almost 80% of those older than 85 years.[47] Although the disorder is prevalent in the developed countries of the world, it is almost nonexistent in many African nations and underdeveloped countries. This suggests that dietary factors (*e.g.,* lack of fiber content), a decrease in physical activity, and poor bowel habits (*e.g.,* neglecting the urge to defecate), along with the effects of aging, contribute to the development of the disease.

In the colon, the longitudinal muscle does not form a continuous layer, as it does in the small bowel. Instead, there are three separate longitudinal bands of muscle called the *teniae coli.* In a manner similar to the small intestine, bands of circular muscle constrict the large intestine. At each of these constrictive points (approximately every 2.5 cm), the circular muscle contracts, sometimes constricting the lumen of the bowel so that it is almost occluded (see Fig. 39-6). The combined contraction of the circular muscle and the lack of a continuous longitudinal muscle layer cause the intestine to bulge outward into pouches called *haustra.* Diverticula develop between the longitudinal muscle bands of the haustra, in the area where the blood vessels pierce the circular muscle layer to bring blood to the mucosal layer. An increase in intraluminal pressure in the haustra provides the force for creating these herniations. The increase in pressure is thought to be related to the volume of the colonic contents. The scantier the contents, the more vigorous are the contractions, and the greater is the pressure in the haustra.

Most persons with diverticular disease remain asymptomatic. The disease often is found when x-ray studies are done for other purposes. When symptoms do occur, they often are attributed to irritable bowel syndrome or other causes. Ill-defined lower abdominal discomfort, a change in bowel habits (*e.g.,* diarrhea, constipation), bloating, and flatulence are common.

Diverticulitis is a complication of diverticulosis in which there is inflammation and gross or microscopic perforation of the diverticulum. One of the most common complaints of diverticulitis is pain in the lower left quadrant, accompanied by nausea and vomiting, tenderness in the lower left quadrant, a slight fever, and an elevated white blood cell count. These symptoms usually last for several days, unless complications occur, and usually are caused by localized inflammation of the diverticula with perforation and development of a small, localized abscess. Complications include perforation with peritonitis, hemorrhage, and bowel obstruction. Fistulas can form, usually involving the bladder (*i.e.,* vesicosigmoid fistula), but sometimes involving the skin, perianal area, or small bowel. Pneumaturia (*i.e.,* air in the urine) is a sign of vesicosigmoid fistula.

The diagnosis of diverticular disease is based on history and presenting clinical manifestations. The disease may be confirmed by barium enema x-ray studies, CT scans, and ultrasonographic studies. CT scans are the safest and most cost-effective method.[47] Because of the risk for peritonitis, barium enema studies should be avoided in persons who are suspected of having acute diverticulitis. Flat abdominal radiographs may be used to detect complications associated with acute diverticulitis.

The usual treatment for diverticular disease is to prevent symptoms and complications. This includes increasing the bulk in the diet and bowel retraining so that the person has at least one bowel movement each day. The increased bulk promotes regular defecation and increases colonic con-

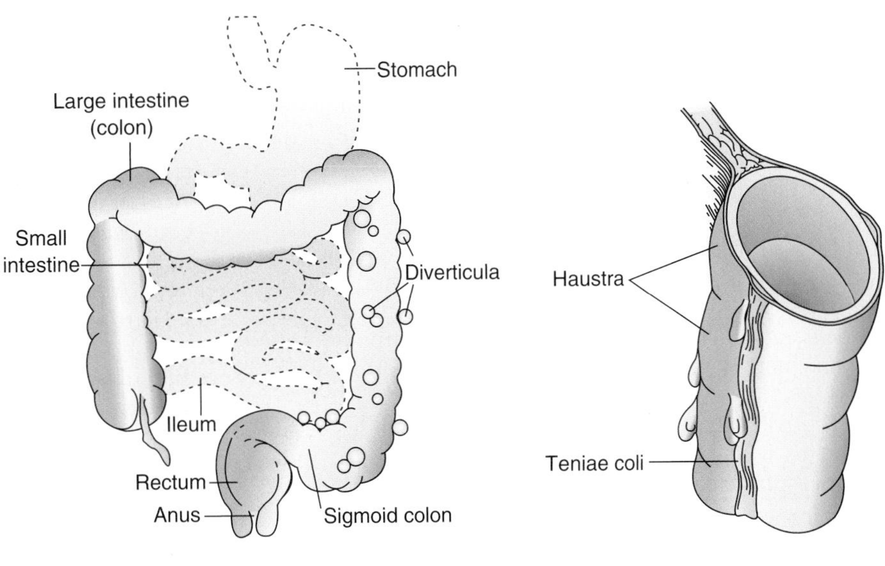

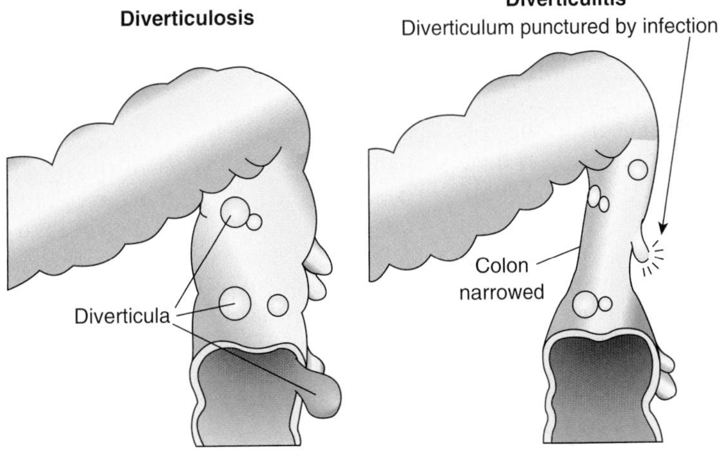

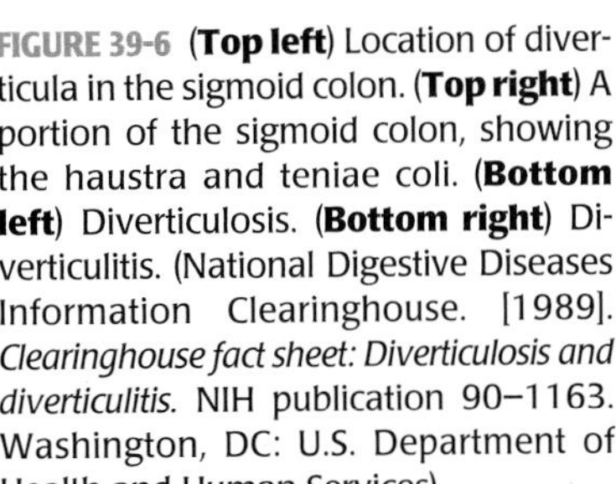

FIGURE 39-6 (**Top left**) Location of diverticula in the sigmoid colon. (**Top right**) A portion of the sigmoid colon, showing the haustra and teniae coli. (**Bottom left**) Diverticulosis. (**Bottom right**) Diverticulitis. (National Digestive Diseases Information Clearinghouse. [1989]. *Clearinghouse fact sheet: Diverticulosis and diverticulitis.* NIH publication 90–1163. Washington, DC: U.S. Department of Health and Human Services)

tents and colon diameter, thereby decreasing intraluminal pressure. Acute diverticulitis is treated by withholding solid food and administering a broad-spectrum antibiotic. Surgical treatment is reserved for complications.

APPENDICITIS

Acute appendicitis is extremely common. It is seen most frequently in the 5- to 30-year-old age group, but it can occur at any age. The appendix becomes inflamed, swollen, and gangrenous, and it eventually perforates if not treated. Although the cause of appendicitis is unknown, it is thought to be related to intraluminal obstruction with a fecalith (*i.e.*, hard piece of stool) or to twisting.

Appendicitis usually has an abrupt onset, with pain referred to the epigastric or periumbilical area. This pain is caused by stretching of the appendix during the early inflammatory process. At approximately the same time that the pain appears, there are one or two episodes of nausea. Initially, the pain is vague, but over a period of 2 to 12 hours, it gradually increases and may become colicky. When the inflammatory process has extended to involve the serosal layer of the appendix and the peritoneum, the pain becomes localized to the lower right quadrant. There usually is an elevation in temperature and a white blood cell count greater than 10,000/mm^3, with 75% or more polymorphonuclear cells. Palpation of the abdomen usually reveals a deep tenderness in the lower right quadrant, which is confined to a small area approximately the size of the fingertip. It usually is located at approximately the site of the inflamed appendix. The person with appendicitis often is able to place his or her finger directly over the tender area. Rebound tenderness, which is pain that occurs when pressure is applied to the area and then released, and spasm of the overlying abdominal muscles are common.

Diagnosis is usually based on history and findings on physical examination. Ultrasonography or CT may be used to confirm the diagnosis.[49] Treatment consists of surgical removal of the appendix. Complications include peritonitis, localized periappendiceal abscess formation, and septicemia.

ALTERATIONS IN INTESTINAL MOTILITY

The movement of contents through the gastrointestinal tract is controlled by neurons located in the submucosal and myenteric plexuses of the gut (see Chapter 38). The axons from the cell bodies in the myenteric plexus innervate the circular and longitudinal smooth muscle layers of the gut. These neurons receive impulses from local receptors located in the mucosal and muscle layers of the gut and extrinsic input from the parasympathetic and sympathetic nervous systems. As a general rule, the parasympathetic nervous system tends to increase the motility of the bowel, whereas sympathetic stimulation tends to slow its activity.

The colon has sphincters at both ends: the ileocecal sphincter, which separates it from the small intestine, and the anal sphincter, which prevents the movement of feces to the outside of the body. The colon acts as a reservoir for fecal material. Normally, approximately 400 mL of water, 55 mEq of sodium, 30 mEq of chloride, and 15 mEq of bicarbonate are absorbed each day in the colon. At the same time, approximately 5 mEq of potassium is secreted into the lumen of the colon. The amount of water and electrolytes that remains in the stool reflects the absorption or secretion that occurs in the colon. The average adult ingesting a typical American diet evacuates approximately 200 to 300 g of stool each day.

Diarrhea

The usual definition of *diarrhea* is excessively frequent passage of stools. Diarrhea can be acute or chronic. Diarrhea is considered to be chronic when the symptoms persist for 3 weeks in children or adults and 4 weeks in infants. In developing countries, diarrhea is a common cause of mortality among children less than 5 years of age, with an estimated 2 million deaths annually.[50] Although diarrheal diseases are less prevalent in the United States than in other countries, they place a burden on the health care system. Approximately 1.5 million children are seen in outpatient clinics, and 220,000 are hospitalized each year for acute gastroenteritis.[50]

The complaint of diarrhea is a general one and can be related to a number of pathologic and nonpathologic factors. Diarrhea can be acute or chronic and can be caused by infectious organisms, food intolerance, drugs, or intestinal disease. Acute diarrheas that last less than 4 days are predominantly caused by infectious agents and follow a self-limited course.[51] Chronic diarrheas are those that persist for longer than 3 to 4 weeks. They often are caused by conditions such as inflammatory bowel disease, irritable bowel syndrome, malabsorption syndrome, endocrine disorders (hyperthyroidism, diabetic autonomic neuropathy), or radiation colitis.

Diarrhea commonly is divided into two types, large volume and small volume, based on the characteristics of the diarrheal stool. Large-volume diarrhea results from an increase in the water content of the stool, and small-volume diarrhea results from an increase in the propulsive activity of the bowel. Some of the common causes of small- and large-volume diarrhea are summarized in Chart 39-1. Often, diarrhea is a combination of these two types.

Large-Volume Diarrhea. Large-volume diarrhea can be classified as secretory or osmotic, according to the cause of the increased water content in the feces. Water is pulled into the colon along an osmotic gradient (*i.e.*, osmotic di-

DISORDERS OF GASTROINTESTINAL MOTILITY

- The luminal contents move down the gastrointestinal tract as a result of peristaltic movements regulated by a complex interaction of electrical, neural, and hormonal control mechanisms.
- The enteric nervous system that is incorporated into the wall of the gut controls the basic movement of the gastrointestinal tract, with input from the autonomic nervous system.
- Local irritation and the composition and constituents of gastrointestinal contents influence motility through the submucosal afferent neurons of the enteric nervous system. Gastrointestinal wall distention, chemical irritants, osmotic gradients, and bacterial toxins exert many of their effects on gastrointestinal motility through these afferent pathways.
- Autonomic influences generated by factors such as medications, trauma, and emotional experiences interact with the enteric nervous system to alter gastrointestinal motility.

CHART 39-1

Causes of Large- and Small-Volume Diarrhea

Large-Volume Diarrhea

Osmotic diarrhea
- Saline cathartics
- Lactase deficiency

Secretory diarrhea
- Acute infectious diarrhea
- Failure to absorb bile salts
- Fat malabsorption
- Chronic laxative abuse
- Carcinoid syndrome
- Zollinger-Ellison syndrome
- Fecal impaction

Small-Volume Diarrhea

Inflammatory bowel disease
- Crohn disease
- Ulcerative colitis

Infectious disease
- Shigellosis
- Salmonellosis

Irritable colon

arrhea) or is secreted into the bowel by the mucosal cells (*i.e.,* secretory diarrhea). The large-volume form of diarrhea usually is a painless, watery type without blood or pus in the stools.

In osmotic diarrhea, water is pulled into the bowel by the hyperosmotic nature of its contents. It occurs when osmotically active particles are not absorbed. In persons with lactase deficiency, the lactose in milk cannot be broken down and absorbed. Magnesium salts, which are contained in milk of magnesia and many antacids, are poorly absorbed and cause diarrhea when taken in sufficient quantities. Another cause of osmotic diarrhea is decreased transit time, which interferes with absorption. Osmotic diarrhea usually disappears with fasting.

Secretory diarrhea occurs when the secretory processes of the bowel are increased. Most acute infectious diarrheas are of this type. Enteric organisms cause diarrhea by several ways. Some are noninvasive but secrete toxins that stimulate fluid secretion (*e.g., Vibrio cholerae,* pathogenic *E. coli,* and rotavirus).[52–54] Others (*e.g., Shigella, Salmonella, Yersinia,* and *Campylobacter*) invade and destroy intestinal epithelial cells, thereby altering fluid transport so that secretory activity continues while absorption activity is halted.[52] Diarrhea with vomiting and fever suggests food poisoning, often caused by staphylococcal enterotoxin. Secretory diarrhea also occurs when excess bile acids remain in the intestinal contents as they enter the colon. This often happens with disease processes of the ileum because bile salts are absorbed there. It also may occur with bacterial overgrowth in the small bowel, which interferes with bile absorption. Some tumors, such as those of the Zollinger-Ellison syndrome and carcinoid syndrome, produce hormones that cause increased secretory activity of the bowel.

Small-Volume Diarrhea. Small-volume diarrhea commonly is associated with acute or chronic inflammation or intrinsic disease of the colon, such as ulcerative colitis or Crohn disease. Small-volume diarrhea usually is evidenced by frequency and urgency and colicky abdominal pain. It commonly is accompanied by tenesmus (*i.e.,* painful straining at stool), fecal soiling of clothing, and awakening during the night with the urge to defecate.

Diagnosis and Treatment. The diagnosis of diarrhea is based on complaints of frequent stools and a history of accompanying factors such as concurrent illnesses, medication use, and exposure to potential intestinal pathogens. Disorders such as inflammatory bowel disease should be considered. If the onset of diarrhea is related to travel outside the United States, the possibility of traveler's diarrhea must be considered.

Although most acute forms of diarrhea are self-limited and require no treatment, diarrhea can be particularly serious in infants and small children, persons with other illnesses, the elderly, and even previously healthy persons if it continues for any length of time. Thus, the replacement of fluids and electrolytes is considered to be a primary therapeutic goal in the treatment of diarrhea. Oral replacement therapy (ORT) can be used in situations of uncomplicated diarrhea that can be treated at home. First applied to the treatment of diarrhea in developing countries, ORT can be regarded as a case of reverse technology, in which the protocols originally implemented in these countries has changed health care in industrialized countries as well.[50] Complete ORT solutions contain carbohydrate, sodium, potassium, chloride, and base to replace that lost in the diarrheal stool.[50,55,56] Commonly used beverages such as apple juice and cola drinks, which have increased osmolarity due to their high carbohydrate content and low electrolyte content, are not recommended. The effectiveness of ORT is based on the coupled transport of sodium and glucose or other actively transported small organic molecules (see Chapter 38). ORT can be particularly effective in treating dehydration associated with diarrheal diseases in infants and small children. Bottled ORT solutions are available but can be costly, particularly in cases in which large amounts of replacement fluids are needed. The cost can represent a sizable burden for socioeconomically disadvantaged families. Less expensive premeasured packets and recipes for preparing replacement solutions are available. The use of ORT for treatment of diarrhea in infants and small children is often labor intensive, requiring frequent feeding, sometimes using a spoon.[52] More important, the diarrhea does not promptly cease after ORT has been instituted; this can be discouraging for parents and caregivers who desire early results from their efforts. When oral rehydration is not feasible or adequate, intravenous fluid replacement may be needed.

Evidence suggests that feeding should be continued during diarrheal illness, particularly in children.[50,54,55] It is recommended that children who require rehydration therapy because of diarrhea be fed an age-appropriate diet. Starch and simple proteins are thought to provide cotransport molecules with little osmotic activity, increasing fluid and electrolyte uptake by intestinal cells. It has been shown that unrestricted diets do not worsen the course or symptoms of mild diarrhea and can decrease stool output.[50,56] Although there is little agreement on which foods are best, fatty foods and foods high in simple sugars are best avoided. The traditional BRAT diet of bananas, rice, applesauce, and toast usually works well.[54]

Drugs used in the treatment of diarrhea include diphenoxylate (Lomotil) and loperamide (Imodium), which are opium-like drugs. These drugs decrease gastrointestinal motility and stimulate water and electrolyte absorption. Adsorbents, such as kaolin and pectin, adsorb irritants and toxins from the bowel. These ingredients are included in many over-the-counter antidiarrheal preparations because they adsorb toxins responsible for certain types of diarrhea. Bismuth subsalicylate (Pepto-Bismol) can be used to reduce the frequency of unformed stools and increase stool consistency, particularly in cases of traveler's diarrhea. The drug is thought to inhibit intestinal secretion caused by enterotoxigenic *E. coli* and cholera toxins. Diarrheal medications should not be used in persons with bloody diarrhea, high fever, or signs of toxicity for fear of worsening the disease. Antibiotics should be reserved for use in persons with identified enteric pathogens.

Constipation

Constipation can be defined as the infrequent passage of stools. The difficulty with this definition arises from the many individual variations of function that are normal. What is considered normal for one person (*e.g.*, two or three bowel movements per week) may be considered evidence of constipation by another. The problem increases with age; there is a sharp rise in health care visits for constipation after 65 years of age.

Constipation can occur as a primary problem or as a problem associated with another disease condition. Some common causes of constipation are failure to respond to the urge to defecate, inadequate fiber in the diet, inadequate fluid intake, weakness of the abdominal muscles, inactivity and bed rest, pregnancy, and hemorrhoids. Diseases associated with chronic constipation include neurologic diseases such as spinal cord injury, Parkinson's disease, and multiple sclerosis; endocrine disorders such as hypothyroidism; and obstructive lesions in the gastrointestinal tract. Drugs such as narcotics, anticholinergic agents, calcium channel blockers, diuretics, calcium (antacids and supplements), iron supplements, and aluminum antacids tend to cause constipation. Elderly people with long-standing constipation may develop dilation of the rectum, colon, or both. This condition allows large amounts of stool to accumulate with little or no sensation. Constipation, in the context of a change in bowel habits, may be a sign of colorectal cancer.

Diagnosis of constipation usually is based on a history of infrequent stools, straining with defection, the passing of hard and lumpy stools, or the sense of incomplete evacuation with defecation.[57,58] Constipation as a sign of another disease condition should be ruled out. The treatment of constipation usually is directed toward relieving the cause. A conscious effort should be made to respond to the defecation urge. A time should be set aside after a meal, when mass movements in the colon are most likely to occur, for a bowel movement. Adequate fluid intake and bulk in the diet should be encouraged. Moderate exercise is essential, and persons on bed rest benefit from passive and active exercises. Laxatives and enemas should be used judiciously. They should not be used on a regular basis to treat simple constipation because they interfere with the defecation reflex and actually may damage the rectal mucosa.

Fecal Impaction

Fecal impaction is the retention of hardened or putty-like stool in the rectum and colon, which interferes with normal passage of feces. If not removed, it can cause partial or complete bowel obstruction. It may occur in any age group but is more common in incapacitated elderly persons. Fecal impaction may result from painful anorectal disease, tumors, or neurogenic disease; use of constipating antacids or bulk laxatives; a low-residue diet; drug-induced colonic stasis; or prolonged bed rest and debility. In children, a habitual neglect of the urge to defecate because it interferes with play may promote impaction.[59]

The manifestations may be those of severe constipation, but frequently there is a history of watery diarrhea, fecal soiling, and fecal incontinence. This is caused by increased secretory activity of the bowel, representing the body's attempt to break up the mass so that it can be evacuated. The abdomen may be distended, and there may be blood and mucus in the stool. The fecal mass may compress the urethra, giving rise to urinary incontinence. Fecal impaction should be considered in an elderly or immobilized person who develops watery stools with fecal or urinary incontinence.

Digital examination of the rectum is done to assess for the presence of a fecal mass. The mass may need to be broken up and dislodged manually or with the use of a sigmoidoscope. Oil enemas often are used to soften the mass before removal. The best treatment is prevention.

Intestinal Obstruction

Intestinal obstruction designates an impairment of movement of intestinal contents in a cephalocaudal direction. The causes can be categorized as mechanical or paralytic obstruction. Strangulation with necrosis of the bowel may occur and lead to perforation, peritonitis, and sepsis.

Mechanical obstruction can result from a number of conditions, intrinsic or extrinsic, that encroach on the patency of the bowel lumen (Fig. 39-7). Major inciting causes include external hernia (*i.e.*, inguinal, femoral, or umbilical) and postoperative adhesions. Less common causes are strictures, tumor, foreign bodies, intussusception, and volvulus.

Intussusception involves the telescoping of bowel into the adjacent segment. It is the most common cause of intestinal obstruction in children younger than 2 years of age.[60] The most common form is intussusception of the terminal ileum into the right colon, but other areas of the bowel may be involved. In most cases, the cause of the disorder is unknown. The condition can also occur in adults when an intraluminal mass or tumor acts as a traction force and pulls the segment along as it telescopes into the distal segment. Volvulus refers to a complete twisting of the bowel on an axis formed by its mesentery (Fig. 39-8). Me-

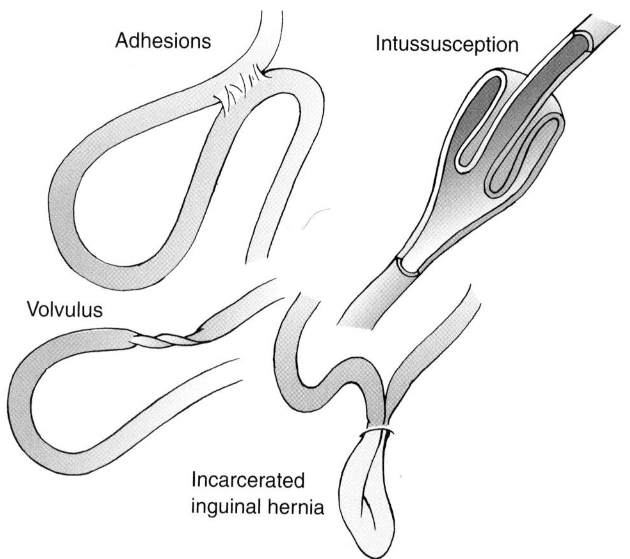

FIGURE 39-7 Causes of mechanical bowel obstruction.

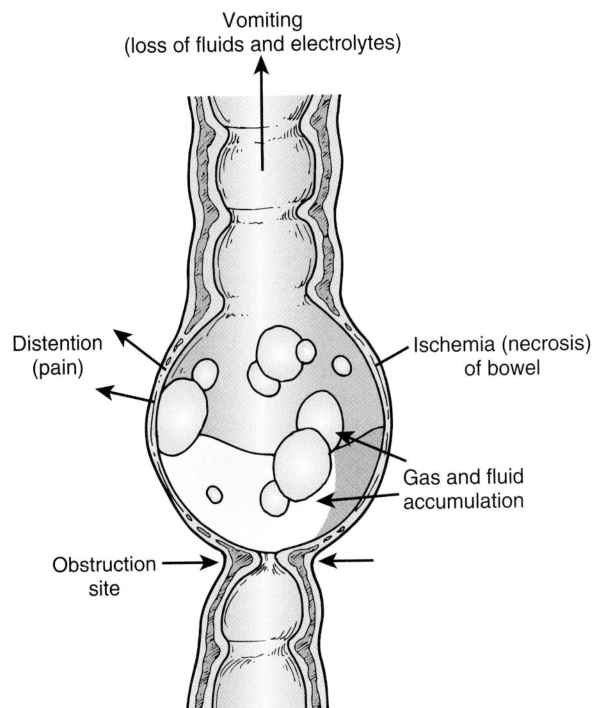

FIGURE 39-8 Pathophysiology of intestinal obstruction.

chanical bowel obstruction may be a simple obstruction, in which there is no alteration in blood flow, or a strangulated obstruction, in which there is impairment of blood flow and necrosis of bowel tissue.

Paralytic, or adynamic, obstruction results from neurogenic or muscular impairment of peristalsis. Paralytic ileus is seen most commonly after abdominal surgery. It also accompanies inflammatory conditions of the abdomen, intestinal ischemia, pelvic fractures, and back injuries. It occurs early in the course of peritonitis and can result from chemical irritation caused by bile, bacterial toxins, electrolyte imbalances as in hypokalemia, and vascular insufficiency.

The major effects of both types of intestinal obstruction are abdominal distention and loss of fluids and electrolytes (see Fig. 39-8). Gases and fluids accumulate in the area; if untreated, the distention resulting from bowel obstruction tends to perpetuate itself by causing atony of the bowel and further distention. Distention is further aggravated by the accumulation of gases. Approximately 70% of these gases are derived from swallowed air. As the process continues, the distention moves proximally (*i.e.,* toward the mouth), involving additional segments of bowel. Either form of obstruction eventually may lead to strangulation (*i.e.,* interruption of blood flow), gangrenous changes, and, ultimately, perforation of the bowel. The increased pressure in the intestine tends to compromise mucosal blood flow, leading to necrosis and movement of blood into the luminal fluids. This promotes rapid growth of bacteria in the obstructed bowel. Anaerobes grow rapidly in this favorable environment and produce a lethal endotoxin.

The manifestations of intestinal obstruction depend on the degree of obstruction and its duration. With acute obstruction, the onset usually is sudden and dramatic. With chronic conditions, the onset often is more gradual. The cardinal symptoms of intestinal obstruction are pain, absolute constipation, abdominal distention, and vomiting. With mechanical obstruction, the pain is severe and colicky, in contrast to the continuous pain and silent abdomen of paralytic ileus. There also is borborygmus (*i.e.,* rumbling sounds made by propulsion of gas in the intestine); audible, high-pitched peristalsis; and peristaltic rushes. Visible peristalsis may appear along the course of the distended intestine. Extreme restlessness and conscious awareness of intestinal movements are experienced along with weakness, perspiration, and anxiety. Should strangulation occur, the symptoms change. The character of the pain shifts from the intermittent colicky pain caused by the hyperperistaltic movements of the intestine to a severe and steady type of pain. Vomiting and fluid and electrolyte disorders occur with both types of obstruction.

Diagnosis of intestinal obstruction usually is based on history and physical findings. Plain film radiography of the abdomen may be used to detect the presence of a gas-filled bowel. CT scans and ultrasound may also be used to detect the presence of mechanical obstruction.

Treatment depends on the cause and type of obstruction. Most cases of adynamic obstruction respond to decompression of the bowel through nasogastric suction and correction of fluid and electrolyte imbalances. Strangulation and complete bowel obstruction require surgical intervention.

Peritonitis

Peritonitis is an inflammatory response of the serous membrane that lines the abdominal cavity and covers the visceral organs. It can be caused by bacterial invasion or chemical irritation. Most commonly, enteric bacteria enter the peritoneum because of a defect in the wall of one of the abdominal organs. The most common causes of peritonitis are perforated peptic ulcer, ruptured appendix, perforated diverticulum, gangrenous bowel, pelvic inflammatory disease, and gangrenous gallbladder. Other causes are abdominal trauma and wounds. Generalized peritonitis, although no longer the overwhelming problem it once was, is still a leading cause of death after abdominal surgery.

The peritoneum has several characteristics that increase its vulnerability to or protect it from the effects of peritonitis. One weakness of the peritoneal cavity is that it is a large, unbroken space that favors the dissemination of contaminants. For the same reason, it has a large surface that permits rapid absorption of bacterial toxins into the blood. The peritoneum is particularly well adapted for producing an inflammatory response as a means of controlling infection. It tends, for example, to exude a thick, sticky, and fibrinous substance that adheres to other structures, such as the mesentery and omentum, and that seals off the perforated viscus and aids in localizing the process. Localization is enhanced by sympathetic stimulation that limits intestinal motility. Although the diminished or absent peristalsis that occurs tends to give rise to associated problems, it does inhibit the movement of contaminants throughout the peritoneal cavity.

One of the most important manifestations of peritonitis is the translocation of extracellular fluid into the peritoneal cavity (through weeping or serous fluid from the inflamed peritoneum) and into the bowel as a result of bowel obstruction. Nausea and vomiting cause further losses of fluid. The fluid loss may encourage development of hypovolemia and shock. The onset of peritonitis may be acute, as with a ruptured appendix, or it may have a more gradual onset, as occurs in pelvic inflammatory disease. Pain and tenderness are common symptoms. The pain usually is more intense over the inflamed area. The person with peritonitis usually lies still because any movement aggravates the pain. Breathing often is shallow to prevent movement of the abdominal muscles. The abdomen usually is rigid and sometimes described as boardlike because of reflex muscle guarding. Vomiting is common. Fever, an elevated white blood cell count, tachycardia, and hypotension are common. Hiccups may develop because of irritation of the phrenic nerve. Paralytic ileus occurs shortly after the onset of widespread peritonitis and is accompanied by abdominal distention. Peritonitis that progresses and is untreated leads to toxemia and shock.

Treatment. Treatment measures for peritonitis are directed toward preventing the extension of the inflammatory response, correcting the fluid and electrolyte imbalances that develop, and minimizing the effects of paralytic ileus and abdominal distention. Surgical intervention may be needed to remove an acutely inflamed appendix or close the opening in a perforated peptic ulcer. Oral fluids are forbidden. Nasogastric suction, which entails the insertion of a tube placed through the nose into the stomach or intestine, is used to decompress the bowel and relieve the abdominal distention. Fluid and electrolyte replacement is essential. These fluids are prescribed on the basis of frequent blood chemistry determinations. Antibiotics are given to combat infection. Narcotics often are needed for pain relief.

ALTERATIONS IN INTESTINAL ABSORPTION

Malabsorption is the failure to transport dietary constituents, such as fats, carbohydrates, proteins, vitamins, and minerals, from the lumen of the intestine to the extracellular fluid compartment for transport to the various parts of the body. It can selectively affect a single component, such as vitamin B_{12} or lactose, or its effects can extend to all the substances absorbed in a specific segment of the intestine. When one segment of the intestine is affected, another may compensate. For example, the ileum may compensate for malabsorption in the proximal small intestine by absorbing substantial amounts of fats, carbohydrates, and amino acids. Similarly, the colon, which normally absorbs water, sodium, chloride, and bicarbonate, can compensate for small intestine malabsorption by absorbing additional end products of bacterial carbohydrate metabolism.

The conditions that impair one or more steps involved in digestion and absorption of nutrients can be divided into three broad categories: intraluminal maldigestion, disorders of transepithelial transport, and lymphatic obstruction. Intraluminal maldigestion involves a defect in processing of nutrients in the intestinal lumen. The most common causes are pancreatic insufficiency, hepatobiliary disease, and intraluminal bacterial growth. Disorders of transepithelial transport are caused by mucosal lesions that impair uptake and transport of available intraluminal nutrients across the mucosal surface of the intestine. They include disorders such as celiac disease and Crohn disease. Lymphatic obstruction interferes with the transport of the products of fat digestion to the systemic circulation after they have been absorbed by the intestinal mucosa. The process can be interrupted by congenital defects, neoplasms, trauma, and selected infectious diseases.

Malabsorption Syndrome

Persons with intestinal malabsorption usually have symptoms directly referable to the gastrointestinal tract that include diarrhea, steatorrhea, flatulence, bloating, abdominal pain, and cramps. Weakness, muscle wasting, weight loss, and abdominal distention often are present. Weight loss often occurs despite normal or excessive caloric intake. Steatorrheic stools contain excess fat. The fat content causes bulky, yellow-gray, malodorous stools that float in the toilet and are difficult to dispose of by flushing. In a person consuming a diet containing 80 to 100 g of fat each day, excretion of 7 to 9 g of fat indicates steatorrhea.

Along with loss of fat in the stools, there is failure to absorb the fat-soluble vitamins. This can lead to easy bruising and bleeding (*i.e.,* vitamin K deficiency), bone pain, a predisposition to the development of fractures and tetany (*i.e.,* vitamin D and calcium deficiency), macrocytic anemia, and glossitis (*i.e.,* folic acid deficiency). Neuropathy, atrophy of the skin, and peripheral edema may be present. Table 39-2 describes the signs and symptoms of impaired absorption of dietary constituents.

Celiac Disease

Celiac disease, also known as *celiac sprue* and *gluten-sensitive enteropathy*, is an immune-mediated disorder triggered by ingestion of gluten-containing grains (including wheat, barley, rye). Until recently, the disorder was considered to be relatively uncommon in the United States, with an estimated prevalence of 1 per 3000 population. However, increased awareness and newer and more accurate serologic tests have led to the realization that the condition is much more common, affecting 1 in every 120 to 300 persons in both Europe and North America.[61,62] The highest reported prevalence is in Western Europe and in places where Europeans migrated, mainly North America and Australia. The condition is rare among people from purely African-Caribbean, Chinese, or Japanese background.

The disease results from an inappropriate T-cell–mediated immune response against ingested α-gliadin (a component of gluten protein) in genetically predisposed

TABLE 39-2 Sites of and Requirements for Absorption of Dietary Constituents and Manifestations of Malabsorption

Dietary Constituent	Site of Absorption	Requirements	Manifestations
Water and electrolytes	Mainly small bowel	Osmotic gradient	Diarrhea Dehydration Cramps
Fat	Upper jejunum	Pancreatic lipase Bile salts Functioning lymphatic channels	Weight loss Steatorrhea Fat-soluble vitamin deficiency
Carbohydrates			
Starch	Small intestine	Amylase Maltase Isomaltase α-dextrins	Diarrhea Flatulence Abdominal discomfort
Sucrose	Small intestine	Sucrase	
Lactose	Small intestine	Lactase	
Maltose	Small intestine	Maltase	
Fructose	Small intestine		
Protein	Small intestine	Pancreatic enzymes (*e.g.*, trypsin, chymotrypsin, elastin)	Loss of muscle mass Weakness Edema
Vitamins			
A	Upper jejunum	Bile salts	Night blindness Dry eyes Corneal irritation
Folic acid	Duodenum and jejunum	Absorptive; may be impaired by some drugs (*i.e.*, anticonvulsants)	Cheilosis Glossitis Megaloblastic anemia
B_{12}	Ileum	Intrinsic factor	Glossitis Neuropathy Megaloblastic anemia
D	Upper jejunum	Bile salts	Bone pain Fractures Tetany
E	Upper jejunum	Bile salts	Uncertain
K	Upper jejunum	Bile salts	Easy bruising and bleeding
Calcium	Duodenum	Vitamin D and parathyroid hormone	Bone pain Fractures Tetany
Iron	Duodenum and jejunum	Normal pH (hydrochloric acid secretion)	Iron-deficiency anemia Glossitis

people. The genetic component is supported by the approximate 10% prevalence of the disease among first-degree relatives.[61–64] More than 95% of people with celiac disease exhibit the HLA class II allele HLA-DQ2, which preferentially presents gluten-derived gliadin peptides on its antigen-presenting grove to stimulate intestinal mucosal T cells.[61,62] Persons with the disease have increased levels of antibodies to a variety of antigens, including transglutaminase, endomysium, and gliadin. The resultant immunologic response produces an intense inflammatory reaction that results in loss of absorptive villi from the small intestine. When the resulting lesions are extensive, they may impair absorption of macronutrients (*i.e.*, proteins, carbohydrates, fats) and micronutrients (*i.e.*, vitamins and minerals). Small bowel involvement is most prominent in the proximal part of the small intestine where the exposure to gluten is greatest.

The classic form of celiac disease presents in infancy and manifests as failure to thrive, diarrhea, abdominal distention, and occasionally, severe malnutrition. Beyond infancy, the manifestations tend to be less dramatic. Older children may present with constitutional short stature and dental enamel defects. Women compromise about 75% of newly diagnosed adult celiac disease. In adults, gastrointestinal symptoms may manifest as diarrhea, constipation, or other symptoms of malabsorption such as bloating, flatus, or belching. A small percentage (<10%) of adults with gluten-sensitive enteropathy may present with dermatitis herpetiformis. This skin condition, which is characterized by lesions that are very similar to those of herpes simplex, may be misdiagnosed as atypical psoriasis or nonspecific dermatitis.

The diagnosis of celiac disease is based on clinical manifestations and confirmed by serum immunoglobulin

A (IgA) antiendomysial antibody tests and intestinal biopsy. IgA antiendomysial antibody tests have been shown to be 85% to 100% sensitive for celiac disease. Usually, additional laboratory tests are done to determine whether the disorder has resulted in nutritional disorders such as iron-deficiency anemia.

The primary treatment of celiac disease consists of removal of gluten and related proteins from the diet. Gluten is the primary protein in wheat, barley, and rye. Oats, which are nontoxic, may be contaminated with wheat. Many gluten-free breads, cereals, cookies, and other products are available. Meats, vegetables, fruits, and dairy products are free of gluten as long as they are not contaminated during processing. Complete exclusion of dietary gluten generally results in rapid and complete healing of the intestinal mucosa.

NEOPLASMS

Epithelial cell tumors of the intestines are a major cause of morbidity and mortality worldwide. The colon, including the rectum, is the site of more primary neoplasms than any other organ in the body.[8] Although the small intestine accounts for approximately 75% of the length of the gastrointestinal tract, it is an uncommon site of benign or malignant tumors.

Adenomatous Polyps

By far the most common types of neoplasms of the intestine are adenomatous polyps. A gastrointestinal polyp can be described as a mass that protrudes into the lumen of the gut.[8,22] Polyps can be subdivided according to their attachment to the bowel wall (sessile [raised mucosal nodules] or pedunculated [attached by a stalk]); their histopathologic appearance (hyperplastic or adenomatous); and their neoplastic potential (benign or malignant).[22]

Adenomatous polyps (adenomas) are benign neoplasms that arise from the mucosal epithelium of the intestine. They are composed of neoplastic cells that have proliferated in excess of those needed to replace the cells that normally are shed from the mucosal surface (Fig. 39-9). The pathogenesis of adenoma formation involves neoplastic alteration in the replication of the crypt epithelial cells. There may be diminished apoptosis (see Chapter 5), persistence of cell replication, and failure of cell maturation and differentiation of the cells that migrate to the surface of the crypts.[22] Normally, DNA synthesis ceases as the cells reach the upper two thirds of the crypts, after which they mature, migrate to the surface, and become senescent. They then become apoptotic and are shed from the surface.[22] Adenomas arise from a disruption in this sequence, such that the epithelial cells retain their proliferative ability throughout the entire length of the crypt. Alterations in cell differentiation can lead to dysplasia and progression to the development of invasive carcinoma.

More than half of all adenomatous polyps are located in the rectosigmoid colon and can be detected by rectal examination or sigmoidoscopy.[22] The remainder are evenly distributed throughout the rest of the colon. Adenomas can range in size from a barely visible nodule to a large, sessile mass. They can be classified as tubular, villous, or tubulovillous adenomas.

Tubular adenomas, which constitute approximately 65% of benign large bowel adenomas, typically are smooth-surfaced spheres, usually less than 2 cm in diameter, that are attached to the mucosal surface by a stalk.[22] Although most tubular adenomas display little epithelial dysplasia,

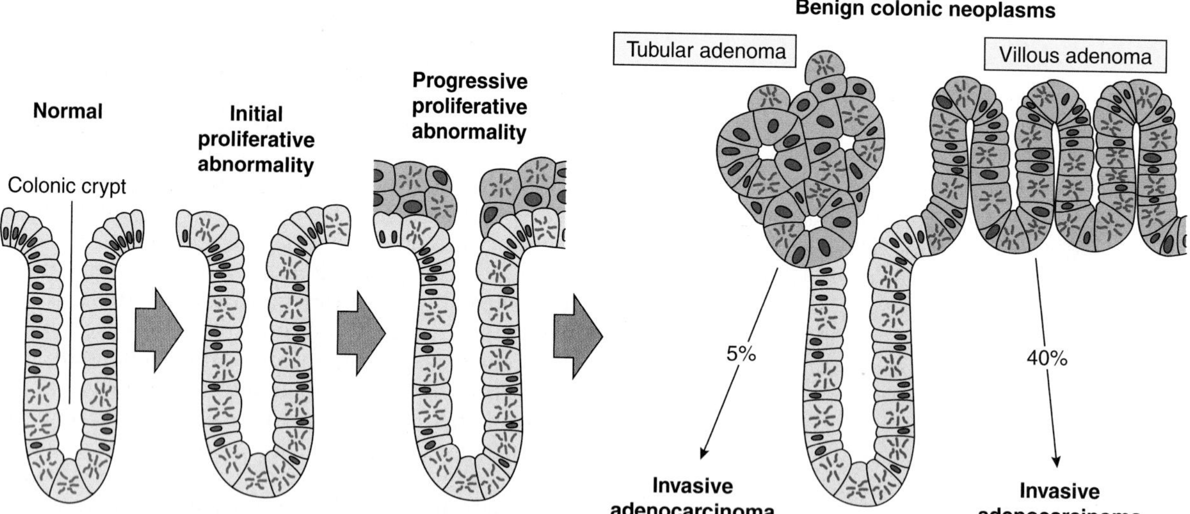

FIGURE 39-9 The histogenesis of adenomatous polyps of the colon. The initial proliferative abnormality of the colonic mucosa, the extension of the mitotic zone in the crypts, leads to accumulation of mucosal cells. The formation of adenomas may reflect epithelial–mesenchymal interactions. (From Rubin E., Farber J.L. [1999]. *Pathology* [3rd ed., p. 739]. Philadelphia: Lippincott-Raven) (Artist: Dmitri Karetnikov)

approximately 20% show a range of dysplastic changes, from mild nuclear changes to frank invasive carcinoma. *Villous adenomas* constitute 10% of adenomas of the colon.[22] They are found predominantly in the rectosigmoid colon. They typically are broad-based, elevated lesions, with a shaggy, cauliflower-like surface. In contrast to tubular adenomas, villous adenomas are more likely to contain malignant cells. When invasive carcinoma develops, there is no stalk to isolate the tumor, and invasion is directly into the wall of the colon. *Tubulovillous adenomas* manifest both tubular and villous architecture. They are intermediate between tubular and villous adenomas in terms of invasive carcinoma risk.

Most cases of colorectal cancer begin as benign adenomatous colonic polyps (Fig. 39-10). The frequency of polyps increases with age, and the prevalence of adenomatous polyps, which is approximately 20% to 30% before 40 years of age, rises to 40% to 50% after age 60 years.[22] Men and women are equally affected. The peak incidence of adenomatous polyps precedes by some years the peak for colorectal cancer. Programs that provide careful follow-up for persons with adenomatous polyps and removal of all suspect lesions have substantially reduced the incidence of colorectal cancer.[22]

Colorectal Cancer

Colorectal cancer is the third most common cancer in men and women and the second leading cause of cancer death in the United States. The annual incidence of colorectal cancer in the United States is approximately 148,300 (affecting 72,600 males and 75,700 females), with 56,600 deaths (in 27,800 males and 28,800 females).[65] The death rate for colorectal cancer has been steadily declining since the early 1980s. This may be due to decreased number of cases because more of the cases are found earlier and because treatments have improved.

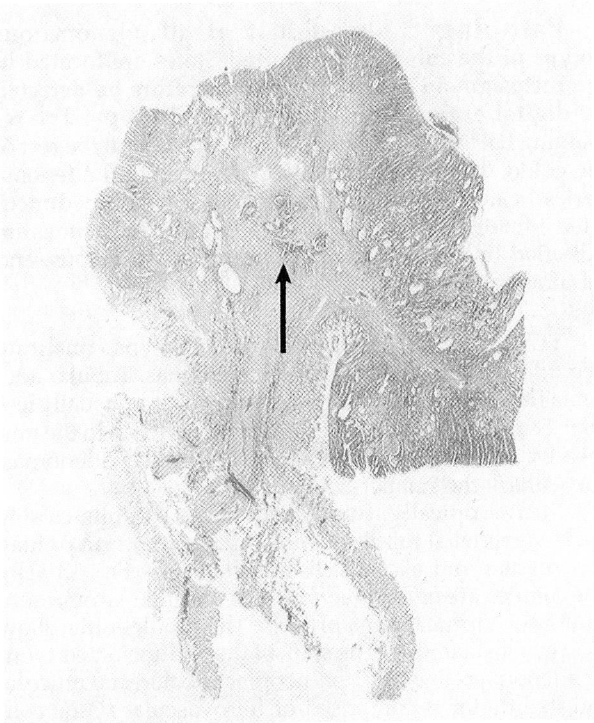

FIGURE 39-10 Adenocarcinoma arising from a pedunculated adenomatous polyp. A low-grade micrograph shows irregular neoplastic glands *(arrow)* invading the stalk. (From Rubin E., Farber J.L. [1999]. *Pathology* [3rd ed., p. 738]. Philadelphia: Lippincott-Raven)

The cause of cancer of the colon and rectum is largely unknown. Its incidence increases with age, as evidenced by the fact that approximately 90% of persons who develop this form of cancer are older than 50 years of age.[65] Its incidence is increased among persons with a family history of cancer, persons with Crohn disease or ulcerative colitis, and those with familial adenomatous polyposis of the colon. Persons with a familial risk—those who have two or more first- or second-degree relatives (or both) with colorectal cancer—make up approximately 20% of all persons with colorectal cancer.[66] Familial adenomatous polyposis is a rare autosomal dominant trait linked to a mutation in the long arm of chromosome 5. Persons with the disorder develop multiple adenomatous polyps of the colon at an early age.[8,66] Carcinoma of the colon is inevitable, often by 40 years of age, unless a total colectomy is performed.

Diet also is thought to play a role.[65] Attention has focused on dietary fat intake, refined sugar intake, fiber intake, and the adequacy of such protective micronutrients as vitamins A, C, and E in the diet. It has been hypothesized that a high level of fat in the diet increases the synthesis of bile acids in the liver, which may be converted to potential carcinogens by the bacterial flora in the colon. Bacterial organisms in particular are suspected of converting bile acids to carcinogens; their proliferation is enhanced by a high dietary level of refined sugars. Dietary fiber is thought to increase stool bulk and thereby dilute and remove potential carcinogens. Refined diets often contain reduced amounts of vitamins A, C, and E, which may act as oxygen free radical scavengers.

Reports indicate that aspirin may protect against colorectal cancer.[67] An analysis of the incidence of colorectal cancer in the Nurses Health Study showed a decreased incidence of colorectal cancer among women who took four to six aspirin per week.[68] Although the mechanism of aspirin's action is unknown, it may be related to its effect on the synthesis of prostaglandins, one or more of which may be involved in signal systems that influence cell proliferation or tumor growth. Aspirin and other NSAIDs inhibit COX-1 and COX-2, both of which are involved in prostaglandin synthesis. Analysis of COX-2 expression shows that it is elevated in up to 90% of sporadic colon cancers and 40% of colonic adenomas, but is not elevated in normal colonic epithelium.[69] There has been recent interest in what has been termed *chemoprevention* or the use of oral agents such as aspirin or other NSAIDs, particularly the COX-2 selective NSAIDs, in the prevention of colorectal cancer. Supplemental folate and calcium, selected vitamins, and postmenopausal hormone replacement therapy (estrogen) also have been proposed as potential chemoprotective agents.[69] All of these agents will require more extensive study before they can be recommended for long-term chemoprevention of colorectal cancer.

Usually, cancer of the colon and rectum is present for a long time before it produces symptoms. Bleeding is a highly significant early symptom, and it usually is the one that causes persons to seek medical care. Other symptoms include a change in bowel habits, diarrhea or constipation, and sometimes a sense of urgency or incomplete emptying of the bowel. Pain usually is a late symptom.

The prognosis for persons with colorectal cancer depends largely on the extent of bowel involvement and on the presence of metastasis at the time of diagnosis. Colorectal cancer commonly is divided into four categories according to the Dukes classification or its variant.[12] A stage I tumor is limited to invasion of the mucosal and submucosal layers of the colon and has a 5-year survival rate of 80% to 100%.[12] A stage II tumor invades the entire wall of the colon, but without lymph node involvement, and has a 5-year survival rate of 50% to 70%.[12] With a stage III tumor, in which there is invasion of the serosal layer and regional lymph node involvement, the 5-year survival rate is 30% to 50%.[12] Stage IV colorectal cancer involves far-advanced metastasis and has a much poorer prognosis.

Screening, Diagnosis, and Treatment. The single most important prognostic indicator of colorectal cancer is the extent (stage) of the tumor at time of diagnosis. Therefore, the challenge is to discover the tumors at their earliest stages. Among the methods used for the detection of colorectal cancers are stool occult blood tests and digital rectal examination, usually done during routine physical examinations; x-ray studies using barium (*e.g.,* barium enema); and flexible sigmoidoscopy and colonoscopy.[65,70] Digital rectal examinations are most helpful in detecting neoplasms of the rectum. Rectal examination should be considered a routine part of a good physical examination. The American Cancer Society recommends that all asymptomatic men and women older than 40 years of age should have a digital rectal examination performed annually as a part of their physical examination, and that those older than 50 years should have an annual stool test for occult blood and a flexible sigmoidoscopy examination done every 5 years, as recommended by their physician.[65] People with increased risk for colorectal cancer should be screened earlier and more often. Colonoscopy is recommended whenever a screening test is positive.

Almost all cancers of the colon and rectum bleed intermittently, although the amount of blood is small and usually not apparent in the stools. It therefore is feasible to screen for colorectal cancers using commercially prepared tests for occult blood in the stool. This method uses a guaiac-impregnated filter paper. The technique involves preparing two slides per day from different portions of the same stool for 3 to 4 days while the patient follows a high-fiber diet that is free of meat and ascorbic acid. Although the diet is not particularly appealing, this stool test has been shown to be a relatively reliable and inexpensive method of screening for colorectal cancer. Persons with a positive stool occult blood test should be referred to their physicians for further study. Usually, a physical examination, rectal examination, barium enema, and sigmoidoscopy or colonoscopy are done.

Flexible sigmoidoscopy involves examination of the rectum and sigmoid colon with a hollow, lighted tube that is inserted through the rectum. The procedure is performed without sedation and is well tolerated. Approximately 40% of cancers and polyps are out of the reach of the sigmoidoscope, emphasizing the need for fecal occult blood tests. Polyps can be removed, or tissue can be obtained for biopsy during the procedure.

Colonoscopy provides a means for direct visualization of the rectum and colon. The colonoscope consists of a flexible, 4 cm in diameter glass fiber bundle that contains approximately 250,000 glass fibers and has a lens at either end to focus and magnify the image. Light from an external source is transmitted by the fiberoptic viewing bundle. Instruments are available that afford direct examination of the sigmoid colon or the entire colon. This method is used for screening persons at high risk for developing cancer of the colon (*e.g.,* those with ulcerative colitis) and for those with symptoms. Colonoscopy also is useful for obtaining a biopsy and for removing polyps. Although this method is one of the most accurate for detecting early colorectal cancers, it is not suitable for mass screening because it is expensive and time consuming and must be done by a person who is highly trained in the use of the instrument.

The only recognized treatment for cancer of the colon and rectum is surgical removal.[70] Preoperative radiation therapy may be used and has in some cases demonstrated increased 5-year survival rates. Postoperative adjuvant chemotherapy with 5-fluorouracil (5-FU), 5-FU plus levamisole (an antihelmintic agent that appears to modulate the cellular immune response); or 5-FU with leucovorin (a folic acid derivative) may be used. Radiation therapy and chemotherapy are used as palliative treatment methods.

In summary, disorders of the small and large intestines include irritable bowel syndrome, inflammatory bowel disease, diverticular disease, disorders of motility (*i.e.,* diarrhea, constipation, fecal impaction, and intestinal obstruction), alterations in intestinal absorption, and colorectal cancer.

Irritable bowel syndrome is a functional disorder characterized by a variable combination of chronic and recurrent intestinal symptoms not explained by structural or biochemical abnormalities. The term *inflammatory bowel disease* is used to designate two inflammatory conditions: Crohn disease, which affects the small and large bowel, and ulcerative colitis, which affects the colon and rectum. Both are chronic diseases characterized by remissions and exacerbations of diarrhea, weight loss, fluid and electrolyte disorders, and systemic signs of inflammation.

Infectious forms of enterocolitis include viral (*e.g.,* rotavirus), bacterial (*e.g., C. difficile* and *E. coli* O157:H7), and protozoal (*E. histolytica*) infections. Diverticular disease includes diverticulosis, which is a condition in which the mucosal layer of the colon herniates through the muscularis layer, and diverticulitis, in which there is inflammation and gross or microscopic perforation of the diverticulum.

Diarrhea and constipation represent disorders of intestinal motility. Diarrhea, characterized by excessively frequent passage of stools, can be divided into large-volume diarrhea, characterized by an increased water content in the feces, and small-volume diarrhea, associated with intrinsic bowel disease and frequent passage of small stools. Constipation can be defined as the infrequent passage of stools; it commonly is caused by failure to respond to the urge to defecate, inadequate fiber or fluid intake, weakness of the abdominal muscles, inactivity and bed rest, pregnancy, hemorrhoids, and gastrointestinal disease. Fecal impaction is the retention of hardened or putty-like stool in the rectum and colon, which interferes with normal passage of feces. Intestinal obstruction designates an impairment of movement of intestinal contents in a cephalocaudal direction as the result of mechanical or paralytic mechanisms. Peritonitis is an inflammatory response of the serous membrane that lines the abdominal cavity and covers the visceral organs. It can be caused by bacterial invasion or chemical irritation resulting from perforation of the viscera or abdominal organs.

Malabsorption results from the impaired absorption of nutrients and other dietary constituents from the intestine. It can involve a single dietary constituent, such as vitamin B_{12}, or extend to involve all of the substances absorbed in a particular part of the small intestine. Malabsorption can result from disease of the small bowel and disorders that impair digestion and in some cases obstruct the lymph flow by which fats are transported to the general circulation.

Colorectal cancer, the second most common fatal cancer, is seen most commonly in persons older than 50 years of age. Most, if not all, cancers of the colon and rectum arise in preexisting adenomatous polyps. Programs that provide careful follow-up for persons with adenomatous polyps and removal of all suspect lesions have substantially reduced the incidence of colorectal cancer.

REVIEW EXERCISES

A 40-year-old man reports to his health care provider complaining of "heartburn" that occurs after eating and also wakes him up at night. He is overweight and admits to enjoying fatty foods and lying down on the sofa and watching TV in the evening. He also complains that lately he has been having a cough and some wheezing. A diagnosis of gastroesophageal reflux disease (GERD) was made.

A. Explain the cause of "heartburn" and why it becomes worse after eating.

B. Persons with GERD are advised to lose weight, avoid eating fatty foods, remain sitting after eating, and sleep with the head slightly elevated. Explain the possible relationship between these situations and the occurrence of reflux.

C. Explain the possible relationship between GERD and the respiratory symptoms this man is having.

A 36-year-old woman, who has been taking aspirin for back pain, experiences a sudden episode of tachycardia and feeling faint, accompanied by the vomiting of a coffee-ground emesis and the passing of a tarry stool. She relates that she hasn't had any signs of a "stomach ulcer" such as pain or heartburn.

A. Relate the mucosal protective effects of prostaglandins to the development of peptic ulcer associated with aspirin or NSAID use.

B. Explain the apparent suddenness of the bleeding and the fact that the woman did not experience pain as a warning signal.

C. Among the results of her initial laboratory tests is an elevated BUN level. Explain the reason for the elevated BUN.

A 29-year-old woman has been diagnosed with Crohn disease. Her medical history reveals that the woman began having symptoms of the disease at 24 years of age and that her mother died of complications of the disease at 54 years of age. She complains of diarrhea and chronic cramping abdominal pain.

A. Define the term *inflammatory bowel disease* and compare the pathophysiology and manifestations of Crohn disease and ulcerative colitis.

B. Describe the possible association between genetic and environmental factors in the pathogenesis of Crohn disease.

C. Relate the use of the monoclonal antibody infliximab to the pathogenesis of the inflammatory lesions that occur in Crohn disease.

References

1. National Digestive Diseases Information Clearing House (NDDIC). *Digestive disease statistics.* [On-line]. Available: http://www.digestive.niddk.nih.gov/statistics/statistics.htm (accessed 1/14/2004).
2. Lindley C. (2001). Nausea and vomiting. In Young L.Y., Koda-Kimble M.A. (Eds.), *Applied therapeutics: The clinical use of drugs* (7th ed., pp. 6-1–6-17). Philadelphia: Lippincott Williams & Wilkins.
3. Grélot L., Miller A.D. (1994). Vomiting: Its ins and outs. *NIPS 9,* 142–147.
4. Rockey D.C. (1999). Occult gastrointestinal bleeding. *New England Journal of Medicine 341,* 38–46.
5. Guyton A.C., Hall J.E. (2000). *Textbook of medical physiology* (10th ed., pp. 728–737). Philadelphia: W.B. Saunders.
6. Mittal R.K. (1998). The spectrum of diaphragmatic hernia. *Hospital Practice* November 15, 65–79.
7. Spieker M.R. (2000). Evaluating dysphagia. *American Family Physician 61,* 3639–3648.
8. Crawford J.M., Kumar V. (2003). The oral cavity and the gastrointestinal tract. In Kumar V., Cotran R.S., Robbins S.L. (Eds.), *Robbins basic pathology* (6th ed., pp. 549–554, 555–563, 572–577). Philadelphia: W.B. Saunders.
9. Mittal R.K., Balaban D.H. (1997). The esophagogastric junction. *New England Journal of Medicine 336,* 924–931.

10. Orlando R.C. (2002). Pathogenesis of gastroesophageal reflux disease. *Gastroenterology Clinics of North America 31,* S35–S44.
11. Katzka D.A., Rustgi A.K. (2000). Gastroesophageal reflux disease and Barrett's esophagus. *Medical Clinics of North America 84,* 1137–1161.
12. McQuaid K.R. (2003). Alimentary tract. In Tierney L.M., McPhee S.J., Papadakis M. (Eds.), *Current medical diagnosis and treatment* (42nd ed., pp. 551–566, 567–582, 617–623). New York: Lange Medical Books/McGraw-Hill.
13. Alexander J.A., Hunt L.W., Patel A.M. (1999). Prevalence, pathophysiology, and treatment of patients with asthma and gastroesophageal reflux disease. *Mayo Clinic Proceedings 75,* 1055–1063.
14. Patterson P.E., Harding S.M. (1999). Gastroesophageal reflux disorders and asthma. *Current Opinion in Pulmonary Medicine 5,* 63–67.
15. Spechler S.J. (2002). Barrett's esophagus. *New England Journal of Medicine 346*(11), 836–842.
16. Scott M., Gelhot A.R. (1999). Gastroesophageal reflux disease: Diagnosis and management. *American Family Physician 59,* 1161–1169, 1199.
17. Mason D.B. (2000). Gastroesophageal reflux in children. *Nursing Clinics of North America 35,* 15–36.
18. Orenstein S., Peters J., Khan S., et al. (2004). The esophagus. In Behrman R.E., Kliegman R.M., Jenson H.B. (Eds.), *Nelson textbook of pediatrics* (17th ed., pp. 1222–1224). Philadelphia: W.B. Saunders.
19. Enzinger P.C., Mayer R.J. (2003). Esophageal cancer. *New England Journal of Medicine 349*(23), 2241–2252.
20. Fromm D. (1987). Mechanisms involved in gastric mucosal resistance to injury. *Annual Review of Medicine 38,* 119.
21. Wolfe M.M., Lichtenstein D.R., Singh G. (1999). Gastrointestinal toxicity of nonsteroidal antiinflammatory drugs. *New England Journal of Medicine 340,* 1888–1899.
22. Hamilton S.R., Farber J.L., Rubin E. (1999). The gastrointestinal tract. In Rubin E., Farber J.L. (Eds.), *Pathology* (3rd ed., pp. 688–695, 727–746). Philadelphia: Lippincott-Raven.
23. Suerbaum S., Michetti P. (2002). Helicobacter pylori infections. *New England Journal of Medicine 347*(15), 1175–1186.
24. Shiotani A., Nurgalieva Z.Z., Yamaoka Y., Graham D.Y. (2000). *Helicobacter pylori. Medical Clinics of North America 84,* 1125–1136.
25. Fass R. (1995). Zollinger-Ellison syndrome: Diagnosis and management. *Hospital Practice* November 15, 73–80.
26. Scarapelli D.G. (1999). The pancreas. In Rubin E., Farber J.L. (Eds.), *Pathology* (3rd ed., pp. 855–856). Philadelphia: Lippincott-Raven.
27. Zuckerman G.R., Cort D., Schuman R.B. (1988). Stress ulcer syndrome. *Journal of Intensive Care Medicine 3,* 21.
28. Konopad E., Noseworthy T. (1988). Stress ulceration: A serious complication in critically ill patients. *Heart and Lung 17,* 339.
29. American Cancer Society. (2004). *Overview: Stomach cancer.* [On-line.] Available: http://www.cancer.org.
30. Viera A.J., Hoag S., Shaughnessy J. (2002). Management of irritable bowel syndrome. *American Family Physician 66*(10), 1867–1874.
31. Hassler W.L. (2002). The irritable bowel syndrome. *Medical Clinics of North America 86,* 1524–1551.
32. Olden K.W. (2003). Irritable bowel syndrome: An overview of diagnosis and pharmacologic treatment. *Cleveland Clinic Journal of Medicine 70*(Suppl. 2), S3–S17.
33. Thompson W.G., Longstreth G.E., Drossman D.A., et al. (Committee on Functional Bowel Disorders and Functional Abdominal Pain, Multinational Working Teams to Develop Diagnostic Criteria for Functional Gastrointestinal Disorders (ROME II), University of Ottawa, Canada). (1999). Functional bowel disorders and functional abdominal pain. *Gut 45* (Suppl. 2), 1143–1147.
34. Stotland B.R., Stein R.B., Lichtenstein G.R. (2000). Advances in inflammatory bowel disease. *Medical Clinics of North America 84,* 1107–1123.
35. Bridget S., Lee J.C., Bjarnason I., et al. (2002). In siblings with similar genetic susceptibility for inflammatory bowel disease, smokers tend to develop Crohn's disease and nonsmokers develop ulcerative colitis. *Gut 51*(1), 21–25.
36. Podolsky D.K. (2002). Inflammatory bowel disease. *New England Journal of Medicine 347*(6), 417–429.
37. Chinyu S., Lichtenstein G.R. (2002). Recent developments in inflammatory bowel disease. *Medical Clinics of North America 86,* 1497–1523.
38. Hanauer S.B., Present D.H. (2003). The state of the art in the management of inflammatory bowel disease. *Reviews in Gastrointestinal Disorders 3*(2), 81–92.
39. Knutson D., Greenberg G., Cronau H. (2003). Management of Crohn's disease: A practical approach. *American Family Physician 68*(4), 707–714.
40. Lewis C. (1999). Crohn's disease: New drug may help when others fail. FDA Consumer Magazine. [On-Line]. Available: http://www.fda.gov/fdac/features/1999_crohn.html.
41. Bass D.M. (2004). Rotavirus and other agents of viral gastroenteritis. In Behrman R.E., Kliegman R.M., Jenson H.B. (Eds.), *Nelson textbook of pediatrics* (17th ed., pp. 1081–1083). Philadelphia: W.B. Saunders.
42. Mylonakis E., Ryan E.T., Claderswood S.B. (2001). *Clostridium difficile*–associated diarrhea: A review. *Archives of Internal Medicine 161,* 525–533.
43. Yassen S.F., Young-Fadok T.M., Zein N.N., Pardi D.S. (2001). *Clostridium difficile*–associated diarrhea and colitis. *Mayo Clinic Proceedings 76,* 725–730.
44. Greenwald D.A., Brandt L.J. (1997). Recognizing *E. coli* O157:H7 infection. *Hospital Practice 32,* 123–140.
45. Goldsmith R.S. (2003). Infectious diseases: Protozoal and helminthic. In Tierney L.M., McPhee S.J., Papadakis M. (Eds.), *Current medical diagnosis and treatment* (42nd ed., pp. 1415–1420). New York: Lange Medical Books/McGraw-Hill.
46. Genta R.M., Connor D.H. (1999). Infectious and parasitic diseases. In Rubin E., Farber J.L. (Eds.), *Pathology* (3rd ed., pp. 452–455). Philadelphia: Lippincott-Raven.
47. Ferzoco L.B., Raptopoulos V., Silen W. (1998). Acute diverticulitis. *New England Journal of Medicine 338,* 1521–1526.
48. Van Ness M., Peller C. (1991). Acute diverticular disease: Diagnosis and management. *Hospital Practice 26*(3A), 83–91.
49. Paulson E.K., Kalady M.F., Pappas T.N. (2003). Suspected appendicitis. *New England Journal of Medicine 348*(3), 236–242.
50. King C.K., Glass R., Brewer J.S., Duggan C. (2003). Managing acute gastroenteritis among children: Oral rehydration, maintenance, and nutritional therapy. *MMWR Morbidity and Mortality Weekly Report 52*(RR-16), 1–16.
51. Schiller L.R. (2000). Diarrhea. *Medical Clinics of North America 84,* 1259–1275.
52. Field M., Rao M.C., Chang E.B. (1989). Intestinal electrolyte transport and diarrheal disease (part 2). *New England Journal of Medicine 321,* 879–883.
53. Field M. (2003). Intestinal ion transport and the pathophysiology of diarrhea. *Journal of Clinical Investigation 111,* 931–943.
54. Ghishan F.K. (2004). Chronic diarrhea. In Berman R.E., Kliegman R.M., Jenson H.B. (Eds.), *Nelson textbook of pediatrics* (17th ed., pp. 1276–1281). Philadelphia: W.B. Saunders.
55. Limbos M.A., Lieberman J.M. (1995). Management of acute diarrhea in children. *Contemporary Pediatrics 12*(12), 68–88.
56. American Academy of Pediatrics, Subcommittee on Acute Gastroenteritis. (1996). Practice parameter: The manage-

ment of acute gastroenteritis in young children. *Pediatrics 97*, 424–435.

57. Wald A. (2000). Constipation. *Medical Clinics of North America 84*, 1231–1246.
58. Lembo A., Camilleri M. (2003). Chronic constipation. *New England Journal of Medicine 349*(14), 1360–1368.
59. Wrenn K. (1989). Fecal impaction. *New England Journal of Medicine 321*, 658–662.
60. Wyllie R. (2000). Ileus, adhesions, intussusception, and closed-loop obstruction. In Bierman R.E., Kliegman R.M., Jenson H.B. (Eds.), *Nelson textbook of pediatrics* (17th ed., pp. 1241–1243). Philadelphia: W.B. Saunders.
61. Farrell R.J., Kelly C. (2002). Celiac sprue. *New England Journal of Medicine 346*(3), 180–188.
62. Nelson D.A. (2002). Gluten-sensitive enteropathy (celiac disease): More common than you think. *American Family Physician 66*(12), 2259–2266.
63. Fasano A. (2003). Celiac disease—How to handle a clinical chameleon. *New England Journal of Medicine 348*(25), 2568–2569.
64. Garcia-Carega M., Kerner J.A. (2004). Malabsorption disorders. In Bierman R.E., Kliegman R.M., Jenson H.B. (Eds.), *Nelson textbook of pediatrics* (16th ed., pp. 1264–1266). Philadelphia: W.B. Saunders.
65. American Cancer Society. (2004). Colorectal cancer. [On-line]. Available: http://www.cancer.org.
66. Guttmacher A.E., de la Chapelle A. (2003). Hereditary colorectal cancer. *New England Journal of Medicine 348*(10), 919–932.
67. Giovannucci E., Egan K.M., Hunter D.J., et al. (1995). Aspirin and the risk of colorectal cancer in women. *New England Journal of Medicine 333*, 609–614.
68. Marcus A.J. (1995). Aspirin as prophylaxis against colorectal cancer. *New England Journal of Medicine 333*, 656–657.
69. Pasi J.A., Mayer R.J. (2000). Chemoprevention of colorectal cancer. *New England Journal of Medicine 342*, 1960–1966.
70. Engstrom P.F. (2001). Colorectal cancer. In Lenhard R.E., Osteen R.T., Gansler T. (Eds.), *American Cancer Society's clinical oncology* (pp. 362–372). Atlanta: American Cancer Society.

CHAPTER

40

Disorders of Hepatobiliary and Exocrine Pancreas Function

The liver, the gallbladder, and exocrine pancreas are classified as accessory organs of the gastrointestinal tract. In addition to producing digestive secretions, the liver and the pancreas have other important functions. The endocrine pancreas, for example, supplies the insulin and glucagon needed in cell metabolism, whereas the liver synthesizes glucose, plasma proteins, and blood clotting factors and is responsible for the degradation and elimination of drugs and hormones, among other functions. This chapter focuses on functions and disorders of the liver, the biliary tract and gallbladder, and the exocrine pancreas.

The Liver and Hepatobiliary System

After completing this section of the chapter, you should be able to meet the following objectives:

- Describe the lobular structures of the liver
- Trace the movement of blood flow into, through, and out of the liver
- Describe the function of the liver in terms of carbohydrate, protein, and fat metabolism
- State the origin of ammonia and describe the function of the liver in terms of its detoxification
- Characterize the function of the liver in terms of bilirubin elimination and describe the difference between unconjugated and conjugated hyperbilirubinemia
- Relate the mechanism of bile formation and elimination to the development of cholestasis
- List four laboratory tests used to assess liver function and relate them to impaired liver function

The liver is the largest visceral organ in the body, weighing approximately 1.3 kg (3 lb) in the adult. It is located below the diaphragm and occupies much of the right hypochondrium (Fig. 40-1). The liver is surrounded by a tough fibroelastic capsule called *Glisson's capsule*. The falciform ligament, which extends from the peritoneal surface of the anterior abdominal wall between the umbilicus and diaphragm, divides the liver into two lobes, a large right lobe and a small left lobe. There are two additional lobes on the visceral surface of the liver: the caudate

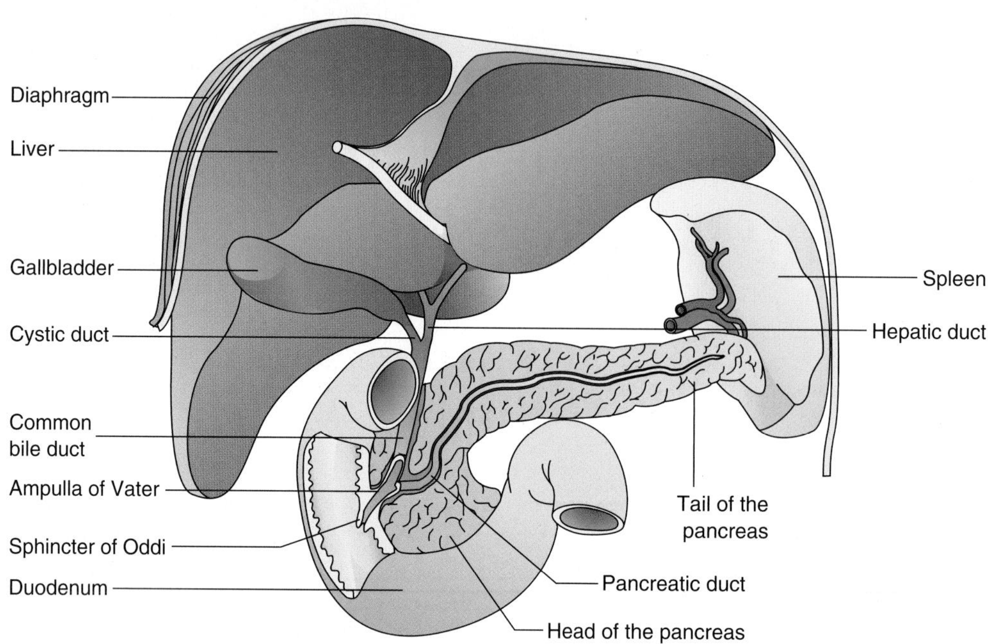

FIGURE 40-1 The liver and biliary system, including the gallbladder and bile ducts.

and quadrate lobes. Except for the portion that is in the epigastric area, the liver is contained within the rib cage and in healthy persons cannot normally be palpated.

The liver is unique among the abdominal organs in having a dual blood supply—the hepatic artery and the portal vein. Approximately 300 mL of blood per minute enters the liver through the hepatic artery; another 1050 mL/minute enters by way of the valveless portal vein, which carries blood from the stomach, the small and the large intestines, the pancreas, and the spleen[1] (Fig. 40-2). Although the blood from the portal vein is incompletely saturated with oxygen, it supplies approximately 60% to 70% of the

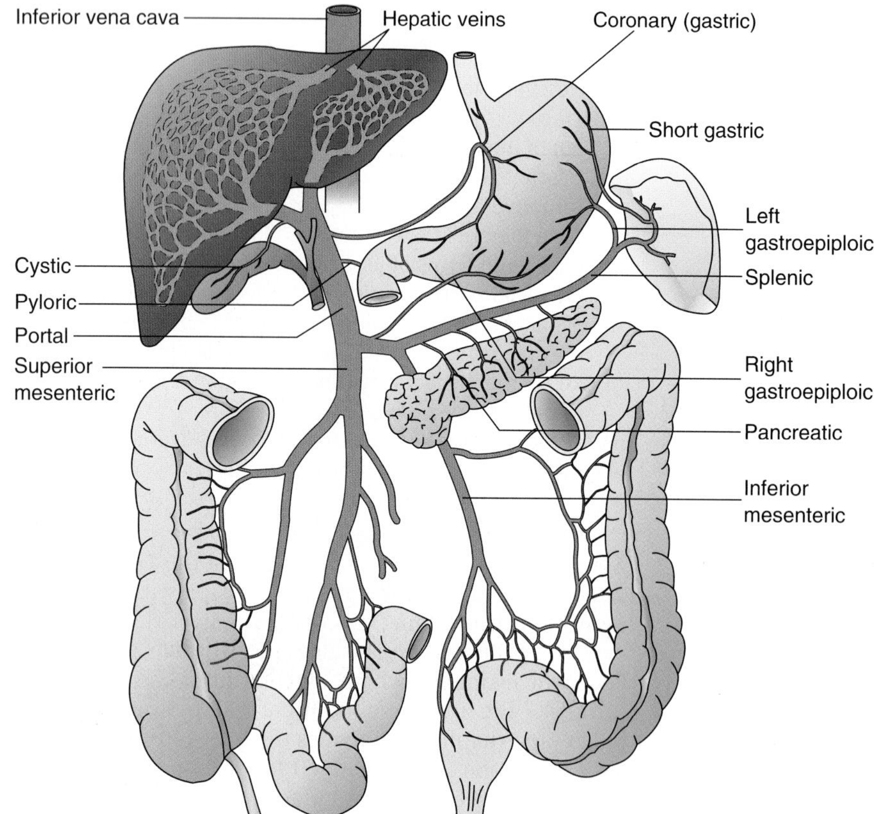

FIGURE 40-2 The portal circulation. Blood from the gastrointestinal tract, spleen, and pancreas travels to the liver by way of the portal vein before moving into the vena cava for return to the heart.

oxygen needs of the liver. The venous outflow from the liver is carried by the valveless hepatic veins, which empty into the inferior vena cava just below the level of the diaphragm. The pressure difference between the hepatic vein and the portal vein normally is such that the liver stores approximately 450 mL of blood.[1] This blood can be shifted back into the general circulation during periods of hypovolemia and shock. In congestive heart failure, in which the pressure in the vena cava increases, blood backs up and accumulates in the liver.

The *lobules* are the functional units of the liver. Each lobule is a cylindrical structure that measures approximately 0.8 to 2 mm in diameter and several millimeters long. There are approximately 50,000 to 100,000 lobules in the liver.[1] Each lobule is organized around a central vein that empties into the hepatic veins and from there into the vena cava. The terminal bile ducts and small branches of the portal vein and hepatic artery are located at the periphery of the lobule. Plates of hepatic cells radiate centrifugally from the central vein like spokes on a wheel (Fig. 40-3). These hepatic plates are separated by wide, thin-walled channels, called *sinusoids,* that extend from the periphery of the lobule to its central vein. The sinusoids are supplied by blood from the portal vein and hepatic artery. Because the plates of hepatic cells are no more than two layers thick, every cell is exposed to the blood that travels through the sinusoids. Thus, the hepatic cells can remove substances from the blood or can release substances into the blood as it moves through the sinusoids.

The venous sinusoids are lined with two types of cells: the typical endothelial cells and Kupffer's cells. *Kupffer's cells* are reticuloendothelial cells that are capable of removing and phagocytizing old and defective blood cells, bacteria, and other foreign material from the portal blood as it flows through the sinusoid. This phagocytic action removes the enteric bacilli and other harmful substances that filter into the blood from the intestine.

The lobules also are supplied by small tubular channels, called *bile canaliculi,* that lie between the cell membranes of adjacent hepatocytes. The bile produced by the hepatocytes flows into the canaliculi and then to the periphery of the lobules, which drain into progressively larger ducts, until it reaches the right and left hepatic ducts. The intrahepatic and extrahepatic bile ducts often are collectively referred to as the *hepatobiliary tree.* The hepatic and cystic ducts unite to form the common bile duct (see Fig. 40-1). The common bile duct, which is approximately 10 to 15 cm long, descends and passes behind the pancreas and enters the descending duodenum. The pancreatic duct joins the common duct at a short dilated tube called the *hepatopancreatic ampulla* (ampulla of Vater), which empties into the duodenum through the duodenal papilla. Muscle tissue at the junction of the papilla, sometimes called the *sphincter of Oddi,* regulates the flow of bile into the duodenum. When this sphincter is closed, bile moves back into the common duct and gallbladder.

METABOLIC FUNCTIONS OF THE LIVER

The liver is one of the most versatile and active organs in the body. It produces bile; metabolizes hormones and drugs; synthesizes proteins, glucose, and clotting factors;

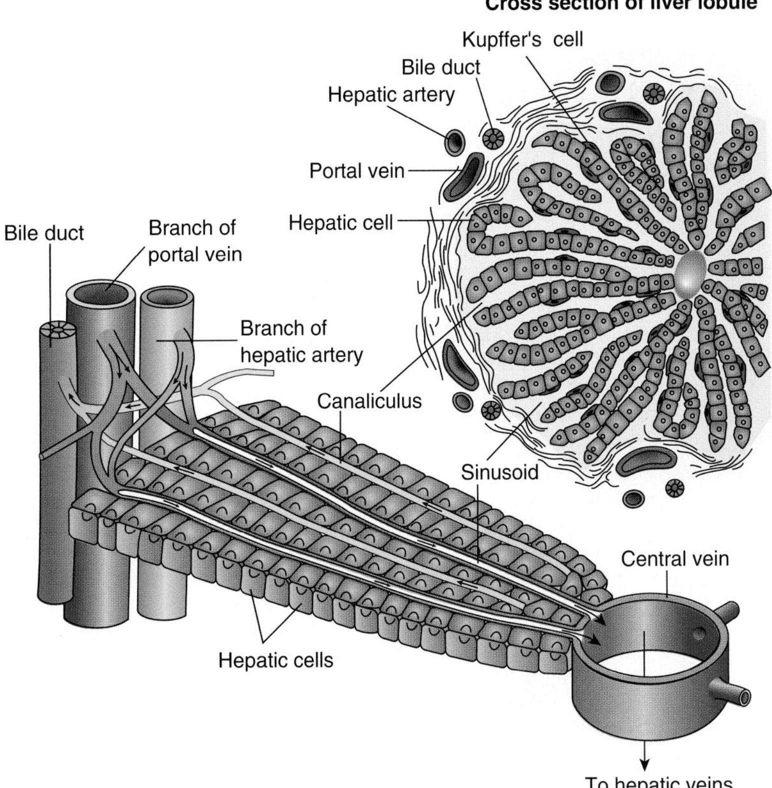

FIGURE 40-3 A section of liver lobule showing the location of the hepatic veins, hepatic cells, liver sinusoids, and branches of the portal vein and hepatic artery.

stores vitamins and minerals; changes ammonia produced by deamination of amino acids to urea; and converts fatty acids to ketones. The liver degrades excess nutrients and converts them into substances essential to the body. It builds carbohydrates from proteins, converts sugars to fats that can be stored, and interchanges chemical groups on amino acids so that they can be used for a number of purposes. In its capacity for metabolizing drugs and hormones, the liver serves as an excretory organ. In this respect, the bile, which carries the end products of substances metabolized by the liver, is much like the urine, which carries the body wastes filtered by the kidneys. The functions of the liver are summarized in Table 40-1.

Carbohydrate Metabolism

The liver plays an essential role in carbohydrate metabolism and glucose homeostasis (Fig. 40-4). The liver stores excess glucose as glycogen and releases it into the circulation when blood glucose levels fall. The liver also synthesizes glucose from amino acids, glycerol, and lactic acid as a means of maintaining blood glucose during periods of fasting or increased need. The liver also converts excess carbohydrates to triglycerides for storage in adipose tissue.

Protein Synthesis and Conversion of Ammonia to Urea

The liver is an important site for protein synthesis and degradation. It produces the proteins for its own cellular needs and secretory proteins that are released into the circulation. The most important of these secretory proteins is albumin. Albumin contributes significantly to the plasma colloidal osmotic pressure (see Chapter 33) and to the binding and transport of numerous substances, including some hormones and drugs, fatty acids, bilirubin, and other anions. The liver also produces other important proteins, such as fibrinogen and the blood clotting factors.

Through a variety of anabolic and catabolic processes, the liver is the major site of amino acid interconversion (Fig. 40-5). These processes involve two major reactions: transamination and deamination. In *transamination,* an amino group (NH_2) is transferred to an acceptor substance. As a result of transamination, amino acids can participate in the intermediary metabolism of carbohydrates and lipids. During periods of fasting or starvation, amino acids are used for producing glucose (*i.e.,* gluconeogenesis). Most of the nonessential amino acids are synthesized in the liver by transamination. The process of transamination

TABLE 40-1 Functions of the Liver and Manifestations of Altered Function

Function	Manifestations of Altered Function
Production of bile salts	Malabsorption of fat and fat-soluble vitamins
Elimination of bilirubin	Elevation in serum bilirubin and jaundice
Metabolism of steroid hormones	
Sex hormones	Disturbances in gonadal function, including gynecomastia in the male
Glucocorticoids	Signs of increased cortisol levels (*i.e.,* Cushing's syndrome)
Aldosterone	Signs of hyperaldosteronism (*e.g.,* sodium retention and hypokalemia)
Metabolism of drugs	Decreased drug metabolism Decreased plasma binding of drugs owing to a decrease in albumin production
Carbohydrate metabolism	Hypoglycemia may develop when glycogenolysis and gluconeogenesis are impaired
Stores glycogen and synthesizes glucose from amino acids, lactic acid, and glycerol	Abnormal glucose tolerance curve may occur because of impaired uptake and release of glucose by the liver
Fat metabolism	
Formation of lipoproteins	Impaired synthesis of lipoproteins
Conversion of carbohydrates and proteins to fat	
Synthesis, recycling, and elimination of cholesterol	Altered cholesterol levels
Formation of ketones from fatty acid	
Protein metabolism	
Deamination of proteins	
Formation of urea from ammonia	Elevated blood ammonia levels
Synthesis of plasma proteins	Decreased levels of plasma proteins, particularly albumin, which contributes to edema formation
Synthesis of clotting factors (fibrinogen, prothrombin, factors V, VII, IX, X)	Bleeding tendency
Storage of minerals and vitamins	Signs of deficiency of fat-soluble and other vitamins that are stored in the liver
Filtration of blood and removal of bacteria and particulate matter by Kupffer's cells	Increased exposure of the body to colonic bacteria and other foreign matter

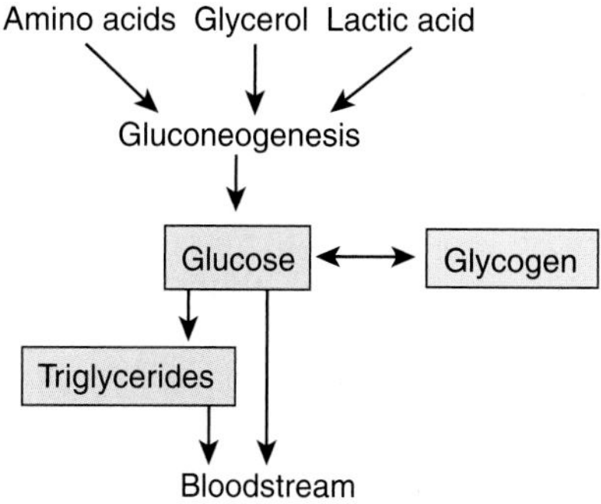

FIGURE 40-4 Hepatic pathways for storage and synthesis of glucose and conversion of glucose to fatty acids.

is catalyzed by *aminotransferases,* enzymes that are found in high amounts in the liver.

Oxidative *deamination* involves the removal of the amino groups from the amino acids and conversion of amino acids to ketoacids and ammonia. This occurs mainly by transamination, in which the amino groups are removed and then transferred to another acceptor substance. The acceptor substance can then transfer the amino group to still another substance or release it as ammonia. Ammonia is very toxic to body tissues, particularly neurons. The ammonia that is released during deamination is removed from the blood almost immediately and converted to urea. Essentially all urea formed in the body is synthesized by the urea cycle in the liver and is then excreted by the kidneys.[2] Although urea is mostly excreted by the kidneys, some diffuses into the intestine, where it is converted to ammonia by enteric bacteria. The intestinal production of ammonia also results from bacterial deamination of unabsorbed amino acids and protein derived from the diet, exfoliated cells, or blood in the gastrointestinal tract. Ammonia produced in the intestine is absorbed into the portal circulation and transported to the liver, where it is converted to urea before being released into the systemic circulation. Intestinal production of ammonia is increased after ingestion of high-protein foods and gastrointestinal bleeding. In advanced liver disease, urea synthesis often is impaired, leading to an accumulation of blood ammonia.

Pathways of Lipid Metabolism

Although most cells of the body metabolize fat, certain aspects of lipid metabolism occur mainly in the liver, including oxidation of fatty acids to supply energy for other body functions; the synthesis of large quantities of cholesterol, phospholipids, and most lipoproteins; and the formation of triglycerides from carbohydrates and proteins (Fig. 40-6). To derive energy from neutral fats, the fat must first be split into glycerol and fatty acids, and then the fatty acids split by *beta oxidation* into two-carbon acetyl-

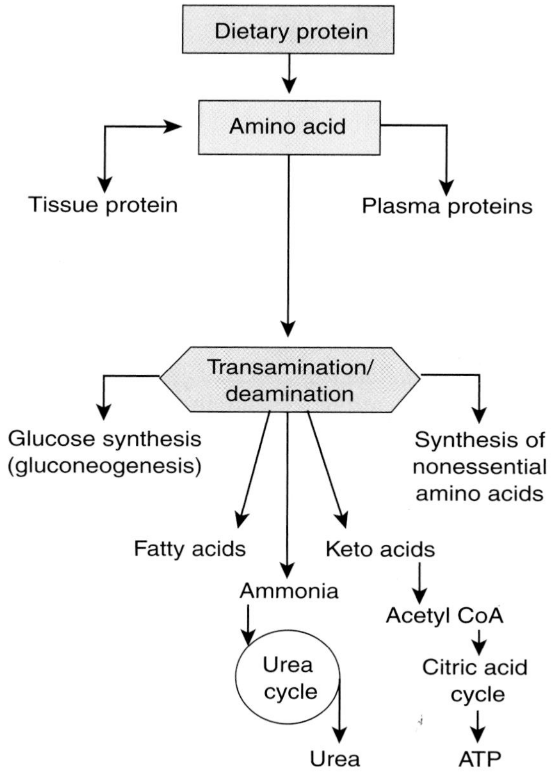

Dietary protein
Amino acid
Tissue protein
Plasma proteins
Transamination/ deamination
Glucose synthesis (gluconeogenesis)
Synthesis of nonessential amino acids
Fatty acids
Keto acids
Ammonia
Acetyl CoA
Urea cycle
Citric acid cycle
Urea
ATP

FIGURE 40-5 Hepatic pathways for conversion of amino acids to proteins, nucleic acids, ketone bodies, and glucose. The urea cycle converts ammonia generated by the deamination of amino acids to urea.

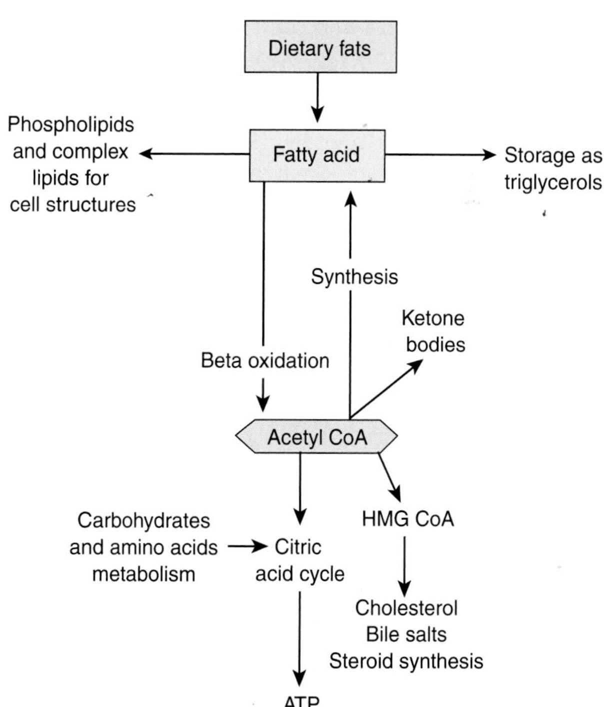

FIGURE 40-6 Hepatic pathways for fat metabolism. Beta oxidation breaks fatty acids into two carbon acetyl-coenzyme A (acetyl-CoA) units that are used in the citric acid cycle to generate adenosine triphosphate (ATP) or are used in the synthesis of ketone bodies and cholesterol.

coenzyme A (acetyl-CoA) units. Acetyl-CoA is readily channeled into the citric acid cycle to produce adenosine triphosphate (ATP). Because the liver cannot use all the acetyl-CoA that is formed, it converts the excess into acetoacetic acid, a highly soluble ketoacid that is released into the bloodstream and transported to other tissues, where it is used for energy. During periods of starvation, ketones become a major source of energy as fatty acids released from adipose tissue are converted to ketones by the liver.

Acetyl-CoA units from fat metabolism also are used to synthesize cholesterol and bile acids in the liver. Cholesterol has several fates in the liver. It can be esterified and stored; it can be exported bound to lipoproteins; or it can be converted to bile acids. The rate-limiting step in cholesterol synthesis is that which is catalyzed by 3-hydroxy-3-methylglutaryl-coenzyme A reductase (HMG-CoA reductase). The HMG-CoA reductase inhibitors, or statins (*e.g.*, fluvastatin, lovastatin, pravastatin, atorvastatin), that are used to treat high cholesterol levels act by inhibiting this step in cholesterol synthesis (see Chapter 24).

Almost all the fat synthesis in the body from carbohydrates and proteins occurs in the liver. As fat is synthesized in the liver, it is transported as triglycerides in the lipoproteins to adipose tissue to be stored.

BILE PRODUCTION AND CHOLESTASIS

The secretion of bile is essential for digestion of dietary fats and absorption of fats and fat-soluble vitamins from the intestine. The liver produces approximately 600 to 1200 mL of yellow-green bile daily.[1] Bile contains water, bile salts, bilirubin, cholesterol, and certain products of organic metabolism. Of these, only bile salts, which are formed from cholesterol, are important in digestion. The other components of bile depend on the secretion of sodium, chloride, bicarbonate, and potassium by the bile ducts.

The liver forms approximately 0.6 g of bile salts daily.[1] Bile salts serve an important function in digestion; they aid in emulsifying dietary fats, and they are necessary for the formation of the micelles that transport fatty acids and fat-soluble vitamins to the surface of the intestinal mucosa for absorption. Approximately 94% of bile salts that enter the intestine are reabsorbed into the portal circulation by an active transport process that takes place in the distal ileum. From the portal circulation, the bile salts pass into the liver, where they are recycled. Normally, bile salts travel this entire circuit approximately 18 times before being expelled in the feces.[1] This system for recirculation of bile salts and other substances is called the *enterohepatic circulation.*

Cholestasis

Cholestasis represents a decrease in bile flow through the intrahepatic canaliculi and a reduction in secretion of water, bilirubin, and bile acids by the hepatocytes. As a result, the materials normally transferred to the bile, including bilirubin, cholesterol, and bile acids, accumulate in the blood.[3,4] The condition may be caused by intrinsic liver disease, in which case it is referred to as *intrahepatic cholestasis,* or by obstruction of the large bile ducts, a condition known as *extrahepatic cholestasis.*

A number of mechanisms are implicated in the pathogenesis of cholestasis. Primary biliary cirrhosis and primary sclerosing cholangitis are caused by disorders of the small intrahepatic canaliculi and bile ducts. In the case of extrahepatic obstruction, such as that caused by conditions such as cholelithiasis, common duct strictures, or obstructing neoplasms, the effects begin with increased pressure in the large bile ducts. Genetic disorders involving the transport of bile into the canaliculi also can result in cholestasis.

The morphologic features of cholestasis depend on the underlying cause. Common to all types of obstructive and hepatocellular cholestasis is the accumulation of bile pigment in the liver. Elongated green-brown plugs of bile are visible in the dilated bile canaliculi. Rupture of the canaliculi leads to extravasation of bile and subsequent degenerative changes in the surrounding hepatocytes. Prolonged obstructive cholestasis leads not only to fatty changes in the hepatocytes but also to destruction of the supporting connective tissue, giving rise to bile lakes filled with cellular debris and pigment.[3] Unrelieved obstruction leads to biliary tract fibrosis and ultimately to end-stage biliary cirrhosis.

Pruritus is the most common presenting symptom in persons with cholestasis, probably related to an elevation in plasma bile acids. Skin xanthomas (focal accumulations of cholesterol) may occur, the result of hyperlipidemia and impaired excretion of cholesterol. A characteristic laboratory finding is an elevated serum alkaline phosphatase level, an enzyme present in the bile duct epithelium and canalicular membrane of hepatocytes. Other manifestations of reduced bile flow relate to impaired intestinal absorption, including nutritional deficiencies of fat-soluble vitamins A, D, and K.

BILIRUBIN ELIMINATION AND JAUNDICE

Bilirubin is the substance that gives bile its color. It is formed from senescent red blood cells. In the process of degradation, the hemoglobin from the red blood cell is broken down to form biliverdin, which is rapidly converted to free bilirubin (Fig. 40-7). Free bilirubin, which is insoluble in plasma, is transported in the blood attached to plasma albumin. Even when it is bound to albumin, this bilirubin is still called *free bilirubin.* As it passes through the liver, free bilirubin is released from its albumin carrier molecule and moved into the hepatocytes. Inside the hepatocytes, free bilirubin is converted to conjugated bilirubin, making it soluble in bile. Conjugated bilirubin is secreted as a constituent of bile, and in this form, it passes through the bile ducts into the small intestine. In the intestine, approximately one half of the bilirubin is converted into a highly soluble substance called *urobilinogen* by the intestinal flora. Urobilinogen is either absorbed into the portal circulation or excreted in the feces. Most of the urobilinogen that is absorbed is returned to the liver to be re-excreted into the bile. A small amount of urobilinogen, approximately 5%, is absorbed into the general circulation and then excreted by the kidneys.

Usually, only a small amount of bilirubin is found in the blood; the normal level of total serum bilirubin is 0.1 to 1.2 mg/dL. Laboratory measurements of bilirubin usually

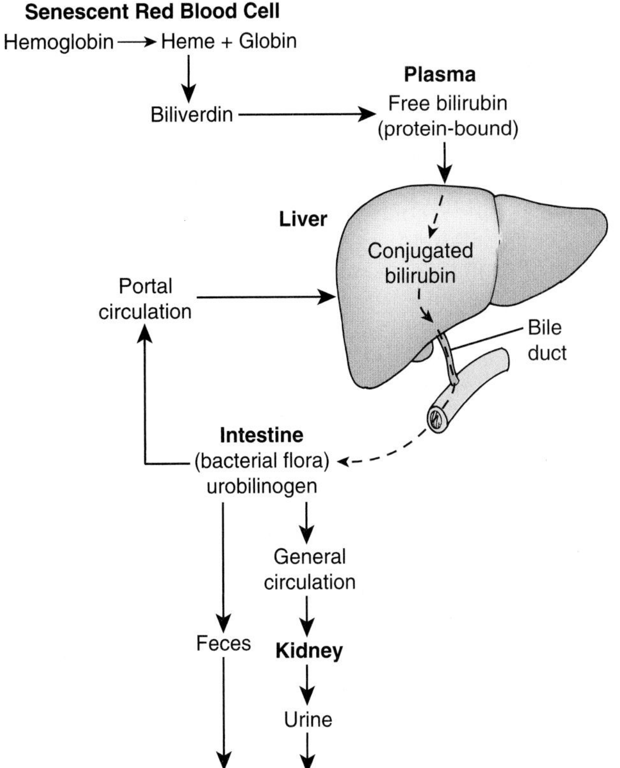

FIGURE 40-7 The process of bilirubin formation, circulation, and elimination.

measure the free and the conjugated bilirubin as well as the total bilirubin. These are reported as the direct (conjugated) bilirubin and the indirect (unconjugated or free) bilirubin.

Jaundice

Jaundice (*i.e.*, icterus) results from an abnormally high accumulation of bilirubin in the blood, as a result of which there is a yellowish discoloration to the skin and deep tissues. Jaundice becomes evident when the serum bilirubin levels rise above 2 to 2.5 mg/dL.[3,4] Because normal skin has a yellow cast, the early signs of jaundice often are difficult to detect, especially in persons with dark skin. Bilirubin has a special affinity for elastic tissue. The sclera of the eye, which contains considerable elastic fibers, usually is one of the first structures in which jaundice can be detected (Fig. 40-8).

The four major causes of jaundice are excessive destruction of red blood cells, impaired uptake of bilirubin by the liver cells, decreased conjugation of bilirubin, and obstruction of bile flow in the canaliculi of the hepatic lobules or in the intrahepatic or extrahepatic bile ducts. From an anatomic standpoint, jaundice can be categorized as prehepatic, intrahepatic, and posthepatic. Chart 40-1 lists the common causes of prehepatic, hepatic, and posthepatic jaundice.

The major cause of prehepatic jaundice is excessive hemolysis of red blood cells. Hemolytic jaundice occurs when red blood cells are destroyed at a rate in excess of the liver's ability to remove the bilirubin from the blood. It may follow a hemolytic blood transfusion reaction or may occur in diseases such as hereditary spherocytosis, in which the red cell membranes are defective, or in hemolytic disease of the newborn (see Chapter 16). Neonatal hyperbilirubinemia results from an increased production of bilirubin in newborn infants and their limited ability to excrete it.[5] Premature infants are at particular risk because their red cells have a shorter life span and higher turnover rate. In prehepatic jaundice, there is mild jaundice, the unconjugated bilirubin is elevated, the stools are of normal color, and there is no bilirubin in the urine.

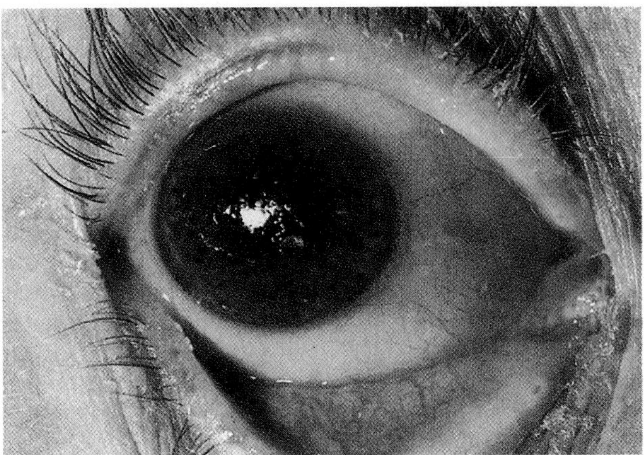

FIGURE 40-8 Jaundice. A patient with hepatic failure displays a yellow sclera. (Rubin E., Farber J.L. [1999]. *Pathology* [3rd ed., p. 762]. Philadelphia: Lippincott-Raven)

CHART 40-1

Causes of Jaundice

Prehepatic (Excessive Red Blood Cell Destruction)

Hemolytic blood transfusion reaction
Hereditary disorders of the red blood cell
- Sickle cell anemia
- Thalassemia
- Spherocytosis

Acquired hemolytic disorders
Hemolytic disease of the newborn
Autoimmune hemolytic anemias

Intrahepatic

Decreased bilirubin uptake by the liver
Decreased conjugation of bilirubin
Hepatocellular liver damage
- Hepatitis
- Cirrhosis
- Cancer of the liver

Drug-induced cholestasis

Posthepatic (Obstruction of Bile Flow)

Structural disorders of the bile duct
Cholelithiasis
Congenital atresia of the extrahepatic bile ducts
Bile duct obstruction caused by tumors

Intrahepatic or hepatocellular jaundice is caused by disorders that directly affect the ability of the liver to remove bilirubin from the blood or to conjugate it, so that it can be eliminated in the bile. Gilbert's disease is inherited as a dominant trait and results in a reduced removal of bilirubin from the blood; the disorder is benign and fairly common. Affected persons have no symptoms other than a slightly elevated unconjugated bilirubin and mild jaundice. Conjugation of bilirubin is impaired whenever liver cells are damaged, when transport of bilirubin into liver cells becomes deficient, or when the enzymes needed to conjugate the bile are lacking. Liver diseases such as hepatitis and cirrhosis are the most common causes of intrahepatic jaundice. Drugs such as the anesthetic agent halothane, oral contraceptives, estrogen, anabolic steroids, isoniazid, and chlorpromazine may also be implicated in this type of jaundice. Intrahepatic or hepatocellular jaundice usually interferes with all phases of bilirubin metabolism—uptake, conjugation, and excretion. Both the conjugated and unconjugated bilirubin are elevated, the urine often is dark because of bilirubin in the urine, and the alkaline phosphatase is slightly elevated. Alkaline phosphatase is produced by the bile duct epithelium and canalicular membranes of hepatocytes and excreted with the bile; when bile flow is obstructed, the blood alkaline phosphatase level becomes elevated.

Posthepatic or obstructive jaundice, also called *cholestatic jaundice,* occurs when bile flow is obstructed between the liver and the intestine, with the obstruction located at any point between the junction of the right or left hepatic duct and the point where the bile duct opens into the intestine. Among the causes are strictures of the bile duct, gallstones, and tumors of the bile duct or the pancreas. Conjugated bilirubin levels usually are elevated; the stools are clay colored because of the lack of bilirubin in the bile; the urine is dark; the levels of serum alkaline phosphatase are markedly elevated; and the aminotransferase levels are slightly increased. Blood levels of bile acids often are elevated in obstructive jaundice. As the bile acids accumulate in the blood, pruritus develops. A history of pruritus preceding jaundice is common in obstructive jaundice.

TESTS OF HEPATOBILIARY FUNCTION

The history and physical examination, in most instances, provide clues about liver function. Diagnostic tests help to evaluate liver function and the extent of liver damage. Laboratory tests commonly are used to assess liver function and confirm the diagnosis of liver disease.

Liver function tests, including serum levels of liver enzymes, are used to assess injury to liver cells, the liver's ability to synthesize proteins, and the excretory functions of the liver.[6] Elevated serum enzyme tests usually indicate liver injury earlier than other indicators of liver function. The key enzymes are alanine aminotransferase (ALT) and aspartate aminotransferase (AST), which are present in liver cells. ALT is liver specific, whereas AST is derived from organs other than the liver. In most cases of liver damage, there are parallel rises in ALT and AST. The most dramatic rise is seen in cases of acute hepatocellular injury, as occurs with viral hepatitis, hypoxic or ischemic injury, acute toxic injury, or Reye's syndrome.

The liver's synthetic capacity is reflected in measures of serum protein levels and prothrombin time (*i.e.,* synthesis of coagulation factors). Hypoalbuminemia due to depressed synthesis may complicate severe liver disease. Deficiencies of coagulation factor V and vitamin K–dependent factors (II, VII, IX, and X) may occur.

Serum bilirubin, γ-glutamyltransferase (GGT), and alkaline phosphatase measure hepatic excretory function. Alkaline phosphatase is present in the membranes between liver cells and the bile duct and is released by disorders affecting the bile duct.[6] GGT is thought to function in the transport of amino acids and peptides into liver cells; it is a sensitive indicator of hepatobiliary disease. Measurement of GGT may be helpful in diagnosing alcohol abuse.[6]

Ultrasonography provides information about the size, composition, and blood flow of the liver. It has largely replaced cholangiography in detecting stones in the gallbladder or biliary tree. Computed tomography (CT) scanning provides information similar to that obtained by ultrasound. Magnetic resonance imaging (MRI) has proved to be useful in some disorders. Selective angiography of the celiac, superior mesenteric, or hepatic artery may be used to visualize the hepatic or portal circulation. A liver biopsy affords a means of examining liver tissue without surgery. There are several methods for obtaining liver tissue: percutaneous liver biopsy, which uses a suction, cutting, or spring-loaded cutting needle; laparoscopic liver biopsy; and fine-needle biopsy, which is performed under ultrasound or CT guidance.[7] The type of method used is based on the number of specimens needed and the amount of tissue required for evaluation. Laparoscopic liver biopsy provides the means for examining abdominal masses, evaluating ascites of unknown cause, and staging liver cancers.

In summary, the hepatobiliary system consists of the liver, gallbladder, and bile ducts. The liver is the largest and, in its functions, one of the most versatile organs in the body. It is located between the gastrointestinal tract and the systemic circulation; venous blood from the intestine flows through the liver before it is returned to the heart. In this way, nutrients can be removed for processing and storage, and bacteria and other foreign matter can be removed by Kupffer's cells before the blood is returned to the systemic circulation.

The liver synthesizes fats, glucose, and plasma proteins. Other important functions of the liver include the deamination of amino acids, conversion of ammonia to urea, and interconversion of amino acids and other compounds that are important to the metabolic processes of the body. The liver produces approximately 600 to 1200 mL of yellow-green bile daily. Bile serves as an excretory vehicle for bilirubin, cholesterol, and certain products of organic metabolism, and it contains bile salts that are essential for digestion of fats and absorption of fat-soluble vitamins. The liver also removes, conjugates, and secretes bilirubin into the bile. Jaundice occurs when bilirubin accumulates in the blood. It can occur because of excessive red blood cell destruction, failure of the liver to remove and conjugate the bilirubin, or obstructed biliary flow.

Liver function tests, including serum aminotransferase levels, are used to assess injury to liver cells. Serum bilirubin, GGT, and alkaline phosphatase are used as a measure of hepatic excretory function. Ultrasonography, CT scans, and MRI are used to evaluate liver structures. Angiography may be used to visualize the hepatic or portal circulation, and a liver biopsy may be used to obtain tissue specimens for microscopic examination.

Disorders of Hepatic and Biliary Function

After completing this section of the chapter, you should be able to meet the following objectives:

- ✦ State the three ways by which drugs and other substances are metabolized or inactivated in the liver and provide examples of liver disease related to the toxic effects of drugs and chemical agents
- ✦ Compare hepatitis A, B, C, D, and E in terms of source of infection, incubation period, acute disease manifestations, development of chronic disease, and the carrier state
- ✦ Define chronic hepatitis and compare the pathogenesis of chronic autoimmune and chronic viral hepatitis
- ✦ Characterize the metabolism of alcohol by the liver and state metabolic mechanisms that can be used to explain liver injury
- ✦ Summarize the three patterns of injury that occur with alcohol-induced liver disease.
- ✦ Describe the pathogenesis of intrahepatic biliary tract disease
- ✦ Characterize the liver changes that occur with cirrhosis
- ✦ Describe the physiologic basis for portal hypertension and relate it to the development of ascites, esophageal varices, and splenomegaly
- ✦ Relate the functions of the liver to the manifestations of liver failure
- ✦ Characterize etiologies of hepatocellular cancer and state the reason for the poor prognosis in persons with this type of cancer

The structures of the hepatobiliary system are subject to many of the same pathologic conditions that affect other body systems: injury from drugs and toxins; infection, inflammation, and immune responses; metabolic disorders; and neoplasms. This section focuses on alterations in liver function due to drug-induced injury; viral and autoimmune hepatitis; intrahepatic biliary tract disorders; alcohol-induced liver disease; cirrhosis, portal hypertension, and liver failure; and cancer of the liver.

DRUG-INDUCED LIVER DISEASE

By virtue of its many enzyme systems that are involved in biochemical transformations and modifications, the liver has an important role in the metabolism of many drugs and chemical substances. The liver is particularly important in terms of metabolizing lipid-soluble substances that cannot be directly excreted by the kidneys. Because the liver is central to metabolic disposition of virtually all drugs and foreign substances, drug-induced liver toxicity is a potential complication of many medications.

Drug and Hormone Metabolism

Two major types of reactions are involved in the hepatic detoxification and metabolism of drugs and other chemicals: phase 1 reactions, which involve chemical modification or inactivation of a substance, and phase 2 reactions, which involve conversion of lipid-soluble substances to water-soluble derivatives.[8,9] Often, the two types of reactions are linked. Many phase 1 reactants are not soluble and must therefore undergo a subsequent phase 2 reaction to be eliminated. These reactions, which are called *biotransformations,* are important considerations in drug therapy.

Phase 1 reactions result in chemical modification of reactive drug groups by oxidation, reduction, hydroxylation, or other chemical reactions. Most drug-metabolizing enzymes are located in the lipophilic membranes of the smooth endoplasmic reticulum of liver cells (see Chapter 4). When these membranes are broken down and separated in the laboratory, they reform into vesicles called *microsomes.* The enzymes in these membranes are often referred to as *microsomal enzymes.* The enzymes involved in most phase 1 oxidation-reduction processes are products of a gene superfamily that has nearly 300 members.[8] These genes code for a group of microsomal isoenzymes that make up the cytochrome (CYP) P450 system. (The name cytochrome P450 is derived from the spectral properties [absorb light at 450 nm] of the hematoproteins that participate in oxidation-reduction processes.) The gene products of many of the *CYP* genes have been identified and traced to the metabolism of specific drugs and to potential interactions among drugs. Each family of genes is responsible for certain drug-metabolizing processes, and each member of the family undertakes specific drug-metabolizing functions. For example, the *CYP3* gene family contains an A subfamily and several genes numbered 1, 2, 3, and so forth. The primary enzyme for the metabolism of erythromycin in humans is CYP 3A4.[8]

Many gene members of the CYP system can have their activity induced or suppressed as they undergo the task of metabolizing drugs. For example, drugs such as alcohol and barbiturates can induce certain members to increase enzyme production, accelerating drug metabolism and decreasing the pharmacologic action of the drug and of coadministered drugs that use the same member of the CYP system. In the case of drugs metabolically transformed to reactive intermediates, enzyme induction may exacerbate drug-mediated tissue toxicity. Enzymes in the cytochrome system also can be inhibited by drugs. For example, imidazole-containing drugs such as cimetidine (a histamine-2 receptor–blocking drug that is used to reduce gastric acid secretion) and ketoconazole (an antifungal agent) effectively inhibit the metabolism of testosterone.[8] Environmental pollutants also are capable of inducing *CYP* gene activity. For example, exposure to benzo[*a*]pyrene, which is present in tobacco smoke, charcoal-broiled meat, and other organic pyrolysis products, is known to induce members of the cytochrome CYP family and alter the rates of metabolism of some drugs.

Phase 2 reactions, which involve the conversion of lipid-soluble derivatives to water-soluble substances, may follow phase 1 reactions or proceed independently. Conjugation, catalyzed by endoplasmic reticulum enzymes that couple the drug with an activated endogenous compound to render it more water soluble, is one of the most common phase 2 reactions. Although many water-soluble drugs and endogenous substances are excreted unchanged in the urine or bile, lipid-soluble substances tend to accumulate in the body unless they are converted to less active compounds or water-soluble metabolites. In general, the conjugates are more soluble than the parent compound and are pharmacologically inactive. Because the endogenous substrates used in the conjugation process are obtained from the diet, nutrition plays a critical role in phase 2 reactions.

An alternative CYP P450–dependent conjugation pathway is important in detoxifying reactive metabolic intermediates. This pathway uses a thiol or sulfur-containing substance called *glutathione,* which is used in conjugating drugs that form potentially harmful electrophilic groups.[9] Glutathione is depleted in the detoxification process and must be constantly replenished by compounds from the diet or by cysteine-containing drugs such as *N*-acetylcysteine.[8] The glutathione pathway is central to the detoxification of a number of compounds, including the over-the-counter pain medication acetaminophen (*e.g.,* Tylenol). Acetaminophen metabolism involves a phase 2 reaction. Normally, the capacity of the phase 2 reactants is much greater than that required for metabolizing recommended doses of the drug. However, in situations of acetaminophen overdose, the capacity of the phase 2 system is exceeded, and the drug is transformed into toxic metabolites that can cause necrosis of the liver if allowed to accumulate. In this situation, the glutathione pathway plays a critical role in the detoxification of these metabolites. Because the glutathione stores are rapidly depleted, the drug *N*-acetylcysteine, which serves as a glutathione substitute, is used as an antidote for acetaminophen overdose.[9] Chronic alcohol ingestion decreases glutathione stores and increases the risk for acetaminophen toxicity.

In addition to its role in metabolism of drugs and chemicals, the liver also is responsible for hormone inactivation or modification. Insulin and glucagon are inactivated by proteolysis or deamination. Thyroxine and triiodothyronine are metabolized by reactions involving deiodination. Steroid hormones such as the glucocorticoids are first inactivated by a phase 1 reaction and then conjugated by a phase 2 reaction.

Drug-Induced Liver Disease

As the major drug-metabolizing and detoxifying organ in the body, the liver is subject to potential damage from the enormous array of pharmaceutical and environmental chemicals. Many of the widely used therapeutic drugs, including over-the-counter "natural" products, can cause hepatic injury. Of the numerous remedies, medicinal agents, chemicals, and herbal remedies in existence, more than 600 are recognized as being capable of producing hepatic injury.[10] Numerous host factors contribute to the susceptibility to drug-induced liver disease, including genetic predisposition, age differences, underlying chronic liver disease, diet and alcohol consumption, and the use of multiple interacting drugs. For some reason, women generally predominate among persons with drug-induced liver disease. According to a recent study, women accounted for 79% of reactions to acetaminophen and 73% of idiosyncratic drug reactions.[11] Early identification of drug-induced liver disease is important because withdrawal of the drug is curative in most cases.

Drugs and chemicals can exert their effects by causing hepatocyte injury and death or by cholestatic liver damage due to injury of biliary drainage structures.[12] Drug reactions can be predictable based on the drug's chemical structure and metabolites or unpredictable (idiosyncratic) based on individual characteristics of the person receiving the drug.

Direct Hepatotoxic Injury. Some drugs are known to have toxic effects on the liver based on their chemical structure and the way they are metabolized in the liver. Direct hepatic damage often is age and dose dependent. Direct hepatotoxic reactions usually are a recognized characteristic of certain drugs. They usually result from drug metabolism and the generation of toxic metabolites. Because of the greater activity of the drug-metabolizing enzymes in the central zones of the liver, these agents typically cause centrilobular necrosis. Examples of drugs that cause direct hepatotoxicity are acetaminophen, isoniazid, and phenytoin, as well as a number of chemical agents, including carbon tetrachloride. Acetaminophen toxicity produces the most common form of acute liver failure, accounting for 39% of cases in a recent survey of tertiary care centers.[11] The injury is characterized by marked elevations in ALT and AST values with minimally elevated alkaline phosphatase. Bilirubin levels invariably are increased, and the prognosis often is worse when hepatocellular necrosis is accompanied by jaundice.

Idiosyncratic Reactions. In contrast to direct hepatotoxic drug reactions, idiosyncratic reactions are unpredictable, not related to dose, and sometimes accompanied by features suggesting an allergic reaction. In some cases, the reaction results directly from a metabolite that is produced only in certain persons based on a genetic predisposition. For example, certain people are capable of rapid acetylation of isoniazid, an antituberculosis drug. These people have increased likelihood of toxic reactions resulting from acetyl hydrazine, which is transformed to a toxic metabolite.[9]

Cholestatic Reactions. Cholestatic drug reactions result in decreased secretion of bile or obstruction of the biliary tree. Acute intrahepatic cholestasis is one of the most frequent types of idiosyncratic drug reactions. Among the drugs credited with causing cholestatic drug reactions are estradiol, chlorpromazine, an antipsychotic drug, and some of the antibiotics, including amoxicillin/clavulanic acid, erythromycin, and nafcillin. Typically, cholestatic drug reactions are characterized by early onset of jaundice and pruritus, with little alteration in the person's general feeling of well-being. Most instances of acute drug-induced cholestasis subside once the drug is withdrawn.

Chronic Hepatitis. Some drugs produce a more indolent form of liver damage that closely resembles autoimmune hepatitis. Early identification of drug-related chronic hepatitis often is difficult; cirrhosis may develop before the hepatitis is diagnosed. Identifying the responsible drug that caused the liver damage may be difficult retrospectively if the person has been consuming alcohol or taking several drugs.

HEPATITIS

Hepatitis refers to inflammation of the liver. It can be caused by autoimmune disorders or reactions to drugs and toxins; by infectious disorders such as malaria, infectious mononucleosis, salmonellosis, and amebiasis that cause primary infections of extrahepatic tissues and secondary hepatitis; and by hepatotropic viruses that primarily affect liver cells or hepatocytes.

Acute Viral Hepatitis

The known hepatotropic viruses include hepatitis A virus (HAV), hepatitis B virus (HBV), the hepatitis B–associated delta virus (HDV), hepatitis C virus (HCV), and hepatitis E virus (HEV). Although all of these viruses cause acute hepatitis, they differ in the mode of transmission and incubation period; mechanism, degree, and chronicity of liver damage; and ability to evolve to a carrier state. The presence of viral antigens and antigen antibodies can be determined through laboratory tests. Epidemiologic studies have indicated that some cases of infectious hepatitis are due to other viruses. A viral agent similar to HCV has been cloned and identified as hepatitis G virus (HGV). Evidence of HGV has been found in 1% to 4% of blood donors in the United States. However, HGV does not appear to cause liver disease or exacerbations of liver disease.[3]

There are two mechanisms of liver injury in viral hepatitis: direct cellular injury and induction of immune responses against the viral antigens. The mechanisms of injury have been most closely studied in HBV. It is thought that the extent of inflammation and necrosis depends on the individual's immune response. Accordingly, a prompt immune response during the acute phase of the infection would be expected to cause cell injury but at the same time eliminate the virus. Thus, people who respond with fewer symptoms and a marginal immune response are less likely to eliminate the virus, and hepatocytes expressing the viral antigens persist, leading to the chronic or carrier state. Fulminant hepatitis would be explained in terms of an accelerated immune response with severe liver necrosis.

The clinical course of viral hepatitis involves a number of syndromes, including asymptomatic infection with only serologic evidence of disease; acute hepatitis; the carrier state without clinically apparent disease or with chronic hepatitis; chronic hepatitis with or without progression to cirrhosis; or fulminating disease (>1% to 3%) with rapid onset of liver failure. Not all hepatotropic viruses provoke each of the clinical syndromes.

The manifestations of acute hepatitis can be divided into three phases: the prodromal or preicterus period, the icterus period, and the convalescent period. The manifestations of the prodromal period vary from abrupt to insidious, with general malaise, myalgia, arthralgia, easy fatigability, and severe anorexia out of proportion to the degree of illness. Gastrointestinal symptoms such as nausea, vomiting, and diarrhea or constipation may occur. Abdominal pain is usually mild and is felt on the right side. Chills and fever may mark an abrupt onset. In persons who smoke, there may be a distaste for smoking that parallels the anorexia. Serum levels of AST and ALT show variable increases during the preicterus phase of acute hepatitis and precede a rise in bilirubin that accompanies the onset of the icterus or jaundice phase of infection. The icterus phase, if it occurs, usually follows the prodromal phase by 5 to 10 days. Jaundice is less likely to occur with HCV infection. The prodromal symptoms may become worse with the onset of jaundice, followed by progressive clinical improvement. Severe pruritus and liver tenderness are common during the icterus period. The convalescent phase is characterized by an increased sense of well-being, return of appetite, and disappearance of jaundice. The acute illness usually subsides gradually over a 2- to 3-week period, with complete clinical recovery by approximately 9 weeks in hepatitis A and 16 weeks in uncomplicated hepatitis B.

Infection with HBV and HCV can produce a *carrier state* in which the person does not have symptoms but harbors the virus and can therefore transmit the disease. Evidence also indicates a carrier state for HDV infection. There is no carrier state for HAV infection. There are two types of carriers: healthy carriers who have few or no ill effects, and those with chronic disease who may or may not have symptoms. Factors that increase the risk for becoming a

DISEASES OF THE LIVER

- Diseases of the liver can affect the hepatocytes or the biliary drainage system.
- Diseases of hepatocytes impair the metabolic and synthetic functions of the liver, causing disorders in carbohydrate, protein, and fat metabolism; metabolism and removal of drugs, hormones, toxins, ammonia, and bilirubin from the blood; and the interconversion of amino acids and synthesis of proteins. Elevations in serum aminotransferase levels signal the presence of hepatocyte damage.
- Diseases of the biliary drainage system obstruct the flow of bile and interfere with the elimination of bile salts and bilirubin, producing cholestatic liver damage because of the backup of bile into the lobules of the liver. Elevations in bilirubin and alkaline phosphatase signal the presence of cholestatic liver damage.

carrier are age at time of infection and immune status. The carrier state for infections that occur early in life, as in infants of HBV-infected mothers, may be as high as 90% to 95%, compared with 1% to 10% of infected adults.[3] Other persons at high risk for becoming carriers are those with impaired immunity, those who have received multiple transfusions or blood products, those who are on hemodialysis, and drug addicts.

Hepatitis A. Hepatitis A is caused by the small, unenveloped, RNA-containing HAV. It usually is a benign, self-limited disease, although it can cause acute fulminant hepatitis and death from liver failure in rare cases. The onset of symptoms usually is abrupt and includes fever, malaise, nausea, anorexia, abdominal discomfort, dark urine, and jaundice. The likelihood of having symptoms is related to age.[13,14] Children younger than 5 years often are asymptomatic. The illness in older children and adults usually is symptomatic, and jaundice occurs in approximately 90% of cases. Symptoms usually last approximately 2 months but can last longer. HAV does not cause chronic hepatitis or induce a carrier state.

Hepatitis A has a brief incubation period (15 to 45 days) and usually is transmitted by the fecal–oral route.[13,14] The virus replicates in the liver, is excreted in the bile, and is shed in the stool. The fecal shedding of HAV occurs up to 2 weeks before the development of symptoms and ends as the immunoglobulin M (IgM) levels rise.[3] The disease often occurs sporadically or in epidemics. Drinking contaminated milk or water and eating shellfish from infected waters are fairly common routes of transmission. At special risk are persons traveling abroad who have not previously been exposed to the virus. Because young children are asymptomatic, they play an important role in the spread of the disease. Institutions housing large numbers of persons (usually children) sometimes are stricken with an epidemic of hepatitis A. Oral behavior and lack of toilet training promote viral infection among children attending preschool day care centers, who then carry the virus home to older siblings and parents. Hepatitis A usually is not transmitted by transfusion of blood or plasma derivatives, presumably because its short period of viremia usually coincides with clinical illness, so that the disease is apparent, and blood donations are not accepted.

Serologic Markers. Antibodies to HAV (anti-HAV) appear early in the disease and tend to persist in the serum (Fig. 40-9). The IgM antibodies (see Chapter 19) usually appear during the first week of symptomatic disease and begin to decline in a few months. Their presence coincides with a decline in fecal shedding of the virus. Peak levels of IgG antibodies occur after 1 month of illness and may persist for years; they provide long-term protective immunity against reinfection. The presence of IgM anti-HAV is indicative of acute hepatitis A, whereas IgG anti-HAV merely documents past exposure.

Vaccination. A hepatitis A vaccine is available.[15] Vaccination is intended to replace the use of immune globulin in persons at high risk for HAV exposure. These include international travelers to regions where sanitation is poor

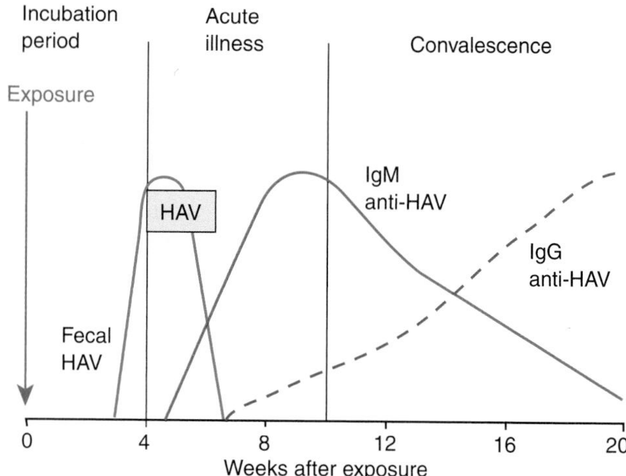

FIGURE 40-9 The sequence of fecal shedding of the hepatitis A virus (HAV), HAV viremia, and HAV antibody (IgM and IgG anti-HAV) changes in hepatitis A.

and endemic HAV infections are high, children living in communities with high rates of HAV infection, homosexually active men, and users of illicit drugs. Persons with preexisting chronic liver disease also may benefit from immunization. A public health benefit also may be derived from vaccinating persons with increased potential for transmitting the disease (*e.g.*, food handlers). The Centers for Disease Control and Prevention (CDC) recently recommended vaccination of children in states, counties, and communities with high rates of infection.[15] Because the vaccine is of little benefit in prevention of hepatitis in persons with known HAV exposure, immune globulin (IgG) is recommended for these persons.

Hepatitis B. Hepatitis B is caused by a double-stranded DNA virus (HBV).[3,16] The complete virion, also called a *Dane particle,* consists of an outer envelope and an inner nucleocapsid that contains HBV DNA and DNA polymerase (Fig. 40-10). Hepatitis B can produce acute hepatitis, chronic hepatitis, progression of chronic hepatitis to cirrhosis, fulminant hepatitis with massive hepatic necrosis, and the carrier state. It also participates in the development of hepatitis D (delta hepatitis).

HBV infects more than 350 million people worldwide.[3,16,17] Approximately 1.2 million persons in the United States have chronic HBV infection and are sources of HBV transmission to others.[18] At particular risk for becoming carriers are infants born to hepatitis B–infected mothers. However, since the late 1980s, the incidence of acute hepatitis B has declined steadily, especially among vaccinated children.[18] The decline was much lower among adults, indicating a need for vaccination programs that target high-risk populations.

Hepatitis B has a longer incubation period and represents a more serious health problem than hepatitis A. The HBV usually is transmitted through inoculation with infected blood or serum. However, the viral antigen can be found in most body secretions and can be spread by oral or sexual contact. In the United States, most persons with hep-

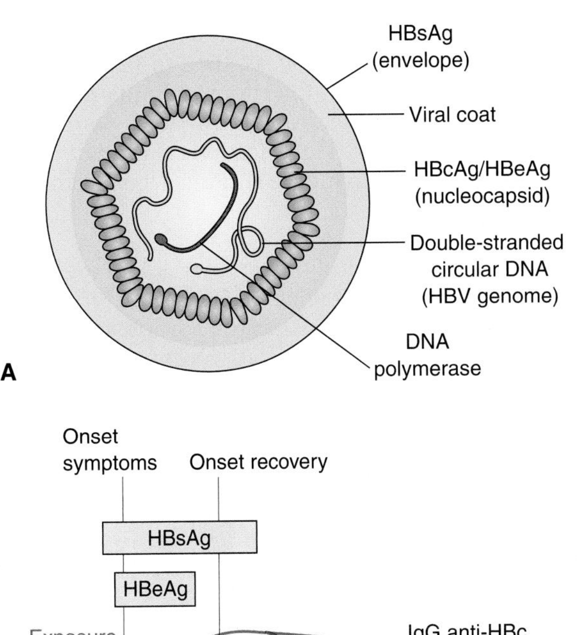

FIGURE 40-10 (**A**) The hepatitis B virus. (**B**) The sequence of hepatitis B virus (HBV) viral antigens (HBsAg, HbeAg), HBV DNA, and HBV antibody (IgM, IgG, anti-HBc, and anti-HBs) changes in acute resolving hepatitis B.

atitis B acquire the infection as adults or adolescents. The disease is highly prevalent among injecting drug users, persons with multiple sex partners, and men who have sex with men.[18] Health care workers are at risk owing to blood exposure and accidental needle injuries. Although the virus can be spread through transfusion or administration of blood products, routine screening methods have appreciably reduced transmission through this route. The risk for hepatitis B in infants born to HBV-infected mothers ranges from 10% to 85%, depending on the mother's HBV core antigen (HBeAg) status. Infants who become infected have a 90% risk for becoming chronic carriers, and up to 25% will die of chronic liver disease as adults.[19]

Serologic Markers. Three well-defined antigens are associated with the virus: two core antigens, HBcAg and HBeAg, which are contained in the nucleocapsid, and a third, surface antigen, HBsAg, which is found in the outer envelope of the virus (see Fig. 40-10). Each of these antigens evokes specific antibodies: anti-HBs, anti-HBc, and anti-HBe. These antigens and their antibodies serve as serologic markers for following the course of the disease.

The *HBsAg* is the viral antigen measured most routinely in blood. It is produced in abundance by infected liver cells and released into the serum. HBsAg is the earliest serologic marker to appear; it appears before the onset of symptoms and is an indicator of acute or chronic infection. The HBsAg level begins to decline after the onset of the illness and usually is undetectable in 3 to 6 months. Persistence beyond 6 months indicates continued viral replication, infectivity, and risk for chronic hepatitis. *Anti-HBs,* a specific antibody to HBsAg, occurs in most individuals after clearance of HBsAg. There often is a delay in appearance of anti-HBs after clearance of HBsAg. During this period of serologic gap, called the *window period,* infectivity has been demonstrated. Development of anti-HBs signals recovery from HBV infection, noninfectivity, and protection from future HBV infection. Anti-HBs is the antibody present in persons who have been successfully immunized for HBV.

The HBeAg is thought to be a cleavage product of the viral core antigen; it may be found in the serum as a soluble protein and is an active marker for the disease and shedding of complete virions into the bloodstream. It appears during the incubation period, shortly after the appearance of HBsAg, and is found only in the presence of HBsAg. HBeAg usually disappears before HBsAg. The antibody to HBeAg, *anti-HBe,* begins to appear in the serum at about the time that HBeAg disappears, and its appearance signals the onset of resolution of the acute illness. The clinical usefulness of the antigen and its antibody lies in their predictive value as markers for infectivity.

The *HBcAg* does not circulate in the blood; therefore, it is not a useful marker for the disease. Although the antigen is not found in the blood, its antibodies (anti-HBc) are the first to be detected. They appear toward the end of the incubation period and persist during the acute illness and for several months to years after that. The initial HBcAg antibody is IgM; it serves as a marker for recent infection and is followed in 6 to 18 months by IgG antibodies. These antibodies are not protective and are detectable in the presence of chronic disease.

The presence of viral DNA (HBV DNA) in the serum is the most certain indicator of hepatitis B infection. It is transiently present during the presymptomatic period and for a brief time during the acute illness. The presence of DNA polymerase, the enzyme used in viral replication, usually is transient but may persist for years in persons who are chronic carriers and is an indication of continued infectivity.

Vaccination. Hepatitis B vaccine provides long-term protection against HBV infection. Hepatitis immune globulin may be effective for unvaccinated persons who are exposed to the infection if given within 7 days of exposure. Hepatitis vaccination is recommended for preexposure and postexposure prophylaxis.

The hepatitis B vaccine is produced by recombinant DNA technology.[20] The CDC recommends vaccination of all children aged 0 to 18 years as a means of preventing HBV transmission.[21] The vaccine also is recommended for all persons who are at high risk for exposure to the virus, health care workers exposed to blood (required by Occupational Health and Safety Administration regulations), clients and staff of institutions for the developmentally disabled, patients on hemodialysis, recipients of certain blood products, household contacts and sexual partners of HBV carriers, adoptees from countries where HBV is endemic, international travelers, injecting drug users, sexually active homosexual and bisexual men, heterosexual men and women having sex with multiple partners, and inmates of long-term correctional agencies. It is recommended that persons with end-stage renal disease be vaccinated before they require hemodialysis and that universal hepatitis B vaccination of teenagers be implemented in communities where injecting drug use, pregnancy among teenagers, and sexually transmitted diseases are common. The CDC also recommends that all pregnant women be routinely tested for HBsAg during an early prenatal visit and that infants born to HBsAg-positive mothers receive appropriate doses of hepatitis immune globulin and hepatitis B vaccine.[19]

Hepatitis C. Hepatitis C is the most common cause of chronic hepatitis, cirrhosis, and hepatocellular cancer in the world. In the United States, there are approximately 3.9 million persons infected with the virus.[22] Most of these people are chronically infected and unaware of their infection because they are not clinically ill. Infected persons serve as a source of infection to others and are at risk for chronic liver disease during the first two or more decades after initial infection.

Formerly known as *non-A, non-B hepatitis,* hepatitis C is caused by a single-stranded RNA virus (HCV) that is distantly related to the viruses that cause yellow fever and dengue fever. There are at least 6 genotypes and more than 50 subtypes of the virus.[22–24] Genotype 1, which is associated with more severe liver disease, accounts for 70% to 75% of cases in the United States. It is likely that the wide diversity of genotypes contributes to the pathogenicity of the virus, allowing it to escape the actions of host immune mechanisms and antiviral medications, and to the difficulties in developing a preventative vaccine.[22,23]

Before 1990, the main route of transmission was through contaminated blood transfusions or blood products. With implementation of HCV testing in blood banks, the risk for HCV infection from blood transfusion is almost nonexistent.[22] Currently, injecting drug use is thought to be the single most important risk factor for HCV infection. There also is concern that transmission of small amounts of blood during tattooing, acupuncture, and body piercing may facilitate the transmission of HCV. Although the virus may also be transmitted through sexual contact or through vertical transmission from mother to infant, the incidence of such transmission is uncertain.[22] Occupational exposure through incidents such as unintentional needle sticks can result in infection. However, the prevalence of HCV among health care, emergency medical, and public safety workers who are exposed to blood in the workplace is reported to be no greater than in the general public.

The incubation period for HCV infection ranges from 15 to 150 days (average, 50 days). Clinical symptoms with acute hepatitis C tend to be milder than those seen in persons with other types of viral hepatitis. Children and adults who acquire the infection usually are asymptomatic, or have a nonspecific clinical disease characterized by fatigue, malaise, anorexia, and weight loss. Jaundice is uncommon, and only 25% to 30% of symptomatic adults have jaundice.[25] These symptoms usually last for 2 to 12 weeks. Unlike hepatitis A and B viral infections, fulminant hepatic failure is rare, and only a few cases have been reported. The most alarming aspects of HCV infection are its high rate of persistence and ability to induce chronic hepatitis and cirrhosis.

Serologic Markers. Both antibody and viral tests are available for detecting the presence of hepatitis C infection (Fig. 40-11). Antibody testing has the advantage of being readily available and having a relatively lower cost. False-negative results can occur in immunocompromised people and early in the course of the disease before antibodies develop. Direct measurement of HCV in the serum remains the most accurate test for infection. The viral tests are highly sensitive and specific, but more costly than antibody tests. With newer antibody testing methods, infection often can be detected as early as 6 to 8 weeks after exposure, and as early as 1 to 2 weeks with viral tests that use the polymerase chain reaction (PCR) testing methods (see Chapter 18). Unlike hepatitis A and B, antibodies to HCV are not protective, but they serve as markers for the disease. At present, there is no vaccine that protects against HCV infection.

Hepatitis D. Hepatitis D virus, or the delta hepatitis agent, is a defective RNA virus. It can cause acute or chronic hepatitis. Infection depends on concomitant infection with hepatitis B, specifically the presence of HBsAg. Acute hepatitis D occurs in two forms: coinfection that occurs simultaneously with acute hepatitis B, and a superinfection in which hepatitis D is superimposed on chronic hepatitis B or hepatitis B carrier state.[26] The delta agent often increases the severity of HBV infection. It can convert mild HBV infection into severe, fulminating hepatitis, cause acute hepatitis in asymptomatic carriers, or increase the tendency for progression to chronic hepatitis and cirrhosis.

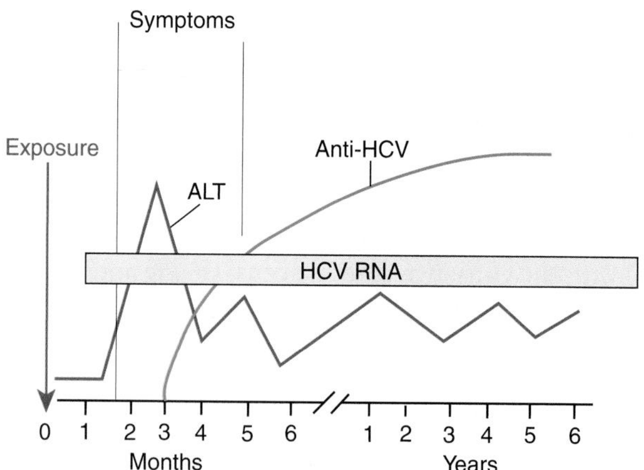

FIGURE 40-11 The sequence of serologic changes in chronic hepatitis C with persistence of hepatitis C virus (HCV) RNA and exacerbations and remissions of clinical symptoms designated by changes in serum alanine amino transferase (ALT) levels.

The routes of transmission of hepatitis D are similar to those for hepatitis B. In the United States, infection is restricted largely to persons at high risk for HBV infection, particularly injecting drug users and persons receiving clotting factor concentrates. The greatest risk is in HBV carriers; these persons should be informed about the dangers of HDV superinfection.

Hepatitis D is diagnosed by detection of antibody to HDV (anti-HDV) in the serum or HDV RNA in the serum. There is no specific treatment for hepatitis D. Because the infection is linked to hepatitis B, prevention of hepatitis D should begin with prevention of hepatitis B through vaccination.

Hepatitis E. Hepatitis E virus is an unenveloped, single-stranded RNA virus. It is transmitted by the fecal–oral route and causes manifestations of acute hepatitis that are similar to hepatitis A. It does not cause chronic hepatitis or the carrier state. Its distinguishing feature is the high mortality rate (approximately 20%) among pregnant women, owing to the development of fulminant hepatitis. The infection occurs primarily in developing areas such as India, other Southeast Asian countries, parts of Africa, and Mexico. The only reported cases in the United States have been in persons who have recently been in an endemic area.

Chronic Hepatitis

Chronic hepatitis is defined as chronic inflammatory reaction of the liver of more than 3 to 6 months' duration. It is characterized by persistently elevated serum aminotransferase levels and characteristic histologic findings on liver biopsy. The causes of chronic hepatitis include HBV, HCV, HDV, autoimmune hepatitis, and drug-induced hepatitis.

Chronic Viral Hepatitis. Chronic viral hepatitis is the principal cause of chronic liver disease, cirrhosis, and hepatocellular cancer worldwide and now ranks as the chief reason for liver transplantation in adults.[27] Of the hepatotropic viruses, only three are known to cause chronic hepatitis—HBV, HCV, and HDV.

The clinical features of chronic viral hepatitis are highly variable and not predictive of outcome. The most common symptoms are fatigue, malaise, loss of appetite, and occasional bouts of jaundice. Elevation of serum aminotransferase concentrations depends on the level of disease activity.

Chronic hepatitis B accounts for 5% to 10% of chronic liver disease and cirrhosis in the United States.[27] Hepatitis B is less likely than hepatitis C to progress to chronic infection. Chronic hepatitis B is characterized by the persistence of HBV DNA and usually by HBeAg in the serum, indicating active viral replication. Many persons are asymptomatic at the time of diagnosis, and elevated serum aminotransferase levels are the first sign of infection. Chronic hepatitis D depends on concurrent infection with HBV.

Chronic hepatitis C accounts for most cases of chronic viral hepatitis. HCV infection becomes chronic in 75% to 80% of cases.[22] Chronic HCV infection often smolders over a period of years, silently destroying liver cells. Most persons with chronic hepatitis C are asymptomatic, and diagnosis usually follows a finding of elevated serum aminotransferase levels, a tender liver, or complaints of fatigue or nonspecific weakness. Because the course of acute hepatitis C often is mild, many persons do not recall the events of the acute infection.

Treatment. There are no simple and effective treatment methods for chronic viral hepatitis. Persons with chronic hepatitis B who have evidence of active viral replication may be treated with a course of recombinant interferon-alfa-2b.[27,28] The nucleoside analog lamivudine may be used as a substitute for interferon-alfa. Lamivudine can be given orally and usually is well tolerated, even after being given for prolonged periods. However, 15% to 30% of responders experience a mild relapse during therapy as the virus becomes resistant to the drug.[27] Moreover, hepatitis activity may resume once the drug is discontinued, suggesting that long-term therapy may be required. In persons with concurrent hepatitis D infection, recombinant interferon-alfa-2a may lead to normalization of aminotransferase levels, histologic improvement, and elimination of HDV RNA from the serum in approximately 50% of cases, but relapse is common after the therapy is stopped.[27] Lamivudine is not effective in chronic hepatitis D.

Many persons with chronic HCV can now be cured with a combination of the new pegylated forms of interferon (alfa-2b or alfa-2a) plus ribavirin.[21,29] Peginterferons were developed by adding a polyethylene glycol (PEG) moiety to an interferon molecule, resulting in a prolonged serum half-life and the ability to administer the compound once weekly rather than three times a week.[29] Ribavirin, a nucleoside analog, may be added to the treatment regimen. Treatment with peginterferon and ribavirin is costly, and the side effects, which include flulike symptoms, are almost universal. More serious side effects, which include psychiatric symptoms (depression), thyroid dysfunction, and bone marrow depression, are less common. Although most persons with HCV infection are candidates for treatment, many have other health problems that are contraindications for therapy.[22,29]

Liver transplantation is a treatment option for end-stage liver disease due to viral hepatitis. Liver transplantation has been more successful in persons with hepatitis C than those with hepatitis B. Although the transplanted liver often is reinfected, the disease seems to progress more slowly.

Autoimmune Hepatitis. Chronic autoimmune hepatitis is a chronic inflammatory liver disease of unknown origin, but it is associated with circulating autoantibodies and high serum gamma globulin levels. Autoimmune hepatitis accounts for only approximately 10% of chronic hepatitis in the United States, a decrease from previously reported rates that probably reflects not a true change in incidence but better methods of detecting viral pathogens. The pathogenesis of the disorder is one of a genetically predisposed person exposed to an environmental agent that triggers an autoimmune response directed at liver cell antigens.[30] The resulting immune response produces a necrotizing inflammatory response that eventually leads to destruction of liver cells and development of cirrhosis. The factors surrounding the genetic predisposition and the triggering events that lead to the autoimmune response are unclear. Autoimmune hepatitis is mainly a disease of young women, although it can occur at any age and in men or women.

Clinical manifestations of the disorder cover a spectrum that extends from no apparent symptoms to the signs accompanying liver failure. In asymptomatic cases, the disorder may be discovered when abnormal serum enzyme levels are discovered during performance of routine screening tests.

The differential diagnosis includes measures to exclude other causes of liver disease, including hepatitis B and C. A characteristic laboratory finding is that of a marked elevation in serum gamma globulins. A biopsy is used to confirm the diagnosis. Corticosteroid drugs and immunosuppressant drugs are the treatment of choice for this type of hepatitis. Liver transplantation may be the only treatment for end-stage disease.

INTRAHEPATIC BILIARY DISORDERS

Intrahepatic biliary diseases disrupt the flow of bile through the liver, causing cholestasis and biliary cirrhosis. Among the causes of intrahepatic biliary disease are primary biliary cirrhosis, primary sclerosing cholangitis, and secondary biliary cirrhosis.

Primary Biliary Cirrhosis

Primary biliary cirrhosis involves inflammation and scarring of small intrahepatic bile ducts, portal inflammation, and progressive scarring of liver tissue.[31,32] The disease is seen most commonly in women 40 to 60 years of age and accounts for 2% to 5% of cases of cirrhosis. Familial occurrences of the disease are found between parents and children and among siblings. Abnormalities of cell-mediated and humoral immunity suggest an autoimmune mechanism. Antimitochondrial antibodies are found in 98% of persons with the disease, but their role in the pathogenesis of the disease is unclear.[32] Up to 84% of persons with primary biliary cirrhosis have at least one other autoimmune disorder, such as scleroderma, Hashimoto's thyroiditis, rheumatoid arthritis, or Sjögren's syndrome.

The disorder is characterized by an insidious onset and progressive scarring and destruction of liver tissue. The liver becomes enlarged and takes on a green hue because of the accumulated bile. The earliest symptoms are unexplained pruritus or itching, weight loss, and fatigue, followed by dark urine and pale stools. Jaundice is a late manifestation of the disorder, as are other signs of liver failure. Serum alkaline phosphatase levels are elevated in persons with primary biliary cirrhosis.

Treatment is largely symptomatic. Bile acid–binding drugs are used as a treatment for itching. Some persons have responded to ultraviolet B light, methyltestosterone, cimetidine, phenobarbital, and prednisone. There is no generally accepted treatment for the underlying disease. Clinical trials using ursodiol, a drug that increases bile flow and decreases the toxicity of bile contents, have shown a decreased rate of clinical deterioration with drug treatment.[27,32] Colchicine, which acts to prevent leukocyte migration and phagocytosis, and methotrexate, a drug with immunosuppressive properties, have had some reported benefit in improving symptoms. However, liver transplantation remains the only treatment for advanced disease. Primary biliary cirrhosis does not recur after liver transplantation if appropriate immunosuppression is used.[31,32]

Primary Sclerosing Cholangitis

Cholangitis involves inflammation of hepatic bile ducts. Primary sclerosing cholangitis is a chronic cholestatic disease of unknown origin that causes destruction and fibrosis of intrahepatic and extrahepatic bile ducts.[33] Bile flow is obstructed (*i.e.,* cholestasis), and the bile retention destroys hepatic structures. The disease commonly is associated with inflammatory bowel disease, occurs more often in men than women, and is seen most commonly in the third to fifth decades of life. Primary sclerosing cholangitis, although much less common than alcoholic cirrhosis, is the fourth leading indication for liver transplantation in adults in the United States.[33]

Most persons with the disorder are initially asymptomatic, with the disorder being detected during routine liver function tests that reveal elevated levels of serum alkaline phosphatase or GGT. Alternatively, some persons present with progressive fatigue, jaundice, and pruritus. The later stages of the disease are characterized by cirrhosis, portal hypertension, and liver failure.[33] Ten-year survival rates range from 50% to 75%. Other than measures aimed at symptom relief, the only treatment is liver transplantation.

Secondary Biliary Cirrhosis

Secondary biliary cirrhosis results from prolonged obstruction of the extrabiliary tree. The most common cause is cholelithiasis. Other causes of secondary biliary cirrhosis are malignant neoplasms of the biliary tree or head of the pancreas and strictures of the common duct caused by previous surgical procedures. Extrahepatic biliary cirrhosis may benefit from surgical procedures designed to relieve the obstruction.

ALCOHOL-INDUCED LIVER DISEASE

The spectrum of alcoholic liver disease includes fatty liver disease, alcoholic hepatitis, and cirrhosis. Alcoholic cirrhosis causes 100,000 to 200,000 deaths annually and is the fifth leading cause of death in the United States.[3] Most deaths from alcoholic cirrhosis are attributable to liver failure, bleeding esophageal varices, or kidney failure. It has been estimated that there are 10 million alcoholics in the United States. Only approximately 10% to 15% of alcoholics develop cirrhosis, however, suggesting that other conditions such as genetic and environmental factors contribute to its occurrence.[3]

Metabolism of Alcohol

Alcohol is absorbed readily from the gastrointestinal tract; it is one of the few substances that can be absorbed from the stomach. As a substance, alcohol fits somewhere between a food and a drug. It supplies calories but cannot be broken down or stored as protein, fat, or carbohydrate. As a food, alcohol yields 7.1 kcal/g, compared with the 4 kcal/g produced by metabolism of an equal amount of carbohydrate.[34] Between 80% and 90% of the alcohol a person drinks is metabolized by the liver. The rest is excreted through the lungs, kidneys, and skin.

Alcohol metabolism proceeds simultaneously by three pathways: the alcohol dehydrogenase (ADH) system, located in the cytoplasm of the hepatocytes; the microsomal ethanol-oxidizing system (MEOS), located in the endoplasmic reticulum; and catalase, located in the peroxisomes[35] (see Chapter 4). The ADH and MEOS pathways produce specific metabolic and toxic disturbances, and all three pathways result in the production of acetaldehyde, a very toxic metabolite.[36]

The MEOS pathway, which is located in the smooth endoplasmic reticulum, produces acetaldehyde and free radicals. Prolonged and excessive alcohol ingestion results in enzyme induction and increased activity of the MEOS. One of the most important enzymes of the MEOS, a member of the CYP P450 system, also oxidizes a number of other compounds, including various drugs (*e.g.,* acetaminophen, isoniazid), toxins (*e.g.,* carbon tetrachloride, halothane), vitamins A and D, and carcinogenic agents (*e.g.,* aflatoxin, nitrosamines). Increased activity of this system enhances the susceptibility of persons with heavy alcohol consumption to the hepatotoxic effects of industrial toxins, anesthetic agents, chemical carcinogens, vitamins, and the pain-reliever acetaminophen.[37]

The metabolic end products of alcohol metabolism (*e.g.,* acetaldehyde, free radicals) are responsible for a variety of metabolic alterations that can cause liver injury. Acetaldehyde, for example, has multiple toxic effects on liver cells and liver function. Age and sex play a role in metabolism of alcohol and production of harmful metabolites. The ADH system is depressed by testosterone. Thus, women tend to produce greater amounts of acetaldehyde and are more predisposed to alcohol-induced liver damage than men.[37] Age also appears to affect the alcohol-metabolizing abilities of the liver and the resistance to hepatotoxic effects. Liver injury is related to the average amount of daily consumption and the duration of alcohol abuse. In general, a daily intake of less than 80 g of alcohol in men and 40 g in women seldom results in liver disease.[37]

Alcohol metabolism requires a cofactor, nicotinamide adenine dinucleotide (NAD), that is necessary for many other metabolic processes, including the metabolism of pyruvates, urates, and fatty acids. Because alcohol competes for the use of NAD, it tends to disrupt other metabolic functions of the liver. The preferential use of NAD for alcohol metabolism can result in increased production and accumulation of lactic acid in the blood. By reducing the availability of NAD, alcohol also impairs the liver's ability to form glucose from amino acids and other glucose precursors. Alcohol-induced hypoglycemia can develop when excessive alcohol ingestion occurs during periods of depleted liver glycogen stores. This may become a particular problem for the alcoholic who has been vomiting and has not eaten for several days.

Alcoholic Liver Disease

The metabolism of alcohol leads to chemical attack on certain membranes of the liver, but whether the damage is caused by acetaldehyde or other metabolites is unknown. Acetaldehyde is known to impede the mitochondrial electron transport system, which is responsible for oxidative metabolism and generation of ATP; as a result, the hydrogen ions that are generated in the mitochondria are shunted into lipid synthesis and ketogenesis. Abnormal accumulations of these substances are found in hepatocytes (*i.e.,* fatty liver) and blood. Binding of acetaldehyde to other molecules impairs the detoxification of free radicals and synthesis of proteins. Acetaldehyde also promotes collagen synthesis and fibrogenesis. The lesions of hepatocellular injury tend to be most prevalent in the centrilobular area that surrounds the central vein where the pathways for alcohol metabolism are concentrated. This is the part of the lobule that has the lowest oxygen tension; it is thought that the low oxygen concentration in this area of the liver may contribute to the damage.

Even after alcohol intake has stopped and all alcohol has been metabolized, the processes that damage liver cells may continue for many weeks and months. Clinical and chemical effects often become worse before the disease resolves. The accumulation of fat usually disappears within a few weeks, and cholestasis and inflammation also subside with time. However, fibrosis and scarring remain. The liver lobules become distorted as new liver cells regenerate and form nodules.

Although the mechanism by which alcohol exerts its toxic effects on liver structures is somewhat uncertain, the changes that develop can be divided into three stages: fatty changes, alcoholic hepatitis, and cirrhosis.[3,4]

Fatty liver is characterized by the accumulation of fat in hepatocytes, a condition called *steatosis* (Fig. 40-12). The liver becomes yellow and enlarges owing to excessive fat accumulation. The pathogenesis of fatty liver is not completely understood and can depend on the amount of alcohol consumed, dietary fat content, body stores of fat, hormonal status, and other factors. There is evidence that ingestion of large amounts of alcohol can cause fatty liver changes even with an adequate diet. For example, young, nonalcoholic volunteers had fatty liver changes after 2 days of consuming 18 to 24 oz of alcohol, even though adequate carbohydrates, fats, and proteins were included in the diet.[38] The fatty changes that occur with ingestion of alcohol usually do not produce symptoms and are reversible after the alcohol intake has been discontinued.

Alcoholic hepatitis is the intermediate stage between fatty changes and cirrhosis. It often is seen after an abrupt increase in alcohol intake and is common in "spree" drinkers. Alcoholic hepatitis is characterized by inflammation and necrosis of liver cells. This stage usually is characterized by hepatic tenderness, pain, anorexia, nausea, fever, jaundice, ascites, and liver failure, but some individuals may be asymptomatic. The condition is always serious and sometimes fatal. The immediate prognosis correlates with severity of liver cell injury. In some cases, the disease progresses rapidly to liver failure and death. The mortality rate

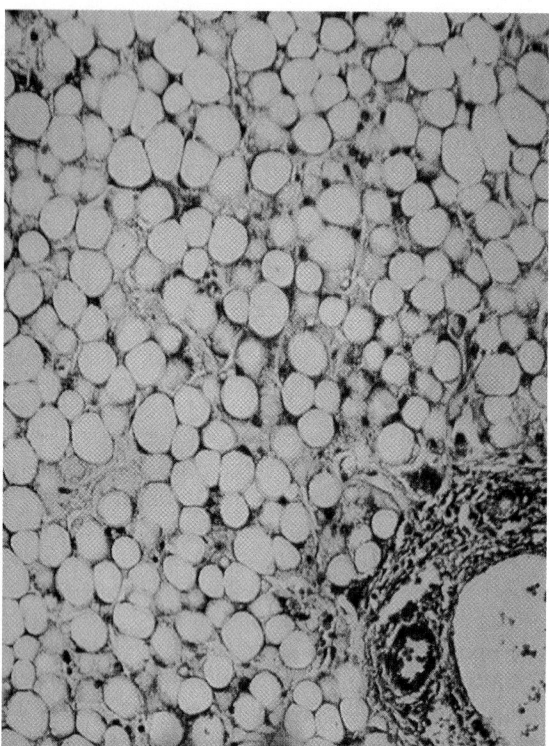

FIGURE 40-12 Alcoholic fatty liver. A photomicrograph shows the cytoplasm of almost all the hepatocytes to be distended by fat, which displaces the nucleus to the periphery. Note the absence of inflammation and fibrosis. (Rubin E., Farber J.L. [1999]. *Pathology* [3rd ed., p. 791]. Philadelphia: Lippincott-Raven)

in the acute stage ranges from 10% to 30%.[4] In persons who survive and continue to drink, the acute phase often is followed by persistent alcoholic hepatitis with progression to cirrhosis in a matter of 1 to 2 years.[4]

Alcoholic cirrhosis is the end result of repeated bouts of drinking-related liver injury and designates the onset of end-stage alcoholic liver disease. The gross appearance of the early cirrhotic liver is one of fine, uniform nodules on its surface. The condition has traditionally been called *micronodular* or *Laennec cirrhosis.* With more advanced cirrhosis, regenerative processes cause the nodules to become larger and more irregular in size and shape. As this happens, the nodules cause the liver to become relobulized through the formation of new portal tracts and venous outflow channels. The nodules may compress the hepatic veins, curtailing blood flow out of the liver and producing portal hypertension, extrahepatic portosystemic shunts, and cholestasis.

Nonalcoholic Fatty Liver Disease

The term *nonalcoholic fatty liver disease* is often used to describe fatty liver disease with its potential for progression to cirrhosis and end-stage liver disease arising from causes other than alcohol.[39,40] The condition can range from simple steatosis to steatohepatitis. Although steatosis alone does not appear to be progressive, approximately 20% of persons with steatohepatitis progress to cirrhosis over a decade.[39] Obesity, type 2 diabetes, the metabolic syndrome, and hyperlipidemia are coexisting conditions frequently associated with fatty liver disease (see Chapter 43). The condition is also associated with other nutritional abnormalities, surgical conditions, drugs, and occupational exposure to toxins. Both rapid weight loss and parenteral nutrition may lead to nonalcoholic fatty liver disease. Jejunoileal bypass, a surgical procedure used for weight loss, has largely been abandoned for this reason. The pathogenesis of nonalcoholic liver disease is thought to involve both hepatic fat accumulation and oxidative stress associated with formation of free radicals. The accumulation of toxic levels of free fatty acids increases the oxidative formation of free radicals, including hydrogen peroxide and superoxide (see Chapter 5). Abnormal lipid peroxidation ensues, followed by direct hepatocyte injury, release of toxic byproducts, inflammation, and fibrosis.

CIRRHOSIS, PORTAL HYPERTENSION, AND LIVER FAILURE

The most serious consequences of many liver diseases reside in their ability to cause cirrhosis, portal hypertension, and/or liver disease.

Cirrhosis

Cirrhosis represents the end stage of chronic liver disease in which much of the functional liver tissue has been replaced by fibrous tissue. It is characterized by diffuse fibrosis and conversion of normal liver architecture into structurally abnormal nodules.[3,4] The fibrous tissue replaces normally functioning liver tissue and forms constrictive bands that disrupt flow in the vascular channels and biliary duct systems of the liver. The disruption of vascular channels predisposes to portal hypertension and its complications; obstruction of biliary channels and exposure to the destructive effects of bile stasis; and loss of liver cells, leading to liver failure. Although cirrhosis usually is associated with alcoholism, it can develop in the course of other disorders, including viral hepatitis, toxic reactions to drugs and chemicals, biliary obstruction, and cardiac disease. Cirrhosis also accompanies metabolic disorders that cause the deposition of minerals in the liver. Two of these disorders are hemochromatosis (*i.e.,* iron deposition) and Wilson's disease (*i.e.,* copper deposition).

The manifestations of cirrhosis are variable, ranging from asymptomatic hepatomegaly to hepatic failure. Often there are no symptoms until the disease is far advanced. The most common signs and symptoms of cirrhosis are weight loss (sometimes masked by ascites), weakness, and anorexia. Diarrhea frequently is present, although some persons may complain of constipation. Hepatomegaly and jaundice also are common signs of cirrhosis. There may be abdominal pain because of liver enlargement or stretching of Glisson's capsule. This pain is located in the epigastric area or in the upper right quadrant and is described as dull, aching, and causing a sensation of fullness.

The late manifestations of cirrhosis are related to portal hypertension and liver cell failure. Splenomegaly, ascites, and portosystemic shunts (*i.e.*, esophageal varices, anorectal varices, and caput medusae) result from portal hypertension. Other complications include bleeding due to decreased clotting factors, thrombocytopenia due to splenomegaly, gynecomastia and a feminizing pattern of pubic hair distribution in men because of testicular atrophy, spider angiomas, palmar erythema, and encephalopathy with asterixis and neurologic signs.

Portal Hypertension

Portal hypertension is characterized by increased resistance to flow in the portal venous system and sustained portal vein pressure above 12 mm Hg (normal, 5 to 10 mm Hg).[4,41] Normally, venous blood returning to the heart from the abdominal organs collects in the portal vein and travels through the liver before entering the vena cava. Portal hypertension can be caused by a variety of conditions that increase resistance to hepatic blood flow, including prehepatic, posthepatic, and intrahepatic obstructions (with *hepatic* referring to the liver lobules rather than the entire liver).[4] Prehepatic causes of portal hypertension include portal vein thrombosis and external compression due to cancer or enlarged lymph nodes that produce obstruction of the portal vein before it enters the liver.

Posthepatic obstruction refers to any obstruction to blood flow through the hepatic veins beyond the liver lobules, either within or distal to the liver. It is caused by conditions such as thrombosis of the hepatic veins, veno-occlusive disease, and severe right-sided heart failure that impede the outflow of venous blood from the liver. *Budd-Chiari syndrome* refers to congestive disease of the liver caused by occlusion of the portal veins and their tributaries. The principal cause of the Budd-Chiari syndrome is thrombosis of the hepatic veins, in association with diverse conditions such as polycythemia vera, hypercoagulability states associated with malignant tumors, pregnancy, bacterial infection, metastatic disease of the liver, and trauma. *Hepatic veno-occlusive disease* is a variant of the Budd-Chiari syndrome seen most commonly in persons treated with certain cancer chemotherapeutic drugs, hepatic irradiation, or bone marrow transplantation, possibly because of graft-versus-host disease.[4]

PORTAL HYPERTENSION

- Venous blood from the gastrointestinal tract empties into the portal vein and travels through the liver before moving into the general venous circulation.
- Obstruction of blood flow in the portal vein produces an increase in the hydrostatic pressure within the peritoneal capillaries, contributing to the development of ascites, splenic engorgement with sequestration and destruction of blood cells and platelets, and shunting of blood to collateral venous channels causing varicosities of the hemorrhoidal and esophageal veins.

Intrahepatic causes of portal hypertension include conditions that cause obstruction of blood flow within the liver. In alcoholic cirrhosis, which is the major cause of portal hypertension, bands of fibrous tissue and fibrous nodules distort the architecture of the liver and increase the resistance to portal blood flow, which leads to portal hypertension.

Complications of portal hypertension arise from the increased pressure and dilatation of the venous channels behind the obstruction (Fig. 40-13). In addition, collateral channels open that connect the portal circulation with the systemic circulation. The major complications of the increased portal vein pressure and the opening of collateral channels are ascites, splenomegaly, and the formation of portosystemic shunts.

Ascites. Ascites occurs when the amount of fluid in the peritoneal cavity is increased, and is a late-stage manifestation of cirrhosis and portal hypertension.[42] It is not uncommon for persons with advanced cirrhosis to present

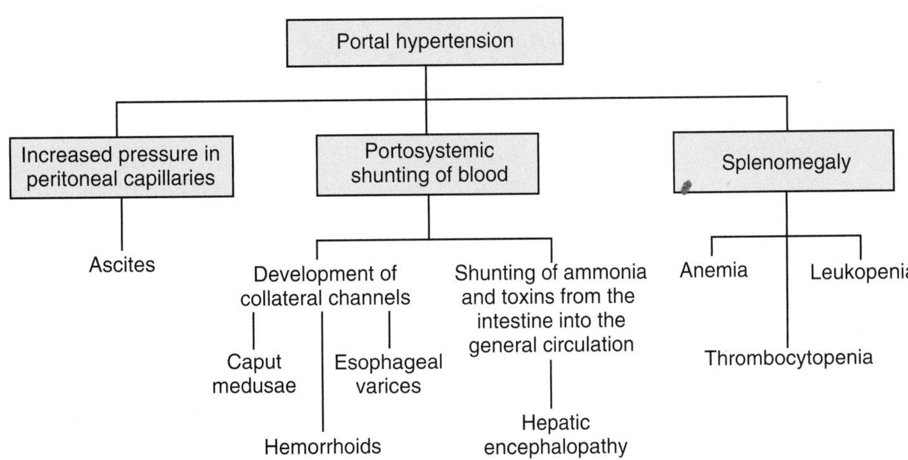

FIGURE 40-13 Mechanisms of disturbed liver function related to portal hypertension.

with an accumulation of 15 L or more of ascitic fluid. Those who gain this much fluid often experience abdominal discomfort, dyspnea, and insomnia. Some persons may have difficulty walking or living independently.[43]

Although the mechanisms responsible for the development of ascites are not completely understood, several factors seem to contribute to fluid accumulation, including an increase in capillary pressure due to portal hypertension and obstruction of venous flow through the liver, salt and water retention by the kidney, and decreased colloidal osmotic pressure due to impaired synthesis of albumin by the liver. Diminished blood volume (*i.e.,* underfill theory) and excessive blood volume (*i.e.,* overfill theory) have been used to explain the increased salt and water retention by the kidney. According to the underfill theory, a contraction in the effective blood volume constitutes an afferent signal that causes the kidney to retain salt and water. The effective blood volume may be reduced because of loss of fluid into the peritoneal cavity or because of vasodilatation caused by the presence of circulating vasodilating substances. The overfill theory proposes that the initial event in the development of ascites is renal retention of salt and water caused by disturbances in the liver itself. These disturbances include failure of the liver to metabolize aldosterone, causing an increase in salt and water retention by the kidney. Another likely contributing factor in the pathogenesis of ascites is a decreased colloidal osmotic pressure, which limits reabsorption of fluid from the peritoneal cavity (see Chapter 33).

Treatment of ascites usually focuses on dietary restriction of sodium and administration of diuretics. Water intake also may need to be restricted. Because of the many limitations in sodium restriction, the use of diuretics has become the mainstay of treatment for ascites. Two classes of diuretics are used: a diuretic that acts in the distal part of the nephron to inhibit aldosterone-dependent sodium reabsorption, and a loop diuretic such as furosemide. Oral potassium supplements often are given to prevent hypokalemia. The upright position is associated with the activation of the renin-angiotensin-aldosterone system; therefore, bed rest may be recommended for persons with a large amount of ascites.[44] Large-volume paracentesis (removal of 5 L or more of ascitic fluid) may be done in persons with massive ascites and pulmonary compromise. Because the removal of fluid produces a decrease in vascular volume along with increased plasma renin activity and aldosterone-mediated sodium and water reabsorption by the kidneys, a volume expander such as albumin usually is administered to maintain the effective circulating volume.[27] A transjugular intrahepatic portosystemic shunt may be inserted in persons with refractory ascites (discussed later).[27]

Spontaneous bacterial peritonitis is a complication in persons with both cirrhosis and ascites. The infection is serious and carries a high mortality rate even when treated with antibiotics. Presumably, the peritoneal fluid is seeded with bacteria from the blood or lymph or from passage of bacteria through the bowel wall. Symptoms include fever and abdominal pain. Other symptoms include worsening of hepatic encephalopathy, diarrhea, hypothermia, and shock. It is diagnosed by a neutrophil count of 250 cells/mm^3 or higher and a protein concentration of 1 g/dL or less in the ascitic fluid.[27]

Splenomegaly. The spleen enlarges progressively in portal hypertension because of shunting of blood into the splenic vein. The enlarged spleen often gives rise to sequestering of significant numbers of blood elements and development of a syndrome known as *hypersplenism.* Hypersplenism is characterized by a decrease in the life span and a subsequent decrease in all the formed elements of the blood, leading to anemia, thrombocytopenia, and leukopenia. The decreased life span of the blood elements is thought to result from an increased rate of removal because of the prolonged transit time through the enlarged spleen.

Portosystemic Shunts. With the gradual obstruction of venous blood flow in the liver, the pressure in the portal vein increases, and large collateral channels develop between the portal and systemic veins that supply the lower rectum and esophagus and the umbilical veins of the falciform ligament that attaches to the anterior wall of the abdomen. The collaterals between the inferior and internal iliac veins may give rise to hemorrhoids. In some persons, the fetal umbilical vein is not totally obliterated; it forms a channel on the anterior abdominal wall (Fig. 40-14). Dilated veins around the umbilicus are called *caput medusae.* Portopulmonary shunts also may develop and cause blood to bypass the pulmonary capillaries, interfering with blood oxygenation and producing cyanosis.

Clinically, the most important collateral channels are those connecting the portal and coronary veins that lead to reversal of flow and formation of thin-walled varicosities in the submucosa of the esophagus (Fig. 40-15). These thin-walled *esophageal varices* are subject to rupture, producing massive and sometimes fatal hemorrhage. Impaired hepatic synthesis of coagulation factors and decreased platelet levels (*i.e.,* thrombocytopenia) due to splenomegaly may further complicate the control of esophageal bleeding. Esophageal varices develop in approximately 65% of persons with advanced cirrhosis and cause massive hemorrhage and death in approximately half of them.[3]

Treatment of portal hypertension and esophageal varices is directed at prevention of initial hemorrhage, management of acute hemorrhage, and prevention of recurrent variceal hemorrhage. Pharmacologic therapy is used to lower portal venous pressure and prevent initial hemorrhage. β-Adrenergic–blocking drugs (*e.g.,* propranolol) commonly are used for this purpose. These agents reduce portal venous pressure by decreasing splanchnic blood flow and thereby decreasing blood flow in collateral channels. Long-acting nitrates may be used to decrease the risk for variceal rebleeding in people who cannot tolerate β-blockers.

Several methods are used to control acute hemorrhage, including administration of octreotide or vasopressin, balloon tamponade, endoscopic injection sclerotherapy, vessel ligation, or esophageal transection. Octreotide, a long-acting synthetic analog of somatostatin, reduces splanchnic and hepatic blood flow and portal pressures in persons with cirrhosis. The drug, which is given intravenously, provides control of variceal bleeding in up to

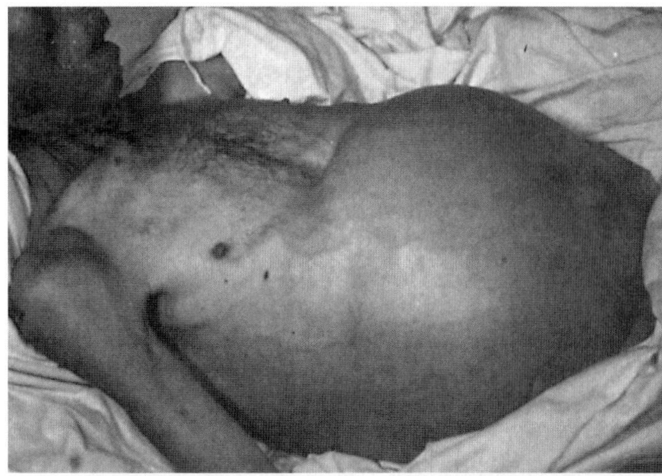

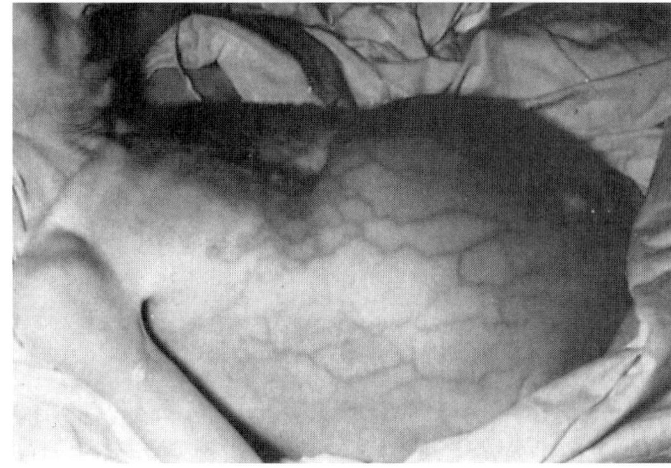

FIGURE 40-14 Collateral abdominal veins on the anterior abdominal wall in a patient with alcoholic liver disease as recorded by black and white photography (**top**) and infrared photography (**bottom**). (Schiff L. [1982]. *Diseases of the liver.* Philadelphia: J.B. Lippincott)

80% of cases. Vasopressin, a hormone from the posterior pituitary, is a nonselective vasoconstrictor that also can be used to control variceal bleeding. Because octreotide has fewer side effects and appears to be more effective than vasopressin, it has become the drug of choice for pharmacologic management of acute variceal bleeding.[45] Balloon tamponade provides compression of the varices and is accomplished through the insertion of a tube with inflatable gastric and esophageal balloons. After the tube has been inserted, the balloons are inflated; the esophageal balloon compresses the bleeding esophageal veins, and the gastric balloon helps to maintain the position of the tube. During endoscopic sclerotherapy, the varices are injected with a sclerosing solution that obliterates the vessel lumen.

Prevention of recurrent hemorrhage focuses on lowering portal venous pressure and diverting blood flow away from the easily ruptured collateral channels. Two procedures may be used for this purpose: the surgical creation of a portosystemic shunt or transjugular intrahepatic portosystemic shunt (TIPS). *Surgical portosystemic shunt* procedures involve the creation of an opening between the portal vein and a systemic vein. These shunts have a considerable complication rate, and TIPS has evolved as the preferred treatment for refractory portal hypertension. The TIPS procedure involves insertion of an expandable metal stent between a branch of the hepatic vein and the portal vein using a catheter inserted through the internal jugular vein. A limitation of the procedure is that stenosis and thrombosis of the stent occurs in most cases over time, with consequent risk for rebleeding. A complication that is associated with the creation of a portosystemic shunt is hepatic encephalopathy, which is thought to result when ammonia and other neurotoxic substances from the gut pass directly into the systemic circulation without going through the liver.

Liver Failure

The most severe clinical consequences of liver disease is hepatic failure. It may result from sudden and massive liver destruction, as in fulminant hepatitis, or be the result of progressive damage to the liver, as occurs in alcoholic cirrhosis. Whatever the cause, 80% to 90% of hepatic functional capacity must be lost before liver failure occurs.[3] In many cases, the progressive decompensating effects of the disease are hastened by intercurrent conditions such as gastrointestinal bleeding, systemic infection, electrolyte disturbances, or superimposed diseases such as heart failure.

The manifestations of liver failure reflect the various synthesis, storage, metabolic, and elimination functions of the liver (Fig. 40-16). *Fetor hepaticus* refers to a characteristic

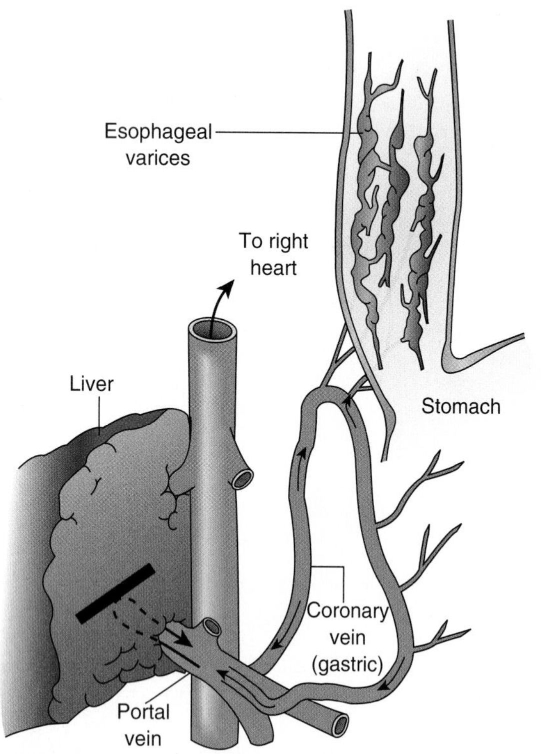

FIGURE 40-15 Obstruction of blood flow in the portal circulation, with portal hypertension and diversion of blood flow to other venous channels, including the gastric and esophageal veins.

musty, sweetish odor of the breath in the patient in advanced liver failure, resulting from the metabolic byproducts of the intestinal bacteria.

Hematologic Disorders. Liver failure can cause anemia, thrombocytopenia, coagulation defects, and leukopenia. Anemia may be caused by blood loss, excessive red blood cell destruction, and impaired formation of red blood cells. A folic acid deficiency may lead to severe megaloblastic anemia. Changes in the lipid composition of the red cell membrane increase hemolysis. Because factors V, VII, IX, X, prothrombin, and fibrinogen are synthesized by the liver, their decline in liver disease contributes to bleeding disorders. Malabsorption of the fat-soluble vitamin K contributes further to the impaired synthesis of these clotting factors. Thrombocytopenia often occurs as the result of splenomegaly. The person with liver failure is subject to purpura, easy bruising, hematuria, and abnormal menstrual bleeding, and is vulnerable to bleeding from the esophagus and other segments of the gastrointestinal tract.

Endocrine Disorders. The liver metabolizes the steroid hormones. Endocrine disorders, particularly disturbances in gonadal (sex hormone) function, are common accompaniments of cirrhosis and liver failure. Women may have menstrual irregularities (usually amenorrhea), loss of libido, and sterility. In men, testosterone levels usually fall, the testes atrophy, and loss of libido, impotence, and gynecomastia occur. A decrease in aldosterone metabolism

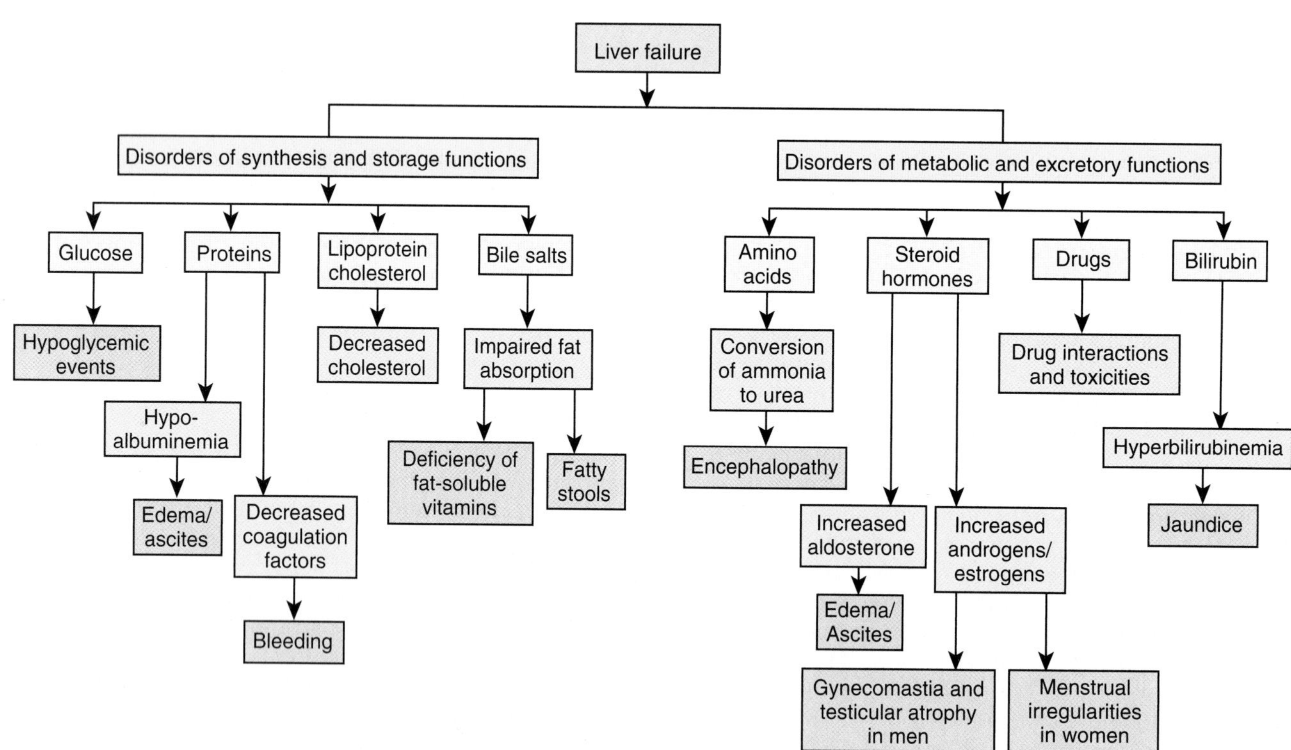

FIGURE 40-16 Alterations in liver function and manifestations of liver failure.

may contribute to salt and water retention by the kidney, along with a lowering of serum potassium resulting from increased elimination of potassium.

Skin Disorders. Liver failure brings on numerous skin disorders. These lesions, called variously *vascular spiders, telangiectases, spider angiomas,* and *spider nevi,* are seen most often in the upper half of the body. They consist of a central pulsating arteriole from which smaller vessels radiate. Palmar erythema is redness of the palms, probably caused by increased blood flow from higher cardiac output. Clubbing of the fingers may be seen in persons with cirrhosis. Jaundice usually is a late manifestation of liver failure.

Hepatorenal Syndrome. The hepatorenal syndrome refers to a functional renal failure sometimes seen during the terminal stages of liver failure with ascites.[46] It is characterized by progressive azotemia, increased serum creatinine levels, and oliguria. Although the basic cause is unknown, a decrease in renal blood flow is believed to play a part. Ultimately, when renal failure is superimposed on liver failure, azotemia and elevated levels of blood ammonia occur; this condition is thought to contribute to hepatic encephalopathy and coma.

Hepatic Encephalopathy. Hepatic encephalopathy refers to the totality of central nervous system manifestations of liver failure. It is characterized by neural disturbances ranging from a lack of mental alertness to confusion, coma, and convulsions. A very early sign of hepatic encephalopathy is a flapping tremor called *asterixis.* Various degrees of memory loss may occur, coupled with personality changes such as euphoria, irritability, anxiety, and lack of concern about personal appearance and self. Speech may be impaired, and the patient may be unable to perform certain purposeful movements. The encephalopathy may progress to decerebrate rigidity and then to a terminal deep coma.

Although the cause of hepatic encephalopathy is unknown, the accumulation of neurotoxins, which appear in the blood because the liver has lost its detoxifying capacity, is believed to be a factor. Hepatic encephalopathy develops in approximately 10% of persons with portosystemic shunts.

One of the suspected neurotoxins is ammonia. A particularly important function of the liver is the conversion of ammonia, a byproduct of protein and amino acid metabolism, to urea. The ammonium ion is produced in abundance in the intestinal tract, particularly in the colon, by the bacterial degradation of luminal proteins and amino acids. Normally, these ammonium ions diffuse into the portal blood and are transported to the liver, where they are converted to urea before entering the general circulation. When the blood from the intestine bypasses the liver or the liver is unable to convert ammonia to urea, ammonia moves directly into the general circulation and from there to the cerebral circulation. Hepatic encephalopathy may become worse after a large protein meal or gastrointestinal tract bleeding. Narcotics and tranquilizers are poorly metabolized by the liver, and administration of these drugs may cause central nervous system depression and precipitate hepatic encephalopathy.

A nonabsorbable antibiotic, such as neomycin, may be given to eradicate bacteria from the bowel and thus prevent this cause of ammonia production. Another drug that may be given is lactulose. It is not absorbed from the small intestine but moves directly to the large intestine, where it is catabolized by colonic bacteria to small organic acids that cause production of large, loose stools with a low pH. The low pH favors the conversion of ammonia to ammonium ions, which are not absorbed by the blood. The acid pH also inhibits the degradation of amino acids, proteins, and blood.

Treatment

The treatment of liver failure is directed toward eliminating alcohol intake when the condition is caused by alcoholic cirrhosis; preventing infections; providing sufficient carbohydrates and calories to prevent protein breakdown; correcting fluid and electrolyte imbalances, particularly hypokalemia; and decreasing ammonia production in the gastrointestinal tract by controlling protein intake. In many cases, liver transplantation remains the only effective treatment.

Liver transplantation rapidly is becoming a realistic form of treatment for many persons with irreversible chronic liver disease, fulminant liver failure, primary biliary cirrhosis, chronic active hepatitis, sclerosing cholangitis, and certain metabolic disorders that result in end-stage liver disease. Currently, 1-year survival rates approach 90%, and a 3-year survival rate of 80% is achieved at many transplant centers in the United States.[47] In addition to longer survival, many liver recipients are now experiencing improved quality of life, including return to active employment. Unfortunately, the shortage of donor organs severely limits the number of transplantations that are done, and many persons die each year while waiting for a transplant. During the past several years, a number of innovative ways, including split liver transplantation and living donor transplantation, have emerged as a way of dealing with the donor shortage.[47]

CANCER OF THE LIVER

Primary liver tumors are relatively rare in the United States, accounting for approximately 0.5% to 2% of all cancers.[3] The American Cancer Society estimates that more than 18,920 new cases of primary liver and intrahepatic cancer will be diagnosed during 2004, and more than 14,270 people will die of the disease during the same period.[48] In contrast to many other cancers, the number of people who develop liver cancer and die of it is increasing. Liver cancer accounts for 20% to 40% of all cancers in many other countries. The global distribution of hepatocellular carcinoma is strongly linked to HBV infection. In the Western world, where HBV is less common, 85% to 95% of hepatocellular carcinomas are associated with cirrhosis.

There are two major types of primary liver cancer: hepatocellular carcinoma, which arises from the liver cells (Fig. 40-17), and cholangiocarcinoma, which is a primary cancer of bile duct cells.[3] Hepatocellular cancer is one of the few cancers for which an underlying etiology can be identified in most cases and is unique because it usually occurs in a background of chronic liver disease.[49] Among the factors identified as etiologic agents in liver cancer are chronic viral hepatitis (HBV, HCV, HDV), cirrhosis, long-term exposure to environmental agents such as aflatoxin, and drinking water contaminated with arsenic. Just how these etiologic agents contribute to the development of liver cancer is still unclear. With HBV and HCV, both of which become integrated into the host DNA, repeated cycles of cell death and regeneration afford the potential for development of cancer-producing mutations. Aflatoxins, produced by food spoilage molds in certain areas endemic for hepatocellular carcinoma, are particularly potent carcinogenic agents.[3,50] They are activated by hepatocytes and their products incorporated into the host DNA with the potential for causing cancer-producing mutations. A particularly susceptible site for aflatoxin is the *Tp53* tumor suppressor gene (see Chapter 8).

The manifestations of hepatocellular cancer often are insidious in onset and masked by those related to cirrhosis or chronic hepatitis. The initial symptoms include weakness, anorexia, weight loss, fatigue, bloating, a sensation of abdominal fullness, and a dull, aching abdominal pain. Ascites, which often obscures weight loss, is common. Jaundice, if present, usually is mild. There may be a rapid increase in liver size and worsening of ascites in persons with preexisting cirrhosis. Usually, the liver is enlarged when these symptoms appear. Serum α-fetoprotein, a serum protein present during fetal life, normally is barely detectable in the serum after the age of 2 years, but it is present in 90% of cases of hepatocellular carcinoma.[3] Diagnostic methods include ultrasound, CT scans, and MRI. Liver biopsy is used to confirm the diagnosis.

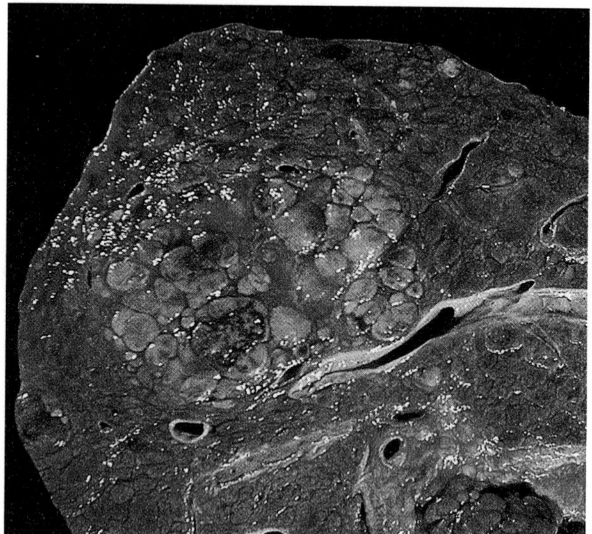

FIGURE 40-17 Hepatocellular carcinoma. Cross-section of a cirrhotic liver showing a poorly circumscribed, nodular area of yellow, partially hemorrhagic carcinoma. (Rubin E., Farber J.L. [1999]. *Pathology* [3rd ed., p. 826]. Philadelphia: Lippincott-Raven)

Cholangiocarcinoma occurs much less frequently than hepatocellular carcinoma. The etiology, clinical features, and prognosis vary considerably with the part of the biliary tree that is the site of origin. Cholangiocarcinoma is not associated with the same risk factors as hepatocellular carcinoma. Instead, most of the risk factors revolve around long-standing inflammation and injury of the bile duct epithelium. Cholangiocarcinoma often presents with pain, weight loss, anorexia, and abdominal swelling or awareness of a mass in the right hypochondrium. Tumors affecting the central or distal bile ducts may present with jaundice.

Primary cancers of the liver usually are far advanced at the time of diagnosis; the 5-year survival rate is approximately 7%.[48] The treatment of choice is subtotal hepatectomy, if conditions permit. Chemotherapy and radiation therapy are largely palliative. Although liver transplantation may be an option for people with well-compensated cirrhosis and small tumors, it often is impractical because of the shortage of donor organs.

Metastatic tumors of the liver are much more common than primary tumors. Common sources include colorectal cancer and spread from the breast, lung, or urogenital cancers. In addition, tumors of neuroendocrine origin spread to the liver. It often is difficult to distinguish primary from metastatic tumors with the use of CT scans, MRI, or ultrasonography. Usually, the diagnosis is confirmed by biopsy.

In summary, the liver is subject to most of the disease processes that affect other body structures, such as vascular disorders, inflammation, metabolic diseases, toxic injury, and neoplasms. As the major drug-metabolizing and detoxifying organ in the body, the liver is subject to potential damage from an enormous array of pharmaceutical and environmental chemicals. Drugs and chemicals can exert their effects by causing hepatocyte injury and death or by cholestatic liver damage due to injury of biliary drainage structures. Drug reactions can be predictable based on the drug's chemical structure and metabolites, or unpredictable (idiosyncratic) based on individual characteristics of the person receiving the drug. Early identification of drug-induced liver disease is important because withdrawal of the drug is curative in most cases.

Hepatitis is characterized by inflammation of the liver. Acute viral hepatitis is caused by hepatitis viruses A, B, C, D, and E. Although all these viruses cause acute hepatitis, they differ in terms of mode of transmission, incubation period, mechanism, degree and chronicity of liver damage, and the ability to evolve to a carrier state. HBV, HCV, and HDV have the potential for progression to the carrier state, chronic hepatitis, and hepatocellular carcinoma.

Intrahepatic biliary diseases disrupt the flow of bile through the liver, causing cholestasis and biliary cirrhosis. Among the causes of intrahepatic biliary diseases are primary biliary cirrhosis, primary sclerosing cholangitis, and secondary biliary cirrhosis. Because alcohol competes for use of intracellular cofactors normally needed by the liver for other metabolic processes, it tends to disrupt the metabolic functions of the liver. The spectrum of alcoholic liver disease includes fatty liver disease, alcoholic hepatitis, and cirrhosis.

Cirrhosis represents the end stage of chronic liver disease in which much of the functional liver tissue has been replaced by fibrous tissue. The fibrous tissue replaces normally functioning liver tissue and forms constrictive bands that disrupt flow in the vascular channels and biliary duct systems of the liver. The disruption of vascular channels predisposes to portal hypertension and its complications, loss of liver cells, and eventual liver failure. Portal hypertension is characterized by increased resistance to flow and increased pressure in the portal venous system; the pathologic consequences of the disorder include ascites, the formation of collateral channels between the portal and systemic veins (*e.g.,* esophageal varices). Liver failure represents the end stage of a number of liver diseases and occurs when less than 10% of liver tissue is functional. The manifestations of liver failure reflect the various functions of the liver, including hematologic disorders, disruption of endocrine function, skin disorders, hepatorenal syndrome, and hepatic encephalopathy.

Cancers of the liver include metastatic and primary neoplasms. Primary hepatic neoplasms are rare, accounting for less than 2% of cancers, and those involving the hepatocytes or liver cells are commonly associated with underlying diseases of the liver such as cirrhosis and chronic hepatitis. Liver cancer usually is usually far advanced at the time of diagnosis.

Disorders of the Gallbladder and Exocrine Pancreas

After completing this section of the chapter, you should be able to meet the following objectives:

- ✦ Explain the function of the gallbladder in regulating the flow of bile into the duodenum
- ✦ Describe the formation of gallstones
- ✦ Describe the clinical manifestations of acute and chronic cholecystitis
- ✦ Characterize the effects of choledocholithiasis and cholangitis on bile flow and the potential for hepatic and pancreatic complications
- ✦ Cite the possible causes and describe the manifestations and treatment of acute pancreatitis
- ✦ Describe the manifestations of chronic pancreatitis
- ✦ State the reason for the poor prognosis in pancreatic cancer

DISORDERS OF THE GALLBLADDER AND EXTRAHEPATIC BILE DUCTS

The so-called hepatobiliary system consists of the gallbladder; the left and right hepatic ducts, which come together to form the common hepatic duct; the cystic duct, which extends to the gallbladder; and the common bile duct, which is formed by the union of the common hepatic duct and the cystic duct (Fig. 40-18). The common bile duct

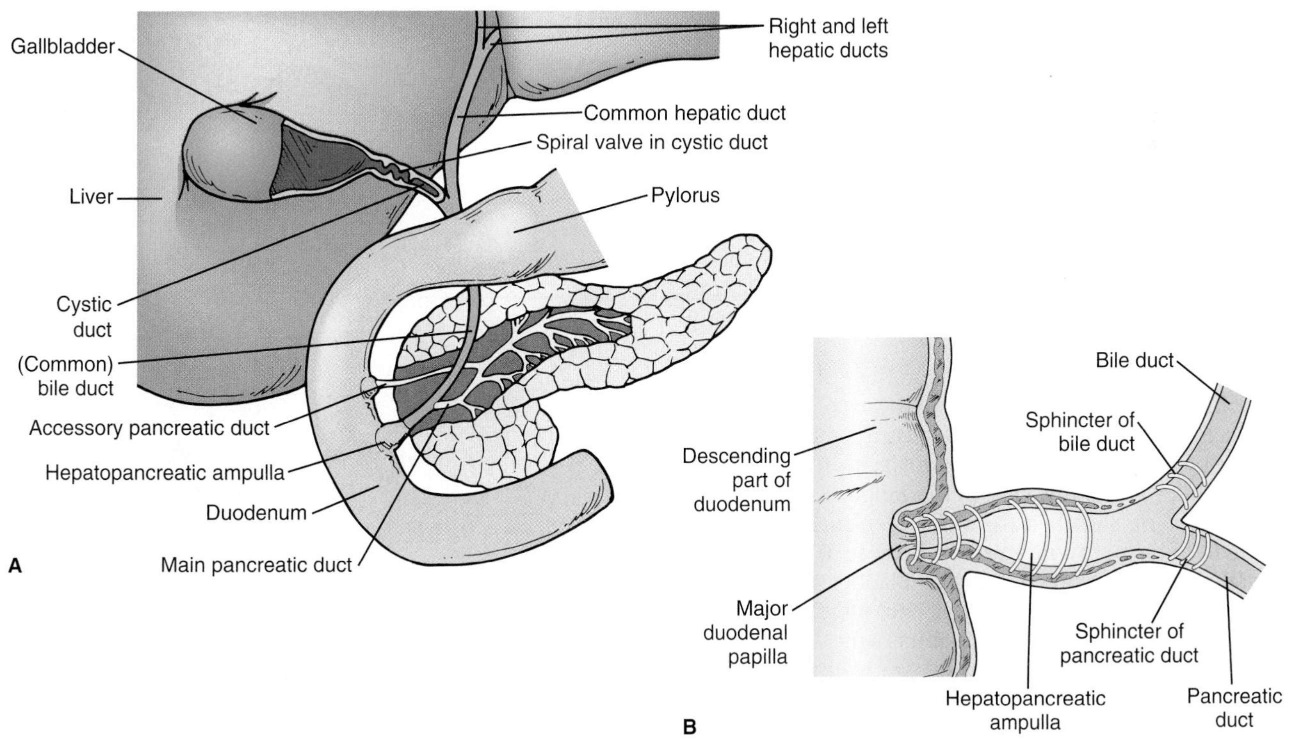

FIGURE 40-18 **(A)** Extrahepatic bile passages, gall bladder, and pancreatic ducts. **(B)** Entry of bile duct and pancreatic duct into the hepatopancreatic ampulla, which opens into the duodenum.

descends posterior to the first part of the duodenum, where it comes in contact with the main pancreatic duct. These ducts unite to form the hepatopancreatic ampulla. The circular muscle around the distal end of the bile duct is thickened to form the sphincter of the bile duct (see Fig. 40-18).

The gallbladder is a distensible, pear-shaped, muscular sac located on the ventral surface of the liver. It has an outer serous peritoneal layer, a middle smooth muscle layer, and an inner mucosal layer that is continuous with the linings of the bile duct. The function of the gallbladder is to store and concentrate bile.

Entrance of food into the intestine causes the gallbladder to contract and the sphincter of the bile duct to relax, such that bile stored in the gallbladder moves into the duodenum. The stimulus for gallbladder contraction is primarily hormonal. Products of food digestion, particularly lipids, stimulate the release of a gastrointestinal hormone called *cholecystokinin* from the mucosa of the duodenum. Cholecystokinin provides a strong stimulus for gallbladder contraction. The role of other gastrointestinal hormones in bile release is less clearly understood.

Passage of bile into the intestine is regulated largely by the pressure in the common duct. Normally, the gallbladder regulates this pressure. It collects and stores bile as it relaxes and the pressure in the common bile duct decreases, and it empties bile into the intestine as the gallbladder contracts, producing an increase in common duct pressure. After gallbladder surgery, the pressure in the common duct changes, causing the common duct to dilate. The flow of bile then is regulated by the sphincters in the common duct.

Two common disorders of the biliary system are cholelithiasis (*i.e.,* gallstones) and inflammation of the gallbladder (cholecystitis) or common bile duct (cholangitis). At least 10% of adults have gallstones.[51,52] Approximately twice as many women as men have gallstones, and there is an increased prevalence with age—after 60 years of age, 10% to 15% among men and 20% to 40% among women.[53]

Cholelithiasis

Cholelithiasis, or gallstones, is caused by precipitation of substances contained in bile, mainly cholesterol and bilirubin. Bile contains bile salts, cholesterol, bilirubin, lecithin, fatty acids, and water and the electrolytes normally found in the plasma. The cholesterol found in bile has no known function; it is assumed to be a byproduct of bile salt formation, and its presence is linked to the excretory function of bile. Normally insoluble in water, cholesterol is rendered soluble by the action of bile salts and lecithin, which combine with it to form micelles. In the gallbladder, water and electrolytes are absorbed from the liver bile, causing the bile to become more concentrated. Because neither lecithin nor bile salts are absorbed in the gallbladder, their concentration increases along with that of cholesterol; in this way, the solubility of cholesterol is maintained.

The bile of which gallstones are formed usually is supersaturated with cholesterol or bilirubinate. Approximately 80% of gallstones are composed primarily of cholesterol; the other 20% are black or brown pigment stones consisting of calcium salts with bilirubin.[51] Many stones have a mixed composition. Figure 40-19 shows a gallbladder with numerous cholesterol gallstones.

Three factors contribute to the formation of gallstones: abnormalities in the composition of bile, stasis of bile, and inflammation of the gallbladder. The formation of cholesterol stones is associated with obesity and occurs more frequently in women, especially women who have had multiple pregnancies or who are taking oral contraceptives. All of these factors cause the liver to excrete more cholesterol into the bile. Estrogen reduces the synthesis of bile acid in women. Gallbladder sludge (thickened gallbladder mucoprotein with tiny trapped cholesterol crystals) is thought to be a precursor of gallstones. Sludge frequently occurs with pregnancy, starvation, and rapid weight loss.[51] Drugs that lower serum cholesterol levels, such as clofibrate, also cause increased cholesterol excretion into the bile. Malabsorption disorders stemming from ileal disease or intestinal bypass surgery, for example, tend to interfere with the absorption of bile salts, which are needed to maintain the solubility of cholesterol. Inflammation of the gallbladder alters the absorptive characteristics of the mucosal layer, allowing excessive absorption of water and bile salts. Cholesterol gallstones are extremely common among Native Americans, which suggests that a genetic component may have a role in gallstone formation. Pigment stones containing bilirubin are seen in persons with hemolytic disease (*e.g.,* sickle cell disease) and hepatic cirrhosis.

Many persons with gallstones have no symptoms. Gallstones cause symptoms when they obstruct bile flow. Small stones (*e.g.,* <8 mm in diameter) pass into the common duct, producing symptoms of indigestion and biliary

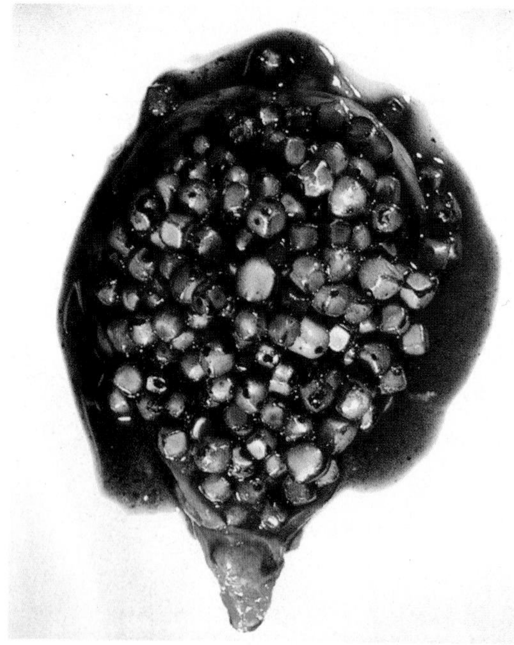

FIGURE 40-19 Cholesterol gallstones. The gallbladder has been opened to reveal numerous yellow cholesterol gallstones (Rubin E., Farber J.L. [1999]. *Pathology* [3rd ed., p. 791]. Philadelphia: Lippincott-Raven)

colic. Larger stones are more likely to obstruct flow and cause jaundice. The pain of biliary colic usually is abrupt in onset and increases steadily in intensity until it reaches a climax in 30 to 60 minutes. The upper right quadrant, or epigastric area, is the usual location of the pain, often with referred pain to the back, above the waist, the right shoulder, and the right scapula or the midscapular region. A few persons experience pain on the left side. The pain usually persists for 2 to 8 hours and is followed by soreness in the upper right quadrant.

Acute and Chronic Cholecystitis

The term *cholecystitis* refers to inflammation of the gallbladder. Both the acute and chronic forms of cholecystitis are associated with cholelithiasis. Acute cholecystitis may be superimposed on chronic cholecystitis.

Acute cholecystitis almost always is associated with complete or partial obstruction. It is believed that the inflammation is caused by chemical irritation from the concentrated bile, along with mucosal swelling and ischemia resulting from venous congestion and lymphatic stasis. The gallbladder usually is markedly distended. Bacterial infections may arise secondary to the ischemia and chemical irritation. The bacteria reach the injured gallbladder through the blood, lymphatics, or bile ducts or from adjacent organs. Among the common pathogens are staphylococci and enterococci. The wall of the gallbladder is most vulnerable to the effects of ischemia, as a result of which mucosal necrosis and sloughing occur. The process may lead to gangrenous changes and perforation of the gallbladder.

Chronic cholecystitis results from repeated episodes of acute cholecystitis or chronic irritation of the gallbladder by stones. It is characterized by varying degrees of chronic inflammation. Gallstones almost always are present. Cholelithiasis with chronic cholecystitis may be associated with acute exacerbations of gallbladder inflammation, common duct stones, pancreatitis, and, rarely, carcinoma of the gallbladder.

Manifestations. The signs and symptoms of acute cholecystitis vary with the severity of obstruction and inflammation. Pain, initially similar to that of biliary colic, is characteristic of acute cholecystitis. It often is precipitated by a fatty meal and may initiate with complaints of indigestion. It does not, however, subside spontaneously and responds poorly or only temporarily to potent analgesics. When the inflammation progresses to involve the peritoneum, the pain becomes more pronounced in the right upper quadrant. The right subcostal region is tender, and the muscles that surround the area spasm. Approximately 75% of patients have vomiting, and approximately 25% have jaundice.[51] Fever and an abnormally high white blood cell count attest to inflammation. Total serum bilirubin, aminotransferase, and alkaline phosphatase levels usually are elevated.

The manifestations of chronic cholecystitis are more vague than those of acute cholecystitis. There may be intolerance to fatty foods, belching, and other indications of discomfort. Often, there are episodes of colicky pain with obstruction of biliary flow caused by gallstones. The gallbladder, which in chronic cholecystitis usually contains stones, may be enlarged, shrunken, or of normal size.

Diagnosis and Treatment. The methods used to diagnose gallbladder disease include ultrasonography and cholescintigraphy (nuclear scanning).[52] Ultrasonography is widely used in diagnosing gallbladder disease and has largely replaced the oral cholecystogram in most medical centers. It can detect stones as small as 1 to 2 cm, and its overall accuracy in detecting gallbladder disease is high. In addition to stones, ultrasonography can detect wall thickening, which indicates inflammation. It also can rule out other causes of right upper quadrant pain such as tumors. Cholescintigraphy, also called a *gallbladder scan,* relies on the ability of the liver to extract a rapidly injected radionuclide, technetium-99m, bound to one of several iminodiacetic acids, that is excreted into the bile ducts. Serial scanning images are obtained within several minutes of the injection of the tracer and every 10 to 15 minutes during the next hour. The gallbladder scan is highly accurate in detecting acute cholecystitis.

Gallbladder disease usually is treated by removing the gallbladder. The gallbladder stores and concentrates bile, and its removal usually does not interfere with digestion. Laparoscopic cholecystectomy has become the treatment of choice for symptomatic gallbladder disease.[52] The procedure involves insertion of a laparoscope through a small incision near the umbilicus, and surgical instruments are inserted through several stab wounds in the upper abdomen. Although the procedure requires more time than the older open surgical procedure, it usually requires only 1 night in the hospital. A major advantage of the procedure is that patients can return to work in 1 to 2 weeks, compared with 4 to 6 weeks after open cholecystectomy.

Choledocholithiasis and Cholangitis

Choledocholithiasis refers to stones in the common duct and *cholangitis* to inflammation of the common duct. Common duct stones usually originate in the gallbladder, but can form spontaneously in the common duct. The stones frequently are clinically silent unless there is obstruction.

The manifestations of choledocholithiasis are similar to those of gallstones and acute cholecystitis. There is a history of acute biliary colic and right upper abdominal pain, with chills, fever, and jaundice associated with episodes of abdominal pain. Bilirubinuria and an elevated serum bilirubin are present if the common duct is obstructed.

Complications include acute suppurative cholangitis accompanied by pus in the common duct. It is characterized by the presence of an altered sensorium, lethargy, and septic shock.[51] Acute suppurative cholangitis represents an endoscopic or surgical emergency. Common duct stones also can obstruct the outflow of the pancreatic duct, causing a secondary pancreatitis.

Diagnosis and Treatment. Ultrasonography, CT scans, and radionuclide imaging may be used to demonstrate dilatation of bile ducts and impaired blood flow. Endoscopic ultrasonography and magnetic resonance cholangiography are used for detecting common duct stones. Both percutaneous transhepatic cholangiography (PTC) and endoscopic retrograde cholangiopancreatography (ERCP) provide a direct means for determining the cause, location, and extent of obstruction. PTC involves the injection of dye directly into the biliary tree. It requires the insertion of a thin, flexible needle through a small incision in the skin with advancement into the biliary tree. ERCP involves the passage of an endoscope into the duodenum and the passage of a catheter into the hepatopancreatic ampulla. ERCP can be used to enlarge the opening of the sphincter of the pancreatic duct, which may allow the lodged stone to pass, or an instrument may be inserted into the common duct to remove the stone.

Common duct stones in persons with cholelithiasis usually are treated by stone extraction followed by laparoscopic cholecystectomy. Antibiotic therapy, with an agent that penetrates the bile, is used to treat the infection. Emergency decompression of the common duct, usually by ERCP, may be necessary for persons who are septic or fail to improve with antibiotic treatment.

Cancer of the Gallbladder

Cancer of the gallbladder is the fifth most common cancer of the gastrointestinal tract. It is slightly more common in women and occurs most often in the seventh decade of life. The onset of symptoms usually is insidious, and they resemble those of cholecystitis; the diagnosis often is made unexpectedly at the time of gallbladder surgery. About 80% to 85% of persons with gallbladder cancer have cholelithiasis.[52] Because of its ability to produce chronic irritation of the gallbladder mucosa, it is believed that cholelithiasis plays a role in the development of gallbladder cancer. It is seldom resectable at the time of diagnosis, and the mean 5-year survival rate has remained a dismal 1% for many years.[3]

DISORDERS OF THE EXOCRINE PANCREAS

The pancreas lies transversely in the posterior part of the upper abdomen. The head of the pancreas is at the right of the abdomen; it rests against the curve of the duodenum in the area of the hepatopancreatic ampulla and its entrance into the duodenum. The body of the pancreas lies beneath the stomach. The tail touches the spleen. The pancreas is virtually hidden because of its posterior position; unlike many other organs, it cannot be palpated. Because of the position of the pancreas and its large functional reserve, symptoms from conditions such as cancer of the pancreas do not usually appear until the disorder is far advanced.

The pancreas is both an endocrine and exocrine organ. Its function as an endocrine organ is discussed in Chapter 43. The exocrine pancreas is made up of lobules that consist of acinar cells, which secrete digestive enzymes into a system of microscopic ducts. These ducts empty into the main pancreatic duct, which extends from left to right through the substance of the pancreas. The main pancreatic duct and the bile duct unite to form the hepatopancreatic ampulla, which empties into the duodenum. The sphincter of the pancreatic duct controls the flow of pancreatic secretions into the duodenum (see Fig. 40-18).

The pancreatic secretions contain proteolytic enzymes that break down dietary proteins, including trypsin, chymotrypsin, carboxypolypeptidase, ribonuclease, and deoxyribonuclease. The pancreas also secretes pancreatic amylase, which breaks down starch, and lipases, which hydrolyze neutral fats into glycerol and fatty acids. The pancreatic enzymes are secreted in the inactive form and become activated in the intestine. This is important because the enzymes would digest the tissue of the pancreas itself if they were secreted in the active form. The acinar cells secrete a trypsin inhibitor, which prevents trypsin activation. Because trypsin activates other proteolytic enzymes, the trypsin inhibitor prevents subsequent activation of those other enzymes.

Two types of pancreatic disease are discussed in this chapter: acute and chronic pancreatitis and cancer of the pancreas.

Acute Pancreatitis

Acute pancreatitis is a severe, life-threatening disorder associated with the escape of activated pancreatic enzymes into the pancreas and surrounding tissues. These enzymes cause fat necrosis, or autodigestion, of the pancreas and produce fatty deposits in the abdominal cavity with hemorrhage from the necrotic vessels. Although a number of factors are associated with the development of acute pancreatitis, most cases result from gallstones (stones in the common duct) or alcohol abuse.[53–55] In the case of biliary tract obstruction due to gallstones, pancreatic duct obstruction or biliary reflux is believed to activate the enzymes in the pancreatic duct system. The precise mechanisms whereby alcohol exerts its action are largely unknown. Alcohol is known to be a potent stimulator of pancreatic secretions, and it also is known to cause partial obstruction of the sphincter of the pancreatic duct. Acute pancreatitis also is associated with hyperlipidemia, hyperparathyroidism, infections (particularly viral), abdominal and surgical trauma, and drugs such as steroids and thiazide diuretics.

The onset of acute pancreatitis usually is abrupt and dramatic, and it may follow a heavy meal or an alcoholic binge. The most common initial symptom is severe epigastric and abdominal pain that radiates to the back. The pain is aggravated when the person is lying supine; it is less severe when the person is sitting and leaning forward. Abdominal distention accompanied by hypoactive bowel sounds is common. An important disturbance related to acute pancreatitis is the loss of a large volume of fluid into the retroperitoneal and peripancreatic spaces and the abdominal cavity. Tachycardia, hypotension, cool and clammy skin, and fever often are evident. Signs of hypocalcemia may develop, probably as a result of the precipitation of serum calcium in the areas of fat necrosis. Mild jaundice may appear after the first 24 hours because of biliary obstruction.

Total serum amylase is the test used most frequently in the diagnosis of acute pancreatitis. Serum amylase levels rise within the first 24 hours after onset of symptoms and remain elevated for 48 to 72 hours. The serum lipase level also is elevated during the first 24 to 48 hours, but remains elevated for 5 to 14 days. Urinary clearance of amylase is increased. Because the serum amylase level may be elevated as a result of other serious illnesses, the urinary level of amylase is often measured. The white blood cell count may be increased, and hyperglycemia and an elevated serum bilirubin level may be present. Plain radiographs of the abdomen may be used for detecting gallstones or abdominal complications. CT scans and dynamic contrast-enhanced CT of the pancreas are used to detect necrosis and fluid accumulation.

Complications include acute respiratory distress syndrome and acute tubular necrosis. Hypocalcemia occurs in approximately 25% of patients. Age older than 55 years, elevated white blood cell count (>16,000 cells/μL), and elevated levels of blood glucose (>200 mg/dL), serum lactate dehydrogenase (>350 IU/L), and AST (>250 IU/L) at the time of diagnosis are associated with a poorer prognosis, as are a decrease in hematocrit and serum calcium, increased fluid sequestration (>6 L), arterial oxygen tension less than 60 mm Hg, and a base deficit greater than 4 mEq/L that develop within the first 48 hours.[54]

The treatment consists of measures directed at pain relief, "putting the pancreas to rest," and restoration of lost plasma volume. Antibiotic prophylaxis is used to prevent infection of necrotic pancreatic tissue. Meperidine (Demerol), rather than morphine, usually is given for pain relief because it causes fewer spasms of the sphincter of the pancreatic duct. Papaverine, nitroglycerin, barbiturates, or anticholinergic drugs may be given as supplements to provide smooth muscle relaxation. Oral foods and fluids are withheld, and gastric suction is instituted to treat distention of the bowel and prevent further stimulation of the secretion of pancreatic enzymes. Intravenous fluids and electrolytes are administered to replace those lost from the circulation and to combat hypotension and shock. Intravenous colloid solutions are given to replace the fluid that has become sequestered in the abdomen and retroperitoneal space. Percutaneous peritoneal lavage has been tried as an early treatment of acute pancreatitis with encouraging results. If a pancreatic abscess develops, it must be drained, usually through the flank.

A pseudocyst is a collection of pancreatic fluid in the peritoneal cavity enclosed in a layer of inflammatory tissue (Fig. 40-20). Autodigestion or liquefaction of pancreatic tissue may be the cause. The pseudocyst most often is connected to a pancreatic duct, so that it continues to increase in mass. The symptoms depend on its location; for example, jaundice may occur when a cyst develops near the head of the pancreas, close to the common duct. Pseudocysts may resolve or, if they persist, may require surgical intervention.

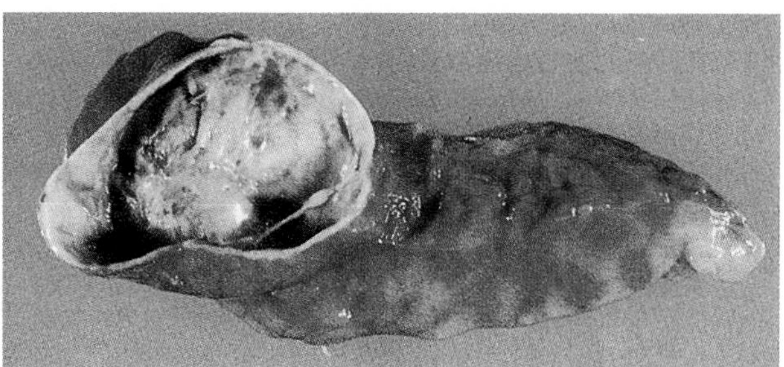

FIGURE 40-20 Pancreatic pseudocyst. A cystic cavity arises from the head of the pancreas. (Rubin E., Farber J.L. [1999]. *Pathology* [3rd ed., p. 847]. Philadelphia: Lippincott-Raven)

Chronic Pancreatitis

Chronic pancreatitis is characterized by progressive destruction of the pancreas. It can be divided into two types: chronic calcifying pancreatitis and chronic obstructive pancreatitis.[56] In chronic calcifying pancreatitis, calcified protein plugs (*i.e.,* calculi) form in the pancreatic ducts. This form is seen most often in alcoholics. Alcohol damages pancreatic cells directly and also increases the concentration of proteins in the pancreatic secretions, which eventually leads to formation of protein plugs.[57] Other causes of chronic pancreatitis are cystic fibrosis and chronic obstructive pancreatitis owing to stenosis of the sphincter of the pancreatic duct. In obstructive pancreatitis, lesions are more prominent in the head of the pancreas. The disease usually is caused by cholelithiasis and sometimes is relieved by removal the stones.

Chronic pancreatitis is manifested in episodes that are similar, albeit of lesser severity, to those of acute pancreatitis. Patients have persistent, recurring episodes of epigastric and upper left quadrant pain; the attacks often are precipitated by alcohol abuse or overeating. Anorexia, nausea, vomiting, constipation, and flatulence are common. Eventually, the disease progresses to the extent that endocrine and exocrine pancreatic functions become deficient. At this point, signs of diabetes mellitus and the malabsorption syndrome (*e.g.,* weight loss, fatty stools [steatorrhea]) become apparent.

Treatment consists of measures to treat coexisting biliary tract disease. A low-fat diet usually is prescribed. The signs of malabsorption may be treated with pancreatic enzymes. When diabetes is present, it is treated with insulin. Alcohol is forbidden because it frequently precipitates attacks. Because of the frequent episodes of pain, narcotic addiction is a potential problem in persons with chronic pancreatitis. Surgical intervention sometimes is needed to relieve the pain and usually focuses on relieving any obstruction that may be present. In advanced cases, a subtotal or total pancreatectomy may be necessary.[51]

Cancer of the Pancreas

Pancreatic cancer is now the fourth leading cause of death in the United States, with more than 28,000 deaths attributed to the neoplasm each year.[58] Considered to be one of the most deadly malignancies, pancreatic cancer is associated with a death : incidence ratio of approximately 0.99. The risk for pancreatic cancer increases after the age of 50 years, with most cases occurring between the ages of 60 and 80 years. The incidence and mortality rates for both male and female African Americans are higher than for whites.

The cause of pancreatic cancer is unknown. Smoking appears to be a major risk factor.[58,59] The incidence of pancreatic cancer is twice as high among smokers than nonsmokers. The second most important factor appears to be diet. There appears to be an association of pancreatic cancer with an increasing total calorie intake and a high intake of fat, meat, salt, dehydrated foods, fried foods, refined sugars, soy beans, and nitrosamines. Data from animal studies indicate that nitrosamines and tobacco smoke are carcinogenic in the pancreas. A protective effect has been ascribed to a diet containing dietary fiber, vitamin C, fresh fruits and vegetables, and no preservatives. Diabetes and chronic pancreatitis also are associated with pancreatic cancer, although neither the nature nor the sequence of the possible cause-and-effect relation has been established.[59,60] Genetic alterations appear to play a role. There appears to be an association between pancreatic cancer and certain genetic disorders, including nonpolyposis colon cancer, familial breast cancer with the *BRCA2* gene mutation (see Chapter 8), ataxia-telangiectasia syndrome, familial atypical multiple mole–melanoma syndrome, and hereditary pancreatitis.[58] There has been a recent focus on the molecular genetics of pancreatic cancer, and more insights into the genetic mechanisms involved in pancreatic cancer undoubtedly will be forthcoming.

Cancer of the pancreas usually has an insidious onset. Pain, jaundice, and weight loss constitute the classic presentation of the disease. The most common pain is a dull epigastric pain often accompanied by back pain, often worse in the supine position, and relieved by sitting forward. Duodenal obstruction with nausea and vomiting is a late sign.

Because of the proximity of the pancreas to the common duct and the hepatopancreatic ampulla, cancer of the head of the pancreas tends to obstruct bile flow; this causes distention of the gallbladder and jaundice. Jaundice frequently is the presenting symptom of a person with cancer of the head of the pancreas, and it usually is accompanied by complaints of pain and pruritus. Cancer of the body of the pancreas usually impinges on the celiac ganglion, causing pain. The pain usually worsens with ingestion of food or with assumption of the supine position. Cancer of the tail of the pancreas usually has metastasized before symptoms appear.

Ultrasonography and CT scanning are the most frequently used diagnostic methods to confirm the disease. Intravenous and oral contrast-enhanced spiral CT is the preferred method for imaging the pancreas. Percutaneous fine-needle aspiration cytology of the pancreas has been one of the major advances in the diagnosis of pancreatic cancer. Unfortunately, the smaller and more curable tumors are most likely to be missed by this procedure. ERCP may be used for evaluation of persons with suspected pancreatic cancer and obstructive jaundice.

Most cancers of the pancreas have metastasized by the time of diagnosis. Surgical resection of the tumor is done when the tumor is localized, or as a palliative measure. Radiation therapy may be useful when the disease is not resectable but appears to be localized. The use of irradiation and chemotherapy for pancreatic cancer continues to be investigated. Pain control is one of the most important aspects in the management of persons with end-stage pancreatic cancer.

In summary, the biliary tract serves as a passageway for the delivery of bile from the liver to the intestine. This tract consists of the bile ducts and gallbladder. The most common causes of biliary tract disease are cholelithiasis and cholecystitis. Three factors contribute to the development of cholelithiasis: abnormalities in the composition of bile, stasis of bile, and inflammation of the gallbladder. Cholelithiasis predisposes to obstruction of bile flow, causing biliary colic and acute or chronic cholecystitis. Cancer of the gallbladder is the fifth most common cancer of the gastrointestinal tract. it is usually associated with cholelithiasis and has a poor 5-year survival rate.

The pancreas is an endocrine and exocrine organ. Diabetes mellitus is the most common disorder of the endocrine pancreas, and it occurs independently of disease of the exocrine pancreas. The exocrine pancreas produces digestive enzymes that are secreted in an inactive form and transported to the small intestine through the main pancreatic duct, which usually empties into the hepatopancreatic ampulla and then into the duodenum through the sphincter of the pancreatic duct. The most common diseases of the exocrine pancreas are acute and chronic forms of pancreatitis, and cancer. Acute and chronic types of pancreatitis are associated with biliary reflux and chronic alcoholism. Acute pancreatitis is a dramatic and life-threatening disorder in which there is autodigestion of pancreatic tissue. Chronic pancreatitis causes progressive destruction of the endocrine and exocrine pancreas. It is characterized by episodes of pain and epigastric distress that are similar to but less severe than those that occur with acute pancreatitis. Cancer of the pancreas is the fourth leading cause of death in the United States.

REVIEW EXERCISES

A 24-year-old woman reports to her health care provider with complaints of yellow discoloration to her skin, loss of appetite, and a feeling of upper gastric discomfort. She denies the use of intravenous drugs and has not received blood products. She cannot recall eating uncooked shellfish or drinking water that might be contaminated. She has a daughter who attends day care.

A. What tests could be used to confirm a diagnosis of hepatitis A?

B. What is the most common mode of transmission for hepatitis A? It is suggested that the source of her infection could be through the day care that her daughter attends. Explain.

C. What methods could be used to protect other family members from getting the disease?

A 56-year-old man with a history of heavy alcohol consumption and a previous diagnosis of alcoholic cirrhosis and portal hypertension is admitted to the emergency room with acute gastrointestinal hemorrhage and signs of circulatory shock.

A. Relate the development of esophageal varices to portal hypertension in persons with cirrhosis of the liver.

B. Many persons with bleeding esophageal varices have accompanying blood coagulation problems. Explain.

C. What are the possible treatment measures for this man, both in terms of controlling the current bleeding episode and preventing further bleeding episodes?

A 46-year-old woman presents in the emergency room with sudden onset of vomiting and severe right epigastric pain that developed after eating a fatty evening meal. Although there is no evidence of jaundice to her skin, the sclera of her eyes is noted to have a yellowish discoloration. Palpation reveals tenderness in the right upper quadrant with associated muscle guarding and rebound pain. Right upper quadrant abdominal ultrasound confirms the presence of gallstones. The woman is treated conservatively with pain and antiemetic medications. She is subsequently scheduled for a laparoscopic cholecystectomy.

A. Relate this woman's signs and symptoms to gallstones and their effect on gallbladder function.

B. Explain the initial appearance of jaundice in the sclera of the eyes as opposed to the skin. Which of the two laboratory tests for bilirubin would you expect to be elevated—direct (conjugated) or indirect (unconjugated or free)?

C. What effect will removal of the gallbladder have on the storage and release of bile into the intestine, particularly as it relates to meals?

References

1. Guyton A., Hall J.E. (2000). *Textbook of medical physiology* (10th ed., pp. 781–802). Philadelphia: W.B. Saunders.
2. Rose S. (1998). *Gastrointestinal and hepatic pathophysiology.* Madison, CT: Fence Creek Publishing.
3. Crawford J.M. (2003). The liver and biliary tract. In Kumar V., Cotran R.S., Robbins S.L. (Eds.), *Robbins pathologic basis of disease* (7th ed., pp. 592–627). Philadelphia: W.B. Saunders.
4. Rubin E., Farber J.L. (1999). The liver and biliary system. In Rubin E., Farber J.L. (Eds.), *Pathophysiology* (3rd ed., pp. 757–838). Philadelphia: Lippincott-Raven.
5. Denery P.A., Seidman D.S., Stevenson D.K. (2001). Neonatal hyperbilirubinemia. *New England Journal of Medicine 344,* 581–590.
6. Pratt D.S., Kaplan M.M. (2000). Evaluation of abnormal liver-enzyme results in asymptomatic patients. *New England Journal of Medicine 342,* 1266–1271.
7. Bravo A., Sheth S.G., Chopra S. (2001). Liver biopsy. *New England Journal of Medicine 344,* 495–500.
8. Katzung B.G. (2001). *Basic and clinical pharmacology* (8th ed., pp. 51–63). New York: Lange Medical Books/McGraw-Hill.
9. Lee W.M. (1995). Drug-induced hepatotoxicity. *New England Journal of Medicine 333,* 1118–1127.
10. Lewis J.H. (2000). Drug-induced liver disease. *Medical Clinics of North America 84,* 1275–1311.
11. Ostapowicz G., Fontana F.J., Schiøtz F.V., et al. (2002). Results of a prospective study of acute liver failure at 17 tertiary care centers in the United States. *Annals of Internal Medicine 137,* 947–954.
12. Lee W.M. (2003). Drug-induced hepatotoxicity. *New England Journal of Medicine 349*(5), 474–485.
13. Marsano L.S. (2003). Hepatitis. *Primary Care 30,* 81–107.
14. Kemmer N.M., Miskovsky E.P. (2000). Hepatitis A. *Infectious Disease Clinics of North America 14,* 605–615.
15. Advisory Committee on Immunization Practices. (1999). Prevention of hepatitis A through active and passive immunization. *Morbidity and Mortality Weekly Report 48* (RR-12), 1–25.
16. Lee W.M. (1997). Hepatitis B virus infection. *New England Journal of Medicine 337,* 1733–1745.
17. Befeler A.S., DiBisceglie A.M. (2000). Hepatitis B. *Infectious Disease Clinics of North America 14,* 617–632.
18. Centers for Disease Control. (2003). Incidence of acute hepatitis B–United States, 1990–2002. *Morbidity and Mortality Weekly Report 52*(52), 1252–1254.
19. Advisory Committee on Immunization Practices. (1991). Hepatitis B: A comprehensive strategy for eliminating transmission in the United States through Universal Childhood Vaccination. *Morbidity and Mortality Weekly Report 40*(RR-13), 1–25.
20. Lemon S.M., Thomas D.L. (1997). Vaccines to prevent viral hepatitis. *New England Journal of Medicine 336,* 196–203.
21. Advisory Committee on Immunization Practices. (1999). Notice to readers update: Recommendations to prevent hepatitis B transmission—United States. *Morbidity and Mortality Weekly Report 48*(2), 33–34.
22. National Institutes of Health. (2002). National Institutes of Health Consensus Development Conference Statement: Management of Hepatitis C. *Gastroenterology 123,* 476–482.
23. Lauer G.M., Walker R.D. (2001). Hepatitis C infection. *New England Journal of Medicine 345*(1), 41–52.
24. Liang T.J., Reheman B., Seeff L.B., Hoffnagle J.H. (2000). Pathogenesis, natural history, treatment, and prevention of hepatitis C. *Annals of Internal Medicine 132,* 296–305.
25. Cheney C.P., Chopra S., Graham C. (2000). Hepatitis C. *Infectious Disease Clinics of North America 14,* 633–659.
26. Hoffnagle J.H. (1989). Type D (delta) hepatitis. *Journal of the American Medical Association 261,* 1321–1325.
27. Friedman S. (2003). Liver, biliary tract and pancreas. In Tierney L.M., McPhee S.J., Papadakis M.A. (Eds.), *Current medical diagnosis and treatment* (42nd ed., 631–641, 644–651, 657–666). New York: Lange Medical Books/McGraw-Hill.
28. Davis G.L. (2002). Update on the management of chronic hepatitis B. *Reviews in Gastroenterological Disorders 2*(3), 10–115.
29. Russo M.W., Zacks S.L., Fried M.W. (2003). Management of newly diagnosed hepatitis C infection. *Cleveland Clinic Journal of Medicine 70*(Suppl. 4), S14–S20.
30. Krawitt E.L. (1996). Autoimmune hepatitis. *New England Journal of Medicine 334,* 897–902.
31. Talwalker J.A. (2003). Primary biliary cirrhosis. *Lancet 362,* 53–61.
32. Kaplan M.M. (1996). Primary biliary cirrhosis. *New England Journal of Medicine 335,* 1570–1580.
33. Lee Y-M., Kaplan M.M. (1995). Primary sclerosing cholangitis. *New England Journal of Medicine 332,* 924–932.
34. Lieber C.S. (2000). Alcohol: Its metabolism and interaction with nutrients. *Annual Review of Nutrition 20,* 395–430.
35. Alchord J.L. (1995). Alcohol and the liver. *Scientific American Science and Medicine 2*(2), 16–25.

36. Lieber C.S. (1994). Alcohol and the liver: 1994 update. *Gastroenterology 106,* 1085–1105.
37. Lieber C.S. (1988). Biochemical and molecular basis for alcohol-induced injury to the liver and other tissues. *New England Journal of Medicine 319,* 1639–1650.
38. Rubin E., Lieber C.S. (1968). Alcohol-induced hepatic injury in non-alcoholic volunteers. *New England Journal of Medicine 278,* 869–876.
39. Angulo P. (2002). Nonalcoholic fatty liver disease. *New England Journal of Medicine 346*(16), 1221–1231.
40. Yu A.S., Keeffe E.B. (2002). Nonalcoholic fatty liver disease. *Reviews in Gastrointestinal Disorders 2*(1), 11–19.
41. Trevillyan J., Carroll P.J. (1997). Management of portal hypertension and esophageal varices in alcoholic cirrhosis. *American Family Physician 55,* 1851–1858.
42. Roberts L.R., Kamath P.S. (1996). Ascites and hepatorenal syndrome: Pathophysiology and management. *Mayo Clinic Proceedings 71,* 874–881.
43. Epstein M. (1995). Renal sodium retention in liver disease. *Hospital Practice 30*(9), 33–41.
44. Garcia N., Sanyal A.J. (2001). Minimizing ascites: Complications of cirrhosis signals clinical deterioration. *Postgraduate Medicine 109*(2), 91–103.
45. Hegab A.M., Luketic V.A. (2001). Bleeding esophageal varices. *Postgraduate Medicine 109*(2), 75–89.
46. Brigalia A.E., Anania F.A. (2002). Hepatorenal syndrome: Definition, pathophysiology, and intervention. *Critical Care Clinics 18,* 345–373.
47. Weimer R.H., Rakela J., Ishitani M.B., et al. (2003). Recent advances in liver transplantation. *Mayo Clinic Proceedings 78*(2), 197–210.
48. American Cancer Society. (2004). *What are the key statistics on liver cancer?* (updated January 30, 20001). [On-line]. Available: http://www.cancer.org.
49. Bisceglie A.M. (1999). Malignant neoplasms of the liver. In Schiff E.R., Sorrell M.F., Maddrey W.C. (Eds.), *Schiff's diseases of the liver* (8th ed., pp. 1281–1300). Philadelphia: Lippincott Williams & Wilkins.
50. Hamnett R.J.H., Gollan J.L. (2001). Liver cancer. In Lenhard R.E., Osteen R.T., Gansler T. (Eds.), *American Cancer Society's clinical oncology* (pp. 395–405). Atlanta: American Cancer Society.
51. Crawford J.M. (2003). The biliary tract. In Kumar V., Cotran R.S., Collins T. (Eds.), *Basic pathology* (7th ed., pp. 628–633). Philadelphia: W.B. Saunders.
52. Vogt D.P. (2002). Gallbladder disease. *Cleveland Clinic Journal of Medicine 69*(12), 977–984.
53. Steinberg W., Jenner S. (1994). Acute pancreatitis. *New England Journal of Medicine 330,* 1198–1210.
54. Baron T.H., Morgan D.E. (1999). Acute necrotizing pancreatitis. *New England Journal of Medicine 340,* 1412–1417.
55. Cartmell M.T., Kingsnorth A.N. (2000). Acute pancreatitis. *Hospital Medicine 61,* 382–385.
56. Steer M.L., Waxman L., Freeman S. (1995). Chronic pancreatitis. *New England Journal of Medicine 332,* 1482–1490.
57. Isla A.M. (2000). Chronic pancreatitis. *Hospital Medicine 61,* 386–389.
58. Lillemoe K.D. (2000). Pancreatic cancer: State-of-the-art care. *CA: A Cancer Journal for Clinicians 50,* 241–268.
59. Warshaw A.I., Castillo C.F. (1992). Pancreatic carcinoma. *New England Journal of Medicine 326,* 455–465.
60. Wanebo H.J., Vezeridis M.P. (1996). Pancreatic cancer in perspective. *Cancer 76,* 580–587.

UNIT X

Endocrine Function

By the end of the Middle Ages, a great storehouse of anatomic knowledge existed; however, this repository had been culled from a combination of incomplete observations, religious beliefs, extrapolation from animal structures, and philosophical guesswork. Scientists slavishly adhered to these teachings, many of which were the products of the early Greeks (such as Aristotle and Galen), even though personal experience provided them with contradictory evidence.

The endocrine system fell victim to the outdated theories postulated long before. Even when some of its parts were discovered, their importance went unrecognized. For example, the pituitary gland, first noted in 1524 by Jacob Berengar of Carpi, was considered to be necessary to the cooling function of the brain. The brain was thought to secrete *pituita*, phlegm (mucus), and discharge it from the nose as part of its cooling process. The gland received its name from Andreas Vesalius, who referred to it in his text *De Fabrica* (1543) as *glandula pituitam cerebri excipiens*, or the gland that receives the phlegm from the brain. It was not until the late 19th and early 20th centuries that the field of endocrinology had its beginnings. It was then that the importance of the pituitary gland was finally realized, and it was called the master endocrine gland.

CHAPTER 41

Mechanisms of Endocrine Control

Glenn Matfin
Julie A. Kuenzi
Safak Guven

The endocrine system is involved in all of the integrative aspects of life, including growth, sex differentiation, metabolism, and adaptation to an ever-changing environment. This chapter focuses on general aspects of endocrine function, organization of the endocrine system, hormone receptors and hormone actions, and regulation of hormone levels.

The Endocrine System

After completing this section of the chapter, you should be able to meet the following objectives:

- Characterize a hormone
- State a difference between the synthesis of protein hormones and that of steroid hormones
- Describe mechanisms of hormone transport and inactivation
- State the function of a hormone receptor and state the difference between cell surface hormone receptors and intracellular hormone receptors
- Describe the role of the hypothalamus in regulating pituitary control of endocrine function
- State the major difference between positive and negative feedback control mechanisms
- Describe methods used in diagnosis of endocrine disorders

The endocrine system uses chemical substances called *hormones* as a means of regulating and integrating body functions. The endocrine system participates in the regulation of digestion, use, and storage of nutrients; growth and development; electrolyte and water metabolism; and reproductive functions. Although the endocrine system once was thought to consist solely of discrete endocrine glands, it is now known that a number of other tissues release chemical messengers that modulate body processes. The functions of the endocrine system are closely linked with those of the nervous system and the immune system. For example, neurotransmitters such as epinephrine can act as neurotransmitters or as hormones. The functions of the immune system also are closely linked with those of the endocrine system. The immune system responds to foreign agents by means of chemical messengers (cytokines, such as interleukins, interferons) and complex receptor mechanisms (see Chapter 19). The immune system also is extensively regulated by hormones such as the adrenal corticosteroid hormones.

HORMONES

Hormones generally are thought of as chemical messengers that are transported in body fluids. They are highly specialized organic molecules produced by endocrine organs that exert their action on specific target cells. Hormones do not initiate reactions but function as modulators of cellular and systemic responses. Most hormones are present in body fluids at all times, but in greater or lesser amounts depending on the needs of the body.

A characteristic of hormones is that a single hormone can exert various effects in different tissues or, conversely, a single function can be regulated by several hormones. For example, estradiol, which is produced by the ovary, can act on the ovarian follicles to promote their maturation, on the uterus to stimulate its growth and maintain the cyclic changes in the uterine mucosa, on the mammary gland to stimulate ductal growth, on the hypothalamic-pituitary system to regulate the secretion of gonadotropins and prolactin, on the bone to maintain skeletal integrity, and on general metabolic processes to affect adipose tissue distribution. Lipolysis, which is the release of free fatty acids from adipose tissue, is an example of a single function that is regulated by several hormones, including the catecholamines, glucagon, and secretin, but also by the cytokine, tumor necrosis factor-α (TNF-α). Table 41-1 lists the major functions and sources of body hormones.

Paracrine and Autocrine Actions

In the past, hormones were described as chemical substances that were released into the bloodstream and transported to distant target sites, where they exerted their action. Although many hormones travel by this mechanism, some hormones and hormone-like substances never enter the bloodstream but instead act locally in the vicinity in which they are released. When they act locally on cells other than those that produced the hormone, the action is called *paracrine*. The action of sex steroids on the ovary is a paracrine action. Hormones also can exert an *autocrine* action on the cells from which they were produced. For example, the release of insulin from pancreatic beta cells can inhibit its release from the same cells.

Eicosanoids and Retinoids

A group of compounds that have a hormone-like action are the eicosanoids, which are derived from polyunsaturated fatty acids in the cell membrane. Among these, *arachidonic acid* is the most important and abundant precursor of the various eicosanoids. The most important of the eicosanoids are the prostaglandins, leukotrienes, and thromboxanes. These fatty acid derivatives are produced by most body cells, are rapidly cleared from the circulation, and are thought to act mainly by paracrine and autocrine mechanisms. Eicosanoid synthesis often is stimulated in response to hormones, and eicosanoids serve as mediators of hormone action.

Retinoids (*e.g.*, retinoic acid) also are derived from fatty acids and have an important role in regulating nuclear receptor action.

HORMONES

- Hormones function as chemical messengers, moving through the blood to distant target sites of action, or acting more locally as paracrine or autocrine messengers that incite more local effects.
- Most hormones are present in body fluids at all times, but in greater or lesser amounts depending on the needs of the body.
- Hormones exert their actions by interacting with high-affinity receptors, which in turn are linked to one or more effector systems in the cell. Some hormone receptors are located on the surface of the cell and act through second messenger mechanisms, and others are located in the cell, where they modulate the synthesis of enzymes, transport proteins, or structural proteins.

Structural Classification

Hormones have diverse structures ranging from single amino acids to complex proteins and lipids. Hormones usually are divided into four categories according to their structures: (1) amines and amino acids; (2) peptides, polypeptides, proteins, and glycoproteins; (3) steroids; and (4) fatty acid derivatives (Table 41-2). The first category, the amines, includes norepinephrine and epinephrine, which are derived from a single amino acid (*i.e.,* tyrosine), and the thyroid hormones, which are derived from two iodinated tyrosine amino acid residues. The second category, the peptides, polypeptides, proteins, and glycoproteins, can be as small as thyrotropin-releasing hormone (TRH), which contains three amino acids, and as large and complex as growth hormone (GH) and follicle-stimulating hormone (FSH), which have approximately 200 amino acids. Glycoproteins are large peptide hormones associated with a carbohydrate (*e.g.,* FSH). The third category comprises the steroid hormones, which are derivatives of cholesterol. The fourth category, the fatty acid derivatives, includes the eicosanoids and retinoids.

Synthesis and Transport

The mechanisms for hormone synthesis vary with hormone structure. Protein and peptide hormones are synthesized and stored in granules or vesicles in the cytoplasm of the cell until secretion is required. The lipid-soluble steroid hormones are released as they are synthesized.

Protein and peptide hormones are synthesized in the rough endoplasmic reticulum in a manner similar to the synthesis of other proteins (see Chapter 4). The appropriate amino acid sequence is dictated by messenger RNA (mRNA) from the nucleus. Usually, synthesis involves the production of a precursor hormone, which is modified by the addition of peptides or sugar units. These precursor hormones often contain extra peptide units that ensure proper folding of the molecule and insertion of essential linkages. If extra amino acids are present, as in insulin, the precursor hormone is called a *prohormone*. After synthesis and sequestration in the endoplasmic reticulum, the protein and peptide hormones move into the Golgi complex, where they are packaged in granules or vesicles. It is in the Golgi complex that prohormones are converted into hormones.

Steroid hormones are synthesized in the smooth endoplasmic reticulum, and steroid-secreting cells can be identified by their large amounts of smooth endoplasmic

TABLE 44-1 Major Action and Source of Selected Hormones

Source	Hormone	Major Action
Hypothalamus	Releasing and inhibiting hormones Corticotropin-releasing hormone (CRH) Thyrotropin-releasing hormone (TRH) Growth hormone-releasing hormone (GHRH) Gonadotropin-releasing hormone (GnRH)	Controls the release of pituitary hormones
	Somatostatin	Inhibits GH and TSH
Anterior pituitary	Growth hormone (GH)	Stimulates growth of bone and muscle, promotes protein synthesis and fat metabolism, decreases carbohydrate metabolism
	Adrenocorticotropic hormone (ACTH)	Stimulates synthesis and secretion of adrenal cortical hormones
	Thyroid-stimulating hormone (TSH)	Stimulates synthesis and secretion of thyroid hormone
	Follicle-stimulating hormone (FSH)	Female: stimulates growth of ovarian follicle, ovulation Male: stimulates sperm production
	Luteinizing hormone (LH)	Female: stimulates development of corpus luteum, release of oocyte, production of estrogen and progesterone Male: stimulates secretion of testosterone, development of interstitial tissue of testes
	Prolactin	Prepares female breast for breast-feeding
Posterior pituitary	Antidiuretic hormone (ADH)	Increases water reabsorption by kidney
	Oxytocin	Stimulates contraction of pregnant uterus, milk ejection from breasts after childbirth
Adrenal cortex	Mineralocorticosteroids, mainly aldosterone	Increases sodium absorption, potassium loss by kidney
	Glucocorticoids, mainly cortisol	Affects metabolism of all nutrients; regulates blood glucose levels, affects growth, has antiinflammatory action, and decreases effects of stress
	Adrenal androgens, mainly dehydroepiandrosterone (DHEA) and androstenedione	Have minimal intrinsic androgenic activity; they are converted to testosterone and dihydrotestosterone in the periphery
Adrenal medulla	Epinephrine Norepinephrine	Serve as neurotransmitters for the sympathetic nervous system
Thyroid (follicular cells)	Thyroid hormones: triiodothyronine (T_3), thyroxine (T_4)	Increase the metabolic rate; increase protein and bone turnover; increase responsiveness to catecholamines; necessary for fetal and infant growth and development
Thyroid C cells	Calcitonin	Lowers blood calcium and phosphate levels
Parathyroid glands	Parathyroid hormone (PTH)	Regulates serum calcium
Pancreatic islet cells	Insulin	Lowers blood glucose by facilitating glucose transport across cell membranes of muscle, liver, and adipose tissue
	Glucagon	Increases blood glucose concentration by stimulation of glycogenolysis and glyconeogenesis
	Somatostatin	Delays intestinal absorption of glucose
Kidney	1,25-Dihydroxyvitamin D	Stimulates calcium absorption from the intestine
Ovaries	Estrogen	Affects development of female sex organs and secondary sex characteristics
	Progesterone	Influences menstrual cycle; stimulates growth of uterine wall; maintains pregnancy
Testes	Androgens, mainly testosterone	Affect development of male sex organs and secondary sex characteristics; aid in sperm production

TABLE 41-2 Classes of Hormones Based on Structure

Amines and Amino Acids	Peptides, Polypeptides, and Proteins	Steroids	Fatty Acid Compounds
Dopamine	Corticotropin-releasing hormone (CRH)	Aldosterone	Eicosanoids
Epinephrine	Growth hormone–releasing hormone (GHRH)	Glucocorticoids	Retinoids
Norepinephrine	Thyrotropin-releasing hormone (TRH)	Estrogens	
Thyroid hormone	Adrenocorticotropic hormone (ACTH)	Testosterone	
	Follicle-stimulating hormone (FSH)	Progesterone	
	Luteinizing hormone (LH)	Androstenedione	
	Thyroid-stimulating hormone (TSH)	1,25-Dihydroxyvitamin D	
	Growth hormone (GH)	Dihydrotestosterone (DHT)	
	Antidiuretic hormone (ADH)	Dehydroepiandrosterone (DHEA)	
	Oxytocin		
	Insulin		
	Glucagon		
	Somatostatin		
	Calcitonin		
	Parathyroid hormone (PTH)		
	Prolactin		

reticulum. Certain steroids serve as precursors for the production of other hormones. In the adrenal cortex, for example, progesterone and other steroid intermediates are enzymatically converted into aldosterone, cortisol, or androgens (see Chapter 42).

Hormones that are released into the bloodstream circulate as either free, unbound molecules or as hormones attached to transport carriers (Fig. 41-1). Peptide hormones and protein hormones usually circulate unbound in the blood. Steroid hormones and thyroid hormone are carried by specific carrier proteins synthesized in the liver. The extent of carrier binding influences the rate at which hormones leave the blood and enter the cells. The half-life of a hormone—the time it takes for the body to reduce the concentration of the hormone by one half—is positively correlated with its percentage of protein binding. Thyroxine, which is more than 99% protein bound, has a half-life of 6 days. Aldosterone, which is only 15% bound, has a half-life of only 25 minutes. Drugs that compete with a hormone for binding with transport carrier molecules increase hormone action by increasing the availability of the active unbound hormone. For example, aspirin competes with thyroid hormone for binding to transport proteins; when the drug is administered to persons with excessive levels of circulating thyroid hormone, such as during thyroid crisis, serious effects may occur because of the dissociation of free hormone from the binding proteins.

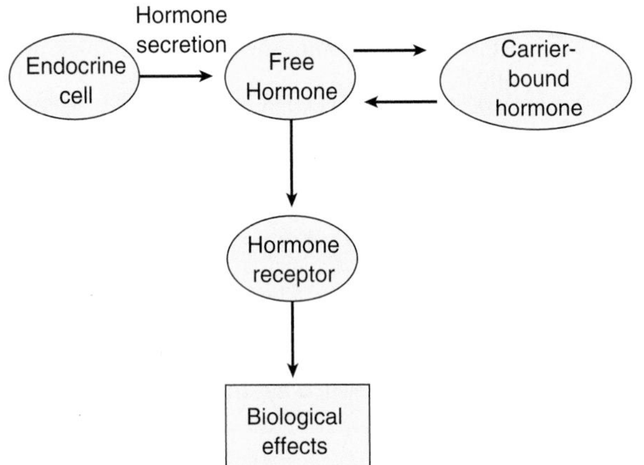

FIGURE 41-1 Relationship of free and carrier-bound hormone.

Metabolism and Elimination

Metabolism of hormones and their precursors can generate more or less active products or it can degrade them to inactive forms. In some cases, hormones are eliminated in the intact form. Hormones secreted by endocrine cells must be inactivated continuously to prevent their accumulation. Intracellular and extracellular mechanisms participate in the termination of hormone function. Some hormones are enzymatically inactivated at receptor sites where they exert their action. The catecholamines, which have a very short half-life, are degraded by catechol-*O*-methyl transferase (COMT) and monoamine oxidase (MAO). Because of their short half-life, their production is measured by some of their metabolites. In general, peptide hormones also have a short life span in the circulation. Their major mechanism of degradation is through binding to cell surface receptors, with subsequent uptake and degradation by peptide-splitting enzymes in the cell membrane or inside the cell. Steroid hormones are bound to protein carriers for transport and are inactive in the bound state. Their activity depends on the availability of transport carriers. Unbound adrenal and gonadal steroid hormones are conjugated in the liver, which renders them inactive, and then excreted in the bile or urine. Thyroid hormones also are transported by carrier molecules. The free hormone is rendered inactive by the removal of amino acids (*i.e.*, deamination) in the tissues, and the hormone is conjugated in the liver and eliminated in the bile.

Mechanisms of Action

Hormones produce their effects through interaction with high-affinity receptors, which in turn are linked to one or more effector systems within the cell. These mechanisms involve many of the cell's metabolic activities, ranging from ion transport at the cell surface to stimulation of nuclear transcription of complex molecules. The rate at which hormones react depends on their mechanism of action. The neurotransmitters, which control the opening of ion channels, have a reaction time of milliseconds. Thyroid hormone, which functions in the control of cell metabolism and synthesis of intracellular signaling molecules, requires days for its full effect to occur.

Receptors. Hormone receptors are complex molecular structures that are located either on the surface or inside target cells. The function of these receptors is to recognize a specific hormone and translate the hormonal signal into a cellular response. The structure of these receptors varies in a manner that allows target cells to respond to one hormone and not to others. For example, receptors in the thyroid are specific for thyroid-stimulating hormone (TSH), and receptors on the gonads respond to the gonadotropic hormones.

The response of a target cell to a hormone varies with the *number* of receptors present and with the *affinity* of these receptors for hormone binding. A variety of factors influence the number of receptors that are present on target cells and their affinity for hormone binding.

There are approximately 2000 to 100,000 hormone receptor molecules per cell. The number of hormone receptors on a cell may be altered for any of several reasons. Antibodies may destroy or block the receptor proteins. Increased or decreased hormone levels often induce changes in the activity of the genes that regulate receptor synthesis. For example, decreased hormone levels often produce an increase in receptor numbers by means of a process called *up-regulation;* this increases the sensitivity of the body to existing hormone levels. Likewise, sustained levels of excess hormone often bring about a decrease in receptor numbers by *down-regulation,* producing a decrease in hormone sensitivity. In some instances, the reverse effect occurs, and an increase in hormone levels appears to recruit its own receptors, thereby increasing the sensitivity of the cell to the hormone. The process of up-regulation and down-regulation of receptors is regulated largely by inducing or repressing the transcription of receptor genes.

The affinity of receptors for binding hormones also is affected by a number of conditions. For example, the pH of the body fluids plays an important role in the affinity of insulin receptors. In ketoacidosis, a lower pH reduces insulin binding.

Some hormone receptors are located on the surface of the cell and act through second messenger mechanisms, and others are located within the cell, where they modulate the synthesis of enzymes, transport proteins, or structural proteins. The receptors for thyroid hormones, which are found in the nucleus, are thought to be directly associated with controlling the activity of genes located on one or more of the chromosomes. Chart 41-1 lists examples of hormones that act through the two types of receptors.

Surface Receptors. Because of their low solubility in the lipid layer of cell membranes, peptide hormones and catecholamines cannot readily cross the cell membrane. Instead, these hormones interact with surface receptors in a manner that incites the generation of an intracellular signal or message. The intracellular signal system is termed the *second messenger,* and the hormone is considered to be the first messenger (Fig. 41-2). For example, the first messenger glucagon binds to surface receptors on liver cells to incite glycogen breakdown by way of the second messenger system.

The most widely distributed second messenger is cyclic adenosine monophosphate (cAMP). cAMP is formed from cellular adenosine triphosphate (ATP) by the enzyme adenylate cyclase, a membrane-bound enzyme that is located on the inner aspect of the cell membrane. Adenylate cyclase is functionally coupled to various cell surface receptors by the regulatory actions of G proteins (see Chapter 4, Fig. 4-11). A second messenger similar to cAMP is cyclic guanosine monophosphate (cGMP), derived from guanine triphosphate (GTP). As a result of binding to specific cell receptors, many peptide hormones incite a series of enzymatic reactions that produce an almost immediate increase in cAMP. Some hormones act to decrease cAMP levels and have an opposite effect.

In some cells, binding of hormones or neurotransmitters to surface receptors acts directly rather than through a second messenger to open ion channels in the cell membrane. The influx of ions serves as an intracellular signal to convey the hormonal message to the cell interior. In many instances, activation of hormone receptors results in the opening of calcium channels. The increasing cytoplasmic concentration of calcium may result in direct activation of

CHART 41-1

Hormone–Receptor Interactions

Second Messenger Interactions

Glucagon
Insulin
Epinephrine
Parathyroid hormone (PTH)
Thyroid-stimulating hormone (TSH)
Adrenocorticotropic hormone (ACTH)
Follicle-stimulating hormone (FSH)
Luteinizing hormone (LH)
Antidiuretic hormone (ADH)
Secretin

Intracellular Interactions

Estrogens
Testosterone
Progesterone
Adrenal cortical hormones
Thyroid hormones

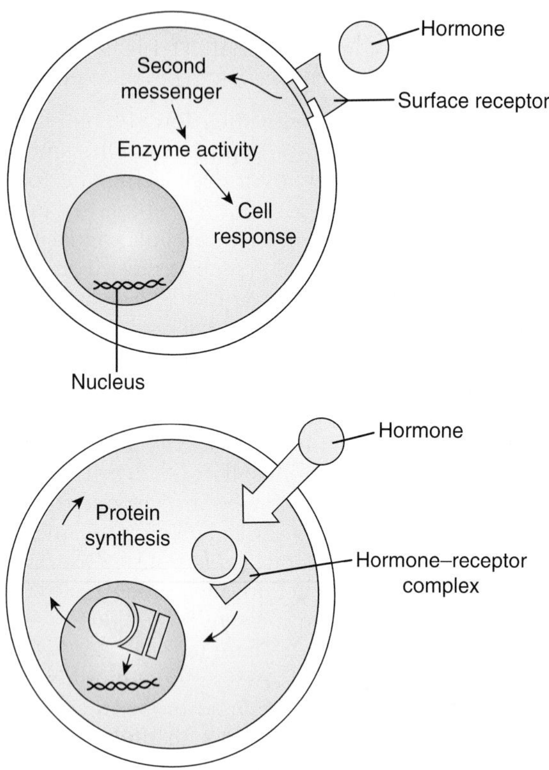

FIGURE 41-2 The two types of hormone–receptor interactions: the surface receptor (**top**) and the intracellular receptor (**bottom**).

calcium-dependent enzymes or calcium–calmodulin complexes with their attendant effects.

Cytokine receptors are part of the large class of receptors that also mediate the actions of GH and leptin. These receptors have an extracellular domain that binds ligand, a transmembrane component, and an intracellular domain that associates (when activated) with cytoplasmic tyrosine kinases (such as Janus kinases [JAKs]), that mediate downstream signaling (see Chapter 19).

Intracellular Receptors. A second type of receptor mechanism is involved in mediating the action of hormones such as the steroid and thyroid hormones (see Fig. 41-2). These hormones are lipid soluble and pass freely through the cell membrane. They then attach to intracellular receptors and form a hormone–receptor complex that travels to the cell nucleus. The hormone–messenger complex binds to hormone response elements (HRE) that then activates or suppresses intracellular mechanisms such as gene activity, with subsequent production or inhibition of messenger RNA and protein synthesis.

An example of this type of mechanism is the interaction of the peroxisomal proliferator-activated receptor (PPAR) that binds to the HRE (in association with a retinoid X receptor, RXR) and activates genes involved in glucose and lipid metabolism (see Chapter 43, Fig. 43-9). Agents that are agonists for the PPAR include the PPAR-γ agonists (the thiazolidinediones, *e.g.*, rosiglitazone and pioglitazone) and the PPAR-α agonists (the fibrates, *e.g.*, fenofibrate and gemfibrozil), which are important new therapies for type 2 diabetes (see Chapter 43), dyslipidemia (see Chapter 24), and the metabolic syndrome (see Chapter 47).

CONTROL OF HORMONE LEVELS

Hormone secretion varies widely over a 24-hour period. Some hormones, such as GH and adrenocorticotropic hormone (ACTH), have diurnal fluctuations that vary with the sleep–wake cycle. Others, such as the female sex hormones, are secreted in a complicated cyclic manner. The levels of hormones such as insulin and antidiuretic hormone (ADH) are regulated by feedback mechanisms that monitor substances such as glucose (insulin) and water (ADH) in the body. The levels of many of the hormones are regulated by feedback mechanisms that involve the hypothalamic-pituitary-target cell system.

Hypothalamic-Pituitary Regulation

The hypothalamus and pituitary (*i.e.*, hypophysis) form a unit that exerts control over many functions of several endocrine glands as well as a wide range of other physiologic functions. These two structures are connected by blood flow in the hypophyseal portal system, which begins in the hypothalamus and drains into the anterior pituitary gland, and by the nerve axons that connect the supraoptic and paraventricular nuclei of the hypothalamus with the posterior pituitary gland (Fig. 41-3). The pituitary is enclosed in the bony sella turcica ("Turkish saddle") and is bridged over by the diaphragma sellae. Embryologically, the anterior pituitary gland developed from glandular tissue and the posterior pituitary developed from neural tissue.

Hypothalamic Hormones. The synthesis and release of anterior pituitary hormones are largely regulated by the action of releasing or inhibiting hormones from the hypothalamus, which is the coordinating center of the brain for endocrine, behavioral, and autonomic nervous system function. It is at the level of the hypothalamus that emotion, pain, body temperature, and other neural input are communicated to the endocrine system (Fig. 41-4). The posterior pituitary hormones, ADH and oxytocin, are synthesized in the cell bodies of neurons in the hypothalamus that have axons that travel to the posterior pituitary. The release and function of ADH are discussed in Chapter 33.

The hypothalamic hormones that regulate the secretion of anterior pituitary hormones include GH-releasing hormone (GHRH), somatostatin, dopamine, thyrotropin-releasing hormone (TRH), corticotropin-releasing hormone (CRH), and gonadotropin-releasing hormone (GnRH). With the exception of GH and prolactin, most of the pituitary hormones are regulated by hypothalamic stimulatory hormones. GH secretion is stimulated by GHRH; thyroid-stimulating hormone (TSH) by TRH; ACTH by CRH; and luteinizing hormone (LH) and FSH by GnRH. Somatostatin functions as an inhibitory hormone for GH and TSH. Prolactin secretion is inhibited by dopamine; thus, persons receiving antipsychotic drugs that block dopamine often have increased prolactin levels.

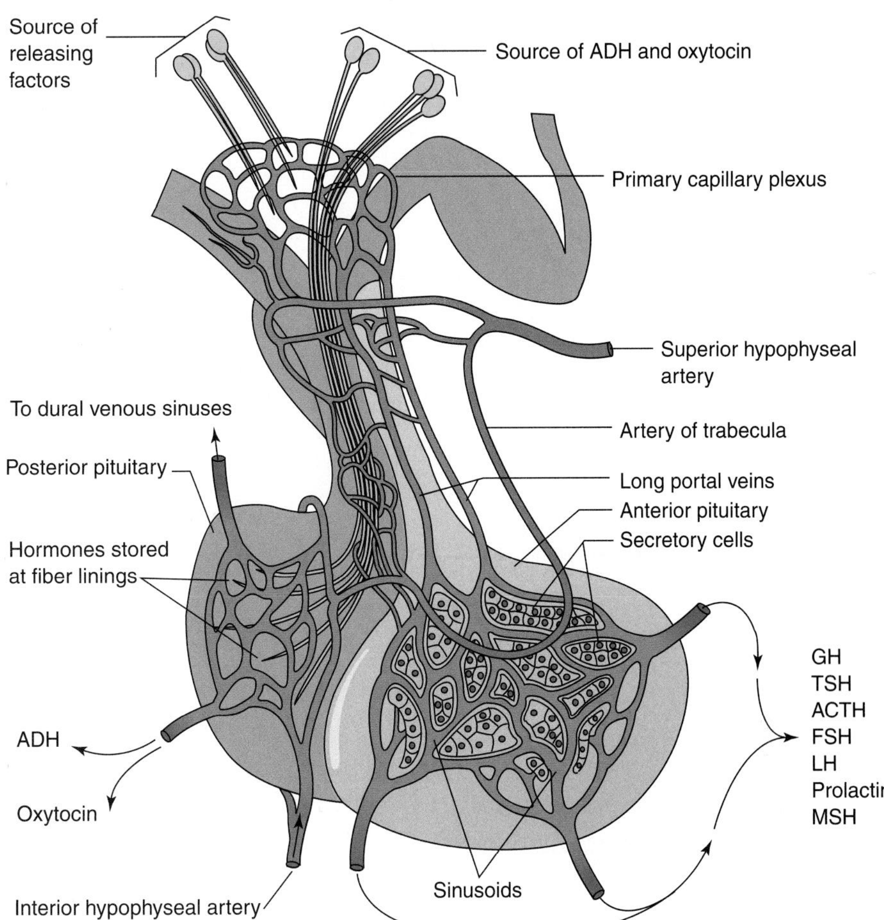

FIGURE 41-3 The hypothalamus and the anterior and posterior pituitary. The hypothalamic releasing or inhibiting hormones are transported to the anterior pituitary by way of the portal vessels. ADH and oxytocin are produced by nerve cells in the supraoptic and paraventricular nuclei of the hypothalamus and then transported through the nerve axon to the posterior pituitary, where they are released into the circulation.

The activity of the hypothalamus is regulated by both hormonally mediated signals (*e.g.*, negative feedback signals) and neuronal input from a number of sources. Neuronal signals are mediated by neurotransmitters such as acetylcholine, dopamine, norepinephrine, serotonin, γ-aminobutyric acid (GABA), and opioids. Cytokines that are involved in immune and inflammatory responses, such as the interleukins, also are involved in the regulation of hypothalamic function. This is particularly true of the hormones involved in the hypothalamic-pituitary-adrenal axis. Thus, the hypothalamus can be viewed as a bridge by which signals from multiple systems are relayed to the pituitary gland.

Pituitary Hormones. The pituitary gland has been called the *master gland* because its hormones control the functions of many target glands and cells. The anterior pituitary gland contains five cell types: (1) thyrotrophs, which produce thyrotropin, also known as TSH; (2) corticotrophs, which produce corticotrophin, also called adrenocorticotropic hormone (ACTH); (3) gonadotrophs, which produce the gonadotropins LH and FSH; (4) somatotrophs, which produce GH; and (5) lactotrophs, which produce prolactin. Hormones produced by the anterior pituitary control body growth and metabolism (GH), function of the thyroid gland (TSH), glucocorticoid hormone levels (ACTH), function of the gonads (FSH and LH), and breast growth and milk production (prolactin). Melanocyte-stimulating hormone (MSH), which is involved in the control of pigmentation of the skin, is produced by the pars intermedia of the pituitary gland. The functions of many of these hormones are discussed in other parts of this book (*e.g.*, thyroid hormone, GH, and the corticosteroids in Chapter 42, the sex hormones in Chapters 45 and 47, and ADH from the posterior pituitary in Chapter 33).

Feedback Regulation

The level of many of the hormones in the body is regulated by negative feedback mechanisms. The function of this type of system is similar to that of the thermostat in a heating system. In the endocrine system, sensors detect a change in the hormone level and adjust hormone secretion so that body levels are maintained within an appropriate range. When the sensors detect a decrease in hormone levels, they initiate changes that cause an increase in hormone production; when hormone levels rise above the set point of the system, the sensors cause hormone production and release to decrease. For example, an increase in thyroid hormone is detected by sensors in the hypothalamus or anterior pituitary gland, and this causes a reduction in the

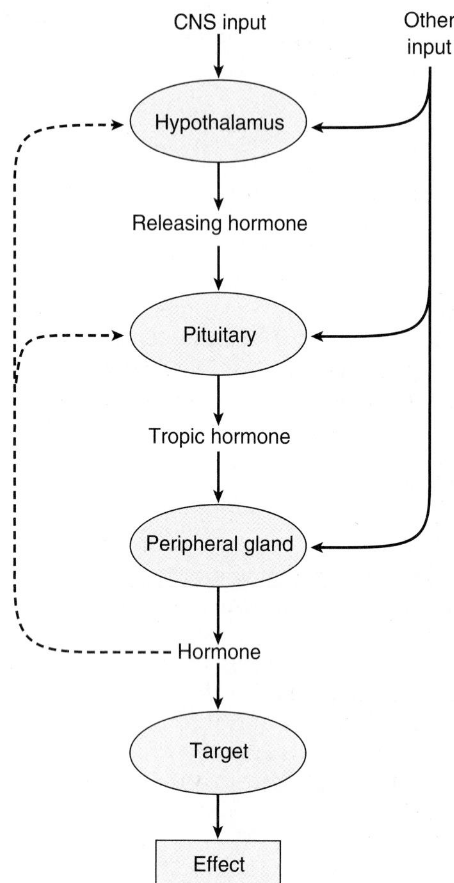

FIGURE 41-4 Hypothalamic–pituitary control of hormone levels. The *dashed line* represents feedback control.

secretion of TSH, with a subsequent decrease in the output of thyroid hormone from the thyroid gland. The feedback loops for the hypothalamic-pituitary feedback mechanisms are illustrated in Figures 41-4 and 41-5.

Exogenous forms of hormones (given as drug preparations) can influence the normal feedback control of hormone production and release. One of the most common examples of this influence occurs with the administration of the corticosteroid hormones, which causes suppression of the hypothalamic-pituitary-target cell system that regulates the production of these hormones.

Although the levels of most hormones are regulated by negative feedback mechanisms, a small number are under positive feedback control, in which rising levels of a hormone cause another gland to release a hormone that is stimulating to the first. There must, however, be a mechanism for shutting off the release of the first hormone, or its production would continue unabated. An example of such a system is that of the female ovarian hormone estradiol. Increased estradiol production during the follicular stage of the menstrual cycle causes increased gonadotropin (FSH) production by the anterior pituitary gland. This stimulates further increases in estradiol levels until the demise of the follicle, which is the source of estradiol, results in a fall in gonadotropin levels.

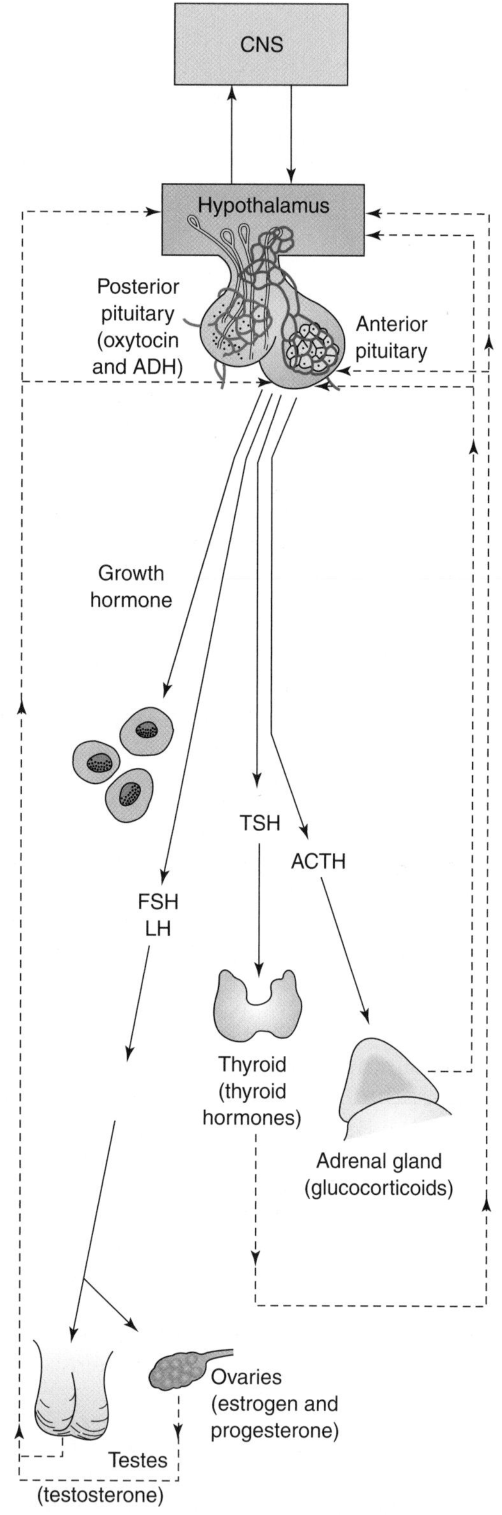

FIGURE 41-5 Control of hormone production by hypothalamic–pituitary–target cell feedback mechanism. Hormone levels from the target glands regulate the release of hormones from the anterior pituitary by means of a negative feedback system. The *dashed line* represents feedback control.

In addition to positive and negative feedback mechanisms that monitor changes in hormone levels, some hormones are regulated by the level of the substance they regulate. For example, insulin levels normally are regulated in response to blood glucose levels, and those of aldosterone in response to body levels of sodium and potassium. Other factors such as stress, environmental temperature, and nutritional status can alter feedback regulation of hormone levels.

DIAGNOSTIC TESTS

Several techniques are available for assessing endocrine function and hormone levels. One technique measures the effect of a hormone on body function. Measurement of blood glucose, for example, reflects insulin levels and is an indirect method of assessing insulin availability. The most common method is to measure hormone levels directly.

Blood Tests

Hormones circulating in the plasma were first detected by bioassays using the intact animal or a portion of tissue from the animal. At one time, female rats or male frogs were used to test women's urine for the presence of human chorionic gonadotropin, which is produced by the placenta during pregnancy. Most bioassays lack the precision, sensitivity, and specificity to measure low concentrations of hormones in plasma, and they are inconvenient to perform.

Blood hormone levels provide information about hormone levels at a specific time. For example, blood insulin levels can be measured along with blood glucose after administration of a challenge dose of glucose to measure the time course of change in blood insulin levels.

Real progress in measuring plasma hormone levels came more than 40 years ago with the use of competitive binding and the development of radioimmunoassay (RIA) methods. RIA uses a radiolabeled form of the hormone and a hormone antibody that has been prepared by injecting an appropriate animal with a purified form of the hormone. The unlabeled hormone in the sample being tested competes with the radiolabeled hormone for attachment to the binding sites of the antibody. Measurement of the radiolabeled hormone–antibody complex then provides a means of arriving at a measure of the hormone level in the sample. Because hormone binding is competitive, the amount of radiolabeled hormone–antibody complex that is formed decreases as the amount of unlabeled hormone in the sample is increased. Newer techniques of RIA have been introduced, including the immunoradiometric assay (IRMA). IRMA uses two antibodies instead of one. These two antibodies are directed against two different parts of the molecule, and therefore IRMA assays are more specific. RIA has several disadvantages, including limited shelf life of the radiolabeled hormone and the cost of disposal of radioactive waste.

Nonradiolabeled methods have been developed in which the antigen of the hormone being measured is linked to an enzyme-activated label (*e.g.*, fluorescent label, chemiluminescent label) or latex particles that can be agglutinated with an antigen and measured. The enzyme-linked immunosorbent assay (ELISA) uses antibody-coated plates and an enzyme-labeled reporter antibody. Binding of the hormone to the enzyme-labeled reporter antibody produces a colored reaction that can be measured using a spectrophotometer.

Other blood tests that are routinely done in endocrine disorders include measurement of various autoantibodies. For example, anti–thyroid peroxidase (anti-TPO) antibodies are measured during the initial diagnostic workup and subsequent follow-up of patients with Hashimoto's thyroiditis. Other endocrine disorders that use autoantibody testing include type 1 diabetes, Graves' disease, autoimmune hypoparathyroidism, and autoimmune Addison's disease.

Urine Tests

Measurements of urinary hormone or hormone metabolite excretion often are done on a 24-hour urine sample and provide a better measure of hormone levels during that period than hormones measured in an isolated blood sample. The advantages of a urine test include the relative ease of obtaining urine samples and the fact that blood sampling is not required. The disadvantage is that reliably timed urine collections often are difficult to obtain. For example, a person may be unable to urinate at specific timed intervals, and urine samples may be accidentally discarded or inaccurately preserved. Because many urine tests involve the measure of a hormone metabolite rather than the hormone itself, drugs or disease states that alter hormone metabolism may interfere with the test result. Some urinary hormone metabolite measurements include hormones from more than one source and are of little value in measuring hormone secretion from a specific source. For example, urinary 17-ketosteroids are a measure of both adrenal and gonadal androgens.

Stimulation and Suppression Tests

Stimulation tests are used when hypofunction of an endocrine organ is suspected. A tropic or stimulating hormone can be administered to test the capacity of an endocrine organ to increase hormone production. The capacity of the target gland to respond is measured by an increase in the appropriate hormone. For example, the function of the hypothalamic-pituitary-thyroid system can be evaluated through stimulation tests using TRH and measuring TSH response. Failure to increase TSH levels after a TRH stimulation test suggests an inadequate capacity to produce TSH by the pituitary (*i.e.*, the pituitary is dysfunctional in some way).

Suppression tests are used when hyperfunction of an endocrine organ is suspected. Usually when an organ or tissue is functioning autonomously (*i.e.*, it is not responding to the normal negative feedback control mechanisms, and continues to secrete excessive amounts of hormone), a suppression test may be useful to confirm this situation. For example, when a GH- secreting tumor is suspected, the GH response to a glucose load is measured as part of the diagnostic workup. Normally, a glucose load would suppress GH levels. However, in adults with GH-secreting tumors (a condition known as acromegaly), GH levels do not suppress (and paradoxically increase in 50% of cases).

Genetic Tests

The diagnosis of genetic diseases, using deoxyribonucleic acid (DNA) analysis, is rapidly becoming a routine part of endocrine practice. Completion of the human genome sequence has revealed the presence of about 30,000 to 40,000 genes. The considerable interest in the field of genomics (*i.e.*, examination of the DNA) and transcriptomics (*i.e.*, examination of the mRNA) has been complemented by advances in proteomics (*i.e.*, examination of the proteome, which is all of the proteins expressed by a cell or tissue type). It is proposed that in comparison to the size of the genome, the proteome is far larger, with several hundred thousand to several million different protein forms possible. Analysis of the proteins produced by normal and abnormal endocrine cells, tissues, and organs will lead to a better understanding of the pathophysiology of endocrine conditions. This may also lead to selective targeting for new drug development.

The cloning of many endocrine system genes has had an enormous impact on everyday clinical practice. For example, identification of a gene for a given disorder (*e.g.*, the *RET* protooncogene in certain multiple endocrine neoplasia syndromes) means that faster diagnosis and more appropriate management of the affected individual can occur, but also that screening of family members for kindred harboring a known mutation can be undertaken.

Imaging

Imaging studies are important in the diagnosis and follow-up of endocrine disorders. Imaging modalities related to endocrinology can be divided into isotopic and nonisotopic. Isotopic imaging includes radioactive scanning of the thyroid (*e.g.*, using radioiodine), parathyroids (*e.g.*, using sestamibi), and adrenals (*e.g.*, using metaiodobenzylguanidine [MIBG] to detect pheochromocytoma). Nonisotopic imaging includes magnetic resonance imaging (MRI, which is the preferred choice for pituitary and hypothalamic imaging) and computed tomography (CT) scanning (which is preferred for adrenal lesions and abdominal endocrine lesions). Ultrasound scanning provides excellent and reproducible anatomic images for thyroid, parathyroid, and neighboring structures. Thyroid ultrasound is recommended for managing thyroid nodules and can aid in visualization of the nodule for biopsy (fine-needle aspiration [FNA]), which is necessary to help distinguish benign from malignant etiology. Selective venography is usually accompanied by venous sampling to determine hormonal output from a gland or organ (e.g., adrenal, pituitary, and kidney). Positron-emission tomography (PET) scanning is being used more widely for evaluation of endocrine tumors. Dual-energy x-ray absorptiometry (DEXA) is used routinely for the diagnosis and monitoring of osteoporosis and metabolic bone diseases.

In summary, the endocrine system acts as a communication system that uses chemical messengers, or hormones, for the transmission of information from cell to cell and from organ to organ. Hormones act by binding to receptors that are specific for the different types of hormones. Many of the endocrine glands are under the regulatory control of other parts of the endocrine system. The hypothalamus and the pituitary gland form a complex integrative network that joins the nervous system and the endocrine system; this central network controls the output from many of the other glands in the body.

Endocrine function can be assessed directly by measuring hormone levels, or indirectly by assessing the effects that a hormone has on the body (*e.g.*, assessment of insulin function through blood glucose). Imaging techniques are increasingly used to visualize endocrine structures, and genetic techniques are used to determine the presence of genes that contribute to the development of endocrine disorders.

REVIEW EXERCISES

People that are being treated with exogenous forms of corticosteroid hormones often experience diminished levels of ACTH and endogenously produced cortisol.

A. Explain, using information regarding the hypothalamic-pituitary feedback control of cortisol production by the adrenal cortex.

Bibliography

Belchetz P., Hammond P. (2003). *Mosby's colour atlas and text of diabetes and endocrinology*. New York: Mosby.

Greenspan F.S., Gardner D.G. (Eds.). (2004). *Basic and clinical endocrinology* (7th ed.). New York: Lange Medical Books/McGraw-Hill.

Griffin J.E., Sergio R.O. (Eds.). (2000). *Textbook of endocrine physiology* (4th ed.). New York: Oxford University Press.

Larsen P.R., Kronenberg H.M., Melmed S., et al. (Eds.). (2003). *Williams textbook of endocrinology* (10th ed.). Philadelphia: W.B. Saunders.

Lavin N. (Ed.) (2002). *Manual of endocrinology and metabolism* (3rd ed.). New York: Lippincott, Williams & Wilkins.

CHAPTER 42

Disorders of Endocrine Control of Growth and Metabolism

Glenn Matfin
Julie A. Kuenzi
Safak Guven

The endocrine system affects all aspects of body function, including growth and development, energy metabolism, muscle and adipose tissue distribution, sexual development, fluid and electrolyte balance, and inflammation and immune responses. This chapter focuses on disorders of pituitary function, growth and growth hormone, thyroid function, and adrenocortical function.

General Aspects of Altered Endocrine Function

After completing this section of the chapter, you should be able to meet the following objectives:

- ✦ Describe the mechanisms of endocrine hypofunction and hyperfunction
- ✦ Differentiate primary, secondary, and tertiary endocrine disorders

HYPOFUNCTION AND HYPERFUNCTION

Disturbances of endocrine function usually can be divided into two categories: hypofunction and hyperfunction. Hypofunction of an endocrine gland can occur for a variety of reasons. Congenital defects can result in the absence or impaired development of the gland or in the absence of an enzyme needed for hormone synthesis. The gland may be destroyed by a disruption in blood flow, infection, inflammation, autoimmune disorder, or neoplastic growth. There may be a decline in function with aging, or the gland may atrophy as the result of drug therapy or for unknown reasons. Some endocrine-deficient states are associated with receptor defects: hormone receptors may be absent, the receptor binding of hormones may be defective, or the cellular responsiveness to the hormone may be impaired. It is suspected that in some cases a gland may produce a biologically inactive hormone or that an active hormone may be destroyed by circulating antibodies before it can exert its action.

Hyperfunction usually is associated with excessive hormone production. This can result from excessive stimulation and hyperplasia of the endocrine gland or from a hormone-producing tumor of the gland. An ectopic tumor can produce hormones; for example, certain bronchogenic tumors produce hormones such as antidiuretic hormone (ADH) and adrenocorticotropic hormone (ACTH).

PRIMARY, SECONDARY, AND TERTIARY DISORDERS

Endocrine disorders in general can be divided into primary, secondary, and tertiary groups. *Primary defects* in endocrine function originate in the target gland responsible for producing the hormone. In *secondary disorders* of endocrine function, the target gland is essentially normal, but its function is altered by defective levels of stimulating hormones or releasing factors from the pituitary system. For example, adrenalectomy produces a primary deficiency of adrenal corticosteroid hormones. Removal or destruction of the pituitary gland eliminates ACTH stimulation of the adrenal cortex and brings about a secondary deficiency. A *tertiary disorder* results from hypothalamic dysfunction (as may occur with craniopharyngiomas or cerebral irradiation); thus, both the pituitary and target organ are understimulated.

In summary, endocrine disorders are the result of hypofunction or hyperfunction of an endocrine gland. They can occur as a primary defect in hormone production by a target gland or as a secondary or tertiary disorder resulting from a defect in the hypothalamic-pituitary system that controls a target gland's function.

Pituitary and Growth Disorders

After completing this section of the chapter, you should be able to meet the following objectives:

- Discuss the classification of pituitary tumors
- Describe the clinical features and causes of hypopituitarism
- State the effects of a deficiency in growth hormone
- Differentiate genetic short stature from constitutional short stature
- State the mechanisms of short stature in hypothyroidism, poorly controlled diabetes mellitus, treatment with adrenal glucocorticosteroid hormones, malnutrition, and psychosocial dwarfism
- List three causes of tall stature
- Relate the functions of growth hormone to the manifestations of acromegaly and adult-onset growth hormone deficiency
- Explain why children with isosexual precocious puberty are tall-statured children but short-statured adults

The anterior lobe of the pituitary gland produces ACTH, thyroid-stimulating hormone (TSH), growth hormone (GH), the gonadotrophic hormones (follicle-stimulating hormone [FSH] and luteinizing hormone [LH]), and prolactin[1] (see Chapter 41, Fig. 41-3). Four of these, ACTH, TSH, LH, and FSH control the secretion of hormones from other endocrine glands. ACTH controls the release of cortisol from the adrenal gland, TSH controls the secretion of thyroid hormone from the thyroid gland, LH regulates sex hormone levels, and FSH regulates fertility.

PITUITARY TUMORS

Pituitary tumors can be divided into primary or secondary tumors (*i.e.*, metastatic lesions). Tumors of the pituitary can be further divided into functional tumors that secrete pituitary hormones and nonfunctional tumors that do not secrete hormones. They can range in size from small lesions that do not enlarge the gland (microadenomas, <10 mm) to large, expansive tumors (macroadenomas, >10 mm) that erode the sella turcica and impinge on surrounding cranial structures.[1] Small, nonfunctioning tumors are found in approximately 25% of adult autopsies. Benign adenomas account for most of the functioning anterior pituitary tumors. Carcinomas of the pituitary are less common tumors. Functional adenomas can be subdivided according to cell type and the type of hormone secreted (Table 42-1).

TABLE 42-1 Frequency of Adenomas of the Anterior Pituitary

Cell Type	Hormone	Frequency (%)
Lactotrope	Prolactin (PRL)	32
Somatotrope	Growth hormone (GH)	21
Lactotrope/somatotrope	Mixed PRL/GH	6
Corticotrope	Adrenocorticotropic hormone (ACTH)	13
Gonadotrope	Follicle-stimulating hormone (FSH)	<4
	Luteinizing hormone (LH)	<4
Thyrotrope	Thyroid-stimulating hormone (TSH)	<4
Nonfunctional tumors		25

HYPOPITUITARISM

Hypopituitarism, which is characterized by a decreased secretion of pituitary hormones, is a condition that affects many of the other endocrine systems.[1] Typically, 70% to 90% of the anterior pituitary must be destroyed before hypopituitarism becomes clinically evident. The cause may be congenital or result from a variety of acquired abnormalities (Chart 42-1). The manifestations of hypopituitarism usually occur gradually, but it can present as an acute and life-threatening condition. Patients usually complain of being chronically unfit, with weakness, fatigue, loss of appetite, impairment of sexual function, and cold intolerance. However, ACTH deficiency (secondary adrenal failure) is the most serious endocrine deficiency, leading to weakness, nausea, anorexia, fever, and postural hypotension. Hypopituitarism is associated with increased morbidity and mortality.

Anterior pituitary hormone loss tends to follow a typical sequence, especially with progressive loss of pituitary reserve due to tumors or previous pituitary radiation therapy (which may take 10 to 20 years to produce hypopituitarism). The sequence of loss of pituitary hormones can be remembered by the mnemonic "*Go Look For The Adenoma*," for *G*H (GH secretion typically is first to be lost), *L*H (results in sex hormone deficiency), *F*SH (causes infertility), *T*SH (leads to secondary hypothyroidism), and *A*CTH (usually the last to become deficient, results in secondary adrenal insufficiency).

Treatment of hypopituitarism includes treating any identified underlying cause. Hormone deficiencies should be treated as dictated by baseline hormone levels and by more sophisticated pituitary testing when appropriate (and safe). Cortisol replacement is started when ACTH deficiency is present, thyroid replacement when TSH deficiency is detected, and sex hormone replacement when LH and FSH are deficient. GH replacement is being used increasingly to treat GH deficiency.[1–3]

CHART 42-1

Causes of Hypopituitarism

- Tumors and mass lesions—pituitary adenomas, cysts, metastatic cancer, and other lesions
- Pituitary surgery or radiation
- Infiltrative lesions and infections—hemochromatosis, lymphocytic hypophysitis
- Pituitary infarction—infarction of the pituitary gland after substantial blood loss during childbirth (Sheehan's syndrome)
- Pituitary apoplexy—sudden hemorrhage into the pituitary gland
- Genetic diseases—rare congenital defects of one or more pituitary hormones
- Empty sella syndrome—an enlarged sella turcica that is not entirely filled with pituitary tissue
- Hypothalamic disorders—tumors and mass lesions (*e.g.,* craniopharyngiomas and metastatic malignancies), hypothalamic radiation, infiltrative lesions (*e.g.,* sarcoidosis), trauma, infections

ASSESSMENT OF HYPOTHALAMIC-PITUITARY FUNCTION

The assessment of hypothalamic-pituitary function has been made possible by many newly developed imaging and radioimmunoassay methods. Assessment of the baseline status of the hypothalamic-pituitary target cell hormones involves measuring the following (ideally performed at 8:00 AM): (1) serum cortisol, (2) serum prolactin, (3) serum thyroxine and TSH, (4) serum testosterone (male) or serum estrogen (female) and serum LH and FSH, (5) serum GH and insulin-like growth factor-1, and (6) plasma osmolality and urine osmolality. Imaging studies (*e.g.,* magnetic resonance imaging [MRI] of the hypothalamus and pituitary) also should be performed as required. When further information regarding pituitary function is required, combined hypothalamic-pituitary function tests are undertaken (although these are performed less often today).[1] These tests consist mainly of hormone stimulation tests (*e.g.,* rapid ACTH stimulation test) or suppression tests (*e.g.,* GH suppression test).

It often is important to test pituitary function, especially if pituitary adenomas are discovered and surgery or radiation treatment is being considered. Diagnostic methods include both static and dynamic testing, as well as radiologic assessment as required. Any of the systems discussed previously may be affected by either deficiency or excess of the usual hormones secreted.

GROWTH AND GROWTH HORMONE DISORDERS

Several hormones are essential for normal body growth and maturation, including growth hormone (GH), insulin, thyroid hormone, and androgens.[3] In addition to its actions on carbohydrate and fat metabolism, insulin plays an essential role in growth processes. Children with diabetes, particularly those with poor control, often fail to grow normally even though GH levels are normal. When levels of thyroid hormone are lower than normal, bone growth and epiphyseal closure are delayed. Androgens such as testosterone and dihydrotestosterone exert anabolic growth effects through their actions on protein synthesis. Glucocorticoids at excessive levels inhibit growth, apparently because of their antagonistic effect on GH secretion.

Growth Hormone

Growth hormone, also called *somatotropin,* is a 191–amino acid polypeptide hormone synthesized and secreted by special cells in the anterior pituitary called *somatotropes.* For many years, it was thought that GH was produced primarily during periods of growth. However, this has proved to be incorrect because the rate of GH production in adults is almost as great as in children. GH is necessary for growth and contributes to the regulation of metabolic functions (Fig. 42-1). All aspects of cartilage growth are stimulated by GH; one of the most striking effects of GH is on linear

GROWTH HORMONE

- Growth hormone (GH), which is produced by somatotropes in the anterior pituitary, is necessary for linear bone growth in children. It also stimulates cells to increase in size and divide more rapidly; it enhances amino acid transport across cell membranes and increases protein synthesis; and it increases the rate at which cells use fatty acids and decreases the rate at which they use carbohydrates.
- The effects of GH on cartilage growth require insulin-like growth factors (IGFs), also called *somatomedins,* which are produced mainly by the liver.
- In children, GH deficiency interferes with linear bone growth, resulting in short stature or dwarfism. In a rare condition called *Laron-type dwarfism,* GH levels are normal or elevated, but there is a hereditary defect in IGF production.
- GH excess in children results in increased linear bone growth, or gigantism. In adults, GH excess results in overgrowth of the cartilaginous parts of the skeleton, enlargement of the heart and other organs of the body, and metabolic disturbances resulting in altered fat metabolism and impaired glucose tolerance.

bone growth, resulting from its action on the epiphyseal growth plates of long bones. The width of bone increases because of enhanced periosteal growth; visceral and endocrine organs, skeletal and cardiac muscle, skin, and connective tissue all undergo increased growth in response to GH. In many instances, the increased growth of visceral and endocrine organs is accompanied by enhanced functional capacity. For example, increased growth of cardiac muscle is accompanied by an increase in cardiac output.

In addition to its effects on growth, GH facilitates the rate of protein synthesis by all of the cells of the body; it enhances fatty acid mobilization and increases the use of fatty acids for fuel; and it maintains or increases blood glucose levels by decreasing the use of glucose for fuel. GH has an initial effect of increasing insulin levels. However, the predominant effect of prolonged GH excess is to increase glucose levels despite an insulin increase. This is because GH induces a resistance to insulin in the peripheral tissues, inhibiting the uptake of glucose by muscle and adipose tissues.[1]

Many of the effects of GH depend on a family of peptides called *insulin-like growth factors* (IGF), also called *somatomedins,* which are produced mainly by the liver.[3] GH cannot directly produce bone growth; instead, it acts indirectly by causing the liver to produce IGF. These peptides act on cartilage and bone to promote their growth. At least four IGFs have been identified; of these, IGF-1

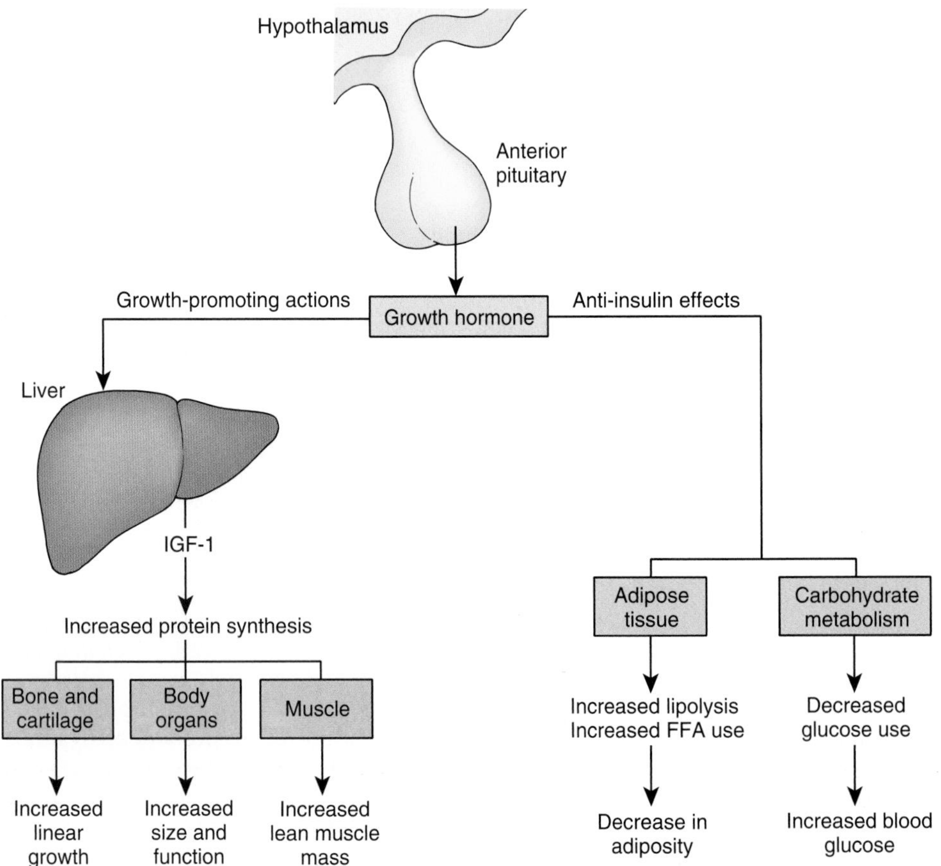

FIGURE 42-1 Growth-promoting and anti-insulin effects of growth hormone. IGF-1, insulin-like growth factor 1.

(somatomedin C) appears to be the more important in terms of growth, and it is the one that usually is measured in laboratory tests. The IGFs have been sequenced and have structures that are similar to that of proinsulin. This undoubtedly explains the insulin-like activity of the IGFs and the weak action of insulin on growth. IGF levels are themselves influenced by a family of at least six binding factors called *IGF-binding proteins* (IGFBPs).

GH is carried unbound in the plasma and has a half-life of approximately 20 to 50 minutes. The secretion of GH is regulated by two hypothalamic hormones: GH-releasing hormone (GHRH), which increases GH release, and somatostatin, which inhibits GH release. A third hormone, the recently identified ghrelin, also may be important. These hypothalamic influences (*i.e.,* GHRH and somatostatin) are tightly regulated by neural, metabolic, and hormonal factors. The secretion of GH fluctuates over a 24-hour period, with peak levels occurring 1 to 4 hours after onset of sleep (*i.e.,* during sleep stages 3 and 4 [see Chapter 15]). The nocturnal sleep bursts, which account for 70% of daily GH secretion, are greater in children than in adults.

GH secretion is stimulated by hypoglycemia, fasting, starvation, increased blood levels of amino acids (particularly arginine), and stress conditions such as trauma, excitement, emotional stress, and heavy exercise. GH is inhibited by increased glucose levels, free fatty acid release, cortisol, and obesity. Impairment of secretion, leading to growth retardation, is not uncommon in children with severe emotional deprivation.

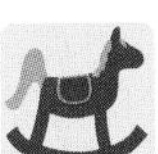

Short Stature in Children

Short stature is a condition in which the attained height is well below the fifth percentile or linear growth is below normal for age and sex. Short stature, or growth retardation, has a variety of causes, including chromosomal abnormalities such as Turner's syndrome (see Chapter 7), GH deficiency, hypothyroidism, and panhypopituitarism.[3] Other conditions known to cause short stature include protein-calorie malnutrition, chronic diseases such as renal failure and poorly controlled diabetes mellitus, malabsorption syndromes, and certain therapies such as corticosteroid administration. Emotional disturbances can lead to functional endocrine disorders, causing psychosocial dwarfism. The causes of short stature are summarized in Chart 42-2.

Accurate measurement of height is an extremely important part of the physical examination of children. Completion of the developmental history and growth charts is essential. Growth curves and growth velocity studies also are needed. Diagnosis of short stature is not made on a single measurement, but is based on actual height and on velocity of growth and parental height.[3]

The diagnostic procedures for short stature include tests to exclude nonendocrine causes. If the cause is hormonal, extensive hormonal testing procedures are initiated. Usually, GH and IGF-1 levels are determined (IGFBP-3 levels also are useful). Tests can be performed using insulin (to induce hypoglycemia), levodopa, and arginine, all of which stimulate GH secretion so that GH reserve can be evaluated.[2,3] Because administration of pharmacologic agents can result in false-negative responses, two or more tests usually are performed. If a prompt rise in GH is realized, the child is considered normal. Physiologic tests of GH reserve (*e.g.,* GH response to exercise) also can be performed. Levels of IGF-1 usually reflect those of GH and may be used to indicate GH deficiency. Radiologic films are used to assess bone age, which most often is delayed. Lateral skull x-rays may be used to evaluate the size and shape of the sella turcica (*i.e.,* depression in the sphenoid bone that contains the pituitary gland) and to determine whether a pituitary tumor exists. However, MRI or computed tomography (CT) scans of the hypothalamic-pituitary area are recommended if a lesion is clinically suspected. After the cause of short stature has been determined, treatment can be initiated.

CHART 42-2

Causes of Short Stature

Variants of Normal

Genetic or "familial" short stature
Constitutional short stature

Low Birth Weight (e.g., intrauterine growth retardation)

Endocrine Disorders

Growth hormone (GH) deficiency
- Primary GH deficiency
  - Idiopathic GH deficiency
  - Pituitary agenesis
- Secondary GH deficiency (panhypopituitarism)
- Biologically inactive GH production
- Deficient IGF-1 production in response to normal or elevated GH (Laron-type dwarfism)

Hypothyroidism
Diabetes mellitus in poor control
Glucocorticoid excess
- Endogenous (Cushing's disease)
- Exogenous (glucocorticoid drug treatment)

Abnormal mineral metabolism (*e.g.,* pseudohypoparathyroidism)

Chronic Illness and Malnutrition

Chronic organic or systemic disease (*e.g.,* asthma, especially when treated with glucocorticoids; heart or renal disease)
Nutritional deprivation
Malabsorption syndrome

Functional Endocrine Disorders (Psychosocial Dwarfism)

Chromosomal Disorders (e.g., Turner's Syndrome)

Skeletal Abnormalities (e.g., achondroplasia)

Unusual Syndromes

Genetic and Constitutional Short Stature. Two forms of short stature, genetic short stature and constitutional short stature, are not disease states but rather are variations from population norms. Genetically short children tend to be well proportioned and to have a height close to the midparental height of their parents. The midparental height for boys can be calculated by adding 13 cm (5 inches) to the height of the mother, adding the father's height, and dividing the total by two. For girls, 13 cm (5 inches) is subtracted from the father's height, the result is added to the mother's height, and the total is divided by two. Ninety-five percent of normal children are within 8.5 cm of the midparental height.

Constitutional short stature is a term used to describe children (particularly boys) who have moderately short stature, thin build, delayed skeletal and sexual maturation, and absence of other causes of decreased growth. *Catch-up growth* is a term used to describe an abnormally high growth rate that occurs as a child approaches normal height for age. It occurs after the initiation of therapy for GH deficiency and hypothyroidism and the correction of chronic diseases.[3]

Psychosocial Dwarfism. Psychosocial dwarfism involves a functional hypopituitarism and is seen in some emotionally deprived children. These children usually present with poor growth, potbelly, and poor eating and drinking habits. Typically, there is a history of disturbed family relationships in which the child has been severely neglected or disciplined. Often, the neglect is confined to one child in the family. GH function usually returns to normal after the child is removed from the constraining environment. The prognosis depends on improvement in behavior and catch-up growth. Family therapy usually is indicated, and foster care may be necessary.

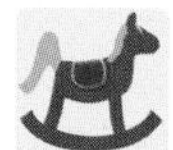

Growth Hormone Deficiency in Children

There are several forms of GH deficiency that present in childhood. Children with idiopathic GH deficiency lack the hypothalamic GHRH but have adequate somatotropes, whereas children with pituitary tumors or agenesis of the pituitary lack somatotropes. The term *panhypopituitarism* refers to conditions that cause a deficiency of all of the anterior pituitary hormones. In a rare condition called *Laron-type dwarfism,* GH levels are normal or elevated, but there is a hereditary defect in IGF production that can be treated directly with IGF-1 replacement.[4]

Congenital GH deficiency is associated with normal birth length, followed by a decrease in growth rate that can be identified by careful measurement during the first year and that becomes obvious by 1 to 2 years of age. Persons with classic GH deficiency have normal intelligence, short stature, obesity with immature facial features, and some delay in skeletal maturation (Fig. 42-2). Puberty often is delayed, and males with the disorder have microphallus (abnormally small penis), especially if the condition is accompanied by gonadotropin-releasing hormone (GnRH) deficiency. In the neonate, GH deficiency can lead to hypoglycemia and seizures; if adrenocorticotropic hormone (ACTH) deficiency also is present, the hypoglycemia often is more severe. Acquired GH deficiency develops in later childhood; it may be caused by a hypothalamic-pituitary tumor, particularly if it is accompanied by other pituitary hormone deficiencies.

When short stature is caused by a GH deficiency, GH replacement therapy is the treatment of choice. GH is species specific, and only human GH is effective in humans. GH previously was obtained from human cadaver pituitaries but now is produced by recombinant DNA technology and is available in adequate supply. In 1985, the National Hormone and Pituitary Program halted the distribution of human GH derived from cadaver pituitaries in the United States after receiving reports that several recipients died of Creutzfeldt-Jakob disease[2,3] (see Chapter 53). The disease, which is caused by a prion protein, was thought to be transmitted by cadaver GH preparations. GH is administered subcutaneously in multiple weekly doses during the period of active growth and can be continued into adulthood.[2,3]

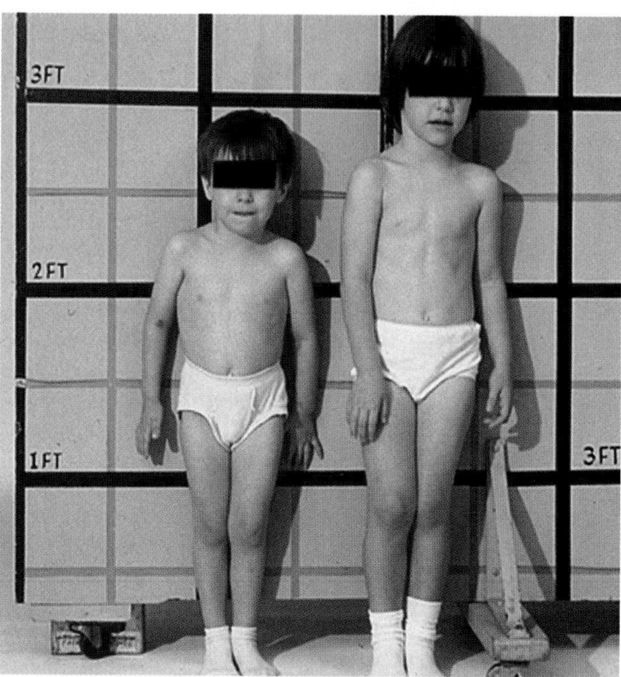

FIGURE 42-2 Child with GH deficiency. A 5.5-year-old boy (**left**) with growth hormone deficiency was significantly shorter than his fraternal twin sister (**right**), with discrepancy beginning early in childhood. Notice his chubby immature appearance compared with his sister. (Shulman D., Bercu B. [2000]. *Atlas of clinical endocrinology, neuroendocrinology, and pituitary diseases* [edited by S. Korenman]. Philadelphia: Current Medicine)

Children with short stature due to Turner's syndrome and chronic renal insufficiency also are treated with GH. GH therapy may be considered for children with short stature but without GH deficiency. Several studies suggest that short-term treatment with GH increases the rate of growth in these children. Although the effect of GH on adult height is not great, it can result in improved psychological well-being. There are concerns about misuse of the drug to produce additional growth in children with normal GH function who are of near-normal height. Guidelines for use of the hormone continue to be established.[2,3]

Growth Hormone Deficiency in Adults

There are two categories of GH deficiency in adults: (1) GH deficiency that was present in childhood, and (2) GH deficiency that developed during adulthood, mainly as the result of hypopituitarism resulting from a pituitary tumor or its treatment. GH levels also can decline with aging, and there has been interest in the effects of declining GH levels in elderly persons (described as *somatopause*). GH replacement obviously is important in the growing child; however, the role in adults (especially for somatopause) is being assessed. Some of the differences between childhood and adult-onset GH deficiency are described in Table 42-2.

Several studies have shown that cardiovascular mortality is increased in GH-deficient adults. Increased arterial intima–media thickness and a higher prevalence of atherosclerotic plaques and endothelial dysfunction have been reported in both childhood and adult GH deficiency. The GH deficiency syndrome is associated with a cluster of cardiovascular risk factors, including central adiposity (increased waist-to-hip ratio), increased visceral fat, insulin resistance, and dyslipidemia. These features also are associated with the *metabolic syndrome* (see Chapter 43). In addition to these so-called traditional cardiovascular risk factors, nontraditional cardiovascular risk factors (*e.g.*, C-reactive protein and interleukin-6, which are markers of the inflammatory pathway) also are elevated. GH therapy can improve many of these factors.[2,3,5]

The diagnosis of GH deficiency in adults is made by finding subnormal serum GH responses to two provocative stimuli (this is the "official" response; however, in reality, at least one stimulation test is needed). Measurements of the serum IGF-1 or basal GH do not distinguish reliably between normal and subnormal GH secretion in adults. Insulin-induced hypoglycemia is the gold standard test for GH reserve. The L-dopa test probably is the next best test. Other stimulation tests involve the use of arginine or arginine plus GHRH, clonidine (an α-adrenergic agonist), glucagon, or GHRH.

The approval of several recombinant human GH preparations (*e.g.*, Humatrope, Genotropin) for treating adults with GH deficiency allows physicians in the United States and elsewhere to prescribe this treatment. In the United States, persons with GH deficiency acquired as an adult must meet at least two criteria for therapy: a poor GH response to at least two standard stimuli, and hypopituitarism due to pituitary or hypothalamic damage. Difficulties can occur with the diagnosis of adult-onset GH deficiency, determining the GH dosage to be given, and monitoring the GH therapy.[1,2]

GH replacement therapy may lead to increased lean body mass and decreased fat mass, increased bone mineral density, increased glomerular filtration rate, decreased lipid levels, increased exercise capacity, and improved sense of well-being in GH-deficient adults. The most common side effects of GH treatment in adults with hypopituitarism are peripheral edema, arthralgias and myalgias, carpal tunnel syndrome, paresthesias, and decreased glucose tolerance. Side effects appear to be more common in people who are older and heavier and are overtreated, as judged by a high serum IGF-1 concentration during therapy. Women seem to tolerate higher doses better then men.

TABLE 42-2 Differences Between Childhood and Adult-Onset Growth Hormone Deficiency

Characteristic	Childhood Onset	Adult Onset
Adult height	↓	NL
Body fat	↑	↑
Lean body mass	↓↓	↓
Bone mineral density	↓	NL, ↓
Insulin-like growth factor (IGF)-1	↓↓	NL, ↓
IGF binding protein-3	↓	NL
Low-density lipoprotein cholesterol	↑	↑
High-density lipoprotein cholesterol	NL, ↓	↓

NL, normal

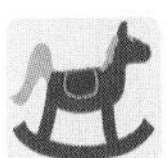

Tall Stature in Children

Just as there are children who are short for their age and sex, there also are children who are tall for their age and sex.[6] Normal variants of tall stature include genetic tall stature and constitutional tall stature. Children with exceptionally tall parents tend to be taller than children with shorter parents. The term *constitutional tall stature* is used to describe a child who is taller than his or her peers and is growing at a velocity that is within the normal range for bone age. Other causes of tall stature are genetic or chromosomal disorders such as Marfan's syndrome or XYY syndrome (see Chapter 7). Endocrine causes of tall stature include sexual precocity because of early onset of estrogen and androgen secretion and excessive GH.

Exceptionally tall children (*i.e.*, genetic tall stature and constitutional tall stature) can be treated with sex hormones—estrogens in girls and testosterone in boys—to effect early epiphyseal closure. Such treatment is undertaken only after full consideration of the risks involved. To be effective, such treatment must be instituted 3 to 4 years before expected epiphyseal fusion.[3,6]

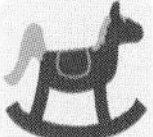

Growth Hormone Excess in Children

Growth hormone excess occurring before puberty and the fusion of the epiphyses of the long bones results in *gigantism* (Fig. 42-3). Excessive secretion of GH by somatotrope adenomas causes gigantism in the prepubertal child. It occurs when the epiphyses are not fused and high levels of IGF stimulate excessive skeletal growth. Fortunately, the condition is rare because of early recognition and treatment of the adenoma.

Growth Hormone Excess in Adults

When GH excess occurs in adulthood or after the epiphyses of the long bones have fused, the condition is referred to as *acromegaly*. Acromegaly results from excess levels of GH that stimulate the hepatic secretion of IGF-1, which causes most of the clinical manifestations of acromegaly. The annual incidence of acromegaly is 3 to 4 cases per 1 million people, with a mean age at the time of diagnosis of 40 to 45 years.[1,7,8]

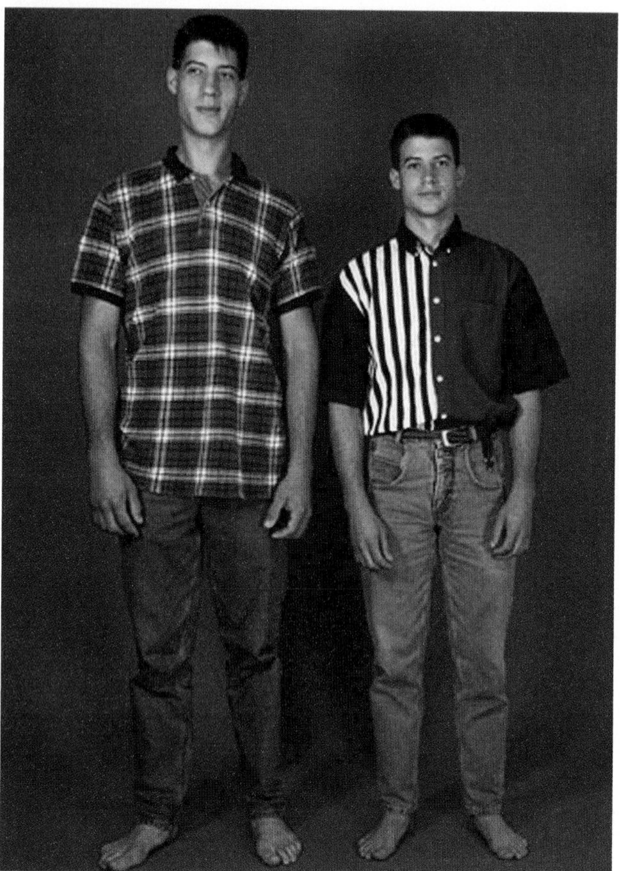

FIGURE 42-3 Primary gigantism. A 22-year-old man with gigantism due to excess growth hormone is shown to the left of his identical twin. (Gagel R.F., McCutcheon I.E. [1999]. Images in Clinical Medicine. *New England Journal of Medicine 340*, 524. Copyright © 2003. Massachusetts Medical Society)

The most common cause (95%) of acromegaly is a somatotrope adenoma. Approximately 75% of persons with acromegaly have a somatotrope macroadenoma at the time of diagnosis, and most of the remainder have microadenomas. The other causes of acromegaly (<5%) are excess secretion of GHRH by hypothalamic tumors, ectopic GHRH secretion by nonendocrine tumors such as carcinoid tumors or small cell lung cancers, and ectopic secretion of GH by nonendocrine tumors.[1,7,8]

The disorder usually has an insidious onset, and symptoms often are present for a considerable period before a diagnosis is made. When the production of excessive GH occurs after the epiphyses of the long bones have closed, as in the adult, the person cannot grow taller, but the soft tissues continue to grow. Enlargement of the small bones of the hands and feet and of the membranous bones of the face and skull results in a pronounced enlargement of the hands and feet, a broad and bulbous nose, a protruding lower jaw, and a slanting forehead. The teeth become splayed, causing a disturbed bite and difficulty in chewing. The cartilaginous structures in the larynx and respiratory tract also become enlarged, resulting in a deepening of the voice and tendency to develop bronchitis. Vertebral changes often lead to kyphosis, or hunchback. Bone overgrowth often leads to arthralgias and degenerative arthritis of the spine, hips, and knees. Virtually every organ of the body is increased in size. Enlargement of the heart and accelerated atherosclerosis may lead to an early death.

The metabolic effects of excess levels of GH include alterations in fat and carbohydrate metabolism. GH causes increased release of free fatty acids from adipose tissue, leading to increased concentration of free fatty acids in body fluids. In addition, GH enhances the formation of ketones and the utilization of free fatty acids for energy in preference to use of carbohydrates and proteins. GH exerts multiple effects on carbohydrate metabolism, including decreased glucose uptake by tissues such as skeletal muscle and adipose tissue, increased glucose production by the liver, and increased insulin secretion. Each of these changes results in GH-induced insulin resistance (see Chapter 43). This leads to glucose intolerance, which stimulates the beta cells of the pancreas to produce additional insulin. Long-term elevation of GH results in overstimulation of the beta cells, causing them literally to "burn out." Impaired glucose tolerance occurs in as many as 50% to 70% of persons with acromegaly; overt diabetes mellitus subsequently can result.

The pituitary gland is located in the pituitary fossa of the sphenoid bone (*i.e.*, sella turcica), which lies directly below the optic nerve. Almost all persons with acromegaly have a recognizable adenohypophysial tumor. Enlargement of the pituitary gland eventually causes erosion of the surrounding bone, and because of its location, this can lead to headaches, visual field defects resulting from compression of the optic nerve (classically bitemporal hemianopia), and palsies of cranial nerves III, IV, and VI. Compression of other pituitary structures can cause secondary hypothyroidism, hypogonadism, and adrenal insufficiency. The hypogonadism can result from direct damage to the hypothalamic or pituitary system, or indirectly from the hyperprolactinemia that can occur due to prevention of the prolactin inhibitory factor (dopamine) from reaching pituitary lactotrophs (cells which secrete prolactin) due to damage by the pituitary tumor.

Other manifestations include excessive sweating with an unpleasant odor, oily skin, heat intolerance, moderate weight gain, muscle weakness and fatigue, menstrual irregularities, and decreased libido. Hypertension is relatively common. Sleep apnea syndrome is present in up to 90% of patients. The pathogenesis of the sleep apnea syndrome is obstructive in the majority of patients, owing to increased pharyngeal soft tissue accumulation. Paresthesias may develop because of nerve entrapment and compression caused by excess soft tissue and accumulation of subcutaneous fluid (especially carpal tunnel syndrome). Acromegaly also is associated with an increased risk for colonic polyps and colorectal cancer. The mortality rate of patients with acromegaly is two to three times the expected rate, mostly from cardiovascular diseases and cancer. The cardiovascular disease results from the combination of cardiomyopathy, hypertension, insulin resistance and hyperinsulinemia, and hyperlipidemia.

Acromegaly often develops insidiously, and only a small number of persons seek medical care because of changes in appearance. The diagnosis of acromegaly is facilitated by the typical features of the disorder—enlargement of the hands and feet and coarsening of facial features. Laboratory tests to detect elevated levels of GH not suppressed by a glucose load are used to confirm the diagnosis. MRI and CT scans can detect and localize the pituitary lesions. Because most of the effects of GH are mediated by IGF-1, IGF-1 levels may provide information about disease activity.

The treatment goals for acromegaly focus on the correction of metabolic abnormalities, and include normalization of the GH response to an oral glucose load; normalization of IGF-1 levels to age- and sex-matched control levels; removal or reduction of the tumor mass, relieving the central pressure effects; improvement of adverse clinical features; and normalization of the mortality rate.[7–9] Pituitary tumors can be removed surgically using the transsphenoidal approach or, if that is not possible, a transfrontal craniotomy. Radiation therapy may be used, but remission (reduction in GH levels) may not occur for several years after therapy. Radiation therapy also significantly increases the risk for hypopituitarism, hypothyroidism, hypoadrenalism, and hypogonadism.

Medical therapy is usually given in an adjunctive role.[1,7,8] Octreotide acetate, an analog of somatostatin that produces feedback inhibition of GH, has been effective in the medical management of acromegaly. However, the medication must be given subcutaneously three times per week for effective dosing. Newer, longer-acting analogs of somatostatin are now available, including Sandostatin LAR, which is a sustained-release formulation of octreotide that effectively inhibits GH secretion for 30 days after a single intramuscular injection of 20 to 30 mg. Lanreotide also is available in a long-acting formulation that has comparable efficacy to octreotide when injected intramuscularly two to three times per month. Bromocriptine, a long-acting dopamine agonist, reduces GH levels and has been used with some success in the medical management of acromegaly. However, high doses often are required, and side effects may be troublesome. Several newly available dopamine agonists (*e.g.*, cabergoline, quinagolide) also can be considered as an alternative or adjunctive therapy.[7,8,10] Growth hormone receptor antagonists (*e.g.*, pegvisomant) are analogs of human GH that have been structurally altered. GH receptor antagonists bind to GH receptors on the cell surfaces, where they block the binding of endogenous GH and thus interfere with GH signal transduction. This results in a decrease in serum IGF-1 levels.[7,8,11]

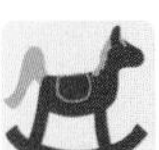

ISOSEXUAL PRECOCIOUS PUBERTY

Precocious sexual development may be idiopathic or may be caused by gonadal, adrenal, or hypothalamic disease.[12,13] Isosexual precocious puberty is defined as early activation of the hypothalamic-pituitary-gonadal axis, resulting in the development of appropriate sexual characteristics and fertility. Classically, sexual development was considered precocious and warranting investigation when it occurred before 8 years of age for girls and before 9 years of age for boys. However, these criteria were revised recently based on an office pediatric study of more than 17,000 American girls.[14] Precocious puberty is now defined as the appearance of secondary sexual development before the age of 7 years in white girls and 6 years in African-American girls.[13] In boys of either race, the age lower limit remains 9 years; however, it is recognized that puberty can develop earlier in boys with obesity (an increasingly common problem).[13] Benign and malignant tumors of the central nervous system (CNS) can cause precocious puberty. These tumors are thought to remove the inhibitory influences normally exerted on the hypothalamus during childhood. CNS tumors are found more often in boys with precocious puberty than in girls. In girls, most cases are idiopathic.

Diagnosis of precocious puberty is based on physical findings of early thelarche (*i.e.*, beginning of breast development), adrenarche (*i.e.*, beginning of augmented adrenal androgen production), and menarche (*i.e.*, beginning of menstrual function) in girls. The most common sign in boys is early genital enlargement. Radiologic findings may indicate advanced bone age. Persons with precocious puberty usually are tall for their age as children but short as adults because of the early closure of the epiphyses. MRI or CT should be used to exclude intracranial lesions.

Depending on the cause of precocious puberty, the treatment may involve surgery, medication, or no treatment. The treatment of choice is administration of a long-acting GnRH agonist. Constant levels of the hormone cause a decrease in pituitary responsiveness to GnRH, leading to decreased secretion of gonadotropic hormones and sex steroids. Parents often need education, support, and anticipatory guidance in dealing with their feelings and the child's physical needs and in relating to a child who appears older than his or her years.[12,13]

In summary, pituitary tumors can result in deficiencies or excesses of pituitary hormones. Hypopituitarism, which is characterized by a decreased secretion of pituitary hormones, is a condition that affects many of the other endocrine systems. Depending on the extent of the disorder, it can result in decreased levels of GH, thyroid hormones, adrenal corticosteroid hormones, and testosterone in the male and of estrogens and progesterone in the female.

A number of hormones are essential for normal body growth and maturation, including GH, insulin, thyroid hormone, and androgens. GH exerts its growth effects through a group of IGFs. GH also exerts an effect on metabolism and is produced in the adult and in the child. Its metabolic effects include a decrease in peripheral use of carbohydrates and an increased mobilization and use of fatty acids.

In children, alterations in growth include short stature, isosexual precocious puberty, and tall stature. Short stature is a condition in which the attained height is well below the fifth percentile or the linear growth velocity is below normal for a child's age or sex. Short stature can occur as a variant of normal growth (*i.e.*, genetic short stature or constitutional short stature) or as the result of endocrine disorders, chronic illness, malnutrition, emotional disturbances, or chromosomal disorders. Short stature resulting from GH deficiency can be treated with human GH preparations. In adults, GH deficiency represents a deficiency carried over from childhood or one that develops during adulthood as the result of a pituitary tumor or its treatment. GH levels also can decline with aging, and there has been interest in the effects of declining GH levels in elderly persons (described as *somatopause*).

Tall stature refers to the condition in which children are tall for their age and sex. It can occur as a variant of normal growth (*i.e.*, genetic tall stature or constitutional tall stature) or as the result of a chromosomal abnormality or GH excess. GH excess in adults results in acromegaly, which involves proliferation of bone, cartilage, and soft tissue along with the metabolic effects of excessive hormone levels. Isosexual precocious puberty defines a condition of early activation of the hypothalamic-pituitary-gonadal axis (*i.e.*, before 6 years of age in black girls and 7 years in white girls, and before 9 years of age in boys of either race), resulting in the development of appropriate sexual characteristics and fertility. It causes tall stature during childhood but results in short stature in adulthood because of the early closure of the epiphyses.

Thyroid Disorders

After completing this section of the chapter, you should be able to meet the following objectives:

- Characterize the synthesis, transport, and regulation of thyroid hormone
- Diagram the hypothalamic-pituitary-thyroid feedback system
- Describe tests in the diagnosis and management of thyroid disorders
- Relate the functions of thyroid hormone to hypothyroidism and hyperthyroidism
- Describe the effects of congenital hypothyroidism
- Characterize the manifestations and treatment of myxedematous coma and thyroid storm

CONTROL OF THYROID FUNCTION

The thyroid gland is a shield-shaped structure located immediately below the larynx in the anterior middle portion of the neck. It is composed of a large number of tiny, saclike structures called *follicles* (Fig. 42-4). These are the functional units of the thyroid. Each follicle is formed by a single layer of epithelial (follicular) cells and is filled with a secretory substance called *colloid,* which consists largely of a glycoprotein–iodine complex called *thyroglobulin.*

The thyroglobulin that fills the thyroid follicles is a large glycoprotein molecule that contains 140 tyrosine amino acids. In the process of thyroid synthesis, iodine is attached to these tyrosines. Both thyroglobulin and iodide are secreted into the colloid of the follicle by the follicular cells.

The thyroid is remarkably efficient in its use of iodide (I^-). A daily absorption of 150 to 200 μg of dietary iodine (I) is sufficient to form normal quantities of thyroid hormone. In the process of removing it from the blood and storing it for future use, iodide is pumped into the follicular cells against a concentration gradient. Iodide is transported across the basement membrane of the thyroid cells by an intrinsic membrane protein called the Na^+/I^-

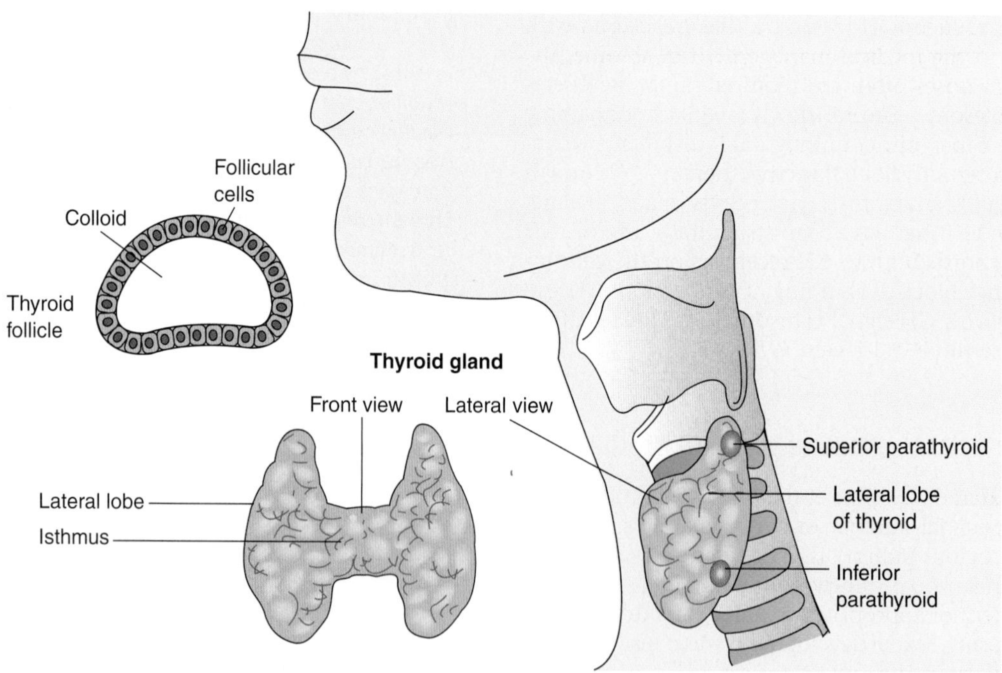

FIGURE 42-4 The thyroid gland and the follicular structure.

symporter (NIS).[15] At the apical border, a second I^- transport protein called pendrin moves iodine into the colloid, where it is involved in hormonogenesis. The NIS derives its energy from Na^+-K^+-ATPase, which drives the process. As a result, the concentration of iodide in the normal thyroid gland is approximately 40 times that in the blood.

The NIS is stimulated by both TSH and the TSH receptor-stimulating antibody found in Graves' disease. Pendrin, encoded by the Pendred's syndrome gene (PDS), is a transporter of chloride and iodide. Mutations in the PDS gene have been found in patients with goiter and congenital deafness (Pendred's syndrome).

Once inside the follicle, most of the iodide is oxidized by the enzyme thyroid peroxidase (TPO) in a reaction that facilitates combination with a tyrosine molecule to form monoiodotyrosine and then diiodotyrosine (Fig. 42-5). Two diiodotyrosine residues are coupled to form thyroxine (T_4), or a monoiodotyrosine and a diiodotyrosine are coupled to form triiodothyronine (T_3). Only T_4 (90%) and T_3 (10%) are released into the circulation. There is evidence that T_3 is the active form of the hormone and that T_4 is converted to T_3 before it can act physiologically.

Thyroid hormones are bound to thyroid-binding globulin and other plasma proteins for transport in the blood. Only the free hormone enters cells and regulates the pituitary feedback mechanism. Protein-bound thyroid hormone forms a large reservoir that is slowly drawn on as free thyroid hormone is needed. There are three major thyroid-binding proteins: thyroid hormone–binding globulin (TBG), thyroxine-binding prealbumin (TBPA), and albumin. More than 99% of T_4 and T_3 is carried in the bound form. TBG carries approximately 70% of T_4 and T_3; TBPA binds approximately 10% of circulating T_4 and lesser amounts of T_3; and albumin binds approximately 15% of circulating T_4 and T_3.

A number of disease conditions and pharmacologic agents can decrease the amount of binding protein in the plasma or influence the binding of hormone. Congenital TBG deficiency is an X-linked trait that occurs in 1 of every 2500 live births. Corticosteroid medications and systemic disease conditions such as protein malnutrition, nephrotic syndrome, and cirrhosis decrease TBG concentrations. Medications such as phenytoin, salicylates, and diazepam can affect the binding of thyroid hormone to normal concentrations of binding proteins.

The secretion of thyroid hormone is regulated by the hypothalamic-pituitary-thyroid feedback system (Fig. 42-6). In this system, thyrotropin-releasing hormone (TRH), which is produced by the hypothalamus, controls the release of TSH from the anterior pituitary gland. TSH increases the overall activity of the thyroid gland by increasing thyroglobulin breakdown and the release of thyroid hormone from follicles into the bloodstream, activating the iodide pump (by increasing NIS activity), increasing the oxidation of iodide and the coupling of iodide to tyrosine, and increasing the number and the size of the follicle cells. The effect of TSH on the release of thyroid hormones occurs within approximately 30 minutes, but the other effects require days or weeks.

Increased levels of thyroid hormone act in the feedback inhibition of TRH or TSH. High levels of iodide (*e.g.*, from iodide-containing cough syrup or kelp tablets) also cause a temporary decrease in thyroid activity that lasts for several weeks, probably through a direct inhibition of TSH on the thyroid. Cold exposure is one of the strongest stimuli for increased thyroid hormone production and probably is mediated through TRH from the hypothalamus. Various emotional reactions also can affect the output of TRH and TSH and therefore indirectly affect secretion of thyroid hormones.

Actions of Thyroid Hormone

All the major organs in the body are affected by altered levels of thyroid hormone. Thyroid hormone has two major functions: it increases metabolism and protein synthesis, and it is necessary for growth and development in children,

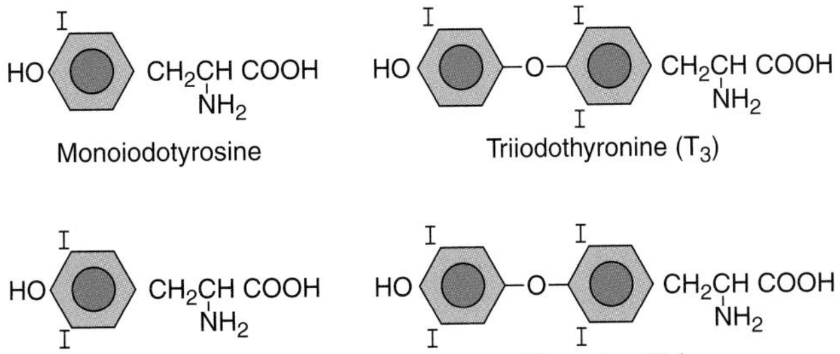

Tyrosine

Monoiodotyrosine

Triiodothyronine (T_3)

Diiodotyrosine

Thyroxine (T_4)

FIGURE 42-5 Chemistry of thyroid hormone production.

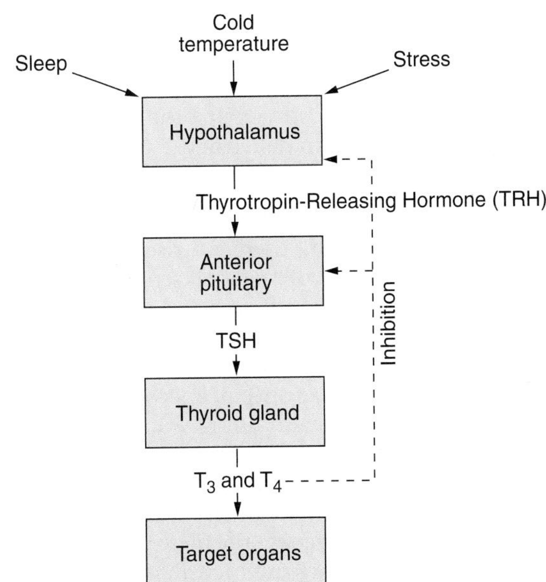

FIGURE 42-6 The hypothalamic-pituitary-thyroid feedback system, which regulates the body levels of thyroid hormone.

THYROID HORMONE

- Thyroid hormone increases the metabolism and protein synthesis in nearly all of the tissues of the body.
- It also is necessary for brain development and growth in infants and small children. Infants born with decreased or absent thyroid function have impaired mental and physical development.
- When hypothyroidism occurs in older children or adults, it produces a decrease in metabolic rate, an accumulation of a hydrophilic mucopolysaccharide substance (myxedema) in the connective tissues throughout the body, and an elevation in serum cholesterol.
- Hyperthyroidism has an effect opposite that of hypothyroidism. It produces an increase in metabolic rate and oxygen consumption, increased use of metabolic fuels, and increased sympathetic nervous system responsiveness.

including mental development and attainment of sexual maturity. Circulating T_4 is converted to T_3 in the periphery. In the cell, T_3 binds to a nuclear receptor, resulting in transcription of specific thyroid hormone responsive genes.[15]

Metabolic Rate. Thyroid hormone increases the metabolism of all body tissues except the retina, spleen, testes, and lungs. The basal metabolic rate can increase by 60% to 100% above normal when large amounts of T_4 are present. As a result of this higher metabolism, the rate of glucose, fat, and protein use increases. Lipids are mobilized from adipose tissue, and the catabolism of cholesterol by the liver is increased. Blood levels of cholesterol are decreased in hyperthyroidism and increased in hypothyroidism. Muscle proteins are broken down and used as fuel, probably accounting for some of the muscle fatigue that occurs with hyperthyroidism. The absorption of glucose from the gastrointestinal tract is increased. Because vitamins are essential parts of metabolic enzymes and coenzymes, an increase in metabolic rate "speeds up" the use of vitamins and tends to cause vitamin deficiency.

Cardiovascular Function. Cardiovascular and respiratory functions are strongly affected by thyroid function. With an increase in metabolism, there is a rise in oxygen consumption and production of metabolic end products, with an accompanying increase in vasodilatation. Blood flow to the skin, in particular, is augmented as a means of dissipating the body heat that results from the higher metabolism. Blood volume, cardiac output, and ventilation all are increased as a means of maintaining blood flow and oxygen delivery to body tissues. Heart rate and cardiac contractility are enhanced as a means of maintaining the needed cardiac output. On the other hand, blood pressure is likely to change little because the increase in vasodilatation tends to offset the increase in cardiac output.

Gastrointestinal Function. Thyroid hormone enhances gastrointestinal function, causing an increase in motility and production of gastrointestinal secretions that often results in diarrhea. An increase in appetite and food intake accompanies the higher metabolic rate that occurs with increased thyroid hormone levels. At the same time, weight loss occurs because of the increased use of calories.

Neuromuscular Effects. Thyroid hormone has marked effects on neural control of muscle function and tone. Slight elevations in hormone levels cause skeletal muscles to react more vigorously, and a drop in hormone levels causes muscles to react more sluggishly. In the hyperthyroid state, a fine muscle tremor is present. The cause of this tremor is unknown, but it may represent an increased sensitivity of the neural synapses in the spinal cord that control muscle tone.

In the infant, thyroid hormone is necessary for normal brain development. The hormone enhances cerebration; in the hyperthyroid state, it causes extreme nervousness, anxiety, and difficulty in sleeping.

Evidence suggests a strong interaction between thyroid hormone and the sympathetic nervous system. Many of the signs and symptoms of hyperthyroidism suggest overactivity of the sympathetic division of the autonomic nervous system, such as tachycardia, palpitations, and sweating. Tremor, restlessness, anxiety, and diarrhea also may reflect autonomic nervous system imbalances. Drugs that block sympathetic activity have proved to be valuable adjuncts in the treatment of hyperthyroidism because of their ability to relieve some of these undesirable symptoms.

Tests of Thyroid Function

Various tests aid in the diagnosis of thyroid disorders.[15,16] Measures of T_3, T_4, and TSH have been made available through immunoassay methods. The free T_4 test measures the unbound portion of T_4 that is free to enter cells to produce its effects. The resin uptake test is an inverse test of TBG. The test involves adding radiolabeled T_3 or T_4 to a serum sample and allowing it to compete with the T_3 or T_4 in the sample for binding sites on TBG. The mixture is then added to a thyroid hormone–binding resin and the resin assayed for uptake of the labeled T_3 or T_4. A high resin test result indicates that the serum sample contains low amounts of TBG or high T_4 levels. TSH levels are used to differentiate between primary and secondary thyroid disorders. T_3, T_4, and free T_4 levels are low in primary hypothyroidism, and the TSH level is elevated. The assessment of thyroid autoantibodies (*e.g.,* anti–thyroid peroxidase [anti-TPO] antibodies in Hashimoto's thyroiditis) is important in the diagnostic workup and consequent follow-up of thyroid patients.

The radioiodine (^{123}I) uptake test measures the ability of the thyroid gland to remove and concentrate iodine from the blood. Thyroid scans (*i.e.,* ^{123}I, ^{99m}Tc-pertechnetate) can be used to detect thyroid nodules and determine the functional activity of the thyroid gland. Ultrasonography can be used to differentiate cystic from solid thyroid lesions, and CT and MRI scans are used to demonstrate tracheal compression or impingement on other neighboring structures. Fine-needle aspiration (FNA) biopsy of a thyroid nodule has proved to be the best method for differentiation of benign from malignant thyroid disease.

TABLE 42-3 Manifestations of Hypothyroid and Hyperthyroid States

Level of Organization	Hypothyroidism	Hyperthyroidism
Basal metabolic rate	Decreased	Increased
Sensitivity to catecholamines	Decreased	Increased
General features	Myxedematous features Deep voice Impaired growth (child)	Exophthalmos Lid lag Decreased blinking
Blood cholesterol levels	Increased	Decreased
General behavior	Mental retardation (infant) Mental and physical sluggishness Somnolence	Restlessness, irritability, anxiety Hyperkinesis Wakefulness
Cardiovascular function	Decreased cardiac output Bradycardia	Increased cardiac output Tachycardia and palpitations
Gastrointestinal function	Constipation Decreased appetite	Diarrhea Increased appetite
Respiratory function	Hypoventilation	Dyspnea
Muscle tone and reflexes	Decreased	Increased, with tremor and fibrillatory twitching
Temperature tolerance	Cold intolerance	Heat intolerance
Skin and hair	Decreased sweating Coarse and dry skin and hair	Increased sweating Thin and silky skin and hair
Weight	Gain	Loss

Alterations in Thyroid Function

An alteration in thyroid function can represent a hypofunctional or a hyperfunctional state. The manifestations of these two altered states are summarized in Table 42-3. Disorders of the thyroid may be due to a congenital defect in thyroid development, or they may develop later in life, with a gradual or sudden onset.

Goiter is an increase in the size of the thyroid gland. It can occur in hypothyroid, euthyroid, and hyperthyroid states. Goiters may be diffuse, involving the entire gland without evidence of nodularity, or they may contain nodules. Diffuse goiters usually become nodular. Goiters may be toxic, producing signs of extreme hyperthyroidism, or thyrotoxicosis, or they may be nontoxic. Diffuse nontoxic and multinodular goiters are the result of compensatory hypertrophy and hyperplasia of follicular epithelium from some derangement that impairs thyroid hormone output.

The degree of thyroid enlargement usually is proportional to the extent and duration of thyroid deficiency. Multinodular goiters produce the largest thyroid enlargements and often are associated with thyrotoxicosis. When sufficiently enlarged, they may compress the esophagus and trachea, causing difficulty in swallowing, a choking sensation, and inspiratory stridor. Such lesions also may compress the superior vena cava, producing distention of the veins of the neck and upper extremities, edema of the eyelids and conjunctiva, and syncope with coughing.

HYPOTHYROIDISM

Hypothyroidism can occur as a congenital or an acquired defect. Congenital hypothyroidism develops prenatally and is present at birth. Acquired hypothyroidism develops later in life because of primary disease of the thyroid gland or secondary to disorders of hypothalamic or pituitary origin.

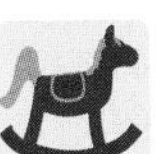

Congenital Hypothyroidism

Congenital hypothyroidism is a common cause of preventable mental retardation. It affects approximately 1 of 5000 infants. Hypothyroidism in the infant may result from a congenital lack of the thyroid gland or from abnormal biosynthesis of thyroid hormone or deficient TSH secretion. With congenital lack of the thyroid gland, the infant usually appears normal and functions normally at birth because hormones have been supplied in utero by the mother. The manifestations of untreated congenital hypothyroidism are referred to as *cretinism*. However, the term does not apply to the normally developing infant in whom replacement thyroid hormone therapy was instituted shortly after birth.

Thyroid hormone is essential for normal brain development and growth, almost half of which occurs during the first 6 months of life. If untreated, congenital hypothyroidism causes mental retardation and impairs growth. Long-term studies show that closely monitored T_4 supplementation begun in the first 6 weeks of life results in normal intelligence. Fortunately, neonatal screening tests have been instituted to detect congenital hypothyroidism during early infancy. Screening usually is done in the hospital nursery. In this test, a drop of blood is taken from the infant's heel and analyzed for T_4 and TSH.

Transient congenital hypothyroidism has been recognized more frequently since the introduction of neonatal screening. It is characterized by high TSH levels and low thyroid hormone levels. The fetal and infant thyroids are sensitive to iodine excess. Iodine crosses the placenta and mammary glands and is readily absorbed by infant skin. Transient hypothyroidism may be caused by maternal or infant exposure to substances such as povidone-iodine used as a disinfectant (*i.e.,* vaginal douche or skin disinfectant, in the nursery). Antithyroid drugs, such as propylthiouracil and methimazole, can cross the placenta and block fetal thyroid function.

Congenital hypothyroidism is treated by hormone replacement. Evidence indicates that it is important to normalize T_4 levels as rapidly as possible because a delay is accompanied by poorer psychomotor and mental development. Dosage levels are adjusted as the child grows. Infants with transient hypothyroidism usually can have the replacement therapy withdrawn at 6 to 12 months. When early and adequate treatment regimens are followed, the risk for mental retardation in infants detected by screening programs essentially is nonexistent.

Acquired Hypothyroidism and Myxedema

Hypothyroidism in older children and adults causes a general slowing down of metabolic processes and myxedema. Myxedema implies the presence of a nonpitting mucous type of edema caused by an accumulation of a hydrophilic mucopolysaccharide substance in the connective tissues throughout the body. The hypothyroid state may be mild, with only a few signs and symptoms, or it may progress to a life-threatening condition called *myxedematous coma.* It can result from destruction or dysfunction of the thyroid gland (*i.e.,* primary hypothyroidism), or it can be a secondary disorder caused by impaired pituitary function or a tertiary disorder caused by a hypothalamic dysfunction.

Primary hypothyroidism is much more common than secondary (and tertiary) hypothyroidism. It may result from thyroidectomy (*i.e.,* surgical removal) or ablation of the gland with radiation. Certain goitrogenic agents, such as lithium carbonate (*i.e.,* used in the treatment of manic-depressive states), and the antithyroid drugs propylthiouracil and methimazole in continuous dosage can block hormone synthesis and produce hypothyroidism with goiter. Large amounts of iodine (*i.e.,* ingestion of kelp tablets or iodide-containing cough syrups, or administration of iodide-containing radiographic contrast media or the cardiac drug amiodarone [which contains 75 mg of iodine per 200-mg tablet]) also can block thyroid hormone production and cause goiter, particularly in persons with autoimmune thyroid disease. Iodine deficiency, which can cause goiter and hypothyroidism, is rare in the United States because of the widespread use of iodized salt and other iodide sources.

The most common cause of hypothyroidism is Hashimoto's thyroiditis, an autoimmune disorder in which the thyroid gland may be totally destroyed by an immunologic process.[17] It is the major cause of goiter and hypothyroidism in children and adults. Hashimoto's thyroiditis is predominantly a disease of women, with a female-to-male ratio of 5:1. The course of the disease varies. At the onset, only a goiter may be present. In time, hypothyroidism usually becomes evident. Although the disorder usually causes hypothyroidism, a hyperthyroid state may develop midcourse in the disease. The transient hyperthyroid state is caused by leakage of preformed thyroid hormone from damaged cells of the gland. Subacute thyroiditis, which can occur in up to 10% of pregnancies postpartum (postpartum thyroiditis), also can result in hypothyroidism.

Hypothyroidism affects almost all of the organ systems in the body. The manifestations of the disorder are related largely to two factors: the hypometabolic state resulting from thyroid hormone deficiency, and myxedematous involvement of body tissues. Although the myxedema is most obvious in the face and other superficial parts, it also affects many of the body organs and is responsible for many of the manifestations of the hypothyroid state (Fig. 42-7).

The hypometabolic state associated with hypothyroidism is characterized by a gradual onset of weakness and fatigue, a tendency to gain weight despite a loss of appetite, and cold intolerance. As the condition progresses, the skin becomes dry and rough and acquires a pale yellowish cast, which primarily results from carotene deposition, and the hair becomes coarse and brittle. There can be loss of the lateral one third of the eyebrows. Gastrointestinal motility is decreased, producing constipation, flatulence, and abdominal distention. Nervous system involvement is manifested in mental dullness, lethargy, and impaired memory.

As a result of myxedematous fluid accumulation, the face takes on a characteristic puffy look, especially around the eyes. The tongue is enlarged, and the voice is hoarse and husky. Myxedematous fluid can collect in the interstitial spaces of almost any organ system. Pericardial or pleural effusion may develop. Mucopolysaccharide deposits in the heart cause generalized cardiac dilatation, bradycardia, and

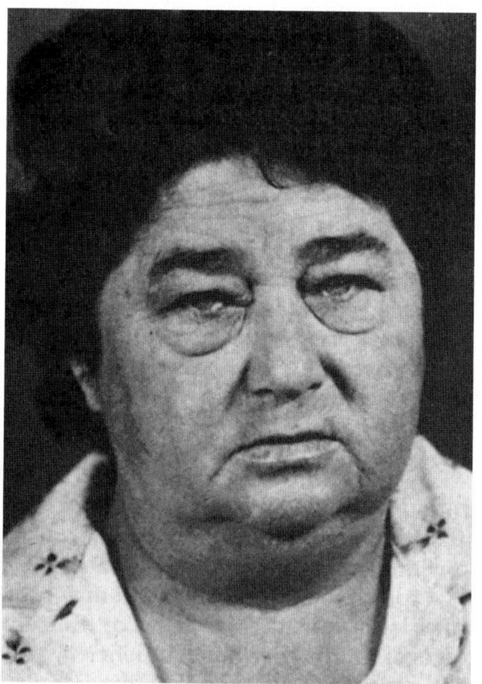

FIGURE 42-7 Patient with myxedema. Courtesy of Dr. Herbert Langford. (From Guyton A. [1981]. *Medical physiology* [6th ed., p. 941]. Philadelphia: W.B. Saunders. Reprinted by permission)

other signs of altered cardiac function. The signs and symptoms of hypothyroidism are summarized in Table 42-3.

Diagnosis of hypothyroidism is based on history, physical examination, and laboratory tests. A low serum T_4 and elevated TSH levels are characteristic of primary hypothyroidism. The tests for antithyroid antibodies should be done when Hashimoto's thyroiditis is suspected (antithyroid peroxidase [anti-TPO] antibody titer measurement is the preferred test). A TRH stimulation test may be helpful in differentiating pituitary (secondary hypothyroidism) from hypothalamic (tertiary hypothyroidism) disease.

Hypothyroidism is treated by replacement therapy with synthetic preparations of T_3 or T_4. Most people are treated with T_4. Serum TSH levels are used to estimate the adequacy of T_4 replacement therapy. When the TSH level is normalized, the T_4 dosage is considered satisfactory (for primary hypothyroidism only). A "go low and go slow" approach should be considered in the treatment of elderly patients with hypothyroidism because of the risk for inducing acute coronary syndromes in the susceptible individual.

Myxedematous Coma

Myxedematous coma is a life-threatening, end-stage expression of hypothyroidism. It is characterized by coma, hypothermia, cardiovascular collapse, hypoventilation, and severe metabolic disorders that include hyponatremia, hypoglycemia, and lactic acidosis. The pathophysiology of myxedema coma involves three major aspects: (1) carbon dioxide retention and hypoxia, (2) fluid and electrolyte imbalance, and (3) hypothermia.[15] It occurs most often in elderly women who have chronic hypothyroidism from a spectrum of causes. The fact that it occurs more frequently in winter months suggests that cold exposure may be a precipitating factor. The severely hypothyroid person is unable to metabolize sedatives, analgesics, and anesthetic drugs, and buildup of these agents may precipitate coma.

Treatment includes aggressive management of precipitating factors; supportive therapy, such as management of cardiorespiratory status, hyponatremia, and hypoglycemia; and thyroid replacement therapy. If hypothermia is present (a low-reading thermometer should be used), active rewarming of the body is contraindicated because it may induce vasodilation and vascular collapse. Prevention is preferable to treatment and entails special attention to high-risk populations, such as women with a history of Hashimoto's thyroiditis. These persons should be informed about the signs and symptoms of severe hypothyroidism and the need for early medical treatment.

HYPERTHYROIDISM

Thyrotoxicosis is the clinical syndrome that results when tissues are exposed to high levels of circulating thyroid hormone.[15,18,19] In most instances, thyrotoxicosis is due to hyperactivity of the thyroid gland, or hyperthyroidism.[15,18] The most common cause of hyperthyroidism is Graves' disease, which is accompanied by ophthalmopathy (or dermopathy) and diffuse goiter.[15,18,19] Other causes of hyperthyroidism are multinodular goiter, adenoma of the thyroid, and, occasionally, ingestion of excessive thyroid hormone.[18] Iodine-containing agents can induce hyperthyroidism as well as hypothyroidism. Thyroid crisis, or storm, is an acutely exaggerated manifestation of the thyrotoxic state.

Many of the manifestations of hyperthyroidism are related to the increase in oxygen consumption and use of metabolic fuels associated with the hypermetabolic state as well as to the increase in sympathetic nervous system activity that occurs.[18] The fact that many of the signs and symptoms of hyperthyroidism resemble those of excessive sympathetic nervous system activity suggests that thyroid hormone may heighten the sensitivity of the body to the catecholamines or that it may act as a pseudocatecholamine. With the hypermetabolic state, there are frequent complaints of nervousness, irritability, and fatigability. Weight loss is common despite a large appetite. Other manifestations include tachycardia, palpitations, shortness of breath, excessive sweating, muscle cramps, and heat intolerance. The person appears restless and has a fine muscle tremor. Even in persons without exophthalmos (*i.e.,* bulging of the eyeballs seen in ophthalmopathy), there is an abnormal retraction of the eyelids and infrequent blinking such that they appear to be staring. The hair and skin usually are thin and have a silky appearance. About 15% of elderly individuals with new-onset atrial fibrillation have thyrotoxicosis.[18] The signs and symptoms of hyperthyroidism are summarized in Table 42-3.

The treatment of hyperthyroidism is directed toward reducing the level of thyroid hormone. This can be accomplished with eradication of the thyroid gland with radioactive iodine, through surgical removal of part or all of the gland, or with the use of drugs that decrease thyroid function and thereby the effect of thyroid hormone on the peripheral tissues. Eradication of the thyroid with radioactive iodine is used more frequently than surgery. The β-adrenergic–blocking drugs (*e.g.,* propranolol, metoprolol, atenolol, and nadolol are preferred) are administered to block the effects of the hyperthyroid state on sympathetic nervous system function. They are given in conjunction with antithyroid drugs such as propylthiouracil and methimazole. These drugs prevent the thyroid gland from converting iodine to its organic (hormonal) form and block the conversion of T_4 to T_3 in the tissues. Iodinated contrast agents (iopanoic acid and ipodate sodium) may be given orally to block thyroid hormone synthesis and release as well as the peripheral conversion of T_4 and T_3. These agents may be used in treatment of thyroid storm or in persons who are intolerant of propylthiouracil or methimazole.

Graves' Disease

Graves' disease is a state of hyperthyroidism, goiter, and ophthalmopathy (or, less commonly, dermopathy).[15,18,19] The onset usually is between the ages of 20 and 40 years, and women are five times more likely to develop the disease than men. Graves' disease is an autoimmune disorder characterized by abnormal stimulation of the thyroid gland by thyroid-stimulating antibodies (thyroid-stimulating immunoglobulins [TSI]) that act through the normal TSH receptors. It may be associated with other autoimmune disorders such as myasthenia gravis and pernicious anemia. The disease is associated with human leukocyte antigen (HLA)-DR3 and HLA-B8, and a familial tendency is evident.

The ophthalmopathy, which occurs in up to one third of persons with Graves' disease, is thought to result from a cytokine-mediated activation of fibroblasts in orbital tissue behind the eyeball.[15–20] Humoral autoimmunity also is important; an ophthalmic immunoglobulin may exacerbate lymphocytic infiltration of the extraocular muscles. The ophthalmopathy of Graves' disease can cause severe eye problems, including paralysis of the extraocular muscles; involvement of the optic nerve, with some visual loss; and corneal ulceration because the lids do not close over the protruding eyeball (due to the exophthalmos). The ophthalmopathy usually tends to stabilize after treatment of the hyperthyroidism. However, ophthalmopathy can worsen acutely after radioiodine treatment. Some physicians prescribe glucocorticoids for several weeks surrounding the radioiodine treatment if the person had signs of ophthalmopathy. Others do not use radioiodine therapy under these circumstances, but prefer antithyroid therapy with drugs (which may decrease the immune activation in the condition). Unfortunately, not all of the ocular changes are reversible with treatment. Ophthalmopathy also can be aggravated by smoking, which should be strongly discouraged. Figure 42-8 depicts a woman with Graves' disease.

Thyroid Storm

Thyroid storm, or crisis, is an extreme and life-threatening form of thyrotoxicosis, rarely seen today because of improved diagnosis and treatment methods.[15,18] When it does occur, it is seen most often in undiagnosed cases or in persons with hyperthyroidism who have not been adequately treated. It often is precipitated by stress such as an infection (usually respiratory), by diabetic ketoacidosis, by physical or emotional trauma, or by manipulation of a hyperactive thyroid gland during thyroidectomy. Thyroid storm is manifested by a very high fever, extreme cardiovascular effects (*i.e.,* tachycardia, congestive failure, and angina), and severe CNS effects (*i.e.,* agitation, restlessness, and delirium). The mortality rate is high.

Thyroid storm requires rapid diagnosis and implementation of treatment. Peripheral cooling is initiated with cold packs and a cooling mattress. For cooling to be effective, the shivering response must be prevented. General supportive measures to replace fluids, glucose, and electrolytes are essential during the hypermetabolic state. A β-adrenergic–blocking drug, such as propranolol, is given to block the undesirable effects of T_4 on cardiovascular function. Glucocorticoids are used to correct the relative adrenal insufficiency resulting from the stress imposed by the hyperthyroid state and to inhibit the peripheral conversion of T_4 to T_3. Propylthiouracil or methimazole may be given to block thyroid synthesis. Aspirin increases the level of free thyroid hormones by displacing the hormones from their protein carriers and should not be used for treatment of fever during thyroid storm. The iodide-containing radiographic contrast medium sodium ipodate also can be useful for blocking thyroid hormone production.

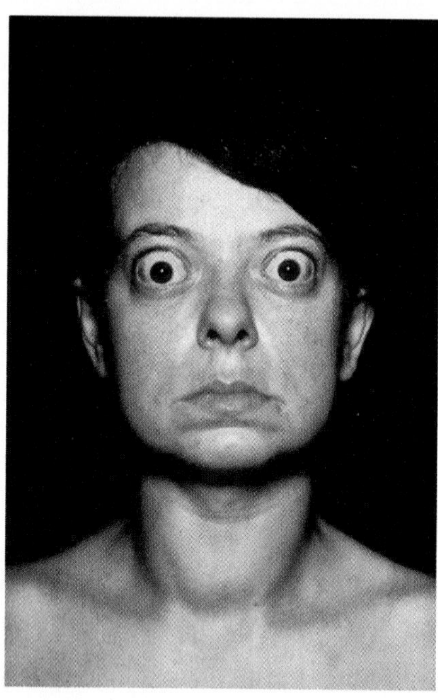

FIGURE 42-8 Graves' disease. A young woman with hyperthyroidism presented with a mass in the neck and exophthalmos. (Rubin E., Farber J.L. [1999]. *Pathology* [3rd ed., p. 1167]. Philadelphia: Lippincott-Raven)

In summary, thyroid hormones play a role in the metabolic process of almost all body cells and are necessary for normal physical and mental growth in the infant and young child. Alterations in thyroid function can manifest as a hypothyroid or a hyperthyroid state. Hypothyroidism can occur as a congenital or an acquired defect. Congenital hypothyroidism leads to mental retardation and impaired physical growth unless treatment is initiated during the first months of life. Acquired hypothyroidism leads to a decrease in metabolic rate and an accumulation of a mucopolysaccharide substance in the intercellular spaces; this substance attracts water and causes a mucous type of edema called *myxedema.* Hyperthyroidism causes an increase in metabolic rate and alterations in body function similar to those produced by enhanced sympathetic nervous system activity. Graves' disease is characterized by the triad of hyperthyroidism, goiter, and ophthalmopathy (or dermopathy).

Disorders of Adrenal Cortical Function

After completing this section of the chapter, you should be able to meet the following objectives:

- Describe the function of the adrenal cortical hormones and their feedback regulation
- State the underlying cause of the adrenogenital syndrome
- Relate the functions of the adrenal cortical hormones to Addison's disease (*i.e.,* adrenal insufficiency) and Cushing's syndrome (*i.e.,* cortisol excess)

CONTROL OF ADRENAL CORTICAL FUNCTION

The adrenal glands are small, bilateral structures that weigh approximately 5 g each and lie retroperitoneally at the apex of each kidney (Fig. 42-9). The medulla or inner portion of the gland secretes epinephrine and norepinephrine and is part of the sympathetic nervous system. The cortex forms the bulk of the adrenal gland and is responsible for secreting three types of hormones: the glucocorticoids, the mineralocorticoids, and the adrenal sex hormones.[21] Because the sympathetic nervous system also secretes epinephrine and norepinephrine, adrenal medullary function is not essential for life, but adrenal cortical function is. The total loss of adrenal cortical function is fatal in 4 to 14 days if untreated. This section of the chapter describes the synthesis and function of the adrenal cortical hormones and the effects of adrenal cortical insufficiency and excess.

Biosynthesis, Transport, and Metabolism

More than 30 hormones are produced by the adrenal cortex. Of these hormones, aldosterone is the principal mineralocorticoid, cortisol (hydrocortisone) is the major glucocorticoid, and androgens are the chief sex hormones. All of the adrenal cortical hormones have a similar structure in that all are steroids and are synthesized from acetate and cholesterol. Each of the steps involved in the synthesis of the various hormones requires a specific enzyme (Fig. 42-10). The secretion of the glucocorticoids and the adrenal androgens is controlled by the ACTH secreted by the anterior pituitary gland.

Cortisol and the adrenal androgens are secreted in an unbound state and bind to plasma proteins for transport in the circulatory system. Cortisol binds largely to corticosteroid-binding globulin and to a lesser extent to albumin. Aldosterone circulates mostly bound to albumin. It has been suggested that the pool of protein-bound hormones may extend the duration of their action by delaying metabolic clearance.

The main site for metabolism of the adrenal cortical hormones is the liver, where they undergo a number of metabolic conversions before being conjugated and made water soluble. They are then eliminated in either the urine or the bile.

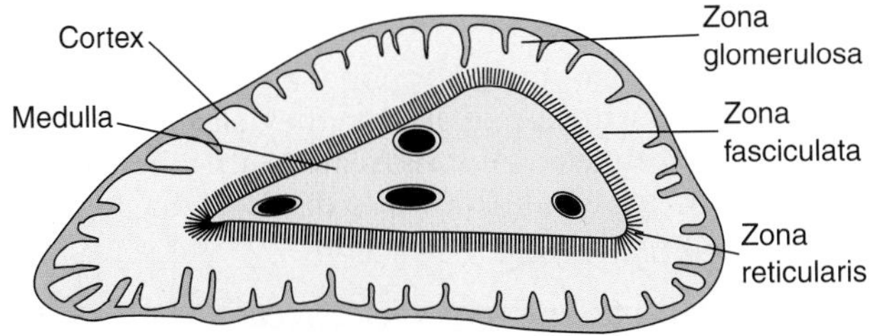

FIGURE 42-9 The adrenal gland, showing the medulla (site of epinephrine and norepinephrine synthesis) and the three layers of the cortex. The zona glomerulosa is the outer layer of the cortex and is primarily responsible for mineralocorticoid production. The middle layer, the zona fasciculata, and the inner layer, the zona reticularis, produce the glucocorticoids and the adrenal sex hormones.

Adrenal Sex Hormones

The adrenal sex hormones are synthesized primarily by the zona reticularis and the zona fasciculata of the cortex (see Fig. 42-9). These sex hormones probably exert little effect on normal sexual function. There is evidence, however, that the adrenal sex hormones (the most important of which is dehydroepiandrosterone [DHEA]) contribute to the pubertal growth of body hair, particularly pubic and axillary hair in women. They also may play a role in the steroid hormone economy of the pregnant woman and the fetal-placental unit. Dehydroepiandrosterone sulfate (DHEAS) is increasingly being used in the treatment of both Addison's disease (to be discussed) and adults who have decreased levels of DHEAS. Adrenal androgens are physiologically important in women with Addison's disease, and replacement with 25 to 50 mg of DHEAS daily should be considered.[22] Because the testes produce these hormones, there is no rationale for using it in men. The levels of DHEAS decline to approximately one sixth the levels of a 20-year-old by 60 years of age (*adrenopause*). The significance if this is unknown, but replacement may improve general well-being and sexuality, and have other important effects in women. The value of routine replacement of DHEAS during adrenopause is largely unproved.

Mineralocorticoids

The mineralocorticoids play an essential role in regulating potassium and sodium levels and water balance. They are produced in the zona glomerulosa, the outer layer of cells of the adrenal cortex. Aldosterone secretion is regulated by the renin-angiotensin mechanism and by blood levels of potassium. Increased levels of aldosterone promote sodium retention by the distal tubules of the kidney while increasing urinary losses of potassium. The influence of aldosterone on fluid and electrolyte balance is discussed in Chapter 33.

Glucocorticoids

The glucocorticoid hormones, mainly cortisol, are synthesized in the zona fasciculata and the zona reticularis of the adrenal gland. The blood levels of these hormones are regulated by negative feedback mechanisms of the hypothalamic-pituitary-adrenal (HPA) system (Fig. 42-11). Just as other pituitary hormones are controlled by releasing factors from the hypothalamus, corticotropin-releasing hormone (CRH) is important in controlling the release of ACTH. Cortisol levels increase as ACTH levels rise and decrease as ACTH levels fall. There is considerable diurnal variation in ACTH levels, which reach their peak in the early morning (around 6:00 to 8:00 AM) and decline as the day progresses (Fig. 42-12). This appears to be due to rhythmic activity in the CNS, which causes bursts of CRH secretion and, in turn, ACTH secretion. This diurnal pattern is reversed in people who work during the night and sleep during the day. The rhythm also may be changed by physical and psychological stresses, endogenous depression, manic-depressive psychosis, and liver disease or other conditions that affect cortisol metabolism. One of the earliest signs of Cushing's syndrome, a disorder of cortisol excess, is the loss of diurnal variation in CRH and ACTH

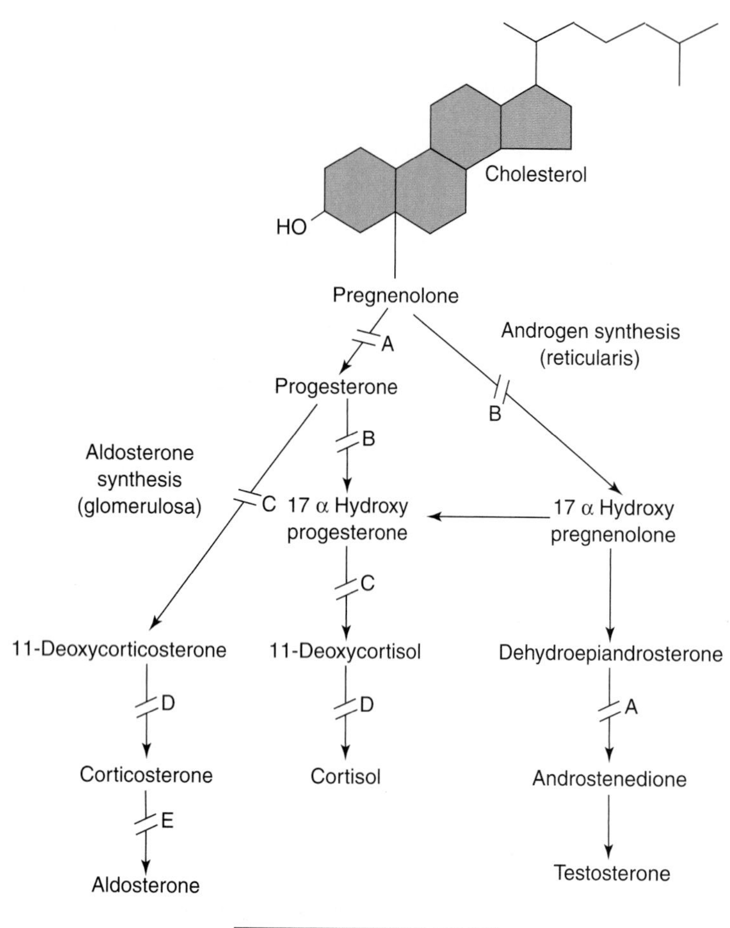

FIGURE 42-10 Predominant biosynthetic pathways of the adrenal cortex. Critical enzymes in the biosynthetic process include 11-beta-hydroxylase and 21-hydroxylase. A deficiency in one of these enzymes blocks the synthesis of hormones dependent on that enzyme and routes the precursors into alternative pathways.

secretion. This is why late-night (between 11:00 PM and midnight) serum or salivary cortisol levels can be inappropriately elevated, aiding in the diagnosis of Cushing's syndrome.[21]

The glucocorticoids perform a necessary function in response to stress and are essential for survival. When produced as part of the stress response, these hormones aid in regulating the metabolic functions of the body and in controlling the inflammatory response. The actions of cortisol are summarized in Table 42-4. Many of the antiinflammatory actions attributed to cortisol result from the administration of pharmacologic levels of the hormone.

Metabolic Effects. Cortisol stimulates glucose production by the liver, promotes protein breakdown, and causes mobilization of fatty acids. As body proteins are broken down, amino acids are mobilized and transported to the liver, where they are used in the production of glucose (*i.e.*, gluconeogenesis). Mobilization of fatty acids converts cell metabolism from the use of glucose for energy to the use of fatty acids instead. As glucose production by the liver rises and peripheral glucose use falls, a moderate resistance to insulin develops. In persons with diabetes and those who are diabetes prone, this has the effect of raising the blood glucose level.

Psychological Effects. The glucocorticoid hormones appear to be involved directly or indirectly in emotional behavior. Receptors for these hormones have been identified in brain tissue, which suggests that they play a role in the regulation of behavior. Persons treated with adrenal cortical hormones have been known to display behavior ranging from mildly aberrant to psychotic.

Immunologic and Inflammatory Effects. Cortisol influences multiple aspects of immunologic function and inflammatory responsiveness. Large quantities of cortisol are required for an effective antiinflammatory action. This is achieved by the administration of pharmacologic rather than physiologic doses of synthetic cortisol. The increased cortisol blocks inflammation at an early stage by decreasing capillary permeability and stabilizing the lysosomal

ADRENAL CORTICAL HORMONES

- The adrenal cortex produces three types of steroid hormones: the mineralocorticoids (principally aldosterone), which function in sodium, potassium, and water balance; the glucocorticoids (principally cortisol), which aid in regulating the metabolic functions of the body and in controlling the inflammatory response, and are essential for survival in stress situations; and the adrenal sex hormones (principally androgens), which serve mainly as a source of androgens for women.
- The manifestations of primary adrenal cortical insufficiency are related mainly to mineralocorticoid deficiency (impaired ability to regulate salt and water elimination) and glucocorticoid deficiency (impaired ability to regulate blood glucose and control the effects of the immune and inflammatory responses).
- Adrenal cortical excess results in derangements in glucose metabolism, disorders of sodium and potassium regulation (increased sodium retention and potassium loss), impaired ability to respond to stress because of inhibition of inflammatory and immune responses, increased gastric acid secretion with gastric ulceration and bleeding, and signs of increased androgen levels such as hirsutism.

membranes so that inflammatory mediators are not released. Cortisol suppresses the immune response by reducing humoral and cell-mediated immunity. With this lessened inflammatory response comes a reduction in fever. During the healing phase, cortisol suppresses fibroblast activity and thereby lessens scar formation. Cortisol also inhibits prostaglandin synthesis, which may account in large part for its antiinflammatory actions.

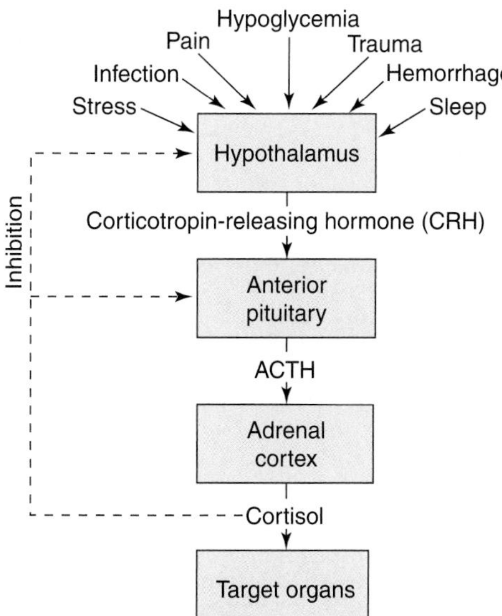

FIGURE 42-11 The hypothalamic-pituitary-adrenal (HPA) feedback system that regulates glucocorticoid (cortisol) levels. Cortisol release is regulated by ACTH. Stress exerts its effects on cortisol release through the HPA system and the corticotropin-releasing hormone (CRH), which controls the release of ACTH from the anterior pituitary gland. Increased cortisol levels incite a negative feedback inhibition of ACTH release.

Pharmacologic Suppression of Adrenal Function

A highly significant aspect of long-term therapy with pharmacologic preparations of the adrenal cortical hormones is adrenal insufficiency on withdrawal of the drugs. The deficiency results from suppression of the HPA system. Chronic suppression causes atrophy of the adrenal gland, and the abrupt withdrawal of drugs can cause acute adrenal insufficiency. Recovery to a state of normal adrenal function may be prolonged, requiring up to 12 months or more.

Tests of Adrenal Function

Several diagnostic tests can be used to evaluate adrenal cortical function and the HPA system.[21] Blood levels of cortisol, aldosterone, and ACTH can be measured using immunoassay methods. A 24-hour urine specimen measuring the excretion of various metabolic end products of the adrenal hormones and the male androgens provides information about alterations in the biosynthesis of the adrenal cortical hormones. The 24-hour urinary free cortisol, late-night (between 11:00 PM and midnight) serum or salivary cortisol levels, and the overnight 1-mg dexamethasone suppression test (see later) are excellent screening tests for Cushing's syndrome.[21,23,24]

Suppression and stimulation tests afford a means of assessing the state of the HPA feedback system. For example, a test dose of ACTH can be given to assess the response of the adrenal cortex to stimulation. Similarly, administration of dexamethasone, a synthetic glucocorticoid drug, provides a means of measuring negative feedback suppression of ACTH. Adrenal tumors and ectopic ACTH-producing tumors usually are unresponsive to ACTH suppression by dexamethasone. CRH tests can be used to diagnose a pituitary ACTH-secreting tumor (*i.e.,* Cushing's disease), especially when combined with inferior petrosal venous sampling (this allows the blood drainage of the pituitary to be sampled directly). Metyrapone blocks the final step in cortisol synthesis, resulting in the production of 11-dehydroxycortisol, which does not inhibit ACTH. This test measures the ability of the pituitary to release ACTH. The gold standard test for assessing the HPA axis is the insulin hypoglycemic stress test.

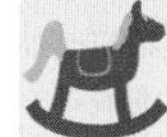

CONGENITAL ADRENAL HYPERPLASIA

Congenital adrenal hyperplasia (CAH), or the adrenogenital syndrome, describes a congenital disorder caused by an autosomal recessive trait in which a deficiency exists in any of the enzymes necessary for the synthesis of cortisol[25] (see Fig. 42-10). A common characteristic of all types of CAH is a defect in the synthesis of cortisol that results in increased levels of ACTH and adrenal hyperplasia. The increased levels of ACTH overstimulate the pathways for production of adrenal androgens. Mineralocorticoids may be produced in excessive or insufficient amounts, depending

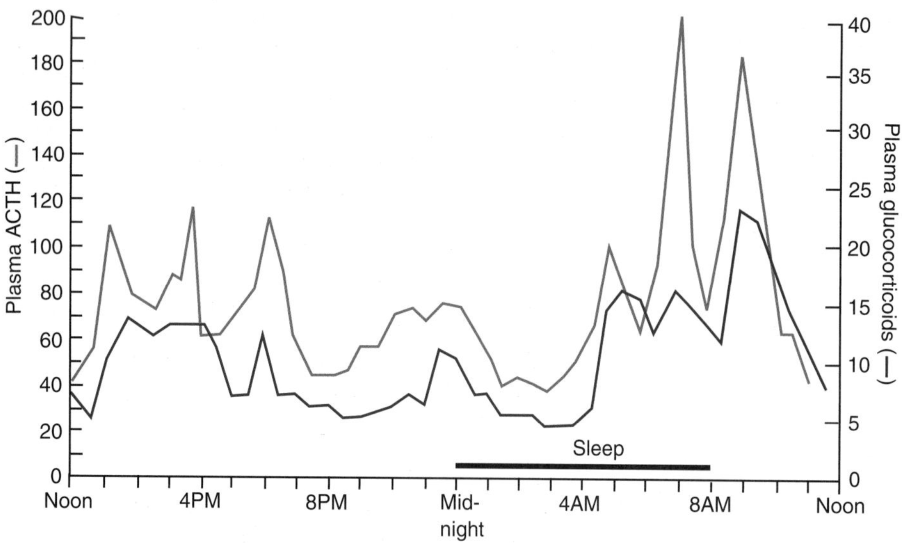

FIGURE 42-12 Pulsatile changes in the concentration of adrenocorticotropic hormone (ACTH) and glucocorticoids over a 24-hour period. The amplitude of the pulses of ACTH and glucocorticoids is lower in the evening hours and then increases greatly during the early morning hours. This is due to the diurnal oscillation of the hypothalamic-pituitary axis. (Modified from Krieger D.T. [1979]. Rhythms of CRF, ACTH and corticosteroids. In Krieger D.T. [Ed.], *Endocrine rhythms* [pp. 123–142]. New York: Raven)

on the precise enzyme deficiency. Infants of both sexes are affected. Males seldom are diagnosed at birth unless they have enlarged genitalia or lose salt and manifest adrenal crisis. In female infants, an increase in androgens is responsible for creating the virilization syndrome of ambiguous genitalia with an enlarged clitoris, fused labia, and urogenital sinus (Fig. 42-13). In male and female children, other secondary sex characteristics are normal, and fertility is unaffected if appropriate therapy is instituted.

The two most common enzyme deficiencies are 21-hydroxylase (accounting for >90% of cases) and 11-β-hydroxylase deficiency. The clinical manifestations of both deficiencies are largely determined by the functional properties of the steroid intermediates and the completeness of the block in the cortisol pathway.

A spectrum of 21-hydroxylase deficiency states exists, ranging from simple virilizing CAH to a complete salt-losing enzyme deficiency.[25,26] Simple virilizing CAH impairs the synthesis of cortisol, and steroid synthesis is shunted to androgen production. Persons with these deficiencies usually produce sufficient aldosterone or aldosterone intermediates to prevent signs and symptoms of

TABLE 42-4 Actions of Cortisol

Major Influence	Effect on Body
Glucose metabolism	Stimulates gluconeogenesis Decreases glucose use by the tissues
Protein metabolism	Increases breakdown of proteins Increases plasma protein levels
Fat metabolism	Increases mobilization of fatty acids Increases use of fatty acids
Anti-inflammatory action (pharmacologic levels)	Stabilizes lysosomal membranes of the inflammatory cells, preventing the release of inflammatory mediators Decreases capillary permeability to prevent inflammatory edema Depresses phagocytosis by white blood cells to reduce the release of inflammatory mediators Suppresses the immune response Causes atrophy of lymphoid tissue Decreases eosinophils Decreases antibody formation Decreases the development of cell-mediated immunity Reduces fever Inhibits fibroblast activity
Psychic effect	May contribute to emotional instability
Permissive effect	Facilitates the response of the tissues to humoral and neural influences, such as that of the catecholamines, during trauma and extreme stress

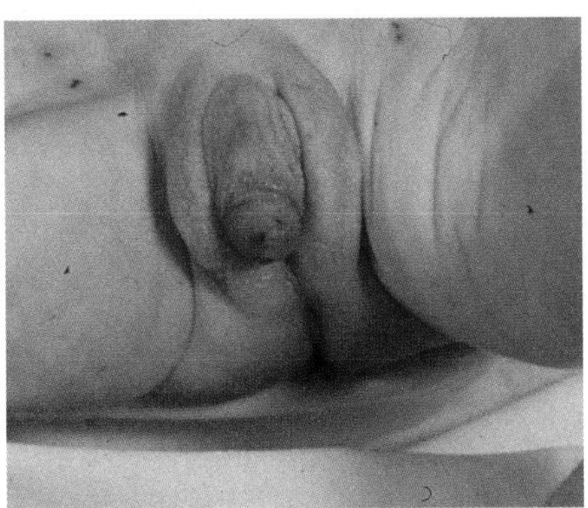

FIGURE 42-13 A female infant with congenital adrenal hyperplasia demonstrating virilization of the genitalia with hypertrophy of the clitoris and partial fusion of labioscrotal folds. (Rubin E., Farber J.L. [1999]. *Pathology* [3rd ed., p. 1186]. Philadelphia: Lippincott-Raven)

mineralocorticoid deficiency. The salt-losing form is accompanied by deficient production of aldosterone and its intermediates. This results in fluid and electrolyte disorders after the fifth day of life (including hyponatremia, hyperkalemia, vomiting, dehydration, and shock).

The 11-β-hydroxylase deficiency is rare and manifests a spectrum of severity. Affected persons have excessive androgen production and impaired conversion of 11-deoxycorticosterone to corticosterone. The overproduction of 11-deoxycorticosterone, which has mineralocorticoid activity, is responsible for the hypertension that accompanies this deficiency. Diagnosis of the adrenogenital syndrome depends on the precise biochemical evaluation of metabolites in the cortisol pathway and on clinical signs and symptoms. Genetic testing is also invaluable; however, correlation between the phenotype and genotype is not always straightforward.[25,26]

Medical treatment of adrenogenital syndrome includes oral or parenteral cortisol replacement. Fludrocortisone acetate, a mineralocorticoid, also may be given to children who are salt losers. Depending on the degree of virilization, reconstructive surgery during the first 2 years of life is indicated to reduce the size of the clitoris, separate the labia, and exteriorize the vagina. Advances in surgical techniques have led to earlier use of single-stage surgery—between 2 and 6 months of life in girls with 21-hydroxylase deficiency, a time when the tissues are maximally pliable and psychological trauma to the child is minimized.[25] Surgery has provided excellent results and does not usually impair sexual function.

ADRENAL CORTICAL INSUFFICIENCY

There are two forms of adrenal insufficiency: primary and secondary[27] (see Table 42-5 for distinguishing features). Primary adrenal insufficiency, or Addison's disease, is caused by destruction of the adrenal gland. Secondary adrenal insufficiency results from a disorder of the HPA system.

Primary Adrenal Cortical Insufficiency

In 1855, Thomas Addison, an English physician, provided the first detailed clinical description of primary adrenal insufficiency, now called *Addison's disease*. The use of this term is reserved for primary adrenal insufficiency in which adrenal cortical hormones are deficient and ACTH levels are elevated because of lack of feedback inhibition.

Addison's disease is a relatively rare disorder in which all the layers of the adrenal cortex are destroyed. Autoimmune destruction is the most common cause of Addison's disease in the United States. Before 1950, tuberculosis was the major cause of Addison's disease in the United States, and it continues to be a major cause of the disease in countries where it is more prevalent. Rare causes include metastatic carcinoma, fungal infection (particularly histoplasmosis), cytomegalovirus infection, amyloid disease, and hemochromatosis. Bilateral adrenal hemorrhage may occur in persons taking anticoagulants, during open heart surgery, and during birth or major trauma. Adrenal insufficiency can be caused by acquired immunodeficiency syndrome, in which the adrenal gland is destroyed by a variety of opportunistic infectious agents.

Addison's disease, like type 1 diabetes mellitus, is a chronic metabolic disorder that requires lifetime hormone replacement therapy. The adrenal cortex has a large reserve capacity, and the manifestations of adrenal insufficiency usually do not become apparent until approximately 90%

TABLE 42-5 Clinical Findings of Adrenal Insufficiency

Finding	Primary	Secondary/Tertiary
Anorexia and weight loss	Yes (100%)	Yes (100%)
Fatigue and weakness	Yes (100%)	Yes (100%)
Gastrointestinal symptoms, nausea, diarrhea	Yes (50%)	Yes (50%)
Myalgia, arthralgia, abdominal pain	Yes (10%)	Yes (10%)
Orthostatic hypotension	Yes	Yes
Hyponatremia	Yes (85%–90%)	Yes (60%)
Hyperkalemia	Yes (60%–65%)	No
Hyperpigmentation	Yes (>90%)	No
Secondary deficiencies of testosterone, growth hormone, thyroxine, antidiuretic hormone	No	Yes
Associated autoimmune conditions	Yes	No

of the gland has been destroyed. These manifestations are related primarily to mineralocorticoid deficiency, glucocorticoid deficiency, and hyperpigmentation resulting from elevated ACTH levels. Although lack of the adrenal androgens (*i.e.,* DHEAS) exerts few effects in men because the testes produce these hormones, women have sparse axillary and pubic hair.

Mineralocorticoid deficiency causes increased urinary losses of sodium, chloride, and water, along with decreased excretion of potassium. The result is hyponatremia, loss of extracellular fluid, decreased cardiac output, and hyperkalemia. There may be an abnormal appetite for salt. Orthostatic hypotension is common. Dehydration, weakness, and fatigue are common early symptoms. If loss of sodium and water is extreme, cardiovascular collapse and shock ensue. Because of a lack of glucocorticoids, the person with Addison's disease has poor tolerance to stress. This deficiency causes hypoglycemia, lethargy, weakness, fever, and gastrointestinal symptoms such as anorexia, nausea, vomiting, and weight loss.

Hyperpigmentation results from elevated levels of ACTH. The skin looks bronzed or suntanned in exposed and unexposed areas, and the normal creases and pressure points tend to become especially dark. The gums and oral mucous membranes may become bluish-black. The amino acid sequence of ACTH is strikingly similar to that of melanocyte-stimulating hormone; hyperpigmentation occurs in more than 90% of persons with Addison's disease and is helpful in distinguishing the primary and secondary forms of adrenal insufficiency.

The daily regulation of the chronic phase of Addison's disease usually is accomplished with oral replacement therapy, with higher doses being given during periods of stress. The pharmacologic agent that is used should have both glucocorticoid and mineralocorticoid activity. Mineralocorticoids are needed only in primary adrenal insufficiency. Hydrocortisone usually is the drug of choice. In mild cases, hydrocortisone alone may be adequate. Fludrocortisone (a mineralocorticoid) is used for persons who do not obtain a sufficient salt-retaining effect from hydrocortisone. DHEAS replacement also may be helpful in the female patient.[22,27]

Because persons with the disorder are likely to have episodes of hyponatremia and hypoglycemia, they need to have a regular schedule for meals and exercise. Persons with Addison's disease also have limited ability to respond to infections, trauma, and other stresses. Such situations require immediate medical attention and treatment. All persons with Addison's disease should be advised to wear a medical alert bracelet or medal.

Secondary Adrenal Cortical Insufficiency

Secondary adrenal insufficiency can occur as the result of hypopituitarism or because the pituitary gland has been surgically removed. Tertiary adrenal insufficiency results from a hypothalamic defect. However, a far more common cause than either of these is the rapid withdrawal of glucocorticoids that have been administered therapeutically. These drugs suppress the HPA system, with resulting adrenal cortical atrophy and loss of cortisol production. This suppression continues long after drug therapy has been discontinued and can be critical during periods of stress or when surgery is performed.

Acute Adrenal Crisis

Acute adrenal crisis is a life-threatening situation.[27] If Addison's disease is the underlying problem, exposure to even a minor illness or stress can precipitate nausea, vomiting, muscular weakness, hypotension, dehydration, and vascular collapse. The onset of adrenal crisis may be sudden, or it may progress over a period of several days. The symptoms may occur suddenly in children with salt-losing forms of the adrenogenital syndrome. Massive bilateral adrenal hemorrhage causes an acute fulminating form of adrenal insufficiency. Hemorrhage can be caused by meningococcal septicemia (*i.e.,* Waterhouse-Friderichsen syndrome), adrenal trauma, anticoagulant therapy, adrenal vein thrombosis, or adrenal metastases.

Adrenal insufficiency is treated with hormone replacement therapy that includes a combination of glucocorticoids and mineralocorticoids. For acute adrenal insufficiency, the *five S's* of management should be followed: (1) *S*alt replacement, (2) *S*ugar (dextrose) replacement, (3) *S*teroid replacement, (4) *S*upport of physiologic functioning, and (5) *S*earch for and treat the underlying cause (*e.g.,* infection). Extracellular fluid volume should be restored with several liters of 0.9% saline and 5% dextrose. Corticosteroid replacement is accomplished through the intravenous administration of either dexamethasone or hydrocortisone. Dexamethasone is preferred acutely for two reasons: it is long acting (12 to 24 hours), and it does not interfere with measurement of serum or urinary steroids during subsequent corticotropin (ACTH) stimulation tests. Thereafter, hydrocortisone often is given either intravenously or intramuscularly at 6-hour intervals and then tapered over 1 to 3 days to maintenance levels. Oral hydrocortisone replacement therapy can be resumed once the saline infusion has been discontinued and the person is taking food and fluids by mouth. Mineralocorticoid therapy is not required when large amounts of hydrocortisone are being given, but as the dose is reduced, it usually is necessary to add fludrocortisone. Corticosteroid replacement therapy is monitored using heart rate and blood pressure measurements, serum electrolyte values, and titration of plasma renin activity into the upper-normal range.

GLUCOCORTICOID HORMONE EXCESS (CUSHING'S SYNDROME)

The term *Cushing's syndrome* refers to the manifestations of hypercortisolism from any cause.[21,23,24] Three important forms of Cushing's syndrome result from excess glucocorticoid production by the body. One is a pituitary form, which results from excessive production of ACTH by a tumor of the pituitary gland. This form of the disease was the one originally described by Cushing; therefore; it is called *Cushing's disease.* The second form is the adrenal form, caused by a benign or malignant adrenal tumor. The third form is ectopic Cushing's, caused by a nonpituitary ACTH-secreting tumor. Certain extrapituitary malignant tumors such as small cell carcinoma of the lung may secrete ACTH or, rarely, CRH, and produce Cushing's syndrome. Cushing's syndrome also can result from long-term therapy with one of the potent pharmacologic preparations of glucocorticoids; this form is called *iatrogenic Cushing's syndrome.*

The major manifestations of Cushing's syndrome represent an exaggeration of the many actions of cortisol (see Table 42-4). Altered fat metabolism causes a peculiar deposition of fat characterized by a protruding abdomen; subclavicular fat pads or "buffalo hump" on the back; and a round, plethoric "moon face" (Fig. 42-14). There is muscle weakness, and the extremities are thin because of protein breakdown and muscle wasting. In advanced cases, the skin over the forearms and legs becomes thin, having the appearance of parchment. Purple striae, or stretch marks, from stretching of the catabolically weakened skin and subcutaneous tissues are distributed over the breast, thighs, and abdomen. Osteoporosis may develop because of destruction of bone proteins and alterations in calcium metabolism, resulting in back pain, compression fractures of the vertebrae, and rib fractures. As calcium is mobilized from bone, renal calculi may develop.

Derangements in glucose metabolism are found in approximately 75% of patients, with clinically overt diabetes mellitus occurring in approximately 20%. The glucocorticoids possess mineralocorticoid properties; this causes hypokalemia as a result of excessive potassium excretion and hypertension resulting from sodium retention. Inflammatory and immune responses are inhibited, resulting in increased susceptibility to infection. Cortisol increases gastric acid secretion, which may provoke gastric ulceration and bleeding. An accompanying increase in androgen levels causes hirsutism, mild acne, and menstrual irregularities in women. Excess levels of the glucocorticoids may give rise to extreme emotional lability, ranging from mild euphoria and absence of normal fatigue to grossly psychotic behavior.

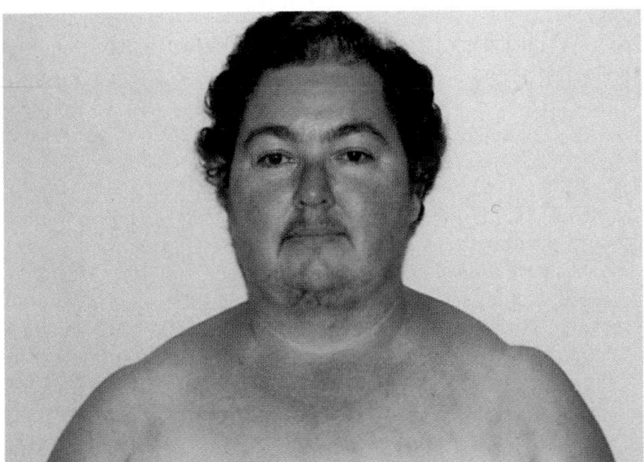

FIGURE 42-14 Cushing's syndrome. A woman who suffered from a pituitary adenoma that produced ACTH exhibits a moon face, buffalo hump, increased facial hair, and thinning of the scalp hair. (Rubin E., Farber J.L. [1999]. *Pathology* [3rd ed., p. 1193]. Philadelphia: Lippincott-Raven)

Diagnosis of Cushing's syndrome depends on the finding of cortisol hypersecretion. The determination of 24-hour excretion of cortisol in urine provides a reliable and practical index of cortisol secretions. One of the prominent features of Cushing's syndrome is loss of the diurnal pattern of cortisol secretion. This is why late-night (between 11:00 PM and midnight) serum or salivary cortisol levels can be inappropriately elevated, aiding in the diagnosis of Cushing's syndrome.[21,23,24] The overnight 1-mg dexamethasone suppression test is also used as a screening tool for Cushing's syndrome.

Other tests include measurement of the plasma levels of ACTH.[21,23,24] ACTH levels should be normal or elevated in ACTH-dependent Cushing's syndrome (Cushing's disease and ectopic ACTH), and low in non–ACTH-dependent Cushing's syndrome (adrenal tumors). Various suppression or stimulation tests of the HPA system are performed to further delineate the cause. MRI or CT scans afford a means for locating adrenal or pituitary tumors.

Untreated, Cushing's syndrome produces serious morbidity and even death. The choice of surgery, irradiation, or pharmacologic treatment is determined largely by the cause of the hypercortisolism. The goal of treatment for Cushing's syndrome is to remove or correct the source of hypercortisolism without causing permanent pituitary or adrenal damage. Transsphenoidal removal of a pituitary adenoma or hemihypophysectomy is the preferred method of treatment for Cushing's disease. This allows removal of only the tumor rather than the entire pituitary gland. After successful removal, the person must receive cortisol replacement therapy for 6 to 12 months or until adrenal function returns. Patients also may receive pituitary radiation therapy, but the full effects of treatment may not be realized for 3 to 12 months. Unilateral or bilateral adrenalectomy may be done in the case of adrenal adenoma. When possible, ectopic ACTH-producing tumors are removed. Pharmacologic agents that block steroid synthesis (*i.e.,* etomidate, mitotane, ketoconazole, metyrapone, and aminoglutethimide) may be used to treat persons with ectopic tumors or adrenal carcinomas that cannot be resected.[21,23] Many of these patients also require *Pneumocystis carinii* pneumonia prophylaxis because of the profound immunosuppression caused by the excessive glucocorticoid levels.

INCIDENTAL ADRENAL MASS

An incidentaloma is a mass lesion found unexpectedly in an adrenal gland by an imaging procedure (done for other reasons), most commonly CT (but also MRI and ultrasonography). They have been increasingly recognized since the early 1980s. The prevalence of adrenal incidentalomas at autopsy is approximately 10 to 100 per 1000. In CT series, 0.4% to 0.6% are the usual figures published. Incidentalomas also can occur in other organs (*e.g.,* pituitary, thyroid).[28] The two most important questions are (1) is the mass malignant, and (2) is the mass hormonally active (*i.e.,* is it functioning)?

Primary adrenal carcinoma is quite rare, but other cancers, particularly lung cancers, commonly metastasize to the adrenal gland (other cancers include breast, stomach, pancreas, colon, and kidney tumors, melanomas, and lymphomas). The size and imaging characteristics of the mass may help determine whether the tumor is benign or malignant. The risk for cancer is high in adrenal masses larger than 6 cm. Many experts recommend surgical removal of masses larger than 4 cm, particularly in younger patients.[29]

In summary, the adrenal cortex produces three types of hormones: mineralocorticoids, glucocorticoids, and adrenal sex hormones. The mineralocorticoids, along with the renin-angiotensin mechanism, aid in controlling body levels of sodium and potassium. The glucocorticoids have antiinflammatory actions and aid in regulating glucose, protein, and fat metabolism during periods of stress. These hormones are under the control of the HPA system. The adrenal sex hormones exert little effect on daily control of body function, but they probably contribute to the development of body hair in women. The adrenogenital syndrome describes a genetic defect in the cortisol pathway resulting from a deficiency of one of the enzymes needed for its synthesis. Depending on the enzyme involved, the disorder causes virilization of female infants and, in some instances, fluid and electrolyte disturbances because of impaired mineralocorticoid synthesis.

Chronic adrenal insufficiency can be caused by destruction of the adrenal gland (Addison's disease) or by dysfunction of the HPA system. Adrenal insufficiency requires replacement therapy with cortical hormones. Acute adrenal insufficiency is a life-threatening situation. Cushing's syndrome refers to the manifestations of excessive cortisol levels. This syndrome may be a result of pharmacologic doses of cortisol, a pituitary or adrenal tumor, or an ectopic tumor that produces ACTH. The clinical manifestations of Cushing's syndrome reflect the very high level of cortisol that is present.

An incidentaloma is a mass lesion found unexpectedly in an adrenal gland (and other glands) by an imaging procedure done for other reasons. Incidentalomas are being recognized with increasing frequency, emphasizing the need for correct diagnosis and treatment.

REVIEW EXERCISES

A 59-year-old man is referred to a neurologist for evaluation of headaches. Subsequent MRI imaging studies revealed a large suprasellar mass (2.5 × 2.4 cm), consistent with a pituitary tumor. His history is positive for hypertension, and on direct inquiry, he believes that his hands are slightly larger than previously, with increased sweating. Family history is negative, as are weight change, polyuria and polydipsia, visual disturbance, and erectile dysfunction. Subsequent laboratory findings reveal a baseline serum growth hormone (GH) of 8.7 ng/mL (normal is 0–5 ng/mL), which is unsuppressed following oral glucose tolerance testing; glucose intolerance; and increased insulin-like growth factor-1 (IGF-1) on two occasions (1044 and 1145 μg/L [upper limit of normal is 480]). Other indices of pituitary function are within the normal range.

A. What diagnosis would this man's clinical features, MRI, and laboratory findings suggest?

B. What is the reason for asking the patient about weight change, polyuria and polydipsia, visual disturbance, and erectile dysfunction?

C. How would you explain his impaired glucose tolerance?

D. What are the possible local effects of a large pituitary tumor?

A 76-year-old woman presents with weight gain, subjective memory loss, dry skin, and cold intolerance. On examination, she is found to have a multinodular goiter. Laboratory findings reveal a low serum T_4 and elevated TSH.

A. What diagnosis would this woman's history, physical, and laboratory tests suggest?

B. Explain the possible relationship between the diagnosis and her weight gain, dry skin, cold intolerance, and subjective memory loss.

C. What type of treatment would be indicated?

A 45-year-old woman presents with a history of progressive weakness, fatigue, weight loss, nausea, and increased skin pigmentation (especially of creases, pressure areas, and nipples). Her blood pressure is 120/78 mm Hg when supine and 105/52 mm Hg when standing. Laboratory findings revealed a serum sodium level of 120 mEq/L (normal is 135 to 145 mEq/L); potassium level of 5.9 mEq/L (normal is 3.5 to 5.0 mEq/L); low plasma cortisol levels, and high ACTH levels.

A. What diagnosis would this woman's clinical features and laboratory findings suggest?

B. Would her diagnosis be classified as a primary or secondary endocrine disorder?

C. What is the significance of her darkened skin?

D. What type of treatment would be indicated?

References

1. Aron D.C., Findling J.W., Tyrrell J.B. (2004). Hypothalamus and pituitary gland. In Greenspan F.S., Gardner D.G. (Eds.), *Basic and clinical endocrinology* (7th ed., pp. 106–175). New York: Lange Medical Books/McGraw-Hill.
2. AACE Growth Hormone Task Force (2003). AACE medical guidelines for clinical practice for growth hormone use in adults and children—2003 update. *Endocrine Practice 9,* 64–76.
3. Styne D. (2004). Growth. In Greenspan F.S., Gardner D.G. (Eds.), *Basic and clinical endocrinology* (7th ed., pp. 176–214). New York: Lange Medical Books/McGraw-Hill.
4. Laron Z. (1995). Laron syndrome (primary GH resistance) from patient to laboratory to patient. *Journal of Clinical Endocrinology and Metabolism 80,* 1526–1531.
5. Sesmilo G., Biller B.M., Levadot J., et al. (2000). Effects of GH administration on inflammatory and other cardiovascular

risk markers in men with GH deficiency. *Annals of Internal Medicine 133,* 111–122.

6. Root A. (2001). The tall, rapidly growing infant, child, and adolescent. *Current Opinion in Endocrinology and Diabetes 8,* 6–16.
7. Katznelson L. (2002) Acromegaly: current concepts. *Endocrinology Rounds 10,* 1–6. Available www.endocrinologyrounds.org.
8. Merza Z. (2003). Modern treatment of acromegaly. *Postgraduate Medical Journal 79,* 189–194.
9. Giustina A., Barkan A., Casanaeva F.F., et al. (2000). Criteria for cure of acromegaly: A consensus statement. *Journal of Clinical Endocrinology and Metabolism 85,* 526–529.
10. Abs R., Verhelst J., Maitero D., et al. (1998). Cabergoline in the treatment of acromegaly: a study in 64 patients. *Journal of Clinical Endocrinology and Metabolism 83,* 374–378.
11. Utiger R.D. (2000). Treatment of acromegaly. *New England Journal of Medicine 342,* 1210–1211.
12. Lebrethon M.C., Bourguignon J.P. (2001). Central and peripheral isosexual precocious puberty. *Current Opinion in Endocrinology and Diabetes 8,* 17–22.
13. Styne D. (2004). Puberty. In Greenspan F.S., Gardner D.G. (Eds.), *Basic and clinical endocrinology* (7th ed., pp. 608–636). New York: Lange Medical Books/McGraw-Hill.
14. Kaplowitz P.B., Oberfield S.E. (1999). Reexamination of the age limit for defining when puberty is precocious in girls in the United States: Implications for evaluation and treatment. *Pediatrics 104,* 936–941.
15. Greenspan F.S. (2004). The thyroid gland. In Greenspan F.S., Gardner D.G. (Eds.), *Basic and clinical endocrinology* (7th ed., pp. 215–294). New York: Lange Medical Books/McGraw-Hill.
16. Dayan C.M. (2001). Interpretation of thyroid function tests. *Lancet 357,* 619–624.
17. Pearce E.N., Farwell A.P., Braverman L.E. (2003). Thyroiditis. *New England Journal of Medicine 348,* 2646–2655.
18. Cooper D.S. (2003). Hyperthyroidism. *Lancet 362,* 459–468.
19. McKenna T.J. (2001). Graves' disease. *Lancet 357,* 1793–1796.
20. Bahn R. (2003). Pathophysiology of Graves' ophthalmopathy: The cycle of disease. *Journal of Clinical Endocrinology and Metabolism 88,* 1939–1946.
21. Aron D.C., Findling J.W., Tyrrell J.B. (2004). Glucocorticoids and adrenal androgens. In Greenspan F.S., Gardner D.G. (Eds.), *Basic and clinical endocrinology* (7th ed., pp. 362–413). New York: Lange Medical Books/McGraw-Hill.
22. Ackermann J.C., Silverman B.L. (2001). Dehydroepiandrosterone replacement for patients with adrenal insufficiency. *Lancet 357,* 1381–1382.
23. Boscaro M. (2001). Cushing's syndrome. *Lancet 357,* 783–791.
24. Raff H., Findling J.W. (2003). A physiological approach to the diagnosis of Cushing's syndrome. *Annals of Internal Medicine 138,* 980–991.
25. Speiser P.W., White P.C. (2003). Congenital adrenal hyperplasia. *New England Journal of Medicine 349,* 776–788.
26. Boos, C.J., Rumsby, G., Matfin, G. (2002) Multiple tumors associated with late onset congenital hyperplasia due to aberrant splicing of adrenal 21-hydroxylase gene. *Endocrine Practice 8,* 470–473.
27. Arlt W., Allolio B. (2003). Adrenal insufficiency. *Lancet 361,* 1881–1893.
28. Aron D.C. (Ed). (2000). Endocrine incidentalomas. *Endocrinology and Metabolism Clinics of North America 29,* 1–230.
29. Grumbach M.M., Biller B.M.K., Braunstein G.D., et al. (2003). Management of the clinically inapparent adrenal mass ("incidentaloma"). *Annals of Internal Medicine 138,* 424–429.

CHAPTER 43

Diabetes Mellitus and the Metabolic Syndrome

Safak Guven
Julie A. Kuenzi
Glenn Matfin

Diabetes mellitus is a chronic health problem affecting more than 17 million people in the United States.[1] Approximately 11 million of these people have been diagnosed, leaving about 6 million undiagnosed. There are 800,000 new cases of diabetes per year; almost all of these are type 2 diabetes. The disease affects people in all age groups and from all walks of life. It is more prevalent among African Americans (13%) and Hispanic Americans (10.2%) compared with whites (6.2%).[1] Diabetes is a significant risk factor in coronary heart disease and stroke, and it is the leading cause of blindness and end-stage renal disease, as well as a major contributor to lower extremity amputations.

The metabolic syndrome, which is characterized by risk of developing diabetes mellitus and cardiovascular disease, is becoming an increasingly recognized disorder, with an age-adjusted prevalence of 23.7%.[2] Using 2000 census data, it is estimated that about 47 million U.S. residents have the metabolic syndrome.

Hormonal Control of Blood Glucose

After completing this section of the chapter, you should be able to meet the following objectives:

- Characterize the actions of insulin with reference to glucose, fat, and protein metabolism
- Explain what is meant by *counterregulatory hormones* and describe the actions of glucagon, epinephrine, growth hormone, and the adrenal cortical hormones in regulation of blood glucose levels

The body uses glucose, fatty acids, and other substrates as fuel to satisfy its energy needs. Although the respiratory and circulatory systems combine efforts to furnish the body with the oxygen needed for metabolic purposes, it is the liver, in concert with the endocrine pancreas, that controls the body's fuel supply (Fig. 43-1).

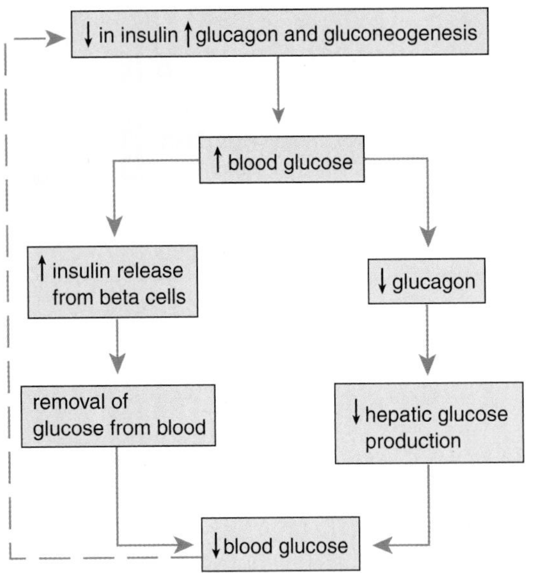

FIGURE 43-1 Hormonal and hepatic regulation of blood glucose.

The pancreas is made up of two major tissue types: the acini and the islets of Langerhans (Fig. 43-2). The acini secrete digestive juices into the duodenum, and the islets of Langerhans secrete hormones into the blood. Each islet is composed of beta cells that secrete insulin and amylin, alpha cells that secrete glucagon, and delta cells that secrete somatostatin. Insulin lowers the blood glucose concentration by facilitating the movement of glucose into body tissues. Glucagon maintains blood glucose by increasing the release of glucose from the liver into the blood. Somatostatin inhibits the release of insulin and glucagon. Somatostatin also decreases gastrointestinal activity after ingestion of food. By decreasing gastrointestinal activity, somatostatin is thought to extend the time during which food is absorbed into the blood, and by inhibiting insulin and glucagon, it is thought to extend the use of absorbed nutrients by the tissues.[3]

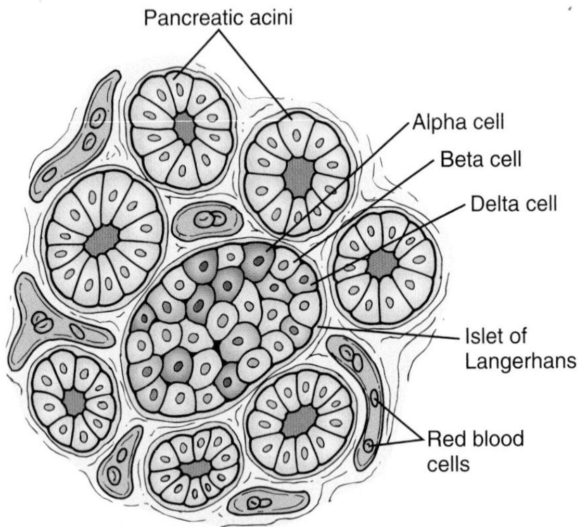

FIGURE 43-2 Islet of Langerhans in the pancreas. (Guyton A.C., Hall J.E. [1996]. *Textbook of medical physiology* [9th ed., p. 972]. Philadelphia: W.B. Saunders)

BLOOD GLUCOSE

Body tissues obtain glucose from the blood. In nondiabetic individuals, fasting blood glucose levels are tightly regulated between 80 and 90 mg/dL. After a meal, blood glucose levels rise, and insulin is secreted in response to this rise in glucose. Approximately two thirds of the glucose that is ingested with a meal is removed from the blood and stored in the liver as glycogen. Between meals, the liver releases glucose as a means of maintaining blood glucose within its normal range.

Glucose is an optional fuel for tissues such as muscle, adipose tissue, and the liver, which largely use fatty acids and other fuel substrates for energy. Glucose that is not needed for energy is stored as glycogen or converted to fat. When tissues such as those in the liver and skeletal muscle become saturated with glycogen, the additional glucose is converted into fatty acids and then stored as triglycerides in fat cells. When blood glucose levels fall below normal, as they do between meals, glycogen is broken down by a process called *glycogenolysis,* and glucose is released. Glycogen stored in the liver can be released into the bloodstream. Although skeletal muscle has glycogen stores, it lacks the enzyme glucose-6-phosphatase that allows glucose to be broken down sufficiently to pass through the cell membrane and enter the bloodstream, limiting its usefulness to the muscle cell. In addition to mobilizing its glycogen stores, the liver synthesizes glucose from amino acids, glycerol, and lactic acid in a process called *gluconeogenesis.* Glucose metabolism is discussed more fully in Chapter 11.

In contrast to other body tissues such as the liver and skeletal muscle, which use fatty acids and other substrates for fuel, the brain and nervous system rely almost exclusively on glucose for their energy needs. Because the brain can neither synthesize nor store more than a few minutes' supply of glucose, normal cerebral function requires a continuous supply from the circulation. Severe and prolonged hypoglycemia can cause brain death, and even moderate hypoglycemia can result in substantial brain dysfunction. The body maintains a system of counterregulatory mechanisms to counteract hypoglycemia-producing situations and ensure brain function and survival. The physiologic mechanisms that prevent or correct hypoglycemia include the actions of the counterregulatory hormones: glucagon, the catecholamines, growth hormone, and the glucocorticoids.

GLUCOSE-REGULATING HORMONES

Insulin

Although several hormones are known to increase blood glucose levels, insulin is the only hormone known to have a direct effect in lowering blood glucose levels. The actions of insulin are threefold: (1) it promotes glucose uptake by target cells and provides for glucose storage as glycogen, (2) it prevents fat and glycogen breakdown, and (3) it

TABLE 43-1 Actions of Insulin and Glucagon on Glucose, Fat, and Protein Metabolism

	Insulin	Glucagon
Glucose		
Glucose transport	Increases glucose transport into skeletal muscle and adipose tissue	
Glycogen synthesis	Increases glycogen synthesis	Promotes glycogen breakdown
Gluconeogenesis	Decreases gluconeogenesis	Increases gluconeogenesis
Fats		
Triglyceride synthesis	Increases triglyceride synthesis	
Triglyceride transport into adipose tissue	Increases fatty acid transport into adipose cells	Enhances lipolysis in adipose tissue, liberating fatty acids and glycerol for use in gluconeogenesis
Activation of adipose cell lipase	Inhibits adipose cell lipase Activates lipoprotein lipase in capillary walls	Activates adipose cell lipase
Proteins		
Amino acid transport	Increases active transport of amino acids into cells	Increases transport of amino acids into hepatic cells
Protein synthesis	Increases protein synthesis by increasing transcription of messenger RNA and accelerating protein synthesis by ribosomal RNA	Increases breakdown of proteins into amino acids for use in gluconeogenesis
Protein breakdown	Decreases protein breakdown by enhancing the use of glucose and fatty acids as fuel	Increases conversion of amino acids into glucose precursors

inhibits gluconeogenesis and increases protein synthesis (Table 43-1). Insulin acts to promote fat storage by increasing the transport of glucose into fat cells. It also facilitates triglyceride synthesis from glucose in fat cells and inhibits the intracellular breakdown of stored triglycerides. Insulin also inhibits protein breakdown and increases protein synthesis by increasing the active transport of amino acids into body cells; and it inhibits gluconeogenesis, or the building of glucose from new sources, mainly amino acids. When sufficient glucose and insulin are present, protein breakdown is minimal because the body is able to use glucose and fatty acids as a fuel source. In children and adolescents, insulin is needed for normal growth and development.

Insulin is produced by the pancreatic beta cells in the islets of Langerhans. The active form of the hormone is composed of two polypeptide chains—an A chain and a B chain (Fig. 43-3). Active insulin is formed in the beta cells from a larger molecule called *proinsulin.* In converting proinsulin to insulin, enzymes in the beta cell cleave proinsulin at specific sites to form two separate substances: active insulin and a

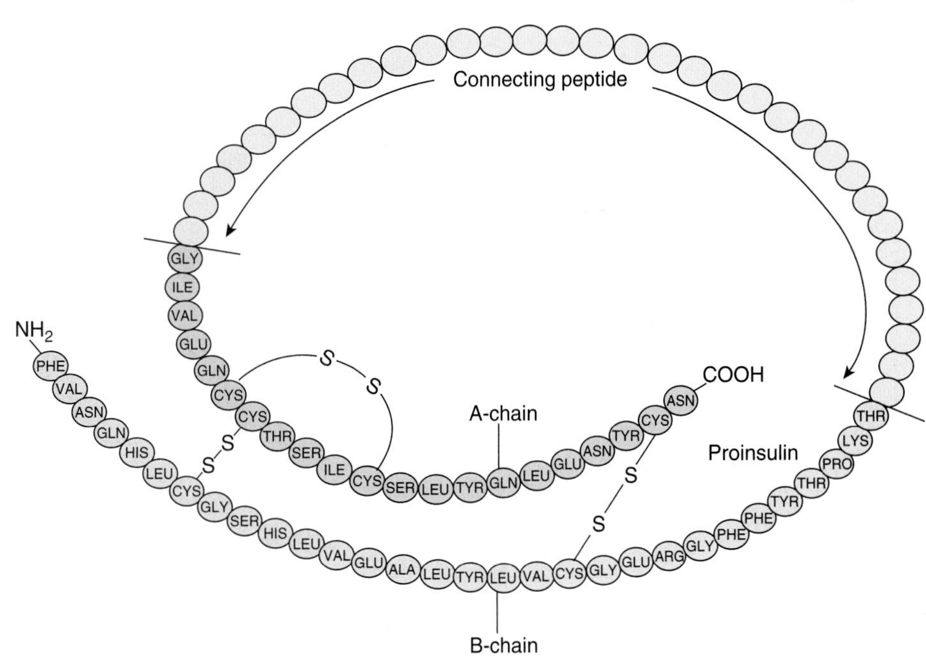

FIGURE 43-3 Structure of proinsulin. With removal of the connecting peptide (C-peptide), proinsulin is converted to insulin.

biologically inactive C-peptide (connecting peptide) chain that joined the A and B chains before they were separated. Active insulin and the inactive C-peptide chain are packaged into secretory granules and released simultaneously from the beta cell. The C-peptide chains can be measured clinically, and this measurement can be used to study beta cell activity. *Amylin* is a 37-amino acid peptide that is cosecreted with insulin from the pancreatic beta cells in response to glucose and other beta-cell stimulators.[4] Studies indicate that amylin acts as a neuroendocrine hormone, with several effects that complement the actions of insulin in regulating postprandial blood glucose levels. These include a suppression of glucagon secretion and a slowing of the rate at which glucose is delivered to the small intestine for absorption.

The release of insulin from the pancreatic beta cells is regulated by blood glucose levels, increasing as blood glucose levels rise and decreasing when blood glucose levels decline. Blood glucose enters the beta cell by means of the glucose transporter, is phosphorylated by an enzyme called *glucokinase,* and is metabolized to form the adenosine triphosphate (ATP) needed to close the potassium channels and depolarize the cell. Depolarization, in turn, results in opening of the calcium channels and insulin secretion[4] (Fig. 43-4). Secretion of insulin occurs in an oscillatory or pulsatile fashion. After exposure to glucose, which is a nutrient secretagogue, a first-phase release of stored preformed insulin occurs, followed by a second-phase release of newly synthesized insulin (Fig. 43-5). Diabetes may result from dysregulation or deficiency in any of the steps involved in this process (*e.g.,* impaired function of the glucose transporters, intracellular metabolic defects, glucokinase deficiency). Serum insulin levels begin to rise within minutes after a meal, reach a peak in approximately 3 to 5 minutes, and then return to baseline levels within 2 to 3 hours.

Insulin secreted by the beta cells enters the portal circulation and travels directly to the liver, where approximately 50% is used or degraded. Insulin, which is rapidly bound to peripheral tissues or destroyed by the liver or kidneys, has a half-life of approximately 15 minutes once it is released into the general circulation. To initiate its effects on target tissues, insulin binds to a membrane receptor. The insulin receptor is a combination of four subunits—a pair of larger α subunits that extend outside the cell membrane and are involved in insulin binding, and a smaller pair of β subunits that are predominantly inside the cell membrane and contain a kinase enzyme that becomes activated during insulin binding (Fig. 43-6). Activation of the kinase enzyme results in autophosphorylation of the β subunit itself. Phosphorylation of the β subunit in turn

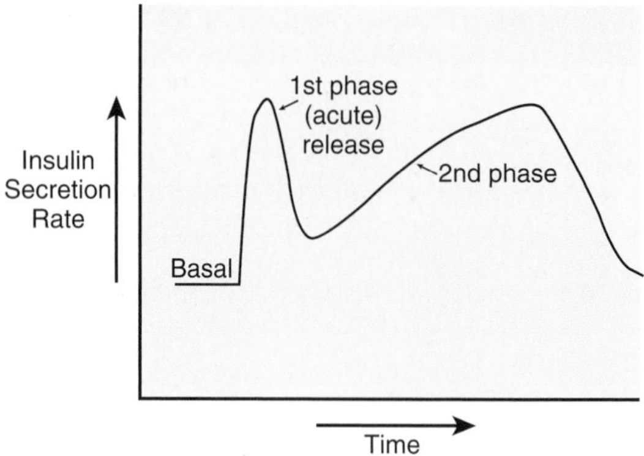

FIGURE 43-5 Biphasic insulin response to a constant glucose stimulus. The peak of the first phase in humans is 3 to 5 minutes; the second phase begins at 2 minutes and continues to increase slowly for at least 60 minutes or until the stimulus stops. (From Ward W.K., Beard J.C., Halter J.B., Pfeifer M.A., Porte D. Jr. [1984]. Pathology of insulin secretion in non-insulin-dependent diabetes mellitus. *Diabetes Care 7,* 491–502. Reprinted with permission from The American Diabetes Association. Copyright © 1984 American Diabetes Association)

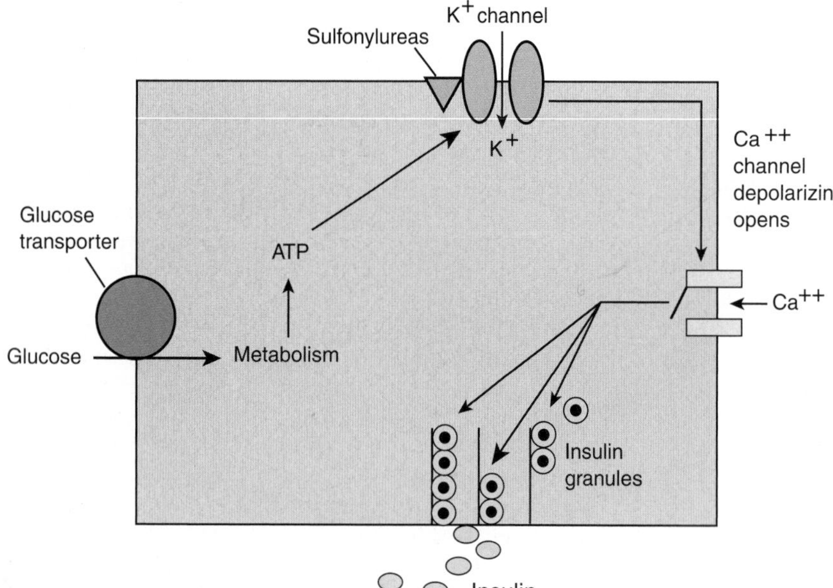

FIGURE 43-4 One model of control of release of insulin by the pancreatic beta cells and the action of the sulfonylurea agents. In the resting beta cell with low ATP levels, potassium diffuses through the ATP-gated channels maintaining the resting membrane potential. As blood glucose rises and is transported into the beta cell via the glucose transporter, ATP rises causing the potassium channels to close and depolarization to occur. Depolarization results in opening of the voltage-gated calcium channels, which results in insulin secretion. (Modified from Karam J.H. [1992]. Type II diabetes and syndrome X. *Endocrine and Metabolic Clinics of North America 21,* 339)

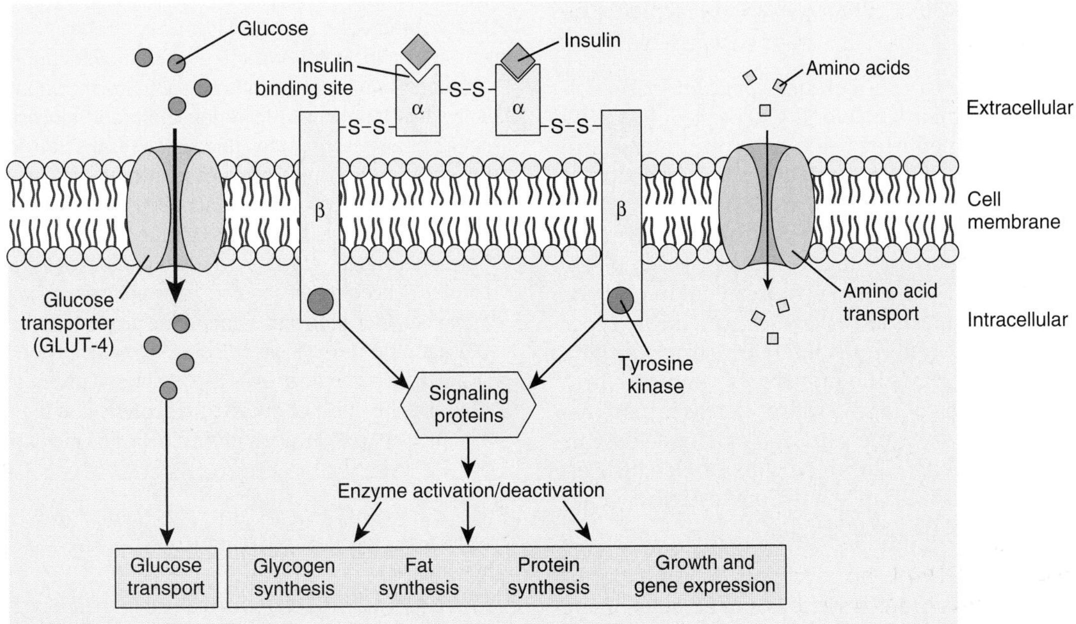

FIGURE 43-6 Insulin receptor. Insulin binds to the α subunits of the insulin receptor, which increases glucose transport and causes autophosphorylation of the β subunit of the receptor, which induces tyrosine kinase activity. Tyrosine phosphorylation, in turn, activates a cascade of intracellular signaling proteins that mediate the effects of insulin on glucose, fat, and protein metabolism.

activates some enzymes and inactivates others, thereby directing the desired intracellular effect of insulin on glucose, fat, and protein metabolism.

Because cell membranes are impermeable to glucose, they require a special carrier, called a *glucose transporter,* to move glucose from the blood into the cell. These transporters move glucose across the cell membrane at a faster rate than would occur by diffusion alone. Considerable research has revealed a family of glucose transporters termed *GLUT-1, GLUT-2,* and so forth.[4] GLUT-4 is the insulin-dependent glucose transporter for skeletal muscle and adipose tissue. It is sequestered inside the membrane of these cells and thus is unable to function as a glucose transporter until a signal from insulin causes it to move from its inactive site into the cell membrane, where it facilitates glucose entry. GLUT-2 is the major transporter of glucose into beta cells and liver cells. It has a low affinity for glucose and acts as a transporter only when plasma glucose levels are relatively high, such as after a meal. GLUT-1 is present in all tissues. It does not require the actions of insulin and is important in transport of glucose into the nervous system.

Glucagon

Glucagon, a polypeptide molecule produced by the alpha cells of the islets of Langerhans, maintains blood glucose between meals and during periods of fasting. Like insulin, glucagon travels through the portal vein to the liver, where it exerts its main action. Unlike insulin, glucagon produces an increase in blood glucose. The most dramatic effect of glucagon is its ability to initiate *glycogenolysis* or the breakdown of liver glycogen as a means of raising blood glucose, usually within a matter of minutes. Glucagon also increases the transport of amino acids into the liver and stimulates their conversion into glucose, a process called *gluconeogenesis.* Because liver glycogen stores are limited, gluconeogenesis is important in maintaining blood glucose levels over time (see Table 43-1). Other actions of glucagon occur only when the hormone is present in high concentrations, usually well above those normally present in the blood. At high concentrations, glucagon activates adipose cell lipase, making fatty acids available for use as energy.[2] At very high concentrations, glucagon can increase the strength of the heart, increase blood flow to some tissues, including the kidneys, enhance bile secretion, and inhibit gastric acid secretion.

As with insulin, glucagon secretion is regulated by blood glucose. A decrease in blood glucose concentration to a hypoglycemic level produces an immediate increase in glucagon secretion, and an increase in blood glucose to hyperglycemic levels produces a decrease in glucagon secretion. High concentrations of amino acids, as occur after a protein meal, also can stimulate glucagon secretion. In this way, glucagon increases the conversion of amino acids to glucose as a means of maintaining the body's glucose levels. Glucagon levels also increase during strenuous exercise as a means of preventing a decrease in blood glucose.

Other Hormones

Other hormones that can affect blood glucose include the catecholamines, growth hormone, and the glucocorticoids. These hormones, along with glucagon, are sometimes called counterregulatory hormones because they counteract the storage functions of insulin in regulating blood glucose levels during periods of fasting, exercise, and other situations that either limit glucose intake or deplete glucose stores.

Catecholamines. The catecholamines, *epinephrine* and *norepinephrine,* help to maintain blood glucose levels during periods of stress. Epinephrine inhibits insulin release and promotes glycogenolysis by stimulating the conversion of muscle and liver glycogen to glucose. Muscle glycogen cannot be released into the blood; nevertheless, the mobilization of these stores for muscle use conserves blood glucose for use by other tissues such as the brain and the nervous system. During periods of exercise and other types of stress, epinephrine inhibits insulin release from the beta cells and thereby decreases the movement of glucose into muscle cells. The catecholamines also increase lipase activity and thereby increase mobilization of fatty acids; this process conserves glucose. The blood glucose–elevating effect of epinephrine is an important homeostatic mechanism during periods of hypoglycemia.

Growth Hormone. Growth hormone has many metabolic effects. It increases protein synthesis in all cells of the body, mobilizes fatty acids from adipose tissue, and antagonizes the effects of insulin. Growth hormone decreases cellular uptake and use of glucose, thereby increasing the level of blood glucose. The increased blood glucose level stimulates further insulin secretion by the beta cells. The secretion of growth hormone normally is inhibited by insulin and increased levels of blood glucose. During periods of fasting, when both blood glucose levels and insulin secretion fall, growth hormone levels increase. Exercise, such as running and cycling, and various stresses, including anesthesia, fever, and trauma, increase growth hormone levels.

Chronic hypersecretion of growth hormone, as occurs in acromegaly (see Chapter 42), can lead to glucose intolerance and the development of diabetes mellitus. In people who already have diabetes, moderate elevations in growth hormone levels that occur during periods of stress and periods of growth in children can produce the entire spectrum of metabolic abnormalities associated with poor regulation, despite optimized insulin treatment.

Glucocorticoid Hormones. The glucocorticoid hormones, which are synthesized in the adrenal cortex along with other corticosteroid hormones, are critical to survival during periods of fasting and starvation. They stimulate gluconeogenesis by the liver, sometimes producing a 6- to 10-fold increase in hepatic glucose production. These hormones also moderately decrease tissue use of glucose. In predisposed persons, the prolonged elevation of glucocorticoid hormones can lead to hyperglycemia and the development of diabetes mellitus. In people with diabetes, even transient increases in cortisol can complicate control.

There are several steroid hormones with glucocorticoid activity; the most important of these is cortisol, which accounts for approximately 95% of all glucocorticoid activity (see Chapter 42). Cortisol levels increase during periods of stress, such as that produced by infection, pain, trauma, surgery, prolonged and strenuous exercise, and acute anxiety. Hypoglycemia is a potent stimulus for cortisol secretion.

In summary, energy metabolism is controlled by a number of hormones, including insulin, glucagon, epinephrine, growth hormone, and the glucocorticoids. Of these hormones, only insulin has the effect of lowering the blood glucose level. Insulin's blood glucose–lowering action results from its ability to increase the transport of glucose into body cells and to decrease hepatic production and release of glucose into the bloodstream. Other hormones–glucagon, epinephrine, growth hormone, and the glucocorticoids–maintain or increase blood glucose concentrations and are referred to as *counterregulatory hormones.* Glucagon and epinephrine promote glycogenolysis. Glucagon and the glucocorticoids increase gluconeogenesis. Growth hormone decreases the peripheral use of glucose. Insulin has the effect of decreasing lipolysis and the use of fats as a fuel source; glucagon and epinephrine increase fat use.

Diabetes Mellitus

After completing this section of the chapter, you should be able to meet the following objectives:

- ✦ Compare the distinguishing features of type 1 and type 2 diabetes mellitus, list causes of other specific types of diabetes, and cite the criteria for gestational diabetes
- ✦ Define prediabetes
- ✦ Relate the physiologic functions of insulin to the manifestations of diabetes mellitus
- ✦ Define the metabolic syndrome and describe its associations
- ✦ Discuss the role of diet and exercise in the management of diabetes mellitus
- ✦ Characterize the actions of oral hypoglycemic agents in terms of the lowering of blood glucose
- ✦ Describe the clinical manifestations of diabetic ketoacidosis and their physiologic significance
- ✦ Describe the clinical condition resulting from the hyperosmolar hyperglycemic state
- ✦ Name and describe the types (according to duration of action) of insulin
- ✦ Relate the actions of the oral hypoglycemic agents to alterations in glucose metabolism that occur in persons with type 2 diabetes
- ✦ Describe the clinical manifestations of insulin-induced hypoglycemia and state how these may differ in elderly people
- ✦ Describe alterations in physiologic function that accompany diabetic peripheral neuropathy, retinopathy, and nephropathy
- ✦ Describe the causes of foot ulcers in people with diabetes mellitus
- ✦ Explain the relation between diabetes mellitus and infection

The term *diabetes* is derived from a Greek word meaning "going through" and *mellitus* from the Latin word for "honey" or "sweet." Reports of the disorder can be traced back to the first century AD, when Aretaeus the Cappadocian described the disorder as a chronic affliction characterized by intense thirst and voluminous, honey-sweet urine: "the melting down of flesh into urine." It was the discovery of insulin by Banting and Best in 1922 that transformed the once-fatal disease into a manageable chronic health problem.[5]

Diabetes is a disorder of carbohydrate, protein, and fat metabolism resulting from an imbalance between insulin availability and insulin need. It can represent an absolute insulin deficiency, impaired release of insulin by the pancreatic beta cells, inadequate or defective insulin receptors, or the production of inactive insulin or insulin that is destroyed before it can carry out its action. A person with uncontrolled diabetes is unable to transport glucose into fat and muscle cells; as a result, the body cells are starved, and the breakdown of fat and protein is increased.

CLASSIFICATION AND ETIOLOGY

Although diabetes mellitus clearly is a disorder of insulin availability, it probably is not a single disease. A revised system for the classification of diabetes was developed in 1997 by the Expert Committee on the Diagnosis and Classification of Diabetes Mellitus.[6] The intent of this revision, which replaces the 1979 classification system, was to move away from focusing on the type of pharmacologic treatment used in management of diabetes to one based on disease etiology. The revised system continues to include type 1 and type 2 diabetes, but uses Arabic rather than Roman numerals and eliminates the use of "insulin-dependent" and "non–insulin-dependent" diabetes mellitus (Table 43-2). Type 2 diabetes currently accounts for about 90% to 95% of the cases of diabetes. Included in the classification system are the categories of gestational diabetes

TABLE 43-2 Etiologic Classification of Diabetes Mellitus

Type	Subtypes	Etiology of Glucose Intolerance
I. Type 1*	Beta cell destruction usually leading to absolute insulin deficiency	
	A. Immune mediated	Autoimmune destruction of beta cells
	B. Idiopathic	Unknown
II. Type 2*	May range from predominantly insulin resistance with relative insulin deficiency to a predominantly secretory defect with insulin resistance	
III. Other specific types	A. Genetic defects in beta cell function, *e.g.*, glucokinase	Regulates insulin secretion due to defect in glucokinase generation
	B. Genetic defects in insulin action, *e.g.*, leprechaunism, Rabson-Mendenhall syndrome	Pediatric syndromes that have mutations in insulin receptors
	C. Diseases of exocrine pancreas, *e.g.*, pancreatitis, neoplasms, cystic fibrosis	Loss or destruction of insulin-producing beta cells
	D. Endocrine disorders, *e.g.*, acromegaly, Cushing's syndrome	Diabetogenic effects of excess hormone levels
	E. Drug or chemical induced, *e.g.*, Vacor, glucocorticosteroids, thiazide diuretics, interferon-alfa	Toxic destruction of beta cells Insulin resistance Impaired insulin secretion Production of islet cell antibodies
	F. Infections, *e.g.*, congenital rubella, cytomegalovirus	Beta cell injury followed by autoimmune response
	G. Uncommon forms of immune-mediated diabetes, *e.g.*, "stiff man syndrome"	Autoimmune disorder of central nervous system with immune-mediated beta cell destruction
	H. Other genetic syndromes sometimes associated with diabetes, *e.g.*, Down syndrome, Klinefelter's syndrome, Turner's syndrome	Disorders of glucose tolerance related to defects associated with chromosomal abnormalities
IV. Gestational diabetes mellitus (GDM)	Any degree of glucose intolerance with onset or first recognition during pregnancy	Combination of insulin resistance and impaired insulin secretion

*Patients with any form of diabetes may require insulin treatment at some stage of the disease. Such use of insulin, does not, of itself, classify the patient.

(Adapted from The Expert Committee on the Diagnosis and Classification of Diabetes Mellitus. [2004]. Report of the Expert Committee on the Diagnosis and Classification of Diabetes Mellitus. *Diabetes Care 27,* S5–S10. Reprinted with permission from the American Diabetes Association. Copyright © 2004 American Diabetes Association.)

TABLE 43-3 Expert Committee on the Diagnosis and Classification of Diabetes Mellitus Using Fasting Plasma Glucose (FPG) and Oral Glucose Tolerance Test (OGTT)

Test	Normoglycemic	Impaired FPG (IFG)*	Impaired GT (IGT)*	Diabetes Mellitus†
FPG‡	<100 mg/dL (5.6 mmol/L)	100–125 mg/dL (5.6–6.9 mmol/L)		≥126 mg/dL (7.0 mmol/L)
2-h OGTT§	<140 mg/dL (7.8 mmol/L)		140–199 mg/dL (7.8–11.1 mmol/L)	≥200 mg/dL (11.1 mmol/L)
Other				Symptoms of diabetes mellitus and casual plasma glucose ≥200 mg/dL

*IFG and IGT are prediabetic states and can occur in isolation or together in a given subject.
†In the absence of unequivocal hyperglycemia with acute metabolic decompensation, these criteria should be confirmed by repeat testing on a separate day.
‡Fasting is defined as no caloric intake for at least 8 hours.
§OGTT with 2-h measurement of venous plasma or serum glucose following a 75-g carbohydrate load.
(Developed from data in American Diabetes Association. [2004]. Diagnosis and classification of diabetes mellitus. *Diabetes Care 27*[Suppl. 1], S5–10.)

mellitus (*i.e.,* diabetes that develops during pregnancy) and other specific types of diabetes, many of which occur secondary to other conditions (*e.g.,* Cushing's syndrome, hematochromatosis, pancreatitis, acromegaly).

The revised classification system also includes a system for diagnosing diabetes according to stages of glucose intolerance[6] (Table 43-3). The revised criteria have retained the former category of *impaired glucose tolerance* (IGT) and have added a new category of *impaired fasting plasma glucose* (IFG). The categories of IFG and IGT refer to metabolic stages intermediate between normal glucose homeostasis and diabetes, and are labeled together as *prediabetes.* A fasting plasma glucose (FPG) of less than 100 mg/dL or a 2-hour oral glucose tolerance test (OGTT) result of less than 140 mg/dL is considered normal. IFG is defined as FPG of 100 mg/dL to 125 mg/dL. IGT reflects abnormal plasma glucose measurements (≥140 mg/dL but <200 mg/dL) 2 hours after an oral glucose load.[6] IFG and IGT (*i.e.,* prediabetes) is associated with increased risk for atherosclerotic heart disease and increased risk for progression to type 2 diabetes. Approximately 5% of people with IFG and IGT progress to diabetes each year. Calorie restriction and weight reduction are important in overweight people with prediabetes.[7] Persons with an FPG of 126 mg/dL or higher or a 2-hour OGTT of 200 mg/L or higher are considered to have *provisional diabetes.*[6] The criteria in Chart 43-1 are used to confirm the diagnosis of diabetes in persons with provisional diabetes.

Type 1 Diabetes Mellitus

Type 1 diabetes mellitus is characterized by destruction of the pancreatic beta cells.[8] Type 1 diabetes is subdivided into two types: type 1A, immune-mediated diabetes, and type 1B, idiopathic diabetes. In the United States and Europe, approximately 10% of people with diabetes mellitus have type 1 diabetes, with 95% of them having type 1A, immune-mediated diabetes.

Type 1A diabetes is characterized by autoimmune destruction of beta cells. This type of diabetes, formerly called *juvenile diabetes,* occurs more commonly in young persons but can occur at any age. Type 1 diabetes is a catabolic disorder characterized by an absolute lack of insulin, an elevation in blood glucose, and a breakdown of body fats and proteins. The absolute lack of insulin in people with type 1 diabetes mellitus means that they are particularly prone to the development of ketoacidosis. One of the actions of insulin is the inhibition of *lipolysis* (*i.e.,* fat breakdown) and release of free fatty acids (FFAs) from fat cells. In the absence of insulin, ketosis develops when these fatty acids are released from fat cells and converted to ketones in the liver.

Because of the loss of the first-phase insulin (preformed insulin) response, all people with type 1A diabetes require

CHART 43-1

Criteria for Diagnosis of Diabetes Mellitus

1. Symptoms of diabetes plus casual plasma glucose concentration >200 mg/dL (11.1 mmol/L). *Casual* is defined as any time of the day without regard to time since last meal. The classic symptoms of diabetes include polyuria, polydipsia, and unexplained weight loss.

   or
2. Fasting plasma glucose ≥126 mg/dL (7.0 mmol/L). *Fasting* is defined as no caloric intake for at least 8 h.

   or
3. 2-h postload glucose ≥200 mg/dL (11.1 mmol/L) during oral glucose tolerance test (OGTT). The test should be performed as described by the World Health Organization, using a glucose load containing the equivalent of 75 g anhydrous glucose dissolved in water.

In the absence of unequivocal hyperglycemia, these criteria should be confirmed by repeat testing on a different day. The third measure (OGTT) is not recommended for routine use. (Developed from data in American Diabetes Association. [2004]. Diagnosis and classification of diabetes mellitus. *Diabetes Care 27*[Suppl. 1], S5–10.)

DIABETES MELLITUS

- Diabetes mellitus is a disorder of carbohydrate, fat, and protein metabolism brought about by impaired beta cell synthesis or release of insulin, or the inability of tissues to use glucose.
- Type 1 diabetes results from loss of beta cell function and an absolute insulin deficiency.
- Type 2 diabetes results from impaired ability of the tissues to use insulin (insulin resistance) accompanied by a relative lack of insulin or impaired release of insulin in relation to blood glucose levels (beta cell dysfunction).

exogenous insulin replacement to reverse the catabolic state, control blood glucose levels, and prevent ketosis. The rate of beta cell destruction is quite variable, being rapid in some individuals and slow in others. The rapidly progressive form commonly is observed in children, but also may occur in adults. The slowly progressive form usually occurs in adults and is sometimes referred to as *latent autoimmune diabetes in adults* (LADA). LADA may constitute up to 10% of adults who are currently classified as having type 2 diabetes.

It has been suggested that type 1A, immune-mediated diabetes results from a genetic predisposition (*i.e.*, diabetogenic genes), a hypothetical triggering event that involves an environmental agent that incites an immune response, and immunologically mediated beta cell destruction. Much evidence has focused on the inherited major histocompatibility complex (MHC) genes that encode three human leukocyte antigens (HLA-DP, HLA-DQ, and HLA-DR) found on the surface of body cells (see Chapter 19). Susceptibility to type 1 diabetes also has been associated with HLA-DR3 and HLA-DR4.[4] It appears that what is inherited as part of the HLA genotype in people with type 1 diabetes is a susceptibility to an abnormal immune response that affects the beta cells. On the other hand, resistance to the development of type 1 diabetes has been traced to other HLA subtypes: DR11, DR15, and DQB1. In addition to the major susceptibility gene for type 1 diabetes in the MHC region on chromosome 6, an insulin gene regulating beta cell replication and function has been identified on chromosome 11.

Type 1 diabetes–associated autoantibodies may exist for years before the onset of hyperglycemia. There are two major types of autoantibodies: insulin autoantibodies (IAAs), and islet cell autoantibodies and antibodies directed at other islet autoantigens, including glutamic acid decarboxylase (GAD) and the protein tyrosine phosphatase IA-2.[9] Testing for antibodies to GAD or IA-2 and for IAAs using sensitive radiobinding assays can identify more than 85% of cases of new or future type 1 diabetes with 98% specificity.[10] The appearance of IAAs may precede that of antibodies to GAD or IA-2, and IAAs may be the only antibodies detected at diagnosis in young children. Therefore, it is recommended that determination of IAAs be included in primary testing of children younger than 10 years of age to maximize sensitivity. Strategies for full evaluation of the risk for developing future type 1 diabetes should include determination of at least three of the four best-established markers, IAAs, islet cell autoantibodies, and antibodies to GAD and IA-2, as well as a test of the first-phase insulin response. These people also may have other autoimmune disorders such as Graves' disease, rheumatoid arthritis, and Addison's disease.

The fact that type 1 diabetes is thought to result from an interaction between genetic and environmental factors has led to research into methods directed at prevention and early control of the disease. These methods include the identification of genetically susceptible persons and early intervention in newly diagnosed persons with type 1 diabetes. After the diagnosis of type 1 diabetes, there often is a short period of beta cell regeneration, during which symptoms of diabetes disappear and insulin injections are not needed. This is sometimes called the *honeymoon period*. Immune interventions (immunomodulation) designed to interrupt the destruction of beta cells before development of type 1 diabetes are being investigated in various trials, including the Diabetes Prevention Trial-1 (DPT-1). Unfortunately, none of the interventions studied to date to prevent complete and irreversible beta cell failure have shown any clinical utility. Effects of modulation of various environmental influences such as infant diet and breast-feeding remains unclear.[11]

The term *idiopathic type 1B diabetes* is used to describe those cases of beta cell destruction in which no evidence of autoimmunity is present. Only a small number of people with type 1 diabetes fall into this category; most are of African or Asian descent. Type 1B diabetes is strongly inherited. People with the disorder have episodic ketoacidosis due to varying degrees of insulin deficiency with periods of absolute insulin deficiency that may come and go.

Type 2 Diabetes Mellitus and the Metabolic Syndrome

Type 2 diabetes mellitus is a heterogeneous condition that describes the presence of hyperglycemia in association with *relative* insulin deficiency. In contrast to type 1 diabetes in which *absolute* insulin deficiency is present, type 2 diabetes can be associated with high, normal, or low insulin levels. However, in the presence of insulin resistance, the insulin cannot function effectively, and hyperglycemia can result. Type 2 diabetes is therefore a disorder of both insulin levels (beta cell dysfunction) and insulin function (insulin resistance).[12] Type 2 diabetes (unlike type 1) is not associated with HLA markers or autoantibodies.

Most people with type 2 diabetes are older and overweight; however, type 2 diabetes is becoming a more common occurrence in obese adolescents.[13,14] The metabolic abnormalities that contribute to hyperglycemia in people with type 2 diabetes include (1) impaired beta cell function and insulin secretion, (2) peripheral insulin resistance, and (3) increased hepatic glucose production.[12]

Insulin resistance initially produces an increase in beta cell secretion of insulin (resulting in hyperinsulinemia) as the body attempts to maintain a normoglycemic state. In time, however, the insulin response declines because of increasing beta cell dysfunction. This results initially in elevated postprandial blood glucose levels. Eventually, fasting blood glucose levels also rise until frank type 2 diabetes occurs. During the evolutionary phase, an individual with type 2 diabetes may eventually develop *absolute* insulin deficiency because of progressive beta cell failure. As with persons with type 1 diabetes, these persons require insulin therapy to survive. Because most persons with type 2 diabetes do not have an absolute insulin deficiency, they are less prone to develop ketoacidosis as compared with people with type 1 diabetes (the presence of circulating insulin in most type 2 diabetics suppresses ketone body formation).

Beta Cell Dysfunction. Specific causes of beta cell dysfunction in patients with prediabetes and type 2 diabetes may include: (1) an initial decrease in the beta cell mass (this may be related to genetic factors responsible for beta cell differentiation and function, and environmental factors such as the presence of maternal diabetes during pregnancy or in utero factors such as the presence of intrauterine growth retardation), (2) increased beta cell apoptosis/decreased regeneration, (3) long-standing insulin resistance leading to beta cell exhaustion, (4) chronic hyperglycemia can induce beta cell desensitization termed *glucotoxicity,* (5) chronic elevation of free fatty acids can cause toxicity to beta cells termed *lipotoxicity,* and (6) amyloid deposition in the beta cell can cause dysfunction.[12] According to one study, beta cell function was reduced 50% at diagnosis of type 2 diabetes, and its progressive decrease (by approximately 4% per year) profoundly influenced the subsequent response to treatment (meaning that combination treatment with several agents is usually the norm to maintain glycemic goals).

Insulin Resistance and the Metabolic Syndrome. There is increasing evidence to suggest that insulin resistance not only contributes to the hyperglycemia in persons with type 2 diabetes, but may also play a role in other metabolic abnormalities. These include high levels of plasma triglycerides and low levels of high-density lipoproteins (HDLs), hypertension, systemic inflammation (as detected by C-reactive protein [CRP] and other mediators), abnormal fibrinolysis, abnormal function of the vascular endothelium, and macrovascular disease (coronary artery, cerebrovascular, and peripheral arterial disease). This constellation of abnormalities often is referred to as the *insulin resistance syndrome, syndrome X,* or the preferred term, *metabolic syndrome.*[13] In clinical practice, the Third Report of the National Cholesterol Education Program Expert Panel on Detection, Evaluation, and Treatment of High Blood Cholesterol in Adults (NCEP ATP III) definition of metabolic syndrome is widely used[15] (Chart 43-2). Insulin resistance and increased risk for developing type 2 diabetes are also seen in women with polycystic ovary syndrome[16] (see Chapter 47).

A major factor in persons with the metabolic syndrome that leads to type 2 diabetes is central obesity. Approximately 80% of persons with type 2 diabetes are overweight. Obese people have increased resistance to the action of insulin and impaired suppression of glucose production by the liver, resulting in both hyperglycemia and hyperinsulinemia.[12] The type of obesity is an important consideration in the development of type 2 diabetes. It has been found that people with upper body obesity (central obesity) are at greater risk for developing type 2 diabetes and metabolic disturbances than persons with lower body obesity (see Chapter 11). The increased insulin resistance has been attributed to increased visceral (intraabdominal) obesity detected on computed tomography scan.[17] Waist circumference, which is a measure of central obesity, has been shown to correlate well with insulin resistance. The new terminology that is emerging for persons with obesity and type 2 diabetes is *diabesity*. Therefore, a diagnosis of the metabolic syndrome using the NCEP ATP III criteria (see Chart 43-2) should be considered for persons with IFG or type 2 diabetes. For management, weight loss with initial 5% to 10% of body weight should be incorporated into their treatment plan as well as addressing the diabetes and other related metabolic abnormalities. Over time, insulin resistance may improve with weight loss, to the extent that many people with type 2 diabetes can be managed with a weight-reduction program and exercise.[7]

It has been theorized that the insulin resistance and increased glucose production in obese people with type 2 diabetes may stem from an increased concentration of free fatty acids (FFAs).[12] Visceral obesity is especially important because it is accompanied by increases in fasting and postprandial FFA concentrations. This has several consequences: (1) acutely, FFAs act at the level of the beta cell to stimulate insulin secretion, which, with excessive and chronic stimulation, causes beta cell failure (lipotoxicity); (2) they act at the level of the peripheral tissues to cause insulin resistance and glucose underutilization by inhibiting glucose uptake and glycogen storage through a reduction in

CHART 43-2

NCEP ATP III Criteria for a Diagnosis of Metabolic Syndrome*

Three or more of the following:

- Abdominal obesity: waist circumference >35 inches in women or >40 inches in men
- Triglycerides ≥150 mg/dL
- High-density lipoproteins (HDL) <50 mg/dL in women or <40 mg/dL in men
- Blood pressure >130/85 mm Hg
- Fasting plasma glucose >110 mg/dL†

*Developed from: Grundy S.M., Panel Chair. (2001). Third Report of the National Cholesterol Education Program (NCEP) Expert Panel on Detection, Evaluation, and Treatment of High Blood Cholesterol in Adults (Adult Treatment Panel III). (NIH Publication No. 01-3670.) Bethesda, MD: National Institutes of Health.

†In view of the recent changes in the definition of abnormal glucose levels (American Diabetes Association. [2004]. Diagnosis and classification of diabetes mellitus. *Diabetes Care 27*[Suppl. 1], S5–10), an FPG value >100 mg/dL should now be used in the diagnosis of the metabolic syndrome.

muscle glycogen synthetase activity; (3) the accumulation of FFAs and triglycerides reduce hepatic insulin sensitivity, leading to increased hepatic glucose production and hyperglycemia, especially fasting plasma glucose levels. Thus, an increase in FFA that occurs in obese individuals (especially visceral obesity) with a genetic predisposition to type 2 diabetes may eventually lead to beta cell dysfunction/failure, increased insulin resistance, and hepatic glucose production (Fig. 43-7). A further consequence is the diversion of excess FFAs to nonadipose tissues, including liver, skeletal muscle, heart, and pancreatic beta cells.[12] The uptake of FFAs from the portal blood can lead to hepatic triglyceride accumulation and nonalcoholic fatty liver disease (see Chapter 40).

A proposed link to the insulin resistance associated with obesity is an adipose cell secretion (adipocytokine) called *adiponectin*.[18] Adiponectin is secreted by adipose tissue and circulates in the blood. It has been shown that decreased levels of adiponectin coincide with insulin resistance in animal models and patients with obesity and type 2 diabetes. Moreover, there is evidence that the expression of adiponectin mRNA might be partially regulated by peroxisome proliferator–activated receptor-γ, a nuclear receptor that leads to the regulation of genes controlling FFA levels and glucose metabolism (discussed under the thiazolidinedione oral antidiabetic agents). In skeletal muscle, adiponectin has been shown to decrease tissue triglyceride content by increasing the utilization of fatty acids as a fuel source. Because its level is low in the metabolic syndrome, the replenishment of adiponectin may be considered as an alternative treatment of insulin resistance in the future.[18,19]

The fact that lifestyle plays an important role in the pathogenesis of type 2 diabetes has led to an increased emphasis on prevention. The findings of the Diabetes Prevention Program (DPP), a research project involving 27 centers in the United States, found that diet and exercise dramatically delay the onset of type 2 diabetes.[20] Participants randomly assigned to an intensive lifestyle modification program (low-fat diet and exercising 150 minutes a week) with a 7% weight loss, reduced their risk for developing type 2 diabetes by 58%. The study also found that participants assigned to treatment with the oral diabetic drug metformin reduced their risk for developing diabetes by 31%.[20]

Other Specific Types

The category of other specific types of diabetes, formerly known as *secondary diabetes,* describes diabetes that is associated with certain other conditions and syndromes. Such diabetes can occur with pancreatic disease or the removal of pancreatic tissue and with endocrine diseases, such as acromegaly, Cushing's syndrome, or pheochromocytoma. Endocrine disorders that produce hyperglycemia do so by increasing the hepatic production of glucose or decreasing the cellular use of glucose. Several specific types of diabetes are associated with monogenetic defects in beta cell function. These specific types of diabetes, which resemble type 2 diabetes but occur at an earlier age (usually before 25 years of age), are referred to as *maturity-onset diabetes of the young* (MODY).[4]

Environmental agents that have been associated with altered pancreatic beta cell function include viruses (*e.g.,* mumps, congenital rubella, coxsackievirus) and chemical toxins. Among the suspected chemical toxins are the nitrosamines, which sometimes are found in smoked and cured meats. The nitrosamines are related to streptozocin, which is used to induce diabetes in experimental animals, and to the rat poison Vacor, which can produce diabetes when ingested by humans.

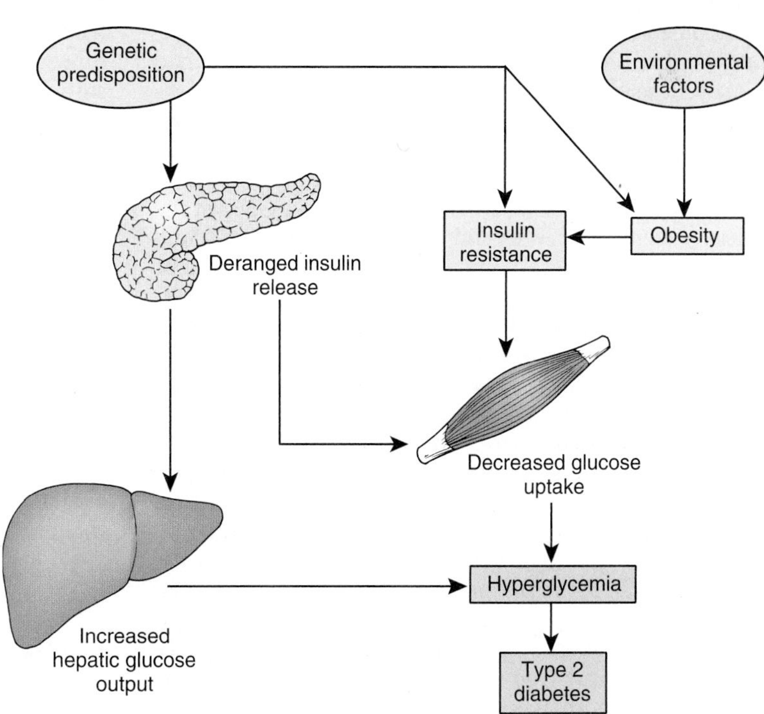

FIGURE 43-7 Pathogenesis of type 2 diabetes mellitus.

Several diuretics—thiazides and loop diuretics—elevate blood glucose. These diuretics increase potassium loss, which is thought to impair insulin release. Other drugs known to cause hyperglycemia are diazoxide, glucocorticoids, levodopa, oral contraceptives, sympathomimetics, phenothiazines, phenytoin, and total parenteral nutrition (*i.e.,* hyperalimentation). Drug-related increases in blood glucose usually are reversed after the drug has been discontinued.

The advent of potent antiretroviral therapy (especially protease inhibitors) for the treatment of human immunodeficiency virus (HIV) and acquired immunodeficiency syndrome (AIDS) has significantly improved survival. However, these patients are now developing metabolic derangements similar to the features seen in the metabolic syndrome (insulin resistance, high levels of plasma triglycerides, low levels of high-density lipoproteins [HDLs], hypertension, obesity, systemic inflammation [as detected by C-reactive protein (CRP) and other mediators], abnormal fibrinolysis, abnormal endothelial dysfunction, and macrovascular disease).[21] In addition, changes in fat distribution (peripheral lipoatrophy and visceral obesity), sometimes referred to as *lipodystrophy,* often occur (see Chapter 22). These people should be aggressively treated to prevent cardiovascular complications resulting from the abnormal risk factors.[21]

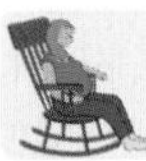

Gestational Diabetes

Gestational diabetes mellitus (GDM) refers to any degree of glucose intolerance that is detected first during pregnancy. It occurs to various degrees in 1% to 14% of all pregnancies, depending on the population and diagnostic tests used.[22] It most frequently affects women with a family history of diabetes; with glycosuria; with a history of stillbirth or spontaneous abortion, fetal anomalies in a previous pregnancy, or a previous large- or heavy-for-date baby; and who are obese, of advanced maternal age, or have had five or more pregnancies.

All pregnant women should undergo risk assessment for diabetes during their first prenatal visit. Those with significant risk should undergo plasma glucose testing as soon as feasible. If they are found not found to have GDM at the initial screening, they should be retested between 24 and 28 weeks of gestation. Women with average risk should be tested at 24 to 28 weeks of gestation. Women with an FPG of more than 126 mg/dL or casual glucose of more than 200 mg/dL meet the threshold for diabetes, if confirmed on a subsequent day, and do not need to undergo oral glucose tolerance testing.[22] Women with high or average GDM risk who do not demonstrate this degree of hyperglycemia on FPG testing should undergo further screening using the oral glucose tolerance test. This screening test consists of 50 g of glucose given without regard to the last meal and followed in 1 hour by a venous blood sample for glucose concentration. If the plasma glucose level is greater than 140 mg/dL, then a 100-g 3-hour glucose tolerance test is indicated to establish the diagnosis of GDM[22] (Table 43-4). On the other hand, women who are younger than 25 years of age, were of normal body weight before pregnancy, have no family history of diabetes or poor obstetric outcome, and are not members of a high-risk ethnic or racial group (*e.g.,* Hispanic, Native American, Asian, African American) may not need to be screened.

TABLE 43-4 Diagnosis of Gestational Diabetes Mellitus With a 100-g Glucose Load

100-g Glucose Load	mg/dL (mmol/L)
Fasting	95 (5.3)
1 hour	180 (10.0)
2 hour	155 (8.6)
3 hour	140 (7.8)

Two or more of the venous plasma concentrations must be met or exceeded for a positive diagnosis. The test should be done in the morning after an overnight fast of between 8 and 14 h and after at least 3 days of unrestricted diet (>150 g carbohydrate/day) and unlimited physical activity. The subject should remain seated and should not smoke throughout the test. (Developed from data in American Diabetes Association. [2004]. Diagnosis and classification of diabetes mellitus. *Diabetes Care 27*[Suppl 1], S5–10.)

Diagnosis and careful medical management are essential because women with GDM are at higher risk for complications of pregnancy, mortality, and fetal abnormalities.[4] Fetal abnormalities include macrosomia (*i.e.,* large body size), hypoglycemia, hypocalcemia, polycythemia, and hyperbilirubinemia.

Treatment of GDM includes close observation of mother and fetus because even mild hyperglycemia has been shown to be detrimental to the fetus.[22] Maternal fasting and postprandial blood glucose levels should be measured regularly. Fetal surveillance depends on the degree of risk for the fetus. The frequency of growth measurements and determinations of fetal distress depends on available technology and gestational age. All women with GDM require nutritional guidance because nutrition is the cornerstone of therapy. The nutrition plan should provide the necessary nutrients for maternal and fetal health, result in normoglycemia and proper weight gain, and prevent ketosis.[4] If dietary management alone does not achieve a fasting blood glucose level no greater than 105 mg/dL or a 2-hour postprandial blood glucose no greater than 120 mg/dL, the Third International Workshop on GDM recommends therapy with human insulin.[22] Oral antidiabetic agents may be teratogenic and are not recommended in pregnancy. Self-monitoring of blood glucose levels is essential.

Women with GDM are at increased risk for developing diabetes 5 to 10 years after delivery. Women in whom GDM is diagnosed should be followed after delivery to detect diabetes early in its course. These women should be evaluated during their first postpartum visit with a 2-hour oral glucose tolerance test with a 75-g glucose load.

CLINICAL MANIFESTATIONS

Diabetes mellitus may have a rapid or an insidious onset. In type 1 diabetes, signs and symptoms often arise suddenly. Type 2 diabetes usually develops more insidiously;

its presence may be detected during a routine medical examination or when a patient seeks medical care for other reasons.

The most commonly identified signs and symptoms of diabetes are referred to as the *three polys:* (1) polyuria (*i.e.,* excessive urination), (2) polydipsia (*i.e.,* excessive thirst), and (3) polyphagia (*i.e.,* excessive hunger). These three symptoms are closely related to the hyperglycemia and glycosuria of diabetes. Glucose is a small, osmotically active molecule. When blood glucose levels are sufficiently elevated, the amount of glucose filtered by the glomeruli of the kidney exceeds the amount that can be reabsorbed by the renal tubules; this results in glycosuria accompanied by large losses of water in the urine. Thirst results from the intracellular dehydration that occurs as blood glucose levels rise and water is pulled out of body cells, including those in the thirst center. Cellular dehydration also causes dryness of the mouth. This early symptom may be easily overlooked in people with type 2 diabetes, particularly in those who have had a gradual increase in blood glucose levels. Polyphagia usually is not present in people with type 2 diabetes. In type 1 diabetes, it probably results from cellular starvation and the depletion of cellular stores of carbohydrates, fats, and proteins.

Weight loss despite normal or increased appetite is a common occurrence in people with uncontrolled type 1 diabetes. The cause of weight loss is twofold. First, loss of body fluids results from osmotic diuresis. Vomiting may exaggerate the fluid loss in ketoacidosis. Second, body tissue is lost because the lack of insulin forces the body to use its fat stores and cellular proteins as sources of energy. In terms of weight loss, there often is a marked difference between type 2 diabetes and type 1 diabetes. Weight loss is a frequent phenomenon in people with uncontrolled type 1 diabetes, whereas many people with uncomplicated type 2 diabetes have problems with obesity.

Other signs and symptoms of hyperglycemia include recurrent blurred vision, fatigue, paresthesias, and skin infections. In type 2 diabetes, these often are the symptoms that prompt a person to seek medical treatment. Blurred vision develops as the lens and retina are exposed to hyperosmolar fluids. Lowered plasma volume produces weakness and fatigue. Paresthesias reflect a temporary dysfunction of the peripheral sensory nerves. Chronic skin infections are common in people with type 2 diabetes. Hyperglycemia and glycosuria favor the growth of yeast organisms. Pruritus and vulvovaginitis resulting from candidal infections are common initial complaints in women with diabetes. Balanitis secondary to candidal infections can occur in men.

DIAGNOSTIC TESTS

The diagnosis of diabetes mellitus in nonpregnant adults is based on fasting plasma glucose levels, casual plasma glucose tests, or the results of a glucose challenge test (see Table 43-3). Testing for diabetes should be considered in all individuals 45 years of age and older. Testing should be considered at a younger age in people who are obese, have a first-degree relative with diabetes, are members of a high-risk group, have delivered an infant weighing more than 9 pounds or have been diagnosed with GDM, have hypertension or hyperlipidemia, or have met the criteria for IGT or IFG (*i.e.,* prediabetes) on previous testing.[23]

Blood Tests

Blood glucose measurements are used in both the diagnosis and management of diabetes. Diagnostic tests include the fasting plasma glucose, casual plasma glucose, and glucose tolerance test. Laboratory and capillary or "finger stick" glucose tests are used for glucose management in people with diagnosed diabetes. Glycosylated hemoglobin (A1C, previously termed HbA_{1c}) provides a measure of glucose control over time. Table 43-5 shows the correlation between mean plasma glucose levels and A1C values for people with diabetes.[24]

Fasting Blood Glucose Test. The fasting plasma glucose has been suggested as the preferred diagnostic test because of ease of administration, convenience, patient acceptability, and cost.[23] Glucose levels are measured after food has been withheld for at least 8 hours. An FPG level below 100 mg/dL is considered normal (see Table 43-3). A level between 100 mg/dL and 126 mg/dL is significant and is defined as impaired fasting glucose. If the FPG level is 126 mg/dL or higher on two occasions, diabetes is diagnosed.

Casual Blood Glucose Test. A casual plasma glucose is one that is done without regard to the time of the last meal. A casual plasma glucose concentration that is unequivocally elevated (≥200 mg/dL) in the presence of classic symptoms of diabetes such as polydipsia, polyphagia, polyuria, and blurred vision is diagnostic of diabetes mellitus at any age.

Glucose Tolerance Test. The oral glucose tolerance test is an important screening test for diabetes. The test measures the body's ability to store glucose by removing it from the blood. In men and women, the test measures the plasma glucose response to 75 g of concentrated glucose solution at selected intervals, usually 1 hour and 2 hours. In pregnant women, a glucose load of 100 g is given (see the Gestational Diabetes section) with an additional 3-hour plasma glucose determination. In people with normal glucose tolerance, blood glucose levels return to normal within 2 to 3 hours after ingestion of a glucose load, in which case, it can be assumed that sufficient insulin is present to allow

TABLE 43-5 Correlation Between Hemoglobin A1C Level and Mean Plasma Glucose Levels

Hemoglobin AIC (%)	Mean Plasma Glucose mg/dL (mmol/L)
6	135 (7.5)
7	170 (9.5)
8	205 (11.5)
9	240 (13.5)
10	275 (13.5)
11	310 (17.5)
12	345 (19.5)

glucose to leave the blood and enter body cells. Because a person with diabetes lacks the ability to respond to an increase in blood glucose by releasing adequate insulin to facilitate storage, blood glucose levels rise above those observed in normal people and remain elevated for longer periods (see Table 43-3).

Capillary Blood Tests and Self-Monitoring of Capillary Blood Glucose Levels. Technologic advances have provided the means for monitoring blood glucose levels by using a drop of capillary blood. This procedure has provided health professionals with a rapid and economical means for monitoring blood glucose and has given people with diabetes a way of maintaining near-normal blood glucose levels through self-monitoring of blood glucose. These methods use a drop of capillary blood obtained by pricking the finger or forearm with a special needle or small lancet. Small trigger devices make use of the lancet virtually painless. The drop of capillary blood is placed on or absorbed by a reagent strip, and glucose levels are determined electronically using a glucose meter.

Laboratory tests that use plasma for measurement of blood glucose give results that are 10% to 15% higher than the finger stick method, which uses whole blood.[25] Many blood glucose monitors approved for home use and some test strips now calibrate blood glucose readings to plasma values. It is important that people with diabetes know whether their monitors or glucose strips provide whole blood or plasma test results.

Glycated Hemoglobin Testing. Glycated hemoglobin, also referred to as glycohemoglobin, glycosylated hemoglobin, HbA_{1c}, or A1C (the preferred term), is a term used to describe hemoglobin into which glucose has been incorporated. Hemoglobin normally does not contain glucose when it is released from the bone marrow. During its 120-day life span in the red blood cell, hemoglobin normally becomes glycated to form hemoglobins A_{1a} and A_{1b} (2% to 4%) and A_{1c} (termed A1C, 4% to 6%). In uncontrolled diabetes or diabetes with hyperglycemia, there is an increase in the level of A1C. Based on the Diabetes Control and Complications Trial (DCCT) and United Kingdom Prospective Diabetic Study (UKPDS), it is recommended that persons with diabetes lower their A1C to 7.0% or even achieve a normal glycemic level of less than 6.0%.[25] Because glucose entry into the red blood cell is not insulin dependent, the rate at which glucose becomes attached to the hemoglobin molecule depends on blood glucose. Glycosylation is essentially irreversible, and the level of A1C present in the blood provides an index of blood glucose levels over the previous 6 to 12 weeks.

Urine Tests

The ease, accuracy, and convenience of self-administered blood glucose monitoring techniques have made urine testing for glucose obsolete for most people with diabetes. These tests only reflect urine glucose levels and are influenced by such factors as the renal threshold for glucose, fluid intake and urine concentration, urine testing methodologies, and some drugs. Because of these factors, the ADA recommends that all people who use insulin should self-monitor their blood glucose, not urine glucose. Unlike glucose tests, urine ketone determinations remain an important part of monitoring diabetic control, particularly in people with type 1 diabetes who are at risk for developing ketoacidosis and in pregnant diabetic women to check the adequacy of nutrition and glucose control.[25]

DIABETES MANAGEMENT

The desired outcomes of glycemic control in both type 1 and type 2 diabetes is normalization of blood glucose as a means of preventing short- and long-term complications. Treatment plans involve nutrition therapy, exercise, and antidiabetic agents. People with type 1 diabetes require insulin therapy from the time of diagnosis. Weight loss and dietary management may be sufficient to control blood glucose levels in people with type 2 diabetes. However, they require follow-up care because insulin secretion from the beta cells may decrease or insulin resistance may persist, in which case oral antidiabetic agents are prescribed. Among the methods used to achieve these goals are education in self-management and problem solving. Individual treatment goals should take into account the person's age and other disease conditions, the person's capacity to understand and carry out the treatment regime, and socioeconomic factors that might influence compliance with the treatment plan. Optimal control of type 2 diabetes is associated with prevention or delay of chronic diabetes complications.[26]

Dietary Management

Dietary management usually is prescribed to meet the specific needs of each person with diabetes. Goals and principles of diet therapy differ between type 1 and type 2 diabetes, as well as for lean and obese people. Integral to diabetes management is a prescribed plan for nutrition therapy.[27] Therapy goals include maintenance of near-normal blood glucose levels, achievement of optimal lipid levels, adequate calories to maintain and attain reasonable weights, prevention and treatment of chronic diabetes complications, and improvement of overall health through optimal nutrition.

For a person with type 1 diabetes, the usual food intake is assessed and used as a basis for adjusting insulin therapy to fit with the person's lifestyle. Eating consistent amounts and types of food at specific and routine times is encouraged. Home blood glucose monitoring is used to fine-tune the plan. Newer forms of therapy, such as multiple daily insulin injections and the use of an insulin pump, provide many options. Most people with type 2 diabetes are overweight. Nutrition therapy goals focus on achieving glucose, lipid, and blood pressure goals, and weight loss if indicated. Mild to moderate weight loss (5% to 10% of total body weight) has been shown to improve diabetes control, even if desirable weight is not achieved.

A coordinated team effort, including the person with diabetes, is needed to individualize the nutrition plan. The diabetic diet has undergone marked changes over the years, particularly in the recommendations for distribution of calories among carbohydrates, proteins, and fats. There no longer is a specific diabetic or ADA diet but rather a dietary prescription based on nutrition assessment and treatment goals. Information is assessed regarding metabolic parameters and medical history of factors such as renal impairment and gastrointestinal autonomic neuropathy. Evaluating the effectiveness of the meal plan requires monitoring metabolic parameters such as blood glucose, A1C, lipids, blood pressure, body weight, and quality of life. Self-management education is essential to facilitate understanding of the associations among food, exercise, medication, and blood glucose.

The registered dietitian plays an essential role in the diabetes care team and is able to select from a variety of methods such as carbohydrate counting, food exchanges, healthy food choices, glycemic index, and total available glucose to tailor the meal plan to meet individual needs. Simpler recommendations have been associated with improved client understanding and dietary adherence. Carbohydrate counting uses product label information that is easily available to people with diabetes.[28] Regardless of food source, total grams of carbohydrate are counted, placing an emphasis on the nutrient that most affects blood glucose control.

Nutrition therapy also is tailored to control of other dietary components. Because diabetes is a risk factor for cardiovascular disease, it is recommended that less than 10% of daily calories should be obtained from saturated fat and that dietary cholesterol be limited to 300 mg or less. Periodic fasting lipid panels may identify concomitant lipid disorders. If lipid disorders are identified, appropriate modifications according to the Third Report of the National Cholesterol Education Program (NECP ATP III) on detection, evaluation, and treatment of high blood cholesterol should be followed.[15] For example, with a low-density lipoprotein cholesterol elevation, a diet with less than 7% of total calories from saturated fat, with 25% to 35% of daily calories obtained from fat, and with a cholesterol intake of less than 200 mg/day is recommended. For people with diabetic nephropathy, some studies suggest lowering the intake of protein to 10% of daily calories. Recommendations for dietary sodium are the same as for the general population: 2400 to 3000 mg/day as a baseline; less than 2400 mg/day if mild to moderate hypertension is present; and less than 2000 if severe hypertension or nephropathy exists. The ADA provides literature with more detailed information on diet therapy and patient education. Included is the method of calculating individual meal plans. Registered dietitians are valuable resources to the nurse, physician, and person with diabetes and should be included in nutritional planning.

Exercise

The benefits of exercise include cardiovascular fitness and psychological well-being. For many people with type 2 diabetes, the benefits of exercise include a decrease in body fat, better weight control, and improvement in insulin sensitivity.[7,20,29] Exercise is so important in diabetes management that a planned program of regular exercise usually is considered an integral part of the therapeutic regimen for every person with diabetes. In general, sporadic exercise has only transient benefits; a regular exercise or training program is the most beneficial. It is better for cardiovascular conditioning and can maintain a muscle-to-fat ratio that enhances peripheral insulin receptivity.

In people with insulin-treated diabetes, the beneficial effects of exercise are accompanied by an increased risk for hypoglycemia. Although muscle uptake of glucose increases significantly, the ability to maintain blood glucose levels is hampered by failure to suppress the absorption of injected insulin and activate the counterregulatory mechanisms that maintain blood glucose. Not only is there an inability to suppress insulin levels, but insulin absorption also may increase. This increased absorption is more pronounced when insulin is injected into the subcutaneous tissue of the exercised muscle, but it occurs even when insulin is injected into other body areas. Even after exercise ceases, insulin's lowering effect on blood glucose continues. In some people with type 1 diabetes, the symptoms of hypoglycemia occur many hours after cessation of exercise. This may occur because subsequent insulin doses (in people using multiple daily insulin injections) are not adjusted to accommodate the exercise-induced decrease in blood glucose. The cause of hypoglycemia in people who do not administer a subsequent insulin dose is unclear. It may be related to the fact that the liver and skeletal muscles increase their uptake of glucose after exercise as a means of replenishing their glycogen stores, or that the liver and skeletal muscles are more sensitive to insulin during this time. People with insulin-treated diabetes should be aware that delayed hypoglycemia can occur after exercise and that they may need to alter their diabetes medication dose, their carbohydrate intake, or both.

Although of benefit to people with diabetes, exercise must be weighed on the risk–benefit scale. Before beginning an exercise program, persons with diabetes should undergo an appropriate evaluation for macrovascular and microvascular disease.[29] The goal of exercise is safe participation in activities consistent with an individual's lifestyle. As with nutrition guidelines, exercise recommendations need to individualized. Considerations include the potential for hypoglycemia, hyperglycemia, ketosis, cardiovascular ischemia, and dysrhythmias (particularly silent ischemic heart disease); exacerbation of proliferative retinopathy; and lower extremity injury. For those with chronic diabetes, the complications of vigorous exercise can be harmful and can cause eye hemorrhage and other problems. For people with type 1 diabetes who exercise during periods of poor control (*i.e.,* when blood glucose is elevated, exogenous insulin levels are low, and ketonemia exists), blood glucose and ketone rise to even higher levels because the stress of exercise is superimposed on preexisting insulin deficiency and increased counterregulatory hormone activity.

Oral Antidiabetic Agents

There are two categories of antidiabetic agents: oral medications and insulin. Because people with type 1 diabetes are deficient in insulin, they are in need of exogenous insulin replacement therapy from the start. People with type 2 diabetes have increased hepatic glucose production; decreased peripheral utilization of glucose; decreased utilization of ingested carbohydrates; and over time, impaired insulin secretion from the pancreas (Fig. 43-8). The oral antidiabetic agents used in the treatment of type 2 diabetes attack each one of these areas and sometimes more.[30–32] In order to optimize the beneficial effects from each agent and improve compliance, the new approach in the pharmaceutical armamentarium is to have combination drugs such as rosiglitazone and metformin or a sulfonylurea and metformin. If good glycemic control cannot be achieved with a combination of oral agents, insulin can be used with the oral agents or by itself.

Oral antidiabetic agents approved by the U.S. Food and Drug Administration (FDA) fall into four categories: beta cell stimulator agents (sulfonylureas, repaglinide, and nateglinide), biguanides, α-glucosidase inhibitors, and thiazolidinediones (TZDs)[30–32] (see Fig. 43-8).

Sulfonylureas. The sulfonylureas were discovered accidentally in 1942, when scientists noticed that one of the sulfonamide drugs being developed at the time caused hypoglycemia. These drugs reduce blood glucose by stimulating the release of insulin from beta cells in the pancreas and increasing the sensitivity of peripheral tissues to insulin. These agents are effective only when some residual beta cell function remains. Sulfonylurea receptors in beta cells of the pancreas are linked to potassium–adenosine triphosphate (ATP) channels; when the drug attaches to the receptors, these channels close, and a coupled reaction leads to an influx of calcium. The influx of calcium triggers secretion of insulin from the beta cells (see Fig. 43-4).

The sulfonylureas are used in the treatment of type 2 diabetes and cannot be substituted for insulin in people with type 1 diabetes, who have an absolute insulin deficiency. Slight modifications in the basic structure of the members of this drug group produce agents that have similar qualitative actions but markedly different potencies. The sulfonylureas traditionally are grouped into first- and second-generation agents (Table 43-6). These agents differ

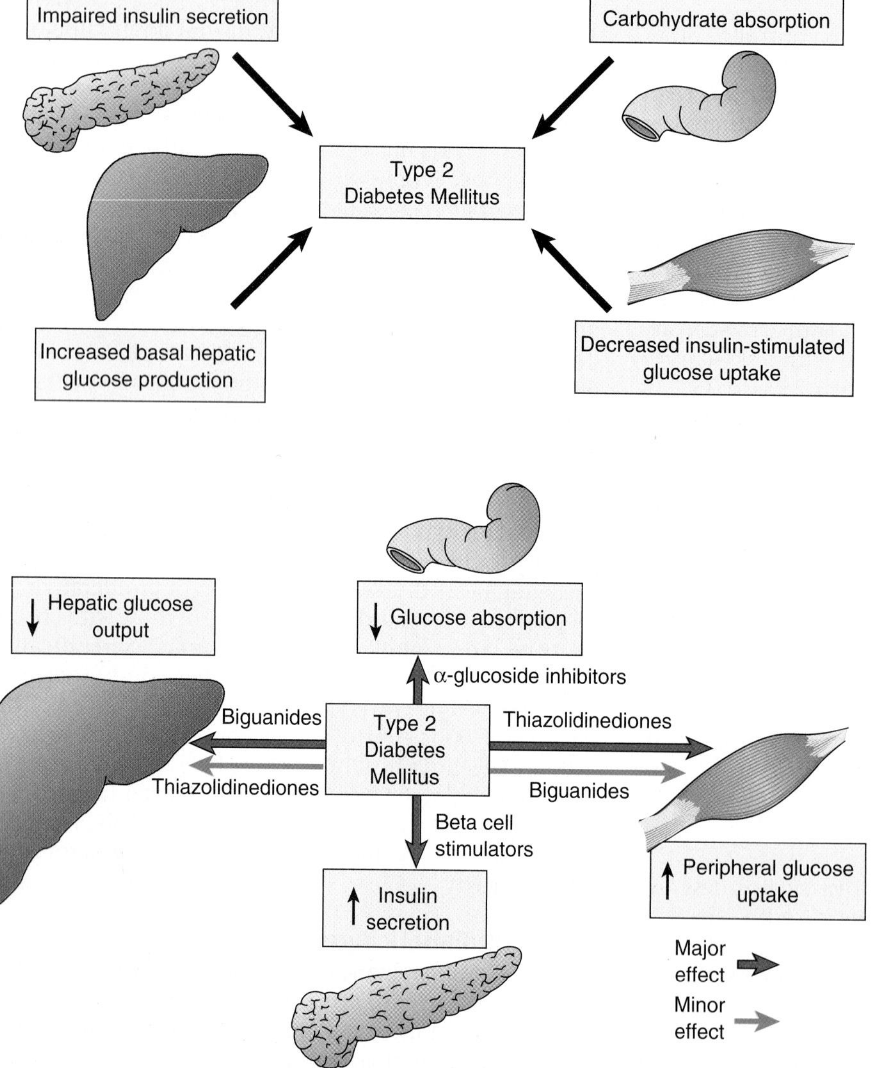

FIGURE 43-8 **(Top)** Mechanisms of elevated blood glucose in type 2 diabetes. **(Bottom)** Action sites of oral hypoglycemic agents and mechanisms of lowering blood glucose in type 2 diabetes mellitus.

TABLE 43-6 Oral Antidiabetic Agents*

Pharmacologic Agent	Daily Dosage (mg)	Duration of action (h)	Dosing Schedule	Mechanism of Action
Beta cell stimulators				Stimulates release of insulin from beta cells in the pancreas
Sulfonylureas (first generation)				
Chlorpropamide (generic)	100–500	60	1 time/day	
Sulfonylureas (second generation)				
Glipizide (Glucotrol)	2.5–40	6–24	1–2 times/day 30 min before meal	
Glyburide (DiaBeta, Micronase)	1.25–20	16–24	1–2 times/day with meal	
Glimepiride (Amaryl)	1–8	18–24	1 time/day with first meal	
Nonsulfonylureas				
Repaglinide (Prandin)	0.5–16	5	15–30 min before meal	
Nateglinide (Starlix)	60–360	3–4	1–30 min before meal	
Biguanide				Decreases production and release of glucose by the liver
Metformin (Glucophage, Glucophage XR)	500–2000	7–12	1–3 times/day with food	
Alpha glucosidase inhibitors				Delays the breakdown and absorption of carbohydrates from the intestine
Acarbose (Precose)	25–300	4–6	1–3 times/day first bite food	
Miglitol (Glyset)	25–300	4–6	1–3 times/day with food	
Thiazolidinediones				Sensitizes body cells to the action of insulin
Rosiglitazone (Avandia)	4–8	16–24	1–2 times/day with or without food	
Pioglitazone (Actos)	15–45	16–24	1 time/day without food	

*List may not be inclusive.

in dosage and duration of action. The second-generation drugs (glyburide, glipizide, glimepiride) are considerably more potent than the first-generation drugs (tolbutamide, acetohexamide, tolazamide, chlorpropamide). The second-generation agents are used more widely than the first-generation agents.

Because the sulfonylureas increase insulin levels and the rate at which glucose is removed from the blood, it is important to recognize that they can cause hypoglycemic reactions. This problem is more common in elderly people with impaired hepatic and renal function who are taking the longer-acting sulfonylureas.

Repaglinide and Nateglinide. Repaglinide (Prandin) and nateglinide (Starlix) are nonsulfonylurea beta cell stimulators that require the presence of glucose for their main action. These agents exert their action by closing the ATP-dependent potassium channel in the beta cells (see Fig. 43-4). Insulin release is glucose dependent and diminishes at low glucose levels. These agents, which are rapidly absorbed from the gastrointestinal tract, are taken shortly before meals (repaglinide 15 to 30 minutes and nateglinide 15 to 30 minutes). Both repaglinide and nateglinide can produce hypoglycemia; thus, proper timing of meals in relation to drug administration is important.

Biguanides. The biguanides are older oral antidiabetic drugs. Metformin (Glucophage) is the most significant agent in this group. Phenformin, the earlier form of the drug, was used extensively in the 1960s but was removed from the U.S. market in 1977 because of the occurrence of lactic acidosis in people treated with it. After more than a decade of use in Europe as well as Canada and other countries, metformin was approved by the FDA in 1995. Unlike its precursor, phenformin, metformin rarely results in lactic acidosis (0.03 cases per 1000 patients). Metformin inhibits hepatic glucose production and increases the sensitivity of peripheral tissues to the actions of insulin. Because metformin does not stimulate insulin secretion, it does not produce hypoglycemia as a side effect. Secondary benefits of metformin therapy include weight loss and improved lipid profiles. Whereas the primary action of the sulfonylurea drugs is to increase insulin secretion, metformin exerts its beneficial effects on glycemic control through increased peripheral use of glucose and mainly by decreasing hepatic glucose production. To decrease the risk for lactic acidosis, metformin is contraindicated in people with elevated serum creatinine levels (a test of renal function), clinical and laboratory evidence of hepatic disease, and any condition associated with hypoxemia or dehydration. Metformin sometimes is combined with other oral agents such as a sulfonylurea or with insulin to improve blood glucose control.[30–32]

α-Glucosidase Inhibitors. In patients with type 2 diabetes, sulfonylureas, biguanides, or both may have beneficial effects on fasting plasma glucose levels. However, postprandial hyperglycemia persists in more than 60% of these patients and probably accounts for sustained increases in A1C levels. An alternative approach to the problem of postprandial hyperglycemia is the use of drugs such as acarbose

(Precose) and miglitol (Glyset), inhibitors of α-glucosidase, which is a small intestine brush border enzyme that breaks down complex carbohydrates. By delaying the breakdown of complex carbohydrates, the α-glucosidase inhibitors delay the absorption of carbohydrates from the gut and blunt the postprandial increase in plasma glucose and insulin levels. Although not a problem with monotherapy or combination therapy with a biguanide, hypoglycemia may occur with concurrent sulfonylurea treatment. If hypoglycemia does occur, it should be treated with glucose (dextrose) and not sucrose (table sugar), whose breakdown may be blocked by the action of the α-glucosidase inhibitors.

Thiazolidinediones. The TZDs (or glitazones) are the only class of drugs that directly target insulin resistance, a fundamental defect in the pathophysiology of type 2 diabetes. The TZDs improve glycemic control by increasing insulin sensitivity in the insulin-responsive tissues—liver, skeletal muscle, and fat—allowing the tissues to respond to endogenous insulin more efficiently without increased output from already dysfunctional beta cells.[12,32] A secondary effect is the suppression of hepatic glucose production. Rosiglitazone (Avandia) and pioglitazone (Actos) were approved by the FDA in 1999. Another TZD, troglitazone, was approved in 1997, but because of hepatic safety concerns, it is no longer available, having been withdrawn worldwide in March 2000. Subsequent postmarketing analysis of both rosiglitazone and pioglitazone has shown no indication of similar liver dysfunction. Rosiglitazone and pioglitazone both are approved for use as monotherapy and in combination therapy. Because of the previous problem with liver toxicity in this class of drugs, liver enzymes should be measured according to the current guidelines.

The mechanism of action of the TZDs is complex and not fully understood. The action of the TZDs is associated with binding to a nuclear receptor, the *peroxisome proliferator–activated receptor-γ* (PPAR-γ; Fig. 43-9).[32] Binding of the TZDs to the PPAR-γ receptor begins a cascade of events that lead to regulation of genes involved in lipid and glucose metabolism. These include insulin-responsive genes such as the *GLUT-4,* lipoprotein lipase, and resistin genes. The result is an increase in the number of *GLUT-4* transporters and increased insulin-mediated uptake of glucose in the peripheral tissues. Newly described proteins produced by adipocytes, called *adiponectin* and *resistin,* may be a part of the missing link in explaining insulin resistance in persons with type 2 diabetes. Resistin suppresses insulin's ability to stimulate glucose uptake by adipose cells. The TZDs seem to decrease insulin resistance, in part, by suppressing the production of resistin by adipocytes.[33] Additional effects of TZDs are numerous, and include correction of many of the abnormal metabolic features associated with type 2 diabetes. This includes a decrease in FFA and triglycerides, microalbuminuria, blood pressure, inflammatory mediators (*e.g.,* fibrinogen and C-reactive protein), and procoagulation factors.[32] The TZDs also have the potential for preventing beta cell exhaustion by reducing FFAs and blood glucose levels.

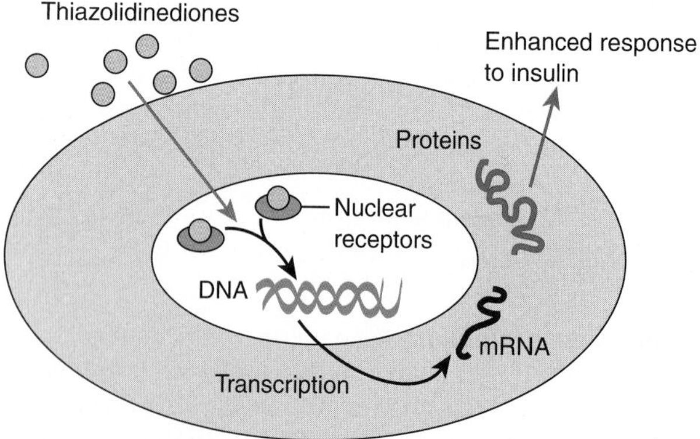

FIGURE 43-9 Action of the thiazolidinediones on activation of the PPARγ receptor that regulates gene transcription of proteins that regulate glucose uptake and reduce fatty acid release.

Amylin. A synthetic version of the human hormone amylin (pramlintide acetate [Symlin]) has recently been developed for use in the treatment of insulin-dependent diabetes and is now in clinical trials.[34] It is the first in a new class of amylin-receptor agonists. Amylin, which is normally co-secreted with insulin, is thought to suppress glucagon secretion, slow gastric emptying, and reduce the range of after-meal variations in blood glucose levels. The drug, which is administered by injection, is not a substitute for insulin but is complementary to its action.

Insulin

Type 1 diabetes mellitus always requires treatment with insulin, and many people with type 2 diabetes eventually require insulin therapy. Insulin is destroyed in the gastrointestinal tract and must be administered by injection. Insulin preparations are categorized according to onset, peak, and duration of action. An inhaled form of insulin is in the clinical trial stage.

During the past several decades, many pharmaceutical companies have entered the insulin-manufacturing market. After much research, human insulin has become available, providing an alternative to previous forms of insulin that were obtained from bovine and porcine sources. The manufacture of human insulin uses recombinant DNA technology. Beef insulin differs from human insulin by three amino acids, and pork insulin differs by only one amino acid. Many people with diabetes develop antibodies to beef and pork insulin. Improvements in the purification techniques for insulin extracted from animal pancreases have made it possible to reduce or eliminate many of the contaminants that could incite antibody formation. However, synthetic human insulin is widely available and generally used. A change from pork or beef to human insulin should be carefully monitored because hypoglycemia can occur owing to increased receptivity to the human insulin.

There are three principal types of insulin: short acting, intermediate acting, and long acting (Table 43-7). The short-acting insulins fall into two categories: short acting and ultra-short acting. Insulin injection (Regular) is a short-acting soluble crystalline insulin whose effects begin within 30 minutes after subcutaneous injection and generally last for 5 to 8 hours. The ultra–short-acting insulins (insulin lispro [Humalog] and insulin aspart [NovoLog])

TABLE 43-7 Activity Profile of Human Insulin Preparations in the United States*

Type (Human Insulin)	Onset	Peak (hrs)	Duration (hrs)
Lispro insulin solution (Humalog)	5–15 min	1–1.5	3.0–4.0
Insulin aspart injection (Novalog)	5–15 min	1–1.5	3.0–4.0
Insulin injection (Regular Insulin)	0.5–1.0 h	2.0–4.0	5.0–8.0
Isophane insulin suspension (NPH) or insulin zinc suspension (Lente)	2.0–4.0 h	4.0–10.0	18.0–24.0
70/30 (70% NPH/30% regular) premixed	0.5–1.0 h	Peak 1 @ 3.0 and peak 2 @ 4.0–10.0	10–18.0
75/25 (75% NPH/25% Humalog) premixed	15 min	Peak 1 @ 0.5–1.5 and peak 2 @ 5.0–6.0	22.0
Extended insulin zinc suspension (Ultralente)	4.0–8.0 h	8–12.0 (may have second peak)	18.0–36.0
Insulin glargine (Lantus)†	4.0–8.0 h	No peak	Up to 24

*List may not be inclusive.
†Lantus insulin should never be mixed with or administered using the same syringe used to administer any other type of insulin.

are produced by recombinant technology with an amino acid substitution. These insulins have a more rapid onset, peak, and shorter duration of action than short-acting Regular insulin. The ultra–short-acting insulins, which are used in combination with an intermediate- or long-acting insulin, are usually administered immediately before a meal. Intermediate-acting insulins (NPH and Lente) have a slower onset and duration of action. Because the intermediate-acting insulins require several hours to reach therapeutic levels, their use in type 1 diabetes requires supplementation with an ultra–short- or short-acting insulin. The long-acting Ultralente insulin has an even longer onset and duration of action than the intermediate-acting insulins. As with intermediate-acting insulins, it is used in combination with the shorter-acting insulins. Glargine (Lantus) is a new long-acting human insulin analog. It has a slower, more prolonged absorption than NPH insulin and provides a relatively constant concentration over 24 hours. Glargine is usually taken as a single dose and is used in combination with preprandial injections of a short-acting insulin. All forms of insulin have the potential of producing hypoglycemia or "insulin reaction" as a side effect (discussed later).

Two intensive treatment regimens—multiple daily injection (MDI) and continuous subcutaneous infusion of insulin (CSII)—closely simulate the normal pattern of insulin secretion by the body. With each method, a basal insulin level is maintained, and bolus doses of short-acting insulin are delivered before meals.

The MDI treatment regimen uses long-acting or intermediate-acting insulin administered once or twice daily to maintain the basal insulin level. Boluses of short-acting insulin are used before meals. The development of convenient injection devices (*e.g.*, pen injector) has made it easier for people with diabetes to comply with the multiple doses of short-acting insulin that are administered before meals.

With the CSII (insulin pump) method, the basal insulin requirements are met by continuous infusion of subcutaneous insulin, the rate of which can be varied to accommodate diurnal variations. The CSII technique involves the self-insertion of a small needle or plastic catheter into the subcutaneous tissue of the abdomen. Tubing from the catheter is connected to a syringe set into a small infusion pump worn on a belt or in a jacket pocket. The computer-operated pump then delivers one or more set basal amounts of insulin. In addition to the basal amount delivered by the pump, a bolus amount of insulin may be delivered when needed (*e.g.*, before a meal) by pushing a button.

Self-monitoring of blood glucose levels is a necessity when using the CSII method of management. Each basal and bolus dose is determined individually and programmed into the infusion pump computer. Although the pump's safety has been proved, strict attention must be paid to signs of hypoglycemia. However, investigations have found CSII therapy to be associated with a marked and sustained reduction in the rate of severe hypoglycemia. Ketotic episodes caused by pump failure, catheter clogging, and infections at the needle site also are possible complications.

Candidate selection is crucial to the successful use of the insulin pump. Only people who are highly motivated to do frequent blood glucose tests and make daily insulin adjustments are candidates for this method of treatment.[34] Use of an insulin pump requires an intensive therapy program that is best implemented with the support of a diabetes health care team. The diabetologist, nurse educator, and dietitian are key team members; a social worker or psychologist and exercise physiologist are helpful additions to the team.

Pancreas or Islet Cell Transplantation

Pancreas or islet cell transplantation is not a lifesaving procedure. It does, however, afford the potential for significantly improving the quality of life. The most serious problems are the requirement for immunosuppression and the need for diagnosis and treatment of rejection. Investigators are looking for methods of transplanting islet cells and protecting the cells from destruction without the use of immunosuppressive drugs.

ACUTE COMPLICATIONS

The three major acute complications of diabetes are diabetic ketoacidosis, hyperosmolar hyperglycemic state, and hypoglycemia.

Diabetic Ketoacidosis

Diabetic ketoacidosis (DKA) occurs when ketone production by the liver exceeds cellular use and renal excretion. DKA most commonly occurs in a person with type 1 diabetes, in whom the lack of insulin leads to mobilization of fatty acids from adipose tissue because of the unsuppressed adipose cell lipase activity that breaks down triglycerides into fatty acids and glycerol. The increase in fatty acid levels leads to ketone production by the liver (Fig. 43-10). It can occur at the onset of the disease, often before the disease has been diagnosed. For example, a mother may bring a child into the clinic or emergency department with reports of lethargy, vomiting, and abdominal pain, unaware that the child has diabetes. Stress increases the release of gluconeogenic hormones and predisposes the person to the development of ketoacidosis. DKA often is preceded by physical or emotional stress, such as infection, pregnancy, or extreme anxiety. In clinical practice, ketoacidosis also occurs with the omission or inadequate use of insulin.

The three major metabolic derangements in DKA are hyperglycemia, ketosis, and metabolic acidosis. The definitive diagnosis of DKA consists of hyperglycemia (blood glucose levels >250 mg/dL), low serum bicarbonate (<15 mEq/L), and low pH (<7.3), with ketonemia (positive at 1:2 dilution) and moderate ketonuria.[37] Hyperglycemia leads to osmotic diuresis, dehydration, and a critical loss of electrolytes. Hyperosmolality of extracellular fluids from hyperglycemia leads to a shift of water and potassium from the intracellular to the extracellular compartment. Extracellular sodium concentration frequently is low or normal despite enteric water losses because of the intracellular–extracellular fluid shift. This dilutional effect is referred to as *pseudohyponatremia.* Serum potassium levels may be normal or elevated, despite total potassium depletion resulting from protracted polyuria and vomiting. Metabolic acidosis is caused by the excess ketoacids that require buffering by bicarbonate ions; this leads to a marked decrease in serum bicarbonate levels.

Compared with an insulin reaction, DKA usually is slower in onset, and recovery is more prolonged. The person typically has a history of 1 or 2 days of polyuria, polydipsia, nausea, vomiting, and marked fatigue, with eventual stupor that can progress to coma. Abdominal pain and tenderness may be experienced without abdominal disease. The breath has a characteristic fruity smell because of the presence of the volatile ketoacids. Hypotension and tachycardia may be present because of a decrease in blood volume. A number of the signs and symptoms that occur in DKA are related to compensatory mechanisms. The heart rate increases as the body compensates for a decrease in blood volume, and the rate and depth of respiration increase (*i.e.,* Kussmaul's respiration) as the body attempts to prevent further decreases in pH. Metabolic acidosis is discussed further in Chapter 34.

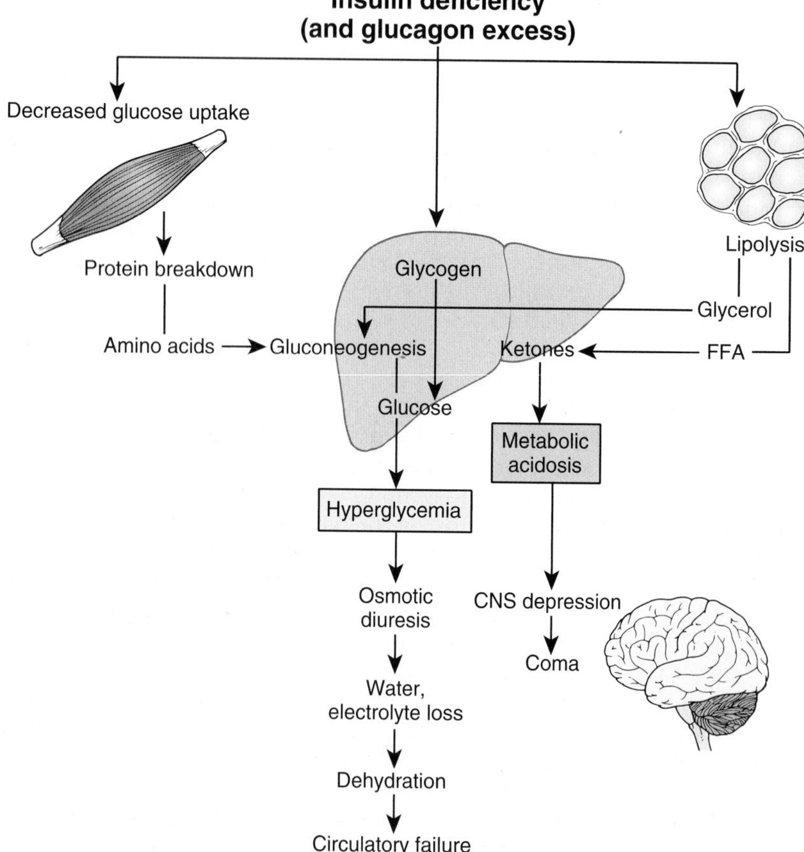

FIGURE 43-10 Mechanisms of diabetic ketoacidosis. Diabetic ketoacidosis is associated with very low insulin levels and extremely high levels of glucagon, catecholamines, and other counterregulatory hormones. Increased levels of glucagon and the catecholamines lead to mobilization of substrates for gluconeogenesis and ketogenesis by the liver. Gluconeogenesis in excess of that needed to supply glucose for the brain and other glucose-dependent tissues produces a rise in blood glucose levels. Mobilization of free fatty acids (FFA) from triglyceride stores in adipose tissue leads to accelerated ketone production and ketosis.

The goals in treating DKA are to improve circulatory volume and tissue perfusion, decrease serum glucose, correct the acidosis, and correct electrolyte imbalances. These objectives usually are accomplished through the administration of insulin and intravenous fluid and electrolyte replacement solutions. Because insulin resistance accompanies severe acidosis, low-dose insulin therapy is used. An initial loading dose of regular insulin often is given intravenously, followed by continuous low-dose infusion. Frequent laboratory tests are used to monitor blood glucose and serum electrolyte levels and to guide fluid and electrolyte replacement. It is important to replace fluid and electrolytes and correct pH while bringing the blood glucose concentration to a normal level. Too rapid a drop in blood glucose may cause hypoglycemic symptoms and cerebral edema. A sudden change in the osmolality of extracellular fluid occurs when blood glucose is lowered too rapidly, and this can cause cerebral edema. Serum potassium levels often fall as acidosis is corrected and extracellular potassium moves into the intracellular compartment; at this time, it may be necessary to add potassium to the intravenous infusion. Identification and treatment of the underlying cause, such as infection, also are important. With the better understanding of the pathogenesis of DKA and more uniform agreement on diagnosis and treatment, the mortality rate has been reduced to less than 5%.

Hyperosmolar Hyperglycemic State

The hyperosmolar hyperglycemic state (HHS) is characterized by hyperglycemia (blood glucose >600 mg/dL), hyperosmolarity (plasma osmolarity >310 mOsm/L) and dehydration, the absence of ketoacidosis, and depression of the sensorium.[37] HHS may occur in various conditions, including type 2 diabetes, acute pancreatitis, severe infection, myocardial infarction, and treatment with oral or parenteral nutrition solutions. It is seen most frequently in people with type 2 diabetes. Two factors appear to contribute to the hyperglycemia that precipitates the condition: an increased resistance to the effects of insulin and an excessive carbohydrate intake.

In hyperosmolar states, the increased serum osmolarity has the effect of pulling water out of body cells, including brain cells. The condition may be complicated by thromboembolic events arising because of the high serum osmolality. The most prominent manifestations are dehydration, neurologic signs and symptoms, and excessive thirst. The neurologic signs include grand mal seizures, hemiparesis, Babinski's reflexes, aphasia, muscle fasciculations, hyperthermia, hemianopia, nystagmus, and visual hallucinations. The onset of HHS often is insidious, and because it occurs most frequently in older people, it may be mistaken for a stroke.

The treatment of HHS requires judicious medical observation and care because water moves back into brain cells during treatment, posing a threat of cerebral edema. Extensive potassium losses that also have occurred during the diuretic phase of the disorder require correction. Because of the problems encountered in the treatment and the serious nature of the disease conditions that cause HHS, the prognosis for this disorder is less favorable than that for ketoacidosis.

Hypoglycemia

Hypoglycemia, or an insulin reaction, occurs from a relative excess of insulin in the blood and is characterized by below-normal blood glucose levels.[38] It occurs most commonly in people treated with insulin injections, but prolonged hypoglycemia also can result from some oral hypoglycemic agents.

Hypoglycemia usually has a rapid onset and progression of symptoms. The signs and symptoms of hypoglycemia can be divided into two categories: those caused by altered cerebral function and those related to activation of the autonomic nervous system. Because the brain relies on blood glucose as its main energy source, hypoglycemia produces behaviors related to altered cerebral function. Headache, difficulty in problem solving, disturbed or altered behavior, coma, and seizures may occur. At the onset of the hypoglycemic episode, activation of the parasympathetic nervous system often causes hunger. The initial parasympathetic response is followed by activation of the sympathetic nervous system; this causes anxiety, tachycardia, sweating, and constriction of the skin vessels (*i.e.*, the skin is cool and clammy).

There is wide variation in the manifestation of signs and symptoms; not every person with diabetes manifests all or even most of the symptoms. The signs and symptoms of hypoglycemia are more variable in children and in elderly people. Elderly people may not display the typical autonomic responses associated with hypoglycemia but frequently develop signs of impaired function of the central nervous system, including mental confusion. Some people develop hypoglycemic unawareness. Unawareness of hypoglycemia should be suspected in people who do not report symptoms when their blood glucose concentrations are less than 50 to 60 mg/dL. This occurs most commonly in people who have a longer duration of diabetes and A1C levels within the normal range.[38] Some medications, such as β-adrenergic–blocking drugs, interfere with the sympathetic response normally seen in hypoglycemia.

Many factors precipitate an insulin reaction in a person with type 1 diabetes, including error in insulin dose, failure to eat, increased exercise, decreased insulin need after removal of a stress situation, medication changes, and a change in insulin site. Alcohol decreases liver gluconeogenesis, and people with diabetes need to be cautioned about its potential for causing hypoglycemia, especially if it is consumed in large amounts or on an empty stomach.

The most effective treatment of an insulin reaction is the immediate administration of 15 to 20 g of glucose in concentrated carbohydrate source, which can be repeated as necessary. Monosaccharides such as glucose, which can be absorbed directly into the bloodstream, work best for this purpose. Complex carbohydrates can be administered after the acute reaction has been controlled to sustain blood glucose levels. It is important not to overtreat hypoglycemia and cause hyperglycemia.

Alternative methods for increasing blood glucose may be required when the person having the reaction is unconscious or unable to swallow. A small amount of glucose gel (available in most pharmacies) may be inserted into the buccal pouch when glucagon is unavailable. Glucagon may be given intramuscularly or subcutaneously. Glucagon acts by hepatic glycogenolysis to raise blood sugar. The liver contains only a limited amount of glycogen (approximately 75 g); glucagon is ineffective in people whose glycogen stores have been depleted. Some people report becoming nauseated after glucagon administration, which also could be in response to the severe hypoglycemia. In situations of severe or life-threatening hypoglycemia, it may be necessary to administer glucose (20 to 50 mL of a 50% solution) intravenously.

COUNTERREGULATORY MECHANISMS AND THE SOMOGYI EFFECT AND DAWN PHENOMENON

The Somogyi effect describes a cycle of insulin-induced posthypoglycemic episodes. In 1924, Joslin and associates noticed that hypoglycemia was associated with alternate episodes of hyperglycemia.[39] It was not until 1959 that Somogyi presented the results of his 20 years of studies, which confirmed the observation that "hypoglycemia begets hyperglycemia." In people with diabetes, insulin-induced hypoglycemia produces a compensatory increase in blood levels of catecholamines, glucagon, cortisol, and growth hormone. These counterregulatory hormones cause blood glucose to become elevated and produce some degree of insulin resistance. The cycle begins when the increase in blood glucose and insulin resistance is treated with larger insulin doses. The hypoglycemic episode often occurs during the night or at a time when it is not recognized, rendering the diagnosis of the phenomenon more difficult.

Research suggests that even rather mild insulin-associated hypoglycemia, which may be asymptomatic, can cause hyperglycemia in those with type 1 diabetes through the recruitment of counterregulatory mechanisms, although the insulin action does not wane. A concomitant waning of the effect of insulin (*i.e.*, end of the duration of action), when it occurs, exacerbates posthypoglycemic hyperglycemia and accelerates its development. These findings may explain the labile nature of the disease in some people with diabetes. Measures to prevent hypoglycemia and the subsequent activation of counterregulatory mechanisms include a redistribution of dietary carbohydrates and an alteration in insulin dose or time of administration.[40]

The dawn phenomenon is characterized by increased levels of fasting blood glucose or insulin requirements, or both, between 5:00 and 9:00 AM without antecedent hypoglycemia. It occurs in people with type 1 or type 2 diabetes. It has been suggested that a change in the normal circadian rhythm for glucose tolerance, which usually is higher during the later part of the morning, is altered in people with diabetes.[41] Growth hormone has been suggested as a possible factor. When the dawn phenomenon occurs alone, it may produce only mild hyperglycemia, but when it is combined with the Somogyi effect, it may produce profound hyperglycemia.

CHRONIC COMPLICATIONS

The chronic complications of diabetes include disorders of the microvasculature (*i.e.*, neuropathies, nephropathies, and retinopathies), macrovascular complications, and foot ulcers. The microvascular complications occur in the insulin-independent tissues of the body—tissues that do not require insulin for glucose entry into the cell. This probably means that intracellular glucose concentrations in many of these tissues approach or equal those in the blood. The level of chronic glycemia is the best-established concomitant factor associated with diabetic complications.[42] The Diabetes Control and Complications Trial (DCCT), which was conducted with 1441 people with type 1 diabetes, has demonstrated that the incidence of retinopathy, nephropathy, and neuropathy can be reduced by intensive diabetic treatment.[43] Similar results have been demonstrated by the UKPDS in people with type 2 diabetes.[25,44]

Theories of Pathogenesis

The interest among researchers in explaining the causes and development of chronic lesions in a person with diabetes has led to a number of theories. Several of these theories have been summarized to prepare the reader for understanding specific chronic complications.

Polyol Pathway. A polyol is an organic compound that contains three or more hydroxyl (OH) groups. The polyol pathway refers to the intracellular mechanisms responsible for changing the number of hydroxyl units on a glucose molecule. In the sorbitol pathway, glucose is transformed first to sorbitol and then to fructose. This process is activated

CHRONIC COMPLICATIONS OF DIABETES

- The chronic complications of diabetes result from elevated blood glucose levels and associated impairment of lipid and other metabolic pathways.
- Diabetic nephropathy, which is a leading cause of end-stage renal disease, is associated with the increased work demands and microalbuminuria imposed by poorly controlled blood glucose levels.
- Diabetic retinopathy, which is a leading cause of blindness, is closely linked to elevations in blood glucose and hyperlipidemia seen in persons with uncontrolled diabetes.
- Diabetic peripheral neuropathies, which affect both the somatic and autonomic nervous systems, result from the demyelinating effect of long-term uncontrolled diabetes.
- Macrovascular disorders such as coronary heart disease, stroke, and peripheral vascular disease reflect the combined effects of unregulated blood glucose levels, elevated blood pressure, and hyperlipidemia.
- The chronic complications of diabetes are best prevented by measures aimed at tight control of blood glucose levels, maintenance of normal lipid levels, and control of hypertension.

by the enzyme aldose reductase.[42] Although glucose is converted readily to sorbitol, the rate at which sorbitol can be converted to fructose and then metabolized is limited. Sorbitol is osmotically active, and it has been hypothesized that the presence of excess intracellular amounts may alter cell function in those tissues that use this pathway (*e.g.*, lens, kidneys, nerves, blood vessels). In the lens, for example, the osmotic effects of sorbitol cause swelling and opacity. Increased sorbitol also is associated with a decrease in myoinositol and reduced adenosine triphosphatase activity. The reduction of these compounds may be responsible for the peripheral neuropathies caused by Schwann cell damage. Aldose reductase inhibitors are in development to try to reduce complications resulting from this pathway; however, to date, none has been successful for a variety of reasons.[42]

Formation of Advanced Glycation End Products. Glycoproteins, or what could be called *glucose proteins,* are normal components of the basement membrane in smaller blood vessels and capillaries. These glycoproteins are also termed *advanced glycation end products* (AGEs). It has been suggested that the increased intracellular concentration of glucose associated with uncontrolled blood glucose levels in diabetes favors the formation of AGEs. These abnormal glycoproteins are thought to produce structural defects in the basement membrane of the microcirculation and to contribute to eye, kidney, and vascular complications. Some of the altered cellular functions resulting from AGEs are due to binding to specific receptors for AGEs (RAGEs).[42]

Problems With Tissue Oxygenation. Proponents of the tissue oxygenation theories suggest that many of the chronic complications of diabetes arise because of a decrease in oxygen delivery in the small vessels of the microcirculation. Among the factors believed to contribute to this inadequate oxygen delivery is a defect in red blood cell function that interferes with the release of oxygen from the hemoglobin molecule. In support of this theory is the finding of a two- to threefold increase in A1C in some people with diabetes. In A1C, a glycoprotein is substituted for valine in the β chain, causing a high affinity for oxygen. The concentration of the red blood cell glycolytic intermediate, 2,3-diphosphoglycerate (2,3-DPG), declines during the acidotic and recovery phases of DKA; 2,3-DPG reduces hemoglobin's affinity for oxygen. An increase in A1C and a decrease in 2,3-DPG increase the hemoglobin's affinity for oxygen, and less oxygen is released for tissue use.

Protein Kinase C. Diacylglycerol (DAG) and protein kinase C (PKC) are critical intracellular signaling molecules that can regulate many vascular functions, including permeability, vasodilator release, endothelial activation, and growth factor signaling.[42] Levels of DAG and PKC are elevated in diabetes. Activation of PKC in blood vessels of the retina, kidney, and nerves can produce vascular damage. A PKC inhibitor is currently in clinical trials for diabetic retinopathy and neuropathy.[42]

Neuropathies

Although the incidence of peripheral neuropathies is high among people with diabetes, it is difficult to document exactly how many people are affected by these disorders because of the diversity in clinical manifestations and because the condition often is far advanced before it is recognized. Results of the DCCT study show that intensive therapy can reduce the incidence of clinical neuropathy by 60% compared with conventional therapy.[43]

Two types of pathologic changes have been observed in connection with diabetic peripheral neuropathies. The first is a thickening of the walls of the nutrient vessels that supply the nerve, leading to the assumption that vessel ischemia plays a major role in the development of these neural changes. The second finding is a segmental demyelinization process that affects the Schwann cell. This demyelinization process is accompanied by a slowing of nerve conduction.

It appears that the diabetic peripheral neuropathies are not a single entity. The clinical manifestations of these disorders vary with the location of the lesion. Although there are several methods for classifying the diabetic peripheral neuropathies, a simplified system divides them into the somatic and autonomic nervous system neuropathies (Chart 43-3).

Somatic Neuropathy. A distal symmetric polyneuropathy, in which loss of function occurs in a stocking-glove pattern, is the most common form of peripheral neuropathy. Somatic sensory involvement usually occurs first and usually is bilateral, symmetric, and associated with diminished

CHART 43-3

Classification of Diabetic Peripheral Neuropathies

Somatic

- Polyneuropathies (bilateral sensory)
  - Paresthesias, including numbness and tingling
  - Impaired pain, temperature, light touch, two-point discrimination, and vibratory sensation
  - Decreased ankle and knee-jerk reflexes
- Mononeuropathies
  - Involvement of a mixed nerve trunk that includes loss of sensation, pain, and motor weakness
- Amyotrophy
  - Associated with muscle weakness, wasting, and severe pain of muscles in the pelvic girdle and thigh

Autonomic

- Impaired vasomotor function
  - Postural hypotension
- Impaired gastrointestinal function
  - Gastric atony
  - Diarrhea, often postprandial and nocturnal
- Impaired genitourinary function
  - Paralytic bladder
  - Incomplete voiding
  - Erectile dysfunction
  - Retrograde ejaculation
- Cranial nerve involvement
  - Extraocular nerve paralysis
  - Impaired pupillary responses
  - Impaired special senses

perception of vibration, pain, and temperature, particularly to the lower extremities. In addition to the discomforts associated with the loss of sensory or motor function, lesions in the peripheral nervous system predispose a person with diabetes to other complications. The loss of feeling, touch, and position sense increases the risk for falling. Impairment of temperature and pain sensation increases the risk for serious burns and injuries to the feet.

Painful diabetic neuropathy involves the somatosensory neurons that carry pain impulse. This disorder, which causes hypersensitivity to light touch and occasionally severe "burning pain," particularly at night, can become physically and emotionally disabling.[45]

Autonomic Neuropathy. The autonomic neuropathies involve disorders of sympathetic and parasympathetic nervous system function, There may be disorders of vasomotor function, decreased cardiac responses, impaired motility of the gastrointestinal tract, inability to empty the bladder, and sexual dysfunction.[45] Defects in vasomotor reflexes can lead to dizziness and syncope when the person moves from the supine to the standing position (see Chapter 25). Incomplete emptying of the bladder predisposes to urinary stasis and bladder infection and increases the risk for renal complications.

In the male, disruption of sensory and autonomic nervous system function may cause sexual dysfunction (see Chapter 45). Diabetes is the leading physiologic cause of erectile dysfunction, and it occurs in both type 1 and type 2 diabetes. Of the 7.8 million men with diabetes in the United States, 30% to 60% have erectile dysfunction.[46]

Disorders of Gastrointestinal Motility. Gastrointestinal motility disorders are common in persons with longstanding diabetes. Although the pathogenesis of these disorders is poorly understood, neuropathy and metabolic abnormalities secondary to hyperglycemia are thought to play an important role.[47] The symptoms vary in severity and include constipation, diarrhea and fecal incontinence, nausea and vomiting, and upper abdominal discomfort referred as *dyspepsia*. The presence and severity of these symptoms do not correlate well with the disturbances of gastrointestinal motility.

Gastroparesis (delayed emptying of stomach) is commonly seen in persons with diabetes.[47] The disorder is characterized by complaints of epigastric discomfort, nausea, postprandial vomiting, bloating, and early satiety. Abnormal gastric emptying also jeopardizes the regulation of the blood glucose level. Diagnostic measures include the use of endoscopy or a barium radiography to exclude mechanical obstruction due to peptic ulcer disease or cancer. Gastric emptying tests using a radionuclide-labeled solid meal such as chicken liver can be used to confirm the presence of gastroparesis. Management includes the use of prokinetic agents (*e.g.*, metoclopramide, erythromycin) as well as antiemetic agents. Gastric pacing is a clinical research tool proposed as an alternative for severe, refractory gastroparesis.[48] Strict control of blood glucose is important because hyperglycemia may slow gastric emptying, even in the absence of diabetic neuropathy.

Diarrhea is another common symptom seen mostly in persons with poorly controlled type 1 diabetes and autonomic neuropathy.[49] The pathogenesis is thought to be multifactorial. Diabetic diarrhea is typically intermittent, watery, painless, and nocturnal and may be associated with fecal incontinence. Management includes the use of antidiarrheal agents (loperamide, diphenoxylate). Clonidine (an α_2-adrenergic agonist)[50] and octreotide (a long-acting somatostatin analog)[51] have been used with some success in persons with rapid transit. Antibiotics are used for those with small bowel bacterial overgrowth secondary to slow transit. As with gastroparesis, strict control of blood glucose is important.

Nephropathies

Diabetic nephropathy is the leading cause of end-stage renal disease (ESRD), accounting for 40% of new cases.[1] In the United States, 40% of all people who seek renal replacement therapy (see Chapter 36) have diabetes.[52] The complication affects people with both type 1 and type 2 diabetes. According to the reports of the U.S. Renal Data System, the increase in ESRD since the early 1980s has been predominantly among people with type 2 diabetes.[53]

The term *diabetic nephropathy* is used to describe the combination of lesions that often occur concurrently in the diabetic kidney. The most common kidney lesions in people with diabetes are those that affect the glomeruli. Various glomerular changes may occur in people with diabetic nephropathy, including capillary basement membrane thickening, diffuse glomerular sclerosis, and nodular glomerulosclerosis (see Chapter 35). Changes in the capillary basement membrane take the form of thickening of basement membranes along the length of the glomeruli. Diffuse glomerulosclerosis consists of thickening of the basement membrane and the mesangial matrix. Nodular glomerulosclerosis, also called *intercapillary glomerulosclerosis* or *Kimmelstiel-Wilson disease,* is a form of glomerulosclerosis that involves the development of nodular lesions in the glomerular capillaries of the kidneys, causing impaired blood flow with progressive loss of kidney function and, eventually, renal failure. Nodular glomerulosclerosis is thought to occur only in people with diabetes. Changes in the basement membrane in diffuse glomerulosclerosis and Kimmelstiel-Wilson syndrome allow plasma proteins to escape in the urine, causing proteinuria and the development of hypoproteinemia, edema, and others signs of impaired kidney function.

Not all people with diabetes develop clinically significant nephropathy; for this reason, attention is focusing on risk factors for the development of this complication. Among the suggested risk factors are genetic and familial predisposition, elevated blood pressure, poor glycemic control, smoking, hyperlipidemia, and microalbumuria.[52,54,55] Diabetic nephropathy occurs in family clusters, suggesting a familial predisposition, although this does not exclude the possibility of environmental factors shared by siblings. The risk for development of ESRD also is greater among Native Americans, Hispanics (especially Mexican Americans), and African Americans.[52,54] Kidney enlargement, nephron hypertrophy, and hyperfiltration occur early in the disease, suggesting increased work of the kidneys in reabsorbing excessive amounts of glucose. One of the first manifestations of diabetic nephropathy is an increase in urinary albumin excretion (*i.e.,* microalbuminuria), which is easily assessed by laboratory methods. Microalbuminuria is defined as a urine protein loss between 30 and 300 mg/day; or between 30 and 300 µg/mg creatinine on albumin-to-creatinine ratio (A/C ratio) from a spot urine collection.[52] It is recommended that the A/C ratio be the preferred screen for microalbuminuria.[52] The risk for microalbuminuria increases abruptly with A1C levels above 8.1%[55] (Fig. 43-11). Both systolic and diastolic hypertension accelerates the progression of diabetic nephropathy. Even moderate lowering of blood pressure can decrease the risk for ESRD.[52,53,56] Smoking increases the risk for ESRD in both diabetic and nondiabetic people. People with type 2 diabetes who smoke have a greater risk for microalbuminuria, and their rate of progression to ESRD is approximately twice as rapid as in those who do not smoke.[54]

Measures to prevent diabetic nephropathy or its progression in persons with diabetes include achievement of glycemic control; maintenance of blood pressure less than 130/80 mm Hg, or less than 125/75 mm Hg in the presence of significant proteinuria; prevention or reduction in the level of proteinuria (using angiotensin-converting enzyme [ACE] inhibitors or angiotensin-receptor blockers [ARBs], or protein restriction in selected patients); treatment of hyperlipidemia; and smoking cessation in people who smoke.[52,54,56,57]

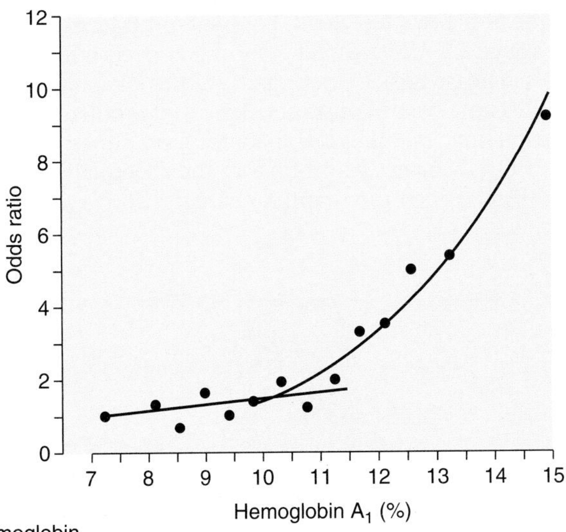

FIGURE 43-11 Relationship between mean hemoglobin A_1 and the risk for microalbuminuria in patients with type 2 diabetes mellitus. (Krolewski A.S., Laffel L.M.B., Krolewski M., et al. [1995]. Glycosylated hemoglobin and the risk for microalbuminuria in patients with insulin-dependent diabetes mellitus. *New England Journal of Medicine 332*(19), 1251–1255)

Retinopathies

Diabetes is the leading cause of acquired blindness in the United States. Although people with diabetes are at increased risk for development of cataracts and glaucoma, retinopathy is the most common pattern of eye disease. Diabetic retinopathy is estimated to be the most frequent cause of newly diagnosed blindness among Americans between the ages of 20 and 74 years.[58] Diabetic retinopathy is characterized by abnormal retinal vascular permeability, microaneurysm formation, neovascularization and associated hemorrhage, scarring, and retinal detachment[58,59] (see Chapter 54). Twenty years after the onset of diabetes, nearly all people with type 1 diabetes and more than 60% of people with type 2 diabetes have some degree of retinopathy. Pregnancy, puberty, and cataract surgery can accelerate these changes.[58,59]

Although there has been no extensive research on risk factors associated with diabetic retinopathy, they appear to be similar to those for other complications. Among the suggested risk factors associated with diabetic retinopathy are poor glycemic control, elevated blood pressure, and hyperlipidemia. The strongest case for control of blood glucose comes from the UKPDS study, which demonstrated a reduction in retinopathy with improved glucose control.[25]

Because of the risk for retinopathy, it is important that people with diabetes have regular dilated eye examinations. They should have an initial examination for retinopathy shortly after the diagnosis of diabetes is made. The recommendation for follow-up examinations is based on the type of examination that was done and the findings of that examination. People with persistently elevated glucose levels or proteinuria should be examined yearly.[58] Women who are planning a pregnancy should be counseled on the risk for development or progression of diabetic retinopathy. Women with diabetes who become pregnant should be followed closely throughout pregnancy. This does not apply to women who develop GDM because such women are not at risk for development of diabetic retinopathy.

People with macular edema, moderate to severe nonproliferative retinopathy, or any proliferative retinopathy should receive the care of an ophthalmologist. Methods used in the treatment of diabetic retinopathy include the destruction and scarring of the proliferative lesions with laser photocoagulation. The Diabetic Retinopathy Study provides evidence that photocoagulation may delay or prevent visual loss in more than 50% of eyes with proliferative retinopathy.

Macrovascular Complications

Diabetes mellitus is a major risk factor for coronary artery disease, cerebrovascular disease, and peripheral vascular disease (see Chapter 24). The prevalence of these macrovascular complications is increased twofold to fourfold in people with diabetes. Approximately 50% to 75% of all type 2 diabetics will die of a macrovascular problem.

Multiple risk factors for macrovascular disease, including obesity, hypertension, hyperglycemia, hyperinsulinemia, hyperlipidemia, altered platelet function, endothelial dysfunction, systemic inflammation (as evidenced by increased CRP), and elevated fibrinogen levels, frequently are found in people with diabetes. There appear to be differences between type 1 and type 2 diabetes in terms of duration of disease and the development of macrovascular disease. In people with type 2 diabetes, macrovascular disease may be present at the time of diagnosis. Indeed, approximately 50% of type 2 diabetics have some form of complication at presentation (either microvascular or macrovascular). In type 1 diabetes, the attained age and the duration of diabetes appear to correlate with the degree of macrovascular disease. The reason for these discrepancies has been attributed to the associated cardiovascular risk factors that are part of the metabolic syndrome.[60]

Aggressive management of cardiovascular risk factors should include smoking cessation, control of hypertension, lipid lowering, diabetes control, and antiplatelet agents (aspirin, clopidogrel, or both) if not contraindicated[23] (see Chapter 24). If treatment is warranted for peripheral vascular disease, the peroneal arteries between the knees and ankles commonly are involved in diabetics, making revascularization difficult.

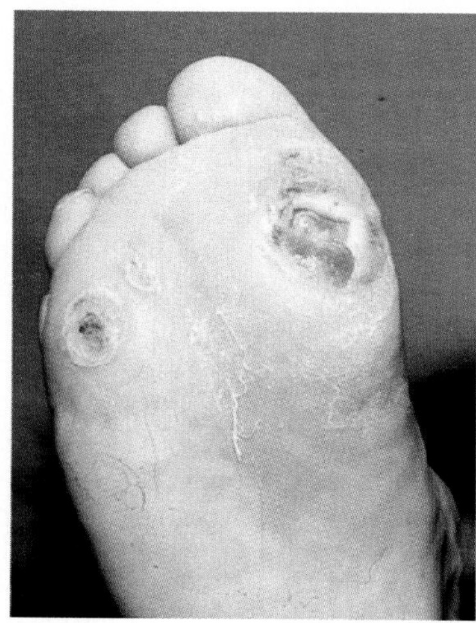

FIGURE 43-12 Neuropathic ulcers occur on pressure points in areas with diminished sensation in diabetic polyneuropathy. Pain is absent (and therefore the ulcer may go unnoticed). (Bates B.B. [1995]. *A guide to physical examination and history taking* [6th ed.]. Philadelphia: J.B. Lippincott)

Diabetic Foot Ulcers

Foot problems are common among people with diabetes and may become severe enough to cause ulceration, infection, and, eventually, a need for amputation. Foot problems have been reported as the most common complication leading to hospitalization among people with diabetes. In a controlled study of 854 outpatients with diabetes followed in a general medical clinic, foot problems accounted for 16% of hospital admissions over a 2-year period and 23% of total hospital days.[61] In people with diabetes, lesions of the feet represent the effects of neuropathy and vascular insufficiency. Approximately 60% to 70% of people with diabetic foot ulcers have neuropathy without vascular disease, 15% to 20% have vascular disease, and 15% to 20% have neuropathy and vascular disease.[61]

Distal symmetric neuropathy is a major risk factor for foot ulcers. People with sensory neuropathies have impaired pain sensation and often are unaware of the constant trauma to the feet caused by poorly fitting shoes, improper weight bearing, hard objects or pebbles in the shoes, or infections such as athlete's foot. Neuropathy prevents people from detecting pain; they are unable to adjust their gait to avoid walking on an area of the foot where pressure is causing trauma and necrosis. Motor neuropathy with weakness of the intrinsic muscles of the foot may result in foot deformities, which lead to focal areas of high pressure. When the abnormal focus of pressure is coupled with loss of sensation, a foot ulcer can occur. Common sites of trauma are the back of the heel, the plantar metatarsal area, or the great toe, where weight is borne during walking (Fig. 43-12).

All persons with diabetes should receive a full foot examination at least once a year. This examination should include assessment of protective sensation, foot structure and biomechanics, vascular status, and skin integrity.[3,61] Evaluation of neurologic function should include a somatosensory test using either the Semmes-Weinstein monofilament or vibratory sensation. The Semmes-Weinstein monofilament is a simple, inexpensive device for testing sensory status (Fig. 43-13). The monofilament is held in the hand or attached to a handle at one end. When the unattached or unsupported end of the monofilament is pressed against the skin until it buckles or bends slightly, it delivers 10 g of pressure at the point of contact.[61] The test consists of having the person being tested report at which of two moments he or she is being touched by the monofilament. For example, the examiner will call out "one" and then "two" and briefly touch the monofilament to the site at one of the two test times. Between 4 and 10 sites per foot are touched. An incorrect response at even one site indicates increased risk for neuropathy and foot complications.

Because of the constant risk for foot problems, it is important that people with diabetes wear shoes that have been fitted correctly and inspect their feet daily, looking for blisters, open sores, and fungal infection (*e.g.*, athlete's

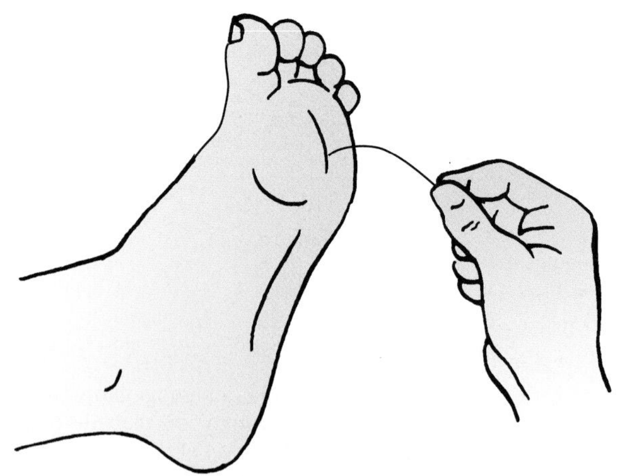

FIGURE 43-13 Use of a monofilament in testing for impaired sensation in the foot of a person with diabetes.

foot) between the toes. If their eyesight is poor, a family member should do this for them. In the event a lesion is detected, prompt medical attention is needed to prevent serious complications. Specially designed shoes have been demonstrated to be effective in preventing relapses in people with previous ulcerations.[61] Smoking should be avoided because it causes vasoconstriction and contributes to vascular disease. Because cold produces vasoconstriction, appropriate foot coverings should be used to keep the feet warm and dry. Toenails should be cut straight across to prevent ingrown toenails. The toenails often are thickened and deformed, requiring the services of a podiatrist.

Persons with diabetes mellitus develop more extensive and rapidly progressive peripheral vascular disease than do nondiabetic individuals. Cardiovascular risk factors should be addressed in patients with diabetic ulcers and peripheral vascular disease. Ulcers, which are resistant to standard therapy, may respond to the application of growth factors. Growth factors provide a means by which cells communicate with each other and can have profound effects on cell proliferation, migration, and extracellular matrix synthesis. Becaplermin, a topical preparation of recombinant human platelet-derived growth factor (PDGF), is used in treatment of neuropathic lower extremity ulcers.

INFECTIONS

Although not specifically an acute or a chronic complication, infections are a common concern of people with diabetes. Certain types of infections occur with increased frequency in people with diabetes: soft tissue infections of the extremities, osteomyelitis, urinary tract infections and pyelonephritis, candidal infections of the skin and mucous surfaces, dental caries and periodontal disease, and tuberculosis.[62] Controversy exists about whether infections are more common in people with diabetes or whether infections seem more prevalent because they often are more serious in people with diabetes.

Suboptimal response to infection in a person with diabetes is caused by the presence of chronic complications, such as vascular disease and neuropathies, and by the presence of hyperglycemia and altered neutrophil function. Sensory deficits may cause a person with diabetes to ignore minor trauma and infection, and vascular disease may impair circulation and delivery of blood cells and other substances needed to produce an adequate inflammatory response and effect healing. Pyelonephritis and urinary tract infections are relatively common in persons with diabetes, and it has been suggested that these infections may bear some relation to the presence of a neurogenic bladder or nephrosclerotic changes in the kidneys. Hyperglycemia and glycosuria may influence the growth of microorganisms and increase the severity of the infection. Diabetes and elevated blood glucose levels also may impair host defenses such as the function of neutrophils and immune cells. Polymorphonuclear leukocyte function, particularly adherence, chemotaxis, and phagocytosis, are depressed in persons with diabetes, particularly those with poor glycemic control.

In summary, diabetes mellitus is a disorder of carbohydrate, protein, and fat metabolism resulting from an imbalance between insulin availability and insulin need. The disease can be classified as type 1 diabetes, in which there is destruction of beta cells and an absolute insulin deficiency, or type 2 diabetes, in which there is a lack of insulin availability or effectiveness (*i.e.*, beta cell dysfunction or insulin resistance). Type 1 diabetes can be further subdivided into type 1A immune-mediated diabetes, which is thought to be caused by autoimmune mechanisms, and type 1B idiopathic diabetes, for which the cause is unknown. Other specific types of diabetes include secondary forms of carbohydrate intolerance, which occur secondary to some other condition, such as pancreatic disorders, that destroys beta cells, or endocrine diseases such as Cushing's syndrome, which cause increased production of glucose by the liver and decreased use of glucose by the tissues. GDM develops during pregnancy, and although glucose tolerance often returns to normal after childbirth, it indicates an increased risk for development of diabetes. A prediabetes state also exists and is composed of IFG, IGT, or both. The metabolic syndrome represents a constellation of metabolic abnormalities characterized by obesity, insulin resistance, high triglycerides levels and low HDL levels, hypertension and cardiovascular disease, insulin resistance, and increased risk for development of type 2 diabetes.

The diagnosis of diabetes mellitus is based on clinical signs of the disease, fasting blood glucose levels, casual plasma glucose measurements, and results of the glucose tolerance test. Self-monitoring provides a means of maintaining near-normal blood glucose levels through frequent testing of blood glucose and adjustment of insulin dosage. Glycosylation involves the irreversible attachment of glucose to the hemoglobin molecule; the measurement of A1C provides an index of blood glucose levels over several months.

The treatment of diabetes includes diet, exercise, and, in many cases, the use of an antidiabetic agent. Dietary management focuses on maintaining a well-balanced diet, controlling calories to achieve and maintain an optimum weight, and regulating the distribution of carbohydrates, proteins, and fats. Two types of antidiabetic agents are used in the management of diabetes: injectable insulin and oral diabetic drugs. Type 1, and sometimes type 2, diabetes requires treatment with injectable insulin. Oral diabetic drugs include the beta cell stimulating agents, biguanides, α-glucosidase inhibitors, and TZDs. These drugs require a functioning pancreas and may be used in the treatment of type 2 diabetes. The benefits of exercise include cardiovascular fitness and psychological well-being. Many people with type 2 diabetes benefit from a decrease in body fat, better weight control, and an improvement in insulin sensitivity. In people with type 1 diabetes, the benefits of exercise are accompanied by a risk for hypoglycemia.

The metabolic disturbances associated with diabetes affect almost every body system. The acute complications of diabetes include DKA, HHS, and hypoglycemia. The chronic complications of diabetes affect the microvascular system (including the retina, kidneys, and peripheral nervous system) and the macrovascular system (coronary, cerebrovascular, and peripheral arteries). The diabetic foot is usually a combination of both microvascular and macrovascular dysfunction. Infection is also a frequent cofactor in the diabetic foot.

REVIEW EXERCISES

A 6-year-old boy is admitted to the emergency room with nausea, vomiting, and abdominal pain. He is very lethargic; his skin is warm, dry, and flushed; his pulse is rapid; and he has a sweet smell to his breath. His parents relate that he has been very thirsty during the past several weeks, his appetite has been poor, and he has been urinating frequently. His initial plasma glucose is 420 mg/dL, and a urine test for ketones is strongly positive.

A. What is the most likely cause of this boy's elevated blood glucose and ketonuria? Explain his presenting signs and symptoms in terms of the elevated blood glucose and metabolic acidosis.

B. What type of treatment will this boy require?

A 53-year-old accountant presents for his routine yearly examination; his history indicates that he was found to have a fasting glucose of 120 mg/dL on two prior occasions. Currently, he is asymptomatic. He has no other medical problems and does not use any medications. He neither smokes nor drinks alcohol. His father had type 2 diabetes at age 60 years. His physical examination reveals a blood pressure of 125/80 mm Hg, BMI (body mass index) of 32 kg/m^2, and waist circumference of 45 inches. Laboratory study results are as follows: CBC, TSH, and ALT are within normal limits. The lipid panel shows an HDL of 30 mg/dL, LDL of 136 mg/dL, and triglycerides of 290 mg/dL (normal <165 mg/dL).

A. What is this man's probable diagnosis?

B. Based on this man's blood glucose level and the ADA diabetes classification system, what diabetic status would you place this man in? Does he need a 75-g oral glucose tolerance test (OGTT) for further assessment of his IFG?

C. His OGTT test results reveals a 2 hr glucose value of 175 mg/dL. What is the diagnosis? What type of treatment would be appropriate for this man?

Acknowledgments

We would like to thank Tan Attila, MD, for his contributions regarding diabetic gastroparesis and nonalcoholic fatty liver disease.

References

1. American Diabetes Association. (2004). Diabetes facts and figures. [On-line]. Available: http://www.diabetes.org.
2. Ford E.S., Giles W.H., Dietz W.H. (2002). Prevalence of the metabolic syndrome among US adults: Findings from the Third National Health and Nutrition Examination Survey. *Journal of the American Medical Association 287*(3), 356–359.
3. Guyton A., Hall J.E. (2000). *Medical physiology* (10th ed., pp. 884–898). Philadelphia: W.B. Saunders.
4. Masharani U, Karam J.H., German M.S. (2004). Pancreatic hormones and diabetes. In Greenspan F.S., Gardner D.G. *Basic and clinical endocrinology* (7th ed., pp. 658–746). New York: Lange Medical Books/McGraw-Hill.
5. Goldfine I.R., Youngren J.F. (1998). Contributions of the *American Journal of Physiology* to the discovery of insulin. *American Journal of Physiology 274,* E207–E209.
6. Expert Committee on the Diagnosis and Classification of Diabetes Mellitus. (1997). Report of the Expert Committee on the Diagnosis and Classification of Diabetes Mellitus. *Diabetes Care 20,* 1183–1199.
7. Tataranni C., Bogardus C. (2001). Changing habits to delay diabetes. *New England Journal of Medicine 344,* 1390–1391.
8. Atkinson M.A., Eisenbarth G.S. (2001). Type 1 diabetes: New perspectives on disease pathogenesis and treatment. *Lancet 358,* 221–229.
9. Atkinson M.A. (2000). The $64,000 question in diabetes continues. *Lancet 356,* 4–5.
10. Bingley P.J., Bonifacio E., Ziegler A.G., et al. (2001). Proposed guidelines for screening for risk of type 1 diabetes. *Diabetes Care 24,* 398.
11. Atkinson M., Gale E.A.M. (2003). Infant diets and type 1 diabetes. *Journal of the American Medical Association 290,* 1771–1772.
12. Gerich J.E. (2003). Contributions of insulin-resistance and insulin-secretory defects to the pathogenesis of type 2 diabetes. *Mayo Clinic Proceedings 78,* 447–456.
13. Meigs J.B., Avruch J. (2003). The Metabolic syndrome. *Endocrinology Rounds 5,* 1–6. [On-line]. Available: www.endocrinologyrounds.org.
14. Freemark M. (2003). Pharmacological approaches to the prevention of type 2 diabetes in high risk pediatric patients. *Journal of Clinical Endocrinology and Metabolism 88,* 3–13.
15. Grundy S.M., Panel Chair. (2001). Third Report of the National Cholesterol Education Program (NCEP) Expert Panel on Detection, Evaluation, and Treatment of High Blood Cholesterol in Adults (Adult Treatment Panel III). (NIH Publication No. 01-3670.) Bethesda, MD: National Institutes of Health.
16. Welt C.K. (2003). Insulin resistance in polycystic ovary syndrome. *Endocrinology Rounds 7,* 1–6. [On-line]. Available: www.endocrinologyrounds.org.
17. Guven S., El-Bershawi A., Sonnenberg G.E., et al. (1999). Persistent elevation in plasma leptin level in ex-obese with normal body mass index: Relation to body composition and insulin sensitivity. *Diabetes 48,* 347–352.
18. Yamauchi T., Kamon J., Waki H., et. al. (2001). The fat-derived hormone adiponectin reverses insulin resistance associated with both lipoatrophy and obesity. *Nature Medicine 7*(8), 941–946.
19. Kissebah A.H., Sonneberg G.F., Myklebust J., et al. (2000). Quantitative trait loci on chromosomes 3 and 17 influence phenotypes of metabolic syndrome. *Proceedings of the National Academy of Science U S A 97*(26), 14478–14483.
20. American Diabetes Association (2004). Prevention or delay of type 2 diabetes. *Diabetes Care 27,* S47–54.
21. Kuritzkes D.R., Currier J. (2003). Cardiovascular risk factors and antiretroviral therapy. *New England Journal of Medicine 348,* 679–680.
22. American Diabetes Association. (2004). Gestational diabetes mellitus. *Diabetes Care 27*(Suppl. 1), S88–S90.
23. American Diabetes Association. (2004). Standards of medical care for patients with diabetes mellitus. *Diabetes Care 27*(Suppl. 1), S15–S35.
24. American Diabetes Association. (2004). Tests of glycemia in diabetes. *Diabetes Care 27*(Suppl. 1), S91–S93.
25. UKPDS Group. (1998). Intensive blood-glucose control with sulfonylureas or insulin compared with conventional treat-

ment and risk of complications in patients with type 2 diabetes (UKPDS 33). *Lancet 352,* 837–853.

26. Shichiri M., Kishikquq H., Ohkubo Y., Wake N. (2000). Long-term results of Kumamoto Study on optimal diabetes control in type 2 diabetes patients. *Diabetes Care 23*(Suppl. 2), B21–B29.
27. American Diabetes Association. (2004). Evidence-based nutrition principles and recommendations for the treatment and prevention of diabetes and related complications [Position Statement]. *Diabetes Care 27*(Suppl 1), S36–S47.
28. Gillespie S., Kulkairni K., Daly A. (1998). Using carbohydrate counting in diabetes clinical practice. *Journal of the American Dietetic Association 98,* 897–905.
29. American Diabetes Association. (2004). Physical activity: exercise and diabetes mellitus. *Diabetes Care 27*(Suppl. 1), S55–S59.
30. Nathan D.M. (2002). Initial management of glycemia in type 2 diabetic mellitus. *New England Journal of Medicine 347,* 1342–1349.
31. Chan J.L., Abrahamson M.J. (2003). Pharmacological management of type 2 diabetes. *Mayo Clinic Proceedings 78,* 459–467.
32. Zangeneh F., Kudva Y.C., Basu A. (2003). Insulin sensitizers. *Mayo Clinic Proceedings 78,* 471–479.
33. Flier J.S. (2001). The missing link in diabetes. *Nature 409,* 292–293.
34. Buse J.B., Weyer C., Maggs D.G. (2002). Amylin replacement with pramlintide in type 1 and type 2 diabetes: A physiological approach to overcome barriers with insulin therapy. *Clinical Diabetes 20*(3), 137–143.
35. American Diabetes Association. (2004). Continuous subcutaneous insulin infusion. *Diabetes Care 27*(Suppl. 1), S110.
36. American Diabetes Association. (2004). Pancreas transplantation for patients with type 1 diabetes. *Diabetes Care 27*(Suppl. 1), S105.
37. American Diabetes Association. (2004). Hyperglycemic crises in patients with diabetes mellitus. *Diabetes Care 27*(Suppl. 1), S94–S102.
38. Karam J.H., Masharani U. (2004). Hypoglycemic disorders. In Greenspan F.S., Gardner D.G. (Eds.), *Basic and clinical endocrinology* (7th ed., pp. 747–765). New York: Lange Medical Books/McGraw-Hill.
39. Somogyi M. (1957). Exacerbation of diabetes in excess insulin action. *American Journal of Medicine 26,* 169–191.
40. Bolli G.B., Gotterman I.S., Campbell P.J. (1984). Glucose counterregulation and waning of insulin in the Somogyi phenomenon (posthypoglycemic hyperglycemia). *New England Journal of Medicine 311,* 1214–1219.
41. Bolli G.B., Gerich J.E. (1984). The dawn phenomenon: A common occurrence in both non-insulin and insulin dependent diabetes mellitus. *New England Journal of Medicine 310,* 746–750.
42. Sheetz M.J., King G.L. (2002). Molecular understanding of hyperglycemia's adverse effects for diabetic complications. *JAMA 288,* 2579–2588.
43. The Diabetes Control and Complications Trial Research Group. (1993). The effect of intensified treatment of diabetes on the development and progression of long-term complications in insulin-dependent diabetes mellitus. *New England Journal of Medicine 329,* 955–977.
44. Stratton I.M., Adler A.I., Neil H.A., et al. (2000). Association of glycaemia with macrovascular and microvascular complications in type 2 diabetes (UKPDS 35) group: Prospective observational study. *British Medical Journal 321,* 405–412.
45. Vinik A.I. (1999). Diabetic neuropathy: Pathogenesis and therapy. *American Journal of Medicine 107*(Suppl. 2B), 17S–26S.
46. AACE Male Sexual Dysfunction Taskforce. (2003). AACE medical guidelines for clinical practice for the evaluation and treatment of male sexual dysfunction: a couple's problem—2003 update. *Endocrine Practice 9,* 77–95.
47. Camilleri M., Prather C.M. (1998). Gastric motor physiology and motor disorders. In *Sleisenger and Fordtran's gastrointestinal and liver disease* (6th ed., pp. 572–586). Philadelphia. W.B. Saunders.
48. McCallum R.W., Chen J.D., Lin Z., et al. (1998). Gastric pacing improves emptying and symptoms in patients with gastroparesis. *Gastroenterology 114,* 456–461.
49. Lysy J., Israeli E., Goldin E. (1999). The prevalence of chronic diarrhea among diabetic patients. *American Journal of Gastroenterology 94,* 2165–2170.
50. Fedorak R.N., Field M., Chang E.B. (1985). Treatment of diabetic diarrhea with clonidine. *Annals of Internal Medicine 102,* 197–199.
51. Walker J.J., Kaplan D.S. (1993). Efficacy of the somatostatin analog octreotide in the treatment of two patients with refractory diabetic diarrhea. *American Journal of Gastroenterology 88,* 765–767.
52. American Diabetes Association. (2004). Diabetic nephropathy. *Diabetes Care 27*(Suppl. 1), S79–S83.
53. Renal Data System. (1998, April). *USRDS 1998 annual data report.* NIH publication 98:3176. Bethesda, MD: National Institute of Diabetes and Digestive and Kidney Diseases.
54. Ritz E., Orth S.R. (1999). Nephropathy in patients with type 2 diabetes mellitus. *New England Journal of Medicine 341,* 1127–1133.
55. Krolewski A.S., Laffel L.M.B., Krolewski M., et al. (1995). Glycosylated hemoglobin and the risk of microalbuminemia in patients with insulin-dependent diabetes mellitus. *New England Journal of Medicine 332,* 1251–1255.
56. Barnett A.H. (2003). Adopting more aggressive strategies for the management of renal disease in type 2 diabetes. *Practical Diabetes International 20,* 186–190.
57. Chobanian A.V., Bakris G.L., Black H.R., et al. (2003). The seventh report of the joint national committee on prevention, detection, evaluation, and treatment of high blood pressure: The JNC 7 Report. *Journal of the American Medical Association 289,* 2560–2572.
58. American Diabetes Association. (2004). Diabetic retinopathy. *Diabetes Care 27*(Suppl. 1), S84–S87.
59. Aiello L.P., Gardner T.W., King G.L., et al. (1998). Diabetic retinopathy (Technical Review). *Diabetes Care 21,* 143–156.
60. American College of Endocrinology. (2003). ACE position statement on the insulin resistance syndrome. *Endocrine Practice 9,* 237–252.
61. American Diabetes Association. (2004). Preventative foot care in people with diabetes. *Diabetes Care 27*(Suppl. 1), S63–S64.
62. Joshi N., Caputo G.M., Weitekamp M.R., Karchmer A.W. (1999). Infections in patients with diabetes mellitus. *New England Journal of Medicine 341,* 1906–1912.

Genitourinary and Reproductive Function

UNIT XI

There is a long history of misunderstanding and myths about human reproduction, especially the female reproductive system. Early on, the uterus was deemed the most important structure of the female reproductive anatomy. One of the first representations of the uterus appears in ancient Egyptian hieroglyphs (c. 2900 BC). Its importance was a direct result of the understanding that it was from the uterus that a child was born. That a woman was the carrier of the next generation was enough to establish her importance to society. However, society also imposed harsh restrictions on women that made it difficult, if not impossible, for further understanding. Until the Renaissance, custom and manners dictated that a woman's body could not be represented unless it was fully clothed.

To a regrettable extent, the associations made in ancient times that surmised a destiny for women based on the anatomy peculiar to their sex still affect how women are viewed today. The Greek philosopher Plato (427?–347? BC) postulated that the unused womb became "indignant" and wandered around the body, inhibiting the body's "spirits," or life force, and causing disease. The reasonings of Aristotle (384–322 BC) were equally fanciful. It was he, believing as others of the time did that women were irrational and prone to emotional outbursts, who provided the nomenclature for the womb, naming it *hystera* (ustera). Their concept that emotional excitability or instability was the domain of women is confirmed by another word that was coined by the Greeks: hysteria.

CHAPTER

44

The Male Genitourinary System

Glenn Matfin

The male genitourinary system is composed of the paired gonads, or testes, genital ducts, accessory organs, and penis (Fig. 44-1). The dual function of the testes is to produce male sex androgens (*i.e.,* male sex hormones), mainly testosterone, and spermatozoa (*i.e.,* male germ cells). The internal accessory organs produce the fluid constituents of semen, and the ductile system aids in the storage and transport of spermatozoa. The penis functions in urine elimination and sexual function. This chapter focuses on the structure of the male reproductive system, spermatogenesis and control of male reproductive function, neural control of sexual function, and changes in function that occur at puberty and as a result of the aging process.

Structure of the Male Reproductive System

After completing this section of the chapter, you should be able to meet the following objectives:

- ✦ Characterize the embryonic development of the male reproductive organs and genitalia
- ✦ Describe the structure and function of the testes and scrotum, the genital ducts, accessory organs, and penis

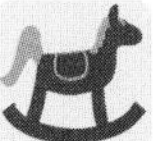

EMBRYONIC DEVELOPMENT

The sex of a person is determined at the time of fertilization by the sex chromosomes. In the early stages of embryonic development, the tissues from which the male and female reproductive organs develop are undifferentiated. Until approximately the seventh week of gestation, it is impossible to determine whether the embryo is male or female unless the chromosomes are studied. Until this time, the male and female genital tracts consist of two wolffian ducts, from which the male genitalia develop, and two müllerian ducts, from which the female genital structures develop. During this period of gestation, the gonads (*i.e.,* ovaries and testes) also are undifferentiated.[1–3]

Between the sixth and eighth weeks of gestation, the testes begin development under the influence of the Y chromosome. Differentiation of the indifferent gonad into a testis is initiated by the actions of a single gene on the short arm of the Y chromosome. This gene is called the *s*ex-determining *r*egion of the *Y* chromosome *(SRY).*[1] In the presence of the *SRY* gene, the embryonic gonads develop into testes, and in its absence, the gonads develop into ovaries.

During this time, the testicular cells of the male embryo begin producing an antimüllerian hormone (AMH) and testosterone. The AMH suppresses the müllerian ducts and prevents development of the uterus and fallopian tubes in the male. Testosterone stimulates the wolffian ducts to develop into the epididymis, vas deferens, and seminal vesicles. Testosterone also is the precursor of a third hormone, dihydrotestosterone (DHT), which functions in the formation of the male urethra, prostate, and external genitalia. The conversion of testosterone to DHT, predominantly in the peripheral tissues, is performed by the enzyme 5-α reductase. Although testosterone and DHT share the same nuclear androgen receptor, they have

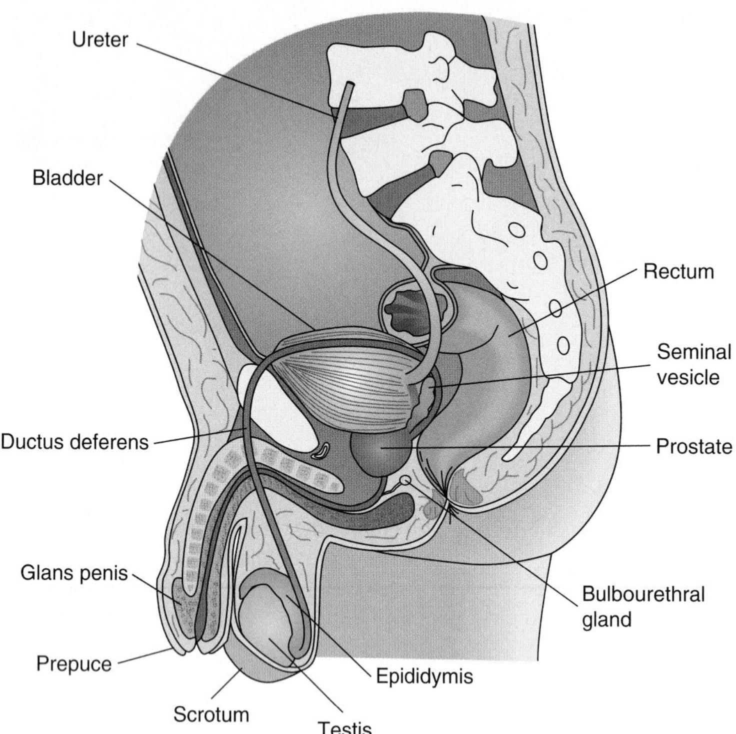

FIGURE 44-1 The structures of the male reproductive system, including the testes, the scrotum, and the excretory ducts.

marked differences in tissue activity (DHT has most effects on the external genitalia, including the prostate, but is also subsequently important for facial and body hair, and temporal hair recession). In the absence of testosterone (and DHT), a male embryo with an XY chromosomal pattern develops female genitalia.[1]

TESTES AND SCROTUM

The testes, or male gonads, are two egg-shaped structures located outside the abdominal cavity in the scrotum. The adult male testes are approximately 15 to 25 mL in volume (>4 mL indicates pubertal onset), with 80% of this volume being cells involved in spermatogenesis and 20% in testosterone production. Embryologically, the testes develop in the abdominal cavity and then descend through the inguinal canal into a pouch of peritoneum (which becomes the tunica vaginalis) in the scrotum. Testicular descent occurs in two stages: (1) between 7 and 12 weeks of fetal life, AMH is responsible for descent to the inguinal region; and (2) during the seventh to ninth months of fetal life, testosterone is responsible for descent into the scrotum. As they descend, the testes pull their arteries, veins, lymphatics, nerves, and conducting excretory ducts with them. These structures are encased by the cremaster muscle and layers of fascia that constitute the spermatic cord (Fig. 44-2A). After descent of the testes, the inguinal canal closes almost completely. Failure of this canal to close predisposes to the development of an inguinal hernia later in life (see Fig. 44-2B). An inguinal hernia or "rupture" is a protrusion of the parietal peritoneum and part of the intestine through an abnormal opening from the abdominal cavity. A loop of small bowel may become incarcerated in an inguinal hernia (strangulated hernia), in which case the lumen may become obstructed, and the vascular supply compromised.

The testes are enclosed in a double-layered membrane, the tunica vaginalis, which is derived embryologically from the abdominal peritoneum[2,3] (see Fig. 44-2). An outer covering, the tunica albuginea, is a tough, white, fibrous sheath that resembles the sclera of the eye. The tunica albuginea protects the testes and gives them their ovoid shape. The cremaster muscles, which are bands of skeletal muscle arising from the internal oblique muscles of the trunk, elevate the testes. The testes receive their arterial blood supply from the long testicular arteries, which branch from the aortic artery. The testicular veins, which drain the testes, arise from a venous network called the *pampiniform plexus* that surrounds the testicular artery. The testes are innervated by fibers from both divisions of the autonomic nervous system. Associated sensory nerves transmit pain impulses, resulting in excruciating pain, especially when the testes are hit forcibly.

The scrotum, which houses the testes, is made up of a thin outer layer of skin that forms rugae, or folds, and is continuous with the perineum and outer skin of the groin. Under the outer skin lies a thin layer of fascia and smooth muscle (*i.e.,* dartos muscle). This layer contains a septum that separates the two testes. The dartos muscle responds to changes in temperature. When it is cold, the muscle contracts, bringing the testes closer to the body, and the scrotum becomes shorter and heavily wrinkled. When it is warmer, the muscle relaxes, allowing the scrotum to fall away from the body.

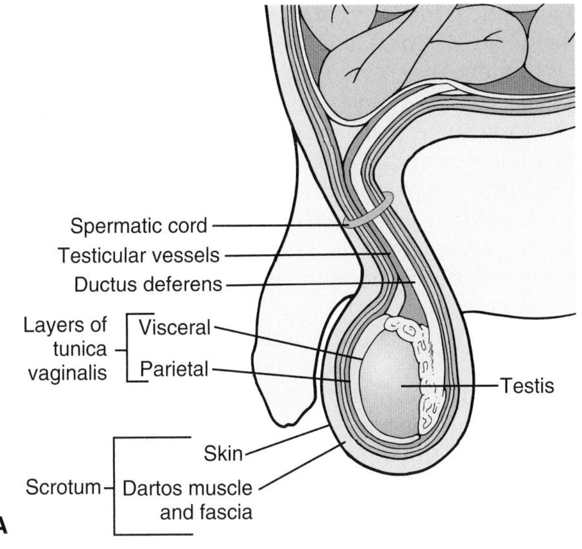

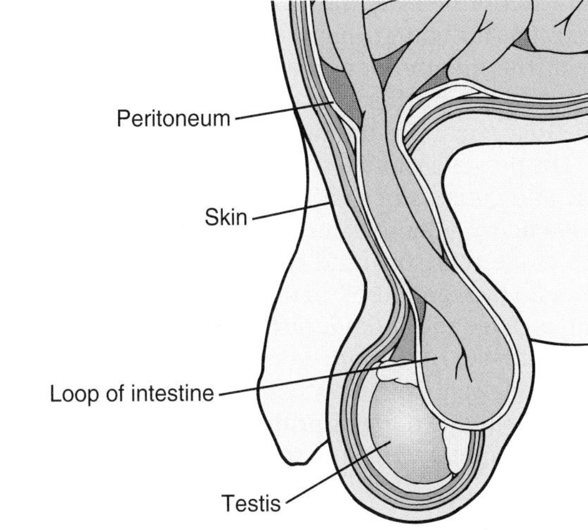

FIGURE 44-2 (**A**) Anterior view of the spermatic cord and inguinal canal and coverings of the spermatic cord and testes. (**B**) Indirect inguinal hernia. (Adapted from Moore K.L., Agur A.M. [2002]. *Essentials of clinical anatomy* [2nd ed., pp. 130, 138]. Philadelphia: Lippincott Williams & Wilkins)

The location of the testes in the scrotum is important for sperm production, which is optimal at 2°C to 3°C below body temperature. Two systems maintain the temperature of the testes at a level consistent with sperm production. One is the pampiniform plexus of testicular veins that surround the testicular artery. This plexus absorbs heat from the arterial blood, cooling it as it enters the testes. The other is the cremaster muscles, which respond to decreases in testicular temperature by moving the testes closer to the body. Prolonged exposure to elevated temperatures, as a result of prolonged fever or the dysfunction of thermoregulatory mechanisms, can impair spermatogenesis. Some tight-fitting undergarments hold the testes against the body and are thought to contribute to a decrease in sperm counts and infertility by interfering with the thermoregulatory function of the scrotum. Cryptorchidism, the failure of the testes to descend into the scrotum, also exposes the testes to the higher temperature of the body (see Chapter 45).

MALE REPRODUCTIVE SYSTEM

- The male genitourinary system functions in both urine elimination and reproduction.
- The testes function in both production of male germ cells (spermatogenesis) and secretion of the male sex hormone, testosterone.
- The ductile system (epididymides, vas deferens, and ejaculatory ducts) transports and stores sperm, and assists in their maturation; and the accessory glands (seminal vesicles, prostate gland, and bulbourethral glands) prepare the sperm for ejaculation.
- Sperm production requires temperatures that are 2°C to 3°C below body temperature. The position of the testes in the scrotum and the unique blood flow cooling mechanisms provide this environment.
- The urethra, which is enclosed in the penis, is the terminal portion of the male genitourinary system. Because it conveys both urine and semen, it serves both urinary and reproductive functions.

GENITAL DUCT SYSTEM

Internally, the testes are composed of several hundred compartments or lobules (Fig. 44-3). Each lobule contains one or more coiled seminiferous tubules. These tubules are the site of sperm production. As the tubules lead into the efferent ducts, the seminiferous tubules become the rete testis.

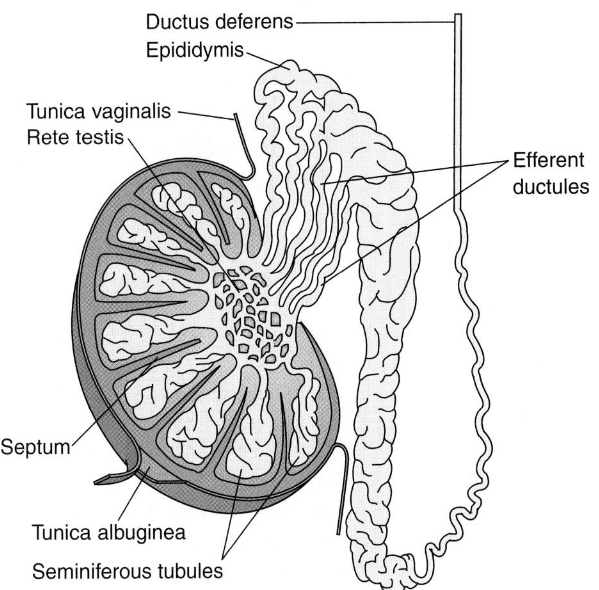

FIGURE 44-3 The parts of the testes and epididymis.

From the rete testis, 10,000 to 20,000 efferent ducts emerge to join the epididymis, which is the final site for sperm maturation. Because the spermatozoa are not motile at this stage of development, peristaltic movements of the ductal walls of the epididymis aid in their movement. The spermatozoa continue their migration through the ductus deferens, also called the *vas deferens*. The ampulla of the vas deferens serves as a storage reservoir for sperm. Sperm are stored in the ampulla until they are released through the penis during ejaculation (Fig. 44-4). Spermatozoa can be stored in the genital ducts for as long as 42 days and still maintain their fertility. Surgical disconnection of the vas deferens in the scrotal area (*e.g.*, vasectomy) serves as an effective method of male contraception. Because sperm are stored in the ampulla, men can remain fertile for 4 to 5 weeks after performance of a vasectomy.

ACCESSORY ORGANS

The male accessory organs consist of the seminal vesicles, the prostate gland, and the bulbourethral glands. Spermatozoa are transported through the reproductive structures by movement of the seminal fluid, which is combined with secretions from the genital ducts and accessory organs. The spermatozoa plus the secretions from the genital ducts and accessory organs make up the semen (from the Latin word meaning *seed*).

The seminal vesicles consist of two highly tortuous tubes that secrete fluid for the semen. Each of the paired seminal vesicles is lined with secretory epithelium containing an abundance of fructose, prostaglandins, and several other proteins. The fructose secreted by the seminal vesicles provides the energy for sperm motility. The prostaglandins are thought to assist in fertilization by making the cervical mucus more receptive to sperm and by causing reverse peristaltic contractions in the uterus and fallopian tubes to move the sperm toward the ovaries.

Each seminal vesicle joins its corresponding vas deferens to form the ejaculatory duct, which enters the posterior part of the prostate and continues through until it ends in the prostatic portion of the urethra. During the emission phase of coitus, each vesicle empties fluid into the ejaculatory duct, adding bulk to the semen. Approximately 70% of the ejaculate originates in the seminal vesicles.

The prostate is a fibromuscular and glandular organ lying just inferior to the bladder. The prostate gland secretes a thin, milky, alkaline fluid containing citric acid, calcium, acid phosphate, a clotting enzyme, and a profibrinolysin. During ejaculation, the capsule of the prostate contracts, and the added fluid increases the bulk of the semen. Both vaginal secretions and the fluid from the vas deferens are strongly acidic. Because sperm mobilization occurs at a pH of 6.0 to 6.5, the alkaline nature of the prostatic secretions is essential for successful fertilization of the ovum. The bulbourethral or Cowper's glands lie on either side of the membranous urethra and secrete an alkaline mucus, which further aids in neutralizing acids from the urine that remain in the urethra.

The prostate gland also functions in the elimination of urine and consists of a thin, fibrous capsule that encloses the circularly oriented smooth muscle fibers and collagenous tissue that surround the urethra where it joins the bladder. The segment of urethra that traverses the prostate gland is called the *prostatic urethra*. It is lined by a thin, longitudinal layer of smooth muscle that is continuous with the bladder wall. The smooth muscle incorporated with the prostate gland is derived primarily from the longitudinal bladder musculature. This smooth muscle represents the

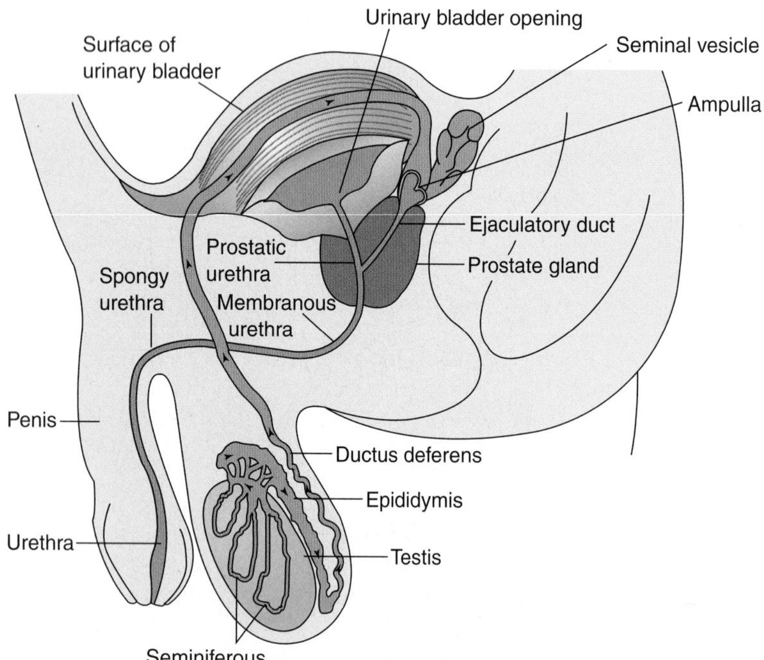

FIGURE 44-4 The excretory ducts of the male reproductive system and the path that sperm follows as it leaves the testis and travels to the urethra.

true involuntary sphincter of the male posterior urethra. Because the prostate surrounds the urethra, enlargement of the gland can produce urinary obstruction.

The prostate gland is made up of many secretory glands arranged in three concentric areas surrounding the prostatic urethra, into which they open. The component glands of the prostate include the small mucosal glands associated with the urethral mucosa, the intermediate submucosal glands that lie peripheral to the mucosal glands, and the large main prostatic glands that are situated toward the outside of the gland. It is the overgrowth of the mucosal glands that causes benign prostatic hyperplasia in older men (see Chapter 45).

PENIS

The penis is the external genital organ through which the urethra passes. Anatomically, the external penis consists of a shaft that ends in a tip called the *glans* (Fig. 44-5). The loose skin of the penis shaft folds to cover the glans, forming the prepuce, or foreskin. The glans of the penis contains many sensory nerves, making this the most sensitive portion of the penile shaft. It is the foreskin that is removed during circumcision.

The cylindrical body or shaft of the penis is composed of three masses of erectile tissue held together by fibrous strands and covered with a thin layer of skin. The two lateral masses of tissue are called the *corpora cavernosa*. The third, ventral mass is called the *corpus spongiosum*. The corpora cavernosa and corpus spongiosum are cavernous sinuses that normally are relatively empty but become engorged with blood during penile erection.

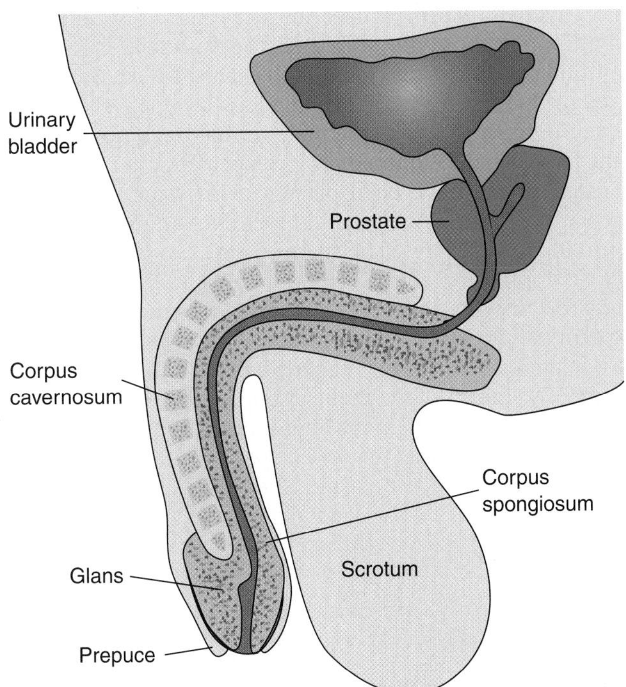

FIGURE 44-5 Sagittal section of the penis, showing the prepuce, glans, corpus cavernosum, and corpus spongiosum.

In summary, the male reproductive system consists of a pair of gonads (*i.e.*, testes), a system of excretory ducts (*i.e.*, seminiferous tubules and efferent ducts), the accessory organs (*i.e.*, epididymis, seminal vesicles, prostate, and Cowper's glands), and the penis. The sex of a person is determined by the sex chromosomes at the time of fertilization. During the seventh week of gestation, the XY chromosome pattern (and the *SRY* gene) in the male embryo is responsible for the development of the testes; with the subsequent production of AMH and testosterone, development of the internal and external male genital structures occurs. Before this period of embryonic development, the tissues from which the male and female reproductive structures develop are undifferentiated. In the absence of testosterone production (and its derivative DHT), the male embryo with an XY chromosomal pattern develops female genitalia.

Spermatogenesis and Hormonal Control of Male Reproductive Function

After completing this section of the chapter, you should be able to meet the following objectives:

- Describe the process of spermatogenesis
- State the functions of testosterone
- Draw a diagram illustrating the secretion, site of action, and feedback control of gonadotropin-releasing hormone, luteinizing hormone, follicle-stimulating hormone and inhibin
- Describe the function of follicle-stimulating hormone in terms of spermatogenesis
- Describe the classification and clinical features of male hypogonadism

During childhood, the gonads remain essentially quiescent. At puberty, the male gonads and testes begin to mature and to carry out spermatogenesis and hormone production. At approximately 10 or 11 years of age, the adenohypophysis, or anterior pituitary, under the control of the hypothalamus, begins to secrete the gonadotropins that stimulate testicular function and cause the interstitial cells of Leydig to begin producing testosterone. Approximately the same time, hormonal stimulation induces mitotic activity of the germ cells that develop in sperm. After cell maturation has begun, the testes begin to enlarge rapidly as the individual tubules grow. Full maturity and spermatogenesis usually are attained by 15 or 16 years of age.

SPERMATOGENESIS

Spermatogenesis refers to the generation of spermatozoa or sperm. It begins at an average age of 13 years and continues throughout the reproductive years of a man's life. Spermatogenesis occurs in the seminiferous tubules of the testes (see Fig 44-3). These tubules, if placed end to end, would measure approximately 750 feet. The outer layer of the seminiferous tubules is made up of connective tissue and smooth muscle; the inner lining is composed of Sertoli's cells, which are embedded with sperm in various stages of development (Fig 44-6). Sertoli's cells secrete a special fluid that contains nutrients to bathe and nourish the immature germ cells; they provide digestive enzymes that play a role in spermiation (*i.e.,* converting the spermatocytes to sperm); and they are thought to play a role in shaping the head and tail of the sperm. Sertoli's cells also secrete several hormones, including AMH, which is secreted by the testes during fetal life to inhibit development of fallopian tubes; estradiol, the principal feminizing sex hormone, which seems to be required in the male for spermatogenesis; and inhibin, which controls the function of Sertoli's cells through feedback inhibition of follicle-stimulating hormone (FSH) from the anterior pituitary gland.[4–6] For spermatogenesis to occur, FSH binds to specific receptors in Sertoli's cells. Testosterone is also required (the intratesticular concentration of testosterone is 100-fold greater than serum levels).[4]

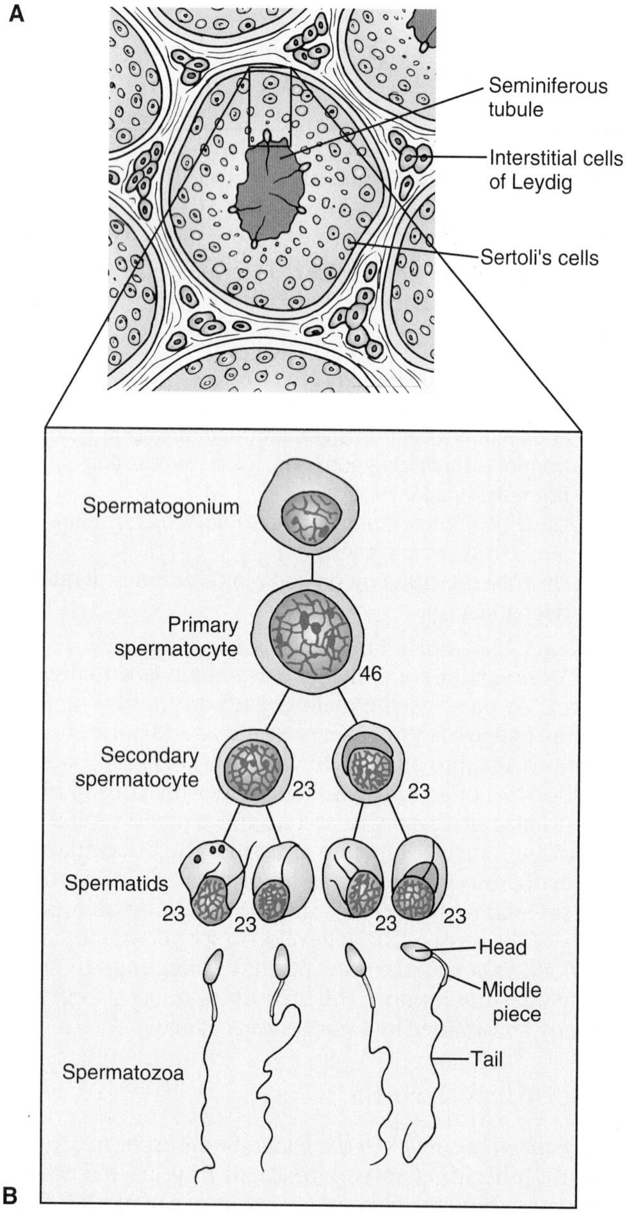

FIGURE 44-6 The various stages of spermatogenesis. (**A**) Cross section of seminiferous tubule and (**B**) stages of development of spermatozoa.

In the first stage of spermatogenesis, small and unspecialized diploid germinal cells located immediately adjacent to the tubular wall, called the *spermatogonia,* undergo rapid mitotic division and provide a continuous source of new germinal cells. As these cells multiply, the more mature spermatogonia divide into two daughter cells, which grow and become the primary spermatocytes—the precursors of sperm. Over several weeks, large primary spermatocytes divide by a process called *meiosis* to form two smaller secondary spermatocytes. Each of the secondary spermatocytes divides to form two spermatids, each containing 23 chromosomes. Meiosis is a unique form of cell division that occurs only in the gonads. It consists of two consecutive nuclear divisions with formation of four daughter cells, each containing a single set of 23 chromosomes rather than a pair of 46 chromosomes, as occurs during mitotic cell division in other body cells (see Chapter 6).

The spermatid elongates into a spermatozoon, or mature sperm cell, with a head and tail (see Fig. 44-6B). The outside of the anterior two thirds of the head, called the *acrosome,* contains enzymes necessary for penetration and fertilization of the ovum. The to-and-fro flagellar motion of the tail imparts movement to the sperm. The energy for this process is supplied by the mitochondria in the tail. Normal sperm move in a straight line at a velocity of 1 to 4 mm/minute. This allows them to move through the female genital tract. When the sperm grow to full size, they move to the epididymis to mature further and gain mobility. A small quantity of sperm can be stored in the epididymis, but most are stored in the vas deferens or the ampulla of the vas deferens. With excessive sexual activity, storage may be no longer than a few days. The sperm can live for many weeks in the male genital tract; however, in the female genital tract, their life expectancy is 1 or 2 days. Frozen sperm have been preserved for years. The entire process of spermatogenesis and sperm maturation takes approximately 90 days. The sperm count in a normal ejaculate is approximately 100 million to 400 million. Infertility may occur when insufficient numbers of motile, healthy sperm are present. A "fertile sample" on semen analysis is associated with a count higher than 20 million/mL, more than 50% motility, normal morphology, and a volume of 1.5 to 6 mL.[7] However, new reproductive technology techniques mean that as few as 20 sperm in the semen may be effective (intracytoplasmic sperm injection [ICSI]; see Chapter 47).

HORMONAL CONTROL OF MALE REPRODUCTIVE FUNCTION

Testosterone and Other Male Sex Hormones

The male sex hormones are called *androgens.* The testes secrete several male sex hormones, including *testosterone, dihydrotestosterone,* and *androstenedione.* Testosterone, which is the most abundant of these hormones, is considered the main testicular hormone. The adrenal cortex also produces androgens, although in much smaller quantities (<5% of the total male androgens) than those produced in the testes. The testes also secrete small quantities of estradiol and estrone.[5,6]

Testosterone is produced and secreted by the interstitial Leydig's cells in the testes. Under the influence of luteinizing hormone (LH), Leydig's cells produce approximately 6 mg/day of testosterone (peak at 4:00 to 8:00 AM).[5] It is metabolized in the liver and excreted by the kidneys. In the bloodstream, testosterone exists in a free (unbound) or a bound form. The bound form is attached to plasma proteins, including albumin and the sex hormone–binding globulin (SHBG) produced by the liver. Only approximately 2% of circulating testosterone is unbound and therefore able to enter the cell and exert its metabolic effects. Much of the testosterone that becomes fixed to the tissues is converted by the action of 5-α reductase to DHT, especially in certain target tissues such as the prostate gland. Some of the actions of testosterone depend on this conversion, whereas others do not.[5] Testosterone also can be aromatized or converted to estradiol in the peripheral tissues.

Testosterone (and DHT) exerts a variety of biologic effects in the male (Chart 44-1). In the male embryo, testosterone is essential for the appropriate differentiation of the internal and external genitalia, and it is necessary for descent of the testes in the fetus. Testosterone is essential to the development of primary and secondary male sex characteristics during puberty and for the maintenance of these characteristics during adult life.[6] It causes growth of pubic, chest, and facial hair; it produces changes in the larynx that result in the male bass voice; and it increases the thickness of the skin and the activity of the sebaceous glands, predisposing to acne.

All or almost all of the actions of testosterone and other androgens result from increased protein synthesis in target tissues. Androgens function as anabolic agents in males and females to promote metabolism and musculoskeletal growth. Testosterone and the androgens have a great effect on the development of increasing musculature during puberty, with boys averaging approximately a 50% increase in muscle mass compared with girls.

CHART 44-1

Main Actions of Testosterone

- Induces differentiation of the male genital tract during fetal development
- Induces development of primary and secondary sex characteristics
  - Gonadal function
  - External genitalia and accessory organs
  - Male voice timbre
  - Male skin characteristics
  - Male hair distribution
- Anabolic effects
  - Promotes protein metabolism
  - Promotes musculoskeletal growth
  - Influences subcutaneous fat distribution
- Promotes spermatogenesis (in FSH-primed tubules) and maturation of sperm
- Stimulation of erythropoiesis

Androgens and Athletic Performance. Because of the great effect that testosterone and other androgens have on body musculature, synthetic androgens sometimes are used by athletes to improve their appearance and muscle performance.[5] Frequently, these agents are taken in doses that far exceed physiologic levels. This practice has been strongly discouraged because of potential harmful effects. Among the undesired or harmful effects of supraphysiologic doses of androgens are acne, decreased testicular size, and azoospermia. These effects may persist for months after use of the agents has ceased. Because testosterone can be aromatized to estradiol in the peripheral tissues, androgens can induce gynecomastia. The undesired effects of androgens depend on the type and dose administered. Virtually all androgens produced for human and veterinary purposes have been taken by athletes. Occasionally, athletes take several medications simultaneously in an attempt to increase the overall effect on performance, or to counter a side effect of one medication. For example, an athlete may take human chorionic gonadotropin (hCG) for its LH-like action to counteract the decrease in testicular size resulting from high-dose androgen abuse, and take an antiestrogen to counteract the gynecomastia from administration of high doses of hCG and androgens. Alkylated androgens at high doses can cause hepatocellular and intrahepatic cholestasis that occasionally results in severe jaundice and liver damage. Alkylated androgens also may lower high-density lipoprotein (HDL) and may increase low-density lipoprotein (LDL) levels. The behavioral effects of anabolic-androgenic steroids are also important. Increased and decreased libido, increased aggression, and a variety of psychotic symptoms have been described. In preadolescents who have not yet achieved their full height, increased androgen levels can cause premature closure of the epiphyseal growth plates.

Attention has also focused on androgen precursors, including oral androstenedione and dehydroepiandrosterone (DHEA) products that are available over the counter and often are marketed as a safe natural alternative to androgens for building muscle.[5,8] Androstenedione and DHEA exert only weak androgenic activity, but their main purpose is to act as a key precursor for testosterone after peripheral conversion. For example, androstenedione normally is produced by the adrenal gland and converted to testosterone through the action of 17β-hydroxysteroid dehydrogenase, which is found in most body tissues. However, the interconversion of androstenedione is complex. In addition to being a precursor for testosterone, androstenedione may be converted into estrogens directly. The testosterone that is produced also can be converted to estradiol. A randomized, controlled study measured the short-term effect of androstenedione supplementation on serum hormone levels and muscle development during an 8-week resistance training program in young normotestosterogenic men.[9] The results from this study indicated that androstenedione supplementation did not significantly increase serum testosterone levels or skeletal muscle adaptation. It did, however, elevate serum levels of estrone and estradiol, suggesting that a significant proportion of the ingested androstenedione underwent conversion to these estrogens. Although this study was carefully controlled in terms of drug dose, it is known that many athletes take doses that exceed the clinically recommended amount. Whether large doses of these over-the-counter products can produce some of the serious side effects seen with standard anabolic steroids is largely unknown.

Detection of androgen usage in athletes can be confirmed by one of several tests, depending on the compound being tested. Other drugs can be used in addition to androgens to enhance performance. These include stimulants, erythropoietin, growth hormone, insulin, and creatine.[10]

Action of the Hypothalamic and Anterior Pituitary Hormones

The hypothalamus and the anterior pituitary gland play an essential role in promoting spermatogenic activity in the testes and maintaining the endocrine function of the testes by means of the gonadotropic hormones. The synthesis and release of the gonadotropic hormones from the pituitary gland are regulated by gonadotropin-releasing hormone (GnRH), which is synthesized by the hypothalamus and secreted into the hypothalamo-hypophysial portal circulation (Fig. 44-7).

Two gonadotropic hormones are secreted by the pituitary gland: FSH and luteinizing hormone (LH). In the male, LH also is called *interstitial cell–stimulating hormone.*

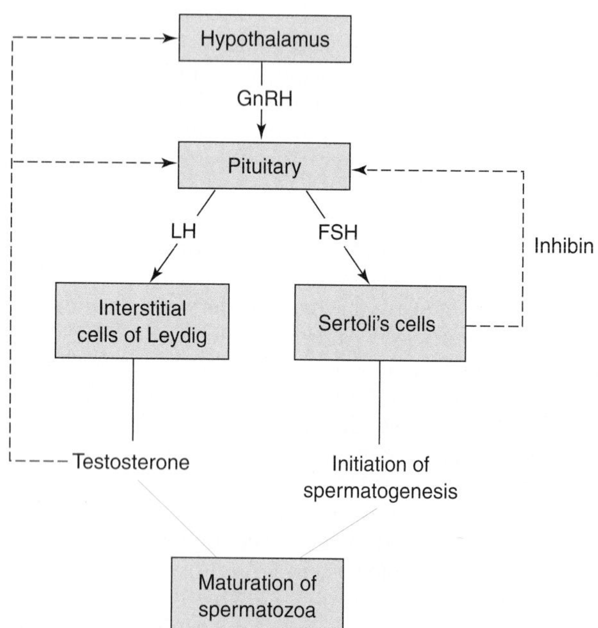

FIGURE 44-7 Hypothalamic–pituitary feedback control of spermatogenesis and testosterone levels in the male. The *dashed line* represents negative feedback.

The production of testosterone by the interstitial cells of Leydig is regulated by LH (see Fig. 44-7). FSH binds selectively to Sertoli's cells surrounding the seminiferous tubules, where it functions in the initiation of spermatogenesis. Under the influence of FSH, Sertoli's cells produce androgen-binding protein, plasminogen activator, and inhibin. Androgen-binding protein binds testosterone and serves as a carrier of testosterone in Sertoli's cells and as a storage site for testosterone. Although FSH is necessary for the initiation of spermatogenesis, full maturation of the spermatozoa requires testosterone (the intratesticular concentration of testosterone is 100-fold greater than serum levels). Androgen-binding protein also serves as a carrier of testosterone from the testes to the epididymis. Plasminogen activator, which converts plasminogen to plasmin, functions in the final detachment of mature spermatozoa from Sertoli's cells.

Circulating levels of the gonadotropic hormones are regulated in a negative feedback manner by testosterone. High levels of testosterone suppress LH secretion through a direct action on the pituitary and an inhibitory effect on the hypothalamus. FSH is thought to be inhibited by a substance called *inhibin,* produced by Sertoli's cells. Inhibin suppresses FSH release from the pituitary gland. The pituitary gonadotropic hormones and Sertoli's cells in the testes form a classic negative feedback loop in which FSH stimulates inhibin and inhibin suppresses FSH.[5,6] Unlike the cyclic hormonal pattern in the female, in the male, FSH, LH, and testosterone secretion and spermatogenesis occur at relatively unchanging rates during adulthood.

Hypogonadism

Androgen deficiency may be suspected by certain clinical features (*e.g.,* fatigue, depression, decreased libido); however, the diagnosis needs confirming by appropriate laboratory testing. A measure of free testosterone (*i.e.,* testosterone not bound [especially to SHBG], and therefore available for binding to, and activating, androgen receptors) is preferred and is low in hypogonadism.

Hypogonadism can be primary (*i.e.,* testicular failure due to problem in testes) or secondary (*i.e.,* failure resulting from lack of stimulation, through gonadotropins [LH and FSH], from the pituitary). Tertiary hypogonadism also occurs and is due to lack of stimulation of LH and FSH secretion from the pituitary as a result of decreased or absent GnRH secretion from the hypothalamus. In men, primary hypogonadism is characterized by low androgens and sperm and results from a lack of negative feedback at the hypothalamic-pituitary level and high gonadotropins (*i.e.,* low testosterone and high LH and FSH). This is termed *hyper*gonadotrophic *hypog*onadism (hyper hypog). Secondary (and tertiary) hypogonadism is characterized by low androgens and sperm and results from a lack of secretion of gonadotropins from the hypothalamic-pituitary level and low gonadotropins (*i.e.,* low testosterone and low LH and FSH). This is termed *hypog*onadotrophic *hypog*onadism (hypog hypog).

The clinical features of male hypogonadism depends on whether the impairment involves only spermatogenesis (FSH increase reflects Sertoli's cell damage) or testosterone secretion is also impaired (LH increase reflects Leydig's cell damage). There are only two clinical manifestations of impaired spermatogenesis: subfertility or infertility and decreased testicular size (80% of testicular size is related to sperm production and 20% to testosterone production). In contrast, there are several possible clinical manifestations of impaired testosterone secretion, which are determined by its time of onset. Onset occurring in the adult includes fatigue; depression; decreased sexual desire and activity; erectile dysfunction (ED); loss of secondary sex characteristics; changes in body composition (including loss of muscle mass, increase in fat mass); osteoporosis; and subfertility or infertility.[7]

Diagnosis of hypogonadism includes two measurements (approximately 20 minutes apart) of free testosterone levels (ideally at 8.00 AM when the testosterone level is at its peak) in the ambulatory male (the two samples may be pooled together for subsequent analysis). If the free testosterone level is low, the LH and FSH levels are measured. Subsequently high LH and FSH levels indicate a primary hypogonadism (hypergonadotrophic hypogonadism); low or inappropriately normal LH and FSH indicate a secondary or tertiary hypogonadism (hypogonadotrophic hypogonadism). Sperm analysis should be considered in both types of hypogonadism. In men with hypogonadotrophic hypogonadism, other pituitary hormones should be assessed and a pituitary magnetic resonance imaging (MRI) study done. In cases of hypergonadotrophic hypogonadism, a karyotype analysis is indicated because Klinefelter's syndrome is the most common chromosomal abnormality associated with male hypogonadism (see Chapter 7). The usual karyotype is 47,XXY, although mosaicism or variants can also present with similar phenotype (the normal male is 46,XY and the normal female is 46,XX). Males with Klinefelter's syndrome characteristically have small, firm testes (unlike many other cases in which the testicular consistency is soft). Other common causes of primary hypogonadism are listed in Chart 44-2.

Treatment of androgen deficiency with testosterone should only be administered to men who are hypogonadal, as evidenced by a distinctly subnormal serum testosterone concentration. The principal goal of testosterone therapy is to restore the serum testosterone concentration to the normal range.

In summary, the function of the male reproductive system is under the negative feedback control of the hypothalamus and the anterior pituitary gonadotropic hormones FSH and LH. Spermatogenesis is initiated by FSH, and the production of testosterone is regulated by LH. Testosterone, the major male sex hormone, is produced by the interstitial Leydig's cells in the testes. In addition to its role in the differentiation of the internal and external genitalia in the male embryo, testosterone is essential for the development of secondary male characteristics during puberty, the maintenance of these characteristics during adult life, and spermatozoa maturation. Hypogonadism can be classified into primary (gonadal problem), secondary (pituitary problem), or tertiary (hypothalamic problem).

CHART 44-2

Common Causes of Primary Gonadal Failure

Chromosomal abnormalities (*e.g.,* Klinefelter's syndrome)
Disorders of androgen biosynthesis
Cryptorchidism
Alkylating and antineoplastic agents
Other medications (*e.g.,* ketoconazole and glucocorticoids)
Infections—mumps orchitis (gonadal failure is a much more common manifestation when mumps occurs after puberty)
Radiation (direct and indirect testicular radiation)
Environmental toxins
Trauma
Testicular torsion
Autoimmune damage
Chronic systemic diseases (many of these can result in both primary and secondary hypogonadism, *e.g.,* cirrhosis, hemochromatosis, chronic renal failure, and AIDS)
Idiopathic

Neural Control of Sexual Function and Aging Changes

After completing this section of the chapter, you should be able to meet the following objectives:

- Describe the autonomic nervous system control of erection, emission, and ejaculation
- Describe changes in the male reproductive system that occur with aging

In the male, the stages of the sexual act involve erection, emission, ejaculation, and detumescence. The physiology of the sexual act involves a complex interaction between spinal cord reflexes, higher neural centers, the vascular system, and the endocrine system.

NEURAL CONTROL

The most important source of impulse stimulation for initiating the male sexual act is the glans penis, which contains a highly organized sensory system. Afferent impulses from sensory receptors in the glans penis pass through the pudendal nerve to ascending fibers in the spinal cord by way of the sacral plexus. Stimulation of other perineal areas, such as the anal epithelium, the scrotum, and the testes, can transmit signals to higher brain centers, such as the limbic system and cerebral cortex, through the cord, adding to sexual satisfaction.

The psychic element to sexual stimulation, such as thinking sexual thoughts, can cause erection and ejaculation. Although psychic involvement and higher-center functions contribute to the sex act, they are not necessary for sexual performance. Genital stimulation can produce erection and ejaculation in some men with complete transection of the spinal cord (see Chapter 51).

Erection involves the shunting of blood into the corpus cavernosum. It is controlled by the sympathetic, parasympathetic, and nonsympathetic-nonparasympathetic systems. Nitric oxide is the locally released nonsympathetic-nonparasympathetic mediator that produces relaxation of vascular smooth muscle. In the flaccid or detumescent state, sympathetic discharge through α-adrenergic receptors maintains contraction of the arteries that supply the penis and vascular sinuses of the corpora cavernosa and corpus spongiosum (Fig. 44-8). Parasympathetic stimulation produces erection by inhibiting sympathetic neurons that cause detumescence and by stimulating the release of nitric oxide to effect a rapid relaxation of the smooth muscle in the sinusoidal spaces of the corpus cavernosum. During sexual stimulation, parasympathetic impulses also cause the urethral and bulbourethral glands to secrete mucus to aid in lubrication. Parasympathetic innervation is effected through the pelvic nerve and sacral segments of the spinal cord. Sympathetic innervation exits the spinal cord at the L1 and L2 levels. Erectile dysfunction can be caused by disease or dysfunction of the brain, spinal cord, cavernous or pudendal nerves, or terminal nerve endings or receptors[11–13] (see Chapter 45).

Emission and ejaculation, which constitute the culmination of the male sexual act, are a function of the sympathetic nervous system. As with erection, emission and ejaculation are mediated through spinal cord reflexes. With increasing intensity of the sexual stimulus, reflex centers of the spinal cord begin to emit sympathetic impulses that leave the cord at the L1 and L2 level and pass through the hypogastric plexus to the genital organs to initiate emission, which is the forerunner of ejaculation. Emission causes the sperm to move from the epididymis to the urethra. Efferent impulses from the spinal cord produce contraction of smooth muscle in the vas deferens and ampulla that move sperm forward and close the internal urethral sphincter to prevent retrograde ejaculation into the bladder.

Ejaculation represents the expulsion of the sperm from the urethra. It involves contraction of the seminal vesicles and prostate gland, which add fluid to the ejaculate and propel it forward. Ejaculation is accompanied by contraction of the ischiocavernous and bulbocavernous muscles at the base of the penis. The filling of the internal urethra elicits signals that are transmitted through the pudendal nerves from the spinal cord, giving the sudden feeling of fullness of genital organs. Rhythmic increases in pressure in the urethra cause the semen to be propelled to the exterior, resulting in ejaculation. At the same time, rhythmic contractions of the pelvic and trunk muscles produce thrusting movements of the pelvis and penis, which help propel the ejaculate into the vagina.

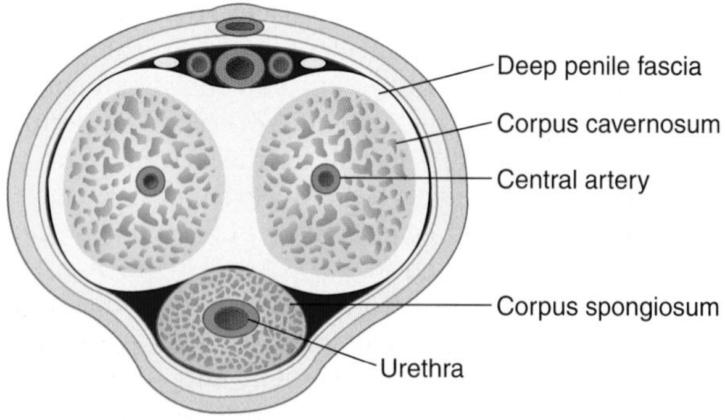

FIGURE 44-8 Erectile tissue of the penis.

The period of emission and ejaculation is called *male orgasm*. After ejaculation, erection ceases within 1 to 2 minutes. A man usually ejaculates approximately 2 to 5 mL of semen. The ejaculate may vary with frequency of intercourse. It is less with frequent ejaculation and may increase two to four times its normal amount during periods of abstinence. The semen that is ejaculated is 98% fluid and approximately 2% sperm.

The role of circulating androgens in sexual function remains unclear.[11–13] It is apparent that sexual desire and performance depend on some threshold level of testosterone; however, this level varies from man to man. Studies of hypogonadal and castrated men show a variety of sexual behavior, ranging from complete loss of libido to normal sexual activity. It may be that the role of testosterone in male sexuality is in the area of sexual interest and motivation, with individual intrapsychic factors playing a significant role.

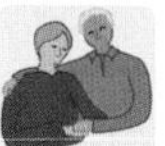

AGING CHANGES

Like other body systems, the male reproductive system undergoes degenerative changes as a result of the aging process; it becomes less efficient with age. The declining physiologic efficiency of male reproductive function occurs gradually and involves the endocrine, circulatory, and neuromuscular systems. Compared with the marked physiologic change in aging females, the changes in the aging male are more gradual and less drastic. Gonadal and reproductive failure usually are not related directly to age because a man remains fertile into advanced age; 80- and 90-year-old men have been known to father children.

As the male ages, his reproductive system becomes measurably different in structure and function from that of the younger male. Male sex hormone levels, particularly of testosterone, decrease with age, with the decline starting later on the average than in women. The term *andropause* has been used to describe an ill-defined collection of symptoms in aging men, typically those older than 50 years, who have a relative or absolute hypogonadism associated with aging.[5–7,14,15] The existence and significance of andropause has important public health implications given that there are currently approximately 35 million American men over the age of 65 years, with the number expected to double over the next 30 years. One study reported a prevalence of hypogonadism (defined as serum testosterone <325 ng/dL [normal is between 300 and 1000 ng/dL]) in each decade as follows: 12% of men in their 50s, 19% in their 60s, 28% in their 70s, and 49% of men in their 80s.[16] This number increases dramatically if a measure of free testosterone is used: 9%, 34%, 68%, and 91% of men in their 50s, 60s, 70s, and 80s, respectively, had hypogonadism.[16]

The sex hormones play a part in the structure and function of the reproductive system and other body systems from conception to old age; they affect protein synthesis, salt and water balance, bone growth, and cardiovascular function (with low testosterone levels having adverse effects on atherosclerosis and possibly explaining the higher incidence of heart disease in men).[17] Decreasing levels of testosterone affect sexual energy, muscle strength, and the genital tissues. The testes become smaller and lose their firmness. The seminiferous tubules, which produce spermatozoa, thicken and begin a degenerative process that finally inhibits sperm production, resulting in a decrease of viable spermatozoa. The prostate gland enlarges, and its contractions become weaker. The force of ejaculation decreases because of a reduction in the volume and viscosity of the seminal fluid. The seminal vesicle changes little from childhood to puberty. The pubertal increases in the fluid capacity of the gland remain throughout adulthood and decline after 60 years of age. After age 60 years, the walls of the seminal vesicles thin, the epithelium decreases, and the muscle layer is replaced by connective tissue. Age-related changes in the penis consist of fibrotic changes in the trabeculae in the corpus spongiosum, with progressive sclerotic changes in arteries and veins. Sclerotic changes also follow in the corpora cavernosa, with the condition becoming generalized in 55- to 60-year-old men.

As a sexual partner, the aging male exhibits some differences in responsiveness and activity from his younger counterpart. Masters and Johnson studied the significant aging changes in the physiology of the sex act.[18] They observed that frequency of intercourse, intensity of sensation, speed of attaining erection, and force of ejaculation are all reduced.

Erectile dysfunction (ED; see Chapter 45) in the elderly male often is directly related to the general physical condition of the person.[11–13] ED has largely replaced the term "impotence." It is defined as the persistent inability to achieve and maintain an erection sufficient to permit satisfactory sexual intercourse. It has been estimated that the disorder affects up to 30 million men in the United States. Aging is a major etiologic factor in this condition. However, even among younger men (those in their 40s), nearly 40% report at least occasional difficulty obtaining or maintaining an erection. This figure approaches 70% in 70-year-olds. However, men older than the age of 50 years are less likely to suffer from ED if they avoid cigarettes, junk food, and TV—and spend more time at the gym![19] In a large study of 31,742 men aged 50 to 93 with no history of prostate cancer, 33% overall reported ED in the past 3 months. That number increased steadily with age: 26% of men aged 50 to 59, 40% aged 60 to 69, and 61% older than 70 reported ED. Men who were most physically active (3 hours of running per week or the equivalent) had a 30% lower risk for ED when compared with men who reported little or no physical activity. Conversely, watching more than 20 hours per week of TV, smoking, and being overweight were associated with increased risk for ED.[19]

Diseases that accompany aging can have direct bearing on male reproductive function. Various cardiovascular, respiratory, hormonal, neurologic, and hematologic disorders can be responsible for secondary impotence. For example, vascular disease affects male potency because it may impair blood flow to the pudendal arteries or their tributaries, resulting in loss of blood volume with subsequent poor distention of the vascular spaces of erectile tissue. Other diseases affecting potency include hypertension, diabetes, cardiac disease, and malignancies of the reproductive organs. In addition, certain medications can have an effect on sexual function.

One of the greatest inhibitors of sexual functioning in older men is the loss of self-esteem and the development of a negative self-image. The emphasis on youth pervades much of our society. The image of success for a man often involves qualities of masculinity and sexual attractiveness. When queried about success, men often mention such things as work, managing money well, participating in sports or other activities, discussing politics or world events, advising younger persons, and being attractive to women. When a man feels good about himself and expresses self-confidence, sexual attractiveness is communicated regardless of age. Many older men live in environments that are not sensitive to the importance of helping them maintain a positive self-image. Premature cessation of the aforementioned esteem-building activities can contribute to loss of libido and zest for life in the elderly man.

Testosterone and other synthetic androgens may be used in older males with low androgen levels to improve muscle strength and vigor. Preliminary studies of androgen replacement in aging males with low androgen levels show an increase in lean body mass and a decrease in bone turnover. Before testosterone replacement therapy is initiated, all men should be screened for prostate cancer. Testosterone is available as an injectable form that is administered every 2 to 3 weeks, or as a transdermal patch or gel. Side effects of replacement therapy may include acne, gynecomastia, and reduced HDL levels. Replacement therapy also may contribute to a worsening of sleep apnea in men who are troubled by this problem.[5–8]

At the present time, it is not recommended that routine treatment of elderly men with testosterone should be undertaken. A trial of testosterone administration, however, might be warranted in an elderly man whose serum testosterone concentration is less than 200 ng/dL and who has manifestations of testosterone deficiency.[15] If treatment is undertaken, the man should be screened before treatment and monitored during therapy for evidence of testosterone-dependent diseases.

In summary, the sex act involves erection, emission, ejaculation, and detumescence. The physiology of these functions involves a complex interaction among autonomic-mediated spinal cord reflexes, higher neural centers, and the vascular system. Erection is mediated by the parasympathetic nervous system, and emission and ejaculation by the sympathetic nervous system. Like other body systems, the male reproductive system undergoes changes as a result of the aging process. The changes occur gradually and involve parallel changes in endocrine, circulatory, and neuromuscular function. Testosterone levels decrease (andropause), the size and firmness of the testes decrease, sperm production declines, and the prostate gland enlarges. There usually is a decrease in frequency of intercourse, intensity of sensation, speed of attaining erection, and force of ejaculation. However, sexual thought, interest, and activity usually continue into old age.

REVIEW EXERCISES

In the absence of the *SRY* gene on the Y chromosome, a developing embryo with an XY genotype will develop female genitalia.

A. Explain.

Men who have had a vasectomy remain fertile for 4 to 5 weeks after the procedure has been done.

A. Explain.

A 55-year-old man presents with various vague symptoms (fatigue, depression). On examination, he is noted to have small soft testes (8 mL bilaterally), marked gynecomastia, and scanty body hair. He is obese at 122 kg with a body mass index (BMI) of 34.2. Investigations reveal a low free testosterone level and elevated gonadotropins (LH and FSH).

A. What is the endocrine diagnosis related to his phenotypic and biochemical manifestations?

B. What other clinical features are associated with this diagnosis?

References

1. Conte F.A., Grumbach M.M. (2004). Abnormalities of sexual determination and differentiation. In Greenspan F.S., Gardner D.G. (Eds.), *Basic and clinical endocrinology* (7th ed., pp. 564–607). New York: Lange Medical Books/McGraw-Hill.
2. Tanglio E.A. (2000). Embryology of the genitourinary system. In Tanagho E.A., McAnnich J.W. (Eds.), *Smith's general urology* (15th ed., pp. 17–28). New York: Lange Medical Books/McGraw-Hill.
3. Moore K.L., Persaud T.V.N. (1998). *The developing human: Clinically oriented embryology* (6th ed., pp. 323–330). Philadelphia: W.B. Saunders.
4. Guyton A.C., Hall J. (2000). *Textbook of medical physiology* (10th ed., pp. 916–928). Philadelphia: W.B. Saunders.
5. Griffin J.E., Wilson J.D. (2003). Disorders of the testes and the male reproductive tract. In Larsen P.R., Kronenberg H.M., Melmed S., et al. (Eds.), *Williams textbook of endocrinology* (10th ed., pp. 2143–2154). Philadelphia: W.B. Saunders.
6. Braunstein G.D. (2004). Testes. In Greenspan F.S., Gardner D.G. (Eds.), *Basic and clinical endocrinology* (7th ed., pp. 478–510). New York: Lange Medical Books/McGraw-Hill.
7. AACE Hypogonadism Taskforce (2002). AACE medical guidelines for clinical practice for the evaluation and treatment of hypogonadism in adult male patients—2002 update. *Endocrine Practice 8,* 439–456.
8. Bagatell C.J., Bremner W.J. (1996). Androgens in men: Uses and abuses. *New England Journal of Medicine 334,* 707–714.
9. King D.S., Sharp R.L., Vukovich M.D., et al. (1999). Effect of oral androstenedione on serum testosterone and adaptations to resistance training in young men. *Journal of the American Medical Association 281,* 202–228.
10. Jenkins P. (2002). Doping in sport. *Lancet 360,* 99–100.
11. Lue T.F. (2000). Erectile dysfunction. *New England Journal of Medicine 342,* 1802–1813.
12. AACE Male Sexual Dysfunction Taskforce (2003). AACE medical guidelines for clinical practice for the evaluation and treatment of male sexual dysfunction: A couple's problem—2003 update. *Endocrine Practice 9,* 77–95.
13. Matfin G. (2003). Erectile dysfunction. *Sexuality, Reproduction and Menopause 1,* 40–45.
14. Muller M., Grobbee D.E., Thijssen J.H.H., et al. (2003). Sex hormones and male health: Effects on components of the frailty syndrome. *Trends in Endocrinology and Metabolism 14,* 289–296.
15. Yialamas M.A., Hayes F.J. (2003). Androgens and the aging male. *Endocrinology Rounds 2,* 1–6. [On-line.] Available: www.endocrinologyrounds.org.
16. Harman S.M., Metter E.J., Tobin J., et al. (2001). Longitudinal effects of aging on serum total and free testosterone levels in healthy men. *Journal of Clinical Endocrinology and Metabolism 86,* 724–731.
17. Channer K.S., Jones T.H. (2003). Cardiovascular effects of testosterone: Implications of the 'male menopause'? *Heart 89,* 121–122.
18. Masters W.H., Johnson V. (1970). *Human sexual inadequacy* (pp. 337–338). Boston: Little, Brown.
19. Bacon C.G., Mittleman M.A., Kawachi I., et al. (2003). Sexual function in men older than 50 years of age: Results from the Health Professionals follow-up study. *Annals of Internal Medicine 139,* 161–168.

CHAPTER

45

Disorders of the Male Genitourinary System

Glenn Matfin

The male genitourinary system is subject to structural defects, inflammation, and neoplasms, all of which can affect urine elimination, sexual function, and fertility. This chapter discusses disorders of the penis, the scrotum and testes, and the prostate.

Disorders of the Penis

After completing this section of the chapter, you should be able to meet the following objectives:

- State the difference between hypospadias and epispadias
- Cite the significance of phimosis
- Describe the anatomic changes that occur with Peyronie's disease
- Explain the physiology of penile erection and relate it to erectile dysfunction and priapism
- Describe the appearance of balanitis xerotica obliterans
- List the signs of penile cancer

The penis is the external male genital organ through which the urethra passes to the exterior of the body. It is involved in urinary and sexual function. Disorders of the penis include congenital and acquired defects, inflammatory conditions, and neoplasms.

CONGENITAL AND ACQUIRED DISORDERS

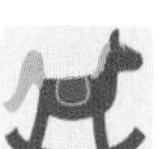

Hypospadias and Epispadias

Hypospadias and epispadias are congenital disorders of the penis resulting from embryologic defects in the development of the urethral groove and penile urethra (Fig. 45-1). In hypospadias, which affects approximately 1 in 300 male infants, the termination of the urethra is on the ventral surface of the penis.[1–3] It is common to categorize hypospadias as glandular (involving the glans penis), penile, or perineoscrotal. The etiology in most cases is unknown; however, known causes (single-gene defects, chromosomal abnormalities, and maternal progestational drug ingestion in early pregnancy) account for only about one fourth of cases. The testes are undescended in 10% of boys born with hypospadias and chordee (*i.e.,* ventral bowing of the penis), and inguinal hernia also may accompany the disorder. In the newborn with severe hypospadias and cryptorchidism

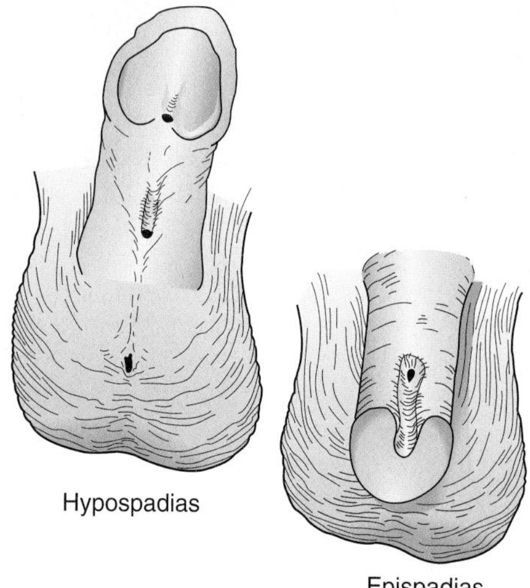

FIGURE 45-1 Hypospadias and epispadias.

(undescended testes), the differential diagnosis should consider ambiguous genitalia and masculinization that is seen in females with congenital adrenal hyperplasia (see Chapter 42). Because many chromosomal aberrations result in ambiguity of the external genitalia, chromosomal studies often are recommended for male infants with hypospadias and cryptorchidism.[1]

Surgery is the treatment of choice for hypospadias.[1] Circumcision is avoided because the foreskin is used for surgical repair. Factors that influence the timing of surgical repair include anesthetic risk, penile size, and the psychological effects of the surgery on the child. In mild cases, the surgery is done for cosmetic reasons only. In more severe cases, repair becomes essential for normal sexual functioning and to prevent the psychological sequelae of having malformed genitalia. In contrast to the practices of several decades ago, when surgical repair often was delayed until the child was 2 to 6 years of age, surgical repair is now done between the ages of 6 and 12 months.

Epispadias, in which the opening of the urethra is on the dorsal surface of the penis, is a less common defect. Although epispadias may occur as a separate entity, it often is associated with exstrophy of the bladder, a condition in which the abdominal wall fails to cover the bladder. The treatment depends on the extent of the developmental defect.

Phimosis and Paraphimosis

Phimosis refers to a tightening of the prepuce or penile foreskin that prevents its retraction over the glans. Embryologically, the foreskin begins to develop during the eighth week of gestation as a fold of skin at the distal edge of the penis that eventually grows forward over the base of the glans.[2] By the 16th week of gestation, the prepuce and the glans are adherent. Only a small percentage of newborns have a fully retractable foreskin. With growth, a space develops between the glans and foreskin, and by 3 years of age, approximately 90% of male children have retractable foreskins.

Because the foreskin of many boys cannot be fully retracted in early childhood, it is important that the area be cleaned thoroughly. There is no need to retract the foreskin forcibly because this could lead to infection, scarring, or paraphimosis. As the child grows, the foreskin becomes retractable, and the glans and foreskin should be cleaned routinely. If symptomatic phimosis occurs after childhood, it can cause difficulty with voiding or sexual activity. Circumcision is then the treatment of choice. Phimosis is also one of the most important predisposing factors for penile cancer.

In a related condition called *paraphimosis,* the foreskin is so tight and constricted that it cannot cover the glans. A tight foreskin can constrict the blood supply to the glans and lead to ischemia and necrosis. Many cases of paraphimosis result from the foreskin being retracted for an extended period, as in the case of catheterized uncircumcised males.

Balanitis and Balanoposthitis

Balanitis is an acute or chronic inflammation of the glans penis. *Balanoposthitis* refers to inflammation of the glans and prepuce. It usually is encountered in males with phimosis or a large, redundant prepuce that interferes with cleanliness and predisposes to bacterial growth in the accumulated secretions and smegma (*i.e.,* debris from the desquamated epithelia). If left untreated, the condition may cause ulcerations of the mucosal surface of the glans; these ulcerations may lead to inflammatory scarring of the phimosis and further aggravate the condition.

Acute superficial balanoposthitis is characterized by erythema of the glans and prepuce. An exudate in the form of malodorous discharge may be present. Extension of the erythema and edema may result in phimosis. The condition may result from infection, trauma, or irritation. Infective balanoposthitis may be caused by a wide variety of organisms. Chlamydiae and mycoplasmas have been identified as causative organisms in this disease. Gonococcal balanitis may develop as a complication of infection in uncircumcised men. The inflammatory reaction is nonspecific, and correct identification of the specific agent requires microbial smears and cultures.

Balanitis due to candidal infection may be a presenting feature or result from poorly controlled diabetes mellitus. Noninfectious causes of balanitis also occur. These include circinate balanitis, which is seen in reactive arthritis (see Chapter 59). Lesions are superficial, painless ulcers that heal without scarring.

Balanitis xerotica obliterans is a chronic, sclerosing, atrophic process of the glans penis that occurs in uncircumcised males. It is clinically and histologically similar to the lichen sclerosus that is seen in females. Typically, the lesions consist of whitish plaques on the surface of the glans penis and the prepuce. The foreskin is thickened and fibrous and is not retractable. Although balanitis xerotica obliterans is considered a benign condition, it has been associated with several reports of penile cancer and is now recognized as a precancerous state. Treatment measures include circumcision and topical or intralesional injections of corticosteroids.[4]

Spermatocele

A spermatocele is a painless, sperm-containing cyst that forms at the end of the epididymis. It is located above and posterior to the testis, is attached to the epididymis, and is separate from the testes. Spermatoceles may be solitary or multiple and usually are less than 1 cm in diameter. They are freely movable and should transilluminate. Spermatoceles rarely cause problems, but a large one may become painful and require excision.

Varicocele

A varicocele is characterized by varicosities of the pampiniform plexus, a network of veins supplying the testes (see Fig. 45-5). The left side is more commonly affected (85% to 95%) because the left internal spermatic vein inserts into the left renal vein at a right angle, whereas the right spermatic vein usually enters the inferior vena cava. Incompetent valves are more common in the left internal spermatic veins, causing a reflux of blood back into the veins of the pampiniform plexus. The force of gravity resulting from the upright position also contributes to venous dilatation. If the condition persists, there may be damage to the elastic fibers and hypertrophy of the vein walls, as occurs in formation of varicose veins in the leg. Sperm concentration and motility are decreased in 65% to 75% of men with varicocele.[24]

Varicoceles rarely are found before puberty, and the incidence is highest in men between 15 and 35 years of age. Symptoms of varicocele include an abnormal feeling of heaviness in the left scrotum, although many varicoceles are asymptomatic. Usually, the varicocele is readily diagnosed on physical examination with the patient in the standing and recumbent positions. Typically, the varicocele disappears in the lying position because of venous decompression into the renal vein. Scrotal palpation of a varicocele has been compared to feeling a "bag of worms." Small varicoceles sometimes are difficult to identify. Valsalva's maneuver (*i.e.,* forced expiration against a closed glottis) may be used to accentuate small varicosities.[24] A handheld Doppler stethoscope is used while the patient performs Valsalva's maneuver. If the varicocele is present, a distinct venous rush is heard because of the sudden occurrence of retrograde blood flow. Other diagnostic aids include real-time ultrasonography, radioisotope scanning, spermatic venography, and scrotopenography.

Treatment options include surgical ligation or sclerosis using a percutaneous transvenous catheter under fluoroscopic guidance. Both can be performed as outpatient procedures. The benefits of the percutaneous technique include a slightly lower recurrence rate and more rapid return to full physical activity. It has been suggested that men with abnormalities in their semen and a varicocele show some degree of improvement in fertility after obliteration of the dilated veins.[24,25] However, the effectiveness of varicocele treatment in men from subfertile couples is still debated, especially when other assisted reproductive techniques (*e.g.,* intracytoplasmic sperm injection [ICSI]) may be effective with as few as 20 sperm[25] (see Chapter 47). Aside from improving fertility, other reasons for surgery include the relief of the sensation of heaviness and cosmetic improvement.

Testicular Torsion

Testicular torsion is a twisting of the spermatic cord that suspends the testis (Fig. 45-6). It is the most common acute scrotal disorder in the pediatric and young adult population. Testicular torsion can be divided into two distinct clinical entities, depending on the level of spermatic cord involvement: extravaginal and intravaginal torsion.[22,26]

Extravaginal torsion, which occurs almost exclusively in neonates, is the less common form of testicular torsion.[22] It occurs when the testicle and the fascial tunicae that surround it rotate around the spermatic cord at a level well above the tunica vaginalis. The torsion probably occurs during fetal or neonatal descent of the testes before the tunica adheres to the scrotal wall. At birth or shortly thereafter, a firm, smooth, painless scrotal mass is identified. The scrotal skin appears red, and some edema is present. Differential diagnosis is relatively easy because testicular tumors, epididymitis, and orchitis are exceedingly rare in neonates; a hydrocele is softer and can be transilluminated, and physical examination can exclude the presence of hernia. The use of surgical treatment (orchiopexy and orchiectomy) is controversial. There are multiple animal studies indicating that failure to remove the torsed testes may produce an autoimmune response that affects the normal testis.[22,26]

Intravaginal torsion is considerably more common than extravaginal torsion. It occurs when the testis rotates on the long axis in the tunica vaginalis. In most cases, congenital abnormalities of the tunica vaginalis or spermatic cord exist. The tunica vaginalis normally surrounds the testes and epididymis, allowing the testicle to rotate freely in the tunica. Although anomalies of suspension vary, the epididymal attachment may be loose enough to permit torsion between the testis and the epididymis. More commonly, the testis rotates around the distal spermatic cord. Because this abnormality is developmental, bilateral anomalies are common.

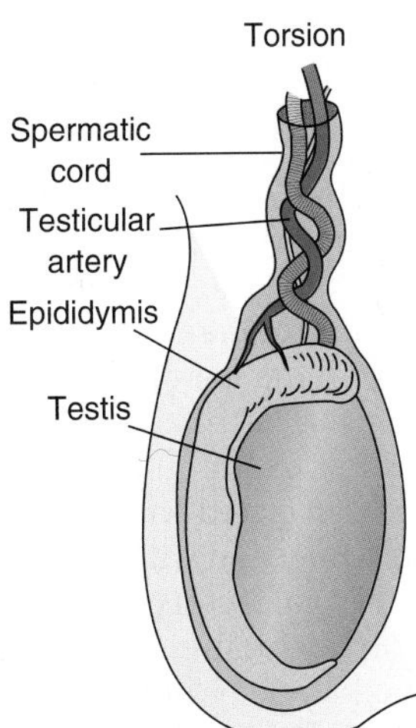

FIGURE 45-6 Testicular torsion with twisting of the spermatic cord that suspends the testis and the spermatic vessels that supply the testis with blood.

Intravaginal torsion occurs most frequently between the ages of 8 and 18 years and rarely is seen after 30 years of age. Patients usually present in severe distress within hours of onset and often have nausea, vomiting, and tachycardia. The affected testis is large and tender, with pain radiating to the inguinal area. Extensive cremaster muscle contraction causes a thickening of the spermatic cord.

Testicular torsion must be differentiated from epididymitis, orchitis, and trauma to the testis. On physical examination, the testicle often is high in the scrotum and in an abnormal orientation. These changes are caused by the twisting and shortening of the spermatic cord. The degree of scrotal swelling and redness depends on the duration of symptoms. The testes are firm and tender. The cremasteric reflex, normally elicited by stroking the medial aspect of the thigh and observing testicular retraction, frequently is absent.[26] Color Doppler ultrasonography is increasingly used in the evaluation of suspected testicular torsion.[24,26]

Intravaginal testicular torsion is a true surgical emergency, and early recognition and treatment are necessary if the testicle is to be saved. Detorsion within six hours usually results in 100% viability of the testicle; this decreases to 20% at 12 hours and to 0% at 24 hours.[22] Treatment includes surgical detorsion and orchiectomy.[27] Orchiectomy is carried out when the testis is deemed nonviable after surgical detorsion. Testicular salvage rates are directly related to the duration of torsion.[27] Because the opposite testicle usually is affected by the same abnormal attachments, prophylactic fixation of that testis often is performed.

INFECTION AND INFLAMMATION

Epididymitis

Epididymitis is an inflammation of the epididymis, the elongated cordlike structure that lies along the posterior border of the testis, whose function is the storage, transport, and maturation of spermatozoa. There are two major types of epididymitis: sexually transmitted infections associated with urethritis and primary nonsexually transmitted infections associated with urinary tract infections and prostatitis. Most cases of epididymitis are caused by bacterial pathogens.

In primary nonsexual infections, the pressure associated with voiding or physical strain may force pathogen-containing urine from the urethra or prostate up the ejaculatory duct and through the vas deferens and into the epididymis. Infections also may reach the epididymis through the lymphatics of the spermatic cord. In rare cases, organisms from other foci of infection reach the epididymis through the bloodstream. In prepubertal children, the disorder usually is associated with congenital urinary tract abnormalities and infection with gram-negative rods. In postpubertal boys, several factors may predispose to developing epididymitis, including sexual activity, heavy physical exertion, and bicycle or motorcycle riding. Sexually transmitted acute epididymitis occurs mainly in young men without underlying genitourinary disease and is most commonly caused by *Chlamydia trachomatis* and *Neisseria gonorrhoeae* (singly or in combination). In men older than 35 years of age, epididymitis often is associated with pathogens such as *Escherichia coli, Pseudomonas,* and gram-positive cocci.

Epididymitis is characterized by unilateral pain and swelling, accompanied by erythema and edema of the overlying scrotal skin that develops over a period of 24 to 48 hours. Initially, the swelling and induration are limited to the epididymis. However, the distinction between the testis and epididymis becomes less evident as the inflammation progresses, and the testis and epididymis become one mass. In contrast to patients with testicular torsion, patients with epididymitis usually have a normal cremasteric reflex. There may be tenderness over the groin (spermatic cord) or in the lower abdomen. Fever and complaints of dysuria occur in approximately one half of cases. Whether urethral discharge is present depends on the organism causing the infection; it usually accompanies gonorrheal infections, is common in chlamydial infections, and is less common in infections caused by gram-negative organisms.

Laboratory findings usually reveal an elevated white blood cell count. Urinalysis and urine culture are important in the diagnosis of epididymitis, with bacteriuria and pyuria suggestive of the disorder; however, urinalysis may be normal. The cause of epididymitis can be differentiated by Gram's stain examination or culture of a midstream urine specimen or a urethral specimen. If the diagnosis remains uncertain, a Doppler ultrasound may be useful, revealing increased blood flow to the affected testis.

Treatment during the acute phase (which usually lasts for 3 to 4 days) includes bed rest, scrotal elevation and support, and antibiotics.[26] Bed rest with scrotal support improves lymphatic drainage. The choice of antibiotics is determined by age, physical findings, urinalysis, Gram's stain results, cultures, and sexual history.[28] Oral analgesics and antipyretics usually are indicated. Sexual activity or physical strain may exacerbate the infection and worsen the symptoms, and should be avoided. If a sexually transmitted disease is suspected as an etiology, it is important to ensure that the sexual partner receives treatment[28] (see Chapter 48).

Orchitis

Orchitis is an infection of the testes. It can be precipitated by a primary infection in the genitourinary tract or can be spread to testes through the bloodstream or the lymphatics. Epididymitis with subsequent infection of the testis is commonly related to genitourinary tract infections (cystitis, urethritis, genitoprostatitis) that travel to the epididymis and testis through the vas deferens or the lymphatics of the spermatic cord.

Orchitis can develop as a complication of a systemic infection, such as parotitis (*i.e.,* mumps), scarlet fever, or pneumonia. Probably the best known of these complications is orchitis caused by the mumps virus.[29] Mumps orchitis is the most common complication of mumps infection in the postpubertal male, occurring in approximately 20% to 35% of adolescent boys and young men with mumps. The onset of mumps orchitis is sudden; it usually occurs approximately 3 to 4 days after the onset of the parotitis and is characterized by fever, painful enlargement of the testes, and small hemorrhages into the tunica albuginea. Unlike epididymitis, the urinary symptoms are absent. The symptoms usually run their course in 7 to 10 days. Microscopically, an acute inflammatory response is seen in the seminiferous tubules, with proliferation of neutrophils, lymphocytes, and histiocytes causing distention of the tubules. The residual effects seen after the acute phase include hyalinization of the seminiferous tubules and atrophy of the testes (seen in half of affected men). Spermatogenesis is irreversibly impaired in approximately 30% of testes damaged by mumps orchitis. If both testes are involved (which occurs in fewer than 15% of cases), permanent sterility can result, but is rare. Androgenic hormone function is usually maintained in these cases.[29]

NEOPLASMS

Tumors can develop in the scrotum or the testes. Benign scrotal tumors are common and often do not require treatment. Carcinoma of the scrotum is rare and usually is associated with exposure to carcinogenic agents. Almost all solid tumors of the testes are malignant.

Scrotal Cancer

Cancer of the scrotum was the first cancer directly linked to a specific occupation when, in the 1800s, it was associated with chimney sweeps.[30] Studies have linked this cancer to exposure to tar, soot, and oils. Most squamous cell cancers of the scrotum are linked to poor hygiene and chronic inflammation. Exposure to ultraviolet A radiation (*e.g.*, PUVA) or HPV also has been associated with the disease. The mean age of presentation with the disease is 60 years, often preceded by 20 to 30 years of chronic irritation.

In the early stages, cancer of the scrotum may appear as a small tumor or wartlike growth that eventually ulcerates. The thin scrotal wall lacks the tissue reactivity needed to block the malignant process; more than one half of the cases seen involve metastasis to the lymph nodes. Because this tumor does not respond well to chemotherapy or irradiation, the treatment includes wide local excision of the tumor with inguinal and femoral node dissection.[31] Prognosis correlates with lymph node involvement.

Testicular Cancer

Testicular cancer accounts for 1% of all male cancers and 3% of male urogenital cancers. Although relatively rare, it is the most common cause of cancer in the 15- to 35-year-old age group.[17,32,33] In the past, testicular cancer was a leading cause of death among males entering their most productive years. However, since the late 1970s, advances in therapy have transformed an almost invariably fatal disease into one that is highly curable. With the exception of men with advanced metastatic disease at the time of presentation or those who relapse after primary chemotherapy, most men with these tumors are cured with available therapy (>90% of all newly diagnosed patients will be cured). The prognosis and extent of treatment required for testicular cancer are related to the stage of the disease at the time of presentation.

Although the cause of testicular cancer is unknown, several predisposing influences may be important: cryptorchidism, genetic factors, human immunodeficiency virus (HIV) infection, and disorders of testicular development.[20] The strongest association has been with cryptorchid testis. Approximately 10% of testicular tumors are associated with cryptorchidism. The higher the location of the undescended testis, the greater the risk.[22] One fourth of these tumors occur in the contralateral, normally descended testicle—hence the need for regular follow-up of these individuals. Genetic predisposition also appears to be important. Family clustering of the disorder has been described, although a well-defined pattern of inheritance has not been established. An increased incidence of testicular germ cell tumors, particularly seminomas, has been described in HIV-infected men. Men with disorders of testicular development, including those with Klinefelter's syndrome and testicular feminization, have a higher risk for germ cell tumors.

Approximately 95% of malignant tumors arising in the testis are germ cell tumors.[22,33] Germ cell tumors can be classified as seminomas and nonseminomas based on their origin in primordial germ cells and their ability to differentiate in vivo. Because these tumors derive from germ cells in the testis, they are multipotential (able to differentiate into different tissue types) and often secrete polypeptide hormones or enzymes representing earlier stages of development.

Seminomas account for approximately 50% of germ cell tumors and are most frequent in the fourth decade of life.[33] They almost never occur in infants or small children.[22] Seminomas are thought to arise from the seminiferous epithelium of the testes and are the type of germ cell tumor most likely to produce a uniform population of cells.

The nonseminoma tumors include embryonal carcinoma, teratoma, choriocarcinoma, and yolk cell carcinoma derivatives. Nonseminoma tumors usually contain more than one cell type and are less differentiated than seminomas. Embryonal carcinomas are the least differentiated of the tumors, with totipotential capacity to differentiate into other nonseminomatous cell types. They occur most commonly in the 20- to 30-year-old age group. Choriocarcinoma is a rare and highly malignant form of testicular cancer that is identical to tumors that arise in placental tissue. Yolk sac tumors mimic the embryonic yolk sac histologically. They are the most common type of testicular tumors in infants and children up to 3 years of age and in this age group have a very good prognosis.[22] Teratomas are composed of somatic cell types from two or more germ-line layers (ectoderm, mesoderm, or endoderm). They constitute less than 2% to 3% of germ cell tumors and can occur at any age from infancy to old age. They usually behave as benign tumors in children; in adults, they often contain minute foci of cancer cells.

Often, the first sign of testicular cancer is a slight enlargement of the testicle that may be accompanied by some degree of discomfort. This may be an ache in the abdomen or groin or a sensation of dragging or heaviness in the scrotum. Frank pain may be experienced in the later stages, when the tumor is growing rapidly and hemorrhaging occurs. Testicular cancer can spread when the tumor may be barely palpable. The presenting manifestations of testicular cancer can be attributed to metastasis in approximately 10% of cases. Signs of metastatic spread include swelling of the lower extremities, back pain, neck mass, cough, hemoptysis, or dizziness. Gynecomastia (breast enlargement) may result from human chorionic gonadotropin (hCG)-producing tumors and occurs in about 5% of men with germ cell tumors.

Early diagnosis of testicular cancer is important because a delay in seeking medical attention often results in presentation with a later stage of the disease and decreased treatment effectiveness. Recognition of the importance of prompt diagnosis and treatment has resulted in the development of a procedure for testicular self-examination and an emphasis on public education programs about this type of cancer. The American Cancer Society strongly advocates that every young adult male examine his testes at least once each month as a means of early detection of testicular cancer. The examination should be done after a warm bath or shower, when the scrotal skin is relaxed. To do this self-examination, each testicle is examined with the fingers of both hands by rolling the testicle between the thumb and fingers to check for the presence of any lumps. If any lump, nodule, or enlargement is noted, it should be brought immediately to the attention of a physician.

The diagnosis of testicular cancer requires a thorough urologic history and physical examination. A painless testicular mass may be cancer. Conditions that produce an intrascrotal mass similar to testicular cancer include epididymitis, orchitis, hydrocele, or hematocele. The examination for masses should include palpation of the testes and surrounding structures, transillumination of the scrotum, and abdominal palpation. Testicular ultrasonography can be used to differentiate testicular masses. The intravenous pyelogram may be used to evaluate kidney structure. CT scans and MRI are used in assessing metastatic spread.

Tumor markers, assayed by immunoassay methods that measure protein antigens produced by malignant cells, provide information about the existence of a tumor and the type of tumor present. These markers may detect tumors that are too small to be found on physical examination or radiographs. Three tumor markers are useful in evaluating the tumor response: α-fetoprotein, a glycoprotein that normally is present in fetal serum in large amounts; hCG, a hormone that normally is produced by the placenta in pregnant women; and lactate dehydrogenase (LDH), a cellular enzyme normally found in muscle, liver, kidney, and brain. During embryonic development, the totipotential germ cells of the testes travel down normal differentiation pathways and produce different protein products. The reappearance of these protein markers in the adult suggests activity of the undifferentiated cells in a testicular germ cell tumor.

The clinical staging (TNM classification) for testicular cancer is as follows: stage I, tumor confined to testes, epididymis, or spermatic cord; stage II, tumor spread to retroperitoneal lymph nodes below the diaphragm; and stage III, metastases outside the retroperitoneal nodes or above the diaphragm (see Chapter 8). Staging procedures include CT scans of the chest, abdomen, and pelvis; ultrasonography for detection of bulky inferior nodal metastases; and occasionally lymphangiography. Radiographic methods are used to detect metastatic spread.

The basic treatment of all testicular cancers includes orchiectomy, which is done at the time of diagnostic exploration. The widely used surgical procedure is the unilateral radical orchiectomy through an inguinal incision. Surgical therapy is advantageous because it enables precise staging of the disease. Recommendations for further therapy (*e.g.*, retroperitoneal lymph node dissection, chemotherapy, radiation therapy) are based on the pathologic findings from the surgical procedure.

Treatment after orchiectomy depends on the histologic characteristics of the tumor and the clinical stage of the disease. Seminomas are highly radiosensitive; the treatment of stage I or II seminoma is irradiation of the retroperitoneal and homolateral lymph nodes to the level of the diaphragm. Patients with bulky retroperitoneal or distant metastases often are treated with multiagent chemotherapy. Seminoma is probably the most curable of all solid tumors. Men with nonseminomatous tumors usually are managed with observation, chemotherapy, or retroperitoneal lymph node dissection. Rigorous follow-up in all men with testicular cancer is necessary to detect recurrences, most of which occur within 2 years after the end of treatment.[32,33] Testicular cancer is a disease in which even recurrence is highly treatable. With appropriate treatment, the prognosis for men with testicular cancer is excellent. The 5-year survival rate for patients with stage I and II disease exceeds 95%.[32,33] Even patients with more advanced disease have excellent chances for long-term survival. Patients subsequently cured of testicular cancer are also at increased risk for the development of other cancers later in life.[32]

Therapy for testicular cancer can have potentially adverse effects on sexual functioning. Men who have retroperitoneal lymph node dissection may experience retrograde ejaculation or failure to ejaculate because of severing of the sympathetic plexus. Infertility may result from retrograde ejaculation or as a result of retroperitoneal lymph node dissection or the toxic effects of chemotherapy or radiotherapy on the germ cells in the remaining testis.[32,33] Sperm banking should be considered for men undergoing these treatments.

In summary, disorders of the scrotum and testes include cryptorchidism (*i.e.,* undescended testicles), hydrocele, hematocele, spermatocele, varicocele, and testicular torsion. Inflammatory conditions can involve the scrotal sac, epididymis, or testes. Tumors can arise in the scrotum or the testes. Scrotal cancers usually are associated with exposure to petroleum products such as tar, pitch, and soot. Testicular cancers account for 1% of all male cancers and 3% of cancers of the male genitourinary system. With current treatment methods, a large percentage of men with these tumors can be cured. Testicular self-examination is recommended as a means of early detection of this form of cancer.

Disorders of the Prostate

After completing this section of the chapter, you should be able to meet the following objectives:

- Compare the pathology and symptoms of acute bacterial prostatitis, chronic bacterial prostatitis, and chronic prostatitis/pelvic pain syndrome.
- Describe the urologic manifestations and treatment of benign prostatic hyperplasia
- List the methods used in the diagnosis and treatment of prostatic cancer

The prostate is a firm, glandular structure that surrounds the urethra. It produces a thin, milky, alkaline secretion that aids sperm motility by helping to maintain an optimum pH. The contraction of the smooth muscle in the gland promotes semen expulsion during ejaculation.

INFECTION AND INFLAMMATION

Prostatitis refers to a variety of inflammatory disorders of the prostate gland, some bacterial and some not. It may occur spontaneously, as a result of catheterization or instrumentation, or secondary to other diseases of the male genitourinary system. As an outcome of 1995 and 1998 consensus conferences, the National Institutes of Health has established a classification system with four categories of prostatitis syndromes: acute bacterial prostatitis, chronic bacterial prostatitis, chronic prostatitis/pelvic pain syndrome, and asymptomatic inflammatory prostatitis.[34] Men with asymptomatic inflammatory prostatitis have no subjective symptoms and are detected incidentally on biopsy or examination of prostatic fluid.

One U.S.-based community study (58,955 visits by men >18 years of age to office-based physicians) estimated that 9% of men have a diagnosis of chronic prostatitis at any one time.[35]

Acute Bacterial Prostatitis

Acute bacterial prostatitis often is considered a subtype of urinary tract infection. The most likely etiology of acute bacterial prostatitis is an ascending urethral infection or reflux of infected urine into the prostatic ducts. The most common organism is *E. coli.* Other frequently found species include *Pseudomonas, Klebsiella,* and *Proteus.* Less frequently, the infection is caused by *Staphylococcus aureus, Streptococcus faecalis, Chlamydia* species, or anaerobes such as *Bacteroides* species. [36,37]

The manifestations of acute bacterial prostatitis include fever and chills, malaise, myalgia, arthralgia, frequent and urgent urination, dysuria, and urethral discharge. Dull, aching pain often is present in the perineum, rectum, or sacrococcygeal region. The urine may be cloudy and malodorous because of urinary tract infection. Rectal examination reveals a swollen, tender, warm prostate with scattered soft areas. Prostatic massage produces a thick discharge with white blood cells that grows large numbers of pathogens on culture.

Treatment of acute bacterial prostatitis depends on the severity of symptoms. It usually includes antibiotics, bed rest, adequate hydration, antipyretics, analgesics (often narcotics) or spasmolytic drugs to alleviate pain, and stool softeners. Men who are extremely ill, such as those with sepsis, may require hospitalization. A suprapubic catheter may be indicated if voiding is difficult or painful.

Acute prostatitis usually responds to appropriate antimicrobial therapy chosen in accordance with the sensitivity of the causative agents in the urethral discharge. Depending on the urine culture results, antibiotic therapy usually is continued for at least 4 weeks. Because acute prostatitis often is associated with anatomic abnormalities, a thorough urologic examination usually is performed after treatment is completed.

A persistent fever indicates the need for further investigation for an additional site of infection or a prostatic abscess. CT scans and transrectal ultrasonography of the prostate are useful in the diagnosis of prostatic abscesses. Prostatic abscesses, which are relatively uncommon since the advent of effective antibiotic therapy, are found more commonly in males with diabetes mellitus. Because prostatic abscesses usually are associated with bacteremia, prompt drainage by transperitoneal or transurethral incision followed by appropriate antimicrobial therapy usually is indicated.[36]

Chronic Bacterial Prostatitis

In contrast to acute bacterial prostatitis, chronic bacterial prostatitis is a subtle disorder that is difficult to treat. Men with the disorder typically have recurrent urinary tract infections with persistence of the same strain of pathogenic bacteria in prostatic fluid and urine. Organisms responsible for chronic bacterial prostatitis usually are the gram-negative enterobacteria (*E. coli, Proteus,* or *Klebsiella*) or *Pseudomonas.* Occasionally, a gram-positive organism such as *S. faecalis* is the causative organism. Infected prostatic calculi may develop and contribute to the chronic infection.

The symptoms of chronic prostatitis are variable and include frequent and urgent urination, dysuria, perineal discomfort, and low back pain. Occasionally, myalgia and arthralgia accompany the other symptoms. Secondary epididymitis sometimes is associated with the disorder. Many men experience relapsing lower or upper urinary tract infections because of recurrent invasion of the bladder by the prostatic bacteria. Bacteria may exist in the prostate gland even when the prostatic fluid is sterile. The most accurate method of establishing a diagnosis is by localizing cultures. This method is based on sequential collections of the first part of the voided urine (urethral specimen), midstream specimen (bladder specimen), the expressed prostatic secretion (obtained by prostatic massage), and the urine voided after prostatic massage. The last two specimens are considered prostatic urine. A positive expressed prostatic specimen establishes the diagnosis of bacterial prostatitis, excluding nonbacterial prostatitis.

Even after an accurate diagnosis has been established, treatment of chronic prostatitis often is difficult and frustrating.[35] Unlike their action in the acutely inflamed prostate, antibacterial drugs penetrate poorly into the chronically inflamed prostate. Long-term therapy (3 to 4 months) with an appropriate low-dose oral antimicrobial agent often is used to treat the infection. Adding α_1-adrenergic blocking drugs (*e.g.,* prazosin, terazosin, doxazosin, and tamsulosin) to antibacterial drugs may significantly improve symptoms and reduce recurrence.[35] Transurethral prostatectomy may be indicated when the infection is not cured or adequately controlled by medical therapy, particularly when prostate stones are present.

Chronic Prostatitis/Chronic Pelvic Pain Syndrome

Chronic prostatitis/pelvic pain syndrome is both the most common and least understood of the prostatitis syndromes.[38] The category is divided into two types, inflammatory and noninflammatory, based on the presence of leukocytes in the prostatic fluid. The inflammatory type was previously referred to as *nonbacterial prostatitis,* and the noninflammatory type as *prostatodynia.*

Inflammatory Prostatitis. A large group of men with prostatitis have pains along the penis, testicles, and scrotum; painful ejaculation; low back pain; rectal pain along the inner thighs; urinary symptoms; decreased libido; and impotence—but they have no bacteria in the urinary system. Men with nonbacterial prostatitis often have inflammation of the prostate with an elevated leukocyte count and abnormal inflammatory cells in their prostatic secretions. The cause of the disorder is unknown, and efforts to prove the presence of unusual pathogens (*e.g.,* mycoplasmas, chlamydiae, trichomonads, viruses) have been largely unsuccessful. It also is thought that nonbacterial prostatitis may be an autoimmune disorder.

Noninflammatory Prostatitis. Men with noninflammatory prostatitis or prostatodynia have symptoms resembling those of nonbacterial prostatitis but have negative urine culture results and no evidence of prostatic inflammation (*i.e.,* normal leukocyte count). The cause of noninflammatory prostatitis is unknown, but because of the absence of inflammation, the search for the cause of symptoms has been directed toward extraprostatic sources. In some cases, there is an apparent functional obstruction of the bladder neck near the external urethral sphincter; during voiding, this results in higher than normal pressures in the prostatic urethra that cause intraprostatic urine reflux and chemical irritation of the prostate by urine. In other cases, there is an apparent myalgia (*i.e.,* muscle pain) associated with prolonged tension of the pelvic floor muscles. Emotional stress also may play a role.

Treatment. Treatment methods for chronic prostatitis/pelvic pain syndrome are highly variable and require further study. Antibiotic therapy is used when an occult infection is suspected. Treatment often is directed toward symptom control. Sitz baths and nonsteroidal antiinflammatory agents may provide some symptom relief. In men with irritative urination symptoms, anticholinergic agents (*e.g.,* oxybutynin) or α-adrenergic blocking agents may be beneficial. Reassurance can be helpful. It is important that these men know that the condition is neither infectious or contagious, nor is it known to cause cancer.[35,38]

HYPERPLASIA AND NEOPLASMS

Benign Prostatic Hyperplasia

Benign prostatic hyperplasia (BPH) is an age-related, nonmalignant enlargement of the prostate gland (Fig. 45-7). It is characterized by the formation of large, discrete lesions in the periurethral region of the prostate rather than the peripheral zones, which commonly are affected by prostate cancer (Fig. 45-8). BPH is one of the most common diseases of aging men. It has been reported that more than 50% of men older than 60 years of age have BPH.[39] Between 15% and 30% of these men will develop lower urinary tract symptoms.

The exact cause of the BPH is unknown. Potential risk factors include age, family history, race, ethnicity, dietary fat and meat consumption, and hormonal factors. The incidence of BPH increases with advanced age, is highest in African Americans, and is lowest in native Japanese. Men with a family history of BPH are reported to have had larger prostates that those of control subjects, and higher rates of BPH were found in monozygotic twins than in dizygotic twins.

Both androgens (testosterone and dihydrotestosterone) and estrogens appear to contribute to the development of BPH. The prostate consists of a network of glandular elements embedded in smooth muscle and supporting tissue, with testosterone being the most important factor for prostatic growth. Dihydrotestosterone (DHT), the biologically active metabolite of testosterone, is thought to be the

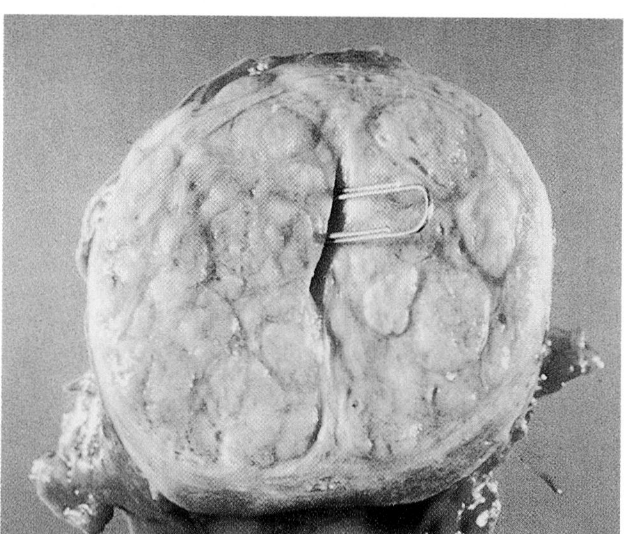

FIGURE 45-7 Nodular hyperplasia of the prostate. Cut surface of a prostate enlarged by nodular hyperplasia shows numerous, well-circumscribed nodules of prostatic tissue. The prostatic urethra (*paper clip*) has been compressed to a narrow slit. (Rubin E., Farber J.L. [1999]. *Pathology* [3rd ed., p. 955]. Philadelphia: Lippincott-Raven)

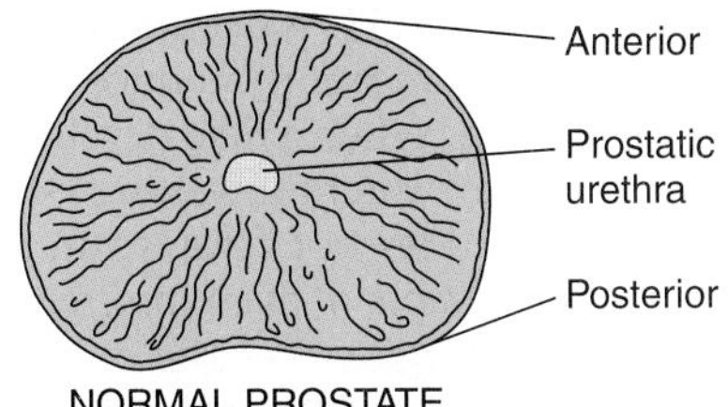

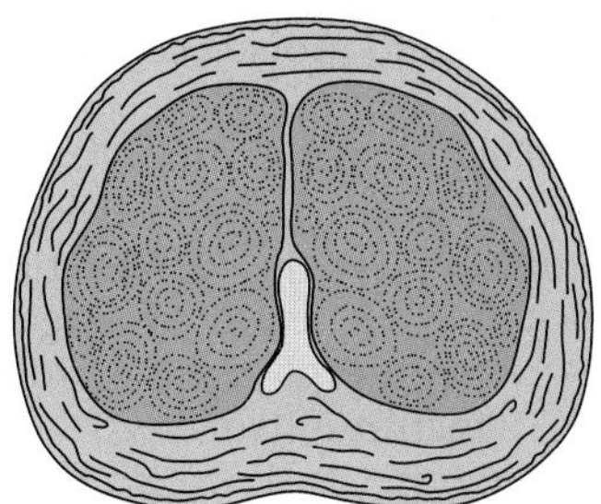

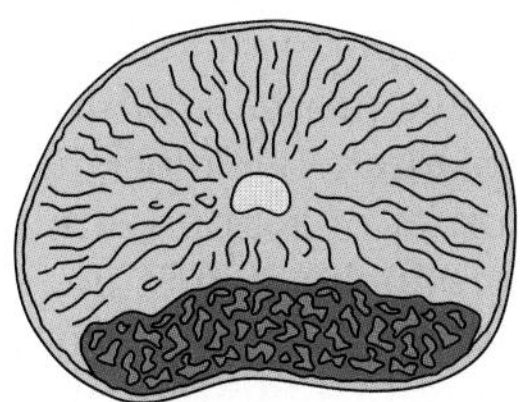

FIGURE 45-8 Normal prostate, nodular benign prostatic hypertrophy, and cancer of the prostate. (Rubin E., Farber J.L. [1999]. *Pathology* [3rd ed., p. 954]. Philadelphia: Lippincott-Raven) (Artist: Dimitri Karetnikov)

HYPERPLASIA AND CANCER OF THE PROSTATE

- The prostate gland surrounds the urethra and periurethral enlargement causes manifestations of urinary obstruction.
- Benign prostatic hyperplasia is an age-related enlargement of the prostate gland with formation of large, discrete lesions in the periurethral region of the prostate. These lesions compress the urethra and produce symptoms of dysuria or difficulty urinating.
- Prostatic cancer begins in the peripheral zones of the prostate gland and usually is asymptomatic until the disease is far advanced and the tumor has eroded the outer prostatic capsule and spread to adjacent pelvic tissues or metastasized.

ultimate mediator of prostatic hyperplasia, with estrogen serving to sensitize the prostatic tissue to the growth-producing effects of DHT. Free plasma testosterone enters prostatic cells, where at least 90% is converted into DHT by the action of 5α-reductase. The discovery that DHT is the active factor in BPH is the rationale for use of 5α-reductase inhibitors (*e.g.*, finasteride and dutasteride) in the treatment of the disorder. Although the exact source of estrogen is uncertain, small amounts of estrogen are produced in the male. It has been postulated that a relative increase in estrogen levels that occurs with aging may facilitate the action of androgens in the prostate despite a decline in testicular output of testosterone. Other hormonal factors that have been implicated include increased intraprostate levels of insulin-like growth factor-1 (IGF-1).[39]

The anatomic location of the prostate at the bladder neck contributes to the pathophysiology and symptomatology of BPH. There are two prostatic components to the obstructive properties of BPH and development of lower urinary tract symptoms: dynamic and static.[39] The static component of BPH is related to an increase in prostatic size and gives rise to symptoms such as a weak urinary stream, postvoid dribbling, frequency of urination, and nocturia. The dynamic component of BPH is related to prostatic smooth muscle tone. α_1-Adrenergic receptors are the main receptors for the smooth muscle component of the prostate. The recognition of the role of α_1-adrenergic receptor on neuromuscular function in the prostate is the basis for use of α_1-adrenergic receptor blockers in treating BPH. A third component, detrusor instability and impaired bladder contractility, may contribute to the symptoms of BPH independent of the outlet obstruction created by an enlarged prostate[39] (see Chapter 37). It has been suggested that some of the symptoms of BPH might be related to a decompensating or aging bladder rather than being primarily related to outflow obstruction. An example is the involuntary contraction that results in urgency and an attempt to void that occurs because of small bladder volume.[39]

The clinical significance of BPH resides in its tendency to compress the urethra and cause partial or complete obstruction of urinary outflow. As the obstruction increases, acute retention may occur with overdistention of the bladder. The residual urine in the bladder causes increased frequency of urination and a constant desire to empty the bladder, which becomes worse at night. With marked bladder distention, overflow incontinence may occur with the slightest increase in intraabdominal pressure. The resulting obstruction to urinary flow can give rise to urinary tract infection, destructive changes of the bladder wall, hydroureter, and hydronephrosis. Hypertrophy and changes in bladder wall structure develop in stages. Initially, the hypertrophied fibers form trabeculations and then herniations, or sacculations; finally, diverticula develop as the herniations extend through the bladder wall (see Chapter 37, Fig. 37-4). Because urine seldom is completely emptied from them, these diverticula are readily infected. Back pressure on the ureters and collecting system of the kidneys promotes hydroureter, hydronephrosis, and danger of eventual renal failure.

Diagnosis. It is now thought that the single most important factor in the evaluation and treatment of BPH is the man's own experiences related to the disorder. The American Urological Association Symptom Index consists of seven questions about symptoms regarding incomplete emptying, frequency, intermittency, urgency, weak stream, straining, and nocturia.[40] Each question is rated with a score of 0 (mild) to 7 (severe). A maximum score of 35 indicates severe symptoms. Total scores below 7 are considered mild; those between 8 and 20, moderate; and scores over 20, severe. A final question relates to quality of life due to urinary problems.

In 1994, the Agency for Health Care Policy and Research published clinical practice guidelines for management of BPH.[41] These guidelines suggest that the initial evaluation of men for a diagnosis of BPH includes history, physical examination, digital rectal examination (DRE), urinalysis, blood tests for serum creatinine and prostate-specific antigen (PSA), and urine flow rate. Blood and urine analyses are used as adjuncts to determine BPH complications. Urinalysis is done to detect bacteria, white blood cells, or microscopic hematuria in the presence of infection and inflammation. The serum creatinine test is used as an estimate of the glomerular filtration rate and renal function. The PSA test is used to screen for prostatic cancer. These evaluation measures, along with the symptom index, are used to describe the extent of obstruction, determine whether other diagnostic tests are needed, and establish the need for treatment.

The DRE is used to examine the external surface of the prostate. Enlargement of the prostate due to BPH usually produces a large, palpable prostate with a smooth, rubbery surface. Hardened areas of the prostate gland suggest cancer and should undergo biopsy. An enlarged prostate found during a DRE does not always correlate with the degree of urinary obstruction. Some men can have greatly enlarged prostate glands with no urinary obstruction, but others may have severe symptoms without a palpable enlargement of the prostate.

Residual urine measurement may be made by ultrasonography or postvoiding catheterization for residual urine volume. Residual urine values greater than 100 mL are considered high. Uroflowmetry provides an objective measure of urine flow rate. The patient is asked to void with a relatively full bladder (at least 150 mL) into a device that electronically measures the force of the stream and urine flow rate. A urinary flow rate of greater than 14 mL/second is considered normal, and less than 10 mL/second is indicative of obstruction.

Transabdominal or transrectal diagnostic ultrasonography can be used to evaluate the kidneys, ureters, and bladder. Urethrocystoscopy is indicated in men with a history of hematuria, stricture disease, urethral injury, or prior lower urinary tract surgery. It is used to evaluate the length and diameter of the urethra, the size and configuration of the prostate, and bladder capacity. It also detects the presence of trabeculations, bladder stones, and small bladder cancers. CT scans, MRI studies, and radionuclide scans are reserved for rare instances of tumor detection.

Treatment. Treatment of BPH is determined by the degree of symptoms that the condition produces and complications due to obstruction. When a man develops mild symptoms related to BPH, a "watchful waiting" stance often is taken. The condition does not always run a predictable course; it may remain stable or even improve.

Until the 1980s, surgery was the mainstay of treatment to alleviate urinary obstruction due to BPH. Currently, there is an emphasis on less invasive methods of treatment, including use of pharmacologic agents. However, when more severe signs of obstruction develop, surgical treatment is indicated to provide comfort and avoid serious renal damage.

Pharmacologic management includes the use of 5α-reductase inhibitors and α_1-adrenergic blocking drugs.[39] The 5α-reductase inhibitors, such as finasteride, reduce prostate size by blocking the effect of androgens on the prostate. Finasteride causes atrophy of the prostate glandular epithelial cells, which results in a 20% to 30% reduction in volume. The onset is slow (3–6 months), but long lasting. The side effects of finasteride are minimal but include erectile dysfunction (4%–16%) and decreased libido (1%–10%).[39] The presence of α-adrenergic receptors in prostatic smooth muscle has prompted the use of α_1-adrenergic blocking drugs (prazosin, terazosin, doxazosin, and tamsulosin) to relieve prostatic obstruction and increase urine flow. All α_1-adrenergic blocking drugs in current use have a rapid onset of action (within weeks) and similar effectiveness, producing a 40% increase in maximum urine flow rate with good symptom improvement.[39] Combination of 5α-reductase inhibitors and α_1-adrenergic blocking agents appears to be more effective than either monotherapy.

Herbal therapies have been used for many years by men for the treatment of BPH and lower urinary tract symptoms. Several studies have looked at the effects of these agents, including the extract of the Saw Palmetto berry. Improvements in peak urine flow rates and nocturia can occur compared with placebo, but the durability of these effects is unproved. The long-term toxicity and mechanism of action of these agents remain unclear.[39] Standardization of these products is also worrisome (as with all herbal therapies).

The surgical removal of an enlarged prostate can be accomplished by the transurethral, suprapubic, or perineal approach. The transurethral prostatectomy (TURP) is the most commonly used technique in the United States. With this approach, an instrument is introduced through the urethra, and prostate tissue is removed using a resectoscope and electrocautery. Immediate complications of TURP include the inability to urinate, postoperative hemorrhage or clot retention, and urinary tract infection. Late complications of TURP include erectile dysfunction, incontinence, and bladder neck contractures. Retrograde ejaculation is another problem that may occur because of resection of bladder neck tissue.

Several alternative procedures for treatment of BPH have been developed. A new surgical approach is the transurethral incision of the prostate (TUIP). This procedure involves making one or two incisions in the bundle of smooth muscle where the prostate gland is attached to the bladder. The gland is split to reduce pressure on the urethra. TUIP is helpful for smaller prostate glands that cause obstruction. Many different techniques of laser surgery are available. Two main energy sources have been used, neodymium: yttrium-aluminum-garnet (Nd:YAG) and holmium-YAG.[39]

Other new and experimental techniques that can be used to treat BPH include transurethral vaporization, transurethral microwave therapy, transurethral needle ablation, high-intensity focused ultrasound, and transurethral ultrasound-guided laser-induced prostatectomy. Most of these procedures are minimally invasive, and each has advantages and disadvantages when considered as an alternative measure in treatment of BPH.

A balloon dilation approach for removing the obstruction is another new technique. Transrectal ultrasonography is used to monitor balloon dilation of the prostate. Although the procedure may improve symptom score and flow rates, the effects usually are transitory.

For men who have heart or lung disease or a condition that precludes major surgery, a stent may be used to widen and maintain the patency of the urethra. A stent is a device made of tubular mesh that is inserted under local or regional anesthesia. Within several months, the lining of the urethra grows to cover the inside of the stent.

Prostatic Cancer

Prostatic cancer is the most common nonskin cancer in the United States, is second to lung cancer as a cause of cancer-related death in American men, and is the seventh leading cause of death in the United States.[42] The American Cancer Society estimates that during 2003, approximately 220,900 men in the United States were diagnosed with prostate cancer, and 28,900 men died of the disorder.[17] The increase in diagnosed cases is thought to reflect earlier diagnosis because of the widespread use of PSA testing since the early 1990s. The incidence of prostate cancer varies markedly from country to country and varies among races in the same country.[43,44] African-American men have the highest reported incidence of prostate cancer at all ages. Prostate cancer also tends to be diagnosed at a later stage in African-American men. Asians and Native-American men have the lowest rate.[44] Prostate cancer also is a disease of aging. The incidence increases rapidly after 50 years of age; more than 85% of all prostate cancers are diagnosed in men older than 65 years of age.[44]

The precise cause of prostatic cancer is unclear. As with other cancers, it appears that the development of prostate cancer is a multistep process involving genes that control cell differentiation and growth.[43] Several risk factors, such as age, race, heredity, and environmental influences (such as a high-fat diet), are suspected of playing a role.[42–44] Male hormone levels also play a role. There is insufficient evidence linking socioeconomic status, infectious agents, smoking, vasectomy, sexual behavior, or BPH to the pathogenesis of prostate cancer.

The incidence of prostate cancer appears to be higher in relatives of men with prostate cancer. It has been estimated that men who have an affected first-degree relative (*e.g.*, father, brother) and an affected second-degree relative (*e.g.*, grandfather, uncle) have an eightfold increase in risk.[44] It has been suggested that dietary patterns, including increased dietary fats, may alter the production of sex hormones and growth factors and increase the risk for prostate cancer.[43,44] Supporting the role of dietary fats as a risk factor for prostate cancer has been the observation that the diet of Japanese men, who have a low rate of prostate cancer, is much lower in fat content than that of U.S. men, who have a much higher incidence.

Several factors appear to be protective against the development of prostate cancer. These include dietary factors such as lycopene, selenium, and vitamin E.[43,44] In a recent study, chemoprevention (using drugs to prevent disease) with the 5α-reductase inhibitor finasteride was shown to decrease the risk of developing prostate cancer in men without BPH.[42] The role of these putative, protective agents remains to be clarified.

In terms of hormonal influence, androgens are believed to play a role in the pathogenesis of prostate cancer.[42,44] Evidence favoring a hormonal influence includes the presence of steroid receptors in the prostate, the requirement of sex hormones for normal growth and development of the prostate, and the fact that prostate cancer almost never develops in men who have been castrated. The response of prostatic cancer to estrogen administration or androgen deprivation further supports a correlation between the disease and testosterone levels. Other hormonal factors that have been implicated in prostate cancer include increased levels of IGF-1.[44]

Prostatic adenocarcinomas, which account for 98% of all primary prostatic cancers, are commonly multicentric and located in the peripheral zones of the prostate (see Fig. 45-8). The high frequency of invasion of the prostatic capsule by adenocarcinoma relates to its subcapsular location. Invasion of the urinary bladder is less frequent and occurs later in the clinical course. Metastasis to the lung reflects lymphatic spread through the thoracic duct and dissemination from the prostatic venous plexus to the inferior vena cava. Bony metastases, particularly to the vertebral column, ribs, and pelvis, produce pain that often presents as a first sign of the disease.

Most men with early-stage prostate cancer are asymptomatic. The presence of symptoms often suggests locally advanced or metastatic disease. Depending on the size and location of prostatic cancer at the time of diagnosis, there may be changes associated with the voiding pattern similar to those found in BPH. These include urgency, frequency, nocturia, hesitancy, dysuria, hematuria, or blood in the ejaculate. On DRE, the prostate is nodular and fixed. Bone metastasis often is characterized by low back pain. Pathologic fractures can occur at the site of metastasis. Men with metastatic disease may experience weight loss, anemia, or shortness of breath.

Screening. Because early cancers of the prostate usually are asymptomatic, screening tests are important. The screening tests currently available are DRE, PSA testing, and transrectal ultrasonography. PSA is a glycoprotein secreted into the cytoplasm of benign and malignant prostatic cells that is not found in other normal tissues or tumors. However, a positive PSA test indicates only the possible presence of prostate cancer. It also can be positive in cases of BPH and prostatitis. It has been reported that one third of men with elevated PSA levels have prostate cancer determined by biopsy, and two thirds do not.[45] Measures to increase the specificity of PSA testing in terms of predicting prostate cancer are being developed and evaluated. For example, because PSA levels increase with age, age-specific ranges have been established.[46] PSA velocity (a change of PSA level over time) and PSA density (*i.e.,* PSA level/prostate volume as measured by rectal ultrasonography) are being evaluated as methods of predicting the presence of prostate cancer in men with a positive PSA test result.[46]

The American Cancer Society and the American Urological Association recommend that men 50 years of age or older should undergo annual measurement of PSA and rectal examination for early detection of prostate cancer.[47] Men at high risk for prostate cancer, such as blacks and those with a strong family history, should undergo annual screening beginning at 45 years of age.[47] However, some controversy regarding the widespread use of PSA for screening remains. In 2002, the American College of Physicians and the U.S. Preventive Services Task Force emphasized the lack of reliable evidence for the benefits of screening.[48] Informed decision making regarding screening with PSA is warranted.

A new approach, transrectal ultrasonography, may detect cancers that are too small to be detected by physical examination. This method is not used for first-line detection because of its expense, but it may benefit men who are at high risk for development of prostate cancer.

Diagnosis. The diagnosis of prostate cancer is based on history and physical examination and confirmed through biopsy methods. Transrectal ultrasonography is used to guide a biopsy needle and document the exact location of the biopsied tissue. It also is used for providing staging information. Newly developed small probes for transrectal MRI have been shown to be effective in detecting the presence of cancer in the prostate. Radiologic examination of the bones of the skull, ribs, spine, and pelvis can be used to reveal metastases, although radionuclide bone scans are more sensitive. Excretory urograms are used to delineate changes due to urinary tract obstruction and renal involvement.

Staging. Cancer of the prostate, like other forms of cancer, is graded and staged (see Chapter 8). Prostatic adenocarcinoma commonly is classified using the Gleason grading system.[20] Well-differentiated tumors are assigned a grade of 1, and poorly differentiated tumors a grade of 5. The American Joint Committee on Cancer in 2002 updated the TNM system for staging.[49] Primary stage tumors (T1) are asymptomatic and discovered on histologic examination of prostatic tissue specimens; T2 tumors are palpable on digital examination but are confined to the prostate gland; T3 tumors have extended beyond the prostate; and T4 tumors have pushed beyond the prostate to involve adjacent structures. Regional lymph node (N) and distant metastasis (M) are described as Nx or Mx (cannot be assessed), N0 or M0 (not present), and N1 or M1 (present).[49]

Two tumor markers, PSA and serum acid phosphatase, are important in the staging and management of prostatic cancer. In untreated cases, the level of PSA correlates with the volume and stage of disease. A rising PSA after treatment is consistent with progressive disease, whether it is locally recurring or metastatic. Measurement of PSA is used to detect recurrence after total prostatectomy. Because the prostate is the source of PSA, levels should drop to zero after surgery; a rising PSA indicates recurring disease. Serum acid phosphatase is less sensitive than PSA and is used less frequently. However, it is more predictive of metastatic disease and may be used for that purpose.

Treatment. Cancer of the prostate is treated by surgery, radiation therapy, and hormonal manipulations.[50] Chemotherapy has shown limited effectiveness in the treatment of prostate cancer. Treatment decisions are based on tumor grade and stage and on the age and health of the man. Expectant therapy (watchful waiting) may be used if the tumor is not producing symptoms, is expected to grow slowly, and is small and contained in one area of the prostate. This approach is particularly suited for men who are elderly or have other health problems. Most men with an anticipated survival time of longer than 10 years are considered for surgical or radiation therapy.[50] Radical prostatectomy involves complete removal of the seminal vesicles, prostate, and ampullae of the vas deferens. Refinements in surgical techniques (nerve-sparing prostatectomy) have allowed maintenance of continence in most men and erectile function in selected cases. Radiation therapy can be delivered by a variety of techniques, including external beam radiation therapy and transperineal implantation of radioisotopes.

Metastatic disease often is treated with androgen deprivation therapy. Androgen deprivation may be induced at several levels along the pituitary-gonadal axis using a variety of methods or agents. Orchiectomy or estrogen therapy often is effective in reducing symptoms and extending survival. The GnRH analogs (*e.g.,* leuprolide, buserelin, nafarelin, triptorelin, and goserelin) block luteinizing hormone (LH) and follicle-stimulating hormone (FSH) release from the pituitary and reduce testosterone levels without orchiectomy or estrogen therapy. When given continuously (as opposed to pulsatile, which is the normal physiologic secretory rhythm) and in therapeutic doses, these drugs desensitize GnRH receptors in the pituitary, thereby preventing the release of LH. However, because these agents are GnRH *agonists,* LH and FSH initially rise and cause testosterone levels to increase. This can cause a clinical flare, which can be especially important in certain circumstances, such as if spinal cord compression due to metastatic disease is present.[50] This clinical flare can be decreased by pretreatment with antiandrogens. The nonsteroidal antiandrogens (*i.e.,* flutamide, nilutamide, and bicalutamide) block the uptake and actions of androgens in the target tissues. Complete androgen blockade can be achieved by combining an antiandrogen with a GnRH agent or orchiectomy. In men with metastatic prostate cancer, treatment with a combination of a GnRH agonist and flutamide seems to increase survival, particularly in those with minimal disease. Although testosterone is the main circulating androgen, the adrenal gland also secrets androgens. Inhibitors of adrenal androgen synthesis (*i.e.,* ketoconazole, and aminoglutethimide) may be used for treating men with advanced prostatic cancer who present with spinal cord compression, bilateral ureteral obstruction, or disseminated intravascular clotting. This is because these men need rapid decreases in their testosterone levels (*i.e.,* ketoconazole can produce chemical castration within 24 hours). Palliative care includes adequate pain control and focal irradiation of symptomatic or unstable bone disease. In men with advanced prostate cancer, the bisphosphonates (*e.g.,* etidronate, pamidronate, zoledronate, alendronate, risedronate), which act mainly by inhibiting osteoclastic activity (see Chapter 58), have several potential uses in prostate cancer. These include (1) preventing osteopenia that accompanies the use of androgen deprivation therapy, (2) preventing and delaying skeletal complications (*e.g.,* the need for local radiation treatment, fractures) in patients with metastatic bone involvement, (3) decreasing bone pain, and (4) treating hypercalcemia of malignancy.

In summary, the prostate is a firm, glandular structure that surrounds the urethra. Inflammation of the prostate occurs as an acute or a chronic process. Chronic prostatitis probably is the most common cause of relapsing urinary tract infections in men. BPH is a common disorder in men older than 50 years of age. Because the prostate encircles the urethra, BPH exerts its effect through obstruction of urinary outflow from the bladder. Advances in the treatment of BPH include laser surgery, balloon dilatation, prostatic stents, and pharmacologic treatment using 5α-reductase inhibitors such as finasteride, which reduce prostate size by blocking the effects of androgen on the prostate, and α_1-adrenergic receptor blockers, which inhibit contraction of prostatic smooth muscle.

Prostatic cancer is the most common nonskin cancer in the United States and is second to lung cancer as a cause of cancer-related death in men. A recent increase in diagnosed cases is thought to reflect earlier diagnosis because of widespread use of PSA testing. The incidence of prostate cancer increases with age and is greater in African Americans of all ages. Most prostate cancers are asymptomatic and are incidentally discovered on rectal examination. Screening for prostate cancer has become recognized as a method for early identification of prostate cancer. The American Cancer Society suggests that every man 50 years of age or older should have a rectal examination and PSA test done as part of his annual physical examination. Cancer of the prostate, like other forms of cancer, is graded according to the histologic characteristics of the tumor and staged clinically using the TNM system. Treatment, which is based on the extent of the disease, includes surgery, radiation therapy, and hormonal manipulation.

REVIEW EXERCISES

A 64-year-old man presents to his family physician with erectile dysfunction. He is on multiple medications for his "heart disease." An initial physical examination is unremarkable.

A. What additional information should be obtained?

B. Given his medical history, what are possible factors contributing to his problem?

A 23-year-old man presents in the emergency room in severe distress. His left testicle is large and tender and he has pain radiating to the inguinal area.

A. What would be a tentative diagnosis for this man?

B. Why would this problem necessitate immediate diagnosis and surgical intervention?

A 72-year-man had a radical prostatectomy for localized prostate cancer. After surgery, his PSA level was undetectable. He presents 5 years later having been "lost to follow-up." He complains of difficulty walking due to pain in his hip and lower back. His PSA level is now markedly elevated.

A. What initial investigations are warranted?

B. What therapies are available for this complication?

References

1. Behrman R., Kleigman R.M., Jenson H.B. (2004). *Nelson textbook of pediatrics* (16th ed., pp. 1812–1815, 1817–1818). Philadelphia: Saunders.
2. Moore K.L., Persaud T.V.N. (1998). *The developing human: Clinically oriented embryology* (6th ed., pp. 338–339). Philadelphia: W.B. Saunders.
3. Conte F.A., Grumbach M.M. (2004). Abnormalities of sexual determination and differentiation. In Greenspan F.S., Gardner D.G. (Eds.), *Basic and clinical endocrinology* (7th ed., pp. 564–607). New York: Lange Medical Books/McGraw-Hill.
4. Edwards S. (1996). Balanitis and balanoposthitis: A review. *Genitourinary Medicine 72,* 155–159.
5. Fitkin J., Ho G.T. (1999). Peyronie's disease: Current management. *American Family Physician 60,* 549–554.
6. McAninch J.W. (2000). Disorders of the penis and male urethra. In Tanagho E.A., McAninch J.W. (Eds.), *Smith's general urology* (15th ed., pp. 663–675). New York: Lange Medical Books/McGraw-Hill.
7. Backhaus B.O., Muller S.C., Albers P. (2003) Corporoplasty for advanced Peyronie's disease using venous and/or dermis patch grafting: new surgical technique and long-term patient satisfaction. *Journal of Urology 169,* 981–984.
8. AACE Male Sexual Dysfunction Taskforce (2003). AACE medical guidelines for clinical practice for the evaluation and treatment of male sexual dysfunction: A couple's problem—2003 update. *Endocrine Practice 9,* 77–95.
9. Matfin G. (2003). Erectile dysfunction. *Sexuality, Reproduction and Menopause 1,* 40–45.
10. NIH Consensus Development Panel on Impotence. (1993). NIH Consensus Conference: Impotence. *Journal of the American Medical Association 270,* 83–90.

11. Lue T.F. (2000). Erectile dysfunction. *New England Journal of Medicine 342,* 1802–1813.
12. Bacon C.G., Mittleman M.A., Kawachi I., et al. (2003). Sexual function in men older than 50 years of age: Results from the Health Professionals follow-up study. *Annals of Internal Medicine 139,* 161–168.
13. Feldman H.A., Goldstein J., Hatzichristou D.G., et al. (1994). Impotence and its medical and psychosocial effects. Results of the Massachusetts Male Aging Study. *Journal of Urology 151,* 54–61.
14. Harmon W.J., Nehra A. (1997). Priapism: Diagnosis and treatment. *Mayo Clinic Proceedings 72,* 350–355.
15. Bruno D., Wigfall D.R., Zimmerman S.A., et al. (2001). Genitourinary complications of sickle cell disease. *Journal of Urology 166,* 803–811.
16. Kachhi P.N., Henderson S.O. (2000). Priapism after androstenedione intake for athletic performance enhancement. *Annals of Emergency Medicine 35,* 391–393.
17. Jemal A., Murray T., Samuels A., et al. (2003). Cancer statistics. *CA—A Cancer Journal for Clinicians 53,* 5–26.
18. Krieg R., Hoffman R. (1999). Current management of unusual genitourinary cancers: Part 1. Penile cancer. *Oncology 13,* 1347–1352.
19. Presti J.C., Herr H.W. (2000). Genital tumors. In Tanagho E.A., McAninch J.W. (Eds.), *Smith's general urology* (15th ed., pp. 430–434). New York: Lange Medical Books/McGraw-Hill.
20. Cotran R.S., Kumar V., Collins T. (1999). *Robbins pathologic basis of disease* (6th ed., pp. 1015–1016, 1018–1024, 1029–1033). Philadelphia: W.B. Saunders.
21. Docimo S.G., Silver R.I., Cromie W. (2000). The undescended testicle: Diagnosis and management. *American Family Physician 62,* 2037–2048.
22. Pillai S.B., Besner G.E. (1998). Pediatric testicular problems. *Pediatric Clinics of North America 45,* 813–818.
23. Kapur P., Caty M.G., Glick P.L. (1998). Pediatric hernias and hydroceles. *Pediatric Clinics of North America 45,* 773–789.
24. McAninch J.W. (2000). Disorders of the testis, scrotum, and spermatic cord. In Tanagho E.A., McAninch J.W. (Eds.), *Smith's general urology* (15th ed., pp. 684–693). New York: Lange Medical Books/McGraw-Hill.
25. Templeton A. (2003) Varicocele and infertility. *Lancet 361,* 1838–1839.
26. Galejs L.E., Kass E.J. (1999) Diagnosis and treatment of acute scrotum. *American Family Physician 59,* 817–824.
27. Sessions A.E., Rabinowitz R., Hulbert W.C., et al. (2003). Testicular torsion: direction, degree, duration, and disinformation. *Journal of Urology 169,* 663–665.
28. Centers for Disease Control and Prevention. (2002). Sexually transmitted diseases treatment guidelines. *Morbidity and Mortality Weekly Report 51*(No.RR-6), 1–118.
29. Gershon A.A. (2001) Mumps. In Braunwald E. (Ed.), *Harrison's principles of internal medicine* (15th Ed., pp 1147–1148). New York: McGraw-Hill.
30. Mebcow M.M. (1975). Percivall Pott (1713–1788): 200th anniversary of first report of occupation-induced cancer of the scrotum in chimney sweepers (1745). *Urology 6,* 745.
31. Lowe F.C. (1992). Squamous cell carcinoma of the scrotum. *Urologic Clinics of North America 19,* 297–405.
32. Vaughn D.J., Gignac G.A., Meadows A.T. (2002) Long-term medical care of testicular cancer survivors. *Annals of Internal Medicine 136,* 463–470.
33. Motzer R.J., Bosl G.J. (2001) Testicular Cancer. In Braunwald E. (Ed.), *Harrison's principles of internal medicine* (15th Ed., pp. 1147–1148). New York: McGraw-Hill.
34. Krieger J.N., Nyberg L., Nickel J.C. (1999). NIH consensus definition and classification of prostatitis. *Journal of the American Medical Association 282,* 721–725.
35. Stern J., Schaeffer A. (2003) Chronic prostatitis. *Clinical Evidence Concise 9,* 181–182.
36. McRae S.N., Shortliffe L.M.D. (2000). Bacterial infections of the genitourinary system. In Tanagho E.A., McAninch J.W. (Eds.), *Smith's general urology* (15th ed., pp. 254–259). New York: Lange Medical Books/McGraw-Hill.
37. Stevermer J.J., Easley S.K. (2000). Treatment of prostatitis. *American Family Physician 61,* 3015–3026.
38. Collins M.M., MacDonald R., Wilt T.J. (2000). Diagnosis and treatment of chronic abacterial prostatitis: A systemic review. *Annals of Internal Medicine 133,* 367–381.
39. Thorpe A., Neal D. (2003) Benign prostatic hyperplasia. *Lancet 361,* 1359–1367.
40. Barry M.J., et al. (1992). The American Urological Association Index of Benign Prostatic Hypertrophy. *Journal of Urology 148,* 1549–1557.
41. Agency of Health Care Policy and Research. (1994). *Clinical practice guidelines for benign prostatic hyperplasia.* AHCPR publication no. 94-0582. Rockville, MD: U.S. Department of Health and Human Services.
42. Scardino P.T. (2003) The prevention of prostate cancer: the dilemma continues. *New England Journal of Medicine 349,* 297–299.
43. Nelson W.G., De Manzo A.M., Isaacs W.B. (2003) Prostate cancer. *New England Journal of Medicine 349,* 366–381.
44. Gronberg H. (2003). Prostate cancer epidemiology. *Lancet 361,* 859–864.
45. Woolf S.H. (1995). Screening for prostate cancer with prostate specific antigen: An examination of the evidence. *New England Journal of Medicine 333,* 1401–1405.
46. Balk S.P., Ko Y.J., Bubley G.J. (2003) Biology of prostate-specific antigen. *Journal of Clinical Oncology 21,* 383–391.
47. American Cancer Society. (2003). Prostate cancer resource center. [On-line]. Available: http://www.cancer.org.
48. U.S. Preventive Services Task Force (2002). Screening for prostate cancer: Recommendations and rationale. *Annals of Internal Medicine 137,* 915–916.
49. American Joint Committee on Cancer (2002). AJCC Cancer Staging Manual/American Joint Committee on Cancer (6th Ed., pp. 310–311). New York: Springer-Verlag.
50. Scher H.I. (2001) Hyperplastic and malignant diseases of the prostate. In Braunwald E. (Ed.), *Harrison's principles of internal medicine* (15th Ed., pp. 608–616). New York: McGraw-Hill.

CHAPTER

46

The Female Reproductive System

Patricia McCowen Mehring

The female genitourinary system consists of internal paired ovaries, uterine tubes, uterus, vagina, external mons pubis, labia majora, labia minora, clitoris, urethra, and perineal body. Although the female urinary structures are anatomically separate from the genital structures, their anatomic proximity provides a means for cross-contamination and shared symptomatology between the two systems (Fig. 46-1). This chapter focuses on the internal and external genitalia. It includes a discussion of hormonal and physical changes that occur throughout the life cycle in response to the gonadotropic hormones. The reader is referred to a specialty text for a discussion of pregnancy.

Reproductive Structures

After completing this section of the chapter, you should be able to meet the following objectives:

- Describe the anatomic relation of the structures of the external genitalia
- Name the three layers of the uterus and describe their function
- Cite the location of the ovaries in relation to the uterus, fallopian tubes, broad ligaments, and ovarian ligaments
- Explain the function of the fallopian tubes
- State the function of endocervical secretions

EXTERNAL GENITALIA

The external genitalia are located at the base of the pelvis in the perineal area and include the mons pubis, labia majora, labia minora, clitoris, and perineal body. The urethra and anus, although not genital structures, usually are considered in a discussion of the external genitalia. The external genitalia, also known collectively as the *vulva,* are diagrammed in Figure 46-2.

The *mons pubis* is a rounded, skin-covered fat pad located anterior to the symphysis pubis. Puberty stimulates an increase in the amount of fat and the development of darker and coarser hair over the mons. Normal pubic hair distribution in the female follows an inverted triangle with the base centered over the mons. Hair color and texture varies from person to person and among racial groups. There is an abundance of sebaceous glands in the skin that can become infected owing to normal variations in glandular secretions or poor hygiene. The mons pubis is the most common site of pubic lice infestation in the female. The *labia majora* (singular, labium majus) are analogous to the male scrotum. These structures are the outermost lips of the vulva, beginning anteriorly at the base of the mons pubis and ending posteriorly at the anus. The labia majora are composed of folds of skin and fat and become covered with hair at the onset of puberty. Before puberty, the labia majora have a skin covering similar to that covering the

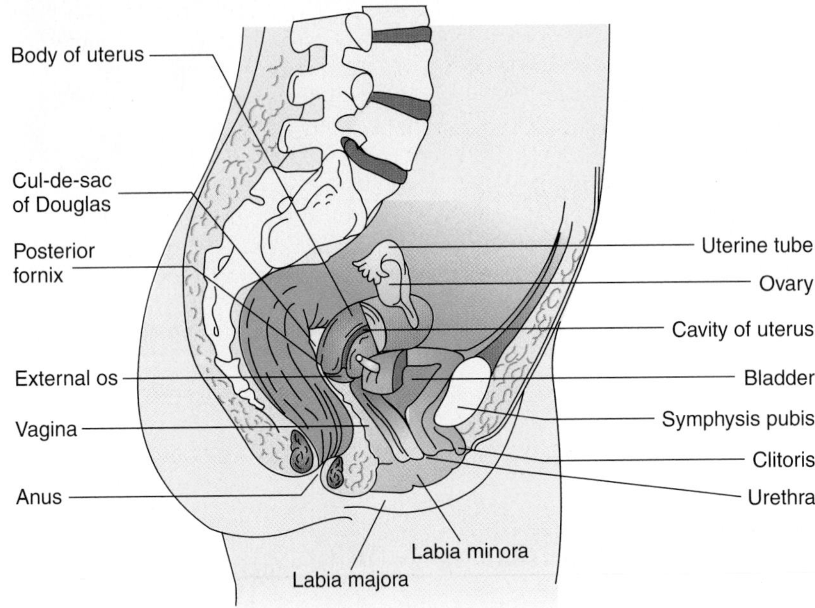

FIGURE 46-1 Female reproductive system as seen in sagittal section.

abdomen. With sufficient hormonal stimulation, the labia of a mature woman close over the urethral and vaginal openings; this can change after childbirth or surgery.

The *labia minora* (singular, labium minus) are located between the labia majora. These delicate cutaneous structures are smaller than the labia majora and are composed of skin, fat, and some erectile tissue. Unlike the skin of the labia majora, that of the labia minora is hairless and usually light pink. The labia minora begin anteriorly at the hood of the clitoris and end posteriorly at the base of the vagina. During sexual arousal, the labia minora become distended with blood; with resolution, the labia throb and then return to normal size. The sebaceous glands secrete an odoriferous fluid in the presence or absence of sexual arousal. The clitoris is located below the clitoral hood, or prepuce, which is formed by the joining of the two labia minora. The female clitoris is an erectile organ, rich in vascular and nervous supply. Analogous to the male penis, it is a highly sensitive organ that becomes distended during sexual stimulation.

The area between labia minora is called the *vestibule.* Located in the vestibule are the urethral and vaginal openings and Bartholin's lubricating glands. The *urethra,* or urinary meatus, is the external opening of the internal urinary

Mons pubis
Prepuce
Clitoris
Labium minus
Urinary meatus
Orifice of vagina
Labium majus
Hymen
Obstetrical perineum
Anus

FIGURE 46-2 External genitalia of the female.

THE FEMALE GENITOURINARY SYSTEM

- The female reproductive system, which consists of the external and internal genitalia, has both sexual and reproductive functions.
- The external genitalia (labia majora, labia minora, clitoris, and vestibular glands) surround the openings of the urethra and vagina. Although the female urinary and genital structures are anatomically separate, their close proximity provides a means for cross-contamination and shared symptomatology.
- The internal genitalia of the female reproductive system are specialized to participate in sexual intercourse (the vagina), to produce and maintain the female egg cells (the ovaries), to transport these cells to the site of fertilization (the fallopian tubes), to provide a favorable environment for development of the offspring (the uterus), and to produce the female sex hormones (the ovaries).

bladder. The urethra is located posterior to the clitoris and usually is closer to the vaginal opening than to the clitoris. The urethral opening is the site of *Skene's glands,* which have a lubricating function. The vaginal orifice, commonly known as the *introitus,* is the opening between the external and internal genitalia. The size and shape of the opening are determined by a connective tissue membrane called the *hymen* that surrounds the introitus. The opening may be oval, circular, or sievelike and may be partially or completely occluded. Occlusion may occur because of the presence of an intact or partially intact hymen. Contrary to popular notion, an intact hymen does not indicate virginity because this tissue can be stretched without tearing. At puberty, an intact hymen may require surgical intervention to permit discharge of menstrual fluids.

The *perineal body* is that tissue located posterior to the vaginal opening and anterior to the anus. It is composed of fibrous connective tissue and is the site of insertion of several perineal muscles.

INTERNAL GENITALIA

Vagina

Connecting the internal and external genitalia is a fibromuscular tube called the *vagina.* The vagina, which is essentially free of sensory nerve fibers, is located behind the urinary bladder and urethra and anterior to the rectum. The uterine cervix projects into the vagina at its upper end, forming recesses called *fornices* (Fig. 46-3). The vagina functions as a route for discharge of menses and other secretions. It also serves as an organ of sexual fulfillment and reproduction.

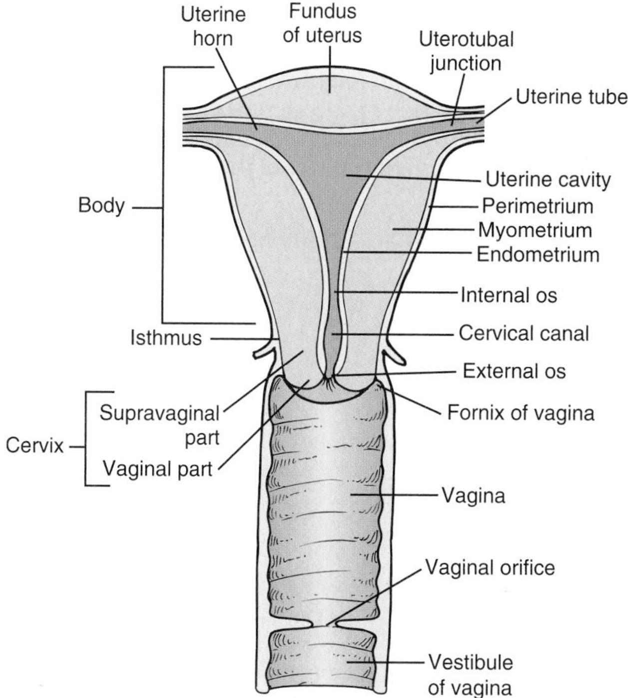

FIGURE 46-3 Median section of the vagina and uterus.

The membranous vaginal wall forms two longitudinal folds and several transverse folds, or rugae. The vagina is lined with mucus-secreting stratified squamous epithelial cells. Vaginal tissue usually is moist, with a pH maintained within the bacteriostatic range of 3.8 to 4.2.

The epithelial cells of the vagina, like other tissues of the reproductive system, respond to changing levels of the ovarian sex hormones. Estrogen stimulates the proliferation and maturation of the vaginal mucosa; this results in a thickening of the vaginal mucosa and an increased glycogen content of the epithelial cells. The glycogen is fermented to lactic acid by the lactobacilli (*i.e., Döderlein's bacilli*) that are part of the normal vaginal flora, accounting for the mildly acid pH of vaginal fluid. The vaginal ecology can be disrupted at many levels, rendering it susceptible to infection. Pregnancy and the use of oral contraceptive agents increase the amount of estrogen in the system. Diabetes or a prediabetic state may increase the glycogen content of the cells. The use of systemic antibiotics may decrease the number of lactobacilli in the vagina.

Decreased estrogen stimulation after menopause causes the vaginal mucosa to become thin and dry, often resulting in dyspareunia (*i.e.,* painful intercourse), atrophic vaginitis, and occasionally in vaginal bleeding. Estrogen levels can be estimated by means of vaginal scrapings obtained during a routine pelvic examination. The scrapings are used for a test, known as the *maturation index,* which examines the cellular structure and configuration of the vaginal epithelial cells. The maturation index determines the ratio of parabasal (least mature), intermediate, and superficial (most mature) cells. Typically, this index is 0-40-60 during the reproductive years. With diminished estrogen levels, there is a shift to the left, producing an index of 30-40-30 during the perimenopausal period and an index of 75-25-0 during the postmenopausal period.

Uterus and Cervix

The uterus is a thick-walled muscular organ. This pear-shaped, hollow structure is located between the bladder and the rectum. The uterus can be divided into three parts: the portion above the insertion of the fallopian tubes, called the *fundus;* the lower, constricted part, called the *cervix;* and the portion between the fundus and the cervix, called the *body of the uterus* (see Fig. 46-3). The uterus is supported on both sides by four sets of ligaments: the *broad ligaments,* which run laterally from the body of the uterus to the pelvic side walls; the *round ligaments,* which run from the fundus laterally into each labium majus; the *uterosacral ligaments,* which run from the uterocervical junction to the sacrum; and the *cardinal* or *transverse cervical* ligaments.

The wall of the uterus is composed of three layers: the perimetrium, the myometrium, and the endometrium. The *perimetrium* is the outer serous covering that is derived from the abdominal peritoneum. This outer layer merges with the peritoneum that covers the broad ligaments. Anteriorly, the perimetrium is reflected over the bladder wall, forming the vesicouterine pouch; posteriorly, it extends to form the *cul-de-sac,* or *pouch of Douglas* (see Fig. 46-1). Because of the proximity of the perimetrium to the urinary bladder, infection of this organ often causes uterine symptoms, particularly during pregnancy.

The middle layer, or myometrium, which is composed of smooth muscle fibers, forms the major portion of the uterine wall. It is continuous with the smooth muscle layer of the fallopian tubes and the vagina and extends into all the supporting ligaments with the exception of the broad ligaments. The inner fibers of the myometrium run in various directions, giving it an interwoven appearance. Contractions of these muscle fibers help to expel menstrual flow and the products of conception during miscarriage or childbirth. When pain accompanies the contractions associated with menses, it is called *dysmenorrhea.* The myometrium has an amazing ability to change length during pregnancy and labor, increasing the uterine capacity from 90 to 1000 g to accommodate gestation.[1]

The *endometrium,* the inner layer of the uterus, is continuous with the lining of the fallopian tubes and vagina. The endometrium is made up of a basal and a superficial layer. The superficial layer is shed during menstruation and regenerated by cells of the basal layer. Ciliated cells promote the movement of tubal and uterine secretions out of the uterine cavity into the vagina.

The round *cervix* is the neck of the uterus that projects into the vagina. The cervix is a firm structure, composed of a connective tissue matrix of glands and muscular tissue elements, which become soft and pliable under the influence of hormones produced during pregnancy. Glandular tissue provides a rich supply of protective mucus that changes in character and quantity during the menstrual cycle and during pregnancy. The cervix is richly supplied with blood from the uterine artery and can be a site of significant blood loss during delivery.

The opening of the cervix, the os, forms a pathway between the uterus and the vagina. The vaginal opening is called the *external os* and the uterine opening, the *internal os* (see Fig. 46-3). The space between these two openings is the endocervical canal. Secretions from the columnar epithelium of the endocervix protect the uterus from infection, alter receptivity to sperm, and form a mucoid "plug" during pregnancy. The endocervical canal provides a route for menstrual discharge and sperm entrance.

Fallopian Tubes

The *fallopian,* or uterine, tubes are slender, cylindrical structures attached bilaterally to the uterus and supported by the upper folds of the broad ligament. The end of the fallopian tube nearest the ovary forms a funnel-like opening with fringed, finger-like projections, called *fimbriae,* which pick up the ovum after its release into the peritoneal cavity after ovulation (see Figure 46-4). The fallopian tubes are formed of smooth muscle and lined with a ciliated, mucus-producing epithelial layer. The beating of the cilia, along with contractile movements of the smooth muscle, propels the nonmobile ovum toward the uterus. If coitus has occurred recently, fertilization normally occurs in the middle to outer portion of the fallopian tube. Besides providing a passageway for ova and sperm, the fallopian tubes provide for drainage of tubal secretions into the uterus.

Ovaries

By the third month of fetal life, the *ovaries* have fully developed and descended to their permanent pelvic position. Remnants of the primitive genital system provide lateral supporting attachments to the uterus; in the mature female, these supporting structures evolve into the round and suspensory ligaments. Remnants that do not evolve may form cysts, which may become symptomatic later in life.

Oogenesis is the process of generation of ova by mitotic division that begins at the sixth week of fetal life. These primitive germ cells ultimately provide the 1 to 2 million oocytes that are present in the ovaries at birth. At puberty, this number is reduced through cell death to approximately 300,000.

The neonate's ovaries are smooth, pale, and elongated. They become shorter, thicker, and heavier before the onset of menarche, which is initiated by pituitary influence. The initial hormonal stimulus for this development is believed to come from ovarian rather than systemic estrogen.

In the adult, the ovaries are flat, almond-shaped structures that are 3 to 5 cm long and weigh 2 to 3 g. They are located on either side of the uterus below the fimbriated ends of the two oviducts, or fallopian tubes. The ovaries are attached to the posterior surface of the broad ligament and

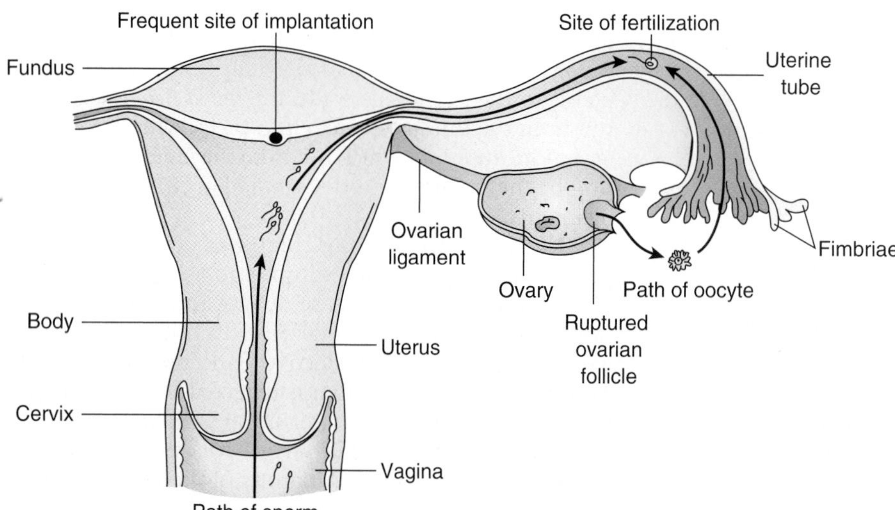

FIGURE 46-4 Schematic drawing of female reproductive organs, showing the path of the oocyte as it moves from the ovary into the fallopian (uterine) tube; the path of sperm is also shown, as is the usual site of fertilization.

to the uterus by the ovarian ligament. They are covered with a thin layer of surface epithelium that is continuous with the lining of the peritoneum. The integrity of this covering is periodically broken at the time of ovulation.

The ovaries, like the male testes, have a dual function: they store the female germ cells, or ova, and produce the female sex hormones, estrogen and progesterone. Unlike the male gonads, which produce sperm throughout a man's reproductive life, the female gonads contain a fixed number of ova at birth that diminishes throughout a woman's life.

Structurally, the mature ovary is divided into a highly vascular inner medulla, which contains supporting connective tissue, and an outer cortex of stroma and epithelial follicles (*i.e.*, vesicles), which contain the primary oocytes, or germ cells. After puberty, the pituitary gonadotropic hormones—follicle-stimulating hormone (FSH) and luteinizing hormone (LH)—stimulate the primordial follicles to develop into *mature graafian follicles*. The graafian follicle produces estrogen, which begins to stimulate the development of the endometrium in the uterus. Although several follicles begin to develop during each ovulatory cycle, only one or two complete the entire developmental process and rupture to release a mature ovum. After ovulation, the follicle becomes luteinized; as the corpus luteum, it produces estrogen and progesterone to support the endometrium until conception occurs or the cycle begins again.

In summary, the female reproductive system consists of internal paired ovaries, uterine tubes, uterus, vagina, external mons pubis, labia majora, labia minora, clitoris, urethra, and perineal body. The genitourinary system as a whole serves sexual and reproductive functions throughout the life cycle. The uterus is a thick-walled, muscular organ. The wall of the uterus is composed of three layers: the outer perimetrium; the myometrium or muscle layer, which is continuous with the myometrium of the fallopian tubes and the vagina; and the inner lining or endometrium, which is continuous with the lining of the fallopian tubes and vagina. The gonads, or ovaries, which are internal in the female (unlike the testes in the male), have the dual function of storing the female germ cells, or ova, and producing the female sex hormones. Through the regulation and release of sex hormones, the ovaries influence the development of secondary sexual characteristics, regulation of menstrual cycles, maintenance of pregnancy, and advent of menopause.

Menstrual Cycle

After completing this section of the chapter, you should be able to meet the following objectives:

- Describe the feedback control of estrogen and progesterone levels by means of gonadotropin-releasing hormone, LH, FSH, and ovarian follicle function
- List the actions of estrogen and progesterone
- Describe the four functional compartments of the ovary
- Relate FSH and LH levels to the stages of follicle development and to estrogen and progesterone production
- Describe the endometrial changes that occur during the menstrual cycle
- Describe the composition of normal cervical mucus and the changes that occur during the menstrual cycle
- Describe the physiology of normal menopause

Between menarche (*i.e.*, first menstrual bleeding) and menopause (*i.e.*, last menstrual bleeding), the female reproductive system undergoes cyclic changes called the *menstrual cycle*. This includes the maturation and release of oocytes from the ovary during ovulation and periodic vaginal bleeding resulting from the shedding of the endometrial lining. It is not necessary for a woman to ovulate to menstruate; anovulatory cycles do occur. The menstrual cycle produces changes in the breasts, uterus, skin, ovaries, and perhaps other, unidentified tissues. The maintenance of the cycle affects biologic and sociologic aspects of a woman's life, including fertility, reproduction, sexuality, and femaleness.

HORMONAL CONTROL

Normal menstrual function results from interactions among the central nervous system, hypothalamus, anterior pituitary, ovaries, and associated target tissues. Although each part of the system is essential to normal function, the ovaries are primarily responsible for controlling the cyclic changes and the length of the menstrual cycle. In most women in the middle reproductive years, menstrual bleeding occurs every 25 to 35 days, with a median length of 28 days.

The hormonal control of the menstrual cycle is complex. There is evidence that a certain minimum body weight (48 kg) and fat content (16% to 24%) are necessary for menarche to occur and for the menstrual cycle to be maintained. This is supported by the observation of amenorrhea in women with anorexia nervosa, chronic disease, and malnutrition and in those who are long-distance runners. In women with anorexia nervosa, gonadotropin and estradiol secretion, including LH release and responsiveness to the hypothalamic gonadotropin-releasing hormone (GnRH), can revert to prepubertal levels. With resumption of weight gain and attainment of sufficient body fat, the normal hormonal pattern usually

MENSTRUAL CYCLE

- The menstrual cycle begins at menarche and continues until menopause. It includes the maturation and release of oocytes from the ovary during ovulation and periodic vaginal bleeding resulting from the shedding of the endometrial lining.
- The menstrual cycle is controlled by rhythmic synthesis and release of ovarian hormones (the estrogens and progesterone) under feedback control from the hypothalamic gonadotropin-releasing hormone and the anterior pituitary gonadotropic follicle-stimulating and luteinizing hormones.

is reinstated (see Chapter 11). Obesity or significant weight gain also is associated with oligomenorrhea or amenorrhea and infertility, although the mechanism is not well understood.

Hypothalamic and Pituitary Hormones

Growth, prepubertal maturation, the reproductive cycle, and sex hormone secretion in males and females are regulated by FSH and LH from the anterior pituitary gland (Fig. 46-5). Because these hormones promote the growth of cells in the gonads (ovaries and testes) as a means of stimulating the production of sex hormones, they are called the *gonadotropic hormones*. The secretion of LH and FSH is stimulated by GnRH from the hypothalamus. In addition to LH and FSH, the anterior pituitary secretes a third hormone called *prolactin*. The primary function of prolactin is the stimulation of lactation in the postpartum period. During pregnancy, prolactin, along with other hormones such as estrogen, progesterone, insulin, and cortisol, contributes to breast development in preparation for lactation. Although prolactin does not appear to play a physiologic role in ovarian function, hyperprolactinemia leads to hypogonadism. This may include an initial shortening of the luteal phase with subsequent anovulation, oligomenorrhea or amenorrhea, and infertility. The hypothalamic control of prolactin secretion is primarily inhibitory, and dopamine is the most important inhibitory factor. Hyperprolactinemia may occur as an adverse effect of drug treatment using phenothiazine derivatives (*i.e.*, antipsychotic drugs that block dopamine receptors).

Ovarian Hormones

The ovaries produce estrogens, progesterone, and androgens. Ovarian hormones are secreted in a cyclic pattern as a result of the interaction between the hypothalamic GnRH and the pituitary gonadotropic hormones, FSH and LH. The steroid sex hormones enter cells by passive diffusion, bind to specific receptor proteins in the cytoplasm, and then move to the nucleus, where they bind to specific sites on the chromosomes. These hormones exert their effects through gene–hormone interactions, which stimulate the synthesis of specific messenger ribonucleic acid (mRNA). In addition, estrogen appears to have the ability to influence cell activity through other nongenomic mechanisms. These nongenomic effects take place in cells that have no steroid receptors, possibly mediated by other membrane receptors. This may explain in part some of the nonreproductive effects of estrogen. An example of a nongenomic cardioprotective effect would be the antioxidant activity of estrogen in preventing endothelial injury that can lead to platelet adherence.[2] The number of hormonal receptor sites on a cell is not fixed; evidence suggests that they are constantly being removed and replaced. An increase or a decrease in the number of receptors can serve as a mechanism for regulating hormonal activity. For example, estrogen may induce the development of an increased number of estrogen receptors in some tissues and may stimulate the synthesis of progesterone receptors in others. In contrast, progesterone may cause a reduction in the number of estrogen and progesterone receptors.

The recent discovery of a second type of estrogen receptor (ER_2) that is different in structure, tissue distribution, and expression from ER_1 helps to expand our understanding of the mechanism of action of estrogen in the body. The ER_2 appears to be an activator of estrogen response, whereas the ER_1 appears to modulate or inhibit the action of estrogen.[3] Likewise, the progesterone receptor has two major forms (A and B), expressed by a single gene, but produced differently in a complex system of transcription regulation.

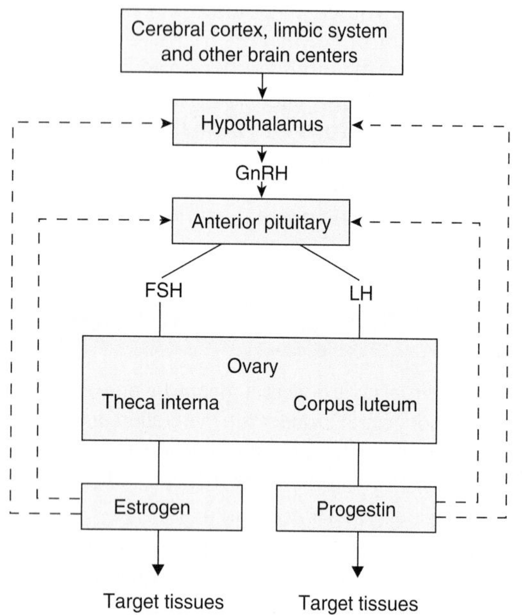

FIGURE 46-5 Hypothalamic-pituitary feedback control of estrogen and progesterone levels in the female.

Estrogens. Estrogens are a family of structurally related female sex hormones synthesized and secreted by cells in the ovaries and, in small amounts, by cells in the adrenal cortex. Androgens can be converted to estrogens peripherally, especially in fat tissue. Three estrogens occur naturally in humans: estrone (E_1), estradiol (E_2), and estriol (E_3). Of these, estradiol is the most biologically potent and the most abundantly secreted product of the ovary. Estrogens are secreted throughout the menstrual cycle. Two peaks occur: one before ovulation and one in the middle of the luteal phase. Estrogens are transported in the blood bound to specific plasma globulins (which can also bind testosterone), inactivated and conjugated in the liver, and then excreted in the bile.

Estrogens are necessary for the normal female physical maturation. In concert with other hormones, estrogens provide for the reproductive processes of ovulation, implantation of the products of conception, pregnancy, parturition, and lactation by stimulating the development and maintaining the growth of the accessory organs. In the absence of androgens, estrogens stimulate the intrauterine development of the vagina, uterus, and fallopian tubes from the embryonic müllerian system. They also stimulate the stromal development and ductal growth of the breasts at puberty, are responsible for the accelerated pubertal skeletal growth phase and for closure of the epiphyses of the long bones, contribute to the growth of axillary and pubic hair, and alter the distribution of body fat to produce the typical female body contours, including the accumulation of body fat around the hips and breasts. Larger quantities of estrogen stimulate pigmentation of the skin in the nipple, areolar, and genital regions.

In addition to their effects on the growth of uterine muscle, estrogens play an important role in the development of the endometrial lining. During anovulatory cycles, continued exposure to estrogens for prolonged periods leads to abnormal hyperplasia of the endometrium and abnormal bleeding patterns. When estrogen production is poorly coordinated during the normal menstrual period, inappropriate bleeding and shedding of the endometrium also can occur (see Chapter 47).

Estrogens have a number of important extragenital metabolic effects. They are responsible for maintaining the normal structure of skin and blood vessels in women. Estrogens decrease the rate of bone resorption by antagonizing the effects of parathyroid hormone on bone; for this reason, osteoporosis is a common problem in estrogen-deficient postmenopausal women. In the liver, estrogens increase the synthesis of transport proteins for thyroxine, estrogen, testosterone, and other hormones. Estrogens also affect the composition of the plasma lipoproteins. They produce an increase in high-density lipoproteins (HDLs), a slight reduction in low-density lipoproteins (LDLs), and a reduction in cholesterol levels (see Chapter 24).

Estrogens have additional cardioprotective actions, including direct antiatherosclerotic effects on the arterial wall (augmentation of vasodilating and antiplatelet aggregation factors such as nitric oxide and prostacyclin), vasodilation through endothelium-independent mechanisms, antioxidant activity, reduced levels of angiotensin-converting enzyme and renin, reduction of homocysteine levels, improved peripheral glucose metabolism with subsequent decreased circulating insulin levels, and direct effects on cardiac function (*i.e.,* increased left ventricular diastolic filling and stroke volume output). Estrogens increase plasma triglyceride levels and enhance the coagulability of blood by effecting increased circulating levels of plasminogen and factors II, VII, IX, and X.

Estrogens appear to have both neurotropic and neuroprotective effects on cognitive function and memory. Observational studies indicate possible prevention of Alzheimer's disease through antiinflammatory mechanisms to prevent vascular injury, increased cerebral blood flow, and altered brain activation. Estrogens promote dendritic branching and enhance presynaptic and postsynaptic signal transmission through increased production of neurotransmitters and receptors.[4]

The estrogens cause moderate retention of sodium and water. Most women retain sodium and water and gain weight just before menstruation. This occurs because the estrogens facilitate the movement of intravascular fluids into the extracellular spaces, producing edema and increased sodium and water retention by the kidneys because of the decreased plasma volume. The actions of estrogens are summarized in Table 46-1.

Progesterone. Although the word *progesterone* refers to a substance that maintains pregnancy, progesterone is secreted as part of the normal menstrual cycle. The corpus luteum of the ovary secretes large amounts of progesterone after ovulation, and the adrenal cortex secretes small amounts. The hormone circulates in the blood attached to a specific plasma protein. It is metabolized in the liver and conjugated for excretion in the bile.

The local effects of progesterone on reproductive organs include the glandular development of the lobular and alveolar tissue of the breasts and the cyclic glandular development of the endometrium. Progesterone also can compete with aldosterone at the level of the renal tubule,

TABLE 46-1 Actions of Estrogens

General Function	Specific Actions
Growth and development	
Reproductive organs	Stimulate development of vagina, uterus, and fallopian tubes in utero and of secondary sex characteristics during puberty
Skeleton	Accelerate growth of long bones and closure of epiphyses at puberty
Reproductive processes	
Ovulation	Promote growth of ovarian follicles
Fertilization	Alter the cervical secretions to favor survival and transport of sperm
	Promote motility of sperm within the fallopian tubes by decreasing mucus viscosity
Implantation	Promote development of endometrial lining in the event of pregnancy
Vagina	Proliferate and cornify vaginal mucosa
Cervix	Increase mucus consistency
Breasts	Stimulate stromal development and ductal growth
General metabolic effects	
Bone resorption	Decrease rate of bone resorption
Plasma proteins	Increase production of thyroid and other binding globulins
Lipoproteins	Increase high-density and slightly decrease low-density lipoproteins

causing a decrease in sodium reabsorption, with a resultant increase in secretion of aldosterone by the adrenal cortex, as occurs in pregnancy. Although the mechanism is uncertain, progesterone increases basal body temperature and is responsible for the increase in body temperature that occurs with ovulation. Smooth muscle relaxation under the influence of progesterone plays an important role in maintaining pregnancy by decreasing uterine contractions and is responsible for many of the common discomforts of pregnancy, such as edema, nausea, constipation, flatulence, and headaches. The increased progesterone present during pregnancy and the luteal phase of the menstrual cycle enhances the ventilatory response to carbon dioxide, leading to a measurable change in arterial and alveolar carbon dioxide (PCO_2) levels.

Androgens. The normal female produces androgens, estrogens, and progesterone. Approximately 25% of these androgens are secreted from the ovaries, 25% from the adrenal cortex, and 50% from ovarian or adrenal precursors. In the female, androgens contribute to normal hair growth at puberty and may have other important metabolic effects.

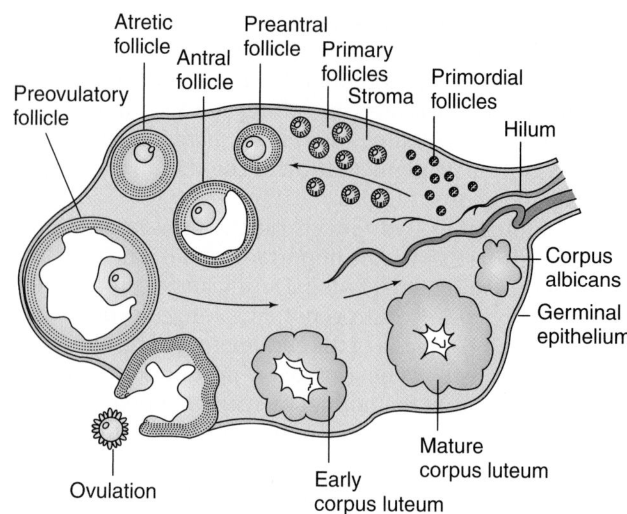

FIGURE 46-6 Schematic diagram of an ovary, showing the sequence of events in the origin, growth, and rupture of an ovarian follicle and the formation and retrogression of a corpus luteum. The atretic follicles are those that show signs of degeneration and death.

OVARIAN FOLLICLE DEVELOPMENT AND OVULATION

The tissues of the adult ovary can be conveniently divided into four compartments, or units: the stroma, or supporting tissue; the interstitial cells; the follicles; and the corpus luteum. The *stroma* is the connective tissue substance of the ovary in which the follicles are distributed. The *interstitial cells* are estrogen-secreting cells that resemble the Leydig's cells, or interstitial cells, of the testes.

Beginning at puberty, a cyclic rise in the anterior pituitary hormones FSH and LH stimulates the development of several graafian, or mature, follicles. Follicles at all stages of development can be found in both ovaries, except in menopausal women (Fig. 46-6). Most follicles exist as primary follicles, each of which consists of a round oocyte surrounded by a single layer of flattened, epithelium-derived granulosa cells and a basement membrane. The primary follicles constitute an inactive pool of follicles from which all the ovulating follicles develop. Under the influence of endocrine stimulation, 6 to 12 primary follicles develop into secondary follicles once every ovulatory cycle. During the development of the secondary follicle, the primary oocyte increases in size, and the granulosa cells proliferate to form a multilayered wall around it. During this time, a membrane called the *zona pellucida* develops and surrounds the oocyte, and small pockets of fluid begin to appear between the granulosa cells. Blood vessels, however, do not penetrate the basement membrane; the granulosa cell layer remains avascular until after ovulation has occurred.

As the follicles mature, FSH stimulates the development of the cell layers. Cells from the surrounding stromal tissue align themselves to form a cellular wall called the *theca*. The cells of the theca become differentiated into two layers: an inner theca interna, which lies adjacent to the follicular cells; and an outer theca externa. As the follicle enlarges, a single large cavity, or *antrum,* is formed, and a portion of the granulosa cells and the oocyte are displaced to one side of the follicle by the fluid that accumulates. The secondary oocyte remains surrounded by a crown of granulosa cells, the corona radiata. As the follicle ripens, ovarian estrogen is produced by the granulosa cells. Selection of a dominant follicle occurs with the conversion to an estrogen microenvironment. The lesser follicles, although continuing to produce some estrogen, atrophy or become atretic. The dominant follicle accumulates a greater mass of granulosa cells, and the theca becomes richly vascular, giving the follicle a hyperemic appearance. High levels of estrogen exert a negative feedback effect on FSH, inhibiting multiple follicular development and causing an increase in LH levels. This represents the follicular stage of the menstrual cycle. As estrogen suppresses FSH, the actions of LH predominate, and the mature follicle (measuring approximately 20 mm) bursts; the oocyte, along with the corona radiata, is ejected from the follicle. The ovum normally is then picked up and transported through the fallopian tube toward the uterus.

After ovulation, the follicle collapses, and the luteal stage of the menstrual cycle begins. The granulosa cells are invaded by blood vessels and yellow lipochrome-bearing cells from the theca layer. A rapid accumulation of blood and fluid forms a mass called the *corpus luteum.* Leakage of this blood onto the peritoneal surface that surrounds the ovary is thought to contribute to the *mittelschmerz (i.e.,* middle [or intermenstrual] pain) of ovulation. During the luteal stage, progesterone is secreted from the corpus luteum. If fertilization does not take place, the corpus luteum atrophies and is replaced by white scar tissue called the *corpus albicans;* the hormonal support of the endometrium is withdrawn, and menstruation occurs. In the event of fertilization, a hormone called *human chorionic gonadotropin* is produced by the trophoblastic cells in the blastocyst. This hormone prevents luteal regression. The corpus luteum remains functional for 3 months and provides hormonal support for pregnancy until the placenta is fully functional. Figure 46-7 shows the hormonal changes that occur during the development of the ovarian follicle and ovulation.

ENDOMETRIAL CHANGES

The endometrium consists of two distinct layers, or zones, that are responsive to hormonal stimulation: a basal layer and a functional layer. The *basal layer* lies adjacent to the myometrium and is not sloughed during menstruation. The *functional layer* arises from the basal layer and undergoes proliferative changes and menstrual sloughing. It can be subdivided into two components: a thin, superficial, compact layer and a deeper spongiosa layer that makes up most of the secretory and fully developed endometrium. The endometrial cycle can be divided into three phases: the proliferative, or preovulatory, phase, during which the glands and stroma of the superficial layer grow rapidly under the influence of estrogen; the secretory, or postovulatory, phase, during which progesterone produces glandular dilation and active mucus secretion and the endometrium becomes highly vascular and edematous; and the menstrual phase, during which the superficial layer degenerates and sloughs off.

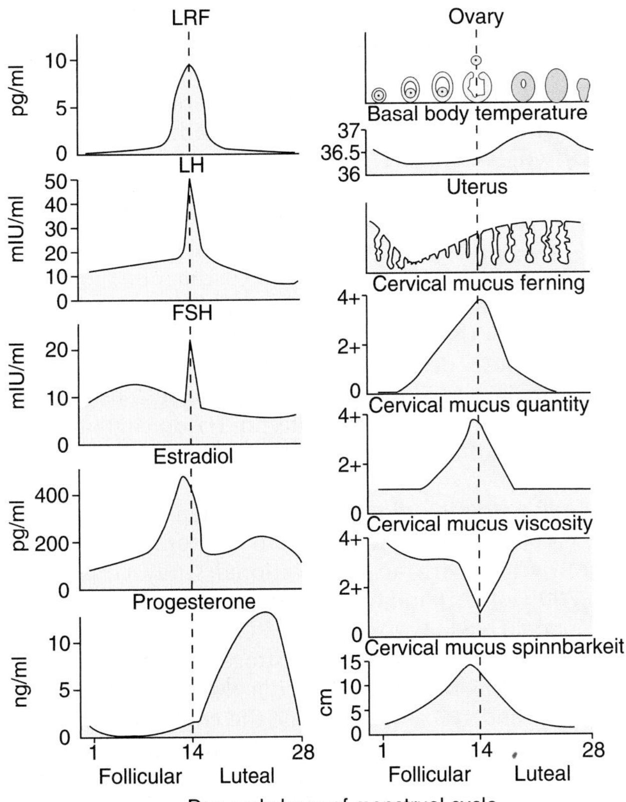

FIGURE 46-7 Hormonal and morphologic changes during the normal menstrual cycle. (Hershman J.M. [1982]. *Endocrine pathophysiology* [2nd ed.]. Philadelphia: Lea & Febiger)

CERVICAL MUCUS CHANGES

Cervical mucus is a complex, heterogeneous secretion produced by the glands of the endocervix. It is composed of 92% to 98% water and 1% inorganic salts, mainly sodium chloride. The mucus also contains simple sugars, polysaccharides, proteins, and glycoproteins. Its pH usually is alkaline, ranging from 6.5 to 9.0. Its characteristics are strongly influenced by serum levels of estrogen and progesterone. Estrogen stimulates the production of large amounts of clear, watery mucus through which sperm can penetrate most easily. Progesterone, even in the presence of estrogen, reduces the secretion of mucus. During the luteal phase of the menstrual cycle, mucus is scant, viscous, and cellular (see Fig. 46-7).

Two methods are used to examine the properties of cervical mucus and correlate them with hormonal activity. *Spinnbarkeit* is the property that allows cervical mucus to be stretched or drawn into a thread. Spinnbarkeit can be estimated by stretching a sample of cervical mucus between two glass slides and measuring the maximum length of the thread before it breaks. At midcycle, spinnbarkeit usually exceeds 10 cm. A second method of estimating hormonal levels is *ferning,* or arborization. Ferning refers to the characteristic microscopic pattern that results from the crystallization of the inorganic salts in the cervical mucus when it is dried. As the estrogen levels increase, the composition of the cervical mucus changes, so that dried mucus begins to demonstrate ferning in the later part of the follicular phase. The absence of ferning can indicate inadequate estrogen stimulation of the endocervical glands or inhibition of the endocervical glands by increased secretion of progesterone. Persistent ferning throughout the menstrual cycle suggests anovulatory cycles or insufficient progesterone secretion.

MENOPAUSE

Menopause is the cessation of menstrual cycles. Like menarche, it is more of a process than a single event. Most women stop menstruating between 48 and 55 years of age. *Perimenopause* (the years immediately surrounding menopause) precedes menopause by approximately 4 years and is characterized by menstrual irregularity and other menopausal symptoms. *Climacteric* is a more encompassing term that refers to the entire transition to the nonreproductive period of life. Premature ovarian failure describes the approximately 1% of women who experience menopause before the age of 40 years. A woman who has not menstruated for a full year or who has an FSH level greater than 30 mIU/mL is considered menopausal.

Functional Changes

Menopause results from the gradual cessation of ovarian function and the resultant diminished levels of estrogen. Although estrogens derived from the adrenal cortex continue to circulate in a woman's body, they are insufficient to maintain the secondary sexual characteristics in the same manner as ovarian estrogens. As a result, body hair, skin elasticity, and subcutaneous fat decrease. The breasts become pendulous with decrease in tissue mass, leaving only the ducts, fat, and connective tissue. The ovaries and uterus diminish in size; and the cervix and vagina become pale and friable.

Problems that can arise as a result of urogenital atrophy include vaginal dryness, urinary stress incontinence, urgency, nocturia, vaginitis, and urinary tract infection. The woman may find intercourse painful and traumatic, although some type of vaginal lubrication may be helpful. A metaanalysis of studies published between 1969 and 1995 concluded that estrogen therapy is effective in the treatment of symptoms of genitourinary atrophy, including urinary tract infection (UTI).[4]

Systemically, a woman may experience significant vasomotor instability secondary to the decrease in estrogens and the relative increase in other hormones, including FSH, LH, GnRH, dehydroepiandrosterone, androstenedione, epinephrine, corticotropin, β-endorphin, growth hormone, and calcitonin gene-related peptide. This instability may give rise to "hot flashes," palpitations, dizziness, and headaches as the blood vessels dilate. Despite the association with these biochemical changes, the underlying cause of hot flashes is unknown.[5] Tremendous variation exists in the onset, frequency, severity, and length of time that women experience hot flashes. When they occur at night and are accompanied by significant perspiration, they are referred to as *night sweats*. Insomnia or frequent awakening because of vasomotor symptoms can lead to sleep deprivation. A woman may experience irritability, anxiety, and depression as a result of these uncontrollable and unpredictable events.

In addition to changes that closely follow the cessation of ovarian function, there are changes that over many years influence the health and well-being of postmenopausal women. Consequences of long-term estrogen deprivation include osteoporosis due to an imbalance in bone remodeling (*i.e.,* bone resorption occurs at a faster rate than bone formation) and an increased risk for cardiovascular disease (atherosclerosis is accelerated), which is the leading cause of death in women after menopause. Other potential health threats, which reflect both aging and cessation of ovarian function, are loss of vision due to macular degeneration and cognitive impairment.

Hormone Therapy

During the past four to five decades, hormone therapy (HT) became increasingly prescribed for postmenopausal women. Initially, hormone therapy was used only for symptom management and later for prevention of osteoporosis. During the 1990s, hormone therapy evolved to the status of *replacement* for a vital hormone lost due to an endocrine organ failure (menopause). It was routinely offered to all postmenopausal women based on mounting evidence of preventive benefits in numerous areas. During this time, data from observational studies demonstrated a 50% reduction in coronary heart disease mortality rates in women using HT. This was considered highly significant because heart disease is the leading cause of death in women after menopause. Other demonstrated advantages to HT included a reduced risk for Alzheimer's disease (leading cause of lost independence and institutionalization),[6] decreased risk for colon cancer (third leading cause of cancer death among women),[7] less tooth loss,[8] and lower incidence of macular degeneration (leading cause of legal blindness in the United States).[9]

The type of HT prescribed was determined by whether the woman had an intact uterus. Women with an intact uterus received a combination of estrogen and progesterone, and those who had previously had their uterus removed received estrogen only. The addition of progesterone to HT was the established protocol for women with an intact uterus because the association between unopposed estrogen and the development of endometrial cancer was noted in the 1970s. Unopposed estrogen can lead to the development of endometrial hyperplasia, which in some cases can increase a woman's risk for endometrial cancer. HT that involves the use of both estrogen and progesterone is not associated with endometrial cancer. When used cyclically, progesterone is added for 12 to 14 days to mature any endometrium that has developed in response to the estrogen. Progesterone withdrawal results in endometrial shedding (*i.e.,* a cyclic bleeding episode). When used continuously, a small amount of progesterone is added to the daily estrogen regimen. This continuous exposure to progesterone inhibits endometrial development. Eventually, the combined continuous estrogen progesterone therapy (CCEPT) results in no bleeding; however, it can be associated with irregular bleeding and spotting until the lining becomes atrophic. Prevention of endometrial hyperplasia either by shedding the endometrial buildup or by preventing its development minimizes the risk for endometrial cancer. This protection must now be considered when weighing the risks and benefits of HT. When the estrogen-only arm of the Women's Health Initiative (to be discussed) is complete, it will provide statistics comparing the risk–benefit profile of estrogen therapy versus CCEPT.

With the current shift to evidence-based medicine, randomized controlled trials (RCTs) were undertaken to confirm the earlier findings using an experimental model and to demonstrate that the intervention (HT) was in fact responsible for the outcome and not other variables. Several RCTs have now demonstrated that HT does not prevent and can increase the likelihood of a cardiovascular event.[10–12] Other studies looking at the effect of HT on cognition and Alzheimer's disease have failed to show benefit.[13,14]

Women's Health Initiative. The Women's Health Initiative (WHI) was planned as an 8- to 10-year nationwide research effort with an observational study component (93,700 women) and a multicentered, prospective, RCT component (68,000 women). The RCT component included three arms: HT (estrogen alone, estrogen plus progestin, and placebo), a low-fat diet, and calcium plus vitamin D. The HT arm was undertaken to examine the effect of estrogen or estrogen plus progestin on the prevention of heart disease and any associated change in risk for breast and colon cancer. Because the women in the study were generally healthy, the independent Data and Safety Monitoring Committee chose conservative safety criteria for early termination of the study. The study enrolled 16,608 women aged 50 to 79 years with an intact uterus in the estrogen-plus-progestin arm, and it was stopped after 5.2 years of data analysis when the risk for breast cancer crossed the predetermined safety boundary and a global index suggested that the risks of HT outweigh its benefits. Results demonstrated that instead of lowering the risk for heart disease, the women using estrogen plus progestin had increased risks for coronary events (29%), stroke (40%), and pulmonary embolism (100%). On the positive side, there was a 37% reduction in colon cancer and a 34% reduction in hip fractures among the women using HT.[12] The estrogen-only (ET) arm was not stopped.

When the National Heart, Lung and Blood Institute (NHLBI) of the National Institute of Health (NIH) prematurely stopped one arm of the WHI in July 2002, the published data resulted in revised recommendations from the U.S. Food and Drug Administration (FDA) and numerous professional organizations regarding the use of HT in women.

Studies of Breast Cancer Risk. The association with breast cancer has long been the other area of concern with HT, and the data are not clear here despite more than 50 years of study. When evaluating the many studies reporting estimated risks for breast cancer associated with ET and HT, most of the confidence intervals cross the relative risk of 1 and therefore are not statistically significant.[15] However, new studies linking estrogen and breast cancer continue to make front-page news, and consequently the worry persists. WHI added to this concern by demonstrating a 26% increased risk for invasive breast cancer in the women using CCEPT.[12] In actual numbers, this represented an additional 8 cases of breast cancer per 10,000 women using HT. For an individual woman, the added risk is quite small. However, when extrapolated to the estimated 6 million American women using HT, it represents a significant public health concern. Although the rate of breast cancer in WHI was not higher than previously reported in other studies, it has added weight given the type and size of the study.

Another large European study recruited more than 1 million women aged 50 to 64 years and analyzed the 80% who were postmenopausal for breast cancer incidence (2.6 years average follow-up) and mortality (4.1 years average follow-up). Approximately half the women had used HT at some time. Results of this observational study revealed increased risk (relative risk [RR], 1.66) among current users of HT, with the largest increase associated with CCEPT (RR, 1.88), slightly less with ET (RR, 1.33), and the risk declining after discontinuation to return to baseline within 5 years.[16]

Current theory postulates that these studies are in fact detection studies rather than incidence studies because it is known that breast cancer cells can be present in the body for up to 8 to 10 years before being clinically detected by any means currently available. If unknown cancer cells exist in the breast, estrogen may accelerate the growth of those cells to a point at which the cancer can then be detected. This would explain why some studies show a positive correlation between estrogen and breast cancer and others do not. Increases in breast cancer detection may in fact be a positive because it can then be treated. Mortality studies to date show a lower death rate among women using hormones at the time of breast cancer diagnosis compared with those not using HT. At present, there is insufficient evidence to support estrogen as the cause (initiator) of breast cancer. The lack of biologic plausibility for causation will continue to support the drive to find better ways for early detection of breast cancer. This would assist women in assessing their own risk-to-benefit ratio, taking into account their individual circumstances, when making decisions about HT.

Current Recommendations. Although the average age of menopause has not changed substantially since 1900, life expectancy has increased dramatically. Today, the average woman will live almost one third of her life after menopause. Menopause now represents only the end of reproductive capability. Estrogen's role in many other bodily functions has been well documented, but its replacement after the ovary ceases production has become highly controversial. Current recommendations for HT, in light of the findings of the WHI and pending other RCT data, are to avoid HT for primary or secondary prevention of coronary heart disease; develop an individual risk profile for every woman contemplating HT and provide information regarding known risks; use HT only in those women who require relief from menopausal symptoms that affect quality of life; consider lower-than-standard doses and alternative routes of administration; limit the use of HT to the shortest duration consistent with goals, benefits, and risks for treatment in each woman; and because of risks associated with HT products that are FDA-approved for the prevention of postmenopausal osteoporosis, consider alternative therapies if the woman is not symptomatic.[17] The U.S. Preventive Services Task Force has recommended against the routine use of HT for preventing chronic conditions in general.[17]

The results of the WHI have led to an increased interest in alternative methods for management of postmenopausal symptoms, including the use of bio-identical hormones. Bio-identical hormone therapy uses "natural" substances derived from plant oils that are similar in structure to human steroid hormones,[18] and "phytoestrogens," substances occurring in nature with estrogen-like properties such as isoflavones (soy, red clover). To date, these agents, although widely used, have not demonstrated effectiveness in controlled trials.

Because the risk for osteoporosis remains high, there is a continued search for methods to prevent or decrease the rate of bone loss in postmenopausal women. At present, therapies with demonstrated effectiveness in treating osteoporosis include bisphosphonates, calcitonin, raloxifene (a selective estrogen receptor modulator [SERM] that works only on certain estrogen receptors, but not others), calcium, fluoride, and parathyroid hormone (see Chapter 58).

Societal mores influence behaviors. A society that emphasizes youthfulness, fitness, and vigor may not look on aging as a positive process, and menopause is regarded as a hallmark of advancing age. A woman who focuses her energy on beauty and youth may feel frustrated or depressed by the natural aging process. A woman who values her other, nonphysical attributes may welcome advancing age as a time when she may more fully develop as a person.

In summary, between the menarche and menopause, the female reproductive system undergoes cyclic changes called the *menstrual cycle.* The normal menstrual function results from complex interactions among the hypothalamus, which produces GnRH; the anterior pituitary gland, which synthesizes and releases FSH, LH, and prolactin; the ovaries, which synthesize and release estrogens, progesterone, and androgens; and associated target tissues, such as the endometrium and the vaginal mucosa. Although each component of the system is essential for normal functioning, the ovarian hormones are largely responsible for controlling the cyclic changes and length of the menstrual cycle. Estrogens are necessary for normal female physical maturation, for growth of ovarian follicles, for generation of a climate that is favorable to fertilization and implantation of the ovum, and for promoting the development of the endometrium in the event of pregnancy. Estrogens also have a number of extragenital effects, including prevention of bone resorption and regulation of the composition of cholesterol-carrying lipoproteins (HDL and LDL) in the blood. The functions of progesterone include the glandular development of the lobular and alveolar tissue of the breasts, the cyclic glandular development of the endometrium, and maintenance of pregnancy. Androgens contribute to hair distribution in the female and may have important metabolic effects.

Menopause is the cessation of menstrual cycles. Systemically, a woman may experience significant vasomotor instability and "hot flashes" secondary to the decrease in estrogens and the relative increase in other hormones, including FSH, LH, GnRH, dehydroepiandrosterone, and androstenedione. The long-term effects of estrogen deprivation include osteoporosis due to an imbalance in bone remodeling (*i.e.,* bone resorption occurs at a faster rate than bone formation) and an increased risk for cardiovascular disease (atherosclerosis is accelerated), which is the leading cause of death in women after menopause. Hormone therapy, which was regarded as a hormone replacement therapy for postmenopausal women during the late 20th century, has come under scrutiny as a result of the WHI, which indicates that CCEPT may increase the risk for cardiovascular disease (continuous estrogen and progestin) and breast cancer.

Breasts

After completing this section of the chapter, you should be able to meet the following objectives:

- Describe the anatomy of the female breast
- Describe the influence of hormones on breast development
- Characterize the changes in breast structure that occur with pregnancy and lactation

Although anatomically separate, the breasts are functionally related to the female genitourinary system in that they respond to the cyclic changes in sex hormones and produce milk for infant nourishment. The breasts also are important for their sexual function and for cosmetic appearance. Breast cancer represents the most common malignancy among women in the United States. The high rate of breast cancer has drawn even greater attention to the importance of the breasts throughout the life span.

STRUCTURE AND FUNCTION

The breasts, or mammary tissues, are located between the third and seventh ribs of the anterior chest wall and are supported by the pectoral muscles and superficial fascia. They are specialized glandular structures that have an abundant shared nervous, vascular, and lymphatic supply (Fig. 46-8). What are commonly called breasts are two parts of a single anatomic breast. This contiguous nature of breast tissue is important in health and illness. Men and women alike are born with rudimentary breast tissue, with the ducts lined with epithelium. In women, the pituitary release of FSH, LH, and prolactin at puberty stimulates the ovary to produce and release estrogen. This estrogen stimulates the growth and proliferation of the ductile system. With the onset of ovulatory cycles, progesterone release stimulates the growth and development of ductile and alveolar secretory epithelium. By adolescence, the breasts have developed characteristic fat deposition patterns and contours.

Structurally, the breast consists of fat, fibrous connective tissue, and glandular tissue. The superficial fibrous connective tissue is attached to the skin, a fact that is important in the visual observation of skin movement over the breast during breast self-examination. The breast mass is supported by the fascia of the pectoralis major and minor muscles and by the fibrous connective tissue of the breast. Fibrous tissue ligaments, called *Cooper's ligaments,* extend from the outer boundaries of the breast to the nipple area in a radial manner, like the spokes on a wheel (see Fig. 46-8). These ligaments further support the breast and form septa that divide the breast into 15 to 25 lobes. Each lobe consists of grapelike clusters, alveoli or glands, which are interconnected by ducts. The alveoli are lined with secretory cells capable of producing milk or fluid under the proper hormonal conditions (Fig. 46-9). The route of descent of milk and other breast secretions is from alveoli to duct, to intralobar duct, to lactiferous duct and reservoir, to nipple. Breast milk is produced secondary to complex hormonal changes associated with pregnancy. Fluid is produced and reabsorbed during the menstrual cycle. The breasts respond to the cyclic changes in the menstrual cycle with fullness and discomfort.

The nipple is made up of epithelial, glandular, erectile, and nervous tissue. Areolar tissue surrounds the nipple and is recognized as the darker, smooth skin between the nipple and the breast. The small bumps or projections on the areolar surface, known as *Montgomery's tu-*

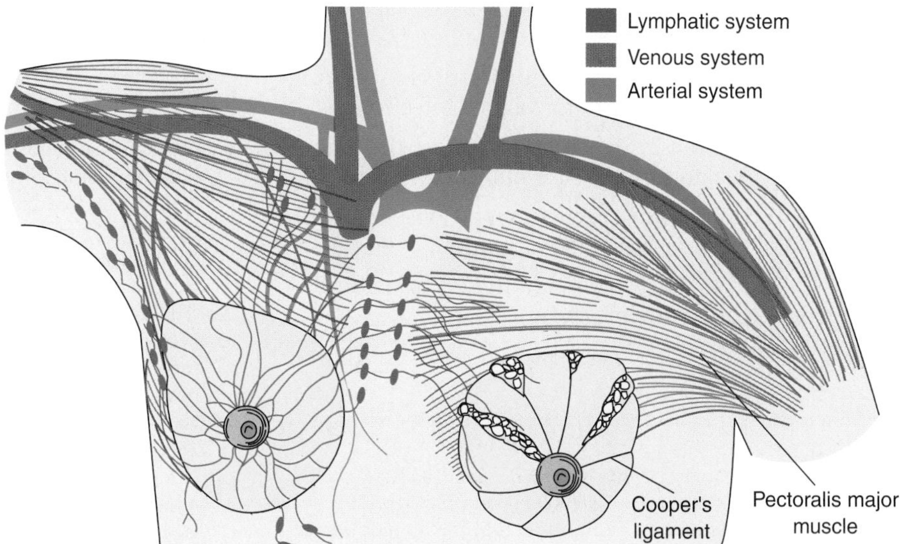

FIGURE 46-8 The breasts, showing the shared vascular and lymphatic supply as well as the pectoral muscles.

bercles, are sebaceous glands that keep the nipple area soft and elastic. At puberty and during pregnancy, increased levels of estrogen and progesterone cause the areola and nipple to become darker and more prominent and Montgomery's glands to become more active. The erectile tissue of the nipple is responsive to psychological and tactile stimuli, which contributes to the sexual function of the breasts.

There are many individual variations in breast size and shape. The shape and texture vary with hormonal, genetic, nutritional, and endocrine factors and with muscle tone, age, and pregnancy. A well-developed set of pectoralis muscles supports the breast mass higher on the chest wall. Poor posture, significant weight loss, and lack of support may cause the breasts to droop.

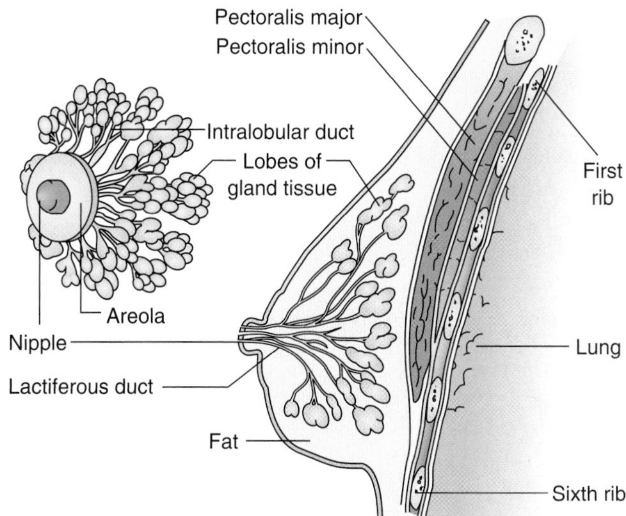

FIGURE 46-9 The breast, showing the glandular tissue and ducts of the mammary glands.

Pregnancy

During pregnancy, the breasts are significantly altered by increased levels of estrogen and progesterone. Estrogen stimulates increased vascularity of the breasts and the growth and extension of the ductile structures, causing "heaviness" of the breasts. Progesterone causes marked budding and growth of the alveolar structures. The alveolar epithelium assumes a secretory state in preparation for lactation. The progesterone-induced changes that occur during pregnancy may confer some protection against cancer. Cellular changes that occur in the alveolar lining are thought to change the susceptibility of these cells to estrogen-mediated changes later in life.

Lactation

During lactation, milk is secreted by alveolar cells, which are under the influence of the anterior pituitary hormone prolactin. Milk ejection from the ductile system occurs in response to the release of oxytocin from the posterior pituitary. The suckling of the infant provides the stimulus for milk ejection. Suckling produces feedback to the hypothalamus, stimulating the release of oxytocin from the posterior pituitary. Oxytocin causes contraction of the myoepithelial cells lining the alveoli and ejection of milk into the ductal system. A woman may have breast leakage for 3 months to 1 year after the termination of breast-feeding as breast tissue and hormones regress to the nonlactating state. Overzealous breast stimulation with or without pregnancy can likewise cause breast leakage.

In summary, the breast is a complex structure of variable size, consistency, and composition. Although anatomically distinct, the breasts are functionally related to the female genitourinary system in that they respond to cyclic changes in sex hormones and produce milk for infant nourishment.

REVIEW EXERCISES

Diabetes mellitus and treatment with broad-spectrum antibiotics increase the risk for vaginal infections.

A. Explain how these two conditions change the vaginal ecology, making it more susceptible to infection.

Most oral contraceptive agents use low doses of estrogen and progestin to prevent conception.

A. Use Figure 46-4 to explain how these oral agents prevent ovulation and pregnancy.

References

1. Pernoll M.L. (2001). *Benson & Pernoll's handbook of obstetrics and gynecology* (10th ed., p. 31). New York: McGraw-Hill.
2. Revelli A., Massobrio M., Tesarik J. (1998). Nongenomic actions of steroid hormones in reproductive tissue. *Endocrine Review 19,* 3–17.
3. Gruber C.J., Tschugguel W., Schneeberger C., Huber J.C. (2002). Production and actions of estrogens. *New England Journal of Medicine 346*(5), 340–352.
4. Maloney C. (2002). Estrogen and recurrent UTI in postmenopausal women. *American Journal of Nursing 102*(8), 47–52.
5. Dormire S.L. (2003). What we know about managing menopausal hot flashes: navigating without a compass. *Journal of Obstetric, Gynecologic, and Neonatal Nursing 32*(4), 455–464.
6. Seifer D.B., Kennard E.A. (1999). *Menopause: Endocrinology and management* (p. 100). Totowa, NJ: Humana Press.
7. Nanda K., Bostoc L.A., Hasselblad V., Simmel D.L. (1999). Hormone replacement therapy and the risk of colorectal cancer: A meta-analysis. *Obstetrics and Gynecology 93,* 880–888.
8. Grodstein F., Colditz G.A., Stampfer M.J. (1996). Postmenopausal hormone use and tooth loss: A prospective study. *Journal of the American Dental Association 127,* 370–377.
9. The Eye Disease Case Control Study Group. (1992). Risk factors for neurovascular age-related macular degeneration. *Archives of Ophthalmology 110,* 1701–1708.
10. Hulley S., Grady D., Bush T., et al. (1998). Randomized trial of estrogen plus progestin for secondary prevention of coronary heart disease in postmenopausal women: Heart and Estrogen/progestin Replacement Study (HERS) Research Group. *JAMA 280,* 605–613.
11. Grady D., Herrington D., Bittner V., et al. (2002). Cardiovascular disease outcomes during 6.8 years of hormone therapy: Heart and Estrogen/progestin Replacement Study Follow-up (HERS-II). *JAMA 288,* 49–57.
12. Writing Group for the Women's Health Initiative Investigators. (2002). Risks and benefits of estrogen and progestin in healthy postmenopausal women: Principal results from the Women's Health Initiative randomized controlled trial. *JAMA 288,* 321–333.
13. Grady D., Yaffe K., Kristof M., et al. (2002). Effect of postmenopausal hormone therapy on cognitive function: The Heart and Estrogen/progestin Replacement Study. *American Journal of Medicine 113,* 543–548.
14. Mulnard R.A., Cotman C.W., Kawas C., et al. (2000). Estrogen replacement therapy for treatment of mild to moderate Alzheimer disease: a randomized controlled trial. Alzheimer Disease Cooperative Study. *JAMA 283,* 1007–1015.
15. Speroff L. (2000). Postmenopausal estrogen-progestin therapy and breast cancer: A clinical response to an epidemiologic report. *Contemporary Obstetrics/Gynecology 3,* 103–121.
16. Beral V. (2003). Current combined HT use doubles risk of breast cancer. *Lancet 362*(9383), 419–427.
17. Berg A.O.Chairman. (2003). Postmenopausal hormone replacement therapy for the primary prevention of chronic conditions: Recommendations and rationale of the US Preventive Task Force. *American Family Physician* 67(2), 358–364.
18. Francisco L. (2003). Is bio-identical hormone therapy fact or fairy tale? *Nurse Practitioner 28*(7), 39–47.

CHAPTER 47

Disorders of the Female Reproductive System

Patricia McCowen Mehring

Disorders of the female genitourinary system have widespread effects on physical and psychological function, affecting sexuality and reproductive function. The reproductive structures are located close to other pelvic structures, particularly those of the urinary system, and disorders of the reproductive system may affect urinary function. This chapter focuses on infection and inflammation, benign conditions, and neoplasms of the female reproductive structures; disorders of pelvic support and uterine position; and alterations in menstruation. An overview of infertility also is included.

Disorders of the External Genitalia and Vagina

After completing this section of the chapter, you should be able to meet the following objectives:

- ✦ Compare the abnormalities associated with vulvitis, Bartholin's cyst, epidermal cysts, nevi, nonneoplastic epithelial disorders, vulvodynia, and cancer of the vulva
- ✦ State the role of Döderlein's bacilli in maintaining the normal ecology of the vagina
- ✦ Describe the conditions that predispose to vaginal infections and the methods used to prevent and treat these infections
- ✦ Cite the association between diethylstilbestrol and adenocarcinoma of the vagina

DISORDERS OF THE EXTERNAL GENITALIA

Vulvitis and Folliculitis

Vulvitis is characterized by inflammation and pruritus (itching) of the vulva. It is not considered a specific disease but typically accompanies other local and systemic disorders. The cause often is an irritating vaginal discharge. *Candida albicans,* a yeast, is the most common cause of chronic vulvar pruritus, particularly in women with diabetes mellitus. Vulvitis also may be a component of sexually transmitted diseases (STDs) such as herpes genitalis and human papillomavirus (HPV) infection (*i.e.,* condyloma). Local dermatologic reactions to chemical irritants, such as laundry products, perfumed soaps or sprays, and spermicides, or to allergens such as poison ivy, also can cause inflammation. Vulvar itching also may be caused by atrophy that is part of the normal aging process.

Management of vulvitis focuses on appropriate treatment of underlying causes and comfort measures to relieve the irritation. These include keeping the area clean and dry; using warm sitz baths with baking soda, wet dressings, or Burow's solution soaks (a mild astringent); or applying a mild hydrocortisone cream for the immediate relief of symptoms.

Folliculitis is an infection that involves the hair follicles of the mons or labia majora. The infection, characterized by small red papules or pustules surrounding the hair shaft, is relatively common because of the density of bacteria in this area and the occlusive nature of clothing covering the genitalia. Treatment includes thorough cleaning of the area with germicidal soap, followed by the application of a mild antibacterial ointment (*e.g.,* Neosporin or Polysporin).

Bartholin's Gland Cyst and Abscess

Bartholin's cyst is a fluid-filled sac that results from the occlusion of the duct system in Bartholin's gland. When the cyst becomes infected, the contents become purulent; if the infection goes untreated, an abscess can result. The obstruction that causes cyst and abscess formation most commonly follows a bacterial, chlamydial, or gonococcal infection. Cysts can attain the size of an orange and frequently recur (Fig. 47-1). Abscesses can be extremely tender and painful.

Asymptomatic cysts require no treatment. The treatment of symptomatic cysts consists of the administration of appropriate antibiotics, local application of moist heat, and incision and drainage. Cysts that frequently are abscessed or are large enough to cause blockage of the introitus may require surgical intervention (*i.e.,* marsupialization, a procedure that involves removal of a wedge of vulvar skin and the cyst wall).[1]

Epidermal Cysts

Epidermal cysts (*i.e.,* sebaceous or inclusion cysts) are common semisolid tumors of the vulva. These small nodules are lined with stratified squamous epithelium and contain cellular debris with a sebaceous appearance and odor. Epidermal cysts may be solitary or multiple and have a yellow appearance when stretched or compressed. They usually resolve spontaneously, and treatment is unnecessary unless they become infected or significantly enlarged.

Nevi

Nevi (moles) occur on the vulva as elsewhere on the body. They can be singular or multiple, flat or raised, and may vary in degree of pigmentation from flesh colored to dark brown or black. Nevi are asymptomatic but should be observed for changes that could indicate cancer. Nevi may resemble melanomas or basal cell carcinomas, and excisional biopsy is recommended when doubt exists (see Chapter 61).

Nonneoplastic Epithelial Disorders

Nonneoplastic epithelial disorders of the vulva (formerly vulvar dystrophy) are characterized by white lesions of the

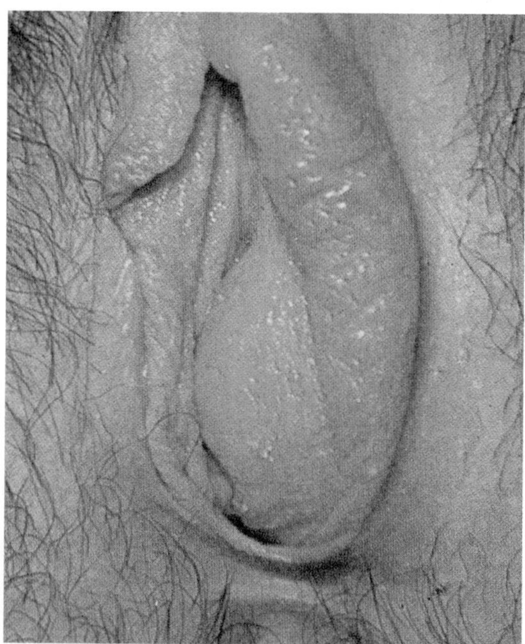

FIGURE 47-1 Bartholin's gland cyst. The 4-cm lesion is located to the right of and posterior to the vaginal introitus. (Rubin E., Farber J.L. [1999]. *Pathology* [3rd ed., p. 970]. Philadelphia: Lippincott-Raven)

vulva accompanied by itching or irritation. The lesions can be further categorized as lichen sclerosus, squamous cell hyperplasia, or other dermatoses, depending on clinical and histologic characteristics.

Lichen sclerosus patches are hypopigmented, plaque-like areas that may progress to parchment-thin epithelium with focal areas of ecchymosis and superficial ulceration secondary to scratching. Atrophy and agglutination of the labia minora with eventual stenosis of the introitus is common when this condition becomes chronic. Perirectal involvement is not uncommon.[2]

Squamous cell hyperplasia presents as thickened, gray-white plaques with an irregular surface. Presumed to be a response of the genital skin to some type of irritant, this diagnosis is used only when HPV, fungal infections, or other known causative conditions have been excluded.[3] Pruritus is the most common presenting complaint, but unlike lichen sclerosus, hyperplasia is generally not symmetric and often presents as a focal area involving the labia majora.

Current treatment of lichen sclerosus favors the use of potent topical corticosteroids (clobetasol or halobetasol).[3] Hyperplastic areas respond well to a combination corticosteroid (*e.g.*, betamethasone valerate) and antipruritic cream (*e.g.*, crotamiton) and to the removal of any irritants (*e.g.*, detergents, perfumes). Lichen sclerosus frequently recurs, and lifetime maintenance therapy may be required. Hyperplastic areas that occur in the field of lichen sclerosus may be sites of malignant change and warrant close follow-up and possible biopsy.

Vulvodynia

Vulvodynia is a syndrome of unexplained vulvar pain, also referred to as *vulvar pain syndrome* or *burning vulva syndrome*. It is a chronic disorder characterized by burning, stinging, irritation, and rawness. Several forms or subsets of vulvodynia have been identified, including cyclic vulvaginitis, vulvar dermatoses, vulvar vestibular syndrome, and vulvar dysesthesia. Because vulvodynia is a multifaceted condition, certain subsets may coexist with others.

Cyclic vulvodynia demonstrates episodic flares that occur only before menses or after coitus. *Vulvar dermatoses* are manifested by pruritus, and in some cases, pain develops progressively during the perimenopausal or postmenopausal period. Vulvar dermatoses include thick and scaly (*e.g.*, papulosquamous) lesions. Erosions may occur from excessive scratching.

Vulvar vestibulitis syndrome (VVS) is characterized by pain at onset of intercourse (*i.e.*, insertional dyspareunia), localized point tenderness near the vaginal opening, and sensitivity to tampon placement, tight-fitting pants, bicycling, or prolonged sitting. It is the leading cause of dyspareunia in women younger than 50 years of age. VVS can be primary (present from first contact) or secondary (developing after a period of comfortable sexual relations). Etiology is unknown but VVS can evolve from chronic vulvar inflammation or trauma. Nerve fibers to the vestibular epithelium become highly sensitized, causing neurons in the dorsal horn to respond abnormally, which transforms the sensation of touch in the vestibule into pain (allodynia).[4] Surgical vestibulectomy can become necessary for symptom relief when medical management fails.

Vulvar dysesthesia, also known as *idiopathic* or *essential vulvodynia,* involves severe, constant, widespread burning that interferes with daily activities. No abnormalities are found on examination, but there is diffuse and variable hypersensitivity and altered sensation to light touch. The quality of pain shares many of the features of neuropathic pain, particularly complex regional pain syndrome (see Chapter 50) or pudendal neuralgia. Although the cause of the neuropathic pain is unknown, it has been suggested that it may result from myofascial restrictions affecting sacral and pelvic floor nerves. Surface electromyography-assisted pelvic floor muscle rehabilitation has been shown to be an effective and long-term cure for dysesthetic vulvodynia.[5]

Possible causes for other forms of vulvodynia include candidal hypersensitivity related to chronic recurrent yeast infections; chemical irritation or drug effects, especially prolonged use of topical steroid creams; the irritating effects of elevated urinary levels of calcium oxalate; immunoglobulin A deficiency; and dermatoses such as lichen sclerosus, lichen planus, or squamous cell hyperplasia. Herpes simplex virus may be related to episodic vulvodynia, and long-term viral suppressive therapy may be of benefit to women with known herpes simplex virus infection who experience multiple outbreaks each year. Previous links to HPV infection have not been supported by studies, and the finding of subclinical HPV infection in women with vulvodynia now is thought to be a secondary or unrelated phenomenon.

Treatment of this chronic, often debilitating problem is aimed at symptom relief and elimination of suspected underlying problems. Careful history taking and physical assessment are essential for the differential diagnosis and treatment. Regimens can include long-term vaginal or oral antifungal therapy, avoidance of potential irritants, cleaning with water only or a gentle soap, sitz baths with baking soda, emollients such as vitamin E or vegetable oil for lubrication, low-oxalate diet plus calcium citrate supplements (calcium binds oxalate in the bowel, and citrate inhibits the formation of oxalate crystals), topical anesthetic or steroid ointments, physical therapy, and surgery. The tricyclic antidepressants are often used to treat the neuropathic pain associated with vulvar dysesthesia. Psychosocial support often is needed because this condition can cause strain in sexual, family, and work relationships. Vulvodynia often needs to be managed from a multidimensional, chronic pain perspective.[5]

Cancer of the Vulva

Carcinoma of the vulva accounts for approximately 4% of all cancers of the female genitourinary system. This translates to approximately 4000 U.S. cases of vulvar cancer in 2003, resulting in 800 deaths.[6] Vulvar cancer appears to exist as two separate diseases affecting different age groups. Invasive carcinoma occurs most frequently in women who are 60 years of age or older, and its incidence has remained relatively stable since the early 1980s. The mean age for carcinoma in situ is 20 years younger than for invasive carcinoma (45 to 50 years), and the incidence of vulvar cancer in women younger than 50 years of age has increased from 2% to 21% during the past 20 years.[7]

Approximately 90% of vulvar malignancies are squamous cell carcinomas. Less common types of cancer found on the vulva include adenocarcinoma in the form of extramammary Paget disease (intraepithelial or invasive) or carcinoma of Bartholin's gland, basal cell carcinoma, and malignant melanoma.[6]

Vulvar intraepithelial neoplasia (VIN), which is a precursor lesion of squamous cell carcinoma, represents a spectrum of neoplastic changes that range from minimal cellular atypia to invasive cancer. VIN appears to be caused by the oncogenic (cancer-promoting) potential of certain strains of HPV (subtypes 16 and 18) that are sexually transmitted and is associated with the type of vulvar cancer found in younger women.[7] VIN lesions may take many forms. The lesions may be singular or multicentric, macular, papular, or plaquelike. VIN frequently is multicentric, and approximately 50% are associated with squamous neoplasms in the vagina and cervix.[2] Microscopically, VIN presents as a proliferative process characterized by cells with abnormal epithelial maturation, nuclear enlargement, and nuclear atypia. The same system that is used for grading cervical cancer is used for vulvar cancer.[2,3] The extent of replacement of epithelial cells by abnormal cells determines the grade of involvement (VIN I, II, or III). Full-thickness replacement, VIN III, is synonymous with carcinoma in situ. Spontaneous resolution of VIN lesions has occurred. The risk for progression to invasive cancer increases in older women and in immunosuppressed women.

A second form of vulvar cancer, which is seen more often in older women, is generally preceded by vulvar nonneoplastic epithelial disorders (VNED) such as chronic vulvar irritation or lichen sclerosus. The pruritus associated with VNED causes an itch–scratch cycle that can lead to squamous cell hyperplasia. If left untreated, the hyperplasia progresses to atypia (differentiated VIN), and many of these women develop invasive cell carcinoma after 6 to 7 years.[7] The etiology of this type of VIN is infrequently associated with HPV.

The initial lesion of squamous cell vulvar carcinoma may appear as an inconspicuous thickening of the skin, a small raised area or lump, or an ulceration that fails to heal. It may be single or multiple and vary in color from white to velvety red or black. The lesions may resemble eczema or dermatitis and may produce few symptoms, other than pruritus, local discomfort, and exudation. A recurrent, persistent, pruritic vulvitis may be the only complaint. The symptoms frequently are treated with various home remedies before medical treatment is sought. The lesion may become secondarily infected, causing pain and discomfort. The malignant lesion gradually spreads superficially or as a deep furrow involving all of one labial side. Because there are many lymph channels around the vulva, the cancer metastasizes freely to the regional lymph nodes. The most common extension is to the superficial inguinal, deep femoral, and external iliac lymph nodes. Overall incidence of lymph node metastasis is approximately 30%.[7]

Early diagnosis is important in the treatment of vulvar carcinoma. Because malignant lesions can vary in appearance and commonly are mistaken for other conditions, biopsy and treatment often are delayed. Any vulvar lesion that is increasing in size or has an unusual warty appearance should be biopsied.[7] Treatment is primarily wide surgical excision of the lesion for noninvasive cancer and radical excision or vulvectomy with node resection for invasive cancer. Postoperative groin and pelvic radiation is recommended when groin lymph nodes are involved. Nonsurgical treatment options such as photodynamic therapy or topical immunotherapy are currently under investigation for patients with early-stage vulvar cancer.[8]

The 5-year survival rate for women with lesions less than 3 cm in diameter and minimal node involvement is approximately 90% after surgical treatment. Follow-up visits every 3 months for the first 2 years after surgery and every 6 months thereafter are important to detect recurrent disease or a second primary cancer. The 5-year survival rate for patients who have larger lesions in conjunction with pelvic lymphadenopathy drops to 30% to 55% after surgical treatment. Outlook for survival diminishes with increasing nodal involvement.[6]

GYNECOLOGIC CANCERS

- Cancers of the vulva, cervix, endometrium, and ovaries represent a spectrum of malignancies.
- Cancers of the vulva and cervix are mainly squamous cell carcinomas. Certain types of sexually transmitted human papillomaviruses are risk factors for cervical intraepithelial neoplasia, which can be a precursor lesion of invasive carcinoma.
- Endometrial cancers, which are seen most frequently in women 55 to 65 years of age, are strongly associated with conditions that produce excessive estrogen stimulation and endometrial hyperplasia.
- Ovarian cancer is the second most common female cancer and the most lethal. The most significant risk factors for ovarian cancers are the length of time that a woman's ovarian cycles are not suppressed by pregnancy, lactation, or oral contraceptive use, and family history.

DISORDERS OF THE VAGINA

The normal vaginal ecology depends on the delicate balance of hormones and bacterial flora. Normal estrogen levels maintain a thick, protective squamous epithelium that contains glycogen. Döderlein's bacilli, part of the normal vaginal flora, metabolize glycogen, and in the process produce the lactic acid that normally maintains the vaginal pH below 4.5. Disruptions in these normal environmental conditions predispose to infection.

Vaginitis

Vaginitis is inflammation of the vagina; it is characterized by vaginal discharge and burning, itching, redness, and swelling of vaginal tissues. Pain often occurs with urination and sexual intercourse. Vaginitis may be caused by chemical irritants, foreign bodies, or infectious agents. The causes of vaginitis differ in various age groups. In premenarchal girls, most vaginal infections have nonspecific causes, such as poor hygiene, intestinal parasites, or the presence of foreign bodies. *C. albicans, Trichomonas vaginalis,* and bacterial vaginosis are the most common causes of vaginitis in the childbearing years, and some of these organisms can be transmitted sexually[2,3,9] (see Chapter 48). In postmenopausal women, atrophic vaginitis is the most common form.

Atrophic vaginitis is an inflammation of the vagina that occurs after menopause or removal of the ovaries and their estrogen supply. Estrogen deficiency results in a lack of regenerative growth of the vaginal epithelium, rendering these tissues more susceptible to infection and irritation. Döderlein's bacilli disappear, and the vaginal secretions become less acidic. The symptoms of atrophic vaginitis include itching, burning, and painful intercourse. These symptoms usually can be reversed by local application of estrogen.[2,3]

Every woman has a normal vaginal discharge during the menstrual cycle, but it should not cause burning or itching or have an unpleasant odor. These symptoms suggest inflammation or infection. Because these symptoms are common to the different types of vaginitis, precise identification of the organism is essential for proper treatment. A careful history should include information about systemic disease conditions, the use of drugs such as antibiotics that foster the growth of yeast, dietary habits, stress, and other factors that alter the resistance of vaginal tissue to infections. A physical examination usually is done to evaluate the nature of the discharge and its effects on the genital structures.

Microscopic examination of a saline wet-mount smear (prepared by placing a sample of vaginal mucus in one to two drops of normal saline) is the primary means of identifying the organism responsible for the infection. A small amount of 10% potassium hydroxide (KOH) is added to a second specimen on the slide to aid in the identification of *C. albicans*. KOH destroys the cellular material, causing the epithelial cells to become increasingly transparent so that the hyphae and buds that are characteristic of *Candida* become much easier to see. Culture methods may be needed when the organism is not apparent on the wet-mount preparation.[3]

The prevention and treatment of vaginal infections depend on proper hygiene habits and accurate diagnosis and treatment of ongoing infections. Measures to prevent infection include development of daily hygiene habits that keep the genital area clean and dry, maintenance of normal vaginal flora and healthy vaginal mucosa, and avoidance of contact with organisms known to cause vaginal infections. Perfumed products, such as feminine deodorant sprays, douches, bath powders, soaps, and even toilet paper, can be irritating and may alter the normal vaginal flora. Tight clothing prevents the dissipation of body heat and evaporation of skin moisture and promotes favorable conditions for irritation and the growth of pathogens. Nylon and other synthetic undergarments, pantyhose, and swimsuits hold body moisture next to the skin and harbor infectious organisms, even after they have been washed. Cotton undergarments that withstand hot water and bleach (*i.e.,* a fungicide) may be preferable for women to prevent such infections. Swimsuits and other garments that cannot withstand hot water or bleaching should be hung in the sunlight to dry. Women should be taught to wipe the perineal area from front to back to avoid bringing rectal contamination into the vagina. Avoiding sexual contact whenever an infection is known to exist or suspected should limit that route of transmission.

Cancer of the Vagina

Primary cancers of the vagina are extremely rare. They account for approximately 3% of all cancers of the female reproductive system. Like vulvar carcinoma, carcinoma of the vagina is largely a disease of older women. Approximately half of women are 60 years of age or older at the time of diagnosis. The exception to that is the clear cell adenocarcinoma associated with diethylstilbestrol (DES) exposure in utero, which is associated with an average age at diagnosis of 19 years. Vaginal cancers may result from local extension of cervical cancer, from exposure to sexually transmitted HPV, or rarely from local irritation such as occurs with prolonged use of a pessary.[10]

Approximately 85% to 90% of vaginal cancers are squamous cell carcinomas, with other common types being adenocarcinomas (5% to 10%), sarcomas (2% to 3%), and melanomas (2% to 3%).[10] Squamous cell carcinomas begin in the epithelium and progress over many years from precancerous changes called vaginal intraepithelial neoplasia (VAIN). Maternal ingestion of DES in early pregnancy has been associated with the development of clear cell adenocarcinoma in female offspring who were exposed in utero. Between 1938 and 1971, DES, a nonsteroidal synthetic estrogen, commonly was prescribed to prevent miscarriage.[11] The incidence of clear cell adenocarcinoma of the vagina is low, approximately 0.1%, in young women who were exposed to DES in utero. Although only a small percentage of girls exposed to estrogen actually develop clear cell adenocarcinoma, 75% to 90% of them develop benign adenosis (*i.e.,* ectopic extension of cervical columnar epithelium into the vagina, which normally is stratified squamous epithelium), which may predispose to cancer. Most DES-exposed daughters are now between 40 and 60 years of age, so they are just entering the postmenopausal period when this malignancy develops in women who were not exposed to DES. Because the upper age limit for this type of cancer is unknown, there is no age at which a DES-exposed daughter can be considered risk free.[12]

The most common symptom of vaginal carcinoma is abnormal bleeding. Other signs or symptoms include an abnormal vaginal discharge, a palpable mass, or pain during intercourse. Ten to twenty percent of women are asymptomatic, with the cancer being discovered during a routine pelvic examination. The anatomic proximity of the vagina to other pelvic structures (*e.g.,* urethra, bladder, rectum) permits early spread to these areas. Pelvic pain, dysuria, and constipation can be associated symptoms. Vaginal squamous cell carcinoma most often is detected in the upper posterior one third of the vagina, with adenocarcinoma more often found on the lower anterior and lateral vaginal vault. Women should continue to have vaginal cytology studies

(Papanicolaou's test [Pap smear]) every 3 to 5 years after hysterectomy to exclude development of vaginal cancer if the hysterectomy was performed for a reproductive cancer. Diagnosis requires biopsy of suspicious lesions or areas.

Treatment of vaginal cancer must take into consideration the type of cancer; the size, location, and spread of the lesion; and the woman's age. Local excision, laser vaporization, or a loop electrode excision procedure (LEEP) can be considered with stage 0 squamous cell cancer. Radical surgery and radiation therapy are both curative with more advanced cancers. When there is upper vaginal involvement, radical surgery may be required. This includes a total hysterectomy, pelvic lymph node dissection, partial vaginectomy, and placement of a graft from the buttock to the area from which the vagina was excised. Vaginal reconstruction often is possible to allow for sexual intercourse. The ovaries usually are preserved unless they are diseased. Extensive lesions and those located in the middle or lower vaginal area usually are treated by radiation therapy, which can be intracavitary, interstitial, or external beam. The prognosis depends on the stage of the disease, the involvement of lymph nodes, and the degree of mitotic activity of the tumor. With appropriate treatment and follow-up, the 5-year survival rate for squamous cell and adenocarcinoma ranges from 96% for stage 0 and 73% when confined to the vagina (stage I), to 36% for those with extensive spread (stages III and IV).[10]

In summary, the surface of the vulva is affected by disorders that affect skin on other parts of the body. These disorders include inflammation (*i.e.,* vulvitis and folliculitis), epidermal cysts, and nevi. Although these disorders are not serious, they can be distressing because they produce severe discomfort and itching. Bartholin's cysts are the result of occluded ducts in Bartholin's glands. They often are painful and can become infected. Nonneoplastic epithelial disorders are characterized by thinning or hyperplastic thickening of vulvar tissues. Vulvodynia is a chronic vulvar pain syndrome with several classifications and variable treatment results. Cancer of the vulva, which accounts for 4% of all female genitourinary cancers, is associated with HPV infections in younger women and lichen sclerosus in older women.

The normal vaginal ecology depends on the delicate balance of hormones and bacterial flora. Normal estrogen levels maintain a thick protective squamous epithelium that contains glycogen. Döderlein's bacilli, which are part of the normal vaginal flora, metabolize glycogen and, in the process, produce the lactic acid that normally maintains the vaginal pH below 4.5. Disruptions in these normal environmental conditions predispose to vaginal infections. Vaginitis or inflammation of the vagina is characterized by vaginal discharge and burning, itching, redness, and swelling of vaginal tissues. It may be caused by chemical irritants, foreign bodies, or infectious agents. Primary cancers of the vagina are relatively uncommon, accounting for 3% of all cancers of the female reproductive system. Daughters of women treated with DES to prevent miscarriage are at increased risk for development of adenocarcinoma of the vagina.

Disorders of the Cervix and Uterus

After completing this section of the chapter, you should be able to meet the following objectives:

- Describe the importance of the cervical transformation zone in the development of cervical cancer
- Compare the lesions associated with nabothian cysts and cervical polyps
- List the complications of untreated cervicitis
- Compare the age distribution and risk factors for cervical and endometrial cancer
- Characterize the development of cervical cancer, from the appearance of atypical cells to the development of invasive cervical cancer
- Relate the importance of Papanicolaou's test in early detection and decreased incidence of deaths from cervical cancer
- Describe the methods used in the treatment of cervical cancer
- Compare the pathology and manifestations of endometriosis and adenomyosis
- Cite the major early symptom of endometrial cancer
- Compare intramural and subserosal leiomyomas

DISORDERS OF THE UTERINE CERVIX

The cervix is composed of two distinct types of tissue. The exocervix, or visible portion, is covered with stratified squamous epithelium, which also lines the vagina. The endocervical canal is lined with columnar epithelium. The junction of these two tissue types (*i.e.,* squamocolumnar junction) appears at various locations on the cervix at different points in a woman's life (Fig. 47-2). During periods of high estrogen production, particularly fetal existence, menarche, and the first pregnancy, the cervix everts or turns outward, exposing the columnar epithelium to the vaginal environment. The combination of estrogen and low vaginal pH leads to a gradual transformation from columnar to squamous epithelium—a process called *metaplasia* (see Chapter 5). The dynamic area of change where metaplasia takes place is called the *transformation zone.* The process of transformation is increased by trauma and infections occurring during the reproductive years.[2,12] As the squamous epithelium expands and obliterates the surface columnar papillae, it covers and obstructs crypt openings, with trapping of mucus in the deeper crypts (glands) to form retention cysts, called *nabothian cysts.* These are benign cysts that require no treatment unless they become so numerous that they cause cervical enlargement. The nabothian cyst farthest away from the external cervical os indicates the outer aspect of the transformation zone.

The transformation zone is a critical area for the development of cervical cancer. During metaplasia, the newly developed squamous epithelial cells are vulnerable to development of dysplasia and genetic change if exposed to carcinogenic agents (*i.e.,* cancer-producing substances). *Dysplasia* means disordered growth or development. Although initially a reversible cell change, untreated dysplasia can

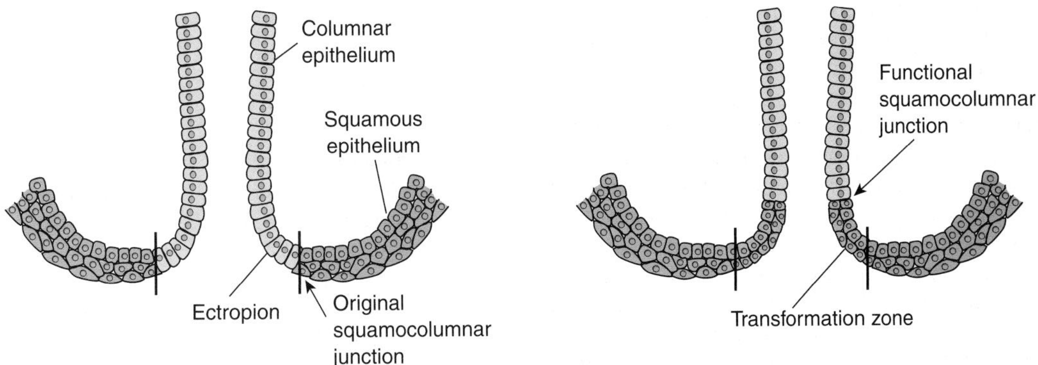

FIGURE 47-2 The transformation zone of the cervix. (Rubin E., Farber J.L. [1999]. *Pathology* [3rd. ed., p. 978]. Philadelphia: Lippincott-Raven)

develop into carcinoma. The transformation zone is the area of the cervix that must be sampled to have an adequate Pap smear and the area most carefully examined during colposcopy.

Cervicitis and Cervical Polyps

Cervicitis is an acute or chronic inflammation of the cervix. Acute cervicitis may result from the direct infection of the cervix or may be secondary to a vaginal or uterine infection. It may be caused by a variety of infective agents, including *C. albicans, T. vaginalis, Neisseria gonorrhoeae, Gardnerella vaginalis, Chlamydia trachomatis, Ureaplasma urealyticum,* and herpes simplex virus. *C. trachomatis* is the organism most commonly associated with mucopurulent cervicitis. Chronic cervicitis represents a low-grade inflammatory process. It is common in parous women and may be a sequela to minute lacerations that occur during childbirth, instrumentation, or other trauma. The organisms usually are of a nonspecific type, often staphylococcal, streptococcal, or coliform bacteria.

With acute cervicitis, the cervix becomes reddened and edematous. Irritation from the infection results in copious mucopurulent drainage and leukorrhea. The symptoms of chronic cervicitis are less well defined: the cervix may be ulcerated or normal in appearance; it may contain nabothian cysts; the cervical os may be distorted by old lacerations or everted to expose areas of columnar epithelium; and a mucopurulent drainage may be present.

Untreated cervicitis may extend to include the development of pelvic cellulitis, low back pain, painful intercourse, cervical stenosis, dysmenorrhea, and further infection of the uterus or fallopian tubes. Depending on the causative agent, acute cervicitis is treated with appropriate antibiotic therapy. Diagnosis of chronic cervicitis is based on vaginal examination, colposcopy, cytologic (Pap) smears, and occasionally biopsy to exclude malignant changes. The treatment usually involves cryosurgery or cauterization, which causes the tissues to slough and leads to eradication of the infection. Colposcopically guided laser vaporization of abnormal epithelium is the newest but most expensive treatment for cervicitis.

Polyps are the most common lesions of the cervix. They can be found in women of all ages, but their incidence is higher during the reproductive years. Polyps are soft, velvety red lesions; they usually are pedunculated and often are found protruding through the cervical os. They usually develop as a result of inflammatory hyperplasia of the endocervical mucosa. Polyps typically are asymptomatic but may have associated postcoital bleeding. Most are benign, but they should be removed and examined by a pathologist to exclude the possibility of malignant change.

Cancer of the Cervix

Cervical cancer is readily detected and, if detected early, is the most easily cured of all the cancers of the female reproductive system. According to the American Cancer Society, an estimated 12,200 cases of invasive cervical cancer were diagnosed in 2003, with approximately 4100 deaths from cervical cancer during the same period.[13] By comparison, there were four times as many new cases of cervical carcinoma in situ (*i.e.,* precancerous lesion) diagnosed, indicating that a large number of potentially invasive cancers are cured by early detection and effective treatment. The death rate has steadily declined over the past 50 years with the introduction of more sensitive and readily available screening methods (*e.g.,* Pap smear, colposcopy, cervicography), consistent use of a standardized grading system that guides treatment, and more effective treatment methods. However, the mortality rate is more than twice as high for black women as for white women. The 5-year survival rate for all patients with cervical cancer is 71%. For women with localized disease, the 5-year survival rate is 92%, but only 56% of cancers are discovered at that stage in white women and 46% in African Americans.[13]

Risk Factors and Pathogenesis. Carcinoma of the cervix is considered an STD. It is rare among celibate women. Risk factors include early age at first intercourse, multiple sexual partners, a promiscuous male partner, smoking, and a history of STDs.[13–15] A preponderance of evidence suggests a causal link between HPV infection and cervical cancer. Certain strains of HPV have been identified in invasive carcinoma of the cervix, whereas others are associated more often with dysplasia or carcinoma in situ. The strongest link is with HPV types 16, 18, 31, 33, 35, 39, 45, 52, 56, 58, and 59.[1,2] Because these viruses are spread by sexual contact, their association with cervical cancer provides a tempting hypothesis to explain the relation between sexual practices and cervical cancer. HPV is discussed further in Chapter 48. Other factors such as smoking, nutrition, and coexisting sexual infections such as *C. trachomatis,* herpes simplex virus type 2 (HSV-2), and human immunodeficiency virus (HIV) may play a contributing role in determining whether a woman with HPV infection develops cervical cancer.[2,14]

One of the most important advances in the early diagnosis and treatment of cancer of the cervix was made possible by the observation that this cancer arises from precursor lesions, which begin with the development of atypical cervical cells. These atypical cells gradually progress to carcinoma in situ and to invasive cancer of the cervix. Atypical cells differ from normal cervical squamous epithelium. There are changes in the nuclear and cytoplasmic parts of the cell and more variation in cell size and shape (*i.e.,* dysplasia). Carcinoma in situ is localized to the epithelial layer, whereas invasive cancer of the cervix spreads to deeper layers.[2]

A system of grading devised to describe the dysplastic changes of cancer precursors uses the term *cervical intraepithelial neoplasia* (CIN). This histologic terminology system divides the precursors according to the extent of involvement of the epithelial thickness of the cervix. (Table 47-1). It was presumed that CIN represented a single, progressive disease process. Current understanding of the pathogenesis of cervical cancer precursors now suggests two distinct biologic entities: a productive viral infection (HPV), which can regress spontaneously (mild dysplasia or CIN 1), and a true neoplastic process confined to the epithelium (CIN 2 or 3). CIN histologic terminology has been largely replaced with cytopathology terms for these two biologic entities: low-grade squamous intraepithelial lesion (LSIL) and high-grade squamous intraepithelial lesion (HSIL).[2]

The precursor lesions can exist in a reversible form, which may regress spontaneously, persist, or progress and undergo malignant change. Studies of the natural history of these precursor lesions have yielded variable rates of progression and regression. Generally, only a small percentage of lesions progress to invasive carcinoma. HSIL has a much greater potential for progressing than does LSIL. De novo development of HSIL has also been demonstrated, challenging the concept that LSIL is always a precursor to HSIL. Cancers of the cervix have a long latent period; untreated dysplasia gradually progresses to carcinoma in situ, which may remain static for 7 to 10 years before it becomes invasive. After the preinvasive period, growth may be rapid, and survival rates decline significantly depending on the extent of disease at the time of diagnosis.[2]

The atypical cellular changes that precede frank neoplastic changes consistent with cancer of the cervix can be recognized by a number of direct and microscopic techniques, including Pap smear, colposcopy, and cervicography. Currently, Pap smears are used for cervical cancer screening. The purpose of the Pap smear is to detect the presence of abnormal cells on the surface of the cervix or in the endocervix. Following an extensive review of the literature, the American Cancer Society (ACS) in late 2002 released revised guidelines for cervical cancer screening[16] (Chart 47-1). The U.S. Preventive Services Task Force (USPSTF) screening guidelines were also updated in 2002.[17] Although many clinicians and women themselves are reluctant to move away from yearly Pap smears, the evidence about the natural progression of cervical cancer supports the position that this is the more cost-effective approach to screening.

It has been estimated that approximately 20% of women with intraepithelial lesions have normal Pap smear results.[16] Care must be taken to obtain an adequate smear from the transformation zone that includes endocervical cells and to ensure that the cytologic examination is done by a competent laboratory. New techniques of specimen collection, slide preparation and processing, and computer-assisted evaluation of Pap smears are being evaluated and offer hope of improved accuracy in diagnosis of precancerous cervical changes.

The presence of normal endometrial cells in a cervical cytologic sample during the luteal phase of the menstrual cycle or during the postmenopausal period has been associated with endometrial disease and warrants further evaluation with endometrial biopsy. This demonstrates that

TABLE 47-1 Classification Systems for Papanicolaou Smears

Dysplasia/Neoplasia	CIN	Bethesda System
Benign	Benign	Negative for intraepithelial lesion or malignancy
Benign with inflammation	Benign with inflammation	Negative for intraepithelial lesion or malignancy, ASC-US
Mild dysplasia	CIN 1	Low-grade SIL, ASC-H
Moderate dysplasia	CIN 2	High-grade SIL
Severe dysplasia and carcinoma in situ	CIN 3	
Invasive cancer	Invasive cancer	Invasive cancer

CIN, cervical intraepithelial neoplasia; SIL, squamous intraepithelial lesion; ASC-US, atypical squamous cells of undetermined significance; ASC-H, cannot rule out high-grade SIL.
Adapted from information in Rubin E., Farber J.L. (1999). *Pathology* (3rd ed., p 982). Philadelphia: Lippincott-Raven; Solomon D., Davey D., Kurman R., et al., Forum Group Members and Bethesda 2001 Workshop. (2002). The 2001 Bethesda System. *Journal of the American Medical Association 287*(16), 2114–2119.

CHART 47-1

Guidelines for Cervical Cancer Screening Using the Papanicolaou (Pap) Smear

- Screening should begin 3 years after first vaginal intercourse or after age 21, whichever comes first.
- Women 30 years of age and older may be screened at longer intervals after three consecutive normal/negative cytology results.
- Screening may be discontinued in women aged 65 years and older if they had adequate screening with normal Pap smears and are not otherwise at increased risk for cervical cancer.
- Women who have had a total hysterectomy with removal of the cervix do not need screening unless the surgery was performed to treat cervical cancer or a precancerous condition.
- If a woman has risk factors, such as HPV infection, DES exposure in utero, or strong family history of cervical cancer, more frequent Pap smears may be recommended.

Adapted from Smith R.A., Cokkinides V., von Eschenbach A.C., et al. (2002). American Cancer Society guideline for early detection of cervical neoplasia and cancer. *CA: A Cancer Journal for Clinicians 52*(1), 8–22; U.S. Preventive Services Task Force. (2002). Recommendations for Screening for Cervical Cancer. [On-line]. Available: http://www.AHRQ.gov.

shedding of even normal cells at an inappropriate time may indicate disease. Because adenocarcinoma of the cervix is being detected more frequently, especially in women younger than 35 years of age, a Pap smear result of atypical glandular cells (AGCs) warrants further evaluation by endocervical or endometrial curettage, hysteroscopy, or, ultimately, a cone biopsy if the abnormality cannot be located or identified through other means.[2,3]

The accepted format for reporting cervical and vaginal cytologic diagnoses, called *The Bethesda System* (TBS), was developed during a National Cancer Institute Workshop in 1989 and updated in 1991 and 2001 (see Table 47-1).[18] TBS 2001 Terminology includes the following components: specimen type (conventional vs. liquid based); specimen adequacy (satisfactory or unsatisfactory for evaluation); general categorization (negative for intraepithelial lesion or malignancy versus epithelial cell abnormality); and interpretation/result (negative for intraepithelial lesion or malignancy: includes the presence of organisms and other nonneoplastic findings, versus epithelial cell abnormalities: squamous cell or glandular cell).[18] In 2002, a task force composed of Bethesda 2001 group members and representatives of the American Society of Colposcopy and Cervical Pathology (ASCCP) provided additional guidance regarding Pap specimen adequacy and management.[19] The minimally abnormal Pap smear (*i.e.*, atypical squamous cells [ASC], or low-grade squamous intraepithelial lesion [LSIL]) presents the greatest challenge to clinicians.

Current guidelines indicate that the management of women with atypical squamous cells (ASC) depends on whether the Pap test is subcategorized as "of undetermined significance" (ASC-US) or as "cannot exclude high-grade squamous intraepithelial lesion [HSIL]" (ASC-H). The uncertain significance of ASC-US often is related to inflammation, atrophy, or other temporary or reversible processes. Even squamous intraepithelial lesions (SILs) regress spontaneously in approximately 60% of patients, and costly evaluation or aggressive treatment may not be warranted. Follow-up with repeat Pap smears at 4- to 6-month intervals for a total of three tests is the preferred conservative approach for women with ASC-US. Referral for colposcopy is generally recommended for women with ASC-H, LSIL, or HSIL or if compliance with follow-up observation is uncertain; women who have had suspicious findings on exam, previous abnormal Pap results, history of STDs or high-risk sexual behaviors; and women who are long-term or heavy smokers or are immunocompromised. Colposcopy, with endocervical curettage, or directed biopsy may be used to confirm the presence of a lesion so that treatment can be selected.[2,3,14,15]

DNA testing for high-risk strains of HPV provides an additional means of determining which women may be acceptable candidates for conservative management and those who may be at greatest risk for developing cervical cancer. Adjunct HPV DNA testing is an acceptable tool to determine which women with ASC-US may benefit from immediate referral for colposcopy. Research is ongoing in this area, but at this time, HPV DNA typing is not recommended for primary screening.[14–17,19] A vaccine to prevent infection with the HPV subtype 16 has shown promising results in preliminary trials and offers hope that we may someday have the means to prevent cervical cancer.[14]

Clinical Course. Diagnosis of cervical cancer requires pathologic confirmation. Pap smear results demonstrating SIL often require further evaluation by colposcopy. This is a vaginal examination that is done using a colposcope, an instrument that affords a well-lit and magnified stereoscopic view of the cervix. During colposcopy, the cervical tissue may be stained with an iodine solution (*i.e.*, Schiller's test) or acetic acid solution to accentuate topographic or vascular changes that can differentiate normal from abnormal tissue. A biopsy sample may be obtained from suspect areas and examined microscopically.

An alternate diagnostic tool in areas where colposcopy is not readily available is cervicography, a noninvasive photographic technique that provides permanent objective documentation of normal and abnormal cervical patterns. Acetic acid (5%) is applied to the cervix, a cervicography camera is used to take photographs, and the projected cervicogram (*i.e.*, slide after film developing) can be sent for expert evaluation. In one study, the cervicogram was found to give a greater yield of CIN than Pap smear alone in patients with previous abnormal pap smears.[20]

Before the availability of colposcopy, many women with abnormal Pap smears required surgical cone biopsy for further evaluation. Cone biopsy involves the removal of a cone-shaped wedge of cervix, including the entire transformation zone and at least 50% of the endocervical canal. Postoperative hemorrhage, infection, cervical stenosis, infertility, and incompetent cervix are possible sequelae that warrant avoidance of this procedure unless it is truly necessary. Diagnostic conization still is indicated when a lesion is partly or completely beyond colposcopic view or when colposcopically directed biopsy fails to explain the cytologic findings.

The LEEP or large loop excision of the transformation zone (LLETZ), a refinement of loop diathermy techniques dating back to the 1940s, is quickly becoming the first-line management tool for SIL. This outpatient procedure allows for the simultaneous diagnosis and treatment of dysplastic lesions found on colposcopy. It uses a thin, rigid, wire loop electrode attached to a generator that blends high-frequency, low-voltage current for cutting and a modulated higher voltage for coagulation. In skilled hands, this wire can remove the entire transformation zone, providing adequate treatment for the lesion while obtaining a specimen for further histologic evaluation. The width and depth of the tissue excised are controlled by the size and shape of the loop and the speed and pressure that is applied during the procedure. This can help avoid the problems that can occur after surgical cone biopsy (*e.g.*, stenosis, incompetent cervix). Bleeding can be minimized by fulguration of the base with electrocoagulation or by applying a thin layer of Monsel's gel (*i.e.*, chemical cautery). Although long-term results are not available, this procedure, which requires only local anesthesia, appears to provide a lower-cost, office-based alternative to cone biopsy.

Early treatment of cervical cancer involves removal of the lesion by one of various techniques. Biopsy or local cautery may be therapeutic in and of itself. Electrocautery, cryosurgery, or carbon dioxide laser therapy may be used to treat moderate to severe dysplasia that is limited to the exocervix (*i.e.*, squamocolumnar junction clearly visible). Therapeutic conization becomes necessary if the lesion extends into the endocervical canal and can be done surgically or with LEEP in the physician's office.[3]

Depending on the stage of involvement of the cervix, invasive cancer is treated with radiation therapy, surgery, or both. External beam irradiation and intracavitary cesium irradiation (*i.e.*, insertion of a closed metal cylinder containing cesium) can be used in the treatment of cervical cancer. Intracavitary radiation provides direct access to the central lesion and increases the tolerance of the cervix and surrounding tissues, permitting curative levels of radiation to be used. External beam radiation eliminates metastatic disease in pelvic lymph nodes and other structures and shrinks the cervical lesion to optimize the effects of intracavitary radiation. Surgery can include extended hysterectomy (*i.e.*, removal of the uterus, fallopian tubes, ovaries, and upper portion of the vagina) without pelvic lymph node dissection, radical hysterectomy with pelvic lymph node dissection, or pelvic exenteration (*i.e.*, removal of all pelvic organs, including the bladder, rectum, vulva, and vagina). The choice of treatment is influenced by the stage of the disease as well as the woman's age and health.[3]

DISORDERS OF THE UTERUS

Endometritis

Inflammation or infection of the endometrium is an ill-defined entity that produces variable symptoms. The presence of plasma cells is required for diagnosis. Endometritis can occur as a postpartum or postabortal infection, with gonococcal or chlamydial salpingitis, or after instrumentation or surgery, or it can be associated with an intrauterine device or tuberculosis.[3] Causative organisms, in addition to *N. gonorrhoeae, Chlamydia,* and *Mycobacterium tuberculosis,* include *Escherichia coli, Proteus, Pseudomonas, Klebsiella, Bacteroides,* and *Mycoplasma* species. Abnormal vaginal bleeding, mild to severe uterine tenderness, fever, malaise, and foul-smelling discharge have been associated with endometritis, but the clinical picture is variable. Treatment involves oral or intravenous antibiotic therapy, depending on the severity of the condition.

Endometriosis

Endometriosis is the condition in which functional endometrial tissue is found in ectopic sites outside the uterus. The site may be the ovaries, posterior broad ligaments, uterosacral ligaments, pouch of Douglas (cul-de-sac), pelvis, vagina, vulva, perineum, or intestines (Fig 47-3). Rarely, endometrial implants have been found in the nostrils, umbilicus, lungs, and limbs.

The cause of endometriosis is unknown. There appears to have been an increase in its incidence in the developed Western countries during the past four to five decades. Approximately 10% to 15% of premenopausal women have some degree of endometriosis. The incidence may be higher in women with infertility (15% to 70%) or women younger than 20 years of age with chronic pelvic pain (47% to 73%).[21] It is more common in women who have postponed childbearing. Risk factors for endometriosis may include early menarche; regular periods with shorter cycles (<27 days), longer duration (>7 days), or heavier flow; increased menstrual pain; and other first-degree relatives with the condition.

Several theories attempt to account for endometriosis. One theory suggests that menstrual blood containing fragments of endometrium is forced upward through the fallopian tubes into the peritoneal cavity. Retrograde menstruation is not an uncommon phenomenon, and it is unknown why endometrial cells implant and grow in some women but not in others. Another proposal is that dormant, immature cellular elements, spread over a wide area during embryonic development, persist into adult life and that the ensuing metaplasia accounts for the development of ectopic endometrial tissue. Another theory suggests that the endometrial tissue may metastasize through the lymphatics or vascular system. Altered cellular immunity and genetic components also have been studied as contributing factors to the development of endometriosis.[2,3]

The gross pathologic changes that occur in endometriosis differ with location and duration. In the ovary, the endometrial tissue may form cysts (*i.e.*, endometriomas filled with old blood that resembles chocolate syrup [chocolate cysts]). Rupture of these cysts can cause peritonitis and

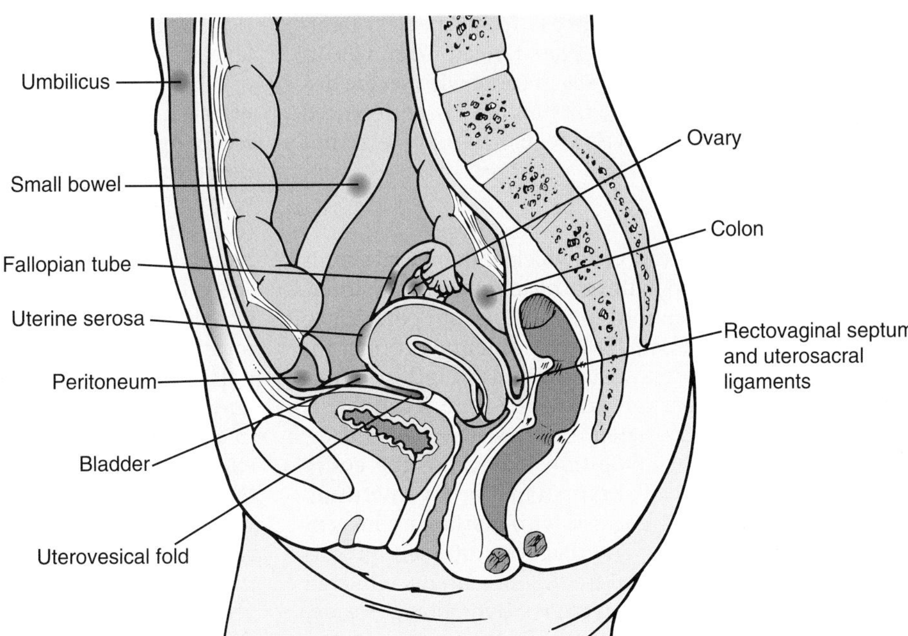

FIGURE 47-3 Common locations of endometriosis within the pelvis and abdomen.

adhesions. Elsewhere in the pelvis, the tissue may take the form of small hemorrhagic lesions that may be black, bluish, red, clear, or opaque. Some may be surrounded by scar tissue. These ectopic implants respond to hormonal stimulation in the same way normal endometrium does, becoming proliferative, then secretory, and finally undergoing menstrual breakdown. Bleeding into the surrounding structures can cause pain and the development of significant pelvic adhesions. Extensive fibrotic tissue can develop and occasionally causes bowel obstruction.

Endometriosis may be difficult to diagnose because its symptoms mimic those of other pelvic disorders. The severity of the symptoms does not always reflect the extent of the disease. The classic triad of dysmenorrhea, dyspareunia, and infertility strongly suggests endometriosis. Accurate diagnosis can be accomplished only through laparoscopy. This minimally invasive surgery allows direct visualization of pelvic organs to determine the presence and extent of endometrial lesions. Imaging techniques including ultrasound and magnetic resonance imaging (MRI) can be useful tools in evaluating endometriomas. CA-125 is a serum marker that may be elevated in the presence of endometriosis. It has limitations as a screening tool but can be useful in monitoring response to therapy and recurrence.[21]

Treatment goals for endometriosis are pain management or restoration of fertility. Treatment modalities fall into three categories: pain relief, endometrial suppression, and surgery. In young women, simple observation and antiprostaglandin analgesics (*i.e.*, nonsteroidal anti-inflammatory drugs) may be sufficient treatment. The use of hormones to induce physiologic amenorrhea is based on the observation that pregnancy affords temporary relief by inducing atrophy of the endometrial tissue. This can be accomplished through administration of progesterone, oral contraceptive pills, danazol (a synthetic androgen), or long-acting gonadotropin-releasing hormone analogs that inhibit the pituitary gonadotropins and suppress ovulation.[3,22]

Surgery is the most definitive therapy for many women with endometriosis. In the past, laparoscopic cautery was limited to mild endometriosis without significant adhesions. More extensive treatment required laparotomy. With the advent of carbon dioxide, potassium-titanyl-phosphate (KTP), neodymium–yttrium-aluminum-garnet (Nd-YAG), argon, and holmium-YAG lasers, in-depth treatment of endometriosis or pelvic adhesions can be accomplished by means of laparoscopy. Advantages of laser surgery include better hemostasis, more precision in vaporizing lesions with less damage to surrounding tissue, and better access to areas that are not well visualized or would be difficult to reach with cautery. Each type of laser has distinct properties that allow it to be useful for tissue vaporization under different conditions. The KTP laser is particularly useful for endometriosis because of its flexible fiberoptic delivery system, which allows tissue incision and vaporization in addition to photocoagulation, and its green beam, which makes visualization and fine focusing easier. Carbon dioxide permits the operator to excise easily with extreme accuracy and control and causes less peripheral tissue damage than other wavelengths. The Nd-YAG laser allows for a contact mode that avoids direct application of laser energy to tissues. Lasers are expensive instruments and require skill to use effectively. Some hospitals and surgeons have turned to other therapies in an effort to conserve financial resources. Electrosurgical, thermal, and ultrasonic ablation techniques are under investigation.[23] Radical treatment involves total hysterectomy and bilateral salpingo-oophorectomy (*i.e.*, removal of the fallopian tubes and ovaries) when the symptoms are unbearable or the woman's childbearing is completed.

Treatment offers relief but not cure. Recurrence of endometriosis is not uncommon, regardless of the treatment (except for radical surgery). Recurrence rates appear to correlate with severity of disease. With medical treatment, recurrence rates after 7 years ranged from 34% in women with mild disease to 74% in those with severe disease. Recurrence rates of 20% to 40% have been reported within 5 years after surgery.[24] Pregnancy may delay but does not preclude recurrence.

Adenomyosis

Adenomyosis is the condition in which endometrial glands and stroma are found within the myometrium, interspersed between the smooth muscle fibers. In contrast to endometriosis, which usually is a problem of young, infertile women, adenomyosis typically is found in multiparous women in their late fourth or fifth decade. It is thought that events associated with repeated pregnancies, deliveries, and uterine involution may cause the endometrium to be displaced throughout the myometrium. Adenomyosis frequently coexists with uterine myomas or endometrial hyperplasia. The diagnosis of adenomyosis often occurs as an incidental finding in a uterus removed for symptoms suggestive of myoma or hyperplasia. Heavy, painful periods with clots and painful intercourse are common complaints of women with adenomyosis. Although in the past the diagnosis was made primarily through careful history and the pelvic examination findings of an enlarged, boggy uterus, magnetic resonance imaging is now considered an excellent diagnostic tool for confirming this condition. Color Doppler ultrasound can be used to distinguish vascular patterns that may differentiate adenomyosis from uterine fibroids.[25] Adenomyosis resolves with menopause. Conservative therapy using oral contraceptives or gonadotropin-releasing hormone (GnRH) agonists is the first choice for treatment. Hysterectomy (with preservation of the ovaries in premenopausal women) is considered when this approach fails.

Endometrial Cancer

Endometrial cancer is the most common cancer found in the female pelvis; it occurs more than twice as often as cervical cancer. In 2003, the American Cancer Society estimated that approximately 40,100 women were diagnosed with endometrial cancer and 6800 died of the disorder.[13] Endometrial cancer occurs more frequently in older women (peak ages of 55 to 65 years), with only a 2% to 5% incidence among women younger than 40 years of age.

Prolonged estrogen stimulation with excessive growth (*i.e.*, hyperplasia) of endometrium has been identified as a major risk factor for the development of type I (endometrioid) endometrial cancer. Obesity, anovulatory cycles, conditions that alter estrogen metabolism, estrogen-secreting neoplasms, and unopposed estrogen therapy all increase the risk for endometrial cancer.[2,3,13]

Estrogens are synthesized in body fats from adrenal and ovarian androgen precursors. Endometrial hyperplasia and endometrial cancer appear to be related to obesity. Ovulatory dysfunction that causes infertility at any age or occurs with declining ovarian function in perimenopausal women also can result in unopposed estrogen and increase the risk for endometrial cancer. Diabetes mellitus, hypertension, and polycystic ovary syndrome are conditions that alter estrogen metabolism and elevate estrogen levels.

Endometrial cancer risk also is increased in women with estrogen-secreting granulosa cell tumors and in those receiving unopposed estrogen therapy. A sharp rise in endometrial cancer was seen in the 1970s among middle-aged women who had received unopposed estrogen therapy (*i.e.*, estrogen therapy without progesterone) for menopausal symptoms. It was later determined that it was not the estrogen exposure that increased the risk for cancer, but that the hormone was administered without progesterone. It is the presence of progesterone in the second half of the menstrual cycle that matures the endometrium and the withdrawal of progesterone that ultimately results in endometrial sloughing. Long-term unopposed estrogen exposure without periodic addition of progesterone allows for continued endometrial growth. Hyperplasia may develop, with or without the presence of atypical cells, and can progress to carcinoma if left untreated. Hyperplasia usually regresses after treatment with cyclic progesterone. Sequential oral contraceptives (estrogen alone for 15 days followed by 7 days of combined estrogen and progestin) were withdrawn from the market in the 1970s because of potential risk for endometrial hyperplasia. In contrast, combination oral contraceptives (estrogen and progestin in each pill) effectively prevent hyperplasia and decrease the risk for cancer by 50%.[3] Tamoxifen, a drug that blocks estrogen receptor sites and is used in treatment of breast cancer, exerts a weak estrogenic effect on the endometrium and represents another exogenous risk factor for endometrial cancer.

A small subset of women in whom endometrial cancer develops do not exhibit increased estrogen levels or preexisting hyperplasia (type II or serous carcinoma). These women usually acquire the disease at an older age. These tumors arise from clones of cancer-initiated mutant cells and are more poorly differentiated. This type of endometrial cancer usually has a poorer prognosis than that associated with prolonged estrogen stimulation and endometrial hyperplasia.[2]

Endometrial cancer is the most commonly inherited gynecologic cancer. Women with a family history of hereditary nonpolyposis colon cancer (HNPCC) may have an inherited mutation that has been identified as mismatch repair genes. This autosomal dominant disease carries an 80% risk of developing cancer of some type for those who inherit the mutation. In the normal population, the lifetime risk for developing endometrial cancer is 1.6%, compared with 60% with the inherited mismatch repair defect.[3] A detailed family history for cancer can be the best means of identifying those who would benefit from genetic counseling.

Clinical Course. The major symptom of endometrial hyperplasia or overt endometrial cancer is abnormal, painless bleeding. In menstruating women, this takes the form of bleeding between periods or excessive, prolonged menstrual flow. In postmenopausal women, any bleeding is abnormal and warrants investigation. Abnormal bleeding is an early warning sign of the disease, and because endometrial cancer tends to be slow growing in its early stages, the chances of cure are good if prompt medical care is sought. Later signs of uterine cancer may include cramping, pelvic discomfort, postcoital bleeding, lower abdominal pressure, and enlarged lymph nodes.

Although the Pap smear can identify a small percentage of endometrial cancers, it is not a good screening test for this gynecologic cancer. Endometrial biopsy (*i.e.,* tissue sampling obtained in an office procedure by direct aspiration of the endometrial cavity) is far more accurate; 80% to 90% of endometrial cancers are identified if adequate tissue is obtained. Dilatation and curettage (D & C), which consists of dilating the cervix and scraping the uterine cavity, is the definitive procedure for diagnosis because it provides a more thorough evaluation. Transvaginal ultrasonography used to measure the endometrial thickness is being evaluated as an initial test for postmenopausal bleeding because it is less invasive than endometrial biopsy and less costly than D & C when biopsy is not possible.

The prognosis for endometrial cancer depends on the clinical stage of the disease when it is discovered and its histologic grade and type. Surgery and radiation therapy are the most successful methods of treatment for endometrial cancer. When used alone, radiation therapy has a 20% lower cure rate than surgery for stage I disease. It may be the best option, however, in women who are not good surgical candidates. Total abdominal hysterectomy with bilateral salpingo-oophorectomy plus sampling of regional lymph nodes and peritoneal washings for cytologic evaluation of occult disease is the treatment of choice whenever possible. Postoperative radiation therapy may be added in cases of advanced disease for more complete treatment and to prevent recurrence or metastasis, although the benefits of this as adjuvant therapy are still controversial. The 5-year relative survival rates are 96%, 64%, and 26% if the cancer is diagnosed at local, regional, and distant stages, respectively.[13]

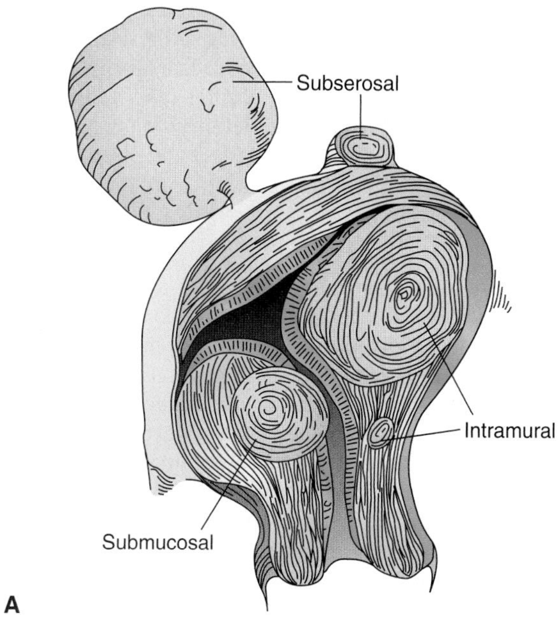

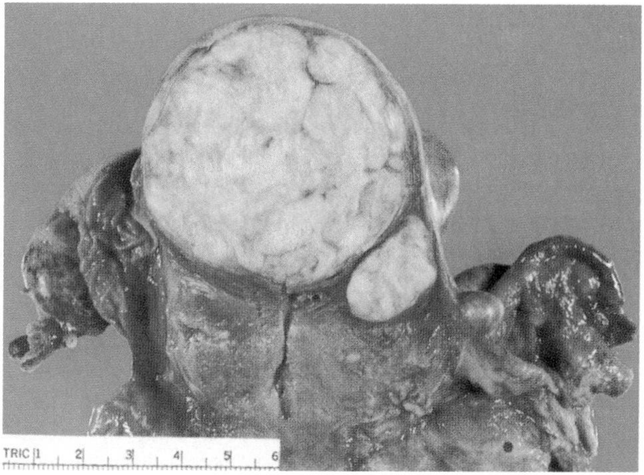

FIGURE 47-4 (**A**) Submucosal, intramural, and subserosal leiomyomas. (**A** redrawn from Green T.H. [1977]. *Gynecology: Essentials of clinical practice* [3rd ed.]. Boston: Little, Brown.) (**B**) A bisected uterus displays a prominent, sharply circumscribed, fleshy tumor. (Rubin E., Farber J.L. [1999]. *Pathology* [3rd ed., p. 999]. Philadelphia: Lippincott-Raven)

Leiomyomas

Leiomyomas are benign neoplasms of smooth muscle origin. They also are known as *myomas* and sometimes are called *fibroids*. These are the most common form of pelvic tumor and are believed to occur in one of every four or five women older than 35 years of age. They are seen more often and their rate of growth is more rapid in black women than in white women. Leiomyomas usually develop in the corpus of the uterus; they may be submucosal, subserosal, or intramural (Fig. 47-4). Intramural fibroids are embedded in the myometrium. They are the most common type of fibroid and present as a symmetric enlargement of the nonpregnant uterus. Subserosal tumors are located beneath the perimetrium of the uterus. These tumors are recognized as irregular projections on the uterine surface; they may become pedunculated, displacing or impinging on other genitourinary structures and causing hydroureter or bladder problems. Submucosal fibroids displace endometrial tissue and are more likely to cause bleeding, necrosis, and infection than either of the other types.

Leiomyomas are asymptomatic approximately half of the time and may be discovered during a routine pelvic examination, or they may cause menorrhagia (excessive menstrual bleeding), anemia, urinary frequency, rectal pressure/constipation, abdominal distention, and infrequently pain. Their rate of growth is variable, but they may increase in size during pregnancy or with exogenous estrogen stimulation (*i.e.,* oral contraceptives or menopausal estrogen replacement therapy). Interference with pregnancy is rare unless the tumor is submucosal and interferes with implantation or obstructs the cervical outlet. These tumors may outgrow their blood supply, become infarcted, and undergo degenerative changes. Most leiomyomas regress with menopause, but if bleeding, pressure on the bladder, pain, or other problems persist, hysterectomy may be required. Myomectomy (removal of just the tumors) can be done to preserve the uterus for future childbearing. Cesarean section may be recommended if the uterine cavity is entered during myomectomy. GnRH (*e.g.*, leuprolide [Lupron]) may be used to suppress leiomyoma growth before surgery. Uterine artery embolization done by an interventional radiologist is a nonsurgical therapy for management of heavy bleeding.[26]

In summary, disorders of the cervix and uterus include inflammatory conditions (*i.e.*, cervicitis and endometritis), cancer (*i.e.*, cervical and endometrial cancer), endometriosis, and leiomyomas. Cervicitis is an acute or chronic inflammation of the cervix. Acute cervicitis may result from the direct infection of the cervix or may be secondary to a vaginal or uterine infection. It may be caused by a variety of infective agents. Chronic cervicitis represents a low-grade inflammatory process resulting from trauma or nonspecific infectious agents. Cervical cancer is readily detected, and if detected early, it is the most easily cured of all the cancers of the female reproductive system. It arises from precursor lesions that can be detected on a Pap smear; the condition can be cured if detected and treated early.

Endometritis represents an ill-defined inflammation or infection of the endometrium that produces variable symptoms. Endometriosis is the condition in which functional endometrial tissue is found in ectopic sites outside the uterus such as the ovaries, broad ligaments, pouch of Douglas (cul-de-sac), pelvis, vagina, vulva, perineum, or intestines. It causes dysmenorrhea, dyspareunia, and infertility. Adenomyosis is the condition in which endometrial glands and stroma are found in the myometrium, interspersed between the smooth muscle fibers. Endometrial cancer is the most common cancer found in the female pelvis; it occurs more than twice as often as cervical cancer. Prolonged estrogen stimulation with hyperplasia of the endometrium has been identified as a major risk factor for endometrial cancer.

Leiomyomas are benign uterine wall neoplasms of smooth muscle origin. They can develop in the corpus of the uterus and can be submucosal, subserosal, or intramural. Submucosal fibroids displace endometrial tissue and are more likely to cause bleeding, necrosis, and infection than either of the other types.

Disorders of the Fallopian Tubes and Ovaries

After completing this section of the chapter, you should be able to meet the following objectives:

- List the common causes and symptoms of pelvic inflammatory disease
- State the causative factors associated with tubal pregnancy
- Describe the symptoms of a tubal pregnancy
- State the underlying cause of ovarian cysts
- Differentiate benign ovarian cyst and polycystic ovary syndrome (previously called *Stein-Leventhal syndrome*)
- List the hormones produced by the three types of functioning ovarian tumors
- State the reason that ovarian cancer may be difficult to detect in an early stage

PELVIC INFLAMMATORY DISEASE

Pelvic inflammatory disease (PID) is an inflammation of the upper reproductive tract that involves the uterus (endometritis), fallopian tubes (salpingitis), or ovaries (oophoritis). Most women with acute salpingitis have *N. gonorrhoeae* or *C. trachomatis* identified in the reproductive tract. PID is a polymicrobial infection, and the cause varies by geographic location and population. In addition to the primary causative agents already mentioned, *Mycoplasma hominis, Ureaplasma urealyticum, Bacteroides, Peptostreptococcus, E. coli, Haemophilus influenzae,* and *Streptococcus agalactiae* may be involved.[27] The organisms ascend through the endocervical canal to the endometrial cavity, and then to the tubes and ovaries. The endocervical canal is slightly dilated during menstruation, allowing bacteria to gain entrance to the uterus and other pelvic structures. After entering the upper reproductive tract, the organisms multiply rapidly in the favorable environment of the sloughing endometrium and ascend to the fallopian tube.

Factors that predispose women to the development of PID include an age of 16 to 24 years, unmarried status, nulliparity, history of multiple sexual partners, and previous history of PID. Although the use of an intrauterine contraceptive device (IUD) has been associated with a threefold to fivefold increased risk for development of PID, studies have shown that women with only one sexual partner who are at low risk for acquiring STDs have no significant risk for development of PID from using an IUD.

Clinical Course

The symptoms of PID include lower abdominal pain, which may start just after a menstrual period; purulent cervical discharge; adnexal tenderness; and an exquisitely painful cervix. New-onset breakthrough bleeding on oral contraceptives, Depo-Provera, or Norplant has recently been associated with PID. Fever (>101°F), increased erythrocyte sedimentation rate, and an elevated white blood cell count (>10,000 cells/mL) commonly are seen, even though the woman may not appear acutely ill. A newer test involves measurement of C-reactive protein in the blood. Elevated C-reactive protein levels equate with inflammation. Laparoscopy is the gold standard for diagnosis of PID, but clinical criteria have a positive predictive value of 65% to 90% compared with laparoscopy.[27] Minimal criteria for a presumptive diagnosis of PID require only the presence of lower abdominal, adnexal, and cervical motion tenderness.

Treatment may involve hospitalization with intravenous administration of antibiotics. If the condition is diagnosed early, outpatient antibiotic therapy may be sufficient. Antibiotic regimens should be selected according to STD treatment guidelines, which are published every 4 years by the Centers for Disease Control and Prevention (CDC).[28] Treatment is aimed at preventing complications, which can include pelvic adhesions, infertility, ectopic pregnancy, chronic abdominal pain, and tubo-ovarian abscesses. Accurate diagnosis and appropriate antibiotic therapy may decrease the severity and frequency of PID sequelae. The CDC recommends empiric treatment with a presumptive diagnosis of PID, while waiting for confirmation by culture or other definitive test results.

ECTOPIC PREGNANCY

Although pregnancy is not discussed in detail in this text, it is reasonable to mention ectopic pregnancy because it represents a true gynecologic emergency and should be considered when a woman of reproductive age presents with the complaint of pelvic pain. Ectopic pregnancy occurs when a fertilized ovum implants outside the uterine cavity. The most common site for ectopic pregnancy is the fallopian tube (Fig. 47-5). According to the CDC, between 1970 and 1992, the number of ectopic pregnancies increased from 17,800 to 108,800, and the rate of occurrence among women aged 15 to 44 years rose from 4.5 to 19.7 per 1000 reported pregnancies (*i.e.*, live births, abortions, and ectopic pregnancies).[29] Although ectopic pregnancy is the leading cause of maternal mortality in the first trimester and accounts for 9% of all maternal deaths in the United States, the death rate has steadily declined as a result of improved diagnostic methods. Earlier detection reduces the risk for tubal rupture, which could result in intraabdominal hemorrhage, major complications, future infertility, or death.[30]

The cause of ectopic pregnancy is delayed ovum transport, which may result from decreased tubal motility or distorted tubal anatomy (*i.e.*, narrowed lumen, convolutions, or diverticula). Factors that may predispose to the development of an ectopic pregnancy include PID, therapeutic abortion, tubal ligation or tubal reversal, previous ectopic pregnancy, intrauterine exposure to DES, infertility, and the use of fertility drugs to induce ovulation. Contraceptive failure with progestin-only birth control pills or the "morning-after pill" also has been associated with ectopic pregnancy.

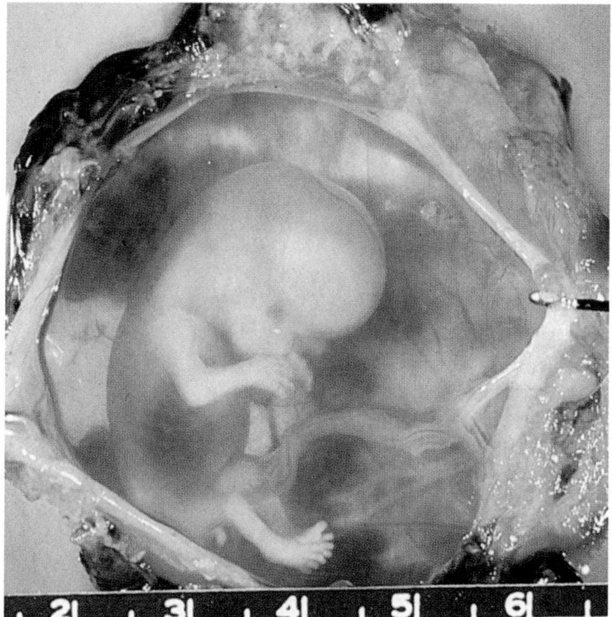

FIGURE 47-5 Ectopic pregnancy. An enlarged fallopian tube has been opened to disclose a minute fetus. (Rubin E., Farber J.L. [1999]. *Pathology* [3rd ed., p. 1001]. Philadelphia: Lippincott-Raven)

Clinical Course

The site of implantation in the tube (*e.g.*, isthmus, ampulla) may determine the onset of symptoms and the timing of diagnosis. As the tubal pregnancy progresses, the surrounding tissue is stretched. The pregnancy eventually outgrows its blood supply, at which point the pregnancy terminates or the tube itself ruptures because it can no longer contain the growing pregnancy. Symptoms can include lower abdominal discomfort—diffuse or localized to one side—which progresses to severe pain caused by rupture, spotting, syncope, referred shoulder pain from bleeding into the abdominal cavity, and amenorrhea.

Physical examination usually reveals adnexal tenderness; an adnexal mass is found in only 50% of cases. Although rarely used today, culdocentesis (*i.e.*, needle aspiration from the cul-de-sac) may reveal blood if rupture has occurred. Quantitative β-human chorionic gonadotropin (hCG) pregnancy tests may detect lower-than-normal hCG production. Pelvic ultrasound studies after 5 weeks' gestation may demonstrate an empty uterine cavity or presence of the gestational sac outside the uterus. In a comparison of various protocols for diagnosing ectopic pregnancy, ultrasound followed by serial hCG levels was found to yield the best results.[30] Definitive diagnosis may require laparoscopy. Differential diagnosis for this type of pelvic pain includes ruptured ovarian cyst, threatened or incomplete abortion, PID, acute appendicitis, and degenerating fibroid.

Treatment usually is surgical: a laparoscopic salpingostomy to remove the ectopic pregnancy if the fallopian tube has not ruptured or salpingectomy to remove the tube if it has. In salpingostomy, a linear incision is made in the tube and allowed to heal closed without suturing to decrease scar tissue formation; this procedure preserves fertility but requires careful surgical technique to minimize the risk for recurrent ectopic pregnancies. Laparoscopic treatment of ectopic pregnancy is well tolerated and more cost effective than laparotomy because of shorter convalescence and the reduced need for postoperative analgesia. When possible, it is the preferred method of treatment. In laparotomy, an open incision is made into the abdominopelvic cavity; this procedure becomes necessary when there is uncontrolled internal bleeding, when the ectopic site cannot be visualized through the laparoscope, or when the surgeon is not trained in operative laparoscopy.

Methotrexate, a chemotherapeutic agent, has been successfully used to eliminate residual ectopic pregnancy tissue after laparoscopy, in cases in which the pregnancy is diagnosed early and is unruptured, or in which surgery is contraindicated. There are several methotrexate regimens and no standardized protocol as yet. Overall success rate for women treated with intramuscular methotrexate has been reported as 89%, with the multidose regimen being most successful.[31] The drug is given for 1 to 8 days and is better tolerated when given orally or in a single injection. Adverse effects can include oral lesions, transient elevation of liver enzyme levels, and anemia. Close follow-up with weekly monitoring of hCG levels is necessary until the pregnancy is completely resolved.[32]

CANCER OF THE FALLOPIAN TUBE

Although a common site of metastases, primary cancer of the fallopian tube is rare, accounting for less than 1% of all female genital tract cancers. Fewer than 3000 cases have been reported worldwide. Most primary tubal cancers are papillary adenocarcinomas, and these tumors develop bilaterally in 30% of patients with advanced disease.

Symptoms are uncommon, but intermittent serosanguineous vaginal discharge, abnormal vaginal bleeding, and colicky low abdominal pain have been reported. An adnexal mass may be present; however, the preoperative diagnosis in most cases is leiomyoma or ovarian tumor. Management is similar to that for ovarian cancer and usually includes total hysterectomy, bilateral salpingo-oophorectomy, and pelvic lymph node dissection. More extensive procedures may be warranted, depending on the stage of the disease. Two thirds of patients are diagnosed at stage I or II. The 5-year survival rate in these cases is approximately 60%, but drops to 10% if metastasis has occurred.[2]

BENIGN OVARIAN CYSTS AND TUMORS

The ovaries have a dual function: they produce germ cells, or ova, and they synthesize the female sex hormones. Disorders of the ovaries frequently cause menstrual and fertility problems. Benign conditions of the ovaries can present as primary lesions of the ovarian structures or as secondary disorders related to hypothalamic, pituitary, or adrenal dysfunction.

Ovarian Cysts

Cysts are the most common form of ovarian tumor. Many are benign. A follicular cyst is one that results from occlusion of the duct of the follicle. Each month, several follicles begin to develop and are blighted at various stages of development. These follicles form cavities that fill with fluid, producing a cyst. The dominant follicle normally ruptures to release the egg (*i.e.*, ovulation) but occasionally persists and continues growing. Likewise, a luteal cyst is a persistent cystic enlargement of the corpus luteum that is formed after ovulation and does not regress in the absence of pregnancy. Functional cysts are asymptomatic unless there is substantial enlargement or bleeding into the cyst. This can cause considerable discomfort or a dull, aching sensation on the affected side. The cyst may become twisted or may rupture into the intraabdominal cavity (Fig. 47-6). These cysts usually regress spontaneously.

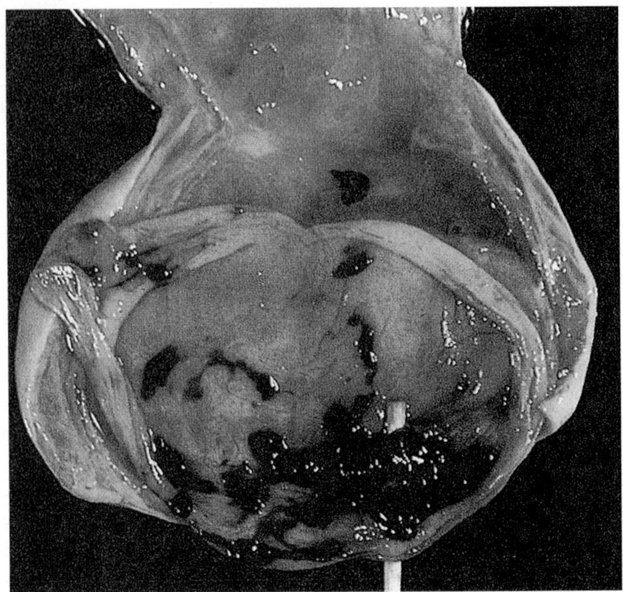

FIGURE 47-6 Follicle cyst of the ovary. The rupture of this thin-walled cyst has been opened and the rupture site indicated with a dowel stick. (Rubin E., Farber J.L. [1999]. *Pathology* [3rd ed., p. 1002]. Philadelphia: Lippincott-Raven)

Polycystic Ovary Syndrome. Ovarian dysfunction associated with infrequent or absent menses in obese, infertile women was first reported in the 1930s by Stein and Leventhal, for whom the syndrome was originally named. Polycystic ovary syndrome (PCOS) is characterized by numerous cystic follicles or follicular cysts. Once thought to be relatively rare, it appears that this clinical entity is one of the most common endocrine disorders among women in the reproductive years.[33–35]

PCOS is characterized by varying degrees of hirsutism, obesity, and infertility, and often is associated with hyperinsulinemia or insulin resistance. This syndrome has been the subject of considerable research. Chronic anovulation, causing amenorrhea or irregular menses, is now thought to be the underlying cause of the bilaterally enlarged "polycystic" ovaries. Hence, the appearance of the ovary is a sign, not the disease itself.[33] The precise etiology of this condition is still being debated. A possible genetic basis has been suggested with an autosomal dominant mode of inheritance and premature balding as the phenotype in males.[34]

Most women with PCOS have elevated luteinizing hormone (LH) levels with normal estrogen and follicle-stimulating hormone (FSH) production. Elevated levels of testosterone, dehydroepiandrosterone sulfate (DHAS), or androstenedione are not uncommon, and these women occasionally have hyperprolactinemia or hypothyroidism. Persistent anovulation results in an estrogen environment that alters the hypothalamic release of GnRH. Increased sensitivity of the pituitary to GnRH results in increased LH secretion and suppression of FSH. This altered LH:FSH ratio often is used as a diagnostic criterion for this condition, but it is not universally present. The presence of some FSH allows for new follicular development; however, full maturation is not attained, and ovulation does not occur. The elevated LH level also results in increased androgen production, which in turn prevents normal follicular development and contributes to the vicious cycle of anovulation.[33] The association between hyperandrogenism and insulin resistance is now well recognized. Evidence suggests that the hyperinsulinemia may lead to the excess androgen production, and several reports have shown that normal ovulation and sometimes pregnancy have occurred when women with hyperandrogenism were treated with insulin-sensitizing drugs.[36,37]

The diagnosis can be suspected from the clinical picture. Although there is no consensus about which laboratory tests should be used, laboratory evaluation to exclude hyperprolactinemia, late-onset adrenal hyperplasia, and adrenogenic-secreting tumors of the ovary and adrenal gland is commonly done. Because insulin resistance is common and may affect treatment, fasting blood glucose and insulin levels are often measured to evaluate for hyperinsulinemia.[34,35] Confirmation with ultrasonography or laparoscopic visualization of the ovaries is not required.

The overall goal of treatment is to suppress insulin-facilitated, LH-driven androgen production. Although numerous medications and protocols are available, the choice depends on the manifestations that are bothersome to the woman and on her stage in reproductive life. If fertility is not desired, oral contraceptives or cyclic progesterone can induce regular menses and prevent the development of endometrial hyperplasia caused by unopposed estrogen. Chronic anovulation can increase a woman's risk for endometrial cancer, cardiovascular disease, and hyperinsulinemia, leading to diabetes mellitus. Treatment is essential for anyone with this condition.

When fertility is desired, the condition usually is treated by the administration of the hypothalamic-pituitary–stimulating drug clomiphene citrate or injectable gonadotropins to induce ovulation. These drugs must be used carefully because they can induce extreme enlargement of the ovaries. Metformin, an insulin-sensitizing drug, may be used before or concurrent with ovulation-inducing medications.[37] Use of this drug has been associated with reductions in androgen and LH levels. When medication is ineffective, laser surgery to puncture the multiple follicles may restore normal ovulatory function, although adhesion formation is a potential problem. Weight loss also may be beneficial in restoring normal ovulation when obesity is present.

Benign and Functioning Ovarian Tumors

Serous cystadenoma and mucinous cystadenoma are the most common benign ovarian neoplasms. Some of these adenomas, however, are considered to have low malignant potential. They are asymptomatic unless their size is sufficient to cause abdominal enlargement. Endometriomas are the "chocolate cysts" that develop secondary to ovarian endometriosis (see the endometriosis section earlier in this chapter). Ovarian fibromas are connective tissue tumors composed of fibrocytes and collagen. They range in size from 6 to 20 cm. Cystic teratomas, or dermoid cysts, are derived from primordial germ cells and are composed of various combinations of well-differentiated ectodermal, mesodermal, and endodermal elements. Not uncommonly, they contain sebaceous material, hair, or teeth. Treatment for all ovarian tumors is surgical excision. Ovarian tissue that is not affected by the tumor can be left intact if frozen-section analysis does not reveal malignancy. When ovarian tumors are very large, as is frequently the case with serous or mucinous cystadenomas, the entire ovary must be removed.

The three types of functioning ovarian tumors are estrogen secreting, androgen secreting, and mixed estrogen-androgen secreting. These tumors may be benign or cancerous. One such tumor, the granulosa cell tumor, is associated with excess estrogen production. When it develops during the reproductive period, the persistent and uncontrolled production of estrogen interferes with the normal menstrual cycle, causing irregular and excessive bleeding, endometrial hyperplasia, or amenorrhea and fertility problems. When it develops after menopause, it causes postmenopausal bleeding, stimulation of the glandular tissues of the breast, and other signs of renewed estrogen production. Androgen-secreting tumors (*i.e.,* Sertoli-Leydig cell tumor or androblastoma) inhibit ovulation and estrogen production. They tend to cause hirsutism and development of masculine characteristics, such as baldness, acne, oily skin, breast atrophy, and deepening of the voice. The treatment is surgical removal of the tumor.

Ovarian Cancer

Ovarian cancer is the second most common female genitourinary cancer and the most lethal. In 2003, 25,400 new cases of ovarian cancer were reported in the United States, two thirds of which were in advanced stages of the disease. Most of these women die of the disease (14,300 women in 2003).[13] The incidence of ovarian cancer increases with age, being greatest between 65 and 84 years of age. Ovarian cancer is difficult to diagnose, and up to 75% of women have metastatic disease before the time of discovery.

The most significant risk factor for ovarian cancer appears to be ovulatory age—the length of time during a woman's life when her ovarian cycle is not suppressed by pregnancy, lactation, or oral contraceptive use. The incidence of ovarian cancer is much lower in countries where women bear numerous children than in the United States. Family history also is a significant risk factor for ovarian cancer. Women with two or more first- or second-degree relatives who have had *site-specific ovarian cancer* have up to a 50% risk for development of the disease. There are two other types of inherited risk for ovarian cancer: *breast-ovarian cancer syndrome,* in which both breast and ovarian cancer occur among first- and second-degree relatives, and *family cancer syndrome* or *Lynch syndrome II* (a subtype of hereditary nonpolyposis colon cancer [HNPCC]), in which male or female relatives have a history of colorectal, endometrial, ovarian, pancreatic, or other types of cancer.[2,38,39] The breast cancer (BRCA) susceptibility genes, *BRCA1* and *BRCA2,* which are tumor suppressor genes (see Chapter 8), are incriminated in approximately 10% of hereditary ovarian cancers despite being identified as "breast cancer genes." Susceptibility to ovarian cancer is transmitted as an autosomal dominant characteristic; therefore, a mutated gene from either parent is sufficient to cause the problem. Most men who pass on the *BRCA* mutations do not themselves manifest male breast cancer.[40] A high-fat Western diet and use of powders containing talc in the genital area are other factors that have been linked to the development of ovarian cancer.

Chemoprevention strategies that have been suggested include long-term oral contraceptive use, nonsteroidal antiinflammatory drugs (NSAIDs), acetaminophen, or retinoids.[41] Each of these agents acts in a slightly different way. The NSAIDs are thought to exert their protective effects through growth inhibition and increased apoptosis (programmed cell death) of ovarian cancer cell lines. The structure of the acetaminophen bears a similarity to the sex hormones, suggesting a potential sex steroid–antagonist property. Support for the use of retinoids comes from experimental data in which retinoic acid was shown to induce the differentiation of cultured ovarian cancer cells. Undoubtedly, continued laboratory studies and clinical trials will provide further evidence of the effectiveness of these chemoprevention agents. Surgical strategies that have reduced the risk for developing ovarian cancer include prophylactic removal of both tubes and ovaries (BSO) and bilateral tubal ligation. These strategies have generally been reserved for women at highest risk, and those who undergo surgical intervention must be counseled that there is still a small risk for developing peritoneal cancer.[41]

Cancer of the ovary is complex because of the diversity of tissue types that originate in the ovary. As a result of this diversity, there are several types of ovarian cancers. Malignant neoplasms of the ovary can be divided into three categories: epithelial tumors, germ cell tumors, and gonadal stromal tumors. Epithelial tumors account for approximately 90% of cases. These different cancers display various degrees of virulence, depending on the type of tumor and degree of differentiation involved. A well-differentiated cancer of the ovary may have produced symptoms for many months and may still be found operable at the time of surgery. A poorly differentiated tumor may have been clinically evident for only a few days but found to be widespread and inoperable. Often, no correlation exists between the duration of symptoms and the extent of the disease.

Clinical Course. Most cancers of the ovary produce no symptoms, or the symptoms are so vague that the woman seldom seeks medical care until the disease is far advanced. These vague discomforts include abdominal distress, flatulence, and bloating, especially after ingesting food. These gastrointestinal manifestations may precede other symptoms by months. Many women take antacids or bicarbonate of soda for a time before consulting a physician. The physician also may dismiss the woman's complaints as being caused by other conditions, further delaying diagnosis and treatment. It is not fully understood why the initial symptoms of ovarian cancer are manifested as gastrointestinal disturbances. It is thought that biochemical changes in the peritoneal fluids may irritate the bowel or that pain originating in the ovary may be referred to the abdomen and be interpreted as a gastrointestinal disturbance. Clinically evident ascites (*i.e.,* fluid in the peritoneal cavity) is seen in approximately one fourth of women with malignant ovarian tumors and is associated with a worse prognosis.

No good screening tests or other early methods of detection exist for ovarian cancer. The serum tumor marker CA-125 is a cell surface antigen; its level is elevated in 80% to 90% of women with stage II to IV nonmucinous ovarian epithelial cancers. The result is negative, however, for as many as 50% of women with stage I disease. In a postmenopausal woman with a pelvic mass, an elevated CA-125 has a positive predictive value of greater than 70% for cancer. It also can be used in monitoring therapy and recurrences when preoperative levels have been elevated. Despite its role in diagnostic evaluation and follow-up, CA-125 is not cancer or tissue specific for ovarian cancer. Levels also are elevated in the presence of endometriosis, uterine fibroids, pregnancy, liver disease, and other benign conditions and with cancer of the endometrium, cervix, fallopian tube, and pancreas. Because it lacks sensitivity and specificity, CA-125 has limited value as a single screening test. Clinical trials to identify more sensitive and specific ovarian cancer tumor markers are under way.[42]

Transvaginal ultrasonography (TVS) has been used to evaluate ovarian masses for malignant potential. As a screening test, it has demonstrated 80% to 90% sensitivity and 83% to 95% specificity. Because the lifetime risk for development of ovarian cancer is 1 in 70 women with family history of the disease, the cost of universal screening for ovarian cancer using the available technology has been estimated at $2.7 million to diagnose one case of ovarian cancer.[39] The National Institutes of Health Consensus Panel convened in 1995 recommended no widespread screening of women for ovarian cancer. CA-125 with TVS is suggested only for women who are part of a family with hereditary ovarian cancer syndrome (*i.e.,* two or more affected first-degree relatives), or less than 1% of all women.[43] Several large national studies are under way to determine the benefit of widespread population-based screening for ovarian cancer.[38,39] Molecular biologic studies have identified tumor suppressor genes that may play a role in the cause of ovarian cancer. Further evaluation in this area is ongoing and may eventually lead to identification of appropriate screening techniques for ovarian cancer.

When ovarian cancer is suspected, surgical evaluation is required for diagnosis, complete and accurate staging, and cytoreduction and debulking procedures to reduce the size of the tumor. At the time of surgery, the uterus, fallopian tubes, ovaries, and omentum are removed; the liver, diaphragm, retroperitoneal and aortic lymph nodes, and peritoneal surface are examined and biopsies are taken as needed. Cytologic washings are done to test for cancerous cells in the peritoneal fluid. Recommendations regarding treatment beyond surgery and prognosis depend on the stage of the disease. Women with limited disease (*i.e.,* well-differentiated stage Ia or Ib) usually do not require adjuvant treatment; women with intermediate disease (*i.e.,* stage Ib or II) or advanced disease (*i.e.,* stage III or IV) can benefit from chemotherapy with cisplatin and cyclophosphamide. When this combination therapy fails, salvage chemotherapy with newer drugs such as paclitaxel (Taxol) may prolong survival. Irradiation no longer plays a major role in treatment of ovarian cancer because of the difficulty in irradiating the entire abdomen without causing life-threatening damage to vital organs.

The lack of accurate screening tools and the resistant nature of ovarian cancers significantly affects success of treatment and survival. The 5-year survival rate is 80% to 90% for women whose ovarian cancer is detected and treated early; however, only 25% of all cases are detected at the localized stage. Overall, the 5-year survival rate is 50.4%.[44,45]

In summary, PID is an inflammation of the upper reproductive tract that involves the uterus (endometritis), fallopian tubes (salpingitis), or ovaries (oophoritis). It is most commonly caused by *N. gonorrhoeae* or *C. trachomatis.* Accurate diagnosis and appropriate antibiotic therapy are aimed at preventing complications such as pelvic adhesions, infertility, ectopic pregnancy, chronic abdominal pain, and tubo-ovarian abscesses.

Ectopic pregnancy occurs when a fertilized ovum implants outside the uterine cavity; the common site is the fallopian tube. Causes of ectopic pregnancy are delayed ovum transport resulting from complications of PID, therapeutic abortion, tubal ligation or tubal reversal, previous ectopic pregnancy, or other conditions such as use of fertility drugs to induce ovulation. It represents a true gynecologic emergency, often necessitating surgical intervention. Cancer of the fallopian tube is rare; the diagnosis is difficult, and the condition usually is well advanced when diagnosed.

Disorders of the ovaries include benign cysts, functioning ovarian tumors, and cancer of the ovary; they usually are asymptomatic unless there is substantial enlargement or bleeding into the cyst, or the cyst becomes twisted or ruptures. Polycystic ovarian disease is characterized by numerous cystic follicles or follicular cysts; it causes various degrees of hirsutism, obesity, and infertility. Benign ovarian tumors consist of endometriomas, which are chocolate cysts that develop secondary to ovarian endometriosis; ovarian fibromas, which are connective tissue tumors composed of fibrocytes and collagen; and cystic teratomas or dermoid cysts, which are derived from primordial germ cells and are composed of various combinations of well-differentiated ectodermal, mesodermal, and endodermal elements. Functioning ovarian tumors are of three types: estrogen secreting, androgen secreting, and mixed estrogen–androgen secreting, and may be benign or cancerous. Cancer of the ovary is the second most common female genitourinary cancer and the most lethal. It can be divided into three categories: epithelial tumors, germ cell tumors, and gonadal stromal tumors. There are no effective screening methods for ovarian cancer, and often the disease is well advanced at the time of diagnosis.

Disorders of Pelvic Support and Uterine Position

After completing this section of the chapter, you should be able to meet the following objectives:

- Characterize the function of the supporting ligaments and pelvic floor muscles in maintaining the position of the pelvic organs, including the uterus, bladder, and rectum
- Describe the manifestations of cystocele, rectocele, and enterocele
- Explain how uterine anteflexion, retroflexion, and retroversion differ from normal uterine position
- Describe the cause and manifestations of uterine prolapse

DISORDERS OF PELVIC SUPPORT

The uterus and the pelvic structures are maintained in proper position by the uterosacral ligaments, round ligaments, broad ligament, and cardinal ligaments. The two cardinal ligaments maintain the cervix in its normal position. The uterosacral ligaments normally hold the uterus in a forward position (Fig. 47-7). The broad ligament suspends the uterus, fallopian tubes, and ovaries in the pelvis.

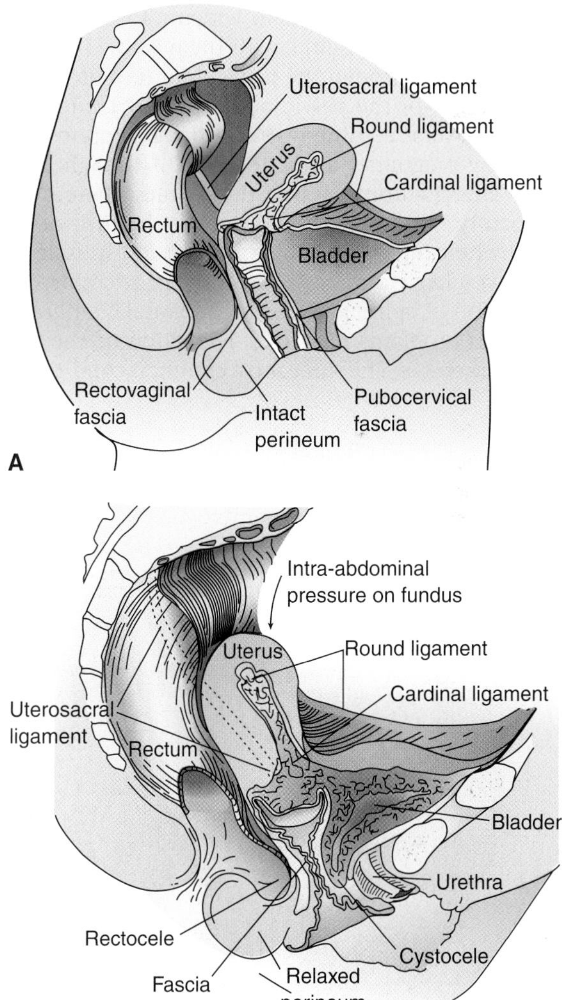

FIGURE 47-7 (**A**) Normal support of the uterus and vagina. (**B**) Relaxation of pelvic support structures with descent of the uterus as well as formation of cystocele and rectocele. (Rock J.A., Thompson J.D. [1992]. *Te Linde's operative gynecology* [7th ed.]. Philadelphia: J.B. Lippincott)

The vagina is encased in the semirigid structure of the strong supporting fascia. The muscular floor of the pelvis is a strong, slinglike structure that supports the uterus, vagina, urinary bladder, and rectum (Fig. 47-8). In the female anatomy, nature is faced with the problems of supporting the pelvic viscera against the force of gravity and increases in intraabdominal pressure associated with coughing, sneezing, defecation, and laughing while at the same time allowing for urination, defecation, and normal reproductive tract function, especially the delivery of an infant. Three supporting structures are provided for the abdominal pelvic diaphragm. The bony pelvis provides support and protection for parts of the digestive tract and genitourinary structures, and the peritoneum holds the pelvic viscera in place. The main support for the viscera, however, is the pelvic diaphragm, made up of muscles and connective tissue that stretch across the bones of the pelvic outlet. The openings that must exist for the urethra, rectum, and vagina cause an inherent weakness in the pelvic diaphragm. Congenital or acquired weakness of the pelvic diaphragm results in widening of these openings, particularly the vagina, with the possible herniation of pelvic viscera through the pelvic floor (*i.e.,* prolapse).

Relaxation of the pelvic outlet usually comes about because of overstretching of the perineal supporting tissues during pregnancy and childbirth. Although the tissues are stretched only during these times, there may be no difficulty until later in life, such as the fifth or sixth decade, when further loss of elasticity and muscle tone occurs. Even in a woman who has not borne children, the combination of aging and postmenopausal changes may give rise to problems related to relaxation of the pelvic support structures. The three most common conditions associated with this relaxation are cystocele, rectocele, and uterine prolapse. These may occur separately or together.

Cystocele

Cystocele is a herniation of the bladder into the vagina. It occurs when the normal muscle support for the bladder is weakened, and the bladder sags below the uterus. The vaginal wall stretches and bulges downward because of the force of gravity and the pressure from coughing, lifting, or straining at stool. The bladder herniates through the anterior vaginal wall, and a cystocele forms (see Fig. 47-7).

The symptoms include an annoying bearing-down sensation, difficulty in emptying the bladder, frequency and urgency of urination, and cystitis. Stress incontinence may occur at times of increased abdominal pressure, such as during squatting, straining, coughing, sneezing, laughing, or lifting.

Rectocele and Enterocele

Rectocele is the herniation of the rectum into the vagina. It occurs when the posterior vaginal wall and underlying rectum bulge forward, ultimately protruding through the introitus as the pelvic floor and perineal muscles are weakened. The symptoms include discomfort because of the protrusion of the rectum and difficulty in defecation (see Fig. 47-7). Digital pressure (*i.e.,* splinting) on the bulging posterior wall of the vagina may become necessary for defecation.

The area between the uterosacral ligaments just posterior to the cervix may weaken and form a hernial sac into which the small bowel protrudes when the woman is standing. This defect, called an *enterocele,* may extend into the rectovaginal septum. It may be congenital or acquired

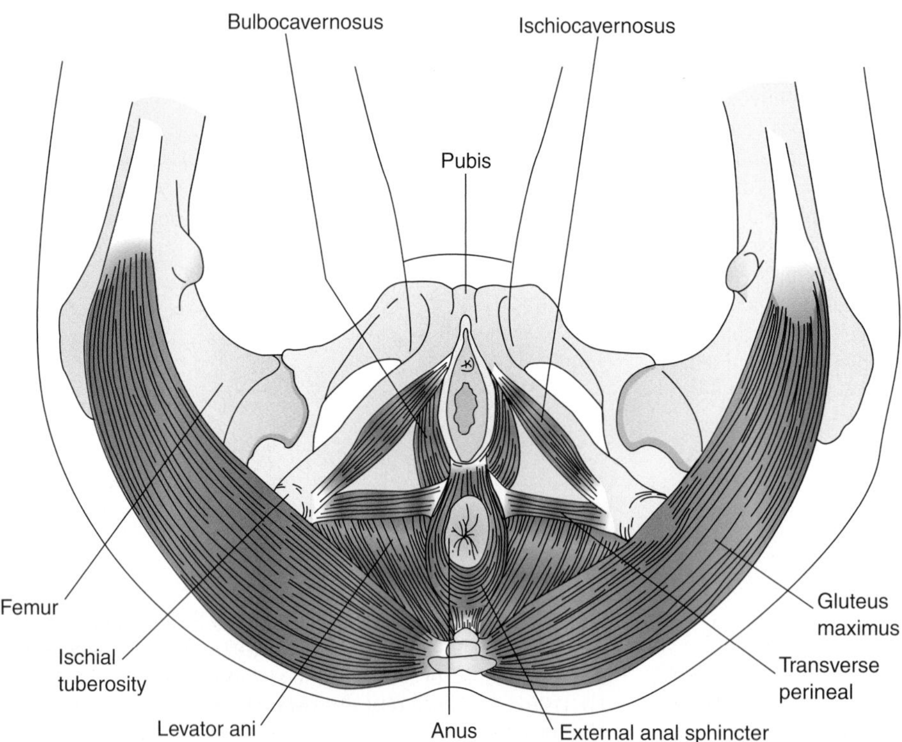

FIGURE 47-8 Muscles of the pelvic floor (female perineum).

through birth trauma. Enterocele can be asymptomatic or cause a dull, dragging sensation and occasionally causes low backache.

Uterine Prolapse

Uterine prolapse is the bulging of the uterus into the vagina that occurs when the primary supportive ligaments (*i.e.*, cardinal ligaments) are stretched. Prolapse is ranked as first, second, or third degree, depending on how far the uterus protrudes through the introitus. First-degree prolapse shows some descent, but the cervix has not reached the introitus. In second-degree prolapse, the cervix or part of the uterus has passed through the introitus. The entire uterus protrudes through the vaginal opening in third-degree prolapse (*i.e.*, procidentia).

The symptoms associated with uterine prolapse result from irritation of the exposed mucous membranes of the cervix and vagina and the discomfort of the protruding mass. Prolapse often is accompanied by perineal relaxation, cystocele, or rectocele. Like cystocele, rectocele, and enterocele, it occurs most commonly in multiparous women because childbearing is accompanied by injuries to pelvic structures and uterine ligaments. It also may result from pelvic tumors and neurologic conditions, such as spina bifida and diabetic neuropathy, that interrupt the innervation of pelvic muscles. A pessary may be inserted to hold the uterus in place and may stave off surgical intervention in women who want to have children or in older women for whom the surgery may pose a significant health risk.

Treatment of Pelvic Support Disorders

Most of the disorders of pelvic relaxation require surgical correction. These are elective surgeries and usually are deferred until after the childbearing years. The symptoms associated with the disorders often are not severe enough to warrant surgical correction. In other cases, the stress of surgery is contraindicated because of other physical disorders; this is particularly true of older women, in whom many of these disorders occur.

There are a number of surgical procedures for the conditions that result from relaxation of pelvic support structures. Removal of the uterus through the vagina (vaginal hysterectomy) with appropriate repair of the vaginal wall (colporrhaphy) often is done when uterine prolapse is accompanied by cystocele or rectocele. A vesicourethral suspension may be done to alleviate the symptoms of stress incontinence. Repair may involve abdominal hysterectomy along with anteroposterior repair. Kegel exercises, which strengthen the pubococcygeus muscle, may be helpful in cases of mild cystocele or rectocele or after surgical repair to help maintain the improved function.

VARIATIONS IN UTERINE POSITION

Variations in the position of the uterus are common. Some variations are innocuous; others, which may be the result of weakness and relaxation of the perineum, give rise to various problems that compromise the structural integrity of the pelvic floor, particularly after childbirth.

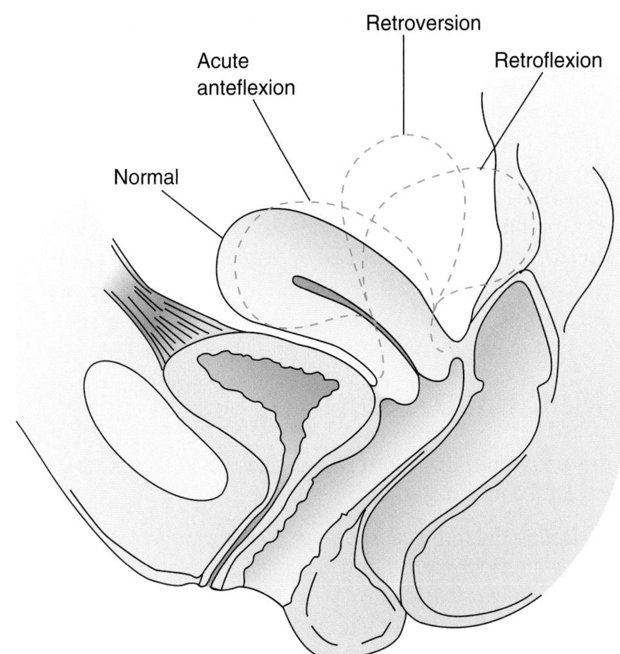

FIGURE 47-9 Variations in uterine position.

The uterus usually is flexed approximately 45 degrees anteriorly, with the cervix positioned posteriorly and downward in the anteverted position. When the woman is standing, the angle of the uterus is such that it lies practically horizontal, resting lightly on the bladder. Asymptomatic, normal variations in the axis of the uterus in relation to the cervix (*i.e.*, flexion) and physiologic displacements that arise after pregnancy or with pathology of the cul-de-sac include anteflexion, retroflexion, and retroversion (Fig. 47-9). An anteflexed uterus is flexed forward on itself. Retroflexion is flexion backward at the isthmus. Retroversion describes the condition in which the uterus inclines posteriorly while the cervix remains tilted forward. Simple retroversion of the uterus is the most common displacement, found in 30% of normal women. It usually is a congenital condition caused by a short anterior vaginal wall and relaxed uterosacral ligaments; together, these force the uterus to fall back into the cul-de-sac. Retroversion also can follow certain diseases, such as endometriosis and PID, which produce fibrous tissue adherence with retraction of the fundus posteriorly. Large leiomyomas also may cause the uterus to move into a posterior position. Dyspareunia with deep penetration or low back pain with menses can be associated with retroversion. Most symptoms in these women are caused by the associated condition (*e.g.*, adhesions, fibroids) rather than congenital retroversion.

In summary, alterations in pelvic support frequently occur because of weaknesses and relaxation of the pelvic floor and perineum. Cystocele and rectocele involve herniation of the bladder or rectum into the vagina. Uterine prolapse occurs when the uterus bulges into the vagina. Pelvic relaxation disorders typically result from overstretching of the perineal supporting muscles during pregnancy and childbirth. The loss of elasticity in these structures that is a normal accompaniment of aging contributes to these problems. Variations in uterine position are common; they include anteflexion, retroflexion, and retroversion. These disorders, which often are innocuous, can be the result of a congenital shortness of the vaginal wall, development of fibrous adhesions secondary to endometriosis or PID, or displacement caused by large uterine leiomyomas.

Menstrual Disorders

After completing this section of the chapter, you should be able to meet the following objectives:

- Define the terms *amenorrhea, hypomenorrhea, oligomenorrhea, menorrhagia, metrorrhagia,* and *menometrorrhagia*
- State the function of alterations in estrogen and progesterone levels as a cause of dysfunctional menstrual cycles
- Differentiate between primary dysmenorrhea and secondary dysmenorrhea
- Characterize the manifestations of the premenstrual syndrome, its possible causes, and the methods of treatment

DYSFUNCTIONAL MENSTRUAL CYCLES

Although unexplained uterine bleeding can occur for many reasons, such as pregnancy, abortion, bleeding dyscrasias, and neoplasms, the most frequent cause in the nonpregnant female is what is commonly called *dysfunctional menstrual cycles* or *bleeding*. Dysfunctional cycles may take the form of *amenorrhea* (absence of menstruation), *hypomenorrhea* (scanty menstruation), *oligomenorrhea* (infrequent menstruation, periods more than 35 days apart), *polymenorrhea* (frequent menstruation, periods less than 27 days apart), *menorrhagia* (excessive menstruation), or *metrorrhagia* (bleeding between periods). *Menometrorrhagia* is heavy bleeding during and between menstrual periods.

Dysfunctional menstrual cycles are related to alterations in the hormones that support normal cyclic endometrial changes. Estrogen deprivation causes retrogression of a previously built-up endometrium and bleeding. Such bleeding often is irregular in amount and duration, with the flow varying with the time and degree of estrogen stimulation and with the degree of estrogen withdrawal. A lack of progesterone can cause abnormal menstrual bleeding; in its absence, estrogen induces development of a much thicker endometrial layer with a richer blood supply. The absence of progesterone results from the failure of any of the developing ovarian follicles to mature to the point of ovulation, with the subsequent formation of the corpus luteum and production and secretion of progesterone.

Periodic bleeding episodes alternating with amenorrhea are caused by variations in the number of functioning ovarian follicles present. If sufficient follicles are present and active and if new follicles assume functional capacity, high levels of estrogen develop, causing the endometrium to proliferate for weeks or even months. In time, estrogen withdrawal and bleeding develop. This can occur for two reasons: an absolute estrogen deficiency may develop when several follicles simultaneously degenerate, or a relative deficiency may develop as the needs of the enlarged endometrial tissue mass exceed the capabilities of the existing follicles, even though estrogen levels remain constant. Estrogen and progesterone deficiency are associated with the absence of ovulation, hence the term *anovulatory bleeding.* Because the vasoconstriction and myometrial contractions that normally accompany menstruation are caused by progesterone, anovulatory bleeding seldom is accompanied by cramps, and the flow frequently is heavy. Anovulatory cycles are common among adolescents during the first several years after menarche, when ovarian function is becoming established, and among perimenopausal women, whose ovarian function is beginning to decline.

Dysfunctional menstrual cycles can originate as a primary disorder of the ovaries or as a secondary defect in ovarian function related to hypothalamic-pituitary stimulation. The latter can be initiated by emotional stress, marked variation in weight (*i.e.,* sudden gain or loss), or nonspecific endocrine or metabolic disturbances. Organic causes of irregular menstrual bleeding include endometrial polyps, submucosal myoma (*i.e.,* fibroid), blood dyscrasia, infection, endometrial cancer, polycystic ovarian disease, and pregnancy.

The treatment of dysfunctional bleeding depends on what is identified as the probable cause. The minimum evaluation should include a detailed history with emphasis on bleeding pattern and a physical examination. Endocrine studies (FSH : LH ratio, prolactin, testosterone, DHAS), β-hCG pregnancy test, ultrasound of the endometrium with or without saline infusion, endometrial biopsy, D & C with or without hysteroscopy, and progesterone withdrawal tests may be needed for diagnosis. Organic causes

DYSFUNCTIONAL MENSTRUAL CYCLES

- The pattern of menstrual bleeding tends to be fairly consistent in most healthy women with regard to frequency, duration, and amount of flow.
- Dysfunctional bleeding in postpubertal women can take the form of absent or scanty periods, infrequent periods, excessive and irregular periods, excessive bleeding during periods, and bleeding between periods.
- When the basic pattern of bleeding is changed it is most often due to a lack of ovulation and disturbances in the pattern of hormone secretion.
- When the basic pattern is undisturbed and there are superimposed episodes of bleeding or spotting, the etiology is more likely to be related to organic lesions or hematologic disorders.

generally require surgical intervention. D & C can be therapeutic as well as diagnostic. Endometrial ablation (thinning or elimination of the basalis layer of the endometrium from which the monthly buildup generates) has become a primary management strategy for heavy bleeding and can be accomplished with heat, cold, light, microwaves, chemicals, and radiofrequency as energy sources.[46] Approximately 80% to 90% of women will have a significant reduction in their menorrhagia, with 25% to 40% experiencing amenorrhea.[3] If organic problems are excluded and alterations in hormone levels are the primary cause, treatment may include the use of oral contraceptives, cyclic progesterone therapy, or long-acting progesterone injections.

AMENORRHEA

There are two types of amenorrhea: primary and secondary. Primary amenorrhea is the failure to menstruate by 16 years of age, or by 14 years of age if failure to menstruate is accompanied by absence of secondary sex characteristics. Secondary amenorrhea is the cessation of menses for at least 6 months in a woman who has established normal menstrual cycles. Primary amenorrhea usually is caused by gonadal dysgenesis, congenital mullerian agenesis, testicular feminization, or a hypothalamic-pituitary-ovarian axis disorder. Causes of secondary amenorrhea include ovarian, pituitary, or hypothalamic dysfunction; intrauterine adhesions (*i.e.*, Asherman's syndrome); infections (*e.g.*, tuberculosis, schistosomiasis); pituitary tumor; anorexia nervosa; or strenuous physical exercise, which can alter the critical body fat–to-muscle ratio needed for menses to occur.[47]

Diagnostic evaluation resembles that for dysfunctional uterine bleeding, with the possible addition of a computed tomographic scan to exclude a pituitary tumor. Treatment is based on correcting the underlying cause and inducing menstruation with cyclic progesterone or combined estrogen-progesterone regimens.

DYSMENORRHEA

Dysmenorrhea is pain or discomfort with menstruation. Although not usually a serious medical problem, it causes some degree of monthly disability for a significant number of women. There are two forms of dysmenorrhea: primary and secondary. Primary dysmenorrhea is menstrual pain that is not associated with a physical abnormality or pathology.[48] It usually occurs with ovulatory menstruation beginning 6 months to 2 years after menarche. Symptoms may begin 1 to 2 days before menses, peak on the first day of flow, and subside within several hours to several days. Severe dysmenorrhea may be associated with systemic symptoms such as headache, nausea, vomiting, diarrhea, fatigue, irritability, dizziness, and syncope. The pain typically is described as dull, lower abdominal aching or cramping, spasmodic or colicky in nature, often radiating to the lower back, labia majora, or upper thighs.

Secondary dysmenorrhea is menstrual pain caused by specific organic conditions, such as endometriosis, uterine fibroids, adenomyosis, pelvic adhesions, IUDs, or PID. Laparoscopy often is required for diagnosis of secondary dysmenorrhea if medication for primary dysmenorrhea is ineffective.

Treatment of primary dysmenorrhea is directed at symptom control. Although analgesic agents such as aspirin and acetaminophen may relieve minor uterine cramping or low back pain, prostaglandin synthetase inhibitors, such as ibuprofen, naproxen, mefenamic acid, and indomethacin, are more specific for dysmenorrhea and are the treatment of choice if contraception is not desired. Several cyclooxygenase II (COX II) inhibitors (valdecoxib, celecoxib, rofecoxib) also carry the indication for dysmenorrhea. Ovulation suppression and symptomatic relief of dysmenorrhea can be instituted simultaneously with the use of oral contraceptives. Relief of secondary dysmenorrhea depends on identifying the cause of the problem. Medical or surgical intervention may be needed to eliminate the problem.

PREMENSTRUAL SYNDROME

The *premenstrual syndrome* (PMS) is a distinct clinical entity characterized by a cluster of physical and psychological symptoms limited to 3 to 14 days preceding menstruation and relieved by onset of the menses. According to surveys, 80% of women experience premenstrual emotional or physical changes, with 20% to 40% of the adult female population in the United States indicating that these mild to moderate monthly symptoms cause some difficulty; only 2% to 5% report extreme or severe symptoms that negatively affect their life.[49] How many of these women have symptoms that are severe enough to warrant treatment is unknown. The incidence of PMS seems to increase with age. It is less common in women in their teens and twenties, and most of the women seeking help for the problem are in their mid-thirties. There is some dispute about whether PMS occurs more frequently in women who have not had children or in those who have had children. The disorder is not culturally distinct; it affects non-Westerners and Westerners.

The physical symptoms of PMS include painful and swollen breasts, bloating, abdominal pain, headache, and backache. Psychologically, there may be depression, anxiety, irritability, and behavioral changes. In some cases, there are puzzling alterations in motor function, such as clumsiness and altered handwriting. Women with PMS may report one or several symptoms, with symptoms varying from woman to woman and from month to month in the same patient. Signs and symptoms associated with this disorder are summarized in Table 47-2. PMS can significantly affect a woman's ability to perform at normal levels. She may lose time from or function ineffectively at work. Family responsibilities and relationships may suffer. Students have had lower grades during the premenstrual period. More crimes are committed by females during the premenstrual phase of the cycle, and more lives are lost to suicide during this period. The term *premenstrual dysphoric disorder* (PMDD) is a psychiatric diagnosis that has been developed to distinguish those women whose symptoms are severe enough to interfere significantly with activities

TABLE 47-2 Symptoms of Premenstrual Syndrome (PMS) by System

Body System	Symptoms
Cerebral	Irritability, anxiety, nervousness, fatigue, and exhaustion; increased physical and mental activity; lability; crying spells; depressions; inability to concentrate
Gastrointestinal	Craving for sweets or salts, lower abdominal pain, bloating, nausea, vomiting, diarrhea, constipation
Vascular	Headache, edema, weakness, or fainting
Reproductive	Swelling and tenderness of the breasts, pelvic congestion, ovarian pain, altered libido
Neuromuscular	Trembling of the extremities, changes in coordination, clumsiness, backache, leg aches
General	Weight gain, insomnia, dizziness, acne

of daily living. A minimum of 5 of the 11 symptom groups described in the DSM-IV must be present to establish the diagnosis of PMDD. Presence of a single symptom is sufficient for the diagnosis of PMS.[48,50]

Although the causes of PMS are poorly documented, they probably are multifactorial. Like dysmenorrhea, it is only recently that PMS has been recognized as a bona fide disorder rather than merely a psychosomatic illness. There has been a tendency to link the disorder with endocrine imbalances such as hyperprolactinemia, estrogen excess, and alteration in the estrogen-to-progesterone ratio. Prolactin concentration affects sodium and water retention, is higher in the luteal phase than in the follicular phase, and can be increased by estrogens, stress, hypoglycemia, pregnancy, and oral contraceptives.[51] Estrogens stimulate anxiety and nervous tension, and increased progesterone levels may produce depression. The role of hormonal factors in the cause of PMS is supported by two well-established phenomena. First, women who have undergone a hysterectomy but not an oophorectomy may have cyclic symptoms that resemble PMS. Second, PMS symptoms are rare in postmenopausal women. Research has failed to confirm these theories.

Other hypotheses suggest that increased aldosterone may contribute to symptoms associated with fluid retention (*e.g.*, headache, bloating, breast tenderness, weight gain); that pyridoxine (vitamin B_6) deficiency may lead to estrogen excess or decreased production of the neurotransmitters dopamine and serotonin, which may contribute to PMS symptoms; or that decreased prostaglandin E_1 concentrations can lead to abnormal sensitivity to prolactin, with associated fluid retention, irritability, and depression. In addition, increased appetite, binge eating, fatigue, and depression have been associated with altered endorphin activity and subclinical hypoglycemia.[51] There also is evidence that learned beliefs about menstruation can contribute to the production of PMS or at least affect the woman's response to the symptoms.

The most recent theory to emerge suggests a relationship between normal gonadal fluctuations and central neurotransmitter activity, particularly serotonin. It is unclear whether decreased levels of serotonin are present during the luteal phase and only susceptible women respond with varying degrees of premenstrual symptoms, or whether women with PMDD have a neurotransmitter abnormality.[3,48,50]

Diagnosis focuses on identification of the symptom clusters by means of prospective charting for at least 3 months. Several validated tools are available for recording symptoms; however, any calendar used for this purpose must include information regarding specific symptoms, severity, timing in relation to the menstrual cycle, and baseline level of symptoms in the follicular phase.[3] A complete history and physical examination are necessary to exclude other physical causes of the symptoms. Depending on the symptom pattern, blood studies, including thyroid hormones, glucose, and prolactin assays, may be done. Psychosocial evaluation is helpful to exclude emotional illness that is merely exacerbated premenstrually.

In the past, the treatment of PMS has been largely symptomatic. Attempts have been made to effect weight loss and reduce fluid retention through the use of diuretics. Tranquilizer drugs were used to treat mood changes, and pain was treated with mild analgesics. Treatment still is directed to some extent toward somatic complaints. Relief of somatic pain does not, however, totally resolve PMS suffering. The latest approach is to recommend an integrated program of personal assessment by diary, regular exercise, avoidance of caffeine, and a diet low in simple sugars and high in lean proteins. Additional therapeutic regimens include vitamin or mineral supplements (particularly pyridoxine, vitamin E, and magnesium), natural progesterone supplements, low-dose monophasic oral contraceptives, GnRH agonists, bromocriptine for prolactin suppression, danazol (a synthetic androgen), spironolactone (an aldosterone antagonist and steroidogenesis inhibitor), evening primrose oil (which contains linoleic acid, a precursor of prostaglandin E_1), and lithium for marked functional impairment from affective symptoms.[49–51] Few treatments have been adequately evaluated in randomized, controlled trials. The use of selective serotonin reuptake inhibitors, however, has demonstrated significant improvement in overall symptoms compared with placebo, whether used continuously or only in the luteal phase.[52]

The daily use of prescribed relaxation techniques during the premenstrual period can improve physical and emotional symptoms.[51] Management of PMS/PMDD includes education and support directed toward lifestyle changes. Drug therapy should be used cautiously until well-controlled studies establish criteria for use and effective treatment results. The placebo effect may account for symptom relief in a significant number of women. It is unlikely that a single cause or treatment for PMS will be found. Evaluation and management should focus on identifying and controlling the individual symptom clusters when possible.

In summary, menstrual disorders include dysfunctional menstrual cycles, dysmenorrhea, and PMS. Dysfunctional menstrual cycles occur when the hormonal support of the endometrium is altered. Estrogen deprivation causes retrogression of a previously built-up endometrium and bleeding. A lack of progesterone can cause abnormal menstrual bleeding; in its absence, estrogen induces development of a much thicker endometrial layer with a richer blood supply. The absence of progesterone results from the failure of any of the developing ovarian follicles to mature to the point of ovulation, with the subsequent formation of the corpus luteum and production and secretion of progesterone. Dysfunctional menstrual cycles produce amenorrhea, oligomenorrhea, metrorrhagia, or menorrhagia. Dysmenorrhea is characterized by pain or discomfort during menses. It can occur as a primary or secondary disorder. Primary dysmenorrhea is not associated with other disorders and begins soon after menarche. Secondary dysmenorrhea is caused by a specific organic condition, such as endometriosis or pelvic adhesions. It occurs in women with previously painless menses. PMS represents a cluster of physical and psychological symptoms that precede menstruation by 1 to 2 weeks. PMDD describes the most severe, disabling form of PMS. The true incidence and nature of PMS has been recognized only recently, and its cause and methods for treatment are still under study.

Disorders of the Breast

After completing this section of the chapter, you should be able to meet the following objectives:

- Describe changes in breast function that occur with galactorrhea, mastitis, and ductal ectasia
- Describe the manifestations of fibrocystic disease and state why it is often referred to as a "catchall" for breast irregularities
- Cite the risk factors for breast cancer, the importance of breast self-examination, and recommendations for mammography
- Describe the methods used in the diagnosis and treatment of breast cancer

Most breast disease may be described as benign or cancerous. Breast tissue is never static; the breast is constantly responding to changes in hormonal, nutritional, psychological, and environmental stimuli that cause continual cellular changes. Benign breast conditions are nonprogressive; some forms of benign disease, however, increase the risk for malignant disease. In light of this, strict adherence to a dichotomy of benign versus malignant disease may not always be appropriate. This dichotomy, however, is useful for the sake of simplicity and clarity.

GALACTORRHEA

Galactorrhea is the secretion of breast milk in a nonlactating breast. Galactorrhea may result from vigorous nipple stimulation during lovemaking, exogenous hormones, internal hormonal imbalance, or local chest infection or trauma. A pituitary tumor may produce large amounts of prolactin and cause galactorrhea. Galactorrhea occurs in men and women and usually is benign. Observation may be continued for several months before diagnostic hormonal screening.

MASTITIS

Mastitis is inflammation of the breast. It most frequently occurs during lactation but may also result from other conditions.

In the lactating woman, inflammation results from an ascending infection that travels from the nipple to the ductile structures. The most common organisms isolated are *Staphylococcus* and *Streptococcus*.[3] The offending organisms originate from the suckling infant's nasopharynx or the mother's hands. During the early weeks of nursing, the breast is particularly vulnerable to bacterial invasion because of minor cracks and fissures that occur with vigorous suckling. Infection and inflammation cause obstruction of the ductile system. The breast area becomes hard, inflamed, and tender if not treated early. Without treatment, the area becomes walled off and may abscess, requiring incision and drainage. It is advisable for the mother to continue breastfeeding during antibiotic therapy to prevent this.

Mastitis is not confined to the postpartum period; it can occur as a result of hormonal fluctuations, tumors, trauma, or skin infection. Cyclic inflammation of the breast occurs most frequently in adolescents, who commonly have fluctuating hormone levels. Tumors may cause mastitis secondary to skin involvement or lymphatic obstruction. Local trauma or infection may develop into mastitis because of ductal blockage of trapped blood, cellular debris, or the extension of superficial inflammation.

The treatment of mastitis symptoms may include application of heat or cold, excision, aspiration, mild analgesics, antibiotics, and a supportive brassiere or breast binder.

DUCTAL DISORDERS

Ductal ectasia manifests in older women as a spontaneous, intermittent, usually unilateral, grayish-green nipple discharge. Palpation of the breast increases the discharge. Ectasia occurs during or after menopause and is symptomatically associated with burning, itching, pain, and a pulling sensation of the nipple and areola. The disease results in inflammation of the ducts and subsequent thickening. The treatment requires removal of the involved ductal mass.

Intraductal papillomas are benign epithelial tissue tumors that range in size from 2 mm to 5 cm. Papillomas usually manifest with a bloody nipple discharge. The tumor may be palpated in the areolar area. The papilloma is probed through the nipple, and the involved duct is removed.

FIBROADENOMA AND FIBROCYSTIC DISEASE

Fibroadenoma is seen in premenopausal women, most commonly in the third and fourth decade. The clinical findings include a firm, rubbery, sharply defined round mass. On palpation, the mass "slides" between the fingers and is easily movable. These masses usually are singular; only 15% are multiple or bilateral. Fibroadenoma is asymptomatic and usually found by accident. It is not thought to be precancerous. Treatment involves simple excision.

The term *fibrocystic breast disease* is the most frequent lesion of the breast. It is most common in women 30 to 50 years of age and is rare in postmenopausal women not receiving hormone replacement.[53] Fibrocystic disease usually presents as nodular (*i.e.,* "shotty"), granular breast masses that are more prominent and painful during the luteal or progesterone-dominant portion of the menstrual cycle. Discomfort ranges from heaviness to exquisite tenderness, depending on the degree of vascular engorgement and cystic distention.

Fibrocystic disease encompasses a wide variety of lesions and breast changes. Microscopically, fibrocystic disease refers to a constellation of morphologic changes manifested by (1) cystic dilation of terminal ducts, (2) relative increase in fibrous tissue, and (3) variable proliferation of terminal duct epithelial elements.[54] Autopsy studies have demonstrated some degree of fibrocystic change in 60% to 80% of adult women in the United States.[54] Symptomatic fibrocystic disease, in which large, clinically detectable cysts are present, is much less common, occurring in approximately 10% of adult women between 35 and 50 years of age.[54] Although fibrocystic disease often has been thought to increase the risk for breast cancer, only certain variants in which proliferation of the epithelial components is demonstrated represent a true risk. Fibrocystic disease with giant cysts and proliferative epithelial lesions with atypia are more common in women who are at increased risk for developing breast cancer. The nonproliferative form of fibrocystic disease that does not carry an increased risk for development of cancer is more common.

Diagnosis of fibrocystic disease is made by physical examination, biopsy (*i.e.,* aspiration or tissue sample), and mammography. The presence of diffuse radiographic densities, lumpy breasts, or premenstrual breast pain correlate poorly with the presence or degree of fibrocystic change. Instead, a diagnosis of fibrocystic disease should be based on the results of a microscopic examination of a biopsy specimen. Fine-needle aspiration may be used, but if a suspect mass that was nonmalignant on cytologic examination does not resolve over several months, it should be removed surgically. Any discrete mass or lump on the breast should be viewed as possible carcinoma, and cancer should be excluded before instituting the conservative measures used to treat fibrocystic disease. The use of mammography for diagnosis in high-risk groups younger than 35 years of age on a routine basis is still controversial. Mammography may be helpful in establishing the diagnosis, but increased breast tissue density in women with fibrocystic disease may make an abnormal or cancerous mass difficult to discern among the other structures. Hand-held ultrasonography can be useful in clarifying inconclusive mammographic densities.

Treatment of fibrocystic breast disease usually is symptomatic. Aspirin, mild analgesics, and local application of heat or cold may be recommended. Some physicians attempt to aspirate prominent or persistent cysts and send any fluid obtained to the laboratory for cytologic analysis. Women are advised to avoid foods that contain xanthines (*e.g.,* coffee, cola, chocolate, and tea) in their daily diets, particularly premenstrually. Vitamin E may be helpful in reducing mastalgia (breast pain), and women should be encouraged to wear a good supporting brassiere. Danazol can be used for women with severe pain, although the potential for adverse effects warrants trying other methods first.[3]

BREAST CANCER

Cancer of the breast is the most common female cancer. One in eight women in the United States will have breast cancer in her lifetime. In 2003, breast cancer affected 211,300 American women and killed an estimated 40,200 women.[13] Although the breast cancer mortality rate has shown a slight decline, it is second only to lung cancer as a cause of cancer-related deaths in women. An additional 400 deaths occurred from breast cancer in males.[13] Incidence rates for carcinoma in situ have increased dramatically since the mid-1970s because of recommendations regarding mammography screening. The decline in the breast cancer mortality rate since 1989 is due to this earlier diagnosis as well as improvements in cancer treatments.[13]

Risk factors for breast cancer include sex, increasing age, personal or family history of breast cancer (*i.e.,* at highest risk are those with multiple affected first-order relatives), history of benign breast disease (*i.e.,* primary "atypical" hyperplasia), and hormonal influences that promote breast maturation and may increase the chance of cell mutation (*i.e.,* early menarche, late menopause, and no term pregnancies or first child after 30 years of age).[13] Most women with breast cancer have no identifiable risk factors.

Approximately 10% of all breast cancers are hereditary, with genetic mutations causing up to 80% of breast cancers in women younger than 50 years of age.[55] Two breast cancer susceptibility genes—*BRCA1* on chromosome 17 and *BRCA2* on chromosome 13—may account for most inherited forms of breast cancer (see Chapter 8). *BRCA1* is known to be involved in tumor suppression. A woman with known mutations in *BRCA1* has a lifetime risk of 56%

to 85% for breast cancer and an increased risk for ovarian cancer. *BRCA2* is another susceptibility gene that carries an elevated cancer risk similar to that with *BRCA1*.[48,55] A task force organized by the National Institutes of Health and the National Genome Research Institute has proposed a set of provisional consensus recommendations for monitoring known carriers of *BRCA1* and *BRCA2* mutations. The task force recommended that known carriers should begin monthly breast self-examination (BSE) at 18 years of age and begin having annual mammograms at 25 years of age.[55] Prophylactic surgery, in the form of bilateral mastectomy, bilateral oophorectomy, or both, may decrease the risk for developing cancer. These controversial surgeries can have physical and psychological side effects that warrant careful consideration before proceeding.[55]

Detection

Cancer of the breast may manifest clinically as a mass, a puckering, nipple retraction, or unusual discharge. Many cancers are found by women themselves through BSE—sometimes when only a thickening or subtle change in breast contour is noticed. The variety of symptoms and potential for self-discovery underscore the need for regular, systematic self-examination. BSE should be done routinely by women older than 20 years of age. Premenopausal women should conduct the examination right after menses. This time is most appropriate in relation to cyclic breast changes that occur in response to fluctuations in hormone levels. Postmenopausal women and women who have had a hysterectomy should perform the examination on the same day of every month. Examination should be done in the shower or bath or at bedtime. The most important aspect of BSE is to devise a regular, systematic, convenient, and consistent method of examination. As an adjunct to BSE, women should have a clinical examination by a trained health professional at least every 3 years between 20 and 40 years of age, and annually after 40 years of age.

Mammography is the only effective screening technique for the early detection of clinically inapparent lesions. Although recent studies have brought into question the value of mammography,[56–58] in 2002, the United States Preventive Services Task Force (USPSTF) issued new guidelines concluding that there were sufficient data to justify recommending mammography every 1 to 2 years in women older than 40 years.[59] A generally slow-growing form of cancer, breast cancer may have been present for 2 to 9 years before it reaches 1 cm, the smallest mass normally detected by palpation. Mammography can disclose lesions as small as 1 mm and the clustering of calcifications that may warrant biopsy to exclude cancer. The American Cancer Society recommends annual evaluation for women after 40 years of age.[60] Mammography has a sensitivity of 80% to 85% for the detection of breast cancer even when performed by the most capable institutions.[61] Approximately 40% of breast cancers can be detected only by palpation and another 40% only by mammography.[13] The most comprehensive approach to screening is a combination of BSE, clinical evaluation by a health professional, and mammography.

Diagnosis and Classification

Procedures used in the diagnosis of breast cancer include physical examination, mammography, ultrasonography, percutaneous needle aspiration, stereotactic needle biopsy (*i.e.*, core biopsy), and excisional biopsy. Figure 47-10 illustrates the appearance of breast cancer on mammography. Breast cancer often manifests as a solitary, painless, firm, fixed lesion with poorly defined borders. It can be found anywhere in the breast but is most common in the upper outer quadrant. Because of the variability in presentation, any suspect change in breast tissue warrants further investigation. The diagnostic use of mammography enables additional definition of the clinically suspect area (*e.g.*, appearance, character, calcification). Placement of a wire marker under radiographic guidance can ensure accurate surgical biopsy of nonpalpable suspect areas. Ultrasonography is useful as a diagnostic adjunct to differentiate cystic from solid tissue in women with nonspecific thickening.

Fine-needle aspiration is a simple in-office procedure that can be performed repeatedly in multiple sites and with minimal discomfort. It can be accomplished by stabilizing a palpable mass between two fingers or in conjunction with handheld sonography to define cystic masses or fibrocystic changes and to provide specimens for cytologic examination. Fine-needle aspiration can identify the presence of malignant cells, but it cannot differentiate in situ from infiltrating cancers. Stereotactic needle biopsy is an outpatient procedure done with the guidance of a mammography machine. After the lesion is localized radiologically, a large-bore needle is mechanically thrust quickly into the area, removing a core of tissue. Discomfort is similar to that with ear piercing, and even when multiple cores are obtained, healing occurs quite rapidly. Cells are available for histologic evaluation with 96% accuracy in detecting cancer. This procedure is less costly than excisional biopsy. Excisional biopsy to remove the entire lump provides the only definitive diagnosis of breast cancer and often is therapeutic without additional surgery. Magnetic resonance imaging (MRI) techniques, positron-emission tomography, and computer-based or digital mammography are being evaluated as additional diagnostic modalities for breast cancer and may be recommended to supplement conventional mammography in women with a strong family history of cancer or known carriers of *BRCA1* or *BRCA2*.[55]

Tumors are classified histologically according to tissue characteristics and staged clinically according to tumor size, nodal involvement, and presence of metastasis. It is recommended that estrogen and progesterone receptor analysis be performed on surgical specimens. Information about the presence or absence of estrogen and progesterone receptors can be used in predicting tumor responsiveness to hormonal manipulation. High levels of both receptors improve the prognosis and increase the likelihood of remission.

Treatment

The treatment methods for breast cancer are controversial. They may include surgery, chemotherapy, radiation therapy, and hormonal manipulation. Radical mastectomy (*i.e.*, removal of the entire breast, underlying muscles, and

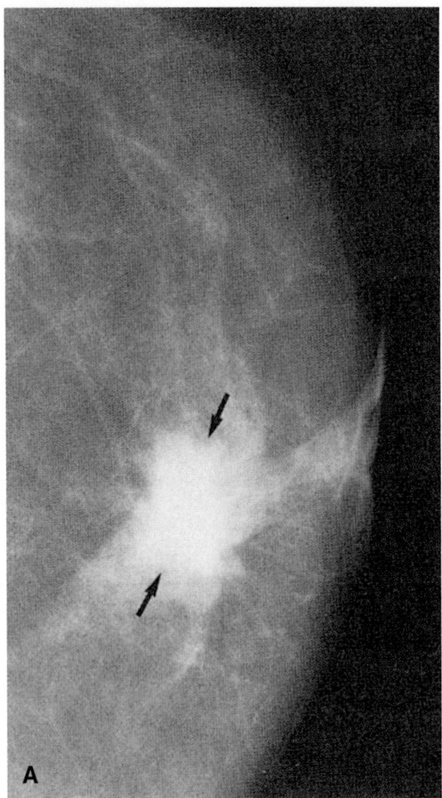

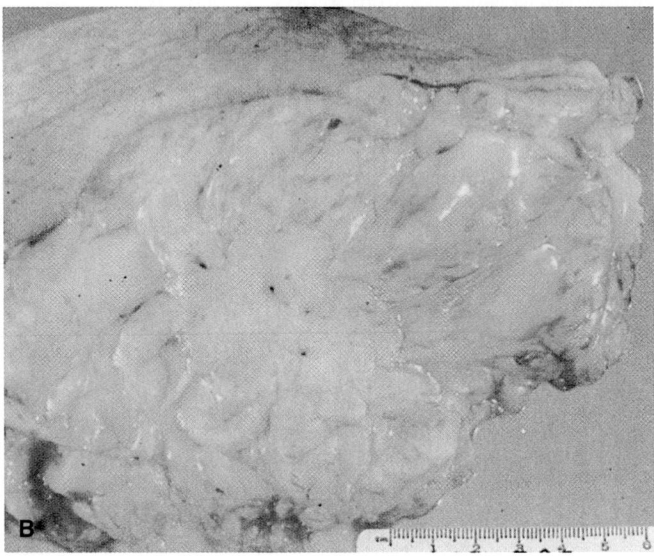

FIGURE 47-10 Carcinoma of the breast. (**A**) Mammogram. An irregularly shaped, dense mass (*arrows*) is seen in this otherwise fatty breast. (**B**) Mastectomy specimen. The irregular white, firm mass in the center is surrounded by fatty tissue. (Rubin E., Farber J.L. [1999]. *Pathology* [3rd ed., p. 1042]. Philadelphia: Lippincott-Raven)

all axillary nodes) rarely is used today as a primary surgical therapy unless breast cancer is advanced at the time of diagnosis. Modified surgical techniques (*i.e.,* mastectomy plus axillary dissection or lumpectomy for breast conservation) accompanied by chemotherapy or radiation therapy have achieved outcomes comparable with those obtained with radical surgical methods and constitute the preferred treatment methods.

The prognosis is related more to the extent of nodal involvement than to the extent of breast involvement. Greater nodal involvement requires more aggressive postsurgical treatment, and many cancer specialists believe that a diagnosis of breast cancer is not complete until dissection and testing of the axillary lymph nodes has been accomplished. A newer technique for evaluating lymph node involvement is a sentinel lymph node (SLN) biopsy. A radioactive substance or dye is injected into the region of the tumor. In theory, the dye is carried to the first (sentinel) node to receive lymph from the tumor.[62] This would therefore be the node most likely to contain cancer cells if the cancer has spread. If the sentinel node biopsy is positive, more nodes are removed. If it is negative, further lymph node evaluation may not be needed. Successful identification of the SLN occurs 92% to 98% of the time, and when blue dye and isotope are used together, SLN has a positive predictive value approaching 100% and a negative predictive value near 95%.[3]

Adjuvant systemic therapy refers to the administration of chemotherapy or hormonal therapy to women without detectable metastatic disease. The goal of this therapy depends on nodal involvement, menopausal status, and hormone receptor status. Adjuvant systemic therapy has been widely studied and has demonstrated benefits in reducing rates of recurrence and death from breast cancer.[3] Tamoxifen is a nonsteroidal antiestrogen that binds to estrogen receptors and blocks the effects of estrogens on the growth of malignant cells in the breast. Studies have shown decreased cancer recurrence, decreased mortality rates, and increased 5-year survival rates in women with estrogen receptor–positive tissue samples who have been treated with the drug. Autologous bone marrow transplantation and peripheral stem cell transplantation are experimental therapies that may be used for treatment of advanced disease or in women at increased risk for recurrence. Immunotherapy, using a drug called trastuzumab (Herceptin), is used to stop the growth of breast tumors that express the HER2/neu receptor on their cell surface. The HER2/neu receptor binds an epidermal growth factor that contributes to cancer cell growth. Trastuzumab is a recombinant DNA-derived monoclonal antibody that binds to the HER2/neu receptor, thereby inhibiting proliferation of tumor cells that overexpress the receptor gene.[62]

The 5-year survival rate for localized cancer is 97%; with nodal involvement, it is approximately 78%; and it is approximately 23% with distant metastasis.[13] Five-year survival rates by age at diagnosis range from 81% for women younger than 45 years to 87% for women older than 65 years of age.[12]

Paget Disease

Paget disease accounts for 1% of all breast cancers. The disease presents as an eczemoid lesion of the nipple and areola (Fig. 47-11). Paget disease usually is associated with an infiltrating, intraductal carcinoma. When the lesion is limited to the nipple only, the rate of axillary metastasis is approximately 5%. Complete examination is required and includes a mammogram and biopsy. Treatment depends on the extent of spread.

In summary, the breasts are subject to benign and malignant disease. Mastitis is inflammation of the breast, occurring most frequently during lactation. Galactorrhea is an abnormal secretion of milk that may occur as a symptom of increased prolactin secretion. Ductal ectasia and intraductal papilloma cause abnormal drainage from the nipple. Fibroadenoma and fibrocystic disease are characterized by abnormal masses in the breast that are benign. By far the most important disease of the breast is breast cancer, which is a significant cause of death in women. BSE and mammography afford a woman the best protection against breast cancer. They provide the means for early detection of breast cancer and, in many cases, allow early treatment and cure.

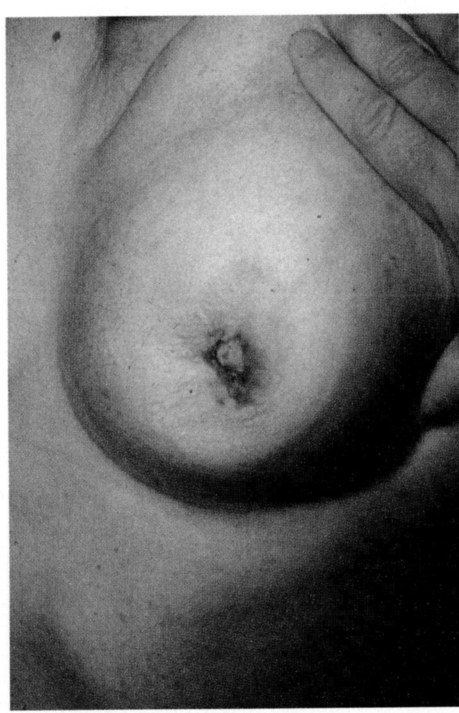

FIGURE 47-11 Paget disease of the nipple. An erythematous, scaly, and weeping "eczema" involves the nipple. (Rubin E., Farber J.L. [1999]. *Pathology* [3rd ed., p. 1043]. Philadelphia: Lippincott-Raven)

Infertility

After completing this section of the chapter, you should be able to meet the following objectives:

- Provide a definition of infertility
- List male and female factors that contribute to infertility
- Briefly describe methods used in the treatment of infertility

Infertility is the inability to conceive a child after 1 year of unprotected intercourse. It affects approximately 15% of couples in the United States. Primary infertility refers to situations in which there has been no prior conception. Secondary infertility is infertility that occurs after one or more previous pregnancies. Sterility is the inability to father a child or to become pregnant because of congenital anomalies, disease, or surgical intervention. Approximately 1% to 2% of U.S. couples are affected by sterility.

The complexity of the process that must occur to achieve a pregnancy is taken for granted by most couples. For some couples, pregnancy occurs far too easily, whereas for others, no amount of money, hard work, love, patience, or medical resources seems to be able to bring about this amazing, desired event. Although a full discussion of the diagnosis and treatment of infertility is beyond the scope of this book, an overview of the areas in which problems can occur is presented.

The causes of infertility are almost equally divided among male factors (30% to 40%), female factors (30% to 40%), and combined factors (30% to 40%). In approximately 10% to 25% of infertile couples, the cause remains unknown even after a full workup.

MALE FACTORS

For pregnancy to occur, the male must be able to provide sperm in sufficient quantity, delivered to the upper end of the vagina, with adequate motility to traverse the female reproductive tract. The male contribution to this process is assessed by means of a semen analysis, which evaluates volume of semen (normally 2 to 5 mL), sperm density (20 million/mL), motility (50% good progressive), viability (50%), morphology (60% normal), and viscosity (full liquefaction within 20 minutes). The specimen is best collected by masturbation into a sterile container after 3 days of abstinence. Because of variability in specimens, abnormal results should lead to a repeat test before the need for treatment is presumed.

Azoospermia is the absence of sperm; *oligospermia* refers to decreased numbers of sperm; and *asthenospermia* refers to poor motility of sperm. Tests of sperm function include cervical mucus penetration tests (*e.g.,* postcoital test, Penetrak), sperm penetration assay (*i.e.,* Hamster Zona Free Ovum test), and sperm antibody testing. None of these tests are included in the routine infertility evaluation.

The causes of male infertility include varicocele, ejaculatory dysfunction, hyperprolactinemia, hypogonadotropic hypogonadism, infection, immunologic problems (*i.e.*, antisperm antibodies), obstruction, and congenital anomalies. Risk factors for sperm problems include a history of mumps orchitis, cryptorchidism (*i.e.*, undescended testes), testicular torsion, hypospadias, previous urologic surgery, infection, and exposure to known gonadotoxins.[48] Treatment depends on the cause and may include surgery, medication, or the use of artificial insemination to deliver a more concentrated specimen directly to the cervical canal or uterine fundus. Artificial insemination with donor sperm can be offered if the male is sterile and if this alternative is acceptable to the husband and wife.

FEMALE FACTORS

The female contribution to pregnancy is more complex, requiring production and release of a mature ovum capable of being fertilized; production of cervical mucus that assists in sperm transport and maintains sperm viability in the female reproductive tract; patent fallopian tubes with the motility potential to pick up and transfer the ovum to the uterine cavity; development of an endometrium that is suitable for the implantation and nourishment of a fertilized ovum; and a uterine cavity that allows for growth and development of a fetus. Each of these factors is discussed briefly, along with an overview of diagnostic tests and treatment.

Ovulatory Dysfunction

In a normally menstruating female, ovulatory cycles begin several months to a year after menarche. Release of FSH from the pituitary causes the development of several primordial follicles in the ovary. At some point, a dominant follicle is selected, and the remaining follicles undergo atresia. When the dominant follicle has become large enough to contain a mature ovum (16 to 20 mm in diameter) and is producing sufficient estradiol to ensure adequate proliferation of the endometrium, production of LH increases (*i.e.*, the LH surge), and the increased LH level induces release of the ovum from within the follicle (*i.e.*, ovulation).

After ovulation, under the influence of LH, the former follicle luteinizes and begins producing progesterone in addition to estradiol. The progesterone stimulates the development of secretory endometrium, which has the capability to nourish a fertilized ovum if one should implant.

The presence of progesterone after ovulation causes a rise in the woman's basal body temperature (BBT). This thermogenic property of progesterone provides the basis for the simplest, most inexpensive beginning test of ovulatory function—the measurement of BBT. Women should be able to detect at least a 0.4°F rise in their BBT (at rest) after ovulation that should be maintained throughout the luteal phase. This biphasic temperature pattern demonstrates that ovulation has taken place, where in the cycle it occurred, and the length of the luteal phase. BBT can be influenced by many other factors, including restless sleep, alcohol intake, drug use, fever due to illness, and change in usual rising time. However, as an initial step in the infertility investigation, it can provide useful information to direct other forms of testing.

Endometrial biopsy, the removal of a sample of the endometrium during an office procedure, provides histologic evidence of secretory endometrium and the level of maturation of the lining. In a normal cycle, the luteal phase should be 14 days long. Without pregnancy and the subsequent secretion of hCG, the corpus luteum begins to degenerate 7 to 10 days after the LH surge. The luteal phase of the cycle is so consistent that a pathologist can tell by evaluating a section of endometrium that it is representative of a particular day of the luteal phase. The pathologist's assessment of maturation is compared with the arrival of the next menses. If a discrepancy of more than 2 days exists, the woman is said to have a luteal phase defect (LPD). This diagnosis indicates that, although ovulation is occurring, endometrial development is insufficient and implantation may not be possible. Pregnancy requires fertilization and implantation. LPD also can be suggested by an abnormal serum progesterone level 7 days after ovulation. It can be treated directly with supplemental progesterone after ovulation or with the use of clomiphene citrate to stimulate increased pituitary production of FSH and LH.

Anovulation (no ovulation) and oligoovulation (irregular ovulation) are other forms of ovulatory dysfunction. These problems can be identified by the tests for LPD previously described but are more often identified and treated based on a history of menstrual irregularity. Ovulatory problems can be primary problems of the ovary or secondary problems related to endocrine dysfunction. When disturbances in ovulation are confirmed, it is reasonable to evaluate other endocrine functions before initiating treatment. If the results of tests for pituitary hormones (*e.g.*, FSH, LH, prolactin), thyroid studies, and tests of adrenal function (*e.g.*, DHAS, androstenedione) are normal, ovulatory dysfunction is primary and should respond to treatment. Abnormalities in any of the other endocrine areas should be further evaluated as needed and treated appropriately. Hyperprolactinemia responds well to bromocriptine, but pituitary microadenoma may need to be excluded first. Hypothyroidism requires thyroid replacement, and hyperthyroidism requires suppressive therapy and, sometimes, surgical intervention with thyroid replacement later. Adrenal suppression can be instituted with dexamethasone, a glucocorticoid analog. Normal ovulatory function may resume without further intervention; if not, treatment can be concurrent with management of other endocrine problems.

Cervical Mucus Problems

High preovulatory levels of estradiol stimulate the production of large amounts of clear, stretchy cervical mucus that aids the transport of sperm into the uterine cavity and helps to maintain an environment that keeps the sperm viable for up to 72 hours. Insufficient estrogen production (*i.e.*, inherent or secondary to treatment with clomiphene citrate, an antiestrogen), cervical abnormalities from disease or invasive procedures (*e.g.*, DES exposure, stenosis, conization), and cervical infection (*e.g.*, chlamydial infection, mycoplasmal infection, gonorrhea) can adversely affect the production of healthy cervical mucus.

A postcoital test (Sims-Huhner) involves evaluation of the cervical mucus 1 to 8 hours after intercourse within the 48 hours before ovulation. A sample of cervical mucus is obtained using a special syringe and evaluated grossly for amount, clarity, and stretch (*i.e.,* spinnbarkeit) and microscopically for cellularity, number and quality of motile sperm, and the presence of ferning after the sample has air-dried on the slide. To obtain good-quality mucus, it is essential to obtain the sample within the 48 hours before ovulation. Tests may have to be repeated in the same cycle or in subsequent cycles to ensure appropriate timing. This can be a source of stress and frustration, as well as added cost to the couple. Intrauterine insemination (IUI) with the husband's sperm can bypass the cervical mucus and may be offered empirically as an alternative to postcoital testing.

If inadequate estrogen effect is seen (poor-quality mucus), supplemental oral estrogen can be given in the first 9 days of the next cycle, and the test can be repeated. Administration of mucolytic expectorants (1 teaspoon four times daily, starting on day 10 and continuing until ovulation is confirmed) also may improve the quality of the mucus. If mucus is good but sperm are inadequate in number or motility, further evaluation of the male may be needed. The man and woman can be tested for antisperm antibodies when repeated postcoital tests reveal that the sperm are all dead or agglutinated; however, IUI is the only effective treatment for sperm antibodies and may be offered without the need for further testing.

Cervical cultures for gonorrhea, chlamydial infection, and mycoplasmal infection should be obtained and treatment instituted as needed. Prophylactic treatment with antibiotics can be provided before IUI or other procedures that pass through the cervical canal as a more cost-effective alternative to obtaining cervical cultures.

Uterine Cavity Abnormalities

Alterations in the uterine cavity can occur because of DES exposure, submucosal fibroids, cervical polyps, bands of scar tissue, or congenital anomalies (*e.g.,* bicornuate septum, single horn). These defects may be suspected from the patient's history or pelvic examination but require hysterosalpingography (*i.e.,* x-ray study in which dye is placed through the cervix to outline the uterine cavity and demonstrate tubal patency) or hysteroscopy (*i.e.,* study in which a lighted fiberoptic endoscope placed through the cervix under general anesthesia allows direct visualization of the uterine cavity) for confirmation. Treatment is surgical when possible.

Tubal Factors

Tubal patency is required for fertilization and can be disrupted secondary to PID, ectopic pregnancy (*i.e.,* after salpingectomy or salpingostomy), large myomas, endometriosis, pelvic adhesions, and previous tubal ligation. Hysterosalpingography can reveal the location and type of any blockage, such as fimbrial, cornual, or hydrosalpinx. Microsurgical repair sometimes is possible.

Even when tubal patency is demonstrated, tubal disease may make ovum pickup impossible. Contrary to popular belief, the ovum is not extruded directly into the fallopian tube. The tube must be free to move to engulf the ovum after release. Pelvic adhesions from previous infection, surgery, or endometriosis can interfere with the tube's mobility. Laparoscopic evaluation of the pelvis is needed for diagnosis. Laser ablation or cautery can be used to lyse adhesions and remove endometriosis through the laparoscope or, if severe, by means of laparotomy.

ASSISTED REPRODUCTIVE TECHNOLOGIES

In vitro fertilization (IVF) was developed in 1978 for women with significantly damaged or absent tubes to provide them with an opportunity for pregnancy where none normally existed. The ovaries are superstimulated to produce multiple follicles using clomiphene citrate, human menopausal menotropins (*e.g.,* Pergonal, Repronex), pure FSH (*e.g.,* Gonal-F, Follistim, Bravelle), or a combination of these drugs. Follicular maturation is monitored by means of ultrasonography and assay of serum estradiol levels. When preovulatory criteria are met, an injection of hCG is given to simulate an LH surge; 35 hours later, the follicles are aspirated laparoscopically or, more often, by the ultrasound-guided transvaginal route. The follicular fluid is evaluated microscopically for the presence of ova. When found, they are removed and placed into culture media in an incubator.

The eggs are inseminated with sperm from the husband that have been prepared by a washing technique that removes the semen, begins the capacitation process, and allows the strongest sperm to be used for fertilization. When very low numbers of normal motile sperm are available, microsurgical techniques can be used to assist with fertilization. Earlier procedures such as *partial zona dissection* (PZD), which involves the creation of a small opening in the layer (*i.e.,* zona pellucida) that surrounds the egg, and *subzonal insertion,* whereby several sperm are inserted into the space just beneath the protective layer, are rarely used today. The most definitive form of micromanipulation is a procedure called *intracytoplasmic sperm injection* (ICSI), whereby a single spermatozoa is injected directly into the cytoplasm of the egg.

Between 12 and 24 hours after insemination, the ova are evaluated for signs of fertilization. If signs are present, the ova are returned to the incubator, and 48 to 72 hours after egg retrieval, the fertilized eggs are placed back into the woman's uterus by means of a transcervical catheter. A procedure similar to PZD can be performed just before embryo transfer to help the fertilized egg escape from the zona pellucida. This "assisted hatching" improves the chances of implantation. In an effort to reduce the number of multiple births resulting from this type of technology, the embryos may be grown to the blastocyst stage and transferred back to the uterus on the fifth day after fertilization. Because many embryos will not advance to the blastocyst stage in vitro, this therapy usually is limited to those women who have produced a significant number of embryos.

Hormonal supplementation of the luteal phase often is used to increase the possibility of implantation. The overall live delivery rate in 2000 for women using their own eggs, as reported by the Society for Assisted Reproductive Technology and the American Society for Reproductive Medicine, was 31.6% per egg retrieval.[63] Indications for IVF have been expanded to include male factors (*i.e.,* severe oligospermia or asthenospermia), immunologic infertility, severe endometriosis, and idiopathic infertility (*i.e.,* infertility of unknown cause). The substantial risk for multiple births with IVF procedures has been reduced with the availability of cryopreservation, which allows freezing of excess embryos and limits the number of fresh embryos transferred. The live delivery rate in 2000 after frozen embryo transfer was 20.3%.[63]

An outgrowth of IVF technology is gamete intrafallopian transfer (GIFT), which uses similar ovarian stimulation protocols and egg retrieval procedures but uses laparoscopy to place ovum and sperm directly into the fallopian tube. This procedure requires at least one patent fallopian tube and was developed primarily to increase the pregnancy rate in women with idiopathic infertility. The basic premises are that if a transportation problem is interfering with ovum pickup, GIFT could solve that problem, and that implantation may result more often if fertilization occurs in the body. Because of the added expense involving laparoscopy and the limited indications, GIFT procedures are used infrequently. In 2000, GIFT represented less than 1% of all ART procedures performed, and statistics were not reported separately.[63]

Other ART include zygote intrafallopian transfer (ZIFT) and tubal embryo transplant (TET). With ZIFT, the zygote is placed laparoscopically into the fallopian tube after the traditional IVF procedure. With TET, the embryos are transferred into the fallopian tubes transcervically using ultrasound guidance or by means of hysteroscopy. The theoretic advantages of these procedures involve tubal factors that may facilitate implantation. As with GIFT, these procedures accounted for only 1% of all assisted reproductive technology (ART) procedures performed in 2000 and statistics were not reported separately.[63]

By 2003, more than 1 million infants had been born worldwide using some type of ART, with almost 100,000 births being made possible with the use of intracytoplasmic sperm injection. Future research will focus on understanding and improving the implantation process.

In summary, infertility is the inability to conceive a child after 1 year of unprotected intercourse. Male factors are related to number and motility of sperm and their ability to penetrate the cervical mucus and the ovum. Causes of male infertility include varicocele, ejaculatory dysfunction, hyperprolactinemia, hypogonadotropic hypogonadism, infection, immunologic problems (*i.e.,* antisperm antibodies), obstruction, and congenital anomalies. Risk factors for sperm disorders include a history of mumps orchitis, cryptorchidism (undescended testes), testicular torsion, hypospadias, previous urologic surgery, infection, and exposure to known gonadotoxins.

The female contribution to pregnancy is more complex, requiring production and release of a mature ovum capable of being fertilized; production of cervical mucus that assists in sperm transport and maintains sperm viability in the female reproductive tract; patent fallopian tubes with the mobility potential to pick up and transfer the ovum to the uterine cavity; development of an endometrium that is suitable for the implantation and nourishment of a fertilized ovum; and a uterine cavity that allows for growth and development of a fetus.

Evaluation and treatment of infertility can be lengthy and highly stressful for the couple. Options for therapy continue to expand, but newer ART modalities are expensive, and financial resources can be strained while couples seek to fulfill their sometimes elusive dream of having a child.

REVIEW EXERCISES

A 32-year-old woman has been told that the report of her annual Pap test revealed the presence of mild dysplasia.

A. What questions should this woman ask as a means of becoming informed about the significance of these findings?

B. In obtaining additional information about the results of her Pap test, the woman is informed that dysplastic changes are consistent with CIN 1 classification.

1. Does this mean that the woman has cervical cancer?
2. How would these findings translate into the *Bethesda System* for grading cervical cytology?
3. Cervical cancer is often referred to as a sexually transmitted disease. Explain.
4. What type of follow-up care would be indicated?

A 30-year-old woman consults her gynecologist because of amenorrhea, and she has been unable to become pregnant. Her physical exam reveals an obese woman with hirsutism. The physician tells the woman that she might have a condition known as polycystic ovary disease and that further laboratory tests are indicated.

A. Among tests ordered are a fasting blood glucose, LH, FSH, and dehydroepiandrosterone levels. What information can these tests provide that would help in establishing a diagnosis of polycystic ovarian syndrome?

B. What is the probable cause of this woman's amenorrhea, hirsutism, and failure to become pregnant?

C. What type of treatment might be used to help this woman become pregnant?

A 45-year-old woman makes an appointment to see her physician because of a painless lump in her breast that she discovered while doing her routine monthly breast exam.

A. What tests should be done to confirm the presence or absence of breast cancer?

B. During the removal of breast cancer, a sentinel node biopsy is often done to determine whether the cancer has spread to the lymph nodes. Explain how this procedure is done and its value in determining lymph node spread.

C. Following surgical removal of breast cancer, tamoxifen may used as an adjuvant systemic therapy for women without detectable metastatic disease. The presence or absence of estrogen receptors in the cytoplasm of tumor cells is important in determining the selection of an agent for use in adjuvant therapy. Explain.

References

1. Hill A.D., Lense J.J. (1998). Office management of Bartholin gland cysts and abscesses. *American Family Physician 57,* 1611–1620.
2. Kurman R.J. (2002). *Blaustein's pathology of the female genital tract* (5th ed., pp. 53–55, 99, 109, 168, 216–222, 253–256, 327, 336, 746–749, 502–503, 637–639, 801, 802). New York: Springer-Verlag.
3. Scott J.R., Gibbs R.S., Karlan B.Y., Haney A.F. (2003). *Danforth's obstetrics and gynecology* (9th ed., pp. 585, 586, 591, 606–608, 653–662, 713–720, 727, 839, 898, 899, 906, 913, 927, 941–949, 953–963). Philadelphia: Lippincott Williams & Wilkins.
4. Stewart E.G. (2003). Treatment options for vulvar vestibulitis. *Contemporary OB/GYN 1,* 47–61.
5. Edwards L. (2003). New concepts in vulvodynia. *American Journal of Obstetrics and Gynecology 189*(3, S-1): S24–30.
6. Cancer Reference Information. (2003). *Vulvar cancer.* The American Cancer Society. [On-line]. Available: http:/www.cancer.org/docroot/CRI. Accessed October 1, 2003.
7. Canavan T.P., Cohen D. (2002). Vulvar cancer. *American Family Physician 66,* 1269–1274.
8. Tyring S.K. (2003). Vulvar squamous cell carcinoma: guidelines for early diagnosis and treatment. *American Journal of Obstetrics and Gynecology 189*(3, S-1), S17–23.
9. Sweet R.L., Gibbs R.S. (2002). *Infectious diseases of the female genital tract* (4th ed., pp. 337–340). Philadelphia: Lippincott Williams & Wilkins.
10. Cancer Reference Information. (2003). *Vaginal cancer.* The American Cancer Society. [On-line]. Available: http:/www.cancer.org/docroot/CRI. Accessed October 1, 2003.
11. Hammes B., Laitman C.J. (2003). Diethylstilbestrol (DES) update: Recommendations for the identification and management of DES-exposed individuals. *Journal of Midwifery and Women's Health 48*(1): 19–29.
12. Crum C.P., Lester S.C., Cotran R.S. (2003). The female genital system and breast. In Kumar V., Cotran R.S., Robbins S.L. (Eds.), Robbins basic pathology (7th ed., pp. 679–717). Philadelphia: W.B. Saunders.
13. American Cancer Society. (2003). *Cancer facts and figures 2003.* New York: Author.
14. Snyder U. (2003). March/April 2003: A look at cervical cancer. *Medscape Ob/Gyn & Women's Health 8*(1); posted 4/25/2003. [On-line.] Available: http://www.medscape.com/viewarticle/452727. Accessed November 7, 2003.
15. Choma K.K. (2003). ASC-US HPV testing. *American Journal of Nursing 103*(2):42–50.
16. Saslow D., Runowicz C.D., Solomon D., et al. (2002). American Cancer Society guideline for the early detection of cervical neoplasia and cancer. *CA: A Cancer Journal for Clinicians 52*(6), 342–362.
17. U.S. Preventive Services Task Force. (2003). Screening for cervical cancer: Recommendations and rationale. *American Journal of Nursing 103*(11), 101–109.
18. Solomon D., Davey D., Kurman R., et al., for the Forum Group Members and the Bethesda 2001 Workshop. (2002). The 2001 Bethesda System. *Journal of the American Medical Association 287*(16), 2114–2119.
19. Wright T., Cox, T., Massad L.S., et al., for the 2001 ASCCP-Sponsored Consensus Conference. (2002). 2001 Consensus guidelines for the management of women with cervical cytological abnormalities. *Journal of the American Medical Association 287*(16), 2120–2129.
20. Eskridge C., Begneaud W.P., Landwehr C. (1998). Cervicography combined with repeat Papanicolaou test as triage for low grade cytologic abnormalities. *Obstetrics and Gynecology 92,* 351–355.
21. Spaczynski R.Z., Duleba A.J. (2003). Diagnosis of endometriosis. *Seminars in Reproductive Medicine 21*(2), 193–207.
22. Gambone J.C., Mittman B.S., Munro M.G., et al., for the Chronic Pelvic Pain/Endometriosis Working Group. (2002). Consensus statement for the management of chronic pelvic pain and endometriosis: proceedings of an expert-panel consensus process. *Fertility and Sterility 78*(5), 961–972.
23. Feste J.R., Schattman G.L. (2000). Laparoscopy and endometriosis: Preventing complications and improving outcomes. In *Changing perspectives: A new outlook on gynecologic disorders. Symposia proceedings 2000* (p. 40–42). Medical Education Collaborative.
24. American College of Obstetricians and Gynecologists. (1999). Medical management of endometriosis. ACOG Practice Bulletin no. 11. In *2001 Compendium of selected publications* (pp. 982, 986). Washington, DC: Author.
25. Johnson K. (2003). Differentiating adenomyosis and fibroids. *Medscape OB/Gyn & Women's Health* 8(2). [On-line] Available: https://www.medscape.com/viewarticle/459772. Accessed November 20, 2003.
26. Pron G., Bennett J., Common A., et al., for the Ontario Uterine Fibroid Embolization Collaborative Group. (2003). The Ontario Uterine Fibroid Embolization Trial. 2. Uterine fibroid reduction and symptom relief after uterine artery embolization for fibroids. *Fertility and Sterility 799*(1), 120–127.
27. Mott A.M. (2000). Prevention and management of pelvic inflammatory disease by primary care providers. *American Journal of Nurse Practitioners 8,* 7–13.
28. Centers for Disease Control and Prevention. (2002). 2002 Guidelines for treatment of sexually transmitted diseases. *Morbidity and Mortality Weekly Report 51*(RR06), 1–80.
29. Centers for Disease Control and Prevention. (1995). Current trends for ectopic pregnancy—United States, 1990–1992. *Morbidity and Mortality Weekly Report 44*(RR-3), 46–48.
30. Gracie C.R., Barnhart K.T. (2001). Diagnosing ectopic pregnancy: Decision analysis comparing six strategies. *Obstetrics & Gynecology 97*(3), 464–470.
31. Barnhart K.T., Gosman G., Ashby R., Sammel M. (2003). The medical management of ectopic pregnancy: a meta-analysis comparing "single dose" and "multidose" regimens. *Obstetrics & Gynecology 101*(4), 778–784.
32. Tenore J.L. (2000). Ectopic pregnancy. *American Family Physician 61,* 1080–1088.
33. Speroff L., Glass R.H., Kase N.G. (1999). *Clinical gynecologic endocrinology and infertility* (6th ed., pp. 497–503), Philadelphia: Lippincott Williams & Wilkins.
34. Mark T.L., Menta A.E. (2003). Polycystic ovary syndrome: Pathogenesis and treatment over the short and long term. *Cleveland Clinic Journal of Medicine 70*(1), 31–45.
35. Richardson M.B. (2003). Current perspectives in polycystic ovary syndrome. *American Family Physician 68*(4), 697–704.
36. Nestler J.E., Stovall D., Ahkter N., et al. (2002). Strategies for the use of insulin-sensitizing drugs to treat infertility in

women with polycystic ovary syndrome. *Fertility and Sterility 17*(2), 20915.
37. Costello M.F., Eden J.A., (2003). A systematic review of the reproductive system effects of metformin in patients with polycystic ovary syndrome. *Fertility and Sterility 79*(1), 1–13.
38. Harris L.L. (2002). Ovarian cancer: Screening for early detection. *American Journal of Nursing 102*(10), 46–52.
39. Rubin S.C., Sutton G.P. (2001). *Ovarian cancer* (2nd ed., pp. 167–177). Philadelphia: Lippincott Williams & Wilkins.
40. Frank T.S. (1998). Identifying women with inherited risk for ovarian cancer: Who and why? *Contemporary OB/Gyn 12,* 27–50.
41. Barnes M.N., Grizzle W.E., Grubbs C.J, Partridge E.E. (2002). Paradigms for primary prevention of ovarian carcinoma. *CA: A Cancer Journal for Clinicians 52*(4), 216–225.
42. Petricoin E.F. III, Ardekani A.M., Hitt B.A., et al. (2002). Use of proteomic patterns in serum to identify ovarian cancer. *Lancet 359,* 572–577.
43. National Institutes of Health Consensus Development Panel on Ovarian Cancer. (1995). Ovarian cancer: Screening and follow-up. *Journal of the American Medical Association 273,* 491–497.
44. Cancer Reference Information. (2003). *Ovarian cancer.* The American Cancer Society. [On-line.] Available: http://www.cancer.org/docroot/CRI. Accessed December 6, 2003.
45. National Cancer Institute. (2000). *SEER Cancer statistics review 1973–1997* (pp. 122, 370). [On-line]. Available: http://www.seer.cancer.gov.
46. Feitozoa S.S., Gebhart J.B., Gostour B.S., et al. (2003). Efficacy of thermal balloon ablation in patients with abnormal uterine bleeding. *American Journal of Obstetrics and Gynecology 189,* 453–457.
47. American College of Obstetricians and Gynecologists. (2000). Management of anovulatory bleeding. ACOG Practice Bulletin no. 14. In *2001 Compendium of selected publications* (pp. 961–968). Washington, DC: Author.
48. Mishell D.R., Goodwin T.M., Brenner P.F. (2002). *Management of common problems in obstetrics and gynecology* (4th ed., 236, 253, 260, 278, 395, 428, 431–435). Williston, VT: Blackwell Science.
49. Hudson T. (2002). Premenstrual syndrome, part 1. *Female Patient 27,* 38–40.
50. Kovacs P. (2002). Evaluation and recognition of premenstrual dysphoric disorder. *Clinical Advisor 5*(4), 110–118.
51. Moline M.L., Zendell S.M. (2000). Evaluating and managing premenstrual syndrome. *Medscape Women's Health 5*(2). [On-line]. Available: http://www.medscape.com/Medscape WomensHealth/journal/2000/v05,n02.
52. Dimmock P.W., Wyatt K.M., Jones P.W., O'Brien P.M.S. (2000). Efficacy of selective serotonin-reuptake inhibitors in premenstrual syndrome: A systemic review. *Lancet 356,* 1131–1136.
53. Giuliano A.E. (2001). Benign breast disorders. In Tierney L.M., McPhee S.J., Papadakis M.A. (Eds.), *Current medical diagnosis and treatment* (40th ed., pp. 706–707). New York: Lange Medical Books/McGraw-Hill.
54. Rubin E., Farber J.L., (1999). *Pathology* (3rd ed., 1033–1035). Philadelphia: Lippincott-Raven.
55. Zimmerman V.L. (2002). BRCA gene mutations and cancer. *American Journal of Nursing 102*(8): 28–36.
56. Gotzsche P.C., Olsen O. (2000). Is screening for breast cancer with mammography justifiable? *Lancet 355,* 129–134.
57. Olsen O., Gotzsche P.C. (2001). Cochrane review on screening for breast cancer with mammography. *Lancet 358,* 1340–1342.
58. Miller A.B., To T., Baines C.J., Wall C. (2002). The Canadian National Breast Screening Study. 1. Breast cancer mortality after 11 to 16 years of follow-up. *Annuals of Internal Medicine 137,* 305–312.
59. Humphrey L.L., Helfand M, Chan B.K.S., Woolf S.H. (2002). Breast cancer screening: A summary of the evidence for the U.S. Preventive Service Task Force. *Annals of Internal Medicine 137,* 347–360.
60. Smith R.A., Saslow D, Sawyers K.A., et al. American Cancer Society guidelines for breast cancer screening updated 2003. *CA: A Cancer Journal for Clinicians 53,* 134–137.
61. Harvey S.C., Geller B., Oppenheimer R.G., et al. (2003). Increase in cancer detection and recall rates with independent double interpretation of screening mammography. *American Journal of Roentgenology 180,* 1461–1467.
62. Hortobagyi G.N. (1998). Treatment of breast cancer. *New England Journal of Medicine 339,* 974–984.
63. CDC's Reproductive Health Information Source. (2003). *2000 Assisted reproductive technology success rates.* Centers for Disease Control and Prevention. [On-line.] Available: http://www.cdc.gov/reproductivehealth/ART. Accessed December 5, 2003.

CHAPTER 48

Sexually Transmitted Diseases

Patricia McCowen Mehring

The incidence and types of sexually transmitted diseases (STDs), as reported in the professional literature and public health statistics, are increasing. The incidence of disease is based on clinical reports, however, and many STDs are not reportable or not reported. The agents of transmission include bacteria, chlamydiae, viruses, fungi, protozoa, parasites, and unidentified microorganisms (see Chapter 18). Portals of entry include the mouth, genitalia, urinary meatus, rectum, and skin. All STDs are more common in persons who have more than one sexual partner, and it is not uncommon for a person to be concurrently infected with more than one type of STD. This chapter discusses the manifestations of STDs in men and women in terms of infections of the external genitalia, vaginal infections, and infections that have systemic effects and genitourinary manifestations. Human immunodeficiency virus (HIV) infection is presented in Chapter 22.

Infections of the External Genitalia

After completing this section of the chapter, you should be able to meet the following objectives:

- ✦ Define what is meant by a sexually transmitted disease (STD)
- ✦ Give a reason why the reported incidence of STDs may not accurately reflect the true incidence
- ✦ List common portals of entry for STDs
- ✦ Name the organisms responsible for condylomata acuminata, genital herpes, molluscum contagiosum, chancroid, granuloma inguinale, and lymphogranuloma venereum
- ✦ State the significance of condylomata acuminata
- ✦ Explain the recurrent infections in genital herpes

Some STDs primarily affect the mucocutaneous tissues of the external genitalia. These include human papillomavirus (HPV) infection, genital herpes, molluscum contagiosum, chancroid, granuloma inguinale, and lymphogranuloma venereum (LGV).

HUMAN PAPILLOMAVIRUS (CONDYLOMATA ACUMINATA)

Condylomata acuminata, or *genital warts,* are caused by HPV. Although recognized for centuries, HPV-induced genital warts have become one of the fastest-growing STDs of the past decade. The Centers for Disease Control and Prevention (CDC) estimates that 20 million Americans carry the virus and that up to 5.5 million new cases are diagnosed each year.[1] The true prevalence of HPV is difficult to determine because it is not a reportable disease in all states, it can be a transient infection, of short duration, with only a small number of women exposed remaining persistently infected, and most infections remain subclinical without developing overt lesions or abnormal cytologic changes.[2–4]

A 1998 American Medical Association consensus conference on external genital warts identified four specific types of warts: *condylomata acuminata* (cauliflower-shaped lesions that tend to appear on moist skin surfaces such as the vaginal introitus or anus); *keratotic warts* (display a thick, horny layer; develop on dry, fully keratinized skin such as the penis, scrotum, or labia majora); *papular warts* (smooth surface, typically develop on fully keratinized

SEXUALLY TRANSMITTED DISEASE

- Sexually transmitted diseases (STDs) are spread by sexual contact and involve both male and female partners. Portals of entry include the mouth, genitalia, urinary meatus, rectum, and skin. All STDs are more common in persons who have more than one sexual partner, and it is not uncommon for a person to be concurrently infected with more than one type of STD.
- In general, STDs due to bacterial pathogens can be successfully treated and the pathogen eliminated by antimicrobial therapy. However, many of these pathogens are developing antibiotic resistance.
- STDs due to viral pathogens such as the human papillomavirus (HPV) and genital herpes simplex virus infections (HSV-1 and HSV-2) are not eliminated by current treatment modalities and persist with risk of recurrence (HSV infections) or increased cancer risk (HPV).
- Untreated, STDs such as chlamydial infection and gonorrhea can spread to involve the internal genital organs with risk of complications and infertility.
- Intrauterine or perinatally transmitted STDs can have potentially fatal or severely debilitating effects on a fetus or an infant.

skin); and *flat warts* (macular, sometimes faintly raised, usually invisible to the naked eye, occur on either fully or partially keratinized skin). Flat warts sometimes can be visualized by applying a 5% acetic acid solution to opacify the lesions ("acetowhitening"). However, this procedure is no longer routinely used because of the high number of both false-positive and false-negative results with this technique. Biopsy may be required to differentiate warts from other hyperkeratotic or precancerous lesions.

A relation between HPV and genital neoplasms has become increasingly apparent since the mid-1970s. With newer technologies, HPV DNA has been identified in almost all of cervical cancers worldwide and in approximately 50% to 80% of vaginal, vulvar, and anogenital carcinomas.[4] One hundred types of HPV have been identified, more than 30 of which affect the anogenital area. Of the high-risk types, type 16 and type 18 appear to be the most virulent and are associated with most invasive squamous cell cancers. Types 31, 33, 35, 39, 45, 51, 52, 56, and 58 are less common but also have demonstrated some malignant potential in squamous intraepithelial lesions. In contrast, types 6 and 11 are found in most external genital warts but usually are benign, with only a low potential for dysplasia. Only a subset of women infected with HPV develop cancer. There may be variants of even the most virulent HPV, type 16, with differing oncogenic potential. Cofactors that may increase the risk for cancer include smoking, immunosuppression, and exposure to hormonal alteration (*e.g.*, pregnancy, oral contraceptives).[2–4] The association with premalignant and malignant changes has increased the concern about diagnosis and treatment of this viral infection.

HPV infection begins with viral inoculation into a stratified squamous epithelium, where infection stimulates the replication of the squamous epithelium, producing the various HPV-proliferative lesions. The incubation period for HPV-induced genital warts ranges from 6 weeks to 8 months. Subclinical infection occurs more frequently than visible genital warts among men and women. Infection often is indirectly diagnosed on the cervix by Papanicolaou testing (Pap smear), colposcopy, or biopsy. Both spontaneous resolution and infection with new HPV types are common. Although reinfection from sexual partners has been considered as a reason for the high prevalence of this disease, it is now thought that reinfection with the same HPV type is infrequent. Instead, it is thought that HPV may be a lifelong infection.

Genital condylomas should be considered in any woman who presents with the primary complaint of vulvar pruritus or who has had an abnormal Pap smear. Microscopic examination of a wet-mount slide preparation and cultures are used to exclude associated vaginitis. Careful inspection of the vulva, with magnification as needed, will generally reveal the characteristic lesions, and specimens for biopsy can be taken from questionable areas. Colposcopic examination of the cervix and vagina may be advised as a follow-up measure when there is an abnormal Pap smear or when HPV lesions are identified on the vulva. Evaluation and treatment of sexual partners may be suggested, although this may be difficult considering that warts often do not become clinically apparent for several years after exposure.

The recent development and controlled trial of a vaccine to protect against HPV type 16 may eventually reduce the risk for cervical cancer associated with this strain of HPV.[5] However, currently there is no treatment to eradicate the virus once a person has become infected. Thus, treatment goals are aimed at elimination of symptomatic warts, surveillance for malignancy and premalignant changes, and education and counseling to decrease psychosocial distress.[6] Prevention of HPV transmission through condom use has not been adequately demonstrated.

The CDC identifies several pharmacologic treatments for symptomatic removal of visible genital warts, including patient-applied therapies (podofilox and imiquimod) and provider-administered therapies (podophyllin and trichloroacetic acid).[7] Podophyllin, a topical cytotoxic agent, has long been used for treatment of visible external growths. Multiple applications may be required for resolution of lesions. The amount of drug used and the surface area treated should be limited with each treatment session to avoid systematic absorption and toxicity. This treatment is contraindicated in pregnancy for the same reason. An alternative therapy is the topical application of a solution of trichloroacetic acid. This weak destructive agent produces an initial burning in the affected area, followed in several days by a sloughing of the superficial tissue. Several applications 1 to 2 weeks apart may be necessary to eradicate the lesion. Podofilox is a topical patient-applied antimitotic agent that results in visible necrosis of wart tissue. It is applied twice a day for 3 days, followed by 4 days of nontreatment for a total of four cycles. The safety of podofilox during pregnancy has not been established. Imiquimod cream is a new type of therapeutic agent that stimulates the body's immune system (*i.e.,* production of interferon-α and other cytokines). This cream is applied at home three times a week for up to 16 weeks. It must be washed off 6 to 10 hours after application to avoid excessive skin reaction. It is a category B drug and therefore potentially safe for use in pregnancy. Interferon, in the form of a topical application or as an intralesional injection, has not shown an advantage over other available forms of treatment and, because of its cost, should be reserved for recurrent or refractory lesions.[4] Sexual abstinence is suggested during any type of treatment to enhance healing.

Genital warts also may be removed using cryotherapy, surgical excision, laser vaporization, or electrocautery. Because it can penetrate deeper than other forms of therapy, cryotherapy (*i.e.,* freezing therapy) often is the treatment of choice for cervical HPV lesions. Laser surgery can be used to remove large or widespread lesions of the cervix, vagina, or vulva, or lesions that have failed to respond to other first-line methods of treatment. Electrosurgical treatment has become more widespread for these types of lesions because it is more readily available in outpatient settings and is much less expensive than laser.

GENITAL HERPES

Herpesviruses are large, encapsulated viruses that have a double-stranded genome. There are nine types of herpesviruses, belonging to three groups, that cause infections in humans: neurotropic α-group viruses, including herpes simplex virus type 1 (HSV-1, usually associated with cold sores) and HSV-2 (usually associated with genital herpes); varicella-zoster virus (causes chickenpox and shingles); and lymphotropic β-group viruses, including cytomegalovirus (causes cytomegalic inclusion disease), Epstein-Barr virus (causes infectious mononucleosis and Burkitt's lymphoma), and human herpesvirus type 8 (the apparent cause of Kaposi's sarcoma).[8]

Genital herpes is caused by the herpes simplex virus. Because herpesvirus infection is not reportable in all states, reliable data on its true incidence (estimated number of new cases every year) and prevalence (estimated number of people currently infected) are lacking. From the late 1970s to early 1990s, genital herpes prevalence increased 30%. Incidence rates have been relatively stable since 1990, with an estimated 1 million new cases occurring each year. Recent estimates in the United States indicate that 45 million people (one in five adolescents or adults) are infected with genital herpes.[1] Women have a greater mucosal surface area exposed in the genital area and therefore are at greater risk for acquiring the infection.

HSV-1 and HSV-2 are genetically similar; both cause a similar set of primary and recurrent infections, and both can cause genital lesions. Both viruses replicate in the skin and mucous membranes at the site of infection (oropharynx or genitalia), where they cause vesicular lesions of the epidermis and infect the neurons that innervate the area. HSV-1 and HSV-2 are *neurotropic* viruses, meaning that they grow in neurons and share the biologic property of latency. Latency refers to the ability to maintain disease potential in the absence of clinical signs and symptoms. In genital herpes, the virus ascends through the peripheral nerves to the sacral dorsal root ganglia (Fig. 48-1). The virus can remain dormant in the dorsal root ganglia, or it can reactivate, in which case the viral particles are transported back down the nerve root to the skin, where they multiply and cause a lesion to develop. During the dormant or latent period, the virus replicates in a different manner so that the immune system or available treatments have no effect on it. It is not known what reactivates the virus. It may be that the body's defense mechanisms are altered. Numerous studies have shown that host responses to infection influence initial development of the disease, severity of infection, development and maintenance of latency, and frequency of HSV recurrences.

HSV is transmitted by contact with infectious lesions or secretions. HSV-1 is transmitted by oral secretions, and infections frequently occur in childhood. HSV-1 may be spread to the genital area by autoinoculation after poor hand washing or through oral intercourse. At least 15% of new cases of genital herpes are caused by HSV-1,[9] and it has been estimated that among sexually active adults, new genital HSV-1 infections are as common as new orogenital HSV-1 infections.[3] HSV-2 usually is transmitted by sexual contact but can be passed to an infant during childbirth if the virus is actively being shed from the genital tract. Most cases of HSV-2 infection are subclinical, manifesting as truly asymptomatic or symptomatic but unrecognized infections. These subclinical infections can occur in people who have never had a symptomatic outbreak or between

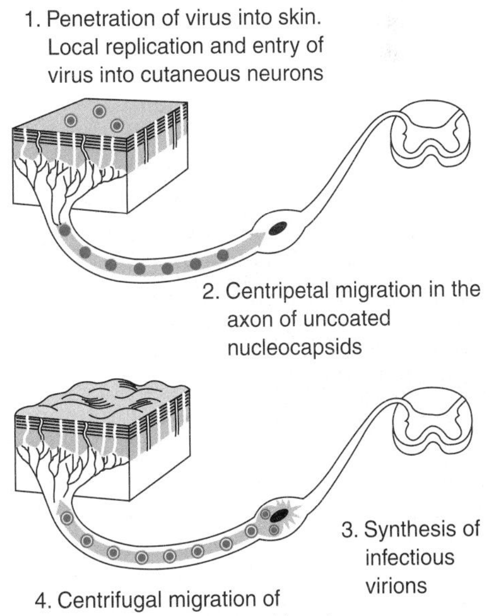
1. Penetration of virus into skin. Local replication and entry of virus into cutaneous neurons
2. Centripetal migration in the axon of uncoated nucleocapsids
3. Synthesis of infectious virions
4. Centrifugal migration of infectious virions to epidermis

FIGURE 48-1 Pathogenesis of primary mucocutaneous herpes simplex virus infection. (Corey L., Spear P.G. [1986]. Infections with herpes simplex viruses. Pt. 1. *New England Journal of Medicine 314,* 686)

recognized clinical recurrences. Fifty to 80% of genital herpes cases are spread through asymptomatic shedding by people who do not realize they have the infection.[9] This "unknown" transmission of the virus to sex partners explains why this infection has reached epidemic proportions throughout the world. Because HSV is readily inactivated at room temperature and by drying, aerosol and fomite spread are unusual means of transmission.[10]

The incubation period for HSV is 2 to 10 days. Genital HSV infection may manifest as a primary, nonprimary, or recurrent infection. *Primary infections* are infections that occur in a person who is seronegative for antibody to HSV-1 or HSV-2. *Initial nonprimary infections* refer to the first clinical episode in a person who is seropositive for antibodies to the opposite HSV type (usually genital herpes in someone seropositive to HSV-1). *Recurrent infections* refer to the second or subsequent outbreak due to the same virus type. HSV-2 is responsible for greater than 90% of recurrent genital herpes infections.[6] Many "severe" presumed primary cases are actually first-recognized recurrences in persons with long-standing infection. Presence of antibodies to one type of HSV may decrease the symptomatic response to the initial infection with the other virus. Correct classification requires clinical correlation with viral isolation and type-specific serologic testing.[3]

The initial symptoms of primary genital herpes infections include tingling, itching, and pain in the genital area, followed by eruption of small pustules and vesicles. These lesions rupture on approximately the fifth day to form wet ulcers that are excruciatingly painful to touch and can be associated with dysuria, dyspareunia, and urine retention. Involvement of the cervix, vagina, urethra, and inguinal lymph nodes is common in women with primary infections. In men, the infection can cause urethritis and lesions of the penis and scrotum. Rectal and perianal infections are possible with anal contact. Systemic symptoms associated with primary infections include fever, headache, malaise, muscle ache, and lymphadenopathy. Primary infections may be debilitating enough to require hospitalization, particularly in women.

Untreated primary infections typically are self-limited and last for approximately 2 to 4 weeks. The symptoms usually worsen for the first 10 to 12 days. This period is followed by a 10- to 12-day interval during which the lesions crust over and gradually heal. Nonprimary episodes of genital herpes manifest with less severe symptoms that usually are of shorter duration and have fewer systemic manifestations. Except for the greater tendency of HSV-2 to recur, the clinical manifestations of HSV-2 and genital HSV-1 are similar. Recurrent HSV infection results from reactivation of the virus stored in the dorsal root ganglia of the infected dermatomes. An outbreak may be preceded by a prodrome of itching, burning, or tingling at the site of future lesions. Because the person has already developed immune lymphocytes from the primary infection, recurrent episodes have fewer lesions, fewer systemic symptoms, less pain, and a shorter duration (7 to 10 days). Frequency and severity of recurrences vary from person to person. Numerous factors, including emotional stress, lack of sleep, overexertion, other infections, vigorous or prolonged coitus, and premenstrual or menstrual distress have been identified as triggering mechanisms.

Diagnosis of genital herpes is based on the symptoms, appearance of the lesions, and identification of the virus from cultures taken from the lesions. Depending on the laboratory, a preliminary culture report takes from 2 to 5 days, and a final negative report takes from 10 to 12 days to establish. The stability of the virus in transport media is good for 48 to 72 hours, making mail transport possible. The likelihood of obtaining a positive culture decreases with each day that has elapsed after a lesion develops. The chance of obtaining a positive culture from a crusted lesion is slight, and patients suspected of having genital herpes should be instructed to have a culture within 48 hours of development of new lesions. Type-specific (HSV-1 and HSV-2) serologic tests are available for determining past infection. Because almost all HSV-2 infections are sexually acquired, the presence of type-specific HSV-2 antibodies usually indicates anogenital infection, whereas the presence of HSV-1 antibodies does not distinguish between anogenital and orolabial infections. The CDC recommends that serologic assays for HSV-2 be available for persons who request them but does not recommend they be used for screening of the general population.[5]

There is no known cure for genital herpes, and the methods of treatment are largely symptomatic. The antiviral drugs acyclovir, valacyclovir, and famciclovir have become the cornerstone for management of genital herpes. By interfering with viral DNA replication, these drugs decrease the frequency of recurrences, shorten the duration of active lesions, reduce the number of new lesions formed, and decrease viral shedding with primary infections. Valacyclovir, the active component of acyclovir, and famciclovir have greater bioavailability, which enables improved dosing schedules and increased compliance. Episodic intervention reduces the duration of viral shedding and the healing time for recurrent lesions. Continuous antiviral suppressive therapy may be advised when more than six outbreaks occur within 1 year. These drugs are well tolerated, with few adverse effects. This long-term suppressive therapy does not limit latency, and reactivation of the disease frequently occurs after the drug is discontinued. In 2002, the U.S. Food and Drug Administration (FDA) approved long-term suppressive therapy with valacyclovir for the prevention of HSV-2 transmission to an uninfected sexual partner. Topical treatment with antibacterial soaps, lotions, dyes, ultrasonography, and ultraviolet light has been tried with little success. Sometimes, symptomatic relief can be obtained with cool compresses (*i.e.,* Burow's soaks), sitz baths, topical anesthetic agents, and oral analgesic drugs.

Good hygiene is essential to prevent secondary HSV infection. Fastidious hand washing is recommended to avoid hand-to-eye spread of the infection. HSV infection of the eye is the most frequent cause of corneal blindness in the United States. To prevent spread of the disease, intimate contact should be avoided until lesions are completely healed.

Current information indicates that the risk for neonatal infection is very low when the mother has developed type-specific antibodies, which are then protective to the neonate. Newborns at highest risk are those born to women who shed the virus and have not developed antibodies from previous infections. Disseminated neonatal infection has high mortality and morbidity. Active infection during labor may necessitate cesarean delivery, ideally before membranes rupture. Recommendations from the American College of Obstetricians and Gynecologists direct care providers to obtain cultures when a woman has active lesions during pregnancy. Vaginal delivery is acceptable if visible lesions are not present at the onset of labor.[3]

MOLLUSCUM CONTAGIOSUM

Molluscum contagiosum is a common viral disease of the skin that gives rise to multiple umbilicated papules. The disease is mildly contagious; it is transmitted by skin-to-skin contact, fomites, and autoinoculation. Lesions are domelike and have a dimpled appearance. A curdlike material can be expressed from the center of the lesion. Necrosis and secondary infection are possible. Diagnosis is based on the appearance of the lesion and microscopic identification of intracytoplasmic molluscum bodies. Molluscum is a benign and self-limited disease.

Spontaneous regression of mature lesions followed by continued emergence of new lesions is common with molluscum, and in the absence of therapy, this cycle may persist for 6 months to 5 years. Recurrence is frequent after treatment; therefore, the goal of therapy is to hasten the resolution of individual lesions and reduce the likelihood of further spread.[11] When indicated, treatment consists of removing the top of the papule with a sterile needle or scalpel, expressing the contents of each lesion, and applying alcohol or silver nitrate to the base. Electrodesiccation, cryosurgery, laser ablation, and surgical biopsy are alternative treatments but seldom are needed unless lesions are large or extend over a wide area. A new approach to therapy is the application of imiquimod 1% cream to lesions. This self-applied therapy is the first to show efficacy in patients with immunosuppressive diseases such as acquired immunodeficiency syndrome (AIDS).[11]

CHANCROID

Chancroid (*i.e.,* soft chancre) is a disease of the external genitalia and lymph nodes. The causative organism is the gram-negative bacterium *Haemophilus ducreyi,* which causes acute ulcerative lesions with profuse discharge. This disease has become uncommon in the United States, with only 67 reported cases in 2002.[1] It typically occurs in discrete outbreaks rather than as an endemic disease in this country. It is more prevalent in Southeast Asia, the West Indies, and North Africa. As a highly infectious disease, chancroid usually is transmitted by sexual intercourse or through skin and mucous membrane abrasions. Autoinoculation may lead to multiple chancres.

Lesions begin as macules, progress to pustules, and then rupture. This painful ulcer has a necrotic base and jagged edges. In contrast, the syphilitic chancre is nontender and indurated. Subsequent discharge can lead to further infection of self or others. On physical examination, lesions and regional lymphadenopathy (*i.e.,* buboes) may be found. Secondary infection may cause significant tissue destruction. Diagnosis usually is made clinically but may be confirmed through culture. Gram stain rarely is used today because it is insensitive and nonspecific. Polymerase chain reaction (PCR) methods may soon be available commercially for definitive identification of *H. ducreyi* (see Chapter 18 for an explanation of PCR methods). The organism has shown resistance to treatment with sulfamethoxazole alone and to tetracycline. The CDC recommends treatment with azithromycin, erythromycin, or ceftriaxone.[7]

GRANULOMA INGUINALE

Granuloma inguinale (*i.e.,* granuloma venereum) is caused by a gram-negative bacillus, *Calymmatobacterium donovani,* which is a tiny, encapsulated intracellular parasite. This disease is almost nonexistent in the United States. It is found most frequently in India, Brazil, the West Indies, and parts of China, Australia, and Africa.

Granuloma inguinale causes ulceration of the genitalia, beginning with an innocuous papule. The papule progresses through nodular or vesicular stages until it begins to break down as pink, granulomatous tissue. At this final stage, the tissue becomes thin and friable and bleeds easily. There are complaints of swelling, pain, and itching. Extensive inflammatory scarring may cause late sequelae, such as lymphatic obstruction with the development of enlarged and elephantoid external genitalia. The liver, bladder, bone, joint, lung, and bowel tissue may become involved. Genital complications include tubo-ovarian abscess, fistula, vaginal stenosis, and occlusion of vaginal or anal orifices. Lesions may become neoplastic.

Diagnosis is made through the identification of Donovan bodies (*i.e.,* large mononuclear cells filled with intracytoplasmic gram-negative rods) in tissue smears, biopsy samples, or culture. A 3-week period of treatment with doxycycline, tetracycline, erythromycin, or gentamicin is used in treating the disorder.[7]

LYMPHOGRANULOMA VENEREUM

Lymphogranuloma venereum is an acute and chronic venereal disease caused by *Chlamydia trachomatis* types L1, L2, and P3. The disease, although found worldwide, has a low incidence outside the tropics. Most cases reported in the United States are in men.

The lesions of LGV can incubate for a few days to several weeks and thereafter cause small, painless papules or vesicles that may go undetected. An important characteristic of the disease is the early (1 to 4 weeks later) development of large, tender, and sometimes fluctuant inguinal lymph nodes called *buboes*. There may be flulike symptoms with joint pain, rash, weight loss, pneumonitis, tachycardia, splenomegaly, and proctitis. In later stages of the disease, a small percentage of affected persons develop elephantiasis of the external genitalia, caused by lymphatic obstruction or fibrous strictures of the rectum or urethra from inflammation and scarring. Urethral involvement may cause pyuria and dysuria. Cervicitis is a common manifestation of primary LGV, and could extend to perimetritis or salpingitis, which are known to occur in other chlamydial infections.[10] Anorectal structures may be compromised to the point of incontinence. Complications of LGV may be minor or extensive, involving compromise of whole systems or progression to a cancerous state.

Diagnosis usually is accomplished by means of a complement fixation test for LGV-specific *Chlamydia* antibodies. High titers for this antibody differentiate this group from other chlamydial subgroups. Treatment involves 3 weeks of doxycycline, tetracycline, or erythromycin.[7] Surgery may be required to correct sequelae such as strictures or fistulas or to drain fluctuant lymph nodes.

In summary, STDs that primarily affect the external genitalia include HPV (condyloma acuminata), genital herpes (HSV-2), molluscum contagiosum, chancroid, granuloma inguinale, and LGV. The lesions of these infections occur on the external genitalia of male and female sexual partners. Of concern is the relation between HPV and genital neoplasms. Genital herpes is caused by a neurotropic virus (HSV-2) that ascends through the peripheral nerves to reside in the sacral dorsal root ganglia. The herpesvirus can be reactivated, producing recurrent lesions in genital structures that are supplied by the peripheral nerves of the affected ganglia. There is no permanent cure for herpes infections. Molluscum contagiosum is a benign and self-limited infection that is only mildly contagious. Chancroid, granuloma inguinale, and LGV produce external genital lesions with various degrees of inguinal lymph node involvement. These diseases are uncommon in the United States.

Vaginal Infections

After completing this section of the chapter, you should be able to meet the following objectives:

- State the difference between wet-mount slide and culture methods of diagnosis of STDs
- Compare the signs and symptoms of infections caused by *Candida albicans, Trichomonas vaginalis,* and bacterial vaginosis

Candidiasis, trichomoniasis, and bacterial vaginosis are vaginal infections that can be sexually transmitted. Although these infections can be transmitted sexually, the male partner usually is asymptomatic.

CANDIDIASIS

Also called *yeast infection, thrush,* and *moniliasis, candidiasis* is the second leading cause of vulvovaginitis in the United States. Approximately 75% of reproductive-age women in the United States experience one episode in their lifetime; 40% to 45% experience two or more infections.[10]

The causative organism is *Candida,* a genus of yeast-like fungi. The species most commonly identified is *Candida albicans,* but other candidal species, such as *Candida glabrata* and *Candida tropicalis,* have caused symptoms. These organisms are present in 20% to 55% of healthy women without causing symptoms, and alteration of the host vaginal environment usually is necessary before the organism can cause pathologic effects.[10] Although vulvovaginal candidiasis usually is not transmitted sexually, it is included in the CDC STD treatment guidelines because it often is diagnosed in women being evaluated for STDs.[7] The possibility of sexual transmission has been recognized for many years; however, candidiasis requires a favorable environment for growth. The gastrointestinal tract also serves as a reservoir for this organism, and candidiasis can develop through autoinoculation in women who are not sexually active. Although studies have documented the presence of *Candida* on the penis of male partners of women with vulvovaginal candidiasis, few men develop balanoposthitis that requires treatment.

Causes for the overgrowth of *C. albicans* include antibiotic therapy, which suppresses the normal protective bacterial flora; high hormone levels owing to pregnancy or the use of oral contraceptives, which cause an increase in vaginal glycogen stores; and diabetes mellitus or HIV infection because they compromise the immune system. Food allergies, hypothyroidism, endocrine disorders, dietary influences, tight-fitting clothing, and douching also have been suggested as possible contributors to the development of vulvovaginal candidiasis. However, there is little evidence to support these etiologies.

In obese persons, *Candida* may grow in skin folds underneath the breast tissue, the abdominal flap, and the inguinal folds. Vulvar pruritus accompanied by irritation, dysuria, dyspareunia, erythema, and an odorless, thick, cheesy vaginal discharge are the predominant symptoms of the infection. Accurate diagnosis is made by identification of budding yeast filaments (*i.e.*, hyphae) or spores on a wet-mount slide using 20% potassium hydroxide (Fig. 48-2). The pH of the discharge, which is checked

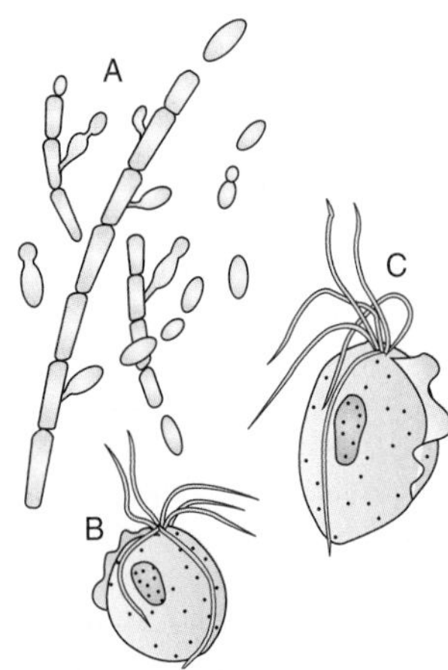

FIGURE 48-2 Organisms that cause vaginal infections. **(A)** *Candida albicans* (blastospores and pseudohyphae). **(B,C)** *Trichomonas vaginalis.*

with litmus paper, typically is less than 4.5. When the wet-mount technique is negative but the clinical manifestations are suggestive of candidiasis, a culture may be necessary.

Antifungal agents such as clotrimazole, miconazole, butoconazole, and terconazole, in various forms, are effective in treating candidiasis. These drugs, with the exception of terconazole, are available without prescription for use by women who have had a previously confirmed diagnosis of candidiasis. Oral fluconazole has been shown to be as safe and effective as the standard intravaginal regimens.[7] Gentian violet solution (1%) applied to the vagina by swabs or tampon (not recommended in pregnant women), boric acid vaginal suppositories, or boric acid soaks to the vulva are treatment adjuncts. Tepid sodium bicarbonate baths, clothing that allows adequate ventilation, and the application of cornstarch to dry the area may increase comfort during treatment. Chronic vulvovaginal candidiasis, defined as four or more mycologically confirmed episodes within 1 year, affects approximately 5% of women and is difficult to manage. Subsequent prophylaxis (maintenance therapy) often is required for long-term management of this problem.[12]

Candidiasis can be confused with Döderlein cytolysis—an excess of lactobacilli—that can present with a similar clinical picture. In the case of Döderlein cytolysis, wet-mount and culture techniques show only excessive lactobacilli, but no yeast. Treatment of Döderlein cytolysis involves use of a sodium bicarbonate douche two to three times each week to raise the vaginal pH and decrease the symptoms.

TRICHOMONIASIS

An anaerobic protozoan that can be transmitted sexually, *Trichomonas vaginalis* is shaped like a turnip and has three or four anterior flagella (see Fig. 48-2). Trichomonads can reside in the paraurethral glands of both sexes. Males harbor the organism in the urethra and prostate and are asymptomatic. Although 10% to 25% of women are asymptomatic, trichomoniasis is a common cause of vaginitis when some imbalance allows the protozoan to proliferate. Five million cases of trichomoniasis were diagnosed in 1999.[1] This extracellular parasite feeds on the vaginal mucosa and ingests bacteria and leukocytes. The infection causes a copious, frothy, malodorous, green or yellow discharge. There commonly is erythema and edema of the affected mucosa, with occasional itching and irritation. Sometimes, small hemorrhagic areas, called *strawberry spots,* appear on the cervix.

Diagnosis is made microscopically by identification of the protozoan on a wet-mount slide preparation. The pH of the discharge usually is greater than 6.0. Special culture media are available for diagnosis, but are costly and not needed for diagnosis.

Because the organism resides in other urogenital structures besides the vagina, systemic treatment is recommended. The treatment of choice is oral metronidazole (Flagyl), a medication that is effective against anaerobic protozoans.[7] Metronidazole is chemically similar to disulfiram (Antabuse), a drug used in the treatment of alcohol addiction that causes nausea, vomiting, flushing of the skin, headache, palpitations, and lowering of the blood pressure when alcohol is ingested. Alcohol should be avoided during and for 24 to 48 hours after treatment. Gastrointestinal disturbances and a metallic taste in the mouth are potential adverse effects of the drug. Metronidazole has not been proved safe for use during pregnancy and is used only after the first trimester for fear of potential teratogenic effects. Sexual partners should be treated to avoid reinfection, and abstinence is recommended until the full course of therapy is completed.

BACTERIAL VAGINOSIS (NONSPECIFIC VAGINITIS)

Considerable controversy exists regarding the organisms responsible for a vaginal infection that produces a characteristic fishy- or ammonia-smelling discharge yet fails to produce an inflammatory response that is characteristic of most infections. A number of terms have been used to describe the nonspecific vaginitis that cannot be attributed to one of the accepted pathogenic organisms, such as *T. vaginalis* or *C. albicans*.

In 1955, Gardner and Dukes isolated an organism from women with this type of vaginitis and proposed the name *Haemophilus vaginalis,* apparently because the gram-negative organism required blood for growth.[13] In 1963, gram-positive isolates were found, and the organism was renamed *Corynebacterium vaginale.* Because the organism did not meet all the criteria of corynebacteria, it was renamed *Gardnerella vaginalis* in 1980, after its original discoverer, and admitted to a taxonomic genus of its own. The development of a special agar on which *G. vaginalis* could be cultured led to the discovery that 40% to 70% of women harbor this organism as part of their normal vaginal flora. Further study revealed that abnormal discharge frequently contained highly motile, crescent-shaped rods called *Mobiluncus* and many more anaerobic than aerobic bacteria. It has been suggested that the presence of anaerobes, which produce ammonia or amines from amino acids, favors the growth of *G. vaginalis* by raising vaginal pH. Because of the presence of anaerobic bacteria and the lack of an inflammatory response, a new term, *bacterial vaginosis* (BV), was proposed.[10] Bacterial vaginosis is characterized by absence of the normal lactobacillus species in the vagina and an overgrowth of other organisms, including *G. vaginalis, Mobiluncus* species, *Mycoplasma hominis,* and numerous anaerobes.[6]

Bacterial vaginosis is the most prevalent form of vaginal infection seen by health care professionals. Its relation to sexual activity is not clear. Sexual activity is believed to be a catalyst rather than a primary mode of transmission, and endogenous factors play a role in the development of symptoms. The predominant symptom of bacterial vaginosis is a thin, grayish-white discharge that has a foul, fishy odor. Burning, itching, and erythema usually are absent because the bacteria has only minimal inflammatory potential. Bacterial vaginosis may be carried asymptomatically by men and women.

The diagnosis is made when at least three of the following characteristics are present: homogeneous discharge, production of a fishy, amine odor when a 10% potassium hydroxide solution is dropped onto the secretions, vaginal pH above 4.5 (usually 5.0 to 6.0), and appearance of characteristic "clue cells" on wet-mount microscopic studies. *Clue cells* are squamous epithelial cells covered with masses of coccobacilli, often with large clumps of organisms floating free from the cell. Because *G. vaginalis* can be a normal vaginal flora, cultures should not be done routinely. They are of limited clinical value because it is believed that the condition is caused by a combination of *G. vaginalis* and anaerobic bacteria.

The mere presence of *G. vaginalis* in an asymptomatic woman is not an indication for treatment. When indicated, treatment is aimed at eradicating the anaerobic component of bacterial vaginosis to reestablish the normal balance of the vaginal flora. The CDC recommends oral metronidazole. Alternative therapies include metronidazole vaginal gel, clindamycin vaginal cream, or oral clindamycin. Treatment of sexual partners is not recommended.[7]

Pelvic inflammatory disease (PID), preterm labor, premature rupture of membranes, chorioamnionitis, and postpartum endometritis have been linked to the organisms associated with bacterial vaginosis. Oral or cream clindamycin formulations can be used for treatment during the first trimester of pregnancy; oral or vaginal metronidazole can be used after the first trimester for treatment failures. Routine screening for bacterial vaginosis is not advocated, but all pregnant women with BV should be treated.

In summary, candidiasis, trichomoniasis, and bacterial vaginosis are common vaginal infections that become symptomatic because of changes in the vaginal ecosystem. Only trichomoniasis is spread through sexual contact. Trichomoniasis is caused by an anaerobic protozoan. The infection incites the production of a copious, frothy, yellow or green, malodorous discharge. Candidiasis, also called a *yeast infection,* is the form of vulvovaginitis with which women are most familiar. *Candida* can be present without producing symptoms; usually some host factor, such as altered immune status, contributes to the development of vulvovaginitis. It can be treated with over-the-counter medications. Bacterial vaginosis is the most common cause of vaginal discharge. It is a nonspecific type of infection that produces a characteristic fishy-smelling discharge. The infection is thought to be caused by the combined presence of *G. vaginalis* and anaerobic bacteria. The anaerobe raises the vaginal pH, thereby favoring the growth of *G. vaginalis.*

Vaginal-Urogenital-Systemic Infections

After completing this section of the chapter, you should be able to meet the following objectives:

- Compare the signs and symptoms of gonorrhea in the male and female
- Describe the three stages of syphilis
- State the genital and nongenital complications that can occur with chlamydial infections, gonorrhea, and syphilis
- State the treatment for chlamydial urogenital infections, gonorrhea, nonspecific urogenital infections, and syphilis

Some STDs infect male and female genital and extragenital structures. Among the infections of this type are chlamydial infections, gonorrhea, and syphilis. Many of these infections also pose a risk to infants born to infected mothers. Some infections, such as syphilis, may be spread to the infant while in utero; others, such as chlamydial and gonorrheal infections, can be spread to the infant during the birth process.

CHLAMYDIAL INFECTIONS

Chlamydia trachomatis is an obligate intracellular bacterial pathogen that is closely related to gram-negative bacteria. It resembles a virus in that it requires tissue culture for isolation, but like a bacteria, it has RNA and DNA and is susceptible to some antibiotics. *C. trachomatis* causes a wide variety of genitourinary infections, including nongonococcal urethritis in men and PID in women. The closely related organisms *Chlamydia pneumoniae* and *Chlamydia psittaci* cause mild and severe pneumonia, respectively. *C. trachomatis* can be serologically subdivided into types A, B, and C, which are associated with trachoma and chronic keratoconjunctivitis; types D through K, which are associated with genital infections and their complications; and types L1, L2, and L3, which are associated with LGV. *C. trachomatis* can cause significant ocular disease in neonates; it is a leading cause of blindness in underdeveloped countries. In these countries, the organism is spread primarily by flies, fomites, and nonsexual personal contact. In industrial countries, the organism is spread almost exclusively by sexual contact and therefore affects primarily the genitourinary structures.

Chlamydial infection is the most prevalent STD in the United States, with an incidence estimated to be more than twice that of gonorrhea. As of December 2000, chlamydia infections are reportable in all 50 states and the District of Columbia. According to CDC estimates, chlamydial infections occur at a rate of 3 million new cases each year, predominantly among individuals younger than 25 years of age. Rates for chlamydial infections have risen significantly over the past 15 years due to an increase in screening programs, improved sensitivity of diagnostic tests, and improved surveillance and reporting systems. Reported rates are higher in women largely because of screening efforts, although actual occurrence rates are thought to be the same for men and women.[14] Significant declines in prevalence have been noted in areas where screening programs have been initiated.[15] In the United States, costs associated with managing chlamydial infections and their complications exceed $2 billion annually.[1]

Chlamydiae exist in two forms: elementary bodies, which are the infectious particles capable of entering uninfected cells, and the initiator or reticulate bodies, which multiply by binary fission to produce the inclusions identified in stained cells. The 48-hour growth cycle starts with attachment of the elementary body to the susceptible host cell, after which it is ingested by a process that resembles phagocytosis (Fig. 48-3). Once inside the cell, the elementary body is organized into the reticulate body, the metabolically active form of the organism that is capable of reproduction. The reticulate body is not infectious and cannot survive outside the body. The reticulate bodies divide in the cell for up to 36 hours and then condense to form new elementary bodies, which are released when the infected cell bursts.

The signs and symptoms of chlamydial infection resemble those produced by gonorrhea. The most significant difference between chlamydial and gonococcal salpingitis is that chlamydial infections may be asymptomatic or subclinically nonspecific. In women, chlamydial infections may cause urinary frequency, dysuria, and vaginal discharge. The most common symptom is a mucopurulent cervical discharge. The cervix itself frequently hypertrophies and becomes erythematous, edematous, and extremely friable. Seventy-five percent of women and 50% of men with chlamydial infection have no symptoms; therefore, most cases are undiagnosed, unreported, and untreated.[1] This can lead to greater fallopian tube damage and increase the reservoir for further chlamydial infections. Approximately 40% of women with an untreated chlamydial infection develop PID, and 1 in 5 of these women becomes infertile. Research has identified a possible link between three specific serotypes of chlamydiae and an increased risk for cervical cancer. The mechanism by which this occurs is unclear.[16]

In men, chlamydial infections cause urethritis, including meatal erythema and tenderness, urethral discharge, dysuria, and urethral itching. Prostatitis and epididymitis with subsequent infertility may develop. The most serious complication that can develop with nongonococcal urethritis is Reiter's syndrome, a systemic condition characterized by urethritis, conjunctivitis, arthritis, and mucocutaneous lesions (see Chapter 59).

Routine screening for sexually active adolescents and young adults has been suggested by the CDC and the U.S. Preventive Services Task Force (USPSTF) in an effort to minimize these serious sequelae of asymptomatic infection. Between 25% and 50% of infants born to mothers with cervical chlamydial infections develop ocular disease (*i.e.,* inclusion conjunctivitis), and 10% to 20% develop chlamydial pneumonitis.

Diagnosis of chlamydial infections takes several forms. The identification of polymorphonuclear leukocytes on Gram stain of male discharge or cervical discharge is presumptive evidence. The direct fluorescent antibody test and the enzyme-linked immunosorbent assay that use antibodies against an antigen in the *Chlamydia* cell wall are rapid tests that are highly sensitive and specific. The positive predictive value of these tests is excellent among high-risk groups, but false-positive results occur more often in populations with lower rates. Nucleic acid amplification tests (NAATs) do not require viable organisms for detection and can produce a positive signal from as little as a single copy of the target DNA or RNA. Commercial tests differ in their amplification methods and their target nucleic acid sequences. Tests such as polymerase chain reaction (PCR), ligase chain reaction (LCR), or transcription-mediated amplification (TMA) have demonstrated specificities of nearly 100% (same as culture) and sensitivities of 90% to 95%. Sensitivity of cell culture has been estimated at 70% to 85% for endocervical specimens and 50% to 75% for male urethral specimens. Because NAATs can be performed on urine and swab specimens from the distal vagina as well as the traditional endocervical and urethral specimens, this easy, convenient means of accurate detection has become the diagnostic method of choice.[6,14,15] Nucleic acid hybridization assays detect *C. trachomatis* and *N. gonorrhoeae* in a single test. This type of test does not differentiate between the

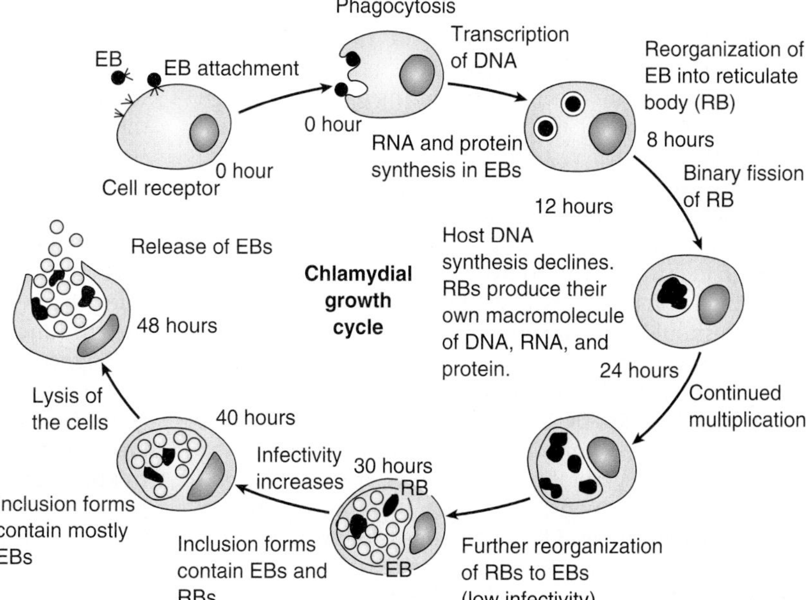

FIGURE 48-3 Chlamydial growth cycle. EB, elementary body; RB, reticulate body. (Thompson S.E., Washington A.E. [1983]. Epidemiology of sexually transmitted *Chlamydia trachomatis* infections. *Epidemiologic Reviews 5,* 96–123)

two organisms, and a positive result requires follow-up testing to obtain organism-specific results.[14] Cost often is a factor in determining which type of testing to use.

The CDC recommends the use of azithromycin or doxycycline in the treatment of chlamydial infection; penicillin is ineffective. Erythromycin or amoxicillin is the preferred choice in pregnancy.[7] Antibiotic treatment of both sexual partners simultaneously is recommended. Abstinence from sexual activity is encouraged to facilitate cure. Rescreening all women with chlamydial infection 3 to 4 months after treatment has been recommended to rule out recurrence.[7]

GONORRHEA

Gonorrhea is a reportable disease caused by the bacterium *N. gonorrhoeae.* In 1999, there were 360,076 reported cases of gonorrhea in the United States. Of these reported cases, more than 90% involved persons between 15 and 44 years of age, with the heaviest concentration among young adults (15 to 24 years of age).[1] There are an estimated 600,000 new cases every year.[7] Although the incidence of gonorrhea has declined steadily from its peak in 1975, there was an increase in occurrence between 1997 and 1998. Improved screening efforts, as well as greater use of more sensitive nonculture methods of testing, may have contributed to this increase. Higher rates of occurrence among homosexual men were documented in several states, leading to a concern that a rise in unsafe sexual behavior may be occurring because of the availability of highly active antiretroviral agents for treatment of HIV infection.[17]

The gonococcus is a pyogenic (*i.e.,* pus-forming), gram-negative diplococcus that evokes inflammatory reactions characterized by purulent exudates. Humans are the only natural host for *N. gonorrhoeae.* The organism grows best in warm, mucus-secreting epithelia. The portal of entry can be the genitourinary tract, eyes, oropharynx, anorectum, or skin.

Transmission usually is by heterosexual or homosexual intercourse. Autoinoculation of the organism to the conjunctiva is possible. Neonates born to infected mothers can acquire the infection during passage through the birth canal and are in danger of developing gonorrheal conjunctivitis, with resultant blindness, unless treated promptly. An amniotic infection syndrome characterized by premature rupture of the membranes, premature delivery, and increased risk for infant morbidity and mortality has been identified as an additional complication of gonococcal infections in pregnancy. Genital gonorrhea in young children should raise the possibility of sexual abuse.

The infection commonly manifests 2 to 7 days after exposure. It typically begins in the anterior urethra, accessory urethral glands, Bartholin's or Skene's glands, and the cervix. If untreated, gonorrhea spreads from its initial sites upward into the genital tract. In males, it spreads to the prostate and epididymis; in females, it commonly moves to the fallopian tubes. Pharyngitis may follow orogenital contact. The organism also can invade the bloodstream (*i.e.,* disseminated gonococcal infection), causing serious sequelae such as bacteremic involvement of joint spaces, heart valves, meninges, and other body organs and tissues.

Persons with gonorrhea may be asymptomatic and may unwittingly spread the disease to their sexual partners. Men are more likely to be symptomatic than women. In men, the initial symptoms include urethral pain and a creamy, yellow, sometimes bloody discharge. The disorder may become chronic and affect the prostate, epididymis, and periurethral glands. Rectal infections are common in homosexual men. In women, recognizable symptoms include unusual genital or urinary discharge, dysuria, dyspareunia, pelvic pain or tenderness, unusual vaginal bleeding (including bleeding after intercourse), fever, and proctitis. Symptoms may occur or increase during or immediately after menses because the bacterium is an intracellular diplococcus that thrives in menstrual blood but cannot survive long outside the human body. There may be infections of the uterus and development of acute or chronic infection of the fallopian tubes (*i.e.,* salpingitis), with ultimate scarring and sterility.

Diagnosis is based on the history of sexual exposure and symptoms. It is confirmed by identification of the organism on Gram stain or culture. A Gram stain usually is an effective means of diagnosis in symptomatic men (*i.e.,* those with discharge). In women and asymptomatic men, a culture usually is preferred because the Gram stains often are unreliable. A specimen should be collected from the appropriate site (*i.e.,* endocervix, urethra, anal canal, or oropharynx), plated onto selective Thayer-Martin media, and placed in a carbon dioxide environment. *N. gonorrhoeae* is a fastidious organism with specific nutrient and environmental needs. Optimal growth requires a pH of 7.4, a temperature of 35.5°C, and an atmosphere that contains 2% to 10% carbon dioxide.[3] The accuracy of culture results is affected if transport is delayed or growth requirements are not available. Culture detects more than 95% of male urethral gonorrhea and 80% to 90% of cervical, rectal, and pharyngeal infections.[6] An enzyme immunoassay for detecting gonococcal antigens (Gonozyme) is available but has several requirements that limit its usefulness. Detection by means of amplified DNA probes (PCR, LCR, TMA) is possible using urine and urethral swab specimens. The sensitivity of these probes is similar to that of culture, and they may be cost effective in high-risk populations.

Testing for other STDs, particularly syphilis and chlamydial infections, is suggested at the time of examination. Pregnant women are routinely screened at the time of their first prenatal visit; high-risk populations should have repeat cultures during the third trimester. Neonates are routinely treated with various antibacterial agents applied to the conjunctiva within 1 hour of birth to protect against undiagnosed gonorrhea and other diseases.

Penicillin-resistant strains of *N. gonorrhoeae* are prevalent worldwide, and strains with other kinds of antibiotic resistance continue to evolve and spread. The current treatment recommendation to combat tetracycline- and penicillin-resistant strains of *N. gonorrhoeae* is ceftriaxone in a single injection or cefixime, ciprofloxacin, ofloxacin, or levofloxacin in a single oral dose. All are equally effective and should be followed with azithromycin or doxycycline for chlamydiae. Quinolone-resistant strains are now common in Asia, the Pacific islands including Hawaii, and California; hence, the CDC recommends avoiding the use of fluoroquinolones in those areas. All sex partners within 60 days before discovery of the infection should be contacted, tested, and treated. Test of cure is not required with observed single-dose therapy. Patients are instructed to refrain from intercourse until therapy is completed and symptoms are no longer present.[7]

SYPHILIS

Syphilis is a reportable disease caused by a spirochete, *Treponema pallidum*. After declining every year from 1990 to 2000, the rate of primary and secondary syphilis increased between 2001 and 2002 by 12.4%. In 2002, 6862 cases of syphilis were reported in the United States (2.4 per 100,000 population). Increased rates were found only in men, and syphilis transmission occurred over a wider geographic area then in the past.[18] Syphilis continues to affect minority populations disproportionately. Although the rate for blacks declined by 10% over the previous year, it was still 8.2 times the rate reported in whites. The rate for Hispanics and Asian/Pacific islanders increased 20%, primarily among men. The National Plan to Eliminate Syphilis was launched in 1999 with a goal of reducing primary and secondary syphilis to fewer than 1000 cases and increasing the number of syphilis-free counties to 90% by 2005. Initial efforts, focused on the South and minority populations, have been credited with the decreases in those areas in 2002. Federal funding is available to support this effort.[18]

T. pallidum is spread by direct contact with an infectious, moist lesion, usually through sexual intercourse. Bacteria-laden secretions may transfer the organism during kissing or intimate contact. Skin abrasions provide another possible portal of entry. There is rapid transplacental transmission of the organism from the mother to the fetus after 16 weeks' gestation, so that active disease in the mother during pregnancy can produce congenital syphilis in the fetus. Untreated syphilis can cause prematurity, stillbirth, and congenital defects and active infection in the infant. Once treated for syphilis, a pregnant woman usually is followed throughout pregnancy by repeat testing of serum titers.

The clinical disease is divided into three stages: primary, secondary, and tertiary. Primary syphilis is characterized by the appearance of a chancre at the site of exposure. Chancres typically appear within 3 weeks of exposure but may incubate for 1 week to 3 months. The primary chancre begins as a single, indurated, button-like papule up to several centimeters in diameter that erodes to create a clean-based ulcerated lesion on an elevated base. These lesions usually are painless and located at the site of sexual contact. Primary syphilis is readily apparent in males, where the lesion is on the penis or scrotum. Although chancres can develop on the external genitalia in females, they are more common on the vagina or cervix, and primary syphilis therefore may go untreated. There usually is an accompanying regional lymphadenopathy. The disease is highly contagious at this stage, but because the symptoms are mild, it frequently goes unnoticed. The chancre usually heals within 3 to 12 weeks, with or without treatment.

The timing of the second stage of syphilis varies even more than that of the first, lasting from 1 week to 6 months. The symptoms of a rash (especially on the palms and soles), fever, sore throat, stomatitis, nausea, loss of appetite, and inflamed eyes may come and go for a year but usually last for 3 to 6 months. Secondary manifestations may include alopecia and genital condylomata lata. Condylomata lata are elevated, red-brown lesions that may ulcerate and produce a foul discharge. They are 2 to 3 cm in diameter, contain many spirochetes, and are highly infectious.

After the second stage, syphilis frequently enters a latent phase that may last the lifetime of the person or progress to tertiary syphilis at some point. Persons can be infective during the first 1 to 2 years of latency.

Tertiary syphilis is a delayed response of the untreated disease. It can occur as long as 20 years after the initial infection. Only approximately one third of those with untreated syphilis progress to the tertiary stage of the disease, and symptoms develop in approximately one half of these. Approximately one third undergo spontaneous cure, and the remaining one third continue to have positive serologic tests but do not develop structural lesions.[19] When syphilis does progress to the symptomatic tertiary stage, it commonly takes one of three forms: development of localized destructive lesions called *gummas*, development of cardiovascular lesions, or development of central nervous system lesions. The syphilitic gumma is a peculiar, rubbery, necrotic lesion that is caused by noninflammatory tissue necrosis. Gummas can occur singly or multiply and vary in size from microscopic lesions to large, tumorous masses. They most commonly are found in the liver, testes, and bone. Central nervous system lesions can produce dementia, blindness, or injury to the spinal cord, with ataxia and sensory loss (*i.e.*, tabes dorsalis). Cardiovascular manifestations usually result from scarring of the medial layer of the thoracic aorta with aneurysm formation. These aneurysms produce enlargement of the aortic valve ring with aortic valve insufficiency.

T. pallidum does not produce endotoxins or exotoxins but evokes a humoral immune response that provides the basis for serologic tests. Two types of antibodies—nonspecific and specific—are produced. The nonspecific antibodies can be detected by flocculation tests such as the Venereal Disease Research Laboratory (VDRL) test or the rapid plasma reagin (RPR) test. Because these tests are nonspecific, positive results can occur with diseases other than syphilis. The tests are easy to perform, rapid, and inexpensive and frequently are used as screening tests for syphilis. Results become positive 4 to 6 weeks after infection or 1 to 3 weeks after the appearance of the primary lesion. Because these tests are quantitative, they can be used to measure the degree of disease activity or treatment effectiveness. The VDRL titer usually is high during the secondary stage of the disease and becomes less so during the tertiary stage. A falling titer during treatment suggests a favorable response. The fluorescent treponemal antibody absorption test or microhemagglutinin test is used to detect specific antibodies to *T. pallidum*. These qualitative tests are used to determine whether a positive result on a nonspecific test such as the VDRL is attributable to syphilis. The test results remain positive for life.

T. pallidum cannot be cultured. The diagnosis of syphilis is based on serologic tests or dark-field microscopic examination with identification of the spirochete in specimens collected from lesions. Because the disease's incubation period may delay test sensitivity, serologic tests usually are repeated after 6 weeks if the initial test results were negative.

The treatment of choice for syphilis is penicillin. Because of the spirochetes' long generation time, effective tissue levels of penicillin must be maintained for several weeks. Long-acting injectable forms of penicillin are used. Tetracycline or doxycycline is used for treatment in persons who are sensitive to penicillin. Pregnant patients should be desensitized and treated with penicillin because erythromycin does not treat fetal infection. Sexual partners should be evaluated and treated prophylactically even though they may show no sign of infection. All treated individuals should be reexamined clinically and serologically 6 and 12 months after completing therapy; more frequent monitoring (3-month intervals) is suggested for individuals with HIV infection.[7]

In summary, the vaginal-urogenital-systemic STDs—chlamydial infections, gonorrhea, and syphilis—can severely involve the genital structures and manifest as systemic infections. Gonorrheal and chlamydial infections can cause a wide variety of genitourinary complications in men and women, and both can cause ocular disease and blindness in neonates born to infected mothers. Syphilis is caused by a spirochete, *T. pallidum*. It can produce widespread systemic effects and is transferred to the fetus of infected mothers through the placenta.

REVIEW EXERCISES

A 25-year-old woman has been told that her Pap test indicates infection with HPV type 16.

A. What are the possible implications of infection with HPV type 16?

B. How might she have acquired this infection?

C. What treatments are currently available for treatment of this infection?

A 35-year-old woman presents with vulvar pruritus, dysuria, dyspareunia, and an odorless, thick, cheeselike vaginal discharge. She has diabetes mellitus and has recently recovered from a respiratory tract infection, which required antibiotic treatment.

A. Given that these manifestations are consistent with *Candida* infection, what tests might be used to confirm the diagnosis?

B. What risk factors does this woman have that predispose to this type of vaginitis?

C. How might this infection be treated?

References

1. Centers for Disease Control and Prevention. (2000). *Tracking the hidden epidemics: Trends in STDs in the United States*. [Online]. Available: http://www.cdc.gov/nchstp/dstd/dstdp.html. Accessed December 10, 2003.
2. Kurman R.J. (2002). *Blaustein's pathology of the female genital tract* (5th ed., pp. 258–276). New York: Springer.
3. Sweet R.L., Gibbs R.S. (2002). *Infectious diseases of the female genital tract* (5th ed., pp. 155–164). Baltimore: Williams & Wilkins.
4. Gunter J. (2003). Genital and perianal warts: New treatment opportunities for human papillomavirus infection. *American Journal of Obstetrics and Gynecology 189*(3), S3–11.
5. Koutsky L.A., Ault K.A., Wheeler C.M. (2002). A controlled trial of human papilloma virus type 16 vaccine. *New England Journal of Medicine 347,* 1645–1651.
6. Handsfield H.H. (2001). *Color atlas and synopsis of sexually transmitted diseases* (pp. 13, 23, 71, 87, 163). New York: McGraw-Hill.
7. Centers for Disease Control and Prevention. (2002). Sexually transmitted diseases: Treatment guidelines 2002. *MMWR Morbidity and Mortality Weekly Report 51*(RR-6), 1–118.
8. Cotran R.S., Kumar V., Collins T. (1999). *Robbins pathologic basis of disease* (6th ed., pp. 359–361). Philadelphia: W.B. Saunders.
9. Mark H.D., Hanahan A.P., Stender S.C. (2003). Herpes simplex virus type 2: An update. *Nurse Practitioner 28*(11), 34–41.
10. Holmes K.K., Per-Anders M., Sparling P.F., et al. (1999). *Sexually transmitted diseases* (3rd ed., pp., 287, 290, 424, 563–564, 629, 820–821). New York: McGraw-Hill.
11. Turing S.K. (2003). Molluscum contagiosum: The importance of early diagnosis and treatment. *American Journal of Obstetrics and Gynecology 189*(3), S12–16.
12. Ringdahl E.N. (2000). Treatment of recurrent vulvovaginal candidiasis. *American Family Physician 61,* 3306–3317.
13. Gardner H.L., Dukes C.D. (1955). *Haemophilus vaginalis* vaginitis. *American Journal of Obstetrics and Gynecology 69,* 962.
14. U.S. Department of Health and Human Services. (2002). Screening tests to detect *Chlamydia trachomatis* and *Neisseria gonorrhea* infections. *MMWR Morbidity and Mortality Weekly Report 51*(RR15), 1–27.
15. U.S. Preventive Services Task Force. (2002). Screening for *Chlamydia* infection: Recommendations and rationale. *American Journal of Nursing 102*(10), 87–93.
16. Antilla T., Saiku P., Koskela P., et al. (2001). Serotypes of *Chlamydia trachomatis* and risk for development of cervical squamous cell carcinoma. *Journal of the American Medical Association 285,* 47–51.
17. Centers for Disease Control and Prevention. (2000). Gonorrhea—United States, 1998. *MMWR Morbidity and Mortality Weekly Report 49,* 538.
18. Centers for Disease Control and Prevention. (2003). Primary and secondary syphilis—United States, 2002. *MMWR Morbidity and Mortality Weekly Report 52*(46), 1117–1120.
19. Chapin K. (1999). Probing the STDs. *American Journal of Nursing 99*(7), 24AAA–24DDD.

UNIT

XII

Neural Function

For centuries, the nervous system was ignored or even deemed unimportant. Aristotle (384–322 BC), the great Greek philosopher, decreed that the heart was the seat of the soul, whereas the brain—which he assumed was composed largely of water—simply cooled it. Although Galen (AD 130–200) was able to show that the spinal cord was essential to many sensations and movements, his experiments were conducted only on animals. Not until the 1500s, when the Flemish anatomist Andreas Vesalius (1514–1564) dissected "the heads of executed criminals . . . still warm," was the overarching importance of the human brain and spinal cord established.

Investigations continued with scientists debating whether the brain should be considered as a whole or as consisting of separate areas, each responsible for specific functions. Progress in brain research took an impressive, if accidental, leap in 1841, when an explosion at a railroad work site in Vermont shot an iron rod into the left cheek of Phineas Gage, through his brain, and out the top of his head. Gage survived the accident, but it became clear to all who knew him that he had changed greatly. Formerly a conscientious, hardworking man, he became fitful, obstinate, foul-mouthed, and capricious. Gage died in 1860, and an autopsy showed destruction of the left lobe of his brain and damage to his right lobe. Scientists concluded that his personality change was the result of the grievous damage to the frontal lobes, an observation that supported the then-emerging concept that different parts of the brain serve different functions.

CHAPTER 49

Organization and Control of Neural Function

Edward W. Carroll and Robin L. Curtis

The nervous system, in coordination with the endocrine system, provides the means by which cell and tissue functions are integrated into a solitary, surviving organism. It controls skeletal muscle movement and helps to regulate cardiac and visceral smooth muscle activity. The nervous system enables the reception, integration, and perception of sensory information; it provides the substratum necessary for intelligence, anticipation, and judgment; and it facilitates adjustment to an ever-changing external environment. No part of the nervous system functions independently from other parts. In humans, who are thinking and feeling creatures, the effects of emotion can exert a strong influence on neural and hormonal control of body function. However, alterations in neural and endocrine function, particularly at the biochemical level, also can exert a strong influence on psychological behavior.

This chapter is divided into six parts: nervous tissue cells, neuronal communication, the development and organization of the nervous system, the spinal cord, the brain, and the autonomic nervous system.

Nervous Tissue Cells

After completing this section of the chapter, you should be able to meet the following objectives:

- Differentiate between the central and peripheral nervous systems
- List the three parts of a neuron and describe their structure and function
- Name the supporting cells in the central nervous system and peripheral nervous system and state their functions
- Describe the energy requirements of nervous tissue

All portions of the nervous system can be divided into two basic components: the central nervous system (CNS) and the peripheral nervous system (PNS). The CNS consists of the brain and spinal cord, which are protected by the skull and vertebral column, whereas the PNS is found outside these structures. Inherent in the basic design of the nervous system is the provision for the concentration of computational and control functions in the CNS. In this design, the PNS functions as an input–output system for relaying information to the CNS and for transmitting output messages that control effector organs, such as muscles and glands.

Nervous tissue contains two types of cells: neurons and supporting cells. The neurons are the functional cells of the nervous system. They exhibit membrane excitability and conductivity and secrete neurotransmitters and hormones, such as epinephrine and antidiuretic hormone. The supporting cells, such as Schwann cells in the PNS and the glial cells in the CNS, protect the nervous system and provide metabolic support for the neurons.

THE STRUCTURAL ORGANIZATION OF THE NERVOUS SYSTEM

- The nervous system is divided into two parts: the central nervous system (CNS), consisting of the brain and spinal cord, which are located in the skull and spinal column, and the peripheral nervous system, which is located outside these structures.
- The nervous system contains two major types of cells: neurons, which are functioning cells of the nervous system, and supporting cells, which protect the nervous system and supply metabolic support.
- The neurons consist of a cell body with cytoplasm-filled processes, the dendrites, and the axons.
- There are two types of neurons: afferent neurons or sensory neurons, which carry information to the CNS, and efferent neurons or motoneurons, which carry information from the CNS to the effector organs.

NEURONS

Neurons, which are the functioning cells of the nervous system, have three distinct parts: the cell body and its cytoplasm-filled processes, the dendrites and axons (Fig. 49-1). These processes form the functional connections, or synapses, with other nerve cells, with receptor cells, or with effector cells. Axonal processes are particularly designed for rapid communication with other neurons and the many body structures innervated by the nervous system. Afferent, or sensory, neurons transmit information from the PNS to the CNS. Efferent neurons, or motoneurons, carry information away from the CNS. Interspersed between the afferent and efferent neurons is a network of interconnecting neurons (interneurons or internuncial neurons) that modulate and control the body's response to changes in the internal and external environments.

The cell body, or soma, of a neuron contains a large, vesicular nucleus with one or more distinct nucleoli and a well-developed rough endoplasmic reticulum. A neuron's nucleus has the same DNA and genetic code content present in other cells of the body, and its nucleolus, which is composed of portions of several chromosomes, produces RNA associated with protein synthesis. The cytoplasm contains large masses of ribosomes that are prominent in most neurons. These acidic RNA masses, which are involved in protein synthesis, stain as dark Nissl bodies with basic histologic stains (see Fig. 49-1).

Dendrites (*i.e.*, "treelike") are multiple, branched extensions of the nerve cell body; they conduct information toward the cell body and are the main source of information for the neuron. The dendrites and cell body are studded with synaptic terminals that communicate with axons and dendrites of other neurons.

Axons are long efferent processes that project from the cell body and carry impulses away from the cell. Most neurons have only one axon; however, axons may exhibit multiple branchings that result in many axonal terminals. The cytoplasm of the cell body extends to fill the dendrites and the axon. Proteins and other materials used by the axon are synthesized in the cell body and then flow down the axon through its cytoplasm.

The cell body of the neuron is equipped for a high level of metabolic activity. This is necessary because the cell body must synthesize the cytoplasmic and membrane constituents required to maintain the function of the axon and its terminals. Some of these axons extend for a distance of 1 to 1.5 m and have a volume that is 200 to 500 times greater than the cell body itself. Two axonal transport systems, one slow and one rapid, move molecules from the cell body through the cytoplasm of the axon to its terminals. Replacement proteins and nutrients slowly diffuse from the cell body, where they are synthesized, down the axon, moving at the rate of approximately 1 mm/day. Other molecules, such as some neurosecretory granules or their precursors, are conveyed by a rapid, energy-dependent active transport system, moving at the rate of approximately 400 mm/day. Often, membrane-bound vesicles containing neurosecretory granules (*e.g.*, neurotransmitters, neuro-

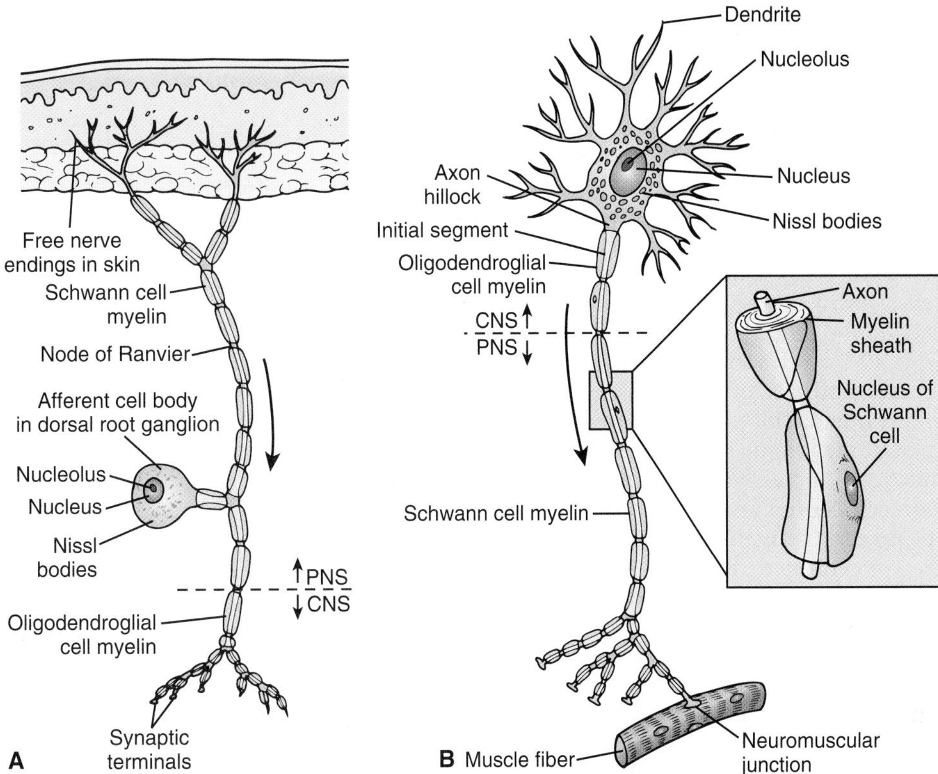

FIGURE 49-1 (**A**) Afferent and (**B**) efferent neurons, showing the soma or cell body, dendrites, and axon. *Arrows* indicate the direction for conduction of action potentials.

modulators, and neurohormones) are moved to the axon synaptic terminals by the active transport process. For example, rapid axonal transport carries antidiuretic hormones and oxytocin from hypothalamic neurons through their axons to the posterior pituitary, where the hormones are released into the blood. A reverse rapid (*i.e.*, retrograde) axonal transport system moves materials, including target cell messenger molecules, from axonal terminals back to the cell body.

SUPPORTING CELLS

Supporting cells of the nervous system, the Schwann and satellite cells of the PNS and the several types of glial cells of the CNS, give the neurons protection and metabolic support. The supporting cells segregate the neurons into isolated metabolic compartments, which are required for normal neural function. Astrocytes and the tightly joined endothelial cells of the capillaries in the CNS contribute to what is called the *blood–brain barrier*. This term is used to emphasize the impermeability of the nervous system to large or potentially harmful molecules.

Recent information suggests that many glial cells have functions other than protection and support. Evidence suggests that Schwann cells release developmental signals in embryonic nervous tissue that are crucial for the survival of neonatal neurons. Postnatally, Schwann cells synthesize and release self-regulating autocrine substances that bind to receptors on their cell surface, enabling them to survive without axons. The survival of Schwann cells is essential for the successful regeneration of damaged peripheral nerves. Schwann cells and astrocytes respond to neuronal activity by elevating their internal calcium (Ca^{2+}) ion concentrations, triggering the release of glial neurotransmitters and thus influencing feedback regulation of neuronal function and synaptic activity.

The many-layered myelin wrappings of Schwann cells of the PNS and the oligodendroglia of the CNS produce the myelin sheaths that serve to increase the velocity of nerve impulse conduction in axons. Myelin has a high lipid content, which gives it a whitish color, and the name *white matter* is given to the masses of myelinated fibers of the spinal cord and brain. Besides its role in increasing conduction velocity, the myelin sheath is essential for the survival of larger neuronal processes, perhaps by the secretion of neurotrophic compounds.

In some pathologic conditions, such as multiple sclerosis in the CNS and Guillain-Barré syndrome in the PNS, the myelin may degenerate or be destroyed. This degeneration leaves a section of the axonal process without myelin while leaving the nearby Schwann or oligodendroglial cells intact. Unless remyelination takes place, the axon eventually dies.

Supporting Cells of the Peripheral Nervous System

Schwann cells and satellite cells are the two types of supporting cells in the PNS. Normally, the nerve cell bodies in the PNS are collected into ganglia, such as the dorsal root and autonomic ganglia. Each of the cell bodies and processes of the peripheral nerves is separated from the connective tissue framework of the ganglion by a single layer of flattened capsular cells called *satellite cells*. Satellite cells secrete a basement membrane that protects the cell body from the diffusion of large molecules.

The processes of larger afferent and efferent neurons are surrounded by the cell membrane and cytoplasm of Schwann cells, which are close relatives of the satellite cells. During myelination, the Schwann cell wraps around each nerve process several times in a "jelly roll" fashion (Fig. 49-2). Schwann cells line up along the neuronal process, and each of these cells forms its own discrete myelin segment. The end of each myelin segment attaches to the cell membrane of the axon by means of intercellular junctions. Successive Schwann cells are separated by short extracellular fluid gaps called the *nodes of Ranvier,* where the myelin is missing and voltage-gated sodium channels are concentrated (Fig. 49-3). The nodes of Ranvier increase nerve conduction by allowing the impulse to jump from node to node through the extracellular fluid in a process called *saltatory conduction* (from the Latin *saltare,* "to jump"). In this way, the impulse can travel more rapidly than it could if it were required to move systematically along the entire nerve process. This increased conduction velocity greatly reduces reaction time, or time between the application of a stimulus and the subsequent motor response. The short reaction time is especially important in peripheral nerves with long distances (sometimes 1 to 1.5 m) for conduction between the CNS and distal effector organs.

Each of the Schwann cells along a peripheral nerve is encased in a continuous tube of basement membrane, which in turn is surrounded by a multilayered sheath of loose connective tissue known as the *endoneurium* (Fig. 49-4). These endoneurial sheaths, which are essential to the regeneration of peripheral nerves, provide a collagenous tube through which a regenerating axon can again reach its former target. The endoneurial sheath does not penetrate the CNS. The absence of the endoneurial sheaths is thought to be a major factor in the limited axonal regeneration of CNS nerves compared with those of the PNS.

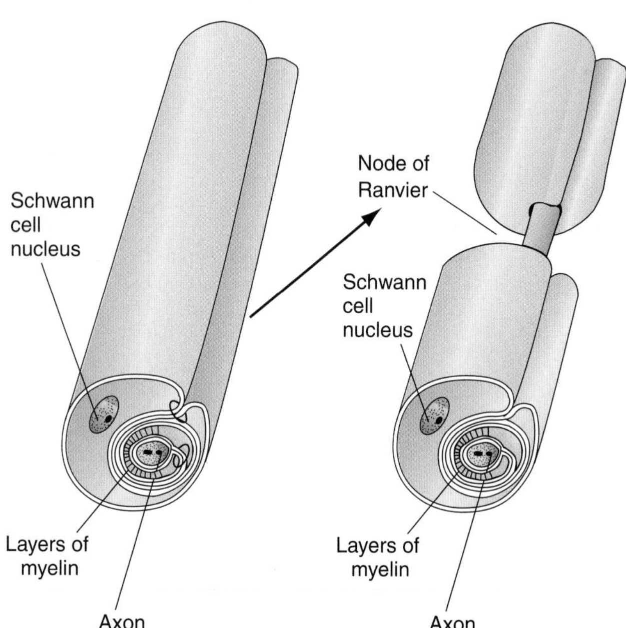

FIGURE 49-2 The Schwann cell migrates down a larger axon to a bare region, settles down, and encloses the axon in a fold of its plasma membrane. It then rotates around and around, wrapping the axon in many layers of plasma membrane, with most of the Schwann cell cytoplasm squeezed out. The resultant thick, multiple-layered coating around the axon is called myelin.

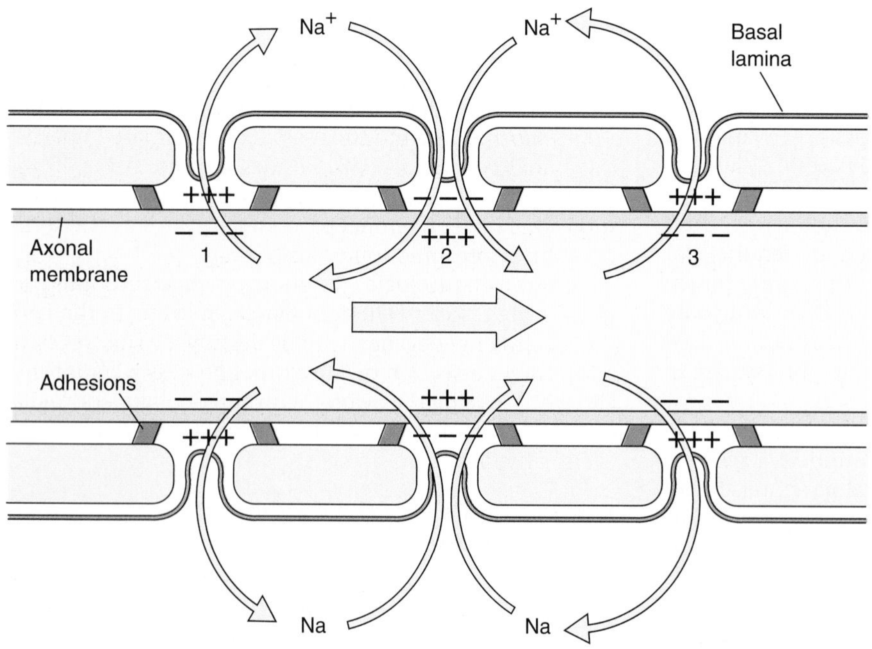

FIGURE 49-3 Schematic drawing of a longitudinal section of a myelinated axon in the peripheral nervous system. Schwann cells insulate the axon, decreasing flow through the membrane. Action potentials occur at the nodes of Ranvier, which are unmyelinated areas of the basal lamina between the Schwann cells. The impulses jump from node to node in a process called saltatory conduction, which greatly increases the velocity of conduction. (1) represents the trailing hyperpolarized region behind the action potential, (2) the hypopolarized region at the action potential, and (3) the leading hyperpolarized area ahead of the action potential. The Schwann cell adhesions (*red*) to the plasma membrane of the axon block the leakage of current under the myelin.

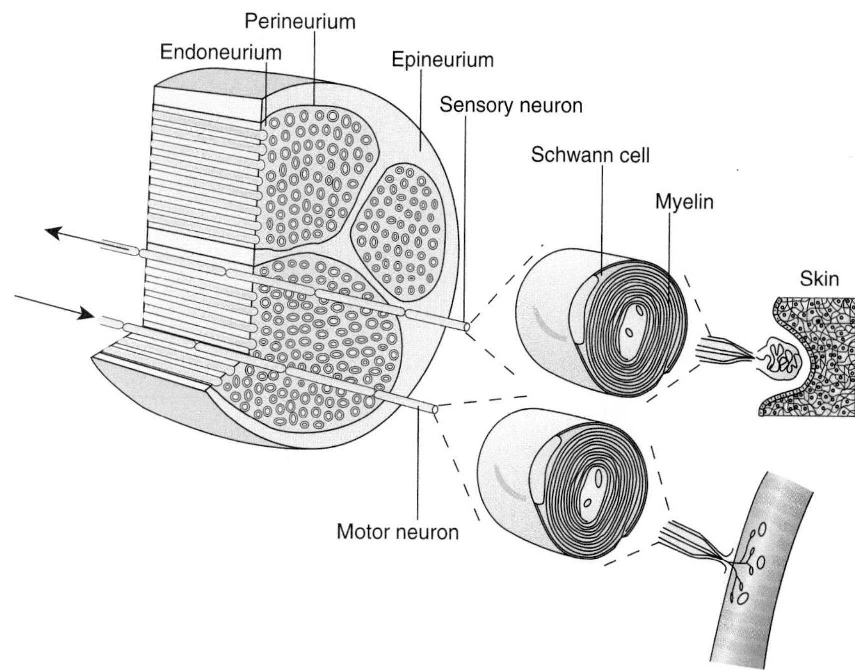

FIGURE 49-4 Section of a peripheral nerve containing axons of both afferent (sensory) and efferent (motor) neurons. (Modified from Cormack D.H. [1987]. *Ham's histology* [9th ed., p. 374]. Philadelphia: J.B. Lippincott)

Endoneurial sheaths are bundled with blood vessels into small bundles or clusters of nerves called *fascicles*. In the nerve, the fascicles consisting of bundles of nerve fibers are surrounded by another protective covering called the *perineurium*. Usually, several fascicles are further surrounded by the heavy, protective *epineurial sheath* of the peripheral nerve. The protective layers that surround the peripheral nerve processes are continuous with the connective tissue capsule of the sensory nerve endings and the connective tissue that surrounds the effector structures, such as the skeletal muscle cell. Centrally, the connective tissue layers continue along the dorsal and ventral roots of the nerve and fuse with the meninges that surround the spinal cord and brain.

Myelin formation is essentially the same in both the PNS and CNS; both contain myelin basic protein, and both involve the winding of plasma membranes around the nerve fiber. During the wrapping of myelin, the cytoplasm between two adjacent inner leaflets of the plasma membrane is expelled. The two adjacent inner leaflets and any remaining cytoplasm appear as a dark line called the *major dense line*. Likewise, during the wrapping of the plasma membranes to form myelin, adjacent outer plasma membrane leaflets become opposed, creating the interperiod or *minor dense line*. Linking proteins, *proteolipid protein* (PLP) found only in the CNS and *protein 0* (P_0) found only in the PNS, help stabilize adjacent plasma membranes of the myelin sheath.

Supporting Cells of the Central Nervous System

Supporting cells of the CNS consist of the oligodendroglia, astroglia, microglia, and ependymal cells. *Oligodendroglial* cells form the myelin in the CNS. Instead of forming a myelin covering for a single axon, these cells reach out with several processes, each wrapping around and forming a multilayered myelin segment around several different axons (Fig. 49-5). The coverings of axons in the CNS function in increasing the velocity of nerve conduction, similar to the peripheral myelinated fibers.

A second type of glial cell, the *astroglia,* is particularly prominent in the gray matter of the CNS. These large cells have many processes, some reaching to the surface of the capillaries, others reaching to the surface of the nerve cells, and still others filling most of the intercellular space within the CNS. The astrocytic linkage between the blood vessels and the neurons may provide a transport mechanism for the exchange of oxygen, carbon dioxide, and metabolites. Astrocytes also have an important role in sequestering cations such as calcium and potassium from the intercellular fluid. Astrocytes can fill their cytoplasm with microfibrils (*i.e.*, fibrous astrocytes), and masses of these cells form the special type of scar tissue called *gliosis* that develops in the CNS when tissue is destroyed.

A third type of glial cell, the *microglia,* is a small phagocytic cell that is available for cleaning up debris after cellular damage, infection, or cell death. The fourth type of cell, the *ependymal* cell, forms the lining of the neural tube cavity, the ventricular system. In some areas, these cells combine with a rich vascular network to form the *choroid plexus,* where production of the cerebrospinal fluid (CSF) takes place.

METABOLIC REQUIREMENTS OF NERVOUS TISSUE

Nervous tissue has a high rate of metabolism. Although the brain constitutes only 2% of the body's weight, it receives approximately 15% of the resting cardiac output

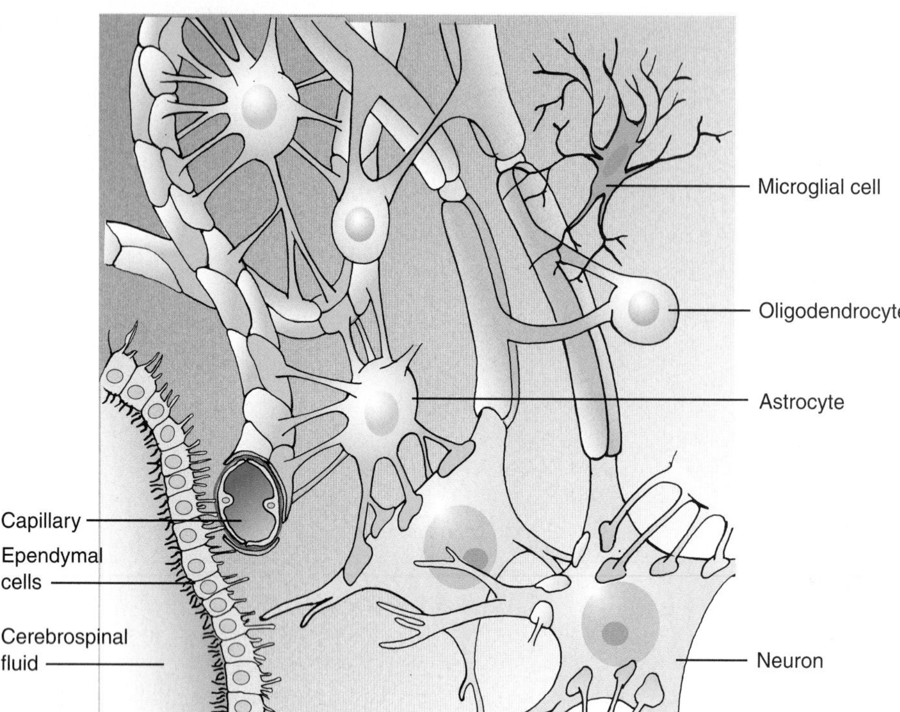

FIGURE 49-5 The supporting cells of the central nervous system (CNS). Diagrammatic view of relationships between the glial elements (astrocyte, oligodendrocyte, microglial cell, and the ependymal cells), the capillaries, the cerebral spinal fluid, and the cell bodies of CNS neurons.

and consumes 20% of its oxygen. Despite its substantial energy requirements, the brain can neither store oxygen nor effectively engage in anaerobic metabolism. An interruption in the blood or oxygen supply to the brain rapidly leads to clinically observable signs and symptoms. Without oxygen, brain cells continue to function for approximately 10 seconds. Unconsciousness occurs almost simultaneously with cardiac arrest, and the death of brain cells begins within 4 to 6 minutes. Interruption of blood flow also leads to the accumulation of metabolic byproducts that are toxic to neural tissue.

Glucose is the major fuel source for the nervous system, but neurons have no provision for storing glucose. Ketones can provide for limited temporary energy requirements; however, these sources are rapidly depleted. Unlike muscle cells, neurons have no glycogen stores and must rely on glucose from the blood or the glycogen stores of supporting glial cells. Persons receiving insulin for diabetes may experience signs of neural dysfunction and unconsciousness (*i.e.,* insulin reaction or shock) when blood glucose drops because of insulin excess (see Chapter 43).

In summary, nervous tissue is composed of two types of cells: neurons and supporting cells. Neurons are composed of three parts: a cell body, which controls cell activity; the dendrites, which conduct information toward the cell body; and the axon, which carries impulses from the cell body. The supporting cells consist of Schwann and satellite cells of the PNS and the glial cells of the CNS. Supporting cells protect and provide metabolic support for the neurons and aid in segregating them into isolated compartments, which is necessary for normal neuronal function. The function of the nervous system demands a high amount of metabolic energy. Glucose is the major fuel for the nervous system. The brain comprises only 2% of body weight but receives 15% of the resting cardiac output.

Nerve Cell Communication

After completing this section of the chapter, you should be able to meet the following objectives:

- Describe the functional importance of ion channels and relate this to the different phases of an action potential
- Discuss the differences between electrical and chemical synapses
- Describe the interaction of the presynaptic and postsynaptic terminals
- Relate excitatory and inhibitory postsynaptic potentials with respect to the processes of spatial and temporal summation of membrane potentials
- Briefly describe how neurotransmitters are synthesized, stored, released, and inactivated

Neurons are characterized by the ability to communicate with other neurons and body cells through electrical signals called *impulses.* An impulse, or action potential, represents the movement of electrical charge along the axon membrane. This phenomenon, sometimes called *conductance,* is based on the rapid flow of charged ions through the plasma membrane. In excitable tissue, ions such as sodium, potassium, and calcium move through the membrane channels and carry the electrical charges involved in the initiation and transmission of such impulses.

ACTION POTENTIALS

Cell membranes of excitable tissue, including neurons, contain ion channels that are responsible for generating action potentials (see Chapter 4). These membrane channels are guarded by voltage-dependent gates that open and close with changes in the membrane potential. Separate voltage-gated channels exist for the sodium, potassium, and calcium ions. Each type of ion channel has a characteristic membrane potential that opens and closes its channels. Also present are ligand-gated channels that respond to chemical messengers such as neurotransmitters, mechanically gated channels that respond to physical changes in the cell membrane, and light-gated channels that respond to fluctuations in light levels.

Nerve signals are transmitted by action potentials, which are abrupt, pulsatile changes in the membrane potential that last a few ten-thousandths to a few thousandths of a second. Action potentials can be divided into three phases: the resting or polarized state, depolarization, and repolarization (Fig. 49-6).

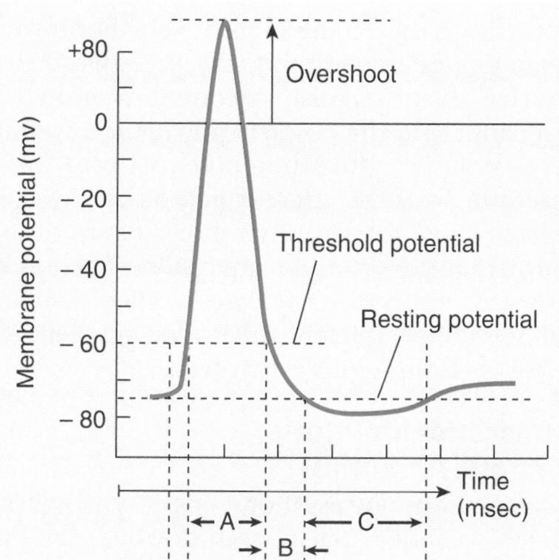

FIGURE 49-6 Time course of the action potential recorded at one point of an axon with one electrode inside and one on the outside of the plasma membrane. The rising part of the action potential is called the spike. The rising phase plus approximately the first half of the repolarization phase is equal to the absolute refractory period (**A**). The portion of the repolarization phase that extends from the threshold to the resting membrane potential represents the relative refractory period (**B**). The remaining portion of the repolarization phase to the resting membrane potential is equal to the negative after potential (**C**). Hyperpolarization is equal to the positive relative refractory period.

The resting phase is the undisturbed period of the action potential during which the nerve is not transmitting impulses. During this period, the membrane is said to be *polarized* because of the large separation of charge (*i.e.*, positive on the outside and negative on the inside). The resting membrane potential for large nerve fibers is approximately –90 mV. However, in small neurons and in many neurons in the CNS, the resting membrane potential is often as little as –40 to –60 mV. The resting phase of the membrane potential continues until some event causes the membrane to increase its permeability to sodium.

A threshold potential represents the membrane potential at which neurons or other excitable tissues are stimulated to fire. In large nerve fibers, the sodium channels open at approximately –60 mV, which is the threshold for initiation of an action potential. When the threshold potential is reached, the gatelike structures in the ion channels open. Below the threshold potential, these gates remain tightly closed. These gates are either fully open or fully closed. Under ordinary circumstances, the threshold stimulus is sufficient to open many ion channels, triggering massive depolarization of the membrane (the action potential).

Depolarization is characterized by the flow of electrically charged ions. During the depolarization phase, the membrane suddenly becomes permeable to sodium ions; the rapid inflow of sodium ions produces local currents that travel through the adjacent cell membrane, causing the sodium channels in this part of the membrane to open. In neurons, sodium ion gates remain open for approximately one fourth of a millisecond. During this phase of the action potential, the inner face of the membrane becomes positive (approximately +30 to +45 mV).

Repolarization is the phase during which the polarity of the resting membrane potential is reestablished. This is accomplished with closure of the sodium channels and opening of the potassium channels. The outflow of positively charged potassium ions across the cell membrane returns the membrane potential to negativity. The sodium–potassium pump gradually reestablishes the resting ionic concentrations on each side of the membrane. Membranes of excitable cells must be sufficiently repolarized before they can be reexcited. During repolarization, the membrane remains refractory (*i.e.*, does not fire) until repolarization is approximately one-third complete. This period, which lasts approximately one half of a millisecond, is called the *absolute refractory period.* During one portion of the recovery period, the membrane can be excited, although only by a stronger-than-normal stimulus. This period is called the *relative refractory period.*

SYNAPTIC TRANSMISSION

Neurons communicate with each other through structures known as *synapses.* Two types of synapses are found in the nervous system: electrical and chemical.

Electrical synapses permit the passage of current-carrying ions through small openings called *gap junctions* that penetrate the cell junction of adjoining cells and allow current to travel in either direction. The gap junctions allow an action potential to pass directly and quickly from one neuron to another. They may link neurons having close functional relationships into circuits.

The most common type of synapse is the *chemical synapse*. Chemical synapses involve special presynaptic and postsynaptic membrane structures, separated by a synaptic cleft (Fig. 49-7). Presynaptic terminals secrete one and often several chemical messenger molecules (*i.e.,* neurotransmitters or neuromodulators) into the synaptic cleft. Neurotransmitters diffuse into the synaptic cleft and unite with receptors on the postsynaptic membrane; this causes excitation or inhibition of the postsynaptic neuron by producing either hypopolarization or hyperpolarization of the postsynaptic membrane. Hypopolarization increases the excitability of the postsynaptic neuron by bringing the membrane potential closer to the threshold potential so that a smaller subsequent stimulus is needed to cause the neuron to fire. Hyperpolarization, on the other hand, brings the membrane potential further from the threshold and has the opposite effect. It has an inhibitory effect and decreases the likelihood that an action potential will be generated.

In contrast to an electrical synapse, a chemical synapse serves as a rectifier, permitting only one-way communication. One-way conduction is a particularly important characteristic of chemical synapses. It is this specific transmission of signals to discrete and highly localized areas of the nervous system that allows it to perform the myriad functions of sensation, motor control, and memory.

Chemical synapses are the slowest component in progressive communication through a sequence of neurons, such as in a spinal reflex. In contrast to the conduction of electrical action potentials, each successive event at the chemical synapse—transmitter secretion, diffusion across the synaptic cleft, interaction with postsynaptic receptors, and generation of a subsequent action potential in the postsynaptic neuron—consumes time. On the average, conduction across a chemical synapse requires approximately 0.3 milliseconds.

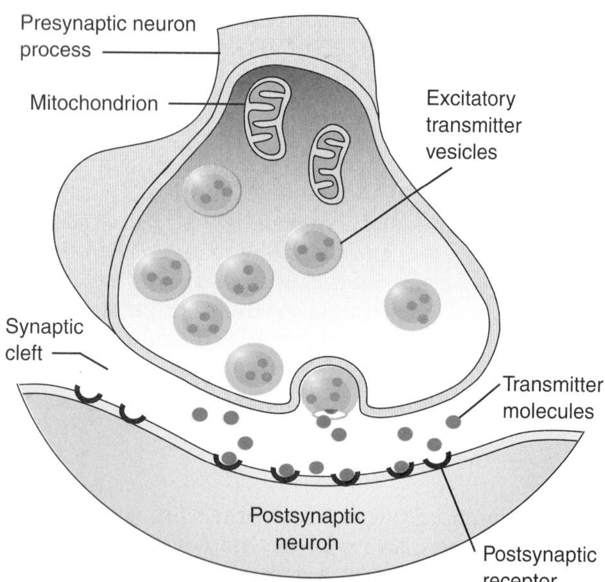

FIGURE 49-7 A synapse showing the synaptic vesicles in the presynaptic neuron, release of the transmitter, and binding of the transmitter to the receptors on the membrane surface of the postsynaptic neuron.

A neuron's cell body and dendrites are covered by thousands of synapses, any or many of which can be active at any moment. Because of the interaction of this rich synaptic input, each neuron resembles a little integrator, in which circuits of many neurons interact with one another. It is the complexity of these interactions and the subtle integrations involved in producing behavioral responses that give the system its intelligence. This complexity also makes the prediction of stimulus–response associations difficult without a millisecond-to-millisecond knowledge of the excitatory and inhibitory activity that takes place on the surfaces of each neuron in a functional circuit. It is amazing that predictions are possible at all considering the number of these tiny integrators. Even more astounding is that the basic microcircuitry present in the nervous system is reproduced reliably during the development of each new organism.

Chemical synapses exhibit several relationships. Axons can synapse with dendrites (axodendritic), with the cell body (axosomatic), or to the axon (axoaxonic). Dendrites can synapse with axons (dendroaxonic), other dendrites (dendrodendritic), or the soma of other neurons (dendrosomatic). Synapses between the nerve cell body and axons (somatoaxonic synapses) also have been observed. Synapses occurring between the soma of neighboring neurons (somasomatic) are uncommon, except between some efferent nuclei. The mechanism of communication between the presynaptic and the postsynaptic neuron is similar in all types of synapses; the action potential sweeps into the axonal terminals of the afferent neuron and triggers the rapid release of neurotransmitter molecules from the axonal, or presynaptic, surface. Conversion of action potentials into neurotransmitter release is called *coupling,* and although it is not completely understood, it is believed that the release of calcium ions is involved.

Excitatory and Inhibitory Postsynaptic Potentials

Many CNS neurons possess thousands of synapses on their dendritic or somatic surfaces, each of which can produce partial excitation or inhibition of the postsynaptic neuron. When the combination of a neurotransmitter with a receptor site causes partial depolarization of the postsynaptic membrane, it is called an *excitatory postsynaptic potential* (EPSP). In other synapses, the combination of a transmitter with a receptor site is inhibitory in the sense that it causes the local nerve membrane to become hyperpolarized and less excitable. This is called an *inhibitory postsynaptic potential* (IPSP).

Action potentials do not begin in the membrane adjacent to the synapse. They begin in the initial segment of the axon, near the *axon hillock* (see Fig. 49-1), that lies just before the first myelin segment. The initial segment of the axon is more excitable than the rest of the neuron. The local currents resulting from an EPSP (sometimes called a *generator potential*) are usually insufficient to reach threshold and cause depolarization of the axon's initial segment. However, if several EPSPs occur simultaneously, the area of depolarization can become large enough and the currents at the initial segment can become strong enough to exceed the threshold potential and initiate an action potential. This summation of depolarized areas is called *spatial summation.* EPSPs also can summate and cause an action potential if they occur in rapid succession. This temporal aspect of the occurrence of two or more EPSPs is called *temporal summation.*

IPSPs also can undergo spatial and temporal summation with each other and with EPSPs, reducing the effectiveness of the latter by a roughly algebraic summation. If the sum of EPSPs and IPSPs keeps the depolarization at the initial segment below threshold levels, no action potential occurs.

Spatial and temporal summation during synaptic activity serves as a sensitive and complicated switch that requires the right combination of incoming activity before the cell can elicit an action potential. The occurrence and frequency of action potentials in axons is in an all-or-none language (*i.e.,* digital language), which varies only as to the presence or absence of such impulses and their frequency. Action potentials permit rapid communication over long distances. However, it is the capacity for integration of excitatory and inhibitory synaptic bombardment of the soma and dendrites that gives the neuron and the nervous system the capability for complexity, memory, and intelligence.

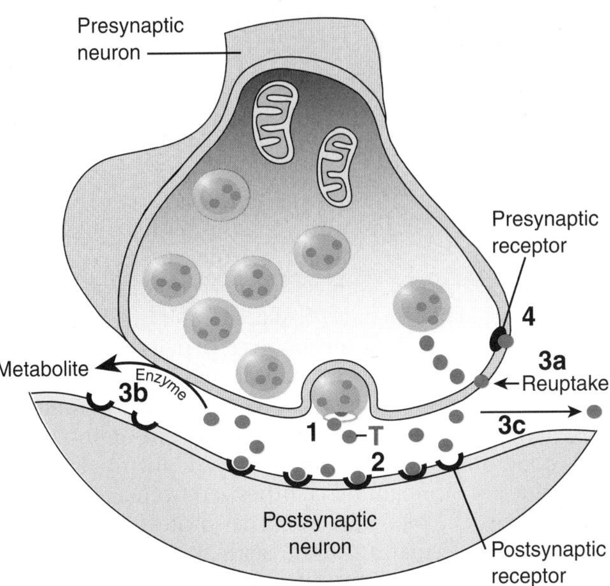

FIGURE 49-8 Schematic illustration of (1) neurotransmitter (T) release; (2) binding of transmitter to postsynaptic receptor; termination of transmitter action by (3a) reuptake of transmitter into the presynaptic terminal, (3b) enzymatic degradation, or (3c) diffusion away from the synapse; and (4) binding of transmitter to presynaptic receptors for feedback regulation of transmitter release.

MESSENGER MOLECULES

Neurotransmitters are the chemical messenger molecules of the nervous system. The process of neurotransmission involves the synthesis, storage, and release of a neurotransmitter; the reaction of the neurotransmitter with a receptor; and termination of the receptor action (Fig. 49-8). Newer research methods, including staining techniques and the use of radiolabeled antibodies, have allowed scientists to study and gain answers in each of these areas.

Both the nervous system and the endocrine system use chemical molecules as messengers. As more information is obtained about the chemical messengers of these systems, the distinction between them becomes less evident. Many neurons, such as those in the adrenal medulla, secrete transmitters into the bloodstream, and it has been found that other neurons possess receptor sites for hormones. Many hormones have turned out to be neurotransmitters. Vasopressin (also known as *antidiuretic hormone*), a peptide hormone released from the posterior pituitary gland, acts as a hormone in the kidney and as a neurotransmitter for nerve cells in the hypothalamus. More than a dozen of these cell-to-cell and bloodborne messengers can relay signals in the nervous system or the endocrine system.

Neurotransmitters are synthesized in the cytoplasm of the axon terminal. The synthesis of transmitters may require one or more enzyme-catalyzed steps (*e.g.,* one for acetylcholine and three for norepinephrine). Neurons are limited as to the type of transmitter they can synthesize by their enzyme systems.

After synthesis, the neurotransmitter molecules are stored in the axon terminal in tiny, membrane-bound sacs called *synaptic vesicles*. Thousands of vesicles may be present in a single terminal, each containing 10,000 to 100,000 transmitter molecules. The vesicle protects the neurotransmitters from enzyme destruction in the nerve terminal. The arrival of an impulse at a nerve terminal causes the vesicles to move to the cell membrane and release their transmitter molecules into the synaptic space.

Neurotransmitters exert their actions through specific proteins, called *receptors,* embedded in the postsynaptic membrane. These receptors are tailored precisely to match the size and shape of the transmitter. In each case, the interaction between a transmitter and receptor results in a specific physiologic response. The action of a transmitter is determined by the type of receptor to which it binds. For example, acetylcholine is excitatory when it is released at a myoneural junction, and it is inhibitory when it is released at the sinoatrial node in the heart. Receptors are named according to the type of neurotransmitter with which they interact. For example, a *cholinergic receptor* is a receptor that binds acetylcholine.

Rapid removal of a transmitter, once it has exerted its effects on the postsynaptic membrane, is necessary to maintain precise control of neural transmission. A released transmitter can undergo one of three fates: it can be broken down into inactive substances by enzymes; it can be taken back up into the presynaptic neuron in a process called *reuptake;* or it can diffuse away into the intercellular fluid until its concentration is too low to influence postsynaptic excitability. Acetylcholine, for example, is rapidly broken down by acetylcholinesterase into acetic acid and choline, with the choline being taken back into the presynaptic neuron for reuse in acetylcholine synthesis. The catecholamines are largely taken back into the neuron in an unchanged form for reuse. Catecholamines also can be degraded by enzymes in the synaptic space or in the nerve terminals.

Neurotransmitters are small molecules that incorporate a positively charged nitrogen atom; they include several peptides, amino acids, and monoamines. Peptides are low-molecular-weight molecules made up of two or more amino acids. They include substance P and the endorphins and enkephalins, which are involved in pain sensation and perception (see Chapter 50). Amino acids are the building blocks of proteins and are present in body fluids. A monoamine is an amine molecule containing one amino group (NH_2). Serotonin, dopamine, norepinephrine, and epinephrine are monoamines synthesized from amino acids. Fortunately, the blood–brain barrier protects the nervous system from circulating amino acids and other molecules with potential neurotransmitter activity.

Much needs to be learned about the role of amino acids and peptides as neurotransmitters. For example, several amino acids (especially glutamic acid and aspartic acid) appear to exert powerful excitatory effects on synaptic transmission; they are often called *excitatory amino acids.* Glycine, another amino acid, is known to have strong inhibitory effects. One of the most common inhibitory transmitters is γ-aminobutyric acid (GABA). This amino acid is unique in that it is synthesized almost exclusively in the brain and spinal cord. It has been established that almost one third of the synapses use GABA. Adding to the already complicated nature of neurotransmitters, it is puzzling that the same amino acid can function as both a neurotransmitter and as a building block for protein synthesis.

The actions of most neurotransmitters are localized in specific clusters of neurons with axons that project to highly specific brain regions. As more has been learned about the location and mechanism of action of the various neurotransmitters, many disease conditions clearly have their origin in altered neurotransmitter physiology. Occasionally, there is evidence of degeneration or dysfunction of the neurons producing the neurotransmitters; in other cases, there is an apparent alteration in the postsynaptic response to the neurotransmitter. For example, the neurons containing dopamine are concentrated in regions of the midbrain known as the *substantia nigra* and *ventral tegmentum.* Many of these dopamine-containing neurons project their axons to areas of the forebrain thought to be involved in regulation of emotional behavior. Other dopamine fibers terminate in regions near the middle of the brain called the *corpus striatum.* The latter fibers are thought to play an essential role in the performance of complex motor movements. Degeneration of the dopamine fibers in this area of the brain leads to the tremor and rigidity that are characteristic of Parkinson's disease. Some forms of mental illness, such as schizophrenia, are thought to involve abnormal release of or response to neurotransmitters in the brain. Pharmacologic methods of supplying neurotransmitters (*e.g.*, in Parkinson's disease) or modifying their actions (*e.g.*, with psychoactive drugs) are used to treat some of these disorders. Undoubtedly, more specific treatment methods will become available as more is learned about the transmission of neural information.

Other classes of messenger molecules, known *neuromodulators,* also may be released from axon terminals. Neuromodulator molecules react with presynaptic or postsynaptic receptors to alter the release of or response to neurotransmitters. Neuromodulators may act on postsynaptic receptors to produce slower and longer-lasting changes in membrane excitability. This alters the action of the faster-acting neurotransmitter molecules by enhancing or decreasing their effectiveness. By combining with autoreceptors on its own presynaptic membrane, a transmitter can act as a neuromodulator to augment or inhibit further nerve activity. In some nerves, such as the peripheral sympathetic nerves, a messenger molecule can have both transmitter and modulator functions. For example, norepinephrine can activate an α_1-adrenergic postsynaptic receptor to produce vasoconstriction, or stimulate an α_2-adrenergic presynaptic receptor to inhibit further norepinephrine release.

Neurohumoral mediators reach their target cells through the bloodstream and produce an even slower action than the neuromodulators. Neurotrophic or nerve growth factors are required to maintain the long-term survival of the postsynaptic cell and are secreted by axon terminals independent of action potentials. Examples include lower motoneurons (LMNs) to muscle cell trophic factors and neuron-to-neuron trophic factors in the sequential synapses of CNS sensory neurons. Trophic factors from target cells that enter the axon and are necessary for the long-term survival of presynaptic neurons have also been demonstrated. Target cell-to-neuron trophic factors probably have great significance in establishing specific neural connections during normal embryonic development.

In summary, neurons are characterized by the ability to communicate with other neurons and body cells through electrical signals called *action potentials.* The cell membranes of neurons contain ion channels that are responsible for generating action potentials. These channels are guarded by voltage-dependent gates that open and close with changes in the membrane potential. Action potentials are divided into three parts: the resting membrane potential, during which the membrane is polarized but no electrical activity occurs; the depolarization phase, during which sodium channels open, allowing rapid inflow of the sodium ions that generate the electrical impulse; and the repolarization phase, during which the membrane is permeable to potassium ions, allowing for the efflux of potassium ions and the return to the resting membrane potential.

The membrane threshold represents the membrane potential at which the sodium channels open, heralding the onset of an action potential. Once initiated, an action potential travels rapidly along the cell's axonal membrane to trigger transmitter release from the next neuron in the sequence.

Synapses are structures that permit communication between neurons. Two types of synapses have been identified: electrical and chemical. Electrical synapses consist of gap junctions between adjacent cells that allow action potentials to move rapidly from one cell to another. Chemical synapses involve special presynaptic and postsynaptic structures, separated by a synaptic cleft. They rely on chemical messengers, released from the presynaptic neuron, that cross the synaptic cleft and then interact with receptors on the postsynaptic neuron.

Neurotransmitters are chemical messengers that control neural function; they selectively cause excitation or inhibition of action potentials. Three major types of neurotransmitters are known: amino acids such as glutamic acid and GABA, peptides such as the endorphins and enkephalins, and monoamines such as epinephrine and norepinephrine. Neurotransmitters interact with cell membrane receptors to produce either excitatory or inhibitory actions. Neuromodulators are chemical messengers that react with membrane receptors to produce slower and longer-acting changes in membrane permeability. Neurotrophic or growth factors, also released from presynaptic terminals, are required to maintain the long-term survival of postsynaptic neurons.

Developmental Organization of the Nervous System

After completing this section of the chapter, you should be able to meet the following objectives:

- Cite the significance of the hierarchy of control levels of the CNS
- Use the segmental approach to explain the development of the nervous system and the organization of the postembryonic nervous system
- Define the terms *afferent, efferent, ganglia, association neuron, cell column,* and *tract*
- State the origin and destination of nerve fibers contained in the dorsal and ventral roots
- State the structures innervated by general somatic afferent, special visceral afferent, general visceral afferent, special somatic afferent, general visceral efferent, pharyngeal efferent, and general somatic efferent neurons

The development of the nervous system can be traced far back into evolutionary history. During its development, newer functional features and greater complexity resulted from the modification and enlargement of more primitive structures. Survival of the species depended on the rapid reaction to environmental danger, to potential food sources, or to a sexual partner.

The front, or rostral, end of the CNS became specialized for sensing the external environment and controlling reactions to it. In time, the ancient organization, which is largely retained in the spinal cord segments, was expanded in the forward segments of the nervous system. Of these, the most forward segments have undergone the most radical modification and have developed into the forebrain: the diencephalon and the cerebral hemispheres. The dominance of the front end of the CNS is reflected in a hierarchy of control levels: brain stem over spinal cord, and forebrain over brain stem. Throughout evolution, newer functions were added to the surface of functionally more ancient systems. As newer functions became concentrated at the rostral end of the nervous system, they also became more vulnerable to injury.

Three basic principles underlie the functioning of the nervous system: no portion of the nervous system functions independently of the other parts; newer systems control older systems; and the newer systems are more vulnerable to injury. These principles provide a basis for understanding the many manifestations of injuries and diseases of the nervous system.

EMBRYONIC DEVELOPMENT

The nervous system appears very early in embryonic development (week 3). This early development is essential because it influences the development and organization of many other body systems, including the axial skeleton, skeletal muscles, and sensory organs such as the eyes and ears. During later fetal life and afterward, the nervous system provides communication, signal processing, integrative, and memory functions. The early induction and later, lifelong communication functions of the nervous system are at the center of the integrity, survival, and individuality of each person.

THE DEVELOPMENTAL ORGANIZATION OF THE NERVOUS SYSTEM

- Embryologically, the nervous system begins its development as a hollow tube, the cephalic portion of which becomes the brain and the more caudal part the spinal cord.
- In the process of development, the basic organizational pattern of the body is that of a longitudinal series of segments, each repeating the same basic fundamental organizational pattern: a body wall or soma containing the axial skeleton and a neural tube, which develops into the nervous system.
- On cross section, the embryonic neural tube develops into a central canal surrounded by gray matter or cellular portion (cell columns) and the white matter, or tract system of the central nervous system (CNS).
- As the nervous system develops, it becomes segmented, with a repeating pattern of afferent neuron axons forming the dorsal roots of each succeeding segmental nerve, and the exiting efferent neurons forming the ventral roots of each succeeding segmental nerve.
- The nerve cells in the gray matter are arranged longitudinally in cell columns, with afferent sensory neurons located in the dorsal columns and efferent motor neurons located in the ventral columns.
- The axons of the cell column neurons project out into the white matter of the CNS, forming the longitudinal tract systems.

During the second week of development, embryonic tissue consists of two layers, the endoderm and the ectoderm. At the beginning of week 3, the ectoderm begins to invaginate and migrates between the two layers, forming a third layer called the *mesoderm* (Fig. 49-9). Mesoderm along the entire midline of the embryo forms a specialized rod of embryonic tissue called the *notochord.* The notochord and adjacent mesoderm provide the necessary induction signal for the overlying ectoderm to differentiate and form a thickened structure called the *neural plate,* the primordium of the nervous system. Within the neural plate an axial groove (*i.e.,* neural groove) develops that sinks into the underlying mesoderm; its walls fuse across the top, forming an ectodermal tube called the *neural tube.* This process, called *closure,* occurs during the later third and fourth weeks of gestation and is vital to the survival of the embryo. During development, the neural tube develops into the CNS, while the notochord becomes the foundation around which the vertebral column ultimately develops. The surface ectoderm separates from the neural tube and fuses over the top to become the outer layer of skin. Initial closure of the neural tube begins at the cervical and high thoracic levels and zippers rostrally toward the cephalic end of the embryo and caudally toward the sacrum. Complete closure occurs at the rostral-most end of brain (*i.e.,* anterior neuropore) at about day 24 to 26, and at about day 26 to 28 in the lumbosacral region (*i.e.,* posterior neuropore).

As the neural tube closes, ectodermal cells called *neural crest cells* migrate away from the dorsal surface of the neural tube to become the progenitors of the neurons and supporting cells of the PNS (see Fig. 49-9). During this period of embryonic development, the production of nerve cell adhesion molecules (N-CAMs) is programmed to decrease, allowing the neural crest cells to migrate, and the production of fibronectin molecules, which form the pathways that guide their migration, is programmed to increase. Some of these cells gather into clusters to form the *dorsal root ganglia* at the sides of each spinal cord segment and the *cranial ganglia* in most brain segments. Neurons of these ganglia become the afferent or sensory neurons of the PNS. Other neural crest cells become the pigment cells of the skin or contribute to the formation of the meninges, many structures of the face, and the peripheral ganglion cells of the autonomic nervous system, including those of the adrenal cortex.

During development, the more rostral portions of the embryonic neural tube—approximately 10 segments—undergo extensive modification and enlargement to form the brain (Fig. 49-10). In the early embryo, 3 swellings, or primary vesicles, develop, subdividing these 10 segments into the prosencephalon, or forebrain, containing the first 2 segments; the mesencephalon, or midbrain, which develops from segment 3; and the rhombencephalon, or hindbrain, which develops from segments 4 to 10.

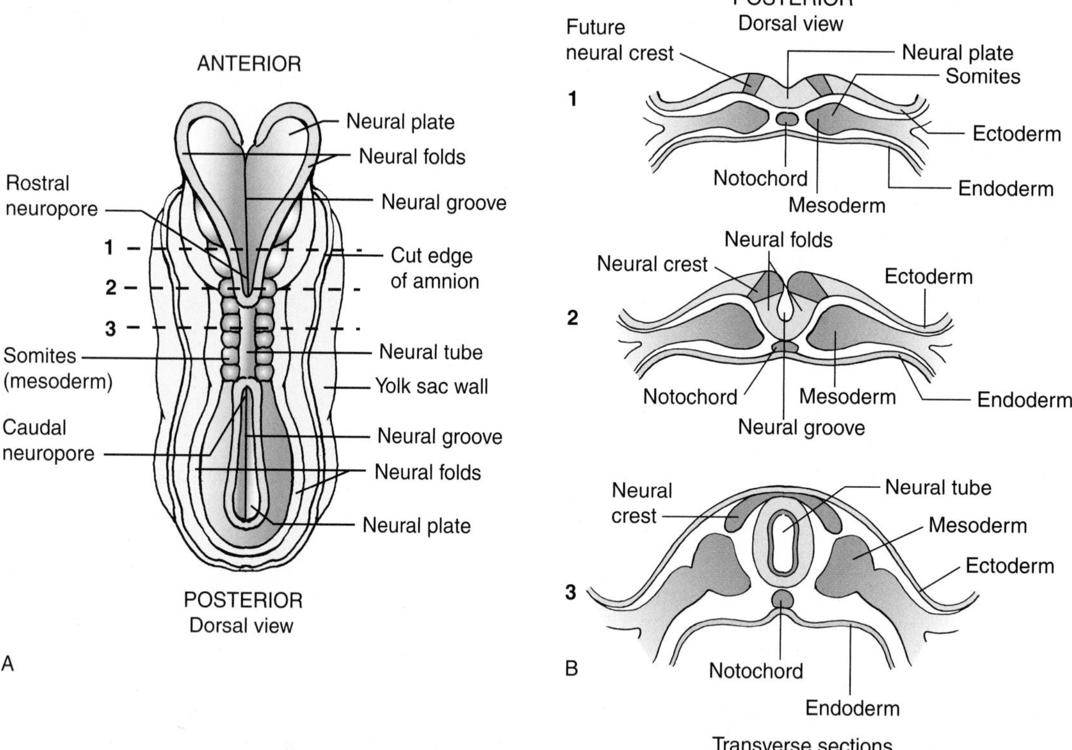

FIGURE 49-9 Folding of the neural tube. (**A**) Dorsal view of a six somite embryo (22–23 days) showing the neural folds, groove, and the fused neural tube. The anterior neuropore closes at about day 26 and the posterior neuropore at about day 28. (**B**) Three cross-sections taken at the levels indicated in (**A**). The sections indicate where the neural tube is just beginning to form.

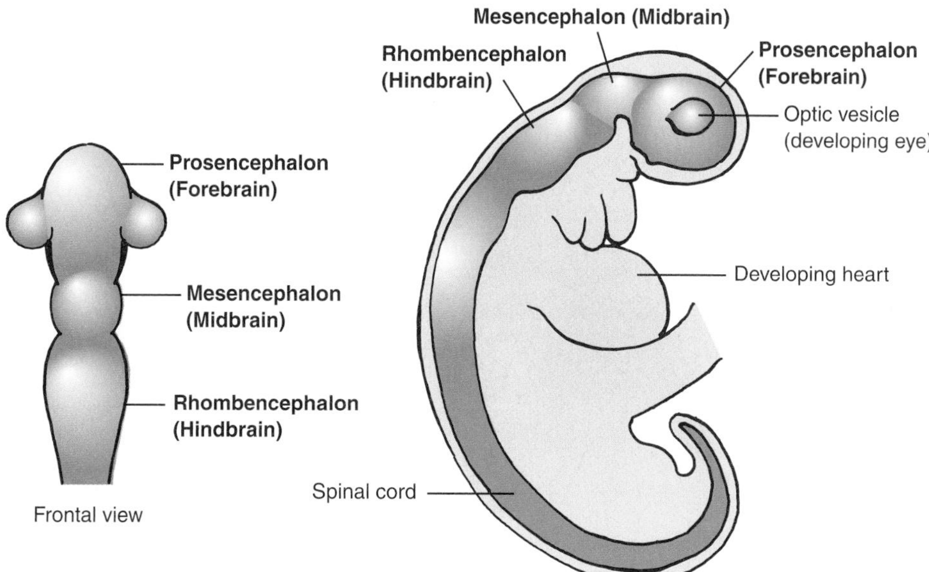

FIGURE 49-10 A lateral and frontal view of 5-week-old embryo showing the brain vesicles and three embryonic divisions of the brain and brain stem.

The brain stem is formed from modifications of the 10 rostral segments of the wall of the neural tube. In the prosencephalon or forebrain, two pairs of lateral outpouchings develop: the optic cup, which becomes the optic nerve and retina, and the telencephalic vesicles, which become the cerebral hemispheres. Within the prosencephalon, the hollow central canal expands to become enlarged CSF-filled cavities, the first and second (lateral) ventricles. The remaining diencephalic portion of the neural tube develops into the thalamus and hypothalamus. The neurohypophysis (posterior pituitary) grows as a midline ventral outgrowth at the junctions of segments 1 and 2. A dorsal outgrowth, the pineal body, develops between segments 2 and 3.

All brain segments, except segment 2, retain some portion of the basic segmental organization of the nervous system. The evolutionary development of the brain is reflected in the cranial and upper cervical paired segmental nerves. This reflects the original pattern of a segmented neural tube, each segment of which has multiple paired branches containing a grouping of component axons. One segment would have paired branches to body muscles and another set to visceral structures, and so on. The classic pattern of spinal nerve organization, which consists of a pair of dorsal and a pair of ventral roots, is a later evolutionary development that has not occurred in the cranial nerves. Consequently, the cranial nerves, which are arbitrarily numbered 1 through 12, retain the ancient pattern, with more than one cranial nerve branching from a single segment. The truly segmental nerve pattern of the cranial nerves is altered because all branches from segment 2 and most of the branches from segment 1 are missing. Cranial nerve II, also called the *optic nerve,* is not a segmental nerve. It is a brain tract connecting the retina (modified brain) with the first forebrain segment from which it developed.

Soma and Viscera. All body tissues and organs have developed from the three embryonic layers (*i.e.,* endoderm, ectoderm, and mesoderm) that were present during the third week of embryonic life. The body is organized into the soma and viscera (Fig. 49-11). The *soma,* or body wall, includes all of the structures derived from the embryonic ectoderm, such as the epidermis of the skin and the CNS. Mesodermal connective tissues of the soma include the dermis of the skin, skeletal muscle, bone, and outer lining of the body cavity (*i.e.,* parietal pleura and peritoneum). The nervous system innervates all somatic structures plus the internal structures making up the viscera. *Viscera* include the great vessels derived from the intermediate mesoderm, the urinary system, and the gonadal structures; it also includes the inner lining of the body cavities, such as the visceral pleura and peritoneum, and the mesodermal tissues that surround the endoderm-lined gut and its derivative organs (*e.g.,* lungs, liver, pancreas).

SEGMENTAL ORGANIZATION

The early pattern of segmental development is presented as a framework for understanding the nervous system. Developmentally, the basic organizational pattern of the body is that of a longitudinal series of segments, each repeating the same fundamental pattern (Fig. 49-12). Although the early muscular, skeletal, vascular, and excretory systems and the nerves that supply the somatic and visceral structures have the same segmental pattern, it is the nervous system that most clearly retains this organization in postnatal life. The CNS and its associated peripheral nerves consist of approximately 43 segments, 33 of which form the spinal cord and spinal nerves, and 10 of which form the brain and its cranial nerves.

Each segment of the CNS is accompanied by bilateral pairs of bundled nerve fibers, or roots—a ventral pair and a dorsal pair. The paired dorsal roots connect a pair of dorsal root ganglia and their corresponding CNS segment. The dorsal root ganglia contain many afferent nerve cell bodies, each having two axon-like processes—one that ends in

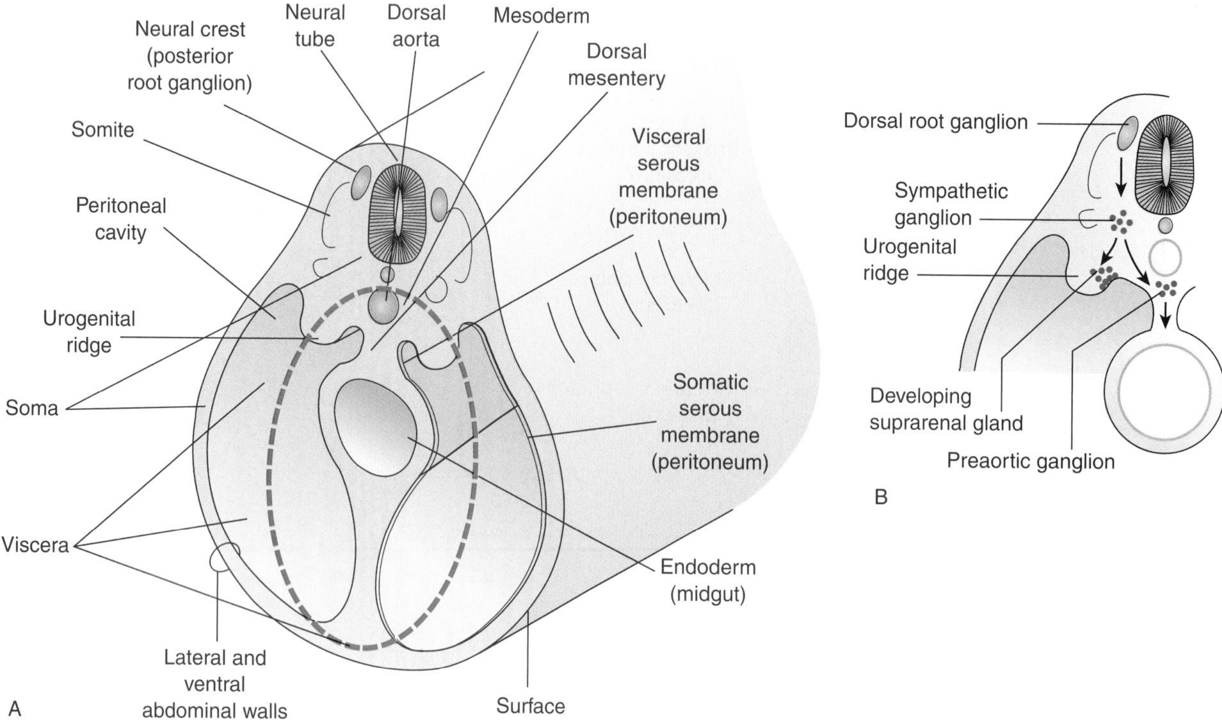

FIGURE 49-11 (**A**) Cross-section of a human embryo, illustrating the development of the somatic and visceral structures. (**B**) The derivatives of the neural crest: the dorsal root ganglia, sympathetic trunk ganglia, and preaortic ganglia, as well as the adrenal medulla and the enteric or organ plexus.

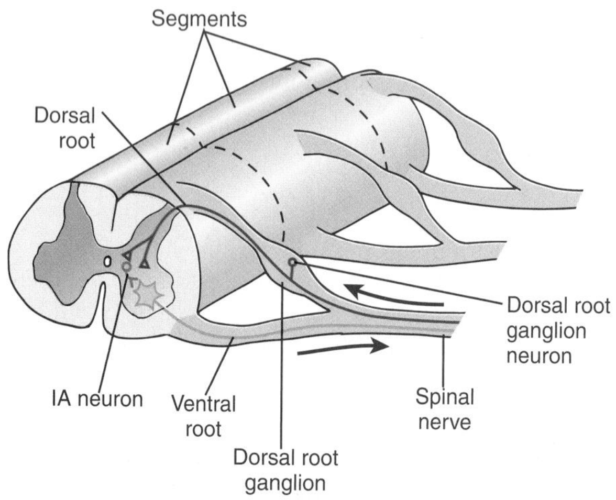

FIGURE 49-12 In this diagram of three segments of the spinal cord, three dorsal roots enter the dorsal lateral surface of the cord, and three ventral roots exit. The dorsal root ganglion contains dorsal root ganglion cells, whose axons bifurcate: one process enters the spinal cord in the dorsal root, and the other extends peripherally to supply the skin and muscle of the body. The ventral root is formed by axons from motoneurons in the spinal cord. (Adapted from Conn P.M. [1995]. *Neuroscience in medicine* [p. 199]. Philadelphia: J.B. Lippincott)

a peripheral receptor and the other that enters the central neural segment. These axon-like processes that enter the central neural segment communicate with neurons called *input association* (IA) *neurons*. Somatic afferent (SA) neurons transmit information from the soma to somatic IA (SIA) neurons, and visceral afferent (VA) neurons transmit information from the viscera to visceral IA (VIA) neurons. The paired ventral roots of each segment are bundles of axons that provide efferent output to effector sites such as the muscles and glandular cells of the body segment.

On cross-section, the hollow embryonic neural tube can be divided into a central canal, or ventricle, containing CSF, and the wall of the tube. The latter develops into an inner gray cellular portion, which is functionally divided into longitudinal columns of neurons called the *cell columns*. These cell columns contain nerve cell bodies surrounded by a superficial white matter region containing the longitudinal tract systems of the CNS. These tract systems are composed of many nerve cell processes. The dorsal half of the gray matter in the spinal cord is called the *dorsal horn*. It contains sensory IA neurons that receive afferent information from the dorsal roots. The ventral portion, or ventral horn, contains efferent neurons that communicate by way of the ventral roots with effector cells of the body segment. Many CNS neurons develop axons that grow longitudinally as tract systems that communicate between neighboring and distal segments of the neural tube.

Cell Columns

The organizational structure of the nervous system can be best explained and simplified as a pattern in which functionally specific PNS and CNS neurons are repeated as parallel cell columns running lengthwise along the nervous system. In this organizational pattern, afferent neurons, dorsal horn cells, and ventral horn cells are organized as a bilateral series of 11 cell columns. A box of 22 colored beverage straws can be used as a model to represent the cell columns. In this model, the right and left sides are each represented in mirror fashion by a set of 11 colored straws. If these straws were cut crosswise (equivalent to a transverse section through the nervous system) at several places along their length, the spatial relations among the different colored straws would be repeated in each section.

The cell columns on each side can be further grouped according to their location in the PNS: four in the dorsal ganglia that contain sensory neurons; four in the dorsal horn containing sensory IA neurons; and three in the ventral horn that contain motoneurons (Fig. 49-13A). Each column of dorsal root ganglia projects to its particular column of IA neurons in the dorsal horn. IA neurons distribute afferent information to local reflex circuitry and to more rostral and elaborate segments of the CNS. The ventral horns contain output association (OA) neurons and LMNs. These LMNs provide the final circuitry for organizing efferent nerve activity.

Between the IA neurons and the OA neurons are networks of small internuncial neurons (interneurons) arranged in complex circuits. Internuncial neurons provide the discreteness, appropriateness, and intelligence of responses to stimuli. Most of the billions of CNS cells in the spinal cord and brain gray matter are internuncial neurons.

Dorsal Horn Cell Columns. Four columns of afferent (sensory) neurons in the dorsal root ganglia directly innervate four corresponding columns of IA neurons in the dorsal horn. These columns are categorized as special and general afferents: special somatic afferent, general somatic afferent, special visceral afferent, and general visceral afferent.

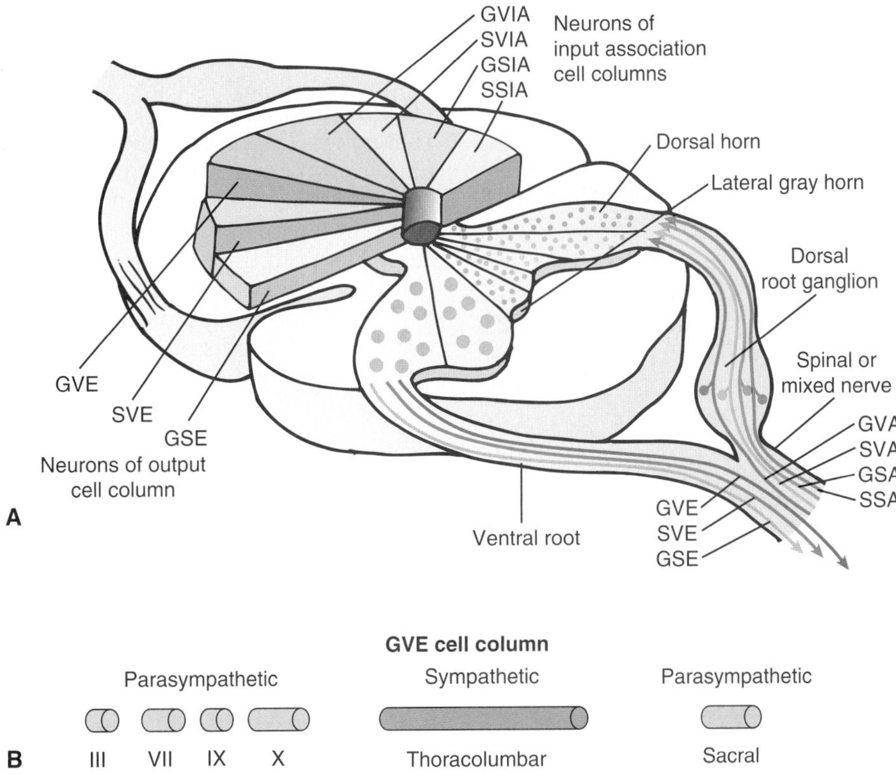

FIGURE 49-13 **(A)** Cell columns of the central nervous system. The cell columns in the dorsal horn contain input association (IA) neurons for the general visceral afferent (GVA), special visceral afferent (SVA), special sensory afferent (SSA), and general somatic afferent (GSA) neurons with cell bodies in the dorsal root ganglion. The cell columns in the ventral horn contain the general visceral efferent (GVE), pharyngeal efferent (PE), and general somite efferent (GSE) neurons and their output association (OA) neurons. **(B)** Schematic of the GVE cell column showing both parasympathetic and sympathetic components. The column is not continuous but is interrupted in the brain stem because only the nuclei of cranial nerves III, VII, IX, and X contain preganglionic parasympathetic neurons. The column again is interrupted until levels T1 to L1 or L2 where the preganglionic neurons of the sympathetic portion are found in the lateral horn of the spinal cord. Another gap is evident until the sacral portion of the parasympathetic nervous system.

Special somatic afferent fibers are concerned with internal sensory information such as joint and tendon sensation (*i.e.*, proprioception). Neurons in the special SIA column cells relay their information to local reflexes concerned with posture and movement. These neurons also relay information to the cerebellum, contributing to coordination of movement, and to the forebrain, contributing to experience. Afferents innervating the labyrinth and derived auditory end organs of the inner ear also belong to the special somatic afferent category.

General somatic afferents innervate the skin and other somatic structures and respond to stimuli such as those that produce pressure or pain. General SIA column cells relay the sensory information to protective and other reflex circuits and project the information to the forebrain, where it is perceived as painful, warm, cold, and the like.

Special visceral afferent cells innervate specialized gut-related receptors, such as the taste buds and receptors of the olfactory mucosa. Their central processes communicate with special VIA column neurons that project to reflex circuits producing salivation, chewing, swallowing, and other responses. Forebrain projection fibers from these association cells provide sensations of taste and smell.

General visceral afferent neurons innervate visceral structures such as the gastrointestinal tract, urinary bladder, and heart and great vessels; they project to the general VIA column, which relays information to vital reflex circuits in the brain and sends information to the forebrain regarding visceral sensations such as stomach fullness, bladder pressure, and sexual experience.

Ventral Horn Cell Columns. The ventral horn contains three longitudinal cell columns: general visceral efferent, pharyngeal efferent, and general somatic efferent. Each of these cell columns contains OA and efferent neurons. The OA neurons coordinate and integrate the function of the efferent motoneuron cells of its column.

General visceral efferent (GVE) neurons transmit the efferent output of the autonomic nervous system (ANS) and are called *preganglionic neurons*. These neurons are structurally and functionally divided into either the sympathetic or the parasympathetic nervous systems. Their axons project through the segmental ventral roots to innervate smooth and cardiac muscle and glandular cells of the body, most of which are in the viscera. In the viscera, three additional neural crest–derived cell columns are present on each side of the body. These become the postganglionic neurons of the autonomic nervous system. In the sympathetic nervous system, the columns are represented by paravertebral ganglia (sympathetic chain) and the prevertebral series of ganglia (*e.g.*, celiac ganglia) associated with the dorsal aorta (to be discussed). For the parasympathetic system, these become the enteric plexus in the wall of the gut-derived organs and a series of ganglia in the head. Figure 49-13B is a schematic of the potential GVE cell column as it exists throughout the brain stem and spinal cord. This figure shows the four clusters of neurons in the brain stem that represent the parasympathetic outputs of cranial nerves III, VII, IX, and X. Also indicated is the continuation of the GVE cell column as the thoracolumbar portion of the sympathetic nervous system as well as the sacral portion of the parasympathetic nervous system.

Pharyngeal efferent neurons innervate branchial arch skeletal muscles: the muscles of mastication, of facial expression, and of the pharynx and larynx. Pharyngeal efferent neurons also innervate muscles responsible for moving the head.

The *general somatic efferent* neurons supply somite-derived muscles of the body and head, which include the skeletal muscles of the body, limbs, tongue, and extrinsic eye muscles. These efferent neurons transmit the commands of the CNS to peripheral effectors, the skeletal muscles. They are the "final common pathway neurons" in the sequence leading to motor activity. They are often called *LMNs* because they are under the control of higher levels of the CNS, including precise control by upper motoneurons (UMNs).

Peripheral Nerves. With rare exceptions, peripheral nerves, including the cranial nerves, contain afferent and efferent processes of more than one of the four afferent and three efferent cell columns. This provides the basis for assessing the function of any peripheral nerve. The functional components of each of the cranial nerves and spinal nerve roots are presented in Table 49-1.

Longitudinal Tracts

The gray matter of the cell columns in the CNS is surrounded by bundles of myelinated axons (*i.e.*, white matter) and unmyelinated axons that travel longitudinally along the length of the neural axis. This white matter can be divided into three layers: an inner, a middle, and an outer layer (Fig. 49-14). The inner layer, or *archilayer*, contains short fibers that project for a maximum of approximately five segments before reentering the gray matter. Fibers in the middle layer, or *paleolayer*, project to six or more segments. Archilayer and paleolayer fibers have many branches, or collaterals, that enter the gray matter of intervening segments. In the outer layer, or *neolayer*, are found large-diameter axons that can travel the entire length of the nervous system (Table 49-2). *Suprasegmental* is a term that refers to higher levels of the CNS, such as the brain stem and cerebrum and structures above a given CNS segment. Paleolayer and neolayer fibers have suprasegmental projections.

The longitudinal layers are arranged in bundles, or fiber tracts, that contain axons that have the same destination, origin, and function (Fig. 49-15). These longitudinal tracts are named systematically to reflect their origin and destination; the origin is named first, and the destination is named second. For example, the spinothalamic tract originates in the spinal cord and terminates in the thalamus. The corticospinal tract originates in the cerebral cortex and ends in the spinal cord.

The Inner Layer. Lying immediately superficial to the deep gray matter, the inner layer of white matter contains the axons of neurons that connect neighboring segments of the nervous system. Axons of this layer permit the pool of motoneurons of several segments to work together as a functional unit. They also allow the afferent neurons of

TABLE 49-1 The Segmental Nerves and Their Components

Segment and Nerve	Component	Innervation	Function
1. Forebrain			
I. Olfactory	SVA	Receptors in olfactory mucosa	Reflexes, olfaction (smell)
2. II. Optic nerve		Optic nerve and retina (part of brain system, not a peripheral nerve)	
3. Midbrain			
V. Trigeminal (V_1) ophthalmic division	SSA	Muscles: upper face: forehead, upper lid	Facial expression, proprioception
	GSA	Skin, subcutaneous tissue; conjunctiva; frontal/ethmoid sinuses	Somesthesia Reflexes (blink)
III. Oculomotor	GVE	Iris sphincter Ciliary muscle	Pupillary constriction Accommodation
	GSE	Extrinsic eye muscles	Eye movement, lid movement
4. Pons			
V. Trigeminal (V_2) maxillary division	SSA	Muscles: facial expression	Proprioception Reflexes (sneeze), somesthesia
	GSA	Skin, oral mucosa, upper teeth, hard palate, maxillary sinus	
V. Trigeminal (V_3) mandibular division	SSA	Lower jaw, muscles: mastication	Proprioception, jaw jerk
	GSA	Skin, mucosa, teeth, anterior ⅔ of tongue	Reflexes, somesthesia
	PE	Muscles: mastication tensor tympani tensor veli palatini	Mastication: speech Protects ear from loud sound Tenses soft palate
IV. Trochlear	GSE	Extrinsic eye muscle	Moves eye down and in
5. Caudal Pons			
VIII. Vestibular, cochlear (vestibulocochlear)	SSA	Vestibular end organs Organ of Corti	Reflexes, sense of head position Reflexes, hearing
VII. Facial nerve, intermedius portion	GSA	External auditory meatus	Somesthesia
	GVA	Nasopharynx	Gag reflex: sensation
	SVA	Taste buds of anterior ⅔ of tongue	Reflexes: gustation (taste)
	GVE	Nasopharynx Lacrimal, sublingual, submandibular glands	Mucous secretion, reflexes Lacrimation, salivation
Facial nerve	PE	Muscles: facial expression, stapedius	Facial expression Protects ear from loud sounds
VI. Abducens	GSE	Extrinsic eye muscle	Lateral eye deviation
6. Middle Medulla			
IX. Glossopharyngeal	SSA	Stylopharyngeus muscle	Proprioception
	GSA	Posterior external ear	Somesthesia
	SVA	Taste buds of posterior ⅓ of tongue	Gustation (taste)
	GVA	Oral pharynx	Gag reflex: sensation
	GVE	Parotid gland; pharyngeal mucosa	Salivary reflex: mucous secretion
	PE	Stylopharyngeus muscle	Assists swallowing
7,8,9,10. Caudal Medulla			
X. Vagus	SSA	Muscles: pharynx, larynx	Proprioception
	GSA	Posterior external ear	Somesthesia
	SVA	Taste buds, pharynx, larynx	Reflexes, gustation
	GVA	Visceral organs (esophagus to midtransverse colon, liver, pancreas, heart, lungs)	Reflexes, sensation
	GVE	Visceral organs as above	Parasympathetic efferent
	PE	Muscles: pharynx, larynx	Swallowing, phonation, emesis
XIII. Hypoglossal	GSE	Muscles of tongue	Tongue movement, reflexes
Spinal Segments			
C1–C4 Upper Cervical XI. Spinal accessory nerve	PE	Muscles: sternocleidomastoid, trapezius	Head, shoulder movement
Spinal nerves	SSA	Muscles of neck	Proprioception, DTRs
	GSA	Neck, back of head	Somesthesia
	GSE	Neck muscles	Head, shoulder movement

(continued)

TABLE 49-1 The Segmental Nerves and Their Components (Continued)

Segment and Nerve	Component	Innervation	Function
C5–C8 Lower Cervical	SSA	Upper limb muscles	Proprioception, DTRs
	GSA	Upper limbs	Reflexes, somesthesia
	GSE	Upper limb muscles	Movement, posture
T1–L2 Thoracic, Upper Lumbar	SSA	Muscles: trunk, abdominal wall	Proprioception
	GSA	Trunk, abdominal wall	Reflexes, somesthesia
	GVA	All of viscera	Reflexes and sensation
	GVE	All of viscera	Sympathetic reflexes, vasomotor control, sweating, piloerection
	GSE	Muscles: trunk, abdominal wall, back	Movement, posture, respiration
L2–S1 Lower Lumbar, Upper Sacral	SSA	Lower limb muscles	Proprioception, DTRs
	GSA	Lower trunk, limbs, back	Reflexes, somesthesia
	GSE	Muscles: trunk, lower limbs, back	Movement, posture
S2–S4 Lower Sacral	SSA	Muscles: pelvis, perineum	Proprioception
	GSA	Pelvis, genitalia	Reflexes, somesthesia
	GVA	Hindgut, bladder, uterus	Reflexes, sensation
	GVE	Hindgut, visceral organs	Visceral reflexes, defecation, urination, erection
S5–Co2 Lower Sacral, Coccygeal	SSA	Perineal muscles	Proprioception
	GSA	Lower sacrum, anus	Reflexes, somesthesia
	GSE	Perineal muscles	Reflexes, posture

Afferent (sensory) components: SSA, special somatic afferent; GSA, general somatic afferent; SVA, special visceral afferent; GVA, general visceral afferent.
Efferent (motor) components: GVE, general visceral efferent (autonomic nervous system); PE, pharyngeal efferent; GSE, general somatic efferent; DTRs, deep tendon reflexes.

one segment to trigger reflexes that activate motor units in neighboring and in the same segments. As to evolutionary development, this is the oldest of the three layers, and it is sometimes called the *archilayer*. It is the first of the longitudinal layers to become functional, and its circuitry may be limited to reflex types of movements, including reflex movements of the fetus (*i.e.,* quickening) that begin during the fifth month of intrauterine life.

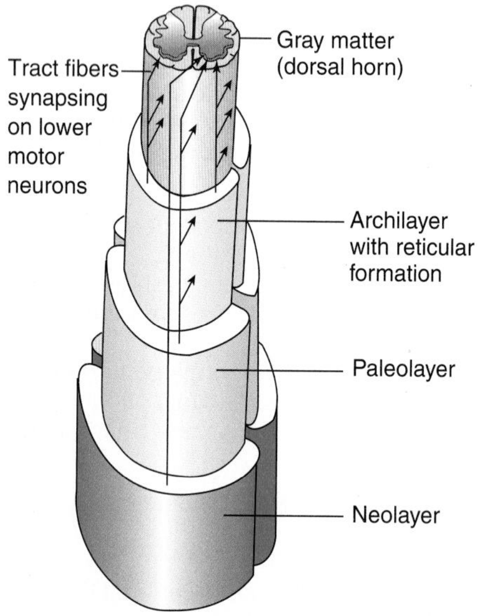

FIGURE 49-14 The three concentric subdivisions of the tract systems of the white matter. Migration of neurons into the archilayer converts it into the reticular formation of the white matter.

The inner layer of the white matter differs from the other two layers in one important aspect. Many neurons in the embryonic gray matter migrate out into this layer, resulting in a rich mixture of neurons and local fibers called the *reticular formation*. The circuitry of most reflexes is contained in the reticular formation. In the brain stem, the reticular formation becomes quite large and contains major portions of vital reflexes, such as those controlling respiration, cardiovascular function, swallowing, and vomiting. A functional system called the *reticular activating system* operates in the lateral portions of the reticular formation of the medulla, pons, and especially the midbrain. Information derived from all sensory modalities, including those of the somesthetic, auditory, visual, and visceral afferent nerves, bombards the neurons of this system.

The reticular activating system has descending and ascending portions. Descending portions communicate with all spinal segmental levels through paleolevel reticulospinal tracts and serve to facilitate many cord-level reflexes. For example, they speed reaction time and stabilize postural reflexes. The ascending portion accelerates brain activity, particularly thalamic and cortical activity. This is reflected by the appearance of awake brain-wave patterns. Sudden stimuli result in protective and attentive postures and increased awareness.

The Middle Layer. The middle layer of the white matter contains most of the major fiber tract systems required for

TABLE 49-2 Characteristics of the Concentric Subdivisions of the Longitudinal Tracts in the White Matter of the Central Nervous System

Characteristics	Archilayer Tracts	Paleolayer Tracts	Neolayer Tracts
Segmental span	Intersegmental (<5 segments)	Suprasegmental (≥5 segments)	Suprasegmental
Number of synapses	Multisynaptic	Multisynaptic but fewer than archilayer tracts	Monosynaptic with target structures
Conduction velocity	Very slow	Fast	Fastest
Examples of functional systems	Flexor withdrawal reflex circuitry	Spinothalamic tracts	Corticospinal tracts

sensation and movement. It contains the ascending spinoreticular and spinothalamic tracts. This layer consists of larger-diameter and longer suprasegmental fibers, which ascend to the brain stem and are largely functional at birth. These tracts are quite old from an evolutionary standpoint, and as such, this layer is sometimes called the *paleolayer.* It facilitates many primitive functions, such as the auditory startle reflex, which occurs in response to loud noises. This reflex consists of turning the head and body toward the sound, dilating the pupils of the eyes, catching of the breath, and quickening of the pulse.

The Outer Layer. The outer layer of the tract systems is the newest of the three layers with respect to evolutionary development, and it is sometimes called the *neolayer.* It becomes functional approximately the second year of life, and it includes the pathways needed for bladder training. Myelination of these suprasegmental tracts, which include many pathways required for delicate and highly coordinated skills, is not complete until approximately the fifth year of life. This includes the development of tracts needed for fine manipulative skills, such as the finger–thumb coordination required for using tools and the toe movements needed for acrobatics. Neolayer tracts are the most recently evolved systems and, being more superficial on the brain and spinal cord, are the most vulnerable to injury. When neolayer tracts are damaged, the paleolayer and archilayer tracts often remain functional, and rehabilitation methods can result in effective use of the older systems. Delicacy and refinement may be lost, but basic function remains. For example, when the corticospinal system, an important neolayer system that permits the fine manipulative control required for writing, is damaged, the remaining paleolayer systems, if intact, permit the grasping and holding of objects. The hand can still be used to perform its basic function, but the individual manipulation of the fingers is permanently lost.

Collateral Communication Pathways. Axons in the archilayer and paleolayer characteristically possess many

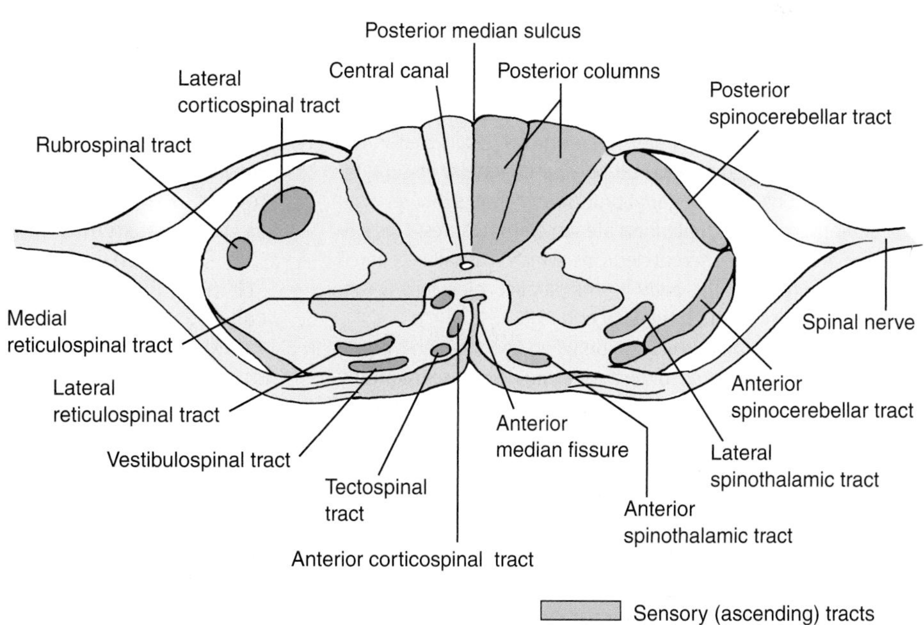

FIGURE 49-15 Transverse section of the spinal cord showing selected sensory and motor tracts. The tracts are bilateral but are only indicated on one half of the cord.

collateral branches that move into the gray cell columns or synapse with fibers of the reticular formation as the axon passes each succeeding CNS segment. Should a major axon be destroyed at some point along its course, these collaterals provide multisynaptic alternative pathways that bypass the local damage. Neolayer tracts do not possess these collaterals but instead project mainly to the target neurons with which they communicate. Because of this, damage to the neolayer tracts causes permanent loss of function. Damage to the archilayer or paleolayer systems is usually followed by a slow return of function, presumably through the collateral connections.

In summary, development of the nervous system can be traced far back into evolutionary history. The CNS develops from the ectoderm of the early embryo by formation of a hollow tube that closes along its longitudinal axis and sinks below the surface. This hollow tube forms the ventricles of the brain and spinal canal, and the sidewall develops to form the brain stem and spinal cord. The brain stem and spinal cord are subdivided into the dorsal horn, which contains neurons that receive and process incoming or afferent information, and the ventral horn, which contains efferent motoneurons that handle the final stages of output processing. The PNS develops from ectodermal cells called *neural crest cells* that migrate away from the dorsal surface of the forming neural tube.

Throughout life, the organization of the nervous system retains many patterns established during early embryonic life. This segmental pattern of early embryonic development is retained in the fully developed nervous system. Each of the 43 or more body segments is connected to corresponding CNS or neural tube segments by segmental afferent and efferent neurons. Afferent neuronal processes enter the CNS through the dorsal root ganglia and the dorsal roots. Afferent neurons of the dorsal root ganglia are of four types: general somatic afferent, special somatic afferent, general visceral afferent, and special visceral afferent. Each of these afferent neurons synapses with its appropriate IA neurons in the cell columns of the dorsal horn (*e.g.,* general somatic afferents synapse with neurons in the general somatic afferent IA cell column). Efferent fibers from motoneurons in the ventral horn exit the CNS in the ventral roots. General somatic efferent neurons are LMNs that innervate somite-derived skeletal muscles, and general visceral efferent neurons are preganglionic fibers that synapse with postganglionic fibers that innervate visceral structures. This pattern of afferent and efferent neurons, which is usually repeated in each segment of the body, forms parallel cell columns running lengthwise through the CNS and PNS.

Longitudinal communication between CNS segments is provided by neurons that send the axons into nearby segments by means of the innermost layer of the white matter, the ancient archilayer system of fibers. These cells provide coordination between neighboring segments. Neurons have invaded this layer, and the mix of these cells and axons is called the *reticular formation.* The reticular formation is the location of many important reflex circuits of the spinal cord brain stem. Paleolayer tracts, located outside this layer, provide the longitudinal communication between more distant segments of the nervous system; this layer includes most of the important ascending and descending tracts. The recently evolved neolayer systems, which become functional during infancy and childhood, travel in the outer layer of the white matter and provide the means for very delicate and discriminative function. The outer position of the neolayer tracts and their lack of collateral and redundant pathways make them the most vulnerable to injury.

The Spinal Cord

After completing this section of the chapter, you should be able to meet the following objectives:

- Describe the longitudinal and transverse structures of the spinal cord
- Trace an afferent and efferent neuron from its site in the periphery through its entrance into or exit from the spinal cord
- Explain muscle tone and posture using the myotatic or stretch reflex

In the adult, the spinal cord is found in the upper two thirds of the spinal canal of the vertebral column (Fig. 49-16). It extends from the foramen magnum at the base of the skull to a cone-shaped termination, the conus medullaris, usually at the level of the first or second lumbar vertebra (L1 or L2) in the adult. The dorsal and ventral roots of the more caudal portions of the cord elongate during development and angle downward from the cord, forming what is called the *cauda equina* (from the Latin for "horse's tail"). The filum terminale, which is composed of nonneural tissues and the pia mater, continues caudally and attaches to the second sacral vertebra (S2).

The spinal cord is somewhat oval on transverse section. Internally, the gray matter has the appearance of a butterfly or the letter "H" on cross-section (see Fig. 49-16). Some neurons that make up the gray matter of the cord have processes or axons that leave the cord, enter the peripheral nerves, and supply tissues such as autonomic ganglia or skeletal muscles. The white matter of the cord that surrounds the gray matter contains nerve fiber tracts or descending axons that transmit information between segments of the cord or from higher levels of the CNS, such as the brain stem or cerebrum.

The extensions of the gray matter that form the letter "H" are called the *horns.* Those that extend posteriorly are called the *dorsal horns,* and those that extend anteriorly are called the *ventral horns.* Dorsal horns contain IA neurons that receive afferent impulses through the dorsal roots and other connecting neurons. Ventral horns contain OA neurons and the efferent LMNs that leave the cord through the ventral roots.

The spinal cord contains many small internuncial neurons that surround the efferent motoneurons and synapse with the cell body or dendrites of the efferent cells. Action potentials of these internuncial neurons exert excitatory or inhibitory effects on the LMNs. Although some CNS systems communicate directly with the LMNs,

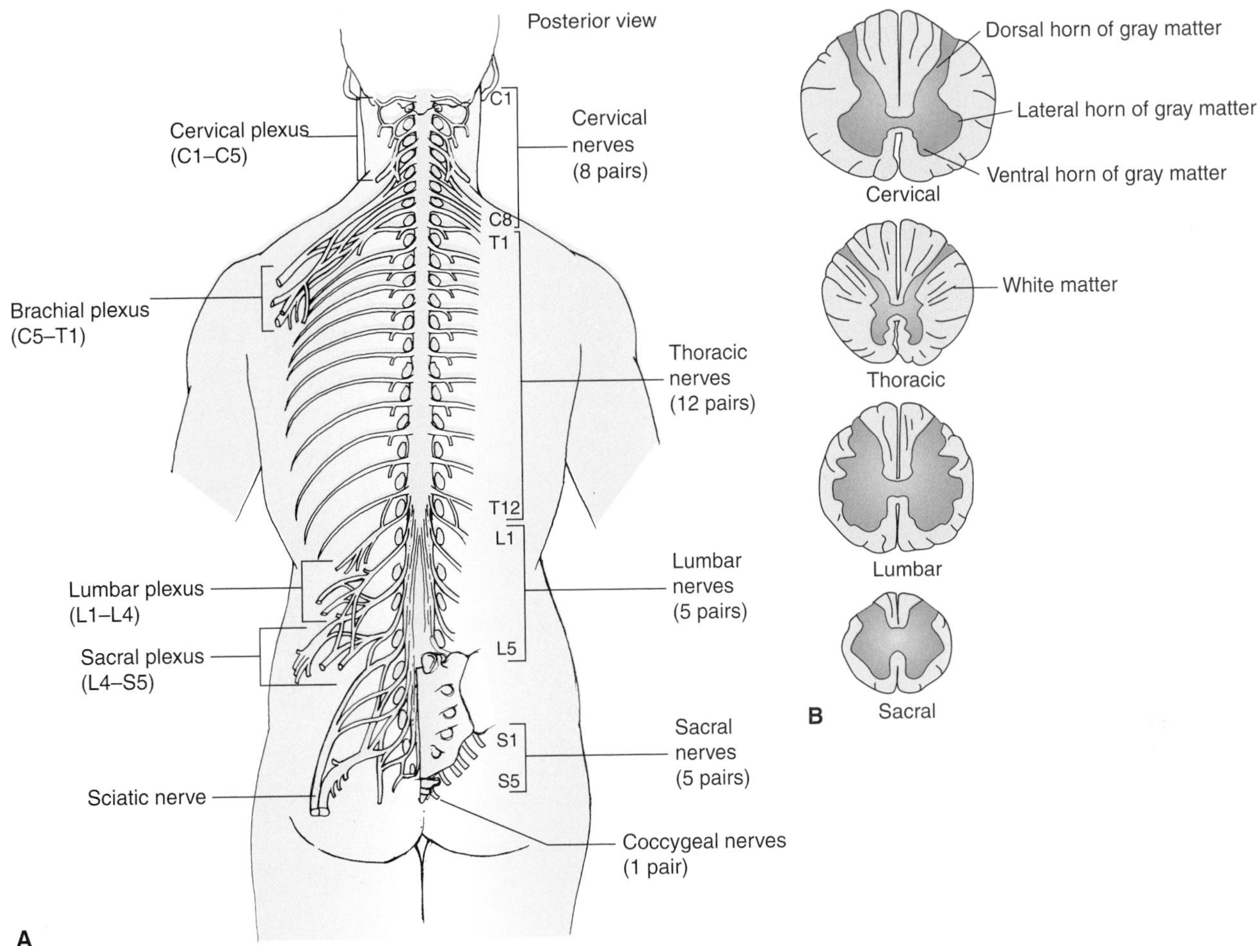

FIGURE 49-16 (**A**) Dorsal view of the spinal cord including portions of the major spinal nerves and some of the components of the major nerve plexuses. (**B**) Cross-sectional views of the spinal cord, showing regional variations in gray matter and increasing white matter as the cord ascends.

most LMN activity is controlled by systems communicating through excitatory or inhibitory internuncial neurons. These internuncial neurons represent the final stage of communication between elaborate CNS neuronal circuits and the skeletal muscle cells of the motor unit.

The central portion of the cord, which connects the dorsal and ventral horns, is called the *intermediate gray matter*. The intermediate gray matter surrounds the central canal. In the thoracic area, the small, slender projections that emerge from the intermediate gray matter are called the *intermediolateral columns* of the horns. These columns contain the visceral OA neurons and the efferent neurons of the sympathetic nervous system.

The gray matter is proportional to how much tissue is innervated by a given segment of the cord (see Fig. 49-16). Larger amounts of gray matter are present in the lower lumbar and upper sacral segments, which supply the lower extremities, and in the fifth cervical segment to the first thoracic segment, which supply the upper limbs. The white matter in the spinal cord also increases progressively toward the brain because ever more ascending fibers are added and the number of descending axons is greater.

The spinal cord and the dorsal and ventral roots are covered by a connective tissue sheath, the pia mater, which also contains the blood vessels that supply the white and gray matter of the cord (Fig. 49-17). On the lateral sides of the spinal cord, extensions of the pia mater, the denticulate ligaments, attach the sides of the spinal cord to the bony walls of the spinal canal. Thus, the cord is suspended by both the denticulate ligaments and the segmental nerves. A fat- and vessel-filled epidural space intervenes between the spinal dura mater and the inner wall of the spinal canal. Each vertebral body has two pedicles that extend posteriorly and support the laterally oriented transverse processes of the neural laminae, which arch medially and fuse to continue as the spinal processes.

Fibrocartilaginous discs fill the spaces between the vertebral bodies and are stabilized with tough ligaments. A gap, the intervertebral foramen, occurs between each two succeeding pedicles, allowing for the exit of the segmental nerves and passage of blood vessels. The spinal cord lies in the protective confines of this series of concentric flexible tissue and body sheaths. Supporting structures of the spinal cord are discussed further in Chapter 51.

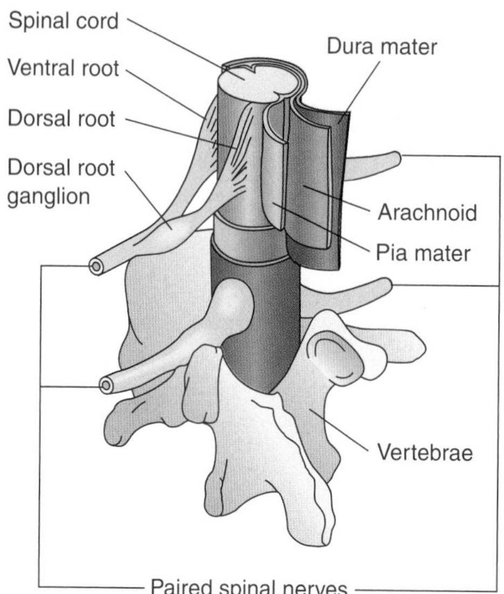

FIGURE 49-17 Spinal cord and meninges.

Early in fetal life, the spinal cord extends the entire length of the vertebral column, and the spinal nerves exit through the intervertebral foramina (openings) near their level of origin. Because the vertebral column and spinal dura grow faster than the spinal cord, a disparity develops between each succeeding cord segment and the exit of its dorsal and ventral nerve roots through the corresponding intervertebral foramina. In the newborn, the cord terminates at vertebral level L2 or L3. In the adult, the cord usually terminates in the inferior border of L1. In addition, the arachnoid and its enclosed subarachnoid space, which is filled with CSF, do not close down on the filum terminale until they reach the second sacral vertebra. This results in the formation of a pocket of CSF, the *dural cisterna spinalis,* which extends from approximately L2 to S2. Because this area contains an abundant supply of CSF and the spinal cord does not extend this far, the area is often used for sampling the CSF. A procedure called a *spinal tap,* or puncture, can be done by inserting a special needle into the dural sac at L3 or L4. The spinal roots, which are covered with pia mater, are in little danger of trauma from the needle used for this purpose.

SPINAL NERVES

The peripheral nerves that carry information to and from the spinal cord are called *spinal nerves.* Usually, 32 or more pairs of spinal nerves are present (*i.e.,* 8 cervical, 12 thoracic, 5 lumbar, 5 sacral, and 2 or more coccygeal); each pair is named for the segment of the spinal cord from which it exits. Because the first cervical spinal nerve exits the spinal cord just above the first cervical vertebra (C1), the nerve is given the number of the bony vertebra just below it. The numbering is changed for all lower levels, however. An extracervical nerve, the C8 nerve, exits above the T1 vertebra, and each subsequent nerve is numbered for the vertebra just above its point of exit (see Fig. 49-18).

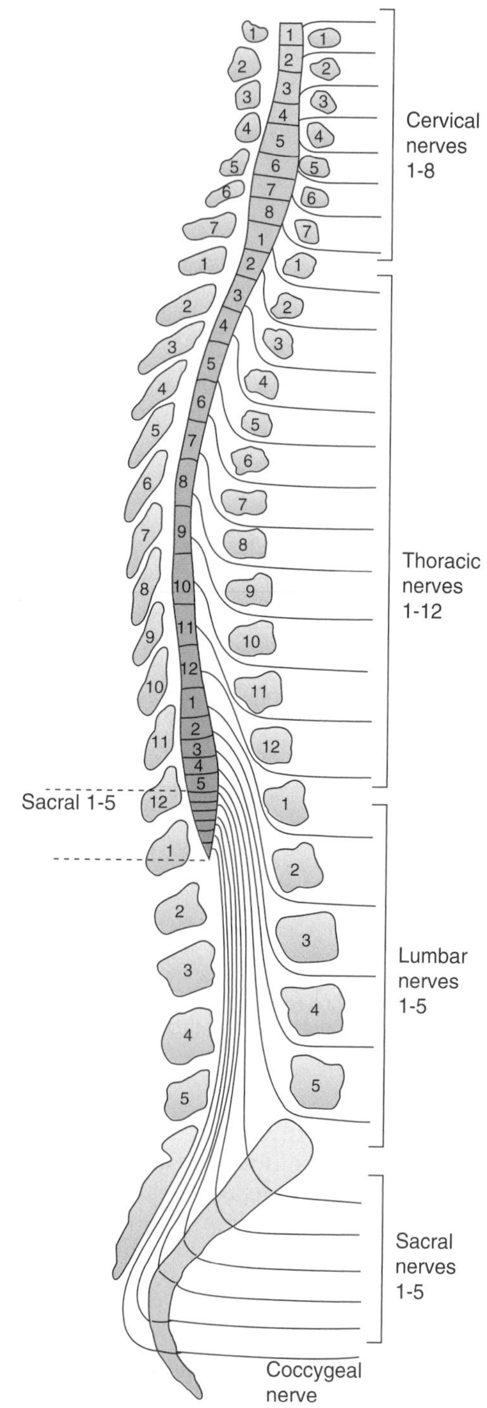

FIGURE 49-18 Relation of segments of the spinal cord and spinal nerves to the vertebral column. (Barr M.L., Kiernan J.A. [1998]. *The human nervous system: An anatomic viewpoint* [5th ed., p. 65]. Philadelphia: J.B. Lippincott)

Each spinal cord segment communicates with its corresponding body segment through the paired segmental spinal nerves (see Fig. 49-12). Each spinal nerve, accompanied by the blood vessels supplying the spinal cord, enters the spinal canal through an intervertebral foramen, where it divides into two branches, or roots. One branch enters the dorsolateral surface of the cord (*i.e.,* dorsal root), carrying the axons of afferent neurons into the CNS. The other branch leaves the ventrolateral surface of the cord (*i.e.,* ventral root), carrying the axons of efferent neurons into the periphery. These two branches or roots fuse at the intervertebral foramen, forming the mixed spinal nerve—"mixed" because it has both afferent and efferent axons.

The observation that afferent fibers travel in the dorsal or posterior root while efferent fibers leave through the ventral root is known as the *Bell-Magendie law*. This observation holds true for all but a few pain and temperature fibers of certain pelvic viscera. In these afferent fibers, the dorsal root ganglia are still in their normal location; however, some of the fibers enter the ventral root instead of the dorsal root. Clinically, this is observed when sectioning of the dorsal roots to alleviate pain will not completely eliminate pelvic pain.

After emerging from the vertebral column, the spinal nerve divides into two branches or *rami* (singular, *ramus*): a small dorsal primary ramus and a larger ventral primary ramus (Fig. 49-19). Thoracic and upper lumbar spinal nerves also produce a third branch, the ramus communicans, which contains sympathetic axons supplying the blood vessels, the genitourinary system, and the gastrointestinal system. The dorsal ramus contains sensory fibers from the skin and motor fibers to muscles of the back. The anterior primary ramus contains motor fibers that innervate the skeletal muscles of the anterior body wall and the legs and arms.

Spinal nerves do not go directly to skin and muscle fibers; instead, they form complicated nerve networks called *plexuses* (see Fig. 49-16). A plexus is a site of intermixing nerve branches. Many spinal nerves enter a plexus and connect with other spinal nerves before exiting from the plexus. Nerves emerging from a plexus form progressively smaller branches that supply the skin and muscles of the various parts of the body. The PNS contains four major plexuses: the cervical plexus, the brachial plexus, the lumbar plexus, and the sacral plexus.

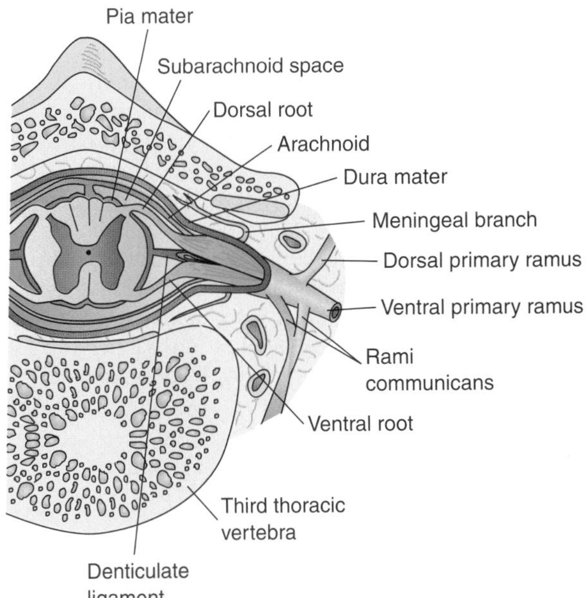

FIGURE 49-19 Cross-section of vertebral column at the level of the third thoracic vertebra, showing the meninges, the spinal cord, and the origin of a spinal nerve and its branches or rami.

SPINAL REFLEXES

A *reflex* is a highly predictable relationship between a stimulus and an elicited motor response. Its anatomic basis consists of an afferent neuron, the connection or synapse with CNS interneurons that communicate with the effector neuron, and the effector neuron that innervates a muscle or organ. Reflexes are essentially "wired in" to the CNS in that normally they are always ready to function; with training, most reflexes can be modulated to become parts of more complicated movements. A reflex may involve neurons in a single cord segment (*i.e.,* segmental reflexes), several or many segments (*i.e.,* intersegmental reflexes), or structures in the brain (*i.e.,* suprasegmental reflexes). Two important types of spinal motor reflexes are discussed in this chapter: the myotatic reflex and the withdrawal reflex.

Myotatic or Stretch Reflex

The myotatic (*myo* from the Greek for "muscle," *tatic* from the Greek for "stretch") or stretch reflex controls muscle tone and helps maintain posture. Specialized sensory nerve terminals in skeletal muscles and tendons relay information on muscle stretch and joint tension to the CNS. This information, which drives postural reflex mechanisms, also is relayed to the thalamus and the sensory cortex and is experienced as *proprioception,* the sense of body movement and position. To provide this information, the muscles and their tendons are supplied with two types of sensory receptors: muscle spindle receptors and Golgi tendon organs (Fig. 49-20). The *muscle spindles* are stretch receptors that are distributed throughout the belly of a muscle and transmit information about muscle length and rate of stretch. The *Golgi tendon organs* are found in muscle tendons and transmit information about muscle tension or force of contraction at the junction of the muscle and the tendon that attaches to bone. A likely role of the tendon organs is to equalize the contractile forces of the separate muscle groups, spreading the load over all the fibers to prevent the local muscle damage that might occur when small numbers of fibers are overloaded.

Essentially all skeletal muscles contain many muscle spindles. The muscle spindles consist of a group of specialized miniature skeletal muscle fibers called *intrafusal fibers* that are encased in a connective tissue capsule and attached to muscle fibers (*i.e.,* extrafusal fibers) of a skeletal muscle (see Fig. 49-20). An afferent Ia sensory neuron, which spirals around the intrafusal fibers, transmits information to the spinal cord. The extrafusal fibers and the intrafusal fibers are innervated by motoneurons that reside in the ventral horns of the spinal cord. Extrafusal fibers are innervated by large alpha motoneurons that produce contraction of the muscle. The intrafusal fibers are innervated by gamma

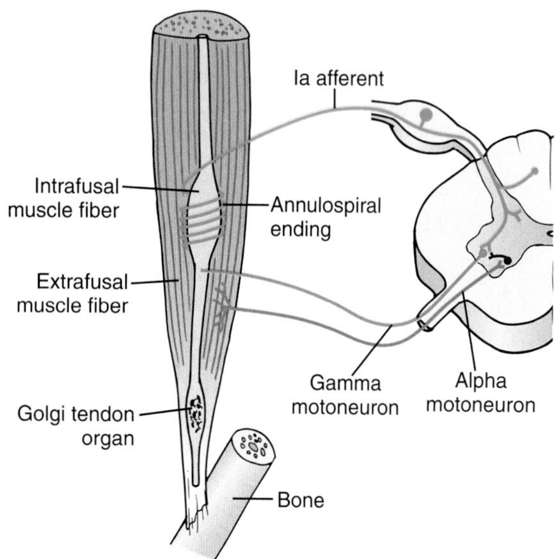

FIGURE 49-20 Spinal cord innervation of muscle spindle and Golgi tendon organ. Cell bodies from both the alpha motoneurons that innervate the extrafusal muscle fibers and the gamma fibers that innervate the intrafusal fibers reside in the ventral horns of the spinal cord and are activated by the same afferent systems.

motoneurons that adjust the length of the intrafusal fibers to match that of the extrafusal fibers.

The intrafusal muscle fibers in a spindle function as "skinniness" receptors. When a skeletal muscle is stretched, the spindle and its intrafusal fibers are stretched and therefore become more slender. Increased stretching of the intrafusal fibers results in an increased firing rate of its afferent fibers. The rate of firing is proportional to the degree of spindle stretch and therefore of extrafusal muscle length. Axons of the spindle afferent neurons enter the spinal cord through the several branches of the dorsal root. Some branches end in the segment of entry; some ascend in the spinal cord, sending collateral branches into the dorsal horn of the adjacent segments influencing intersegmental reflex function; and others ascend in the dorsal column of the cord to the medulla of the brain stem and cerebellum. The segmental branches make connections, along with other branches, that pass directly to the anterior gray matter of the spinal cord and establish monosynaptic contact with each of the LMNs that have motor units in the muscle containing the spindle receptor. This produces an opposing muscle contraction. The knee-jerk reflex that occurs when the knee is tapped with a reflex hammer tests for the intactness of the myotatic reflex arc in the quadriceps muscle. Another segmental branch of the same afferent neuron innervates an internuncial neuron that is inhibitory to motor units of antagonistic muscle groups. Inhibition of these muscle units helps in opposing muscle stretch. The intersegmental reflexes are particularly important in coordinating hand, leg, neck, and limb movements.

The ascending fibers from the stretch reflex ultimately provide information about muscle length to the cerebellum and cerebral cortex. The role of afferent spindle fibers is to inform the CNS of the status of muscle length. When a skeletal muscle lengthens or shortens against tension, a feedback mechanism needs to be available for readjustment such that the spindle apparatus remains sensitive to moment-to-moment changes in muscle stretch, even while changes in muscle length are occurring. This is accomplished by the gamma motoneurons that adjust spindle

CLINICAL APPLICATION

Assessment of Deep Tendon Reflexes

The status of the stretch reflex can be determined by assessing muscle tone and deep tendon reflexes. Clinically, muscle tone is evaluated by asking a person to relax while supporting the limb except at the joint that is being examined. The distal part of the extremity is then moved passively around the joint. Normally, there is a mild resistance to movement. A method for assessing muscle stretch excitability is to tap the tendon of a muscle briskly with a reflex hammer, which is normally immediately followed by a sudden contraction or *muscle jerk*, as illustrated. The stretch reflex has been "tricked" by the sudden tug on the tendon. A synchronous burst of afferent Ia nerve activity from the many spindles in the muscle results in essentially simultaneous firing of a large number of lower motoneuron units. The stretch reflex was tricked into responding, as though the muscle had been suddenly stretched. These muscle jerk reflexes are called *deep tendon reflexes* (DTRs). They usually are checked at the wrists, elbows, knees, and Achilles tendons.

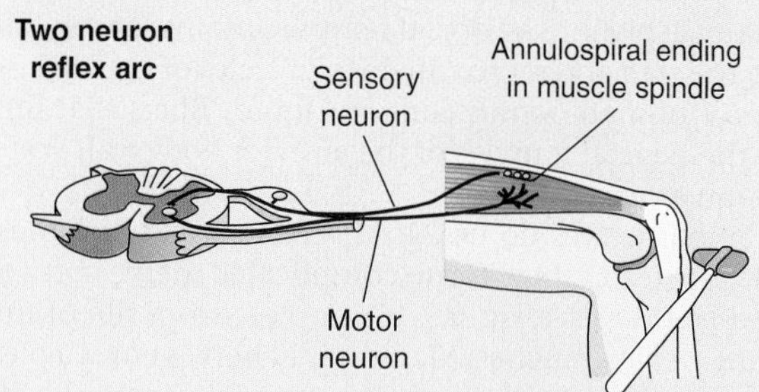

Testing the stretch reflex with a reflex hammer.

The DTRs can provide much information in a brief period. A normal-range DTR indicates that the afferent peripheral process in the peripheral muscle and nerves is normal; the dorsal root ganglion function is normal; the dorsal root function is normal; and the dorsal, intermediate, and ventral horns are functioning appropriately, as are the ventral root and lower motoneuron cell body and axon. It also means that the neuromuscular synapse is functioning normally; the muscle fibers are capable of normal contraction; and suprasegmental input is normal. Using this method of assessment, it is possible to test the function of many spinal nerves and spinal cord segments and some of the cranial nerves and brain stem segments in a short time. If abnormality of excitability is detected, further tests are required to determine the nature and location of the pathologic process.

fiber length to match the length of the extrafusal muscle fiber. Descending fibers of motor pathways synapse with and simultaneously activate both alpha and gamma motoneurons so that the sensitivity of the spindle fibers is coordinated with muscle movement.

In the muscles that are supporting body weight, the stretch reflex operates continuously, producing a continuous resistance to passive stretch called *muscle tone.* An abnormal increase or decrease in muscle tone suggests that the stretch reflex is not functioning normally or that the excitability of the alpha LMNs innervating the muscle is abnormal. Reduced excitability of the stretch reflex results in decreased muscle tone, or *hypotonia,* ranging from postural weakness to total flaccid paralysis. It can result from decreased function of the descending facilitory systems controlling the gamma LMNs that innervate the muscle or damage to the stretch reflex or peripheral nerves innervating the muscle. *Hypertonia,* or spasticity, is an abnormal increase in muscle tone. It can result from increased excitation or loss of inhibition of the spindle's gamma LMNs or changes in the segmental spinal cord circuitry controlling the stretch reflex. The result is strong facilitation of transmission in the monosynaptic reflex pathway from Ia sensory fibers supplying the alpha LMNs. Hypertonicity is characterized by hyperactive tendon reflexes and an increase in resistance to rapid muscle stretch. It commonly occurs with UMN lesions such as those that exist after spinal shock in persons with spinal cord injury (see Chapter 51).

The CNS, through its coordinated control of the muscle's alpha LMNs and the spindle's gamma LMNs, can suppress the stretch reflex. This occurs during centrally programmed movements such as pitching a baseball, permitting the muscle to produce its greatest range of motion. Without this programmed adjustability of the stretch reflex, any movement is immediately opposed and prevented. All reflex and learned movement patterns involve programmed control of gamma efferents, resulting in continuous readjustments of stretch reflex sensitivity in agonists, antagonists, and synergists as the movement progresses. The status of the stretch reflex can be determined by assessing muscle tone and deep tendon reflexes.

Inverse Myotatic Reflex

The *inverse myotatic reflex,* most prominent in antigravity extensor muscles, reduces the strength of alpha LMN–driven muscle contraction when the force generated by the muscle threatens the integrity of the muscle or tendon. This protective reflex, consisting of two or more synapses in its path, has a very high threshold and activates inhibitory interneurons in the ventral horn that decrease the firing rate of alpha LMNs. Type II muscle spindle afferents in the Golgi tendon apparatus and nociceptive afferents from the connective tissue of muscle and tendon units drive this high-threshold protective reflex. The inverse myotatic reflex also has a contralateral component. If, for example, the inverse myotatic reflex produced relaxation of the quadriceps in one leg, the contralateral component would produce contraction in the quadriceps of the other leg. The inverse myotatic reflex provides postural stability to ambulatory movements. For example, when the inverse myotatic reflex produces relaxation of antigravity muscles (with flexion) of one leg as we walk, the contralateral component produces contraction and extension of the opposite leg.

In persons with spastic paralysis, the inverse myotatic reflex becomes hyperactive and produces what is called the *clasp-knife reaction.* If an examiner were passively to flex the lower limb of such a person at the knee, increasing resistance would be encountered. This resistance would continue to increase until, at some point, it would abruptly cease and the leg could then be passively flexed. Similar signs are seen in spastic upper limbs.

Withdrawal Reflex

The withdrawal reflex is stimulated by a damaging (nociceptive) stimulus and quickly moves the body part away from the offending stimulus, usually by flexing a limb part. The withdrawal reflex is a powerful reflex, taking precedence over other reflexes associated with locomotion. Any of the major joints may be involved, depending on the site of afferent stimulation. All the joints of an extremity (*e.g.,* finger, wrist, elbow, shoulder) typically are involved. This complex, polysynaptic reflex also shifts postural support to the opposite side of the body with a crossed extensor reflex and simultaneously alerts the forebrain to the offending stimulus event (Fig. 49-21). The withdrawal reflex also can produce contraction of muscles other than the extremities. For example, irritation of the abdominal viscera may cause contraction of the abdominal muscles.

In summary, in the adult, the spinal cord is in the upper two thirds of the spinal canal of the vertebral column. On transverse section, the spinal cord has an oval shape. Internally, the gray matter has the appearance of a butterfly or letter "H." The dorsal horns contain the IA neurons and receive afferent information from dorsal root and other connecting neurons. The ventral horns contain the OA neurons and efferent LMNs that leave the cord by the ventral roots.

Thirty-two pairs of spinal nerves (*i.e.,* 8 cervical, 12 thoracic, 5 lumbar, 5 sacral, and 2 or more coccygeal) are present. Each pair communicates with its corresponding body segments. The spinal nerves and the blood vessels that supply the spinal cord enter the spinal canal through an intervertebral foramen. After entering the foramen, they divide into two branches, or roots, one of which enters the dorsolateral surface of the cord (*i.e.,* dorsal root), carrying the axons of afferent neurons into the CNS. The other root leaves the ventrolateral surface of the cord (*i.e.,* ventral root), carrying the axons of efferent neurons into the periphery. These two roots fuse at the intervertebral foramen, forming the mixed spinal nerve.

A reflex provides a highly reliable relation between a stimulus and a motor response. Its anatomic basis consists of an afferent neuron, the connection or synapse with CNS neurons that communicate with the effector neuron, and the effector neuron that innervates a muscle or organ. Reflexes are essentially "wired in" to the CNS in that normally they are always ready to function; with training, most reflexes can be modulated to become parts of more complicated movements.

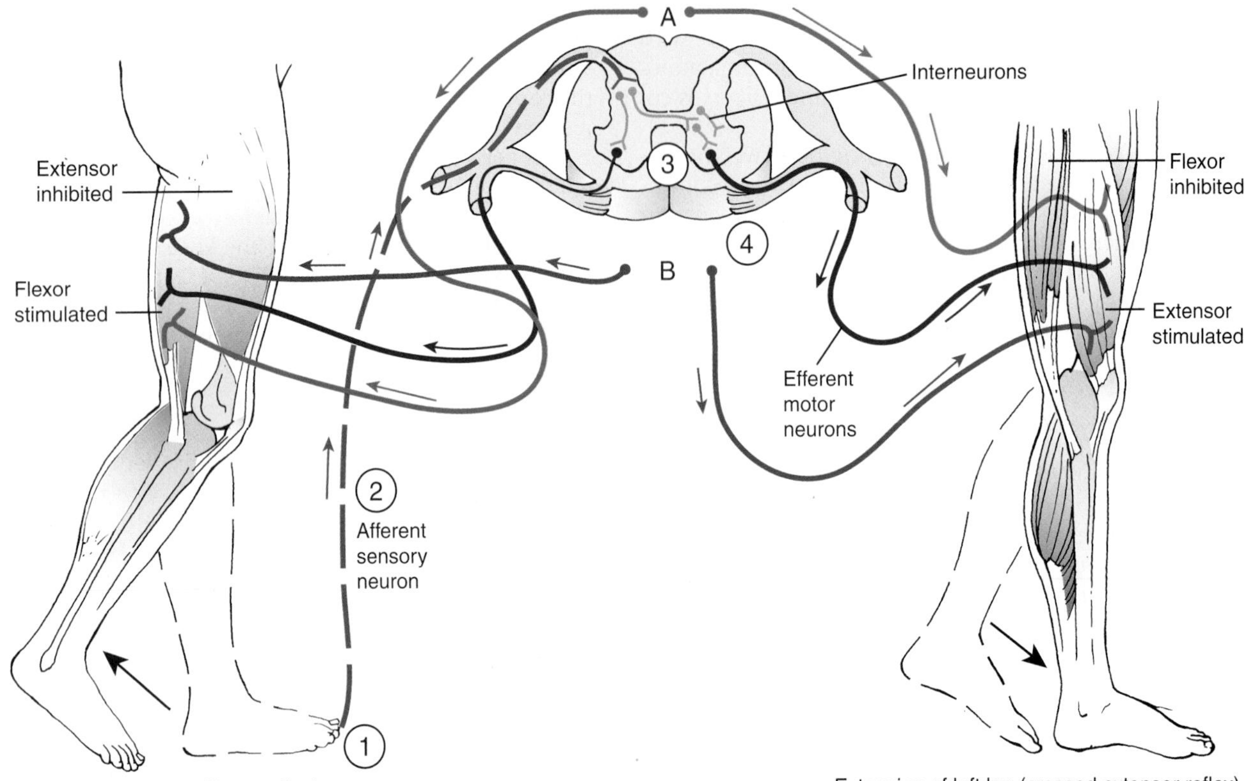

FIGURE 49-21 Crossed extensor reflex. Ipsilateral and contralateral circuitry, including interneurons, are shown for one spinal segment: (1) stepping on a painful object, (2) excitation of afferent sensory neurons, (3) integration of spinal cord circuitry, and (4) excitation of efferent motor neurons. Lower motoneuron outputs from more rostral (**A**) and more caudal (**B**) segments are also indicated. These outputs are via ascending and descending interneurons. Inhibitory circuits are not shown.

Two important types of spinal motor reflexes are the myotatic or stretch reflex and the withdrawal reflex. The myotatic reflex controls muscle tone and is important in maintaining posture, whereas the withdrawal reflex is stimulated by any tissue-threatening or damaging stimulus and quickly moves the body part away from the offending stimulus. Hundreds of reflexes exist, including those involved in stepping, gagging, swallowing, and inspiration. These are polysynaptic and complex, except for the disynaptic inverse myotatic reflex and monosynaptic stretch reflex.

The Brain

After completing this section of the chapter, you should be able to meet the following objectives:

- List the structures of the hindbrain, midbrain, and forebrain and describe their functions
- Name the cranial nerves and cite their location and function
- State the characteristics of the dominant and nondominant hemispheres of the brain
- Describe the characteristics of the CSF and trace its passage through the ventricular system
- Contrast and compare the blood–brain and CSF–brain barriers

Based on its embryonic development, the brain is divided into three regions: the hindbrain, the midbrain, and the forebrain (Fig. 49-22A). The hindbrain includes the medulla oblongata, the pons, and its dorsal outgrowth, the cerebellum. Midbrain structures include two pairs of dorsal enlargements, the superior and inferior colliculi. The forebrain, which consists of two hemispheres and is covered by the cerebral cortex, contains central masses of gray matter, the basal ganglia, and the rostral end of the neural tube, the diencephalon with its adult derivatives—the thalamus and hypothalamus.

An important concept is that the more rostral, recently developed parts of neural tube gain dominance or control over regions and functions at lower levels. They do not replace the more ancient circuitry but merely dominate it. After damage to the more vulnerable parts of the forebrain, as occurs with brain death, a brain stem–controlled organism remains that is capable of breathing and may survive if the environmental temperature is regulated and nutrition and other aspects of care are provided. However, all aspects

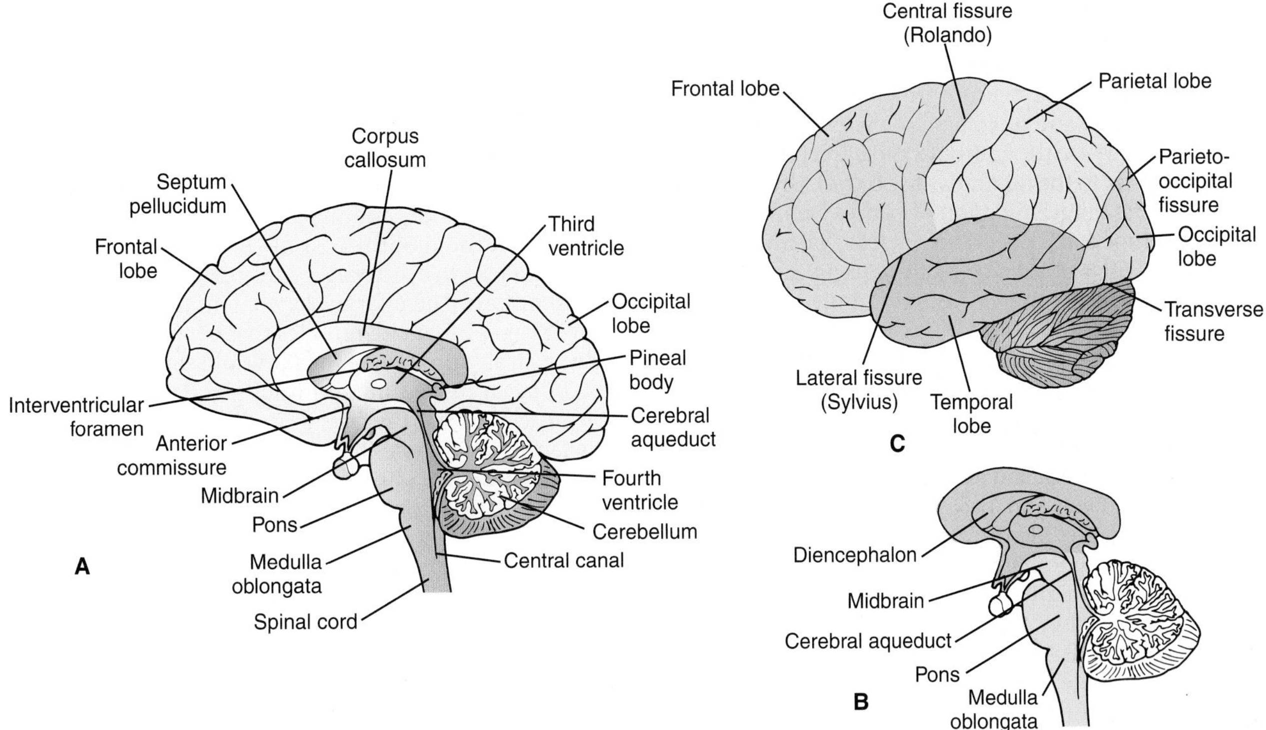

FIGURE 49-22 **(A)** Midsagittal section of the brain, showing the structures of the forebrain, midbrain, and hindbrain. **(B)** Diencephalon, brainstem, and the cerebral aqueduct connecting the 3rd and 4th ventricles. **(C)** Lateral view of the cerebral hemispheres.

of intellectual function, experience, perception, and memory are usually permanently lost. The organization of content in this section moves from the more ancient circuitry of the hindbrain to the more dominant and recently developed structures of the forebrain.

HINDBRAIN

The term *brain stem* is often used to include the hindbrain, pons, and midbrain (see Fig. 49-22B). These regions of the neural tube have the organization of spinal cord segments, except that more of the longitudinal cell columns are present, reflecting the increased complexity of the cranial segmental nerves. In the brain stem, the structure and function of the reticular formation have been greatly expanded. In the pons and medulla, the reticular formation contains networks controlling basic breathing, eating, and locomotion functions. Higher-level integration of these functions occurs in the midbrain. The reticular formation is surrounded on the outside by the long tract systems that connect the forebrain with lower parts of the CNS.

Medulla

The *medulla oblongata* represents the caudal five segments of the brain part of the neural tube; the cranial nerve branches entering and leaving it have functions similar to the spinal segmental nerves. Although the ventral horn areas in the medulla are quite small, the dorsal horn areas are enlarged, processing a large amount of the information pouring through the cranial nerves. The segmental peripheral nerve components of the medulla can be divided into those leaving the neural tube ventromedially (*i.e.,* hypoglossal and abducens cranial nerves) or dorsolaterally (*i.e.,* vagus, spinal accessory, glossopharyngeal, and vestibulocochlear cranial nerves). Because pathologic signs and symptoms reflect the spatial segregation of brain stem components, neurologic syndromes resulting from trauma, tumors, aneurysms, and cerebrovascular accidents are often classified as ventral or dorsolateral syndromes.

The general somatic efferent LMNs of the lower segments of the medulla supply the extrinsic and intrinsic muscles of the tongue by means of the *hypoglossal nerve,* or *cranial nerve XII* (see Table 49-1). Damage to the hypoglossal nerve results in weakness or paralysis of tongue muscles. When the tongue is protruded, it deviates toward the damaged and therefore weaker side because of the greater protrusion strength on the normal side. Axons of the hypoglossal nerve exit the medulla adjacent to two long, longitudinal ridges along the medial undersurface of the medulla. These ridges, called the *pyramids,* contain the corticospinal fibers, most of which cross to descend in the lateral column to the opposite side of the spinal cord. Lesions of the ventral surface of the caudal medulla result in the syndrome of alternating hypoglossal hemiplegia. These lesions are characterized by signs of ipsilateral (*i.e.,* same side) denervation of the tongue and contralateral (*i.e.,* opposite side) weakness or paralysis of both the upper and lower extremities.

The *vagus nerve,* or *cranial nerve X,* has several afferent (sensory) and efferent (motor) components. General somatic afferent neurons innervate the external ear, whereas special visceral afferent neurons innervate the pharyngeal taste buds. Sensory and motor components of the nerve innervate the pharynx, the gastrointestinal tract (from the laryngeal pharynx to the midtransverse colon), the heart, the spleen, and the lungs. Initiation of many essential reflexes and normal functions depends on intact vagal innervation. For example, 80% of the fibers of the vagus are afferents, some of which are involved in vomiting and hiccup reflexes and in ongoing feedback during swallowing and speech. The unilateral loss of vagal function can result in slowed gastrointestinal motility, a permanently husky voice, and deviation of the uvula away from the damaged side. Bilateral loss of vagal function can seriously damage reflex maintenance of cardiovascular and respiratory reflexes. Swallowing may become difficult and, occasionally, paralysis of laryngeal structures causes life-threatening airway obstruction.

The sternocleidomastoid, a powerful head-turning muscle, and the trapezius muscle, which elevates the shoulders, are innervated by the *spinal accessory nerve,* or *cranial nerve XI,* with LMNs in the upper four cervical spinal segments. Intermediate rootlets from these segmental levels combine and enter the cranial cavity through the foramen magnum and exit the jugular foramen with cranial nerves IX and X. Loss of spinal accessory nerve function results in drooping of the shoulder on the damaged side and weakness when turning the head to the opposite side.

The dorsolateral *glossopharyngeal nerve,* or *cranial nerve IX,* contains the same components as the vagus nerve but for a more rostral segment of the gastrointestinal tract and the pharynx. This nerve provides the special visceral sensory innervation of the taste buds of the oral pharynx and the back of the tongue; the afferent innervation of the oral pharynx and the baroreceptors of the carotid sinus; the efferent innervation of the otic ganglion, which controls the salivary function of the parotid gland; and the efferent innervation of the stylopharyngeus muscles of the pharynx. This cranial nerve is seldom damaged, but when it is, anesthesia of the ipsilateral oral pharynx develops along with dry mouth resulting from reduced salivation.

The special sensory afferent *vestibulocochlear nerve,* or *cranial nerve VIII,* formerly called the *auditory nerve,* is attached laterally at the junction of the medulla oblongata and the pons, often called the *caudal pons.* It consists of two distinct fiber divisions, the cochlear and vestibular divisions, both of which are sensory. Cell bodies in the cochlea of the inner ear produce fibers of the cochlear division. These fibers transmit impulses related to the sense of hearing. The vestibular division arises from two ganglia that innervate cell bodies in the utricle, saccule, and semicircular canals and transmits impulses related to head position and movement of the body through space. Irritation of the cochlear division results in tinnitus (*i.e.,* ringing of the ears); destruction of the nerve results in nerve deafness. Injury to the vestibular division leads to vertigo, nystagmus, and some postural instability (see Chapter 55).

Another segmental branch of the caudal pons, the *facial nerve,* or *cranial nerve VII,* and its intermediate component (the intermedius) contain both afferent and efferent functional components. The nervus intermedius, containing the general somatic afferent, special visceral afferent, general visceral afferent, and general visceral efferent neurons, innervates the nasopharynx and taste buds of the palate. It also innervates the anterior two thirds of the tongue, the submandibular and sublingual salivary glands, the lacrimal glands, and mucous membranes of the nose and roof of the mouth. Loss of this branch of the facial nerve can lead to eye dryness with risk for corneal scarring and blindness. The pharyngeal efferent LMNs of the facial nerve proper innervate muscles that control facial expression, such as wrinkling of the brow and smiling. Unilateral loss of facial nerve function results in flaccid paralysis of the muscles of half the face, a condition called *Bell's palsy.* The facial nerve passes through a bony tunnel behind the middle ear cavity. Sometimes, Bell's palsy has been attributed to inflammatory reactions involving the facial nerve in or near this bony tunnel. Because such injuries result from pressure caused by edematous tissue, the integrity of the endoneurial sheath is retained, and regeneration with full recovery of all muscles usually occurs within several months.

Another segmental nerve branch of the caudal pons, the *abducens nerve,* or *cranial nerve VI,* sends LMNs out ventrally on either side of the pyramids and then forward into the orbit to innervate the lateral rectus muscle of the eye. As the name suggests, the abducens nerve abducts the eye (lateral or outward rotation); peripheral damage to this nerve results in medial strabismus, which is a weakness or loss of eye abduction (see Chapter 54).

Pons

The pons (from the Latin for "bridge") develops from the fifth neural tube segment. Internally, the central canal of the spinal cord, which is enlarged in the pons and rostral medulla, forms the fourth ventricle (see Fig. 49-22). An enlarged area on the ventral surface of the pons contains the pontine nuclei, which receive information from all parts of the cerebral cortex. The axons of these neurons form a massive bundle that swings around the lateral side of the fourth ventricle to enter the cerebellum. In the pons, the reticular formation is large and contains the circuitry for masticating food and manipulating the jaws during speech.

The *trigeminal nerve,* or *cranial nerve V,* which has sensory and motor subdivisions (see Table 49-1), exits the brain stem laterally on the forward surface of the pons. The trigeminal is the main sensory nerve conveying the modalities of pain, temperature, touch, and proprioception to the superficial and deep regions of the face. Regions innervated include the skin of the anterior scalp and face, the conjunctiva and orbit, the meninges, the paranasal sinuses, and the mouth, including the teeth and the anterior two thirds of the tongue. Lower motor neurons of the trigeminal nerve innervate skeletal muscles involved with mastication and contribute to swallowing and speech, movements of the soft palate, and tension of the tympanic membrane through the tensor tympani muscle. The tensor tympani has a protective reflex function, dampening movement of the middle ear ossicles during high-intensity sound.

CEREBELLUM

The cerebellum is located in the posterior fossa of the cranium superior to the pons (see Fig. 49-22). It is separated from the cerebral hemispheres by a fold of dura mater, the tentorium cerebelli. The cerebellum consists of a small, unpaired median portion, called the *vermis,* and two large lateral masses, the *cerebellar hemispheres.* In contrast to the brain stem with its external white matter and internal gray nuclei, the cerebellum, like the cerebrum, has an outer cortex of gray matter overlying the white matter. Next to the fourth ventricle, several masses of gray matter, called the *deep cerebellar nuclei,* border the roof of the fourth ventricle. Cells of the cerebellar cortex and deep nuclei interact, and axons from the latter send information to many regions, particularly to the motor cortex by means of a thalamic relay. Synergistic (*i.e.,* temporal and spatial smoothing) functions of the cerebellum participate in all movements of limbs, trunk, head, larynx, and eyes, whether the movement is part of a voluntary movement or of a highly learned semiautomatic or automatic movement. During highly skilled movements, the motor cortex sends signals to the cerebellum, informing it about the movement that is to be performed. The cerebellum makes continuous adjustments, resulting in smoothness of movement, particularly during delicate maneuvers. Highly skillful movement requires extensive motor training, and considerable evidence suggests many of these learned movement patterns involve cerebellar circuits.

The cerebellum receives proprioceptor input from the vestibular system; feedback from the muscles, tendons, and joints; and indirect signals from the somesthetic, visual, and auditory systems that provide background information for ongoing movement. Sensory and motor information from a given area of the body is sent to the same area in the cerebellum. In this way, the cerebellum can assess continuously the status of each body part—position, rate of movement, and forces such as gravity that are opposing movement. The cerebellum compares what is actually happening with what is intended to happen. It then transmits the appropriate corrective signals back to the motor system, instructing it to increase or decrease the activity of the participating muscle groups so that smooth and accurate movements can be performed.

Another function of the cerebellum is the dampening of muscle movement. All body movements are essentially pendular (*i.e.,* swinging back and forth). As movement begins, momentum develops and must be overcome before the movement can be stopped. This momentum would cause movements to overshoot if they were not dampened. In the intact cerebellum, automatic signals stop movement precisely at the intended point. The cerebellum analyzes proprioceptive information to predict the future position of moving parts, their rapidity of movement, and the projected time course of the movement. This allows the cerebellum to inhibit agonist muscles and excite antagonist muscles when movement approaches the intended target.

MIDBRAIN

The midbrain develops from the fourth segment of the neural tube, and its organization is similar to that of a spinal segment. Internally, the central canal is reestablished as the cerebral aqueduct, connecting the fourth ventricle with the third ventricle (see Fig. 49-22). Two general somatic efferent cranial nerves, the oculomotor nerve, or cranial nerve III, and the trochlear nerve, or cranial nerve IV, exit the midbrain.

Two prominent bundles of nerve fibers, the *cerebral peduncles,* pass along the ventral surface of the midbrain. These fibers include the corticospinal tracts and are the main motor pathways between the forebrain and the pons. On the dorsal surface, four "little hills," the *superior* and *inferior colliculi,* are areas of cortical formation. The inferior colliculus is involved in directional turning and, to some extent, in experiencing the direction of sound sources, whereas the superior colliculi are essential to the reflex mechanisms that control conjugate eye movements when the visual environment is surveyed.

The ventral central gray matter (*i.e.,* ventral horn) of the midbrain contains the LMNs that innervate most of the skeletal muscles that move the optic globe and raise the eyelids. These axons leave the midbrain through the *oculomotor nerve,* or *cranial nerve III.* This nerve also contains the parasympathetic LMNs that control pupillary constriction and ciliary muscle focusing of the lens (see Table 49-1). Damage to the ventrally exiting cranial nerve III and to the adjacent cerebral peduncle, which contains the corticospinal axon system on one side, results in paralysis of eye movement combined with contralateral hemiplegia.

A small group of cells in the ventral part of the caudal central gray matter contains the *trochlear nerve,* or *cranial nerve IV,* which innervates the superior oblique eye muscle. This muscle moves the upper part of the eye downward and toward the nose when the eye is adducted, or turned inward. The trochlear nerve exits the dorsal surface of the midbrain and decussates (crosses over) before exiting the brain stem. Lesions of the trochlear nerve affect downward gaze on the side opposite the denervated muscle, producing diplopia, or double vision. Walking downstairs becomes particularly difficult. Because the superior oblique muscle has inward rotation of the optic globe as its major function, persons with trochlear nerve damage usually carry their heads tilted to the side of damage.

Forebrain

The most rostral part of the brain, the forebrain consists of the telencephalon, or "end brain," and the diencephalon, or "between brain." The diencephalon forms the core of the forebrain, and the telencephalon forms the cerebral hemispheres.

DIENCEPHALON

Three of the most forward brain segments form an enlarged dorsal horn and ventral horn with a narrow, deep, enlarged central canal—the third ventricle—separating the two sides. This region is called the *diencephalon.* The dorsal horn part of the diencephalon is the thalamus and subthalamus, and the ventral horn part is the hypothalamus (Fig. 49-23). The optic nerve, or cranial nerve II, and retina are outgrowths of the diencephalon. The structure and function of the optic nerve are presented in Chapter 54.

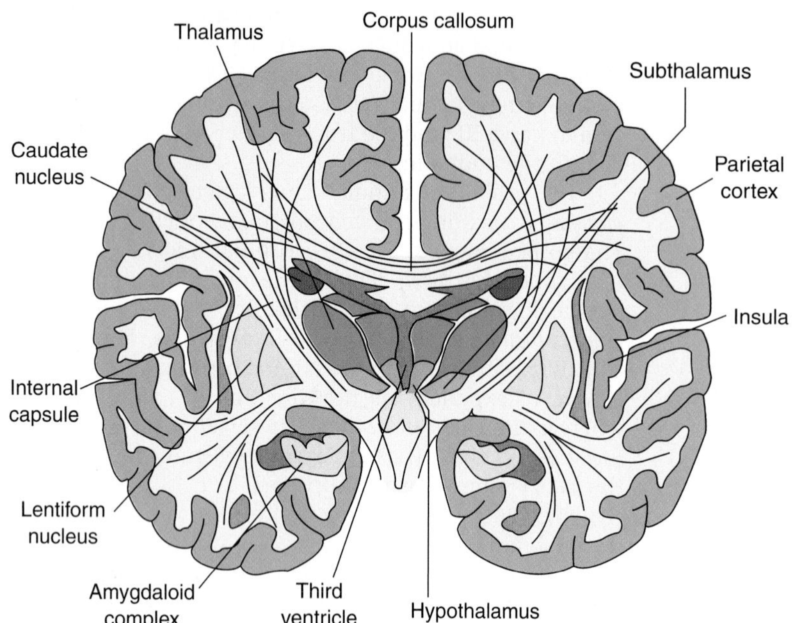

FIGURE 49-23 Frontal section of the brain passing through the third ventricle, showing the thalamus, subthalamus, hypothalamus, internal capsule, corpus callosum, basal ganglia (caudate nucleus, lenticular nucleus), amygdaloid complex, insula, and parietal cortex.

The thalamus consists of two large, egg-shaped masses, one on either side of the third ventricle. It is divided into several major parts, and each part is divided into distinct nuclei, which are the major relay stations for information going to and from the cerebral cortex. All sensory pathways have direct projections to thalamic nuclei, which convey the information to restricted areas of the sensory cortex. Coordination and integration of peripheral sensory stimuli occur in the thalamus, along with some crude interpretation of highly emotion-laden auditory experiences that not only occur but also can be remembered. For example, a person can recover from a deep coma in which cerebral cortex activity is minimal and remember some of what was said at the bedside.

The thalamus also plays a role in relaying critical information regarding motor activities to and from selected areas of the motor cortex. Two neuronal circuits are significant in this regard. One is the pathway from the cerebral cortex to the pons and cerebellum and then, by way of the thalamus, back to the motor cortex. The second is the feedback circuit that travels from the cortex to the basal ganglia, then to the thalamus, and from the thalamus back to the cortex. The subthalamus also contains movement control systems related to the basal ganglia.

Through its connections with the ascending reticular activating system, the thalamus processes neural influences that are basic to cortical excitatory rhythms (*i.e.,* those recorded on the electroencephalogram), to essential sleep–wake cycles, and to the process of attending to stimuli. Besides their cortical connections, the thalamic nuclei have connections with each other and with neighboring nonthalamic brain structures such as the limbic system. Through their connections with the limbic system, some thalamic nuclei are involved in the relation between stimuli and the emotional responses they evoke.

Inferior to the thalamus, and representing the ventral horn portion of the diencephalon, is the hypothalamus. It also borders the third ventricle and includes a ventral extension, the neurohypophysis (*i.e.,* posterior pituitary). The hypothalamus is the area of master-level integration of homeostatic control of the body's internal environment. Maintenance of blood gas concentration, water balance, food consumption, and major aspects of endocrine and autonomic nervous system control require hypothalamic function.

The internal capsule is a broad band of projection fibers that lies between the thalamus medially and the basal ganglia laterally (see Fig. 49-23). It contains all of the fibers that connect the cerebral cortex with deeper structures, including the basal ganglia, thalamus, midbrain, pons, medulla, and spinal cord.

Cerebral Hemispheres

The two cerebral hemispheres are lateral outgrowths of the diencephalon. Internally, the cerebral hemispheres contain the lateral ventricles (*i.e.,* ventricles I and II), which are connected with the third ventricle of the diencephalon by a small opening called the *interventricular foramen* (*i.e.,* foramen of Monro). Axons of the olfactory nerve, or cranial nerve I, terminate in the most ancient portion of the cerebrum—the olfactory bulb, where initial processing of olfactory information occurs. Projection axons from the olfactory bulb relay information through the olfactory tracts to the thalamus and to other parts of the cerebral cortex (*i.e.,* orbital cortex), where olfactory-related reflexes and olfactory experience occur.

The *corpus callosum* is a massive commissure, or bridge, of myelinated axons that connects the cerebral cortex of the two sides of the brain. Two smaller commissures, the anterior and posterior commissures, connect the two sides of the more specialized regions of the cerebrum and diencephalon.

The surfaces of the hemispheres are lateral (side), medial (area between the two sides of the brain), and basal (ventral). The cerebral cortex is the recently evolved six-layered neocortex. Many ridges and grooves are present on the surface of the hemispheres. A *gyrus* is the ridge between two grooves, and the groove is called a *sulcus* or *fissure*. The cerebral cortex is arbitrarily divided into lobes named after the bones that cover them: the frontal, parietal, temporal, and occipital lobes.

Basal Ganglia

A section through the cerebral hemispheres reveals the surface of the cerebral cortex, a subcortical layer of white matter made up of masses of myelinated axons and deep masses of gray matter: the basal ganglia that border the lateral ventricle. The basal ganglia lie on either side of the internal capsule, just lateral to the thalamus. Each basal ganglia consists of the comma-shaped *caudate* (tailed) nucleus, the shield-shaped *putamen*, and the *globus pallidus* (*i.e.*, "pale globe"). The term *striatum* (*i.e.*, "striped body") refers to the caudate plus the putamen. Together, the globus pallidus and putamen make up the *lentiform* (lens-shaped) *nucleus*.

The basal ganglia supply axial and proximal unlearned and learned postures and movements, which enhance and add gracefulness to UMN-controlled manipulative movements. These background movement functions are called *associated movements*. Intact and functional basal ganglia provide arm swinging during walking and running. Basal ganglia also are involved in follow-through movements that accompany throwing a ball or swinging a club. As with the motor cortex, the nuclei on the left side control movement on the right side of the body, and vice versa. Circuits connecting the premotor cortex and supplementary motor cortex, the basal ganglia, and parts of the thalamus provide associated movements that accompany highly skilled behaviors. Parkinson's disease, Huntington's chorea, and some forms of cerebral palsy, among other dysfunctions involving the basal ganglia, result in a frequent or continuous release of abnormal postural or axial and proximal movement patterns. If damage to the basal ganglia is localized to one side, the movements occur on the opposite side of the body. These automatic movement patterns stop only in sleep, but in some conditions, the movements are so violent that getting to sleep becomes difficult.

Frontal Lobe

The frontal lobe extends from the frontal pole to the central sulcus (*i.e.*, fissure) and is separated from the temporal lobe by the lateral sulcus. Each frontal lobe can be subdivided rostrally into the frontal pole and laterally into the superior, middle, and inferior gyri, which continue on the undersurface over the eyes as the orbital cortex. These areas are associated with the medial thalamic nuclei, which also are related to the limbic system. Functionally, the prefrontal cortex is thought to be involved in anticipation and prediction of consequences of behavior. This "future-oriented" region is particularly depressed by many drugs, including alcohol.

The precentral gyrus (area 4), next to the central sulcus, is the *primary motor cortex* (Fig. 49-24). This area of the cortex provides precise movement control for distal flexor muscles of the hands and feet and of the phonation apparatus required for speech. Just rostral to the precentral gyrus is a region of the frontal cortex called the *premotor* or *motor association cortex*. This region (area 8 and rostral area 6) is involved in the planning of complex learned movement patterns, and damage to these areas results in dyspraxia or apraxia. Such people can manipulate a screwdriver, for instance, but cannot use it to loosen a screw. The primary motor cortex and the association motor cortex are connected with lateral thalamic nuclei, through which they receive feedback information from the basal ganglia and cerebellum. On the medial surface of the hemisphere, the premotor area includes a *supplementary motor cortex* involved in the control of bilateral movement patterns requiring great dexterity.

Parietal Lobe

The parietal lobe of the cerebrum lies behind the central sulcus (*i.e.*, postcentral gyrus) and above the lateral sulcus.

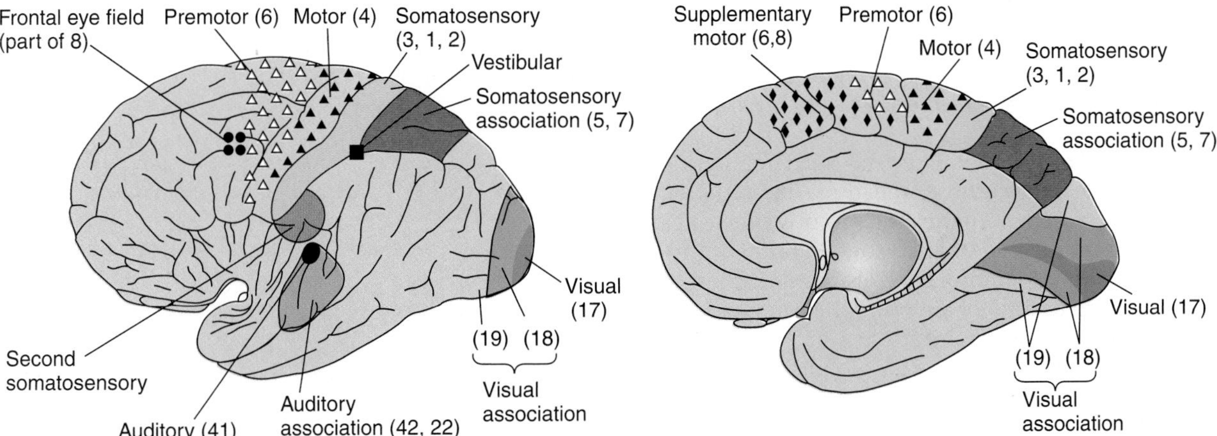

FIGURE 49-24 Motor and sensory areas of the cerebral cortex. (**Left**) The lateral view of the left (dominant) side is drawn as though the lateral sulcus had been pried open, exposing the insula. (**Right**) The diagram represents the areas in a brain that has been sectioned in the median plane. (Reproduced by permission from Nolte J. [1981]. *The human brain.* St. Louis: C.V. Mosby)

A strip of cortex bordering the central sulcus is called the *primary somatosensory cortex* (areas 3, 1, and 2) because it receives very discrete sensory information from the lateral nuclei of the thalamus. Just behind the primary sensory cortex is the *somesthetic association cortex* (areas 5 and 7), which is connected with the thalamic nuclei and with the primary sensory cortex. This region is necessary for somesthetic perception (*i.e.*, appreciation of the meaningfulness [gnosis] of integrated sensory information from various sensory systems), especially concerning perception of "where" the stimulus is in space and in relation to body parts. Localized lesions of this region can result in the inability to recognize the meaningfulness of an object (*i.e.*, agnosia). With the person's eyes closed, a screwdriver can be felt and described as to shape and texture. Nevertheless, the person cannot integrate the sensory information required to identify it as a screwdriver (*i.e.*, astereognosis). Somesthetic functions of the sensory cortex are discussed further in Chapter 50.

Temporal Lobe

The temporal lobe lies below the lateral sulcus and merges with the parietal and occipital lobes. It includes the temporal pole and three primary gyri: the superior, middle, and inferior gyri. It is separated from the limbic areas on the ventral surface by the collateral or rhinal sulcus. Area 41, the primary auditory cortex, involves the part of the superior temporal gyrus that extends into the lateral sulcus (see Fig. 49-22). This area is particularly important in discrimination of sounds entering opposite ears. It receives auditory input projections by way of the inferior colliculus of the midbrain and a ventrolateral thalamic nucleus. The more exposed part of the superior temporal gyrus involves the auditory association or perception area (area 22). The gnostic aspects of hearing (*e.g.*, the meaning of a certain sound pattern) require that this area functions properly. Remaining portions of the temporal cortex are less defined functionally but apparently are important in long-term memory recall. This is particularly true with respect to perception and memory of complex sensory patterns such as geometric figures and faces (*i.e.*, recognition of "what" or "who" the stimulus is). Irritation or stimulation can result in vivid hallucinations of long-past events. These higher-order temporal and parietal cortical regions are connected with a large, recently evolved dorsal lateral thalamic nuclear complex.

The cortices of the frontal, parietal, and temporal lobes, surrounding the older cortex of the insula, located deep in the lateral fissure, represent the most recently evolved parts of the cerebral cortex. These areas contain primary and association functions for motor control and somesthesias for the lips and tongue and for audition; they are particularly involved in speech mechanisms.

Occipital Lobe

The occipital lobe lies posterior to the temporal and parietal lobes and is arbitrarily separated from them. The medial surface of the occipital lobe contains a deep sulcus extending from the limbic lobe to the occipital pole, the *calcarine sulcus*, which is surrounded by the primary visual cortex (area 17). Stimulation of this cortex causes the experience of bright lights (phosphenes) in the visual field. Just superior and inferior and extending onto the lateral side of the occipital pole is the *visual association cortex* (areas 18 and 19). This area is closely connected with the primary visual cortex and with complex nuclei of the thalamus. Integrity of the association cortex is required for gnostic visual function, by which the meaningfulness of visual experience, including experiences of color, motion, depth perception, pattern, form, and location in space, takes place.

The neocortical areas of the parietal lobe, between the somesthetic and the visual cortices, have a function in relating the texture, or "feel," and location of an object with its visual image. Between the auditory and visual association areas, the *parietooccipital region* is necessary for relating the meaningfulness of a sound and image to an object or person.

Limbic System

The medial aspect of the cerebrum is organized into concentric bands of cortex, the *limbic system* (*limbic* = borders), which surrounds the connection between the lateral and third ventricles. The innermost band just above and below the cut surface of the corpus callosum is folded out of sight but is an ancient, three-layered cortex ending as the hippocampus in the temporal lobe. Just outside the folded area is a band of transitional cortex, which includes the cingulate and the parahippocampal gyri (Fig. 49-25). This limbic lobe has reciprocal connections with the medial and the intralaminar nuclei of the thalamus, with the deep nuclei of the cerebrum (*e.g.*, amygdaloid nuclei, septal nuclei), and with the hypothalamus. Overall, this region of the brain is involved in emotional experience and in the control of emotion-related behavior. Stimulation of specific areas in this system can lead to feelings of dread, high anxiety, or exquisite pleasure. It also can result in violent

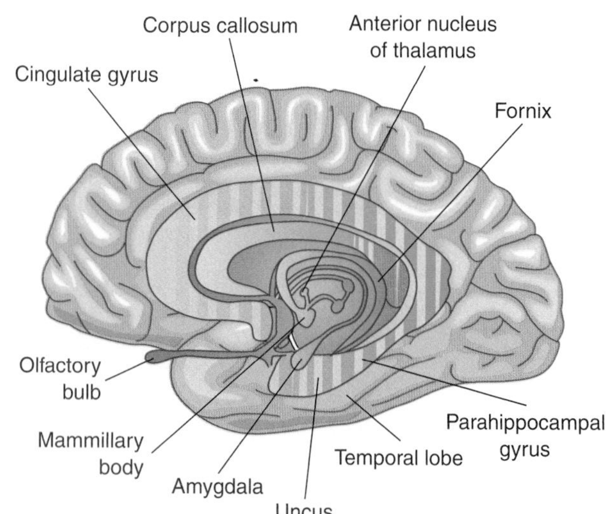

FIGURE 49-25 The limbic system includes the limbic cortex (cingulate gyrus, parahippocampal gyrus, uncus) and associated subcortical structures (thalamus, hypothalamus, amygdala).

behaviors, including attack, defense, or explosive and emotional speech.

Cerebral Dominance

Cerebral dominance refers to the fact that control of certain learned forms of behavior is exerted primarily by one of the two cerebral hemispheres. Handedness, perception of language, performance of speech, and appreciation of spatial relations are primarily expressions of one or the other hemisphere. By convention, speech is used to designate the dominant hemisphere. The dominant hemisphere has a major role in verbal and analytic abilities; the nondominant hemisphere has a lesser role in these functions and a major role in nonverbal and spatial abilities. Although it is assumed that the dominance of speech and handedness are assigned to the same hemisphere, this is not always the case. In clinical practice, communication dominance is the determinant of cerebral dominance. In most persons, even left-handed persons, the left hemisphere is the dominant hemisphere for speech. Because of substantial overlap, the concept of strict lateralization may not be appropriate other than in primary sensory areas.

The interhemispheric communication pathways are largely undeveloped at birth. The communication between the two hemispheres increases with age and is well developed by the second or third year of life. Cerebral dominance probably develops gradually throughout childhood. This explains why a child with an injury to the normally dominant hemisphere can often be trained to become left-handed and proficient in speech, but an older person with similar deficits finds such learning difficult or impossible.

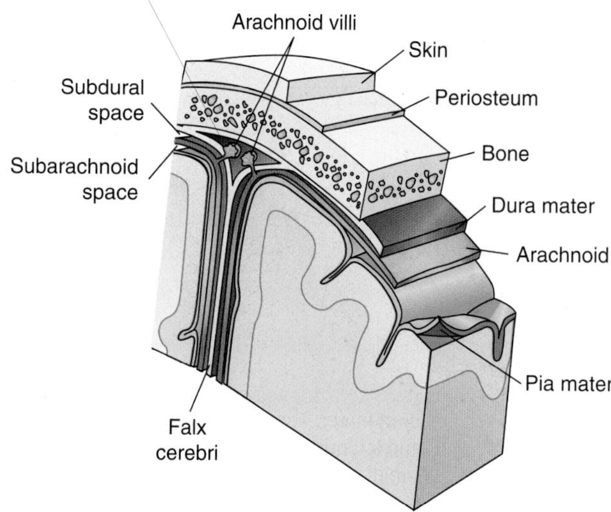

FIGURE 49-26 The cranial meninges. Arachnoid villi, shown within the superior sagittal sinus, are one site of cerebrospinal fluid absorption into the blood.

MENINGES

Inside the skull and vertebral column, the brain and spinal cord are loosely suspended and protected by several connective tissue sheaths called the *meninges* (Fig. 49-26). All surfaces of the spinal cord, brain, and segmental nerves are covered with a delicate connective tissue layer called the *pia mater* (Latin for "delicate mother"). Surface blood vessels and those that penetrate the brain and spinal cord are encased in this protective tissue layer. A second, very delicate, nonvascular, and waterproof layer, called the *arachnoid,* encloses the entire CNS (Fig. 49-27). The arachnoid layer is named for its spider web appearance. Cerebrospinal fluid is contained in the subarachnoid space. Immediately outside the arachnoid is a continuous sheath of strong connective tissue, the *dura mater* (*i.e.*, "tough mother"), which provides the major protection for the brain and spinal cord. The cranial dura often splits into two layers, with the outer layer serving as the periosteum of the inner surface of the skull.

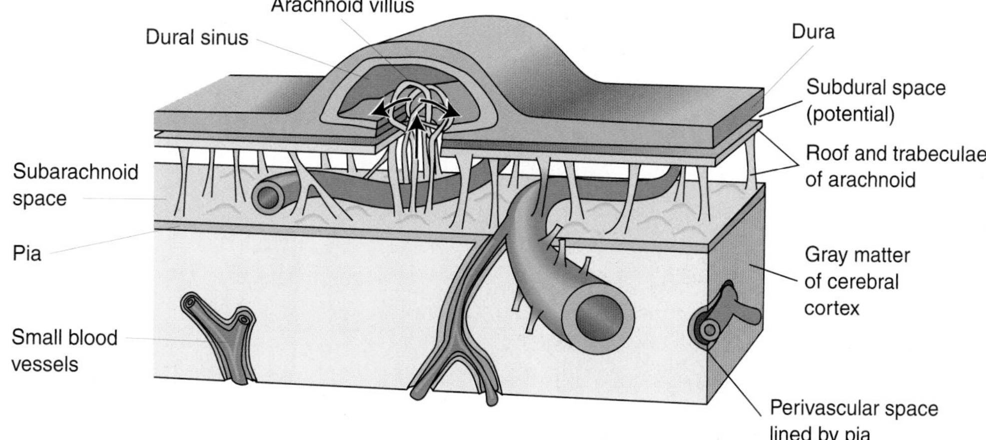

FIGURE 49-27 Schematic diagram of the three connective tissue membranes (pia, arachnoid, and dura) constituting the meninges of the central nervous system. Cerebrospinal fluid is resorbed (*arrows*) by way of the arachnoid villi projecting into the dural sinuses. (From Cormack D.H. [1987]. *Ham's histology* [9th ed., p. 367]. Philadelphia: J.B. Lippincott)

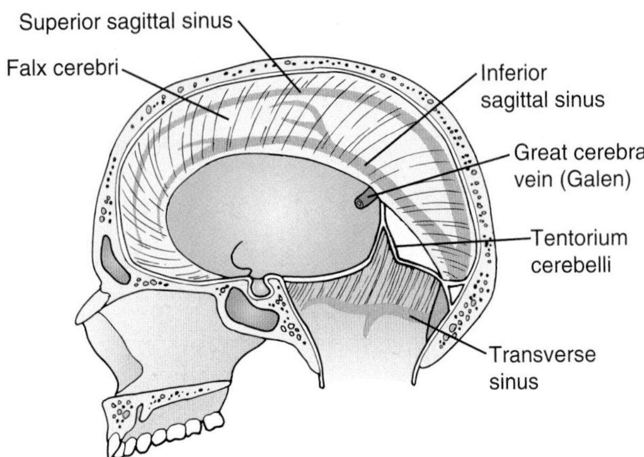

FIGURE 49-28 Cranial dura mater. The skull is open to show the falx cerebri and the right and left portions of the tentorium cerebelli, as well as some of the cranial venous sinuses.

The inner layer of the dura forms two major folds: a longitudinal fold called the *falx cerebri* separates the cerebral hemispheres and fuses with a second transverse fold called the *tentorium cerebelli* (Fig. 49-28). The tentorium cerebelli acts as a hammock, supporting the occipital lobes above the cerebellum. It also forms a tough septum, separating the anterior and middle cranial fossae, which contain the cerebral hemispheres, from the posterior fossa, found interiorly and containing the brain stem and cerebellum. The tentorium attaches to the petrous portion of the temporal bone and the dorsum sellae of the cranial floor, with a semicircular gap, or incisura, formed at the midline to permit the midbrain to pass forward from the posterior fossa. This compartmentalization is the basis for the commonly used terms *supratentorial* (*i.e.*, above the tentorium) and *infratentorial* (*i.e.*, below the tentorium). The cerebral hemispheres and the diencephalon are supratentorial structures, and the pons, cerebellum, and medulla are infratentorial structures.

The tentorium and falx cerebri normally support and protect the brain, which floats in the CSF within the enclosed space. During extreme trauma, however, the sharp edges of these folds can damage the brain. Space-occupying lesions such as enlarging tumors or hematomas can squeeze the brain against these edges or through the incisura of the tentorium (*i.e.*, herniation). As a result, brain tissue can be compressed, contused, or destroyed, often causing permanent deficits (see Chapter 52).

VENTRICULAR SYSTEM AND CEREBROSPINAL FLUID

The ventricular system is a series of CSF-filled cavities in the brain (Fig. 49-29). Cerebrospinal fluid provides a supporting and protective fluid in which the brain and spinal cord float. CSF helps maintain a constant ionic environment that serves as a medium for diffusion of nutrients, electrolytes, and metabolic end products into the extracellular fluid surrounding CNS neurons and glia. Filling the ventricles, the CSF supports the mass of the brain. Because it fills the subarachnoid space surrounding the CNS, a physical force delivered to either the skull or spine is to some extent diffused and cushioned.

The lining of the ventricles and central canal of the spinal cord is called the *ependyma.* There is a tremendous expansion of the ependyma in the roof of the lateral, third, and fourth ventricles. The CSF is produced by tiny reddish masses of specialized capillaries from the pia mater, called the *choroid plexus,* that project into the ventricles. CSF is an ultrafiltrate of blood plasma, composed of 99% water with other constituents, making it close to the composition of the brain extracellular fluid (Table 49-3). Humans secrete approximately 500 mL of CSF each day. However, only approximately 150 mL is in the ventricular system at any one time, meaning that the CSF is continuously being absorbed.

The CSF produced in the ventricles must flow through the interventricular foramen, the third ventricle, the cere-

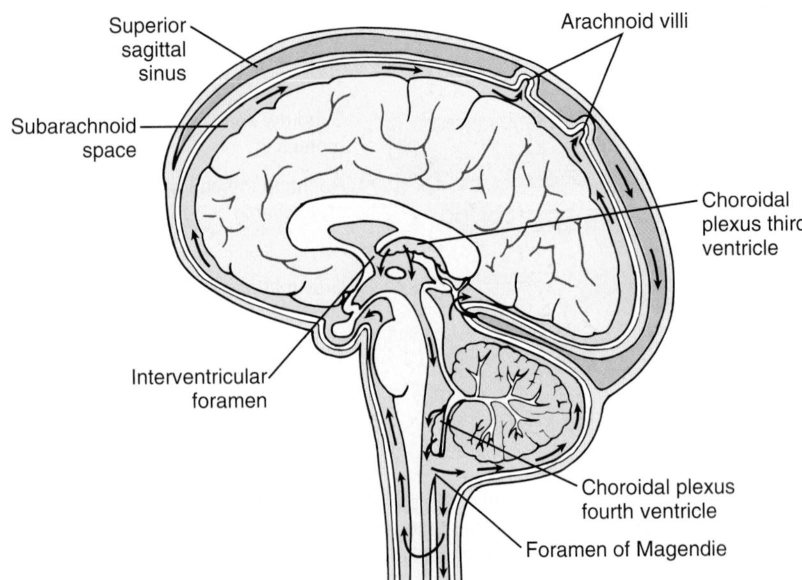

FIGURE 49-29 The flow of cerebrospinal fluid from the time of its formation from blood in the choroid plexuses until its return to the blood in the superior sagittal sinus. Plexuses in the lateral ventricles are not illustrated.

TABLE 49-3 Composition of Cerebrospinal Fluid Compared With Plasma

Substance	Plasma	Cerebrospinal Fluid
Protein mg/dL	6000.00	20.00
Na^+ mEq/L	145.00	141.00
CL^- mEq/L	101.00	124.00
K^+ mEq/L	4.50	2.90
HCO_3^- mEq/L	25.00	24.00
pH	7.4	7.32
Glucose mg/dl	92.00	61.00

bral aqueduct, and the fourth ventricle to exit from the neural tube. Three openings, or foramina, allow the CSF to pass into the subarachnoid space. Two of these, the foramina of Luschka, are located at the lateral corners of the fourth ventricle. The third, the medial foramen of Magendie, is in the midline at the caudal end of the fourth ventricle (see Fig. 49-29). Approximately 30% of the CSF passes down into the subarachnoid space that surrounds the spinal cord, mainly on its dorsal surface, and moves back up to the cranial cavity along its ventral surface.

Reabsorption of CSF into the vascular system occurs along the sides of the superior sagittal sinus in the anterior and middle fossa. To reach this area, the CSF must pass along the sides and ventral surface of the medulla and pons and then through the tentorial incisura or opening that surrounds the midbrain. Some CSF exits the posterior fossa ventrally, along the sides of the basilar artery rostrally, and through a CSF cistern between the midbrain peduncles (*i.e.,* basilar cistern). The major part of the flow continues along the sides of the hypothalamus to the region of the optic chiasm and then laterally and superiorly along the lateral fissure and over the parietal cortex to the superior sagittal sinus region. Here, the waterproof arachnoid has protuberances, the arachnoid villi, that penetrate the inner dura and venous walls of the superior sagittal sinus.

Reabsorption of CSF into the vascular system occurs through a pressure gradient. The normal CSF pressure is approximately 130 H_2O (10 mm Hg) in the lateral recumbent position, although it may be as low as 65 mm H_2O to as high as 195 mm H_2O, even in healthy persons. The microstructure of the arachnoid villi is such that if the CSF pressure falls below approximately 50 mm H_2O, the passageways collapse, and reverse flow is blocked. Arachnoid villi function as one-way valves, permitting CSF outflow into the blood but not allowing blood to pass into the arachnoid spaces.

BLOOD–BRAIN AND CEREBROSPINAL FLUID–BRAIN BARRIERS

Maintenance of a chemically stable environment is essential to the function of the brain. In most regions of the body, extracellular fluid undergoes small fluctuations in pH and concentrations of hormones, amino acids, and potassium ions during routine daily activities such as eating and exercising. If the brain were to undergo such fluctuations, the result would be uncontrolled neural activity because some substances such as amino acids act as neurotransmitters, and ions such as potassium influence the threshold for neural firing. Two barriers, the blood–brain barrier and the CSF–brain barrier, provide the means for maintaining the stable chemical environment of the brain. Only water, carbon dioxide, and oxygen enter the brain with relative ease; the transport of other substances between the brain and the blood is slow.

Blood–Brain Barrier

The blood–brain barrier depends on the unique characteristics of the brain capillaries. Endothelial cells of brain capillaries are joined by continuous tight junctions. In addition, most brain capillaries are surrounded by a basement membrane and by the processes of supporting cells of the brain, called *astrocytes* (Fig. 49-30). The blood–brain barrier permits passage of essential substances while excluding unwanted materials. Reverse transport systems remove materials from the brain. Large molecules such as proteins and peptides are largely excluded from crossing the blood–brain barrier. Acute cerebral lesions, such as trauma and infection, increase the permeability of the blood–brain barrier and alter brain concentrations of proteins, water, and electrolytes.

The blood–brain barrier prevents many drugs from entering the brain. Most highly water-soluble compounds are excluded from the brain, especially molecules with high ionic charge such as many of the catecholamines. In contrast, many lipid-soluble molecules cross the lipid layers of the blood–brain barrier with ease. Some drugs, such as the antibiotic chloramphenicol, are highly lipid soluble

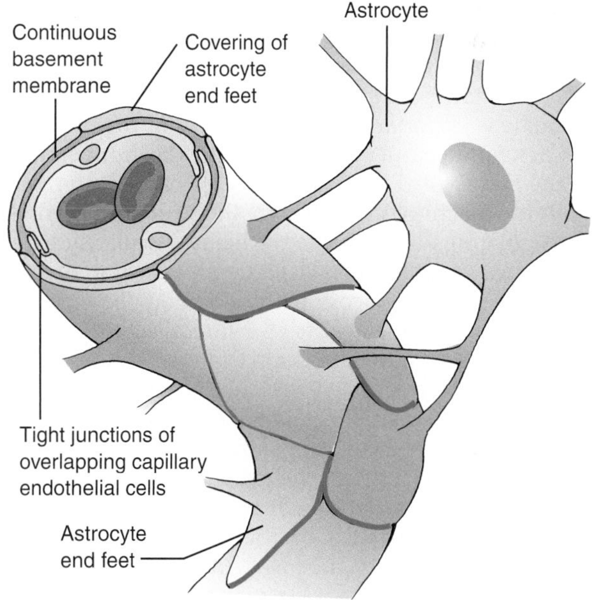

FIGURE 49-30 The three components of the blood–brain barrier: the astrocyte and astrocytic feet that encircle the capillary, the capillary basement membrane, and the tight junctions that join the overlapping capillary endothelial cells.

and therefore enter the brain readily. Other medications have a low solubility in lipids and enter the brain slowly or not at all. Alcohol, nicotine, and heroin are very lipid soluble and rapidly enter the brain. Some substances that enter the capillary endothelium are converted by metabolic processes to a chemical form incapable of moving into the brain.

The cerebral capillaries are much more permeable at birth than in adulthood, and the blood–brain barrier develops during the early years of life. In severely jaundiced infants, bilirubin can cross the immature blood–brain barrier, producing kernicterus and brain damage (see Chapter 15). In adults, the mature blood–brain barrier prevents bilirubin from entering the brain, and the nervous system is not affected.

Cerebrospinal Fluid–Brain Barrier and Arachnoid–Cerebrospinal Fluid Barrier

The ependymal cells covering the choroid plexus are linked together by tight junctions, forming a blood–CSF barrier to diffusion of many molecules from the blood plasma of choroid plexus capillaries to the CSF. Water is transported through the choroid epithelial cells by osmosis. Oxygen and carbon dioxide move into the CSF by diffusion, resulting in partial pressures roughly equal to those of plasma. The high sodium and low potassium contents of the CSF are actively regulated and kept relatively constant. Lipids and nonpeptide hormones diffuse through the barrier rather easily, but most large molecules, such as proteins, peptides, many antibiotics, and other medications, do not normally get through. The choroid epithelium uses energy in the form of adenosine triphosphate (ATP) to secrete actively many components into the CSF, including proteins, sodium ions, and a number of micronutrients, such as vitamins C and B_6 (pyridoxine) and folate. Because the resultant CSF has a relatively high sodium content, the negatively charged chloride and bicarbonate diffuse into the CSF along an ionic gradient. The choroid cells also generate bicarbonate from carbon dioxide in the blood. This bicarbonate is important to the regulation of the pH of the CSF. Arachnoid barrier cells prevent the CSF from contacting the blood-filled dural sinuses. This barrier essentially covers the arachnoid villi that are the structures involved in recirculating CSF back into the blood vascular system.

Mechanisms exist that facilitate the transport of other molecules such as glucose without energy expenditure. Ammonia, a toxic metabolite of neuronal activity, is converted to glutamine by astrocytes. Glutamine moves by facilitated diffusion through the choroid epithelium into the plasma. This exemplifies a major function of the CSF, that of providing a means of removal of toxic waste products from the CNS. Because the brain and spinal cord have no lymphatic channels, the CSF serves this function.

Several specific areas of the brain do not have a blood–CSF barrier. One area is at the caudal end of the fourth ventricle (*i.e.*, area postrema), where specialized receptors for the carbon dioxide level of the CSF influence respiratory function. Another area consists of the walls of the third ventricle, which permit hypothalamic neurons to monitor blood glucose levels. This mechanism permits hypothalamic centers to respond to these blood glucose levels, contributing to hunger and eating behaviors. Most of the cells lining the third ventricle are ependymal cells; however, modified ependymal cells called *tanycytes* (Greek for "stretched out") are also present. Processes of tanycytes extend through the glial limitans lining the third ventricle to terminate on blood vessels, neurons, or glial cells of the neurophil (Fig. 49-31). The glial limitans consists of astrocytic end plates that provide an additional barrier between the CSF and brain. Evidence suggests that tanycytes may have important neuroendocrine functions besides their function as barrier cells. For example, tanycytes express high levels of the enzyme needed to convert thyroxine (T_4) into its more potent triiodothyronine (T_3) form.

In summary, during development, the most rostral part of the embryonic neural tube develops to form the brain. The brain can be divided into three parts: hindbrain, midbrain, and forebrain. The hindbrain, consisting of the medulla oblongata, pons, and cerebellum, contains the neuronal circuits for the eating, breathing, and locomotive functions required for survival. Cranial nerves XII, XI, X, IX, VIII, VII, VI, and V are located in the hindbrain. Cranial nerves III and IV arise from the midbrain. The forebrain is the most rostral part of the brain; it consists of the diencephalon and the telencephalon. The dorsal horn part of the diencephalon comprises the thalamus and subthalamus, and the ventral horn part is the hypothalamus. The cerebral hemispheres are the lateral outgrowths of the diencephalon. Although there may be considerable overlap, one of the hemispheres is the more dominant hemisphere; it has

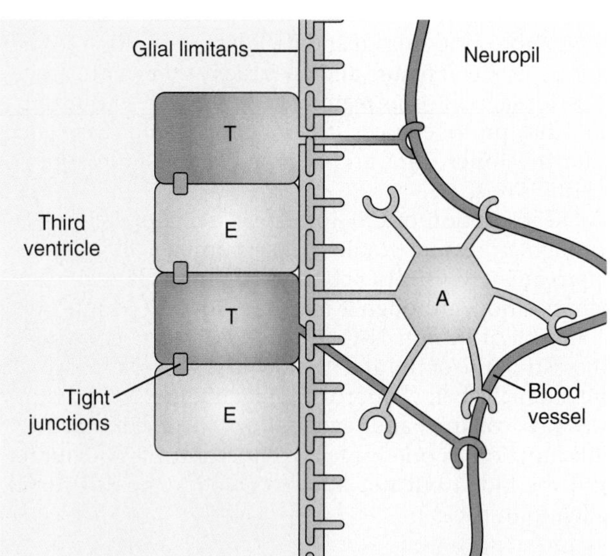

FIGURE 49-31 Ependymal cells (*E*) and tanycytes (*T*) lining the third ventricle. As indicated, tanycytes extend into the neuropil to contact blood vessels. They may also contact neurons or glial cells. An astrocyte (*A*) is shown forming the blood–brain barrier around a blood vessel; other processes of astrocytes form the glial limitans, thus isolating the cerebrospinal fluid in the ventricle from the substance of the brain. Tight or occluding junctions are found between adjacent tanycytes and ependymal cells. (Courtesy of Edward W. Carroll)

a major role in verbal and analytic abilities. The less dominant hemisphere has a major role in nonverbal and spatial abilities.

The cerebral hemispheres are arbitrarily divided into lobes—the frontal, parietal, temporal, and occipital lobes—named after the bones of the skull that cover them. Contained within the frontal lobe are the prefrontal premotor area and primary motor cortex; the primary sensory cortex and somesthetic association area are in the parietal cortex; the primary auditory cortex and the auditory association area are in the temporal lobe; and the primary visual cortex and association visual cortex are in the occipital lobe. The limbic system, which is involved in emotional experience and release of emotional behaviors, is located in the medial aspect of the cerebrum. These cortical areas are reciprocally connected with underlying thalamic nuclei through the internal capsule. Thalamic involvement is essential for normal forebrain function.

The brain is enclosed and protected by the pia mater, arachnoid, and dura mater. The protective CSF in which the brain and spinal cord float isolates them from minor and moderate trauma. Cerebrospinal fluid is secreted into the ventricles, circulates through the ventricular system, passes outside to surround the brain, and is reabsorbed into the venous system through the arachnoid villi. The CSF–brain barrier, the arachnoid–CSF barrier, and the blood–brain barrier protect the brain from substances in the blood that would disrupt brain function.

THE AUTONOMIC NERVOUS SYSTEM (ANS)

- The ANS functions at the subconscious level and is responsible for maintaining homeostatic functions of the body.
- The ANS has two divisions: the sympathetic and parasympathetic systems. Although the two divisions function in concert, they are generally viewed as having opposite and antagonistic actions.
- The sympathetic division functions in maintaining vital functions and responding when there is a critical threat to the integrity of the individual—the "fight-or-flight" response.
- The parasympathetic nervous system is concerned with conservation of energy, resource replenishment, and maintenance of organ function during periods of minimal activity.
- The outflow of both divisions of the ANS consists of a two-neuron pathway: a preganglionic and a postganglionic neuron. Acetylcholine is the neurotransmitter for the preganglionic neurons for both ANS divisions, as well as the postganglionic neurons of the parasympathetic nervous system. Norepinephrine and epinephrine are the neurotransmitters for the sympathetic postganglionic neurons.

The Autonomic Nervous System

After completing this section of the chapter, you should be able to meet the following objectives:

- State the function of the autonomic nervous system
- Compare the anatomic location and functions of the sympathetic and parasympathetic nervous systems
- Describe neurotransmitter synthesis, release, and degradation and receptor function in the sympathetic and parasympathetic nervous systems

The ability to maintain homeostasis and perform the activities of daily living in an ever-changing physical environment is largely vested in the autonomic nervous system (ANS). This portion of the nervous system functions at the subconscious level and is involved in regulating, adjusting, and coordinating vital visceral functions such as blood pressure and blood flow, body temperature, respiration, digestion, metabolism, and elimination. The ANS is strongly affected by emotional influences and is involved in many of the expressive aspects of behavior. Blushing, pallor, palpitations of the heart, clammy hands, and dry mouth are several emotional expressions mediated through the ANS. Biofeedback and relaxation exercises have been used for modifying the subconscious functions of the ANS.

As with the somatic nervous system, the ANS is represented in both the CNS and the PNS. Traditionally, the ANS has been defined as a general efferent system innervating visceral organs. The efferent outflow from the ANS has two divisions: the sympathetic nervous system and the parasympathetic nervous system. The afferent input to the ANS is provided by visceral afferent neurons, usually not considered a part of the ANS.

The functions of the sympathetic nervous system include maintaining body temperature and adjusting blood flow and blood pressure to meet the changing needs of the body that occur with activities of daily living, such as moving from the supine to the standing position. The sympathoadrenal system also can discharge as a unit when there is a critical threat to the integrity of the individual—the so-called fight-or-flight response. During a stress situation, the heart rate accelerates; blood pressure rises; blood flow shifts from the skin and gastrointestinal tract to the skeletal muscles and brain; blood sugar increases; the bronchioles and pupils dilate; the sphincters of the stomach and intestine and the internal sphincter of the urethra constrict; and the rate of secretion of exocrine glands involved in digestion diminishes. Emergency situations often require vasoconstriction and shunting of blood away from the skin and into the muscles and brain, a mechanism that, should a wound occur, provides for a reduction in blood flow and preservation of vital functions needed for survival. Sympathetic function is often summarized as catabolic in that its actions predominate during periods of pronounced energy expenditure, such as when survival is threatened.

In contrast to the sympathetic nervous system, the functions of the parasympathetic nervous system are concerned with conservation of energy, resource replenishment and storage (*i.e.*, anabolism), and maintenance of organ function during periods of minimal activity. The parasympathetic nervous system slows heart rate, stimulates gastrointestinal function and related glandular secretion, promotes bowel and bladder elimination, and constricts the pupil, protecting the retina from excessive light during periods when visual function is not vital to survival. The two divisions of the ANS are usually viewed as having opposite and antagonistic actions (*i.e.,* if one activates, the other inhibits a function). Exceptions are functions, such as sweating and regulation of arteriolar blood vessel diameter, controlled by a single division of the ANS, in this case the sympathetic nervous system.

The sympathetic and parasympathetic nervous systems are continually active. The effect of this continual or basal (baseline) activity is referred to as *tone.* The tone of an effector organ or system can be increased or decreased and is usually regulated by a single division of the ANS. For example, vascular smooth muscle tone is controlled by the sympathetic nervous system. Increased sympathetic activity produces local vasoconstriction from increased vascular smooth muscle tone, and decreased activity results in vasodilatation due to decreased tone. In structures such as the sinoatrial node and atrioventricular node of the heart, which are innervated by both divisions of the ANS, one division predominates in controlling tone. In this case, the tonically active parasympathetic nervous system exerts a constraining or braking effect on heart rate, and when parasympathetic outflow is withdrawn, the heart rate increases. The increase in heart rate that occurs with vagal withdrawal can be further augmented by sympathetic stimulation. Table 49-4 describes the responses of effector organs to sympathetic and parasympathetic impulses.

AUTONOMIC EFFERENT PATHWAYS

The outflow of both divisions of the ANS follows a two-neuron pathway. The first motoneuron, called the *preganglionic neuron,* lies in the intermediolateral cell column in the ventral horn of the spinal cord or its equivalent location in the brain stem. The second motoneuron, called the *postganglionic neuron,* synapses with a preganglionic neuron in an autonomic ganglion in the PNS. The two divisions of the ANS differ as to location of preganglionic cell bodies, relative length of preganglionic fibers, general function, nature of peripheral responses, and preganglionic and postganglionic neuromediators (see Table 49-4). This two-neuron outflow pathway and the interneurons in the autonomic ganglia that add further modulation to ANS function are features distinctly different from the arrangement in somatic motor innervation (Fig. 49-32).

Most visceral organs are innervated by both sympathetic and parasympathetic fibers. Exceptions include structures such as blood vessels and sweat glands that have input from only one division of the ANS. The fibers of the sympathetic nervous system are distributed to effectors throughout the body, and as a result, sympathetic actions tend to be more diffuse than those of the parasympathetic nervous system, in which there is a more localized distribution of fibers. The preganglionic fibers of the sympathetic nervous system may traverse a considerable distance and pass through several ganglia before synapsing with postganglionic neurons, and their terminals contact many postganglionic fibers. In some ganglia, the ratio of preganglionic to postganglionic cells may be 1:20; because of this, the effects of sympathetic stimulation are diffuse. Considerable overlap exists, and one ganglion cell may be supplied by several preganglionic fibers. In contrast to the sympathetic nervous system, the parasympathetic nervous system has its postganglionic neurons located very near or in the organ of innervation. Because the ratio of preganglionic to postganglionic communication is often 1:1, the effects of the parasympathetic nervous system are much more circumscribed.

Sympathetic Nervous System

The neurons of the sympathetic nervous system are located primarily in the thoracic and upper lumbar segments (T1

TABLE 49-4 Characteristics of the Sympathetic and Parasympathetic Nervous Systems

Characteristic	Sympathetic Outflow	Parasympathetic Outflow
Location of preganglionic cell bodies	T1–T12, L1 and L2	Cranial nerves: III, VII (intermedius), IX, X; sacral segments 2, 3, and 4
Relative length of preganglionic fibers	Short—to paravertebral chain of ganglia or to aortic prevertebral of ganglia	Long—to ganglion cells near or in the innervated organ
General function	Catabolic—mobilizes resources in anticipation of challenge for survival (preparation for "fight-or-flight" response)	Anabolic—concerned with conservation, renewal, and storage of resources
Nature of peripheral response	Generalized	Localized
Transmitter between preganglionic terminals and postganglionic neurons	ACh	ACh
Transmitter of postganglionic neuron	ACh (sweat glands and skeletal muscle vasodilator fibers); norepinephrine (most synapses); norepinephrine and epinephrine (secreted by adrenal gland)	ACh

ACh, acetylcholine.

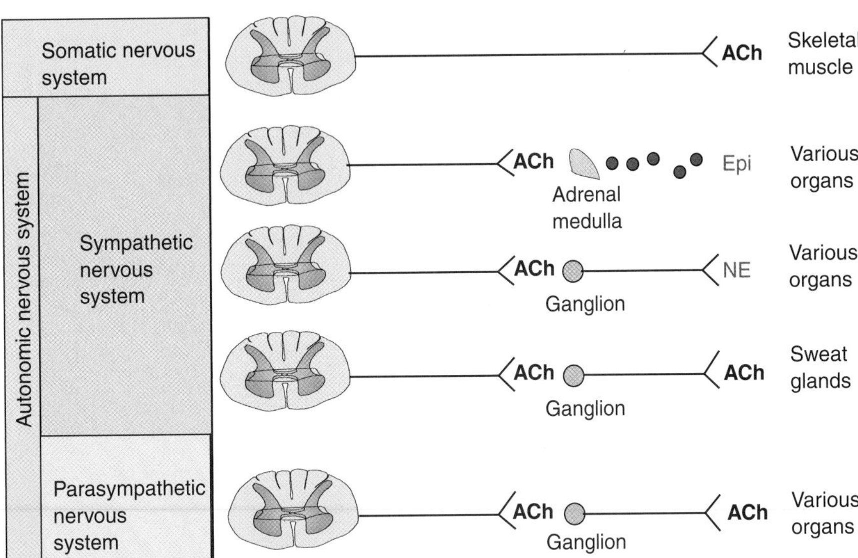

FIGURE 49-32 Comparison of the neurotransmission in the somatic and autonomic nervous systems. In the somatic nervous system, all motor neurons release acetylcholine (ACh) as their neurotransmitter. In the autonomic nervous system, both sympathetic and parasympathetic preganglionic neurons release ACh as their neurotransmitter. Parasympathetic postganglionic neurons release ACh at the site of organ innervation. Most postganglionic neurons of the sympathetic nervous system release norepinephrine (NE) at the site of organ innervation. The principal neurotransmitter released by the adrenal gland is epinephrine (Epi), which travels to the site of organ innervation by way of the bloodstream. The postganglionic neurons innervating the sweat gland are sympathetic fibers that use ACh as their neurotransmitter.

to L2) of the spinal cord; hence, the sympathetic nervous system is often called the *thoracolumbar division* of the ANS. These preganglionic neurons, located primarily in the ventral horn intermediolateral cell column, have axons that are largely myelinated and relatively short. The postganglionic neurons of the sympathetic nervous system are located in the paravertebral ganglia of the sympathetic chain of ganglia that lie on either side of the vertebral column, or in prevertebral sympathetic ganglia such as the celiac ganglia (Fig. 49-33). Besides postganglionic efferent neurons, the sympathetic ganglia contain neurons of the internuncial, short-axon type, similar to those associated with complex circuitry in the brain and spinal cord. Many of these inhibit and others modulate preganglionic-to-postganglionic transmission. The full significance of these modulating circuits awaits further investigation.

The axons of the preganglionic neurons leave the spinal cord through the ventral root of the spinal nerves (T1 to L2), enter the ventral primary rami, and leave the spinal nerve through white rami of the rami communicantes to reach the paravertebral ganglionic chain (Fig. 49-34). In the sympathetic chain of ganglia, preganglionic fibers may synapse with neurons of the ganglion they enter, pass up or down the chain and synapse with one or more ganglia, or pass through the chain and move outward through a splanchnic nerve to terminate in prevertebral ganglia (*i.e.*, celiac, superior mesenteric, or inferior mesenteric) scattered along the dorsal aorta and its branches.

Preganglionic fibers from the thoracic segments of the cord pass upward to form the cervical chain connecting the inferior, middle, and superior cervical sympathetic ganglia with the rest of the sympathetic chain at lower levels. Postganglionic sympathetic axons of the cervical and lower lumbosacral chain ganglia spread further through nerve plexuses along continuations of the great arteries. Cranial structures, particularly blood vessels, are innervated by the spread of postganglionic axons along the external and internal carotid arteries into the face and the cranial cavity. The sympathetic fibers from T1 usually continue up the sympathetic chain into the head; those from T2 pass into the neck; those from T1 to T5 travel to the heart; those from T3, T4, T5, and T6 proceed to the thoracic viscera; those from T7, T8, T9, T10, and T11 pass to the abdominal viscera; and those from T12, L1, and L2 pass to the kidneys and pelvic organs. Many preganglionic fibers from the fifth to the last thoracolumbar segment pass through the paravertebral ganglia to continue as the splanchnic nerves. Most of these fibers do not synapse until they reach the celiac or superior mesenteric ganglion; others pass to the adrenal medulla.

The adrenal medulla, which is part of the sympathetic nervous system, contains postganglionic sympathetic neurons that secrete sympathetic neurotransmitters directly into the bloodstream. Some postganglionic fibers, all of which are unmyelinated, exit the paravertebral ganglionic chain and reenter the segmental nerve through unmyelinated branches, called *gray rami*. These segmental nerves are then distributed to all parts of the body wall in the spinal nerve branches. These fibers innervate the sweat glands, piloerector muscles of the hair follicles, all blood vessels of the skin and skeletal muscles, and the CNS itself.

Parasympathetic Nervous System

The preganglionic fibers of the parasympathetic nervous system, also called the *craniosacral division* of the ANS, originate in some segments of the brain stem and sacral segments of the spinal cord (see Fig. 49-33). The central regions of origin are the midbrain, pons, medulla oblongata, and sacral part of the spinal cord. The midbrain outflow passes through the oculomotor nerve (cranial nerve III) to the ciliary ganglion that lies in the orbit behind the eye; it supplies the pupillary sphincter muscle of each eye and the ciliary muscles that control lens thickness for accommodation. From the caudal pontine outflow originate the preganglionic fibers of the intermedius component of the facial nerve (cranial nerve VII) complex. This outflow synapses in the submandibular ganglia, which sends postganglionic fibers to supply the submandibular and sublingual

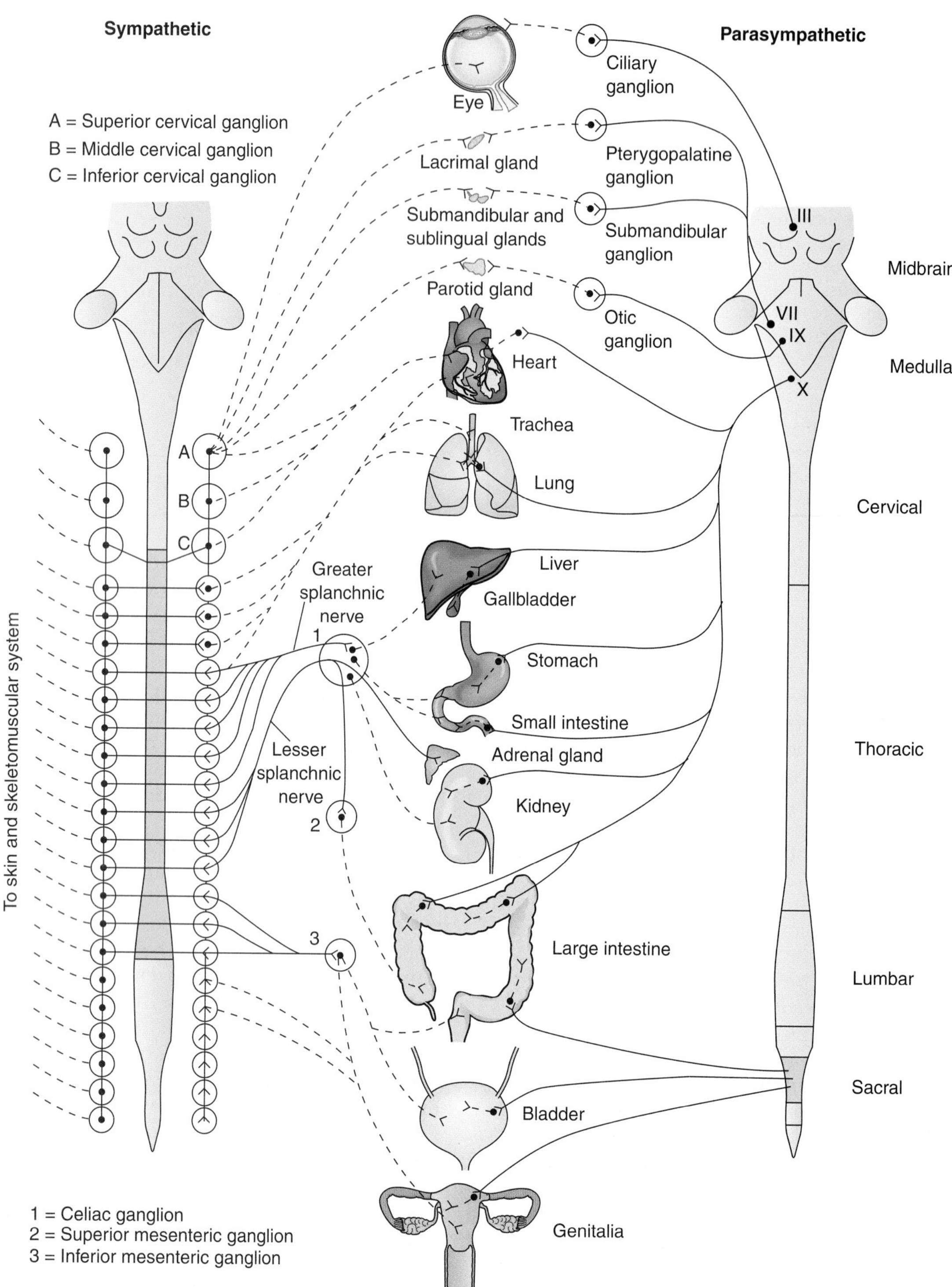

FIGURE 49-33 The autonomic nervous system. The involuntary organs are depicted with their parasympathetic innervation (craniosacral) indicated on the right and sympathetic innervation (thoracolumbar) on the left. Preganglionic fibers are *solid lines;* postganglionic fibers are *dashed lines.* For purposes of illustration, the sympathetic outflow to the skin and skeletomuscular system is shown separately (to the far left); effectors include sweat glands, pilomotor muscles and blood vessels of the skin, and blood vessels of the skeletal muscles and bones. (Modified from Hemer L. [1983]. *The human brain and spinal cord: Functional neuroanatomy and dissection guide.* New York: Springer-Verlag)

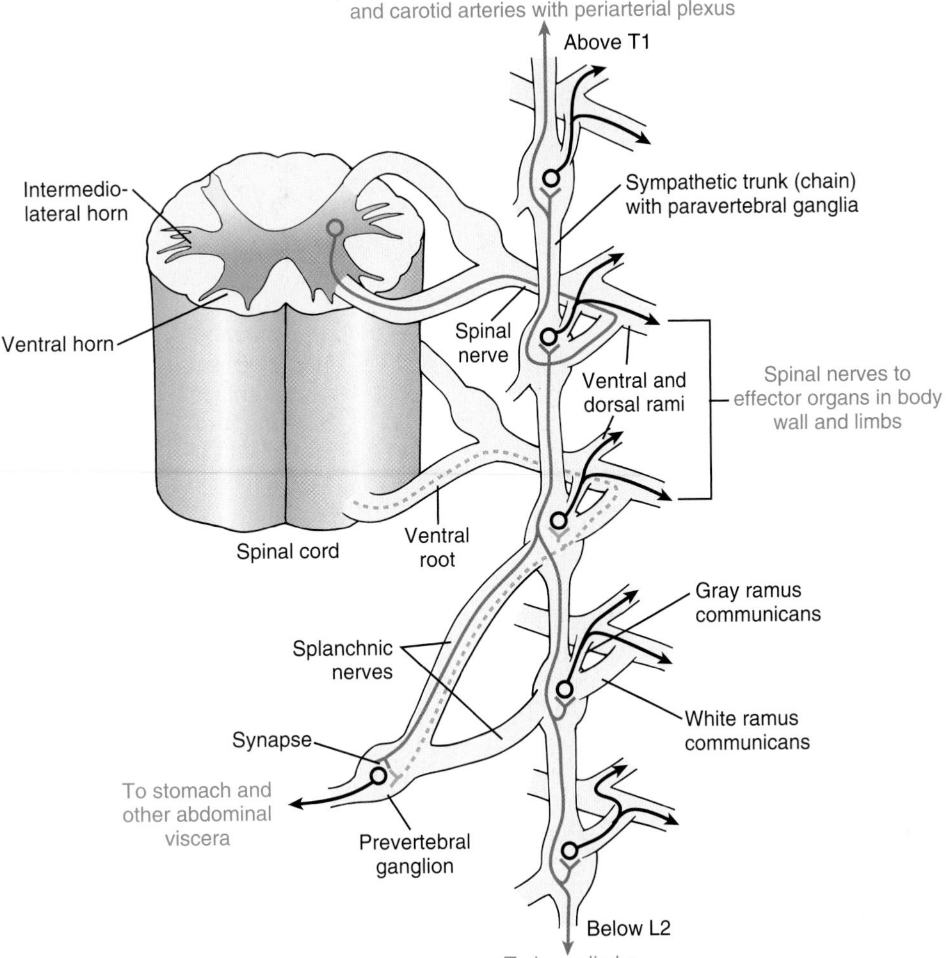

FIGURE 49-34 Sympathetic pathways. Sympathetic fibers (*blue*) leave the spinal cord by way of the ventral root of the spinal nerves, enter the ventral primary rami, and pass through the white rami to the prevertebral or paravertebral ganglia of the sympathetic chain, where they synapse with postganglionic neurons (*black*). Some postganglionic fibers from the paravertebral ganglia reenter the segmental nerves through the gray rami and are then distributed in the spinal nerve branches that innervate the effector organs (*e.g.*, sweat glands and arrector pili muscles of skin and vascular smooth muscle of blood vessels). Other postganglionic neurons (*red dotted lines*) travel directly to their destination in the various effector organs.

glands. In addition, preganglionic fibers are distributed to the pterygopalatine ganglia to synapse on postganglionic neurons. These postganglionic fibers emanating from the pterygopalatine ganglia supply the lacrimal and nasal glands. The medullary outflow develops from cranial nerves VII, IX, and X. Fibers in the glossopharyngeal nerve (cranial nerve IX) synapse in the otic ganglia, which supply the parotid salivary glands. Approximately 75% of parasympathetic efferent fibers are carried in the vagus nerve (cranial nerve X). The vagus nerve provides parasympathetic innervation for the heart, trachea, lungs, esophagus, stomach, small intestine, proximal half of the colon, liver, gallbladder, pancreas, kidneys, and upper portions of the ureters.

Sacral preganglionic axons leave the S2 to S4 segmental nerves by gathering into the pelvic nerves, also called the *nervi erigentes*. The pelvic nerves leave the sacral plexus on each side of the cord and distribute their peripheral fibers to the bladder, uterus, urethra, prostate, distal portion of the transverse colon, descending colon, and rectum. Sacral parasympathetic fibers also supply the venous outflow from the external genitalia to facilitate erectile function.

Excepting cranial nerves III, VII, and IX, which synapse in discrete ganglia, the long parasympathetic preganglionic fibers pass uninterrupted to short postganglionic fibers within the organ wall. In the walls of these organs, postganglionic neurons send axons to smooth muscle and glandular cells that modulate their functions.

The gastrointestinal tract has its own intrinsic network of ganglionic cells found between the smooth muscle layers, called the *enteric* (or *intramural*) *plexus,* which controls local peristaltic movements and secretory functions. This network of parasympathetic postganglionic neurons and interneurons runs from the lower two thirds of the esophagus to the internal anal sphincter. Local afferent sensory neurons respond to mechanical and chemical stimuli and communicate these influences to motor fibers in the enteric plexus. The number of neurons in the enteric neural network (10^8) is so large that it approximates that of the spinal cord. It is thought that this enteric nervous system is capable of independent function without control from CNS fibers. The CNS has a modulating role, by way of preganglionic innervation of the plexus, converting local peristalsis to longer-distance movements, thereby speeding the transit of intestinal contents.

CENTRAL INTEGRATIVE PATHWAYS

General visceral afferent fibers accompany the sympathetic and parasympathetic outflow into the spinal and cranial nerves, bringing chemoreceptor, pressure, organ capsule stretch, and nociceptive information from organs of the viscera to the brain stem, thoracolumbar cord, and sacral cord. Local reflex circuits relating visceral afferent and autonomic efferent activity are integrated into a hierarchic control system in the spinal cord and brain stem. Progressively greater complexity in the responses and greater precision in their control occur at each higher level of the nervous system. Most visceral reflexes contain contributions from the LMNs that innervate skeletal muscles as part of their response patterns. The distinction between purely visceral and somatic reflex hierarchies becomes less and less meaningful at the higher levels of hierarchic control and behavioral integration.

For most autonomic-mediated functions, the hypothalamus serves as the major control center. The hypothalamus, having connections with the cerebral cortex, the limbic system, and the pituitary gland, is in a prime position to receive, integrate, and transmit information to other areas of the nervous system. Neurons concerned with thermoregulation, thirst, and feeding behaviors are also found in the hypothalamus. The hypothalamus also is the site for integrating neuroendocrine function. Hypothalamic releasing and inhibiting hormones control the secretion of anterior pituitary hormones (*i.e.,* thyroid-stimulating hormone, corticotropin, growth hormone, luteinizing hormone, follicle-stimulating hormone, and prolactin). The supraoptic nuclei of the hypothalamus are involved in water metabolism through synthesis of antidiuretic hormone and its release from the posterior pituitary gland (see Chapter 33). Oxytocin, which causes contraction of the pregnant uterus and milk letdown during breast-feeding, is synthesized in the hypothalamus and released from the posterior pituitary gland similar to that of antidiuretic hormone.

The organization of many life-support reflexes occurs in the reticular formation of the medulla and pons. These areas of reflex circuitry, often called *centers,* produce complex combinations of autonomic and somatic efferent functions required for the respiration, gag, cough, sneeze, swallow, and vomit reflexes, and for the more purely autonomic control of the cardiovascular system. At the hypothalamic level, these reflexes are integrated into more general response patterns such as rage, defensive behavior, eating, drinking, voiding, and sexual function. Forebrain and especially limbic system control of these behaviors involves inhibiting or facilitating release of the response patterns according to social pressures during learned emotion-provoking situations.

Reflex adjustments of cardiovascular and respiratory function occur at the level of the brain stem. A prominent example is the carotid sinus baroreflex. Increased blood pressure in the carotid sinus results in increased discharge from afferent fibers that travel by way of the ninth cranial nerve to cardiovascular centers in the brain stem. These centers increase the activity of descending efferent vagal fibers that slow heart rate, while inhibiting sympathetic fibers that increase heart rate and blood vessel tone. Striking features of ANS function are the rapidity and intensity with which it can change visceral function. Within 3 to 5 seconds, it can increase heart rate to approximately twice its resting level. Bronchial smooth muscle tone is largely controlled by parasympathetic fibers carried in the vagus nerve. These nerves produce mild to moderate constriction of the bronchioles.

Other important ANS reflexes are located at the level of the spinal cord. As with other spinal reflexes, these reflexes are modulated by input from higher centers. When a loss of communication exists between the higher centers and the spinal reflexes, as occurs in spinal cord injury, these reflexes function in an unregulated manner (see Chapter 51). This results in uncontrolled sweating, vasomotor instability, and reflex bowel and bladder function.

AUTONOMIC NEUROTRANSMISSION

The generation and transmission of impulses in the ANS occur in the same manner as in other neurons. There are self-propagating action potentials with transmission of impulses across synapses and other tissue junctions by way of neurohumoral transmitters. However, the somatic motoneurons that innervate skeletal muscles divide into many branches, with each branch innervating a single muscle fiber; in contrast, the distribution of postganglionic fibers of the ANS forms a diffuse neural plexus at the site of innervation. The membranes of the cells of many smooth muscle fibers are connected by conductive protoplasmic bridges, called *gap junctions,* that permit rapid conduction of impulses through whole sheets of smooth muscle, often in repeating waves of contraction. Autonomic neurotransmitters released near a limited portion of these fibers provide a modulating function extending to many effector cells. Smooth muscle layers of the gut and of the bladder wall are examples. Sometimes, isolated smooth muscle cells are individually innervated by the ANS, such as the piloerector cells that elevate the hair on the skin during cold exposure.

The main neurotransmitters of the autonomic nervous system are acetylcholine and the catecholamines, epinephrine and norepinephrine. Acetylcholine is released at all preganglionic synapses in the autonomic ganglia of both sympathetic and parasympathetic nerve fibers and from postganglionic synapses of all parasympathetic nerve endings. It also is released at sympathetic nerve endings that innervate the sweat glands and cholinergic vasodilator fibers found in skeletal muscle. Norepinephrine is released at most sympathetic nerve endings. The adrenal medulla, which is a modified prevertebral sympathetic ganglion, produces epinephrine along with small amounts of norepinephrine. Dopamine, which is an intermediate compound in the synthesis of norepinephrine, also acts as a neurotransmitter. It is the principal inhibitory transmitter of internuncial neurons in the sympathetic ganglia. It also has vasodilator effects on renal, splanchnic, and coronary blood vessels when given intravenously and is sometimes used in the treatment of shock (see Chapter 28).

Many neurons secreting peptide molecules have been identified in ANS ganglia, especially in the enteric plexus and in postganglionic ANS terminals of the sympathetic and parasympathetic systems. Many of these are secreted by internuncial neurons or as additional transmitters or "cotransmitters" by preganglionic and postganglionic neurons. Binding at postsynaptic neuropeptide receptors usually does not result in action potentials; instead, it alters the membrane potential or receptor numbers, producing long-term (minutes to hours) changes in responsiveness to the neurotransmitter. For example, dual secretion of norepinephrine and neuropeptide Y in some sympathetic vasoconstrictor terminals results in longer vasomotor constriction. Similarly, some parasympathetic postganglionic acetylcholine-secreting neurons can secrete vasoactive intestinal peptide as a cotransmitter that potentiates postsynaptic actions. Many neuropeptides involved in peripheral ANS function are under active investigation, including substance P, cholecystokinin, somatostatin, and neurotensin.

Acetylcholine and Cholinergic Receptors

Acetylcholine is synthesized in the cholinergic neurons from choline and acetyl coenzyme A (acetyl CoA; Fig. 49-35). After acetylcholine is secreted by the cholinergic nerve endings, it is rapidly broken down by the enzyme acetylcholinesterase. The choline molecule is transported back into the nerve ending, where it is used again in the synthesis of acetylcholine.

Receptors that respond to acetylcholine are called *cholinergic receptors*. Two types of cholinergic receptors are known: muscarinic and nicotinic. Muscarinic receptors are present on the innervational targets of postganglionic fibers of the parasympathetic nervous system and the sweat glands, which are innervated by the sympathetic nervous system. Nicotinic receptors are found in autonomic ganglia and the end plates of skeletal muscle. Acetylcholine is excitatory to most muscarinic and nicotinic receptors, except those in the heart and lower esophagus, where it has an inhibitory effect. The drug atropine is an antimuscarinic or muscarinic cholinergic-blocking drug that prevents the action of acetylcholine at excitatory and inhibitory muscarinic receptor sites. Because it is a muscarinic-blocking drug, it exerts little effect at nicotinic receptor sites.

Catecholamines and Adrenergic Receptors

The catecholamines, which include norepinephrine, epinephrine, and dopamine, are synthesized in the axoplasm of sympathetic nerve terminal endings from the amino acid tyrosine (see Fig. 49-35). During catecholamine synthesis, tyrosine is hydroxylated (*i.e.*, has a hydroxyl group added) to form DOPA, and DOPA is decarboxylated (*i.e.*, has a carboxyl group removed) to form dopamine. Dopamine in turn is hydroxylated to form norepinephrine. In the adrenal gland, an additional step occurs during which norepinephrine is methylated (*i.e.*, a methyl group is added) to form epinephrine.

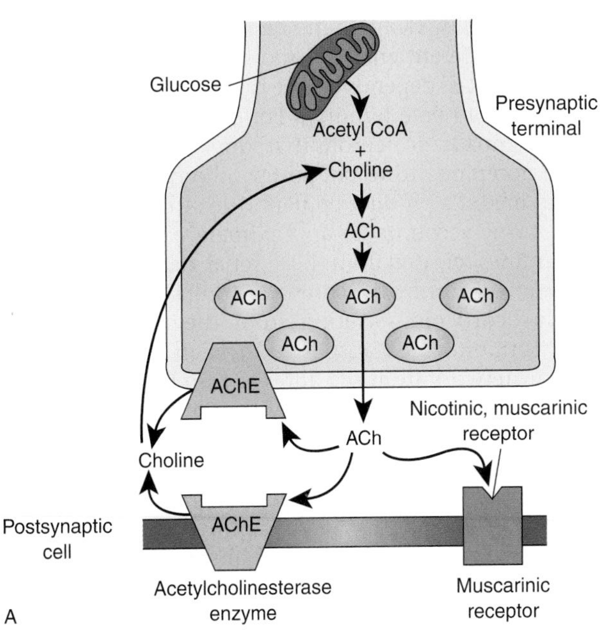

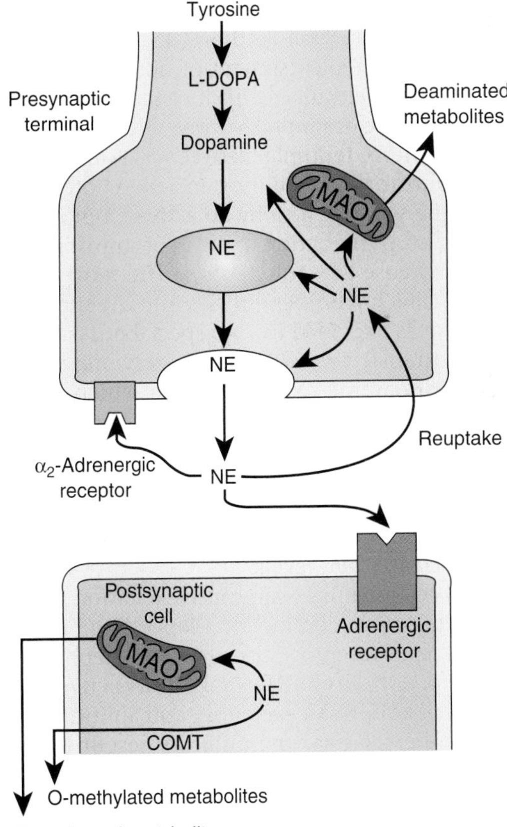

FIGURE 49-35 Schematic illustration of cholinergic parasympathetic (**A**) and noradrenergic sympathetic (**B**) neurotransmitter synthesis, release, receptor binding, neurotransmitter degradation, and metabolite transport back into the presynaptic neuron (acetylcholine) and reuptake (norepinephrine). (Adapted from Rhoades R.A., Tanner G.A. [1996]. *Medical physiology.* Boston: Little, Brown)

Each step in sympathetic neurotransmitter synthesis requires a different enzyme, and the type of neurotransmitter produced depends on the types of enzymes that are available in a nerve terminal. For example, the postganglionic sympathetic neurons that supply blood vessels synthesize norepinephrine, but postganglionic neurons in the adrenal medulla produce epinephrine or norepinephrine. Epinephrine accounts for approximately 80% of the catecholamines released from the adrenal gland. The synthesis of epinephrine by the adrenal medulla is influenced by the glucocorticoid secretion from the adrenal cortex. These hormones are transported through an intraadrenal vascular network from the adrenal cortex to the adrenal medulla, where they cause the sympathetic neurons to increase their production of epinephrine through increased enzyme activity. Thus, any stress situation sufficient to evoke increased levels of glucocorticoids also increases epinephrine levels. As the catecholamines are synthesized, they are stored in vesicles. The final step of norepinephrine synthesis occurs in these vesicles. When an action potential reaches an axon terminal, the neurotransmitter molecules are released from the storage vesicles. The storage vesicles provide a means for concentrated storage of the catecholamines and protect them from the cytoplasmic enzymes that degrade the neurotransmitters.

Besides neuronal synthesis, a second major mechanism exists for the replenishment of norepinephrine in sympathetic nerve terminals. This mechanism consists of the active recapture or reuptake of the released neurotransmitter into the nerve terminal. Between 50% and 80% of the norepinephrine released during an action potential is removed from the synaptic area by an active reuptake process. This process stops the action of the neurotransmitter and allows it to be reused by the neuron. The remainder of the released catecholamines diffuses into the surrounding tissue fluids or is degraded by two special enzymes: catechol-*O*-methyltransferase, which is diffusely present in all tissues, and monoamine oxidase (MAO), which is found in the nerve endings. Some drugs, such as the tricyclic antidepressants, are thought to increase the level of catecholamines at the site of nerve endings in the brain by blocking the reuptake process. Others, such as the MAO inhibitors, decrease the enzymatic degradation of the neurotransmitters and increase their levels.

Catecholamines can cause excitation or inhibition of smooth muscle contraction, depending on the site, dose, and type of receptor present. Norepinephrine has potent excitatory activity and low inhibitory activity. Epinephrine is potent as both an excitatory and an inhibitory agent.

The excitatory or inhibitory responses of organs to sympathetic neurotransmitters are mediated by interaction with special structures in the cell membrane called *receptors*. In 1948, Ahlquist proposed the designations α and β for the receptor sites where catecholamines produce their excitatory (α) and inhibitory (β) effects.

In vascular smooth muscle, excitation of α receptors causes vasoconstriction, and excitation of β receptors causes vasodilatation. Endogenously and exogenously administered norepinephrine produces marked vasoconstriction of the blood vessels in the skin, kidneys, and splanchnic circulation that are supplied with α receptors. The β receptors are most prevalent in the heart, the blood vessels of skeletal muscle, and the bronchioles. Blood vessels in skeletal muscle have α and β receptors. In these vessels, high levels of norepinephrine produce vasoconstriction; low levels produce vasodilatation. The low levels are thought to have a diluting effect on norepinephrine levels in the arteries of these blood vessels so that the β effect predominates. With respect to vessels having few receptors, such as those that supply the brain, norepinephrine has little effect.

α-Adrenergic receptors have been further subdivided into α_1 and α_2 receptors, and β-adrenergic receptors into β_1 and β_2 receptors. β_1-Adrenergic receptors are found primarily in the heart and can be selectively blocked by β_1 receptor–blocking drugs. β_2-Adrenergic receptors are found in the bronchioles and in other sites that have β-mediated functions. The α_1 receptors are found primarily in postsynaptic effector sites; they mediate responses in vascular smooth muscle. The α_2 receptors are mainly located presynaptically and can inhibit the release of norepinephrine from sympathetic nerve terminals. The α_2 receptors are abundant in the CNS and are thought to influence the central control of blood pressure.

The various classes of adrenergic receptors provide a mechanism by which the same adrenergic neurotransmitter can have many selective effects on different effector cells. This mechanism also permits neurotransmitters carried in the bloodstream, whether from neuroendocrine secretion by the adrenal gland or from subcutaneously or intravenously administered drugs, to produce the same effects.

The catecholamines produced and released from sympathetic nerve endings are called *endogenous neuromediators*. Sympathetic nerve endings also can be activated by exogenous forms of these neuromediators, which reach the nerve endings by way of the bloodstream after being injected into the body or administered orally. These drugs mimic the action of the neuromediators and are said to have a *sympathomimetic action*. Other drugs can selectively block the receptor sites on the neurons and temporarily prevent the neurotransmitter from exerting its action.

In summary, the ANS regulates, adjusts, and coordinates the visceral functions of the body. The ANS, which is divided into the sympathetic and parasympathetic systems, is an efferent system. It receives its afferent input from visceral afferent neurons. The ANS has CNS and PNS components. The outflow of the sympathetic and parasympathetic nervous system follows a two-neuron pathway, which consists of a preganglionic neuron in the CNS and a postganglionic neuron located outside the CNS. Sympathetic fibers leave the CNS at the thoracolumbar level, and the parasympathetic fibers leave at the craniosacral level. Usually, the sympathetic and parasympathetic nervous systems have opposing effects on visceral function—if one excites, the other inhibits. The hypothalamus serves as the major control center for most ANS functions; local reflex circuits relating visceral afferent and autonomic efferent activity are integrated in a hierarchic control system in the spinal cord and brain stem.

The main neurotransmitters for the ANS are acetylcholine and the catecholamines, epinephrine and norepinephrine. Acetylcholine is the transmitter for all preganglionic neurons, for postganglionic parasympathetic neurons, and for selected postganglionic sympathetic neurons. The catecholamines are the neurotransmitters for most postganglionic sympathetic neurons. Neurotransmitters exert their target action through specialized cell surface receptors—cholinergic receptors that bind acetylcholine and adrenergic receptors that bind the catecholamines. The cholinergic receptors are divided into nicotinic and muscarinic receptors, and adrenergic receptors are divided into α and β receptors. Different receptors for the same transmitter at various sites in the same tissue or in other tissues result in differences in tissue responses to the same transmitter. This arrangement also permits the use of pharmacologic agents that act at specific receptor types.

REVIEW EXERCISES

An event such as cardiac arrest, which produces global ischemia of the brain, can produce a selective loss of recent memory and cognitive skills while preserving the more vegetative and life-sustaining functions such as breathing.

A. Use principles related to the development of the nervous system and hierarchy of control to explain why.

Usually, spinal cord injury or disease produces both sensory and motor deficits. An exception is infection by the poliomyelitis virus, which produces weakness and paralysis without loss of sensation in the affected extremities.

A. Explain using information on the organization of nervous system into cell columns.

The brief tapping of the area over a tendon with a reflex hammer produces what is called a *deep tendon reflex*. This procedure is one of the more commonly used methods for assessing the integrity of the peripheral and central nervous systems.

A. Explain how this simple diagnostic procedure can provide information about the integrity of the afferent and efferent peripheral nerves, the cell columns, and the longitudinal tract systems.

The functions of the sympathetic nervous system are often described in relation to the fight-or-flight response. Using this description, explain the physiologic advantage for the following distribution of sympathetic nervous system receptors:

A. The presence of β_2 receptors on the blood vessels that provide blood flow to the skeletal muscles during "flight" and α_1 receptors on the resistance vessels that control blood pressure.

B. The presence of acetylcholine receptors on the sweat glands that allow for evaporative loss of body heat during "flight" and the presence of α_1 receptors that constrict the skin vessels that control blood flow to the skin.

C. The presence of β_2 receptors that produce relaxation in the detrusor muscle of the bladder during "fight" or "flight" and the α_1 receptors that produce contraction of the smooth muscle in the internal sphincter of the bladder.

Bibliography

Alberts B., Johnson A., Lewis J., et al. (2002). *Molecular biology of the cell* (4th ed., pp. 1227–1236). New York: Garland Science.

Araque A., Parpura V., Sanzgiri, R.P., Haydon P.G. (1999). Tripartite synapses: Glia, the unacknowledged partner. *Trends in Neuroscience 22,* 208–215.

Bear M.F., Connors B.W., Paradiso M.A. (1996). *Neuroscience: Exploring the brain.* Philadelphia: Lippincott-Raven.

Brodal P. (1998). *The central nervous system: Structure and function* (2nd ed.). New York: Oxford University Press.

Carlson B.M. (1994). *Human embryology and developmental biology* (pp. 204–240). St. Louis: C.V. Mosby.

Cochard L.R. (2002). *Netter's atlas of human embryology* (pp. 51–81). Teterboro, NJ: Icon Learning Systems.

Dambska M., Wisniewski K.E. (1999). *Normal and pathologic development of the human brain and spinal cord.* London: John Libbey & Company.

Gartner L.P., Hiatt J.L. (2001). *Color textbook of histology* (2nd ed., pp. 183–217). Philadelphia: W.B. Saunders.

Guyton A.C., Hall J.E. (2000). *Textbook of medical physiology* (10th ed.). Philadelphia: W.B. Saunders.

Haines D.E. (Ed.). (1997). *Fundamental neuroscience* (pp. 115–121, 126–127, 146–148, 443–454). New York: Churchill Livingstone.

Jessen K.R., Mirsky R. (1999). Schwann cells and their precursors emerge as major regulators of nerve development. *Trends in Neuroscience 22,* 402–410.

Kierszenbaum A.L. (2002). *Histology and cell biology: An introduction to pathology* (pp. 199–225). St. Louis: Mosby.

Kandel E.R., Schwartz J.H., Jessell T.M. (2000). *Principles of neural science* (4th ed.). New York: McGraw-Hill.

Matthews G.G. (1998). *Neurobiology: Molecules, cells, and systems.* Malden, MA: Blackwell Science.

Moore K.L., Dalley A.F. (1999). *Clinically oriented anatomy* (4th ed., pp. 872–898). Philadelphia: Lippincott Williams & Wilkins.

Moore K.L., Persaud T.V.N. (2003). *The developing human: Clinically oriented embryology* (7th ed., pp. 59–76, 427–463). Philadelphia: W.B. Saunders.

Parent A. (1996). *Carpenter's human neuroanatomy* (9th ed., pp. 186–192, 268–292, 748–756). Baltimore: Williams & Wilkins.

Sadler T.W. (2000). *Langman's medical embryology* (8th ed., pp. 83–111, 345–381, 411–458). Philadelphia: Lippincott Williams & Wilkins.

Sanes D.H., Reh T.A., Harris W.A. (2000). *Development of the nervous system.* San Diego: Academic Press.

Tortora G.J., Grabowski S.R. (2003). *Principles of anatomy and physiology* (10th ed.). Hoboken, NJ: John Wiley & Sons.

Wong-Riley M.T.T. (2000). *Neuroscience secrets.* Philadelphia: Hanley & Belfus.

Zigmond M.J., Bloom E.F., Landis S.C., et al. (1999). *Fundamental neuroscience.* San Diego: Academic Press.

CHAPTER

50

Somatosensory Function, Pain, and Headache

Elizabeth C. Devine

Sensory mechanisms provide individuals with a continuous stream of information about their bodies, the outside world, and the interactions between the two. The somatosensory component of the nervous system provides an awareness of body sensations such as touch, temperature, limb position, and pain. Other sensory components of the nervous system include the special senses of vision, hearing, smell, and taste, which are discussed in other chapters. The sensory receptors for somatosensory function consist of discrete nerve endings in the skin and other body tissues. Between 2 and 3 million sensory neurons deliver a steady stream of encoded information. Only a small proportion of this information reaches awareness; most provides input essential for a myriad of reflex and automatic mechanisms that keep us alive and manage our functioning.

This chapter is organized into two distinct parts. The first part describes the organization and control of somatosensory function, and the second focuses on pain as a somatosensory modality.

Organization and Control of Somatosensory Function

After completing this section of the chapter, you should be able to meet the following objectives:

- Describe the four major classes of somatosensory modalities
- Describe the organization of the somatosensory system in terms of first-, second-, and third-order neurons
- Characterize the structure and function of the dorsal root ganglion neurons in terms of sensory receptors, conduction velocities, and spinal cord projections
- Compare the discriminative pathway with the anterolateral pathway, and explain the clinical usefulness of this distinction
- Describe the sensory homunculus in the cerebral cortex
- Compare the tactile, thermal, and position sense modalities in terms of receptors, adequate stimuli, ascending pathways, and central integrative mechanisms
- Describe the role of clinical examination in assessing somatosensory function

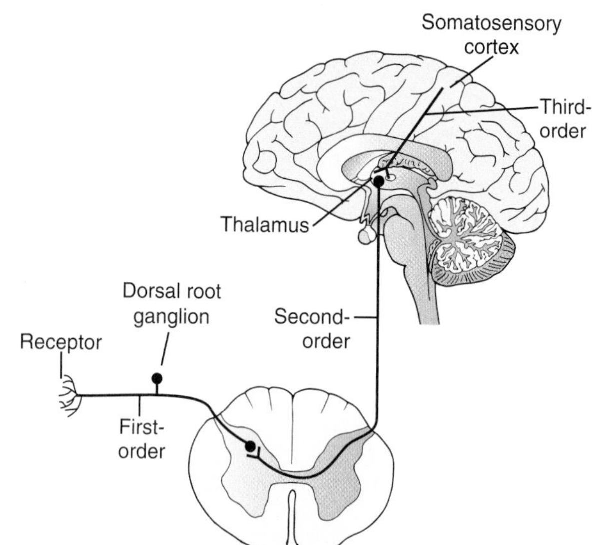

FIGURE 50-1 Arrangement of first-order, second-order, and third-order neurons of the somatosensory system.

The somatosensory system is designed to provide the central nervous system (CNS) with information about the body. Sensory neurons can be divided into three types that vary in distribution and the type of sensation detected: general somatic, special somatic, and general visceral afferent neurons. *General somatic afferent neurons* have branches with widespread distribution throughout the body and with many distinct types of receptors that result in sensations such as pain, touch, and temperature. *Special somatic afferent neurons* have receptors located primarily in muscles, tendons, and joints. These receptors sense position and movement of the body. *General visceral afferent neurons* have receptors on various visceral structures and sense fullness and discomfort.

SENSORY SYSTEMS

Sensory systems can be conceptualized as a serial succession of neurons consisting of first-order, second-order, and third-order neurons. *First-order neurons* transmit sensory information from the periphery to the CNS. *Second-order neurons* communicate with various reflex networks and sensory pathways in the spinal cord and travel directly to the thalamus. *Third-order neurons* relay information from the thalamus to the cerebral cortex (Fig. 50-1).

This organizing framework corresponds with the three primary levels of neural integration in the somatosensory system: the sensory units, which contain the sensory receptors; the ascending pathways; and the central processing centers in the thalamus and cerebral cortex. Sensory information usually is relayed in a cephalad direction by the three orders of neurons; along the way, it also is processed. Many interneurons process and modify the sensory information at the level of the second- and third-order neurons, and many more participate before coordinated and appropriate learned-movement responses occur. The number of participating neurons increases exponentially from the primary through the secondary and the secondary through the tertiary levels.

The Sensory Unit

The somatosensory experience arises from information provided by a variety of receptors distributed throughout the body. There are four major modalities of sensory experience: discriminative touch, which is required to identify the size and shape of objects and their movement across the skin; temperature sensation; sense of movement of the limbs and joints of the body; and nociception, or pain sense.

Each of the somatosensory modalities is mediated by a distinct system of receptors and pathways to the brain; however, all somatosensory information from the limbs

> **THE SOMATOSENSORY SYSTEM**
>
> - The somatosensory system relays information about four major modalities: touch, temperature, pain, and body position.
> - The system is organized segmentally into dermatomes, with each segment supplied by a single dorsal root ganglion that contains the neuronal cell bodies for the sensory units of the segment.
> - Somatosensory information is sequentially transmitted over three types of neurons: first-order neurons, which transmit information from sensory receptors to dorsal horn neurons; second-order CNS association neurons, which communicate with various reflex circuits and transmit information to the thalamus; and third-order neurons, which forward the information from the thalamus to the sensory cortex.

and trunk shares a common class of sensory neurons called *dorsal root ganglion neurons.* Somatosensory information from the face and cranial structures is transmitted by the trigeminal sensory neurons, which function in the same manner as the dorsal root ganglion neurons. The cell body of the dorsal root ganglion neuron, its peripheral branch (which innervates a small area of periphery), and its central axon (which projects to the CNS) form a *sensory unit.* Individual dorsal root ganglion neurons respond selectively to specific types of stimuli because of their specialized peripheral terminals, or receptors.

The fibers of different dorsal root ganglion neurons conduct impulses at varying rates, ranging from 0.5 to 120 m/second. This rate depends on the diameter of the nerve fiber. There are three types of nerve fibers that transmit somatosensory information: types A, B, and C. Type A fibers, which are myelinated, have the fastest rate of conduction. They are further divided into type Aα, type Aβ, and type Aδ fibers.[1,2] Type A fibers convey cutaneous pressure and touch sensation, cold sensation, mechanical pain, and heat pain. Type B fibers, which also are myelinated, transmit information from cutaneous and subcutaneous mechanoreceptors. The unmyelinated type C fibers have the smallest diameter and the slowest rate of conduction. They convey warm-hot sensation and mechanical and chemical as well as heat- and cold-induced pain sensation. Type Aα and Aδ fibers transmit information about muscle length and tendon stretch (discussed in Chapter 49).

Dermatomal Pattern of Dorsal Root Innervation

The somatosensory innervation of the body, including the head, retains a basic segmental organizational pattern that was established during embryonic development. Thirty-three paired spinal (*i.e.,* segmental) nerves provide sensory and motor innervation of the body wall, the limbs, and the viscera (see Chapter 49). Sensory input to each spinal cord segment is provided by sensory neurons with cell bodies in the dorsal root ganglia.

The region of the body wall that is supplied by a single pair of dorsal root ganglia is called a *dermatome.* These dorsal root ganglion–innervated strips occur in a regular sequence moving upward from the second coccygeal segment through the cervical segments, reflecting the basic segmental organization of the body and the nervous system (Fig. 50-2). The cranial nerves that innervate the head send their axons to equivalent nuclei in the brain stem. Neighboring dermatomes overlap one another sufficiently so that a loss of one dorsal root or root ganglion results in reduced but not total loss of sensory innervation of a dermatome (Fig. 50-3). Dermatome maps are helpful in interpreting the level and extent of sensory deficits that are the result of segmental nerve and spinal cord damage.

Spinal Circuitry and Ascending Neural Pathways

On entry into the spinal cord, the central axons of the somatosensory neurons branch extensively and project to

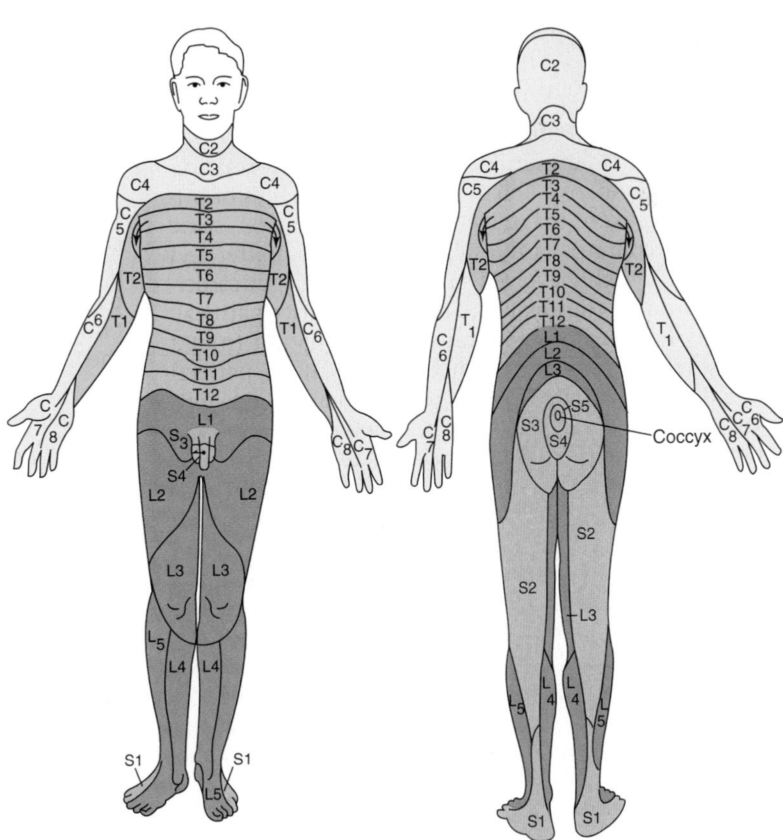

FIGURE 50-2 Cutaneous distribution of spinal nerves (dermatomes). (Barr, M. [1993]. *The human nervous system.* New York: Harper & Row)

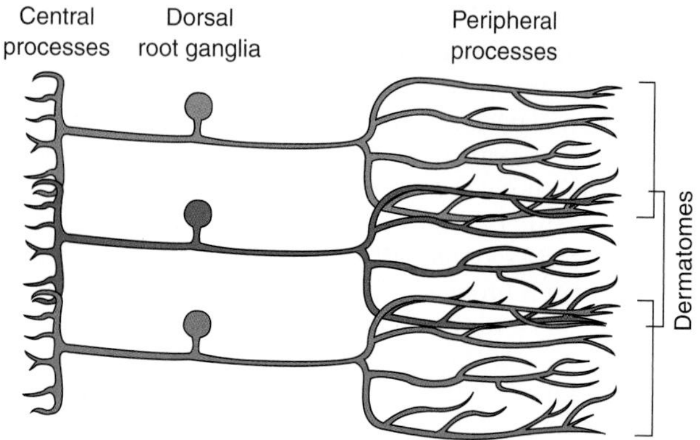

FIGURE 50-3 The dermatomes formed by the peripheral processes of adjacent spinal nerves overlap on the body surface. The central processes of these fibers also overlap in their spinal distribution.

nuclei in the spinal cord gray matter. Some branches become involved in local spinal cord reflexes and directly initiate motor reflexes (*e.g.*, flexor-withdrawal reflex). Two parallel pathways, the *discriminative pathway* and the *anterolateral pathway*, carry the information from the spinal cord to the thalamic level of sensation, each taking a different route through the CNS. The discriminative pathway crosses at the base of the medulla, and the anterolateral pathway crosses within the first few segments of entering the spinal cord. These pathways relay information to the brain for three purposes: perception, arousal, and motor control. Having a two-pathway system has several advantages. It adds richness to the sensory input by allowing the sensory information to be handled in two different ways, and it ensures that if one pathway is damaged, the other still can provide input.

The Discriminative Pathway. The discriminative pathway is used for the rapid transmission of sensory information such as discriminative touch. It contains branches of primary afferent axons that travel up the ipsilateral (*i.e.*, same side) dorsal columns of the spinal cord white matter and synapse with highly evolved somatosensory input association neurons in the medulla. The discriminative pathway uses only three neurons to transmit information from a sensory receptor to the somatosensory strip of parietal cerebral cortex of the opposite side of the brain: (1) the primary dorsal root ganglion neuron, which projects its central axon to the dorsal column nuclei; (2) the dorsal column neuron, which sends its axon through a rapid conducting tract, called the *medial lemniscus*, that crosses at the base of the medulla and travels to the thalamus on the opposite side of the brain, where basic sensation begins; and (3) the thalamic neuron, which projects its axons through the somatosensory radiation to the primary sensory cortex[1] (Fig. 50-4). The medial lemniscus is joined by fibers from the sensory nucleus of the trigeminal nerve (cranial nerve V) that supplies the face. Sensory information arriving at the sensory cortex by this route can be discretely localized and discriminated in terms of intensity.

One of the distinct features of the discriminative pathway is that it relays precise information regarding spatial orientation. This is the only pathway taken by the sensa-

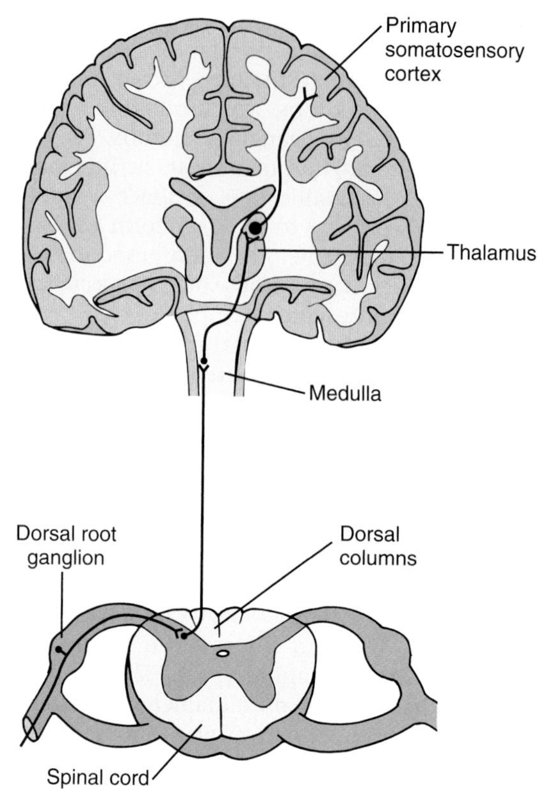

FIGURE 50-4 Discriminative pathway. This pathway is an ascending system for rapid transmission of sensations that relate joint movement (kinesthesis), body position (proprioception), vibration, and delicate touch. Primary afferents travel up the dorsal columns of the spinal cord white matter and synapse with somatosensory input association neurons in the medulla. Secondary neurons project through the brain stem to the thalamus and synapse with tertiary neurons, which relay the information to the primary somatosensory cortex on the opposite side of the brain.

tions of muscle and joint movement, vibration, and delicate discriminative touch, as is required to differentiate correctly the location of touch on the skin at two neighboring points (*i.e.*, two-point discrimination). One of the important functions of the discriminative pathway is to integrate the input from multiple receptors. The sense of shape and size of an object in the absence of visualization, called *stereognosis*, is based on precise afferent information from muscle, tendon, and joint receptors. For example, a screwdriver is perceived as being different from a knife in terms of its texture (tactile sensibility) and shape based on the relative position of the fingers as they move over the object. This complex interpretive perception requires that the discriminative system must be functioning optimally and that higher-order parietal association cortex processing and prior learning must have occurred. If the discriminative somatosensory pathway is functional but the parietal association cortex has become discretely damaged, the person can correctly describe the object but does not recognize that it is a screwdriver. This deficit is called *astereognosis*.

The Anterolateral Pathway. The anterolateral pathways (anterior and lateral spinothalamic pathways) consist of bilateral multisynaptic slow-conducting tracts (see Chapter 49, Fig. 49-15). These pathways provide for transmission of sensory information such as pain, thermal sensations, crude touch, and pressure that does not require discrete localization of signal source or fine discrimination of intensity. The fibers of the anterolateral pathway originate in the dorsal horns at the level of the segmental nerve, where the dorsal root neurons enter the spinal cord. They cross in the anterior commissure, within a few segments of origin, to the opposite anterolateral pathway, where they ascend upward toward the brain. The fibers of the spinothalamic tracts synapse with several nuclei in the thalamus, but en route they give off numerous branches that travel to the reticular activating system of the brain stem. These projections provide the basis for increased wakefulness or awareness after strong somatosensory stimulation and for the generalized startle reaction that occurs with sudden and intense stimuli. They also stimulate autonomic nervous system responses, such as a rise in blood pressure and heart rate, dilation of the pupils, and the pale, moist skin that results from constriction of the cutaneous blood vessels and activation of the sweat glands.

There are two subdivisions in the anterolateral pathway: the *neospinothalamic tract* and the *paleospinothalamic tract*[1] (Fig. 50-5). The neospinothalamic tract, which carries bright pain, consists of a sequence of at least three neurons with long axons. It provides for relatively rapid transmission of sensory information to the thalamus. The paleospinothalamic tract, which is phylogenetically older than the neospinothalamic system, consists of bilateral, multisynaptic slow-conducting tracts that transmit sensory signals that do not require discrete localization of signal source or discrimination of fine gradations in intensity. This slower-conducting pathway also projects into the intralaminar nuclei of the thalamus, which have close connections with the limbic cortical systems. This circuitry gives touch its affective or emotional aspects, such as the particular unpleasantness of heavy pressure and the peculiar pleasantness of the tickling and gentle rubbing of the skin.

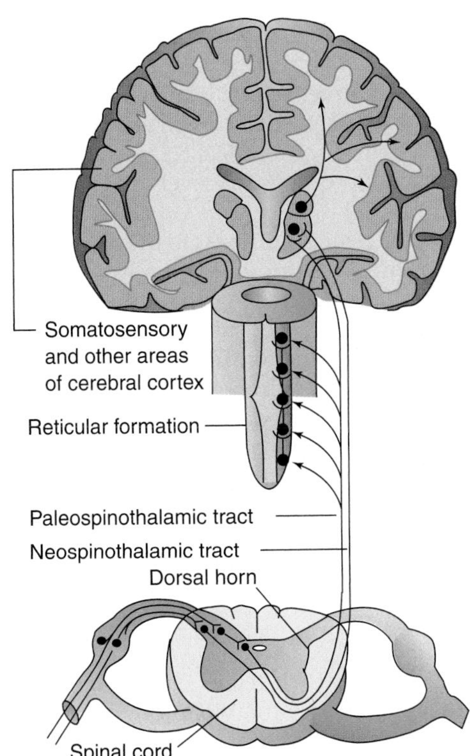

FIGURE 50-5 Neospinothalamic and paleospinothalamic subdivisions of the anterolateral sensory pathway. The neospinothalamic tract runs to the thalamic nuclei and has fibers that project to the somatosensory cortex. The paleospinothalamic tract sends collaterals to the reticular formation and other structures, from which further fibers project to the thalamus. These fibers influence the hypothalamus and the limbic system as well as the cerebral cortex.

Central Processing of Somatosensory Information

Perception, or the final processing of somatosensory information, involves awareness of the stimuli, localization and discrimination of their characteristics, and interpretation of their meaning. As sensory information reaches the thalamus, it begins to enter the level of consciousness. In the thalamus, the sensory information is roughly localized and perceived as a crude sense. The full localization, discrimination of the intensity, and interpretation of the meaning of the stimuli require processing by the somatosensory cortex.

The somatosensory cortex is located in the parietal lobe, which lies behind the central sulcus and above the lateral sulcus (Fig. 50-6). The strip of parietal cortex that borders the central sulcus is called the *primary somatosensory cortex* because it receives primary sensory information by way of direct projections from the thalamus. A distorted map of the body and head surface, called the *sensory homunculus,* reflects the density of cortical neurons devoted to sensory input from afferents in corresponding

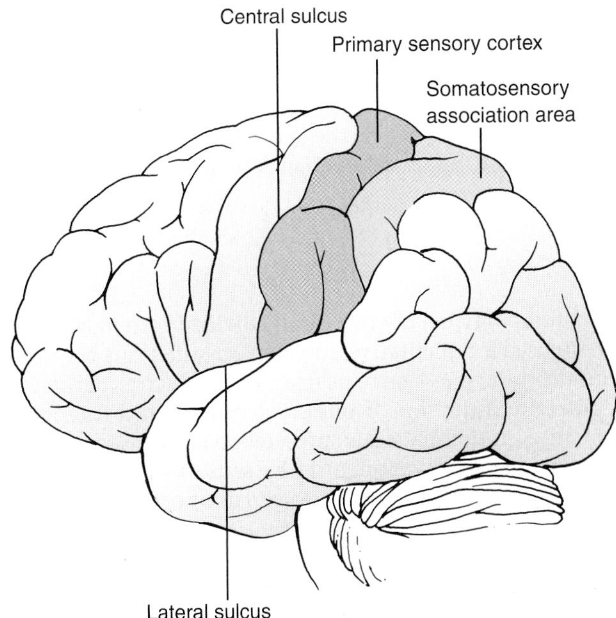

FIGURE 50-6 Primary somatosensory and association somatosensory cortex.

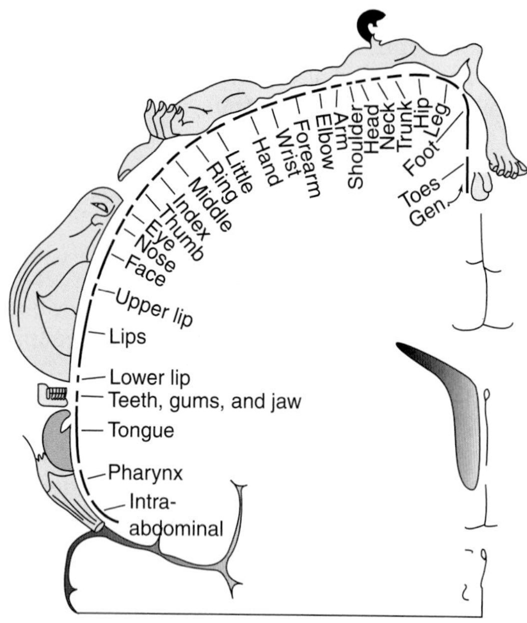

FIGURE 50-7 Homunculus, as determined by stimulation studies on the human cortex during surgery. (Penfield E., Rasmussen T. [1955]. *The cerebral cortex of man.* New York: Macmillan. Copyright © by Macmillan Publishing Co., Inc., renewed 1978 by Theodore Rasmussen)

peripheral areas. As depicted in Figure 50-7, most of the cortical surface is devoted to areas of the body such as the thumb, forefinger, lips, and tongue, where fine touch and pressure discrimination are essential for normal function.

Parallel to and just behind the primary somatosensory cortex (*i.e.,* toward the occipital cortex) lie the somatosensory association areas, which are required to transform the raw material of sensation into meaningful learned perception. Most of the perceptive aspects of body sensation, or somesthesia, require the function of this parietal association cortex. The perceptive aspect, or meaningfulness, of a stimulus pattern involves the integration of present sensation with past learning. For instance, a person's past learning plus present tactile sensation provides the perception of sitting on a soft chair rather than on a hard bicycle seat.

SENSORY MODALITIES

Somatosensory experience can be divided into *modalities,* a term used for qualitative, subjective distinctions between sensations such as touch, heat, and pain. Such experiences require the function of sensory receptors and forebrain structures in the thalamus and cerebral cortex. Sensory experience also involves quantitative sensory discrimination or the ability to distinguish between different levels of sensory stimulation.

The receptive endings of different afferent neurons are particularly sensitive to specific forms of physical and chemical energy. They can initiate action potentials to many forms of energy at high energy levels, but they usually are highly tuned to be differentially sensitive to low levels of a particular energy type. For instance, a receptive ending may be particularly sensitive to a small increase in local skin temperature. Stimulating the ending with a mild electric current or strong pressure also can result in action potentials. The amount of energy required, however, is much greater than it is for a change in temperature. Other afferent sensory terminals are most sensitive to slight indentations of the skin, and their signals are subjectively interpreted as touch. Cool versus warm, sharp versus dull pain, and delicate touch versus deep pressure are all based on different populations of afferent neurons or on central integration of simultaneous input from several differently tuned afferents. For example, the sensation of itch results from a combination of high activity in pain- and touch-sensitive afferents, and the sensation of tickle requires a gently moving tactile stimulus over cool skin.

When information from different primary afferents reaches the forebrain, where subjective experience occurs, the qualitative differences between warmth and touch are called *sensory modalities*. Although the receptor-detected information is relayed to the thalamus and cortex over separate pathways, the experience of a modality, such as cold versus warm, is uniquely subjective.

Stimulus Discrimination

The ability to discriminate the location of a somesthetic stimulus is called *acuity* and is based on the sensory field in a dermatome innervated by an afferent neuron. High acuity (*i.e.,* the ability to make fine discriminations of location) requires a high density of innervation by afferent neurons. For example, acuity is high on the thumb but lower on the back of the hand. High acuity also requires a projection system through the CNS to the forebrain that preserves distinctions between levels of activity in neighboring sensory fields. Receptors or receptive endings of primary afferent neurons differ as to the intensity at which they begin to fire. This threshold usually is lower than the stimulus threshold required for first brain-level perception of subjective sensation (*i.e.,* subjective threshold). For instance, when a single hair on the back of the hand is bent progressively, some bending occurs before action potentials appear in the primary afferent neuron (*i.e.,* afferent threshold). The hair must be bent further and the action potentials must increase in frequency before a person is able reliably to detect the bending of the hair (*i.e.,* subjective sensation threshold). For highly developed discriminative systems, under ideal conditions, these thresholds may correspond closely.

Tactile Sensation

The tactile system, which relays sensory information regarding touch, pressure, and vibration, is considered the basic somatosensory system. Loss of temperature or pain sensitivity leaves the person with no awareness of deficiency. However, if the tactile system is lost, total anesthesia (*i.e.,* numbness) of the involved body part results.

Touch sensation results from stimulation of tactile receptors in the skin and in tissues immediately beneath the skin, pressure from deformation of deeper tissues, and vibration from rapidly repetitive sensory signals. There are at least six types of specialized tactile receptors in the skin and deeper structures: free nerve endings,[1,2] Meissner's corpuscles, Merkel's disks, pacinian corpuscles, hair follicle end-organs, and Ruffini's end-organs (Fig. 50-8).

Free nerve endings are found in skin and many other tissues, including the cornea. They detect touch and pressure. *Meissner's corpuscle* is an elongated encapsulated nerve ending that is present in nonhairy parts of the skin. It is particularly abundant in the fingertips, lips, and other areas where the sense of touch is highly developed. *Merkel's disks* are dome-shaped receptors found in nonhairy areas and in hairy parts of the skin. In contrast to Meissner's corpuscles, which adapt within a fraction of a second, Merkel's disks transmit an initial strong signal that diminishes in strength but is slow in adapting. For this reason, Meissner's corpuscles are particularly sensitive to the movement of very light objects over the surface of the skin and to low-frequency vibration. Merkel's disks are responsible for giving steady-state signals that allow for continuous determination of touch against the skin.

The *pacinian corpuscle* is located immediately beneath the skin and deep in the fascial tissues of the body. This type of receptor, which is stimulated by rapid movements of the tissues and adapts within a few hundredths of a second, is important in detecting tissue vibration. The *hair follicle end-organ* consists of afferent unmyelinated fibers entwined around most of the length of the hair follicle. These receptors, which are rapidly adapting, detect movement on the surface of the body. *Ruffini's end-organs* are found in the skin and deeper structures, including the joint capsules. These receptors, which have multibranched encapsulated endings, have very little adaptive capacity and are important for signaling continuous states of deformation, such as heavy and continuous touch and pressure.

Almost all the specialized touch receptors, such as Merkel's disks, Meissner's corpuscles, hair follicle end-organs, pacinian corpuscles, and Ruffini's end-organs, transmit their signals in large myelinated nerve fibers (*i.e.*, type Aα, β) that have transmission velocities ranging from 25 to 70 m/second. Most free nerve endings transmit signals by way of small myelinated fibers (*i.e.*, type Aδ) with conduction velocities of 10 to 30 m/second.

The sensory information for tactile sensation enters the spinal cord through the dorsal roots of the spinal nerves. All tactile sensation that requires rapid transmission is transmitted through the discriminative pathway to the thalamus by way of the dorsal column and medial lemniscus. This includes touch sensation requiring a high degree of localization or fine gradations of intensity, vibratory sensation, and sensation that signals movement against the skin. In addition to the ascending discriminative pathway, tactile sensation uses the more primitive and crude anterolateral pathway. The afferent axons that carry tactile information up the dorsal columns have many branches or collaterals, and some of these synapse in the dorsal horn near the level of dorsal root entry. After several synapses, axons are projected up both sides of the anterolateral aspect of the spinal cord to the thalamus. Few fibers travel all the way to the thalamus. Most synapse on reticular formation neurons that then send their axons on toward the thalamus. The lateral nuclei of the thalamus are capable of contributing a crude, poorly localized sensation from the opposite side of the body. From the thalamus, some projections travel to the somatosensory cortex, especially to the side opposite the stimulus.

Because of these multiple routes, total destruction of the anterolateral pathway seldom occurs. The only time this crude alternative system becomes essential is when the discriminative pathway is damaged. Then, despite projection of the anterolateral system information to the somatosensory cortex, only a poorly localized, high-threshold sense of touch remains. Such persons lose all sense of joint and muscle movement, body position, and two-point discrimination.

Thermal Sensation

Thermal sensation is discriminated by three types of receptors: cold receptors, warmth receptors, and pain receptors. The cold and warmth receptors are located immediately under the skin at discrete but separate points, each serving an area of approximately 1 mm^2. In some areas, there are

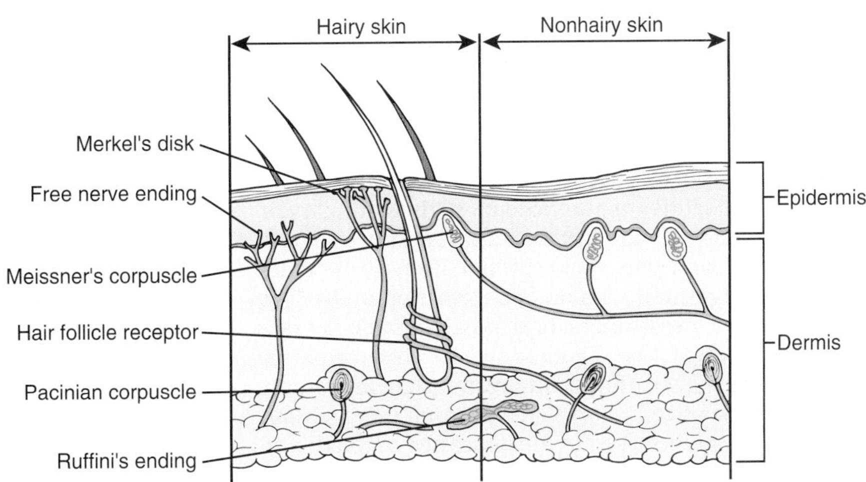

FIGURE 50-8 Somatic sensory receptors in the skin. Hairy and nonhairy skin have a variety of sensory receptors within the skin. (Adapted from Bear M.F., Connors B.W., Paradiso M.A. [1996]. *Neuroscience: Exploring the brain* [p. 311]. Philadelphia: Williams & Wilkins)

more cold receptors than warmth receptors. For example, the lips have 15 to 25 cold receptors per square centimeter, compared with 3 to 5 in the same-sized area of the finger.[1] There are correspondingly fewer warmth receptors in these areas. The different gradations of heat and cold result from the relative degrees of stimulation of the different types of nerve endings. The thermal receptors are very sensitive to differences between the temperature of skin and temperature of objects that are touched. Warmth receptors respond proportionately to increases in skin temperature above resting values of 34°C and cold receptors to temperatures below 34°C.[2] The thermal pain receptors are stimulated only by extremes of temperature such as "freezing cold" (temperatures below 5°C) and "burning hot" (temperatures above 45°C) sensations.[2] With the exception of pain receptors, thermal receptors tend to adapt rapidly during the first few minutes and then more slowly during the next 30 minutes or so. However, these receptors do not appear to adapt completely, as evidenced by the experience of an intense sense of heat on entering a tub of hot water or the extreme degree of cold initially sensed when going outside on a cold day.

Thermal afferents, with receptive thermal endings in the skin, send their central axons into the segmental dorsal horn of the spinal cord. On entering the dorsal horn, thermal signals are processed by second-order input association neurons. These association neurons activate projection neurons whose axons then cross to the opposite side of the cord and ascend in the multisynaptic, slow-conducting anterolateral system to the opposite side of the brain. Thalamic and cortical somatosensory regions for temperature are mixed with those for tactile sensibility.

Conduction of thermal information through peripheral nerves is quite slow compared with the rapid tactile afferents that travel through the discriminative system. If a person places a foot in a tub of hot water, the tactile sensation occurs well in advance of the burning sensation. The foot has been removed from the hot water by the local withdrawal reflex well before the excessive heat is perceived by the forebrain. Local anesthetic agents block the small-diameter afferents that carry thermal sensory information before they block the large-diameter axons that carry discriminative touch information.

Position Sensation

Position sense refers to the sense of limb and body movement and position without using vision. It is mediated by input from proprioceptive receptors (muscle spindle receptors and Golgi tendon organs) found primarily in muscles, tendons, and joint capsules (see Chapter 49). There are two submodalities of proprioception: the stationary or static component (limb position sense) and the dynamic aspects of position sense (kinesthesia). Both of these depend on constant transmission of information to the CNS regarding the degree of angulation of all joints and the rate of change in angulation. In addition, stretch-sensitive receptors in the skin (Ruffini's end-organs, pacinian corpuscles, and Merkel's cells) also signal postural information. Signals from these receptors are processed through the dorsal column–medial lemniscus pathway. In addition to the transmission of signals from the periphery to the cerebral cortex, the signals are processed in the thalamus before reaching the cerebral cortex. Lesions affecting the posterior column impair position sense. The vestibular system also plays an essential role in position sense. The vestibular system's role and the diseases affecting it and thus impairing position sense are discussed in Chapter 55.

CLINICAL ASSESSMENT OF SOMATOSENSORY FUNCTION

Clinically, neurologic assessment of somatosensory function can be done by testing the integrity of spinal segmental nerves. A pinpoint pressed against the skin of the sole of the foot that results in a withdrawal reflex and a complaint of skin pain confirms the functional integrity of the afferent terminals in the skin, the entire pathway through the peripheral nerves of the foot, leg, and thigh to the sacral (S1) dorsal root ganglion, and through the dorsal root into the spinal cord segment. It confirms that the somatosensory input association cells receiving this information are functioning and that the reflex circuitry of the cord segments (L5 to S2) is functioning. In addition, the lower motor neurons of the L4 to S1 ventral horn can be considered operational, and their axons through the ventral roots, the mixed peripheral nerve, and the motor neuron to the muscles producing the withdrawal response can be considered intact and functional. The communication between the lower motor neuron and the muscle cells is functional, and these muscles have normal responsiveness and strength.

Testing is done at each segmental level, or dermatome, moving upward along the body and neck from coccygeal segments through the high cervical levels to test the functional integrity of all the spinal nerves. Similar dermatomes cover the face and scalp, and these, although innervated by cranial segmental nerves, are tested in the same manner.

The observation of a normal withdrawal reflex rules out peripheral nerve disease, disorders of the dorsal root and ganglion, diseases of the myoneural junction, and severe muscle diseases. Normal reflex function also indicates that many major descending CNS tract systems are functioning within normal limits. If the person is able to report the pinprick sensation and accurately identify its location, many ascending systems through much of the spinal cord and brain also are functioning normally, as are basic intellect and speech mechanisms.

The integrity of the discriminative dorsal column–medial lemniscus pathway compared with the anterolateral tactile pathways is tested with the person's eyes closed by gently brushing the skin with a wisp of cotton, touching an area with one or two sharp points, touching corresponding parts of the body on each side simultaneously or in random sequence, and passively bending the person's finger one way and then another in random order. If only the anterolateral pathway is functional, the tactile threshold is markedly elevated, two-point discrimination and proprioception are missing, and the patient has difficulty discriminating which side of the body received stimulation.

In summary, the somatosensory component of the nervous system provides an awareness of body sensations such as touch, temperature, position sense, and pain. There are three primary levels of neural integration in the somatosensory system: the sensory units containing the sensory receptors, the ascending pathways, and the central processing centers in the thalamus and cerebral cortex. A sensory unit consists of a single dorsal root ganglion neuron, its receptors, and its central axon that terminates in the dorsal horn of the spinal cord or medulla. The part of the body innervated by the somatosensory afferent neurons of one set of dorsal root ganglia is called a *dermatome.* Ascending pathways include the discriminative pathway, which crosses at the base of the medulla, and the anterolateral pathway, which crosses within the first few segments of entering the spinal cord. Perception, or the final processing of somatosensory information, involves centers in the thalamus and somatosensory cortex. In the thalamus, the sensory information is crudely localized and perceived. The full localization, discrimination of the intensity, and interpretation of the meaning of the stimuli require processing by the somatosensory cortex. A distorted map of the body and head surface, called the *sensory homunculus,* reflects the density of cortical neurons devoted to sensory input from afferents in corresponding peripheral areas.

The tactile system relays the sensations of touch, pressure, and vibration. It uses two anatomically separate pathways to relay touch information to the opposite side of the forebrain: the dorsal column discriminative pathway and the anterolateral pathway. Delicate touch, vibration, position, and movement sensations use the discriminative pathway to reach the thalamus, where third-order relay occurs to the primary somatosensory strip of parietal cortex. Crude tactile sensation is carried by the bilateral slow-conducting anterolateral pathway. Temperature sensations of warm-hot and cool-cold are the result of stimulation to thermal receptors of sensory units projecting to the thalamus and cortex through the anterolateral system on the opposite side of the body. Proprioception is the sense of limb and body movement and position without using vision. Proprioceptive information is processed through the rapidly transmitting dorsal column–medial lemniscus pathway. Testing of the ipsilateral dorsal column (discriminative touch) system or the contralateral temperature projection systems permits diagnostic analysis of the level and extent of damage in spinal cord lesions.

Pain

After completing this section of the chapter, you should be able to meet the following objectives:

- Differentiate among the specificity, pattern, gate control, and neuromatrix theories of pain
- Characterize the response of nociceptors to stimuli that produce pain
- State the difference between the Aδ- and C-fiber neurons in the transmission of pain information
- Trace the transmission of pain signals with reference to the neospinothalamic, paleospinothalamic, and reticulospinal pathways, including the role of chemical mediators and factors that modulate pain transmission
- Describe the function of endogenous analgesic mechanisms as they relate to transmission of pain information
- Compare pain threshold and pain tolerance
- Differentiate acute pain from chronic pain in terms of mechanisms, manifestations, and treatment
- Describe the mechanisms of referred pain, and list the common sites of referral for cardiac and other types of visceral pain
- Describe three methods for assessing pain
- Describe the proposed mechanisms of pain relief associated with the use of heat, cold, transcutaneous electrical nerve stimulation, and acupuncture and acupressure
- State the mechanisms whereby nonnarcotic and narcotic analgesics, tricyclic antidepressants, and antiseizure drugs relieve pain

Pain is an "unpleasant sensory and emotional experience associated with actual and potential tissue damage, or described in terms of such damage."[3] The early work by Sir Charles Sherrington[4] introduced the important concept that pain perception and reaction to pain can be separated. This is particularly important for clinical pain because suffering is more heavily influenced by the reaction to pain than by actual pain intensity. Attention, motivation, past experience, and the meaning of the situation can influence the individual's reaction to pain. Thus, pain involves anatomic structures, physiologic behaviors, and psychological, social, cultural, and cognitive factors.

Pain is a common symptom that varies widely in intensity and spares no age group. When pain is extremely severe, it disrupts a person's customary behavior and can consume all of a person's attention. It can be equally devastating for infants and children, young and middle-aged adults, the young-old, and the old-old. Both acute pain and chronic pain can be major health problems. Acute pain often results from injury, surgery, or invasive medical procedures. It also can be a presenting symptom for some infections (*e.g.,* pharyngitis, appendicitis, and otitis media). Chronic pain can be symptomatic of a wide range of health problems (*e.g.,* arthritis, back injury, or cancer). In recent epidemiologic surveys, approximately 46% of adults reported having chronic pain.[5] Results from the National Health Interview Survey revealed that 13.7% of the population limits daily activities because of chronic pain conditions.[6]

The experience of pain depends on both sensory stimulation and perception. The perception of pain can be heavily influenced by the endogenous analgesia system that modulates the sensation of pain. This is perhaps most dramatically illustrated by the phenomenon of soldiers injured in battle or athletes injured during a game who do not perceive major injuries as painful until they leave the battlefield or the game.

Pain can be either nociceptive or neuropathic in origin. When nociceptors (pain receptors) are activated in response to actual or impending tissue injury, *nociceptive pain* is the consequence. *Neuropathic pain,* on the other hand, arises from direct injury to nerves. Tissue and nerve injury can result in a wide range of symptoms. These include pain from noninjurious stimuli to the skin (*allodynia*), extreme sensitivity to pain (*hyperalgesia*), and the absence of pain from stimuli that normally would be painful (*analgesia*). The latter, although not painful, can be extremely serious (*e.g.,* in diabetic persons with peripheral neuropathy) because the normally protective early warning system for the presence of tissue injury is absent.

PAIN THEORIES

Traditionally, two theories have been offered to explain the physiologic basis for the pain experience. The first, *specificity theory,* regards pain as a separate sensory modality evoked by the activity of specific receptors that transmit information to pain centers or regions in the forebrain where pain is experienced.[7] The second theory includes a group of theories collectively referred to as *pattern theory.* It proposes that pain receptors share endings or pathways with other sensory modalities, but that different patterns of activity (*i.e.,* spatial or temporal) of the same neurons can be used to signal painful and nonpainful stimuli.[7] For example, light touch applied to the skin would produce the sensation of touch through low-frequency firing of the receptor; intense pressure would produce pain through high-frequency firing of the same receptor. Both theories focus on the neurophysiologic basis of pain, and both probably apply. Specific nociceptive afferents have been identified; however, almost all afferent stimuli, if driven at a very high frequency, can be experienced as painful.

Gate control theory, a modification of specificity theory, was proposed by Melzack and Wall in 1965 to meet the challenges presented by the pattern theories. This theory postulated the presence of neural gating mechanisms at the segmental spinal cord level to account for interactions between pain and other sensory modalities.[8] The original gate control theory proposed a spinal-cord–level network of transmission or projection cells and internuncial neurons that inhibits the transmission cells, forming a segmental-level gating mechanism that could block projection of pain information to the brain.

According to the gate control theory, the internuncial neurons involved in the gating mechanism are activated by large-diameter, faster-propagating fibers that carry tactile information. The simultaneous firing of the large-diameter tactile fibers has the potential for blocking the transmission of impulses from the small-diameter myelinated and unmyelinated pain fibers. Pain therapists have long known that pain intensity can be temporarily reduced during active tactile stimulation. For example, repeated sweeping of a soft-bristled brush on the skin (*i.e.,* brushing) over or near a painful area may result in pain reduction for several minutes to several hours.

Pain modulation is now known to be a much more complex phenomenon than that proposed by the original gate control theory. Tactile information is transmitted by small- and large-diameter fibers. Major interactions between sensory modalities, including the so-called gating phenomenon, occur at several levels of the CNS rostral to the input segment. Perhaps the most puzzling aspect of locally applied stimuli, such as brushing, that can block the experience of pain is the relatively long-lasting effect (minutes to hours) of such treatments. This prolonged effect has been difficult to explain on the basis of specificity theories, including the gate control theory. Other important factors include the effect of endogenous opioids and their receptors at the segmental and brain stem levels, descending feedback modulation, altered sensitivity, learning, and culture. Despite this complexity, the Melzack and Wall gate-control theory has served a useful purpose. It excited interest in pain and stimulated research and clinical activity related to the pain-modulating systems.

More recently, Melzack developed the *neuromatrix theory* to address further the brain's role in pain as well as the multiple dimensions and determinants of pain.[9] This theory is particularly useful in understanding chronic pain and phantom limb pain, in which there is not a simple one-to-one relationship between tissue injury and pain experience. The neuromatrix theory proposes that the brain contains a widely distributed neural network, called the *body-self neuromatrix,* that contains somatosensory, limbic, and thalamocortical components. Genetic and sensory influences determine the synaptic architecture of an individual's neuromatrix that integrates multiple sources of input and yields the neuro-signature pattern that evokes the sensory, affective, and cognitive dimensions of pain experience and behavior. These multiple sources include somatosensory inputs; other sensory inputs affecting interpretation of the situation; phasic and tonic inputs from the brain addressing such things as attention, expectation, culture, and personality; intrinsic neural inhibitory modulation; and various components of stress-regulation systems. This theory may open entire new areas of research, such as investigating the role that cortisol plays in chronic pain, the effect estrogen has on pain mediated through the release of peripheral cytokines, and the reported increase in chronic pain that occurs with age.

PAIN MECHANISMS AND PATHWAYS

Pain usually is viewed in the context of tissue injury. The term *nociception,* which means "pain sense," comes from the Latin word *nocere* ("to injure"). Nociceptive stimuli are objectively defined as stimuli of such intensity that they cause or are close to causing tissue damage. Researchers often use the withdrawal reflex (*e.g.,* the reflexive withdrawal of a body part from a tissue-damaging stimulus) to determine when a stimulus is nociceptive. Stimuli used include pressure from a sharp object, strong electric current to the skin, or application of heat or cold of approximately 10°C above or below normal skin temperature. At low levels of intensity, these noxious stimuli do not activate nociceptors (pain receptors), but they typically are perceived as painful only when the intensity reaches a level where tissue damage occurs or is imminent.

The mechanisms of pain are many and complex. As with other forms of somatosensation, the pathways are composed of first-, second-, and third-order neurons (Fig. 50-9).

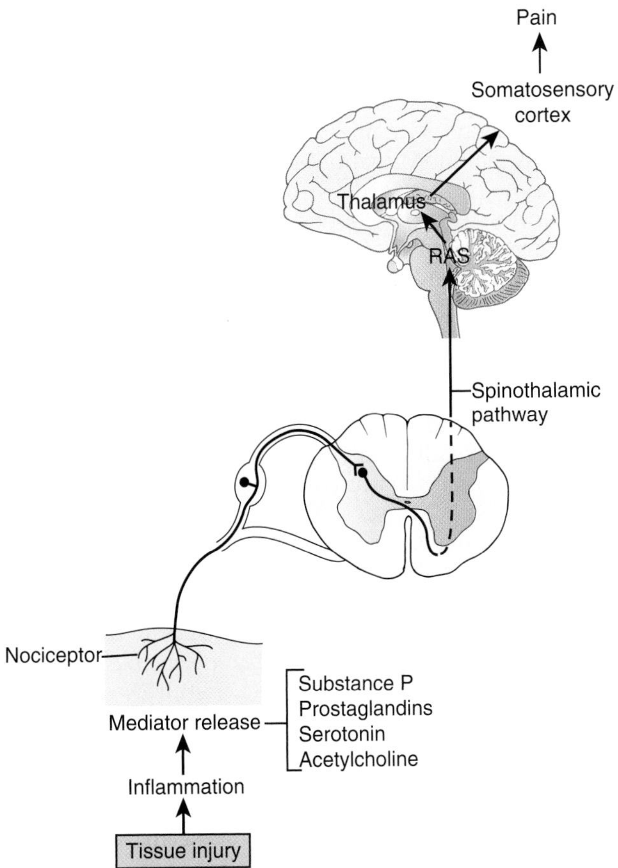

FIGURE 50-9 Mechanism of acute pain. Tissue injury leads to release of inflammatory mediators with subsequent nociceptor stimulation. Pain impulses are then transmitted to the dorsal horn of the spinal cord, where they make contact with second-order neurons that cross to the opposite side of the cord and ascend via the spinothalamic tract to the reticular activating system (RAS) and thalamus. The localization and meaning of pain occurs at the level of the somatosensory cortex.

The first-order neurons and their receptive endings detect stimuli that threaten the integrity of innervated tissues. Second-order neurons are located in the spinal cord and process nociceptive information. Third-order neurons project pain information to the brain. The thalamus and somatosensory cortex integrate and modulate pain as well as the person's subjective reaction to the pain experience.

Pain Receptors and Mediators

Nociceptors, or pain receptors, are sensory receptors that are activated by noxious insults to peripheral tissues. Structurally, the receptive endings of the peripheral pain fibers are free nerve endings. These receptive endings, which are widely distributed in the skin, dental pulp, periosteum, meninges, and some internal organs, translate the noxious stimuli into action potentials that are transmitted by a dorsal root ganglion to the dorsal horn of the spinal cord.

Nociceptive action potentials are transmitted through two types of afferent nerve fibers: myelinated Aδ fibers and unmyelinated C fibers.[1,2] The larger Aδ fibers have considerably greater conduction velocities, transmitting impulses at a rate of 10 to 30 m/second. The C fibers are the smallest of all peripheral nerve fibers; they transmit impulses at the rate of 0.5 to 2.5 m/second. Pain conducted by Aδ fibers traditionally is called *fast pain* or first pain and typically is elicited by mechanical or thermal stimuli. C-fiber pain often is described as *slow-wave pain* or second pain because it is slower in onset and longer in duration. It typically is incited by chemical stimuli or by persistent mechanical or thermal stimuli. The slow postexcitatory potentials generated in C fibers are now believed to be responsible for central sensitization to chronic pain.

Stimulation of Nociceptors. Unlike other sensory receptors, nociceptors respond to several forms of stimulation, including mechanical, thermal, and chemical. Some receptors respond to a single type of stimuli (mechanical or thermal), and others, called *polymodal receptors,* respond to all three types of stimuli (mechanical, thermal, and chemical). Mechanical stimuli can arise from intense pressure applied to skin or from the violent contraction or extreme stretch of a muscle. Both extremes of heat and cold can stimulate nociceptors. Chemical stimuli arise from a number of sources, including tissue trauma, ischemia, and inflammation. A wide range of chemical mediators are released from injured and inflamed tissues, including hydrogen and potassium ions, prostaglandins, leukotrienes, histamine, bradykinin,

PAIN SENSATION

- Pain is both a protective and an unpleasant physical and emotionally disturbing sensation originating in pain receptors that respond to a number of stimuli that threaten tissue integrity.
- There are two pathways for pain transmission:
  - The pathway for fast, sharply discriminated pain that moves directly from the receptor to the spinal cord using myelinated Aδ fibers and from the spinal cord to the thalamus using the neospinothalamic tract
  - The pathway for slow, continuously conducted pain that is transmitted to the spinal cord using unmyelinated C fibers and from the spinal cord to the thalamus using the more circuitous and slower-conducting paleospinothalamic tract
- The central processing of pain information includes transmission to the somatosensory cortex, where pain information is perceived and interpreted, the limbic system, where the emotional components of pain are experienced, and to brain stem centers, where autonomic nervous system responses are recruited.
- Modulation of the pain experience occurs by way of the endogenous analgesic center in the midbrain, the pontine noradrenergic neurons, and the nucleus raphe magnus in the medulla, which sends inhibitory signals to dorsal horn neurons in the spinal cord or trigeminal nerve.

acetylcholine, and serotonin. These chemical mediators produce their effects by directly stimulating nociceptors or sensitizing them to the effects of nociceptive stimuli; perpetuating the inflammatory responses that lead to the release of chemical agents that act as nociceptive stimuli; or inciting neurogenic reflexes that increase the response to nociceptive stimuli. For example, bradykinin, histamine, serotonin, and potassium activate and also sensitize nociceptors.[10,11] Adenosine triphosphate, acetylcholine, and platelets act alone or in concert to sensitize nociceptors through other chemical agents such as prostaglandins. Aspirin and other nonsteroidal analgesic drugs are effective in controlling pain because they block the enzyme needed for prostaglandin synthesis.

Nociceptive stimulation that activates C fibers can cause a response known as *neurogenic inflammation* that produces vasodilation and an increased release of chemical mediators to which nociceptors respond.[11] This mechanism is thought to be mediated by a dorsal root neuron reflex that produces retrograde transport and release of chemical mediators, which in turn causes increasing inflammation of peripheral tissues. This reflex can set up a vicious cycle, which has implications for persistent pain and hyperalgesia.[10]

Mediators in the Spinal Cord. In the spinal cord, the transmission of impulses between the nociceptive neurons and the dorsal horn neurons is mediated by chemical neurotransmitters released from central nerve endings of the nociceptive neurons. Some of these neurotransmitters are amino acids (*e.g.*, glutamate), others are amino acid derivatives (*e.g.*, norepinephrine), and still others are low-molecular-weight peptides composed of two or more amino acids. The amino acid glutamate is a major excitatory neurotransmitter released from the central nerve endings of the nociceptive neurons. Substance P, a neuropeptide, also is released in the dorsal horn by C fibers in response to nociceptive stimulation. Substance P elicits slow excitatory potentials in dorsal horn neurons. Unlike glutamate, which confines its action to the immediate area of the synaptic terminal, some neuropeptides released in the dorsal horn can diffuse some distance because they are not inactivated by reuptake mechanisms. In persistent pain, this may help to explain the excitability and unlocalized nature of many painful conditions. Neuropeptides such as substance P also appear to prolong and enhance the action of glutamate. If these neurotransmitters are released in large quantities or over extended periods, they can lead to secondary hyperalgesia, a condition in which the second-order neurons are overly sensitive to low levels of noxious stimulation. Understanding how chemical mediators function in nociception is an active area of research that has implications for the development of new treatments for pain.

Spinal Cord Circuitry and Pathways

On entering the spinal cord through the dorsal roots, the pain fibers bifurcate and ascend or descend one or two segments before synapsing with association neurons in the dorsal horn. From the dorsal horn, the axons of association projection neurons cross through the anterior commissure to the opposite side and then ascend upward in the previously described neospinothalamic and paleospinothalamic pathways.

The faster-conducting fibers in the neospinothalamic tract are associated mainly with the transmission of sharp-fast pain information to the thalamus. In the thalamus, synapses are made, and the pathway continues to the contralateral (*i.e.*, opposite) parietal somatosensory area to provide the precise location of the pain. Typically, the pain is experienced as bright, sharp, or stabbing in nature.

The paleospinothalamic tract is a slower-conducting, multisynaptic tract concerned with the diffuse, dull, aching, and unpleasant sensations that commonly are associated with chronic and visceral pain. This information travels through the small, unmyelinated C fibers. Fibers of this system also project up the contralateral anterolateral pathway to terminate in several thalamic regions, including the intralateral nuclei, which project to the limbic system. It is associated with the emotional or affective-motivational aspects of pain. Spinoreticular fibers from this pathway project bilaterally to the reticular formation of the brain stem. This component of the paleospinothalamic system facilitates avoidance reflexes at all levels. It also contributes to an increase in the electroencephalographic activity associated with alertness and indirectly influences hypothalamic functions associated with sudden alertness, such as increased heart rate and blood pressure. This may explain the tremendous arousal effects of certain pain stimuli.

Dorsal horn (second-order) neurons are divided primarily into two types: wide-dynamic-range (WDR) neurons that respond to low-intensity stimuli, and nociceptive-specific neurons that respond only to noxious or nociceptive stimuli. When stimuli are increased to a noxious level, the WDR neurons respond more intensely. After more severe damage to peripheral sensory afferents, Aδ and C fibers respond more intensely as they are increasingly stimulated. When C fibers are repetitively stimulated at a rate of once per second, each stimulus produces a progressively increasing response from WDR neurons. This phenomenon of amplification of transmitted signals has been called *windup* and may explain why pain sensation appears to increase with repeated stimulation. Windup and sensitization of dorsal horn neurons have implications for appropriate and early, or even preemptive, pain therapy to avoid the possibility of spinal cord neurons becoming hypersensitive or subject to firing spontaneously.[10,12]

Brain Centers and Pain Perception

Information from tissue injury is carried from the spinal cord to brain centers in the thalamus where the basic sensation of hurtfulness, or pain, occurs. In the neospinothalamic system, interconnections between the lateral thalamus and the somatosensory cortex are necessary to add precision, discrimination, and meaning to the pain sensation. The paleospinothalamic system projects diffusely from the intralaminar nuclei of the thalamus to large areas of the limbic cortex. These connections probably are associated with the hurtfulness and the mood-altering and attention-narrowing effect of pain.

Recent research using magnetoencephalography has demonstrated cortical representation of first and second pain sensation in humans. In healthy adults, nociceptive Aδ afferent stimulation is related to activation in the contralateral primary somatosensory cortex in the parietal lobe, whereas C afferent stimulation is related to activation of the secondary somatosensory cortices and the anterior cingulated cortex, which is part of the limbic system. With both afferents, there is activation of the bilateral secondary somatosensory cortices in the posterior parietal lobes.[13]

Central Pathways for Pain Modulation

A major advance in understanding pain was the discovery of neuroanatomic pathways that arise in the midbrain and brain stem, descend to the spinal cord, and modulate ascending pain impulses. One such pathway begins in an area of the midbrain called the *periaqueductal gray* (PAG) region. Through research, it was found that electrical stimulation of the midbrain PAG regions produced a state of analgesia that lasted for many hours. This stimulation-induced analgesia was found to be remarkably specific and was not associated with changes in either the levels of consciousness or the reactions to auditory and visual stimuli.[2] Subsequently, opioid receptors were found to be highly concentrated in this and other regions of the CNS where electrical stimulation produced analgesia. Because of these findings, the PAG area of the midbrain often is referred to as the *endogenous analgesia center.*[1]

The PAG area receives input from widespread areas of the CNS, including the cerebral cortex, hypothalamus, brain stem reticular formation, and spinal cord by way of the paleospinothalamic and neospinothalamic tracts. This region is intimately connected to the limbic system, which is associated with emotional experience. The neurons of the PAG have axons that descend into an area in the rostral medulla called the *nucleus raphe magnus* (NRM). The axons of these NRM neurons project to the dorsal horn of the spinal cord, where they terminate in the same layers as the entering primary pain fibers (Fig. 50-10). In the spinal cord, these descending pathways inhibit pain transmission by dorsal horn projection neurons.[2] Serotonin has been identified as a neurotransmitter in the NRM medullary nuclei. It has been shown that tricyclic antidepressant drugs, such as amitriptyline, which enhance the effects of serotonin by blocking its presynaptic uptake, have been found to be effective in the management of certain types of chronic pain.[14] Additional inhibitory spinal projections arise from noradrenergic neurons in the pons and medulla, which also receive input from the PAG.[2] The discovery that norepinephrine can block pain transmission led to studies directed at the combined administration of opioids and clonidine, a central-acting α-adrenergic agonist for pain relief.

Endogenous Analgesic Mechanisms

There is evidence that opioid receptors and endogenously synthesized opioid peptides, which are morphine-like substances, are found on the peripheral processes of primary afferent neurons, in human synovia, and in many regions of the CNS.[15] Three families of endogenous opioid peptides have been identified—the enkephalins, endorphins, and dynorphins. Each family is derived from a distinct precursor polypeptide and has a characteristic anatomic distribution. Although each family usually is located in different groups of neurons, occasionally more than one family is present in the same neuron. For example, proenkephalin peptides are present in areas of the spinal cord and PAG that are related to perception of pain, in the hippocampus and other areas of the brain that modulate emotional behavior, in structures in the basal ganglia that modulate motor control, and in brain stem neurons that regulate autonomic nervous system responses.

Although the endogenous opioid peptides appear to function as neurotransmitters, their full significance in pain control and other physiologic functions is not completely understood. Laboratory studies, although somewhat inconsistent, have found that opioid agonists inhibit the opening of calcium channels in dorsal root and trigeminal ganglion neurons as well as on primary afferent neurons. Because it is calcium ions that cause neurotransmitter release at the synapse, such calcium blockage would inhibit synaptic transmission of pain impulses. Other studies are focusing on the effect of opioids on sodium and potassium channels that influence the transmission of pain impulses.[15]

Probably of greater importance in understanding mechanisms of pain control has been the characterization of receptors that bind the endogenous opioid peptides. The identification of these receptors has facilitated a more thorough understanding of the actions of available opioid drugs, such as morphine, and it also has facilitated ongoing research into the development of newer preparations; for example, development of an opioid that acted exclusively on the peripheral opioid receptors of sensory neurons could eliminate many of the undesirable, centrally mediated side effects, such as respiratory depression.[15]

PAIN THRESHOLD AND TOLERANCE

Pain threshold and tolerance affect an individual's response to a painful stimulus. Although the terms often are used interchangeably, pain threshold and pain tolerance have distinct meanings. *Pain threshold* is closely associated with the point at which a stimulus is perceived as painful. *Pain tolerance* relates more to the total pain experience; it is defined as the maximum intensity or duration of pain that a person is willing to endure before the person wants something done about the pain. Psychological, familial, cultural, and environmental factors significantly influence the amount of pain a person is willing to tolerate. The threshold to pain is fairly uniform from one person to another, whereas pain tolerance is extremely variable.[10] Separation and identification of the role of each of these two aspects of pain continue to pose fundamental problems for the pain management team and for pain researchers.

TYPES OF PAIN

The most widely accepted classifications of pain are according to source or location, referral, and duration (acute or chronic). Classification based on associated medical diag-

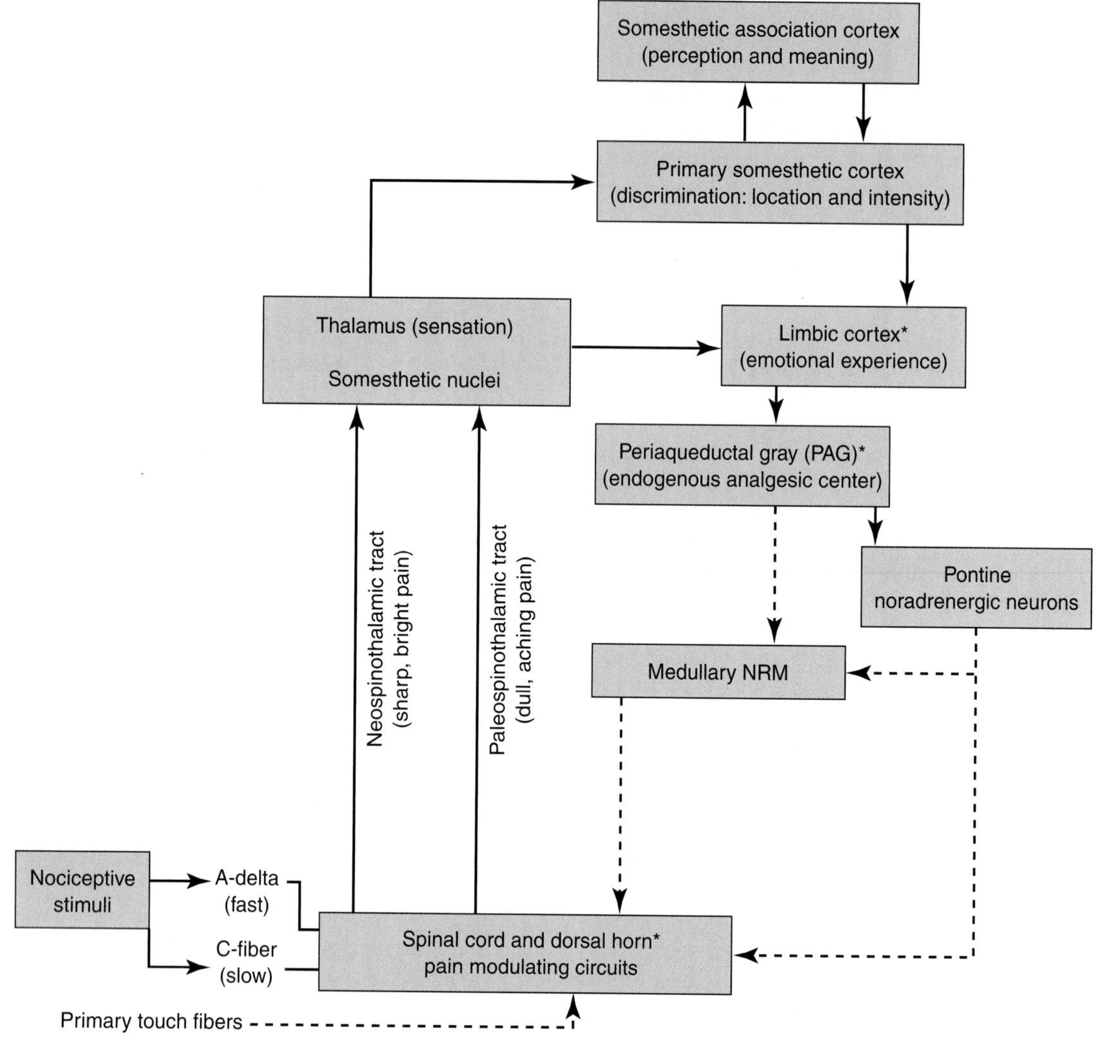

FIGURE 50-10 Primary pain pathways. The transmission of incoming nociceptive impulses is modulated by dorsal horn circuitry that receives input from peripheral touch receptors and from descending pathways that involve the limbic cortical systems (orbital frontal cortex, amygdala, and hypothalamus), periaqueductal endogenous analgesic center in the midbrain, pontine noradrenergic neurons, and the nucleus raphe magnus (NRM) in the medulla. *Dashed lines* indicate inhibition or modulation.

nosis (*e.g.*, surgery, trauma, cancer, sickle cell disease, fibromyalgia) is useful in planning appropriate interventions.

Cutaneous and Deep Somatic Pain

Cutaneous pain arises from superficial structures, such as the skin and subcutaneous tissues. A paper cut on the finger is an example of easily localized superficial, or cutaneous, pain. It is a sharp, bright pain with a burning quality and may be abrupt or slow in onset. It can be localized accurately and may be distributed along the dermatomes. Because there is an overlap of nerve fiber distribution between the dermatomes, the boundaries of pain frequently are not as clearcut as the dermatomal diagrams indicate.

Deep somatic pain originates in deep body structures, such as the periosteum, muscles, tendons, joints, and blood vessels. This pain is more diffuse than cutaneous pain. Various stimuli, such as strong pressure exerted on bone, ischemia to a muscle, and tissue damage, can produce deep somatic pain. This is the type of pain a person experiences from a sprained ankle. Radiation of pain from the original site of injury can occur. For example, damage to a nerve root can cause a person to experience pain radiating along its fiber distribution.

Visceral Pain

Visceral, or splanchnic, pain has its origin in the visceral organs and is one of the most common pains produced by disease. Although similar to somatic pain in many ways, both the neurologic mechanisms and the perception of visceral pain differ from somatic pain. One of the most important differences between surface pain and visceral pain is the type of damage that causes pain. For example, "a surgeon

TYPES OF PAIN

- Pain can be classified according to location (cutaneous or deep and visceral), duration (acute or chronic), and site of referral.
- Cutaneous pain is a sharp, burning pain that has its origin in the skin or subcutaneous tissues.
- Deep pain is a more diffuse and throbbing pain that originates in structures such as the muscles, bones, and tendons and radiates to the surrounding tissues.
- Visceral pain is a diffuse and poorly defined pain that results from stretching, distention, or ischemia of tissues in a body organ.
- Acute pain is a self-limiting pain that lasts less than 6 months.
- Chronic pain is persistent pain that lasts longer than 6 months, lacks the autonomic and somatic responses associated with acute pain, and is accompanied by loss of appetite, sleep disturbances, depression, and other debilitating responses.
- Referred pain is pain that originates at a visceral site but is perceived as originating in part of the body wall that is innervated by neurons entering the same segment of the nervous system.

can cut the bowel entirely in two in a patient who is awake without causing significant pain."[1] In contrast, strong contractions, distention, or ischemia affecting the walls of the viscera can induce severe pain. Also, visceral pain is not evoked from all viscera (*e.g.*, the liver, lung parenchyma).[16] Another difference is the diffuse and poorly localized nature of visceral pain—its tendency to be referred to other locations and to be accompanied by symptoms associated with autonomic reflexes (*e.g.*, nausea).[17] There are several explanations for this. There is a low density of nociceptors in the viscera as compared with the skin. There is functional divergence of visceral input within the central nervous system, which occurs when many second-order neurons respond to stimulus from a single visceral afferent. There is also convergence between somatic and visceral afferents in the spinal cord and in the supraspinal centers and possibly also between visceral afferents (*e.g.*, bladder, uterus, cervix, and vagina).[17]

Visceral afferents are predominately small, unmyelinated pain fibers that terminate in the dorsal horn of the spinal cord and express peptide neurotransmitters such as substance P.[16] There are thought to be two classes of nociceptive receptors that innervate the viscera: high-threshold and intensity-coding receptors.[16,17] High-threshold receptors have a high threshold for stimulation and respond only to stimuli within the noxious range. Intensity-coding receptors have a lower threshold for stimulation and an encoding function that incorporates the intensity of the stimulus into the magnitude of their discharge. Acute visceral pain, such as pain produced by intense contraction of a hollow organ, is thought to be triggered initially by high-threshold receptors. More extended forms of visceral stimulation, such as that caused by hypoxia and inflammation, often result in sensitization of the receptors. Once sensitized, these receptors begin to respond to otherwise innocuous stimuli (*e.g.*, motility and secretory activity) that normally occur in the viscera. This sensitization may resolve more slowly than the initial injury, and thus visceral pain may persist longer than expected based on the initial injury.[16]

Visceral nociceptive afferents from the thorax and abdomen travel along the cranial and spinal nerve pathways of the autonomic nervous system. For many years, it was believed that the spinothalamic and spinoreticular tracts carried visceral nociceptive information. More recently, additional pathways have been identified: the dorsal column pathway, the spino(trigemino)-parabrachio-amygdaloid pathway, and the spinohypothalamic pathway.[16] Identification of new pathways are sometimes quite important clinically. For example, knowledge of the dorsal column pathway has led to new surgical approaches to visceral pain due to pelvic cancer pain, such as midline myelotomy.[17]

Referred Pain

Referred pain is pain that is perceived at a site different from its point of origin but innervated by the same spinal segment. It is hypothesized that visceral and somatic afferent neurons converge on the same dorsal horn projection neurons (Fig. 50-11). For this reason, it can be difficult for the brain to identify correctly the original source of pain. Pain that originates in the abdominal or thoracic viscera is diffuse and poorly localized and often perceived at a site far removed from the affected area. For example, the pain associated with myocardial infarction commonly is referred to the left arm, neck, and chest.

Referred pain may arise alone or concurrent with pain located at the origin of the noxious stimuli. This lack of correspondence between the location of the pain and the location of the painful stimuli can make diagnosis difficult.

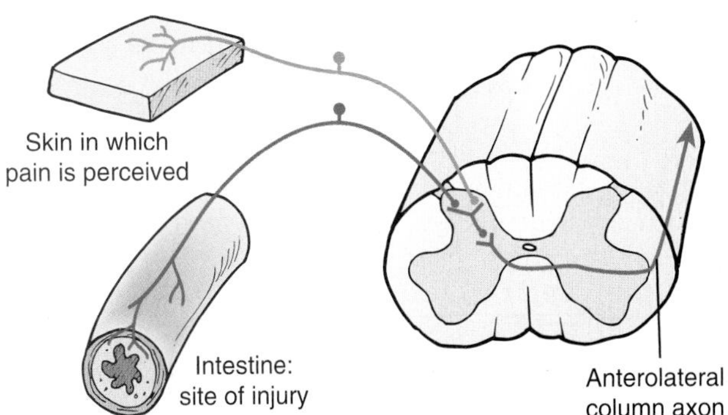

FIGURE 50-11 Convergence of cutaneous and visceral inputs onto the same second-order projection neuron in the dorsal horn of the spinal cord. Although virtually all visceral inputs converge with cutaneous inputs, most cutaneous inputs do not converge with other sensory inputs.

Although the term *referred* usually is applied to pain that originates in the viscera and is experienced as if originating from the body wall, it also may be applied to pain that arises from somatic structures. For example, pain referred to the chest wall could be caused by nociceptive stimulation of the peripheral portion of the diaphragm, which receives somatosensory innervation from the intercostal nerves. An understanding of pain referral is of great value in diagnosing illness. The typical pattern of pain referral can be derived from our understanding that the afferent neurons from visceral or deep somatic tissue enter the spinal cord at the same level as the afferent neurons from the cutaneous areas to which the pain is referred (Fig. 50-12).

The sites of referred pain are determined embryologically with the development of visceral and somatic structures that share the same site for entry of sensory information into the CNS and then move to more distant locations. For example, a person with peritonitis may complain of pain in the shoulder. Internally, there is inflammation of the peritoneum that lines the central part of the diaphragm. In the embryo, the diaphragm originates in the neck, and its central portion is innervated by the phrenic nerve, which enters the cord at the level of the third to fifth segments (C3 to C5). As the fetus develops, the diaphragm descends to its adult position between the thoracic and abdominal cavities, while maintaining its embryonic pattern of innervation. Thus, fibers that enter the spinal cord at the C3 to C5 level carry information from both the neck area and the diaphragm, and the diaphragmatic pain is interpreted by the forebrain as originating in the shoulder or neck area.

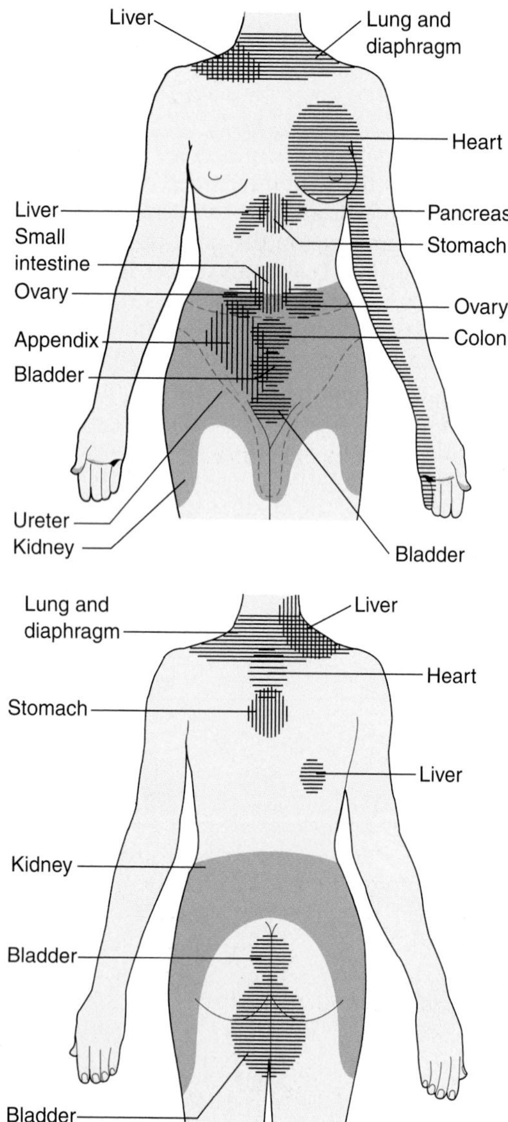

FIGURE 50-12 Areas of referred pain. (**Top**) Anterior view. (**Bottom**) Posterior view.

Although the visceral pleura, pericardium, and peritoneum are said to be relatively free of pain fibers, the parietal pleura, pericardium, and peritoneum do react to nociceptive stimuli. Visceral inflammation can involve parietal and somatic structures, and this may give rise to diffuse local or referred pain. For example, irritation of the parietal peritoneum resulting from appendicitis typically gives rise to pain directly over the inflamed area in the lower right quadrant. Such stimuli can evoke pain referred to the umbilical area.

Muscle spasm, or *guarding,* occurs when somatic structures are involved. Guarding is a protective reflex rigidity; its purpose is to protect the affected body parts (*e.g.,* an abscessed appendix or a sprained muscle). This protective guarding may cause blood vessel compression and give rise to the pain of muscle ischemia, causing local and referred pain.

Acute and Chronic Pain

It is common to classify pain according to its duration. Pain research of the past three decades has emphasized the importance of differentiating acute pain from chronic pain. The diagnosis and therapy for each is distinctive because they differ in cause, function, mechanisms, and psychological sequelae (Table 50-1).

Acute Pain. The classic definition of acute pain is pain that lasts less than 6 months. This somewhat arbitrary cutoff point reflects the notion that acute pain is the result of a tissue-damaging event, such as trauma or surgery, and usually is self-limited, ending when the injured tissues heal. The purpose of acute pain is to serve as a warning system. Besides alerting the person to the existence of actual or impending tissue damage, it prompts a search for professional help. The pain's location, radiation, intensity, and duration, as well as those factors that aggravate or relieve it, provide essential diagnostic clues.

Acute pain can lead to anxiety and secondary reflex musculoskeletal spasms, which in turn tend to worsen the pain.[18] Interventions that alleviate the pain usually alleviate the anxiety and musculoskeletal spasms as well. Inadequately treated pain can provoke physiologic responses that alter circulation and tissue metabolism and produce physical manifestations, such as tachycardia, reflective of increased sympathetic activity. Inadequately treated acute pain tends to decrease mobility and respiratory move-

TABLE 50-1 Characteristics of Acute and Chronic Pain

Characteristic	Acute Pain	Chronic Pain
Onset	Recent	Continuous or intermittent
Duration	Short duration (<6 months)	6 months or more
Autonomic responses	Consistent with sympathetic fight-or-flight response* Increased heart rate Increased stroke volume Increased blood pressure Increased pupillary dilation Increased muscle tension Decreased gut motility Decreased salivary flow (dry mouth)	Absence of autonomic responses
Psychological component	Associated anxiety	Increased irritability Associated depression Somatic preoccupation Withdrawal from outside interests Decreased strength of relationships
Other types of response		Decreased sleep Decreased libido Appetite changes

*Responses are approximately proportional to intensity of the stimulus.

ments such as deep breathing and coughing to the extent that it may complicate or delay recovery.

Chronic Pain. Chronic pain classically has been defined as pain lasting 6 months or longer. In practice, however, one does not wait an arbitrary 6 months before deciding that the pain is chronic; rather, one considers the normal expected healing time for the underlying cause of the pain. The International Association for the Study of Pain defines chronic pain as that which persists beyond the expected normal time of healing.[18] Chronic pain can be quite variable. It may be unrelenting and extremely severe, as in metastatic bone pain. It can be relatively continuous with or without periods of escalation, as with some forms of back pain. Some conditions with recurring episodes of acute pain are particularly problematic because they have characteristics of both acute and chronic pain. These include the pain associated with sickle cell crisis or migraine headaches.

Chronic pain is a leading cause of disability in the United States. Unlike acute pain, persistent chronic pain usually serves no useful function. To the contrary, it imposes physiologic, psychological, familial, and economic stresses and may exhaust a person's resources. In contrast to acute pain, psychological and environmental influences may play an important role in the development of behaviors associated with chronic pain. Chronic pain often is associated with loss of appetite, sleep disturbances, and depression.[19] The physiology of chronic pain is poorly understood.

Persons with chronic pain may not exhibit the somatic, autonomic, or affective behaviors often associated with acute pain. With chronic pain, it is particularly important to heed the person's own description of the pain because the expected psychophysiologic responses may or may not be present. As painful conditions become prolonged and continuous, autonomic nervous system responses decrease. Decreased pain tolerance, which may result from the depletion of serotonin and endorphins, and depression are common in individuals with chronic pain. The link between depression and decreased pain tolerance may be explained by the similar manner in which both respond to changes in the biologic pathways of serotonergic and noradrenergic systems.[20] Tricyclic antidepressants and other medications with serotonergic and noradrenergic effects have been shown to relieve a variety of chronic pain syndromes (*e.g.,* peripheral neuropathic pain, facial pain, and fibrositis), lending credence to the theory that chronic pain and depression share a common biologic pathway.[19]

ASSESSMENT OF PAIN

Careful assessment of pain assists clinicians in diagnosing, managing, and relieving the patient's pain. Assessment includes such things as the nature, severity, location, and radiation of the pain. As with other disease states, it is preferable to eliminate the cause of the pain rather than simply to treat the symptom. A careful history often provides information about the triggering factors (*i.e.,* injury, infection, or disease) and the site of nociceptive stimuli (*i.e.,* peripheral receptor or visceral organ). Although the observation of facial expression and posture may provide additional information, the *Clinical Practice Guideline No. 1. Acute Pain Management: Operative and Medical Procedures and Trauma* (released in 1992 by the Agency for

Health Care Policy and Research [AHCPR], currently the Agency for Healthcare Research and Quality, Public Health Service, U.S. Department of Health and Human Services) emphasizes that "the single most reliable indicator of the existence and intensity of acute pain—and any resultant affective discomfort or distress—is the patient's self report."[21] A comprehensive pain history should include pain onset; description, localization, radiation, intensity, quality, and pattern of the pain; anything that relieves or exacerbates it; and the individual's personal reaction to the pain.

Unlike many other bodily responses, such as temperature and blood pressure, the nature, severity, and distress of pain cannot be measured objectively. To overcome this problem, various methods have been developed for quantifying a person's pain. Most of these are based on the patient's report. They include numeric pain intensity, visual analog, and verbal descriptor scales. Most pain questionnaires assess a single aspect of pain such as pain intensity. For example, a *numeric pain intensity* scale would have patients select which number best represents the intensity of their pain, where 0 represents no pain and 10 represents the most intense pain imaginable. A *visual analog* scale also can be used; it is a straight line, often 10 cm in length, with a word description (*e.g.,* "no pain" or "the most intense pain imaginable") at each of the ends of the line representing the continuum of pain intensity. Patients are asked to choose a point on the continuum that represents the intensity of their pain. The response can be quantified by measuring the line to determine the distance of the mark, measured in millimeters, from the "no pain" end of the line. *Verbal descriptor* scales consist of several numerically ranked choices of words such as none = 0, slight = 1, mild = 2, moderate = 3, and severe = 4. The word chosen is used to determine the numeric representation of pain severity on an ordinal scale.

Some pain questionnaires are multidimensional (*e.g.,* the McGill Pain Questionnaire) in that they include several sections or sets of questions that are scored into subscales that quantify various aspects of pain. The McGill Pain Questionnaire[22] is divided into four parts. The first part uses a drawing of the body on which the person indicates the location of pain. The second part uses a list of 20 words to describe the sensory, affective, evaluative, and other qualities of pain, with the selected words being given a numeric score (*e.g.,* words implying the least pain are assigned a value of 1, moderate pain a value of 2, and so on). The third part asks the person to select words such as *brief, momentary,* and *constant* to describe the pattern of pain. The fourth part of the instrument evaluates the present pain intensity on a scale with scores from 0 to 5. The Memorial Pain Assessment Card, another multidimensional instrument, can be used to determine the intensity of pain, mood, and effectiveness of analgesia.[20]

MANAGEMENT OF PAIN

The therapeutic approaches to acute and chronic pain differ markedly. In acute pain, therapy is directed at providing pain relief by interrupting the nociceptive stimulus. Because the pain is self-limited, in that it resolves as the injured tissues heal, long-term therapy usually is not needed. Chronic pain management is much more complex and is based on multiple considerations, including life expectancy.

Acute Pain

Acute pain should be aggressively managed and pain medication provided before the pain becomes severe. This allows the person to be more comfortable and active and to assume a greater role in directing his or her own care. Part of the reluctance of health care workers to provide adequate relief for acute pain has been fear of addiction. However, addiction to opioid medications is thought to be virtually nonexistent when these drugs are prescribed for acute pain. Usually, less medication is needed when the drug is given before the pain becomes severe and the pain pathways become sensitized.

The AHCPR guidelines, which address pain from surgery, medical procedures, and trauma, emphasize the need for (1) a collaborative, interdisciplinary approach to pain control, which includes members of the health care team and input from the patient and the patient's family when appropriate; (2) an individualized, proactive pain control plan developed before surgery (if possible) by patients and providers; (3) the assessment and frequent reassessment of the patient's pain, facilitated by a pain management log or flow sheet; (4) the use of drug and nondrug therapies to control or prevent pain; and (5) a formal, institutional approach to management of acute pain with clear lines of responsibility.[20]

Chronic Pain

Management of chronic pain requires early attempts to prevent pain and adequate therapy for acute bouts of pain. Specific treatment depends on the cause of the pain, the natural history of the underlying health problem, and the life expectancy of the individual. If the organic illness causing the pain cannot be cured, then noncurative methods of pain control become the cornerstone of treatment. Treatment methods for chronic pain can include neural blockade, electrical modalities (*e.g.,* transcutaneous electrical nerve stimulation), physical therapy, cognitive behavioral interventions, and nonnarcotic and narcotic medications. Nonnarcotic medications such as tricyclic antidepressants, antiseizure medications, and nonsteroidal antiinflammatory drugs (NSAIDs) serve as useful adjuncts to opioids for the treatment of different types of chronic pain. Chronic pain is best handled by a multidisciplinary team that includes specialists in areas such as anesthesiology, nursing, physical therapy, social services, and surgery.

Cancer is a common cause of chronic pain. The goal of chronic cancer pain management should be pain alleviation and prevention. Preemptive therapy tends to reduce sensitization of pain pathways and provides for more effective pain control. In 1994, the AHCPR published Clinical Practice Guideline No. 9, *Management of Cancer Pain.*[20] This guideline highlights the fact that pain control remains a significant problem despite the advances in understanding and management of cancer pain. The report emphasizes that pain control merits high priority because pain diminishes activity, appetite, and sleep and can further weaken a person already debilitated with cancer. It also emphasizes that pain interferes with productive employment, enjoying recreation, and taking an active part in family life. As with the AHCPR acute pain guideline, the cancer pain guideline also emphasizes the need for a collaborative multidisciplinary approach to cancer pain management. Clinically useful interventions are described in the guideline. Some of these (*e.g.,* analgesics, adjuvant drugs, cognitive or behavioral strategies, physical modalities, and nerve blocks) are used for many forms of chronic pain. Depending on the form and stage of the cancer, other treatments such as palliative radiation, antineoplastic therapies, and palliative surgery may help to control the pain. The AHCPR guideline also stresses that written patient education materials at an appropriate reading level should be provided. The World Health Organization has created an analgesic ladder for cancer pain that assists clinicians in choosing the appropriate analgesic.[23]

Nonpharmacologic Treatment

A number of nonpharmacologic methods of pain control often are used in pain management. These include cognitive-behavioral interventions, physical agents such as heat and cold, and electroanalgesia. Often, these methods are used in addition to analgesics rather than as the only form of pain management.

Cognitive-Behavioral Interventions. Cognitive-behavioral interventions, which often are helpful for individuals experiencing acute as well as chronic pain, include relaxation, distraction, cognitive reappraisal, imagery, meditation, and biofeedback. If the person is having surgery or a painful procedure, it is ideal to teach these techniques before the pain begins (*e.g.,* before surgery). If the person is already in severe pain, the use of cognitive-behavioral interventions should be based on the person's ability to master the technique as well as his or her response to the intervention. For example, it would be a more appropriate adjunct to analgesics for a terminally ill person in severe pain to use self-selected relaxing music rather than trying to teach that person an intervention requiring more attention (*e.g.,* meditation or cognitive reappraisal).

Relaxation is one of the best-evaluated cognitive-behavioral approaches to pain relief. The relaxation method need not be complex. Relatively simple strategies, such as slow rhythmic breathing and brief jaw relaxation procedures, have been successful in decreasing self-reported pain and analgesic use.

Distraction (*i.e.,* focusing a person's attention on stimuli other than painful stimuli or negative emotions) does not eliminate pain, but it can make pain more tolerable. It may serve as a type of sensory shielding whereby attention to pain is sacrificed to pay attention to other stimuli that are easily perceived. Examples of distraction include counting, repeating phrases or poems, and engaging in activities that require concentration, such as projects, activities, work, conversation, or describing pictures. Television, adventure movies, music, and humor also can provide distraction. *Cognitive reappraisal* is a form of self-distraction or cognitive control in which individuals focus their attention on the positive aspects of the experience and away from their pain. Individuals using distraction may not appear to be in severe pain. Nonetheless, it is inappropriate to assume that a person who copes with pain by using distraction does not have pain. Prescribed analgesics should not be denied to patients simply because they appear to be coping with their pain without medication. Appropriate assessment is needed to determine the patient's level of pain and what other interventions for pain may be needed.

Imagery consists of using one's imagination to develop a mental picture. In pain management, therapeutic guided imagery (*i.e.,* goal-directed imaging) is used. It can be used alone or in conjunction with other cognitive behavioral interventions (*e.g.,* relaxation or biofeedback) to develop sensory images that may decrease the perceived intensity of pain. It also can be used to lessen anxiety and reduce muscle tension. *Meditation* also can be used, but it requires practice and the ability to concentrate to be effective.

Biofeedback is used to provide feedback to a person concerning the current status of some body function (*e.g.,* finger temperature, temporal artery pulsation, blood pressure, or muscle tension). It involves a process of learning designed to make the person aware of certain of his or her own body functions for the purpose of modifying these functions at a conscious level. Interest in biofeedback increased with the possibility of using this treatment modality in the management of migraine and tension headaches or for other pain that has a muscle tension component.

Physical Agents. Heat and cold are physical agents that are used to provide pain relief. The choice of physical agent depends on the type of pain being treated and, in many cases, personal preference.

Heat has long been used to relieve pain. Heat dilates blood vessels and increases local blood flow; it also can influence the transmission of pain impulses and increase collagen extensibility. An increase in local circulation can reduce the level of nociceptive stimulation by reducing local ischemia caused by muscle spasm or tension, increase the removal of metabolites and inflammatory mediators that act as nociceptive stimuli, and help to reduce swelling and relieve pressure on local nociceptive endings. The heat sensation is carried to the posterior horn of the spinal cord and may exert its effect by modulating projection of pain transmission. It also may trigger the release of endogenous opioids. Heat also alters the viscosity of collagen fibers in ligaments, tendons, and joint structures so that they are more easily extended and can be stretched further before the nociceptive endings are stimulated. Thus, heat often is applied before therapy aimed at stretching joint structures and increasing range of motion. Care must be taken not to use excessive heat. When excessive heat is used, the heat itself becomes a noxious stimulus, which results in actual or impending tissue damage and pain. In certain conditions, the use of heat is controversial, and in some conditions (*e.g.,* peripheral vascular disease) in which increased blood flow or metabolism would be detrimental, the use of heat is contraindicated.

Like heat, the application of *cold* may produce a dramatic reduction in pain. Cold exerts its effect on pain through circulatory and neural mechanisms. The initial response to local application of cold is sudden local vasoconstriction. This initial vasoconstriction is followed by alternating periods of vasodilatation and vasoconstriction during which the body "hunts" for its normal level of blood flow to prevent local tissue damage. This gives rise to the so-called *hunting reflex* whereby the circulation to the cooled area undergoes alternating periods of pallor caused by ischemia and flushing caused by hyperemia.[24] The vasoconstriction is caused by local stimulation of sympathetic fibers and direct cooling of blood vessels, and the hyperemia by local autoregulatory mechanisms. In situations of acute injury, cold is used to produce vasoconstriction and prevent extravasation of blood into the tissues; pain relief results from decreased swelling and decreased stimulation of nociceptive endings. The vasodilatation that follows can be useful in removing substances that stimulate nociceptive endings.

Cold also can have a marked and dramatic effect on pain that results from the spasm-induced accumulation of metabolites in muscle. In terms of pain modulation, cold may reduce afferent activity reaching the posterior horn of the spinal cord by modulating sensory input. The application of cold is a noxious stimulus and may influence the release of endogenous opioids from the PAG area. Cold packs should be flexible to conform to body parts easily, adequately wrapped to protect the skin, and applied no more than 15 to 20 minutes at a time. Cold should be used only with great caution in anyone whose circulation is compromised.

Stimulus-Induced Analgesia. Stimulus-induced analgesia is one of the oldest known methods of pain relief. Historical references to the use of electricity to decrease or control pain date back to AD 46, when a Roman physician, Scribonius Largus, described how the stimulus from an electric eel was able to provide pain relief for headache and gout.[25] Electrical stimulation methods of pain relief include transcutaneous electrical nerve stimulation (TENS) and electrical acupuncture. TENS refers to the transmission of electrical energy across the surface of the skin to the peripheral nerve fibers. TENS units have been developed that are convenient, easily transported, and relatively economical to use. Most are approximately the size of a transistor radio or cigarette package. These battery-operated units deliver an electrical current to a target site.

The system usually consists of three parts: a pair of electrodes, lead wires, and a stimulator. The electrical stimulation is delivered in a pulsed waveform that can be varied in terms of pulse amplitude, width, and rate. The type of stimulation used varies with the type of pain being treated. Electrode placement is determined by the physiologic pathways and an understanding of the pain mechanisms involved. Electrodes may be placed on either side of a painful area, over an affected dermatome, over an affected peripheral nerve where it is most superficial, or over a nerve trunk. For example, the electrodes commonly are placed medial and lateral to the incision when treating postoperative pain.

There probably is no single explanation for the physiologic effects of TENS. Each specific type of stimulator may have different sites of action and may be explained by more than one theory. The gate control theory was proposed as one possible mechanism. According to this theory, pain information is transmitted by small-diameter Aδ and C fibers. Large-diameter afferent A fibers and small-diameter fibers carry tactile information mediating touch, pressure, and kinesthesia. TENS may function on the basis of differential firing of impulses in the large fibers that carry nonpainful information. Accordingly, increased activity in these larger fibers purportedly modulates transmission of painful information to the forebrain. A second possible explanation is that the high-frequency stimulation (50 to 60 Hz) produced by some units simply acts as a counterirritant.[26] A third possible explanation is that stimulators that produce strong rhythmic contractions may act through the release of endogenous analgesics such as the endorphins and enkephalins that suppress or modulate pain transmission. A fourth, and probably the best, explanation for quick analgesia with brief, intense stimulation is that it acts as a conduction block.[27,28] TENS has the advantage that it is noninvasive, easily regulated by the person or health professional, and effective in some forms of acute and chronic pain. Its use can be taught before surgery, affording a reduction in postoperative analgesic medication and, possibly, preventing the development of persistent pain.

Acupuncture. The practice of acupuncture involves introducing needles into specific points on the surface of the body. Charts are available that describe the points of needle placement that are used to relieve pain at certain anatomic sites. In addition to needles, sometimes palpation is used. The practice of acupuncture dates back thousands of years to ancient China, when the stimulation was achieved by using needles made of bone, stone, or bamboo. Annually, approximately 1 million individuals in the United States receive acupuncture, and pain is the major complaint for which they receive it.[29] Acupuncture is widely available in pain clinics even though large, high-quality, randomized studies on the effects of acupuncture for chronic pain are not plentiful. Various theories of how acupuncture achieves analgesia have been proposed, including the gate control theory and the neurohumoral theory, involving the cascade of endorphins and monoamines. This possible physiologic basis for pain relief from acupuncture alone or acupuncture with electrical stimulation has been demonstrated by reversing pain control through the use of the morphine antagonist naloxone.[29]

Pharmacologic Treatment

Analgesics have been used for many years to relieve pain of short duration, enabling the person to achieve mobility after surgery, for example, when exercises such as coughing and deep breathing may be required. With acute pain, and even more so with chronic pain, the use of analgesics is only one aspect of a comprehensive pain management program. An analgesic drug is a medication that acts on the nervous system to decrease or eliminate pain without inducing loss of consciousness. Analgesic drugs do not cure the underlying cause of the pain, but their appropriate use may prevent acute pain from progressing to chronic pain. The AHCPR cancer pain guideline classifies pain medications into three categories: aspirin, other NSAIDs, and acetaminophen; opioid analgesics; and adjuvant analgesics.[20]

The ideal analgesic would be effective, nonaddictive, and inexpensive. In addition, it would produce minimal adverse effects and not affect the person's level of consciousness. Although long-term treatment with opioids can result in opioid tolerance (*i.e.*, more drug being needed to achieve the same effect) and physical dependence, this should not be confused with addiction. Long-term drug-seeking behavior is rare in persons who are treated with opioids only during the time that they require pain relief. The unique needs and circumstances presented by each person in pain must be addressed to achieve satisfactory pain management.

Nonnarcotic Analgesics. Common nonnarcotic oral analgesic medications include aspirin, other NSAIDs, and acetaminophen. Aspirin, or acetylsalicylic acid, acts centrally and peripherally to block the transmission of pain impulses. It also has antipyretic and antiinflammatory properties. The actions of aspirin and other NSAIDs is through the inhibition of the cyclooxygenase (COX) enzymes, which mediates the biosynthesis of prostaglandins. Prostaglandins (particularly, prostaglandin E_2) exert their effect through peripheral sensitization of nociceptors to chemical mediators such as bradykinin and histamine.[30] The NSAIDs also decrease the sensitivity of blood vessels to bradykinin and histamine, affect lymphokine production by T lymphocytes, reverse vasodilation, and decrease the release of inflammatory mediators from granulocytes, mast cells, and basophils. Acetaminophen is an alternative to the NSAIDs. Although usually considered equivalent to aspirin as an analgesic and antipyretic agent, it lacks antiinflammatory properties.

Opioid Analgesics. The term *opioid* or *narcotic* is used to refer to a group of medications, natural or synthetic, with morphine-like actions. The older term *opiate* was used to designate drugs derived from opium—morphine, codeine, and many other semisynthetic congeners of morphine. Opioids are used for relief of short-term pain and for more long-term use in conditions such as cancer pain. When given for temporary relief of severe pain, such as that occurring after surgery, there is much evidence that opioids given routinely before the pain starts or becomes extreme are far more effective than those administered in a sporadic manner. Persons who are treated in this manner seem to require fewer doses and are able to resume regular activities sooner.

Opioids also are used for persons with limited life expectancy. Too often, because of undue concern about the possibility of addiction, many chronic pain sufferers with a short life expectancy receive inadequate pain relief. Most pain experts agree that it is appropriate to provide the level of opioid necessary to relieve the severe, intractable pain of persons whose life expectancy is limited. Addiction is not considered a problem in patients with cancer.[34] In persons with chronic cancer pain, morphine remains the most useful strong opioid. The World Health Organization has recommended that oral morphine be part of the essential medication list and be made available throughout the world as the medication of choice for cancer pain.[23] Oral forms of morphine are well absorbed from the gastrointestinal tract and have a half-life of approximately 2.5 hours and a duration of action of 4 to 6 hours. Liquid forms of the medication usually are given at 4-hour intervals to maintain an adequate blood level for analgesia, while minimizing the potential for toxic side effects. Controlled-release forms of the drug also are available.

Although the analgesic and psychopharmacologic properties of morphine have been known for centuries, the knowledge that the brain contains its own endogenous opioid-like chemicals, the *endorphins (enkephalins, endorphins,* and *dynorphins*), has only become known within the last 40 to 50 years. It has been hypothesized that part of the pain-relieving properties of exogenous opioids such as morphine involves the release of these endogenous opioids.[30]

The opioid analgesics are characterized by their interaction with three types of opioid receptors, designated mu (μ, for "morphine"), delta (δ), and kappa (κ).[30] Each receptor type has been cloned, and subtypes have been identified using receptor-binding and molecular studies. Morphine and most opioids that are used clinically exert their effects through the mu receptor. Kappa receptor opioids are effective analgesics, but their side effects have proved troublesome, and the clinical impact of delta receptor opioids has been negligible.

It is well documented that the mu receptors modulate both the therapeutic effect of analgesia and the side effects of respiratory depression, miosis, reduced gastrointestinal motility (causing constipation), feelings of well-being or euphoria, and physical dependence. The mu receptors are found at presynaptic and postsynaptic sites in the spinal dorsal horn and in the ascending pathways of the brain stem, thalamus, and cortex as well as the descending inhibitory system that modulates pain at the spinal cord. Their spinal location has been exploited clinically by direct application of opioid analgesics to the spinal cord, which provides regional anesthesia while minimizing the unwanted respiratory depression, nausea and vomiting, and sedation that occur with systemically administered drugs that act at the brain level. Mu receptors are also found in peripheral sensory neurons following inflammation. This location supports the exploration and eventual clinical use of locally applied opioids (*e.g.*, intraarticular instillation of opioids after knee surgery).

As more information becomes available regarding the opioids and their receptors, it seems likely that pain medications can be developed that act selectively at certain receptor sites, providing more effective pain control while producing fewer adverse effects and affording less danger of addiction. For example, it might be possible to develop opioid drugs that produce effective analgesia but not undesirable adverse effects, such as respiratory depression and the most common complication, constipation.

One of the problems with the need for long-term use of opioids, as in relief of cancer pain, is the development of tolerance or the need for larger and larger doses to achieve the same level of pain relief. Clinicians have long noted two important phenomena that suggest the possibility of multiple mu opioid receptor subtypes and support the importance of research in this area.[34] First, there are often noteworthy differences in patient responses to mu opioids. Patient-specific responses to these drugs include both the extent of relief obtained and the side-effect profiles observed. Second, patients who become tolerant to one mu opioid are often far less tolerant to another mu opioid. The difference in tolerance across mu opioids is called *incomplete cross-tolerance*.[33]

Some clinicians use opioid rotation to improve analgesia once opioid tolerance becomes problematic. It is important to note that the standard equianalgesic conversion tables are based primarily on single-dose studies and as such do not account for incomplete cross-tolerance. When opioid rotation is used with patients demonstrating a tolerance to opioids, it is recommended that the new opioid be started at a fraction of the dosage that is predicted to be equivalent to the current opioid dosage.[33]

Adjuvant Analgesics. Adjuvant analgesics include medications such as tricyclic antidepressants, antiseizure medications, and neuroleptic anxiolytic agents. The fact that the pain suppression system has nonendorphin synapses raises the possibility that potent, centrally acting, nonopiate medications may be useful in relieving pain. Serotonin has been shown to play an important role in producing analgesia. The tricyclic antidepressant medications (*i.e.,* imipramine, amitriptyline, and doxepin) that block the removal of serotonin from the synaptic cleft have been shown to produce pain relief in some persons. These medications are particularly useful in some chronic painful conditions, such as postherpetic neuralgia.

Certain antiseizure medications, such as carbamazepine (Tegretol) and phenytoin (Dilantin), have analgesic effects in some pain conditions. These medications, which suppress spontaneous neuronal firing, are particularly useful in the management of pain that occurs after nerve injury. Other agents, such as the corticosteroids, may be used to decrease inflammation and nociceptive stimuli responsible for pain.

Surgical Intervention

If surgery removes the problem causing the pain, such as a tumor pressing on a nerve or an inflamed appendix, it can be curative. In other instances, surgery is used for symptom management rather than for cure. However, with rare exceptions, noninvasive analgesic approaches should precede invasive palliative approaches.[20] Surgery for severe, intractable pain of peripheral or central origin has met with some success. It can be used to remove the cause or block the transmission of intractable pain from phantom limb pain, severe neuralgia, inoperable cancer of certain types, and causalgia.

In summary, pain is an elusive and complex phenomenon; it is a symptom common to many illnesses. It is a highly individualized experience that is shaped by a person's culture and previous life experiences, and it is difficult to measure. Traditionally, there have been two principal theories of pain: specificity and pattern theories. Scientifically, pain is viewed within the context of nociception. Nociceptors are receptive nerve endings that respond to noxious stimuli. Pain receptors respond to mechanical, thermal, and chemical stimuli. Nociceptive neurons transmit impulses to the dorsal horn neurons using chemical neurotransmitters. The neospinothalamic and the paleospinothalamic paths are used to transmit pain information to the brain. Several neuroanatomic pathways, as well as endogenous opioid peptides, modulate pain in the CNS.

Pain can be classified according to location, referral, and duration as well as associated medical diagnoses. Pain can arise from cutaneous, deep somatic, or visceral locations. Referred pain is pain perceived at a site different from its origin. Acute pain is self-limiting pain that ends when the injured tissue heals, whereas chronic pain is pain that lasts much longer than the anticipated healing time for the underlying cause of the pain. Pain threshold, pain tolerance, age, sex, and other factors affect an individual's reaction to pain.

Treatment modalities for pain include the use of physiologic, cognitive, and behavioral measures; heat and cold; stimulation-induced analgesic methods; and pharmacologic agents singly or in combination. It is becoming apparent that even with chronic pain, the most effective approach is early treatment or even prevention. After pain is present, the greatest success in pain assessment and management is achieved with the use of an interdisciplinary approach.

Alterations in Pain Sensitivity and Special Types of Pain

After completing this section of the chapter, you should be able to meet the following objectives:

- Define allodynia, hypoesthesia, hyperesthesia, paresthesias, hyperpathia, analgesia, and hypoalgesia
- Describe the cause and characteristics and treatment of neuropathic pain, trigeminal neuralgia, postherpetic neuralgia, and complex regional pain syndrome
- Cite possible mechanisms of phantom limb pain

ALTERATIONS IN PAIN SENSITIVITY

Sensitivity and perception of pain vary among persons and in the same person under different conditions and in different parts of the body. Irritation, mild hypoxia, and mild compression of a peripheral nerve often result in hyperexcitability of the sensory nerve fibers or cell bodies. This is experienced as unpleasant hypersensitivity (*i.e., hyperesthesia*) or increased painfulness (*i.e., hyperalgesia*). Possible causes of increased sensitivity to noxious stimuli include a decrease in the threshold of nociceptors, an increase in pain produced by suprathreshold stimuli, and the windup phenomenon. Primary hyperalgesia occurs at the site of injury. Secondary hyperalgesia occurs in nearby uninjured tissue.

Hyperpathia is a syndrome in which the sensory threshold is raised, but when it is reached, continued stimulation, especially if repetitive, results in a prolonged and unpleasant experience. This pain can be explosive and radiates through a peripheral nerve distribution. It is associated with pathologic changes in peripheral nerves, such as localized ischemia. Spontaneous, unpleasant sensations called *paresthesias* occur with more severe irritation (*e.g.,* the pins-and-needles sensation that follows temporary compression of a peripheral nerve). The general term *dysesthesia* is given to distortions (usually unpleasant) of somesthetic sensation that typically accompany partial loss of sensory innervation.

More severe pathologic processes can result in reduced or lost tactile (*e.g., hypoesthesia, anesthesia*), temperature (*e.g., hypothermia, athermia*), and pain sensation (*i.e., hypalgesia*). *Analgesia* is the absence of pain on noxious stimulation or the relief of pain without loss of consciousness. The inability to sense pain may result in trauma, infection, and even loss of a body part or parts. Inherited insensitivity to pain may take the form of congenital indifference or congenital insensitivity to pain. In the former, transmission of nerve impulses appears normal, but appreciation of painful stimuli at higher levels appears to be absent. In the latter, a peripheral nerve defect apparently exists such that transmission of painful nerve impulses does not result in perception of pain. Whatever the cause, persons who lack the ability to perceive pain are at constant risk for tissue damage because pain is not serving its protective function.

Allodynia (Greek *allo,* "other," and *odynia,* "painful") is the term used for the puzzling phenomenon of pain that follows a non-noxious stimulus to apparently normal skin. This term is intended to refer to instances in which otherwise normal tissues may be abnormally innervated or may be referral sites for other loci that give rise to pain with non-noxious stimuli. It can result from increased responsiveness within the spinal cord (central sensitization) or a reduction in the threshold for nociceptor activation (peripheral sensitization). With central sensitization, activity in non-nociceptive nerve fibers can produce pain. With peripheral sensitization, tissue damage and inflammation (referred to as the "inflammatory soup") may cause the area to become hypersensitive, in which case a normally subthreshold stimulus is sufficient to trigger the sensation of pain.[12]

One type of allodynia involves *trigger points,* which are highly localized points on the skin or mucous membrane that can produce immediate intense pain at that site or elsewhere as a result of light tactile stimulation. Myofascial trigger points are foci of exquisite tenderness found in many muscles and can be responsible for pain projected to sites remote from the points of tenderness. Trigger points are widely distributed in the back of the head and neck and in the lumbar and thoracic regions. These trigger points cause reproducible myofascial pain syndromes in specific muscles. These pain syndromes are the major source of pain in clients at chronic pain treatment centers.

SPECIAL TYPES OF PAIN

Neuropathic Pain

When peripheral nerves are affected by injury or disease, it can lead to unusual and sometimes intractable sensory disturbances. These include numbness, paresthesias, and pain. Depending on the cause, few or many axons can be damaged, and the condition can be unilateral or bilateral. Causes of neuropathic pain can be categorized according to the extent of peripheral nerve involvement. Conditions that can lead to pain by causing damage to peripheral nerves in a single area include nerve entrapment, nerve compression from a tumor mass, and various neuralgias (*e.g.,* trigeminal, postherpetic, and post-traumatic). Conditions that can lead to pain by causing damage to peripheral nerves in a wide area include diabetes mellitus, long-term alcohol use, hypothyroidism, renal insufficiency, and drug treatment with neurotoxic agents.[36] Injury to a nerve also can lead to a multisymptom, multisystem syndrome called *complex regional pain syndrome* (previously known as *causalgia* or *reflex sympathetic dystrophy*). Nerve damage associated with amputation is believed to be a cause of phantom limb pain.

Neuropathic pain can vary with the extent and location of disease or injury. There may be allodynia or pain that is stabbing, jabbing, burning, or shooting. The pain may be persistent or intermittent. The diagnosis depends on the mode of onset, the distribution of abnormal sensations, the quality of the pain, and other relevant medical conditions (*e.g.,* diabetes, hypothyroidism, alcohol use, rash, or trauma). Injury to peripheral nerves sometimes results in pain that persists beyond the time required for the tissues to heal. Peripheral pathologic processes (*e.g.,* neural degeneration, neuroma formation, and generation of abnormal spontaneous neural discharges from the injured sensory neuron) and neural plasticity (*i.e.,* changes in CNS function) are the primary working hypotheses to explain persistent neuropathic pain.

Treatment methods include measures aimed at restoring or preventing further nerve damage (*e.g.,* surgery to resect a tumor causing nerve compression, improving glycemic control for diabetic patients with painful neuropathies), and interventions for the palliation of pain. Although many adjuvant analgesics are used for neuropathic pain, pain control often is difficult. The initial approach in seeking adequate pain control is to try these drugs in sequence and then in combination. The adjuvant analgesics can be divided into three general classes according to the pain they are used to treat: burning, tingling, or aching pain; stabbing or shooting pain; and neurogenic pain. For pain that is burning, tingling or aching, tricyclic antidepressants, antiarrhythmics (*e.g.,* mexiletine), and the α_2-adrenergic agonist clonidine frequently are used. For the stabbing or shooting pain of neuralgias, antiseizure medications or baclofen, a drug used in treatment of spasticity, may be used.[36]

Poor pain control or unacceptable side effects may lead to a trial with other medications. If there has been a poor response to the adjuvant analgesics, opioids also can be used. However, concerns about side effects and the remote possibility of addiction must be considered. When opioids are used, the use of long-acting opioids with a plan for breakthrough pain is desirable because it addresses the typically continuous nature of neuropathic pain. Using long-acting opioids also avoids the hepatotoxic effect of high doses of acetaminophen that could result from frequent and long-term treatment of severe pain with the oral combination opioid preparations. Nonpharmacologic therapies also are used for neurogenic pain. Electrical stimulation of the peripheral nerve or spinal cord can be used for radiculopathies and neuralgias. As a last resort, neurolysis or neurosurgical blockade sometimes is used.

Neuralgia

Neuralgia is characterized by severe, brief, often repetitive attacks of lightning-like or throbbing pain. It occurs along the distribution of a spinal or cranial nerve and usually is precipitated by stimulation of the cutaneous region supplied by that nerve.

Trigeminal Neuralgia. Trigeminal neuralgia, or *tic douloureux,* is one of the most common and severe neuralgias. It is manifested by facial tics or grimaces and stabbing, paroxysmal attacks of pain that usually are limited to the unilateral sensory distribution of one or more branches of the trigeminal nerve, most often the maxillary or mandibular divisions. Although intermittent, the pain often is excruciating and may be triggered or precipitated by stimuli such as touch, movement, drafts, and eating or talking. Spontaneous remissions for weeks or months may occur. However, as the disease progresses, the remissions become shorter and a dull pain may persist between episodes. Although the cause of the disorder is controversial, recent evidence suggests a structural cause such as the presence of an anomalous artery or vein impinging on the trigeminal nerve root.

Diagnosis is based on pain distribution and the absence of other neurologic manifestations. Multiple sclerosis should be ruled out in a young person presenting with symptoms of the disorder. The drug most helpful for treatment of the disorder is carbmazepine, an antiseizure drug. Surgical release of the vessels, dural structures, or scar tissues impinging on the trigeminal nerve root often provides lasting relief of symptoms. Gamma radiosurgery to the trigeminal root is another noninvasive approach that provides relief with essentially no side effects other than facial paresthesias in a few cases. In elderly patients, or those with limited life expectancy, radiofrequency destruction of the peripheral branches of the trigeminal nerve is sometimes preferred because it is easy to perform, has few complications, and provides symptomatic relief for a period of time.

Postherpetic Neuralgia. Herpes zoster (also called *shingles*) is caused by the same herpesvirus that causes varicella (*i.e.,* chickenpox) and is thought to represent a localized recurrent infection by the varicella virus that has remained latent in the dorsal root ganglia since the initial attack of chickenpox. During the acute attack of herpes zoster, the reactivated virus travels from the ganglia to the skin of the corresponding dermatomes, causing neuritis and dermatomal pain, with subsequent development of a localized vesicular eruption of the skin (see Chapter 61). Nearly all patients with acute herpes zoster have pain and 10% to 70% of these develop postherpetic neuralgia, the risk being highest in the elderly.[36]

The pain associated with acute herpes zoster and postherpetic neuralgia results from injury to the peripheral nerves and altered central nervous system processing. There is inflammation of the dorsal root ganglion, hemorrhagic necrosis, and neuronal loss. There is a proportionately greater injury and loss of large nerve fibers, and regenerated nerves tend to have a smaller diameter. After injury, the affected peripheral nerves discharge spontaneously, have lower activation thresholds for discharge, and display exaggerated responses to stimuli. Because there is a relative loss of large fibers with age, elderly persons are particularly prone to suffering because of the shift in the proportion of large- to small-diameter nerve fibers. Normally, the pain of acute herpes zoster tends to resolve spontaneously. Postherpetic neuralgia describes the presence of pain more than 1 month after the onset of herpes zoster.

Early treatment of shingles with high doses of systemic corticosteroids and an oral antiviral drug such as acyclovir or valacyclovir, medications that inhibit herpesvirus DNA replication, may reduce the incidence of postherpetic neuralgia. Initially, postherpetic neuralgia can be treated with a topical anesthetic agent such as lidocaine or lidocaine with prilocaine. A tricyclic antidepressant medication, such as amitriptyline or desipramine, may be used for pain relief. Regional nerve blockade (*i.e.,* stellate ganglion, epidural, local infiltration, or peripheral nerve block) has been used with limited success. Topical capsaicin preparations have been used with mixed results because many persons are intolerant of the burning sensation that precedes anesthesia after application.[37]

Complex Regional Pain Syndrome

The *complex regional pain syndrome*, formerly known as *reflex sympathetic dystrophy,* is a regional, neurotrophic pain problem that affects one or more limbs. Recently, the International Association for the Study of Pain established the terminology for the syndrome and subdivided it into two types: type 1 and type 2.[37] With the exception of one distinguishing feature, which is the presence of a major peripheral nerve injury in persons with complex regional pain syndrome 2, the two types are identical. Both are characterized by allodynia, hyperalgesia, or spontaneous pain along the distribution of a single peripheral nerve along with a history of edema and abnormalities of skin blood flow in the painful region. Characteristically, the pain is severe and burning with or without deep aching. Usually, the pain can be elicited with the slightest movement or touch to the affected area, increases with repetitive stimulation, and lasts even after the stimulation has stopped. The pain can be exacerbated by emotional upsets or any increased peripheral sympathetic nerve stimulation. All the variations of complex regional pain syndromes include sympathetic components. These are characterized by vascular and trophic (*e.g.,* dystrophic or atrophic) changes to the skin, soft tissue, and bone and can include rubor or pallor, sweating or dryness, edema (often sharply demarcated), skin atrophy, and, with time, patchy osteoporosis.

The pathophysiology of the complex regional pain syndromes remains obscure. In 1916, Leriche proposed that increased local sympathetic outflow in response to heightened afferent activity was the cause of symptoms such as pain, redness, heat, and edema. Although abnormalities in sympathetic activity are observed, local sensitivity due to an increase in the number or sensitivity of peripheral axonal adrenoceptors, rather than increased outflow of catecholamines, appears to be the cause. Increased vascular sensitivity to catecholamines may lead to the decreased cutaneous blood flow observed in the later stages of the disease. Other likely mechanisms include neurogenic inflammation caused by the activation of neuromediators, such as substance P and calcitonin gene-related peptide, and histamine, which also mediates inflammation and vasodilatation of microvessels.[38]

According to the clinical practice guideline proposed by the Reflex Sympathetic Dystrophy Syndrome Association of America, the cornerstone of treatment is promoting normal use of the affected part to the extent possible.[39] Initially, oral analgesics (including the adjuvant analgesics), TENS, and physical activity are used. If this does not lead to improvement, treatment by sympathetic blockade may provide relief from pain; it also determines the extent to which the pain is sympathetically maintained. If the block successfully treats the pain, then sympathectomy may be an effective treatment. If not, electrical stimulation of the spinal cord or narcotics may be considered.

Phantom Limb Pain

Phantom limb pain, a type of neurologic pain, follows amputation of a limb or part of a limb. As many as 70% of amputees experience phantom pain.[40] The pain often begins as sensations of tingling, heat and cold, or heaviness, followed by burning, cramping, or shooting pain. It may disappear spontaneously or persist for many years. One of the more troublesome aspects of phantom pain is that the person may experience painful sensations that were present before the amputation, such as that of a painful ulcer or bunion.

Several theories have been proposed as to the causes of phantom pain.[40] One theory is that the end of a regenerating nerve becomes trapped in the scar tissue of the amputation site. It is known that when a peripheral nerve is cut, the scar tissue that forms becomes a barrier to regenerating outgrowth of the axon. The growing axon often becomes trapped in the scar tissue, forming a tangled growth (*i.e.*, neuroma) of small-diameter axons, including primary nociceptive afferents and sympathetic efferents. It has been proposed that these afferents show increased sensitivity to innocuous mechanical stimuli and to sympathetic activity and circulating catecholamines. A related theory moves the source of phantom limb pain to the spinal cord, suggesting that the pain is due to the spontaneous firing of spinal cord neurons that have lost their normal sensory input from the body. In this case, a closed self-exciting neuronal loop in the posterior horn of the spinal cord is postulated to send impulses to the brain, resulting in pain. Even the slightest irritation to the amputated limb area can initiate this cycle. Other theories propose that the phantom limb pain may arise in the brain itself. In one hypothesis, the pain is caused by changes in the flow of signals through somatosensory areas of the brain. In other words, there appears to be plasticity even in the adult CNS. Treatment of phantom limb pain has been accomplished by the use of sympathetic blocks, TENS of the large myelinated afferents innervating the area, hypnosis, and relaxation training.

In summary, pain may occur with or without an adequate stimulus, or it may be absent in the presence of an adequate stimulus—either of which describes a pain disorder. There may be analgesia (absence of pain), hyperalgesia (increased sensitivity to pain), hypoalgesia (a decreased sensitivity to painful stimuli), hyperpathia (an unpleasant and prolonged response to pain), hyperesthesia (an abnormal increase in sensitivity to sensation), hypoesthesia (an abnormal decrease in sensitivity to sensations), paresthesia (abnormal touch sensation such as tingling or "pins and needles" in the absence of external stimuli), or allodynia (pain produced by stimuli that do not normally cause pain).

Neuropathic pain may be due to trauma or disease of neurons in a focal area or in a more global distribution (*e.g.*, from endocrine disease or neurotoxic medications). Neuralgia is characterized by severe, brief, often repetitiously occurring attacks of lightning-like or throbbing pain that occurs along the distribution of a spinal or cranial nerve and usually is precipitated by stimulation of the cutaneous region supplied by that nerve. Trigeminal neuralgia, or tic douloureux, is one of the most common and severe neuralgias. It is manifested by facial tics or grimaces. Postherpetic neuralgia is chronic pain that can occur after herpes zoster, an infection of the dorsal root ganglia and corresponding areas of innervation by the herpes zoster virus. Complex regional pain syndrome is an extremely painful condition that may follow sudden and traumatic deformation of peripheral nerves. Phantom limb pain, a neurologic pain, can occur after amputation of a limb or part of a limb.

Headache and Associated Pain

After completing this section of the chapter, you should be able to meet the following objectives:

- State the importance of distinguishing between primary and secondary types of headache
- Differentiate between the periodicity of occurrence and manifestations of migraine headache, cluster headache, tension-type headache, and headache due to temporomandibular joint syndrome
- Characterize the nonpharmacologic and pharmacologic methods used in treatment of headache
- Cite the most common cause of temporomandibular joint pain

HEADACHE

Headache is a very common health problem, with more than 90% of adults reporting having a headache at least once. Seventy-six percent of women and 57% of men report at least one headache a month.[41] Twenty-five percent of adults report having recurrent severe headaches, and 4% report having daily or nearly daily headaches.[42] Although head and facial pain have characteristics that distinguish them from other pain disorders, they also share many of the same features.

Headache is caused by a number of conditions. Some headaches represent primary disorders, and others occur secondary to other disease conditions in which head pain is a symptom. The most common types of primary and chronic headaches are migraine headache, tension-type headache, cluster headache, and chronic daily headache. Although most causes of secondary headache are benign, some are indications of serious disorders such as meningitis, brain tumor, or cerebral aneurysm. The sudden onset of a severe, intractable headache in an otherwise healthy person is more likely related to a serious intracranial disorder, such as subarachnoid hemorrhage or meningitis, than to a chronic headache disorder. Headaches that disturb sleep, exertional headaches (*e.g.*, triggered by physical or sexual activity or a Valsalva maneuver), and headaches accompanied by neurologic symptoms such as drowsiness, visual or limb disturbances, or altered mental status also are suggestive of underlying serious intracranial lesions or other pathology. Other red flags for secondary headache disorder include fundamental change or progression in headache pattern or a new headache in individuals younger than 5 or older than 50 years of age or in individuals with cancer, immunosuppression, or pregnancy.[42]

The diagnosis and classification of headaches often is difficult. It requires a comprehensive history and physical examination to exclude secondary causes. The history should include factors that precipitate headache, such as foods and food additives, missed meals, and association with the menstrual period. A careful medication history is essential because many medications can provoke or aggravate headaches. Alcohol also can cause or aggravate headache. A headache diary in which the person records his or her headaches and concurrent or antecedent events may be helpful in identifying factors that contribute to headache onset. Appropriate laboratory and imaging studies of the brain may be done to rule out secondary headaches.

In 2004, the International Headache Society (IHS) published the second edition of classification of headache disorders. The classification system is divided into three sections: (1) primary headaches, (2) headaches secondary to other medical conditions, and (3) cranial neuralgias and facial pain[43] (see Chart 50-1 for a summary of the components of the system).

CHART 50-1

Classification of Headache Disorders

1. Migraine
   - 1.1. Migraine without aura
   - 1.2. Migraine with aura
   - 1.3. Childhood periodic syndromes that are common precursors of migraine
   - 1.4. Retinal migraine
   - 1.5. Complications of migraine
   - 1.6. Probable migraine
2. Tension-type headache
   - 2.1. Infrequent episodic tension-type headache
   - 2.2. Frequent episodic tension-type headache
   - 2.3. Chronic tension-type headache
   - 2.4. Probable tension-type headache
3. Cluster headache and other trigeminal autonomic cephalalgias
4. Other primary headaches
5. Headache attributed to head and/or neck trauma
6. Headache attributed to cranial or cervical vascular disorder
7. Headache attributed to nonvascular intracranial disorder
8. Headache attributed to a substance or its withdrawal
9. Headache attributed to infection
10. Headache attributed to disorder of homeostasis
11. Headache or facial pain attributed to disorder of cranium, neck, eyes, ears, nose, sinuses, teeth, mouth, or other facial or cranial structures
12. Headache attributed to psychiatric disorder
13. Cranial neuralgias and central causes of facial pain
14. Other headache, cranial neuralgia, central or primary facial pain

(Adapted from Headache Classification Subcommittee of the International Headache Society [2004]. The International Classification of headache disorders [2nd ed.]. *Cephalalgia 24*[Suppl. 1], 1–152)

Migraine Headache

Migraine headaches affect approximately 20 million persons in the United States. They occur in about 18% of women and 6% of men and result in considerable time lost from work and other activities.[44] Migraine headaches tend to run in families and are thought to be inherited as an autosomal dominant trait with incomplete penetrance.[41] It is noteworthy that the genetic influence is stronger for migraine with aura than for migraine without aura.[44]

There are two categories of migraine headache—migraine without aura, which accounts for approximately 85% of migraines, and migraine with aura, which accounts for most of the remaining migraines. Migraine without aura is a pulsatile, throbbing, unilateral headache that typically lasts 1 to 2 days and is aggravated by routine physical activity. The headache is accompanied by nausea and vomiting, which often are disabling, and sensitivity to light and sound. Visual disturbances occur quite commonly and consist of visual hallucinations such as stars, sparks, and flashes of light. Migraine with aura has similar symptoms, but with the addition of visual or neurologic symptoms that precede the headache. The aura usually develops over a period of 5 to 20 minutes and lasts less than an hour. Although only a small percentage of persons with migraine experience an aura before an attack, many persons without aura have prodromal symptoms, such as fatigue and irritability, that precede the attack by hours or even days.

Subtypes of migraine include ophthalmoplegic migraine, hemiplegic migraine, aphasic migraine, and retinal migraine, in which transient visual and motor deficits occur. Ophthalmoplegic migraine is characterized by diplopia, due to a transient paralysis of the muscles that control eye movement (usually the third cranial nerve), and localized pain around the eye. Migraine headache also can present as a mixed headache, including symptoms typically associated with tension-type headache, sinus headache, or chronic daily headache. This is called *transformed migraine* and is difficult to classify. Although nasal symptoms are not one of the diagnostic criteria for migraine, they frequently accompany migraine and are probably due to cranial parasympathetic activation. Sinus pain may indicate either a headache due to sinus inflammation or migraine. In a recent study, 96% of those self-diagnosed with sinus headache, in fact, met the IHS criteria for migraine or migrainous headache.[45]

Migraine headaches occur in children as well as adults.[46,47] Before puberty, migraine headaches are equally distributed between sexes. The essential diagnostic criterion for migraine in children is the presence of recurrent headaches separated by pain-free periods. Diagnosis is based on at least three of the following symptoms or associated findings: abdominal pain, nausea or vomiting, throbbing headache, unilateral location, associated aura (visual, sensory, motor), relief during sleep, and a positive family history.[47] Symptoms vary widely among children, from those that interrupt activities and cause the child to seek relief in a dark environment to those detectable only by direct questioning. A common feature of migraine in children is intense nausea and vomiting. The vomiting may be associated with abdominal pain and fever; thus, migraine may be confused with other conditions such as appendicitis. More than half of children with migraine undergo spontaneous prolonged remission after their 10th birthday. Because headaches in children can be a symptom of other, more serious disorders, including intracranial lesions, it is important that other causes of headache that require immediate treatment be ruled out.

Migraines are believed to result from a primary disorder in the brain related to episodic changes in neural hyperexcitability that results in dilation of blood vessels, which in turn, results in pain and further nerve activation.[44] Possible reasons for this neural hyperexcitability may rest with dysfunction of an ion channel in the brain stem or diencephalic nuclei that modulate sensory input and exert neural influences on cranial vessels. In persons with familial hemiplegic migraine, for example, a mutation in one of the subunits of a voltage-gated calcium channel has been identified.[48]

The pathophysiological mechanisms of the pain associated with migraines remain poorly understood. Although many alternate theories exist, it is well established that during a migraine, the trigeminal nerve becomes activated.[49] Activation of the trigeminal sensory fibers may lead to the release of neuropeptides, causing painful neurogenic inflammation within the meningeal vasculature characterized by plasma protein extravasation, vasodilation, and mast cell degranulation.[49] Another possible mechanism implicates neurogenic vasodilation of meningeal blood vessels as a key component of the inflammatory processes that occur during migraine. Activation of trigeminal sensory fibers evokes a neurogenic dural vasodilation mediated by calcitonin gene-related peptide. It also has been observed that calcitonin gene-related peptide level is elevated during migraine and is normalized after successful treatment with sumatriptan.[49] Supporting the neurogenic basis for migraine is the frequent presence of premonitory symptoms before the headach[illegible]s; the presence of focal neurologic disturbances [illegible]t be explained in terms of cerebral blood fl[illegible]us accompanying symptoms, inclu[illegible] constitutional dysfunction.[41]

Hormonal variations, particularly in estrogen levels, play a role in the pattern of migraine attacks. For many women, migraine headaches coincide with their menstrual periods. The greater predominance of migraine headaches in women is thought to be related to the aggravating effect of estrogen on the migraine mechanism.[41] Dietary substances, such as monosodium glutamate, aged cheese, and chocolate, also may precipitate migraine headaches. The actual triggers for migraine are the chemicals in the food, not allergens.[50]

Treatment. The treatment of migraine headaches includes preventative and abortive nonpharmacologic and pharmacologic treatment. In 2002, the American College of Physicians–American Society of Internal Medicine and the American Academy of Family Physicians produced a set of evidence-based guidelines for the nonpharmacologic and pharmacologic management and prevention of migraine headaches in primary care settings.[51]

Nonpharmacologic treatment includes the avoidance of migraine triggers, such as foods, that precipitate an attack. Many persons with migraines benefit from maintaining regular eating and sleeping habits. Measures to control stress, which also can precipitate an attack, also are important. During an attack, many persons find it helpful to retire to a quiet, darkened room until symptoms subside.

Pharmacologic treatment involves both abortive therapy for acute attacks and preventive therapy. A wide range of medications is used to treat the acute symptoms of migraine headache. Based on clinical trials, first-line agents include acetylsalicylic acid; combinations of acetaminophen, acetylsalicylic acid, and caffeine and NSAIDs analgesics (*e.g.*, naproxen sodium, ibuprofen); serotonin receptor agonists (*e.g.*, sumatriptan, naratriptan, rizatriptan, zolmitriptan); ergotamine derivatives (*e.g.*, dihydroergotamine); and antiemetic medications (*e.g.*, prochlorperazine, metoclopramide). Nonoral routes of administration may be preferred in individuals who develop severe pain rapidly or upon awakening or in those with severe nausea and vomiting. Both sumatriptan and dihydroergotamine have been approved for intranasal administration. For intractable migraine headache, dihydroergotamine may be administered parenterally with an antiemetic (metoclopramide or prochlorperazine) or opioid analgesic (transnasal butorphanol).[52] Frequent use of abortive headache medications may cause rebound headache.

Preventative pharmacologic treatment may be necessary if migrainous headaches are disabling, if they occur more than two or three times a month, if abortive treatment is being used more than two times a week, or if the individual has hemiplegic migraine, migraine with prolonged aura, or migrainous infarction.[51] In most cases, preventative treatment must be taken daily for months to years. First-line agents include β-adrenergic blocking medications (*e.g.*, propranolol, timolol, atenolol), antidepressants (amitriptyline), and antiseizure medications (divalproex sodium, sodium valproate).[51] When a decision to discontinue preventive therapy is made, the medications should be gradually withdrawn.

Other effective medications are available, but they can have serious side effects in some individuals. For example, because of the risk for coronary vasospasm, the 5-HT_1 receptor agonists should not be given to persons with coronary artery disease. Ergotamine preparations can cause uterine contractions and should not be given to pregnant women. They also can cause vasospasm and should be used with caution in persons with peripheral vascular disease.

Cluster Headache

Cluster headaches are relatively uncommon headaches occurring in about 1 in 1000 individuals, affecting men (80% to 85%) more frequently than women, and typically beginning in the third decade of life and rarely beginning beyond age 70 years.[50] These headaches tend to occur in clusters over weeks or months, followed by a long, headache-free remission period. Cluster headache is a type of primary neurovascular headache that typically includes severe, unrelenting, unilateral pain located, in order of decreasing frequency, in the orbital, retroorbital, temporal, supraorbital, and infraorbital region. The pain is of rapid onset and builds to a peak in approximately 10 to 15 minutes, lasting for 15 to 180 minutes. The pain behind the eye radiates to the ipsilateral trigeminal nerve (*e.g.,* temple, cheek, gum). The headache frequently is associated with one or more symptoms such as restlessness or agitation, conjunctival redness, lacrimation, nasal congestion, rhinorrhea, forehead and facial sweating, miosis, ptosis, and eyelid edema. Because of their location and associated symptoms, cluster headaches are often mistaken for sinus infections or dental problems.[50]

The underlying pathophysiologic mechanisms of cluster headaches are not completely known. Although recently it has been noted that heredity, through an autosomal dominant gene, plays some role in the pathogenesis of cluster headache, the likely pathophysiologic mechanisms include the interplay of vascular, neurogenic, metabolic, and humoral factors. Activation of the trigeminovascular system and the cranial autonomic parasympathetic reflexes is thought to explain the pain and autonomic symptoms. The hypothalamus is believed to play a key role. The possible role of the regulating centers in the anterior hypothalamus is implicated from observations of circadian rhythm changes and neuroendocrine disturbances (*e.g.,* changes in cortisol, prolactin, and testosterone) that occur in both active periods and during clinical remission. The hypothalamic gray matter also has been implicated. Positron-emission tomography has demonstrated increased blood flow as well as structural changes in the hypothalamic gray area on the painful side during an attack. Magnetic resonance imaging has demonstrated dilated intracranial arteries on the painful side. Loss of vascular tone is believed to result from a defect in the sympathetic perivascular innervation.[53]

Treatment. Because of the relatively short duration and self-limited nature of cluster headache, oral preparations typically take too long to reach therapeutic levels. The most effective treatments are those that act quickly (*e.g.,* oxygen inhalation and subcutaneous sumatriptan). Intranasal lidocaine also may be effective.[41] Oxygen inhalation may be indicated for home use. Prophylactic medications for cluster headaches include ergotamine, verapamil, methysergide, lithium carbonate, corticosteroids, sodium valproate, and indomethacin.

Tension-Type Headache

The most common type of headache is tension-type headache. Unlike migraine and cluster headaches, tension-type headache usually is not sufficiently severe that it interferes with daily activities. Tension-type headaches frequently are described as dull, aching, diffuse, nondescript headaches, occurring in a hatband distribution around the head, and not associated with nausea or vomiting or worsened by activity. They can be infrequent, episodic, or chronic.

The exact mechanisms of tension-type headache are not known, and the hypotheses of causation are contradictory. One popular theory is that tension-type headache results from sustained tension of the muscles of the scalp and neck; however, some research has found no correlation between muscle contraction and tension-type headache. Many authorities now believe that tension-type headaches are forms of migraine headache.[41] It is thought that migraine headache may be transformed gradually into chronic tension-type headache. Tension-type headaches also may be caused by oromandibular dysfunction, psychogenic stress, anxiety, depression, and muscular stress. They also may result from overuse of analgesics or caffeine. Daily use of caffeine, whether in beverages or medications, can produce addiction, and a headache can develop in such persons who go without caffeine for several hours.[50]

Treatment. Tension-type headaches often are more responsive to nonpharmacologic techniques, such as biofeedback, massage, acupuncture, relaxation, imagery, and physical therapy, than other types of headache. For persons with poor posture, a combination of range-of-motion exercises, relaxation, and posture improvement may be helpful.[50]

The medications of choice for acute treatment of tension-type headaches are analgesics, including acetylsalicylic acid, acetaminophen, and NSAIDs. Persons with infrequent tension-type headache usually self-medicate using over-the-counter analgesics to treat the acute pain, and do not require prophylactic medication. These agents should be used cautiously because rebound headaches can develop when the medications are taken regularly.

Because the "dividing lines" between tension-type headache, migraine, and chronic daily headache often are vague, addition of medications as well as the entire range of migraine medications may be tried in refractory cases. Other medications used concomitantly with analgesics include sedating antihistamines (*e.g.,* promethazine and diphenhydramine), antiemetics (*e.g.,* metoclopramide and prochlorperazine), or sedatives (*e.g.,* butalbital). Prophylactic treatment for chronic tension-type headaches can include antidepressants (*e.g.,* amitriptyline) and selective serotonin reuptake inhibitors (SSRIs) (*e.g.,* paroxetine, venlafaxine, and fluoxetine).[54]

Chronic Daily Headache

The term *chronic daily headache* (CDH) is used to refer to headaches that occur 15 days or more a month, including those due to medication overuse.[55] Little is known about the prevalence and incidence of CDH. Diagnostic criteria for CDH are not provided in the International Headache Society [illegible]sification System. The cause of CDH is unknown, although there are several hypotheses. They include transformed migraine headache, evolved tension-type headache, new daily persistent headache, and post-traumatic headache. In many persons, CDH retains certain characteristics of migraine, whereas in others, it resembles chronic tension-type headache. CDH may be associated with chronic and episodic tension-type headache. New daily persistent headache may have a fairly rapid onset, with no history of migraine, tension-type headache, trauma, or psychological stress. Although overuse of symptomatic medications (*e.g.*, analgesics, ergotamine) has been related to CDH, there is a group of patients in whom CDH is unrelated to excessive use of medications.

Treatment. For patients with CDH, a combination of pharmacologic and behavioral interventions may be necessary. As with tension-type headaches, nonpharmacologic techniques, such as biofeedback, massage, acupuncture, relaxation, imagery, and physical therapy, may be helpful. Measures to reduce or eliminate medication overuse may be helpful. Most of the medications used for prevention of CDH have not been examined in well-designed, double-blind studies.

TEMPOROMANDIBULAR JOINT PAIN

A common cause of head pain is temporomandibular joint (TMJ) syndrome. It usually is caused by an imbalance in joint movement because of poor bite, bruxism (*i.e.*, teeth grinding), or joint problems such as inflammation, trauma, and degenerative changes.[56] The pain almost always is referred and commonly presents as facial muscle pain, headache, neck ache, or earache. Referred pain is aggravated by jaw function. Headache associated with this syndrome is common in adults and children and can cause chronic pain problems.

Treatment of TMJ pain is aimed at correcting the problem, and in some cases, this may be difficult. The initial therapy for TMJ should be directed toward relief of pain and improvement in function. Pain relief often can be achieved with use of the NSAIDs. Muscle relaxants may be used when muscle spasm is a problem. In some cases, the selected application of heat or cold, or both, may provide relief. Referral to a dentist who is associated with a team of therapists, such as a psychologist, physical therapist, or pain specialist, may be indicated.[56]

In summary, head pain is a common disorder that is caused by a number of conditions. Some headaches represent primary disorders, and others occur secondary to another disease state in which head pain is a symptom. Primary headache disorders include migraine headache, tension-type headache, cluster headache, and chronic daily headache. Although most causes of secondary headache are benign, some are indications of serious disorders such as meningitis, brain tumor, or cerebral aneurysm. TMJ syndrome is one of the major causes of headaches. It usually is caused by an imbalance in joint movement because of poor bite, teeth grinding, or joint problems such as inflammation, trauma, and degenerative changes.

Pain in Children and Older Adults

After completing this section of the chapter, you should be able to meet the following objectives:

- State how the pain response may differ in children and older adults
- Explain how pain assessment may differ in children and older adults
- Explain how pain treatment may differ in children and older adults

Pain frequently is underrecognized and undertreated in both children and the elderly. In addition to the common obstacles to adequate pain management, such as concern about the effects of analgesia on respiratory status and the potential for addiction to opioids, there are additional deterrents to adequate pain management in children and the elderly. With regard to both children and the elderly, there are stereotypic beliefs that they feel less pain than other patients.[57–59] These beliefs may affect a clinician's opinion about the need for pain control. In very young children and confused elderly, there are several additional factors. These include the extreme difficulty of assessing the location and intensity of pain in individuals who are cognitively immature or cognitively impaired, and the argument that even if they feel pain, they do not remember it. Research during the past few decades has added a great deal to the body of knowledge about pain in children and the elderly. It also has provided valuable data to refute previously held misconceptions and has changed markedly the practices of health professionals.[57–59]

Human responsiveness to painful stimuli begins in the neonatal period and continues through the life span. Although the specific and localized behavioral reactions are less marked in the younger neonate or the more cognitively impaired individual, protective or withdrawal reflexes in response to nociceptive stimuli are clearly demonstrated. Pain pathways, cortical and subcortical centers, and neurochemical responses associated with pain transmission are developed and functional by the last trimester of pregnancy. Premature infants in intensive care units demonstrate protective withdrawal to a heel stick after repeated episodes. As infants mature and children grow, their responses to pain become more complex and reflective of their maturing cognitive and developmental processes. Children do feel pain and have been shown to report pain reliably and accurately at as young as 3 years of age. They also remember pain, as evidenced in studies of children with cancer, whose distress during painful procedures increases over time without intervention.

Among adults, the prevalence of pain in the general population increases with age: 32% of those between 18 and 34 years of age report daily pain, whereas 55% of Americans aged 65 and older report daily pain. Among the elderly, the most common self-attributed causes of pain are getting older (88%) and arthritis (69%).[60] In long-term care facilities, it has been estimated that 80% of individuals experience pain on a regular basis.[61] Research is inconsistent about whether there are age-related changes in pain perception. Some apparent age-related differences in pain may be due to differences in willingness to report the pain rather than actual differences in pain. The elderly may be reluctant to report pain so as not to be a burden or out of fear of the diagnoses, tests, medications, or costs that may result from an attempt to diagnose or treat their pain.

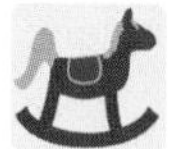

PAIN IN CHILDREN

Pain Assessment

Depending on the age of the child, assessment of pain in children can be somewhat complicated. With children 8 years of age or older, numeric scales (*i.e.,* 1 to 10) and word graphic scales (*i.e.,* "none," "a little," "most I have ever experienced") can be used. With children 3 to 8 years old, scales with faces of actual children or cartoon faces can be used to obtain a report of pain. Another supplementary strategy for assessing a child's pain is to use a body outline and ask the child to indicate where the hurt is located. Particular care must be taken in assessing children's reports of pain because their reports may be influenced by a variety of factors, including age, anxiety and fear levels, and parental presence. In very young children, infants, and neonates, as well as in children with disabilities that impair cognition or communication, clinicians must rely on physiologic parameters or age- and development-appropriate behavioral pain scales.

Nurses and physicians have reported that they rely most often on physiologic parameters such as heart rate, respiratory rate, and behavior expressions rather than the child's self-report of pain.[62] Relying on indicators of sympathetic nervous system activity and behaviors can be problematic because they can be caused by things other than pain (*e.g.,* anxiety and activity) and do not always accompany pain, particularly chronic pain. If a child is able to report pain, pain experts recommend that health professionals consider the child's report of pain as the gold standard and a primary component of their assessment, in addition to their assessment of the child's behavior and physiologic parameters. When children are too cognitively immature or are otherwise unable to report pain, behavior and physiologic parameters must be used. When there is no obvious source of pain, such as a typically painful procedure being performed, clinicians might try comfort measures or analgesics in an attempt to identify the source of distress.

Pain Management

The management of children's pain basically falls into two categories: pharmacologic and nonpharmacologic. In terms of pharmacologic interventions, many of the analgesics used in adults can be used safely and effectively in children and adolescents. However, it is critical when using specific medications to determine that the medication has been approved for use with children and that it is dosed appropriately according to the child's weight and level of physiologic development.

Age-related differences in physiologic functioning, notably in neonates, will affect drug action. Neonates have decreased fat and muscle and increased water, which increases the duration of action for some water-soluble drugs; neonates also have decreased concentration of plasma proteins, which increases the unbound concentration of protein-binding drugs. The hepatic drug metabolizing pathways of neonates and infants are also immature, leading to decreased clearance of drugs metabolized in the liver. In addition, they have decreased glomerular filtration rates, leading to delayed clearance of renally excreted drugs and their active metabolites.[63] Children ages 2 to 6 years have an increased hepatic mass compared with adults, leading to increased metabolic clearance of similar drugs.[63]

As with any person in pain, the type of analgesic used should be matched to the type and intensity of pain; and whether the patient is a child or adult, the management of chronic pain may require a multidisciplinary team. The overriding principle in all pediatric pain management is to treat each child's pain on an individual basis and to match the analgesic agent with the cause and the level of pain. A second principle involves maintaining the balance between the level of side effects and pain relief such that pain relief is obtained with as little opioid and sedation as possible. One strategy toward this end is to time the administration of analgesia so that a steady blood level is achieved and, as much as possible, pain is prevented. This requires that the child receive analgesia on a regular dosing schedule, rather than on an "as needed basis."

Nonpharmacologic strategies can be very effective in reducing the overall amount of pain and amount of analgesia used. In addition, some nonpharmacologic strategies can reduce anxiety and increase the child's level of self-control during pain. In full-term infants, ingesting 2 mL of a sucrose solution has been found to relieve the pain from a heel stick.[64] Children as young as 4 years of age can use TENS,[65] and they can be taught to use simple distraction and relaxation and other techniques such as application of heat and cold.[66] Other nonpharmacologic techniques can be taught to the child to provide psychological preparation for a painful procedure or surgery. These include positive self-talk, imagery, play therapy, modeling, and rehearsal. The nonpharmacologic interventions must be developmentally appropriate, and if possible, the child and parent should be taught these techniques when the child is not in pain (*e.g.,* before surgery or a painful procedure) so that it is easier to practice the technique. Research has provided health professionals with a wide variety of pharmacologic and nonpharmacologic options to treat a child's pain. The application of this research is critical if effective and safe pain care is to be provided.

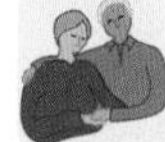

PAIN IN OLDER ADULTS

Pain Assessment

The assessment of pain in the elderly can range from relatively simple in a well-informed, alert, cognitively intact individual with pain from a single source and no comorbidities to extraordinarily difficult in a frail individual with severe dementia and many concurrent health problems.

When possible, a patient's report of pain is the gold standard, but outward signs of pain should be considered as well. Accurately diagnosing pain when the individual has many health problems or some decline in cognitive function can be particularly challenging. In recent years, there has been increased awareness of the need to address issues of pain in individuals with dementia. The Assessment for Discomfort in Dementia Protocol is one example of the efforts to improve assessment and pain management in these individuals. It includes behavioral criteria for assessing pain and recommended interventions for pain. Its use has been shown to improve pain management.[59]

Pain Management

Treatment of pain in the elderly can be complicated. The elderly may have physiologic changes that affect the pharmacokinetics of medications prescribed for pain management. These changes include decreased blood flow to organs, delayed gastric motility, reduced kidney function, and decreased albumin related to poor nutrition. These changes may affect the choice of medications or dosing (*e.g.*, using a lower initial dose of tricyclic antidepressants).[68] Also, the elderly often have many coexisting health problems, leading to polypharmacy. Whenever multiple medications are being taken, there is an increased risk for drug interactions and noncompliance because of the complexity of the treatment regimen. When prescribing pharmacologic and nonpharmacologic methods of pain management, care must be taken to consider the cause of the pain, the patient's health status, concurrent therapies, and the patient's mental status. Careful monitoring and treatment of side effects is critical.

In summary, children experience and remember pain, and even fairly young children are able to report their pain accurately and reliably. Recognition of this has changed the clinical practice of health professionals involved in the assessment of children's pain. Pain management in children is improving as exaggerated fears and misconceptions concerning the risks for addiction and side effects in children treated with opioids also are dispelled. Pharmacologic (including opioids) and nonpharmacologic pain management interventions have been shown to be effective in children. Nonpharmacologic techniques must be based on the developmental level of the child and should be taught to both children and parents.

Pain is a common symptom in the elderly. Assessment, diagnosis, and treatment of pain in the elderly can be complicated. The elderly may be reluctant or cognitively unable to report their pain. Diagnosis and treatment can be complicated by comorbidities and age-related changes in cognitive and physiologic function.

REVIEW EXERCISES

A 25-year-old man is admitted to the emergency department with acute abdominal pain that began in the epigastric area and has now shifted to the lower right quadrant of the abdomen. There is localized tenderness and guarding or spasm of the muscle over the area. His heart rate and blood pressure are elevated, and his skin is moist and cool from perspiring. He is given a tentative diagnosis of appendicitis and referred for surgical consultation.

A. Describe the origin of the pain stimuli and the neural pathways involved in the pain that this man is experiencing.

B. Explain the neural mechanisms involved in the spasm of the overlying abdominal muscles.

C. What is the significance of his cool, moist skin and increased heart rate and blood pressure?

A 65-year-old woman with breast cancer is receiving hospice care in her home. She is currently receiving a long-acting opioid analgesic supplemented with a short-acting combination opioid and nonnarcotic medication for breakthrough pain.

A. Explain the difference between the mechanisms and treatment of acute and chronic pain.

B. Describe the action of opioid drugs in the treatment of pain.

A 42-year-old woman presents with sudden stabbing-type facial pain that arises near the right side of her mouth and then shoots toward the right ear, eye, and nostril. She is holding her hand to protect her face because the pain is "triggered by touch, movement, and drafts." Her initial diagnosis is trigeminal neuritis.

A. Explain the distribution and mechanisms of the pain, particularly the triggering of the pain by stimuli applied to the skin.

B. What are possible treatment methods for this woman?

A 21-year-old woman presents in the student health center with complaints of a throbbing pain on the left side of her head, nausea and vomiting, and extreme sensitivity to light, noise, and head movement. She also tells you she had a similar headache 3 months ago that lasted for 2 days and states that she thinks she is developing migraine headaches like her mother. She is concerned because she has been unable to attend classes and has exams next week.

A. Are this woman's history and symptoms consistent with migraine headaches?

B. Use the distribution of the trigeminal nerve and the concept of neurogenic inflammation to explain this woman's symptoms.

References

1. Guyton A., Hall J.E. (2000). *Textbook of medical physiology* (10th ed., pp. 552–563). Philadelphia: W.B. Saunders.
2. Kandel E.R., Schwartz J.H., Jessell T.M. (2000). *Principles of neural science* (4th ed., pp. 430–450). New York: McGraw-Hill.
3. Ready L.B. (Chair) (1992). *International Association for the Study of Pain Task Force on Chronic Pain.* Seattle: IASP Publications.

4. Sherrington C. (1947). *The integrative action of the nervous system.* New Haven: Yale University Press.
5. Elliott A.M., Smith B.H., Penny K.I., et al. (1999). The epidemiology of chronic pain in the community. *Lancet 354,* 1248–1252.
6. Lister B.J. (1996). Dilemmas in the treatment of chronic pain. *American Journal of Medicine 101*(Suppl. 1A), 2S–4S.
7. Bonica J.J. (1991). History of pain concepts and pain theory. *Mount Sinai Journal of Medicine 58,* 191–202.
8. Melzack R., Wall P.D. (1965). Pain mechanisms: A new theory. *Science 150,* 971–979.
9. Melzack R. (1999). From the gate to the neuromatrix. *Pain 6*(Suppl.), S121–S126.
10. Cross S.A. (1994). Pathophysiology of pain. *Mayo Clinic Proceedings 69,* 375–383.
11. Julius D., Basbaum A.I. (2001). Molecular mechanisms of nociception. *Nature 413,* 203–210.
12. Markenson J.A. (1996). Mechanisms of chronic pain. *American Journal of Medicine 101*(Suppl. 1A), 6S–18S.
13. Ploner M., Gross J., Timmerman L., Schnitzler A. (2002). Cortical representation of first and second pain sensation in humans. *Proceedings of the National Academy of Sciences of the United States of America 99,* 12444–12448.
14. Fields H.L., Heinricher M.M., Mason P. (1991). Neurotransmitters in nociceptive modulatory circuits. *Review of Neuroscience 14,* 219–245.
15. Stein C. (2003). Opioid receptors on peripheral sensory neurons. In Machelska H., Stein C. (Eds.), *Immune mechanisms of pain and analgesia* (pp. 69–76). New York: Kluwer Academic/Plenum.
16. Cervero F., Laird J.M. (1999). Visceral pain. *Lancet 353,* 2145–2148.
17. Al-Chaer E.D., Traub R.J. (2002). Biological basis of visceral pain: recent developments. *Pain 96,* 221–225.
18. Grichnick K., Ferrante F.M. (1991). The difference between acute and chronic pain. *Mount Sinai Journal of Medicine 58,* 217–220.
19. Ruoff G.E. (1996). Depression in the patient with chronic pain. *Journal of Family Practice 43*(6 Suppl.), S25–S33.
20. Jacox A., Carr D.B., Payne R., et al. (1994). *Clinical practice guideline no. 9. Management of cancer pain.* AHCPR Publication No. 94-0592. Rockville, MD: Agency for Health Care Policy and Research, Public Health Service, U.S. Department of Health and Human Services.
21. Acute Pain Management Guideline Panel. (1992). *Clinical practice guideline no. 1. Acute pain management: Operative or medical procedures and trauma.* AHCPR Publication No. 92-0032. Rockville, MD: Agency for Health Care Policy and Research, Public Health Service, U.S. Department of Health and Human Services.
22. Melzack R. (1975). The McGill Pain Questionnaire: Major properties and scoring methods. *Pain 1,* 277–299.
23. World Health Organization. (1990). *Cancer pain relief and palliative care: Report of the WHO Expert Committee* (Technical Report Series. 804). Geneva, Switzerland: Author.
24. Shepard J.T., Rusch N.J., Vanhoutte P.M. (1983). Effect of cold on the blood vessel walls. *General Pharmacology 14*(1), 61–64.
25. Hymes A. (1984). A review of the historical area of electricity. In Mannheimer J.S., Lampe G.N. (Eds.), *Clinical transcutaneous electrical stimulation* (pp. 1–5). Philadelphia: F.A. Davis.
26. Anderson S.A. (1979). Pain control by sensory stimulation. In Bonica J.J., Liebeskind J.C., Albe-Fessard D.G. (Eds.), *Advances in pain research and therapy* (pp. 569–585). New York: Raven Press.
27. Ignelzi R.J., Nyquist J.K. (1979). Excitability changes in peripheral nerve fibers after repetitive electrical stimulation: Implications for pain modulation. *Journal of Neurosurgery 51,* 824–833.
28. Wolf S.L. (1984). Neurophysiologic mechanisms of pain modulation: Relevance to TENS. In Mannheimer J.S., Lampe G.N. (Eds.), *Clinical transcutaneous electrical stimulation* (pp. 41–55). Philadelphia: F.A. Davis.
29. Ezzo J., Berman B., Hadhazy A., et al. (2000). Is acupuncture effective for the treatment of chronic pain: A systematic review. *Pain 86,* 217–225.
30. Way W.L., Field H.L., Schumacher M.A. (2001). Opioid analgesics and antagonists. In Katzung H. (Ed.), *Basic and clinical pharmacology* (8th ed., pp. 512–531). New York: Lange Medical Books/McGraw-Hill.
31. Inturrisi C.E. (2002). Clinical pharmacology of opioids for pain. *Clinical Journal of Pain 18*(Suppl. 4), S3–S13.
32. Kurz A., Sessler D. (2003). Opioid-induced bowel dysfunction: Pathophysiology and potential new therapies. *Drugs 63,* 649–671.
33. Pasternak G.W. (2001). The pharmacology of Mu analgesics: From patients to genes. *Neuroscientist 7,* 220–231.
34. Melzack R. (1990). The tragedy of needless pain. *Scientific American 262*(2), 2–8.
35. Swerdlow M., Stjerward J. (1982). Cancer pain relief: An urgent problem. *World Health Forum 3,* 325–330.
36. Kost R.G., Straus S.E. (1996). Postherpetic neuralgia: Pathogenesis, treatment and prevention. *New England Journal of Medicine 335,* 32–42.
37. Stanton-Hicks M., Baron R., Boas R., Gordh T., Harden N., Hendler N., et al. (1998). Complex regional pain syndromes: Guidelines for therapy. *Clinical Journal of Pain 14*(2), 155–166.
38. Pham T., Lafforgue P. (2003). Reflex sympathetic dystrophy syndrome and neuromediators. *Joint Bone Spine 70,* 12–17.
39. Reflex Sympathetic Dystrophy Syndrome Association of America. (2000). Clinical practice guideline for treatment of reflex sympathetic dystrophy syndrome. [On-line]. Available: http://www.rsds.org/cpgeng.htm.
40. Melzack R. (1992). Phantom limb. *Scientific American 226,* 120–126.
41. Saper J.R. (1999). Headache disorders. *Medical Clinics of North America 83,* 663–670.
42. Kaniecki R. (2003). Headache assessment and management. *JAMA 289,* 1430–1433.
43. Headache Classification Subcommittee of the International Headache Committee (2004). The International Classification of headache disorders (2nd ed.). *Cephalalgia 24*(Suppl. 1), 1–152.
44. Mathew N.T. (2001). Pathophysiology, epidemiology, and impact of migraine. *Clinical Cornerstone 4,* 1–17.
45. Cady R., Schreiber, C. (2003). Sinus headache or migraine? Considerations in making a differential diagnosis. *Headache 43,* 305.
46. Annequin D., Tourniare B., Massoui H. (2000). Migraine and headache in childhood and adolescence. *Pediatric Clinics of North America 47,* 617–631.
47. Behrman R.E., Kliegman R.M., Jensen H.B. (2000). *Nelson textbook of pediatrics* (16th ed., pp. 1832–1834). Philadelphia: W.B. Saunders.
48. Goadsby P.J., Lipton R.B., Farrari M.D. (2002). Migraine—Current understanding and treatment. *New England Journal of Medicine 346*(4), 257–270.
49. Williamson D.H., Hargreaves R.J. (2001). Neurogenic inflammation in the context on migraine. *Microscopy Research and Technique 53,* 167–178.
50. Kunkel R.S. (2000). Managing primary headache syndromes. *Patient Care* January 30. [On-line]. Available: www.patientcareonline.com.

51. Snow V., Weiss K., Wall E.M., Mottur-Pilson C. (2002). Pharmacologic management of acute attacks of migraine and prevention of migraine headache. *Annals of Internal Medicine 137,* 840–849.
52. Silberstein S.D. (2000). Practice parameter: Evidence-based guidelines for migraine headache. *Neurology 55,* 754–763.
53. Ekbom K., Hardebo J.E. (2002). Cluster headache aetiology, diagnosis and management. *Drugs 62,* 61–69.
54. Millea, P.J., Brodie, J.J. (2002). Tension-type headache. *American Family Physician 66,* 797–804.
55. Silberstein S.D., Lipton R.B. (2000). Chronic daily headache. *Current Opinion in Neurology 13,* 277–283.
56. Okeson J.P. (1996). Temporomandibular disorders in the medical practice. *Journal of Family Practice 43,* 347–356.
57. Broome M., Richtsmeier A., Maikler V., Alexander M. (1996). Pediatric pain practices: A survey of health professionals. *Journal of Pain and Symptom Management 4,* 315–319.
58. McCaffery M., Bebee A. (1994). *Pain: Clinical manual for nursing practice.* St Louis: Mosby.
59. Kovach C.R., Weissman, D.E., Griffie J., et al. (1999). Assessment and treatment of discomfort for people with late-stage dementia. *Journal of Pain and Symptom Management 18,* 412–419.
60. Gallup survey. Conducted by the Gallup Organization from May 21 to June 9, 1999. Supported by the Arthritis Foundation and Merk & Company, Inc. (http://www.arthritis.org/conditions/speakingofpain/factsheet.asp. Accessed on 8-1-03).
61. Ferrell B.A., Ferrell B.R., Osterweil D. (1990). Pain in the nursing home. *Journal of the American Geriatric Society 38,* 409–414.
62. Watt-Watson J., Donovan M. (1992). *Nursing management of the patient in pain.* Philadelphia: J.B. Lippincott.
63. Berde C.B., Sethna N.F. (2002). Analgesics for the treatment of pain in children. *New England Journal of Medicine 347,* 1094–1103.
64. Haouari N., Wood C., Griffiths G., Levene, M. (1995). The analgesic effect of sucrose in full term infants: A randomized controlled trial. *British Medical Journal 310,* 1498–1500.
65. Merkel S.I., Gutstein H.B., Malviya S. (1999). Use of transcutaneous electrical nerve stimulation in a young child with pain from open perineal lesions. *Journal of Pain and Symptom Management 18,* 376–381.
66. Vessey J., Carlson K., McGill J. (1995). Use of distraction with children during an acute pain experience. *Nursing Research 43,* 369–372.
67. Morrison R.S., Siu A.L. (2000). A comparison of pain and its treatment in advanced dementia and cognitively intact patients with hip fracture. *Journal of Pain and Symptom Management 19,* 240–248.
68. Irving G.A., Wallace M.S. (1997). *Pain management for the practicing physician.* Philadelphia: Churchill Livingstone.

CHAPTER

51

Disorders of Motor Function

Carol M. Porth and Robin L. Curtis

Effective motor function requires that muscles move and that the mechanics of their movement be programmed in a manner that provides for smooth and coordinated movement. In some cases, purposeless and disruptive movements can be almost as disabling as relative or complete absence of movement.

Control of Motor Function

After completing this section of the chapter, you should be able to meet the following objectives:

- Define a motor unit and characterize its mechanism of controlling muscle movement
- Define the function of the following muscle types: extensors, flexors, adductors, abductors, rotators, agonists, antagonists, and synergists
- Describe the distribution of upper and lower motoneurons in relation to the central nervous system
- Differentiate between upper and lower motoneuron lesions in terms of spinal cord reflex function and muscle tone

Movement begins in utero at approximately 21 weeks of gestation with the quickening of the fetus, and the capability for some coordinated movement is present at birth. Maturation of the spinal cord and brain circuitry during the first year or two of life allows the child to defy the force of gravity and learn to sit, then stand, and, in rapid sequence, master the skills of walking, running, jumping, and climbing.

MOTOR FUNCTION

Motor function, whether it involves walking, running, or precise finger movements, requires movement and maintenance of posture. Posture can be described as the relative position of various parts of the body with respect to one another (limb extension, flexion) or to the environment (standing, supine).[1] Posture also can be described as the active muscular resistance to the displacement of the body by gravity or acceleration. The structures that control posture and movement are located throughout the neuromuscular system. The system consists of the neuromuscular unit, which includes the motoneurons, the myoneural junction, and the muscle fibers; the spinal cord, which contains the basic reflex circuitry for posture and movement; and the descending pathways from the brain stem circuits, the cerebellum, basal ganglia, and the motor cortex.

Muscle Groups

Skeletal muscle is composed of muscle cells, or fibers, which contain the interacting actin and myosin filaments that generate the contractile force required for movement (see Chapter 4). In terms of function, muscles can be classified as extensors, muscles that increase the angle of a joint, or flexors, muscles that decrease the angle of a joint. In the legs, groups of extensor muscles work together to resist gravity and function to maintain the upright posture and provide locomotion power. In general, flexor muscle groups assist gravity, participate in withdrawal reflexes, and provide the more delicate aspects of manipulation. Other muscle groups work roughly in pairs: adductors versus abductors, which move a part toward or away from the midline of the body, and rotators, which work in pairs to rotate a part of the limb, the trunk, or the head around each part's longitudinal axis. Many muscles participate in more than one of these functions.

MOTOR SYSTEMS

- Motor systems require upper motoneurons (UMNs) that project from the motor cortex to the brain stem or spinal cord, where they directly or indirectly innervate the lower motoneurons (LMNs) of the contracting muscles; sensory feedback from the involved muscles that is continuously relayed to the cerebellum, basal ganglia, and sensory cortex; and a functioning neuromuscular junction that links nervous system activity with muscle contraction.
- The pyramidal motor system originating in the motor cortex provides control of delicate muscle movement, and the extrapyramidal system originating in the basal ganglia provides the background for the more crude, supportive movement patterns.
- The efficiency of the movement by the motor system depends on a background of muscle tone provided by the stretch reflex and vestibular system input to maintain stable postural support.

Coordinated movement requires the action of two or more muscle groups: agonists, which promote a movement; antagonists, which oppose it; and synergists, which assist the agonist muscles by stabilizing a joint or contributing additional force to the movement. Some simple types of movement require only a burst of energy from an agonist muscle group. Other types of movement, such as self-terminated actions, require a smooth sequence of coordinated agonist and antagonist movements to stop and stabilize the end of the movement. Agonist and antagonist contractions are programmed by higher brain centers to fit the situation. Simple movements are programmed before they start so that the movement proceeds from start to finish without modification. Self-terminated movements are more complex; they are programmed to start and then are modified as they proceed.

The Motor Unit

The neurons that control motor function are referred to as *motoneurons* or sometimes as *alpha motoneurons*. A motor unit consists of one motoneuron and the group of muscle fibers it innervates in a muscle. The motoneurons supplying a motor unit are located in the ventral horn of the spinal cord and are called *lower motoneurons* (LMNs). The synapse between a LMN and the muscle fibers of a motor unit is called the *neuromuscular junction*. Upper motoneurons (UMNs), which exert control over LMNs, project from the motor strip in the cerebral cortex to the ventral horn and are fully contained within the central nervous system (CNS) (Fig. 51-1).

Axons of the LMNs exit the spinal cord at each segment to innervate skeletal muscle cells, including those of the limbs, back, abdomen, and chest. Each LMN undergoes multiple branching, making it possible for a single LMN to innervate 10 to 2000 muscle cells. In general, large muscles—those containing hundreds or thousands of muscle cells and providing gross motor movement—have large motor units. This sharply contrasts with those that control the hand, tongue, and eye movements, for which the motor units are small and permit very discrete control.

Basic to the understanding of motor control is the concept of the *motor unit*—the LMN and the muscle fibers it innervates—functioning as a unit. All muscles contain thousands of muscle fibers and are innervated by fewer LMNs. When the LMN develops an action potential, all of the muscle fibers in the motor unit it innervates develop action potentials, causing them to contract simultaneously. Thus, a LMN and the muscle fibers it innervates function as a single unit—the basic unit of motor control. All neural-controlled motor functions involve the differential use of combinations of motor units in agonist and antagonist muscles around a joint, manipulating the resultant joint angle. Movement involves some joints being held stable and the angle of other joints being changed.

Most skeletal muscle groups fall into two categories based on differences in the chemistry of their contractile proteins and their source of energy.[2] The first type, the *slow-twitch fibers*, have many mitochondria, depend on blood-borne oxygen for energy, and are slow to fatigue. The second type, the *fast-twitch fibers*, depend on muscle

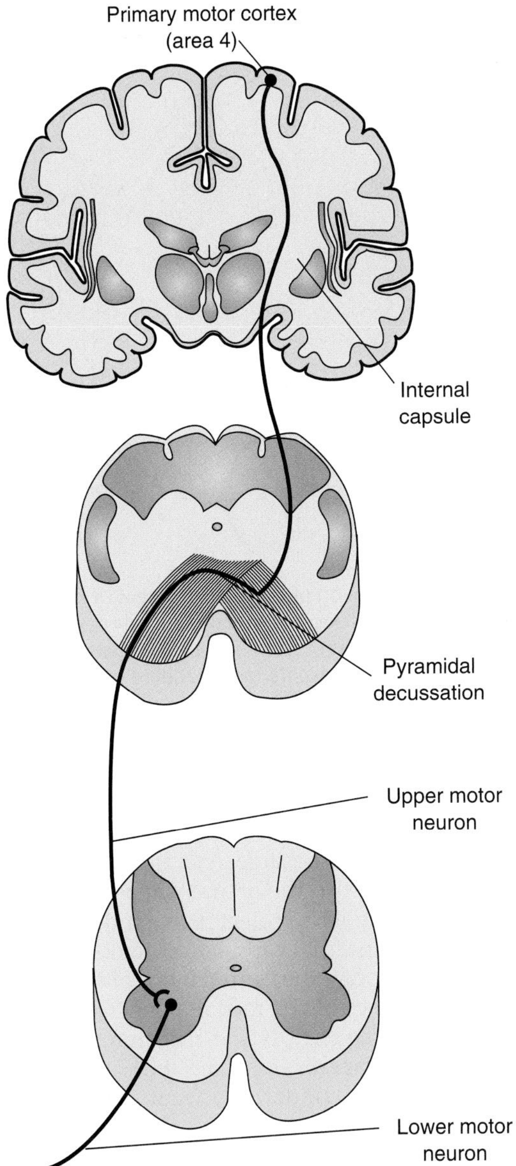

FIGURE 51-1 The corticospinal tract. The long axons of motoneurons originating in the primary motor cortex descend through the telencephalon through the internal capsule and traverse the brain stem in a ventral path through the cerebral peduncles and the pyramids. The axons cross in the lower medulla (pyramidal decussation) to the opposite side and continue as the corticospinal tract in the spinal cord, where they synapse on motoneurons and interneurons in the ventral horns. (Modified from Kandel E.R., Schwartz J.H. [1985]. *Principles of neural science* [2nd ed.]. New York: Elsevier)

glycogen stores that can be rapidly depleted. The fast-twitch fibers are further divided into fast-twitch fatigable and fast-twitch fatigue-resistant fibers. The antigravity postural muscles that use slow-twitch fibers are slow to fatigue. Muscles used for more rapid movements, such as jumping and throwing, are rich in large, powerful, but rapidly fatiguing fast-twitch motor units.

Most muscles contain motor units with both slow-twitch and fast-twitch fibers, but the proportions may vary with muscle function. For example, postural muscles and delicate distal flexor muscles are predominantly slow-twitch fibers, whereas the large, proximal limb muscles such as the gas-trocnemius are mixed, with many fast-twitch fatigable and fast-twitch fatigue-resistant fiber motor units that can provide brief, high power.

The muscle fibers for each motor unit are uniform as to muscle fiber type (*e.g.*, slow-twitch and fast-twitch). The group of LMNs in the spinal cord ventral horn that have muscle fibers in a particular muscle is called a *motoneuron pool*. When reflex or descending systems activate such a pool, the first motor units to fire are the slow-twitch units. With stronger activation, the fast-twitch fatigue-resistant units begin firing, and then the fast-twitch fatigable units.

The motor system is designed to minimize participation of the forebrain in details of movements, permitting the forebrain to specialize in the planning and motor learning required for precise control of motor function. The recruitment order of slow-twitch, then fast-twitch fatigue-resistant, and finally fast-twitch fatigable motor units provides the automatic sequence for increasing muscle contraction power and for the initial, delicate control of movement.

The Motor Cortex

Delicate, skillful, intentional movement of distal and especially flexor muscles of the limbs and the speech apparatus is initiated and controlled from the motor cortex located in the posterior part of the frontal lobe. It consists of the primary, premotor, and supplementary motor cortex[2,3] (Fig. 51-2). These areas receive information from the thalamus and the somatosensory cortex and, indirectly, from the cerebellum and basal ganglia. The primary motor cortex (area 4), also called the *motor strip,* is located on the rostral surface and adjacent portions of the central sulcus. The primary motor cortex controls discrete muscle movement sequences and is the first level of descending control for precise movements. Discrete lesions in the most posterior part of the primary motor cortex can result in profound weakness in specific distal flexor muscle groups and permanent inability to perform delicate manipulative motor patterns on the opposite side of the body or face. Lesions restricted to the more anterior part of the motor strip result in weakness of larger limb, girdle, and axial muscles.

The premotor cortex (areas 6 and 8), which is located just anterior to the primary motor cortex, sends some fibers into the corticospinal tract but mainly innervates the primary motor strip. A movement pattern to accomplish a particular objective, such as throwing a ball or picking up a fork, is programmed by the prefrontal association cortex and associated thalamic nuclei. The "program" for the movement pattern includes the muscle contraction sequences for complex distal manipulation and for the larger preparative and supportive actions of whole-limb and limb girdle muscles.

The supplementary motor cortex, which contains representations of all parts of the body, is located on the medial surface of the hemisphere (areas 6 and 8) in the premotor region. It is intimately involved in the performance of complex, skillful movements that involve both sides of

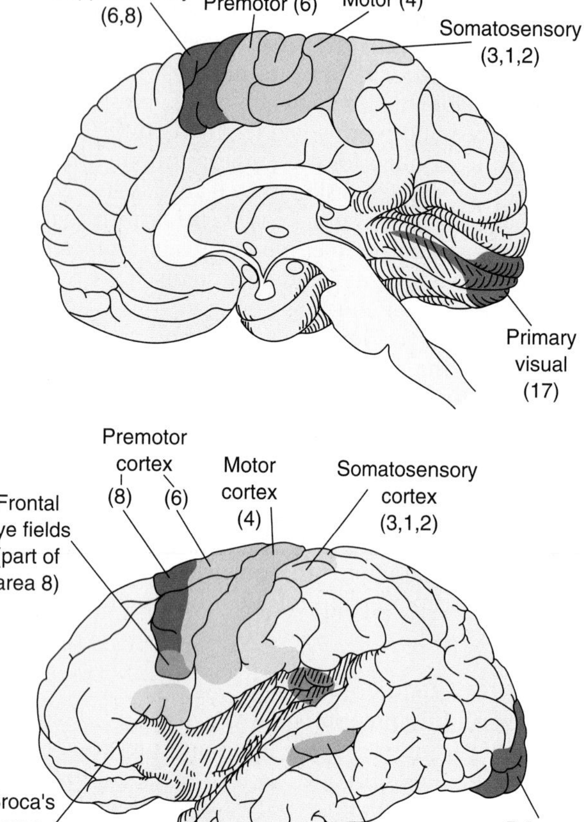

FIGURE 51-2 Primary motor cortex. (**Top**) The location of the primary, premotor, and supplementary cortex on the medial surface of the brain. (**Bottom**) The location of the primary and premotor cortex on the lateral surface of the brain. (Courtesy of Carole Russell Hilmer, C.M.I.)

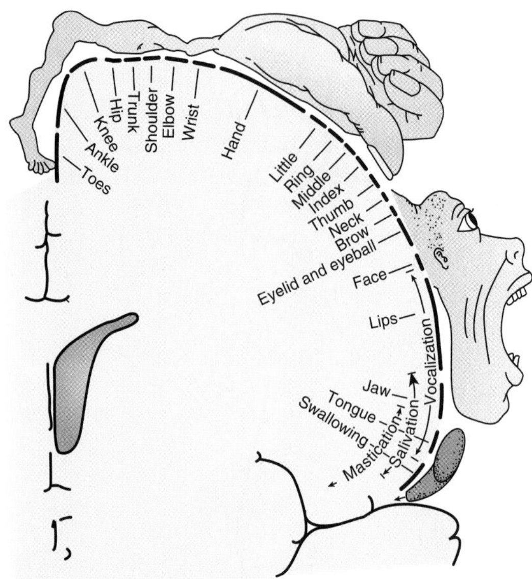

FIGURE 51-3 Representation of the relative extent of motor cortical area 4 devoted to muscles of the various body regions. Medial surface is at the left, lateral fissure is at the right, with pharyngeal and laryngeal muscle representation extending toward the insula. (Penfield E., Rasmussen T. [1968]. *The cerebral cortex in man: A clinical study of localization of function.* New York: Macmillan)

the body. Bilateral lesions cause long-lasting loss of movements involving both hands or both feet.

The neurons in the primary motor cortex are arranged in a somatotopic array or distorted map of the body called the *motor homunculus* (Fig. 51-3). This map, which shows the degree of representation of the neurons that control voluntary movement of a particular body part, was published by Penfield and Rasmussen in 1950.[4] The mapping was done by electrically stimulating the brain of persons who were undergoing brain surgery. The body parts that require the greatest dexterity have the largest cortical areas devoted to them. More than one half of the primary motor cortex is concerned with controlling the muscles of the hands, of facial expression, and of speech.[2]

Motor Pathways

The primary motor cortex is very thick. It contains many layers of pyramid-shaped output neurons that project to the same side of the cortex (*i.e.,* premotor and somatosensory areas), project to the opposite side of the cortex, or descend to subcortical structures such as the basal ganglia and thalamus. The large pyramidal cells located in the fifth layer project to the brain stem and spinal cord. The axons of these UMNs project through the subcortical white matter and internal capsule to the deep surface of the brain stem, through the ventral bulge of the pons, and to the ventral surface of the medulla, where they form a ridge or pyramid (see Fig. 51-1). At the junction between the medulla and cervical spinal cord, 80% or more of the UMN axons cross the midline to form the lateral corticospinal tract in the lateral white matter of the spinal cord. This tract extends throughout the spinal cord, with roughly 50% of the fibers terminating in the cervical segments, 20% in the thoracic segments, and 30% in the lumbosacral segments. Most of the remaining uncrossed fibers travel down the ventral column of the cord, mainly to cervical levels, where they cross and innervate contralateral LMNs.

Monosynaptic innervation of LMNs by UMNs of the primary motor cortex only occurs for the most distal muscles involved with delicate manipulative skills, such as those of the hands and fingers, tongue, mouth, and pharynx. For LMNs of other muscles, the connection is multisynaptic and less discrete. As the UMN axons pass along their long pathways, collateral branches move out and innervate regions of the basal ganglia, the thalamus, the brain stem, and nuclei that project into the cerebellum. The cerebellum matches the temporal smoothness aspect of the ongoing movement against very rapid proprioceptive feedback from the actual movement and sends error signals back to the thalamus and motor cortex for corrective modifications of the ongoing movement. Similarly, sensory feedback to the basal ganglia results in error-correcting feedback for supportive and background aspects of the movement. Slower sensory feedback from the somatosensory cortex permits error correction on the next trial. Ongoing error correction becomes less and less important for well-learned movements that can proceed without sensory feedback.

Traditionally, motor tracts have been classified as belonging to one of two motor systems: the pyramidal and extrapyramidal systems. According to this classification system, the pyramidal system consists of the motor pathways originating in the motor cortex and terminating in the corticobulbar fibers in the brain stem and the corticospinal fibers in the spinal cord. The corticospinal fibers traverse the ventral surface of the medulla in a bundle called the *pyramid* before decussating or crossing to the opposite side of the brain at the medulla–spinal cord junction, hence the name *pyramidal system.* Other fibers from the cortex and basal ganglia also project to the brain stem reticular formation and reticulospinal systems, following a more ancient pathway to LMNs of proximal and extensor muscles. These fibers do not decussate in the pyramids, hence the name *extrapyramidal system.* Disorders of the pyramidal tracts (*e.g.,* stroke) are characterized by spasticity and paralysis and those affecting the extrapyramidal tracts (*e.g.,* Parkinson disease) by involuntary movements, muscle rigidity, and immobility without paralysis. As increased knowledge regarding motor pathways has merged, it has become evident that the extrapyramidal and pyramidal systems are extensively interconnected and cooperate in the control of movement.[1] Thus, this classification is used less frequently than in the past.

DISORDERS OF MOTOR FUNCTION

Disorders of motor function include skeletal muscle weakness and paralysis, which result from lesions in the voluntary motor pathways, including the UMNs of the corticospinal and corticobulbar tracts or the LMNs that leave the CNS and travel by way of the peripheral nerve to the muscle. Muscle tone, which is a necessary component of muscle movement, is a function of the muscle spindle (myotatic) system (see Chapter 49) and the extrapyramidal system, which monitors and buffers input to the LMNs by way of the multisynaptic pathways.

DISORDERS OF MUSCLE TONE

Muscle tone is the normal tension in a muscle as evidenced by the resistance to passive movement around a joint. Disorders of skeletal muscle tone are characteristic of many nervous system pathologies. Any interruption of the myotatic reflex circuit by peripheral nerve injury, pathology of the neuromuscular junction and of skeletal muscle fibers, damage to the corticospinal system, or injury to the spinal cord or spinal nerve root results in disturbance of muscle tone. Muscle tone may be described as less than normal (hypotonia), absent (flaccidity), or excessive (hypertonia, rigidity, spasticity, or tetany). Rigidity and spasticity are extremes of hypertonia that include other distinguishing features.

PARESIS AND PARALYSIS

The suffix *plegia* comes from the Greek word for a blow, a stroke, or paralysis. Terms used to describe the extent and anatomic location of motor damage are *paralysis,* meaning loss of movement, and *paresis,* implying weakness or incomplete loss of muscle function. *Monoparesis* or *monoplegia* results from the destruction of pyramidal UMN innervation of one limb; *hemiparesis* or *hemiplegia,* both limbs on one side; *diparesis* or *diplegia* or *paraparesis* or *paraplegia,* both upper or lower limbs; and *tetraparesis* or *tetraplegia,* also called *quadriparesis* or *quadriplegia,* all four limbs (Fig. 51-4). Paresis or paralysis can be further designated as of UMN or LMN origin.

Upper Motoneuron Lesions

A UMN lesion can involve the motor cortex, the internal capsule, or other brain structures through which the corticospinal or corticobulbar tracts descend, or the spinal cord. When the lesion is at or above the level of the pyramids, paralysis affects structures on the opposite side of the body. In UMN disorders involving injury to the L1 level or above, there is an immediate, profound weakness and loss of fine, skilled voluntary lower limb movement, reduced bowel and bladder control, and diminished sexual functioning, followed by an exaggeration of muscle tone. With UMN damage above C5, upper limb movement also is affected.

With UMN lesions, the LMN spinal reflexes remain intact, but communication and control from higher brain centers are lost. Descending excitatory influences from the pyramidal system and some descending inhibitory influences from other cortical regions are lost after injury, resulting in immediate weakness accompanied by the loss of control of delicate, skilled movements. After several weeks, this weakness becomes converted to hypertonicity or spasticity, which is manifested by an initial increased resistance

SPASTIC VERSUS FLACCID PARALYSIS

- Afferent input from stretch receptors located in muscles and joints is incorporated into spinal cord reflexes that control muscle tone. The activity of the spinal cord reflexes that control muscle tone is constantly monitored and regulated by input from higher brain centers.
- Upper motor neuron lesions that interrupt communication between the spinal cord reflexes and higher brain centers result in unregulated reflex activity, increased muscle tone, and spastic paralysis.
- Lower motor neuron lesions that interrupt communication between the muscle and the spinal cord reflex result in a loss of reflex activity, decreased or absent muscle tone, and flaccid paralysis.

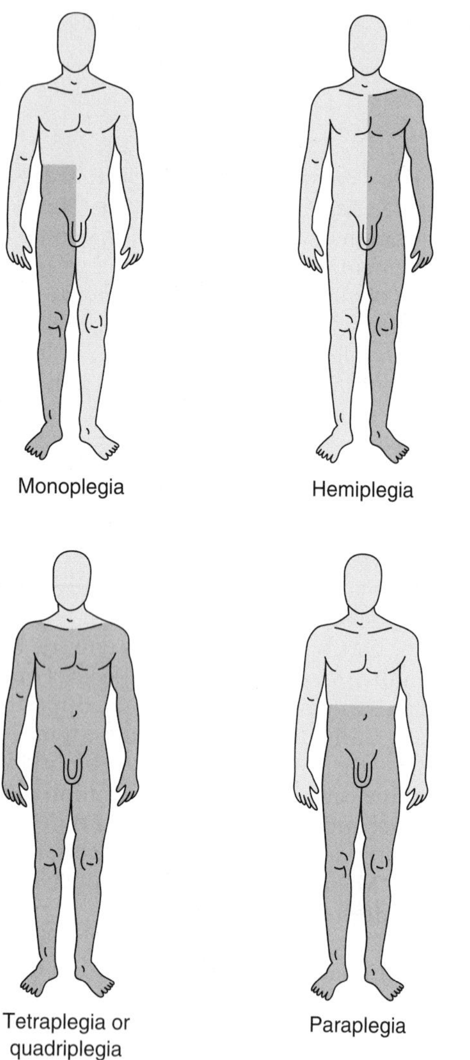

FIGURE 51-4 Areas of the body affected by monoplegia, hemiplegia, tetraplegia or quadriplegia, and paraplegia. The *shaded area* shows the extent of motor and sensory loss. (Hickey J.V. [1997]. *The clinical practice of neurological and neurosurgical nursing* [3rd ed.]. Philadelphia: J.B. Lippincott)

(stiffness) to the passive movement of a joint at the extremes of range of motion followed by a sudden or gradual release of resistance. The spasticity often is greatest in the flexor muscles of the upper limbs and extensor muscles of the lower limbs. Sometimes, a lesion of the pyramidal tract is less severe and results in a relatively minor degree of weakness. In this case, the finer and more skilled movements are most severely impaired.

Clonus is the rhythmic contraction and alternate relaxation of a limb that is caused by suddenly stretching a muscle and gently maintaining it in the stretched position. It is seen in the hypertonia of spasticity associated with UMN lesions. It is caused by an oscillating stimulation of the muscle spindles that occurs when the spindle fibers are activated by an initial muscle stretch. This results in reflex contraction of the muscle and unloading of the spindle fibers with decreased afferent activity. The reduced spindle fiber activity causes the muscle to relax, which causes the spindle fiber to stretch again, and the cycle starts over.

Lower Motoneuron Lesions

In contrast to UMN lesions, in which the spinal reflexes remain intact, LMN disorders disrupt communication between the muscle and all neural input from spinal cord reflexes, including the stretch reflex, which maintains muscle tone.

Infection or irritation of the cell body of the LMN or its axon can lead to hyperexcitability, which causes spontaneous contractions of the muscle units. These can be observed as twitching and squirming movements on the muscle surface, a condition called *fasciculations*. Toxic agents, such as the tetanus toxin, produce extreme hyperexcitability of the LMN, which results in continuous firing at maximum rate. The resultant sustained contraction of the muscles is called *tetany*. Tetany of muscles on both sides of a joint produces immobility or tetanic paralysis. When a virus, such as the poliomyelitis virus, attacks an LMN, it first irritates the LMN, causing fasciculations to occur. These fasciculations often are followed by death of LMNs. Weakness and severe muscle wasting or denervation atrophy result. If muscles are totally denervated, total weakness and total loss of reflexes, called *flaccid paralysis,* occurs.

With complete LMN lesions, the muscles of the affected limbs, bowel, bladder, and genital areas become atonic, and it is impossible to elicit contraction by stretching the tendons. One of the outstanding features of LMN lesions is the profound development of muscle atrophy. Damage to a LMN with or without spinal cord damage, often called *peripheral nerve injury,* may occur at any level of the spinal cord. For example, a C7 peripheral nerve injury leads to LMN hand weakness only. Usually, injury to the spinal cord at the T12 level or below results in LMN injury and flaccid paralysis to all areas below the level of injury. This occurs because the spinal cord ends at the T12 to L1 level, and from this level, the spinal roots of the LMNs continue caudally in the vertebral canal as part of the cauda equina.

In summary, motor function involves the neuromuscular unit, spinal cord circuitry, brain stem neurons, the cerebellum, the basal ganglia, and the motor cortex. A motor unit consists of one LMN and the group of muscle fibers it innervates in the muscle. Delicate, skillful, intentional movement of distal and especially flexor muscles of the limbs and the speech apparatus is initiated and controlled from the motor cortex located in the posterior frontal lobe. It consists of the primary, premotor, and supplementary motor cortex. These areas receive information from the thalamus and somatosensory cortex and, indirectly, from the cerebellum and basal ganglia. The UMNs in the motor cortex send their axons through the subcortical white matter and internal capsule and the deep surface of the brain stem traversing the ventral surface to the opposite side of the medulla, where they form a pyramid before crossing the midline to form the lateral corticospinal tract in the spinal cord. If the UMN system is severely damaged, delicate and skillful movement is lost, but crude movements still can be made using extrapyramidal systems.

Alterations in musculoskeletal function include weakness resulting from lesions of voluntary UMN pathways of the corticobulbar and corticospinal tracts and the LMNs of the peripheral nerves. Muscle tone is maintained through the combined function of the muscle spindle system and the extrapyramidal system that monitors and buffers UMN innervation of the LMNs. Hypotonia is a condition of less-than-normal muscle tone, and hypertonia or spasticity is a condition of excessive tone. Paresis refers to weakness in muscle function, and paralysis refers to a loss of muscle movement. UMN lesions produce spastic paralysis, and LMN lesions produce flaccid paralysis. Damage to the UMNs of the corticospinal and corticobulbar tracts is a common component of stroke.

Skeletal Muscle and Peripheral Nerve Disorders

After completing this section of the chapter, you should be able to meet the following objectives:

- Describe muscle atrophy and differentiate between disuse and degenerative atrophy
- Describe the pathology associated with Duchenne muscular dystrophy
- Relate the clinical manifestations of myasthenia gravis to its cause
- Trace the steps in regeneration of an injured peripheral nerve
- Describe the manifestation of peripheral nerve root injury due to a ruptured intervertebral disk
- Compare the cause and manifestations of peripheral mononeuropathies with peripheral polyneuropathies

SKELETAL MUSCLE DISORDERS

Disorders of skeletal muscle groups involve atrophy and dystrophy. Atrophy describes a decrease in muscle mass. Muscular dystrophy is a primary disorder of muscle tissue and is characterized by a defect in the muscle fibers.

Muscle Atrophy

Maintenance of muscle strength requires relatively frequent movements against resistance. Reduced use results in muscle atrophy, which is characterized by a reduction in the diameter of the muscle fibers because of a loss of protein filaments. When a normally innervated muscle is not used for long periods, the muscle cells shrink in diameter, and although the muscle cells do not die, they lose much of their contractile protein and become weakened. This is called *disuse atrophy,* and it occurs with conditions such as immobilization and chronic illness.

The most extreme examples of muscle atrophy are found in persons with disorders that deprive muscles of their innervation. This form is called *denervation atrophy.* During early embryonic development, outgrowing skeletal nerves innervate partially mature muscle cells. If the developing muscle cells are not innervated, they do not mature and eventually die. In the process of innervation, randomly contracting muscle cells become enslaved by the innervating neurons, and from then on, the muscle cell contracts only when stimulated by that particular neuron. If the LMN dies or its axon is destroyed, the skeletal muscle cell is again free of neural domination. When this happens, it begins to have temporary spontaneous contractions, called *fibrillations,* of its own. It also begins to lose its contractile proteins and, after several months, if not reinnervated, it degenerates.

If a peripheral motoneuron is crushed and its endoneurial tube remains intact, regenerating axons can grow down the connective tissue tube to reinnervate the muscle cell. If the nerve is cut, however, scar tissue between the cut ends of the endoneurial tube reduces the likelihood of reinnervation by the original axon, and muscle cell loss is likely to occur. If some intact LMN axons remain in the muscle, nearby denervated muscle cells apparently emit what is called a *trophic signal,* probably a chemical messenger, that signals intact axons to sprout and send outgrowing collaterals into the denervated area and recapture control of some of the denervated muscle fibers. The degree of axonal regeneration that occurs after injury to an LMN depends on the amount of scar tissue that develops at the site of injury and how quickly reinnervation occurs. If reinnervation occurs after the muscle cell has degenerated, no recovery is possible. Peripheral nerve section usually results in some loss of muscle cell function, which is experienced as weakness. Collateral sprout reinnervation results in enlarged motor units and therefore in a reduction in the precision of muscle control after recovery.

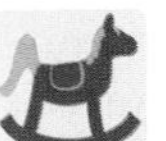

Muscular Dystrophy

Muscular dystrophy is a term applied to a number of genetic disorders that produce progressive deterioration of skeletal muscles because of mixed muscle cell hypertrophy, atrophy, and necrosis. They are primary diseases of muscle tissue and probably do not involve the nervous system. As the muscle undergoes necrosis, fat and connective tissue replace the muscle fibers, which increases muscle size and results in muscle weakness. The increase in muscle size resulting from connective tissue infiltration is called *pseudohypertrophy.* The muscle weakness is insidious in onset but continually progressive, varying with the type of disorder.

The most common form of the disease is *Duchenne muscular dystrophy,* which occurs once in every 3500 live male births.[5] Duchenne muscular dystrophy is inherited as a recessive single-gene defect on the X chromosome and is transmitted from the mother to her male offspring (see Chapter 7). A spontaneous (mutation) form may occur in females. Another form of dystrophy, *Becker muscular dystrophy,* is similarly X-linked but manifests later in childhood or adolescence and has a slower course.

The Duchenne muscular dystrophy mutation results in a defective form of a very large protein associated with the muscle cell membrane, called *dystrophin,* which fails to provide the normal attachment site for the contractile proteins. As a result, there is necrosis of muscle fibers, a continuous effort at repair and regeneration, and progressive necrosis (Fig. 51-5).

Clinical Course. Children with Duchenne muscular dystrophy are usually asymptomatic at birth and during infancy.[6] Early gross movements such as rolling, sitting, and standing are usually achieved at the proper age. The postural muscles of hip and shoulder are usually the first to be affected. Signs of muscle weakness usually become evident beginning at 2 to 3 years, when frequent falling begins to occur. Imbalances between agonist and antagonist muscles lead to abnormal postures and the development of contractures and joint immobility. Scoliosis is common. Wheelchairs usually are needed at approximately 7 to 12 years of age.[6] The function of the distal muscles usually is preserved well enough that the child can continue to use eating utensils and a computer keyboard. The function of the extraocular nerves also is well preserved, as is the function of the muscles controlling urination and defecation. Incontinence is an uncommon and late event. Respiratory muscle involvement results in weak and ineffective cough, frequent respiratory infections, and decreasing respiratory reserve. Cardiomyopathy is a common feature of the disease. The severity of cardiac involvement, however, does not necessarily correlate with skeletal muscle weakness. Some patients die early of severe cardiomyopathy, whereas others maintain adequate cardiac function until the terminal stages of the disease. Death from respiratory and cardiac muscle involvement usually occurs in young adulthood.

Observation of the child's voluntary movement and a complete family history provide important diagnostic data for the disease. Serum levels of the enzyme creatine kinase, which leaks out of damaged muscle fibers, can be used to assist the diagnosis. Muscle biopsy, which shows a mixture of muscle cell degeneration and regeneration and reveals fat and scar tissue replacement, is diagnostic of the disorder. Echocardiography, electrocardiography, and chest radiography are used to assess cardiac function. A specific molecular genetic diagnosis is possible by demonstrating defective dystrophin through the use of immunohistochemical staining of sections of muscle biopsy tissue or by DNA analysis from the peripheral blood. The same methods of DNA analysis may be used on blood samples to establish carrier status in female relatives at risk, such as sisters and cousins. Prenatal diagnosis is possible as early as 12 weeks' gestation by sampling chorionic villi for DNA analysis[6] (see Chapter 7).

Management of the disease is directed toward maintaining ambulation and preventing deformities. Passive stretching, correct or counter posturing, and splints help to prevent deformities. Precautions should be taken to avoid respiratory infections. Although there have been exciting advances in identifying the gene and gene product involved in Duchenne muscular dystrophy, there is no known cure.

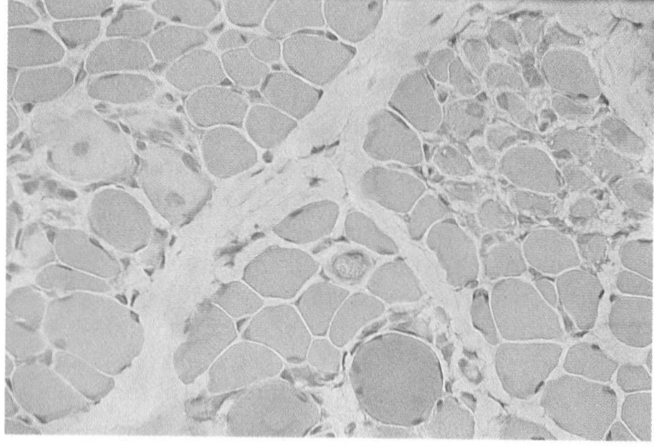

FIGURE 51-5 Duchenne muscular dystrophy: Hematoxylin and eosin stain. A section of the vastus lateralis muscle shows necrotic muscle fibers, some of them invaded by macrophages. The endomysial septa are thickened, indicating fibrosis. (Rubin E., Farber J.L [1999]. *Pathology* [3rd ed., p. 1422]. Philadelphia: Lippincott-Raven).

DISORDERS OF THE NEUROMUSCULAR JUNCTION

The neuromuscular junction serves as a synapse between a motor neuron and a skeletal muscle fiber.[7] It consists of the axon terminals of a motor neuron and a specialized region of the muscle membrane called the motor *end plate*. The transmission of impulses at the neuromuscular junction is mediated by the release of the neurotransmitter acetylcholine from the axon terminals. Acetylcholine binds to specific receptors in the end-plate region of the muscle fiber surface to cause muscle contraction (Fig. 51-6). Acetylcholine is active in the neuromuscular junction only for a brief period, during which an action potential is generated in the innervated muscle cell. Some of the transmitter diffuses out of the synapse, and the remaining transmitter is rapidly inactivated by an enzyme called *acetylcholinesterase*. The rapid inactivation of acetylcholine allows repeated muscle contractions and gradations of contractile force.

A number of drugs and agents can alter neuromuscular function by changing the release, inactivation, or receptor binding of acetylcholine. Curare acts on the postjunctional membrane of the motor end plate to prevent the depolarizing effect of the neurotransmitter. Blocking of neuromuscular transmission by curare-type drugs is used during many types of surgical procedures to facilitate relaxation of involved musculature. Drugs such as physostigmine and neostigmine inhibit the action of acetylcholinesterase and allow acetylcholine released from the motoneuron to accumulate. These drugs are used in the treatment of myasthenia gravis.

Toxins from the botulism organism (*Clostridium botulinum*) produce paralysis by blocking acetylcholine release.[7] Spores from the botulism organism may be found in soil-grown foods that are not cooked at temperatures of at least 100°C in home canning procedures. A pharmacologic preparation of the botulism toxin (botulism toxin type A [Botox]) has become available for use in treating eyelid and eye movement disorders such as blepharospasm and

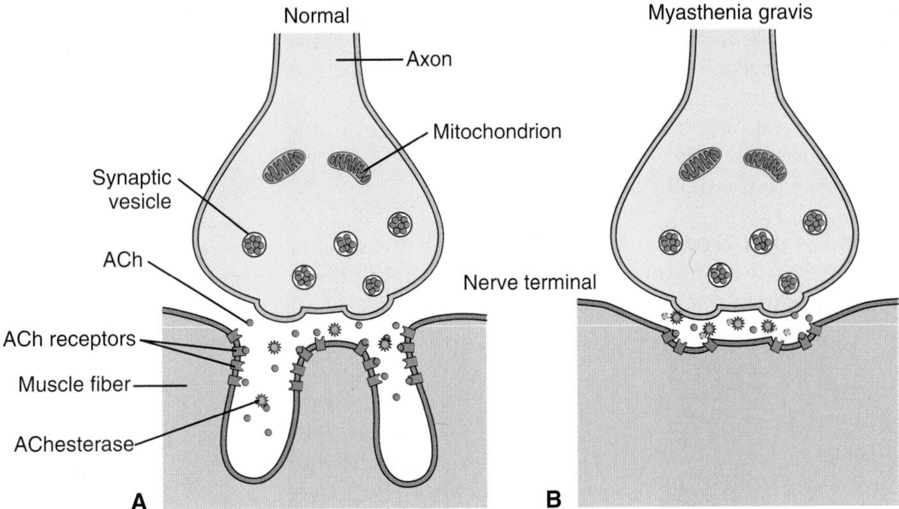

FIGURE 51-6 Neuromuscular junction. (**A**) Acetylcholine (ACh) released from the motoneurons in the myoneural junction crosses the synaptic space to reach receptors that concentrated in the folds of the endplate of the muscle fiber. Once released, ACh is rapidly broken down by the enzyme acetylcholinesterase (AChesterase). (**B**) Decrease in ACh receptors in myasthenia gravis.

strabismus. It also is used for treatment of spasmodic torticollis, spasmodic dysphonias (laryngeal dystonia), and other dystonias. The drug is injected into the target muscle using the electrical activity recorded from the tip of a special electromyographic injection needle to guide the injection. The treatment is not permanent and usually needs to be repeated approximately every 3 months.

The organophosphates (*e.g.,* malathion, parathion) that are used in some insecticides bind acetylcholinesterase to prevent the breakdown of acetylcholine. They produce excessive and prolonged acetylcholine action with a depolarization block of cholinergic receptors, including those of the neuromuscular junction.[8] The organophosphates are well absorbed from the skin, lungs, gut, and conjunctiva of the eye, making them particularly effective as insecticides but also potentially dangerous to humans. Malathion and certain other organophosphates are rapidly metabolized to inactive products in humans and are considered safe for sale to the general public. The sale of other insecticides, such as parathion, which is not effectively metabolized to inactive products, has been banned. Other organophosphate compounds (*e.g.,* soman) were developed as "nerve gases"; if absorbed in high enough concentrations, they have lethal effects from depolarization block and loss of respiratory muscle function.

Myasthenia Gravis

Myasthenia gravis is a disorder of transmission at the neuromuscular junction that affects communication between the motoneuron and the innervated muscle cell. The disease may occur at any age, but the peak incidence occurs between 20 and 30 years of age, and the disease is approximately three times more common in women than men. A smaller, second peak occurs in later life and affects men more often than women.[9]

Now recognized as an autoimmune disease, the disorder is caused by an antibody-mediated loss of acetylcholine receptors in the neuromuscular junction (see Fig. 51-6).[5] Although the exact mechanism that triggers the autoimmune response is unclear, it is thought that T cells have a key role. Approximately 75% of persons with myasthenia gravis also have thymic abnormalities, such as a thymoma (*i.e.,* thymus tumor) or thymic hyperplasia (*i.e.,* increased thymus weight from an increased number of thymus cells).[9] The Lambert-Eaton myasthenic syndrome is a special type of myasthenic syndrome that develops in association with neoplasms, particularly small cell carcinoma of the lung (see Chapter 8). Neonatal myasthenia gravis, caused by placental transfer of the acetylcholine receptor antibody, occurs in about 10% of infants born to mothers with the disease. Spontaneous resolution of symptoms usually occurs within a few months of birth.

In persons with myasthenia gravis who have fewer acetylcholine receptors in the postsynaptic membrane, each release of acetylcholine from the presynaptic membrane results in a lower-amplitude end-plate potential. This results in both muscle weakness and fatigability with sustained effort. Most commonly affected are the eye and periorbital muscles. Either ptosis due to eyelid weakness or diplopia due to weakness of the extraocular muscles is an initial symptom in approximately 50% of persons with the disease.[10] The disease may progress from ocular muscle weakness to generalized weakness, including respiratory muscle weakness. Chewing and swallowing may be difficult, and persons with the disease often choose to eat soft puddings and cereals rather than meats and hard fruit. Weakness in limb movement usually is more pronounced in proximal than in distal parts of the extremity, so that climbing stairs and lifting objects are difficult. As the disease progresses, the muscles of the lower face are affected, causing speech impairment. When this happens, the person often supports the chin with one hand to assist in speaking. In most persons, symptoms are least evident when arising in the morning, but they grow worse with effort and as the day proceeds.

Persons with myasthenia gravis may experience a sudden exacerbation of symptoms and weakness known as *myasthenia crisis.* Myasthenia crisis occurs when muscle weakness becomes severe enough to compromise ventilation to the extent that ventilatory support and airway protection are needed. This usually occurs during a period of stress, such as infection, emotional upset, pregnancy, alcohol ingestion, cold, or after surgery. It also can result from inadequate or excessive doses of the anticholinesterase drugs used in treatment of the disorder.

Diagnosis and Treatment. The diagnosis of myasthenia gravis is based on history and physical examination, the anticholinesterase test, nerve stimulation studies, and an assay for acetylcholine receptor antibodies. The anticholinesterase test uses a drug that inhibits acetylcholinesterase, the enzyme that breaks down acetylcholine. Edrophonium (Tensilon), a short-acting acetylcholinesterase inhibitor, commonly is used for the test. The drug, which is administered intravenously, decreases the breakdown of acetylcholine in the neuromuscular junction. When weakness is caused by myasthenia gravis, a dramatic transitory improvement in muscle function occurs. Electrophysiologic studies can be done to demonstrate a decremental muscle response to repetitive 2- or 3-Hz stimulation of motor nerves. An advance in diagnostic methods for myasthenia gravis is single-fiber electromyography, which is available in many medical centers. Single-fiber electromyography detects delayed or failed neuromuscular transmission in muscle fibers supplied by a single nerve fiber.[9,10] An immunoassay test can be used to detect the presence of acetylcholine receptor antibodies circulating in the blood.

Treatment methods include the use of pharmacologic agents; immunosuppressive therapy, including corticosteroid drugs; management of myasthenic crisis; thymectomy; and plasmapheresis or intravenous immunoglobulin.[9] Medications that may exacerbate myasthenia gravis, such as the aminoglycoside antibiotics, should be avoided.[11] Pharmacologic treatment with reversible anticholinesterase drugs inhibits the breakdown of acetylcholine at the neuromuscular junction by acetylcholinesterase. Pyridostigmine and neostigmine are the drugs of choice. Corticosteroid drugs, which suppress the immune response, are used in cases of a poor response to anticholinesterase drugs and thymectomy. Immunosuppressant drugs (*e.g.*, azathioprine, cyclosporine) also may be used, often in combination with plasmapheresis.

Plasmapheresis removes antibodies from the circulation and provides short-term clinical improvement. It is used primarily to stabilize the condition of persons in myasthenic crisis or for short-term treatment in persons undergoing thymectomy. Intravenous immunoglobulin also produces improvement in persons with myasthenia gravis. Although the effect is temporary, it may last for weeks to months. The indications for its use are similar to those for plasmapheresis. The mechanism of action of intravenous immunoglobulin is unknown. Intravenous immunoglobulin therapy is very expensive, which limits its use.

Thymectomy, or surgical removal of the thymus, may be used as a treatment for myasthenia gravis. Because the mechanism whereby surgery exerts its effect is unknown, the treatment is controversial. Thymectomy is performed in persons with thymoma, regardless of age, and in persons 50 to 60 years of age or older with recent onset of moderate disease.

PERIPHERAL NERVE DISORDERS

The peripheral nervous system consists of the motor and sensory branches of the cranial and spinal nerves, the peripheral parts of the autonomic nervous system, and the peripheral ganglia. A peripheral neuropathy is any primary disorder of the peripheral nerves. The result usually is muscle weakness, with or without atrophy and sensory changes. The disorder can involve a single nerve (mononeuropathy) or multiple nerves (polyneuropathy).

Unlike the nerves of the CNS, peripheral nerves are fairly strong and resilient. They contain a series of connective tissue sheaths that enclose their nerve fibers. An outer fibrous sheath called the *epineurium* surrounds the medium-sized to large nerves; inside, a sheath called the *perineurium* invests each bundle of nerve fibers, and within each bundle, a delicate sheath of connective tissue known as the *endoneurium* surrounds each nerve fiber (see Chapter 49, Fig. 49-4). Small peripheral nerves lack the epineurial covering. In its endoneurial sheath, each nerve fiber is invested by a segmented sheath of Schwann cells. The Schwann cells produce the myelin sheath that surrounds the peripheral nerves. Each Schwann cell, however, can myelinate only one segment of a single axon—the one that it covers—so that myelination of an entire axon requires the participation of a long line of these cells.

Peripheral Nerve Injury and Repair

Neurons exemplify the general principle that the more specialized the function of a cell type, the less able it is to regenerate. In neurons, cell division ceases by the time of birth, and from then on, the cell body of a neuron is unable to divide and replace itself. Although the entire neuron cannot be replaced, it often is possible for the dendritic and axonal cell processes to regenerate as long as the cell body remains viable.

When a peripheral nerve is destroyed by a crushing force or by a cut that penetrates the nerve, the portion of the nerve fiber that is separated from the cell body rapidly undergoes degenerative changes, whereas the central stump and cell body of the nerve often are able to survive (Fig. 51-7). Because the cell body synthesizes the material required for nourishing and maintaining the axon, it is likely that the loss of these materials results in the degeneration of the separated portion of the nerve fibers.

After injury, the Schwann cells that are distal to the site of damage also are able to survive, but their myelin degenerates in a process called *wallerian degeneration.* The Schwann cells assist other phagocytic cells in the area in the cleanup of the debris caused by the degenerating axon and myelin. As they remove the debris, the Schwann cells multiply and fill the empty endoneurial tube. At this point, nothing further happens, unless a regenerating nerve fiber penetrates into the endoneurial tube, in which case the Schwann cells reform the myelin segments around the fiber.

Meanwhile, the cell body of the neuron responds to the loss of part of its nerve fiber by shifting into a phase of

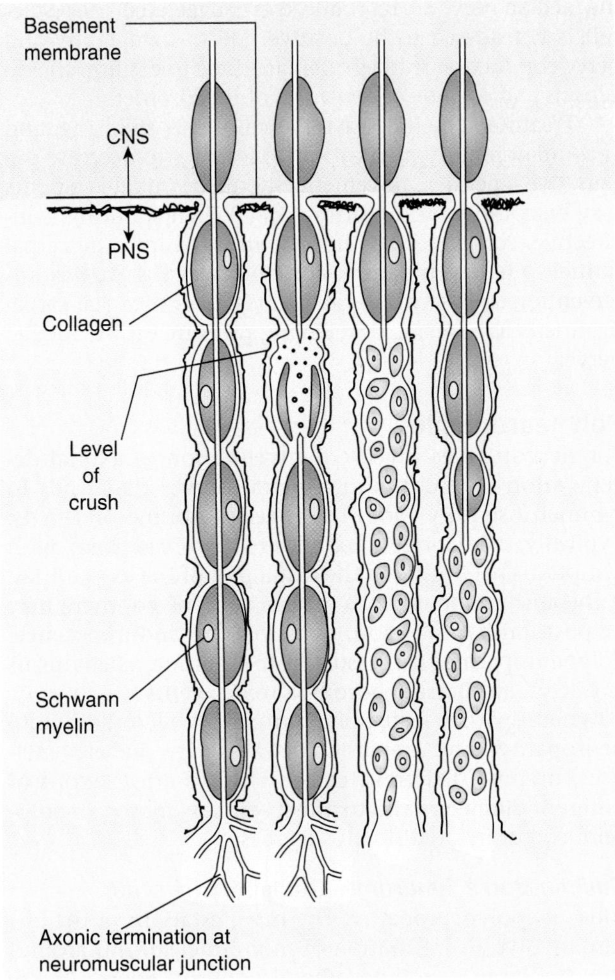

FIGURE 51-7 Sequential stages in efferent axon degeneration and regeneration within its endoneurial tube, following peripheral nerve crush injury.

greatly increased protein and lipid synthesis. It does this by dispersing masses of ribosomes, which stain as Nissl granules. They cease to be stainable and disappear in a process called *chromatolysis*. In the process, the nucleus moves away from the axonal side of the cell body, as though displaced by the active synthetic apparatus of the cells. These changes reach their height within approximately 10 days of injury and continue until regrowth of the nerve fiber ceases.

In the process of regeneration, the injured nerve fiber develops one or more new branches from the proximal nerve stump that grow into the developing scar tissue. If a crushing injury has occurred and the endoneurial tube is intact through the trauma area, the outgrowing fiber will grow back down this tube to the structure that was originally innervated by the neuron. If, however, the injury involves the severing of a nerve, the outgrowing branch must come in contact with its original endoneurial tube if it is to be reunited with its original target structure. The rate of outgrowth of regenerating nerve fibers is approximately 1 to 2 mm/day; the recovery of conduction to a target structure depends on regrowth into the appropriate endoneurial tube and on the distance involved. It can take weeks or months for the regrowing fiber to reach the end-organ and for communicative function to be reestablished. More time is required for the Schwann cells to form new myelin segments and for the axon to recover its original diameter and conduction velocity.

The successful regeneration of a nerve fiber in the peripheral nervous system depends on many factors. If a nerve fiber is destroyed relatively close to the neuronal cell body, the chances are that the nerve cell will die, and if it does, it will not be replaced. If a crushing type of injury has occurred, partial or often full recovery of function occurs. Cutting-type trauma to a nerve is an entirely different matter. Connective scar tissue forms rapidly at the wound site, and when it does, only the most rapidly regenerating axonal branches are able to get through to the intact distal endoneurial tubes. A number of scar-inhibiting agents have been used in an effort to reduce this hazard, but they have met with only moderate success. In another attempt to improve nerve regeneration, various types of tubular implants have been placed to fill longer gaps in the endoneurial tube.

Perhaps the most difficult problem is the alignment of the proximal and distal endoneurial tubes so that a regenerating fiber can return down its former tube and innervate its former organ. This problem is similar to realigning a large telephone cable that has been cut so that all the wires are reconnected exactly as before the separation. Microscopic alignment of the cut edges during microsurgical repair results in improved success. If an efferent nerve fiber that formerly innervated a skeletal muscle regrows down an endoneurial tube formerly occupied by an afferent fiber and reaches the former sensory area, then its cell body eventually dies. A sensory fiber that grows down an endoneurial tube that connects with a skeletal muscle fiber undergoes the same fate. If, however, these fibers grow down endoneurial tubes that innervate the appropriate type of target organ, reinnervation and function may return, even though the fibers have changed places. Under the best of conditions, a 50% regeneration to the appropriate organ is considered a success after a peripheral nerve has been severed. Even so, considerable function can return with that amount of innervation.

Mononeuropathies

Mononeuropathies usually are caused by localized conditions such as trauma, compression, or infections that affect a single spinal nerve, plexus, or peripheral nerve trunk. Fractured bones may lacerate or compress nerves; excessively tight tourniquets may injure nerves directly or produce ischemic injury; and infections such as herpes zoster may affect a single segmental afferent nerve distribution. Recovery of nerve function usually is complete after compression lesions and incomplete or faulty after nerve transection.

Carpal Tunnel Syndrome. Carpal tunnel syndrome is an example of a compression-type mononeuropathy that is relatively common. The syndrome affects an estimated 3% of adult Americans and is approximately three times more common in women than men.[12] It is caused by compression of the median nerve as it travels with the flexor tendons through a canal made by the carpal bones and transverse carpal ligament (Fig. 51-8). The condition can be caused by a variety of conditions that produce a reduction in the capacity of the carpal tunnel (*i.e.*, bony or ligament changes) or an increase in the volume of the tunnel contents (*i.e.*, inflammation of the tendons, synovial swelling, or tumors).[13] Carpal tunnel syndrome can be a feature of many systemic diseases such as rheumatoid arthritis, hyperthyroidism, acromegaly, and diabetes mellitus.[12,14] The condition can result from wrist injury; it can occur during pregnancy and use of birth control drugs; and it is seen in persons with repetitive use of the wrist (*i.e.*, flexion-extension movements and stress associated with pinching and gripping motions).

Carpal tunnel syndrome is characterized by pain, paresthesia, and numbness of the thumb and first two and one-half digits of the hand; pain in the wrist and hand, which worsens at night; atrophy of abductor pollicis muscle; and weakness in precision grip. All of these abnormalities may contribute to clumsiness of fine motor activity.

Diagnosis usually is based on sensory disturbances confined to median nerve distribution, a positive Tinel's sign, and a positive Phalen's sign. *Tinel's sign* describes the development of a tingling sensation radiating into the palm of the hand that is elicited by light percussion over the median nerve at the wrist.[12] The *Phalen test* is performed by having the person hold the wrist in complete flexion for approximately a minute; if numbness and paresthesia along the median nerve are reproduced or exaggerated, the test result is considered to be positive. Electromyography and nerve conduction studies often are done to confirm the diagnosis and exclude other causes of the disorder.

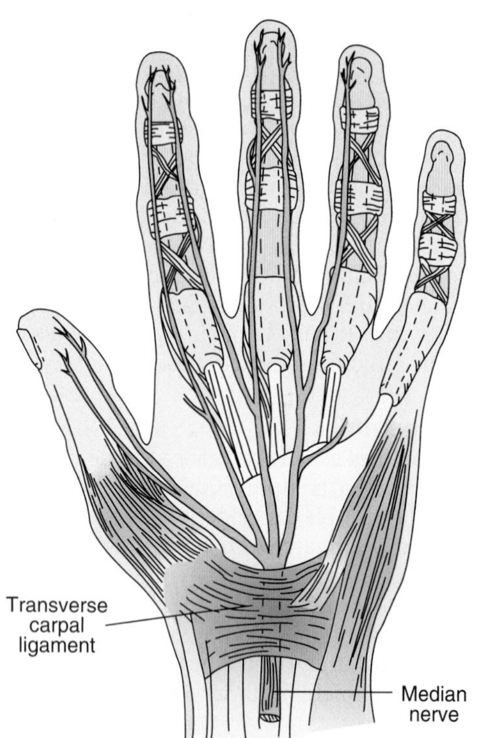

FIGURE 51-8 Carpal tunnel syndrome: compression of the median nerve by the transverse carpal ligament. (Courtesy Carole Russell Hilmer, C.M.I.)

Treatment includes avoidance of use, splinting, and anti-inflammatory medications. Measures to decrease the causative repetitive movements should be initiated. Splints may be confined to nighttime use. When splinting is ineffective, corticosteroids may be injected into the carpal tunnel to reduce inflammation and swelling. Surgical intervention consists of operative division of the volar carpal ligaments as a means of relieving pressure on the medial nerve.

Polyneuropathies

Polyneuropathies involve demyelination or axonal degeneration of multiple peripheral nerves that leads to symmetric sensory, motor, or mixed sensorimotor deficits. Typically, the longest axons are involved first, with symptoms beginning in the distal part of the extremities. If the autonomic nervous system is involved, there may be postural hypotension, constipation, and impotence. Polyneuropathies can result from immune mechanisms (*e.g.*, Guillain-Barré syndrome), toxic agents (*e.g.*, arsenic polyneuropathy, lead polyneuropathy, alcoholic polyneuropathy), and metabolic diseases (*e.g.*, diabetes mellitus, uremia). Different causes tend to affect axons of different diameters and to affect sensory, motor, or autonomic neurons to different degrees.

Guillain-Barré Syndrome. Guillain-Barré syndrome is a subacute polyneuropathy. The manifestations of the disease involve an infiltration of mononuclear cells around the capillaries of the peripheral neurons, edema of the endoneurial compartment, and demyelination of ventral spinal roots. Guillain-Barré syndrome affects approximately 3500 persons in the United States and Canada each year.[15] Approximately 80% to 90% of persons with the disease achieve a spontaneous recovery.

The cause of Guillain-Barré syndrome probably has an immune component. Controlled epidemiologic studies have linked it to infection with *Campylobacter jejuni* in addition to other viruses, including cytomegalovirus and Epstein-Barr virus.[16,17] A widely studied outbreak of the disorder followed the swine flu vaccination program of 1976 and 1977.[18]

The disorder is characterized by progressive ascending muscle weakness of the limbs, producing a symmetric flaccid paralysis. Symptoms of paresthesia and numbness often accompany the loss of motor function. The rate of disease progression varies, and there may be disproportionate involvement of the upper or lower extremities. Paralysis may progress to involve the respiratory muscles; approximately 30% of persons with the disorder require ventilatory assistance.[15] Autonomic nervous system involvement that causes postural hypotension, arrhythmias, facial flushing, abnormalities of sweating, and urinary retention is common.

Guillain-Barré syndrome usually is a medical emergency. There may be a rapid development of ventilatory failure and autonomic disturbances that threaten circulatory function. Treatment includes support of vital functions and prevention of complications such as skin breakdown and thrombophlebitis. Clinical trials have shown the effectiveness of plasmapheresis in decreasing morbidity and shortening the course of the disease. Treatment is most effective if initiated early in the course of the disease. High-dose intravenous immunoglobulin therapy also has proved effective.[15]

Back Pain and Herniated Intervertebral Disk

Back pain can result from a number of interrelated problems involving the structures of the vertebral column, the spinal nerve roots, or the muscles and ligamentous structures of the back. Perhaps the most common are musculoligamentous injuries and age-related degenerative changes in the intervertebral disks and facet joints.[19] Low back pain affects men and women equally, with onset most often between ages of 30 and 50 years. It is the most common cause of work-related disability. Risk factors include heavy lifting, twisting, bodily vibration, obesity, and poor conditioning, although low back pain is common even in persons without these risk factors.

Although back problems commonly are attributed to a herniated disk, most acute back problems are caused by other, less serious conditions. It has been reported that 90% of persons with acute lower back problems of less than 3 months' duration recover spontaneously.[20,21] The diagnostic challenge is to identify those persons who require more extensive evaluation for more serious problems such as tumors, compression fractures, or disk herniation.

Treatment of back pain usually is conservative and consists of analgesic medications and education on how to protect the back. Muscle relaxants may be used on a short-term basis. Bed rest does not increase the speed of recovery, and sometimes delays recovery.[19,21] Instruction in the correct mechanics for lifting and methods of protecting the back is important. Conditioning exercises of the trunk muscles, particularly the back extensors, may be recommended for persons with acute low back pain, particularly if the problem persists.

Herniated Intervertebral Disk. The intervertebral disk is considered the most critical component of the load-bearing structures of the spinal column. The intervertebral disk consists of a soft, gelatinous center called the *nucleus pulposus,* which is encircled by a strong, ringlike collar of fibrocartilage called the *annulus fibrosus*. The structural components of the disk make it capable of absorbing shock and changing shape while allowing movement. With dysfunction, the nucleus pulposus can be squeezed out of place and herniate through the annulus fibrosus, a condition referred to as a *herniated* or *slipped disk* (Fig. 51-9A and B).

The intervertebral disk can become dysfunctional because of trauma, the effects of aging, or degenerative disorders of the spine. Trauma accounts for 50% of disk herniations. It results from activities such as lifting while in the flexed position, slipping, falling on the buttocks or back, or suppressing a sneeze. With aging, the gelatinous center of the disk dries out and loses much of its elasticity, causing it to fray and tear. Degenerative processes such as osteoarthritis or ankylosing spondylitis predispose to malalignment of the vertebral column.

The cervical and lumbar regions are the most flexible area of the spine and most often involved in disk herniations. Usually, herniation occurs at the lower levels of the lumbar spine, where the mass being supported and the bending of the vertebral column are greatest. Approximately 90% to 95% of lumbar herniations occur in the L4 or L5 to S1 regions. With herniations of the cervical spine, the most frequently involved levels are C6 to C7 and C5 to C6. Protrusion of the nucleus pulposus usually occurs posteriorly and toward the intervertebral foramen and its contained spinal nerve root, where the annulus fibrosus is relatively thin and poorly supported by either the posterior or anterior ligaments[22] (see Fig. 51-9A).

The level at which a herniated disk occurs is important (see Fig. 51-9C). When the injury occurs in the lumbar area, only the cauda equina is involved. Because these elongated dorsal and ventral roots contain endoneurial tubes of connective tissue, regeneration of the nerve fibers is likely. However, several weeks or months are required for full recovery to occur because of the distance to the innervated muscle or skin of the lower limbs.

The signs and symptoms of a herniated disk are localized to the area of the body innervated by the nerve roots and include both motor and sensory manifestations (Fig. 51-10). Pain is the first and most common symptom of a herniated disk. The nerve roots of L4, L5, S1, S2, and S3 give rise to a syndrome of back pain that spreads down the back of the leg and over the sole of the foot. The pain is usually intensified with coughing, sneezing, straining, stooping, standing, and the jarring motions that occur during walking or riding. Slight motor weakness may occur, although major weakness is rare. The most common sensory deficits from spinal nerve root compression are paresthesias and numbness, particularly of the leg and foot. Knee and ankle reflexes also may be diminished or absent.

A herniated disk must be differentiated from other causes such as traumatic injury or fracture of the vertebral column, tumor, infection, cauda equina syndrome (see Spinal Cord Injury), or other conditions that cause back pain.[20] Diagnostic measures include history and physical examination. Neurologic assessment includes testing of muscle strength and reflexes. The straight-leg test is done in the supine position and is performed by passively raising the person's leg. Normally, it is possible to raise the leg approximately 90 degrees without causing discomfort of the hamstring muscles. The test result is positive if pain is produced when the leg is raised to 60 degrees or less. Other diagnostic methods include radiographs of the back, magnetic resonance imaging (MRI), myelography, and computed tomography (CT).[23]

Treatment usually is conservative and consists of analgesic medications and education on how to protect the back. Pain relief usually can be provided using nonsteroidal anti-inflammatory drugs, although short-term use of opioid pain medications may be required for severe pain. Muscle relaxants such as diazepam, cyclobenzaprine, carisoprodol, or methocarbamol may be used on a short-term basis.

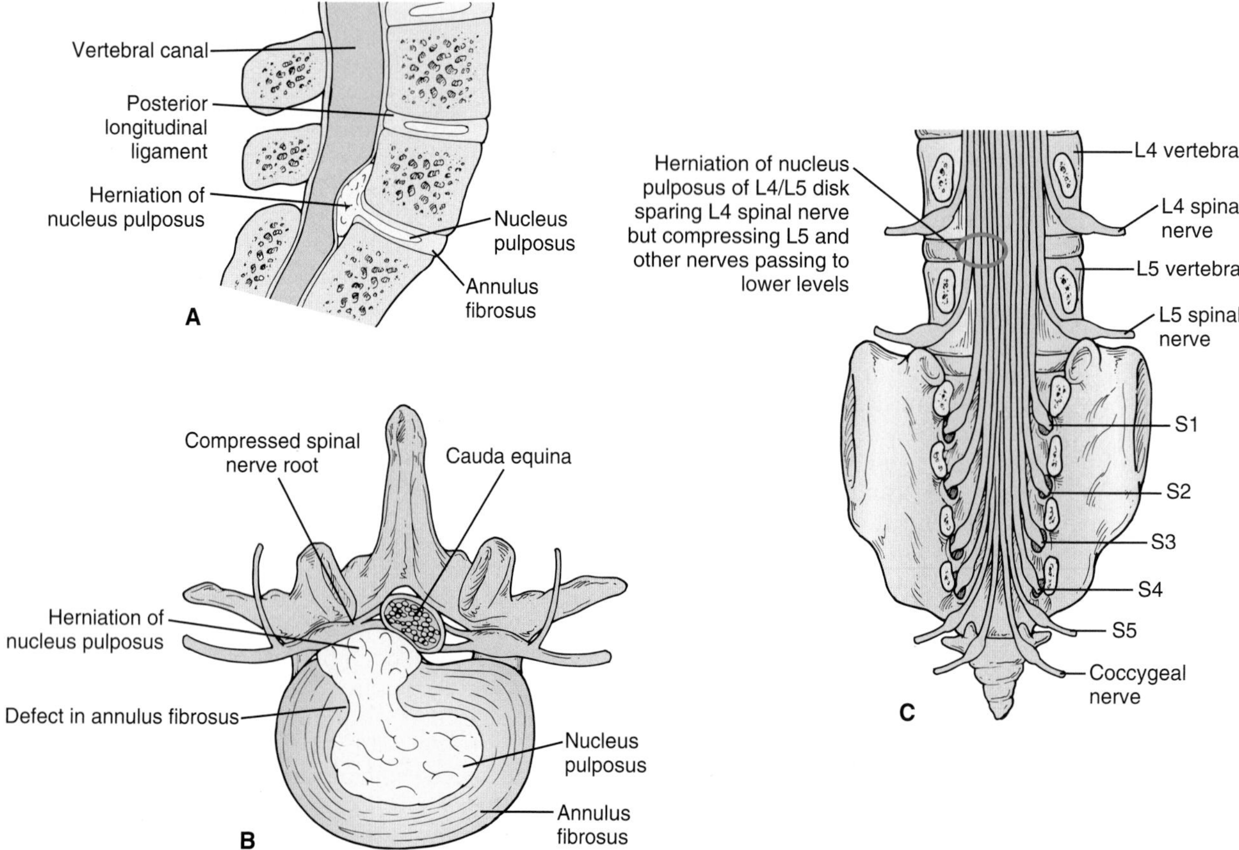

FIGURE 51-9 Herniated intervertebral disk. (**A**) Longitudinal section. (**B**) Cross-section. (**C**) Location of L4–5 and S1–5 spinal nerves with site of L4/5 herniation of nucleus pulposus indicated. (Modified from Moore K.L. Dalley A.F. [1999]. *Clinically oriented anatomy* (4th ed., p. 452). Philadelphia: Lippincott Williams & Wilkins)

Conditioning exercises of the trunk muscles, particularly the back extensors, may be recommended. Surgical treatment may be indicated when there is documentation of herniation by an imaging procedure, consistent pain, or consistent neurologic deficit that has failed to respond to conservative therapy.

In summary, the motor unit consists of the LMN, the neuromuscular junction, and the skeletal muscle that the nerve innervates. Disorders of the neuromuscular unit include muscular dystrophy, myasthenia gravis, and peripheral nerve disorders. *Muscular dystrophy* is a term used to describe a number of disorders that produce progressive deterioration of skeletal muscle. Muscle necrosis is followed by fat and connective tissue replacement. One form, Duchenne muscular dystrophy, is inherited as a X-linked trait and transmitted by the mother to her male offspring. Myasthenia gravis is a disorder of the neuromuscular junction resulting from a deficiency of functional acetylcholine receptors, which causes weakness of the skeletal muscles. Because the disease affects the neuromuscular junction, there is no loss of sensory function. The most common manifestations are weakness of the eye muscles, with ptosis and diplopia. Usually, the proximal muscles and extremities are involved, making it difficult to climb stairs and lift objects.

Disorders of peripheral nerves include mononeuropathies and polyneuropathies. Mononeuropathies involve a single spinal nerve, plexus, or peripheral nerve trunk. Carpal tunnel syndrome, a mononeuropathy, is caused by compression of the medial nerve that passes through the carpal tunnel in the wrist. Polyneuropathies involve multiple peripheral nerves and produce symmetric sensory, motor, and mixed sensorimotor deficits. Guillain-Barré syndrome is a subacute polyneuropathy of uncertain origin. It causes progressive ascending motor, sensory, and autonomic nervous system manifestations. Respiratory involvement may occur and necessitate mechanical ventilation.

Acute back pain is most commonly the result of conditions such as muscle strain with treatment that focuses on measures to improve activity tolerance. A herniated intervertebral disk is characterized by protrusion of the nucleus pulposus into the spinal canal with irritation or compression of the nerve root. Usually, herniation occurs at the lower levels of the lumbar and sacral (L4 or L5 to S1) and cervical (C6 to C7 and C5 to C6) regions of the spine. The signs and symptoms of a herniated disk are localized to the area of the body innervated by the affected nerve roots and include pain and both motor and sensory manifestations.

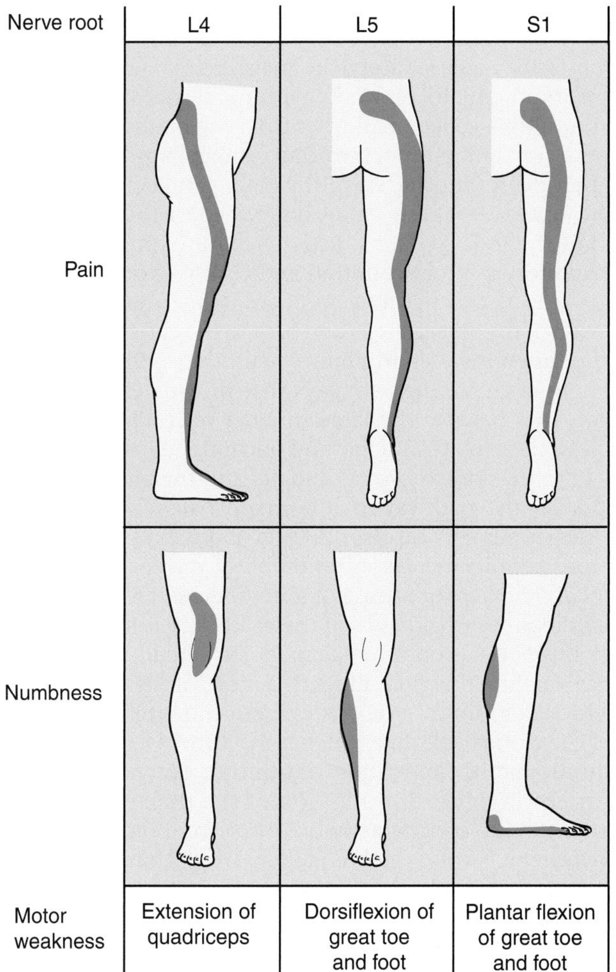

Nerve root
L4
L5
S1
Pain
Numbness
Motor weakness
Extension of quadriceps
Dorsiflexion of great toe and foot
Plantar flexion of great toe and foot

FIGURE 51-10 Dermatomes of the leg (L1 through S5) where pain and numbness would be experienced with spinal root irritation.

Disorders of the Basal Ganglia and Cerebellum

After completing this section of the chapter, you should be able to meet the following objectives:

- Describe the functional organization of the basal ganglia and communication pathways with the thalamus and cerebral cortex
- State the possible mechanisms responsible for the development of Parkinson disease and characterize the manifestations and treatment of the disorder
- Relate the functions of the cerebellum to production of vestibulocerebellar ataxia, decomposition of movement, and cerebellar tremor

DISORDERS OF THE BASAL GANGLIA

The basal ganglia are a group of deep, interrelated subcortical nuclei that play an essential role in control of movement. The basal ganglia receive indirect input from the cerebellum and from all sensory systems, including vision, and direct input from the motor cortex. They function in the organization of inherited and highly learned and rather automatic movement programs, especially those affecting the trunk and proximal limbs. The movements are released when commanded by the motor cortex, contributing gracefulness to cortically initiated and controlled skilled movements. The function of the basal ganglia is not limited to motor functions. They also are involved in cognitive and perception functions.

Disorders of the basal ganglia comprise a complex group of motor disturbances characterized by involuntary movements, alterations in muscle tone, and disturbances in body posture. Unlike disorders of the motor cortex and corticospinal (pyramidal) tract, lesions of the basal ganglia disrupt movement but do not cause paralysis.

Functional Organization of the Basal Ganglia

The structural components of the basal ganglia include the caudate nucleus, putamen, and the globus pallidus in the forebrain.[24] The caudate and putamen are collectively referred to as the *striatum,* and the putamen and the globus pallidus form a wedge-shaped region called the *lentiform nucleus.* Two other structures, the *subthalamic nucleus* of the diencephalon and the *substantia nigra* of the midbrain, are considered part of the basal ganglia (Fig. 51-11). The dorsal part of the substantia nigra contains cells that use dopamine as a neurotransmitter and are rich in a black pigment called *melanin.* The high concentration of melanin gives the structure a black color, hence the name *substantia nigra.* The axons of the substantia nigra form the *nigrostriatal pathway,* which supplies dopamine to the striatum. The dopamine released from the substantia nigra regulates the overall excitability of the striatum and the release of other neurotransmitters.

The basal ganglia have input structures that receive afferent information from outside structures, internal circuits

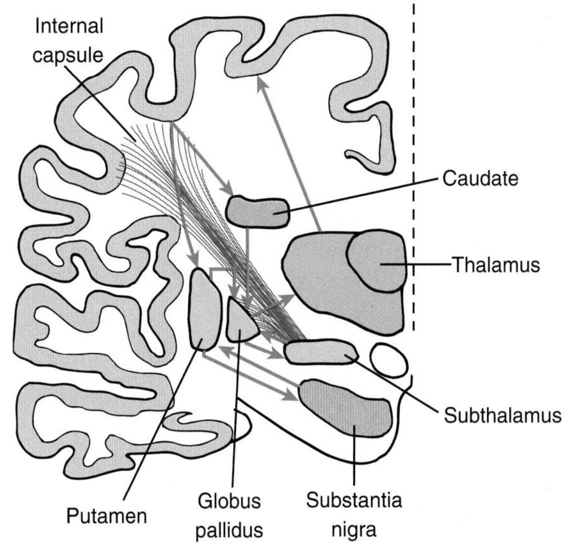

FIGURE 51-11 Basal ganglia.

that connect the various structures of the basal ganglia, and output structures that deliver information to other brain centers. The neostriatum represents the major input structure for the basal ganglia. Virtually all areas of the cortex and afferents from the thalamus project to the neostriatum. The output areas of the basal ganglia, including the lateral globus pallidus, have ascending and descending components. The major ascending input is transmitted to thalamic nuclei, which process all incoming information that is transmitted to the cerebral cortex. Descending output is directed to the midbrain, brain stem, and spinal cord. The output functions of the basal ganglia are mainly inhibitory. Looping circuits from specific cortical areas pass through the basal ganglia to modulate the excitability of specific thalamic nuclei and control the cortical activity involved in highly learned, automatic, and stereotyped motor functions.

Each region of the cerebral cortex is interconnected with a corresponding region of the ventral row of thalamic nuclei. For the motor and premotor cortex, these nuclei are the ventral lateral (VL) and the ventral anterior (VA) nuclei. The cortex-to-thalamus (corticothalamic) and thalamus-to-cortex (thalamocortical) feedback circuitries are excitatory and, if unmodulated, would produce hyperactivity of the cortical area, causing stiffness and rigidity of the face, body, and limbs, and, if alternating, a continuous tremor (*i.e.,* tremor at rest). The excitability of the thalamic nuclei in this reciprocal circuit is regulated by other thalamic afferents, many of which depress thalamic excitability.

For many semiautomatic stereotyped movements, thalamic excitability is modulated through inhibition by the basal ganglia. The basal ganglia form a major component of an inhibitory loop from each specific cortical region. Discrete inhibitory cortex-to-basal ganglia and thalamus-to-cortex loops modulate the function of all cerebral cortex regions. These modulatory loops exist for the prefrontal, limbic, premotor, motor, sensory, and parietal higher-order areas of the cerebral cortex. Abnormalities of the modulatory loop that influence motor function have such dramatic results that the role of the basal ganglia often has been relegated to that of the modulation of movement patterns.

The most is known about the inhibitory basal ganglia loop involved in modulating cortical motor control. This loop regulates release of stereotyped movement patterns that add efficiency and gracefulness to precise and delicate cortically controlled movements. These movements include inherited patterns that add efficiency, balance, and gracefulness to motion, such as the swinging of the arms during walking and running and the highly learned automatic postural and follow-through movements of throwing a ball or swinging a bat. The basic repertoire of many of these complex movement patterns is built into brain stem circuitry under gene control. Individual differences limit the extent to which learning and practice can enhance their perfection. Thus, not everyone can become an accomplished ballerina or gymnast.

There are four functional pathways involving the basal ganglia: (1) a dopamine pathway from the substantia nigra to the striatum; (2) a gamma-aminobutyric acid (GABA) pathway from the striatum to the globus pallidus and substantia nigra; (3) acetylcholine-secreting neurons, which are important in networks within the neostriatum; and (4) multiple general pathways from the brain stem that secrete norepinephrine, serotonin, enkephalin, and several other neurotransmitters in the basal ganglia and the cerebral cortex.[24] These pathways provide a balance of inhibitory and excitatory activity. GABA functions as an inhibitory neurotransmitter, and GABAergic neurons participate in the negative feedback loop from the cortex through the basal ganglia and back to the cortex. Dopamine also functions as an inhibitory neurotransmitter. There are multiple glutamine pathways that provide excitatory signals that balance the large number of inhibitory signals transmitted by GABAergic and dopaminergic neurons.

In the cortex-to-basal ganglia and thalamus-to-cortex loop are two pathways that normally balance each other.[24] One permits cortical disinhibition of the thalamus, and the other permits increased inhibition of the thalamus. *Cortical disinhibition* or release of a stereotyped movement pattern requires withdrawal of the inhibitory influence of the globus pallidus on the thalamus. The circuit involves cortical facilitation (glutaminergic action) of the neostriatum, which is inhibitory (GABAergic) to the internal segment of the globus pallidus, which is inhibitory (GABAergic) to the thalamus. Activation of a motor cortex movement pattern involves disinhibition of the thalamus, thereby potentiating cortical activity. The second *thalamic inhibition* circuit involves globus pallidus inhibition (GABAergic) and cortical facilitation of the subthalamic nucleus, which is excitatory (glutaminergic) to the internal segment of the globus pallidus. Increased activity in this circuit increases the inhibitory function of the globus pallidus. Pathologic movement regulation results from damaged function of one or both of these circuits. For example, destruction of the subthalamic nucleus by a stroke results in loss of thalamic inhibition, with a consequent release of violent, flailing (ballistic) limb movements on the contralateral side of the body.

An additional modulating circuit involves a *neostriatal inhibitory projection* (GABAergic) on the substantia nigra. The substantia nigra projects dopaminergic axons back on the neostriatum. A deficiency in the dopaminergic projection of this modulating circuit is implicated in Parkinson syndrome. The function of the neostriatum also involves local cholinergic interneurons, and its destruction is thought to be related to the choreiform movements of Huntington's chorea, another basal ganglia-related syndrome (see Chapter 53). Precisely how these transmitter-related abnormalities affect the functional microcircuitry of the basal ganglia circuit remains to be elucidated. However, some progress has been made in supplying decreased or missing transmitters, reducing at least temporarily the severity of several of these disorders.

Movement Disorders

Considerable progress has been made in understanding the mechanisms underlying the major movement disorders of the basal ganglia. They include the hypokinetic disorders, which are characterized by rigidity and bradykinesia (impaired initiation of movement), and the hyperkinetic disorders, which are characterized by excessive and often uncontrolled movement.[24]

Hypokinetic Disorders. Hyperfunction of the basal ganglia inhibitory loop results in excessive inhibition of cortical function, producing *bradykinesia* or *hypokinesis*. The results are slowness in beginning movement, a reduced range and force of the movement ("poverty of movement"), reduced or absent emotional responses, including emotion-related facial expressions, and a loss of the balance and grace-producing movements and postures associated with skilled motion. An example of hypokinesis is seen in severely affected persons with Parkinson syndrome. These disorders are usually accompanied by muscular rigidity and tremor.

Basal ganglia–derived rigidity involves a strong resistance to movement that decreases to stiffness after the movement gets underway. In some instances, forcing a rigid joint to turn is met with a series of sudden releases followed by renewed resistance, a phenomenon called *cogwheel rigidity*.

Tremor is caused by involuntary, oscillating contractions of opposing muscle groups around a joint. It usually is fairly uniform in frequency and amplitude. Certain tremors are considered physiologic in that they are transitory and normally occur under conditions of increased muscle tone, as in highly emotional situations, or they may be related to muscle fatigue or reduced body temperature (*i.e.*, shivering). Toxic tremors are produced by hyperexcitability related to conditions such as thyrotoxicosis. The tremor of Parkinson disease is caused by degenerative changes in the basal ganglia. *Tics* involve sudden and irregularly occurring contractions of whole muscles or major portions of a muscle. These are particularly evident in the muscles of the face, but can occur elsewhere.

Hyperkinetic Disorders. Hyperkinetic disorders are characterized by excessive motor activity. They are caused by reduced function of the basal ganglia inhibitory loop, which results in *hyperkinesis*, or release of movement patterns at inappropriate times or sometimes continuously. Descending pathways to the LMNs involved in basal ganglia–related movement disorders involve the corticospinal systems and other descending systems. Because these movement patterns are not under cortical control, they often are referred to as *involuntary movements*. The involuntary movements may take several forms, including choreiform movements, athetoid movements, ballismus movements, dystonias, and dyskinesias (Table 51-1). Various types of involuntary movements often occur in combination, and some appear to have the same underlying cause. For example, chorea and ballismus may be simply distal (chorea) and proximal (ballismus) forms of the same underlying disorder.[24] The movements are manifested on the side of the body opposite to basal ganglia damage and are usually lost during sleep, although they may make getting to sleep difficult.

Choreiform movements are sudden, jerky, and irregular but are coordinated and graceful. They can involve the distal limb, face, tongue, or swallowing muscles. Choreiform movements are accentuated by movement and by environmental stimulation; they often interfere with normal movement patterns. The word *chorea* originated from the Greek word meaning "to dance." There may be grimacing movements of the face, raising of the eyebrows, rolling of the eyes, and curling, protrusion, and withdrawal of the tongue. In the limbs, the movements largely are distal;

TABLE 51-1 Involuntary Movement Disorders Associated With Extrapyramidal Disorders

Movement Disorder	Characteristics
Tremor	Rhythmic oscillating contractions or movements of whole muscles or major portions of a muscle. They can occur as resting tremors, which are prominent at rest and decrease or disappear with movement; intention tremors, which increase with activity and become worse when the target is reached; and postural tremors, which appear when the affected part is maintained in a stabilized position.
Tics	Irregularly occurring brief, repetitive, stereotyped, coordinated movements such as winking, grimacing, or shoulder shrugging
Chorea	Brief, rapid, jerky, and irregular movements that are coordinated and graceful. The face, head, and distal limbs are most commonly involved. They often interfere with normal movement patterns.
Athetosis	Continuous, slow, wormlike, twisting and turning motions of a limb or body that most commonly involve the face and distal extremities and are often associated with spasticity
Ballismus	Involve violent sweeping, flinging-type limb movements, especially on one side of the body (hemiballismus)
Dystonia	Abnormal maintenance of posture results from a twisting, turning motion of the limbs, neck, or trunk. Motions are similar to athetosis but involve larger portions of the body. They can result in grotesque and twisted postures.
Dyskinesias	Rhythmic, repetitive, bizarre movements that chiefly involve the face, mouth, jaw, or tongue, causing grimacing, pursing of the lips, protrusion of the tongue, opening and closing of the mouth, and deviations of the jaw. The limbs are affected less often.

(From Bates B. [1991]. *A guide to physical examination and history taking* [5th ed., pp. 554–556]. Philadelphia: J.B. Lippincott) there may be piano playing–type movements with alternating extension and flexion of the fingers. The shoulders may be elevated and depressed or rotated. Movements of the face or limbs may occur alone or, more commonly, in combination.

Athetoid movements are relatively continuous, wormlike, twisting and turning motions of the joints of a limb or body. These result from continuous and prolonged contraction of agonist and antagonistic muscle groups. These are normal, smooth, and useful movements, except in extrapyramidal diseases, when they occur continuously in a nonrhythmic, often irregular sequence.

The term *ballismus* originated from a Greek word meaning "to jump around." Ballistic movements are violent, sweeping, flinging motions, especially of the limbs on one side of the body (hemiballismus). They may occur as the result of a small vascular accident involving the subthalamic nucleus on the opposite side of the brain.

Dystonia refers to the abnormal maintenance of a posture resulting from a twisting, turning movement of the limbs, neck, or trunk. These postures often result from simultaneous contraction of agonist and antagonist muscles. Long-sustained simultaneous hypertonia across a joint can result in degenerative changes and permanent fixation in unusual postures. These effects can occur as a side effect of some antipsychotic medications. *Spasmodic torticollis,* the most common type of dystonia, affects the muscles of the neck and shoulder. The condition, which is caused by bilateral and simultaneous contraction of the neck and shoulder muscles, results in unilateral head turning or head extension, sometimes limiting rotation. Elevations of the shoulder commonly accompany the spasmodic movements of the head and neck. Immobility of the cervical vertebrae eventually can lead to degenerative fixation in the twisted posture. Torsional spasm involving the trunk also can occur.

Dyskinesias are rhythmic, repetitive, bizarre movements. They frequently involve the face, mouth, jaw, and tongue, causing grimacing, pursing of the lips, or protrusion of the tongue. The limbs are affected less often. Tardive dyskinesia is an untoward reaction that can develop with long-term use of some of the antipsychotic medications.

Parkinson Disease

Parkinson disease is a degenerative disorder of basal ganglia function that results in variable combinations of tremor, rigidity, and bradykinesia. The disorder is characterized by progressive destruction of the nigrostriatal pathway, with subsequent reduction in striatal concentrations of dopamine. Up to 1 million people in the United States are affected by the disease.[25] It usually begins after 50 years of age, affecting 1% of the population older than 65 years of age.[26]

The clinical syndrome arising from the degenerative changes in basal ganglia function often is referred to as *parkinsonism*. Parkinson disease, the most common form of parkinsonism, is named after James Parkinson, a British physician who first described the disease in a paper he published in 1817 on the "shaking palsy."[27] In Parkinson disease, also known as idiopathic parkinsonism, dopamine depletion results from degeneration of the dopamine nigrostriatal system. Parkinsonism can also develop as a postencephalitic syndrome, as a side effect of therapy with antipsychotic drugs that block dopamine receptors, as a toxic reaction to a chemical agent, or as an outcome of severe carbon monoxide poisoning. Symptoms of parkinsonism also may accompany conditions such as cerebral vascular disease, brain tumors, repeated head trauma, or degenerative neurologic diseases that structurally damage the nigrostriatal pathway.

Postencephalitic parkinsonism was a particular problem in the 1930s and 1940s as a result of an outbreak of lethargic encephalitis (sleeping sickness) that occurred in 1914 to 1918.[28] Drug-induced parkinsonism can follow the administration of antipsychotic drugs in high doses (*e.g.,* phenothiazines, butyrophenones). These drugs block dopamine receptors and dopamine output by the cells of the substantia nigra. Of interest in terms of research was the development of Parkinson disease in several persons who had attempted to make a narcotic drug and instead synthesized a compound called MPTP (1-methyl-phenyl-2, 3,6-tetrahydropyridine).[28] This compound selectively destroys the dopaminergic neurons of the substantia nigra. This incident prompted investigations into the role of toxins that are produced by the body as a part of metabolic processes and those that enter the body from outside sources in the pathogenesis of Parkinson disease. One theory is that the auto-oxidation of catecholamines such as dopamine during melanin synthesis injures neurons in the substantia nigra. There is increasing evidence that the development of Parkinson disease may be related to oxidative metabolites of this process and the inability of neurons to render these products harmless. MPTP is an inhibitor of the mitochondrial electron transport system that functions in the inactivation of these metabolites, suggesting that it may produce Parkinson disease in a manner similar to the naturally occurring disease.[25,29]

Recent discovery of inherited forms of Parkinson disease suggest that genetic factors may play a role in the pathogenesis of early-onset Parkinson disease. Eight genetic loci for monogenic forms of Parkinson disease or dopa-responsive parkinsonism have been identified.[30] Mutations in the parkin gene (*Park2*) have been identified in a high percentage of family members with early-onset Parkinson disease (*i.e.,* persons who developed symptoms before 45 years of age).[31,32] A second gene mutation involves the α-synuclein gene (*Park1*).[30,32] α-Synuclein is a member of a small family of proteins that are expressed preferentially in the substantia nigra. Although mutations in this gene appear to be a rare cause of Parkinson disease, α-synuclein has received much attention because it is one of the major components of the Lewy bodies (intracytoplasmic inclusions found in the substantia nigra neurons) that are found in brain tissue of persons with Parkinson disease.[29,32]

Manifestations. The cardinal manifestations of Parkinson disease are tremor, rigidity, and bradykinesia or slowness of movement.[25,30] Other advanced-stage parkinsonian manifestations are falls, fluctuations in motor function, neuropsychiatric disorders, and sleep problems.

Tremor is the most visible manifestation of the disorder. The tremor affects the distal segments of the limbs, mainly the hands and feet; head, neck, face, lips, and tongue; or jaw. It is characterized by rhythmic, alternating flexion and contraction movements (4 to 6 beats per minute) that resemble the motion of rolling a pill between the thumb and forefinger. The tremor usually is unilateral, occurs when the limb is supported and at rest, and disappears with movement and sleep. The tremor eventually progresses to involve both sides of the body. Although the most noticeable sign of Parkinson disease, tremor usually is the least disabling manifestation of the disorder.

Rigidity is defined as resistance to movement of both flexors and extensors throughout the full range of motion. It is most evident during passive joint movement, and involves jerky, cogwheel–type or ratchet-like movements that require considerable energy to perform. Flexion contractions may develop as a result of the rigidity. As with tremor, rigidity usually begins unilaterally but progresses to involve both sides of the body.

Bradykinesia is characterized by slowness in initiating and performing movements and difficulty in sudden, unexpected stopping of voluntary movements. Unconscious associative movements occur in a series of disconnected steps rather than in a smooth, coordinated manner. This is the most disabling of the symptoms of Parkinson disease. Persons with Parkinson disease have difficulty initiating walking and difficulty turning. While walking, they may freeze in place and feel as if their feet are glued to the floor, especially when moving through a doorway or preparing to turn. When they walk, they lean forward to maintain their center of gravity and take small, shuffling steps without swinging their arms, and they have difficulty in changing their stride (Fig. 51-12). Loss of postural reflexes predispose them to falling, often backward. Emotional and voluntary facial movements become limited and slow as the disease progresses, and facial expression becomes stiff and masklike. There is loss of the blinking reflex and a failure to express emotion. The tongue, palate, and throat muscles become rigid; the person may drool because of difficulty in moving the saliva to the back of the mouth and swallowing it. The speech becomes slow and monotonous, without modulation, and poorly articulated.

Because the basal ganglia also influence the autonomic nervous system, persons with Parkinson disease often have excessive and uncontrolled sweating, sebaceous gland secretion, and salivation. Autonomic symptoms, such as lacrimation, dysphagia, orthostatic hypotension, thermal regulation, constipation, impotence, and urinary incontinence, may be present, especially late in the disease. Other advanced-stage parkinsonian manifestations are falls, fluctuations in motor function, neuropsychiatric disorders, and sleep disorders.

Dementia is an important feature associated with Parkinson disease. It occurs in approximately 20% of persons with the disease and develops late in the course of the disease.[31] The mental state of some persons with Parkinson disease may be indistinguishable from that seen in Alzheimer's disease. It has been suggested that many of the brain changes in both diseases may result from degeneration of acetylcholine-containing neurons in a region of the brain called the *nucleus basalis of Meynert,* which is the main source of cholinergic innervation of the cerebral cortex. Persons with Parkinson disease also have other neurochemical disturbances that can account for some of the features of dementia.

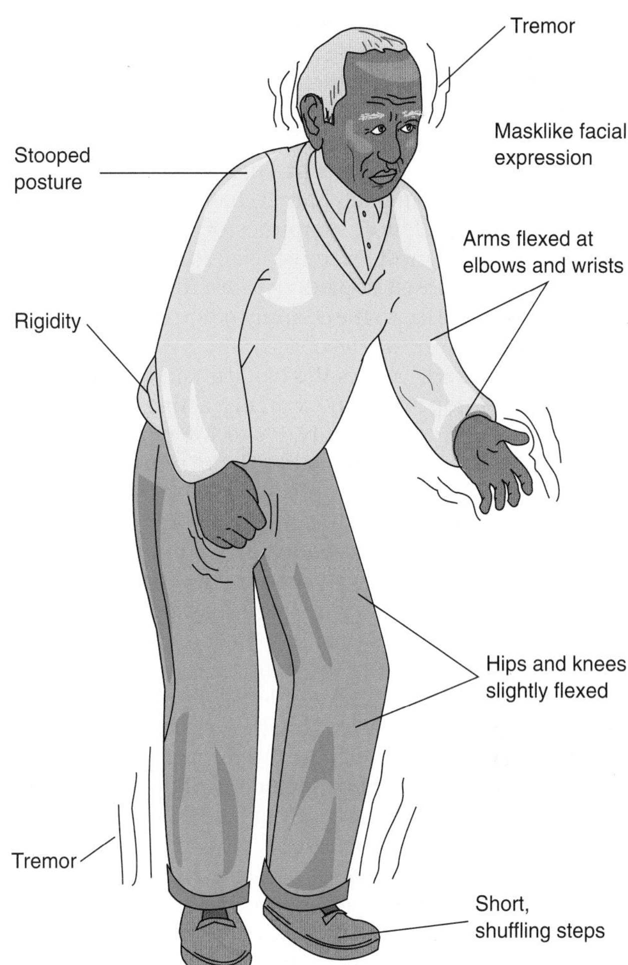

FIGURE 51-12 The clinical features of Parkinson disease. (Timby B.K., Smith N.E. [2003]. *Introductory medical–surgical nursing* [8th ed. p. 626]. Philadelphia: Lippincott Williams & Wilkins)

Treatment. The approach to treatment of parkinsonism must be highly individualized. It includes nonpharmacologic, pharmacologic, and, when indicated, surgical methods. Nonpharmacologic interventions offer group support, education, daily exercise, and adequate nutrition. Botulinum toxin injections may be used in the treatment of dystonias such as eyelid spasm and limb dystonias that frequently are associated with Parkinson disease.[28]

Pharmacologic treatment usually is determined by the severity of symptoms. Antiparkinson drugs act by increasing the functional ability of the underactive dopaminergic system, or they reduce the excessive influence of excitatory cholinergic neurons. Drugs that increase dopamine levels include levodopa and levodopa with the decarboxylase inhibitor (carbidopa), amantadine, bromocriptine, pergolide, and selegiline. Because dopamine transmission is disrupted in Parkinson disease, there is a preponderance of cholinergic activity, which may be treated with anticholinergic drugs.

Dopamine does not cross the blood–brain barrier. Administration of levodopa, a precursor of dopamine that does cross the blood–brain barrier, has yielded significant improvement in clinical symptoms of Parkinson disease and remains the most effective drug for treatment. The evidence of decreased dopamine levels in the striatum in Parkinson disease led to the administration of large doses of the synthetic compound levodopa, which is absorbed from the intestinal tract, crosses the blood–brain barrier, and is converted to dopamine by centrally acting dopa decarboxylase. Unfortunately, only 1% to 3% of administered levodopa enters the brain unaltered; the remainder is metabolized outside the brain, predominantly by decarboxylation to dopamine, which cannot cross the blood–brain barrier. However, when levodopa is given in combination with carbidopa, a decarboxylase inhibitor, the peripheral metabolism of levodopa is reduced, plasma levels of levodopa are higher, the plasma half-life is longer, more dopa is available for entry into the brain, and a smaller dose is needed. A later adverse effect of levodopa treatment is the "on–off phenomenon," in which frequent, abrupt, and unpredictable fluctuations in motor performance occur during the day. These fluctuations include periods of dyskinesia (the "on" response) and periods of bradykinesia (the "off" response). Some fluctuations reflect the timing of drug administration, in which case the on response coincides with peak drug levels and the off response with low drug levels.

Amantadine was introduced as an antiviral agent for prophylaxis of A_2 influenza and was unexpectedly found to cause symptomatic improvement in persons with parkinsonism. Although the exact mechanism of action remains to be elucidated, it may augment release of dopamine from the remaining intact dopaminergic terminals in the nigrostriatal pathway of persons with Parkinson disease. It is used to treat persons with mild symptoms, but no disability. Bromocriptine, pergolide, pramipexole, and ropinirole are dopamine agonists that act directly to stimulate dopamine receptors. These drugs are used as adjunctive therapy in Parkinson disease. They often are used for persons who have become refractory to levodopa or have developed an on–off phenomenon.

Selegiline is a monoamine oxidase type B inhibitor that inhibits the metabolic breakdown of dopamine. Selegiline may be used as adjunctive treatment to reduce mild on–off fluctuations in the responsiveness of persons who are receiving levodopa. It has been proposed that in inhibiting dopamine metabolism and the generation of destructive metabolites, selegiline also may delay the progression of the disease.

Anticholinergic drugs (*e.g.*, trihexyphenidyl, benztropine) are thought to restore a "balance" between reduced dopamine and uninhibited cholinergic neurons in the striatum. They are more useful in alleviating tremor and rigidity than bradykinesia. The anticholinergic drugs lessen the tremors and rigidity and afford some improvement of function. However, their potency seems to decrease over time, and increasing the dosage merely increases side effects such as blurred vision, dry mouth, bowel and bladder problems, and some mental changes.

Surgical treatment includes thalamotomy or pallidectomy that is performed using stereotactic surgery. With these procedures, part of the thalamus or globus pallidum in the basal ganglia is destroyed using an electrical stimulator or supercooled tip of a metal probe (cryothalamotomy). Brain mapping is done during the surgery to identify and prevent injury to sensory and motor tracts. Surgery is generally confined to one side of the brain and is usually restricted to persons who have failed to respond satisfactorily to drug therapy. Surgical transplantation of adrenal medullary tissue or fetal substantia nigra tissue is still experimental.

Increased neuronal activity of the subthalamic nuclei and the pars interna of the globus pallidus are thought to account for motor dysfunction in patients with Parkinson disease. Another surgical procedure involves the implantation of electrodes for deep brain stimulation into areas of the brain that are thought to account for rest tremors (thalamus) or motor dysfunction in Parkinson disease (subthalamic nuclei or the pars interna of the globus pallidus).[33] Electrical stimulation has the advantage of being reversible and of causing minimal or no damage to the brain.

DISORDERS OF THE CEREBELLUM

The functions of the cerebellum, or "little brain," are essential for smooth, coordinated, skillful movement. The cerebellum does not initiate activity, but it is responsible for smoothing the temporal and spatial aspects of rapid movement anywhere in the body. It influences the motor systems by evaluating disparities between intention and action and by adjusting the operation of motor centers in the brain while a movement is in progress as well as during repetition of the movement.[34]

The signs of cerebellar dysfunction can be grouped into three classes: vestibulocerebellar disorders, cerebellar ataxia or decomposition of movement, and cerebellar tremor. These disorders occur on the side of cerebellar damage, whether because of congenital defect, vascular accident, or growing tumor. The abnormality of movement occurs whether the eyes are open or closed. Visual monitoring of movement cannot compensate for cerebellar defects.

Damage to the part of the cerebellum associated with the vestibular system leads to difficulty or inability to maintain a steady posture of the trunk, which normally requires constant readjusting movements. This is seen as an unsteadiness of the trunk, called *truncal ataxia,* and it can be so severe that standing is not possible. The ability to fix the eyes on a target also can be affected. Constant conjugate readjustment of eye position, called *nystagmus,* results and makes reading extremely difficult, especially when the eyes are deviated toward the side of cerebellar damage.

Cerebellar ataxia and tremor are different aspects of defects in the smooth, continuously correcting functions. Cerebellar dystaxia or, if severe, ataxia includes a decomposition of movement; each succeeding component of a complex movement occurs separately instead of being blended into a smoothly proceeding action. Because ethanol specifically affects cerebellar function, persons who are inebriated often walk with a staggering and unsteady gait. Rapid alternating movements such as supination–pronation–supination of the hands are jerky and performed slowly (dysdiadochokinesia). Reaching to touch a target breaks down into small sequential components, each going too far, followed by overcorrection. The finger moves jerkily toward the target, misses, corrects in the other direction, and misses again, until the target is finally reached. This is called *over-and-under reaching,* and the general term is *dysmetria.*

Cerebellar tremor is a rhythmic back-and-forth movement of a finger or toe that worsens as the target is approached. The tremor results from the inability of the damaged cerebellar system to maintain ongoing fixation of a body part and to make smooth, continuous corrections in the trajectory of the movement; overcorrection occurs, first in one direction and then the other. Often, the tremor of an arm or leg can be detected during the beginning of an intended movement. The common term for cerebellar tremor is *intention tremor.* Cerebellar function as it relates to tremor can be assessed by asking a person to touch one heel to the opposite knee, to gently move the toes along the back of the opposite shin, or to move the hand so as to touch the nose with a finger.

Cerebellar function also can affect the motor skills of chewing and swallowing (dysphagia) and of speech (dysarthria). Normal speech requires smooth control of respiratory muscles and highly coordinated control of the laryngeal, lip, and tongue muscles. Cerebellar dysarthria is characterized by slow, slurred speech of continuously varying loudness. Rehabilitative efforts directed by speech therapists include learning to slow the rate of speech and to compensate as much as possible through the use of less-affected muscles.

In summary, alterations in coordination of muscle movements and abnormal muscle movements result from disorders of the cerebellum and basal ganglia. The basal ganglia organize basic movement patterns into more complex patterns and release them when commanded by the motor cortex, contributing gracefulness to cortically initiated and controlled skilled movements. Disorders of the basal ganglia are characterized by involuntary movements, alterations in muscle tone, and disturbances in posture. These disorders include tremor, tics, hemiballismus, chorea, athetosis, dystonias, and dyskinesias.

Parkinsonism, a disorder of the basal ganglia, is characterized by destruction of the nigrostriatal pathway, with a subsequent reduction in striatal concentrations of dopamine. This results in an imbalance between the inhibitory effects of dopaminergic basal ganglia functions and an increase in the excitatory cholinergic functions. The disorder is manifested by combinations of slowness of movement (*i.e.,* bradykinesia), increased muscle tonus and rigidity, rest tremor, gait disturbances, and impaired autonomic postural responses. The disease usually is slowly progressive over several decades, but the rate of progression varies from 2 to 30 years. The tremor often begins in one or both hands and then becomes generalized. Postural changes and gait disturbances continue to become more pronounced, resulting in significant disability.

The function of the cerebellum is essential for smooth, coordinated movements. Cerebellar disorders include vestibulocerebellar dysfunction, cerebellar ataxia, and cerebellar tremor.

Upper Motoneuron Disorders

After completing this section of the chapter, you should be able to meet the following objectives:

- Relate the pathologic UMN and LMN changes that occur in amyotrophic lateral sclerosis to the manifestations of the disease
- Explain the significance of demyelination and plaque formation in multiple sclerosis
- Describe the manifestations of multiple sclerosis
- Relate the structures of the vertebral column to mechanisms of spinal cord injury
- Explain how loss of UMN function contributes to the muscle spasms that occur after recovery from spinal cord injury
- State the effects of spinal cord injury on ventilation and communication, the autonomic nervous system, cardiovascular function, sensorimotor function, and bowel, bladder, and sexual function

AMYOTROPHIC LATERAL SCLEROSIS

Amyotrophic lateral sclerosis (ALS), also known as *Lou Gehrig's disease* after the famous New York Yankees baseball player, is a devastating neurologic disorder that selectively affects motor function. There are approximately 5000 new cases of ALS in the United States each year.[35] ALS is primarily a disorder of middle to late adulthood, affecting persons between 55 and 60 years of age, with men developing the disease nearly twice as often as women. The disease typically follows a progressive course, with a mean survival period of 2 to 5 years from the onset of symptoms.

ALS affects motoneurons in three locations: the anterior horn cells of the spinal cord; the motor nuclei of the brain stem, particularly the hypoglossal nuclei; and the UMNs of the cerebral cortex. The fact that the disease is more extensive in the distal parts of the affected tracts in the lower spinal cord rather than the proximal parts suggests that affected neurons first undergo degeneration at their distal terminals and that the disease proceeds in a centripetal direction until ultimately the parent nerve cell dies. A remarkable feature of the disease is that the entire sensory system, the regulatory mechanisms of control and coordination of movement, and the intellect remain intact. The neurons for ocular motility and the parasympathetic neurons in the sacral spinal cord also are spared.

The death of LMNs leads to denervation, with subsequent shrinkage of musculature and muscle fiber atrophy. It is this fiber atrophy, called *amyotrophy,* which appears in the name of the disease. The loss of nerve fibers in lateral columns of the white matter of the spinal cord, along with fibrillary gliosis, imparts a firmness or sclerosis to this CNS tissue; the term *lateral sclerosis* designates these changes.

The cause of LMN and UMN destruction in ALS is uncertain. Five to 10% of cases are familial; the others are believed to be sporadic, with no family history of the disease. Recently, mutation to a gene encoding superoxide dismutase 1 (*SOD1*) was mapped to chromosome 21. This enzyme functions in the prevention of free radical formation (see Chapter 5). The mutation accounts for 20% of familial ALS, with the remaining 80% being caused by mutations in other genes.[36] Five percent of persons with sporadic ALS also have *SOD1* mutations. Possible targets of *SOD1*-induced toxicity include the neurofilament proteins, which function in the axonal transport of molecules necessary for the maintenance of axons.[36] Another suggested mechanism of pathogenesis in ALS is exotoxic injury through activation of glutamate-gated ion channels, which are distinguished by their sensitivity to *N*-methyl-D-aspartic acid (see Chapter 52). The possibility of glutamate excitotoxicity in the pathogenesis of ALS was suggested by the finding of increased glutamine levels in the cerebrospinal fluid of patients with sporadic ALS.[36] Although autoimmunity has been suggested as a cause of ALS, the disease does not respond to the immunosuppressant agents that normally are used in treatment of autoimmune disorders.

The symptoms of ALS may be referable to UMN or LMN involvement. Manifestations of UMN lesions include weakness, spasticity or stiffness, and impaired fine motor control.[35,37] Dysphagia (difficulty swallowing), dysarthria (impaired articulation of speech), and dysphonia (difficulty making the sounds of speech) may result from brain stem LMN involvement or from dysfunction of UMNs descending to the brain stem. Manifestations of LMN destruction include fasciculations, weakness, muscle atrophy, and hyporeflexia. Muscle cramps involving the distal legs often are an early symptom. The most common clinical presentation is slowly progressive weakness and atrophy in distal muscles of one upper extremity. This is followed by regional spread of clinical weakness, reflecting involvement of neighboring areas of the spinal cord. Eventually, UMNs and LMNs involving multiple limbs and the head are affected. In the more advanced stages, muscles of the palate, pharynx, tongue, neck, and shoulders become involved, causing impairment of chewing, swallowing, and speech. Dysphagia with recurrent aspiration and weakness of the respiratory muscles produces the most significant acute complications of the disease. Death usually results from involvement of cranial and respiratory musculature.

Currently, there is no cure for ALS. Rehabilitation measures assist persons with the disorder to manage their disability, and respiratory and nutritional support allows persons with the disorder to survive longer than would otherwise have been the case. An antiglutamate drug, riluzole, is the only drug approved by the U.S. Food and Drug Administration (FDA) for treatment of ALS. The drug is designed to decrease glutamate accumulation and slow the progression of the disease. In two therapeutic trials, the drug prolonged survival by 3 to 6 months.[36]

DEMYELINATING DISORDERS

Multiple Sclerosis

Multiple sclerosis (MS), a demyelinating disease of the CNS, is the most common nontraumatic cause of neurologic disability among young and middle-aged adults. Approximately two thirds of persons with MS experience their first symptoms between 20 and 40 years of age. Sometimes, a diagnosis may be delayed until the fourth or fifth decade because symptoms were short lasting or were not bothersome enough to warrant medical attention. In these cases, a detailed medical history usually reveals that symptoms did appear previously. In approximately 80% of the cases, the disease is characterized by exacerbations and remissions over many years in several different sites in the CNS.[38] Initially, there is normal or near-normal neurologic function between exacerbations. As the disease progresses, there is less improvement between exacerbations and increasing neurologic dysfunction.

Epidemiologic Features. The prevalence of MS varies considerably around the world. The disease is more prevalent in the colder northern latitudes; it is more common in the northern Atlantic states, the Great Lakes region, and the Pacific Northwest than in the southern parts of the United States. Other high-incidence areas include northern Europe, Great Britain, southern Australia, and New Zealand.[5,38] Estimates of the total number of cases of MS in the United States range from 250,000 to 350,000.[5,39,40] The incidence among women is almost double that among men. Migration studies have shown that persons who move from a high-risk area tend to retain the risk of their birthplace if they move after 15 years of age, or adopt the risk of their new home if they migrate as children.[5]

Genetic Factors. Although MS is not directly inherited, there is a familial predisposition in some cases, suggesting a genetic influence on susceptibility. Also, the severity and course of the disease may be influenced by genetic factors. The risk for developing MS is 15 times greater when the disease is present in a first-degree relative.[5] The concordance rate for monozygotic twins is approximately 30%, compared with 5% for dizygotic twins.[38] There also is a strong association between MS and certain human leukocyte antigens (HLAs; see Chapter 19). The presence of the HLA-DR2 allele substantially increases the risk for development of MS.[38] Presumably, class II HLA genes regulate the autoimmune response.[5]

Pathophysiology. The pathophysiology of MS involves the demyelination of nerve fibers in the white matter of the brain, spinal cord, and optic nerve. In the CNS, myelin is formed by the oligodendrocytes, chiefly those lying among the nerve fibers in the white matter. This function is equivalent to that of the Schwann cells in the peripheral nervous system (see Chapter 49). The properties of the myelin sheath—high electrical resistance and low capacitance—permit it to function as an electrical insulator. Demyelinated nerve fibers display a variety of conduction abnormalities, ranging from decreased conduction velocity to conduction blocks, resulting in a variety of symptoms that depend on the location and duration of the lesion.

The lesions of MS consist of hard, sharp-edged demyelinated or sclerotic patches that are macroscopically visible throughout the white matter of the CNS[5] (Fig. 51-13). These lesions, which represent the end result of acute myelin breakdown, are called *plaques*. The lesions have a predilection for the optic nerves, periventricular white matter, brain stem, cerebellum, and spinal cord white matter.[38] In an active plaque, there is evidence of ongoing myelin breakdown. The sequence of myelin breakdown is not well understood, although it is known that the lesions contain small amounts of myelin basic proteins and increased amounts of proteolytic enzymes, macrophages, lymphocytes, and plasma cells. Oligodendrocytes are decreased in number and may be absent, especially in older lesions. Acute, subacute, and chronic lesions often are seen at multiple sites throughout the CNS.

Magnetic resonance imaging has shown that the lesions of MS may occur in two stages: a first stage that involves the sequential development of small inflammatory lesions, and a second stage during which the lesions extend and consolidate and when demyelination and gliosis (scar formation) occur. It is not known whether the inflammatory process, present during the first stage, is directed against the myelin or against the oligodendrocytes that produce myelin. Remyelination of the nervous system was considered to be impossible until the late 1990s. Evidence now suggests that remyelination can occur in the CNS if the process that initiated the demyelination is halted before the oligodendrocyte dies.[41]

Multiple sclerosis generally is believed to be an immune-mediated disorder that occurs in genetically susceptible individuals. However, the sequence of events that initiates the process is largely unknown. The demyelination process in MS is marked by prominent lymphocytic invasion in the lesion. The infiltrate in plaques contains both $CD8^+$ and $CD4^+$ T cells as well as macrophages. Both macrophages and cytotoxic $CD8^+$ T cells are thought to induce oligodendrocyte injury. There also is evidence of antibody-mediated damage involving myelin oligodendroglial protein.[5]

Manifestations and Clinical Course. The interruption of neural conduction in the demyelinated nerves is manifested by a variety of symptoms, depending on the location and extent of the lesion. Areas commonly affected by MS are the optic nerve (visual field), corticobulbar tracts (speech and swallowing), corticospinal tracts (muscle strength), cerebellar tracts (gait and coordination), spinocerebellar tracts (balance), medial longitudinal fasciculus (conjugate gaze function of the extraocular eye muscles), and posterior cell columns of the spinal cord (position and vibratory sensation). Typically, an otherwise healthy person presents with an acute or subacute episode of paresthesias, optic neuritis (*i.e.,* visual clouding or loss of vision in part of the visual field with pain on movement of the globe), diplopia, or specific types of gaze paralysis.

Paresthesias are evidenced as numbness, tingling, a burning sensation, or pressure on the face or involved extremities; symptoms can range from annoying to severe. *Lhermitte's symptom* is an electric shock–like tingling down the back and onto the legs that is produced by flexion of the neck. Pain from spasticity also may be a factor that can be aided by appropriate stretching exercises. Although pain may not be a prominent symptom, approximately 80% of persons with MS experience some pain in the course of the disease. Other common symptoms are abnormal gait, bladder and sexual dysfunction, vertigo, nystagmus, fatigue, and speech disturbance. These symptoms usually last for several days to weeks, and then completely or partially resolve. After a period of normal or relatively normal function, new symptoms appear. Psychological manifestations, such as mood swings, may represent an emotional reaction to the nature of the disease or, more likely, involvement of the white matter of the cerebral cortex. Depression, euphoria, inattentiveness, apathy, forgetfulness, and loss of memory may occur.

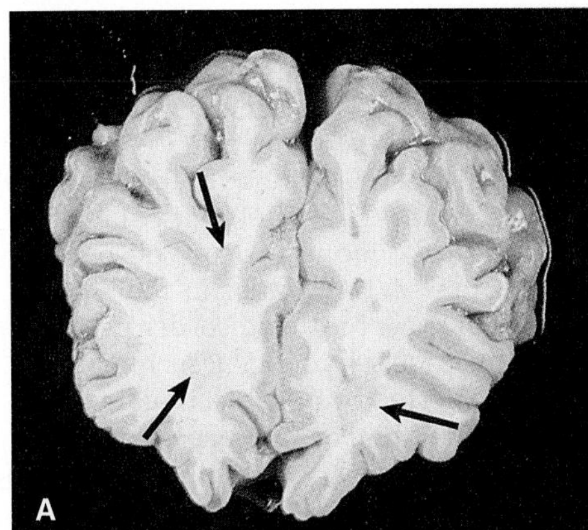

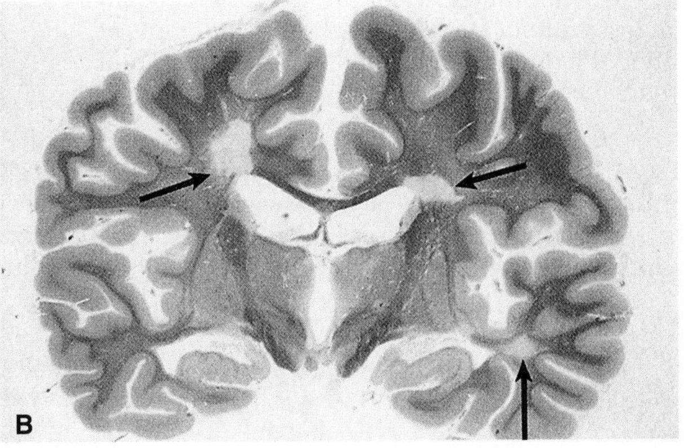

FIGURE 51-13 Multiple sclerosis. (**A**) In this unfixed brain, the plaques of multiple sclerosis in the white matter (*arrows*) assume the darker color of the cerebral cortex. (**B**) A coronal section of the brain from a patient with long-standing multiple sclerosis, which has been stained for myelin, shows discrete areas of demyelination (*arrows*) with characteristic involvement of the superior angles of the lateral ventricles. (Rubin E., Farber J.L [1999]. *Pathology* [3rd ed., p. 1497]. Philadelphia: Lippincott-Raven).

Fatigue is one of the most common problems for persons with MS. Fatigue often is described as a generalized low-energy feeling not related to depression and different from weakness. Fatigue has a harmful impact on activities of daily living and sustained physical activity. Interventions such as spacing activities and setting priorities often are helpful.

The course of the disease may fall into one of four categories: relapsing-remitting, secondary progressive, primary progressive, or progressive relapsing.[41,42] The *relapsing-remitting* form of the disease is characterized by episodes of acute worsening with recovery and a stable course between relapses. *Secondary progressive disease* involves a gradual neurologic deterioration with or without superimposed acute relapses in a person with previous relapsing-remitting disease. *Primary progressive disease* is characterized by nearly continuous neurologic deterioration from onset of symptoms. The *progressive relapsing* category of disease involves gradual neurologic deterioration from the onset of symptoms but with subsequent superimposed relapses.

Diagnosis. The diagnosis of MS is based on established clinical and, when necessary, laboratory criteria. Advances in cerebrospinal fluid analysis and MRI have greatly simplified the procedure. A definite diagnosis of MS requires evidence of one of the following patterns: two or more episodes of exacerbation separated by 1 month or more and lasting more than 24 hours, with subsequent recovery; a clinical history of clearly defined exacerbations and remissions, with or without complete recovery, followed by progression of symptoms over a period of at least 6 months; or slow and stepwise progression of signs and symptoms over a period of at least 6 months.[43] Primary progressive MS may be suggested by a progressive course that lasts longer than 6 months. A person who has not had a relapse or progression of symptoms is described as having stable MS.

Magnetic resonance imaging can be used as an adjunct to clinical diagnosis. MRI studies can detect the multiplicity of lesions even when CT scans appear normal. A computer-assisted method of MRI can measure lesion size. Many new areas of myelin abnormality are asymptomatic. Serial MRI studies can be done to detect asymptomatic lesions, monitor the progress of existing lesions, and evaluate the effectiveness of treatment. Although MRI can be used to provide evidence of disseminated lesions in persons with the disease, normal findings do not exclude the diagnosis.[43] Electrophysiologic evaluations (*e.g.,* evoked potential studies) and CT scans may assist in the identification and documentation of lesions.

Although no laboratory test can be used to diagnose MS, examination of the cerebrospinal fluid is helpful. A large percentage of patients with MS have elevated immunoglobulin G (IgG) levels, and some have oligoclonal patterns (*i.e.,* discrete electrophoretic bands) even with normal IgG levels. Total protein or lymphocyte levels may be mildly elevated in the cerebrospinal fluid. These test results can be altered in a variety of inflammatory neurologic disorders and are not specific for MS.

Treatment. Most treatment measures for MS are directed at modifying the course and managing the primary symptoms of the disease. The variety of symptoms, unpredictable course, and lack of specific diagnostic methods have made the evaluation and treatment of MS difficult. Persons who are minimally affected by the disorder require no specific treatment. The person should be encouraged to maintain as healthy a lifestyle as possible, including good nutrition and adequate rest and relaxation. Physical therapy may help maintain muscle tone. Every effort should be made to avoid excessive fatigue, physical deterioration, emotional stress, viral infections, and extremes of environmental temperature, which may precipitate an exacerbation of the disease.

The pharmacologic agents used in the treatment of MS fall into four categories: (1) those used to treat acute symptoms of the disease, (2) those used to modify the course of the disease, (3) those used to interrupt progressive disease, and (4) those used to treat the symptoms of the disorder.[42] Corticosteroids are the mainstay of treatment for acute relapses of MS. These agents are thought to reduce the inflammation, improve nerve conduction, and have important immunologic effects. Long-term administration does not, however, appear to alter the course of the disease and can have harmful side effects. Adrenocorticotropic hormone (ACTH) also may be used in treatment of MS. Plasmapheresis has proved beneficial in some cases.

The agents used to modify the course of the disease include interferon-beta and glatiramer acetate.[40] Both agents have shown some benefit in reducing exacerbations in persons with relapsing-remitting MS. Interferon-beta is a cytokine that acts as an immune enhancer. Two forms of recombinant interferon have been approved by the FDA for treatment of MS—interferon-beta-1a and interferon-beta-1b. Both types of interferon are administered by injection, and both are usually well tolerated. The most common side effects are flulike symptoms for 24 to 48 hours after each injection, and these usually subside after 2 to 3 months of treatment. Glatiramer acetate is a synthetic polypeptide that simulates parts of the myelin basic protein. Although the exact mechanism of action is unknown, the drug seems to block myelin-damaging T cells by acting as a myelin decoy. The drug is given daily by subcutaneous injection.

Progressive MS may be treated with immunosuppressive drugs such as methotrexate, cyclophosphamide, mitoxantrone, and cyclosporine.[44] Among the medications used to relieve symptoms associated with MS are dantrolene (Dantrium), baclofen (Lioresal), or diazepam (Valium) for spasticity; cholinergic drugs for bladder problems; and antidepressant drugs for depression.

SPINAL CORD INJURY

Spinal cord injury (SCI) represents damage to the neural elements of the spinal cord. SCI is primarily a disorder of young adults, with about 53% of cases occurring among persons in the 16- to 30-year age group. The most common cause of SCI is motor vehicle accidents, followed by falls, violence (primarily gunshot wounds), and recreational sporting activities.[45] Life expectancy for persons with SCI continues to increase, but is somewhat below life expectancy for those without SCI. Mortality rates are significantly higher during the first year after injury than during subsequent years, particularly for severely injured persons.[45]

Most SCIs involve damage to the vertebral column or supporting ligaments as well as the spinal cord. Because of extensive tract systems that connect sensory afferent neurons and LMNs with high brain centers, SCIs commonly involve both sensory and motor function.

Injury to the Vertebral Column

Injuries to the vertebral column include fractures, dislocations, and subluxations. A fracture can occur at any part of the bony vertebrae, causing fragmentation of the bone. It most often involves the pedicle, lamina, or processes (*e.g.,* facets). Dislocation or subluxation (partial dislocation) injury causes the vertebral bodies to become displaced, with one overriding another and preventing correct alignment of the vertebral column. Damage to the ligaments or bony vertebrae may make the spine unstable. In an unstable spine, further unguarded movement of the spinal column can impinge on the spinal canal, causing compression or overstretching of neural tissue.

Most injuries result from some combination of compressive force or bending movement.[46] Flexion injuries occur when forward bending of the spinal column exceeds the limits of normal movement. Typical flexion injuries result, for example, when the head is struck from behind, as in a fall with the back of the head as the point of impact. Extension injuries occur with excessive forced bending (*i.e.,* hyperextension) of the spine backward. A typical extension injury involves a fall in which the chin or face is the point of impact, causing hyperextension of the neck. Injuries of flexion and extension occur more commonly in the cervical spine (C4 to C6) than in any other area. Limitations imposed by the ribs, spinous processes, and joint capsules in the thoracic and lumbar spine make this area less flexible and less susceptible to flexion and extension injuries than the cervical spine.

A compression injury, causing the vertebral bones to shatter, squash, or even burst, occurs when there is spinal loading from a high-velocity blow to the top of the head or when landing forcefully on the feet or buttocks[46] (Fig. 51-14A). This typically occurs at the cervical level (*e.g.,* diving injuries) or in the thoracolumbar area (*e.g.,* falling from a distance and landing on the buttocks). Compression injuries may occur when the vertebrae are weakened by conditions such as osteoporosis and cancer with bone metastasis. Axial rotation injuries can produce highly unstable injuries. Maximal axial rotation occurs in the cervical region, especially between C1 and C2 and at the lumbosacral joint[46] (see Fig. 51-14B). Coupling of vertebral motions is common in injury when two or more individual motions occur (*e.g.,* lateral bending and axial rotation).

Acute Spinal Cord Injury

Spinal cord injury involves damage to the neural elements of the spinal cord. The damage may result from direct trauma to the cord from penetrating wounds or indirect injury resulting from vertebral fractures, fracture-dislocations, or subluxations of the spine. The spinal cord may be contused, not only at the site of injury but also above and below the trauma site[46] (Fig. 51-15). Traumatic injury may be complicated by blood flow to the cord, with resulting infarction.

Sudden complete transection of the spinal cord results in complete loss of motor, sensory, reflex, and autonomic function below the level of injury. This immediate response to spinal cord injury is often referred to as *spinal cord shock.* It is characterized by flaccid paralysis with loss of tendon reflexes below the level of injury, absence of

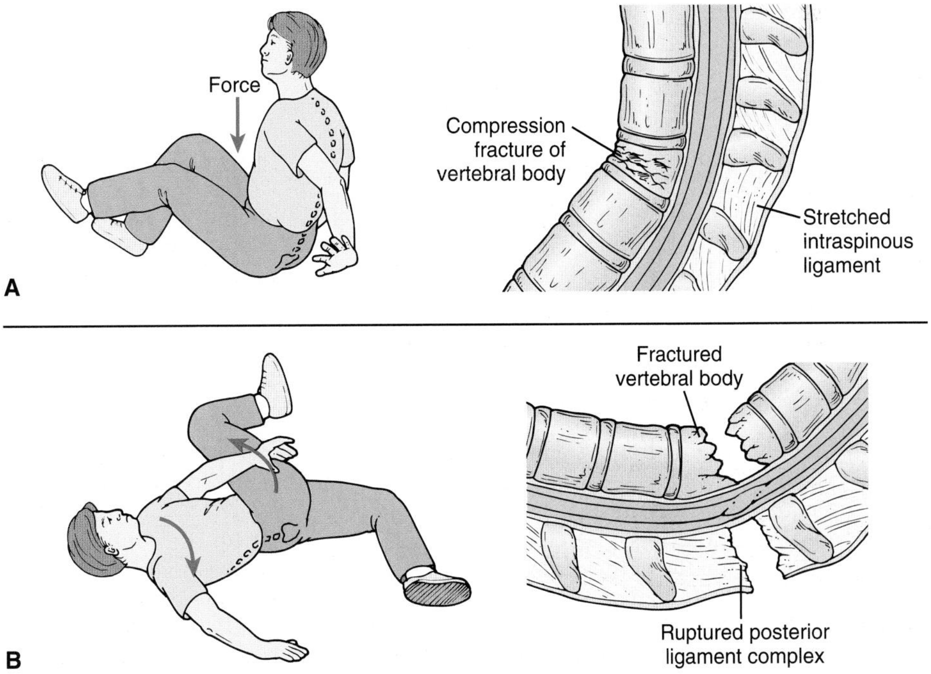

FIGURE 51-14 (**A**) Compression vertebral fracture secondary to axial loading as occurs when a person falls from a height and lands on the buttocks. (**B**) Rotational injury, in which there is concurrent fracture and tearing of the posterior ligamentous complex, is caused by extreme lateral flexion or twisting of the head or neck. (Modified from Hickey J.V. [2003]. *The clinical practice of neurological and neurosurgical nursing.* [5th ed., pp. 411–412]. Philadelphia: Lippincott Williams & Wilkins)

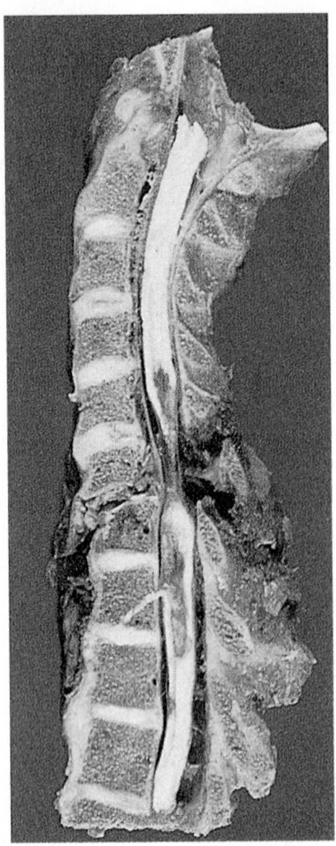

FIGURE 51-15 Cervical contusion. Hyperflexion injury caused forward angulation of the cervical cord, with fracture of the anterior lip of the underlying vertebral body. The cord is angulated over the superior-posterior ridge of the fixed underlying cervical body. (Rubin E., Farber J.L. [1999]. *Pathology* [3rd ed., p. 1465]. Philadelphia: Lippincott-Raven).

somatic and visceral sensations below the level of injury, and loss of bowel and bladder function. Loss of systemic sympathetic vasomotor tone may result in vasodilation, increased venous capacity, and hypotension. These manifestations occur regardless of whether the level of the lesion eventually will produce spastic (UMN) or flaccid (LMN) paralysis. The basic mechanisms accounting for transient spinal shock are unknown. Spinal shock may last for hours, days, or weeks. Usually, if reflex function returns by the time the person reaches the hospital, the neuromuscular changes are reversible. This type of reversible spinal shock may occur in football-type injuries, in which jarring of the spinal cord produces a concussion-like syndrome with loss of movement and reflexes, followed by full recovery within days. In persons in whom the loss of reflexes persists, hypotension and bradycardia may become critical but manageable problems. In general, the higher the level of injury, the greater is the effect.

Pathophysiology. The pathophysiology of acute SCI can be divided into two types: primary and secondary.[47–49] The *primary neurologic injury* occurs at the time of mechanical injury and is irreversible. It is characterized by small hemorrhages in the gray matter of the cord, followed by edematous changes in the white matter that lead to necrosis of neural tissue. This type of pathology results from the forces of compression, stretch, and shear associated with fracture or compression of the spinal vertebrae, dislocation of vertebrae (*e.g.,* flexion, extension, subluxation), and contusions due to jarring of the cord in the spinal canal. Penetrating injuries produce lacerations and direct trauma to the cord and may occur with or without spinal column damage. Lacerations occur when there is cutting or tearing of the spinal cord, which injures nerve tissue and causes bleeding and edema.

Secondary injuries follow the primary injury and promote the spread of injury. Although there is considerable debate about the pathogenesis of secondary injuries, the tissue destruction that occurs ends in progressive neurologic damage. After SCI, several pathologic mechanisms come into play, including vascular damage, neuronal injury that leads to loss of reflexes below the level of injury, and release of vasoactive agents and cellular enzymes. Vascular pathology (*i.e.,* vessel trauma and hemorrhage) can lead to ischemia, increased vascular permeability, and edema. Blood flow to the spinal cord may be further compromised by spinal shock that results from a loss of vasomotor tone and neural reflexes below the level of injury. The release of vasoactive substances (*i.e.,* norepinephrine, serotonin, dopamine, and histamine) from the wound tissue causes vasospasm and impedes blood flow in the microcirculation, producing further necrosis of blood vessels and neurons. The release of proteolytic and lipolytic enzymes from injured cells causes delayed swelling, demyelination, and necrosis in the neural tissue in the spinal cord.

Management. The goal of management of acute SCI is to reduce the neurologic deficit and prevent any additional loss of neurologic function. The specific steps in resuscitation and initial evaluation can be carried out at the trauma site or in the emergency room, depending on the urgency of the situation.[46,50] Most traumatic injuries to the spinal column render it unstable, mandating measures such as immobilization with collars and backboards and limiting the movement of persons at risk for or with known SCI. Every person with multiple trauma or head injury, including victims of traffic and sporting accidents, should be suspected of having sustained an acute SCI.[46,50]

The nature of the injury determines further methods of stabilization and treatment. In unstable injuries of the cervical spine, cervical traction improves or restores spinal alignment, decompresses neural structures, and facilitates recovery. Fractures and dislocations of the thoracic and lumbar vertebrae may be initially stabilized by restricting the person to bed rest and turning him or her in a log-rolling manner to keep the spine rigid. Gunshot or stab wounds of the spinal column may not produce structural instability and require immobilization. The goal of early surgical intervention for an unstable spine is to provide internal skeletal stabilization so that early mobilization and rehabilitation can occur.

One of the more important aspects of early SCI care is the prevention and treatment of spinal or systemic shock and the hypoxia associated with compromised respiration. Correcting hypotension or hypoxia is essential to maintaining circulation to the injured cord.[49–51] The use of high-dose methylprednisolone has been shown to improve the outcome from SCI when given shortly after injury. Methylprednisolone is a short-acting corticosteroid that has been used extensively in the treatment of inflammatory and allergic disorders.[52,53] In acute SCI, it is thought to stabilize cell membranes, enhance impulse generation, improve blood flow, and inhibit free radical formation.

Types and Classification of Spinal Cord Injury

Alterations in body function that result from SCI depend on the level of injury and the amount of cord involvement. *Tetraplegia,* sometimes referred to as *quadriplegia,* is the impairment or loss of motor or sensory function (or both) after damage to neural structures in the cervical segments of the spinal cord.[54] It results in impairment of function in the arms, trunk, legs, and pelvic organs (see Fig. 51-4). *Paraplegia* refers to impairment or loss of motor or sensory function (or both) in the thoracic, lumbar, or sacral segments of the spinal cord from damage of neural elements in the spinal canal. With paraplegia, arm functioning is spared, but depending on the level of injury, functioning of the trunk, legs, and pelvic organs may be involved. Paraplegia includes conus medullaris and cauda equina injuries (discussed later).

Further definitions of SCI describe the extent of neurologic damage as *complete* or *incomplete.* Complete SCI implies there is an absence of motor and sensory function below the level of injury. Complete cord injuries can result from severance of the cord, disruption of nerve fibers although they remain intact, or interruption of blood supply to that segment, resulting in complete destruction of neural tissue and UMN or LMN paralysis. Approximately 3% of persons with signs of complete injuries on initial examination experience some recovery within 24 hours.[48]

Incomplete SCI implies there is some residual motor or sensory function below the level of injury.[48] The prognosis for return of function is better in an incomplete injury because of preservation of axonal function. Incomplete injuries may manifest in a variety of patterns but can be organized into certain patterns or "syndromes" that occur more frequently and reflect the predominant area of the cord that is involved. Types of incomplete lesions include the central cord syndrome, anterior cord syndrome, Brown-Séquard syndrome, and conus medullaris syndrome.

Central Cord Syndrome. A condition called *central cord syndrome* occurs when injury is predominantly in the central gray or white matter of the cord[46] (Fig. 51-16). Because the corticospinal tract fibers are organized with those controlling the arms located more centrally and those controlling the legs located more laterally, some external axonal transmission may remain intact. Motor function of the upper extremities is affected, but the lower extremities may not be affected or may be affected to a lesser degree, with some sparing of sacral sensation. Bowel, bladder, and sexual functions usually are affected to various degrees and may parallel the degree of lower extremity involvement. This syndrome occurs almost exclusively in the cervical cord, rendering the lesion a UMN lesion with spastic paralysis. Central cord damage is more frequent in elderly persons with narrowing or stenotic changes in the spinal canal that are related to arthritis. Damage also may occur in persons with congenital stenosis.

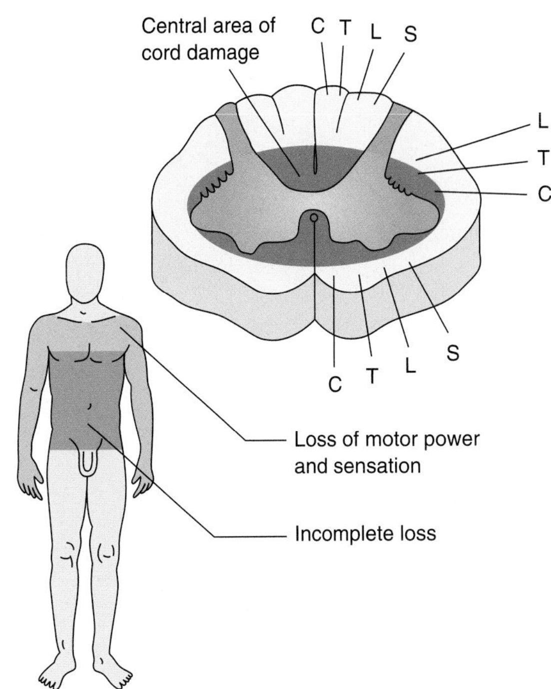

FIGURE 51-16 Central cord syndrome. A cross-section of the cord shows central damage and the associated motor and sensory loss. (C, cervical; T, thoracic; L, lumbar; S, sacral). (Hickey J.V. [1997]. *The clinical practice of neurological and neurosurgical nursing.* [3rd ed.]. Philadelphia: J.B. Lippincott)

Anterior Cord Syndrome. Anterior cord syndrome usually is caused by damage from infarction of the anterior spinal artery, resulting in damage to the anterior two thirds of the cord[46] (Fig. 51-17). The deficits result in loss of motor function provided by the corticospinal tracts and loss of pain and temperature sensation from damage to the lateral spinothalamic tracts. The posterior one third of the cord is relatively unaffected, preserving the dorsal column axons that convey position, vibration, and touch sensation.

Brown-Séquard Syndrome. A condition called *Brown-Séquard syndrome* results from damage to a hemisection of the anterior and posterior cord[46] (Fig. 51-18). The effect is a loss of voluntary motor function from the corticospinal tract, proprioception loss from the ipsilateral side of the body, and contralateral loss of pain and temperature sensation from the lateral spinothalamic tracts for all levels below the lesion.

Conus Medullaris Syndrome. The conus medullaris syndrome involves damage to the conus medullaris or the sacral cord (*i.e.,* conus) and lumbar nerve roots in the neural canal. Functional deficits resulting from this type of injury usually result in flaccid bowel, bladder, and sexual function. Sacral segments occasionally show preserved

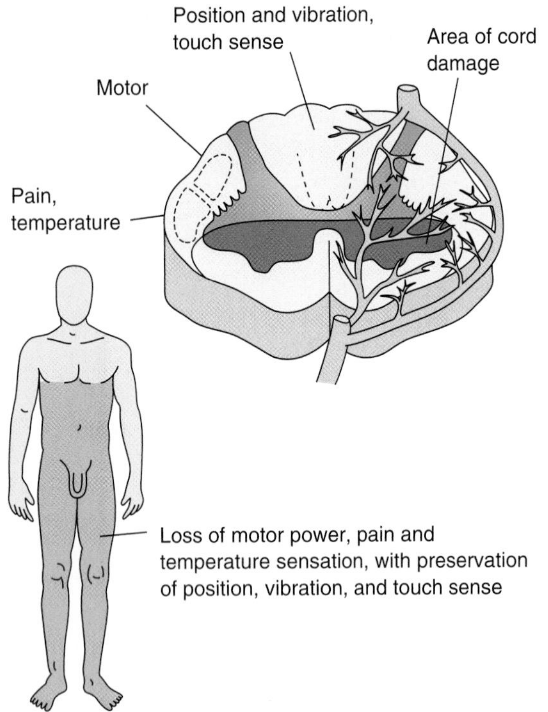

FIGURE 51-17 Anterior cord syndrome. Cord damage and associated motor and sensory loss are illustrated. (Hickey J.V. [1997]. *The clinical practice of neurological and neurosurgical nursing.* [3rd ed.]. Philadelphia: J.B. Lippincott)

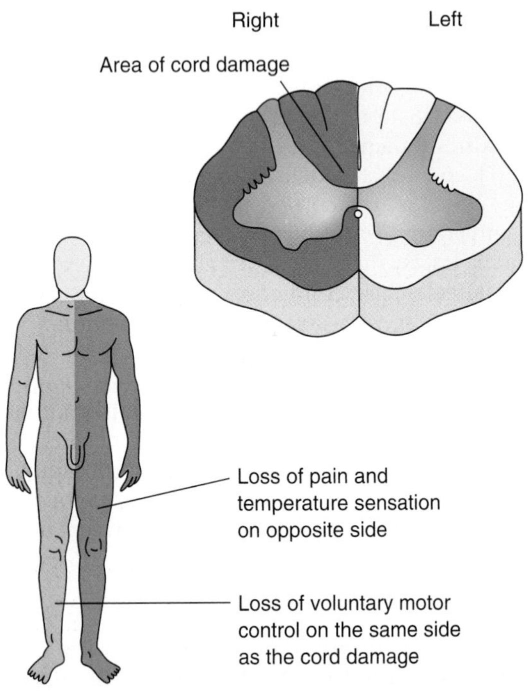

FIGURE 51-18 Brown-Séquard syndrome. Cord damage and associated motor and sensory loss are illustrated. (Hickey J.V. [1997]. *The clinical practice of neurological and neurosurgical nursing.* [3rd ed.]. Philadelphia: J.B. Lippincott)

reflexes if only the conus is affected. Motor function in the legs and feet may be impaired without significant sensory impairment. Damage to the lumbosacral nerve roots in the spinal canal usually results in LMN and sensory neuron damage known as *cauda equina syndrome.* Functional deficits present as various patterns of asymmetric flaccid paralysis, sensory impairment, and pain.

Disruption of Functional Abilities

Functional abilities after SCI are subject to various degrees of somatosensory and skeletal muscle function loss and altered reflex activity based on the level of cord injury and extent of cord damage (Table 51-2).

Motor and Somatosensory Function. Motor function in cervical injuries ranges from complete dependence to independence with or without assistive devices in activities of mobility and self-care. The functional levels of cervical injury are related to C5, C6, C7, or C8 innervation. At the C5 level, deltoid and biceps function is spared, allowing full head, neck, and diaphragm control with good shoulder strength and full elbow flexion. At the C6 level, wrist dorsiflexion by the way of wrist extensors is functional, allowing tenodesis, which is the natural bending inward and flexion of the fingers when the wrist is extended and bent backward. Tenodesis is a key movement because it can be used to pick up objects when finger movement is absent. A functional C7 injury allows full elbow flexion and extension, wrist plantar flexion, and some finger control. At the C8 level, finger flexion is added.

Thoracic cord injuries (T1 to T12) allow full upper extremity control with limited to full control of intercostal and trunk muscles and balance. Injury at the T1 level allows full fine motor control of the fingers. Because of the lack of specific functional indicators at the thoracic levels, the level of injury usually is determined by sensory level testing.

Functional capacity in the L1 through L5 nerve innervations allows hip flexors, hip abductors (L1 to L3), movement of the knees (L2 to L5), and ankle dorsiflexion (L4 to L5). Sacral (S1 to S5) innervation allows for full leg, foot, and ankle control and innervation of perineal musculature for bowel, bladder, and sexual function.

Reflex Activity. Spinal cord reflexes are fully integrated within the spinal cord and can function independent of input from higher centers. Altered spinal reflex activity following SCI is essentially determined by the level of injury and whether UMNs or LMNs are affected. With UMN injuries at T12 and above, the cord reflexes remain intact, whereas communication pathways with higher centers have been interrupted. This results in spasticity of involved skeletal muscle groups and of smooth and skeletal muscles that control bowel, bladder, and sexual function. In LMN injuries at T12 or below, the reflex circuitry itself has been damaged at the level of the spinal cord or spinal nerve, resulting in a decrease or absence of reflex function. The LMN injuries cause flaccid paralysis of involved skeletal muscle groups and the smooth and skeletal muscles that control bowel, bladder, and sexual function. However, injuries near the T12 level may result in mixed UMN and

TABLE 51-2 Functional Abilities by Level of Cord Injury

Injury Level	Segmental Sensorimotor Function	Dressing, Eating	Elimination	Mobility*
C1	Little or no sensation or control of head and neck; no diaphragm control; requires continuous ventilation	Dependent	Dependent	Limited. Voice or sip-n-puff controlled electric wheelchair
C2 to C3	Head and neck sensation; some neck control. Independent of mechanical ventilation for short periods	Dependent	Dependent	Same as for C1
C4	Good head and neck sensation and motor control; some shoulder elevation; diaphragm movement	Dependent; may be able to eat with adaptive sling	Dependent	Limited to voice, mouth, head, chin, or shoulder-controlled electric wheelchair
C5	Full head and neck control; shoulder strength; elbow flexion	Independent with assistance	Maximal assistance	Electric or modified manual wheelchair, needs transfer assistance
C6	Fully innervated shoulder; wrist extension or dorsiflexion	Independent or with minimal assistance	Independent or with minimal assistance	Independent in transfers and wheelchair
C7 to C8	Full elbow extension; wrist plantar flexion; some finger control	Independent	Independent	Independent; manual wheelchair
T1 to T5	Full hand and finger control; use of intercostal and thoracic muscles	Independent	Independent	Independent; manual wheelchair
T6 to T10	Abdominal muscle control, partial to good balance with trunk muscles	Independent	Independent	Independent; manual wheelchair
T11 to L5	Hip flexors, hip abductors (L1–3); knee extension (L2–4); knee flexion and ankle dorsiflexion (L4–5)	Independent	Independent	Short distance to full ambulation with assistance
S1 to S5	Full leg, foot, and ankle control; innervation of perineal muscles for bowel, bladder, and sexual function (S2–4)	Independent	Normal to impaired bowel and bladder function	Ambulate independently with or without assistance

*Assistance refers to adaptive equipment, setup, or physical assistance.

LMN deficits (*e.g.,* spastic paralysis of the bowel and bladder with flaccid muscle tone).

After the period of spinal shock in a UMN injury, isolated spinal reflex activity and muscle tone that is not under the control of higher centers return. This may result in hypertonia and spasticity of skeletal muscles below the level of injury.[46] These spastic movements are involuntary instead of voluntary, a distinction that needs to be explained to persons with SCI and their families. The antigravity muscles, the flexors of the arms and extensors of the legs, are predominantly affected. Spastic movements are usually heightened initially after injury, reaching a peak and then becoming stable in approximately 1.5 to 2 years.[46]

The stimuli for reflex muscle spasm arise from somatic and visceral afferent pathways that enter the cord below the level of injury. The most common of these stimuli are muscle stretching, bladder infections or stones, fistulas, bowel distention or impaction, pressure areas or irritation of the skin, and infections. Because the stimuli that precipitate spasms vary from person to person, careful assessment needs to be done to identify the factors that precipitate spasm in each person. Passive range-of-motion exercises to stretch the spastic muscles help to prevent spasm induced by muscle stretching such as occurs with a change in body position.

Spasticity in and of itself is not detrimental and may even facilitate maintenance of muscle tone to prevent muscle wasting, improve venous return, and aid in mobility. Spasms become detrimental when they impair safety; they reduce the ability to make functional gains in mobility and activities of daily living. Spasms also may cause trauma to bones and tissues, leading to joint contractures and skin breakdown.

Respiratory Muscle Function. Ventilation requires movement of the expiratory and inspiratory muscles, all of which receive innervation from the spinal cord. The main muscle of ventilation, the diaphragm, is innervated by segments C3 to C5 through the phrenic nerves. The intercostal muscles, which function in elevating the rib cage and are needed for coughing and deep breathing, are innervated by spinal segments T1 through T7. The major muscles of expiration are the abdominal muscles, which receive their innervation from levels T6 to T12.

Although the ability to inhale and exhale may be preserved at various levels of SCI, functional deficits in ventilation are most apparent in the quality of the breathing cycle and the ability to oxygenate tissues, eliminate carbon dioxide, and mobilize secretions. Cord injuries involving C1 to C3 result in a lack of respiratory effort, and affected patients require assisted ventilation. Although a C3 to C5 injury allows partial or full diaphragmatic function, ventilation is diminished because of the loss of intercostal muscle function, resulting in shallow breaths and a weak cough. Below the C5 level, as less intercostal and abdominal musculature is affected, the ability to take a deep breath and cough is less impaired. Maintenance therapy consists of muscle training to strengthen existing muscles for endurance and mobilization of secretions. The ability to speak is compromised with assisted ventilation, whether continuous or intermittent. Thus, ensuring adequate communication of needs is also essential.

Disruption of Autonomic Nervous System Function

In addition to its effects on skeletal muscle function, SCI interrupts autonomic nervous system function below the site of injury. This includes sympathetic outflow from the thoracic and lumbar cord and parasympathetic outflow from the sacral cord. Because of their site of exit from the CNS, the cranial nerves, such as the vagus, are unaffected. Dependent on the level of injury, the spinal reflexes that control autonomic nervous system function are largely isolated from the rest of the CNS. Afferent sensory input that enters the spinal cord is unaffected, as is the efferent motor output from the cord. Lacking is the regulation and integration of reflex function by centers in the brain and brain stem. This results in a situation in which the autonomic reflexes below the level of injury are uncontrolled, whereas those above the level of injury function in a relatively controlled manner.

The sympathetic nervous system regulation of circulatory function and thermoregulation present some of the most severe problems in SCI. The higher the level of injury and the greater the surface area affected, the more profound are the effects on circulation and thermoregulation. Persons with injury at the T6 level or above experience problems in regulating vasomotor tone; those with injuries below the T6 level usually have sufficient sympathetic function to maintain adequate vasomotor function. The level of injury and its corresponding problems may vary among persons, and some dysfunctional effects may be seen at levels below T6. With lower lumbar and sacral injuries, sympathetic function remains essentially unaltered.

Vasovagal Response. The vagus nerve (cranial nerve X), which is unaffected in SCI, normally exerts a continuous inhibitory effect on heart rate. Vagal stimulation that causes a marked bradycardia is called the *vasovagal response.* Visceral afferent input to the vagal centers in the brain stem of persons with tetraplegia or high-level paraplegia can produce marked bradycardia when unchecked by a dysfunctional sympathetic nervous system. Severe bradycardia and even asystole can result when the vasovagal response is elicited by deep endotracheal suctioning or rapid position change. Preventive measures, such as hyperoxygenation before, during, and after suctioning, are advised. Rapid position changes should be avoided or anticipated, and anticholinergic drugs should be immediately available to counteract severe episodes of bradycardia.

Autonomic Dysreflexia. Autonomic dysreflexia, also known as *autonomic hyperreflexia,* represents an acute episode of exaggerated sympathetic reflex responses that occur in persons with injuries at T6 and above, in which CNS control of spinal reflexes is lost (Fig. 51-19). It does not occur until spinal shock has resolved and autonomic reflexes return, most often within the first 6 months after injury. It is most unpredictable during the first year after injury but can occur throughout the person's lifetime.

Autonomic dysreflexia is characterized by vasospasm, hypertension ranging from mild (20 mm Hg above baseline) to severe (as high as 240/120 mm Hg or higher), skin pallor, and gooseflesh associated with the piloerector response.[55] Because baroreceptor function and parasympathetic control of heart rate travel by way of the cranial nerves, these responses remain intact. Continued hypertension produces a baroreflex-mediated vagal slowing of the heart rate to bradycardic levels. There is an accompanying baroreflex-mediated vasodilatation with flushed skin and profuse sweating above the level of injury, headache ranging from dull to severe and pounding, nasal stuffiness, and feelings of anxiety. A person may experience one, several, or all of the symptoms with each episode.

The stimuli initiating the dysreflexic response include visceral distention, such as a full bladder or rectum; stimulation of pain receptors, as occurs with pressure ulcers, ingrown toenails, dressing changes, and diagnostic or operative procedures; and visceral contractions, such as ejaculation, bladder spasms, or uterine contractions. In many cases, the dysreflexic response results from a full bladder.

Autonomic dysreflexia is a clinical emergency, and without prompt and adequate treatment, convulsions, loss of consciousness, and even death can occur. The major components of treatment include monitoring blood pressure while removing or correcting the initiating cause or stimulus. The person should be placed in an upright position, and all support hose or binders should be removed to promote venous pooling of blood and reduce venous return, thereby decreasing blood pressure. If the stimuli have been removed or the stimuli cannot be identified and the upright position is established, but the blood pressure remains elevated, drugs that block autonomic function are administered. Prevention of the type of stimuli that trigger the dysreflexic event is advocated.

Postural Hypotension. Postural, or orthostatic, hypotension usually occurs in persons with injuries at T4 to T6 and above and is related to the interruption of descending control of sympathetic outflow to blood vessels in the extremities and abdomen. Pooling of blood, along with gravitational forces, impairs venous return to the heart, and there is a subsequent decrease in cardiac output when the person is placed in an upright position. The signs of orthostatic hypotension include dizziness, pallor, excessive sweating above the level of the lesion, complaints of blurred vision, and possibly fainting. Postural hypoten-

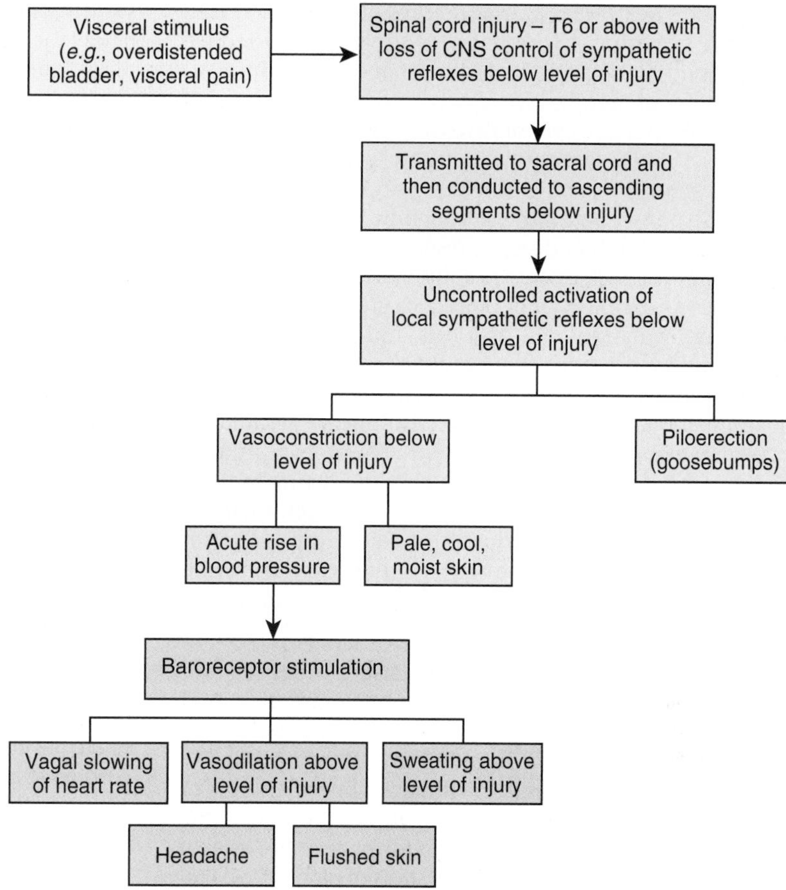

FIGURE 51-19 Mechanisms of autonomic hyperreflexia.

sion usually is prevented by slow changes in position and measures to promote venous return.

Bladder, Bowel, and Sexual Function. Among the most devastating consequences of SCI is the loss of bowel, bladder, and sexual function.[56] Loss of bladder function results from disruption of neural pathways between the bladder and the reflex voiding center at the S2 to S4 level (*i.e.,* an LMN lesion) or between the reflex voiding center and higher brain centers for communication and coordinated sphincter control (*i.e.,* a UMN lesion). Persons with UMN lesions or spastic bladders lack awareness of bladder filling (*i.e.,* storage) and voluntary control of voiding (*i.e.,* evacuation). In LMN lesions or flaccid bladder dysfunction, lack of awareness of bladder filling and lack of bladder tone render the person unable to void voluntarily or involuntarily (see Chapter 37).

Bowel elimination is a coordinated function involving the enteric nervous system, the autonomic nervous system, and the CNS. Persons with SCI above S2 to S4 develop spastic functioning of the defecation reflex and loss of voluntary control of the external anal sphincter. Damage to the cord at the S2 to S4 level causes flaccid functioning of the defecation reflex and loss of anal sphincter tone. Even though the enteric nervous system innervation of the bowel remains intact, without the defecation reflex, peristaltic movements are ineffective in evacuating stool.

Sexual function, as in bladder and bowel control, is mediated by the S2 to S4 segments of the spinal cord. The genital sexual response in SCI, which is manifested by an erection in men and vaginal lubrication in women, may be initiated by mental or touch stimuli, depending on the level of injury. The T11 to L2 cord segments have been identified as the mental-stimuli, or psychogenic, sexual response area, where autonomic nerve pathways in communication with the forebrain leave the cord and innervate the genitalia. The S2 to S4 cord segments have been identified as the sexual-touch reflex center. In T10 or higher injuries (UMN lesion), reflex sexual response to genital touch may occur freely. However, a sexual response to mental stimuli (T11 to L2) does not occur because of the spinal lesion blocking the communication pathway. In an injury at T12 or below (LMN lesion), the sexual reflex center may be damaged, and there may be no response to touch.

In men, the lack of erectile ability or inability to experience penile sensations or orgasm is not a reliable indicator of fertility, which should be evaluated by an expert. In women, fertility is parallel to menses; usually, it is delayed 3 months to 5 months after injury. There are hazards to pregnancy, labor, and birth control devices relative to SCI that require knowledgeable health care providers.

Disruption of Other Functions

Temperature Regulation. The central mechanisms for thermoregulation are located in the hypothalamus (see Chapter 10). In response to cold, the hypothalamus stimulates vasoconstrictor responses in peripheral blood vessels, particularly those of the skin. This results in decreased loss of body heat. Heat production results from increased metabolism, voluntary activity, or shivering. To reduce heat, hypothalamus-stimulated mechanisms produce vasodilatation of skin blood vessels to dissipate heat, and sweating to increase evaporative heat losses.

After SCI, the communication between the thermoregulatory centers in the hypothalamus and the sympathetic effector responses below the level of injury is disrupted; the ability to control blood vessel responses that conserve or dissipate heat is lost, as are the abilities to sweat and shiver. Higher levels of injury tend to produce greater disturbances in thermoregulation. In tetraplegia and high paraplegia, there are few defenses against changes in the environmental temperature, and body temperature tends to assume the temperature of the external environment, a condition known as *poikilothermy*. Persons with lower-level injuries have various degrees of thermoregulation. Disturbances in thermoregulation are chronic and may cause continual loss of body heat. Treatment consists of education in the adjustment of clothing and awareness of how environmental temperatures affect the person's ability to accommodate these changes.

Deep Vein Thrombosis and Edema. Persons with SCI are at high risk for development of deep vein thrombosis (DVT) and pulmonary emboli (PE), particularly during the 2 to 3 weeks following injury.[57] Fatal PE has been reported in 1% to 2% of all persons with SCI within the first 3 months of injury.[46] The high risk for DVT in acute SCI patients is due to immobility, decreased vasomotor tone below the level of injury, and hypercoagulability and stasis of blood flow. Prevention strategies include the use of low-molecular-weight heparin, thigh-high graduated compression stockings, sequential compression boots, and early mobilization.[46,57] Electrical stimulation applied to the lower limbs has been reported to provide some benefit by achieving muscular contraction and improving venous flow. Local pain, a common symptom of DVT, is often absent because of sensory deficits. Thus, a regular schedule of visual inspection for local signs of DVT (*e.g.*, swelling) is important. Testing of persons at high risk for DVT includes plethysmography and duplex ultrasonography.

Edema is also a common problem in persons with SCI. The development of edema is related to decreased peripheral vascular resistance, decreased muscle tone in the paralyzed limbs, and immobility that causes increased venous pressure and abnormal pooling of blood in the abdomen, lower limbs, and upper extremities. Edema in the dependent body parts usually is relieved by positioning to minimize gravitational forces or by using compression devices (*e.g.*, support stockings, binders) that encourage venous return.

Skin Integrity. The entire surface of the skin is innervated by cranial or spinal nerves organized into dermatomes that show cutaneous distribution. The CNS and autonomic nervous system also play a vital role in skin function. The sympathetic nervous system, through control of vasomotor and sweat gland activity, influences the health of the skin by providing adequate circulation, excretion of body fluids, and temperature regulation. The lack of sensory warning mechanisms and voluntary motor ability below the level of injury, coupled with circulatory changes, place the spinal cord–injured person at major risk for disruption of skin integrity (see Chapter 24). Significant factors associated with disruption of skin integrity are pressure, shearing forces, and localized trauma and irritation. Relieving pressure, allowing adequate circulation to the skin, and skin inspection are primary ways of maintaining skin integrity. Of all the complications after SCI, skin breakdown is the most preventable.

Future Directions in Repair of the Injured Spinal Cord

There is a continued effort to determine new and innovative strategies for repairing the injured spinal cord. At present, these strategies focus on promoting the regrowth of interrupted nerve fiber tracts, using nerve growth–stimulating factors or molecules that suppress inhibitors of neuronal extension; bridging spinal cord lesions with scaffolds that are impregnated with nerve growth factors, which promote axon growth and reduce the barriers caused by scar tissue; repairing damaged myelin and restoring nerve fiber conductivity in the lesion area; and enhancing CNS plasticity by promoting compensatory growth of spared, intact nerve fibers above and below the level of injury.[58] Although these strategies may not allow for complete repair of the spinal cord so as to recreate what was present before the injury, even small successes may be useful for someone with SCI. For a person with an injury in the cervical region, "a return of function over even one spinal segment would improve the quality of life, while return to function over three or four segments would transform it."[59]

In summary, UMN lesions are those involving neurons completely contained in the CNS. Amyotrophic lateral sclerosis is a progressive and devastating neurologic disorder that selectively affects motor function. It affects LMNs in the spinal cord as well as UMNs in the brain stem and cerebral cortex. Multiple Sclerosis is a slowly progressive demyelinating disease of the CNS. The most common symptoms are paresthesias, optic neuritis, and motor weakness. The disease is usually characterized by exacerbations and remissions. Initially, near-normal function returns between exacerbations. Spinal cord injury is a disabling neurologic condition most commonly caused by motor vehicle accidents, falls, and sports injuries. Dysfunctions of the nervous system after SCI comprise various degrees of sensorimotor loss and altered reflex activity based on the level of injury and extent of cord damage. Depending on the level of injury, the physical problems of SCI include spinal shock; ventilation and communication problems; autonomic nervous system dysfunction that predisposes to the vasovagal response, autonomic hyperreflexia, impaired body temperature regulation, and postural hypotension; impaired muscle pump and venous innervation leading to edema of dependent areas of the body and risk for deep vein thrombosis; altered sensorimotor integrity that contributes to uncontrolled muscle spasms, altered pain responses, and threat to skin integrity; alterations in bowel and bladder elimination; and impaired sexual function.

REVIEW EXERCISES

A 32-year-old woman presents with complaints of drooping eyelids, difficulty chewing and swallowing, and weakness of her arms and legs that is less severe in the morning but becomes worse as the day progresses. She complains that climbing stairs and lifting objects is becoming increasingly difficult. Clinical examination confirms weakness of the eyelid and jaw muscles. She is told that she may have myasthenia gravis and is scheduled for a test using the short-acting acetylcholinesterase inhibitor edrophonium (Tensilon).

A. Explain the pathogenesis of this woman's symptoms as it relates to myasthenia gravis.

B. Explain how information from the administration of the acetylcholinesterase inhibitor edrophonium can be used to assist in the diagnosis of the disorder.

A 20-year-old man suffered spinal cord injury at the C2 to C3 level as the result of a motorcycle accident.

A. Explain the effects of this man's injury on ventilation and communication; sensorimotor function; autonomic nervous system function; bowel, bladder, and sexual function; and temperature regulation.

B. Autonomic dysreflexia, which is a threat to persons with spinal cord injury at T6 or above, is manifested by hypertension, often to extreme levels, and bradycardia; constriction of skin vessels below the level of injury; and severe headache and nasal stuffiness. Explain the origin of the elevated blood pressure and bradycardia. The condition does not occur until after shock has resolved and usually occurs only in persons with injuries at T6 and above. Explain.

References

1. Jones G.M. (2000). Posture. In Kandel E.R., Schwartz J.H., Jessell T.M. (Eds.). *Principles of neural science* (4th ed., pp. 816–831). New York: McGraw-Hill.
2. Guyton A., Hall J.E. (2000). *Medical physiology* (10th ed., pp. 634–637, 973). Philadelphia: W.B. Saunders.
3. Conn M.P. (1995). *Neuroscience in medicine* (pp. 312–317). Philadelphia: J.B. Lippincott.
4. Penfield W., Rasmussen T. (1950). *The cerebral cortex of man.* New York: Macmillan.
5. Burns D.K., Kumar V. (2003). *Robbins basic pathology* (7th ed., pp. 809–849). Philadelphia: W.B. Saunders.
6. Sarnat H.B. (2004). Muscular dystrophies. In Behrman R.E., Kliegman R.M., Jenson H.B. (Eds.), *Nelson textbook of pediatrics* (17th ed., pp. 1873–1877). Philadelphia: W.B. Saunders.
7. Meiss R.A. (2003). Skeletal muscle and smooth muscle. In Rhoads R.A., Tanner G.A. (Eds.), *Medical physiology* (2nd ed., pp. 152–176). Philadelphia: Lippincott Williams & Wilkins.
8. Katzung B.G. (2001). *Basic and clinical pharmacology* (8th ed., pp. 92–102). New York: Lange Medical Books/McGraw-Hill.
9. Vincent A., Palace J., Hilton-Jones D. (2001). Myasthenia gravis. *Lancet* 357, 2122–2128.
10. Drachman D.B. (1994). Myasthenia gravis. *New England Journal of Medicine 330,* 1797–1810.
11. Wittbrodt E.T. (1997). Drugs and myasthenia gravis. *Archives of Internal Medicine 157,* 399–408.
12. Viera A.J. (2003). Management of carpal tunnel syndrome. *American Family Physician 68*(2), 265–272.
13. Hickey J.V. (2003). *Neurological and neurosurgical nursing* (5th ed., pp. 419–465, 469–480). Philadelphia: Lippincott-Raven.
14. Katz J.N., Simmons B.P. (2002). Carpal tunnel syndrome. *New England Journal of Medicine 346*(23), 1807–1812.
15. Asbury A.K., Hauser S.L. (2001). Guillain-Barré syndrome. In Braunwald E., Fauci A., Kasper D.L., et al. (Eds.), *Harrison's principles of internal medicine* (15th ed., pp. 2507–2509). New York: McGraw-Hill.
16. Winer J.B. (2011). Guillain-Barré syndrome. *Molecular Pathology 51,* 381–385.
17. Rees J.H., Saudain S.E., Gregson N.A., Hughes R.A.C. (1995). *Campylobacter jejuni* infection and Guillain-Barré syndrome. *New England Journal of Medicine 333,* 1374–1379.
18. Langmuir A.D., Bregman D.J., Nathanson N., Victor M. (1984). An epidemic and clinical evaluation of Guillain-Barré syndrome reported in association of swine influenza vaccines. *American Journal of Epidemiology 119,* 841–879.
19. Deyo R.A., Weinstein J.N. (2001). Low back pain. *New England Journal of Medicine 344*(5), 363–370.
20. Acute Low Back Problems Guideline Panel. (1994). *Acute low back problems in adults: Assessment and treatment.* AHCPR publication no. 95-0642. Rockville, MD: Agency for Health Care Policy and Research, Public Health Service, U.S. Department of Health and Human Services.
21. Deyo R.A. (1998). Low-back pain. *Scientific American 283,* 49–53.
22. Moore K.L. Dalley A.F. (1999). *Clinically oriented anatomy* (4th ed., 452–453). Philadelphia: Lippincott Williams & Wilkins.
23. Bratton R.L. (1999). Assessment and management of acute low back pain. *American Family Physician 60,* 2299–2308.
24. DeLong M.R. (2000). The basal ganglia. In Kandel E.R., Schwartz J.H., Jessell T.M. (Eds.), (2001). *Principles of neural science* (4th ed., pp. 853–867). New York. McGraw-Hill.
25. Lang A.E., Lozano A.M. (1998). Parkinson disease (Part 1 and Part 2). *New England Journal of Medicine 339*(15, 16), 1044–1052, 1130–1143.
26. Colcher A., Simuni T. (1999). Clinical manifestations of Parkinson disease. *Medical Clinics of North America 83,* 327–347.
27. Parkinson J. (1817). *An essay on the shaking palsy.* London: Sherwood, Nelley & Jones.
28. Youdim M.B.H., Riederer P. (1997). Understanding Parkinson disease. *Scientific American 276,* 52–59.
29. Rubin E., Farber J.L. (1999). *Pathology* (3rd ed., pp. 1496–1498, 1502–1505). Philadelphia: Lippincott-Raven.
30. Guttman M., Kish S.J., Furukawa Y. (2003). Current concepts in the diagnosis and management of Parkinson disease. *Canadian Medical Association Journal 168*(3), 293–301.
31. Lücking C.B., Dürr A., Bonifati V., et al. (European Consortium on Genetic Susceptibility in Parkinson Disease Genetic Study Group). (2000). Association between early-onset Parkinson disease and mutations in the Parkin gene. *New England Journal of Medicine 342,* 1560–1567.
32. Steece-Collier K., Maries E., Kordower J.H. (2002). Etiology of Parkinson disease: Genetics and environment revisited. *Proceedings National Academy of Science 99*(22), 1772–1774.
33. The Deep-Brain Stimulation for Parkinson Disease Group. (2001). Deep-brain stimulation of the subthalamic nucleus and of the pars interna of the globus pallidus in Parkinson disease. *New England Journal of Medicine 345*(13), 956–963.

34. Ghez C. (2000). The cerebellum. In Kandel E.R., Schwartz J.H., Jessell T.M. (Eds.), (2001). *Principles of neural science* (4th ed., pp. 832–852). New York. McGraw-Hill.
35. Mackin G.A. (1999). Optimizing care of patients with ALS. *Postgraduate Medicine 105*(4), 143–146.
36. Rowland L.P., Shneider N.A. (2001). Amyotropic lateral sclerosis. *New England Journal of Medicine 344,* 1688–1700.
37. Walling A.D. (1999). Amyotropic lateral sclerosis: Lou Gehrig's disease. *American Family Practitioner 59*(6), 1489–1496.
38. Noseworthy J.H., Lucchinetti C., Rodriguez M., Weinshenker B.G. (2000). Multiple sclerosis. *New England Journal of Medicine 343*(18), 938–952.
39. Anderson D.W., Ellenberg J.H., Leventhal C.M., et al. (1992). Revised estimate of multiple sclerosis in the United States. *Annals of Neurology 31,* 333–336.
40. Keegan B.M., Noseworthy J.H. (2002). Multiple sclerosis. *Annual Review of Medicine 53,* 285–302.
41. Lublin F.D., Reingold S.C. (1996). Defining the clinical course of multiple sclerosis: Results of an international survey. *Neurology 46,* 907–911.
42. Rudick R.A., Cohen J.A., Weinstock-Guttman B., et al. (1997). Management of multiple sclerosis. *New England Journal of Medicine 337,* 1604–1611.
43. Brod S.A., Lindsey W., Wolinsky J.S. (1996). Multiple sclerosis: Clinical presentation, diagnosis and treatment. *American Family Physician 54,* 1301–1311.
44. Goodin D.S. et al. (2002). Disease modifying therapies in multiple sclerosis: Subcommittee of Neurology and MS Council for Clinical Practice Guidelines. *Neurology 58,* 169.
45. National Spinal Cord Injury Statistical Center. (2003). Spinal cord injury: Facts and figures at a glance. Birmingham: University of Alabama. [On-line]. Available: http://www.spinalcord.uab.edu.
46. Hickey J.V. (2003). *The clinical practice of neurological and neurosurgical nursing* (5th ed. pp. 407–480). Philadelphia: Lippincott Williams & Wilkins.
47. McDonald J.W. (2002). Spinal cord injury. *Lancet 359,* 417–425.
48. Buckley D.A., Guanci M.K. (1999). Spinal cord trauma. *Nursing Clinics of North America 34,* 661–687.
49. Chiles B.W., Cooper P.R. (1996). Acute spinal cord injury. *New England Journal of Medicine 334,* 514–520.
50. Fehling M.G., Louw D. (1996). Initial stabilization and medical management of acute spinal cord injury. *American Family Physician 42,* 155–162.
51. Atkinson P.P., Atkinson J.L.D. (1996). Spinal shock. *Mayo Clinic Proceedings 71,* 384–389.
52. Tator C.H., Fehlings M.G. (1999). Review of clinical trials in neuroprotection in acute spinal cord injury. *Neurosurgical Focus 6*(1), 1–14.
53. Bracken M.B., Shepard M.J., Collins W.F., et al. (1997). Administration of methylprednisolone for 24 or 48 hours or tirilazad mesylate for 48 hours in the treatment of acute spinal cord injury: Results of the Third National Acute Spinal Cord Injury Study. *Journal of the American Medical Association 277,* 1597–1604.
54. American Spinal Injury Association. (1992). *Standards of neurological and functional classification of spinal cord injury.* Chicago: American Spinal Cord Injury Association.
55. Blackner J. (2003). Rehabilitation medicine: Autonomic dysreflexia. *Canadian Medical Association Journal 169*(9), 931–935.
56. Benevento B.T., Sipski M.L. (2002). Neurogenic bladder, neurogenic bowel, and sexual dysfunction in people with spinal cord injury. *Physical Therapy 62*(6), 601–612.
57. Aito S., Pieri A., Marcelli F., Cominelli E. (2002). Primary prevention of deep venous thrombosis and pulmonary embolism in acute spinal cord injured patients. *Spinal Cord 40,* 300–303.
58. Schwab M.E. (2002). Repairing the injured spinal cord. *Science 295,* 1029–1031.
59. Fawcett J. (2002). Repair of spinal cord injuries: Where are we, where are we going? *Spinal Cord 40,* 615–623.

CHAPTER

52

Disorders of Brain Function

Diane Book

Anatomically and functionally, the brain is the most complex structure in the body. It controls our ability to think, our awareness of things around us, and our interactions with the outside world. Brain functions are diverse and highly localized within the brain. Therefore, unlike other organs that have a global function, the brain is much more vulnerable to focal lesions. For example, an isolated renal infarct would not be expected to have a significant effect on kidney function, whereas an infarct of comparable size in the brain could have serious impact on an isolated brain function, such as complete paralysis on one side of the body.

Mechanisms and Manifestations of Brain Injury

After completing this section of the chapter, you should be able to meet the following objectives:

- Differentiate cerebral hypoxia from cerebral ischemia and focal from global ischemia
- Characterize the role of excitatory amino acids as a common pathway for neurologic disorders
- State the determinants of intracranial pressure and describe compensatory mechanisms used to prevent large changes in intracranial pressure when there are changes in brain, blood, and cerebrospinal fluid volumes

- Explain the causes of tentorial herniation of the brain and its consequences
- Compare the causes of communicating and noncommunicating hydrocephalus
- Compare cytotoxic, vasogenic, and interstitial cerebral edema
- Differentiate primary and secondary brain injuries due to head trauma
- Describe the mechanism of brain damage in coup–contrecoup injuries
- List the constellation of symptoms involved in the postconcussion syndrome
- Differentiate among the location, manifestations, and morbidity of epidural, subdural, and intracerebral hematoma
- Define consciousness and trace the rostral-to-caudal progression of consciousness in terms of pupillary changes, respiration, and motor function as the effects of brain dysfunction progress to involve structures in the diencephalon, midbrain, pons, and medulla
- State two criteria for the diagnosis of brain death

The brain is protected from external forces by the rigid confines of the skull and the cushioning afforded by the cerebrospinal fluid (CSF). The metabolic stability required by its electrically active cells is maintained by a number of regulatory mechanisms, including the blood–brain barrier and autoregulatory mechanisms that ensure its blood supply. Nonetheless, the brain remains remarkably vulnerable to injury by ischemia, trauma, tumors, degenerative processes, and metabolic derangements.

MECHANISMS OF INJURY

Injury to brain tissue can result from a number of conditions, including trauma, tumors, stroke, metabolic derangements, and degenerative disorders. Brain damage resulting from these disorders involves several common pathways, including the effects of ischemia, excitatory amino acid injury, cerebral edema, and injury due to increased intracranial pressure (ICP). In many cases, the mechanisms of injury are interrelated.

Hypoxic and Ischemic Injury

The energy requirements of the brain are provided mainly by adenosine triphosphate (ATP); the ability of the cerebral circulation to deliver oxygen in sufficiently high concentrations to facilitate metabolism of glucose and generate ATP is essential to brain function. Although the brain makes up only 2% of the body weight, it receives one sixth of the resting cardiac output and accounts for 20% of the oxygen consumption.[1,2] Thus, deprivation of oxygen or blood flow can have a deleterious effect on brain structures.

By definition, hypoxia denotes a deprivation of oxygen with maintained blood flow, whereas ischemia is a situation of greatly reduced or interrupted blood flow. The brain tends to have different sensitivities to the two conditions. Whereas hypoxia interferes with the delivery of oxygen, ischemia interferes with delivery of oxygen and glucose as well as the removal of metabolic wastes. Hypoxia usually is seen in conditions such as exposure to reduced atmospheric pressure, carbon monoxide poisoning, severe anemia, and failure to oxygenate the blood. Because hypoxia indicates decreased oxygen levels in all brain tissue, it produces a generalized depressant effect on the brain. Contrary to popular belief, neurons are capable of substantial anaerobic metabolism and are fairly tolerant of pure hypoxia; it commonly produces euphoria, listlessness, drowsiness, and impaired problem solving. Unconsciousness and convulsions may occur when hypoxia is sudden and severe. However, the effects of severe hypoxia (*i.e.*, anoxia) on brain function seldom are seen because the condition rapidly leads to cardiac arrest and ischemia.

Ischemia can be focal, as in stroke, or global, as in cardiac arrest. Persons with global ischemia have no collateral circulation during the ischemic event. In contrast, collateral circulation provides blood flow to uninvolved brain areas during focal ischemia. The collateral perfusion may even provide sufficient substrates to the focal ischemic region to maintain a low level of metabolic activity, thereby preserving membrane integrity. At the same time, the delivery of glucose under these anaerobic conditions may result in additional lactic acid production and worsening of lactic acidosis.[2]

Global Ischemia. Global ischemia occurs when blood flow is inadequate to meet the metabolic needs of the entire brain, as in cardiac arrest or circulatory shock. The result is a spectrum of neurologic disorders reflecting global brain dysfunction. Unconsciousness occurs within seconds of severe global ischemia, such as that resulting from complete cessation of blood flow, as in cardiac arrest, or with marked decrease in blood flow, as in serious cardiac dysrhythmias. If circulation is restored immediately, consciousness is regained quickly. However, if blood flow is not promptly restored, severe pathologic changes take place. Energy sources, glucose and glycogen, are exhausted in 2 to 4 minutes, and cellular ATP stores are depleted in 4 to 5 minutes. Approximately 50% to 75% of the total energy requirement of neuronal tissue is spent on mechanisms for maintenance of ionic gradients across the cell membrane (*e.g.*, sodium–potassium pump), resulting in fluxes of sodium, potassium, and calcium ions[3] (Table 52-1). Excessive influx of sodium results in neuronal and interstitial edema. The influx of calcium initiates a cascade of events, including release of intracellular and nuclear enzymes that cause cell destruction. When ischemia is sufficiently severe or prolonged, infarction or death of all the cellular elements of the brain occurs.

The pattern of global ischemia reflects the anatomic arrangement of the cerebral vessels and the sensitivity of various brain tissues to oxygen deprivation[4] (Fig. 52-1). Selective neuronal sensitivity to a lack of oxygen is most apparent in the Purkinje cells of the cerebellum and neurons in Sommer's sector of the hippocampus. The anatomic arrangement of the cerebral blood vessels predisposes to two types of injury: watershed infarcts and laminar necrosis.

Watershed infarcts are concentrated in anatomically vulnerable border zones between the overlapping territo-

TABLE 52-1 Pathophysiologic Consequences of Impaired Cerebral Perfusion

Consequences	Timing
Depletion of oxygen	10 sec
Depletion of glucose	2–4 min
Conversion to anaerobic metabolism	2–4 min
Exhaustion of cellular ATP	4–5 min
Consequences	
Efflux of potassium	
Influx of sodium	
Influx of calcium	

(Adapted from Richmond T.S. [1997]. Cerebral resuscitation after global brain ischemia: Linking research to practice. *AACN Clinical Issues* 8 [2], 173)

ries supplied by the major cerebral arteries, notably the middle, anterior, and posterior cerebral arteries. The overlapping territory at the distal ends of these vessels forms extremely vulnerable areas in terms of ischemia, called watershed zones. During events such as severe hypotension, these distal territories undergo a profound lowering of blood flow, predisposing to ischemia and infarction of brain tissues. As a consequence, areas of the cortex that are supplied by the major cerebral arteries usually regain function on recovery of adequate blood flow; however, infarctions may occur in the watershed boundary strips, resulting in focal neurologic deficits.[4]

Laminar necrosis occurs in areas supplied by the penetrating arteries. The gray matter of the cerebral cortex receives its major blood supply through short penetrating arteries that emerge at right angles from larger vessels in the pia mater and then form a cascade as they repeatedly branch, forming a rich capillary network. An abrupt loss of arterial blood pressure markedly diminishes flow through these capillary channels. Because of the branching arrangement of these vessels, the necrosis that develops is laminar and is most severe in the deeper layers of the cortex.

Although the threshold for ischemic neuronal injury is unknown, there is a period during which neurons can survive if blood flow is reestablished. Unfortunately, brain injury may not be reversible if the duration of ischemia is such that the threshold of injury has been reached. Even after circulation has been reestablished, damage to blood vessels and changes in blood flow can prevent return of adequate tissue perfusion. This period of postischemic hypoperfusion is thought to be associated with mechanisms such as desaturation of venous blood, capillary and venular clotting, or sludging of blood flow.[2] Because of sludging, blood viscosity increases, and there is increased resistance to blood flow. There is also evidence of compromised flow to immediate vasomotor paralysis of the surface conducting blood vessels due to extracellular acidosis, followed by ischemic vasoconstriction.

Hypermetabolism due to increased circulating catecholamines also has been implicated as a contributing factor in postischemic hypoperfusion. Catecholamine release results in an increased cerebral metabolic rate and increased need for all energy-producing substrates, which the damaged brain is unable to sustain.

The neurologic deficits that result from global ischemic injury vary widely. If the period of nonflow or low flow is minimal, the neurologic damage usually is minimal to nonexistent. When the period is extensive or resuscitation is lengthy, the early neurologic clinical picture is that of fixed and dilated pupils, abnormal motor posturing, and coma. If the brain recovers, there is gradual improvement in neurologic status, although cognitive and focal deficits usually persist and can prevent a return to preischemic levels of functioning.

An exception to this time frame is the circumstance of cold-water drowning in which the person, especially a child, is submerged in cold water for longer than 10 minutes.[5] Hypothermia develops and reduces the cerebral

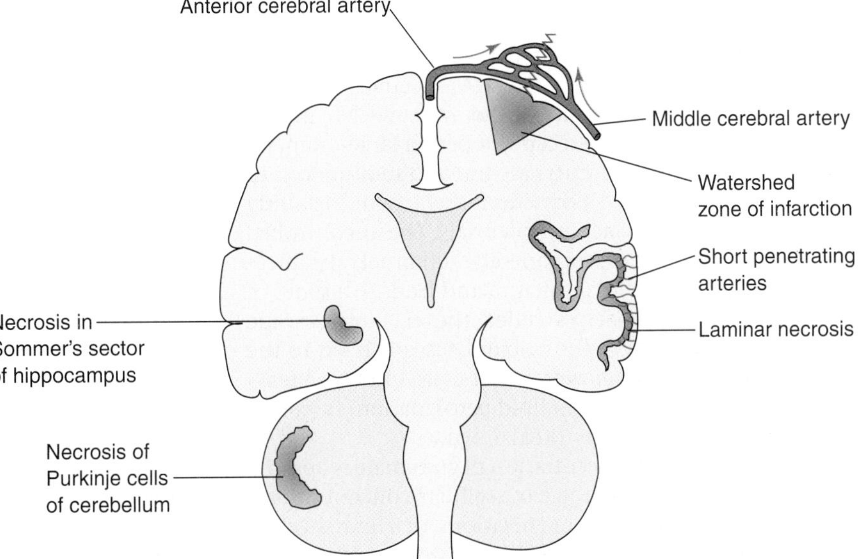

FIGURE 52-1 Consequences of global ischemia. A global insult induces lesions that reflect the vascular architecture (watershed infarcts, laminar necrosis) and the sensitivity of individual neuronal systems (pyramidal cells of Sommer's section, Purkinje cells). (Courtesy of Dmitri Karetnikov, artist). (Rubin E., Farber J.L. [1999]. *Pathology* [3rd ed., p. 1470]. Philadelphia: Lippincott-Raven)

metabolic requirements for oxygen; it subsequently serves as a protective mechanism for the neurons. In this case, recovery can be rapid and remarkable, and resuscitation efforts should not be discontinued precipitously.

Treatment of global ischemia is aimed at providing oxygen to the troubled brain and decreasing the metabolic needs of brain tissue during the nonflow state. Methods that decrease brain temperature as a means of decreasing brain metabolism have shown promise.[3] Normovolemic hemodilution may be used to overcome sludging of cerebral blood flow during reperfusion. Because both hypoglycemia and hyperglycemia adversely affect the outcome in persons with global ischemia, control of blood glucose within a range of 100 to 200 mg/dL has been advocated.[3,6] Although several pharmacologic agents have been advocated as a means of preventing brain damage in global ischemia, none has proved highly effective. In the past, barbiturates were used as a means of decreasing brain metabolism. However, the beneficial effects of barbiturates are minimal unless they are administered before the anticipated ischemia (*e.g.*, before neurosurgery).[2] Recent interest has focused on inducing hypothermia and on pharmacologic agents that could minimize injury from free radicals and excitatory amino acids.

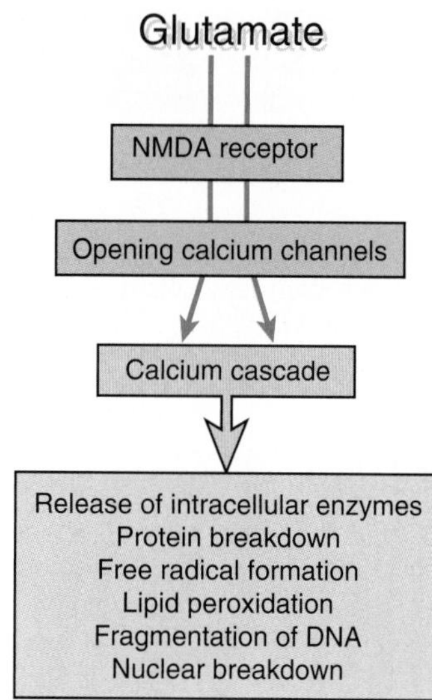

FIGURE 52-2 The role of the glutamate-NMDA receptor in brain cell injury.

Injury From Excitatory Amino Acids

In many neurologic disorders, injury to neurons may be caused by overstimulation of receptors for specific amino acids such as glutamate and aspartate that act as excitatory neurotransmitters.[7] These neurologic conditions range from acute insults such as stroke, hypoglycemic injury, and trauma to chronic degenerative disorders such as Huntington's disease and possibly Alzheimer's dementia. The term excitotoxicity has been coined for the final common pathway for neuronal cell injury and death associated with excessive activity of the excitatory neurotransmitters and their receptor-mediated functions.

Glutamate is the principal excitatory neurotransmitter in the brain, and its interaction with specific receptors is responsible for many higher-order functions, including memory, cognition, movement, and sensation.[7] Many of the actions of glutamate are coupled with receptor-operated ion channels. One subtype in particular, called the glutamate N-methyl-D-aspartate (NMDA) receptor, has been implicated in causing central nervous system (CNS) injury. This subtype of glutamate receptor opens a large-diameter calcium channel that permits calcium and sodium ions to enter the cell and allows potassium ions to exit, resulting in prolonged (seconds) action potentials. The uncontrolled opening of NMDA receptor–operated channels produces an increase in intracellular calcium and leads to a series of calcium-mediated processes called the calcium cascade (Fig. 52-2). Activation of the calcium cascade leads to the release of intracellular enzymes that cause protein breakdown, free radical formation, lipid peroxidation, fragmentation of DNA, and nuclear breakdown.

The intracellular concentration of glutamate is approximately 16 times that of the extracellular concentration.[7] Normally, extracellular concentrations of glutamate are tightly regulated, with excess amounts removed and actively transported into astrocytes and neurons. During prolonged ischemia, these transport mechanisms become immobilized, causing extracellular glutamate to accumulate. In the case of cell injury and death, intracellular glutamate is released from the damaged cells, causing injury to surrounding cells. The uncontrolled opening of NMDA receptor–operated channels by glutamate produces an increase in intracellular calcium and leads to the calcium cascade. Activation of the calcium cascade eventually causes cell death within several hours after exposure to glutamate.

The effects of acute glutamate toxicity do not necessarily lead to cell death; they are reversible if excess glutamate can be removed or if its effects can be blocked. Drugs called neuroprotectants are being developed to interfere with the glutamate–NMDA pathway and thus reduce brain cell injury. These pharmacologic strategies may protect viable brain cells from irreversible damage in the setting of excitotoxicity. Pharmacologic strategies that are being explored include those that inhibit the synthesis or release of excitatory amino acid transmitters; block the NMDA receptors; stabilize the membrane potential to prevent initiation of the calcium cascade using lidocaine and certain barbiturates; and specifically block certain intracellular proteases, endonucleases, and lipases that are known to be cytotoxic.[8,9] The drug riluzole, which acts presynaptically to inhibit glutamate release, currently is being used in the treatment of amyotrophic lateral sclerosis (see Chapter 51). Nimodipine, a calcium channel blocker that acts at the level of the NMDA receptor–operated channels, is being investigated for use in subarachnoid hemorrhage and acquired immunodeficiency syndrome dementia.[7] In the setting of ischemic stroke, multiple mechanisms of pharmacologic action, including NMDA receptor blockade, nitric oxide potentiation, and potassium channel opening, are being studied.[10]

Central nervous system neurons can be divided into two major categories: macroneurons and microneurons. Macroneurons are large cells with long axons that leave the local network of intercommunicating neurons to send action potentials to other regions of the nervous system at distances of centimeters to meters (*e.g.,* upper motoneurons that communicate with lower motoneurons that control leg movement). Microneurons are very small cells that are intimately involved in local circuitry. Their axons transmit action potentials to other members of the same local network. In contrast to macroneurons, which number in the thousands, microneurons account for most of the many billions of CNS neurons.

Many macroneurons use glutamate as a neurotransmitter in their excitatory communication with microneurons. It is the microneuron network that provides the analytic, integrative, and learning circuitry that is the basis for the higher-order function of the CNS. The microneurons of the cerebral cortex and hippocampus are particularly vulnerable to excessive stimulation of the glutamate NMDA receptors and the neurotoxic effects of increased intracellular calcium levels. Because of their increased vulnerability, many of the small interneurons that make up essential parts of the complex control and memory functions of the brain are selectively damaged, even if the remainder of the brain survives the insult. This pattern may account for the long-term effects of brain insult, which frequently include subtle and noticeable reductions in cognitive and memory functions.

Increased Intracranial Volume and Pressure

The brain is enclosed in the rigid confines of the skull, or cranium, making it particularly susceptible to increases in ICP. Increased ICP is a common pathway for brain injury from different types of insults and agents. Excessive ICP can obstruct cerebral blood flow, destroy brain cells, displace brain tissue as in herniation, and otherwise damage delicate brain structures.

The cranial cavity contains blood (approximately 10%), brain tissue (approximately 80%), and CSF (approximately 10%) in the rigid confines of a nonexpandable skull.[11] Each of these three volumes contributes to the ICP, which normally is maintained within a range of 0 to 15 mm Hg when measured in the lateral ventricles. The volumes of each of these components can vary slightly without causing marked changes in ICP. This is because small increases in the volume of one component can be compensated for by a decrease in the volume of one or both of the other two components.[12] This association is called the *Monro-Kellie hypothesis*. Normal fluctuations in ICP occur with respiratory movements and activities of daily living such as straining, coughing, and sneezing.

Abnormal variation in intracranial volume with subsequent changes in ICP can be caused by a volume change in any of the three intracranial components. For example, an increase in tissue volume can result from a brain tumor, brain edema, or bleeding into brain tissue. An increase in blood volume develops when there is vasodilatation of cerebral vessels or obstruction of venous outflow. Excess production, decreased absorption, or obstructed circulation of CSF affords the potential for an increase in the CSF component. When the change in volume is caused by a brain tumor, it tends to occur slowly and usually is localized to the immediate area, whereas the increase resulting from head injury usually develops rapidly.

According to the modified Monro-Kellie hypothesis, reciprocal compensation occurs among the three intracranial compartments.[11] Of the three intracranial volumes, tissue volume is relatively restricted in its ability to undergo change; CSF and blood volume are best able to compensate for changes in ICP. Initial increases in ICP are buffered by a translocation of CSF to the spinal subarachnoid space and increased reabsorption of CSF. The compensatory ability of the blood compartment is limited by the small amount of blood that is in the cerebral circulation. The cerebral blood vessels contain less than 10% of the intracranial volume, most of which is contained in the low-pressure venous system. As the volume-buffering capacity of this compartment becomes exhausted, venous pressure increases, and cerebral blood volume and ICP rise. Also, cerebral blood flow is highly controlled by autoregulatory mechanisms, which affect its compensatory capacity. Conditions such as ischemia and an elevated partial pressure of carbon dioxide (PCO_2) in the blood produce a compensatory vasodilation of the cerebral blood vessels. A decrease in PCO_2 has the opposite effect; for this reason, hyperventilation, which results in a decrease in PCO_2 levels, is sometimes used in the treatment of ICP.

Cerebral Compliance and the Impact of Intracranial Pressure. The impact of increases in blood, brain tissue, or CSF volumes on ICP varies among individuals and depends on the amount of increase that occurs, the effectiveness of compensatory mechanisms, and the compliance of brain tissue. Compliance represents the ratio of change in volume to the resulting change in pressure (compliance = change in volume/change in pressure).[11] The effects of intracranial volume changes (horizontal axis) on ICP changes (vertical axis) are depicted in Figure 52-3.[11] The shape of the curve demonstrates effects of intracranial volume changes on ICP. The ICP remains constant from point A to point B when volume is added to the intracranial space. Because the compensatory mechanisms are adequate, compliance is high in this area of the curve, and there is little change in ICP. From points B to C, the compensatory mechanisms become less efficient; compliance decreases, and ICP begins to rise. At points C to D, the compensatory mechanisms have been exceeded such that even small changes in volume produce large changes in ICP.

Impact of Intracranial Pressure on Cerebral Perfusion Pressure. The cerebral perfusion pressure (CPP), which represents the difference between the mean arterial blood pressure (MABP) and the ICP (CPP = MABP − ICP), is the pressure perfusing the brain.[11] CPP is determined by the pressure gradient between the internal carotid artery and the subarachnoid veins. The MABP and ICP are monitored frequently in persons with brain conditions that increase ICP and impair brain perfusion. Normal CPP ranges from 70 to 100 mm Hg. Brain ischemia develops at levels below 40 mm Hg.[11] When the pressure in the cranial cavity

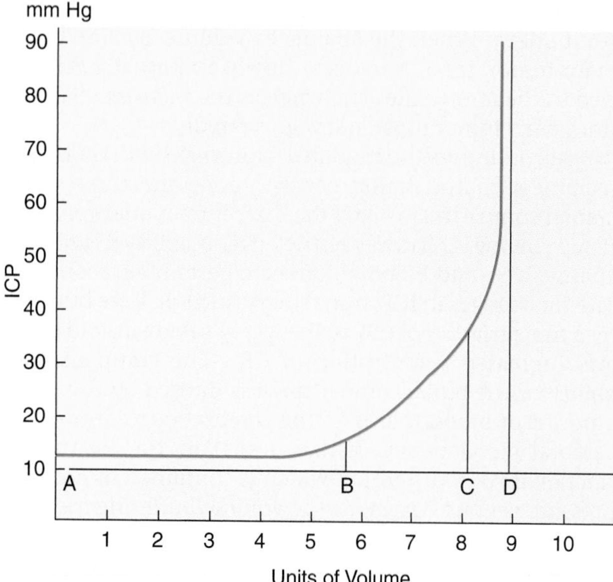

FIGURE 52-3 Pressure–volume curve. From point A to just before B, the ICP remains constant although there is an addition of volume (compliance is high). At point B, even though the ICP is within normal limits, compliance begins to change, as evidenced by the slight rise in ICP. From points B to C, the ICP rises with an increase in volume (low compliance). From points C to D, ICP rises significantly with each minute increase in volume (compliance is lost). (Hickey J.V. [1996]. *Neurological and neurosurgical nursing* [4th ed., p. 296]. Philadelphia: Lippincott-Raven)

approaches or exceeds the MABP, tissue perfusion becomes inadequate, cellular hypoxia results, and, if the pressure is maintained, neuronal death may occur. The highly specialized cortical neurons are the most sensitive to oxygen deficit; a decrease in the level of consciousness is one of the earliest and most reliable signs of increased ICP. The continued cellular hypoxia leads to general neurologic deterioration; the level of consciousness may deteriorate from alertness through confusion, lethargy, obtundation, stupor, and coma.

One of the late reflexes seen with a marked increase in ICP is the CNS ischemic response, which is triggered by ischemia of the vasomotor center in the brain stem. Neurons in the vasomotor center respond directly to ischemia by producing a marked increase in MABP, sometimes to levels as high as 270 mm Hg, accompanied by a widening of the pulse pressure and reflex slowing of the heart rate. These three signs, sometimes called the Cushing reflex, are important but late indicators of increased ICP.[13] The ischemic reflex is a last-ditch effort by the nervous system to maintain the cerebral circulation. The Cushing reflex seldom is seen in modern clinical settings since the advent of ICP monitoring.

Brain Herniation

The brain is protected by the nonexpandable skull and supporting septa, the falx cerebri and the tentorium cerebelli, that divide the intracranial cavity into fossae or compartments that normally protect against excessive movement. The falx cerebri is a sickle-shaped septum that separates the two hemispheres. The tentorium cerebelli divides the cranial cavity into anterior and posterior fossae (Fig. 52-4A). This inflexible dural sheath extends posteriorly from the bony petrous ridges and anterior to the clinoid process, sloping downward and outward from its medial edge to attach laterally to the occipital bone. Extending posteriorly into the center of the tentorium is a large semicircular opening called the incisura or tentorial notch. The temporal lobe rests on the tentorial incisura, and the midbrain occupies the anterior portion of the tentorial notch. The cerebellum is closely opposed to the dorsum of the midbrain and fills the posterior part of the notch. Other important anatomic associations exist among the anterior cerebral, internal carotid, posterior communicating, and posterior and superior cerebellar arteries, and the incisura (see Fig. 52-4B). The oculomotor nerve (cranial nerve III) emerges from the mediolateral surface of each peduncle just caudal to the tentorium.

Brain herniation represents a displacement of brain tissue under the falx cerebri or through the tentorial notch or incisura of the tentorium cerebelli. It occurs when an elevated ICP in one brain compartment causes displacement of the cerebral tissue toward an area of lower ICP. The different types of herniation syndromes are based on the area of the brain that has herniated and the structure under which it has been pushed (see Fig. 52-4C). They commonly are divided into two broad categories, supratentorial and infratentorial, based on whether they are located above or below the tentorium.

Supratentorial Herniations. Three major patterns of supratentorial herniation were described by Plum and Posner in their classic work: cingulate, central transtentorial, and uncal transtentorial.[14] Table 52-2 describes the key structures and clinical signs of these three types of herniations. Of the three, cingulate herniation poses the less serious threat in terms of clinical outcomes.[11] Transtentorial herniations result in two distinct syndromes: an uncal syndrome and a central syndrome. Clinically, they display distinct patterns early in their course, but both merge in a similar pattern once they begin to involve the midbrain level and below (brain stem structures).

Cingulate herniation involves displacement of the cingulate gyrus and hemisphere beneath the sharp edges of the falx cerebri to the opposite side of the brain. Displacement of the falx can compress the local brain tissue and blood supply from the anterior cerebral artery, causing ischemia and edema, which further increase ICP levels. Unilateral or bilateral leg weakness is an early sign of impending cingulate herniation.

Central transtentorial herniations involve the downward displacement of the cerebral hemispheres, basal ganglia, diencephalon, and midbrain through the tentorial incisura. The diencephalon may be compressed tightly against the midbrain with such force that edema and hemorrhage result. It may or may not be associated with uncal or lateral herniation. In the early diencephalic stage, there is clouding of consciousness, bilaterally small pupils (approximately 2 mm in diameter) with a full range of con-

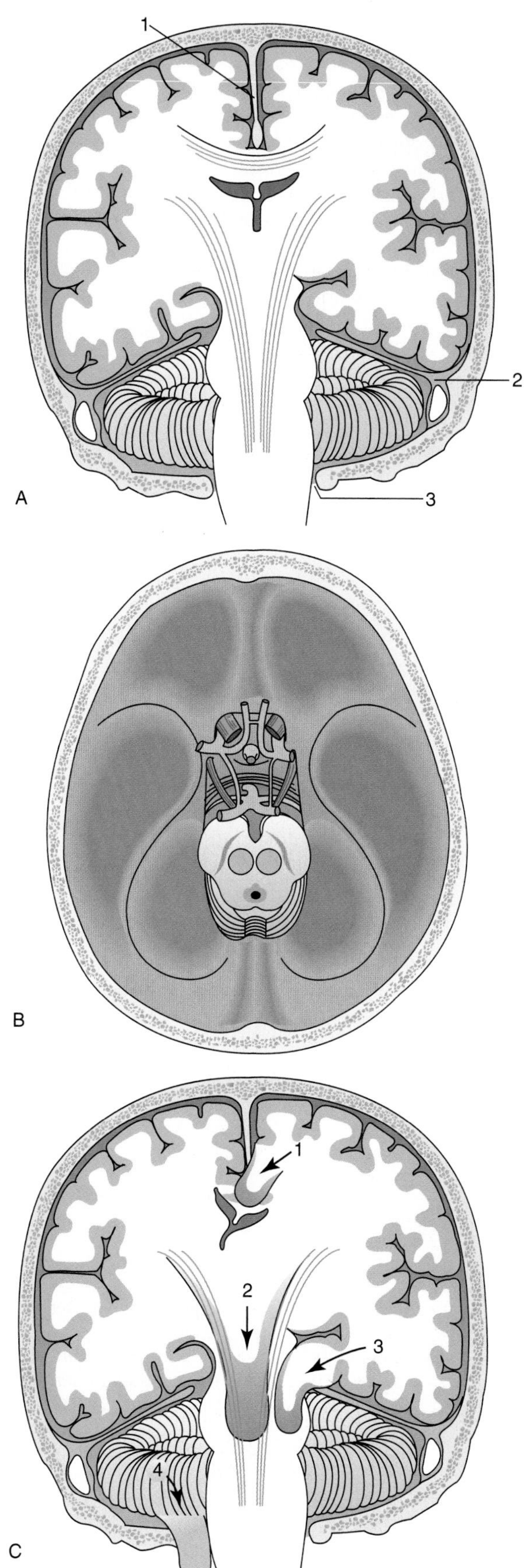

striction, and motor responses to pain that are purposeful or semipurposeful (localizing) and often asymmetric. The clouding of consciousness, which is often a first sign of central herniations, is caused by pressure on the reticular activating system (RAS) in the upper midbrain, which is responsible for wakefulness. As the herniation progresses to the late diencephalic stage, painful stimulation results in decorticate posturing, which may be asymmetric (Fig. 52-5), and there is waxing and waning of respirations with periods of apnea (Cheyne-Stokes respirations). With midbrain involvement, the pupils are fixed and midsize (approximately 5 mm in diameter), and reflex adduction of the eyes is impaired; pain elicits cerebrate posturing; and respirations change from Cheyne-Stokes to neurogenic hyperventilation, in which the frequency may exceed 40 breaths per minute because of uninhibited stimulation of the inspiratory and expiratory centers. Progression to involve the lower pons and upper medulla produces fixed, midpoint (3 to 5 mm) pupils with loss of reflex abduction and adduction of the eyes, and absence of motor responses or only leg flexion on painful stimuli. Once the area of herniation has progressed beyond the diencephalon and into the midbrain and brain stem, the process is generally irreversible and the prognosis poor.[11]

Uncal herniation occurs when a lateral mass pushes the brain tissue centrally and forces the medial aspect of the temporal lobe, which contains the uncus and hippocampal gyrus, under the edge of the tentorial incisura, into the posterior fossa. As a result, the diencephalon and midbrain are compressed and displaced laterally to the opposite side of the tentorium. Cranial nerve III (oculomotor nerve) and the posterior cerebral artery frequently are caught between the uncus and the tentorium. The oculomotor nerve controls pupillary constriction; entrapment of this nerve results in ipsilateral pupillary dilatation, which usually is an early sign of uncal herniation. Consciousness may be unimpaired because the RAS has not yet been affected. However, after any signs of herniation or brain stem compression appear, deterioration may proceed rapidly—making it important to recognize the distinguishing early features of uncal herniations.

As uncal herniations progress, there are changes in motor strength and coordination of voluntary movements because of compression of the descending motor pathways. It is not unusual for initial changes in motor function to occur on the side of the damage because of compression of the contralateral cerebral peduncles. This may result in a false localizing sign of hemiparesis on the same side as cranial nerve III, rather than on the opposite side, where the motor nerves have crossed over, as would be expected. As

FIGURE 52-4 Supporting septa of the brain and patterns of herniation. (**A**) The falx cerebri [1], tentorium cerebelli [2], foramen magnum [3]. (**B**) The location of the incisura or tentorial notch in relation to the cerebral arteries and oculomotor nerve. (**C**) Herniation of the cingulate gyrus under the falx cerebri [1], central transtentorial herniation [2], uncal herniation of the temporal lobe into the tentorial notch [3], and infratentorial herniation of the cerebellar tonsils [4]. (Courtesy of Carole Hilmer, C.M.I.)

TABLE 52-2 Key Structures and Clinical Signs of Cingulate, Central, and Uncal Herniation

Herniation Syndrome	Key Structures Involved	Key Clinical Signs
Cingulate	Anterior cerebral artery	Leg weakness
Central transtentorial	Reticular activating system Corticospinal tract	Altered level of consciousness Decorticate posturing Rostral–caudal deterioration
Uncal	Cerebral peduncle Oculomotor nerve Posterior cerebral artery Cerebellar tonsil Respiratory center	Hemiparesis Ipsilateral pupil dilatation Visual field loss Respiratory arrest

the condition progresses, bilateral positive Babinski responses and respiratory changes (*e.g.*, Cheyne-Stokes respirations, ataxic patterns) occur. Decorticate and decerebrate posturing may develop, followed by dilated, fixed pupils, flaccidity, and respiratory arrest.

Infratentorial Herniation. Infratentorial herniation results from increased pressure in the infratentorial compartment. It often progress rapidly and can cause death because it is likely to involve the lower brain stem centers that control vital cardiopulmonary functions. Herniation may occur superiorly (upward) through the tentorial incisura or inferiorly (downward) through the foramen magnum.

Upward displacement of brain tissue can cause blockage of the aqueduct of Sylvius and lead to hydrocephalus and coma. Downward displacement of the midbrain through the tentorial notch or the cerebellar tonsils through the foramen magnum can interfere with medullary functioning and cause cardiac or respiratory arrest. In cases of preexisting ICP elevations, herniation may occur when the pressure is released from below, such as in a lumbar puncture. If the CSF pathway is blocked and fluid cannot leave the ventricles, the volume expands, and fluid is displaced downward through the tentorial notch. The expanding volume causes all function at a given level to cease as destruction progresses in a rostral-to-caudal direction. The result of this displacement is brain stem ischemia and hemorrhage extending from the diencephalon to the pons. If the lesion expands rapidly, displacement and obstruction occur quickly, leading to irreversible infarction and hemorrhage.

Cerebral Edema

Cerebral edema, or brain swelling, is an increase in tissue volume secondary to abnormal fluid accumulation. There are two types of brain edema: vasogenic and cytotoxic.[1,15] Vasogenic edema occurs when integrity of blood–brain barrier is disrupted, allowing fluid to escape into the extracellular fluid that surrounds brain cells. Cytotoxic edema involves the actual swelling of brain cells themselves. Brain edema may or may not increase ICP. The impact of brain edema depends on the brain's compensatory mechanisms and the extent of the swelling.

Vasogenic Edema. Vasogenic edema occurs with conditions that impair the function of the blood–brain barrier and allow transfer of water and protein from the vascular into the interstitial space. It occurs in conditions such as tumors, prolonged ischemia, hemorrhage, brain injury,

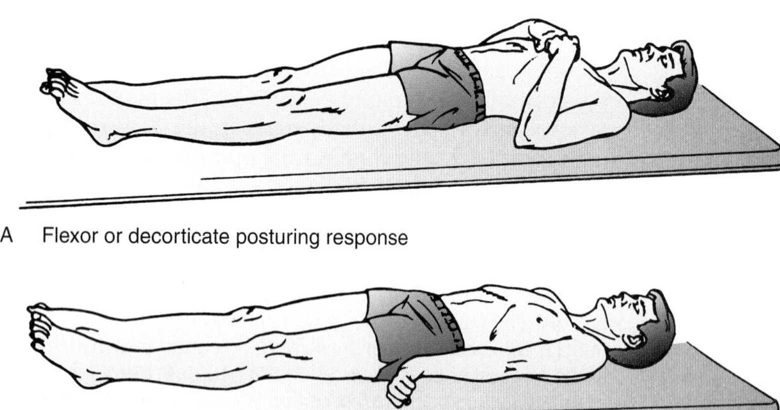

FIGURE 52-5 Abnormal posturing. (**A**) Decorticate rigidity. In decorticate rigidity, the upper arms are held at the sides, with elbows, wrists, and fingers flexed. The legs are extended and internally rotated. The feet are plantar flexed. (**B**) Decerebrate rigidity. In decerebrate rigidity, the jaws are clenched and neck extended. The arms are adducted and stiffly extended at the elbows with the forearms pronated, wrists and fingers flexed. (From Fuller J., Schaller-Ayers J. [1994]. *Health assessment: A nursing approach.* [2nd ed.]. Philadelphia: J.B. Lippincott)

and infectious processes (*e.g.*, meningitis). Vasogenic edema occurs primarily in the white matter of the brain, possibly because the white matter is more compliant than the gray matter. Vasogenic edema can displace a cerebral hemisphere and can be responsible for various types of herniation. The functional manifestations of vasogenic edema include focal neurologic deficits, disturbances in consciousness, and severe intracranial hypertension.

Cytotoxic Edema. Cytotoxic edema involves an increase in intracellular fluid. It can result from hypoosmotic states such as water intoxication or severe ischemia that impair the function of the sodium–potassium membrane pump. Ischemia also results in the inadequate removal of anaerobic metabolic end products such as lactic acid, producing extracellular acidosis. If blood flow is reduced to low levels for extended periods or to extremely low levels for a few minutes, cellular edema can cause the cell membrane to rupture, allowing the escape of intracellular contents into the surrounding extracellular fluid. This leads to damage of neighboring cells. The altered osmotic conditions result in water entry and cell swelling. Major changes in cerebral function, such as stupor and coma, occur with cytotoxic edema. The edema associated with ischemia may be severe enough to produce cerebral infarction with necrosis of brain tissue.

Treatment. Although cerebral edema is viewed as a pathologic process, it does not necessarily disrupt brain function unless it increases the ICP. The localized edema surrounding a brain tumor often responds to corticosteroid therapy (*e.g.*, dexamethasone), but use of these drugs for generalized edema is controversial. The mechanism of action of the corticosteroid drugs in the treatment of cerebral edema is unknown, but in therapeutic doses, they seem to stabilize cell membranes and scavenge free radicals. Osmotic diuretics (*e.g.*, mannitol) may be useful in the acute phase of vasogenic and cytotoxic edema when hypoosmolarity is present.

Hydrocephalus

Enlargement of the CSF compartment occurs with hydrocephalus, which is defined as an abnormal increase in CSF volume in any part or all of the ventricular system. The two causes of hydrocephalus are decreased absorption of CSF and overproduction of CSF. There are two types of hydrocephalus: noncommunicating and communicating.

Noncommunicating or obstructive hydrocephalus occurs when obstruction in the ventricular system prevents the CSF from reaching the arachnoid villi. CSF flow can be obstructed by congenital malformations, from tumors encroaching on the ventricular system, and by inflammation or hemorrhage. The ependyma (*i.e.*, lining of ventricles and CSF-filled spaces) is especially sensitive to viral infections, particularly during embryonic development; ependymitis is believed to be the cause of congenital aqueductal stenosis.[4]

Communicating hydrocephalus results from impaired reabsorption of CSF from the arachnoid villi into the venous system. Decreased absorption can result from a block in the CSF pathway to the arachnoid villi or a failure of the villi to transfer the CSF to the venous system. It can occur if too few villi are formed, if postinfective (meningitis) scarring occludes them, or if the villi become obstructed with fragments of blood or infectious debris. Adenomas of the choroid plexus can cause an overproduction of CSF. This form of hydrocephalus is much less common than that resulting from decreased absorption of CSF.

Similar pathologic patterns occur with noncommunicating and communicating types of hydrocephalus. The cerebral hemispheres become enlarged, and the ventricular system is dilated beyond the point of obstruction. The gyri on the surface of the brain become less prominent, and the white matter is reduced in volume. The presence and extent of the ICP is determined by fluid accumulation and the type of hydrocephalus, the age at onset, and the rapidity and extent of pressure rise. Acute hydrocephalus usually is manifested by increased ICP. Slowly developing hydrocephalus is less likely to produce an increase in ICP, but it may produce deficits such as progressive dementia and gait changes. Computed tomographic (CT) scans are used to diagnose all types of hydrocephalus. The usual treatment is a shunting procedure, which provides an alternative route for return of CSF to the circulation.

When hydrocephalus develops in utero or before the cranial sutures have fused in infancy, the ventricles expand beyond the point of obstruction, the cranial sutures separate, the head expands, and there is bulging of the fontanels (Fig. 52-6). Because the skull is able to expand, signs of increased ICP usually are absent, and intelligence usually is spared. Seizures are common, and in severe cases, optic nerve atrophy leads to blindness. Weakness and uncoordinated movement are common. Surgical placement of a shunt allows for diversion of excess CSF fluid, preventing extreme enlargement of the head. Before surgical shunting procedures were available, the weight and size of the enlarged head made ambulation difficult.

In contrast to hydrocephalus that develops in utero or during infancy, head enlargement does not occur in adults, and increases in ICP depend on whether the condition developed rapidly or slowly. Acute-onset hydrocephalus in adults usually is marked by symptoms of increased ICP, including headache, vomiting, and papilledema or lateral rectus palsy from pressure effects on the cranial nerves. If the obstruction is not relieved, mental deterioration eventually occurs. The pressure of CSF is not always elevated, and the syndrome of low-pressure hydrocephalus may go undetected. Treatment includes surgical shunting for noncommunicating hydrocephalus. In communicating hydrocephalus, attempts to clear the arachnoid villi of exudate may be made, and if these are unsuccessful, surgical shunting may be required.

HEAD INJURY

The brain is enclosed in the protective confines of the rigid bony skull. Although the skull affords protection for the tissues of the CNS, it also provides the potential for development of ischemic and traumatic brain injuries. This is because it cannot expand to accommodate the increase in volume that occurs when there is swelling or bleeding in its

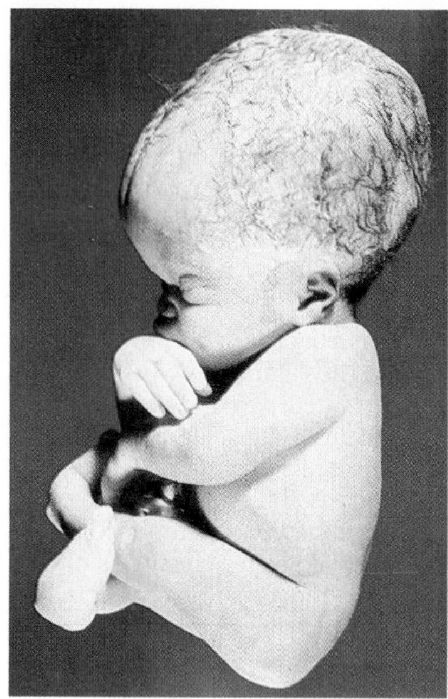

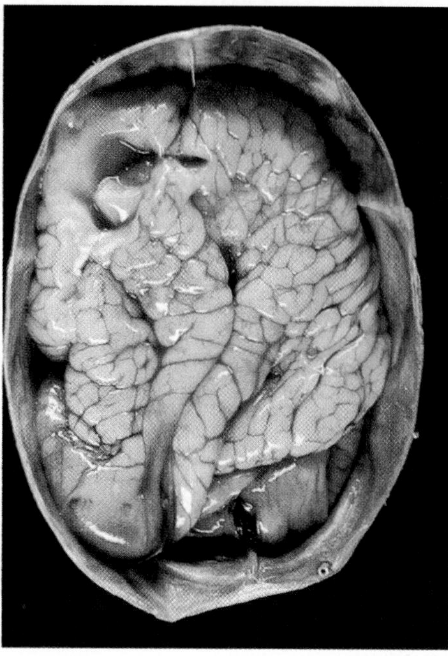

FIGURE 52-6 Congenital hydrocephalus. (**A**) Hydrocephalus occurring before the fusion of the cranial sutures causes pronounced enlargement of the head. (**B**) Removal of the calvarium demonstrates an atrophic and collapsed cerebral cortex. (Rubin E., Farber J.L. [1999]. *Pathology* [3rd ed., p. 1454]. Philadelphia: Lippincott-Raven)

confines. The bony structures themselves can cause injury to the nervous system. Fractures of the skull can compress sections of the nervous system, or they can splinter and cause penetrating wounds.

The term head injury is used to describe all structural damage to the head and has become synonymous with brain injury.[16,17] In the United States, head injury is the leading cause of death among persons younger than 24 years of age. The main causes of head injury are road accidents, falls, and assaults, and the most common cause of fatal head injuries is road accidents involving vehicles and pedestrians.[18]

Head injuries can involve both closed injuries and open wounds. Skull fractures can be divided into three groups: simple, depressed, and basilar. A simple or linear skull fracture is a break in the continuity of bone. A comminuted skull fracture refers to a splintered or multiple fracture line. When bone fragments are embedded into the brain tissue, the fracture is said to be depressed. A fracture of the bones that form the base of the skull is called a basilar skull fracture.

Radiologic examination usually is needed to confirm the presence and extent of a skull fracture. This evaluation is important because of the possible damage to the underlying tissues. The ethmoid cribriform plate, through which the olfactory fibers enter the skull, represents the most fragile portion of the neurocranium and is shattered in basal skull fractures. A frequent complication of basilar skull fractures is leakage of CSF from the nose (rhinorrhea) or ear (otorrhea); this occurs because of the proximity of the base of the skull to the nose and ear. This break in protection of the brain becomes a probable source of infection of the meninges or of brain substance. There may be lacerations to the vessels of the dura, with resultant intracranial bleeding. Skull fractures can damage the cranial nerves (I, II, III, VII, VIII) as they exit the cranial vault.

Types of Brain Injuries

The effects of traumatic head injuries can be divided into two categories: primary or direct injuries, in which damage is caused by impact; and secondary injuries, in which damage results from the subsequent brain swelling, infection, or cerebral hypoxia. The direct brain injuries include diffuse axonal injury and the focal lesions of laceration, contusion, and hemorrhage. Secondary brain injuries are often diffuse or multifocal, including concussion, infection, and hypoxic brain injury. Although the skull and CSF provide protection for the brain, they also can contribute to trauma. When the mechanical forces inducing head injury cause bouncing of the brain in the closed confines of the rigid skull, a coup–contrecoup injury occurs. Because the brain floats freely in the CSF, blunt force to the head can cause the brain to accelerate in the skull and then to decelerate abruptly on hitting the inner confines of the skull. The direct contusion of the brain at the site of external force is referred to as a coup injury, whereas the opposite side of the brain receives the contrecoup injury from rebound against the inner skull surfaces (Fig. 52-7). As the brain strikes the rough surface of the cranial vault, brain tissue, blood vessels, nerve tracts, and other structures are bruised and torn, resulting in contusions and hematomas.

Ischemia is considered the most common cause of secondary brain injury. It can result from the hypoxia and hypotension that occur during the resuscitation process or from the impairment of regulatory mechanisms by which cerebrovascular responses maintain an adequate blood flow and oxygen supply.[19,20] Insults that occur immediately after injury or in the course of resuscitation efforts are important determinants of the outcome from severe brain injury. More than 25% of patients with severe head injury sustain one or more secondary insults in the time between injury and resuscitation, indicating the need for

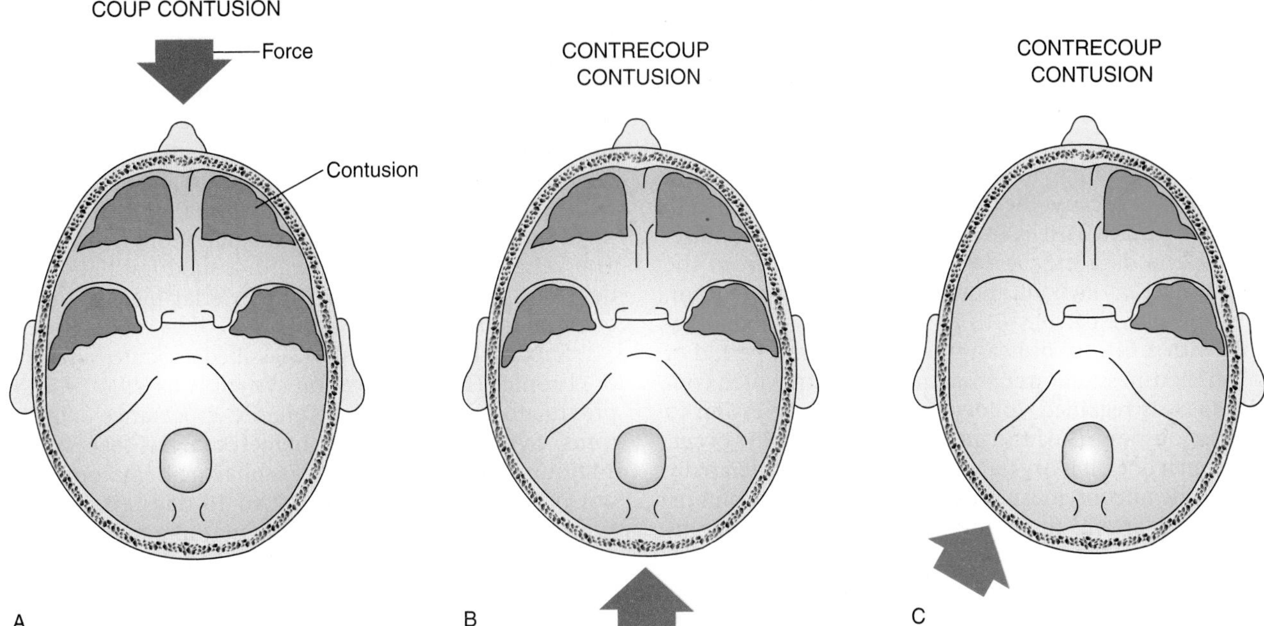

FIGURE 52-7 Mechanisms of cerebral contusion in coup–contrecoup injuries. (**A**) A focal area of cerebral injury (coup contusion) at the point of impact. The cerebral hemispheres float in the cerebrospinal fluid. (**B**) Rapid deceleration or, less commonly, acceleration, causes the cortex to forcefully impact into the anterior and middle fossa causing injury to the side of the brain opposite the site of injury (contrecoup contusion). (**C**) The position of a contrecoup contusion is determined by the direction of force and the intracranial anatomy. (Courtesy of Dmitri Karetnikov, artist). (Rubin E., Farber J.L. [1999]. *Pathology* [3rd ed., p. 1461]. Philadelphia: Lippincott-Raven)

improved airway management and circulatory status.[19] The significance of secondary injuries depends on the extent of damage caused by the primary injury. Certain secondary injuries have been discussed, such as increased ICP, cerebral edema, and brain herniation.

In mild head injury, there may be momentary loss of consciousness without demonstrable neurologic symptoms or residual damage, except for possible residual amnesia. Microscopic changes usually can be detected in the neurons and glia within hours of injury, but brain imaging is normal. Concussion is defined as a momentary interruption of brain function with or without loss of consciousness. Although recovery usually takes place within 24 hours, mild symptoms, such as headache, irritability, insomnia, and poor concentration and memory, may persist for months. This is known as the postconcussion syndrome. Because these complaints are vague and subjective, they sometimes are regarded as being of psychological origin. Postconcussion syndrome can have a significant effect on activities of daily living and return to employment. Persons with postconcussion syndrome may need cognitive retraining or psychological support.

In moderate head injury, many small hemorrhages and some swelling of brain tissue occur. These contusions often are distributed along the rough, irregular inner surface of the brain and are more likely to occur in the frontal or temporal lobes, resulting in cognitive and motor deficits. Moderate head injury is characterized by a longer period of unconsciousness and may be associated with focal manifestations such as hemiparesis, aphasia, and cranial nerve palsy. In this type of injury, the contusions often can be visualized on CT scan.

Severe head injury involves more extensive damage to brain structures and a deeper level of coma than moderate head injury. In severe head injury, primary damage to the brain often is instantaneous and irreversible, resulting from shearing and pressure forces that cause diffuse axonal injury, disruption of blood vessels, and tissue damage. It often is accompanied by neurologic deficits such as hemiplegia. Severe head injuries often occur with injury to other parts of the body such as the extremities, chest, and abdomen. Blood may extravasate into the brain; if the contusion is severe, the blood may accumulate, as in intracranial hemorrhage. Similarly, when laceration of the brain directly under the area of injury occurs, especially if the skull is fractured, hemorrhage may be sufficiently extensive to form a hematoma.

Hematomas

Hematomas result from vascular injury and bleeding. Depending on the anatomic position of the ruptured vessel, bleeding can occur in any of several compartments, including the epidural, subdural, and subarachnoid spaces or into the brain itself (intracerebral hematoma).

Epidural Hematoma. Epidural hematomas usually are caused by head injury in which the skull is fractured. An epidural (extradural) hematoma is one that develops between the inner table of the bones of the skull and the dura (Fig. 52-8). It usually results from a tear in an artery, most often the middle meningeal, usually in association with a skull fracture.[1] Because bleeding is arterial in origin, rapid compression of the brain occurs from the expanding hematoma. Epidural hematoma is more common in a young person because the dura is not so firmly attached to the skull surface as it is in an older person; as a consequence, the dura can be easily stripped away from the inner surface of the skull, allowing the hematoma to form.

Typically, a person with an epidural hematoma presents with a history of head injury and a brief period of unconsciousness followed by a lucid period in which consciousness is regained, followed by rapid progression to unconsciousness. The lucid interval does not always occur, but when it does, it is of great diagnostic value. With rapidly developing unconsciousness, there are focal symptoms related to the area of the brain involved. These symptoms can include ipsilateral (same side) pupil dilatation and contralateral (opposite side) hemiparesis from uncal herniation. If the hematoma is not removed, the condition progresses, with increased ICP, tentorial herniation, and death. However, prognosis is excellent if the hematoma is removed before loss of consciousness occurs.

Subdural Hematoma. A subdural hematoma develops in the area between the dura and the arachnoid (subdural space) and usually is the result of a tear in the small bridging veins that connect veins on the surface of the cortex to dural sinuses. The bridging veins pass from the pial vessels through the CSF-filled subarachnoid space, penetrate the arachnoid and the dura, and empty into the intradural sinuses.[4] These veins are readily snapped in head injury when the brain moves suddenly in relation to the cranium (Fig. 52-9). Bleeding can occur between the dura and arachnoid (*i.e.,* subdural hematoma) or into the CSF-filled subarachnoid space (*i.e.,* subarachnoid hematoma). The venous source of bleeding in a subdural hematoma develops more slowly than the arterial bleeding in an epidural hematoma.

Subdural hematomas are classified as acute, subacute, or chronic. This classification system is based on the approximate time intervals before the appearance of symptoms. Symptoms of acute hematoma are seen within 24 hours of the injury, whereas subacute hematoma does not produce symptoms until 2 to 10 days after injury. Symptoms of chronic subdural hematoma may not arise until several weeks after the injury. These classifications are based partially on pathologic considerations.

Acute subdural hematomas progress rapidly and have a high mortality rate because of the severe secondary injuries related to edema and increased ICP. The high mortality rate has been associated with uncontrolled ICP increase, loss of consciousness, decerebrate posturing, and delay in surgical removal of the hematoma. The clinical picture is similar to that of epidural hematoma, except that there usually is no lucid interval. Morbidity and mortality rates are higher with acute subdural hematoma than with epidural and intracerebral hematoma. By contrast, in subacute hematoma, there may be a period of improvement in the level of consciousness and neurologic symptoms, only to be followed by deterioration if the hematoma is not removed.

Symptoms of chronic subdural hematoma develop weeks after a head injury, so much later that the person may not remember having had a head injury. Chronic subdural hematoma is more common in older persons because brain atrophy causes the brain to shrink away from the dura and stretch fragile bridging veins. These veins rupture, causing slow seepage of blood into the subdural space. Fibroblastic activity causes the hematoma to become encapsulated. The sanguinous fluid within this encapsulated area has high os-

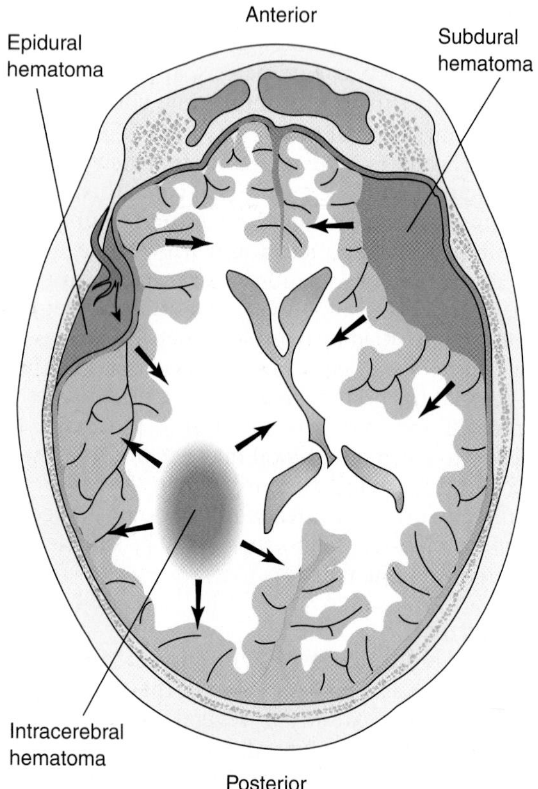

FIGURE 52-8 Location of epidural, subdural, and intracerebral hematomas.

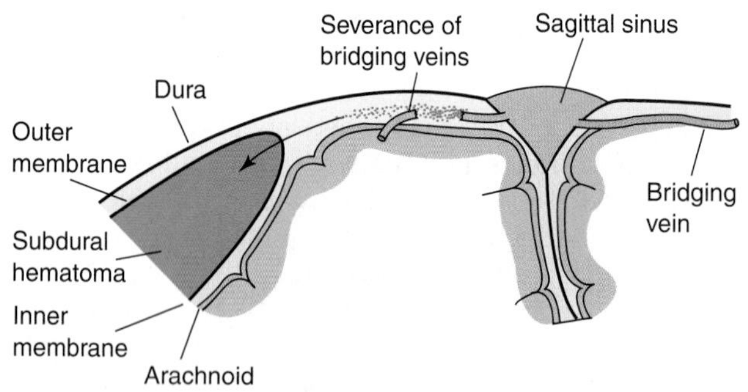

FIGURE 52-9 Mechanism of bleeding in subdural hematoma. (Courtesy of Dmitri Karetnikov, artist). (Rubin E., Farber J.L. [1999]. *Pathology* [3rd ed., p. 1460]. Philadelphia: Lippincott-Raven)

motic pressure and draws in fluid from the surrounding subarachnoid space; the mass increases in size, exerting pressure on the cranial contents. In some instances, the clinical picture is less defined, with the most prominent symptom being a decreasing level of consciousness indicated by drowsiness, confusion, headache, and apathy.

Traumatic Intracerebral Hematomas. Traumatic intracerebral hematomas may be single or multiple. They can occur in any lobe of the brain but are most common in the frontal or temporal lobes. They may occur in association with the severe motion that the brain undergoes during head injury, or a contusion can coalesce into a hematoma. Intracerebral hematomas occur more frequently in older persons and alcoholics whose brain vessels are more friable.

The signs and symptoms produced by an intracerebral hematoma depend on its size and location within the brain. Signs of increased ICP can be manifested if the hematoma is large and encroaching on vital structures. A hematoma in the temporal lobe can be dangerous because of the potential for lateral herniation.

Treatment of an intracerebral hematoma can be medical or surgical. For a large hematoma with a rapidly deteriorating neurologic condition, surgery to evacuate the clot usually is indicated. Surgery may not be needed in someone who is neurologically stable despite neurologic deficits; in this case, the hematoma may resolve much like a contusion.

MANIFESTATIONS OF GLOBAL BRAIN INJURY

Global brain injury, whether due to head trauma, stroke, or other pathologies, is manifested by alterations in sensory and motor function and by changes in the level of consciousness. In contrast to focal injury, which causes alterations in sensory function or motor function, global injury tends to result in altered levels of consciousness. Severe injury that seriously compromises brain function may result in brain death.

The cerebral hemispheres are the most susceptible to damage, and the most frequent sign of brain dysfunction is altered level of consciousness and change in behavior. As the brain structures in the diencephalon, midbrain, pons, and medulla are affected, additional respiratory, pupillary and eye movement reflexes, and motor signs become evident (Table 52-3). Hemodynamic and respiratory instability are the last signs to occur because their regulatory centers are located low in the medulla.

In progressive brain deterioration, the person's neurologic capabilities appear to deteriorate in stepwise fashion. Similarly, as neurologic function returns, there appears to be stepwise progress to higher levels of consciousness. Deterioration of brain function from supratentorial lesions tends to follow a rostral-to-caudal stepwise progression, which is observed as the brain initially compensates for injury and subsequently decompensates with loss of autoregulation and cerebral perfusion. Infratentorial (brain stem) lesions may lead to an early, sometimes abrupt disturbance in consciousness without any orderly rostrocaudal progression of neurologic signs.

Altered Levels of Consciousness

All forms of brain injury and pathology can lead to altered levels of consciousness. Consciousness is the state of awareness of self and the environment and of being able to become oriented to new stimuli.[6] It has traditionally been divided into two components: (1) arousal and wakefulness, and (2) content and cognition. The content and cognition aspects of consciousness are determined by a functioning cerebral cortex. Arousal and wakefulness requires the concurrent functioning of both cerebral hemispheres and an intact RAS in the brain stem.

Anatomic and Physiologic Basis of Consciousness. The reticular formation is a diffuse, primitive system of interlacing nerve cells and fibers in the brain stem that receive input from multiple sensory pathways (Fig. 52-10). Anatomically, the reticular formation constitutes the central core of the brain stem, extending from the medulla through the pons to the midbrain, which is continuous caudally with the spinal cord and rostrally with the subthalamus, the hypothalamus, and the thalamus.[21] Fibers from the RAS also project to the autonomic nervous system and motor systems. The hypothalamus plays a predominant role in maintaining homeostasis through integration of somatic, visceral, and endocrine functions. Inputs from the reticular formation, vestibulospinal projections, and other motor

TABLE 52-3 Key Signs in Rostral-to-Caudal Progression of Brain Lesions

Level of Brain Injury	Key Clinical Signs
Diencephalon	Impaired consciousness; small, reactive pupils; intact oculocephalic reflex; decorticate posturing; Cheyne-Stokes respirations
Midbrain	Coma, fixed, midsize pupils; impaired oculocephalic reflex; neurogenic hyperventilation; decerebrate posturing
Pons	Coma, fixed, irregular pupils; dysconjugate gaze; impaired cold caloric stimulation; loss of corneal reflex; hemiparesis/quadriparesis; decerebrate posturing; apneustic respirations
Medulla	Coma, fixed pupils, flaccidity, loss of gag and cough reflexes, ataxic/apneic respirations

BRAIN INJURY AND LEVELS OF CONSCIOUSNESS

- Consciousness is a global function that depends on a diffuse neural network that includes activity of the reticular activating system (RAS) and both cerebral hemispheres.
- Impaired consciousness implies diffuse brain injury to the RAS at any level (medulla through thalamus) or both cerebral hemispheres simultaneously.
- In contrast, local brain injury causes focal neurologic deficit but does not disrupt consciousness.

systems are integrated to provide a continuously adapting background of muscle tone and posture to facilitate voluntary motor actions. Reticular formation neurons that function in regulation of cardiovascular, respiratory, and other visceral functions are intermingled with those that maintain other reticular formation functions.

Ascending fibers of the reticular formation, known as the ascending RAS, transmit activating information to all parts of the cerebral cortex. The flow of information in the ascending RAS activates the hypothalamic and limbic structures that regulate emotional and behavioral responses such as those that occur in response to pain and loud noises, and they exert facilitory effects on cortical neurons. Without cortical activation, a person is less able to detect specific stimuli, and the level of consciousness is reduced. The pathways for the ascending RAS travel through the midbrain, and lesions of the midbrain can interrupt RAS activity, leading to altered levels of consciousness and coma.

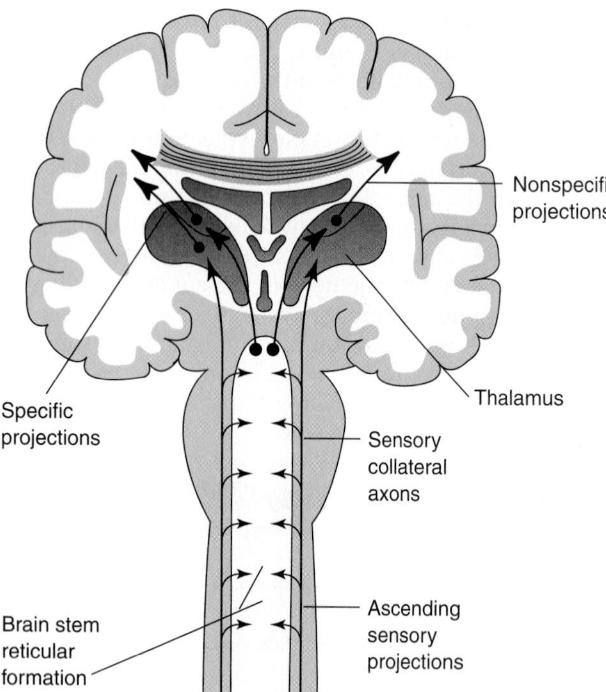

FIGURE 52-10 The brain stem reticular formation and reticular activating system. Ascending sensory tracts send axon collateral fibers to the reticular formation. These give rise to fibers synapsing in the nonspecific nuclei of the thalamus. From there the nonspecific thalamic projections influence widespread areas of the cerebral cortex and limbic system. (Rhoades R.A., Tanner G.A. [1996]. *Medical physiology.* Boston: Little, Brown)

Any deficit in level of consciousness, from mild confusion to stupor or coma, indicates injury to either the RAS or to both cerebral hemispheres concurrently. For example, consciousness may decline owing to severe systemic metabolic derangements that affect both hemispheres, or from head trauma causing shear injuries to white matter of both the RAS and the cerebral hemispheres. Brain injuries that affect a hemisphere unilaterally and also spare the RAS, such as cerebral infarction, usually do not cause impaired consciousness.

Altered Levels of Consciousness. Levels of consciousness reflect an orientation to person, place, and time. A fully conscious person is totally aware of her or his surroundings.[6] Levels of consciousness exist on a continuum that includes consciousness, confusion, delirium, obtundation, stupor, and coma (Table 52-4).

The earliest signs of diminution in level of consciousness are inattention, mild confusion, disorientation, and blunted responsiveness. With further deterioration, the delirious person becomes markedly inattentive and variably lethargic or agitated. The person may progress to become obtunded and may respond only to vigorous or noxious stimuli.

Because of its simplicity of application, the Glasgow Coma Scale has gained almost universal acceptance as a method for assessing the level of consciousness in persons with brain injury[22,23] (Table 52-5). Numbered scores are given to responses of eye opening, verbal utterances, and motor responses. The total score is the sum of the best response in each category.

Other Manifestations of Deteriorating Brain Function

Additional elements in the initial neurologic evaluation of a person with brain injury include checking for abnormalities in the size of the pupils and their reaction to light, weakness and asymmetry of motor function, and evidence of decortication or decerebration posturing.

Pupillary Reflexes and Eye Movements. Although the pupils may initially respond briskly to light, they become unreactive and dilated as brain function deteriorates. A bilateral loss of the pupillary light response is indicative of lesions of the brain stem. A unilateral loss of the pupillary light response may be due to a lesion of the optic or oculomotor pathways. The oculocephalic reflex (doll's-head eye movement) can be used to determine whether the brain stem centers for eye movement are intact (Fig. 52-11). If the oculocephalic reflex is inconclusive, and if there are no contraindications, the oculovestibular (*i.e.,* cold caloric test, in which cold water is instilled into the ear canal) may be used to elicit nystagmus (see Chapter 55).

TABLE 52-4 Descending Levels of Consciousness and Their Characteristics

Level of Consciousness	Characteristics
Confusion	Disturbance of consciousness characterized by impaired ability to think clearly, and to perceive, respond to, and remember current stimuli; also disorientation
Delirium	State of disturbed consciousness with motor restlessness, transient hallucinations, disorientation, and sometimes delusions
Obtundation	Disorder of decreased alertness with associated psychomotor retardation
Stupor	A state in which the person is not unconscious but exhibits little or no spontaneous activity
Coma	A state of being unarousable and unresponsive to external stimuli or internal needs; often determined by the Glasgow Coma Scale

(Data from Bates D. [1993]. The management of medical coma. *Journal of Neurology, Neurosurgery, and Psychiatry* 56, 590)

Decorticate and Decerebrate Posturing. With the early onset of unconsciousness, there is some combative movement and purposeful movement in response to pain. As coma progresses, noxious stimuli can initiate rigidity and abnormal postures if the motor tracts are interrupted at specific levels. These abnormal postures are called decortication and decerebration.[11] Decorticate (flexion) posturing is characterized by flexion of the arms, wrists, and fingers, with abduction of the upper extremities, internal rotation, and plantar flexion of the lower extremities (Fig. 52-5A). Decorticate posturing results from lesions of the cerebral hemisphere or internal capsule. Decerebrate (extensor) posturing results from increased muscle excitability (see Fig. 52-5B). It is characterized by rigidity of the arms with palms of the hands turned away from the body and with stiffly extended legs and plantar flexion of the feet. This response occurs when lesions of the diencephalon extend to involve the midbrain and upper brain stem. Both decerebrate and decorticate posturing are poor prognostic signs.

Respiratory Responses. Early respiratory changes include yawning and sighing, with progression to Cheyne-Stokes breathing. With progression continuing to the midbrain,

TABLE 52-5 The Glasgow Coma Scale

Test	Score*
Eye Opening (E)	
Spontaneous	4
To call	3
To pain	2
None	1
Motor Response (M)	
Obeys commands	6
Localizes pain	5
Normal flexion (withdrawal)	4
Abnormal flexion (decorticate)	3
Extension (decerebrate)	2
None (flaccid)	1
Verbal Response (V)	
Oriented	5
Confused conversation	4
Inappropriate words	3
Incomprehensible sounds	2
None	1

*GCS Score = E + M + V. Best possible score = 15; worst possible score = 3.

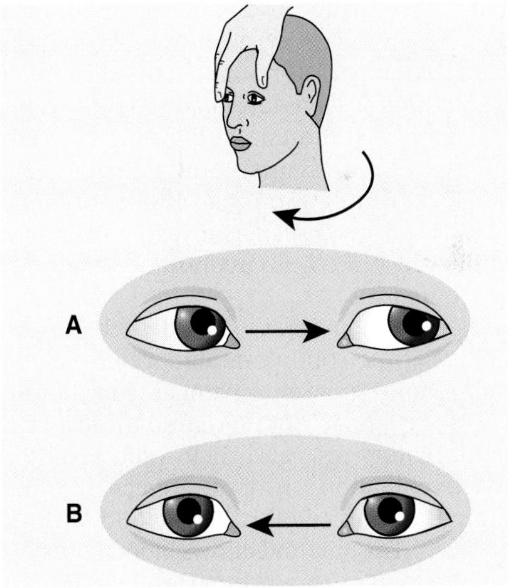

FIGURE 52-11 Doll's head response. The *doll's-head eye response* demonstrates the always-present vestibular static reflexes without forebrain interference or suppression. Severe damage to the forebrain or to the brain stem rostral to the pons often results in loss of rostral control of these static vestibular reflexes. If the person's head is moved from side to side or up and down, the eyes will move in conjugate gaze to the opposite side (**A**), much like those of a doll with counterweighted eyes. If the doll's-head phenomenon is observed, brain stem function at the level of the pons is considered intact (in a comatose person). In the unconscious person without intact brain stem function and vestibular static reflexes, the eyes stay in midposition (fixed) or turn in the same direction (**B**) as the head is turned.

respirations change to neurogenic hyperventilation, in which the frequency of respirations may exceed 40 breaths per minute because of uninhibited stimulation of inspiratory and expiratory centers. With medullary involvement, respirations become ataxic (*i.e.*, totally uncoordinated and irregular). Apnea may occur because of a lack of responsiveness to carbon dioxide stimulation. Complete ventilatory assistance is often required at this point.

Brain Death

Brain death is defined as the irreversible loss of function of the brain, including the brain stem.[24] Irreversibility implies that brain death cannot be reversed. Some conditions such as drug and metabolic intoxication can cause cessation of brain functions that is completely reversible, even when they produce clinical cessation of brain functions and electroencephalogram (EEG) silence. This needs to be excluded before declaring that a person is brain dead.

With advances in scientific knowledge and technology that have provided the means for artificially maintaining ventilatory and circulatory function, the definition of death has had to be continually reexamined. In 1995, the Quality of Standards Subcommittee of the American Academy of Neurology published the clinical parameters for determining brain death and procedures for testing persons older than 18 years of age.[25] According to these parameters, "brain death is the absence of clinical brain function when the proximate cause is known and demonstrably irreversible."[25] Clinical examination must disclose at least the absence of responsiveness, brain stem reflexes, and respiratory effort. Brain death is a clinical diagnosis, and a repeat evaluation at least 6 hours later is recommended.[25] Longer periods of observation of absent brain activity are required in cases of children, drug overdose (*e.g.*, barbiturates, other CNS depressants), drug toxicity (*e.g.*, neuromuscular blocking drugs, aminoglycoside antibiotics), and neuromuscular diseases such as myasthenia gravis, hypothermia, and shock. Medical circumstances may require use of confirmatory tests.

Medical documentation should include cause and irreversibility of the condition, absence of brain stem reflexes and motor responses to pain, absence of respiration with a PCO_2 of 60 mm Hg or more, and the justification for use of confirmatory tests and their results. Apnea is confirmed after ventilation with pure oxygen 10 minutes before withdrawal from the ventilator, followed by passive flow of oxygen. This method allows blood levels of carbon dioxide to rise to a PCO_2 of 60 mm Hg after a 10-minute period of apnea, without hazardously lowering the oxygen content of the blood. If respiratory reflexes are intact, the hypercarbia that develops should stimulate ventilatory effort within 30 seconds. Spontaneous breathing efforts indicate that the brain stem is functioning. Confirmatory tests of brain death include conventional angiography (*i.e.*, no intracerebral filling at the level of the carotid bifurcation or circle of Willis), transcranial Doppler ultrasonography, technetium-99m hexamethylpropyleneamine oxime brain scan (*i.e.*, no uptake of isotope in brain parenchyma), somatosensory evoked potentials, and EEG. In the United States, EEG testing is often used to establish brain death. EEG testing should reveal no electrical activity during at least 30 minutes of recording that adheres to the minimal technical criteria for EEG recording in suspected brain death as adopted by the American Electroencephalographic Society, including 16-channel EEG instruments.

Persistent Vegetative State

Advances in the care of brain-injured persons during the past several decades have resulted in survival of many persons who previously would have died. Unfortunately, most persons in prolonged coma who survive evolve to what often is called the persistent vegetative state. The vegetative state is characterized by loss of all cognitive functions and the unawareness of self and surroundings. Reflex and vegetative functions remain, including sleep–wake cycles.[26] Persons in the vegetative state must be fed and require full nursing care.

The criteria for diagnosis of vegetative state include the absence of awareness of self and environment and an inability to interact with others; the absence of sustained or reproducible voluntary behavioral responses; lack of language comprehension; sufficiently preserved hypothalamic and brain stem function to maintain life; bowel and bladder incontinence; and variably preserved cranial nerve (*e.g.*, pupillary, gag) and spinal cord reflexes.[26] The diagnosis of persistent vegetative state requires that the condition has continued for at least 1 month.

In summary, many of the agents that cause brain damage do so through common pathways, including hypoxia or ischemia, accumulation of excitatory neurotransmitters, increased ICP, and cerebral edema. Deprivation of oxygen (*i.e.*, hypoxia) or blood flow (*i.e.*, ischemia) can have deleterious effects on the brain structures. Ischemia can be focal, as in stroke, or global. Global ischemia occurs when blood flow is inadequate to meet the metabolic needs of the brain, as in cardiac arrest.

The term head injury is used to describe all structural damage to the head and has become synonymous with brain injury. The effects of traumatic head injuries can be divided into two categories: primary or secondary injuries. Primary injuries result from direct impact, resulting in skull fracture, concussion, or contusion. In secondary injuries, damage results from the subsequent brain swelling; epidural, subdural, or intracerebral hematoma formation; infection; cerebral hypoxia; and ischemia. Even if there is no break in the skull, a blow to the head can cause severe and diffuse brain damage. Such closed injuries vary in severity and can be classified as focal or diffuse. Diffuse injuries include concussion and diffuse axonal injury. Focal injuries include contusion, laceration, and hemorrhage.

Brain injury is manifested by alterations in sensory and motor function and by changes in the level of consciousness. Consciousness is a state of awareness of self and environment. It exists on a normal continuum of wakefulness and sleep and a pathologic continuum of wakefulness and coma. In progressive brain injury, coma may follow a rostral-to-caudal progression with characteristic changes in levels of consciousness, respiratory activity, pupillary and oculovestibular reflexes, and muscle tone occurring as the diencephalon through the medulla are affected.

Brain death is defined as the irreversible loss of function of the brain, including that of the brain stem. Clinical examination must disclose at least the absence of responsiveness, brain stem reflexes, and respiratory effort. The vegetative state is characterized by loss of all cognitive functions and the unawareness of self and surroundings, whereas reflex and vegetative functions remain intact.

Cerebrovascular Disease

After completing this section of the chapter, you should be able to meet the following objectives:

- List the major vessels in the cerebral circulation and state the contribution of the internal carotid arteries, the vertebral arteries, and the circle of Willis to the cerebral circulation
- Describe the autoregulation of cerebral blood flow
- Explain the substitution of "brain attack" for stroke in terms of making a case for early diagnosis and treatment
- Differentiate the pathologies of ischemic and hemorrhagic stroke
- Explain the significance of transient ischemic attacks, the ischemic penumbra, and watershed zones of infarction and how these conditions relate to ischemic stroke
- Cite the most common cause of subarachnoid hemorrhage and state the complications associated with subarachnoid hemorrhage
- Describe the alterations in cerebral vasculature that occur with arteriovenous malformations
- Describe the progression of motor deficits and problems with speech and language that occur as a result of stroke

Cerebrovascular disease encompasses a number of disorders involving vessels in the cerebral circulation. These disorders include stroke and transient ischemic attacks (TIAs), aneurysmal subarachnoid hemorrhage, and arteriovenous malformations.

CEREBRAL CIRCULATION

Cerebral Blood Vessels

The blood flow to the brain is supplied by the two internal carotid arteries anteriorly and the vertebral arteries posteriorly (Fig. 52-12). The internal carotid artery, a terminal branch of the common carotid artery, branches into several arteries: ophthalmic, posterior communicating, anterior choroidal, anterior cerebral, and middle cerebral (Fig. 52-13). Most of the arterial blood in the internal carotid arteries is distributed through the anterior and middle cerebral arteries. The anterior cerebral arteries supply the medial surface of the frontal and parietal lobes and the anterior half of the thalamus, the corpus striatum, part of the corpus callosum, and the anterior limb of the internal capsule. The genu and posterior limb of the internal capsule and medial globus pallidus are fed by the anterior choroidal branch of the internal carotid artery. The middle cerebral artery passes laterally, supplying the lateral basal ganglia and the insula, and then emerges on the lateral cortical surface, supplying the inferior frontal gyrus, the motor and premotor frontal cortex concerned with delicate face and hand control. It is the major vascular source for the language cortices (frontal and superior temporal), the primary and association auditory cortex (superior temporal gyrus), and primary and association somesthetic cortex for the face and hand (postcentral gyrus, parietal). The middle cerebral artery is functionally

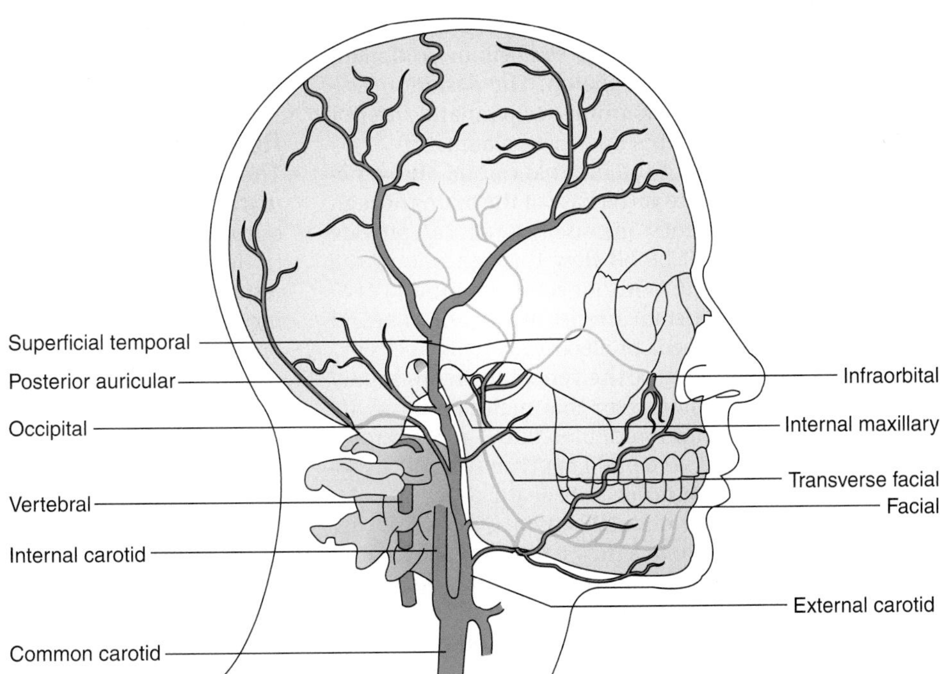

FIGURE 52-12 Branches of the right external carotid artery. The internal carotid artery ascends to the base of the brain. The right vertebral artery is also shown as it ascends through the transverse foramina of the cervical vertebrae.

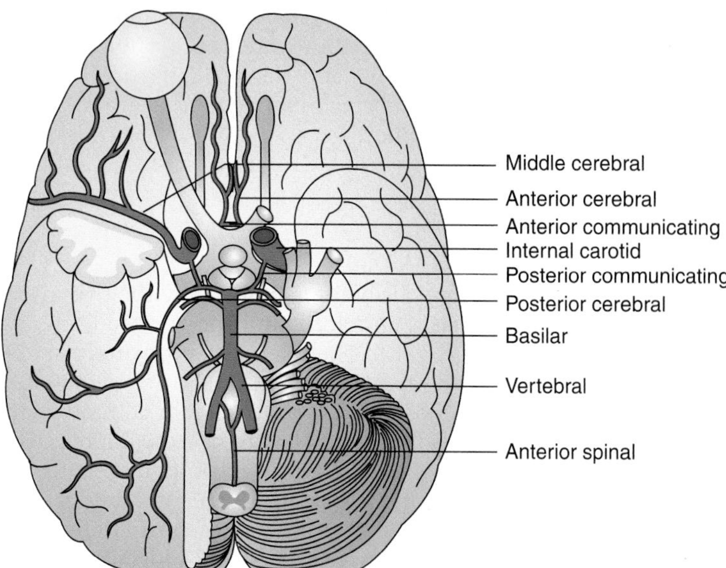

FIGURE 52-13 The circle of Willis as seen at the base of a brain removed from the skull.

a continuation of the internal carotid; emboli of the internal carotid most frequently become lodged in branches of the middle cerebral artery. The consequences of ischemia of these areas may be most devastating, resulting in damage to the fine manipulative skills of the face or upper limb and to receptive and expressive communication functions (*e.g.*, aphasia).

The two vertebral arteries arise from the subclavian artery and enter the foramina in the transverse spinal processes at the level of the sixth cervical vertebra and continue upward through the foramina of the upper six vertebrae; they wind behind the atlas and enter the skull through the foramen magnum and unite to form the basilar artery, which then diverges to terminate in the posterior cerebral arteries. Branches of the basilar and vertebral arteries supply the medulla, pons, cerebellum, midbrain, and caudal part of the diencephalon. The posterior cerebral arteries supply the remaining occipital and inferior regions of the temporal lobes and the thalamus.

The distal branches of the internal carotid and vertebral arteries communicate at the base of the brain through the circle of Willis; this anastomosis of arteries can provide continued circulation if blood flow through one of the main vessels is disrupted. Without collateral input, cessation of blood flow in cerebral arteries may result in neural damage as metabolic needs of electrically active cells exceed nutrient supply. Because the vertebral arteries supply the structures in the brain stem that maintain basic life support reflexes, interruption of blood flow in the carotid arteries with preserved vertebral supply may result in severe coma, although not necessarily death.

The cerebral blood is drained by two sets of veins that empty into the dural venous sinuses: the deep (great) cerebral venous system and the superficial venous system. In contrast to the superficial cerebral veins that travel through the pia mater on the surface of the cerebral cortex, the deep system is well protected. These vessels connect directly to the sagittal sinuses in the falx cerebri by way of bridging veins. They travel through the CSF-filled subarachnoid space and penetrate the arachnoid and then the dura to reach the dural venous sinuses. This system of sinuses returns blood to the heart primarily by way of the internal jugular veins. Alternate routes for venous flow also exist; for example, venous blood may exit through the emissary veins that pass through the skull and through veins that traverse various foramina to empty into extracranial veins.

The intracranial venous system has no valves. The direction of flow depends on gravity or the relative pressure in the venous sinuses compared with that of the extracranial veins. Increases in intrathoracic pressure, as can occur with coughing or performance of Valsalva's maneuver, produce a rise in central venous pressure that is reflected back into the internal jugular veins and to the dural sinuses. This briefly raises the ICP.

Regulation of Cerebral Blood Flow

The blood flow to the brain is maintained at approximately 750 mL/minute or one sixth of the resting cardiac output.[13] The regulation of blood flow to the brain is controlled largely by autoregulatory or local mechanisms that respond to the metabolic needs of the brain. Cerebral autoregulation has been classically defined as the ability of the brain to maintain constant cerebral blood flow despite changes in systemic arterial pressure. This allows the cerebral cortex to adjust cerebral blood flow locally to satisfy its metabolic needs. The autoregulation of cerebral blood flow is efficient within a MABP range of approximately 60 to 140 mm Hg.[13] Although total cerebral blood flow remains relatively stable throughout marked changes in cardiac output and arterial blood pressure, regional blood flow may vary markedly in response to local changes in metabolism. If blood pressure falls below 60 mm Hg, cerebral blood flow becomes severely compromised, and if it rises above the upper limit of autoregulation, blood flow increases rapidly and overstretches the cerebral vessels. In persons with hypertension, this autoregulatory range shifts to a higher level.

At least three metabolic factors affect cerebral blood flow: carbon dioxide, hydrogen ion, and oxygen concentration. Increased carbon dioxide provides a potent stimulus for vasodilatation—a doubling of the PCO_2 in the blood results in a doubling of cerebral blood flow. Increased hydrogen ion concentrations also increase cerebral blood flow, serving to wash away the neurally depressive acidic materials.[13] Profound extracellular acidosis induces vasomotor paralysis, in which case cerebral blood flow may depend entirely on the systemic arterial blood pressure. Decreased oxygen concentration also increases cerebral blood flow.

The deep cerebral blood vessels appear to be completely controlled by autoregulation. However, the superficial and major cerebral blood vessels are innervated by the sympathetic nervous system. Under normal physiologic conditions, local regulatory and autoregulatory mechanisms override the effects of sympathetic stimulation. However, when local mechanisms fail, sympathetic control of cerebral blood pressure becomes important.[13] For example, when the arterial pressure rises to very high levels during strenuous exercise or in other conditions, the sympathetic nervous system constricts the large and intermediate-sized superficial blood vessels as a means of protecting the smaller, more easily damaged vessels. Sympathetic reflexes are believed to cause vasospasm in the intermediate and large arteries in some types of brain damage, such as that caused by rupture of a cerebral aneurysm.

STROKE (BRAIN ATTACK)

Stroke is the syndrome of acute focal neurologic deficit from a vascular disorder that injures brain tissue. Stroke remains one of the leading causes of mortality and morbidity in the United States. Each year, 700,000 Americans are afflicted with stroke, and approximately 167,661 of these persons die; many survivors are left with at least some degree of neurologic impairment.[27] The term brain attack has been promoted to highlight that time-dependent tissue damage occurs and to raise awareness of the need for rapid emergency treatment, similar to that with heart attack.

There are two main types of strokes: ischemic and hemorrhagic. Ischemic strokes are caused by an interruption of blood flow in a cerebral vessel and are the most common type of stroke, accounting for 70% to 80% of all strokes. The less common hemorrhagic strokes are caused by bleeding into brain tissue. This type of stroke usually is from a blood vessel rupture caused by hypertension, aneurysms, arteriovenous malformations, head injury, or blood dyscrasias and has a much higher fatality rate than ischemic strokes.

Risk Factors

Among the major risk factors for stroke are age, sex, race, family history, hypertension, smoking, diabetes mellitus, asymptomatic carotid stenosis, sickle cell disease, hyperlipidemia, and atrial fibrillation.[28] Other less well-documented risk factors include obesity, physical inactivity, alcohol and drug abuse, hypercoagulability disorders, hormone replacement therapy, and oral contraceptive use.[28] The incidence of stroke increases with age, with a 1% per year increased risk for persons 65 to 74 years of age; the incidence of stroke is approximately 19% greater in men than women; and African Americans have a 60% greater risk for death and disability from stroke than whites.[29] Heart disease, particularly atrial fibrillation and other conditions that predispose to clot formation on the wall of the heart or valve leaflets or to paradoxical embolism through right-to-left shunting, predisposes to cardioembolic stroke. Polycythemia, sickle cell disease (during sickle cell crisis), and blood disorders predispose to clot formation in the cerebral vessels. Alcohol can contribute to stroke in several ways: induction of cardiac arrhythmias and defects in ventricular wall motion that lead to cerebral embolism, induction of hypertension, enhancement of blood coagulation disorders, and reduction of cerebral blood flow.[30] Cocaine use causes both ischemic and hemorrhagic strokes by inducing vasospasm, enhanced platelet activity, and increased blood pressure, heart rate, body temperature, and metabolic rate. Cocaine stroke victims range in age from newborn (*i.e.*, from maternal cocaine use) to old age.[31]

Elimination or control of risk factors for cerebrovascular disease (*e.g.*, use of tobacco, control of blood lipids and blood sugar, reduction of hypertension) offers the best opportunity to prevent cerebral ischemia from cerebral atherosclerosis. Early detection and treatment offer significant advantages over waiting until a serious event has occurred.

STROKE/BRAIN ATTACK

- Stroke is an acute focal neurologic deficit from an interruption of blood flow in a cerebral vessel (ischemic stroke, the most common type) due to thrombi or emboli or to bleeding into the brain tissue (hemorrhagic stroke).
- The term *brain attack* as a description for stroke is intended to alert people to the need for immediate treatment at the first sign of a stroke.
- During the evolution of an ischemic stroke, there usually is a central core of dead or dying cells surrounded by an ischemic band of minimally perfused cells called a *penumbra*. Whether the cells of the penumbra continue to survive depends on the successful timely return of adequate circulation.
- The realization that there is a window of opportunity during which ischemic but viable brain tissue can be salvaged has led to the use of thrombolytic agents in the early treatment of ischemic stroke.

Ischemic Stroke

Ischemic strokes are caused by cerebrovascular obstruction by thrombosis or emboli (Fig. 52-14). Various methods have been used to classify ischemic cerebrovascular disease.

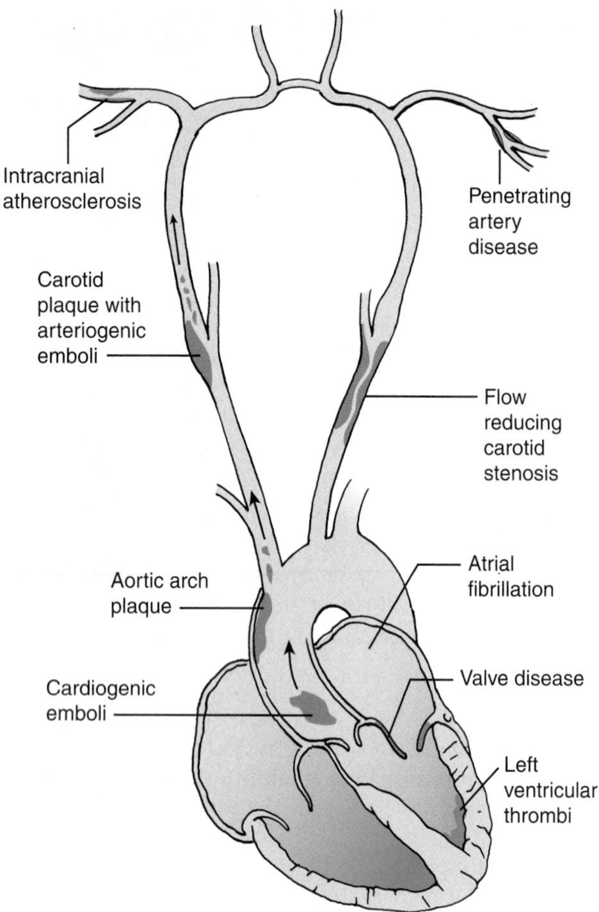

FIGURE 52-14 The most frequent sites of arterial and cardiac abnormalities causing ischemic stroke. (From Albers G.W., Easton D., Sacco R.L., Teal P. [1999]. Antithrombotic and thrombotic therapy for ischemic stroke. *Chest 114*(5), 684S)

A common classification system identifies five stroke subtypes and their frequency; 20% large artery atherosclerotic disease (both thrombosis and arterial emboli); 25% small vessel or penetrating artery disease (so-called lacunar stroke); 20% cardiogenic embolism; 30% cryptogenic stroke (undetermined cause); and 5% other, unusual causes[32] (*i.e.*, migraine, vessel dissection, coagulopathy).

Ischemic Penumbra in Evolving Stroke. During the evolution of a stroke, there usually is a central core of dead or dying cells, surrounded by an ischemic band or area of minimally perfused cells called the penumbra (*i.e.*, halo). Brain cells of the penumbra receive marginal blood flow, and their metabolic activities are impaired; although the area undergoes an "electrical failure," the structural integrity of the brain cells is maintained.[33] Whether the cells of the penumbra continue to survive depends on the successful timely return of adequate circulation, the volume of toxic products released by the neighboring dying cells, the degree of cerebral edema, and alterations in local blood flow. If the toxic products result in additional death of cells in the penumbra, the core of dead or dying tissue enlarges, and the volume of surrounding ischemic tissue increases.

Transient Ischemic Attacks. Transient ischemic attacks (TIAs) are characterized by focal ischemic cerebral neurologic deficits that last for less than 24 hours (usually less than 1 to 2 hours).[34] TIA or "ministroke" is equivalent to "brain angina" and reflects a temporary disturbance in focal cerebral blood flow, which reverses before infarction occurs, analogous to angina in relation to heart attack. The term TIA and the qualification of a deficit resolving within 24 hours were defined before the mechanisms of ischemic cell damage and the penumbra were known. A more accurate definition now is a deficit lasting less than 1 hour, and it may best be described as a zone of penumbra without central infarction. The causes of TIAs are the same as those of ischemic stroke and include atherosclerotic disease of cerebral vessels and emboli. TIAs are important because they may provide warning of impending stroke. In fact, the risk for stroke after a TIA is similar to the risk after a first stroke and is maximal immediately after the event: 4% to 8% risk for stroke within 1 month, 12% to 13% risk during the first year, and 24% to 29% risk over 5 years.[35] Diagnosis of TIA before a stroke may permit surgical or medical intervention that prevents an eventual stroke and the associated neurologic deficits.[35]

Large Vessel (Thrombotic) Stroke. Thrombi are the most common cause of ischemic strokes, usually occurring in atherosclerotic blood vessels. In the cerebral circulation, atherosclerotic plaques are found most commonly at arterial bifurcations. Common sites of plaque formation include larger vessels of the brain, notably the origins of the internal carotid and vertebral arteries, and junctions of the basilar and vertebral arteries. Cerebral infarction can result from an acute local thrombosis and occlusion at the site of chronic atherosclerosis, with or without embolization of the plaque material distally, or from critical perfusion failure distal to a stenosis (watershed). These infarcts often affect the cortex, causing aphasia or neglect, visual field defects, or transient monocular blindness (amaurosis fugax). In most cases of stroke, a single cerebral artery and its territories are affected. Usually, thrombotic strokes are seen in older persons and frequently are accompanied by evidence of atherosclerotic heart or peripheral arterial disease. The thrombotic stroke is not associated with activity and may occur in a person at rest.

Small Vessel Stroke (Lacunar Infarct). Lacunar infarcts are small (1.5 to 2 cm) to very small (3 to 4 mm) infarcts located in the deeper, noncortical parts of the brain or in the brain stem. They are found in the territory of single deep penetrating arteries supplying the internal capsule, basal ganglia, or brain stem. They result from occlusion of the smaller penetrating branches of large cerebral arteries, commonly the middle cerebral and posterior cerebral arteries. In the process of healing, lacunar infarcts leave behind small cavities, or lacunae (lakes). They are thought to result from arteriolar lipohyalinosis or microatheroma, commonly in the settings of chronic hypertension or diabetes. Six basic causes of lacunar infarcts have been proposed: embolism, hypertension, small vessel occlusive disease, hematologic abnormalities, small intracerebral hemorrhages, and vasospasm. Because of their size and location, lacunar infarcts usually do not cause cortical deficits like aphasia or apraxia. Instead, they produce classic recognizable "lacunar syndromes" such as pure motor hemiplegia, pure sensory hemiplegia, and dysarthria with the clumsy hand syndrome. Because CT scans are not sensitive enough to detect these tiny infarcts, diagnosis used to depend on clinical features alone. The use of magnetic resonance imaging (MRI) has allowed frequent visualization of small vessel infarcts and is obligatory to confirm such a lesion.

Cardiogenic Embolic Stroke. An embolic stroke is caused by a moving blood clot that travels from its origin to the brain. It usually affects the larger proximal cerebral vessels, often lodging at bifurcations. The most frequent site of embolic strokes is the middle cerebral artery, reflecting the large territory of this vessel and its position as the terminus of the carotid artery. Although most cerebral emboli originate from a thrombus in the left heart, they also may originate in an atherosclerotic plaque in the carotid arteries. The embolus travels quickly to the brain and becomes lodged in a smaller artery through which it cannot pass. Embolic stroke usually has a sudden onset with immediate maximum deficit.

Various cardiac conditions predispose to formation of emboli that produce embolic stroke, including rheumatic heart disease, atrial fibrillation, recent myocardial infarction, ventricular aneurysm, mobile aortic arch atheroma, and bacterial endocarditis. More recently, the use of transesophageal echocardiography, which better images the interatrial septum, has implicated a patent foramen ovale as a source for paradoxical venous emboli to the arterial system. Advances in the diagnosis and treatment of heart disease can be expected to alter favorably the incidence of embolic stroke.

Hemorrhagic Stroke

The most frequently fatal stroke is a spontaneous hemorrhage into the brain substance.[36–38] With rupture of a blood vessel, hemorrhage into the brain tissue occurs, resulting in edema, compression of the brain contents, or spasm of the adjacent blood vessels (Fig. 52-15). The most common predisposing factors are advancing age and hypertension. Other causes of hemorrhage are aneurysm, trauma, erosion of the vessels by tumors, arteriovenous malformations, blood coagulation disorders, vasculitis, and drugs. A cerebral hemorrhage occurs suddenly, usually when the person is active. Vomiting commonly occurs at the onset, and headache often occurs. Focal symptoms depend on which vessel is involved. In the most common situation, hemorrhage into the basal ganglia results in contralateral hemiplegia, with initial flaccidity progressing to spasticity. The hemorrhage and resultant edema exert great pressure on the brain substance, and the clinical course progresses rapidly to coma and frequently to death.

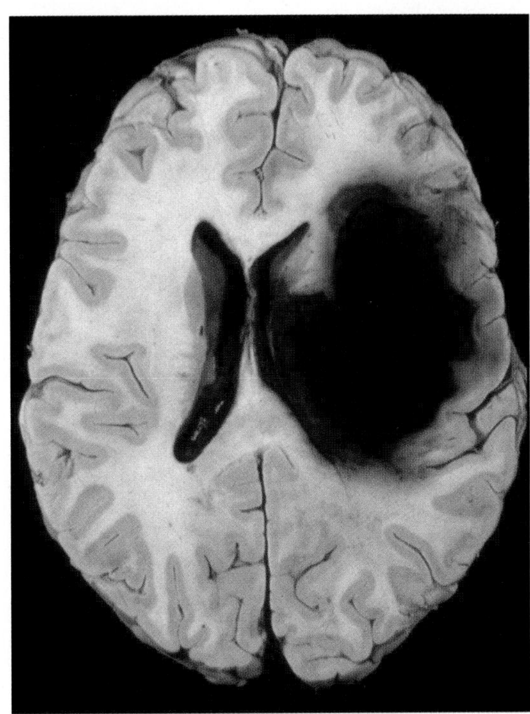

FIGURE 52-15 Cerebral hemorrhage. A spontaneous cerebral hemorrhage began near the external capsule and produced a hematoma that threatened rupture of a lateral ventricle. (Rubin E., Farber J.L. [1999]. *Pathology* [3rd ed., p. 1469]. Philadelphia: Lippincott-Raven)

Manifestations of Acute Stroke

The specific manifestations of stroke or TIA are determined by the cerebral artery that is affected, by the area of brain tissue that is supplied by that vessel, and by the adequacy of the collateral circulation. Symptoms of stroke/TIA always are sudden in onset and focal, and usually are one-sided. The most common symptom is weakness of the face and arm, sometimes also of the leg. Other frequent stroke symptoms are unilateral numbness, vision loss in one eye (amaurosis fugax) or to one side (hemianopia), language disturbance (aphasia), slurred speech (dysarthria), and sudden, unexplained imbalance or ataxia. In the event of TIA, symptoms rapidly resolve spontaneously, although the underlying mechanisms are the same as for stroke. The specific stroke signs depend on the specific vascular territory compromised (Table 52-6). As a generalization, carotid ischemia causes monocular visual loss or aphasia (dominant hemisphere) or hemineglect (nondominant hemisphere), contralateral sensory or motor loss, or other discrete cortical signs such as apraxia and agnosia. Vertebrobasilar ischemia induces ataxia, diplopia, hemianopia, vertigo, cranial nerve deficits, contralateral hemiplegia, sensory deficits (either contralateral or crossed, *i.e.,* contralateral body and ipsilateral face), and arousal defects. Discrete subsets of these vascular syndromes usually occur, depending on which branches of the involved artery are blocked.

Diagnosis and Treatment

Diagnosis. Accurate diagnosis of acute stroke is based on a complete history and thorough physical and neurologic examination. A careful history, including documentation of previous TIAs, the time of onset and pattern and rapidity of system progression, the specific focal symptoms (to

TABLE 52-6 Signs and Symptoms of Stroke by Involved Cerebral Artery

Cerebral Artery	Brain Area Involved	Signs and Symptoms*
Anterior cerebral	Infarction of the medial aspect of one frontal lobe if lesion is distal to communicating artery; bilateral frontal infarction if flow in other anterior cerebral artery is inadequate	Paralysis of contralateral foot or leg; impaired gait; paresis of contralateral arm; contralateral sensory loss over toes, foot, and leg; problems making decisions or performing acts voluntarily; lack of spontaneity, easily distracted; slowness of thought; aphasia depends on the hemisphere involved; urinary incontinence; cognitive and affective disorders
Middle cerebral	Massive infarction of most of lateral hemisphere and deeper structures of the frontal, parietal, and temporal lobes; internal capsule; basal ganglia	Contralateral hemiplegia (face and arm); contralateral sensory impairment; aphasia; homonymous hemianopia; altered consciousness (confusion to coma); inability to turn eyes toward paralyzed side; denial of paralyzed side or limb (hemiattention); possible acalculia, alexia, finger agnosia, and left–right confusion; vasomotor paresis and instability
Posterior cerebral	Occipital lobe; anterior and medial portion of temporal lobe	Homonymous hemianopia and other visual defects such as color blindness, loss of central vision, and visual hallucinations; memory deficits, perseveration (repeated performance of same verbal or motor response)
	Thalamus involvement	Loss of all sensory modalities; spontaneous pain; intentional tremor; mild hemiparesis; aphasia
	Cerebral peduncle involvement	Oculomotor nerve palsy with contralateral hemiplegia
Basilar and vertebral	Cerebellum and brain stem	Visual disturbance such as diplopia, dystaxia, vertigo, dysphagia, dysphonia

*Depend on hemisphere involved and adequacy of collaterals.

determine the likely vascular territory), and any coexisting diseases, can help to determine the type of stroke that is involved. The diagnostic evaluation should aim to determine the presence of hemorrhage or ischemia, identify the stroke or TIA mechanism (large vessel or small vessel atherothrombotic, cardioembolic, other or cryptogenic, hemorrhagic), characterize the severity of clinical deficits, and unmask the presence of risk factors.

Imaging studies document the brain infarction and the anatomy and pathology of the related blood vessels. CT scans and MRI have become essential tools in diagnosing stroke, differentiating cerebral hemorrhage from ischemia, and excluding intracranial lesions that mimic stroke clinically. CT scans are a necessary screening tool in the acute setting for rapid identification of hemorrhage but are insensitive to ischemia within 24 hours and to any brain stem or small infarcts. MRI is superior for imaging ischemic lesions in all territories. Newer MRI techniques such as perfusion- and diffusion-weighted imaging can reveal cerebral ischemia immediately after onset and identify areas of potentially reversible damage (*i.e.,* penumbra). Arteriography can demonstrate the site of the vascular abnormality and afford visualization of most intracranial vascular areas. Although angiography still is required for invasive treatments and for maximal sensitivity, magnetic resonance angiography (MRA) has largely replaced angiography as a screening tool for vascular lesions.

Two other types of imaging, positron-emission tomography and single-photon emission computed tomography, are nuclear studies used to assess the distribution of blood flow and metabolic activity of the brain. These tests rarely are used in routine stroke management because of limited availability and are applied more often in clinical research of cerebral ischemia. The introduction of several Doppler ultrasonographic techniques has facilitated the noninvasive evaluation of the cerebral circulation, especially for detection of carotid stenosis. Emitted signals may be uninterrupted (*i.e.,* continuous-wave Doppler), sampling all vessels in the depth of field, or intermittent (*i.e.,* pulsed-wave Doppler), sampling flow at any depth. Use of these methods has increased because of low cost, ease of application, safety features, continuous technical advances, improved imaging quality, and increased reliability.[33]

Treatment. The treatment of acute ischemic stroke changed markedly since the early 1990s, with an emphasis on salvaging brain tissue and minimizing long-term disability. The realization that there is a window of opportunity during which ischemic but viable brain tissue can be salvaged has led to the use of reperfusion techniques and neuroprotective strategies in the early treatment of ischemic stroke. Although the results of emergent treatment of hemorrhagic stroke have been less dramatic, continued efforts to reduce disability have been promising.

Emergent treatments for ischemic stroke involving neuroprotection include drugs that limit the calcium cascade (see Fig. 52-2) and treatments like hypothermia that decrease brain metabolic demands in the setting of ischemia. All are being actively tested in clinical trials. Reperfusion techniques include catheter-directed mechanical clot disruption, augmentation of CPP during acute stroke, and thrombolytic drugs, administered either intravenously or intraarterially. The use of thrombolytics for stroke was first investigated in the late 1960s, but it was quickly abandoned because of hemorrhagic complications resulting from treatment many hours beyond the time window of penumbral cell viability and because exclusion of persons with hemorrhagic stroke was difficult before CT scanning was available. The interest in thrombolytic therapy has increased because of the development of new thrombolytic agents and the availability of rapid diagnostic scanning methods that are able to differentiate between ischemic and hemorrhagic stroke.

Thrombolytic agents include streptokinase, urokinase, recombinant tissue-type plasminogen activator (tPA), and p-anisoylated lys-plasminogen-streptokinase activator complex[39] (see Chapter 15). The first and only agent approved by the U.S. Food and Drug Administration (FDA) for treatment of acute ischemic stroke is tPA, which was approved in 1996. A subcommittee of the Stroke Council of the American Heart Association has developed guidelines for the use of tPA for acute stroke.[40,41] These guidelines recommend that in persons with suspected stroke, the diagnosis of hemorrhagic stroke be excluded through the use of CT scanning before administration of thrombolytic therapy, which must be administered within 3 hours of onset of symptoms. The major risk of treatment with thrombolytic agents is intracranial hemorrhage of the infarcted brain. A number of conditions, including therapeutic levels of oral anticoagulant medications, a history of gastrointestinal bleeding, previous stroke or head injury within 3 months, surgery within the past 14 days, and a blood pressure greater than 200/120 mm Hg, are considered contraindications to thrombolytic therapy.[41]

The successful treatment of stroke depends on education of the public, paramedics, and health care professionals about the need for early diagnosis and treatment. As with heart attack, the message should be "do not wait to decide if the symptoms subside but seek immediate treatment." Effective medical and surgical procedures may preserve brain function and prevent disability.

Poststroke treatment is aimed at preventing complications and recurrent stroke and promoting the fullest possible recovery of function. During the acute phase, proper positioning and range-of-motion exercises are essential. Early rehabilitation efforts include all members of the rehabilitation team—physician, nurse, speech therapist, physical therapist, and occupational therapist—and the family. Much research is ongoing into the determinants and mechanisms of stroke recovery.

Stroke-Related Deficits

Deficits from stroke include motor and sensory deficits, language and speech problems, and higher cognitive deficits. Motor deficits are most common, followed by deficits of language, sensation, and cognition.

Motor Deficits. After a stroke affecting the corticospinal tract such as the motor cortex, posterior limb of the internal capsule, basis pontis, or medullary pyramids, there is profound weakness on the contralateral side (hemiparesis) (Fig. 52-16). Involvement at the level of the motor cortex is most often in the territory of the middle cerebral artery, usually with a sparing of the leg, which is supplied by the anterior cerebral artery. Subcortical lesions of the corticospinal tracts will cause equal weakness of the face, arm, and leg. Within 6 to 8 weeks, the initial weakness and flaccidity is replaced by hyperreflexia and spasticity. Spasticity involves an increase in the tone of affected muscles and usually an element of weakness. The flexor muscles usually are more strongly affected in the upper extremities and the extensor muscles more strongly affected in the lower extremities. There is a tendency toward foot drop; outward rotation and circumduction of the leg with gait; flexion at the wrist, elbow, and fingers; lower facial paresis; slurred speech; an upgoing toe to plantar stimulation (Babinski sign); and dependent edema in the affected extremities. A slight corticospinal lesion may be indicated only by clumsiness in carrying out fine coordinated movements rather than obvious weakness. Passive range-of-motion exercises help to maintain the joint function and to prevent edema, shoulder subluxation (*i.e.,* incomplete dislocation), and muscle atrophy and may help to reestablish motor patterns. If no voluntary movement or movement on command appears within a few months, significant function usually will not return to that extremity.

Dysarthria and Aphasia. Two key aspects of verbal communication are speech and language. Speech involves the mechanical act of articulating language, the "motor act" of verbal expression; whereas language involves the written or spoken use of symbolic formulations, such as words or numbers.[42] Dysarthria is a disorder of speech, manifest as the imperfect articulation of speech sounds or changes in voice pitch or quality. It results from a stroke affecting the muscles of the pharynx, palate, tongue, lips, or mouth and does not relate to the content of speech. A person with dysarthria may demonstrate slurred speech while still retaining language ability or may have a concurrent language problem as well. Aphasia is a general term that encompasses varying degrees of inability to comprehend, integrate, and express language. Aphasia may be localized to the dominant cerebral cortex or thalamus, usually the left side in 95% of people who are right handed and 70% of people who are left handed. In children, language dominance can readily shift to the unaffected hemisphere, resulting in more transient language deficits after stroke. A stroke in the territory of the middle cerebral artery is the most common aphasia-producing stroke.

Aphasia can be categorized as receptive or expressive, or as fluent or nonfluent. Fluency relates to the ease and spontaneity of conversational speech and is more strictly defined by the rate of speech. This has been classified as (fluent = many words, nonfluent = few words). Expressive or nonfluent aphasia is characterized by an inability to communicate spontaneously or translate thoughts or ideas into meaningful speech or writing. Speech production is limited, effortful, and halting and often may be poorly articulated because of a concurrent dysarthria. The person may be able, with difficulty, to utter or write two or three words, especially those with an emotional overlay. Comprehension is normal, and the person seems to be aware of his or her deficits but is unable to correct them. This often leads to frustration, anger, and depression. Expressive,

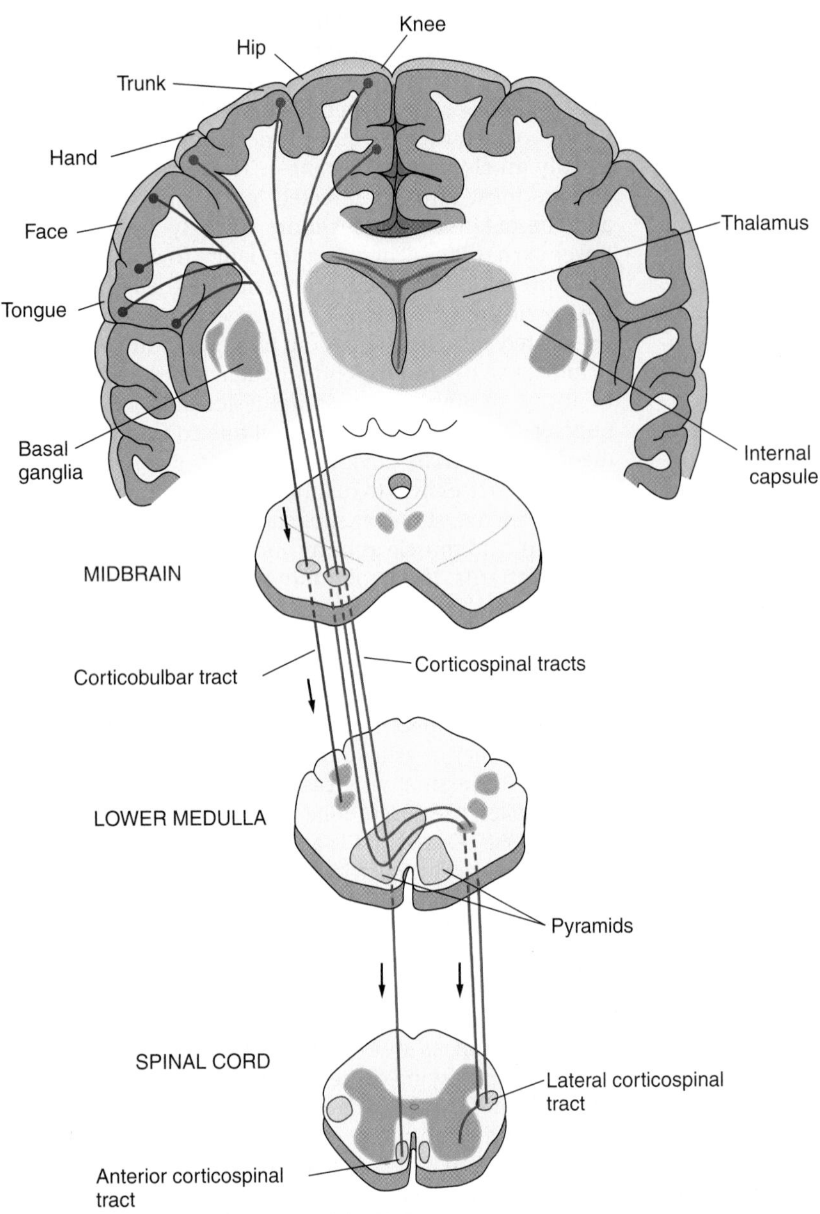

FIGURE 52-16 Motor pathways: corticospinal and corticobulbar tracts (Bickley L.S. [2003]. *Bates' guide to physical examination and history taking* [8th ed., p. 543]. Philadelphia: Lippincott Williams & Wilkins)

nonfluent aphasia is associated with lesions of Broca's area of the dominant frontal lobe (areas 44 and 45).

Fluent speech requires little or no effort, is articulate, and is of increased quantity. The term fluent refers only to the ease and rate of verbal output, and does not relate to the content of speech or the ability of the person to comprehend what is being said. There are three categories of fluent aphasia: Wernicke's, anomic, and conductive aphasia. Wernicke's aphasia is characterized by an inability to comprehend the speech of others or to comprehend written material. Lesions of the posterior temporal or lower parietal lobe (areas 22 and 39) are associated with receptive, fluent aphasia. Anomic aphasia is speech that is nearly normal except for a difficulty with finding singular words. Conduction aphasia is manifest as impaired repetition and speech riddled with letter substitutions, despite good comprehension and fluency. Conduction aphasia (*i.e.*, disconnection syndrome) results from destruction of the fiber system under the insula that connects Wernicke's and Broca's areas.

Cognitive and Other Deficits. Stroke can also cause cognitive, sensory, visual, and behavioral deficits. One distinct cognitive syndrome is that of hemineglect or hemiinattention. Usually from strokes affecting the nondominant (right) hemisphere, hemineglect is the inability to attend to and react to stimuli coming from the contralateral (left) side of space. Patients may not visually track, orient, or reach to the neglected side. They may neglect to use the limbs on that side, despite normal motor function, and may not shave, wash, or comb that side. Such persons are unaware of this deficit, which is another form of their neglect. Other cognitive deficits include apraxia (impaired ability to carry out previously learned motor activities despite normal sensory and motor function), agnosia (impaired recognition with normal sensory function), memory loss, behavioral syndromes, and depression. Sensory deficits affect the body contralateral to the lesion and can manifest as numbness, tingling paresthesias, or distorted sensations such as dysesthesia and neuropathic pain. Visual disturbances from stroke are diverse, but most common are hemianopia from a lesion of the optic radiations between the lateral geniculate body and the temporal or occipital lobes, or monocular blindness from occlusion of the ipsilateral central retinal artery, a branch of the internal carotid.

Aneurysmal Subarachnoid Hemorrhage

Aneurysmal subarachnoid hemorrhage represents bleeding into the subarachnoid space caused by a ruptured cerebral aneurysm. Bleeding into the subarachnoid space can extend well beyond the site of origin, flooding the basal cistern, ventricles, and spinal subarachnoid space.[41–43] An aneurysm is a bulge at the site of a localized weakness in the muscular wall of an arterial vessel. Most cerebral aneurysms are small saccular aneurysms called berry aneurysms (Fig. 52-17). They usually occur in the anterior circulation and are found at bifurcations and other junctions of vessels such as those in the circle of Willis (Fig. 52-18). They are thought to arise from a congenital defect in the media of the involved vessels. Their incidence is higher in persons with certain disorders, including polycystic kidney disease, fibromuscular dysplasia, coarctation of aorta, and arteriovenous malformations of the brain.[1] Other causes of cerebral aneurysms are atherosclerosis, hypertension, and bacterial infections.

Rupture of a cerebral aneurysm results in subarachnoid hemorrhage.[43–45] The probability of rupture increases with the size of the aneurysm; aneurysms larger than 10 mm in diameter have a 50% chance of bleeding per year. Rupture often occurs with acute increases in ICP. Of the various environmental factors that may predispose to aneurysmal subarachnoid hemorrhage, cigarette smoking and hypertension appear to constitute the greatest threat. Intracranial aneurysms are rare in children, and the mean age for subarachnoid hemorrhage is approximately 50 years. The mortality and morbidity rates with aneurysmal subarachnoid hemorrhage are high, with only one third of persons recovering without major disability.[11]

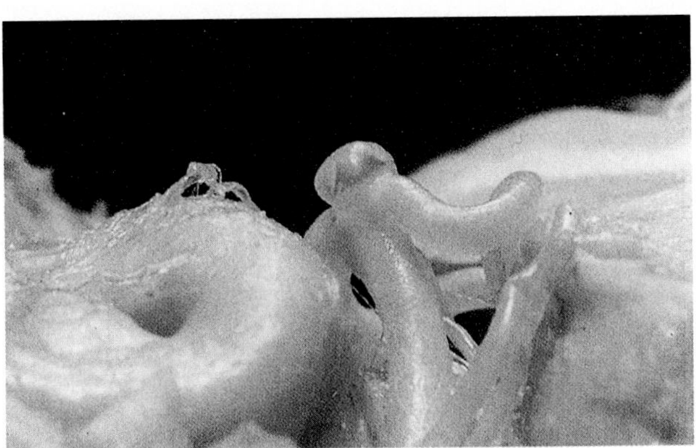

FIGURE 52-17 Berry aneurysm. A thin-walled aneurysm protrudes from the arterial bifurcation in the circle of Willis. (Rubin E., Farber J.L. [1999]. *Pathology* [3rd ed., p. 1466]. Philadelphia: Lippincott-Raven)

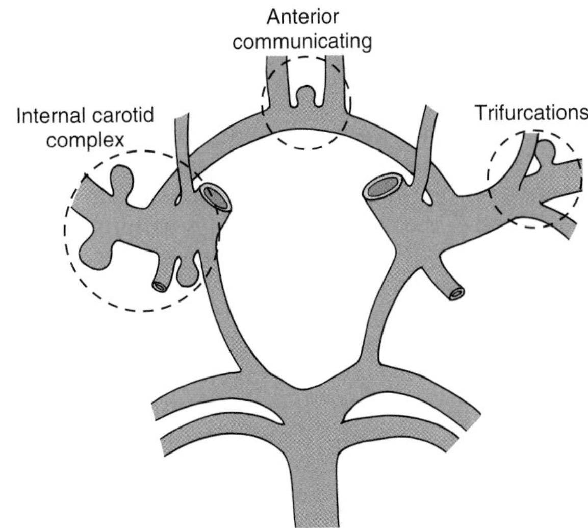

FIGURE 52-18 Common sites of berry aneurysms.

The signs and symptoms of cerebral aneurysms can be divided into two phases: those presenting before rupture and bleeding and those presenting after rupture and bleeding. Most small aneurysms are asymptomatic; intact aneurysms frequently are found at autopsy as an incidental finding.[1] Large aneurysms may cause chronic headache, neurologic deficits, or both. Approximately 50% of persons with subarachnoid hemorrhage have a history of atypical headaches occurring days to weeks before the onset of hemorrhage, suggesting the presence of a small leak.[43,44] These headaches are characterized by sudden onset and often are accompanied by nausea, vomiting, and dizziness. Persons with these symptoms may be mistakenly diagnosed as having tension or migraine headaches.

The onset of subarachnoid aneurysmal rupture often is heralded by a sudden and severe headache, described as "the worst headache of my life." If the bleeding is severe, the headache may be accompanied by collapse and loss of consciousness. Vomiting may accompany the presenting symptoms. Other manifestations include signs of meningeal irritation such as nuchal rigidity (neck stiffness) and photophobia (light intolerance); cranial nerve deficits, especially cranial nerve II, and sometimes III and IV (diplopia and blurred vision); stroke syndrome (focal motor and sensory deficits); cerebral edema and increased ICP; and pituitary dysfunction (diabetes insipidus and hyponatremia). Hypertension, a frequent finding, and cardiac dysrhythmias result from massive release of catecholamines triggered by the subarachnoid hemorrhage.

The complications of aneurysmal rupture include rebleeding, vasospasm with cerebral ischemia, hydrocephalus, hypothalamic dysfunction, and seizure activity. Rebleeding and vasospasm are the most serious and most difficult to treat. Rebleeding, which has its highest incidence on the first day after the initial rupture, results in further and usually catastrophic neurologic deficits.

Vasospasm is a dreaded complication of aneurysmal rupture. The condition is difficult to treat and is associated with a high incidence of morbidity and mortality. Although the description of aneurysm-associated vasospasm is relatively uniform, its proposed mechanisms are controversial. Usually, the condition develops within 3 to 10 days (peak, 7 days) after aneurysm rupture and involves a focal narrowing of the cerebral artery or arteries that can be visualized on arteriography or by transcranial doppler. The neurologic status gradually deteriorates as blood supply to the brain in the region of the spasm is decreased; this usually can be differentiated from the rapid deterioration seen in rebleeding. Vasospasm is treated by attempting to maintain adequate CPP through the use of vasoactive drugs or administration of large amounts of intravenous fluids to increase intravascular volume and produce hemodilution. There is risk for rebleeding from this therapy. Early surgery may provide some protection from vasospasm. Endovascular techniques, including balloon dilatation, have been developed to treat spasmodic arterial segments mechanically. Nimodipine, a drug that blocks calcium channels and selectively acts on cerebral blood vessels, may be used to prevent or treat vasospasm.

Another complication of aneurysm rupture is the development of hydrocephalus. It is caused by plugging of the arachnoid villi with products from lysis of blood in the subarachnoid space. Hydrocephalus is diagnosed by serial CT scans showing increasing size of the ventricles and by the clinical signs of increased ICP. Hydrocephalus may respond to osmotic diuretics, but if neurologic deterioration is significant, surgical placement of a shunt is indicated.

The diagnosis of subarachnoid hemorrhage and intracranial aneurysms is made by clinical presentation, CT scan, lumbar puncture, and angiography. Lumbar puncture may reveal the presence of blood in the CSF, whereas CT may demonstrate the location and extent of subarachnoid blood. To identify the aneurysm at the source of bleeding, conventional angiography, MRA, and helical (spiral) CT angiography are used. Conventional catheter angiography is the definitive diagnostic tool for detecting the aneurysm. MRA is noninvasive and does not require the intravascular administration of contrast, but is less sensitive. Helical CT angiography does require intravenous contrast, but can be used in persons after clipping when the use of MRI may be contraindicated.

The course of treatment after aneurysm rupture depends on the extent of neurologic deficit. Persons with mild to no neurologic deficits may undergo cerebral arteriography and early surgery, usually within 24 to 72 hours. Surgery involves craniotomy and inserting a specially designed silver clip that is tightened around the neck of the aneurysm. This procedure offers protection from rebleeding and may permit removal of the hematoma. Some persons with subarachnoid hemorrhage are managed medically for 10 days or more in an attempt to improve their clinical status before surgery. The use of endovascular techniques such as balloon embolization and platinum coil electrothrombosis is emerging as an alternative to surgery, particularly in surgically inaccessible aneurysms or poor surgical candidates.

Arteriovenous Malformations

Arteriovenous malformations are a complex tangle of abnormal arteries and veins linked by one or more fistulas[46,47] (Fig. 52-19). These vascular networks lack a capillary bed, and the small arteries have a deficient muscularis layer. Arteriovenous malformations are thought to arise from failure in development of the capillary network in the embryonic brain. As the child's brain grows, the malformation acquires additional arterial contributions that enlarge to form a tangled collection of thin-walled vessels that shunt blood directly from the arterial to the venous circulation. Arteriovenous malformations typically present before 40 years of age and affect men and women equally. Rupture of vessels in the malformation causing hemorrhagic stroke accounts for approximately 2% of all strokes.[46]

The hemodynamic effects of arteriovenous malformations are twofold. First, blood is shunted from the high-pressure arterial system to the low-pressure venous system without the buffering advantage of the capillary network. The draining venous channels are exposed to high levels of pressure, predisposing them to rupture and hemorrhage. Second, the elevated arterial and venous pressures divert blood away from the surrounding tissue, impairing tissue perfusion. Clinically, this is evidenced by slowly progressive neurologic deficits. The major clinical manifestations of arteriovenous malformations are intracerebral and subarachnoid hemorrhage, seizures, headache, and progressive neurologic deficits. Headaches often are severe, and persons with the disorder may describe them as throbbing and synchronous with their heartbeat. Other, focal symptoms depend on the location of the lesion and include visual symptoms (*i.e.*, diplopia and hemianopia), hemiparesis, mental deterioration, and speech deficits. Learning disorders have been documented in 66% of adults with arteriovenous malformations.[46]

Definitive diagnosis often is obtained through cerebral angiography. Treatment methods include surgical excision, endovascular occlusion, and radiation therapy. Be-

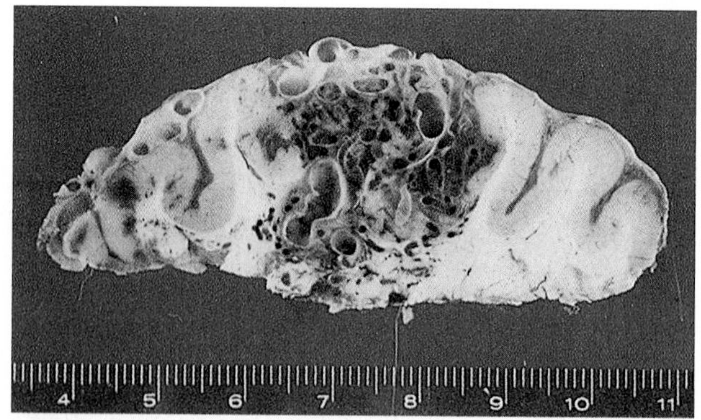

FIGURE 52-19 Arteriovenous malformation. Abnormal blood vessels replace the cortical gray matter and extend deeply into the underlying white matter. (Rubin E., Farber J.L. [1999]. *Pathology* [3rd ed., p. 1466]. Philadelphia: Lippincott-Raven)

cause of the nature of the malformation, each of these methods is accompanied by some risk for complications. If the arteriovenous malformation is accessible, surgical excision usually is the treatment of choice. Endovascular treatment involves the insertion of microcatheters into the cerebral circulation for delivery of embolic materials (*e.g.*, microballoons, sclerosing agents, microcoils, or quick-drying glue) into the arteriovenous malformation vessels.[46,48] Radiation therapy (also known as radiosurgery) may involve the use of a gamma knife, proton beam, or linear accelerator.

In summary, a stroke, or "brain attack," is an acute focal neurologic deficit caused by a vascular disorder that injures brain tissue. It is the third leading cause of death in the United States and a major cause of disability. There are two main types of stroke: ischemic and hemorrhagic. Ischemic stroke, which is the most common type, is caused by cerebrovascular obstruction by a thrombus or emboli. Hemorrhagic stroke, which is associated with greater morbidity and mortality, is caused by the rupture of a blood vessel and bleeding into the brain. The acute manifestations of stroke depend on the location of the blood vessel that is involved and can include motor, sensory, language, speech, and cognitive disorders. Early diagnosis and treatment with thrombolytic agents can prevent disabling brain injury from ischemic stroke. Treatment of long-term neurologic deficits from stroke is primarily symptomatic, involving the combined efforts of the health care team, the patient, and the family.

A subarachnoid hemorrhage involves bleeding into the subarachnoid space. Most subarachnoid hemorrhages are the result of a ruptured cerebral aneurysm. Presenting symptoms include headache, nuchal rigidity, photophobia, and nausea. Complications include rebleeding, vasospasm, and hydrocephalus.

Arteriovenous malformations are congenital abnormal communications between arterial and venous channels that result from failure in development of the capillary network in the embryonic brain. The vessels in the arteriovenous malformations may enlarge to form a space-occupying lesion, become weak and predispose to bleeding, and divert blood away from other parts of the brain; they can cause brain hemorrhage, seizures, headache, and other neurologic deficits.

Infections and Neoplasms

After completing this section of the chapter, you should be able to meet the following objectives:

- List the sequence of events that occur with meningitis
- Describe the symptoms of encephalitis
- List the major categories of brain tumors and interpret the meaning of benign and malignant as related to brain tumors
- Describe the general manifestations of brain tumors
- List the methods used in diagnosis and treatment of brain tumors

INFECTIONS

Infections of the CNS may be classified according to the structure involved: the meninges, meningitis; the brain parenchyma, encephalitis; the spinal cord, myelitis; and the brain and spinal cord, encephalomyelitis. They also may be classified by the type of invading organism: bacterial, viral, or other. In general, the pathogens enter the CNS through the bloodstream by crossing the blood–brain barrier or by direct invasion through skull fracture or a bullet hole, or, rarely, by contamination during surgery or lumbar puncture.

Meningitis

Meningitis is an inflammation of the pia mater, the arachnoid, and the CSF-filled subarachnoid space. Inflammation spreads rapidly because of CSF circulation around the brain and spinal cord. The inflammation usually is caused by an infection, but chemical meningitis can occur. There are two types of acute infectious meningitis: acute purulent meningitis (usually bacterial) and acute lymphocytic (usually viral) meningitis.[1] Factors responsible for the severity of meningitis include virulence factors of the pathogen, host factors, brain edema, and the presence of permanent neurologic sequelae.

Bacterial Meningitis. Most cases of bacterial meningitis are caused by *Streptococcus pneumoniae* (pneumococcus), *Haemophilus influenzae*, or *Neisseria meningitidis* (the meningococcus), except in neonates (infected most by group B streptococcus). The incidence of *H. influenzae* in children younger than 5 years has declined dramatically during recent years because of vaccination against *H. influenzae*. Epidemics of meningococcal meningitis occur in settings such as the military, where the recruits must reside in close contact. The very young and the very old are at highest risk for pneumococcal meningitis. Other pathogens in adults are gram-negative bacilli and staphylococci. Risk factors associated with contracting meningitis include head trauma with basilar skull fractures, otitis media, sinusitis or mastoiditis, neurosurgery, dermal sinus tracts, systemic sepsis, or immunocompromise. Despite the use of antibiotics, morbidity and mortality rates remain high for bacterial meningitis. The mortality rate for bacterial meningitis in adults remains at approximately 25%, whereas 61% of infants who survive gram-negative bacillary meningitis have developmental and neurologic sequelae.[49]

In the pathophysiology of bacterial meningitis, the bacterial organisms replicate and undergo lysis in the CSF, releasing endotoxins or cell wall fragments. These substances initiate the release of inflammatory mediators, which set off a complex sequence of events permitting pathogens, neutrophils, and albumin to move across the capillary wall into the CSF. As the pathogens enter the subarachnoid space, they cause inflammation, characterized by a cloudy, purulent exudate. Thrombophlebitis of the bridging veins and dural sinuses may develop, followed by congestion and infarction in the surrounding tissues. Ultimately, the meninges thicken, and adhesions form. These adhesions may impinge on the cranial nerves, giving rise to cranial nerve palsies, or may impair the outflow of CSF, causing hydrocephalus.

The most common symptoms of acute bacterial meningitis are fever and chills; headache; stiff neck; back, abdominal, and extremity pains; and nausea and vomiting. Other signs include seizures, cranial nerve palsies, and focal cerebral signs.[50] Meningococcal meningitis causes a petechial rash with palpable purpura in most people. These petechiae vary from pinhead size to large ecchymoses or even areas of skin gangrene that slough if the person survives. Other types of meningitis also may produce a petechial rash. Persons infected with *H. influenzae* or *S. pneumoniae* may present with difficulty in arousal and seizures, whereas those with *N. meningitidis* infection may present with delirium or coma.[50] The development of brain edema, hydrocephalus, or increased cerebral blood flow can increase ICP.

Meningeal signs (*e.g.*, photophobia and nuchal rigidity), such as those seen in subarachnoid hemorrhage, also may be present. Two assessment techniques can help determine whether meningeal irritation is present. Kernig's sign is resistance to extension of the knee while the person is lying with the hip flexed at a right angle. Brudzinski's sign is elicited when flexion of the neck induces flexion of the hip and knee. These postures reflect resistance to the painful stretching of the inflamed meninges from the lumbar level to the head. Cranial nerve damage (especially the eighth nerve, with resulting deafness) and hydrocephalus may occur as complications of pyogenic meningitis.

Diagnosis of bacterial meningitis is based on the history and physical examination, along with laboratory data. Lumbar puncture (*i.e.*, spinal tap) findings, which are necessary for accurate diagnosis, include a cloudy and purulent CSF under increased pressure. The CSF typically contains large numbers of polymorphonuclear neutrophils (up to 90,000/mm^3), increased protein content, and reduced sugar content. Bacteria can be seen on smears and can easily be cultured with appropriate media. Occasionally, previous antibiotic use limits culture sensitivities, in which case latex agglutination can be used, or polymerase chain reaction (PCR) testing for *N. meningitidis*, *H. influenzae*, and *Listeria species*.

Treatment includes antibiotics and corticosteroids. Optimal antibiotic treatment requires that the drug have a bactericidal effect in the CSF. Because bactericidal therapy often results in rapid lysis of the pathogen, treatment can promote the release of biologically active cell wall products into the CSF. The release of these cell wall products can increase the production of inflammatory mediators that have the potential for exacerbating the abnormalities of the blood–brain barrier and the inflammatory process. Because of evidence linking the inflammatory mediators to the pathogenesis of bacterial meningitis, adjunctive corticosteroid therapy usually is administered with or just before the first dose of antibiotics in infants and children. Growing evidence also supports the adjunctive use of corticosteroid therapy in adults.[51]

Persons who have been exposed to someone with meningococcal meningitis should be treated prophylactically with antibiotics.[52] Effective polysaccharide vaccines are available to protect against meningococcal groups A, C, Y, and W-135. These vaccines are recommended for military recruits and college students, who are at increased risk for invasive meningococcal disease.

Viral Meningitis. Viral meningitis manifests in much the same way as bacterial meningitis, but the course is less severe, and the CSF findings are markedly different. There are lymphocytes in the fluid rather than polymorphonuclear cells, the protein content is only moderately elevated, and the sugar content usually is normal. The acute viral meningitides are self-limited and usually require only symptomatic treatment, except for herpes simplex virus (HSV) type 2, which responds to intravenous acyclovir. Viral meningitis can be caused by many different viruses, most often Enteroviruses, including coxsackie, poliovirus, and echovirus virus. Others include Epstein-Barr virus, mumps, HSV, and West Nile virus. In many cases, the virus cannot be identified.

Encephalitis

Encephalitis represents a generalized infection of the parenchyma of the brain or spinal cord. It usually is caused by a virus, but it also may be caused by bacteria, fungi, and other organisms. The nervous system is subjected to invasion by many viruses, such as arbovirus, poliovirus, and rabies virus. The mode of transmission may be the bite of a mosquito (arbovirus), a rabid animal (rabies virus), or ingestion (poliovirus). A common cause of encephalitis in the United States is herpes simplex virus. Less frequent causes of encephalitis are toxic substances such as ingested lead and vaccines for measles and mumps. Encephalitis caused by human immunodeficiency virus infection is discussed in Chapter 22.

The pathologic picture of encephalitis includes local necrotizing hemorrhage, which ultimately becomes generalized, with prominent edema. There is progressive degeneration of nerve cell bodies. The histologic picture, although rather general, demonstrates some specific characteristics. For example, the poliovirus selectively destroys the cells of the anterior horn of the spinal cord.

Like meningitis, encephalitis is characterized by fever, headache, and nuchal rigidity, but more often patients also experience neurologic disturbances, such as lethargy, disorientation, seizures, focal paralysis, delirium, and coma. Diagnosis of encephalitis is made by clinical history and presenting symptoms, in addition to traditional CSF studies.

BRAIN TUMORS

Brain tumors account for 2% of all cancer deaths. The American Cancer Society estimates that there were 18,300 new cases and more than 13,100 deaths from brain and CNS cancers in 2001.[53] Metastasis to the brain from other sites is even more common. One estimate suggests that more than 100,000 people per year die with symptomatic intracranial metastasis.[54] In children, primary brain tumors are second only to leukemia as a cause of death from cancer, with 2,200 primary brain tumors being diagnosed each year. The mortality rate among this age group approaches 45%.[55]

Types of Tumors

The term brain tumor refers to a collection of intracranial neoplasms, each with its own histology, site of origin, prognosis, and treatment.[54,56,57] For most neoplasms, the term malignant is used to describe the tumor's lack of cell differentiation, its invasive nature, and its ability to metastasize. However, the terms benign and malignant do not apply to brain tumors in the same sense they do to tumors in other parts of the body. In the brain, however, even a well-differentiated and histologically benign tumor may grow and cause death because of its location. Also, tumors within the brain are rarely benign because surgery rarely cures.[56] Most histologically benign tumors infiltrate the normal brain tissue, preventing total resection and allowing for tumor recurrence. Furthermore, brain tumors seldom metastasize, except within the CNS itself.[56] Because of difficulty with pathologic discrimination and absence of metastasis, the clinical staging systems used for other cancers are not used for describing brain tumors. Instead, the terms low-grade tumors and high-grade tumors are often used.[56]

Brain tumors can be divided into three basic types: primary intracranial tumors of neuroepithelial tissue (*e.g.*, neurons, neuroglia), primary intracranial tumors that originate in the skull cavity but are not derived from the brain tissue itself (*e.g.*, meninges, pituitary gland, pineal gland, primary CNS lymphoma), and metastatic tumors. Collectively, neoplasms of astrocytic origin are the most common type of primary brain tumor in adults, followed by primary CNS lymphoma.

Glial Tumors. Glial tumors are divided into two main categories: astrocytic and oligodendroglial. For purposes of classification, astrocytic tumors can be subdivided into fibrillary (infiltrating) astrocytic tumors and pilocytic astrocytomas.

Fibrillary or diffuse astrocytomas account for 80% of adult primary brain tumors. They are most common in middle age, with the anaplastic astrocytomas having a peak incidence in the sixth decade. Although they usually are found in the cerebral hemispheres, they also can occur in the cerebellum, brain stem, or spinal cord. Astrocytomas of the cerebral hemispheres commonly are divided into three grades of increasing pathologic anaplasia and rapidity of progression: well-differentiated lesions, designated astrocytomas; intermediate-grade tumors, termed anaplastic astrocytomas; and the least differentiated and most aggressive, designated glioblastoma multiforme. Clinically, infiltrating astrocytic tumors present with symptoms of increased ICP (*e.g.*, headache) or focal abnormalities related to their position (seizures).

Pilocytic astrocytomas are distinguished from other astrocytomas by their cellular appearance and their benign behavior. Typically, they occur in children and young adults and usually are located in the cerebellum, but they also can be found in the floor and walls of the third ventricle, in the optic chiasm and nerves, and occasionally in the cerebral hemispheres. The prognosis of persons with pilocytic astrocytomas is influenced primarily by their location. The prognosis is usually better for persons with surgically resectable tumors, such as those located in the cerebellar cortex, than for persons with less accessible tumors, such as those involving the hypothalamus or brain stem.

Oligodendrogliomas are tumors of the oligodendrocytes or their precursors, or they have histologic features representing both oligodendrocytes and astrocytes.[56] They represent approximately 5% of glial tumors and are most common in middle life. The prognosis of persons with oligodendrogliomas is less predictable than for persons with infiltrating astrocytomas. It depends on the histologic grade of the tumor and its location. The oligodendroglial tumors are prone to spontaneous hemorrhage owing to their delicate vasculature.[54]

Ependymomas. Ependymomas are derived from the single layer of epithelium that lines the ventricles and spinal canal. Although they can occur at any age, they are most likely to occur in the first two decades of life and most frequently affect the fourth ventricle; they constitute 5% to 10% of brain tumors in this age group. The spinal cord is the most common site for ependymomas occurring in middle age. The clinical features depend on the location of the neoplasm. Intracranial tumors are often associated with hydrocephalus and evidence of increased ICP.

Meningiomas. Meningiomas develop from the meningothelial cells of the arachnoid and are outside the brain. They usually have their onset in the middle or later years of life and constitute approximately 20% of primary brain tumors in this age group. Meningiomas are slow growing, well circumscribed, and often highly vascular tumors. They usually are benign, and complete removal is possible if the tumor does not involve vital structures.

Primary CNS Lymphomas. Primary CNS lymphoma has increased in incidence by a factor of 10 in the past two decades. These deep, periventricular and diffuse tumors are especially common in immunocompromised patients and are associated with the Epstein-Barr virus and derived from large B cells. Most are malignant, and recurrence is common despite treatment. Behavioral and cognitive changes, which are the most common presenting symptoms, occur in about 65% of patients; hemiparesis, aphasia, and visual-field deficits in about 50%; and seizures in 15% to 20%.[54]

Etiology

The etiology of brain tumors is largely unknown. Although a large number of studies have examined the relationship between environmental and occupational factors, only two have shown a relationship to brain cancer: ionizing radiation and immunosuppression.[56] Irradiation given to treat intracranial and extracranial cancers, including prophylactic irradiation for leukemia, increases the incidence of gliomas. Immunosuppression, either congenital or acquired (*e.g.*, immunosuppression to prevent organ rejection, HIV), increases the risk of primary CNS lymphomas. There may also be a hereditary factor. A few inherited disorders predispose to the development of brain tumors. For example, neurofibromatosis (see Chapter 7) is associated with primary brain tumors. Some childhood tumors, such as medulloblastoma, are considered to be of embryonic origin.

Manifestations

Intracranial tumors give rise to focal disturbances in brain function and increased ICP. Focal disturbances occur because of brain compression, tumor infiltration, disturbances in blood flow, and brain edema.

Tumors may be located intraaxially (*i.e.,* within brain tissue) or extraaxially (*i.e.,* outside brain tissue, within the cranium). Disturbances in brain function usually are greatest with fast-growing, infiltrative, intraaxial tumors because of compression, infiltration, and necrosis of brain tissue. Extraaxial tumors, such as meningiomas, may reach a large size without producing signs and symptoms. Cysts may form in tumors and contribute to brain compression. Cerebral edema usually is of the vasogenic type, which develops around brain tumors and is characterized by increased brain water and expanded extracellular fluid. The edema is thought to result from increased permeability of tumor capillary endothelial cells.

Because the volume of the intracranial cavity is fixed, brain tumors cause a generalized increase in ICP when they reach sufficient size. Tumors can obstruct the flow of CSF in the ventricular cavities and produce hydrocephalic dilatation of the proximal ventricles and atrophy of the cerebral hemispheres. Complete compensation of ventricular volumes can occur with very slow-growing tumors, but with rapidly growing tumors, increased ICP is an early sign. Depending on the location of the tumor, brain displacement and herniation of the uncus or cerebellum may occur. The clinical manifestations of brain tumors depend on the size and location of the tumor. General signs and symptoms include headache, nausea, vomiting, mental changes, papilledema, visual disturbances (*e.g.,* diplopia), alterations in sensory and motor function, and seizures.

The brain itself is insensitive to pain. The headache that accompanies brain tumors results from compression or distortion of pain-sensitive dural or vascular structures. It may be felt on the same side of the head as the tumor but more commonly is diffuse. In the early stages, the headache is mild and occurs in the morning upon awakening and improves with head elevation. The headache becomes more constant as the tumor enlarges and often is worsened by coughing, bending, or sudden movements of the head.

Vomiting occurs with or without nausea, may be projectile, and is a common symptom of increased ICP and brain stem compression. Direct stimulation of the vomiting center, which is located in the medulla, may contribute to the vomiting that occurs with brain tumors. The vomiting is often associated with headache. Papilledema (edema of the optic disc) results from increased ICP and obstruction of the CSF pathways. It is associated with decreased visual acuity, diplopia, and deficits in the visual fields. Visual defects associated with papilledema often are the reason that persons with brain tumor seek medical care.

Personality and mental changes are common with brain tumors. Persons with brain tumors often are irritable initially and later become quiet and apathetic. They may become forgetful, seem preoccupied, and appear to be psychologically depressed. Because of the mental changes, a psychiatric consultation may be sought before a diagnosis of brain tumor is made.

Focal signs and symptoms are determined by the location of the tumor. Tumors arising in the frontal lobe may grow to large size, increase the ICP, and cause signs of generalized brain dysfunction before focal signs are recognized. Tumors that impinge on the visual system cause visual loss or visual field defects long before generalized signs develop. Certain areas of the brain have a relatively low threshold for seizure activity. Temporal lobe tumors often produce seizures as their first symptom. Hallucinations of smell or hearing and déjà vu phenomena are common focal manifestations of temporal lobe tumors. Brain stem tumors commonly produce upper and lower motoneuron signs, such as weakness of facial muscles and ocular palsies that occur with or without involvement of sensory or long motor tracts. Cerebellar tumors often cause ataxia of gait.

Diagnosis and Treatment

Diagnostic procedures for brain tumor include physical and neurologic examinations, visual field and funduscopic examination, CT scans and MRI, skull x-ray films, technetium pertechnetate brain scans, electroencephalography, and cerebral angiography.[54,56] Physical examination is used to assess motor and sensory function. Because the visual pathways travel through many areas of the cerebral lobes, detection of visual field defects can provide information about the location of tumors. A funduscopic examination is done to detect papilledema. Although CT scanning is used as a screening test, MRI scans are more sensitive than CT for detecting mass lesions. Skull x-ray films are used to detect calcified areas in a neoplasm or erosion of skull structures due to tumors. Approximately 75% of persons with a brain tumor have an abnormal electroencephalogram; in some cases, the results of the test can be used to localize the tumor. Cerebral angiography can be used to locate a tumor and visualize its vascular supply, information that is important when planning surgery. MRA can be used to distinguish vascular masses from tumors.

The three general methods for treatment of brain tumors are surgery, irradiation, and chemotherapy. Surgery is part of the initial management of virtually all brain tumors; it establishes the diagnosis and achieves tumor removal in many cases. The development of microsurgical neuroanatomy, the operating microscope, and advanced stereotactic and ultrasonographic technology; the fusion of imaging systems with resection techniques; and the intraoperative monitoring of evoked potentials or EEG have improved the effectiveness of surgical resection. However, removal may be limited by the location of the tumor and its invasiveness. Stereotactic surgery uses three-dimensional coordinates and CT and MRI to localize a brain lesion precisely. Ultrasonographic technology has been used for localizing and removing tumors. The ultrasonic aspirator, which combines a vibrating head with suction, permits atraumatic removal of tumors from cranial nerves and important cortical areas. Intraoperative monitoring of evoked potentials is an important adjunct to some types of surgery.

For example, evoked potentials can be used to monitor auditory, visual, speech, or motor responses during surgery done under local anesthesia.

Most malignant brain tumors respond to external irradiation. Irradiation can increase longevity and sometimes can allay symptoms when tumors recur. The treatment dose depends on the tumor's histologic type, radioresponsiveness, and anatomic site and on the level of tolerance of the surrounding tissue. A newer technique called gamma knife combines stereotactic localization of tumor with radiosurgery, allowing delivery of high-dose radiation to deep tumors, sparing surrounding brain. Radiation therapy is avoided in treating children younger than 2 years of age because of the long-term effects, which include developmental delay, panhypopituitarism, and secondary tumors.

The use of chemotherapy for brain tumors is somewhat limited by the blood–brain barrier. Chemotherapeutic agents can be administered intravenously, intraarterially, intrathecally (*i.e.*, into the spinal canal), or intraventricularly. A promising area of improved delivery of chemotherapeutic agents is the use of biodegradable anhydrous wafers impregnated with a drug and implanted into the tumor at the time of surgery. These wafers are constructed so they release the drug over a period of many months.

In summary, infections of the CNS may be classified according to the structures involved (*e.g.*, meningitis, encephalitis) or the type of organism causing the infection. The damage caused by infection may predispose to hydrocephalus, seizures, or other neurologic defects.

Brain tumors account for 2% of all cancer deaths and are the second most common type of cancer in children. Brain tumors can arise primarily from intracranial structures, and tumors from other parts of the body often metastasize to the brain. Primary brain tumors can arise from any structure in the cranial cavity. Most begin in brain tissue, but the pituitary, the pineal region, and the meninges also are sites of tumor development. Brain tumors cause focal disturbances in brain function and increase the ICP. Focal disturbances result from brain compression, tumor infiltration, disturbances in blood flow, and cerebral edema. The clinical manifestations of brain tumor depend on the size and location of the tumor. General signs and symptoms include headache, nausea, vomiting, mental changes, papilledema, visual disturbances, alterations in motor and sensory function, and seizures. Diagnostic tests include physical examination, visual field testing and funduscopic examination, CT scans, MRI studies, skull x-ray films, brain scans, electroencephalography, and cerebral angiography. Treatment includes surgery, irradiation, and chemotherapy.

Seizure Disorders

After completing this section of the chapter, you should be able to meet the following objectives:

- Explain the difference between a seizure and epilepsy
- State four or more causes of seizures other than epilepsy
- Differentiate between the origin of seizure activity in partial and generalized forms of epilepsy and compare the manifestations of simple partial seizures with those of complex partial seizures and major and minor motor seizures
- Characterize status epilepticus

A seizure represents the abnormal behavior caused by an electrical discharge from neurons in the cerebral cortex. A seizure is a discrete clinical event with associated signs and symptoms that vary according to the site of neuronal discharge in the brain. Manifestations of seizure generally include sensory, motor, autonomic, or psychic phenomenon. A convulsion refers to the specific seizure type of a motor seizure involving the entire body. Approximately 2 million persons in the United States are subject to recurrent seizures.[58] Seizure activity is the most common disorder encountered in pediatric neurology, and among adults, its incidence is exceeded only by cerebrovascular disorders. In most persons, the first seizure episode occurs before 20 years of age. After 20 years of age, a seizure is caused most often by a structural change, trauma, tumor, or stroke.

A seizure is not a disease but a symptom of underlying CNS dysfunction. Seizures may occur during almost

SEIZURES

- Seizures are paroxysmal motor, sensory, or cognitive manifestations of spontaneous, abnormally synchronous electrical discharges from collections of neurons in the cerebral cortex.
- Seizures are thought to result directly or indirectly from changes in excitability of single neurons or groups of neurons.
- The site of seizure generation and the extent to which the abnormal neural activity is conducted to other areas of the brain determine the type and manifestations of the seizure activity.
- Partial seizures originate in a small group of neurons in one hemisphere with secondary spread of seizure activity to other parts of the brain. Simple partial seizures usually are confined to one hemisphere and do not involve loss of consciousness. Complex partial seizures begin in a localized area, spread to both hemispheres, and involve impairment of consciousness.
- Generalized seizures show simultaneous disruption of normal brain activity in both hemispheres from the onset. They include unconsciousness and varying bilateral degrees of symmetric motor responses with evidence of localization to one hemisphere. Absence seizures are generalized nonconvulsive seizure events that are expressed mainly by brief periods of unconsciousness. Tonic-clonic seizures involve unconsciousness along with both tonic and clonic muscle contractions.

all serious illnesses or injuries affecting the brain, including infections, tumors, drug abuse, vascular lesions, congenital deformities, and brain injury. A seizure represents the clinical manifestations of an abnormal, uncontrolled electrical discharge from a group of neurons. Seizures are one feature of epileptic syndromes. Epilepsy refers to the syndromes of associated seizure types, EEG patterns, exam findings, hereditary patterns, and precipitating factors. Patients with an epileptic syndrome may have several seizure types. The current classification system endorsed by the International League Against Epilepsy identifies both seizure type (generalized or partial), and epilepsy syndromes.

ETIOLOGY: PROVOKED AND UNPROVOKED SEIZURES

Many theories have been proposed to explain the cause of the abnormal brain electrical activity that occurs with seizures. Seizures may be caused by alterations in cell membrane permeability or distribution of ions across the neuronal cell membranes. Another cause may be decreased inhibition of cortical or thalamic neuronal activity or structural changes that alter the excitability of neurons. Neurotransmitter imbalances such as an acetylcholine excess or γ-aminobutyric acid (GABA, an inhibitory neurotransmitter) deficiency have been proposed as causes.

Clinically, seizures may be categorized as unprovoked (primary or idiopathic) or provoked (secondary or acute symptomatic).[58–61] Unprovoked or idiopathic seizures are those for which no identifiable cause can be determined, and are thought to be genetic. Most unprovoked seizures occur in the setting of an epileptic syndrome. These patients usually require chronic administration of antiepileptic medications to limit seizure recurrences. Provoked or symptomatic seizures include febrile seizures, seizures precipitated by systemic metabolic conditions, and those that follow a primary insult to the CNS. Most provoked seizures are best prevented by treatment of the underlying cause. For example, the most common subgroup is that of febrile seizures in children.[62] In susceptible children, a high fever, usually over 104°F, will provoke a generalized seizure. Treatment includes aggressive use of antipyretics to prevent seizures during a febrile illness. Transient systemic metabolic disturbances may precipitate seizures. Examples include electrolyte imbalances, hypoglycemia, hypoxia, hypocalcemia, uremia, alkalosis, and rapid withdrawal of sedative drugs. Specific CNS injuries such as toxemia of pregnancy, water intoxication, meningoencephalitis, trauma, cerebral hemorrhage and stroke, and brain tumors may precipitate a seizure. In all cases of provoked seizures, treatment of the immediate underlying cause often results in their resolution.

CLASSIFICATION

The International Classification of Epileptic Seizures determines seizure type by clinical symptoms and EEG activity. It divides seizures into two broad categories: partial seizures, in which the seizure begins in a specific or focal area of one cerebral hemisphere, and generalized seizures, which begin simultaneously in both cerebral hemispheres[63,64] (Chart 52-1). Further classification of epileptic syndromes characterizes the underlying diseases that cause the seizures, and divides seizures into idiopathic (suspected to be genetic), symptomatic (resulting from some CNS injury), and cryptogenic (presumed to be symptomatic of some unidentified cause).[61] The system also has categories for seizures of undetermined origin such as neonatal seizures and a category of special syndromes such as febrile seizures.

Partial Seizures

Partial or focal seizures are the most common type of seizure among newly diagnosed cases in all groups older than 10 years of age. Partial seizures can be subdivided into three major groups: simple partial (consciousness is not impaired), complex partial (impairment of consciousness), and secondarily generalized partial seizures. These categories are based primarily on current neurophysiologic theories related to seizure propagation and the extent of involvement of the brain's hemispheres.

Simple Partial Seizures. Simple partial seizures usually involve only one hemisphere and are not accompanied by

CHART 52-1

Classification of Epileptic Seizures

Partial Seizures

Simple partial seizures (no impairment of consciousness)
- With motor symptoms
- With sensory symptoms
- With autonomic signs
- With psychic symptoms

Complex partial seizures (impairment of consciousness)
- Simple partial onset followed by impaired consciousness
- Impairment of consciousness at onset

Partial seizures evolving to secondarily generalized seizures
- Simple partial leading to generalized seizures
- Complex partial leading to generalized seizures

Unclassified Seizures

Classification not possible because of inadequate or incomplete data

Generalized Seizures

Absence seizures (typical or atypical)
Atonic seizures
Myoclonic seizures
Clonic seizures
Tonic
Tonic-clonic seizures

(Adapted from Commission on Classification and Terminology of the International League Against Epilepsy [1981]. Proposal for revised clinical and electroencephalographic classification of epileptic seizures. *Epilepsia* 22, 489)

loss of consciousness or responsiveness. These seizures also have been referred to as elementary partial seizures, partial seizures with elementary symptoms, or focal seizures. The 1981 Commission on Classification and Terminology of the International League Against Epilepsy classified simple partial seizures according to motor signs, sensory symptoms, autonomic manifestations, and psychic symptoms.[63]

The observed clinical signs and symptoms depend on the area of the brain where the abnormal neuronal discharge is taking place. If the motor area of the brain is involved, the earliest symptom is motor movement corresponding to the location of onset on the contralateral side of the body. The motor movement may remain localized or may spread to other cortical areas, with sequential involvement of body parts in an epileptic-type "march," known as a Jacksonian seizure. If the sensory portion of the brain is involved, there may be no observable clinical manifestations. Sensory symptoms correlating with the location of seizure activity on the contralateral side of the brain may involve somatic sensory disturbance (*e.g.,* tingling and crawling sensations) or special sensory disturbance (*i.e.,* visual, auditory, gustatory, or olfactory phenomena). When abnormal cortical discharge stimulates the autonomic nervous system, flushing, tachycardia, diaphoresis, hypotension or hypertension, or pupillary changes may be evident.

The term prodrome or aura traditionally has meant a sensory warning sign of impending seizure activity or the onset of seizure that affected persons could describe because they were conscious. The aura itself now is considered part of the seizure. Because only a small area of the brain is involved and consciousness is maintained, an aura is considered a simple partial seizure. Simple partial seizures may progress to complex partial seizures or generalized tonic-clonic seizures that result in unconsciousness. Therefore, the aura in simple partial seizure may be considered a warning sign of impending complex partial seizures.

Complex Partial Seizures. Complex partial seizures involve impairment of consciousness and often arise from the temporal lobe. The seizure begins in a localized area of the brain but may progress rapidly to involve both hemispheres. These seizures also may be referred to as temporal lobe seizures or psychomotor seizures.

Complex partial seizures often are accompanied by automatisms. Automatisms are repetitive, nonpurposeful activity such as lip smacking, grimacing, patting, or rubbing clothing. Confusion during the postictal state (after a seizure) is common. Hallucinations and illusional experiences such as déjà vu (familiarity with unfamiliar events or environments) or jamais vu (unfamiliarity with a known environment) have been reported. There may be overwhelming fear, uncontrolled forced thinking or a flood of ideas, and feelings of detachment and depersonalization. A person with a complex partial seizure disorder sometimes is misunderstood and believed to require hospitalization for a psychiatric disorder.

Secondarily Generalized Partial Seizures. These seizures are focal at onset but then become generalized as the ictal neuronal discharge spreads, involving deeper structures of the brain, such as the thalamus or the reticular formation. Discharges spread to both hemispheres, resulting in progression to tonic-clonic seizure activity. These seizures may start as simple or complex partial seizures and may be preceded by an aura. The aura, often a stereotyped peculiar sensation that precedes the seizure, is the result of partial seizure activity. A history of an aura is clinically useful to identify the seizure as partial and not generalized in onset. However, absence of an aura does not reliably exclude a focal onset because many partial seizures generalize too rapidly to generate an aura.

Generalized-Onset Seizures

Generalized-onset seizures are the most common type in young children. These seizures are classified as primary or generalized when clinical signs, symptoms, and supporting EEG changes indicate involvement of both hemispheres at onset. The clinical symptoms include unconsciousness and involve varying bilateral degrees of symmetric motor responses without evidence of localization to one hemisphere.

These seizures are divided into four broad categories: absence seizures (typical and atypical), atonic (akinetic) seizures, myoclonic seizures, and major motor (formerly grand mal) seizures, characterized by tonic, clonic, or tonic-clonic activity.[59,61]

Absence Seizures. Absence seizures are generalized, nonconvulsive epileptic events and are expressed mainly as disturbances in consciousness. Formerly referred to as petit mal seizures, absence seizures typically occur only in children and cease in adulthood or evolve to generalized motor seizures. Children may present with a history of school failure that predates the first evidence of seizure episodes. Although typical absence seizures have been characterized as a blank stare, motionlessness, and unresponsiveness, motion occurs in many cases of absence seizures. This motion takes the form of automatisms such as lip smacking, mild clonic motion (usually in the eyelids), increased or decreased postural tone, and autonomic phenomena. There often is a brief loss of contact with the environment. The seizure usually lasts only a few seconds, and then the person is able to resume normal activity immediately. The manifestations often are so subtle that they may pass unnoticed. Because automatisms and unresponsiveness are common to complex partial seizures, the latter often are mistakenly labeled as "petit mal" seizures.

Atypical absence seizures are similar to typical absence seizures except for greater alterations in muscle tone and less abrupt onset and cessation. In practice, it is difficult to distinguish typical from atypical absence seizures without benefit of supporting EEG findings. However, it is important to distinguish between complex partial and absence seizures because the drugs of choice are different. Medications that are effective for partial seizures may increase the frequency of absence seizures.

Atonic Seizures. In akinetic or atonic seizures, there is a sudden, split-second loss of muscle tone leading to slackening of the jaw, drooping of the limbs, or falling to the ground. These seizures also are known as drop attacks.

Myoclonic Seizures. Myoclonic seizures involve brief involuntary muscle contractions induced by stimuli of cerebral origin. A myoclonic seizure involves bilateral jerking of muscles, generalized or confined to the face, trunk, or one or more extremities. Tonic seizures are characterized by a rigid, violent contraction of the muscles, fixing the limbs in a strained position. Clonic seizures consist of repeated contractions and relaxations of the major muscle groups.

Tonic-Clonic Seizures. Tonic-clonic seizures, formerly called grand mal seizures, are the most common major motor seizure. Frequently, a person has a vague warning (probably a simple partial seizure) and experiences a sharp tonic contraction of the muscles with extension of the extremities and immediate loss of consciousness. Incontinence of bladder and bowel is common. Cyanosis may occur from contraction of airway and respiratory muscles. The tonic phase is followed by the clonic phase, which involves rhythmic bilateral contraction and relaxation of the extremities. At the end of the clonic phase, the person remains unconscious until the RAS begins to function again. This is called the postictal phase. The tonic-clonic phases last approximately 60 to 90 seconds.

Unclassified Seizures

Unclassified seizures are those that cannot be placed in one of the previous categories. These seizures are observed in the neonatal and infancy periods. Determination of whether the seizure is focal or generalized is not possible. Unclassified seizures are difficult to control with medication.

DIAGNOSIS AND TREATMENT

The diagnosis of seizure disorders is based on a thorough history and neurologic examination, including a full description of the seizure. The physical examination and laboratory studies help exclude any metabolic disease (*e.g.*, hyponatremia) that could precipitate seizures. Skull radiographs and CT or MRI scans are used to identify structural defects. One of the most useful diagnostic tests is the EEG, which is used to record changes in the brain's electrical activity. It is used to support the clinical diagnosis of epilepsy, to provide a guide for prognosis, and to assist in classifying the seizure disorder.

The first rule of treatment is to protect the person from injury during a seizure, preserve brain function by aborting or preventing seizure activity, and treat any underlying disease. Persons with epilepsy should be advised to avoid situations that could be dangerous or life threatening if seizures occur. Treatment of the underlying disorder may reduce the frequency of seizures.

After the underlying disease is treated, the aim of treatment is to bring the seizures under control with the least possible disruption in lifestyle and minimum side effects from medication. Since the late 1970s, the therapy for epilepsy has changed drastically because of an improved classification system, the ability to measure serum anticonvulsant levels, and the availability of potent new anticonvulsant drugs. With proper drug management, 60% to 80% of persons with epilepsy can obtain good seizure control.

Anticonvulsant Medications

More than 20 drugs are available in the United States for the treatment of epilepsy. This group includes six antiepileptic drugs that were approved for use in the United States since 1996.

Drugs used as first-line therapy for seizure disorders are carbamazepine, phenytoin, ethosuximide, valproate, phenobarbital, primidone, and clonazepam.[60,61,65] Carbamazepine and phenytoin are the drugs of choice in treating partial seizures. They also are used for tonic-clonic seizures resulting from partial seizures. Ethosuximide is the drug of choice for absence seizures, but it is not effective for tonic-clonic seizures that progress from partial seizures. Valproate is helpful for persons with many of the minor motor seizures and tonic-clonic seizures. Valproate and ethosuximide can be used together. Phenobarbital is used for tonic-clonic seizures, as is primidone. Primidone also is prescribed for simple and complex partial seizures. Absence and myoclonic seizures can be treated with clonazepam. Atonic seizures are highly resistant to therapy. Each of the new drugs—gabapentin, lamotrigine, felbamate, topiramate, levetiracetam, tiagabine, and oxcarbazepine—is approved for use in adults who have partial seizures alone or with secondarily generalized (grand mal) seizures.

Women of childbearing age require special consideration concerning fertility, contraception, and pregnancy. Many of the drugs interact with oral contraceptives; some affect hormone function or decrease fertility. All such women should be advised to take folic acid supplementation. For women with epilepsy who become pregnant, antiseizure drugs increase the risk for congenital abnormalities and other perinatal complications.

Whenever possible, a single drug should be used in epilepsy therapy. Monotherapy eliminates drug interactions and additive side effects. Determining the proper dose of the anticonvulsant drug is often a long and tedious process, which can be very frustrating for the person with epilepsy. Consistency in taking the medication is essential. Anticonvulsant drugs never should be discontinued abruptly; the dose should be decreased slowly to prevent seizure recurrence. The most frequent cause of recurrent seizures is patient noncompliance with drug regimens. Ongoing education and support are extremely important in the management of seizures. The psychosocial implications of a diagnosis of epilepsy continue to have a large impact on those affected with the disorder.

The neurologist and primary care physician must work together when a person on anticonvulsant medication becomes ill and must take additional medications. Some drugs act synergistically, and others interfere with the actions of anticonvulsant medications. This situation needs to be carefully monitored to avoid overmedication or interference with successful seizure control.

Surgical Therapy

Surgical treatment may be an option for persons with epilepsy that is refractory to drug treatment.[66] With the use of modern neuroimaging and surgical techniques, a single epileptogenic lesion can be identified and removed without leaving a neurologic deficit. The most common surgery consists of removal of the amygdala and an anterior part of the hippocampus and entorhinal cortex, as well as a small part of the temporal pole, leaving the lateral temporal neocortex intact. Another surgical procedure involves partial removal of the corpus callosum to prevent spread of a unilateral seizure to a generalized seizure. Modern epilepsy surgery requires a multidisciplinary team of highly skilled surgeons and specialists working together in an epilepsy center. Most procedures require only a few hours in the operating room and a few days' stay in the hospital after surgery. Although surgery for epilepsy is still in its early stages, it is increasingly considered a treatment modality for persons with medically intractable epilepsy.

GENERALIZED CONVULSIVE STATUS EPILEPTICUS

Seizures that do not stop spontaneously or occur in succession without recovery are called status epilepticus. There are as many types of status epilepticus as there are types of seizures. Tonic-clonic status epilepticus is a medical emergency and, if not promptly treated, may lead to respiratory failure and death.

The disorder occurs most frequently in the young and old. Morbidity and mortality rates are highest in elderly persons and persons with acute symptomatic seizures, such as those related to anoxia or cerebral infarction.[67] Approximately one third of patients have no history of a seizure disorder, and in another one third, status epilepticus occurs as an initial manifestation of epilepsy.[67] If status epilepticus is caused by neurologic or systemic disease, the cause needs to be identified and treated immediately because the seizures probably will not respond until the underlying cause has been corrected.

Treatment consists of appropriate life-support measures. Medications are given to control seizure activity. Intravenously administered diazepam or lorazepam is considered first-line therapy for the condition. The prognosis is related to the underlying cause as well as the duration of the seizures themselves.

In summary, seizures are caused by spontaneous, uncontrolled, paroxysmal, transitory discharges from cortical centers in the brain. Seizures may occur as a reversible symptom of another disease condition or as a recurrent condition called epilepsy. Epileptic seizures are classified as partial or generalized seizures. Partial seizures have evidence of local onset, beginning in one hemisphere. They include simple partial seizures, in which consciousness is not lost, and complex partial seizures, which begin in one hemisphere but progress to involve both. Generalized seizures involve both hemispheres and include unconsciousness and rapidly occurring, widespread, bilateral symmetric motor responses. They include minor motor seizures such as absence and akinetic seizures, and major motor or grand mal seizures. Control of seizures is the primary goal of treatment and is accomplished with anticonvulsant medications. Anticonvulsant medications interact with each other and need to be monitored closely when more than one drug is used.

REVIEW EXERCISES

A 20-year-man is an unbelted driver involved in a motor vehicle accident and presents in coma.

A. What are the clinical signs of coma?

B. Where does the source of coma localize in the brain?

C. Which complications of traumatic head injury might lead to coma?

D. What are the key treatment options to manage elevated intracranial pressure?

A 65-year-old woman presents with a 1-hour history of right-sided weakness and aphasia. An immediate CT scan of the brain is normal.

A. Where in the brain is the pathology?

B. What are the indications to administer intravenous tissue plasminogen activator?

C. What are the possible causes of this stroke, and what diagnostic tests would reveal the cause?

A child is taken to the emergency room with lethargy, fever, and a stiff neck on examination.

A. What findings on initial lumbar puncture indicate bacterial versus viral meningitis?

B. In the case of bacterial meningitis, what are the most likely organisms?

A 60-year-old man develops involuntary shaking of his right arm, which spreads to the face, then he collapses with whole-body shaking and loss of consciousness. After 1 minute, the shaking stops, and he is confused and disoriented.

A. What type of seizure is suggested by the clinical manifestations?

B. Assuming this is his first seizure, what diagnostic tests should be performed to identify a cause for the seizure?

C. If he has a long history of similar recurrent seizures, what treatments should be instituted? What treatments should be considered if he has failed multiple adequate trials of anticonvulsant medications?

References

1. Burns D.K., Kumar V. (2003). The nervous system. In Kumar V., Cotran R.S. Robbins S.L. (Eds.), *Robbins basic pathology* (7th ed., pp. 809–849). Philadelphia: W.B. Saunders.
2. Meyer F.B. (1992). Brain metabolism, blood flow, and ischemic thresholds. In Awad I.A. (Ed.), *Neurosurgical topics: Cerebrovascular occlusive disease and brain ischemia* (pp. 1–24). Cleveland: American Association of Neurological Surgeons.
3. Richmond T.S. (1997). Cerebral resuscitation after global brain ischemia: Linking research to practice. *AACN Clinical Issues 8*, 171–181.
4. Rubin E., Farber J.L. (1999). *Pathology* (3rd ed., pp. 1470–1473, 1509–1512). Philadelphia: Lippincott-Raven.

5. Martin T.G. (1986). Drowning and near-drowning. *Hospital Medicine 22*(7), 53.
6. Sieber F.E., Traystman R.J. (1992). Special issues: Glucose and the brain. *Critical Care Medicine 20,* 104–116.
7. Lipton S.A., Rosenberg P.A. (1994). Excitatory amino acids as a final common pathway in neurologic disorders. *New England Journal of Medicine 330,* 613–622.
8. Feurerstein G., Hunter J., Barone F.C. (1992). Calcium blockers and neuroprotection. In Marangos P.J., Lal H. (Eds.), *Advances in neuroprotection: Emerging strategies in neuroprotection* (p. 129). Boston: Birkhauser.
9. Sauer D., Massiu L., Allegrini P.R., et al. (1992). Excitotoxicity, cerebral ischemia, and neuroprotection by competitive NMDA receptor antagonists. In Marangos P.J., Lal H. (Eds.), *Advances in neuroprotection: Emerging strategies in neuroprotection* (pp. 93–105). Boston: Birkhauser.
10. Albers G.W., Clark W.M., DeGraba T.J. (1998). *The evolving paradigm of neuronal protection following stroke.* Monograph. Englewood, CO: Postgraduate Institute for Medicine.
11. Hickey J.V. (2003). *The clinical practice of neurological and neurosurgical nursing* (5th ed., pp. 295–327, 159–184). Philadelphia: Lippincott-Raven.
12. Lang E.W., Chestnut R.M. (1995). Intracranial pressure and cerebral perfusion pressure in severe head injury. *New Horizons 3,* 400–409.
13. Guyton A.C., Hall J.E. (2000). *Textbook of medical physiology* (10th ed., pp. 192, 671–722). Philadelphia: W.B. Saunders.
14. Plum F., Posner J.B. (1980). The diagnosis of stupor and coma (3rd ed.). Philadelphia: F.A. Davis.
15. Xiao F. (2002). Bench to bedside: Brain edema and cerebral resuscitation: The present and the future. *Academy of Emergency Medicine 9,* 933–946.
16. Ghajar J. (2000). Traumatic brain injury. *Lancet 356,* 923–929.
17. White R.J., Likavec M.J. (1992). The diagnosis and initial management of head injury. *New England Journal of Medicine 327,* 1507–1511.
18. Jennett B. (1996). Epidemiology of head injury. *Journal of Neurology, Neurosurgery, and Psychiatry 60,* 362–369.
19. Chestnut R.M. (1995). Secondary brain insults after head injury: Clinical perspectives. *New Horizons 3,* 366–375.
20. Teasdale G.M. (1995). Head injury. *Journal of Neurology, Neurosurgery, and Psychiatry 58,* 526–539.
21. Rhoades R.A., Tanner G.A. (2003). *Medical physiology* (2nd ed., pp. 132–133). Philadelphia: Lippincott Williams & Wilkins.
22. Ingersoll G.L., Leyden D.B. (1987). The Glasgow Coma Scale for patients with head injuries. *Critical Care Nursing 7*(5), 26–32.
23. Teasdale G.M. (2000). Revisiting the Glasgow Coma Scale and Coma Score. *Intensive Care Medicine 26,* 153–154.
24. Wijdicks E.F.M. (2001). The diagnosis of brain death. *New England Journal of Medicine 344,* 1215–1221.
25. Quality Standards Subcommittee of American Academy of Neurology. (1995). Practice parameters for determining brain death in adults. *Neurology 45,* 1012–1014.
26. Quality Standards Subcommittee of American Academy of Neurology. (1995). Practice parameters: Assessment and management of patients with persistent vegetative state. *Neurology 45,* 1015–1018.
27. American Stroke Association. (2003). *Heart disease and stroke statistics—2003 update.* Dallas, TX: American Heart Association.
28. Goldstein L.B., Chairperson, Stroke Council of American Heart Association: (2001). Primary prevention of ischemic stroke: A statement for health care professionals. *Circulation 103,* 163–182.
29. American Stroke Association. (1999). *The latest news about stroke.* Dallas, TX: American Heart Association.
30. Gorelick P.B. (1987). Alcohol and stroke. *Current Concepts in Cerebrovascular Disease 21*(5), 21.
31. Blank-Reid C. (1996). How to have a stroke at an early age: The effects of crack, cocaine and other illicit drugs. *Journal of Neuroscience Nursing 28*(1), 19–27.
32. Albers W.A. (Chair). (1998). Antithrombotic and thrombolytic therapy for ischemic stroke. *Chest 114,* 683S–698S.
33. Zambramski J.M., Anson J.A. (1992). Diagnostic evaluation of ischemic cerebrovascular disease. In Awad I.A. (Ed.), *Neurosurgical topics: Cerebrovascular occlusive disease and brain ischemia* (pp. 73–101). Cleveland: American Association of Neurological Surgeons.
34. Johnston S.C. (2002). Transient ischemic attack. *New England Journal of Medicine 347,* 1687–1692.
35. Gregory W. (Chair AD Hoc Committee on Guidelines for Management of Transient Ischemic Attacks, Stroke Council, American Heart Association). (1999). Supplement to the guidelines for transient ischemic attacks. *Stroke 30,* 2502–2511.
36. Qureshi A.I., Tuhrim S., Broderick J.P., et al. (2001). Spontaneous intracerebral hemorrhage. *New England Journal of Medicine 344,* 1450–1460.
37. Fewel M.E., Thompson M.G., Hoff J.T. (2003). Spontaneous intracerebral hemorrhage: A review. *Neurosurgical Focus 15,* 1–17.
38. Broderick J.P., Adams H.P., Barson W., et al. (1999). American Heart Association Scientific Statement: Guidelines to the management of spontaneous intracerebral hemorrhage. *Stroke 30,* 905–915.
39. Brott T., Bogousslavsy J. (2000). Treatment of acute ischemic stroke. *New England Journal of Medicine 343,* 709–721.
40. Adams H.P. (Chair). (1994). Guidelines for the management of patients with acute ischemic stroke: A statement for healthcare professionals from a Special Writing Group of the Stroke Council, American Heart Association. *Stroke 25,* 1901–1914.
41. Adams H.P. (Chair). (1996). Guidelines for thrombolytic therapy of acute stroke: A supplement to the guidelines for the management of patients with acute ischemic stroke: A statement for healthcare professionals from the Special Writing Group of the Stroke Council, American Heart Association. *Circulation 94,* 1167–1174.
42. Bronstein K.S., Popovich J.M., Stewart-Amidei C. (1991). *Promoting stroke recovery: A research based approach for nurses* (p. 200). St. Louis: C.V. Mosby.
43. Schievink W.I. (1997). Intracranial aneurysms. *New England Journal of Medicine 336,* 28–39.
44. Mayberg M.R. (Chair). (1994). Guidelines for the management of aneurysmal subarachnoid hemorrhage: A statement for healthcare professionals from a Special Writing Group of the Stroke Council, American Heart Association. *Stroke 25,* 2315–2327.
45. Sawin P.D., Loftus C.M. (1997). Diagnosis of spontaneous subarachnoid hemorrhage. *American Family Physician 55,* 145–155.
46. Arteriovenous Malformations Study Group. (1999). Arteriovenous malformations of the brain in adults. *New England Journal of Medicine 340,* 1812–1818.
47. Fleetwood I.G., Steinberg G.K. (2002). Arteriovenous malformations. *Lancet 359,* 893.
48. Ogilvy C.S. (Chair, Special Writing Group of the Stroke Council, American Heart Association). (2001). Recommendations for management of intracranial arteriovenous malformations. *Stroke 32,* 1458–1471.
49. Tunkel A.R., Scheld W.M. (1997). Issues in management of bacterial meningitis. *American Family Physician 56,* 1355–1365.
50. Quagliarello V.J., Scheld W.M. (1997). Treatment of bacterial meningitis. *New England Journal of Medicine 336,* 708–716.

51. De Gans J., Van De Beek D. (2002). Dexamethasone in adults with bacterial meningitis. *New England Journal of Medicine 349,* 1549–1556.
52. Mehta N., Levin M. (2000). Management and prevention of meningococcal disease. *Hospital Practice 35*(8), 75–86.
53. American Cancer Society. (2003). Cancer facts & figures: 2003. [On-line]. Available: http://www3.cancer.org.
54. DeAngelo L.M. (2001). Brain tumors. *New England Journal of Medicine 344,* 114–123.
55. Kuttesch J.F., Jr., Ater J.L. (2004). Brain tumors in childhood. In Behrman R.E., Kliegman R.M., Jenson H.B. (Eds.). *Nelson textbook of medicine* (17th ed., pp. 1702–1711). Philadelphia: W.B. Saunders.
56. DeAngelis L.M., Posner J.B. (2001). Cancer of the central nervous system and pituitary gland. In Lenhard R.E., Osteen R.T., Gansler T. (Eds.), *The American Cancer Society's clinical oncology* (pp. 655–703). Atlanta GA, American Cancer Society.
57. Behin A., Hoang-Xuan K., Carpenter A.F., Delattre J-Y. (2003). Primary brain tumors in adults. *Lancet 361,* 323–331.
58. Browne T.R., Holmes G.L. (2001). Epilepsy. *New England Journal of Medicine 344,* 1145–1151.
59. Chang B.S., Lowenstein D.H. (2003). Mechanisms of disease: Epilepsy. *New England Journal of Medicine 349,* 1257–1266.
60. Mosewich R.K., So E.L. (1996). The clinical approach to classification of seizures and epileptic syndromes. *Mayo Clinic Proceedings 71,* 405–441.
61. Benbadis S. (2001). Epileptic seizures and syndromes. Neurology Clinics: *Epilepsy 19*(2), 251–270.
62. Johnston M.V. (2004). Seizures in childhood. In Behrman R.E., Kliegman R.M., Jenson H.B. (Eds.), *Nelson textbook of medicine* (17th ed., pp. 1993–2009). Philadelphia: W.B. Saunders.
63. Commission on Classification and Terminology of the International League Against Epilepsy. (1981). Proposal for revised clinical and electroencephalographic classification of epileptic seizures. *Epilepsia 22,* 489–501.
64. Commission on Classification and Terminology of the International League Against Epilepsy. (1989). Proposal for revised classification of epilepsies and epileptic syndromes. *Epilepsia 30,* 389–399.
65. Nguyen D.K., Spencer S.S. (2003). Recent advances in the treatment of epilepsy. *Archives of Neurology 60,* 929–935.
66. Engel J. (1996). Surgery for seizures. *New England Journal of Medicine 334,* 647–652.
67. Cascino G.D. (1996). Generalized convulsive status epilepticus. *New England Journal of Medicine 71,* 787–792.

CHAPTER

53

Disorders of Thought, Mood, and Memory

Sandra Kawczynski Pasch

Psychiatric disorders are characterized by changes in a person's thoughts, mood, or behaviors that preclude ordinary functioning in one or more spheres of life. Throughout the course of history, persons in the healing professions have tried to uncover the causes and find effective treatments for diseases that alter the way in which people experience the world and behave in it. Over the centuries, the pendulum has swung between those practitioners who espouse the view that mental disease arises from inadequate interpersonal relationships and those who espouse the view that mental disease arises from alterations in brain structure or activity. In the late 20th century, and now in the early years of the 21st century, the conversation between these two apparently divergent philosophies continues, perhaps to conclude with a new synthesis of nurture versus nature and therefore new and effective therapies for those with mental illness.

The purpose of this chapter is to review the evolution in understanding of the pathogenesis and treatment of mental illness, to relate the anatomy of the brain and its integrated regional functions to the causes, manifestations, and treatment of selected thought, mood, and cognitive disorders.

Evolution in Understanding of Mental Illness

After completing this section of the chapter, you should be able to meet the following objectives:

- Define the terms *biologic psychiatry* and *psychosocial psychiatry* and compare them in terms of their definitions of the origins of mental disease

- Describe the changes in the treatment of mental illness over the past three centuries
- Explain the role that heredity plays in the epidemiology and development of mental illness

HISTORICAL PERSPECTIVES

Psychiatry was not an organized specialty before the end of the 18th century, but mental disorders are as old as the human race. Artifacts and cave drawings from a half million years ago indicate that what we have come to call psychotic disorders were known then. Over the ages, the explanations of mental disorders have ranged from possession by gods and demons, to the breaking of taboos, to the idea that a harmful substance had entered the body. Persons with psychiatric disorders were treated with prayers, magic, and exorcisms. In some communities, the mentally ill were viewed with fear and often turned out of their homes, villages, and towns. In other communities, families took care of the mentally ill, but often these people were neglected or locked up in barns or cellars.[1]

The history of our understanding of psychiatric illnesses reveals a tension between two schools of thought as to the origin of mental disease. The pendulum has swung between these two apparently opposite viewpoints across the centuries. One view of psychiatric illness is that mental disorders are due to anatomic, developmental, and functional disorders of the brain, and is called *biologic psychiatry*. Another view is that mental disorders are due to impaired psychological development, a consequence of poor child rearing or environmental stress, and is called *psychosocial psychiatry*.[1] These differences of emphasis in terms of the pathogenesis of mental illness are important because the prevailing theory about the origins of mental disease influences what therapies for psychiatric illness predominate.

Early biologic psychiatry in the late 1800s to early 1900s emphasized the correlation of neurologic symptoms with postmortem microscopic study of anatomic changes in the brain. Although this research was of immense importance in terms of regional localization of brain functions (*e.g.*, Wernicke's aphasia), it provided little help to the clinical psychiatrist of the time. Emil Kraepelin, a German psychiatrist, was the first to begin to classify psychiatric disorders by systematically studying the natural history of the disease. The intent was to be able to predict outcomes. In the sixth edition of his textbook, *Psychiatrie* (1899), Kraepelin laid the groundwork for the *Diagnostic and Statistical Manual of Mental Disorders* (DSM; the current 4th edition [revised] is abbreviated DSM-IV-TR) of the American Psychiatric Association. He divided all mental disorders into 13 groups, including psychoses, which he divided into two distinct groups: those with an affective component, which he called *manic-depressive psychosis,* and those without, which he called *dementia praecox*.[1]

In the mid-20th century, the psychoanalytic view of mental disorders took hold, reaching its zenith in the 1950s and 1960s. Psychiatric illness was explained as the result of unconscious conflicts over events in an individual's past. Alterations in nurture, not nature, became the underlying cause of psychiatric illness.

In the last half of the 20th century, biologic psychiatry became important once again. During the 1970s, techniques of neuroimaging became available that allowed the neuroscientist to visualize brain structures and function.[1] The results of genetic studies examining the correlation between family relationships and incidence of psychiatric illness, in particular the studies of monozygotic and dizygotic twins, suggested that depression and schizophrenia had a strong genetic component. The introduction of chlorpromazine (*i.e.,* Thorazine) as a treatment for schizophrenia revolutionized psychiatry because although it did not cure psychosis, it did control the symptoms of the disease, increasing the potential for more traditional therapies to work and allowing previously institutionalized individuals to lead much more normal lives. It also suggested strongly that mental illness had a biologic foundation. Chlorpromazine soon was followed by other drugs for psychosis and depression.

This move to biologic psychiatry, however, has not excluded the healing value of the therapist–client relationship. It appears that pharmacotherapy in conjunction with psychotherapy is of greater healing power than either alone. Perhaps the distinction drawn between biologic and psychosocial disease is arbitrary. Indeed, experiments indicate that learning and sensory stimulation or deprivation can in fact weaken or strengthen synaptic connections, which in turn could change brain function and thus behavior.[2]

Treatment of Mental Illness

Asylums have existed since the Middle Ages, but until the end of the 18th century, their only function was custodial. One of the oldest asylums was the Priory of St. Mary of Bethlehem, founded in London in the 13th century. Its name was eventually shortened to *Bedlam,* a term that has become synonymous with madness. The asylum as a therapeutic establishment did not become an important concept until the end of the 18th century.[1]

At this time, madness was viewed as an excessive irritation of the nerves; therefore, establishing a calming environment was crucial. These asylums often had a very rigid schedule of daily activities meant to focus the patient and afford mental rest. It was also during this time that practitioners attempted to systematize the techniques known to establish a therapeutic relationship between the doctor and the patient.

In the 1800s, the number of patients in asylums was, at the most, in the hundreds. By the mid-1900s, the number was in the thousands. Unfortunately, by the early 1900s, asylums had become little more than warehouses for the chronically mentally ill.[3] Whether this was due to the failure of asylums as a therapeutic environment or to the increased number of persons housed in them, overwhelming the available resources, remains a matter of debate. The reason for the increased numbers of persons in the asylum in the 19th century also is debated. Was there an increased incidence of mental illness, or did society become increasingly intolerant of deviant behavior?

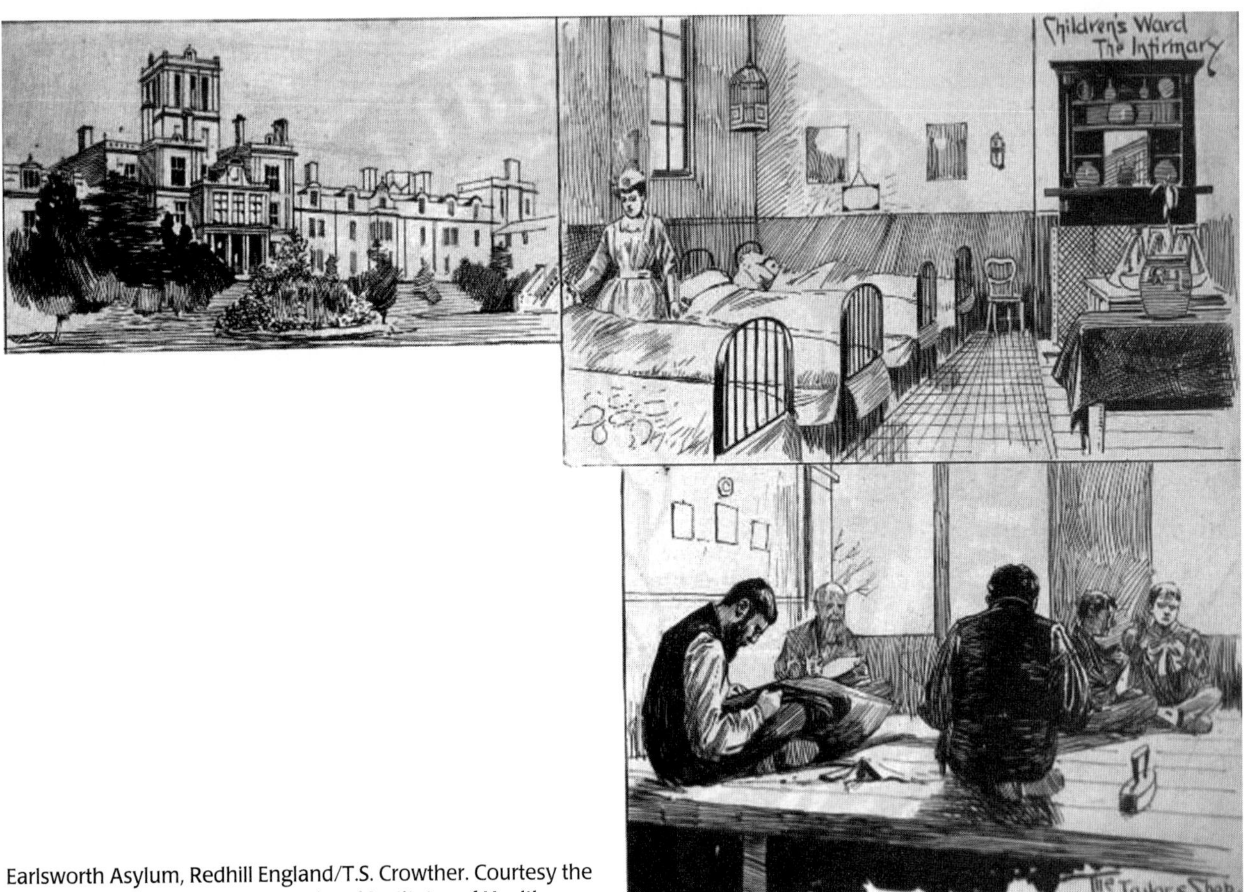

Earlsworth Asylum, Redhill England/T.S. Crowther. Courtesy the National Library of Medicine, National Institutes of Health.

This debate exploded in the 1960s, during which time several writers suggested that there was no such thing as mental illness but rather a medicalizing of deviance and that psychiatric institutions were evil. Schizophrenia in this view was a gifted and creative state of consciousness, not an illness. This antipsychiatry attitude, coupled with the advent of psychopharmacology, laid the foundations for the deinstitutionalization of the mentally ill and the move to community psychiatry. Unfortunately, deinstitutionalization was neither carefully planned nor adequately funded, leaving many mentally ill homeless and without proper care.[1]

THE ROLE OF HEREDITY IN MENTAL ILLNESS

Who we are and how we express ourselves through behavior depend on the complex influences of genetic and environmental factors on neural development and function. Since the early 1990s, the scientific knowledge base in genetics has grown exponentially and has created new tools to study the role of genetic inheritance in the development of mental illness. Research into the complexities of the regulation of gene expression can only deepen our understanding of the etiology of mental disorders, increase our ability to treat the disorders with more precisely targeted psychotherapeutic drugs, and ultimately lead to the discovery of ways to prevent the development of psychiatric illness.

Epidemiologic studies of twins, of adopted children, and of family histories or pedigrees have shed light on the debate over the relative influence of nurture versus nature in the development of mental illness. Twin studies compared the incidence of mental illness among monozygotic (identical) twins, dizygotic (fraternal) twins, and their siblings. If a disease were at all genetically determined, higher rates of coexistence of the disorder (concordance) would be expected among monozygotic twins as compared with dizygotic twins, nontwin siblings, or the general population. Adoption studies questioned whether children with a genetic history of mental illness, adopted by parents with no history of psychiatric illness, had a greater risk for developing mental illness than children with no genetic history of mental illness who were adopted by parents with a psychiatric illness. Also, if a mental illness has a genetic component, it would be expected that higher numbers of persons in a family would have the disorder than would be found in the general population.[4–6] The overwhelming conclusions of these studies have been that both genetic vulnerability and environmental influences play significant roles in the development of mental illness.

For example, studies of twins have shown a 45% concordance for schizophrenia among monozygotic twins, compared with 15% for dizygotic twins or other siblings.[7]

With bipolar depression, there is an 80% concordance in monozygotic twins, compared with 10% for siblings. In monozygotic twins living apart, the concordance rate for affective disorders is 40% to 60%.[8] Even the concordance rates among siblings for these two disorders is suggestive of a genetic influence because schizophrenia has approximately a 1% incidence and depression a 5% incidence among the general population.[7,8] The rate of occurrence of either disorder also is higher in the biologic families of adopted children than in the adoptive families. The incidence of suicide is six times higher among biologic relatives of adoptees with depressive illness than among the biologic relatives of adoptees without depression.

Although the evidence for a genetic basis for mental illness is compelling, the fact that the concordance among monozygotic twins is not 100% indicates that other factors may be involved in the development of a mental illness. It certainly is highly likely that mental illnesses are polygenic and multifactorial rather than simply inherited through transmission of a classic disordered dominant or recessive mendelian trait (see Chapter 6). In addition, mental disorders exhibit variable expressivity. It is possible that a person with the disease genotype needs to have the right environmental stressors (*i.e.*, viral illness, physical or emotional abuse, substance abuse) to express the disease phenotype, or that there are gene–gene interactions that influence the extent to which a mental illness is manifested.[4]

In summary, psychiatric disorders are characterized by alterations in thought, mood, or behavior that may interfere with a person's ability to engage in ordinary social interactions and may in some instances require temporary or long-term institutionalization. Our understanding of the pathogeneses of mental disease is still in its infancy, and the historical debate about the relative importance of nurture and nature in the development of mental illness continues. It is likely that the cause of mental illness is multifactorial and includes a dynamic interplay among genetic predisposition, alterations in early neurodevelopment, and dysfunctional social interactions in a family.

Anatomic and Neurochemical Basis of Behavior

After completing this section of the chapter, you should be able to meet the following objectives:

- Name the cerebral cortical structures and structures from the primitive brain involved in thought and emotion
- Describe the major functions of each brain structure in terms of thought processes, learning, and emotion
- Describe the cortical pathways by which learning and the development of memory occur
- Define the terms *synapse, synaptic transmission,* and *neuromediators*
- Name the major neuromediators in the brain, their major location and source in the brain, and the possible involvement of each in the manifestations of mental illness

BEHAVIORAL ANATOMY OF THE BRAIN

There is increasing scientific evidence that anatomic and biochemical alterations in the brain play a critical role in the behaviors observed in mental illness. The brain is extraordinarily complex, divided into several distinct groups of functional neurons that also are highly interconnected and thus able to influence each other's activity.[9] The information processing happens within nanoseconds. However, for persons with brain injury or degenerative changes, information processing and cognitive function may be impaired.

Cerebral Cortical Structures

The cerebral cortex covers the outermost part of the brain. The cortex, which contains the centers for elaboration of thought, voluntary motor and sensory function, speech, and memory patterns, has extensive connections with deeper parts of the brain. The thalamus, in particular, forms important connections with the cerebral cortex. Thalamic excitation is necessary for almost all cortical activity. Thus, the loss of function is much greater when the thalamus is damaged along with the cortex than when the damage is limited to the cortex. Table 53-1 summarizes the cerebral cortical structures and their functions.

The Prefrontal Cortex. The frontal lobe is the largest lobe and often is referred to as the chief administrator of the brain (Fig. 53-1). It is responsible for planning, problem solving, intellectual insight, judgment, and expression of emotion. It is the function of the prefrontal areas to keep tract of many bits of information simultaneously and then to recall this information as it is needed for subsequent intellectual tasks. Before the discovery of modern drugs to treat psychiatric conditions, some patients were treated surgically with a procedure, called a *prefrontal lobotomy,* that severed the connections between the prefrontal areas of the brain and the remainder of the brain.[10] Subsequent studies of these patients revealed a lack of ability to solve complex problems, to link sequential tasks together, and to learn to do parallel tasks at the same time. Their social responses were inappropriate, and their levels of aggression were decreased to the point at which they lost all ambition. They were still able to perform at their previous level of motor function, talk, and comprehend language, but they were unable to carry through with any long-term trains of thought.

The Temporal Lobe. The temporal lobe integrates and interprets somatic, visual, and auditory information that is critical for recognition of the familiar as well as for appropriate interpretation of and response to social contexts. The temporal lobe also contains the area of the brain (*Wernicke's area*) that is responsible for language comprehension. It is one of the more important areas of the brain in terms of intellect because almost all intellectual functions are language based.

TABLE 53-1 Selected Functions of Several Brain Regions

Frontal Lobe	Temporal Lobe	Parietal Lobe	Occipital Lobe
Abstract vs. concrete reasoning Motivation–volition Concentration Decision making Purposeful behavior Memory and historical sense of self Sequencing Making meaning of language Speech organization Speech production (Broca's area) Aspects of emotional response—blunting	Visual-spatial recognition Attention Motivation Emotional modulation and interpretation Impulse and aggression control Interpretation and meaning of social context Aspects of sexual action and meaning	Sensory integration and spatial relations Bodily awareness Filtration of background stimuli Personality factors and symptom denial Memory and nonverbal memory Concept formation	Vision Possible information holding area

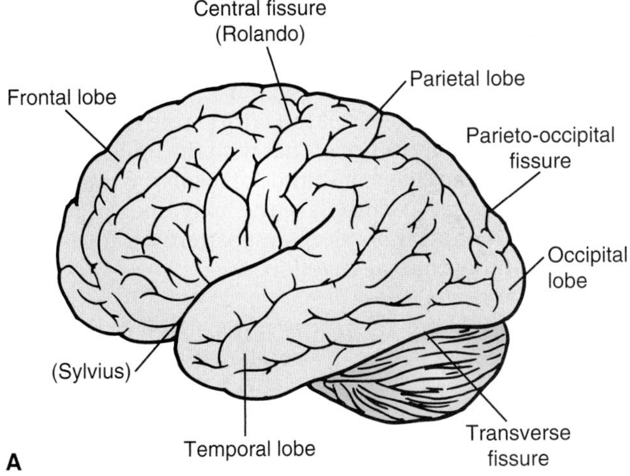

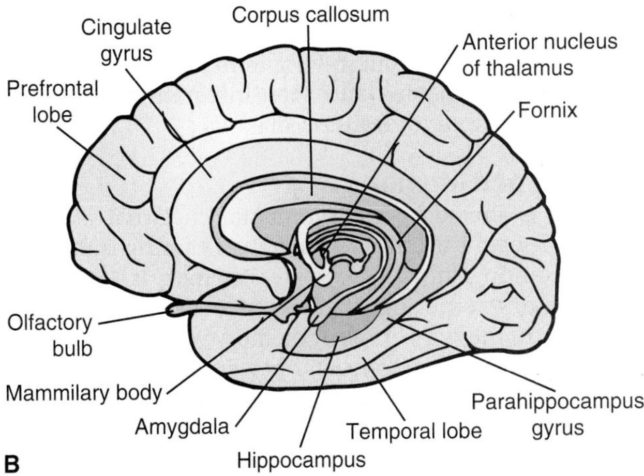

FIGURE 53-1 (**A**) Lateral aspects of the cerebral hemispheres, including the frontal, temporal, parietal, and occipital lobes. (**B**) The structure of the limbic cortex, which include the limbic cortex (cingulate gyrus, parahippocampal gyrus, hippocampus) and associated subcortical structures (thalamus, hypothalamus, amygdala).

Part of appropriate social response is the accurate interpretation of emotions and the ability to respond with the level of emotionality and language deemed socially congruent. Impulse control, the management of aggression and sexual expression, including the culturally determined stereotypy of what it means to be male or female in a given society, also are temporal lobe functions. Emotion originates in the amygdala of the limbic system (discussed later), but the modulation and "fine-tuning" of that emotion into an appropriate level of intensity occurs in the temporal lobe.

Parietal Lobe. The parietal lobe is essential in the integration and processing of sensory (visual, tactile, and auditory) input. It is in the parietal lobe that sensory experiences first begin to coalesce into the cognitions we experience as thinking in the frontal lobes. The coordination of spatial awareness occurs in the parietal lobe and involves not only visual content but also the ability to experience, claim, and care for all of one's body. Another important parietal lobe function is to filter out extraneous information. The ability to filter out background and extraneous noise and sensations is critical to normal daily functioning.

Occipital Lobe. The occipital lobe is the most posterior of the lobes and is responsible for receiving visual information from the eyes. The visual association cortex of the occipital lobe is important for the interpretation of visual experiences, including depth perception and location in space.

Association Areas. A large part of the cerebral cortex forms association areas that add perception and meaning to incoming sensory information. The most important of these are the parieto-occipitotemporal association area, the prefrontal association area, and the limbic association area (Fig. 53-2).

The *parieto-occipitotemporal association area* lies in the large parieto-occipital cortical space bounded by the somatosensory cortex, the visual cortex, and the auditory cortex (see Chapter 49). This association area computes the coordinates of incoming visual, auditory, and somatosensory information, providing information about the

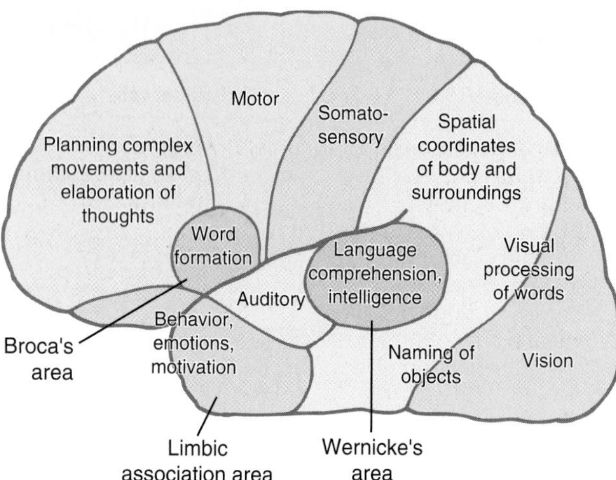

FIGURE 53-2 Map of specific functional areas in the cerebral cortex, showing especially Wernicke's and Broca's areas of language comprehension and speech production, which in 95% of all people is located in the left hemisphere. (Adapted from Guyton A.C., Hall J.E. [2000]. *Textbook of medical physiology* [10th ed., p. 655]. Philadelphia: W.B. Saunders).

location of body parts and their relationship to the environment. It also contains the major area for comprehending language, processing visual language (reading), and naming objects.

The *prefrontal association area* functions in close connection with the motor cortex to plan and execute complex motor movements. This area uses input from sensory receptors in muscles and joints as well as sensory input from the skin and vestibular system. The prefrontal association area is also important in carrying out thought processes that involve input from multiple sensory modalities. It is often described as being the area for short-term "working memories" that are used to analyze each new thought as it is entering the brain. A special area of the frontal cortex, called *Broca's area,* provides the neural circuitry for word formation.

The *limbic association area* is found in the anterior pole of the temporal lobe and in the cingulated gyrus on the medial aspect of the brain. It is concerned primarily with behavior, emotions, and motivation.

The Limbic System

The limbic system is a complex group of neurons that regulate our emotional behavior. It includes several discrete structures in the deep part of the brain, including the hippocampus, the parahippocampal gyrus, cingulate gyrus, amygdala, and a bridgelike structure called the *fornix,* which is a bundle of nerve fibers connecting the hippocampus with the hypothalamus (see Fig. 53-1). Higher and lower brain centers communicate with the limbic system to link thoughts and autonomic nervous system responses to emotions.

The hippocampus, along with its adjacent temporal and parietal lobe structures, has numerous indirect connections with many portions of the cerebral cortex as well as other parts of the limbic system. The hippocampus plays a major role in the encoding, consolidation, and retrieval of memories. Almost all types of sensory information activate some part of the hippocampus. In turn, the hippocampus distributes information to the anterior thalamus, hypothalamus, and other parts of the limbic system. The hippocampus also groups and schematizes input in preparation for memory encoding. It plays a significant role in converting short-term memory to long-term memory. Hippocampal atrophy has been noted in diseases in which memory problems play an important role, such as Alzheimer's disease.

The amygdala is located deep in the medial temporal lobe. It receives neuronal signals from the temporal and occipital lobes of the cortex and has many bidirectional connections with the hypothalamus as well as other parts of the limbic system. Through these connections, the amygdala helps a person relate to the surrounding environment and then pattern appropriate behavior. Because of the many connections, the amygdala has been called the "window" through which a person sees the world. The amygdala is important in emotional function and regulation and modulation of affective responses in social settings. Sexual arousal, aggression, and fear also are functions of the amygdala.

The hypothalamus, although not strictly an anatomic part of the limbic system, plays a critical role in it because of the extensive connections it has with the limbic system. The hypothalamus has a multitude of regulatory functions related to basic survival needs of the body, such as regulation of body temperature, sleep–rest patterns, hunger, sexual drive, and hormonal secretion.

PHYSIOLOGY OF PERCEPTION, THOUGHT, AND MEMORY

Perception is the final stage of information processing. It is the conscious awareness of sensory stimuli and results in behavioral responses to that sensation. Information from the senses is received by the thalamus and then projected to the somatosensory cortex and prefrontal association area. The prefrontal association area keeps track of where information has been put in long-term memory and is responsible for retrieving and then integrating memories with sensory input for decision making.

Learning and Memory

Behavior is altered by environmental cues that are processed through learning and memory. Learning is the process of acquiring knowledge, whereas memory is the process of storing and retrieving what has been learned. There are two forms of memory: implicit memory, which is involved in learning reflexive motor and perceptual skills; and explicit memory, which is involved with processing the factual knowledge of persons, places, and things and its meaning.[11] Psychiatric patients and brain-injured persons not only experience specific cortical dysfunctions but also may experience difficulty in the proposed pathways for learning and memory. These difficulties are likely to influence their behavior and may have an impact on the design of effective interventions.

Thought processes probably involve a pattern of stimuli from many parts of the nervous system at the same time and in a definite sequence. Each thought requires simultaneous input from portions of the cerebral cortex, the thalamus, the limbic system, and the reticular formation in the brain stem. The prefrontal association cortex processes information from many areas of the brain and is necessary to achieve thinking. It has the ability to keep track of bits of information and recall them simultaneously from working memory. This allows us to plan, set goals, and solve problems. Thoughts are expressed in the form of language through the functions of Broca's area for word formation and Wernicke's area for language comprehension.

Physiologically, thought and memories are the result of synaptic transmission between neurons. During the process, new or reactivated pathways transmit neural circuits, sometimes called *memory traces,* through the brain.[10] Although we often think of memories as being positive recollections of past experiences, the greatest share of memories are probably negative encounters that the brain disregards as adverse or unimportant information. It is the basal regions of the limbic system that determine whether information is important and whether to store the thought as a memory trace or to suppress it. This aspect of memory selection is vital to the brain. Without it, the constant inundation of sensory information would exceed the capacity of the brain within minutes.

Memories can last minutes, hours, months, or years. For the purpose of classification, memory can be classified as short-term, intermediate-term, or long-term. Short-term memory is typically confined to the remembering of information for a period of several seconds to minutes (*e.g.,* 7 to 10 digits of a telephone number). It is thought that these memories involve nerve signals that travel around and around a temporary memory trace.[11] Intermediate-term memory involves the remembering of information for a period that may last many minutes or weeks. These memories become lost unless memory traces are established. Long-term memory, which lasts for years, is generally thought to result from actual structural changes in the synapses. For example, there might be an increase in the presynaptic structures responsible for the neurotransmitter synthesis or release.

DISORDERS OF PERCEPTION

Two disorders of information processing, hallucinations and delusional thinking, are common symptoms of many psychiatric disorders. These symptoms may also occasionally occur in healthy persons, they may accompany other health problems, or they may be a side effect of drugs.

Hallucinations

Within the realm of perception reside the input of sensory information from the outside world and the processing of this information into meaning. All sensory information from the external world is transmitted to the thalamus; from there, it is relayed to various parts of the brain and then transformed into meaningful experience. For example, visual stimuli from the retina are transmitted to centers in the thalamus through the optic nerve; from there, they are relayed to the primary visual cortex in the occipital lobe and then to the visual association cortex, where they gain meaning (see Chapter 54).

Hallucinations can be described as "sensory perceptions that occur without external stimulation of the relevant sensory organ."[12] Hallucinations should be differentiated from illusions, which are misinterpreted sensory perceptions that are stimulated by actual external stimuli. The pathophysiology of hallucinations can occur at several levels. The disorder may originate at the end organ, occur during sensory transmission, or be based on abnormal cortical reception, perception, or interpretation.

Hallucinations can be classified in several ways, such as by the structure or function involved, the etiology, or the affected sense perception. One functional method categorizes hallucinations as *release hallucinations* and *ictal hallucinations.*[12] Release hallucinations occur when a normal sensory input is blocked, and as a replacement, stored images are experienced; whereas ictal hallucinations are produced by abnormal neuronal discharges. Visual ictal hallucinations tend to be brief, stereotyped in content, and geometric in design. These are the type of hallucinations that occur during the aura in people with epilepsy. Hallucinations that are classified according to etiology may occur as the result of disorders of brain structure or function (brain tumors, epilepsy, metabolic disorders), drug reactions, sensory deprivation, or psychotic disorders. The type and content of hallucinations often provides insight into their etiology.

The most commonly used classification is based on the sensory perception involved (*e.g.,* visual, auditory, olfactory, tactile). Within this method, hallucinatory experiences involving the visual system are the most clearly categorized. Several types of visual hallucinations are normal life experiences (*e.g.,* images seen in a dream). Also, several ophthalmologic stimuli are accompanied by visual hallucinations. Ocular phosphenes, which are produced by vigorous rubbing of the eye, are a form of visual hallucination. The Charles Bonnet syndrome is an organic disorder occurring in the elderly that is characterized by complex visual hallucinations. It is associated with loss of vision and is seen in older adults with preserved intellectual functions.[13] In one study, 10% of persons (mean age of 75 years) with severe visual disability experienced visual hallucinations.[14] These persons retained insight into the problem and needed only reassurance that their hallucinations did not represent mental illness. Visual hallucinations associated with psychiatric disorders tend to be complex, may be enhanced by auditory hallucinations, and often lead to delusional beliefs.

Auditory hallucinations include misperceptions of sounds such as ringing and buzzing noises, musical sounds, and voices. Although they commonly occur in psychiatric disorders, particularly schizophrenia, they also occur in other disorders. Musical hallucinations featuring the perception of music without an external stimulus can be seen in disorders ranging from deafness to temporal lobe pathology. When associated with brain pathology, the lesion is usually on the right side of the brain. Auditory hallucinations are commonly reported as an aura of epilepsy.

Tinnitus, the perception of ringing, buzzing, or whistling sounds, is often the result of disorders of the inner ear (see Chapter 55). Withdrawal states, particularly from alcohol, are known to cause auditory hallucinations. A variety of psychiatric disorders are accompanied by auditory hallucinations, such as the sound of voices. Often, the source of the sound, which is sensed as occurring within the head, is difficult to localize. The voice often comments on the person's behavior and echoes their thoughts. Voices are rarely described as supportive; they are most often described as critical and negative in tone. Strategies of distraction used by persons hearing voices include listening to music, especially through headphones, or snapping rubber bands on their wrists. Additionally, keeping a record helps identify hallucinatory precipitants and thus helps individuals avoid those situations that act as precipitants.[15]

Hallucinations involving smell and taste are often the result of damage to the olfactory bulb. Tumors at the base of the brain that extend into the olfactory cortex can produce olfactory hallucinations. Persons with migraine headaches may also experience an aura consisting of olfactory or gustatory hallucinations. Somatosensory hallucinations, such as phantom limb pain, are discussed in Chapter 50.

Delusions

Delusions are characterized by a false belief and the persistent, unshakable acceptance of the false belief. In contrast to hallucinations, which are abnormalities of perception, delusions are abnormalities of thought. Delusions commonly incorporate input from multiple sensory systems, whereas hallucinations are confined to a single sensory modality.

Delusions are formed from and colored by an individual's background, including personal, family, and social experiences; educational background; and cultural (including religious) influences. Delusional thinking may include, among others, delusions of persecution (*e.g.,* believing one's self or property is being threatened), influence (*e.g.,* believing thoughts can move through radio or atomic rays), ill health, grandeur (*e.g.,* believing oneself to be a great person, such as the King of England), poverty, and possession (*e.g.,* believing one's body is possessed by God or some great power).

The causes and mechanisms underlying delusional thinking are unclear. It has been suggested that delusional thinking is the product of repeated stress, rather than a disorder based on a single, acute situational problem.[12] Interestingly, delusions have been associated with conditions that produce sensory deprivation, such as hearing loss. In one study that used a case-control method, elderly persons with late-life psychoses that included paranoid symptomatology were four times more likely to have hearing impairments compared with control subjects.[16]

ROLE OF NEUROMEDIATORS

Many of the new advances in the understanding and treatment of mental illness are derived from an increased understanding of how nerve cells in the brain communicate with one another. Nerve cells of discrete brain regions communicate with each other rapidly and over long distances by electrochemical signals that are propagated along the length of each neuron. The point at which two neurons meet is called a *synapse,* and the process by which the signal from one neuron to another is communicated is called *synaptic transmission* or *neurotransmission* (see Chapter 49). Chemical substances called *neurotransmitters* or *neuromediators* are released from the axonal terminal of one neuron (presynaptic cell), cross the synapse, bind to receptors on the postsynaptic cells, and cause excitatory or inhibitory actions.[17]

Neurotransmission involves several discrete steps: (1) the synthesis of a transmitter substance, (2) the storage and release of the transmitter, (3) binding of the transmitter to receptors on the postsynaptic membrane, and (4) removal of the transmitter from the synaptic cleft. The classic neurotransmitters include small-molecule transmitters and neuroactive peptides. These molecules typically are stored in vesicles in the presynaptic axonal terminal and released by the process of exocytosis[18] (see Chapter 49, Fig. 49-8).

The substances generally agreed to be neurotransmitters and implicated in mental illness include acetylcholine, the biogenic amines (dopamine, epinephrine, norepinephrine, and serotonin), and amino acids (gamma-aminobutyric acid [GABA], glutamate, glycine, and aspartate). Table 53-2 summarizes the major source and effect of each neurotransmitter.

Emergence of Psychotropic Medications

The treatment of many psychiatric disorders is based on pharmacologic interventions that alter neurotransmitter or receptor properties of the brain. In the 1950s, a French neurosurgeon, Henri Laborit, was searching for a drug that would reduce the effects of preoperative anxiety-induced histamine release in his patients. Through trial and error, he found chlorpromazine to be the most effective calming agent and recommended the drug to his psychiatric colleagues. It was subsequently found that high doses of chlorpromazine were efficacious in calming agitated persons with schizophrenia and bipolar disorders. It eventually became clear that chlorpromazine was not simply a tranquilizer but also had some specific antipsychotic effects. Chlorpromazine and related drugs in the phenothiazine class attenuated or abolished delusions, hallucinations, and disordered thinking.

There are now four major groups of antipsychotic agents used to treat schizophrenia, divided into two major categories: the typical and the atypical antipsychotics. The typical antipsychotics include the phenothiazines (e.g. chlorpromazine), butyrophenones (haloperidol), and thioxanthene (Navane). The atypical antipsychotics, exemplified first by clozapine, are more effective in treating the negative symptoms of schizophrenia (discussed later) and produce fewer extrapyramidal effects. Both categories of drugs exert their effect by blocking dopamine receptors, although the atypical antipsychotics have a more refined blockade action. The atypical antipsychotics also exert some of their effects through blockade of serotonin (5-HT) receptors.

TABLE 53-2 The Source and Effect of Brain Neuromediators

Neuromediator	Major Source in the Brain	Effect and Implications for Mental Illness
Acetylcholine (Ach)	Formed in many synapses of the brain; in high concentration in basal ganglia and motor cortex Derived from choline	Can be excitatory or inhibitory, depending on the area of the brain Underactivity implicated in Alzheimer's disease
Dopamine (DA)	Substantia nigra and ventral segmental area in the midbrain Derived from tyrosine	Usually excitatory Involved in motivation, thought, and emotional regulation Overactivity thought to be involved in schizophrenia and other psychotic disorders
Norepinephrine (NE) and epinephrine (E)	Locus ceruleus in brain stem Derived from dopamine	Can be excitatory or inhibitory, depending on the area of the brain Noradrenergic pathways to cerebral cortex, limbic system, and brain stem Underactivity thought to be involved in some depressions
Serotonin (5-HT)	Raphe nucleus in the brain stem Derived from tryptophan	Involved in the regulation of attention and complex cognitive functions Pathways to cerebral cortex, limbic system, and brain stem Underactivity thought to be involved in some depressions and obsessive-compulsive disorder
γ-Aminobutyric acid (GABA), glutamate, aspartate, and glycine	No single major source	GABA and glycine usually are inhibitory; glutamate is excitatory Implicated in anxiety disorders

Psychopharmacology has been particularly productive in developing highly effective treatments for affective disorders. Antidepressants alleviate depressive symptoms by increasing the activity of norepinephrine and serotonin at postsynaptic membrane receptors. The most widely used antidepressants can be divided into four major categories: the monoamine oxidase inhibitors (MAOIs), the tricyclic compounds, the serotonin reuptake inhibitors (SRIs), and the novel, or atypical, antidepressants. MAOIs increase the concentration of serotonin and norepinephrine by reducing the degradation of these neurotransmitters by monoamine oxidase. Tricyclics block the reuptake of serotonin and norepinephrine by the presynaptic membrane, whereas the SRIs inhibit the reuptake of serotonin. Formulations of the SRIs vary and target different neurotransmitters. These include the selective serotonin reuptake inhibitors (SSRIs), the serotonin antagonist and reuptake inhibitors (SARIs), and the serotonin norepinephrine reuptake inhibitors (SNRIs). The atypical antidepressants affect serotonergic and noradrenergic neurotransmission.

The therapeutic effect of the antipsychotic and antidepressant drugs probably is not entirely due to increasing or decreasing the neural levels of one or more neurotransmitters. For example, the clinical effect of the antidepressants typically is slow (weeks), even though the drugs rapidly block receptors. This suggests that the real mechanism of these drugs may be due to their effects on expression of receptors at the cellular membrane or on other intracellular pathways that regulate protein synthesis.[19]

NEUROIMAGING

Abnormalities in brain structure and function can contribute to the manifestations of mental illness. Since the early 1970s, imaging techniques have been developed that allow practitioners and researchers to map brain anatomy in exquisite detail and to estimate brain activity by measuring brain blood flow and metabolic rate. These imaging studies have suggested intriguing correlations between brain pathologies and psychiatric manifestations that provide clues to the pathogenesis of mental disorders. Brain imaging techniques, however, remain research tools and have not yet been applied clinically, which means that imaging cannot be used to make a diagnosis of mental illness. The techniques include computed tomography (CT) scans, magnetic resonance imaging (MRI), positron-emission tomography (PET), and single photon emission computed tomography (SPECT).

A CT scan of the brain provides a three-dimensional view of brain structures that can differentiate fine densities. Abnormalities in a CT scan are not diagnostic of any particular mental illness; however, they suggest a brain-based problem. Structural abnormalities of the brain have been measured in people with schizophrenia, mood disorders, and dementias. MRI is used primarily for diagnosis of structural changes in the brain, although newer techniques are able to measure brain function as well. Unlike CT, MRI is able to distinguish between gray and white matter. The basis of PET is the variable brain tissue uptake of an infused radioactive substance (Fig. 53-3). The tissue uptake of the

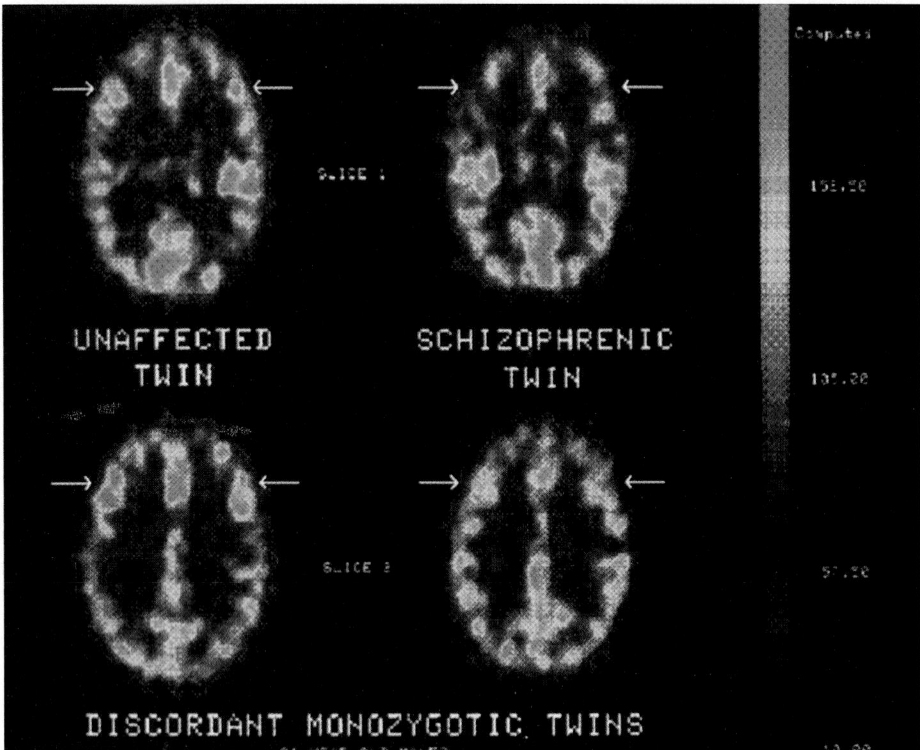

FIGURE 53-3 PET scan showing differences in frontal lobe activity of a pair of twins, one with a mental disorder of schizophrenia, and one who does not have the disorder. (From Boyd M.A. [2002]. *Psychiatric nursing: Contemporary practice.* [2nd ed., p. 98]. Philadelphia: Lippincott Williams & Wilkins. Courtesy Drs. K.F. Berman and D.R. Weinberger, Clinical Brain Disorders Branch, National Institutes of Mental Health)

substance depends on tissue type and metabolic activity. Labeled drugs can be infused to study neurotransmitter receptor activity or concentration in the brain. SPECT is similar to PET but is less expensive and uses more stable substances and different detectors to visualize blood flow patterns. This is useful for diagnosis of cerebrovascular accidents and brain tumors.[19,20]

In summary, the symptoms of mental illness arise from alterations in neural functioning or from destruction of neurons in the brain. Because the brain integrates the processes of learning, memory, and emotions, the manifestations of mental disease may be primarily cognitive impairment, emotional impairment, or a combination of both. Psychiatric patients and brain-injured persons not only experience specific cortical dysfunctions but also may experience difficulty in the proposed pathways for learning and memory. These difficulties are likely to influence behavior and may have an impact on the design of effective interventions.

Many of the new advances in the understanding and treatment of mental illness and symptoms such as hallucinations, mood disruptions, and cognitive dysfunctions are derived from an increased understanding of how nerve cells in the brain communicate with one another. Neurotransmission involves several discrete steps: (1) the synthesis of a transmitter substance, (2) the storage and release of the transmitter, (3) the binding of the transmitter to receptors on the postsynaptic membrane, and (4) the removal of the transmitter from the synaptic cleft. The substances generally agreed to be neurotransmitters and implicated in mental illness include acetylcholine, the biogenic amines, and amino acids.

New diagnostic tools, such as increasingly sophisticated neuroimaging techniques, may help to develop more precise correlations between behavior, thought, and mood disorders and microscopic alterations in brain structure and neuron function. In addition, an increased understanding of the complex interactions among the different parts of the brain will assist in the development of more effective psychotherapies and more efficacious psychotropic drugs.

Disorders of Thought and Volition

After completing this section of the chapter, you should be able to meet the following objectives:

- Define the term *schizophrenia*
- Describe the epidemiology of schizophrenia
- Describe the manifestations of schizophrenia, both positive and negative symptoms, and their underlying neuropathophysiology
- Cite the diagnostic criteria for schizophrenia according to the DSM-IV-TR classification
- Describe the treatment for the positive and negative manifestations of schizophrenia

SCHIZOPHRENIA

Schizophrenia refers to the disconnection between thought and language that occurs in this disease. Although the word *schizophrenia* means "splitting of the mind," it should not be confused with "split personality." Schizophrenia accounts for 25% of all hospital admissions,[21] and it is estimated that between 20% and 25% of the homeless have some form of severe and persistent mental illness, such as schizophrenia.[22] The onset of the disorder typically occurs between 17 and 25 years of age. The peak age of onset for males is between late teens and 25 years of age, and for females, between 25 and 35 years of age. Ninety percent of those in treatment are between 15 and 55 years of age. Onset before age 10 or after age 60 years is rare. Men and women seem to be affected equally, but the age of onset is later in women than in men. Risk factors for schizophrenia include having a close relative with schizotypal personality disorder or schizophrenia (first-degree relatives of a person with schizophrenia have a 10-fold greater prevalence of the illness than the population at large), winter/spring birth date, second-trimester prenatal influenza infection, and early history of attentional deficits.[23,24]

Manifestations

Schizophrenia is a psychotic disorder with many subtypes characterized by positive or negative symptoms. *Positive symptoms* are those that reflect the presence of abnormal behaviors and include disorganized, incomprehensible speech; delusions (*e.g.*, that one is being controlled by an outside force); hallucinations (hearing voices is the most common); and grossly disorganized or catatonic behavior. Alterations in speech patterns can include using invented words (neologisms), derailment (loose associations), tangentiality (inability to stick to the original point), incoherence (loss of logical connections), or word salad (groups of disconnected words) (Fig. 53-4). Frequently, persons with schizophrenia lose the ability to sort appropriately and interpret incoming stimuli, which impairs the ability to respond appropriately to the environment. An enhancement or a blunting of the senses is very common in the early stages of schizophrenia. Sounds may be experienced as louder and more intrusive; colors may be brighter and sharper. In addition, the person with schizophrenia often experiences sensory overload owing to a loss of the ability to screen external sensory stimuli.[23–26]

Delusions and hallucinations may be a natural outgrowth of the inability of the person with schizophrenia to interpret and respond appropriately to stimuli. Delusions are false ideas believed by the affected person that cannot be corrected by reason. They range from simply believing that people are watching them to beliefs that they are being controlled and manipulated by others. Delusions of being a historical figure (*e.g.*, Jesus Christ or the President) also are common. Sometimes, the delusions include a belief that the affected person is able to control others with his or her thoughts.[25]

Hallucinations are very common in schizophrenia, especially the auditory type. In these cases, the individual sees and hears things that are not in the external world but nevertheless are very real phenomena to the person experiencing them. Hallucinations may represent the end of the spectrum of increasing intensity of sensual stimuli. Auditory hallucinations range from simple repetitive sounds to many voices speaking at once. Sometimes, the voices are pleasant, but much more often, they accuse and curse. When visual hallucinations occur, they usually are in conjunction with auditory hallucinations.[23–25,27]

FIGURE 53-4 A schizophrenic woman expresses her incoherent thinking, combined with neologisms, in this drawing. (From Sadock B.J., Sadock V.A. [2003]. Kaeplan and Sadock's *synopsis of psychiatry.* [9th ed., p. 494]. Philadelphia: Lippincott Williams & Wilkins. Courtesy of Heniz E. Lehaman)

The *negative symptoms* of schizophrenia reflect the absence of normal social and interpersonal behaviors and include alogia (tendency to speak very little), avolition (lack of motivation for goal-oriented activity), apathy, affective flattening (lack of emotional expression), and anhedonia (an inability to experience pleasure in things that ordinarily are pleasurable). Some persons with schizophrenia have a blunted response to pain. Negative symptoms often are severe and persistent between acute episodes of illness.[23,26]

Paranoid schizophrenia manifests with persecutory or grandiose delusions. Auditory hallucinations are common. Interactions with others are rigid, intense, and controlled. Paranoid schizophrenia often has a sudden onset, and negative symptoms are not prominent. The prognosis of this form of schizophrenia seems to be better, with less evidence of disturbance in the anatomy of the brain and less cognitive deficits than in those types in which negative symptoms predominate.[28]

Disorganized schizophrenia is characterized by a disintegration of the personality and a predominance of negative symptoms. Socially, the person is withdrawn and inept. Speech often is disorganized and incoherent. Personal grooming is neglected and because behavior is aimless, the person with this disorder often is not able to complete activities of daily living. The person also may have cognitive and psychomotor deficits. In general, the prognosis is not as good as that for the paranoid schizophrenic type.[28]

Catatonic schizophrenia was common decades ago, but is now rare in the United States and Europe.[29] This disorder is characterized by intense psychomotor disturbance (retardation or excitement), extreme negativism, and peculiar voluntary movements such as grimacing, posturing, and echolalia (repeating what is said by another) or echopraxia (imitating the movements of others).[28]

Neurophysiology of Symptoms

The pathogenesis of schizophrenia is unknown. However, abnormalities in brain structure that are characteristic of this disorder are present at the first episode and in unmedicated persons. This suggests that the anatomic alterations are not the result of progressive brain deterioration due to repeated psychotic episodes or to effects of psychotropic drugs, but rather are caused by abnormalities in neurodevelopment in intrauterine and early postnatal life. The lateral and third ventricles are enlarged, the thalamus and hippocampus are somewhat smaller, and the left hemisphere is both smaller and smoother than that of persons without the illness. These changes are accompanied by a change in brain volume. Schizophrenia also is characterized by hypofrontality (reduced metabolic activity in the frontal cortex), although marked decreases in activity can be seen in almost every area of the brain, depending on the individual and the particular symptoms being experienced at the time of the scan (see Fig. 53-3).

It is not known at what age these differences might be visible with imaging because children usually are not subjected to imaging techniques without a specific event indicating a clinical need for the procedure. Nevertheless, adolescents and young adults who are at high risk for development of schizophrenia because of a strong family history have enlarged ventricles and smaller medial temporal lobes.[30]

An additional anatomic finding is an increased density of dopamine (D_2) receptor sites, particularly in the basal ganglia. With the additional information that effective antipsychotic drugs are dopamine antagonists and that dopamine-releasing agents such as amphetamine can cause psychosis, the "dopamine hypothesis" was developed; it proposes that the symptoms of schizophrenia are due to dopaminergic overactivity. However, this hypothesis cannot explain types of schizophrenia in which negative symptoms predominate or explain the residual symptoms of an acute psychotic episode. In addition, it is possible that the increased density of dopamine receptors found in some studies is related to the effects of antipsychotic drugs. In contrast, there is emerging evidence of a presynaptic dopaminergic autoreceptor abnormality such that there is a dysregulation or hyperresponsiveness of the neurons.[30]

Other transmitters implicated in the development of schizophrenia include a decreased activity of serotonin through the 5-HT_{2A} receptor and a decreased activity of glutamate through dysfunction of its *N*-methyl-D-aspartate receptor (see Chapter 52). Norepinephrine and GABA have also been identified in the pathophysiology of schizophrenia.[30]

Diagnostic Criteria

According to the DSM-IV-TR classification system, a diagnosis of schizophrenia requires that two or more of the following symptoms must be present for a significant portion of 1 month: delusions, hallucinations, disorganized speech, grossly disorganized or catatonic behavior, or negative symptoms.[31] In addition, one or more areas of functioning must be significantly impaired compared with premorbid abilities, and continuous signs of the disturbance must persist for at least 6 months.[31]

Treatment

The goals of treatment for schizophrenia are to induce a remission, prevent a recurrence, and restore behavioral, cognitive, and psychosocial function to premorbid levels. Initially, in some cases, the goal may be primarily to reduce agitation and the risk of physical harm. Both pharmacotherapy and psychotherapy are essential components in the treatment of persons with schizophrenia. The positive symptoms of schizophrenia (delusion, hallucinations, agitation, and thought broadcasting) are most likely to respond to drug therapy. Both typical and atypical antipsychotic drugs address these positive symptoms. The negative symptoms of schizophrenia respond more favorably to the atypical antipsychotic drugs (*e.g.,* olanzapine, ziprasidone). Often, antipsychotics are combined with benzodiazepines or antiparkinsonian agents during the acute phase of treatment to reduce the risk for extrapyramidal effects from large doses of antipsychotic agents. Psychotherapy (individual and group) is particularly important after the acute phase of therapy to help patients gain insight into the illness, to enhance their socialization skills, and to support and educate them in the maintenance of pharmacotherapy.

SCHIZOPHRENIA

- Schizophrenia is a psychotic disorder of thought and language that is characterized by disorganized speech, delusions, visual and auditory hallucinations, and possible catatonic behavior.
- The positive symptoms of schizophrenia include delusions, or false beliefs, and hallucinations, or abnormal sensory perceptions, that occur without external visual or auditory input.
- The negative symptoms of schizophrenia reflect the absence of the normal social and interpersonal relationships such as lack of motivation, apathy, and affective flattening of emotional expression.

In summary, schizophrenia is a mental illness classified as a disorder of thought and volition. Schizophrenia and its various subtypes are psychotic mental alterations in which thought and language become disconnected. It is characterized by both positive symptoms and negative symptoms. Positive symptoms are abnormal behaviors (*e.g.,* incomprehensible speech), delusions, and auditory or visual hallucinations. Negative symptoms are abnormal social and interpersonal behaviors (*e.g.,* lack of emotional expression) and an inability to experience pleasure. The onset of the disorder typically occurs between the ages of 17 and 25 years, with an equal incidence in men and women. Risk factors for schizophrenia include having a close relative with schizotypal personality disorder or schizophrenia. The pathogenesis of schizophrenia is unknown, although neuroimaging reveals several anatomic and functional changes in regions of the brain. Abnormalities in neurotransmission have been implicated, including changes in concentration and activity of the neurotransmitters dopamine, serotonin, norepinephrine, GABA, and glutamate. Treatment includes both psychotherapy and antipsychotic drugs.

Disorders of Mood

After completing this section of the chapter, you should be able to meet the following objectives:

- Define the terms *unipolar depression* and *bipolar depression*
- Describe the epidemiology of unipolar and bipolar depression
- Describe the manifestations of unipolar depression, bipolar depression, and mania and the underlying neuropathophysiology of each
- Cite the diagnostic criteria for depression according to the DSM-IV-TR classification
- Describe the treatment modalities for depression

DEPRESSION

Depression is a disorder of emotion rather than a disturbance of thought. It is a common and highly underdiagnosed and undertreated illness. Major depression, which affects approximately 20% of the population, is classified as either unipolar (characterized by a persistent unpleasant mood) or bipolar (characterized by alternating periods of depression and mania). The prevalence of unipolar depression among women is double that of men, while the prevalence of bipolar disorder is more equally distributed between men and women. Men more often have the manic phase in the initial episode, whereas women more often have the depressed phase as the initial episode. Approximately 20% to 40% of adolescents who present with major depression develop bipolar disorder within 5 years.[32,33] The average age of onset of bipolar disorder is the middle to late 20s and for unipolar depression, the mid-30s; however, the age of onset of both disorders has been decreasing. In addition, the incidence of depression appears to be increasing. Prevalence of depression is higher in individuals from families with a history of mood disorders than in the population at large, indicating a genetic component to the etiology. Mood disorders are thought to occur with equal prevalence among races, although it is more frequently misdiagnosed as schizophrenia among nonwhite populations.[32,34] Bipolar depression appears more frequently in the higher socioeconomic groups, although there is no correlation between major depression and socioeconomic status.[35–38]

As with schizophrenia, genetic factors appear to play an important role in the development of mood disorders. Several studies have identified genetic loci that might contribute to the vulnerability to depression in families and individuals. However, the expression of affective disorders is not 100% in vulnerable families, which strongly suggests that environmental factors also play a critical role in the development of mood disorders.[9]

Manifestations

Depression is classified as a mood disorder and is characterized by the following: depressed mood, anhedonia (inability to experience pleasure), feelings of worthlessness or excessive guilt, decreased concentration, psychomotor agitation or retardation, insomnia or hypersomnia, decreased libido, change in weight or appetite, and thoughts of death or suicidal ideation. Depression can vary in intensity and often is recurrent. The earlier and more frequent the onset of symptoms, the more likely it is that the affected individual will require medications for symptom relief. Depression in the elderly often appears with an element of confusion and often is left untreated. A first episode of depression that occurs after 65 years of age can be a precursor to dementia and should precipitate both assessment and treatment of the depression as well as a thorough evaluation for dementia. Early intervention often greatly retards the progression of dementia, maintaining the individual's independence and quality of life.

Unipolar Depression. Unipolar depression has various subclassifications distinguished by symptom patterns. Depression with melancholic features is characterized by depression that is worse in the morning, insomnia with early morning awakening, anorexia with significant weight loss, psychomotor retardation or agitation, excessive or inappropriate guilt, loss of interest in activity, inability to respond to pleasurable stimuli, and a complete loss of capacity for joy. The symptoms of atypical depression are the opposite of melancholic depression; it is characterized by a depression that becomes worse as the day progresses, overeating, and hypersomnia (excessive sleep). Depression with psychotic features involves the presence of delusions or hallucinations that may or may not be mood congruent. The classification of depression with catatonic features is applied when symptoms include excessive mobility or motoric immobility, extreme negativism, repetitive speech, and peculiar voluntary movements. The chronic specifier is applied if symptoms of major depression persist for 2 years or longer. A postpartum specifier is included if the onset is within 4 weeks of childbirth. Dysthymic disorder, a type of unipolar depression that is not classified as a major depression, is characterized by a persistent but mild depression that lasts longer than 2 years.[35–37]

Bipolar Depression. Bipolar depression, or manic-depressive illness, also has multiple subclassifications, all of which are usually characterized by episodes of elation and irritability (mania) with or without episodes of depression.[37,39] Although the occurrence of mania without associated depression (unipolar mania) can occur, it is rare. Mania can be precipitated by antidepressant medications in persons with bipolar disorder.

The manifestations of mania include decreased need for food and sleep, labile mood, irritability, racing thoughts, high distractibility, rapid and pressured speech, inflated self-esteem, and excessive involvement with pleasurable activities, some of which may be high risk. In its minor forms, the subjective experience of mania can be quite pleasurable to the individual, with a heightened sense of well-being and increased alertness.[40] The severity of manic symptoms runs the gamut from a condition called *cyclothymia,* in which mood fluctuates between mild elation and depression and severe delusional mania.[39] Mania may begin abruptly within hours or days or develop over a few weeks. Mixed states with features of both mania and depression present at the same time often are not well recognized. Bipolar episodes, left untreated, become more severe with age. Rapid cycling is said to occur when an individual has four or more shifts in mood from normal within a 1-year period. Women are more likely than men to be rapid cyclers.[41]

Kindling is a hypothesized phenomenon in which a stressor creates an electrophysiologic vulnerability to future stressful events by causing long-lasting changes in neuronal function. This may be the basis for the phenomenon of rapid cycling in bipolar depression. The more frequently a person has a shift in mood, cycling into either mania or depression, the easier it becomes to have another episode. There now is evidence that many psychiatric disorders, not just bipolar, are subject to this phenomenon. The better the control of the illness and the fewer cycles an individual has, the better his or her quality of life is likely to be.[42]

MOOD DISORDERS

- Mood disorders, which include unipolar depression and bipolar depression, represent a disturbance in emotion rather than thought.
- Depression is characterized by feelings of worthlessness and guilt, decreased concentration, alterations in sleep and appetite, and possible suicidal ideation.
- Bipolar depression is characterized by alternating periods of depression and mania during which there is a decreased need for food and sleep, racing thoughts, irritability, and high distractibility.

Neurophysiology of Symptoms

In some cases of familial unipolar and bipolar depression, PET and MRI studies have demonstrated a reduction in the volume of gray matter in the prefrontal cortex, with an associated decrease in activity in the region. Clinical studies have suggested that this area of the brain is important for mood states and has extensive connections with the limbic system. Physiologically, there is evidence of decreased functioning in the frontal and temporal lobes, although it is not known whether this is a cause or an effect of depression because the activity returns to normal with the resolution of the symptoms[38,43,44] (Fig. 53-5). The amygdala tends to have increased blood flow and oxygen consumption during depression.[38] Unlike those areas where function returns to normal with the resolution of depression, the amygdala continues to be excessively active for 12 to 24 months after the resolution of depression. It is hypothesized that relapse into depression is more likely to occur if medications are decreased or stopped before the amygdala returns to normal functioning. Neurologic disorders of the limbic system and basal ganglia are also involved in the development of mood disorders.[33]

A number of neurotransmitters, serotonin and norepinephrine in particular, are implicated in depression.[35,37,45] The biogenic amine hypothesis suggests that decreased levels of these hormones in the synaptic cleft, due either to decreased presynaptic release or decreased postsynaptic sensitivity, is the underlying pathology in depression. The hypothesis is derived from the fact that drugs that depleted brain serotonin and norepinephrine caused depression, and drugs that increased brain levels of norepinephrine and serotonin decreased depression. Dopamine activity has also been implicated in mood disorders—with decreased dopamine activity found in depression, and increased dopamine activity in mania.[32] It has become increasingly clear, however, that a simple decrease in the concentration of amines in neuronal synapses cannot entirely explain the complexities of depression. Neuromodulatory systems in the brain interact with each other in complex ways. For example, cholinergic and GABA-ergic pathways also may play a role in the development of depression because both of these pathways influence the activity of brain norepinephrine neurons.[35,37,45]

Disturbances in the function of the hypothalamic-pituitary-adrenal (HPA) axis also may play a critical role in depression. In the general population, cortisol levels usually are flat from late in the afternoon until a few hours before dawn, when they begin to rise. In persons with depression, cortisol levels spike erratically over the 24 hours of the day. Cortisol levels return to the normal pattern as depression resolves. In 40% of those diagnosed with depression, hypersecretion of cortisol is resistant to feedback inhibition by dexamethasone, indicating a dysfunction of the HPA axis.[45] About 5% to 10% of persons with depression have a decrease in thyroid function; in which case, the person is less likely to have a vigorous response to medical intervention.[32]

Circadian rhythms also are an area of serious research interest.[42] A specific type of depression known as *seasonal affective disorder* (SAD) is triggered for persons in the win-

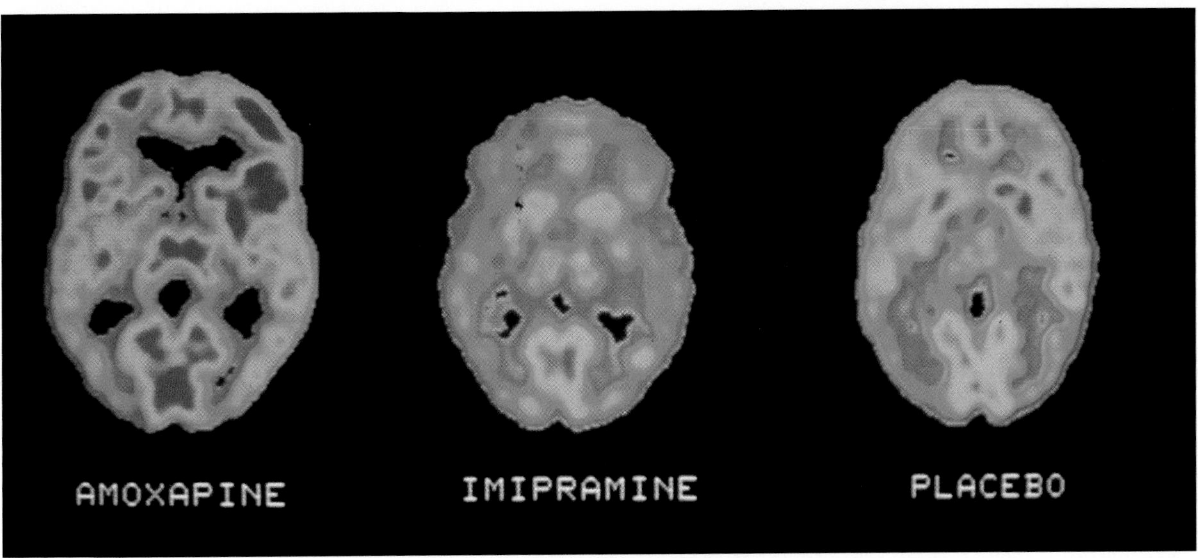

FIGURE 53-5 Acute effects of antidepressant medications in patients with affective disorder showing widespread effects on the cortex that vary dramatically with the medication used. Positron-emission tomography is useful in revealing specific patterns of metabolic change in the brain and in providing clues to the mechanisms of antidepressant response (Courtesy of Monte S. Buchsbaum, MD. The Mount Sinai Medical Center and School of Medicine, New York, NY)

ter by the shortening of daylight hours as fall commences, with symptoms of depression usually resolving in the spring when daylight hours again lengthen.

Alteration in the sleep–wake cycle is common in many mental illnesses and often is one of the prodromal signs of relapse. Researchers have found that the normal sleep cycle is reversed in depression. Persons with depression often have what is called *dream pressure sleep*. The depressed individual falls into light and dream-state sleep early in the sleep cycle and reaches deep stage 4 sleep only late in the sleep cycle. This finding helps explain why many inpatients report they did not sleep all night and the staff reports that the patient was asleep all night. Although the sleep cycle usually reverts to normal after the resolution of the depression, it may not be completely normal for weeks to months. Decreasing or halting medications before the sleep disturbances resolve may lead to a relapse of depressive symptoms.

Circadian rhythm considerations are critical in symptom management for persons with bipolar depression. One of the fastest ways to precipitate a manic episode is for the individual to stay up all night. It is not unusual for a first manic episode to occur when someone "pulls an all-nighter" studying for final examinations. Persons with bipolar disorder should have a fairly rigid schedule for sleeping and awakening if cycling is to be minimized. Although exercise is important, the person with bipolar disorder should exercise before mid-afternoon to prevent the normal increase in metabolic rate from disrupting the sleep cycle.

Diagnostic Criteria

The DSM-IV-TR diagnostic criteria for a major depressive episode include the simultaneous presence of five or more of the aforementioned symptoms during a 2-week period, and these must represent a change from previous functioning.[31] Depression must be differentiated from grief reactions, medication side effects, and sequelae of medical illnesses. Bipolar disorder is diagnosed on the basis of the pattern of occurrence of manic, hypomanic, and depressed episodes over time that are not due to medications or other therapies. The frequency, duration, and severity of the manic or depressive periods are unique to each individual.[35,37] Mania, particularly in its severe delusional forms, also needs to be differentiated from schizophrenia or drug-induced states.

Treatment

Effective treatments exist for unipolar and bipolar illnesses, including antidepressant drugs, electroconvulsive therapy, lithium, anticonvulsants, and psychotherapy.[35–37,46] The antidepressants most often used are SRIs, which inhibit the reuptake of serotonin; atypical antidepressants; MAOIs, which block the degradation of norepinephrine and serotonin; and tricyclic compounds, which block the reuptake of norepinephrine and serotonin. Electroconvulsive therapy, a procedure that electrically stimulates a generalized seizure, is a highly effective treatment for depression, with 70% to 90% of clients showing a good response.

Lithium and several anticonvulsant agents are used in the treatment of bipolar depression. Lithium's exact mechanism of action is unknown. It is known to block the enzymatic breakdown of inositol triphosphate (IP_3), increasing its intracellular concentration. IP_3 is an important regulator of intracellular calcium levels. The anticonvulsants agents, carbamazepine and valproate, also have proved efficacious in the treatment of bipolar depression, although the mechanism by which the drugs work is not completely understood.

Psychotherapy is an important component of therapy for persons and families with major depressive disorders. Individuals and families can learn how to deal with stressful life events and heal disrupted interpersonal relationships.

Many people who have bipolar disorder do not believe they need treatment, particularly during the manic phase of the illness, and tend to self-medicate with alcohol or recreational drugs. It is not unusual for people with bipolar depression to be diagnosed with substance abuse. When in the manic phase, they often feel exceptionally creative and talented. When helping people make the decision to enter treatment, it is important that they understand the treatment will not stop their creativity.

In summary, depression is a disorder of emotion rather than of thought and is classified as unipolar, characterized by a persistent unpleasant mood, or bipolar, characterized by alternating periods of depression and mania. Depression is characterized by an inability to experience pleasure, feelings of worthlessness and excessive guilt, alterations in sleeping patterns and appetite, and thoughts of death or suicidal ideation. Mania is characterized by elation, irritability, high distractibility, and, often, engagement in high-risk pleasurable activities. As with schizophrenia, genetic factors appear to play an important role in the development of mood disorders. Neuroimaging techniques have revealed several anatomic and functional abnormalities in different regions of the brain. Abnormalities in neurotransmission also have been implicated in the development and maintenance of depression, including changes in concentration and activity of the neurotransmitters norepinephrine, serotonin, acetylcholine, and GABA. Treatment includes antidepressant drugs and psychotherapy.

Anxiety Disorders

After completing this section of the chapter, you should be able to meet the following objectives:

- Define the terms *panic disorder, generalized anxiety disorder, social phobia,* and *obsessive-compulsive disorder*
- Describe the epidemiology of panic disorder, generalized anxiety disorder, social phobia, and obsessive-compulsive disorder
- Describe the manifestations of panic disorder, generalized anxiety disorder, social phobia, and obsessive-compulsive disorder and the underlying neuropathophysiology of each
- Cite the diagnostic criteria for panic disorder, generalized anxiety disorder, social phobia, and obsessive-compulsive disorder according to the DSM-IV-TR classification
- Describe the treatment for panic disorder, generalized anxiety disorder, social phobia, and obsessive-compulsive disorder

Anxiety disorders are extremely common, and the intensity of disability experienced by the person living with anxiety varies widely. Anxiety disorders affect approximately 15% of all individuals, women more often than men.

The common feature of anxiety disorders is increased fearfulness that sometimes is intense. The basic symptoms that are common to all anxiety disorders occur with the activation of the sympathetic cascade through the HPA axis. The core issue with anxiety disorders is that these symptoms occur without a precipitating potentially dangerous event. Anxiety disorders have a higher rate of occurrence among family members, but there is not yet any clearly delineated genetic process. According to the DSM-IV-TR classification system, anxiety is subdivided into five types, depending on clinical characteristics and response to pharmacologic agents. These five types include panic disorder, post-traumatic stress disorder (PTSD), generalized anxiety disorder, social phobia, and obsessive-compulsive disorder (OCD). See Chapter 9 for the discussion of PTSD.

PANIC DISORDER

Epidemiologic studies suggest that panic disorder has a lifetime prevalence of between 1.5% and 3%. First-degree relatives of persons with panic disorder have a 3- to 21-fold higher risk for developing panic disorder than unrelated persons.[32] Panic disorder is characterized by neurologic symptoms (dizziness or lightheadedness, paresthesias, fainting), cardiac symptoms (tachycardia, chest pain, palpitations), respiratory symptoms (shortness of breath, feeling of smothering or choking), and psychological symptoms (feelings of impending doom, fear of dying, and a sense of unreality). The attacks, which are unexpected and not related to external events, usually last 15 to 30 minutes, but sometimes continue for an hour. Depression may coexist in 40% to 80% of persons with panic disorder.[32]

Responses to medications suggest that multiple mechanisms and neurotransmitters are involved in initiating the panic attack. Norepinephrine, serotonin, and GABA are the three neurotransmitters most associated with this disorder.[32] Persons experiencing panic attacks have been

ANXIETY DISORDERS

- Anxiety disorders constitute a group of disorders that are characterized by intense episodes of fearfulness with symptoms related to activation of the sympathetic nervous system through the hypothalamic-pituitary-adrenal axis.
- Generalized anxiety disorder is characterized by excessive, uncontrollable worry.
- Obsessive-compulsive disorder is characterized by repetitive thoughts and compulsions.
- Panic disorder is characterized by an experience of intense fear with neurologic, cardiac, respiratory, and psychological symptoms.
- Social phobia is an intense fear reaction to social interaction.

found to have somewhat lower levels of serotonin than do persons with no known mental illness, but the mechanism for that decrease is not known. The SSRIs are effective in the treatment of panic, but full response to medication can easily take 12 or more weeks. The tricyclic antidepressants also may be helpful, but their risk with overdose may limit their use in the treatment of panic in an effort to reduce suicides.[47,48]

Responses to yohimbine and clonidine indicate that the adrenergic system clearly is involved. Yohimbine, an α_2-adrenergic receptor blocker, precipitates panic attacks in persons who are susceptible to the attacks but not in others. This suggests that alterations in the adrenergic system may be part of the etiology of this disorder. The administration of clonidine, an α_2-adrenergic agonist, has been shown to block the panic-inducing effect of yohimbine. However, clonidine has not proved to be an efficacious treatment for panic disorder.[49]

Gamma-aminobutyric acid is the third neurotransmitter system hypothesized to be involved in panic disorder. It has been suggested that persons experiencing panic disorder may have excess inverse agonists to GABA, which is generally an inhibitory transmitter. The benzodiazepines, which act on GABA receptor sites, are effective in the treatment of panic. One of the risks is that of addiction among persons who may have a propensity for substance misuse. There has been some out-of-class use of the GABA-ergic anticonvulsants in the treatment of panic disorder.[49]

Many individuals may require the use of more than one class of medication for the management of panic attacks. However, treatment is most effective when psychotherapy focused on cognitive and behavioral changes is included as part of a comprehensive program. If inadequately treated, persons with panic disorder frequently develop phobias, particularly agoraphobia, which can be so debilitating that the person cannot leave his or her house.[47,49,50]

GENERALIZED ANXIETY DISORDER

In 1980, generalized anxiety disorder was first recognized as a separate entity from panic disorder in the DSM-III. Since then, the diagnostic criteria have been sharpened in an attempt to improve the ability of practitioners to discriminate the disorder. The central characteristic of generalized anxiety disorder is prolonged (more than 6 months) excessive worry that is not easily controlled by the person. The characteristics of the disorder include muscle tension, autonomic hyperactivity, and vigilance and scanning (exaggerated startle response, inability to concentrate). Drugs that are particularly effective in treating this disorder are the benzodiazepines (chlordiazepoxide, diazepam). These drugs increase the activity of the $GABA_A$ receptor, which increases the flow of chloride ions across the cell membrane, hyperpolarizing the membrane and thus inhibiting the firing of target cells.[35,49]

Other medications used in the treatment of generalized anxiety disorder include antidepressants (tricyclic antidepressants [TCAs], SSRIs, and atypical antidepressants) and β-blockers.[29,32]

OBSESSIVE-COMPULSIVE DISORDER

Obsessive-compulsive disorder is characterized by obsessions (repeated thoughts) and compulsions (repeated acts), which are attempts to reduce the anxiety associated with the obsessions.[51,52] These obsessions are time consuming or distressing to the individual. Usually, the person experiencing the symptoms recognizes that the rituals are unreasonable. For instance, the person may have to recheck the stove many times before she is able to leave for work or may have to check the stairwells repeatedly at work for debris to ensure that no one is injured. Between 2% and 3% of the world's population has OCD. This disorder is found with equal frequency among men and women, and there is a higher prevalence among family members. The average age of onset is approximately 20 years, although the disorder also may occur in children and, undiagnosed, may appear as behavior problems and angry outbursts that can seem impulsive and may be confused with attention deficit or hyperactivity disorders.[51,53]

There is evidence from CT and MRI studies that patients with OCD have bilaterally smaller caudates.[32] There also appear to be consistent physiologic changes represented by increased activity in the anterior cingulate and the caudate. Some studies have suggested increased activity in the thalamus and the putamen as well as a decrease in serotonin activity.[53] Treatment of OCD involves a combination of medication (SSRIs or certain tricyclic antidepressants) and psychotherapy. This disorder is particularly amenable to cognitive behavioral therapy. Studies indicate that there are physiologic changes in affected areas in response to this psychotherapeutic intervention.[51,52]

SOCIAL ANXIETY DISORDER

Social anxiety disorder is a generalized or specific, intense, irrational, and persistent fear of being scrutinized or negatively evaluated by others. Diagnostic criteria include the development of symptoms of anxiety when the person is exposed to the feared social situation, recognition by the person that the fear is irrational, avoidance by the person of the social situation, and interference of the anxiety or avoidance behavior with the person's normal routine. The fear must not be related to any physiologic effects of a substance and must be present for at least 6 months.[35,49,54]

Social phobia is a fairly common disorder with a lifetime prevalence of 3% to 13%, with a slight tendency to occur more often in women than in men. Typically, the onset is between 11 and 19 years of age. The major adverse effects of social anxiety disorder are felt in employment and school, causing a loss of earning power and socioeconomic status. In addition, approximately one half of persons with social phobia also have a drug or alcohol problem. Several drugs have proved efficacious for the treatment of social phobia, including SSRIs, benzodiazepines, and MAOIs. β-Adrenergic blockers are useful in specific social performance situations. Social phobia also has been particularly responsive to behavioral and cognitive therapies.[35,49,54]

In summary, anxiety disorders include generalized anxiety, panic disorder, OCD, and social phobia. A common characteristic of the disorders is an intense fear that occurs in the absence of a precipitating dangerous event. The symptoms of anxiety disorders suggest an inappropriate and intense activation of the sympathetic nervous system. Panic disorder is characterized by neurologic, cardiac, respiratory, and psychological symptoms. The central characteristic of generalized anxiety disorder is excessive worry not easily controlled by the person and lasting more than 6 months. OCD is characterized by repetitive thoughts and acts. Social anxiety disorder is a generalized or specific, intense, irrational, and persistent fear of being scrutinized or negatively evaluated by others.

Disorders of Memory and Cognition: Dementias

After completing this section of the chapter, you should be able to meet the following objectives:

- State the criteria for a diagnosis of dementia
- Compare the causes associated with Alzheimer's disease, vascular dementia, Pick's disease, Creutzfeldt-Jakob disease, Wernicke-Korsakoff syndrome, and Huntington's disease
- Describe the changes in brain tissue that occur with Alzheimer's disease
- Use the three stages of Alzheimer's disease to describe its progress
- Cite the difference between Wernicke's disease and the Korsakoff component of the Wernicke-Korsakoff syndrome
- State the pros and cons for the presymptomatic use of genetic testing for Huntington's disease

Dementia is a syndrome of intellectual deterioration severe enough to interfere with occupational or social performance. It may involve disturbances in memory, language use, perception, and motor skills and may interrupt the ability to learn necessary skills, solve problems, think abstractly, and make judgments. Dementia can be caused by any disorder that permanently damages large association areas of the cerebral hemispheres or subcortical areas subserving memory and learning. The dementias include Alzheimer's disease, multi-infarct dementia, Pick's disease, Creutzfeldt-Jakob disease, Wernicke-Korsakoff syndrome, and Huntington's chorea.

Depression is the most common treatable illness that may masquerade as dementia, and it must be excluded when a diagnosis of dementia is considered. This is important because cognitive functioning usually returns to baseline levels after depression is treated.

ALZHEIMER'S DISEASE

Dementia of the Alzheimer's type occurs in middle or late life and accounts for 50% to 70% of all cases of dementia. The disorder affects approximately 4 million Americans and may be the fourth leading cause of death in the United States.[55] The risk for developing Alzheimer's disease increases with age, and the prevalence doubles for every 5 years beyond age 65 years.[56] As the elderly population in the United States continues to increase, the number of persons with Alzheimer's-type dementia also is expected to increase.

Pathophysiology

Alzheimer's disease is characterized by cortical atrophy and loss of neurons, particularly in the parietal and temporal lobes (Fig. 53-6). With significant atrophy, there is ventricular enlargement (*i.e.*, hydrocephalus) from the loss of brain tissue.

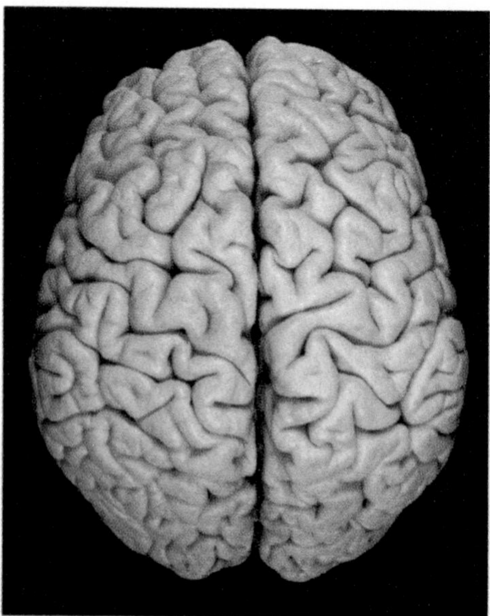

A

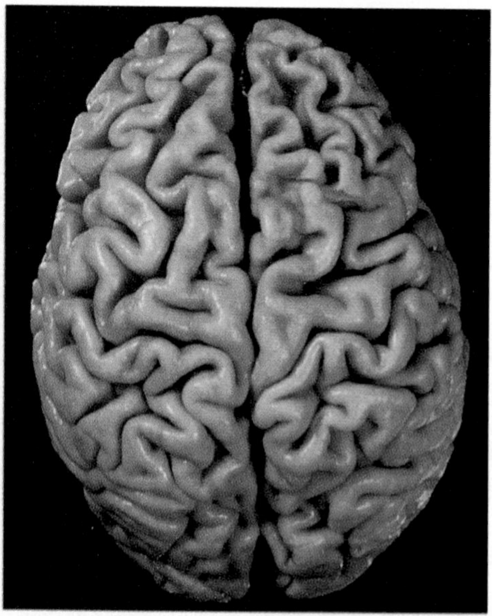

B

FIGURE 53-6 Alzheimer's disease. (**A**) Normal brain. (**B**) The brain of a patient with Alzheimer's disease shows cortical atrophy, characterized by slender gyri and prominent sulci. (Rubin E., Farber J.L. [1999]. *Pathology* [3rd ed., p. 1511]. Philadelphia: Lippincott-Raven)

The major microscopic features of Alzheimer's disease are the presence of amyloid-containing neuritic plaques and neurofibrillary tangles. The neurofibrillary tangles, found in the cytoplasm of abnormal neurons, consist of fibrous proteins that are wound around each other in a helical fashion. These tangles are resistant to chemical or enzymatic breakdown, and they persist in brain tissue long after the neuron in which they arose has died and disappeared. The senile plaques are patches or flat areas composed of clusters of degenerating nerve terminals arranged around a central core of amyloid β-peptide (BAP).[57] These plaques are found in areas of the cerebral cortex that are linked to intellectual function. BAP is a fragment of a much larger membrane-spanning amyloid precursor protein (APP). The function of APP is unclear, but it appears to be associated with the cytoskeleton of nerve fibers. Normally, the degradation of APP involves cleavage in the middle of the BAP portion of the molecule, with both fragments being lost in the extracellular fluid. In Alzheimer's disease, the APP molecule is cut at both ends of the BAP segment, thereby releasing an intact BAP molecule that accumulates in neuritic plaques as amyloid fibrils.[57]

Some plaques and tangles can be found in the brains of older persons who do not show cognitive impairment. The number and distribution of the plaques and tangles appear to contribute to the intellectual deterioration that occurs with Alzheimer's disease. In persons with the disease, the plaques and tangles are found throughout the neocortex and in the hippocampus and amygdala, with relative sparing of the primary sensory cortex.[58] Hippocampal function in particular may be compromised by the pathologic changes that occur in Alzheimer's disease. The hippocampus is crucial to information processing, acquisition of new memories, and retrieval of old memories. The development of neurofibrillary tangles in the entorhinal cortex and superior portion of the hippocampal gyrus interferes with cortical input and output, thereby isolating the hippocampus from the remainder of the cortex and rendering it functionless.

Neurochemically, Alzheimer's disease has been associated with a decrease in the level of choline acetyltransferase activity in the cortex and hippocampus. This enzyme is required for the synthesis of acetylcholine, a neurotransmitter that is associated with memory. The reduction in choline acetyltransferase is quantitatively related to the numbers of neuritic plaques and severity of dementia.

Several drugs have been shown to be effective in slowing the progression of the disease by potentiating the available acetylcholine. The drugs—tacrine, donepezil, rivastigmine, and galantamine—inhibit acetylcholinesterase, preventing the metabolism of endogenous acetylcholine. Thus far, such therapy has not halted disease progression, but it can establish a meaningful plateau in decline.

It is likely that Alzheimer's disease is caused by several factors that interact differently in different persons. Progress on the genetics of inherited early-onset Alzheimer's disease shows that mutations in at least three genes—the *APP* gene on chromosome 21; presenilin-1 (*PS1*), a gene on chromosome 14; and presenilin-2 (*PS2*), a gene on chromosome 1—can cause Alzheimer's disease in certain families.[57,59,60] The *APP* gene is associated with an autosomal dominant form of early-onset Alzheimer's disease, and can be tested clinically. Persons with Down syndrome (trisomy 21) develop the pathologic changes of Alzheimer's disease and a comparable decline in cognitive functioning at a relatively young age. Virtually all persons with Down syndrome who survive past 50 years of age develop the full-blown pathologic features of dementia. Because the *APP* gene is located on chromosome 21, it is thought that the additional dosage of the gene product in trisomy 21 predisposes to accumulation of BAP.[57] There is some indication that PS1 and PS2 mutant proteins alter the processing of APP.[57] A fourth gene, an allele of the apolipoprotein E gene, *APOE e4,* has been identified as a risk factor for late-onset Alzheimer's disease.

Manifestations

Alzheimer's-type dementia follows an insidious and progressive course. The hallmark symptoms are loss of short-term memory and a denial of such memory loss, with eventual disorientation, impaired abstract thinking, apraxias, and changes in personality and affect. Three stages of Alzheimer's dementia have been identified, each characterized by progressive degenerative changes (Chart 53-1). The *first stage,* which may last for 2 to 4 years, is characterized by short-term memory loss that often is difficult to differentiate from the normal forgetfulness that occurs in the elderly, and usually is reported by caregivers and denied by the patient. Although most elderly have trouble retrieving from memory incidental information and proper names, persons

CHART 53-1

Stages of Alzheimer's Disease

Stage 1

Memory loss
Lack of spontaneity
Subtle personality changes
Disorientation to time and date

Stage 2

Impaired cognition and abstract thinking
Restlessness and agitation
Wandering, "sundown syndrome"
Inability to carry out activities of daily living
Impaired judgment
Inappropriate social behavior
Lack of insight, abstract thinking
Repetitive behavior
Voracious appetite

Stage 3

Emaciation, indifference to food
Inability to communicate
Urinary and fecal incontinence
Seizures

(From Matteson M.A., McConnell E.S. [1988]. *Gerontological nursing* [p. 251]. Philadelphia: J.B. Lippincott)

with Alzheimer's disease randomly forget important and unimportant details. They forget where things are placed, get lost easily, and have trouble remembering appointments and performing novel tasks. Mild changes in personality, such as lack of spontaneity, social withdrawal, and loss of a previous sense of humor, occur during this stage.

As the disease progresses, the person with Alzheimer's disease enters the *second* or *confusional stage* of dementia. This stage may last several years and is marked by a more global impairment of cognitive functioning. During this stage, there are changes in higher cortical functioning needed for language, spatial relationships, and problem solving. Depression may occur in persons who are aware of their deficits. There is extreme confusion, disorientation, lack of insight, and inability to carry out the activities of daily living. Personal hygiene is neglected, and language becomes impaired because of difficulty in remembering and retrieving words. Wandering, especially in the late afternoon or early evening, becomes a problem. The *sundown syndrome,* which is characterized by confusion, restlessness, agitation, and wandering, may become a daily occurrence late in the afternoon. Some persons may become hostile and abusive toward family members. Persons who enter this stage become unable to live alone and should be assisted in making decisions about supervised placement with family members or friends or in a community-based facility.

Stage 3 is the terminal stage. It usually is relatively short (1 to 2 years) compared with the other stages, but it has been known to last for as long as 10 years.[61] The person becomes incontinent, apathetic, and unable to recognize family or friends. It usually is during this stage that the person is institutionalized.

Diagnosis and Treatment

Alzheimer's disease is essentially a diagnosis of exclusion. There are no peripheral biochemical markers or tests for the disease. The diagnosis can be confirmed only by microscopic examination of tissue obtained from a cerebral biopsy or at autopsy. The diagnosis is based on clinical findings. Guidelines for the early recognition and assessment of Alzheimer's disease have been published by the Agency for Health Care Policy and Research (AHCPR).[61] A diagnosis of Alzheimer's disease requires the presence of dementia established by clinical examination and documented by results of a Mini-Mental State Examination, Blessed Dementia Test, or similar mental status test; no disturbance in consciousness; onset between ages 40 and 90 years, most often after age 65 years; and absence of systemic or brain disorders that could account for the memory or cognitive deficits.[62] Brain imaging, CT scan, or MRI is done to exclude other brain disease. Metabolic screening should be done for known reversible causes of dementia such as vitamin B_{12} deficiency, thyroid dysfunction, and electrolyte imbalance.

There is no curative treatment for Alzheimer's dementia. Drugs are used primarily to slow the progression and to control depression, agitation, or sleep disorders. Two major goals of care are maintaining the person's socialization and providing support for the family. Self-help groups that provide support for family and friends have become available, with support from the Alzheimer's Disease and Related Disorders Association. Day care and respite centers are available in many areas to provide relief for caregivers and appropriate stimulation for the patient.

Although there is no current drug therapy that is curative for Alzheimer's disease, some show promise in terms of slowing the progress of the disease. The use of pharmacologic agents such as tacrine, donepezil, rivastigmine, and galantamine has been approved for symptomatic therapy in Alzheimer's disease.[63] There also is interest in the use of agents such as antioxidants (*e.g.,* vitamin E, ginkgo), anti-inflammatory agents, and estrogen replacement therapy in women to prevent or delay the onset of the disease.

OTHER TYPES OF DEMENTIA

Vascular Dementia

Dementia associated with cerebrovascular disease does not result directly from atherosclerosis, but rather is caused by multiple infarctions throughout the brain—hence the name vascular or *multi-infarct dementia.* Approximately 20% to 25% of dementias are vascular in origin, and the incidence is closely associated with hypertension. Other contributing factors are arrhythmias, myocardial infarction, peripheral vascular disease, diabetes mellitus, and smoking. The usual onset is between the ages of 55 and 70 years. The disease differs from Alzheimer's dementia in its presentation and tissue abnormalities. The onset may be gradual or abrupt, the course usually is stepwise progression, and there should be focal neurologic symptoms related to local areas of infarction.

Pick's Disease

Pick's disease is a rare form of dementia characterized by atrophy of the frontal and temporal areas of the brain. The neurons in the affected areas contain cytoplasmic inclusions called *Pick bodies.* The average age at onset of Pick's disease is 38 years. The disease is more common in women than men. Behavioral manifestations may be noticed earlier than memory deficits, taking the form of a striking absence of concern and care, a loss of initiative, echolalia (*i.e.,* automatic repetition of anything said to the person), hypotonia, and incontinence. The course of the disease is relentless, with death ensuing within 2 to 10 years. The immediate cause of death usually is infection.

Creutzfeldt-Jakob Disease

Creutzfeldt-Jakob disease is a rare transmissible form of dementia thought to be caused by an infective protein agent called a *prion*[64] (see Chapter 18). Similar diseases occur in animals, including scrapie in sheep and goats and bovine spongiform encephalitis (BSE; mad cow disease) in cows. The pathogen is resistant to chemical and physical methods commonly used for sterilizing medical and surgical equipment. The disease reportedly has been transmitted through corneal transplants and human growth hormone obtained from cadavers. The National Hormone and Pituitary Program halted the distribution of human pituitary hormone in 1985 after reports that three young persons who had received the hormone had died of Creutzfeldt-Jakob disease.[65]

Creutzfeldt-Jakob disease causes degeneration of the pyramidal and extrapyramidal systems and is distinguished most readily by its rapid course. Affected persons usually are demented within 6 months of onset. The disease is uniformly fatal, with death often occurring within months, although a few persons may survive for several years.[65] The early symptoms consist of abnormalities in personality and visual-spatial coordination. Extreme dementia, insomnia, and ataxia follow as the disease progresses.[64]

Wernicke-Korsakoff Syndrome

Wernicke-Korsakoff syndrome most commonly results from chronic alcoholism. Wernicke's disease is characterized by acute weakness and paralysis of the extraocular muscles, nystagmus, ataxia, and confusion. The affected person also may have signs of peripheral neuropathy. The person has an unsteady gait and complains of diplopia. There may be signs attributable to alcohol withdrawal such as delirium, confusion, and hallucinations. This disorder is caused by a deficiency of thiamine (vitamin B_1), and many of the symptoms are reversed when nutrition is improved with supplemental thiamine.

The Korsakoff component of the syndrome involves the chronic phase with severe impairment of recent memory. There often is difficulty in dealing with abstractions, and the person's capacity to learn is defective. Confabulation (*i.e.*, recitation of imaginary experiences to fill in gaps in memory) probably is the most distinctive feature of the disease. Polyneuritis also is common. Unlike Wernicke's disease, Korsakoff's psychosis does not improve significantly with treatment.

Huntington's Disease

Huntington's disease is a hereditary disorder characterized by chronic progressive chorea, psychological changes, and dementia. Although the disease is inherited as an autosomal dominant disorder, the age of onset most commonly is in the fourth and fifth decades.[1] By the time the disease has been diagnosed, the person often has passed the gene on to his or her children. Approximately 10% of the Huntington's cases involve juvenile onset.[66] Children with the disease rarely live to adulthood.

Huntington's disease produces localized death of brain cells. The first and most severely affected neurons are of the caudate nucleus and putamen of the basal ganglia. The neurochemical changes that occur with the disease are complex. The neurotransmitter GABA is an inhibitory neurotransmitter in the basal ganglia. Postmortem studies have shown a decrease of GABA and GABA receptors in the basal ganglia of persons dying of Huntington's disease. Likewise, the levels of acetylcholine, an excitatory neurotransmitter in the basal ganglia, are reduced in persons with Huntington's disease. The dopaminergic pathway of the nigrostriatal system, which is affected in parkinsonism, is preserved in Huntington's disease, suggesting that an imbalance in dopamine and acetylcholine may contribute to manifestations of the disease.

Depression and personality changes are the most common early psychological manifestations; memory loss often is accompanied by impulsive behavior, moodiness, antisocial behavior, and a tendency toward emotional outbursts.[67] Other early signs of the disease are lack of initiative, loss of spontaneity, and inability to concentrate. Fidgeting or restlessness may represent early signs of dyskinesia, followed by choreiform and some dystonic posturing. Eventually, progressive rigidity and akinesia (rather than chorea) develop in association with dementia. Symptoms of juvenile onset include dystonias and seizures.

There is no cure for Huntington's disease. The treatment is largely symptomatic. Drugs may be used to treat the dyskinesias and behavioral disturbances. Study of the genetics of Huntington's disease led to the discovery that the gene for the disease is located on chromosome 4.[57] The discovery of a marker probe for the gene locus has enabled testing that can predict whether a person will develop the disease.

In summary, cognitive disorders can be caused by any disorder that permanently damages large cortical or subcortical areas of the hemispheres, including Alzheimer's disease, vascular dementia, Pick's disease, Creutzfeldt-Jakob disease, Wernicke-Korsakoff syndrome, and Huntington's disease. Multi-infarct dementia is associated with vascular disease, and Pick's disease with atrophy of the frontal and temporal lobes. Creutzfeldt-Jakob disease is a rare transmissible form of dementia. Wernicke-Korsakoff syndrome most often results from chronic alcoholism. Huntington's disease is a hereditary disorder characterized by chronic and progressive chorea, psychological change, and dementia.

By far the most common cause of dementia (50% to 70%) is Alzheimer's disease. The condition is a major health problem among the elderly. It is characterized by cortical atrophy and loss of neurons, the presence of neuritic plaques, granulovacuolar degeneration, and cerebrovascular deposits of amyloid. The disease follows an insidious and progressive course that begins with memory impairment and terminates in an inability to recognize family or friends and the loss of control over bodily functions. The particular tragedy of Alzheimer's disease and other related dementias is that they dissolve the mind and rob the victim of humanity. Simultaneously, these disorders devastate the lives of spouses and other family members, who must endure an insidious loss of the person and a valued relationship.

REVIEW EXERCISES

A 45-year-old woman was brought to the emergency room after being picked up by the police. She was wandering in and out of traffic saying someone was after her and was recognized as a homeless person. Her appearance is dirty and disheveled, and she is wearing several layers of clothing although it is July. She smacks her lips and at times does not seem to understand questions. Periodically she laughs for no apparent reason and often repeats the words of her questioner. She has a 20-year history of schizophrenia with multiple admissions.

A. List the positive and negative signs she exhibits as well as others not listed.

B. What are the brain areas and transmitters responsible for these signs?

C. What are the DSM-IV-TR criteria that would have led to her diagnosis?

A 35-year-old woman was recently admitted with suicidal tendencies shortly after a diagnosis of major depression. She had lost 40 pounds in the past 6 months. She appears tired and supplies only short answers to questions. She complains of dizziness and informs the nurse that it is not her business to discuss her suicidal thoughts. Her husband says she relies heavily on alcohol.

A. Describe some of her manifestations. Why is she using alcohol?

B. Provide an explanation for her tiredness.

C. What areas of the brain and transmitters are involved in depression? How is it different from mania?

D. What is the possible role of thyroid and adrenal hormones?

A 40-year-old woman is seen in the emergency room in a state of severe panic. She has had panic attacks for several months and had not sought treatment until her husband came home and found her sitting in the bedroom unable to move. She had been there all day and had soiled her clothing. In the emergency room she appeared frightened and paced in one area. She had difficulty understanding questions and cooperated as long as she could pace. The husband relates that his wife had been under much stress in her job and had recently lost some important clients.

A. What are some manifestations of her panic?

B. What is the biologic cause of anxiety disorders—the brain structures and neurotransmitters?

C. Describe the physiologic manifestations of a panic attack.

References

1. Shorter E. (1997). *A history of psychiatry: From the era of the asylum to the age of Prozac.* New York: John Wiley & Sons.
2. Kandel E.R. (2000). Cellular mechanisms of learning and biological basis of individuality. In Kandel E.R., Schwartz J.H., Jessel T.M. (Eds.), *Principles of neural science* (4th ed., pp. 1247–1277). New York: McGraw-Hill.
3. Grob G.N. (1994). *The mad among us: A history of the care of America's mentally ill.* New York: Macmillan.
4. Plomin R. (1996). Beyond nature vs. nurture. In Hall L.L. (Ed.), *Genetics and mental illness: Evolving issues for research and society* (pp. 29–50). New York: Plenum Press.
5. Hyman S.E. (1999). Looking to the future: The role of genetics and molecular biology in research on mental illness. In Weissman S., Sabshin M., Eist H. (Eds.), *Psychiatry in the new millennium* (pp. 97–117). Washington, DC: American Psychiatric Press.
6. Taylor C.J.A., Macdonald A.M., Murray R.M. (1992). The genetics of psychiatric syndromes. In Weller M., Eysenck M. (Eds.), *The scientific basis of psychiatry* (2nd ed., pp. 270–300). Philadelphia: W.B. Saunders.
7. Gottesman I.I. (1996). Blind men and elephants: Genetic and other perspectives on schizophrenia. In Hall L.L. (Ed.), *Genetics and mental illness: Evolving issues for research and society* (pp. 51–77). New York: Plenum Press.
8. Tsuang M.T., Faraone S.V. (1996). The inheritance of mood disorders. In Hall L.L. (Ed.), *Genetics and mental illness: Evolving issues for research and society* (pp. 79–109). New York: Plenum Press.
9. Mohr W.K. (2003). *Johnson's psychiatric-mental health nursing* (5th ed.). Philadelphia: Lippincott Williams & Wilkins.
10. Guyton A.G., Hall J.E. (2001). *Textbook of medical physiology* (10th ed., pp. 663–677). Philadelphia: W.B. Saunders.
11. Kandel E.R., Kupfermann I., Iverson S. (2000). Learning and memory. In Kandel E.R., Schwartz J.H., Jessell T.M. (Eds.), *Principles of neural science* (4th ed., 1227–1246). New York: McGraw-Hill.
12. Benson D.F., Gorman D.G. (1996). Hallucinations and delusional thinking. In Fogel B.S., Schiffer R.B. (Eds.), *Neuropsychiatry* (pp. 307–323). Baltimore: Williams & Wilkins.
13. Mojica T.R., Baily P.P. (2000). Hallucinations in the vision-impaired elderly: The Charles Bonnet syndrome. *Nurse Practitioner 25*(8), 74–76.
14. Teunisse R.J., Cruysberg J.R., Hoefnagels W.H., et al. (1996). Visual hallucinations in psychologically normal people: Charles Bonnet's syndrome. *Lancet 347,* 794–797.
15. National Empowerment Center. [On-line.] Available: http://www.power2u.org/selfhep/voices.html. Retrieved 11/17/03.
16. Almedia O.P., Howard R.J., Levy R. (1995). Psychotic states arising in late life (late paraphrenia): The role of risk factors. *British Journal of Psychiatry 166,* 215–228.
17. Kandel E.R., Siegelbaum S.A. (2000). Overview of synaptic transmission. In Kandel E.R., Schwartz J.H., Jessel T.M. (Eds.), *Principles of neural science* (4th ed., pp. 175–185). New York: McGraw-Hill.
18. Kandel E.R. (2000). Neurotransmitters. In Kandel E.R., Schwartz J.H., Jessel T.M. (Eds.), *Principles of neural science* (4th ed., pp. 280–296). New York: McGraw-Hill.
19. Trimble M.R. (1996). *Biological psychiatry* (2nd ed., pp. 116–141, 325–378). West Sussex, England: John Wiley & Sons.
20. Callicott J.H., Weinberger D.R. (1999). Functional brain imaging: Future perspectives for clinical practice. In Weissman S., Sabshin M., Eist H. (Eds.), *Psychiatry in the new millennium* (pp. 119–135). Washington, DC: American Psychiatric Press.
21. Dr. Joseph F. Smith Medical Library. [On-line.] Available: http://www.chclibrary.org/micromed/64440.html. Retrieved 11/16/03.
22. *National Coalition of Homeless fact sheet.* [On-line.] Available: http://www.nationalhomeless.org/mental.html. Retrieved 11/16/03.
23. Kandel E.R. (2000). Disorders of thought and volition: Schizophrenia. In Kandel E.R., Schwartz J.H., Jessel T.M. (Eds.), *Principles of neural science* (4th ed., pp. 1188–1207). New York: McGraw-Hill.
24. Marken P.A., Stanislav S.W. (2001). Schizophrenia. In Koda-Kimble M.A., Young L.L. (Eds.), *Applied therapeutics* (7th ed., pp. 76-1–76-40). Philadelphia: Lippincott Williams & Wilkins.
25. Torrey E.F. (1988). *Surviving schizophrenia: A family manual.* New York: Harper & Row.
26. Turner T. (1997). ABC of mental health: Schizophrenia. *British Medical Journal 315,* 108–111.

27. Andreasen N.C. (1997). Linking mind and brain in the study of mental illnesses: A project for a scientific psychopathology. *Science 275,* 1585–1593.
28. Fortinash K.M. (2000). The schizophrenias. In Fortinash K.M., Holoday-Worret P.A. (Eds.), *Psychiatric mental health nursing* (2nd ed., pp. 294–328). St. Louis: Mosby.
29. Boyd M.A. (2002). *Psychiatric nursing: Contemporary practice* (2nd ed., pp. 419, 487, 494, 498). Philadelphia: Lippincott Williams & Wilkins.
30. Harrison P.J. (1999). The neuropathology of schizophrenia: A critical review of the data and their interpretation. *Brain 122,* 593–624.
31. American Psychiatric Association. (2000). *Diagnostic and statistical manual of mental disorders (DSM-IV-TR) classification system* (4th ed.). Washington, DC: Author.
32. Sadock B.J., Sadock V.A. (2003). *Kaplan & Sadock's synopsis of psychiatry: behavioral sciences/clinical psychiatry* (9th ed., pp. 536–539, 594, 606–617, 1278). Philadelphia: Lippincott Williams & Wilkins.
33. Brent D.A., Birmaher B. (2002). Adolescent depression. *New England Journal of Medicine 347,* 667–671.
34. *Surgeon General's report.* [On-line.] Available: http://www.mentalhealth.org/cre/ch3_appropriateness.asp. Retrieved 11/18/03.
35. Kandel E.R. (2000). Disorders of mood: Depression, mania, and anxiety disorders. In Kandel E.R., Schwartz J.H., Jessel T.M. (Eds.), *Principles of neural science* (4th ed., pp. 1209–1225). New York: McGraw-Hill.
36. Finley P.R., Laird L.K., Benefield W.H., Jr. (2001). Mood disorders I: Major depressive disorders. In Koda-Kimble M.A., Young L.L. (Eds.), *Applied therapeutics* (7th ed., 77-1–77-36). Philadelphia: Lippincott Williams & Wilkins.
37. Love R.C., Borovicka M.D. (2001). Mood disorders II: Bipolar disorders. In Koda-Kimble M.A., Young L.L., (Eds.), *Applied therapeutics* (7th ed., pp. 78-1–78-18). Philadelphia: Lippincott Williams & Wilkins.
38. Doris A., Ebmeier K., Shajahan P. (1999). Depressive illness. *Lancet 354,* 1369–1375.
39. Manning J.S., Connor P.D., Sahai A. (1998). The bipolar spectrum: A review of current concepts and implications for the management of depression in primary care. *Archives of Family Medicine 7*(1), 63–71.
40. Daly I. (1997). Mania. *Lancet 349,* 1157–1160.
41. Kilzieh N., Akiskal H.S. (1999). Rapid-cycling bipolar disorder: An overview of research and clinical experience. *Psychiatric Clinics of North America 22,* 585–607.
42. Haber J., Krainovich-Miller B., McMahon A., Price-Hoskins P. (1997). *Comprehensive psychiatric nursing* (5th ed., pp. 609–610). St. Louis: Mosby.
43. Soares J.C., Mann J.J. (1997). The anatomy of mood disorders: Review of structural neuroimaging studies. *Biological Psychiatry 41,* 86–106.
44. Videbech P. (2000). PET measurements of brain glucose metabolism and blood flow in major depressive disorder: A critical review. *Acta Psychiatrica Scandinavica 101,* 11–20.
45. McAllister-Williams R.H., Ferrier I.N., Young A.H. (1998). Mood and neuropsychological function in depression: The role of corticosteroids and serotonin. *Psychological Medicine 28,* 573–584.
46. Williams J.W., Mulrow C.D., Chiquette E., et al. (2000). A systematic review of newer pharmacotherapies for depression in adults: Evidence report summary. Clinical guideline, part 2. *Annals of Internal Medicine 132,* 743–756.
47. Saeed S.A., Bruce T.J. (1998). Panic disorder: Effective treatment options. *American Family Physician 57,* 2412–2415, 2419–2420.
48. Roy-Byrne P.P., Cowley D.S. (1998). Search for pathophysiology of panic disorder. *Lancet 352,* 1646–1647.
49. Grimsley S.R. (1995). Anxiety disorders. In Young L.L., Koda-Kimble M.A. (Eds.), *Applied therapeutics: The clinical use of drugs* (6th ed., pp. 73-1–73-28). Vancouver, WA: Applied Therapeutics.
50. Gorman J.M., Kent J.M., Sullivan G.M., Coplan J.D. (2000). Neuroanatomical hypothesis of panic disorder, revised. *American Journal of Psychiatry 157,* 493–505.
51. Eddy M.F., Walbroehl G.S. (1998). Recognition and treatment of obsessive-compulsive disorder. *American Family Physician 57,* 1623–1628, 1632–1634.
52. Gedenk M., Nepps P. (1997). Obsessive-compulsive disorder: Diagnosis and treatment in the primary care setting [Medical practice]. *Journal of the American Board of Family Practice 10,* 349–356.
53. Tibbo P., Warneke L. (1999). Obsessive-compulsive disorder in schizophrenia: Epidemiologic and biologic overlap. *Journal of Psychiatry and Neuroscience 24,* 15–24.
54. Bruce T.J., Saeed S.A. (1999). Social anxiety disorder: A common, underrecognized mental disorder. *American Family Physician 60,* 2311–2322.
55. Morrison-Borgorad M., Phelps C., Buckholtz N. (1996). Alzheimer disease research comes of age. *Journal of the American Medical Association 277,* 837–840.
56. U.S. Health and Human Services. (2003). *2001–2002 Alzheimer's disease progress report.* U.S. Department of Health and Human Services National Institute of Health. NIH publication number 03-533.
57. Rubin E., Farber J.L. (1999). *Pathology* (3rd ed., pp. 2470–2473). Philadelphia: Lippincott-Raven.
58. Cotran R.S., Kumar V., Collins T. (1999). *Robbins' pathologic basis of disease* (6th ed., pp. 1343–1349). Philadelphia: W.B. Saunders.
59. van Duijn C.M. (1996). Epidemiology of the dementias: Recent developments and new approaches. *Journal of Neurology, Neurosurgery, and Psychiatry 60,* 478–488.
60. Lendon C.L., Ashall F., Goate A.M. (1996). Exploring the etiology of Alzheimer's disease using molecular genetics. *Journal of the American Medical Association 277,* 825–831.
61. U.S. Department of Health and Human Services. (1996). *Recognition and initial assessment of Alzheimer's disease and related disorders.* AHCPR publication no. 97-0702. Washington, DC: Public Health Service, Agency for Health Care Policy and Research.
62. Morris J.C. (1997). Alzheimer's disease: A review of clinical assessment and management issues. *Geriatrics 52*(Suppl. 2), S22–S25.
63. Mayeux R., Sano M. (1999). Treatment of Alzheimer's disease. *New England Journal of Medicine 341,* 1670–1679.
64. Prusiner S.B. (2001). Shattuck lecture: Neurodegenerative diseases and prions. *New England Journal of Medicine 344,* 1516–1526.
65. Rappaport E.B. (1987). Iatrogenic Creutzfeldt-Jakob disease. *Neurology 37,* 1520–1522.
66. *Juvenile Huntington's disease* [On-line.] Available: http://www.geocities.com/hdsarmc/juvenile_hd.htm. Retrieved 11/16/03.
67. Martin J., Gusella J. (1987). Huntington's disease: Pathogenesis and management. *New England Journal of Medicine 315,* 1267–1276.

UNIT XIII

Special Sensory Function

Of all the ancient civilizations, it was the Greeks who led the way in understanding the body and its workings. One of the earliest Greek anatomists was Alcmaeon of Croton (c. 500 BC). Through his animal dissections, Alcmaeon came to recognize many structures and was the first to mention the eye in his writings. He described the optic nerve and decided that three things were necessary for vision—external light, the "fire" in the eye (he assumed there must be fire in the eye because a blow to the eye produces sparks, or stars), and the liquid in the eyeball.

The Greeks also developed early surgical procedures, among them techniques for the removal of cataracts. However, it was the Roman encyclopedist, Aulus Cornelius Celsus (1st century AD), whose most important surviving works are concerned with medicine, who provided a vivid description of the procedure:

The needle is to be sharp enough to penetrate, yet not too fine; and this to be inserted straight through . . . at a spot between the pupil of the eye and the angle adjacent to the temple, away from the middle of the cataract, in such a way that no vein is wounded. The needle, however, should not be inserted timidly. When the spot is reached, the needle is to be sloped against the colored area [lens] itself and rotated gently, guiding it little by little below the pupil; when the cataract has passed below the pupil, it is pressed upon more firmly in order that it may settle below.

CHAPTER

54

Disorders of Visual Function

Edward W. Carroll
Carol M. Porth
Robin L. Curtis

About 70% of all sensory receptors are in the eyes. The photoreceptors sense and encode the patterns made by light in our surroundings. Neural pathways carry the coded information from the eyes to the brain where the signals gain meaning, fashioning images of the world around us.

Almost 17.3 million persons in the United States have some degree of visual impairment; of these, 1.1 million are legally blind.[1] The prevalence of vision impairment increases with age. An estimated 26% of persons 75 years of age and older report visual impairment severe enough to interfere with recognizing a friend across the room or reading newspaper print even when wearing glasses. At the other end of the age spectrum, an estimated 95,100 children younger than 18 years of age are severely visually impaired.[1]

Alterations in vision can result from disorders of the eyelids and optic globe (conjunctiva, cornea, and uvea), intraocular pressure (glaucoma), lens (cataract), vitreous humor and retina, visual pathways and visual cortex, and extraocular muscles and eye movement.

VISION

- Vision is a special sensory function that incorporates the visual receptor functions of the eyeball, the optic nerve, and visual pathways that carry and distribute sensory information from the optic globe to the central nervous system, and the primary and visual association cortices that translate the sensory signals into visual images.
- The eyeball is a hollow spherical structure that functions in the reception of the light rays that provide the stimuli for vision. The refractive surface of the cornea and accommodative properties of the lens serve to focus the light signals from near and far objects on the photoreceptors in the retina.
- Visual information is carried to the brain by axons of the retinal cells that form the optic nerve. The two optic nerves fuse in the optic chiasm, where axons of the nasal retina of each eye cross to the contralateral side and travel with axons of the ipsilateral temporal retina to form the fibers of the optic radiations that travel to the visual cortex.
- Binocular vision depends on the coordination of three pairs of extraocular nerves that provide for the conjugate eye movements, with optical axes of the two eyes maintained parallel with one another as the eyes rotate in their sockets.

Disorders of the Accessory Structures of the Eye

After completing this section of the chapter, you should be able to meet the following objectives:

- State the cause of eyelid weakness
- Define *entropion* and *ectropion*
- Explain the differences between marginal blepharitis, a hordeolum, and a chalazion as to causes and manifestations
- State the causes and treatment of dry eye

The optic globe, commonly called the *eyeball,* is a remarkable, mobile, nearly spherical structure contained in a pyramid-shaped cavity of the skull called the *orbit* (Fig. 54-1). Only the anterior one fifth of the orbit is occupied by the eyeball; the remainder is filled with muscles, nerves, the lacrimal gland, and adipose tissue that supports the normal position of the optic globe. Exposed surfaces of the eyes are protected by the eyelids, which are mucous membrane–lined skin flaps that provide a means for shutting out most light. Tears bathe the anterior surface of the eye; they prevent friction between it and the lid, maintain hydration of the cornea, and protect the eye from irritation by foreign objects.

Three distinct layers form the wall of the eyeball: the sclera or outer supporting layer, the choroid or middle vascular layer, and the retina, which is composed of the neuronal retinal layer and the outer pigmented layer (Fig. 54-2).

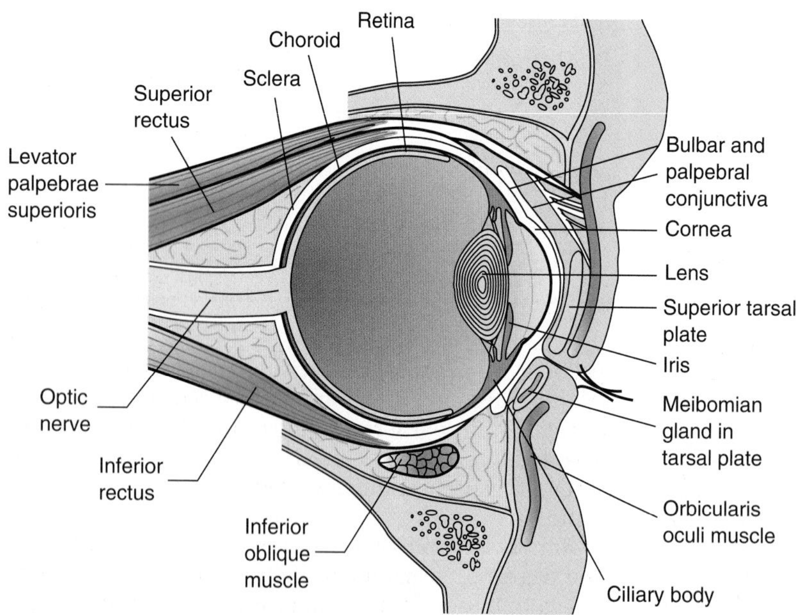

FIGURE 54-1 Lateral view of the eye and its appendages.

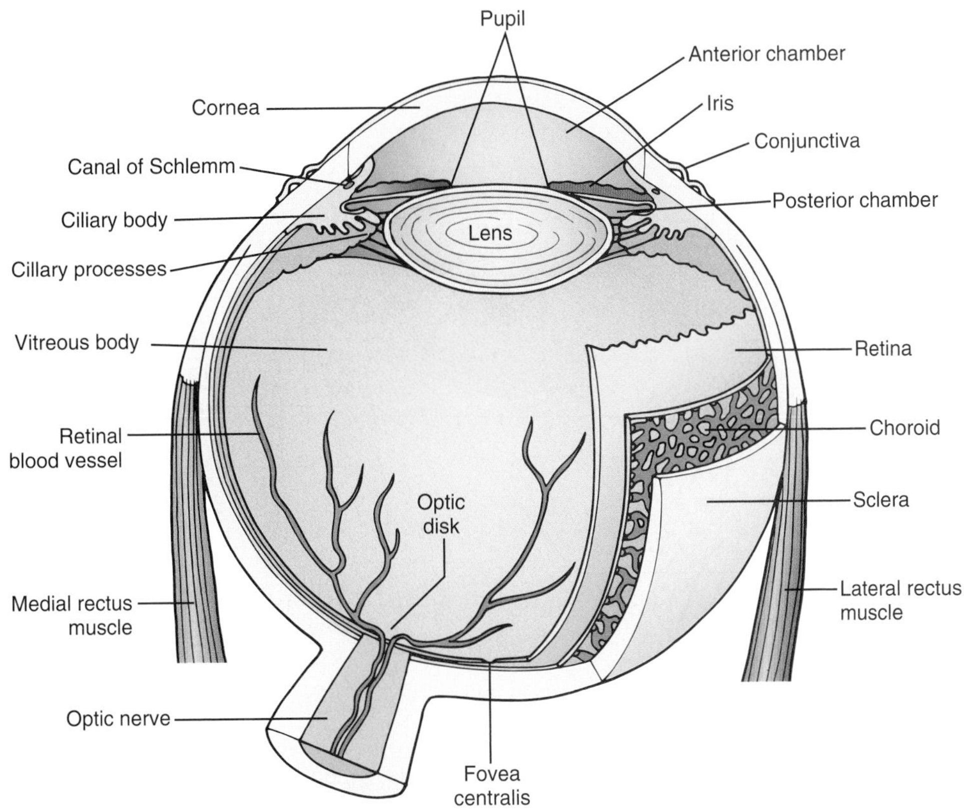

FIGURE 54-2 Transverse section of the eyeball.

The outer layer of the eyeball consists of a tough, opaque, white, fibrous layer called the *sclera.* It is strong yet elastic, and maintains the shape of the globe. The sclera is continuous with the cornea anteriorly and with the cranial dural sheath that surrounds and protects the optic nerve posteriorly.

DISORDERS OF THE EYELIDS

The upper and lower eyelids, the *palpebrae,* are modified folds of skin that protect the eyeball. The palpebral fissure is the oval opening between the upper and lower eyelids. At the corners of the eye, where the upper and lower lids meet, is an angle called the *canthus;* the lateral canthus is the outer, or temporal, angle, and the medial canthus is the inner, or nasal, angle. In each lid, a tarsus, or plate of dense connective tissue, gives the lid its shape (see Fig. 54-1). Each tarsus contains modified sebaceous glands, called *meibomian glands,* the ducts of which open onto the eyelid margins. Sebaceous secretions of the meibomian glands enable airtight closure of the lids and prevent rapid evaporation of tears.

Two striated muscles, the levator palpebrae superioris and the orbicularis oculi, provide for movement of the eyelids (Fig. 54-3). The levator palpebrae, which is innervated by the oculomotor cranial nerve (cranial nerve [CN] III), raises the upper lid. Encircling the eye is the orbicularis oculi muscle, which is supplied by the facial nerve (CN VII). When this muscle contracts, it closes the eyelids.

Eyelid Weakness

Drooping of the eyelid is called *ptosis.* It can result from weakness of the levator muscle that elevates the upper lid in conjunction with the unopposed action of the orbicularis oculi that forcefully closes the eyelids. Weakness of the orbicularis oculi causes an open eyelid, but not ptosis. Neurologic causes of eyelid weakness include damage to the innervating cranial nerves or to the nerves' central nuclei in the midbrain and the caudal pons.

Normally, the edges of the eyelids, or palpebrae, are in such a position that the palpebral conjunctiva that lines the eyelids is not exposed and the eyelashes do not rub against the cornea. Turning in of the lid is called *entropion.* It is usually caused by scarring of the palpebral conjunctiva or degeneration of the fascial attachments to the lower lid that occurs with aging. Corneal irritation may occur as the eyelashes turn inward. *Ectropion* refers to eversion of the lower lid. The condition is usually bilateral and caused by relaxation of the orbicularis oculi muscle because of CN VII weakness or the aging process. Ectropion causes tearing and ocular irritation and may lead to inflammation of the cornea.

Entropion and ectropion can be treated surgically. Electrocautery penetration of the lid conjunctiva also can be used to treat mild forms of ectropion. After electrocautery,

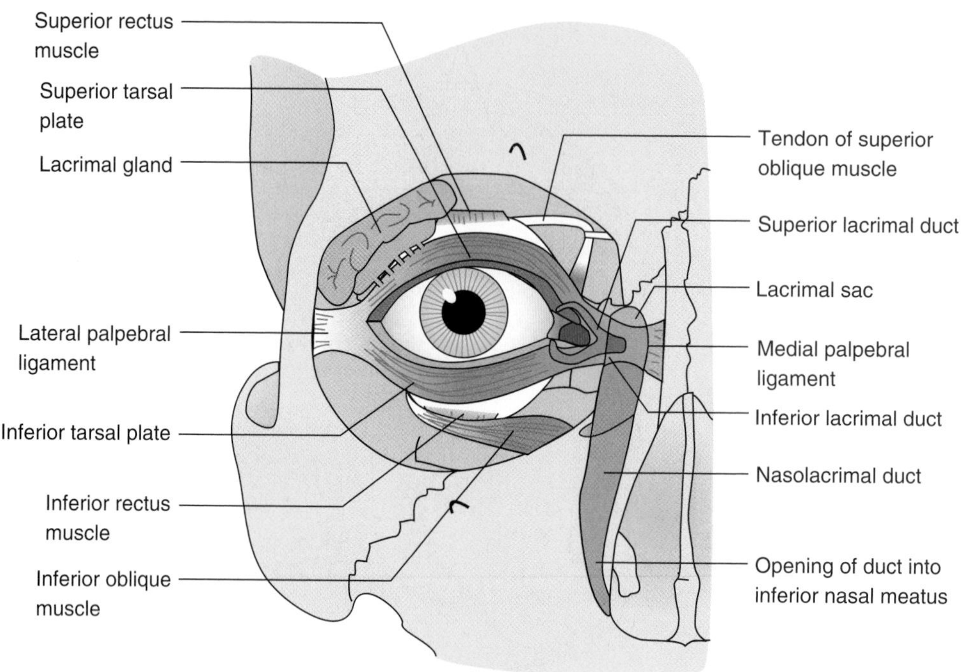

FIGURE 54-3 The eye and its appendages: anterior view.

contraction of the resulting scar tissue usually draws the lid up to its normal position.

Eyelid Inflammation

Blepharitis is a common bilateral inflammation of the anterior or posterior structures of eyelid margins. *Anterior blepharitis* involves the eyelid skin, eyelashes, and associated glands. Two main types of anterior blepharitis occur: seborrheic and staphylococcal.[2,3] The seborrheic form is usually associated with seborrhea (*i.e.,* dandruff) of the scalp or brows. Staphylococcal blepharitis may be caused by *Staphylococcus epidermidis* or *Staphylococcus aureus,* in which case the lesions are often ulcerative. The chief symptoms of anterior blepharitis are irritation, burning, redness, and itching of the eyelid margins. Treatment includes careful cleaning with a wet applicator or clean washcloth to remove the scales. When the disorder is associated with a microbial infection, an antibiotic ointment is prescribed.

Posterior blepharitis is inflammation of the eyelids that involves the meibomian glands. It may result from a bacterial infection, particularly with staphylococci, or dysfunction of the meibomian glands, in which there is a strong association with acne rosacea.[2,3] The meibomian glands and their orifices are inflamed, with dilation of the glands, plugging of the orifices, and abnormal secretions. The lid margins are often rolled inward to produce mild entropion, and the tears may be frothy and abnormally greasy from the meibomian secretions. Treatment of posterior blepharitis is determined by associated conjunctival and corneal changes. Long-term, low-dose systemic antibiotic therapy guided by results of bacterial cultures, along with short-term topical steroids, may be needed.

A *hordeolum,* or *stye,* is caused by infection of the sebaceous glands of the eyelid and can be internal or external (Fig. 54-4A). The main symptoms are pain, redness, and swelling. The treatment is similar to that of abscesses in other parts of the body. Heat, such as a warm compress, is applied, and antibiotic ointment may be used. Incision or expression of the infectious contents of the abscess may be necessary.

A *chalazion* is a granulomatous inflammation of a meibomian gland that may follow an internal hordeolum. It is characterized by a small nontender nodule on the upper or lower lid (see Fig. 54-4B). The conjunctiva around the chalazion is red and elevated. If the chalazion is large enough, it may press on the eyeball and distort vision. Treatment consists of surgical excision.

DISORDERS OF THE LACRIMAL SYSTEM

The lacrimal system includes the major lacrimal gland, which produces the tears; the puncta and tear sac, which collect the tears; and the nasolacrimal duct, which empties the tears into the nasal cavity. The lacrimal gland lies in the orbit, superior and lateral to the eyeball (see Fig. 54-3). Approximately 12 small ducts connect the lacrimal gland to the superior conjunctival fornix. Tears contain approximately 98% water, 1.5% sodium chloride, and small amounts of potassium, albumin, and glucose. The function of tears is to make a smooth optical surface by abolishing minute surface irregularities. Tears also wet and protect the delicate surface of the cornea and conjunctiva. They flush and remove irritating substances and microorganisms, and they provide the cornea with necessary nutrient substances. Tears also contain lysozymes and immunoglobulin A (IgA), IgG, and IgE, which synergistically act to protect against infection. Although IgA predominates, IgE concentrations are increased in some allergic conditions.

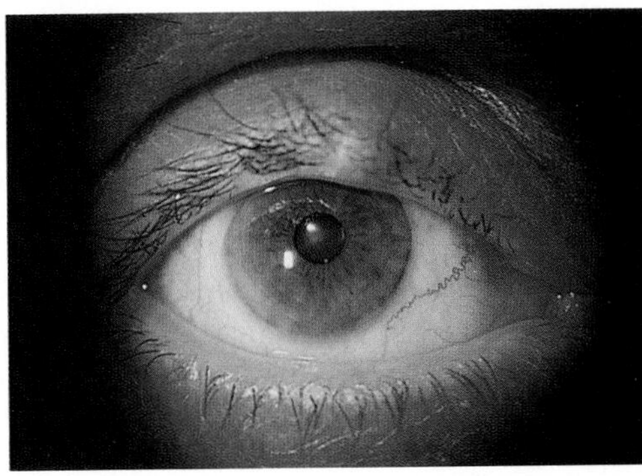

A

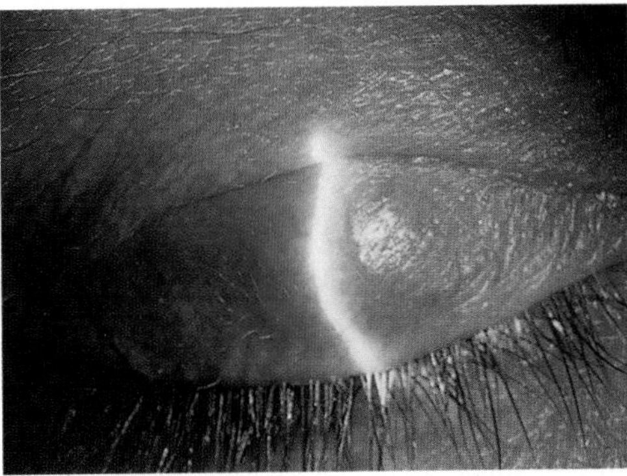

B

FIGURE 54-4 (**A**) Stye (acute hordeolum). (**B**) Chalazion. (Bickley L.S. (2003). *Bates' guide to physical examination and history taking* (8th ed., p. 178). Philadelphia: Lippincott Williams & Wilkins)

Dry Eyes

The thin film of tears that covers the cornea is essential in preventing drying and damage of the outer layer of the cornea. This tear film is composed of three layers: the superficial lipid layer, derived from the meibomian glands and thought to retard evaporation; the aqueous layer, secreted by the lacrimal glands; and the mucinous layer, which overlies the cornea and epithelial cells. Because the epithelial cell membranes are hydrophobic and cannot be wetted by aqueous solutions alone, the mucinous layer plays an essential role in wetting these surfaces. Periodic blinking of the eyes is needed to maintain a continuous tear film over the ocular surface.

Several conditions reduce the functioning of the lacrimal glands. With aging, the lacrimal glands diminish their secretion, and as a result, many older persons awaken from a night's sleep with highly irritated eyes. Dry eyes also result from loss of reflex lacrimal gland secretion because of congenital defects, infection, irradiation, damage to the parasympathetic innervation of the gland, and medications such as antihistamines and drugs with an anticholinergic action. Wearing contact lenses contributes to eye dryness through decreased blinking. *Sjögren's syndrome* is a systemic disorder in which lymphocytes and plasma cells infiltrate the lacrimal and parotid glands. The disorder is associated with diminished salivary and lacrimal secretions, resulting in keratoconjunctivitis sicca (dry eye syndrome) and xerostomia (*i.e.,* dry mouth). The syndrome occurs mainly in women near menopause and is often associated with connective tissue disorders such as rheumatoid arthritis.

Persons with dry eyes complain of a dry or gritty sensation in the eye, burning, itching, inability to produce tears, photosensitivity, redness, pain, and difficulty in moving the eyelids. Dry eyes and the absence of tears can cause keratinization of the cornea and conjunctival epithelium. In severe cases, corneal ulcerations can occur. Consequent corneal scarring can cause blindness.

The treatment of dry eyes includes frequent instillation of artificial tear solutions into the conjunctival sac. More prolonged duration of action can be obtained from topical preparations containing methylcellulose or polyvinyl alcohol. An ointment is useful for prolonged lubrication. Overall, these artificial tear preparations are safe and without side effects. However, the preservatives necessary to maintain their sterility can be irritating to the cornea.[2,5]

Dacryocystitis

Dacryocystitis is an infection of the lacrimal sac. It occurs most often in infants and in persons older than 54 years of age.[2] It is usually unilateral and most often occurs secondary to obstruction of the nasolacrimal duct. Often, the cause of the obstruction is unknown, although there may be a history of severe trauma to the midface. The symptoms include tearing and discharge, pain, swelling, and tenderness. The treatment includes application of warm compresses and antibiotic therapy. In chronic forms of the disorder, surgical repair of the tear duct may be necessary.

In infants, dacryocystitis is usually caused by failure of the nasolacrimal ducts to open spontaneously before birth. When a duct fails to open, a secondary dacryocystitis may develop. These infants are usually treated with gentle massage of the tear sac, instillation of antibiotic drops into the conjunctival sac, and, if that fails, probing of the tear duct.

In summary, the eyelids serve to protect the eye. Ptosis refers to drooping of the upper lid, which is caused by injury to CN III. Entropion, which refers to turning in the upper eyelid and eyelashes, is discomforting and causes corneal irritation. Ectropion, or eversion of the lower eyelid, causes tearing and may lead to corneal inflammation. Marginal blepharitis is the most common disorder of the eyelids. It commonly is caused by a staphylococcal infection or seborrhea (*i.e.,* dandruff).

The lacrimal system includes the major lacrimal gland, which produces the tears, the puncta and tear sac, which collect the tears, and the nasolacrimal duct, which empties the tears into the nasal cavity. Tears protect the cornea from drying and irritation. Impaired tear production or conditions that prevent blinking and the spread of tears produce drying of the eyes and predispose them to corneal irritation and injury. Dacryocystitis is an infection of the lacrimal sac.

Disorders of the Conjunctiva, Cornea, and Uveal Tract

After completing this section of the chapter, you should be able to meet the following objectives:

- Compare symptoms associated with red eye caused by conjunctivitis, corneal irritation, and acute glaucoma
- List at least four causes of red eye
- Describe the appearance of corneal edema
- Characterize the manifestations, treatment, and possible complications of bacterial, *Acanthamoeba,* and herpes keratitis
- Describe the structures of the uveal tract
- Describe tests used in assessing the pupillary reflex and cite the possible causes of abnormal pupillary reflexes

DISORDERS OF THE CONJUNCTIVA

The conjunctiva is a thin layer of mucous membrane that lines the anterior surface of both eyelids as the *palpebral conjunctiva* and folds back over the anterior surface of the optic globe as the *ocular* or *bulbar conjunctiva.* The ocular conjunctiva covers only the sclera or white portion of the optic globe, not the cornea. When both eyes are closed, the conjunctiva lines the closed conjunctival sac. Although the conjunctiva protects the eye by preventing foreign objects from entering beyond the conjunctival sac, its main function is the production of a lubricating mucus that bathes the eye and keeps it moist.

Conjunctivitis, or inflammation of the conjunctiva (*i.e.,* red eye or pink eye), is one of the most common forms of eye disease.[4,5] It may result from bacterial or viral infection, allergens, chemical agents, physical irritants, or radiant energy. Infections may extend from areas adjacent to the conjunctiva or may be blood-borne, such as in measles or chickenpox. Newborns can contract conjunctivitis during the birth process. Infectious forms of conjunctivitis are often bilateral and may involve other family members and close associates. Unilateral disease suggests sources of irritation such as foreign bodies or chemical irritation.

Depending on the cause, conjunctivitis can vary in severity from a mild hyperemia (redness) with tearing to severe conjunctivitis with purulent drainage. The conjunctiva is extremely sensitive to irritation and inflammation. Important symptoms of conjunctivitis are a foreign body sensation, a scratching or burning sensation, itching, and photophobia. Severe pain suggests corneal rather than conjunctival disease. Itching is common in allergic conditions. A discharge, or exudate, may be present with all types of conjunctivitis and may cause transient blurring of vision. It is usually watery when the conjunctivitis is caused by allergy, a foreign body, or viral infection and mucopurulent in the presence of bacterial or fungal infection. A characteristic of many forms of conjunctivitis is papillary hypertrophy. This occurs because the palpebral conjunctiva is bound to the tarsus by fine fibrils. As a result, inflammation that develops between the fibrils causes the conjunctiva to be elevated in mounds called *papillae.* When the papillae are small, the conjunctiva has a smooth, velvety appearance. Red papillary conjunctivitis suggests bacterial or chlamydial conjunctivitis. In allergic conjunctivitis, the papillae often become flat topped, polygonal, and milky in color and have a cobblestone appearance.

The diagnosis of conjunctivitis is based on history, physical examination, and microscopic and culture studies to identify the cause. Because a red eye may be the sign of several eye conditions, it is important to differentiate between redness caused by conjunctivitis and that caused by more serious eye disorders, such as corneal lesions and acute glaucoma. In contrast to corneal lesions and acute glaucoma, conjunctivitis produces injection (*i.e.,* enlargement and redness) of the peripheral conjunctival blood vessels rather than those radiating around the corneal limbus. Conjunctivitis also produces only mild discomfort, as compared with the moderate to severe discomfort associated with corneal lesions or the severe and deep pain associated with acute glaucoma. Infectious forms of conjunctivitis are usually bilateral and may involve other family members and associates. Unilateral disease suggests sources of irritation such as foreign bodies or chemical irritation.

Allergic Conjunctivitis

Allergic conjunctivitis encompasses a spectrum of conjunctival conditions usually characterized by itching. The most common of these is seasonal allergic rhinoconjunctivitis, or hay fever. Seasonal allergic conjunctivitis is an IgE-mediated hypersensitivity reaction precipitated by small airborne allergens such as pollens.[6] It typically causes bilateral tearing, itching, and redness of the eyes.

The treatment of seasonal allergic rhinoconjunctivitis includes allergen avoidance, the use of cold compresses, oral antihistamines, and vasoconstrictor eye drops. Allergic conjunctivitis also has been successfully treated with topical mast cell stabilizers, histamine H_1 receptor antagonists, and topical nonsteroidal antiinflammatory drugs.[6] All three types of agents are well tolerated and have a rapid onset of action. In severe cases, a short course of topical corticosteroids may be required to afford symptomatic relief.

Infectious Conjunctivitis

The agents of infectious conjunctivitis include bacteria, viruses, and chlamydiae. Infections may spread from areas adjacent to the conjunctiva or may be blood-borne, such as in measles or chickenpox. Newborns can contract conjunctivitis during the birth process.

Bacterial Conjunctivitis. Bacterial conjunctivitis may present as a hyperacute, acute, or chronic infection. *Hyperacute conjunctivitis* is a severe, sight-threatening ocular infection. The infection has an abrupt onset and is characterized by a copious amount of yellow-green drainage. The symptoms, which typically are progressive, include conjunctival redness and chemosis, lid swelling, and tender, swollen preaurical lymph nodes. The most common causes of hyperacute purulent conjunctivitis are *Neisseria gonorrhoeae* and *Neisseria meningitidis,* with *N. gonorrhoeae* being the most common.[3–5] Gonococcal ocular infections left untreated result in corneal ulceration with ultimate perforation, and sometimes permanent loss of vision. Diagnostic methods include immediate Gram staining of ocular specimens and special cultures for *Neisseria* species. Treatment includes systemic antibiotics supplemented with ocular antibiotics. Because of the increasing prevalence of penicillin-resistant *N. gonorrhoeae,* antibiotic choice should be determined by current information regarding antibiotic sensitivity.

Acute bacterial conjunctivitis typically presents with burning, tearing, and mucopurulent or purulent discharge. Common agents of bacterial conjunctivitis are *Streptococcus pneumoniae, S. aureus,* and *Haemophilus influenzae.*[4] The eyelids are sticky, with possible excoriation of the lid margins. Treatment may include local application of antibiotics. The disorder is usually self-limited, lasting approximately 10 to 14 days if untreated. Scrupulous eyelid hygiene and prompt adequate treatment of infected persons and their contacts are effective.

Chronic bacterial conjunctivitis most commonly is caused by *Staphylococcus* species, although other bacteria may be involved. It is often associated with blepharitis and bacterial colonization of eyelid margins. The symptoms of chronic bacterial conjunctivitis vary and can include itching, burning, foreign body sensation, and morning eyelash crusting. Other symptoms include flaky debris and erythema along the lid margins, eyelash loss, and eye redness. Some people with chronic bacterial conjunctivitis also have recurrent styes and chalazia of the lid margins. Treatment includes good eyelid hygiene and application of topical antibiotics.

Viral Conjunctivitis. Etiologic agents of viral conjunctivitis include adenoviruses, herpesviruses, and enteroviruses. *Adenovirus type 3* infection is usually associated with pharyngitis, fever, and malaise.[4,5] It causes generalized hyperemia, copious tearing, and minimal exudate. Children are affected more often than adults. Swimming pools contaminated because of inadequate chlorination are common sources of infection. Infections due to adenovirus types 4 and 7 are often associated with acute respiratory disease. These viruses are rapidly disseminated when large groups mingle with infected individuals (*e.g.,* military recruits). Adenovirus type 8 epidemics are associated with contamination of ophthalmic products and equipment. No specific treatment for this type of viral conjunctivitis exists; it usually lasts 7 to 14 days. Preventive measures include scrupulous eyelid hygiene and avoiding shared use of eyedroppers, eye makeup, goggles, and towels.

Herpes simplex virus conjunctivitis is characterized by unilateral infection, irritation, mucoid discharge, pain, and mild photophobia. Herpetic vesicles may develop on the eyelids and lid margins. Although the infection is usually caused by the type 1 herpesvirus, it also can be caused by the type 2 virus that causes genital herpes. It is often associated with herpes simplex virus keratitis, in which the cornea shows discrete epithelial lesions. Treatment involves the use of systemic or local antiviral agents. Topical antiviral agents such as vidarabine, trifluridine, or idoxuridine usually provide prompt relief.[4] Local corticosteroid preparations increase the activity of the herpes simplex virus, apparently by enhancing the destructive effect of collagenase on the collagen of the cornea. The use of these medications should be avoided in those suspected of having herpes simplex conjunctivitis or keratitis.

Chlamydial Conjunctivitis. Chlamydial conjunctivitis is usually a benign suppurative conjunctivitis transmitted by the type of *Chlamydia trachomatis* (serotypes D through K) that causes venereal infections (see Chapter 48). It is spread by contaminated genital secretions and occurs in newborns of mothers with *C. trachomatis* infections of the birth canal. It also can be contracted through swimming in unchlorinated pools. The incubation period varies from 5 to 12 days, and the disease may last for several months if untreated. The infection is usually treated with appropriate oral antibiotics.

A more serious form of infection is caused by a different strain of *C. trachomatis* (serotypes A through C). This form of chlamydial infection affects the conjunctiva and causes ulceration and scarring of the cornea. It is the leading cause of preventable blindness in the world. Although the agent is widespread, it is seen mostly in developing countries, particularly those of Africa, Asia, and the Middle East.[7] It is transmitted by direct human contact, contaminated objects (fomites), and flies.

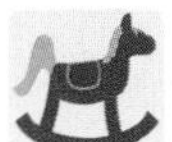

Ophthalmia Neonatorum

Ophthalmia neonatorum is a form of conjunctivitis that occurs in newborns younger than 1 month of age and is usually contracted during or soon after vaginal delivery. Many causes are known, including *N. gonorrhoeae, Pseudomonas,* and *C. trachomatis.*[8] Epidemiologically, these infections reflect those sexually transmitted diseases most common in a particular area. Once the most common form of conjunctivitis in the newborn, gonococcal ophthalmia neonatorum has an incidence of 0.3% of live births in the United States; *C. trachomatis* has an incidence of 8.2% of live births.[8] Drops of 0.5% erythromycin or 1% silver nitrate are applied immediately after birth to prevent gonococcal ophthalmia. Silver nitrate instillation may cause mild, self-limited conjunctivitis.

Signs of ophthalmia neonatorum include redness and swelling of the conjunctiva, swelling of the eyelids, and discharge, which may be purulent. The conjunctivitis caused by silver nitrate occurs within 6 to 12 hours of birth and clears within 24 to 48 hours.[8] The incubation period for *N. gonorrhoeae* is 2 to 5 days and for *C. trachomatis,* 5 to 14 days. Infection should be suspected when conjunctivitis develops 48 hours after birth.[7] Ophthalmia neonatorum is a potentially blinding condition, and it can cause serious and potentially systemic manifestations. It requires immediate diagnosis and treatment.

DISORDERS OF THE CORNEA

At the anterior part of the eyeball, the outer covering of the eye is modified to form the transparent cornea, which bulges anteriorly from its junction with the sclera (Fig. 54-5). A major part of the refraction (*i.e.,* bending) of

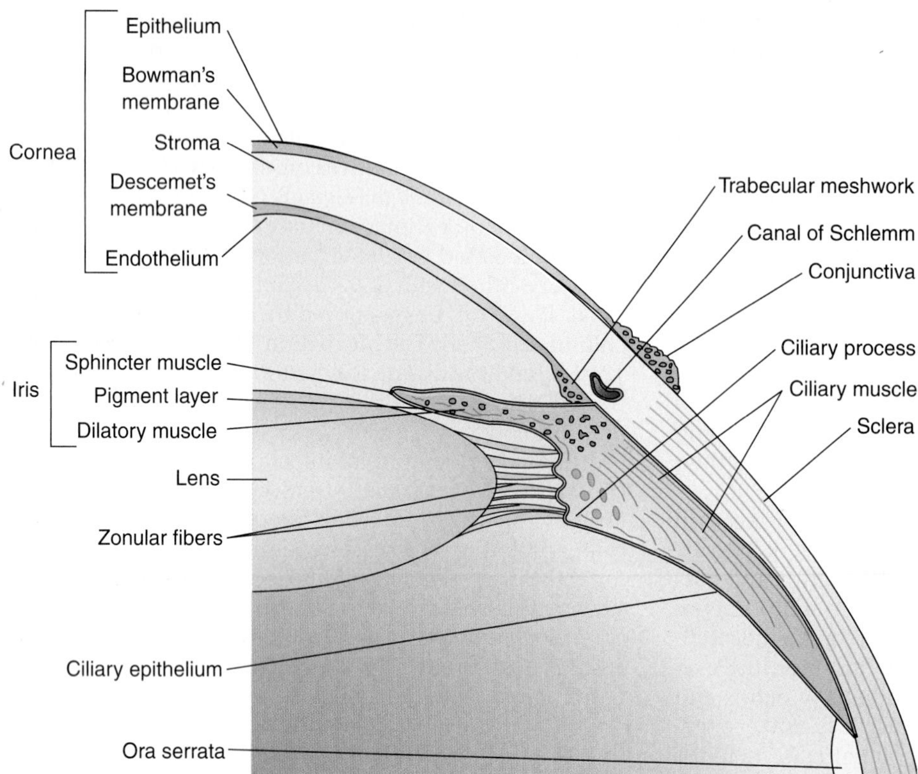

FIGURE 54-5 Anterior chamber angle and surrounding structures.

light rays and focusing of vision occurs in the cornea. Three layers of tissue form the cornea: an extremely thin outer epithelial layer, which is continuous with the bulbar conjunctiva; a middle layer called the *substantia propria* or *stroma;* and an inner endothelial layer, which lies next to the aqueous humor of the anterior chamber. The substantia propria is composed of regularly arranged collagen bundles embedded in a mucopolysaccharide matrix. This organization of the collagen fibers, which makes the substantia propria transparent, is necessary for light transmission. Hydration within a limited range is necessary to maintain the spacing of the collagen fibers and transparency.

The cornea is avascular and obtains its nutrient and oxygen supply by diffusion from blood vessels of the adjacent sclera, from the aqueous humor at its deep surface, and from tears. The corneal epithelium is heavily innervated by sensory neurons (trigeminal nerve [CN V], ophthalmic division [CN V_1]). Epithelial damage causes discomfort that ranges from a foreign body sensation and burning of the eyes to severe, stabbing or knifelike, incapacitating pain. Reflex lacrimation is common. Disorders of the cornea include trauma and infections, abnormal corneal deposits, and arcus senilis.

Corneal Trauma

Trauma that causes abrasions of the cornea can be extremely painful, but if minor, the abrasions usually heal in a few days. The epithelial layer can regenerate, and small defects heal without scarring. If the stroma is damaged, healing occurs more slowly, and the danger of infection is increased. Injuries to Bowman's membrane and the stromal layer heal with scar formation and permanent opacification. Opacities of the cornea impair the transmission of light. A minor scar can severely distort vision because it disturbs the refractive surface.

The integrity of the epithelium and the endothelium is necessary to maintain hydration of the cornea within a limited range. Damage to either structure leads to edema and loss of transparency. Among the causes of corneal edema is the prolonged and uninterrupted wearing of hard contact lenses, which can deprive the epithelium of oxygen, disrupting its integrity. The edema disappears spontaneously when the cornea contacts the atmosphere. Corneal edema also occurs after a sudden rise in intraocular pressure. With corneal edema, the cornea appears dull, uneven, and hazy. Visual acuity decreases, and iridescent vision (*i.e.,* rainbows around lights) occurs. Iridescent vision results from epithelial and subepithelial edema, which splits white light into its component parts, with blue in the center and red on the outside.

Keratitis

Keratitis refers to inflammation of the cornea. It can be caused by infections, hypersensitivity reactions, ischemia, defects in tearing, trauma, and interruption in sensory innervation, as occurs with local anesthesia. Scar tissue formation due to keratitis is the leading cause of blindness and impaired vision throughout the world. Most of this vision loss is preventable if the condition is diagnosed early and appropriate treatment is begun.

Diagnosis of keratitis is based on history of trauma, medication use, and signs and symptoms associated with corneal irritation and disease.[9] Because the cornea has many pain fibers, superficial or deep corneal abrasions cause discomfort, photophobia, and lacrimation. The discomfort may range from a foreign body sensation to severe pain. Defective vision results from the changes in transparency and curvature of the cornea that occur. Because of the discomfort involved, examination of the eye is often eased by instillation of a local anesthetic agent. Fluorescein staining can be used to outline an ulcerated area. The biomicroscope (slit lamp) is used for proper examination of the cornea. In cases of an infectious etiology, scrapings from the ulcer are obtained for staining and culture studies.

Keratitis can be divided into two types: nonulcerative, in which all the layers of the epithelium are affected but the epithelium remains intact, and ulcerative, in which parts of the epithelium, stroma, or both are destroyed. Nonulcerative or interstitial keratitis is associated with many diseases, including syphilis, tuberculosis, and lupus erythematosus. It also may result from a viral infection entering through a small defect in the cornea. Treatment is usually symptomatic.

Causes of ulcerative keratitis include infectious agents such as those causing conjunctivitis (*e.g., Staphylococcus, S. pneumoniae, Chlamydia*), exposure trauma, and use of extended-wear contact lenses. Bacterial keratitis is aggressive and demands immediate care. Exposure trauma may result from deformities of the lid, paralysis of the lid muscles, or severe exophthalmos. Mooren's ulcer is a chronic, painful, indolent ulcer that occurs in the absence of infection. It is usually seen in older persons and may affect both eyes. Although the cause is unknown, an autoimmune origin is suspected.

Acanthamoeba is a free-living protozoan that thrives in contaminated water. *Acanthamoeba keratitis* is an increasingly serious and sight-threatening complication of wearing a soft contact lens, particularly when homemade saline solutions are used for cleaning.[9] It also may occur in non–contact lens wearers after exposure to contaminated water or soil. It is characterized by pain that is disproportionate to the clinical manifestations, redness of the eye, and photophobia. The disorder commonly is misdiagnosed as herpes keratitis. Diagnosis is confirmed by scrapings and culture with specially prepared medium. In the early stages of infection, epithelial débridement may be beneficial. Treatment includes intensive use of topical antibiotics. However, the organism may encyst within the corneal stroma, making treatment more difficult. Keratoplasty may be necessary in advanced disease to arrest the progression of the infection.

Herpes Simplex Keratitis. Herpes simplex virus (HSV) keratitis is the most common cause of corneal ulceration in the United States. Most cases are caused by HSV type 1 infections. However, in neonatal infections acquired during passage through the birth canal, approximately 80% are caused by HSV type 2. The disease can occur as a primary or recurrent infection.[9] Primary infections cause follicular conjunctivitis and blepharitis, characterized by a rounded cobblestone pattern of avascular lesions. Epithelial keratitis may develop. After the initial primary infection, the virus may persist in a quiescent or latent state that remains in the trigeminal ganglion and possibly in the cornea without causing signs of infection. During childhood, mild primary herpes simplex virus infection may go unnoticed.

Recurrent infection may be precipitated by various poorly understood, stress-related factors that reactivate the virus. Involvement is usually unilateral. The first symptoms are irritation, photophobia, and tearing. Some reduction in vision may occur when the lesion affects the central part of the cornea. Because corneal anesthesia occurs early in the disease, the symptoms may be minimal, and the person may delay seeking medical care. A history of fever blisters or other herpetic infection is often noted, but corneal lesions may be the only sign of recurrent herpes infection. Most typically, the corneal lesion involves the epithelium and has a typical branching pattern. These epithelial lesions heal without scarring.

Herpetic lesions that involve the stromal layer of the cornea produce increasingly severe corneal opacities. They are thought to have an immune rather than an infectious cause. The most common cause of corneal blindness in the Western world is stromal scarring from herpes simplex keratitis.[9]

The treatment of HSV keratitis focuses on eliminating viral replication within the cornea while minimizing the damaging effects of the inflammatory process. It involves the use of epithelial debridement and drug therapy. Debridement is used to remove the virus from the corneal epithelium. Topical antiviral agents such as trifluridine (Viroptic) drops, idoxuridine (IDU) drops, or vidarabine (Vira-A) ointment are used to promote healing. Corticosteroid drugs increase viral replication. With a few exceptions, their use is usually contraindicated.

Varicella Zoster Ophthalmicus. Herpes zoster or shingles is a relatively common infection caused by herpesvirus type 3, the same virus that causes varicella (chickenpox).[10] It occurs when the varicella virus, which has remained dormant in the neurosensory ganglia since the primary infection, is reactivated. Herpes ophthalmicus, which represents 10% to 25% of all cases of herpes zoster, occurs when reactivation of the latent virus occurs in the ganglia of the ophthalmic division of the trigeminal nerve.[9,10] Immunocompromised persons, particularly those with human immunodeficiency disease (HIV) infection, are at higher risk for developing herpes zoster ophthalmicus than those with a normally functioning immune system.

Herpes zoster ophthalmicus usually presents with malaise, fever, headache, and burning and itching of the periorbital area. These symptoms commonly precede the eruption by 1 or 2 days. The rash, which is initially vesicular, becomes pustular and then crusting (see Chapter 61). Involvement of the tip of the nose and lid margins indicates a high likelihood of ocular involvement. Ocular signs include conjunctivitis, keratitis, and anterior uveitis, often with elevated intraocular pressure. Persons with corneal disease present with varying degrees of decreased vision, pain, and light insensitivity.

Treatment includes the use of high-dose oral antiviral drugs (acyclovir, valacyclovir). Initiation of treatment within the first 72 hours after the appearance of the rash reduces the incidence of ocular complications but not the postherpetic neuralgia (see Chapter 50).

Abnormal Corneal Deposits

The cornea frequently is the site for deposition of abnormal metabolic products. In hypercalcemia, calcium salts can precipitate in the cornea, producing a cloudy band keratopathy. Cystine crystals are deposited in cystinosis, cholesterol esters in hypercholesterolemia, and a golden ring of copper (*i.e.,* Kayser-Fleischer ring) in hepatolenticular degeneration due to Wilson's disease. Pharmacologic agents, such as chloroquine, can result in crystal deposits in the cornea.

Arcus senilis is an extremely common, bilateral, benign corneal degeneration that may occur at any age but is more common in the elderly. It consists of a grayish-white infiltrate, approximately 2 mm wide, that occurs at the periphery of the cornea. It represents an extracellular lipid infiltration and commonly is associated with hyperlipidemia. Arcus senilis does not produce visual symptoms, and there is no treatment for the disorder.

Corneal Transplantation

Advances in ophthalmologic surgery permit corneal transplantation using a cadaver cornea. Unlike kidney or heart transplantation procedures, which are associated with considerable risk for rejection of the transplanted organ, the use of cadaver corneas entails minimal danger of rejection because this tissue is not exposed to the vascular system and therefore the immunologic defense system. Instead, the success of this type of transplantation operation depends on the prevention of scar tissue formation, which would limit the transparency of the transplanted cornea.

DISORDERS OF THE UVEAL TRACT

The middle vascular layer, or uveal tract, is an incomplete ball with gaps at the pupil and the optic nerve (see Fig. 54-3). The pigmented uveal tract has three distinct regions: the choroid, ciliary body, and iris. The *choroid* is a highly vascular, dark-brown membrane that forms the posterior five sixths of the uveal tract. Its blood vessels provide nourishment for the other layers of the eyeball. Its brown pigment, produced by melanocytes, absorbs light within the eyeball and light that penetrates the retina. The light absorptive function prevents the scattering of light and is important for visual acuity, particularly with high background illumination levels. The *ciliary body* is a thickened ring of tissue that encircles the lens. It has smooth muscle and secretory functions. Its smooth muscle function contributes to changes in lens shape and its secretory function to the production of aqueous humor.

The iris is an adjustable diaphragm that permits changes in pupil size and in the light entering the eye. The posterior surface of the iris is formed by a two-layer epithelium continuous with those layers covering the ciliary body. The anterior layer contains the dilator or radial muscles of the iris. Just anterior to these muscles is a layer of highly vascular connective tissue. Embedded in this layer are concentric rings of smooth muscle that compose the sphincter muscle of the pupil. The anterior layer of the iris forms an irregular anterior surface, containing many fibroblasts and melanocytes. Eye color differences result from the density of the pigment. The amount of pigment decreases from that found in dark brown eyes through shades of brown and gray to that found in blue eyes.

Several mutations affect the pigment of the uveal tract, including albinism. *Albinism* is a genetic (autosomal recessive trait) deficiency of tyrosinase, the enzyme needed for the synthesis of melanin by the melanocytes. Tyrosinase-negative albinism, also called *classic albinism,* is characterized by an absence of tyrosinase; affected persons have white hair, pink skin, and light blue eyes. In these persons, excessive light penetrates the unpigmented iris and choroid, and, to some extent, the anterior sclera. Their photoreceptors are flooded with excess light, and visual acuity is markedly reduced. Excess stimulation of the photoreceptors at normal or high illumination levels is experienced as painful photophobia.

Uveitis

Inflammation of the entire uveal tract, which supports the lens and neural components of the eye, is called *uveitis*. It is one of several inflammatory disorders of ocular tissue with clinical features in common and an immunologically based cause.[5] A serious consequence of uveitis can be the involvement of the underlying retina. Parasitic invasion of the choroid can result in local atrophic changes that usually involve the retina; examples include toxoplasmosis and histoplasmosis. Sarcoid deposition in the form of small nodules results in irregularities of the underlying retinal surface.

THE PUPIL AND PUPILLARY REFLEXES

Changes in pupil size are controlled by contraction or relaxation of the dilator sphincter muscle of the iris. The pupillary reflex, which controls the size of the pupillary opening, is controlled by the autonomic nervous system, with the parasympathetic nervous system producing pupillary constriction or *miosis* and the sympathetic nervous system producing pupillary dilation or *mydriasis*. The sphincter muscle that produces pupillary constriction is innervated by postganglionic parasympathetic neurons of the ciliary ganglion and other scattered ganglion cells between the scleral and choroid layers. Part of the oculomotor (CN III) nucleus is called the *Edinger-Westphal nucleus.*[11] This autonomic nucleus, found in the midbrain, provides the preganglionic innervation for these parasympathetic axons. Pupillary dilation is provided by sympathetic innervation under excitatory descending control from the hypothalamus. Innervation is derived from preganglionic neurons in the upper thoracic cord, which send axons along the sympathetic chain to synapse with postganglionic neurons in the superior cervical ganglion. Postganglionic fibers travel along the surfaces of the carotid and smaller arteries to reach the eye.

The pupillary reflex is controlled by a region in the midbrain called the *pretectum*. Pretectal areas on each side of the brain are connected, explaining the binocular aspect of the light reflex. The afferent stimuli for pupillary constriction arise in the ganglionic cells of the retina and are transmitted to the *pretectal nuclei* at the junction of the thalamus and the midbrain, and from there to preganglionic neurons in the oculomotor (CN III) nuclei (Fig. 54-6).

Normal function of the pupillary reflex mechanism can be tested by shining a penlight into one eye of the person being tested. To avoid a change in pupil size due to accommodation, the person is asked to stare into the distance. A rapid constriction of the pupil exposed to light should occur; this is called the *direct pupillary light reflex.* Because the reflex is normally bilateral, the contralateral pupil also should constrict, a reaction called the *consensual pupillary light reflex.* The circuitry of the light reflex is partially separated from the main visual pathway. This is illustrated by the fact that the pupillary reflex remains unaffected when lesions to the optic radiations or the visual cortex occur. The cortically blind person retains direct and consensual light reflexes.

Integrity of the dual autonomic control of pupillary diameter is vulnerable to trauma, tumor enlargement, or vascular disease. With diffuse damage to the forebrain involving the thalamus and hypothalamus, the pupils are typically small but respond to light. Damage to the CN III nucleus or nerve eliminates innervation of four of the six extraocular muscles and the levator muscle of the upper lid, and it results in permanent pupillary dilation in the affected eye. Lesions affecting the cervical spinal cord or the ascending sympathetic ganglionic chain in the neck or internal carotid artery (e.g., Horner's syndrome) can interrupt the sympathetic control of the iris dilator muscle, resulting in permanent pupillary constriction. Tumors of the orbit that compress structures behind the eye can eliminate all pupillary reflexes, usually before destroying the optic nerve.

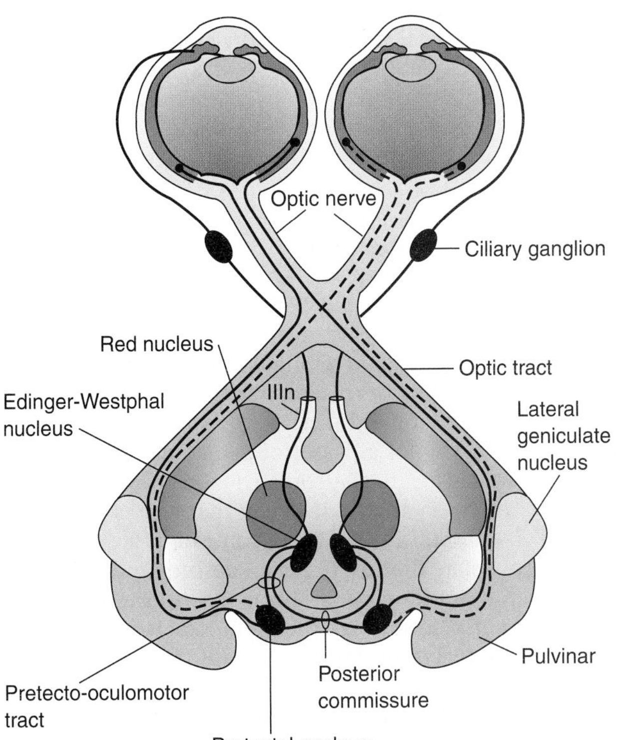

FIGURE 54-6 Diagram of the path of the pupillary light reflex. (Reproduced with permission from Walsh F.B., Hoyt W.F. [1969]. *Clinical neuro-ophthalmology* [3rd ed., vol. 1]. Baltimore: Williams & Wilkins)

Pupillary size can also be differentially affected by pharmacologic agents. Bilateral pupillary constriction is characteristic of opiate usage. Pupillary dilation results when topical parasympathetic blocking agents such as atropine are applied and sympathetic pupillodilatory function is left unopposed. These medications are used by ophthalmologists to facilitate the examination of the transparent media and fundus of the eye. Miotic drugs (*e.g.,* pilocarpine), which are used in the treatment of narrow-angle glaucoma, produce pupil constriction and in that manner facilitate aqueous humor circulation.

In summary, the conjunctiva lines the inner surface of the eyelids and covers the optic globe to the junction of the cornea and sclera. Conjunctivitis, also called *red eye* or *pink eye,* may result from bacterial or viral infection, allergens, chemical agents, physical agents, or radiant energy. It is important to differentiate between redness caused by conjunctivitis and that caused by more serious eye disorders, such as acute glaucoma or corneal lesions.

Keratitis, or inflammation of the cornea, can be caused by infections, hypersensitivity reactions, ischemia, trauma, or defects in tearing. Trauma or disease that involves the stromal layer of the cornea heals with scar formation and permanent opacification. These opacities interfere with the transmission of light and may impair vision.

The uveal tract is the middle vascular layer of the eye. It contains melanocytes that prevent diffusion of light through the wall of the optic globe. Inflammation of the uveal tract (uveitis) can affect visual acuity.

The pupillary reflex, which controls the size of the pupil, is controlled by the autonomic nervous system. The parasympathetic nervous system controls pupillary constriction, and the sympathetic nervous system controls pupillary dilation.

Intraocular Pressure and Glaucoma

After completing this section of the chapter, you should be able to meet the following objectives:

- Describe the formation and outflow of aqueous humor from the eye and relate to the development of glaucoma
- Compare closed-angle and open-angle glaucoma
- Explain why glaucoma leads to blindness

Glaucoma includes a group of conditions that produce an elevation in intraocular pressure. If left untreated, the pressure may increase sufficiently to cause ischemia and degeneration of the optic nerve, leading to progressive blindness. An estimated 60 million people worldwide currently have glaucoma. About 6 million people worldwide are blind from glaucoma, including 100,000 Americans, making it the leading cause of blindness in the United States.[12] African Americans are three to four times more likely to have open-angle glaucoma as whites, and even greater racial disparities exist in terms of blindness from the disease. The condition is often asymptomatic, and a significant loss of peripheral vision may occur before medical attention is sought.

CONTROL OF INTRAOCULAR PRESSURE

The intraocular pressure is largely regulated by the aqueous humor, which occupies the anterior segment of the optic globe. The aqueous humor serves to maintain the intraocular pressure and provides for the nutritive needs of the lens and posterior cornea. It contains a low concentration of protein and high concentrations of ascorbic acid, glucose, and amino acids. It also mediates the exchange of respiratory gases.

The aqueous humor is produced by the ciliary epithelium in the posterior chamber and flows between the anterior surface of the lens and posterior surface of the iris, through the pupil and into the anterior chamber. Aqueous humor, which is an ultrafiltrate of plasma, is secreted at an average rate of 2 to 3 microliters per minute.[13] Essentially all of the aqueous humor is secreted by the ciliary processes, which are linear folds that project from the ciliary body into the space behind the iris where the lens ligaments and ciliary muscle attach to the eyeball.

Aqueous humor leaves through the iridocorneal angle between the iris and the sclera. Here it filters through the trabecular meshwork and enters the canal of Schlemm for return to the venous circulation (see Fig. 54-5). The canal of Schlemm is actually a thin-walled vein that extends circumferentially around the eye. Its endothelial membrane is so porous that even large protein molecules up to the size of a red blood cell can pass from the posterior chamber into the canal of Schlemm.

The interior pressure of the eye must exceed atmospheric pressure to prevent the eyeball from collapsing. Hydrostatic pressure of the aqueous humor results from a balance of several factors: the rate of secretion, the resistance to flow between the iris and the ciliary body, and the resistance to resorption at the trabeculated region of the sclera at the iridocorneal angle. Normally, the rate of aqueous production is equal to the rate of aqueous outflow, and the intraocular pressure is maintained within a normal range of 9 to 21 mm Hg. However, data suggest that the value may be closer to 12 ±1 mm Hg in young, healthy adults during daylight hours. The mean value increases by approximately 1 mm Hg per decade after 40 years of age.[14]

GLAUCOMA

Glaucoma is an optic neuropathy characterized by optic disk cupping and visual field loss. It usually results from an increase in intraocular pressure that results from abnormalities in the balance between aqueous production and outflow. The most common cause is an interference with aqueous outflow from the anterior chamber, rather than overproduction of aqueous humor. Glaucoma is commonly classified as angle-closure (*i.e.,* narrow-angle) or open-angle (*i.e.,* wide-angle) glaucoma, depending on the location of the compromised aqueous humor production or circulation. Glaucoma may occur as a congenital or an acquired condition, and it may manifest as a primary or secondary disorder. Primary glaucoma occurs without evidence of preexisting ocular or systemic disease. Secondary glaucoma can result from inflammatory processes that affect the eye, from tumors, or from the blood cells of trauma-produced hemorrhage that obstruct the outflow of aqueous humor.

In glaucoma, temporary or permanent impairment of vision results from pressure-induced degenerative changes in the retina and optic nerve and from corneal edema and opacification. Damage to optic nerve axons in the region of the optic nerve can be recognized on ophthalmoscopic examination. The normal optic disk has a central depression called the *optic cup.* With progressive atrophy of axons caused by increased intraocular pressure, pallor of the optic disk develops, and the size and depth of the optic cup increase. Because changes in the optic cup precede the visual field loss, regular ophthalmoscopic examination is important for detecting eye changes that occur with increased intraocular pressure. Stereoscopic viewing during slit-lamp examination improves the accuracy of evaluation.[15]

Advances in computer technology allow detection and quantification of visual changes due to glaucoma. These tests of vision include color vision analysis, blue-on-yellow visual field testing and testing of contrast sensitivity, dark adaptation, and other tests of retinal function. In the future, these tests are likely to be used in detecting visual field defects not currently detected by standard means.

Angle-Closure Glaucoma

Angle-closure glaucoma results from occlusion of the anterior chamber angle by the iris (Fig. 54-7). It is most likely to develop in eyes with preexisting narrow anterior chambers. An acute attack is often precipitated by pupillary dilation, which causes the iris to thicken, blocking the circulation between the posterior and anterior chambers.[5,12,15] Approximately 5% to 10% of all cases of glaucoma fall into this category. Angle-closure glaucoma usually occurs as the result of an inherited anatomic defect that causes a shallow anterior chamber. It is seen more commonly in people of Far-Eastern, Asian, or Inuit (Eskimo) descent and in people with hypermetropic eyes.[12,15] This defect is exaggerated by the anterior displacement of the peripheral iris that occurs in older persons because of the increase in lens size that occurs with aging.

The depth of the anterior chamber can be evaluated by transillumination or by a technique called *gonioscopy.* Gonioscopy uses a special contact lens and mirrors or prisms to view and measure the angle of the anterior chamber. The transillumination method uses only a penlight. The light source is held at the temporal side of the

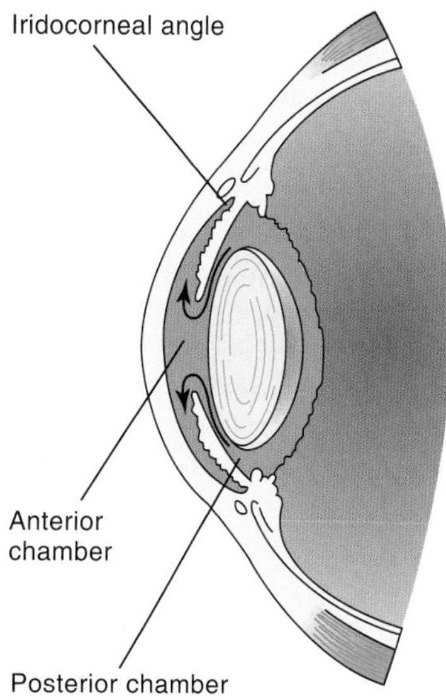

FIGURE 54-7 Narrow anterior chamber.

eye and directed horizontally across the iris. In persons with a normal-sized anterior chamber, the light passes through the chamber to illuminate both halves of the iris. In persons with a narrow anterior chamber, only the half of the iris adjacent to the light source is illuminated.

Symptoms of acute angle-closure glaucoma are related to sudden, intermittent increases in intraocular pressure. These occur after prolonged periods in the dark, emotional upset, and other conditions that cause extensive and prolonged dilation of the pupil. Administration of pharmacologic agents such as atropine that cause pupillary dilation (mydriasis) also can precipitate an acute episode of increased intraocular pressure in persons with the potential for angle-closure glaucoma. Attacks of increased intraocular pressure are manifested by ocular pain and blurred or iridescent vision caused by corneal edema.[12] The pupil may be enlarged and fixed. Symptoms are often spontaneously relieved by sleep and conditions that promote pupillary constriction. With repeated or prolonged attacks, the eye becomes reddened, and edema of the cornea may develop, giving the eye a hazy appearance. A unilateral, often excruciating, headache is common. Nausea and vomiting may occur, causing the headache to be confused with migraine.

Some persons with congenitally narrow anterior chambers never develop symptoms, and others develop symptoms only when they are elderly. Because of the dangers of vision loss, those with narrow anterior chambers should be warned about the significance of blurred vision, halos, and ocular pain. Sometimes, decreased visual acuity and an unreactive pupil may be the only clue to angle-closure glaucoma in the elderly.

The treatment of acute angle-closure glaucoma is primarily surgical. It involves creating an opening between the anterior and posterior chambers with laser or incisional iridectomy to allow aqueous humor to bypass the pupillary block. The anatomic abnormalities responsible for angle-closure glaucoma are usually bilateral, and prophylactic surgery is often performed on the other eye.

Open-Angle Glaucoma

Primary open-angle glaucoma is the most common form of glaucoma. It tends to manifest after 35 years of age, with an incidence of 0.5% to 2% among persons 40 years of age and older. The condition is characterized by an abnormal increase in intraocular pressure that occurs without obstruction at the iridocorneal angle, hence the name *open-angle glaucoma*. Instead, it usually occurs because of an abnormality of the trabecular meshwork that controls the flow of aqueous humor into the canal of Schlemm.[12,16]

Primary open-angle glaucoma is usually asymptomatic and chronic, causing progressive damage to the optic nerve and visual field loss unless it is appropriately treated. Elevated intraocular pressure is the major risk factor for open-angle glaucoma, but it is not the only diagnostic factor. Some people maintain a higher intraocular pressure without evidence of optic nerve or visual field loss. It is suggested that these people be described as glaucoma suspects or ocular hypertensives.[15]

The etiology of primary open-angle glaucoma remains unclear. There is question as to whether damage to the optic nerve is the result of excessive intraocular pressure, decreased blood flow to the optic nerve, or both factors. The only known causative risk factors are elevated intraocular pressure and insults to the eye, including trauma, uveitis, and corticosteroid therapy. Risk factors for this disorder include: an age of 40 years and older, black race, a positive first-degree family history, diabetes mellitus, and myopia.[15] In some persons, the use of moderate amounts of topical or inhaled corticosteroid medications can cause an increase in intraocular pressure. Sensitive persons also may sustain an increase in intraocular pressure with the use of systemic corticosteroid drugs.

Diagnostic methods include applanation tonometry (measurement of intraocular pressure), ophthalmoscopic visualization of the optic nerve, and central visual field testing. Measurement of intraocular pressures provides a means of assessing glaucoma risk. Because the condition is usually asymptomatic, persons at risk for open-angle glaucoma should have regular direct ophthalmoscopic examinations, on both eyes, concentrating on the optic disk. Optic disk changes frequently are noted before visual field defects become apparent.

The elevation in intraocular pressure in persons with open-angle glaucoma is usually treated pharmacologically or, in cases where pharmacologic treatment fails, by increasing aqueous outflow through a surgically created pathway. Drugs used in the long-term management of glaucoma fall into five classes: β-adrenergic antagonists, prostaglandin analogs, adrenergic agonists, carbonic anhydrase inhibitors, and cholinergic agonists.[17] Most glaucoma drugs are applied topically. However, systemic side effects may occur.

Topical β-adrenergic antagonists are usually the drugs of first choice for lowering intraocular pressure. The β-adrenergic antagonists are thought to lower intraocular pressure by decreasing aqueous humor production in the ciliary body. β-adrenergic antagonists decrease the production of aqueous humor by approximately one third.[17] Prostaglandins are locally acting hormones, found in most tissues. At low concentrations, prostaglandin $F_{2\alpha}$ increases uveoscleral outflow through the iris root and ciliary body, either by decreasing the extracellular matrix or by relaxing the ciliary musculature. A topical prostaglandin analog, latanoprost (Xalatan), is the only drug of this class currently available in the United States.[17]

Adrenergic agonists cause an early decrease in production of aqueous humor by constricting the vessels supplying the ciliary body. Nonselective adrenergic agents such as epinephrine stimulate both α and β receptors and tend to cause more systemic side effects such as tachycardia than nonselective drugs. Apraclonidine, an α-adrenergic agonist, reduces intraocular pressure by decreasing aqueous humor formation. Dipivefrin is a prodrug converted to epinephrine in the eye and seldom causes side effects.

Carbonic anhydrase inhibitors reduce the secretion of aqueous humor by the ciliary epithelium. Until recently, these drugs had to be taken orally, and systemic side effects were common. A topical carbonic anhydrase inhibitor (dorzolamide), which acts locally, is now available. Acetylcholine is the postganglionic neuromediator for the parasympathetic system; it increases aqueous outflow through contraction of the ciliary muscle and pupillary constriction (miosis). Cholinergic drugs exert their effects by increasing the effects of acetylcholine. Acetylcholine is broken down by the enzyme acetylcholinesterase. The most commonly used miotic drug is pilocarpine, which functions as a direct cholinergic agonist. Echothiophate, another miotic agent, acts indirectly by inhibiting the breakdown of acetylcholine by acetylcholinesterase.

When a reduction in intraocular pressure cannot be maintained through pharmacologic methods, surgical treatment may become necessary. Until recently, the main surgical treatment for open-angle glaucoma was a filtering procedure in which an opening was created between the anterior chamber and the subconjunctival space. An argon or neodymium–yttrium-aluminum-garnet (Nd:YAG) laser technique, in which multiple spots are applied 360 degrees around the trabecular meshwork, has been developed.[12] The microburns resulting from the laser treatment scar rather than penetrate the trabecular meshwork, a process thought to enlarge the outflow channels by increasing the tension exerted on the trabecular meshwork. Cryotherapy, diathermy, and high-frequency ultrasound may be used in some cases to destroy the ciliary epithelium and reduce aqueous humor production.

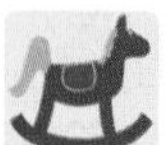

Congenital and Infantile Glaucoma

There are several types of childhood glaucoma including congenital glaucoma that is present at birth and infantile glaucoma that develops during the first 2 to 3 years of life. As with glaucoma in adults, childhood glaucoma can occur as a primary or secondary disorder.

Congenital glaucoma is caused by a disorder in which the anterior chamber retains its fetal configuration, with aberrant trabecular meshwork extending to the root of the iris, or is covered by a membrane. In general, it has a much poorer prognosis than infantile glaucoma. Primary infantile glaucoma occurs in approximately 1 in 10,000 live births but accounts for 2% to 15% of persons in institutions for the blind.[18] It is bilateral in 65% to 80% of cases and occurs more commonly in males than females. About 10% of cases have a familial origin, and the rest are either sporadic or possibly multifactorial with reduced penetrance. The familial cases are usually transmitted as an autosomal dominant trait with potentially high penetrance. Recent studies suggest a mutation in chromosome 2 (2p21 region). This gene is expressed in the tissues of the anterior chamber of the eye and its protein product plays an important role in the metabolism of molecules that are used in signaling pathways during the terminal stages of anterior chamber development.[18]

The earliest symptoms of congenital or infantile glaucoma are excessive lacrimation and photophobia. Affected infants tend to be fussy, have poor eating habits, and rub their eyes frequently. Diffuse edema of the cornea usually occurs, giving the eye a grayish-white appearance. Chronic elevation of the intraocular pressure before the age of 3 years causes enlargement of the entire globe (*i.e.*, buphthalmos). Early surgical treatment is necessary to prevent blindness.

In summary, glaucoma is a leading cause of blindness in the United States. It is characterized by conditions that cause an increase in intraocular pressure and that, if untreated, can lead to atrophy of the optic disk and progressive blindness. The aqueous humor is formed by the ciliary epithelium in the posterior chamber and flows through the pupil to the angle formed by the cornea and the iris. Here, it filters through the trabecular meshwork and enters the canal of Schlemm for return to the venous circulation. Glaucoma results from overproduction or the impeded outflow of aqueous humor from the anterior chamber of the eye.

Two major forms of glaucoma exist: angle closure and open angle. Angle-closure glaucoma is caused by a narrow anterior chamber and blockage of the outflow channels at the angle formed by the iris and the cornea. This occurs when the iris becomes thickened during pupillary dilation. Open-angle glaucoma is caused by microscopic obstruction of the trabecular meshwork. Open-angle glaucoma is usually asymptomatic, and considerable loss of the visual field often occurs before medical treatment is sought. Routine screening by applanation tonometry provides one of the best means for early detection of glaucoma before vision loss has occurred. Congenital glaucoma is caused by a disorder in which the anterior chamber retains its fetal configuration, with aberrant trabecular meshwork extending to the root of the iris, or is covered by a membrane. It occurs in approximately 1 in 10,000 live births but accounts for 2% to 15% of persons in institutions for the blind.

Disorders of the Lens and Lens Function

After completing this section of the chapter, you should be able to meet the following objectives:

- ✦ Describe the changes in eye structure that occur with cataract

- Cite risk factors associated with cataract
- Characterize the visual changes that occur with cataract
- Describe the treatment of persons with cataracts

The function of the eye is to transform light energy into nerve signals that can be transmitted to the cerebral cortex for interpretation. Optically, the eye is similar to a camera. It contains a lens system that inverts an image, an aperture (*i.e.*, the pupil) for controlling light exposure, and a retina that corresponds to the film and records the image.

DISORDERS OF REFRACTION AND ACCOMMODATION

The lens is an avascular, transparent, biconvex body, the posterior side of which is more convex than the anterior side. A thin, highly elastic lens capsule is attached to the surrounding ciliary body by delicate suspensory radial ligaments called *zonules,* which hold the lens in place (see Fig. 54-5). In providing for a change in lens shape, the tough elastic sclera acts as a bow, and the zonule and the lens capsule act as the bowstring. The suspensory ligaments and lens capsule are normally under tension, causing the lens to have a flattened shape for distant vision. Contraction of the muscle fibers of the ciliary body narrows the diameter of the ciliary body, relaxes the fibers of the suspensory ligaments, and allows the lens to relax to a more spherical or convex shape for near vision.

When light passes from one medium to another, its velocity is decreased or increased, and the direction of light transmission is changed. This change in direction of light rays is called *refraction.* When light rays pass through the center of a lens, their direction is not changed; however, other rays passing peripherally through a lens are bent (Fig. 54-8). The refractive power of a lens is usually described as the distance (in meters) from its surface to the point at which the rays come into focus (*i.e.*, focal length). Usually, this is reported as the reciprocal of this distance (*i.e.*, diopters).[13] For example, a lens that brings an object into focus at 0.5 m has a refractive power of 2 diopters (1.0/0.5 = 2.0). With a fixed-power lens, the closer an object is to the lens, the further behind the lens is its focus point. The closer the object, the stronger and more precise the focusing system must be.

In the eye, the major refraction of light begins at the convex corneal surface. Further refraction occurs as light moves from the posterior corneal surface to the aqueous humor, from the aqueous humor to the anterior lens surface, from the anterior lens surface to the posterior lens surface, and from the posterior lens surface to the vitreous humor.

Disorders of Refraction

A perfectly shaped optic globe and cornea result in optimal visual acuity, producing a sharp image in focus at all points on the retinal surface in the posterior part, or fundus, of the eye (see Fig. 54-8). Unfortunately, individual differences in formation and growth of the eyeball and cornea frequently result in inappropriate focal image formation. If the anteroposterior dimension of the eyeball is

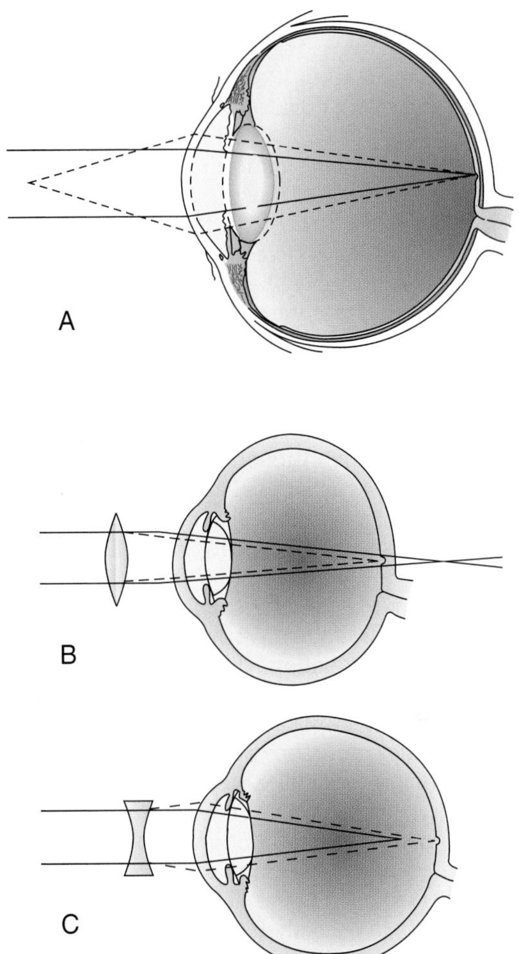

FIGURE 54-8 (**A**) Accommodation. The *solid lines* represent rays of light from a distant object, and the *dotted lines* represent rays from a near object. The lens needs to be flatter for the former and more convex for the latter. In each case, the rays of light are brought to a focus on the retina. (**B**) Hyperopia corrected by a biconvex lens, shown by the *dotted lines.* (**C**) Myopia corrected by a biconcave lens, shown by the *dotted lines.*

too short, the image is focused posterior to (behind) the retina. This is called *hyperopia* or *farsightedness.* In such cases, the accommodative changes of the lens can bring distant images into focus, but near images become blurred. Hyperopia is corrected by appropriate biconvex lenses. If the anteroposterior dimension of the eyeball is too long, the focus point for an infinitely distant target is anterior to the retina. This condition is called *myopia* or *nearsightedness* (see Fig. 54-8). Persons with myopia can see close objects without problems because accommodative changes in their lens bring near objects into focus, but distant objects are blurred. Myopia can be corrected with an appropriate biconcave lens. Radial keratotomy, a form of refractive corneal surgery, can be performed to correct the defect. This surgical procedure involves the use of radial incisions to alter the corneal curvature.

Refractive defects of the corneal surface do not permit the formation of a sharp image. Nonuniform curvature of the refractive medium (*e.g.*, horizontal vs. vertical plane) is called *astigmatism*. Astigmatism is usually the result of a defect in the cornea, but it can result from defects in the lens or the retina. Spherical aberration, another refractive error, involves a cornea with nonspherical surfaces. Lens correction is available for both refractive errors.

Disorders of Accommodation

Because the retina is at a fixed distance from the lens, adjustability in the refractive power of the lens is needed so that a clear image is maintained as gaze is shifted from afar to a near object. The process by which the refractory power of the lens is increased and the diverging light rays are bent more sharply is called *accommodation*. Accommodation requires convergence of the eyes, pupillary constriction, and thickening of the lens through contraction of the ciliary muscle. Contraction of the ciliary muscles is controlled mainly by the parasympathetic fibers of the oculomotor cranial nerve (CN III). In near vision, pupillary constriction (*i.e., miosis*) improves the clarity of the retinal image. This must be balanced against the resultant decrease in light intensity reaching the retina. During changes from near to far vision, pupillary dilation partially compensates for the reduced size of the retinal image by increasing the light entering the pupil. A third component of accommodation involves the reflex narrowing of the palpebral opening during near vision and widening during far vision.

Paralysis of the ciliary muscle, with loss of accommodation, is called *cycloplegia*. Pharmacologic cycloplegia is sometimes necessary to aid ophthalmoscopic examination of the fundus of the eye, especially in small children who are unable to hold a steady fixation during the examination. Lens shape is totally controlled by the pretectal region and the parasympathetic pathways through the oculomotor nerve to the ciliary muscle. Accommodation is lost with destruction of this pathway.

The term *presbyopia* refers to changes in vision that occur because of aging. The lens consists of transparent fibers arranged in concentric layers, of which the external layers are the newest and softest. No loss of lens fibers occurs with aging; instead, additional fibers are added to the outermost portion of the lens. As the lens ages, it thickens, and its fibers become less elastic, so that the range of focus or accommodation is diminished to the point at which reading glasses become necessary for near vision.

CATARACTS

A cataract is a lens opacity that interferes with the transmission of light to the retina. It has been estimated that 13 million persons in the United States 40 years of age or older are visually disabled because of cataracts.[1] Cataracts are the most common cause of age-related visual loss in the world; they are found in approximately 50% of those between 65 and 74 years of age and in 70% of those older than 75 years.[1] Cataract surgery is the most common surgical procedure covered by Medicare, with more than 1 million procedures performed annually. More than 90% of persons undergoing cataract surgery experience visual improvement if there is no ocular comorbidity.[19]

Causes and Types of Cataracts

The cause of cataract development is thought to be multifactorial, with different factors being associated with different types of opacities. The pathogenesis of cataracts is not completely understood. Several risk factors have been proposed, including the effects of aging, genetic influences, environmental and metabolic influences, drugs, and injury.[20] Metabolically induced cataracts are caused by disorders of carbohydrate metabolism (diabetes) or inborn errors of metabolism.[21] In a condition called *Lowe's syndrome*, abnormal synthesis of lens proteins leads to opacification. Long-term exposure to sunlight (ultraviolet B radiation) and heavy smoking has been associated with increased risk for cataract formation.[20] Occasionally, cataracts occur as a developmental defect (*i.e.*, congenital cataracts) or secondary to trauma or diseases.

Cataracts can result from several drugs. Corticosteroid drugs have been implicated as causative agents in cataract formation. Both systemic and inhaled corticosteroids have been cited as risk factors.[22,23] Other drugs associated with cataracts include the phenothiazines, amiodarone, and strong miotic ophthalmic drugs such as phospholine iodine.[20] Frequent examination of lens transparency should accompany the use of these and any other medications with potential cataract-forming effects.

Traumatic Cataract. Traumatic cataracts are most often caused by foreign body injury to the lens or blunt trauma to the eye. Foreign body injury that interrupts the lens capsule allows aqueous and vitreous humor to enter the lens and initiate cataract formation. Other causes of traumatic cataract are overexposure to heat (*e.g.*, glassblower's cataract) or to ionizing radiation. The radiation dose necessary to cause a cataract varies with the amount and type of energy; younger lenses are most vulnerable.

Congenital Cataract. A congenital cataract is one that is present at birth. Among the causes of congenital cataracts are genetic defects, toxic environmental agents, and viruses such as rubella.[8] A maternal rubella infection during the first trimester of pregnancy can cause congenital cataract. Cataracts and other developmental defects of the ocular apparatus depend on the total dose and the embryonic stage at the time of exposure. During the last trimester of pregnancy, genetically or environmentally influenced malformation of the superficial lens fibers can occur. Congenital lens opacities may occur in children of diabetic mothers.

Most congenital cataracts are not progressive and are not dense enough to cause significant visual impairment. However, if the cataracts are bilateral and the opacity is significant, lens extraction should be done on one eye by the age of 2 months to permit the development of vision and prevent nystagmus. If the surgery is successful, the contralateral lens should be removed soon after.

Senile Cataract. Cataract is the most common cause of age-related vision loss in the world.[24] With normal aging, the nucleus and the cortex of the lens enlarge as new fibers are formed in the cortical zones of the lens. In the nucleus, the old fibers become more compressed and dehydrated. Metabolic changes also occur. Lens proteins become more insoluble, and concentrations of calcium, sodium, potassium, and phosphate increase. During the early stages of cataract formation, a yellow pigment and vacuoles accumulate in the lens fibers. The unfolding of protein molecules, cross-linking of sulfhydryl groups, and conversion of soluble to insoluble proteins lead to the loss of lens transparency. The onset is usually gradual, and the only symptoms are increasingly blurred vision and visual distortion.

Manifestations

The manifestations of cataract depend on the extent of opacity and whether the defect is bilateral or unilateral. With the exception of traumatic or congenital cataract, most cataracts are bilateral. Age-related cataracts, which are the most common type, are characterized by increasingly blurred vision and visual distortion. Vision for far and near objects decreases. Dilation of the pupil in dim light improves vision. With nuclear cataracts (those involving the lens nucleus), the refractive power of the anterior segment often increases to produce an acquired myopia. Persons with hyperopia may experience a "second sight" or improved reading acuity until increasing opacity reduces acuity. Central lens opacities may divide the visual axis and cause an optical defect in which two or more blurred images are seen. Posterior subcapsular cataracts are located in the posterior cortical layer and usually involve the central visual axis. In addition to decreased visual acuity, cataracts tend to cause light entering the eye to be scattered, thereby producing glare or the abnormal presence of light in the visual field.

Diagnosis and Treatment

Diagnosis of cataract is based on ophthalmoscopic examination and the degree of visual impairment on the Snellen vision test. On ophthalmoscopic examination, cataracts may appear as a gross opacity filling the pupillary aperture or as an opacity silhouetted against the red background of the fundus. A Snellen test acuity of 20/50 is a common requirement for drivers of motor vehicles. Other tests of potential vision (*e.g.*, the ability to see well after surgery), such as electrophysiologic testing in which the response to visual stimuli is measured electronically, may be done.

There is no effective medical treatment for cataract. Use of strong bifocals, magnification, appropriate lighting, and visual aids may be used as the cataract progresses. Surgery is the only treatment for correcting cataract-related vision loss. Surgery usually involves lens extraction and intraocular lens implantation. It is commonly performed on an outpatient basis with the use of local anesthesia. The use of extracapsular surgery, which leaves the posterior capsule of the lens intact, has significantly improved the outcomes of cataract surgery. The cataract lens is usually removed using phacoemulsification techniques.[20,23] Phacoemulsification involves ultrasonic fragmentation of the lens into fine pieces, which then are aspirated from the eye.

One of the greatest advances in cataract surgery has been the development of reliable intraocular implants. Until recently, only monofocal intraocular lenses that correct for distance vision were available, and eyeglasses were needed for near vision. This has been remedied by the introduction of multifocal lenses.

In summary, the lens is a biconvex, avascular, colorless, and almost transparent structure suspended behind the iris. The shape of the lens is controlled by the ciliary muscle, which contracts and relaxes the zonule fibers, thus changing the tension on the lens capsule and altering the focus of the lens. Refraction, which refers to the ability to focus an object on the retina, depends on the size and shape of the eyeball and the cornea and on the focusing ability of the lens. Errors in refraction occur when the visual image is not focused on the retina because of individual differences in the size or shape of the eyeball or cornea. In hyperopia, or farsightedness, the image falls behind the retina. In myopia, or nearsightedness, the image falls in front of the retina. Accommodation is the process by which a clear image is maintained as the gaze is shifted from afar to a near object. It requires convergence of the eyes, pupillary constriction, and thickening of the lens through contraction of the ciliary muscle. Presbyopia is a change in the lens that occurs because of aging such that the lens becomes thicker and less able to change shape and accommodate for near vision.

A cataract is a lens opacity. It can occur as the result of congenital influences, metabolic disturbances, infection, injury, and aging. The most common type of cataract is the senile cataract that occurs with aging. Treatment of a totally opaque or mature cataract is surgical extraction. An intraocular lens implant may be inserted during the surgical procedure to replace the removed lens; otherwise, thick convex lenses or contact lenses are used to compensate for the loss of lens function.

Disorders of the Vitreous and Retina

After completing this section of the chapter, you should be able to meet the following objectives:

- Relate the phagocytic function of the retinal pigment epithelium to the development of retinitis pigmentosa
- Cite the manifestations and long-term visual effects of papilledema and central artery and central venous occlusions
- Describe the pathogenesis of background and proliferative diabetic retinopathies and their mechanisms of visual impairment
- Discuss the cause of retinal detachment
- Explain the pathology and visual changes associated with macular degeneration

The posterior segment, comprising five sixths of the eyeball, contains the transparent vitreous humor and the neural retina. The posterior aspect of the retina, the fundus, is visualized through the pupil with an ophthalmoscope.

S OF THE VITREOUS

mor (*i.e.,* vitreous body) is a colorless, amor- gic gel that fills the posterior cavity of the eye. f approximately 99% water, some salts, glycoproteins, proteoglycans, and dispersed collagen fibrils. The vitreous is attached to the ciliary body and the peripheral retina in the region of the ora serrata and to the periphery of the optic disk.

Disease, aging, and injury can disturb the factors that maintain the water of the vitreous humor in suspension, causing liquefaction of the gel to occur. With the loss of gel structure, fine fibers, membranes, and cellular debris develop. When this occurs, floaters (images) can often be noticed as these substances move within the vitreous cavity during head movement. Blood vessels may grow from the surface of the retina or optic nerve into the posterior surface of the vitreous, and cause bleeding into the vitreous cavity.

In a procedure called a *vitrectomy,* the removal and replacement of the vitreous with a balanced saline solution can restore sight in some persons with vitreous opacities resulting from hemorrhage or vitreoretinal membrane formations that cause legal blindness. Using this procedure, a small probe with a cutting tip is used to remove the opaque vitreous and membranes. The procedure is difficult and requires complex instrumentation. It is of no value if the retina is not functional.

DISORDERS OF THE RETINA

The function of the retina is to receive visual images, partially analyze them, and transmit this modified information to the brain.[11] It is composed of two layers: the outer, melanin-containing layer and the inner neural layer. The light-sensitive neural retina covers the inner aspect of the eyeball. A non–light-sensitive portion of the retina, along with the retinal pigment epithelium, continues anteriorly to form the posterior surface of the iris. A wavy border called the *ora serrata* exists at the junction between the light-sensitive and the non–light-sensitive retinas. Separating the vascular portion of the choroid from the single layer of pigmented cells is a thin layer of elastic tissue, *Bruch's membrane,* which contains collagen fibrils in its superficial and deep portions. Cells of the pigmented layer receive their nourishment by diffusion from the choroid vessels. Tight junctions between the endothelial cells of the retinal blood vessels combine to form a blood–retina barrier.

Disorders of the retina and its function include derangements of the pigment epithelium (*e.g.,* retinitis pigmentosa); ischemic conditions caused by disorders of the retinal blood supply; disorders of the retinal vessels such as retinopathies that cause hemorrhage and the development of opacities; separation of the pigment and sensory layers of the retina (*i.e.,* retinal detachment); retinopathy of prematurity; and abnormalities of Bruch's membrane and choroid (*e.g.,* macular degeneration). Because the retina has no pain fibers, most diseases of the retina are painless.

The Neural Retina

The neural retina is composed of three layers of neurons: a posterior layer of photoreceptors, a middle layer of bipolar cells, and an inner layer of ganglion cells that communicate with the photoreceptors (Fig. 54-9). A pattern of light on the retina falls on a massive array of photoreceptors. These photoreceptors synapse with bipolar and other interneurons before action potentials in ganglion cells relay the message to specific regions of the brain and the brain stem associated with vision. For rods, this micro-

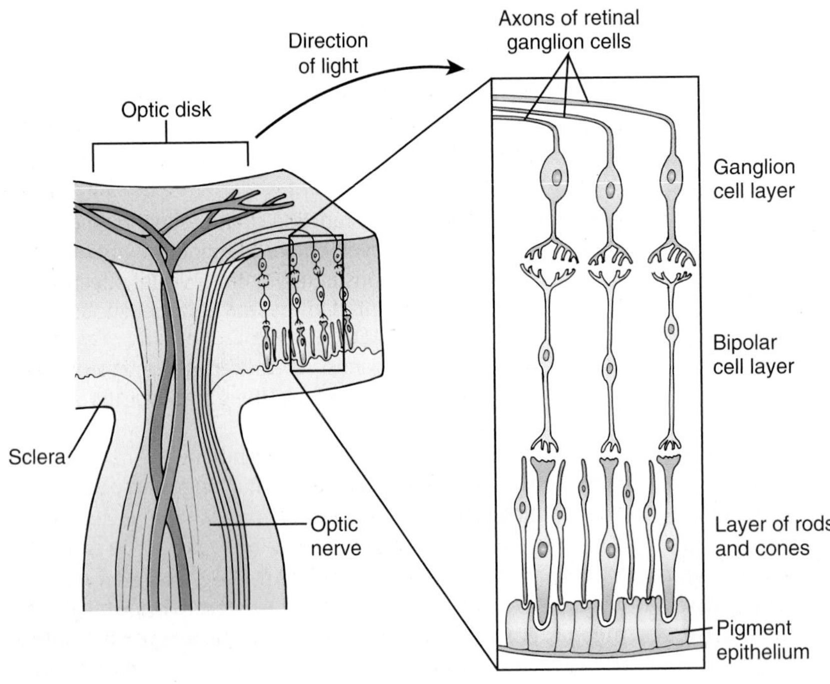

FIGURE 54-9 Organization of the human retina. The visual pathway begins with photoreceptors (rods and cones) in the retina. The responses of the photoreceptors are transmitted by the bipolar cells to the ganglion cell layer of the retina.

circuitry involves the convergence of signals from many rods on a single ganglion cell. This arrangement maximizes spatial summation and the detection of stimulated (light vs. dark) receptors. The interneurons, composed of horizontal and amacrine cells, have cell bodies in the bipolar layer, and they play an important role in modulating retinal function. A superficial marginal layer contains the axons of the ganglion cells as they collect and leave the eye by way of the optic nerve (see Fig. 54-9). These fibers lie beside the vitreous humor. Light must pass through the transparent inner layers of the sensory retina before it reaches the photoreceptors.

Photoreceptors

Two types of photoreceptors are present in the retina: rods, capable of black–white discrimination, and cones, capable of color discrimination.[11] Both types of photoreceptors are thin, elongated, mitochondria-filled cells with a single, highly modified cilium (Fig. 54-10). The cilium has a short base, or inner segment, and a highly modified outer segment. The plasma membrane of the outer segment is tightly folded to form membranous disks (rods) or conical shapes (cones) containing visual pigment. These disks are continuously synthesized at the base of the outer segment and shed at the distal end. Discarded membranes are phagocytized by the retinal pigment cells. If this phagocytosis is disrupted, as in retinitis pigmentosa, the sensory retina degenerates.

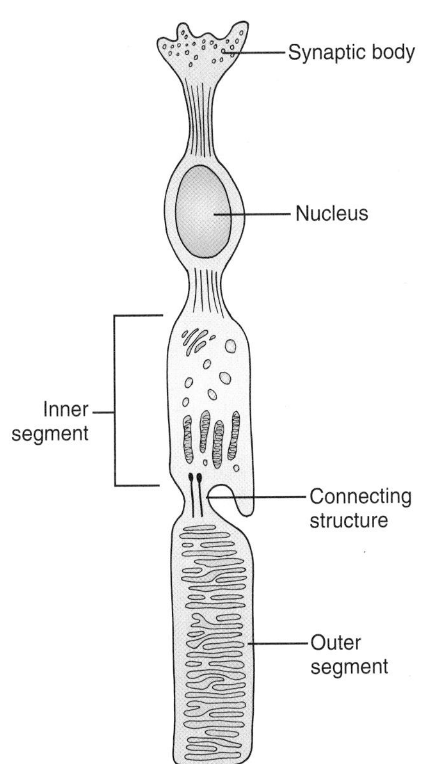

FIGURE 54-10 Retinal rod, showing its component parts and the distribution of its organelles. Its outer segment contains the disks (rods). The connecting structure joins the outer and inner segments. The inner segment contains the mitochondria, the ribosomal endoplasmic reticulum, the free ribosomes, and the Golgi saccules. The synaptic body forms the site where the photo receptors synapse with other nerve cells.

Rods. Photoreception involves the transduction of light energy into an altered ionic membrane potential of the rod cell. Light passing through the eye penetrates the nearly transparent neural elements to produce decomposition of the photochemical substance (visual pigment) called *rhodopsin* in the outer segment of the rod. Light that is not trapped by a rhodopsin molecule is absorbed by the retinal pigment melanin or the more superficial choroid melanin. Rhodopsin consists of a protein called *opsin* and a vitamin A–derived pigment called *retinal.* During light stimulation, rhodopsin is broken down into its component parts, opsin and retinal; retinal subsequently is converted into vitamin A. The reconstitution of rhodopsin occurs during total darkness; vitamin A is transformed into retinal, and then opsin and retinal combine to form rhodopsin. Considerable stores of vitamin A are present in the retinal pigment cells and in the liver; therefore, a vitamin A deficiency must be present for weeks or months to affect the photoreceptive process. Reduced sensitivity to light, a symptom of vitamin A deficiency, initially affects night vision; however, this is quickly reversed by injection or ingestion of the vitamin.

Rod-based vision is particularly sensitive to detecting light, especially moving light stimuli, at the expense of clear pattern discrimination. Rod vision is particularly adapted for night and low-level illumination. Dark adaptation is the process by which rod sensitivity increases to the optimum level. This requires approximately 4 hours in total or near-total darkness and involves only rods or scotopic vision (night vision). During daylight or high-intensity bombardment, the concentration of vitamin A increases, and the concentration of the photopigment retinal decreases. During dark adaptation, increased synthesis of retinal from vitamin A results in a higher concentration of rhodopsin for capture of light energy.

Cones and Color Sensitivity. Cone receptors that are selectively sensitive to different wavelengths of light provide the basis for color vision. Three types of cones, or cone-color systems, respond to the blue, green, and red portions of the visible electromagnetic spectrum. This selectivity reflects the presence of one of three color-sensitive molecules to which the photochemical substance (visual pigment) is bound. The decomposition and reconstitution processes of the cone visual pigments are believed to be similar to that of the rods. The color a person perceives depends on which set of cones or combination of sets of cones is stimulated in a given image.

Cones do not have the dark adaptation of rods. Consequently, the dark-adapted eye is a rod receptor eye with only black-gray-white experience (*scotopic* or *night vision*). The light-adapted eye (*photopic vision*) adds the capacity for color discrimination. Rhodopsin has its maximum sensitivity in the blue-green region of the electromagnetic spectrum. If red lenses are worn in daylight, the red cones (and green cones to some extent) are in use, whereas the rods and blue cones are essentially in the dark, and therefore dark adaptation proceeds. This method is used by military and night-duty airport control tower personnel to allow adaptation to take place before they go on duty in the dark.

Macula and Fovea. An area approximately 1.5 mm in diameter near the center of the retina, called the *macula lutea* (*i.e.*, "yellow spot"), is especially adapted for acute and detailed vision.[11] This area is composed entirely of cones. In the central portion of the macula, the *fovea centralis* (foveola), blood vessels, and innermost layers are displaced to one side instead of resting on top of the cones (Fig. 54-11). This allows light to pass unimpeded to the cones without passing through several layers of the retina. Of the approximately 6.4 million cones found in the retina, 200,000 cones are located in the fovea. The density of cones drops off rapidly away from the fovea. Rods are not present in the fovea, but their numbers increase as the cones decrease in density toward the periphery of the retina. An estimated 110 to 125 million rods are found in the retina.

Many cones are connected one-to-one with ganglion cells. Retinal microcircuitry for cones emphasizes the detection of edges. This type of circuitry favors high acuity. A concentration of acuity-favoring cones at the fovea supports the use of this part of the retina for fine analysis of focused central vision. It is not until the age of 4 years that the fovea is fully developed.

Color Blindness. Color blindness is a misnomer for a condition in which persons appear to confuse or mismatch colors or experience reduced acuity for color discrimination. Such persons are often unaware of their defect until they attempt to discriminate between red and green traffic lights or show difficulty matching colors. Most often the result of genetic factors, the deficit can result from the defective function of one or more of the three color-cone mechanisms. The deficiency is usually partial but can be complete. Rarely are two of the color mechanisms missing; when this occurs, usually red and green are missing. Persons with no color mechanisms are rare. For them, the world is experienced entirely as black, gray, and white.

The genetically color-blind person has never experienced the full range of normal color vision and is unaware of what he or she is missing. Color discrimination is necessary for everyday living, and color-blind persons, knowingly or unknowingly, make color discriminations based on other criteria, such as brightness or position. For example, the red light of a traffic signal is always the upper light, and the green is the lower light. Color-blind persons experience difficulties when brightness differences are small and discrimination must be based on hue and saturation qualities.

The genes responsible for color blindness affect receptor mechanisms rather than central acuity. The gene for the red and green mechanisms is sex linked (*i.e.*, on the X chromosomes), resulting in a much higher incidence among males of red, green, or red-green color blindness; however, the gene affecting the blue mechanism is autosomal. Acquired color defects are more complex but follow a general rule: disease of the more peripheral retina affects blue discrimination, and disease of the more central retina affects red and green discrimination because blue cones are not present in the central fovea.

Retinitis Pigmentosa. Retinitis pigmentosa (RP) is a group of hereditary diseases that cause slow degenerative changes in the retinal photoreceptors.[25,26] There are several modes

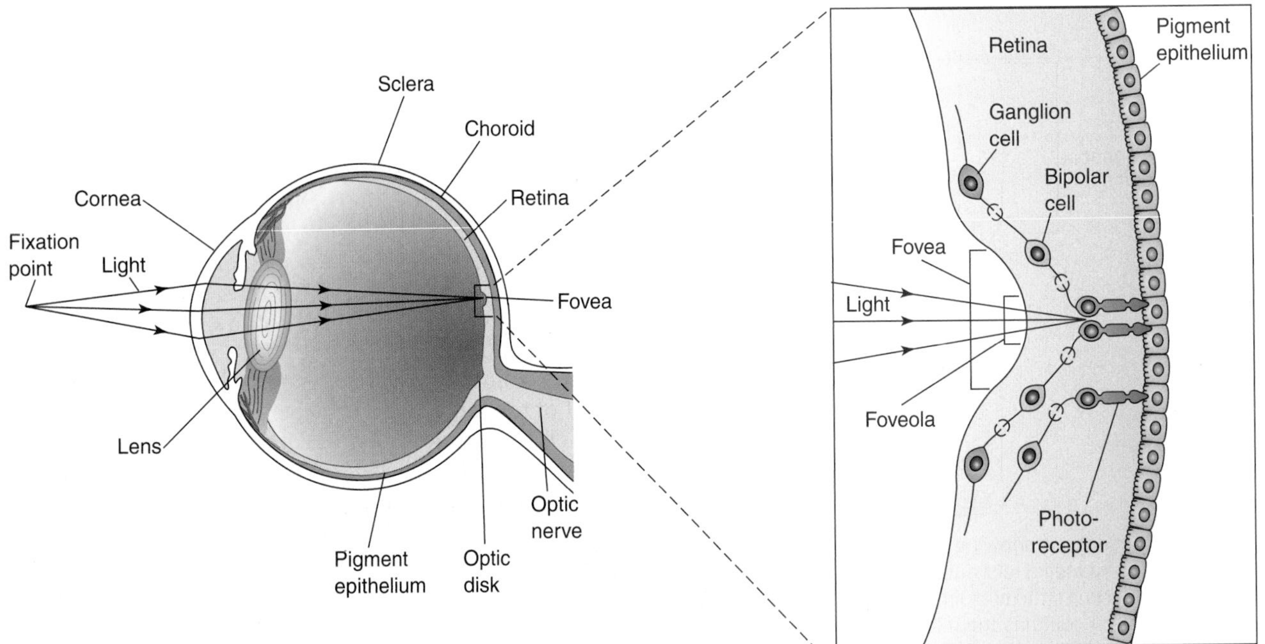

FIGURE 54-11 Location of fovea in the retina. (Kandel E.R., Schwartz J.H., Jessell T.M. [1991]. *Principles of neural science* [3rd ed.]. New York: Elsevier)

of inheritance, including autosomal dominant, autosomal recessive, sex linked, and sporadic. With the advances of gene technology, there are now 36 known or predicted RP genes.[25] The most common group of these mutated genes are those encoding proteins in the visual cascade of the photoreceptor outer segment.

In typical cases, known as rod-cone RP, the rods are the predominantly affected photoreceptor cells. This generally produces a number of characteristic clinical symptoms including night blindness, which is usually an early symptom, and bilateral symmetric loss of mid-peripheral fields. Although there is relative preservation of macular vision, the visual field defects gradually increase both centrally and peripherally. With progression, cone photoreceptor cells are also affected, and day vision and central visual acuity are compromised. The rate of visual failure is variable. Some people are severely visually handicapped before the age of 20, whereas others experience few symptomatic visual deficits even after age 70.[26]

DISORDERS OF THE RETINAL BLOOD SUPPLY

- The blood supply for the retina is derived from the central retinal artery, which supplies blood flow for the entire inside of the retina, and from vessels in the choroid, which supply the rods and cones.
- Central retinal occlusion interrupts blood flow to the inner retina and results in unilateral blindness.
- The retinopathies, which are disorders of the retinal vessels, interrupt blood flow to the visual receptors, leading to visual impairment.
- Retinal detachment separates the visual receptors from the choroid, which provides their major blood supply.

Disorders of Retinal Blood Supply

The blood supply for the retina is derived from two sources: the choriocapillaris of the choroid and the branches of the central retinal artery (Fig. 54-12). Oxygen and other nutritional substances needed by the retina and its component parts (pigment cells, rods and cones) are supplied by diffusion from blood vessels in the choroid. Because the choriocapillary layer provides the only blood supply for the fovea centralis (*i.e.*, foveola), detachment of this part of the sensory retina from the pigment epithelium causes irreparable visual loss.

The bipolar, horizontal, amacrine, and ganglion cells, and the ganglion cell axons that gather at the optic disk, are supplied by branches of the central retinal artery.[27] The central artery of the retina is a branch of the ophthalmic artery. It enters the globe through the optic disk. Branches of this artery radiate over the entire retina, except the central fovea, which is surrounded by, but is not crossed by, arterial branches. The central retinal artery is an end artery meaning that it does not anastomose with other arteries. This is critical because an infarct in this artery will totally deprive distal structures of their vascular supply. Retinal veins follow a distribution parallel to the arterial branches and carry venous blood to the central vein of the retina, which exits the back of the eye through the optic disk.

Funduscopic examination of the eye with an ophthalmoscope provides an opportunity to examine the retinal blood vessels and other aspects of the retina (Fig. 54-13). Because the retina is an embryonic outgrowth of the brain

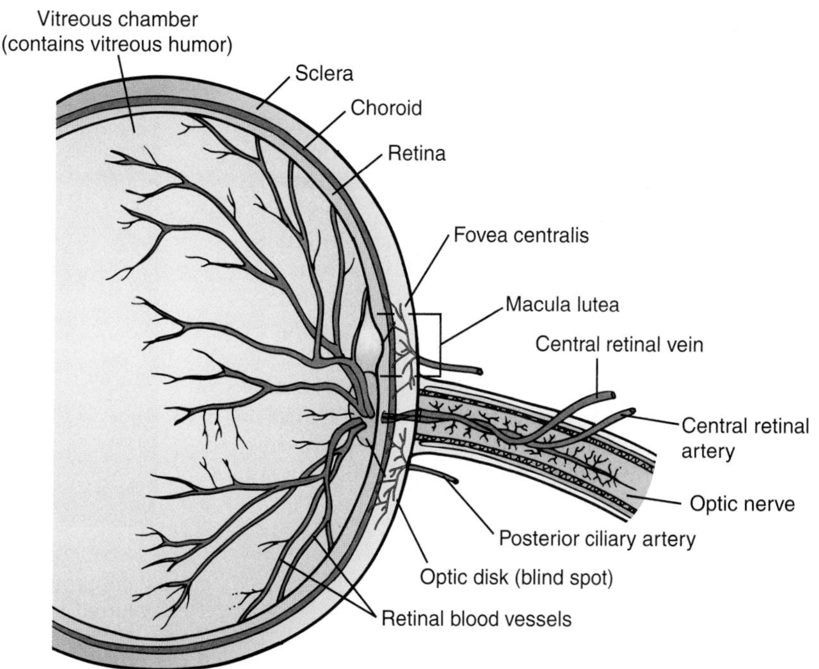

FIGURE 54-12 Retinal circulation.

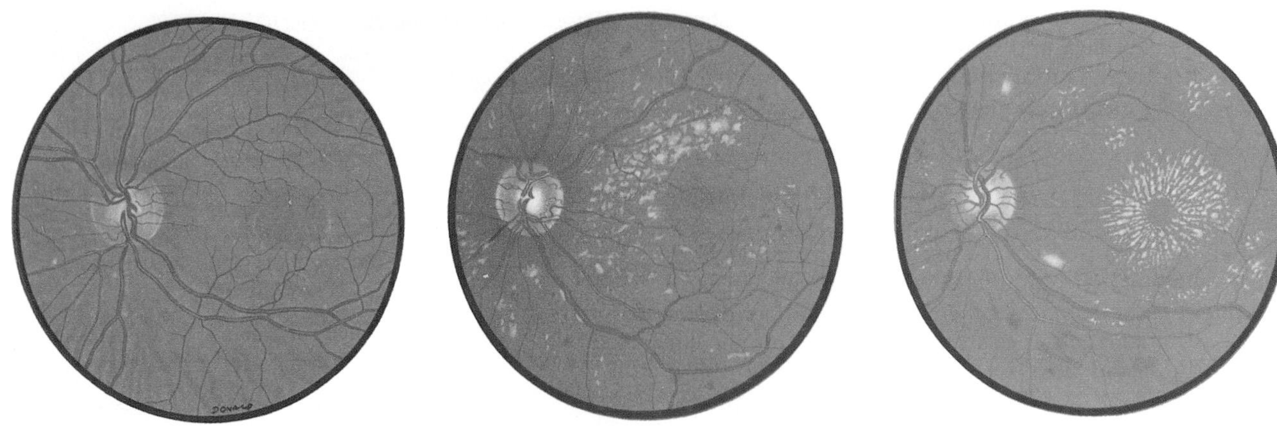

FIGURE 54-13 Fundus of the eye as seen in retinal examination with an ophthalmoscope: (**left**) normal fundus; (**middle**) diabetic retinopathy—combination of microaneurysms, deep hemorrhages, and hard exudates of background retinopathy; (**right**) hypertensive retinopathy with purulent exudates. Some exudates are scattered, while others radiate from the fovea to form a macular star. (Bates B. [1995]. *A guide to physical examination and history taking.* (pp. 208, 210). Philadelphia: J.B. Lippincott)

and the blood vessels are to a considerable extent representative of brain blood vessels, the ophthalmoscopic examination of the fundus of the eye permits the study and diagnosis of metabolic and vascular diseases of the brain and of pathologic processes that are specific to the retina.

Functioning of the retina, like that of other cellular portions of the central nervous system (CNS), depends on an oxygen supply from the vascular system. One of the earliest signs of decreased perfusion pressure in the head region is a graying-out or blackout of vision, which usually precedes loss of consciousness. This can occur during large increases in intrathoracic pressure, which interfere with the return of venous blood to the heart, as occurs with Valsalva's maneuver; with systemic hypotension; and during sudden postural movements (e.g., postural hypotension).

Ischemia of the retina occurs during general circulatory collapse. If a person survives cardiopulmonary arrest, for instance, permanently decreased visual acuity can occur as a result of edema and the ischemic death of retinal neurons. This is followed by primary optic nerve atrophy proportional to the extent of ganglionic cell death. The ophthalmic artery, the source of the central retinal artery, takes its origin from the internal carotid artery.[27]

Intermittent retinal ischemia can accompany internal carotid or common carotid stenosis. *Amaurosis fugax* is characterized by transient episodes of monocular visual loss lasting 5 to 10 minutes.[27] Persons with the disorder often describe a curtain coming down from above or across their vision, usually with complete return of vision within seconds or minutes. Besides the vision loss, contralateral hemiplegia or sensory deficits may accompany the episodes. The condition, commonly due to emboli, is most often the result of carotid artery disease.[27]

Papilledema. The central retinal artery enters the eye through the optic papilla in the center of the optic nerve. An accompanying vein exits the eye along the same path. The entrance and exit of the central artery and vein of the retina through the tough scleral tissue at the optic papilla can be compromised by any condition causing persistent increased intracranial pressure. The most common of these conditions are cerebral tumors, subdural hematomas, hydrocephalus, and malignant hypertension.

Usually, the thin-walled, low-pressure veins are the first to collapse, with the consequent backup and slowing of arterial blood flow. Under these conditions, capillary permeability increases, and leakage of fluid results in edema of the optic papilla, called *papilledema.* The interior surface of the papilla is normally cup shaped and can be evaluated through an ophthalmoscope. With papilledema, sometimes called *choked disk,* the optic cup is distorted by protrusion into the interior of the eye (Fig. 54-14). Because this sign does not occur until the intracranial pressure is significantly elevated, compression damage to the optic nerve fibers passing through the lamina cribrosa may have

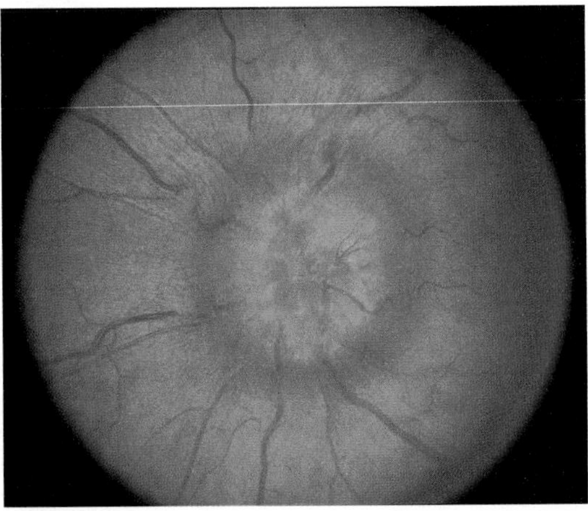

FIGURE 54-14 Chronic papilledema. The optic nerve head is congested and protrudes anteriorly toward the interior of the eye. It has blurred margins, and vessels within it are poorly seen. (Rubin E., Farber J.L. [1999]. *Pathology* [3rd ed., p. 1558]. Philadelphia: Lippincott-Raven)

begun. As a warning sign, papilledema occurs quite late. Unresolved papilledema results in the destruction of the optic nerve axons and blindness.

Central Retinal Artery Occlusion. Complete occlusion of the central artery of the retina results in sudden unilateral blindness. This is an uncommon disorder of older persons and most often is caused by embolism or atherosclerosis. Because the retina has a dual blood supply, the survival of retinal structures is possible if blood flow can be reestablished within approximately 90 minutes.[27] If blood flow is not restored, the infarcted retina swells and opacifies. Because the receptors of the central fovea are supplied with blood from the choroid, they survive (*i.e.,* macular sparing). A cherry-red spot, indicating a healthy fovea, is surrounded by the pale white, opacified retina.[31] Although the nerve fibers of the optic disk are adequately supplied by the choroid, the disk becomes pale after death of the ganglion cells and their axonal processes (*i.e.,* optic nerve fibers), resulting in optic nerve atrophy.

Occlusions of branches of the central artery, called *branch arterial occlusions,* are essentially retinal strokes. These occur mainly from emboli and local infarction in the neural retina. The opacification that follows is often slowly resolved, and retinal transparency is restored. Local blind spots or scotomas may occur after destruction of local elements of the retina. Loss of the axons of destroyed ganglion cells results in some optic nerve atrophy.

Central Retinal Vein Occlusion. Occlusion of the central retinal vein results in venous dilation, stasis, and reduced flow through the retinal veins. It is usually monocular and causes painless rapid deterioration of visual acuity because of an accompanying increase in capillary wall fragility and a lack of arterial inflow.[27] Superficial and deep hemorrhages may occur throughout the retina.

Among the causes of central retinal vein obstruction are hypertension, diabetes mellitus, and conditions such as sickle cell anemia that slow venous blood flow. The reduction in blood flow results in neovascularization with fibrovascular invasion of the space between the retina and the vitreous humor. Besides obstructing normal visual function, the new vessels are fragile and prone to hemorrhage. Escaped blood may fill the space between the retina and vitreous, producing the appearance of a sudden veil over the visual field. The blood can find its way into the aqueous humor (*i.e.,* hemorrhagic glaucoma). Photocoagulation of the spreading new blood vessels with high-intensity light or laser beam is used to prevent blindness and eye pain. As the hemorrhage is resolved, degenerating blood products can produce contraction of the vitreous and formation of fibrous tissue within it, causing tears and detachment of the retina.

Much more common are local vein occlusions with regional and focal capillary microhemorrhages that produce the same but more restricted pathologic effects. These microhemorrhages result in the formation of rings of yellow exudate composed of lipid and lipoprotein blood breakdown products. Microhemorrhages deep in the neural retina are somewhat restricted by the vertical organization of the neural elements and result in dot hemorrhages. Microhemorrhages in the layer of ganglionic cell axon bundles result in the appearance of cotton-wool spots on the fundus.

Retinopathies

Disorders of the retinal vessels result in microaneurysms, neovascularization, hemorrhage, and formation of retinal opacities. *Microaneurysms* are outpouchings of the retinal vasculature. On ophthalmoscopic examination, they appear as minute, unchanging red dots associated with blood vessels. These microaneurysms tend to leak plasma, resulting in localized edema that gives the retina a hazy appearance. Microaneurysms can be identified with certainty using fluorescein angiography; the fluorescein dye is injected intravenously, and the retinal vessels subsequently are photographed using a special ophthalmoscope and fundus camera. The microaneurysms may bleed, but areas of hemorrhage and edema tend to clear spontaneously. However, they reduce visual acuity if they encroach on the macula and cause degeneration before they are absorbed.

Neovascularization involves the formation of new blood vessels. They can develop from the choriocapillaris, extending between the pigment layer and the sensory layer, or from the retinal veins, extending between the sensory retina and the vitreous cavity and sometimes into the vitreous. These new blood vessels are fragile, leak protein, and are likely to bleed. Neovascularization occurs in many conditions that impair retinal circulation, including stasis because of hyperviscosity of blood or decreased flow, vascular occlusion, sickle cell disease, sarcoidosis, diabetes mellitus, and retinopathy of prematurity. Although the cause of neovascularization is uncertain, research links the process with a vascular endothelial growth factor (VEGF) produced by the lining of blood vessels.[28,29] The vitreous humor is thought to contain a substance that normally inhibits neovascularization, and this factor apparently is suppressed under conditions in which the new blood vessels invade the vitreous cavity. It is likely that other growth factors and signaling systems are also involved.

Hemorrhage can be preretinal, intraretinal, or subretinal. Preretinal hemorrhages occur between the retina and the vitreous. These hemorrhages are usually large because the blood vessels are only loosely restricted; they may be associated with a subarachnoid or subdural hemorrhage and are usually regarded as a serious manifestation of the disorder. They usually reabsorb without complications unless they penetrate into the vitreous. Intraretinal hemorrhages occur because of abnormalities of the retinal vessels, diseases of the blood, increased pressure in the retinal vessels, or vitreous traction on the vessels. Systemic causes include diabetes mellitus, hypertension, and blood dyscrasias. Subretinal hemorrhages are those that develop between the choroid and pigment layer of the retina. A common cause of subretinal hemorrhage is neovascularization. Photocoagulation may be used to treat microaneurysms and neovascularization.

Light normally passes through the transparent inner portions of the sensory retina before reaching the photoreceptors. Opacities such as hemorrhages, exudate, cotton-wool patches, and edema can produce a localized loss of transparency observable with an ophthalmoscope. Exudates are opacities resulting from inflammatory processes. The development of exudates often results in the destruction of the underlying retinal pigment and choroid layer. Deposits are localized opacities consisting of lipid-laden macrophages or accumulated cellular debris. Cotton-wool patches are retinal opacities with hazy, irregular outlines. They occur in the nerve fiber layer and contain cell organelles. Cotton-wool patches are associated with retinal trauma, severe anemia, papilledema, and diabetic retinopathy.

Diabetic Retinopathy. Diabetic retinopathy is the third leading cause of blindness for all ages in the United States. It ranks first as the cause of newly reported cases of blindness in persons between the ages of 20 and 74 years. During the first two decades of the disease, nearly all persons with type 1 diabetes and more than 60% of persons with type 2 diabetes have retinopathy.[30]

Diabetic retinopathy can be divided into two types: *nonproliferative* (*i.e.*, background) and *proliferative*.[31] Background or nonproliferative retinopathy is confined to the retina. It involves thickening of the retinal capillary walls and microaneurysm formation (Fig. 54-15). Ruptured capillaries cause small intraretinal hemorrhages, and microinfarcts may cause cotton-wool exudates. A sensation of glare (because of the scattering of light) is a common complaint. The most common cause of decreased vision in persons with background retinopathy is macular edema.[28,29] It represents fluid accumulation in the retina stemming from a breakdown in the blood–retina barrier.

Proliferative diabetic retinopathy represents a more severe retinal change than background retinopathy. It is characterized by formation of fragile blood vessels (*i.e.*, neovascularization) at the disk and elsewhere in the retina. These vessels grow in front of the retina along the posterior surface of the vitreous or into the vitreous. They threaten vision in two ways. First, because they are abnormal, they often bleed easily, leaking blood into the vitreous cavity and decreasing visual acuity. Second, the blood vessels attach firmly to the retinal surface and posterior surface of the vitreous, such that normal movement of the

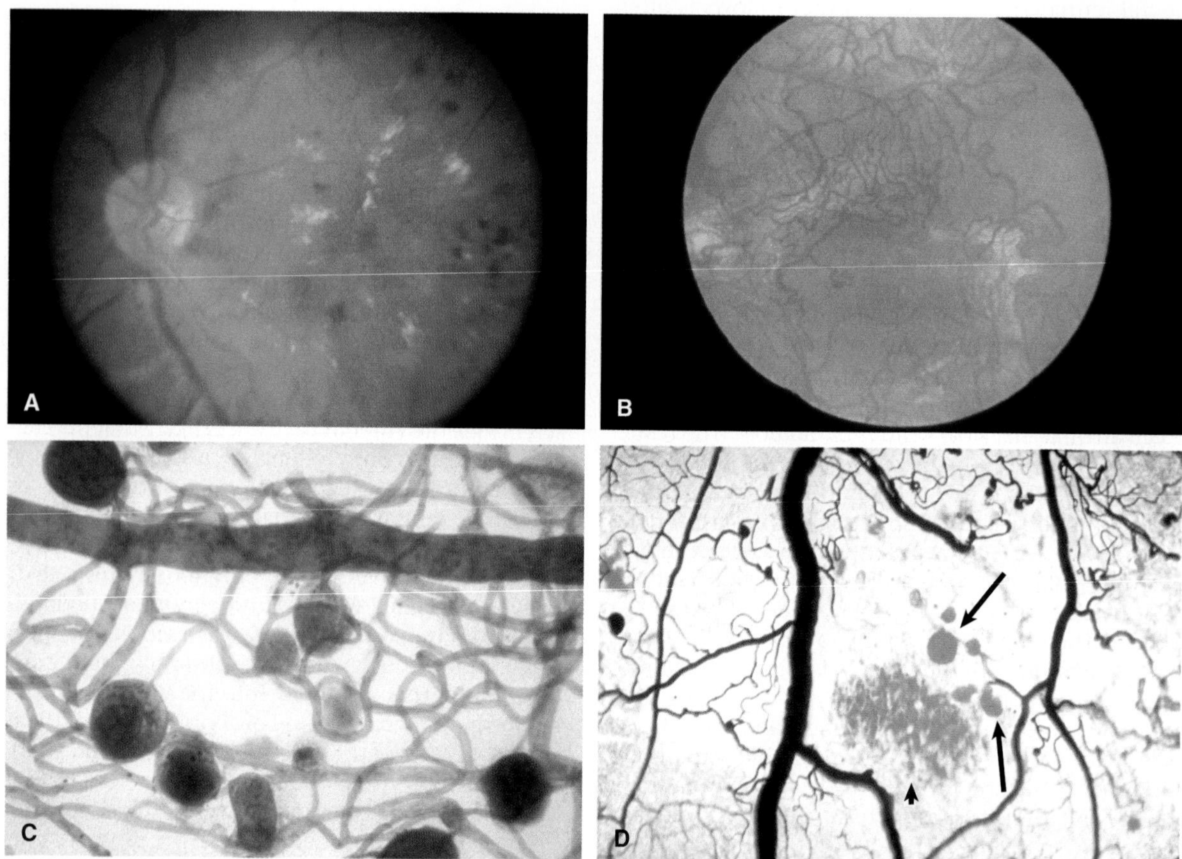

FIGURE 54-15 Diabetic retinopathy. (**A**) View of the ocular fundus in a patient with background diabetic retinopathy. Several yellowish "hard" exudates, which are rich in lipids, are evident, together with several relatively small retinal hemorrhages. (**B**) A vascular frond has extended anterior to the retina in the eye with proliferative retinopathy. (**C**) Numerous microaneurysms are present in this flat preparation of a diabetic retina. (**D**) This flat preparation from a diabetic is stained with periodic acid–Schiff (PAS) after the retinal vessels had been perfused with India ink. Microaneurysms (*arrows*) and an exudate (*arrowhead*) are evident in a region of retinal nonperfusion. (Rubin E., Farber J.L. [1999]. *Pathology* [3rd ed., p. 1553]. Philadelphia: Lippincott-Raven)

vitreous may exert a pull on the retina, causing retinal detachment and progressive blindness. Because early proliferative diabetic retinopathy is likely to be asymptomatic, it must be identified early, before bleeding occurs and obscures light transmission or leads to fibrosis and retinal detachment.

The cause of diabetic retinopathy is uncertain. Many studies have demonstrated that hyperglycemia, hypertension, and hyperlipidemia contribute to the pathogenesis of the disorder.[30] Either directly or indirectly, these conditions are thought to contribute to the growth of abnormal retinal blood vessels secondary to ischemia. These blood vessels grow in an attempt to supply oxygenated blood to hypoxic retinal. It has been suggested that conditions such as leukostasis may play a role. Leukocytes have a large cell volume, high cytoplasmic rigidity, a natural tendency to adhere to the vascular endothelium, and a capacity to generate toxic superoxide radicals and proteolytic enzymes. In diabetics, the leukocytes tend to be less deformable, and a greater number are activated, indicating that they may be involved in retinal capillary underperfusion, endothelial cell damage, and vascular leakage.[28,29] As a result of the occluded capillaries, retinal ischemia stimulates a pathologic neovascularization mediated by angiogenic factors such as VEGF. Whereas leukocytes have been implicated in the pathogenesis of diabetic retinopathy, other blood components such as platelets and red blood cells are probably also involved.

The American Diabetes Association, American College of Physicians, and American Academy of Ophthalmology have developed screening guidelines for diabetic retinopathy.[30] These guidelines recommend that persons with type 1 diabetes should have an initial dilated and comprehensive eye examination by an ophthalmologist or optometrist within 3 to 5 years after the onset of diabetes. Usually, screening is not indicated before the start of puberty. Persons with type 2 diabetes should have an initial comprehensive examination shortly after diagnosis. Subsequent examinations for persons with either type 1 or type 2 diabetes should be repeated annually. The ocular examination by the ophthalmologist should include acuity measurements, slit-lamp biomicroscopy, and direct and indirect ophthalmoscopy of the retina through fully dilated pupils. When indicated, color fundus photographs and fluorescein angiograms should be done. When planning pregnancy, women with preexisting diabetes should be counseled about the risk for developing retinopathy or progression of existing retinopathy. Women who become pregnant should have a comprehensive eye examination just before or soon after conception and at least every 3 months throughout pregnancy.

Preventing diabetic retinopathy from developing or progressing is considered the best approach to preserving vision. Growing evidence suggests that careful control of blood glucose levels in persons with diabetes mellitus may retard the onset and progression of retinopathy. The Diabetes Control and Complications Trial Research Group demonstrated that intensive management of persons with type 1 diabetes to maintain blood glucose levels at near-normal levels reduced the risk for retinopathy by 76% in persons with no retinopathy and slowed the progress by 54% in persons with early disease.[33] There also is need for intensive management of hypertension[34] and hyperlipidemia, both which have been shown to increase the risk for diabetic retinopathy.[30]

Photocoagulation using an argon laser provides the major direct treatment modality for diabetic retinopathy.[31,32] Treatment strategies include laser photocoagulation applied directly to leaking microaneurysms and grid photocoagulation with a checkerboard pattern of laser burns applied to diffuse areas of leakage and thickening.[31] Because laser photocoagulation destroys the proliferating vessels and the ischemic retina, it reduces the stimulus for further neovascularization. However, photocoagulation of neovascularization near the disk is not recommended.[31] Vitrectomy has proved effective in removing vitreous hemorrhage and severing vitreoretinal membranes that develop.

Because of the limitations of current treatment measures, new pharmacologic therapies are being developed, targeting the underlying biochemical mechanisms that cause diabetic retinopathy. Among the pharmacologic therapies being explored are those related to the control of the growth factors and signaling systems that participate in the abnormal proliferation of retinal vessels.[28,29]

Hypertensive Retinopathy. Long-standing systemic hypertension results in the compensatory thickening of arteriolar walls, which effectively reduces capillary perfusion pressure. Ordinarily, a retinal blood vessel is transparent and seen as a red line; in venules, the red cells resemble a string of boxcars. On ophthalmoscopy, arteries in persons with long-standing hypertension appear paler than veins because they have thicker walls. The thickened arterioles in chronic hypertension become opaque and have a copper-wiring appearance. Edema, microaneurysms, intraretinal hemorrhages, exudates, and cotton-wool spots all are observed (see Fig. 54-12). Malignant hypertension involves swelling of the optic disk because of the local edema produced by escaped fluid. If the condition is permitted to progress long enough, serious visual deficits result.

Protective thickening of arteriolar walls cannot occur with sudden increases in blood pressure. Therefore, hemorrhage is likely to occur. Trauma to the optic globe or the head, sudden high blood pressure in preeclampsia, and some types of renal disease may be accompanied by edema of the retina and optic disk and by an increased likelihood of hemorrhage.

Atherosclerosis of Retinal Vessels. In atherosclerosis, the lumen of the arterioles becomes narrowed. As a result, the retinal arteries become tortuous and narrowed. At sites where the arteries cross and compress veins, the red cell column of the vein appears distended. Exudate accumulates on arteriolar walls as "fluffy" white plaques (cotton-wool patches). These patches are damaged axons that on cross-section resemble crystalloid bodies. Deep and superficial hemorrhages are common. Atheromatous plaques of the central artery are associated with increased danger of stasis, thrombi of the central veins, and occlusion.

Retinal Detachment

Retinal detachment involves the separation of the sensory retina from the pigment epithelium (Fig. 54-16). It occurs when traction on the inner sensory layer or a tear in this layer allows fluid, usually vitreous, to accumulate between the two layers.[31] Retinal detachment that results from breaks in the sensory layer of the retina is called *rhegmatogenous detachment* (*rhegma* in Greek, meaning "rent" or "hole"). The vitreous normally adheres to the retina at the optic disk, macula, and periphery of the retina. When the vitreous shrinks, it separates from the retina at the posterior pole of the eye (posterior vitreous detachment). However, at the periphery, the vitreous pulls on the attached retina, which can lead to tearing of the retina. Vitreous fluid can enter the tear and contribute to further separation of the retina from its overlying pigment layer.

Persons with high grades of myopia may have abnormalities in the peripheral retina that predispose to sudden detachment. Intraocular surgery such as cataract extraction may produce traction on the peripheral retina that causes eventual detachment months or even years after surgery. Detachment may result from exudates that separate the two retinal layers. Exudative retinal detachment may be caused by intraocular inflammation, intraocular tumors, or certain systemic diseases. Inflammatory processes include posterior scleritis, uveitis, or parasitic invasion. Retinal detachment also can follow trauma immediately or at some later time.

Detachment of the neural retina from the retinal pigment layer separates the receptors from their major blood supply, the choroid. If retinal detachment continues for some time, permanent destruction and blindness of that part of the retina occur. The bipolar and ganglion cells may survive because their blood supply, by way of the retinal arteries, remains intact. Without receptors, however, there is no visual function. The primary symptom of retinal detachment is loss of vision. Sometimes, flashing lights or sparks, followed by small floaters or spots in the field of vision, occur as the retina pulls away from the posterior pole of the eye. No pain is associated with this retinal detachment. As detachment progresses, the person perceives a dark curtain progressing across the visual field. Because the process begins in the periphery and spreads circumferentially and posteriorly, initial visual disturbances may involve only one quadrant of the visual field. Large peripheral detachments may occur without involvement of the macula, so that visual acuity remains unaffected. The tendency, however, is for detachments to enlarge until the entire retina is detached.

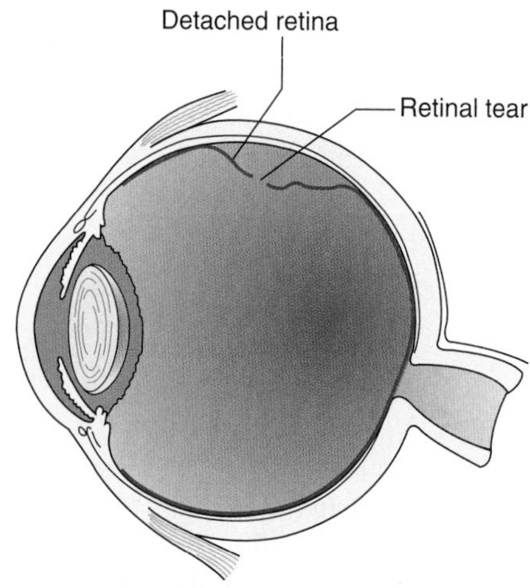

FIGURE 54-16 Detached retina.

Diagnosis is based on the ophthalmoscopic appearance of the retina. Treatment is aimed at closing retinal tears and reattaching the retina. Rhegmatogenous detachment usually requires surgical treatment. Scleral buckling or pneumatic retinopexy is the most commonly used surgical technique.[31] Scleral buckling is the primary surgical procedure performed to reattach the retina. The procedure requires careful location of the retinal break and treatment with diathermy, cryotherapy, or laser to produce chorioretinal adhesions that seal the retinal tears so that the vitreous can no longer leak into the subretinal space. With scleral buckling, a piece of silicone (*i.e.,* the buckle) is sutured and infolded into the sclera, physically indenting the sclera so that it contacts the separated pigment and retinal layers. Pneumatic retinopexy involves the intraocular injection of an expandable gas instead of a piece of silicone to form the indentation. An overall reattachment rate of 90% is reported, but the visual results depend on the preoperative status of the macula.[31] The most common cause of failure after surgical treatment for detached retina is the development of membranes on the retina.

Macular Degeneration

Macular degeneration is characterized as loss of central vision due to destructive changes of the yellow-pigmented area surrounding the central fovea. Age-related macular degeneration is the most common cause of reduced vision in the United States. It is the leading cause of blindness among persons older than 75 years and of newly reported cases of blindness among those older than 65 years of age.[1] The cause of age-related macular degeneration is poorly understood. In addition to older age, identifiable risk factors include female sex, white race, cigarette smoking, and low dietary intake of carotenoids. Increasing evidence suggests that genetic factors may also play a role.[35]

There are two types of age-related macular degeneration: an atrophic nonexudative or "dry" form and an exudative or "wet" form. Both types are progressive, but differ in manifestations, prognosis, and management. Although most people with age-related macular degeneration manifest nonproliferative changes only, most people who experience severe vision loss do so from the development of the exudative form of the disease.[31]

Nonexudative age-related macular degeneration is characterized by various degrees of atrophy and degeneration of the outer retina, Bruch's membrane, and the choriocapillaris. It does not involve leakage of blood or serum; hence, it is called *dry age-related macular degeneration.* On ophthalmoscopic examination, there are visible changes in the retinal pigmentary epithelium and pale yellow spots, called *drusen,* that may occur individually or in groups throughout the macula. Histopathologically, most drusen contain remnants of materials representative of focal detachment of the pigment epithelium. With time, the drusen enlarge, coalesce, and increase in number. The level of associated visual impairment is variable and may be minimal. Most people with macular drusen do not experience significant loss of central vision; and the atrophic changes may stabilize or progress slowly. However, people with the nonexudative form of age-related macular degeneration need to be followed closely because the exudative stage may develop suddenly at any time.

The exudative form of macular degeneration is characterized by the formation of a choroidal neovascular membrane that separates the pigmented epithelium from the neuroretina. These new blood vessels have weaker walls than normal and are prone to leakage; therefore, this condition is called *wet age-related macular degeneration.* The leakage of serous or hemorrhagic fluid into the subretinal space causes separation of the pigmented epithelium from the neurosensory retina.

Even though some subretinal neovascular membranes may regress spontaneously, the natural course of exudative macular degeneration is toward irreversible loss of central vision. Persons with late-stage disease often find it difficult to see at long distances (*e.g.,* in driving), do close work (*e.g.,* reading), see faces clearly, or distinguish colors. However, they may not be severely incapacitated because the peripheral retinal function usually remains intact. With the help of low-vision aids, many of them are able to continue many of their normal activities. The early stages of subretinal neovascularization may be difficult to detect ophthalmoscopically. Therefore, there is need to be alert for recent or sudden changes in central vision, blurred vision, or scotoma in persons with evidence of age-related macular degeneration.

Although there is no treatment for the nonexudative form of macular degeneration, argon laser photocoagulation may be useful in treating the neovascularization that occurs with the exudative form.[36,37] Another method used to halt neovascularization is photodynamic therapy. It is a nonthermal process leading to localized production of reactive oxygen species that mediate cellular, vascular, and immunologic injury and destruction of new blood vessels. There has been recent interest in the effect of supplemental antioxidants (high-dose vitamin C, vitamin E, and beta-carotene) and zinc for persons at risk for developing macular degeneration.[38]

While rare, macular degeneration can occur as a hereditary condition in young persons and sometimes in adults. The genetic form of macular dystrophy, *Stargardt's disease,* becomes manifest in the middle of the first to second decade of life and is inherited as a classic recessive trait, requiring mutations in both alleles of a single disease-related gene.[39] The gene codes for an ABCR (ATP-binding cassette transporter—retina) transporter molecule located in the retina that functions in the transport of retinal lipids and peptides. It is thought that mutations in this gene allow degraded material to accumulate and interfere with retinal function.

In summary, the retina covers the inner aspect of the posterior two thirds of the eyeball and is continuous with the optic nerve. It contains the neural receptors for vision, and it is here that light energy of different frequencies and intensities is converted to graded local potentials, which then are converted to action potentials and transmitted to visual centers in the brain. The photoreceptors normally shed portions of their outer segments. These segments are phagocytized by cells in the pigment epithelium. Failure of phagocytosis, as occurs in one form of retinitis pigmentosa, results in degeneration of the pigment layer and blindness.

The retina receives its blood from two sources: the choriocapillaris, which supplies the pigment layer and the outer portion of the sensory retina adjacent to the choroid, and the branches of the retinal artery, which supply the inner half of the retina. Retinal blood vessels are normally apparent through the ophthalmoscope. Disorders of retinal vessels can result from many local and systemic disorders, including diabetes mellitus and hypertension. They cause vision loss through changes that result in hemorrhage, production of opacities, and separation of the pigment epithelium and sensory retina. Retinal detachment involves separation of the sensory receptors from their blood supply; it causes blindness unless reattachment is accomplished promptly. Macular degeneration is characterized as loss of central vision due to destructive changes of the yellow-pigmented area surrounding the central fovea. Age-related macular degeneration is the most common cause of reduced vision in the United States.

Disorders of Neural Pathways and Cortical Centers

After completing this section of the chapter, you should be able to meet the following objectives:

- Characterize what is meant by a *visual field defect*
- Explain the use of perimetry in the diagnosis of a visual field defect
- Define the terms *hemianopia, quadrantanopia, heteronymous hemianopia,* and *homonymous hemianopia* and relate to disorders of the optic pathways
- Describe visual defects associated with disorders of the visual cortex and visual association areas

Full visual function requires the normally developed brain-related functions of photoreception and the pupillary reflex. These functions depend on the integrity of all visual pathways, including retinal circuitry and the pathway from the optic nerve to the visual cortex and other visual regions of the brain and brain stem.

OPTIC PATHWAYS

Visual information is carried to the brain by axons of the retinal ganglion cells, which form the optic nerve. Sur-

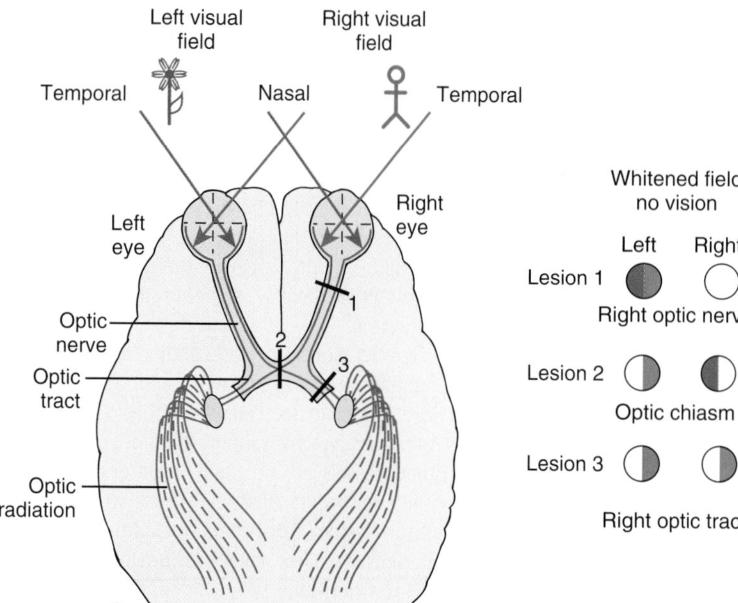

FIGURE 54-17 Diagram of optic pathways. The *red lines* indicate the right visual field and the *blue lines* the left visual field. Note the crossing of fibers from the medial half of each retina at the optic chiasm. Lesion 1 (right optic nerve) produces unilateral blindness. Lesion 2 (optic chiasm) may involve only those fibers that originate in the nasal half of each retina and cross to the opposite side in the optic chiasm; visual loss involves the temporal half of each field (bitemporal hemianopia). Lesion 3 (right optic tract) interrupts fibers (and vision) originating on the same side of both eyes (homonymous) with loss of vision from half of each field (hemianopia).

rounded by pia mater, cerebrospinal fluid (CSF), arachnoid, and the dura mater, the optic nerve represents an outgrowth of the brain rather than a peripheral nerve. The optic nerve extends from the back of the optic globe through the orbit and the optic foramen, into the middle fossa, and on to the optic chiasm at the base of the brain[11] (Fig. 54-17). Axons from the nasal portion of the retina remain medial, and those from the temporal retina remain lateral in the optic nerve.

The two optic nerves meet and fuse in the optic chiasm, beyond which they are continued as the optic tracts. In the optic chiasm, axons from the nasal retina of each eye cross to the opposite side and join with the axons of the temporal retina of the contralateral eye to form the optic tracts. Thus, one optic tract contains fibers from both eyes that transmit information from the same visual field.

VISUAL CORTEX

The primary visual cortex (area 17) surrounds the calcarine fissure, which lies in the occipital lobe. It is at this level that visual sensation is first experienced (Fig. 54-18). Immediately surrounding area 17 are the visual association cortices (areas 18 and 19) and several other association cortices.[11] These association cortices, with their thalamic nuclei, must be functional for added meaningfulness of visual perception. This higher-order aspect of the visual experience depends on previous learning.

Circuitry in the primary visual cortex and the visual association areas is extremely discrete with respect to the location of retinal stimulation. For example, specific neurons respond to the particular orientation of a moving edge, specific colors, or familiar shapes. This elaborate organization of the visual cortex, with its functionally separate and multiple representations of the same visual field, provides the major basis for visual sensation and perception. Because of this discrete circuitry, lesions of the visual cortex must be large to be detected clinically.

VISUAL FIELDS

The *visual field* refers to the area that is visible during fixation of vision in one direction. Because visual system deficits are often expressed as visual field deficits rather than as direct measures of neural function, the terminology for normal and abnormal visual characteristics usually is based on visual field orientation.

Most of the visual field is *binocular,* or seen by both eyes. This binocular field is subdivided into central and pe-

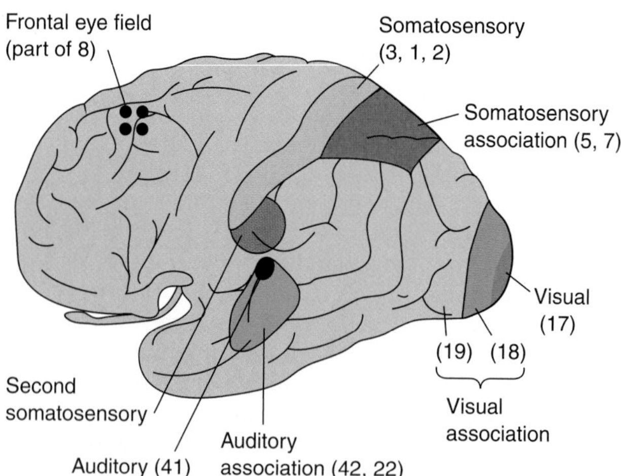

FIGURE 54-18 Lateral view of the cortex illustrating the location of the visual, visual association, auditory, and auditory association areas.

ripheral portions. Central portions of the retina provide high visual acuity and correspond to the field focused on the central fovea; the peripheral and surrounding portion provides the capacity to detect objects, particularly moving objects. Beyond the visual field shared by both eyes, the left lateral periphery of the visual field is seen exclusively by the left nasal retina, and the right peripheral field is seen by the right nasal retina.

As with a camera, the simple lens system of the eye inverts the image of the external world on each retina. In addition, the right and left sides of the visual field also are reversed. The right binocular visual field is seen by the left retinal halves of each eye: the nasal half of the right eye and the temporal half of the left eye.

Once the level of the retina is reached, the nervous system plays a consistent role. The upper half of the visual field is received by the lower half of the retinas of both eyes. Representations of this upper half of the field are carried in the lower half of each optic nerve: they synapse in the lower half of the lateral geniculate nucleus (LGN) of each side of the brain. Neurons in this part of the LGN send their axons through the inferior half of the optic radiation, looping into the temporal lobe to terminate in the lower half of the primary visual cortex on each side of the brain.

Because of the lateral separation of the two eyes, each eye contributes a different image of the world to the visual field. This is called *binocular disparity*. Disparity between the laterally displaced images seen by the two eyes provides a powerful source of three-dimensional depth perception for objects within a distance of 30 m. Beyond that distance, binocular disparity becomes insignificant: depth perception is based on other cues (*e.g.*, the superimposition of the image of near objects over that of far objects, and the faster movement of near objects than of far objects).

Visual Field Defects

Visual field defects result from damage to the visual pathways or the visual cortex. Perimetry or visual field testing, in which the visual field of each eye is measured and plotted in an arc, is used to identify defects and determine the location of lesions.

Retinal Defects. All of us possess a hole, or scotoma, in our visual field, of which we are unaware. Because the optic disk, where the optic nerve fibers exit the retina, does not contain photoreceptors, the corresponding location in the visual field constitutes a blind spot. Local retinal damage caused by small vascular lesions (*i.e.*, retinal stroke) and other localized pathologies can produce additional blind spots. As with the normal blind spot, persons are usually not aware of the existence of scotomata in their visual fields unless they encounter problems seeing objects in certain restricted parts of the visual field.

Absences near or in the center of the bilateral visual field can be annoying and even disastrous. Although the hole is not recognized as such, the person finds that a part of a printed page appears or disappears, depending on where the fixation point is held. Most persons learn to position their eyes to use the remaining central foveal vision for high-acuity tasks. Defects in the peripheral visual field, including the monocular peripheral fields, are less annoying but potentially more dangerous. The person who is unaware of the defect, when walking or driving an automobile, does not see cars or bicyclists until their image reaches the functional visual field—sometimes too late to avert an accident. With careful education, a person can learn to shift the gaze constantly to obtain visual coverage of important parts of the visual field. If the damage is at the retinal or optic nerve level, only the monocular field of the damaged eye becomes a problem. A lesion affecting the central foveal vision of one eye can result in complaints of eyestrain during reading and other close work because only one eye really is being used. Localized damage to the optic tracts, LGN, optic radiation, or primary visual cortex affects corresponding parts of the visual fields of both eyes.

Disorders of the Optic Pathways

The visual pathway extends from the front to the back of the head. It is much like a telephone line between distant points in that damage at any point along the pathway results in functional defects (see Fig. 54-17). Among the disorders that can interrupt the visual pathway are vascular lesions, trauma, and tumors. For example, normal visual system function depends on vascular adequacy in the ophthalmic artery and its branches; the central artery of the retina; the anterior and middle cerebral arteries, which supply the intracranial optic nerve, chiasm, and optic tracts; and the posterior cerebral artery, which supplies the LGN, optic radiation, and visual cortex. The adequacy of posterior cerebral artery function depends on that of the vertebral and basilar arteries that supply the brain stem. Vascular insufficiency in any one of these arterial systems can seriously affect vision. Examination of visual system function is of particular diagnostic use because lesions at various points along the pathway have characteristic symptoms that assist in the localization of the pathology.

Visual field defects of each eye and of the two eyes together are useful in localizing lesions affecting the system. Blindness in one eye is called *anopia*. If half of the visual field for one eye is lost, the defect is called *hemianopia;* loss of a quarter field is called *quadrantanopia*. Enlarging pituitary tumors can produce longitudinal damage through the optic chiasm with loss of the medial fibers of the optic nerve representing both nasal retinas and both temporal visual half-fields. Loss of the temporal or peripheral visual fields on both sides results in a narrow binocular field, commonly called *tunnel vision*. The loss of different half-fields in the two eyes is called a *heteronymous loss,* and the abnormality is called *heteronymous hemianopia*. Destruction of one or both lateral halves of the chiasm is common with multiple aneurysms of the circle of Willis. In this condition, the function of one or both temporal retinas is lost, and the nasal fields of one or both eyes are lost. The loss of the temporal fields (nasal retina) of both eyes is called *bitemporal heteronymous anopia*. With both eyes open, the person with bilateral defects still has the full binocular visual field.

Loss of the optic tract, LGN, full optic radiation, or complete visual cortex on one side results in loss of the corresponding visual half-fields in each eye. *Homonymous* means "the same" for both eyes. In left-side lesions, the right visual field is lost for each eye and is called *complete right homonymous hemianopia.* Partial injury to the left optic tract, LGN, or optic radiation can result in the loss of one fourth of the visual field in both eyes. This is called *homonymous quadrantanopia,* and depending on the lesion, it can involve the upper (superior) or lower (inferior) fields. Because the optic radiation fibers for the superior fourth of the visual field traverse the temporal lobe, superior quadrantanopia is more common. The LGN, optic radiation, and visual cortex all receive their major blood supply from the posterior cerebral artery; unilateral occlusion of this artery results in complete loss of the opposite field (*i.e.,* homonymous hemianopia). Bilateral occlusion of these arteries results in total cortical blindness.

Disorders of the Visual Cortex

Discrete damage to the binocular portion of the primary visual cortex also can result in scotomata in the corresponding visual fields. If the visual loss is in the central high-acuity part of the field, severe loss of visual acuity and pattern discrimination occurs. The central high-acuity portion of the visual field is located at the occipital pole. This region can be momentarily compressed against the occipital bone (*i.e.,* contrecoup) after severe trauma to the frontal part of the cranium. Mechanical trauma to the cortex results in firing of neurons, experienced as flashes of light or "seeing stars." Destruction of the polar visual cortex causes severe loss of visual acuity and pattern discrimination. Such damage is permanent and cannot be corrected with lenses.

The bilateral loss of the entire primary visual cortex, called *cortical blindness,* eliminates all visual experience. Crude analysis of visual stimulation at reflex levels, such as eye-orienting and head-orienting responses to bright moving lights, pupillary reflexes, and blinking at sudden bright lights, may be retained even though vision has been lost. Extensive damage to the visual association cortex (areas 18 and 19) that surrounds an intact primary visual cortex results in a loss of the learned meaningfulness of visual images (*i.e.,* visual agnosia). The patient can see the patterns of color, shapes, and movement, but no longer can recognize formerly meaningful stimuli. Familiar objects can be described but not named or reacted to meaningfully. However, if other sensory modalities, such as hearing and touch, can be applied, full recognition occurs. This disorder represents a problem of recognition rather than intellect.

Testing of Visual Fields

Crude testing of the binocular visual field and the visual field of each individual eye (*i.e.,* monocular vision) can be accomplished without specialized equipment. In the confrontation method, the examiner stands or sits 2 to 3 feet in front of the person to be tested and instructs the person to focus on an object such as a penlight with one eye closed. The object is moved from the center toward the periphery of the person's visual field and from the periphery toward the center, and the person is instructed to report the presence or absence of the object. By moving the object through the vertical, horizontal, and oblique aspects of the visual field, a crude estimate can be made of the visual field. Large field defects can be estimated by the confrontation method, and it may be the only way for testing young children and uncooperative adults.

Accurate determination of the presence, size, and shape of smaller holes, or scotomata, in the visual field of a particular eye can be demonstrated only by perimetry. This is done by having the person look with one eye toward a central spot directly in front of the eye while the head is stabilized by a chin rest or bite board. A small dot of light or a colored object is moved back and forth in all areas of the visual field. The person reports whether the stimulus is visible and, if a colored stimulus is used, what the perceived color is. A hemispheric support is used to control and standardize the movement of the test object, and a plot of radial coordinates of the visual field is made. Perimetry provides a means of determining alterations from normal and, with repeated testing, a way of following the progress of the disease or treatment.

In summary, visual information is carried to the brain by axons of the retinal ganglion cells that form the optic nerve. The two optic nerves meet and fuse in the optic chiasm. The axons of each nasal retina cross in the chiasm and join the uncrossed fibers of the temporal retina of the opposite eye in the optic tract to form the optic tracts. The fibers of each optic tract then synapse in the LGN, and from there, travel by way of the optic radiations to the primary visual cortex in the calcarine area of the occipital lobe. Damage to the visual pathways or visual cortex leads to visual field defects that can be identified through visual field testing or perimetry and used to determine the lesion's location. Damage to the visual association cortex can result in the phenomenon of seeing an object, but with loss of learned recognition (*i.e.,* visual agnosia).

Disorders of Eye Movement

After completing this section of the chapter, you should be able to meet the following objectives:

- Describe the function and innervation of the extraocular muscles
- Recognize the use of smooth pursuit, saccadic, and vergence conjugate gaze movements in self or others
- Cite the function of optic tremor in terms of visual function
- Explain the difference between paralytic and nonparalytic strabismus
- Define *amblyopia* and explain its pathogenesis
- Explain the need for early diagnosis and treatment of eye movement disorders in children

Normal vision depends on the coordinated action of the entire visual system and a number of central control systems. It is through these mechanisms that an object is simultaneously imaged on the fovea of both eyes and perceived as a single image. Strabismus and amblyopia are two disorders that affect this highly integrated system. Although strabismus may develop in later life, it is seen most commonly in children, among whom its incidence is approximately 4%.[40]

EXTRAOCULAR EYE MUSCLES AND THEIR INNERVATION

Each eyeball can rotate around its vertical axis (lateral or medial rotation in which the pupil moves away from or toward the nose), its horizontal left-to-right axis (vertical elevation or depression, in which the pupil moves up or down), and longitudinal horizontal axis in which the top of the pupil moves toward or away from the nose.

Three pairs of extraocular muscles—the superior and inferior recti, the medial and lateral recti, and the superior and inferior obliques—control the movement of each eye (Fig. 54-19). The four rectus muscles are named according to where they insert into the sclera on the medial, lateral, inferior, and superior surfaces of each eye. The two oblique muscles insert on the lateral posterior quadrant of the eyeball—the superior oblique on the upper surface and the inferior oblique on the lower. Each of the three sets of muscles in each eye is reciprocally innervated so that one muscle relaxes when the other contracts. Reciprocal contraction of the medial and lateral recti moves the eye from side to side (adduction and abduction); the superior and inferior recti move the eye up and down (elevation and depression). The oblique muscles rotate (intorsion and extorsion) the eye around its optic axis. A seventh muscle, the levator palpebrae superioris, elevates the upper lid.

The extraocular muscles are innervated by three cranial nerves. The abducens nerve (CN VI) innervates the lateral rectus, the trochlear nerve (CN IV) innervates the superior oblique, and the oculomotor nerve (CN III) innervates the remaining four muscles. The extraocular muscles are among the most rapidly contracting and precisely controlled skeletal muscles in the entire body. This reflects the high nerve-to-muscle ratio, with one lower motoneuron (LMN) innervating 2 to 10 muscle fibers. Table 54-1 describes the function and innervation of the extraocular muscles.

The CN VI (abducens) nucleus, in the caudal pons, innervates the lateral rectus muscle, which rotates the ipsilateral (same side) eye laterally (abduction). The long pathway of CN VI along the floor of the cranial cavity from the pons to the orbit makes it vulnerable to damage from severe injury or fracture of the cranial base. Partial or complete damage to this nerve results in weakness or complete paralysis of the muscle. Medial gaze is normal, but the affected eye fails to rotate laterally with an attempted gaze toward the affected side, a condition called *medial strabismus*.

The CN IV (trochlear) nucleus, at the junction of the pons and midbrain, innervates the contralateral or opposite side superior oblique muscle, which rotates the top of the globe inward toward the nose, a movement called *intorsion*. In combination with other muscles, it also contributes strength to movement of the innervated eye downward and outward. The superior oblique muscle neurons cross over the roof of the midbrain, drop vertically through the roof of the cavernous sinus, and then enter the orbit. This short pathway is rarely damaged, and signs of dysfunction are usually the result of a small brain stem stroke affecting the CN IV nucleus or from damage to the midbrain-level vertical gaze networks.

The CN III (oculomotor) nucleus, which extends through a considerable part of the midbrain, contains clusters of LMNs for each of the five eye muscles it innervates: inferior rectus, ipsilateral superior rectus, inferior oblique, medial rectus, and levator palpebrae superioris. The medial rectus, superior rectus, and inferior rectus rotate the eye in the directions shown in Table 54-1. The action of the inferior rectus is antagonistic to the superior rectus. Because of its plane of attachment to the globe, the inferior oblique rotates the eye in the frontal plane (*i.e., torsion*), pulling the top of the eye laterally (*i.e., extorsion*). The levator palpebrae superioris elevates the upper lid and is involved only in vertical gaze eye movements. As the eyes rotate upward, the upper lid is reflexively retracted, and in

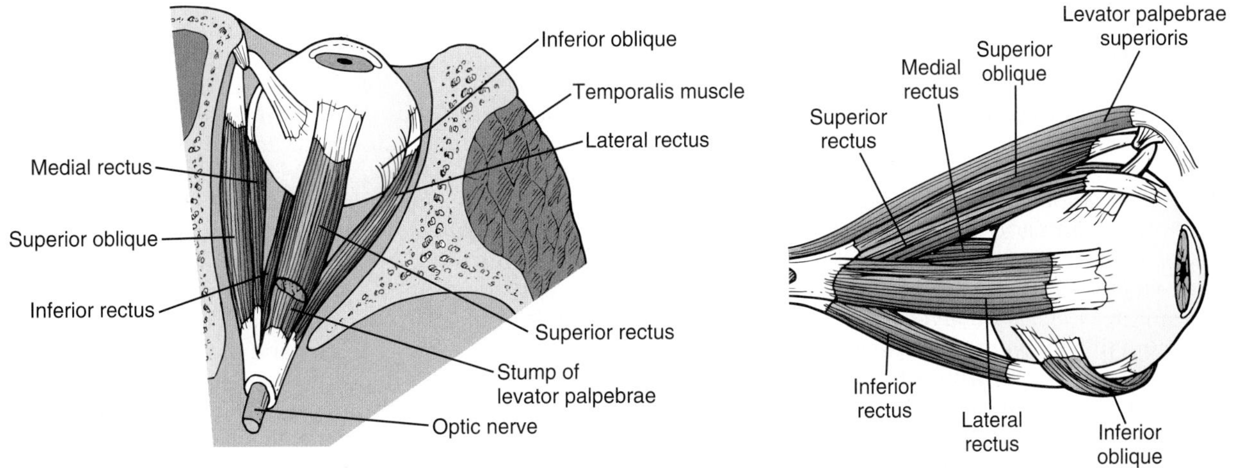

FIGURE 54-19 Extraocular eye muscles of the right eye.

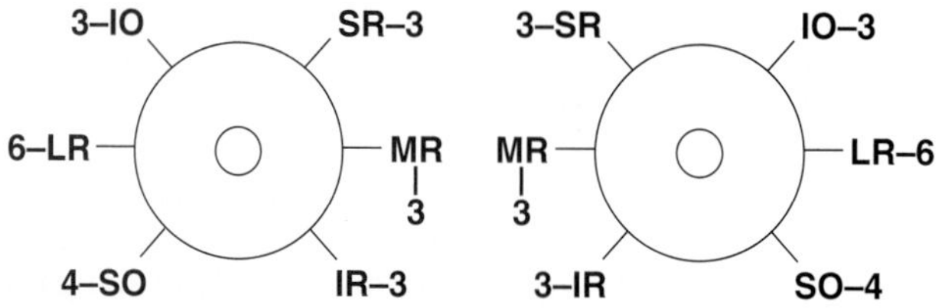

3–IO SR–3 3–SR IO–3
6–LR MR MR LR–6
3 3
4–SO IR–3 3–IR SO–4

TABLE 54-1 Eye in Primary Position: Extrinsic Ocular Muscle Actions

Muscle*	Innervation	Primary	Secondary	Tertiary
MR: medial rectus	III	Adduction		
LR: lateral rectus	VI	Abduction		
SR: superior rectus	III	Elevation	Intorsion	Adduction
IR: inferior rectus	III	Depression	Extorsion	Adduction
SO: superior oblique	IV	Intorsion	Depression	Abduction
IO: inferior oblique	III	Extorsion	Elevation	Abduction

*In the schema of the functional roles of the six extraocular muscles, the major directional force applied by each muscle is indicated on the top. These muscles are arranged in functionally opposing pairs per eye and in parallel opposing pairs for conjugate movements of the two eyes. The numbers associated with each muscle indicate the cranial nerve innervation: 3, oculomotor (III) cranial nerve; 4, trochlear (IV) cranial nerve; 6, abducens (VI) cranial nerve.

the downward gaze, the upper lid is lowered, restricting the exposure of the conjunctiva to air and reducing the effects of drying.

Eye movements include lateral gaze, vertical gaze, oblique gaze, and torsional gaze. Lateral gaze movements are in the horizontal plane and are controlled by lateral gaze centers. These gaze centers consist of interneurons in the abducens (CN VI) nucleus on the side of abduction. Vertical gaze upward or downward is controlled by a vertical gaze center of interneurons in and near the oculomotor (CN III) nucleus. Oblique gaze involves a combination of lateral and vertical gaze controls. Torsional gaze movements involve ocular rotation around the optical axis of the eyes, and although they occur frequently, they are more difficult to observe. The torsional gaze center involves interneurons in the bilaterally located trochlear (CN IV) nucleus on both sides. Each of these control centers maintains a moderate level of tonic activity (*i.e.*, low level of "spontaneous" action potentials) in each opposing pair of muscles. This maintains a neutral position of eye posture. More motor units are automatically recruited when an eye deviates from this neutral position. When released from a directional signal, the eyes automatically return to the neutral position.

Communication between the eye muscle nuclei of each side occurs primarily through the posterior commissure at the rostral end of the midbrain. Longitudinal communication among the three nuclei occurs along a fiber tract called the *medial longitudinal fasciculus* (MLF), which extends from the midbrain to the upper part of the spinal cord. Each pair of eye muscles is reciprocally innervated, by way of the MLF or other associated pathways, so that as one muscle contracts, the other relaxes. For example, the LMNs of CN VI produce lateral rotation (*i.e.*, abduction) of the left eye. Simultaneously, interneurons of the left CN VI, which communicate with the right CN III by way of the MLF, move the right eye medially (adduction). These MLF-linked communication paths are vulnerable to damage in the caudal midbrain and pons. Damage to the pontine MLF on one side results in a loss of this linkage such that lateral deviation in the ipsilateral eye no longer is linked to adduction on the contralateral side (*i.e.*, internuclear ophthalmoplegia). If the MLF is damaged bilaterally, the linkage is lost for lateral gaze in either direction.

Eye Movements and Gaze

Conjugate movements are those in which the optical axes of the eyes are kept parallel, sharing the same visual field. *Gaze* refers to the act of looking steadily in one direction. Eye movements can be categorized into five classes of movements: smooth pursuit movements, saccadic movements, optic tremor, vergence movement, and nystagmus. Although the conjugate reflexes are essential to efficient visual function during head movement or target movement, their circuitry is so deeply embedded in CNS function that they are present and can be elicited when the eyes are closed, during sleep, and in deep coma, and they function normally and accurately in congenitally blind persons.

Smooth Pursuit Movements. Smooth pursuit movements are tracking movements that serve to maintain an object at a fixed point in the center of the visual fields of both eyes. The object may be moving and the eyes following, or the object may be stationary and the head of the observer moving. Normal eye posture is a conjugate gaze directed straight forward with the head held in a forward-looking posture. Smooth pursuit movements normally begin from this position. In fact, holding a strongly deviated gaze becomes tiring after about 30 seconds, and most people will make head and body rotation adjustments to bring the eyes to a central position within that time.

Voluntary pursuit movements are tested by asking the person to follow a finger or another object as it is moved slowly through the visual field. Successful conjugate following requires a functional optic system communicating to the superior colliculus and to the primary visual cortex.

Saccadic Eye Movements. Saccadic eye movements are sudden, jerky conjugate movements that quickly change the fixation point. During reading, the fixation pattern involves a focus on a word or short series of words and then a sudden jump of the eyes to a new fixation point on the next word or phrase. These shifts in fixation points are saccadic movements. During the saccade, a person does not experience the blur of the rapidly moving visual field. The mechanism by which visual experience is momentarily shut off is not understood. Saccadic movements are automatic reflex movements that, in most situations, operate at the brain stem level.

Saccadic shifts of a gaze toward the source of a sudden, unexpected visual, auditory, tactile, or painful stimulus are a component of the startle pattern. This is functionally a visual grasping reflex, redirecting conjugate gaze in the direction of the startle stimulus. This reflex occurs in the absence of the cortical portion of the visual system (cortical blindness). The auditory startle reaction (startle reflex) involves rapid saccadic movements in the direction of a auditory stimulus. It is present in the neonate and in persons with impaired cortical auditory apparatus.

The frontal eye fields of the premotor cortex are important for voluntary saccadic movements such as reading. If this frontal premotor area is not functional, a person can describe objects in the visual field but cannot voluntarily search the visual environment.

Eye Tremor. An eye tremor refers to involuntary, rhythmic, oscillatory eye movements, occurring approximately 10 times per second. Small-range optical tremors are a normal and useful independent function of each eye. One function of the fine optic tremor is to constantly move a bright image onto a new bank of cones, permitting previously stimulated receptors quickly to recover from adaptation.

Vergence Eye Movements. Vergence movements are those that move the eyes in opposite directions to keep the image of an object precisely positioned on the fovea of each eye. Convergence and divergence, which assist in maintaining a binocularly fixed image in near vision, have a major role in accurate depth perception. The vergence system is driven by retinal disparity (*i.e.,* differential placement of an object's image on each retina). A nearby target (<30 feet) moving in the same dimension as the optical axis elicits a reflex mechanism that provides redirection of the optical axes of each eye away from parallel (*i.e.,* in opposite directions) in the horizontal plane (*i.e.,* vergence gaze). This process permits a continued binocular focus on the near target. Perception of depth is a higher-order function of the cortical visual system and is based on one or more of several classes of stimuli, such as superimposition and relative movement.

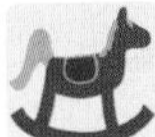

STRABISMUS

Strabismus, or squint, refers to any abnormality of eye coordination or alignment that results in loss of binocular vision (Fig. 54-20). When images from the same spots in visual space do not fall on corresponding points of the two retinas, diplopia, or double vision, occurs.

In standard terminology, the disorders of eye movement are described according to the direction of movement. Esotropia refers to medial deviation, exotropia refers to lateral deviation, hypertropia refers to upward deviation, hypotropia refers to downward deviation, and cyclotropia refers to torsional deviation. The term *concomitance* refers to equal deviation in all directions of gaze. A nonconcomitant strabismus is one that varies with the direction of gaze. Strabismus may be divided into paralytic (nonconcomitant) forms, in which there is weakness or paralysis of one or more of the extraocular muscles, and nonparalytic (concomitant) forms, in which there is no primary muscle impairment. Strabismus is called *intermittent,* or *periodic,* when there are periods in which the eyes are parallel. It is monocular when the same eye always deviates and the fellow eye fixates. Figure 54-21 illustrates abnormalities in eye movement associated with esotropia and exotropia.

Strabismus affects approximately 4% of children younger than 6 years of age.[40,41] Because 30% to 50% of these children sustain permanent secondary loss of vision, or amblyopia, if the condition is left untreated, early diagnosis and treatment are essential.[42,43]

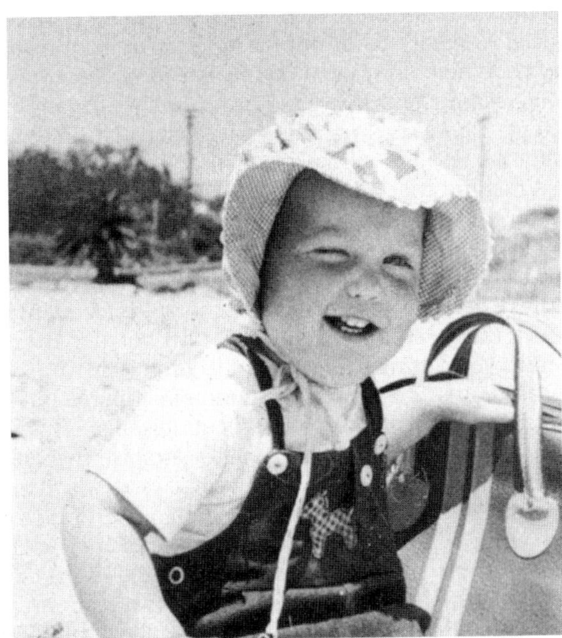

FIGURE 54-20 Photograph of a child with intermittent exotropia squinting in the sunlight. (Vaughn D.G., Asbury T., Riordon-Eva P. [1995]. *General ophthalmology* [p. 239]. Stamford, CT: Appleton & Lange)

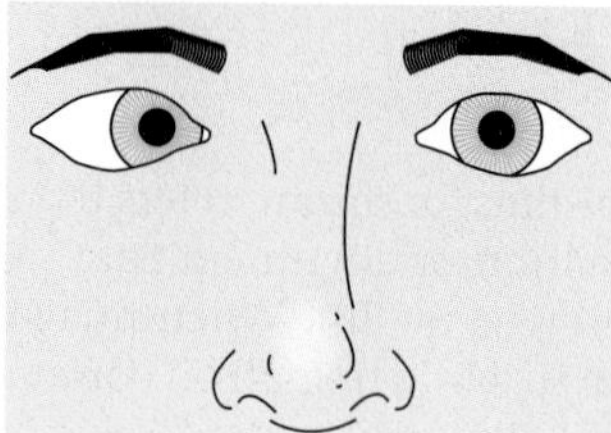

A Primary position: right esotropia

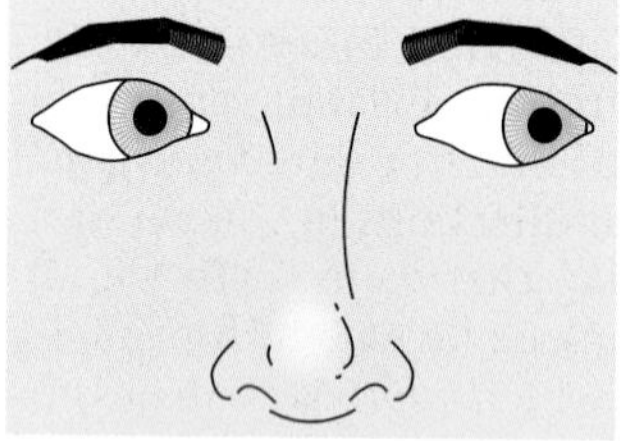

B Left gaze: no deviation

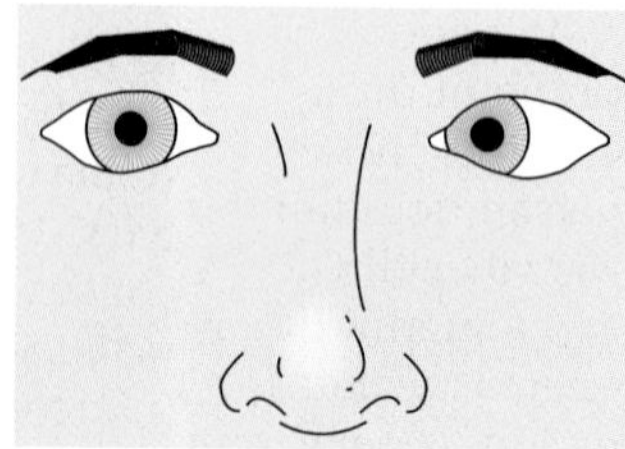

C Right gaze: left esotropia

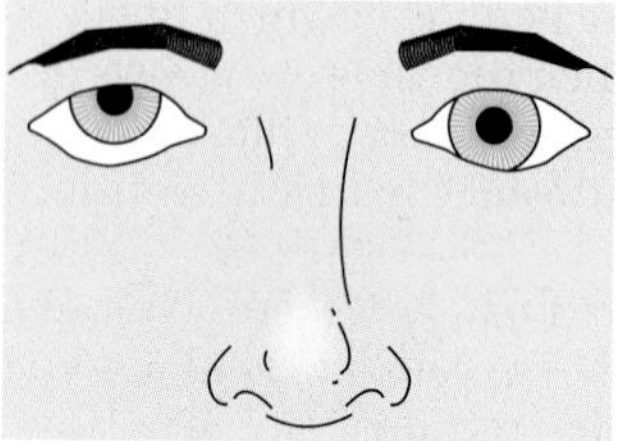

D Right hypertropia

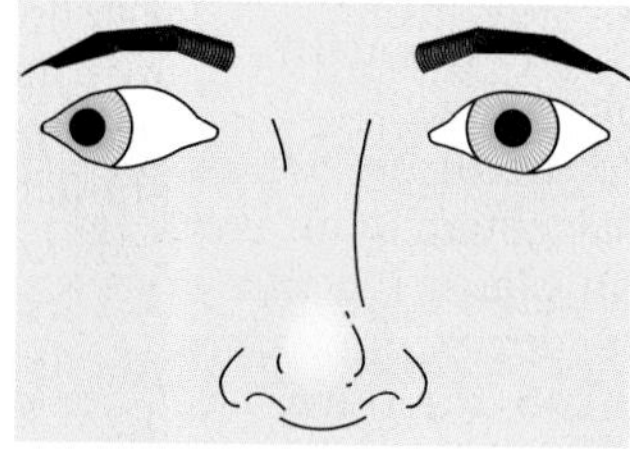

E Right exotropia

FIGURE 54-21 Paralytic strabismus associated with paralysis of the right lateral rectus muscle: (**A**) primary position (looking straight ahead) of the eyes; (**B**) left gaze with no deviation; and (**C**) right gaze with left esotropia. (**D**) Primary position of the eyes with weakness of the right inferior rectus and right hypertropia; and (**E**) primary position of the eyes with weakness of the right medial rectus and right exotropia.

Paralytic Strabismus

Paralytic strabismus results from paresis (*i.e.*, weakness) or plegia (*i.e.*, paralysis) of one or more of the extraocular muscles. When the normal eye fixates, the affected eye is in the position of primary deviation. A manifestation of esotropia is a weakness of one of the lateral rectus muscles, usually the result of weakness of the abducens nerve (CN VI). When the affected eye fixates, the unaffected eye is in a position of secondary deviation. The secondary deviation of the unaffected eye is greater than the primary deviation of the affected eye. This is because the affected eye requires an excess of innervational impulse to maintain fixation; the excess impulses also are distributed to the unaffected eye, causing overaction of its muscles.[40]

Paralytic strabismus is uncommon in children but accounts for nearly all cases of adult strabismus; it can be caused by many conditions. Paralytic strabismus is seen most commonly in adults who have had cerebral vascular accidents and may occur as the first sign of a tumor or inflammatory condition involving the CNS. One type of muscular dystrophy exerts its effects on the extraocular muscles. Initially, eye movements in all directions are weak, with later progression to bilateral optic immobility. Weakness of eye movement and lid elevation is often the first evidence of myasthenia gravis. The pathway of the oculomotor (CN III), trochlear (CN IV), and abducens (CN VI) nerves through the cavernous sinus and the back of the orbit make them vulnerable to basal skull fracture and tumors of the cavernous sinus (*e.g.*, cavernous sinus syndrome) or orbit (*e.g.*, orbital syndrome).[44] In infants, paralytic strabismus can be caused by birth injuries affecting the extraocular muscles or the cranial nerves supplying these muscles. It also can result from congenital anomalies of the muscles. In general, paralytic strabismus in an adult with previously normal binocular vision causes diplopia. This does not occur in persons who have never developed binocular vision.

Nonparalytic Strabismus

In nonparalytic strabismus, there is no extraocular muscle weakness or paralysis, and the angle of deviation is always the same in all fields of gaze. With persistent deviation, secondary abnormalities may develop because of overaction or underaction of the muscles in some fields of gaze. Nonparalytic esotropia is the most common type of strabismus. The disorder may be accommodative, nonaccommodative, or a combination of the two. Accommodative strabismus is caused by disorders such as uncorrected hyperopia, in which the esotropia occurs with accommodation. Onset of this type of esotropia characteristically occurs between 18 months and 4 years of age because accommodation is not well developed until that time. The disorder most often is monocular but may be alternating. Approximately 50% of the cases of esotropia are accommodative. The causes of nonaccommodative strabismus are obscure. This disorder may be related to faulty muscle insertion, fascial abnormalities, or faulty innervation. Research suggests that idiopathic strabismus may have a genetic basis; siblings often present with similar disorders.

Diagnosis and Treatment

All infants and children should be examined for visual alignment. Alignment of the visual axis occurs in the first 3 months of life.[45] All infants should have consistent, synchronized eye movement by 5 to 6 months of age. Infants who have reached this age and whose eyes are not aligned at all times during waking hours should be examined by a qualified practitioner.

Rapid assessment of extraocular muscle function is accomplished by three methods. The first occurs in a darkened room with the child staring straight ahead. A penlight is then pointed at the midpoint between the two eyes, and a bright dot of reflected light can be seen on the cornea of each eye. With normal eye alignment, the reflected light should appear at the same spot on the cornea of each eye. Nonparallelism of the two eyes indicates muscle imbalance because of weakness or paralysis of the deviant eye. In a second method, the child is asked to follow the movement of a small object (*e.g.*, a pencil point, lighted penlight) as it is moved through the extremes of what are called the *six cardinal positions of gaze.* In extreme lateral gaze, normal subjects can show a few quick beats of a jerky or nystagmoid movement. Nystagmoid movement is abnormal if it is prolonged or present in any other eye posture. The third method, called the *cover–uncover test,* eliminates binocular fusion as a factor in maintaining parallelism between the eyes and is used to determine which eye is used for fixation. The child's attention is directed toward a fixed object such as a small picture or tongue blade. A light should not be used because it may not stimulate accommodation. If a mild weakness is present, the eye with blocked vision drifts into a resting position, the extent of which depends on the relative strength of the muscles. The eye should snap back when the card is removed. This test is always done for near and far fixation. Visual acuity is evaluated to obtain a comparison of the two eyes. A tumbling E chart (or similar test chart) can be used for young children.[46]

Treatment of strabismus is directed toward the development of normal visual acuity, correction of the deviation, and superimposition of the retinal images to provide binocular vision. Nonsurgical and surgical methods can be used. In children, early treatment is important; the ideal age to begin is 6 months. Nonsurgical treatment includes occlusive patching, pleoptics (*i.e.*, eye exercises), and prism glasses. Because prolonged occlusive patching leads to loss of useful vision in the covered eye, patching is alternated between the affected and unaffected eye. This improves the vision in the affected eye without sacrificing vision in the unaffected eye. Prism glasses compensate for an abnormal alignment of an optic globe. Occasionally, long-acting miotics in weak strengths (*e.g.*, echothiophate iodide solution [Phospholine Iodide] or pilocarpine [Pilocarpine HS]) are used to cause pharmacologic accommodation in place of or in combination with corrective lenses.[41] Surgical procedures may be used to strengthen or weaken an extraocular muscle by altering its length or attachment site.

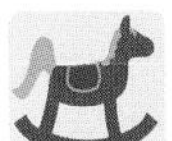

AMBLYOPIA

Amblyopia describes a condition of diminished vision (uncorrectable by lenses) in which no detectable organic lesion of the eye is present.[40,47,48] This condition is sometimes called *lazy eye.* Types of amblyopia include deprivation occlusion, strabismus, and refractive and organic amblyopia. It is caused by visual deprivation (*e.g.*, cataracts, severe ptosis) or abnormal binocular interactions (*e.g.*, strabismus, anisometropia) during visual immaturity. Normal development of the thalamic and cortical circuitry necessary for binocular visual perception requires simultaneous binocular use of each fovea during a critical period early in life (0 to 5 years). In infants with unilateral cataracts that are dense, central, and larger than 2 mm in diameter, this time is before 2 months of age.[40] In conditions causing abnormal binocular interactions, one image is suppressed to provide clearer vision. In esotropia, vision of the deviated eye is suppressed to prevent diplopia. A similar situation exists in anisometropia, in which the refractive indexes of the two eyes are different. Although the eyes are correctly aligned, they are unable to focus together, and the image of one eye is suppressed. In animal experiments, monocular deprivation results in reduced synaptic density in the LGN and the primary visual cortical areas that process information from the affected eye or eyes.[47]

The reversibility of amblyopia depends on the maturity of the visual system at the time of onset and the duration of the abnormal experience. If esotropia is involved, some persons alternate eyes and do not experience diplopia. With late adolescent or adult onset, this habit pattern must be unlearned after correction.

Peripheral vision is less affected than central foveal vision in amblyopia. Suppression becomes more evident with high illumination and high contrast. It is as if the affected eye did not possess central vision and the person learns to fixate with the nonfoveal retina. If bilateral congenital blindness or near blindness (*e.g.*, from cataracts) occurs and remains uncorrected during infancy and early childhood, the person remains without pattern vision and has only overall field brightness and color discrimination. This is essentially bilateral amblyopia.

The treatment of children with the potential for development of amblyopia must be instituted well before the age of 6 years to avoid the suppression phenomenon. Surgery for congenital cataracts and ptosis should be done early. Severe refractive errors should be corrected. In strabismus, alternately blocking vision in one eye and then the other forces the child to use both eyes for form discrimination. The duration of occlusion of vision in the good eye must be short (2 to 5 hours per day) and closely monitored, or deprivation amblyopia can develop in the good eye as well. Although amblyopia is not likely to occur after 8 or 9 years of age, some plasticity in central circuitry is evident even in adulthood. For example, after refractive correction for long-standing astigmatism in adults, visual acuity improves slowly, requiring several months to reach normal levels.

In summary, binocular vision depends on three pairs of extraocular muscles—the medial and lateral recti, which move the eye from side to side; the superior and inferior recti, which move the eye up and down; and the superior and inferior obliques, which rotate the eye around its optical axis. The extraocular muscles are innervated by three pairs of cranial nerves: (1) the trochlear nerve (CN IV), which innervates the superior oblique and turns the eye downward and laterally; (2) the abducens nerve (CN VI), which innervates the lateral rectus and moves the eye laterally; and (3) the oculomotor nerve (CN III), which innervates the medial rectus and turns the eye medially, the superior rectus, which elevates the eye and rolls it upward, the inferior rectus, which depresses the eye and rolls it downward, and the inferior oblique, which elevates the eye and turns it laterally.

For full visual function, it is necessary that the two eyes point toward the same fixation point and the two images become fused. Binocular fusion is controlled by ocular reflex mechanisms that adjust the orientation of each eye to produce a single image. The term *conjugate gaze* refers to the use of both eyes to look steadily in one direction. During conjugate eye movements, the optical axes of the two eyes are maintained parallel with each other as the eyes rotate upward, downward, or from side to side in their sockets. Smooth pursuit movements are tracking movements that serve to maintain an object at a fixed point in the center of the visual fields of both eyes. Saccadic eye movement consists of small jumping movements that represent rapid shifts in conjugate gaze orientation. Vergence movements (convergence and divergence) are necessary for maintaining the focus on a near image.

Strabismus refers to abnormalities in the coordination of eye movements with loss of binocular eye alignment. This inability to focus a visual image on corresponding parts of the two retinas results in diplopia. Esotropia refers to medial deviation, exotropia refers to lateral deviation, hypertropia refers to upward deviation, hypotropia refers to downward deviation, and cyclotropia refers to torsional deviation. Paralytic strabismus is caused by weakness or paralysis of the extraocular muscles. Nonparalytic strabismus results from the inappropriate length or insertion of the extraocular muscles or from accommodation disorders. Amblyopia (*i.e.*, lazy eye) is a condition of diminished vision that cannot be corrected by lenses and in which no detectable organic lesion in the eye can be observed. It results from inadequately developed CNS circuitry because of visual deprivation (*e.g.*, cataracts) or abnormal binocular interactions (*e.g.*, strabismus, anisometropia) during visual immaturity.

REVIEW EXERCISES

The mother of a 3-year-old boy notices that his left eye is red and watering when she picks him up from day care. He keeps rubbing his eye as though it itches. The next morning, however, she notices that both eyes are red, swollen, and watering. She takes him to the pediatrician in the morning and is told that he has "pink eye." She is told that the infection should go away by itself.

A. What part of the eye is involved?

B. What type of conjunctivitis do you think this child has: bacterial, viral, or allergic?

C. Why didn't the pediatrician order an antibiotic?

D. Is the condition contagious? What measures should the mother take to prevent its spread?

During a routine eye exam to get new glasses because she had been having difficulty with her distant vision, a 75-year-old woman is told that she is developing cataracts.

A. What type of visual changes occur as the result of a cataract?

B. What can the woman do to prevent the cataracts from getting worse?

C. What treatment may she eventually need?

A 50-year-old woman is told by her eye doctor that her intraocular pressure is slightly elevated and that although there is no evidence of damage to her eyes at this time, she is at risk for developing glaucoma and should have regular eye exams.

A. Describe the physiologic mechanisms involved in the regulation of intraocular pressure.

B. What are the risk factors for development of glaucoma?

C. Explain how an increase in intraocular pressure produces its damaging effects.

The parents of a newborn infant have been told that their son has congenital cataracts in both eyes and will require cataract surgery so that he does not lose his sight.

A. Explain why the infant is at risk for losing his sight if the cataracts are not removed.

B. When should this procedure be done to prevent loss of vision?

References

1. Leonard R. (1999). *Statistics on visual impairment: A resource manual.* Lighthouse International. [On-line]. Available: http://www.lighthouse.org.
2. Sullivan J.H., Shetlar D.J., Whitcher J.P. (2004). Lids, lacrimal apparatus & tears. In Riordan-Eva P. *Vaughan & Ashbury's general ophthalmology* (16th ed., pp. 80–99). New York: Lange Medical Books/McGraw-Hill.
3. Morrow G.L., Abbott R.L. (1998). Conjunctivitis. *American Family Physician 57*(4), 735–746.
4. Leibowitz H.M. (2000). The red eye. *New England Journal of Medicine 343*(5), 345–351.
5. Riordan-Eva P. (2003). Eye. In Tierney L.M., McPhee S.J., Papadakis M.A. (Eds.), *Current medical diagnosis and treatment* (42nd ed., pp. 146–177). New York: Lange Medical Books/McGraw-Hill.

6. Collum L.M.T., Kilmartin D.J. (2001). Acute allergic conjunctivitis. In Abelson MB. *Allergic diseases of the eye* (pp. 112–131). Philadelphia: W.B. Saunders.
7. Klintworth G.K. (1999). The eye. In Rubin E., Farber J.L. (Eds.), *Pathology* (3rd ed., pp. 1537–1543). Philadelphia: Lippincott-Raven.
8. Olitsky S.E., Nelson L. (2004). Disorders of the eye. In Behrman R.E., Kliegman R.M., Jenson H.B. (Eds.), *Nelson textbook of pediatrics* (17th ed., pp. 2099–2102, 2105–2111). Philadelphia: W.B. Saunders.
9. Biswell R. (2004). Cornea. In Riordan-Eva P. *Vaughan & Ashbury's general ophthalmology* (16th ed., pp. 129–153). New York: Lange Medical Books/McGraw-Hill.
10. Shaikh S., Ta C. (2002). Evaluation and management of herpes zoster ophthalmicus. *American Family Physician 66,* 1723–1732.
11. Kandel E.R., Schwartz J.H., Jessell T.M. (2000). *Principles of neural science* (4th ed., pp. 523–547). New York: McGraw-Hill.
12. Riordan-Eva P. (2004). Glaucoma. In Riordan-Eva P. *Vaughan & Ashbury's general ophthalmology* (16th ed., pp. 212–229). New York: Lange Medical Books/McGraw-Hill.
13. Guyton A.C., Hall J.E. (2000). *Textbook of medical physiology* (10th ed., pp. 575–576). Philadelphia: W.B. Saunders.
14. Martin X.D. (1992). Normal intraocular pressure in man. *Ophthalmologica 205,* 57–63.
15. Coleman A.L. (1999). Glaucoma. *Lancet 354*(9192), 1803–1810.
16. Distellhorst J.S., Hughes G.M. (2003). Open-angle glaucoma. *American Family Physician 67,* 1937–1950.
17. Alward W.L.M. (1998). Medical management of glaucoma. *New England Journal of Medicine 339,* 1299–1307.
18. Kipp M.A. (2003). Childhood glaucoma. *Pediatric Clinics of North America 50,* 89–104.
19. Quillen D.A. (1999). Common causes of vision loss in elderly patients. *American Family Physician 60,* 99–108.
20. Harper R.A., Shock J.P. (2004). Lens. In Riordan-Eva P. *Vaughan & Ashbury's general ophthalmology* (16th ed., pp. 212–229). New York: Lange Medical Books/McGraw-Hill.
21. Schmitt C., Hockwin O. (1990). The mechanisms of cataract formation. *Journal of Inherited Metabolic Disease 13,* 501–508.
22. Chylack L.T. (1997). Cataracts and inhaled corticosteroids. *New England Journal of Medicine 337*(1), 44–48.
23. Jobling A.J., Augusteyn R.C. (2002). What causes steroid cataracts? A review of steroid-induced posterior subcapsular cataracts. *Clinical and Experimental Optometry 852,* 61–75.
24. Solomon B., Donnenfeld E.D. (2003). Recent advances and future frontiers in treating Age-related cataracts. *JAMA 290*(2), 248–251.
25. Phelan J.K. (2000). A brief review of retinitis pigmentosa and the identified retinitis pigmentosa genes. *Molecular Vision 6,* 116–124.
26. Albert D.M., Dryja T.P. (1999). The eye. In Cotran R.S., Kumar V., Collins T. (Eds.), *Robbins pathologic basis of disease* (6th ed., pp. 1359–1377). Philadelphia: W.B. Saunders.
27. Poole T.R.G., Graham E.M. (2004). Ocular disorders associated with systemic disease. In Riordan-Eva P. *Vaughan & Ashbury's general ophthalmology* (16th ed., pp. 307–342). New York: Lange Medical Books/McGraw-Hill.
28. Fong D.S., Aiello L., Gardner T.W., et al. (2003). Diabetic retinopathy. *Diabetes Care 26*(1), 226–229.
29. Cuilla T.A., Amador A.G., Zinman B. (2003). Diabetic retinopathy and diabetic macular edema. *Diabetes Care 26,* 2653–2664.
30. Donaldson M., Dockson P. (2003). Medical treatment of diabetic neuropathy. *Eye 17,* 550–562.
31. Hardy R.A., Shetlar D.J. (2004). Retina. In Riordan-Eva P. *Vaughan & Ashbury's general ophthalmology* (16th ed., pp. 189–211). New York: Lange Medical Books/McGraw-Hill.
32. Ferris F.L., Davis M.D., Aiello L.M. (1999). Treatment of diabetic retinopathy. *New England Journal of Medicine 341,* 667–678.
33. Diabetes Control and Complications Trial Research Group. (1993). The effect of intensive treatment of diabetes on the development and progression of long-term complications in insulin-dependent diabetes mellitus. *New England Journal of Medicine 329,* 977–986.
34. Adler A.I., Stratton I.M., Neil A.W., et al. (2000). Association of systolic blood pressure with macrovascular and microvascular complications of type 2 diabetes (UKPDS 36): Prospective observational study. *British Medical Journal 321,* 412–419.
35. Fine S.L., Berger J.W., MacGuire M., Ho A.C. (2000). Age-related macular degeneration. *New England Journal of Medicine 342,* 483–492.
36. Chopdar A., Chakravarthy U., Verma D. (2003). Age-related macular degeneration. *British Medical Journal 326,* 484–488.
37. Gottlieb J.L. (2002). Age-related macular degeneration. *JAMA 288*(18), 2233–2236.
38. Lewis R.A., Lupski J.R. (2000). Macular degeneration: The emerging genetics. *Hospital Practice 35*(6), 41–58.
39. Jampol L.M., Ferris F.L. (2001). Antioxidants and zinc to prevent progression of age-related macular degeneration. *JAMA 286*(19), 2466–2468.
40. Fredrick D.P., Asbury T. (2004). Strabismus. In Riordan-Eva P. *Vaughan & Ashbury's general ophthalmology* (16th ed., pp. 230–249). New York: Lange Medical Books/McGraw-Hill.
41. Mills M.D. (1999). The eye in childhood. *American Family Physician 60,* 907–918.
42. Lavrich J.B., Nelson L.B. (1993). Diagnosis and management of strabismus disorders. *Pediatric Clinics of North America 40,* 737–751.
43. Ticho B.H. (2003). Strabismus. *Pediatric Clinics of North America 50,* 173–188.
44. Kline L.B., Bajandas F.J. (1996). *Neuro-ophthalmology review manual* (Chapters 4–7). Thorofare, NJ: Slack.
45. Broderick P. (1998). Pediatric vision screening for the family physician. *American Family Practitioner 58*(3), 691–704.
46. Scheiman M. (1997). *Understanding and managing vision defects* (pp. 26–27). Thorofare, NJ: Slack.
47. Mittelman D. (2003). Amblyopia. *Pediatric Clinics of North America 50,* 189–196.
48. Simon J.W., Kaw P. (2001). Commonly missed diagnoses in childhood eye exams. *American Family Physician 64,* 623–628.

CHAPTER

55

Disorders of Hearing and Vestibular Function

Susan A. Fontana and Carol M. Porth

The ears are paired organs consisting of an external and middle ear, which function in capturing, transmitting, and amplifying sound, and an inner ear that contains the receptive organs that are stimulated by sound waves (*i.e.*, hearing) or head position and movement (*i.e.*, vestibular function). Otitis media, or inflammation of the middle ear, is a common disorder of childhood. Hearing loss is one of the most common disabilities experienced by persons in the United States, particularly among the elderly. Vertigo, a disorder of vestibular function, is also a common cause of disability among the elderly. This chapter is divided into two parts: the first focuses on disorders of the ear and auditory function and the second on disorders of the inner ear and vestibular function.

Disorders of Auditory Function

After completing this section of the chapter, you should be able to meet the following objectives:

- ✦ List the structures of the external, middle, and inner ear and cite their function
- ✦ Describe two common disorders of the outer ear
- ✦ Relate the functions of the eustachian tube to the development of middle ear problems, including acute otitis media and otitis media with effusion
- ✦ Describe anatomic variations as well as risk factors that make infants and young children more prone to develop acute otitis media
- ✦ List three common symptoms of acute otitis media
- ✦ Describe the disease process associated with otosclerosis and relate it to the progressive conductive hearing loss that occurs
- ✦ Characterize tinnitus
- ✦ Differentiate between conductive, sensorineural, and mixed hearing loss and cite the more common causes of each
- ✦ Describe methods used in the diagnosis and treatment of hearing loss
- ✦ Define the term *presbycusis* and describe factors that contribute to its development

- ✦ Characterize the causes of hearing loss in infants and children and describe the need for early diagnosis and treatment

THE EXTERNAL EAR

The external ear consists of the auricle, which collects sound, and the external acoustic meatus or ear canal, which conducts the sound to the tympanic membrane[1,2] (Fig. 55-1). The auricle, or pinna, is composed of elastic cartilage covered with thin skin, and an occasional hair. Its rim is somewhat thicker, and its fleshy earlobe lack surrounding cartilage. The funnel shape of the auricle concentrates high-frequency sound entering from the lateral-forward direction into the ear canal. This shape also helps to prevent front–back confusion of sound sources. The external acoustic meatus, or ear canal, is a short (2 to 3 cm in adults) S-shaped canal. A thin layer of skin containing fine hairs, sebaceous glands, and ceruminous glands lines the ear canal. Ceruminous glands secrete cerumen, or earwax, which has certain antimicrobial properties and is thought to serve a protective function.

The anterior portion of the auricle and external part of the ear canal are innervated by branches of the trigeminal nerve (cranial nerve [CN] V). The posterior portions of the auricle and the wall of the ear canal are innervated by auricular branches of the facial (CN VII), glossopharyngeal (CN IX), and vagus (CN X) nerves. Because of the vagal innervation, the insertion of a speculum or an otoscope into the external ear canal can stimulate coughing or vomiting reflexes, particularly in young children.

The tympanic membrane, which separates the external ear from the middle ear, has three layers: an outer layer of thin skin continuous with the lining of the external ear canal, a middle layer of tough collagenous fibers mixed with fibrocytes and some elastic fibers, and an inner epithelial layer continuous with the lining of the middle ear. It is attached in a manner that allows it to vibrate freely when audible sound waves enter the external auditory canal.

When viewed through an otoscope, the tympanic membrane appears as a shallow, almost circular cone pointing inward toward its apex, the umbo (Fig. 55-2). Light usually is reflected from the pars tensa at approximately the 4-o'clock position. Landmarks include the lightened stripe over the handle of the malleus; the umbo at the end of the handle; the pars tensa, which constitutes most of the drum; and the pars flaccida, the small area above the malleus attachment. The tympanic membrane is semitransparent, and a small, whitish cord, which traverses the middle ear from back to front, can be seen just under its upper edge. This is the *chorda tympani,* a branch of the intermedius component of the facial nerve (CN VII).

Disorders of the External Ear

The function of the external ear is disturbed when sound transmission is obstructed by impacted cerumen, inflammation (*i.e.,* otitis externa), or drainage from the external ear (otorrhea).

Impacted Cerumen. Cerumen, or earwax, is a protective secretion produced by the ceruminous glands of the skin that lines the ear canal. Although the ear normally is self-cleaning, the cerumen can accumulate and narrow the

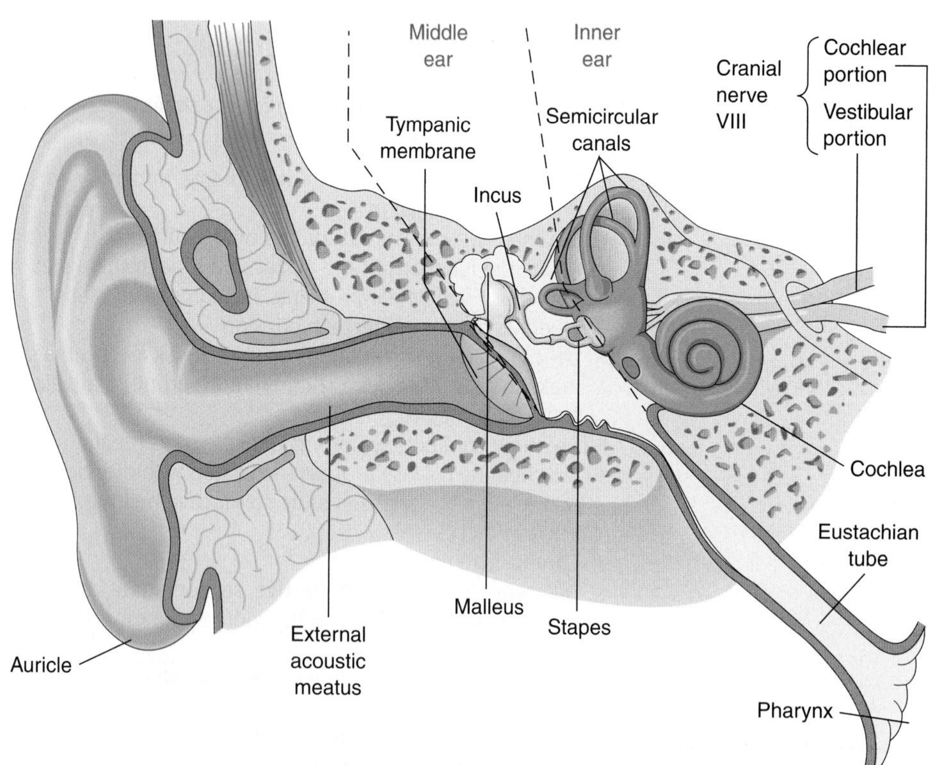

FIGURE 55-1 External, middle, and internal subdivisions of the ear.

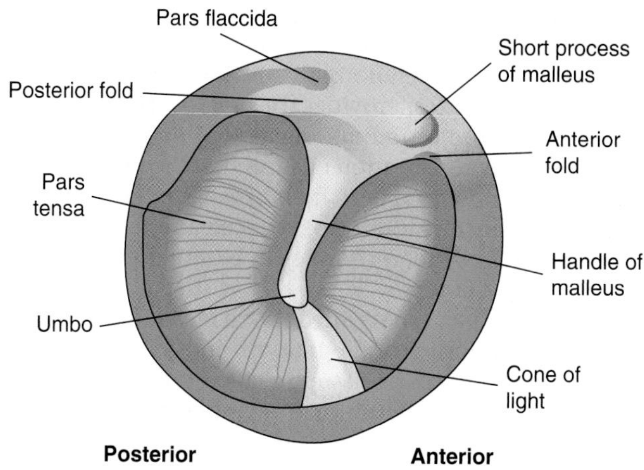

FIGURE 55-2 Right eardrum.

canal. Impaction is a common cause of reversible hearing loss.[3] Impacted cerumen usually produces no symptoms until the canal becomes completely occluded, at which point the person experiences a feeling of fullness, loss of hearing, tinnitus (*i.e.*, ringing in the ears), or coughing because of vagal stimulation.

In most cases, cerumen can be removed by gentle irrigation using a bulb syringe and warm tap water. Warm water is used to avoid inducing a feeling of disequilibrium owing to the vestibular caloric response. The ear canal should be dried thoroughly after irrigation to avoid introducing an infection. Irrigation should be avoided in an only-hearing ear or one that is postsurgical, prone to infection, or suspect for perforation of the tympanic membrane. Alternatively, health care professionals may remove cerumen using an otoscope and a wire loop or blunt cerumen curette.

Cerumen that has become hardened or impacted can be softened by instillation of a few drops of a ceruminolytic agent available commercially (*e.g.*, dilute hydrogen peroxide solution) or by prescription. Typically, these agents are instilled in the affected ear one or two times daily for up to 4 days before irrigation. Ceruminolytic agents should not be used in ears that may have a perforated tympanic membrane.

Otitis Externa. Otitis externa is an inflammation of the external ear that can vary in severity from a mild eczematoid dermatitis to severe cellulitis. It can be caused by infectious agents, irritation (*e.g.*, wearing earphones), or allergic reactions. Predisposing factors include moisture in the ear canal after swimming (*i.e.*, swimmer's ear) or bathing and trauma resulting from scratching or attempts to clean the ear. Most infections are caused by gram-negative bacteria (*e.g.*, *Pseudomonas, Proteus*) or fungi that grow in the presence of excess moisture.[4] Otitis externa commonly occurs in the summer and is manifested by itching, redness, tenderness, and narrowing of the ear canal because of swelling. Inflammation of the pinna or canal makes movement of the ear painful. There may be watery or purulent drainage and intermittent hearing loss.

Treatment usually includes the use of ear drops containing an appropriate antimicrobial agent in combination with a corticosteroid to reduce inflammation. An antifungal agent may also be used. Protection of the ear from additional moisture and avoidance of trauma from scratching are important. Preventing recurrences is important, particularly in persons who swim frequently. Instillation of a dilute alcohol, acetic acid, or Burow's otic solution (available in over-the-counter ear drops) immediately after swimming usually is an effective prophylaxis.

THE MIDDLE EAR AND EUSTACHIAN TUBE

The middle ear, or tympanic cavity, is a small, mucosa-lined cavity within the petrous portion of the temporal bone (Fig. 55-3). It is bounded laterally by the tympanic membrane and medially by a bony wall with two openings, the superior oval (vestibular window) and the round (cochlear window). The middle ear is connected anteriorly with the nasopharynx by the *eustachian tube,* also called the pharyngotympanic tube. Posteriorly, it is connected with small air pockets in the temporal bone called *mastoid air spaces* or *cells.*

Three tiny bones, the auditory ossicles, are suspended from the roof of the middle ear cavity and connect the tympanic membrane with the oval window (see Fig. 55-3). They are connected by synovial joints and are covered with the epithelial lining of the cavity.[1,2] The *malleus* ("hammer") has its handle firmly fixed to the upper portion of the tympanic membrane. The head of the malleus articulates with the *incus* ("anvil"), which articulates with the *stapes* ("stirrup"), which is inserted and sealed into the oval window by an annular ligament. Arrangement of the ear ossicles is such that their lever movements transmit vibrations from the tympanic membrane to the oval window and from there to the fluid in the inner ear. Two tissue-covered openings in the medial wall, the oval and the round windows, provide

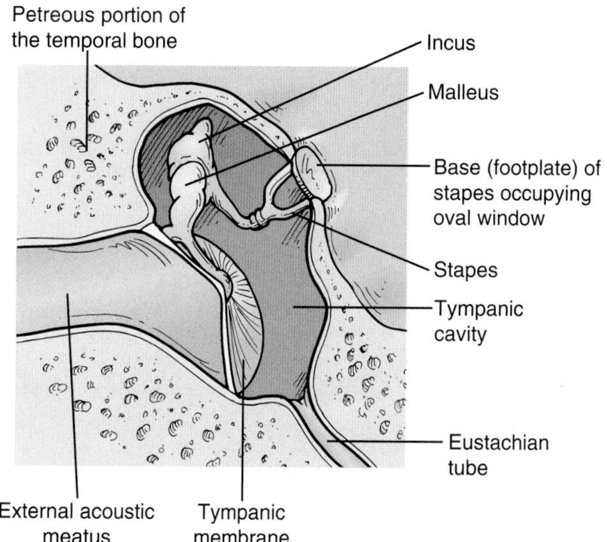

FIGURE 55-3 Anterior view of the ossicles in the middle ear.

DISORDERS OF THE MIDDLE EAR

- The middle ear is a small, air-filled compartment in the temporal bone. It is separated from the outer ear by the tympanic membrane; communication between the nasopharynx and the middle ear occurs through the eustachian tube; and tiny bony ossicles that span the middle ear transmit sound to the sensory receptors in the inner ear.
- Otitis media (OM) refers to inflammation of the middle ear, usually associated with an acute infection (acute OM) or an accumulation of fluid (OME). It commonly is associated with disorders of eustachian tube function.
- The function of the middle ear is to conduct sound waves from the external to the inner ear. Impaired conduction of sound waves and hearing loss occur when the tympanic membrane has been perforated; air in the middle ear has been replaced with fluid (OME); or the function of the bony ossicles has been impaired (otosclerosis).

for the transmission of sound waves between the air-filled middle ear and the fluid-filled inner ear. It is the piston-like action of the stapes footplate that sets up compression waves in the inner ear fluid.

Eustachian Tube Dysfunction

The eustachian tube, which connects the nasopharynx with the middle ear, is located in a gap in the bone between the anterior and medial walls of the middle ear (Fig. 55-4). The eustachian tube serves three basic functions: (1) ventilation of the middle ear, along with equalization of middle ear and ambient pressures; (2) protection of the middle ear from unwanted nasopharyngeal sound waves and secretions; and (3) drainage of middle ear secretions into the nasopharynx.[4,5] The nasopharyngeal entrance to the eustachian tube, which usually is closed, is opened by the action of the trigeminal (CN V)–innervated *tensor veli palatini muscles* (Fig. 55-5). Opening of the eustachian tube, which normally occurs with swallowing and yawning reflexes, provides the mechanism for equalizing the pressure of the middle ear with that of the atmosphere. This equalization ensures that the pressures on both sides of the tympanic membrane are the same, so that sound transmission is not reduced and rupture does not result from sudden changes in external pressure, as occurs during plane travel.

The eustachian tube is lined with a mucous membrane that is continuous with the pharynx and the mastoid air cells. Infections from the nasopharynx can travel from the nasopharynx along the mucous membrane of the eustachian tube to the middle ear, causing acute otitis media. Toward the nasopharynx, the eustachian tube becomes lined by columnar epithelium with mucus-secreting cells. Hypertrophy of the mucus-secreting cells is thought to contribute to the mucoid secretions that develop during certain types of otitis media.

Abnormalities in eustachian tube function are important factors in the pathogenesis of middle ear infections. There are two important types of eustachian tube dysfunction: abnormal patency and obstruction (see Fig. 55-5). The *abnormally patent tube* does not close or does not close completely. In infants and children with an abnormally patent tube, air and secretions often are pumped into the eustachian tube during crying and nose blowing.

Obstruction can be functional or mechanical. *Functional obstruction* results from the persistent collapse of the eustachian tube due to a lack of tubal stiffness or poor function of the tensor veli palatini muscle that controls the opening of the eustachian tube. It is common in infants and young children because the amount and stiffness of the cartilage supporting the eustachian tube are less than in older children and adults. Changes in the craniofacial base also render the tensor muscle less efficient for opening the eustachian tube in this age group. In addition, craniofacial disorders, such as a cleft palate, alter the

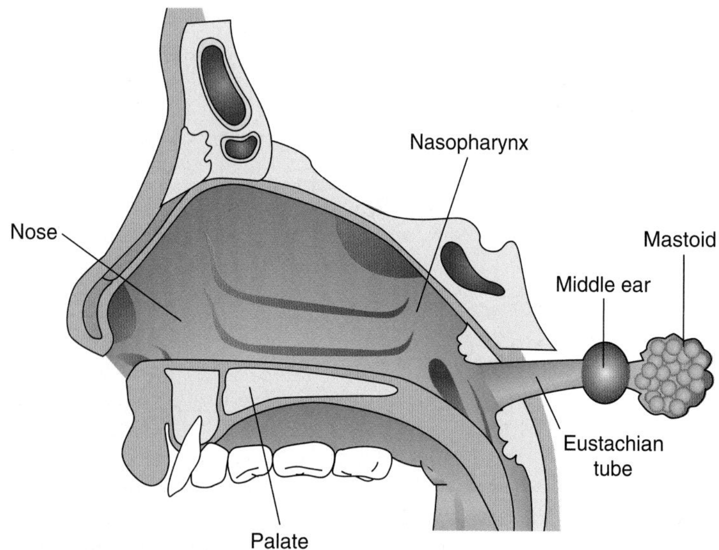

FIGURE 55-4 Nasopharynx–eustachian tube–mastoid air cell system. (Bluestone C.D. [1981]. Recent advances in pathogenesis, diagnosis, and management of otitis media. *Pediatric Clinics of North America 28*[4], 36. Reproduced with permission)

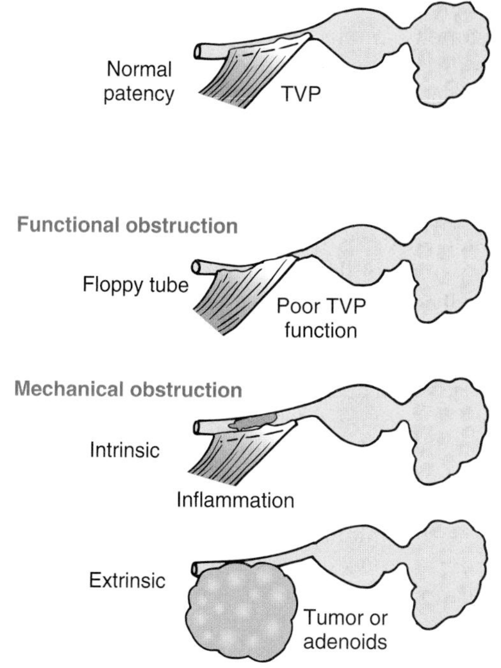

FIGURE 55-5 Pathophysiology of the eustachian tube. TVP, tensor veli palatini. (Bluestone C.D. [1981]. Recent advances in the pathogenesis, diagnosis, and management of otitis media. *Pediatric Clinics of North America 28*[4], 737. With permission from Elsevier Science)

attachment of the tensor muscles, producing functional obstruction of the eustachian tube.

Mechanical obstruction results from internal obstruction or external compression of the eustachian tube. Ethnic differences in the structure of the palate may increase the likelihood of obstruction. The most common internal obstruction is caused by swelling and secretions resulting from allergy and viral respiratory infections. External compression by prominent or enlarged adenoidal tissue surrounding the opening of the eustachian tube may make drainage less effective. Tumors also may obstruct drainage. With obstruction, air in the middle ear is absorbed, causing a negative pressure and the transudation of serous capillary fluid into the middle ear.

Barotrauma

Barotrauma represents injury resulting from the inability to equalize the barometric stress on the middle ear imposed by air travel or, less commonly, by underwater diving. It occurs most often during air travel when there is a sudden change in atmospheric pressure. The pressure in the middle ear parallels atmospheric pressure; it decreases at high altitudes and increases at lower altitudes. The problem occurs during rapid airplane descent, when the negative pressure in the middle ear tends to cause the eustachian tube to collapse. If air cannot pass back through the eustachian tube, hearing loss and discomfort develop.

This most often occurs in persons who travel while suffering from an upper respiratory tract infection. Autoinflation measures such as yawning, swallowing, and chewing gum facilitate opening of the eustachian tube, which equalizes air pressure in the middle ear. Intranasal (*e.g.*, phenylephrine HCl) or systemic decongestants may be used to prevent symptoms. Acute negative middle ear pressure that persists on the ground is treated with decongestants and attempts at autoinflation. More severe hearing loss or discomfort may require that the person consult an otolaryngologist. Myringotomy (*i.e.*, surgical incision in the tympanic membrane) provides immediate relief and may be used in cases of acute otalgia and hearing loss. Placement of ventilation tubes may be considered for persons with repeated episodes of barotrauma related to frequent air travel.

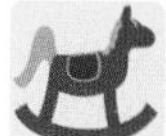

Otitis Media

Otitis media (OM) is an infection of the middle ear that is associated with a collection of fluid. Although OM may occur in any age group, it is the most common diagnosis made by health care providers who care for children.[6–10] Infants and young children are at highest risk for OM, with the peak occurrence between 6 and 20 months of age.[11] The occurrence of the disease tends to decrease as a function of age, with a marked decline after 6 years of age. The incidence is higher in boys, non–breast-fed infants, those who use pacifiers beyond infancy, children in large day care settings, children exposed to tobacco smoke, those with siblings or parents with a significant history of OM, those with allergic rhinitis, and children with congenital or acquired immune deficiencies (*e.g.*, acquired immunodeficiency syndrome). The incidence of OM also is higher among children with craniofacial anomalies (*e.g.*, cleft palate, Down syndrome) and among Canadian and Alaskan Eskimos and Native Americans. It is more common during the winter months, reflecting the seasonal patterns of upper respiratory tract infections.

There are two reasons for the increased risk for OM in infants and young children: the eustachian tube is shorter, more horizontal, and wider in this age group than in older children and adults; and infection can spread more easily through the eustachian canal of infants who spend most of their day lying supine. Bottle-fed infants have a higher incidence of OM than breast-fed infants, probably because they are held in a more horizontal position during feeding, and swallowing while in the horizontal position facilitates the reflux of milk into the middle ear. Breast-feeding also provides for the transfer of protective maternal antibodies to the infant.

Otitis media may present as acute otitis media (AOM), recurrent OM, or OM with effusion (OME) or fluid in the middle ear.

Acute Otitis Media. Acute OM is characterized by the presence of fluid in the middle ear in combination with signs and symptoms of an acute or systemic infection. Acute otitis media can fail to resolve despite antibiotic treatment (persistent OM), or it may resolve and then recur (recurrent OM). It is estimated that AOM resolves spontaneously without treatment in approximately 60% of children.[11]

Most cases of AOM follow an upper respiratory tract infection that has been present for several days. The mucosal lining of the middle ear is continuous with the eustachian tube and nasopharynx, and most middle ear infections enter through the eustachian tube (see Fig. 55-4). AOM may be of either bacterial or viral origin. *Streptococcus pneumoniae, Haemophilus influenzae,* and *Moraxella catarrhalis* are the three major bacterial pathogens isolated from the middle ear in children with AOM.[7–12] There may be more than one type of bacteria present in some children. *S. pneumoniae* causes the largest proportion (40% to 50%) of cases generated by a single organism, and it is the least likely to resolve without treatment.[8,11] Emergence of a multidrug-resistant strain of *S. pneumoniae* (DRSP) has led to increased numbers of treatment failures.[13] Children may be considered as at either high or low risk for DRSP. Children who are at high risk for DRSP include those younger than 2 years of age, those who attend day care, and those who have received antibiotics in the past 3 months.[8,11]

The role of viruses as etiologic agents in AOM is controversial. Viruses have been identified as a single pathogen in only a few middle ear aspirates obtained from children with AOM. Viruses may promote bacterial infection by impairing eustachian tube function and other host defenses.[11] The respiratory syncytial virus is the virus most frequently associated with AOM. Parainfluenza and influenza viruses are other common viral pathogens in AOM. As with bacterial infections, more than one type of respiratory virus may be present in the middle ear fluid of children with AOM.[14]

Manifestations. Acute OM is characterized by otalgia (earache), fever (temperature up to 104°F), and hearing loss. Children older than 3 years of age may have rhinorrhea or running nose, vomiting, and diarrhea. In contrast, younger children often have nonspecific signs and symptoms that manifest as ear tugging, irritability, nighttime awakening, and poor feeding. Ear pain usually increases as the effusion accumulates behind the tympanic membrane. Perforation of the tympanic membrane may occur acutely, allowing purulent material from the eustachian tube to drain into the external auditory canal. This may prevent spread of the infection into the temporal bone or intracranial cavity. Spontaneous perforation with discharge occurs most frequently in children of high-risk ethnic groups.

Diagnosis. Diagnosis of AOM is made by associated signs and symptoms and otoscopic examination. In persons with AOM, a bulging yellow or red tympanic membrane with subsequent obliteration of the bony landmarks and cone of light is observed. Gentle movement of the pinna can help to differentiate OM from otitis externa. This maneuver does not produce pain in AOM but causes severe discomfort in otitis externa. Although diagnosis of AOM often can be made by otoscopic examination alone, pneumatic otoscopy usually is performed to document middle ear effusion and immobility of the tympanic membrane.[15] The use of the pneumatic otoscope permits the introduction of air into the ear canal for the purpose of determining tympanic membrane flexibility. The movement of the tympanic membrane is decreased in some cases of AOM and absent in chronic middle ear infection.

The diagnosis of AOM can be confirmed using tympanometry or acoustic reflectometry. *Tympanometry* is helpful in detecting effusion in the middle ear or high negative middle ear pressure. A tympanogram is obtained by inserting a small probe into the external auditory canal; a tone of fixed characteristics is then presented through the probe, and the mobility of the tympanic membrane is measured electronically while the external canal pressure is artificially varied. The tympanogram provides a determination of the degree of negative pressure present in the middle ear. It detects disease when present but is less reliable when disease is absent. *Acoustic reflectometry* is used to reflect sound waves from the middle ear and provides information as to whether an effusion is absent or present. Increased reflected sound correlates with an increased likelihood of effusion. This technique is most useful in children older than 3 months, and its success depends on user technique.

Tympanocentesis may be done to relieve pain from an effusion or to obtain an organism for culture and sensitivity testing. The procedure involves the insertion of a needle through the inferior part of the tympanic membrane. Because of the cost, effort, and lack of availability, it is not routinely used in management of AOM.[12] In selected cases of refractory or recurrent middle ear disease, tympanocentesis can serve to improve diagnostic accuracy, guide treatment, and avoid unnecessary medical or surgical interventions. In instances in which the tympanic membrane has perforated with resultant drainage into the external ear, a culture c an be made and microbiologic studies done to identify a microorganism.

Treatment. The treatment of AOM includes the judicious use of antibiotic therapy in high-risk children, especially those younger than 2 years of age who are at increased risk for intracranial complications and speech and language impairment.[8,11] The dramatic emergence of DRSP in the United States has led to increased treatment failures for AOM. Current recommendations suggest that if there is a lack of improvement in symptoms by day 3 of the initial antibiotic therapy, a switch to an antibiotic that targets resistant pathogens is recommended.[16] Older children who have no fever or a low-grade fever usually do not require antibiotic treatment provided follow-up evaluation of symptoms occurs within 1 to 3 days. Regardless of whether antibiotic therapy is indicated, supportive therapy that includes analgesics, antipyretics, and local heat often is helpful. If the tympanic membrane is bulging and painful because of the accumulation of purulent drainage, a myringotomy may be done to relieve the pressure, thus reducing pain and hearing loss. In addition, this procedure prevents the ragged opening that can follow spontaneous rupture of the tympanic membrane.

Residual middle ear effusions are part of the continuum of AOM and persist regardless of whether antibiotics have been used. The effusion usually clears spontaneously within 1 to 3 months and does not require further treatment unless it persists beyond this period.

Recurrent Otitis Media. Recurrent OM is defined as three new AOM episodes within 6 months or four episodes in 1 year that occur with almost every upper respiratory tract infection. Reinforcement of environmental controls, such as avoidance of passive tobacco smoke, is important. Children with recurrent OM should be evaluated to rule out any anatomic variations (*e.g.*, enlarged adenoids) and immunologic abnormalities. Children with immunoglobulin G subclass deficiencies (see Chapter 21) and poor responses to polysaccharide vaccines are more likely to develop recurrent OM.[11]

Traditionally, prophylactic antibiotics or antibiotics given at one half the therapeutic dose may be given once daily for up to 6 months during winter and spring. Although children with recurrent OM respond well to such treatment, increasing concern regarding the emergence of bacterial resistance has emerged as a rationale for more judicious use of prophylactic antibiotics. Another approach to prevent recurrent OM is immunization with pneumococcal and influenza vaccines. Referral for placement of tympanostomy tubes is another alternative, particularly for children who have experienced five or more OM episodes within a 12-month period.

Otitis Media With Effusion. Otitis media with effusion is a condition in which the tympanic membrane is intact and there is an accumulation of fluid in the middle ear without signs or symptoms of infection. The type of effusion often is described as serous, nonsuppurative, or secretory, but these terms may not be correct in all cases. The duration of the effusion may range from less than 3 weeks to more than 3 months. The similarity between OME and AOM is that hearing loss may be present in both conditions. The major distinction is that signs and symptoms of infection are lacking in OME, although some children may complain of a feeling of ear fullness. Distinguishing between OME and AOM often is difficult because of the variability and overlap of symptoms, particularly in young children.

Diagnosis is based on otoscopic examination, which frequently reveals opacification of the tympanic membrane, making it difficult to visualize the effusion and, thus, characterize the type. If the tympanic membrane is translucent, a yellow or bluish fluid may be seen, as may an air–fluid level or bubbles, or both. Pneumatic otoscopy often reveals decreased mobility of the tympanic membrane, with a shape that is either retracted or convex. Alternatively, fullness or bulging may be noted.

Most cases of persistent middle ear effusion resolve spontaneously within a 3-week to 3-month period. The management options for this duration include observation only, antibiotic therapy, or combination antibiotic and corticosteroid therapy. Topical and systemic decongestants usually are of little value in clearing middle ear effusion. Because there is concern over hearing loss and its effect on learning and speech, a hearing evaluation may be indicated and usually is done after 6 weeks.

If the effusion persists for 3 months or longer and is accompanied by hearing loss of 20 decibels (dB) or greater in children of normal development, tympanostomy tube placement may be indicated.[11] The tubes usually are placed under general anesthesia. The ears of children with tubes must be kept out of water. Spontaneous extrusion of tubes usually occurs after 5.5 to 7 months.[17] Complications of tube placement include recurrent otorrhea; persistent perforation, scarring, and atrophy of the tympanic membrane; and cholesteatoma.

Complications. Since the advent of antimicrobial therapy, the intracranial suppurative complications of OM have been uncommon. However, extratemporal complications, including those affecting the middle ear, mastoid, and adjacent structures of the temporal bone, continue to occur.

Hearing loss, which is a common complication of OM, usually is conductive and temporary based on the duration of the effusion. Hearing loss that is associated with fluid collection usually resolves when the effusion clears. Permanent hearing loss may occur as the result of damage to the tympanic membrane or other middle ear structures. Cases of sensorineural hearing loss are rare. Persistent and episodic conductive hearing loss in children may impair their cognitive, linguistic, and emotional development.[8,9] Children younger than 3 years of age with recurrent OME are at increased risk for impaired language development.[8] Additional studies indicate that before 3 years of age, time spent with middle ear effusion correlates with decreased cognitive development as measured by standardized inventories.[18] However, the degree and duration of hearing loss required to produce such effects are unknown.

Perforation of the tympanic membrane can occur spontaneously or result from surgical interventions. Temporary perforations are created for surgical treatment of AOM (myringotomy) or for tube placement. Usually, the perforations heal spontaneously. Antimicrobial treatment for AOM with acute perforation is the same as for AOM without perforation.[13] When chronic drainage is present, cultures usually are performed and the antimicrobial regimen adjusted accordingly. Otic drops also may be instilled in the external ear to prevent or treat an external canal infection.[13] Healing of the tympanic membrane usually follows resolution of the middle ear infection.

Adhesive OM involves an abnormal healing reaction in an inflamed middle ear. It produces irreversible thickening of the mucous membranes and may cause impaired movement of the ossicles and possibly conductive hearing loss. Tympanosclerosis involves the formation of whitish plaques and nodular deposits on the submucosal surface of the tympanic membrane, with possible adherence of the ossicles and conductive hearing loss.

A *cholesteatoma* is a saclike mass containing silvery-white debris of keratin, which is shed by the squamous epithelial lining of the tympanic membrane.[19] As the lining of the epithelium sheds and desquamates, the lesion expands and erodes the surrounding tissues. The lesion, which is associated with chronic middle ear infection, is insidiously progressive, and erosion may involve the temporal bone, causing intracranial complications. Although often thought of as a complication of otitis media, a cholesteatoma may also occur as a congenital condition. Symptoms commonly include painless drainage from the ear and hearing loss. Treatment involves microsurgical techniques to remove the cholesteatomatous material.

The mastoid antrum and air cells constitute a portion of the temporal bone and may become inflamed as an extension of acute or chronic OM. The disorder causes necrosis of the mastoid process and destruction of the bony intercellular matrix, which are visible by radiologic examination. Mastoid tenderness and drainage of exudate through a perforated tympanic membrane can occur. Chronic mastoiditis can develop as the result of chronic middle ear infection. The usefulness of antibiotics for this condition is limited. Mastoid or middle ear surgery, along with other medical treatment, may be indicated. The incidence of mastoiditis has markedly decreased compared with the preantimicrobial era. It remains uncertain whether this decrease is due to antimicrobial treatment, changes in the natural history of OM, changes in organism virulence, or increased host resistance.[20]

Intracranial complications, although rare, can develop if the infection spreads through vascular channels, by direct extension, or through preformed pathways such as the round window. These complications are seen more often with chronic suppurative OM and mastoiditis. They include meningitis, focal encephalitis, brain abscess, lateral sinus thrombophlebitis or thrombosis, labyrinthitis, and facial nerve paralysis. Any child who develops persistent headache, tinnitus, stiff neck, or visual or other neurologic symptoms should be investigated for possible intracranial complications.

Otosclerosis

Otosclerosis refers to the formation of new spongy bone around the stapes and oval window, which results in progressive deafness[21] (see Fig. 55-3). In most cases, the condition is familial and follows an autosomal dominant pattern with variable penetrance. Otosclerosis may begin at any time in life but usually does not appear until after puberty, most frequently between the ages of 20 and 30 years. The disease process accelerates during pregnancy.

Otosclerosis begins with resorption of bone in one or more foci. During active bone resorption, the bone structure appears spongy and softer than normal (*i.e.,* osteospongiosis). The resorbed bone is replaced by an overgrowth of new, hard, sclerotic bone. The process is slowly progressive, involving more areas of the temporal bone, especially in front of and posterior to the stapes footplate. As it invades the footplate, the pathologic bone increasingly immobilizes the stapes, reducing the transmission of sound. Pressure from the otosclerotic bone on inner ear structures or the vestibulocochlear nerve (CN VIII) may contribute to the development of tinnitus, sensorineural hearing loss, and vertigo.

The symptoms of otosclerosis involve an insidious hearing loss. Initially, the affected person is unable to hear a whisper or someone speaking at a distance. In the earliest stages, the bone conduction by which the person's own voice is heard remains relatively unaffected. At this point, the person's own voice sounds unusually loud, and the sound of chewing becomes intensified. Because of bone conduction, most of these persons can hear fairly well on the telephone, which provides an amplified signal. Many are able to hear better in a noisy environment, probably because the masking effect of background noise causes other persons to speak louder.

The treatment of otosclerosis can be medical or surgical. A carefully selected, well-fitting hearing aid may allow a person with conductive deafness to lead a normal life. Sodium fluoride has been used with some success in the medical treatment of osteospongiosis. Because much of the conductive hearing loss associated with otosclerosis is caused by stapedial fixation, surgical treatment involves stapedectomy with stapedial reconstruction using the patient's own stapes or a stapedial prosthesis. The argon laser may be used in the surgical procedure.

DISORDERS OF THE INNER EAR

The inner ear contains the receptors for hearing.[1,2,22] It contains a labyrinth or system of intercommunicating channels and the receptors for hearing and position sense. Structurally, it consists of an outer bony labyrinth located in the temporal bone and an inner, fluid-filled membranous labyrinth (Fig. 55-6). Two separate fluids are found in the inner ear. The *perilymph* or *periotic fluid* separates the bony labyrinth from the membranous labyrinth, and the *endolymph* or *otic fluid* fills the membranous labyrinth. The composition of the perilymph is similar to that of the CSF, and a tubular perilymphatic duct connects the perilymph with the CSF in the arachnoid space of the posterior fossa. The endolymph has a potassium content that is similar to that of intracellular fluid. A small-diameter tubular extension, the endolymphatic sac, connects this system with the subdural space near the jugular foramen, providing an exit for the slowly circulating endolymph.

The bony labyrinth occupies a volume with a diameter less than the size of a dime. It is divided into a series of perilymph-filled interconnected cavities: the cochlea, the semicircular canals, the utricle, and the saccule. The receptors for hearing are contained in the cochlea, and those for head position sense are contained in the semicircular canals, the utricle, and the saccule. The vestibule is the central egg-shaped cavity of the bony labyrinth that lies posterior to the cochlea and anterior to the semicircular canals. The oval window that connects the inner ear with the middle ear is located in its lateral wall.

The cochlea is enclosed in a bony tube shaped like a snail shell that winds around a central bone column called the *modiolus.* A membranous triangular cochlear duct stretches across the cochlea, separating it into two parallel tubes, each containing perilymph: the *scala vestibuli* and the *scala tympani* (Fig. 55-7). One side of the cochlear duct, the *basilar membrane,* stretches under tension laterally from the modiolus to an elastic spiral ligament. A second side, the *vestibular membrane* (*i.e.,* Reissner's membrane), is a delicate double layer of squamous epithelial cells. The third side consists of a well-vascularized epithelium, the *stria vascularis,* which is the source of the endolymph. The cochlear duct separates the scala vestibuli and the scala tympani from the base of the cochlea throughout its two and one-half spiral turns to its apex. An opening at the

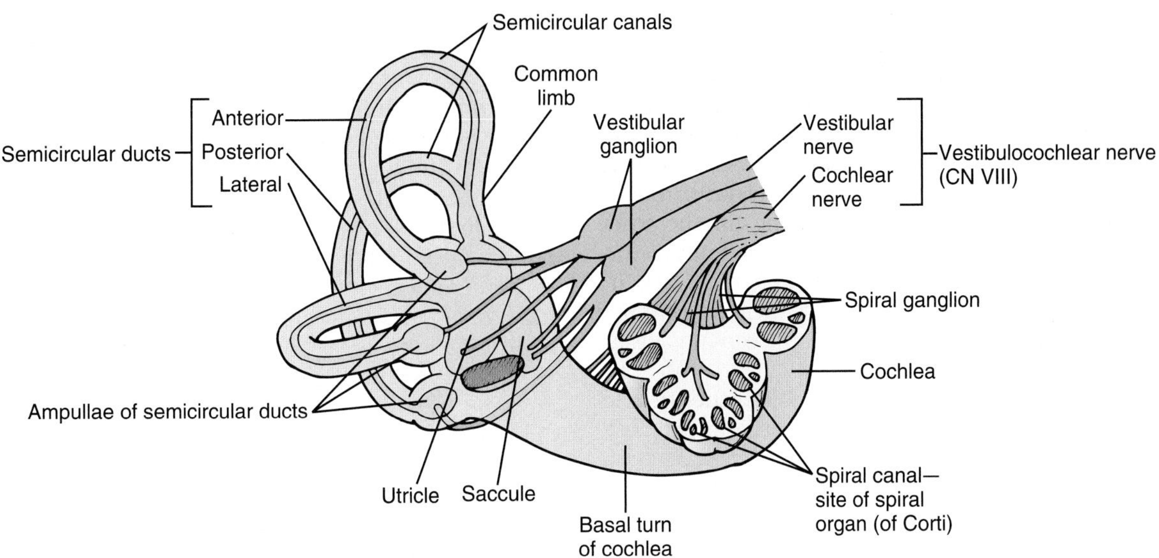

FIGURE 55-6 Schematic lateral view of the bony and membranous labyrinths showing the membranous labyrinth in a closed system of ducts and chambers filled with endolymph and bathed in perilymph with the bony labyrinth. Observe the parts of membranous labyrinth: the cochlear duct, the saccule and utricle within the vestibule, and the semicircular ducts within the semicircular canals. (From Moore K.L., Dalley A.F. [1999]. *Clinically oriented anatomy* [4th ed., p. 1102]. Philadelphia: Lippincott Williams & Wilkins)

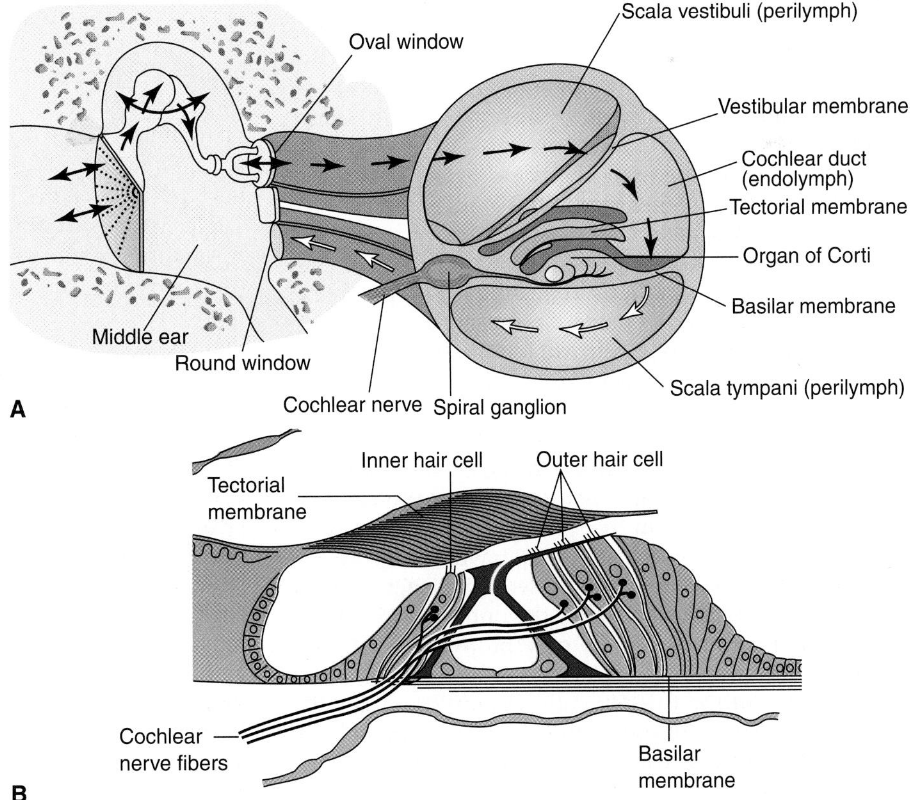

FIGURE 55-7 (**A**) Path taken by sound waves reaching the inner ear. (**B**) Spiral organ of Corti has been removed from the cochlear duct and greatly enlarged to show the inner and outer hair cells, the basilar membrane, and cochlear nerve fibers.

apex, called the *helicotrema,* permits fluid waves to move between the two scalae.

Unlike light, which can be transmitted through a vacuum such as outer space, sound is a pressure disturbance originating from a vibrating object and propagated by the molecules of an elastic medium. Sound waves, delivered by the stapes footplate to the perilymph, travel throughout the fluid of the inner ear, including up the scala vestibuli, to the apex of the cochlea. Because fluids are incompressible, each time the fluid adjacent to the oval window is forced medially by the stapes, the membrane in the round window bulges out into the middle ear and acts as a pressure valve.

As the pressure wave descends through the flexible vestibular membrane, it sets the entire basilar membrane into vibrations. The basilar membrane becomes progressively more massive from base to its distal apex and resonates to higher frequencies near the base and to lower frequencies toward the apex as the fluid pressure wave travels up the cochlear spiral. This "tuned" aspect of the basilar membrane results in increased amplitude of displacement at the resonant locations, responding to a particular sound frequency and greater firing of cochlear neurons innervating this region. This mechanism provides the major basis for the discrimination of sound frequency.

Perched on the basilar membrane and extending along its entire length is an elaborate arrangement of columnar epithelium called the *organ of Corti* (see Fig. 55-7). Continuous rows of hair cells separated into inner and outer rows can be found within the columnar arrangement. The cells have hairlike cilia that protrude through openings in an overlying supporting reticular membrane into the endolymph of the cochlear duct. A gelatinous mass, the tectorial membrane, extends from the medial side of the duct to enclose the cilia of the outer hair cells. The traveling compression waves moving from base to apex through the periotic fluid distort the organ of Corti, causing the hairs to bend against the less flexible tectorial membrane. Each inner hair cell is innervated by several nerve fibers and the outer hair cells, by many cochlear afferent neuron terminals.

Selective destruction of hair cells in a particular segment of the cochlea can lead to hearing loss of particular tones. The outer rows of hair cells appear to provide the signals on which the experience of loudness, a correlate of the sound's physical intensity, is based.

Neural Pathways

Afferent fibers from the organ of Corti have their cell bodies in the spiral ganglion in the central portion of the cochlea. Nerve fibers from the spiral ganglion (*i.e.,* vestibulocochlear or auditory nerve [CN VIII]) travel to the cochlear nuclei in the caudal pons. Many secondary nerve fibers from the cochlear nuclei pass to the opposite side of the pons. These secondary fibers may project to such cell groups as the trapezoid or the superior olivary nucleus, or rostrally toward the inferior colliculus of the midbrain. Ipsilateral (same side) projections and interconnections between the nuclei of the two sides occur throughout the central auditory system. Consequently, impulses from either ear are transmitted through the auditory pathways to both sides of the brain stem.

From the inferior colliculus, the auditory pathway passes to the medial geniculate nucleus of the thalamus, where all the fibers synapse. Considerable evidence supports the capability of this level of organization to provide crude auditory experience, including crude tone and intensity discrimination and the directionality of a sound source. From the medial geniculate nucleus, the auditory tract spreads through the auditory radiation to the primary auditory cortex (area 41), located mainly in the superior temporal gyrus and insula (see Chapter 49, Fig. 49-24). This area and its corresponding higher-order thalamic nucleus are required for high-acuity loudness discrimination and precise discrimination of pitch. The auditory association cortex (areas 42 and 22) borders the primary cortex on the superior temporal gyrus. This area and its associated higher-order thalamic nuclei are necessary for auditory gnosis, or the meaningfulness of sound, to occur. Experience and the precise analysis of momentary auditory information are integrated during this process.

Tinnitus

Tinnitus (from the Latin *tinniere,* meaning "to ring") is the perception of abnormal ear or head noises, not produced by an external stimulus.[23–25] Although it often is described as "ringing of the ears," it may also assume a hissing, roaring, buzzing, or humming sound. Tinnitus may be constant, intermittent, and unilateral or bilateral. It has been estimated that 37 million people in the United States have the disorder. Nearly 10 million of these are estimated to have severe or troubling tinnitus.[24] The condition affects males and females equally, is most prevalent between 40 and 70 years of age, and occasionally affects children.[23]

Although tinnitus is subjective, for clinical purposes it is subdivided into objective and subjective tinnitus. *Objective tinnitus* refers to those rare cases in which the sound is detected or potentially detectable by another observer. Typical causes of objective tinnitus include vascular abnormalities or neuromuscular disorders. In some vascular disorders, for example, sounds generated by turbulent blood flow (*e.g.,* arterial bruits or venous hums) are conducted to the auditory system. Vascular disorders typically produce a pulsatile form of tinnitus.

Subjective tinnitus refers to noise perception when there is no noise stimulation of the cochlea. A number of causes and conditions have been associated with subjective tinnitus. Intermittent periods of mild, high-pitched tinnitus lasting for several minutes are common in normal-hearing persons. Impacted cerumen is a benign cause of tinnitus, which resolves after the earwax is removed. Medications such as aspirin and stimulants such as nicotine and caffeine can cause transient tinnitus. Conditions associated with more persistent tinnitus include noise-induced hearing loss, presbycusis (sensorimotor hearing loss that occurs with aging), hypertension, atherosclerosis, head injury, and cochlear or labyrinthine infection or inflammation.

The physiologic mechanism underlying subjective tinnitus is largely unknown. It seems likely that there are several mechanisms, including abnormal firing of auditory receptors, dysfunction of cochlear neurotransmitter function or ionic balance, damage to the auditory nerve, or alterations in central processing of the signal.

Because tinnitus is a symptom, the diagnosis relies heavily on the person's description of the problem, including onset, frequency, description, and location of the tinnitus; perceived cause; and extent to which the person is bothered by the problem.[26] A history of medication or stimulant use and dietary factors that may cause tinnitus should be obtained. Tinnitus often accompanies hearing disorders, and tests of auditory function usually are done. Causes of objective tinnitus, such as serious vascular abnormalities, should be ruled out.

Treatment measures are designed to treat the symptoms rather than effect a cure.[23–25] They include elimination of drugs or other substances such as caffeine, some cheeses, red wine, and foods containing monosodium glutamate that are suspected of causing tinnitus. The use of an externally produced sound (noise generators or tinnitus-masking devices) may be used to mask or inhibit the tinnitus. Medications, including antihistamines, anticonvulsant drugs, calcium channel blockers, benzodiazepines, and antidepressants, have been used for tinnitus alleviation, but most are not effective, and many produce undesirable side effects. For persistent tinnitus, psychological interventions may be needed to help the person deal with the stress and distraction associated with the condition. Tinnitus retraining therapy, which includes directive counseling and extended use of low-noise generators to facilitate auditory adaptation to the tinnitus, has met with considerable success. Surgical intervention (*i.e.*, cochlear nerve section, vascular decompression) is a last resort for persons in which all other interventions have failed and in whom the disorder is disabling.

DISORDERS OF THE CENTRAL AUDITORY PATHWAYS

The auditory pathways in the brain involve communication between the two sides of the brain at many levels. As a result, strokes, tumors, abscesses, and other focal abnormalities seldom produce more than a mild reduction in auditory acuity on the side opposite the lesion. For intelligibility of auditory language, lateral dominance becomes important. On the dominant side, usually the left side, the more medial and dorsal portion of the auditory association cortex is of crucial importance. This area is called *Wernicke's area,* and damage to it is associated with auditory receptive aphasia (and agnosia of speech). Persons with damage to this area of the brain can speak intelligibly and read normally but are unable to understand the meaning of major aspects of audible speech.

Irritative foci that affect the auditory radiation or the primary auditory cortex can produce roaring or clicking sounds, which appear to come from the auditory environment of the opposite side (*i.e.,* auditory hallucinations). Focal seizures that originate in or near the auditory cortex often are immediately preceded by the perception of ringing or other sounds preceded by a prodrome (*i.e.,* aura). Damage to the auditory association cortex, especially if bilateral, results in deficiencies of sound recognition and memory (*i.e.,* auditory agnosia). If the damage is in the dominant hemisphere, speech recognition can be affected (*i.e.,* sensory or receptive aphasia).

HEARING LOSS

Nearly 30 million Americans have hearing loss.[27,28] It affects persons of all age groups. One of every 1000 infants born in the United States is completely deaf, and more than 3 million children have hearing loss. Between 25% and 40% of people older than 65 years of age have hearing loss.[29]

Hearing is a specialized sense that provides the ability to perceive vibration of sound waves. Functions of the ear include receiving sound waves, distinguishing their frequency, translating this information into nerve impulses, and transmitting these impulses to the CNS. The compression waves that produce sound have frequency and intensity. *Frequency* indicates the number of waves per unit time (reported in cycles per second [cps] or hertz [Hz]). The human ear is most sensitive to waves in the frequency range of 1000 to 3000 Hz. Most persons cannot hear compression waves that have a frequency higher than 20,000 Hz. Waves of higher frequency are called *ultrasonic waves,* meaning that they are above the audible range. In the audible frequency range, the subjective experience correlated with sonic frequency is the pitch of a

HEARING LOSS

- Hearing is a special sensory function that incorporates the sound-transmitting properties of the external ear canal, the eardrum that separates the external and middle ear, the bony ossicles of the middle ear, the sensory receptors of the cochlea in the inner ear, the neural pathways of the vestibulocochlear or auditory nerve, and the primary auditory and auditory association cortices.
- Hearing loss represents impairment of the ability to detect and perceive sound.
- It can range from mild, affecting sounds of different tones and intensities, to moderate or profound.
- Hearing loss can be caused by conductive disorders, in which auditory stimuli are not transmitted through the structures of the outer and middle ears to the sensory receptors in the inner ear; by sensorineural disorders that affect the inner ear, auditory nerve, or auditory pathways; or by a combination of conductive and sensorineural disorders.

sound. Waves below 20 to 30 Hz are experienced as a rattle or drum beat rather than a tone.

Wave intensity is represented by amplitude or units of sound pressure. By convention, the intensity (in power units, or ergs per square centimeter) of a sound is expressed as the ratio of intensities between the sound and a reference value. A 10-fold increase in sound pressure is called a bel, after Alexander Graham Bell. Because this representation is too crude to be of use, the decibel (dB), or one tenth of a bel, is used. For purposes of hearing evaluation, the threshold for perception of sound at a given frequency in persons with normal hearing is set at 0 dB.[30]

Hearing loss is qualified as mild, moderate, severe, or profound. "Hard of hearing" is defined as hearing loss greater than 20 to 25 dB in adults and greater than 15 dB in children. Profound deafness is defined as hearing loss greater than 100 dB[31] or 70 dB in children.[32] There are many causes of hearing loss or deafness. Most fit into the categories of conductive, sensorineural, or mixed deficiencies that involve a combination of conductive and sensorineural function deficiencies of the same ear.[30] Chart 55-1 summarizes common causes of hearing loss. Hearing loss may be genetic or nongenetic, sudden or progressive, unilateral or bilateral, partial or complete, reversible or irreversible. Age and suddenness of onset provide important clues as to the cause of hearing loss.

CHART 55-1

Common Causes of Conductive and Sensorineural Hearing Loss

Conductive Hearing Loss

- External ear conditions
  - Impacted earwax or foreign body
  - Otitis externa
- Middle ear conditions
  - Trauma
  - Otitis media (acute and with effusion)
  - Otosclerosis
  - Tumors

Sensorineural Hearing Loss

- Trauma
  - Head injury
  - Noise
- Central nervous system infections (*e.g.*, meningitis)
- Degenerative conditions
  - Presbycusis
- Vascular
  - Atherosclerosis
  - Sudden deafness
- Ototoxic drugs (*e.g.*, aminoglycosides, salicylates, loop diuretics)
- Tumors
  - Vestibular schwannoma (acoustic neuroma)
  - Meningioma
  - Metastatic tumors
- Idiopathic
  - Ménière's disease

Mixed Conductive and Sensorineural Hearing Loss

- Middle ear conditions
  - Barotrauma
  - Cholesteatoma
  - Otosclerosis
- Temporal bone fractures

Conductive Hearing Loss

Conductive hearing loss occurs when auditory stimuli are not adequately transmitted through the auditory canal, tympanic membrane, middle ear, or ossicle chain to the inner ear. Temporary hearing loss can occur as the result of impacted cerumen in the outer ear or fluid in the middle ear. Foreign bodies, including pieces of cotton and insects, may impair hearing. More permanent causes of hearing loss are thickening or damage of the tympanic membrane or involvement of the bony structures (ossicles and oval window) of the middle ear due to otosclerosis or Paget's disease (see Chapter 58).

Sensorineural Hearing Loss

Sensorineural, or perceptive, hearing loss occurs with disorders that affect the inner ear, auditory nerve, or auditory pathways of the brain. With this type of deafness, sound waves are conducted to the inner ear, but abnormalities of the cochlear apparatus or auditory nerve decrease or distort the transfer of information to the brain. Tinnitus often accompanies cochlear nerve irritation. Abnormal function resulting from damage or malformation of the central auditory pathways and circuitry is included in this category.

Sensorineural hearing loss may have a genetic cause or may result from intrauterine infections such as maternal rubella, or developmental malformations of the inner ear. Genetic hearing loss may result from mutation in a single gene (monogenetic) or from a combination of mutations in different genes and environmental factors (multifactorial). It has been estimated that 50% of profound deafness in children has a monogenetic basis.[30,31] The inheritance pattern for monogenetic hearing loss is autosomal recessive in approximately 75% of cases.[32] Hearing loss may begin before development of speech (prelingual) or after speech development (postlingual). Most prelingual forms are present at birth. Genetic forms of hearing loss also can be classified as being part of a syndrome in which other abnormalities are present, or as nonsyndromic, in which deafness is the only abnormality.

Sensorineural hearing loss also can result from trauma to the inner ear, tumors that encroach on the inner ear or sensory neurons, vascular disorders with hemorrhage, or thrombosis of vessels that supply the inner ear. Other causes of sensorineural deafness are infections and drugs. Sudden sensorineural hearing loss represents an abrupt loss of hearing that occurs instantaneously or on awakening. It most commonly is caused by viral infections, circulatory disorders, or rupture of the labyrinth membrane that can occur during tympanotomy.[33]

Environmentally induced deafness can occur through direct exposure to excessively intense sound, as in the workplace or at a concert. This is a particular problem in older adults who were working in noisy environments before the mid-1960s, when there were no laws mandating use of devices for protective hearing. This type of deafness was once called *boilermaker's deafness* because of the intense reverberating sound to which riveters were exposed when putting together boiler tanks. Sustained or repeated exposure to noise pollution at sound intensities greater than 100 to 120 dB can cause corresponding mechanical damage to the organ of Corti on the "tuned" basilar membrane. If damage is severe, permanent sensorineural deafness to the offending sound frequencies results. Wearing earplugs or ear protection is important under many industrial conditions and for musicians and music listeners exposed to high sound amplification. Noise pollution often is characterized by high-intensity sounds of a specific frequency that cause corresponding damage to the organ of Corti. Temporary threshold shift is a reversible hearing loss that occurs in individuals who attend loud concerts and hear ringing sounds after the event.

A number of infections can cause hearing loss. Deafness or some degree of hearing impairment is the most common serious complication of bacterial meningitis in infants and children, reportedly resulting in sensorineural hearing loss in 5% to 35% of persons who survive the infection.[30] The mechanism causing hearing impairment seems to be a suppurative labyrinthitis or neuritis resulting in the loss of hair cells and damage to the auditory nerve. Untreated suppurative OM also can extend into the inner ear and cause sensorineural hearing loss through the same mechanisms. Congenital and acquired syphilis can cause unilateral or bilateral sensorineural hearing loss. Hypothyroidism is a potential cause of sensorineural hearing loss in older persons.

Among the neoplasms that impair hearing are *acoustic neuromas*. Acoustic neuromas are benign Schwann cell tumors affecting CN VIII. These tumors usually are unilateral and cause hearing loss by compressing the cochlear nerve or interfering with blood supply to the nerve and cochlea. Other neoplasms that can affect hearing include meningiomas and metastatic brain tumors. The temporal bone is a common site of metastases. Breast cancer may metastasize to the middle ear and invade the cochlea.

Drugs that damage inner ear structures are labeled *ototoxic*. Vestibular symptoms of ototoxicity include lightheadedness, giddiness, and dizziness; if toxicity is severe, cochlear symptoms consisting of tinnitus or hearing loss occur. Hearing loss is sensorineural and may be bilateral or unilateral, transient or permanent. Several classes of drugs have been identified as having ototoxic potential, including the aminoglycoside antibiotics and some other basic antibiotics, antimalarial drugs, some chemotherapeutic drugs, loop diuretics, and salicylates (*e.g.*, aspirin). The symptoms of drug-induced hearing loss may be transient, as often is the case with salicylates and diuretics, or they may be permanent. The risk for ototoxicity depends on the total dose of the drug and its concentration in the bloodstream. It is increased in persons with impaired kidney functioning and in those previously or currently treated with another potentially ototoxic drug.

Diagnosis and Treatment

Although approximately 10% of Americans have some degree of hearing loss, including one third of persons older than 65 years of age, hearing loss often is underdiagnosed. While visual impairments are readily accepted and vigorously treated, loss of hearing often is denied, minimized, or ignored. In a society that favors youth, glasses and contact lens are considered normal and even fashionable, whereas hearing aids often are regarded as a sign of "graceless aging."[31]

Diagnosis of hearing loss is aided by careful history of associated otologic factors such as otalgia, otorrhea, tinnitus, and self-described hearing difficulties; physical examination to detect the presence of conditions such as otorrhea, impacted cerumen, or injury to the tympanic membrane; and hearing tests.[28,29] A history of occupational and noise exposure is important, as is the use of medications with ototoxic potential. Testing for hearing loss includes a number of methods, including a person's reported ability to hear an observer's voice, use of a tuning fork to test air and bone conduction, audioscopes, and auditory brain stem evoked responses (ABRs).

Tuning forks are used to differentiate conductive and sensorineural hearing loss. A 512-Hz or higher-frequency tuning fork is used because frequencies below this level elicit a tactile response. The Weber test evaluates conductive hearing loss by lateralization of sound. It is done by placing the lightly vibrating tuning fork on the forehead or vertex of the head. In persons with conductive losses, the sound is louder on the side with the hearing loss, but in persons with sensorineural loss, it radiates to the side with the better hearing. The Rinne test compares air and bone conduction. The test is done by alternately placing the tuning fork on the mastoid bone and in front of the ear canal. In conductive losses, bone conduction exceeds air conduction; in sensorineural losses, the opposite occurs.

Audioscopes can be used to assess a person's ability to hear pure tones at 1000 to 2000 Hz (usual speech frequencies). If a person cannot hear these tones, referral for a full audiogram should be done. The audiogram is an important method of analyzing a person's hearing and is generally considered the gold standard for diagnosis of hearing loss. It is done by an audiologist and requires highly specialized sound production and control equipment. Pure tones of controlled intensity are delivered, usually to one ear at a time, and the minimum intensity needed for hearing to be experienced is plotted as a function of frequency.

The ABR is a noninvasive method that permits functional evaluation of certain defined parts of the central auditory pathways. Electroencephalographic (EEG) electrodes and high-gain amplifiers are required to produce a record of the brain wave activity elicited during repeated acoustic stimulations of either or both ears. ABR recording involves subjecting the ear to loud clicks and using a computer to pick up nerve impulses as they are processed in the midbrain. With this method, certain of the early waves that come from discrete portions of the pons and midbrain auditory pathways can be correlated with specific sensorineural abnormalities. Imaging studies such as computed tomography scans and magnetic resonance imaging can be done to determine the site of a lesion and the extent of damage.[27]

Treatment. Untreated hearing loss can have many consequences. Social isolation and depressive disorders are common in hearing-impaired elderly. Hearing-impaired people may avoid social situations in which background noise makes conversation difficult to hear. Safety issues, both in and out of the home, may become significant. Treatment of hearing loss ranges from simple removal of impacted cerumen in the external auditory canal to surgical procedures such as those used to reconstruct the tympanic membrane. For other people, particularly the frail elderly, hearing aids remain an option. Cochlear implants also are an option for some people.

Hearing aids remain the mainstay of treatment for many persons with conductive and sensorineural hearing loss. With the advent of microcircuitry, hearing aids are now being designed with computer chips that allow multiple programs to be placed in a single hearing aid. The various programs allow the user to select a specific setting for different listening situations. The development of microcircuitry has also made it possible for hearing aids to be miniaturized to the point that, in many cases, they can be placed deep in the ear where they take advantage of the normal shape of the external ear and ear canal. Although modern hearing aids have improved greatly, they cannot replicate the hearing person's ability to hear both soft and loud noises. They also fail to filter out distorted or background noise consistently. Many persons who are fitted with hearing aids use them inconsistently, often because of social embarrassment, increase in background noise, or the sound of their own voice being transmitted through the hearing aid.[34] Other aids for the hearing impaired include alert and signal devices, assisted-listening devices from telephone companies, and dogs trained to respond to various sounds.

Most important, hearing impairment produces a loss of the important communicative function of auditory language, leading to social isolation. Although many assistance devices are available to persons with hearing loss, understanding on the part of family and friends is perhaps the most important.[31] The interpretation of speech involves both visual and auditory clues. It is important that people speaking to persons with hearing impairment face the person and articulate so that lip reading cues can be used. Adequate lighting is important. Distractions such as background noise can make communication difficult and should be avoided when possible.

Surgically implantable cochlear prostheses for the profoundly deaf have been developed and are available for use in adults and children 2 years of age or older.[35] These prostheses are inserted into the scala tympani of the cochlea and work by providing direct stimulation to the auditory nerve, bypassing the stimulation that typically is provided by transducer cells but that is absent or nonfunctional in a deaf cochlea. For the implant to work, the auditory nerve must be functional. Whereas early implants used a single electrode, current implants use multielectrode placement, enhancing speech perception. Much of the progress in implant performance has been achieved through improvements in the speech processors that convert sound into electrical stimuli. Advances in the development of the multichannel implant have improved performance such that cochlear implants have been established as an effective option for adults and children with profound hearing impairment.[36,37] Most persons who are deafened after learning speech derive substantial benefit when cochlear implants are used in conjunction with lip reading; some are able to understand selected types of speech without lip reading; and some are able to communicate by telephone.

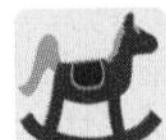

Hearing Loss in Infants and Children

Even mild or unilateral hearing loss can have a detrimental effect on the language development and hearing-associated learning of the young child. Although estimates vary dependent on the group surveyed and testing methods used, from 1 to 2 per 1000 newborns have moderate (30 to 50 dB), severe (50 to 70 db), or profound (≥70 dB) sensorineural hearing loss.[11] An additional 1 to 2 per 1000 may have milder or unilateral impairments. When considering less severe or transient conductive hearing loss that is commonly associated with middle ear disease in young children, the numbers are even greater.

The cause of hearing impairment in children depends on whether the hearing loss is conductive or sensorineural. Most cases of conductive hearing loss is caused by middle ear infections. Causes of sensorineural hearing impairment include genetic, infectious, traumatic, and ototoxic factors. Genetic causes are probably responsible for as many as 50% of sensorineural hearing loss in children. The most common infectious cause of congenital sensorineural hearing loss is cytomegalovirus (CMV), which infects 1 in 100 newborns in the United States each year; of these, about 1200 to 2000 have sensorineural hearing loss.[11] Of particular concern is the fact that congenital CMV can cause both symptomatic and asymptomatic hearing loss in the newborn. Some children with congenital CMV infection, who were asymptomatic as newborns, have suddenly lost residual hearing at 4 to 5 years of age.[11] Postnatal causes of sensorineural hearing loss include β streptococcal sepsis in the newborn and bacterial meningitis. *Streptococcus pneumoniae* is the most common cause of bacterial meningitis that results in sensorineural hearing loss after the neonatal period; this cause may become less frequent with the routine administration of the conjugate pneumococcal vaccine. Other causes of sensorineural hearing loss are toxins and trauma. Early in pregnancy, the embryo is particularly sensitive to toxic substances, including ototoxic drugs such as the aminoglycosides and loop diuretics. Trauma, particularly head trauma, may cause sensorineural hearing loss.

Because hearing impairment can have a major impact on the development of a child, early identification through screening programs is strongly advocated. The American Academy of Pediatricians (AAP) and the Joint Commission on Infant Hearing (JCIH) recently published a position paper calling for universal screening of all infants by physiologic measurements before 3 months of age, with proper intervention no later than 6 months of age.[37,38] Many states have now enacted legislation supporting the position paper; as result, newborn hearing screening programs have been implemented in newborn nurseries throughout the United States.[39] The currently recommended screening techniques are either the evoked otoacoustic emissions (EOAE) or the ABR. Both methodologies are noninvasive, relatively quick (<5 minutes), and easy to perform. The EOAE measures sound waves generated in the inner ear (cochlea) in response to clicks or tone bursts emitted and recorded by a minute microphone placed in the external ear canals of the infant. The ABR uses three electrodes pasted to the infant's scalp to measure the EEG waves generated by clicks. Because many children become hearing impaired after the neonatal period and are not identified by neonatal screening programs, the AAP Joint Commission on Infant Hearing Impairment recommends that all infants with risk factors for delayed onset of progressive hearing loss receive ongoing audiologic and medical monitoring for 3 years and at appropriate intervals thereafter.

Once hearing loss has been identified, a full developmental and speech and language evaluation is needed. Parenteral involvement and counseling are essential. Children with sensorineural hearing loss should be evaluated for possible hearing aid use by a pediatric audiologist.[40] Hearing aids may be fitted for infants as young as 2 months of age. The use of surgically implanted cochlear implants in children with profound hearing loss has currently been approved for use in children 2 years of age and older.[35,36,41] At present, more than 25,000 children worldwide have received cochlear implants. One limitation is that the earliest age for implantation in children in the United States is no earlier than 2 years of age, which is beyond the critical period of auditory input for the acquisition of oral language. Because of the increased risk for pneumococcal meningitis, children who undergo implants should receive age-appropriate immunization against pneumococcal disease.[11] At present, the best educational approach to children with significant hearing loss is open to controversy. Some members of the hearing-impaired community have objected to the use of cochlear implants in children, maintaining that the child can develop adequate communication skills using more conventional strategies such as sign language and lip reading.

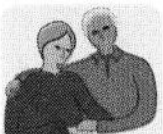

Hearing Loss in the Elderly

The term *presbycusis* is used to describe degenerative hearing loss that occurs with advancing age. Approximately 23% of persons between 65 and 75 years of age and 40% of the population older than 75 years of age are affected.[42] Men are affected earlier and experience a greater loss than women.

The degenerative changes that impair hearing may begin in the fifth decade of life and may not be clinically apparent until later.[43] Onset may be associated with chronic noise exposure or vascular disorders.[43] The disorder involves loss of neuroepithelial (hair) cells, neurons, and the stria vascularis.[30] High-frequency sounds are affected more than low-frequency sounds because high and low frequencies distort the base of the basilar membrane, but only low frequencies affect the distal (apical) region. Through the years, permanent mechanical damage to the organ of Corti is more likely to occur near the base of the cochlea, where the high sonic frequencies are discriminated.

Although hearing loss is a common problem in the elderly, many older persons are not appropriately assessed for hearing loss. When assessing an older person's ability to hear, it is important to ask both the person and the family about awareness of hearing loss. The ability to hear high-frequency sounds usually is lost first. Loss of high-frequency discrimination is characterized by difficulty in understanding words in noisy environments, in hearing a speaker in an adjacent room, or in hearing a speaker whose back is turned. Hearing loss may be estimated by having the person report hearing of softly whispered, normally spoken, or shouted words. In the English language, vowels are low-frequency sounds, whereas consonants are of higher frequency. A ticking watch also may be used to test for the higher frequencies.

In summary, hearing is a specialized sense whose external stimulus is the vibration of sound waves. Our ears receive sound waves, distinguish their frequencies, translate this information into nerve impulses, and transmit them to the CNS. Anatomically, the auditory system consists of the outer ear, middle ear, and inner ear, the auditory pathways, and the auditory cortex. The middle ear is a tiny air-filled cavity in the temporal bone. A connection exists between the middle ear and the nasopharynx. This connection, called the *eustachian tube,* allows equalization of pressure between the middle ear and the atmosphere. The inner ear contains the receptors for hearing.

Disorders of the auditory system include infections of the external and middle ear, otosclerosis, and conduction and sensorineural deafness. Otitis externa is an inflammatory process of the external ear. The middle ear is a tiny, air-filled cavity located in the temporal bone. The eustachian tube connects the middle ear to the nasopharynx and allows for equalization of pressure between the middle ear and the atmosphere. Infections can travel from the nasopharynx to the middle ear along the eustachian tube, causing OM or inflammation of the middle ear. The eustachian tube is shorter and more horizontal in infants and young children, and infections of the middle ear are a common problem in these age groups.

Otitis media is an infection of the middle ear that is associated with a collection of fluid. OM may present as AOM, recurrent OM, or OME. AOM usually follows an upper respiratory tract infection and is characterized by otalgia, fever, and hearing loss. The effusion that accompanies OM can persist for weeks or months, interfering with hearing and impairing speech development. Otosclerosis is a familial disorder of the otic capsule. It causes bone resorption followed by excessive replacement with sclerotic bone. The disorder eventually causes immobilization of the stapes and conduction deafness.

Deafness, or hearing loss, can develop as the result of a number of auditory disorders. It can be conductive, sensorineural, or mixed. Conduction deafness occurs when transmission of sound waves from the external to the inner ear is impaired. Sensorineural deafness can involve cochlear structures of the inner ear or the neural pathways that transmit auditory stimuli. Sensorineural hearing loss can result from genetic or congenital disorders, trauma, infections, vascular disorders, tumors, or ototoxic drugs. Hearing loss in infants and young children impairs language and speech development. Treatment of hearing loss includes the use of hearing aids and, in some cases of profound deafness, implantation of a cochlear prosthesis.

Disorders of Vestibular Function

After completing this section of the chapter, you should be able to meet the following objectives:

- Explain the function of the vestibular system with respect to postural reflexes and maintaining a stable visual field despite marked changes in head position
- Relate the function of the vestibular system to nystagmus and vertigo
- Differentiate the structures of peripheral and central vestibular function
- Characterize the physiologic cause of motion sickness
- Compare the manifestations and pathologic processes associated with benign positional vertigo and Ménière's disease
- Differentiate the manifestations of peripheral and central vestibular disorders

THE VESTIBULAR SYSTEM AND VESTIBULAR REFLEXES

The vestibular receptive organs, which are located in the inner ear, and their central nervous system connections contribute to the reflex activity necessary for effective posture and movement in a physical world governed by momentum and a gravitational field. Because the vestibular apparatus is part of the inner ear and located in the head, it is head position and acceleration that are sensed. The vestibular system serves two general and related functions. It maintains and assists recovery of stable body and head position through control of postural reflexes, and it maintains a stable visual field despite marked changes in head position.

Peripheral Vestibular Apparatus

The vestibular system consists of the peripheral vestibular apparatus and its CNS connections. The peripheral apparatus of the vestibular system, which is contained in the bony labyrinth of the inner ear next to and continuous with the cochlea of the auditory system, is divided into five prominent structures: three semicircular canals, a utricle, and a saccule (Fig. 55-8). Receptors in these structures are differentiated into the angular acceleration-deceleration receptors of the semicircular canals and the linear acceleration-deceleration and static gravitational receptors of the utricle and saccule.

DISORDERS OF THE VESTIBULAR SYSTEM

- The receptors concerned with the sense of balance and position in space are located in fluid (endolymph)-filled semicircular canals of the vestibular system of the inner ear.
- The vestibular system has extensive interconnections with neural pathways controlling vision, hearing, and autonomic nervous system function. Disorders of the vestibular system are characterized by vertigo, nystagmus, tinnitus, nausea and vomiting, and autonomic nervous system manifestations.
- Disorders of vestibular function can result from repeated stimulation of the vestibular system such as during car, air, and boat travel (motion sickness); acute infection of the vestibular pathways (acute vestibular neuritis); dislodgement of otoliths that participate in the receptor function of the vestibular system (benign positional vertigo); or distention of the endolymphatic compartment of the inner ear (Ménière's disease).

The three semicircular canals, each subtending approximately two thirds of a circle, are arranged at right angles to one another, with the horizontal duct tilted approximately 12 degrees above the normal horizontal plane of the head. The horizontal canals in the inner ears on the two sides of the head are in the same plane, whereas the superior (anterior) duct of one side is parallel with the inferior (posterior) duct on the other side, and the two function as a pair. Each canal is filled with endolymph and has a swelling at the base called the *ampulla.* Each ampulla contains a hair cell sensory surface raised into a crest, or crista, at right angles to the duct (see Fig. 55-8). The hair bundles extend into a flexible gelatinous mass, called the *cupula,* which essentially closes off fluid flow through the semicircular ducts.

When the head begins to rotate around the axis of a semicircular canal (*i.e.,* undergoes angular acceleration), the momentum of the endolymph causes an increase in pressure on one side of the cupula. This is similar to the lagging behind of the water in a glass that is suddenly rotated, except that the endolymph cannot flow past the cupula. Instead, the endolymph applies a differential pressure to the two sides of the cupula, bending the hair bundles. Because all the hair bundles in each semicircular canal share a common orientation, angular acceleration in one direction depolarizes hair cells and excites afferent neurons, whereas acceleration in the opposite direction hyperpolarizes the receptor cells and diminishes afferent nerve activity. Thus, the semicircular canals of the vestibular system provide a mechanism for signaling the angular acceleration during turning and tilting motions of the head, rotatory body movements, and turning movements during active and passive locomotion.

Both the utricle and saccule are widened membranous sacs in the bony vestibule. The utricle connects the ends of each semicircular duct, whereas the saccule communicates with the utricle through a small duct and with the

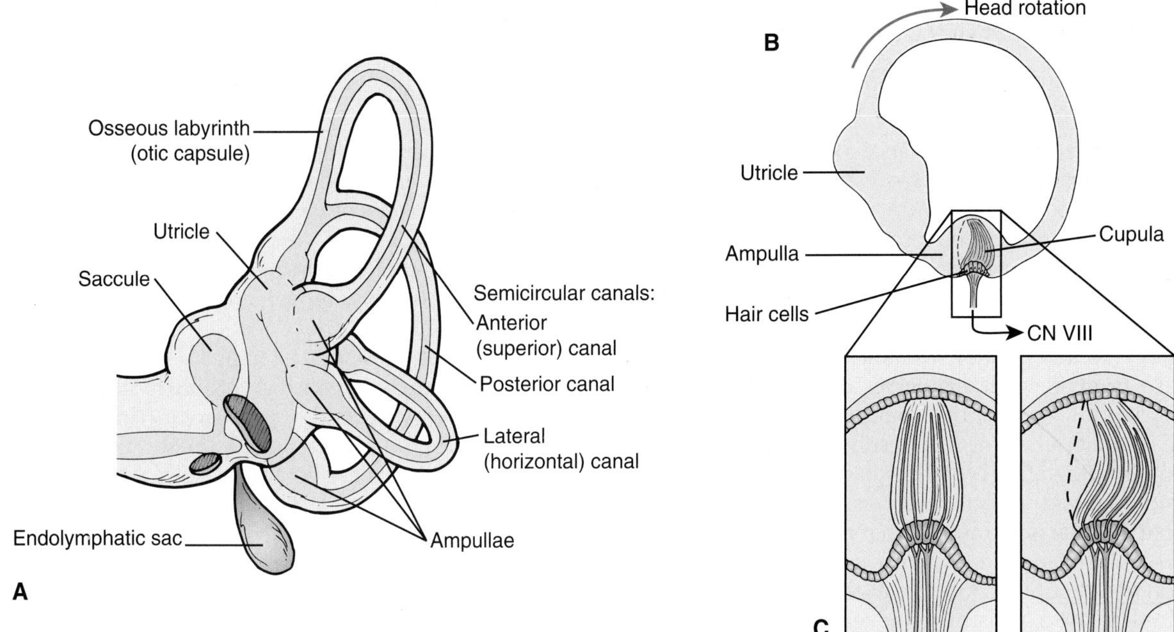

FIGURE 55-8 (**A**) The osseous and membranous labyrinth of the left ear. (**B**) Location of the ampulla. (**C**) The cupula and movement of hair bundles with head movement.

cochlear duct of the auditory apparatus through the ductus reuniens. The utricle and saccule house equilibrium receptors called *maculae* that respond to the pull of gravity and report on changes in head position. Located at right angles to the macula of the utricle, the macula of the saccule is oriented in the vertical plane. Small patches of hair cells are located in the floor of the utricle (*utricular macula*), in the sidewall of the saccule (*saccular macula*). Each hair cell has several microvilli and one true cilium, called a *kinocilium.* At the apical end of each inner hair cell is a projecting bundle of rodlike structures called *stereocilia.* The stereocilia of the hair cells in both utricular and saccular macula are embedded in a flattened gelatinous mass, the *otolithic membrane,* which is studded with tiny stones (calcium carbonate crystals) called *otoliths* (Fig. 55-9). Although small, the density of the otoliths increases the membrane's weight and its resistance to change in motion. When the head is tilted, the gelatinous mass shifts its position because of the pull of the gravitational field, bending the stereocilia of the macular hair cells. Although each hair cell becomes more or less excitable depending on the direction in which the cilia are bending, the hair cells are oriented in all directions, making these sense organs sensitive to static or changing head position in relation to the gravitational field.

Besides their static tilt reception function, the utricle and saccule provide linear acceleration and deceleration reception. Differential movement between the head and the otolithic membranes provides the basis for compensatory reflex bracing of neck, trunk, and limbs. This happens when the head is accelerated linearly, such as during the initial or terminal phase of an elevator ride or during automobile acceleration or deceleration. The utricle and saccule also provide the input data on which the air-righting reflexes are based. A cat dropped from an upside-down position lands on its feet and would do so even if blindfolded. Most vestibular reflexes, including air-righting, are functional at birth. If a neonate is supported in the prone position and the support is momentarily (and with great care) removed, the trunk and all four limbs are extended as falling begins. In the supine position, the trunk is flexed and the limbs are flexed as the fall progresses. However, the head-on-body vestibular reflexes of the infant are not sufficiently operational during the first 6 weeks or so after

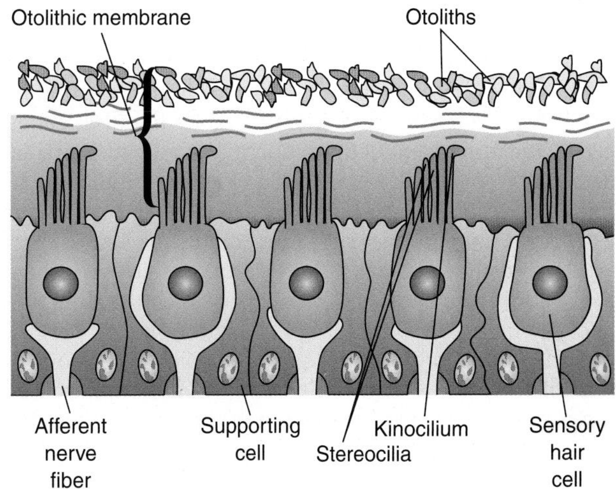

FIGURE 55-9 The relation of the otoliths to the sensory cells in the macula of the utricle and saccule. (Adapted from Selkurt F.D. [Ed.] [1982]. *Basic physiology for the health sciences* [2nd ed.]. Boston: Little, Brown)

birth to maintain head posture. This is why the neonate's head must be supported when the neonate is lifted in the supine position.

Neural Pathways

Ganglion cells, homologous with dorsal root ganglion cells, form afferent ganglia: the *superior vestibular ganglion,* which innervates the hair cells of the utricular macula and the cristae of the superior and horizontal semicircular ducts; and the *inferior vestibular ganglion,* which innervates the saccular macula and the cristae of the inferior semicircular duct (see Fig. 55-6). The central axons of these ganglion cells become the superior and inferior vestibular nerves.

Impulses from the vestibular nerves initially pass to one of two destinations: the vestibular nuclear complex in the brain stem or the cerebellum. The vestibular nuclei, which form the main integrative center for balance, also receive input from visual and somatic receptors, particularly from proprioceptors in the neck muscles that report the angle or inclination of the head. The vestibular nuclei integrate this information and then send impulses to the brain stem centers that control the extrinsic eye movements (CN III, IV, and VI) and reflex movements of the neck, limb, and trunk muscles (via the vestibulospinal tracts). These reflexes include the vestibuloocular reflexes that keep the eyes still as the head moves and the vestibulospinal reflexes that enable the skeletomotor system to make the quick adjustments needed to maintain or regain balance.

Neurons of the vestibular nuclei also project to the thalamus, the temporal cortex, the somesthetic area of the parietal cortex, and the chemoreceptor trigger zone. The thalamic and cortical projections provide the basis for the subjective experiences of position in space and of rotation. Connections with the chemoreceptor trigger zone stimulate the vomiting center in the brain. This accounts for the nausea and vomiting that often are associated with vestibular disorders.

Nystagmus

The term *nystagmus* is used to describe the involuntary rhythmic and oscillatory eye movements that preserve eye fixation on stable objects in the visual field during angular and rotational movements of the head.[22] These vestibular-controlled eye movements are initiated by impulses generated by the movement of the endolymph in the semicircular ducts. This movement is transmitted to the vestibular nuclei and relayed to the appropriate extraocular motor nuclei for controlling conjugate eye movement.

The vestibuloocular reflexes produce slow compensatory conjugate eye rotations that occur in the direction precisely opposite to ongoing head rotation and provide for continuous, ongoing reflex stabilization of the binocular fixation point. This reflex can be demonstrated by holding a pencil vertically in front of the eyes and moving it from side to side through a 10-degree arc at a rate of approximately five times per second. At this rate of motion, the pencil appears blurred because a different and more complex reflex, smooth pursuit, cannot compensate quickly enough. However, if the pencil is maintained in a stable position and the head is moved back and forth at the same rate, the image of the pencil is clearly defined. The eye movements are the same in both cases. The reason that the pencil image remains clear in the second situation is because the vestibuloocular reflexes keep the image of the pencil on the retinal fovea. When compensatory vestibuloocular reflexes carry the conjugate eye rotations to their physical limit, a very rapid conjugate movement moves the eyes in the direction of head rotation to a new fixation point, followed by a slow vestibuloocular reflex as the head continues to rotate past the new fixation point. This pattern of slow–fast–slow movements is called *nystagmus* (Fig. 55-10). Clinically, the direction of nystagmus is named for the fast phase of nystagmus.

Nystagmus can be classified according to the direction of eye movement: horizontal, vertical, rotary (torsional), or mixed. If head rotation is continued, friction between endolymph and semicircular duct walls results in endolymph

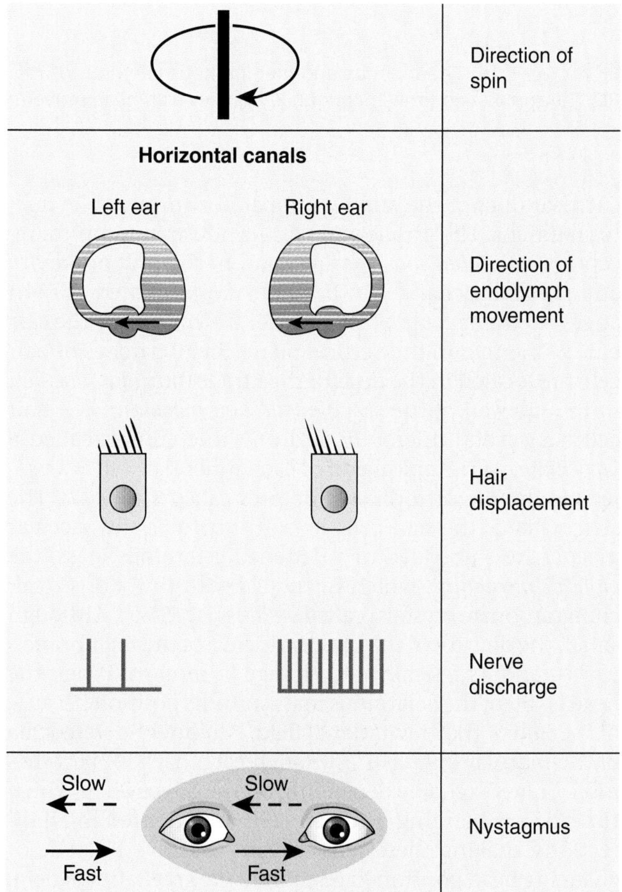

FIGURE 55-10 Effect of spinning a subject clockwise. On acceleration, the endolymph in the horizontal canals will lag behind with respect to movement of the canal wall. The hairs of cristae will be displaced to the left. In the left semicircular canal, hair displacement is away from the kinocilium, leading to decreased nerve discharges below the resting level. On the right, hair displacement is toward the kinocilium, leading to an increase in nerve discharge above the resting level. (Sekurt F.E. [1982]. *Basic physiology for the health professions* [2nd ed., p. 140]. Boston: Little, Brown)

rotating at the same velocity as the head, and nystagmus adapts to a stable eye posture. If rotation is suddenly stopped, vestibular nystagmus reappears in the direction precisely opposite to the angular accelerating nystagmus. This results because the inertia of the endolymph is again bending ampullar hair cells of a now stationary ampulla.

Nystagmus eye movements can be tested by caloric stimulation (see Chapter 52) or rotation (discussed later). Nystagmus always is abnormal if it occurs spontaneously or is sustained. Nystagmus due to CNS pathology, in contrast to vestibular end organ or vestibulocochlear nerve sources, seldom is accompanied by vertigo. If present, the vertigo is of mild intensity.

Postural Reflexes

Sudden changes in balance or orientation, such as falling to the right or left or backward or forward, result in powerful reflexes needed to maintain equilibrium and posture. The vestibulospinal tract provides for the control of the muscle tone of axial muscles, including the dorsal back muscles. A rapidly conducting lateral vestibulospinal tract descends in or within the spinal cord to provide powerful vestibular control of the lower motoneurons of the upper and lower limbs. As the head begins to tip (*i.e.,* rotate) on the neck or moves as part of general body tipping, the vestibular system activates the appropriate extensor muscles of the neck, trunk, and limbs, opposing the direction of the tilt. These powerful reflex adjustments in muscle tone assist in maintaining stable head and therefore body postural support during static posture and during passive or active movement.

All the vestibular nuclei receive input from the cerebellum and the vestibular nerve. The cerebellar connections of the vestibular system are necessary for adjustments of temporally smooth, coordinated movements to ongoing head movement, tilt, or angular acceleration. For instance, accurate grasping can occur during a fall, indicating cerebellar adjustments based on vestibular information during the performance of a smooth, accurate movement.

Vestibular reflexes are powerful, and considerable learning is required to inhibit or greatly modify them, as is necessary for acrobatic pilots, divers, and gymnasts. Dancers and skaters who engage in rapid spinning movements also learn to use or at least partially inhibit these reflexes.

VERTIGO

Disorders of vestibular function are characterized by a condition called *vertigo,* in which an illusion of motion occurs. With vertigo, the person may be stationary and the environment in motion (*i.e.,* objective vertigo), or the person may be in motion and the environment stationary (*i.e.,* subjective vertigo). Persons with vertigo frequently describe a sensation of spinning, "to-and-fro" motion, or falling.

Vertigo should be differentiated from light-headedness, faintness, unsteadiness, or syncope (loss of consciousness) [44–46] (Table 55-1). Presyncope, which is characterized by a feeling of light-headedness or "blacking out," is commonly caused by postural hypotension (see Chapter 25) or a stenotic lesion in the cerebral circulation that limits blood flow. An inability to maintain normal gait may be described as dizziness despite the absence of objective vertigo. The unstable gait may be caused by disorders of sensory input (*e.g.,* proprioception), peripheral neuropathy, gait problems, or disorders other than vestibular function and usually is corrected by touching a stationary object such as the wall or a table.

Vertigo or dizziness can result from central or peripheral vestibular disorders. Approximately 85% of persons with vertigo have a peripheral vestibular disorder, whereas only 15% have a central disorder.[45] Vertigo due to peripheral vestibular disorders tends to be severe in intensity and episodic or brief in duration. In contrast, vertigo due to central vestibular causes tends to be mild and constant and chronic in duration.

MOTION SICKNESS

Motion sickness is a form of normal physiologic vertigo. It is caused by repeated rhythmic stimulation of the vestibular system, such as is encountered in car, air, or boat

TABLE 55-1 Differences in Pathology and Manifestations of Dizziness Associated With Benign Positional Vertigo, Presyncope, and Disequilibrium State

Type of Disorder	Pathology	Symptoms
Benign positional vertigo	Disorder of otoliths	Vertigo initiated by a change in head position, usually lasts less than a minute
Presyncope	Orthostatic hypotension	Light-headedness and feeling faint on assumption of standing position
Disequilibrium	Sensory (*e.g.,* vision, proprioception) deficits	Dizziness and unsteadiness when walking, especially when turning; relieved by additional proprioceptive stimulation such as touching wall or table

travel. Vertigo, malaise, nausea, and vomiting are the principal symptoms. Autonomic signs, including lowered blood pressure, tachycardia, and excessive sweating, may occur. Hyperventilation, which commonly accompanies motion sickness, produces changes in blood volume and pooling of blood in the lower extremities, leading to postural hypotension and sometimes to syncope. Some persons experience a variant of motion sickness, complaining of sensing the rocking motion of the boat after returning to ground. This usually resolves after the vestibular system becomes accustomed to the stationary influence of being back on land.

Motion sickness can usually be suppressed by supplying visual signals that more closely match the motion signals being supplied to the vestibular system. For example, looking out the window and watching the environment move when experiencing motion sickness associated with car travel provides the vestibular system with the visual sensation of motion, but reading a book provides the vestibular system with the miscue that the environment is stable. Motion sickness usually decreases in severity with repeated exposure. Anti–motion sickness drugs also may be used to reduce or ameliorate the symptoms. These drugs work by suppressing the activity of the vestibular system.

DISORDERS OF PERIPHERAL VESTIBULAR FUNCTION

The peripheral vestibular system consists of a set of paired inner ear sensory organs, each sending messages to brain centers that interpret signals related to the body's position in space and control eye movement. Disorders of peripheral vestibular function occur when these signals are distorted, as in benign paroxysmal positional vertigo, or are unbalanced by unilateral involvement of one of the vestibular organs, as in Ménière's disease. The inner ear is vulnerable to injury caused by fracture of the petrous portion of the temporal bones; by infection of nearby structures, including the middle ear and meninges; and by blood-borne toxins and infections. Damage to the vestibular system can occur as an adverse effect of certain drugs or from allergic reactions to foods. The aminoglycosides (*e.g.,* streptomycin, gentamicin) have a specific toxic affinity for the vestibular portion of the inner ear. Alcohol can cause transient episodes of vertigo. The cause of peripheral vertigo remains unknown in approximately half of the cases.

Severe irritation or damage of the vestibular end organs or nerves results in severe balance disorders reflected by instability of posture, dystaxia, and falling accompanied by vertigo. With irritation, falling is away from the affected side; with destruction, it is toward the affected side. Adaptation to asymmetric stimulation occurs within a few days, after which the signs and symptoms diminish and eventually are lost. After recovery, there usually is a slightly reduced acuity for tilt, and the person walks with a somewhat broadened base to improve postural stability. The neurologic basis for this adaptation to unilateral loss of vestibular input is not understood. After adaptation to the loss of vestibular input from one side, the loss of function of the opposite vestibular apparatus produces signs and symptoms identical to those resulting from unilateral rather than bilateral loss. Within weeks, adaptation is again sufficient for locomotion and even for driving a car. Such a person relies heavily on visual and proprioceptive input and has severe orientation difficulty in the dark, particularly when traversing uneven terrain.

Benign Paroxysmal Positional Vertigo

Benign paroxysmal positional vertigo (BPPV) is the most common cause of pathologic vertigo and usually develops after the fourth decade. It is characterized by brief periods of vertigo, usually lasting less than 1 minute, that are precipitated by a change in head position.[44,47] The most prominent symptom of BPPV is vertigo that occurs in bed when the person rolls into a lateral position. It also commonly occurs when the person is getting in and out of bed, bending over and straightening up, or extending the head to look up. It also can be triggered by amusement rides that feature turns and twists.

BPPV is thought to result from damage to the delicate sensory organs of the inner ear, the semicircular ducts, and otoliths (see Fig. 55-9). In persons with BPPV, the calcium carbonate particles (otoliths) from the utricle become dislodged and become free-floating debris in the endolymph of the posterior semicircular duct, which is the most dependent part of the inner ear.[47] Movement of the free-floating debris causes this portion of the vestibular system to become more sensitive, such that any movement of the head in the plane parallel to the posterior duct may cause vertigo and nystagmus. There usually is a several-second delay between head movement and onset of vertigo, representing the time it takes to generate the exaggerated endolymph activity. Symptoms usually subside with continued movement, probably because the movement causes the debris to be redistributed throughout the endolymph system and away from the posterior semicircular canal.

Diagnosis is based on tests that involve the use of a change in head position to elicit vertigo and nystagmus.[47,48] BPPV often is successfully treated with drug therapy to control vertigo-induced nausea. Nondrug therapies using habituation exercises and canalith repositioning are successful in many people.[47] Canalith repositioning involves a series of maneuvers in which the head is moved to different positions in an effort to reposition the free-floating debris in the endolymph of the semicircular canals.

Acute Vestibular Neuronitis

Acute vestibular neuronitis is characterized by an acute onset (usually hours) of vertigo, nausea, and vomiting lasting several days and not associated with auditory or other neurologic manifestations. Most persons experience gradual improvement over 1 to 2 weeks, but some develop recurrent episodes.[49,50] A large percentage report an upper respiratory tract illness 1 to 2 weeks before onset of symptoms, suggesting a viral origin. The condition also can occur in persons with herpes zoster oticus. In some persons, attacks of acute vestibulopathy recur over months or years.

There is no way to determine whether a person who experiences a first attack will have repeated attacks.

Ménière's Disease

Ménière's disease is a disorder of the inner ear due to distention of the endolymphatic compartment of the inner ear, causing a triad of hearing loss, vertigo, and tinnitus.[51–55] The primary lesion appears to be in the endolymphatic sac, which is thought to be responsible for endolymph filtration and excretion. A number of pathogenic mechanisms have been postulated, including an increased production of endolymph, decreased production of perilymph accompanied by a compensatory increase in volume of the endolymphatic sac, and decreased absorption of endolymph caused by malfunction of the endolymphatic sac or blockage of endolymphatic pathways.

Ménière's disease is characterized by fluctuating episodes of tinnitus, feelings of ear fullness, and violent rotary vertigo that often renders the person unable to sit or walk. There is a need to lie quietly with the head fixed in a comfortable position, avoiding all head movements that aggravate the vertigo. Symptoms referable to the autonomic nervous system, including pallor, sweating, nausea, and vomiting, usually are present. The more severe the attack, the more prominent are the autonomic manifestations. A fluctuating hearing loss occurs with a return to normal after the episode subsides. Initially, the symptoms tend to be unilateral, resulting in rotatory nystagmus caused by an imbalance in vestibular control of eye movements. Because initial involvement usually is unilateral and because the sense of hearing is bilateral, many persons with the disorder are not aware of the full extent of their hearing loss. However, as the disease progresses, the hearing loss stops fluctuating and progressively worsens, with both ears tending to be affected so that the prime disability becomes one of deafness.[53] The episodes of vertigo diminish and then disappear, although the person may be unsteady, especially in the dark.

The cause of Ménière's disease is unknown. A number of conditions, such as trauma, infection (*e.g.*, syphilis), and immunologic, endocrine (adrenal-pituitary insufficiency and hypothyroidism), and vascular disorders have been proposed as possible causes of Ménière's disease.[53,54] The most common form of the disease is an idiopathic form thought to be caused by a single viral injury to the fluid transport system of the inner ear. One area of investigation has been the relation between immune disorders and Ménière's disease.

Methods used in the diagnosis of Ménière's disease include audiograms, vestibular testing by electronystagmography, and petrous pyramid radiographs. The administration of hyperosmolar substances, such as glycerin and urea, often produces acute temporary hearing improvement in persons with Ménière's disease and sometimes is used as a diagnostic measure of endolymphatic hydrops. The diuretic furosemide also may be used for this purpose.

The management of Ménière's disease focuses on attempts to reduce the distention of the endolymphatic space and can be medical or surgical. Pharmacologic management consists of suppressant drugs (*e.g.*, prochlorperazine, promethazine, diazepam), which act centrally to decrease the activity of the vestibular system. Diuretics are used to reduce endolymph fluid volume. Histamine analogs, which directly reduce inner ear fluid mainly by decreasing cochlear blood flow, are being studied.[52] A low-sodium diet is recommended in addition to these medications. The steroid hormone prednisone may be used to maintain satisfactory hearing and resolve dizziness. Gentamicin therapy has been used for ablation of the vestibular system.[53,54,56] Persons who are candidates for intratympanic gentamicin infusion include those who have frequent attacks of Ménière's disease, disease that involves one ear, good contralateral vestibular function, or normal or near-normal balance between episodes. This treatment is mainly effective in controlling vertigo and does not alter the underlying pathology.

Surgical methods include the creation of an endolymphatic shunt in which excess endolymph from the inner ear is diverted into the subarachnoid space or the mastoid (endolymphatic sac surgery) and vestibular nerve section. Advances in vestibular nerve section have facilitated the monitoring of CN VII and CN VIII potentials. These methods are used to prevent hearing damage. In unilateral cases, vestibular nerve section has a success rate of 90% to 95% in terms of providing complete relief of vertigo at 2 years after surgery.[53,54] The surgery, however, involves an intracranial procedure with possible postoperative morbidity.

DISORDERS OF CENTRAL VESTIBULAR FUNCTION

Abnormal nystagmus and vertigo can occur as a result of CNS lesions involving the cerebellum and lower brain stem. Central causes of vertigo include brain stem ischemia, tumors, and multiple sclerosis.[57] When brain stem ischemia is the cause of vertigo, it usually is associated with other brain stem signs such as diplopia, ataxia, dysarthria, or facial weakness. Compression of the vestibular nuclei by cerebellar tumors invading the fourth ventricle results in progressively severe signs and symptoms. In addition to abnormal nystagmus and vertigo, vomiting and a broad-based and dystaxic gait become progressively more evident. The central demyelinating effects of multiple sclerosis can present with vertigo up to 10% of the time, and up to one third of persons with multiple sclerosis experience vertigo and nystagmus some time in the course of the disease.[57]

Centrally derived nystagmus usually has equal excursion in both directions (*i.e.*, pendular). In contrast to peripherally generated nystagmus, CNS-derived nystagmus is relatively constant rather than episodic, can occur in any direction rather than being primarily in the horizontal or torsional (rotatory) dimensions, often changes direction through time, and cannot be suppressed by visual fixation. Repeated induction of nystagmus results in rapid diminution or "fatigue" of the reflex with peripheral abnormalities, but fatigue is not characteristic of central lesions. Abnormal nystagmus can make reading and other tasks that require precise eye positional control difficult.

DIAGNOSTIC TESTS OF VESTIBULAR FUNCTION

Diagnosis of vestibular disorders is based on a description of the symptoms, a history of trauma or exposure to agents that are destructive to vestibular structures, and physical examination. Tests of eye movements (*i.e.*, nystagmus) and muscle control of balance and equilibrium often are used. The tests of vestibular function focus on the horizontal semicircular reflex because it is the easiest reflex to stimulate rotationally and calorically and to record using electronystagmography.

Electronystagmography

Electronystagmography (ENG) is a precise and objective diagnostic method of evaluating nystagmus eye movements. Electrodes are placed lateral to the outer canthus of each eye and above and below each eye. A ground electrode is placed on the forehead. With ENG, the velocity, frequency, and amplitude of spontaneous or induced nystagmus and the changes in these measurements brought by a loss of fixation, with the eyes open or closed, can be quantified. The advantages of ENG are that it is easily administered, is noninvasive, does not interfere with vision, and does not require head restraint.[58]

Caloric Stimulation

Caloric testing involves elevating the head 30 degrees and irrigating each external auditory canal separately with 30 to 50 mL of ice water. The resulting changes in temperature, which are conducted through the petrous portion of the temporal bone, set up convection currents in the endolymph that mimic the effects of angular acceleration. In an unconscious person with a functional brain stem and intact oculovestibular reflexes, the eyes exhibit a jerk nystagmus lasting 2 to 3 minutes, with the slow component toward the irrigated ear followed by rapid movement away from the ear (see Chapter 52, Fig. 52-11). With impairment of brain stem function, the response becomes perverted and eventually disappears. An advantage of the caloric stimulation method is the ability to test the vestibular apparatus on one side at a time. The test should never be done on persons who do not have an intact eardrum or who have blood or fluid collected behind the eardrum.

Rotational Tests

Rotational testing involves rotation using a rotatable chair or motor-driven platform. Unlike caloric testing, rotational testing depends only on the inner ear and is unrelated to conditions of the external ear or temporal bone. A major disadvantage of the method is that both ears are tested simultaneously.

Motor-driven platforms can be precisely controlled, and multiple graded stimuli can be delivered in a relatively short period. For rotational testing, the person is seated in a chair mounted on the motor-driven platform. Testing usually is performed in the dark without visual influence and with selected light stimuli. Eye movements are monitored using ENG. The Bárány chair, a rotatable chair that is much like a barber's chair, can be used for assessing postrotational vestibular reflexes. The person is strapped into the chair with the head positioned so that the plane of one pair of semicircular ducts is in the horizontal plane (*i.e.*, plane of rotation); each of the three primary planes of the ducts is tested in turn. The person is rotated until a steady rate of rotation is achieved. The chair is suddenly stopped, and the ensuing postrotational reflex nystagmus and the compensatory movements of the body and limbs are observed. Vestibular reflexes are very powerful, and extreme caution is needed when rotational tests are used to evaluate these reflexes.

Romberg Test

The Romberg test is used to demonstrate disorders of static vestibular function. The person being tested is requested to stand with feet together and arms extended forward so that the degree of sway and arm stability can be observed. The person then is asked to close his or her eyes. When visual clues are removed, postural stability is based on proprioceptive sensation from the joints, muscles, and tendons and from static vestibular reception. Deficiency in vestibular static input is indicated by greatly increased sway and a tendency for the arms to drift toward the side of deficiency.

If vestibular input is severely deficient, the subject falls toward the deficient side. Care must be taken because defects of proprioceptive projection to the forebrain also result in some arm drift and postural instability toward the deficient side. Only if two-point discrimination and vibratory sensation from the lower and upper limbs are bilaterally normal can the deficiency be attributed to the vestibular system.

TREATMENT OF VESTIBULAR DISORDERS

Pharmacologic Methods

Depending on the cause, vertigo may be treated pharmacologically. There are two types of drugs used in the treatment of vertigo.[59] First, the drugs used to suppress the illusion of motion include drugs such as antihistamines (*e.g.*, meclizine, cyclizine, dimenhydrinate, and promethazine) and anticholinergic drugs (*e.g.*, scopolamine, atropine) that suppress the vestibular system. Although the antihistamines have long been used in treating vertigo, little is known about their mechanism of action. The second type includes drugs used to relieve the nausea and vomiting that commonly accompany the condition. Antidopaminergic drugs (*e.g.*, phenothiazines) and benzodiazepines commonly are used for this purpose.

Vestibular Rehabilitation Exercises

Vestibular rehabilitation, a relatively new treatment modality for peripheral vestibular disorders, has met with considerable success.[60–62] It commonly is done by physical therapists and uses a home exercise program that incorporates habituation exercises, balance retraining exercises, and a general conditioning program.[60] The habituation exercises take advantage of physiologic fatigue of the neurovegetative response to repetitive movement or positional stimulation and are done to decrease motion-provoked vertigo, light-headedness, and unsteadiness. The exercises are selected to provoke the vestibular symptoms. The person moves quickly into the position that causes symptoms, holds the position until the symptoms subside (*i.e.,* fatigue of the neurovegetative response), relaxes, and then repeats the exercise for a prescribed number of times. The exercises usually are repeated twice daily. The habituation effect is characterized by decreased sensitivity and duration of symptoms. It may occur in as little as 2 weeks or take as long as 6 months.[62]

Balance-retraining exercises consist of activities directed toward improving individual components of balance that may be abnormal. General conditioning exercises, a vital part of the rehabilitation process, are individualized to the person's preferences and lifestyle. They should consist of motion-oriented activity that the person is interested in and should be done on a regular basis, usually four to five times per week.[62]

In summary, the vestibular system plays an essential role in the equilibrium sense, which is closely integrated with the visual and proprioceptive (position) senses. Receptors in the semicircular canals, utricle, and saccule of vestibular system, located in the inner ear, respond to changes in linear and angular acceleration of the head. The vestibular nerve fibers travel in CN VIII to the vestibular nuclei at the junction of the medulla and pons; some fibers pass through the nuclei to the cerebellum. Cerebellar connections are necessary for temporally smooth, coordinated movements during ongoing head movements, tilt, and angular acceleration. The vestibular nuclei also connect with nuclei of the oculomotor (CN III), trochlear (CN IV), and abducens (CN VI) nerves that control eye movement. *Nystagmus* is a term used to describe vestibular-controlled eye movements that occur in response to angular and rotational movements of the head. The vestibulospinal tract, which provides for the control of muscle tone in the axial muscles, including those of the back, provide the support for maintaining balance. Neurons of the vestibular nuclei also project to the thalamus, to the temporal cortex, and to the somesthetic area of the parietal cortex. The thalamic and cortical projections provide the basis for the subjective experiences of position in space and of rotation and vertigo.

Vertigo, an illusory sensation of motion of either oneself or one's surroundings, tinnitus, and hearing loss are common manifestations of vestibular dysfunction, as are autonomic manifestations such as perspiration, nausea, and vomiting. Common disorders of the vestibular system include motion sickness, BPPV, and Ménière's disease.

Benign paroxysmal positional vertigo is a condition believed to be caused by free-floating particles in the posterior semicircular canal. It presents as a sudden onset of dizziness or vertigo that is provoked by certain changes in head position. Ménière's disease, which is caused by an overaccumulation of endolymph, is characterized by severe, disabling episodes of tinnitus, feelings of ear fullness, and violent rotary vertigo. The diagnosis of vestibular disorders is based on a description of the symptoms, a history of trauma or exposure to agents destructive to vestibular structures, and tests of eye movements (*i.e.,* nystagmus) and muscle control of balance and equilibrium. Among the methods used in treatment of the vertigo that accompanies vestibular disorders are habituation exercises and antivertigo drugs. These drugs act by diminishing the excitability of neurons in the vestibular nucleus.

REVIEW EXERCISES

A mother notices that her 13-month-old child is fussy and tugging at his ear and that he refuses to eat his breakfast. When she takes his temperature it is 100°F. Although the child attends day care, the mother has kept him home and made an appointment with the child's pediatrician. In the physician's office, the child's temperature is 100.2°F, he is somewhat irritable, and he has a clear nasal drainage. His left tympanic membrane shows normal landmarks and motility on pneumatic otoscopy. His right tympanic membrane is erythematous, and there is decreased motility on pneumatic otoscopy.

A. What risk factors are present that predispose this child to the development of acute otitis media?

B. Are his signs and symptoms typical of otitis media in a child of his age?

C. What are the most likely pathogens? What treatment would be indicated?

D. Later in the week, the mother notices that the child does seem to hear as well as he did before developing the infection. Is this a common occurrence, and should the mother be concerned about transient hearing loss in a child of this age?

A granddaughter is worried that her grandfather is "losing his hearing." Lately, he has been staying away from social gatherings that he always enjoyed, saying everybody mumbles. He is defiant in maintaining that there is nothing wrong with his hearing. However, he does complain that his ears have been ringing a lot lately.

A. What are common manifestations of hearing loss in the elderly?

B. What type of evaluation would be appropriate for determining whether this man has a hearing loss and the extent of his hearing loss?

C. What are some things that the granddaughter might do so that her grandfather could hear her better when she is talking to him?

A 70-year-old man complains that he gets this terrible feeling "like the room is moving around" and becomes nauseated when he rolls over in bed or bends over suddenly. It usually goes away once he has been up for awhile. He has been told that his symptoms are consistent with benign paroxysmal positional vertigo.

A. What is the pathophysiology associated with this man's vertigo?

B. Why do the symptoms subside once he has been up for awhile?

C. What methods are available for treatment of the disorder?

References

1. Moore K.L., Dallen A.F. (1999). *Clinically oriented anatomy* (4th ed., 962–976). Philadelphia: Lippincott Williams & Wilkins.
2. Rhoades R.A., Tanner G.A. (2003). *Medical physiology* (2nd ed., pp. 77–89). Philadelphia: Lippincott Williams & Wilkins.
3. Grossan M. (2000). Safe, effective techniques for cerumen removal. *Geriatrics 55,* 83–86.
4. Jackler R.K., Kaplan M.J. (2003). Diseases of the ear. In Tierney L.M., McPhee S.J., Papadakis M.A. (Eds.), *Current medical diagnosis and treatment* (42nd ed., pp. 178–192). New York: Lange Medical Books/McGraw-Hill.
5. Licameli G.R. (2002). The eustachian tube: Update on anatomy, development and function. *Otolaryngology Clinics of North America 35,* 803–809.
6. Bluestone C.D., Klein J. (1995). *Otitis media in infants and children.* Philadelphia: W.B. Saunders.
7. Hendley J.O. (2002). Otitis media. *New England Journal of Medicine 347*(15), 1169–1174.
8. Weber S.M., Grundast K.M. (2003). Modern management of otitis media. *Pediatric Clinics of North America,* 399–411.
9. Perkins J.A. (2002). Medical and surgical management of otitis media in children. *Otolaryngology Clinics of North America 35,* 811–825.
10. Swanson J.A., Hoecker J.L. (1996). Otitis media in young children. *Mayo Clinic Proceedings 71,* 179–183.
11. Haddad J. Jr. (2004). The ear. In Behrman R.E., Kliegman R.M., Jenson H.B. (Eds.), *Nelson textbook of pediatrics* (17th ed., pp. 2127–2152). Philadelphia: W.B. Saunders.
12. Pichichero M.E. (2000). Acute otitis media: Part II. Treatment in an era of increasing antibiotic resistance. *American Family Physician 61,* 2410–2415.
13. McCracken G.H. Jr. (1998). Treatment of acute otitis media in an era of increasing microbial resistance. *Pediatric Infectious Disease Journal 17,* 576–579.
14. Heikkinen T., Thint M., Chonmaitree T. (1999). Prevalence of various respiratory viruses in the middle ear during acute otitis media. *New England Journal of Medicine 340,* 260–264.
15. Rothman R., Owens T., Simel D.L. (2003). Does this child have acute otitis media? *JAMA 290*(13), 1633–1640.
16. Dowell S.F., Butler J.C., Giebink G.S., et al. (1999). Acute otitis media: Management and surveillance in an era of pneumococcal resistance—a report from the Drug Resistant *Streptococcus pneumoniae* Therapeutic Working Group. *Pediatric Infectious Disease Journal 18*(1), 1–9.
17. Heald M.M., Matkin N.D., Merideth K.E. (1990). Pressure-equalization (PE) tubes in treatment of otitis media: National survey of otolaryngologists. *Otolaryngology—Head and Neck Surgery 102,* 334–338.
18. Teele D.W., Klein J.O., Chase C., et al. (1990). Otitis media in infancy and intellectual development, school achievement, speech, and language at age 7 years. Greater Boston Otitis Media Study Group. *Journal of Infectious Diseases 162,* 685–694.
19. Shohet J.A., deJong A.L. (2002). The management of pediatric cholesteatoma. *Otolaryngology Clinics of North America 35,* 841–851.
20. Culpepper L., Froom J. (1997). Routine antimicrobial treatment of acute otitis media: Is it necessary? *Journal of the American Medical Association 278,* 1643–1645.
21. Rubin E., Farber J.L. (1999). *Pathology* (3rd ed., pp. 1331–1332). Philadelphia: Lippincott Williams & Wilkins.
22. Kandel E.R., Schwartz J.H., Jessel T.M. (2000). *Principles of neural science* (pp. 591–624, 801–815). New York: McGraw-Hill.
23. Fortune D.S. (1999). Tinnitus: Current evaluation and management. *Medical Clinics of North America 83,* 153–162.
24. Noell C.A., Meyerhoff W.L. (2003). Tinnitus: Diagnosis and treatment of this elusive symptom. *Geriatrics 58*(2), 28–34.
25. Lockwood A.H., Salvi R.J., Burckard R.F. (2002). Tinnitus. *New England Journal of Medicine 347*(12), 904–910.
26. Schwaber M.K. (2003). Medical evaluation of tinnitus. *Otolaryngology Clinics of North America 36,* 287–292.
27. Weissman J.L. (1996). Hearing loss. *Radiology 199,* 593–611.
28. Isaacson J.E., Vora N.M. (2003). Differential diagnosis and treatment of hearing loss. *American Family Physician 68*(6), 1125–1132.
29. Yueh B., Shapiro N., MacLean C.H., Shekelle P.G. (2003). Screening and management of hearing loss in primary care: Scientific review. *JAMA 289*(15), 1976–1985.
30. Nadol J.G. (1993). Hearing loss. *New England Journal of Medicine 329,* 1092–1101.
31. Shohet J.A., Bent T. (1998). Hearing loss: The invisible disability. *Postgraduate Medicine 104*(3), 81–83, 87–90.
32. Willems P.J. (2000). Genetic causes of hearing loss. *New England Journal of Medicine 342,* 1101–1109.
33. Yamasoba T., Kikuchi S., O'uchi T., et al. (1993). Sudden sensorineural hearing loss associated with slow blood flow of the vertebrobasilar system. *Annals of Otorhinolaryngology 102,* 873–877.
34. Committee on Disabilities of the Group for the Advancement of Psychiatry. (1997). Issues to consider in deaf and hard-of-hearing patients. *American Family Physician 56*(8), 2057–2068.
35. NIH Consensus Development Panel on Cochlear Implants in Adults and Children. (1995). Cochlear implants in adults and children. *Journal of the American Medical Association 274,* 1955–1961.
36. Francis H.W., Niparko J.K. (2003). Cochlear implantation update. *Pediatric Clinics of North America 50,* 341–361.
37. Task Force on Newborn and Infant Hearing of the American Academy of Pediatrics. (1999). Newborn and infant hearing loss: Detection and intervention. *Pediatrics 103,* 527–530.
38. Joint Commission on Infant Hearing. (2000). Year 2000 position statement: Principles and Guidelines for early hearing detection and intervention programs. *Pediatrics 106,* 798–817.
39. Kenna M.A. (2003). Neonatal hearing screening. *Pediatric Clinics of North America 50,* 301–313.
40. Johnson K.C. (2002). Audiologic assessment of children with suspected hearing loss. *Otolaryngology Clinics of North America 35,* 711–732.
41. Rubinstein J.T. (2002). Paediatric cochlear implantation: Prosthetic hearing and language development. *Lancet 360,* 483–485.
42. Saeed S., Ramsden R. (1994). Hearing loss. *Practitioner 238,* 454–460.
43. Gates G.A. (Chairperson). (1989). Invitational Geriatric Otorhinolaryngology Workshop: Presbycusis. *Otolaryngology—Head and Neck Surgery 100,* 266–271.
44. Baloh R.W. (1999). The dizzy patient: Presence of vertigo points to vestibular cause. *Postgraduate Medicine 105*(5), 161–172.

45. Derebery J.M. (1999). The diagnosis and treatment of dizziness. *Medical Clinics of North America 83,* 163–176.
46. Ruckenstein M.J. (2001). The dizzy patient: How you can help. *Consultant 41*(1), 29–33.
47. Furman J.M., Cass S.P. (1999). Benign paroxysmal positional vertigo. *New England Journal of Medicine 341,* 1590–1596.
48. Parnes L.S., Agrawal S.K., Atlas J. (2003). Diagnosis and management of benign paroxysmal positional vertigo (BPPV). *Canadian Medical Association Journal 169*(7), 681–693.
49. Hotson J.R., Baloh R.W. (1998). Acute vestibular syndrome. *New England Journal of Medicine 339,* 680–685.
50. Baloh R.W. (2003). Vestibular neuritis. *New England Journal of Medicine 348*(11), 1027–1032.
51. Paparella M.M., Djalilian H.R. (2002). Etiology, pathophysiology of symptoms and pathogenesis of Ménière's disease. *Otolaryngology Clinics of North America 35,* 529–545.
52. Dickins J.R.E., Graham S.S. (1990). Ménière's disease: 1983–1989. *American Journal of Otology 11,* 51–65.
53. Saeed S.R. (1998). Fortnightly review: Diagnosis and treatment of Ménière's disease. *British Medical Journal 316,* 368–372.
54. Hollis L., Bottrill I. (1999). Ménière's disease. *Hospital Medicine (London) 60,* 574–578.
55. Brooks C.B. (1996). The pharmacological treatment of Ménière's disease. *Clinical Otolaryngology 21,* 3–11.
56. Odkvist L.M., Bergenius J., Moller C. (1997). When and how to use gentamicin in the treatment of Ménière's disease. *Acta Otolaryngologica Supplement 526,* 54–57.
57. Derebery M.J. (1999). The diagnosis and treatment of dizziness. *Medical Clinics of North America 83,* 163–176.
58. Baloh R.W. (1989). Modern vestibular function testing. *Western Journal of Medicine 150,* 59–67.
59. Rascol O., Hain T.C., Brefel C., et al. (1995). Antivertigo drugs and drug-induced vertigo. *Drugs 50,* 777–789.
60. Horak F.B., Jones-Rycewicz C., Black F.W., et al. (1992). Effects of vestibular rehabilitation on dizziness and imbalance. *Otolaryngology—Head and Neck Surgery 106,* 175–180.
61. Smith-Whellock M., Shepard N.T., Telian S.A. (1991). Physical therapy program for vestibular rehabilitation. *American Journal of Otology 12,* 218–225.
62. Brandt T. (2000). Management of vestibular disorders. *Journal of Neurology 247,* 491–499.

UNIT

XIV

Musculoskeletal and Integumentary Function

Some of the most significant investigations of the skeleton and muscles took place during the Renaissance—a time that celebrated the human body and lifted the knowledge of the body and its workings out of medieval murkiness.

The first comprehensive description of musculature was presented by Andreas Vesalius (1514–1564), a professor of anatomy and surgery at Padua. The product of his scrupulous dissections was the masterwork *De Humani Corporis Fabrica* (On the Structure of the Human Body), the second volume of which dealt with muscles and their structure. The work was beautifully illustrated with elegantly poised cadavers set against backgrounds of medieval Italy. Vesalius' effort successfully challenged many of the long-held pronouncements of Galen. The studies of artist Leonardo da Vinci (1452–1519) sought not to dispute or confirm previous teachings but to learn of the "divine form" so that it could be better rendered. A physician of the time wrote that "in order that he might be able to paint the various joints and muscles as they bend and extend according to the laws of nature, he [Leonardo] dissected in medical schools the corpses of criminals, indifferent to this inhuman and nauseating work." Although da Vinci was primarily a painter studying anatomy for the sake of art, there is little doubt that had his anatomic drawings been published during his lifetime or shortly after, science would have been advanced by years.

CHAPTER

56

Structure and Function of the Musculoskeletal System

Without the skeletal system, movement in the external environment would not be possible. The bones of the skeletal system serve as a framework for the attachment of muscles, tendons, and ligaments. The skeletal system protects and maintains soft tissues in their proper position, provides stability for the body, and maintains the body's shape. The bones act as a storage reservoir for calcium, and the central cavity of some bones contains the hematopoietic connective tissue in which blood cells are formed.

The skeletal system consists of the axial and appendicular skeleton. The axial skeleton, which is composed of the bones of the skull, thorax, and vertebral column, forms the axis of the body. The appendicular skeleton consists of the bones of the upper and lower extremities, including the shoulder and hip. For our purposes, the skeletal system is considered to include the bones and cartilage of the axial and appendicular skeleton, as well as the connective tissue structures (*i.e.*, ligaments and tendons) that connect the bones and join muscles to bone.

Characteristics of Skeletal Tissue

After completing this section of the chapter, you should be able to meet the following objectives:

- Cite the common components of cartilage and bone
- Compare the properties of the intercellular collagen and elastic fibers of skeletal tissue
- Cite the characteristics and name at least one location of elastic cartilage, hyaline cartilage, and fibrocartilage
- Name and characterize the function of the four types of bone cells
- State the function of parathyroid hormone, calcitonin, and vitamin D in terms of bone formation and metabolism
- State the location and function of the periosteum and the endosteum

Two types of connective tissue are found in the skeletal system: cartilage and bone. Each of these connective tissue types consists of living cells, nonliving intercellular protein fibers, and an amorphous (shapeless) ground substance. The tissue cells are responsible for secreting and maintaining the intercellular substances in which they are housed. These substances provide the structural characteristics of the tissue. For example, the intercellular matrix of bone is impregnated with calcium salts, providing the hardness that is characteristic of this tissue.

Two main types of intercellular fibers are found in skeletal tissue: collagenous and elastic. Collagen is an inelastic and insoluble fibrous protein. Because of its molecular configuration, collagen has great tensile strength; the breaking point of collagenous fibers found in human tendons is reached with a force of several hundred kilograms per square centimeter. Fresh collagen is colorless, and tissues that contain large numbers of collagenous fibers generally appear white. The collagen fibers in tendons and ligaments give these structures their white color. Elastin is the major component of elastic fibers that allows them to stretch several times their length and rapidly return to their original shape when the tension is released. Ligaments and structures that must undergo repeated stretching contain a high proportion of elastic fibers.

THE SKELETAL SYSTEM

- The skeletal system consists of the bones of the skull, thorax, and vertebral column, which form the axial skeleton, and the bones of the upper and lower extremities, which form the appendicular skeleton.
- Two types of connective tissue are found in the skeletal system: (1) cartilage, a semirigid and slightly flexible structure that plays an essential role in prenatal and childhood development of the skeleton and as a surface for the articulating ends of skeletal joints; and (2) bones, which provide for the firm structure of the skeleton and serve as a reservoir for calcium and phosphate storage.
- Both bone and cartilage are composed of living cells and a nonliving intercellular matrix that is secreted by the living cells.
- Bone matrix is maintained by three types of cells: osteoblasts, which synthesize and secrete the constituents of bone; osteoclasts, which resorb surplus bone and are required for bone remodeling; and the osteocytes, which make up the osteoid tissue of bone.

CARTILAGE

Cartilage is a firm but flexible type of connective tissue consisting of cells and intercellular fibers embedded in an amorphous, gel-like material. It has a smooth and resilient surface and a weight-bearing capacity exceeded only by that of bone.

Cartilage is essential for growth before and after birth. It is able to undergo rapid growth while maintaining a considerable degree of stiffness. In the embryo, most of the axial and appendicular skeleton is formed first as a cartilage model and is replaced by bone. In postnatal life, cartilage continues to play an essential role in the growth of long bones and persists as articular cartilage in the adult.

There are three types of cartilage: elastic cartilage, hyaline cartilage, and fibrocartilage. *Elastic cartilage* contains some elastin in its intercellular substance. It is found in areas, such as the ear, where some flexibility is important. Pure cartilage is called *hyaline cartilage* (from a Greek word meaning "glass") and is pearly white. It is the type of cartilage seen on the articulating ends of fresh soup bones found in the supermarket. *Fibrocartilage* has characteristics that are intermediate between dense connective tissue and hyaline cartilage. It is found in the intervertebral disks, in areas where tendons are connected to bone, and in the symphysis pubis.

Hyaline cartilage is the most abundant type of cartilage. It forms much of the cartilage of the fetal skeleton and the epiphyseal plates of growing children. In adults, it forms the cartilage that joins the ribs to the sternum and vertebrae, the cartilage that supports the respiratory airways, and the articulating surface of moving joints.

Cartilage cells, which are called *chondrocytes,* are located in lacunae. These lacunae are surrounded by an uncalcified, gel-like intercellular matrix of collagen fibers and ground substance. Cartilage is devoid of blood vessels and nerves. The free surfaces of most hyaline cartilage, with the exception of articular cartilage, are covered by a layer of fibrous connective tissue called the *perichondrium.*

It has been estimated that approximately 65% to 80% of the wet weight of cartilage is water held in its gel structure. Because cartilage has no blood vessels, this tissue fluid allows the diffusion of gases, nutrients, and wastes between the chondrocytes and blood vessels outside the cartilage. Diffusion cannot take place if the cartilage matrix becomes impregnated with calcium salts, and cartilage dies if it becomes calcified.

BONE

Bone is connective tissue in which the intercellular matrix has been impregnated with inorganic calcium salts so that it has great tensile and compressible strength but is light enough to be moved by coordinated muscle contractions. The intercellular matrix is composed of two types of substances—organic matter and inorganic salts. The organic matter, including bone cells, blood vessels, and nerves, constitutes approximately one third of the dry weight of bone; the inorganic salts make up the other two thirds.

The organic matter consists primarily of collagen fibers embedded in an amorphous ground substance. The inorganic matter consists of hydroxyapatite, an insoluble macrocrystalline structure of calcium phosphate salts, and small amounts of calcium carbonate and calcium fluoride. Bone may also take up lead and other heavy metals, thereby removing these toxic substances from the circulation. This can be viewed as a protective mechanism. The antibiotic tetracycline is readily bound to calcium deposited in newly formed bones and teeth. When tetracycline is given during pregnancy, it can be deposited in the teeth of the fetus, causing discoloration and deformity. Similar changes can occur if the drug is given for long periods to children younger than 6 years of age.

Types of Bone

There are two types of mature bones: cancellous and compact bone (Fig. 56-1). Both types are formed in layers and are therefore called *lamellar bone.* Cancellous (spongy) bone is found in the interior of bones and is composed of *trabeculae,* or *spicules,* of bone that form a lattice-like pattern. These lattice-like structures are lined with osteogenic cells and filled with red or yellow bone marrow. Cancellous bone is relatively light, but its structure is such that it has considerable tensile strength and weight-bearing properties. Compact (cortical) bone, which forms the outer shell of a bone, has a densely packed calcified intercellular matrix that makes it more rigid than cancellous bone. The relative quantity of compact and cancellous bone varies in different types of bones throughout the body and in different parts of the same bone, depending on the need for strength and lightness. Compact bone is the major component of tubular bones. It is also found along the lines of stress on long bones and forms an outer protective shell on other bones.

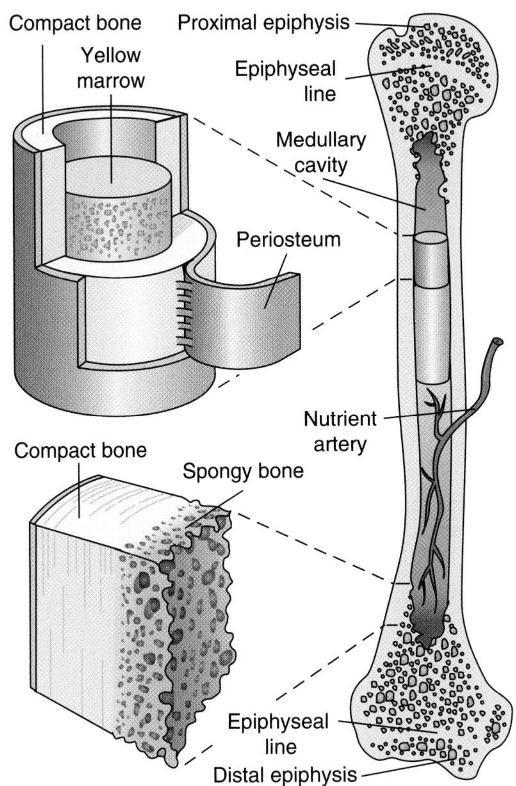

FIGURE 56-1 A long bone shown in longitudinal section.

Bone Cells

Four types of bone cells participate in the formation and maintenance of bone tissue: osteogenic cells, osteoblasts, osteocytes, and osteoclasts (Table 56-1).

Osteogenic Cells. The undifferentiated osteogenic cells are found in the periosteum, endosteum, and epiphyseal plate of growing bone. These cells differentiate into osteoblasts and are active during normal growth; they may also be activated in adult life during healing of fractures and other injuries. Osteogenic cells also participate in the continual replacement of worn-out bone tissue.

Osteoblasts. The osteoblasts, or bone-building cells, are responsible for the formation of the bone matrix. Bone formation occurs in two stages: ossification and calcification. Ossification involves the formation of osteoid, or prebone. Calcification of bone involves the deposition of calcium salts in the osteoid tissue. The osteoblasts synthesize collagen and other proteins that make up osteoid tissue. They also participate in the calcification process of the osteoid tissue, probably by controlling the availability of calcium and phosphate. Osteoblasts secrete the enzyme *alkaline phosphatase,* which is thought to act locally in bone tissue to raise calcium and phosphate levels to the point at which precipitation occurs. The activity of the osteoblasts undoubtedly contributes to the rise in serum levels of alkaline phosphatase that follows bone injury and fractures.

Osteocytes. The osteocytes are mature bone cells that are actively involved in maintaining the bony matrix. Death of the osteocytes results in the resorption of this matrix. The osteocytes lie in a small lake filled with extracellular fluid, called a *lacuna,* and are surrounded by a calcified intercellular matrix. Extracellular fluid-filled passageways permeate the calcified matrix and connect with the lacunae of adjacent osteocytes. These passageways are called *canaliculi.* Because diffusion does not occur through the calcified matrix of bone, the canaliculi serve as communicating channels for the exchange of nutrients and metabolites between the osteocytes and the blood vessels on the surface of the bone layer.

The osteocytes, together with their intercellular matrix, are arranged in layers, or lamellae. In compact bone, 4 to 20 lamellae are arranged concentrically around a central haversian canal, which runs essentially parallel to the long axis of the bone. Each of these units is called a *haversian system,* or *osteon.* The haversian canals contain blood vessels that carry nutrients and wastes to and from the canaliculi (Fig. 56-2). The blood vessels from the periosteum enter the bone through tiny openings called *Volkmann's canals* and connect with the haversian systems. Cancellous bone is also composed of lamellae, but its trabeculae usually are not penetrated by blood vessels. Instead, the bone cells of cancellous bone are nourished by diffusion from the endosteal

TABLE 56-1 Function of Bone Cells

Type of Bone Cell	Function
Osteogenic cells	Undifferentiated cells that differentiate into osteoblasts. They are found in the periosteum, endosteum, and epiphyseal growth plate of growing bones.
Osteoblasts	Bone-building cells that synthesize and secrete the organic matrix of bone. Osteoblasts also participate in the calcification of the organic matrix.
Osteocytes	Mature bone cells that function in the maintenance of bone matrix. Osteocytes also play an active role in releasing calcium into the blood.
Osteoclasts	Bone cells responsible for the resorption of bone matrix and the release of calcium and phosphate from bone.

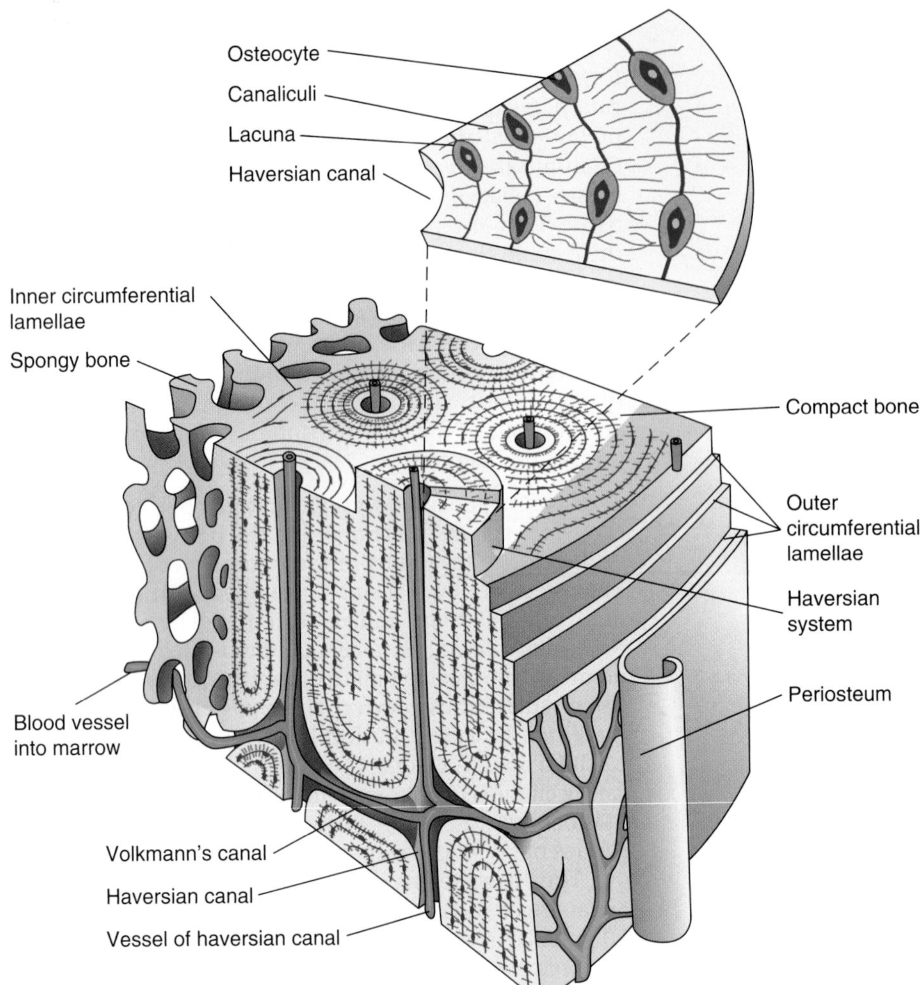

FIGURE 56-2 Haversian systems as seen in a wedge of compact bone tissue. The periosteum has been peeled back to show a blood vessel entering one of Volkmann's canals. **(Top)** Osteocytes lying within lacunae; canaliculi permit interstitial fluid to reach each lacuna.

surface through canaliculi, which interconnect their lacunae and extend to the bone surface.

Osteoclasts. Osteoclasts are bone cells that function in the resorption of bone, removing the mineral content and the organic matrix. Osteoclasts originate from bone marrow granulocyte/macrophage progenitor cells. They have receptors for parathyroid hormone (PTH), calcitonin, osteoclast-stimulating factor, and other growth and inhibiting factors. PTH is thought to increase the number and resorptive activity of the osteoclasts. The mechanism whereby the osteoclasts exert their resorptive effect on bone is unclear. It has been suggested that they may secrete acids that remove calcium from the bone matrix as well as proteolytic enzymes that digest and degrade the organic components of the bone matrix.

Periosteum and Endosteum

Bones are covered, except at their articular ends, by a membrane called the *periosteum* (see Fig. 56-1). The periosteum has an outer fibrous layer and an inner layer that contains the osteogenic cells needed for bone growth and development. The periosteum contains blood vessels and acts as an anchorage point for vessels as they enter and leave the bone. The endosteum is the membrane that lines the spaces of spongy bone, the marrow cavities, and the haversian canals of compact bone. It is composed mainly of osteogenic cells. These osteogenic cells contribute to the growth and remodeling of bone and are necessary for bone repair.

HORMONAL CONTROL OF BONE FORMATION AND METABOLISM

The process of bone formation and mineral metabolism is complex. It involves the interplay between the actions of PTH, calcitonin, and vitamin D. Other hormones, such as cortisol, growth hormone, thyroid hormone, and the sex hormones, also influence bone formation directly or indirectly. The actions of PTH, calcitonin, and vitamin D are summarized in Table 56-2.

Parathyroid Hormone

PTH is one of the important regulators of calcium and phosphate levels in the blood. The hormone is secreted by the parathyroid glands. There are two pairs of parathyroid glands located on the dorsal surface of the thyroid gland.

TABLE 56-2 Actions of Parathyroid Hormone, Calcitonin, and Vitamin D

Actions	Parathyroid Hormone	Calcitonin	Vitamin D
Intestinal absorption of calcium	Increases indirectly through increased activation of vitamin D	Probably not affected	Increases
Intestinal absorption of phosphate	Increases	Probably not affected	Increases
Renal excretion of calcium	Decreases	Increases	Probably increases, but less effect than PTH
Renal excretion of phosphate	Increases	Increases	Increases
Bone resorption	Increases	Decreases	1,25-$(OH)_2D_3$ increases
Bone formation	Decreases	Uncertain	24,25-$(OH)_2D_3$ increases (?)
Serum calcium levels	Produces a prompt increase	Decreases with pharmacologic doses	No effect
Serum phosphate levels	Prevents an increase	Decreases with pharmacologic doses	No effect

PTH prevents serum calcium levels from falling below and serum phosphate levels from rising above normal physiologic concentrations. The secretion of PTH is regulated by negative feedback according to serum levels of ionized calcium (see Chapter 33). PTH, which is released from the parathyroid gland in response to a decrease in plasma calcium, restores the concentration of the calcium ion to just above the normal set point. This inhibits further secretion of the hormone. Other factors, such as serum phosphate and arterial blood pH, indirectly influence parathyroid secretion by altering the amount of calcium that is complexed to phosphate or bound to albumin.

PTH maintains serum calcium levels by initiation of calcium release from bone, by conservation of calcium by the kidney, by enhanced intestinal absorption of calcium through activation of vitamin D, and by reduction of serum phosphate levels (Fig. 56-3). PTH also increases the movement of calcium and phosphate from bone into the extracellular fluid. Calcium is immediately released from the canaliculi and bone cells; a more prolonged release of calcium and phosphate is mediated by increased osteoclast activity. In the kidney, PTH stimulates tubular reabsorption of calcium while reducing the reabsorption of phosphate. The latter effect ensures that increased release of phosphate from bone during mobilization of calcium does not produce an elevation in serum phosphate levels. This is important because an increase in calcium and phosphate levels could lead to crystallization in soft tissues. PTH increases intestinal absorption of calcium because of its ability to stimulate activation of vitamin D by the kidney.

Calcitonin

Whereas PTH increases blood calcium levels, the hormone calcitonin lowers blood calcium levels. Calcitonin, sometimes called *thyrocalcitonin,* is secreted by the parafollicular, or C, cells of the thyroid gland.

Calcitonin inhibits the release of calcium from bone into the extracellular fluid. It is thought to act by causing calcium to become sequestered in bone cells and by inhibiting osteoclast activity. Calcitonin also reduces the renal tubular reabsorption of calcium and phosphate; the decrease in serum calcium level that follows administration of pharmacologic doses of calcitonin may be related to this action.

The major stimulus for calcitonin synthesis and release is a rise in serum calcium. The role of calcitonin in overall mineral homeostasis is uncertain. There are no clearly definable syndromes of calcitonin deficiency or excess, which suggests that calcitonin does not directly alter calcium metabolism. It has been suggested that the physiologic actions of calcitonin are related to the postprandial handling and processing of dietary calcium. This theory proposes that after meals, calcitonin maintains parathyroid secretion at

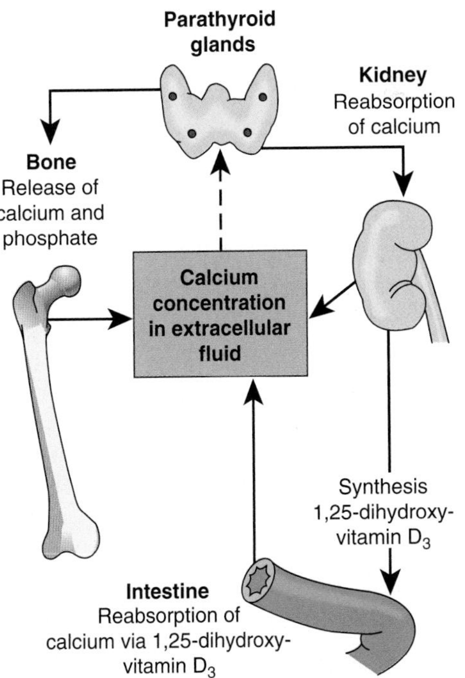

FIGURE 56-3 Actions and feedback regulation (*dashed line*) of parathyroid hormone.

a time when it normally would be reduced by calcium entering the blood from the digestive tract. Although excess or deficiency states associated with alterations in physiologic levels of calcitonin have not been observed, it has been shown that pharmacologic doses of the hormone reduce osteoclastic activity. Because of this action, calcitonin has proved effective in the treatment of Paget's disease (see Chapter 58). The hormone is also used to reduce serum calcium levels during hypercalcemic crises.

Salmon calcitonin, which differs from human calcitonin in 9 of 32 amino acids, is 100 times more potent than human calcitonin. The higher potency may be related to higher affinity for receptor sites and slower degradation by peripheral tissues. Calcitonin used clinically is often a synthetic preparation containing the amino acid sequence of salmon calcitonin.

Vitamin D

Vitamin D and its metabolites are not vitamins but steroid hormones. There are two forms of vitamin D: vitamin D_2 (ergocalciferol) and vitamin D_3 (cholecalciferol). The two forms differ by the presence of a double bond, but they have identical biologic activity. The term vitamin D is used to indicate both forms.

Vitamin D has little or no activity until it has been metabolized to compounds that mediate its activity. Figure 56-4 depicts sources of vitamin D and pathways for activation. The first step of the activation process occurs in the liver, where vitamin D is hydroxylated to form the metabolite 25-hydroxyvitamin D_3 [25-$(OH)D_3$]. From the liver, 25-$(OH)D_3$ is transported to the kidneys, where it undergoes conversion to 1,25-dihydroxyvitamin D_3 [1,25-$(OH)_2D_3$] or 24,25-dihydroxyvitamin D_3 [24,25-$(OH)_2D_3$].

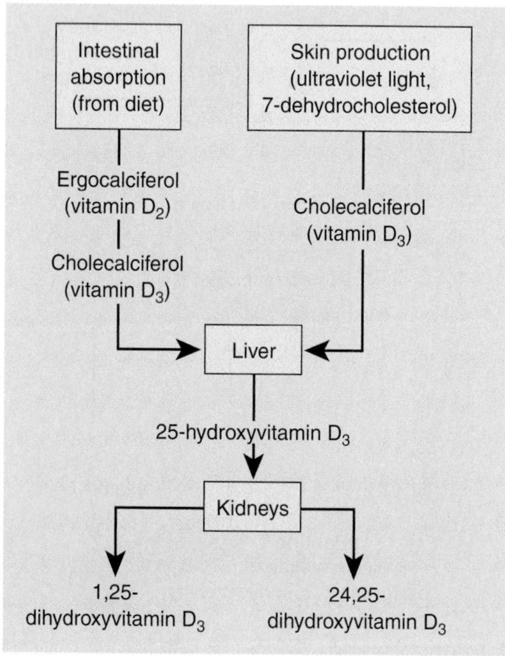

FIGURE 56-4 Sources and pathway for activation of vitamin D.

Other metabolites of vitamin D have been and still are being discovered.

There are two sources of vitamin D: intestinal absorption and skin production. Intestinal absorption occurs mainly in the jejunum and includes vitamin D_2 and vitamin D_3. The most important dietary sources of vitamin D are fish, liver, and irradiated milk. Because vitamin D is fat soluble, its absorption is mediated by bile salts and occurs by means of the lymphatic vessels. In the skin, ultraviolet radiation from sunlight spontaneously converts 7-dehydrocholesterol provitamin D_3 to vitamin D_3. A circulating vitamin D–binding protein provides a mechanism to remove vitamin D from the skin and make it available to the rest of the body.

With adequate exposure to sunlight, the amount of vitamin D that can be produced by the skin is usually sufficient to meet physiologic requirements. The importance of sunlight exposure is evidenced by population studies that report lower vitamin D levels in countries, such as England, that have less sunlight than the United States. Elderly persons who are housebound or institutionalized frequently have low vitamin D levels. The deficiency often goes undetected until there are problems such as pseudofractures or electrolyte imbalances. Seasonal variations in vitamin D levels probably reflect changes in sunlight exposure.

The most potent of the vitamin D metabolites is 1,25-$(OH)_2D_3$. The main action of this metabolite is regulation of calcium and phosphate homeostasis, in conjunction with PTH. Vitamin D increases intestinal absorption of calcium and it functions in the regulation of bone formation and mineralization. The actions of vitamin D on bone include an increase in osteoclast number and activity and an increase in osteoblast differentiation. Intestinal absorption and bone resorption serve to maintain calcium and phosphorous levels, a factor that is essential for bone mineralization. The major pathologic complication of a vitamin D deficiency is rickets in children and osteomalacia in adults (see Chapter 58).

The regulation of vitamin D activity is influenced by several hormones. PTH and prolactin stimulate 1,25-$(OH)_2D_3$ production by the kidney. States of hyperparathyroidism are associated with increased levels of 1,25-$(OH)_2D_3$, and hypoparathyroidism leads to lowered levels of this metabolite. Prolactin may have an ancillary role in regulating vitamin D metabolism during pregnancy and lactation. Calcitonin inhibits 1,25-$(OH)_2D_3$ production by the kidney. In addition to hormonal influences, changes in the concentration of ions such as calcium, phosphate, hydrogen, and potassium exert an effect on 1,25-$(OH)_2D_3$ and 24, 25-$(OH)_2D_3$ production. Under conditions of deprivation of phosphate and calcium, 1,25-$(OH)_2D_3$ levels are increased, whereas hyperphosphatemia and hypercalcemia decrease the levels of metabolite.

In summary, skeletal tissue is composed of two types of connective tissue: cartilage and bone. These skeletal structures are composed of similar tissue types; each has living cells and nonliving intercellular fibers and ground substance that is secreted by the cells. Cartilage is a firm, flexible type of skeletal tissue that is essential for growth before and after birth. There are three types of cartilage: elastic, hyaline, and fibrocartilage. Hyaline cartilage, which is the most abundant type, forms the costal cartilages that join the ribs to the sternum and vertebrae, many of the cartilages of the respiratory tract, and the articular cartilages.

The characteristics of the various skeletal tissue types are determined by the intercellular matrix. In bone, this matrix is impregnated with calcium salts to provide hardness and strength. There are four types of bone cells: osteocytes, or mature bone cells; osteoblasts, or bone-building cells; osteoclasts, which function in bone resorption; and osteogenic cells, which differentiate into osteoblasts. Densely packed compact bone forms the outer shell of a bone, and lattice-like cancellous bone forms the interior. The periosteum, the membrane that covers bones, contains blood vessels and acts as an anchorage point for vessels as they enter and leave the bone. The endosteum is the membrane that lines the spaces of spongy bone, the marrow cavities, and the haversian canals of compact bone.

The process of bone formation and mineral metabolism involves the interplay among the actions of PTH, calcitonin, and vitamin D. PTH acts to maintain serum levels of ionized calcium; it increases the release of calcium and phosphate from bone, the conservation of calcium and elimination of phosphate by the kidney, and the intestinal reabsorption of calcium through vitamin D. Calcitonin inhibits the release of calcium from bone and increases renal elimination of calcium and phosphate, thereby serving to lower serum calcium levels. Vitamin D functions as a hormone in regulating calcium and phosphate homeostasis. It increases absorption of calcium from the intestine and promotes the actions of PTH on bone.

Skeletal Structures

After completing this section of the chapter, you should be able to meet the following objectives:

- ✦ Characterize the structure of bones based on their shape and list the structures of long bones
- ✦ State the characteristics of tendons and ligaments
- ✦ State the difference between synarthrodial and diarthrodial joints
- ✦ Describe the source of blood supply to a diarthrodial joint
- ✦ Explain why pain is often experienced in all the joints of an extremity when only a single joint is affected by a disease process
- ✦ Describe the structure and function of a bursa
- ✦ Explain the pathology associated with a torn meniscus of the knee

CLASSIFICATION OF BONES

Bones are classified by shape as long, short, flat, and irregular. Long bones are found in the upper and lower extremities. Short bones are irregularly shaped bones located in the ankle and the wrist. Except for their surface, which is compact bone, these bones are spongy throughout. Flat bones are composed of a layer of spongy bone between two layers of compact bone. They are found in areas such as the skull and rib cage, where extensive protection of underlying structures is needed, or, as in the scapula, where a broad surface for muscle attachment must be provided. Irregular bones, because of their shapes, cannot be classified in any of the previous groups. This group includes bones such as the vertebrae and the bones of the jaw.

A typical long bone has a shaft, or *diaphysis,* and two ends, called *epiphyses*. Long bones usually are narrow in the midportion and broad at the ends so that the weight they bear can be distributed over a wider surface. The shaft of a long bone is formed mainly of compact bone roughly hollowed out to form a marrow-filled medullary canal. The ends of long bones are covered with articular cartilage that rests on a bony plate, the subchondral bone.

In growing bones, the part of the bone shaft that funnels out as it approaches the epiphysis is called the *metaphysis* (Fig. 56-5). It is composed of bony trabeculae that have cores of cartilage. In the child, the epiphysis is separated from the metaphysis by the cartilaginous growth plate. After puberty, the metaphysis and epiphysis merge, and the growth plate is obliterated.

Bone marrow occupies the medullary cavities of the long bones throughout the skeleton and the cavities of cancellous bone in the vertebrae, ribs, sternum, and flat bones of the pelvis. The cellular composition of the bone marrow varies with age and skeletal location. Red bone marrow contains developing red blood cells and is the site of blood cell formation. Yellow bone marrow is composed largely of adipose cells. At birth, nearly all of the marrow is red and hematopoietically active. As the need for red blood cell production decreases during postnatal growth, red marrow is gradually replaced with yellow bone marrow in most of the bones. In the adult, red marrow persists in the vertebrae, ribs, sternum, and ilia.

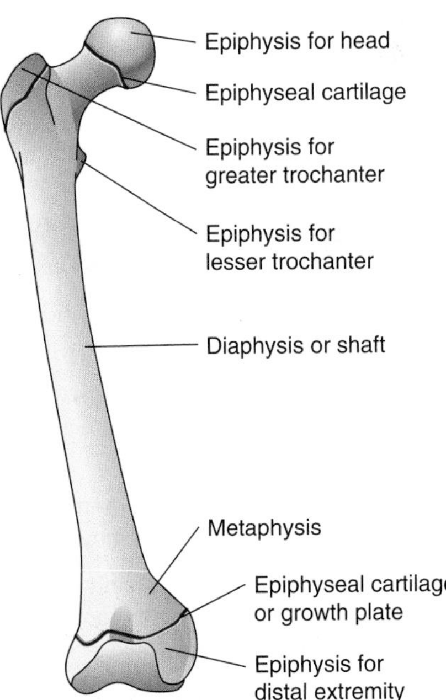

FIGURE 56-5 A femur, showing epiphyseal cartilages for the head, metaphysis, trochanters, and distal end of the bone.

TENDONS AND LIGAMENTS

In the skeletal system, tendons and ligaments are dense connective tissue structures that connect muscles and bones. Tendons connect muscles to bone, and ligaments connect the movable bones of joints. Tendons can appear as cord-like structures or as flattened sheets, called *aponeuroses,* such as in the abdominal muscles.

The dense connective tissue found in tendons and ligaments has a limited blood supply and is composed largely of intercellular bundles of collagen fibers arranged in the same direction and plane. This type of connective tissue provides great tensile strength and can withstand tremendous pull in the direction of fiber alignment. At the sites where tendons or ligaments are inserted into cartilage or bone, a gradual transition from pure dense connective tissue to bone or cartilage occurs. In cartilage, this transitional tissue is called *fibrocartilage.*

Tendons that may rub against bone or other friction-generating surfaces are enclosed in double-layered sheaths. An outer connective tissue tube is attached to the structures surrounding the tendon, and an inner sheath encloses the tendon and is attached to it. The space between the inner and outer sheath is filled with a fluid similar to synovial fluid.

ARTICULATIONS (JOINTS)

Articulations, or joints, are areas where two or more bones meet. The term *arthro* is the prefix used to designate a joint. For example, *arthrology* is the study of joints, and *arthroplasty* is the repair of a joint. There are two classes of joints, based on movement and the presence of a joint cavity: synarthroses and diarthroses.

Synarthroses

Synarthroses are joints that lack a joint cavity and move little or not at all. There are three types of synarthroses: synostoses, synchondroses, and syndesmoses. *Synostoses* are nonmovable joints in which the surfaces of the bones are joined by dense connective tissue or bone. The bones of the skull are joined by synostoses; they are joined by dense connective tissue in children and young adults and by bone in older persons. *Synchondroses* are joints in which bones are connected by hyaline cartilage and have limited motion. The ribs are attached to the sternum by this type of joint. *Syndesmoses* permit a certain amount of movement; they are separated by a fibrous disk and joined by interosseous ligaments. The symphysis pubis of the pelvis and the bodies of the vertebrae that are joined by intervertebral disks are examples of syndesmoses.

Diarthroses

Diarthrodial joints (*i.e.,* synovial joints) are freely movable joints. Most joints in the body are of this type. Although they are classified as freely movable, their movement ranges from almost none (*e.g.,* sacroiliac joint), to simple hinge movement (*e.g.,* interphalangeal joint), to movement in many planes (*e.g.,* shoulder or hip joint). The bony surfaces of these joints are covered with thin layers of articular cartilage, and the cartilaginous surfaces of these joints slide past each other during movement. As discussed in Chapter 59, diarthrodial joints are the joints most frequently affected by rheumatic disorders.

In a diarthrodial joint, the articulating ends of the bones are not connected directly but are indirectly linked by a strong fibrous capsule (*i.e.,* joint capsule) that surrounds the joint and is continuous with the periosteum (Fig. 56-6). This capsule supports the joint and helps to hold the bones in place. Additional support may be provided by ligaments that extend between the bones of the joint.

The joint capsule consists of two layers: an outer fibrous layer and an inner membrane, the synovium. The synovium surrounds the tendons that pass through the joints and the free margins of other intraarticular structures such as ligaments and menisci. The synovium forms folds that surround the margins of articulations but do not cover the weight-bearing articular cartilage. These folds permit stretch-

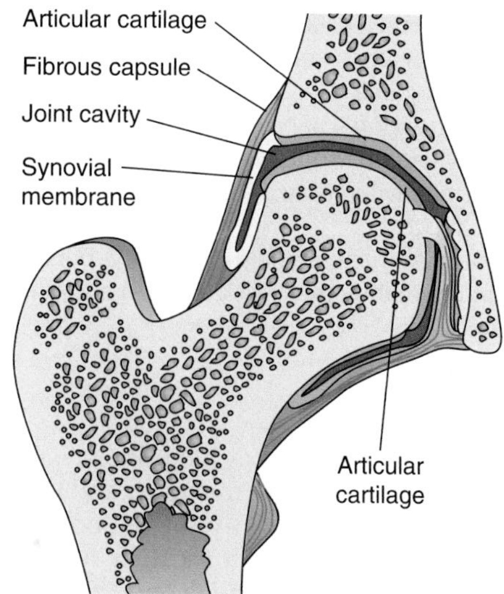

FIGURE 56-6 Diarthrodial joint, showing the articular cartilage, fibrous joint capsule, joint cavity, and synovial membrane.

SKELETAL JOINTS

- Articulations, or joints, are sites where two or more bones meet to hold the skeleton together and give it mobility.
- There are two types of joints: synarthroses, which are immovable joints, and diarthroses, which are freely movable joints.
- All limb joints are synovial diarthroidal joints, which are enclosed in a joint cavity containing synovial fluid.
- The articulating surfaces of synovial joints are covered with a layer of avascular cartilage that relies on oxygen and nutrients contained in the synovial fluid.
- Regeneration of articular cartilage of synovial joints is slow, and healing of injuries often is slow and unsatisfactory.

ing of the synovium so that movement can occur without tissue damage.

The synovium secretes a slippery fluid with the consistency of egg white called *synovial fluid.* This fluid acts as a lubricant and facilitates the movement of the articulating surfaces of the joint. Normal synovial fluid is clear or pale yellow, does not clot, and contains fewer than 100 cells/mm^3. The cells are predominantly mononuclear cells derived from the synovium. The composition of the synovial fluid is altered in many inflammatory and pathologic joint disorders. Aspiration and examination of the synovial fluid play an important role in the diagnosis of joint diseases.

The articular cartilage is an example of hyaline cartilage and is unique in that its free surface is not covered with perichondrium. It has only a peripheral rim of perichondrium, and calcification of the portion of cartilage abutting the bone may limit or preclude diffusion from blood vessels supplying the subchondral bone. Articular cartilage is apparently nourished by the diffusion of substances contained in the synovial fluid bathing the cartilage. Regeneration of most cartilage is slow; it is accomplished primarily by growth that requires the activity of perichondrium cells. In articular cartilage, which has no perichondrium, superficial injuries heal slowly.

Blood Supply and Innervation

The blood supply to a joint arises from blood vessels that enter the subchondral bone at or near the attachment of the joint capsule and form an arterial circle around the joint. The synovial membrane has a rich blood supply, and constituents of plasma diffuse rapidly between these vessels and the joint cavity. Because many of the capillaries are near the surface of the synovium, blood may escape into the synovial fluid after relatively minor injuries. Healing and repair of the synovial membrane usually are rapid and complete. This is important because synovial tissue is injured in many surgical procedures that involve the joint.

The nerve supply to joints is provided by the same nerve trunks that supply the muscles that move the joints. These nerve trunks also supply the skin over the joints. As a rule, each joint of an extremity is innervated by all the peripheral nerves that cross the articulation; this accounts for the referral of pain from one joint to another. For example, hip pain may be perceived as pain in the knee.

The tendons and ligaments of the joint capsule are sensitive to position and movement, particularly stretching and twisting. These structures are supplied by the large sensory nerve fibers that form proprioceptor endings (see Chapter 49). The proprioceptors function reflexively to adjust the tension of the muscles that support the joint and are particularly important in maintaining muscular support for the joint. For example, when a weight is lifted, there is a proprioceptor-mediated reflex contraction and relaxation of appropriate muscle groups to support the joint and protect the joint capsule and other joint structures. Loss of proprioception and reflex control of muscular support leads to destructive changes in the joint.

The synovial membrane is innervated only by autonomic fibers that control blood flow. It is relatively free of pain fibers, as evidenced by the fact that surgical procedures on the joint are often done under local anesthesia. The joint capsule and the ligaments have pain receptors; these receptors are more easily stimulated by stretching and twisting than other joint structures. Pain arising from the capsule tends to be diffuse and poorly localized.

Bursae

In some diarthrotic joints, the synovial membrane forms closed sacs that are not part of the joint. These sacs, called *bursae,* contain synovial fluid. Their purpose is to prevent friction on a tendon. Bursae occur in areas where pressure is exerted because of close approximation of joint structures (Fig. 56-7). Such conditions occur where tendons are deflected over bone or where skin must move freely over

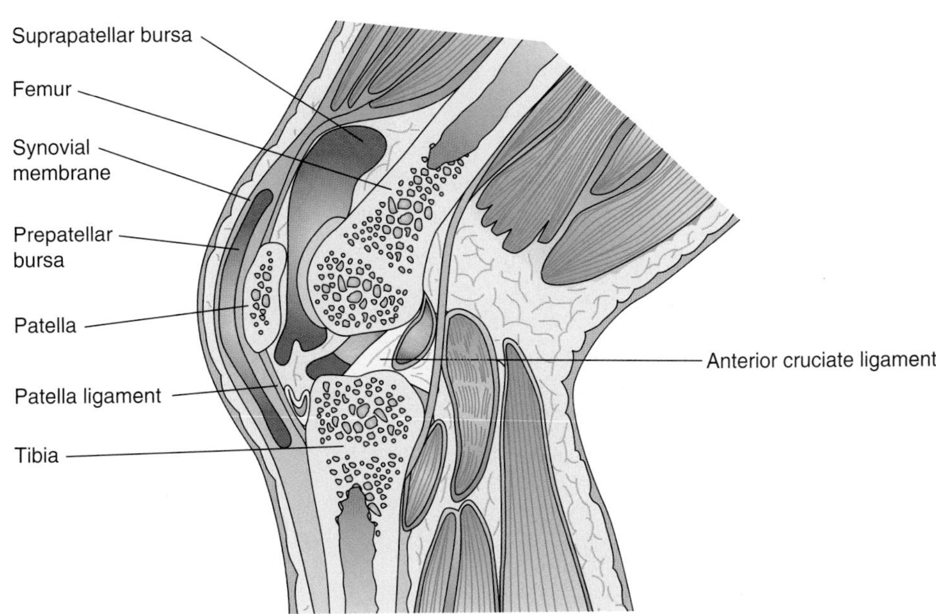

FIGURE 56-7 Sagittal section of knee joint, showing prepatellar and suprapatellar bursae.

bony tissue. Bursae may become injured or inflamed, causing discomfort, swelling, and limitation in movement of the involved area. A bunion is an inflamed bursa of the metatarsophalangeal joint of the great toe.

Intra-articular Menisci

Intra-articular menisci are fibrocartilaginous structures that develop from portions of the articular disk that occupied the space between articular cartilage surfaces during fetal development. Menisci may extend part way through the joint and have a free inner border, as at the lateral and medial articular surfaces of the knee, or they may extend through the joint, separating it into two separate cavities, as in the sternoclavicular joint. The menisci of the knee joint may be torn as the result of an injury (see Chapter 57).

In summary, bones are classified on the basis of their shape as long, short, flat, or irregular. Long bones are found in the upper and lower extremities; short bones in the ankle and wrist; flat bones in the skull and rib cage; and irregular bones in the vertebrae and jaw. Tendons and ligaments are dense connective skeletal tissues that connect muscles and bones. Tendons connect muscles to bones, and ligaments connect the movable bones of joints.

Articulations, or joints, are areas where two or more bones meet. Synarthroses are joints in which bones are joined together by fibrous tissue, cartilage, or bone; they lack a joint cavity and have little or no movement. Diarthrodial, or synovial, joints are freely movable. The surfaces of the articulating ends of bones in diarthrodial joints are covered with a thin layer of articular cartilage, and they are enclosed in a fibrous joint capsule. The joint capsule consists of two layers: an outer fibrous layer and an inner membrane, the synovium. The synovial fluid, which is secreted by the synovium into the joint capsule, acts as a lubricant and facilitates movement of the joint's articulating surfaces. Bursae, which are closed sacs containing synovial fluid, prevent friction in areas where tendons are deflected over bone or where skin must move freely over bony tissue.

Menisci are fibrocartilaginous structures that develop from portions of the articular disk that occupied the space between the articular cartilages during fetal development. The menisci may have a free inner border, or they may extend through the joint, separating it into two cavities. The menisci in the knee joint may be torn as a result of injury.

REVIEW EXERCISES

Often, pain from injury to the knee is experienced as pain in the hip.

A. Explain why this might occur.

Persons with end-stage kidney disease have a deficiency of activated vitamin D.

A. Explain why this occurs and what effect it would have on their bones.

Recent studies have revealed that estrogen deficiency, as well as normal aging, may produce a decrease in osteoblast activity.

A. Explain how this would contribute to the development of osteoporosis.

Bibliography

DeLuca H.F. (1988). The vitamin D story: A collaborative effort of basic science and clinical medicine. *FASEB Journal 2*, 236–242.

Gartner L.P., Hiatt J. (2001). *Color textbook of histology* (2nd ed., pp. 139–154). Philadelphia: W.B. Saunders.

Guyton A.C., Hall J.E. (2000). *Textbook of medical physiology* (10th ed., pp. 899–912). Philadelphia: W.B. Saunders.

Junqueira L.C., Carneiro J., Kelly O. (1995). *Basic histology* (8th ed., pp. 124–151). Los Altos, CA: Lange Medical Publications.

Moore K.L., Dalley A.F. (1999). *Clinically oriented anatomy* (4th ed). Philadelphia: Lippincott Williams & Wilkins.

Rhoades R.A., Tanner G.A. (2003). *Medical physiology* (2nd ed. pp. 638–648). Philadelphia: Lippincott Williams & Wilkins.

Schiller A.L., Teitelbaum S.L. (1999). Bones and joints. In Rubin E., Farber J.L. (Eds.), *Pathology* (3rd ed., pp. 1337–1344). Philadelphia: Lippincott-Raven.

CHAPTER

57

Disorders of Skeletal Function: Trauma, Infections, and Neoplasms

Kathleen E. Gunta and Marilyn King Hightower

The musculoskeletal system includes the bones, joints, and muscles of the body together with associated structures such as ligaments and tendons. This system, which constitutes more than 70% of the body, is subject to a large number of disorders. These disorders affect persons in all age groups and walks of life, causing pain and disability. The discussion in this chapter focuses on the effects of trauma, infections, ischemia, and neoplasms on musculoskeletal structures such as bones, muscles, tendons, and ligaments.

Injury and Trauma of Musculoskeletal Structures

After completing this section of the chapter, you should be able to meet the following objectives:

- Describe the physical agents responsible for soft tissue trauma
- Differentiate among the three types of soft tissue injuries
- Compare muscle strains and ligamentous sprains
- Describe the healing process of soft tissue injuries
- Differentiate open from closed fractures
- List the signs and symptoms of a fracture
- Explain the measures used in treatment of fractures
- Describe the fracture healing process
- Differentiate the early complications of fractures from later complications of fracture healing

A broad spectrum of musculoskeletal injuries result from numerous physical forces, including blunt tissue trauma, disruption of tendons and ligaments, and fractures of bony structures. Many of the forces that cause injury to the musculoskeletal system are typical for a particular environmental setting, activity, or age group. Trauma resulting from high-speed motor vehicle accidents is ranked as the number one killer of adults younger than 45 years of age.[1] Motorcycle accidents are especially common in young men, with fractures of the distal tibia, midshaft femur, and radius occurring most often.

Trauma in children is usually the result of an accident. Childhood falls cause approximately 3 million emergency department visits each year,[2] and bicycle-related injuries, most of them involving the 5- to 14-year-old age group, account for another 50,000 visits.[1] More than 775,000 children younger than 15 years of age are treated each year in hospital emergency departments for sports injuries. About 80% of these injuries occur in football, basketball, baseball, and soccer.[2] Most injuries are strains and sprains. Teenage athletes get injured at about the same rate as professionals. Unfortunately, this is due, in part, to the increasing level of competition.[3]

Falls are the most common cause of injury in people 65 years of age and older. Current statistics indicate that 30% of persons in this age group experience at least one fall each year.[4] Impaired vision and hearing, dizziness, and unsteadiness of gait contribute to falls in the older person. Among older adults, the majority of fractures are caused by falls.[5] These falls often are compounded by osteoporosis, or bone atrophy, which makes fractures more likely.[5] Fractures of the vertebrae, proximal humerus, and hip are particularly common in this age group. These injuries reduce mobility and independence and increase the risk for premature death.

ATHLETIC INJURIES

Athletic injuries are either acute injuries or overuse injuries. Acute injuries are caused by sudden trauma and include injuries to soft tissues (contusion, strains, and sprains) and to bone (fractures). Overuse injuries have been described as chronic injuries, including stress fractures that result from constant high levels of physiologic stress without sufficient recovery time.[6] They commonly occur in the elbow ("Little League elbow" or "tennis elbow") and in tissue where tendons attach to the bone, such as the heel, knee, and shoulder. Contact sports pose a greater threat for injury to the neck, spine, and growth plates in children and adolescents, who have not yet reached maturity. Injuries can be prevented by proper training, use of safety equipment, and competition according to skill and size rather than chronologic age. Adequate warm-up time, hydration, and proper nutrition are also key factors in injury prevention.[3]

SOFT TISSUE INJURIES

Most skeletal injuries are accompanied by soft tissue (muscle, tendon, or ligament) injuries. These injuries include contusions, hematomas, and lacerations. They are discussed here because of their association with musculoskeletal injuries.

A *contusion* is an injury to soft tissue that results from direct trauma and is usually caused by striking a body part against a hard object. With a contusion, the skin overlying the injury remains intact. Initially, the area becomes ecchymotic (*i.e.,* black and blue) because of local hemorrhage; later, the discoloration gradually changes to brown and then to yellow as the blood is reabsorbed. A large area of local hemorrhage is called a *hematoma.* Hematomas cause pain as blood accumulates and exerts pressure on nerve endings. The pain increases with movement or when pressure is applied to the area. The pain and swelling of a hematoma take longer to subside than those accompanying a contusion. A hematoma may become infected because of bacterial growth. Unlike a contusion, which does not drain, a hematoma may eventually split the skin because of increased pressures and produce drainage.

Treatment of a contusion and a hematoma consists of elevating the affected part and applying cold for the first 24 hours to reduce the bleeding into the area. A hematoma may need to be aspirated. After the first 24 hours, heat or cold should be applied intermittently for 20 minutes at a time.

A *laceration* is an injury in which the skin is torn or its continuity is disrupted. The seriousness of a laceration depends on the size and depth of the wound and on whether there is contamination from the object that caused the injury. Puncture wounds from nails or rusted material provide the setting for growth of anaerobic bacteria such as those that cause tetanus and gas gangrene.

Lacerations are usually treated by wound closure, which is done after the area is sufficiently cleaned; the closed wound is covered with a sterile dressing. It is important to minimize contamination of the wound and to control bleeding. Contaminated wounds and open fractures are copiously irrigated and débrided, and the skin usually is left open to heal to prevent the development of an anaerobic infection or a sinus tract. Antimicrobial agents are selectively used based on the suspected nature of the contaminants.

JOINT (MUSCULOTENDINOUS) INJURIES

Joints, or articulations, are sites where two or more bones meet. Joints (*i.e.,* diarthrodial) are supported by tough bundles of collagenous fibers called *ligaments* that attach to the joint capsule and bind the articular ends of bones together, and by *tendons* that join muscles to the periosteum of the articulating bones. Joint injuries involve mechanical overloading or forcible twisting or stretching.

JOINT INJURIES

- Joints are the weakest part of the skeletal system and common sites for injury due to mechanical overloading or forcible twisting or stretching.
- Injury can include damage to the tendons, which connect muscle to bone; ligaments, which hold bones together; or the cartilage that covers the articular surface.
- Healing of the dense connective tissue involved in joint injuries requires time to restore the structures so that they are strong enough to withstand the forces imposed on the joint. Ligamentous injuries may require surgical intervention with approximation of many fibrous strands to facilitate healing.
- Injuries involving the articular cartilage may predispose to later joint disease.

Strains and Sprains

Strains. A *strain* is a stretching injury to a muscle or a musculotendinous unit caused by mechanical overloading. This type of injury may result from an unusual muscle contraction or an excessive forcible stretch. Although there usually is no external evidence of a specific injury, pain, stiffness, and swelling exist. The most common sites for muscle strains are the lower back and the cervical region of the spine. The elbow and the shoulder are also supported by musculotendinous units that are subject to strains. Foot strain is associated with the weight-bearing stresses of the feet; it may be caused by inadequate muscular and ligamentous support, overweight, or excessive exercise such as standing, walking, or running.

In the lumbar and cervical spine regions, muscle strains are more common than sprains. Mechanical low back pain is becoming increasingly common in the adolescent athlete. Overuse, especially hyperextension of the lumbar spine in such sports as track, wrestling, gymnastics, and diving, can tear the muscles, fascia, and ligaments. Careful diagnosis is necessary because chronic low back pain may indicate a stress fracture. Fractures near the top and bottom surface of the vertebrae can occur when the growing lumbar spine is overstressed, causing the disks to push into the spinal nerve roots. Early detection and treatment are important to prevent complications and disability. Treatment of back strains consists of bed rest, traction, application of heat, and massage. Cold should be used during the first 24 hours to reduce pain and swelling of the affected area. Exercises, correct posture, and good body mechanics help to reduce the risk for reinjury.

Sprains. A *sprain,* which involves the ligamentous structures (strong bands of connective tissue) surrounding the joint, resembles a strain, but the pain and swelling subside more slowly. It usually is caused by abnormal or excessive movement of the joint. With a sprain, the ligaments may be incompletely torn or, as in a severe sprain, completely torn or ruptured (Fig. 57-1). The signs of sprain are pain, rapid swelling, heat, disability, discoloration, and limitation of function. Any joint may be sprained, but the ankle joint is most commonly involved, especially in fast moving injuries in which an ankle or knee can be suddenly twisted. Most ankle sprains occur in the lateral ankle when the foot is turned inward under a person, forcing the ankle into inversion beyond the structural limits. Other common sites of sprain are the knee (the collateral ligament and anterior cruciate ligament) and elbow (the ulnar side). As with a strain, the soft tissue injury that occurs with a sprain is not evident on the radiograph. Wrist sprains most often occur with a fall on an outstretched hand. Occasionally, however, a chip of bone is evident when the entire ligament, including part of its bony attachment, has been ruptured or torn from the bone.

Healing. Healing of the dense connective tissues in tendons and ligaments is similar to that of other soft tissues.[7] If properly treated, injuries usually heal with the restoration of the original tensile strength. Repair is accomplished by fibroblasts from the inner tendon sheath or, if the tendon has no sheath, from the loose connective tissue that surrounds the tendon. Capillaries infiltrate the injured area during the initial healing process and supply the fibroblasts with the materials they need to produce large amounts of collagen. Formation of the long collagen bundles occurs within the first 2 weeks, and although tensile strength increases steadily thereafter, it is not sufficient to permit strong tendon pulls for 6 to 8 weeks.[7] During the healing process, there is a danger that muscle contraction will pull the injured ends apart, causing the tendon to heal in the lengthened position. There is also a danger that adhesions will develop in areas where tendons pass through fibrous channels, such as in the distal palm of the hands, rendering the tendon useless.

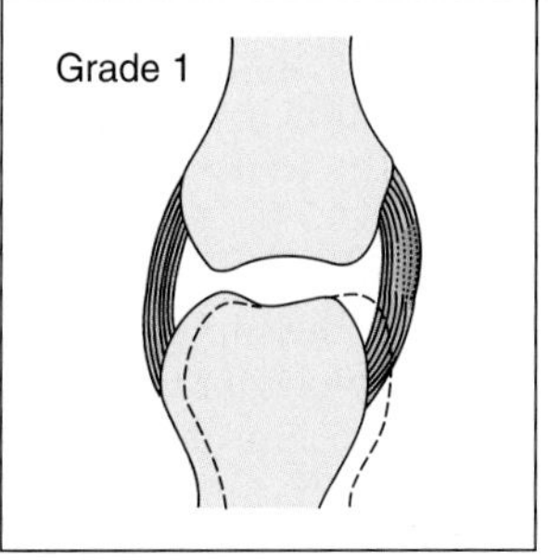

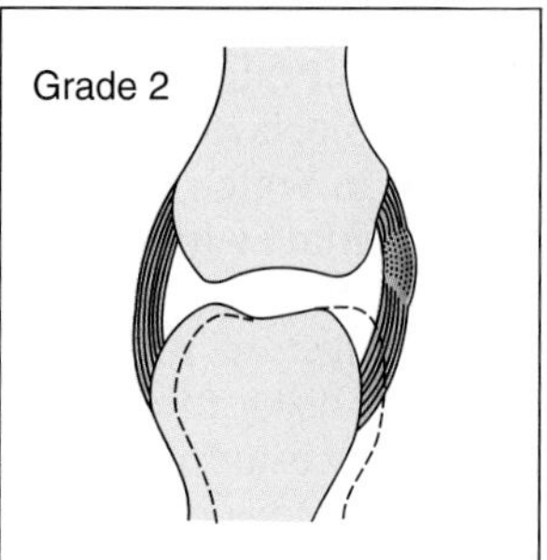

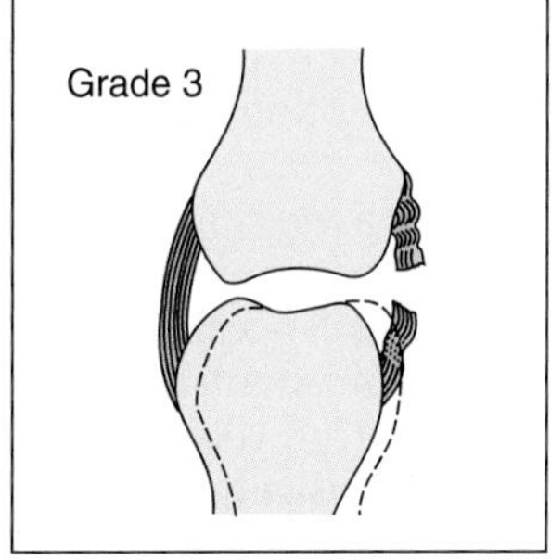

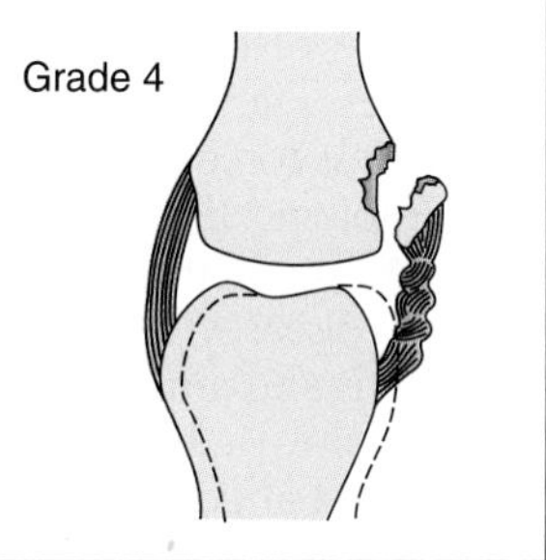

FIGURE 57-1 Degrees of sprain on the medial side of the right knee: grade 1, mild sprain of the medial collateral ligament; grade 2, moderate sprain with hematoma formation; grade 3, severe sprain with total disruption of the ligament; and grade 4, severe sprain with avulsion of the medial femoral condyle at the insertion of the medial collateral ligament. (Adapted from Spickler L.L. [1983]. Knee injuries of the athlete. *Orthopedic Nursing 2* [5], 12–13)

Treatment. The treatment of muscle strains and ligamentous sprains is similar in several ways. For an injured extremity, elevation of the part followed by local application of cold may be sufficient. Compression, accomplished through the use of adhesive wraps or a removable splint, helps reduce swelling and provides support. A cast is applied for severe sprains, especially those severe enough to warrant surgical repair. Immobilization for a muscle strain is continued until the pain and swelling have subsided. In a sprain, the affected joint is immobilized for several weeks. Immobilization may be followed by graded active exercises. Early diagnosis, treatment, and rehabilitation are essential in preventing chronic ligamentous instability.

Dislocations

A dislocation involves the displacement or separation of the bone ends of a joint with loss of articulation. It usually follows a severe trauma that disrupts the holding ligaments. Dislocations are seen most often in the shoulder and acromioclavicular joints. A subluxation is a partial dislocation in which the bone ends in the joint are still in partial contact with each other.

Dislocations can be congenital, traumatic, or pathologic. Congenital dislocations occur in the hip and knee. Traumatic dislocations occur after falls, blows, or rotational injuries. For example, car accidents often cause dislocations of the hip and accompanying acetabular fractures because of the direction of impact. This is true of persons wearing seat belts and those who are unrestrained. In the shoulder and patella, dislocations may become recurrent, especially in athletes. They recur with the same motion but require less and less force each time.

Pathologic dislocation in the hip is a late complication of infection, rheumatoid arthritis, paralysis, and neuromuscular diseases. Dislocations of the phalangeal joints are not serious and are usually reduced by manipulation. Less common sites of dislocation, seen mainly in young adults, are the wrist and midtarsal region. They usually are the result of direct force, such as a fall on an outstretched hand.

Diagnosis of a dislocation is based on history, physical examination, and radiologic findings. The symptoms are pain, deformity, and limited movement. With recurrent dislocations, the person often experiences apprehension during tests of joint rotation, fearing that the joint will slip out of place.

The treatment depends on the site, mechanism of injury, and associated injuries such as fractures. Dislocations that do not reduce spontaneously usually require manipulation or surgical repair. Various surgical procedures also can be used to prevent redislocation of the patella, shoulder, or acromioclavicular joints. Immobilization is necessary for several weeks after reduction of a dislocation to allow healing of the joint structures. In dislocations affecting the knee, alternatives to surgery are isometric quadriceps-strengthening exercises and a temporary brace.

Loose Bodies

Loose bodies are small pieces of bone or cartilage within a joint space. These can result from trauma to the joint or may occur when cartilage has worn away from the articular surface, causing a necrotic piece of bone to separate and become free floating. The symptoms are painful catching and locking of the joint. Loose bodies are commonly seen in the knee, elbow, hip, and ankle. The loose body repeatedly gets caught in the crevice of a joint, pinching the underlying healthy cartilage; unless the loose body is removed, it may cause osteoarthritis and restricted movement. The treatment consists of removal using operative arthroscopy.

Shoulder and Rotator Cuff Injuries

The shoulder is a complex series of joints that produce extraordinary range of motion. The extreme mobility is accomplished at the expense of instability. This instability, combined with its relatively exposed position, makes the shoulder extremely vulnerable to injuries such as sprains and dislocations and degenerative processes such as rotator cuff disorders.

The shoulder is composed of three bones: the scapula, the clavicle, and the humerus (Fig 57-2). The scapula is a thin bone that articulates widely and closely with the chest wall.[8] It also articulates with the humerus by way of a small, shallow glenoid cavity and with the clavicle at the acromion process. Clavicle fractures are among the most common fractures of childhood.[9] The typical mechanism of fracture is a fall on the point of the shoulder.

Three articulations form the shoulder joint: the acromioclavicular, glenohumeral, and sternoclavicular joints. The stability of these joints is provided by a series of muscles and tendons. Sprains of the acromioclavicular joint usually occur as a result of a blow to the top of the shoulder but are known to occur with a fall to the lateral or posterior aspects of the shoulder.[9] The most common site of shoulder dislocation occurs in the glenohumeral joint.[9,10] Most acute dislocations involve anterior displacement of the humeral head with respect to the glenoid, the result of the shoulder being abducted and forcefully extended and rotated. Other mechanisms include a fall on an outstretched arm or a blow to the posterior shoulder.

Motion of the arm involves the coordinated movement of muscles of the rotator cuff (supraspinous, teres minor, infraspinatus, subscapularis) and their musculotendinous attachments. These muscles are separated from the overlying coracoacromial arch by two bursae, the subdeltoid and subcoracoid. These two bursae, sometimes referred to as the *subacromial bursa,* often communicate and are affected by lesions of the rotator cuff.

The rotator cuff is not unlike other muscle groups of the body in that its risk for injury increases when it is required to perform a high-stress function in an unconditioned state. Rotator cuff injuries and impingement disorders can result from a number of causes, including

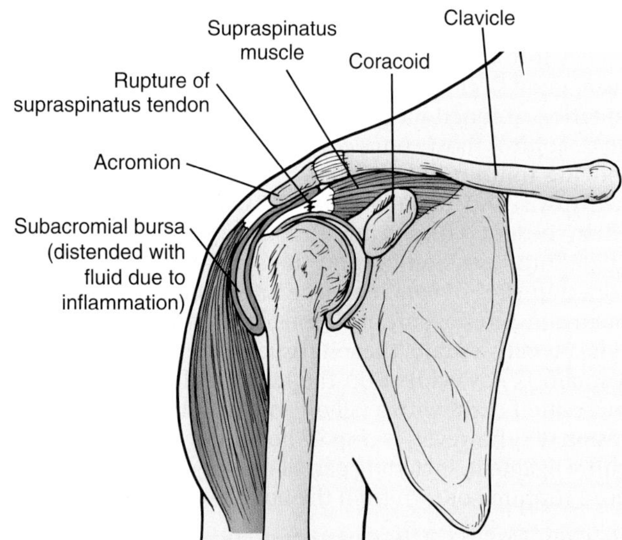

FIGURE 57-2 Structures of the shoulder showing the location of common rotator cuff injuries. The supraspinatus muscle is the most commonly injured part of the rotator cuff. (Adapted from Moore K.L., Dalley A.F. *Clinically Oriented Anatomy* [4th ed., p. 698]. Philadelphia: Lippincott Williams & Wilkins)

excessive use, a direct blow, or stretch injury, usually involving throwing or swinging, as with baseball pitchers or tennis players. Complete tears or rupture of the rotator cuff usually occur in young persons after severe trauma (see Fig. 57-2). Overuse and degenerative disorders have a slower onset and are seen in older persons with minor or no trauma. The tendons of the rotator cuff fuse together near their insertions into the tuberosites of the humerus to form the musculotendinous cuff. Degeneration of these tendons can result from a number factors, including repetitive microtrauma, impairment of vascularity as a result of age, or shoulder instability with secondary overload of the cuff. Degeneration is most severe near the tendon insertion, with the supraspinous being affected most often. Chronic irritation of the musculotendinous unit can lead to tendinitis with scarring and thickening of the tendon and with secondary inflammation of the overlying bursae.[8] Thickening of these tissues decreases the distance between the cuff and the overlying coracoacromial arch. Pain and impingement may be noted when motions of the arm squeeze and pinch these tissues between the humerus and the overlying arch. Severe tendinitis also can cause either a partial or complete rotator cuff tear.

Several physical examination maneuvers are used to define shoulder pathology.[11] The history and mechanism of injury are important. In addition to standard radiographs, arthrography, computed tomography (CT), or magnetic resonance imaging (MRI) may be used. Arthroscopic examination under anesthesia is obtained for diagnostic purposes and operative arthroscopy to repair severe tears. Conservative treatment with antiinflammatory agents, corticosteroid injections, and physical therapy often is undertaken. A period of rest is followed by a customized exercise and rehabilitation program to improve strength, flexibility, and endurance.

Knee Injuries

The knee is a common site of injury, particularly sport-related injuries in which the knee is subjected to abnormal twisting and compression forces. These forces can result in injury to the menisci, patellar subluxation and dislocation, and chondromalacia. Knee injuries in young adulthood and both knee and hip injuries in middle age substantially increase the risk for osteoarthritis in the same joint later in life.

Meniscus Injuries. The menisci are C-shaped plates of fibrocartilage that are superimposed between the condyles of the femur and tibia. There are two menisci in each knee, a lateral and medial meniscus (Fig. 57-3). The menisci are thicker at their external margins and taper to thin, unattached edges at their interior margin. They are firmly attached at their ends to the intercondylar area of the tibia and are supported by the coronary and transverse ligaments of the knee. The menisci play a major role in load bearing and shock absorption. They also help to stabilize the knee by deepening the tibial socket and maintaining the femur and tibia in proper position. In addition, the meniscus assists in joint lubrication and serves as source of nutrition for articular cartilage in the knee.

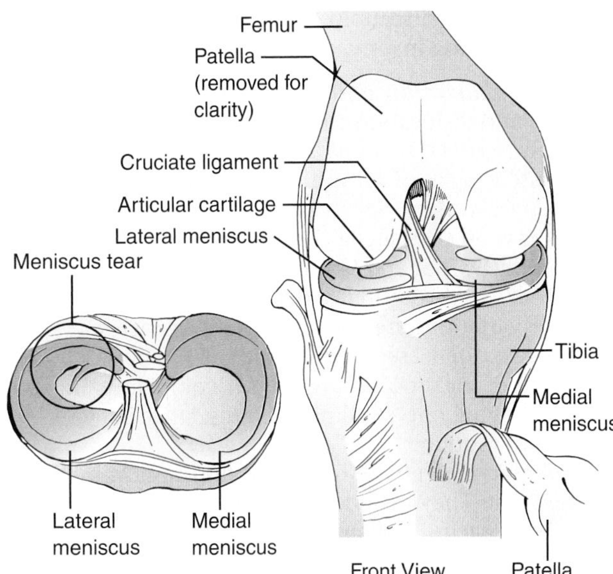

FIGURE 57-3 The knee, showing the lateral and medial meniscus (with the patella removed for clarity). Insert (**lower left**) shows meniscus tear.

Any action of the knee that causes injury to the knee ligaments can also cause a meniscal tear.[12] Meniscus injury commonly occurs as the result of a rotational injury from a sudden or sharp pivot or a direct blow to the knee, as in hockey, basketball, or football. The type and location of the meniscal tear are determined by the magnitude and direction of the force that acts on the knee and the position of the knee at the time of injury. Meniscus tears can be described by their appearance (*e.g.*, parrot-beak, bucket handle) or their location (*e.g.*, posterior horn, anterior horn). The injured knee is edematous and painful, especially with hyperflexion and hyperextension. A loose fragment may cause knee instability and locking.

Diagnosis is made by examination and confirmed by methods such as arthroscopy and radiologic, CT scans, and radionuclide imaging. MRI has proved particularly useful in the diagnosis of meniscal tears.[12] Initial treatment of meniscal injuries may be conservative. The knee may be placed in a removable knee immobilizer. Isometric quadriceps exercises may be prescribed. Activity usually is restricted until complete motion is recovered. Arthroscopic meniscectomy may be performed when there is recurrent or persistent locking, recurrent effusion, or disabling pain.

There is evidence that loss of meniscal function is associated with progressive deterioration of knee function.[13] Damaged articular cartilage has a limited capacity to heal because of its avascular nature and inadequate mobilization of regenerative cells. Meniscal reconstruction procedures have been developed to preserve these functions before development of significant degenerative changes occur, thus preventing a total joint replacement later in life. Among the reconstruction methods used is replacement of the damaged meniscus with a meniscal transplant (fresh, frozen, or cryopreserved allografts).[13,14] Use of a synthetic collagen scaffold that allows fibrochondrocyte ingrowth is being investigated.[13]

Patellar Subluxation and Dislocations. Recurrent subluxation and dislocation of the patella (*i.e.*, knee cap) are common injuries in young adults. They account for approximately 10% of all athletic injuries and are more common in women. Sports such as skiing or tennis may cause stress on the patella. These sports involve external rotation of the foot and lower leg with knee flexion, a position that exerts rotational stresses on the knee. Congenital knee variations are also a predisposing factor.

There is often a sensation of the patella "popping out" when the dislocation occurs.[8] Other complaints include the knee giving out, swelling, crepitus, stiffness, and loss of range of motion.

Treatment can be difficult, but nonsurgical methods are used first. They include immobilization with the knee extended, bracing, administration of antiinflammatory agents, and isometric quadriceps-strengthening exercises. Surgical intervention often is necessary.

Chondromalacia. Chondromalacia, or softening of the articular cartilage, is seen most commonly on the undersurface of the patella and occurs most frequently in young adults.[8] It can be the result of recurrent subluxation of the patella or overuse in strenuous athletic activities. Persons with this disorder typically complain of pain, particularly when climbing stairs or sitting with the knees bent. Occasionally, the person experiences weakness of the knee.

Treatment consists of rest, isometric exercises, and application of ice after exercise. Part of the patella may be surgically removed in severe cases. In less severe cases, the soft portion is shaved using a saw inserted through an arthroscope. Articular cartilage maintenance and repair is a complex process, currently under investigation. Polypeptide growth factors that direct cells to divide, differentiate, migrate, and produce matrix appear to have a role in the preservation and degradation of the articular cartilage matrix. Growth factors such as insulin-like growth factor (IGF), bone morphogenic proteins (BMP), and transforming growth factor-β (TGF-β) have been shown to affect chondrocyte growth and metabolism.[15]

FRACTURES

Fracture, or discontinuity of the bone, is the most common type of bone lesion. Normal bone can withstand considerable compression and shearing forces and, to a lesser extent, tension forces. A fracture occurs when more stress is placed on the bone than it is able to absorb. Grouped according to cause, fractures can be divided into three major categories: fractures caused by sudden injury, fatigue or stress fractures, and pathologic fractures. The most common fractures are those resulting from sudden injury. The force causing the fracture may be direct, such as a fall or blow, or indirect, such as a massive muscle contraction or trauma transmitted along the bone. For example, the head of the radius or clavicle can be fractured by the indirect forces that result from falling on an outstretched hand. A fatigue fracture results from repeated wear on a bone. Pain associated with overuse injuries of the lower extremities, especially posterior medial tibial pain, is one of the most common symptoms that physically active persons, such as runners, experience. Stress fractures in the tibia may be confused with "shin splints," a nonspecific term for pain in the lower leg from overuse in walking and running, because they frequently do not appear on x-ray films until 2 weeks after the onset of symptoms.

A pathologic fracture occurs in bones that already are weakened by disease or tumors. Fractures of this type may occur spontaneously with little or no stress. The underlying disease state can be local, as with infections, cysts, or tumors, or it can be generalized, as in osteoporosis, Paget disease, or cancer metastasis.

Classification

Fractures usually are classified according to location, type, and direction or pattern of the fracture line (Fig. 57-4).

Location. A long bone is divided into three parts: proximal, midshaft, and distal (see Fig. 57-4). A fracture of the long bone is described in relation to its position in the bone. Other descriptions are used when the fracture affects the head or neck of a bone, involves a joint, or is near a prominence such as a condyle or malleolus.

Types. The type of fracture is determined by its communication with the external environment, the degree of break in continuity of the bone, and the character of the fracture pieces. A fracture can be classified as open or closed. When the bone fragments have broken through the skin,

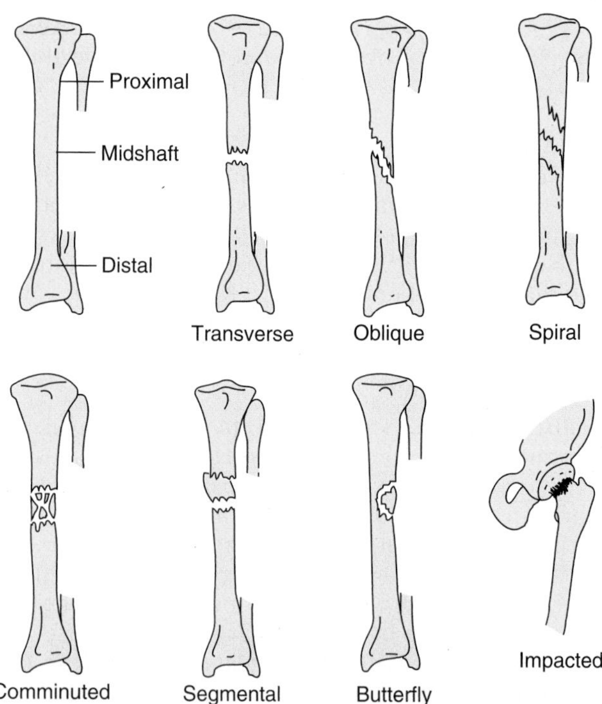

FIGURE 57-4 Classification of fractures. Fractures are classified according to location (proximal, midshaft, or distal), the direction of fracture line (transverse, oblique, spiral), and type (comminuted, segmental, butterfly, or impacted).

the fracture is called an *open* or *compound fracture*.[8] Open fractures often are complicated by infection, osteomyelitis, delayed union, or nonunion. In a closed fracture, there is no communication with the outside skin.

The degree of a fracture is described in terms of a partial or complete break in the continuity of bone. A *greenstick fracture,* which is seen in children, is an example of a partial break in bone continuity and resembles that seen when a young sapling is broken. This kind of break occurs because children's bones, especially until approximately 10 years of age, are more resilient than the bones of adults.

A fracture is also described by the character of the fracture pieces. A *comminuted fracture* has more than two pieces. A *compression fracture,* as occurs in the vertebral body, involves two bones that are crushed or squeezed together. A fracture is called *impacted* when the fracture fragments are wedged together. This type usually occurs in the humerus, often is less serious, and usually is treated without surgery.

Patterns. The direction of the trauma or mechanism of injury produces a certain configuration or pattern of fracture. *Reduction* is the restoration of a fractured bone to its normal anatomic position. The pattern of a fracture indicates the nature of the trauma and provides information about the easiest method for reduction. *Transverse fractures* are caused by simple angular forces. A *spiral fracture* results from a twisting motion, or torque. A transverse fracture is not likely to become displaced or lose its position after it is reduced. On the other hand, spiral, oblique, and comminuted fractures often are unstable and may change position after reduction.

Manifestations

The signs and symptoms of a fracture include pain, tenderness at the site of bone disruption, swelling, loss of function, deformity of the affected part, and abnormal mobility. The deformity varies according to the type of force applied, the area of the bone involved, the type of fracture produced, and the strength and balance of the surrounding muscles.

In long bones, three types of deformities—angulation, shortening, and rotation—are seen. Severely angulated fracture fragments may be felt at the fracture site and often push up against the soft tissue to cause a tenting effect on the skin. Bending forces and unequal muscle pulls cause angulation. Shortening of the extremity occurs as the bone fragments slide and override each other because of the pull of the muscles on the long axis of the extremity (Fig. 57-5). Rotational deformity occurs when the fracture fragments rotate out of their normal longitudinal axis; this can result from rotational strain produced by the fracture or unequal pull by the muscles that are attached to the fracture fragments. A crepitus or grating may be felt as the bone fragments rub against each other. In the case of an open fracture, there is bleeding from the wound where the bone protrudes. Blood loss from a pelvic fracture or multiple long bone fractures can cause hypovolemic shock in a trauma victim.

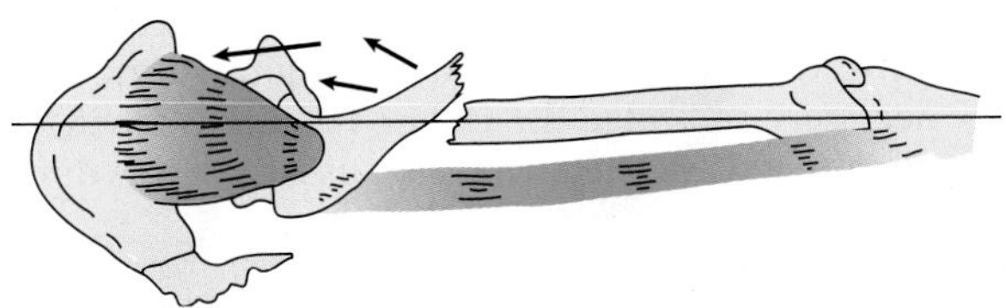

FIGURE 57-5 Displacement and overriding of fracture fragments of a long bone (femur) caused by severe muscle spasm.

Shortly after the fracture has occurred, nerve function at the fracture site may be temporarily lost. The area may become numb, and the surrounding muscles may become flaccid. This condition has been called *local shock.* During this period, which may last for a few minutes to half an hour, fractured bones may be reduced with little or no pain. After this brief period, the pain returns and, with it, muscle spasms and contractions occur in the surrounding muscles.

The early complications of fractures are associated with loss of skeletal continuity, injury from bone fragments, pressure from swelling and hemorrhage, involvement of nerve fibers, or development of fat emboli. The extent of early complications depends on the severity of the fracture and the area of the body that is involved. For example, bone fragments from a skull fracture may cause injury to brain tissue, or multiple rib fractures may lead to a flail chest and respiratory insufficiency. With flail chest, the chest wall on the fractured side becomes so unstable that it may move in the opposite direction as the person breathes (*i.e.,* in during inspiration and out during expiration).

Healing

Bone healing occurs in a manner similar to soft tissue healing. It is, however, a more complex process and takes longer. Although the exact mechanisms of bone healing are open to controversy, five stages of the healing process have been identified: (1) hematoma formation, (2) cellular proliferation, (3) callus formation, (4) ossification, and (5) remodeling[16] (Fig. 57-6). The degree of response during each of these stages is in direct proportion to the extent of trauma.

Hematoma Formation. Hematoma formation occurs during the first 48 to 72 hours after fracture. It develops as blood from torn vessels in the bone fragments and surrounding soft tissue leaks between and around the fragments of the

FRACTURE HEALING

- Fractures are caused by forces that disrupt the continuity of bone.
- Fracture healing depends on the extent of the injury, the ability to align the bone fragments, and immobilizing the fracture site so that healing can take place.
- Bone healing occurs by replacement of injured bone cells. It involves formation of a hematoma that provides the foundation for blood vessel and fibroblast infiltration, proliferation of bone repair cells (osteoblasts), callus formation, ossification of the callus, and remodeling of the fracture site.

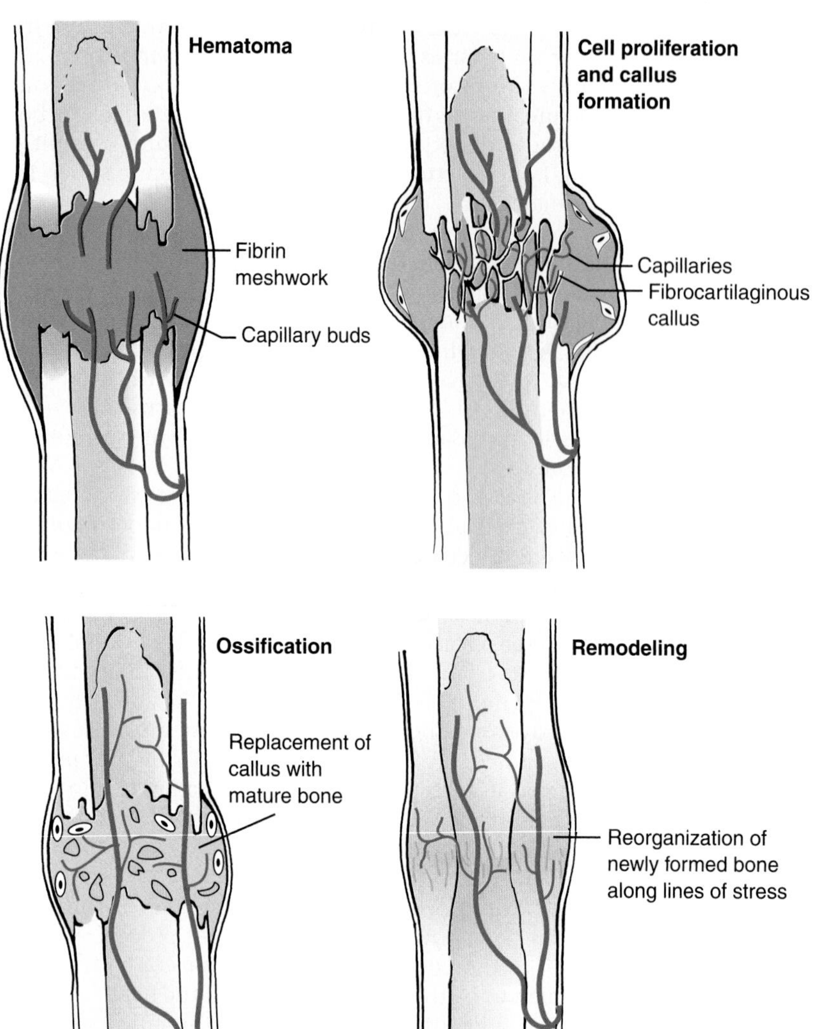

FIGURE 57-6 The stages of bone healing. The hematoma stage provides the fibrin meshwork and capillary buds needed for subsequent cellular invasion. Cellular proliferation and callus formation represent the stages during which osteoblasts enter the area and form the fibrocartilaginous callus that joins the bone fragments. The ossification stage involves the mineralization of the fibrocartilaginous callus; and the remodeling stage, the reorganization of mineralized bone along the lines of mechanical stress.

fractured bone. Evidence suggests that the function of the hematoma is to be a source of signaling molecules that initiate the cellular events essential to fracture healing.[17] As the result of hematoma formation, clotting factors remain in the injured area to initiate the formation of a fibrin meshwork, which serves as a framework for the ingrowth of fibroblasts and new capillary buds. Granulation tissue, the result of fibroblasts and new capillaries, gradually invades and replaces the clot. When a large hematoma develops, healing is delayed because macrophages, platelets, oxygen, and nutrients for callus formation are prevented from entering the area.

Cellular Proliferation. Three layers of bone structure are involved in the cellular proliferation that occurs during bone healing: the periosteum, or outer covering of the bone; the endosteum, or inner covering; and the medullary canal, which contains the bone marrow. During this process, the osteoblasts, or bone-forming cells, multiply and differentiate into a fibrocartilaginous callus. The fibrocartilaginous callus is softer and more flexible than callus. Cellular proliferation begins distal to the fracture, where there is a greater supply of blood. After a few days, a fibrocartilage "collar" becomes evident around the fracture site. The collar edges on either side of the fracture eventually unite to form a bridge, which connects the bone fragments.

Callus Formation. During the early stage of callus formation, the fracture becomes "sticky" as osteoblasts continue to move in and through the fibrin bridge to help keep it firm. Cartilage forms at the level of the fracture, where there is less circulation. In areas of the bone with muscle insertion, periosteal circulation is better, bringing in the nutrients necessary to bridge the callus. The bone calcifies as mineral salts are deposited. This stage usually occurs during the third to fourth week of fracture healing.

Ossification. Ossification involves the final laying down of bone. This is the stage at which the fracture has been bridged and the fracture fragments are firmly united. Mature bone replaces the callus, and the excess callus is gradually resorbed by the osteoclasts. The fracture site feels firm and immovable and appears united on the radiograph. At this point, it is safe to remove the cast.

Remodeling. Remodeling involves resorption of the excess bony callus that develops in the marrow space and encircles the external aspect of the fracture site. The remodeling process is directed by mechanical stress and direction of weight bearing. It continues according to Wolff's law—bone responds to mechanical stress by becoming thicker and stronger in relation to its function.

Healing Time. Healing time depends on the site of the fracture, the condition of the fracture fragments, hematoma formation, and other local and host factors. In general, fractures of long bones, displaced fractures, and fractures with less surface area heal more slowly. Function usually returns within 6 months after union is complete. However, return to complete function may take longer. Stress fractures usually require less time to heal, usually 2 to 4 weeks, during which time a reduction in activity and protection of the area are needed.

Factors that influence bone healing are specific to the person, the type of injury sustained, and local factors that disrupt healing (Chart 57-1). Individual factors that may delay bone healing are the patient's age; current medications; debilitating diseases, such as diabetes and rheumatoid arthritis; local stress around the fracture site; circulatory problems and coagulation disorders; and poor nutrition.

Diagnosis and Treatment

Diagnosis is the first step in the care of fractures and is based on history and physical manifestations. X-ray examination is used to confirm the diagnosis and direct the treatment. The ease of diagnosis varies with the location and severity of the fracture. In the trauma patient, the presence of other, more serious injuries may make diagnosis more difficult. A thorough history includes the mechanism, time, and place of the injury; first recognition of symptoms; and any treatment initiated. A complete history is important because a delay in seeking treatment or a period of weight bearing on a fracture may cause further injury or displacement of the fracture. When a fracture is suspected, the injured part always should be splinted before it is moved.[8] This is essential for preventing further injury.

There are three objectives for treatment of fractures: reduction of the fracture, immobilization, and preservation and restoration of the function of the injured part.

Reduction. Reduction is directed at alignment of the bones in the angular and rotational planes, restoration of proper length, and restoration of apposition of the bone ends.[8]

This can be accomplished by closed manipulation or surgical (open) reduction. Closed manipulation uses methods such as manual pressure and traction. Fractures are held in reduction by external or internal fixation devices. Surgical reduction involves the use of various types of hardware to accomplish internal fixation of the fracture fragments (Fig. 57-7).

Immobilization. Immobilization prevents movement of the injured parts and is the single most important element in obtaining union of the fracture fragments. Immobilization can be accomplished through the use of external devices, such as splints, casts, traction, or external fixation devices; or by internal fixation devices inserted during surgical reduction of the fracture.

Splints are made from many different materials. Metal splints or air splints may be used during transport to a health care facility as a temporary measure until the fracture has been reduced and another form of immobilization instituted. Plaster of Paris splints, which are molded to fit the extremity, work well. Splinting should be done if there is any suspicion of a fracture because motion of the fracture

CHART 57-1

Factors Affecting Fracture Healing

- Nature of the injury or the severity of the trauma, including fracture displacement, edema, and arterial occlusion with crushing injuries
- Degree of fibrocartilaginous bridge formation that develops during bone healing
- Amount of bone loss (*e.g.*, it may be too great for the healing to bridge the gap)
- Type of bone that is injured (*e.g.*, cancellous bone heals faster than cortical bone)
- Degree of immobilization that is achieved (*e.g.*, movement disrupts the fibrin bridge and cartilage forms instead of bone)
- Local infection, which retards or prevents healing
- Local malignancy, which must be treated before healing can proceed
- Bone necrosis, which prevents blood flow into the fracture site

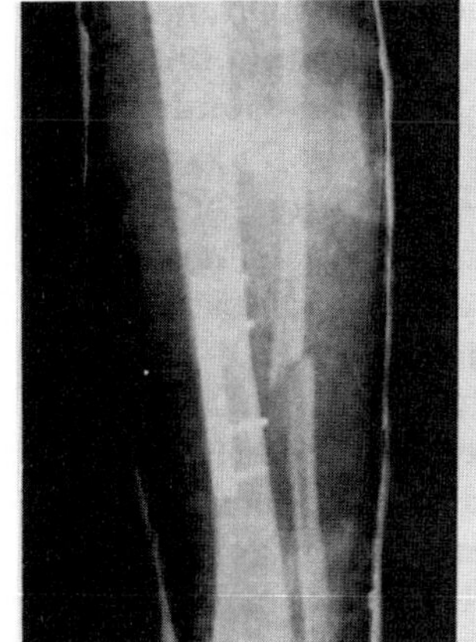
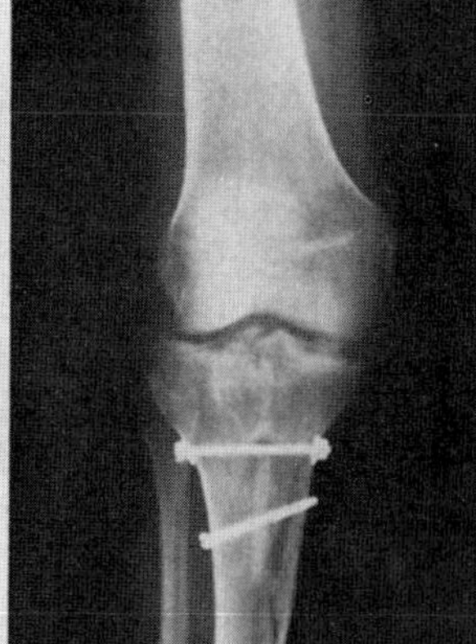

FIGURE 57-7 (**Left**) Internal fixation of the tibia with compression plate. (**Right**) Internal fixation of an intraarticular fracture of the upper tibia with a screw and bolt. (Adapted with permission from Farrell J. [1986]. *Illustrated guide to orthopaedic nursing* [3rd ed.]. Philadelphia: J.B. Lippincott)

site can cause pain, bleeding, more soft tissue damage, and nerve or blood vessel compression. If the fracture has sharp fragments, movement can cause perforation of the skin and conversion of a closed fracture into an open one. When a splint is applied to an extremity, it should extend from the joint above the fracture site to the joint below it.

Casts, which are made of plaster or synthetic material such as fiberglass, are commonly used to immobilize fractures of the extremities. They often are applied with a joint in partial flexion to prevent rotation of the fracture fragments. Without this flexion, the extremity, which is essentially a cylinder, tends to rotate within the cylindrical structure of the cast. A brace may be used after a cast is removed or instead of a cast, as with a tibial stress fracture. The application of a cast carries the risk for impaired circulation to the extremity because of blood vessel compression. A cast applied shortly after a fracture may not be large enough to accommodate the swelling that inevitably occurs in the hours that follow. After a cast is applied, the peripheral circulation must be observed carefully until this danger has passed. If the circulation becomes inadequate, the parts that are exposed at the distal end of the cast (*i.e.,* the toes with a leg cast and the fingers with an arm cast) usually become cold and cyanotic or pale. An increase in pain may occur initially, followed by paresthesia (*i.e.,* tingling or abnormal sensation) or anesthesia as the sensory neurons that supply the area are affected. There is a decrease in the amplitude or absence of the pulse in areas where the arteries can be palpated. Capillary refill time, which is assessed by applying pressure to the fingernail and observing the rate of blood return, is prolonged to longer than 3 seconds. This condition demands immediate measures, such as splitting the cast, to restore the circulation and prevent permanent damage to the extremity. A casted extremity should be elevated above the level of the heart for the first 24 hours to minimize swelling.

Traction is another method for achieving immobility and maintaining alignment of the bone ends and maintaining the reduction, particularly if the fracture is unstable or comminuted. Traction is a pulling force applied to an extremity or part of the body while a counterforce, or countertraction, pulls in the opposite direction. The five goals of traction therapy are to correct and maintain the skeletal alignment of entire bones or joints; reduce pressure on a joint surface; correct, lessen, or prevent deformities such as contractures and dislocations; decrease muscle spasm; and immobilize the fracture site to promote healing. Traction may be used as a temporary measure before surgery or as a primary treatment method. There are three types of traction: manual traction, skin traction, and skeletal traction. *Manual traction* consists of a steady, firm pull that is exerted by the hands. It is a temporary measure used to manipulate a fracture during closed reduction, for support of a neck injury during transport when a cervical spine fracture is suspected, or for reduction of a dislocated joint. *Skin traction* is a pulling force applied to the skin and soft tissue. It is accomplished by strips of adhesive flannel or foam secured to the injured part. *Skeletal traction* is a pulling force applied directly to the bone. Pins, wires, or tongs are inserted through the skin and subcutaneous tissue into the bone distal to the fracture site. Skeletal traction provides an excellent pull and can be used for long periods with large amounts of weight. It is commonly used for fractures of the femur, the humerus, and the cervical spine (*e.g.,* Crutchfield tongs applied to the skull).

With *external fixation devices,* pins or screws are inserted directly into the bone above and below the fracture site. They are secured to a metal frame and adjusted to align the fracture. This method of treatment is used primarily for open fractures, infections such as osteomyelitis and septic joints, unstable closed fractures, and limb lengthening.

Limb-lengthening systems, such as the Ilizarov external fixator (Fig. 57-8), are used to lengthen or widen bones, correct angular or rotational defects, or immobilize fractures.[18] The apparatus is applied with a surgical technique called a *corticotomy,* which is a percutaneous osteotomy that preserves the periosteal and endosteal tissues. A circular external apparatus is attached to bone by tensioned Kirschner wires. The corticotomy site is gradually distracted or pulled apart by approximately 1 mm/day until the desired length is achieved. The continuous distraction activates regeneration of bone, soft tissue, nerves, and blood vessels. New bone forms (*i.e.,* osteogenesis) in the distraction gap. This newly formed bone can fill posttraumatic defects or those formed after resection for osteomyelitis, consolidate nonunions, regenerate bone in limb lengthening, correct deformities, and eliminate the need for bone grafting. The apparatus is left on until the desired length is achieved and consolidation is complete.

Preservation and Restoration of Function. During the period of immobilization required for fracture healing, the preservation and restoration of the function of muscles and joints are an ongoing process in the unaffected and affected extremities. Exercises designed to preserve function, maintain muscle strength, and reduce joint stiffness should be started early. Active range of motion, in which the person moves the extremity, is done on unaffected extremities, and isometric, or muscle-tensing, exercises are done on the affected extremities. In some instances, an electrical muscle stimulator is applied directly to the skin to stimulate isometric muscle contraction as a means of preventing disuse atrophy. After the fracture has healed, a program of physical therapy may be necessary. However, the most important factor in restoring function is the person's own active exercises.

Muscles tend to atrophy during immobilization because of lack of use. Joints stiffen as muscles and tendons contract and shorten. The degree of muscle atrophy and joint stiffness depends on several factors. In adults, the degree of atrophy and muscle stiffness is directly related to the length of immobilization, with longer periods of immobility resulting in greater stiffness. Children have a natural tendency to move on their own, and this movement maintains muscle and joint function. They usually have less atrophy and recover sooner after the source of immobilization has been removed. Associated soft tissue injury, infection, and preexisting joint disease increase the risk for stiffness. Although limbs are immobilized in a functional position, casts are removed as soon as fracture healing has taken place so that joint stiffness does not occur.

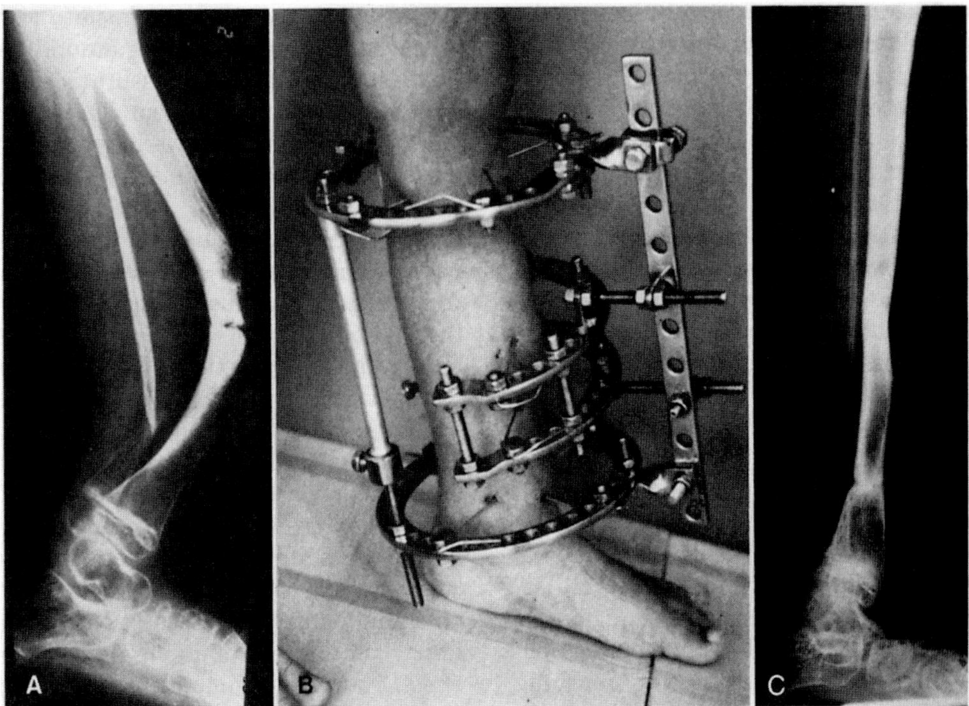

FIGURE 57-8 Ilizarov device used to treat a tibial fracture with anterolateral bow and medullary sclerosis: before (**A**), with Ilizarov device in place (**B**), and 3-year follow-up lateral roentgenograph (**C**). (Paley D., Catagni M., Argnani F. et al. [1992]. Treatment of congenital pseudoarthrosis of the tibia using Ilizarov technique. *Clinical Orthopaedics and Related Research, 280,* 84)

Impaired Healing

Union of a fracture has occurred when the fracture is solid enough to withstand normal stresses and it is clinically and radiologically safe to remove the external fixation. In children, fractures usually heal within 4 to 6 weeks; in adolescents, they heal within 6 to 8 weeks; and in adults, they heal within 10 to 18 weeks. The increased rate of healing among children compared with adults may be related to the increased cellularity and vascularity of the child's periosteum.[19] A number of factors can contribute to impaired bone healing, including the nature and extent of the injury, the health of the person with the fracture and his or her responses to injury, the adequacy of initial treatment, and pharmacologic factors. For large bone defects caused by trauma or a tumor, bone regeneration may need enhancement. Various growth factors, such bone morphologic protein (BMP), are thought to induce bone formation and repair bone defects.[20]

Malunion is healing with deformity, angulation, or rotation that is visible on x-ray films. Early, aggressive treatment, especially of the hand, can prevent malunion and result in earlier alignment and return of function. It is caused by inadequate reduction or alignment of the fracture.

Delayed union is the failure of a fracture to unite within the normal period (*e.g.,* 20 weeks for a fracture of the tibia or femur in an adult). Intraarticular fractures (those through a joint) may heal more slowly and may eventually produce arthritis. *Nonunion* is failure to produce union and cessation of the processes of bone repair. It is seen most often in the tibia, especially with open fractures or crushing injuries. It is characterized by mobility of the fracture site and pain on weight bearing. Muscle atrophy and loss of range of motion may occur. Nonunion usually is established 6 to 12 months after the time of the fracture. The complications of fracture healing are summarized in Table 57-1.

Treatment methods for impaired bone healing encompass surgical interventions, including bone grafts, bracing, external fixation, or electrical stimulation of the bone ends. The treatment for delayed union consists of determining and correcting the cause of the delay. Electrical stimulation is thought to stimulate the osteoblasts to lay down a network of bone. Three types of commercial bone growth stimulators are available: a noninvasive model, which is placed outside the cast; a semi-noninvasive model, in which pins are inserted around the fracture site; and a totally implantable type, in which a cathode coil is wound around the bone at the fracture site and operated by a battery pack implanted under the skin. The Ilizarov method of circular external fixation is used to treat nonunions, especially those that are infected.

COMPLICATIONS OF FRACTURES AND OTHER MUSCULOSKELETAL INJURIES

The complications of fractures and other orthopedic injuries are associated with loss of skeletal continuity, injury from bone fragments, pressure from swelling and

TABLE 57-1 Complications of Fracture Healing

Complication	Manifestations	Contributing Factors
Delayed union	Failure of fracture to heal within predicted time as determined by x-ray	Large displaced fracture Inadequate immobilization Large hematoma Infection at fracture site Excessive loss of bone Inadequate circulation
Malunion	Deformity at fracture site Deformity or angulation on x-ray	Inadequate reduction Malalignment of fracture at time of immobilization
Nonunion	Failure of bone to heal before the process of bone repair stops Evidence on x-ray Motion at fracture site Pain on weight bearing	Inadequate reduction Mobility at fracture site Severe trauma Bone fragment separation Soft tissue between bone fragments Infection Extensive loss of bone Inadequate circulation Malignancy Bone necrosis Noncompliance with restrictions

hemorrhage (*e.g.,* fracture blisters, compartment syndrome), involvement of nerve fibers (*e.g.,* reflex sympathetic dystrophy and causalgia), or development of fat emboli.

Fracture Blisters

Fracture blisters are skin bullae and blisters representing areas of epidermal necrosis with separation of epidermis from the underlying dermis by edema fluid. They occur when the intracompartmental pressure is too high to be relieved by normal means. They are seen with more severe, twisting types of injuries (*e.g.,* motor vehicle accidents and falls from heights), but can also occur after excessive joint manipulation, dependent positioning, and heat application, or from peripheral vascular disease. They can be solitary, multiple, or massive depending on the extent of injury. Most fracture blisters occur in the ankle, elbow, foot, knee, or areas where there is little soft tissue between the bone and the skin. The development of fracture blisters reportedly is reduced by early surgical intervention in persons requiring operative repair.[21] This probably reflects the early operative release of the fracture hematoma, reapproximation of the disrupted soft tissues, ligation of bleeding vessels, and fixation of bleeding fracture surfaces. Prevention of fracture blisters is important because they pose an additional risk for infection. They also constitute a warning sign of compartment syndrome.

Compartment Syndrome

Compartment syndrome is the result of increased pressure in a limited anatomic space that compromises circulation and threatens the viability and function of the nerves and muscles (see Chapter 24). It can be acute or chronic. Acute compartment syndrome can occur after a fracture or crushing injury when excessive swelling around the site of injury results in increased pressure (>30 mm Hg) in a closed compartment. This increase in pressure occurs because fascia, which covers and separates muscles, is inelastic and unable to stretch and compensate for the extreme swelling. The most common sites are the four compartments of the lower leg (*i.e.,* deep posterior, superficial posterior, lateral, and anterior compartments) and the dorsal and volar compartments of the forearm.

The condition is characterized by pain that is out of proportion to original injury or physical findings.[22,23] Nerve compression may cause changes in sensation (*e.g.,* paresthesias such as burning or tingling or loss of sensation), diminished reflexes, and eventually the loss of motor function. Symptoms usually begin within a few hours, but can be delayed up to 64 hours.[23] Compression of blood vessels may cause muscle ischemia and loss of function. Muscles and nerves may be permanently damaged if the pressure is not relieved. In contrast to the diminished or absent pulses that occur when ischemia is caused by a tight bandage or cast, the arterial pulses often are normal in compartment syndrome. Pallor and loss of the pulse, when they occur, are late findings. It may be difficult to diagnose compartment syndrome in children, unresponsive persons, and those with hypotension.

Treatment of compartment syndrome is directed at reducing the compression of blood vessels and nerves. Constrictive dressings and casts are loosened. Intracompartmental pressure can be measured by means of a catheter or needle inserted into the compartment. A fasciotomy, or transection of the fascia that is restricting the muscle compartment, may be required when the pressure in the area rises above 30 mm Hg, which is roughly equal to the perfusion pressure in the capillary beds. Delay in diagnosis and treatment of compartment syndrome can lead to irreversible nerve and muscle damage.

Chronic compartment syndrome occurs most often in young adults after activity that involves repetitive strain on lower extremities, such as long-distance running or marching. Although the exact mechanism is unclear, exercise causes an increase in compartment size and intramuscular pressure that results in tissue ischemia and pain.[24] The compartment is stretched and becomes inflamed. The fascia is scarred, less elastic, and unable to compensate for further compartment volume. Pain is experienced during activity. Tissue pressure measurements usually are done. Conservative measures, such as shoe orthotics, stretching exercises, and activity modification, are attempted. A fasciotomy is done for persistent symptoms.

Crush syndrome a third type of compartment syndrome accompanied by systemic manifestations resulting from severe muscle ischemia with multicompartmental involvement.[25] Prolonged compression of skeletal muscle or severe tissue trauma can lead to muscle necrosis and infection. Myoglobinuria occurs as proteins are broken down in damaged muscle cells. Potassium is also released. This can result in third space fluid loss, acidosis, renal failure, and circulatory shock (see Chapter 28).

Reflex Sympathetic Dystrophy and Causalgia

Reflex sympathetic dystrophy and causalgia represent soft tissue complications of musculoskeletal injuries that cause pain out of proportion to the injury and autonomic nervous system dysfunction manifested by hyperhidrosis (increased sweating) and vasomotor instability (either flushed and warm or cold and pale).[21,26] The disorder often produces long-term disability and chronic pain syndromes (see Chapter 50).

Pain, which is the prominent symptom of the disorder, is described as severe, aching, or burning. It usually increases in intensity with movement and with noxious and nonnoxious stimuli. The pathophysiologic cause of the pain is unclear, but it is thought to have a sympathetic nervous system component. Muscle wasting, thin and shiny skin, and abnormalities of the nails and bone can occur. Decreased muscle strength and disuse can lead to contractures and osteoporosis.

Treatment focuses on pain management and prevention of disability. Physical therapy interventions such as hot/cold baths and elevation of the limb are used to maximize range of motion and minimize pain. Medications include antiinflammatory agents, vasodilators, and antidepressant medications. Sympathetic nerve blocks may be used.

Fat Embolism Syndrome

The fat embolism syndrome (FES) refers to a constellation of clinical manifestations resulting from the presence of fat droplets in the small blood vessels of the lung or other organs after a long bone fracture or other major trauma.[21,27–30] The main clinical features of fat embolism syndrome are respiratory failure, cerebral dysfunction, and skin and mucosal petechiae. Cerebral manifestations include encephalopathy, seizures, and focal neurologic deficits.

Clinically, the incidence of fat embolization is related to fractures and surgery of bones containing the most marrow (*i.e.*, long bones and the bones of the pelvis). An increase in intramedullary pressure in the femur is the most important pathogenic factor in the development of emboli. The use of conventional cement for fracture fixation of joint arthroplasty also increases the risk for FES.[31,32] Although fat embolization occurs with fractures or operative fixation of fractures, FES occurs only in a small percentage of cases (0.5% to 3%), supporting the hypothesis that factors other than mechanical obstruction by fat globules may be necessary in the development of FES.[28]

There are two theories about the mechanisms leading to the FES: mechanical and biochemical. The mechanical theory is that fat globules are released from the bone marrow or subcutaneous tissue at the fracture site into the venous system through torn veins and are lodged in the lungs, brain, or other organs.[21] The biochemical theory postulates that the fat emboli develop intravascularly secondary to an alteration in lipid stability caused by increased release of tissue lipases, catecholamines, glucagon, or other steroid hormones in response to the stress of injury.[21] The mechanical and biochemical theories are not mutually exclusive. Fat emboli also may be caused by exogenous sources of fat, such as blood transfusions, sickle cell disease, intravenous fat emulsions, or bone marrow transplantation.

Initial symptoms of FES begin to develop within a few hours to 3 to 4 days after injury and do not appear beyond 1 week after the injury. The first symptoms include a subtle change in behavior and signs of disorientation resulting from emboli in the cerebral circulation combined with respiratory depression. There may be complaints of substernal chest pain and dyspnea accompanied by tachycardia and a low-grade fever. Diaphoresis, pallor, and cyanosis become evident as respiratory function deteriorates. A petechial rash that does not blanch with pressure often occurs 2 to 3 days after the injury. This rash usually is found on the anterior chest, axillae, neck, and shoulders. It also may appear on the soft palate and conjunctiva. The rash is thought to be related to embolization of the skin capillaries or thrombocytopenia.

Three degrees of severity are seen: subclinical, overt clinical, and fulminating. Although the subclinical and overt clinical forms of FES respond well to treatment, the fulminating form often is fatal. There are three possible outcomes when fat emboli enter the pulmonary circulation: (1) small emboli can mold to vessel caliber, pass through the lung, and enter the systemic circulation, where they are trapped in the tissues or eliminated through the kidney; (2) the fat particles can be broken down by alveolar cells and eliminated through sputum; or (3) local lipolysis can occur with the release of free fatty acids.[27] Free fatty acids cause direct injury to the alveolar capillary membrane, which leads to hemorrhagic interstitial pneumonitis with disruption of surfactant production and development of the adult respiratory distress syndrome. The fat globules also become coated with platelets, causing thrombocytopenia. Serotonin released by the sequestered platelets causes bronchospasm and vasodilatation.

An important part of the treatment of fat emboli is early diagnosis. Arterial blood gases should be assayed immediately after recognition of clinical manifestations. A lung scan may be done. Carotid ultrasonography or an MRI can detect brain embolism. Transesophageal echocardiography can be used to show the sequence of the embolic event.[33]

Treatment is directed toward correcting hypoxemia and maintaining adequate fluid balance. Mechanical ventilation may be required. Corticosteroid drugs are administered to decrease the inflammatory response of lung tissues, decrease the edema, stabilize the lipid membranes to reduce lipolysis, and combat the bronchospasm. Corticosteroids are also given prophylactically to high-risk persons. The only preventive approach to FES is early stabilization of the fracture.

In summary, many external physical agents can cause trauma to the musculoskeletal system. Particular factors, such as environment, activity, or age, can place a person at greater risk for injury. Some soft tissue injuries, such as contusions, hematomas, and lacerations, are relatively minor and easily treated. Muscle strains and ligamentous sprains are caused by mechanical overload on the connective tissue. They heal more slowly than the minor soft tissue injuries and require some degree of immobilization. Healing of soft tissue begins within 4 to 5 days of the injury and is primarily the function of fibroblasts, which produce collagen. Joint dislocation is caused by trauma to the supporting structures. Repeated trauma to the joint can cause articular softening (*i.e.*, chondromalacia) or the separation of small pieces of bone or cartilage, called *loose bodies*, in the joint.

Fractures occur when more stress is placed on a bone than the bone can absorb. The nature of the stress determines the type of fracture and the character of the resulting bone fragments. Healing of fractures is a complex process that takes place in five stages: hematoma formation, cellular proliferation, callus formation, ossification, and remodeling. For satisfactory healing to take place, the affected bone has to be reduced and immobilized. Immobilization is accomplished with the use of external devices, such as splints, casts, traction, or an external fixation apparatus, or with a surgically implanted internal fixation device. The complications associated with fractures can occur early due to soft tissue and nerve damage, or later when the healing process of the fracture is interrupted. The early complications of fractures and other orthopedic injuries are associated with swelling and hemorrhage (fracture blisters and compartment syndrome), involvement of nerve fibers (reflex sympathetic dystrophy and causalgia), and development of fat emboli. Impaired healing of a fracture can cause malunion with deformity, angulation, or rotation; delayed healing in which the healing process is prolonged; or nonunion, in which the fracture fails to heal.

Bone Infections

After completing this section of the chapter, you should be able to meet the following objectives:

- Explain the implications of bone infection
- Differentiate among osteomyelitis due to spread from a contaminated wound, hematogenous osteomyelitis, and osteomyelitis due to vascular insufficiency in terms of etiologies, manifestations, and treatment
- Cite the characteristics of chronic osteomyelitis
- Describe the most common sites of tuberculosis of the bone

Bone infections, including acute and chronic osteomyelitis, are known for their ability to cause pain, disability, and deformity. Despite the common use of antibiotics, they remain difficult to treat and eradicate. A resurgence of tuberculosis is occurring in industrialized parts of world, attributed in part to immigrants from Third World countries and the greater numbers of immunosuppressed people.

OSTEOMYELITIS

Osteomyelitis represents an acute or chronic pyogenic infection of the bone. The term *osteo* refers to bone, and *myelo* refers to the marrow cavity, both of which are involved in this disease. The infection can be caused by direct extension or contamination of an open fracture or wound (contiguous invasion); seeding through the bloodstream (hematogenous spread); or skin infections in persons with vascular insufficiency. Osteomyelitis can occur as an acute, subacute, or chronic condition.

The specific agents isolated in bacterial osteomyelitis are often associated with the age of the person or the inciting condition (*e.g.*, trauma or surgery). *Staphylococcus aureus* is responsible for most cases of acute hematogenous osteomyelitis.[16,34–36] *Staphylococcus epidermidis, S. aureus, Pseudomonas aeruginosa, Serratia marcescens,* and *Escherichia coli* are commonly isolated in persons with chronic osteomyelitis.[36] *S. aureus* has two characteristics that favor its ability to produce osteomyelitis: (1) it has the ability to

BONE INFECTIONS

- Bone infections may be caused by a wide variety of microorganisms introduced during injury, during operative procedures, or from the bloodstream.
- Once localized in bone, the microorganisms proliferate, produce cell death, and spread within the bone shaft, inciting a chronic inflammatory response with further destruction of bone.
- Bone infections are difficult to treat and eradicate. Measures to prevent infection include careful cleaning and débridement of skeletal injuries and strict operating room protocols.

produce a collagen-binding adhesion molecule that allows it to adhere to the connective tissue elements of bone; and (2) it has the ability to be internalized and survive in osteoblasts, making the microorganism more resistant to antibiotic therapy.[35]

Hematogenous Osteomyelitis

Hematogenous osteomyelitis originates with infectious organisms that reach the bone through the bloodstream. Acute hematogenous osteomyelitis occurs predominantly in children.[36] In adults, it is seen most commonly in debilitated patients and in those with a history of chronic skin infections, chronic urinary tract infections, and intravenous drug use and in those who are immunologically suppressed. Intravenous drug users are at risk for infections with *Streptococcus* and *Pseudomonas*.

Pathogenesis. The pathogenesis of hematogenous osteomyelitis differs in children and adults. In children, the infection usually affects the long bones of the appendicular skeleton. It starts in the metaphyseal region close to the growth plate, where termination of nutrient blood vessels and sluggish blood flow favor the attachment of blood-borne bacteria. With advancement of the infection, purulent exudate collects in the rigidly enclosed bony tissue. Because of the bone's rigid structure, there is little room for swelling, and the purulent exudate finds its way beneath the periosteum, shearing off the perforating arteries that supply the cortex with blood, thereby leading to necrosis of cortical bone. The necrotic bone that is formed may separate from the viable surrounding bone to form devascularized fragments, called *sequestra*.[16] Eventually, the purulent drainage may penetrate the periosteum and skin to form a draining sinus. In young children (1 year and younger), the adjacent joint is often involved because the periosteum is not firmly attached to the cortex.[16] From age 1 year to puberty, subperiosteal abscesses are more common. As the process continues, periosteal new bone formation and reactive bone formation in the marrow tend to wall the infection. *Involucrum* refers to a lesion in which bone formation forms a sheath around the necrotic sequestrum. It is seen most commonly in cases of chronic osteomyelitis (discussed later).

In adults, the long bone microvasculature no longer favors seeding, and hematogenous infection rarely affects the appendicular skeleton. Instead, vertebrae, sternoclavicular and sacroiliac joints, and the symphysis pubis are involved. Infection typically first involves subchondral bone, then spreads to the joint space. During vertebral osteomyelitis, this causes sequential destruction of the end plate, adjoining disk, and contiguous vertebral body. Infection less commonly begins in the joint and spreads to the adjacent bone. There is a tendency for infectious organisms to seed sites of previous, often minor injury.

Manifestations. The signs and symptoms of acute hematogenous osteomyelitis are those of bacteremia accompanied by symptoms referable to the site of the bone lesion. Bacteremia is characterized by chills, fever, and malaise. There often is pain on movement of the affected extremity, loss of movement, and local tenderness followed by redness and swelling. X-ray studies may appear normal initially, but they show evidence of periosteal elevation and increased osteoclastic activity after an abscess has formed. Changes are evident on a bone scan 10 to 14 days before any changes are seen on x-ray films.[36]

Treatment. The treatment of hematogenous osteomyelitis begins with identification of the causative organism through blood and bone aspiration cultures.[36] Antibiotics are given first parenterally and then orally. The amount of time that the affected limb needs to be rested and pain control measures used is based on the person's symptoms. Débridement and surgical drainage also may be necessary.

Contiguous Spread Osteomyelitis

Osteomyelitis secondary to a contiguous focus of infection may occur as a result of direct inoculation from an exogenous source or from an adjacent extraskeletal site. The most common cause is the direct contamination of bone from an open wound. It may be the result of an open fracture, a gunshot wound, or a puncture wound. Inadequate irrigation or débridement, introduction of foreign material into the wound, and extensive tissue injury increase the bone's susceptibility to infection.

Iatrogenic bone infections are those inadvertently brought about by surgery or other treatments. These infections include complications of pin tract infection in skeletal traction, septic (infected joints) in joint replacement surgery, and wound infections after surgery. Measures to prevent these infections include preparation of the skin to reduce bacterial growth before surgery or insertion of traction devices or wires; strict operating room protocols; prophylactic use of antibiotics immediately before and for 24 hours after surgery and as a topical wound irrigation; and maintenance of sterile technique after surgery when working with drainage tubes and dressing changes.

Pathogenesis. The pathogenesis of osteomyelitis resulting from contiguous spread of infection differs from hematogenous infection in that virtually any traumatized bone may be involved. Although healthy bone is highly resistant to infection, injury from local inflammation and trauma may devitalize bone and tissue, providing an inert matrix upon which microorganisms introduced during trauma thrive.

Manifestations. Osteomyelitis after trauma or bone surgery usually is associated with persistent or recurrent fevers, increased pain at the operative or trauma site, and poor incisional healing, which often is accompanied by continued wound drainage and wound separation. Prosthetic joint infections present with joint pain, fever, and cutaneous drainage.

Diagnosis and Treatment. Diagnosis requires both confirming the infection and identifying the offending microorganism with culture and sensitivity studies. The diagnosis of skeletal infection entails use of various imaging strategies, including conventional radiology, nuclear imaging studies, CT scans, and MRI.[36] Bone biopsy may be used to identify the causative microorganisms.

Treatment includes the use of antibiotics and selective use of surgical interventions. Antibiotics should be administered prophylactically to persons undergoing bone surgery. For persons with osteomyelitis, early antibiotic treatment, before there is extensive destruction of bone, produces the best results. The choice of antibiotics and method of administration depend on the microorganisms causing the infection. Antibiotic beads (*e.g.*, vancomycin, tobramycin, or other broad-spectrum antibiotic) can be embedded into the cement as part of the procedure for an infected hip arthroplasty or for a wound infection after spinal cord injury.[37] In acute osteomyelitis that does not respond to antibiotic therapy, surgical decompression is used to release intramedullary pressure and remove drainage from the periosteal area. The use of bioabsorbable tobramycin-impregnated bone graft substitute is effective in post-traumatic infected bone defects or nonunions.[38]

Chronic Osteomyelitis

Chronic osteomyelitis usually occurs in adults. Generally, these infections occur secondary to an open wound, most often to the bone or surrounding tissue. Chronic osteomyelitis has long been recognized as a disease. However, the incidence has decreased in the past century because of improvements in surgical techniques and broad-spectrum antibiotic therapy. Chronic osteomyelitis includes all inflammatory processes of bone, excluding those in rheumatic diseases that are caused by microorganisms. It may be the result of delayed or inadequate treatment of acute hematogenous osteomyelitis or osteomyelitis caused by direct contamination of bone. Acute osteomyelitis is considered to have become chronic when the infection persists beyond 6 to 8 weeks or when the acute process has been adequately treated and is expected to resolve but does not. Chronic osteomyelitis can persist for years; it may appear spontaneously, after a minor trauma, or when resistance is lowered.

The hallmark feature of chronic osteomyelitis is the presence of infected dead bone, a *sequestrum,* that has separated from the living bone. A sheath of new bone, called the *involucrum,* forms around the dead bone (Fig. 57-9). Radiologic techniques such as x-ray films, bone scans, and sinograms are used to identify the infected site. Chronic osteomyelitis or infection around a total joint prosthesis can be difficult to diagnose because the classic signs of infection are not apparent and the blood leukocyte count may not be elevated. A subclinical infection may exist for years. Bone scans are used in conjunction with bone biopsy for a definitive diagnosis.[39]

The treatment of chronic bone infections begins with wound cultures to identify the microorganism and its sensitivity to antibiotic therapy. The goal in selecting antimicrobial treatment for osteomyelitis is to use the drug with the highest bactericidal activity and least toxicity and at the lowest cost. Intravenous therapy is usually needed for up to 6 weeks.[36]

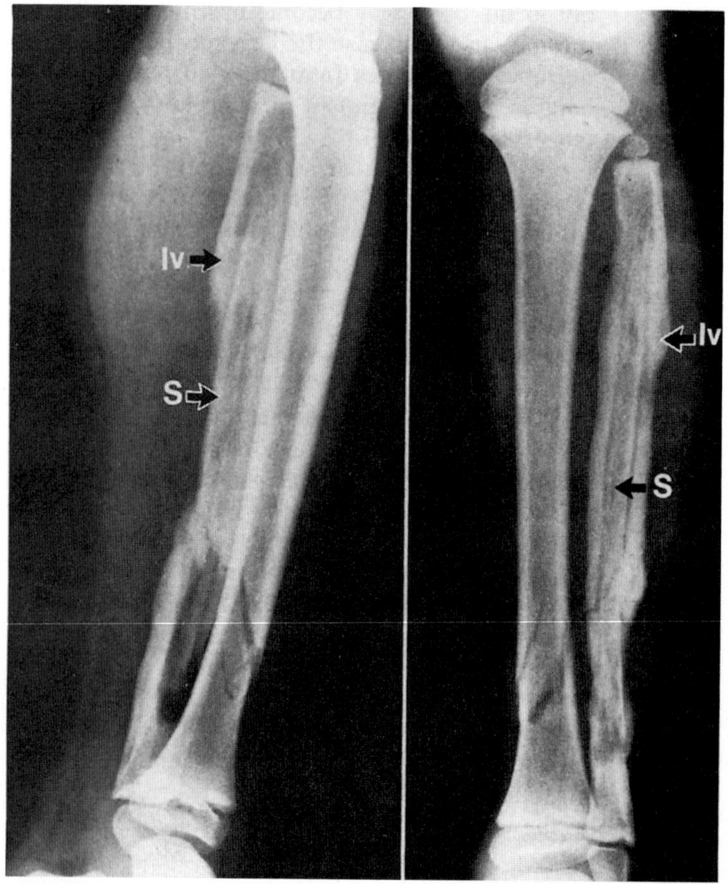

FIGURE 57-9 Hematogenous osteomyelitis of the fibula of 3 months' duration. The entire shaft has been deprived of its blood supply and has become a sequestrum (S) surrounded by new immature bone, involucrum (Iv). Pathologic fractures are present in the lower tibia and fibula. (Wilson F.C. [1980]. *The musculoskeletal system.* [2nd ed., p. 150]. Philadelphia: J.B. Lippincott)

Initial antibiotic therapy is followed by surgery to remove foreign bodies (*e.g.*, metal plates, screws) or sequestra and by long-term antibiotic therapy. Immobilization of the affected part usually is necessary, with restriction of weight bearing on a lower extremity. External fixation devices are sometimes used. With this method, chronic refractory osteomyelitis frequently can be cured because the mass regeneration of new bone within the focus of infection serves as a highly vascularized bone graft.[40]

Osteomyelitis With Vascular Insufficiency

In persons with vascular insufficiency, osteomyelitis may develop from a skin lesion. It is most commonly associated with chronic or ischemic foot ulcers in persons with longstanding diabetes or other chronic vascular disorders. It is characterized by local cellulitis with inflammation and necrosis. Treatment depends on the oxygen tension of the involved tissues. Débridement and antibiotic therapy may benefit persons who have good oxygen tension in the infected site. Amputation may be indicated when oxygen tension is inadequate.

TUBERCULOSIS OF THE BONE OR JOINT

Tuberculosis can spread from one part of the body, such as the lungs or the lymph nodes, to the bones and joints. When this happens, it is called *extrapulmonary* or *miliary tuberculosis*. It is caused by *Mycobacterium tuberculosis*. The disease is localized and progressively destructive but not as contagious as primary pulmonary tuberculosis. In approximately 50% of cases, it affects the vertebrae, but it also frequently is seen in the hip and knee.[41] Tuberculosis also can affect the joints and soft tissues. The disease is characterized by bone destruction and abscess formation. Local symptoms include pain, immobility, and muscle atrophy; joint swelling, mild fever, and leukocytosis also may occur. Diagnosis is confirmed by a positive culture. The most important part of the treatment is antituberculosis drug therapy. Conservative treatment is usually as effective as surgery, especially for earlier and milder cases.

Because of improved methods to prevent and treat tuberculosis, its incidence had diminished in recent decades. However, tuberculosis has reemerged as a health problem, affecting one third of the global population and 10 million people in the United States.[42] Tuberculosis has increased because of the spread of disease in communal settings (*e.g.*, jails, shelters, nursing homes), the human immunodeficiency virus epidemic, and the influx of immigrants who have come to the United States from countries where the disease is endemic.[43] The incidence is now decreasing.[44] Death rates have dropped steadily as a result of multiple chemotherapy agents, including multidrug regimens and second-line drugs for atypical mycobacterium.[44]

Unfortunately, the diagnosis of tuberculosis in the bones and joints still may be missed, especially when the musculoskeletal infection is the sole presenting sign. CT scans and MRI can be used as aids for early diagnosis.

In summary, bone infections occur because of the direct or indirect invasion of the skeletal circulation by microorganisms, most commonly *S. aureus*. Tuberculosis of the bone, which is characterized by bone destruction and abscess formation, is caused by spread of the infection from the lungs or lymph nodes. Osteomyelitis, or infection of the bone and marrow, can be an acute or chronic disease. Acute osteomyelitis is seen most often as a result of the direct contamination of bone by a foreign object. Chronic osteomyelitis represents an infection that continues beyond 6 to 8 weeks and may persist for years. The incidence of all types of bone infection has been dramatically reduced since the advent of antibiotic therapy. Iatrogenic infections are those inadvertently brought about by surgery or other treatments.

Osteonecrosis

After completing this section of the chapter, you should be able to meet the following objectives:

- Define *osteonecrosis*
- Cite four major causes of osteonecrosis
- Characterize the blood supply of bone and relate it to the pathologic features of the condition
- Describe the methods used in diagnosis and treatment of the condition

Osteonecrosis, or death of a segment of bone, is a condition caused by the interruption of blood supply to the marrow, medullary bone, or cortex. It is a relatively common disorder and can occur in the medullary cavity of the metaphysis and the subchondral region of the epiphysis, especially in the proximal femur, distal femur, and proximal humerus. It is a common complicating disorder of Legg-Calvé-Perthes disease, slipped capital epiphysis, sickle cell disease, steroid therapy, alcohol abuse, and hip trauma, fracture, or surgery.[45–47] The rates of osteonecrosis among persons treated with corticosteroids range from 5% to 25%. More than 10% of 500,000 joint replacements performed annually in the United States are for treatment of osteonecrosis.[45]

Although bone necrosis results from ischemia, the mechanisms producing the ischemia are varied and include mechanical vascular interruption such as occurs with trauma or a fracture; thrombosis and embolism (*e.g.*, sickle cell disease, nitrogen bubbles caused by inadequate decompression during deep sea diving); and vessel injury (*e.g.*, vasculitis, radiation therapy). In many cases, the cause of the necrosis is uncertain. Other than fracture, the most common causes of bone necrosis are idiopathic (*i.e.*, those of unknown cause) and prior steroid therapy. Chart 57-2 lists disorders associated with osteonecrosis.

Bone has a rich blood supply that varies from site to site. The flow in the medullary portion of bone originates in nutrient vessels from an interconnecting plexus that

CHART 57-2

Causes of Osteonecrosis

- Mechanical disruption of blood vessels
  - Fractures
  - Legg-Calvé-Perthes disease
  - Blount's disease
- Thrombosis and embolism
  - Sickle cell disease
  - Nitrogen bubbles in decompression sickness
- Vessel injury
  - Vasculitis
  - Connective tissue disease
    - Systemic lupus erythematosus
    - Rheumatoid arthritis
  - Radiation therapy
  - Gaucher's disease
- Corticosteroid therapy

supplies the marrow, trabecular bone, and endosteal half of the cortex. The outer cortex receives its blood supply from periosteal, muscular, metaphyseal, and epiphyseal vessels that surround the bone. Some bony sites, such as the head of the femur, have only limited collateral circulation, so that interruption of the flow, such as with a hip fracture, can cause necrosis of a substantial portion of medullary and cortical bone and irreversible damage.

The pathologic features of bone necrosis are the same, regardless of cause. The site of the lesion is related to the vessels involved. There is necrosis of cancellous bone and marrow. The cortex usually is not involved because of collateral blood flow. In subchondral infarcts (*i.e.*, ischemia below the cartilage), a triangular or wedge-shaped segment of tissue that has the subchondral bone plate as its base and the center of the epiphysis as its apex undergoes necrosis. When medullary infarcts occur in fatty marrow, death of bone results in calcium release and necrosis of fat cells with the formation of free fatty acids. Released calcium forms an insoluble "soap" with free fatty acids. Because bone lacks mechanisms for resolving the infarct, the lesions remain for life.

One of the most frequent causes of osteonecrosis is that associated with administration of corticosteroids.[44,45,47] Despite numerous studies, the mechanism of steroid-induced osteonecrosis remains unclear. The condition may develop after the administration of very high, short-term doses; during long-term treatment; or even from intraarticular injection. Although the risk increases with the dose and duration of treatment, it is difficult to predict who will be affected. The interval between corticosteroid administration and onset of symptoms rarely is less than 6 months and may be more than 3 years. There is no satisfactory method for preventing progression of the disease.

The symptoms associated with osteonecrosis are varied and depend on the extent of infarction. Typically, subchondral infarcts cause chronic pain that is initially associated with activity but that gradually becomes more progressive until it is experienced at rest. Subchondral infarcts often collapse and predispose the patient to severe secondary osteoarthritis.

Diagnosis of osteonecrosis is based on history, physical findings, radiographic findings, and results of special imaging studies, including CT scans and technetium-99m bone scans. MRI is particularly effective in the diagnosis of osteonecrosis. Plain radiographs are used to define and classify the course of the disease, particularly of the hip.

Treatment of osteonecrosis depends on the underlying pathology. In some cases, only short-term immobilization, nonsteroidal antiinflammatory drugs, exercises, and limitation in weight bearing are used. Osteonecrosis of the hip is particularly difficult to treat. In persons with early disease, limitation of weight bearing through the use of crutches may allow the condition to stabilize. Although several surgical approaches have been used, the most definitive treatment of advanced osteonecrosis of the knee or hip is total joint replacement. Treatment with hyperbaric oxygenation can also be effective.[48]

In summary, osteonecrosis is a common condition that has long been recognized but is not fully understood. Death of bone is caused by disruption of the blood supply from intravascular or extravascular processes. Sites with poor collateral circulation, such as the femoral head, are most seriously affected. Causative factors include corticosteroids. Symptoms include pain that varies in severity, depending on the extent of infarction. Total joint replacement is the most frequently used treatment for advanced osteonecrosis.

Neoplasms

After completing this section of the chapter, you should be able to meet the following objectives:

- Differentiate between the properties of benign and malignant bone tumors
- Contrast osteogenic sarcoma, Ewing's sarcoma, and chondrosarcoma in terms of the most common age groups and anatomic sites that are affected
- List the primary sites of tumors that frequently metastasize to the bone
- State the three primary goals for treatment of metastatic bone disease

Neoplasms in the skeletal system are referred to as *bone tumors*. Primary malignant tumors of the bone are uncommon, constituting approximately 1% of all adult cancers and 15% of pediatric malignancies.[49] Metastatic disease of the bone, however, is relatively common. Primary bone tumors may arise from any of the skeletal components, including osseous bone tissue, cartilage, and bone marrow. The discussion in this section focuses on primary benign and malignant bone tumors of osseous or cartilaginous origin and metastatic bone disease. Tumors of bone marrow origin (*i.e.*, leukemia and multiple myeloma) are discussed in Chapter 17.

Like other types of neoplasms, bone tumors may be benign or malignant. The benign types, such as osteochondromas, tend to grow rather slowly and usually do not destroy the supporting or surrounding tissue or spread to other parts of the body. Malignant tumors, such as osteosarcoma, grow rapidly and can spread to other parts of the body through the bloodstream or lymphatics. The two major forms of bone cancer in children and young adults are osteosarcoma and Ewing's sarcoma. Both tumor types occur more frequently in the second decade of life.[50] Chondrosarcoma is most common in those 40 years of age and older.[34] The classification of benign and malignant bone tumors is described in Table 57-2.

CHARACTERISTICS OF BONE TUMORS

There are three major symptoms of bone tumors: pain, presence of a mass, and impairment of function (Chart 57-3). Pain is a feature common to almost all malignant tumors, but may or may not occur with benign tumors. For example, a benign bone cyst usually is asymptomatic until a fracture occurs. Pain that persists at night and is not relieved by rest suggests malignancy. A mass or hard lump may be the first sign of a bone tumor. A malignant tumor is suspected when a painful mass exists that is enlarging or eroding the cortex of the bone. The ease of discovery of a mass depends on the location of the tumor; a small lump arising on the surface of the tibia is easy to detect, whereas a tumor that is deep in the medial portion of the thigh may grow to a considerable size before it is noticed. Benign and malignant tumors may cause the bone to erode to the point at which it cannot withstand the strain of ordinary use. In such cases, even a small amount of bone stress or trauma precipitates a pathologic fracture. A tumor may produce pressure on a peripheral nerve, causing decreased sensation, numbness, a limp, or limitation of movement.

TABLE 57-2 Classification of Primary Bone Neoplasms

Tissue Type	Benign Neoplasm	Malignant Neoplasm
Bone	Osteoid osteoma Benign osteoblastoma	Osteosarcoma Parosteal osteogenic sarcoma
Cartilage	Osteochondroma Chondroma Chrondroblastoma Chondromyxoid fibroma	Chondrosarcoma
Lipid	Lipoma	Liposarcoma
Fibrous and fibroosseous tissue	Fibrous dysplasia	Fibrosarcoma Malignant fibrous histiocytoma
Miscellaneous	Giant cell tumor	Malignant giant cell Ewing's sarcoma
Bone marrow		Multiple myeloma Reticulum cell sarcoma

BONE NEOPLASMS

- Neoplasms of the skeletal system can affect bone tissue, cartilage, or bone marrow.
- Benign tumors tend to grow slowly, do not spread to other parts of the body, and exert their effects through the space-occupying nature of the tumor and their ability to weaken bone structures.
- Malignant bone tumors are rare before 10 years of age, have their peak incidence in the teenage years, tend to grow rapidly, and have a high mortality rate.

BENIGN NEOPLASMS

Benign bone tumors usually are limited to the confines of the bone, have well-demarcated edges, and are surrounded by a thin rim of sclerotic bone. The four most common types of benign bone tumors are osteoma, chondroma, osteochondroma, and giant cell tumor.[34] An *osteoma* is a small bony tumor found on the surface of a long bone, flat bone, or the skull. It usually is composed of hard, compact (ivory osteoma), or spongy (cancellous) bone. It may be excised or left alone.

A *chondroma* is a tumor composed of hyaline cartilage. It may arise on the surface of the bone (*i.e.*, ecchondroma)

CHART 57-3

Symptoms of Bone Cancer

- Bone pain in an adult or child that comes on slowly but lasts for as long as a week, is constant or intermittent, and may be worse at night.
- Unexplained swelling or lump on the bones of the arms, legs, thighs, or other parts of the body that is firm and slightly tender and may be felt through the skin. It may interfere with normal movement and can cause the bone to break.

These symptoms are not sure signs of cancer. They also may be caused by other, less serious problems. Only a physician can tell for sure.

(Adapted from U.S. Department of Health and Human Services [1993]. *What you need to know about cancers of the bone.* NIH publication no. 93-1517. Bethesda, MD: U.S. Government Printing Office) or within the medullary cavity (*i.e.,* endochondroma). These tumors may become large and are especially common in the hands and feet. A chondroma may persist for many years and then take on the attributes of a malignant chondrosarcoma. A chondroma usually is not treated unless it becomes unsightly or uncomfortable.

An *osteochondroma* is the most common form of benign tumor in the skeletal system, representing 50% of all benign bone tumors and approximately 15% of all primary skeletal lesions.[34] It grows only during periods of skeletal growth, originating in the epiphyseal cartilage plate and growing out of the bone like a mushroom. An osteochondroma is composed of cartilage and bone and usually occurs singly but may affect several bones in a condition called *multiple exostoses.* Malignant changes are rare, and excision of the tumor is done only when necessary.

A *giant cell tumor,* or *osteoclastoma,* is an aggressive tumor of multinucleated cells that often behaves like a malignant tumor, metastasizing through the bloodstream and recurring locally after excision. It arises most often in people in their 20s to 40s and is found most commonly in the knee, wrist, or shoulder. The tumor begins in the metaphyseal region, grows into the epiphysis, and may extend into the joint surface. Pathologic fractures are common because the tumor destroys the bone substance. Clinically, pain may occur at the tumor site, with gradually increasing swelling. X-ray films show destruction of the bone with expansion of the cortex.

The treatment of giant cell tumors depends on their location. If the affected bone can be eliminated without loss of function, such as the clavicle or fibula, the entire bone or part of it may be removed. When the tumor is near a major joint, such as the knee or shoulder, a local excision is done. Irradiation may be used to prevent recurrence of the tumor.

MALIGNANT BONE TUMORS

In contrast to benign tumors, primary malignant tumors tend to be ill defined, lack sharp borders, and extend beyond the confines of the bone. Primary bone tumors occur in all age groups and may arise in any part of the body. However, certain types of tumors tend to target certain age groups and anatomic sites. For example, most osteogenic sarcomas occur in adolescents and are particularly common around the knee joint. Also, people with certain conditions such as Paget disease are at increased risk for development of bone cancer. Metastatic bone lesions are considerably more common than primary bone tumors.

The diagnosis of bone tumors includes radiologic staging and biopsy. Radiographs give the most general diagnostic information, such as malignant versus benign and primary versus metastatic status. The radiograph demonstrates the region of bone involvement, extent of destruction, and amount of reactive bone formed. Radioisotope scans are used to estimate the local intramedullary extent of the tumor and screen for other skeletal areas of involvement. CT scans further aid diagnosis and anatomic localization and can identify small pulmonary metastases not seen by conventional radiographs. MRI is the most accurate method of evaluating the intramedullary extent of bone tumor and can demarcate the soft structures in relation to neurovascular structures without the use of contrast media. It is best used in conjunction with a CT scan.[50] Radionuclide bone scans are used to assess for metastasis. A biopsy also is done because the definitive treatment of most bone tumors is based on pathologic interpretation of the biopsy specimen.

Osteosarcoma

Osteosarcoma is an aggressive and highly malignant bone tumor. It is the most common primary malignant bone tumor, representing one fifth of all bone tumors. Osteosarcoma is the most common bone tumor in children and the third most common cancer in children and adolescents.[51] Although they can develop in any bone, osteosarcomas most commonly arise the vicinity of knee (*e.g.,* lower femur or upper tibia or fibula). The proximal humerus is the second most common site. The hands, feet, skull, and jaw are less frequent sites for the disease, being affected most frequently in persons older than 25 years of age.[16]

The cause of osteosarcoma is unknown. The tumor has a bimodal distribution, with 75% occurring in persons younger than 20 years of age. A second peak occurs in the elderly with predisposing factors such as Paget disease, bone infarcts, or prior irradiation.[34] The correlation of age and location of most of the tumors with the period of maximum growth suggests some relation to increased osteoblastic activity.[52] In younger persons, the primary tumor most often is located at the anatomic sites associated with maximum growth velocity—the distal femur, proximal tibia, and proximal humerus. Bone tumors in the elderly are more common in the humerus, pelvis, and proximal femur. Paget disease, which is linked to osteosarcoma in adults, also is associated with increased osteoblastic activity. Irradiation from an internal source, such as the radioactive pharmaceutical technetium used in bone scans, or an external source, such as x-ray films, also has been associated with osteosarcoma. There are known genetic factors associated with osteosarcoma. Two genes are reported to increase the susceptibility to the development of osteosarcoma: the retinoblastoma gene (*RB*) and *TP53* gene[50,52,53] (see Chapter 8).

Osteosarcomas are aggressive tumors that grow rapidly; they often are eccentrically placed in the bone and move from the metaphysis of the bone out into the periosteal surface, with subsequent spread to adjacent soft tissues (Fig. 57-10). The tumor infrequently metastasizes to the lymph nodes because the cells are unable to grow in the node. Nodal metastases usually occur only in the late course of disseminated disease. Most often, the tumor cells exit the primary tumor through the venous end of the capillary, and early metastasis to the lung is common. Lung metastases, even if massive, usually are relatively asymptomatic. The prognosis for a person with osteosarcoma depends on the aggressiveness of the disease, radiologic features, presence or absence of pathologic fractures, size of the tumor, and rapidity of tumor growth.

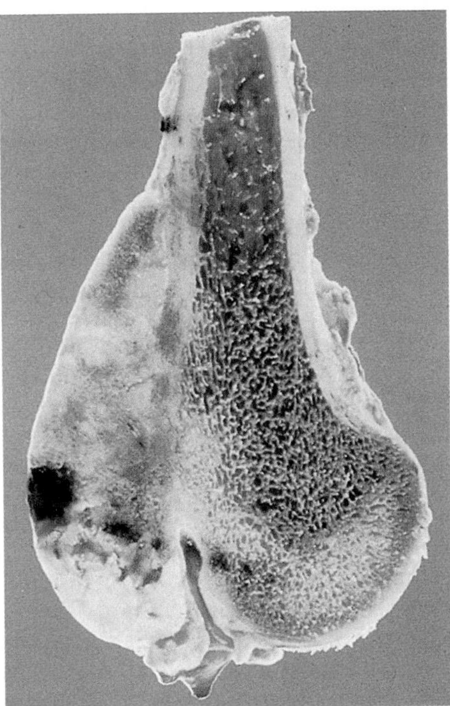

FIGURE 57-10 Juxtacortical osteosarcoma. The lower femur contains a malignant tumor arising from the periosteal surface of the bone and sparing the medullary cavity. (Rubin E., Farber L.F. [1999]. *Pathophysiology* [3rd ed., p. 1386]. Philadelphia: Lippincott-Raven)

The primary clinical feature of osteosarcoma is deep localized pain with nighttime awakening and swelling in the affected bone. Because the pain is often of sudden onset, patients and their families often associate the symptoms with recent trauma.[50] The skin overlying the tumor may be warm, shiny, and stretched, with prominent superficial veins. The range of motion of the adjacent joint may be restricted.

History, physical examination, and radiographic studies are all part of the evaluation of a patient with osteosarcoma. Plain films of the primary site and of the chest are first obtained. MRI, CT scan, and full body scan are required to evaluate the extent of the local disease and to determine the extent of metastasis if present. Radionuclide bone scans are done to evaluate for lung and bone metastasis.[50,51] An open biopsy is required to confirm the diagnosis and to determine the histologic features and cell type of the tumor.[51,52]

Treatment of osteosarcoma is surgery in combination with multiagent chemotherapy used both before and after surgery.[50–54] In the past, treatment usually entailed amputation above the level of the tumor. Limb salvage surgical procedures, using a metal prosthesis or cadaver allograft, are becoming a standard alternative. Studies have shown that limb salvage surgery has no adverse effects on the long-term survival of persons with osteosarcoma. The success of limb salvage appears to depend on the use of a wide surgical margin, improved radiographic imaging studies, multiagent chemotherapy, and more refined surgical reconstructive techniques. Advanced imaging techniques, including serum thallium scans, and the use of angiography assist the surgeon in determining the best type of treatment. Chemotherapy using various drug combinations is the most effective treatment for metastatic osteosarcoma.

Many advances have been made in the limb salvage and reconstructive surgical procedures being used as alternatives to limb amputation. These procedures involve the wide resection of the tumor, the biopsy site, and wide margins of healthy bone. Bone reconstruction is done by either open reduction and internal fixation (ORIF), arthrodesis, or arthroplasty. ORIF uses rods, plates, screws, and either an allograft or autograft of bone. Arthrodesis is a limb salvage procedure that involves fusion of a joint, usually the knee or shoulder. A rod is inserted and secured with locking screws after the removal of the tumor and the surrounding bone and tissue.[51] Arthroplasty involves total replacement of a joint, such as a hip or knee, with a metallic implant. In younger children who undergo arthroplasty, an expandable internal prosthesis is used to allow for bone growth. In the past, this has required surgery every 6 to 12 months to lengthen the prosthesis until full skeletal maturity is achieved.[51] A new type of implant, the Repiphysis expandable implant for skeletally mature children, was recently approved by the U.S. Food and Drug Administration.[55] The Repiphysis contains a polymer that can be melted and manipulated when exposed to an electromagnetic ray. An internal spring then stretches the material as it cools and will lengthen the limb without further invasive surgery.

Amputation is another surgical option. It involves either the removal of expendable bones such as the fibula, ribs, toes, or ulna or the complete removal of the tumor and the affected limb. The primary objective of overall treatment of patients with osteosarcoma is long-term disease-free survival or cure. Preserving limb function is a secondary objective. In cases in which adequate limb salvage surgery cannot be achieved, limb amputation may be necessary.[51,53]

Ewing's Sarcoma

Ewing's sarcoma is a member of a group of small, round cell, undifferentiated tumors thought to be of neural crest origin[50] (see Chapter 49). The family of tumors includes Ewing's sarcoma of the bone and soft tissue and peripheral primitive neuroectodermal tumor (PPNET). Of the tumors in this family, Ewing's sarcoma accounts for most cases. It is the second most common type of primary bone tumor in children and adolescents. It can occur at any age, but is seen most commonly in the early teenage years. This tumor rarely presents in black or Asian children.[52,56]

The most frequent site of Ewing's sarcoma is the femur, usually in the diaphysis. The pelvis represents the second most common site; other sites include the pubis, sacrum, humerus, vertebrae, ribs, skull, and other flat bones. The characteristic pathologic findings of Ewing's sarcoma include densely packed, regularly shaped, small cells with round or oval nuclei. The majority of cells have a characteristic reciprocal translocation of chromosomes 11 and 22.

Manifestations of Ewing's tumor include pain, limitation of movement, and tenderness over the involved bone or soft tissue.[57] It often is accompanied by systemic manifestations such as fever or weight loss, which may serve to confuse the diagnosis. There may be a delay in diagnosis when the pain and swelling associated with the tumor are attributed to a sports injury. Pathologic fractures are common because of bone destruction. The most common sites of metastasis are the lungs, bone marrow, and other bones.

Because Ewing's sarcoma is a difficult diagnosis to establish, the diagnostic biopsy is very important. Clinical evaluations include MRI and CT scans of the primary tumor, chest x-rays, CT of the chest, bone scan, bilateral bone marrow aspiration, and biopsy of the primary tumor site.[50] The extent of disease at diagnosis is the most important prognostic factor. The presence of metastatic disease at diagnosis is a poor prognostic factor irrespective of the site of the primary lesion.

Treatment methods incorporate a combination of multiagent chemotherapy, surgery, and radiation therapy. Multiagent chemotherapy is important because it can shrink the tumor and is generally given before local control measures are initiated. Ewing's tumor is considered to be a radiosensitive tumor, and local control may be achieved through radiation or surgery. Patients with small, nonmetastatic, distally located tumors generally have the best prognosis. Such patients have up to a 75% cure rate.[50]

Chondrosarcoma

Chondrosarcoma, a malignant tumor of cartilage that can develop in the medullary cavity or peripherally, is the second most common form of malignant bone tumor. It occurs primarily in middle or later life and slightly more often in males. The tumor arises from points of muscle attachment to bone, particularly the knee, shoulder, hip, and pelvis. Chondrosarcomas can arise from underlying benign lesions such as osteochondroma, chrondroblastoma, or fibrous dysplasia.[34]

Chondrosarcomas are slow growing, metastasize late, and often are painless. They can remain hidden in an area such as the pelvis for a long time. This type of tumor, like many primary malignancies, tends to destroy bone and extend into the soft tissues beyond the confines of the bone of origin. Chondrosarcomas mainly affect the bones of the trunk, pelvis, or proximal femur and rarely develop in the distal portion of a bone. Irregular flecks and ringlets of calcification often are prominent radiographic findings.

Early diagnosis is important because chondrosarcoma responds well to early radical surgical excision. It usually is resistant to radiation therapy and available chemotherapeutic agents. Not infrequently, these tumors transform into a highly malignant tumor, mesenchymal chondrosarcoma, which requires a more aggressive treatment, including combination chemotherapy.

METASTATIC BONE DISEASE

Skeletal metastases are the most common malignancy of osseous tissue. Metastatic lesions are seen most often in the spine, femur, pelvis, ribs, sternum, proximal humerus, and skull, and are less common in anatomic sites that are further removed from the trunk of the body. Tumors that frequently spread to the skeletal system are those of the breast, lung, prostate, kidney, and thyroid, although any cancer can ultimately involve the skeleton. More than 85% of bone metastases result from primary lesions in the breast, lung, or prostate.[58] The incidence of metastatic bone disease is highest in persons older than 40 years of age. There typically are several bony metastases, with or without metastatic spread to other organs. Solitary lesions are seen most commonly with cancers of the kidney and thyroid. Because of the effectiveness of current cancer treatment modalities, patients with cancer are living longer, and the incidence of clinically apparent skeletal involvement appears to be increasing in the long run. These skeletal metastases cause great pain, increase the risk for fractures, and increase the disability of the patient with cancer.

Metastasis to the bone frequently occurs without involving other organs because the blood flow in the veins of the skeletal system is sluggish. These are thin-walled, valveless veins, and there are many storage sites along the way. The pattern of metastasis often is related to the specific vascular pathway that is involved (*e.g.,* metastases to the shoulder girdle and pelvis occur when prostatic cancers invade the vertebral vein system). If metastasis is limited to the skeletal system, without other major organ involvement, a person can live for many years. Death usually is a consequence of metastasis to vital organs rather than a consequence of the primary tumor.

The major symptom of bone metastasis is pain with evidence of an impending pathologic fracture. It usually develops gradually, over weeks, and is more severe at night. Pain is caused by stretching of the periosteum of the involved bone or by nerve entrapment, as in the nerve roots of the spinal cord by the vertebral body. X-ray examinations are used along with CT or bone scans to detect, diagnose, and localize metastatic bone lesions. Approximately one third of persons with skeletal metastases have positive bone scans without radiologic findings. This is because 50% of the trabecular bone must be destroyed before a lesion is visible on plain radiographs.[59] Arteriography using radiopaque contrast media may be helpful in outlining the tumor margins. A bone biopsy usually is done when there is a question regarding the diagnosis or treatment. A closed-needle biopsy with CT localization is particularly useful with spine lesions. Serum levels of alkaline phosphatase and calcium often are elevated in persons with metastatic bone disease. Hypercalcemia occurs in 10% to 20% of persons with metastatic bone disease because of bone lysis.

The primary goals in treatment of metastatic bone disease are to prevent pathologic fractures and promote survival with maximum functioning, allowing the person to maintain as much mobility and pain control as possible. Treatment methods include chemotherapy, irradiation, and surgical stabilization. The discovery of new and more effective drugs, along with the use of combination protocols, has increased the effectiveness of chemotherapy in treating metastatic bone disease. Local irradiation can effect rapid pain relief within 1 to 2 weeks in more than 50% of patients.[58] Radiation therapy is primarily used as a palliative treatment to alleviate pain and prevent pathologic fractures. Prophylactic internal fixation may be done in a weight-bearing bone threatened by an expanding lesion. Bracing may be ordered for an unstable spine. It is difficult to find a comfortable fit when there is metastasis to the ribs or pelvis. Steroid drugs also may be helpful. The bisphosphonates inhibit osteoclastic activity and subsequent bone-induced osteolysis. Bisphosphonates are used in metastatic bone disease to relieve the symptoms, enable bone healing to occur, and delay complications.

Hypercalcemia occurs in 10% to 20% of persons with metastatic bone disease because of bone lysis.[58] Symptoms include dulling of consciousness, stupor, weakness, muscle flaccidity, and decreased neural excitability. A total serum calcium level greater than 12 mg/dL requires treatment with diuretics and intravenous sodium chloride (see Chapter 33).

Pathologic fractures occur in approximately 10% to 15% of persons with metastatic bone disease. The affected bone appears to be eaten away on x-ray images and, in severe cases, crumbles on impact, much like dried toast. Many pathologic fractures occur in the femur, humerus, and vertebrae. In the femur, fractures occur because the proximal aspect of the bone is under great mechanical stress. Lesions may be treated prophylactically with surgery and radiation therapy to prevent pathologic fractures. Flexible intramedullary rods may be used to stabilize long bones. After a pathologic fracture has occurred, bracing, intramedullary nailing of the femur, and spine stabilization may be done. Because adequate fixation often is difficult in diseased bone, cement (*i.e.*, methylmethacrylate) often is used with internal fixation devices to stabilize the bone. The selection of a treatment modality for prevention or treatment of pathologic fractures depends on the severity of the lesion, the degree of pain, and the life expectancy of the patient. The goal is to provide flexibility, mobility, and pain relief. Surgeons usually treat metastatic lesions aggressively so that patients can function as normally as possible, even if life expectancy is as short as 3 months.[59]

In summary, bone tumors, like any other type of neoplasm, may be benign or malignant. Benign bone tumors grow slowly and usually do not destroy the surrounding tissues. Malignant tumors can be primary or metastatic. Primary bone tumors are rare, grow rapidly, metastasize to the lungs and other parts of the body through the bloodstream, and have a high mortality rate. Metastatic bone tumors usually are multiple, originating primarily from cancers of the breast, lung, and prostate. The incidence of metastatic bone disease probably is increasing because improved treatment methods enable persons with cancer to live longer. Advances in chemotherapy, radiation therapy, and surgical procedures have substantially increased the survival and cure rates for many types of bone cancers. A primary goal in metastatic bone disease is the prevention of pathologic fractures.

REVIEW EXERCISES

A 39-year-old man is in intensive care following a motorcycle crash in which he skidded on across the pavement on his right side. He has fractures of his right femur, pelvis, and several ribs on the right side. His leg was crushed beneath the cycle. He is beginning to lose movement in his leg.

A. What are the priorities in treating his orthopedic injuries? What are the options for stabilizing his leg?

B. What risk factors for complications of fractures are present?

C. What are the symptoms of compartment syndrome and how is it treated?

A 73-year-old woman sustained a comminuted fracture in the mid-diaphysis of her left humerus when her husband lifted her up in bed. She has multiple lucent lesions scattered throughout her proximal humerus, radius, and ulna. She was recently hospitalized for confusion and was found to have diffuse bone metastases. Her bone marrow biopsy showed adenocarcinoma. She has a history of breast cancer 30 years ago, but her most recent mammogram was negative.

A. What would you consider to be the most likely cause of her fracture?

B. What are the most common sites for bone metastasis?

C. Explain the treatment goals for persons with pathologic fractures.

A 14-year-old boy has complained of recent pain and swelling of knee, with some restriction in movement. Although he thinks he may have injured his knee playing football, his mother insists that he be seen by an orthopedic specialist, who raises the possibility that the boy may have an osteosarcoma.

A. Use the theory that osteosarcoma has its origination in sites of maximal growth velocity to explain the site of this boy's possible tumor.

B. What diagnostic tests could be used to establish a diagnosis of osteosarcoma?

C. The boy and his family are concerned that he will require radical surgery with amputation of the leg. How would you explain possible treatment options to him?

References

1. CDC Web-based Injury Statistics Query and Reporting System (wisqars database). National Centers for Disease Control and Prevention, Centers for Disease Control and Prevention. [On-line]. Available: http://www.cdc.gov/ncipc/wisqars/. Accessed 10/4/2003.
2. Arthritis Foundation (2003). *Safe and sorry: A parent's guide to sports injury prevention.* [On-line]. Available: http://www.arthritis.org/resources.

3. American Academy of Orthopaedic Surgeons (2003). *Pay attention to high school sports injuries.* [On-line]. Available: http://orthoinfo.aaos.org.
4. American Academy of Orthopedic Surgeons (2003). *Don't let a fall be your last trip.* [On-line]. Available: http://www.orthoinfo.aaos.org.
5. Bell A.J., Talbot-Stein J.K., Hennessy A. (2000). Characteristics and outcomes of older patients' presenting to the emergency department after a fall: A retrospective analysis. *Medical Journal of Australia 173*(4), 176–177.
6. Hogan K.A., Gross R.H. (2003). Overuse injuries in pediatric athletes. *Orthopedic Clinics of North America 34,* 405–415.
7. Liu S.H., Yang R., Raad A., Lane J.M. (1999). Collagen in tendon, ligament, and bone healing. *Clinical Orthopaedics and Related Research 316,* 265–278.
8. Mercier L.R. (2000). *Practical Orthopedics* (5th ed., pp. 48–74). St. Louis: Mosby.
9. Gomez J.E. (2002). Upper extremity injuries in youth sports. *Pediatric Clinics of North America 49,* 593–626.
10. Hegenroeder A., Chorley J.N. (2004). Sports injuries. In Behrman R.F., Kliegman R.M., Jenson H.B. (Eds.), *Nelson textbook of pediatrics* (17th ed., pp. 2302–2314). Philadelphia: W.B. Saunders.
11. Fongemie A.E., Buss D.D., Rolnick S.J. (2001). Management of shoulder impingement syndrome and rotator cuff tears. *American Family Physician 57*(4), 667–679.
12. Muellner T., Nikolic A., Vecsei V. (1999). Recommendations for the diagnosis of traumatic meniscal injuries in athletes. *Sports Medicine 27,* 337–345.
13. Maitra R.S., Miller M.D., Johnson D.L. (1999). Meniscal reconstruction. I. Indications, techniques, and graft considerations. *American Journal of Orthopedics 28*(4), 213–218.
14. Maitra R.S., Miller M.D., Johnson D.L. (1999). Meniscal reconstruction. II. Outcome, potential complications, and future directions. *American Journal of Orthopedics 28*(5), 280–286.
15. O'Connor W.J., Botti T., Khan S.N., Lane J.M. (2000). The use of growth factors in cartilage repair. *Orthopedic Clinics of North America 31*(3), 399–409.
16. Schiller A.L., Teitelbaum S.L. (1999). Bones and joints. In Rubin E., Farber J.L. *Pathology* (3rd ed., 1337–1390). Philadelphia: Lippincott-Raven.
17. Einhorn T.A. (1998). The cell and molecular biology of fracture healing. *Clinical Orthopaedics and Related Research 355*(Suppl.), S7–S21.
18. Paley D., Catagni M., Argnani F., et al. (1992). Treatment of congenital pseudoarthrosis of the tibia using Ilizarov technique. *Clinical Orthopaedics and Related Research 280,* 81.
19. Hayda R.A., Brighton C.T., Esterhai J.L. (1998). Pathophysiology of delayed healing. *Clinical Orthopaedics and Related Research 355*(Suppl.), S31–S36.
20. Peng H., Wright V., Usas A., et al. (2002). Synergistic enhancement of bone formation and healing of stem cell-expressed VECF and bone morphogenetic protein-4. *Journal of Clinical Investigation 110*(6), 751–759.
21. Hoover T.J., Siefert J.A. (2000). Soft tissue complications of orthopedic emergencies. *Emergency Medicine Clinics of North America 18,* 115–139.
22. Harvey C.V. (2001). Compartment syndrome: When it is least expected. *Orthopedic Nursing 20*(3), 15–26.
23. Swain R., Ross D. (1999). Lower extremity compartment syndrome. *Postgraduate Medicine 105,* 159–168.
24. Mohler L.R., Styf J.R., Pedowitz R., et al. (1997). Intramuscular deoxygenation during exercise in patients who have chronic anterior compartment syndrome of the leg. *Journal of Bone and Joint Surgery [Am] 79*(6), 844–849.
25. Harvey C.V. (2001). Compartmental syndrome: When it's least expected. *Orthopedic Nursing 20*(3), 15–26.
26. Schwartzman R. (2000). New treatments for reflex sympathetic dystrophy. *New England Journal of Medicine 343,* 654–656.
27. Linquist B.G.P., Schoeman H.S., Dommisee G.F., et al. (1987). Fat embolism and the fat embolism syndrome. *Journal of Bone and Joint Surgery [Br] 69,* 128–131.
28. Forteza A.M., Kock S., Romano J.O., et. al. (1999). Transcranial detection of fat emboli. *Stroke 30*(12), 2687–2691.
29. Richards R.R. (1997). Fat emboli syndrome. *Canadian Journal of Surgery 40,* 334–339.
30. Mellor A., Soni M. (2001). Fat embolism. *Anesthesia 56,* 145–154.
31. Pitto R.P., Koessler M., Kuehle J.W. (1999). Comparison of fixation of the femoral component without cement and fixation with the use of a bone vacuum cementing technique for prevention of fat embolization during total hip arthroplasty. *Journal of Bone and Joint Surgery [Am] 81,* 831–843.
32. Aokin SK., Shindo M., Kurosawa T., et al. (1998). Evaluation of potential fat emboli during placement of intramedullary nails after orthopedic fractures. *Chest 113*(1), 178–181.
33. Estebe J.P. (1997). From fat emboli to fat embolism syndrome. *Annals Francaises d Anesthesie et de Reanimation 16*(2), 138–151.
34. Rosenberg A. (1999). Bones, joints, and soft tissue tumors. In Cotran R.S., Kumar V., Collins T. (Eds.), *Robbins pathologic basis of disease* (6th ed., pp. 1231–1233). Philadelphia: W.B. Saunders.
35. Lew D.P., Waldvogel F.A. (1997). Osteomyelitis. *New England Journal of Medicine 336,* 999–1007.
36. Carek P.J., Dickerson L.M., Sack J.L. (2001). Diagnosis and management of osteomyelitis. *American Family Physician 63*(2), 2413–2420.
37. Taggart T., Kerry R.M., Norman P., Stockley I. (2002). The use of vancomycin-impregnated cement beads in the management of infection in prosthetic joints. *Journal of Bone and Joint Surgery [Br] 84,* 70–72.
38. McKee M.D., Wild L.M., Schemitsch E.T.T., Waddell J.P. (2002). The use of antibiotic impregnated osteoconductive bioabsorbable bone substitute in the treatment of long bone defects: Early results of a prospective trial. *Journal of Orthopedic Trauma 16*(9), 622–627.
39. Haas D.W., McAndrew M.P. (1996). Bacterial osteomyelitis in adults: Evolving considerations in diagnosis and treatment. *American Journal of Medicine 101,* 550–561.
40. Green S.A. (1991). Osteomyelitis: The Ilizarov perspective. *Orthopedic Clinics of North America 22,* 515–521.
41. Childs S.G. (1996). Osteoarticular *Mycobacterium tuberculosis. Orthopedic Nursing 15*(3), 28–33.
42. Silber J.S., Whitfield S.B., Anbari K., et al. (2000). Insidious destruction of the hip by *Mycobacterium tuberculosis* and why early diagnosis is critical. *Journal of Arthroplasty 15,* 392–397.
43. CDC (2003). Tuberculosis cases and case rates per 100,000 population: Deaths and death rates per 100,000. 1953–2000. [On-line]. Available: http://cdc.gov.
44. Shembecker A., Babhukars (2002). Chemotherapy for osteoarticular tuberculosis. *Clinical Orthopedics and Related Research 348,* 20–26.
45. Assouline-Dayan Y., Chang C., Greenspan A., et al. (2002). Pathogenesis and history of osteonecrosis. *Seminars in Arthritis and Rheumatism 32*(2), 94–124.
46. Mont M.A., Jones J.C., Einhorn T.A., et al. (1998) Osteonecrosis of the femoral head. *Clinical Orthopaedics and Related Research 355*(Suppl.), S314–S335.
47. Tokmakova K.P., Stanton R.P., Mason D.E. (2003). Factors influencing the development of osteonecrosis in patients treated for slipped capital femoral epiphysis. *Journal of Bone and Joint Surgery [Am] 85*(5): 198–801.

48. Reis N.O., Schwartz D., Miltianu D., et al. (2003). Hyperbaric oxygen therapy as a treatment for stage I avascular necrosis of the femoral head. *Journal of Bone and Joint Surgery [Br] 85*(3), 371–375.
49. Rosen G., Forscher C.A., Mankin H.J., Selch M.T. (2000). Neoplasms of bone and soft tissue. In Bast R.C., Kufe D.W., Pollack R.E., et al. (Eds.), *Cancer medicine* (pp. 1870–1902). Hamilton, Ontario: B.C. Decker.
50. Arndt C.S. (2004). Neoplasms of bone. In Behrman R.E., Kliegman R.M., Jenson H.B. (Eds.), *Nelson textbook of pediatrics* (16th ed., pp. 1714–1723). Philadelphia: W.B. Saunders.
51. Wittig J.D., Bickels J., Priebat J., et. al. (2002). Osteosarcoma: A multidisciplinary approach to diagnosis and treatment. *American Family Physician 65*(6), 1123–1136.
52. Betcher D.L., Simons P.J., McHard K. (2002). Bone tumors. In Baggott C.R., Kelly K.P., Fotchman D., Foley G.V. (Eds.), *Nursing care of children and adolescents with cancer* (3rd ed., pp. 575–588). Philadelphia: W.B. Saunders.
53. Marcus K.D. (2001). Pediatric solid tumors. In Lenhard R.E., Jr., Osteen R.T., Gansler T. (Eds.), *Clinical oncology* (pp. 590–593). Atlanta: American Cancer Society.
54. Arndt C.A.S., Crist W.M. (1999). Common musculoskeletal tumors of childhood and adolescence. *New England Journal of Medicine 431,* 342–352.
55. Neel M.D., Wilkins R.W., Gitelis S. (2002). *Repiphysis limb salvage system for the skeletally immature.* Arlington, TN: Wright Medical Technology.
56. Horowitz M.E., Malawer M.M., Woo S.Y., et al. (1997). Ewing's sarcoma family of tumors: Ewing's sarcoma of bone and soft tissue and the peripheral primitive neuroectodermal tumors. In Pizzo P.A., Poplack K.H. (Eds.), *Principles and practice of pediatric oncology* (3rd ed., pp 831–863). Philadelphia: Lippincott-Raven.
57. Grier H.E. (1997). The Ewing family of tumors. *Pediatric Clinics of North America 44,* 991–1002.
58. O'Keefe R.J., Schwartz E.M., Boyce B.F. (2000). Bone metastasis: An update on bone resorption and therapeutic strategies. *Current Opinion in Orthopedics 11,* 353–359.
59. Rubens R.D., Coleman R.E. (1995). Bone metastases. In Abeloff M.D., Armitage J.O., Lichter A.S., Niederhuber J.E. (Eds.), *Clinical oncology* (pp. 643–666). New York: Churchill Livingstone.

CHAPTER

58

Disorders of Skeletal Function: Developmental and Metabolic Disorders

Marilyn King Hightower and Kathleen E. Gunta

During childhood, skeletal structures grow in length and diameter and sustain a large increase in bone mass. The term *modeling* refers to the formation of the macroscopic skeleton, which ceases at maturity, usually between 18 and 20 years of age. Bone remodeling replaces existing bone and occurs in children and adults. It involves resorption and formation of bone. With aging, bone resorption and formation are no longer perfectly coupled, and there is loss of bone.

Alterations in musculoskeletal structure and function may develop as a result of normal growth and developmental processes or as a result of impairment of skeletal development due to hereditary or congenital influences. Other skeletal disorders can occur later in life as a result of metabolic disorders or neoplastic growth.

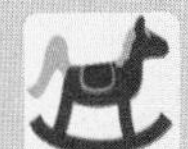

Alterations in Skeletal Growth and Development

After completing this section of the chapter, you should be able to meet the following objectives:

- Describe the function of the epiphyseal growth plate in skeletal growth
- Differentiate between toeing-in and toeing-out
- Describe common torsional deformities that occur in infants and small children, proposed mechanisms of development, diagnostic methods, and treatment
- Define genu varum and genu valgum
- List the problems that occur because of defective tissue synthesis in osteogenesis imperfecta
- Characterize the abnormalities associated with developmental dysplasia of the hip and methods of diagnosis
- Describe the treatment for a newborn with clubfoot
- Define the term *osteochondroses* and describe the pathology and symptomatology of Legg-Calvé-Perthes disease and Osgood-Schlatter disease
- Describe the pathology associated with a slipped capital femoral epiphysis and explain why early treatment is important

- Differentiate between infantile, idiopathic, and neuromuscular scoliosis

BONE GROWTH AND REMODELING

Embryonic Development

The skeletal system develops from the mesodermal and neural crest cells of the developing embryo[1] (see Chapter 49). Development of the vertebrae of the axial skeleton begins at approximately the fourth week in the embryo; during the ninth week, ossification begins with the appearance of ossification centers in the lower thoracic and upper lumbar vertebrae. The paddle-shaped limb buds of the lower extremities make their appearance late in the fourth week of development; the hand pads are developed by days 33 to 36; and the finger rays are evident on days 41 to 43.[1]

Bone Growth in Childhood

During the first two decades of life, the skeleton undergoes general overall growth. The long bones of the skeleton, which grow at a relatively rapid rate, are provided with a specialized structure called the *epiphyseal growth plate.* As long bones grow in length, the deeper layers of cartilage cells in the growth plate multiply and enlarge, pushing the articular cartilage farther away from the metaphysis and diaphysis of the bone.[2,3] As this occurs, the mature and enlarged cartilage cells at the metaphyseal end of the plate become metabolically inactive and are replaced by bone cells (Fig. 58-1). This process allows bone growth to proceed without changing the shape of the bone or causing disruption of the articular cartilage. The cells in the growth plate stop dividing at puberty, at which time the epiphysis and metaphysis fuse.

Several factors can influence the growth of cells in the epiphyseal growth plate. Epiphyseal separation can occur in children as the result of trauma. The separation usually occurs in the zone of the mature enlarged cartilage cells, which is the weakest part of the growth plate. The blood vessels that nourish the epiphysis pass through the growth plate. These vessels are ruptured when the growth plate separates. This can cause cessation of growth and a shortened extremity. The growth plate also is sensitive to nutritional and metabolic changes. Scurvy (*i.e.,* vitamin C deficiency) impairs the formation of the organic matrix of bone, causing slowing of growth at the epiphyseal plate and cessation of diaphyseal growth. In rickets (*i.e.,* vitamin D deficiency), calcification of the newly developed bone on the metaphyseal side of the growth plate is impaired. Thyroid and growth hormones are required for normal growth. Alterations in these and other hormones can affect growth (see Chapter 42).

Growth in the diameter of bones occurs as new bone is added to the outer surface of existing bone along with

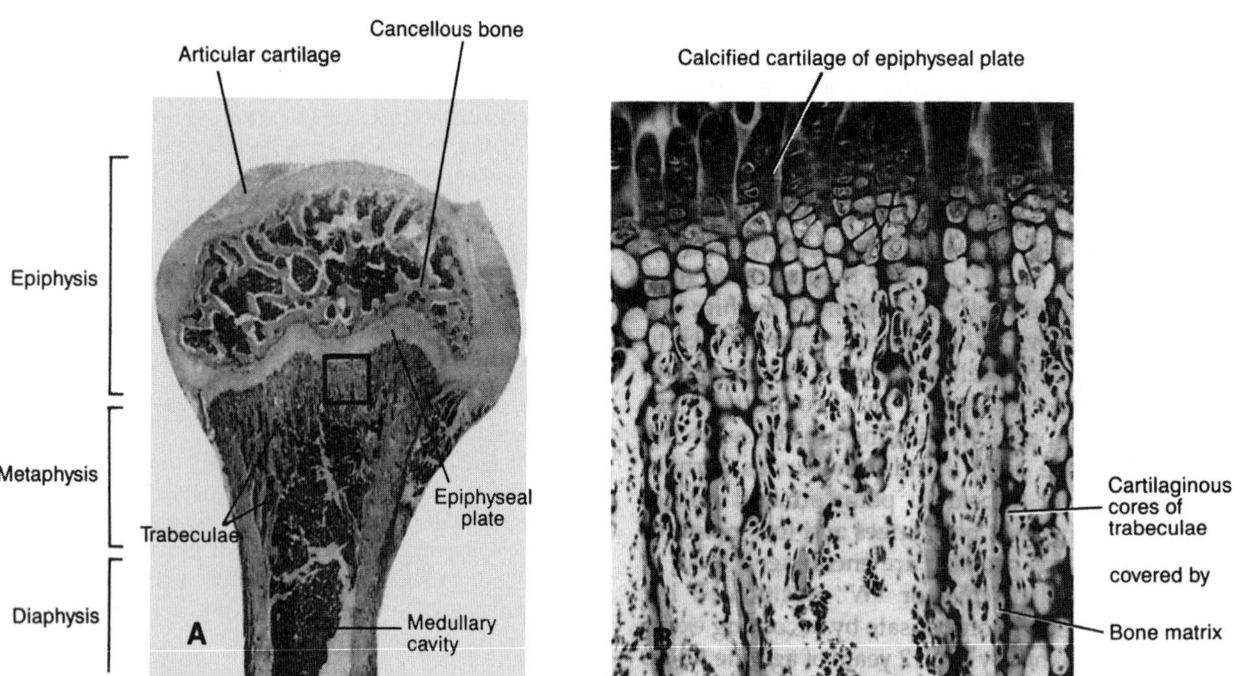

FIGURE 58-1 (**A**) Low-power photomicrograph of one end of a growing long bone (rat). Osteogenesis has spread from the epiphyseal center of ossification so that only the articular cartilage above and the epiphyseal disk below remain cartilaginous. On the diaphyseal side of the epiphyseal plate (disk), metaphyseal trabeculae extend down into the diaphysis. (**B**) Medium-power photomicrograph of the area indicated in **A,** showing trabeculae on the diaphyseal side of the epiphyseal plate (disk). These have cores of calcified cartilage on which bone has been deposited. The cartilaginous cores of the trabeculae were formerly partitions between columns of chondrocytes in the epiphyseal plate (disk). (Cormack D.H. [1987]. *Ham's histology* [9th ed.]. Philadelphia: J.B. Lippincott)

an accompanying resorption of bone on the endosteal or inner surface. Such oppositional growth allows for widening of the marrow cavity while preventing the cortex from becoming too thick and heavy. In this way, the shape of the bone is maintained. As a bone grows in diameter, concentric rings are added to the bone surface, much as rings are added to a tree trunk; these rings form the lamellar structure of mature bone. Osteocytes, which develop from osteoblasts, become buried in the rings. Haversian channels form as periosteal vessels running along the long axis become surrounded by bone (see Fig. 46-2, Chapter 46).

ALTERATIONS DURING NORMAL GROWTH PERIODS

Infants and children undergo changes in muscle tone and joint motion during growth and development. Toeing-in, toeing-out, bowlegs, and knock-knees occur frequently in infancy and childhood.[4] These changes usually cause few problems and are corrected during normal growth processes. The normal folded position of the fetus in utero causes physiologic flexion contractures of the hips and a froglike appearance of the lower extremities (Fig. 58-2). The hips are externally rotated, and the patellae point outward, whereas the feet appear to point forward because of the internal pulling force of the tibiae. During the first year of life, the lower extremities begin to straighten out in preparation for walking. Internal and external rotations become equal, and the hips extend. Flexion contractures of the shoulders, elbows, and knees also are commonly seen in newborns, but they should disappear by 4 to 6 months of age.[5] Musculoskeletal assessment of the newborn is important to identify abnormalities that require early intervention, facilitate treatment, establish baselines for future reference, and educate and counsel parents. There are many clinical deviations that are easily correctable in a newborn. Many others correct spontaneously as the child grows.

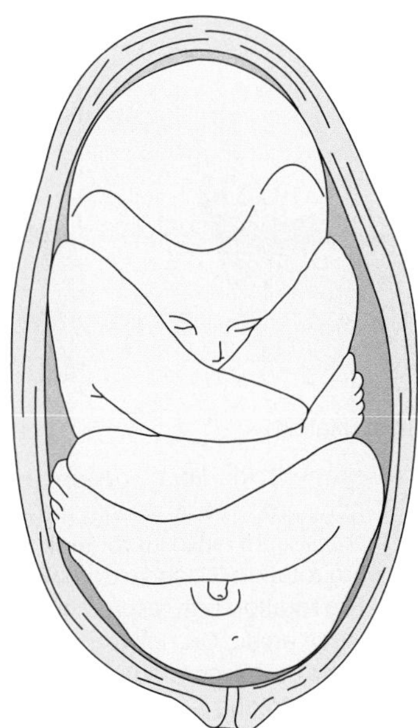

FIGURE 58-2 Position of fetus in utero, with tibial bowing and legs folded. (Dunne K.B., Clarren S.K. [1986]. The origin of prenatal and postnatal deformities. *Pediatric Clinics of North America 33* [6], 1282)

DEVELOPMENTAL SKELETAL DISORDERS

- Many disorders of early infancy are caused by intrauterine positions and resolve as the child grows.
- All infants and toddlers have lax ligaments that predispose to skeletal disorders caused by twisting or torsional forces.
- Bone growth in infants and children occurs at the epiphysis. Separation of the epiphyseal growth plate ruptures the blood vessels that nourish the epiphysis, causing cessation of growth and shortened extremity length.
- Nutritional and metabolic disorders impair the formation of the organic matrix of bone, causing slowing of growth at the epiphyseal plate.

Torsional Deformities

All infants and toddlers have lax ligaments that become tighter with age and assumption of the weight-bearing posture. The hypermobility that accompanies joint laxity, coupled with the torsional, or twisting, forces exerted on the limbs during growth, is responsible for a number of variants seen in young children. Torsional forces caused by intrauterine positions or sleeping and sitting patterns twist the growing bones and can produce the deformities as a child grows and develops.

In infants, the femur normally is rotated to an anteverted position with the femoral head and neck rotated anteriorly with respect to the femoral condyles. Femoral anteversion (*i.e.*, medial rotation) decreases from an average 40 degrees at birth to approximately 15 degrees at maturity. The normal tibia is externally rotated approximately 5 degrees at birth and 15 degrees at maturity. Torsional abnormalities frequently demonstrate a familial tendency.

Toeing-in and Toeing-out. The foot progression angle describes the angle between the axis of the foot and the line of progression. It is determined by watching the child walking and running; although it is usually less noticeable when the child is running or barefoot. Figure 58-3 illustrates the position of the foot in toeing-in and toeing-out.

Toeing-in (*i.e.*, metatarsus adductus) is the most common congenital foot deformity with an incidence of approximately 1 to 2 per 1000, and it affects boys and girls equally.[6] The forefoot commonly is adducted and gives the foot a kidney-shaped appearance, whereas the hindfoot is normal[6] (Fig. 58-4). It can be caused by torsion in the foot, lower leg, or entire leg. Toeing-in due to adduction of the forefoot (*i.e.*, congenital metatarsus adductus) usually is the result of the fetal position maintained in utero. It may occur in one foot or both feet. Diagnostic methods include examination of the plantar aspect of the

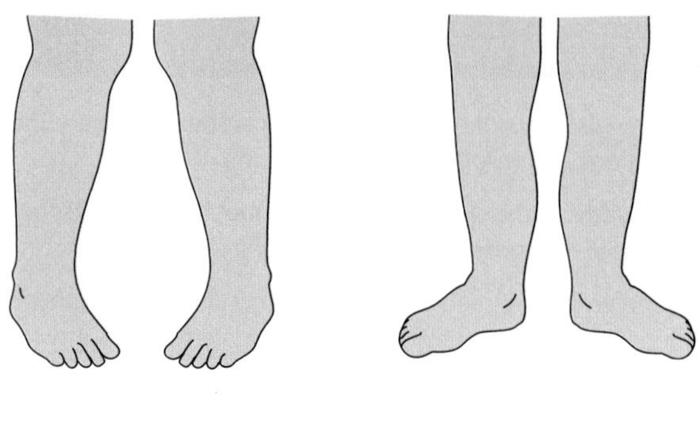

FIGURE 58-3 Position of feet in toeing-in and toeing-out.

foot, noting the overall shape of the foot and the presence or absence of an arch. The presence of a skin crease indicates a congenital deformity (see Fig. 58-4). Metatarsus adductus is graded based on the foot's flexibility while applying pressure to the medial forefoot. The defect is defined as grade I, grade II, or grade III. Grade I is a supple deformity that can be passively manipulated into a straight position and requires no treatment. A grade II deformity only corrects to a straight lateral border, and a grade III deformity is more rigid and may require further treatment.[7] Treatment consisting of serial long leg casting or a brace that pushes the metatarsals (not the hindfoot) into abduction usually is required in a fixed (rigid) deformity (*i.e.*, one in which the forefoot cannot be passively manipulated into a straight position).

Toeing-out is a common problem in children and is caused by external femoral torsion. This occurs when the femur can be externally rotated to approximately 90 degrees but internally rotated only to a neutral position or slightly beyond. Because the femoral torsion persists when a child habitually sleeps in the prone position, an external tibial torsion also may develop. If external tibial torsion is present, the feet point lateral to the midline of the medial plane. External tibial torsion rarely causes toeing-out; it only intensifies the condition. Toeing-out usually corrects itself as the child becomes proficient in walking. Occasionally, a night splint is used.

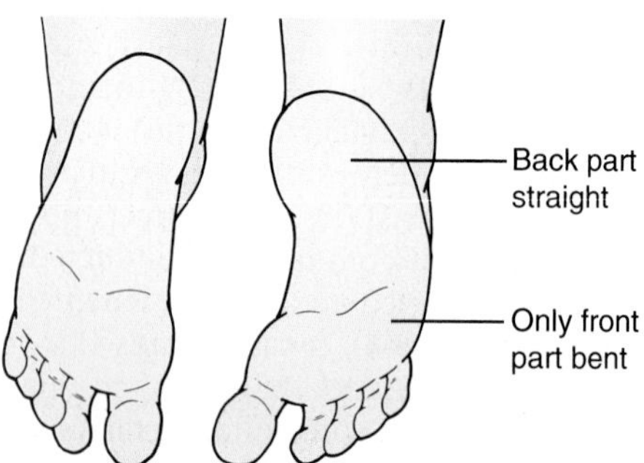

FIGURE 58-4 Shape of foot. The left foot is normal, while the right foot has metatarsus adductus.

Tibial Torsion. Tibial torsion is determined by measuring the thigh–foot angle, which is done with the ankle and knee positioned at 90 degrees (Fig. 58-5A). In this position, the foot normally rotates outward. *Internal tibial torsion* (*i.e.*, bowing of the tibia) is a rotation of the tibia that makes the feet appear to turn inward. It is the most common cause of toeing-in in children younger than 2 years of age. It is present at birth and may fail to correct itself if children sleep on their knees with the feet turned in or sit on in-turned feet. It is thought to be caused by genetic factors and intrauterine compression, such as an unstretched uterus during a first pregnancy or intrauterine crowding with twins or multiple fetuses. Tibial torsion improves naturally with growth, but this may take years.[5,8]

External tibial torsion, a much less common disorder, is associated with calcaneovalgus foot and is caused by a normal variation of intrauterine positioning or a neuromuscular disorder. It is characterized by an abnormally positive thigh–foot angle of 30 to 50 degrees. The condition corrects itself naturally, and treatment is observational. Significant improvement begins during the first year with the onset of ambulation and usually is complete

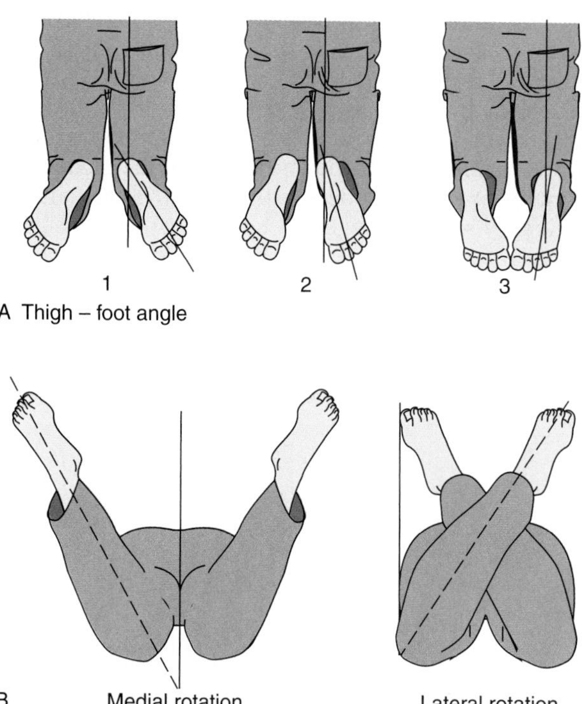

FIGURE 58-5 **(A)** Assessment for tibial torsion using thigh–foot angle. When child is in the prone position with the knee flexed, with normal alignment there is slight external rotation (2); internal tibial torsion produces inward rotation (3); and external tibial torsion, outward rotation (1). **(B)** Hip rotation is measured with child prone and knees flexed at 90-degree angle. On outward rotation the leg produces internal (medial) hip and femoral rotation; on inward rotation the leg produces external hip and femoral rotation. (Adapted from Staheli L.T. [1986]. Torsional deformity. *Pediatric Clinics of North America 33* [6], 1378, and Kliegman R.M., Neider M.I., Super D.M. [Eds.]. [1996]. *Practical strategies in pediatric diagnosis and therapy.* Philadelphia: W.B. Saunders)

by 2 to 3 years of age.[5] The normal adult exhibits 20 degrees of tibial torsion.

Femoral Torsion. *Femoral torsion* refers to abnormal variations in hip rotation. Hip rotation is measured at the pelvic level with the child in the prone position and the knees flexed at a 90-degree angle. In this position, the hip is in a neutral position. Rotating the lower leg outward produces internal or medial femoral rotation; rotating it inward produces external or lateral rotation (see Fig. 58-5B). During measurement of hip rotation, the legs are allowed to fall to full internal rotation by gravity alone; lateral rotation is measured by allowing the legs to fall inward and cross. Hip rotation in flexion and extension also can be measured with computed tomography (CT). By 1 year of age, there are normally approximately 45 degrees of internal rotation and 45 degrees of external rotation.[5]

Internal femoral torsion, also called *femoral anteversion,* is a normal variant commonly seen during the first 6 years of life, especially in 3- and 4-year-old girls.[4] Characteristically, there is 80 to 90 degrees of internal rotation of the hip in the prone position.[5] The condition is thought to be related to increased laxity of the anterior capsule of the hip such that it does not provide the stable pressure needed to correct the anteversion that is present at birth. Children are most comfortable sitting in the "*W*" position with their hips between their knees (Fig. 58-6). It is believed that this position allows the lower leg to act as a lever, producing torsional changes in the femur. When the child stands, the knees turn in and the feet appear to point straight ahead; when the child walks, knees and toes point in. Children with this problem are encouraged to sit cross-legged or in the so-called *tailor position.* If left untreated, the tibiae compensate by becoming externally rotated so that by 8 to 12 years of age, the knees may turn in but the feet no longer do. This can result in patellofemoral malalignment with patellar subluxation or dislocation and pain. A derotational osteotomy may be done in severe cases or if there is functional disability.

External femoral torsion is an uncommon disorder characterized by excessive external rotation of the hip. Bilateral external torsion is usually a benign condition, and treatment is observational. When the disorder is unilateral, slipped capital femoral epiphysis should be excluded, particularly if the condition occurs in an obese child or young adolescent (discussed later).

Genu Varum and Genu Valgum

Genu varum, or *bowlegs,* is an outward bowing of the knees greater than 1 inch when the medial malleoli of the ankles are touching (Fig. 58-7). Most infants and toddlers have some bowing of their legs up to age 2 years. If there is a large separation between the knees (>15 degrees) after 2 years of age, the child may require bracing. The child also should be evaluated for diseases such as rickets or tibia vara (*i.e.,* Blount's disease).

Genu valgum, or *knock-knees,* is a deformity in which there is decreased space between the knees (see Fig. 58-7). The medial malleoli in the ankles cannot be brought in contact with each other when the knees are touching. It is seen most frequently in children between the ages of 3 and 5 years and should resolve by 5 to 8 years of age.[5] The condition usually is the result of lax medial collateral ligaments

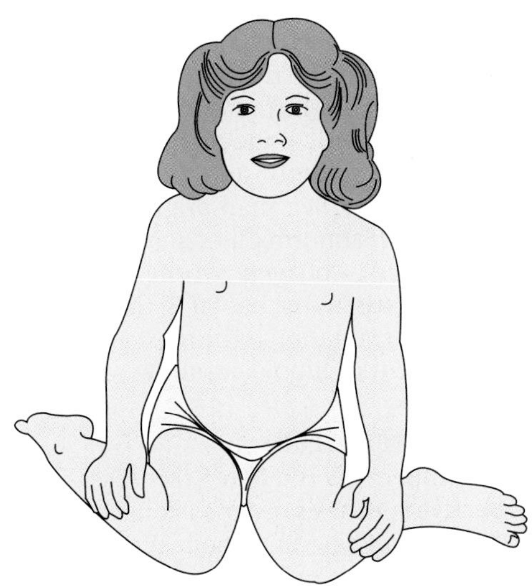

FIGURE 58-6 Typical sitting position of child with femoral anteversion. (Staheli L.T. [1986]. Torsional deformities. *Pediatric Clinics of North America 33* [6], 1382)

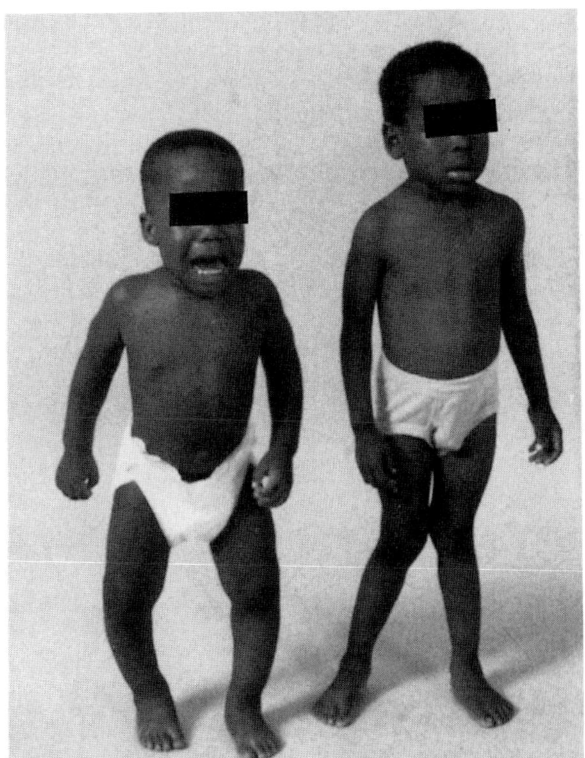

FIGURE 58-7 Normal genu varum (bowlegs) in a toddler *(left)* and genu valgum (knock-knees) in a toddler *(right),* which is often seen in children between 2 and 6 years of age. (From Weinstein S.L., Buckwalter J.A. [1994]. *Turek's orthopaedics* [5th ed.] Philadelphia: J.B. Lippincott)

of the knee and may be exacerbated by sitting in the M position. Genu valgum can be ignored up to age 7 years, unless it is more than 15 degrees, unilateral, or associated with short stature. It usually resolves spontaneously and rarely requires treatment. If genu varum or genu valgum persists and is uncorrected, osteoarthritis may develop in adulthood as a result of abnormal intraarticular stress. Genu varum can cause gait awkwardness and increased risk for sprains and fractures. Uncorrected genu valgum may cause subluxation and recurrent dislocation of the patella, with a predisposition to chondromalacia and joint pain and fatigue.

Idiopathic tibia vara, or *Blount's disease,* is a developmental deformity of the medial half of proximal tibial epiphysis that results in a progressive varus angulation below the knee (Fig. 58-8). It is the most common cause of pathologic genu varum and seen most often in black children, females, obese children, and early walkers.[9,10] Onset can occur early in infancy, or later, during adolescence. Adolescent Blount's disease occurs in the second decade of life, is seen in persons who are above the 95th percentile in height and weight, and is usually unilateral.[7] Long leg braces are used for treatment in early-onset disease. If progression occurs, or onset is late, surgery is done to correct the angulation and prevent further progression.

Flatfoot

Flatfoot (*i.e.,* pes planus) is a deformity characterized by the absence of the longitudinal arch of the foot. Infants normally have a wider and fatter foot than adults. The fat pads that normally are accentuated by pliable muscles create an illusion of fullness often mistaken for flatfeet. Until the longitudinal arch develops at 2 to 3 years of age, all children have flatfeet. The true criterion for flatfoot is that the head of the talus points medially and downward, so that the heel is everted and the forefoot must be inverted (toed-in) for the metatarsal heads to be planted equally on the ground. Weight bearing may cause pain in the longitudinal arch and up the leg.

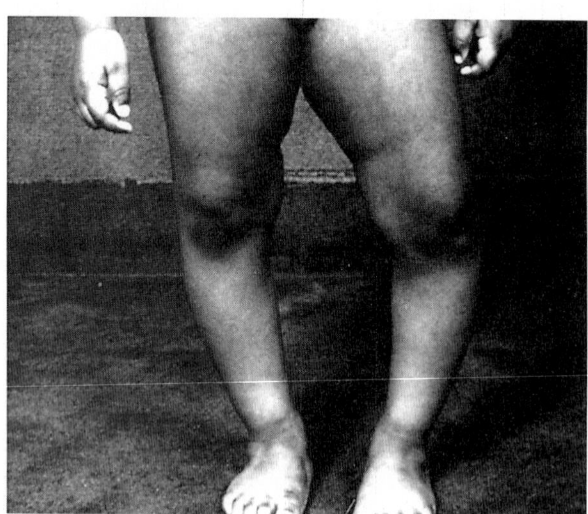

FIGURE 58-8 Rotational deformity of the proximal tibia, especially when unilateral, suggests tibia vera (Blount's disease). (From Weinstein S.L., Buckwalter J.A. [1994]. *Turek's orthopaedics* [5th ed.]. Philadelphia: J.B. Lippincott)

There are two types of flatfeet—flexible and rigid. Most children with flexible (or supple) flatfeet have loose ligaments, allowing the feet to sag when they gain weight. In supple flatfeet, the arch disappears only with weight bearing. No special treatment is needed for flexible flatfeet, and it usually is recommended that children with the disorder wear regular shoes. Recent studies have shown that flexible flat feet are less prone to pain and injury than those of people with normal or high arches.[7] The rigid flatfoot is fixed with no apparent arch in any position. It is seen in conjunction with congenitally tight heel cords, neuromuscular diseases such as cerebral palsy, or juvenile rheumatoid arthritis.

In the adult, treatment of flatfeet is conservative and aimed at relieving fatigue, pain, and tenderness. Supportive, well-fitting shoes with arch supports may be helpful and prevent ligaments from becoming overstretched. Women may complain of pain in the forefoot when wearing poorly fitting high heels. Surgery may be done in cases of severe and persistent symptoms.

HEREDITARY AND CONGENITAL DEFORMITIES

Congenital deformities are abnormalities that are present at birth. They range in severity from mild limb deformities, which are relatively common, to major limb malformations, which are relatively rare. There may be a simple webbing of the fingers or toes (syndactyly), the presence of an extra digit (*i.e.,* polydactyly), or the absence of a bone such as the phalanx, rib, or clavicle. Joint contractures and dislocations produce more severe deformity, as does the absence of entire bones, joints, or limbs. An epidemic of limb deformities occurred from 1957 to 1962 as a result of maternal ingestion of thalidomide.

Congenital deformities are caused by many factors, some unknown. These factors include genetic influences, external agents that injure the fetus (*e.g.,* radiation, alcohol, drugs, viruses), and intrauterine environmental factors. Many of the organic bone matrix components have been identified only recently, and their interactions were found to be more complex than originally thought. Diseases associated with abnormalities in bone matrix include those with deficient collagen synthesis and decreased bone mass. As discussed in Chapter 7, the fourth through the seventh week of gestation is the most vulnerable period for the development of limb deformities.

Osteogenesis Imperfecta

Osteogenesis imperfecta is a hereditary disease characterized by defective synthesis of type I collagen.[11,12] It is one of the most common hereditary bone diseases, with an occurrence rate of approximately 1 case in 10,000 births.[13] Although it usually is transmitted as an autosomal dominant trait, a distinct form of the disorder with multiple lethal defects is thought to be inherited as an autosomal

TABLE 58-1 Types of Osteogenesis Imperfecta

Type	Subtype	Inheritance	Major Features
I	Postnatal fractures, blue sclera	Autosomal dominant	Normal stature, skeletal fragility, hearing impairment, joint laxity, blue sclera
II	Perinatal, lethal	Autosomal recessive	Death in utero, or in days after birth Skeletal deformity with excessive fragility, multiple fractures, blue sclera
III	Progressive deformity	Autosomal dominant (75%) Autosomal recessive (25%)	Growth retardation, multiple fractures, progressive kyphoscoliosis, hearing impairment, blue sclera at birth
IV	Postnatal fractures, normal sclera	Autosomal dominant	Moderate skeletal fragility, short stature

(Developed from Cotran R.S., Kumar V., Collins T. [1999]. *Robbins pathologic basis of disease* [6th ed., p. 1222]. Philadelphia: W.B. Saunders)

recessive trait.[14] In some cases, the defect is caused by a spontaneous mutation.

The clinical manifestations of osteogenesis imperfecta include a spectrum of disorders marked by extreme skeletal fragility. Four major subtypes have been identified[12–14] (Table 58-1). The disorder is characterized by thin and poorly developed bones that are prone to multiple fractures. These children have short limbs and a soft, thin cranium with bifrontal prominences that give a triangular appearance to the face. Other problems associated with defective connective tissue synthesis include short stature, thin skin, blue or gray sclera, abnormal tooth development, hypotonic muscles, loose-jointedness, scoliosis, and a tendency toward hernia formation. Hearing loss due to otosclerosis of the tiny bones in the middle ear is common in affected adults.

The most serious defects occur when the disorder is inherited as a recessive trait (type II). Severely affected fetuses have multiple intrauterine fractures and bowing and shortening of the extremities. Many of these infants are stillborn or die during infancy. Less severe disease occurs when the disorder is inherited as a dominant trait. The skeletal system is not so weakened, and fractures often do not appear until the child becomes active and starts to walk, or even later in childhood. These fractures heal rapidly, although with a poor-quality callus. In some cases, parents may be suspected of child abuse when the child is admitted to the health care facility with multiple fractures. There also is an increased incidence of complications such as hernias and congenital heart abnormalities.

There is no known treatment for correction of the defective collagen synthesis that is characteristic of osteogenesis imperfecta. Instead, treatment modalities focus on preventing and treating fractures. Precise alignment is necessary to prevent deformities. Nonunion is common, especially with repeated fractures. Surgical intervention often is needed to stabilize fractures and correct deformities (*e.g.*, internal fixation of long bones may be done with an intramedullary rod that "grows" with the child). Treatment with bisphosphonate drugs (*e.g.*, alendronate, pamidronate) is effective in improving mobility and decreasing symptoms in many cases.[12]

Developmental Dysplasia of the Hip

Developmental dysplasia of the hip (DDH), formerly known as *congenital dislocation of the hip,* is an abnormality in hip development that leads to a wide spectrum of hip problems in infants and children, including hips that are unstable, malformed, subluxated, or dislocated.[15–17] In less severe cases, the hip joint may be unstable, with excessive laxity of the joint capsule, or subluxated, so that the joint surfaces are separated and there is a partial dislocation (Fig. 58-9). With dislocated hips, the head of the femur is located outside of the acetabulum.

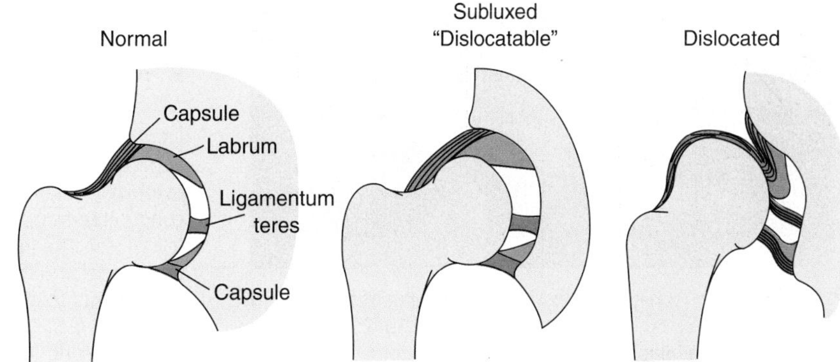

FIGURE 58-9 Normal and abnormal relationships of hip joint structure. (Adapted from Dunn P.M. [1969]. Congenital dislocation of the hip. *Proceedings of the Royal Society of Medicine 62,* 1035–1037)

The results of newborn screening programs have shown that 1 of 100 infants have some evidence of hip instability; however, dislocation of the hip is seen in 1.5 of every 1000 live births.[16] The left hip is involved three times more frequently than the right hip because of the left occipital intrauterine positioning of most infants.[15] In white infants, DDH occurs most frequently in first-born children and is six times more common in female than in male infants.[16] The cause of DDH is multifactorial, with heredity, environmental, and mechanical factors playing a role. A positive family history and generalized laxity of the ligaments are related. The increased frequency in girls is thought to result from their susceptibility to maternal estrogens and other hormones associated with pelvic relaxation. Dislocation also may result from environmental factors such as fetal position, a tight uterus that prevents fetal movement, and breech delivery. Approximately 30% to 50% of children with DDH have a history of breech presentation.[6] The presence of other congenital abnormalities is associated with an increased incidence of DDH. Thus, the hips of children presenting with congenital abnormalities should be examined carefully.

Early diagnosis of DDH is important because treatment is easiest and most effective if begun during the first 6 months of life. Repeated dislocation causes damage to the femoral head and the acetabulum. Clinical examinations to detect dislocation of the hip should be done at birth and every several months during the first year of life. Several examination techniques are used to screen for a dislocatable hip. In infants, signs of dislocation include asymmetry of the hip or gluteal folds, shortening of the thigh so that one knee (on the affected side) is higher than the other, and limited abduction of the affected hip (Fig. 58-10). The asymmetry of gluteal folds is not definitive but indicates the need for further evaluation. The Galeazzi test is a measurement of the length of the femurs that is done by comparing the height at the knees while they are flexed at 90 degrees. Two specific methods of examination are the Ortolani maneuver (for reducible dislocation) and the Barlow test (for the dislocatable hip). The Barlow maneuver involves a manual attempt to dislocate and reduce the abnormal hip while the infant is in the supine position with both knees flexed. With gentle downward pressure being applied to the knees, the knee and thigh are manually abducted as an upward and medial pressure is applied to the proximal thigh (Fig. 58-11). In infants with the disorder, the initial downward pressure on the knee produces a dislocation of the hip, a positive Barlow's sign. This is followed by a palpable or audible click (*i.e.,* Ortolani's sign) as the hip is reduced and moves back into the acetabulum. The sensitivity of these tests is improved significantly with the use of trained and experienced examiners.[18] In an older child, instability of the hip may produce a delay in standing or walking and eventually cause a characteristic waddling gait. When the thumbs are placed over the anterior iliac crest and the hands are placed over the lateral pelvis in examination, the levels of the thumbs are not even; the child is unable to elevate the opposite side of the pelvis (positive Trendelenburg's test). Diagnosis of DDH is confirmed by radiography. Ultrasound is used to diagnose newborns and infants from birth to 4 months of age.

The treatment of a DDH should be individualized and depends on whether the hip is subluxated or dislocated.

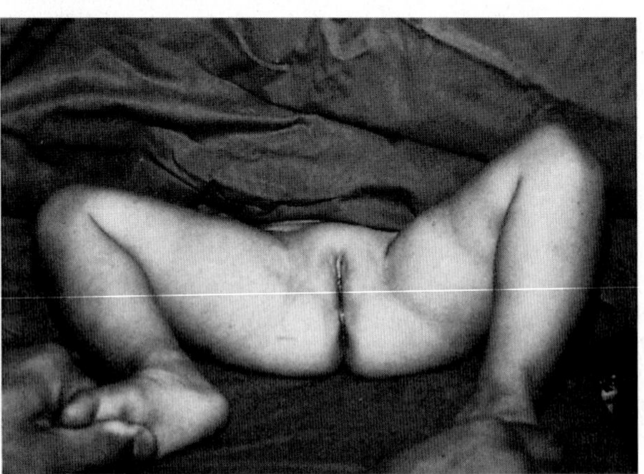

FIGURE 58-10 An 18-month-old girl has congenital dysplasia of the left hip. (From Weinstein S.L., Buckwalter J.A. [1994]. *Turek's orthopaedics* [5th ed.]. Philadelphia: J.B. Lippincott)

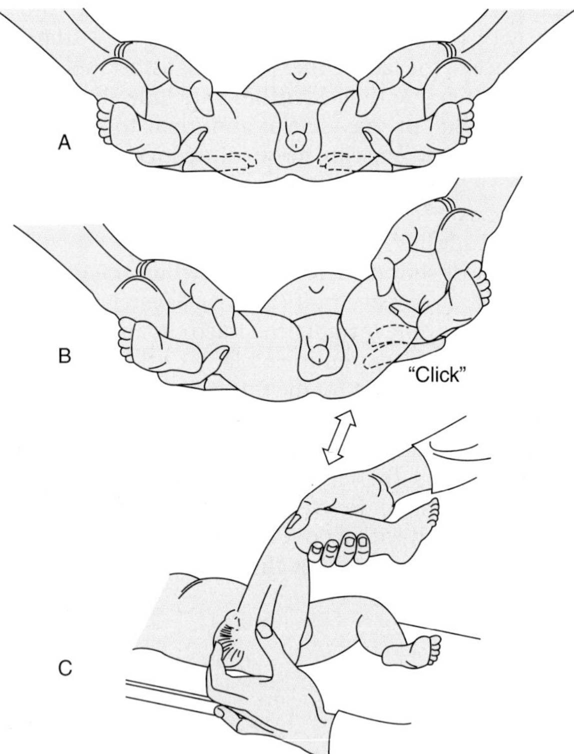

FIGURE 58-11 Examination for developmental dysplasia of the hip. (**A**) In the newborn, both hips can be equally flexed, abducted, and externally rotated without producing a "click." (**B**) A diagnosis of congenital dislocation of the hip may be confirmed by Ortolani's "click" test. The involved hip cannot be abducted as far as the opposite one, and there is a "click" as the hip reduces. (**C**) Telescoping of the femur to aid in the diagnosis of a congenitally dislocated hip. (Hoppenfeld S. [1976]. *Physical examination of the spine and extremities.* New York: Appleton-Century-Crofts)

Mild instability often resolves without treatment. The best results are obtained if the treatment is begun before changes in the hip structure (*e.g.,* 2 to 3 months) prevent it from being reduced by gentle manipulation or abduction devices. The Pavlik harness is used on newborns (up to 6 months) to maintain the femoral head in the acetabulum. The harness allows the child more mobility as the leg is slowly and gently brought into abduction. Infants with dislocated hips caused by anatomic changes and toddlers who may lack development of the acetabular socket require more aggressive treatment, such as open reduction and joint reconstruction. Treatment at any age includes reduction of the dislocation and immobilization of the legs in an abducted position. The most serious complication of any treatment is avascular necrosis of the femoral head as a result of the forced abduction. With children younger than 3 years of age, skin traction is used when reduction cannot be easily obtained. This treatment is followed by several months of immobilization in a hip spica cast, plaster splints, or an abduction splint such as an Ilfeld splint. Older children or adults with an unreduced dislocatable hip may require hip surgery because of damage to the articulating surface of the joint. These persons have considerable problems after surgery because of soft tissue contractures.

Congenital Clubfoot

Clubfoot, or talipes, is a congenital deformity of the foot that can affect one or both feet. Bilateral clubfeet occur in 50% of the cases.[6] Like congenital dislocation of the hip, its occurrence follows a multifactorial inheritance pattern. The condition has an incidence of 1 case per 1000 live births and occurs twice as often in males as in females.[19] Clubfoot is associated with chromosomal abnormalities and may be associated with other congenital syndromes that are transmitted by mendelian inheritance patterns (see Chapter 6). However, it is most commonly idiopathic and found in normal infants in whom no genetic or chromosomal abnormality or other extrinsic cause can be found.

In forefoot adduction, which accounts for approximately 95% of idiopathic cases, the foot is plantar flexed and inverted. This is the so-called *equinovarus type* in which the foot resembles a horse's hoof (Fig. 58-12). The other 5% of cases are of the calcaneovalgus type, or reverse clubfoot, in which the foot is dorsiflexed and everted. The reverse clubfoot can occur as an isolated condition or in association with multiple congenital defects. At birth, the feet of many infants assume one of these two positions, but they can be passively overcorrected or brought back into the opposite position. If the foot cannot be overcorrected, some type of correction may be necessary. Although the exact cause of clubfoot is unknown, three theories are generally accepted: an anomalous development occurs during the first trimester of pregnancy, the leg fails to rotate inward and move from the equinovarus position at approximately the third month, or the soft tissues in the foot do not mature and lengthen. Maternal smoking is associated with occurrence of clubfoot, and the risk increases enormously when combined with a family history.[20]

Treatment of clubfoot is begun as soon as the diagnosis is made. When treatment is initiated during the first few weeks of life, a nonoperative procedure is effective within a short period. Serial manipulations and casting are used to gently correct each component in the forefoot varus, the hindfoot varus, and the equinus. The treatment is continued until the foot is in a normal position with full correction evident clinically and on radiographic studies.

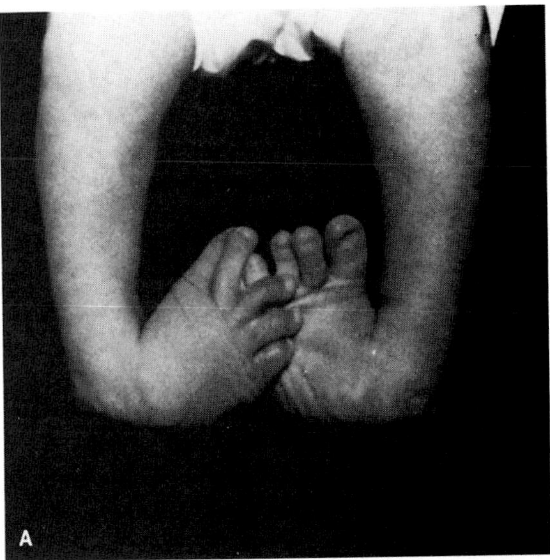

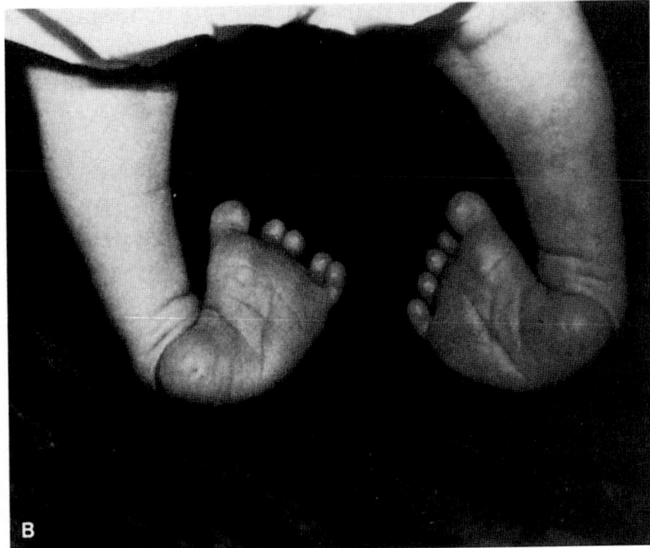

FIGURE 58-12 Severe clubfoot deformity. (**A**) The heel is in severe varus, and the forefoot is adducted and inverted. (**B**) The cavus deformity results from the slightly pronated position of the forefoot in relation to the hindfoot. (From Weinstein S.L., Buckwalter J.A. [1994]. *Turek's orthopaedics* [5th ed.]. Philadelphia: J.B. Lippincott.)

Surgery may be required for severe deformities or when nonoperative treatment methods are unsuccessful. Approximately 30% to 50% of idiopathic deformities are corrected with casts; the others require surgery.[21] An external distractor such as the Ilizarov external fixator may be used to correct the deformity of a relapsed or neglected clubfoot.

JUVENILE OSTEOCHONDROSES

The term *juvenile osteochondroses* is used to describe a group of children's diseases in which one or more growth ossification centers undergoes a period of degeneration, necrosis, or inactivity that is followed by regeneration and usually deformity. The osteochondroses are separated into two groups according to their causes. The first group consists of the true osteonecrotic osteochondroses, so called because the diseases are caused by localized osteonecrosis of an apophyseal or epiphyseal center (*e.g.,* Legg-Calvé-Perthes disease, Freiberg's infraction, Panner's disease, Kienböck's disease). The second group of juvenile osteochondroses is caused by abnormalities in ossification of cartilaginous tissue resulting from a genetically determined normal variation or from trauma (*e.g.,* Osgood-Schlatter disease, Blount's disease, Sever's disease, Scheuermann's disease). The discussion in this section focuses on Legg-Calvé-Perthes disease from the first group and Osgood-Schlatter disease from the second group. Slipped capital femoral epiphysis is a disorder of the growth plate.

Legg-Calvé-Perthes Disease

Legg-Calvé-Perthes disease, or coxa plana, is an osteonecrotic disease of the proximal femoral (capital) epiphysis, which is the growth center for the head of the femur. It occurs in 1 of 1200 children, affecting primarily those between ages 2 and 13 years, with a peak incidence between 4 and 9 years.[5,22] It occurs primarily in boys and is much more common in whites than African Americans. Although no definite genetic pattern has been established, it occasionally affects more than one family member.

The cause of Legg-Calvé-Perthes disease is unknown. The disorder usually is insidious in onset and occurs in otherwise healthy children. It may, however, be associated with acute trauma. Affected children usually have a shorter stature. Undernutrition has been suggested as a causative factor. When girls are affected, they usually have a poorer prognosis than boys because they are skeletally more mature and have a shorter period for growth and remodeling than boys of the same age. Although both legs can be affected, in 85% of cases, only one leg is involved.[8]

The primary pathologic feature of Legg-Calvé-Perthes disease is an avascular necrosis of the bone and marrow involving the epiphyseal growth center in the femoral head. The disorder may be confined to part of the epiphysis, or it may involve the entire epiphysis. In severe cases, there is a disturbance in the growth pattern that leads to a broad, short femoral neck. The necrosis is followed by slow absorption of the dead bone over 2 to 3 years. Although the necrotic trabeculae eventually are replaced by healthy new bone, the epiphysis rarely regains its normal shape. The process occurs in four predictable stages.[22] The *first stage,* which lasts for 1 to 3 weeks, is the synovitis stage, which is characterized by synovial inflammation and increased joint fluid. The *second stage* is the aseptic or avascular stage, during which the ossification center becomes necrotic. This stage may last from several months to a year. Damage to the femoral head is determined by the degree of necrosis that occurs during this stage. The *third stage* is the regenerative or revascularization stage, during which resorption of the necrotic bone takes place. This stage usually lasts 1 to 3 years, during which the necrotic bone is gradually replaced by new immature bone cells and the contour of the bone is remodeled. The *fourth stage,* which is the healed or residual stage, involves the formation and replacement of immature bone cells by normal bone cells.

Legg-Calvé-Perthes disease has an insidious onset with a prolonged course. The main symptoms are pain in the groin, thigh, or knee and difficulty in walking. The child may have a painless limp with limited abduction and internal rotation and a flexion contracture of the affected hip. The age of onset is important because young children have a greater capability for remodeling of the femoral head and acetabulum, and thus less flattening of the femoral head occurs. Early diagnosis is important and is based on correlating physical symptoms with radiographic findings that are related to the stage of the disease.

The goal of treatment is to reduce deformity and preserve the integrity of the femoral head. Conservative and surgical interventions are used in the treatment of Legg-Calvé-Perthes disease. Children younger than 4 years of age with little or no involvement of the femoral head may require only periodic observation. In all other children, some intervention is needed to relieve the force of weight bearing, muscular tension, and subluxation of the femoral head. It is important to maintain the femur in a well-seated position in the concave acetabulum to prevent deformity. This is done by keeping the hip in abduction and mild internal rotation. Treatment involves abduction casts or braces to keep the legs separated in abduction with mild internal rotation. The Atlanta Scottish Rite brace, which does not extend below the knee, is the most widely used orthosis because it provides containment while allowing free knee motion and ambulation without crutches or external support[5,18] (Fig. 58-13). Surgery may be done to contain the femoral head in the acetabulum. This treatment usually is reserved for children older than 6 years of age who at the time of diagnosis have more serious involvement of the femoral head. The best surgical results are obtained when surgery is done early, before the epiphysis becomes necrotic.

Osgood-Schlatter Disease

Osgood-Schlatter disease involves microfractures in the area where the patellar tendon inserts into the tibial tubercle, which is an extension of the proximal tibial epiphysis.[5] This area is particularly vulnerable to injury caused by sudden or continued strain from the patellar tendon during periods of growth, particularly in athletic individuals. It occurs most frequently in boys between the ages of 11 and 15 years and in girls between 8 and 13 years.

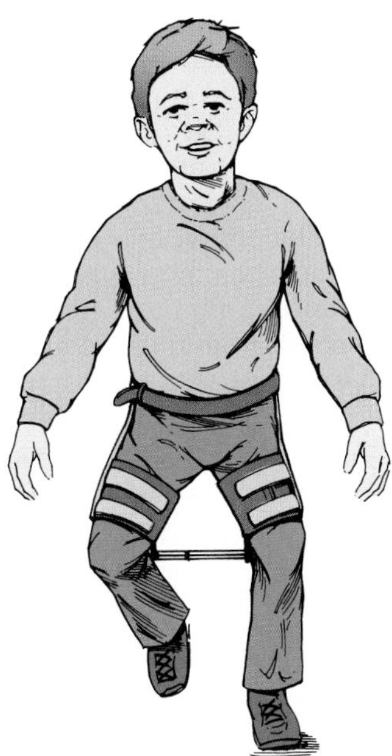

FIGURE 58-13 Scottish Rite brace for Legg-Calvé-Perthes disease produces containment for abduction and allows free knee motion. (Johnson K.B., Oski F.A. [1997]. *Oski's essential pediatrics.* Philadelphia: Lippincott-Raven)

The disorder is characterized by pain in the front of the knee that is associated with inflammation and thickening of the patellar tendon. The pain usually is associated with specific activities such as kneeling, running, bicycle riding, or stair climbing. There is swelling, tenderness, and increased prominence of the tibial tubercle. The symptoms usually are self-limiting. They may recur during growth periods, but usually resolve after closure of the tibial growth plate. In some cases, limitations on activity, tibial bands, or braces to immobilize the knee, anti-inflammatory agents, and application of cold are necessary to relieve the pain. The objective of treatment is to release tension on the quadriceps to permit revascularization and reossification of the tibial tubercle. Complete resolution of symptoms through healing (physical closure) of the tibia tubercle usually requires 12 to 24 months.[5] Occasionally, minor symptoms or an increased prominence of the tibial tubercle may continue into adulthood. In some cases, a high-riding patella can cause dislocation with chondromalacia of the patella and result in degenerative arthritis.

Slipped Capital Femoral Epiphysis

Slipped capital femoral epiphysis, or coxa vara, is a disorder of the growth plate that occurs near the age of skeletal maturity. The condition occurs with an estimated frequency of between 1 in 100,000 and 1 in 800,000 and is the most common disorder of the hip in adolescents.[8] Normally, the proximal capital femoral epiphysis unites with the neck of the femur between 14 and 16 years of age. Before this time (10 to 14 years of age in girls and 10 to 16 years in boys), slippage may occur, with the capital femoral epiphysis remaining in the acetabulum and the femoral neck being rotated anteriorly (although occasionally superiorly).[22] This results in a varus-retroverted femoral head and neck.

The cause of slipped capital femoral epiphysis is obscure, but it may be related to the child's susceptibility to stress on the femoral neck as a result of genetics or structural abnormalities. Boys are affected twice as often as girls, and in approximately one half of cases, the condition is bilateral. Affected children often are overweight with poorly developed secondary sex characteristics or, in some instances, are extremely tall and thin. In many cases, there is a history of rapid skeletal growth preceding displacement of the epiphysis. The condition also may be affected by nutritional deficiencies or endocrine disorders such as hypothyroidism, hypopituitarism, and hypogonadism. Rapid growth after administration of growth hormone has been associated with displacement of the epiphysis.

Children with the condition often complain of referred knee pain accompanied by difficulty in walking, fatigue, and stiffness. The diagnosis is confirmed by radiographic studies in which the degree of slipping is determined and graded according to severity (mild, 0% to 33%; moderate, 34% to 50%; and severe, greater than 50%). Early treatment is imperative to prevent lifelong crippling. Avoidance of weight bearing on the femur and bed rest are essential parts of the treatment. Traction or gentle manipulation under anesthesia is used to reduce the slip. Surgical insertion of pins to keep the femoral neck and head of the femur aligned is a common method of treatment for children with moderate or severe slips. Crutches are used for several months after surgical correction to prevent full weight bearing until the growth plate closes.

Children with the disorder must be followed closely until the epiphyseal plate closes. Long-term prognosis depends on the amount of displacement that occurs. Complications include avascular necrosis, leg shortening, malunion, and problems with the internal fixation. Degenerative arthritis may develop, requiring joint replacement later in life.

SCOLIOSIS

Scoliosis is a lateral deviation of the spinal column that may or may not include rotation or deformity of the vertebrae. It has been estimated that more than 500,000 adults in the United States have scoliosis.[23] It is most commonly seen during adolescence and is eight times more common among girls than boys. Scoliosis can develop as the result of another disease condition, or it can occur without known cause. Idiopathic scoliosis accounts for 75% to 80% of cases of the disorder. The other 20% to 25% of cases result from more than 50 different causes, including poliomyelitis, congenital hemivertebrae, neurofibromatosis, and cerebral palsy. Although minor curves are relatively common (affecting approximately 2% of the population), it has been estimated that less than 0.1% of American schoolchildren have severe idiopathic scoliosis.[24] Earlier studies that indicated a more widespread problem probably were based on inclusion of children with serious systemic diseases such as poliomyelitis.

Types of Scoliosis

Scoliosis is classified as postural or structural. With postural scoliosis, there is a small curve that corrects with bending. It can be corrected with passive and active exercises. Structural scoliosis does not correct with bending. It is a fixed deformity classified according to the cause: congenital, neuromuscular, or idiopathic.

Congenital Scoliosis. Congenital scoliosis is caused by disturbances in vertebral development during the sixth to eighth week of embryologic development. Congenital scoliosis may be divided into failures of formation and failures of segmentation. Failures of formation are the absence of a portion of the vertebra, such as hemivertebra (absence of a whole side of the vertebra) and wedge vertebra (missing only a portion of the vertebra). Failure of segmentation is the absence of the normal separations between the vertebrae.[6] The child may have other anomalies and neurologic complications if the spine is involved. Early diagnosis and treatment of progressive curves are essential for children with congenital scoliosis. Surgical intervention is the treatment of choice for progressive congenital scoliosis.[6]

Neuromuscular Scoliosis. Neuromuscular scoliosis develops from neuropathic or myopathic diseases. Neuropathic scoliosis is seen with cerebral palsy, myelodysplasia, and poliomyelitis. There is often a long, "C"-shaped curve from the cervical to the sacral region. In children with cerebral palsy, severe deformity may make treatment difficult. Myopathic neuromuscular scoliosis develops with Duchenne's muscular dystrophy and usually is not severe.

Idiopathic Scoliosis. Idiopathic scoliosis is a structural spinal curvature for which no cause has been established. The cause is most likely complex and multifactorial. Genetic, neurophysiologic predisposition, abnormal biomechanical forces, connective tissue abnormality, and collagen abnormalities have all been researched as possible causes of idiopathic scoliosis.[25] It seems likely that heredity is involved because mother–daughter pairings are common, and there is a reported prevalence rate of 27% among daughters of women with a scoliotic curve that exceeded 15 degrees.[25] Studies of twins show that monozygotic twins will both present with scoliosis at a rate of 73% and dizygotic twins will both present with scoliosis at a rate of 36%.[25]

Idiopathic scoliosis can be divided into three groups on the basis of age at onset: infantile (birth to 3 years), juvenile (4 to 10 years), and adolescent (11 years and older).[26] The infantile form is rare in the United States. It is seen primarily in the United Kingdom and Europe. It affects males more often than females, and the curvature usually is convex and to the left rather than to the right, as in other forms of scoliosis. Although most forms of juvenile scoliosis regress spontaneously, some progress and are difficult to treat effectively. Juvenile idiopathic scoliosis is uncommon. However, in many children with the diagnosis of adolescent scoliosis, the onset may have occurred when they were juveniles but was not diagnosed until later. Adolescent scoliosis is the most common type, accounts for approximately 80% of cases, and is seen most commonly in girls. An increase in joint laxity, which causes excessive joint motion and is found commonly in girls, has been associated with the development of idiopathic scoliosis. Delayed puberty and menarche are other risk factors for the development of adolescent scoliosis.[27]

Although a scoliosis curve may be present in any area of the spine, the most common curve is a right thoracic curve, which produces a rib prominence on the convex side and hypokyphosis from rotation of the vertebral column around its long axis as the spine begins to curve. A spinal curvature of less than 10 degrees is considered a normal variant, not scoliosis.[23,24] Curves greater than 40 degrees usually are considered severe.

Manifestations

Scoliosis usually is first noticed because of the deformity it causes. A high shoulder, prominent hip, or projecting scapula may be noticed by a parent or in a school-based screening program. In girls, difficulty in hemming or fitting a dress may call attention to the deformity. Idiopathic scoliosis usually is a painless process, although pain may be present in severe cases, usually in the lumbar region. The pain may be caused by pressure on the ribs or on the crest of the ilium. There may be shortness of breath as a result of diminished chest expansion and gastrointestinal disturbances from crowding of the abdominal organs. Adults with less severe deformity may experience mild backache. If scoliosis is left untreated, the curve may progress to an extent that compromises cardiopulmonary function and creates a risk for neurologic complications.

Diagnosis and Treatment

Early diagnosis of scoliosis can be important in the prevention of severe spinal deformity. The cardinal signs of scoliosis are uneven shoulders or iliac crest, prominent scapula on the convex side of the curve, malalignment of spinous processes, asymmetry of the flanks, asymmetry of the thoracic cage, and rib hump or paraspinal muscle prominence when bending forward (Fig. 58-14). A complete physical examination is necessary for children with scoliosis because the defect may be indicative of other, underlying pathology.

School screening programs were instituted with the assumption that early detection and treatment of spinal curves would halt progression of the defect. The Scoliosis Research Society has recommended annual screening for all children between 10 and 14 years of age. The American Academy of Pediatrics has recommended screening during routine health supervision visits at the ages of 10, 12, 14, and 16 years. Scoliosis screening is required by law in many states. The U.S. Preventative Services Task Force examined evidence regarding the effectiveness of routine screening for adolescent idiopathic scoliosis.[23] After reviewing studies regarding the natural history of curve projection, accuracy of screening tests, effectiveness of treatment, potential adverse effects, costs, and burden of suffering, the Task Force issued a statement that "there is insufficient evidence to recommend for or against routine screening of asymptomatic adolescents for idiopathic scoliosis."[28] There is a

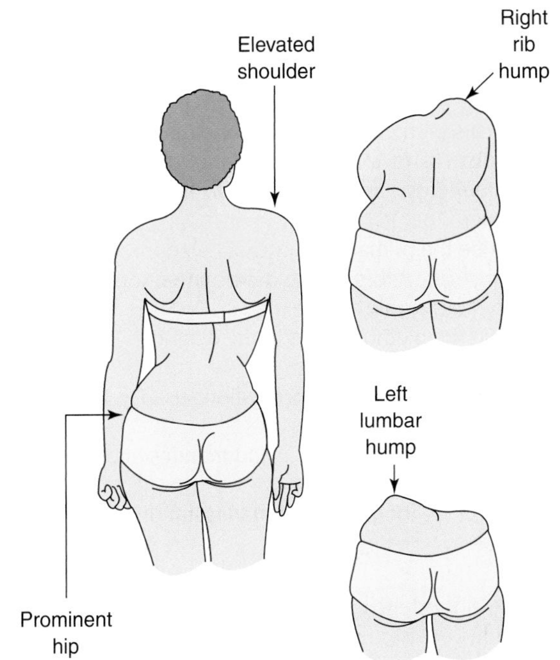

FIGURE 58-14 Scoliosis. Abnormalities to be determined at initial screening examination. (Gore D.R., Passhel R., Sepic S., Dalton A. [1981]. Scoliosis screening: Results of a community project. *Pediatrics* 67 [2]. Copyright 1981 by the American Academy of Pediatrics)

great need for clinical research to demonstrate the effectiveness or ineffectiveness of routine screening. There are times when screening identifies many children as positive who really do not need treatment.[28]

Diagnosis of scoliosis is made by physical examination and confirmed by radiographs. A scoliometer should be used at the apex of the curvature to quantify a prominence; a scoliometer reading of greater than 10 degrees requires referral to a physician. The curve is measured by determining the amount of lateral deviation present on radiographs and is labeled "right" or "left" for the convex portion of the curve. Other radiographic procedures may be done, including CT, magnetic resonance imaging (MRI), and myelography.

The treatment of scoliosis depends on the severity of the deformity and the likelihood of progression. Larger curves are more likely to progress. Age of presentation also is important. Curves that are detected before menarche are more likely to progress than those detected after menarche. For persons with lesser degrees of curvature (10 to 20 degrees), the trend has been away from aggressive treatment and toward a "wait and see" approach, taking advantage of the more sophisticated diagnostic methods that now are available. Treatment is considered for physiologically immature patients with curves between 20 and 30 degrees. Curves between 30 and 40 degrees usually are considered for bracing, and those greater than 40 to 45 degrees are considered for surgery.

A brace may be used to control the progression of the curvature during growth and can provide some correction. A commonly used brace is the Milwaukee brace, which was developed by Blount and Schmitt in the 1940s (Fig. 58-15). This was the first brace to provide some degree of active correction. It involves a pelvic mold, various pads, and two metal upright supports around the throat. It is cumbersome, and compliance with wearing the brace has been shown to be poor. In an effort to improve compliance, a number of new bracing techniques have been developed. They include underarm or thoracolumbosacral orthoses. These orthoses consist of easily concealed, prefabricated forms that are modified to suit the patient.

Surgical intervention with instrumentation and spinal fusion is done in severe cases—when the curvature has progressed to 40 degrees or more at the time of diagnosis or when curves of a lesser degree are compounded with imbalance or rotation of the vertebrae. Unlike bracing, which is intended to halt progression of the curvature, surgical intervention is used to decrease the curve. Instrumentation helps correct the curve and balance, and spinal fusion maintains the spine in the corrected position. Several methods of instrumentation (*i.e.,* rods that attach to the vertebral column and posterior fusion) are used. Combined anterior and posterior surgery is used for more severe curvatures. The newer systems provide better sagittal control and more stable fixation, which allow earlier mobility. Despite great advances in spinal surgery, no one method seems to be the best for all cases.

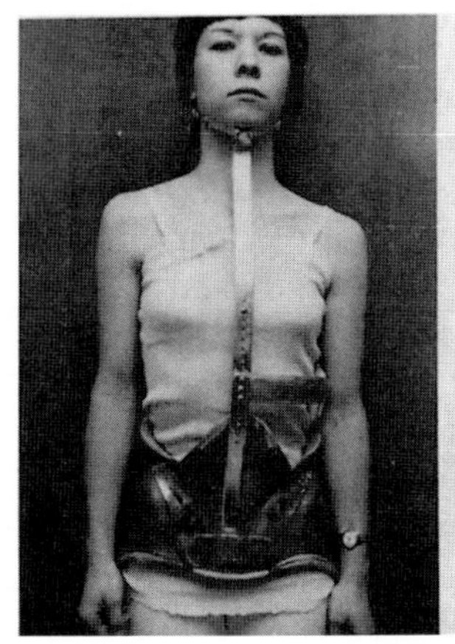
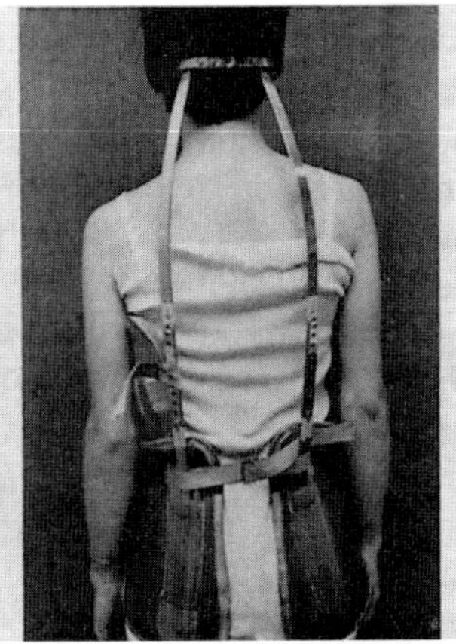
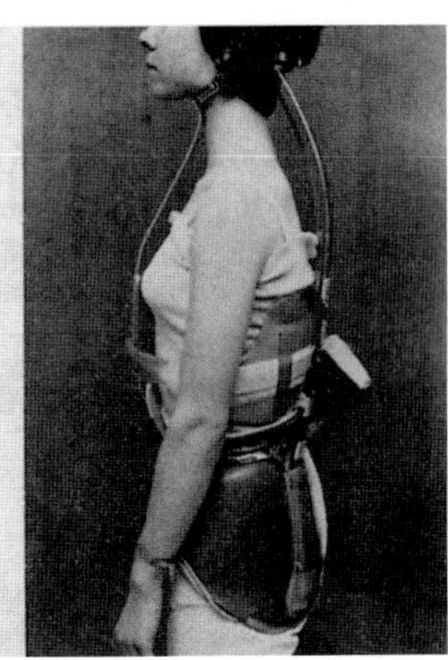

FIGURE 58-15 The Milwaukee brace as seen from front, back, and side. (Farrell J. [1986]. *Illustrated guide to orthopedic nursing* [3rd ed., p. 172]. Philadelphia: J.B. Lippincott)

In summary, skeletal disorders can result from congenital or hereditary influences or from factors that occur during normal periods of skeletal growth and development. Newborn infants undergo normal changes in muscle tone and joint motion, causing torsional conditions of the femur or tibia. Many of these conditions are corrected as skeletal growth and development take place. Osteogenesis imperfecta is a rare autosomal hereditary disorder characterized by defective synthesis of connective tissue, including bone matrix. It results in poorly developed bones that fracture easily. Developmental dysplasia of the hip includes a range of structural abnormalities. Dislocated hips are always treated to prevent changes in the anatomic structure. Other childhood skeletal disorders, such as the osteochondroses, slipped capital femoral epiphysis, and scoliosis, are not corrected by the growth process. These disorders are progressive, can cause permanent disability, and require treatment. Disorders such as congenital dislocation of the hip and congenital clubfoot are present at birth. Both of these disorders are best treated during infancy. Regular examinations during the first year of life are recommended as a means of achieving early diagnosis of such disorders.

Scoliosis is a lateral deviation of the spinal column that may or may not include rotation or deformity of the vertebrae. Scoliosis is classified as postural, which corrects with bending, or structural, which does not. Structural scoliosis is a fixed deformity classified according to the cause: congenital, which results from defects in vertebral development; neuromuscular, which is caused by diseases such as cerebral palsy; and idiopathic, which is the most common form. Curves between 30 and 40 degrees usually are considered for bracing, and those greater than 40 to 45 degrees are considered for surgery. If scoliosis is left untreated, the curve may progress to an extent that compromises cardiopulmonary function and creates a risk for neurologic complications.

Metabolic Bone Disease

After completing this section of the chapter, you should be able to meet the following objectives:

- Name the three factors responsible for maintaining the equilibrium of bone tissue
- Cite the origin of osteoclasts and osteoblasts and describe their functions in bone remodeling
- Describe the function of the RANK ligand/receptor pathway and the osteoprotegerin (OPG)-blocking molecule in the regulation of bone remodeling
- Describe risk factors that contribute to the development of osteoporosis and relate them to the prevention of the disorder
- Describe the primary features of osteoporotic bone
- Identify risk factors for the development of osteoporosis
- Define the female athlete triad
- Explain the methods used in the diagnosis of osteoporosis
- Describe the actions of medications used in the treatment of osteoporosis
- Compare the pathogenesis and manifestations of osteomalacia and rickets
- Characterize the cause and manifestations of Paget disease

Bone remodeling, or the process of bone resorption and formation, is continuous throughout life. There are two types of bone remodeling: structural and internal remodeling. Structural remodeling involves deposition of new bone on the outer aspect of the shaft at the same time that bone is resorbed from the inner aspect of the shaft. It occurs during growth and results in a bone having adult form and shape. Internal remodeling largely involves the replacement of trabecular bone and is continuous during adulthood.

In the adult, approximately 25% of trabecular bone is replaced each year, compared with 3% of compact bone.[29] In the adult skeleton, bone remodeling proceeds in cycles that involve resorption of old bone by osteoclasts and subsequent formation of new bone by osteoblasts (Fig. 58-16). After the bone formation has ceased, the bone is covered by a distinct type of terminally differentiated osteoblast.

The sequence of bone resorption and bone formation is activated by many stimuli, including the actions of parathyroid hormone and calcitonin. It begins with osteoclastic resorption of existing bone, during which the organic (protein matrix) and the inorganic (mineral) components are removed. The sequence proceeds to the formation of new bone by osteoblasts. In the adult, the length of one sequence (*i.e.,* bone resorption and forma-

Quiescent bone surface covered by lining cells

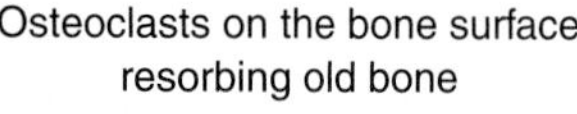

Osteoclasts on the bone surface resorbing old bone

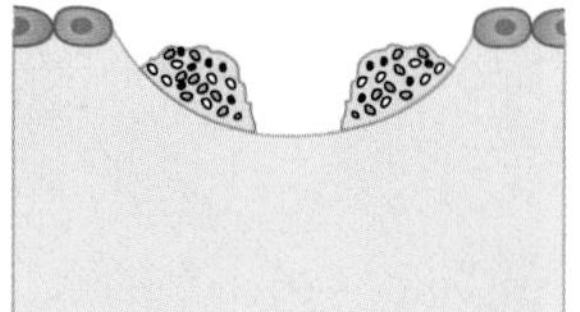

Osteoblasts filling the resorption cavity with osteoid

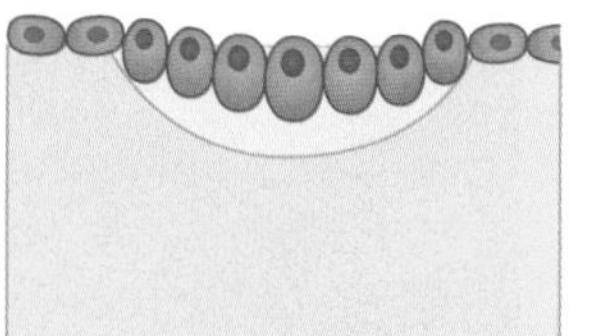

Osteoid becoming mineralized

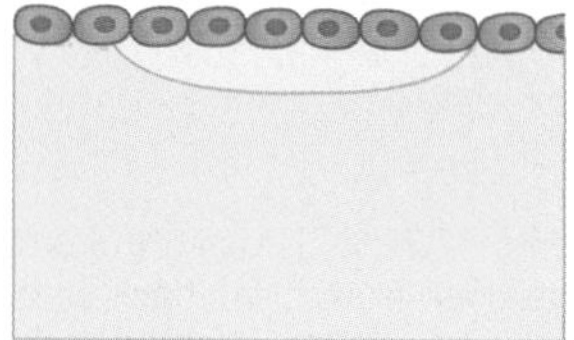

FIGURE 58-16 The process of bone resorption by the osteoclasts and subsequent bone formation by the osteoblasts.

tion) is approximately 4 months. Ideally, the replaced bone should equal the absorbed bone. If it does not, there is a net loss of bone. In the elderly, for example, bone resorption and formation no longer are perfectly coupled, and bone mass is lost.

The three major influences on the equilibrium of bone tissue are mechanical stress, calcium and phosphate levels in the extracellular fluid, and hormones and local growth factors and cytokines, which influence bone resorption and formation. Mechanical stress stimulates osteoblastic activity and formation of the organic matrix. It is important in preventing bone atrophy and in healing fractures. Bone serves as a storage site for extracellular calcium and phosphate ions. Consequently, alterations in the extracellular levels of these ions affect their deposition in bone (see Chapter 33). Vitamin C is required for proper collagen formation. A deficiency of vitamin C can result in a disease called *scurvy*. In the absence of vitamin C, the epiphyseal plates and bony shaft of growing bone are so thin and fragile that they are predisposed to fractures. In the adult, vitamin C deficiency affects bone maintenance rather than growth. Vitamin D is needed for intestinal absorption of calcium and phosphate. Blood levels of calcium and phosphate are regulated by parathyroid hormone and calcitonin. Parathyroid hormone promotes bone resorption, and calcitonin inhibits bone resorption.

Osteoclasts and osteoblasts are derived from progenitor cells in the bone marrow[29] (see Chapter 56). The osteoclasts originate from hematopoietic precursors and osteoblasts from stromal (supporting) cells in the bone marrow. However, the development of osteoclasts from hematopoietic precursors cannot take place unless stromal/osteoblastic cells are present. The effects of systemic hormones and local influences on osteoclast development are mediated by stromal/osteoblastic cells. The differentiation and function of osteoclasts and osteoblasts are regulated by chemical messengers, including colony-stimulating factors and other cytokines (see Chapter 19). Interleukin-6, which is produced in response to systemic hormones such as parathyroid hormone and vitamin D, stimulates the early stages of osteoclast development. Interleukin-6 is thought to be involved in the abnormal bone resorption associated with Paget disease (discussed later). The inhibitory effects of estrogen on bone resorption are thought to be mediated through the inhibition of interleukin-6. With aging, the ability of the bone marrow to produce osteoblastic precursors is decreased.

Recent evidence suggests that an interaction between a chemical messenger called the *RANK ligand,* which is produced by the stromal/osteoblastic cells, and RANK receptors on the macrophage/osteoclastic precursor cell is essential for the differentiation and proliferation of osteoclasts[30,31] (Fig. 58-17). There also is evidence of a blocking molecule called *osteoprotegerin (OPG)* that can prevent the RANK ligand from binding to the RANK receptor, thus inhibiting the formation of osteoclasts. It is now believed that dysregulation of the RANK ligand/receptor pathway plays a prominent role in the pathogenesis of bone diseases such as osteoporosis.

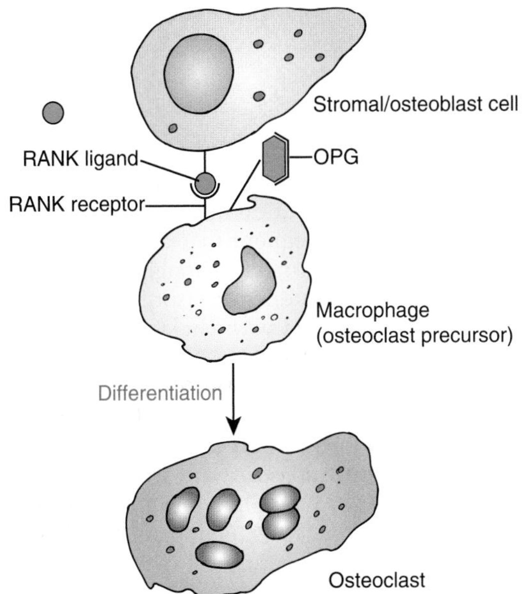

FIGURE 58-17 Molecular mechanisms of RANK ligand/receptor interactions in mediating osteoclast differentiation. The osteoprotegerin (OPG) molecule can block the receptor-mediated action of the RANK ligand. (Adapted from Kumar V., Cotran R.S., Robbins S.L. [2002]. *Robbins basic pathology* [7th ed., p. 759]. Philadelphia: W.B. Saunders)

OSTEOPENIA

Osteopenia is a condition that is common to all metabolic bone diseases. It is characterized by a reduction in bone mass greater than expected for age, race, or sex; and it occurs because of a decrease in bone formation, inadequate bone mineralization, or excessive bone deossification. *Osteopenia* is not a diagnosis but a term used to describe an apparent lack of bone seen on x-ray studies. The major causes of osteopenia are osteoporosis, osteomalacia, malignancies

METABOLIC BONE DISORDERS

- Metabolic bone disorders have their origin in the bone remodeling process that involves an orderly sequence of osteoclastic bone reabsorption, the formation of new bone by the osteoblasts, and mineralization of the newly formed osteoid tissue.
- Osteoporosis represents an increased loss of total bone mass due to an imbalance between bone absorption and bone formation, most often related to the aging process and decreased estrogen levels in postmenopausal women.
- Osteomalacia and rickets represent a softening of bone due to inadequate mineralization of the bone matrix caused by a deficiency of calcium or phosphate.
- Paget disease is a disorder involving excessive bone destruction and repair, resulting in structural deformities of long bones, spine, pelvis, and cranium.

such as multiple myeloma, and endocrine disorders such as hyperparathyroidism and hyperthyroidism.

OSTEOPOROSIS

Osteoporosis is a skeletal disorder characterized by the loss of bone mass and deterioration of the architecture of cancellous bone with a subsequent increase in bone fragility and susceptibility to fractures. Although osteoporosis can occur as the result of an endocrine disorder or malignancy, it most often is associated with the aging process. After maximal bone mass is attained at 30 years of age, the rate of bone resorption exceeds formation, causing a continuous loss of bone mass.[32] It can increase to approximately 1% to 2% per year or more in menopausal women. An estimated 25 million Americans are affected with osteoporosis, and more than 1.5 million sustain fractures related to osteoporosis each year. After menopause, a woman's lifetime risk of osteoporosis fracture is 1 in 3.[33]

Pathogenesis

The pathogenesis of osteoporosis is unclear, but most data suggest an imbalance between bone resorption and formation such that bone resorption exceeds bone formation. Although both of these factors play a role in most cases of osteoporosis, their relative contribution to bone loss may vary dependent on age, sex, nutritional status, and genetic predisposition.

Under normal conditions, bone mass increases steadily during childhood, reaching a peak in the young adult years. The peak bone mass is an important determinant of the subsequent risk for osteoporosis. It is determined in part by genetic factors, hormone (estrogen) levels, exercise, calcium intake and absorption, and environmental factors. Genetic factors are linked, in largest part, to the maximal amount of bone in a given person, referred to as *peak bone mass*. Bone mass positively correlates with the amount of skin pigmentation; whites have the least bone mass, and African Americans have the most. Mexican-American women have bone mass intermediate between non-Hispanic white women and African-American women. Although osteoporosis is uncommon among African-American women, many cases are seen among postmenopausal women with brown and yellow skin.[34] Exercise may prevent or delay the onset of osteoporosis by increasing peak bone mineral density during periods of growth. Poor nutrition or an age-related decrease in intestinal absorption of calcium because of deficient activation of vitamin D may contribute to the development of osteoporosis, particularly in the elderly.

Hormonal factors play a significant role in the development of osteoporosis, particularly in postmenopausal women. Postmenopausal osteoporosis, which is caused by an estrogen deficiency, is manifested by a loss of cancellous bone and a predisposition to fractures of the vertebrae and distal radius. The loss of bone mass is greatest during early menopause when estrogen levels are withdrawing. Several factors appear to influence the increased loss of bone mass associated with an estrogen deficiency. Decreased estrogen levels are associated with an increase in cytokines (*e.g.*, interleukin-1, interleukin-6, and tumor necrosis factor) that stimulate the production of osteoclast precursors. Recent studies indicate that estrogen deficiency also influences osteoclast differentiation via the RANK receptor pathways.[30] Estrogen stimulates the production of OPG and thus inhibits the formation of osteoclasts; it also blunts the responsiveness of osteoclast precursors to the RANK ligand. With menopause and its accompanying estrogen deficiency, this inhibition of osteoclast production is lost.[30] Evidence also suggests that estrogen deficiency, as well as normal aging, may lead to decreased osteoblastic activity and new bone formation. Thus, the bone loss associated with estrogen deficiency may be caused by a combination of increased bone resorption and decreased bone formation. Testosterone deficiency may contribute to bone loss in men with senile osteoporosis, although the effect is not of the same magnitude as that caused by estrogen deficiency.

Age-related changes in bone density occur in all individuals and contribute to the development of osteoporosis in both sexes.[35] After maximal bone mass is attained at about 30 years of age, the rate of bone loss for both sexes is approximately 0.7% per year, and it increases to approximately 1% per year or more in menopausal women.[30] The age-related loss of bone reflects decreased osteoblast activity as well as an increase in osteoclastic activity. The greatest losses occur in areas containing abundant cancellous bone, such as the spine and femoral neck. Hence, these are common sites for fractures in persons with osteoporosis.

Secondary osteoporosis is associated with many conditions, including endocrine disorders, malabsorption disorders, malignancies, alcoholism, and certain medications.[36] Persons with endocrine disorders such as hyperthyroidism, hyperparathyroidism, Cushing's syndrome, or diabetes mellitus are at high risk for development of osteoporosis. Hyperthyroidism causes an acceleration of bone turnover. Some malignancies (*e.g.*, multiple myeloma) secrete osteoclast-activating factor causing significant bone loss. Alcohol is a direct inhibitor of osteoblasts and may also inhibit calcium absorption. Corticosteroid use is the most common form of drug-related osteoporosis, and its long-term use in the treatment of disorders such as rheumatoid arthritis and chronic obstructive lung disease is associated with a high rate of fractures.[37] The prolonged use of medications that increase calcium excretion, such as aluminum-containing antacids, corticosteroids, and anticonvulsants, also is associated with bone loss.[38] Persons with human immunodeficiency virus (HIV) infection or acquired immunodeficiency syndrome (AIDS) who are being treated with antiretroviral therapy may develop a lower bone density and signs of osteoporosis and osteopenia.[39]

Several groups of children and adolescents are at increased risk for decreased bone mass, including premature and low-birth-weight infants who have lower than expected bone mass in the early weeks of life, children who require treatment with corticosteroid drugs (*e.g.*, those with childhood inflammatory diseases and transplant recipients), children with cystic fibrosis, and those with hypogonadal states (*e.g.*, anorexia nervosa and the female athlete triad).[40] Children with cystic fibrosis often have impaired gastrointestinal function that reduces the absorption of calcium and other nutrients, and many also require the frequent use of corticosteroid drugs.

Premature osteoporosis is increasingly being seen in female athletes owing to an increased prevalence of eating disorders and amenorrhea.[40] The *female athlete triad* refers to a pattern of disordered eating that leads to amenorrhea and eventually osteoporosis. Poor nutrition, combined with intense training, can decrease the critical body fat-to-muscle ratio needed for normal menses and estrogen production by the ovary.[41] The lack of estrogen, combined with the lack of calcium and vitamin D from dietary deficiencies, results in a loss of bone density and increased risk for fractures.[41] There is a concern that athletes with low bone mineral density will be at increased risk for fractures during their competitive years. It is unclear whether osteoporosis induced by amenorrhea is reversible. It most frequently affects women engaged in endurance sports, such as running and swimming; in activities where appearance is important, such as figure skating, diving, and gymnastics; or in sports with weight categories, such as horse racing, martial arts, and rowing.[42]

Manifestations

Osteoporotic changes occur in the diaphysis and metaphysis of bone. The diameter of the bone enlarges with age, causing the outer supporting cortex to become thinner. In severe osteoporosis, the bones begin to resemble the fragile structure of a fine porcelain vase. There is loss of trabeculae from cancellous bone and thinning of the cortex to such an extent that minimal stress causes fractures (Fig. 58-18). The changes that occur with osteoporosis have been explained by two distinct disease processes affecting women early and late in life.[34] Type I is caused by early postmenopausal estrogen deficiency and is manifested by loss of trabecular bone, with a predisposition to fractures of the vertebrae and distal radius. Type II (*i.e.*, senile osteoporosis) is caused by a calcium deficiency and is a slower process in which cortical and trabecular bone are lost. Hip fractures, which are seen later in life, result from the second type. The different pathogenic mechanisms and presentations make it difficult to generalize about osteoporosis.

Osteoporosis is usually a silent disorder. Often, the first manifestations of the disorder are those that accompany a skeletal fracture—a vertebral compression fracture or fractures of the hip, pelvis, humerus, or any other bone. Typically, the fractures occur with less force than usual, such as in a gymnast performing a common jump. Women who present with fractures are much more likely to sustain another fracture than are women of the same age without osteoporosis. Wedging and collapse of vertebrae cause a loss of height in the vertebral column and kyphosis, a condition commonly referred to as *dowager's hump*. Usually, there is no generalized bone tenderness. When pain occurs, it is related to fractures. Systemic symptoms such as weakness and weight loss suggest that the osteoporosis may be caused by underlying disease.

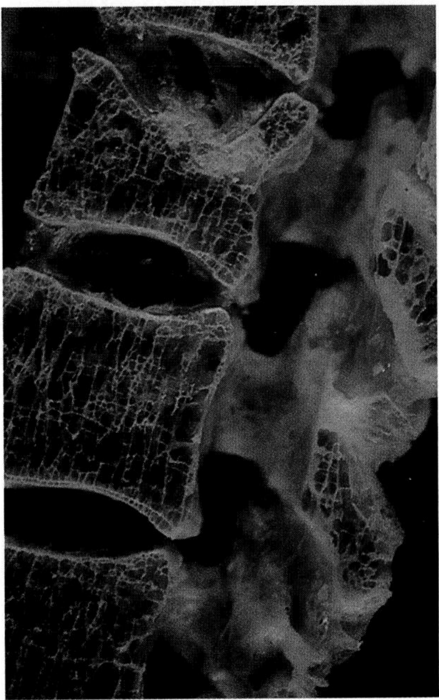

FIGURE 58-18 Osteoporosis. A section of the vertebral column, in which the bone marrow has been washed out, demonstrates a loss of bone tissue and a compression fracture of a vertebral body. (Rubin E., Farber J.L. [1999]. *Pathology* [3rd ed., p. 1367]. Philadelphia: Lippincott-Raven)

Diagnosis and Treatment

An important advance in diagnostic methods used for the identification of osteoporosis has been the use of bone mineral density (BMD) assessment. The clinical method of choice for bone density studies is dual-energy x-ray absorptiometry (DXA) of the spine and hip.[43] Whenever possible, the first four vertebrae should be included. The site with the lowest score should be used to make a diagnosis. In the United States, the National Osteoporosis Foundation sets the diagnostic criterion at 2 standard deviations below peak value. According to these standards, most women would be candidates for treatment by 60 years of age.[34] Measurement of BMD has become increasingly common for early detection and fracture prevention. Measurement of serial heights in older adults is another simple way to screen for osteoporosis. A further advance in the diagnosis of osteoporosis is the refinement of risk factors, permitting better analysis of risk pertaining to particular persons. Women older than 65 years of age who weigh less than 140 pounds at menopause or who have never used estrogens for more than 6 months should be screened for osteoporosis. The simple mnemonic ABONE (*A* = age, *B* = bulk, and *ONE* = never on estrogen) aids in remembering these criteria.[44]

Prevention and early detection of osteoporosis are essential to the prevention of the associated deformities and fractures. It is important to identify persons in high-risk groups so that treatment can begin early. Postmenopausal women of small stature or lean body mass, those with sedentary lifestyles, those with poor calcium intake, and those with diseases that demineralize bone are at greatest risk. Other risk factors include an age of 80 years or greater, maternal history of hip fracture, caffeine intake exceeding two cups of coffee each day, previous hyperthyroidism, current anticonvulsant therapy, and current use of long-acting benzodiazepines. Risk factors for osteoporosis are listed in Chart 58-1.

Regular exercise and adequate calcium intake are important factors in preventing osteoporosis. Weight-bearing exercises such as walking, jogging, rowing, and weight lifting are important in the maintenance of bone mass. Studies have indicated that premenopausal women need more than 1000 mg per day, and postmenopausal women need 1500 mg of calcium daily.[43] This means that adults should drink three to four glasses of milk daily or substitute other foods that are high in calcium. Because most older American women do not consume a sufficient quantity of dairy products to meet their calcium needs, calcium supplementation is recommended. Calcium tablets vary in content of elemental calcium. Calcium carbonate contains 40% elemental calcium but requires normal stomach acidity to be absorbed. Calcium citrate is 21% elemental calcium but can be absorbed in the absence of acidity.[44] There still are conflicting data on recommendations for vitamin D supplementation. Deficient activation of vitamin D may be an important factor in the impaired intestinal absorption of calcium in the elderly. On the basis of this evidence, 1,25-dihydroxyvitamin D_3 is being studied as a treatment for osteoporosis. A daily intake of 400 to 800 IU of vitamin D is recommended because vitamin D optimizes calcium absorption and inhibits parathyroid secretion, which stimulates calcium resorption from bone.[45]

Active treatment of osteoporosis uses four types of antiresorptive agents: gonadal hormones (estrogen), calcitonin, fluorides, and bisphosphonates. Calcitonin can be used to decrease osteoclastic activity. It has some effect on bone pain, but until recently, it was available only as an injectable drug. A nasal spray formulation is now available. The use of sodium fluoride has diminished because of questionable efficacy. There is increasing evidence that the use of parathyroid hormone (PTH) as an anabolic treatment can stimulate bone formation and increase bone density.[46] PTH acts in osteoblast-mediated bone formation.

Although estrogen is one of the most effective interventions for reducing the incidence and progression of osteoporosis in postmenopausal women, the use of hormone therapy (estrogen plus progestin) has come under scrutiny following the recent release of data from the Women's Health Initiative[47,48] (see Chapter 46). A selective estrogen receptor modulator (SERM; raloxifene) that acts only on specific estrogen receptors was recently approved by the U.S. Food and Drug Administration (FDA) for prevention and treatment of osteoporosis in postmenopausal women. The use of phytoestrogens, naturally occurring plant compounds, has gained popularity as an alternative to estrogens; however, information regarding their effect on bone health is conflicting and incomplete.[49]

Biphosphates are effective inhibitors of bone resorption and the most effective agents for prevention and treatment of osteoporosis. The bisphosphonates (*e.g.,* alendronate and risedronate) are analogs of endogenous inorganic pyrophosphate that the body cannot break down. In bone, they bind to hydroxyapatite and prevent bone resorption through the inhibition of osteoclast activity. Bisphosphonates have been shown to reduce the risk for vertebral and hip fractures by up to 60%. The most dramatic impact has been in the reduction of multiple spine fractures, showing that treatment can decrease progression of the disease.

Persons with osteoporosis have many special needs. In treating fractures, it is important to minimize immobility. Surgical intervention is done for stable fracture fixation that allows early restoration of mobility and function; for fractures of the lower extremities, this means early weight bearing. Walking and swimming are encouraged. Unsafe conditions that predispose persons to falls and fractures should be corrected or avoided. Unfortunately, because of an increase in sedentary lifestyles and the continued increase in life expectancy, the incidence of osteoporosis could reach epidemic proportions in the coming decades if better prevention strategies are not implemented.

CHART 58-1

Risk Factors Associated With Osteoporosis

Personal Characteristics

Advanced age
Female
White (fair, thin skin)
Small bone structure
Postmenopausal
Family history

Lifestyle

Sedentary
Calcium deficiency (long-term)
High-protein diet
Excessive alcohol intake
Excessive caffeine intake
Smoking

Drug and Disease Related

Aluminum-containing antacids
Anticonvulsants
Heparin
Corticosteroids or Cushing's disease
Gastrectomy
Diabetes mellitus
Chronic obstructive lung disease
Malignancy
Hyperthyroidism
Hyperparathyroidism
Rheumatoid arthritis

OSTEOMALACIA AND RICKETS

In contrast to osteoporosis, which causes a loss of total bone mass and results in brittle bones, osteomalacia and rickets produce a softening of the bones and do not involve the loss of bone matrix. Approximately 60% of bone is mineral content, approximately 30% is organic matrix, and the remainder is living bone cells. The organic matrix and the inorganic mineral salts are needed for normal bone consistency. If the inorganic mineral salts are removed from fresh bone (by dilute nitric acid), the organic matrix that remains still resembles a bone, but it is so flexible that it can be tied in a knot. When a bone is placed over a hot flame, the organic material is destroyed, and the bone becomes brittle.

Osteomalacia

Osteomalacia is a generalized bone condition in which inadequate mineralization of bone results from a calcium or phosphate deficiency, or both. It is sometimes referred to as the adult form of rickets.

There are two main causes of osteomalacia: insufficient calcium absorption from the intestine because of a lack of calcium, and resistance to the action of vitamin D and phosphate deficiency due to increased renal losses or decreased intestinal absorption. Vitamin D is a fat-soluble vitamin that is absorbed intact through the intestine or produced in the skin with exposure to ultraviolet irradiation (see Chapter 56). Vitamin D that is absorbed from the intestine or synthesized in the skin is inactive. Vitamin D is activated in a two-step process that begins in the liver and is completed in the kidney. Vitamin D deficiency is caused most commonly by reduced vitamin D absorption as a result of biliary tract or intestinal diseases that impair fat and fat-soluble vitamin absorption. Lack of vitamin D in the diet is rare in the United States because many foods are fortified with the vitamin. Anticonvulsant medications, such as phenobarbital and phenytoin, induce hepatic hydroxylases that accelerate breakdown of the active forms of vitamin D.

A form of osteomalacia called *renal rickets* occurs in persons with chronic renal failure. It is caused by the inability of the kidney to activate vitamin D and excrete phosphate and is accompanied by hyperparathyroidism, increased bone turnover, and increased bone resorption (see Chapter 36). Another form of osteomalacia results from renal tubular defects that cause excessive phosphate losses. This form of osteomalacia is commonly referred to as *vitamin D–resistant rickets* and often is a familial disorder.[8] It is inherited as an X-linked dominant gene passed by mothers to one half of their children and by fathers to their daughters only. This form of osteomalacia affects boys more severely than girls. Long-standing primary hyperparathyroidism causes increased calcium resorption from bone and hypophosphatemia, which can lead to rickets in children and osteomalacia in adults. Another cause of phosphate deficiency is the long-term use of antacids, such as aluminum hydroxide, that bind dietary forms of phosphate and prevent their absorption.

The incidence of osteomalacia is high among the elderly because of diets deficient in calcium and vitamin D and often is compounded by the intestinal malabsorption problems that accompany aging. Osteomalacia often is seen in cultures in which the diet is deficient in vitamin D, such as in northern China, Japan, and northern India. Women in these areas have a higher incidence of the disorder than men because of the combined effects of pregnancy, lactation, and more indoor confinement. Osteomalacia occasionally is seen in strict vegetarians, persons who have had a gastrectomy, and those on long-term anticonvulsant, tranquilizer, sedative, muscle relaxant, or diuretic drugs. There also is a greater incidence of osteomalacia in the colder regions of the world, particularly during the winter months, probably because of lessened exposure to sunlight.

The clinical manifestations of osteomalacia are bone pain, tenderness, and fractures as the disease progresses. In severe cases, muscle weakness often is an early sign. The cause of muscle weakness is unclear. The combined effects of gravity, muscle weakness, and bone softening contribute to the development of deformities. There may be a dorsal kyphosis in the spine, rib deformities, a heart-shaped pelvis, and marked bowing of the tibiae and femurs. Osteomalacia predisposes a person to pathologic fractures in the weakened areas, especially in the distal radius and proximal femur. In contrast to osteoporosis, it is not a significant cause of hip fractures. There may be delayed healing and poor retention of internal fixation devices. Osteomalacia usually is accompanied by a compensatory or secondary hyperparathyroidism stimulated by low serum calcium levels. Parathyroid hormone reduces renal absorption of phosphate and removes calcium from the bone. Serum calcium levels are only slightly reduced in osteomalacia.

Diagnostic measures are directed toward identifying osteomalacia and establishing its cause. Diagnostic methods include x-ray studies, laboratory tests, bone scan, and bone biopsy. X-ray findings typical of osteomalacia are the development of transverse lines or pseudofractures called *Looser's zones* or *milkman's fractures*.[8] These apparently are caused by stress fractures that are inadequately healed or by the mechanical inadequacy of penetrating nutrient vessels.[14] A bone biopsy may be done to confirm the diagnosis of osteomalacia in a person with nonspecific osteopenia who shows no improvement after treatment with exercise, vitamin D, and calcium.

The treatment of osteomalacia is directed at the underlying cause. If the problem is nutritional, restoring adequate amounts of calcium and vitamin D to the diet may be sufficient. The elderly with intestinal malabsorption also may benefit from vitamin D. The least expensive and most effective long-term treatment is a diet rich in vitamin D (*i.e.*, fish, dairy products, and margarine) along with careful exposure to the midday sun. Vitamin D is specific for adult osteomalacia and vitamin D–resistant rickets, but large doses usually are needed to overcome the resistance to its calcium-absorption action and to prevent renal loss of phosphate. The biologically active forms of vitamin D, 25-OH vitamin D (calciferol) or 1,25-$(OH)_2$ vitamin D (calcitriol), are available for use in the treatment of osteomalacia resistant to vitamin D (*i.e.*, osteomalacia resulting from chronic liver disease and kidney failure). If osteomalacia is caused by malabsorption, the treatment is directed toward correcting the primary disease. For example, adequate replacement of pancreatic enzymes is of paramount importance in pancreatic insufficiency. In renal tubular disorders, the treatment is directed at the altered renal physiology.

Rickets

Rickets is a disorder of vitamin D deficiency, inadequate calcium absorption, and impaired mineralization of bone in children. Children with rickets manifest inadequate mineralization not only of bone but also of the cartilaginous matrix of the epiphyseal growth plate. Rickets occurs primarily in underdeveloped areas of the world and among immigrants to developed countries. The causes are inadequate exposure to sunlight (*e.g.*, children are often kept clothed and indoors) and prolonged breast-feeding without vitamin D supplementation.[50] Although the vitamin D content of human milk is low, the combination of breast milk and sunlight exposure usually provides sufficient vitamin D. Another cause of rickets is the use of commercial alternative milks (*e.g.*, soy or rice beverages) that are not fortified with vitamin D.[51] A dietary deficiency in calcium and phosphorous may also contribute to the development of rickets. A newly discovered genetic mutation also can cause vitamin D deficiency rickets, a condition that does not respond to simple vitamin supplementation. The mutation results in the absence of a critical enzyme in vitamin D metabolism.[52]

The pathology of rickets is the same as that of osteomalacia seen in adults. Because rickets affects children during periods of active growth, the structural changes seen in the bone are somewhat different. Bones become deformed; ossification at epiphyseal plates is delayed and disordered, resulting in widening of the epiphyseal cartilage plate. Any new bone that does grow is unmineralized.

The symptoms of rickets usually are noticed between 6 months and 3 years of age. The child usually has stunted growth, with a height sometimes far below the normal range. Weight often is not affected so that the children, many of whom present with a protruding abdomen (*i.e.*, rachitic potbelly), have been described as presenting a Buddha-like appearance when sitting. Early symptoms are lethargy and muscle weakness, which may be accompanied by convulsions or tetany related to hypocalcemia. Irritability is common. In severe cases, children lose their skin pigment, acquire flabby subcutaneous tissue, and have poorly developed musculature. The ends of long bones and ribs are enlarged. The thorax may be abnormally shaped, with prominent rib cartilage (*i.e.*, rachitic rosary). The legs exhibit bowleg or knock-knee deformities. The skull is enlarged and soft, and closure of the fontanels is delayed. Teeth are slow to develop, and the child may have difficulty standing.

Rickets is treated with a balanced diet sufficient in calcium, phosphorus, and vitamin D. Exposure to sunlight also is important, especially for premature infants and those on artificial milk feedings. Supplemental vitamin D in excess of normal requirements is given for several months. Maintenance of good posture, positioning, and bracing in older children are used to prevent deformities. After the disease is controlled, deformities may have to be surgically corrected as the child grows.

PAGET DISEASE

Paget disease (*i.e.*, osteitis deformans) is discussed separately because it is not a true metabolic disease. Aside from osteoporosis, it is the second most common bone disorder.[53] Paget disease is a progressive skeletal disorder that involves excessive bone destruction and repair and is characterized by increasing structural changes of the long bones, spine, pelvis, and cranium.[54] The pelvis and upper femur are the areas of the skeleton most involved.[55] The disease usually begins during mid-adulthood and becomes progressively more common thereafter.[14] In children, hyperostosis corticalis deformans juvenilis (a rare inherited disorder), hyperphosphatemia, and diseases that cause diaphyseal stenosis may mimic Paget disease and sometimes are referred to as *juvenile Paget disease*.

The cause of Paget disease is unknown. It may be caused by a virus capable of inciting osteoclastic activity.[13,14] It has been suggested that the virus may induce secretion of interferon-6, which is a potent stimulator of osteoclastic recruitment and resorptive activity.[14] The abnormal osteoclast activity may be the result of both genetic and environmental factors.[56] The disease usually begins insidiously and progresses slowly over many years. An initial osteolytic phase is followed by an osteoblastic sclerotic phase. During the initial osteolytic phase, abnormal osteoclasts proliferate. Bone resorption occurs so rapidly that new bone formation cannot keep up, and the bone is replaced by fibrous tissue. The two processes of destruction and rebuilding occur simultaneously. The bones increase in size and thickness because of accelerated bone resorption followed by abnormal regeneration. Irregular bone formation results in sclerotic and osteoblastic lesions. The result is a thick layer of coarse bone with a rough and pitted outer surface that has the appearance of pumice (Fig. 58-19). Histologically, Paget lesions show increased vascularity and bone marrow fibrosis with intense cellular activity. The bone has a somewhat mosaic-like pattern caused by areas of density outlined by heavy blue lines, called *cement lines*.

Manifestations

The disease varies in severity from a simple lesion to involvement of many bones. It may be present long before it is detected clinically. The clinical manifestations of Paget disease depend on the specific area involved. Approximately 70% of persons with the disorder are totally asymptomatic, and the disease is discovered accidentally.[53] Involvement of the skull causes headaches, intermittent tinnitus, vertigo, and eventual hearing loss. In the spine, collapse of the anterior vertebrae causes kyphosis of the thoracic spine. The femur and tibia become bowed (see Fig. 58-19). Softening of the femoral neck can cause coxa vara (*i.e.*, reduced angle of the femoral neck). Coxa vara, in combination with softening of the sacral and iliac bones, causes a waddling gait. When the lesion affects only one bone, it may cause only mild pain and stiffness. Progressive deossification weakens and distorts the bone structure. The deossification process begins along the inner cortical surfaces and continues until the substance of the bone disappears. Pathologic fractures

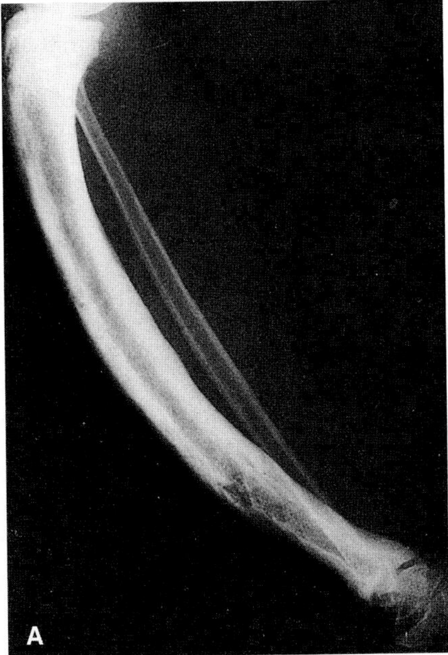

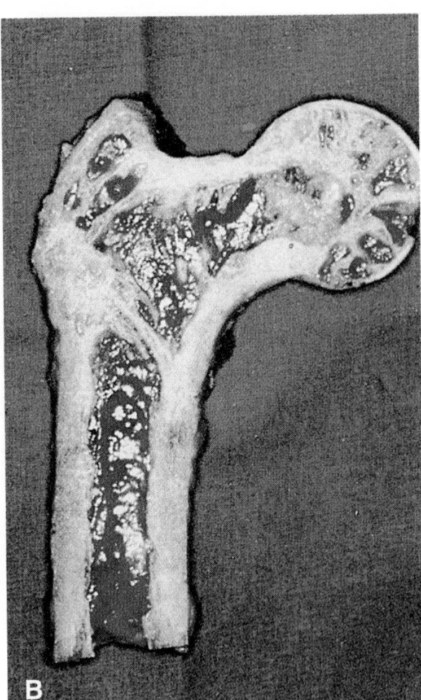

FIGURE 58-19 Paget disease. (**A**) The proximal end of the femur affected by Paget disease shows replacement of the normal cancellous architecture of bone by course thick bundles of trabecular bone. (**B**) The cortical bone is irregularly thickened and exhibits a coarse, granular appearance instead of the normally smooth cortical bone. (Rubin E., Farber L.F. [1999]. *Pathophysiology* [3rd ed., p. 1377]. Philadelphia: Lippincott-Raven)

may occur, especially in the bones subjected to the greatest stress (*e.g.,* upper femur, lower spine, pelvic bones). These fractures often heal poorly, with excessive and poorly distributed callus.

Other manifestations of Paget disease include nerve palsy syndromes from lesions in the upper extremities, mental deterioration, and cardiovascular disease. Cardiovascular disease is the most serious complication and is listed as the most common cause of death in those with advanced generalized Paget disease. It is caused by vasodilation of the vessels in the skin and subcutaneous tissues overlying the affected bones. When one third to one half of the skeleton is affected, the increased blood flow may lead to high-output cardiac failure. Calcific aortic stenosis may occur in severe cases. Ventilatory capacity may be limited by rib and spine involvement.

Osteogenic sarcomas occur in 5% to 10% of persons with severe polyostotic disease.[14] One fifth of all osteogenic sarcomas in persons 50 years of age or older originate in people with Paget disease.[57] The bones most often affected, in order of frequency, are the femur, pelvis, humerus, and tibia. There appears to be a close histopathogenic relationship between Paget disease and the associated sarcoma.[57]

Diagnosis and Treatment

Diagnosis of Paget disease is based on characteristic bone deformities and x-ray changes. Elevated levels of serum alkaline phosphatase and urinary hydroxyproline support the diagnosis, and continued surveillance of these levels may be used to monitor the effectiveness of treatment. Bone scans are used to detect the rapid bone turnover indicative of active disease and to monitor the response to treatment. The scan cannot identify bone activity resulting from malignant lesions. Bone biopsy may be done to differentiate the lesion from osteomyelitis or a primary or metastatic bone tumor.

The treatment of Paget disease is based on the degree of pain and the extent of the disease. Pain can be reduced with nonsteroidal or other antiinflammatory agents. Suppressive agents such as the hormone calcitonin, mithramycin, and bisphosphonates are used to manage pain and prevent further spread of the disease and neurologic defects. Bisphosphonate therapy is the most effective way to control Paget disease.[58] These drugs act by binding directly to bone minerals, inhibiting bone loss by rapidly decreasing bone resorption, followed by a secondary slower decrease in the rate of bone formation.[53] Treatment usually is continued for 3 to 4 months, although recent studies are evaluating shorter courses of treatment. Calcitonin also inhibits bone resorption. It is available in injectable and nasal spray form, but only the injectable form is approved for treatment of Paget disease by the FDA. Persons with Paget disease should receive adequate doses of calcium and vitamin D.

In summary, in addition to its structural function, the skeleton is a homeostatic organ. Metabolic bone diseases such as osteoporosis, osteomalacia, rickets, and Paget disease are the result of a disruption in the equilibrium of bone formation and resorption. Osteoporosis, which is the most common of the metabolic bone diseases, occurs when the rate of bone resorption is greater than that of bone formation. It is seen frequently in postmenopausal women and is the major cause of fractures in persons older than 45 years of age. Osteomalacia and rickets are caused by inadequate mineralization of bone matrix, primarily because of a deficiency of vitamin D. Paget disease results from excessive osteoclastic activity and is characterized by the formation of poor-quality bone. The success rate of the various drugs and hormones that are used to treat metabolic bone diseases varies. Further research is needed to clarify the cause, pathology, and treatment of these diseases.

REVIEW EXERCISES

A newborn girl was found to have developmental dysplasia of the hip (DDH) during a routine screening examination.

A. Describe the anatomic abnormalities that are present in the disorder.

B. Explain the need for early treatment of DDH.

A 12-year-old girl was noted to have asymmetry of the shoulders, scapular height, and pelvic height during routine physical examination. On x-ray examination, she is found to have a 30-degree curvature of the spine.

A. What possible treatments are available for this girl?

B. Describe the physical problems associated with progressive scoliosis.

A 60-year-old postmenopausal woman presents with a compression fracture of the vertebrae. She has also noticed increased backache and loss of height over the past few years.

A. Explain how the lack of estrogen and aging contribute to the development of osteoporosis.

B. What other factors should be considered when assessing the risk for developing osteoporosis?

C. What is the best way to measure bone density?

D. Name the two most important factors in preventing osteoporosis.

E. What medications might be used to treat this woman's condition?

References

1. Moore K.L., Persaud T.V.N. (2003). *The developing human* (6th ed., pp. 382–399). Philadelphia: W.B. Saunders.
2. Cormack D.H. (1993). *Essential histology* (pp. 174–178). Philadelphia: J.B. Lippincott.
3. Gartner L.P., Hiatt J.L. (2001). *Color textbook of histology* (2nd ed., pp. 129–154). Philadelphia: W.B. Saunders.
4. Bruce R.W. (1996). Torsional and angular deformities. *Pediatric Clinics of North America 43,* 867–881.
5. Thompson G.H. (2004). Bone and joint disorders. In Behrman R.E., Kliegman R.M., Jenson H.B. (Eds.), *Nelson textbook of pediatrics* (17th ed., pp. 2251–2290). Philadelphia: W.B. Saunders.
6. Maher A.B., Salmond S.B., Pellino T.A. (2002). *Orthopaedic Nursing* (3rd ed., pp. 552–568, 601–603). Philadelphia: W.B. Saunders.
7. Wall E.J. (2000). Practical primary pediatric orthopedics. *Pediatric Advanced Practice Nursing 35*(1), 95–113.
8. Johnson K.B., Oski F.S. (1997). *Oski's essential pediatrics* (pp. 149–169). Philadelphia: Lippincott-Raven.
9. Schoppee K. (1995). Blount disease. *Orthopedic Nursing 14*(5), 31–34.
10. Pizzutillo P.D. (1994). The pediatric leg and knee. In Weinstein S.L., Buckwalter J.A. (Eds.), *Turek's orthopaedics: Principles and their application* (5th ed., pp. 573–584). Philadelphia: J.B. Lippincott.
11. National Institutes of Health. (1999). Osteoporosis and related bone diseases. Fast facts on osteogenesis imperfecta. [On-line]. Available: http://www.oif.org/tier2/fastfact.htm.
12. Marini J.C. (2004). Osteogenesis imperfecta. In Behrman R.E., Kliegman R.M., Jenson H.B. (Eds.), *Nelson textbook of pediatrics* (17th ed., pp. 2336–2338). Philadelphia: W.B. Saunders.
13. Schiller A.L., Teitelbaum S.L. (1999). Bones and joints. In Rubin E., Farber J.L. (Eds.), *Pathophysiology* (3rd ed., pp. 1352–1380). Philadelphia: Lippincott-Raven.
14. Cotran R.S., Kumar V., Robbins S.L. (1999). *Robbins pathologic basis of disease* (6th ed., pp. 1221–1246). Philadelphia: W.B. Saunders.
15. American Academy of Pediatrics (2000). Clinical practice guideline: Early detection of developmental dysplasia of the hip. *Pediatrics 105,* 896–905.
16. Novacheck T.F. (1996). Developmental dysplasia of the hip. *Pediatrics 43,* 829–848.
17. Eastwood D.M. (2003). Neonatal hip screening. *Lancet 361,* 595–597.
18. Patel H., with the Canadian Task Force on Preventive Health Care. (2001). Preventive health care, 2001 update: Screening and management of developmental dysplasia of the hip in newborns. *Canadian Medical Association Journal 164*(12), 1669–1677.
19. Weinstein S.L. (1994). The pediatric foot. In Weinstein S.L., Buckwalter J.A. (Eds.), *Turek's orthopaedics: Principles and their application* (5th ed., pp. 615–653). Philadelphia: J.B. Lippincott.
20. Honein M., Paulozzi L.J., Moore C.A. (2000). Family history, maternal smoking, and clubfoot: An indication of a gene–environment interaction. *American Journal of Epidemiology 152,* 658–665.
21. Hoffinger S.A. (1996). Evaluation and management of pediatric foot deformities. *Pediatric Clinics of North America 43,* 1091–1101.
22. Koops S., Quanbeck D. (1996). Three common causes of childhood hip pain. *Pediatric Clinics of North America 43,* 1056–1065.
23. U.S. Preventative Services Task Force. (1993). Screening for adolescent idiopathic scoliosis. *Journal of the American Medical Association 269,* 2664–2672.
24. Reamy B.V., Slakey J.B. (2001). Adolescent scoliosis: Review and current comments. *American Family Physician 64*(1), 111–116.
25. Lowwe T.G., Edgar M., Margulles F.Y., et al. (2000). Etiology of idiopathic scoliosis: Current trends in research. *Journal of Bone and Joint Surgery [Am] 82,* 1157–1168.
26. Weinstein S. (1994). The thoracolumbar spine. In Weinstein S.L., Buckwalter J.A. (Eds.), *Turek's orthopaedics: Principles and their application* (5th ed., pp. 447–483). Philadelphia: J.B. Lippincott.
27. Omey M.L., Micheli L.J., Gerbino P.G. (2000). Idiopathic scoliosis and spondylolysis in the female athlete: Tips for treatment. *Clinical Orthopaedics and Related Research 372,* 74–84.
28. Yawn B.P., Yawn R.A., Hodge D., et al. (1999). A population-based study of school scoliosis screening. *JAMA 282,* 1427–1432.
29. Manolagas S.C., Jilka R.L. (1995). Bone marrow, cytokines, and bone remodeling. *New England Journal of Medicine 332,* 305–310.
30. Burns K., Kumar V. (2003). The musculoskeletal system. In Kumar V., Cotran R.S., Robbins S.L. *Basic pathology* (7th ed., pp. 755–771). Philadelphia: W.B. Saunders.
31. Raisz L.G., Rodan G.A. (2003). Pathogenesis of osteoporosis. *Endocrinology Clinics of North America 32,* 15–24.
32. Rodan G.A., Reska H.A. (2003). Osteoporosis and bisphosphonates. *Journal of Bone and Joint Surgery [Am] 85*(Suppl. 3), 8–12.

33. Genant H.K., Guglielmi G., Jergus M. (Eds.). (1998). *Bone densitometry and osteoporosis.* Berlin: Springer-Verlag.
34. Riggs B.L., Melton L.J. (1992). The prevention and treatment of osteoporosis. *New England Journal of Medicine 327,* 620–627.
35. Seeman E. (2003). The structural and biomechanical basis of the gain and loss of bone strength in women and men. *Endocrinology Clinics of North America 32,* 25–38.
36. Stein E., Shane E. (2003). Secondary osteoporosis. *Endocrinology Clinics of North America 32,* 115–134.
37. Saag K.G. (2003). Glucocorticoid-induced osteoporosis. *Endocrinology Clinics of North America 32,* 135–157.
38. Gambert S.R., Schulz B.M., Hamdy B.C. (1995). Osteoporosis: Clinical features, prevention, and treatment. *Endocrinology and Metabolic Clinics of North America 24,* 317–371.
39. Tebas P., Powerly W.G., Claxton S., et al. (2000). Accelerated bone mineral loss in HIV-infected patients receiving potent antiretroviral therapy. *AIDS 14*(4), F63–F67.
40. Dueck C.A., Matt K.S., Manore M.M., Skinner J.S. (1996). Treatment of athletic amenorrhea with a diet and training intervention program. *International Journal of Sport Nutrition 6*(2), 24–40.
41. Otis C.L., Drinkwater B., Johnson M., et al. (1997). American College of Sports Medicine position stand: The female athlete triad. *Medicine and Science in Sports and Exercise 29*(5), i–ix.
42. Hobart J.A., Smucker D.R. (2000). The female athlete triad. *American Family Physician 61,* 3357–3367.
43. Lenchik L., Leid E.S., Hamdy R.C., et al. (2002). Position statement. *Journal of Clinical Densiometry 5*(Suppl), S1–S3.
44. Weinstein L., Ullery B. (2000). Age, weight, and estrogen use determine need for osteoporosis screen. *American Journal of Obstetrics and Gynecology 183,* 547–549.
45. Bukata S.V., Rosier R.N. (2000). Diagnosis and treatment of osteoporosis. *Current Opinion in Orthopedics 11,* 336–340.
46. Crandall C. (2002). Parathyroid hormone for treatment of osteoporosis. *Archives of Internal Medicine 162*(20), 2297–2309.
47. Vogel R.A. (2003). The changing view of hormone replacement therapy. *Reviews in Cardiovascular Medicine 4*(2), 68–71.
48. Cauley J.A., Robbins J., Chen Z., et al. (2003). Effects of estrogen plus progestin on risk of fracture and bone mineral density. *JAMA 290*(13), 1729–1738.
49. National Institutes of Health: Osteoporosis and related bone diseases—National Resource Center (2003). Fact Sheets: Phytoestrogens and Bone Health. [On-line]. Available http://www.osteo.org.
50. Bishop M. (1999). Rickets today—Children still need milk and sunshine. *New England Journal of Medicine 341,* 602–604.
51. Centers for Disease Control. (2001). Severe malnutrition among young children—Georgia, January 1997–June 1999. *MMWR Morbidity and Mortality Weekly Report 50*(12), 224–227.
52. Bouillon R. (1998). The many faces of rickets. *New England Journal of Medicine 131,* 935–942.
53. Schneider D., Hofmann M.T. (2002). Diagnosis and treatment of Paget's disease of bone. *American Family Physician 65*(10), 2069–2072.
54. Ankron M.A., Shapiro J.R. (1998). Paget's disease of bone. *Journal of Bone and Mineral Research 13*(7), 1061–1065.
55. Lewallen D.G. (1999). Hip arthroplasty in patients with Paget's disease. *Clinical Orthopedics 364,* 243–250.
56. Siris E.S. (1998). Paget's disease of bone. *Journal of Bone and Mineral Research 13*(7), 1061–1065.
57. Rosen G., Forxher C.A., Mankin H.J., Selch M.T. (2000). Neoplasms of the bone and soft tissue. In: Bast R.C., Kufe D.W., Pollock R.E., et al. (Eds.), *Cancer medicine* (pp. 1870–1902). Hamilton, Ontario: B.C. Decker.
58. Drake W.M., Kendler D.L., Brown J.P. (2001). Consensus statement on the modern therapy of Paget's disease of bone from a Western Alliance Symposium. Biannual Foothills Meeting on Osteoporosis, Calgary, Alberta, Canada, September 9–10, 2000. *Clinical Therapeutics 23*(4), 620–626.

CHAPTER

59

Disorders of Skeletal Function: Rheumatic Disorders

Debra Bancroft Rizzo

Arthritis is a descriptive term applied to more than 100 rheumatic diseases, ranging from localized, self-limiting conditions to those that are systemic, autoimmune processes. Arthritis affects persons in all age groups and is the second leading cause of disability in the United States.[1,2] Although arthritis cannot be cured, much can be done to control its progress.

The common use of the term *arthritis* oversimplifies the nature of the varied disease processes, the difficulty in differentiating one form of arthritis or rheumatic disease from another, and the complexity of treatment of these usually chronic conditions. These diverse conditions share inflammation of the joint as a prominent or accompanying symptom. In the systemic rheumatic diseases—those affecting body systems in addition to the musculoskeletal system—the inflammation is primary, resulting from an immune response. In rheumatic conditions limited to a single or few diarthrodial joints, the inflammation is secondary, resulting from a degenerative process and the resulting joint irregularities that occur as the bone attempts to remodel itself.

This chapter focuses on systemic autoimmune rheumatic diseases, arthritis associated with spondylitis, osteoarthritis syndromes, metabolic diseases associated with arthritis, and rheumatic disease in children and the elderly. A review of normal joint structures is presented in Chapter 56.

Systemic Autoimmune Rheumatic Diseases

After completing this section of the chapter, you should be able to meet the following objectives:

- Characterize the common features of the different systemic autoimmune rheumatic disorders
- Describe the pathologic changes that may be found in the joint of a person with rheumatoid arthritis
- List the extraarticular manifestations of rheumatoid arthritis

- Describe the immunologic process that occurs in systemic lupus erythematosus
- List four major organ systems that may be involved in systemic lupus erythematosus
- Describe the manifestations of systemic sclerosis

Systemic autoimmune rheumatic diseases are a group of chronic disorders characterized by diffuse inflammatory lesions and degenerative changes in connective tissue. These disorders share similar clinical features and may affect many of the same organs. Rheumatoid arthritis, systemic lupus erythematosus (SLE), polymyalgia rheumatica, temporal arteritis, and juvenile arthritis and dermatomyositis, which share an autoimmune systemic pathogenesis, are discussed in this chapter.

RHEUMATOID ARTHRITIS

Rheumatoid arthritis (RA) is a systemic inflammatory disease that affects 0.3% to 1.5% of the population, with women affected two to three times more frequently than men.[1] Although the disease occurs in all age groups, its prevalence increases with age. The peak incidence among women is between the ages of 40 and 60 years, with the onset at 30 to 50 years of age.

Etiology and Pathogenesis

Although the cause of RA remains uncertain, evidence points to a genetic predisposition and the development of joint inflammation that is immunologically mediated. It has been suggested that the disease is initiated in a genetically predisposed individual by the activation of a T-cell–mediated response to an immunologic trigger, such as a microbial agent. The importance of genetic factors in the pathogenesis of RA is supported by the increased frequency of the disease among first-degree relatives and monozygotic twins. There is also a strong association of human leukocyte antigen (HLA)-DR4 and HLA-DRB1 with RA[1] (see Chapter 19). Thus, certain HLA-DR molecules may predispose to RA by their capacity to bind arthritogenic antigens, which in turn activate helper T cells and initiate the disease.

The pathogenesis of RA can be viewed as an aberrant immune response that leads to synovial inflammation and destruction of the joint architecture. It has been suggested that the disease is initiated by the activation of helper T cells, release of cytokines (*e.g.,* tumor necrosis factor, interleukin-1), and antibody formation. Approximately 70% to 80% of those with the disease have a substance called the *rheumatoid factor* (RF), which is an autologous (self-produced) antibody that reacts with a fragment of immunoglobulin G (IgG) to form immune complexes.[3] RF has been found in the blood, synovial fluid, and synovial membrane of affected individuals. Much of the RF produced by immune cells is present in the inflammatory infiltrate of the synovial tissue.[3]

The role of the autoimmune process in the joint destruction of RA remains obscure. At the cellular level, neutrophils, macrophages, and lymphocytes are attracted to the area. The neutrophils and macrophages phagocytize the immune complexes and, in the process, release lysosomal enzymes capable of causing destructive changes in the joint cartilage (Fig. 59-1). The inflammatory response that follows attracts additional inflammatory cells, setting into motion a chain of events that perpetuates the condition. As the inflammatory process progresses, the synovial cells and subsynovial tissues undergo reactive hyperplasia. Vasodilation and increased blood flow cause warmth and redness. The joint swelling that occurs is the result of the increased capillary permeability that accompanies the inflammatory process.

Characteristic of RA is the development of an extensive network of new blood vessels in the synovial membrane that contributes to the advancement of the rheumatoid

RHEUMATOID ARTHRITIS

- Rheumatoid arthritis is a chronic systemic inflammatory disease with bilateral involvement of diarthrodial joints.
- The initial joint changes involve the synovial cells lining the joint. Inflammatory cells accumulate, and angiogenesis and formation of pannus, which proceed to cover the articular cartilage and isolate it from its nutritional synovial fluid, take place.

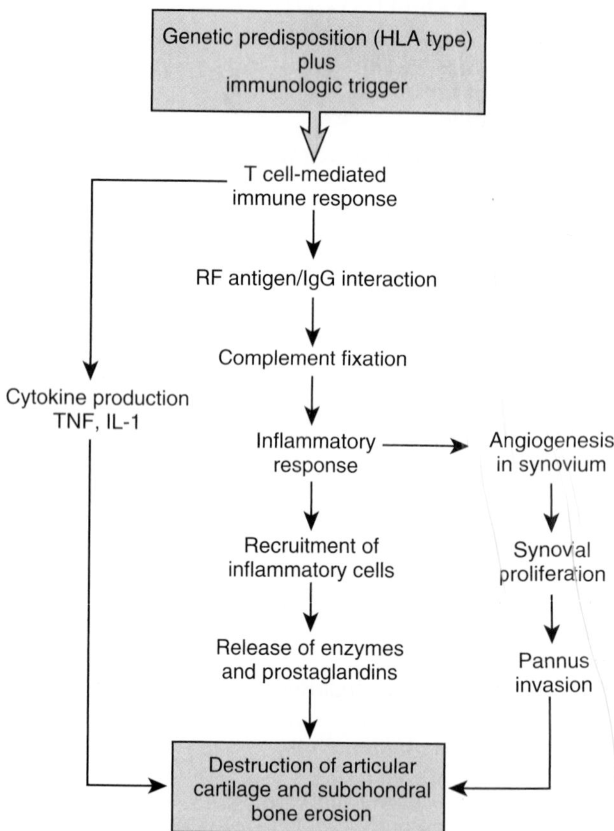

FIGURE 59-1 Disease process in rheumatoid arthritis.

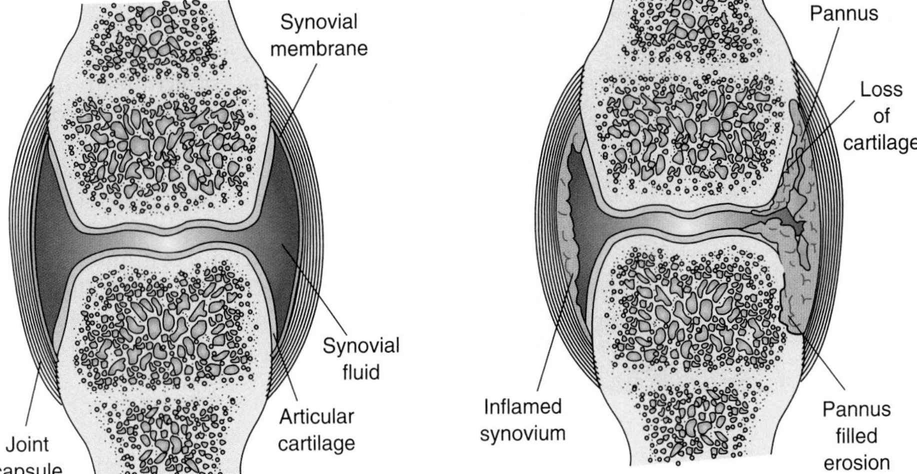

FIGURE 59-2 (**Left**) Normal joint structures. (**Right**) Joint changes in rheumatoid arthritis. The left side denotes early changes occurring within the synovium, and the right side shows progressive disease that leads to erosion and the formation of pannus.

synovitis. This destructive vascular granulation tissue, which is called *pannus,* extends from the synovium to involve the "bare area," a region of unprotected bone at the junction between cartilage and subchondral bone. Pannus is a feature of RA that differentiates it from other forms of inflammatory arthritis[4] (Fig. 59-2). The inflammatory cells found in the pannus have a destructive effect on the adjacent cartilage and bone. Eventually, pannus develops between the joint margins, leading to reduced joint motion and the possibility of eventual ankylosis. With progression of the disease, joint inflammation and the resulting structural changes lead to joint instability, muscle atrophy from disuse, stretching of the ligaments, and involvement of the tendons and muscles. The effect of the pathologic changes on joint structure and function is related to the degree of disease activity, which can change at any time. Unfortunately, the destructive changes are irreversible.

Clinical Manifestations

Rheumatoid arthritis often is associated with extraarticular as well as articular manifestations. It usually has an insidious onset marked by systemic manifestations such as fatigue, anorexia, weight loss, and generalized aching and stiffness. The disease, which is characterized by exacerbations and remissions, may involve only a few joints for brief durations, or it may become relentlessly progressive and debilitating. Approximately 3% of those with the disease have a progressive, unremitting form that does not respond to aggressive therapy.[2]

Joint Manifestations. Joint involvement usually is symmetric and polyarticular. Any diarthrodial joint can be involved. The person may complain of joint pain and stiffness that lasts 30 minutes and frequently for several hours. The limitation of joint motion that occurs early in the disease usually is because of pain; later, it is because of fibrosis. The most frequently affected joints initially are the fingers, hands, wrists, knees, and feet. Later, other diarthrodial joints may become involved. Spinal involvement usually is limited to the cervical region. In the hands, there usually is bilateral and symmetric involvement of the proximal interphalangeal (PIP) and metacarpophalangeal (MCP) joints in the early stages of RA; the distal interphalangeal (DIP) joints rarely are affected. The fingers often take on a spindle-shaped appearance because of inflammation of the PIP joints (Fig. 59-3).

Progressive joint destruction may lead to subluxation (*i.e.,* dislocation of the joint resulting in misalignment of the bone ends) and instability of the joint and in limitation of movement. Swelling and thickening of the synovium can result in stretching of the joint capsule and ligaments. When this occurs, muscle and tendon imbalances develop, and mechanical forces applied to the joints through daily activities produce joint deformities. In the MCP joints, the extensor tendons can slip to the ulnar side of the metacarpal head, causing ulnar deviation of the finger (Fig. 59-4). Subluxation of the MCP joints may develop

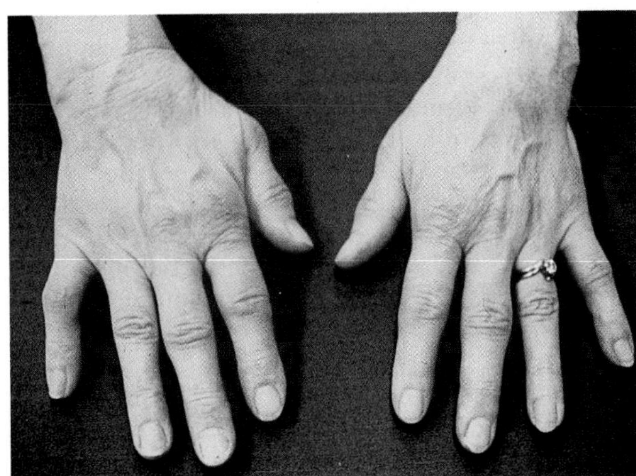

FIGURE 59-3 Inflammation of finger proximal interphalangeal joints in early stages of rheumatoid arthritis, giving the fingers a spindle-shaped appearance. (Reprinted from the ARHP Arthritis Teaching Slide Collection. Used with permission of the American College of Rheumatology.)

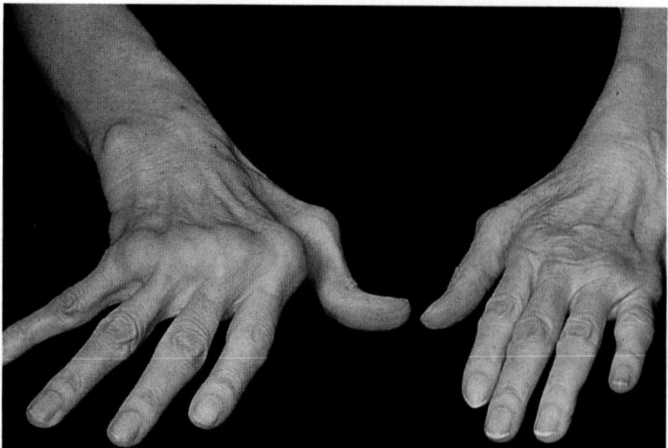

FIGURE 59-4 Subluxation of the metacarpophalangeal joints of the fingers in rheumatoid arthritis (swan neck deformity). (Reprinted from the ARHP Arthritis Teaching Slide Collection. Used with permission of the American College of Rheumatology.)

when this deformity is present. Hyperextension of the PIP joint and partial flexion of the DIP joint is called a *swan neck deformity*. After this condition becomes fixed, severe loss of function occurs because the person can no longer make a fist. Flexion of the PIP joint with hyperextension of the DIP joint is called a *boutonnière deformity*.

The knee is one of the most commonly affected joints and is responsible for much of the disability associated with the disease.[1] Active synovitis may be apparent as visible swelling that obliterates the normal contour over the medial and lateral aspects of the patella. The *bulge sign*, which involves milking fluid from the lateral to the medial side of the patella, may be used to determine the presence of excess fluid when it is not visible. Joint contractures, instability, and genu valgus (knock-knee) deformity are other possible manifestations. Severe quadriceps atrophy can contribute to the disability. A *Baker's cyst* may develop in the popliteal area behind the knee. This is caused by enlargement of the bursa and usually does not cause symptoms unless the cyst ruptures, in which case symptoms mimicking thrombophlebitis appear.

Ankle involvement can limit flexion and extension, which can create difficulty in walking. Involvement of the metatarsophalangeal joints can cause subluxation, hallux valgus, and hammer toe deformities. Neck discomfort is common. In rare cases, long-standing disease can lead to neurologic complications such as occipital headaches, muscle weakness, and numbness and tingling in the upper extremities.

Extraarticular Manifestations. Although characteristically a joint disease, RA can affect a number of other tissues. Extraarticular manifestations probably occur with a fair degree of frequency but usually are mild enough to cause few problems. They are most likely to occur in persons who have the RF.

Because RA is a systemic disease, it may be accompanied by complaints of fatigue, weakness, anorexia, weight loss, and low-grade fever when the disease is active. The erythrocyte sedimentation rate (ESR), which commonly is elevated during inflammatory processes, has been found to correlate with the amount of disease activity.[5] Anemia associated with a low serum iron level or low iron-binding capacity is common.[1] This anemia usually is resistant to iron therapy.

Rheumatoid nodules are granulomatous lesions that develop around small blood vessels. The nodules may be tender or nontender, movable or immovable, and small or large. Typically, they are found over pressure points such as the extensor surfaces of the ulna. The nodules may remain unless surgically removed, or they may resolve spontaneously.

Vasculitis, or inflammation of small and medium-sized arteries, is an uncommon manifestation of RA in persons with a long history of active arthritis and high titers of RF (see Chapter 24). Manifestations include ischemic areas in the nail fold and digital pulp that appear as brown spots. Ulcerations may occur in the lower extremities, particularly around the malleolar areas. In some cases, neuropathy may be the only symptom of vasculitis. The visceral organs, such as the heart, lungs, and gastrointestinal tract, also may be affected.

Other extraarticular manifestations include eye lesions such as episcleritis and scleritis, hematologic abnormalities, pulmonary disease, cardiac complications, infection, and Felty's syndrome (*i.e.*, leukopenia with or without splenomegaly).

Diagnosis and Treatment

The diagnosis of RA is based on findings of the history, physical examination, and laboratory tests. Information should be elicited regarding the duration of symptoms, systemic manifestations, joint stiffness, and family history. The criteria for RA developed by the American Rheumatism Association are useful in establishing the diagnosis[5] (Chart 59-1). At least four of the criteria must be present to make a diagnosis of RA. Although these criteria were developed for use in epidemiologic studies and are designed for classification purposes and not as diagnostic criteria, they can be used as guidelines for diagnosing the illness in individual patients.

In the early stages, the disease often is difficult to diagnose. On physical examination, the affected joints show signs of inflammation, swelling, tenderness, and possibly warmth and reduced motion. The joints have a soft, spongy feeling because of the synovial thickening and inflammation. Body movements may be guarded to prevent pain. Changes in joint structure usually are not visible early in the disease.

The RF test results are not diagnostic for RA, but they can be of value in differentiating rheumatoid arthritis from other forms of arthritis. Between 1% and 5% of healthy persons have the factor, and its presence seems to be more common with advancing age.[1] Also, a person can have RA without the presence of RF. Disease severity and activity tend to correlate with RF levels; patients with high RF levels tend to have a significantly higher frequency of

CHART 59-1

Criteria for Classification of Rheumatoid Arthritis

Four or more of the following conditions must be present to establish a diagnosis of rheumatoid arthritis:

1. Morning stiffness for at least 1 hour and present for at least 6 weeks
2. Simultaneous swelling of three or more joints for at least 6 weeks
3. Swelling of wrist, metacarpophalangeal, or proximal interphalangeal joints for 6 or more weeks
4. Symmetric joint swelling for 6 or more weeks
5. Rheumatoid nodules
6. Serum rheumatoid factor identified by a method that is positive in less than 5% of normal subjects
7. Radiographic changes typical of rheumatoid arthritis on hand or wrist radiographs.

(Adapted from Arnett F.C., Edworthy S.M., Block D.L., et al. [1988]. The American Rheumatism Association 1987 revised criteria for the clarification of rheumatoid arthritis. *Arthritis and Rheumatism 31,* 315–324.)

extraarticular involvement (*e.g.,* rheumatoid nodules, vasculitis, neuropathy).[6] The detection of anti–cyclic citrullinated peptide (CCP) antibodies may be more useful for diagnosing RA because of its higher specificity. Citrulline is an unusual amino acid that is generated by the enzymatic digestion of arginine. Recent research suggests that citrulline-containing proteins may serve as specific targets for the IgG antibody response in RA.[7,8] Anti-CPP antibodies, which have been detected very early in RA, appear to be a good prognostic marker for the disease and discriminate between erosive and nonerosive forms of the disease.[9] Radiologic findings also are not diagnostic in RA because joint erosions often are not seen on radiographic images in the early stages of the disorder. Synovial fluid analysis can be helpful in the diagnostic process. The synovial fluid has a cloudy appearance, the white blood cell count is elevated as a result of inflammation, and the complement components are decreased.

The treatment goals for a person with RA are to reduce pain, minimize stiffness and swelling, maintain mobility, and become an informed health care consumer. The treatment plan includes education about the disease and its treatment, rest, therapeutic exercises, and medications. Because of the chronicity of the disease and the need for continuous, long-term adherence to the prescribed treatment modalities, it is important that the treatment be integrated with the person's lifestyle.

Strategies to aid in symptom control also involve regulating activity by pacing, establishing priorities, and setting realistic goals. Support groups and group education experiences benefit some persons. The home and work environments should be assessed, and interventions should be incorporated as the situation warrants.

Both physical rest and emotional rest are important aspects of care.[1] Physical rest reduces joint stress. Rest of specific joints is recommended to relieve pain. For example, sitting reduces the weight on an inflamed knee, and the use of lightweight splints reduces undue movement of the hand or wrist. Some persons find that discomfort increases with emotional stress; with emotional rest, muscles relax, and discomfort is reduced. Although rest is essential, therapeutic exercises also are important in maintaining joint motion and muscle strength. Range-of-motion exercises involve the active and passive movement of joints. Isometric (muscle-tensing) exercises may be used to strengthen muscles. These exercises are usually taught by a physical therapist and performed daily at home. The difference between normal activity and therapeutic exercise should be emphasized. Aerobic exercise and strengthening exercises can be an important component of the treatment regimen of selected patients. Studies have shown that although persons with RA may have low levels of physical fitness, they can benefit from individualized exercise programs without experiencing joint damage or flare-ups of the disease.[10]

Instruction in the safe use of heat and cold modalities to relieve discomfort and in the use of relaxation techniques also is important. Proper posture, positioning, body mechanics, and the use of supportive shoes can provide further comfort. There often is a need for information about the principles of joint protection and work simplification. Some persons need assistive devices to reduce pain and improve their ability to perform activities of daily living.

The goals of pharmacologic therapy for RA are to reduce pain, decrease inflammation, maintain or restore joint function, and prevent bone and cartilage destruction.[1] Medications used to achieve these goals are classified as those that provide relief of arthritis symptoms and those that have the potential for modifying the course of the disease. The trend in RA management is toward a more aggressive pharmacologic approach earlier in the disease. Ideally, disease modifying antirheumatic drug therapy should be used when the diagnosis of RA is established and before erosive changes appear on radiography.[1] Early treatment is based on the theory that T-cell–dependent pathways, which manifest early in the inflammatory process, are more responsive to treatment than later in the process, when disease progression may be controlled by activated fibroblasts and macrophages.

Nonsteroidal antiinflammatory drugs (NSAIDs) usually are the first choice in the treatment of RA. The NSAIDs inhibit the production of prostaglandins, which have a damaging effect on joint structures. NSAIDs, including salicylates (*e.g.,* aspirin), provide analgesic and antiinflammatory effects. Effectiveness, side effects, cost, and dosing schedules are considered when selecting an NSAID. There is a wide range of responses to the various NSAIDs, and the particular NSAID that works best for any one individual is not always predictable. The incidence of adverse reactions to the NSAIDs (*e.g.,* gastric irritation and bleeding, fluid retention, kidney damage) tends to increase with age and long-term use. A newer class of NSAIDs, the cyclooxygenase-2 (COX-2) inhibitors, has been developed with the goal of decreasing the gastrointestinal adverse effects seen with the traditional NSAIDs.[11] The COX-2 inhibitors (*e.g.*, celecoxib, rofecoxib, and valdecoxib) have been shown to inhibit inflammatory processes, but do not inhibit the protective prostaglandin synthesis in the gastrointestinal tract.

Second-line drug therapy is initiated early in the disease if joint symptoms persist despite use of NSAIDs. Disease-modifying antirheumatic drugs (DMARDs) include gold salts, hydroxychloroquine, sulfasalazine, methotrexate, and azathioprine. Methotrexate has become the drug of choice because of its potency, and it is relatively fast acting (*i.e.*, improvement is seen in 1 month) compared with the slower-acting DMARDs, which can take 3 to 4 months to work. Methotrexate is thought to interfere with purine metabolism, leading to the release of adenosine, a potent antiinflammatory compound. All of the DMARDs can be toxic and require close monitoring for adverse effects, especially those related to bone marrow suppression.[1]

Corticosteroid drugs may be used to reduce discomfort. These agents interrupt the inflammatory and immune cascade at several levels, such as interfering with inflammatory cell adhesion and migration, impairing prostaglandin synthesis, and inhibiting neutrophil superoxide production. To avoid long-term side effects, they are used only in specific situations for short-term therapy at a low dose level.[1] They may be used for unremitting disease with extraarticular manifestations. The corticosteroids do not modify the disease and are unable to prevent joint destruction. Intraarticular corticosteroid injections can provide rapid relief of acute or subacute inflammatory synovitis (after infection is excluded) in a few joints. They should not be repeated more than a few times each year.

Newer antirheumatic drugs include leflunomide, etanercept, infliximab, and adalimumab.[12] Leflunomide is a pyrimidine synthesis inhibitor that blocks the expansion of T cells. Its efficacy is equal to that of methotrexate. Infliximab, etanercept, and adalimumab are biologic response–modifying agents that block tumor necrosis factor-α (TNF-α), one of the key proinflammatory cytokines in rheumatoid arthritis.[13] The anti–TNF-α blockers have shown significant efficacy and favorable safety profiles. These agents have also been shown to inhibit radiologic disease progression and improve functional outcomes.[14]

Another approach to rheumatoid arthritis treatment is combination therapy.[14] This approach is a generally accepted approach and has been shown to be effective in several studies. Individual drugs with different mechanisms of action are given simultaneously to control the disease. The individual drugs are then tapered as symptoms subside and clinical remission is achieved.

Surgery also may be a part of the treatment of rheumatoid arthritis.[1] Synovectomy may be indicated to reduce pain and joint damage when synovitis does not respond to medical treatment. The most common soft tissue surgery is tenosynovectomy (*i.e.*, repair of damaged tendons) of the hand to release nerve entrapments. Total joint replacements (*i.e.*, arthroplasty) may be indicated to reduce pain and increase motion. Arthrodesis (*i.e.*, joint fusion) is indicated only in extreme cases when there is so much soft tissue damage and scarring or infection that a replacement is impossible.

Although the course of rheumatoid arthritis is unpredictable, increasingly effective treatments for the disease have been developed since the late 1990s. Patients with arthritis symptoms are being diagnosed and treated earlier, and criteria have been developed for remission in rheumatoid arthritis.

SYSTEMIC LUPUS ERYTHEMATOSUS

Systemic lupus erythematosus (SLE) is a chronic inflammatory disease that can affect virtually any organ system, including the musculoskeletal system. It is a major rheumatic disease, with a prevalence of approximately 1 case per 2000 persons. Approximately 500,000 persons in the United States have this disease. There is a female predominance of 10 to 1, and this ratio is closer to 30 to 1 during the childbearing years. SLE is more common in African Americans, Hispanics, and Asians than whites, and the incidence in some families is higher than in others.[15]

Etiology and Pathogenesis

The cause of SLE is unknown. It is characterized by the formation of autoantibodies and immune complexes. Persons with SLE appear to have B-cell hyperreactivity and increased production of antibodies against self (*i.e.*, autoantibodies) and nonself antigens. These B cells are polyclonal, each producing a different type of antibody. The autoantibodies can directly damage tissues or combine with corresponding antigens to form tissue-damaging immune complexes. Antibodies have been identified against an array of nuclear and cytoplasmic cell components. Some autoantibodies that have been identified in SLE are antinuclear antibodies (ANAs), including anti–deoxyribonucleic acid (anti-DNA). Other antibodies may be produced against various cells, including red blood cell surface antigens, platelets, coagulation factors, and other antibodies. Autoantibodies against red blood cells can lead to anemia, and those against platelets to thrombocytopenia.

The development of autoantibodies in SLE can result from a combination of factors, including genetic, hormonal, immunologic, and environmental factors.[16] Genetic predisposition is evidenced by the occurrence of familial cases of SLE, especially among identical twins. The increased incidence among African Americans compared with whites also suggests genetic factors. As many as four genes may be involved in the expression of SLE in humans. Genes linked to the HLA-DR and HLA-DQ loci in the class II major histocompatibility complex (MHC) molecules show strong support for a genetic link in the development of SLE.[17] Studies also suggest that an imbalance in sex hormone levels may play a role in the development of the disease, especially because the disease is so prevalent among women. Androgens appear to protect against the development of SLE, whereas estrogens seem to favor its development. It has been suggested that an imbalance in sex hormone levels may lead to heightened helper T-cell and weakened suppressor T-cell immune responses, which could lead to the development of autoantibodies.[1]

Possible environmental triggers include ultraviolet (UV) light, chemicals (*e.g.*, drugs, hair dyes), some foods, and infectious agents.[15] UV light, specifically UVB associated with exposure to the sun or unshielded fluorescent bulbs, may trigger exacerbations. Photosensitivity occurs in approximately one third of patients with SLE.

Certain drugs may provoke a lupus-like disorder in susceptible persons, particularly in the elderly. The most common of these drugs are hydralazine and procainamide. Other drugs, such as quinidine, chlorpromazine, methyldopa, isoniazid, minocycline, and phenytoin, also have been known to produce this syndrome. The disease usually recedes when the drug is discontinued.[1]

Clinical Manifestations

Systemic lupus erythematosus can manifest in a variety of ways. The disease has been called the *great imitator* because it has the capacity for affecting many different body systems, including the musculoskeletal system, the skin, the cardiovascular system, the lungs, the kidneys, the central nervous system (CNS), and the red blood cells and platelets. The onset may be acute or insidious, and the course of the disease is characterized by exacerbations and remissions. Rare cases result in death within weeks or months.

Arthralgias and arthritis are among the most commonly occurring early symptoms of SLE; approximately 90% of all persons with the disease complain of joint pain at some point during the course of their disease.[16] The polyarthritis of SLE initially can be confused with other forms of arthritis, especially rheumatoid arthritis, because of the symmetric arthropathy. However, on radiologic examination, articular destruction rarely is found. Ligaments, tendons, and the joint capsule may be involved, causing varied deformities in approximately 30% of persons with the disease. Flexion contractures, hyperextension of the interphalangeal joint, and subluxation of the carpometacarpal joint contribute to the deformity and subsequent loss of function in the hands. Other musculoskeletal manifestations of SLE include tenosynovitis, rupture of the intrapatellar and Achilles tendons, and avascular necrosis, frequently of the femoral head.

CLINICAL MANIFESTATIONS OF SYSTEMIC LUPUS ERYTHEMATOSUS

- SLE is a chronic autoimmune disorder characterized by production of a wide array of autoantibodies against nuclear and cytoplasmic cell components.
- SLE is often described as the great imitator because it can affect almost any organ system, including the joints of the musculoskeletal system, the skin, kidneys, lungs, nervous system, and the heart.

Skin manifestations can vary greatly and may be classified as acute, subacute, or chronic. The acute skin lesions include the classic malar or "butterfly" rash on the nose and cheeks (Fig. 59-5). This rash is seen in SLE but may be associated with other skin lesions, such as hives or livedo reticularis (*i.e.*, reticular cyanotic discoloration of the skin, often precipitated by cold) and fingertip lesions, such as periungual erythema, nail fold infarcts, and splinter hemorrhages. Hair loss is common. Mucous membrane lesions tend to occur during periods of exacerbation. Sun sensitivity may occur in SLE even after mild sun exposure.

Renal involvement occurs in approximately 50% of persons with SLE. Several forms of glomerulonephritis may occur, including mesangial, focal proliferative, diffuse proliferative, and membranous (see Chapter 35). Interstitial nephritis also may occur. Nephrotic syndrome causes proteinuria with resultant edema in the legs, abdomen, and around the eyes. Renal failure may or may not be preceded by the nephrotic syndrome. Kidney biopsy is the best determinant of renal damage and the extent of treatment needed.

Pulmonary involvement in SLE occurs in 40% to 50% of patients and is manifested primarily by pleural effusions or pleuritis. Less frequently occurring pulmonary problems include acute pneumonitis, pulmonary hemorrhage, chronic interstitial lung disease, and pulmonary embolism.

Pericarditis is the most common of the cardiac manifestations, occurring in up to 30% to 40% of persons with SLE and often accompanied by pleural effusions. Myocarditis affects as many as 25% of those with SLE.

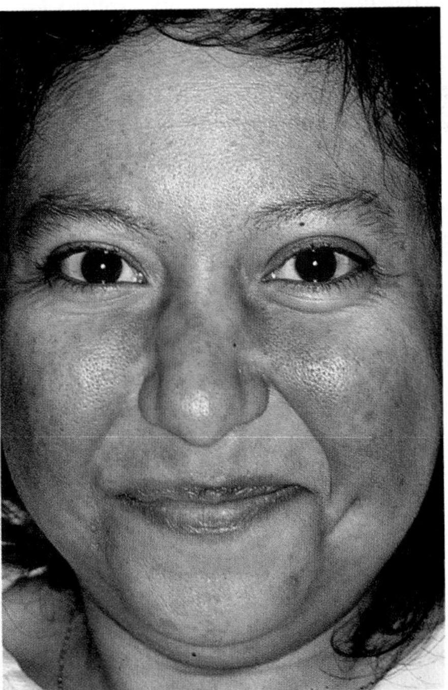

FIGURE 59-5 The butterfly (malar) rash of systemic lupus erythematosus. (Reprinted from the ARHP Arthritis Teaching Slide Collection. Used with permission of the American College of Rheumatology.)

Congenital heart block can occur in infants of mothers with lupus who have a specific type of ANA (anti-Ro) in their serum. Secondary heart disease also is a problem in those with SLE. Hypertension may be associated with lupus nephritis and long-term corticosteroid use. Ischemic heart disease can occur in older patients with longer-duration SLE. Infective carditis is rare but can occur with valvular lesions.[16]

The CNS is involved in 30% to 75% of persons with SLE. The pathologic basis for the CNS symptoms is not entirely clear. It has been ascribed to an acute vasculitis that impedes blood flow, causing strokes or hemorrhage; an immune response involving antineuronal antibodies that attack nerve cells; or production of antiphospholipid antibodies that damage blood vessels and cause blood clots in the brain. Seizures can occur and are more frequent when renal failure is present. Psychotic symptoms, including depression and unnatural euphoria, as well as decreased cognitive functioning, confusion, and altered levels of consciousness, may develop. More research is being done on the role of psychological factors in triggering the onset of SLE.

Hematologic disorders may manifest as hemolytic anemia, leukopenia, lymphopenia, or thrombocytopenia. Lymphadenopathy also may occur in 50% of all patients with SLE.[15] Discoid SLE (*i.e.,* chronic cutaneous lupus) involves plaquelike lesions on the head, scalp, and neck. These lesions first appear as red, swollen patches of skin, and later there can be scarring, depigmentation, and plugging of hair follicles. Ninety percent of patients with discoid lupus have disease that involves only the skin.

Subacute cutaneous lupus erythematosus (SCLE) is a less severe form of lupus. The skin lesions in this condition may resemble psoriasis. These lesions are found in sun-exposed areas such as the face, chest, upper back, and arms. Patients with SCLE may have mild systemic problems, which usually are limited to joint and muscle pains. There is a low incidence of lupus nephritis among those with SCLE.

Diagnosis and Treatment

The diagnosis of SLE can be complicated and difficult. The American College of Rheumatology has defined 11 criteria to be considered in the diagnosis of the disease, but these are intended for use in clinical trials rather than for individual diagnosis.[18] Diagnosis is based on a complete history, physical examination, and analysis of blood work. No single test can diagnose SLE in all persons.

The most common laboratory test performed is the immunofluorescence test for ANA. Ninety-five percent of persons with untreated SLE have high ANA levels. The ANA test is not specific for lupus, and positive ANA results may be found in healthy persons or may be associated with other disorders. The anti-DNA antibody test is more specific for the diagnosis of SLE.[19] Other serum tests may reveal moderate to severe anemia, thrombocytopenia, and leukocytosis or leukopenia. Additional immunologic tests may be done to give support to the diagnosis or to differentiate SLE from other connective tissue diseases.

Treatment of SLE focuses on managing the acute and chronic symptoms of the disease. Communication and trust between health care providers and the person with SLE are the basis for long-term disease management. The goals of treatment include preventing progressive loss of organ function, reducing the possibility of exacerbations, minimizing disability from the disease process, and preventing complications from medication therapy.[20] Treatment with medications may be as simple as a drug to reduce inflammation, such as an NSAID. NSAIDs can control fever, arthritis, and mild pleuritis. An antimalarial drug (*e.g.,* hydroxychloroquine) may be the next medication considered to treat cutaneous and musculoskeletal manifestations of SLE. Corticosteroids are used to treat more significant symptoms of SLE, such as renal and CNS disorders. High-dose corticosteroid treatment is used for acute symptoms, and the drug is tapered to the lowest therapeutic dose as soon as possible to minimize the adverse effects. Immunosuppressive drugs are used in cases of severe disease. Cyclophosphamide, which has been one of the most extensively studied immunosuppressive agents for treatment of SLE, has been found to be beneficial in the treatment of lupus nephritis.[21]

SYSTEMIC SCLEROSIS

Systemic sclerosis, sometimes called *scleroderma,* is an autoimmune disease of connective tissue characterized by excessive collagen deposition in the skin and internal organs such as the lungs, gastrointestinal tract, heart, and kidneys. In this disorder, the skin is thickened through fibrosis, with an accompanying fixation of subdermal structures, including the sheaths or fascia covering tendons and muscles.[22] Systemic sclerosis affects women four times as frequently as men, with a peak incidence in the 35- to 50-year age group.[23] The cause of this rare disorder is poorly understood. There is evidence of both humoral and cellular immune system abnormalities.

Scleroderma presents as two distinct clinical entities: the diffuse or generalized form of the disease and the limited or CREST variant. In the CREST syndrome, hardening of the skin (scleroderma) is limited to the hands and face, whereas the skin changes in diffuse scleroderma also involve the trunk and proximal extremities. Almost all persons with scleroderma develop polyarthritis and Raynaud's phenomenon, a vascular disorder characterized by reversible vasospasm of the arteries supplying the fingers (see Chapter 24).

Diffuse scleroderma is characterized by severe and progressive disease of the skin and the early onset of organ involvement. The typical person has a *stone facies* due to tightening of the facial skin with restricted motion of the mouth. Involvement of the esophagus leads to hypomotility and difficulty swallowing. Malabsorption may develop if the submucosal and muscular atrophy affect the intestine. Pulmonary involvement leads to dyspnea and eventually respiratory failure. Vascular involvement of the kidneys is responsible for malignant hypertension and progressive renal insufficiency. Cardiac problems include pericarditis, heart block, and myocardial fibrosis.

The CREST syndrome is manifest by calcinosis (*i.e.*, calcium deposits in the subcutaneous tissue that erupt through the skin), Raynaud's phenomenon, esophageal dysmotility, sclerodactyly (localized scleroderma of the fingers), and telangiectasia.

Treatment of systemic sclerosis is largely symptomatic and supportive. Studies have indicated that if heart, lung, or kidney involvement is to become severe, it tends to do so early in the disease and is a predictor of shortened survival. Advances in treatment, primarily the use of angiotensin-converting enzyme (ACE) inhibitors in renal involvement, have led to a substantial decrease in the mortality from hypertensive renal disease.[23] There is also some evidence that the ACE inhibitors may be disease modifying.[24]

POLYMYOSITIS AND DERMATOMYOSITIS

Polymyositis and dermatomyositis are chronic inflammatory myopathies. The pathogenesis is multifactorial and includes cellular and humoral immune mechanisms. Systemic manifestations are common, and cardiac and pulmonary complications often adversely affect the outcome. These conditions are characterized by symmetric proximal muscle weakness and occasional muscle pain and tenderness. Treatment for the inflammatory myopathies should seek to control inflammation and prevent long-term damage to muscles, joints, and internal organs. Corticosteroids are the mainstay of treatment for these conditions.

In summary, the systemic autoimmune rheumatic disorders are a group of chronic disorders with overlapping symptoms that are characterized by diffuse inflammatory lesions and degenerative changes in connective tissue. Rheumatoid arthritis is a systemic inflammatory disorder that affects 0.3% to 1.5% of the population. Women are affected more frequently than men. This form of arthritis, the cause of which is unknown, has a chronic course and usually is characterized by remissions and exacerbations. Joint involvement is symmetric and begins with inflammatory changes in the synovial membrane. As joint inflammation progresses, structural changes can occur, leading to joint instability and eventual deformity. Systemic manifestations include weakness, anorexia, weight loss, and low-grade fever. Some extra-articular features include rheumatoid nodules and vasculitis.

Systemic lupus erythematosus is a chronic autoimmune disorder that affects multiple body systems. There is no known cause of SLE, but the disease may result from an immunoregulatory disturbance brought about by a combination of genetic, hormonal, and environmental factors. Some drugs have been shown to induce lupus, especially in the elderly. There is an exaggerated production of autoantibodies, which interact with antigens to produce an inflammatory response that affects many organ systems, including the joints of the musculoskeletal system, the skin, kidneys, lungs, nervous system, and the heart.

Systemic sclerosis (scleroderma) is an autoimmune disorder characterized by excessive fibrosis of the skin, joint structures, gastrointestinal tract, and other internal organs. It can present as the CREST variant with limited involvement of the skin or as a diffuse and progressive disease with early organ involvement. Polymyositis and dermatomyositis are chronic inflammatory myopathies. The pathogenesis is multifactorial and includes cellular and humoral immune mechanisms.

Arthritis Associated With Spondylitis

After completing this section of the chapter, you should be able to meet the following objectives:

- Cite a definition of the seronegative spondyloarthropathies
- Cite the primary features of ankylosing spondylitis
- Describe how the site of inflammation differs in spondyloarthropathies from that in rheumatoid arthritis
- Contrast and compare ankylosing spondylitis, reactive arthritis, and psoriatic arthritis in terms of cause, pathogenesis, and clinical manifestations

SERONEGATIVE SPONDYLOARTHROPATHIES

The *spondyloarthropathies* are an interrelated group of multisystem inflammatory disorders that primarily affect the axial skeleton, particularly the spine. Typically, the inflammation begins at sites where tendon and ligament insert into bone rather than in the synovium. Sacroiliitis is a pathologic hallmark of the disorders. Persons with the spondyloarthropathies may also have inflammation and involvement of the peripheral joints, in which case the signs and symptoms overlap with other inflammatory types of arthritis. Because there is an absence of the RF, these disorders often are referred to as *seronegative spondyloarthropathies*.

The seronegative spondyloarthropathies include ankylosing spondylitis, juvenile ankylosing spondylitis, reactive arthritis, enteropathic arthritis (*i.e.*, inflammatory bowel disease), and psoriatic arthritis. Although they differ in terms of factors such as age and type of onset and extent of joint involvement, there is clinical evidence of overlap between the various seronegative spondyloarthropathies (Table 59-1). In none of these disorders is the cause or pathogenesis well understood. There is a striking association with the HLA-B27 antigen, but the presence of the HLA-B27 antigen by itself is neither necessary nor sufficient for the development of any of the diseases.

Ankylosing Spondylitis

Ankylosing spondylitis is a chronic, systemic inflammatory disease of the joints of the axial skeleton manifested by pain and progressive stiffening of the spine. The disease is more common than once was believed, affecting

TABLE 59-1 Comparison of the Spondyloarthropathies

Characteristic	Ankylosing Spondylitis	Reiter's Syndrome	Psoriatic Arthritis	Inflammatory Bowel Disease
Age at onset	Young adult	Young to middle age	Any age	Any age
Type of onset	Gradual	Sudden	Variable	Gradual
Sacroiliitis	>95%	20%	20%	10%
Peripheral joint involvement	25%	90%	All (about 5% to 7% of those patients with psoriasis)	Occasional
HLA-B27 (in whites)	>90%	75%	<50%	<50%
Eye involvement	25% to 30%	Common	Occasional	Occasional

(Adapted from Arnett F.C., Khan M.A., Willikens R.F. [1989]. A new look at ankylosing spondylitis. *Patient Care 23* [19], 82–101)

approximately 2% to 8% of the HLA-B27–positive white population.[1] Clinical manifestations usually begin in late adolescence or early adulthood and are slightly more common in men than in women. The disease usually evolves more slowly and is less severe in women.

Ankylosing spondylitis produces an inflammatory erosion of the sites where tendons and ligaments attach to bone.[1] Typically, the disease process begins with bilateral involvement of the sacroiliac joints and then moves to the smaller joints of the posterior elements of the spine. The result is ultimate destruction of these joints with ankylosis or posterior fusion of the spine. The vertebrae take on a squared appearance and bone bridges fuse one vertebral body to the next across the intervertebral discs (Fig. 59-6). Progressive spinal changes usually follow an ascending pattern up the spine. Occasionally, large synovial joints (*i.e.*, hips, knees, and shoulders) may be involved. The small peripheral joints usually are not affected. The disease spectrum ranges from an asymptomatic sacroiliitis to a progressive disease that can affect many body systems.

Etiology and Pathogenesis. Although the pathogenesis of ankylosing spondylitis has not been established, the presence of mononuclear cells in acutely involved tissue suggests an immune response. Epidemiologic findings indicate that genetic and environmental factors play a role in the pathogenesis of the disease. The HLA-B27 antigen remains one of the best-known examples of an association between a disease and a hereditary marker.[1] Although approximately 90% of those with ankylosing spondylitis possess the HLA-B27 antigen, and nearly 100% of those who also have uveitis or aortitis have the marker, the HLA-B27 antigen also is present in approximately 8% of the

SERONEGATIVE SPONDYLOARTHROPATHIES

- The seronegative spondyloarthropathies represent a group of related multisystem disorders that lack the RF.
- The inflammatory process associated with the disorders commonly affects the axial skeleton, involving areas where ligaments and tendons attach to bone.
- Although the cause of the disorders is unknown, there is a striking association between the HLA-B27 antigen and development of the spondyloarthropathies.

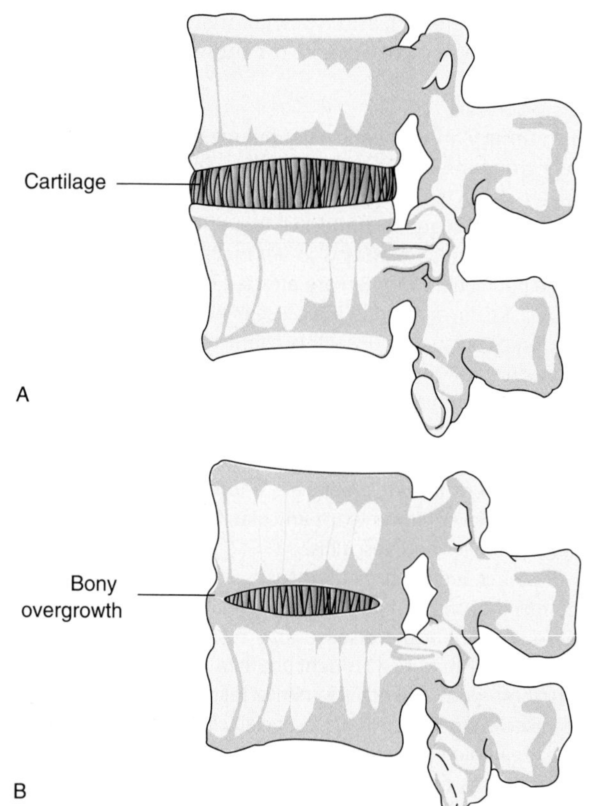

FIGURE 59-6 The bony overgrowth (**B**) of the vertebra characteristic of ankylosing spondylitis is evident when compared with normal vertebra (**A**).

normal population. Several theories have been advanced to account for the association between the HLA-B27 antigen and ankylosing spondylitis. One possibility is that the gene that determines the HLA-B27 antigen may be linked to other genes that determine pathologic autoimmune phenomena or that lead to increased susceptibility to infections or environmental agents. A second theory postulates molecular mimicry; an autoimmune reaction to an antigenic determinant site in the host's tissues may occur as a consequence of an immunologic response to an identical or closely related antigen of a foreign agent, usually an infectious agent[25] (see Chapter 21).

Clinical Manifestations. The person with ankylosing spondylitis typically complains of low back pain, which may be persistent or intermittent. The pain, which becomes worse when resting, particularly when lying in bed, initially may be blamed on muscle strain or spasm from physical activity. Lumbosacral pain also may be present, with discomfort in the buttocks and hip areas. Sometimes, pain can radiate to the thigh in a manner similar to that of sciatic pain. Prolonged stiffness is present in the morning and after periods of rest. Muscle spasm also may contribute to discomfort.[26] Mild physical activity or a hot shower helps reduce pain and stiffness. Sleep patterns frequently are interrupted because of these manifestations. Walking or exercise may be needed to provide the comfort needed to return to sleep.

Loss of motion in the spinal column is characteristic of the disease. The severity and duration of disease activity influence the degree of mobility. Loss of lumbar lordosis occurs as the disease progresses, and this is followed by kyphosis of the thoracic spine and extension of the neck. A spine fused in the flexed position is the end result in severe ankylosing spondylitis. A kyphotic spine makes it difficult for the patient to look ahead and to maintain balance while walking. The image is one of a person bent over looking at the floor and unable to straighten up. X-ray films show a rigid, bamboo-like spine. The heart and lungs are constricted in the chest cavity. Abnormal weight bearing can lead to degeneration and destruction of the hips, necessitating joint replacement procedures. Peripheral arthritis is more common in hips and shoulders. The incidence of hip joint involvement varies from 17% to 36% and potentially is more crippling than involvement in any other joint.[1]

The most common extraskeletal involvement is acute anterior uveitis, which occurs in 25% to 30% of patients sometime in the course of their disease.[1] Systemic features of weight loss, fever, and fatigue may be apparent. Sometimes, the fatigue is a greater problem than pain or stiffness. Osteoporosis can occur, especially in the spine, which contributes to the risk for spinal fracture. Fusion of the costovertebral joints can lead to reduced lung volume.

The disease process varies considerably among individuals. Exacerbations and remissions are common; their unpredictability can create uncertainty in planning daily activities and in setting goals. Fortunately, most of those affected are able to lead productive lives. The prognosis for ankylosing spondylitis in general is good. The first decade of disease predicts the remainder. Severe disease usually occurs early and is marked by peripheral arthritis, especially of the hip.

Diagnosis and Treatment. The diagnosis of ankylosing spondylitis is based on history, physical examination, and x-ray examination. The early and precise diagnosis of ankylosing spondylitis is closely related to a favorable prognosis. Early recognition allows for implementation of a conservative and usually effective treatment program on a lifelong basis.

Several methods are available to assess mobility and detect sacroiliitis. These methods include pressure on the sacroiliac joints with the person in a forward-bending position to elicit pain and muscle spasm, measurement of the distance between the tips of fingers and the floor in a bent-over position with straight knees, and a modified Schöber's test in which contralateral flexion of the back is measured. Although these measures alone do not provide a diagnosis of ankylosing spondylitis or other spondyloarthropathies, they can provide useful measurements for monitoring the disease status. Measurement of chest expansion may be used as an indirect indicator of thoracic involvement, which usually occurs late in the disease course.

Laboratory findings frequently include an elevated ESR. The patient also may have a mild normocytic normochromic anemia. HLA typing is not diagnostic of the disease and should not be used as a routine screening procedure. Radiologic evaluations help differentiate sacroiliitis from other diseases. In early disease, x-ray images may be negative. Vertebrae normally are concave on the anterior border. In ankylosing spondylitis, the vertebrae take on a squared appearance (see Fig. 59-6). Progressive spinal changes usually follow an ascending pattern up the spine.

Treatment is directed at controlling pain and maintaining mobility by suppressing inflammation. Proper posture and positioning are important. This includes sleeping in a supine position on a firm mattress and using one small pillow or no pillow. A bed board may be used to supply additional firmness. Therapeutic exercises are important to assist in maintaining motion in peripheral joints and in the spine. Muscle-strengthening exercises for extensor muscle groups also are prescribed. Heat applications or a shower or bath may be beneficial before exercise to improve ease of movement. Swimming is an excellent general conditioning exercise that avoids joint stress and enhances muscle tone. Immobilizing joints is not recommended. Maintaining ideal weight reduces the stress on weight-bearing joints. Smoking should be discouraged because it can exacerbate respiratory problems. Occupational counseling or job evaluation may be warranted because of postural abnormalities.

Pharmacologic treatment includes the use of NSAIDs to reduce inflammation, relieve pain, and reduce muscle spasm. Phenylbutazone is highly effective, but its use is usually limited to persons with severe disease in whom other agents have failed because of potential bone marrow suppression with long-term use. More recently, promising small-scale studies have been done suggesting that anti–TNF-α agents are efficacious in the treatment of active ankylosing spondylitis.[27]

Reactive Arthropathies

The reactive arthropathies, including Reiter's syndrome and enteropathic arthritis, may be defined as sterile inflammatory joint disorders that are distant in time and place from the initial inciting infective process. The infecting agents cannot be cultured and are not viable once having reached the joints. The list of triggering agents is continuously increasing and may be divided into urogenic, enterogenic, and respiratory tract–associated, along with the idiopathic arthritides. In some cases, the identity of the causative agent is unknown.[28]

Commonly recognized forms of reactive arthritis include those involving *Chlamydia pneumoniae* infection and *Pseudomonas*. Additional and frequently occurring pathogens include *Chlamydia trachomatis, Salmonella, Shigella, Yersinia, Campylobacter,* and *Streptococcus*.[28] Reactive arthritis also has been observed in persons with acquired immunodeficiency syndrome (AIDS). Spondyloarthropathies such as Reiter's syndrome and psoriatic arthritis are more severe and frequent in human immunodeficiency virus (HIV)–infected patients than in the general population. It is thought that the immune response to HIV infection is selective and largely spares the natural killer cells, which may be critical in the pathogenesis of these conditions.[29] This is in contrast to rheumatoid arthritis and SLE, which dramatically improve as immunodeficiency develops. Reactive arthritis may also result from the presence of a foreign substance in the joint tissue, as in silicone implants in the small joints of the hand or feet or after exposure to industrial gases and oils. However, there is no evidence of antigenicity of the causative substance.

In the strictest sense, the definition of reactive arthritis includes a possibility of immunologic sensitization before arthritic development.[28] Similarities exist between reactive arthritis and bacterial arthritis. Several bacteria cause both diseases. When cultured bacteria are isolated from the synovial fluid, the diagnosis is bacterial arthritis. When they cannot be isolated, even though there has been a preceding infection, the diagnosis of reactive arthritis is made.

Reactive arthritis may follow a self-limited course; it may involve recurrent episodes of arthritis; or, in a small number of cases, it may follow a continuous and unremitting course. The treatment is largely symptomatic. NSAIDs are used in treating the arthritic symptoms. Vigorous treatment of possible triggering infections is thought to prevent relapses of reactive arthritis, but in many cases, the triggering infection passes unnoticed or is mild, and the patient contacts a physician only with the onset of definite arthritis. Short antibiotic courses at this time are not effective.

Reiter's Syndrome. Reiter's syndrome is considered to be a clinical manifestation of reactive arthritis that may be accompanied by extraarticular symptoms such as uveitis, bowel inflammation, and carditis. The disease develops in a genetically susceptible host after a bacterial infection due to *Chlamydia trachomatis* in the genitourinary tract or *Salmonella, Shigella, Yersinia,* or *Campylobacter* in the gastrointestinal tract.

The term *Reiter's syndrome* soon may be relegated to history as the pathogenesis becomes better understood. Alternative designations include SARA (sexually associated reactive arthritis) and the BASE syndrome (HLA-B27, arthritis, sacroiliitis, and extraarticular inflammation).[29] Reiter's syndrome was the first rheumatic disease to be recognized in association with HIV infection. Symptoms of arthritis may precede any overt signs of HIV disease. Treatment with agents such as methotrexate and azathioprine may further suppress the immune response and provoke a full expression of AIDS.

Enteropathic Arthritis. Arthritis that is associated with an inflammatory bowel disease usually is considered an enteropathic arthritis because the intestinal disease is directly involved in the pathogenesis. Most cases of enteropathic arthritis are classified among the spondyloarthropathies. These include cases in which the arthritis is associated with inflammatory bowel disease (*i.e.,* ulcerative colitis and Crohn's disease), the reactive arthritides triggered by enterogenic bacteria, some of the undifferentiated spondyloarthropathies, Whipple's disease, and reactions after intestinal bypass surgery.[1] There is no direct relation between the activity of the bowel disease and the degree of arthritis activity.

Psoriatic Arthritis

Psoriatic arthritis is a seronegative inflammatory arthropathy that occurs in 5% to 7% of people with psoriasis. It is a heterogeneous disease with features of the spondyloarthropathies in some persons, rheumatoid arthritis in others, and features of both coexisting in yet others.

The etiology of psoriasis and psoriatic arthritis is unknown. Genetic, environmental, and immunologic factors appear to affect susceptibility and play a role in expression of the psoriatic skin disease and the arthritis. Environmental factors that may play a role in the pathogenesis of the disorder include infectious agents and physical trauma. T-cell–mediated immune responses also seem to play an important role in the skin and joint manifestations of the disease, as indicated by the observation that there is improvement in disease status after treatment with immunosuppressant agents such as cyclosporine.

Although the arthritis can antedate detectable skin rash, the definitive diagnosis of psoriatic arthritis cannot be made without evidence of skin or nail changes typical of psoriasis. Psoriatic arthritis falls into five subgroups: oligoarticular or asymmetric (48%), spondyloarthropathy (24%), polyarticular or symmetric (18%), distal interphalangeal (8%), and arthritis mutilans in which there is osteolysis with telescoping of the fingers and toes (2%).[30] This heterogeneous clinical presentation suggests more than one disease is associated with psoriasis, or various clinical responses to a common cause. At least 20% of those with psoriatic arthritis have an elevated serum level of uric acid. The abnormally elevated serum uric acid level is caused by the rapid skin turnover of psoriasis and the subsequent breakdown of nucleic acid followed by its metabolism to uric acid. This finding may lead to a misdiagnosis of gout. Psoriatic arthritis tends to be slowly progressive, but has a more favorable prognosis than rheumatoid arthritis.

Basic management is similar to the treatment of rheumatoid arthritis. Suppression of the skin disease may be important in helping control the arthritis. Often, affected joints are surprisingly functional and only minimally symptomatic. The biologic response modifiers, specifically the TNF inhibitors (*e.g.*, etanercept and infliximab), have been found to be beneficial in controlling the arthritis as well as the psoriasis in patients with psoriatic arthritis.[30]

In summary, the seronegative arthropathies are a group of rheumatic disorders that lack the rheumatoid factor. The *seronegative spondyloarthropathies* affect the axial skeleton, particularly the spine. Inflammation develops at sites where tendons and ligaments insert into bone. They include ankylosing spondylitis, reactive arthritis, enteropathic arthritis, and psoriatic arthritis. Although there are overlapping features for each of the spondyloarthropathies, identifying etiologic differences and clinical manifestations is important for determining treatment. Ankylosing spondylitis is considered a prototype of this classification category. Bilateral sacroiliitis is the primary feature of ankylosing spondylitis. The disease spectrum ranges from asymptomatic sacroiliitis to a progressive disorder affecting many body systems. The cause remains unknown; however, a strong association between the HLA-B27 antigen and ankylosing spondylitis has been identified. Loss of motion in the spinal column is characteristic of the disease. Peripheral arthritis may occur in some persons. The reactive arthropathies, which include Reiter's syndrome and enteropathic arthritis, are sterile, inflammatory joint disorders that are distant in time and site of an initial inciting infection.

Psoriatic arthritis is a seronegative arthropathy that occurs in 5% to 7% of people with psoriasis. It is a heterogeneous disease with features of the spondyloarthropathies in some persons, rheumatoid arthritis in others, and features of both coexisting in yet others.

Osteoarthritis Syndrome

After completing this section of the chapter, you should be able to meet the following objectives:

- ✦ Compare rheumatoid arthritis and osteoarthritis in terms of joint involvement, level of inflammation, and local and systemic manifestations
- ✦ Describe the pathologic joint changes associated with osteoarthritis
- ✦ Characterize the treatment of osteoarthritis

Osteoarthritis (OA), formerly called *degenerative joint disease,* is the most prevalent form of arthritis and is a leading cause of disability and pain in the elderly. Osteoarthritis is more of a disease process than a specific entity. The term encompasses a heterogeneous collection of syndromes, including osteoarthritis of the hand, knee, hip, foot, and spine.[31] It can occur as a primary idiopathic disorder or as a secondary disorder, although this distinction is not always clear. Idiopathic or primary variants of OA occur as localized or generalized (*i.e.*, involvement of more than three joints) syndromes.[1] Secondary OA has a known underlying cause such as congenital or acquired defects of joint structures, trauma, metabolic disorders, or inflammatory diseases (Chart 59-2).

The joint changes associated with osteoarthritis, which include a progressive loss of articular cartilage and synovitis, result from the inflammation caused when cartilage attempts to repair itself, creating osteophytes or spurs. These changes are accompanied by joint pain, stiffness, limitation of motion, and in some cases joint instability and deformity. Fortunately, changes in the traditional conservative management of this underemphasized condition are occurring. Attitudes regarding the inevitability of the limitations imposed by this condition are changing on the part of health care providers and persons with the disease.

EPIDEMIOLOGY AND RISK FACTORS

Age and gender interact to influence the time of onset and, with race, the pattern of joint involvement in OA. Men are affected more commonly at a younger age than women, but the rate of women affected exceeds that of men by middle age.[1] Heredity influences the occurrence of hand OA in the DIP joint. Hand osteoarthritis is more likely to affect white women, whereas knee osteoarthritis is more common in black women. The incidence of hip osteoarthritis is less among the Chinese than Europeans, perhaps representing the influence of other factors such as

CHART 59-2

Causes of Osteoarthritis

- Postinflammatory disorders
  - Rheumatoid arthritis
  - Septic joint
- Post-traumatic disorders
  - Acute fracture
  - Ligament or meniscal injury
  - Cumulative occupational or recreational trauma
- Anatomic or bony disorders
  - Hip dysplasia
  - Avascular necrosis
  - Paget's disease
  - Slipped capital femoral epiphysis
  - Legg–Calvé–Perthes disease
- Metabolic disorders
  - Calcium crystal deposition
  - Hemochromatosis
  - Acromegaly
  - Wilson's disease
  - Ochronosis
- Neuropathic arthritis
  - Charcot joint
- Hereditary disorders of collagen
- Idiopathic or primary variants

OSTEOARTHRITIS

- Often referred to as "wear-and-tear" arthritis, osteoarthritis is a slowly destructive disorder of the articular cartilage.
- It can present as a primary disease of unknown etiology or as a secondary disorder related to congenital or acquired defects that affect the distribution of joint stress.
- The pathogenesis of osteoarthritis includes the progressive disruption of the smooth surface of the articular cartilage with development of surface cracks that deepen to involve the subchondral bone; followed by complete erosion of the articular cartilage with exposure of ivory-like polished subchondral bone, dislodgment of fragments of free-floating osteocartilaginous bodies, development of bone cysts, and formation of abnormal bony spurs at the joint margins.

occupation, obesity, or heredity. Bone mass may also influence the risk for developing OA. In theory, thinner subchondral bone mass may provide a greater shock-absorbing function than denser bone, allowing less direct trauma to the cartilage.

Obesity is a particular risk factor for OA of the knee in women and a contributory biomechanical factor in the pathogenesis of the disease. Excess fat may have a direct metabolic effect on cartilage beyond the effects of excess joint stress. Weight loss reduces the risk for developing symptomatic arthritis of the knee.[32] Although the radiographic incidence of knee osteoarthritis increases with advancing age, the incidence of symptomatic osteoarthritis of the knee decreases.[32]

PATHOGENESIS

The pathogenesis of OA resides in the homeostatic mechanisms that maintain the articular cartilage. Articular cartilage plays two essential mechanical roles in joint physiology. First, the articular cartilage serves as a remarkably smooth weight-bearing surface. In combination with synovial fluid, the articular cartilage provides extremely low friction during movement of the joint. Second, the cartilage transmits the load down to the bone, dissipating the mechanical stress.[33] The subchondral bone protects the overlying articular cartilage, providing it with a pliable bed and absorbing the energy of the force (Fig. 59-7).

Cartilage is a specialized type of connective tissue. As with other types of tissue, it consists of cells (*i.e.*, chondrocytes) nested in an extracellular matrix. In articular cartilage, the extracellular matrix is composed of water, proteoglycans, collagen, and ground substance. The proteoglycans, which are large macromolecules made up of disaccharides and amino acids, afford elasticity and stiffness, permitting articular cartilage to resist compression. The ground substance constitutes a highly hydrated, semisolid gel. Collagen molecules consist of polypeptide chains that form long fibrous strands. They provide form and tensile strength. The primary function of the collagen fibers is to provide a rigid scaffold to support the chondrocytes and ground substance of cartilage. The hydrated proteoglycan molecules, because of their macromolecular size and charge, are trapped in the collagen meshwork of the extracellular matrix and prevented from expanding to their maximum size. This confers the high interstitial osmotic pressure and fluid volume that is needed for lubrication of the joint.[34] As in the case of adult bone, articular cartilage is not static; it undergoes turnover, and its "worn out" matrix components are continually degraded and replaced. This turnover is maintained by the chondrocytes, which not only synthesize the matrix but also secrete matrix-degrading enzymes. Thus, the health of the chondrocytes determines joint integrity. In osteoarthritis, this integrity can be disturbed by a number of influences.

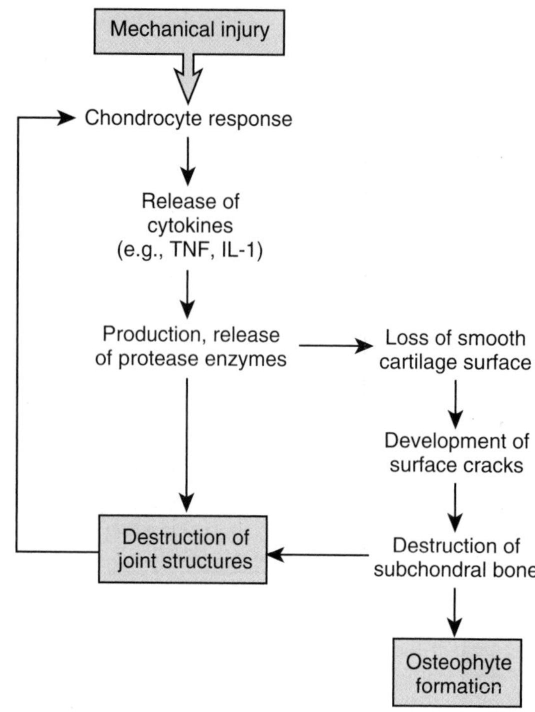

FIGURE 59-7 Disease process in osteoarthritis.

Popularly known as *wear-and-tear* arthritis, OA is characterized by significant changes in both the composition and mechanical properties of cartilage. Early in the course of the disease, the cartilage contains increased water and decreased concentrations of proteoglycans compared with healthy cartilage. In addition, there appears to be a weakening of the collagen network, presumably caused by a decrease in the local synthesis of new collagen and an increase in the breakdown of existing collagen. The articular cartilage injury that occurs in OA is thought to result from the release of cytokines such as interleukin-1 and TNF[1,33] (Fig. 59-8). These chemical messengers stimulate production and release of proteases (enzymes) that are destructive of joint structures.[33] The resulting damage predisposes the chondrocytes to more injury and impairs their ability to repair the damage by producing new collagen and proteo-

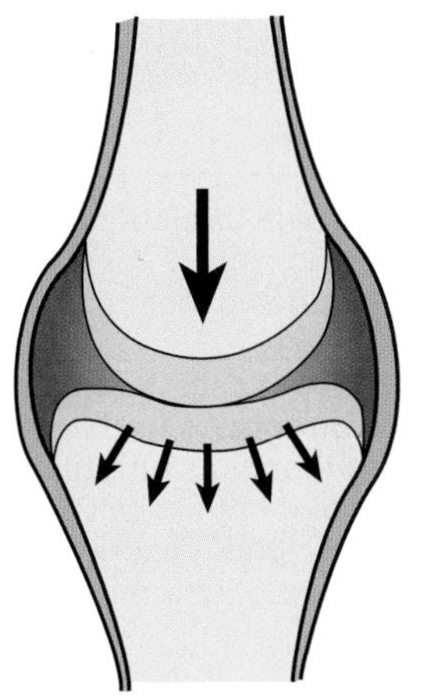

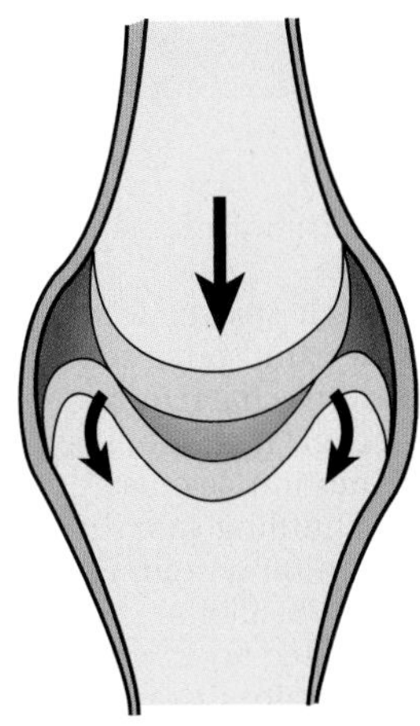

FIGURE 59-8 **(Left)** A joint normally undergoes deformation of the articular cartilage and the subchondral bone when carrying a load. This maximizes the contact area and spreads the force of the load. **(Right)** If the joint does not deform with a load, the stresses are concentrated and the joint breaks down. (Adapted from Brandt K.D. & Radin E. [1987]. The physiology of articular stress: Osteoarthroses. *Hospital Practice* [January 15], 111)

Bone cysts
Osteophyte
Joint space narrows
Erosion of cartilage and bone

FIGURE 59-9 Joint changes in osteoarthritis. The left side denotes early changes and joint space narrowing with cartilage breakdown. The right side shows more severe disease progression with lost cartilage and osteophyte formation.

glycans. The combined effects of inadequate repair mechanisms and imbalances between the proteases and their inhibitors contribute further to disease progression.

The earliest structural changes in OA include enlargement and reorganization of the chondrocytes in the superficial part of the articular cartilage. This is accompanied by edematous changes in the cartilaginous matrix, principally the intermediate layer. The cartilage loses its smooth aspect, and surface cracks or microfractures occur, allowing synovial fluid to enter and widen the crack. As the crack deepens, vertical clefts form and eventually extend through the full thickness of the articular surface and into the subchondral bone.[33] Portions of the articular cartilage eventually become completely eroded, and the exposed surface of the subchondral bone becomes thickened and polished to ivory-like consistency (eburnation). Fragments of cartilage and bone often become dislodged, creating free-floating osteocartilaginous bodies ("joint mice") that enter the joint cavity. Synovial fluid may leak though the defects in the residual cartilage to form cysts within the bone.[33] As the disease progresses, the underlying trabecular bone becomes sclerotic in response to increased pressure on the surface of the joint, rendering it less effective as a shock absorber. Sclerosis, or formation of new bone and cysts, usually occurs at the joint margins forming abnormal bony outgrowths called *osteophytes,* or spurs (Fig. 59-9). As the joint begins to lose its integrity, there is trauma to the synovial membrane, which results in nonspecific inflammation. Compared with RA, however, the changes in the synovium that occur in OA are not as pronounced, nor do they occur as early.

In secondary forms of OA, repetitive impact loading contributes to joint failure, accounting for the high prevalence of OA specific to vocational or avocational sites, such as the shoulders and elbows of baseball pitchers, ankles of ballet dancers, and knees of basketball players. Immobilization also can produce degenerative changes in articular cartilage. Cartilage degeneration due to immobility may result from loss of the pumping action of lubrication that occurs with joint movement. These changes are more marked and appear earlier in areas of contact but occur also in areas not subject to mechanical compression. Although cartilage atrophy is rapidly reversible with activity after a period of immobilization, impact exercise during the period of remobilization can prevent reversal of the atrophy. Therefore, slow and gradual remobilization may be important in preventing cartilage injury. Clinically, it has implications for instructions concerning the recommended level of physical activity after removal of a cast.

CLINICAL MANIFESTATIONS

The manifestations of OA may occur suddenly or insidiously. Initially, pain may be described as aching and may be somewhat difficult to localize. It worsens with use or activity and is relieved by rest. In later stages of disease activity, night pain may be experienced during rest. Pain can occur at rest, several hours after the use of the involved joints. Crepitus and grinding may be evident when the joint is moved. As the disease advances, even minimal activity may cause pain because of the limited range of motion resulting from intraarticular and periarticular structural damage.

The most frequently affected joints are the hips, knees, lumbar and cervical vertebrae, proximal and distal joints of the hand, the first carpometacarpal joint, and the first metatarsophalangeal joints of the feet. Table 59-2 identifies the joints that commonly are affected by OA and the common clinical features correlated with the disease activity of

TABLE 59-2 Clinical Features of Osteoarthritis

Joint	Clinical Features
Cervical spine	Localized stiffness; radicular or nonradicular pain; posterior osteophyte formation may cause vascular compression
Lumbar spine	Low back pain and stiffness; muscle spasm; decreased back motion; nerve root compression causing radicular pain; spinal stenosis
Hip	Most common in older male adults; characterized by insidious onset of pain, localized to groin region or inner aspect of the thigh; may be referred to buttocks, sciatic region, or knee; reduced hip motion; leg may be held in external rotation with hip flexed and adducted; limp or shuffling gait; difficulty getting in and out of chairs
Knee	Localized discomfort with pain on motion; limitation of motion; crepitus; quadriceps atrophy due to lack of use; joint instability; genu varus or valgus; joint effusion
First carpometacarpal joint	Tenderness at base of thumb; squared appearance to joint
Proximal interphalangeal joint—Bouchard's nodes	Same as for distal interphalangeal joint disease
Distal interphalangeal joint—Heberden's nodes	Occurs more frequently in women; usually involves multiple DIPs, lateral flexor deviation of joint, spur formation at joint margins, pain and discomfort after joint use
First metatarsophalangeal joint	Insidious onset; irregular joint contour; pain and swelling aggravated by tight shoes

each particular joint. A single joint or several may be affected. Although a single weight-bearing joint may be involved initially, other joints often become affected because of the additional stress placed on them while trying to protect the original joint. It is not unusual for a person having a knee replacement to discover soon after the surgery is done that the second knee also needs to be replaced. Other clinical features are limitations of joint motion and joint instability. Joint enlargement usually results from new bone formation; the joint feels hard, in contrast to the soft, spongy feeling characteristic of the joint in rheumatoid arthritis. Sometimes, mild synovitis or increased synovial fluid can cause joint enlargement.

DIAGNOSIS AND TREATMENT

The diagnosis of OA usually is determined by history and physical examination, x-ray studies, and laboratory findings that exclude other diseases. Although OA often is contrasted with rheumatoid arthritis for diagnostic purposes, the differences are not always readily apparent. Other rheumatic diseases may be superimposed on OA. Psychological factors, severity of joint disease, and educational level affect the expression of symptoms.[31]

Characteristic radiologic changes initially include medial joint space narrowing, followed by subchondral bony sclerosis, formation of spikes on the tibial eminence, and osteophytes. The results of laboratory studies usually are normal because the disorder is not a systemic disease. The ESR may be slightly elevated in generalized OA or erosive inflammatory variations of the disease. If inflammation is present, there may be a slight increase in the blood cell count. The synovial fluid usually is normal.

Because there is no cure, the treatment of OA is symptomatic and includes physical rehabilitative, pharmacologic, and surgical measures. Physical measures are aimed at improving the supporting structures of the joint and strengthening opposing muscle groups involved in cushioning weight-bearing forces. This includes a balance of rest and exercise, use of splints to protect and rest the joint, use of heat and cold to relieve pain and muscle spasm, and adjusting the activities of daily living. The involved joint should not be further abused, and steps should be taken to protect and rest it. This includes weight reduction (when weight-bearing surfaces are involved) and the use of a cane or walker if the hips and knees are involved. Muscle-strengthening exercises may help protect the joint and decrease pain.[31]

Oral medications are aimed at reducing inflammation or providing analgesia. Popular medications used in the treatment of OA are the NSAIDs, many of which are available without a prescription. Ongoing research may confirm that some NSAIDs impede the repair mechanisms in early cartilage lesions. Because of the growing concern about the side effects of NSAIDs, the newer COX-2–inhibiting agents are often used for the treatment of OA. However, studies have shown that the pain of OA may arise from causes other than an inflamed synovium. These causes include stretching of the joint capsule, ligaments, or nerve endings in the periosteum over osteophytes; nontrabecular microfractures; intraosseous hypertension; bursitis or tendinitis; or muscle spasm. In such cases, the pain may be relieved by an NSAID because of the analgesic action of the drug rather than an antiinflammatory effect.[1] For many persons, acetaminophen may be as effective and less toxic than NSAIDs. The American College of Rheumatology (ACR) recommends the use of acetaminophen as the initial systemic treatment for OA.[35]

Intraarticular corticosteroid injections may be used when other treatment measures have been unsuccessful in adequately relieving symptoms. They are especially helpful in persons who have an effusion of the joint. Injections usually are limited to a total of four, and not more than three, within 1 year because their use is thought to accelerate joint destruction.

Viscosupplementation is a newer concept in treatment and is based on the hypothesis that joint lubrication is abnormal in OA. Hyaluronate is injected into the joint weekly for 3 to 5 weeks. Controlled studies have shown this approach to be as efficacious as NSAIDs.[36] Speculation that other agents (*i.e.*, glucosamine) may be chondroprotective has initiated other studies, but these results have not been confirmed in humans.

Surgery is considered when the person is having severe pain and joint function is severely reduced. Procedures include arthroscopic lavage and débridement, bunion resections, osteotomies to change alignment of the knee and hip joints, and decompression of the spinal roots in osteoarthritic vertebral stenosis. Total hip replacements have provided effective relief of symptoms and improved range of motion for many persons, as have total knee replacements, although the latter procedure has produced less consistent results. Joint replacement is available for the first carpometacarpal joint. Arthrodesis is used in advanced disease to reduce pain; however, this results in loss of motion.

Investigations are underway that use animal models of abrasion of the subchondral bone to permit vascular invasion to stimulate cartilage resorption and replacement with fibrocartilage and that place chondral grafts and progenitor cells under the periosteum.[37] Future management of OA lies in the development of techniques to identify and monitor cartilage lesions at an earlier stage. Potential approaches include bone scanning, magnetic resonance imaging, and arthroscopy.

In summary, OA, the most common form of arthritis, is a localized condition affecting primarily the weight-bearing joints. Risk factors for OA progression include older age, OA in multiple joints, neuropathy, and, for knees, obesity. The disorder is characterized by degeneration of the articular cartilage and subchondral bone. It has been suggested that the cellular events responsible for the development of OA begin with some type of abnormal mechanical insult or stimulus, including hormones and growth factors, drugs, mechanical stresses, and the extracellular environment. Studies also implicate immunologic factors in the perpetuation and acceleration of the osteoarthritic change. As cartilage ages, biochemical events such as collagen fatigue and fracture occur with less stress. Attempts at repair by increased matrix synthesis and cellular proliferation maintain the integrity of the cartilage until failure of reparative processes allows the degenerative changes to progress. Joint enlargement usually results from new bone formation, which causes the joint to feel hard. Pain and stiffness are primary features of the disease. Inflammatory mediators (*e.g.,* prostaglandins) may increase the inflammatory and degenerative response.

Treatment is directed toward the relief of pain and maintenance of mobility while preserving the articular cartilage. Although there is no known cure for OA, appropriate treatment can reduce pain, maintain or improve joint mobility, and limit functional disability.

Metabolic Diseases Associated With Rheumatic States

After completing this section of the chapter, you should be able to meet the following objectives:

- ✦ Relate the metabolism and elimination of uric acid to the pathogenesis of crystal-induced arthropathy
- ✦ State why asymptomatic hyperuricemia is a laboratory finding and not a disease
- ✦ Describe the clinical manifestations, diagnostic measures, and methods used in the treatment of gouty arthritis

Metabolic bone and joint disorders result from biochemical and metabolic disorders that affect the joints. Metabolic and endocrine diseases associated with joint symptoms include amyloidosis, osteogenesis imperfecta, diabetes mellitus, hyperparathyroidism, thyroid disease, AIDS, and hypermobility syndromes. The discussion in this chapter is limited to the crystal-induced arthropathy caused by monosodium urate deposition, or gout.

CRYSTAL-INDUCED ARTHROPATHIES

Crystal deposition in joints produces arthritis. In gout, monosodium urate or uric acid crystals are found in the joint cavity. Another condition in which calcium pyrophosphate dihydrate crystals are found in the joints sometimes is referred to as *pseudogout* or *chondrocalcinosis.* A brief discussion of pseudogout is found in the section on rheumatic diseases in the elderly.

Gout

Gout is actually a group of diseases known as the *gout syndrome.*[38,39] It includes acute gouty arthritis with recurrent attacks of severe articular and periarticular inflammation; tophi or the accumulation of crystalline deposits in articular surfaces, bones, soft tissue, and cartilage; gouty nephropathy or renal impairment; and uric acid kidney stones.

The term *primary gout* is used to designate cases in which the cause of the disorder is unknown or an inborn error in metabolism and is characterized primarily by hyperuricemia and gout. Primary gout is predominantly a disease of men, with a peak incidence in the fourth or sixth decade.[1] In secondary gout, the cause of the hyperuricemia is known, but the gout is not the main disorder. Asymptomatic hyperuricemia is a laboratory finding and not a disease. Most persons with hyperuricemia do not develop gout.

Pathogenesis. The pathogenesis of gout resides in an elevation of the serum uric acid levels. Uric acid is the end product of purine (adenine and guanine from DNA and RNA) metabolism.[33] Two pathways are involved in purine synthesis: (1) a de novo pathway in which purines are synthesized from nonpurine precursors, and (2) the salvage pathway in which purine bases are recaptured from the breakdown of nucleic acids derived from exogenous (dietary) or endogenous sources. The elevation of uric acid and the subsequent development of gout can result from overproduction of purines, decreased salvage of free purine bases, augmented breakdown of nucleic acids as a result of increased cell turnover, or decreased urinary excretion of uric acid. Primary gout, which constitutes 90% of cases, may be a consequence of enzyme defects, which result in an overproduction of uric acid; inadequate elimination of uric acid by the kidney; or a combination of the two.[33] In most cases, the reason is unknown. In secondary gout, the hyperuricemia may be caused by increased breakdown in the production of nucleic acids, as occurs with rapid tumor cell lysis during treatment for lymphoma or leukemia. Other cases of secondary gout result from chronic renal disease. Some of the diuretics, including the thiazides, can interfere with the excretion of uric acid.

An attack of gout occurs when monosodium urate crystals precipitate in the joint and initiate an inflammatory response. Synovial fluid is a poorer solvent for uric acid than plasma and uric acid crystals are even less soluble at temperatures below 37°C. Crystal deposition usually occurs in peripheral areas of the body, such as the great toe, where the temperatures are cooler than other parts of the body. With prolonged hyperuricemia, crystals and microtophi (*i.e.,* small hard nodules with irregular surfaces that contain crystalline deposits of monosodium urate) accumulate in the synovial lining cells and in the joint cartilage. The released crystals are chemotactic to leukocytes and also activate complement. Phagocytosis of urate crystals by polymorphonuclear leukocytes occurs and leads to polymorphonuclear cell death with the release of lysosomal enzymes. As this process continues, the inflammation causes destruction of the cartilage and subchondral bone.

Repeated attacks of acute arthritis eventually lead to chronic arthritis and the formation of the large, hard nodules called tophi[40] (Fig. 59-10). They are found most commonly in the synovium, olecranon bursa, Achilles tendon, subchondral bone, and extensor surface of the forearm and may be mistaken for rheumatoid nodules. Tophi usually do not appear until 10 years or more after the first gout attack. This stage of gout, called *chronic tophaceous gout,* is characterized by more frequent and prolonged attacks, which often are polyarticular.

Clinical Manifestations. The typical acute attack of gout is monoarticular and usually affects the first metatarsophalangeal joint. The tarsal joints, insteps, ankles, heels, knees, wrists, fingers, and elbows also may be initial sites of involvement. Acute gout often begins at night and may be precipitated by excessive exercise, certain medications, foods, alcohol, or dieting. The onset of pain typically is abrupt, and redness and swelling are observed. The attack may last for days or weeks. Pain may be severe enough to be aggravated even by the weight of a bed sheet covering the affected area.

In the early stages of gout after the initial attack has subsided, the person is asymptomatic, and joint abnormalities are not evident. This is referred to as *intercritical gout.* After the first attack, it may be months or years before another attack. As attacks recur with increased frequency, joint changes occur and become permanent.

Diagnosis and Treatment

Diagnosis. Although hyperuricemia is the biochemical hallmark of gout, the presence of hyperuricemia cannot be equated with gout because many persons with this condition never develop gout. A definitive diagnosis of gout can be made only when monosodium urate crystals are in the synovial fluid or in tissue sections of tophaceous deposits. Synovial fluid analysis is useful in excluding other conditions, such as septic arthritis, pseudogout, and rheumatoid arthritis. Diagnostic methods also include measures to determine whether the disorder is related to overproduction or to underexcretion of uric acid. This is done through measurement of serum uric acid levels and collection of a 24-hour urine sample for determination of urate excretion in the urine.[41]

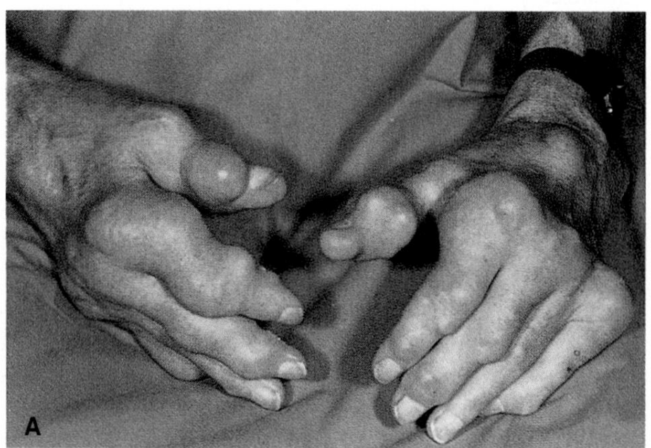

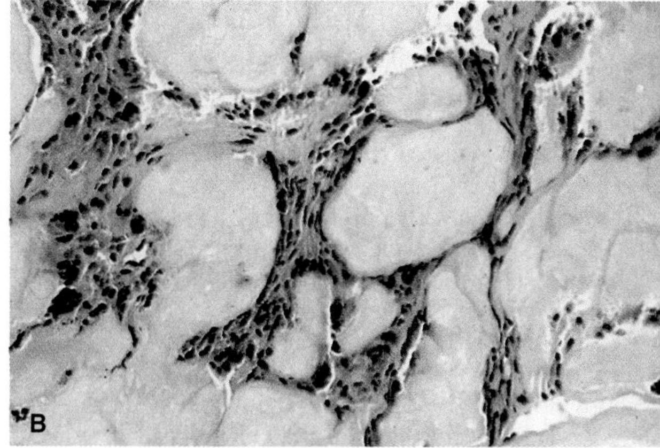

FIGURE 59-10 Gout (**A**) Gouty tophi project from the fingers as rubbery nodules. (**B**) A section from a tophus shows extracellular masses of urate crystals with accompanying foreign-body giant cells. (Rubin E., Farber J.L. [1999]. *Pathology* [3rd ed., p. 1404]. Philadelphia: Lippincott-Raven)

Treatment. The objectives for treatment of gout include the termination and prevention of the acute attacks of gouty arthritis and the correction of hyperuricemia, with consequent inhibition of further precipitation of sodium urate and absorption of urate crystal deposits already in the tissues.

Pharmacologic management of acute gout is directed toward reducing joint inflammation. Hyperuricemia and related problems of tophi, joint destruction, and renal problems are treated after the acute inflammatory process has subsided. NSAIDs, particularly indomethacin and ibuprofen, are used for treating acute gouty arthritis. Alternative therapies include colchicine and intraarticular deposition of corticosteroids. Treatment with colchicine is used early in the acute stage. Colchicine produces its antiinflammatory effects by inhibition of leukocyte migration and phagocytosis. Although the drug usually is given orally, a more rapid response is obtained when colchicine is given intravenously. The acute symptoms of gout usually subside within 48 hours after treatment with oral colchicine has been instituted and within 12 hours after intravenous administration of the drug. The NSAIDs are also effective during the acute stage when used at their maximum dosage and sometimes are preferred to colchicine because they have fewer toxic side effects. Phenylbutazone usually is effective but is used only on a short-term basis because long-term use can cause bone marrow suppression. The corticosteroid drugs are not recommended for treatment of gout unless all other medications have proved unsuccessful. Intraarticular injections of corticosteroid agents may be used when only one joint is involved and the person is unable to take colchicine or NSAIDs.

With the exception of phenylbutazone, the drugs used to treat acute gout have no effect on the serum urate level and are valueless in tophaceous gout and the control of hyperuricemia. After the acute attack has been relieved, the hyperuricemia is treated. Treatment of hyperuricemia is aimed at maintaining normal uric acid levels and is lifelong. One method is to reduce hyperuricemia through the use of allopurinol or a uricosuric agent. Allopurinol inhibits xanthine oxidase, an enzyme needed for the conversion of hypoxanthine to xanthine and xanthine to uric acid.[41] The uricosuric drugs (*e.g.,* probenecid or sulfinpyrazone, a phenylbutazone derivative) prevent the tubular reabsorption of urate and increase its excretion in the urine. The serum urate concentrations are monitored to determine efficacy and dosage. Prophylactic colchicine or NSAIDs may be used between gout attacks.

Although gout can often be effectively controlled by nonpharmacologic methods, many persons with gout have a limited understanding of the disease and therefore a poor compliance with treatment. Thus, education about the disease and its management is fundamental to the treatment and management of gout. Some changes in lifestyle may be needed, such as maintenance of ideal weight, moderation in alcohol consumption, and avoidance of purine-rich foods (*e.g.,* liver, kidney, sardines, anchovies, and sweetbreads) particularly by patients with excessive tophaceous deposits.

In summary, crystal-induced arthropathy is characterized by crystal deposition in the joint. However, hyperuricemia is a laboratory finding and not a disease. Gout is the prototype of this group. Acute attacks of arthritis occur with gout and are characterized by the presence of monosodium urate crystals in the joint. The disorder is accompanied by hyperuricemia, which results from overproduction of uric acid or from the reduced ability of the kidney to rid the body of excess uric acid. Management of acute gout is directed first toward the reduction of joint inflammation; then the hyperuricemia is treated. Hyperuricemia is treated with uricosuric agents, which prevent the tubular reabsorption of urate, or with medication that inhibits the production of uric acid. Although gout is chronic, it can be controlled with appropriate lifestyle changes by most patients.

Rheumatic Diseases in Children and the Elderly

After completing this section of the chapter, you should be able to meet the following objectives:

- ✦ List three types of juvenile rheumatoid arthritis and differentiate among their major characteristics
- ✦ Name one rheumatic disease that affects only the elderly population

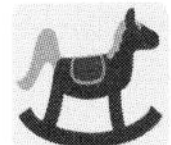

RHEUMATIC DISEASES IN CHILDREN

Children can be affected with almost all of the rheumatic diseases. In addition to disease-specific differences, these conditions affect not only the child but also the family. Growth and development require special attention. Adherence to the treatment program requires intervention with the child and parents. School issues also must be addressed.

Juvenile Rheumatoid Arthritis

Juvenile rheumatoid arthritis (JRA) is a chronic disease that affects approximately 70,000 to 100,000 children younger than 16 years of age in the United States.[1] It is characterized by synovitis and can influence epiphyseal growth by stimulating growth of the affected side. Generalized stunted growth also may occur.

Systemic onset affects approximately 10% of children with JRA.[1] The symptoms of systemic JRA include a daily intermittent high fever, which usually is accompanied by a rash, generalized lymphadenopathy, hepatosplenomegaly, leukocytosis, and anemia. Most of these children also have joint involvement, which develops concurrently with fever and rash. Systemic symptoms usually subside in 6 to 12 months. This form of JRA also can make an initial appearance in adulthood. Infections, heart disease, and adrenal insufficiency may cause death.

A second subgroup of JRA, pauciarticular arthritis, affects no more than four joints. This disease affects approximately 50% of children with JRA.[1] Pauciarticular arthritis affects two distinct groups. The first group generally consists of girls younger than 6 years of age with chronic uveitis. The results of ANA testing in this group usually are positive. The second group, characterized by late-onset arthritis, is made up mostly of boys. The HLA-B27 test results are positive in more than one half of this group. They are affected by sacroiliitis, and the arthritis usually occurs in the lower extremities.

The third subgroup of JRA, accounting for approximately 40% of the total, is polyarticular onset disease.[1] It affects five or more joints during the first 6 months of the disease. This form of arthritis more closely resembles the adult form of the disease than the other two subgroups. Rheumatoid factor sometimes is present and may indicate a more active disease process. Systemic features include a low-grade fever, weight loss, malaise, anemia, stunted growth, slight organomegaly (*e.g.*, hepatosplenomegaly), and adenopathy.[1]

The prognosis for most children with rheumatoid arthritis is good. NSAIDs are the first-line drugs used in treating JRA. Salicylates have been replaced by agents such as naproxen, ibuprofen, and ketoprofen. Second-line agents are low-dose methotrexate and, less often, sulfasalazine. Gold salts, hydroxychloroquine, and D-penicillamine rarely are used.[42] Biologic response modifiers are also being used in juvenile arthritis, with etanercept being the first to receive U.S. Food and Drug Administration (FDA) approval.[43] Other aspects of treatment of children with JRA require careful attention to growth and development and nutritional issues. Children are encouraged to lead as normal a life as possible.

Systemic Lupus Erythematosus

The features of SLE in children are similar to those in adults. The incidence in children is 10 times lower, estimated to occur in 0.6 of 100,000 children. The occurrence in the sexes is almost equal until pubescence, after which it approaches the sex ratio seen in adults. The clinical manifestations of SLE in children reflect the extent and severity of systemic involvement. The best prognostic indicator in children is the extent of renal involvement, which is more common and more severe in children than in adults with SLE. Infectious complications are the most common cause of death (40%) in children with SLE.

Children with SLE may present with constitutional symptoms, including fever, malaise, anorexia, and weight loss. Symptoms of the integumentary, musculoskeletal, central nervous, cardiac, pulmonary, and hematopoietic systems are similar to those of adults. Endocrine abnormalities include Cushing's syndrome from long-term corticosteroid use and autoimmune thyroiditis. Adolescents often experience menstrual disturbances, which tend to resolve with disease remission.

Treatment of SLE in children is similar to that in adults. The use of NSAIDs, corticosteroids, antimalarials, and immunosuppressive agents depends on the symptoms. Corticosteroids may cause stunting of growth and necrosis of femoral heads and other joints. Immunization schedules should be maintained using attenuated rather than live vaccines. Rest periods should be balanced with exercise; children should be encouraged to maintain as normal a schedule as possible.[43] The diversity of the clinical manifestations of SLE in the young requires the establishment of a comprehensive program.

Juvenile Dermatomyositis

Juvenile dermatomyositis (JDMS) is an inflammatory myopathy primarily involving skin and muscle and associated with a characteristic rash. JDMS can affect children of all ages, with a mean age at onset of 8 years. There is an increased incidence among girls. The cause is unknown.

Symmetric proximal muscle weakness, elevated muscle enzymes, evidence of vasculitis, and electromyographic changes confirming an inflammatory myopathy are diagnostic for JDMS. Generalized vasculitis is not seen in the adult form of the disease. The rash may precede or follow the onset of proximal muscle weakness. Periorbital edema, erythema, and eyelid telangiectasia are common.

Calcifications can occur in 30% to 50% of children with JDMS and are by far the most debilitating symptom. The calcifications appear at pressure points or sites of previous trauma. JDMS is treated primarily with corticosteroids to reduce inflammation. Occasionally, immunosuppressives are used in cases of refractory disease.[1] Adjunct therapies include using sun block of at least SPF 36, a calcium-sufficient diet, and vitamin D therapy.

Juvenile Spondyloarthropathies

Ankylosing spondylitis, reactive arthritis, psoriatic arthritis, and spondyloarthropathies associated with ulcerative colitis and regional enteritis can affect children and adults. In children, spondyloarthritis manifests in peripheral joints first, mimicking pauciarticular JRA, with no evidence of sacroiliac or spine involvement for months to years after onset. The spondyloarthropathies are more common in boys and commonly occur in children who have a positive family history. HLA-B27 typing is helpful in diagnosing children because of the unusual presentation of the disease.

Management of the disease involves physical therapy, education, and attention to school and growth and development issues. Medication includes the use of salicylates or other NSAIDs such as tolmetin or indomethacin. More severe disease or symptoms may require systemic corticosteroids.[1] Etanercept and infliximab produce more dramatic improvement of disease activity; however, long-term effects and toxicity are not yet known.[44]

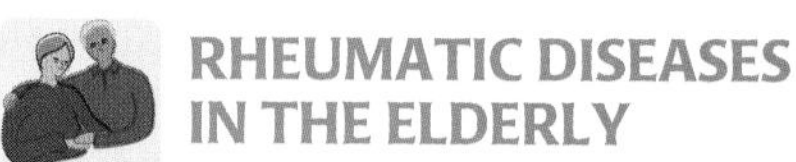

RHEUMATIC DISEASES IN THE ELDERLY

Arthritis is the most common complaint of elderly persons. The pain, stiffness, and muscle weakness affect daily life, often threatening independence and quality of life. Symptoms of the rheumatic diseases also can have an indirect effect and even threaten the duration of life for the elderly. The weakness and gait disturbance that often accompany the rheumatic diseases can contribute to the likelihood of falls and fracture, causing suffering, increased health care costs, further loss of independence, and the potential for a decreased life span.

The elderly cope less well with mild to moderately severe disease that in younger persons is less likely to lead to serious disability for the same degree of impairment. Unfortunately, the elderly and often their health care providers think the problems associated with arthritis are an inevitable consequence of aging and fail to benefit from measures that can improve the quality of life.

Because arthritis is the leading cause of change in the functional status of older adults, a functional approach to the problems of the elderly is appropriate. Inactivity is a societal expectation of the elderly. What activity there is tends to be low impact (*e.g.*, leisurely walking), and deconditioning occurs.

Older patients often have multiple problems complicating diagnosis and management. The diagnosis of an elderly patient with a musculoskeletal problem must consider a wide variety of disorders that usually are regarded as outside the range of typical rheumatic disease. Among these are metastatic malignancy, multiple myeloma, musculoskeletal disorders accompanying endocrine or metabolic disorders, orthopedic conditions, and neurologic disease. The diagnosis may be missed if the assumption is that musculoskeletal problems in the older person are caused by OA.

There is an increased incidence of false-positive test results for rheumatoid factor and ANA in the elderly population with or without rheumatic disease because older persons are better producers of autoantibodies than younger persons. There are differences in the manifestations, diagnosis, and treatment of some of the rheumatic diseases in the elderly. The usual presentation of these conditions was discussed earlier in this chapter. One form of rheumatic disease that has a predilection for the elderly is polymyalgia rheumatica.

Rheumatoid Arthritis

The prevalence of rheumatoid arthritis increases with advancing age, at least until 75 years of age.[45] Seropositive patients are more likely to have had an acute onset with systemic features and higher disease activity. Patients with seronegative, elderly-onset rheumatoid arthritis have a disease that usually follows a mild course. The close resemblance of the manifestations of seronegative rheumatoid arthritis in the elderly to those of polymyalgia rheumatica has led to speculation concerning the relation of these syndromes.[45] It may be that rheumatoid arthritis in the elderly is a broad disorder that includes a number of distinct subsets with characteristic manifestations, courses, and outcomes.

Systemic Lupus Erythematosus

Systemic lupus erythematosus is another condition with different manifestations in the elderly. The disease is accompanied less frequently by renal involvement. However, pleurisy, pericarditis, arthritis, and symptoms closely resembling polymyalgia rheumatica are more common than in younger patients. The characteristics of SLE in the elderly closely resemble those of drug-induced SLE, leading to speculation that the syndrome may result from one of the multiple drugs that are taken by many elderly patients.[46]

Osteoarthritis

Osteoarthritis is by far the most common form of arthritis among the elderly. It is the greatest cause of disability and limitation of activity in older populations. It has been suggested that osteoarthritis begins at a very young age, expressing itself in the elderly only after a long period of latency. Too often, it is accepted by the patient or expected by the physician. Osteoarthritis presents a major management problem, but there is much that can be done. Self-control by maintaining a positive attitude and sense of self-esteem is a frequent coping strategy.[47]

Crystal-Induced Arthropathies

Gout. The incidence of clinical gout increases with advancing age, in part because of the increased involvement of joints after years of continued hyperuricemia. High serum urate levels rarely occur in women before menopause; initial attacks of clinical gout occur around the age of 70 years, or 20 years after menopause.[38] Gouty attacks in elderly women may be precipitated by the use of diuretics. The treatment of gout is often more difficult in the elderly. Although colchicine may be effective in controlling the symptoms of chronic gout, it may cause diarrhea in some patients, limiting its effectiveness in maintenance therapy.

Pseudogout. As part of the tissue-aging process, osteoarthritis develops with associated cartilage degeneration and the shedding of calcium pyrophosphate crystals into the joint cavity. These crystals may produce a low-grade chronic inflammation—the chronic pseudogout syndrome. The accumulation of calcium pyrophosphate and related crystalline deposits in articular cartilage is common in the elderly. There are no medications that can remove the crystals from the joints. Although it may be asymptomatic, presence of the crystals may contribute to more rapid cartilage deterioration. This condition may coexist with severe osteoarthritis.

Polymyalgia Rheumatica

Polymyalgia rheumatica is an inflammatory condition of unknown origin characterized by aching and morning stiffness in the cervical regions and shoulder and pelvic girdle areas.[48] Of the forms of arthritis affecting the elderly, it is one of the more difficult to diagnose and one of the most important to identify. Elderly women are especially at risk. Polymyalgia rheumatica is a common syndrome of older patients, rarely occurring before 50 years of age and usually after 60 years of age. The onset can be abrupt, with the patient going to bed feeling well and awakening with pain and stiffness in the neck, shoulders, and hips.

Diagnosis is based on the pain and stiffness persisting for at least 1 month and an elevated ESR. The diagnosis is confirmed when the symptoms respond dramatically to a small dose of prednisone, a corticosteroid. Biopsies have shown that the muscles are normal, despite the name, but that a nonspecific inflammation affecting the synovial tissue is present. It is possible that a number of patients are erroneously diagnosed as having rheumatoid arthritis or osteoarthritis. For patients with an elevated ESR (0.5 mm), the diagnosis usually is based on a 3-day trial of prednisone treatment.[49] Patients with polymyalgia rheumatica typically exhibit striking clinical improvement approximately the second day. Patients with rheumatoid arthritis also show improvement, although usually days later.

Treatment with NSAIDs provides relief for some patients, but most require continuing therapy with prednisone, with gradual reduction of the dose over the course of 1.5 to 2 years, using the patient's symptoms as the primary guide. Patients need close monitoring during the maintenance phase with prednisone therapy. Because their symptoms are relieved, they often stop taking the prednisone, and their symptoms recur, or doses are missed and the decreased dosage leads to an increase in symptoms. Unless careful assessment reveals the frequency of missed doses, the physician may be misled into increasing the dosage when it is not needed. Because of the side effects of the corticosteroids, the goal is to use the lowest dose of the drug necessary to control the symptoms. Weaning patients off low-dose prednisone therapy after this length of time can be a difficult and extended process.

A certain percentage of patients with polymyalgia rheumatica also have giant cell arteritis (*i.e.,* temporal arteritis), frequently with involvement of the ophthalmic arteries. The two conditions are considered to represent different manifestations of the same disease. Giant cell arteritis, a form of systemic vasculitis, is a systemic inflammatory disease of large and medium-sized arteries (see Chapter 24). The inflammatory response seems to be a T-cell response to an antigen.

Clinical manifestations of giant cell arteritis usually begin insidiously and may exist for some time before being recognized[49] (Chart 59-3). It is potentially dangerous if missed or mistreated, especially if the temporal artery or other vessels supplying the eye are involved, in which case blindness can ensue quickly without treatment. The condition is responsive to appropriate therapy. For those patients at risk, adherence to the medication program is critical, with preservation of sight being the goal. Because this complication can occur so quickly and is relatively asymptomatic, it is vital that the patient understand the importance of taking the correct dose regularly as prescribed. Initial treatment consists of large doses of prednisone. This dosage is continued for 4 to 6 weeks and then decreased gradually.

CHART 59-3

Signs and Symptoms of Giant Cell Arteritis

- Constitutional symptoms
  - Malaise
  - Fatigue
  - Fever (usually low grade)
  - Weight loss
  - Cough
  - Sore throat
- Polymyalgia rheumatica syndrome
  - Limb girdle pain and stiffness
- Manifestations related to vascular involvement
  - New type of headache
  - Scalp tenderness, especially over temporal area
  - Visual loss
  - Diplopia
  - Aortic arch syndrome
- Ischemic optic neuropathy
  - Atrophy
- Claudication of jaw or arm

Localized Musculoskeletal Disorders

The elderly also are prone to localized musculoskeletal syndromes. Years of wear frequently lead to a range of inflammatory disorders, including bursitis and tendinitis. These are known collectively as *impingement syndromes*. An example is a disorder in the shoulder where the rotator cuff rides against the acromion. Tennis elbow (only 5% of those with this problem actually play tennis), or humeral epicondylitis, also is seen frequently among the elderly. Other localized inflammatory conditions of the musculoskeletal system affecting the elderly are fibrositis or fibromyalgia and Dupuytren's contracture.

Management of Rheumatic Diseases in the Elderly

In addition to diagnosis-specific treatment, the elderly require special considerations. Management techniques that rely on modalities other than drugs are particularly important for the elderly. These include splints, walking aids, muscle-building exercise, and local heat. Muscle-strengthening and stretching exercises are particularly effective in the elderly person with age-related losses in muscle function and should be instituted early. Rest, the cornerstone of conservative therapy, is hazardous in the elderly, who can rapidly lose muscle strength.

In terms of medications, the selection of drugs used in the treatment of arthritic disorders and their dosages may need to be considered when prescribing for the elderly. For example, the NSAIDs may be less well tolerated by the elderly, and their side effects are more likely to be serious. In addition to bleeding from the gastrointestinal tract and renal insufficiency, there may be cognitive dysfunction, manifested by forgetfulness, inability to concentrate, sleeplessness, paranoid ideation, and depression.

Joint arthroplasty can also be used for pain relief and increased function. Chronologic age is not a contraindication to surgical treatment of arthritis. In appropriately selected elderly candidates, survival and functional outcome after surgery are equivalent to those in younger age groups. The more sedentary activity level of the elderly makes them even better candidates for joint replacement because they put less stress and demand on the new joint.

In summary, rheumatic diseases that affect children can be similar to the adult diseases, but there also are manifestations unique to the younger population. Children with chronic diseases have to be approached with different priorities than adults. Managing rheumatic diseases in children requires a team approach to address issues of the family, school, growth and development, and coping strategies and requires a comprehensive disease management program.

Arthritis is the most common complaint of the elderly population. The pain, stiffness, and muscle weakness affect daily life, often threatening independence and quality of life. There is a difference in the manifestations, diagnosis, and treatment of some of the rheumatic diseases in the elderly compared with those in the younger population. Osteoarthritis is the most common form of arthritis among the elderly. The prevalence of rheumatoid arthritis and gout increases with advancing age. One form of rheumatic disease that has a predilection for the elderly is polymyalgia rheumatica. A certain percentage of patients with polymyalgia rheumatica also have giant cell arteritis, frequently with involvement of the ophthalmic arteries. If this condition is untreated, it carries a serious threat of blindness.

REVIEW EXERCISES

A 30-year-old woman, recently diagnosed with rheumatoid arthritis (RA), complains of general fatigue and weight loss along with symmetric joint swelling, stiffness, and pain. The stiffness is more prominent in the morning and subsides during the day. Laboratory measures reveal an RA factor of 120 IU/mL (nonreactive, 0–39 IU/mL; weakly reactive, 40–79 IU/mL; reactive, >80 IU/mL).

A. Describe the immunopathogenesis of the joint changes that occur with RA.

B. How do these changes relate to this woman's symptoms?

C. What is the significance of the results of her RA factor test results?

D. How do her complaints of general fatigue and weight relate to the RA disease process?

A 65-year-old obese woman, with a diagnosis of osteoarthritis (OA), has been having increasing pain in her right knee that is made worse with movement and weight bearing and is relieved by rest. Physical examination reveals an enlarged joint with a varus deformity; coarse crepitus is felt over the joint on passive movement.

A. Compare the pathogenesis and articular structures involved in OA with that of RA.

B. What are the origins of the crepitus felt on enlargement of the affected joint, the varus deformity, and the crepitus that is felt on movement of the affected knee?

C. Explain the predilection for involvement of the knee in persons such as this woman.

D. What types of treatment are available for this woman?

A 75-year-old woman is seen by a health care provider because of complaints of fever, malaise, and weight loss. She is having trouble combing her hair, putting on a coat, and getting out of a chair because of the stiffness and pain in her shoulders, hip, and lower back. Because of her age and symptoms, the health care provider suspects the woman has polymyalgia rheumatica.

A. What laboratory test can be used to substantiate the diagnosis?

B. What other diagnostic strategies are used to confirm the diagnosis?

C. How is the disease treated?

References

1. Klippel J.R. (Ed.). (2001). *Primer on the rheumatic diseases* (12th ed., pp. 209–235, 329–351, 239–258, 285–298, 307–324, 534–540). Atlanta: Arthritis Foundation.
2. Harris E.D. (2001). Clinical features of rheumatoid arthritis. In Ruddy S., Harris E.D., Sledge C.B. (Eds.), *Textbook of rheumatology* (6th ed., pp. 967–1000). Philadelphia: W.B. Saunders.
3. Zhang Z., Bridges S.L. (2001). Pathogenesis of rheumatoid arthritis: Role of B lymphocytes. *Annals of Rheumatic Disease 27*(2), 335–353.
4. Robbins L. (Ed.). (2001). *Clinical care in the rheumatic diseases* (2nd ed.). Atlanta: American College of Rheumatology.
5. American College of Rheumatology Subcommittee on Rheumatoid Arthritis Guidelines. (2002). Guidelines for the management of rheumatoid arthritis: 2002 Update. *Arthritis and Rheumatism 46,* 328–346.
6. Ramsburg K. (2000). Rheumatoid arthritis. *American Journal of Nursing 100* (11), 40–43.
7. Terebelo S. (2003). Rheumatoid arthritis, making the diagnosis. *Clinician Reviews 13*(2), 58–64.
8. Lee D.M., Schur P.H. (2003). The detection of anti-cyclic citrullinated peptides (CCP). *Annals of Rheumatic Disease 62,* 870–874.
9. Hill J.A., Southwood S., Sette A., et al. (2003). Cutting edge: The conversion of arginine to citrulline allows for high-affinity interaction between rheumatoid arthritis-associated HLA-DRB1*0401 Class II molecule. *Journal of Immunology 171*(2), 538–541.
10. Stenstrom C.H., Minor M.A. (2003). Evidence for the benefit of aerobic and strengthening exercise in rheumatoid arthritis. *Arthritis Care and Research 49*(3), 428–434.
11. Maetzel A., Krahn M., Naglie G. (2003). The cost effectiveness of rofecoxib and celecoxib in patients with osteoarthritis and rheumatoid arthritis. *Arthritis Care and Research 49*(3), 283–292.
12. Halin J. (2000). Treatment of rheumatoid arthritis: Etanercept, a recent advance. *Journal of the American Academy of Nurse Practitioners 12,* 433–441.
13. Kastanek L. (2002). Using anakinra for adult rheumatoid arthritis. *Nurse Practitioner 27*(4), 62–65.
14. Breedveld F.C. (2002). Paving the way for improved outcomes in RA: The rationale for TNF blockade. In *Biologic DMARDs in the management of rheumatoid arthritis.* CME proceedings (pp. 15–19). Red Bank, NJ: Fallon Medica.
15. Mulvihill K. (2003). Systemic lupus erythematosus. *Advance for Nurse Practitioners* January, 32–37.

16. Edworthy S.M. (2001). Clinical manifestations of systemic lupus erythematosus. In Ruddy S., Harris E.D., Sledge C.B. (Eds.), *Textbook of rheumatology* (6th ed., pp. 1105–1123). Philadelphia: W.B. Saunders.
17. Criscione L.G. (2003). The pathogenesis of systemic lupus erythematosus. *Bulletin on the Rheumatic Diseases 52*(6), 1–7.
18. Tan E.M., Cohen A.S., Fries J.C., et al. (1982). The 1982 revised criteria for the classification of systemic lupus erythematosus. *Arthritis and Rheumatism 25,* 1271–1277.
19. Solomon D.H., Kavanaugh A.J., Shur P.H. (2002). Evidence-based guidelines for the use of immunologic tests: Antinuclear antibody testing. *Arthritis Care and Research 46*(4), 434–444.
20. Pigg J.S., Bancroft D.A. (2000). Management of patients with rheumatic diseases. In Smeltzer S.C., Bare B.C. (Eds.), *Brunner and Suddarth's textbook of medical-surgical nursing* (9th ed., pp. 1405–1433). Philadelphia: Lippincott Williams & Wilkins.
21. Ortman R.A., Klippel J.H. (2000). Update on cyclophosphamide for systemic lupus erythematosus. *Rheumatic Disease Clinics of North America 26,* 363–375.
22. Steen V.D., Medsger T.A. (2000). Severe organ involvement in systemic sclerosis with diffuse scleroderma. *Arthritis and Rheumatism 43,* 2437–2444.
23. Mayes M.D. (2003). Scleroderma epidemiology. *Rheumatic Disease Clinics of North America 29,* 240–254.
24. Lin A.T.H., Clements P.J., Furst D.E. (2003). Update on disease modifying antirheumatic drugs in the treatment of systemic sclerosis. *Rheumatic Disease Clinics of North America 29,* 409–426.
25. Kuon W., Sieper J. (2003). Identification of HLA-B27 restricted peptides in reactive arthritis and other spondyloarthropathies. *Rheumatic Disease Clinics of North America 29,* 595–611.
26. Miceli-Richard C., Heijde D., Dougados M. (2003). Spondyloarthropathy for practicing rheumatologists: Diagnosis, indication for disease-controlling antirheumatic therapy, and evaluation of the response. *Rheumatic Disease Clinics of North America 29,* 449–462.
27. Brandt J., Haibel H., Cornely D., et al. (2000). Successful treatment of active ankylosing spondylitis with the anti-tumor necrosis factor α monoclonal antibody infliximab. *Arthritis and Rheumatism 43,* 1346–1352.
28. Flores D., Marquez J., Garza M., Espinoza L.R. (2003). Reactive arthritis: Newer developments. *Rheumatic Disease Clinics of North America 29,* 37–59.
29. Sigal L.H. (2001). Update on reactive arthritis. *Bulletin on the Rheumatic Diseases 50*(4).
30. Mease P.J. (2003). Current treatment of psoriatic arthritis. *Rheumatic Disease Clinics of North America 29,* 495–511.
31. Loeser R.F. (2003). A stepwise approach to the management of osteoarthritis. *Bulletin on the Rheumatic Diseases 52*(5).
32. Huang M., Chen C., Chen T., et al. (2000). The effects of weight reduction on the rehabilitation of patients with knee osteoarthritis and obesity. *Arthritis Care and Research 13,* 398–405.
33. Burns D.K., Kumar V. (2003). The musculoskeletal system. In Kumar V., Cotran R.S., Robbins S.L. *Robbins basic pathology* (7th ed., pp. 772–775). Philadelphia: W.B. Saunders.
34. Loeser R.F. (2000). Aging and the etiopathogenesis and treatment of osteoarthritis. *Rheumatic Disease Clinics of North America 26*(3), 547–567.
35. American College of Rheumatology Subcommittee on Osteoarthritis Guidelines. (2000). Recommendations for the medical management of osteoarthritis of the hip and knee: 2000 update. *Arthritis and Rheumatology 43,* 1905–1915.
36. Brandt K., Smith G.N., Simon L.S. (2000). Intraarticular injection of hyaluronan as treatment for knee osteoarthritis: What is the evidence? *Arthritis and Rheumatism 43,* 1192–1203.
37. Dieppe P. (2000). The management of osteoarthritis in the third millennium. *Scandinavian Journal of Rheumatology 29,* 279–281.
38. Agudelo C.A., Wise K.M. (2000). Crystal-associated arthritis in the elderly. *Rheumatic Disease Clinics of North America 26,* 527–546.
39. Schlesinger N., Schumacher H.R. (2002). Update on gout. *Arthritis Care and Research 47*(5), 563–565.
40. Schiller A.L., Teitbaum S.L. (1999). Bones and joints. In Rubin E., Farber J.L. (Eds.), *Pathology.* (3rd ed., pp. 1365–1406). Philadelphia: Lippincott-Raven.
41. Perez-Ruiz F., Calabozo M., Pijoan J.I., et al. (2002). Effect of urate lowering therapy on the velocity and size reduction of tophi in chronic gout. *Arthritis Care and Research 47*(4), 356–360.
42. Lomater C., Gerloni V., Gattinara M., et al. (2000). Systemic onset juvenile idiopathic arthritis: A retrospective study of 80 consecutive patients followed for 10 years. *Journal of Rheumatology 27,* 491–496.
43. Milojevic D.S., Ilowite N.T. (2002). Treatment of rheumatic diseases in children: Special considerations. *Rheumatic Disease Clinics of North America 28,* 461–482.
44. Burgos-Vargas R. (2002). The juvenile-onset spondyloarthritides. *Rheumatic Disease Clinics of North America 28,* 531–560.
45. Yaziu Y., Paget S.A. (2000). Elderly-onset rheumatoid arthritis. *Rheumatic Disease Clinics of North America 26,* 517–526.
46. Kammer G.M., Misha N. (2000). Systemic lupus erythematosus in the elderly. *Rheumatic Disease Clinics of North America 26,* 475–492.
47. Rapp S.R., Rejeski W.J., Miller M.E. (2000). Physical function among older adults with knee pain: The role of coping skills. *Arthritis Care and Research 13,* 270–279.
48. Salvarani C., Cantini F., Boiardi L., Hunder G.G. (2002). Polymyalgia rheumatica and giant-cell arteritis. *New England Journal of Medicine 347*(4), 261–271.
49. Evans J.M., Hunder G.C. (2000). Polymyalgia rheumatica and giant cell arteritis. *Rheumatic Disease Clinics of North America 26,* 493–515.

CHAPTER 60

Structure and Function of the Skin

Gladys Simandl

The skin is the largest organ of the body and forms the major barrier between the internal organs and the external environment. The skin accounts for roughly 16% of the body's weight. As the body's first line of defense, the skin is continuously subjected to potentially harmful environmental agents, including solid matter, liquids, gases, sunlight, and microorganisms. Although the skin may become bruised, lacerated, burned, or infected, it has remarkable properties that allow for a continuous cycle of healing, shedding, and cell regeneration.

In its protective role, the skin harbors a constant flora of microorganisms. Relatively harmless strains protect the skin surface from other, more virulent organisms. A thin layer of lipid film covers the skin and contains fatty acids that are bactericidal, protecting against the entry of harmful microorganisms. The skin also serves as an immunologic barrier. The Langerhans' cells detect foreign antigens, playing an important part in allergic skin conditions and skin graft rejections. As a chemical barrier, the skin controls substances entering or leaving the body.

The skin serves several other important functions, including temperature regulation, somatosensory function, and vitamin D synthesis. The skin is richly innervated with pain, temperature, and touch receptors. Skin receptors relay the numerous qualities of touch, such as pressure, sharpness, dullness, and pleasure, to the central nervous system for localization and fine discrimination.

As the outer covering of the body, the skin may demonstrate outwardly what occurs within the body. A number of systemic diseases are manifested by skin disorders (*e.g.*, rash associated with systemic lupus erythematosus and jaundice due to liver disease). In other words, although skin eruptions frequently represent primary diseases of the skin, they may also be a manifestation of systemic disease.

Although broken down into its constituent parts in this chapter, the skin is increasingly being understood as a complex, dynamic, interacting system among the neurologic, immunologic, cutaneous, and endocrine systems.[1] Mind-body influences are bidirectional, and the skin should be considered an "active neuroimmunoendocrine interface, where effector molecules of neuropeptides act as common words used in a dynamic dialogue between brain, immune system, and skin."[2]

Structure of the Skin

After completing this chapter, you should be able to meet the following objectives:

- List and describe the functions of skin
- Describe the changes in a keratinocyte from its inception in the basal lamina to its arrival on the outer surface of the skin
- List the four specialized cells of the epidermis and describe what is known about their functions
- Describe the structure and function of the dermis and subcutaneous layers of skin
- Describe the following skin appendages and their functions: sebaceous gland, eccrine gland, apocrine gland, nails, and hair
- Characterize the skin in terms of sensory and immune functions

FUNCTIONS OF THE SKIN

- The skin is the largest organ of the body.
- As an interface between the internal and external environments, the skin prevents body fluids from leaving the body, protects the body from potentially damaging environmental agents, and serves as an area for heat exchange; in addition, cells of the skin immune system provide protection against invading microorganisms.
- Receptors in the skin relay touch, pressure, temperature, and pain sensation to the central nervous system for localization and discrimination.

There are great variations in skin structure on different parts of the body; therefore, "normal skin" on any one surface of the body is difficult to describe. Variations are found in the properties of the skin, such as the thickness of skin layers, the distribution of sweat glands, and the number and size of hair follicles. For example, the epidermis is thicker on the palms of the hands and soles of the feet (0.8 mm) than elsewhere on the body (0.07 to 0.12 mm). The dermis, on the other hand, is thickest on the back, whereas the subcutaneous fat layer is thickest on the abdomen and buttocks. Hair follicles are densely distributed on the scalp, axillae, and genital areas, but they are sparse on the inner arms and abdomen. The apocrine sweat glands are confined to the axillae and the anogenital area.

Nevertheless, certain structural properties are common to all skin on all areas of the body. The skin is composed of three layers: the epidermis (outer layer), the dermis (inner layer), and the subcutaneous fat layer. The basal lamina (basement membrane) divides the first two layers. The subcutaneous tissue, a layer of loose connective and fatty tissues, binds the dermis to the underlying tissues of the body (Fig. 60-1).

EPIDERMIS

The functions of the skin depend on the properties of its outermost layer, the epidermis. The epidermis covers the body, and it is specialized in areas to form the various skin appendages: hair, nails, and glandular structures.[3–5] The keratinocytes of the epidermis produce a fibrous protein called *keratin,* which is essential to the protective function of skin. In addition to the keratinocytes, the epidermis has three other types of cells that arise from its basal layer: melanocytes that produce a pigment called *melanin,* which is responsible for skin color, tanning, and protecting against ultraviolet radiation; Merkel's cells that provide sensory information; and Langerhans' cells that link the epidermis to the immune system. The epidermis contains openings for two types of glands: sweat glands, which produce watery secretions, and sebaceous glands, which produce an oily secretion called *sebum.*

Keratinocytes

The keratinocyte is the major cell of the epidermis. The epidermis is composed of stratified squamous keratinized epithelium, which, when viewed under the microscope, is seen to consist of five distinct layers, or strata, that represent a progressive differentiation or maturation of the keratinocytes: the stratum germinativum, or basal layer; the stratum spinosum; the stratum granulosum; the stratum lucidum; and the stratum corneum.

The deepest layer, the *stratum germinativum or stratum basale,* consists of a single layer of basal cells that are attached to the basal lamina. The basal cells, which are columnar, undergo mitosis to produce new keratinocytes that move toward the skin surface to replace cells lost during normal skin shedding. Unlike the other layers of the epidermis, the basal cells do not migrate toward the skin surface, but remain stationary in the stratum germinativum.

The next layer, the *stratum spinosum,* is formed as the progeny of the basal cell layer move outward toward the skin surface. The stratum spinosum is two to four layers thick, and its cells become differentiated as they migrate outward. The cells of this layer are commonly referred to as *prickle cells* because they develop a spiny appearance as their cell borders interconnect.

The *stratum granulosum* is only a few cells thick; it consists of granular cells that are the most differentiated cells of the living skin. The cells in this layer are unique in that two opposing functions are occurring simultaneously: while some cells are losing cytoplasm and DNA structures, others continue to synthesize keratin.

The *stratum lucidum,* which lies just superficial to the stratum granulosum, is a thin, transparent layer mostly confined to the palms of the hands and soles of the feet. It consists of transitional cells that retain some of the functions of living skin cells from the layers below but otherwise resemble the cells of the stratum corneum.

The top or surface layer, the *stratum corneum,* consists of dead, keratinized cells. This layer contains the most cell layers and the largest cells of any zone of the epidermis. It ranges from 15 layers thick in areas such as the face to 25 layers or more on the arm. Specialized areas, such as the palms of the hands or soles of the feet, have 100 or more layers.

The keratinocyte that originates in the basal layer changes morphologically as it is pushed toward the outer layer of the epidermis. For example, in the basal layer, the keratinocyte is round. As it is pushed into the stratum spinosum, the keratinocyte becomes multisided. It becomes flatter in the granular layer and is flattened and elongated in the stratum corneum (Fig. 60-2). The migration time of a keratinocyte from the basal layer to the stratum corneum is 20 to 30 days. Keratinocytes also change cytoplasmic structure and composition as they are pushed outward. This transformation from viable cells to the dead cells of the stratum corneum is called *keratinization.*

The movement of the cells to the surface of the skin can best be described as random or nonsynchronized. Keratinocytes pass other keratinocytes, melanocytes, and Langerhans' cells as they migrate in a seemingly random fashion. However, the cells are connected with minute

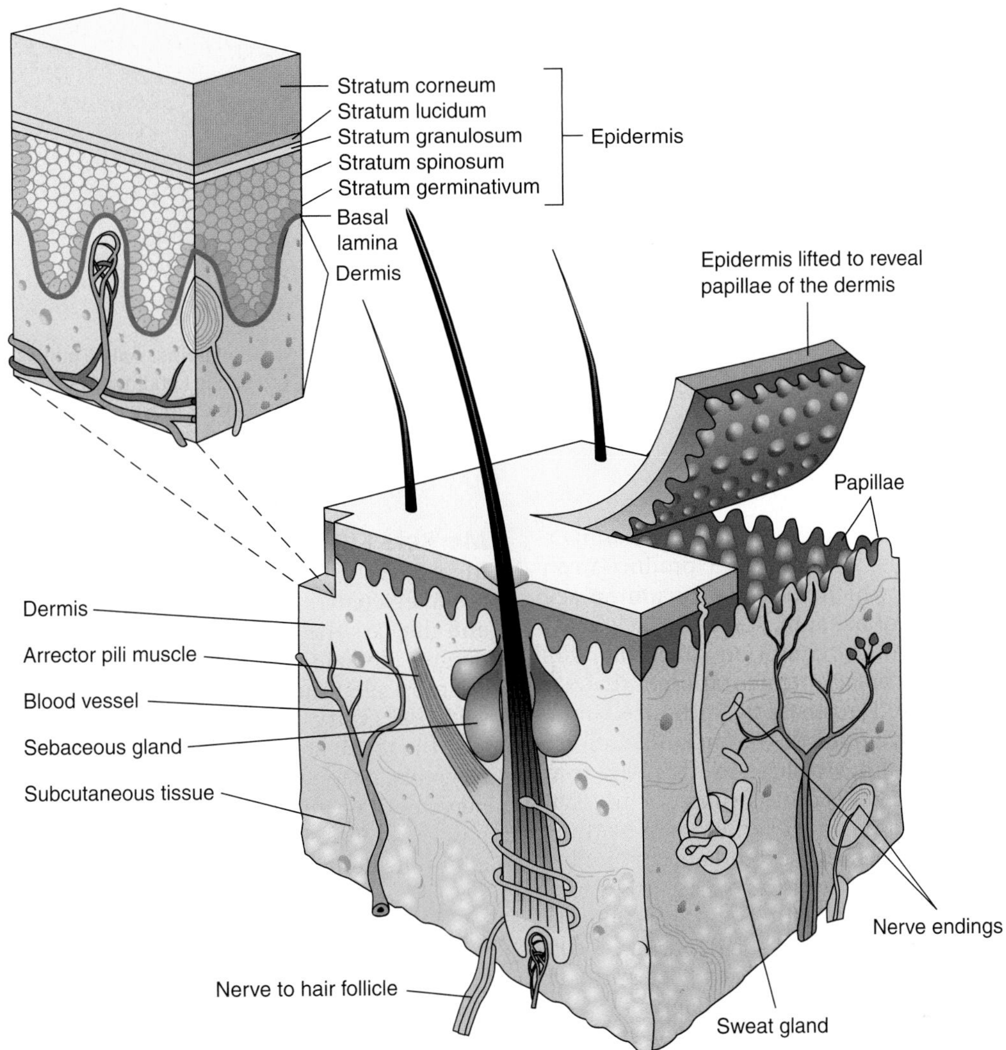

FIGURE 60-1 Three-dimensional view of the skin.

ORGANIZATION OF SKIN STRUCTURES

- The skin has two layers, an outer epidermis and an inner dermis, separated by a basement membrane.
- The epidermis, which is avascular, is composed of four to five layers of stratified squamous keratinized epithelial cells that are formed in the deepest layer of the epidermis and migrate to the skin surface to replace cells that are lost during normal skin shedding.
- The basement membrane is a thin adhesive layer that cements the epidermis to the dermis. This is the layer involved in blister formation.
- The dermis is a connective tissue layer that separates the epidermis from the underlying subcutaneous fat layer. It contains the blood vessels and nerve fibers that supply the epidermis.

points of attachment called *desmosomes*. Desmosomes are actually the terminal end points on the cell wall of a keratinous, fibrous material bound into bundles, called tonofilaments. Desmosomes keep the cells from detaching and provide some structure to the skin while it is in perpetual motion. The basal layer provides the underlying structure and stability for the epidermis.

Keratinocytes function to produce keratin, a complex protein that that forms the surface of the skin and is the structural protein of the hair and nails. Keratinocytes also play an important role in the immunobiology of the skin by communicating and regulating cells of the immune response and secreting cytokines and inflammatory mediators.

Melanocytes

Melanocytes are pigment-synthesizing cells that are located at or in the basal layer. They function to produce pigment granules called *melanin,* the black or brown substance that

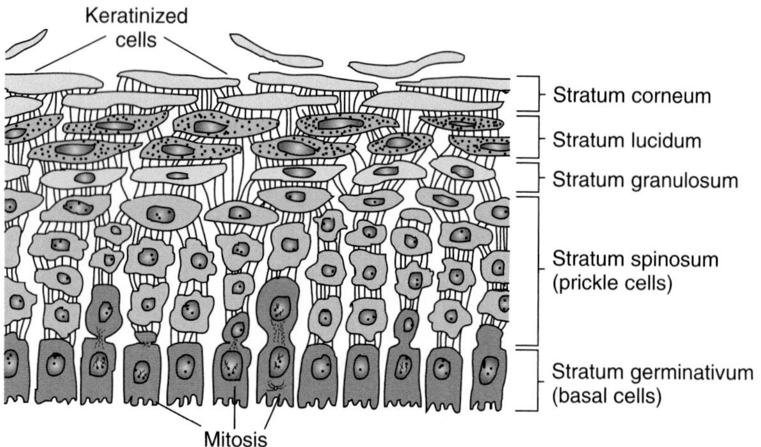

FIGURE 60-2 Epidermal cells. The basal cells undergo mitosis, producing keratinocytes that change their size and shape as they move upward, replacing cells that are lost during normal cell shedding.

gives skin its color. The ability to synthesize melanin depends on the ability of the melanocytes to produce an enzyme called *tyrosinase,* which converts the amino acid tyrosine to a precursor of melanin. A genetic lack of this enzyme results in a clinical condition called *albinism.* Persons with this disorder lack pigmentation in the skin, hair, and iris of the eye. Tyrosinase is synthesized in the rough endoplasmic reticulum of the melanocytes and then routed to membranous vesicles in the Golgi complex called *melanosomes.* Melanin is subsequently synthesized in the melanosomes. Melanocytes have long, cytoplasm-filled extensions that extend among the keratinocytes. Although the melanocytes remain in the basal layer, the melanosomes are transferred to the keratinocytes through these dendritic processes. The dendrite tip containing the melanosome is engulfed by a nearby keratinocyte, and the melanin is transferred (Fig. 60-3). Each melanocyte is capable of supplying several keratinocytes with melanin.

Exposure to the sun's ultraviolet rays increases the production of melanin, causing tanning to occur. The primary function of melanin is to protect the skin from harmful ultraviolet sun rays, which are implicated in skin cancers. Melanin protects by absorbing and scattering the radiation.

The amount of melanin in the keratinocytes determines a person's skin color. Dark-skinned and light-skinned people have the same amount of melanocytes. However, in dark-skinned people, *larger* melanosomes are produced and transferred to the keratinocyte individually. In light skinned people, a number of *smaller* melanosomes are packaged together in a membrane and then transferred to the keratinocyte. The way the melanosomes are packaged is responsible for the pigmentation in darker-skinned persons; darker-skinned people do not have more melanocytes than light-skinned people, but the production and packaging of pigment is different. All people, regardless of skin color, have relatively few or no melanocytes in the epidermis of the palms of the hands or soles of the feet. In light-skinned people, the number of melanocytes decreases with age; the skin becomes lighter and is more susceptible to skin cancer.

Merkel's Cells

Merkel's cells consist of free nerve endings attached to modified epidermal cells. Their origin remains unknown, and they are the least densely populated cells of the epidermis. Merkel's cells are found over the entire body but are most plentiful in the basal layer of the fingers, toes, lips, oral cavity, and outermost sheath of hair follicles (*i.e.,* the touch areas). Merkel's cells function as mechanoreceptors, or touch receptors. Other encapsulated sensory nerve endings (*e.g.,* pacinian corpuscles, Meissner's corpuscles, Ruffini's corpuscles, Krause's end bulbs) are present in the dermis.

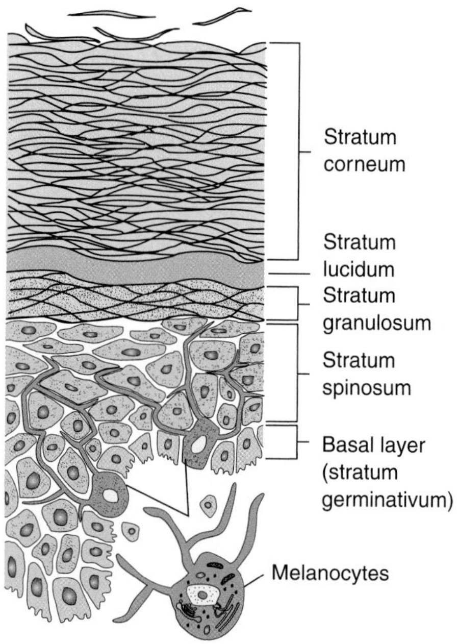

FIGURE 60-3 Melanocytes. The melanocytes, which are located in the basal layer of the skin, produce melanin pigment granules that give skin its color. The melanocytes have threadlike cytoplasmia-filled extensions that are used in passing the pigment granules to the keratinocytes.

Langerhans' Cells

Langerhans' cells are scattered in the suprabasal layers of the epidermis among the keratinocytes. They are few in number (3% to 5%) compared with the keratinocytes. They are derived from precursor cells originating in the bone marrow and continuously repopulate the epidermis. Like melanocytes, they have a dendritic shape and clear cytoplasm. *Birbeck's granules* that often resemble tennis racquets are their most distinguishing characteristic microscopically.

Langerhans' cells are the immunologic cells responsible for recognizing foreign antigens harmful to the body (Fig. 60-4). As such, Langerhans' cells play an important role in defending the body against foreign antigens. Langerhans' cells bind antigen to their surface, process it, and, bearing the processed antigen, migrate from the epidermis into lymphatic vessels and then into regional lymph nodes, where they become known as *dendritic cells.* During their migration in the lymph channels, the Langerhans' cells become potent antigen-presenting cells (see Chapter 19). Langerhans' cells are innervated by sympathetic nerve fibers, which may explain why the skin's immune system is altered under stress. An example of this is the exacerbations of acne seen in persons under stress. Langerhans' cells are antigen-presenting cells, and the keratinocytes produce a number of cytokines that stimulate maturation of skin-localizing T lymphocytes or T cells.

BASAL LAMINA

The basal lamina (basement membrane) is a layer of intercellular and extracellular matrices that serves as an interface between the dermis and the epidermis (Fig. 60-5). It provides for adhesion of the dermis to the epidermis and serves as a selective filter for molecules moving between the two layers. It is also a major site of immunoglobulin and complement deposition in skin disease. The basal lamina is involved in skin disorders that cause bullae or blister formation.

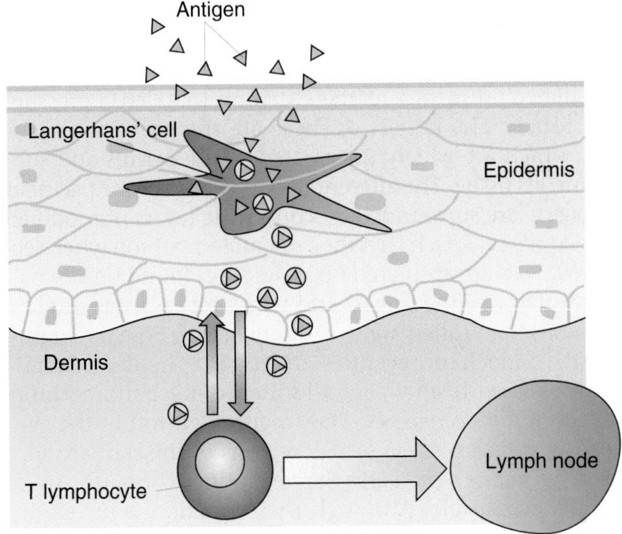

FIGURE 60-4 Langerhans' cells.

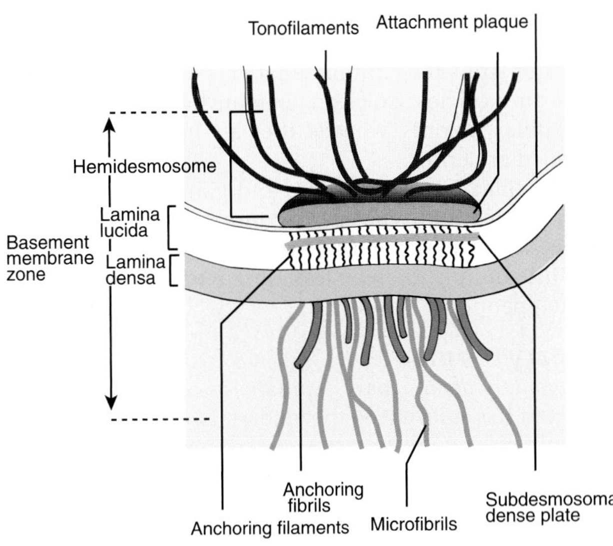

FIGURE 60-5 The dermal–epidermal interface and basement membrane layers. (Adapted from Rubin E., Farber J.L. [1999]. *Pathology* [3rd ed., p. 1244]. Philadelphia: Lippincott-Raven)

Hemidesmosomes, which resemble half-desmosomes, lie immediately at the basal plasma membrane and form the site or source of tonofilaments, which attach the dermis and epidermis. They also may relay signals between the intracellular keratin filament network and the extracellular basement membrane. The basal lamina consists of three distinct zones or layers—the lamina lucida, lamina densa, and lamina fibroreticularis—all of which contribute to the adhesion of the two skin layers. The *lamina lucida* is an electron-lucent layer where the adherence proteins are located. It consists of fine anchoring filaments and a cell adhesion glycoprotein, called *laminin,* that plays a role in organization of the macromolecules in the basement membrane zones and promotes attachment of cells to the extracellular matrix. The *lamina densa* contains an adhesive called *type IV collagen* as well as laminin. It is important in dermal–epidermal attachment. The *lamina fibroreticularis* contains many anchoring microfibrils. These are short, curved structures that insert into the lamina densa and the upper part of the dermis (superficial dermis), where they are known as *anchoring fibrils.* Type VII collagen, another adherent substance, has been found in the anchoring fibrils and plaques. Another component of the lamina fibroreticularis is elastic fiber bundles that extend to the dermis.

DERMIS

The dermis is the connective tissue layer that separates the epidermis from the subcutaneous fat layer. It supports the epidermis and serves as its primary source of nutrition. The two layers of the dermis, the papillary dermis and the reticular dermis, are composed of cells, fibers, ground substances, nerves, and blood vessels. The main component of the dermis is collagen, a group of fibrous proteins. Collagen represents 70% of dry skin weight and serves as the major stress-resistant material of the skin. Collagen is rich in amino acids. Collagen fibers are loosely arranged in the papillary dermis, whereas they are tightly bundled in the reticular dermis.

The pilar (hair) structures and glandular structures are embedded in this layer and continue through the epidermis. In general, a dark dermis is more compact than the white dermis, thereby lessening wrinkling in darker-skinned people.

Papillary Dermis

The *papillary dermis* (pars papillaris) is a thin, superficial layer that lies adjacent to the epidermis. It consists of collagen fibers and ground substance. This layer is densely covered with conical projections called *dermal papillae* (see Fig. 60-1). The basal cells of the epidermis project into the papillary dermis, forming *rete ridges*. Microscopically, the junction between the epidermis and the dermis appears like undulating ridges and valleys. It is believed that the dense structure of the dermal papillae serves to minimize the separation of the dermis and the epidermis. Dermal papillae contain capillaries, end arterioles, and venules that nourish the epidermal layers of the skin. This layer of the dermis is richly vascularized. Lymph vessels and nerve tissue also are found in this layer.

Reticular Dermis

The *reticular dermis* (pars reticularis) is the thicker area of the dermis and forms the bulk of the dermal layer. This is the layer from which the tough leather hides of animals are made. The reticular dermis is characterized by a complex meshwork of three-dimensional collagen bundles interconnected with large elastic fibers and ground substance, a viscid gel that is rich in mucopolysaccharides. The collagen fibers are oriented parallel to the body's surface in any given area. Collagen bundles may be organized lengthwise, as on the abdomen, or in round clusters, as in the heel. The direction of surgical incisions is often determined by this organizational pattern.

Immune Cells. Over time, the reticular dermis has undergone much study. Once thought to be composed primarily of fibroblasts, it is now believed that the main cells of this layer are dendritic cells, called *dermal dendrocytes*. Dermal dendrocytes, having both phagocytic and dendritic properties, are believed to possess antigen-presenting functions and play an important part in the immunobiology of the dermis. In addition, it is possible that dermal dendrocytes may be able either to initiate or respond to immunologic occurrences in the epidermis. Dermal dendrocytes also are thought to be involved in processes such as wound healing, blood clotting, and inflammation.

Immune cells found in the dermis include macrophages, T cells, mast cells, and fibroblasts. Dermal macrophages and venular epithelial cells may present antigen to T cells in the dermis. Most of these T cells are previously activated or memory T cells. T-cell responses to macrophage- or endothelium-associated antigens in the dermis are probably more important in generating an immune response to antigen challenge in previously immunized persons than in initiating a response to a new antigen. The major type of T-cell–mediated immune response in the skin is delayed-type hypersensitivity (see Chapter 21).

Mast cells, which have a prominent role in immunoglobulin E–mediated immediate hypersensitivity, also are present in the dermis. These cells are strategically located at body interfaces such as the skin and mucous membranes and are thought to interact with antigens that come in contact with the skin.

Blood Vessels. The arterial vessels that nourish the skin form two plexuses (*i.e.*, collection of blood vessels), one located between the dermis and the subcutaneous tissue and the other between the papillary and reticular layers of the dermis. The pink color of skin in light skin results primarily from blood seen in the vessels of this plexus. Capillary flow that arises from vessels in this plexus also extends up and nourishes the overlaying epidermis by diffusion. Blood leaves the skin by way of small veins that accompany the subcutaneous arteries. The lymphatic system of the skin, which aids in combating certain skin infections, also is limited to the dermis.

The skin is richly supplied with arteriovenous anastomoses in which blood flows directly between an artery and a vein, bypassing the capillary circulation. These anastomoses are important for temperature regulation. They can open up, letting blood flow through the skin vessels when there is a need to dissipate body heat, and close off, conserving body heat if the environmental temperature is cold.

Innervation. The innervation of the skin is complex. The skin, with its accessory structures, serves as an organ for receiving sensory information from the environment. The dermis is well supplied with sensory neurons as well as nerves that supply the blood vessels, sweat glands, and arrector pili muscles.

The receptors for touch, pressure, heat, cold, and pain are widely distributed in the dermis (see Fig. 50-8, Chapter 50). The papillary layer of the dermis is supplied with free nerve endings that serve as nociceptors (*i.e.*, pain receptors) and thermoreceptors. The dermis also contains encapsulated pressure-sensitive receptors that detect pressure and touch. The largest of these are the *pacinian corpuscles,* which are widely distributed in the dermis and subcutaneous tissue. The afferent nerve endings of the pacinian corpuscle are surrounded by concentric layers of modified Schwann's cells such that they resemble an onion when sectioned. Flat, encapsulated nerve endings found on the palmar surfaces of the fingers and hands and plantar surfaces of the feet are called *Meissner's corpuscles*. These are highly sensitive mechanoreceptors for touch. The deep dermis is supplied with small, spindle-shaped mechanoreceptors called *Ruffini's corpuscles*. They register tension in the supporting collagen fibers. A few regions of the skin are supplied by *Krause's end bulbs,* nerve endings contained in an ill-defined capsule. Although their function is uncertain, they are thought to function as mechanoreceptors.

Because of the variations in function among the different types of nerve endings, it is generally agreed that sensory modalities are not associated with a particular type of receptor. For example, the sensations of pain, touch, and pressure probably result from multiple stimuli. The final sensation may be the result of central summation in the central nervous system, which mediates patterned responses.

Most of the skin's blood vessels are under sympathetic nervous system control. The sweat glands are innervated by cholinergic fibers but controlled by the sympathetic nervous system. Likewise, the sympathetic nervous system controls the arrector pili (pilomotor) muscles that cause elevation of hairs on the skin. Contraction of these muscles tends to cause the skin to dimple, producing "goose bumps."

SUBCUTANEOUS TISSUE

The subcutaneous tissue layer consists primarily of fat and connective tissues that lend support to the vascular and neural structures supplying the outer layers of the skin. There is controversy about whether the subcutaneous tissue should be considered an actual layer of the skin. Because the eccrine glands and deep hair follicles extend to this layer and several skin diseases involve the subcutaneous tissue, the subcutaneous tissue may be considered part of the skin.

SKIN APPENDAGES

The skin houses a variety of appendages, including hair, nails, and sebaceous and sweat glands. The distribution and functions of the appendages vary.

Sweat Glands

There are two types of sweat glands: eccrine and apocrine. *Eccrine sweat glands* are simple tubular structures that originate in the dermis and open directly to the skin surface. They are numerous (several million), vary in density, and are located over the entire body surface. Their purpose is to transport sweat to the outer skin surface to regulate body temperature. *Apocrine sweat glands* are less numerous than eccrine sweat glands. They are larger and located deep in the dermal layer. They open through a hair follicle, even though a hair may not be present, and are found primarily in the axillae and groin. The major difference between these glands and the eccrine glands is that apocrine glands secrete an oily substance. In animals, apocrine secretions give rise to distinctive odors that enable animals to recognize the presence of others. In humans, apocrine secretions are sterile until mixed with the bacteria on the skin surface; then they produce what is commonly known as body odor.

Sebaceous Glands

The sebaceous glands are located over the entire skin surface except for the palms, soles, and sides of the feet. They are part of the *pilosebaceous unit.* They secrete a mixture of lipids, including triglycerides, cholesterol, and wax. This mixture is called *sebum;* it lubricates hair and skin. Sebum is not the same as the surface lipid film. Sebum prevents undue evaporation of moisture from the stratum corneum during cold weather and helps to conserve body heat. Sebum production is under the control of genetic and hormonal influences. Sebaceous glands are relatively small and inactive until an individual approaches adolescence. The glands then enlarge, stimulated by the rise in sex hormones. Gland size directly influences the amount of sebum produced, and the level of androgens influences gland size. The sebaceous glands are the structures that become inflamed in acne (see Chapter 61).

Hair

Hair is a structure that originates from hair follicles in the dermis. Most hair follicles are associated with sebaceous glands, and these structures combine to form the pilosebaceous unit. The entire hair structure consists of the hair follicle, sebaceous gland, hair muscle (arrector pili), and, in some instances, apocrine gland (Fig. 60-6). Hair is a keratinized structure that is pushed upward from the hair follicle. Growth of the hair is centered in the bulb (*i.e.,* base) of the hair follicle, and the hair undergoes changes as it is pushed outward. Hair has been found to go through cyclic phases identified as anagen (the growth phase), catagen (the atrophy phase), and telogen (the resting phase or no growth). Like most animals, human beings shed hair cyclically. However, human hair follicles work independently; therefore, unlike most animals, human beings shed hair asynchronously.

A vascular network at the site of the follicular bulb nourishes and maintains the hair follicle. Melanocytes in the bulb transfer melanosomes to the cells of the bulb matrix much in the same way as in the skin and are therefore responsible for the color of the hair. Similar to the skin, large melanosomes are found in the hair of darker-skinned persons; aggregated and encapsulated melanosomes are found in persons with light skin. Red hair has spherical melanosomes, whereas gray hair is the result of a decreased

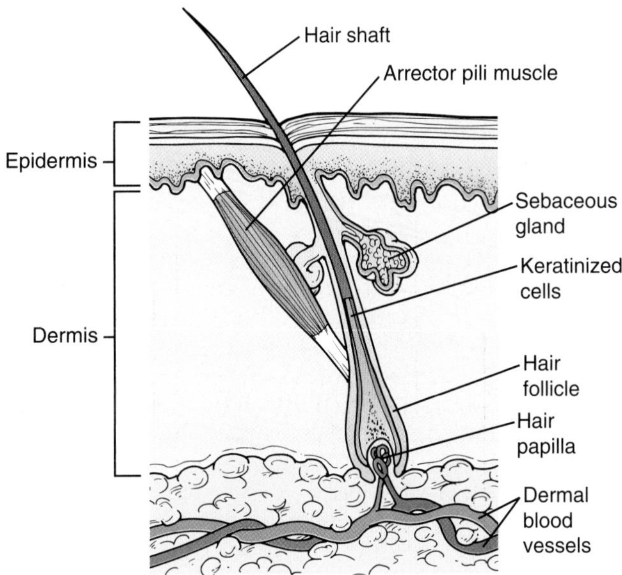

FIGURE 60-6 Parts of a hair follicle.

number of melanosome-producing melanocytes. The arrector pili muscle, located under the sebaceous gland, provides a thermoregulation function by contracting to cause goose bumps, thereby reducing the skin surface area that is available for the dissipation of body heat.

Nails

The nails are hardened keratinized plates, called *fingernails* and *toenails,* that protect the fingers and toes and enhance dexterity. The nails grow out from a curved transverse groove called the *nail groove.* The floor of this groove, called the *nail matrix,* is the germinal region of the nail plate (Fig. 60-7). The underlying epidermis, attached to the nail plate, is called the *nail bed.* Like hair, nails are the end product of dead matrix cells that are pushed outward from the nail matrix. Unlike hair, nails grow continuously rather than cyclically, unless permanently damaged or diseased. The epithelium of the fold of skin that surrounds the nail consists of the usual layers of skin. The stratum corneum forms the *eponychium* or cuticle. The nearly transparent nail plate provides a useful window for viewing the amount of oxygen in the blood, providing a view of the color of the blood in the dermal vessels. Changes or abnormalities of the nail can also serve to help diagnose skin or systemic diseases.

In summary, the skin is primarily an organ of protection. It is the largest organ of the body and forms the major barrier between the internal organs and the external environment. The skin is richly innervated with pain, temperature, and touch receptors; it synthesizes vitamin D and plays an essential role in fluid and electrolyte balance. It contributes to glucose metabolism through its glycogen stores.

The skin is composed of two layers, the epidermis and the dermis, separated by a basal lamina. A layer of subcutaneous tissue binds the dermis to the underlying organs and tissues of the body. The epidermis, the outermost layer of the skin, contains five layers, or strata. The major cells of the epidermis are the keratinocytes, melanocytes, Langerhans' cells, and Merkel's cells. The stratum germinativum, or basal layer, is the source of the cells in all five layers of the epidermis. The keratinocytes, which are the major cells of the epidermis, are transformed from viable keratinocytes to dead keratin as they move from the innermost layer of the epidermis (*i.e.,* stratum germinativum) to the outermost layer (*i.e.,* stratum corneum). The melanocytes are pigment-synthesizing cells that give skin its color. The dermis provides the epidermis with support and nutrition and is the source of blood vessels, nerves, and skin appendages (*i.e.,* hair follicles, sebaceous glands, nails, and sweat glands). Sensory receptors for touch, pressure, heat, cold, and pain are widely distributed in the dermis. The skin serves as a first line of defense against microorganisms and other harmful agents. The epidermis contains Langerhans' cells, which process foreign antigens for presentation to T cells, and the dermis contains macrophages, T cells, mast cells, and fibroblasts.

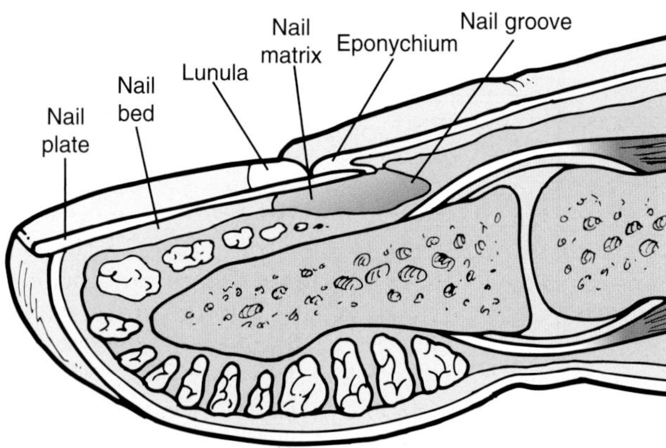

FIGURE 60-7 Parts of a fingernail.

REVIEW EXERCISES

Bullous pemphigoid is a autoimmune blistering disease caused by autoantibodies to constituents of the dermal–epidermal junction.

A. Explain how antibodies that attack glycoproteins, the lamina lucida, and their attachment to the hemidesmosomes can cause blisters to form (hint: see Fig. 60-5).

Allergy tests involve the application of an antigen to the skin, either through a small scratch or intradermal injection.

A. Explain how the body's immune system is able to detect and react to these antigens.

References

1. Lotti, T., Bianchi, B., Ghersetich, I., et al. (2002). Can the brain inhibit inflammation generated in the skin? The lesson of gamma-melanocyte-stimulating hormone. *International Journal of Dermatology 41,* 311–318.
2. Choung, C.M., Nickoloff, B.J., Elias, P.M., et al. (2002). What is the "true" function of the skin? *Experimental Dermatology 11,* 159–187.
3. Hood, A.F., Kwan, T.H., Mihm, M.C., et al. (2002). *Primer of dermatopathology* (3rd ed.). Philadelphia: Lippincott Williams & Wilkins.
4. Harrist T.J., Schapiro B., Quinn T.R., Clark W.H. (1999). The skin. In Rubin E., Farber J.L. (Eds.), *Pathology* (3rd ed., pp. 1237–1246). Philadelphia: Lippincott-Raven.
5. Wysocki A.B. (2000). Skin anatomy, physiology, and pathophysiology. *Nursing Clinics of North America 34,* 777–798.

CHAPTER

61

Alterations in Skin Function and Integrity

Gladys Simandl

The skin is a unique organ in that numerous signs of disease or injury are immediately observable on the skin. The skin serves as the interface between the body's internal organs and the external environment. Therefore, skin disorders represent the culmination of environmental forces and the internal functioning of the body. Sunlight, insects and other arthropods, infectious organisms, chemicals, and physical agents all play a role in the pathogenesis of skin diseases. Although most disorders are intrinsic to skin, many are external manifestations of systemic disease. Thus, skin provides a valuable window for the recognition of many systemic disorders.

The skin also has an elusive property that reflects emotional states. It is through the skin that warmth and other responses are given and received. The skin conveys a sense of health, beauty, integrity, and emotion. Human beings emphasize the body and, in particular, the skin to the degree that even slight imperfections may evoke a wide variety of responses. With the wealth of scientific research and knowledge about the skin, it is increasingly important that people's emotional and psychological responses to their skin conditions be considered.

Manifestations of Skin Disorders

After completing this section of the chapter, you should be able to meet the following objectives:

- Describe the following skin rashes and lesions: macule, patch, papule, plaque, nodule, tumor, wheal, vesicle, bulla, and pustule
- Describe the characteristics and causes of blisters, calluses, and corns
- Cite two physiologic explanations for pruritus
- Describe the causes and treatment of dry skin
- State common variations found in dark-skinned people

No two skin disorders look exactly alike, nor are they necessarily caused by the same agents. The appearance of many skin disorders may be further influenced by excessive itching, infection, or the effects of self-treatment. Skin color also may influence the appearance. Nevertheless, most skin disorders have some common characteristics that can be used to describe their lesions. This section of the chapter covers lesions and rashes, dry skin, pruritus, skin disorders due to mechanical forces, and variations in dark skin.

LESIONS AND RASHES

Rashes are temporary eruptions of the skin, such as those associated with childhood diseases, heat, diaper irritation, or drug-induced reactions. The term *lesion* refers to a traumatic or pathologic loss of normal tissue continuity, structure, or function. The components of a rash often are referred to as *lesions*. Rashes and lesions may range in size from a fraction of a millimeter (*e.g.*, the pinpoint spots of petechiae) to many centimeters (*e.g.*, decubitus ulcer, or pressure sore). They may be blanched (white), erythematous (reddened), hemorrhagic or purpuric (containing blood), or pigmented. Repeated rubbing and scratching can lead to lichenification (thickened and roughened skin characterized by prominent skin markings due to repeated scratching or rubbing) or excoriation (lesion caused by breakage of the epidermis, producing a raw, denuded area). Skin lesions may occur as primary lesions arising in previously normal skin, or they may develop as secondary lesions resulting from other disease conditions. Figure 61-1 illustrates various types of skin lesions.

A *blister* is a vesicle or fluid-filled papule. Blisters of mechanical origin are caused by friction from repeated rubbing on a single area of the skin. Friction blisters most commonly occur on the palmar and plantar surfaces of the hands and feet where the skin is constantly exposed to mechanical trauma, such as shoes and household tools and appliances. Blisters also develop from bullous skin disorders and burns. Histologically, there is degeneration of epidermal cells and a disruption of intercellular junctions that cause the layers of the skin to separate. As a result, fluid accumulates, and a noticeable bleb forms on the skin surface. Friction blisters should be protected by adhesive bandages and gauze to prevent further irritation and rubbing. Breaking the skin of a blister to remove the fluid is inadvisable because of the risk for secondary infections.

A *callus* is a hyperkeratotic plaque of skin due to chronic pressure or friction. It represents a hyperplasia of the dead keratinized cells that make up the cornified or horny layer of the skin. Increased cohesion between cells results in hyperkeratosis and decreased skin shedding. A callus may be filed down but is likely to recur if pressure continues in the localized area.

Corns are small, well-circumscribed, conical keratinous thickenings of the skin. They usually appear on the toes from rubbing or ill-fitting shoes. The corn may be either hard with a central horny core or soft, as commonly seen between the toes. Corns may appear on the hands as an occupational hazard. Corns on the feet often are painful, whereas corns on the hands may be asymptomatic. Corns may be abraded or surgically removed, but they recur if the causative agent is not removed.

SKIN LESIONS

- Skin disorders may present as a primary skin disease or as evidence of disease of other organ systems.
- Skin disorders are characterized by lesions and rashes that vary in size, color, and change in skin structure and integrity.
- The skin is amply supplied with pain and itch receptors that cause varying degrees of pain, pruritus, and discomfort in persons with skin lesions.
- There are normal differences in terms of skin color, texture, and other properties among persons of different ages and ethnic groups that need to be considered when evaluating skin disorders.

PRURITUS

Pruritus, or the sensation of itch, is a common symptom of skin disorders. In some persons, the condition may be so severe that it interrupts sleep and the general quality of life. Although itching commonly occurs with skin disorders, it can also provide a valuable clue to other internal disorders, such as chronic renal disease, diabetes, or biliary disease.

Itch is a sensation that originates in free nerve endings in the skin, is carried by small myelinated type C nerve fibers to the dorsal horn of the spinal cord, and is then transmitted the somatosensory cortex through the spinothalamic tract (see Chapter 50). According to the current theory of itch, which has been demonstrated through micrographic recordings, the afferent fibers that transmit the itch sensation are dedicated type C fibers that are distinct from the

Circumscribed, flat, nonpalpable changes in skin color	Palpable elevated solid masses	Circumscribed superficial elevations of the skin formed by free fluid in a cavity within the skin layers
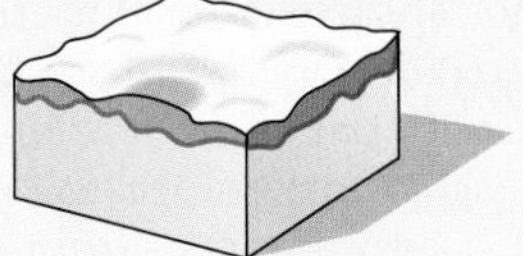	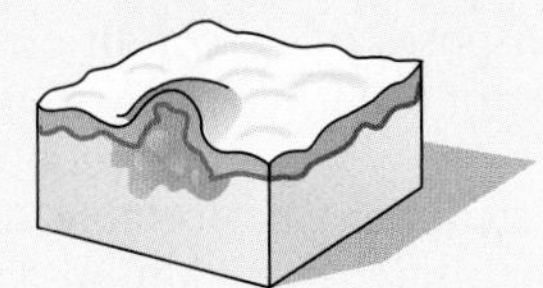	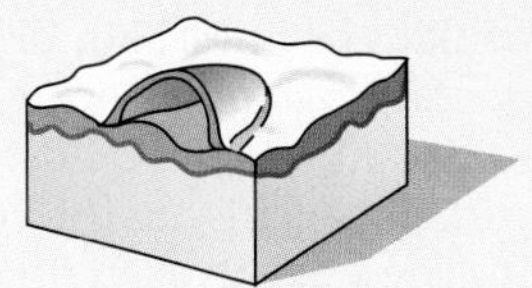
Macule—Small, up to 1 cm. Example: freckle, petechia *Patch*—Larger than 1 cm. Example: vitiligo	*Papule*—Up to 1 cm. Example: elevated nevus *Plaque*—A flat, elevated surface larger than 1 cm, often formed by the coalescence of papules *Nodule*—0.5 cm to 1–2 cm; often deeper and firmer than a papule *Tumor*—Larger than 1–2 cm *Wheal*—A somewhat irregular, relatively transient, superficial area of localized skin edema. Example: mosquito bite, hive	*Vesicle*—Up to 1 cm; filled with serous fluid. Example: herpes simplex *Bulla*—Greater than 1 cm; filled with serous fluid. Example: 2nd-degree burn *Pustule*—Filled with pus. Examples: acne, impetigo

FIGURE 61-1 Primary lesions may arise from previously normal skin. Authorities vary somewhat in their definitions of skin lesions by size. Dimensions given should be considered approximate. (Bates B.B. [1995]. *A guide to physical examination and history taking* [6th ed.]. Philadelphia: J.B. Lippincott)

polymodal nociceptors that are implicated in pain processing.[1] However, the receptors on peripheral nerve endings are unspecialized in that they respond to multiple stimuli such as touch, temperature, pain, and itch. The specificity of itch neurons is therefore based on their spinal connections to a distinct itch pathway, rather than on unique peripheral receptors. Further, this theory postulates a separate "itch center" in the somatosensory cortex.

A variety of mediators stimulate the itch receptors. Warmth, touch, and vibration can act locally to trigger the itch phenomenon. Substances such as histamine, bradykinin, substance P, and bile salts act locally to stimulate the itch sensation. Prostaglandins are modulators of the itch response, lowering the threshold for other mediators. Atopic dermatitis appears to involve an immune-mediated release of cytokines and other proinflammatory mediators.

Scratching, the well-known response to itch, is a spinal reflex response that to varying degrees can be controlled by the individual. Although scratching may temporarily relieve itch, many types of itch are not easily localized and are not relieved by scratching. In many people, excoriations and thickened papular areas develop at the site of repeated scratching or rubbing.

Most treatment measures for pruritus are nonspecific. Measures such as using the entire hand to rub over large areas and keeping the fingernails trimmed often can relieve itch and prevent skin damage. Self-limited or seasonal cases of pruritus may respond to such treatment measures as moisturizing lotions, bath oils, and the use of humidifiers. Because vasodilation tends to increase itching, cold applications may provide relief. Cool showers before bed, light sleep wear, and cool home temperatures also may be helpful. Topical corticosteroids may be helpful in some cases, such as itch related to allergy-mediated urticaria.

Mild cutaneous disorders, such as bug bites, are mediated by histamine; therefore, nonsedating antihistamines tend to be the treatment of choice. However, because most cases of pruritus are not histamine related, management of pruritus should be directed at the underlying cause. For example, systemic antihistamines and corticosteroids may be indicated for persons with severe pruritus or atopic dermatitis. Opioid antagonists may be used for pruritus caused by opioid medications such as morphine. Other modalities that have been used for all cases of pruritus with varying degrees of success are phototherapy, acupuncture,[2] antidepressant therapy, aroma therapy, and behavior modification.[3] In pruritus that has a systemic cause, itching gradually recedes as the primary condition improves.

DRY SKIN

Dry skin, also called *xerosis,* may be a natural occurrence, as in the drying of skin associated with aging, or it may be symptomatic of an underlying systemic disease or skin disorder such as contact dermatitis. Most cases of dry skin are caused by dehydration of the stratum corneum. The effects of aging on skin dryness include a change in the composition of sebaceous gland secretions and a decrease in the secretion of moisture from the sweat glands. Aging is also accompanied by a decrease in skin capillaries and flattening of the dermal rete ridges, resulting in less surface area for exchange of fluids between the dermis, epidermis, and skin surface.

Persons with dry skin often experience severe pruritus and discomfort, most commonly of the extremities. Other commonly involved areas include the back, abdomen, and waist. Dry skin appears rough and scaly; there may be increased wrinkles or lines. Skin drying also predisposes to scratching, cracking and fissuring, and a number of other skin maladies.

Moisturizing agents are the cornerstone of treatment for dry skin. These agents exert their effects by repairing the skin barrier, increasing the water content of the skin, reducing transepidermal water loss, and restoring the lipid barriers' ability to attract, hold, and redistribute water. Moisturizing agents can be classified as emollients, humectants, and occlusives.[4] *Emollients* are fatty acid–containing lotions that replenish the oils on the skin surface, but usually do not leave a residue on the skin. Emollients have a short duration of action and need to be applied frequently. *Humectants* are the additives in lotions, such as alpha-hydroxy acids and urea, that draw out water from the deeper skin layers and hold it on the skin surface. However, the water that is drawn to the skin is transepidermal water, not atmospheric water; thus, continued evaporation from the skin can actually exacerbate dryness. Alpha-hydroxy acids are derived from fruits, hence the abundance of fruit additives in shampoos and lotions in over-the-counter preparations. Urea is a nitrogenous substance that, when combined with lotions, has been quite effective in reducing xerosis. It is a humectant at lower concentrations (10%); but in higher concentrations (20% to 30%), it is mildly keratolytic. Clinical trials of urea have indicated its utility when compared with ammonium lactate (lactic acid) lotion[5] and glycerin.[6] *Occlusives* are thick creams that contain petroleum or some other moisture-proof material. They prevent water loss from the skin. Occlusives are the most effective agents for relieving skin dryness, but because of their greasiness and lack of cosmetic appeal, some people do not wish to use them.

Other lotion or cream additives are corticosteroids or mild anesthetics, such as camphor, menthol, lidocaine, or benzocaine. These agents work by suppressing itching while moisturizing the skin. Using room humidifiers and keeping room temperatures as low as possible to prevent water loss from the skin also may be helpful.

VARIATIONS IN DARK-SKINNED PEOPLE

Some skin disorders common to people of African American, Hispanic, or East Indian descent are not commonly found in European Americans. Similarly, some skin disorders, such as skin cancers, affect light-skinned persons more commonly than dark-skinned persons. Because of these differences, serious skin disorders may be overlooked, and normal variations in darker skin may be mistaken for anomalies.

Skin color is determined by the melanin produced by the melanocytes. Although the number of melanosomes in dark and white skin is the same, black skin produces larger melanin and produces it faster than white skin. Because of their skin color, dark-skinned persons are better protected against skin cancer, premature wrinkling, and aging of the skin that occurs with sun exposure.

Some conditions common in people with dark skin are too much or too little color. Areas of the skin may darken after injury, such as a cut or scrape, or after disease conditions such as acne. These darkened areas may take many months or years to fade. Dry or "ashy" skin also can be a problem for people with dark skin. It often is uncomfortable, and it also is easily noticed because it gives the skin an ashen or grayish appearance. Although using a moisturizer may help relieve the discomfort, it may cause a worsening of acne in predisposed persons.

Normal variations in skin structure and skin tones often make evaluation of dark skin difficult (Table 61-1). The darker pigmentation can make skin pallor, cyanosis, and erythema more difficult to observe. Therefore, verbal histories must be relied on to assess skin changes. The verbal history should include the client's description of her or his normal skin tones. Changes in skin color, in particular hypopigmentation and hyperpigmentation, often accompany disorders of dark skin and are very important signs to observe when diagnosing skin conditions. The appearances of skin disorders common to dark skin are listed in Table 61-2.

In summary, skin lesions and rashes are the most common manifestations of skin disorders. Rashes are temporary skin eruptions. Lesions result from traumatic or pathologic loss of the normal continuity, structure, or function of the skin. Lesions may be vascular in origin; they may occur as primary

TABLE 61-1 Common Normal Variations in Dark Skin

Variation	Appearance
Futcher (Voigt's) line	Demarcation between darkly pigmented and lightly pigmented skin in upper arm; follows spinal nerve distribution; common in black and Japanese populations
Midline hypopigmentation	Line or band of hypopigmentation over the sternum, dark or faint, lessens with age; common in Latin American and black populations
Nail pigmentation	Linear dark bands down nails or diffuse nail pigmentation, brown, blue or blue-black
Oral pigmentation	Blue to blue-gray pigmentation of oral mucosa; gingivae also affected
Palmar changes	Hyperpigmented creases, small hyperkeratotic papules, and tiny pits in creases
Plantar changes	Hyperpigmented macules, can be multiple with patchy distribution, irregular borders, and variance in color

(Developed from information in Rosen T., Martin S. [1981]. *Atlas of black dermatology*. Boston: Little, Brown)

TABLE 61-2 Appearance of Common Disorders of Dark Skin

Disorder	Appearance
Hot-comb alopecia	Well-defined patches of scalp alopecia on crown; extends down; decreased number of follicular orifices, hair loss irreversible; due to use of hot comb with petroleum, more common with Afro hairstyles
Infantile acropustulosis	Crops of vesicopustules for 7 to 10 days, followed by a 2- to 3-week remission before recurrence; pruritus; affects palms and soles of feet in children 2 to 10 months of age; resolves by 3 years of age
Keloids	Firm, smooth, shiny, hairless, elevated scars, sometimes hyperpigmented; often with symptomatic pruritus, tenderness, or pain; extremely common even with simple wounds on ears, neck, jaw, cheeks, upper chest, shoulders, and back (Fig. 20-11, Chapter 20)
Mongolian spot	Very common; ill-defined light blue to slate-gray macule in lumbosacral area; usually disappears but may persist through adulthood
Atopic dermatitis	Follicular lesion development that progresses to a lichenification stage; hyperpigmented lichenifications are interspersed with excoriated pink patches; common in blacks
Pityriasis rosea	Lesions are salmon-pink, dull red, or dark brown; profuse, fine scales, not commonly seen in white skin; postinflammatory pigmentary changes are more common in blacks
Psoriasis	Does not commonly occur in blacks; distribution is similar, but the plaques are bright red, violet, or blue-black; pigment changes may persist after treatment
Tinea versicolor	Common in blacks, increased incidence in tropical climates; hypopigmented or extremely hyper-pigmented patches, gray to dark brown; occurs more often on the face in blacks than in whites
Lichen planus	Papules are deep purple from pigmentary leakage; oral lesions are uncommon; hypertrophic lesions are more common in blacks than in whites

(Developed from information in Rosen T., Martin S. [1981]. *Atlas of black dermatology*. Boston: Little, Brown)

lesions in previously normal skin; or they may develop as secondary lesions resulting from primary lesions. Blisters, calluses, and corns result from rubbing, pressure, and frictional forces applied to the skin. Pruritus and dry skin are symptoms common to many skin disorders. Scratching because of pruritus can lead to excoriation, infection, and other complications. Normal variations in dark skin often make evaluation difficult and result in some disorders being overlooked. Changes in color, especially hypopigmentation or hyperpigmentation, often accompany the skin disorders of dark-skinned people.

Skin Damage Due to Ultraviolet Radiation

After completing this section of the chapter, you should be able to meet the following objectives:

- Describe the three types of ultraviolet radiation and relate them to sunburn, aging skin changes, and the development of skin cancer
- Describe the manifestations and treatment of sunburn
- State the properties of an effective sunscreen

The skin is the protective shield against harmful ultraviolet rays from the sun. The increased production of melanin as a result of exposure to ultraviolet radiation is believed to be the body's protective response. Skin cancers and other skin disorders, such as early wrinkling and aging, have been attributed to the damaging effects of sunlight.

ULTRAVIOLET RAYS

The earth's sunlight is measured in nanometer (one billionth of a meter) wavelengths ranging from approximately 290 nm in the ultraviolet region up to approximately 2500 nm in the infrared region. Ultraviolet radiation accounts for roughly 5% of solar radiation, but the amount of radiation to which humans are exposed has increased because of artificial sources, such as tanning salons, occupational exposure, and thinning of the ozone layer.

Ultraviolet radiation (UVR) is divided into three types: UVC, UVB, and UVA. UVC rays are short (100 to 289 nm) and do not pass through the earth's atmosphere. However, they can be produced artificially and are damaging to the eyes. UVB rays are 290 to 320 nm.[7] These are the rays that are primarily responsible for nearly all the skin effects of sunlight. They are more commonly referred to as *sunburn rays*. UVA rays are 321 to 400 nm. These rays, which can pass through window glass, are more commonly referred

ULTRAVIOLET RADIATION EXPOSURE

- The ultraviolet rays of sunlight have the potential for directly damaging skin cells, accelerating the effect of aging on skin, and producing changes that predispose to development of skin cancer.
- Protection from the sun's harmful rays should include avoidance of sun exposure, use of protective wide-brimmed hats, protective clothing, and use of sunscreens.

to as *suntanning rays*. In general, it takes approximately 1000 times more UVA to match the untoward effects of UVB. Nonetheless, UVA contributes to many skin alterations. Artificial sources of UVA, such as tanning salons and therapeutic solar interventions (PUVA) for certain skin conditions, have been known to produce the same effects as UVB.

The wavelength of sunlight is determined by the ozone layer in the atmosphere. Ozone absorbs wavelengths shorter than 320 nm; the shortest wavelength of sunlight reaching the earth is approximately 290 nm. The diminishing ozone layer is believed to be a critical factor in increased ultraviolet light exposure and the concomitant increased incidence over the past several decades of cancerous skin lesions. Smoke and fog may reduce the intensity of ultraviolet radiation.

When a person is exposed to ultraviolet radiation, the skin cells release vasoactive and injurious chemicals, resulting in vasodilation and sunburn. The melanocytes in the stratum corneum respond to increased exposure to ultraviolet radiation by increasing their melanin content as a means of preventing destruction of the lower skin layers. Components of the immune system in the skin, especially the Langerhans' cells, are also involved. The number of immune cells is decreased and cell activity is lessened by ultraviolet radiation exposure. It is thought that the immune cells are important in removing sun-damaged cells with malignant potential.[8]

SUNBURN

Sunburn is caused by excessive exposure of the epidermal and dermal layers of the skin to ultraviolet radiation, resulting in an erythematous inflammatory reaction. Sunburn ranges from mild to severe. Mild sunburn consists of various degrees of skin redness. Inflammation, blistering, weakness, chills, fever, malaise, and pain accompany more severe forms of sunburn. Scaling and peeling follow any overexposure to sunlight. Dark skin also burns and may appear grayish or gray-black.

Severe sunburns are treated with wet Burow's solution soaks and topical creams and lotions to limit inflammation and pain.[9] Extensive second- and third-degree burns may require hospitalization and specialized burn care techniques, as described later under Burns.

DRUG-INDUCED PHOTOSENSITIVITY

Some drugs are classified as photosensitive drugs because they produce an exaggerated response to ultraviolet light when the drug is taken in combination with sun exposure. Examples include some of the antiinfective agents (sulfonamides, tetracyclines, nalidixic acid), antihistamines (cyproheptadine, diphenhydramine), antipsychotic agents (phenothiazines, haloperidol), diuretics (thiazides, acetazolamide, amiloride), hypoglycemic agents (sulfonylureas), and nonsteroidal antiinflammatory drugs (phenylbutazone, ketoprofen, naproxen).[7]

Drug-induced photosensitivity, such as UVA photosensitivity induced by the psoralens, may be used in treating skin conditions, such as psoriasis, that respond well to ultraviolet radiation exposure.[10] Because an increased incidence of cancerous lesions has been reported in people who have been treated with these agents, their use requires caution and careful surveillance.

SUNSCREENS AND OTHER PROTECTIVE MEASURES

A good tan is sun damage that has already occurred. This statement is a philosophical change that has swept across the world over the past 10 to 20 years in response to the increased incidence of melanoma and nonmelanoma skin cancers.

The ultraviolet rays of sunlight or other sources can now be completely or partially blocked from the skin by sunscreens. There are two primary types of sunscreens available on the market: absorbents and reflectants. Absorbents work primarily in the UVB range, whereas reflectants work across the entire solar spectrum.[7,11] These agents work by protecting the skin from absorbing sunlight or by reflecting sunlight. Many sunscreen agents contain paraaminobenzoic acid (PABA), a chemical blocking agent that protects against UVB. People who are sensitive to benzocaine, procaine, sulfonamides, or thiazide diuretics should not use sunscreens that contain PABA. Broad-spectrum suntan lotions protect against UVA. These products contain a benzophenone such as oxybenzone, dioxybenzone, or avobenzone. Newer agents, such as micronized titanium dioxide and microfine zinc, act by reflecting as well as absorbing sunlight. They protect against most of the ultraviolet spectrum. Sunless suntan creams, such as dihydroxyacetone, produce a tan without exposure to the sun.

Sunscreens are available as lotions, creams, oils, gels, and sprays. They also are incorporated into cosmetics and lip balms. Sunscreens should be used diligently and according to the person's tendency to burn rather than tan. It is recommended that they be applied 30 minutes before sun exposure and reapplied every 2 hours. Water-resistant preparations maintain sunburn protection after being in the water for up to 40 minutes. Early morning and late afternoon sun exposures are less harmful because the ultraviolet rays are longer. Because many skin cancers are correlated with childhood sunburns, children younger than 18 years of age should use sunscreens that have a blocking agent with a Sun Protection Factor (SPF) of at least 15.

The U.S. Food and Drug Administration (FDA) requires an SPF rating on all commercial suntan preparations based on their ability to obstruct ultraviolet radiation absorption. The ratings usually are on a scale of 1 to 30; higher ratings block more sunlight.[11] SPFs are laboratory measured proportions of how much UVR is needed to produce mild erythema in persons with protected versus unprotected skin. For example, an SPF of 8 means that a person needs 8 times as much sun to elicit sunburn. Another way of stating it is an SPF of 8 filters out 88% of UVR. As seen in Table 61-3, an SPF of 16 blocks about 94%

TABLE 61-3 Percentage Reduction in Ultraviolet Radiation (UVR) With Increasing Sun Protection Factor (SPF) Number Showing an Exponential Relationship

SPF Number	Reduction in UVR (%)
2	30
4	75
8	87.5
16	93.75
32	96.88
64	98.14

(From Marks R., Hill D. [2001]. Prevention of skin cancer. In Sober A.J., Haluska F.G. [Eds.], *American Cancer Society atlas of clinical oncology: Skin cancer* [p. 326]. Hamilton, Ontario: B.C. Decker)

of the sun, with little gain in UVB protection as the SPF rises. Hence, the SPF of 15 was set and is recommended for outdoor sun and tanning salon use. Sunscreens are best when applied liberally and often. Resulting sunburns when using sunscreens are due to faulty, hasty, or inadequate use.

Sunscreens may encourage a false sense of security. Prolonged sun exposure as a result of using sunscreens may still increase the chance of getting skin cancers. The use of sunscreens has reduced the occurrence of actinic keratosis and squamous cell cancer. The efficacy of sunscreens as a reducer of melanoma is less clear; however, the benefits of sunscreens by far outweigh the risk of not using them.[12]

Sunscreens should be considered as only one component of an overall program to reduce UV exposure. This program can be recalled by the acronym CHESS: **c**lothing that is sun protective, **h**ats with wide brims all around, **e**yeglass that block UVA and UVB light, **s**unscreen with an SPF of at least 15 that is applied appropriately, and **s**hade, especially between 10:00 AM and 4:00 PM.[7] Shielding the skin with clothing and hats or head coverings helps decrease ultraviolet radiation exposure. Clothing should be tightly woven to avoid penetration of UV rays. Unfortunately, shade does not necessarily protect a person from the sun's rays because ultraviolet rays are reflected from many surfaces. Clouds do not filter UVB; rather, they scatter it through the water droplets. Hence, a person can sunburn on a cloudy day. Sand is a good reflector of sunlight. A person can become sunburned even while sitting under an umbrella on a sandy beach. Water absorbs ultraviolet radiation rather than reflecting it. However, ultraviolet radiation penetrates the upper few inches of clear water. This, combined with the scattered reflection of water, can increase the exposure to ultraviolet radiation.

In summary, there has been an alarming increase in skin cancers since the early 1980s, and repeated exposure to the ultraviolet rays (UVR) of the sun has been implicated as its principal cause. UVR, either from sunlight or artificial sources, also contributes to wrinkling and in early aging of the skin. Sunburn, which is caused by excessive exposure to UVR, is an erythematous inflammatory reaction, ranging from mild to severe. Photosensitive drugs can also produce an exaggerated response to ultraviolet light when they are taken in combination with sun exposure. Sunscreens are protective agents that work by either reflecting sunlight or preventing its absorption.

Primary Disorders of the Skin

After completing this section of the chapter, you should be able to meet the following objectives:

- Describe common pigmentary disorders of the skin
- Relate the behavior of fungi to the production of superficial skin lesions associated with tinea or ringworm
- State the cause and describe the appearance of impetigo and ecthyma
- Compare the viral causes, manifestations, and treatments of verrucae, herpes simplex, and herpes zoster lesions
- Compare acne vulgaris, acne conglobata, and rosacea in terms of appearance and location of lesions
- Describe the pathogenesis of acne vulgaris and relate it to measures used in treating the disorder
- Differentiate allergic and contact dermatitis and atopic and nummular eczema
- Describe the differences and similarities between erythema multiforme minor, Stevens-Johnson syndrome, and toxic epidermal necrolysis
- Define the term *papulosquamous* and use the term to describe the lesions associated with psoriasis, pityriasis rosea, and lichen planus
- Relate the life cycle of *Sarcoptes scabiei* to the skin lesions seen in scabies
- Use knowledge of the life cycles of *Pediculus humanus corporis* and *Pediculus humanus capitis* to explain the lesions associated with body and head lice

Primary skin disorders are those originating in the skin. They include pigmentary skin disorders, infectious processes, acne, rosacea, papulosquamous dermatoses, allergic disorders and drug reactions, and arthropod infestations. Although most of these disorders are not life threatening, they can affect the quality of life.

PIGMENTARY SKIN DISORDERS

Pigmentary skin disorders involve the melanocytes. In some cases, there is an absence of melanin production, as in vitiligo or albinism. In other cases, there is an increase in melanin or some other pigment, as in mongolian spots or melasma. In either case, the emotional impact can be devastating. Because pigmentary changes can result in social ostracism, it is important to treat equally the physiologic, emotional, and social components of these skin disorders.

Vitiligo

Vitiligo is a pigmentary problem of concern to darkly pigmented persons of all races. It also affects white-skinned

PRIMARY SKIN DISORDERS

- Primary skin disorders originate in the skin.
- Pigmentary skin disorders involve increased, decreased, or absent melanocyte function.
- Infectious skin disorders are caused by viruses, bacteria, and fungi that invade the skin, incite inflammatory responses, and otherwise cause rashes and lesions that disrupt the skin surface.
- Acne involves occlusion of the pilosebaceous unit with noninflammatory and inflammatory lesions resulting from occlusion, inflammation due to the irritating effects of sebum, and infection caused by the *P. acnes* organism.
- Allergic and hypersensitivity responses are caused by antigen-antibody responses resulting from sensitization to topical or systemic antigens.
- The papulosquamous dermatoses constitute a group of disorders characterized by scaling papules and plaques that result from uncontrolled keratinocyte proliferation.
- Scabies and lice are arthropod skin infestations that are transmitted from person to person and from animals to humans.

persons, but not as often, and the effects usually are not as socially problematic. The classic sign of vitiligo is the sudden appearance of white patches on the skin. The lesion is a depigmented macule with definite smooth borders on the face, axillae, neck, or extremities (Fig. 61-2). The patches vary in size from small macules to ones involving large skin surfaces. The large macular type is more common. Depigmented areas appear white, pale colored, or sometimes grayish-blue. Histologically, the depigmented areas may contain no melanocytes, greatly altered or decreased amounts of melanocytes; or in some cases, melanocytes that no longer produce melanin. These areas sunburn easily and enlarge over time. Vitiligo often is asymptomatic, although pruritus may occur.

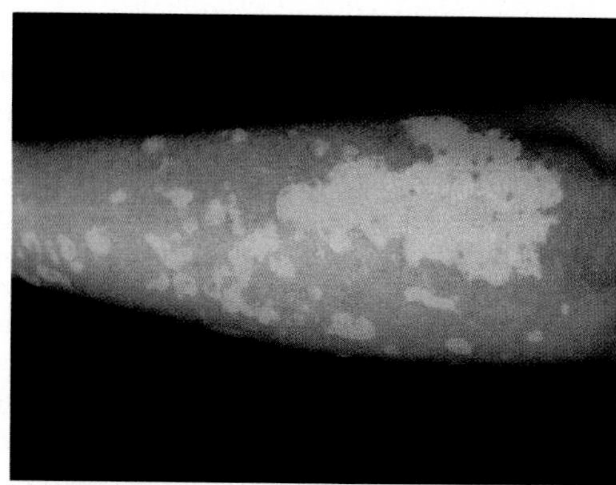

FIGURE 61-2 Vitiligo of the forearm of a black person. (Neutrogena Skin Care Institute.) (Sauer G.C., Hall J.C. [1996]. *Manual of skin diseases* [7th ed.]. Philadelphia: Lippincott-Raven)

Vitiligo appears at any age; roughly half of cases begin before the age of 20. Worldwide, it affects people of all races regardless of gender with an incidence rate of 1% to 2%.[13] The cause is unknown; however, several hypotheses have been postulated, including a hereditary predisposition because up to 38% of people with vitiligo report a family history; an autoimmune process in which there is immunologic destruction of the melanocytes because the disorder often accompanies other autoimmune diseases, such as diabetes mellitus and pernicious anemia; neural mechanisms in which the melanocytes are destroyed by a cytotoxic chemical secreted by nearby nerve endings; a self-destruct phenomenon in which the melanocytes are preprogrammed for self-destruction; a lack of melanocyte growth factors; or a combination of factors in which the origin varies from individual to individual and may be of multiple causes.[14] In some cases, vitiligo has been reportedly precipitated by emotional stress or physical trauma, such as sunburn.

Although there are many treatment regimens for vitiligo, none is curative. Self-tanning lotions, skin stains, and cosmetics are used for camouflage. Self-tanning compounds that contain a chemical such as *dihydroxyacetone* do not need melanocytes to color the skin. Corticosteroids administered topically, intralesionally, and orally have also been used successfully. Broad (large area) and narrow band (focused) UVB has also been used successfully in the treatment of vitiligo. The combination of psoralen and UVA (PUVA) treatment has also been successful in some people with large areas of skin involvement. The incidence of skin cancer thus far has been lower in persons receiving PUVA therapy for vitiligo than in persons receiving it for psoriasis. It may be because people with vitiligo avoid the sun, use sunscreens, and are not taking cytostatic or immunosuppressive drugs.[14]

A variety of skin-grafting techniques have been used in persons unresponsive to other therapies. Successful skin-grafting techniques vary from minigrafting (2 mm full-thickness punch grafts transplanted to involved areas) to grafting melanocytes into involved areas. Micropigmentation (tattooing) has been done on smaller, recalcitrant areas, but it is often difficult to attain a correct color match.

If extensive skin surfaces are involved, the treatment may be reversed and the pigmented areas bleached to match the remainder of the skin color. A melanocytotoxic agent is used to remove remaining melanocytes from skin areas. This process, which is called *depigmentation,* is permanent and irreversible; patients need to be apprised of this and of their need to avoid the sun and use sunscreens for the remainder of their lives.

Albinism

Albinism is a genetic disorder in which there is complete or partial congenital absence of pigment in the skin, hair, and eyes. Although there are more than 10 different types of albinism, the most common type is recessively inherited oculocutaneous albinism, in which there is a normal number of melanocytes, but they lack tyrosinase, the enzyme needed for synthesis of melanin. It affects the skin, hair, and eyes. Individuals have pale or pink skin, white or yellow hair, and light-colored or sometimes pink eyes. Persons with albinism have ocular problems, such as extreme sensitivity to light, refractive errors, lack of stereopsis, and nystagmus. There is no cure for albinism. Treatment efforts for people with albinism are aimed at reducing their risk for cancer through protection from solar radiation and screening for malignant skin changes.

Melasma

Melasma is a disorder characterized by darkened macules on the face. It is common in all skin types but most prominent in brown-skinned people from Asia, India, and South America. It occurs in men but is more common in women, particularly during pregnancy or while using oral contraceptives. It may or may not resolve after giving birth or discontinuing hormonal birth control. Melasma is exacerbated by sun exposure. Treatment measures are palliative, mostly consisting of limiting exposure to the sun and using sunscreens. Bleaching agents, containing 2% to 4% hydroquinone, are standard treatments. Tretinoin cream and azelaic acid have been useful in treating severe cases. Hydroquinone and tretinoin combined (Kligman's formula) has been highly successful, at times combining it with glycolic acid.

INFECTIOUS PROCESSES

The skin is subject to invasion by a number of microorganisms, including fungi, bacteria, and viruses. Normally, the skin flora, sebum, immune responses, and other protective mechanisms guard the skin against infection. Depending on the virulence of the infecting agent and the competence of the host's resistance, infections may result.

Superficial Fungal Infections

Fungi are free-living, saprophytic, plantlike organisms, certain strains of which are considered part of the normal skin flora (see Chapter 18). There are two types of fungi, yeasts and molds. Yeasts, such as *Candida albicans,* grow as single cells and reproduce asexually. Molds grow in long filaments, called hyphae. There are thousands of known species of yeasts and molds, but only about 100 of them cause disease in humans and animals (many cause disease in plants).

Fungal or mycotic infections of the skin are traditionally classified as superficial or deep. The superficial mycoses, more commonly known as *tinea* or *ringworm,* invade only the superficial keratinized tissue (skin, hair, and nails). Deep fungal infections involve the epidermis, dermis, and subcutis. Infections that typically are superficial may exhibit deep involvement in immunosuppressed individuals.

Most of the superficial mycoses (or *dermatophytoses*) are caused by the dermatophytes, a group of closely related fungi classified into three genera: *Microsporum* (*M. audouinii, M. canis, M. gypseum*), *Epidermophyton* (*E. floccosum*), and *Trichophyton* (*T. schoenleinii, T. violaceum, T. tonsurans*). Another way of classifying the dermatophytes is according to their ecologic origin—human, animal, or soil. Anthropophilic species (*M. audouinii, M. tonsurans, T. violaceum*) are parasitic on humans and are spread by other infected humans. Zoophilic species (*M. canis* and *T. mentagrophytes*) cause parasitic infections in animals, some of which can be spread to humans. Geophilic species originate in the soil but may infect animals, which in turn serve to infect humans.

The fungi that cause superficial mycoses live on the dead keratinized cells of the epidermis. They emit an enzyme that enables them to digest keratin, which results in superficial skin scaling, nail disintegration, or hair breakage, depending on the location of the infection. An exception to this is the invading fungus of tinea versicolor, which does not produce a keratolytic enzyme. Deeper reactions involving vesicles, erythema, and infiltration are caused by the inflammation that results from exotoxins liberated by the fungus. Fungi also are capable of producing an allergic or immune response. Superficial fungal infections affect various parts of the body, with the lesions varying according to site and fungal species. Tinea can affect the body (tinea corporis), face and neck (tinea faciale), scalp (tinea capitis), hands (tinea manus), feet (tinea pedis), or nails (tinea unguium).

Diagnosis of superficial fungal infections is primarily done by microscopic examination of skin scrapings for fungal spores, the reproducing bodies of fungi. Potassium hydroxide (KOH) preparations are used to prepare slides of skin scrapings. KOH disintegrates human tissue and leaves behind threadlike filaments, called *hyphae,* that grow from the fungal spores. Cultures also may be done using a dermatophyte test medium or a microculture slide that produces color changes and allows for direct microscopic identification. Wood's light (ultraviolet light) is another method that can assist with the diagnosis of tinea. Some types of fungi (*e.g., M. canis* and *M. audouinii*) fluoresce a yellow-green color when the light is directed onto the affected area.

Superficial fungal infections may be treated with topical or systemic antifungal agents. Treatment usually follows diagnosis confirmed by KOH preparation or culture, particularly if a systemic agent is to be used. Topical agents, both prescription and over-the-counter preparations, are commonly used in the treatment of tinea infections; however, outcome success often is limited because of the lengthy duration of treatment, poor compliance, and high rates of relapse at specific body sites.

The oral systemic antifungal agents include griseofulvin, the azoles, and the allylamines. Griseofulvin is a fungicidal agent derived from a species of *Penicillium* that is used only in the treatment of dermatophytoses. It acts by binding to the keratin of newly forming skin, protecting the skin from new infection. Because its action is to prevent new infection, it must be administered for 2 to 6 weeks to allow for skin replacement. The azoles are a group of synthetic antifungal drugs that act by inhibiting the fungal enzymes needed for the synthesis of ergosterol, which is an essential part of fungal cell membranes. The azoles are classified as either imidazoles or triazoles. The imidazoles consist of ketoconazole, miconazole, and clotrimazole. The latter two drugs are used only in topical therapy. The triazoles include itraconazole and fluconazole, both of which are used for the systemic treatment of fungal infections. Terbinafine, a synthetic allylamine, acts by interrupting ergosterol synthesis, causing the accumulation of a metabolite that is toxic to the fungus. In contrast to griseofulvin, the synthetic agents are fungicidal (*i.e.,* kill the fungus) and therefore are more effective over shorter treatment periods. Some of the oral agents can produce serious side effects, such as hepatic toxicity, or interact adversely with other medications being taken. A number of the synthetic fungicides (*e.g.,* ketoconazole, miconazole, clotrimazole, and terbinafine) are available as topical preparations and produce less severe side effects. Topical corticosteroids may be used in conjunction with antifungal agents to relieve itching and erythema secondary to inflammation.

Tinea of the Body or Face. *Tinea corporis* (ringworm of the body) can be caused by any of the fungi but is most frequently caused by *M. canis* in the United States and by *T. rubrum* worldwide. There has been an increase in *T. tonsurans* as the causative agent in tinea corporis as well. Although tinea corporis affects all ages, children seem most prone to infection. Transmission is most commonly from kittens, puppies, and other children who have infections.

The lesions vary, depending on the fungal agent. The most common types of lesions are oval or circular patches on exposed skin surfaces and the trunk, back, or buttocks (Fig. 61-3). Less common are foot and groin infections. The lesion begins as a red papule and enlarges, often with a central clearing. Patches have raised red borders consisting of vesicles, papules, or pustules. The borders are sharply defined, but lesions may coalesce. Pruritus, a mild burning sensation, and erythema frequently accompany the skin lesion.

Tinea faciale, or ringworm of the face, is an infection caused by *T. mentagrophytes* or *T. rubrum.* Tinea faciale may mimic the annular, erythematous, scaling, pruritic lesions characteristic of tinea corporis. It also may appear as flat erythematous patches.

Topical antifungal agents usually are effective in treating tinea corporis and tinea faciale. Oral antifungal agents may be used in resistant cases.

Tinea of the Scalp. There are two common types of *tinea capitis* (ringworm of the scalp): primary (noninflammatory) and secondary (inflammatory). In the United States, 90% of the cases of noninflammatory tinea capitis are caused by *T. tonsurans,* which does not fluoresce green with Wood's lamp.[15] Children between 3 and 14 years of age are primarily affected, with an alarming increase in the incidence of tinea capitis, particularly among African Americans.[16] Lower incidence rates among adults has been partially attributed to the higher content of fatty acids in the sebum after puberty. Currently, however, there are increasing numbers of adults being diagnosed. Depending on the invading fungus, the lesions of the noninflammatory type can vary from grayish, round, hairless patches to balding spots, with or without black dots on the head. The lesions vary in size and are most commonly seen on the back of the head (Fig. 61-4). Mild erythema, crust, or scale may be present. The individual usually is asymptomatic, although pruritus may exist.

The inflammatory type of tinea capitis is caused by virulent strains of *T. mentagrophytes, T. verrucosum,* and *M. gypseum.* The onset is rapid, and inflamed lesions usually are localized to one area of the head. The inflammation is believed to be a delayed hypersensitivity reaction to the invading fungus. The initial lesion consists of a pustular, scaly, round patch with broken hairs. A secondary bacterial infection is common and may lead to a painful, circumscribed, boggy, and indurated lesion called a *kerion.* The highest incidence is among children and farmers who work with infected animals.

The treatment for both forms of tinea capitis is oral griseofulvin or synthetic antifungals. Griseofulvin is a mainstay of treatment for children because it has fewer side effects than the synthetic antifungals. However, there may be a decrease in this drug's sensitivity given the changes in

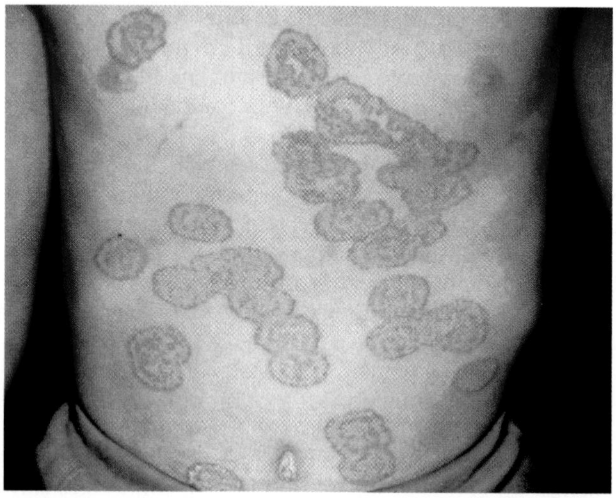

FIGURE 61-3 Tinea of the body caused by *Microsporum canis.* (Sauer G.C., Hall J.C. [1996]. *Manual of skin diseases* [7th ed.]. Philadelphia: Lippincott-Raven)

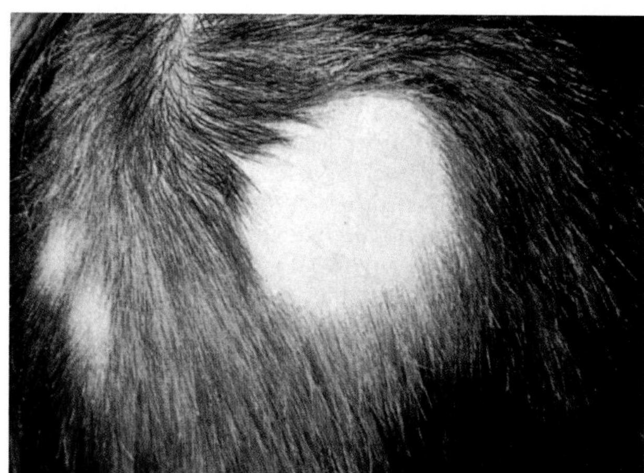

FIGURE 61-4 Tinea of the scalp caused by *Microsporum audouinii.* (Sauer G.C., Hall J.C. [1996]. *Manual of skin diseases* [7th ed.]. Philadelphia: Lippincott-Raven)

is a normal inhabitant of the gastrointestinal tract, mouth, and vagina. The skin problems result from the release of irritating toxins on the skin surface. *C. albicans* is found almost always on the surface of the skin; it rarely penetrates to the deeper layers of the skin, even in immunocompromised people. Some persons are predisposed to candidal infections by conditions such as diabetes mellitus, antibiotic therapy, pregnancy, birth control pill use, poor nutrition, and immunosuppressive diseases. Oral candidiasis may be the first sign of infection with human immunodeficiency virus (HIV).

C. albicans thrives in warm, moist, intertriginous areas of the body. The rash is red with well-defined borders. Patches erode the epidermis, and there is scaling. Mild to severe itching and burning often accompany the infection. Severe forms of infection may involve pustules or vesiculopustules. In addition to microscopy, a candidal infection often can be differentiated from a tinea infection by the presence of satellite lesions. These satellite lesions are maculopapular and are found outside the clearly demarcated borders of the candidal infection. Satellite lesions often are diagnostic of diaper rash complicated by *Candida*. The appearance of candidal infections varies according to the site (Table 61-4).

Diagnosis usually is based on microscopic examination of skin or mucous membrane scrapings placed in a KOH solution. Treatment measures vary according to the location. Preventive measures such as wearing rubber gloves are encouraged for persons with infections of the hands. Intertriginous areas often are separated with clean cotton cloth and allowed to air-dry as a means of decreasing the macerating effects of heat and moisture. Topical and oral antifungal agents, such as clotrimazole, econazole, ketoconazole, miconazole, and others, are used in treatment, depending on the site and the extent of the involvement.

TABLE 61-4 Candidal Infections: Locations and Appearance of Lesions

Variation	Appearance
Breasts, groin, axillae, anus, umbilicus, toe or fingerwebs	Red lesions with well-defined borders and presence of satellite lesions; lesions may be dry or moist
Vagina	Red, oozing lesions with sharply defined borders and inflamed vagina; cervix may be covered with moist, white plaque; cheesy, foul-smelling discharge; presence of pruritus and burning
Glans penis (balanitis)	Red lesions with sharply defined borders; penis may be covered with white plaque; presence of pruritus and burning
Mouth (thrush)	Creamy white flakes on a red, inflamed mucous membrane; papillae on tongue may be enlarged
Nails	Red, painful swelling around nail bed; common in persons who often have their hands in water

Bacterial Infections

Bacteria are considered normal flora of the skin. Most bacteria are not pathogenic, but when pathogenic bacteria invade the skin, superficial or systemic infections may develop. Bacterial skin infections are commonly classified as primary or secondary infections. Primary infections are superficial skin infections such as impetigo or ecthyma. Secondary infections consist of deeper cutaneous infections, such as infected ulcers. Diagnosis usually is based on cultures taken from the infected site. Treatment measures include antibiotic therapy and measures to promote comfort and prevent the spread of infection.

Impetigo. Impetigo is a common, superficial bacterial infection caused by *staphylococci,* group A β-hemolytic *streptococci* (GABHS), or both. Impetigo is common among infants and young children, although older children and adults occasionally contract the disease. Its occurrence is highest during the warm summer months or in warm, moist climates. It is highly communicable in the younger population. Impetigo initially appears as a small vesicle or pustule or as a large bulla on the face or elsewhere on the body. As the primary lesion ruptures, it leaves a denuded area that discharges a honey-colored serous liquid that hardens on the skin surface and dries as a honey-colored crust with a "stuck-on" appearance (Fig. 61-8). New vesicles erupt within hours. Pruritus often accompanies the lesions, and skin excoriations that result from scratching

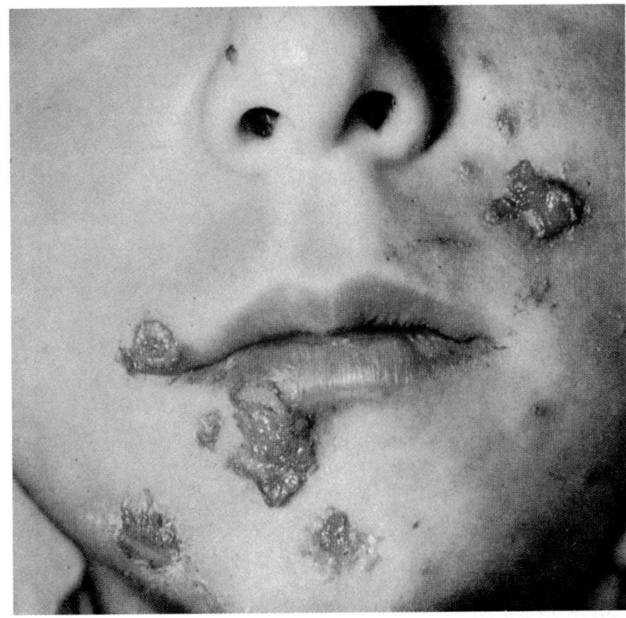

FIGURE 61-8 Impetigo of the face. (Abner Kurten, *Folia Dermatologica.* No. 2. Geigy Pharmaceuticals.) (Sauer G.C., Hall J.C. [1996]. *Manual of skin diseases* [7th ed.]. Philadelphia: Lippincott-Raven)

multiply the infection sites. A possible complication of untreated GABHS impetigo is poststreptococcal glomerulonephritis (see Chapter 35). Topical mupirocin (Bactroban), which has few side effects, may be effective for limited disease. If the area is large or if there is concern about complications, systemic antibiotics are used.

Ecthyma is an ulcerative form of impetigo, usually secondary to minor trauma. It is caused by GABHS, *Staphylococcus aureus,* or *Pseudomonas*. It frequently occurs on the buttocks and thighs of children (Fig. 61-9). The lesions are similar to those of impetigo. A vesicle or pustule ruptures, leaving a skin erosion or ulcer that weeps and dries to a crusted patch, often resulting in scar formation. With extensive ecthyma, there is a low-grade fever and extension of the infection to other organs. Treatment usually involves the use of systemic antibiotics.

A less common form of *S. aureus* infection, called Ritter's disease, manifests with a diffuse, scarlet fever–like rash, followed by skin separation and sloughing (Fig. 61-10). It is also is called *staphylococcal scalded skin syndrome* because the skin looks scalded. Ritter's disease usually affects children younger than 5 years of age; immunosuppressed adults also are at risk. The disorder, considered a deeper skin infection because the superficial layers of the epidermis are separated and shed in sheets, is caused by the hematologic spread of toxins from a focus of infection, such as the nasopharynx or a superficial skin abrasion. The onset of the rash may be preceded by malaise, fever, irritability, and extreme tenderness over the skin. The conjunctiva often is inflamed with purulent drainage. Although the fluid in the unbroken bullae is sterile, cultures usually are obtained from suspected sites of local infection and from the blood. Systemic antibiotics, either oral or parenteral, are used to treat the disorder. Healing usually occurs in 10 to 14 days without scarring.

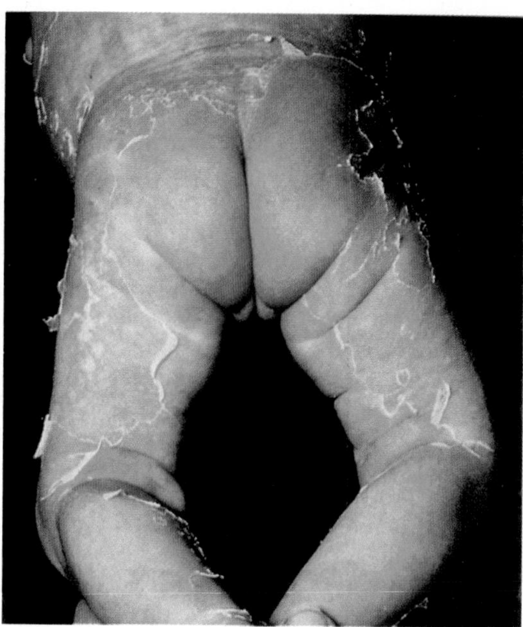

FIGURE 61-10 Staphylococcal scalded-skin syndrome. (Fitzpatrick T.B., Johnson R.A., Polono M.K., et al. [1992]. *Color atlas and synopsis of clinical dermatology* [2nd ed., p. 297]. New York: McGraw-Hill)

Viral Infections

Viruses are intracellular pathogens that rely on live cells of the host for reproduction. They have no organized cell structure but consist of a DNA or RNA core surrounded by a protein coat. The viruses seen in skin lesion disorders tend to be DNA-containing viruses. Viruses invade the keratinocyte, begin to reproduce, and cause cellular proliferation or cellular death. The rapid increase in viral skin diseases has been attributed to the use of corticosteroid drugs, which have immunosuppressive qualities, and the use of antibiotics, which alter the bacterial flora of the skin. As the number of bacterial infections has decreased, there has been a proportional rise in viral skin diseases.

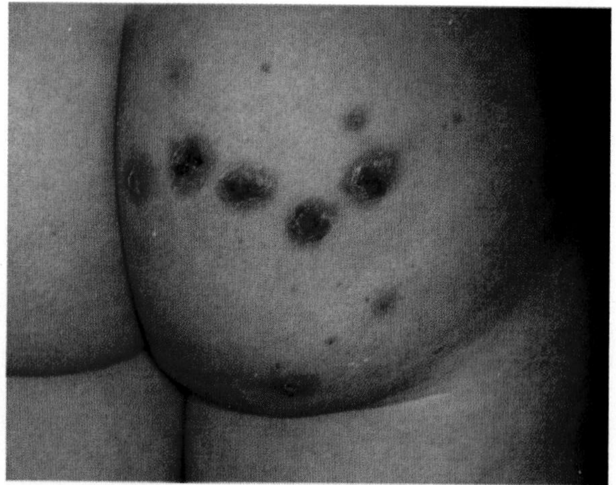

FIGURE 61-9 Ecthyma on the buttocks of a 13-year-old boy. (Glaxo-Wellcome Co.) (Sauer G.C., Hall J.C. [1996]. *Manual of skin diseases* [7th ed.]. Philadelphia: Lippincott-Raven)

Verrucae. Verrucae, or warts, are common benign papillomas caused by DNA-containing human papillomaviruses (HPVs). Although warts vary in appearance depending on their location, they all have a similar histologic appearance (Table 61-5). As benign papillomas, warts represent an exaggeration of the normal skin structures. There is an irregular thickening of the stratum spinosum and greatly increased thickening of the stratum corneum.

There are more than 50 types of HPVs found on the skin and mucous membranes of humans that cause several different kinds of warts, including skin warts and genital warts.[19] Many HPV types that cause genital warts are sexually transmitted; some may increase the risk for genital and cervical cancers. Nongenital warts commonly appear on the hands and feet (Fig. 61-11). They are commonly caused by HPV types 1, 2, 3, and 4 and usually are not precancerous. They are known as common warts, flat warts, and plantar warts. HPV transmission usually occurs through breaks in skin integrity. For example, plantar warts, which occur on the soles of the feet, frequently are transmitted to the abraded, softened heels of children in swimming areas. Common hand warts can be transmitted by biting the cuticles surrounding the nail.

TABLE 61-5 Types and Characteristics of Verrucae (Warts)

Type	Location	Appearance
Verruca vulgaris (common warts)	Anywhere on the skin, usually on the hands	Ragged dome shape with growth above the skin surface
Verruca filiformis	Eyelids, face, neck	Long, fingerlike projections
Verruca plana (flat wart)	Forehead, dorsum of hand	Small, flat tumors; may be barely visible
Verruca plantaris (plantar wart)	Sole of foot	Flat to slightly raised growth extending deep into skin; painful; bleeding occurs with superficial trimming; coalesced plantar warts are referred to as mosaic warts
Condyloma acuminata	Mucous membrane of the penis, female genitalia, perianal areas, and rectum	Large, moist projections with rough surfaces; usually pink or purple

Shaving may cause transmission of warts on the beard or leg areas.

Treatment usually is directed at inducing a "wart-free" period without producing scarring. Warts usually resolve spontaneously when immunity to the virus develops. The immune response, however, may be delayed for years. Because of their appearance or discomfort, people usually desire their removal, rather than waiting for immunity to develop. Removal is usually done by applying a keratolytic agent, such as salicylic acid gel or plaster that breaks down the wart tissue, or by freezing with liquid nitrogen. Intralesional bleomycin injections have been effective for recalcitrant warts. Various types of laser surgery, electrosurgery, and antiviral therapy also have been successful in wart eradication.

Occluding warts with duct tape has been a very effective treatment that is painless and inexpensive. Patients who applied duct tape on warts for 6½ days, removed the tape for 12 hours, then repeated the cycle of taping for up to 2 months had a remarkable cure rate (85%).[20] The mechanism of action for duct tape is unknown, but resolution of other untreated warts on the same person occurred. It was hypothesized that the local irritation of the duct tape may stimulate the immune response. Some dermatologists have been using duct tape occlusion successfully on finger and plantar warts for the past 20 years.[21]

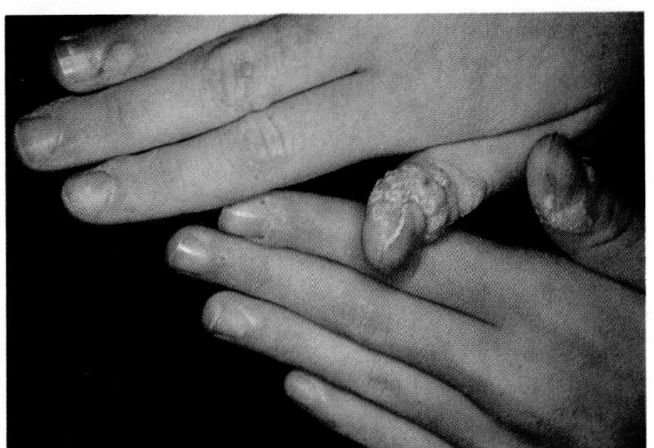

FIGURE 61-11 Common and periungual warts. (Reed & Carnrick Pharmaceuticals.) (Sauer G.C., Hall J.C. [1996]. *Manual of skin diseases* [7th ed.]. Philadelphia: Lippincott-Raven)

Herpes Simplex. Herpes simplex virus (HSV) infections of the skin and mucous membrane (*i.e.,* cold sore or fever blister) are common. Two types of herpesviruses infect humans: type 1 and type 2. HSV-1 usually is confined to the oropharynx, and the organism is spread by respiratory droplets or by direct contact with infected saliva. Genital herpes usually is caused by HSV-2 (see Chapter 48), although HSV-1 also can cause genital herpes. HSV-1 may be transmitted to other parts of the body through the occupational hazards, such as athletics, dentistry, and medicine.

Infection with HSV-1 may present as a primary or recurrent infection. Primary HSV-1 infections usually are asymptomatic. Symptomatic disease occurs most frequently in young children (1 to 5 years of age). Symptoms include fever, sore throat, painful vesicles, and ulcers of the tongue, palate, gingiva, buccal mucosa, and lips. Primary infection results in the production of antibodies to the virus so that recurrent infections are more localized and less severe. After an initial infection, the herpesvirus persists in the trigeminal and other dorsal root ganglia in the latent state. It is likely that many adults were exposed to HSV-1 during childhood and therefore have antibodies to the virus.

The recurrent lesions of HSV-1 usually begin with a burning or tingling sensation. Vesicles and erythema follow and progress to pustules, ulcers, and crusts before healing (Fig. 61-12). Lesions are most common on the lips, face, mouth, nasal septum, and nose. When a lesion is active, HSV-1 is shed and there is risk for transmitting the virus to others. Pain is common, and healing takes place within 10 to 14 days. Precipitating factors may be stress, menses, or injury. In particular, UVB exposure seems to be a frequent trigger for recurrence. Individuals who are immunocompromised may have severe attacks.

There is no cure for oropharyngeal herpes simplex; most treatment measures are palliative. Penciclovir cream, a topical antiviral agent, applied at the first symptom may be used to reduce the duration of an attack. Application of over-the-counter topical preparations containing antihistamines, antipruritics, and anesthetic agents along with aspirin or acetaminophen may be used to relieve pain.

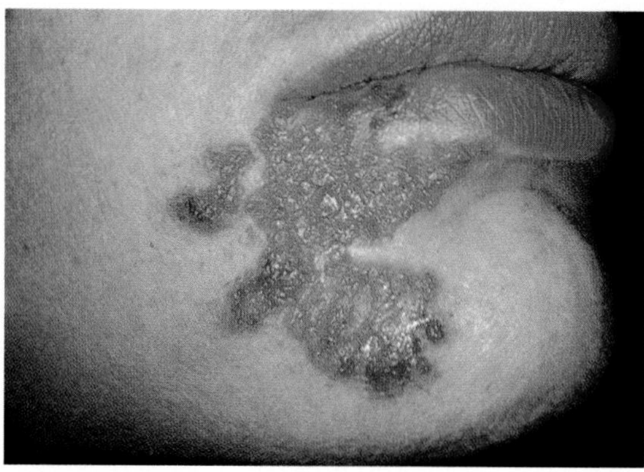

FIGURE 61-12 Recurrent herpes simplex of the face. (Dermik Laboratories, Inc.) (Sauer G.C., Hall J.C. [1996]. *Manual of skin diseases* [7th ed.]. Philadelphia: Lippincott-Raven)

Oral acyclovir, an antiviral drug that inhibits herpesvirus replication, may be used prophylactically to prevent recurrences. The antiviral drugs valacyclovir and famciclovir also may be used for prophylaxis. Sunscreen preparations applied to the lips can prevent sun-induced herpes simplex. Efforts to develop vaccines that would prevent herpes virus infections are in process. They may be the best hope for control of the disease.[22]

Herpes Zoster. Herpes zoster (shingles) is an acute, localized vesicular eruption distributed over a dermatomal segment of the skin. It is caused by the same herpesvirus, varicella-zoster, that causes chickenpox. It is believed to be the result of reactivation of a latent varicella-zoster virus that was dormant in the sensory dorsal root ganglia since a childhood infection. During an episode of herpes zoster, the reactivated virus travels from the ganglia to the skin of the corresponding dermatome. Although herpes zoster is not as contagious as chickenpox, the reactivated virus can be transmitted to nonimmune contacts.

The incidence of herpes zoster increases with age; it occurs 8 to 10 times more frequently in persons older than 60 years of age than in younger persons.[23] An age-related decline in varicella zoster T-cell–mediated immunity is thought to account for the increased viral activation in this age group.[24] The incidence rate is much less among African Americans. Other persons at risk because of impaired T-cell–mediated immunity are those with conditions such as HIV infection or certain malignancies, chronic corticosteroid users, and those undergoing cancer chemotherapy and radiation therapy.

The lesions of herpes zoster typically are preceded by a prodrome consisting of a burning pain, tingling sensation, extreme sensitivity of the skin to touch, and pruritus along the affected dermatome (see Chapter 50). Among the dermatomes, the most frequently involved are the thoracic (55%), cranial (20%), lumbar (15%), and sacral (5%).[25] Prodromal symptoms may be present for 1 to 3 days or longer before the appearance of the rash. During this time, the pain may be mistaken for a number of other conditions such as heart disease, pleurisy, musculoskeletal disorders, or gastrointestinal disorders.

The lesions appear as an eruption of vesicles with erythematous bases that are restricted to skin areas supplied by sensory neurons of a single or associated group of dorsal root ganglia (Fig. 61-13). In immunosuppressed persons, the lesions may extend beyond the dermatome. Eruptions usually are unilateral in the thoracic region, trunk, or face. New crops of vesicles erupt for 3 to 5 days along the nerve pathway. The vesicles dry, form crusts, and eventually fall off. The lesions usually clear in 2 to 3 weeks, although they can persist up to 6 weeks in some elderly persons.

Serious complications can accompany eruptions. Eye involvement can result in permanent blindness and occurs in a large percentage of cases involving the ophthalmic division of the trigeminal nerve (see Chapter 55). Pain can persist for several months after the rash disappears. Post-

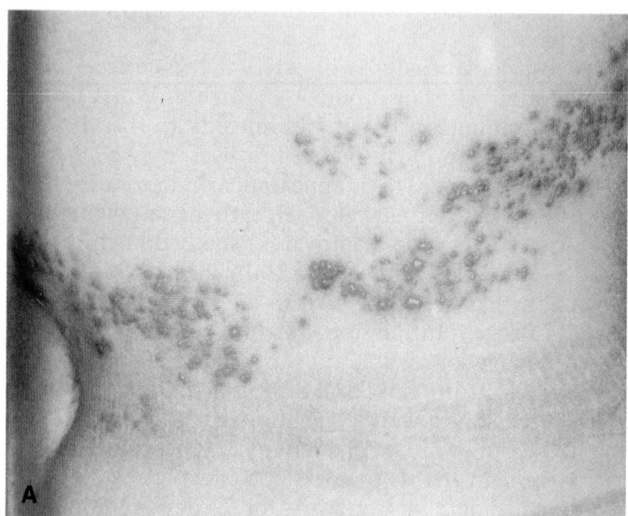

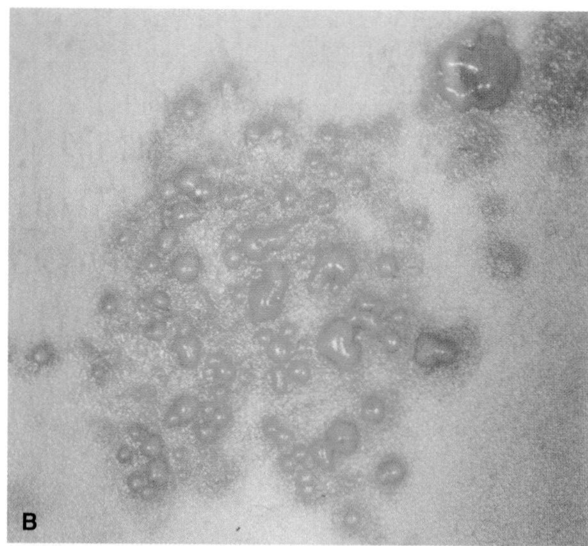

FIGURE 61-13 (**A**) Herpes zoster in a common presentation, with involvement of a single dermatome. (**B**) Herpes zoster is characterized by various sizes of vesicles (vesicles of herpes simplex are uniform in size.) (Habif T.P. [1996]. *Clinical dermatology* [3rd ed., pp. 351, 353]. St. Louis: CV Mosby, with permission from Elsevier Science)

herpetic neuralgia, which is pain that persists longer than 1 to 3 months after the resolution of the rash, is an important complication of herpes zoster.[24] It is seen most commonly in persons who are 50 years of age or older and reportedly affects more than 40% of persons older than 60 years of age.[23] Affected persons complain of sharp, burning pain that often occurs in response to nonnoxious stimuli. Even the slightest pressure of clothing and bed sheets may elicit pain. It usually is a self-limited condition that persists for months, with symptoms abating over time.

The treatment of choice for herpes zoster is the administration of an antiviral agent. Acyclovir, the prototype antiviral drug, may be given orally or intravenously. Other antiviral agents, specifically valacyclovir and famciclovir, appear to be at least or more effective as acyclovir in the relief of pain. The treatment is most effective when started within 72 hours of rash development. When given in the acute vesicular stage, the antiviral drugs have been shown to decrease the amount of lesion development and pain. Bed rest, especially for elderly persons, may be important in the prevention of neuralgia.[25] Narcotic analgesics, tricyclic antidepressants, anticonvulsant drugs, and nerve blocks have been used for management of herpetic pain. Oral corticosteroids sometimes are used to reduce the inflammation that may be contributing to the pain. Local treatment measures include Burow's solution compresses; aqueous alcohol lotions, calamine lotion, and starch shake lotions. Local application of capsaicin cream or lidocaine patches may be used in selected cases. Palliative treatments, such as heat and gentle pressure, may also be helpful.

There is current interest in developing a vaccine for preventing or modifying the course of herpes zoster in the elderly. The intent of a vaccine is to prevent the body's ability to establish and reactivate latent zoster. A major concern regarding childhood vaccination against chickenpox is that it could result in an increase of herpes zoster in later life because of lessened exposure to the virus in vaccinated populations,[26] the rationale being that reexposure to the zoster virus from infected children may protect latently infected individuals boosting their immunity. Thus, it is recommended that vaccination of the elderly should be considered in countries with childhood varicella vaccination programs.[27] Clinical trials are being conducted, with results anticipated toward the end of the decade.

ACNE AND ROSACEA

Acne is a disorder of the pilosebaceous unit (hair follicle and sebaceous gland). The hair follicle is a tubular invagination of the epidermis in which hair is produced (see Fig. 60-6 in Chapter 60). The sebaceous glands empty into the hair follicle, and the pilosebaceous unit opens to the skin surface by means of a widely dilated opening called a *pore*. The sebaceous glands produce a complex lipid mixture called *sebum,* from the Latin word meaning *tallow* or *grease*. Sebum consists of a mixture of free fatty acids, triglycerides, diglycerides, monoglycerides, sterol esters, wax esters, and squalene. Sebum production occurs through what is called a *holocrine process,* in which the sebaceous gland cells that produce the sebum are completely broken down and their lipid contents are emptied through the sebaceous duct into the hair follicle. The amount of sebum produced depends on two factors: the size of the sebaceous gland and the rate of sebaceous cell proliferation. The sebaceous glands are largest on the face, scalp, and scrotum but are present in all areas of the skin except for the soles of the feet and palms of the hands. Sebaceous cell proliferation and sebum production are uniquely responsive to direct hormonal stimulation by androgens. In men, testicular androgens are the main stimulus for sebaceous activity; in women, adrenal and ovarian androgens maintain sebaceous activity.

Acne lesions are divided into noninflammatory and inflammatory lesions. Noninflammatory lesions consist of comedones (whiteheads and blackheads). *Blackheads* are plugs of material that accumulate in sebaceous glands that open to the skin surface. The color of blackheads results from melanin that has moved into the sebaceous glands from adjoining epidermal cells. *Whiteheads* are pale, slightly elevated papules with no visible orifice. Inflammatory lesions consist of papules, pustules, nodules, and, in severe cases, cysts. *Papules* are raised areas less than 5 mm in diameter. *Pustules* have a central core of purulent material. *Nodules* are larger than 5 mm in diameter and may become suppurative or hemorrhagic. Suppurative nodules often are referred to as *cysts* because of their resemblance to inflamed epidermal cysts. The inflammatory lesions are believed to develop from the escape of sebum into the dermis and the irritating effects of the fatty acids contained in the sebum.

Two types of acne occur during different stages of the life cycle: acne vulgaris, which is the most common form among adolescents and young adults, and acne conglobata, which develops later in life. Other types of acne occur in association with various etiologic agents, such as drugs (*e.g.,* steroids, iodides), occupational compounds, cosmetics, and other irritating agents. Treatment measures for these acnes depend on the precipitating agent and the extent of the lesions.

Acne Vulgaris

The prevalence of acne vulgaris during adolescence is approximately 100% because almost all teenagers experience at least a few comedones. The difference is the severity of the condition, rather than incidence. It is the most common skin disorder, affecting 17 million people in the United States.[28] In women, acne may begin earlier and persist until 30 years of age; however, the overall incidence and severity are greater in men. There is a genetic predisposition to acquiring acne, and stress is thought to play an important part in the longer prevalence of the condition among women. The exact link between stress and acne is unknown, but it is believed that stress increases androgen production.

Acne vulgaris lesions form primarily on the face and neck and, to a lesser extent, on the back, chest, and shoulders (Fig. 61-14). The lesions may consist of comedones (whiteheads and blackheads) or inflammatory lesions (pustules, nodules, and cysts). The cause of acne vulgaris remains unknown. It is considered a chronic inflammatory

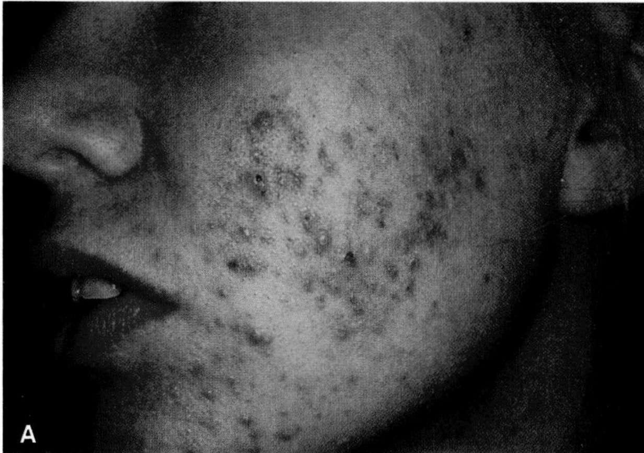

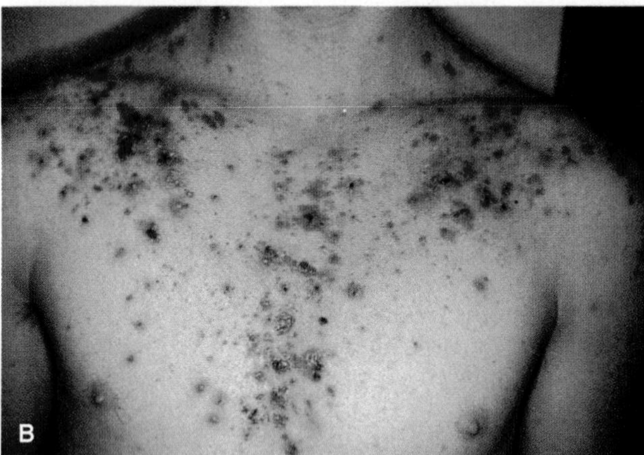

FIGURE 61-14 **(A)** Acne of the face and **(B)** acne of the chest. (Hall J.C. [1999]. *Sauer's manual of skin diseases* [8th ed., p. 118]. Philadelphia: Lippincott Williams & Wilkins)

disease of the pilosebaceous unit. There is a hereditary factor; multiple generations of family members often experience it. Several factors are believed to contribute to acne, including (1) the influence of androgens on sebaceous cell activity, (2) increased proliferation of the keratinizing epidermal cells that form the sebaceous cells, (3) increased sebum production in relation to the severity of the disease, (4) decreased amounts of linoleic acid in the sebum, and (5) the presence of *Propionibacterium acnes*. These factors probably are interrelated. Increased androgen production results in increased sebaceous cell activity, with a resultant plugging of the pilosebaceous ducts. The excessive sebum provides a medium for the growth of *P. acnes*. The *P. acnes* organism contains lipases that break down the free fatty acids that produce the acne inflammation.

Over the years, several factors, such as poor hygiene, acne as an infectious process, diets high in fatty content, and certain foods (*e.g.*, chocolate) have been studied empirically and rejected as causal or contributing factors in the development of acne. Although general hygienic measures are important, obsessive scrubbing can traumatize the skin and worsen the condition.[29] Instead, it is recommended that the affected areas be washed gently and patted dry. Water-based, rather than oil-based, cosmetics and moisturizers should be used. Mechanical trauma, such as squeezing, rubbing, or picking comedones, should be avoided. Even resting the chin, forehead, or cheek on a hand can exacerbate the condition. Hats, sweatbands, and shirt collars can also traumatize the skin and contribute to a worsening of acne. Although rigid dietary restrictions have not been shown to be beneficial in acne management, a balanced diet is recommended. Women should be informed that acne often becomes worse during the week before menses.

Treatment. The treatment of acne focuses on clearing up existing lesions, preventing new lesions from forming, and limiting scar formation. Management includes education regarding the causes of acne and protective skin care measures. Topical or systemic treatment may be used, depending on the extent of involvement and the types of lesions (comedonal or inflammatory). Long-term treatment usually is required. Significant improvement may not be apparent for 3 to 6 weeks after initiation of treatment, and maximum effects may not be apparent for months. An important treatment measure is sensitivity to the client's emotional needs.

Milder forms of acne usually respond to topical application of acne creams, ointments, or lotions. The treatment measures for moderate to severe acne are directed at correcting the defect in epidermal cell proliferation, decreasing sebaceous gland activity, reducing the *P. acnes* population, and limiting the inflammatory process. Often, a combination of comedolytic and antibacterial agents is used.

A number of topical comedolytic and antibacterial agents are available for the treatment of acne. The type of vehicle (cream, gel, or lotion) may be an important consideration in selection of an agent.[30] Persons with drier skin may benefit from creams, whereas persons with oily skin may have better results using a gel or lotion. Many acne creams and lotions containing keratolytic agents such as sulfur, salicylic acid, phenol, and resorcinol are available as over-the-counter preparations. These agents act chemically to break down keratin, loosen comedones, and exert a peeling effect on the skin. With the advent of more effective products, these preparations are used less frequently than in the past.

Benzoyl peroxide is a topical agent that has both antibacterial and comedolytic properties. It is the topical agent most effective in reducing the *P. acnes* population. Bacterial proteins are oxidized by the oxygen free radicals released from the metabolism of benzoyl peroxide on the skin. Because of its mechanism of action, bacterial resistance does not develop to benzoyl peroxide. The irritant effect of the drug also causes vasodilation and increased blood flow, which may hasten resolution of the inflammatory lesions. Azelaic acid, derived from wheat, rye, and barley, has actions similar to benzoyl peroxide. It decreases the proliferation of keratinocytes and has antibacterial actions against *P. acnes*. Azelaic cream is moisturizing and causes only minimal skin irritation.

Tretinoin (Retin-A), an acid derivative of vitamin A, is a topical agent. It acts locally to decrease the cohesiveness of epidermal cells and increase epidermal cell turnover. This is thought to result in an increased extrusion of open comedones and a transformation of closed comedones into open ones. All tretinoin formulations are irritating to the skin, an effect that is increased with sun exposure. Because of the teratogenic effect of oral vitamin A products, pregnant women should not use them. Another form of tretinoin, Retin-A Micro, works by entrapping the drug in microspheres that move into the follicle and serve as reservoirs for drug release. Other retinoid drugs, such as adapalene and tazarotene, have actions similar to tretinoin. Adapalene appears to be as effective as tretinoin but may be less irritating to the skin.[30]

Topically applied antibiotics also are effective in treating mild to moderate acne. Topical tetracycline, erythromycin, and clindamycin are used most commonly. They do not affect existing lesions but prevent future lesions by decreasing the amount of *P. acnes* on the skin, thereby reducing subsequent inflammation formed from the presence of sebaceous fatty acid metabolites. Treatment failure can result from development of antibiotic resistance. Combination drugs such as benzoyl peroxide and erythromycin also have been effective.

Oral low-dose tetracycline has been used effectively for many years. Tetracycline has no effect on sebum production, but it decreases bacterial growth and the amount of free fatty acids produced. Tetracycline requires a sufficient treatment period to establish effective blood levels. Side effects are minimal, which is why the drug has remained so useful. However, it does have teratogenic effects on skeletal and tooth development and should not be given to women who are pregnant, lactating, or children. Tetracycline derivatives, minocycline and doxycycline, are better tolerated than tetracycline. Doxycycline may cause photosensitivity reactions. Erythromycin also is effective in acne treatment, especially when tetracycline and its derivatives cannot be used. Of the antimicrobial drugs, dapsone has been effective in severe cases of cystic acne. However, side effects are many. The drug should be used with caution and close monitoring.

Isotretinoin (Accutane), an orally administered synthetic retinoid or acid form of vitamin A, has revolutionized the treatment of recalcitrant cases of acne and cystic acnes. In carefully planned doses, oral isotretinoin has cleared major cases of acne and initiated long-term remissions of the disease. It is administered for 3- to 4-month treatment periods. Although the exact mode of action is unknown, it decreases sebaceous gland activity, prevents new comedones from forming, reduces the *P. acnes* count through sebum reduction, and has an antiinflammatory effect. Because of its many side effects, it is used only in persons with severe acne. Side effects include dryness of the mouth and other mucous membranes, conjunctivitis, and musculoskeletal system abnormalities. Careful clinical and laboratory monitoring is necessary because the drug can produce elevated serum lipid levels, abnormal liver enzyme test results, and hematologic disorders. Isotretinoin is a teratogen that causes brain, heart, and ear malformations. Women taking isotretinoin are strongly advised not to become pregnant.

Estrogens reduce the size and secretion of the sebaceous gland, but because of the high dosages required, they are contraindicated in men. In women, birth control pills that combine estrogen with a progestin that has low androgenic activity usually are used.[29] Corticosteroid therapy is limited primarily to severe, resistant cases. The therapy results in remarkable healing, but acne usually returns after the therapy has been terminated.

Other treatment measures for acne include surgery, ultraviolet irradiation, cryotherapy (*e.g.,* freezing with carbon dioxide slushes, liquid nitrogen), and intralesional glucocorticosteroid injection. Acne surgery involves the aspiration of comedones with small-bore needles or devices designed to extract comedonal contents. Scarring is a common sequela if surgery is done improperly. Intralesional injection of corticosteroids using a syringe or needleless injector is limited to severe nodulocystic forms of acne. It has been effective in promoting cyst healing but usually has to be repeated frequently.

Acne Conglobata

Acne conglobata occurs later in life and is a chronic form of acne. Comedones, papules, pustules, nodules, abscesses, cysts, and scars occur on the back, buttocks, and chest. Lesions occur to a lesser extent on the abdomen, shoulders, neck, face, upper arms, and thighs. The comedones or cysts have multiple openings; large abscesses, interconnecting sinuses, and inflammatory nodules are not uncommon. Their discharge is odoriferous, serous, and purulent or mucoid. Healing often leaves deep keloidal lesions. Affected persons usually have anemia with increased white blood cell counts, sedimentation rates, and neutrophil counts. The treatment is difficult and stringent. It often includes débridement, systemic corticosteroid therapy, oral retinoids, and systemic antibiotics.

Rosacea

Rosacea is a chronic inflammatory process that occurs in middle-aged and older adults. It is easily confused with acne and may coexist with it. Rosacea is more common in fair-skinned persons and has been called "the curse of the Celts." An early characteristic and diagnostic sign is seen in persons who "flush and blush." From 1990 to 1997, there were 1.1 million outpatient visits for rosacea annually in the United States.[31] Most were white women (69%) with a mean age of 50 plus or minus 17 years.

The cause of rosacea is unknown; however, it is believed to be an inflammatory process accompanied by vascular instability with leakage of fluid and inflammatory mediators into the dermis. It often is accompanied by gastrointestinal symptoms; *Helicobacter pylori* has been implicated as a possible cause.[32]

In the early stage of rosacea development, there are repeated episodes of blushing.[33] The blush eventually becomes a permanent dark-red erythema on the nose and cheeks that sometimes extends to the forehead and chin. This stage often occurs before 20 years of age. Ocular problems occur in at least 50% of persons with rosacea. Prominent symptoms include eyes that are itchy, burning; or dry; a gritty or foreign sensation; and erythema and swelling of the eyelid.[33] As the person ages, the erythema persists, and telangiectasia with or without acne components (*e.g.*, comedones, papules, pustules, nodules, erythema, edema) develops. After years of affliction, acne rosacea may develop into an irregular bullous hyperplasia (thickening of the skin) of the nose, known as *rhinophyma* (Fig. 61-15). Rhinophyma is often considered the end stage of rosacea. The sebaceous follicles and openings of the nose enlarge, and the skin color changes to a purple-red, resulting in hypertrophy of the nose and impaired breathing. Whereas rosacea is more common in women, rhinophyma is more common in men.

Persons with rosacea are heat sensitive. They are instructed to avoid vascular-stimulating agents such as heat, sunlight, hot liquids, foods, and alcohol. Treatment measures are similar to those used for acne vulgaris. Topical metronidazole and azelaic acid have been effective. Rhinophyma can be treated in a number of surgical ways, including electrosurgery, laser ablation, dermabrasion, cryosurgery, and scalpel excision.

ALLERGIC AND HYPERSENSITIVITY DERMATOSES

Allergic and hypersensitivity dermatoses involve the inflammatory response to multiple exogenous and endogenous agents. The disorders that are usually characterized by epidermal edema with separation of epidermal cells include irritant contact dermatitis, allergy contact dermatitis, atopic and nummular eczema, urticaria, and drug-induced skin eruptions.

Contact Dermatitis

Contact dermatitis is a common inflammation of the skin. There are two types of contact dermatitis: irritant and allergic contact dermatitis. The irritant form of contact dermatitis is caused by chemicals (soaps, detergents, organic solvents) that irritate the skin. It can occur from mechanical means such as rubbing (*e.g.*, wool, fiberglass), chemical irritants (*e.g.*, household cleaning products), or environmental irritants (*e.g.*, plants, urine). An example is the skin burn that may occur from contact with cement products. Irritant contact dermatitis ranges from acute to chronic cases. Skin reactions range from mild erythema and scaling to acute necrotic burns.

Allergic contact dermatitis results from a cell-mediated, type IV hypersensitivity response brought about by sensitization to an allergen (see Chapter 21). More than 2000 allergens have been identified as capable of producing an inflammatory skin response. Crude forms of many naturally occurring substances are in general less allergenic than alloys and synthetic products. Additives such as dyes and perfumes account for the major sources of known allergens. Some of the common topical agents causing allergic rashes are antimicrobial agents (especially neomycin), antihistamines, local anesthetic agents (benzocaine), preservatives (*e.g.*, parabens), and adhesive tape. Additional examples are poison ivy and metal alloys found in jewelry. Also of concern is the increased incidence of contact dermatitis from the heavy use of synthetic latex products, specifically latex gloves and condoms used to prevent communicable diseases.

The lesions of allergic contact dermatitis range from a mild erythema with edema to vesicles or large bullae (Fig. 61-16). Secondary lesions from bacterial infection may occur. Lesions can occur almost anywhere on the body, and the many variations of eczema are often classified according to their location (*e.g.*, ear eczema, hand eczema). The location and pattern often help in identifying causative agents. For example, the typical poison ivy lesion consists of vesicles or bullae in a linear pattern (from swiping the plant) on exposed areas. The vesicles and bullae break and weep, leaving an excoriated area.

With both types of contact dermatitis, the location of the lesions is of great benefit in diagnosing the causative agent. Patch testing, in which a small amount of the sus-

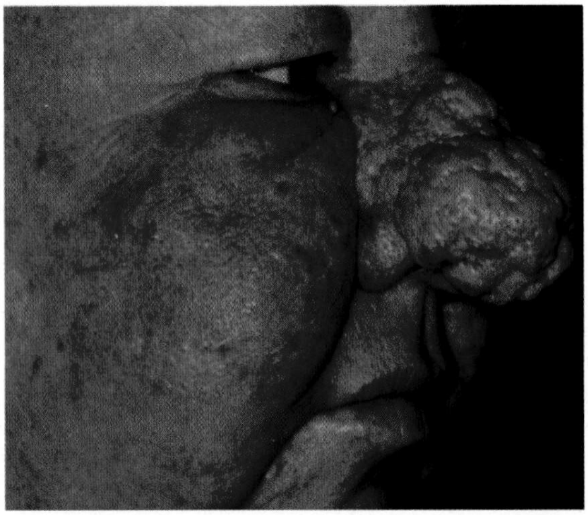

FIGURE 61-15 Chronic rosacea with rhinophyma. (Hoechst Marion Roussel Pharmaceuticals, Inc.) (Sauer G.C., Hall J.C. [1996]. *Manual of skin diseases* [7th ed.]. Philadelphia: Lippincott-Raven)

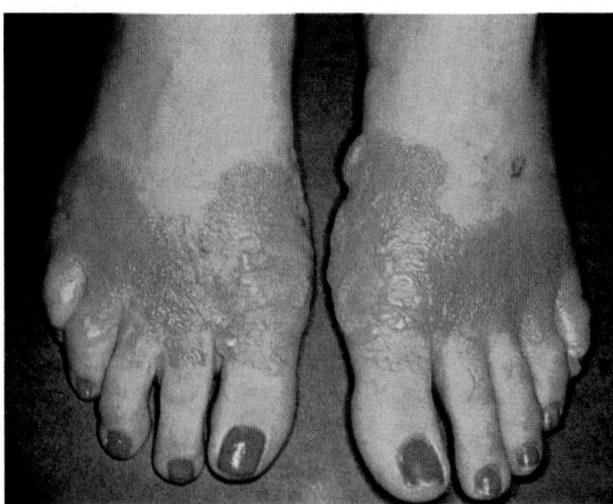

FIGURE 61-16 Contact dermatitis from shoe material. (Glaxo-Wellcome Co.) (Sauer G.C., Hall J.C. [1996]. *Manual of skin diseases* [7th ed.]. Philadelphia: Lippincott-Raven)

pected antigen is applied to the skin, is used to identify the allergens.

Treatment measures for both types of contact dermatitis are aimed at removing the source of the irritant or allergen. This may mean that the person needs to modify his or her behavior. This may be particularly difficult for the person with hand eczema because it may mean changing employment to avoid contact with the irritant or allergen. Minor cases are treated by washing the affected areas to remove further contamination by the irritant or allergen, applying antipruritic creams or lotions, and bandaging the exposed areas. Topical corticosteroids may be helpful in these cases. Systemic treatment regimens differ according to the type of irritant or allergen and the severity of the reaction. Moderate to extreme cases are treated with wet dressings, oral antihistamines, and systemic corticosteroids.

Atopic and Nummular Eczema

Atopic Eczema. Atopic eczema (atopic dermatitis) is a common skin disorder that occurs in two clinical forms, infantile and adult.[34,35] It is associated with a type I hypersensitivity reaction (see Chapter 21). There usually is a family history of asthma, hay fever, or atopic dermatitis, with asthma being a frequent comorbidity. Studies have indicated that there has been a twofold to threefold increase in the prevalence of atopic dermatitis over the past 30 to 50 years in developed countries.[36] Environmental pollutants, as well as food allergies, may contribute to the rise in this disease.

The infantile form of atopic dermatitis is characterized by vesicle formation, oozing, and crusting with excoriations. It usually begins in the cheeks and may progress to involve the scalp, arms, trunk, and legs (Fig. 61-17). The skin of the cheeks may be paler, with extra creases under the eyes, called *Dennie-Morgan folds*. The infantile form may become milder as the child ages, often disappearing by the age of 15 years. However, many individuals have resultant eczematous disorders and rhinitis symptoms that continue throughout life. Adolescents and adults usually have dry, leathery (lichenified), and hyperpigmented or hypopigmented lesions located in the antecubital and popliteal areas. These may spread to the neck, hands, feet, eyelids, and behind the ears. Itching may be severe with both forms. There is marked follicle involvement in darker-skinned persons with lesions that are hypopigmented, hyperpigmented, or both. Secondary infections are common.

Treatment of atopic eczema is designed to target the underlying abnormalities, such as dryness, pruritus, superinfection, and inflammation. It involves allergen control, basic skin care, and medications. Avoiding exposure to environmental irritants and foods that cause exacerbation of the symptoms is recommended. Because dry skin and pruritus often exacerbate the condition, hydration of the skin is essential to treating atopic dermatitis. Daily bathing for 5 to 10 minutes with warm (not hot) water is recommended. Although bathing dries the skin, it is important to maintain a low level of microorganisms to prevent infection. The use of soap should be avoided as much as possible. A moisturizer should be applied immediately after

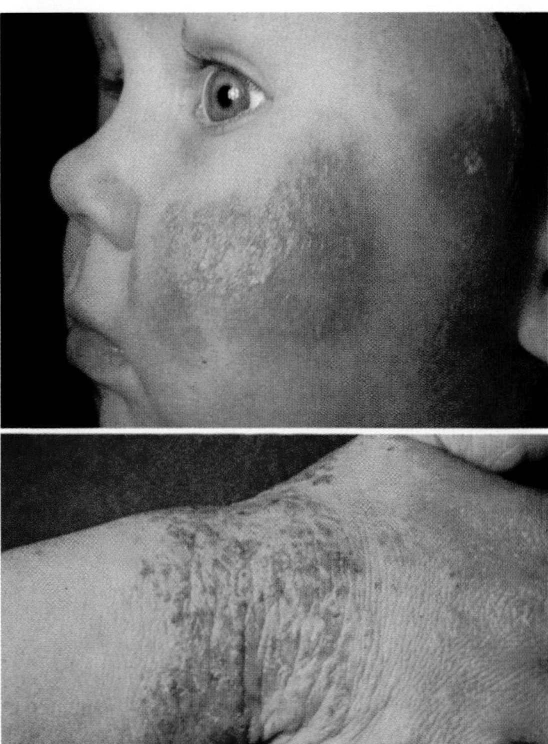

FIGURE 61-17 Atopic eczema on an infant's face and wrist. (Dome Chemicals.) (Sauer G.C., Hall J.C. [1996]. *Manual of skin diseases* [7th ed.]. Philadelphia: Lippincott-Raven)

bathing and before the skin is completely dry. Ointments are superior to creams and lotions, but they are greasy and therefore poorly tolerated.[35] Mild or healing lesions may be treated with lotions containing a mild antipruritic agent. Persons with atopic dermatitis are advised to avoid temperature changes and stress to minimize vascular and sweat responses. Acute weeping lesions are treated with soothing lotions, soaks, or wet dressings. Soaks in sodium bicarbonate or emollient bath preparations such as those containing colloidal oatmeal can be used to treat pruritus. Persistent pruritus can be treated with antihistamines or tricyclic antidepressants. Topical corticosteroids have been the standard of treatment but can cause local and systemic side effects. Because of their side effects, systemic corticosteroids usually are reserved for severe cases.

Topical immune modulators (tacrolimus and pimecrolimus) are demonstrating positive outcomes in atopic dermatitis without the side effect of cortisone therapy (dermal atrophy).[36,37] Immune modulators are immunosuppressive agents that have been used systemically for the prevention of organ rejection. Tacrolimus is believed to control atopic dermatitis by inhibiting activation of cells involved in atopic dermatitis: T lymphocytes, dendritic cells, mast cells, and keratinocytes.[38]

Nummular Eczema. The lesions of nummular eczema (discoid eczema) are coin-shaped (nummular) papulovesicular

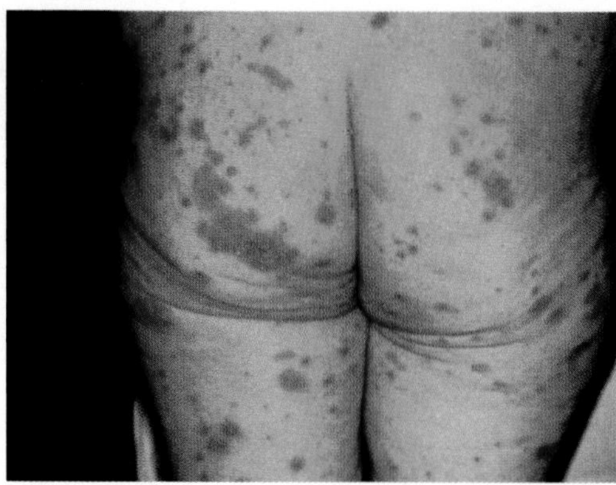

FIGURE 61-18 Nummular eczema of the buttocks. (Johnson & Johnson.) (Sauer G.C., Hall J.C. [1996]. *Manual of skin diseases* [7th ed.]. Philadelphia: Lippincott-Raven)

patches mainly involving the arms and legs (Fig. 61-18). Lichenification and secondary bacterial infections are common. It is not unusual for the initial lesions seemingly to heal, followed by a secondary outbreak of mirror-image lesions on the opposite side of the body. Most nummular eczema is chronic, with weeks to years between exacerbations. Exacerbations are more frequent in the cold winter months. The exact cause of nummular eczema is unknown. There usually is a history of asthma, hay fever, or atopic dermatitis. Ingestion of iodides and bromides usually aggravates the condition. Treatment is palliative. Frequent bathing, foods rich in iodides and bromides, and stress should be reduced, whereas the environmental humidity should be increased. Topical corticosteroids, coal tar preparations, and ultraviolet light treatments are prescribed as necessary.

Urticaria

Urticaria, or hives, is characterized by edematous plaques that are accompanied by intense itching.[39] The lesions typically appear as raised pink or red areas surrounded by a paler halo. They blanch with pressure and vary in size from a few millimeters to centimeters. Thicker lesions that result from massive transudation of fluid into the dermis or subcutaneous tissue are referred to as *angioedema*. Angioedema accompanies urticaria in approximately 40% of cases and when present typically affects the lips, face (particularly the periorbital area), hands, feet, penis, or scrotum. Occasionally, there is swelling of the tongue or pharynx, although the larynx is seldom involved. Another 40% of cases have hives alone, and about 20% of patients have angioedema but not urticaria.[40]

Histamine is the most common mediator of urticaria. Histamine causes hyperpermeability of the microvessels of the skin and surrounding tissue, allowing fluid to leak into the tissues and causing edema and wheal formation. Histamine is contained in the granules of the mast cells. A variety of immunologic, nonimmunologic, physical, and chemical stimuli can cause mast cell degranulation with release of histamine into the surrounding tissues and circulation.

Urticaria can be acute or chronic. Acute urticaria lasts up to 6 weeks; episodes of urticaria persisting longer than 6 weeks are considered chronic. The most common causes of acute urticaria are foods or drinks, medications, insect stings, viral infections, dust mites, and exposure to pollens or chemicals. Food is the most common cause of acute urticaria in children. Although nonsteroidal antiinflammatory drugs, including aspirin, do not normally cause urticaria, they may exacerbate the preexisting disease.

Chronic urticaria primarily affects adults and is twice as common in women as in men. Usually, its cause cannot be determined despite extensive laboratory tests. It appears to be an autoimmune disorder in a substantial number of persons. Approximately 40% to 50% of persons with chronic urticaria have circulating immunoglobulin G (IgG) antibodies to a subunit of the IgE receptor or to the IgE molecule. These antibodies activate basophils and mast cells to release histamine.[40] In rare cases, urticaria is a manifestation of underlying disease, such as certain cancers, collagen diseases, and hepatitis. There is an association between chronic urticaria and autoimmune thyroid disease (*e.g.,* Hashimoto's thyroiditis, Graves' disease, toxic multinodular thyroiditis). A hereditary deficiency of a C1 (complement 1) inhibitor also can cause urticaria and angioedema.

Physical urticarias constitute another form of chronic urticaria. Physical urticarias are intermittent, usually last less than 2 hours, are produced by appropriate stimuli, have distinctive appearances and locations, and are seen most frequently in young adults. Dermographism, or skin writing, is one form of physical urticaria in which wheals appear in response to simple rubbing of the skin (Fig. 61-19). The wheals follow the pattern of the scratch or rubbing, appearing within 10 minutes and dissolving completely within 20 minutes. Other types of physical urticaria are induced by exercise (cholinergic), cold, delayed pressure, sunlight (solar), water (aquagenic), vibration, and heat (external localized). Appropriate challenge tests (*e.g.,* ap-

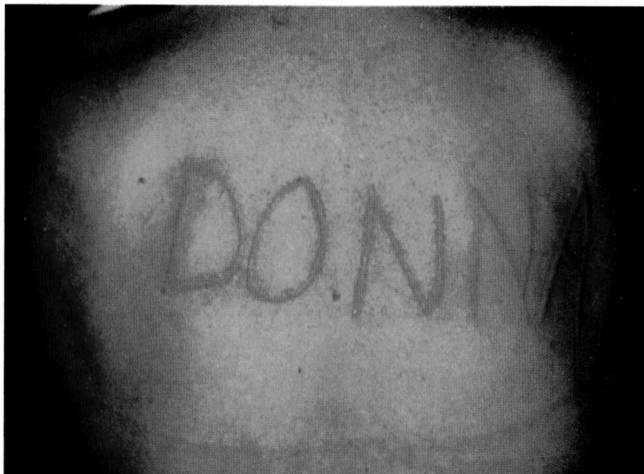

FIGURE 61-19 Dermographism on a patient's back. (Dermik Laboratories, Inc.) (Sauer G.C., Hall J.C. [1996]. *Manual of skin diseases* [7th ed.]. Philadelphia: Lippincott-Raven)

plication of an ice cube to the skin to initiate development of cold urticaria) are used to differentiate physical urticaria from chronic urticaria resulting from other causes.

Most types of urticaria are treated with antihistamines: drugs that block histamine type 1 (H_1) and, less frequently, H_1 in combination with histamine type 2 (H_2). They control urticaria by inhibiting vasodilation and the escape of fluid into the surrounding tissues. Usually, nonsedating antihistamines that alleviate pruritus and decrease the incidence of hives, without producing drowsiness, are used. Leukotriene antagonists (zafirlukast and montelukast) may also be used. Starch or colloid-type (*e.g.,* Aveeno) baths may be used as comfort measures. Persons who experience angioedema of the larynx and pharynx can be counseled to carry a prescription of epinephrine. Oral corticosteroids may be used in the treatment of refractory urticaria. Tricyclic antidepressant drugs, particularly those with antihistamine actions, also may be used.

Drug-Induced Skin Eruptions

Most drugs can cause a localized or generalized skin eruption. Topical drugs usually are responsible for a localized contact dermatitis type of rash, whereas systemic drugs cause generalized skin lesions. Although many drug-induced skin eruptions are morbilliform (*i.e.,* measles-like) or exanthematous, they may mimic almost all skin disorders described in this chapter. Because the lesions vary greatly, the diagnosis depends almost entirely on accurate patient report, including a full drug history. Management of mild cases is aimed at eliminating the offending drug while treating the symptoms. More severe cases require prompt medical attention and treatment with systemic corticosteroids and antihistamines.

Some drug reactions result in epidermal skin detachment and formation of bullous lesions. Three types of drug reactions that result in bullous skin lesions are erythema multiforme minor, Stevens-Johnson syndrome, and toxic epidermal necrolysis. Although erythema multiforme minor may be drug induced, it more frequently occurs after infections, especially with herpes simplex. It is self-limiting, with a small amount of skin detachment at the lesion sites. Stevens-Johnson syndrome and toxic epidermal necrolysis are caused by a hypersensitivity reaction to drugs such as the sulfonamides and anticonvulsants. Although more rare in occurrence, with an incidence of 2 to 3 cases per 1 million people in the United States and Europe, these reactions can be life threatening.[41]

The skin detachment seen with bullous skin lesions is different from the desquamation (*i.e.,* peeling) that occurs with other skin disorders. For example, with scarlet fever, there is peeling of the dead keratinized layer of the stratum corneum. In the bullous disorders, there is full-thickness detachment (*i.e.,* peeling) of the entire epidermis from the dermis. This leaves the person vulnerable to multiple problems, including loss of body fluids and electrolytes, impaired body temperature control, and a greatly increased risk for infection.

The lesions of erythema multiforme minor and Stevens-Johnson syndrome are similar. The primary lesion of both is a round, erythematous papule, resembling an insect bite. Within hours to days, these lesions change into several different patterns. The individual lesions may enlarge and coalesce, producing small plaques, or they may change to concentric zones of color, appearing as "target" or "iris" lesions (Fig. 61-20). The outermost rings of the target lesions usually are erythematous; the central portion usually is opaque white, yellow, or gray (dusky). In the center, small blisters on the dusky purpuric macules may form, giving them their characteristic target-like appearance. Although there is wide distribution of lesions over the body surface area, there is a propensity for them to occur on the face and trunk. With Stevens-Johnson syndrome, there is more skin detachment.

Toxic epidermal necrolysis is the most serious drug reaction, with a mortality rate of 30% to 35%.[42] The person experiences a prodromal period of malaise, low-grade fever, and sore throat. Within a few days, widespread erythema and large, flaccid bullae appear, followed by the loss of the epidermis, leaving a denuded and painful dermis. The skin surrounding the large denuded areas may have the typical target-like lesions seen with Stevens-Johnson syndrome. Often, the lateral pressure causes the surrounding skin to separate easily from the dermis (*Nikolsky's sign*). Usually, the epithelium of mucosal surfaces, especially those of the mouth and eyes, is also involved.

Initially, these three types of bullous skin eruptions are quite similar. The diagnostic boundary for erythema multiforme minor is that it usually occurs after herpes simplex infection and is self-limiting. Precise diagnostic boundaries between Stevens-Johnson syndrome and toxic epidermal necrolysis have not been established. However, there is some general agreement that cases involving less than 10% of the body surface area are called Stevens-Johnson syndrome, and detachment of more than 30% of the epidermis is labeled toxic epidermal necrolysis, with a 10% to 30% overlap of diagnoses.[25]

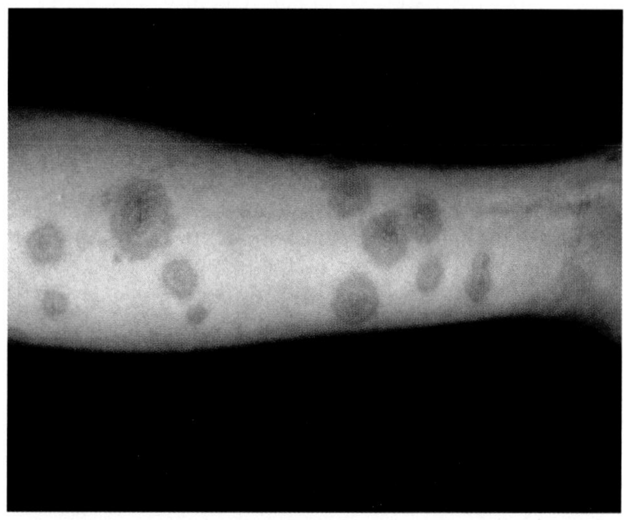

FIGURE 61-20 Erythema-multiforme–like eruption on the patient's arm. Notice the dusky, target-like appearance. (Dermik Laboratories, Inc.) (Sauer G.C., Hall J.C. [1996]. *Manual of skin diseases* [7th ed.]. Philadelphia: Lippincott-Raven)

Treatment of erythema multiforme minor and less severe cases of Stevens-Johnson syndrome includes relief of symptoms using compresses, antipruritic drugs, and topical anesthetics. Corticosteroid therapy may be indicated in moderate cases, although its use is controversial. For severe cases of Stevens-Johnson syndrome and toxic epidermal necrolysis, hospitalization is required for fluid replacement, administration of antibiotics, respiratory care, analgesics, and moist dressings. When large areas of skin are detached, the care is similar to that of thermal burn patients. Intravenous immunoglobulin may hasten the healing response of the skin. Generally, healing is a slow process, taking 6 weeks or more to regenerate skin. The mucous membranes heal more slowly, and follow-up treatment is often needed for ophthalmologic and mucous membrane sequelae. Avoidance of the responsible drug and chemically related compounds is essential.

PAPULOSQUAMOUS DERMATOSES

Papulosquamous dermatoses are a group of skin disorders characterized by scaling papules and plaques. Among the major papulosquamous diseases are psoriasis, pityriasis rosea, and lichen planus, which are discussed in this section of the chapter.

Psoriasis

Psoriasis is a common T-cell–mediated autoimmune disease characterized by circumscribed red, thickened plaques with an overlying silver-white scale. Psoriasis occurs worldwide, although the incidence is lower in warmer, sunnier climates. In the United States, it affects 2.6% or 6 million Americans.[43] The average age of onset is in the fourth decade; its prevalence increases with age. Approximately one third of patients have a genetic history, indicating a hereditary factor. Childhood onset of the disease is more strongly associated with a family history than psoriasis occurring in adults older than 30 years of age. The disease, which can persist throughout life and exacerbate at unpredictable times, is classified as a chronic ailment. A few cases, however, have been known to clear and not recur.

There appears to be an association between psoriasis and arthritis. Psoriatic arthritis occurs in 2% of the United States population and can account for a considerable amount of joint damage[44] (see Chapter 59). It occurs primarily in the hand and finger joints, often including the fingernails, and can be quite disabling.

The primary cause of psoriasis is uncertain. The unintended, yet dramatic, clearing of severe, disabling psoriasis with cyclosporine provided strong evidence that psoriasis may be a T-cell–mediated autoimmune response to an unidentified antigen.[44] It is thought that activated T lymphocytes (mainly CD4 helper cells) produce chemical messengers that stimulate abnormal growth of keratinocytes and dermal blood vessels. Accompanying inflammatory changes are caused by infiltration of neutrophils and monocytes. Skin trauma (*i.e.*, prepsoriasis) is a common precipitating factor in people predisposed to the disease. The reaction of the skin to an original trauma of any type is called the *Köebner reaction.* Stress, infections, trauma, xerosis, and use of medications such as angiotensin-converting enzyme inhibitors, β-adrenergic blocking drugs, lithium, and the antimalarial agent hydroxychloroquine (Plaquenil) may precipitate or exacerbate the condition.

Histologically, psoriasis is characterized by increased epidermal cell turnover with marked epidermal thickening, a process called *hyperkeratosis.* The migration time of the keratinocyte from the basal cell layer of the stratum corneum decreases from the normal 14 days to approximately 4 to 7 days. The granular layer (stratum granulosum) of the epidermis is thinned or absent, and neutrophils are found in the stratum corneum. There also is an accompanying thinning of the epidermal cell layer that overlies the tips of the dermal papillae (suprapapillary plate), and the blood vessels within dermal papillae become tortuous and dilated. These capillary beds show permanent damage even when the disease is in remission or has resolved. The close proximity of the vessels in the dermal papillae to the hyperkeratotic scale accounts for multiple, minute bleeding points that are seen when the scale is lifted.

There are several variants or types of psoriasis, including plaque-type psoriasis, guttate psoriasis, pustular psoriasis (localized and generalized), and erythrodermic psoriasis.[45,46] *Plaque-type psoriasis* (*psoriasis vulgaris*), which is the most common type, is a chronic stationary form of psoriasis. The lesions may occur anywhere on the skin but most often involve the elbows, knees, and scalp (Fig. 61-21). The primary lesions are sharply demarcated thick red plaques with a silvery scale that vary in size and shape. In darker-skinned persons, the plaques may appear purple. There may be excoriation, thickening, or oozing from the lesions. A differential diagnostic finding is that the plaques bleed from minute points when removed, which is known as the *Auspitz sign. Guttate psoriasis* is characterized by teardrop-shaped, pink to salmon, scaly lesions, and it occurs in children and young adults. Its lesions are usually limited to the upper trunk and extremities. This form of psoriasis usually is brought on by a streptococcal infection. It generally responds to treatments such as UVB phototherapy, only to return with recurrent streptococcal infections.[47] *Pustular psoriasis* is characterized by papules or plaques studded with pustules. Localized pustular psoriasis usually is limited to the palms of the hands and soles of the feet. Generalized pustular psoriasis is characterized by more general involvement and may be associated with systemic symptoms such as fever, malaise, and diarrhea. The person may or may not have had preexisting psoriasis. *Erythrodermic psoriasis* is a rare form of psoriasis affecting all body surfaces, including the hands, feet, nails, trunk, and extremities. It is characterized by a process in which the lesions scale and become confluent, leaving much of the body surface a bright red, with continuous skin shedding. Severe itching and pain often accompany it. Severe complications may develop related to loss of body fluids, proteins, and electrolytes and disturbances in temperature regulation. Without treatment, death from sepsis is a well-known complication of erythrodermic psoriasis.[46]

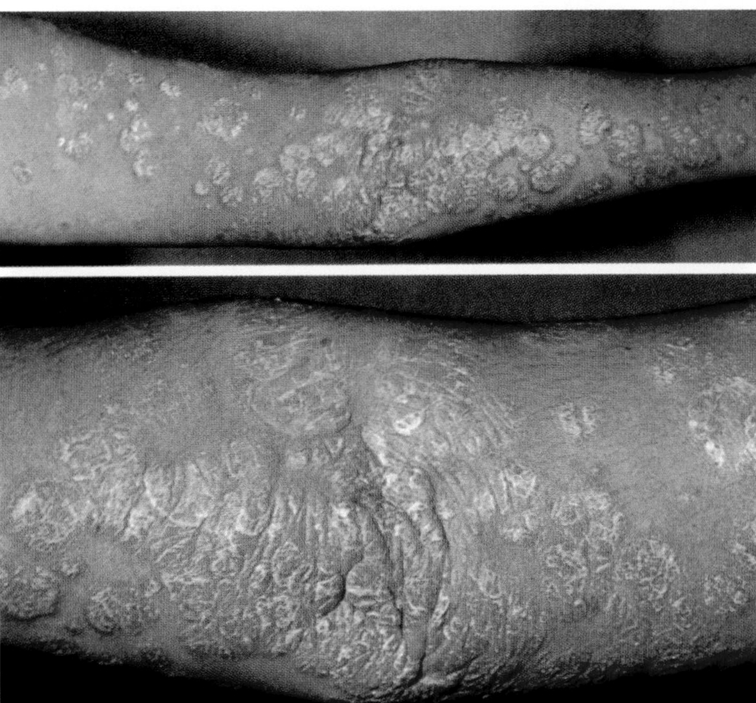

FIGURE 61-21 Psoriasis on the elbows of a 17-year-old girl. (Roche Laboratories.) (Sauer G.C., Hall J.C. [1996]. *Manual of skin diseases* [7th ed.]. Philadelphia: Lippincott-Raven)

Treatment. There is no cure for psoriasis. The goal of treatment is to suppress the signs and symptoms of the disease: hyperkeratosis, epidermal inflammation, and abnormal keratinocyte differentiation. Treatment depends on the severity of the disease as well as the person's age, sex, treatment history, and level of treatment compliance. Treatment measures are divided into topical and systemic approaches. Usually, topical agents are used first in any treatment regimen and when less than 20% of the body surface is involved.[45] Combination therapies that are tailored to the needs of the client are most effective. Also, rotating various therapies may decrease the side effects of any one therapy.

Topical agents include emollients, keratolytic agents, coal tar products, anthralin, corticosteroids, and calcipotriene. Emollients hydrate and soften the psoriatic plaques. Petroleum-based products are more effective than water-based ones, but they are often less acceptable cosmetically to persons with psoriasis. Keratolytic agents are peeling agents. Salicylic acid is the most widely used. It softens and removes plaques. It has been used alone or in conjunction with other topical agents. Coal tar, the byproduct of the processing of coke and gas from coal, is one of the oldest yet more effective forms of treatment. The skin is covered with a film of coal tar for up to several weeks. The exact mechanism of action of the tar products is unknown, but side effects of the treatment are few. Newer preparations of coal tar lotions and shampoos are more aesthetically pleasing, but the odor remains a problem.

Anthralin, a synthesized product of Goa powder from Brazilian araroba tree bark, has remained a topical treatment of choice. It has been effective in resolving lesions in approximately 2 weeks. A disadvantage to anthralin is that it stains the uninvolved skin and clothes brown or purple. A treatment variation, called the *Ingram method,* involves coal tar applications and UVB radiation, followed by anthralin paste application.

Topical corticosteroids are widely used and relatively effective. They are generally more acceptable because they do not stain and are easy to use. Topical corticosteroids are available as low-, medium-, and high-potency preparations. Treatment usually is started with a medium-potency agent. Low-potency drugs usually are used on the face and areas of the body, such as the groin and axillary areas, where the skin tends to be thinner. High-potency preparations are reserved for treatment of thick chronic plaques that do not respond to less potent preparations. Although the corticosteroids are rapidly effective in the treatment of psoriasis, they are associated with flare-ups after discontinuation, and they have many potential side effects. Their effectiveness is increased when used under occlusive dressings, but there is an increase in side effects. *Calcipotriene,* a topical vitamin D derivative, has been effective for the treatment of psoriasis. It inhibits epidermal cell proliferation and enhances cell differentiation. *Tazarotene,* a synthetic retinoid, also has been effective. It is classified as a pregnancy category X drug and should be avoided in women of childbearing age.

Systemic treatments include phototherapy, photochemotherapy, methotrexate, retinoids, corticosteroids, and cyclosporine. The positive effects of sunlight have long been established. Climatotherapy (warm climate and saltwater baths for 4 to 6 weeks) and heliotherapy (sunbathing in a suitable climate) have been effective treatment measures for those who can afford to travel.[46] Phototherapy with UVB is a widely used treatment. Newly developed narrowband UVB radiation is reportedly more effective that broadband UVB.[46]

Photochemotherapy involves using a light-activated form of the drug methoxsalen. Methoxsalen, a psoralen, exerts its actions when exposed to UVA radiation in 320 to 400 nm wavelengths. The combination treatment regimen of psoralen and UVA is known by the acronym PUVA. Methoxsalen is given orally before UVA exposure. Activated by the UVA energy, methoxsalen inhibits DNA synthesis, thereby preventing cell mitosis and decreasing the hyperkeratosis that occurs with psoriasis. Although viewed as one of the safest therapies since its introduction in the 1970s, PUVA increases the risk for squamous cell carcinoma, and it may increase the risk for development of melanoma.

Systemic corticosteroids have been effective in treating severe or pustular psoriasis. However, they can cause severe side effects, including Cushing's syndrome. Intralesional injection of triamcinolone has proved effective in resistant lesions.

The retinoids are another class of systemic psoriasis therapy. These drugs, which are derivatives of vitamin A, are only moderately effective as monotherapy and are associated with numerous mucocutaneous side effects such as hair loss, cheilitis, and thinning of the nails. However, when used as short-term therapy in combination with UVB phototherapy or PUVA, low-dose acitretin has been shown to be effective, allowing substantial clearing of lesions with fewer visits and fewer mucocutaneous side effects.[46] Teratogenicity limits the use of retinoids in women of childbearing potential.

Methotrexate, which is used for cancer treatment, is an antimetabolite that inhibits DNA synthesis and prevents cell mitosis. Oral methotrexate has been effective in treating psoriasis when other approaches have failed. The drug has many side effects, including nausea, malaise, leukopenia, thrombocytopenia, and liver function abnormalities. Cyclosporine is a potent immunosuppressive drug used to prevent rejection of organ transplants. It suppresses inflammation and the proliferation of T cells in persons with psoriasis. Its use is limited to severe psoriasis because of serious side effects, including nephrotoxicity, hypertension, and increased risk for cancers. Intralesional cyclosporine also has been effective. New biologic agents (infliximab, etanercept, and alefacept) that target the activity of T lymphocytes and cytokines responsible for the inflammatory nature of psoriasis have proved effective, not only with the skin lesions, but in halting the effects of the associated arthritis of psoriasis.[47,48] Psoriasis treatment centers have successfully treated patients with recalcitrant cases of psoriasis. These centers have equipment, professionals, and therapists to assist patients in gaining control over the disease process and restoring normality to their lives.

Pityriasis Rosea

Pityriasis rosea is a rash that primarily affects young adults. The origin of the rash is unknown, but it is thought to be caused by an infective agent. Numerous viruses have been investigated, thus far with no conclusive evidence. The incidence is highest in winter. Cases occur in clusters and among persons who are in close contact with each other, indicating an infectious spread. However, there are no data to support communicability. It may be an immune response to any number of agents.

The characteristic lesion is an oval macule or papule with surrounding erythema (Fig. 61-22). The lesion spreads with central clearing, much like tinea corporis. This initial lesion is a solitary lesion called the *herald patch* and is usually on the trunk or neck. As the lesion enlarges and begins to fade away (2 to 10 days), successive crops of lesions appear on the trunk and neck. The lesions on the back have a characteristic "Christmas tree" pattern. The extremities, face, and scalp may be involved. Mild to severe pruritus may occur.

The disease is self-limited and usually disappears within 6 to 8 weeks. Treatment measures are palliative and include topical steroids, antihistamines, and colloid baths. Systemic corticosteroids may be indicated in severe cases.

Lichen Planus

The term *lichen* is of Greek origin and means "tree moss." The term is applied to skin disorders characterized by small (2 to 10 mm), flat-topped papules with irregular, angulated

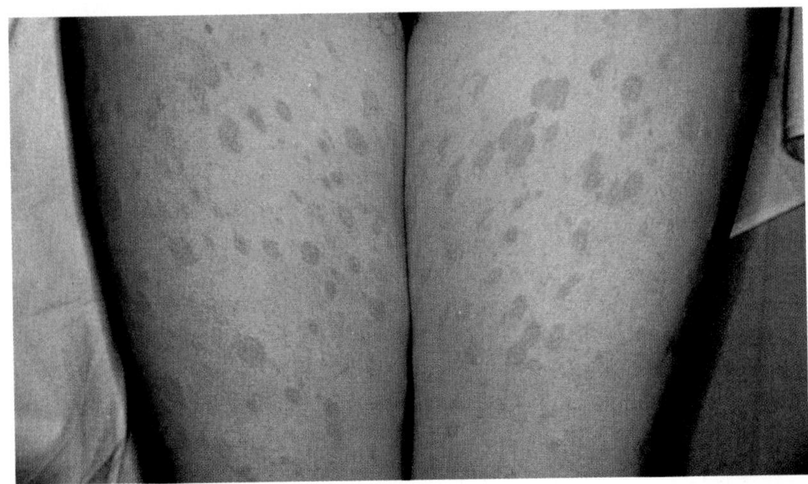

FIGURE 61-22 Pityriasis rosea of the thighs. (Syntex Laboratories.) (Sauer G.C., Hall J.C. [1996]. *Manual of skin diseases* [7th ed.]. Philadelphia: Lippincott-Raven)

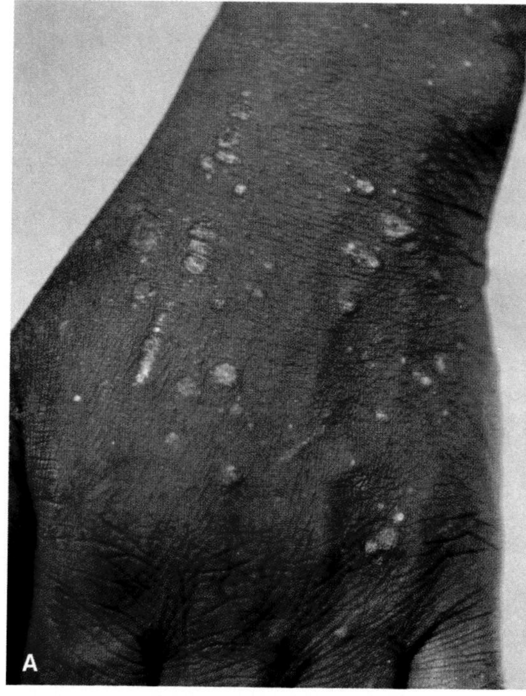

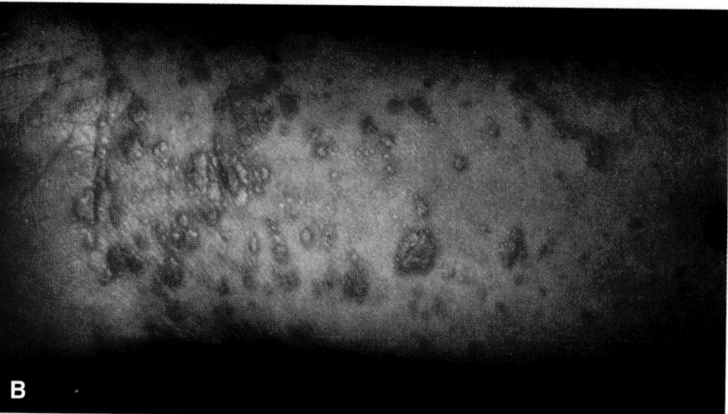

FIGURE 61-23 **(A)** Lichen planus of the dorsum of the hand and wrist. Notice the violaceous color of the papules and the linear Köebner's phenomenon. **(B)** Lichen planus. (E.R. Squibb, Johnson & Johnson.) (Sauer G.C., Hall J.C. [1996]. *Manual of skin diseases* [7th ed.]. Philadelphia: Lippincott-Raven)

borders (Fig. 61-23). Lichen planus is a relatively common chronic, pruritic disease. It involves inflammation and papular eruption of the skin and mucous membranes. There are variations in the pattern of lesions (*e.g.,* annular, linear) and differences in the sites (*e.g.,* mucous membranes, genitalia, nails, scalp). The characteristic lesion is a purple, polygonal papule covered with a shiny, white, lacelike pattern. The lesions appear on the wrist, ankles, and trunk of the body. Most persons who have skin lesions also have oral lesions, appearing as milky white lacework on the buccal mucosa or tongue. Other mucosal surfaces, such as the genital, nasal, laryngeal, otic, gastric, and anal areas, may also be affected.

The etiology of lichen planus is believed to be an abnormal immune response in which epithelial cells are recognized as foreign. The disorder involves the epidermal–dermal junction with damage to the basal cell layer. Lichen planus has been linked in many cases to hepatitis C virus infection or medication use. The most common medication agents include gold, antimalarial agents, thiazide diuretics, β-blockers, nonsteroidal antiinflammatory agents, quinidine, and angiotensin-converting enzyme inhibitors.[49]

Diagnosis is based on the clinical appearance of the lesions and the histopathologic findings from a punch biopsy. For most persons, lichen planus is a self-limited disease. Treatment measures include discontinuation of all medications, followed by treatment with topical corticosteroids and occlusive dressings. Occlusion may be used to enhance the effect of topical medications. Antipruritic agents are helpful in reducing itch. Systemic corticosteroids may be indicated in severe cases. Intralesional corticosteroid injections also may be used. Acitretin, an orally administered retinoid agent, also may be effective. Because retinoids are teratogenic, they should be avoided in women of childbearing age. Cyclosporine, tacrolimus, and other immunosuppressive agents have been helpful.

Lichen Simplex Chronicus

Lichen simplex chronicus is a localized lichenoid, pruritic dermatitis resulting from repeated rubbing and scratching. The term *lichen simplex* denotes that there was no known predisposing skin disorder in the affected person. It is characterized by the occurrence of itchy, reddened, thickened, and scaly patches of dry skin (Fig. 61-24). Persons with the condition may have a single or, less frequently, multiple lesions. The lesions are seen most commonly at the nape of the neck, wrist, ankles, or anal area. The condition usually begins as a small pruritic patch, which after a repetitive cycle of itching and scratching develops into a chronic dermatosis. Because of the chronic itching and scratching, excoriations and lichenification with thickening of the skin develops, often giving the appearance of tree bark. Treatment consists of measures to decrease scratching of the area. A moderate-potency corticosteroid is often prescribed to decrease the itching and subsequent inflammatory process.

ARTHROPOD INFESTATIONS

The skin is susceptible to a variety of disorders as a result of an invasion or infestation by bugs, ticks, or parasites. The type of rash or sometimes singular lesion depends on the causative agent.

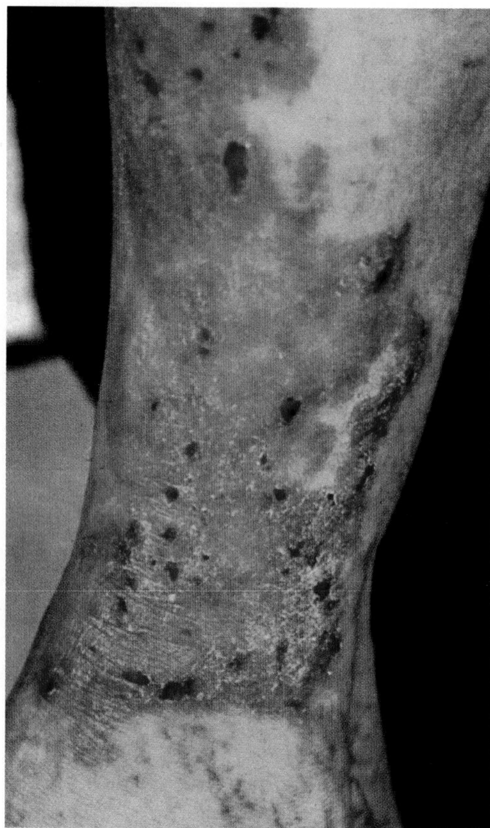

FIGURE 61-24 Localized lichen simplex chronicus of the leg. (Duke Laboratories, Inc.) (Sauer G.C., Hall J.C. [1996]. *Manual of skin diseases* [7th ed.]. Philadelphia: Lippincott-Raven)

Scabies

A mite, *Sarcoptes scabiei,* which burrows into the epidermis, causes scabies. After a female mite is impregnated, she burrows into the skin and lays two to three eggs each day for 4 or 5 weeks. The eggs hatch after 3 to 4 days, and the larvae migrate to the skin surface. At this point, they burrow into the skin only for food or protection. The larvae molt and become nymphs; they molt once more to become adults. After the new adult females are impregnated, the cycle is repeated.

The characteristic lesion is a small burrow (*e.g.,* 2 mm) that may be red to reddish brown. Small vesicles may cover the burrows. The areas most commonly affected are the interdigital web of the finger, flexor surface of the wrist, inner surface of the elbow, axilla, female nipple, penis, belt line, and gluteal crease. Pruritus is common and may result from the burrows, the fecal material of the mite, or both. Excoriations may develop from scratching, leaving the host open to secondary bacterial infections and severe skin lesions if the condition is untreated.

Scabies is transmitted by person-to-person contact, including sexual contact. It also is transmitted by contact with mite-infested sheets in hospitals and nursing homes because the mite can live up to 2 days on sheets or clothing. Scabies affects all people in all socioeconomic classes, although African Americans seem more resistant. Usually more prevalent in times of war and famine, scabies reached pandemic proportions in the 1970s, perhaps as a result of poverty, sexual promiscuity, and worldwide travel. Outbreaks continue to occur, but they are mostly sporadic and localized to nursing homes and families.

Diagnosis is done by skin scrapings. A positive diagnosis relies on the presence of mites, ova, or feces. The treatment is simple and curative. After bathing, permethrin, malathion, or other effective mite-killing agents are applied over the entire skin surface for 12 hours. Repeated applications may be recommended in certain cases, but one treatment usually is sufficient. Care must be taken to ensure that close contacts are treated. Clothes and towels are disinfected with hot water and detergent, or they can be isolated for 2 weeks. If symptoms persist after treatment, the patient should be advised not to retreat the condition without consulting a health care provider. Oral ivermectin, a broad-spectrum antiparasitic agent, has been used for treatment-resistant scabies.[50] A red-brown nodule, thought to be an allergic response from the mite parts left on the skin, may form after treatment.

Pediculosis

Pediculosis is the term for infestation with lice (genus *Pediculus*). Lice are gray, gray-brown, or red-brown, oval, wingless insects that live off the blood of humans and animals. Lice are host specific: lice that live on animals do not transfer to humans, and vice versa. Lice also are host dependent: they cannot live apart from the host beyond a few hours. As with scabies, the incidence of pediculosis increased in the 1970s to pandemic levels, probably because of increases in poverty, sexual activity, and worldwide travel.

Three types of lice affect humans: *Pediculus humanus corporis* (body lice), *Phthirus pubis* (pubic lice), and *Pediculus humanus capitis* (head lice). Although these three types differ biologically, they have similar life cycles. The life cycle of a louse consists of an unhatched egg or "nit," three molt stages, an adult reproductive stage, and death. Before adulthood, lice live off the host and are incapable of reproduction. After fertilization, the female louse lays her eggs along hair shafts. The nits appear pearl gray to brown. Depending on the site, a female louse can lay between 150 and 300 nits in her life. The life span of a feeding louse is 30 to 50 days. Lice are equipped with stylets that pierce the skin. Their saliva contains an anticoagulant that prevents the host's blood from clotting while the louse is feeding. A louse takes up to 1 mL of blood during a feeding.

Pediculosis Corporis. Pediculosis corporis is infestation with *P. humanus corporis,* or body lice. The lice are transferred chiefly through contact with an infested person, clothing, or bedding. The lice live in clothes fibers, coming out only to feed, usually at night, causing nocturnal pruritus. Unlike pubic and head lice, the body louse can survive 10 to 14 days without the host.

The typical lesion is a macule at the site of the bite. Papules and wheals may develop. The infestation is pruritic and evokes scratching that brings about a characteristic linear excoriation. Eczematous patches are found frequently. Secondary lesions may become scaly, hyperpigmented, and leave scars. Areas typically affected are the shoulders, trunk, and buttocks. The presence of nits in the seams of clothes confirms a diagnosis of body lice.

Treatment measures consist of eradicating the louse and nits on the body and on clothing. Dry-cleaning, washing in hot water, or steam pressing clothes are recommended methods. Special attention is given to the seams. Merely storing clothing in plastic bags for 2 weeks also rids clothes of lice. Many health care providers prefer not to treat the body unless nits are in evidence on hair shafts. If treatment is indicated, shampoos or topical preparations containing malathion or other pediculicides are recommended. Care must be taken to ensure that close contacts are treated.

Pediculosis Pubis. Pediculosis pubis, the infestation known as crabs or pubic lice, is a nuisance disease that is uncomfortable and embarrassing. The disease is spread by intimate contact with someone harboring *P. pubis*. The lice and nits are usually found in the pubic area of men and women, where their bites produce itching and erythematous lesions. Occasionally, they may be found in sites of secondary sex characteristics, such as the beard in men or the axilla in both sexes. Symptoms include intense itching and irritation of the skin. Diagnosis is made on the basis of symptoms and microscopic examination. The treatment is the same as for head lice.

Pediculosis Capitis. Pediculosis capitis, or infestation with head lice, primarily affects white-skinned persons; it is relatively unknown in darker-skinned persons. The incidence is higher among girls, although hair length has not been indicated as a contributing factor. Infestations of head lice usually are confined to the nape of the neck and behind the ears. Less frequently, head lice are found on the beard, pubic areas, eyebrows, and body hairs. Although head lice can be transmitted by sharing combs and hats, they usually are spread from hair shaft to hair shaft through close personal contact.[51] A positive diagnosis depends on the presence of firmly attached nits or live adult lice on hair shafts. Pruritus and scratching of the head are the primary indicators that head lice may be present. The scalp may appear red and excoriated from scratching. In severe cases, the hair becomes matted together in a crusty, foul-smelling "cap." An occasional morbilliform rash, which may be misdiagnosed as rubella, may occur with lymphadenopathy.

Head lice are treated with permethrin or malathion shampoos or rinses. Repeated treatments may be needed to eliminate the hatching nits. Dead nits may be removed with a fine-toothed comb or over-the-counter nit removal hair rinses. Over the years, permethrin- and malathion-resistant lice have evolved. There is controversy regarding whether true resistance exists or other factors affect resistance, such as not using the treatment measures correctly, not repeating the treatment measures, or misdiagnosing head lice.[52] There has been a resurgence of older remedies in response, such as asphyxiation with olive oil or petroleum products left on the hair from 24 hours to several months. Rotating therapies also may be helpful. "Bug busting" or removing nits by wet combing the hair every 3 to 4 days for 2 weeks has proved ineffective when used as the only treatment measure.[52]

In summary, primary disorders of the skin include pigmentary skin disorders, infectious processes, inflammatory conditions, immune disorders, allergic reactions, and arthropod infestations. Pigmentary skin disorders include vitiligo, albinism, and melasma. Although the causes of the disorders vary, all involve changes in the amount of melanin produced by the melanocytes. These disorders appear in people of every skin type; however, the manifestations of the disorders vary among light-skinned and dark-skinned persons. Superficial fungal infections are called *dermatophytoses* and are commonly known as *tinea* or *ringworm*. Impetigo, which is caused by staphylococci or β-hemolytic streptococci, is the most common superficial bacterial infection. Viruses are responsible for verrucae (warts), herpes simplex type 1 lesions (cold sores or fever blisters), and herpes zoster (shingles). Noninfectious inflammatory skin conditions, such as acne, lichen planus, psoriasis, and pityriasis rosea, are of unknown origin. They are usually localized to the skin and are rarely associated with specific internal disease. Allergic skin responses involve the body's immune system and are caused by hypersensitivity reactions to allergens, environmental agents, drugs, and other substances. The skin is sensitive to invasion or infestation by bugs or parasites.

Nevi and Skin Cancers

After completing this section of the chapter, you should be able to meet the following objectives:

- Describe the origin of nevi and state their relationship to skin cancers
- Compare the appearance and outcome of basal cell carcinoma, squamous cell carcinoma, and malignant melanoma

NEVI

Nevi, or moles, are common congenital or acquired tumors of the skin that are benign. Almost all adults have nevi, some in greater numbers than others. Nevi can be pigmented or nonpigmented, flat or elevated, and hairy or nonhairy.

Nevocellular nevi are pigmented skin lesions resulting from proliferation of melanocytes in the epidermis or dermis. Nevocellular nevi are tan to deep brown, uniformly pigmented, small papules with well-defined, rounded borders. They are formed initially by melanocytes with their long dendritic extensions that are normally interspersed among the basal keratinocytes[19] (see Fig. 60-3 in Chapter 60). The melanocytes are transformed into round or oval melanin-containing cells that grow in nests or clusters along the dermal–epidermal junction. Because of their location, these lesions are called *junctional nevi* (Fig. 61-25). Eventually, most junctional nevi grow into the surrounding dermis as

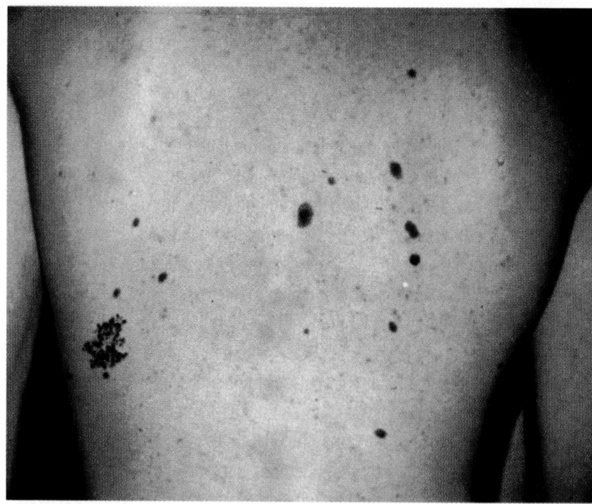

FIGURE 61-25 Junctional nevi of the back of a 16-year-old patient. (Owen Laboratories, Inc.) (Sauer G.C., Hall J.C. [1996]. *Manual of skin diseases* [7th ed.]. Philadelphia: Lippincott-Raven)

nests or cords of cells. *Compound nevi* contain epidermal and dermal components. In older lesions, the epidermal nests may disappear entirely, leaving *dermal nevi*. Compound and dermal nevi usually are more elevated than junctional nevi.

Another form of nevi, *dysplastic nevi,* is important because of their capacity to transform to malignant melanomas. Although the association between nevocellular nevi and malignant melanoma was made more than 175 years ago, it was not until 1978 that the role of dysplastic nevi as a precursor of malignant melanoma was described in detail. Dysplastic nevi are larger than other nevi (often >5 mm in diameter). Their appearance is one of a flat, slightly raised plaque with a pebbly surface, or a target-like lesion with a darker, raised center and irregular border. They vary in shade from brown and red to flesh tones and have irregular borders. A person may have hundreds of these lesions. Unlike other moles or nevi, they occur on both sun-exposed and covered areas of the body. Dysplastic nevi have been documented in multiple members of families prone to development of malignant melanoma.[19]

Because of the possibility of malignant transformation, any mole that undergoes a change warrants immediate medical attention. The changes to observe and report are changes in size, thickness, or color, and itching or bleeding.

SKIN CANCER

There has been an alarming increase in skin cancers over the past several decades. Since the 1970s, the incidence rate of malignant melanoma, the most serious form of skin cancer, has increased significantly, on average 6% per year, from 1973 until the early 1980s. Since 1981, the rate has slowed to roughly 3% per year. In 2003, there were approximately 54,200 new cases and 7,600 deaths from melanoma.[53] There were also approximately 1 million cases in 2002 of highly curable nonmelanoma (basal cell and squamous cell) cancers.

SKIN CANCERS

- An increase in skin cancers over the past several decades has been attributed to increased sun exposure.
- There are three major types of skin cancers: malignant melanomas, which are a rapidly progressive and metastatic form of skin cancer, and the basal cell carcinomas and squamous cell carcinomas, which are highly curable.

The rising incidence of skin cancer has been attributed to increased sun exposure associated with societal and lifestyle shifts in the United States. The thinning of the ozone layer in the earth's stratosphere is thought to be another factor in this incidence rate. Society's emphasis on suntanning also is implicated. People have more leisure time and spend increasing amounts of time in the sun with uncovered skin.

Although the factors linking sun exposure to skin cancer are not completely understood, both total cumulative exposure and altered patterns of exposure are strongly implicated. Basal cell and squamous cell carcinomas are often associated with total cumulative exposure to ultraviolet radiation. Thus, basal cell and squamous cell carcinomas occur more commonly on maximally sun-exposed parts of the body, such as the face and back of the hands and forearms. Melanomas previously occurred more commonly in areas of the body that were exposed to the sun intermittently, such as the back in men and the lower legs in women. However, an increase in melanoma has been noted in sun-exposed areas since the 1950s. It is more common in persons with indoor occupations whose exposure to sun is limited to weekends and vacations.

Malignant Melanoma

Malignant melanoma is a malignant tumor of the melanocytes. It is a rapidly progressing, metastatic form of cancer. As previously mentioned, there has been a dramatic increase in the incidence of malignant melanoma over the past several decades. The increased incidence of melanoma has been credited to increased to sun exposure. The risk is greatest in fair-skinned people, particularly those with blond or red hair who sunburn and freckle easily. Fortunately, the increased risk for melanoma has been associated with a concomitant increase in the 5-year survival rate, from approximately 40% in the 1940s to 90% at present.[54] Public health screening measures, early diagnosis, increased knowledge of precursor lesions, and greater public knowledge of the disease may account for earlier intervention.

Severe, blistering sunburns in early childhood and intermittent intense sun exposures (trips to sunny climates) contribute to increased susceptibility to melanoma in young and middle-aged adults. Roughly 90% of malignant melanomas in whites occur on sun-exposed skin. African

Americans, followed by Hispanics and Asians, have the lowest incidence.[55] Roughly 67% of melanomas occur in darker-skinned persons on non–sun-exposed areas, such as mucous membranes and subungual, palmar, and plantar surfaces. Although sun exposure remains a significant risk factor for melanoma, other potential risk factors have been identified, including atypical mole/dysplastic nevus syndrome, immunosuppression, prior PUVA therapy, and exposure to ultraviolet light at tanning salons. Using statistical analysis, it has been determined that six risk factors independently influence the risk for development of malignant melanoma: family history of malignant melanoma, presence of blond or red hair, presence of marked freckling on the upper back, history of three or more blistering sunburns before 20 years of age, history of 3 or more years of an outdoor job as a teenager, and presence of actinic keratosis. Persons with two of these risk factors had a 3.5-fold increased risk for malignant melanoma, and those with three or more risk factors had a 20-fold increased risk.[55]

Malignant melanomas differ in size and shape. Usually, they are slightly raised and black or brown. Borders are irregular, and surfaces are uneven. Most seem to arise from preexisting nevi or new molelike growths (Fig. 61-26). There may be surrounding erythema, inflammation, and

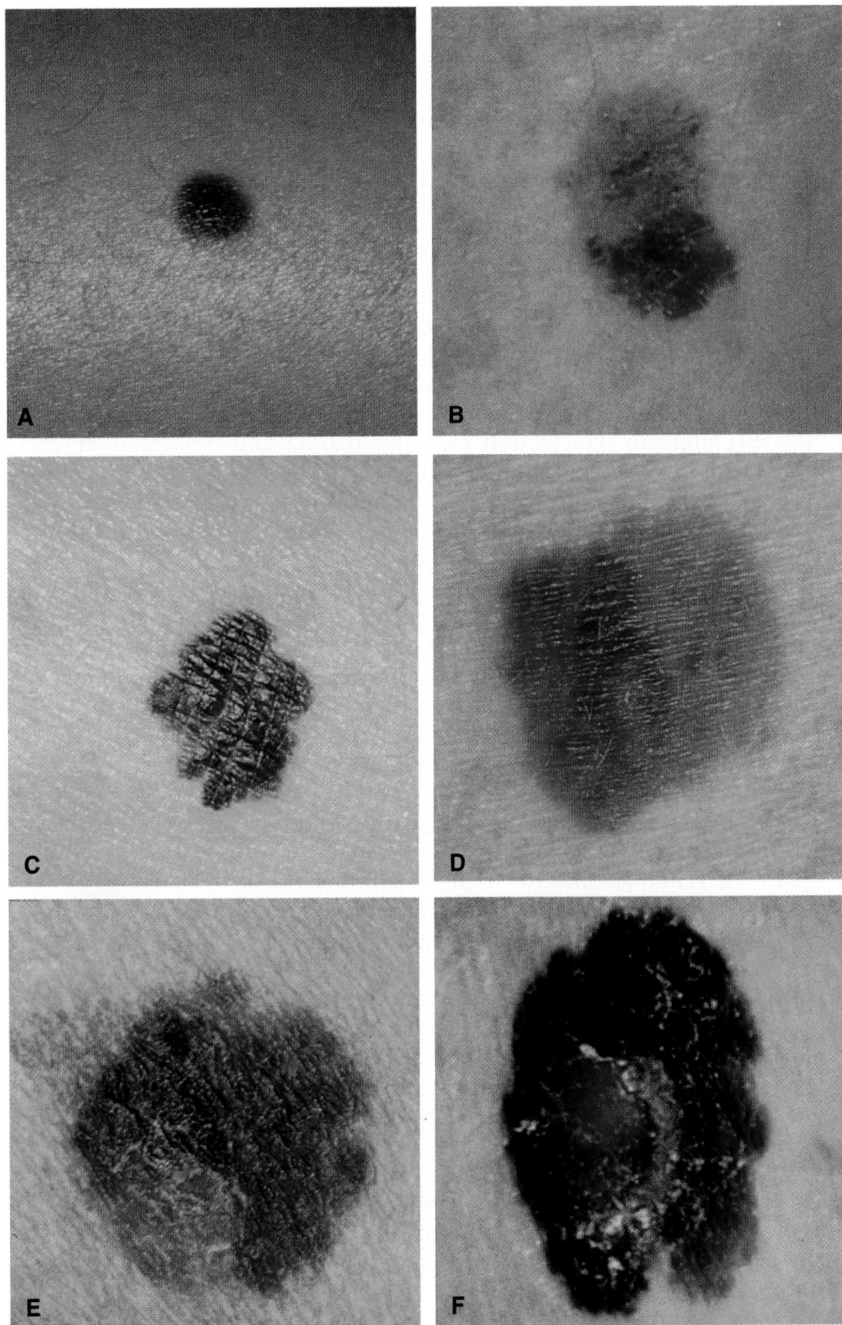

FIGURE 61-26 (**A**) Normal mole with even, round contour and sharply defined borders. (**B**) Changes in appearance of a mole: *asymmetry.* (**C**) Changes in appearance of a mole: *border irregularity.* (**D**) Changes in appearance of a mole: *color and uneven pigmentation.* (**E**) Changes in the appearance of a mole: *diameter* greater than 6 mm. (**F**) Changes in the surface of a mole: *scaliness, oozing, and bleeding.* (American Cancer Society. [1995]. *What you should know about melanoma.* Dallas: American Cancer Society)

tenderness. Periodically, melanomas ulcerate and bleed. Dark melanomas are often mottled with shades of red, blue, and white. These three colors represent three concurrent processes: melanoma growth (blue), inflammation and the body's attempt to localize and destroy the tumor (red), and scar tissue formation (white). Malignant melanomas can appear anywhere on the body. Although they frequently are found on sun-exposed areas, sun exposure alone does not account for their development. In men, they are found frequently on the trunk, head, neck, and arms; in women, they also are found on the legs.

Four types of melanomas have been identified: superficial spreading, nodular, lentigo maligna, and acral lentiginous.[56] *Superficial spreading melanoma* is characterized by a raised-edged nevus with lateral growth. It has a disorderly appearance in color and outline. This lesion tends to have biphasic growth, horizontally and vertically. It typically ulcerates and bleeds with growth. This type of lesion accounts for 70% of all melanomas and is most prevalent in persons who sunburn easily and have intermittent sun exposure. *Nodular melanomas,* which account for 15% to 30% of melanomas, are raised, dome-shaped lesions that can occur anywhere on the body. They are commonly a uniform blue-black color and tend to look like blood blisters. Nodular melanomas tend to rapidly invade the dermis from the start with no apparent horizontal growth phase. *Lentigo maligna* melanomas, which account for 1% to 5% of all melanomas, are slow-growing, flat nevi that occur primarily on sun-exposed areas of elderly persons. Untreated lentigo maligna tends to exhibit horizontal and radial growth for many years before it invades the dermis to become lentigo maligna melanoma. *Acral lentiginous melanoma,* which accounts for 2% to 8% of melanomas, occurs primarily on the palms of the hands, soles of the feet, nail beds, and mucous membranes. It has the appearance of lentigo maligna. Unlike other types of melanomas, it has a similar incidence in all ethnic groups.

Because virtually all the known risks of melanoma are related to susceptibility and magnitude of ultraviolet light exposure, protection from the sun's rays plays a critical role in the prevention of malignant melanoma. Protection includes using a combination regimen of protective clothing, avoidance of midday sun, and regular use of broad-spectrum sunscreen with an SPF of 15 or greater.

Early detection is critical with malignant melanoma. Regular self-examination of the total skin surface in front of a well-lighted mirror provides a method for early detection. It requires that a person undress completely and examine all areas of the body using a full mirror, handheld mirror, and handheld hair dryer (to examine the scalp). An *ABCD* rule has been developed to aid in early diagnosis and timely treatment of malignant melanoma. The acronym stands for **a**symmetry, **b**order irregularity, **c**olor variegation, and **d**iameter greater than 6 mm (¼ inch or pencil eraser size). People should be taught to watch for these changes in existing nevi or the development of new nevi, as well as other alterations such as bleeding or itching.

Diagnosis of melanoma is based on biopsy findings from a lesion. Consistent with other cancerous tumors, melanoma is commonly staged using the TNM (tumor, lymph node, and metastasis) staging system (see Chapter 8) or the Clark system, in which the tumor is rated I to V depending on the depth of tumor invasion.[56] Ulceration and invasion of the tumor into the deeper skin tissue result in poorer prognosis. Although survival rates may vary with individual circumstances, the current survival rate for stage 0 melanoma is 97%; stage I melanoma, 90% to 95%; stage II melanoma, 65% to 70%; stage III melanoma, 45%; and stage IV melanoma, 10%.[57] Early diagnosis and treatment is of extreme importance.

Treatment is usually surgical excision, the extent of which is determined by the thickness of the lesion, invasion of the deeper skin layers, and spread to regional lymph nodes. Deep, wide excisions with elective removal of lymph tissue and the use of skin grafts were once the hallmark of treatment.[58] A current capability allows for mapping lymph flow to a regional lymph node that receives lymphatic drainage from tumor sites on the skin. This lymph node, which is called the *sentinel lymph node,* is then excised for biopsy. If tumor cells have spread from the primary tumor to the regional lymph nodes, the sentinel node will be the first node in which tumor cells appear. Therefore, sentinel biopsy can be used to test for the presence of melanoma cells and to determine whether radical lymph node dissection is necessary. When nodes are positive, consideration is also given to systemic adjuvant therapy.

Other cancer treatment, such as chemotherapy, is indicated when the disease becomes systemic. Interferon has been used for the treatment of melanoma.[59] An area of active research in melanoma therapy involves vaccine development or immunotherapy. Several types of vaccines have been developed and are currently under investigation.[59]

Basal Cell Carcinoma

Basal cell carcinoma, which is a neoplasm of the nonkeratinizing cells of the basal layer of the epidermis, is the most common skin cancer in white-skinned people (Fig. 61-27).

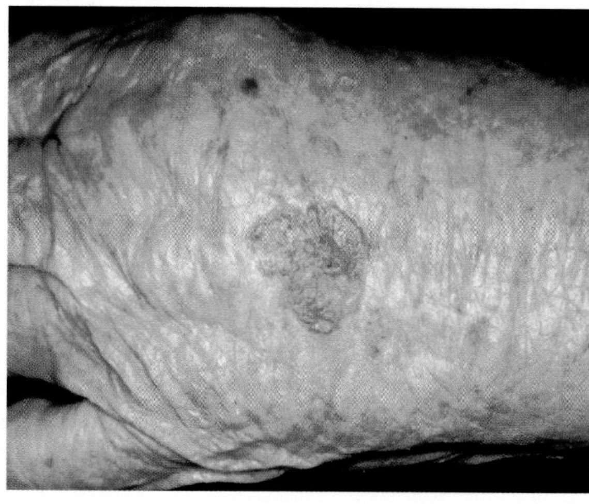

FIGURE 61-27 Basal cell carcinoma and wrinkling of the hand. (Syntex Laboratories.) (Sauer G.C., Hall J.C. [1996]. *Manual of skin diseases* [7th ed.]. Philadelphia: Lippincott-Raven)

Like other skin cancers, basal cell carcinoma has increased in incidence over the past several decades. Fair-skinned persons with a history of significant long-term sun exposure are more susceptible. Black- and brown-skinned persons are affected occasionally. Basal cell carcinoma usually occurs in persons who were exposed to great amounts of sunlight. The lifetime risk for developing basal cell carcinoma in the United States is 30%.[60] The incidence is twice as high among men as women, and peak incidence is at the age of 70 years.[60]

Basal cell carcinoma usually is a nonmetastasizing tumor that extends wide and deep if left untreated. These tumors are most frequently seen on the head and neck, most often occurring on skin that has hair. They do occur on skin surfaces not exposed to the sun, but less frequently. Although there are several histologic types of basal cell carcinoma, nodular ulcerative and superficial basal cell carcinomas are the two most frequently occurring types. *Nodular ulcerative basal cell carcinoma* is the most common.[61] It has a nodulocystic structure that begins as a small, flesh-colored or pink, smooth, translucent nodule that enlarges over time. Telangiectatic vessels frequently are seen beneath the surface. Over the years, a central depression forms that progresses to an ulcer surrounded by the original shiny, waxy border. Basal cell carcinoma in darker-skinned persons usually is darkly pigmented and frequently misdiagnosed as other skin diseases, including melanoma.

The second most common form is *superficial basal cell carcinoma,* which is seen most often on the chest or back. It begins as a flat, nonpalpable, erythematous plaque.[61] The red, scaly areas slowly enlarge, with nodular borders and telangiectatic bases. This type of skin cancer is difficult to diagnose because it mimics other dermatologic problems.

All suspected basal cell carcinomas are biopsied for diagnosis. The treatment depends on the site and extent of the lesion. The most important treatment goal is complete elimination of the lesion. Also important is the maintenance of function and optimal cosmetic effect. Curettage with electrodesiccation, surgical excision, irradiation, and chemosurgery are effective in removing all cancerous cells. Immune-boosting drugs, laser surgery, and retinoids are emerging treatments. Patients should be checked at regular intervals for recurrences.

Squamous Cell Carcinoma

Squamous cell carcinomas are the second most frequent occurring malignant tumors of the outer epidermis. In the United States, there are 200,00 new cases each year.[62] The increase in incidence of squamous cell carcinomas is consistent with increased ultraviolet radiation exposure. There is also a strong occupational hazard link to the development of squamous cell carcinoma: persons exposed to arsenic (*i.e.,* Bowen's disease), industrial tars, coal, and paraffin have an increased likelihood of contracting squamous cell carcinoma. Men are twice as likely to have squamous cell carcinoma as women. Blacks are rarely affected.

There are two types of squamous cell carcinoma: intraepidermal and invasive. *Intraepidermal squamous cell carcinoma* remains confined to the epidermis for a long time. However, at some unpredictable time, it penetrates the basement membrane to the dermis and metastasizes to the regional lymph nodes. It then converts to *invasive squamous cell carcinoma.* The invasive type can develop from intraepidermal carcinoma or from a premalignant lesion (*e.g.,* actinic keratoses). It may be slow growing or fast growing with metastasis.

Squamous cell carcinoma is a red, scaling, keratotic, slightly elevated lesion with an irregular border, usually with a shallow chronic ulcer (Fig. 61-28). The lesions usually lack the pearly rolled border and superficial telangiectases found on basal cell carcinomas.[61] Later lesions grow outward, show large ulcerations, and have persistent crusts and raised, erythematous borders. The lesions occur on sun-exposed areas of the skin, particularly the nose, forehead, helix of the ear, lower lip, and back of the hand. In blacks, the lesions may appear as hyperpigmented nodules and occur more frequently on non–sun-exposed areas. Metastasis is more common with squamous cell carcinoma than with basal cell carcinoma. The overall metastasis rate is 0.5% to 16%. With metastasis, there is a 5-year survival rate of 25%.[62]

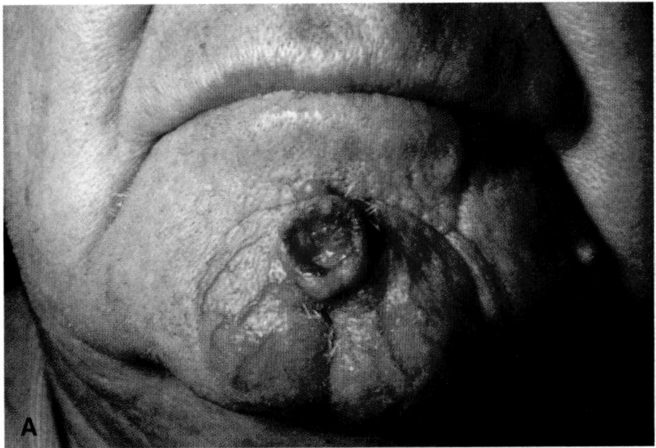

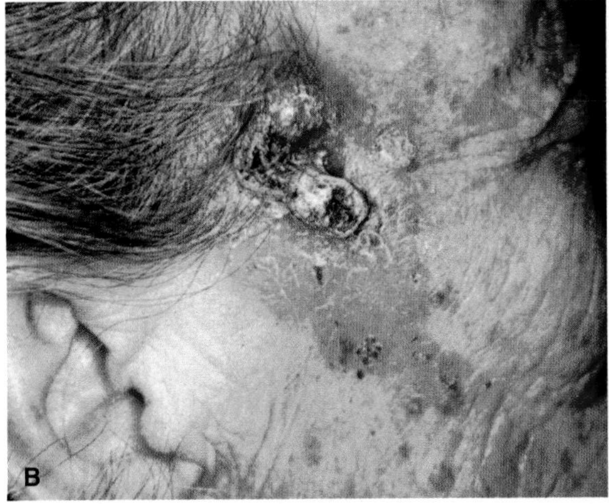

FIGURE 61-28 **(A)** Squamous cell carcinoma of the chin. **(B)** Squamous cell carcinoma and keratosis of aged skin. (Syntex Laboratories, Westwood Pharmaceuticals.) (Sauer G.C., Hall J.C. [1996]. *Manual of skin diseases* [7th ed.]. Philadelphia: Lippincott-Raven)

Treatment measures are aimed at the removal of all cancerous tissue using methods such as electrosurgery, excision surgery, chemosurgery, or radiation therapy. After treatment, the person is observed for the remainder of his or her life for signs of recurrence.

In summary, nevi are moles that usually are benign. Because they may undergo cancerous transformation, any mole that undergoes a change warrants immediate medical attention. There has been an alarming increase in skin cancers over the past few decades. Repeated exposure to the ultraviolet rays of the sun has been implicated as the principal cause of skin cancer. Neoplasms of the skin include malignant melanoma, basal cell carcinoma, and squamous cell carcinoma. Malignant melanoma is a malignant tumor of the melanocytes. It is a rapidly progressing, metastatic form of cancer. Clinically, malignant melanoma of the skin usually is asymptomatic. The most important clinical sign is the change in size, shape, and color of pigmented skin lesions, such as moles. As the result of increased public awareness, early diagnosed melanomas can be cured surgically. Squamous cell carcinoma and basal cell carcinoma are of epidermal origin. Basal cell carcinomas are the most common form of skin cancer among whites. They are slow-growing tumors that rarely metastasize. Squamous cell carcinoma is most common in the elderly. The two types of squamous cell carcinoma are intraepidermal and invasive. Intraepidermal squamous cell carcinoma remains confined to the epidermis for a long time. Invasive squamous cell carcinoma can develop from intraepidermal carcinoma or from premalignant lesions such as actinic keratoses.

Burns

After completing this section of the chapter, you should be able to meet the following objectives:

- Compare the tissue involvement for first-degree, second-degree partial-thickness, second-degree full-thickness, and third-degree burns
- State how the Rule of Nines is used in determining the body surface area involved in a burn
- Cite the determinants for grading burn severity using the American Burn Association classification of burns
- Describe the systemic complications of burns
- Describe major considerations in the treatment of burn injury

The effects and complications of burns serve as a prime example of the essential function that the skin performs as it protects the body from the many damaging elements in the environment while serving to maintain the constancy of the body's internal environment. The massive loss of skin tissue not only predisposes to attack by microorganisms that are present in the environment but also allows for the massive loss of body fluids and their contents, interferes with temperature regulation, challenges the immune system, and imposes excessive demands on the metabolic and reparative processes that are needed to restore the body's interface with the environment.

BURNS

- Burns represent heat-induced injuries of the skin and subcutaneous tissues.
- The extent and depth of injury, the effect on physiologic functioning, and the degree and mechanism of healing are determined by the length of time exposed to the heat source, the temperature of the heating agent, and the amount of surface area that is involved.
- Burns affecting the epidermis heal by regeneration, whereas burns involving the deeper dermal and subcutaneous tissues heal by scar tissue replacement.

More than 1 million Americans experience burns annually. This number represents a dramatic decrease (50%) from the 1990 burn injury estimate of 2 million. There was a concomitant decrease in the number of hospitalizations, from 90,000 to 45,000, in part because of improved burn care, a decreased number of repeat hospitalizations, and improved hospital coding of burn patients. The average size of a burn of a person admitted to the hospital is now 14% of the total body surface area (TBSA). The number of reported large burns (greater than 60% TBSA) has decreased, whereas the number of smaller burns (less than 10% TBSA) has increased.[63] Of the 1 million people who suffer burns, approximately 250,000 are children, 15,000 of them requiring hospitalization, and 1,100 of them dying from fire and burns.[63] Inhalation injury remains the major problem contributing to mortality from burns. Sepsis and pneumonia are other important factors contributing to mortality.

Burns are caused by a number of sources. Flame burns occur because of exposure to direct fire. Scald burns result from hot liquids spilled or poured on the skin surface. In a child, a scald burn may be indicative of child abuse. Chemical burns occur from industrial agents used in occupational sites. Electrical burns occur from contact with live electrical wires in fields or in the home. Electrical burns are usually more extensive because of internal tissue injury and the entrance and exit wounds. Lightning, electromagnetic radiation, and ionizing radiation also can cause skin burns.

CLASSIFICATION

The four classifications for the depth of burn injuries are first-degree, second-degree partial-thickness, second-degree full-thickness, and third-degree burns.[64] The depth of a burn is largely influenced by the length of time exposed to the heat source and the temperature of the heating agent.

First-degree burns (superficial partial-thickness burns) involve only the outer layers of the epidermis. They are red or pink, dry, and painful. There usually is no blister formation. A mild sunburn is an example. The skin maintains its ability to function as a water vapor and bacterial barrier and heals in 3 to 10 days. First-degree burns usually require only palliative treatment, such as pain relief measures and adequate fluid intake. Extensive first-degree burns on infants, the elderly, and persons who receive radiation therapy for cancer may require more care.

Second-degree partial-thickness burns involve the epidermis and various degrees of the dermis. They are painful, moist, red, and blistered. Underneath the blisters is weeping, bright pink or red skin that is sensitive to temperature changes, air exposure, and touch. The blisters prevent the loss of body water and superficial dermal cells. Excluding excision of large burn areas, it is important to maintain intact blisters after injury because they serve as a good bandage and may promote wound healing. These burns heal in approximately 1 to 2 weeks.

Second-degree full-thickness burns involve the entire epidermis and dermis. Structures that originate in the subcutaneous layer, such as hair follicles and sweat glands, remain intact. These burns can be very painful because the pain sensors remain intact. Tactile sensors may be absent or greatly diminished in the areas of deepest destruction. These burns appear as mottled pink, red, or waxy white areas with blisters and edema. The blisters resemble flat, dry tissue paper, rather than the bullous blisters seen with superficial partial-thickness injury. After healing, in approximately 1 month, these burns maintain their softness and elasticity, but there may be the loss of some sensation. Scar formation is usual. These burns heal with supportive medical care aimed at preventing further tissue damage, providing adequate hydration, and ensuring that the granular bed is adequate to support reepithelialization.

Third-degree full-thickness burns extend into the subcutaneous tissue and may involve muscle and bone. Thrombosed vessels can be seen under the burned skin, indicating that the underlying vasculature is involved. Third-degree burns vary in color from waxy white or yellow to tan, brown, deep red, or black. These burns are hard, dry, and leathery. Edema is extensive in the burn area and surrounding tissues. There is no pain because the nerve sensors have been destroyed. However, there is no such thing as a "pure" third-degree burn. Third-degree burns are almost always surrounded by second-degree burns, which are surrounded by an area of first-degree burns. The injury sometimes has an almost target-like appearance because of the various degrees of burn. Full-thickness burns wider than 1.5 inches usually require skin grafts because all the regenerative (*i.e.*, dermal) elements have been destroyed. Smaller injuries usually heal from the margins inward toward the center, the dermal elements regenerating from the healthier margins. However, regeneration may take many weeks and leave a permanent scar, even in smaller burns.

In addition to the depth of the wound, the extent of the burn also is important. Extent is measured by estimating the amount of TBSA involved. Several tools exist for estimating the TBSA. For example, the *Rule of Nines* counts anatomic body parts as multiples of 9% (the head is 9%, each arm 9%, each leg 18%, anterior trunk 18%, posterior trunk 18%), with the perineum 1%. The Lund and Browder chart includes a body diagram table that estimates the TBSA by age and anatomic part.[64] Children are more accurately assessed using this method because it takes into account the difference in relative size of body parts.

The estimates of TBSA are then converted to the American Burn Association Classification of Extent of Injury[64] (Table 61-6). Together, the depth and the extent of the burn indicate the severity of the burn and the need for treatment. Other factors, such as age, location, other injuries, and preexisting conditions, are taken into consideration for a full assessment of burn injury.[65] These factors can increase the severity of the burn assessment and the length of treatment. For example, a first-degree burn is reclassified as a more severe burn if other factors exist, such as burns to the hands, face, and feet; inhalation injury;

TABLE 61-6 American Burn Association Grading System for Burn Severity and Disposition

	Type of Burn		
	Minor	**Moderate**	**Major**
Criteria	<10% TBSA in adult	10%–20% TBSA in adult	>20% TBSA in adult
	<5% TBSA in young (<10 years) or old (>50 years)	5%–10% TBSA in young or old	>10% TBSA in young or old
	<2% Full-thickness burn	2%–5% Full-thickness burn	>5% Full-thickness burn
		High-voltage injury	High-voltage burn
		Suspected inhalation injury	Known inhalation injury
		Circumferential burn	Any significant burn to face, eyes, ears, genitalia, hands, feet, or major joints
		Concomitant medical problem predisposing to infection (*e.g.*, diabetes, sickle cell disease)	Significant associated injuries (*e.g.*, major trauma)
Disposition	Outpatient management	Hospital admission	Referral to burn center

TBSA, total body surface area.
(From American Burn Association. [1990]. Hospital and prehospital resources for optimal care of patients with burn injury: Guidelines for development and operation of burn centers. *Journal of Burn Care and Rehabilitation 11,* 98–104)

electrical burns; other trauma; or existence of psychosocial problems. Genital burns almost always require hospitalization because edema may cause difficulty voiding and the location complicates maintenance of a bacteria-free environment.

SYSTEMIC COMPLICATIONS

Burn victims often are confronted with hemodynamic instability, impaired respiratory function, hypermetabolic response, major organ dysfunction, and sepsis. The magnitude of the response is proportional to the extent of injury, usually reaching a plateau when approximately 60% of the body is burned. The treatment challenge is for immediate resuscitation efforts and for long-term maintenance of physiologic function. Pain and emotional problems are additional problems faced by persons with burns.

Hemodynamic Instability

Hemodynamic instability begins almost immediately with injury to capillaries in the burned area and surrounding tissue. Because of a loss of vascular volume, major burn victims often present in the emergency room in a form of hypovolemic shock (see Chapter 28) known as *burn shock.* The patient has a decrease in cardiac output, increased peripheral vascular resistance, and impaired perfusion of vital organs. Burn shock is proportional to the extent and depth of injury. Fluid is lost from the vascular, interstitial, and cellular compartments. Sodium is lost from the vascular and interstitial fluid compartments, and potassium is lost from the intracellular compartment.

The major hemodynamic derangement results from a rapid shift of plasma from the vascular system into the interstitial fluid compartment, resulting in edema. The loss of plasma fluid and proteins decreases vascular colloidal osmotic pressure and results in additional edema formation in both burned and nonburned areas. Because plasma fluid rather than whole blood is lost from the vascular compartment, there is an increase in hematocrit and a concentration of other blood components. Consequently, damaged red cells in the capillaries may sludge, leading to thrombosis and further impairment of blood flow to vital organs. Because of the increased concentration of coagulation factors, burn victims are at increased risk for development of disseminated intravascular coagulation (see Chapter 15). In persons with hemodynamic instability, adequate fluid resuscitation is essential to survival. The amounts of fluid needed are great. The type and amount of fluid are calculated according to the extent of the burn and the age and weight of the person, balanced with the increased fluid expended through burn sites. In persons receiving adequate fluid resuscitation, cardiac output usually returns to normal in approximately 24 hours.

Respiratory Dysfunction

Smoke inhalation and postburn lung dysfunction are frequent problems in burn victims. Victims often are trapped in a burning structure and inhale significant amounts of smoke, carbon monoxide, and other toxic fumes. Water-soluble gases that are found in smoke from burning plastics and rubber, such as ammonia, sulfur dioxide, and chlorine, react with mucous membranes to form strong acids and alkalis that induce ulceration of the mucous membrane, bronchospasm, and edema. Lipid-soluble gases, such as nitrous oxide and hydrogen chloride, are transported to the lower airways, where they produce damage. These substances damage cell membranes and impair the function of the mucociliary blanket. There also may be thermal injury to the respiratory passages.

Symptoms of inhalation injury include hoarseness, drooling, inability to handle secretions, rales, rhonchi, stridor, hacking cough, and labored and shallow breathing. Serial blood gases show a fall in PO_2. Signs of mucosal injury and airway obstruction often are delayed for 24 to 48 hours after a burn. It is necessary to monitor the patient continually for early signs of respiratory distress. Humidified oxygen is administered to prevent drying and sloughing of the mucosa. Intubation and ventilatory support may be needed. Other pulmonary conditions, such as pneumonia, pulmonary embolism, or pneumothorax, may occur secondary to the burn.

Hypermetabolic Response

The stress of burn injury increases metabolic and nutritional requirements. Secretion of stress hormones such as catecholamines and cortisol is increased in an effort to maintain homeostasis. Heat production is increased in an effort to balance heat losses from the burned area. Hypermetabolism, characterized by increased oxygen consumption, increased glucose use, and protein and fat wasting, is a characteristic response to burn trauma and infection. The hypermetabolic state peaks approximately 7 to 17 days after the burn, and tissue breakdown diminishes as the wounds heal. Nutritional support is essential to recovery from burn injury. Enteral and parenteral hyperalimentation are often used to deliver sufficient nutrients to prevent tissue breakdown and postburn weight loss.

Organ Dysfunction

Burn shock results in impaired perfusion of vital organs. The patient may have impaired function of the kidneys, the gastrointestinal tract, and the nervous system. Although the initial insult often is one of hypovolemic shock and impaired organ perfusion, sepsis may contribute to impaired organ function after the initial resuscitation period.

Renal insufficiency can occur in burn patients as a result of the hypovolemic state, damage to the kidneys at the time of the burn, or drugs that are administered. Immediately after a burn, there is often a short period of relative anuria, followed by a phase of hypermetabolism characterized by increased urine output and nitrogen loss. The effects of burn injury on the gastrointestinal tract include gastric dilation and decreased peristalsis. These effects are compounded by immobility and narcotic analgesics. Burn victims are observed carefully for vomiting and fecal impaction. Acute ulceration of the stomach and duodenum (called *Curling's ulcer*) is a potential complication in burn victims and is thought to be the result of stress and gastric ischemia. It is largely controlled by the prophylactic administration of histamine-2 antagonists or proton-pump inhibitors. Enteral feeding tubes are inserted almost immediately. Tube feeding is intended to mitigate ulcer formation, maintain the integrity of the intestinal mucosa, and provide sufficient calories and protein for the hypermetabolic state. Burn patients are encouraged to begin eating as soon as possible to maintain gastrointestinal integrity.

Neurologic changes can occur from periods of hypoxia. Neurologic damage may result from head injuries, drug or alcohol abuse, carbon monoxide poisoning, fluid volume deficits, and hypovolemia. With an electrical burn, the brain or spine can be directly injured. The responses to physiologic damage may include confusion, memory loss, insomnia, lethargy, and combativeness.

Musculoskeletal effects include fractures that occur at the time of the accident, deep burns extending to the muscles and bone, hypertrophic scarring, and contractures. The hypermetabolic state increases tissue catabolism and severe protein and fat wasting.

Sepsis and Immune Function

A significant complication of the acute phase of burn injury is sepsis. It may arise from the burn wound, pneumonia, urinary tract infection, infection elsewhere in the body, or the use of invasive procedures or monitoring devices. Immunologically, the skin is the body's first line of defense. When the skin is no longer intact, the body is open to bacterial infection. Destruction of the skin also prevents the delivery of cellular components of the immune system to the site of injury. There also is loss of normal protective skin flora and a shift to colonization by more pathogenic flora.

Suppression of the immune system after burn trauma contributes to the development of sepsis. B-cell and T-cell immunity are involved. The cause of immunosuppression is unclear, but undoubtedly multiple factors are involved. It has been suggested that immunosuppression factors are produced by tissues away from the site of injury (*e.g.*, liver, gastrointestinal tract, endocrine system) and by the burned tissue itself. The capillary leak that occurs in the immediate postburn period removes immune cells and immunoglobulins from the circulation. Stress also contributes to immunosuppression through the hypothalamic-pituitary-adrenal axis (see Chapter 9). Persons with prior immunodeficiency, those with chronic debilitating conditions, and known alcoholics are particularly at risk. The very young and the elderly also are at risk for immunosuppression.

Pain

Burn injuries are extremely painful, and pain management must be a major priority in the care of these patients. The degree of pain in the resuscitative and acute phases of care is influenced by the depth and extent of the burn injury. During this stage, pain medications usually are given intravenously because of injury to the skin and because of impaired blood flow to the subcutaneous and intramuscular tissues.

Emotional Trauma

Burns are emotionally devastating because of the impact of disfigurement, pain, and lengthy recovery. These are persons who at one moment were well and were extensively burned the next. Burn patients are faced with enormous physiologic, psychological, and social challenges. Any number of human responses is expected and normal for the person experiencing a major burn. Patients may exhibit responses such as anger, denial, and refusal to cooperate. The patient and family usually need psychological support in addition to all the physiologic forms of life support.

TREATMENT

Regardless of the type of burn, the first step in any burn situation is preventing the causal agent from producing further tissue damage. Copious amounts of water over the burned area are extremely helpful. Immediate submersion is more important than removal of clothing, which may delay cooling the involved areas. Cold (ice) applications are not recommended because ice can further limit blood flow to an area, turning a partial-thickness burn into a full-thickness burn. Depending on the depth and extent of the burn, medical treatment is necessary. Emergency care consists of resuscitation and stabilization with intravenous fluids while maintaining cardiac and respiratory function. Once hospitalized, the treatment regimen includes fluid replacement, maintenance of nutritional demands, antibiotic therapy, maintenance of cardiac and respiratory functions, pain alleviation, and emotional support.

After hemodynamic stability and pulmonary stability have been established, treatment is directed toward initial care of the wound. The wound is cleaned, débrided, and covered with a topical antimicrobial agent. Because of alterations in immune function, protective isolation measures may be instituted.

The sloughed tissue, or *eschar,* produced by the burn is excised as soon as possible. This decreases the chance of infection and allows the skin to regenerate faster. Topical agents (*e.g.*, silver sulfadiazine, sulfacetamide acetate, silver nitrate, and the combination of collagenase ointment and Polysporin powder) are applied to burned areas, which are dressed with various gauzes.[65] Systemic antibiotics seldom are useful at the burn sites because of the loss of the functional components of the skin. The dressings are changed according to the specific practice of the health care provider.

Burns that encircle the entire surface of the body or a body part (*e.g.*, arms, legs, torso) act like tourniquets and can cause major tissue damage to the muscles, tendons, and vasculature under the area of the leathery eschar skin. These burns are called *circumferential burns*. The eschar is incised longitudinally (escharotomy), and sometimes a fasciotomy (surgical incision through the fascia of the muscle) is performed. The timing of these incisions is important. Incision is done after the patient's circulatory condition stabilizes to some degree, thereby limiting some of the massive fluid loss. However, the incisions must occur before the eschar formation can cause hypoxia and necrosis of the tissues and organs under it. This is extremely important when torso burns occur because the pressure placed on a chest can result in inability to breathe and decreased blood return to the heart.

Skin grafts are surgically implanted as soon as possible, often at the same time the burns are débrided, to promote new skin growth, limit fluid loss, and act as a dressing. Skin grafts can be permanent or temporary and split thickness or full thickness. Permanent skin grafts are used over newly excised tissue. Temporary skin grafts are used to cover a burned area until the tissue underneath it has healed.

A *split-thickness skin graft* is one that includes the epidermis and part of the dermis. The thickness of these grafts depends on the donor site and the needs of the burn patient. A split-thickness skin graft can be sent through a skin mesher that cuts tiny slits into the skin, allowing it to expand up to nine times its size. These grafts are used frequently because they can cover large surface areas and there is less autorejection. *Full-thickness skin grafts* include the entire thickness of the dermal layer. They are used primarily for reconstructive surgery or for deep, small areas. The donor site of a full-thickness skin graft requires a split-thickness skin graft to help it heal.

Various sources of skin grafts exist: *autograft* (skin obtained from the person's own body), *homograft* (skin obtained from another human being, alive or recently dead), and *heterograft* (skin obtained from another species, such as pigs). The best choice is autografting when there is enough uninterrupted skin on the person's body. Two-layered synthetic skin grafts (*Apligraf, Integra*) are now available and approved by the FDA.[66] Synthetic skin grafts generally are composed of a layer of silicone, mimicking the properties of the epidermis, and a layer or matrix of fibers. Skin cells attach to the fibers enabling dermal skin growth. Once the dermal skin has regenerated, the silicone layer is removed and a thin epidermal skin graft is applied, thus requiring less skin grafting overall.

REHABILITATION

Treatment measures include positioning, splinting, and physical therapy to prevent contractures and maintain muscle tone. Because the normal body response to disuse is flexion, the contractures that occur with a burn are disfiguring and cause loss of limb or appendage use. Once the wounds have healed sufficiently, elastic pressure garments, sometimes for the full body, often are used to prevent hypertrophic scarring.

Psychological and emotional resources also are provided to burn patients and their families. Rehabilitation can take long periods, considering the numerous hospitalizations, skin grafting procedures, and plastic surgeries. Burn centers across the country specialize in total care for patients and have many of the additional supportive services needed for burn patients. In addition, because of computer technology, patients and families with burn experiences can obtain support, information, and help from a number of Internet sites.

In summary, burns cause damage to skin structures, ranging from first-degree burns, which damage the epidermis, to third-degree full-thickness burns, which extend into the subcutaneous tissue and may involve muscle and bone. The extent of injury is determined by the thickness of the burn and the total body surface area involved. In addition to skin involvement, burn injury can cause hemodynamic instability with hypovolemic shock, inhalation injury with respiratory involvement, a hypermetabolic state, organ dysfunction, immune suppression, sepsis, pain, and emotional trauma. Treatment methods vary with the severity of injury and include immediate resuscitation and maintenance of physiologic function, wound cleaning and débridement, application of antimicrobial agents and dressings, and skin grafting. Efforts are directed toward preventing or limiting disfigurement and disability.

Age-Related Skin Manifestations

After completing this section of the chapter, you should be able to meet the following objectives:

- Differentiate a strawberry hemangioma from a port-wine stain hemangioma in terms of appearance and outcome
- Describe the distinguishing features of rashes associated with the common infectious childhood diseases: roseola infantum, rubeola, rubella, chickenpox, and scarlet fever
- Characterize the physiologic changes of aging skin
- Describe the appearance of skin tags, keratoses, lentigines, and vascular lesions that are commonly seen in the elderly

Many skin problems occur more commonly in certain age groups. Because of aging changes, infants, children, and elderly persons tend to have different skin problems.

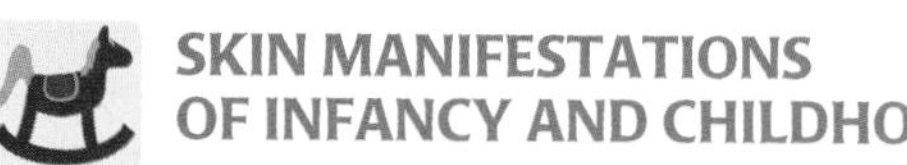

SKIN MANIFESTATIONS OF INFANCY AND CHILDHOOD

Skin Disorders of Infancy

Infancy connotes the image of perfect, unblemished skin. For the most part, this is true. However, several congenital skin lesions, such as mongolian spots, hemangiomas, and nevi, are associated with the early neonatal period.

Vascular and Pigmented Birthmarks. Pigmented and vascular lesions constitute most birthmarks.[67] Pigmented birthmarks represent abnormal migration or proliferation of melanocytes. Mongolian spots are caused by selective pigmentation. They usually occur on the buttocks or sacral area and are seen commonly in Asians and blacks. Nevi or moles are small, tan to brown, uniformly pigmented solid macules. *Nevocellular nevi* are formed initially from aggregates of melanocytes and keratinocytes along the dermal–epidermal border. *Congenital melanocytic nevi* are collections of melanocytes that are present at birth or develop within the first year of life. They present as macular, papular, or plaquelike pigmented lesions of various shades of brown, with a black or blue focus. The texture of the lesions varies, and they may be with or without hair. They usually are found on the hands, shoulders, buttocks, entire arm, or trunk of the body. Some involve large areas of the body in garment-like fashion. They usually grow proportionately with the child. Congenital melanocytic nevi are clinically significant because of their association with malignant melanoma.

Vascular birthmarks are cutaneous anomalies of angiogenesis and vascular development. Two types of vascular birthmarks commonly are seen in infants and small children: bright red, raised strawberry hemangiomas and flat, reddish-purple port-wine stains.

Strawberry hemangiomas begin as small, red lesions that are noticed shortly after birth. Hemangiomas are benign vascular tumors produced by proliferation of the endothelial cells. They are seen in approximately 5% to 10% of 1-year-old children.[68] Female infants are three times as likely as male infants to have hemangiomas, and there is an increased incidence in premature infants. Approximately 35% of these lesions are present at birth, and the remainder develop within a few weeks after birth. Hemangiomas typically undergo an early period of a proliferation during which they enlarge, followed by a period of slow involution during which the growth is reversed until complete resolution. Most strawberry hemangiomas disappear before 5 to 7 years of age without leaving an appreciable scar. Hemangiomas can occur anywhere in the body. Hemangiomas of the airway can be life threatening. Ulceration, the most frequent complication, can be painful and carries the risk for infection, hemorrhage, and scarring.[68]

Port-wine stains are pink or red patches that can occur anywhere on the body and are very noticeable (Fig. 61-29). They represent slow-growing capillary malformations that grow proportionately with the child and persist throughout life. Port-wine stains usually are confined to the skin but may be associated with vascular malformations of the eye or leptomeninges over the cortex, leading to cognitive disorders, seizures, and other neurologic deficits.[68] Cover-up cosmetics are used in an attempt to conceal their disfiguring effects. Laser surgery has revolutionized the treatment of port-wine stains.

Diaper Rash. Because of its newness, infant skin is sensitive to irritation, injury, and extremes of temperature. The contents of soiled diapers, if not changed frequently, can lead to contact dermatitis, bacterial infections, or other skin conditions. Prolonged exposure to a warm, humid environment can lead to prickly heat, and too-frequent bathing can cause dryness that leads to skin problems. Baby lotions are helpful in maintaining skin moisture, whereas baby powder acts as a drying agent. Both are useful aids when used selectively and according to the nature of the skin problem (*i.e.,* excessive moisture or dryness).

The appearance of *diaper rash* ranges from simple (*i.e.,* widely distributed macules on the buttocks and anogenital areas) to severe (*i.e.,* beefy, red, excoriated skin surfaces in the diaper area). Diaper rash is essentially a contact or irritant dermatitis. Although the exact cause is unknown (i.e., ammonia, feces, moisture, or combinations), there is little doubt that moisture is a major contributing factor. Moisture contributes to the maceration of the diapered areas. In cultures in which diapers are not used, diaper rash is nonexistent. The treatment includes measures to minimize or prevent skin wetness, including frequent diaper changes with careful cleaning of the irritated area to remove all waste products. This is particularly important in hot weather. Exposing the irritated area to air is helpful. Protecting the skin with zinc oxide or other ointments also helps.

There is controversy regarding the effects of cloth versus disposable diapers in preventing diaper rash. In the early days of disposable diapers, infants who wore cloth diapers without plastic pants had fewer diaper rashes than those who wore disposable diapers.[69] It has been suggested that this may not be true with the newer disposable diapers that have absorbent gelling material.[69] These superabsorbent diapers have the smallest increase in skin wetness compared with conventional disposable diapers and cloth diapers. When cloth diapers are used, they should be washed in gentle detergent and thoroughly rinsed to remove all traces of waste products. Plastic pants should be discouraged. For intractable, severe cases, the child should be seen by a health care provider for treatment of any secondary infections. Secondary candidal (*i.e.,* yeast) (Fig. 61-30) or other skin manifestations discussed in this

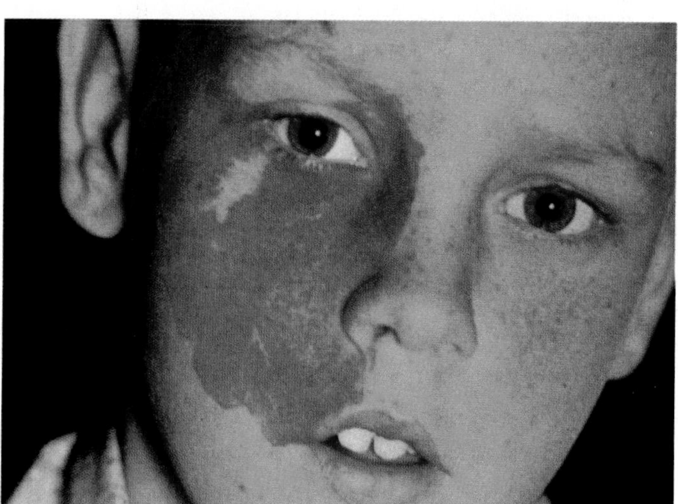

FIGURE 61-29 Port-wine stain on the face of a boy. (Ortho Dermatology Corp.) (Sauer G.C., Hall J.C. [1996]. *Manual of skin diseases* [7th ed.]. Philadelphia: Lippincott-Raven)

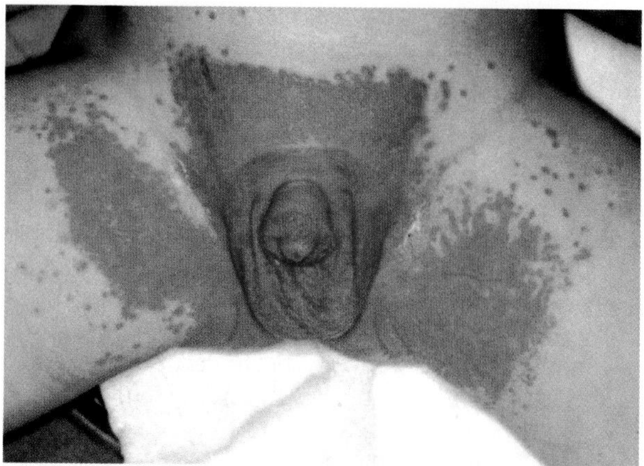

FIGURE 61-30 *Candida* intertrigo after a course of oral antibiotics in a 1-year-old child. (Owen Laboratories, Inc.) (Sauer G.C., Hall J.C. [1996]. *Manual of skin diseases* [7th ed.]. Philadelphia: Lippincott-Raven)

chapter may occur in the diaper area. It is important to differentiate between normal diaper dermatitis and more serious skin problems.

Prickly Heat. *Prickly heat* (heat rash) results from constant maceration of the skin because of prolonged exposure to a warm, humid environment. Maceration leads to mid-epidermal obstruction and rupture of the sweat glands (Fig. 61-31). Although commonly seen during infancy, prickly heat may occur at any age. The treatment includes removing excessive clothing, cooling the skin with warm-water baths, drying the skin with powders, and avoiding hot, humid environments.

Cradle Cap. *Cradle cap* is a greasy crust or scale formation on the scalp. It usually is attributed to infrequent and inadequate washing of the scalp. Cradle cap is treated using mild shampoo and gentle combing to remove the scales.

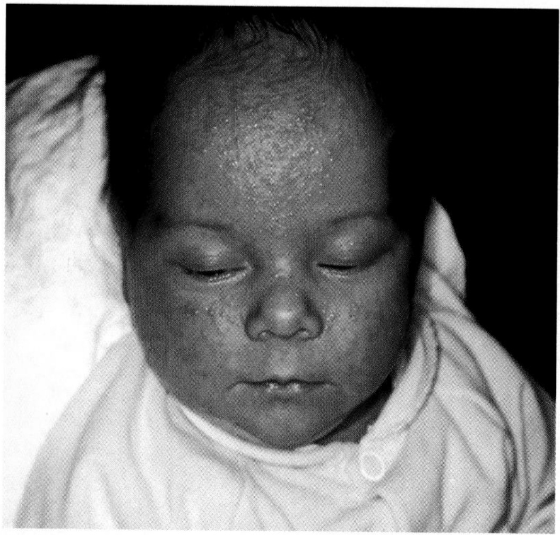

FIGURE 61-31 Prickly heat in a 6-week-old infant. (Hall J.C. [2000]. *Sauer's manual of skin diseases* [8th ed., p. 407]. Philadelphia: Lippincott Williams & Wilkins)

Sometimes, oil can be left on the head for minutes to several hours, softening the scales before scrubbing. Other emulsifying ointments or creams may be helpful in difficult cases. The scalp may need to be rubbed firmly to remove the buildup of keratinized cells. Recalcitrant cases need to be seen by a health care practitioner; serious or chronic forms of seborrheic dermatitis may exist.

Skin Manifestations of Common Infectious Diseases

Infectious childhood diseases that produce rashes include exanthem subitum, rubella, rubeola, varicella, and scarlet fever. Although these diseases are seen less frequently because of successful immunization programs and the use of antibiotics, they still occur.

Roseola Infantum. Roseola infantum (exanthem subitum, or sixth disease) is a contagious disease caused by herpesviruses (HHV) 6 and 7.[65] HHV-6 is the etiologic agent in most cases; hence, it is often referred to as the *sixth disease.* Primary HHV-6 infection occurs early in life, usually between 5 and 15 months of age. Roseola produces a characteristic maculopapular rash covering the trunk and spreading to the appendages. The rash is preceded by an abrupt onset of high fever (≤105°F), inflamed tympanic membranes, and coldlike symptoms usually lasting 3 to 4 days. These symptoms improve at approximately the same time the rash appears. Unlike rubella, no cervical or postauricular lymph node adenopathy occurs. Roseola infantum frequently is mistaken for rubella. Rubella usually can be excluded by the age of the child and the absence of lymph node adenopathy. In general, rubella does not develop in children younger than 6 months of age because they retain some maternal antibodies. Less than half of HHV-6 infections in the United States are clinically recognizable as roseola.[65] Blood antibody titers may be taken to determine the actual diagnosis. In most cases, there are no long-term effects from this disease.

Rubella. *Rubella* (*i.e.,* 3-day measles, or German measles) is a childhood disease caused by the rubella virus (a togavirus). It is characterized by a diffuse, punctate, macular rash that begins on the trunk and spreads to the arms and legs (Fig. 61-32). Mild febrile states occur; usually, the body temperature is less than 100°F. Postauricular, suboccipital, and cervical lymph node adenopathy is common.[65] Coldlike symptoms usually accompany the disease in the form of cough, congestion, and coryza.

Rubella usually has no long-lasting sequelae; however, the transmission of the disease to pregnant women early in their gestation periods may result in congenital rubella syndrome. Among the clinical signs of congenital rubella syndrome are cataracts, microcephaly, mental retardation, deafness, patent ductus arteriosus, glaucoma, purpura, and bone defects. Most states have laws requiring immunization to prevent transmission of rubella. Immunization is accomplished by live-virus injection. A single injection after 12 to 15 months of age has produced a 98% immunity response in immunized children and is considered adequate in the prevention of rubella.[65] Many states require a second preschool or later dose of rubella vaccine to increase im-

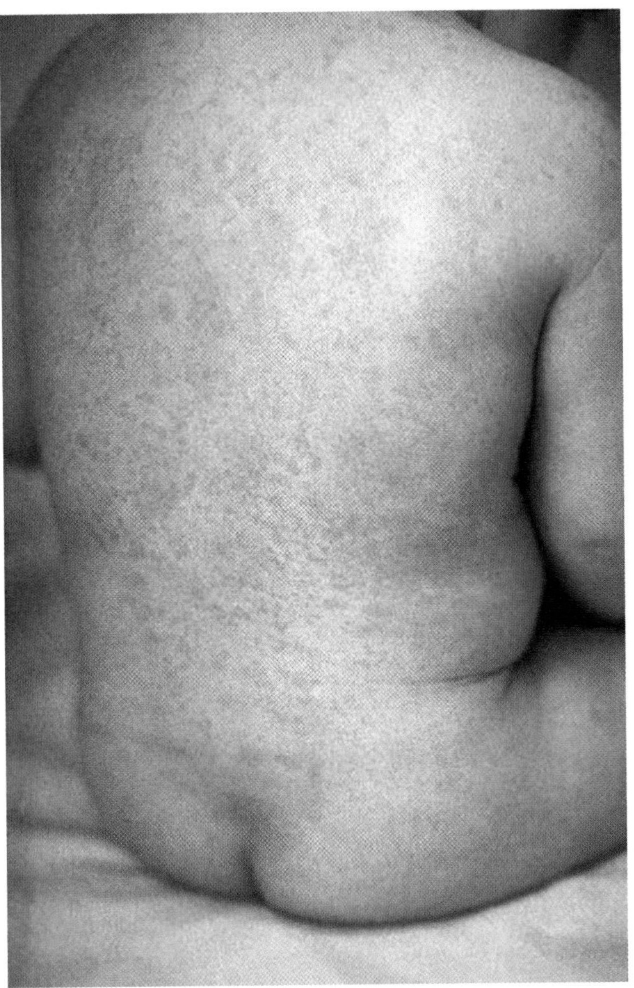

FIGURE 61-32 Rash of rubella on skin of a child's back. (Centers for Disease Control Public Health Image Library).

munity. Cases and outbreaks of rubella occur in the United States, especially among foreign-born unvaccinated adults.

Rubeola. *Rubeola* (measles, hard measles, 7-day measles) is an acute, highly communicable viral disease caused by *Morbillivirus*. The characteristic rash is macular and blotchy; sometimes, the macules become confluent (Fig. 61-33). The rubeola rash usually begins on the face and spreads to the appendages. There are several accompanying symptoms: a temperature of 100°F or greater, *Koplik's spots* (i.e., small, irregular red spots with a bluish white speck in the center) on the buccal mucosa, and mild to severe photosensitivity.[65] The patient commonly has coldlike symptoms, general malaise, and myalgia. In severe cases, the macules may hemorrhage into the skin tissue or onto the outer body surface. This form is called *hemorrhagic measles*. The course of measles is more severe in infants, adults, and malnourished children. The World Health Organization recommends vitamin A treatment for measles in developing countries to reduce morbidity and mortality. There may be severe complications, including otitis media, pneumonia, and encephalitis. Antibody titers are determined for a conclusive diagnosis of rubeola.

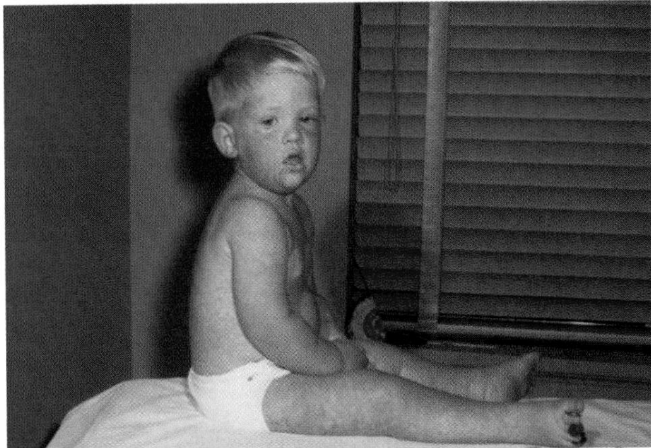

FIGURE 61-33 Child with rubeola displaying the characteristic red blotchy skin during the third day of the rash. (Centers for Disease Control Public Health Image Library)

Measles is a disease preventable by vaccine, and immunization is required by law in the United States. Immunization is accomplished by the injection of a live-virus vaccine. A single injection at 12 to 15 months of age is sufficient to produce initial immunity.[65] A second injection should be given on entry to elementary school.

Varicella. *Varicella* (chickenpox) is a common communicable childhood disease. It is caused by the varicella-zoster virus, which also is the agent in herpes zoster (shingles). The characteristic skin lesion occurs in three stages: macule, vesicle, and granular scab. The macular stage is characterized by development within hours of macules over the trunk of the body, spreading to the limbs, buccal mucosa, scalp, axillae, upper respiratory tract, and conjunctiva[65] (Fig. 61-34). During the second stage, the macules form vesicles with depressed centers. The vesicles break open, and a scab forms during the third stage. Crops of lesions occur successively, so that all three forms of the lesion usually are visible by the third day of the illness.

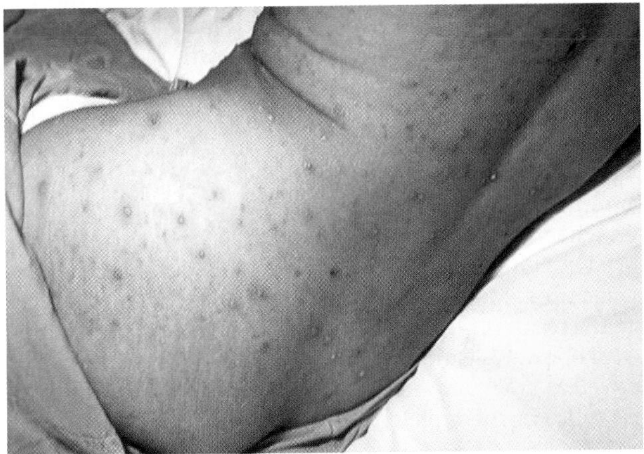

FIGURE 61-34 Blister-like rash on the back of a person with varicella-zoster (*i.e.*, chickenpox). (Centers for Disease Control Public Health Image Library)

Mild to extreme pruritus accompanies the lesions, which can lead to scratching and subsequent development of secondary bacterial infections. Chickenpox also is accompanied by coldlike symptoms, including cough, coryza (*i.e.*, nasal discharge), and sometimes photosensitivity. Mild febrile states usually occur, typically beginning 24 hours before lesion outbreak. Side effects, such as pneumonia, septic complications, and encephalitis, are rare.

Varicella in adults may be more severe, with a prolonged recovery rate and greater chances for development of varicella pneumonitis or encephalitis. Immunocompromised persons may experience a chronic, painful type.

Live attenuated varicella vaccine has been demonstrated to be 95% effective in the preventing of typical varicella and 70% to 90% effective in preventing all disease.[65] The vaccine is available in the United States and required by law in many states.

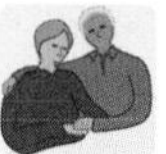

SKIN MANIFESTATIONS AND DISORDERS IN THE ELDERLY

Elderly persons experience a variety of age-related skin disorders and exacerbations of earlier skin problems. Aging skin is believed to involve a complex process of actinic (solar) damage, normal aging, and hormonal influences. Actinic changes primarily involve increased occurrence of lesions on sun-exposed surfaces of the body.

Normal Age-Related Changes

Normal aging consists of changes that occur on areas of the body that have not been exposed to the sun. They include thinning of the dermis and the epidermis, diminution in subcutaneous tissue, a decrease in and thickening of blood vessels, and a decrease in the number of melanocytes, Langerhans' cells, and Merkel's cells. The keratinocytes shrink, but the number of dead keratinized cells at the surface increases. This results in less padding and thinner skin, with color and elasticity changes. The skin also loses its resistance to environmental and mechanical trauma. Tissue repair takes longer.

With aging, there is also less hair and nail growth, and there is permanent hair pigment loss. Hormonally, there is less sebaceous gland activity, although the glands in the facial skin may increase in size. Hair growth reduction also may be hormonally influenced. Although the reason is poorly understood, the skin in most elderly persons older than 70 years of age becomes dry, rough, scaly, and itchy. When there is no underlying pathology, it is called *senile pruritus*. Itching and dryness become worse during the winter, when the need for home heating lowers the humidity.

The aging of skin, however, is not just a manifestation of age itself. Most skin changes associated with the elderly are the result of cumulative actinic or environmental damage. For example, the wrinkled, leathery look of aged skin, as well as odd scars and ecchymotic spots, are due to solar elastotic degenerative change.

Skin Lesions Common Among the Elderly

The most common skin lesions in the elderly are skin tags, keratoses, lentigines, and vascular lesions. Most are actinic manifestations; they occur as a result of exposure to sun and weather over the years.

Skin Tags. Skin tags are soft, brown or flesh-colored papules. They occur on any skin surface, but most frequently the neck, axilla, and intertriginous areas. They range in size from a pinhead to the size of a pea. Skin tags have the normal texture of the skin. They are benign and can be removed with scissors or electrodesiccation for cosmetic purposes.

Keratoses. A *keratosis* is a horny growth or an abnormal growth of the keratinocytes. A *seborrheic keratosis* (*i.e.*, seborrheic wart) is a benign, sharply circumscribed, wartlike lesion that has a stuck-on appearance (Fig. 61-35). Keratoses vary in size up to several centimeters. They are usually round or oval, tan, brown, or black lesions. Less pigmented ones may appear yellow or pink. Keratoses can be found on the face or trunk, as a solitary lesion or sometimes by the hundreds. Seborrheic keratoses are benign, but they must be watched for changes in color, texture, or size, which may indicate malignant transformation to a melanoma.

Actinic keratoses are the most common premalignant skin lesions that develop on sun-exposed areas. The lesions usually are less than 1 cm in diameter and appear as dry, brown scaly areas, often with a reddish tinge. Actinic keratoses often are multiple and more easily felt than seen (Fig. 61-36). They often are indistinguishable from squamous cell carcinoma without biopsy. A hyperkeratotic form also exists that is more prominent and palpable. Often, there is a weathered appearance of the surrounding skin. Slight changes, such as enlargement or ulceration, may indicate malignant transformation. Roughly 20% of actinic keratoses convert to squamous cell carcinomas. However, a current belief is that actinic keratoses do not convert or progress to cancerous cells, but that they are early malignancies.[70,71] Most actinic keratoses are treated with 5-fluorouracil cream, which erodes the lesions.

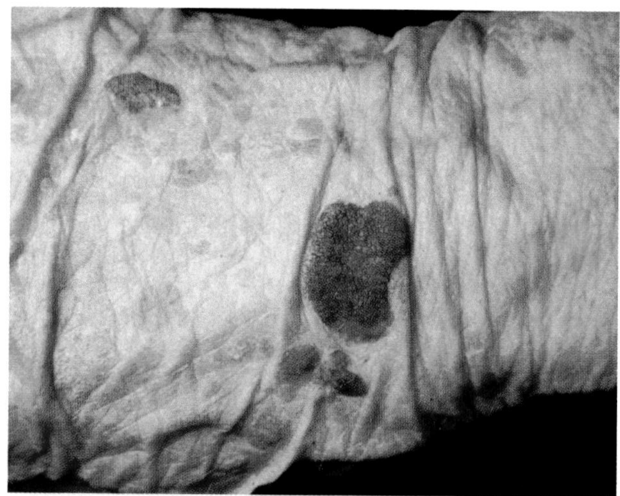

FIGURE 61-35 Large seborrheic keratoses on the hand of an 84-year-old woman. (Sauer G.C., Hall J.C. [1996]. *Manual of skin diseases* [7th ed.]. Philadelphia: Lippincott-Raven)

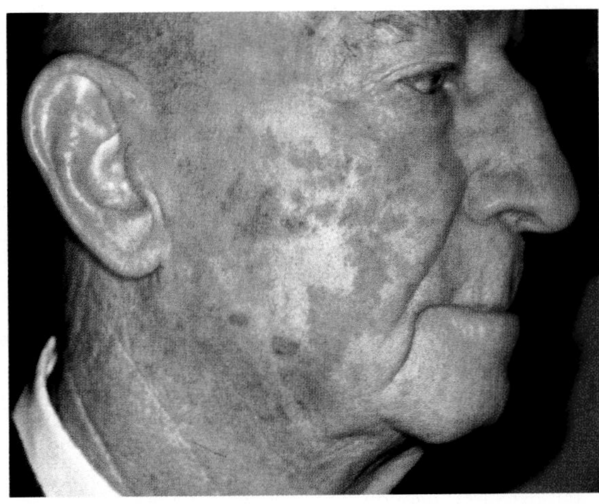

FIGURE 61-36 Multiple actinic keratoses of the face of an 80-year-old man. (Dermik Laboratories, Inc.) (Sauer G.C., Hall J.C. [1996]. *Manual of skin diseases* [7th ed.]. Philadelphia: Lippincott-Raven)

Lentigines. A *lentigo* is a well-bordered brown to black macule, usually less than 1 cm in diameter. *Solar lentigines* are tan to brown, benign spots on sun-exposed areas. They are commonly referred to as liver spots. Creams and lotions containing hydroquinone (*e.g.,* Eldoquin, Solaquin) may be used temporarily to bleach the spots. These agents inhibit the synthesis of new pigment without destroying existing pigment. Higher concentrations are available by prescription. Successful treatment depends on avoiding sun exposure and consistent use of sunscreens. Liquid nitrogen applications have been successful in eradicating senile lentigines.

Lentigo maligna (*i.e.,* Hutchinson's freckle) is a slowly progressive (≤20 years) preneoplastic disorder of melanocytes. It occurs on sun-exposed areas, particularly the face. The lesion is a pigmented macule with a well-defined border and grows to 5 cm or sometimes larger. As it grows over the years, it may become slightly raised and wartlike. If untreated, a true malignant melanoma often develops. Surgery, curettage, and cryotherapy have been effective at removing the lentigines. Careful monitoring for conversion to melanoma is important.

Vascular Lesions. Vascular lesions are vascular tumors with chronically dilated blood vessels. The small blood vessels lie in the middle to upper dermis. *Senile angiomas* (cherry angiomas) are smooth, cherry-red or purple, dome-shaped papules. They usually are found on the trunk. *Telangiectases* are single dilated blood vessels, capillaries, or terminal arteries that appear on areas exposed to sun or harsh weather, such as the cheeks and the nose. The lesions can become large and disfiguring. Pulsed dye lasers have been effective in removing them. *Venous lakes* are small, dark blue, slightly raised papules that have a lake-like appearance. They occur on exposed body parts, particularly the backs of the hands, ears, and lips. They are smooth and compressible. Venous lakes can be removed by electrosurgery, laser therapy, or surgical excision if a person desires.

In summary, some skin problems occur in specific age groups. Common in infants are diaper rash, prickly heat, and cradle cap. Infectious childhood diseases that are characterized by rashes include roseola infantum, rubella, rubeola, varicella, and scarlet fever. Vaccines are available to protect against rubella, rubeola, and varicella. Changes in skin that occur with aging involve a complex process of actinic damage, normal aging, and hormonal influences. With aging, there is thinning of the dermis and the epidermis, diminution in subcutaneous tissue, lessening and thickening of blood vessels, and a slowing of hair and nail growth. Dry skin is common among the elderly, becoming worse during the winter months. Among the skin lesions seen in the elderly are skin tags, keratoses, lentigines, and vascular skin lesions.

REVIEW EXERCISES

The mother of a 7-year-old boy notices that he is scratching his head frequently. On close examination, she notices a grayish round and roughened area, where the hair has broken off. Examination by the child's pediatrician produces a diagnosis of tinea capitis.

A. Explain the cause of the infection and propose possible mechanisms for spread of this infection in school-aged children, particularly during winter months.

B. Referring back to Chapter 18, explain the preference of the superficial mycoses (dermatophytes) for the skin-covered areas of the body.

C. What methods are commonly used in the diagnosis of superficial fungal infections?

A 75-year-old woman presents with severe burning pain and a vesicular rash covering a strip over the rib cage on one side of the chest. She is diagnosed with herpes zoster or shingles.

A. What is the source of this woman's rash and pain?

B. Explain the dermatomal distribution of the lesions.

Psoriasis is a chronically recurring papulosquamous skin disorder, characterized by circumscribed red, thickened plaques with an overlying silver-white scale.

A. Explain the development of the plaques in terms of epidermal cell turnover.

B. Persons with psoriasis are instructed to refrain from rubbing or scratching the lesions. Explain the rationale for these instructions.

C. Among the methods used in treatment psoriasis are the use of topical keratolytic agents and corticosteroid skin preparations. Explain how these two different types of agents exert their effect on the plaque lesions.

During the past several decades, there has been an alarming increase in the incidence of skin cancers, including malignant melanoma, that has been attributed to increased sun exposure.

A. Explain the possible mechanisms whereby ultraviolet radiation promotes the development of malignant skin lesions.

B. Cite two important clinical signs that aid in distinguishing dysplastic nevi from malignant melanoma.

References

1. Stander S., Steinhoff M., Luger T.A. (2002). Pathophysiology of pruritus. In Bieber T., Leung D.Y.M. (Eds.), *Atopic dermatitis* (pp. 183–216). New York: Marcel Dekker.
2. Charlesworth E.N., Beltrani V.S. (2002). Pruritic dermatoses: Overview of etiology and therapy. *American Journal of Medicine 113,* 25S–33S.
3. Buchanan P.I. (2001). Behavior modification: A nursing approach for young children with atopic eczema. *Dermatology Nursing 13,* 15–18, 21–25.
4. Lynde C.W. (2002). Moisturizers: What they are and what they do. *Skin Therapy Letter 6,* 3–8.
5. Ademola J., Frazier C., Kim S.J., et al. (2002). Clinical evaluation of 40% urea and 12% ammonium lactate in the treatment of xerosis. *American Journal of Clinical Dermatology 3*(3), 217–222.
6. Loden M., Andersson A.C., Andersson C., et al. (2001). Instrumental and dermatologist evaluation of the effect of glycerin and urea on dry skin in atopic dermatitis. *Skin Research and Technology 7*(4), 209–213.
7. Ives T.J. (2001). Photosensitivity and burns. In Koda-Kimble M.A., Young L.Y. (Eds.), *Applied therapeutics: The clinical use of drugs* (7th ed., pp. 1–22). Philadelphia: Lippincott Williams & Wilkins.
8. Gilchrest B.A., Eller M.S., Geller A.C., Yaar M. (1999). The pathogenesis of melanoma induced by ultraviolet radiation. *New England Journal of Medicine 340,* 1341–1348.
9. Hall J.C. (1999). *Sauer's manual of skin diseases* (8th ed., p. 295). Philadelphia: Lippincott Williams & Wilkins.
10. Ellsworth A.J. (2001). Skin disorders. In Koda-Kimble M.A., Young L.Y. (Eds.), Applied therapeutics: The clinical use of drugs (7th ed., pp. 1–36). Philadelphia: Lippincott Williams & Wilkins.
11. Epstein J., Kaplan L., Levine N. (2000). The value of sunscreens. *Patient Care 34*(11), 103–107.
12. Marks R., Hill D. (2001). Prevention of skin cancer. In Sober A.J., Haluska F.G. (Eds.), *American Cancer Society atlas of clinical oncology: Skin cancer* (pp. 327–331). Hamilton, Ontario: BC Decker.
13. Taneja A. (2002). Treatment of vitiligo. *Journal of Dermatological Treatment 13,* 19–25.
14. Njoo D.M., Westerhof W. (2001). Vitiligo: Pathogenesis and treatment. *American Journal of Clinical Dermatology 2,* 167–181.
15. Nesbitt L.T. (2000). Treatment of tinea capitis. *International Journal of Dermatology 39,* 261–262.
16. Chen B.K., Friedlander S.F. (2001). Tinea capitis update: A continuing conflict with an old adversary. *Current Opinion in Pediatrics 13,* 331–335.
17. Joish V.N., Armstrong E.P. (2001). Which antifungal agent for onychomycosis? A pharmacoeconomic analysis. *Pharmacoeconomics 19,* 983–1002.
18. Gupta A.K. (1999). The new oral antifungal agents for onychomycosis of the toenails. *Journal of the European Academy of Dermatology and Venereology 13,* 1–13.
19. Cotran R.S., Kumar V., Collins T. (1999). *Robbins pathologic basis of disease* (6th ed., pp. 1174–1177, 1198, 1199, 1208, 1209). Philadelphia: W.B. Saunders.
20. Focht D.R., Spicer C., Fairchok M.P. (2002). The efficacy of duct tape vs cryotherapy in the treatment of verruca vulgaris (the common wart). *Archives of Pediatric & Adolescent Medicine 156,* 971–974.
21. Rudolph R.I. (2003). Warts and duct tape—a good combo! [Comment]. *Archives of Pediatric & Adolescent Medicine 157,* 489.
22. Stanberry L.R., Cunningham A.L., Mindel A., et al. (2000). Prospects for control of herpes simplex virus disease through immunization. *Clinical Infectious Diseases 30,* 549–566.
23. Gilden D.H., Kleinschmidt-DeMasters B.K., LaGuardia J.J., Cohrs R.J. (2000). Neurologic complications of reactivation of varicella-zoster virus. *New England Journal of Medicine 342,* 635–645.
24. Stankus S.J., Dlugopolski M., Packer D. (2000). Management of herpes zoster (shingles) and postherpetic neuralgia. *American Family Physician 61,* 2437–2444, 2447–2448.
25. Odom R.B., James W.D., Berger T.G. (2000). *Andrew's diseases of the skin: Clinical dermatology* (pp. 486, 488, 186). Philadelphia: W.B. Saunders.
26. Edmunds W.J., Brisson M. (2002). The effect of vaccination on the epidemiology of varicella zoster virus. *Journal of Infection 44,* 211–219.
27. Thomas S.L., Wheeler J.G., Hall A.J. (2002). Contacts with varicella or with children and protection against herpes zoster in adults: A case-control study. *Lancet 360,* 678–682.
28. Krowchuk D.P., Lucky A.W. (2001). Managing adolescent acne. *Adolescent Medicine State of the Art Reviews 12,* 355–374.
29. Krowchuk D.P. (2000). Managing acne in adolescents. *Pediatric Clinics of North America 47,* 841–857.
30. Russell J.J. (2000). Topical therapy for acne. *American Family Physician 61,* 357–366.
31. Feldman S.R., Hollar C.B., Gupta A.K., et al. (2001). Women commonly seek care for rosacea: Dermatologists frequently provide the care. *Cutis 68,* 156–160.
32. Szlachcic A. (2002). The link between Helicobacter pylori infection and rosacea. *Journal of the European Academy of Dermatology & Venereology 16,* 328–333.
33. Blount B.W., Pelletter A.L. (2002). Rosacea: A common, yet commonly overlooked, condition. *American Family Physician 66,* 435–442.
34. Correale C.E., Walker C., Craig T.J. (1999). Atopic dermatitis: A review of diagnosis and treatment. *American Family Physician 60,* 1191–1210.
35. Kristal L., Klein P.A. (2000). Atopic dermatitis in infants and children. *Pediatric Clinics of North America 47,* 877–894.
36. Charman C.R., Williams H.C. (2002). Epidemiology. In Bieber T., Leung D.Y.M. (Eds.), *Atopic dermatitis* (pp. 24–25, 29, 34). New York: Marcel Dekker.
37. Leung D.Y., Boguniewicz M. (2003). Advances in allergic skin diseases. *Journal of Allergy & Clinical Immunology 111,* S805–S812.
38. Rico M.J., Lawrence I. (2002). Tacrolimus ointment for the treatment of atopic dermatitis: Clinical and pharmacologic effects. *Allergy & Asthma Proceedings 23,* 191–197.
39. Yates C. (2002). Parameters for the treatment of urticaria and angioedema. *Journal of the American Academy of Nurse Practitioners 14,* 478–483.
40. Kaplan A.P. (2002). Chronic urticaria and angioedema. *New England Journal of Medicine 346,* 175–179.
41. Fritsch P.O., Sidorooff A. (2000). Drug-induced Stevens-Johnson syndrome/toxic epidermal necrolysis. *American Journal of Clinical Dermatology 1,* 349–360.

42. Roujeau J.C., Stern R.S. (1994). Severe adverse cutaneous reactions to drugs. *New England Journal of Medicine 331,* 1272–1284.
43. Koo J.Y. (1999). Current consensus and update on psoriasis therapy: A perspective from the U.S. *Journal of Dermatology 26,* 723–733.
44. Galadari H., Fuchs B., Lebwohl M. (2003). Newly available treatments for psoriatic arthritis and their impact on skin psoriasis. *International Journal of Dermatology 42,* 231–237.
45. Pardasani A.G., Feldman S.R., Clark A.R. (2000). Treatment of psoriasis: An algorithm based approach for primary care physicians. *American Family Physician 61,* 725–733, 736.
46. Lebwohl M. (2003). Psoriasis. *Lancet 363,* 1197–1204.
47. Weinberg J.M., Saini R., Tutrone W.D. (2002). Biologic therapy for psoriasis—the first wave: Infliximab, etanercept, efalizumab, and alefacept. *Journal of Drugs in Dermatology 1,* 303–310.
48. Galadari H., Fuchs B., Lebwohl M. (2003). Newly available treatments for psoriatic arthritis and their impact on skin psoriasis. *International Journal of Dermatology 42,* 231–237.
49. Katta R. (2000). Lichen planus. *American Family Physician 61,* 3319–3324, 3327–3328.
50. Cook A.M., Romanelli F. (2003). Ivermectin for the treatment of resistant scabies. *Annals of Pharmacotherapy 37,* 279–281.
51. Stephens M.B. (2000). Controlling head lice. *Primary Care for Nurse Practitioners* (Sept. 15), 99–107.
52. Burgess I.F., Pollack R.J., Taplin D. (2003). *Cutting through controversy: Special report on the treatment of head lice* (pp. 10, 11). Morristown, NJ: Premier Healthcare Resource.
53. Jemad A., Murray T., Samuels A., et al. (2003). Cancer statistics, 2003. *CA: A Cancer Journal for Clinicians 53,* 5–26.
54. Rigel D.S., Carucci J.A. (2000). Malignant melanoma: Prevention, early detection, and treatment in the 21st century. *CA: A Cancer Journal for Clinicians 50,* 215–236.
55. Mikkilineni R., Weinstock M.A. (2001). Epidemiology (pp. 1–15). In Sober A.J., Haluska F.G., (Eds.), *American Cancer Society atlas of clinical oncology: Skin cancer.* Hamilton, Ontario: B.C. Decker.
56. Urist M.M., Heslin M.J., Miller D.M. (2001). Malignant melanoma. In Lenbard R.E., Osteen R.T., Gansler T. (Eds.), *Clinical oncology* (pp. 553–556). Atlanta: American Cancer Society.
57. Jerant A.F., Johnson J.T., Sheridan C.M., Caffrey T.J. (2000). Early detection and treatment of cancer. *American Family Physician 62,* 357–368, 375–376, 381–382.
58. Lens M.B., Dawes M., Goodacre T., Bishop J.A. (2002). Excision margins in the treatment of primary cutaneous melanoma: A systematic review of randomized controlled trials comparing narrow vs wide excision. *Archives of Surgery 137,* 1101–1105.
59. Yang S., Haluska F.G. (2001). Immunotherapy for melanoma. In Sober A.J., Haluska F.G., (Eds.), *American Cancer Society atlas of clinical oncology: Skin cancer* (pp. 225–252). Hamilton, Ontario: B.C. Decker.
60. Menaker G.M., Chiu D.S. (2001). Basal cell carcinoma. In Sober A.J., Haluska F.G. (Eds.), *American Cancer Society atlas of clinical oncology: Skin cancer* (pp. 60–71). Hamilton, Ontario: B.C. Decker.
61. Carucci J.A., Rigel D.S., Friedman R.J. (2001). Basal cell and squamous cell skin cancer. In Lenbard R.E., Osteen R.T., Gansler T. (Eds.), *Clinical oncology* (pp. 553–556). Atlanta: American Cancer Society.
62. Robinson J.K. (2001). Squamous cell carcinoma. In Sober A.J., Haluska F.G. (Eds.), *American Cancer Society atlas of clinical oncology: Skin cancer.* (pp. 72–84). Hamilton, Ontario: B.C. Decker.
63. American Burn Association. (2003). Burn incidence and treatment in the US: 2000 fact sheet. [On-line]. Available: http://www.ameriburn.org.
64. Morgan E.D., Bledsoe S.C., Barker J. (2000). Ambulatory management of burns. *American Family Physician 62,* 2015–2026, 2029–2030.
65. Behrman R.E., Kliegman R.M., Jensen H.B. (Eds.), (2004). *Nelson textbook of pediatrics* (17th ed., pp. 330–337, 1026–1034, 1069–1072, 1057–1059). Philadelphia: W.B. Saunders.
66. Parenteau N. (1999). Skin: The first tissue-engineered products. *Scientific American 280*(4), 83–84.
67. Dohil M.A., Baugh W.P., Eichenfield L.F. (2000). Vascular and pigmented birthmarks. *Pediatric Clinics of North America 47,* 783–810.
68. Drolet B.A., Esterly N.B., Frieden I.J. (1999). Hemangiomas in children. *New England Journal of Medicine 341,* 173–181.
69. Kazaks E.L., Lane A.T. (2000). Diaper dermatitis. *Pediatric Clinics of North America 47,* 909–918.
70. Lober B.A., Lober C.W. (2000). Actinic keratosis is squamous cell carcinoma. *Southern Medical Journal 93,* 650–655.
71. Cockerell C.J. (2000). Histopathology of incipient intraepidermal squamous cell carcinoma ("actinic keratosis") [Comment]. *Journal of the American Academy of Dermatology 42,* 11–17.

APPENDIX

A

Lab Values

Prefixes Denoting Decimal Factors

Prefix	Symbol	Factor
mega	M	10^{6}
kilo	k	10^{3}
hecto	h	10^{2}
deci	d	10^{-1}
centi	c	10^{-2}
milli	m	10^{-3}
micro	µ	10^{-6}
nano	n	10^{-9}
pico	p	10^{-12}
femto	f	10^{-15}

Hematology

Test	Conventional Units	SI Units
Erythrocyte count (RBC count)	M. 4.2–5.4 × 10^{6}/µL F. 3.6–5.0 × 10^{6}/µL	M. 4.2–5.4 × 10^{12}/L F. 3.6–5.0 × 10^{12}/L
Hematocrit (Hct)	M. 40–50% F. 37–47%	M. 0.40–0.50 F. 0.37–0.47
Hemoglobin (Hb)	M. 14.0–16.5 g/dL F. 12.0–15.0 g/dL	M. 140–165 g/L F. 120–150 g/L
Mean corpuscular hemoglobin (MHC)	27–34 pg/cell	0.40–0.53 fmol/cell
Mean corpuscular hemoglobin concentration (MCHC)	31–35 g/dL	310–350 g/L
Mean corpuscular volume (MCV)	80–100 fL	
Reticulocyte count	1.0–1.5% total RBC	
Leukocyte count (WBC count)	4.8–10.8 × 10^{3}/µL	4.8–10.8 × 10^{9}/L
Basophils	0–2%	
Eosinophils	0–3%	
Lymphocytes	24–40%	
Monocytes	4–9%	
Neutrophils (segmented [Segs])	47–63%	
Neutrophils (bands)	0–4%	

Blood Chemistry*

Test	Conventional Units	SI Units
Alanine aminotransferase (ALT, SGPT, GPT)	0–35 U/L	0–0.58 μkat/L
Alkaline phosphatase	41–133 U/L	0.7–2.2 μkat/L
Ammonia	18–16 μg/dL	11–35 μmol/L
Amylase	20–110 U/L†	0.33–1.83 μkat/L†
Aspartase amino transferase (AST, SGOT, GOT)	0–35 U/L†	0–0.58 μkat/L†
Bicarbonate	24–31 mEq/L	24–31 mmol/L
Bilibrubin (total)	0.1–1.2 mg/dL	2–21 μmol/L
Direct	0.1–0.4 mg/dL	<7 μmol/L
Indirect	0.1–0.7 mg/dL	<12 μmol/L
Blood urea nitrogen (BUN)	8–20 mg/dL	2.9–7.1 mmol/L
Calcium (Ca^{2+})	8.5–10.5 mg/dL	2.1–2.6 mmol/L
Carbon dioxide	24–29 mEq/L	24–29 mmol/L
Chloride	98–106 mEq/L	98–106 mmol/L
Cholesterol (desirable)	<200 mg/dL	<5.2 mmol/L
Creatine kinase (CK, CPK)	32–267 U/L†	0.53–4.45 μkat/L†
Creatine kinase (MB)	<16 IU/L† or 4% of total CK	<0.27 μkat/L†
Creatinine (serum)	0.6–1.2 mg/dL‡	50–100 μmol/L‡
Gamma-glutamyl-transpeptidase (GGT)	9–85 U/L†	0.15–1.42 μkat/L†
Glucose (plasma, fasting)	60–100 mg/dL	3.3–5.6 mmol/L
Glycosylated hemoglobin (HbA_{1c})	3.9–6.9%	
High-density lipoproteins		
(low)	<40 mg/dL	<1.0 mmol/L
(high)	≥60 mg/dL	≥1.56 mmol/L
Lactate dehydrogenase (LDH)	88–230 U/L†	1.46–3.82 μkat/L†
Lipids		
Cholesterol	<200 mg/dL (desirable)	<5.2 mmol/L
Triglycerides	<165 mg/dL	<1.65 g/L
Lipase	0–160 U/L†	0.266 μkat/L†
Low-density lipoproteins (desirable)	<130 mg/dL	<3.37 mmol/L
Magnesium	1.84–3.0 mg/dL	0.75–1.25 mmol/L
Osmolality	275–295 mOsm/kg H_2O	275–295 mmol/kg H_2O
PH (arterial)	7.35–7.45	
Phosphorus (inorganic)	2.5–4.5 mg/dL	0.80–1.45 mmol/L
Potassium	3.5–5.0 mEq/L	3.5–5.0 mmol/L
Prostate specific antigen (PSA)	0–4 ng/mL	0–4 μg/L
Protein total	6.0–8.6 g/dL	60–86 g/L
Albumin	3.8–5.6 g/dL	38–56 g/L
Globulin	2.3–3.5 g/dL	23–35 g/L
A/G ratio	1.0–2.2	1.0–2.2
Triglycerides	<165 mg/dL	<1.65 g/L
Thyroid Tests		
Thyroxine (T_4) total	5.0–11.0 μg/dL	64–142 nmol/L
Thyroxine, free (FT_4)	9–24 pmol/L†	
Triiodothyronine (T_3) total	95–190 ng/dL	1.5–2.9 nmol/L
Thyroid stimulating hormone (TSH)	0.4–6.0 μU/mL	0.4–6.0 mU/L
Thyroglobin	3–42 ng/mL	3–42 μg/L
Sodium	135–145 mEq/L	135–145 mmol/L
Uric acid	M. 2.4–7.4 mg/dL F. 1.4–5.8 mg/dL	M. 140–440 μmol/L F. 80–350 μmol/L

U, units.

*Values may vary with laboratory. The values supplied by the laboratory performing the test should always be used since the ranges may be method specific.

†Laboratory and/or method specific

‡Varies with age and muscle mass

(Values obtained from Tierney L.M., McPhee S.J., Papadakis M.A. [2003]. *Current medical diagnosis and treatment* [41st ed.]. Stamford, CT: Appleton & Lange, pp. 1495–1501; Fischbach F. [2004]. *A manual of laboratory and diagnostic tests* [7th ed.]. Philadelphia: Lippincott Williams & Wilkins, and other sources.)

APPENDIX B

Weblinks

Unit I Concepts of Health and Disease

Medline Plus (health information site of the U.S. National Library of Medicine and National Institutes of Health [NIH]. Includes health topics, drug information, and medical encyclopedia with topics listed in alphabetical order)
http://www.nlm.nih.gov/medlineplus

Health Finder (government site for health information)
http://www.healthfinder.gov

Health Links (source of information on multiple health topics)
http://healthlink.mcw.edu/topics

Virtual Hospital (a digital library of health information)
http://www.vh.org/index.html

Medical Library (links to information by NIH and leading medical societies)
http://www.medem.com/medlb/medlib_entry.cfm

Agency for Health Care Research and Quality (Government site for Clinical Practice Guidelines and Evidence-based Practice)
http://www.ahrq.gov

Virtual Children's Hospital (a digital library of pediatric information)
http://www.vh.org/pediatric/index.html

Maternal Child Health Bureau (information on child health issues listed in alphabetical order)
www.mchb.hrsa.gov

Merck Manual of Geriatrics (information on health problems in the geriatric population)
http://www.merck.com/pubs/mm_geriatrics

Unit II Cell Function and Growth

Virtual Library of Cell Biology (review of biology)
http://vlib.org/Science/Cell_Biology

Cells Alive (review of cell biology, immunology—animation)
http://www.cellsalive.com

Kimball's Biology Pages (online biology textbook with alphabetical index that links the user to desired information)
http://users.rcn.com/jkimball.ma.ultranet/BiologyPages

Genes and Disease. National Center for Biotechnology (information on cancer, immune system [asthma and Crohn's disease], metabolism [atherosclerosis, type 1 diabetes], muscle and bone [Duchenne muscular dystrophy], nervous system [Alzheimer's disease], cellular messengers [baldness, sex determination], and transporters [cystic fibrosis, hemophilia A])
http://www.ncbi.nlm.nih.gov/disease/Metabolism.html

March of Dimes (birth defects information)
http://www.modimes.org

American Cancer Society (information on cancer)
www.cancer.org

American Society of Clinical Oncology (information on cancer)
www.asco.org

National Cancer Institute (information on cancer)
www.nci.nih.gov

Unit III Integrative Body Functions

American Institute of Stress
http://www.stress.org

Hyperthermia: A Hot Weather Hazard for Older People
www.wramc.amedd.army.mil/education/hyperthe.htm

Outdoor Action Guide to Hypothermia And Cold Weather Injuries
www.princeton.edu/~oa/safety/hypocold.shtml

American Dietetic Association
www.eatright.org

National Academies of Sciences (Dietary Reference Intakes: Applications in Dietary Assessment [2001]. Available to read online free.)
www.nap.edu/books/0309071836/html

American Association of Chronic Fatigue Syndrome (AACFS)
www.aacfs.org

President's Council on Physical Fitness
http://aspe.hhs.gov/health/reports/physicalactivity

Unit IV Hematopoietic Function

Emory University Sickle Cell Information Center (source of up-to-date information on sickle cell anemia)
http://www.scinfo.org

National Heart Lung and Blood Institute (information on sickle cell anemia, hemophilia, and other bleeding disorders)
http://www.nhlbi.nih.gov/health/public/blood/index.htm

Karolinska Institute (site for hematology links)
http://www.mic.ki.se/Diseases/c15.html

National Heart Lung and Blood Institute (information on sickle cell anemia and thalassemia)
http://www.nhlbi.nih.gov/health/public/blood/index.htm#scd

Unit V Infection, Inflammation, and Immunity

Centers for Disease Control and Prevention (most recent statistics on infectious diseases)
www.cdc.gov

National Institute of Infectious and Allergic Diseases (a quick reference for infectious diseases, immune disorders, and HIV/AIDS)
http://www.niaid.nih.gov/final/immun/immun.htm

Microbiology and immunology online
http://www.medem.com/medlb/medlib_entry.cfm

HIV/AIDS Information
http://www.aegis.com

Biology Project (website for information on immunology and HIV)
http://www.biology.arizona.edu/default.html

National Library of Medicine HIV/AIDS site
http://sis.nlm.nih.gov/HIV/HIVMain.html

National Institute of Child Health and Human Development (primary Immunodeficiency disorders)
www.nichd.nih.gov/publications/pubs/primaryimmunobooklet.htm

Unit VI Cardiovascular Function

National Cholesterol Education Program
www.nhlbi.nih.gov/about/ncep

American College of Cardiology (source of guidelines for diagnosis and treatment of cardiovascular diseases)
www.acc.org/clinical/statements.htm

American Heart Association (professional and patient education materials)
www.americanheart.org

Cardiovascular Physiology Concepts. (R.E. Kabunde, Ohio University College of Osteopathic Medicine)
http://www.oucom.ohiou.edu/cvphysiology/A017.htm

Unit VII Respiratory Function

National Institute of Allergy and Infectious Diseases (source of information on respiratory disorders)
http://www.niaid.nih.gov/publications/pneumonia.htm

American Lung Association (source of information on respiratory disorders)
http://www.lungusa.org

National Heart, Lung, and Blood Institute (Asthma Guidelines)
http://www.nhlbi.nih.gov/guidelines/asthma/index.htm

Oxygen dissociation curve (interactive)
http://www.ventworld.com/resources/oxydisso/oxydisso.html

Unit VIII Renal Function and Fluids and Electrolytes

Clinical Calculator (calculate body surface area, base excess, calcium equivalents, etc.)
http://www-users.med.cornell.edu/~spon/picu/calc/fenacalc.htm

Acid-base physiology (includes an interactive Henderson equation where you can change H^+ and HCO_3^- values to obtain pH)
http://www.acid-base.com/homepage.html

Fundamentals of acid-base balance
http://www.gasnet.org/acid-base

National Kidney Foundation (information on kidney diseases from A to Z)
http://www.kidney.org

National Kidney Disease Education Program (National Institute Digestive, Diabetes, and Kidney Disease; includes links to websites for kidney diseases)
http://www.nkdep.nih.gov/links.htm

Principles of hemodialysis (animated)
http://www.kidneypatientguide.org.uk/site/HDanim.html

American Foundation for Urologic Disease (information on prostate, urologic, kidney diseases, etc.)
www.afud.org

Unit IX Gastrointestinal Function

American College of Gastroenterology (information on common gastrointestinal disorders)
www.acg.gi.org

National Digestive Diseases Information Clearinghouse
www.niddk.nih.gov/health/digest/nddic.htm

National Institute of Diabetes and Digestive and Kidney Diseases (information on nutrition)
www.niddk.nih.gov

The Diet Channel (source for nutrition content of food)
www.thedietchannel.com

Unit X Endocrine Function

Diagnosing Thyroid Disorders (description of thyroid disorders [including photos], thyroid tests, and case study quiz)
http://www.hsc.missouri.edu/~daveg/thyroid/thyindex.html

Congenital Adrenal Hyperplasia
http://www.hopkinsmedicine.org/pediatricendocrinology/cah/caha.html

Growth, Genetics, and Hormones (Internet journal funded by Genetec)
http://www.gghjournal.com/gghataglance.htm

National Institute Diabetes, Digestive, and Kidney Diseases
http://www.niddk.nih.gov/health/endo/endo.htm

American Diabetes Association (source of professional and patient information on diabetes)
http://www.diabetes.org

Unit XI Genitourinary and Reproductive Function

University of Arizona Overview of Male and Female Reproductive Systems
http://www.blc.arizona.edu/courses/181gh/rick/reproduction/female2.html

Cornell Center for Male Reproductive Medicine
http://www.maleinfertility.org/index.html

American Prostate Society
www.ameripros.org

Erectile Dysfunction
http://www.niddk.nih.gov/health/urolog/pubs/impotnce/impotnce.htm

National Women's Health
http://www.4woman.gov

FDA Office of Women's Health
http://www.fda.gov/womens/default.htm

National Institutes of Health: Women's Health Initiatives
http://www.nhlbi.nih.gov/whi

National Women's Health Resource Center
www.healthywomen.org

Unit XII Neural Function

How Action Potentials Work (animated)
http://www.epub.org.br/cm/n10/fundamentos/pot2_i.htm

American Academy of Neurology (information and practice guidelines)
http://www.aan.com/professionals/practice/guidelines.cfm

Genes and the Brain (genetic basis for brain disorders)
http://www.ncbi.nlm.nih.gov/disease/Brain.html

American Academy of Pain Medicine (position and consensus statements [eg, use of opioids for chronic pain, ethics for pain medicine, quality end-of-life care])
www.painmed.org

American Pain Society (resources for professionals)
www.ampainsoc.org/links

National Institute of Neurological Disorders and Stroke
www.ninds.nih.gov

Unit XIII Special Sensory Function

National Eye Institute (has color images of visual disorders)
http://www.nei.nih.gov

Color vision
http://www.iamcal.com/toys/colors

Marion Downs National Center for Infant Hearing
www.colorado.edu/slhs/mdnc

National Institute on Deafness and Other Communication Disorders
www.nidcd.nih.gov

Unit XIV Musculoskeletal and Integumentary Function

Arthritis Foundation (professional and patient educational materials on arthritis)
http://www.arthritis.org

National Institute of Arthritis and Musculoskeletal and Skin Diseases
http://www.niams.nih.gov

John Hopkins Arthritis
http://www.hopkins-arthritis.som.jhmi.edu

American Academy of Orthopedic Surgeons (fact sheets on orthopedic conditions in adults and children)
http://orthoinfo.aaos.org

University of Iowa (links to orthopedic Internet sites)
http://www.lib.uiowa.edu/hardin/md/rheum.html

Pediatric Orthopedics (information on pediatric orthopedic conditions)
http://www.pediatric-orthopedics.com/home.html

National Institute of Arthritis and Musculoskeletal and Skin Diseases (information on skin diseases such as acne, atopic dermatitis, psoriasis, rosacea, and others)
http://www.niams.nih.gov

American Academy of Dermatology (includes patient education information and photos of some skin disorders)
http://www.aad.org

DermNet—New Zealand Dermatological Society (information on skin diseases)
www.dermnet.org.nz

Glossary

Abduction The act of abducting (moving or spreading away from a position near the midline of the body or the axial line of a limb) or the state of being abducted.

Abrasion The wearing or scraping away of a substance or structure, such as the skin, through an unusual or abnormal mechanical process.

Abscess A collection of pus that is restricted to a specific area in tissues, organs, or confined spaces.

Accommodation The adjustment of the lens (eye) to variations in distance.

Acromion The lateral extension of the spine of the scapula, forming the highest point of the shoulder. (Adjective: acromial)

Acuity The clearness or sharpness of perception, especially of vision.

Adaptation The adjustment of an organism to its environment, physical or psychological, through changes and responses to stress of any kind.

Adduction The act of adducting (moving or drawing toward a position near the midline of the body or the axial line of a limb) or the state of being adducted.

Adhesin The molecular components of the bacterial cell wall that are involved in adhesion processes.

Adrenergic Activated by or characteristic of the sympathetic nervous system or its neurotransmitters (*i.e.,* epinephrine and norepinephrine).

Aerobic Growing, living, or occurring only in the presence of air or oxygen.

Afferent Bearing or conducting inward or toward a center, as an afferent neuron.

Agglutination The clumping together of particles, microorganisms, or blood cells in response to an antigen–antibody reaction.

Agonist A muscle whose action is opposed by another muscle (antagonist) with which it is paired; or a drug or other chemical substance that has affinity for or stimulates a predictable physiologic function.

Akinesia An abnormal state in which there is an absence or poverty of movement.

Allele One of two or more different forms of a gene that can occupy a particular locus on a chromosome.

Alveolus A small saclike structure, as in the alveolus of the lung.

Amine An organic compound containing nitrogen.

Amblyopia A condition of vision impairment without a detectable organic lesion of the eye.

Amorphous Without a definite form; shapeless.

Amphoteric Capable of reacting chemically as an acid or a base.

Ampulla A saclike dilatation of a duct, canal, or any other tubular structure.

Anabolism A constructive metabolic process characterized by the conversion of simple substances into larger, complex molecules.

Anaerobic Growing, living, or occurring only in the absence of air or oxygen.

Analog A part, organ, or chemical having the same function or appearance but differing in respect to a certain component, such as origin or development.

Anaplasia A change in the structure of cells and in their orientation to each other that is characterized by a loss of cell differentiation, as in cancerous cell growth.

Anastomosis The connection or joining between two vessels; or an opening created by surgical, traumatic, or pathologic means.

Androgen Any substance, such as a male sex hormone, that increases male characteristics.

Anergy A state of absent or diminished reaction to an antigen or group of antigens.

Aneuploidy A variation in the number of chromosomes within a cell involving one or more missing chromosomes rather than entire sets.

Aneurysm An outpouching or dilation in the wall of a blood vessel or the heart.

Ankylosis Stiffness or fixation of separate bones of a joint, resulting from disease, injury, or surgical procedure. (Verb: ankylose)

Anorexia Lack or loss of appetite for food. (Adjective: anorexic)

Anoxia An abnormal condition characterized by the total lack of oxygen.

Antagonist A muscle whose action directly opposes that of another muscle (agonist) with which it is paired; or a drug or other chemical substance that can diminish or nullify the action of a neuromediator or body function.

Anterior Pertaining to a surface or part that is situated near or toward the front.

Antigen A substance that generates an immune response by causing the formation of an antibody or reacting with antibodies or T-cell receptors.

Apex The uppermost point, the narrowed or pointed end, or the highest point of a structure, such as an organ.

Aphagia A condition characterized by the refusal or the loss of ability to swallow.

Aplasia The absence of an organ or tissue due to a developmental failure.

Apnea The absence of spontaneous respiration.

Apoptosis A mechanism of programmed cell death, marked by shrinkage of the cell, condensation of chromatin, formation of cytoplasmic blebs, and fragmentation of the cell into membrane-bound bodies eliminated by phagocytosis.

Apraxia Loss of the ability to carry out familiar, purposeful acts or to manipulate objects in the absence of paralysis or other motor or sensory impairment.

Articulation The place of connection or junction between two or more bones of a skeletal joint.

Ascites An abnormal accumulation of serous fluid in the peritoneal cavity.

Asepsis The condition of being free or freed from pathogenic microorganisms.

Astereognosis A neurologic disorder characterized by an inability to identify objects by touch.

Asterixis A motor disturbance characterized by a hand-flapping tremor, which results when the prolonged contraction of groups of muscles lapses intermittently.

Ataxia An abnormal condition characterized by an inability to coordinate voluntary muscular movement.

Athetosis A neuromuscular condition characterized by the continuous occurrence of slow, sinuous, writhing movements that are performed involuntarily. (Adjective: athetoid)

Atopy Genetic predisposition toward the development of a hypersensitivity or an allergic reaction to common environmental allergens.

Atresia The absence or closure of a normal body orifice or tubular organ, such as the esophagus.

Atrophy A wasting or diminution of size, often accompanied by a decrease in function, of a cell, tissue, or organ.

Autocrine A mode of hormone action in which a chemical messenger acts on the same cell that secretes it.

Autosome Any chromosome other than a sex chromosome.

Axillary Of or pertaining to the axilla, or armpit.

Bacteremia The presence of bacteria in the blood.

Bactericide An agent that destroys bacteria. (Adjective: bactericidal)

Bacteriostat An agent that inhibits bacterial growth. (Adjective: bacteriostatic)

Ballismus An abnormal condition characterized by violent flailing motions of the arms and, occasionally, the head, resulting from injury to or destruction of the subthalamic nucleus or its fiber connections.

Baroreceptor A type of sensory nerve ending such as those found in the aorta and the carotid sinus that is stimulated by changes in pressure.

Basal Pertaining to, situated at, or forming the base; or the fundamental or the basic.

Benign Not malignant; or of the character that does not threaten health or life.

Bipolar neuron A nerve cell that has a process at each end—an afferent process and an efferent process.

Bolus A rounded mass of food ready to swallow or such a mass passing through the gastrointestinal tract; or a concentrated mass of medicinal material or other pharmaceutic preparation injected all at once intravenously for diagnostic purposes.

Borborygmus The rumbling, gurgling, or tinkling noise produced by the propulsion of gas through the intestine.

Bruit A sound or murmur heard while auscultating an organ or blood vessel, especially an abnormal one.

Buccal Pertaining to or directed toward the inside of the cheek.

Buffer A substance or group of substances that prevents change in the concentration of another chemical substance.

Bulla A thin-walled blister of the skin or mucous membranes greater than 5 mm in diameter containing serous or seropurulent fluid.

Bursa A fluid-filled sac or saclike cavity situated in places in the tissues at which friction would otherwise develop, such as between certain tendons and the bones beneath them.

Cachexia A condition of general ill health and malnutrition, marked by weakness and emaciation.

Calculus A stony mass formed within body tissues, usually composed of mineral salts.

Capsid The protein shell that envelops and protects the nucleic acid of a virus.

Carcinogen Any substance or agent that causes the development or increases the incidence of cancer.

Carpal Of or pertaining to the carpus, or wrist.

Caseation A form of tissue necrosis in which the tissue is changed into a dry, amorphous mass resembling crumbly cheese.

Catabolism A metabolic process through which living organisms break down complex substances to simple compounds, liberating energy for use in work, energy storage, or heat production.

Catalyst A substance that increases the velocity of a chemical reaction without being consumed by the process.

Catecholamines Any one of a group of biogenic amines having a sympathomimetic action and composed of a catechol molecule and the aliphatic portion of an amine.

Caudal Signifying an inferior position, toward the distal end of the spine.

Cellulitis An acute, diffuse, spreading, edematous inflammation of the deep subcutaneous tissues and sometimes muscle, characterized most commonly by an area of heat, redness, pain, and swelling, and occasionally by fever, malaise, chills, and headache.

Cephalic Of or pertaining to the head, or to the head end of the body.

Cerumen The waxlike secretion produced by vestigial apocrine sweat glands in the external ear canal.

Cheilosis A noninflammatory disorder of the lips and mouth characterized by chapping and fissuring.

Chelate A chemical compound composed of a central metal ion and an organic molecule with multiple bonds, arranged in ring formation, used especially in treatment of metal poisoning.

Chemoreceptor A sensory nerve cell activated by chemical stimuli, as a chemoreceptor in the carotid artery that is sensitive to changes in the oxygen content in the blood and reflexly increases or decreases respiration and blood pressure.

Chemotaxis A response involving cell orientation or cell movement that is either toward (positive chemotaxis) or away from (negative chemotaxis) a chemical stimulus.

Chimeric Relating to, derived from, or being an individual possessing one's own immunologic characteristics and that of another individual; a phenomenon that can occur as the result of procedures such as a bone marrow graft.

Chondrocyte Any one of the mature polymorphic cells that form the cartilage of the body.

Chromatid One of the paired threadlike chromosome filaments, joined at the centromere, that make up a metaphase chromosome.

Chromosome Any one of the structures in the nucleus of a cell containing a linear thread of DNA, which functions in the transmission of genetic information.

Chyme The creamy, viscous, semifluid material produced during digestion of a meal that is expelled by the stomach into the duodenum.

Cilia A minute, hairlike process projecting from a cell, composed of nine microtubules arrayed around a single pair. Cilia beat rhythmically to move the cell around in its environment or they move mucus or fluids over the surface.

Circadian Being, having, pertaining to, or occurring in a period or cycle of approximately 24 hours.

Circumduction The active or passive circular movement of a limb or of the eye.

Cisterna An enclosed space, such as a cavity, that serves as a reservoir for lymph or other body fluids.

Clone One or a group of genetically identical cells or organisms derived from a single parent.

Coagulation The process of transforming a liquid into a semisolid mass, especially of blood clot formation.

Coarctation A condition of stricture or contraction of the walls of a vessel.

Cofactor A substance that must unite with another substance in order to function.

Colic Sharp, intermittent abdominal pain localized in a hollow or tubular organ, resulting from torsion, obstruction, or smooth muscle spasm. (Adjective: colicky)

Collagen The protein substance of the white, glistening, inelastic fibers of the skin, tendons, bone, cartilage, and all other connective tissue.

Collateral Secondary or accessory rather than direct or immediate; or a small branch, as of a blood vessel or nerve.

Complement Any one of the complex, enzymatic serum proteins that are involved in physiologic reactions, including antigen–antibody reaction and anaphylaxis.

Confluent Flowing or coming together; not discrete.

Congenital Present at, and usually before, birth.

Conjugate To pair and fuse in conjugation; or a form of sexual reproduction seen in unicellular organisms in which genetic material is exchanged during the temporary fusion of two cells.

Contiguous In contact or nearly so in an unbroken sequence along a boundary or at a point.

Contralateral Affecting, pertaining to, or originating in the opposite side of a point or reference.

Contusion An injury of a part without a break in the skin, characterized by swelling, discoloration, and pain.

Convolution An elevation or tortuous winding, such as one of the irregular ridges on the surface of the brain, formed by a structure being infolded upon itself.

Corpuscle Any small mass, cell, or body, such as a red or white blood cell.

Costal Pertaining to a rib or ribs.

Crepitus A sound or sensation that resembles a crackling or grating noise.

Cutaneous Pertaining to the skin.

Cyanosis A bluish discoloration, especially of the skin and mucous membranes, caused by an excess of deoxygenated hemoglobin in the blood.

Cytokine Any of a class of polypeptide immunoregulatory substances that are secreted by cells, usually of the immune system, that affect other cells.

Cytology The study of cells, including their origin, structure, function, and pathology.

Decibel A unit for expressing the relative power intensity of electric or acoustic signal power that is equal to one tenth of a bel.

Defecation The evacuation of feces from the digestive tract through the rectum.

Deformation The process of adapting in form or shape; also the product of such alteration.

Degeneration The deterioration of a normal cell, tissue, or organ to a less functionally active form. (Adjective: degenerative)

Deglutition The act or process of swallowing.

Degradation The reduction of a chemical compound to a compound less complex, usually by splitting off one or more groups.

Dehydration The condition that results from excessive loss of water from the body tissues.

Delirium An acute, reversible organic mental syndrome characterized by confusion, disorientation, restlessness, incoherence, fear, and often illusions.

Dendrite One of the branching processes that extends and transmits impulses toward a cell body of a neuron. (Adjective: dendritic)

Depolarization The reduction of a cell membrane potential to a less negative value than that of the potential outside the cell.

Dermatome The area of the skin supplied with afferent nerve fibers of a single dorsal root of a spinal nerve.

Desmosome A small, circular, dense area within the intercellular bridge that forms the site of adhesion between intermediate filaments and cell membranes.

Desquamation A normal process in which the cornified layer of the epidermis is shed in fine scales or sheets.

Dialysis The process of separating colloids and crystalline substances in solution, which involves the two distinct physical processes of diffusion and ultrafiltration; or a medical procedure for the removal of urea and other elements from the blood or lymph.

Diapedesis The outward passage of red or white blood corpuscles through the intact walls of the vessels.

Diaphoresis Perspiration, especially the profuse perspiration associated with an elevated body temperature, physical exertion, exposure to heat, and mental or emotional stress.

Diarthrosis A specialized articulation that permits, to some extent, free joint movement. (Adjective: diarthrodial)

Diastole The dilatation of the heart; or the period of dilatation, which is the interval between the second and the first heart sound and is the time during which blood enters the relaxed chambers of the heart from the systemic circulation and the lungs.

Differentiation The act or process in development in which unspecialized cells or tissues acquire more specialized characteristics, including those of physical form, physiologic function, and chemical properties.

Diffusion The process of becoming widely spread, as in the spontaneous movement of molecules or other particles in solution from an area of higher concentration to an area of lower concentration, resulting in an even distribution of the particles in the fluid.

Diopter A unit of measurement of the refractive power of lenses equal to the reciprocal of the focal length in meters.
Diploid Pertaining to an individual, organism, strain, or cell that has two full sets of homologous chromosomes.
Disseminate To scatter or distribute over a considerable area.
Distal Away from or being the farthest from a point of reference.
Diurnal Of, relating to, or occurring in the daytime.
Diverticulum A pouch or sac of variable size occurring naturally or through herniation of the muscular wall of a tubular organ.
Dorsum The back or posterior. (Adjective: dorsal)
Dysgenesis Defective or abnormal development of an organ or part, typically occurring during embryonic development. (Also called dysgenesia.)
Dyslexia A disturbance in the ability to read, spell, and write words.
Dyspepsia The impairment of the power or function of digestion, especially epigastric discomfort following eating.
Dysphagia A difficulty in swallowing.
Dysphonia Any impairment of the voice that is experienced as a difficulty in speaking.
Dysplasia The alteration in size, shape, and organization of adult cell types.
Eburnation The conversion of bone or cartilage, through thinning or loss, into a hard and dense mass with a worn, polished ivorylike surface.
Ecchymosis A small hemorrhagic spot, larger than a petechia, in the skin or mucous membrane caused by the extravasation of blood into the subcutaneous tissues.
Ectoderm The outermost of the three primary germ layers of the embryo, and from which the epidermis and epidermal tissues, such as nails, hair, and glands of the skin, develop.
Ectopic Relating to or characterized by an object or organ being situated in an unusual place, away from its normal location.
Edema The presence of an abnormal accumulation of fluid in interstitial spaces of tissues. (Adjective: edematous)
Efferent Conveyed or directed away from a center.
Effusion The escape of fluid from blood vessels into a part or tissue, as an exudation or a transudation.
Embolus A mass of clotted blood or other formed elements, such as bubbles of air, calcium fragments, or a bit of tissue or tumor, that circulates in the bloodstream until it becomes lodged in a vessel, obstructing the circulation. (Plural: emboli)
Empyema An accumulation of pus in a cavity of the body, especially the pleural space.
Emulsify To disperse one liquid throughout the body of another liquid, making a colloidal suspension, or emulsion.
Endocytosis The uptake or incorporation of substances into a cell by invagination of its plasma membrane, as in the processes of phagocytosis and pinocytosis.
Endoderm The innermost of the three primary germ layers of the embryo, and from which epithelium arises.
Endogenous Growing within the body; or developing or originating from within the body or produced from internal causes.
Endoscopy The visualization of any cavity of the body with an endoscope.
Enteropathic Relating to any disease of the intestinal tract.
Enzyme A protein molecule produced by living cells that catalyzes chemical reactions of other organic substances without itself being destroyed or altered.
Epiphysis The expanded articular end of a long bone (head) that is separated from the shaft of the bone by the epiphyseal plate until the bone stops growing, the plate is obliterated, and the shaft and the head become united.
Epithelium The covering of the internal and the external surfaces of the body, including the lining of vessels and other small cavities.
Erectile Capable of being erected or raised to an erect position.
Erythema The redness or inflammation of the skin or mucous membranes produced by the congestion of superficial capillaries. (Adjective: erythematous)
Etiology The study or theory of all factors that may be involved in the development of a disease, including susceptibility of an individual, the nature of the disease agent, and the way in which an individual's body is invaded by the agent; or the cause of a disease.
Eukaryotic Pertaining to an organism with cells having a true nucleus; that is, a highly complex, organized nucleus surrounded by a nuclear membrane containing organelles and exhibiting mitosis.
Euploid Pertaining to an individual, organism, strain, or cell with a balanced set or sets of chromosomes, in any number, that is an exact multiple of the normal, basic haploid number characteristic of the species; or such an individual, organism, strain, or cell.
Evisceration The removal of the viscera from the abdominal cavity, or disembowelment; or the extrusion of an internal organ through a wound or surgical incision.
Exacerbation An increase in the severity of a disease as marked by greater intensity in any of its signs and symptoms.
Exfoliation Peeling and sloughing off of tissue cells in scales or layers. (Adjective: exfoliative)
Exocytosis The discharge of cell particles, which are packaged in membrane-bound vesicles, by fusion of the vesicular membrane with the plasma membrane and subsequent release of the particles to the exterior of the cell.
Exogenous Developed or originating outside the body, as a disease caused by a bacterial or viral agent foreign to the body.
Exophthalmos A marked or abnormal protrusion of the eyeball.
Extension A movement that allows the two elements of any jointed part to be drawn apart, increasing the angle between them, as extending the leg increases the angle between the femur and the tibia.
Extrapyramidal Pertaining to motor systems supplied by fibers outside the corticospinal or pyramidal tracts.
Extravasation A discharge or escape, usually of blood, serum, or lymph, from a vessel into the tissues.
Extubation The process of withdrawing a previously inserted tube from an orifice or cavity of the body.
Exudate Fluid, cells, or other substances that have been slowly exuded or have escaped from blood vessels and have been deposited in tissues or on tissue surfaces.
Fascia A sheet or band of fibrous connective tissue that may be separated from other specifically organized structures, as the tendons, the aponeuroses, and the ligaments.
Febrile Pertaining to or characterized by an elevated body temperature, or fever.
Fibrillation A small, local, involuntary contraction of muscle, resulting from spontaneous activation of a single muscle fiber or of an isolated bundle of nerve fibers.

Fibrin A stringy, insoluble protein formed by the action of thrombin on fibrinogen during the clotting process.

Fibrosis The formation of fibrous connective tissue, as in the repair or replacement of parenchymatous elements.

Filtration The process of passing a liquid through or as if through a filter, which is accomplished by gravity, pressure, or vacuum.

Fimbria Any structure that forms a fringe, border, or edge or the processes that resemble such a structure.

Fissure A cleft or a groove, normal or otherwise, on the surface of an organ or a bony structure.

Fistula An abnormal passage or communication from an internal organ to the body surface or between two internal organs.

Flaccid Weak, soft, and lax; lacking normal muscle tone.

Flatus Air or gas in the intestinal tract that is expelled through the anus. (Adjective: flatulent)

Flexion A movement that allows the two elements of any jointed part to be brought together, decreasing the angle between them, as bending the elbow.

Flora The microorganisms, such as bacteria and fungi, both normally occurring and pathological, found in or on an organ.

Focal Relating to, having, or occupying a focus.

Follicle A sac or pouchlike depression or cavity.

Fontanel A membrane-covered opening in bones or between bones, such as the soft spot covered by tough membranes between the bones of an infant's incompletely ossified skull.

Foramen A natural opening or aperture in a membranous structure or bone.

Fossa A hollow or depressed area, especially on the surface of the end of a bone.

Fovea A small pit or depression in the surface of a structure or an organ.

Fundus The base or bottom of an organ or the portion farthest from the mouth of an organ.

Ganglion One of the nerve cell bodies, chiefly collected in groups outside the central nervous system. (Plural: ganglia)

Genotype The entire genetic constitution of an individual, as determined by the particular combination and location of the genes on the chromosomes; or the alleles present at one or more sites on homologous chromosomes.

Glia The neuroglia, or supporting structure of nervous tissue.

Globulin One of a broad group of proteins classified by solubility, electrophoretic mobility, and size.

Gluconeogenesis The formation of glucose from any of the substances of glycolysis other than carbohydrates.

Glycolysis A series of enzymatically catalyzed reactions, occurring within cells, by which glucose is converted to adenosine triphosphate (ATP) and pyruvic acid during aerobic metabolism.

Gonad A gamete-producing gland, as an ovary or a testis.

Gradient The rate of increase or decrease of a measurable phenomenon expressed as a function of a second; or the visual representation of such a change.

Granuloma A small mass of nodular granulation tissue resulting from chronic inflammation, injury, or infection. (Adjective: granulomatous)

Hapten A small, nonproteinaceous substance that is not antigenic by itself but that can act as an antigen when combined with a larger molecule.

Haustrum A structure resembling a recess or sacculation. (Plural: haustra)

Hematoma A localized collection of extravasated blood trapped in an organ, space, or tissue, resulting from a break in the wall of a blood vessel.

Hematopoiesis The normal formation and development of blood cells.

Hemianopia Defective vision or blindness in half of the visual field of one or both eyes.

Heterozygous Having two different alleles at corresponding loci on homologous chromosomes.

Heterogeneous Consisting of or composed of dissimilar elements or parts; or not having a uniform quality throughout. (Noun: heterogeneity)

Histology The branch of anatomy that deals with the minute (microscopic) structure, composition, and function of cells and tissue. (Adjective: histologic)

Homolog Any organ or part corresponding in function, position, origin, and structure to another organ or part, as the flippers of a seal that correspond to human hands. (Adjective: homologous)

Homozygous Having two identical alleles at corresponding loci on homologous chromosomes.

Humoral Relating to elements dissolved in the blood or body fluids.

Hydrolysis The chemical alteration or decomposition of a compound into fragments by the addition of water.

Hypercapnia Excess amounts of carbon dioxide in the blood.

Hyperemia An excess or engorgement of blood in a part of the body.

Hyperesthesia An unusual or pathologic increase in sensitivity of a part, especially the skin, or of a particular sense.

Hyperplasia An abnormal multiplication or increase in the number of normal cells of a body part.

Hypertonic A solution having a greater concentration of solute than another solution with which it is compared, hence exerting more osmotic pressure than that solution.

Hypertrophy The enlargement or overgrowth of an organ that is due to an increase in the size of its cells rather than the number of its cells.

Hypesthesia An abnormal decrease of sensation in response to stimulation of the sensory nerves. (Also called hypoesthesia.)

Hypocapnia A deficiency of carbon dioxide in the blood.

Hypotonic A solution having a lesser concentration of solute than another solution with which it is compared, hence exerting less osmotic pressure than that solution.

Hypoxia An inadequate supply of oxygen to tissue that is below physiologic levels despite adequate perfusion of the tissue by blood.

Iatrogenic Induced inadvertently through the activity of a physician or by medical treatment or diagnostic procedures.

Idiopathic Arising spontaneously or from an unknown cause.

Idiosyncrasy A physical or behavioral characteristic or manner that is unique to an individual or to a group. (Adjective: idiosyncratic)

Incidence The rate at which a certain event occurs (*e.g.*, the number of new cases of a specific disease during a particular period of time in a population at risk).

Inclusion The act of enclosing or the condition of being enclosed; or anything that is enclosed.

Infarction Necrosis or death of tissues due to local ischemia resulting from obstruction of blood flow.

Inotropic Influencing the force or energy of muscular contractions.

In situ In the natural or normal place; or something, such as cancer, that is confined to its place of origin and has not invaded neighboring tissues.

Interferon Any one of a group of small glycoproteins (cytokines) produced in response to viral infection and which inhibit viral replication.

Interleukin Any of several multifunctional cytokines produced by a variety of lymphoid and nonlymphoid cells, including immune cells, that stimulate or otherwise affect the function of lympopoietic and other cells and systems in the body.

Interstitial Relating to or situated between parts or in the interspaces of a tissue.

Intramural Situated or occurring within the wall of an organ.

Intrinsic Pertaining exclusively to a part or situated entirely within an organ or tissue.

In vitro A biologic reaction occurring in an artificial environment, such as a test tube.

In vivo A biologic reaction occurring within the living body.

Involution The act or instance of enfolding, entangling, or turning inward.

Ionize To separate or change into ions.

Ipsilateral Situated on, pertaining to, or affecting the same side of the body.

Ischemia Decreased blood supply to a body organ or part, usually due to functional constriction or actual obstruction of a blood vessel.

Juxtaarticular Situated near a joint or in the region of a joint.

Juxtaglomerular Near to or adjoining a glomerulus of the kidney.

Karyotype The total chromosomal characteristics of a cell; or the micrograph of chromosomes arranged in pairs in descending order of size.

Keratin A fibrous, sulfur-containing protein that is the primary component of the epidermis, hair, and horny tissues. (Adjective: keratinous)

Keratosis Any skin condition in which there is overgrowth and thickening of the cornified epithelium.

Ketosis A condition characterized by the abnormal accumulation of ketones (organic compounds with a carboxyl group attached to two carbon atoms) in the body tissues and fluid.

Kinesthesia The sense of movement, weight, tension, and position of body parts mediated by input from joint and muscle receptors and hair cells. (Adjective: kinesthetic)

Kyphosis An abnormal condition of the vertebral column, characterized by increased convexity in the curvature of the thoracic spine as viewed from the side.

Lacuna A small pit or cavity within a structure, especially bony tissue; or a defect or gap, as in the field of vision.

Lateral A position farther from the median plane or midline of the body or a structure; or situated on, coming from, or directed towards the side.

Lesion Any wound, injury, or pathologic change in body tissue.

Lethargy The lowered level of consciousness characterized by listlessness, drowsiness, and apathy; or a state of indifference.

Ligament One of many predominantly white, shiny, flexible bands of fibrous tissue that binds joints together and connects bones or cartilages.

Ligand A group, ion, or molecule that binds to the central atom or molecule in a chemical complex.

Lipid Any of the group of fats and fatlike substances characterized by being insoluble in water and soluble in nonpolar organic solvents, such as chloroform and ether.

Lipoprotein Any one of the conjugated proteins that is a complex of protein and lipid.

Lobule A small lobe.

Lordosis The anterior concavity in the curvature of the lumbar and cervical spine as observed from the side.

Lumen A cavity or the channel within a tube or tubular organ of the body.

Luteal Of or pertaining to or having the properties of the corpus luteum.

Lysis Destruction or dissolution of a cell or molecule through the action of a specific agent.

Maceration Softening of tissue by soaking, especially in acidic solutions.

Macroscopic Large enough to be visible with the unaided eye or without the microscope.

Macula A small, flat blemish, thickening, or discoloration that is flush with the skin surface. (Adjective: macular)

Malaise A vague feeling of bodily fatigue and discomfort.

Manometry The measurement of tension or pressure of a liquid or gas using a device called a manometer.

Marasmus A condition of extreme protein-calorie malnutrition that is characterized by growth retardation and progressive wasting of subcutaneous tissue and muscle and occurs chiefly during the first year of life.

Matrix The intracellular substance of a tissue or the basic substance from which a specific organ or kind of tissue develops.

Meatus An opening or passage through any body part.

Medial Pertaining to the middle; or situated or oriented toward the midline of the body.

Mediastinum The mass of tissues and organs in the middle of the thorax, separating the pleural sacs containing the two lungs.

Meiosis The division of a sex cell as it matures, so that each daughter nucleus receives one half of the number of chromosomes characteristic of the somatic cells of the species.

Mesoderm The middle layer of the three primary germ layers of the developing embryo, lying between the ectoderm and the endoderm.

Metabolism The sum of all the physical and chemical processes by which living organisms are produced and maintained, and also the transformation by which energy is provided for vital processes and activities.

Metaplasia Change in type of adult cells in a tissue to a form that is not normal for that tissue.

Metastasis The transfer of disease (*e.g.*, cancer) from one organ or part to another not directly connected with it. (Adjective: metastatic)

Miosis Contraction of the pupil of the eye.

Mitosis A type of indirect cell division that occurs in somatic cells and results in the formation of two daughter nuclei containing the identical complements of the number of chromosomes characteristic of the somatic cells of the species.

Molecule The smallest mass of matter that exhibits the properties of an element or compound.

Morbidity A diseased condition or state; the relative incidence of a disease or of all diseases in a population.

Morphology The study of the physical form and structure of an organism; or the form and structure of a particular organism. (Adjective: morphologic)

Mosaicism In genetics, the presence in an individual or in an organism of cell cultures having two or more cell lines that differ in genetic constitution but are derived from a single zygote.

Mutagen Any chemical or physical agent that induces a genetic mutation (an unusual change in form, quality, or some other characteristic) or increases the mutation rate by causing changes in DNA.

Mydriasis Physiologic dilatation of the pupil of the eye.

Myoclonus A spasm of a portion of a muscle, an entire muscle, or a group of muscles.

Myoglobin The oxygen-transporting pigment of muscle consisting of one heme molecule containing one iron molecule attached to a single globin chain.

Myopathy Any disease or abnormal condition of skeletal muscle, usually characterized by muscle weakness, wasting, and histologic changes within muscle tissue.

Myotome The muscle plate or portion of an embryonic somite that develops into a voluntary muscle; or a group of muscles innervated by a single spinal segment.

Necrosis Localized tissue death that occurs in groups of cells or part of a structure or an organ in response to disease or injury.

Neutropenia An abnormal decrease in the number of neutrophilic leukocytes in the blood.

Nidus The point where a morbid process originates, develops, or is located.

Nociception The reception of painful stimuli from the physical or mechanical injury to body tissues by nociceptors (receptors usually found in either the skin or the walls of the viscera).

Nosocomial Pertaining to or originating in a hospital, such as a nosocomial infection; an infection acquired during hospitalization.

Nystagmus Involuntary, rapid, rhythmic movements of the eyeball.

Oncogene A gene that is capable of causing the initial and continuing conversion of normal cells into cancer cells.

Oocyte A primordial or incompletely developed ovum.

Opsonization The process of making cells, such as bacteria, more susceptible to the action of phagocytes.

Oogenesis The process of the growth and maturation of the female gametes, or ova.

Organelle Any one of the various membrane-bound particles of distinctive morphology and function present within most cells, as the mitochondria, the Golgi complex, and the lysosomes.

Orthopnea An abnormal condition in which a person must be in an upright position in order to breathe deeply or comfortably.

Osmolality The concentration of osmotically active particles in solution expressed in osmols or milliosmols per kilogram of solvent.

Osmolarity The concentration of osmotically active particles in solution expressed in osmols or milliosmols per liter of solution.

Osmosis The movement or passage of a pure solvent, such as water, through a semipermeable membrane from a solution that has a lower solute concentration to one that has a higher solute concentration.

Osteophyte A bony project or outgrowth.

Palpable Perceptible by touch.

Papilla A small nipple-shaped projection, elevation, or structure, as the conoid papillae of the tongue.

Papule A small, circumscribed, solid elevation of the skin less than one centimeter in diameter. (Adjective: papular)

Paracrine A mode of hormone action in which a chemical messenger that is synthesized and released from a cell acts on nearby cells of a different type and affects their function.

Paralysis An abnormal condition characterized by the impairment or loss of motor function due to a lesion of the neural or muscular mechanism.

Paraneoplastic Relating to alterations produced in tissue remote from a tumor or its metastases.

Parenchyma The basic tissue or elements of an organ as distinguished from supporting or connective tissue or elements. (Adjective: parenchymal)

Paresis Slight or partial paralysis.

Paresthesia Any abnormal touch sensation, which can be experienced as numbness, tingling, or a "pins and needles" feeling, often in the absence of external stimuli.

Parietal Pertaining to the outer wall of a cavity or organ; or pertaining to the parietal bone of the skull or the parietal lobe of the brain.

Parous Having borne one or more viable offspring.

Pathogen Any microorganism capable of producing disease.

Pedigree A systematic presentation, such as in a table, chart, or list, of an individual's ancestors that is used in human genetics in the analysis of inheritance.

Peptide Any of a class of molecular chain compounds composed of two or more amino acids joined by peptide bonds.

Perfusion The process or act of pouring over or through, especially the passage of a fluid through a specific organ or an area of the body.

Peripheral Pertaining to the outside, surface, or surrounding area of an organ or other structure; or located away from a center or central structure.

Permeable A condition of being pervious, or permitting passage, so that fluids and certain other substances can pass through, as a permeable membrane.

Pervasive Pertaining to something that becomes diffused throughout every part.

Petechia A tiny, perfectly round, purplish red spot that appears on the skin as a result of minute intradermal or submucous hemorrhage. (Plural: petechiae)

Phagocytosis The process by which certain cells engulf and consume foreign material and cell debris.

Phalanx Any one of the bones composing the fingers of each hand and the toes of each foot.

Phenotype The complete physical, biochemical, and physiologic makeup of an individual, as determined by the interaction of both genetic makeup and environmental factors.

Pheresis A procedure in which blood is withdrawn from a donor, a portion (plasma, leukocytes, etc.) is separated and retained, and the remainder is reperfused into the donor. It includes plasmapheresis and leukopheresis.

Pili Hair; or in microbiology, the minute filamentous appendages of certain bacteria. (Singular: pilus)

Plexus A network of intersecting nerves, blood vessels, or lymphatic vessels.

Polygene Any of a group of nonallelic genes that interact to influence the same character in the same way so that the effect is cumulative, usually of a quantitative nature, as size, weight, or skin pigmentation. (Adjective: polygenic)

Polymorph One of several, or many, forms of an organism or cell. (Adjective: polymorphic)

Polyp A small, tumor-like growth that protrudes from a mucous membrane surface.

Polypeptide A molecular chain of more than two amino acids joined by peptide bonds.

Presbyopia A visual condition (farsightedness) that commonly develops with advancing years or old age in which the lens loses elasticity causing defective accommodation and inability to focus sharply for near vision.

Prevalence The number of new and old cases of a disease that are present in a population at a given time or occurrences of an event during a particular period of time.

Prodrome An early symptom indicating the onset of a condition or disease. (Adjective: prodromal)

Prokaryotic Pertaining to an organism, such as bacterium, with cells lacking a true nucleus and nuclear membrane that reproduces through simple fission.

Prolapse The falling down, sinking, or sliding of an organ from its normal position or location in the body.

Proliferation The reproduction or multiplication of similar forms, especially cells.

Pronation Assumption of a position in which the ventral, or front, surface of the body or part of the body faces downward. (Adjective: prone)

Propagation The act or action of reproduction.

Proprioception The reception of stimuli originating from within the body regarding body position and muscular activity by proprioceptors (sensory nerve endings found in muscles, tendons, joints).

Prosthesis An artificial replacement for a missing body part; or a device designed and applied to improve function, such as a hearing aid.

Proteoglycans Any one of a group of polysaccharide-protein conjugates occurring primarily in the matrix of connective tissue and cartilage.

Protooncogene A normal cellular gene that with alteration, such as by mutation, becomes an active oncogene.

Proximal Closer to a point of reference, usually the trunk of the body, than other parts of the body.

Pruritus The symptom of itching, an uncomfortable sensation leading to the urge to rub or scratch the skin to obtain relief. (Adjective: pruritic)

Purpura A small hemorrhage, up to about 1 cm in diameter, in the skin, mucous membrane, or serosal surface; or any of several bleeding disorders characterized by the presence of purpuric lesions.

Purulent Producing or containing pus.

Quiescent Quiet, causing no disturbance, activity, or symptoms.

Reflux An abnormal backward or return flow of a fluid, such as stomach contents, blood, or urine.

Regurgitation A flow of material that is in the opposite direction from normal, as in the return of swallowed food into the mouth or the backward flow of blood through a defective heart valve.

Remission The partial or complete disappearance of the symptoms of a chronic or malignant disease; or the period of time during which the abatement of symptoms occurs.

Resorption The loss of substance or bone by physiologic or pathologic means, for example, the loss of dentin and cementum of a tooth.

Retrograde Moving backward or against the usual direction of flow; reverting to an earlier state or worse condition (degenerating); catabolic.

Retroversion A condition in which an entire organ is tipped backward or in a posterior direction, usually without flexion or other distortion.

Rhabdomyolysis Destruction or degeneration of muscle, associated with myoglobinuria (excretion of myoglobin in the urine).

Rostral Situated near a beak (oral or nasal region).

Sacroiliitis Inflammation in the sacroiliac joint.

Sclerosis A condition characterized by induration or hardening of tissue resulting from any of several causes, including inflammation, diseases of the interstitial substance, and increased formation of connective tissues.

Semipermeable Partially but not wholly permeable, especially a membrane that permits the passage of some (usually small) molecules but not of other (usually larger) particles.

Senescence The process or condition of aging or growing old.

Sepsis The presence in the blood or other tissues of pathogenic microorganisms or their toxins; or the condition resulting from the spread of microorganisms or their products. (Adjective: septic)

Serous Relating to or resembling serum; or containing or producing serum, such as a serous gland.

Shunt To divert or bypass bodily fluid from one channel, path, or part to another; a passage or anastomosis between two natural channels, especially between blood vessels, established by surgery or occurring as an abnormality.

Soma The body of an organism as distinguished from the mind; all of an organism, excluding germ cells; the body of a cell.

Spasticity The condition characterized by spasms or other uncontrolled contractions of the skeletal muscles. (Adjective: spastic)

Spatial Relating to, having the character of, or occupying space.

Sphincter A ringlike band of muscle fibers that constricts a passage or closes a natural orifice of the body.

Stenosis An abnormal condition characterized by the narrowing or stricture of a duct or canal.

Stria A streak or a linear scarlike lesion that often results from rapidly developing tension in the skin; or a narrow bandlike structure, especially the longitudinal collections of nerve fibers in the brain.

Stricture An abnormal temporary or permanent narrowing of the lumen of a duct, canal, or other passage, as the esophagus, because of inflammation, external pressure, or scarring.

Stroma The supporting tissue or the matrix of an organ as distinguished from its functional element, or parenchyma.

Stupor A lowered level of consciousness characterized by lethargy and unresponsiveness in which a person seems unaware of his or her surroundings.

Subchondral Beneath a cartilage.

Subcutaneous Beneath the skin.

Sulcus A shallow groove, depression, or furrow on the surface of an organ, as a sulcus on the surface of the brain, separating the gyri.

Supination Assuming the position of lying horizontally on the back, or with the face upward. (Adjective: supine)

Suppuration The formation of pus, or purulent matter.

Symbiosis Mode of living characterized by close association between organisms of different species, usually in a mutually beneficial relationship.

Sympathomimetic An agent or substance that produces stimulating effects on organs and structures similar to those produced by the sympathetic nervous system.

Syncope A brief lapse of consciousness due to generalized cerebral ischemia.

Syncytium A multinucleate mass of protoplasm produced by the merging of a group of cells.

Syndrome A complex of signs and symptoms that occur together to present a clinical picture of a disease or inherited abnormality.

Synergist An organ, agent, or substance that aids or cooperates with another organ, agent, or substance.

Synthesis An integration or combination of various parts or elements to create a unified whole.

Systemic Pertaining to the whole body rather than to a localized area or regional portion of the body.

Systole The contraction, or period of contraction, of the heart that drives the blood onward into the aorta and pulmonary arteries.

Tamponade Stoppage of the flow of blood to an organ or a part of the body by pathologic compression, such as the compression of the heart by an accumulation of pericardial fluid.

Teratogen Any agent or factor that induces or increases the incidence of developmental abnormalities in the fetus.

Thrombus A stationary mass of clotted blood or other formed elements that remains attached to its place of origin along the wall of a blood vessel, frequently obstructing the circulation. (Plural: thrombi)

Tinnitus A tinkling, buzzing, or ringing noise heard in one or both ears.

Tophus A chalky deposit containing sodium urate that most often develops in periarticular fibrous tissue, typically in individuals with gout. (Plural: tophi)

Torsion The act or process of twisting in either a positive (clockwise) or negative (counterclockwise) direction.

Trabecula A supporting or anchoring stand of connective tissue, such as the delicate fibrous threads connecting the inner surface of the arachnoid to the pia mater.

Transmural Situated or occurring through the wall of an organ.

Transudate A fluid substance passed through a membrane or extruded from the blood.

Tremor Involuntary quivering or trembling movements caused by the alternating contraction and relaxation of opposing groups of skeletal muscles.

Trigone A triangular-shaped area.

Ubiquitous The condition or state of existing or being everywhere at the same time.

Ulcer A circumscribed excavation of the surface of an organ or tissue, which results from necrosis that accompanies some inflammatory, infectious, or malignant processes. (Adjective: ulcerative)

Urticaria A pruritic skin eruption of the upper dermis, usually transient, characterized by wheals (hives) of various shapes and sizes.

Uveitis An inflammation of all or part of the uveal tract of the eye.

Ventral Pertaining to a position toward the belly of the body; or situated or oriented toward the front or anterior of the body.

Vertigo An illusory sensation that the environment or one's own body is revolving.

Vesicle A small bladder or sac, as a small, thin-walled, raised skin lesion, containing liquid.

Visceral Pertaining to the viscera, or internal organs of the body.

Viscosity Pertaining to the physical property of fluids, caused by the adhesion of adjacent molecules, that determines the internal resistance to shear forces.

Zoonosis A disease of animals that may be transmitted to humans from its primary animal host under natural conditions.

Index

Page numbers followed by *c* denote charts; those followed by *f* denote figures; and those followed by *t* denote tables.

B

D

E

I

M

O

P

Q

R

S

T

V

U.W.E.L. LEARNING RESOURCES

PREFIXES

a-, an- without, lack of
apnea (without breath)
anemia (lack of blood)

ab- separation, away from
abductor (leading away from)
aberrant (away from the usual course)

ad- to, toward, near to
adductor (leading toward)
adrenal (near the kidney)

ana- up, again, excessive
anapnea (to breathe again)
anasarca (severe edema)

ante- before, in front of
antecubital (in front of the elbow)
antenatal (occurring before birth)

anti- against, counter
anticoagulant (opposing coagulation)
antisepsis (against infection)

ap-, apo- separation, derivation from
apocrine (type of glandular secretion that contains cast-off parts of the secretory cell)

aut-, auto- self
autoimmune (immunity to self)
autologous (pertaining to self graft or blood transfusion)

bi- two, twice, double
biarticulate (pertaining to two joints)
bifurcation (two branches)

brady- slow
bradyesthesia (slowness or dullness of perception)

cata- down, under, lower, negative, against
catabolism (breaking down)
catalepsy (diminished movement)

circum- around, about
circumflex (winding around)
circumference (surrounding)

contra- against, counter
contraindicated (not indicated)
contralateral (opposite side)

de- away from, down from, remove
dehydrate (remove water)
deaminate (remove an amino group)

dia- through, apart, across, completely
diapedesis (ooze through)
diagnosis (complete knowledge)

dis- apart, reversal, separation
discrete (made up of separated parts)
disruptive (bursting apart)

dys- difficulty, faulty, painful
dysmenorrhea (painful menstruation)
dyspnea (difficulty breathing)

e-, ex- out from, out of
enucleate (remove from)
exostosis (outgrowth of bone)

ec- out from
eccentric (away from center)
ectopic (out of place)

ecto- outside, situated on
ectoderm (outer skin)
ectoretina (outer layer of retina)

em-, en- in, on
empyema (pus in)
encephalon (in the brain)

endo- within, inside
endocardium (within heart)
endometrium (within uterus)

epi- upon, after, in addition
epidermis (on skin)
epidural (upon dura)

eu- well, easily, good
eupnea (easy or normal respiration)
euthyroid (normal thyroid function)

exo- outside
exocolitis (inflammation of outer coat of colon)
exogenous (originating outside)

extra- outside of, beyond
extracellular (outside cell)
extrapleural (outside pleura)

hemi- half
hemialgia (pain affecting only one side of the body)
hemilingual (affecting one side of the tongue)

hyper- extreme, above, beyond
hyperemia (excessive blood)
hypertrophy (overgrowth)

hypo- under, below
hypotension (low blood pressure)
hypothyroidism (underfunction of thyroid)

im-, in- in, into, on
immersion (act of dipping in)
injection (act of forcing fluid into)

im-, in- not
immature (not mature)
inability (not able)

infra- beneath
infraclavicular (below the clavicle)
infraorbital (below the eye)

inter- among, between
intercostal (between the ribs)
intervene (come between)

intra- within, inside
intraocular (within the eye)
intraventricular (within the ventricles)

intro- into, within
introversion (turning inward)
introduce (lead into)

iso- equal, same
isotonia (equal tone, tension, or activity)
isotypical (of the same type)

juxta- near, close by
juxtaglomerular (near an adjoining glomerulus in the kidney)
juxtaspinal (near the spinal column)

macro- large, long, excess
macrocephaly (excessive head size)
macrodystrophia (overgrowth of a part)

mal- bad, abnormal
maldevelopment (abnormal growth or development)
malfunction (to function imperfectly or badly)

mega- large, enlarged, abnormally large size
megaprosopous (having a large face)
megasoma (great size and stature)

meso- middle, intermediate, moderate
mesoderm (middle germ layer of embryo)
mesocephalic (pertaining to a skull with an average breadth–length index)

meta- beyond, after, accompanying
metacarpal (beyond the wrist)
metamorphosis (change of form)

micro- small size or amount
microbe (a minute living organism)
microtiter (a titer of minute quantity)

neo- new, young, recent
neoformation (a new growth)
neonate (newborn)

oligo- few, scanty, less than normal
oligogenic (produced by a few genes)
oligospermia (abnormally low number of spermatozoa in the semen)

para- beside, beyond
paracardiac (beside the heart)
paraurethral (near the urethra)

per- through
perforate (bore through)
permeate (pass through)

peri- around
peribronchia (around the bronchus)
periosteum (around bone)

poly- many, much
polyphagia (excessive eating)
polytrauma (occurrence of multiple injuries)

post- after, behind in time or place
postoperative (after operation)
postpartum (after childbirth)

pre-, pro- in front of, before in time or place
premaxillary (in front of the maxilla)
prognosis (foreknowledge)

pseud-, pseudo- false, spurious
pseudocartilaginous (made up of a substance resembling cartilage)
pseudopregnancy (false pregnancy)

retro- backward, located behind
retrocervical (located behind cervix)
retrograde (going backward)

semi- half, partly
semiflexion (a limb midway between flexion and extension)
semimembranous (composed in part of membrane)

steno- narrow compressed, contracted
stenocoriasis (contraction of the pupil of the eye)
stenopeic (having a narrow slit or opening)